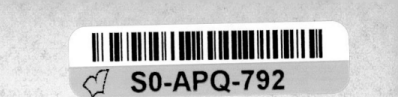

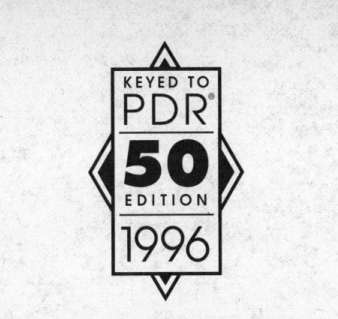

PDR GUIDE TO DRUG INTERACTIONS SIDE EFFECTS INDICATIONS

Interactions Index (White Pages)	.1
Food Interactions Cross-Reference (Blue Pages)	.1199
Side Effects Index (Pink Pages)	.1207
Indications Index (Yellow Pages)	.1451

Editor • Mukesh Mehta, RPh

Index Editors: Paula R. Ajmera, RPh; Ann Ben Larbi; Thomas L. Fleming, RPh; Marion Gray, RPh; Kathryn M. Martin, PharmD; Leila A. Noueihed, RPh; Sarah G. Terzides

Physicians' Desk Reference Staff — Medical Consultant: Ronald Arky, MD, Charles S. Davidson Professor of Medicine and Master, Francis Weld Peabody Society, Harvard Medical School; **President and Chief Operating Officer, Drug Information Services Group:** Thomas F. Rice; **Director of Product Management:** Stephen B. Greenberg; **Senior Product Manager:** Cy S. Caine;**Associate Product Manager:** Howard N. Kanter; **National Sales Manager:** James R. Pantaleo; **Senior Account Manager:** Michael S. Sarajian; **Account Managers:** Dikran N. Barsamian, Donald V. Bruccoleri, Lawrence C. Keary, Jeffrey M. Keller, P. Anthony Pinsonault, Anthony Sorce; **Trade Sales Manager:** Robin B. Bartlett; **Trade Sales Account Executive:** Bill Gaffney; **Direct Marketing Manager:** Robert W. Chapman; **Marketing Communications Manager:** Maryann Malorgio; **Vice President of Production:** Steven R. Andreazza; **Director, Professional Support Services:** Mukesh Mehta, RPh; **Drug Information Specialists:** Thomas Fleming, RPh, Marion Gray, RPh; **Manager, Database Administration:** Lynne Handler; **Contracts and Support Services Director:** Marjorie A. Duffy; **Director of Production:** Carrie Williams; **Production Managers:** Kimberly Hiller-Vivas, Robert Loeser; **Production Coordinators:** Amy B. Douma, Dawn B. McCall; **Senior Format Editor:** Gregory J. Westley; **Format Editor:** Edna V. Berger; **Index Editor:** Jeffrey Schaefer; **Art Associate:** Joan K. Akerlind; **Director of Corporate Communications:** Gregory J. Thomas; **Electronic Publishing Coordinator:** Joanne M. Pearson; **Electronic Publishing Designer:** Kevin J. Leckner; **Art Director:** Richard A. Weinstock; **Digital Photography:** Shawn W. Cahill, Frank J. McElroy, III; **Editor, Special Projects:** David W. Sifton

Copyright (C) 1996 and published by Medical Economics Company at Montvale, NJ 07645-1742. All rights reserved. None of the content of this publication may be reproduced, stored in a retrieval system, resold, redistributed, or transmitted in any form or by any means (electronic, mechanical, photocopying, recording, or otherwise) without the prior written permission of the publisher. PHYSICIANS' DESK REFERENCE®, PDR®, PDR For Nonprescription Drugs®, PDR For Ophthalmology®, Pocket PDR®, PDR Guide to Drug Interactions•Side Effects•Indications®, and The PDR® Family Guide to Prescription Drugs® are registered trademarks used herein under license. PDR® Generics™, The PDR® Family Guide to Women's Health and Prescription Drugs™, The PDR® Family Guide to Nutrition and Health™, PDR® Electronic Library™, PDR® Drug Interactions, Side Effects, Indications Diskettes™, and PDR® Drug REAX™ are trademarks used herein under license.

Officers of Medical Economics: President and Chief Executive Officer: Norman R. Snesil; President and Chief Operating Officer: Curtis B. Allen; Executive Vice President and Chief Financial Officer: J. Crispin Ashworth; Senior Vice President—Corporate Operations: John R. Ware; Senior Vice President—Corporate Business Development: Raymond M. Zoeller; Vice President, Information Services and Chief Information Officer: Edward J. Zecchini

ISBN: 1-56363-132-6

FOREWORD

The *PDR*® family of pharmaceutical references is dedicated to providing you with fast, accurate answers to all your most important prescribing questions. This guide, with its exhaustive indices of interactions, side effects, and indications, is a key way of giving you the comprehensive facts you need as quickly and efficiently as possible.

Extracted from the FDA-approved labeling in *Physicians' Desk Reference*®, *PDR For Nonprescription Drugs*®, and *PDR For Ophthalmology*®, the entries in this guide cover more than 2,400 drug products. With every listing cross-referenced to the underlying text, the book provides you with a quick, reliable means of screening any patient regimen for the source of a drug-related problem.

There are many ways to use this guide:

- To check for potential interactions, turn to the white pages. In this section you'll find an entry for each product described in *PDR* and its companion volumes. Listed are compounds and food items that may interact with the product, as well as the specific brands containing each compound. A brief description of the interaction appears with each compound. (Because product labeling varies in the scope of its interaction reporting, be sure to check the interaction listing for each product in the patient's regimen.)
- If a specific dietary item is suspected of an interaction, turn to the blue pages. There you will find potential drug/food and drug/alcohol interactions cross-referenced alphabetically by the name or type of food. Each entry includes a list of affected drugs and a brief description of each interaction.
- To single-out the most likely source of a side effect, check the pink pages. They contain an alphabetical list of the more than 3,600 distinct reactions cited throughout *PDR* and its companion volumes. Each entry includes an alphabetical list of the brands that have been associated with the problem. To help target the most likely offenders, incidence data are included whenever found in the official labeling.
- If you need to locate an alternative for a problem medication — or simply want to review the full range of options for a particular diagnosis — look up the yellow pages. Here each indication found in *PDR* and its companions is listed alphabetically, with a cross-reference to all brands approved for that particular purpose. For easy comparison, the listings include the generic name and manufacturer of each product. (Only FDA-approved indications are referenced.)

Please note that all entries in the guide are derived directly from the FDA-sanctioned prescribing information published by *PDR*. Therefore the only products listed are those described in *Physicians' Desk Reference* and its companion volumes; and the only facts presented are those that appear in the text of *PDR*.

Although all three *PDR* volumes have been carefully sifted for pertinent facts during compilation of this guide, please remember that the publisher does not guarantee that the entries are totally accurate or complete. Use this guide as a convenient cross-reference; but consult the underlying *PDR* text, as well as the medical literature, when definitive information is needed.

In addition to this guide and its other printed references, *PDR* now offers a variety of electronic prescribing aids:

- *Pocket PDR*® — A handheld personal electronic database of key sections from the prescription-drug listings in *PDR*.
- *PDR*® *Electronic Library*™ — A Windows-compatible CD-ROM with a complete database of *PDR* prescribing information, electronically searchable for instant retrieval. A standard subscription includes *PDR*'s sophisticated prescription-screening program and an exhaustive file of chemical structures, illustrations, and full-color product photographs. Optional enhancements include the complete contents of *The Merck Manual* and *Stedman's Medical Dictionary*, as well as a handy file of patient handouts drawn from *PDR*'s consumer handbook, *The PDR*® *Family Guide to Prescription Drugs*®. The disc is available for use on individual PCs and PC networks.

■ *PDR® Drug REAX™* — A Windows-compatible database of drug interaction information drawn from the peer-reviewed medical literature.

■ *PDR Database Services* — A preformatted text file suitable for integration in large mainframe-based information systems.

In the current cost-conscious healthcare environment, you should also be aware of the newest volume in the *PDR* family of references. Entitled *PDR® Generics™*, this exhaustive pharmaceutical reference includes generic monographs covering virtually all prescription drugs—plus brand/generic unit cost comparisons, average generic prices by package size for all therapeutically equivalent products, and the average wholesale price of all available supplies. Drugs in this volume are indexed by their brand and generic names, therapeutic category, indications, and foreign brand names. Off-label indications are included, and a unique daily cost of therapy guide provides comparative data on the leading medications for a variety of common disorders.

Also new and noteworthy are the *PDR® Nurse's Handbook™*, a specially designed drug reference with complete nursing implications, and the *PDR® Medical Dictionary*, an authoritative reference that combines a complete medical lexicon with *PDR's* unparalleled database of brand and generic drug names.

For more information on any of these important references, please call, toll-free, 1-800-232-7379 or fax 201-573-4956.

SECTION 1

INTERACTIONS INDEX

Cataloged in this section are all interactions found during a review of the labeling published in *PDR, PDR For Nonprescription Drugs*, and *PDR For Ophthalmology*. The list is arranged alphabetically by brand or, when applicable, generic name.

Whenever appropriate, each brand-name heading is followed by a summary of the major pharmaceutical categories with which the product is said to interact. Beneath this summary is an alphabetical list of the compounds in these categories, each followed by a brief notation regarding the results of concurrent administration with the brand in question. After each notation is an alphabetical list of the brands of the compound found in PDR and its companion volumes. Page numbers refer to the 1996 editions of *PDR* and *PDR For Ophthalmology* and the 1995 edition of *PDR For*

Nonprescription Drugs, which is published later each year. A key to the symbols denoting the companion volumes appears in the bottom margin of every other page.

Following the list of interactive drugs is a similar list of foods. Note that interactions with alcohol are listed here as well.

This index lists only interactions cited in official prescribing information as published by *PDR*. Because product labeling varies in the scope of its interaction reporting, the most prudent course is to check each product in the patient's regimen. Note also that cross-sensitivity reactions and effects on laboratory results are not included in the listings.

A AND D MEDICATED DIAPER RASH OINTMENT

(Petrolatum, White, Zinc Oxide) ......✿⊡ 797
None cited in PDR database.

A AND D OINTMENT

(Petrolatum, Lanolin) ....✿⊡ 797
None cited in PDR database.

AMO ENDOSOL (BALANCED SALT SOLUTION)

(Balanced Salt Solution)..................... ◎ 232
None cited in PDR database.

AMO VITRAX VISCOELASTIC SOLUTION

(Sodium Hyaluronate) .... ◎ 232
None cited in PDR database.

AMVISC PLUS

(Sodium Hyaluronate) .... ◎ 329
None cited in PDR database.

A-200 LICE CONTROL SPRAY

(Permethrin) .... ✿⊡ 656
None cited in PDR database.

A-200 LICE KILLING SHAMPOO

(Piperonyl Butoxide).......................... ✿⊡ 657
None cited in PDR database.

A/T/S 2% ACNE TOPICAL GEL AND SOLUTION

(Erythromycin) 1234
May interact with:

Concomitant Topical Acne Therapy (Potential for cumulative irritant effect).

AVC CREAM

(Sulfanilamide) 1500
None cited in PDR database.

AVC SUPPOSITORIES

(Sulfanilamide) 1500
None cited in PDR database.

ABBOKINASE

(Urokinase) 403
May interact with anticoagulants and certain other agents. Compounds in these categories include:

Aspirin (Altered platelet function; aspirin is not recommended for treatment of fever). Products include:

Alka-Seltzer Effervescent Antacid and Pain Reliever ....✿⊡ 701
Alka-Seltzer Extra Strength Effervescent Antacid and Pain Reliever ....✿⊡ 703
Alka-Seltzer Lemon Lime Effervescent Antacid and Pain Reliever ....✿⊡ 703
Alka-Seltzer Plus Cold Medicine ....✿⊡ 705
Alka-Seltzer Plus Cold & Cough Medicine ....✿⊡ 708
Alka-Seltzer Plus Night-Time Cold Medicine ....✿⊡ 707
Alka Seltzer Plus Sinus Medicine ..✿⊡ 707
Arthritis Foundation Safety Coated Aspirin Tablets ....✿⊡ 675
Arthritis Pain Ascriptin ....✿⊡ 631
Maximum Strength Ascriptin ....✿⊡ 630
Regular Strength Ascriptin Tablets ....✿⊡ 629
Arthritis Strength BC Powder..........✿⊡ 609
BC Cold Powder Multi-Symptom Formula (Cold-Sinus-Allergy) ......✿⊡ 609
BC Cold Powder Non-Drowsy Formula (Cold-Sinus) ....✿⊡ 609
BC Powder ....✿⊡ 609
Bayer Children's Chewable Aspirin ....✿⊡ 711
Genuine Bayer Aspirin Tablets & Caplets ....✿⊡ 713
Extra Strength Bayer Arthritis Pain Regimen Formula ....✿⊡ 711
Extra Strength Bayer Aspirin Caplets & Tablets ....✿⊡ 712
Extended-Release Bayer 8-Hour Aspirin ....✿⊡ 712
Extra Strength Bayer Plus Aspirin Caplets ....✿⊡ 713
Extra Strength Bayer PM Aspirin ..✿⊡ 713
Bayer Enteric Aspirin..........................✿⊡ 709
Bufferin Analgesic Tablets and Caplets ....✿⊡ 613
Arthritis Strength Bufferin Analgesic Caplets ....✿⊡ 614
Extra Strength Bufferin Analgesic Tablets ....✿⊡ 615
Cama Arthritis Pain Reliever............✿⊡ 785
Darvon Compound-65 Pulvules 1435
Easprin.. 1914
Ecotrin 2455
Ecotrin Enteric Coated Aspirin Maximum Strength Tablets and Caplets ....✿⊡ 816
Ecotrin Enteric Coated Aspirin Regular Strength Tablets 2455
Empirin Aspirin Tablets ....✿⊡ 854
Empirin with Codeine Tablets............ 1093
Excedrin Extra-Strength Analgesic Tablets & Caplets 732
Fiorinal Capsules 2261
Fiorinal with Codeine Capsules 2262
Fiorinal Tablets 2261
Halfprin 1362
Healthprin Aspirin 2455
Norgesic.. 1496
Percodan Tablets..................................... 939
Percodan-Demi Tablets......................... 940
Robaxisal Tablets.................................... 2071
Soma Compound w/Codeine Tablets 2676
Soma Compound Tablets..................... 2675
St. Joseph Adult Chewable Aspirin (81 mg.) ....✿⊡ 808
Talwin Compound 2335
Ursinus Inlay-Tabs................................✿⊡ 794
Vanquish Analgesic Caplets ....✿⊡ 731

Dalteparin Sodium (Increased risk of hemorrhage). Products include:

Fragmin 1954

Dicumarol (Increased risk of hemorrhage).

No products indexed under this heading.

Enoxaparin (Increased risk of hemorrhage). Products include:

Lovenox Injection.................................... 2020

Heparin Calcium (Increased risk of hemorrhage).

No products indexed under this heading.

Heparin Sodium (Increased risk of hemorrhage). Products include:

Heparin Lock Flush Solution 2725
Heparin Sodium Injection..................... 2726
Heparin Sodium Injection, USP, Sterile Solution 2615
Heparin Sodium Vials............................. 1441

Indomethacin (Altered platelet function). Products include:

Indocin 1680

IMPORTANT NOTE: Always consult each drug listing in the patient's regimen for possible interactions.

Abbokinase Interactions Index 2

Indomethacin Sodium Trihydrate (Altered platelet function). Products include:

Indocin I.V. 1684

Phenylbutazone (Altered platelet function).

No products indexed under this heading.

Warfarin Sodium (Increased risk of hemorrhage). Products include:

Coumadin 926

ABBOKINASE OPEN-CATH

(Urokinase) 405

May interact with:

Aspirin (Concomitant use with aspirin for treatment of fever should be avoided). Products include:

Alka-Seltzer Effervescent Antacid and Pain Reliever .... ▣ 701
Alka-Seltzer Extra Strength Effervescent Antacid and Pain Reliever .... ▣ 703
Alka-Seltzer Lemon Lime Effervescent Antacid and Pain Reliever .... ▣ 703
Alka-Seltzer Plus Cold Medicine .... ▣ 705
Alka-Seltzer Plus Cold & Cough Medicine .... ▣ 708
Alka-Seltzer Plus Night-Time Cold Medicine .... ▣ 707
Alka Seltzer Plus Sinus Medicine .... ▣ 707
Arthritis Foundation Safety Coated Aspirin Tablets .... ▣ 675
Arthritis Pain Ascriptin .... ▣ 631
Maximum Strength Ascriptin .... ▣ 630
Regular Strength Ascriptin Tablets .... ▣ 629
Arthritis Strength BC Powder .... ▣ 609
BC Cold Powder Multi-Symptom Formula (Cold-Sinus-Allergy) .... ▣ 609
BC Cold Powder Non-Drowsy Formula (Cold-Sinus) .... ▣ 609
BC Powder .... ▣ 609
Bayer Children's Chewable Aspirin .... ▣ 711
Genuine Bayer Aspirin Tablets & Caplets .... ▣ 713
Extra Strength Bayer Arthritis Pain Regimen Formula .... ▣ 711
Extra Strength Bayer Aspirin Caplets & Tablets .... ▣ 712
Extended-Release Bayer 8-Hour Aspirin .... ▣ 712
Extra Strength Bayer Plus Aspirin Caplets .... ▣ 713
Extra Strength Bayer PM Aspirin .... ▣ 713
Bayer Enteric Aspirin .... ▣ 709
Bufferin Analgesic Tablets and Caplets .... ▣ 613
Arthritis Strength Bufferin Analgesic Caplets .... ▣ 614
Extra Strength Bufferin Analgesic Tablets .... ▣ 615
Cama Arthritis Pain Reliever .... ▣ 785
Darvon Compound-65 Pulvules 1435
Easprin 1914
Ecotrin 2455
Ecotrin Enteric Coated Aspirin Maximum Strength Tablets and Caplets .... ▣ 816
Ecotrin Enteric Coated Aspirin Regular Strength Tablets 2455
Empirin Aspirin Tablets .... ▣ 854
Empirin with Codeine Tablets 1093
Excedrin Extra-Strength Analgesic Tablets & Caplets 732
Fiorinal Capsules 2261
Fiorinal with Codeine Capsules 2262
Fiorinal Tablets 2261
Halfprin 1362
Healthprin Aspirin 2455
Norgesic 1496
Percodan Tablets 939
Percodan-Demi Tablets 940
Robaxisal Tablets 2071
Soma Compound w/Codeine Tablets 2676
Soma Compound Tablets 2675
St. Joseph Adult Chewable Aspirin (81 mg.) .... ▣ 808
Talwin Compound 2335
Ursinus Inlay-Tabs .... ▣ 794
Vanquish Analgesic Caplets .... ▣ 731

ACCUPRIL TABLETS

(Quinapril Hydrochloride) 1893

May interact with diuretics, potassium sparing diuretics, potassium preparations, tetracyclines, lithium preparations, and certain other agents. Compounds in these categories include:

Amiloride Hydrochloride (Occasional excessive reduction of blood pressure; potential for hyperkalemia). Products include:

Midamor Tablets 1703
Moduretic Tablets 1705

Bendroflumethiazide (Occasional excessive reduction of blood pressure).

No products indexed under this heading.

Bumetanide (Occasional excessive reduction of blood pressure). Products include:

Bumex 2093

Chlorothiazide (Occasional excessive reduction of blood pressure). Products include:

Aldoclor Tablets 1598
Diupres Tablets 1650
Diuril Oral 1653

Chlorothiazide Sodium (Occasional excessive reduction of blood pressure). Products include:

Diuril Sodium Intravenous 1652

Chlorthalidone (Occasional excessive reduction of blood pressure). Products include:

Combipres Tablets 677
Tenoretic Tablets 2845
Thalitone 1245

Demeclocycline Hydrochloride (Reduced absorption of tetracycline by approximately 28% to 37%). Products include:

Declomycin Tablets 1371

Doxycycline Calcium (Reduced absorption of tetracycline by approximately 28% to 37%). Products include:

Vibramycin Calcium Oral Suspension Syrup 1941

Doxycycline Hyclate (Reduced absorption of tetracycline by approximately 28% to 37%). Products include:

Doryx Capsules 1913
Vibramycin Hyclate Capsules 1941
Vibramycin Hyclate Intravenous 2215
Vibra-Tabs Film Coated Tablets 1941

Doxycycline Monohydrate (Reduced absorption of tetracycline by approximately 28% to 37%). Products include:

Monodox Capsules 1805
Vibramycin Monohydrate for Oral Suspension 1941

Ethacrynic Acid (Occasional excessive reduction of blood pressure). Products include:

Edecrin Tablets 1657

Furosemide (Occasional excessive reduction of blood pressure). Products include:

Lasix Injection, Oral Solution and Tablets 1240

Hydrochlorothiazide (Occasional excessive reduction of blood pressure). Products include:

Aldactazide 2413
Aldoril Tablets 1604
Apresazide Capsules 808
Capozide 742
Dyazide 2479
Esidrix Tablets 821
Esimil Tablets 822
HydroDIURIL Tablets 1674
Hydropres Tablets 1675
Hyzaar Tablets 1677
Inderide Tablets 2732
Inderide LA Long Acting Capsules 2734
Lopressor HCT Tablets 832
Lotensin HCT 837
Maxzide 1380
Moduretic Tablets 1705
Oretic Tablets 443
Prinzide Tablets 1737
Ser-Ap-Es Tablets 849
Timolide Tablets 1748
Vaseretic Tablets 1765
Zestoretic 2850
Ziac 1415

Hydroflumethiazide (Occasional excessive reduction of blood pressure). Products include:

Diucardin Tablets 2718

Indapamide (Occasional excessive reduction of blood pressure). Products include:

Lozol Tablets 2022

Lithium Carbonate (Increased serum lithium levels and symptoms of lithium toxicity). Products include:

Eskalith 2485
Lithium Carbonate Capsules & Tablets 2230
Lithonate/Lithotabs/Lithobid 2543

Lithium Citrate (Increased serum lithium levels and symptoms of lithium toxicity).

No products indexed under this heading.

Methacycline Hydrochloride (Reduced absorption of tetracycline by approximately 28% to 37%).

No products indexed under this heading.

Methyclothiazide (Occasional excessive reduction of blood pressure). Products include:

Enduron Tablets 420

Metolazone (Occasional excessive reduction of blood pressure). Products include:

Mykrox Tablets 993
Zaroxolyn Tablets 1000

Minocycline Hydrochloride (Reduced absorption of tetracycline by approximately 28% to 37%). Products include:

Dynacin Capsules 1590
Minocin Intravenous 1382
Minocin Oral Suspension 1385
Minocin Pellet-Filled Capsules 1383

Oxytetracycline Hydrochloride (Reduced absorption of tetracycline by approximately 28% to 37%). Products include:

TERAK Ointment .... ⊙ 209
Terra-Cortril Ophthalmic Suspension 2210
Terramycin with Polymyxin B Sulfate Ophthalmic Ointment 2211
Urobiotic-250 Capsules 2214

Polythiazide (Occasional excessive reduction of blood pressure). Products include:

Minizide Capsules 1938

Potassium Acid Phosphate (Potential for hyperkalemia). Products include:

K-Phos Original Formula 'Sodium Free' Tablets 639

Potassium Bicarbonate (Potential for hyperkalemia). Products include:

Alka-Seltzer Gold Effervescent Antacid .... ▣ 703

Potassium Chloride (Potential for hyperkalemia). Products include:

Chlor-3 Condiment 1004
K-Dur Microburst Release System (potassium chloride, USP) E.R. Tablets 1325
K-Lor Powder Packets 434
K-Norm Extended-Release Capsules 991
K-Tab Filmtab 434
Kolyum Liquid 992
Micro-K 2063
Micro-K LS Packets 2064
NuLYTELY 689
Cherry Flavor NuLYTELY 689
Rum-K Syrup 1005
Slow-K Extended-Release Tablets 851

Potassium Citrate (Potential for hyperkalemia). Products include:

Polycitra Syrup 578
Polycitra-K Crystals 579
Polycitra-K Oral Solution 579
Polycitra-LC 578

Potassium Gluconate (Potential for hyperkalemia). Products include:

Kolyum Liquid 992

Potassium Phosphate, Dibasic (Potential for hyperkalemia).

No products indexed under this heading.

Potassium Phosphate, Monobasic (Potential for hyperkalemia). Products include:

K-Phos Neutral Tablets 639
K-Phos Original Formula 'Sodium Free' Tablets 639

Spironolactone (Occasional excessive reduction of blood pressure; potential for hyperkalemia). Products include:

Aldactazide 2413
Aldactone 2414

Tetracycline Hydrochloride (Reduced absorption of tetracycline by approximately 28% to 37%). Products include:

Achromycin V Capsules 1367

Torsemide (Occasional excessive reduction of blood pressure). Products include:

Demadex Tablets and Injection 686

Triamterene (Occasional excessive reduction of blood pressure; potential for hyperkalemia). Products include:

Dyazide 2479
Dyrenium Capsules 2481
Maxzide 1380

Food Interactions

Diet, high-lipid (Rate and extent of Quinapril absorption are diminished moderately).

ACCUTANE CAPSULES

(Isotretinoin) 2076

May interact with:

Vitamin A (Additive Vitamin A toxicity). Products include:

Aquasol A Vitamin A Capsules, USP 534
Aquasol A Parenteral 534
Materna Tablets 1379
Megadose 512
Nature Made Antioxidant Formula .... ▣ 748
One-A-Day Extras Antioxidant .... ▣ 728
Theragran Antioxidant .... ▣ 623
Zymacap Capsules .... ▣ 772

Food Interactions

Dairy products (Increases oral absorption of isotretinoin).

Food, unspecified (Increases oral absorption of isotretinoin).

ACEL-IMUNE DIPHTHERIA AND TETANUS TOXOIDS AND ACELLULAR PERTUSSIS VACCINE ADSORBED

(Diphtheria & Tetanus Toxoids w/Pertussis Vaccine Combined, Aluminum Phosphate Adsorbed) 1364

May interact with immunosuppressive agents, corticosteroids, cytotoxic drugs, alkylating agents, anticoagulants, and certain other agents. Compounds in these categories include:

Azathioprine (Reduces response to active immunization procedures). Products include:

Imuran 1110

(▣ Described in PDR For Nonprescription Drugs) (⊙ Described in PDR For Ophthalmology)

Betamethasone Acetate (Reduces response to active immunization procedures). Products include:
- Celestone Soluspan Suspension 2347

Betamethasone Sodium Phosphate (Reduces response to active immunization procedures). Products include:
- Celestone Soluspan Suspension 2347

Bleomycin Sulfate (Reduces response to active immunization procedures). Products include:
- Blenoxane 692

Busulfan (Reduces response to active immunization procedures). Products include:
- Myleran Tablets 1143

Carmustine (BCNU) (Reduces response to active immunization procedures). Products include:
- BiCNU 691

Chlorambucil (Reduces response to active immunization procedures). Products include:
- Leukeran Tablets 1133

Cortisone Acetate (Reduces response to active immunization procedures). Products include:
- Cortone Acetate Sterile Suspension 1623
- Cortone Acetate Tablets 1624

Cyclophosphamide (Reduces response to active immunization procedures). Products include:
- Cytoxan 694
- NEOSAR Lyophilized/Neosar 1959

Cyclosporine (Reduces response to active immunization procedures). Products include:
- Neoral 2276
- Sandimmune 2286

Dacarbazine (Reduces response to active immunization procedures). Products include:
- DTIC-Dome 600

Dalteparin Sodium (Caution should be exercised). Products include:
- Fragmin 1954

Daunorubicin Hydrochloride (Reduces response to active immunization procedures). Products include:
- Cerubidine 795

Dexamethasone (Reduces response to active immunization procedures). Products include:
- AK-Trol Ointment & Suspension ...... ◉ 205
- Decadron Elixir 1633
- Decadron Tablets 1635
- Decaspray Topical Aerosol 1648
- Dexacidin Ointment ...... ◉ 263
- Maxitrol Ophthalmic Ointment and Suspension ...... ◉ 224
- TobraDex Ophthalmic Suspension and Ointment 473

Dexamethasone Acetate (Reduces response to active immunization procedures). Products include:
- Dalalone D.P. Injectable 1011
- Decadron-LA Sterile Suspension 1646

Dexamethasone Sodium Phosphate (Reduces response to active immunization procedures). Products include:
- Decadron Phosphate Injection 1637
- Decadron Phosphate Respihaler 1642
- Decadron Phosphate Sterile Ophthalmic Ointment 1641
- Decadron Phosphate Sterile Ophthalmic Solution 1642
- Decadron Phosphate Topical Cream 1644
- Decadron Phosphate Turbinaire 1645
- Decadron Phosphate with Xylocaine Injection, Sterile 1639
- Dexacort Phosphate in Respihaler .. 458
- Dexacort Phosphate in Turbinaire .. 459
- NeoDecadron Sterile Ophthalmic Ointment 1712
- NeoDecadron Sterile Ophthalmic Solution 1713
- NeoDecadron Topical Cream 1714

Dicumarol (Caution should be exercised).
- No products indexed under this heading.

Doxorubicin Hydrochloride (Reduces response to active immunization procedures). Products include:
- Adriamycin PFS 1947
- Adriamycin RDF 1947
- Doxorubicin Astra 540
- Rubex 712

Enoxaparin (Caution should be exercised). Products include:
- Lovenox Injection 2020

Fludrocortisone Acetate (Reduces response to active immunization procedures). Products include:
- Florinef Acetate Tablets 505

Fluorouracil (Reduces response to active immunization procedures). Products include:
- Efudex 2113
- Fluoroplex Topical Solution & Cream 1% 479
- Fluorouracil Injection 2116

Heparin Calcium (Caution should be exercised).
- No products indexed under this heading.

Heparin Sodium (Caution should be exercised). Products include:
- Heparin Lock Flush Solution 2725
- Heparin Sodium Injection 2726
- Heparin Sodium Injection, USP, Sterile Solution 2615
- Heparin Sodium Vials 1441

Hydrocortisone (Reduces response to active immunization procedures). Products include:
- Anusol-HC Cream 2.5% 1896
- Aquanil HC Lotion 1931
- Bactine Hydrocortisone Anti-Itch Cream ...... ▣ 709
- Caldecort Anti-Itch Hydrocortisone Spray ...... ▣ 631
- Cortaid ...... ▣ 836
- CORTENEMA 2535
- Cortisporin Ointment 1085
- Cortisporin Ophthalmic Ointment Sterile 1085
- Cortisporin Ophthalmic Suspension Sterile 1086
- Cortisporin Otic Solution Sterile 1087
- Cortisporin Otic Suspension Sterile 1088
- Cortizone-5 ...... ▣ 831
- Cortizone-10 ...... ▣ 831
- Hydrocortone Tablets 1672
- Hytone 907
- Massengill Medicated Soft Cloth Towelettes 2458
- PediOtic Suspension Sterile 1153
- Preparation H Hydrocortisone 1% Cream ...... ▣ 872
- ProctoCream-HC 2.5% 2408
- VōSoL HC Otic Solution 2678

Hydrocortisone Acetate (Reduces response to active immunization procedures). Products include:
- Analpram-HC Rectal Cream 1% and 2.5% 977
- Anusol HC-1 Anti-Itch Hydrocortisone Ointment ...... ▣ 847
- Anusol-HC Suppositories 1897
- Caldecort ...... ▣ 631
- Carmol HC 924
- Coly-Mycin S Otic w/Neomycin & Hydrocortisone 1906
- Cortaid ...... ▣ 836
- Cortifoam 2396
- Cortisporin Cream 1084
- Epifoam 2399
- Hydrocortone Acetate Sterile Suspension 1669
- Mantadil Cream 1135
- Nupercainal Hydrocortisone 1% Cream ...... ▣ 645
- Ophthocort ...... ◉ 311
- Pramosone Cream, Lotion & Ointment 978
- ProctoCream-HC 2408
- ProctoFoam-HC 2409
- Terra-Cortril Ophthalmic Suspension 2210

Hydrocortisone Sodium Phosphate (Reduces response to active immunization procedures). Products include:
- Hydrocortone Phosphate Injection, Sterile 1670

Hydrocortisone Sodium Succinate (Reduces response to active immunization procedures). Products include:
- Solu-Cortef Sterile Powder 2641

Hydroxyurea (Reduces response to active immunization procedures). Products include:
- Hydrea Capsules 696

Immune Globulin (Human) (Reduces response to active immunization procedures).
- No products indexed under this heading.

Immune Globulin Intravenous (Human) (Reduces response to active immunization procedures).

Lomustine (CCNU) (Reduces response to active immunization procedures). Products include:
- CeeNU 693

Mechlorethamine Hydrochloride (Reduces response to active immunization procedures). Products include:
- Mustargen 1709

Melphalan (Reduces response to active immunization procedures). Products include:
- Alkeran Tablets 1071

Methotrexate Sodium (Reduces response to active immunization procedures). Products include:
- Methotrexate Sodium Tablets, Injection, for Injection and LPF Injection 1275

Methylprednisolone Acetate (Reduces response to active immunization procedures). Products include:
- Depo-Medrol Single-Dose Vial 2600
- Depo-Medrol Sterile Aqueous Suspension 2597

Methylprednisolone Sodium Succinate (Reduces response to active immunization procedures). Products include:
- Solu-Medrol Sterile Powder 2643

Mitotane (Reduces response to active immunization procedures). Products include:
- Lysodren 698

Mitoxantrone Hydrochloride (Reduces response to active immunization procedures). Products include:
- Novantrone 1279

Muromonab-CD3 (Reduces response to active immunization procedures). Products include:
- Orthoclone OKT3 Sterile Solution .. 1837

Mycophenolate Mofetil (Reduces response to active immunization procedures). Products include:
- CellCept Capsules 2099

Prednisolone Acetate (Reduces response to active immunization procedures). Products include:
- AK-CIDE ...... ◉ 202
- AK-CIDE Ointment ...... ◉ 202
- Blephamide Liquifilm Sterile Ophthalmic Suspension 476
- Blephamide Ointment ...... ◉ 237
- Econopred & Econopred Plus Ophthalmic Suspensions ...... ◉ 217
- Poly-Pred Liquifilm ...... ◉ 248
- Pred Forte ...... ◉ 250
- Pred Mild ...... ◉ 253
- Pred-G Liquifilm Sterile Ophthalmic Suspension ...... ◉ 251
- Pred-G S.O.P. Sterile Ophthalmic Ointment ...... ◉ 252
- Vasocidin Ointment ...... ◉ 268

Prednisolone Sodium Phosphate (Reduces response to active immunization procedures). Products include:
- AK-Pred ...... ◉ 204
- Hydeltrasol Injection, Sterile 1665
- Inflamase ...... ◉ 265
- Pediapred Oral Liquid 995
- Vasocidin Ophthalmic Solution ...... ◉ 270

Prednisolone Tebutate (Reduces response to active immunization procedures). Products include:
- Hydeltra-T.B.A. Sterile Suspension 1667

Prednisone (Reduces response to active immunization procedures). Products include:
- Deltasone Tablets 2595

Procarbazine Hydrochloride (Reduces response to active immunization procedures). Products include:
- Matulane Capsules 2131

Tacrolimus (Reduces response to active immunization procedures). Products include:
- Prograf 1042

Tamoxifen Citrate (Reduces response to active immunization procedures). Products include:
- Nolvadex Tablets 2841

Thiotepa (Reduces response to active immunization procedures). Products include:
- Thioplex (Thiotepa For Injection) 1281

Triamcinolone (Reduces response to active immunization procedures). Products include:
- Aristocort Tablets 1022

Triamcinolone Acetonide (Reduces response to active immunization procedures). Products include:
- Aristocort A 0.025% Cream 1027
- Aristocort A 0.5% Cream 1031
- Aristocort A 0.1% Cream 1029
- Aristocort A 0.1% Ointment 1030
- Azmacort Oral Inhaler 2011
- Nasacort Nasal Inhaler 2024

Triamcinolone Diacetate (Reduces response to active immunization procedures). Products include:
- Aristocort Suspension (Forte Parenteral) 1027
- Aristocort Suspension (Intralesional) 1025

Triamcinolone Hexacetonide (Reduces response to active immunization procedures). Products include:
- Aristospan Suspension (Intra-articular) 1033
- Aristospan Suspension (Intralesional) 1032

Vincristine Sulfate (Reduces response to active immunization procedures). Products include:
- Oncovin Solution Vials & Hyporets 1466

Warfarin Sodium (Caution should be exercised). Products include:
- Coumadin 926

ACHROMYCIN V CAPSULES

(Tetracycline Hydrochloride) 1367

May interact with oral anticoagulants, penicillins, antacids, oral contraceptives, and certain other agents. Compounds in these categories include:

Aluminum Carbonate Gel (Impaired absorption of tetracycline). Products include:
- Basaljel 2703

Aluminum Hydroxide (Impaired absorption of tetracycline). Products include:
- ALternaGEL Liquid 1316
- Maximum Strength Ascriptin ...... ▣ 630
- Cama Arthritis Pain Reliever ...... ▣ 785

IMPORTANT NOTE: Always consult each drug listing in the patient's regimen for possible interactions.

Achromycin V Oral

Gaviscon Extra Strength Relief Formula Antacid Tablets.................. ✪ 819
Gaviscon Extra Strength Relief Formula Liquid Antacid .... ✪ 819
Gaviscon Liquid Antacid .... ✪ 820
Gelusil Liquid & Tablets .... ✪ 855
Maalox Heartburn Relief Suspension .... ✪ 642
Maalox Heartburn Relief Tablets.... ✪ 641
Maalox Magnesia and Alumina Oral Suspension .... ✪ 642
Maalox Plus Tablets .... ✪ 643
Extra Strength Maalox Antacid Plus Antigas Liquid and Tablets ✪ 638
Tempo Soft Antacid .... ✪ 835

Aluminum Hydroxide Gel (Impaired absorption of tetracycline). Products include:

ALternaGEL Liquid .... ✪ 659
Aludrox Oral Suspension 2695
Amphojel Suspension 2695
Amphojel Suspension without Flavor 2695
Amphojel Tablets 2695
Arthritis Pain Ascriptin .... ✪ 631
Regular Strength Ascriptin Tablets .... ✪ 629
Gaviscon Antacid Tablets .... ✪ 819
Gaviscon-2 Antacid Tablets .... ✪ 820
Mylanta Liquid 1317
Mylanta Tablets .... ✪ 660
Mylanta Double Strength Liquid 1317
Mylanta Double Strength Tablets .. ✪ 660
Nephrox Suspension .... ✪ 655

Amoxicillin Trihydrate (Interference with bactericidal action of penicillin). Products include:

Amoxil 2464
Augmentin 2468

Ampicillin (Interference with bactericidal action of penicillin). Products include:

Omnipen Capsules 2764
Omnipen for Oral Suspension 2765

Ampicillin Sodium (Interference with bactericidal action of penicillin). Products include:

Unasyn 2212

Ampicillin Trihydrate (Interference with bactericidal action of penicillin).

No products indexed under this heading.

Azlocillin Sodium (Interference with bactericidal action of penicillin).

No products indexed under this heading.

Bacampicillin Hydrochloride (Interference with bactericidal action of penicillin). Products include:

Spectrobid Tablets 2206

Carbenicillin Disodium (Interference with bactericidal action of penicillin).

No products indexed under this heading.

Carbenicillin Indanyl Sodium (Interference with bactericidal action of penicillin). Products include:

Geocillin Tablets 2199

Desogestrel (Reduced efficacy and increased incidence of breakthrough bleeding). Products include:

Desogen Tablets 1817
Ortho-Cept 1851

Dicloxacillin Sodium (Interference with bactericidal action of penicillin).

No products indexed under this heading.

Dicumarol (Depressed plasma prothombin activity; downward adjustment of anticoagulant dosage may be necessary).

No products indexed under this heading.

Dihydroxyaluminum Sodium Carbonate (Impaired absorption of tetracycline).

No products indexed under this heading.

Ethinyl Estradiol (Reduced efficacy and increased incidence of breakthrough bleeding). Products include:

Brevicon 2088
Demulen 2428
Desogen Tablets 1817
Levlen/Tri-Levlen 651
Lo/Ovral Tablets 2746
Lo/Ovral-28 Tablets 2751
Modicon 1872
Nordette-21 Tablets 2755
Nordette-28 Tablets 2758
Norinyl 2088
Ortho-Cept 1851
Ortho-Cyclen/Ortho-Tri-Cyclen 1858
Ortho-Novum 1872
Ortho-Cyclen/Ortho Tri-Cyclen 1858
Ovcon 760
Ovral Tablets 2770
Ovral-28 Tablets 2770
Levlen/Tri-Levlen 651
Tri-Norinyl 2164
Triphasil-21 Tablets 2814
Triphasil-28 Tablets 2819

Ethynodiol Diacetate (Reduced efficacy and increased incidence of breakthrough bleeding). Products include:

Demulen 2428

Levonorgestrel (Reduced efficacy and increased incidence of breakthrough bleeding). Products include:

Levlen/Tri-Levlen 651
Nordette-21 Tablets 2755
Nordette-28 Tablets 2758
Norplant System 2759
Levlen/Tri-Levlen 651
Triphasil-21 Tablets 2814
Triphasil-28 Tablets 2819

Magaldrate (Impaired absorption of tetracycline).

No products indexed under this heading.

Magnesium Hydroxide (Impaired absorption of tetracycline). Products include:

Aludrox Oral Suspension 2695
Arthritis Pain Ascriptin .... ✪ 631
Maximum Strength Ascriptin .... ✪ 630
Regular Strength Ascriptin Tablets .... ✪ 629
Di-Gel Antacid/Anti-Gas .... ✪ 801
Gelusil Liquid & Tablets .... ✪ 855
Maalox Magnesia and Alumina Oral Suspension .... ✪ 642
Maalox Plus Tablets .... ✪ 643
Extra Strength Maalox Antacid Plus Antigas Liquid and Tablets ✪ 638
Mylanta Calcium Carbonate and Magnesium Hydroxide Tablets...... 1318
Mylanta Liquid 1317
Mylanta Tablets .... ✪ 660
Mylanta Double Strength Liquid 1317
Mylanta Double Strength Tablets .. ✪ 660
Phillips' Milk of Magnesia Liquid.... ✪ 729
Rolaids Tablets .... ✪ 843
Tempo Soft Antacid .... ✪ 835

Magnesium Oxide (Impaired absorption of tetracycline). Products include:

Beelith Tablets 639
Bufferin Analgesic Tablets and Caplets .... ✪ 613
Caltrate PLUS .... ✪ 665
Cama Arthritis Pain Reliever .... ✪ 785
Mag-Ox 400 668
Uro-Mag 668

Mestranol (Reduced efficacy and increased incidence of breakthrough bleeding). Products include:

Norinyl 2088
Ortho-Novum 1872

Mezlocillin Sodium (Interference with bactericidal action of penicillin). Products include:

Mezlin 601
Mezlin Pharmacy Bulk Package 604

Nafcillin Sodium (Interference with bactericidal action of penicillin).

No products indexed under this heading.

Norethindrone (Reduced efficacy and increased incidence of breakthrough bleeding). Products include:

Brevicon 2088
Micronor Tablets 1872
Modicon 1872
Norinyl 2088
Nor-Q D Tablets 2135
Ortho-Novum 1872
Ovcon 760
Tri-Norinyl 2164

Norethynodrel (Reduced efficacy and increased incidence of breakthrough bleeding).

No products indexed under this heading.

Norgestimate (Reduced efficacy and increased incidence of breakthrough bleeding). Products include:

Ortho-Cyclen/Ortho-Tri-Cyclen 1858
Ortho-Cyclen/Ortho Tri-Cyclen 1858

Norgestrel (Reduced efficacy and increased incidence of breakthrough bleeding). Products include:

Lo/Ovral Tablets 2746
Lo/Ovral-28 Tablets 2751
Ovral Tablets 2770
Ovral-28 Tablets 2770
Ovrette Tablets 2771

Penicillin G Benzathine (Interference with bactericidal action of penicillin). Products include:

Bicillin C-R Injection 2704
Bicillin C-R 900/300 Injection 2706
Bicillin L-A Injection 2707

Penicillin G Potassium (Interference with bactericidal action of penicillin). Products include:

Pfizerpen for Injection 2203

Penicillin G Procaine (Interference with bactericidal action of penicillin). Products include:

Bicillin C-R Injection 2704
Bicillin C-R 900/300 Injection 2706

Penicillin G Sodium (Interference with bactericidal action of penicillin).

No products indexed under this heading.

Penicillin V Potassium (Interference with bactericidal action of penicillin). Products include:

Pen•Vee K 2772

Sodium Bicarbonate (Impaired absorption of tetracycline). Products include:

Alka-Seltzer Effervescent Antacid and Pain Reliever .... ✪ 701
Alka-Seltzer Extra Strength Effervescent Antacid and Pain Reliever .... ✪ 703
Alka-Seltzer Gold Effervescent Antacid .... ✪ 703
Alka-Seltzer Lemon Lime Effervescent Antacid and Pain Reliever .... ✪ 703
Arm & Hammer Pure Baking Soda .... ✪ 627
Ceo-Two Rectal Suppositories 666
Citrocarbonate Antacid .... ✪ 770
Massengill Disposable Douches ...... ✪ 820
Massengill Liquid Concentrate .... ✪ 820
NuLYTELY 689
Cherry Flavor NuLYTELY 689

Ticarcillin Disodium (Interference with bactericidal action of penicillin). Products include:

Ticar for Injection 2526
Timentin for Injection 2528

Warfarin Sodium (Depressed plasma prothombin activity; downward adjustment of anticoagulant dosage may be necessary). Products include:

Coumadin 926

Food Interactions

Dairy products (Interferes with absorption of oral forms of tetracycline).

Food, unspecified (Interferes with absorption of oral forms of tetracycline).

ACID MANTLE CREME

(Petrolatum, White) .... ✪ 785
None cited in PDR database.

ACI-JEL THERAPEUTIC VAGINAL JELLY

(Acetic Acid, Oxyquinoline Sulfate) 1848
None cited in PDR database.

ACLOVATE CREAM

(Alclometasone Dipropionate) 1069
None cited in PDR database.

ACLOVATE OINTMENT

(Alclometasone Dipropionate) 1069
None cited in PDR database.

ACTHIB

(Haemophilus B Conjugate Vaccine).. **872**
May interact with immunosuppressive agents, alkylating agents, cytotoxic drugs, corticosteroids, and anticoagulants. Compounds in these categories include:

Azathioprine (May reduce the immune response to vaccine). Products include:

Imuran 1110

Betamethasone Acetate (Corticosteroids, when used in greater than physiologic doses, may reduce the immune response to vaccine). Products include:

Celestone Soluspan Suspension 2347

Betamethasone Sodium Phosphate (Corticosteroids, when used in greater than physiologic doses, may reduce the immune response to vaccine). Products include:

Celestone Soluspan Suspension 2347

Bleomycin Sulfate (May reduce the immune response to vaccine). Products include:

Blenoxane 692

Busulfan (May reduce the immune response to vaccine). Products include:

Myleran Tablets 1143

Carmustine (BCNU) (May reduce the immune response to vaccine). Products include:

BiCNU 691

Chlorambucil (May reduce the immune response to vaccine). Products include:

Leukeran Tablets 1133

Cortisone Acetate (Corticosteroids, when used in greater than physiologic doses, may reduce the immune response to vaccine). Products include:

Cortone Acetate Sterile Suspension 1623
Cortone Acetate Tablets 1624

Cyclophosphamide (May reduce the immune response to vaccine). Products include:

Cytoxan 694
NEOSAR Lyophilized/Neosar 1959

Cyclosporine (May reduce the immune response to vaccine). Products include:

Neoral 2276
Sandimmune 2286

Dacarbazine (May reduce the immune response to vaccine). Products include:

DTIC-Dome 600

Dalteparin Sodium (Use with caution). Products include:

Fragmin 1954

Daunorubicin Hydrochloride (May reduce the immune response to vaccine). Products include:

Cerubidine 795

(✪ Described in PDR For Nonprescription Drugs) (◉ Described in PDR For Ophthalmology)

5 **Interactions Index** **Actifed Allergy**

Dexamethasone (Corticosteroids, when used in greater than physiologic doses, may reduce the immune response to vaccine). Products include:

- AK-Trol Ointment & Suspension ◉ 205
- Decadron Elixir 1633
- Decadron Tablets 1635
- Decaspray Topical Aerosol 1648
- Dexacidin Ointment ◉ 263
- Maxitrol Ophthalmic Ointment and Suspension ◉ 224
- TobraDex Ophthalmic Suspension and Ointment 473

Dexamethasone Acetate (Corticosteroids, when used in greater than physiologic doses, may reduce the immune response to vaccine). Products include:

- Dalalone D.P. Injectable 1011
- Decadron-LA Sterile Suspension 1646

Dexamethasone Sodium Phosphate (Corticosteroids, when used in greater than physiologic doses, may reduce the immune response to vaccine). Products include:

- Decadron Phosphate Injection 1637
- Decadron Phosphate Respihaler 1642
- Decadron Phosphate Sterile Ophthalmic Ointment 1641
- Decadron Phosphate Sterile Ophthalmic Solution 1642
- Decadron Phosphate Topical Cream 1644
- Decadron Phosphate Turbinaire 1645
- Decadron Phosphate with Xylocaine Injection, Sterile 1639
- Dexacort Phosphate in Respihaler 458
- Dexacort Phosphate in Turbinaire 459
- NeoDecadron Sterile Ophthalmic Ointment 1712
- NeoDecadron Sterile Ophthalmic Solution 1713
- NeoDecadron Topical Cream 1714

Dicumarol (Use with caution).

- No products indexed under this heading.

Doxorubicin Hydrochloride (May reduce the immune response to vaccine). Products include:

- Adriamycin PFS 1947
- Adriamycin RDF 1947
- Doxorubicin Astra 540
- Rubex 712

Enoxaparin (Use with caution). Products include:

- Lovenox Injection 2020

Fludrocortisone Acetate (Corticosteroids, when used in greater than physiologic doses, may reduce the immune response to vaccine). Products include:

- Florinef Acetate Tablets 505

Fluorouracil (May reduce the immune response to vaccine). Products include:

- Efudex 2113
- Fluoroplex Topical Solution & Cream 1% 479
- Fluorouracil Injection 2116

Heparin Calcium (Use with caution).

- No products indexed under this heading.

Heparin Sodium (Use with caution). Products include:

- Heparin Lock Flush Solution 2725
- Heparin Sodium Injection 2726
- Heparin Sodium Injection, USP, Sterile Solution 2615
- Heparin Sodium Vials 1441

Hydrocortisone (Corticosteroids, when used in greater than physiologic doses, may reduce the immune response to vaccine). Products include:

- Anusol-HC Cream 2.5% 1896
- Aquanil HC Lotion 1931
- Bactine Hydrocortisone Anti-Itch Cream ▣ 709
- Caldecort Anti-Itch Hydrocortisone Spray ▣ 631
- Cortaid ▣ 836
- CORTENEMA 2535
- Cortisporin Ointment 1085
- Cortisporin Ophthalmic Ointment Sterile 1085
- Cortisporin Ophthalmic Suspension Sterile 1086
- Cortisporin Otic Solution Sterile 1087
- Cortisporin Otic Suspension Sterile 1088
- Cortizone-5 ▣ 831
- Cortizone-10 ▣ 831
- Hydrocortone Tablets 1672
- Hytone 907
- Massengill Medicated Soft Cloth Towelettes 2458
- PediOtic Suspension Sterile 1153
- Preparation H Hydrocortisone 1% Cream ▣ 872
- ProctoCream-HC 2.5% 2408
- VōSoL HC Otic Solution 2678

Hydrocortisone Acetate (Corticosteroids, when used in greater than physiologic doses, may reduce the immune response to vaccine). Products include:

- Analpram-HC Rectal Cream 1% and 2.5% 977
- Anusol HC-1 Anti-Itch Hydrocortisone Ointment ▣ 847
- Anusol-HC Suppositories 1897
- Caldecort ▣ 631
- Carmol HC 924
- Coly-Mycin S Otic w/Neomycin & Hydrocortisone 1906
- Cortaid ▣ 836
- Cortifoam 2396
- Cortisporin Cream 1084
- Epifoam 2399
- Hydrocortone Acetate Sterile Suspension 1669
- Mantadil Cream 1135
- Nupercainal Hydrocortisone 1% Cream ▣ 645
- Ophthocort ◉ 311
- Pramosone Cream, Lotion & Ointment 978
- ProctoCream-HC 2408
- ProctoFoam-HC 2409
- Terra-Cortril Ophthalmic Suspension 2210

Hydrocortisone Sodium Phosphate (Corticosteroids, when used in greater than physiologic doses, may reduce the immune response to vaccine). Products include:

- Hydrocortone Phosphate Injection, Sterile 1670

Hydrocortisone Sodium Succinate (Corticosteroids, when used in greater than physiologic doses, may reduce the immune response to vaccine). Products include:

- Solu-Cortef Sterile Powder 2641

Hydroxyurea (May reduce the immune response to vaccine). Products include:

- Hydrea Capsules 696

Immune Globulin (Human) (May reduce the immune response to vaccine).

- No products indexed under this heading.

Lomustine (CCNU) (May reduce the immune response to vaccine). Products include:

- CeeNU 693

Mechlorethamine Hydrochloride (May reduce the immune response to vaccine). Products include:

- Mustargen 1709

Melphalan (May reduce the immune response to vaccine). Products include:

- Alkeran Tablets 1071

Methotrexate Sodium (May reduce the immune response to vaccine). Products include:

- Methotrexate Sodium Tablets, Injection, for Injection and LPF Injection 1275

Methylprednisolone Acetate (Corticosteroids, when used in greater than physiologic doses, may reduce the immune response to vaccine). Products include:

- Depo-Medrol Single-Dose Vial 2600
- Depo-Medrol Sterile Aqueous Suspension 2597

Methylprednisolone Sodium Succinate (Corticosteroids, when used in greater than physiologic doses, may reduce the immune response to vaccine). Products include:

- Solu-Medrol Sterile Powder 2643

Mitotane (May reduce the immune response to vaccine). Products include:

- Lysodren 698

Mitoxantrone Hydrochloride (May reduce the immune response to vaccine). Products include:

- Novantrone 1279

Muromonab-CD3 (May reduce the immune response to vaccine). Products include:

- Orthoclone OKT3 Sterile Solution 1837

Mycophenolate Mofetil (May reduce the immune response to vaccine). Products include:

- CellCept Capsules 2099

Prednisolone Acetate (Corticosteroids, when used in greater than physiologic doses, may reduce the immune response to vaccine). Products include:

- AK-CIDE ◉ 202
- AK-CIDE Ointment ◉ 202
- Blephamide Liquifilm Sterile Ophthalmic Suspension 476
- Blephamide Ointment ◉ 237
- Econopred & Econopred Plus Ophthalmic Suspensions ◉ 217
- Poly-Pred Liquifilm ◉ 248
- Pred Forte ◉ 250
- Pred Mild ◉ 253
- Pred-G Liquifilm Sterile Ophthalmic Suspension ◉ 251
- Pred-G S.O.P. Sterile Ophthalmic Ointment ◉ 252
- Vasocidin Ointment ◉ 268

Prednisolone Sodium Phosphate (Corticosteroids, when used in greater than physiologic doses, may reduce the immune response to vaccine). Products include:

- AK-Pred ◉ 204
- Hydeltrasol Injection, Sterile 1665
- Inflamase ◉ 265
- Pediapred Oral Liquid 995
- Vasocidin Ophthalmic Solution ◉ 270

Prednisolone Tebutate (Corticosteroids, when used in greater than physiologic doses, may reduce the immune response to vaccine). Products include:

- Hydeltra-T.B.A. Sterile Suspension 1667

Prednisone (Corticosteroids, when used in greater than physiologic doses, may reduce the immune response to vaccine). Products include:

- Deltasone Tablets 2595

Procarbazine Hydrochloride (May reduce the immune response to vaccine). Products include:

- Matulane Capsules 2131

Tacrolimus (May reduce the immune response to vaccine). Products include:

- Prograf 1042

Tamoxifen Citrate (May reduce the immune response to vaccine). Products include:

- Nolvadex Tablets 2841

Thiotepa (May reduce the immune response to vaccine). Products include:

- Thioplex (Thiotepa For Injection) 1281

Triamcinolone (Corticosteroids, when used in greater than physiologic doses, may reduce the immune response to vaccine). Products include:

- Aristocort Tablets 1022

Triamcinolone Acetonide (Corticosteroids, when used in greater than physiologic doses, may reduce the immune response to vaccine). Products include:

- Aristocort A 0.025% Cream 1027
- Aristocort A 0.5% Cream 1031
- Aristocort A 0.1% Cream 1029
- Aristocort A 0.1% Ointment 1030
- Azmacort Oral Inhaler 2011
- Nasacort Nasal Inhaler 2024

Triamcinolone Diacetate (Corticosteroids, when used in greater than physiologic doses, may reduce the immune response to vaccine). Products include:

- Aristocort Suspension (Forte Parenteral) 1027
- Aristocort Suspension (Intralesional) 1025

Triamcinolone Hexacetonide (Corticosteroids, when used in greater than physiologic doses, may reduce the immune response to vaccine). Products include:

- Aristospan Suspension (Intra-articular) 1033
- Aristospan Suspension (Intralesional) 1032

Vincristine Sulfate (May reduce the immune response to vaccine). Products include:

- Oncovin Solution Vials & Hyporets 1466

Warfarin Sodium (Use with caution). Products include:

- Coumadin 926

ACTIFED ALLERGY DAYTIME/NIGHTTIME CAPLETS

(Diphenhydramine Hydrochloride, Pseudoephedrine Hydrochloride) ▣ 844

May interact with monoamine oxidase inhibitors, hypnotics and sedatives, tranquilizers, and certain other agents. Compounds in these categories include:

Alprazolam (Increases drowsiness effect). Products include:

- Xanax Tablets 2649

Buspirone Hydrochloride (Increases drowsiness effect). Products include:

- BuSpar 737

Chlordiazepoxide (Increases drowsiness effect). Products include:

- Libritabs Tablets 2177
- Limbitrol 2180

Chlordiazepoxide Hydrochloride (Increases drowsiness effect). Products include:

- Librax Capsules 2176
- Librium Capsules 2178
- Librium Injectable 2179

Chlorpromazine (Increases drowsiness effect). Products include:

- Thorazine Suppositories 2523

Chlorpromazine Hydrochloride (Increases drowsiness effect). Products include:

- Thorazine 2523

Chlorprothixene (Increases drowsiness effect).

- No products indexed under this heading.

Chlorprothixene Hydrochloride (Increases drowsiness effect).

- No products indexed under this heading.

Clorazepate Dipotassium (Increases drowsiness effect). Products include:

- Tranxene 451

IMPORTANT NOTE: Always consult each drug listing in the patient's regimen for possible interactions.

Actifed Allergy

Diazepam (Increases drowsiness effect). Products include:

Dizac 1809
Valium Injectable 2182
Valium Tablets 2183
Valrelease Capsules 2169

Droperidol (Increases drowsiness effect). Products include:

Inapsine Injection...................................... 1296

Estazolam (Increases drowsiness effect). Products include:

ProSom Tablets 449

Ethchlorvynol (Increases drowsiness effect). Products include:

Placidyl Capsules 448

Ethinamate (Increases drowsiness effect).

No products indexed under this heading.

Fluphenazine Decanoate (Increases drowsiness effect). Products include:

Prolixin Decanoate 509

Fluphenazine Enanthate (Increases drowsiness effect). Products include:

Prolixin Enanthate 509

Fluphenazine Hydrochloride (Increases drowsiness effect). Products include:

Prolixin 509

Flurazepam Hydrochloride (Increases drowsiness effect). Products include:

Dalmane Capsules..................................... 2173

Furazolidone (Concurrent administration is not recommended). Products include:

Furoxone 2046

Glutethimide (Increases drowsiness effect).

No products indexed under this heading.

Haloperidol (Increases drowsiness effect). Products include:

Haldol Injection, Tablets and Concentrate 1575

Haloperidol Decanoate (Increases drowsiness effect). Products include:

Haldol Decanoate...................................... 1577

Hydroxyzine Hydrochloride (Increases drowsiness effect). Products include:

Atarax Tablets & Syrup............................. 2185
Marax Tablets & DF Syrup....................... 2200
Vistaril Intramuscular Solution.......... 2216

Isocarboxazid (Concurrent administration is not recommended).

No products indexed under this heading.

Lorazepam (Increases drowsiness effect). Products include:

Ativan Injection... 2698
Ativan Tablets 2700

Loxapine Hydrochloride (Increases drowsiness effect). Products include:

Loxitane 1378

Loxapine Succinate (Increases drowsiness effect). Products include:

Loxitane Capsules 1378

Meprobamate (Increases drowsiness effect). Products include:

Miltown Tablets 2672
PMB 200 and PMB 400 2783

Mesoridazine Besylate (Increases drowsiness effect). Products include:

Serentil.. 684

Midazolam Hydrochloride (Increases drowsiness effect). Products include:

Versed Injection 2170

Molindone Hydrochloride (Increases drowsiness effect). Products include:

Moban Tablets and Concentrate...... 1048

Oxazepam (Increases drowsiness effect). Products include:

Serax Capsules 2810
Serax Tablets... 2810

Perphenazine (Increases drowsiness effect). Products include:

Etrafon 2355
Triavil Tablets 1757
Trilafon.. 2389

Phenelzine Sulfate (Concurrent administration is not recommended). Products include:

Nardil 1920

Prazepam (Increases drowsiness effect).

No products indexed under this heading.

Prochlorperazine (Increases drowsiness effect). Products include:

Compazine 2470

Promethazine Hydrochloride (Increases drowsiness effect). Products include:

Mepergan Injection 2753
Phenergan with Codeine........................... 2777
Phenergan with Dextromethorphan 2778
Phenergan Injection 2773
Phenergan Suppositories........................... 2775
Phenergan Syrup 2774
Phenergan Tablets 2775
Phenergan VC 2779
Phenergan VC with Codeine 2781

Propofol (Increases drowsiness effect). Products include:

Diprivan Injection...................................... 2833

Quazepam (Increases drowsiness effect). Products include:

Doral Tablets 2664

Secobarbital Sodium (Increases drowsiness effect). Products include:

Seconal Sodium Pulvules 1474

Selegiline Hydrochloride (Concurrent administration is not recommended). Products include:

Eldepryl Tablets 2550

Temazepam (Increases drowsiness effect). Products include:

Restoril Capsules 2284

Thioridazine Hydrochloride (Increases drowsiness effect). Products include:

Mellaril 2269

Thiothixene (Increases drowsiness effect). Products include:

Navane Capsules and Concentrate 2201
Navane Intramuscular 2202

Tranylcypromine Sulfate (Concurrent administration is not recommended). Products include:

Parnate Tablets 2503

Triazolam (Increases drowsiness effect). Products include:

Halcion Tablets.. 2611

Trifluoperazine Hydrochloride (Increases drowsiness effect). Products include:

Stelazine 2514

Zolpidem Tartrate (Increases drowsiness effect). Products include:

Ambien Tablets.. 2416

Food Interactions

Alcohol (Increases drowsiness effect).

ACTIFED PLUS CAPLETS

(Acetaminophen, Pseudoephedrine Hydrochloride, Triprolidine Hydrochloride)....................................... ᴿᴰ 845

May interact with monoamine oxidase inhibitors, hypnotics and sedatives, tranquilizers, and certain other agents. Compounds in these categories include:

Alprazolam (Increases drowsiness effect). Products include:

Xanax Tablets 2649

Buspirone Hydrochloride (Increases drowsiness effect). Products include:

BuSpar 737

Chlordiazepoxide (Increases drowsiness effect). Products include:

Libritabs Tablets 2177
Limbitrol 2180

Chlordiazepoxide Hydrochloride (Increases drowsiness effect). Products include:

Librax Capsules 2176
Librium Capsules...................................... 2178
Librium Injectable 2179

Chlorpromazine (Increases drowsiness effect). Products include:

Thorazine Suppositories 2523

Chlorpromazine Hydrochloride (Increases drowsiness effect). Products include:

Thorazine 2523

Chlorprothixene (Increases drowsiness effect).

No products indexed under this heading.

Chlorprothixene Hydrochloride (Increases drowsiness effect).

No products indexed under this heading.

Clorazepate Dipotassium (Increases drowsiness effect). Products include:

Tranxene 451

Diazepam (Increases drowsiness effect). Products include:

Dizac 1809
Valium Injectable 2182
Valium Tablets 2183
Valrelease Capsules 2169

Droperidol (Increases drowsiness effect). Products include:

Inapsine Injection...................................... 1296

Estazolam (Increases drowsiness effect). Products include:

ProSom Tablets 449

Ethchlorvynol (Increases drowsiness effect). Products include:

Placidyl Capsules 448

Ethinamate (Increases drowsiness effect).

No products indexed under this heading.

Fluphenazine Decanoate (Increases drowsiness effect). Products include:

Prolixin Decanoate 509

Fluphenazine Enanthate (Increases drowsiness effect). Products include:

Prolixin Enanthate 509

Fluphenazine Hydrochloride (Increases drowsiness effect). Products include:

Prolixin 509

Flurazepam Hydrochloride (Increases drowsiness effect). Products include:

Dalmane Capsules..................................... 2173

Furazolidone (Concurrent use not recommended). Products include:

Furoxone 2046

Glutethimide (Increases drowsiness effect).

No products indexed under this heading.

Haloperidol (Increases drowsiness effect). Products include:

Haldol Injection, Tablets and Concentrate 1575

Haloperidol Decanoate (Increases drowsiness effect). Products include:

Haldol Decanoate...................................... 1577

Hydroxyzine Hydrochloride (Increases drowsiness effect). Products include:

Atarax Tablets & Syrup............................. 2185
Marax Tablets & DF Syrup....................... 2200

Vistaril Intramuscular Solution.......... 2216

Isocarboxazid (Concurrent use not recommended).

No products indexed under this heading.

Lorazepam (Increases drowsiness effect). Products include:

Ativan Injection... 2698
Ativan Tablets 2700

Loxapine Hydrochloride (Increases drowsiness effect). Products include:

Loxitane 1378

Loxapine Succinate (Increases drowsiness effect). Products include:

Loxitane Capsules 1378

Meprobamate (Increases drowsiness effect). Products include:

Miltown Tablets 2672
PMB 200 and PMB 400 2783

Mesoridazine Besylate (Increases drowsiness effect). Products include:

Serentil.. 684

Midazolam Hydrochloride (Increases drowsiness effect). Products include:

Versed Injection 2170

Molindone Hydrochloride (Increases drowsiness effect). Products include:

Moban Tablets and Concentrate...... 1048

Oxazepam (Increases drowsiness effect). Products include:

Serax Capsules 2810
Serax Tablets... 2810

Perphenazine (Increases drowsiness effect). Products include:

Etrafon 2355
Triavil Tablets 1757
Trilafon.. 2389

Phenelzine Sulfate (Concurrent use not recommended). Products include:

Nardil 1920

Prazepam (Increases drowsiness effect).

No products indexed under this heading.

Prochlorperazine (Increases drowsiness effect). Products include:

Compazine 2470

Promethazine Hydrochloride (Increases drowsiness effect). Products include:

Mepergan Injection 2753
Phenergan with Codeine........................... 2777
Phenergan with Dextromethorphan 2778
Phenergan Injection 2773
Phenergan Suppositories 2775
Phenergan Syrup 2774
Phenergan Tablets 2775
Phenergan VC 2779
Phenergan VC with Codeine 2781

Propofol (Increases drowsiness effect). Products include:

Diprivan Injection...................................... 2833

Quazepam (Increases drowsiness effect). Products include:

Doral Tablets 2664

Secobarbital Sodium (Increases drowsiness effect). Products include:

Seconal Sodium Pulvules 1474

Selegiline Hydrochloride (Concurrent use not recommended). Products include:

Eldepryl Tablets 2550

Temazepam (Increases drowsiness effect). Products include:

Restoril Capsules 2284

Thioridazine Hydrochloride (Increases drowsiness effect). Products include:

Mellaril 2269

Thiothixene (Increases drowsiness effect). Products include:

Navane Capsules and Concentrate 2201
Navane Intramuscular 2202

Tranylcypromine Sulfate (Concurrent use not recommended). Products include:

Parnate Tablets 2503

Triazolam (Increases drowsiness effect). Products include:

Halcion Tablets 2611

Trifluoperazine Hydrochloride (Increases drowsiness effect). Products include:

Stelazine 2514

Zolpidem Tartrate (Increases drowsiness effect). Products include:

Ambien Tablets... 2416

Food Interactions

Alcohol (Increases drowsiness effect).

ACTIFED PLUS TABLETS

(Acetaminophen, Pseudoephedrine Hydrochloride, Triprolidine Hydrochloride) .... ◙ 845

May interact with monoamine oxidase inhibitors, hypnotics and sedatives, tranquilizers, and certain other agents. Compounds in these categories include:

Alprazolam (Increases drowsiness effect). Products include:

Xanax Tablets 2649

Buspirone Hydrochloride (Increases drowsiness effect). Products include:

BuSpar 737

Chlordiazepoxide (Increases drowsiness effect). Products include:

Libritabs Tablets 2177
Limbitrol 2180

Chlordiazepoxide Hydrochloride (Increases drowsiness effect). Products include:

Librax Capsules 2176
Librium Capsules 2178
Librium Injectable 2179

Chlorpromazine (Increases drowsiness effect). Products include:

Thorazine Suppositories........................... 2523

Chlorpromazine Hydrochloride (Increases drowsiness effect). Products include:

Thorazine 2523

Chlorprothixene (Increases drowsiness effect).

No products indexed under this heading.

Chlorprothixene Hydrochloride (Increases drowsiness effect).

No products indexed under this heading.

Clorazepate Dipotassium (Increases drowsiness effect). Products include:

Tranxene 451

Diazepam (Increases drowsiness effect). Products include:

Dizac 1809
Valium Injectable 2182
Valium Tablets 2183
Valrelease Capsules 2169

Droperidol (Increases drowsiness effect). Products include:

Inapsine Injection..................................... 1296

Estazolam (Increases drowsiness effect). Products include:

ProSom Tablets 449

Ethchlorvynol (Increases drowsiness effect). Products include:

Placidyl Capsules 448

Ethinamate (Increases drowsiness effect).

No products indexed under this heading.

Fluphenazine Decanoate (Increases drowsiness effect). Products include:

Prolixin Decanoate 509

Fluphenazine Enanthate (Increases drowsiness effect). Products include:

Prolixin Enanthate 509

Fluphenazine Hydrochloride (Increases drowsiness effect). Products include:

Prolixin 509

Flurazepam Hydrochloride (Increases drowsiness effect). Products include:

Dalmane Capsules 2173

Furazolidone (Concurrent use not recommended). Products include:

Furoxone 2046

Glutethimide (Increases drowsiness effect).

No products indexed under this heading.

Haloperidol (Increases drowsiness effect). Products include:

Haldol Injection, Tablets and Concentrate 1575

Haloperidol Decanoate (Increases drowsiness effect). Products include:

Haldol Decanoate...................................... 1577

Hydroxyzine Hydrochloride (Increases drowsiness effect). Products include:

Atarax Tablets & Syrup............................ 2185
Marax Tablets & DF Syrup....................... 2200
Vistaril Intramuscular Solution................ 2216

Isocarboxazid (Concurrent use not recommended).

No products indexed under this heading.

Lorazepam (Increases drowsiness effect). Products include:

Ativan Injection 2698
Ativan Tablets 2700

Loxapine Hydrochloride (Increases drowsiness effect). Products include:

Loxitane 1378

Loxapine Succinate (Increases drowsiness effect). Products include:

Loxitane Capsules 1378

Meprobamate (Increases drowsiness effect). Products include:

Miltown Tablets 2672
PMB 200 and PMB 400 2783

Mesoridazine Besylate (Increases drowsiness effect). Products include:

Serentil 684

Midazolam Hydrochloride (Increases drowsiness effect). Products include:

Versed Injection 2170

Molindone Hydrochloride (Increases drowsiness effect). Products include:

Moban Tablets and Concentrate 1048

Oxazepam (Increases drowsiness effect). Products include:

Serax Capsules 2810
Serax Tablets.. 2810

Perphenazine (Increases drowsiness effect). Products include:

Etrafon 2355
Triavil Tablets 1757
Trilafon... 2389

Phenelzine Sulfate (Concurrent use not recommended). Products include:

Nardil 1920

Prazepam (Increases drowsiness effect).

No products indexed under this heading.

Prochlorperazine (Increases drowsiness effect). Products include:

Compazine 2470

Promethazine Hydrochloride (Increases drowsiness effect). Products include:

Mepergan Injection 2753
Phenergan with Codeine........................... 2777
Phenergan with Dextromethorphan 2778
Phenergan Injection 2773
Phenergan Suppositories 2775
Phenergan Syrup 2774
Phenergan Tablets 2775
Phenergan VC 2779
Phenergan VC with Codeine 2781

Propofol (Increases drowsiness effect). Products include:

Diprivan Injection..................................... 2833

Quazepam (Increases drowsiness effect). Products include:

Doral Tablets.. 2664

Secobarbital Sodium (Increases drowsiness effect). Products include:

Seconal Sodium Pulvules 1474

Selegiline Hydrochloride (Concurrent use not recommended). Products include:

Eldepryl Tablets 2550

Temazepam (Increases drowsiness effect). Products include:

Restoril Capsules 2284

Thioridazine Hydrochloride (Increases drowsiness effect). Products include:

Mellaril 2269

Thiothixene (Increases drowsiness effect). Products include:

Navane Capsules and Concentrate 2201
Navane Intramuscular 2202

Tranylcypromine Sulfate (Concurrent use not recommended). Products include:

Parnate Tablets 2503

Triazolam (Increases drowsiness effect). Products include:

Halcion Tablets 2611

Trifluoperazine Hydrochloride (Increases drowsiness effect). Products include:

Stelazine 2514

Zolpidem Tartrate (Increases drowsiness effect). Products include:

Ambien Tablets... 2416

Food Interactions

Alcohol (Increases drowsiness effect).

ACTIFED WITH CODEINE COUGH SYRUP

(Codeine Phosphate, Triprolidine Hydrochloride, Pseudoephedrine Hydrochloride) 1067

May interact with central nervous system depressants, monoamine oxidase inhibitors, and certain other agents. Compounds in these categories include:

Alfentanil Hydrochloride (Increased CNS depression). Products include:

Alfenta Injection 1286

Alprazolam (Increased CNS depression). Products include:

Xanax Tablets 2649

Aprobarbital (Increased CNS depression).

No products indexed under this heading.

Buprenorphine (Increased CNS depression). Products include:

Buprenex Injectable 2006

Buspirone Hydrochloride (Increased CNS depression). Products include:

BuSpar 737

Butabarbital (Increased CNS depression).

No products indexed under this heading.

Butalbital (Increased CNS depression). Products include:

Esgic-plus Tablets 1013
Fioricet Tablets 2258
Fioricet with Codeine Capsules 2260

Fiorinal Capsules 2261
Fiorinal with Codeine Capsules 2262
Fiorinal Tablets 2261
Phrenilin 785
Sedapap Tablets 50 mg/650 mg .. 1543

Chlordiazepoxide (Increased CNS depression). Products include:

Libritabs Tablets 2177
Limbitrol 2180

Chlordiazepoxide Hydrochloride (Increased CNS depression). Products include:

Librax Capsules 2176
Librium Capsules 2178
Librium Injectable 2179

Chlorpromazine (Increased CNS depression). Products include:

Thorazine Suppositories 2523

Chlorprothixene (Increased CNS depression).

No products indexed under this heading.

Chlorprothixene Hydrochloride (Increased CNS depression).

No products indexed under this heading.

Clorazepate Dipotassium (Increased CNS depression). Products include:

Tranxene 451

Clozapine (Increased CNS depression). Products include:

Clozaril Tablets.. 2252

Desflurane (Increased CNS depression). Products include:

Suprane 1813

Dezocine (Increased CNS depression). Products include:

Dalgan Injection 538

Diazepam (Increased CNS depression). Products include:

Dizac 1809
Valium Injectable 2182
Valium Tablets 2183
Valrelease Capsules 2169

Droperidol (Increased CNS depression). Products include:

Inapsine Injection..................................... 1296

Enflurane (Increased CNS depression).

No products indexed under this heading.

Estazolam (Increased CNS depression). Products include:

ProSom Tablets 449

Ethchlorvynol (Increased CNS depression). Products include:

Placidyl Capsules..................................... 448

Ethinamate (Increased CNS depression).

No products indexed under this heading.

Fentanyl (Increased CNS depression). Products include:

Duragesic Transdermal System........ 1288

Fentanyl Citrate (Increased CNS depression). Products include:

Sublimaze Injection.................................. 1307

Fluphenazine Decanoate (Increased CNS depression). Products include:

Prolixin Decanoate 509

Fluphenazine Enanthate (Increased CNS depression). Products include:

Prolixin Enanthate 509

Fluphenazine Hydrochloride (Increased CNS depression). Products include:

Prolixin 509

Flurazepam Hydrochloride (Increased CNS depression). Products include:

Dalmane Capsules.................................... 2173

Furazolidone (Enhanced effect of MAO inhibitors). Products include:

Furoxone 2046

IMPORTANT NOTE: Always consult each drug listing in the patient's regimen for possible interactions.

Actifed with Codeine

Glutethimide (Increased CNS depression).

No products indexed under this heading.

Haloperidol (Increased CNS depression). Products include:

Haldol Injection, Tablets and Concentrate 1575

Haloperidol Decanoate (Increased CNS depression). Products include:

Haldol Decanoate.................................... 1577

Hydrocodone Bitartrate (Increased CNS depression). Products include:

Anexsia 5/500 Elixir	1781
Anexia Tablets	1782
Codiclear DH Syrup	791
Deconamine CX Cough and Cold Liquid and Tablets	1319
Duratuss HD Elixir	2565
Hycodan Tablets and Syrup	930
Hycomine Compound Tablets	932
Hycomine	931
Hycotuss Expectorant Syrup	933
Hydrocet Capsules	782
Lorcet 10/650	1018
Lortab	2566
Tussend	1783
Tussend Expectorant	1785
Vicodin Tablets	1356
Vicodin ES Tablets	1357
Vicodin Tuss Expectorant	1358
Zydone Capsules	949

Hydrocodone Polistirex (Increased CNS depression). Products include:

Tussionex Pennkinetic Extended-Release Suspension 998

Hydroxyzine Hydrochloride (Increased CNS depression). Products include:

Atarax Tablets & Syrup	2185
Marax Tablets & DF Syrup	2200
Vistaril Intramuscular Solution	2216

Isocarboxazid (Enhanced effect of MAO inhibitors).

No products indexed under this heading.

Isoflurane (Increased CNS depression).

No products indexed under this heading.

Ketamine Hydrochloride (Increased CNS depression).

No products indexed under this heading.

Levomethadyl Acetate Hydrochloride (Increased CNS depression). Products include:

Orlamm 2239

Levorphanol Tartrate (Increased CNS depression). Products include:

Levo-Dromoran.. 2129

Lorazepam (Increased CNS depression). Products include:

Ativan Injection	2698
Ativan Tablets	2700

Loxapine Hydrochloride (Increased CNS depression). Products include:

Loxitane 1378

Loxapine Succinate (Increased CNS depression). Products include:

Loxitane Capsules 1378

Meperidine Hydrochloride (Increased CNS depression). Products include:

Demerol	2308
Mepergan Injection	2753

Mephobarbital (Increased CNS depression). Products include:

Mebaral Tablets 2322

Meprobamate (Increased CNS depression). Products include:

Miltown Tablets	2672
PMB 200 and PMB 400	2783

Mesoridazine Besylate (Increased CNS depression). Products include:

Serentil 684

Methadone Hydrochloride (Increased CNS depression). Products include:

Methadone Hydrochloride Oral Concentrate	2233
Methadone Hydrochloride Oral Solution & Tablets	2235

Methohexital Sodium (Increased CNS depression). Products include:

Brevital Sodium Vials.............................. 1429

Methotrimeprazine (Increased CNS depression). Products include:

Levoprome 1274

Methoxyflurane (Increased CNS depression).

No products indexed under this heading.

Methyldopa (Diminished antihypertensive effect). Products include:

Aldoclor Tablets	1598
Aldomet Oral	1600
Aldoril Tablets	1604

Methyldopate Hydrochloride (Diminished antihypertensive effect). Products include:

Aldomet Ester HCl Injection 1602

Midazolam Hydrochloride (Increased CNS depression). Products include:

Versed Injection 2170

Molindone Hydrochloride (Increased CNS depression). Products include:

Moban Tablets and Concentrate...... 1048

Morphine Sulfate (Increased CNS depression). Products include:

Astramorph/PF Injection, USP (Preservative-Free)	535
Duramorph	962
Infumorph 200 and Infumorph 500 Sterile Solutions	965
MS Contin Tablets	1994
MSIR	1997
Oramorph SR (Morphine Sulfate Sustained Release Tablets)	2236
RMS Suppositories	2657
Roxanol	2243

Opium Alkaloids (Increased CNS depression).

No products indexed under this heading.

Oxazepam (Increased CNS depression). Products include:

Serax Capsules	2810
Serax Tablets	2810

Oxycodone Hydrochloride (Increased CNS depression). Products include:

Percocet Tablets	938
Percodan Tablets	939
Percodan-Demi Tablets	940
Roxicodone Tablets, Oral Solution & Intensol (Oxycodone)	2244
Tylox Capsules	1584

Pentobarbital Sodium (Increased CNS depression). Products include:

Nembutal Sodium Capsules	436
Nembutal Sodium Solution	438
Nembutal Sodium Suppositories	440

Perphenazine (Increased CNS depression). Products include:

Etrafon	2355
Triavil Tablets	1757
Trilafon	2389

Phenelzine Sulfate (Enhanced effect of MAO inhibitors). Products include:

Nardil 1920

Phenobarbital (Increased CNS depression). Products include:

Arco-Lase Plus Tablets	512
Bellergal-S Tablets	2250
Donnatal	2060
Donnatal Extentabs	2061

Donnatal Tablets .... 2060 Phenobarbital Elixir and Tablets ...... 1469 Quadrinal Tablets 1350

Prazepam (Increased CNS depression).

No products indexed under this heading.

Prochlorperazine (Increased CNS depression). Products include:

Compazine 2470

Promethazine Hydrochloride (Increased CNS depression). Products include:

Mepergan Injection	2753
Phenergan with Codeine	2777
Phenergan with Dextromethorphan	2778
Phenergan Injection	2773
Phenergan Suppositories	2775
Phenergan Syrup	2774
Phenergan Tablets	2775
Phenergan VC	2779
Phenergan VC with Codeine	2781

Propofol (Increased CNS depression). Products include:

Diprivan Injection...................................... 2833

Propoxyphene Hydrochloride (Increased CNS depression). Products include:

Darvon	1435
Wygesic Tablets	2827

Propoxyphene Napsylate (Increased CNS depression). Products include:

Darvon-N/Darvocet-N 1433

Quazepam (Increased CNS depression). Products include:

Doral Tablets 2664

Reserpine (Diminished antihypertensive effect). Products include:

Diupres Tablets	1650
Hydropres Tablets	1675
Ser-Ap-Es Tablets	849

Risperidone (Increased CNS depression). Products include:

Risperdal 1301

Secobarbital Sodium (Increased CNS depression). Products include:

Seconal Sodium Pulvules 1474

Selegiline Hydrochloride (Enhanced effect of MAO inhibitors). Products include:

Eldepryl Tablets 2550

Sufentanil Citrate (Increased CNS depression). Products include:

Sufenta Injection 1309

Temazepam (Increased CNS depression). Products include:

Restoril Capsules 2284

Thiamylal Sodium (Increased CNS depression).

No products indexed under this heading.

Thioridazine Hydrochloride (Increased CNS depression). Products include:

Mellaril 2269

Thiothixene (Increased CNS depression). Products include:

Navane Capsules and Concentrate	2201
Navane Intramuscular	2202

Tranylcypromine Sulfate (Enhanced effect of MAO inhibitors). Products include:

Parnate Tablets 2503

Triazolam (Increased CNS depression). Products include:

Halcion Tablets... 2611

Trifluoperazine Hydrochloride (Increased CNS depression). Products include:

Stelazine 2514

Zolpidem Tartrate (Increased CNS depression). Products include:

Ambien Tablets... 2416

Food Interactions

Alcohol (Increased CNS depression).

ACTIFED SINUS DAYTIME/NIGHTTIME TABLETS AND CAPLETS

(Acetaminophen, Diphenhydramine Hydrochloride, Pseudoephedrine Hydrochloride)..ⓂⒹ 846

May interact with hypnotics and sedatives, monoamine oxidase inhibitors, tranquilizers, and certain other agents. Compounds in these categories include:

Alprazolam (Increases the drowsiness effect). Products include:

Xanax Tablets 2649

Buspirone Hydrochloride (Increases the drowsiness effect). Products include:

BuSpar 737

Chlordiazepoxide (Increases the drowsiness effect). Products include:

Libritabs Tablets	2177
Limbitrol	2180

Chlordiazepoxide Hydrochloride (Increases the drowsiness effect). Products include:

Librax Capsules	2176
Librium Capsules	2178
Librium Injectable	2179

Chlorpromazine (Increases the drowsiness effect). Products include:

Thorazine Suppositories......................... 2523

Chlorpromazine Hydrochloride (Increases the drowsiness effect). Products include:

Thorazine 2523

Chlorprothixene (Increases the drowsiness effect).

No products indexed under this heading.

Chlorprothixene Hydrochloride (Increases the drowsiness effect).

No products indexed under this heading.

Clorazepate Dipotassium (Increases the drowsiness effect). Products include:

Tranxene 451

Diazepam (Increases the drowsiness effect). Products include:

Dizac	1809
Valium Injectable	2182
Valium Tablets	2183
Valrelease Capsules	2169

Droperidol (Increases the drowsiness effect). Products include:

Inapsine Injection...................................... 1296

Estazolam (Increases the drowsiness effect). Products include:

ProSom Tablets 449

Ethchlorvynol (Increases the drowsiness effect). Products include:

Placidyl Capsules 448

Ethinamate (Increases the drowsiness effect).

No products indexed under this heading.

Fluphenazine Decanoate (Increases the drowsiness effect). Products include:

Prolixin Decanoate 509

Fluphenazine Enanthate (Increases the drowsiness effect). Products include:

Prolixin Enanthate 509

Fluphenazine Hydrochloride (Increases the drowsiness effect). Products include:

Prolixin 509

Flurazepam Hydrochloride (Increases the drowsiness effect). Products include:

Dalmane Capsules..................................... 2173

Furazolidone (Effect not specified; concurrent use is not recommended). Products include:

Furoxone 2046

(ⓂⒹ Described in PDR For Nonprescription Drugs) (ⓟ Described in PDR For Ophthalmology)

Interactions Index

Actifed Tablets

Glutethimide (Increases the drowsiness effect).

No products indexed under this heading.

Haloperidol (Increases the drowsiness effect). Products include:

Haldol Injection, Tablets and Concentrate 1575

Haloperidol Decanoate (Increases the drowsiness effect). Products include:

Haldol Decanoate................................... 1577

Hydroxyzine Hydrochloride (Increases the drowsiness effect). Products include:

Atarax Tablets & Syrup......................... 2185
Marax Tablets & DF Syrup.................... 2200
Vistaril Intramuscular Solution.......... 2216

Isocarboxazid (Effect not specified; concurrent use is not recommended).

No products indexed under this heading.

Lorazepam (Increases the drowsiness effect). Products include:

Ativan Injection.. 2698
Ativan Tablets... 2700

Loxapine Hydrochloride (Increases the drowsiness effect). Products include:

Loxitane 1378

Loxapine Succinate (Increases the drowsiness effect). Products include:

Loxitane Capsules 1378

Meprobamate (Increases the drowsiness effect). Products include:

Miltown Tablets 2672
PMB 200 and PMB 400 2783

Mesoridazine Besylate (Increases the drowsiness effect). Products include:

Serentil... 684

Midazolam Hydrochloride (Increases the drowsiness effect). Products include:

Versed Injection 2170

Molindone Hydrochloride (Increases the drowsiness effect). Products include:

Moban Tablets and Concentrate 1048

Oxazepam (Increases the drowsiness effect). Products include:

Serax Capsules 2810
Serax Tablets.. 2810

Perphenazine (Increases the drowsiness effect). Products include:

Etrafon 2355
Triavil Tablets 1757
Trilafon... 2389

Phenelzine Sulfate (Effect not specified; concurrent use is not recommended). Products include:

Nardil 1920

Prazepam (Increases the drowsiness effect).

No products indexed under this heading.

Prochlorperazine (Increases the drowsiness effect). Products include:

Compazine 2470

Promethazine Hydrochloride (Increases the drowsiness effect). Products include:

Mepergan Injection 2753
Phenergan with Codeine....................... 2777
Phenergan with Dextromethorphan 2778
Phenergan Injection 2773
Phenergan Suppositories 2775
Phenergan Syrup 2774
Phenergan Tablets 2775
Phenergan VC... 2779
Phenergan VC with Codeine 2781

Propofol (Increases the drowsiness effect). Products include:

Diprivan Injection................................... 2833

Quazepam (Increases the drowsiness effect). Products include:

Doral Tablets 2664

Secobarbital Sodium (Increases the drowsiness effect). Products include:

Seconal Sodium Pulvules 1474

Selegiline Hydrochloride (Effect not specified; concurrent use is not recommended). Products include:

Eldepryl Tablets 2550

Temazepam (Increases the drowsiness effect). Products include:

Restoril Capsules 2284

Thioridazine Hydrochloride (Increases the drowsiness effect). Products include:

Mellaril 2269

Thiothixene (Increases the drowsiness effect). Products include:

Navane Capsules and Concentrate 2201
Navane Intramuscular 2202

Tranylcypromine Sulfate (Effect not specified; concurrent use is not recommended). Products include:

Parnate Tablets 2503

Triazolam (Increases the drowsiness effect). Products include:

Halcion Tablets.. 2611

Trifluoperazine Hydrochloride (Increases the drowsiness effect). Products include:

Stelazine 2514

Zolpidem Tartrate (Increases the drowsiness effect). Products include:

Ambien Tablets.. 2416

Food Interactions

Alcohol (Increases the drowsiness effect).

ACTIFED SYRUP

(Pseudoephedrine Hydrochloride, Triprolidine Hydrochloride) ....ᴿᴰ 846

May interact with monoamine oxidase inhibitors, hypnotics and sedatives, tranquilizers, and certain other agents. Compounds in these categories include:

Alprazolam (Increases drowsiness effect). Products include:

Xanax Tablets 2649

Buspirone Hydrochloride (Increases drowsiness effect). Products include:

BuSpar 737

Chlordiazepoxide (Increases drowsiness effect). Products include:

Libritabs Tablets 2177
Limbitrol 2180

Chlordiazepoxide Hydrochloride (Increases drowsiness effect). Products include:

Librax Capsules 2176
Librium Capsules 2178
Librium Injectable 2179

Chlorpromazine (Increases drowsiness effect). Products include:

Thorazine Suppositories....................... 2523

Chlorpromazine Hydrochloride (Increases drowsiness effect). Products include:

Thorazine 2523

Chlorprothixene (Increases drowsiness effect).

No products indexed under this heading.

Chlorprothixene Hydrochloride (Increases drowsiness effect).

No products indexed under this heading.

Clorazepate Dipotassium (Increases drowsiness effect). Products include:

Tranxene 451

Diazepam (Increases drowsiness effect). Products include:

Dizac 1809
Valium Injectable 2182
Valium Tablets 2183

Valrelease Capsules 2169

Droperidol (Increases drowsiness effect). Products include:

Inapsine Injection................................... 1296

Estazolam (Increases drowsiness effect). Products include:

ProSom Tablets 449

Ethchlorvynol (Increases drowsiness effect). Products include:

Placidyl Capsules.................................... 448

Ethinamate (Increases drowsiness effect).

No products indexed under this heading.

Fluphenazine Decanoate (Increases drowsiness effect). Products include:

Prolixin Decanoate 509

Fluphenazine Enanthate (Increases drowsiness effect). Products include:

Prolixin Enanthate.................................. 509

Fluphenazine Hydrochloride (Increases drowsiness effect). Products include:

Prolixin 509

Flurazepam Hydrochloride (Increases drowsiness effect). Products include:

Dalmane Capsules................................... 2173

Furazolidone (Concurrent administration is not recommended). Products include:

Furoxone 2046

Glutethimide (Increases drowsiness effect).

No products indexed under this heading.

Haloperidol (Increases drowsiness effect). Products include:

Haldol Injection, Tablets and Concentrate 1575

Haloperidol Decanoate (Increases drowsiness effect). Products include:

Haldol Decanoate.................................... 1577

Hydroxyzine Hydrochloride (Increases drowsiness effect). Products include:

Atarax Tablets & Syrup......................... 2185
Marax Tablets & DF Syrup.................... 2200
Vistaril Intramuscular Solution.......... 2216

Isocarboxazid (Concurrent administration is not recommended).

No products indexed under this heading.

Lorazepam (Increases drowsiness effect). Products include:

Ativan Injection.. 2698
Ativan Tablets... 2700

Loxapine Hydrochloride (Increases drowsiness effect). Products include:

Loxitane 1378

Loxapine Succinate (Increases drowsiness effect). Products include:

Loxitane Capsules 1378

Meprobamate (Increases drowsiness effect). Products include:

Miltown Tablets 2672
PMB 200 and PMB 400 2783

Mesoridazine Besylate (Increases drowsiness effect). Products include:

Serentil... 684

Midazolam Hydrochloride (Increases drowsiness effect). Products include:

Versed Injection 2170

Molindone Hydrochloride (Increases drowsiness effect). Products include:

Moban Tablets and Concentrate 1048

Oxazepam (Increases drowsiness effect). Products include:

Serax Capsules 2810
Serax Tablets.. 2810

Perphenazine (Increases drowsiness effect). Products include:

Etrafon 2355
Triavil Tablets 1757
Trilafon... 2389

Phenelzine Sulfate (Concurrent administration is not recommended). Products include:

Nardil 1920

Prazepam (Increases drowsiness effect).

No products indexed under this heading.

Prochlorperazine (Increases drowsiness effect). Products include:

Compazine 2470

Promethazine Hydrochloride (Increases drowsiness effect). Products include:

Mepergan Injection 2753
Phenergan with Codeine....................... 2777
Phenergan with Dextromethorphan 2778
Phenergan Injection 2773
Phenergan Suppositories 2775
Phenergan Syrup 2774
Phenergan Tablets 2775
Phenergan VC... 2779
Phenergan VC with Codeine 2781

Propofol (Increases drowsiness effect). Products include:

Diprivan Injection................................... 2833

Quazepam (Increases drowsiness effect). Products include:

Doral Tablets 2664

Secobarbital Sodium (Increases drowsiness effect). Products include:

Seconal Sodium Pulvules 1474

Selegiline Hydrochloride (Concurrent administration is not recommended). Products include:

Eldepryl Tablets 2550

Temazepam (Increases drowsiness effect). Products include:

Restoril Capsules 2284

Thioridazine Hydrochloride (Increases drowsiness effect). Products include:

Mellaril 2269

Thiothixene (Increases drowsiness effect). Products include:

Navane Capsules and Concentrate 2201
Navane Intramuscular 2202

Tranylcypromine Sulfate (Concurrent administration is not recommended). Products include:

Parnate Tablets 2503

Triazolam (Increases drowsiness effect). Products include:

Halcion Tablets.. 2611

Trifluoperazine Hydrochloride (Increases drowsiness effect). Products include:

Stelazine 2514

Zolpidem Tartrate (Increases drowsiness effect). Products include:

Ambien Tablets.. 2416

Food Interactions

Alcohol (Increases drowsiness effect).

ACTIFED TABLETS

(Pseudoephedrine Hydrochloride, Triprolidine Hydrochloride) ....ᴿᴰ 844

May interact with monoamine oxidase inhibitors, hypnotics and sedatives, tranquilizers, and certain other agents. Compounds in these categories include:

Alprazolam (Increases drowsiness effect). Products include:

Xanax Tablets 2649

Buspirone Hydrochloride (Increases drowsiness effect). Products include:

BuSpar 737

Chlordiazepoxide (Increases drowsiness effect). Products include:

Libritabs Tablets 2177

IMPORTANT NOTE: Always consult each drug listing in the patient's regimen for possible interactions.

Actifed Tablets **Interactions Index** 10

Limbitrol 2180

Chlordiazepoxide Hydrochloride (Increases drowsiness effect). Products include:

Librax Capsules 2176
Librium Capsules 2178
Librium Injectable 2179

Chlorpromazine (Increases drowsiness effect). Products include:

Thorazine Suppositories 2523

Chlorpromazine Hydrochloride (Increases drowsiness effect). Products include:

Thorazine 2523

Chlorprothixene (Increases drowsiness effect).

No products indexed under this heading.

Chlorprothixene Hydrochloride (Increases drowsiness effect).

No products indexed under this heading.

Clorazepate Dipotassium (Increases drowsiness effect). Products include:

Tranxene 451

Diazepam (Increases drowsiness effect). Products include:

Dizac 1809
Valium Injectable 2182
Valium Tablets 2183
Valrelease Capsules 2169

Droperidol (Increases drowsiness effect). Products include:

Inapsine Injection 1296

Estazolam (Increases drowsiness effect). Products include:

ProSom Tablets 449

Ethchlorvynol (Increases drowsiness effect). Products include:

Placidyl Capsules 448

Ethinamate (Increases drowsiness effect).

No products indexed under this heading.

Fluphenazine Decanoate (Increases drowsiness effect). Products include:

Prolixin Decanoate 509

Fluphenazine Enanthate (Increases drowsiness effect). Products include:

Prolixin Enanthate 509

Fluphenazine Hydrochloride (Increases drowsiness effect). Products include:

Prolixin 509

Flurazepam Hydrochloride (Increases drowsiness effect). Products include:

Dalmane Capsules 2173

Furazolidone (Concurrent administration is not recommended). Products include:

Furoxone 2046

Glutethimide (Increases drowsiness effect).

No products indexed under this heading.

Haloperidol (Increases drowsiness effect). Products include:

Haldol Injection, Tablets and Concentrate 1575

Haloperidol Decanoate (Increases drowsiness effect). Products include:

Haldol Decanoate 1577

Hydroxyzine Hydrochloride (Increases drowsiness effect). Products include:

Atarax Tablets & Syrup 2185
Marax Tablets & DF Syrup 2200
Vistaril Intramuscular Solution 2216

Isocarboxazid (Concurrent administration is not recommended).

No products indexed under this heading.

Lorazepam (Increases drowsiness effect). Products include:

Ativan Injection 2698
Ativan Tablets 2700

Loxapine Hydrochloride (Increases drowsiness effect). Products include:

Loxitane 1378

Loxapine Succinate (Increases drowsiness effect). Products include:

Loxitane Capsules 1378

Meprobamate (Increases drowsiness effect). Products include:

Miltown Tablets 2672
PMB 200 and PMB 400 2783

Mesoridazine Besylate (Increases drowsiness effect). Products include:

Serentil 684

Midazolam Hydrochloride (Increases drowsiness effect). Products include:

Versed Injection 2170

Molindone Hydrochloride (Increases drowsiness effect). Products include:

Moban Tablets and Concentrate 1048

Oxazepam (Increases drowsiness effect). Products include:

Serax Capsules 2810
Serax Tablets 2810

Perphenazine (Increases drowsiness effect). Products include:

Etrafon 2355
Triavil Tablets 1757
Trilafon 2389

Phenelzine Sulfate (Concurrent administration is not recommended). Products include:

Nardil 1920

Prazepam (Increases drowsiness effect).

No products indexed under this heading.

Prochlorperazine (Increases drowsiness effect). Products include:

Compazine 2470

Promethazine Hydrochloride (Increases drowsiness effect). Products include:

Mepergan Injection 2753
Phenergan with Codeine 2777
Phenergan with Dextromethorphan 2778
Phenergan Injection 2773
Phenergan Suppositories 2775
Phenergan Syrup 2774
Phenergan Tablets 2775
Phenergan VC 2779
Phenergan VC with Codeine 2781

Propofol (Increases drowsiness effect). Products include:

Diprivan Injection 2833

Quazepam (Increases drowsiness effect). Products include:

Doral Tablets 2664

Secobarbital Sodium (Increases drowsiness effect). Products include:

Seconal Sodium Pulvules 1474

Selegiline Hydrochloride (Concurrent administration is not recommended). Products include:

Eldepryl Tablets 2550

Temazepam (Increases drowsiness effect). Products include:

Restoril Capsules 2284

Thioridazine Hydrochloride (Increases drowsiness effect). Products include:

Mellaril 2269

Thiothixene (Increases drowsiness effect). Products include:

Navane Capsules and Concentrate 2201
Navane Intramuscular 2202

Tranylcypromine Sulfate (Concurrent administration is not recommended). Products include:

Parnate Tablets 2503

Triazolam (Increases drowsiness effect). Products include:

Halcion Tablets 2611

Trifluoperazine Hydrochloride (Increases drowsiness effect). Products include:

Stelazine 2514

Zolpidem Tartrate (Increases drowsiness effect). Products include:

Ambien Tablets 2416

Food Interactions

Alcohol (Increases drowsiness effect).

ACTIGALL CAPSULES

(Ursodiol) 802

May interact with bile acid sequestering agents, lipid-lowering drugs, estrogens, oral contraceptives, and certain other agents. Compounds in these categories include:

Aluminum Carbonate Gel (Interferes with the action of Actigall by reducing its absorption). Products include:

Basaljel 2703

Aluminum Hydroxide (Interferes with the action of Actigall by reducing its absorption). Products include:

ALternaGEL Liquid 1316
Maximum Strength Ascriptin .... ▣ 630
Cama Arthritis Pain Reliever .... ▣ 785
Gaviscon Extra Strength Relief Formula Antacid Tablets .... ▣ 819
Gaviscon Extra Strength Relief Formula Liquid Antacid .... ▣ 819
Gaviscon Liquid Antacid .... ▣ 820
Gelusil Liquid & Tablets .... ▣ 855
Maalox Heartburn Relief Suspension .... ▣ 642
Maalox Heartburn Relief Tablets .... ▣ 641
Maalox Magnesia and Alumina Oral Suspension .... ▣ 642
Maalox Plus Tablets .... ▣ 643
Extra Strength Maalox Antacid Plus Antigas Liquid and Tablets ▣ 638
Tempo Soft Antacid .... ▣ 835

Aluminum Hydroxide Gel (Interferes with the action of Actigall by reducing its absorption). Products include:

ALternaGEL Liquid .... ▣ 659
Aludrox Oral Suspension 2695
Amphojel Suspension 2695
Amphojel Suspension without Flavor 2695
Amphojel Tablets 2695
Arthritis Pain Ascriptin .... ▣ 631
Regular Strength Ascriptin Tablets .... ▣ 629
Gaviscon Antacid Tablets .... ▣ 819
Gaviscon-2 Antacid Tablets .... ▣ 820
Mylanta Liquid 1317
Mylanta Tablets .... ▣ 660
Mylanta Double Strength Liquid 1317
Mylanta Double Strength Tablets .. ▣ 660
Nephrox Suspension .... ▣ 655

Aluminum Hydroxide Gel, Dried (Interferes with the action of Actigall by reducing its absorption).

Chlorotrianisene (May counteract the effectiveness of Actigall).

No products indexed under this heading.

Cholestyramine (Interferes with the action of Actigall by reducing its absorption; may counteract the effectiveness of Actigall). Products include:

Questran Light 769
Questran Powder 770

Clofibrate (May counteract the effectiveness of Actigall). Products include:

Atromid-S Capsules 2701

Colestipol Hydrochloride (Interferes with the action of Actigall by reducing its absorption; may counteract the effectiveness of Actigall). Products include:

Colestid Tablets 2591

Desogestrel (May counteract the effectiveness of Actigall). Products include:

Desogen Tablets 1817
Ortho-Cept 1851

Dienestrol (May counteract the effectiveness of Actigall). Products include:

Ortho Dienestrol Cream 1866

Diethylstilbestrol (May counteract the effectiveness of Actigall). Products include:

Diethylstilbestrol Tablets 1437

Estradiol (May counteract the effectiveness of Actigall). Products include:

Climara Transdermal System 645
Estrace Cream and Tablets 749
Estraderm Transdermal System 824

Estrogens, Conjugated (May counteract the effectiveness of Actigall). Products include:

PMB 200 and PMB 400 2783
Premarin Intravenous 2787
Premarin with Methyltestosterone .. 2794
Premarin Tablets 2789
Premarin Vaginal Cream 2791
Premphase 2797
Prempro 2801

Estrogens, Esterified (May counteract the effectiveness of Actigall). Products include:

ESTRATAB Tablets (0.3, 0.625, 1.25, 2.5 mg) 2536
Estratest 2539
Menest Tablets 2494

Estropipate (May counteract the effectiveness of Actigall). Products include:

Ogen Tablets 2627
Ogen Vaginal Cream 2630
Ortho-Est 1869

Ethinyl Estradiol (May counteract the effectiveness of Actigall). Products include:

Brevicon 2088
Demulen 2428
Desogen Tablets 1817
Levlen/Tri-Levlen 651
Lo/Ovral Tablets 2746
Lo/Ovral-28 Tablets 2751
Modicon 1872
Nordette-21 Tablets 2755
Nordette-28 Tablets 2758
Norinyl 2088
Ortho-Cept 1851
Ortho-Cyclen/Ortho-Tri-Cyclen 1858
Ortho-Novum 1872
Ortho-Cyclen/Ortho Tri-Cyclen 1858
Ovcon 760
Ovral Tablets 2770
Ovral-28 Tablets 2770
Levlen/Tri-Levlen 651
Tri-Norinyl 2164
Triphasil-21 Tablets 2814
Triphasil-28 Tablets 2819

Ethynodiol Diacetate (May counteract the effectiveness of Actigall). Products include:

Demulen 2428

Fluvastatin Sodium (May counteract the effectiveness of Actigall). Products include:

Lescol Capsules 2267

Gemfibrozil (May counteract the effectiveness of Actigall). Products include:

Lopid Tablets 1917

Levonorgestrel (May counteract the effectiveness of Actigall). Products include:

Levlen/Tri-Levlen 651
Nordette-21 Tablets 2755
Nordette-28 Tablets 2758
Norplant System 2759
Levlen/Tri-Levlen 651
Triphasil-21 Tablets 2814
Triphasil-28 Tablets 2819

Lovastatin (May counteract the effectiveness of Actigall). Products include:

Mevacor Tablets 1699

Interactions Index — Acutrim

Mestranol (May counteract the effectiveness of Actigall). Products include:

Norinyl 2088
Ortho-Novum 1872

Norethindrone (May counteract the effectiveness of Actigall). Products include:

Brevicon 2088
Micronor Tablets 1872
Modicon 1872
Norinyl 2088
Nor-Q D Tablets 2135
Ortho-Novum 1872
Ovcon 760
Tri-Norinyl 2164

Norethynodrel (May counteract the effectiveness of Actigall).

No products indexed under this heading.

Norgestimate (May counteract the effectiveness of Actigall). Products include:

Ortho-Cyclen/Ortho-Tri-Cyclen 1858
Ortho-Cyclen/Ortho Tri-Cyclen 1858

Norgestrel (May counteract the effectiveness of Actigall). Products include:

Lo/Ovral Tablets 2746
Lo/Ovral-28 Tablets 2751
Ovral Tablets 2770
Ovral-28 Tablets 2770
Ovrette Tablets 2771

Polyestradiol Phosphate (May counteract the effectiveness of Actigall).

No products indexed under this heading.

Pravastatin Sodium (Interferes with the action of Actigall by reducing its absorption; may counteract the effectiveness of Actigall). Products include:

Pravachol 765

Probucol (May counteract the effectiveness of Actigall). Products include:

Lorelco Tablets 1517

Quinestrol (May counteract the effectiveness of Actigall).

No products indexed under this heading.

Simvastatin (Interferes with the action of Actigall by reducing its absorption; may counteract the effectiveness of Actigall). Products include:

Zocor Tablets 1775

ACTIMMUNE

(Interferon Gamma-1B) 1056
May interact with:

Bone Marrow Depressants, unspecified (Caution should be exercised when administering with other potentially myelosuppressive agents).

ACTIVASE

(Alteplase, Recombinant) 1058
May interact with oral anticoagulants, platelet inhibitors, and certain other agents. Compounds in these categories include:

Aspirin (Increased risk of bleeding). Products include:

Alka-Seltzer Effervescent Antacid and Pain Reliever .... ⊞ 701
Alka-Seltzer Extra Strength Effervescent Antacid and Pain Reliever .... ⊞ 703
Alka-Seltzer Lemon Lime Effervescent Antacid and Pain Reliever .... ⊞ 703
Alka-Seltzer Plus Cold Medicine .... ⊞ 705
Alka-Seltzer Plus Cold & Cough Medicine .... ⊞ 708
Alka-Seltzer Plus Night-Time Cold Medicine .... ⊞ 707
Alka Seltzer Plus Sinus Medicine .. ⊞ 707
Arthritis Foundation Safety Coated Aspirin Tablets .... ⊞ 675
Arthritis Pain Ascriptin .... ⊞ 631
Maximum Strength Ascriptin .... ⊞ 630
Regular Strength Ascriptin Tablets .... ⊞ 629
Arthritis Strength BC Powder .... ⊞ 609
BC Cold Powder Multi-Symptom Formula (Cold-Sinus-Allergy) ...... ⊞ 609
BC Cold Powder Non-Drowsy Formula (Cold-Sinus) .... ⊞ 609
BC Powder .... ⊞ 609
Bayer Children's Chewable Aspirin .... ⊞ 711
Genuine Bayer Aspirin Tablets & Caplets .... ⊞ 713
Extra Strength Bayer Arthritis Pain Regimen Formula .... ⊞ 711
Extra Strength Bayer Aspirin Caplets & Tablets .... ⊞ 712
Extended-Release Bayer 8-Hour Aspirin .... ⊞ 712
Extra Strength Bayer Plus Aspirin Caplets .... ⊞ 713
Extra Strength Bayer PM Aspirin .. ⊞ 713
Bayer Enteric Aspirin .... ⊞ 709
Bufferin Analgesic Tablets and Caplets .... ⊞ 613
Arthritis Strength Bufferin Analgesic Caplets .... ⊞ 614
Extra Strength Bufferin Analgesic Tablets .... ⊞ 615
Cama Arthritis Pain Reliever .... ⊞ 785
Darvon Compound-65 Pulvules 1435
Easprin 1914
Ecotrin 2455
Ecotrin Enteric Coated Aspirin Maximum Strength Tablets and Caplets .... ⊞ 816
Ecotrin Enteric Coated Aspirin Regular Strength Tablets 2455
Empirin Aspirin Tablets .... ⊞ 854
Empirin with Codeine Tablets 1093
Excedrin Extra-Strength Analgesic Tablets & Caplets 732
Fiorinal Capsules 2261
Fiorinal with Codeine Capsules 2262
Fiorinal Tablets 2261
Halfprin 1362
Healthprin Aspirin 2455
Norgesic 1496
Percodan Tablets 939
Percodan-Demi Tablets 940
Robaxisal Tablets 2071
Soma Compound w/Codeine Tablets 2676
Soma Compound Tablets 2675
St. Joseph Adult Chewable Aspirin (81 mg.) .... ⊞ 808
Talwin Compound 2335
Ursinus Inlay-Tabs .... ⊞ 794
Vanquish Analgesic Caplets .... ⊞ 731

Azlocillin Sodium (Increased risk of bleeding).

No products indexed under this heading.

Carbenicillin Indanyl Sodium (Increased risk of bleeding). Products include:

Geocillin Tablets 2199

Choline Magnesium Trisalicylate (Increased risk of bleeding). Products include:

Trilisate 2000

Diclofenac Potassium (Increased risk of bleeding). Products include:

Cataflam 816

Diclofenac Sodium (Increased risk of bleeding). Products include:

Voltaren Ophthalmic Sterile Ophthalmic Solution .... © 272
Voltaren Tablets 861

Dicumarol (Increased risk of bleeding).

No products indexed under this heading.

Diflunisal (Increased risk of bleeding). Products include:

Dolobid Tablets 1654

Dipyridamole (Increased risk of bleeding). Products include:

Persantine Tablets 681

Fenoprofen Calcium (Increased risk of bleeding). Products include:

Nalfon 200 Pulvules & Nalfon Tablets 917

Flurbiprofen (Increased risk of bleeding). Products include:

Ansaid Tablets 2579

Heparin Calcium (Increased risk of bleeding).

No products indexed under this heading.

Heparin Sodium (Increased risk of bleeding). Products include:

Heparin Lock Flush Solution 2725
Heparin Sodium Injection 2726
Heparin Sodium Injection, USP, Sterile Solution 2615
Heparin Sodium Vials 1441

Ibuprofen (Increased risk of bleeding). Products include:

Advil Cold and Sinus Caplets and Tablets (formerly CoAdvil) .... ⊞ 870
Advil Ibuprofen Tablets and Caplets .... ⊞ 870
Children's Advil Suspension 2692
Arthritis Foundation Ibuprofen Tablets .... ⊞ 674
Bayer Select Ibuprofen Pain Relief Formula .... ⊞ 715
Cramp End Tablets .... ⊞ 735
Dimetapp Sinus Caplets .... ⊞ 775
Haltran Tablets .... ⊞ 771
IBU Tablets 1342
Ibuprohm .... ⊞ 735
Children's Motrin Ibuprofen Oral Suspension 1546
Motrin Tablets 2625
Motrin IB Caplets, Tablets, and Geltabs .... ⊞ 838
Motrin IB Sinus .... ⊞ 838
Motrin Ibuprofen Suspension, Oral Drops, Chewable Tablets, Caplets 1546
Nuprin Ibuprofen/Analgesic Tablets & Caplets .... ⊞ 622
Sine-Aid IB Caplets 1554
Vicks DayQuil SINUS Pressure & PAIN Relief with IBUPROFEN ...... ⊞ 762

Indomethacin (Increased risk of bleeding). Products include:

Indocin 1680

Indomethacin Sodium Trihydrate (Increased risk of bleeding). Products include:

Indocin I.V. 1684

Ketoprofen (Increased risk of bleeding). Products include:

Orudis Capsules 2766
Oruvail Capsules 2766

Magnesium Salicylate (Increased risk of bleeding). Products include:

Backache Caplets .... ⊞ 613
Bayer Select Backache Pain Relief Formula .... ⊞ 715
Doan's Extra-Strength Analgesic .... ⊞ 633
Extra Strength Doan's P.M. .... ⊞ 633
Doan's Regular Strength Analgesic .... ⊞ 634
Mobigesic Tablets .... ⊞ 602

Meclofenamate Sodium (Increased risk of bleeding).

No products indexed under this heading.

Mefenamic Acid (Increased risk of bleeding). Products include:

Ponstel 1925

Mezlocillin Sodium (Increased risk of bleeding). Products include:

Mezlin 601
Mezlin Pharmacy Bulk Package 604

Nafcillin Sodium (Increased risk of bleeding).

No products indexed under this heading.

Naproxen (Increased risk of bleeding). Products include:

Anaprox/Naprosyn 2117

Naproxen Sodium (Increased risk of bleeding). Products include:

Aleve 1975
Anaprox/Naprosyn 2117

Penicillin G Benzathine (Increased risk of bleeding). Products include:

Bicillin C-R Injection 2704

Bicillin C-R 900/300 Injection 2706
Bicillin L-A Injection 2707

Penicillin G Procaine (Increased risk of bleeding). Products include:

Bicillin C-R Injection 2704
Bicillin C-R 900/300 Injection 2706

Phenylbutazone (Increased risk of bleeding).

No products indexed under this heading.

Piroxicam (Increased risk of bleeding). Products include:

Feldene Capsules 1965

Salsalate (Increased risk of bleeding). Products include:

Mono-Gesic Tablets 792
Salflex Tablets 786

Sulindac (Increased risk of bleeding). Products include:

Clinoril Tablets 1618

Ticarcillin Disodium (Increased risk of bleeding). Products include:

Ticar for Injection 2526
Timentin for Injection 2528

Ticlopidine Hydrochloride (Increased risk of bleeding). Products include:

Ticlid Tablets 2156

Tolmetin Sodium (Increased risk of bleeding). Products include:

Tolectin (200, 400 and 600 mg) .. 1581

Warfarin Sodium (Increased risk of bleeding). Products include:

Coumadin 926

ACULAR

(Ketorolac Tromethamine) 474
None cited in PDR database.

ACUTRIM 16 HOUR STEADY CONTROL APPETITE SUPPRESSANT

(Phenylpropanolamine Hydrochloride) .... ⊞ 628

See Acutrim Late Day Strength Appetite Suppressant

ACUTRIM LATE DAY STRENGTH APPETITE SUPPRESSANT

(Phenylpropanolamine Hydrochloride) .... ⊞ 628

May interact with monoamine oxidase inhibitors and certain other agents. Compounds in these categories include:

Furazolidone (Do not use concomitantly). Products include:

Furoxone 2046

Isocarboxazid (Do not use concomitantly).

No products indexed under this heading.

Nasal decongestants, unspecified (Concurrent use is not recommended).

Phenelzine Sulfate (Do not use concomitantly). Products include:

Nardil 1920

Phenylpropanolamine Containing Anoretics (Concurrent use not recommended).

Prescription Drugs, unspecified (Concurrent use not recommended).

Selegiline Hydrochloride (Do not use concomitantly). Products include:

Eldepryl Tablets 2550

Tranylcypromine Sulfate (Do not use concomitantly). Products include:

Parnate Tablets 2503

IMPORTANT NOTE: Always consult each drug listing in the patient's regimen for possible interactions.

ACUTRIM MAXIMUM STRENGTH APPETITE SUPPRESSANT
(Phenylpropanolamine Hydrochloride) ▣ 628
See **Acutrim Late Day Strength Appetite Suppressant**

ADAGEN (PEGADEMASE BOVINE) INJECTION
(Pegademase Bovine) 972
May interact with:

Vidarabine Monohydrate (Concomitant use can substantially alter activities of Adagen).
No products indexed under this heading.

ADALAT CAPSULES (10 MG AND 20 MG)
(Nifedipine) 587
May interact with beta blockers, cardiac glycosides, oral anticoagulants, and certain other agents. Compounds in these categories include:

Acebutolol Hydrochloride (Increased likelihood of congestive heart failure, severe hypotension, or exacerbation of angina). Products include:
Sectral Capsules 2807

Atenolol (Increased likelihood of congestive heart failure, severe hypotension, or exacerbation of angina). Products include:
Tenoretic Tablets 2845
Tenormin Tablets and I.V. Injection 2847

Betaxolol Hydrochloride (Increased likelihood of congestive heart failure, severe hypotension, or exacerbation of angina). Products include:
Betoptic Ophthalmic Solution 469
Betoptic S Ophthalmic Suspension 471
Kerlone Tablets 2436

Bisoprolol Fumarate (Increased likelihood of congestive heart failure, severe hypotension, or exacerbation of angina). Products include:
Zebeta Tablets 1413
Ziac 1415

Carteolol Hydrochloride (Increased likelihood of congestive heart failure, severe hypotension, or exacerbation of angina). Products include:
Cartrol Tablets 410
Ocupress Ophthalmic Solution, 1% Sterile ◉ 309

Cimetidine (Increased peak nifedipine plasma levels). Products include:
Tagamet Tablets 2516

Cimetidine Hydrochloride (Increased peak nifedipine plasma levels). Products include:
Tagamet 2516

Deslanoside (Isolated reports of elevated digoxin levels).
No products indexed under this heading.

Dicumarol (Increased prothrombin time).
No products indexed under this heading.

Digitoxin (Isolated reports of elevated digoxin levels). Products include:
Crystodigin Tablets 1433

Digoxin (Isolated reports of elevated digoxin levels). Products include:
Lanoxicaps 1117
Lanoxin Elixir Pediatric 1120
Lanoxin Injection 1123
Lanoxin Injection Pediatric 1126
Lanoxin Tablets 1128

Esmolol Hydrochloride (Increased likelihood of congestive heart failure, severe hypotension, or exacerbation of angina). Products include:
Brevibloc Injection 1808

Labetalol Hydrochloride (Increased likelihood of congestive heart failure, severe hypotension, or exacerbation of angina). Products include:
Normodyne Injection 2377
Normodyne Tablets 2379
Trandate 1185

Levobunolol Hydrochloride (Increased likelihood of congestive heart failure, severe hypotension, or exacerbation of angina). Products include:
Betagan ◉ 233

Metipranolol Hydrochloride (Increased likelihood of congestive heart failure, severe hypotension, or exacerbation of angina). Products include:
OptiPranolol (Metipranolol 0.3%) Sterile Ophthalmic Solution ◉ 258

Metoprolol Succinate (Increased likelihood of congestive heart failure, severe hypotension, or exacerbation of angina). Products include:
Toprol-XL Tablets 565

Metoprolol Tartrate (Increased likelihood of congestive heart failure, severe hypotension, or exacerbation of angina). Products include:
Lopressor Ampuls 830
Lopressor HCT Tablets 832
Lopressor Tablets 830

Nadolol (Increased likelihood of congestive heart failure, severe hypotension, or exacerbation of angina).
No products indexed under this heading.

Penbutolol Sulfate (Increased likelihood of congestive heart failure, severe hypotension, or exacerbation of angina). Products include:
Levatol 2403

Pindolol (Increased likelihood of congestive heart failure, severe hypotension, or exacerbation of angina). Products include:
Visken Tablets 2299

Propranolol Hydrochloride (Increased likelihood of congestive heart failure, severe hypotension, or exacerbation of angina). Products include:
Inderal 2728
Inderal LA Long Acting Capsules 2730
Inderide Tablets 2732
Inderide LA Long Acting Capsules 2734

Quinidine Gluconate (Decreased plasma level of quinidine). Products include:
Quinaglute Dura-Tabs Tablets 649

Quinidine Polygalacturonate (Decreased plasma level of quinidine).
No products indexed under this heading.

Quinidine Sulfate (Decreased plasma level of quinidine). Products include:
Quinidex Extentabs 2067

Ranitidine Hydrochloride (Produces smaller, non-significant increases in peak nifedipine plasma levels and AUC). Products include:
Zantac 1209
Zantac Injection 1207
Zantac Syrup 1209

Sotalol Hydrochloride (Increased likelihood of congestive heart failure, severe hypotension, or exacerbation of angina). Products include:
Betapace Tablets 641

Timolol Hemihydrate (Increased likelihood of congestive heart failure, severe hypotension, or exacerbation of angina). Products include:
Betimol 0.25%, 0.5% ◉ 261

Timolol Maleate (Increased likelihood of congestive heart failure, severe hypotension, or exacerbation of angina). Products include:
Blocadren Tablets 1614
Timolide Tablets 1748
Timoptic in Ocudose 1753
Timoptic Sterile Ophthalmic Solution 1751
Timoptic-XE 1755

Warfarin Sodium (Increased prothrombin time). Products include:
Coumadin 926

ADALAT CC
(Nifedipine) 589
May interact with beta blockers, cardiac glycosides, oral anticoagulants, narcotic analgesics, and certain other agents. Compounds in these categories include:

Acebutolol Hydrochloride (Combination of nifedipine and beta blocker may increase the likelihood of congestive heart failure, severe hypotension, or exacerbation of angina). Products include:
Sectral Capsules 2807

Alfentanil Hydrochloride (Potential for severe hypotension and/or increased fluid volume requirements cannot be ruled out when nifedipine is co-administered with beta blocker and narcotic analgesic). Products include:
Alfenta Injection 1286

Atenolol (Combination of nifedipine and beta blocker may increase the likelihood of congestive heart failure, severe hypotension, or exacerbation of angina). Products include:
Tenoretic Tablets 2845
Tenormin Tablets and I.V. Injection 2847

Betaxolol Hydrochloride (Combination of nifedipine and beta blocker may increase the likelihood of congestive heart failure, severe hypotension, or exacerbation of angina). Products include:
Betoptic Ophthalmic Solution 469
Betoptic S Ophthalmic Suspension 471
Kerlone Tablets 2436

Bisoprolol Fumarate (Combination of nifedipine and beta blocker may increase the likelihood of congestive heart failure, severe hypotension, or exacerbation of angina). Products include:
Zebeta Tablets 1413
Ziac 1415

Buprenorphine (Potential for severe hypotension and/or increased fluid volume requirements cannot be ruled out when nifedipine is co-administered with beta blocker and narcotic analgesic). Products include:
Buprenex Injectable 2006

Carteolol Hydrochloride (Combination of nifedipine and beta blocker may increase the likelihood of congestive heart failure, severe hypotension, or exacerbation of angina). Products include:
Cartrol Tablets 410
Ocupress Ophthalmic Solution, 1% Sterile ◉ 309

Cimetidine (Both the peak plasma level of nifedipine and AUC may increase in the presence of cimetidine). Products include:
Tagamet Tablets 2516

Cimetidine Hydrochloride (Both the peak plasma level of nifedipine and AUC may increase in the presence of cimetidine). Products include:
Tagamet 2516

Codeine Phosphate (Potential for severe hypotension and/or increased fluid volume requirements cannot be ruled out when nifedipine is co-administered with beta blocker and narcotic analgesic). Products include:
Actifed with Codeine Cough Syrup 1067
Brontex 1981
Deconsal C Expectorant Syrup 456
Deconsal Pediatric Syrup 457
Dimetane-DC Cough Syrup 2059
Empirin with Codeine Tablets 1093
Fioricet with Codeine Capsules 2260
Fiorinal with Codeine Capsules 2262
Isoclor Expectorant 990
Novahistine DH 2462
Novahistine Expectorant 2463
Nucofed 2051
Phenergan with Codeine 2777
Phenergan VC with Codeine 2781
Robitussin A-C Syrup 2073
Robitussin-DAC Syrup 2074
Ryna ▣ 841
Soma Compound w/Codeine Tablets 2676
Tussi-Organidin NR Liquid and S NR Liquid 2677
Tylenol with Codeine 1583

Deslanoside (Potential of elevated digoxin levels).
No products indexed under this heading.

Dezocine (Potential for severe hypotension and/or increased fluid volume requirements cannot be ruled out when nifedipine is co-administered with beta blocker and narcotic analgesic). Products include:
Dalgan Injection 538

Dicumarol (Rare reports of increased prothrombin time).
No products indexed under this heading.

Digitoxin (Potential of elevated digoxin levels). Products include:
Crystodigin Tablets 1433

Digoxin (Potential of elevated digoxin levels). Products include:
Lanoxicaps 1117
Lanoxin Elixir Pediatric 1120
Lanoxin Injection 1123
Lanoxin Injection Pediatric 1126
Lanoxin Tablets 1128

Esmolol Hydrochloride (Combination of nifedipine and beta blocker may increase the likelihood of congestive heart failure, severe hypotension, or exacerbation of angina). Products include:
Brevibloc Injection 1808

Fentanyl (Potential for severe hypotension and/or increased fluid volume requirements cannot be ruled out when nifedipine is co-administered with beta blocker, narcotic analgesic and high dose fentanyl anesthesia). Products include:
Duragesic Transdermal System 1288

Fentanyl Citrate (Potential for severe hypotension and/or increased fluid volume requirements cannot be ruled out when nifedipine is co-administered with beta blocker, narcotic analgesic and high-dose fentanyl anesthesia). Products include:
Sublimaze Injection 1307

(▣ Described in PDR For Nonprescription Drugs) (◉ Described in PDR For Ophthalmology)

Hydrocodone Bitartrate (Potential for severe hypotension and/or increased fluid volume requirements cannot be ruled out when nifedipine is co-administered with beta blocker and narcotic analgesic). Products include:

- Anexsia 5/500 Elixir ... 1781
- Anexia Tablets ... 1782
- Codiclear DH Syrup ... 791
- Deconamine CX Cough and Cold Liquid and Tablets ... 1319
- Duratuss HD Elixir ... 2565
- Hycodan Tablets and Syrup ... 930
- Hycomine Compound Tablets ... 932
- Hycomine ... 931
- Hycotuss Expectorant Syrup ... 933
- Hydrocet Capsules ... 782
- Lorcet 10/650 ... 1018
- Lortab ... 2566
- Tussend ... 1783
- Tussend Expectorant ... 1785
- Vicodin Tablets ... 1356
- Vicodin ES Tablets ... 1357
- Vicodin Tuss Expectorant ... 1358
- Zydone Capsules ... 949

Hydrocodone Polistirex (Potential for severe hypotension and/or increased fluid volume requirements cannot be ruled out when nifedipine is co-administered with beta blocker and narcotic analgesic). Products include:

- Tussionex Pennkinetic Extended-Release Suspension ... 998

Labetalol Hydrochloride (Combination of nifedipine and beta blocker may increase the likelihood of congestive heart failure, severe hypotension, or exacerbation of angina). Products include:

- Normodyne Injection ... 2377
- Normodyne Tablets ... 2379
- Trandate ... 1185

Levobunolol Hydrochloride (Combination of nifedipine and beta blocker may increase the likelihood of congestive heart failure, severe hypotension, or exacerbation of angina). Products include:

- Betagan ... ◉ 233

Levorphanol Tartrate (Potential for severe hypotension and/or increased fluid volume requirements cannot be ruled out when nifedipine is co-administered with beta blocker and narcotic analgesic). Products include:

- Levo-Dromoran ... 2129

Meperidine Hydrochloride (Potential for severe hypotension and/or increased fluid volume requirements cannot be ruled out when nifedipine is co-administered with beta blocker and narcotic analgesic). Products include:

- Demerol ... 2308
- Mepergan Injection ... 2753

Methadone Hydrochloride (Potential for severe hypotension and/or increased fluid volume requirements cannot be ruled out when nifedipine is co-administered with beta blocker and narcotic analgesic). Products include:

- Methadone Hydrochloride Oral Concentrate ... 2233
- Methadone Hydrochloride Oral Solution & Tablets ... 2235

Metipranolol Hydrochloride (Combination of nifedipine and beta blocker may increase the likelihood of congestive heart failure, severe hypotension, or exacerbation of angina). Products include:

- OptiPranolol (Metipranolol 0.3%) Sterile Ophthalmic Solution ... ◉ 258

Metoprolol Succinate (Combination of nifedipine and beta blocker may increase the likelihood of congestive heart failure, severe hypotension, or exacerbation of angina). Products include:

- Toprol-XL Tablets ... 565

Metoprolol Tartrate (Combination of nifedipine and beta blocker may increase the likelihood of congestive heart failure, severe hypotension, or exacerbation of angina). Products include:

- Lopressor Ampuls ... 830
- Lopressor HCT Tablets ... 832
- Lopressor Tablets ... 830

Morphine Sulfate (Potential for severe hypotension and/or increased fluid volume requirements cannot be ruled out when nifedipine is co-administered with beta blocker and narcotic analgesic). Products include:

- Astramorph/PF Injection, USP (Preservative-Free) ... 535
- Duramorph ... 962
- Infumorph 200 and Infumorph 500 Sterile Solutions ... 965
- MS Contin Tablets ... 1994
- MSIR ... 1997
- Oramorph SR (Morphine Sulfate Sustained Release Tablets) ... 2236
- RMS Suppositories ... 2657
- Roxanol ... 2243

Nadolol (Combination of nifedipine and beta blocker may increase the likelihood of congestive heart failure, severe hypotension, or exacerbation of angina).

No products indexed under this heading.

Opium Alkaloids (Potential for severe hypotension and/or increased fluid volume requirements cannot be ruled out when nifedipine is co-administered with beta blocker and narcotic analgesic).

No products indexed under this heading.

Oxycodone Hydrochloride (Potential for severe hypotension and/or increased fluid volume requirements cannot be ruled out when nifedipine is co-administered with beta blocker and narcotic analgesic). Products include:

- Percocet Tablets ... 938
- Percodan Tablets ... 939
- Percodan-Demi Tablets ... 940
- Roxicodone Tablets, Oral Solution & Intensol (Oxycodone) ... 2244
- Tylox Capsules ... 1584

Penbutolol Sulfate (Combination of nifedipine and beta blocker may increase the likelihood of congestive heart failure, severe hypotension, or exacerbation of angina). Products include:

- Levatol ... 2403

Pindolol (Combination of nifedipine and beta blocker may increase the likelihood of congestive heart failure, severe hypotension, or exacerbation of angina). Products include:

- Visken Tablets ... 2299

Propoxyphene Hydrochloride (Potential for severe hypotension and/or increased fluid volume requirements cannot be ruled out when nifedipine is co-administered with beta blocker and narcotic analgesic). Products include:

- Darvon ... 1435
- Wygesic Tablets ... 2827

Propoxyphene Napsylate (Potential for severe hypotension and/or increased fluid volume requirements cannot be ruled out when nifedipine is co-administered with beta blocker and narcotic analgesic). Products include:

- Darvon-N/Darvocet-N ... 1433

Propranolol Hydrochloride (Combination of nifedipine and beta blocker may increase the likelihood of congestive heart failure, severe hypotension, or exacerbation of angina). Products include:

- Inderal ... 2728
- Inderal LA Long Acting Capsules ... 2730
- Inderide Tablets ... 2732
- Inderide LA Long Acting Capsules ... 2734

Quinidine Gluconate (Rare reports of decreased plasma level of quinidine). Products include:

- Quinaglute Dura-Tabs Tablets ... 649

Quinidine Polygalacturonate (Rare reports of decreased plasma level of quinidine).

No products indexed under this heading.

Quinidine Sulfate (Rare reports of decreased plasma level of quinidine). Products include:

- Quinidex Extentabs ... 2067

Ranitidine Hydrochloride (Produces smaller, non-significant increases in peak nifedipine plasma levels and AUC). Products include:

- Zantac ... 1209
- Zantac Injection ... 1207
- Zantac Syrup ... 1209

Sotalol Hydrochloride (Combination of nifedipine and beta blocker may increase the likelihood of congestive heart failure, severe hypotension, or exacerbation of angina). Products include:

- Betapace Tablets ... 641

Sufentanil Citrate (Potential for severe hypotension and/or increased fluid volume requirements cannot be ruled out when nifedipine is co-administered with beta blocker and narcotic analgesic). Products include:

- Sufenta Injection ... 1309

Timolol Hemihydrate (Combination of nifedipine and beta blocker may increase the likelihood of congestive heart failure, severe hypotension, or exacerbation of angina). Products include:

- Betimol 0.25%, 0.5% ... ◉ 261

Timolol Maleate (Combination of nifedipine and beta blocker may increase the likelihood of congestive heart failure, severe hypotension, or exacerbation of angina). Products include:

- Blocadren Tablets ... 1614
- Timolide Tablets ... 1748
- Timoptic in Ocudose ... 1753
- Timoptic Sterile Ophthalmic Solution ... 1751
- Timoptic-XE ... 1755

Warfarin Sodium (Rare reports of increased prothrombin time). Products include:

- Coumadin ... 926

Food Interactions

Diet, high-lipid (High fat meal increases peak plasma nifedipine concentrations by 60%, a prolongation in the time to peak concentration, but no significant change in the AUC; administer on an empty stomach).

ADATOSIL 5000

(Silicone Oil) ... ◉ 274

None cited in PDR database.

ADENOCARD INJECTION

(Adenosine) ... 1021

May interact with xanthine bronchodilators and certain other agents. Compounds in these categories include:

Aminophylline (The effects of adenosine are antagonized).

No products indexed under this heading.

Caffeine-containing medications (The effects of adenosine are antagonized).

Carbamazepine (Potential for higher degrees of heart block). Products include:

- Atretol Tablets ... 573
- Tegretol Chewable Tablets ... 852
- Tegretol Suspension ... 852
- Tegretol Tablets ... 852

Digoxin (The use of adenosine in patients receiving digitalis may be associated with ventricular fibrillation). Products include:

- Lanoxicaps ... 1117
- Lanoxin Elixir Pediatric ... 1120
- Lanoxin Injection ... 1123
- Lanoxin Injection Pediatric ... 1126
- Lanoxin Tablets ... 1128

Dipyridamole (Potentiates the effects). Products include:

- Persantine Tablets ... 681

Dyphylline (The effects of adenosine are antagonized). Products include:

- Lufyllin & Lufyllin-400 Tablets ... 2670
- Lufyllin-GG Elixir & Tablets ... 2671

Theophylline (The effects of adenosine are antagonized). Products include:

- Marax Tablets & DF Syrup ... 2200
- Quibron ... 2053

Theophylline Anhydrous (The effects of adenosine are antagonized). Products include:

- Aerolate ... 1004
- Primatene Dual Action Formula ... 872
- Primatene Tablets ... 873
- Respbid Tablets ... 682
- Slo-bid Gyrocaps ... 2033
- Theo-24 Extended Release Capsules ... 2568
- Theo-Dur Extended-Release Tablets ... 1327
- Theo-X Extended-Release Tablets ... 788
- Uni-Dur Extended-Release Tablets ... 1331
- Uniphyl 400 mg Tablets ... 2001

Theophylline Calcium Salicylate (The effects of adenosine are antagonized). Products include:

- Quadrinal Tablets ... 1350

Theophylline Sodium Glycinate (The effects of adenosine are antagonized).

No products indexed under this heading.

ADENOSCAN

(Adenosine) ... 1024

May interact with beta blockers, cardiac glycosides, calcium channel blockers, adenosine receptor antagonists, and nucleoside transport inhibitors. Compounds in these categories include:

Acebutolol Hydrochloride (Potential for additive or synergistic depressant effects on the SA or AV nodes; adenosine should be used with caution in the presence of these agents; no adverse interactions have been reported when co-administered). Products include:

- Sectral Capsules ... 2807

Aminophylline (Vasoactive effects of adenosine are inhibited by adenosine receptor antagonists such as alkylxanthines).

No products indexed under this heading.

IMPORTANT NOTE: Always consult each drug listing in the patient's regimen for possible interactions.

Amlodipine Besylate (Potential for additive or synergistic depressant effects on the SA or AV nodes; adenosine should be used with caution in the presence of these agents; no adverse interactions have been reported when co-administered). Products include:
- Lotrel Capsules 840
- Norvasc Tablets 1940

Atenolol (Potential for additive or synergistic depressant effects on the SA or AV nodes; adenosine should be used with caution in the presence of these agents; no adverse interactions have been reported when co-administered). Products include:
- Tenoretic Tablets 2845
- Tenormin Tablets and I.V. Injection 2847

Bepridil Hydrochloride (Potential for additive or synergistic depressant effects on the SA or AV nodes; adenosine should be used with caution in the presence of these agents; no adverse interactions have been reported when co-administered). Products include:
- Vascor (200, 300 and 400 mg) Tablets 1587

Betaxolol Hydrochloride (Potential for additive or synergistic depressant effects on the SA or AV nodes; adenosine should be used with caution in the presence of these agents; no adverse interactions have been reported when co-administered). Products include:
- Betoptic Ophthalmic Solution........ 469
- Betoptic S Ophthalmic Suspension 471
- Kerlone Tablets 2436

Bisoprolol Fumarate (Potential for additive or synergistic depressant effects on the SA or AV nodes; adenosine should be used with caution in the presence of these agents; no adverse interactions have been reported when co-administered). Products include:
- Zebeta Tablets 1413
- Ziac 1415

Caffeine (Vasoactive effects of adenosine are inhibited by adenosine receptor antagonists such as alkylxantines). Products include:
- Arthritis Strength BC Powder........ ▣ 609
- BC Powder .... ▣ 609
- Bayer Select Headache Pain Relief Formula .... ▣ 716
- Cafergot........ 2251
- DHCplus Capsules........ 1993
- Darvon Compound-65 Pulvules 1435
- Esgic-plus Tablets 1013
- Aspirin Free Excedrin Analgesic Caplets and Geltabs 732
- Excedrin Extra-Strength Analgesic Tablets & Caplets 732
- Fioricet Tablets........ 2258
- Fioricet with Codeine Capsules 2260
- Fiorinal Capsules 2261
- Fiorinal with Codeine Capsules 2262
- Fiorinal Tablets........ 2261
- Maximum Strength Multi-Symptom Formula Midol .... ▣ 722
- Migralam Capsules 2038
- No Doz Maximum Strength Caplets .... ▣ 622
- Norgesic........ 1496
- Vanquish Analgesic Caplets .... ▣ 731
- Wigraine Tablets & Suppositories .. 1829

Carteolol Hydrochloride (Potential for additive or synergistic depressant effects on the SA or AV nodes; adenosine should be used with caution in the presence of these agents; no adverse interactions have been reported when co-administered). Products include:
- Cartrol Tablets 410
- Ocupress Ophthalmic Solution, 1% Sterile........ ◉ 309

Deslanoside (Potential for additive or synergistic depressant effects on the SA or AV nodes; adenosine should be used with caution in the presence of these agents; no adverse interactions have been reported when co-administered).

No products indexed under this heading.

Digitoxin (Potential for additive or synergistic depressant effects on the SA or AV nodes; adenosine should be used with caution in the presence of these agents; no adverse interactions have been reported when co-administered). Products include:
- Crystodigin Tablets........ 1433

Digoxin (Potential for additive or synergistic depressant effects on the SA or AV nodes; adenosine should be used with caution in the presence of these agents; no adverse interactions have been reported when co-administered). Products include:
- Lanoxicaps 1117
- Lanoxin Elixir Pediatric 1120
- Lanoxin Injection 1123
- Lanoxin Injection Pediatric........ 1126
- Lanoxin Tablets 1128

Diltiazem Hydrochloride (Potential for additive or synergistic depressant effects on the SA or AV nodes; adenosine should be used with caution in the presence of these agents; no adverse interactions have been reported when co-administered). Products include:
- Cardizem CD Capsules 1506
- Cardizem SR Capsules 1510
- Cardizem Injectable 1508
- Cardizem Tablets........ 1512
- Dilacor XR Extended-release Capsules 2018

Dipyridamole (Vasoactive effects of adenosine are potentiated by nucleoside transport inhibited). Products include:
- Persantine Tablets 681

Dyphylline (Vasoactive effects of adenosine are inhibited by adenosine receptor antagonists such as alkylxantines). Products include:
- Lufyllin & Lufyllin-400 Tablets 2670
- Lufyllin-GG Elixir & Tablets 2671

Esmolol Hydrochloride (Potential for additive or synergistic depressant effects on the SA or AV nodes; adenosine should be used with caution in the presence of these agents; no adverse interactions have been reported when co-administered). Products include:
- Brevibloc Injection........ 1808

Felodipine (Potential for additive or synergistic depressant effects on the SA or AV nodes; adenosine should be used with caution in the presence of these agents; no adverse interactions have been reported when co-administered). Products include:
- Plendil Extended-Release Tablets.... 527

Isradipine (Potential for additive or synergistic depressant effects on the SA or AV nodes; adenosine should be used with caution in the presence of these agents; no adverse interactions have been reported when co-administered). Products include:
- DynaCirc Capsules 2256

Labetalol Hydrochloride (Potential for additive or synergistic depressant effects on the SA or AV nodes; adenosine should be used with caution in the presence of these agents; no adverse interactions have been reported when co-administered). Products include:
- Normodyne Injection 2377
- Normodyne Tablets 2379
- Trandate 1185

Levobunolol Hydrochloride (Potential for additive or synergistic depressant effects on the SA or AV nodes; adenosine should be used with caution in the presence of these agents; no adverse interactions have been reported when co-administered). Products include:
- Betagan .... ◉ 233

Metipranolol Hydrochloride (Potential for additive or synergistic depressant effects on the SA or AV nodes; adenosine should be used with caution in the presence of these agents; no adverse interactions have been reported when co-administered). Products include:
- OptiPranolol (Metipranolol 0.3%) Sterile Ophthalmic Solution........ ◉ 258

Metoprolol Succinate (Potential for additive or synergistic depressant effects on the SA or AV nodes; adenosine should be used with caution in the presence of these agents; no adverse interactions have been reported when co-administered). Products include:
- Toprol-XL Tablets 565

Metoprolol Tartrate (Potential for additive or synergistic depressant effects on the SA or AV nodes; adenosine should be used with caution in the presence of these agents; no adverse interactions have been reported when co-administered). Products include:
- Lopressor Ampuls 830
- Lopressor HCT Tablets 832
- Lopressor Tablets 830

Nadolol (Potential for additive or synergistic depressant effects on the SA or AV nodes; adenosine should be used with caution in the presence of these agents; no adverse interactions have been reported when co-administered).

No products indexed under this heading.

Nicardipine Hydrochloride (Potential for additive or synergistic depressant effects on the SA or AV nodes; adenosine should be used with caution in the presence of these agents; no adverse interactions have been reported when co-administered). Products include:
- Cardene Capsules 2095
- Cardene I.V. 2709
- Cardene SR Capsules........ 2097

Nifedipine (Potential for additive or synergistic depressant effects on the SA or AV nodes; adenosine should be used with caution in the presence of these agents; no adverse interactions have been reported when co-administered). Products include:
- Adalat Capsules (10 mg and 20 mg) 587
- Adalat CC 589
- Procardia Capsules........ 1971
- Procardia XL Extended Release Tablets 1972

Nimodipine (Potential for additive or synergistic depressant effects on the SA or AV nodes; adenosine should be used with caution in the presence of these agents; no adverse interactions have been reported when co-administered). Products include:
- Nimotop Capsules 610

Nisoldipine (Potential for additive or synergistic depressant effects on the SA or AV nodes; adenosine should be used with caution in the presence of these agents; no adverse interactions have been reported when co-administered).

No products indexed under this heading.

Penbutolol Sulfate (Potential for additive or synergistic depressant effects on the SA or AV nodes; adenosine should be used with caution in the presence of these agents; no adverse interactions have been reported when co-administered). Products include:
- Levatol 2403

Pindolol (Potential for additive or synergistic depressant effects on the SA or AV nodes; adenosine should be used with caution in the presence of these agents; no adverse interactions have been reported when co-administered). Products include:
- Visken Tablets........ 2299

Propranolol Hydrochloride (Potential for additive or synergistic depressant effects on the SA or AV nodes; adenosine should be used with caution in the presence of these agents; no adverse interactions have been reported when co-administered). Products include:
- Inderal 2728
- Inderal LA Long Acting Capsules 2730
- Inderide Tablets 2732
- Inderide LA Long Acting Capsules .. 2734

Sotalol Hydrochloride (Potential for additive or synergistic depressant effects on the SA or AV nodes; adenosine should be used with caution in the presence of these agents; no adverse interactions have been reported when co-administered). Products include:
- Betapace Tablets 641

Theophylline (Vasoactive effects of adenosine are inhibited by adenosine receptor antagonists such as alkylxantines). Products include:
- Marax Tablets & DF Syrup........ 2200
- Quibron 2053

Theophylline Anhydrous (Vasoactive effects of adenosine are inhibited by adenosine receptor antagonists such as alkylxantines). Products include:
- Aerolate 1004
- Primatene Dual Action Formula...... ▣ 872
- Primatene Tablets .... ▣ 873
- Respbid Tablets 682
- Slo-bid Gyrocaps 2033
- Theo-24 Extended Release Capsules 2568
- Theo-Dur Extended-Release Tablets 1327
- Theo-X Extended-Release Tablets .. 788
- Uni-Dur Extended-Release Tablets.. 1331
- Uniphyl 400 mg Tablets........ 2001

Theophylline Calcium Salicylate (Vasoactive effects of adenosine are inhibited by adenosine receptor antagonists such as alkylxantines). Products include:
- Quadrinal Tablets 1350

Theophylline Sodium Glycinate (Vasoactive effects of adenosine are inhibited by adenosine receptor antagonists such as alkylxantines).

No products indexed under this heading.

(▣ Described in PDR For Nonprescription Drugs) (◉ Described in PDR For Ophthalmology)

Timolol Hemihydrate (Potential for additive or synergistic depressant effects on the SA or AV nodes; adenosine should be used with caution in the presence of these agents; no adverse interactions have been reported when co-administered). Products include:

Betimol 0.25%, 0.5% ◉ 261

Timolol Maleate (Potential for additive or synergistic depressant effects on the SA or AV nodes; adenosine should be used with caution in the presence of these agents; no adverse interactions have been reported when co-administered). Products include:

Blocadren Tablets 1614
Timolide Tablets 1748
Timoptic in Ocudose 1753
Timoptic Sterile Ophthalmic Solution 1751
Timoptic-XE 1755

Verapamil Hydrochloride (Potential for additive or synergistic depressant effects on the SA or AV nodes; adenosine should be used with caution in the presence of these agents; no adverse interactions have been reported when co-administered). Products include:

Calan SR Caplets 2422
Calan Tablets 2419
Isoptin Injectable 1344
Isoptin Oral Tablets 1346
Isoptin SR Tablets 1348
Verelan Capsules 1410
Verelan Capsules 2824

ADIPEX-P TABLETS AND CAPSULES

(Phentermine Hydrochloride) 1048

May interact with monoamine oxidase inhibitors, insulin, and certain other agents. Compounds in these categories include:

Furazolidone (Contraindication; hypertensive crisis may result). Products include:

Furoxone 2046

Guanethidine Monosulfate (Decreased hypotensive effect of guanethidine). Products include:

Esimil Tablets 822
Ismelin Tablets 827

Insulin, Human (Insulin requirement may be altered).

No products indexed under this heading.

Insulin, Human Isophane Suspension (Insulin requirement may be altered). Products include:

Novolin N Human Insulin 10 ml Vials 1795

Insulin, Human NPH (Insulin requirement may be altered). Products include:

Humulin N, 100 Units 1448
Novolin N PenFill Cartridges Durable Insulin Delivery System 1798
Novolin N Prefilled Syringe Disposable Insulin Delivery System 1798

Insulin, Human Regular (Insulin requirement may be altered). Products include:

Humulin R, 100 Units 1449
Novolin R Human Insulin 10 ml Vials 1795
Novolin R PenFill Cartridges Durable Insulin Delivery System 1798
Novolin R Prefilled Syringe Disposable Insulin Delivery System 1798
Velosulin BR Human Insulin 10 ml Vials 1795

Insulin, Human, Zinc Suspension (Insulin requirement may be altered). Products include:

Humulin L, 100 Units 1446
Humulin U, 100 Units 1450
Novolin L Human Insulin 10 ml Vials 1795

Insulin, NPH (Insulin requirement may be altered). Products include:

NPH, 100 Units 1450
Pork NPH, 100 Units 1452
Purified Pork NPH Isophane Insulin 1801

Insulin, Regular (Insulin requirement may be altered). Products include:

Regular, 100 Units 1450
Pork Regular, 100 Units 1452
Pork Regular (Concentrated), 500 Units 1453
Purified Pork Regular Insulin 1801

Insulin, Zinc Crystals (Insulin requirement may be altered). Products include:

NPH, 100 Units 1450

Insulin, Zinc Suspension (Insulin requirement may be altered). Products include:

Iletin I 1450
Lente, 100 Units 1450
Iletin II 1452
Pork Lente, 100 Units 1452
Purified Pork Lente Insulin 1801

Isocarboxazid (Contraindication; hypertensive crisis may result).

No products indexed under this heading.

Phenelzine Sulfate (Contraindication; hypertensive crisis may result). Products include:

Nardil 1920

Selegiline Hydrochloride (Contraindication; hypertensive crisis may result). Products include:

Eldepryl Tablets 2550

Tranylcypromine Sulfate (Contraindication; hypertensive crisis may result). Products include:

Parnate Tablets 2503

Food Interactions

Alcohol (May result in adverse drug interaction).

ADRIAMYCIN PFS

(Doxorubicin Hydrochloride) 1947

May interact with antineoplastics and certain other agents. Compounds in these categories include:

Altretamine (Doxorubicin may potentiate the toxicity of other anticancer therapies). Products include:

Hexalen Capsules 2571

Asparaginase (Doxorubicin may potentiate the toxicity of other anticancer therapies). Products include:

Elspar 1659

Bleomycin Sulfate (Doxorubicin may potentiate the toxicity of other anticancer therapies). Products include:

Blenoxane 692

Busulfan (Doxorubicin may potentiate the toxicity of other anticancer therapies). Products include:

Myleran Tablets 1143

Carboplatin (Doxorubicin may potentiate the toxicity of other anticancer therapies). Products include:

Paraplatin for Injection 705

Carmustine (BCNU) (Doxorubicin may potentiate the toxicity of other anticancer therapies). Products include:

BiCNU 691

Chlorambucil (Doxorubicin may potentiate the toxicity of other anticancer therapies). Products include:

Leukeran Tablets 1133

Cisplatin (Doxorubicin may potentiate the toxicity of other anticancer therapies). Products include:

Platinol 708
Platinol-AQ Injection 710

Cyclophosphamide (Doxorubicin may potentiate the toxicity of other anticancer therapies; serious irreversible myocardial toxicity; exacerbation of cyclophosphamide-induced hemorrhagic cystitis). Products include:

Cytoxan 694
NEOSAR Lyophilized/Neosar 1959

Cyclosporine (Concurrent use may induce coma and/or seizures). Products include:

Neoral 2276
Sandimmune 2286

Cytarabine (Combination therapy results in necrotizing colitis, typhilitis, bloody stools and severe infections). Products include:

Cytosar-U Sterile Powder 2592

Dacarbazine (Doxorubicin may potentiate the toxicity of other anticancer therapies). Products include:

DTIC-Dome 600

Daunorubicin Hydrochloride (Doxorubicin may potentiate the toxicity of other anticancer therapies). Products include:

Cerubidine 795

Estramustine Phosphate Sodium (Doxorubicin may potentiate the toxicity of other anticancer therapies). Products include:

Emcyt Capsules 1953

Etoposide (Doxorubicin may potentiate the toxicity of other anticancer therapies). Products include:

VePesid Capsules and Injection 718

Floxuridine (Doxorubicin may potentiate the toxicity of other anticancer therapies). Products include:

Sterile FUDR 2118

Fluorouracil (Doxorubicin may potentiate the toxicity of other anticancer therapies). Products include:

Efudex 2113
Fluoroplex Topical Solution & Cream 1% 479
Fluorouracil Injection 2116

Flutamide (Doxorubicin may potentiate the toxicity of other anticancer therapies). Products include:

Eulexin Capsules 2358

Hydroxyurea (Doxorubicin may potentiate the toxicity of other anticancer therapies). Products include:

Hydrea Capsules 696

Idarubicin Hydrochloride (Doxorubicin may potentiate the toxicity of other anticancer therapies; concurrent use is contraindicated in patients who have received previous treatment with complete cumulative doses of idarubicin). Products include:

Idamycin 1955

Ifosfamide (Doxorubicin may potentiate the toxicity of other anticancer therapies). Products include:

IFEX 697

Interferon alfa-2A, Recombinant (Doxorubicin may potentiate the toxicity of other anticancer therapies). Products include:

Roferon-A Injection 2145

Interferon alfa-2B, Recombinant (Doxorubicin may potentiate the toxicity of other anticancer therapies). Products include:

Intron A 2364

Levamisole Hydrochloride (Doxorubicin may potentiate the toxicity of other anticancer therapies). Products include:

Ergamisol Tablets 1292

Live Virus Vaccines (Administration of live vaccine to immunocompromised patients, including those undergoing cytotoxic chemotherapy, may be hazardous).

Lomustine (CCNU) (Doxorubicin may potentiate the toxicity of other anticancer therapies). Products include:

CeeNU 693

Mechlorethamine Hydrochloride (Doxorubicin may potentiate the toxicity of other anticancer therapies). Products include:

Mustargen 1709

Megestrol Acetate (Doxorubicin may potentiate the toxicity of other anticancer therapies). Products include:

Megace Oral Suspension 699
Megace Tablets 701

Melphalan (Doxorubicin may potentiate the toxicity of other anticancer therapies). Products include:

Alkeran Tablets 1071

Mercaptopurine (Enhanced hepatotoxicity of 6-mercaptopurine). Products include:

Purinethol Tablets 1156

Methotrexate Sodium (Doxorubicin may potentiate the toxicity of other anticancer therapies). Products include:

Methotrexate Sodium Tablets, Injection, for Injection and LPF Injection 1275

Mitomycin (Mitomycin-C) (Doxorubicin may potentiate the toxicity of other anticancer therapies). Products include:

Mutamycin 703

Mitotane (Doxorubicin may potentiate the toxicity of other anticancer therapies). Products include:

Lysodren 698

Mitoxantrone Hydrochloride (Doxorubicin may potentiate the toxicity of other anticancer therapies). Products include:

Novantrone 1279

Paclitaxel (Doxorubicin may potentiate the toxicity of other anticancer therapies). Products include:

Taxol 714

Phenobarbital (Increases the elimination of doxorubicin). Products include:

Arco-Lase Plus Tablets 512
Bellergal-S Tablets 2250
Donnatal 2060
Donnatal Extentabs 2061
Donnatal Tablets 2060
Phenobarbital Elixir and Tablets 1469
Quadrinal Tablets 1350

Phenytoin (Potential for decreased phenytoin levels with concurrent use). Products include:

Dilantin Infatabs 1908
Dilantin-125 Suspension 1911

Phenytoin Sodium (Potential for decreased phenytoin levels with concurrent use). Products include:

Dilantin Kapseals 1906
Dilantin Parenteral 1910

Procarbazine Hydrochloride (Doxorubicin may potentiate the toxicity of other anticancer therapies). Products include:

Matulane Capsules 2131

Streptozocin (May inhibit the hepatic metabolism; doxorubicin may potentiate the toxicity of other anticancer therapies). Products include:

Zanosar Sterile Powder 2653

Tamoxifen Citrate (Doxorubicin may potentiate the toxicity of other anticancer therapies). Products include:

Nolvadex Tablets 2841

IMPORTANT NOTE: Always consult each drug listing in the patient's regimen for possible interactions.

Adriamycin PFS

Teniposide (Doxorubicin may potentiate the toxicity of other anticancer therapies). Products include:

Vumon 727

Thioguanine (Doxorubicin may potentiate the toxicity of other anticancer therapies). Products include:

Thioguanine Tablets, Tabloid Brand 1181

Thiotepa (Doxorubicin may potentiate the toxicity of other anticancer therapies). Products include:

Thioplex (Thiotepa For Injection) 1281

Vincristine Sulfate (Doxorubicin may potentiate the toxicity of other anticancer therapies). Products include:

Oncovin Solution Vials & Hyporets 1466

ADRIAMYCIN RDF

(Doxorubicin Hydrochloride) 1947

See Adriamycin PFS

ADSORBOTEAR ARTIFICIAL TEAR

(Povidone) .... ◉ 210

None cited in PDR database.

ADVERA SPECIALIZED COMPLETE NUTRITION

(Nutritional Beverage)..........................2220

None cited in PDR database.

ADVIL COLD AND SINUS CAPLETS AND TABLETS (FORMERLY COADVIL)

(Ibuprofen, Pseudoephedrine Hydrochloride)......................................ᴴᴰ 870

May interact with antihypertensives, antidepressant drugs, and aspirin and acetaminophen containing products. Compounds in these categories include:

Acebutolol Hydrochloride (Effects not specified). Products include:

Sectral Capsules 2807

Acetaminophen (Effects not specified). Products include:

Actifed Plus Caplets ....ᴴᴰ 845
Actifed Plus Tablets ....ᴴᴰ 845
Actifed Sinus Daytime/Nighttime Tablets and Caplets ....ᴴᴰ 846
Alka-Seltzer Plus Cold Medicine Liqui-Gels ....ᴴᴰ 706
Alka-Seltzer Plus Cold & Cough Medicine Liqui-Gels..........................ᴴᴰ 705
Alka-Seltzer Plus Night-Time Cold Medicine Liqui-Gels..........................ᴴᴰ 706
Allerest Headache Strength Tablets ....ᴴᴰ 627
Allerest No Drowsiness Tablets......ᴴᴰ 627
Allerest Sinus Pain Formula ....ᴴᴰ 627
Anexsia 5/500 Elixir 1781
Anexia Tablets.. 1782
Arthritis Foundation Aspirin Free Caplets ....ᴴᴰ 673
Arthritis Foundation NightTime Caplets ....ᴴᴰ 674
Bayer Select Headache Pain Relief Formula ....ᴴᴰ 716
Bayer Select Menstrual Multi-Symptom Formula............................ᴴᴰ 716
Bayer Select Night Time Pain Relief Formula.....................................ᴴᴰ 716
Bayer Select Sinus Pain Relief Formula ....ᴴᴰ 717
Benadryl Allergy Sinus Headache Formula Caplets ....ᴴᴰ 849
Comtrex Multi-Symptom Cold Reliever Tablets/Caplets/Liqui-Gels/Liquid...ᴴᴰ 615
Allergy-Sinus Comtrex Multi-Symptom Allergy-Sinus Formula Tablets ....ᴴᴰ 617
Comtrex Non-Drowsy ....ᴴᴰ 618
Contac Day Allergy/Sinus Caplets ᴴᴰ 812
Contac Day & Night ....ᴴᴰ 812
Contac Night Allergy/Sinus Caplets ....ᴴᴰ 812
Contac Severe Cold and Flu Formula Caplets ....ᴴᴰ 814

Contac Severe Cold & Flu Non-Drowsy ....ᴴᴰ 815
Coricidin 'D' Decongestant Tablets ....ᴴᴰ 800
Coricidin Tablets ....ᴴᴰ 800
DHCplus Capsules................................ 1993
Darvon-N/Darvocet-N 1433
Drixoral Cold and Flu Extended-Release Tablets..................................ᴴᴰ 803
Drixoral Cough + Sore Throat Liquid Caps ....ᴴᴰ 802
Drixoral Allergy/Sinus Extended Release Tablets..................................ᴴᴰ 804
Esgic-plus Tablets 1013
Aspirin Free Excedrin Analgesic Caplets and Geltabs 732
Excedrin Extra-Strength Analgesic Tablets & Caplets 732
Excedrin P.M. Analgesic/Sleeping Aid Tablets, Caplets, Liquigels 733
Fioricet Tablets 2258
Fioricet with Codeine Capsules 2260
Hycomine Compound Tablets 932
Hydrocet Capsules 782
Legatrin PM ....ᴴᴰ 651
Lorcet 10/650.. 1018
Lortab 2566
Lurline PMS Tablets 982
Maximum Strength Multi-Symptom Formula Midol ....ᴴᴰ 722
PMS Multi-Symptom Formula Midol ....ᴴᴰ 723
Teen Multi-Symptom Formula Midol ....ᴴᴰ 722
Midrin Capsules 783
Migralam Capsules 2038
Panodol Tablets and Caplets ....ᴴᴰ 824
Children's Panadol Chewable Tablets, Liquid, Infant's Drops....ᴴᴰ 824
Percocet Tablets 938
Percogesic Analgesic Tablets ....ᴴᴰ 754
Phrenilin 785
Pyrroxate Caplets ....ᴴᴰ 772
Sedapap Tablets 50 mg/650 mg .. 1543
Sinarest Tablets ....ᴴᴰ 648
Sinarest Extra Strength Tablets......ᴴᴰ 648
Sinarest No Drowsiness Tablets ....ᴴᴰ 648
Sine-Aid Maximum Strength Sinus Medication Gelcaps, Caplets and Tablets 1554
Sine-Off No Drowsiness Formula Caplets ....ᴴᴰ 824
Sine-Off Sinus Medicine ....ᴴᴰ 825
Singlet Tablets ....ᴴᴰ 825
Sinulin Tablets 787
Sinutab Sinus Allergy Medication, Maximum Strength Tablets and Caplets ....ᴴᴰ 860
Sinutab Sinus Medication, Maximum Strength Without Drowsiness Formula, Tablets & Caplets ....ᴴᴰ 860
Sinutab Sinus Medication, Regular Strength Without Drowsiness Formula ....ᴴᴰ 859
Sudafed Cold and Cough Liquidcaps ....ᴴᴰ 862
Sudafed Severe Cold Formula Caplets ....ᴴᴰ 863
Sudafed Severe Cold Formula Tablets ....ᴴᴰ 864
Sudafed Sinus Caplets......................ᴴᴰ 864
Sudafed Sinus Tablets ....ᴴᴰ 864
Talacen... 2333
TheraFlu..ᴴᴰ 787
TheraFlu Maximum Strength Nighttime Flu, Cold & Cough Medicine...ᴴᴰ 788
TheraFlu Maximum Strength Non-Drowsy Formula Flu, Cold & Cough Medicine ....ᴴᴰ 788
Thera Flu Maximum Strength, Non-Drowsy Formula Flu, Cold and Cough Caplets ....ᴴᴰ 789
Triaminic Sore Throat Formula ......ᴴᴰ 791
Triaminicin Tablets ....ᴴᴰ 793
Children's TYLENOL acetaminophen Chewable Tablets, Elixir, Suspension Liquid 1555
Children's TYLENOL Cold Multi-Symptom Liquid Formula and Chewable Tablets.............................. 1561
Children's TYLENOL Cold Plus Cough Multi Symptom Tablets and Liquid ....ᴴᴰ 681
Infants' TYLENOL acetaminophen Drops and Suspension Drops....... 1555
Infants' TYLENOL Cold Decongestant & Fever-Reducer Drops.......... 1556
TYLENOL Extended Relief Caplets.. 1558

TYLENOL, Extra Strength, Acetaminophen Adult Liquid Pain Reliever 1560
TYLENOL, Extra Strength, acetaminophen Gelcaps, Geltabs, Caplets, Tablets 1559
TYLENOL, Extra Strength, Headache Plus Pain Reliever with Antacid Caplets 1559
TYLENOL, Junior Strength, acetaminophen Coated Caplets, Grape and Fruit Chewable Tablets 1557
TYLENOL Maximum Strength Allergy Sinus Medication Gelcaps and Caplets 1563
TYLENOL Maximum Strength Allergy Sinus NightTime Medication Caplets 1555
TYLENOL Flu Maximum Strength Gelcaps 1565
TYLENOL Flu NightTime, Maximum Strength, Gelcaps 1566
TYLENOL Maximum Strength Flu NightTime Hot Medication Packets 1562
TYLENOL, Maximum Strength, Sinus Medication Geltabs, Gelcaps, Caplets and Tablets 1566
TYLENOL Cold Multi-Symptom Formula Medication Tablets and Caplets 1561
TYLENOL Cold Medication No Drowsiness Formula Gelcaps and Caplets 1562
TYLENOL Cold Multi-Symptom Hot Medication Liquid Packets.............. 1557
TYLENOL Cough Multi-Symptom Medication 1564
TYLENOL Cough Multi-Symptom Medication with Decongestant...... 1565
TYLENOL, Regular Strength, acetaminophen Caplets and Tablets .. 1558
TYLENOL PM, Extra Strength Pain Reliever/Sleep Aid Caplets, Geltabs, Gelcaps.. 1560
TYLENOL Severe Allergy Medication Caplets 1564
Tylenol with Codeine 1583
Tylox Capsules 1584
Unisom With Pain Relief-Nighttime Sleep Aid and Pain Reliever............ 1934
Vanquish Analgesic Caplets ....ᴴᴰ 731
Vicks 44 LiquiCaps Cough, Cold & Flu Relief ....ᴴᴰ 755
Vicks 44M Cough, Cold & Flu Relief ....ᴴᴰ 756
Vicks DayQuil ....ᴴᴰ 761
Vicks Nyquil Hot Therapy..................ᴴᴰ 762
Vicks NyQuil LiquiCaps Multi-Symptom Cold/Flu Relief ....ᴴᴰ 763
Vicks NyQuil Multi-Symptom Cold/Flu Relief - (Original & Cherry Flavor) ....ᴴᴰ 763
Vicodin Tablets 1356
Vicodin ES Tablets 1357
Wygesic Tablets 2827
Zydone Capsules 949

Amitriptyline Hydrochloride (Effects not specified). Products include:

Elavil 2838
Endep Tablets 2174
Etrafon 2355
Limbitrol 2180
Triavil Tablets 1757

Amlodipine Besylate (Effects not specified). Products include:

Lotrel Capsules...................................... 840
Norvasc Tablets 1940

Amoxapine (Effects not specified). Products include:

Asendin Tablets 1369

Aspirin (Effects not specified). Products include:

Alka-Seltzer Effervescent Antacid and Pain Reliever..............................ᴴᴰ 701
Alka-Seltzer Extra Strength Effervescent Antacid and Pain Reliever ....ᴴᴰ 703
Alka-Seltzer Lemon Lime Effervescent Antacid and Pain Reliever ....ᴴᴰ 703
Alka-Seltzer Plus Cold Medicine ....ᴴᴰ 705
Alka-Seltzer Plus Cold & Cough Medicine ....ᴴᴰ 708
Alka-Seltzer Plus Night-Time Cold Medicine ....ᴴᴰ 707

Alka Seltzer Plus Sinus Medicine ..ᴴᴰ 707
Arthritis Foundation Safety Coated Aspirin Tablets ....ᴴᴰ 675
Arthritis Pain Ascriptin ....ᴴᴰ 631
Maximum Strength Ascriptin ....ᴴᴰ 630
Regular Strength Ascriptin Tablets ....ᴴᴰ 629
Arthritis Strength BC Powder........ᴴᴰ 609
BC Cold Powder Multi-Symptom Formula (Cold-Sinus-Allergy) ......ᴴᴰ 609
BC Cold Powder Non-Drowsy Formula (Cold-Sinus)........................ᴴᴰ 609
BC Powder ....ᴴᴰ 609
Bayer Children's Chewable Aspirin ....ᴴᴰ 711
Genuine Bayer Aspirin Tablets & Caplets ....ᴴᴰ 713
Extra Strength Bayer Arthritis Pain Regimen Formula ....ᴴᴰ 711
Extra Strength Bayer Aspirin Caplets & Tablets ....ᴴᴰ 712
Extended-Release Bayer 8-Hour Aspirin ....ᴴᴰ 712
Extra Strength Bayer Plus Aspirin Caplets ....ᴴᴰ 713
Extra Strength Bayer PM Aspirin ..ᴴᴰ 713
Bayer Enteric Aspirin ....ᴴᴰ 709
Bufferin Analgesic Tablets and Caplets ....ᴴᴰ 613
Arthritis Strength Bufferin Analgesic Caplets ....ᴴᴰ 614
Extra Strength Bufferin Analgesic Tablets ....ᴴᴰ 615
Cama Arthritis Pain Reliever..........ᴴᴰ 785
Darvon Compound-65 Pulvules 1435
Easprin... 1914
Ecotrin 2455
Ecotrin Enteric Coated Aspirin Maximum Strength Tablets and Caplets ....ᴴᴰ 816
Ecotrin Enteric Coated Aspirin Regular Strength Tablets 2455
Empirin Aspirin Tablets ....ᴴᴰ 854
Empirin with Codeine Tablets............ 1093
Excedrin Extra-Strength Analgesic Tablets & Caplets 732
Fiorinal Capsules 2261
Fiorinal with Codeine Capsules 2262
Fiorinal Tablets...................................... 2261
Halfprin 1362
Healthprin Aspirin 2455
Norgesic... 1496
Percodan Tablets.................................... 939
Percodan-Demi Tablets........................ 940
Robaxisal Tablets.................................. 2071
Soma Compound w/Codeine Tablets 2676
Soma Compound Tablets 2675
St. Joseph Adult Chewable Aspirin (81 mg.) ....ᴴᴰ 808
Talwin Compound 2335
Ursinus Inlay-Tabs..............................ᴴᴰ 794
Vanquish Analgesic Caplets ....ᴴᴰ 731

Atenolol (Effects not specified). Products include:

Tenoretic Tablets.................................... 2845
Tenormin Tablets and I.V. Injection 2847

Benazepril Hydrochloride (Effects not specified). Products include:

Lotensin Tablets.................................... 834
Lotensin HCT.. 837
Lotrel Capsules...................................... 840

Bendroflumethiazide (Effects not specified).

No products indexed under this heading.

Betaxolol Hydrochloride (Effects not specified). Products include:

Betoptic Ophthalmic Solution............ 469
Betoptic S Ophthalmic Suspension 471
Kerlone Tablets...................................... 2436

Bisoprolol Fumarate (Effects not specified). Products include:

Zebeta Tablets 1413
Ziac 1415

Bupropion Hydrochloride (Effects not specified). Products include:

Wellbutrin Tablets 1204

Captopril (Effects not specified). Products include:

Capoten 739
Capozide 742

(ᴴᴰ Described in PDR For Nonprescription Drugs) (◉ Described in PDR For Ophthalmology)

17 Interactions Index Advil Cold & Sinus

Carteolol Hydrochloride (Effects not specified). Products include:
Cartrol Tablets ... 410
Ocupress Ophthalmic Solution, 1% Sterile ... ◉ 309
Chlorothiazide (Effects not specified). Products include:
Aldoclor Tablets ... 1598
Diupres Tablets ... 1650
Diuril Oral ... 1653
Chlorothiazide Sodium (Effects not specified). Products include:
Diuril Sodium Intravenous ... 1652
Chlorthalidone (Effects not specified). Products include:
Combipres Tablets ... 677
Tenoretic Tablets ... 2845
Thalitone ... 1245
Clonidine (Effects not specified). Products include:
Catapres-TTS ... 675
Clonidine Hydrochloride (Effects not specified). Products include:
Catapres Tablets ... 674
Combipres Tablets ... 677
Deserpidine (Effects not specified).
No products indexed under this heading.
Desipramine Hydrochloride (Effects not specified). Products include:
Norpramin Tablets ... 1526
Diazoxide (Effects not specified). Products include:
Hyperstat I.V. Injection ... 2363
Proglycem ... 580
Diltiazem Hydrochloride (Effects not specified). Products include:
Cardizem CD Capsules ... 1506
Cardizem SR Capsules ... 1510
Cardizem Injectable ... 1508
Cardizem Tablets ... 1512
Dilacor XR Extended-release Capsules ... 2018
Doxazosin Mesylate (Effects not specified). Products include:
Cardura Tablets ... 2186
Doxepin Hydrochloride (Effects not specified). Products include:
Sinequan ... 2205
Zonalon Cream ... 1055
Enalapril Maleate (Effects not specified). Products include:
Vaseretic Tablets ... 1765
Vasotec Tablets ... 1771
Enalaprilat (Effects not specified). Products include:
Vasotec I.V. ... 1768
Esmolol Hydrochloride (Effects not specified). Products include:
Brevibloc Injection ... 1808
Felodipine (Effects not specified). Products include:
Plendil Extended-Release Tablets ... 527
Fluoxetine Hydrochloride (Effects not specified). Products include:
Prozac Pulvules & Liquid, Oral Solution ... 919
Fosinopril Sodium (Effects not specified). Products include:
Monopril Tablets ... 757
Furosemide (Effects not specified). Products include:
Lasix Injection, Oral Solution and Tablets ... 1240
Guanabenz Acetate (Effects not specified).
No products indexed under this heading.
Guanethidine Monosulfate (Effects not specified). Products include:
Esimil Tablets ... 822
Ismelin Tablets ... 827
Hydralazine Hydrochloride (Effects not specified). Products include:
Apresazide Capsules ... 808
Apresoline Hydrochloride Tablets ... 809
Ser-Ap-Es Tablets ... 849
Hydrochlorothiazide (Effects not specified). Products include:
Aldactazide ... 2413
Aldoril Tablets ... 1604
Apresazide Capsules ... 808
Capozide ... 742
Dyazide ... 2479
Esidrix Tablets ... 821
Esimil Tablets ... 822
HydroDIURIL Tablets ... 1674
Hydropres Tablets ... 1675
Hyzaar Tablets ... 1677
Inderide Tablets ... 2732
Inderide LA Long Acting Capsules ... 2734
Lopressor HCT Tablets ... 832
Lotensin HCT ... 837
Maxzide ... 1380
Moduretic Tablets ... 1705
Oretic Tablets ... 443
Prinzide Tablets ... 1737
Ser-Ap-Es Tablets ... 849
Timolide Tablets ... 1748
Vaseretic Tablets ... 1765
Zestoretic ... 2850
Ziac ... 1415
Hydroflumethiazide (Effects not specified). Products include:
Diucardin Tablets ... 2718
Imipramine Hydrochloride (Effects not specified). Products include:
Tofranil Ampuls ... 854
Tofranil Tablets ... 856
Imipramine Pamoate (Effects not specified). Products include:
Tofranil-PM Capsules ... 857
Indapamide (Effects not specified). Products include:
Lozol Tablets ... 2022
Isocarboxazid (Effects not specified).
No products indexed under this heading.
Isradipine (Effects not specified). Products include:
DynaCirc Capsules ... 2256
Labetalol Hydrochloride (Effects not specified). Products include:
Normodyne Injection ... 2377
Normodyne Tablets ... 2379
Trandate ... 1185
Lisinopril (Effects not specified). Products include:
Prinivil Tablets ... 1733
Prinzide Tablets ... 1737
Zestoretic ... 2850
Zestril Tablets ... 2854
Losartan Potassium (Effects not specified). Products include:
Cozaar Tablets ... 1628
Hyzaar Tablets ... 1677
Maprotiline Hydrochloride (Effects not specified). Products include:
Ludiomil Tablets ... 843
Mecamylamine Hydrochloride (Effects not specified). Products include:
Inversine Tablets ... 1686
Methyclothiazide (Effects not specified). Products include:
Enduron Tablets ... 420
Methyldopa (Effects not specified). Products include:
Aldoclor Tablets ... 1598
Aldomet Oral ... 1600
Aldoril Tablets ... 1604
Methyldopate Hydrochloride (Effects not specified). Products include:
Aldomet Ester HCl Injection ... 1602
Metolazone (Effects not specified). Products include:
Mykrox Tablets ... 993
Zaroxolyn Tablets ... 1000
Metoprolol Succinate (Effects not specified). Products include:
Toprol-XL Tablets ... 565
Metoprolol Tartrate (Effects not specified). Products include:
Lopressor Ampuls ... 830
Lopressor HCT Tablets ... 832
Lopressor Tablets ... 830
Metyrosine (Effects not specified). Products include:
Demser Capsules ... 1649
Minoxidil (Effects not specified). Products include:
Loniten Tablets ... 2618
Rogaine Topical Solution ... 2637
Moexipril Hydrochloride (Effects not specified). Products include:
Univasc Tablets ... 2410
Nadolol (Effects not specified).
No products indexed under this heading.
Nefazodone Hydrochloride (Effects not specified). Products include:
Serzone Tablets ... 771
Nicardipine Hydrochloride (Effects not specified). Products include:
Cardene Capsules ... 2095
Cardene I.V. ... 2709
Cardene SR Capsules ... 2097
Nifedipine (Effects not specified). Products include:
Adalat Capsules (10 mg and 20 mg) ... 587
Adalat CC ... 589
Procardia Capsules ... 1971
Procardia XL Extended Release Tablets ... 1972
Nisoldipine (Effects not specified).
No products indexed under this heading.
Nitroglycerin (Effects not specified). Products include:
Deponit NTG Transdermal Delivery System ... 2397
Nitro-Bid IV ... 1523
Nitro-Bid Ointment ... 1524
Nitrodisc ... 2047
Nitro-Dur (nitroglycerin) Transdermal Infusion System ... 1326
Nitrolingual Spray ... 2027
Nitrostat Tablets ... 1925
Transderm-Nitro Transdermal Therapeutic System ... 859
Nortriptyline Hydrochloride (Effects not specified). Products include:
Pamelor ... 2280
Paroxetine Hydrochloride (Effects not specified). Products include:
Paxil Tablets ... 2505
Penbutolol Sulfate (Effects not specified). Products include:
Levatol ... 2403
Phenelzine Sulfate (Effects not specified). Products include:
Nardil ... 1920
Phenoxybenzamine Hydrochloride (Effects not specified). Products include:
Dibenzyline Capsules ... 2476
Phentolamine Mesylate (Effects not specified). Products include:
Regitine ... 846
Pindolol (Effects not specified). Products include:
Visken Tablets ... 2299
Polythiazide (Effects not specified). Products include:
Minizide Capsules ... 1938
Prazosin Hydrochloride (Effects not specified). Products include:
Minipress Capsules ... 1937
Minizide Capsules ... 1938
Propranolol Hydrochloride (Effects not specified). Products include:
Inderal ... 2728
Inderal LA Long Acting Capsules ... 2730
Inderide Tablets ... 2732
Inderide LA Long Acting Capsules ... 2734
Protriptyline Hydrochloride (Effects not specified). Products include:
Vivactil Tablets ... 1774
Quinapril Hydrochloride (Effects not specified). Products include:
Accupril Tablets ... 1893
Ramipril (Effects not specified). Products include:
Altace Capsules ... 1232
Rauwolfia Serpentina (Effects not specified).
No products indexed under this heading.
Rescinnamine (Effects not specified).
No products indexed under this heading.
Reserpine (Effects not specified). Products include:
Diupres Tablets ... 1650
Hydropres Tablets ... 1675
Ser-Ap-Es Tablets ... 849
Sertraline Hydrochloride (Effects not specified). Products include:
Zoloft Tablets ... 2217
Sodium Nitroprusside (Effects not specified).
No products indexed under this heading.
Sotalol Hydrochloride (Effects not specified). Products include:
Betapace Tablets ... 641
Spirapril Hydrochloride (Effects not specified).
No products indexed under this heading.
Terazosin Hydrochloride (Effects not specified). Products include:
Hytrin Capsules ... 430
Timolol Maleate (Effects not specified). Products include:
Blocadren Tablets ... 1614
Timolide Tablets ... 1748
Timoptic in Ocudose ... 1753
Timoptic Sterile Ophthalmic Solution ... 1751
Timoptic-XE ... 1755
Torsemide (Effects not specified). Products include:
Demadex Tablets and Injection ... 686
Tranylcypromine Sulfate (Effects not specified). Products include:
Parnate Tablets ... 2503
Trazodone Hydrochloride (Effects not specified). Products include:
Desyrel and Desyrel Dividose ... 503
Trimethaphan Camsylate (Effects not specified). Products include:
Arfonad Ampuls ... 2080
Trimipramine Maleate (Effects not specified). Products include:
Surmontil Capsules ... 2811
Venlafaxine Hydrochloride (Effects not specified). Products include:
Effexor ... 2719
Verapamil Hydrochloride (Effects not specified). Products include:
Calan SR Caplets ... 2422
Calan Tablets ... 2419
Isoptin Injectable ... 1344
Isoptin Oral Tablets ... 1346
Isoptin SR Tablets ... 1348
Verelan Capsules ... 1410
Verelan Capsules ... 2824

IMPORTANT NOTE: Always consult each drug listing in the patient's regimen for possible interactions.

Advil

Interactions Index

ADVIL IBUPROFEN TABLETS AND CAPLETS

(Ibuprofen) ⊕ 870

May interact with:

Acetaminophen (Concurrent administration should not be undertaken without physician's direction). Products include:

Actifed Plus Caplets ⊕ 845
Actifed Plus Tablets ⊕ 845
Actifed Sinus Daytime/Nighttime Tablets and Caplets ⊕ 846
Alka-Seltzer Plus Cold Medicine Liqui-Gels ⊕ 706
Alka-Seltzer Plus Cold & Cough Medicine Liqui-Gels ⊕ 705
Alka-Seltzer Plus Night-Time Cold Medicine Liqui-Gels ⊕ 706
Allerest Headache Strength Tablets ⊕ 627
Allerest No Drowsiness Tablets ⊕ 627
Allerest Sinus Pain Formula ⊕ 627
Anexsia 5/500 Elixir 1781
Anexia Tablets 1782
Arthritis Foundation Aspirin Free Caplets ⊕ 673
Arthritis Foundation NightTime Caplets ⊕ 674
Bayer Select Headache Pain Relief Formula ⊕ 716
Bayer Select Menstrual Multi-Symptom Formula ⊕ 716
Bayer Select Night Time Pain Relief Formula ⊕ 716
Bayer Select Sinus Pain Relief Formula ⊕ 717
Benadryl Allergy Sinus Headache Formula Caplets ⊕ 849
Comtrex Multi-Symptom Cold Reliever Tablets/Caplets/Liqui-Gels/Liquid ⊕ 615
Allergy-Sinus Comtrex Multi-Symptom Allergy-Sinus Formula Tablets ⊕ 617
Comtrex Non-Drowsy ⊕ 618
Contac Day Allergy/Sinus Caplets ⊕ 812
Contac Day & Night ⊕ 812
Contac Night Allergy/Sinus Caplets ⊕ 812
Contac Severe Cold and Flu Formula Caplets ⊕ 814
Contac Severe Cold & Flu Non-Drowsy ⊕ 815
Coricidin 'D' Decongestant Tablets ⊕ 800
Coricidin Tablets ⊕ 800
DHCplus Capsules 1993
Darvon-N/Darvocet-N 1433
Drixoral Cold and Flu Extended-Release Tablets ⊕ 803
Drixoral Cough + Sore Throat Liquid Caps ⊕ 802
Drixoral Allergy/Sinus Extended Release Tablets ⊕ 804
Esgic-plus Tablets 1013
Aspirin Free Excedrin Analgesic Caplets and Geltabs 732
Excedrin Extra-Strength Analgesic Tablets & Caplets 732
Excedrin P.M. Analgesic/Sleeping Aid Tablets, Caplets, Liquigels 733
Fioricet Tablets 2258
Fioricet with Codeine Capsules 2260
Hycomine Compound Tablets 932
Hydrocet Capsules 782
Legatrin PM ⊕ 651
Lorcet 10/650 1018
Lortab 2566
Lurline PMS Tablets 982
Maximum Strength Multi-Symptom Formula Midol ⊕ 722
PMS Multi-Symptom Formula Midol ⊕ 723
Teen Multi-Symptom Formula Midol ⊕ 722
Midrin Capsules 783
Migraiam Capsules 2038
Panodol Tablets and Caplets ⊕ 824
Children's Panadol Chewable Tablets, Liquid, Infant's Drops ⊕ 824
Percocet Tablets 938
Percogesic Analgesic Tablets ⊕ 754
Phrenilin 785
Pyrroxate Caplets ⊕ 772
Sedapap Tablets 50 mg/650 mg 1543
Sinarest Tablets ⊕ 648
Sinarest Extra Strength Tablets ⊕ 648
Sinarest No Drowsiness Tablets ⊕ 648
Sine-Aid Maximum Strength Sinus Medication Gelcaps, Caplets and Tablets 1554
Sine-Off No Drowsiness Formula Caplets ⊕ 824
Sine-Off Sinus Medicine ⊕ 825
Singlet Tablets ⊕ 825
Sinulin Tablets 787
Sinutab Sinus Allergy Medication, Maximum Strength Tablets and Caplets ⊕ 860
Sinutab Sinus Medication, Maximum Strength Without Drowsiness Formula, Tablets & Caplets ⊕ 860
Sinutab Sinus Medication, Regular Strength Without Drowsiness Formula ⊕ 859
Sudafed Cold and Cough Liquid-caps ⊕ 862
Sudafed Severe Cold Formula Caplets ⊕ 863
Sudafed Severe Cold Formula Tablets ⊕ 864
Sudafed Sinus Caplets ⊕ 864
Sudafed Sinus Tablets ⊕ 864
Talacen 2333
TheraFlu ⊕ 787
TheraFlu Maximum Strength Nighttime Flu, Cold & Cough Medicine ⊕ 788
TheraFlu Maximum Strength Non-Drowsy Formula Flu, Cold & Cough Medicine ⊕ 788
Thera Flu Maximum Strength, Non-Drowsy Formula Flu, Cold and Cough Caplets ⊕ 789
Triaminic Sore Throat Formula ⊕ 791
Triaminicin Tablets ⊕ 793
Children's TYLENOL acetaminophen Chewable Tablets, Elixir, Suspension Liquid 1555
Children's TYLENOL Cold Multi-Symptom Liquid Formula and Chewable Tablets 1561
Children's TYLENOL Cold Plus Cough Multi Symptom Tablets and Liquid ⊕ 681
Infants' TYLENOL acetaminophen Drops and Suspension Drops 1555
Infants' TYLENOL Cold Decongestant & Fever-Reducer Drops 1556
TYLENOL Extended Relief Caplets 1558
TYLENOL, Extra Strength, Acetaminophen Adult Liquid Pain Reliever 1560
TYLENOL, Extra Strength, acetaminophen Gelcaps, Geltabs, Caplets, Tablets 1559
TYLENOL, Extra Strength, Headache Plus Pain Reliever with Antacid Caplets 1559
TYLENOL, Junior Strength, acetaminophen Coated Caplets, Grape and Fruit Chewable Tablets 1557
TYLENOL Maximum Strength Allergy Sinus Medication Gelcaps and Caplets 1563
TYLENOL Maximum Strength Allergy Sinus NightTime Medication Caplets 1555
TYLENOL Flu Maximum Strength Gelcaps 1565
TYLENOL Flu NightTime, Maximum Strength, Gelcaps 1566
TYLENOL Maximum Strength Flu NightTime Hot Medication Packets 1562
TYLENOL, Maximum Strength, Sinus Medication Geltabs, Gelcaps, Caplets and Tablets 1566
TYLENOL Cold Multi-Symptom Formula Medication Tablets and Caplets 1561
TYLENOL Cold Medication No Drowsiness Formula Gelcaps and Caplets 1562
TYLENOL Cold Multi-Symptom Hot Medication Liquid Packets 1557
TYLENOL Cough Multi-Symptom Medication 1564
TYLENOL Cough Multi-Symptom Medication with Decongestant 1565
TYLENOL, Regular Strength, acetaminophen Caplets and Tablets 1558
TYLENOL PM, Extra Strength Pain Reliever/Sleep Aid Caplets, Geltabs, Gelcaps 1560
TYLENOL Severe Allergy Medication Caplets 1564
Tylenol with Codeine 1583
Tylox Capsules 1584
Unisom With Pain Relief-Nighttime Sleep Aid and Pain Reliever 1934
Vanquish Analgesic Caplets ⊕ 731
Vicks 44 LiquiCaps Cough, Cold & Flu Relief ⊕ 755
Vicks 44M Cough, Cold & Flu Relief ⊕ 756
Vicks DayQuil ⊕ 761
Vicks Nyquil Hot Therapy ⊕ 762
Vicks NyQuil LiquiCaps Multi-Symptom Cold/Flu Relief ⊕ 763
Vicks NyQuil Multi-Symptom Cold/Flu Relief - (Original & Cherry Flavor) ⊕ 763
Vicodin Tablets 1356
Vicodin ES Tablets 1357
Wygesic Tablets 2827
Zydone Capsules 949

Aspirin (Concurrent administration should not be undertaken without physician's direction). Products include:

Alka-Seltzer Effervescent Antacid and Pain Reliever ⊕ 701
Alka-Seltzer Extra Strength Effervescent Antacid and Pain Reliever ⊕ 703
Alka-Seltzer Lemon Lime Effervescent Antacid and Pain Reliever ⊕ 703
Alka-Seltzer Plus Cold Medicine ⊕ 705
Alka-Seltzer Plus Cold & Cough Medicine ⊕ 708
Alka-Seltzer Plus Night-Time Cold Medicine ⊕ 707
Alka Seltzer Plus Sinus Medicine ⊕ 707
Arthritis Foundation Safety Coated Aspirin Tablets ⊕ 675
Arthritis Pain Ascriptin ⊕ 631
Maximum Strength Ascriptin ⊕ 630
Regular Strength Ascriptin Tablets ⊕ 629
Arthritis Strength BC Powder ⊕ 609
BC Cold Powder Multi-Symptom Formula (Cold-Sinus-Allergy) ⊕ 609
BC Cold Powder Non-Drowsy Formula (Cold-Sinus) ⊕ 609
BC Powder ⊕ 609
Bayer Children's Chewable Aspirin ⊕ 711
Genuine Bayer Aspirin Tablets & Caplets ⊕ 713
Extra Strength Bayer Arthritis Pain Regimen Formula ⊕ 711
Extra Strength Bayer Aspirin Caplets & Tablets ⊕ 712
Extended-Release Bayer 8-Hour Aspirin ⊕ 712
Extra Strength Bayer Plus Aspirin Caplets ⊕ 713
Extra Strength Bayer PM Aspirin ⊕ 713
Bayer Enteric Aspirin ⊕ 709
Bufferin Analgesic Tablets and Caplets ⊕ 613
Arthritis Strength Bufferin Analgesic Caplets ⊕ 614
Extra Strength Bufferin Analgesic Tablets ⊕ 615
Cama Arthritis Pain Reliever ⊕ 785
Darvon Compound-65 Pulvules 1435
Easprin 1914
Ecotrin 2455
Ecotrin Enteric Coated Aspirin Maximum Strength Tablets and Caplets ⊕ 816
Ecotrin Enteric Coated Aspirin Regular Strength Tablets 2455
Empirin Aspirin Tablets ⊕ 854
Empirin with Codeine Tablets 1093
Excedrin Extra-Strength Analgesic Tablets & Caplets 732
Fiorinal Capsules 2261
Fiorinal with Codeine Capsules 2262
Fiorinal Tablets 2261
Halfprin 1362
Healthprin Aspirin 2455
Norgesic 1496
Percodan Tablets 939
Percodan-Demi Tablets 940
Robaxisal Tablets 2071
Soma Compound w/Codeine Tablets 2676
Soma Compound Tablets 2675
St. Joseph Adult Chewable Aspirin (81 mg.) ⊕ 808
Talwin Compound 2335
Ursinus Inlay-Tabs ⊕ 794
Vanquish Analgesic Caplets ⊕ 731

CHILDREN'S ADVIL SUSPENSION

(Ibuprofen) 2692

May interact with oral anticoagulants, thiazides, lithium preparations, and certain other agents. Compounds in these categories include:

Aspirin (Yields a net decrease in anti-inflammatory activity with lowered blood levels of the non-aspirin drug in animal studies). Products include:

Alka-Seltzer Effervescent Antacid and Pain Reliever ⊕ 701
Alka-Seltzer Extra Strength Effervescent Antacid and Pain Reliever ⊕ 703
Alka-Seltzer Lemon Lime Effervescent Antacid and Pain Reliever ⊕ 703
Alka-Seltzer Plus Cold Medicine ⊕ 705
Alka-Seltzer Plus Cold & Cough Medicine ⊕ 708
Alka-Seltzer Plus Night-Time Cold Medicine ⊕ 707
Alka Seltzer Plus Sinus Medicine ⊕ 707
Arthritis Foundation Safety Coated Aspirin Tablets ⊕ 675
Arthritis Pain Ascriptin ⊕ 631
Maximum Strength Ascriptin ⊕ 630
Regular Strength Ascriptin Tablets ⊕ 629
Arthritis Strength BC Powder ⊕ 609
BC Cold Powder Multi-Symptom Formula (Cold-Sinus-Allergy) ⊕ 609
BC Cold Powder Non-Drowsy Formula (Cold-Sinus) ⊕ 609
BC Powder ⊕ 609
Bayer Children's Chewable Aspirin ⊕ 711
Genuine Bayer Aspirin Tablets & Caplets ⊕ 713
Extra Strength Bayer Arthritis Pain Regimen Formula ⊕ 711
Extra Strength Bayer Aspirin Caplets & Tablets ⊕ 712
Extended-Release Bayer 8-Hour Aspirin ⊕ 712
Extra Strength Bayer Plus Aspirin Caplets ⊕ 713
Extra Strength Bayer PM Aspirin ⊕ 713
Bayer Enteric Aspirin ⊕ 709
Bufferin Analgesic Tablets and Caplets ⊕ 613
Arthritis Strength Bufferin Analgesic Caplets ⊕ 614
Extra Strength Bufferin Analgesic Tablets ⊕ 615
Cama Arthritis Pain Reliever ⊕ 785
Darvon Compound-65 Pulvules 1435
Easprin 1914
Ecotrin 2455
Ecotrin Enteric Coated Aspirin Maximum Strength Tablets and Caplets ⊕ 816
Ecotrin Enteric Coated Aspirin Regular Strength Tablets 2455
Empirin Aspirin Tablets ⊕ 854
Empirin with Codeine Tablets 1093
Excedrin Extra-Strength Analgesic Tablets & Caplets 732
Fiorinal Capsules 2261
Fiorinal with Codeine Capsules 2262
Fiorinal Tablets 2261
Halfprin 1362
Healthprin Aspirin 2455
Norgesic 1496
Percodan Tablets 939
Percodan-Demi Tablets 940
Robaxisal Tablets 2071
Soma Compound w/Codeine Tablets 2676
Soma Compound Tablets 2675
St. Joseph Adult Chewable Aspirin (81 mg.) ⊕ 808
Talwin Compound 2335
Ursinus Inlay-Tabs ⊕ 794
Vanquish Analgesic Caplets ⊕ 731

Aspirin, Enteric Coated (Yields a net decrease in anti-inflammatory activity with lowered blood levels of the non-aspirin drug in animal studies). Products include:

Bayer Enteric Aspirin ⊕ 709
Ecotrin 2455

(⊕ Described in PDR For Nonprescription Drugs)

(◎ Described in PDR For Ophthalmology)

19 **Interactions Index** **Airet**

Bendroflumethiazide (Reduced natriuretic effect).
No products indexed under this heading.

Chlorothiazide (Reduced natriuretic effect). Products include:
Aldoclor Tablets 1598
Diupres Tablets 1650
Diuril Oral 1653

Chlorothiazide Sodium (Reduced natriuretic effect). Products include:
Diuril Sodium Intravenous 1652

Dicumarol (Potential for excessive bleeding).
No products indexed under this heading.

Furosemide (Reduced natriuretic effect). Products include:
Lasix Injection, Oral Solution and Tablets 1240

Hydrochlorothiazide (Reduced natriuretic effect). Products include:
Aldactazide 2413
Aldoril Tablets 1604
Apresazide Capsules 808
Capozide 742
Dyazide 2479
Esidrix Tablets 821
Esimil Tablets 822
HydroDIURIL Tablets 1674
Hydropres Tablets 1675
Hyzaar Tablets 1677
Inderide Tablets 2732
Inderide LA Long Acting Capsules .. 2734
Lopressor HCT Tablets 832
Lotensin HCT 837
Maxzide 1380
Moduretic Tablets 1705
Oretic Tablets 443
Prinzide Tablets 1737
Ser-Ap-Es Tablets 849
Timolide Tablets 1748
Vaseretic Tablets 1765
Zestoretic 2850
Ziac 1415

Hydroflumethiazide (Reduced natriuretic effect). Products include:
Diucardin Tablets 2718

Lithium Carbonate (Reduced renal lithium clearance and elevation of plasma lithium levels). Products include:
Eskalith 2485
Lithium Carbonate Capsules & Tablets 2230
Lithonate/Lithotabs/Lithobid 2543

Lithium Citrate (Reduced renal lithium clearance and elevation of plasma lithium levels).
No products indexed under this heading.

Methotrexate Sodium (Enhanced toxicity of methotrexate). Products include:
Methotrexate Sodium Tablets, Injection, for Injection and LPF Injection 1275

Methyclothiazide (Reduced natriuretic effect). Products include:
Enduron Tablets 420

Polythiazide (Reduced natriuretic effect). Products include:
Minizide Capsules 1938

Warfarin Sodium (Potential for excessive bleeding). Products include:
Coumadin 926

Food Interactions

Food, unspecified (Peak plasma levels are somewhat lower (up to 30%) and the time to reach peak levels is slightly prolonged (up to 30 min.)).

AEROBID INHALER SYSTEM
(Flunisolide) 1005
None cited in PDR database.

AEROBID-M INHALER SYSTEM
(Flunisolide) 1005
None cited in PDR database.

AEROLATE JR. T.D. CAPSULES
(Theophylline Anhydrous) 1004
None cited in PDR database.

AEROLATE SR. T.D. CAPSULES
(Theophylline Anhydrous) 1004
None cited in PDR database.

AEROLATE III T.D. CAPSULES
(Theophylline Anhydrous) 1004
None cited in PDR database.

AFRIN CHERRY SCENTED NASAL SPRAY 0.05%
(Oxymetazoline Hydrochloride) .... ▣ 797
None cited in PDR database.

AFRIN EXTRA MOISTURIZING NASAL SPRAY
(Oxymetazoline Hydrochloride) .... ▣ 797
None cited in PDR database.

AFRIN MENTHOL NASAL SPRAY, 0.05%
(Oxymetazoline Hydrochloride) .... ▣ 797
None cited in PDR database.

AFRIN NASAL SPRAY 0.05% AND NASAL SPRAY PUMP
(Oxymetazoline Hydrochloride) .... ▣ 797
None cited in PDR database.

AFRIN NOSE DROPS 0.05%
(Oxymetazoline Hydrochloride) .... ▣ 797
None cited in PDR database.

AFRIN SALINE MIST
(Sodium Chloride) .... ▣ 798
None cited in PDR database.

AFRIN SINUS
(Oxymetazoline Hydrochloride) .... ▣ 797
None cited in PDR database.

AFTATE FOR ATHLETE'S FOOT
(Tolnaftate) .... ▣ 798
None cited in PDR database.

AFTATE FOR JOCK ITCH
(Tolnaftate) .... ▣ 798
None cited in PDR database.

AIRET SOLUTION FOR INHALATION
(Albuterol Sulfate) 452
May interact with sympathomimetic aerosol bronchodilators, monoamine oxidase inhibitors, tricyclic antidepressants, beta blockers, and certain other agents. Compounds in these categories include:

Acebutolol Hydrochloride (Effect of each other inhibited). Products include:
Sectral Capsules 2807

Albuterol (Concurrent use should be avoided). Products include:
Proventil Inhalation Aerosol 2382
Ventolin Inhalation Aerosol and Refill 1197

Amitriptyline Hydrochloride (Action of albuterol on the vascular system may be potentiated). Products include:
Elavil 2838
Endep Tablets 2174
Etrafon 2355
Limbitrol 2180
Triavil Tablets 1757

Amoxapine (Action of albuterol on the vascular system may be potentiated). Products include:
Asendin Tablets 1369

Atenolol (Effect of each other inhibited). Products include:
Tenoretic Tablets 2845
Tenormin Tablets and I.V. Injection 2847

Betaxolol Hydrochloride (Effect of each other inhibited). Products include:
Betoptic Ophthalmic Solution 469
Betoptic S Ophthalmic Suspension 471
Kerlone Tablets 2436

Bisoprolol Fumarate (Effect of each other inhibited). Products include:
Zebeta Tablets 1413
Ziac 1415

Bitolterol Mesylate (Concurrent use should be avoided). Products include:
Tornalate Solution for Inhalation, 0.2% 956
Tornalate Metered Dose Inhaler 957

Carteolol Hydrochloride (Effect of each other inhibited). Products include:
Cartrol Tablets 410
Ocupress Ophthalmic Solution, 1% Sterile .... ⊙ 309

Clomipramine Hydrochloride (Action of albuterol on the vascular system may be potentiated). Products include:
Anafranil Capsules 803

Desipramine Hydrochloride (Action of albuterol on the vascular system may be potentiated). Products include:
Norpramin Tablets 1526

Doxepin Hydrochloride (Action of albuterol on the vascular system may be potentiated). Products include:
Sinequan 2205
Zonalon Cream 1055

Epinephrine (Do not use concomitantly). Products include:
Bronkaid Mist .... ▣ 717
EPIFRIN .... ⊙ 239
EpiPen 790
Marcaine Hydrochloride with Epinephrine 1:200,000 2316
Primatene Mist .... ▣ 873
Sensorcaine with Epinephrine Injection 559
Sus-Phrine Injection 1019
Xylocaine with Epinephrine Injections 567

Epinephrine Bitartrate (Do not use concomitantly). Products include:
Bronkaid Mist Suspension .... ▣ 718
Sensorcaine-MPF with Epinephrine Injection 559

Epinephrine Hydrochloride (Do not use concomitantly). Products include:
Ana-Kit Anaphylaxis Emergency Treatment Kit 617

Esmolol Hydrochloride (Effect of each other inhibited). Products include:
Brevibloc Injection 1808

Furazolidone (Action of albuterol on the vascular system may be potentiated). Products include:
Furoxone 2046

Imipramine Hydrochloride (Action of albuterol on the vascular system may be potentiated). Products include:
Tofranil Ampuls 854
Tofranil Tablets 856

Imipramine Pamoate (Action of albuterol on the vascular system may be potentiated). Products include:
Tofranil-PM Capsules 857

Isocarboxazid (Action of albuterol on the vascular system may be potentiated).
No products indexed under this heading.

Isoetharine (Concurrent use should be avoided). Products include:
Bronkometer Aerosol 2302
Bronkosol Solution 2302
Isoetharine Inhalation Solution, USP, Arm-a-Med 551

Isoproterenol Hydrochloride (Concurrent use should be avoided). Products include:
Isuprel Hydrochloride Injection 1:5000 2311
Isuprel Hydrochloride Solution 1:200 & 1:100 2313
Isuprel Mistometer 2312

Labetalol Hydrochloride (Effect of each other inhibited). Products include:
Normodyne Injection 2377
Normodyne Tablets 2379
Trandate 1185

Levobunolol Hydrochloride (Effect of each other inhibited). Products include:
Betagan .... ⊙ 233

Maprotiline Hydrochloride (Action of albuterol on the vascular system may be potentiated). Products include:
Ludiomil Tablets 843

Metaproterenol Sulfate (Concurrent use should be avoided). Products include:
Alupent 669
Metaproterenol Sulfate Inhalation Solution, USP, Arm-a-Med 552

Metipranolol Hydrochloride (Effect of each other inhibited). Products include:
OptiPranolol (Metipranolol 0.3%) Sterile Ophthalmic Solution .... ⊙ 258

Metoprolol Succinate (Effect of each other inhibited). Products include:
Toprol-XL Tablets 565

Metoprolol Tartrate (Effect of each other inhibited). Products include:
Lopressor Ampuls 830
Lopressor HCT Tablets 832
Lopressor Tablets 830

Nadolol (Effect of each other inhibited).
No products indexed under this heading.

Nortriptyline Hydrochloride (Action of albuterol on the vascular system may be potentiated). Products include:
Pamelor 2280

Penbutolol Sulfate (Effect of each other inhibited). Products include:
Levatol 2403

Phenelzine Sulfate (Action of albuterol on the vascular system may be potentiated). Products include:
Nardil 1920

Pindolol (Effect of each other inhibited). Products include:
Visken Tablets 2299

Pirbuterol Acetate (Concurrent use should be avoided). Products include:
Maxair Autohaler 1492
Maxair Inhaler 1494

IMPORTANT NOTE: Always consult each drug listing in the patient's regimen for possible interactions.

Airet Interactions Index 20

Propranolol Hydrochloride (Effect of each other inhibited). Products include:
Inderal 2728
Inderal LA Long Acting Capsules 2730
Inderide Tablets 2732
Inderide LA Long Acting Capsules 2734

Protriptyline Hydrochloride (Action of albuterol on the vascular system may be potentiated). Products include:
Vivactil Tablets 1774

Salmeterol Xinafoate (Concurrent use should be avoided). Products include:
Serevent Inhalation Aerosol 1176

Selegiline Hydrochloride (Action of albuterol on the vascular system may be potentiated). Products include:
Eldepryl Tablets 2550

Sotalol Hydrochloride (Effect of each other inhibited). Products include:
Betapace Tablets 641

Terbutaline Sulfate (Concurrent use should be avoided). Products include:
Brethaire Inhaler 813
Brethine Ampuls 815
Brethine Tablets 814
Bricanyl Subcutaneous Injection 1502
Bricanyl Tablets 1503

Timolol Hemihydrate (Effect of each other inhibited). Products include:
Betimol 0.25%, 0.5% ..... ⊙ 261

Timolol Maleate (Effect of each other inhibited). Products include:
Blocadren Tablets 1614
Timolide Tablets 1748
Timoptic in Ocudose 1753
Timoptic Sterile Ophthalmic Solution 1751
Timoptic-XE 1755

Tranylcypromine Sulfate (Action of albuterol on the vascular system may be potentiated). Products include:
Parnate Tablets 2503

Trimipramine Maleate (Action of albuterol on the vascular system may be potentiated). Products include:
Surmontil Capsules 2811

AK-CIDE
(Prednisolone Acetate, Sulfacetamide Sodium) ..... ⊙ 202
None cited in PDR database.

AK-CIDE OINTMENT
(Prednisolone Acetate, Sulfacetamide Sodium) ..... ⊙ 202
None cited in PDR database.

AK-FLUOR INJECTION 10% AND 25%
(Fluorescein Sodium) ..... ⊙ 203
None cited in PDR database.

AKINETON INJECTION
(Biperiden Hydrochloride) 1333
May interact with tricyclic antidepressants, phenothiazines, antihistamines, antipsychotic agents, and certain other agents. Compounds in these categories include:

Acrivastine (Central anticholinergic syndrome). Products include:
Semprex-D Capsules 463
Semprex-D Capsules 1167

Amitriptyline Hydrochloride (Central anticholinergic syndrome). Products include:
Elavil 2838
Endep Tablets 2174
Etrafon 2355
Limbitrol 2180
Triavil Tablets 1757

Amoxapine (Central anticholinergic syndrome). Products include:
Asendin Tablets 1369

Astemizole (Central anticholinergic syndrome). Products include:
Hismanal Tablets 1293

Azatadine Maleate (Central anticholinergic syndrome). Products include:
Trinalin Repetabs Tablets 1330

Bromodiphenhydramine Hydrochloride (Central anticholinergic syndrome).
No products indexed under this heading.

Brompheniramine Maleate (Central anticholinergic syndrome). Products include:
Alka Seltzer Plus Sinus Medicine ..... ◘ 707
Bromfed Capsules (Extended-Release) 1785
Bromfed Syrup ..... ◘ 733
Bromfed Tablets 1785
Bromfed-DM Cough Syrup 1786
Bromfed-PD Capsules (Extended-Release) 1785
Dimetane-DC Cough Syrup 2059
Dimetane-DX Cough Syrup 2059
Dimetapp Elixir ..... ◘ 773
Dimetapp Extentabs ..... ◘ 774
Dimetapp Tablets/Liqui-Gels ..... ◘ 775
Dimetapp Cold & Allergy Chewable Tablets ..... ◘ 773
Dimetapp DM Elixir ..... ◘ 774
Vicks DayQuil Allergy Relief 12-Hour Extended Release Tablets ..... ◘ 760
Vicks DayQuil Allergy Relief 4-Hour Tablets ..... ◘ 760

Chlorpheniramine Maleate (Central anticholinergic syndrome). Products include:
Alka-Seltzer Plus Cold Medicine ..... ◘ 705
Alka-Seltzer Plus Cold Medicine Liqui-Gels ..... ◘ 706
Alka-Seltzer Plus Cold & Cough Medicine ..... ◘ 708
Alka-Seltzer Plus Cold & Cough Medicine Liqui-Gels ..... ◘ 705
Allerest Children's Chewable Tablets ..... ◘ 627
Allerest Headache Strength Tablets ..... ◘ 627
Allerest Maximum Strength Tablets ..... ◘ 627
Allerest Sinus Pain Formula ..... ◘ 627
Allerest 12 Hour Caplets ..... ◘ 627
Ana-Kit Anaphylaxis Emergency Treatment Kit 617
Atrohist Pediatric Capsules 453
Atrohist Plus Tablets 454
BC Cold Powder Multi-Symptom Formula (Cold-Sinus-Allergy) ..... ◘ 609
Cerose DM ..... ◘ 878
Cheracol Plus Head Cold/Cough Formula ..... ◘ 769
Children's Vicks DayQuil Allergy Relief ..... ◘ 757
Children's Vicks NyQuil Cold/Cough Relief ..... ◘ 758
Chlor-Trimeton Allergy Decongestant Tablets ..... ◘ 799
Chlor-Trimeton Allergy Tablets ..... ◘ 798
Comhist 2038
Comtrex Multi-Symptom Cold Reliever Tablets/Caplets/Liqui-Gels/Liquid ..... ◘ 615
Allergy-Sinus Comtrex Multi-Symptom Allergy-Sinus Formula Tablets ..... ◘ 617
Contac Continuous Action Nasal Decongestant/Antihistamine 12 Hour Capsules ..... ◘ 813
Contac Maximum Strength Continuous Action Decongestant/Antihistamine 12 Hour Caplets ..... ◘ 813
Contac Severe Cold and Flu Formula Caplets ..... ◘ 814
Coricidin 'D' Decongestant Tablets ..... ◘ 800
Coricidin Tablets ..... ◘ 800
D.A. Chewable Tablets 951
Deconamine 1320
Dura-Tap/PD Capsules 2867
Dura-Vent/DA Tablets 953
Extendryl 1005
Fedahist Gyrocaps 2401
Fedahist Timecaps 2401
Hycomine Compound Tablets 932
Isoclor Timesule Capsules ..... ◘ 637
Kronofed-A 977
Nolamine Timed-Release Tablets 785
Novahistine DH 2462
Novahistine Elixir ..... ◘ 823
Ornade Spansule Capsules 2502
PediaCare Cold Allergy Chewable Tablets ..... ◘ 677
PediaCare Cough-Cold Chewable Tablets 1553
PediaCare Cough-Cold Liquid 1553
PediaCare NightRest Cough-Cold Liquid 1553
Pediatric Vicks 44m Cough & Cold Relief ..... ◘ 764
Pyrroxate Caplets ..... ◘ 772
Ryna ..... ◘ 841
Sinarest Tablets ..... ◘ 648
Sinarest Extra Strength Tablets ..... ◘ 648
Sine-Off Sinus Medicine ..... ◘ 825
Singlet Tablets ..... ◘ 825
Sinulin Tablets 787
Sinutab Sinus Allergy Medication, Maximum Strength Tablets and Caplets ..... ◘ 860
Sudafed Plus Liquid ..... ◘ 862
Sudafed Plus Tablets ..... ◘ 863
Teldrin 12 Hour Antihistamine/Nasal Decongestant Allergy Relief Capsules ..... ◘ 826
TheraFlu ..... ◘ 787
TheraFlu Maximum Strength Nighttime Flu, Cold & Cough Medicine ..... ◘ 788
Triaminic Allergy Tablets ..... ◘ 789
Triaminic Cold Tablets ..... ◘ 790
Triaminic Nite Light ..... ◘ 791
Triaminic Syrup ..... ◘ 792
Triaminic-12 Tablets ..... ◘ 792
Triaminicin Tablets ..... ◘ 793
Triaminicol Multi-Symptom Cold Tablets ..... ◘ 793
Triaminicol Multi-Symptom Relief ..... ◘ 794
Tussend 1783
Children's TYLENOL Cold Multi-Symptom Liquid Formula and Chewable Tablets 1561
Children's TYLENOL Cold Plus Cough Multi Symptom Tablets and Liquid ..... ◘ 681
TYLENOL Maximum Strength Allergy Sinus Medication Gelcaps and Caplets 1563
TYLENOL Cold Multi-Symptom Formula Medication Tablets and Caplets 1561
TYLENOL Cold Multi-Symptom Hot Medication Liquid Packets 1557
Vicks 44 LiquiCaps Cough, Cold & Flu Relief ..... ◘ 755
Vicks 44M Cough, Cold & Flu Relief ..... ◘ 756

Chlorpheniramine Polistirex (Central anticholinergic syndrome). Products include:
Tussionex Pennkinetic Extended-Release Suspension 998

Chlorpheniramine Tannate (Central anticholinergic syndrome). Products include:
Atrohist Pediatric Suspension 454
Ricobid Tablets and Pediatric Suspension 2038
Rynatan 2673
Rynatuss 2673

Chlorpromazine (Central anticholinergic syndrome). Products include:
Thorazine Suppositories 2523

Chlorprothixene (Central anticholinergic syndrome).
No products indexed under this heading.

Chlorprothixene Hydrochloride (Central anticholinergic syndrome).
No products indexed under this heading.

Clemastine Fumarate (Central anticholinergic syndrome). Products include:
Tavist Syrup 2297
Tavist Tablets 2298
Tavist-1 12 Hour Relief Tablets ..... ◘ 787
Tavist-D 12 Hour Relief Tablets ..... ◘ 787

Clomipramine Hydrochloride (Central anticholinergic syndrome). Products include:
Anafranil Capsules 803

Clorazepate Dipotassium (Central anticholinergic syndrome). Products include:
Tranxene 451

Clozapine (Central anticholinergic syndrome). Products include:
Clozaril Tablets 2252

Cyproheptadine Hydrochloride (Central anticholinergic syndrome). Products include:
Periactin 1724

Desipramine Hydrochloride (Central anticholinergic syndrome). Products include:
Norpramin Tablets 1526

Dexchlorpheniramine Maleate (Central anticholinergic syndrome).
No products indexed under this heading.

Diphenhydramine Citrate (Central anticholinergic syndrome). Products include:
Excedrin P.M. Analgesic/Sleeping Aid Tablets, Caplets, Liquigels 733

Diphenhydramine Hydrochloride (Central anticholinergic syndrome). Products include:
Actifed Allergy Daytime/Nighttime Caplets ..... ◘ 844
Actifed Sinus Daytime/Nighttime Tablets and Caplets ..... ◘ 846
Arthritis Foundation NightTime Caplets ..... ◘ 674
Extra Strength Bayer PM Aspirin ..... ◘ 713
Bayer Select Night Time Pain Relief Formula ..... ◘ 716
Benadryl Allergy Decongestant Liquid Medication ..... ◘ 848
Benadryl Allergy Decongestant Tablets ..... ◘ 848
Benadryl Allergy Liquid Medication ..... ◘ 849
Benadryl Allergy ..... ◘ 848
Benadryl Allergy Sinus Headache Formula Caplets ..... ◘ 849
Benadryl Capsules 1898
Benadryl Dye-Free Allergy Liqui-gel Softgels ..... ◘ 850
Benadryl Dye-Free Allergy Liquid Medication ..... ◘ 850
Benadryl Itch Relief Cream, Children's Formula and Maximum Strength 2% ..... ◘ 851
Benadryl Itch Relief Spray, Children's Formula and Maximum Strength 2% ..... ◘ 851
Benadryl Itch Relief Stick Maximum Strength 2% ..... ◘ 850
Benadryl Itch Stopping Gel, Children's Formula and Maximum Strength 2% ..... ◘ 851
Benadryl Kapseals 1898
Benadryl Injection 1898
Contac Day & Night Cold/Flu Night Caplets ..... ◘ 812
Contac Night Allergy/Sinus Caplets ..... ◘ 812
Extra Strength Doan's P.M. ..... ◘ 633
Legatrin PM ..... ◘ 651
Miles Nervine Nighttime Sleep-Aid ..... ◘ 723
Nytol QuickCaps Caplets ..... ◘ 610
Sleepinal Night-time Sleep Aid Capsules and Softgels ..... ◘ 834
TYLENOL Maximum Strength Allergy Sinus NightTime Medication Caplets 1555
TYLENOL Flu NightTime, Maximum Strength, Gelcaps 1566
TYLENOL Maximum Strength Flu NightTime Hot Medication Packets 1562
TYLENOL PM, Extra Strength Pain Reliever/Sleep Aid Caplets, Geltabs, Gelcaps 1560
TYLENOL Severe Allergy Medication Caplets 1564
Maximum Strength Unisom Sleepgels 1934
Unisom With Pain Relief-Nighttime Sleep Aid and Pain Reliever 1934

(◘ Described in PDR For Nonprescription Drugs) (⊙ Described in PDR For Ophthalmology)

Interactions Index — Aldactazide

Diphenylpyraline Hydrochloride (Central anticholinergic syndrome).

No products indexed under this heading.

Doxepin Hydrochloride (Central anticholinergic syndrome). Products include:

Sinequan 2205
Zonalon Cream 1055

Fluphenazine Decanoate (Central anticholinergic syndrome). Products include:

Prolixin Decanoate 509

Fluphenazine Enanthate (Central anticholinergic syndrome). Products include:

Prolixin Enanthate 509

Fluphenazine Hydrochloride (Central anticholinergic syndrome). Products include:

Prolixin 509

Haloperidol (Central anticholinergic syndrome). Products include:

Haldol Injection, Tablets and Concentrate 1575

Haloperidol Decanoate (Central anticholinergic syndrome). Products include:

Haldol Decanoate.................................... 1577

Imipramine Hydrochloride (Central anticholinergic syndrome). Products include:

Tofranil Ampuls 854
Tofranil Tablets 856

Imipramine Pamoate (Central anticholinergic syndrome). Products include:

Tofranil-PM Capsules.............................. 857

Loratadine (Central anticholinergic syndrome). Products include:

Claritin 2349
Claritin-D 2350

Loxapine Hydrochloride (Central anticholinergic syndrome). Products include:

Loxitane 1378

Loxapine Succinate (Central anticholinergic syndrome). Products include:

Loxitane Capsules 1378

Maprotiline Hydrochloride (Central anticholinergic syndrome). Products include:

Ludiomil Tablets...................................... 843

Meperidine Hydrochloride (Central anticholinergic syndrome). Products include:

Demerol 2308
Mepergan Injection 2753

Mesoridazine Besylate (Central anticholinergic syndrome). Products include:

Serentil 684

Methdilazine Hydrochloride (Central anticholinergic syndrome).

No products indexed under this heading.

Methotrimeprazine (Central anticholinergic syndrome). Products include:

Levoprome 1274

Molindone Hydrochloride (Central anticholinergic syndrome). Products include:

Moban Tablets and Concentrate 1048

Nortriptyline Hydrochloride (Central anticholinergic syndrome). Products include:

Pamelor 2280

Perphenazine (Central anticholinergic syndrome). Products include:

Etrafon 2355
Triavil Tablets 1757
Trilafon.. 2389

Prochlorperazine (Central anticholinergic syndrome). Products include:

Compazine 2470

Promethazine Hydrochloride (Central anticholinergic syndrome). Products include:

Mepergan Injection 2753
Phenergan with Codeine 2777
Phenergan with Dextromethorphan 2778
Phenergan Injection 2773
Phenergan Suppositories 2775
Phenergan Syrup 2774
Phenergan Tablets 2775
Phenergan VC 2779
Phenergan VC with Codeine 2781

Protriptyline Hydrochloride (Central anticholinergic syndrome). Products include:

Vivactil Tablets 1774

Pyrilamine Maleate (Central anticholinergic syndrome syndrome). Products include:

4-Way Fast Acting Nasal Spray (regular & mentholated) .... ⊞ 621
Maximum Strength Multi-Symptom Formula Midol .... ⊞ 722
PMS Multi-Symptom Formula Midol .... ⊞ 723

Pyrilamine Tannate (Central anticholinergic syndrome). Products include:

Atrohist Pediatric Suspension 454
Rynatan 2673

Quinidine Gluconate (Central anticholinergic syndrome). Products include:

Quinaglute Dura-Tabs Tablets 649

Quinidine Polygalacturonate (Central anticholinergic syndrome).

No products indexed under this heading.

Quinidine Sulfate (Central anticholinergic syndrome). Products include:

Quinidex Extentabs 2067

Risperidone (Central anticholinergic syndrome). Products include:

Risperdal 1301

Terfenadine (Central anticholinergic syndrome). Products include:

Seldane Tablets 1536
Seldane-D Extended-Release Tablets 1538

Thioridazine Hydrochloride (Central anticholinergic syndrome). Products include:

Mellaril 2269

Thiothixene (Central anticholinergic syndrome). Products include:

Navane Capsules and Concentrate 2201
Navane Intramuscular 2202

Trifluoperazine Hydrochloride (Central anticholinergic syndrome). Products include:

Stelazine 2514

Trimeprazine Tartrate (Central anticholinergic syndrome). Products include:

Temaril Tablets, Syrup and Spansule Extended-Release Capsules.. 483

Trimipramine Maleate (Central anticholinergic syndrome). Products include:

Surmontil Capsules................................. 2811

Tripelennamine Hydrochloride (Central anticholinergic syndrome). Products include:

PBZ Tablets 845
PBZ-SR Tablets....................................... 844

Triprolidine Hydrochloride (Central anticholinergic syndrome). Products include:

Actifed Plus Caplets .... ⊞ 845
Actifed Plus Tablets .... ⊞ 845
Actifed with Codeine Cough Syrup.. 1067
Actifed Syrup.. ⊞ 846
Actifed Tablets .... ⊞ 844

AKINETON TABLETS (Biperiden Hydrochloride) 1333

See Akineton Injection

AK-PRED (Prednisolone Sodium Phosphate).. ◎ 204

None cited in PDR database.

AK-SPORE OINTMENT (Bacitracin Zinc, Neomycin Sulfate, Polymyxin B Sulfate) .... ◎ 204

None cited in PDR database.

AK-SPORE SOLUTION (Gramicidin, Neomycin Sulfate, Polymyxin B Sulfate) .... ◎ 204

None cited in PDR database.

AKTOB (Tobramycin) .... ◎ 206

None cited in PDR database.

AK-TROL OINTMENT & SUSPENSION (Dexamethasone, Neomycin Sulfate, Polymyxin B Sulfate) .... ◎ 205

None cited in PDR database.

AKORN'S ANTIOXIDANTS (Vitamins with Minerals) .... ◎ 206

None cited in PDR database.

ALBALON SOLUTION WITH LIQUIFILM (Naphazoline Hydrochloride)............ ◎ 231

May interact with monoamine oxidase inhibitors, tricyclic antidepressants, and certain other agents. Compounds in these categories include:

Amitriptyline Hydrochloride (May potentiate the pressor effect of naphazoline). Products include:

Elavil 2838
Endep Tablets 2174
Etrafon 2355
Limbitrol 2180
Triavil Tablets 1757

Amoxapine (May potentiate the pressor effect of naphazoline). Products include:

Asendin Tablets 1369

Clomipramine Hydrochloride (May potentiate the pressor effect of naphazoline). Products include:

Anafranil Capsules 803

Desipramine Hydrochloride (May potentiate the pressor effect of naphazoline). Products include:

Norpramin Tablets 1526

Doxepin Hydrochloride (May potentiate the pressor effect of naphazoline). Products include:

Sinequan 2205
Zonalon Cream 1055

Furazolidone (Severe hypertensive crisis). Products include:

Furoxone 2046

Imipramine Hydrochloride (May potentiate the pressor effect of naphazoline). Products include:

Tofranil Ampuls 854
Tofranil Tablets 856

Imipramine Pamoate (May potentiate the pressor effect of naphazoline). Products include:

Tofranil-PM Capsules.............................. 857

Isocarboxazid (Severe hypertensive crisis).

No products indexed under this heading.

Maprotiline Hydrochloride (May potentiate the pressor effect of naphazoline). Products include:

Ludiomil Tablets...................................... 843

Nortriptyline Hydrochloride (May potentiate the pressor effect of naphazoline). Products include:

Pamelor 2280

Phenelzine Sulfate (Severe hypertensive crisis). Products include:

Nardil 1920

Protriptyline Hydrochloride (May potentiate the pressor effect of naphazoline). Products include:

Vivactil Tablets 1774

Selegiline Hydrochloride (Severe hypertensive crisis). Products include:

Eldepryl Tablets 2550

Tranylcypromine Sulfate (Severe hypertensive crisis). Products include:

Parnate Tablets 2503

Trimipramine Maleate (May potentiate the pressor effect of naphazoline). Products include:

Surmontil Capsules................................. 2811

ALBUMINAR-5, ALBUMIN (HUMAN) U.S.P. 5% (Albumin (Human)) 512

None cited in PDR database.

ALBUMINAR-25, ALBUMIN (HUMAN) U.S.P. 25% (Albumin (Human)) 513

None cited in PDR database.

ALDACTAZIDE (Spironolactone, Hydrochlorothiazide)..............................2413

May interact with potassium preparations, loop diuretics, glucocorticoids, diuretics, insulin, oral hypoglycemic agents, potassium sparing diuretics, cardiac glycosides, ACE inhibitors, thiazides, antigout agents, general anesthetics, lithium preparations, and certain other agents. Compounds in these categories include:

Acarbose (Dosage adjustment of hypoglycemics may be necessary).

No products indexed under this heading.

ACTH (Concomitant administration may result in hypokalemia).

No products indexed under this heading.

Allopurinol (Dosage adjustment may be necessary). Products include:

Zyloprim Tablets 1226

Amiloride Hydrochloride (Concomitant administration has been associated with severe hyperkalemia and may induce dilutional hyponatremia). Products include:

Midamor Tablets 1703
Moduretic Tablets 1705

Benazepril Hydrochloride (Concomitant administration has been associated with severe hyperkalemia). Products include:

Lotensin Tablets...................................... 834
Lotensin HCT.. 837
Lotrel Capsules....................................... 840

Bendroflumethiazide (Concomitant administration has been associated with severe hyperkalemia; concomitant administration may induce dilutional hyponatremia).

No products indexed under this heading.

Betamethasone Acetate (Concomitant administration may result in hypokalemia). Products include:

Celestone Soluspan Suspension 2347

Betamethasone Sodium Phosphate (Concomitant administration may result in hypokalemia). Products include:

Celestone Soluspan Suspension 2347

IMPORTANT NOTE: Always consult each drug listing in the patient's regimen for possible interactions.

Aldactazide **Interactions Index** 22

Bumetanide (Concomitant administration may result in hypokalemia and may induce dilutional hyponatremia). Products include:
Bumex 2093

Captopril (Concomitant administration has been associated with severe hyperkalemia). Products include:
Capoten 739
Capozide 742

Chlorothiazide (Concomitant administration has been associated with severe hyperkalemia and may induce dilutional hyponatremia). Products include:
Aldoclor Tablets 1598
Diupres Tablets 1650
Diuril Oral 1653

Chlorothiazide Sodium (Concomitant administration has been associated with severe hyperkalemia and may induce dilutional hyponatremia). Products include:
Diuril Sodium Intravenous 1652

Chlorpropamide (Dosage adjustment of hypoglycemics may be necessary). Products include:
Diabinese Tablets 1935

Chlorthalidone (Concomitant administration may induce dilutional hyponatremia). Products include:
Combipres Tablets 677
Tenoretic Tablets 2845
Thalitone 1245

Cortisone Acetate (Concomitant administration may result in hypokalemia). Products include:
Cortone Acetate Sterile Suspension 1623
Cortone Acetate Tablets 1624

Deslanoside (Resultant hypokalemia may exaggerate the effects of digitalis therapy).
No products indexed under this heading.

Dexamethasone (Concomitant administration may result in hypokalemia). Products include:
AK-Trol Ointment & Suspension .... ◉ 205
Decadron Elixir 1633
Decadron Tablets 1635
Decaspray Topical Aerosol 1648
Dexacidin Ointment .... ◉ 263
Maxitrol Ophthalmic Ointment and Suspension .... ◉ 224
TobraDex Ophthalmic Suspension and Ointment 473

Dexamethasone Acetate (Concomitant administration may result in hypokalemia). Products include:
Dalalone D.P. Injectable 1011
Decadron-LA Sterile Suspension 1646

Dexamethasone Sodium Phosphate (Concomitant administration may result in hypokalemia). Products include:
Decadron Phosphate Injection 1637
Decadron Phosphate Respihaler 1642
Decadron Phosphate Sterile Ophthalmic Ointment 1641
Decadron Phosphate Sterile Ophthalmic Solution 1642
Decadron Phosphate Topical Cream 1644
Decadron Phosphate Turbinaire 1645
Decadron Phosphate with Xylocaine Injection, Sterile 1639
Dexacort Phosphate in Respihaler .. 458
Dexacort Phosphate in Turbinaire .. 459
NeoDecadron Sterile Ophthalmic Ointment 1712
NeoDecadron Sterile Ophthalmic Solution 1713
NeoDecadron Topical Cream 1714

Digitoxin (Resultant hypokalemia may exaggerate the effects of digitalis therapy). Products include:
Crystodigin Tablets 1433

Digoxin (Resultant hypokalemia may exaggerate the effects of digitalis therapy). Products include:
Lanoxicaps 1117
Lanoxin Elixir Pediatric 1120
Lanoxin Injection 1123
Lanoxin Injection Pediatric 1126
Lanoxin Tablets 1128

Enalapril Maleate (Concomitant administration has been associated with severe hyperkalemia). Products include:
Vaseretic Tablets 1765
Vasotec Tablets 1771

Enalaprilat (Concomitant administration has been associated with severe hyperkalemia). Products include:
Vasotec I.V. 1768

Enflurane (Exercise caution).
No products indexed under this heading.

Ethacrynic Acid (Concomitant administration may result in hypokalemia and may induce dilutional hyponatremia). Products include:
Edecrin Tablets 1657

Fludrocortisone Acetate (Concomitant administration may result in hypokalemia). Products include:
Florinef Acetate Tablets 505

Fosinopril Sodium (Concomitant administration has been associated with severe hyperkalemia). Products include:
Monopril Tablets 757

Furosemide (Concomitant administration may result in hypokalemia and may induce dilutional hyponatremia). Products include:
Lasix Injection, Oral Solution and Tablets 1240

Glipizide (Dosage adjustment of hypoglycemics may be necessary). Products include:
Glucotrol Tablets 1967
Glucotrol XL Extended Release Tablets 1968

Glyburide (Dosage adjustment of hypoglycemics may be necessary). Products include:
DiaBeta Tablets 1239
Glynase PresTab Tablets 2609
Micronase Tablets 2623

Hydrocortisone (Concomitant administration may result in hypokalemia). Products include:
Anusol-HC Cream 2.5% 1896
Aquanil HC Lotion 1931
Bactine Hydrocortisone Anti-Itch Cream .... ▣ 709
Caldecort Anti-Itch Hydrocortisone Spray .... ▣ 631
Cortaid .... ▣ 836
CORTENEMA 2535
Cortisporin Ointment 1085
Cortisporin Ophthalmic Ointment Sterile 1085
Cortisporin Ophthalmic Suspension Sterile 1086
Cortisporin Otic Solution Sterile 1087
Cortisporin Otic Suspension Sterile 1088
Cortizone-5 .... ▣ 831
Cortizone-10 .... ▣ 831
Hydrocortone Tablets 1672
Hytone 907
Massengill Medicated Soft Cloth Towelettes 2458
PediOtic Suspension Sterile 1153
Preparation H Hydrocortisone 1% Cream .... ▣ 872
ProctoCream-HC 2.5% 2408
VōSoL HC Otic Solution 2678

Hydrocortisone Acetate (Concomitant administration may result in hypokalemia). Products include:
Analpram-HC Rectal Cream 1% and 2.5% 977
Anusol HC-1 Anti-Itch Hydrocortisone Ointment .... ▣ 847
Anusol-HC Suppositories 1897
Caldecort .... ▣ 631
Carmol HC 924
Coly-Mycin S Otic w/Neomycin & Hydrocortisone 1906
Cortaid .... ▣ 836
Cortifoam 2396
Cortisporin Cream 1084
Epifoam 2399
Hydrocortone Acetate Sterile Suspension 1669
Mantadil Cream 1135
Nupercainal Hydrocortisone 1% Cream .... ▣ 645
Ophthocort .... ◉ 311
Pramosone Cream, Lotion & Ointment 978
ProctoCream-HC 2408
ProctoFoam-HC 2409
Terra-Cortril Ophthalmic Suspension 2210

Hydrocortisone Sodium Phosphate (Concomitant administration may result in hypokalemia). Products include:
Hydrocortone Phosphate Injection, Sterile 1670

Hydrocortisone Sodium Succinate (Concomitant administration may result in hypokalemia). Products include:
Solu-Cortef Sterile Powder 2641

Hydroflumethiazide (Concomitant administration has been associated with severe hyperkalemia and may induce dilutional hyponatremia). Products include:
Diucardin Tablets 2718

Indapamide (Concomitant administration may induce dilutional hyponatremia). Products include:
Lozol Tablets 2022

Indomethacin (Concomitant administration has been associated with severe hyperkalemia). Products include:
Indocin 1680

Indomethacin Sodium Trihydrate (Concomitant administration has been associated with severe hyperkalemia). Products include:
Indocin I.V. 1684

Insulin, Human (Dosage adjustment of insulin may be necessary).
No products indexed under this heading.

Insulin, Human Isophane Suspension (Dosage adjustment of insulin may be necessary). Products include:
Novolin N Human Insulin 10 ml Vials 1795

Insulin, Human NPH (Dosage adjustment of insulin may be necessary). Products include:
Humulin N, 100 Units 1448
Novolin N PenFill Cartridges Durable Insulin Delivery System 1798
Novolin N Prefilled Syringe Disposable Insulin Delivery System 1798

Insulin, Human Regular (Dosage adjustment of insulin may be necessary). Products include:
Humulin R, 100 Units 1449
Novolin R Human Insulin 10 ml Vials 1795
Novolin R PenFill Cartridges Durable Insulin Delivery System 1798
Novolin R Prefilled Syringe Disposable Insulin Delivery System 1798
Velosulin BR Human Insulin 10 ml Vials 1795

Insulin, Human, Zinc Suspension (Dosage adjustment of insulin may be necessary). Products include:
Humulin L, 100 Units 1446
Humulin U, 100 Units 1450
Novolin L Human Insulin 10 ml Vials 1795

Insulin, NPH (Dosage adjustment of insulin may be necessary). Products include:
NPH, 100 Units 1450
Pork NPH, 100 Units 1452
Purified Pork NPH Isophane Insulin 1801

Insulin, Regular (Dosage adjustment of insulin may be necessary). Products include:
Regular, 100 Units 1450
Pork Regular, 100 Units 1452
Pork Regular (Concentrated), 500 Units 1453
Purified Pork Regular Insulin 1801

Insulin, Zinc Crystals (Dosage adjustment of insulin may be necessary). Products include:
NPH, 100 Units 1450

Insulin, Zinc Suspension (Dosage adjustment of insulin may be necessary). Products include:
Iletin I 1450
Lente, 100 Units 1450
Iletin II 1452
Pork Lente, 100 Units 1452
Purified Pork Lente Insulin 1801

Isoflurane (Exercise caution).
No products indexed under this heading.

Ketamine Hydrochloride (Exercise caution).
No products indexed under this heading.

Lisinopril (Concomitant administration has been associated with severe hyperkalemia). Products include:
Prinivil Tablets 1733
Prinzide Tablets 1737
Zestoretic 2850
Zestril Tablets 2854

Lithium Carbonate (Potential for lithium toxicity). Products include:
Eskalith 2485
Lithium Carbonate Capsules & Tablets 2230
Lithonate/Lithotabs/Lithobid 2543

Lithium Citrate (Potential for lithium toxicity).
No products indexed under this heading.

Metformin Hydrochloride (Dosage adjustment of hypoglycemics may be necessary). Products include:
Glucophage 752

Methohexital Sodium (Exercise caution). Products include:
Brevital Sodium Vials 1429

Methoxyflurane (Exercise caution).
No products indexed under this heading.

Methyclothiazide (Concomitant administration has been associated with severe hyperkalemia and may induce dilutional hyponatremia). Products include:
Enduron Tablets 420

Methylprednisolone Acetate (Concomitant administration may result in hypokalemia). Products include:
Depo-Medrol Single-Dose Vial 2600
Depo-Medrol Sterile Aqueous Suspension 2597

Methylprednisolone Sodium Succinate (Concomitant administration may result in hypokalemia). Products include:
Solu-Medrol Sterile Powder 2643

Metolazone (Concomitant administration may induce dilutional hyponatremia). Products include:
Mykrox Tablets 993
Zaroxolyn Tablets 1000

Moexipril Hydrochloride (Concomitant administration has been associated with severe hyperkalemia). Products include:
Univasc Tablets 2410

(▣ Described in PDR For Nonprescription Drugs) (◉ Described in PDR For Ophthalmology)

Norepinephrine Bitartrate (Reduced vascular responsiveness to norepinephrine). Products include:

Levophed Bitartrate Injection 2315

Polythiazide (Concomitant administration has been associated with severe hyperkalemia and may induce dilutional hyponatremia). Products include:

Minizide Capsules 1938

Potassium Acid Phosphate (Concurrent administration may cause hyperkalemia). Products include:

K-Phos Original Formula 'Sodium Free' Tablets 639

Potassium Bicarbonate (Concurrent administration may cause hyperkalemia). Products include:

Alka-Seltzer Gold Effervescent Antacid .... ⊞ 703

Potassium Chloride (Concurrent administration may cause hyperkalemia). Products include:

Chlor-3 Condiment 1004
K-Dur Microburst Release System (potassium chloride, USP) E.R. Tablets 1325
K-Lor Powder Packets 434
K-Norm Extended-Release Capsules 991
K-Tab Filmtab 434
Kolyum Liquid 992
Micro-K 2063
Micro-K LS Packets 2064
NuLYTELY 689
Cherry Flavor NuLYTELY 689
Rum-K Syrup 1005
Slow-K Extended-Release Tablets 851

Potassium Citrate (Concurrent administration may cause hyperkalemia). Products include:

Polycitra Syrup 578
Polycitra-K Crystals 579
Polycitra-K Oral Solution 579
Polycitra-LC 578

Potassium Gluconate (Concurrent administration may cause hyperkalemia). Products include:

Kolyum Liquid *992

Potassium Phosphate, Dibasic (Concurrent administration may cause hyperkalemia).

No products indexed under this heading.

Potassium Phosphate, Monobasic (Concurrent administration may cause hyperkalemia). Products include:

K-Phos Neutral Tablets 639
K-Phos Original Formula 'Sodium Free' Tablets 639

Prednisolone Acetate (Concomitant administration may result in hypokalemia). Products include:

AK-CIDE .... ◎ 202
AK-CIDE Ointment .... ◎ 202
Blephamide Liquifilm Sterile Ophthalmic Suspension 476
Blephamide Ointment .... ◎ 237
Econopred & Econopred Plus Ophthalmic Suspensions .... ◎ 217
Poly-Pred Liquifilm .... ◎ 248
Pred Forte .... ◎ 250
Pred Mild .... ◎ 253
Pred-G Liquifilm Sterile Ophthalmic Suspension .... ◎ 251
Pred-G S.O.P. Sterile Ophthalmic Ointment .... ◎ 252
Vasocidin Ointment .... ◎ 268

Prednisolone Sodium Phosphate (Concomitant administration may result in hypokalemia). Products include:

AK-Pred .... ◎ 204
Hydeltrasol Injection, Sterile 1665
Inflamase .... ◎ 265
Pediapred Oral Liquid 995
Vasocidin Ophthalmic Solution ...... ◎ 270

Prednisolone Tebutate (Concomitant administration may result in hypokalemia). Products include:

Hydeltra-T.B.A. Sterile Suspension 1667

Prednisone (Concomitant administration may result in hypokalemia). Products include:

Deltasone Tablets 2595

Probenecid (Dosage adjustment may be necessary). Products include:

Benemid Tablets 1611
ColBENEMID Tablets 1622

Propofol (Exercise caution). Products include:

Diprivan Injection 2833

Quinapril Hydrochloride (Concomitant administration has been associated with severe hyperkalemia). Products include:

Accupril Tablets 1893

Ramipril (Concomitant administration has been associated with severe hyperkalemia). Products include:

Altace Capsules 1232

Spirapril Hydrochloride (Concomitant administration has been associated with severe hyperkalemia).

No products indexed under this heading.

Sulfinpyrazone (Dosage adjustment may be necessary). Products include:

Anturane 807

Tolazamide (Dosage adjustment of hypoglycemics may be necessary).

No products indexed under this heading.

Tolbutamide (Dosage adjustment of hypoglycemics may be necessary).

No products indexed under this heading.

Torsemide (Concomitant administration may result in hypokalemia and may induce dilutional hyponatremia). Products include:

Demadex Tablets and Injection 686

Triamcinolone (Concomitant administration may result in hypokalemia). Products include:

Aristocort Tablets 1022

Triamcinolone Acetonide (Concomitant administration may result in hypokalemia). Products include:

Aristocort A 0.025% Cream 1027
Aristocort A 0.5% Cream 1031
Aristocort A 0.1% Cream 1029
Aristocort A 0.1% Ointment 1030
Azmacort Oral Inhaler 2011
Nasacort Nasal Inhaler 2024

Triamcinolone Diacetate (Concomitant administration may result in hypokalemia). Products include:

Aristocort Suspension (Forte Parenteral) 1027
Aristocort Suspension (Intralesional) 1025

Triamcinolone Hexacetonide (Concomitant administration may result in hypokalemia). Products include:

Aristospan Suspension (Intra-articular) 1033
Aristospan Suspension (Intralesional) 1032

Triamterene (Concomitant administration has been associated with severe hyperkalemia and may induce dilutional hyponatremia). Products include:

Dyazide 2479
Dyrenium Capsules 2481
Maxzide 1380

Tubocurarine Chloride (Increased responsiveness to tubocurarine).

No products indexed under this heading.

ALDACTONE

(Spironolactone) 2414

May interact with potassium preparations, diuretics, antihypertensives, potassium sparing diuretics, general anesthetics, ganglionic blocking agents, ACE inhibitors, thiazides, and certain other agents. Compounds in these categories include:

Acebutolol Hydrochloride (Potentiated antihypertensive effects). Products include:

Sectral Capsules 2807

Amiloride Hydrochloride (Potentiated diuretic effects; may cause or aggravate hyponatremia; do not administer concurrently). Products include:

Midamor Tablets 1703
Moduretic Tablets 1705

Amlodipine Besylate (Severe hyperkalemia; potentiated antihypertensive effects). Products include:

Lotrel Capsules 840
Norvasc Tablets 1940

Atenolol (Potentiated antihypertensive effects). Products include:

Tenoretic Tablets 2845
Tenormin Tablets and I.V. Injection 2847

Benazepril Hydrochloride (Severe hyperkalemia; potentiated antihypertensive effects). Products include:

Lotensin Tablets 834
Lotensin HCT 837
Lotrel Capsules 840

Bendroflumethiazide (Potentiated diuretic and antihypertensive effects; may cause or aggravate hyponatremia).

No products indexed under this heading.

Betaxolol Hydrochloride (Severe hyperkalemia; potentiated antihypertensive effects). Products include:

Betoptic Ophthalmic Solution 469
Betoptic S Ophthalmic Suspension 471
Kerlone Tablets 2436

Bisoprolol Fumarate (Severe hyperkalemia; potentiated antihypertensive effects). Products include:

Zebeta Tablets 1413
Ziac 1415

Bumetanide (Potentiated diuretic effects; may cause or aggravate hyponatremia). Products include:

Bumex 2093

Captopril (Severe hyperkalemia; potentiated antihypertensive effects). Products include:

Capoten 739
Capozide 742

Carteolol Hydrochloride (Potentiated antihypertensive effects). Products include:

Cartrol Tablets 410
Ocupress Ophthalmic Solution, 1% Sterile .... ◎ 309

Chlorothiazide (Potentiated diuretic and antihypertensive effects; may cause or aggravate hyponatremia). Products include:

Aldoclor Tablets 1598
Diupres Tablets 1650
Diuril Oral 1653

Chlorothiazide Sodium (Potentiated diuretic and antihypertensive effects; may cause or aggravate hyponatremia). Products include:

Diuril Sodium Intravenous 1652

Chlorthalidone (Potentiated diuretic and antihypertensive effects; may cause or aggravate hyponatremia). Products include:

Combipres Tablets 677
Tenoretic Tablets 2845
Thalitone 1245

Clonidine (Potentiated antihypertensive effects). Products include:

Catapres-TTS 675

Clonidine Hydrochloride (Potentiated antihypertensive effects). Products include:

Catapres Tablets 674
Combipres Tablets 677

Deserpidine (Potentiated antihypertensive effects).

No products indexed under this heading.

Diazoxide (Potentiated antihypertensive effects). Products include:

Hyperstat I.V. Injection 2363
Proglycem 580

Digoxin (Digitalis toxicity). Products include:

Lanoxicaps 1117
Lanoxin Elixir Pediatric 1120
Lanoxin Injection 1123
Lanoxin Injection Pediatric 1126
Lanoxin Tablets 1128

Diltiazem Hydrochloride (Severe hyperkalemia; potentiated antihypertensive effects). Products include:

Cardizem CD Capsules 1506
Cardizem SR Capsules 1510
Cardizem Injectable 1508
Cardizem Tablets 1512
Dilacor XR Extended-release Capsules 2018

Doxazosin Mesylate (Severe hyperkalemia; potentiated antihypertensive effects). Products include:

Cardura Tablets 2186

Enalapril Maleate (Potentiated antihypertensive effects; severe hyperkalemia). Products include:

Vaseretic Tablets 1765
Vasotec Tablets 1771

Enalaprilat (Potentiated antihypertensive effects; severe hyperkalemia). Products include:

Vasotec I.V. 1768

Enflurane (Exercise caution).

No products indexed under this heading.

Esmolol Hydrochloride (Potentiated antihypertensive effects). Products include:

Brevibloc Injection 1808

Ethacrynic Acid (Potentiated diuretic effects; may cause or aggravate hyponatremia). Products include:

Edecrin Tablets 1657

Felodipine (Severe hyperkalemia; potentiated antihypertensive effects). Products include:

Plendil Extended-Release Tablets 527

Fosinopril Sodium (Severe hyperkalemia; potentiated antihypertensive effects). Products include:

Monopril Tablets 757

Furosemide (Potentiated diuretic and antihypertensive effects; may cause or aggravate hyponatremia). Products include:

Lasix Injection, Oral Solution and Tablets 1240

Guanabenz Acetate (Potentiated antihypertensive effects).

No products indexed under this heading.

Guanethidine Monosulfate (Potentiated antihypertensive effects). Products include:

Esimil Tablets 822
Ismelin Tablets 827

IMPORTANT NOTE: Always consult each drug listing in the patient's regimen for possible interactions.

Aldactone

Hydralazine Hydrochloride (Potentiated antihypertensive effects). Products include:

Apresazide Capsules 808
Apresoline Hydrochloride Tablets .. 809
Ser-Ap-Es Tablets 849

Hydrochlorothiazide (Potentiated diuretic and antihypertensive effects; may cause or aggravate hyponatremia). Products include:

Aldactazide 2413
Aldoril Tablets 1604
Apresazide Capsules 808
Capozide 742
Dyazide 2479
Esidrix Tablets 821
Esimil Tablets 822
HydroDIURIL Tablets 1674
Hydropres Tablets 1675
Hyzaar Tablets 1677
Inderide Tablets 2732
Inderide LA Long Acting Capsules .. 2734
Lopressor HCT Tablets 832
Lotensin HCT 837
Maxzide 1380
Moduretic Tablets 1705
Oretic Tablets 443
Prinzide Tablets 1737
Ser-Ap-Es Tablets 849
Timolide Tablets 1748
Vaseretic Tablets 1765
Zestoretic 2850
Ziac 1415

Hydroflumethiazide (Potentiated diuretic and antihypertensive effects; may cause or aggravate hyponatremia). Products include:

Diucardin Tablets 2718

Indapamide (Potentiated diuretic and antihypertensive effects; may cause or aggravate hyponatremia). Products include:

Lozol Tablets 2022

Indomethacin (Severe hyperkalemia). Products include:

Indocin 1680

Indomethacin Sodium Trihydrate (Severe hyperkalemia). Products include:

Indocin I.V. 1684

Isoflurane (Exercise caution).

No products indexed under this heading.

Isradipine (Severe hyperkalemia; potentiated antihypertensive effects). Products include:

DynaCirc Capsules 2256

Ketamine Hydrochloride (Exercise caution).

No products indexed under this heading.

Labetalol Hydrochloride (Potentiated antihypertensive effects). Products include:

Normodyne Injection 2377
Normodyne Tablets 2379
Trandate 1185

Lisinopril (Potentiated antihypertensive effects; severe hyperkalemia). Products include:

Prinivil Tablets 1733
Prinzide Tablets 1737
Zestoretic 2850
Zestril Tablets 2854

Losartan Potassium (Severe hyperkalemia; potentiated antihypertensive effects). Products include:

Cozaar Tablets 1628
Hyzaar Tablets 1677

Mecamylamine Hydrochloride (Potentiated antihypertensive effects; reduce mecamylamine dosage by at least 50 percent). Products include:

Inversine Tablets 1686

Methohexital Sodium (Exercise caution). Products include:

Brevital Sodium Vials 1429

Methoxyflurane (Exercise caution).

No products indexed under this heading.

Methyclothiazide (Potentiated diuretic and antihypertensive effects; may cause or aggravate hyponatremia). Products include:

Enduron Tablets 420

Methyldopa (Potentiated antihypertensive effects). Products include:

Aldoclor Tablets 1598
Aldomet Oral 1600
Aldoril Tablets 1604

Methyldopate Hydrochloride (Potentiated antihypertensive effects). Products include:

Aldomet Ester HCl Injection 1602

Metolazone (Potentiated diuretic and antihypertensive effects; may cause or aggravate hyponatremia). Products include:

Mykrox Tablets 993
Zaroxolyn Tablets 1000

Metoprolol Succinate (Severe hyperkalemia; potentiated antihypertensive effects). Products include:

Toprol-XL Tablets 565

Metoprolol Tartrate (Potentiated antihypertensive effects). Products include:

Lopressor Ampuls 830
Lopressor HCT Tablets 832
Lopressor Tablets 830

Metyrosine (Potentiated antihypertensive effects). Products include:

Demser Capsules 1649

Minoxidil (Potentiated antihypertensive effects). Products include:

Loniten Tablets 2618
Rogaine Topical Solution 2637

Moexipril Hydrochloride (Severe hyperkalemia; potentiated antihypertensive effects). Products include:

Univasc Tablets 2410

Nadolol (Potentiated antihypertensive effects).

No products indexed under this heading.

Nicardipine Hydrochloride (Potentiated antihypertensive effects). Products include:

Cardene Capsules 2095
Cardene I.V. 2709
Cardene SR Capsules 2097

Nifedipine (Severe hyperkalemia; potentiated antihypertensive effects). Products include:

Adalat Capsules (10 mg and 20 mg) 587
Adalat CC 589
Procardia Capsules 1971
Procardia XL Extended Release Tablets 1972

Nisoldipine (Severe hyperkalemia; potentiated antihypertensive effects).

No products indexed under this heading.

Nitroglycerin (Potentiated antihypertensive effects). Products include:

Deponit NTG Transdermal Delivery System 2397
Nitro-Bid IV 1523
Nitro-Bid Ointment 1524
Nitrodisc 2047
Nitro-Dur (nitroglycerin) Transdermal Infusion System 1326
Nitrolingual Spray 2027
Nitrostat Tablets 1925
Transderm-Nitro Transdermal Therapeutic System 859

Norepinephrine Bitartrate (Reduced vascular responsiveness to norepinephrine). Products include:

Levophed Bitartrate Injection 2315

Penbutolol Sulfate (Potentiated antihypertensive effects). Products include:

Levatol 2403

Phenoxybenzamine Hydrochloride (Potentiated antihypertensive effects). Products include:

Dibenzyline Capsules 2476

Phentolamine Mesylate (Potentiated antihypertensive effects). Products include:

Regitine 846

Pindolol (Potentiated antihypertensive effects). Products include:

Visken Tablets 2299

Polythiazide (Potentiated diuretic and antihypertensive effects; may cause or aggravate hyponatremia). Products include:

Minizide Capsules 1938

Potassium Acid Phosphate (May cause hyperkalemia; cardiac irregularities, possibly fatal). Products include:

K-Phos Original Formula 'Sodium Free' Tablets 639

Potassium Bicarbonate (May cause hyperkalemia; cardiac irregularities, possibly fatal). Products include:

Alka-Seltzer Gold Effervescent Antacid .... ⊕ 703

Potassium Chloride (May cause hyperkalemia; cardiac irregularities, possibly fatal). Products include:

Chlor-3 Condiment 1004
K-Dur Microburst Release System (potassium chloride, USP) E.R. Tablets 1325
K-Lor Powder Packets 434
K-Norm Extended-Release Capsules 991
K-Tab Filmtab 434
Kolyum Liquid 992
Micro-K 2063
Micro-K LS Packets 2064
NuLYTELY 689
Cherry Flavor NuLYTELY 689
Rum-K Syrup 1005
Slow-K Extended-Release Tablets 851

Potassium Citrate (May cause hyperkalemia; cardiac irregularities, possibly fatal). Products include:

Polycitra Syrup 578
Polycitra-K Crystals 579
Polycitra-K Oral Solution 579
Polycitra-LC 578

Potassium Gluconate (May cause hyperkalemia; cardiac irregularities, possibly fatal). Products include:

Kolyum Liquid 992

Potassium Phosphate, Dibasic (May cause hyperkalemia; cardiac irregularities, possibly fatal).

No products indexed under this heading.

Potassium Phosphate, Monobasic (May cause hyperkalemia; cardiac irregularities, possibly fatal). Products include:

K-Phos Neutral Tablets 639
K-Phos Original Formula 'Sodium Free' Tablets 639

Prazosin Hydrochloride (Potentiated antihypertensive effects). Products include:

Minipress Capsules 1937
Minizide Capsules 1938

Propofol (Exercise caution). Products include:

Diprivan Injection 2833

Propranolol Hydrochloride (Potentiated antihypertensive effects). Products include:

Inderal 2728
Inderal LA Long Acting Capsules 2730

Inderide Tablets 2732
Inderide LA Long Acting Capsules .. 2734

Quinapril Hydrochloride (Severe hyperkalemia; potentiated antihypertensive effects). Products include:

Accupril Tablets 1893

Ramipril (Severe hyperkalemia; potentiated antihypertensive effects). Products include:

Altace Capsules 1232

Rauwolfia Serpentina (Potentiated antihypertensive effects).

No products indexed under this heading.

Rescinnamine (Potentiated antihypertensive effects).

No products indexed under this heading.

Reserpine (Potentiated antihypertensive effects). Products include:

Diupres Tablets 1650
Hydropres Tablets 1675
Ser-Ap-Es Tablets 849

Sodium Nitroprusside (Potentiated antihypertensive effects).

No products indexed under this heading.

Sotalol Hydrochloride (Severe hyperkalemia; potentiated antihypertensive effects). Products include:

Betapace Tablets 641

Spirapril Hydrochloride (Severe hyperkalemia; potentiated antihypertensive effects).

No products indexed under this heading.

Terazosin Hydrochloride (Potentiated antihypertensive effects). Products include:

Hytrin Capsules 430

Timolol Maleate (Potentiated antihypertensive effects). Products include:

Blocadren Tablets 1614
Timolide Tablets 1748
Timoptic in Ocudose 1753
Timoptic Sterile Ophthalmic Solution 1751
Timoptic-XE 1755

Torsemide (Severe hyperkalemia; potentiated antihypertensive effects). Products include:

Demadex Tablets and Injection 686

Triamterene (Potentiated diuretic effects; may cause or aggravate hyponatremia; do not administer concurrently). Products include:

Dyazide 2479
Dyrenium Capsules 2481
Maxzide 1380

Trimethaphan Camsylate (Potentiated antihypertensive effects; reduce trimethaphan dosage by at least 50 percent). Products include:

Arfonad Ampuls 2080

Verapamil Hydrochloride (Severe hyperkalemia; potentiated antihypertensive effects). Products include:

Calan SR Caplets 2422
Calan Tablets 2419
Isoptin Injectable 1344
Isoptin Oral Tablets 1346
Isoptin SR Tablets 1348
Verelan Capsules 1410
Verelan Capsules 2824

ALDOCLOR TABLETS

(Methyldopa, Chlorothiazide) 1598
May interact with antihypertensives, general anesthetics, corticosteroids, insulin, lithium preparations, oral hypoglycemic agents, non-steroidal anti-inflammatory agents, monoamine oxidase inhibitors, barbiturates, narcotic analgesics, cardiac glycosides, and certain other agents.

Interactions Index — Aldoclor

Compounds in these categories include:

Acarbose (Dosage adjustment of the antidiabetic drug may be required).

No products indexed under this heading.

Acebutolol Hydrochloride (Potentiation of antihypertensive effect). Products include:

Sectral Capsules 2807

ACTH (Hypokalemia may result).

No products indexed under this heading.

Alfentanil Hydrochloride (Aggravates orthostatic hypotension). Products include:

Alfenta Injection 1286

Amlodipine Besylate (Potentiation of antihypertensive effect). Products include:

Lotrel Capsules 840
Norvasc Tablets 1940

Aprobarbital (Aggravates orthostatic hypotension).

No products indexed under this heading.

Atenolol (Potentiation of antihypertensive effect). Products include:

Tenoretic Tablets 2845
Tenormin Tablets and I.V. Injection 2847

Benazepril Hydrochloride (Potentiation of antihypertensive effect). Products include:

Lotensin Tablets 834
Lotensin HCT 837
Lotrel Capsules 840

Bendroflumethiazide (Potentiation of antihypertensive effect).

No products indexed under this heading.

Betamethasone Acetate (Hypokalemia may result). Products include:

Celestone Soluspan Suspension 2347

Betamethasone Sodium Phosphate (Hypokalemia may result). Products include:

Celestone Soluspan Suspension 2347

Betaxolol Hydrochloride (Potentiation of antihypertensive effect). Products include:

Betoptic Ophthalmic Solution........... 469
Betoptic S Ophthalmic Suspension 471
Kerlone Tablets 2436

Bisoprolol Fumarate (Potentiation of antihypertensive effect). Products include:

Zebeta Tablets 1413
Ziac 1415

Buprenorphine (Aggravates orthostatic hypotension). Products include:

Buprenex Injectable 2006

Butabarbital (Aggravates orthostatic hypotension).

No products indexed under this heading.

Butalbital (Aggravates orthostatic hypotension). Products include:

Esgic-plus Tablets 1013
Fioricet Tablets 2258
Fioricet with Codeine Capsules 2260
Fiorinal Capsules 2261
Fiorinal with Codeine Capsules 2262
Fiorinal Tablets 2261
Phrenilin 785
Sedapap Tablets 50 mg/650 mg .. 1543

Captopril (Potentiation of antihypertensive effect). Products include:

Capoten 739
Capozide 742

Carteolol Hydrochloride (Potentiation of antihypertensive effects). Products include:

Cartrol Tablets 410
Ocupress Ophthalmic Solution, 1% Sterile .... ◉ 309

Chlorothiazide Sodium (Potentiation of antihypertensive effect). Products include:

Diuril Sodium Intravenous 1652

Chlorpropamide (Dosage adjustment of the antidiabetic drug may be required). Products include:

Diabinese Tablets 1935

Chlorthalidone (Potentiation of antihypertensive effect). Products include:

Combipres Tablets 677
Tenoretic Tablets 2845
Thalitone 1245

Cholestyramine (Cholestyramine resin has the potential of binding thiazide diuretics and reducing absorption from the gastrointestinal tract). Products include:

Questran Light 769
Questran Powder 770

Clonidine (Potentiation of antihypertensive effect). Products include:

Catapres-TTS 675

Clonidine Hydrochloride (Potentiation of antihypertensive effect). Products include:

Catapres Tablets 674
Combipres Tablets 677

Codeine Phosphate (Aggravates orthostatic hypotension). Products include:

Actifed with Codeine Cough Syrup.. 1067
Brontex 1981
Deconsal C Expectorant Syrup 456
Deconsal Pediatric Syrup 457
Dimetane-DC Cough Syrup 2059
Empirin with Codeine Tablets........... 1093
Fioricet with Codeine Capsules 2260
Fiorinal with Codeine Capsules 2262
Isoclor Expectorant 990
Novahistine DH 2462
Novahistine Expectorant 2463
Nucofed 2051
Phenergan with Codeine 2777
Phenergan VC with Codeine 2781
Robitussin A-C Syrup 2073
Robitussin-DAC Syrup 2074
Ryna .... ◉ 841
Soma Compound w/Codeine Tablets 2676
Tussi-Organidin NR Liquid and S NR Liquid 2677
Tylenol with Codeine 1583

Colestipol Hydrochloride (Colestipole resin has the potential of binding thiazide diuretics and reducing absorption from the gastrointestinal tract). Products include:

Colestid Tablets 2591

Cortisone Acetate (Hypokalemia may result). Products include:

Cortone Acetate Sterile Suspension 1623
Cortone Acetate Tablets 1624

Deserpidine (Potentiation of antihypertensive effect).

No products indexed under this heading.

Deslanoside (Thiazide-induced hypokalemia may cause cardiac arrhythmia and may also sensitize or exaggerate the response of the heart to the toxic effects of digitalis).

No products indexed under this heading.

Dexamethasone (Hypokalemia may result). Products include:

AK-Trol Ointment & Suspension .... ◉ 205
Decadron Elixir 1633
Decadron Tablets 1635
Decaspray Topical Aerosol 1648
Dexacidin Ointment .... ◉ 263
Maxitrol Ophthalmic Ointment and Suspension .... ◉ 224
TobraDex Ophthalmic Suspension and Ointment 473

Dexamethasone Acetate (Hypokalemia may result). Products include:

Dalalone D.P. Injectable 1011
Decadron-LA Sterile Suspension 1646

Dexamethasone Sodium Phosphate (Hypokalemia may result). Products include:

Decadron Phosphate Injection 1637
Decadron Phosphate Respihaler 1642
Decadron Phosphate Sterile Ophthalmic Ointment 1641
Decadron Phosphate Sterile Ophthalmic Solution 1642
Decadron Phosphate Topical Cream 1644
Decadron Phosphate Turbinaire 1645
Decadron Phosphate with Xylocaine Injection, Sterile 1639
Dexacort Phosphate in Respihaler .. 458
Dexacort Phosphate in Turbinaire .. 459
NeoDecadron Sterile Ophthalmic Ointment 1712
NeoDecadron Sterile Ophthalmic Solution 1713
NeoDecadron Topical Cream 1714

Dezocine (Aggravates orthostatic hypotension). Products include:

Dalgan Injection 538

Diazoxide (Potentiation of antihypertensive effects). Products include:

Hyperstat I.V. Injection 2363
Proglycem 580

Diclofenac Potassium (May result in reduced diuretic effect). Products include:

Cataflam 816

Diclofenac Sodium (May result in reduced diuretic effect). Products include:

Voltaren Ophthalmic Sterile Ophthalmic Solution .... ◉ 272
Voltaren Tablets 861

Digitoxin (Thiazide-induced hypokalemia may cause cardiac arrhythmia and may also sensitize or exaggerate the response of the heart to the toxic effects of digitalis). Products include:

Crystodigin Tablets 1433

Digoxin (Thiazide-induced hypokalemia may cause cardiac arrhythmia and may also sensitize or exaggerate the response of the heart to the toxic effects of digitalis). Products include:

Lanoxicaps 1117
Lanoxin Elixir Pediatric 1120
Lanoxin Injection 1123
Lanoxin Injection Pediatric 1126
Lanoxin Tablets 1128

Diltiazem Hydrochloride (Potentiation of antihypertensive effect). Products include:

Cardizem CD Capsules 1506
Cardizem SR Capsules 1510
Cardizem Injectable 1508
Cardizem Tablets 1512
Dilacor XR Extended-release Capsules 2018

Doxazosin Mesylate (Potentiation of antihypertensive effect). Products include:

Cardura Tablets 2186

Enalapril Maleate (Potentiation of antihypertensive effect). Products include:

Vaseretic Tablets 1765
Vasotec Tablets 1771

Enalaprilat (Potentiation of antihypertensive effect). Products include:

Vasotec I.V. 1768

Enflurane (May require reduced dose of anesthetics).

No products indexed under this heading.

Esmolol Hydrochloride (Potentiation of antihypertensive effect). Products include:

Brevibloc Injection 1808

Etodolac (May result in reduced diuretic effect). Products include:

Lodine Capsules and Tablets 2743

Felodipine (Potentiation of antihypertensive effect). Products include:

Plendil Extended-Release Tablets 527

Fenoprofen Calcium (May result in reduced diuretic effects). Products include:

Nalfon 200 Pulvules & Nalfon Tablets 917

Fentanyl (Aggravates orthostatic hypotension). Products include:

Duragesic Transdermal System 1288

Fentanyl Citrate (Aggravates orthostatic hypotension). Products include:

Sublimaze Injection 1307

Fludrocortisone Acetate (Hypokalemia may result). Products include:

Florinef Acetate Tablets 505

Flurbiprofen (May result in reduced diuretic effect). Products include:

Ansaid Tablets 2579

Fosinopril Sodium (Potentiation of antihypertensive effect). Products include:

Monopril Tablets 757

Furazolidone (Concurrent use is contraindicated). Products include:

Furoxone 2046

Furosemide (Potentiation of antihypertensive effect). Products include:

Lasix Injection, Oral Solution and Tablets 1240

Glipizide (Dosage adjustment of the antidiabetic drug may be required). Products include:

Glucotrol Tablets 1967
Glucotrol XL Extended Release Tablets 1968

Glyburide (Dosage adjustment of the antidiabetic drug may be required). Products include:

DiaBeta Tablets 1239
Glynase PresTab Tablets 2609
Micronase Tablets 2623

Guanabenz Acetate (Potentiation of antihypertensive effect).

No products indexed under this heading.

Guanethidine Monosulfate (Potentiation of antihypertensive effect). Products include:

Esimil Tablets 822
Ismelin Tablets 827

Hydralazine Hydrochloride (Potentiation of antihypertensive effect). Products include:

Apresazide Capsules 808
Apresoline Hydrochloride Tablets .. 809
Ser-Ap-Es Tablets 849

Hydrochlorothiazide (Potentiation of antihypertensive effect). Products include:

Aldactazide 2413
Aldoril Tablets 1604
Apresazide Capsules 808
Capozide 742
Dyazide 2479
Esidrix Tablets 821
Esimil Tablets 822
HydroDIURIL Tablets 1674
Hydropres Tablets 1675
Hyzaar Tablets 1677
Inderide Tablets 2732
Inderide LA Long Acting Capsules .. 2734
Lopressor HCT Tablets 832
Lotensin HCT 837
Maxzide 1380
Moduretic Tablets 1705
Oretic Tablets 443
Prinzide Tablets 1737
Ser-Ap-Es Tablets 849
Timolide Tablets 1748
Vaseretic Tablets 1765
Zestoretic 2850
Ziac 1415

IMPORTANT NOTE: Always consult each drug listing in the patient's regimen for possible interactions.

Aldoclor Interactions Index 26

Hydrocodone Bitartrate (Aggravates orthostatic hypotension). Products include:
- Anexsia 5/500 Elixir ... 1781
- Anexia Tablets ... 1782
- Codiclear DH Syrup ... 791
- Deconamine CX Cough and Cold Liquid and Tablets ... 1319
- Duratuss HD Elixir ... 2565
- Hycodan Tablets and Syrup ... 930
- Hycomine Compound Tablets ... 932
- Hycomine ... 931
- Hycotuss Expectorant Syrup ... 933
- Hydrocet Capsules ... 782
- Lorcet 10/650 ... 1018
- Lortab ... 2566
- Tussend ... 1783
- Tussend Expectorant ... 1785
- Vicodin Tablets ... 1356
- Vicodin ES Tablets ... 1357
- Vicodin Tuss Expectorant ... 1358
- Zydone Capsules ... 949

Hydrocodone Polistirex (Aggravates orthostatic hypotension). Products include:
- Tussionex Pennkinetic Extended-Release Suspension ... 998

Hydrocortisone (Hypokalemia may result). Products include:
- Anusol-HC Cream 2.5% ... 1896
- Aquanil HC Lotion ... 1931
- Bactine Hydrocortisone Anti-Itch Cream ... ▣ 709
- Caldecort Anti-Itch Hydrocortisone Spray ... ▣ 631
- Cortaid ... ▣ 836
- CORTENEMA ... 2535
- Cortisporin Ointment ... 1085
- Cortisporin Ophthalmic Ointment Sterile ... 1085
- Cortisporin Ophthalmic Suspension Sterile ... 1086
- Cortisporin Otic Solution Sterile ... 1087
- Cortisporin Otic Suspension Sterile 1088
- Cortizone-5 ... ▣ 831
- Cortizone-10 ... ▣ 831
- Hydrocortone Tablets ... 1672
- Hytone ... 907
- Massengill Medicated Soft Cloth Towelettes ... 2458
- PediOtic Suspension Sterile ... 1153
- Preparation H Hydrocortisone 1% Cream ... ▣ 872
- ProctoCream-HC 2.5% ... 2408
- VōSoL HC Otic Solution ... 2678

Hydrocortisone Acetate (Hypokalemia may result). Products include:
- Analpram-HC Rectal Cream 1% and 2.5% ... 977
- Anusol HC-1 Anti-Itch Hydrocortisone Ointment ... ▣ 847
- Anusol-HC Suppositories ... 1897
- Caldecort ... ▣ 631
- Carmol HC ... 924
- Coly-Mycin S Otic w/Neomycin & Hydrocortisone ... 1906
- Cortaid ... ▣ 836
- Cortifoam ... 2396
- Cortisporin Cream ... 1084
- Epifoam ... 2399
- Hydrocortone Acetate Sterile Suspension ... 1669
- Mantadil Cream ... 1135
- Nupercainal Hydrocortisone 1% Cream ... ▣ 645
- Ophthocort ... ⊙ 311
- Pramosone Cream, Lotion & Ointment ... 978
- ProctoCream-HC ... 2408
- ProctoFoam-HC ... 2409
- Terra-Cortril Ophthalmic Suspension ... 2210

Hydrocortisone Sodium Phosphate (Hypokalemia may result). Products include:
- Hydrocortone Phosphate Injection, Sterile ... 1670

Hydrocortisone Sodium Succinate (Hypokalemia may result). Products include:
- Solu-Cortef Sterile Powder ... 2641

Hydroflumethiazide (Potentiation of antihypertensive effect). Products include:
- Diucardin Tablets ... 2718

Ibuprofen (May result in reduced diuretic effects). Products include:
- Advil Cold and Sinus Caplets and Tablets (formerly CoAdvil) ... ▣ 870
- Advil Ibuprofen Tablets and Caplets ... ▣ 870
- Children's Advil Suspension ... 2692
- Arthritis Foundation Ibuprofen Tablets ... ▣ 674
- Bayer Select Ibuprofen Pain Relief Formula ... ▣ 715
- Cramp End Tablets ... ▣ 735
- Dimetapp Sinus Caplets ... ▣ 775
- Haltran Tablets ... ▣ 771
- IBU Tablets ... 1342
- Ibuprohm ... ▣ 735
- Children's Motrin Ibuprofen Oral Suspension ... 1546
- Motrin Tablets ... 2625
- Motrin IB Caplets, Tablets, and Geltabs ... ▣ 838
- Motrin IB Sinus ... ▣ 838
- Motrin Ibuprofen Suspension, Oral Drops, Chewable Tablets, Caplets ... 1546
- Nuprin Ibuprofen/Analgesic Tablets & Caplets ... ▣ 622
- Sine-Aid IB Caplets ... 1554
- Vicks DayQuil SINUS Pressure & PAIN Relief with IBUPROFEN ... ▣ 762

Indapamide (Potentiation of antihypertensive effect). Products include:
- Lozol Tablets ... 2022

Indomethacin (May result in reduced diuretic effects). Products include:
- Indocin ... 1680

Indomethacin Sodium Trihydrate (May result in reduced diuretic effects). Products include:
- Indocin I.V. ... 1684

Insulin, Human (May alter insulin requirements).
- No products indexed under this heading.

Insulin, Human Isophane Suspension (May alter insulin requirements). Products include:
- Novolin N Human Insulin 10 ml Vials ... 1795

Insulin, Human NPH (May alter insulin requirements). Products include:
- Humulin N, 100 Units ... 1448
- Novolin N PenFill Cartridges Durable Insulin Delivery System ... 1798
- Novolin N Prefilled Syringe Disposable Insulin Delivery System ... 1798

Insulin, Human Regular (May alter insulin requirements). Products include:
- Humulin R, 100 Units ... 1449
- Novolin R Human Insulin 10 ml Vials ... 1795
- Novolin R PenFill Cartridges Durable Insulin Delivery System ... 1798
- Novolin R Prefilled Syringe Disposable Insulin Delivery System ... 1798
- Velosulin BR Human Insulin 10 ml Vials ... 1795

Insulin, Human, Zinc Suspension (May alter insulin requirements). Products include:
- Humulin L, 100 Units ... 1446
- Humulin U, 100 Units ... 1450
- Novolin L Human Insulin 10 ml Vials ... 1795

Insulin, NPH (May alter insulin requirements). Products include:
- NPH, 100 Units ... 1450
- Pork NPH, 100 Units ... 1452
- Purified Pork NPH Isophane Insulin ... 1801

Insulin, Regular (May alter insulin requirements). Products include:
- Regular, 100 Units ... 1450
- Pork Regular, 100 Units ... 1452
- Pork Regular (Concentrated), 500 Units ... 1453
- Purified Pork Regular Insulin ... 1801

Insulin, Zinc Crystals (May alter insulin requirements). Products include:
- NPH, 100 Units ... 1450

Insulin, Zinc Suspension (May alter insulin requirements). Products include:
- Iletin I ... 1450
- Lente, 100 Units ... 1450
- Iletin II ... 1452
- Pork Lente, 100 Units ... 1452
- Purified Pork Lente Insulin ... 1801

Isocarboxazid (Concurrent use is contraindicated).
- No products indexed under this heading.

Isoflurane (May require reduced dose of anesthetics).
- No products indexed under this heading.

Isradipine (Potentiation of antihypertensive effect). Products include:
- DynaCirc Capsules ... 2256

Ketamine Hydrochloride (May require reduced dose of anesthetics).
- No products indexed under this heading.

Ketoprofen (May result in reduced diuretic effects). Products include:
- Orudis Capsules ... 2766
- Oruvail Capsules ... 2766

Ketorolac Tromethamine (May result in reduced diuretic effect). Products include:
- Acular ... 474
- Acular ... ⊙ 277
- Toradol ... 2159

Labetalol Hydrochloride (Potentiation of antihypertensive effect). Products include:
- Normodyne Injection ... 2377
- Normodyne Tablets ... 2379
- Trandate ... 1185

Levorphanol Tartrate (Aggravates orthostatic hypotension). Products include:
- Levo-Dromoran ... 2129

Lisinopril (Potentiation of antihypertensive effect). Products include:
- Prinivil Tablets ... 1733
- Prinzide Tablets ... 1737
- Zestoretic ... 2850
- Zestril Tablets ... 2854

Lithium Carbonate (High risk of lithium toxicity). Products include:
- Eskalith ... 2485
- Lithium Carbonate Capsules & Tablets ... 2230
- Lithonate/Lithotabs/Lithobid ... 2543

Lithium Citrate (High risk of lithium toxicity).
- No products indexed under this heading.

Losartan Potassium (Potentiation of antihypertensive effect). Products include:
- Cozaar Tablets ... 1628
- Hyzaar Tablets ... 1677

Mecamylamine Hydrochloride (Potentiation of antihypertensive effect). Products include:
- Inversine Tablets ... 1686

Meclofenamate Sodium (May result in reduced diuretic effects).
- No products indexed under this heading.

Mefenamic Acid (May result in reduced diuretic effects). Products include:
- Ponstel ... 1925

Meperidine Hydrochloride (Aggravates orthostatic hypotension). Products include:
- Demerol ... 2308
- Mepergan Injection ... 2753

Mephobarbital (Aggravates orthostatic hypotension). Products include:
- Mebaral Tablets ... 2322

Metformin Hydrochloride (Dosage adjustment of the antidiabetic drug may be required). Products include:
- Glucophage ... 752

Methadone Hydrochloride (Aggravates orthostatic hypotension). Products include:
- Methadone Hydrochloride Oral Concentrate ... 2233
- Methadone Hydrochloride Oral Solution & Tablets ... 2235

Methohexital Sodium (May require reduced dose of anesthetics). Products include:
- Brevital Sodium Vials ... 1429

Methoxyflurane (May require reduced dose of anesthetics).
- No products indexed under this heading.

Methyclothiazide (Potentiation of antihypertensive effect). Products include:
- Enduron Tablets ... 420

Methyldopate Hydrochloride (Potentiation of antihypertensive effect). Products include:
- Aldomet Ester HCl Injection ... 1602

Methylprednisolone Acetate (Hypokalemia may result). Products include:
- Depo-Medrol Single-Dose Vial ... 2600
- Depo-Medrol Sterile Aqueous Suspension ... 2597

Methylprednisolone Sodium Succinate (Hypokalemia may result). Products include:
- Solu-Medrol Sterile Powder ... 2643

Metolazone (Potentiation of antihypertensive effect). Products include:
- Mykrox Tablets ... 993
- Zaroxolyn Tablets ... 1000

Metoprolol Succinate (Potentiation of antihypertensive effect). Products include:
- Toprol-XL Tablets ... 565

Metoprolol Tartrate (Potentiation of antihypertensive effect). Products include:
- Lopressor Ampuls ... 830
- Lopressor HCT Tablets ... 832
- Lopressor Tablets ... 830

Metyrosine (Potentiation of antihypertensive effect). Products include:
- Demser Capsules ... 1649

Minoxidil (Potentiation of antihypertensive effect). Products include:
- Loniten Tablets ... 2618
- Rogaine Topical Solution ... 2637

Moexipril Hydrochloride (Potentiation of antihypertensive effect). Products include:
- Univasc Tablets ... 2410

Morphine Sulfate (Aggravates orthostatic hypotension). Products include:
- Astramorph/PF Injection, USP (Preservative-Free) ... 535
- Duramorph ... 962
- Infumorph 200 and Infumorph 500 Sterile Solutions ... 965
- MS Contin Tablets ... 1994
- MSIR ... 1997
- Oramorph SR (Morphine Sulfate Sustained Release Tablets) ... 2236
- RMS Suppositories ... 2657
- Roxanol ... 2243

Nabumetone (May result in reduced diuretic effect). Products include:
- Relafen Tablets ... 2510

(▣ Described in PDR For Nonprescription Drugs) (⊙ Described in PDR For Ophthalmology)

27 Interactions Index Aldomet Injection

Nadolol (Potentiation of antihypertensive effect).
No products indexed under this heading.

Naproxen (May result in reduced diuretic effects). Products include:
Anaprox/Naprosyn ... 2117

Naproxen Sodium (May result in reduced diuretic effects). Products include:
Aleve ... 1975
Anaprox/Naprosyn ... 2117

Nicardipine Hydrochloride (Potentiation of antihypertensive effects). Products include:
Cardene Capsules ... 2095
Cardene I.V. ... 2709
Cardene SR Capsules ... 2097

Nifedipine (Potentiation of antihypertensive effect). Products include:
Adalat Capsules (10 mg and 20 mg) ... 587
Adalat CC ... 589
Procardia Capsules ... 1971
Procardia XL Extended Release Tablets ... 1972

Nisoldipine (Potentiation of antihypertensive effect).
No products indexed under this heading.

Nitroglycerin (Potentiation of antihypertensive effect). Products include:
Deponit NTG Transdermal Delivery System ... 2397
Nitro-Bid IV ... 1523
Nitro-Bid Ointment ... 1524
Nitrodisc ... 2047
Nitro-Dur (nitroglycerin) Transdermal Infusion System ... 1326
Nitrolingual Spray ... 2027
Nitrostat Tablets ... 1925
Transderm-Nitro Transdermal Therapeutic System ... 859

Norepinephrine Bitartrate (May decrease arterial responsiveness to norepinephrine). Products include:
Levophed Bitartrate Injection ... 2315

Opium Alkaloids (Aggravates orthostatic hypotension).
No products indexed under this heading.

Oxaprozin (May result in reduced diuretic effect). Products include:
Daypro Caplets ... 2426

Oxycodone Hydrochloride (Aggravates orthostatic hypotension). Products include:
Percocet Tablets ... 938
Percodan Tablets ... 939
Percodan-Demi Tablets ... 940
Roxicodone Tablets, Oral Solution & Intensol (Oxycodone) ... 2244
Tylox Capsules ... 1584

Penbutolol Sulfate (Potentiation of antihypertensive effects). Products include:
Levatol ... 2403

Pentobarbital Sodium (Aggravates orthostatic hypotension). Products include:
Nembutal Sodium Capsules ... 436
Nembutal Sodium Solution ... 438
Nembutal Sodium Suppositories ... 440

Phenelzine Sulfate (Concurrent use is contraindicated). Products include:
Nardil ... 1920

Phenobarbital (Aggravates orthostatic hypotension). Products include:
Arco-Lase Plus Tablets ... 512
Bellergal-S Tablets ... 2250
Donnatal ... 2060
Donnatal Extentabs ... 2061
Donnatal Tablets ... 2060
Phenobarbital Elixir and Tablets ... 1469
Quadrinal Tablets ... 1350

Phenoxybenzamine Hydrochloride (Potentiation of antihypertensive effect). Products include:
Dibenzyline Capsules ... 2476

Phentolamine Mesylate (Potentiation of antihypertensive effect). Products include:
Regitine ... 846

Phenylbutazone (May result in reduced diuretic effects).
No products indexed under this heading.

Pindolol (Potentiation of antihypertensive effect). Products include:
Visken Tablets ... 2299

Piroxicam (May result in reduced diuretic effects). Products include:
Feldene Capsules ... 1965

Polythiazide (Potentiation of antihypertensive effect). Products include:
Minizide Capsules ... 1938

Prazosin Hydrochloride (Potentiation of antihypertensive effect). Products include:
Minipress Capsules ... 1937
Minizide Capsules ... 1938

Prednisolone Acetate (Hypokalemia may result). Products include:
AK-CIDE ... ◉ 202
AK-CIDE Ointment ... ◉ 202
Blephamide Liquifilm Sterile Ophthalmic Suspension ... 476
Blephamide Ointment ... ◉ 237
Econopred & Econopred Plus Ophthalmic Suspensions ... ◉ 217
Poly-Pred Liquifilm ... ◉ 248
Pred Forte ... ◉ 250
Pred Mild ... ◉ 253
Pred-G Liquifilm Sterile Ophthalmic Suspension ... ◉ 251
Pred-G S.O.P. Sterile Ophthalmic Ointment ... ◉ 252
Vasocidin Ointment ... ◉ 268

Prednisolone Sodium Phosphate (Hypokalemia may result). Products include:
AK-Pred ... ◉ 204
Hydeltrasol Injection, Sterile ... 1665
Inflamase ... ◉ 265
Pediapred Oral Liquid ... 995
Vasocidin Ophthalmic Solution ... ◉ 270

Prednisolone Tebutate (Hypokalemia may result). Products include:
Hydeltra-T.B.A. Sterile Suspension 1667

Prednisone (Hypokalemia may result). Products include:
Deltasone Tablets ... 2595

Propofol (May require reduced dose of anesthetics). Products include:
Diprivan Injection ... 2833

Propoxyphene Hydrochloride (Aggravates orthostatic hypotension). Products include:
Darvon ... 1435
Wygesic Tablets ... 2827

Propoxyphene Napsylate (Aggravates orthostatic hypotension). Products include:
Darvon-N/Darvocet-N ... 1433

Propranolol Hydrochloride (Potentiation of antihypertensive effect). Products include:
Inderal ... 2728
Inderal LA Long Acting Capsules ... 2730
Inderide Tablets ... 2732
Inderide LA Long Acting Capsules .. 2734

Quinapril Hydrochloride (Potentiation of antihypertensive effect). Products include:
Accupril Tablets ... 1893

Ramipril (Potentiation of antihypertensive effect). Products include:
Altace Capsules ... 1232

Rauwolfia Serpentina (Potentiation of antihypertensive effect).
No products indexed under this heading.

Rescinnamine (Potentiation of antihypertensive effect).
No products indexed under this heading.

Reserpine (Potentiation of antihypertensive effect). Products include:
Diupres Tablets ... 1650
Hydropres Tablets ... 1675
Ser-Ap-Es Tablets ... 849

Secobarbital Sodium (Aggravates orthostatic hypotension). Products include:
Seconal Sodium Pulvules ... 1474

Selegiline Hydrochloride (Concurrent use is contraindicated). Products include:
Eldepryl Tablets ... 2550

Sodium Nitroprusside (Potentiation of antihypertensive effect).
No products indexed under this heading.

Sotalol Hydrochloride (Potentiation of antihypertensive effect). Products include:
Betapace Tablets ... 641

Spirapril Hydrochloride (Potentiation of antihypertensive effect).
No products indexed under this heading.

Sufentanil Citrate (Aggravates orthostatic hypotension). Products include:
Sufenta Injection ... 1309

Sulindac (May result in reduced diuretic effects). Products include:
Clinoril Tablets ... 1618

Terazosin Hydrochloride (Potentiation of antihypertensive effect). Products include:
Hytrin Capsules ... 430

Thiamylal Sodium (Aggravates orthostatic hypotension).
No products indexed under this heading.

Timolol Maleate (Potentiation of antihypertensive effect). Products include:
Blocadren Tablets ... 1614
Timolide Tablets ... 1748
Timoptic in Ocudose ... 1753
Timoptic Sterile Ophthalmic Solution ... 1751
Timoptic-XE ... 1755

Tolazamide (Dosage adjustment of the antidiabetic drug may be required).
No products indexed under this heading.

Tolbutamide (Dosage adjustment of the antidiabetic drug may be required).
No products indexed under this heading.

Tolmetin Sodium (May result in reduced diuretic effects). Products include:
Tolectin (200, 400 and 600 mg) .. 1581

Torsemide (Potentiation of antihypertensive effect). Products include:
Demadex Tablets and Injection ... 686

Tranylcypromine Sulfate (Concurrent use is contraindicated). Products include:
Parnate Tablets ... 2503

Triamcinolone (Hypokalemia may result). Products include:
Aristocort Tablets ... 1022

Triamcinolone Acetonide (Hypokalemia may result). Products include:
Aristocort A 0.025% Cream ... 1027
Aristocort A 0.5% Cream ... 1031
Aristocort A 0.1% Cream ... 1029
Aristocort A 0.1% Ointment ... 1030
Azmacort Oral Inhaler ... 2011
Nasacort Nasal Inhaler ... 2024

Triamcinolone Diacetate (Hypokalemia may result). Products include:
Aristocort Suspension (Forte Parenteral) ... 1027
Aristocort Suspension (Intralesional) ... 1025

Triamcinolone Hexacetonide (Hypokalemia may result). Products include:
Aristospan Suspension (Intra-articular) ... 1033
Aristospan Suspension (Intralesional) ... 1032

Trimethaphan Camsylate (Potentiation of antihypertensive effect). Products include:
Arfonad Ampuls ... 2080

Tubocurarine Chloride (Increased responsiveness to tubocurarine).
No products indexed under this heading.

Verapamil Hydrochloride (Potentiation of antihypertensive effect). Products include:
Calan SR Caplets ... 2422
Calan Tablets ... 2419
Isoptin Injectable ... 1344
Isoptin Oral Tablets ... 1346
Isoptin SR Tablets ... 1348
Verelan Capsules ... 1410
Verelan Capsules ... 2824

Food Interactions

Alcohol (Aggravates orthostatic hypotension).

ALDOMET ESTER HCL INJECTION

(Methyldopate Hydrochloride) ... 1602
May interact with general anesthetics, antihypertensives, lithium preparations, monoamine oxidase inhibitors, and certain other agents. Compounds in these categories include:

Acebutolol Hydrochloride (Potentiation of antihypertensive effect). Products include:
Sectral Capsules ... 2807

Amlodipine Besylate (Potentiation of antihypertensive effect). Products include:
Lotrel Capsules ... 840
Norvasc Tablets ... 1940

Atenolol (Potentiation of antihypertensive effect). Products include:
Tenoretic Tablets ... 2845
Tenormin Tablets and I.V. Injection 2847

Benazepril Hydrochloride (Potentiation of antihypertensive effect). Products include:
Lotensin Tablets ... 834
Lotensin HCT ... 837
Lotrel Capsules ... 840

Bendroflumethiazide (Potentiation of antihypertensive effect).
No products indexed under this heading.

Betaxolol Hydrochloride (Potentiation of antihypertensive effect). Products include:
Betoptic Ophthalmic Solution ... 469
Betoptic S Ophthalmic Suspension 471
Kerlone Tablets ... 2436

Bisoprolol Fumarate (Potentiation of antihypertensive effect). Products include:
Zebeta Tablets ... 1413
Ziac ... 1415

Captopril (Potentiation of antihypertensive effect). Products include:
Capoten ... 739
Capozide ... 742

Carteolol Hydrochloride (Potentiation of antihypertensive effect). Products include:
Cartrol Tablets ... 410

IMPORTANT NOTE: Always consult each drug listing in the patient's regimen for possible interactions.

Ocupress Ophthalmic Solution, 1% Sterile ◉ 309

Chlorothiazide (Potentiation of antihypertensive effect). Products include:

Aldoclor Tablets 1598
Diupres Tablets 1650
Diuril Oral 1653

Chlorothiazide Sodium (Potentiation of antihypertensive effect). Products include:

Diuril Sodium Intravenous 1652

Chlorthalidone (Potentiation of antihypertensive effect). Products include:

Combipres Tablets 677
Tenoretic Tablets 2845
Thalitone 1245

Clonidine (Potentiation of antihypertensive effect). Products include:

Catapres-TTS 675

Clonidine Hydrochloride (Potentiation of antihypertensive effect). Products include:

Catapres Tablets 674
Combipres Tablets 677

Deserpidine (Potentiation of antihypertensive effect).

No products indexed under this heading.

Diazoxide (Potentiation of antihypertensive effect). Products include:

Hyperstat I.V. Injection 2363
Proglycem 580

Diltiazem Hydrochloride (Potentiation of antihypertensive effect). Products include:

Cardizem CD Capsules 1506
Cardizem SR Capsules 1510
Cardizem Injectable 1508
Cardizem Tablets 1512
Dilacor XR Extended-release Capsules 2018

Doxazosin Mesylate (Potentiation of antihypertensive effect). Products include:

Cardura Tablets 2186

Enalapril Maleate (Potentiation of antihypertensive effect). Products include:

Vaseretic Tablets 1765
Vasotec Tablets 1771

Enalaprilat (Potentiation of antihypertensive effects). Products include:

Vasotec I.V. 1768

Enflurane (May require reduced dose of anesthetics).

No products indexed under this heading.

Esmolol Hydrochloride (Potentiation of antihypertensive effect). Products include:

Brevibloc Injection 1808

Felodipine (Potentiation of antihypertensive effect). Products include:

Plendil Extended-Release Tablets 527

Fosinopril Sodium (Potentiation of antihypertensive effect). Products include:

Monopril Tablets 757

Furazolidone (Concurrent use is contraindicated). Products include:

Furoxone 2046

Furosemide (Potentiation of antihypertensive effect). Products include:

Lasix Injection, Oral Solution and Tablets 1240

Guanabenz Acetate (Potentiation of antihypertensive effect).

No products indexed under this heading.

Guanethidine Monosulfate (Potentiation of antihypertensive effect). Products include:

Esimil Tablets 822
Ismelin Tablets 827

Hydralazine Hydrochloride (Potentiation of antihypertensive effect). Products include:

Apresazide Capsules 808
Apresoline Hydrochloride Tablets 809
Ser-Ap-Es Tablets 849

Hydrochlorothiazide (Potentiation of antihypertensive effect). Products include:

Aldactazide 2413
Aldoril Tablets 1604
Apresazide Capsules 808
Capozide 742
Dyazide 2479
Esidrix Tablets 821
Esimil Tablets 822
HydroDIURIL Tablets 1674
Hydropres Tablets 1675
Hyzaar Tablets 1677
Inderide Tablets 2732
Inderide LA Long Acting Capsules 2734
Lopressor HCT Tablets 832
Lotensin HCT 837
Maxzide 1380
Moduretic Tablets 1705
Oretic Tablets 443
Prinzide Tablets 1737
Ser-Ap-Es Tablets 849
Timolide Tablets 1748
Vaseretic Tablets 1765
Zestoretic 2850
Ziac 1415

Hydroflumethiazide (Potentiation of antihypertensive effect). Products include:

Diucardin Tablets 2718

Indapamide (Potentiation of antihypertensive effect). Products include:

Lozol Tablets 2022

Isocarboxazid (Concurrent use is contraindicated).

No products indexed under this heading.

Isoflurane (May require reduced dose of anesthetics).

No products indexed under this heading.

Isradipine (Potentiation of antihypertensive effect). Products include:

DynaCirc Capsules 2256

Ketamine Hydrochloride (May require reduced dose of anesthetics).

No products indexed under this heading.

Labetalol Hydrochloride (Potentiation of antihypertensive effect). Products include:

Normodyne Injection 2377
Normodyne Tablets 2379
Trandate 1185

Lisinopril (Potentiation of antihypertensive effects). Products include:

Prinivil Tablets 1733
Prinzide Tablets 1737
Zestoretic 2850
Zestril Tablets 2854

Lithium Carbonate (Potential for lithium toxicity). Products include:

Eskalith 2485
Lithium Carbonate Capsules & Tablets 2230
Lithonate/Lithotabs/Lithobid 2543

Lithium Citrate (Potential for lithium toxicity).

No products indexed under this heading.

Losartan Potassium (Potentiation of antihypertensive effect). Products include:

Cozaar Tablets 1628
Hyzaar Tablets 1677

Mecamylamine Hydrochloride (Potentiation of antihypertensive effect). Products include:

Inversine Tablets 1686

Methohexital Sodium (May require reduced dose of anesthetics). Products include:

Brevital Sodium Vials 1429

Methoxyflurane (May require reduced dose of anesthetics).

No products indexed under this heading.

Methyclothiazide (Potentiation of antihypertensive effect). Products include:

Enduron Tablets 420

Methyldopa (Potentiation of antihypertensive effect). Products include:

Aldoclor Tablets 1598
Aldomet Oral 1600
Aldoril Tablets 1604

Metolazone (Potentiation of antihypertensive effect). Products include:

Mykrox Tablets 993
Zaroxolyn Tablets 1000

Metoprolol Succinate (Potentiation of antihypertensive effect). Products include:

Toprol-XL Tablets 565

Metoprolol Tartrate (Potentiation of antihypertensive effect). Products include:

Lopressor Ampuls 830
Lopressor HCT Tablets 832
Lopressor Tablets 830

Metyrosine (Potentiation of antihypertensive effect). Products include:

Demser Capsules 1649

Minoxidil (Potentiation of antihypertensive effect). Products include:

Loniten Tablets 2618
Rogaine Topical Solution 2637

Moexipril Hydrochloride (Potentiation of antihypertensive effect). Products include:

Univasc Tablets 2410

Nadolol (Potentiation of antihypertensive effect).

No products indexed under this heading.

Nicardipine Hydrochloride (Potentiation of antihypertensive effect). Products include:

Cardene Capsules 2095
Cardene I.V. 2709
Cardene SR Capsules 2097

Nifedipine (Potentiation of antihypertensive effect). Products include:

Adalat Capsules (10 mg and 20 mg) 587
Adalat CC 589
Procardia Capsules 1971
Procardia XL Extended Release Tablets 1972

Nisoldipine (Potentiation of antihypertensive effect).

No products indexed under this heading.

Nitroglycerin (Potentiation of antihypertensive effect). Products include:

Deponit NTG Transdermal Delivery System 2397
Nitro-Bid IV 1523
Nitro-Bid Ointment 1524
Nitrodisc 2047
Nitro-Dur (nitroglycerin) Transdermal Infusion System 1326
Nitrolingual Spray 2027
Nitrostat Tablets 1925
Transderm-Nitro Transdermal Therapeutic System 859

Penbutolol Sulfate (Potentiation of antihypertensive effect). Products include:

Levatol 2403

Phenelzine Sulfate (Concurrent use is contraindicated). Products include:

Nardil 1920

Phenoxybenzamine Hydrochloride (Potentiation of antihypertensive effect). Products include:

Dibenzyline Capsules 2476

Phentolamine Mesylate (Potentiation of antihypertensive effect). Products include:

Regitine 846

Pindolol (Potentiation of antihypertensive effect). Products include:

Visken Tablets 2299

Polythiazide (Potentiation of antihypertensive effect). Products include:

Minizide Capsules 1938

Prazosin Hydrochloride (Potentiation of antihypertensive effect). Products include:

Minipress Capsules 1937
Minizide Capsules 1938

Propofol (May require reduced dose of anesthetics). Products include:

Diprivan Injection 2833

Propranolol Hydrochloride (Potentiation of antihypertensive effect). Products include:

Inderal 2728
Inderal LA Long Acting Capsules 2730
Inderide Tablets 2732
Inderide LA Long Acting Capsules 2734

Quinapril Hydrochloride (Potentiation of antihypertensive effect). Products include:

Accupril Tablets 1893

Ramipril (Potentiation of antihypertensive effect). Products include:

Altace Capsules 1232

Rauwolfia Serpentina (Potentiation of antihypertensive effect).

No products indexed under this heading.

Rescinnamine (Potentiation of antihypertensive effect).

No products indexed under this heading.

Reserpine (Potentiation of antihypertensive effect). Products include:

Diupres Tablets 1650
Hydropres Tablets 1675
Ser-Ap-Es Tablets 849

Selegiline Hydrochloride (Concurrent use is contraindicated). Products include:

Eldepryl Tablets 2550

Sodium Nitroprusside (Potentiation of antihypertensive effect).

No products indexed under this heading.

Sotalol Hydrochloride (Potentiation of antihypertensive effect). Products include:

Betapace Tablets 641

Spirapril Hydrochloride (Potentiation of antihypertensive effect).

No products indexed under this heading.

Terazosin Hydrochloride (Potentiation of antihypertensive effect). Products include:

Hytrin Capsules 430

Timolol Maleate (Potentiation of antihypertensive effect). Products include:

Blocadren Tablets 1614
Timolide Tablets 1748
Timoptic in Ocudose 1753
Timoptic Sterile Ophthalmic Solution 1751
Timoptic-XE 1755

Torsemide (Potentiation of antihypertensive effect). Products include:

Demadex Tablets and Injection 686

Tranylcypromine Sulfate (Concurrent use is contraindicated). Products include:

Parnate Tablets 2503

Trimethaphan Camsylate (Potentiation of antihypertensive effect). Products include:

Arfonad Ampuls 2080

(▣ Described in PDR For Nonprescription Drugs)
(◉ Described in PDR For Ophthalmology)

29 Interactions Index Aldomet Oral

Verapamil Hydrochloride (Potentiation of antihypertensive effect). Products include:
Calan SR Caplets 2422
Calan Tablets 2419
Isoptin Injectable 1344
Isoptin Oral Tablets 1346
Isoptin SR Tablets 1348
Verelan Capsules 1410
Verelan Capsules 2824

ALDOMET ORAL SUSPENSION
(Methyldopa) 1600
May interact with antihypertensives, general anesthetics, lithium preparations, monoamine oxidase inhibitors, and certain other agents. Compounds in these categories include:

Acebutolol Hydrochloride (Potentiation of antihypertensive effect). Products include:
Sectral Capsules 2807
Amlodipine Besylate (Potentiation of antihypertensive effect). Products include:
Lotrel Capsules 840
Norvasc Tablets 1940
Atenolol (Potentiation of antihypertensive effect). Products include:
Tenoretic Tablets 2845
Tenormin Tablets and I.V. Injection 2847
Benazepril Hydrochloride (Potentiation of antihypertensive effect). Products include:
Lotensin Tablets 834
Lotensin HCT 837
Lotrel Capsules 840
Bendroflumethiazide (Potentiation of antihypertensive effect).
No products indexed under this heading.
Betaxolol Hydrochloride (Potentiation of antihypertensive effect). Products include:
Betoptic Ophthalmic Solution 469
Betoptic S Ophthalmic Suspension 471
Kerlone Tablets 2436
Bisoprolol Fumarate (Potentiation of antihypertensive effect). Products include:
Zebeta Tablets 1413
Ziac 1415
Captopril (Potentiation of antihypertensive effect). Products include:
Capoten 739
Capozide 742
Carteolol Hydrochloride (Potentiation of antihypertensive effect). Products include:
Cartrol Tablets 410
Ocupress Ophthalmic Solution, 1% Sterile ◉ 309
Chlorothiazide (Potentiation of antihypertensive effect). Products include:
Aldoclor Tablets 1598
Diupres Tablets 1650
Diuril Oral 1653
Chlorothiazide Sodium (Potentiation of antihypertensive effect). Products include:
Diuril Sodium Intravenous 1652
Chlorthalidone (Potentiation of antihypertensive effect). Products include:
Combipres Tablets 677
Tenoretic Tablets 2845
Thalitone 1245
Clonidine (Potentiation of antihypertensive effect). Products include:
Catapres-TTS 675
Clonidine Hydrochloride (Potentiation of antihypertensive effect). Products include:
Catapres Tablets 674
Combipres Tablets 677
Deserpidine (Potentiation of antihypertensive effect).
No products indexed under this heading.
Diazoxide (Potentiation of antihypertensive effect). Products include:
Hyperstat I.V. Injection 2363
Proglycem 580
Diltiazem Hydrochloride (Potentiation of antihypertensive effect). Products include:
Cardizem CD Capsules 1506
Cardizem SR Capsules 1510
Cardizem Injectable 1508
Cardizem Tablets 1512
Dilacor XR Extended-release Capsules 2018
Doxazosin Mesylate (Potentiation of antihypertensive effect). Products include:
Cardura Tablets 2186
Enalapril Maleate (Potentiation of antihypertensive effect). Products include:
Vaseretic Tablets 1765
Vasotec Tablets 1771
Enalaprilat (Potentiation of antihypertensive effect). Products include:
Vasotec I.V. 1768
Enflurane (May require reduced dose of anesthetics).
No products indexed under this heading.
Esmolol Hydrochloride (Potentiation of antihypertensive effect). Products include:
Brevibloc Injection 1808
Felodipine (Potentiation of antihypertensive effect). Products include:
Plendil Extended-Release Tablets 527
Fosinopril Sodium (Potentiation of antihypertensive effect). Products include:
Monopril Tablets 757
Furazolidone (Concurrent use is contraindicated). Products include:
Furoxone 2046
Furosemide (Potentiation of antihypertensive effect). Products include:
Lasix Injection, Oral Solution and Tablets 1240
Guanabenz Acetate (Potentiation of antihypertensive effect).
No products indexed under this heading.
Guanethidine Monosulfate (Potentiation of antihypertensive effect). Products include:
Esimil Tablets 822
Ismelin Tablets 827
Hydralazine Hydrochloride (Potentiation of antihypertensive effect). Products include:
Apresazide Capsules 808
Apresoline Hydrochloride Tablets 809
Ser-Ap-Es Tablets 849
Hydrochlorothiazide (Potentiation of antihypertensive effect). Products include:
Aldactazide 2413
Aldoril Tablets 1604
Apresazide Capsules 808
Capozide 742
Dyazide 2479
Esidrix Tablets 821
Esimil Tablets 822
HydroDIURIL Tablets 1674
Hydropres Tablets 1675
Hyzaar Tablets 1677
Inderide Tablets 2732
Inderide LA Long Acting Capsules 2734
Lopressor HCT Tablets 832
Lotensin HCT 837
Maxzide 1380
Moduretic Tablets 1705
Oretic Tablets 443
Prinzide Tablets 1737
Ser-Ap-Es Tablets 849
Timolide Tablets 1748
Vaseretic Tablets 1765
Zestoretic 2850
Ziac 1415
Hydroflumethiazide (Potentiation of antihypertensive effect). Products include:
Diucardin Tablets 2718
Indapamide (Potentiation of antihypertensive effect). Products include:
Lozol Tablets 2022
Isocarboxazid (Concurrent use is contraindicated).
No products indexed under this heading.
Isoflurane (May require reduced dose of anesthetics).
No products indexed under this heading.
Isradipine (Potentiation of antihypertensive effect). Products include:
DynaCirc Capsules 2256
Ketamine Hydrochloride (May require reduced dose of anesthetics).
No products indexed under this heading.
Labetalol Hydrochloride (Potentiation of antihypertensive effect). Products include:
Normodyne Injection 2377
Normodyne Tablets 2379
Trandate 1185
Lisinopril (Potentiation of antihypertensive effect). Products include:
Prinivil Tablets 1733
Prinzide Tablets 1737
Zestoretic 2850
Zestril Tablets 2854
Lithium Carbonate (Potential for lithium toxicity). Products include:
Eskalith 2485
Lithium Carbonate Capsules & Tablets 2230
Lithonate/Lithotabs/Lithobid 2543
Lithium Citrate (Potential for lithium toxicity).
No products indexed under this heading.
Losartan Potassium (Potentiation of antihypertensive effect). Products include:
Cozaar Tablets 1628
Hyzaar Tablets 1677
Mecamylamine Hydrochloride (Potentiation of antihypertensive effect). Products include:
Inversine Tablets 1686
Methohexital Sodium (May require reduced dose of anesthetics). Products include:
Brevital Sodium Vials 1429
Methoxyflurane (May require reduced dose of anesthetics).
No products indexed under this heading.
Methyclothiazide (Potentiation of antihypertensive effect). Products include:
Enduron Tablets 420
Methyldopate Hydrochloride (Potentiation of antihypertensive effect). Products include:
Aldomet Ester HCl Injection 1602
Metolazone (Potentiation of antihypertensive effect). Products include:
Mykrox Tablets 993
Zaroxolyn Tablets 1000
Metoprolol Succinate (Potentiation of antihypertensive effect). Products include:
Toprol-XL Tablets 565
Metoprolol Tartrate (Potentiation of antihypertensive effect). Products include:
Lopressor Ampuls 830
Lopressor HCT Tablets 832
Lopressor Tablets 830
Metyrosine (Potentiation of antihypertensive effect). Products include:
Demser Capsules 1649
Minoxidil (Potentiation of antihypertensive effect). Products include:
Loniten Tablets 2618
Rogaine Topical Solution 2637
Moexipril Hydrochloride (Potentiation of antihypertensive effect). Products include:
Univasc Tablets 2410
Nadolol (Potentiation of antihypertensive effect).
No products indexed under this heading.
Nicardipine Hydrochloride (Potentiation of antihypertensive effect). Products include:
Cardene Capsules 2095
Cardene I.V. 2709
Cardene SR Capsules 2097
Nifedipine (Potentiation of antihypertensive effect). Products include:
Adalat Capsules (10 mg and 20 mg) 587
Adalat CC 589
Procardia Capsules 1971
Procardia XL Extended Release Tablets 1972
Nisoldipine (Potentiation of antihypertensive effect).
No products indexed under this heading.
Nitroglycerin (Potentiation of antihypertensive effect). Products include:
Deponit NTG Transdermal Delivery System 2397
Nitro-Bid IV 1523
Nitro-Bid Ointment 1524
Nitrodisc 2047
Nitro-Dur (nitroglycerin) Transdermal Infusion System 1326
Nitrolingual Spray 2027
Nitrostat Tablets 1925
Transderm-Nitro Transdermal Therapeutic System 859
Penbutolol Sulfate (Potentiation of antihypertensive effect). Products include:
Levatol 2403
Phenelzine Sulfate (Concurrent use is contraindicated). Products include:
Nardil 1920
Phenoxybenzamine Hydrochloride (Potentiation of antihypertensive effect). Products include:
Dibenzyline Capsules 2476
Phentolamine Mesylate (Potentiation of antihypertensive effect). Products include:
Regitine 846
Pindolol (Potentiation of antihypertensive effect). Products include:
Visken Tablets 2299
Polythiazide (Potentiation of antihypertensive effect). Products include:
Minizide Capsules 1938
Prazosin Hydrochloride (Potentiation of antihypertensive effect). Products include:
Minipress Capsules 1937
Minizide Capsules 1938
Propofol (May require reduced dose of anesthetics). Products include:
Diprivan Injection 2833
Propranolol Hydrochloride (Potentiation of antihypertensive effect). Products include:
Inderal 2728
Inderal LA Long Acting Capsules 2730
Inderide Tablets 2732
Inderide LA Long Acting Capsules 2734
Quinapril Hydrochloride (Potentiation of antihypertensive effect). Products include:
Accupril Tablets 1893

IMPORTANT NOTE: Always consult each drug listing in the patient's regimen for possible interactions.

Ramipril (Potentiation of antihypertensive effect). Products include:
Altace Capsules 1232

Rauwolfia Serpentina (Potentiation of antihypertensive effect).
No products indexed under this heading.

Rescinnamine (Potentiation of antihypertensive effect).
No products indexed under this heading.

Reserpine (Potentiation of antihypertensive effect). Products include:
Diupres Tablets 1650
Hydropres Tablets 1675
Ser-Ap-Es Tablets 849

Selegiline Hydrochloride (Concurrent use is contraindicated). Products include:
Eldepryl Tablets 2550

Sodium Nitroprusside (Potentiation of antihypertensive effect).
No products indexed under this heading.

Sotalol Hydrochloride (Potentiation of antihypertensive effect). Products include:
Betapace Tablets 641

Spirapril Hydrochloride (Potentiation of antihypertensive effect).
No products indexed under this heading.

Terazosin Hydrochloride (Potentiation of antihypertensive effect). Products include:
Hytrin Capsules 430

Timolol Maleate (Potentiation of antihypertensive effect). Products include:
Blocadren Tablets 1614
Timolide Tablets 1748
Timoptic in Ocudose 1753
Timoptic Sterile Ophthalmic Solution 1751
Timoptic-XE 1755

Torsemide (Potentiation of antihypertensive effect). Products include:
Demadex Tablets and Injection 686

Tranylcypromine Sulfate (Concurrent use is contraindicated). Products include:
Parnate Tablets 2503

Trimethaphan Camsylate (Potentiation of antihypertensive effect). Products include:
Arfonad Ampuls 2080

Verapamil Hydrochloride (Potentiation of antihypertensive effect). Products include:
Calan SR Caplets 2422
Calan Tablets 2419
Isoptin Injectable 1344
Isoptin Oral Tablets 1346
Isoptin SR Tablets 1348
Verelan Capsules 1410
Verelan Capsules 2824

ALDOMET TABLETS
(Methyldopa) 1600
See **Aldomet Oral Suspension**

ALDORIL TABLETS
(Methyldopa, Hydrochlorothiazide) 1604
May interact with corticosteroids, antihypertensives, general anesthetics, insulin, non-steroidal anti-inflammatory agents, barbiturates, narcotic analgesics, monoamine oxidase inhibitors, oral hypoglycemic agents, lithium preparations, cardiac glycosides, and certain other agents. Compounds in these categories include:

Acarbose (Dosage adjustment of the antidiabetic drug may be required).
No products indexed under this heading.

Acebutolol Hydrochloride (Potentiation of antihypertensive effect). Products include:
Sectral Capsules 2807

ACTH (Hypokalemia may result).
No products indexed under this heading.

Alfentanil Hydrochloride (Aggravates orthostatic hypotension). Products include:
Alfenta Injection 1286

Amlodipine Besylate (Potentiation of antihypertensive effect). Products include:
Lotrel Capsules 840
Norvasc Tablets 1940

Aprobarbital (Aggravates orthostatic hypotension).
No products indexed under this heading.

Atenolol (Potentiation of antihypertensive effect). Products include:
Tenoretic Tablets 2845
Tenormin Tablets and I.V. Injection 2847

Benazepril Hydrochloride (Potentiation of antihypertensive effect). Products include:
Lotensin Tablets 834
Lotensin HCT 837
Lotrel Capsules 840

Bendroflumethiazide (Potentiation of antihypertensive effect).
No products indexed under this heading.

Betamethasone Acetate (Hypokalemia may result). Products include:
Celestone Soluspan Suspension 2347

Betamethasone Sodium Phosphate (Hypokalemia may result). Products include:
Celestone Soluspan Suspension 2347

Betaxolol Hydrochloride (Potentiation of antihypertensive effect). Products include:
Betoptic Ophthalmic Solution 469
Betoptic S Ophthalmic Suspension 471
Kerlone Tablets 2436

Bisoprolol Fumarate (Potentiation of antihypertensive effect). Products include:
Zebeta Tablets 1413
Ziac 1415

Buprenorphine (Aggravates orthostatic hypotension). Products include:
Buprenex Injectable 2006

Butabarbital (Aggravates orthostatic hypotension).
No products indexed under this heading.

Butalbital (Aggravates orthostatic hypotension). Products include:
Esgic-plus Tablets 1013
Fioricet Tablets 2258
Fioricet with Codeine Capsules 2260
Fiorinal Capsules 2261
Fiorinal with Codeine Capsules 2262
Fiorinal Tablets 2261
Phrenilin 785
Sedapap Tablets 50 mg/650 mg .. 1543

Captopril (Potentiation of antihypertensive effect). Products include:
Capoten 739
Capozide 742

Carteolol Hydrochloride (Potentiation of antihypertensive effect). Products include:
Cartrol Tablets 410
Ocupress Ophthalmic Solution, 1% Sterile .... ◉ 309

Chlorothiazide (Potentiation of antihypertensive effect). Products include:
Aldoclor Tablets 1598
Diupres Tablets 1650
Diuril Oral 1653

Chlorothiazide Sodium (Potentiation of antihypertensive effect). Products include:
Diuril Sodium Intravenous 1652

Chlorpropamide (Dosage adjustment of the antidiabetic drug may be required). Products include:
Diabinese Tablets 1935

Chlorthalidone (Potentiation of antihypertensive effect). Products include:
Combipres Tablets 677
Tenoretic Tablets 2845
Thalitone 1245

Cholestyramine (Binds the hydrochlorothiazide and reduces its absorption from gastrointestinal tract by up to 85%). Products include:
Questran Light 769
Questran Powder 770

Clonidine (Potentiation of antihypertensive effect). Products include:
Catapres-TTS 675

Clonidine Hydrochloride (Potentiation of antihypertenisve effect). Products include:
Catapres Tablets 674
Combipres Tablets 677

Codeine Phosphate (Aggravates orthostatic hypotension). Products include:
Actifed with Codeine Cough Syrup.. 1067
Brontex 1981
Deconsal C Expectorant Syrup 456
Deconsal Pediatric Syrup 457
Dimetane-DC Cough Syrup 2059
Empirin with Codeine Tablets 1093
Fioricet with Codeine Capsules 2260
Fiorinal with Codeine Capsules 2262
Isoclor Expectorant 990
Novahistine DH 2462
Novahistine Expectorant 2463
Nucofed 2051
Phenergan with Codeine 2777
Phenergan VC with Codeine 2781
Robitussin A-C Syrup 2073
Robitussin-DAC Syrup 2074
Ryna .... ▣ 841
Soma Compound w/Codeine Tablets 2676
Tussi-Organidin NR Liquid and S NR Liquid 2677
Tylenol with Codeine 1583

Colestipol Hydrochloride (Binds the hydrochlorothiazide and reduces its absorption from gastrointestinal tract by up to 43%). Products include:
Colestid Tablets 2591

Cortisone Acetate (Hypokalemia may result). Products include:
Cortone Acetate Sterile Suspension 1623
Cortone Acetate Tablets 1624

Deserpidine (Potentiation of antihypertensive effect).
No products indexed under this heading.

Deslanoside (Hypokalemia may exaggerate cardiac toxicity of digitalis).
No products indexed under this heading.

Dexamethasone (Hypokalemia may result). Products include:
AK-Trol Ointment & Suspension .... ◉ 205
Decadron Elixir 1633
Decadron Tablets 1635
Decaspray Topical Aerosol 1648
Dexacidin Ointment .... ◉ 263
Maxitrol Ophthalmic Ointment and Suspension .... ◉ 224
TobraDex Ophthalmic Suspension and Ointment 473

Dexamethasone Acetate (Hypokalemia may result). Products include:
Dalalone D.P. Injectable 1011
Decadron-LA Sterile Suspension 1646

Dexamethasone Sodium Phosphate (Hypokalemia may result). Products include:
Decadron Phosphate Injection 1637
Decadron Phosphate Respihaler 1642
Decadron Phosphate Sterile Ophthalmic Ointment 1641
Decadron Phosphate Sterile Ophthalmic Solution 1642
Decadron Phosphate Topical Cream 1644
Decadron Phosphate Turbinaire 1645
Decadron Phosphate with Xylocaine Injection, Sterile 1639
Dexacort Phosphate in Respihaler .. 458
Dexacort Phosphate in Turbinaire .. 459
NeoDecadron Sterile Ophthalmic Ointment 1712
NeoDecadron Sterile Ophthalmic Solution 1713
NeoDecadron Topical Cream 1714

Dezocine (Aggravates orthostatic hypotension). Products include:
Dalgan Injection 538

Diazoxide (Potentiation of antihypertensive effect). Products include:
Hyperstat I.V. Injection 2363
Proglycem 580

Diclofenac Potassium (May result in reduced diuretic effect). Products include:
Cataflam 816

Diclofenac Sodium (May result in reduced diuretic effect). Products include:
Voltaren Ophthalmic Sterile Ophthalmic Solution .... ◉ 272
Voltaren Tablets 861

Digitoxin (Hypokalemia may exaggerate cardiac toxicity of digitalis). Products include:
Crystodigin Tablets 1433

Digoxin (Hypokalemia may exaggerate cardiac toxicity of digitalis). Products include:
Lanoxicaps 1117
Lanoxin Elixir Pediatric 1120
Lanoxin Injection 1123
Lanoxin Injection Pediatric 1126
Lanoxin Tablets 1128

Diltiazem Hydrochloride (Potentiation of antihypertensive effect). Products include:
Cardizem CD Capsules 1506
Cardizem SR Capsules 1510
Cardizem Injectable 1508
Cardizem Tablets 1512
Dilacor XR Extended-release Capsules 2018

Doxazosin Mesylate (Potentiation of antihypertensive effect). Products include:
Cardura Tablets 2186

Enalapril Maleate (Potentiation of antihypertensive effect). Products include:
Vaseretic Tablets 1765
Vasotec Tablets 1771

Enalaprilat (Potentiation of antihypertensive effect). Products include:
Vasotec I.V. 1768

Enflurane (May require reduced dose of anesthetics).
No products indexed under this heading.

Esmolol Hydrochloride (Potentiation of antihypertenisve effect). Products include:
Brevibloc Injection 1808

Etodolac (May result in reduced diuretic effect). Products include:
Lodine Capsules and Tablets 2743

Felodipine (Potentiation of antihypertensive effect). Products include:
Plendil Extended-Release Tablets 527

Fenoprofen Calcium (May result in reduced diuretic effects). Products include:
Nalfon 200 Pulvules & Nalfon Tablets 917

(▣ Described in PDR For Nonprescription Drugs) (◉ Described in PDR For Ophthalmology)

Fentanyl (Aggravates orthostatic hypotension). Products include:
- Duragesic Transdermal System ... 1288

Fentanyl Citrate (Aggravates orthostatic hypotension). Products include:
- Sublimaze Injection ... 1307

Fludrocortisone Acetate (Hypokalemia may result). Products include:
- Florinef Acetate Tablets ... 505

Flurbiprofen (May result in reduced diuretic effect). Products include:
- Ansaid Tablets ... 2579

Fosinopril Sodium (Potentiation of antihypertensive effect). Products include:
- Monopril Tablets ... 757

Furazolidone (Concurrent use is contraindicated). Products include:
- Furoxone ... 2046

Furosemide (Potentiation of antihypertensive effect). Products include:
- Lasix Injection, Oral Solution and Tablets ... 1240

Glipizide (Dosage adjustment of the antidiabetic drug may be required). Products include:
- Glucotrol Tablets ... 1967
- Glucotrol XL Extended Release Tablets ... 1968

Glyburide (Dosage adjustment of the antidiabetic drug may be required). Products include:
- DiaBeta Tablets ... 1239
- Glynase PresTab Tablets ... 2609
- Micronase Tablets ... 2623

Guanabenz Acetate (Potentiation of antihypertensive effect).
- No products indexed under this heading.

Guanethidine Monosulfate (Potentiation of antihypertensive effect). Products include:
- Esimil Tablets ... 822
- Ismelin Tablets ... 827

Hydralazine Hydrochloride (Potentiation of antihypertensive effect). Products include:
- Apresazide Capsules ... 808
- Apresoline Hydrochloride Tablets .. 809
- Ser-Ap-Es Tablets ... 849

Hydrocodone Bitartrate (Aggravates orthostatic hypotension). Products include:
- Anexsia 5/500 Elixir ... 1781
- Anexia Tablets ... 1782
- Codiclear DH Syrup ... 791
- Deconamine CX Cough and Cold Liquid and Tablets ... 1319
- Duratuss HD Elixir ... 2565
- Hycodan Tablets and Syrup ... 930
- Hycomine Compound Tablets ... 932
- Hycomine ... 931
- Hycotuss Expectorant Syrup ... 933
- Hydrocet Capsules ... 782
- Lorcet 10/650 ... 1018
- Lortab ... 2566
- Tussend ... 1783
- Tussend Expectorant ... 1785
- Vicodin Tablets ... 1356
- Vicodin ES Tablets ... 1357
- Vicodin Tuss Expectorant ... 1358
- Zydone Capsules ... 949

Hydrocodone Polistirex (Aggravates orthostatic hypotension). Products include:
- Tussionex Pennkinetic Extended-Release Suspension ... 998

Hydrocortisone (Hypokalemia may result). Products include:
- Anusol-HC Cream 2.5% ... 1896
- Aquanil HC Lotion ... 1931
- Bactine Hydrocortisone Anti-Itch Cream ... 709
- Caldecort Anti-Itch Hydrocortisone Spray ... 631
- Cortaid ... 836
- CORTENEMA ... 2535
- Cortisporin Ointment ... 1085
- Cortisporin Ophthalmic Ointment Sterile ... 1085
- Cortisporin Ophthalmic Suspension Sterile ... 1086
- Cortisporin Otic Solution Sterile ... 1087
- Cortisporin Otic Suspension Sterile 1088
- Cortizone-5 ... 831
- Cortizone-10 ... 831
- Hydrocortone Tablets ... 1672
- Hytone ... 907
- Massengill Medicated Soft Cloth Towelettes ... 2458
- PediOtic Suspension Sterile ... 1153
- Preparation H Hydrocortisone 1% Cream ... 872
- ProctoCream-HC 2.5% ... 2408
- VōSoL HC Otic Solution ... 2678

Hydrocortisone Acetate (Hypokalemia may result). Products include:
- Analpram-HC Rectal Cream 1% and 2.5% ... 977
- Anusol HC-1 Anti-Itch Hydrocortisone Ointment ... 847
- Anusol-HC Suppositories ... 1897
- Caldecort ... 631
- Carmol HC ... 924
- Coly-Mycin S Otic w/Neomycin & Hydrocortisone ... 1906
- Cortaid ... 836
- Cortifoam ... 2396
- Cortisporin Cream ... 1084
- Epifoam ... 2399
- Hydrocortone Acetate Sterile Suspension ... 1669
- Mantadil Cream ... 1135
- Nupercainal Hydrocortisone 1% Cream ... 645
- Ophthocort ... ⊙ 311
- Pramosone Cream, Lotion & Ointment ... 978
- ProctoCream-HC ... 2408
- ProctoFoam-HC ... 2409
- Terra-Cortril Ophthalmic Suspension ... 2210

Hydrocortisone Sodium Phosphate (Hypokalemia may result). Products include:
- Hydrocortone Phosphate Injection, Sterile ... 1670

Hydrocortisone Sodium Succinate (Hypokalemia may result). Products include:
- Solu-Cortef Sterile Powder ... 2641

Hydroflumethiazide (Potentiation of antihypertensive effect). Products include:
- Diucardin Tablets ... 2718

Ibuprofen (May result in reduced diuretic effects). Products include:
- Advil Cold and Sinus Caplets and Tablets (formerly CoAdvil) ... 870
- Advil Ibuprofen Tablets and Caplets ... 870
- Children's Advil Suspension ... 2692
- Arthritis Foundation Ibuprofen Tablets ... 674
- Bayer Select Ibuprofen Pain Relief Formula ... 715
- Cramp End Tablets ... 735
- Dimetapp Sinus Caplets ... 775
- Haltran Tablets ... 771
- IBU Tablets ... 1342
- Ibuprohm ... 735
- Children's Motrin Ibuprofen Oral Suspension ... 1546
- Motrin Tablets ... 2625
- Motrin IB Caplets, Tablets, and Geltabs ... 838
- Motrin IB Sinus ... 838
- Motrin Ibuprofen Suspension, Oral Drops, Chewable Tablets, Caplets ... 1546
- Nuprin Ibuprofen/Analgesic Tablets & Caplets ... 622
- Sine-Aid IB Caplets ... 1554
- Vicks DayQuil SINUS Pressure & PAIN Relief with IBUPROFEN ... 762

Indapamide (Potentiation of antihypertensive effect). Products include:
- Lozol Tablets ... 2022

Indomethacin (May result in reduced diuretic effects). Products include:
- Indocin ... 1680

Indomethacin Sodium Trihydrate (May result in reduced diuretic effects). Products include:
- Indocin I.V. ... 1684

Insulin, Human (Insulin requirement may be altered).
- No products indexed under this heading.

Insulin, Human Isophane Suspension (Insulin requirement may be altered). Products include:
- Novolin N Human Insulin 10 ml Vials ... 1795

Insulin, Human NPH (Insulin requirement may be altered). Products include:
- Humulin N, 100 Units ... 1448
- Novolin N PenFill Cartridges Durable Insulin Delivery System ... 1798
- Novolin N Prefilled Syringe Disposable Insulin Delivery System ... 1798

Insulin, Human Regular (Insulin requirement may be altered). Products include:
- Humulin R, 100 Units ... 1449
- Novolin R Human Insulin 10 ml Vials ... 1795
- Novolin R PenFill Cartridges Durable Insulin Delivery System ... 1798
- Novolin R Prefilled Syringe Disposable Insulin Delivery System ... 1798
- Velosulin BR Human Insulin 10 ml Vials ... 1795

Insulin, Human, Zinc Suspension (Insulin requirement may be altered). Products include:
- Humulin L, 100 Units ... 1446
- Humulin U, 100 Units ... 1450
- Novolin L Human Insulin 10 ml Vials ... 1795

Insulin, NPH (Insulin requirement may be altered). Products include:
- NPH, 100 Units ... 1450
- Pork NPH, 100 Units ... 1452
- Purified Pork NPH Isophane Insulin ... 1801

Insulin, Regular (Insulin requirement may be altered). Products include:
- Regular, 100 Units ... 1450
- Pork Regular, 100 Units ... 1452
- Pork Regular (Concentrated), 500 Units ... 1453
- Purified Pork Regular Insulin ... 1801

Insulin, Zinc Crystals (Insulin requirement may be altered). Products include:
- NPH, 100 Units ... 1450

Insulin, Zinc Suspension (Insulin requirement may be altered). Products include:
- Iletin I ... 1450
- Lente, 100 Units ... 1450
- Iletin II ... 1452
- Pork Lente, 100 Units ... 1452
- Purified Pork Lente Insulin ... 1801

Isocarboxazid (Concurrent use is contraindicated).
- No products indexed under this heading.

Isoflurane (May require reduced dose of anesthetics).
- No products indexed under this heading.

Isradipine (Potentiation of antihypertensive effect). Products include:
- DynaCirc Capsules ... 2256

Ketamine Hydrochloride (May require reduced dose of anesthetics).
- No products indexed under this heading.

Ketoprofen (May result in reduced diuretic effects). Products include:
- Orudis Capsules ... 2766
- Oruvail Capsules ... 2766

Ketorolac Tromethamine (May result in reduced diuretic effect). Products include:
- Acular ... 474
- Acular ... ⊙ 277
- Toradol ... 2159

Labetalol Hydrochloride (Potentiation of antihypertensive effect). Products include:
- Normodyne Injection ... 2377
- Normodyne Tablets ... 2379
- Trandate ... 1185

Levorphanol Tartrate (Aggravates orthostatic hypotension). Products include:
- Levo-Dromoran ... 2129

Lisinopril (Potentiation of antihypertensive effect). Products include:
- Prinivil Tablets ... 1733
- Prinzide Tablets ... 1737
- Zestoretic ... 2850
- Zestril Tablets ... 2854

Lithium Carbonate (High risk of lithium toxicity). Products include:
- Eskalith ... 2485
- Lithium Carbonate Capsules & Tablets ... 2230
- Lithonate/Lithotabs/Lithobid ... 2543

Lithium Citrate (High risk of lithium toxicity).
- No products indexed under this heading.

Losartan Potassium (Potentiation of antihypertensive effect). Products include:
- Cozaar Tablets ... 1628
- Hyzaar Tablets ... 1677

Mecamylamine Hydrochloride (Potentiation of antihypertensive effect). Products include:
- Inversine Tablets ... 1686

Meclofenamate Sodium (May result in reduced diuretic effects).
- No products indexed under this heading.

Mefenamic Acid (May result in reduced diuretic effects). Products include:
- Ponstel ... 1925

Meperidine Hydrochloride (Aggravates orthostatic hypotension). Products include:
- Demerol ... 2308
- Mepergan Injection ... 2753

Mephobarbital (Aggravates orthostatic hypotension). Products include:
- Mebaral Tablets ... 2322

Metformin Hydrochloride (Dosage adjustment of the antidiabetic drug may be required). Products include:
- Glucophage ... 752

Methadone Hydrochloride (Aggravates orthostatic hypotension). Products include:
- Methadone Hydrochloride Oral Concentrate ... 2233
- Methadone Hydrochloride Oral Solution & Tablets ... 2235

Methohexital Sodium (May require reduced dose of anesthetics). Products include:
- Brevital Sodium Vials ... 1429

Methoxyflurane (May require reduced dose of anesthetics).
- No products indexed under this heading.

Methyclothiazide (Potentiation of antihypertensive effect). Products include:
- Enduron Tablets ... 420

Methyldopate Hydrochloride (Potentiation of antihypertensive effect). Products include:
- Aldomet Ester HCl Injection ... 1602

Methylprednisolone Acetate (Hypokalemia may result). Products include:
- Depo-Medrol Single-Dose Vial ... 2600
- Depo-Medrol Sterile Aqueous Suspension ... 2597

IMPORTANT NOTE: Always consult each drug listing in the patient's regimen for possible interactions.

Methylprednisolone Sodium Succinate (Hypokalemia may result). Products include:
- Solu-Medrol Sterile Powder 2643

Metolazone (Potentiation of antihypertensive effect). Products include:
- Mykrox Tablets 993
- Zaroxolyn Tablets 1000

Metoprolol Succinate (Potentiation of antihypertensive effect). Products include:
- Toprol-XL Tablets 565

Metoprolol Tartrate (Potentiation of antihypertensive effect). Products include:
- Lopressor Ampuls 830
- Lopressor HCT Tablets 832
- Lopressor Tablets 830

Metyrosine (Potentiation of antihypertensive effect). Products include:
- Demser Capsules 1649

Minoxidil (Potentiation of antihypertensive effect). Products include:
- Loniten Tablets 2618
- Rogaine Topical Solution 2637

Moexipril Hydrochloride (Potentiation of antihypertensive effect). Products include:
- Univasc Tablets 2410

Morphine Sulfate (Aggravates orthostatic hypotension). Products include:
- Astramorph/PF Injection, USP (Preservative-Free) 535
- Duramorph 962
- Infumorph 200 and Infumorph 500 Sterile Solutions 965
- MS Contin Tablets 1994
- MSIR 1997
- Oramorph SR (Morphine Sulfate Sustained Release Tablets) 2236
- RMS Suppositories 2657
- Roxanol 2243

Nabumetone (May result in reduced diuretic effect). Products include:
- Relafen Tablets 2510

Nadolol (Potentiation of antihypertensive effect).
- No products indexed under this heading.

Naproxen (May result in reduced diuretic effects). Products include:
- Anaprox/Naprosyn 2117

Naproxen Sodium (May result in reduced diuretic effects). Products include:
- Aleve 1975
- Anaprox/Naprosyn 2117

Nicardipine Hydrochloride (Potentiation of antihypertensive effect). Products include:
- Cardene Capsules 2095
- Cardene I.V. 2709
- Cardene SR Capsules 2097

Nifedipine (Potentiation of antihypertensive effect). Products include:
- Adalat Capsules (10 mg and 20 mg) 587
- Adalat CC 589
- Procardia Capsules 1971
- Procardia XL Extended Release Tablets 1972

Nisoldipine (Potentiation of antihypertensive effect).
- No products indexed under this heading.

Nitroglycerin (Potentiation of antihypertensive effect). Products include:
- Deponit NTG Transdermal Delivery System 2397
- Nitro-Bid IV 1523
- Nitro-Bid Ointment 1524
- Nitrodisc 2047
- Nitro-Dur (nitroglycerin) Transdermal Infusion System 1326
- Nitrolingual Spray 2027
- Nitrostat Tablets 1925
- Transderm-Nitro Transdermal Therapeutic System 859

Norepinephrine Bitartrate (Decreased arterial responsiveness to norepinephrine). Products include:
- Levophed Bitartrate Injection 2315

Opium Alkaloids (Aggravates orthostatic hypotension).
- No products indexed under this heading.

Oxaprozin (May result in reduced diuretic effect). Products include:
- Daypro Caplets 2426

Oxycodone Hydrochloride (Aggravates orthostatic hypotension). Products include:
- Percocet Tablets 938
- Percodan Tablets 939
- Percodan-Demi Tablets 940
- Roxicodone Tablets, Oral Solution & Intensol (Oxycodone) 2244
- Tylox Capsules 1584

Penbutolol Sulfate (Potentiation of antihypertensive effect). Products include:
- Levatol 2403

Pentobarbital Sodium (Aggravates orthostatic hypotension). Products include:
- Nembutal Sodium Capsules 436
- Nembutal Sodium Solution 438
- Nembutal Sodium Suppositories 440

Phenelzine Sulfate (Concurrent use is contraindicated). Products include:
- Nardil 1920

Phenobarbital (Aggravates orthostatic hypotension). Products include:
- Arco-Lase Plus Tablets 512
- Bellergal-S Tablets 2250
- Donnatal 2060
- Donnatal Extentabs 2061
- Donnatal Tablets 2060
- Phenobarbital Elixir and Tablets 1469
- Quadrinal Tablets 1350

Phenoxybenzamine Hydrochloride (Potentiation of antihypertensive effect). Products include:
- Dibenzyline Capsules 2476

Phentolamine Mesylate (Potentiation of antihypertensive effect). Products include:
- Regitine 846

Phenylbutazone (May result in reduced diuretic effects).
- No products indexed under this heading.

Pindolol (Potentiation of antihypertensive effect). Products include:
- Visken Tablets 2299

Piroxicam (May result in reduced diuretic effects). Products include:
- Feldene Capsules 1965

Polythiazide (Potentiation of antihypertensive effect). Products include:
- Minizide Capsules 1938

Prazosin Hydrochloride (Potentiation of antihypertensive effect). Products include:
- Minipress Capsules 1937
- Minizide Capsules 1938

Prednisolone Acetate (Hypokalemia may result). Products include:
- AK-CIDE .... ⊙ 202
- AK-CIDE Ointment .... ⊙ 202
- Blephamide Liquifilm Sterile Ophthalmic Suspension 476
- Blephamide Ointment .... ⊙ 237
- Econopred & Econopred Plus Ophthalmic Suspensions .... ⊙ 217
- Poly-Pred Liquifilm .... ⊙ 248
- Pred Forte .... ⊙ 250
- Pred Mild .... ⊙ 253
- Pred-G Liquifilm Sterile Ophthalmic Suspension .... ⊙ 251
- Pred-G S.O.P. Sterile Ophthalmic Ointment .... ⊙ 252
- Vasocidin Ointment .... ⊙ 268

Prednisolone Sodium Phosphate (Hypokalemia may result). Products include:
- AK-Pred .... ⊙ 204
- Hydeltrasol Injection, Sterile 1665
- Inflamase .... ⊙ 265
- Pediapred Oral Liquid 995
- Vasocidin Ophthalmic Solution .... ⊙ 270

Prednisolone Tebutate (Hypokalemia may result). Products include:
- Hydeltra-T.B.A. Sterile Suspension 1667

Prednisone (Hypokalemia may result). Products include:
- Deltasone Tablets 2595

Propofol (May require reduced dose of anesthetics). Products include:
- Diprivan Injection 2833

Propoxyphene Hydrochloride (Aggravates orthostatic hypotension). Products include:
- Darvon 1435
- Wygesic Tablets 2827

Propoxyphene Napsylate (Aggravates orthostatic hypotension). Products include:
- Darvon-N/Darvocet-N 1433

Propranolol Hydrochloride (Potentiation of antihypertensive effect). Products include:
- Inderal 2728
- Inderal LA Long Acting Capsules 2730
- Inderide Tablets 2732
- Inderide LA Long Acting Capsules .. 2734

Quinapril Hydrochloride (Potentiation of antihypertensive effect). Products include:
- Accupril Tablets 1893

Ramipril (Potentiation of antihypertensive effect). Products include:
- Altace Capsules 1232

Rauwolfia Serpentina (Potentiation of antihypertensive effect).
- No products indexed under this heading.

Rescinnamine (Potentiation of antihypertensive effect).
- No products indexed under this heading.

Reserpine (Potentiation of antihypertensive effect). Products include:
- Diupres Tablets 1650
- Hydropres Tablets 1675
- Ser-Ap-Es Tablets 849

Secobarbital Sodium (Aggravates orthostatic hypotension). Products include:
- Seconal Sodium Pulvules 1474

Selegiline Hydrochloride (Concurrent use is contraindicated). Products include:
- Eldepryl Tablets 2550

Sodium Nitroprusside (Potentiation of antihypertensive effect).
- No products indexed under this heading.

Sotalol Hydrochloride (Potentiation of antihypertensive effect). Products include:
- Betapace Tablets 641

Spirapril Hydrochloride (Potentiation of antihypertensive effect).
- No products indexed under this heading.

Sufentanil Citrate (Aggravates orthostatic hypotension). Products include:
- Sufenta Injection 1309

Sulindac (May result in reduced diuretic effects). Products include:
- Clinoril Tablets 1618

Terazosin Hydrochloride (Potentiation of antihypertensive effect). Products include:
- Hytrin Capsules 430

Thiamylal Sodium (Aggravates orthostatic hypotension).
- No products indexed under this heading.

Timolol Maleate (Potentiation of antihypertensive effect). Products include:
- Blocadren Tablets 1614
- Timolide Tablets 1748
- Timoptic in Ocudose 1753
- Timoptic Sterile Ophthalmic Solution 1751
- Timoptic-XE 1755

Tolazamide (Dosage adjustment of the antidiabetic drug may be required).
- No products indexed under this heading.

Tolbutamide (Dosage adjustment of the antidiabetic drug may be required).
- No products indexed under this heading.

Tolmetin Sodium (May result in reduced diuretic effects). Products include:
- Tolectin (200, 400 and 600 mg) .. 1581

Torsemide (Potentiation of antihypertensive effect). Products include:
- Demadex Tablets and Injection 686

Tranylcypromine Sulfate (Concurrent use is contraindicated). Products include:
- Parnate Tablets 2503

Triamcinolone (Hypokalemia may result). Products include:
- Aristocort Tablets 1022

Triamcinolone Acetonide (Hypokalemia may result). Products include:
- Aristocort A 0.025% Cream 1027
- Aristocort A 0.5% Cream 1031
- Aristocort A 0.1% Cream 1029
- Aristocort A 0.1% Ointment 1030
- Azmacort Oral Inhaler 2011
- Nasacort Nasal Inhaler 2024

Triamcinolone Diacetate (Hypokalemia may result). Products include:
- Aristocort Suspension (Forte Parenteral) 1027
- Aristocort Suspension (Intralesional) 1025

Triamcinolone Hexacetonide (Hypokalemia may result). Products include:
- Aristospan Suspension (Intra-articular) 1033
- Aristospan Suspension (Intralesional) 1032

Trimethaphan Camsylate (Potentiation of antihypertensive effect). Products include:
- Arfonad Ampuls 2080

Tubocurarine Chloride (Increased responsiveness to tubocurarine).
- No products indexed under this heading.

Verapamil Hydrochloride (Potentiation of antihypertensive effect). Products include:
- Calan SR Caplets 2422
- Calan Tablets 2419
- Isoptin Injectable 1344
- Isoptin Oral Tablets 1346
- Isoptin SR Tablets 1348
- Verelan Capsules 1410
- Verelan Capsules 2824

Food Interactions

Alcohol (Aggravates orthostatic hypotension).

ALEVE
(Naproxen Sodium) 1975
May interact with certain other

(◘ Described in PDR For Nonprescription Drugs) (⊙ Described in PDR For Ophthalmology)

Interactions Index

agents. Compounds in this category include:

Acetaminophen (Concurrent administration is not recommended unless advised by a physician). Products include:

Actifed Plus Caplets ....📖 845
Actifed Plus Tablets ....📖 845
Actifed Sinus Daytime/Nighttime Tablets and Caplets ....📖 846
Alka-Seltzer Plus Cold Medicine Liqui-Gels ....📖 706
Alka-Seltzer Plus Cold & Cough Medicine Liqui-Gels..............................📖 705
Alka-Seltzer Plus Night-Time Cold Medicine Liqui-Gels..............................📖 706
Allerest Headache Strength Tablets ....📖 627
Allerest No Drowsiness Tablets ......📖 627
Allerest Sinus Pain Formula ....📖 627
Anexsia 5/500 Elixir 1781
Anexia Tablets... 1782
Arthritis Foundation Aspirin Free Caplets ....📖 673
Arthritis Foundation NightTime Caplets ....📖 674
Bayer Select Headache Pain Relief Formula ....📖 716
Bayer Select Menstrual Multi-Symptom Formula..............................📖 716
Bayer Select Night Time Pain Relief Formula..............................📖 716
Bayer Select Sinus Pain Relief Formula ....📖 717
Benadryl Allergy Sinus Headache Formula Caplets..............................📖 849
Comtrex Multi-Symptom Cold Reliever Tablets/Caplets/Liqui-Gels/Liquid..............................📖 615
Allergy-Sinus Comtrex Multi-Symptom Allergy-Sinus Formula Tablets ....📖 617
Comtrex Non-Drowsy ....📖 618
Contac Day Allergy/Sinus Caplets 📖 812
Contac Day & Night ....📖 812
Contac Night Allergy/Sinus Caplets ....📖 812
Contac Severe Cold and Flu Formula Caplets ....📖 814
Contac Severe Cold & Flu Non-Drowsy ....📖 815
Coricidin 'D' Decongestant Tablets ....📖 800
Coricidin Tablets ....📖 800
DHCplus Capsules................................... 1993
Darvon-N/Darvocet-N 1433
Drixoral Cold and Flu Extended-Release Tablets..............................📖 803
Drixoral Cough + Sore Throat Liquid Caps ....📖 802
Drixoral Allergy/Sinus Extended Release Tablets..............................📖 804
Esgic-plus Tablets 1013
Aspirin Free Excedrin Analgesic Caplets and Geltabs 732
Excedrin Extra-Strength Analgesic Tablets & Caplets 732
Excedrin P.M. Analgesic/Sleeping Aid Tablets, Caplets, Liquigels 733
Fioricet Tablets... 2258
Fioricet with Codeine Capsules 2260
Hycomine Compound Tablets 932
Hydrocet Capsules 782
Legatrin PM ....📖 651
Lorcet 10/650... 1018
Lortab 2566
Lurline PMS Tablets 982
Maximum Strength Multi-Symptom Formula Midol ....📖 722
PMS Multi-Symptom Formula Midol ....📖 723
Teen Multi-Symptom Formula Midol ....📖 722
Midrin Capsules 783
Migralam Capsules 2038
Panodol Tablets and Caplets ....📖 824
Children's Panadol Chewable Tablets, Liquid, Infant's Drops ....📖 824
Percocet Tablets 938
Percogesic Analgesic Tablets ....📖 754
Phrenilin 785
Pyrroxate Caplets ....📖 772
Sedapap Tablets 50 mg/650 mg .. 1543
Sinarest Tablets ....📖 648
Sinarest Extra Strength Tablets......📖 648
Sinarest No Drowsiness Tablets ....📖 648
Sine-Aid Maximum Strength Sinus Medication Gelcaps, Caplets and Tablets 1554
Sine-Off No Drowsiness Formula Caplets ....📖 824
Sine-Off Sinus Medicine ....📖 825
Singlet Tablets ....📖 825
Sinulin Tablets 787
Sinutab Sinus Allergy Medication, Maximum Strength Tablets and Caplets ....📖 860
Sinutab Sinus Medication, Maximum Strength Without Drowsiness Formula, Tablets & Caplets ....📖 860
Sinutab Sinus Medication, Regular Strength Without Drowsiness Formula ....📖 859
Sudafed Cold and Cough Liquidcaps ....📖 862
Sudafed Severe Cold Formula Caplets ....📖 863
Sudafed Severe Cold Formula Tablets ....📖 864
Sudafed Sinus Caplets..............................📖 864
Sudafed Sinus Tablets ....📖 864
Talacen... 2333
TheraFlu..............................📖 787
TheraFlu Maximum Strength Nighttime Flu, Cold & Cough Medicine ....📖 788
TheraFlu Maximum Strength Non-Drowsy Formula Flu, Cold & Cough Medicine ....📖 788
Thera Flu Maximum Strength, Non-Drowsy Formula Flu, Cold and Cough Caplets ....📖 789
Triaminic Sore Throat Formula ......📖 791
Triaminicin Tablets ....📖 793
Children's TYLENOL acetaminophen Chewable Tablets, Elixir, Suspension Liquid 1555
Children's TYLENOL Cold Multi-Symptom Liquid Formula and Chewable Tablets................................... 1561
Children's TYLENOL Cold Plus Cough Multi Symptom Tablets and Liquid ....📖 681
Infants' TYLENOL acetaminophen Drops and Suspension Drops 1555
Infants' TYLENOL Cold Decongestant & Fever-Reducer Drops 1556
TYLENOL Extended Relief Caplets.. 1558
TYLENOL, Extra Strength, Acetaminophen Adult Liquid Pain Reliever 1560
TYLENOL, Extra Strength, acetaminophen Gelcaps, Geltabs, Caplets, Tablets 1559
TYLENOL, Extra Strength, Headache Plus Pain Reliever with Antacid Caplets 1559
TYLENOL, Junior Strength, acetaminophen Coated Caplets, Grape and Fruit Chewable Tablets 1557
TYLENOL Maximum Strength Allergy Sinus Medication Gelcaps and Caplets 1563
TYLENOL Maximum Strength Allergy Sinus NightTime Medication Caplets 1555
TYLENOL Flu Maximum Strength Gelcaps 1565
TYLENOL Flu NightTime, Maximum Strength, Gelcaps 1566
TYLENOL Maximum Strength Flu NightTime Hot Medication Packets 1562
TYLENOL, Maximum Strength, Sinus Medication Geltabs, Gelcaps, Caplets and Tablets 1566
TYLENOL Cold Multi-Symptom Formula Medication Tablets and Caplets 1561
TYLENOL Cold Medication No Drowsiness Formula Gelcaps and Caplets 1562
TYLENOL Cold Multi-Symptom Hot Medication Liquid Packets.............. 1557
TYLENOL Cough Multi-Symptom Medication 1564
TYLENOL Cough Multi-Symptom Medication with Decongestant 1565
TYLENOL, Regular Strength, acetaminophen Caplets and Tablets .. 1558
TYLENOL PM, Extra Strength Pain Reliever/Sleep Aid Caplets, Geltabs, Gelcaps 1560
TYLENOL Severe Allergy Medication Caplets 1564
Tylenol with Codeine 1583
Tylox Capsules 1584

Unisom With Pain Relief-Nighttime Sleep Aid and Pain Reliever............ 1934
Vanquish Analgesic Caplets ....📖 731
Vicks 44 LiquiCaps Cough, Cold & Flu Relief..............................📖 755
Vicks 44M Cough, Cold & Flu Relief ....📖 756
Vicks DayQuil ....📖 761
Vicks Nyquil Hot Therapy....................📖 762
Vicks NyQuil LiquiCaps Multi-Symptom Cold/Flu Relief..........📖 763
Vicks NyQuil Multi-Symptom Cold/Flu Relief - (Original & Cherry Flavor)..............................📖 763
Vicodin Tablets... 1356
Vicodin ES Tablets 1357
Wygesic Tablets... 2827
Zydone Capsules 949

Aspirin (Concurrent administration is not recommended unless advised by a physician). Products include:

Alka-Seltzer Effervescent Antacid and Pain Reliever ....📖 701
Alka-Seltzer Extra Strength Effervescent Antacid and Pain Reliever ....📖 703
Alka-Seltzer Lemon Lime Effervescent Antacid and Pain Reliever ....📖 703
Alka-Seltzer Plus Cold Medicine ....📖 705
Alka-Seltzer Plus Cold & Cough Medicine ....📖 708
Alka-Seltzer Plus Night-Time Cold Medicine ....📖 707
Alka Seltzer Plus Sinus Medicine ..📖 707
Arthritis Foundation Safety Coated Aspirin Tablets ....📖 675
Arthritis Pain Ascriptin ....📖 631
Maximum Strength Ascriptin ....📖 630
Regular Strength Ascriptin Tablets ....📖 629
Arthritis Strength BC Powder..........📖 609
BC Cold Powder Multi-Symptom Formula (Cold-Sinus-Allergy) ......📖 609
BC Cold Powder Non-Drowsy Formula (Cold-Sinus) ....📖 609
BC Powder ....📖 609
Bayer Children's Chewable Aspirin ....📖 711
Genuine Bayer Aspirin Tablets & Caplets ....📖 713
Extra Strength Bayer Arthritis Pain Regimen Formula ....📖 711
Extra Strength Bayer Aspirin Caplets & Tablets ....📖 712
Extended-Release Bayer 8-Hour Aspirin ....📖 712
Extra Strength Bayer Plus Aspirin Caplets ....📖 713
Extra Strength Bayer PM Aspirin ..📖 713
Bayer Enteric Aspirin ....📖 709
Bufferin Analgesic Tablets and Caplets ....📖 613
Arthritis Strength Bufferin Analgesic Caplets ....📖 614
Extra Strength Bufferin Analgesic Tablets ....📖 615
Cama Arthritis Pain Reliever......📖 785
Darvon Compound-65 Pulvules 1435
Easprin 1914
Ecotrin 2455
Ecotrin Enteric Coated Aspirin Maximum Strength Tablets and Caplets ....📖 816
Ecotrin Enteric Coated Aspirin Regular Strength Tablets .. 2455
Empirin Aspirin Tablets ....📖 854
Empirin with Codeine Tablets.......... 1093
Excedrin Extra-Strength Analgesic Tablets & Caplets 732
Fiorinal Capsules 2261
Fiorinal with Codeine Capsules 2262
Fiorinal Tablets 2261
Halfprin 1362
Healthprin Aspirin 2455
Norgesic... 1496
Percodan Tablets....................................... 939
Percodan-Demi Tablets........................... 940
Robaxisal Tablets....................................... 2071
Soma Compound w/Codeine Tablets 2676
Soma Compound Tablets........................ 2675
St. Joseph Adult Chewable Aspirin (81 mg.)..............................📖 808
Talwin Compound 2335
Ursinus Inlay-Tabs..............................📖 794
Vanquish Analgesic Caplets ....📖 731

Ibuprofen (Concurrent administration is not recommended unless advised by a physician). Products include:

Advil Cold and Sinus Caplets and Tablets (formerly CoAdvil) ....📖 870
Advil Ibuprofen Tablets and Caplets ....📖 870
Children's Advil Suspension 2692
Arthritis Foundation Ibuprofen Tablets ....📖 674
Bayer Select Ibuprofen Pain Relief Formula ....📖 715
Cramp End Tablets..............................📖 735
Dimetapp Sinus Caplets ....📖 775
Haltran Tablets ....📖 771
IBU Tablets... 1342
Ibuprohm..............................📖 735
Children's Motrin Ibuprofen Oral Suspension 1546
Motrin Tablets... 2625
Motrin IB Caplets, Tablets, and Geltabs ....📖 838
Motrin IB Sinus ....📖 838
Motrin Ibuprofen Suspension, Oral Drops, Chewable Tablets, Caplets 1546
Nuprin Ibuprofen/Analgesic Tablets & Caplets ....📖 622
Sine-Aid IB Caplets 1554
Vicks DayQuil SINUS Pressure & PAIN Relief with IBUPROFEN ......📖 762

Naproxen (Concurrent administration is not recommended unless advised by a physician). Products include:

Anaprox/Naprosyn 2117

Food Interactions

Alcohol (Concurrent use should be undertaken with the physician's consultation).

ALFENTA INJECTION

(Alfentanil Hydrochloride) 1286

May interact with central nervous system depressants, certain other agents, and monoamine oxidase inhibitors. Compounds in these categories include:

Alprazolam (Enhances CNS and cardiovascular effects). Products include:

Xanax Tablets 2649

Aprobarbital (Enhances CNS and cardiovascular effects).

No products indexed under this heading.

Buprenorphine (Enhances CNS and cardiovascular effects). Products include:

Buprenex Injectable 2006

Buspirone Hydrochloride (Enhances CNS and cardiovascular effects). Products include:

BuSpar 737

Butabarbital (Enhances CNS and cardiovascular effects).

No products indexed under this heading.

Butalbital (Enhances CNS and cardiovascular effects). Products include:

Esgic-plus Tablets 1013
Fioricet Tablets... 2258
Fioricet with Codeine Capsules 2260
Fiorinal Capsules 2261
Fiorinal with Codeine Capsules 2262
Fiorinal Tablets 2261
Phrenilin 785
Sedapap Tablets 50 mg/650 mg .. 1543

Chlordiazepoxide (Enhances CNS and cardiovascular effects). Products include:

Libritabs Tablets 2177
Limbitrol 2180

Chlordiazepoxide Hydrochloride (Enhances CNS and cardiovascular effects). Products include:

Librax Capsules 2176
Librium Capsules....................................... 2178
Librium Injectable 2179

IMPORTANT NOTE: Always consult each drug listing in the patient's regimen for possible interactions.

Alfenta **Interactions Index** 34

Chlorpromazine (Enhances CNS and cardiovascular effects). Products include:
Thorazine Suppositories 2523
Chlorpromazine Hydrochloride (Enhances CNS and cardiovascular effects). Products include:
Thorazine 2523
Chlorprothixene (Enhances CNS and cardiovascular effects).
No products indexed under this heading.
Chlorprothixene Hydrochloride (Enhances CNS and cardiovascular effects).
No products indexed under this heading.
Cimetidine (Reduces the clearance of alfentanil). Products include:
Tagamet Tablets 2516
Cimetidine Hydrochloride (Reduces the clearance of alfentanil). Products include:
Tagamet 2516
Clorazepate Dipotassium (Enhances CNS and cardiovascular effects). Products include:
Tranxene 451
Clozapine (Enhances CNS and cardiovascular effects). Products include:
Clozaril Tablets 2252
Codeine Phosphate (Enhances CNS and cardiovascular effects). Products include:
Actifed with Codeine Cough Syrup 1067
Brontex 1981
Deconsal C Expectorant Syrup 456
Deconsal Pediatric Syrup 457
Dimetane-DC Cough Syrup 2059
Empirin with Codeine Tablets 1093
Fioricet with Codeine Capsules 2260
Fiorinal with Codeine Capsules 2262
Isoclor Expectorant 990
Novahistine DH 2462
Novahistine Expectorant 2463
Nucofed 2051
Phenergan with Codeine 2777
Phenergan VC with Codeine 2781
Robitussin A-C Syrup 2073
Robitussin-DAC Syrup 2074
Ryna ▣ 841
Soma Compound w/Codeine Tablets 2676
Tussi-Organidin NR Liquid and S NR Liquid 2677
Tylenol with Codeine 1583
Desflurane (Enhances CNS and cardiovascular effects). Products include:
Suprane 1813
Dezocine (Enhances CNS and cardiovascular effects). Products include:
Dalgan Injection 538
Diazepam (Enhances CNS and cardiovascular effects; vasodilation, hypotension, delayed recovery). Products include:
Dizac 1809
Valium Injectable 2182
Valium Tablets 2183
Valrelease Capsules 2169
Droperidol (Enhances CNS and cardiovascular effects). Products include:
Inapsine Injection 1296
Enflurane (Enhances CNS and cardiovascular effects).
No products indexed under this heading.
Erythromycin (Inhibits Alfenta clearance and may increase or prolong respiratory depression). Products include:
A/T/S 2% Acne Topical Gel and Solution 1234
Benzamycin Topical Gel 905
E-Mycin Tablets 1341
Emgel 2% Topical Gel 1093
ERYC 1915
Erycette (erythromycin 2%) Topical Solution 1888
Ery-Tab Tablets 422
Erythromycin Base Filmtab 426
Erythromycin Delayed-Release Capsules, USP 427
Ilotycin Ophthalmic Ointment 912
PCE Dispertab Tablets 444
T-Stat 2.0% Topical Solution and Pads 2688
Theramycin Z Topical Solution 2% 1592
Erythromycin Estolate (Inhibits Alfenta clearance and may increase or prolong respiratory depression). Products include:
Ilosone 911
Erythromycin Ethylsuccinate (Inhibits Alfenta clearance and may increase or prolong respiratory depression). Products include:
E.E.S. 424
EryPed 421
Erythromycin Gluceptate (Inhibits Alfenta clearance and may increase or prolong respiratory depression). Products include:
Ilotycin Gluceptate, IV, Vials 913
Erythromycin Lactobionate (Inhibits Alfenta clearance and may increase or prolong respiratory depression).
No products indexed under this heading.
Erythromycin Stearate (Inhibits Alfenta clearance and may increase or prolong respiratory depression). Products include:
Erythrocin Stearate Filmtab 425
Estazolam (Enhances CNS and cardiovascular effects). Products include:
ProSom Tablets 449
Ethchlorvynol (Enhances CNS and cardiovascular effects). Products include:
Placidyl Capsules 448
Ethinamate (Enhances CNS and cardiovascular effects).
No products indexed under this heading.
Fentanyl (Enhances CNS and cardiovascular effects). Products include:
Duragesic Transdermal System 1288
Fentanyl Citrate (Enhances CNS and cardiovascular effects). Products include:
Sublimaze Injection 1307
Fluphenazine Decanoate (Enhances CNS and cardiovascular effects). Products include:
Prolixin Decanoate 509
Fluphenazine Enanthate (Enhances CNS and cardiovascular effects). Products include:
Prolixin Enanthate 509
Fluphenazine Hydrochloride (Enhances CNS and cardiovascular effects). Products include:
Prolixin 509
Flurazepam Hydrochloride (Enhances CNS and cardiovascular effects). Products include:
Dalmane Capsules 2173
Furazolidone (Severe and unpredictable potentiation of MAO inhibitors has been reported for other opioid analgesics, and rarely with alfentanil; concurrent use should be undertaken very carefully). Products include:
Furoxone 2046
Glutethimide (Enhances CNS and cardiovascular effects).
No products indexed under this heading.
Haloperidol (Enhances CNS and cardiovascular effects). Products include:
Haldol Injection, Tablets and Concentrate 1575
Haloperidol Decanoate (Enhances CNS and cardiovascular effects). Products include:
Haldol Decanoate 1577
Hydrocodone Bitartrate (Enhances CNS and cardiovascular effects). Products include:
Anexsia 5/500 Elixir 1781
Anexia Tablets 1782
Codiclear DH Syrup 791
Deconamine CX Cough and Cold Liquid and Tablets 1319
Duratuss HD Elixir 2565
Hycodan Tablets and Syrup 930
Hycomine Compound Tablets 932
Hycomine 931
Hycotuss Expectorant Syrup 933
Hydrocet Capsules 782
Lorcet 10/650 1018
Lortab 2566
Tussend 1783
Tussend Expectorant 1785
Vicodin Tablets 1356
Vicodin ES Tablets 1357
Vicodin Tuss Expectorant 1358
Zydone Capsules 949
Hydrocodone Polistirex (Enhances CNS and cardiovascular effects). Products include:
Tussionex Pennkinetic Extended-Release Suspension 998
Hydroxyzine Hydrochloride (Enhances CNS and cardiovascular effects). Products include:
Atarax Tablets & Syrup 2185
Marax Tablets & DF Syrup 2200
Vistaril Intramuscular Solution 2216
Isocarboxazid (Severe and unpredictable potentiation of MAO inhibitors has been reported for other opioid analgesics, and rarely with alfentanil; concurrent use should be undertaken very carefully).
No products indexed under this heading.
Isoflurane (Enhances CNS and cardiovascular effects).
No products indexed under this heading.
Ketamine Hydrochloride (Enhances CNS and cardiovascular effects).
No products indexed under this heading.
Levomethadyl Acetate Hydrochloride (Enhances CNS and cardiovascular effects). Products include:
Orlamm 2239
Levorphanol Tartrate (Enhances CNS and cardiovascular effects). Products include:
Levo-Dromoran 2129
Lorazepam (Enhances CNS and cardiovascular effects). Products include:
Ativan Injection 2698
Ativan Tablets 2700
Loxapine Hydrochloride (Enhances CNS and cardiovascular effects). Products include:
Loxitane 1378
Loxapine Succinate (Enhances CNS and cardiovascular effects). Products include:
Loxitane Capsules 1378
Meperidine Hydrochloride (Enhances CNS and cardiovascular effects). Products include:
Demerol 2308
Mepergan Injection 2753
Mephobarbital (Enhances CNS and cardiovascular effects). Products include:
Mebaral Tablets 2322
Meprobamate (Enhances CNS and cardiovascular effects). Products include:
Miltown Tablets 2672
PMB 200 and PMB 400 2783
Mesoridazine Besylate (Enhances CNS and cardiovascular effects). Products include:
Serentil 684
Methadone Hydrochloride (Enhances CNS and cardiovascular effects). Products include:
Methadone Hydrochloride Oral Concentrate 2233
Methadone Hydrochloride Oral Solution & Tablets 2235
Methohexital Sodium (Enhances CNS and cardiovascular effects). Products include:
Brevital Sodium Vials 1429
Methotrimeprazine (Enhances CNS and cardiovascular effects). Products include:
Levoprome 1274
Methoxyflurane (Enhances CNS and cardiovascular effects).
No products indexed under this heading.
Midazolam Hydrochloride (Enhances CNS and cardiovascular effects). Products include:
Versed Injection 2170
Molindone Hydrochloride (Enhances CNS and cardiovascular effects). Products include:
Moban Tablets and Concentrate 1048
Morphine Sulfate (Enhances CNS and cardiovascular effects). Products include:
Astramorph/PF Injection, USP (Preservative-Free) 535
Duramorph 962
Infumorph 200 and Infumorph 500 Sterile Solutions 965
MS Contin Tablets 1994
MSIR 1997
Oramorph SR (Morphine Sulfate Sustained Release Tablets) 2236
RMS Suppositories 2657
Roxanol 2243
Opium Alkaloids (Enhances CNS and cardiovascular effects).
No products indexed under this heading.
Oxazepam (Enhances CNS and cardiovascular effects). Products include:
Serax Capsules 2810
Serax Tablets 2810
Oxycodone Hydrochloride (Enhances CNS and cardiovascular effects). Products include:
Percocet Tablets 938
Percodan Tablets 939
Percodan-Demi Tablets 940
Roxicodone Tablets, Oral Solution & Intensol (Oxycodone) 2244
Tylox Capsules 1584
Pentobarbital Sodium (Enhances CNS and depressant effects). Products include:
Nembutal Sodium Capsules 436
Nembutal Sodium Solution 438
Nembutal Sodium Suppositories 440
Perphenazine (Enhances CNS and cardiovascular effects). Products include:
Etrafon 2355
Triavil Tablets 1757
Trilafon 2389
Phenelzine Sulfate (Severe and unpredictable potentiation of MAO inhibitors has been reported for other opioid analgesics, and rarely with alfentanil; concurrent use should be undertaken very carefully). Products include:
Nardil 1920

Phenobarbital (Enhances CNS and cardiovascular effects). Products include:

Arco-Lase Plus Tablets 512
Bellergal-S Tablets 2250
Donnatal 2060
Donnatal Extentabs............................... 2061
Donnatal Tablets 2060
Phenobarbital Elixir and Tablets 1469
Quadrinal Tablets 1350

Prazepam (Enhances CNS and cardiovascular effects).

No products indexed under this heading.

Prochlorperazine (Enhances CNS and cardiovascular effects). Products include:

Compazine 2470

Promethazine Hydrochloride (Enhances CNS and cardiovascular effects). Products include:

Mepergan Injection 2753
Phenergan with Codeine...................... 2777
Phenergan with Dextromethorphan 2778
Phenergan Injection 2773
Phenergan Suppositories 2775
Phenergan Syrup 2774
Phenergan Tablets 2775
Phenergan VC 2779
Phenergan VC with Codeine 2781

Propofol (Enhances CNS and cardiovascular effects). Products include:

Diprivan Injection.................................. 2833

Propoxyphene Hydrochloride (Enhances CNS and cardiovascular effects). Products include:

Darvon 1435
Wygesic Tablets 2827

Propoxyphene Napsylate (Enhances CNS and cardiovascular effects). Products include:

Darvon-N/Darvocet-N 1433

Quazepam (Enhances CNS and cardiovascular effects). Products include:

Doral Tablets 2664

Risperidone (Enhances CNS and cardiovascular effects). Products include:

Risperdal 1301

Secobarbital Sodium (Enhances CNS and cardiovascular effects). Products include:

Seconal Sodium Pulvules 1474

Selegiline Hydrochloride (Severe and unpredictable potentiation of MAO inhibitors has been reported for other opioid analgesics, and rarely with alfentanil; concurrent use should be undertaken very carefully). Products include:

Eldepryl Tablets 2550

Sufentanil Citrate (Enhances CNS and cardiovascular effects). Products include:

Sufenta Injection 1309

Temazepam (Enhances CNS and cardiovascular effects). Products include:

Restoril Capsules 2284

Thiamylal Sodium (Enhances CNS and cardiovascular effects).

No products indexed under this heading.

Thioridazine Hydrochloride (Enhances CNS and cardiovascular effects). Products include:

Mellaril 2269

Thiothixene (Enhances CNS and cardiovascular effects). Products include:

Navane Capsules and Concentrate 2201
Navane Intramuscular 2202

Tranylcypromine Sulfate (Severe and unpredictable potentiation of MAO inhibitors has been reported for other opioid analgesics, and rarely with alfentanil; concurrent use should be undertaken very carefully). Products include:

Parnate Tablets 2503

Triazolam (Enhances CNS and cardiovascular effects). Products include:

Halcion Tablets 2611

Trifluoperazine Hydrochloride (Enhances CNS and cardiovascular effects). Products include:

Stelazine 2514

Zolpidem Tartrate (Enhances CNS and cardiovascular effects). Products include:

Ambien Tablets...................................... 2416

ALITRAQ SPECIALIZED ELEMENTAL NUTRITION WITH GLUTAMINE

(L-Glutamine, Nutritional Supplement) 2220
None cited in PDR database.

ALKA-MINTS CHEWABLE ANTACID

(Calcium Carbonate) ....✦ 701
May interact with:

Prescription Drugs, unspecified (Antacids may interact with certain unspecified prescription drugs; concurrent use is not recommended).

ALKA-SELTZER EFFERVESCENT ANTACID AND PAIN RELIEVER

(Aspirin, Sodium Bicarbonate, Citric Acid) ....✦ 701
May interact with oral anticoagulants and certain other agents. Compounds in these categories include:

Antiarthritic Drugs, unspecified (Concurrent use is not recommended).

Antidiabetic Drugs, unspecified (Concurrent use is not recommended).

Antigout Drugs, unspecified (Concurrent use is not recommended).

Dicumarol (Concurrent use is not recommended).

No products indexed under this heading.

Prescription Drugs, unspecified (Antacids may interact with certain prescription drugs; concurrent use is not recommended).

Warfarin Sodium (Concurrent use is not recommended). Products include:

Coumadin 926

ALKA-SELTZER GOLD EFFERVESCENT ANTACID

(Citric Acid, Potassium Bicarbonate, Sodium Bicarbonate)..✦ 703
May interact with:

Prescription Drugs, unspecified (Antacids may interact with certain unspecified prescription drugs; check with your doctor).

ALKA-SELTZER LEMON LIME EFFERVESCENT ANTACID AND PAIN RELIEVER

(Aspirin, Sodium Citrate) ....✦ 703
May interact with oral anticoagulants and certain other agents. Compounds in these categories include:

Antiarthritic Drugs, unspecified (Concurrent use is not recommended).

Antidiabetic Drugs, unspecified (Concurrent use is not recommended).

Antigout Drugs, unspecified (Concurrent use is not recommended).

Dicumarol (Concurrent use is not recommended).

No products indexed under this heading.

Prescription Drugs, unspecified (Antacids may interact with certain prescription drugs; concurrent use is not recommended).

Warfarin Sodium (Concurrent use is not recommended). Products include:

Coumadin 926

ALKA-SELTZER EXTRA STRENGTH EFFERVESCENT ANTACID AND PAIN RELIEVER

(Aspirin, Sodium Bicarbonate, Citric Acid) ....✦ 703
May interact with oral anticoagulants and certain other agents. Compounds in these categories include:

Antiarthritic Drugs, unspecified (Concurrent use is not recommended).

Antidiabetic Drugs, unspecified (Concurrent use is not recommended).

Antigout Drugs, unspecified (Concurrent use is not recommended).

Dicumarol (Concurrent use is not recommended).

No products indexed under this heading.

Prescription Drugs, unspecified (Antacids may interact with certain prescription drugs; concurrent use is not recommended).

Warfarin Sodium (Concurrent use is not recommended). Products include:

Coumadin 926

ALKA-SELTZER PLUS COLD MEDICINE

(Chlorpheniramine Maleate, Aspirin, Phenylpropanolamine Bitartrate)..✦ 705
May interact with hypnotics and sedatives, tranquilizers, oral anticoagulants, monoamine oxidase inhibitors, antihypertensives, and certain other agents. Compounds in these categories include:

Acebutolol Hydrochloride (Concurrent use is not recommended). Products include:

Sectral Capsules 2807

Alprazolam (May increase drowsiness effect). Products include:

Xanax Tablets 2649

Amlodipine Besylate (Concurrent use is not recommended). Products include:

Lotrel Capsules...................................... 840
Norvasc Tablets 1940

Antiarthritic Drugs, unspecified (Effect not specified).

Antidiabetic Drugs, unspecified (Effect not specified).

Antigout Drugs, unspecified (Effect not specified).

Atenolol (Concurrent use is not recommended). Products include:

Tenoretic Tablets.................................... 2845
Tenormin Tablets and I.V. Injection 2847

Benazepril Hydrochloride (Concurrent use is not recommended). Products include:

Lotensin Tablets..................................... 834
Lotensin HCT 837
Lotrel Capsules....................................... 840

Bendroflumethiazide (Concurrent use is not recommended).

No products indexed under this heading.

Betaxolol Hydrochloride (Concurrent use is not recommended). Products include:

Betoptic Ophthalmic Solution............ 469
Betoptic S Ophthalmic Suspension 471
Kerlone Tablets...................................... 2436

Bisoprolol Fumarate (Concurrent use is not recommended). Products include:

Zebeta Tablets 1413
Ziac 1415

Buspirone Hydrochloride (May increase drowsiness effect). Products include:

BuSpar 737

Captopril (Concurrent use is not recommended). Products include:

Capoten 739
Capozide 742

Carteolol Hydrochloride (Concurrent use is not recommended). Products include:

Cartrol Tablets 410
Ocupress Ophthalmic Solution, 1% Sterile... © 309

Chlordiazepoxide (May increase drowsiness effect). Products include:

Libritabs Tablets 2177
Limbitrol 2180

Chlordiazepoxide Hydrochloride (May increase drowsiness effect). Products include:

Librax Capsules 2176
Librium Capsules................................... 2178
Librium Injectable 2179

Chlorothiazide (Concurrent use is not recommended). Products include:

Aldoclor Tablets 1598
Diupres Tablets 1650
Diuril Oral 1653

Chlorothiazide Sodium (Concurrent use is not recommended). Products include:

Diuril Sodium Intravenous 1652

Chlorpromazine (May increase drowsiness effect). Products include:

Thorazine Suppositories 2523

Chlorpromazine Hydrochloride (May increase drowsiness effect). Products include:

Thorazine 2523

Chlorprothixene (May increase drowsiness effect).

No products indexed under this heading.

Chlorprothixene Hydrochloride (May increase drowsiness effect).

No products indexed under this heading.

Chlorthalidone (Concurrent use is not recommended). Products include:

Combipres Tablets 677
Tenoretic Tablets 2845
Thalitone 1245

Clonidine (Concurrent use is not recommended). Products include:

Catapres-TTS.. 675

Clonidine Hydrochloride (Concurrent use is not recommended). Products include:

Catapres Tablets 674
Combipres Tablets 677

IMPORTANT NOTE: Always consult each drug listing in the patient's regimen for possible interactions.

Alka-Seltzer Plus — **Interactions Index** — **36**

Clorazepate Dipotassium (May increase drowsiness effect). Products include:
Tranxene ... 451
Deserpidine (Concurrent use is not recommended).
No products indexed under this heading.
Diazepam (May increase drowsiness effect). Products include:
Dizac ... 1809
Valium Injectable ... 2182
Valium Tablets ... 2183
Valrelease Capsules ... 2169
Diazoxide (Concurrent use is not recommended). Products include:
Hyperstat I.V. Injection ... 2363
Proglycem ... 580
Dicumarol (Effect not specified).
No products indexed under this heading.
Diltiazem Hydrochloride (Concurrent use is not recommended). Products include:
Cardizem CD Capsules ... 1506
Cardizem SR Capsules ... 1510
Cardizem Injectable ... 1508
Cardizem Tablets ... 1512
Dilacor XR Extended-release Capsules ... 2018
Doxazosin Mesylate (Concurrent use is not recommended). Products include:
Cardura Tablets ... 2186
Droperidol (May increase drowsiness effect). Products include:
Inapsine Injection ... 1296
Enalapril Maleate (Concurrent use is not recommended). Products include:
Vaseretic Tablets ... 1765
Vasotec Tablets ... 1771
Enalaprilat (Concurrent use is not recommended). Products include:
Vasotec I.V. ... 1768
Esmolol Hydrochloride (Concurrent use is not recommended). Products include:
Brevibloc Injection ... 1808
Estazolam (May increase drowsiness effect). Products include:
ProSom Tablets ... 449
Ethchlorvynol (May increase drowsiness effect). Products include:
Placidyl Capsules ... 448
Ethinamate (May increase drowsiness effect).
No products indexed under this heading.
Felodipine (Concurrent use is not recommended). Products include:
Plendil Extended-Release Tablets ... 527
Fluphenazine Decanoate (May increase drowsiness effect). Products include:
Prolixin Decanoate ... 509
Fluphenazine Enanthate (May increase drowsiness effect). Products include:
Prolixin Enanthate ... 509
Fluphenazine Hydrochloride (May increase drowsiness effect). Products include:
Prolixin ... 509
Flurazepam Hydrochloride (May increase drowsiness effect). Products include:
Dalmane Capsules ... 2173
Fosinopril Sodium (Concurrent use is not recommended). Products include:
Monopril Tablets ... 757
Furazolidone (Concurrent and/or sequential use is not recommended). Products include:
Furoxone ... 2046
Furosemide (Concurrent use is not recommended). Products include:
Lasix Injection, Oral Solution and Tablets ... 1240
Glutethimide (May increase drowsiness effect).
No products indexed under this heading.
Guanabenz Acetate (Concurrent use is not recommended).
No products indexed under this heading.
Guanethidine Monosulfate (Concurrent use is not recommended). Products include:
Esimil Tablets ... 822
Ismelin Tablets ... 827
Haloperidol (May increase drowsiness effect). Products include:
Haldol Injection, Tablets and Concentrate ... 1575
Haloperidol Decanoate (May increase drowsiness effect). Products include:
Haldol Decanoate ... 1577
Hydralazine Hydrochloride (Concurrent use is not recommended). Products include:
Apresazide Capsules ... 808
Apresoline Hydrochloride Tablets ... 809
Ser-Ap-Es Tablets ... 849
Hydrochlorothiazide (Concurrent use is not recommended). Products include:
Aldactazide ... 2413
Aldoril Tablets ... 1604
Apresazide Capsules ... 808
Capozide ... 742
Dyazide ... 2479
Esidrix Tablets ... 821
Esimil Tablets ... 822
HydroDIURIL Tablets ... 1674
Hydropres Tablets ... 1675
Hyzaar Tablets ... 1677
Inderide Tablets ... 2732
Inderide LA Long Acting Capsules ... 2734
Lopressor HCT Tablets ... 832
Lotensin HCT ... 837
Maxzide ... 1380
Moduretic Tablets ... 1705
Oretic Tablets ... 443
Prinzide Tablets ... 1737
Ser-Ap-Es Tablets ... 849
Timolide Tablets ... 1748
Vaseretic Tablets ... 1765
Zestoretic ... 2850
Ziac ... 1415
Hydroflumethiazide (Concurrent use is not recommended). Products include:
Diucardin Tablets ... 2718
Hydroxyzine Hydrochloride (May increase drowsiness effect). Products include:
Atarax Tablets & Syrup ... 2185
Marax Tablets & DF Syrup ... 2200
Vistaril Intramuscular Solution ... 2216
Indapamide (Concurrent use is not recommended). Products include:
Lozol Tablets ... 2022
Isocarboxazid (Concurrent and/or sequential use is not recommended).
No products indexed under this heading.
Isradipine (Concurrent use is not recommended). Products include:
DynaCirc Capsules ... 2256
Labetalol Hydrochloride (Concurrent use is not recommended). Products include:
Normodyne Injection ... 2377
Normodyne Tablets ... 2379
Trandate ... 1185
Levobunolol Hydrochloride (Concurrent use is not recommended). Products include:
Betagan ... ⊚ 233
Lisinopril (Concurrent use is not recommended). Products include:
Prinivil Tablets ... 1733
Prinzide Tablets ... 1737
Zestoretic ... 2850
Zestril Tablets ... 2854
Lorazepam (May increase drowsiness effect). Products include:
Ativan Injection ... 2698
Ativan Tablets ... 2700
Losartan Potassium (Concurrent use is not recommended). Products include:
Cozaar Tablets ... 1628
Hyzaar Tablets ... 1677
Loxapine Hydrochloride (May increase drowsiness effect). Products include:
Loxitane ... 1378
Loxapine Succinate (May increase drowsiness effect). Products include:
Loxitane Capsules ... 1378
Mecamylamine Hydrochloride (Concurrent use is not recommended). Products include:
Inversine Tablets ... 1686
Meprobamate (May increase drowsiness effect). Products include:
Miltown Tablets ... 2672
PMB 200 and PMB 400 ... 2783
Mesoridazine Besylate (May increase drowsiness effect). Products include:
Serentil ... 684
Methyclothiazide (Concurrent use is not recommended). Products include:
Enduron Tablets ... 420
Methyldopa (Concurrent use is not recommended). Products include:
Aldoclor Tablets ... 1598
Aldomet Oral ... 1600
Aldoril Tablets ... 1604
Methyldopate Hydrochloride (Concurrent use is not recommended). Products include:
Aldomet Ester HCl Injection ... 1602
Metipranolol Hydrochloride (Concurrent use is not recommended). Products include:
OptiPranolol (Metipranolol 0.3%) Sterile Ophthalmic Solution ... ⊚ 258
Metolazone (Concurrent use is not recommended). Products include:
Mykrox Tablets ... 993
Zaroxolyn Tablets ... 1000
Metoprolol Succinate (Concurrent use is not recommended). Products include:
Toprol-XL Tablets ... 565
Metoprolol Tartrate (Concurrent use is not recommended). Products include:
Lopressor Ampuls ... 830
Lopressor HCT Tablets ... 832
Lopressor Tablets ... 830
Metyrosine (Concurrent use is not recommended). Products include:
Demser Capsules ... 1649
Midazolam Hydrochloride (May increase drowsiness effect). Products include:
Versed Injection ... 2170
Minoxidil (Concurrent use is not recommended). Products include:
Loniten Tablets ... 2618
Rogaine Topical Solution ... 2637
Moexipril Hydrochloride (Concurrent use is not recommended). Products include:
Univasc Tablets ... 2410
Molindone Hydrochloride (May increase drowsiness effect). Products include:
Moban Tablets and Concentrate ... 1048
Nadolol (Concurrent use is not recommended).
No products indexed under this heading.
Nicardipine Hydrochloride (Concurrent use is not recommended). Products include:
Cardene Capsules ... 2095
Cardene I.V. ... 2709
Cardene SR Capsules ... 2097
Nifedipine (Concurrent use is not recommended). Products include:
Adalat Capsules (10 mg and 20 mg) ... 587
Adalat CC ... 589
Procardia Capsules ... 1971
Procardia XL Extended Release Tablets ... 1972
Nisoldipine (Concurrent use is not recommended).
No products indexed under this heading.
Nitroglycerin (Concurrent use is not recommended). Products include:
Deponit NTG Transdermal Delivery System ... 2397
Nitro-Bid IV ... 1523
Nitro-Bid Ointment ... 1524
Nitrodisc ... 2047
Nitro-Dur (nitroglycerin) Transdermal Infusion System ... 1326
Nitrolingual Spray ... 2027
Nitrostat Tablets ... 1925
Transderm-Nitro Transdermal Therapeutic System ... 859
Oxazepam (May increase drowsiness effect). Products include:
Serax Capsules ... 2810
Serax Tablets ... 2810
Penbutolol Sulfate (Concurrent use is not recommended). Products include:
Levatol ... 2403
Perphenazine (May increase drowsiness effect). Products include:
Etrafon ... 2355
Triavil Tablets ... 1757
Trilafon ... 2389
Phenelzine Sulfate (Concurrent and/or sequential use is not recommended). Products include:
Nardil ... 1920
Phenoxybenzamine Hydrochloride (Concurrent use is not recommended). Products include:
Dibenzyline Capsules ... 2476
Phentolamine Mesylate (Concurrent use is not recommended). Products include:
Regitine ... 846
Pindolol (Concurrent use is not recommended). Products include:
Visken Tablets ... 2299
Polythiazide (Concurrent use is not recommended). Products include:
Minizide Capsules ... 1938
Prazepam (May increase drowsiness effect).
No products indexed under this heading.
Prazosin Hydrochloride (Concurrent use is not recommended). Products include:
Minipress Capsules ... 1937
Minizide Capsules ... 1938
Prochlorperazine (May increase drowsiness effect). Products include:
Compazine ... 2470
Promethazine Hydrochloride (May increase drowsiness effect). Products include:
Mepergan Injection ... 2753
Phenergan with Codeine ... 2777
Phenergan with Dextromethorphan ... 2778
Phenergan Injection ... 2773
Phenergan Suppositories ... 2775
Phenergan Syrup ... 2774
Phenergan Tablets ... 2775
Phenergan VC ... 2779
Phenergan VC with Codeine ... 2781
Propofol (May increase drowsiness effect). Products include:
Diprivan Injection ... 2833

(▣ Described in PDR For Nonprescription Drugs) — (⊚ Described in PDR For Ophthalmology)

Interactions Index

Alka-Seltzer Plus Cold

Propranolol Hydrochloride (Concurrent use is not recommended). Products include:

Inderal 2728
Inderal LA Long Acting Capsules 2730
Inderide Tablets 2732
Inderide LA Long Acting Capsules .. 2734

Quazepam (May increase drowsiness effect). Products include:

Doral Tablets 2664

Quinapril Hydrochloride (Concurrent use is not recommended). Products include:

Accupril Tablets 1893

Ramipril (Concurrent use is not recommended). Products include:

Altace Capsules 1232

Rauwolfia Serpentina (Concurrent use is not recommended).

No products indexed under this heading.

Rescinnamine (Concurrent use is not recommended).

No products indexed under this heading.

Reserpine (Concurrent use is not recommended). Products include:

Diupres Tablets 1650
Hydropres Tablets................................... 1675
Ser-Ap-Es Tablets 849

Secobarbital Sodium (May increase drowsiness effect). Products include:

Seconal Sodium Pulvules 1474

Selegiline Hydrochloride (Concurrent and/or sequential use is not recommended). Products include:

Eldepryl Tablets 2550

Sodium Nitroprusside (Concurrent use is not recommended).

No products indexed under this heading.

Sotalol Hydrochloride (Concurrent use is not recommended). Products include:

Betapace Tablets 641

Spirapril Hydrochloride (Concurrent use is not recommended).

No products indexed under this heading.

Temazepam (May increase drowsiness effect). Products include:

Restoril Capsules 2284

Terazosin Hydrochloride (Concurrent use is not recommended). Products include:

Hytrin Capsules 430

Thioridazine Hydrochloride (May increase drowsiness effect). Products include:

Mellaril 2269

Thiothixene (May increase drowsiness effect). Products include:

Navane Capsules and Concentrate 2201
Navane Intramuscular 2202

Timolol Maleate (Concurrent use is not recommended). Products include:

Blocadren Tablets 1614
Timolide Tablets....................................... 1748
Timoptic in Ocudose 1753
Timoptic Sterile Ophthalmic Solution 1751
Timoptic-XE 1755

Torsemide (Concurrent use is not recommended). Products include:

Demadex Tablets and Injection 686

Tranylcypromine Sulfate (Concurrent and/or sequential use is not recommended). Products include:

Parnate Tablets 2503

Triazolam (May increase drowsiness effect). Products include:

Halcion Tablets 2611

Trifluoperazine Hydrochloride (May increase drowsiness effect). Products include:

Stelazine 2514

Trimethaphan Camsylate (Concurrent use is not recommended). Products include:

Arfonad Ampuls 2080

Verapamil Hydrochloride (Concurrent use is not recommended). Products include:

Calan SR Caplets 2422
Calan Tablets... 2419
Isoptin Injectable 1344
Isoptin Oral Tablets 1346
Isoptin SR Tablets 1348
Verelan Capsules 1410
Verelan Capsules 2824

Warfarin Sodium (Effect not specified). Products include:

Coumadin 926

Zolpidem Tartrate (May increase drowsiness effect). Products include:

Ambien Tablets... 2416

Food Interactions

Alcohol (May increase drowsiness effect).

ALKA-SELTZER PLUS COLD MEDICINE LIQUI-GELS

(Chlorpheniramine Maleate, Pseudoephedrine Hydrochloride, Acetaminophen) .... ⊞ 706

May interact with hypnotics and sedatives, tranquilizers, monoamine oxidase inhibitors, antihypertensives, and certain other agents. Compounds in these categories include:

Acebutolol Hydrochloride (Concurrent use is not recommended). Products include:

Sectral Capsules 2807

Alprazolam (May increase drowsiness effect; consult your doctor). Products include:

Xanax Tablets 2649

Amlodipine Besylate (Concurrent use is not recommended). Products include:

Lotrel Capsules 840
Norvasc Tablets 1940

Atenolol (Concurrent use is not recommended). Products include:

Tenoretic Tablets...................................... 2845
Tenormin Tablets and I.V. Injection 2847

Benazepril Hydrochloride (Concurrent use is not recommended). Products include:

Lotensin Tablets....................................... 834
Lotensin HCT.. 837
Lotrel Capsules 840

Bendroflumethiazide (Concurrent use is not recommended).

No products indexed under this heading.

Betaxolol Hydrochloride (Concurrent use is not recommended). Products include:

Betoptic Ophthalmic Solution............ 469
Betoptic S Ophthalmic Suspension 471
Kerlone Tablets... 2436

Bisoprolol Fumarate (Concurrent use is not recommended). Products include:

Zebeta Tablets 1413
Ziac 1415

Buspirone Hydrochloride (May increase drowsiness effect; consult your doctor). Products include:

BuSpar 737

Captopril (Concurrent use is not recommended). Products include:

Capoten 739
Capozide 742

Carteolol Hydrochloride (Concurrent use is not recommended). Products include:

Cartrol Tablets 410
Ocupress Ophthalmic Solution, 1% Sterile... ⊙ 309

Chlordiazepoxide (May increase drowsiness effect; consult your doctor). Products include:

Libritabs Tablets 2177
Limbitrol 2180

Chlordiazepoxide Hydrochloride (May increase drowsiness effect; consult your doctor). Products include:

Librax Capsules 2176
Librium Capsules..................................... 2178
Librium Injectable 2179

Chlorothiazide (Concurrent use is not recommended). Products include:

Aldoclor Tablets 1598
Diupres Tablets 1650
Diuril Oral 1653

Chlorothiazide Sodium (Concurrent use is not recommended). Products include:

Diuril Sodium Intravenous 1652

Chlorpromazine (May increase drowsiness effect; consult your doctor). Products include:

Thorazine Suppositories 2523

Chlorpromazine Hydrochloride (May increase drowsiness effect; consult your doctor). Products include:

Thorazine 2523

Chlorprothixene (May increase drowsiness effect; consult your doctor).

No products indexed under this heading.

Chlorprothixene Hydrochloride (May increase drowsiness effect; consult your doctor).

No products indexed under this heading.

Chlorthalidone (Concurrent use is not recommended). Products include:

Combipres Tablets 677
Tenoretic Tablets...................................... 2845
Thalitone 1245

Clonidine (Concurrent use is not recommended). Products include:

Catapres-TTS... 675

Clonidine Hydrochloride (Concurrent use is not recommended). Products include:

Catapres Tablets 674
Combipres Tablets 677

Clorazepate Dipotassium (May increase drowsiness effect; consult your doctor). Products include:

Tranxene 451

Deserpidine (Concurrent use is not recommended).

No products indexed under this heading.

Diazepam (May increase drowsiness effect; consult your doctor). Products include:

Dizac 1809
Valium Injectable 2182
Valium Tablets 2183
Valrelease Capsules 2169

Diazoxide (Concurrent use is not recommended). Products include:

Hyperstat I.V. Injection 2363
Proglycem... 580

Diltiazem Hydrochloride (Concurrent use is not recommended). Products include:

Cardizem CD Capsules 1506
Cardizem SR Capsules 1510
Cardizem Injectable 1508
Cardizem Tablets..................................... 1512
Dilacor XR Extended-release Capsules 2018

Doxazosin Mesylate (Concurrent use is not recommended). Products include:

Cardura Tablets 2186

Droperidol (May increase drowsiness effect; consult your doctor). Products include:

Inapsine Injection.................................... 1296

Enalapril Maleate (Concurrent use is not recommended). Products include:

Vaseretic Tablets 1765
Vasotec Tablets 1771

Enalaprilat (Concurrent use is not recommended). Products include:

Vasotec I.V... 1768

Esmolol Hydrochloride (Concurrent use is not recommended). Products include:

Brevibloc Injection.................................. 1808

Estazolam (May increase drowsiness effect; consult your doctor). Products include:

ProSom Tablets 449

Ethchlorvynol (May increase drowsiness effect; consult your doctor). Products include:

Placidyl Capsules.................................... 448

Ethinamate (May increase drowsiness effect; consult your doctor).

No products indexed under this heading.

Felodipine (Concurrent use is not recommended). Products include:

Plendil Extended-Release Tablets.... 527

Fluphenazine Decanoate (May increase drowsiness effect; consult your doctor). Products include:

Prolixin Decanoate 509

Fluphenazine Enanthate (May increase drowsiness effect; consult your doctor). Products include:

Prolixin Enanthate 509

Fluphenazine Hydrochloride (May increase drowsiness effect; consult your doctor). Products include:

Prolixin 509

Flurazepam Hydrochloride (May increase drowsiness effect; consult your doctor). Products include:

Dalmane Capsules................................... 2173

Fosinopril Sodium (Concurrent use is not recommended). Products include:

Monopril Tablets 757

Furazolidone (Concurrent use not recommended; consult your doctor). Products include:

Furoxone 2046

Furosemide (Concurrent use is not recommended). Products include:

Lasix Injection, Oral Solution and Tablets 1240

Glutethimide (May increase drowsiness effect; consult your doctor).

No products indexed under this heading.

Guanabenz Acetate (Concurrent use is not recommended).

No products indexed under this heading.

Guanethidine Monosulfate (Concurrent use is not recommended). Products include:

Esimil Tablets 822
Ismelin Tablets 827

Haloperidol (May increase drowsiness effect; consult your doctor). Products include:

Haldol Injection, Tablets and Concentrate 1575

Haloperidol Decanoate (May increase drowsiness effect; consult your doctor). Products include:

Haldol Decanoate.................................... 1577

Hydralazine Hydrochloride (Concurrent use is not recommended). Products include:

Apresazide Capsules 808

IMPORTANT NOTE: Always consult each drug listing in the patient's regimen for possible interactions.

Alka-Seltzer Plus Cold **Interactions Index** **38**

- Apresoline Hydrochloride Tablets .. 809
- Ser-Ap-Es Tablets ... 849

Hydrochlorothiazide (Concurrent use is not recommended). Products include:
- Aldactazide ... 2413
- Aldoril Tablets ... 1604
- Apresazide Capsules ... 808
- Capozide ... 742
- Dyazide ... 2479
- Esidrix Tablets ... 821
- Esimil Tablets ... 822
- HydroDIURIL Tablets ... 1674
- Hydropres Tablets ... 1675
- Hyzaar Tablets ... 1677
- Inderide Tablets ... 2732
- Inderide LA Long Acting Capsules .. 2734
- Lopressor HCT Tablets ... 832
- Lotensin HCT ... 837
- Maxzide ... 1380
- Moduretic Tablets ... 1705
- Oretic Tablets ... 443
- Prinzide Tablets ... 1737
- Ser-Ap-Es Tablets ... 849
- Timolide Tablets ... 1748
- Vaseretic Tablets ... 1765
- Zestoretic ... 2850
- Ziac ... 1415

Hydroflumethiazide (Concurrent use is not recommended). Products include:
- Diucardin Tablets ... 2718

Hydroxyzine Hydrochloride (May increase drowsiness effect; consult your doctor). Products include:
- Atarax Tablets & Syrup ... 2185
- Marax Tablets & DF Syrup ... 2200
- Vistaril Intramuscular Solution ... 2216

Indapamide (Concurrent use is not recommended). Products include:
- Lozol Tablets ... 2022

Isocarboxazid (Concurrent use not recommended; consult your doctor).
- No products indexed under this heading.

Isradipine (Concurrent use is not recommended). Products include:
- DynaCirc Capsules ... 2256

Labetalol Hydrochloride (Concurrent use is not recommended). Products include:
- Normodyne Injection ... 2377
- Normodyne Tablets ... 2379
- Trandate ... 1185

Levobunolol Hydrochloride (Concurrent use is not recommended). Products include:
- Betagan ... ◉ 233

Lisinopril (Concurrent use is not recommended). Products include:
- Prinivil Tablets ... 1733
- Prinzide Tablets ... 1737
- Zestoretic ... 2850
- Zestril Tablets ... 2854

Lorazepam (May increase drowsiness effect; consult your doctor). Products include:
- Ativan Injection ... 2698
- Ativan Tablets ... 2700

Losartan Potassium (Concurrent use is not recommended). Products include:
- Cozaar Tablets ... 1628
- Hyzaar Tablets ... 1677

Loxapine Hydrochloride (May increase drowsiness effect; consult your doctor). Products include:
- Loxitane ... 1378

Loxapine Succinate (May increase drowsiness effect; consult your doctor). Products include:
- Loxitane Capsules ... 1378

Mecamylamine Hydrochloride (Concurrent use is not recommended). Products include:
- Inversine Tablets ... 1686

Meprobamate (May increase drowsiness effect; consult your doctor). Products include:
- Miltown Tablets ... 2672
- PMB 200 and PMB 400 ... 2783

Mesoridazine Besylate (May increase drowsiness effect; consult your doctor). Products include:
- Serentil ... 684

Methyclothiazide (Concurrent use is not recommended). Products include:
- Enduron Tablets ... 420

Methyldopa (Concurrent use is not recommended). Products include:
- Aldoclor Tablets ... 1598
- Aldomet Oral ... 1600
- Aldoril Tablets ... 1604

Methyldopate Hydrochloride (Concurrent use is not recommended). Products include:
- Aldomet Ester HCl Injection ... 1602

Metipranolol Hydrochloride (Concurrent use is not recommended). Products include:
- OptiPranolol (Metipranolol 0.3%) Sterile Ophthalmic Solution ... ◉ 258

Metolazone (Concurrent use is not recommended). Products include:
- Mykrox Tablets ... 993
- Zaroxolyn Tablets ... 1000

Metoprolol Succinate (Concurrent use is not recommended). Products include:
- Toprol-XL Tablets ... 565

Metoprolol Tartrate (Concurrent use is not recommended). Products include:
- Lopressor Ampuls ... 830
- Lopressor HCT Tablets ... 832
- Lopressor Tablets ... 830

Metyrosine (Concurrent use is not recommended). Products include:
- Demser Capsules ... 1649

Midazolam Hydrochloride (May increase drowsiness effect; consult your doctor). Products include:
- Versed Injection ... 2170

Minoxidil (Concurrent use is not recommended). Products include:
- Loniten Tablets ... 2618
- Rogaine Topical Solution ... 2637

Moexipril Hydrochloride (Concurrent use is not recommended). Products include:
- Univasc Tablets ... 2410

Molindone Hydrochloride (May increase drowsiness effect; consult your doctor). Products include:
- Moban Tablets and Concentrate ... 1048

Nadolol (Concurrent use is not recommended).
- No products indexed under this heading.

Nicardipine Hydrochloride (Concurrent use is not recommended). Products include:
- Cardene Capsules ... 2095
- Cardene I.V. ... 2709
- Cardene SR Capsules ... 2097

Nifedipine (Concurrent use is not recommended). Products include:
- Adalat Capsules (10 mg and 20 mg) ... 587
- Adalat CC ... 589
- Procardia Capsules ... 1971
- Procardia XL Extended Release Tablets ... 1972

Nisoldipine (Concurrent use is not recommended).
- No products indexed under this heading.

Nitroglycerin (Concurrent use is not recommended). Products include:
- Deponit NTG Transdermal Delivery System ... 2397
- Nitro-Bid IV ... 1523
- Nitro-Bid Ointment ... 1524
- Nitrodisc ... 2047
- Nitro-Dur (nitroglycerin) Transdermal Infusion System ... 1326
- Nitrolingual Spray ... 2027
- Nitrostat Tablets ... 1925
- Transderm-Nitro Transdermal Therapeutic System ... 859

Oxazepam (May increase drowsiness effect; consult your doctor). Products include:
- Serax Capsules ... 2810
- Serax Tablets ... 2810

Penbutolol Sulfate (Concurrent use is not recommended). Products include:
- Levatol ... 2403

Perphenazine (May increase drowsiness effect; consult your doctor). Products include:
- Etrafon ... 2355
- Triavil Tablets ... 1757
- Trilafon ... 2389

Phenelzine Sulfate (Concurrent use not recommended; consult your doctor). Products include:
- Nardil ... 1920

Phenoxybenzamine Hydrochloride (Concurrent use is not recommended). Products include:
- Dibenzyline Capsules ... 2476

Phentolamine Mesylate (Concurrent use is not recommended). Products include:
- Regitine ... 846

Pindolol (Concurrent use is not recommended). Products include:
- Visken Tablets ... 2299

Polythiazide (Concurrent use is not recommended). Products include:
- Minizide Capsules ... 1938

Prazepam (May increase drowsiness effect; consult your doctor).
- No products indexed under this heading.

Prazosin Hydrochloride (Concurrent use is not recommended). Products include:
- Minipress Capsules ... 1937
- Minizide Capsules ... 1938

Prochlorperazine (May increase drowsiness effect; consult your doctor). Products include:
- Compazine ... 2470

Promethazine Hydrochloride (May increase drowsiness effect; consult your doctor). Products include:
- Mepergan Injection ... 2753
- Phenergan with Codeine ... 2777
- Phenergan with Dextromethorphan 2778
- Phenergan Injection ... 2773
- Phenergan Suppositories ... 2775
- Phenergan Syrup ... 2774
- Phenergan Tablets ... 2775
- Phenergan VC ... 2779
- Phenergan VC with Codeine ... 2781

Propofol (May increase drowsiness effect; consult your doctor). Products include:
- Diprivan Injection ... 2833

Propranolol Hydrochloride (Concurrent use is not recommended). Products include:
- Inderal ... 2728
- Inderal LA Long Acting Capsules ... 2730
- Inderide Tablets ... 2732
- Inderide LA Long Acting Capsules .. 2734

Quazepam (May increase drowsiness effect; consult your doctor). Products include:
- Doral Tablets ... 2664

Quinapril Hydrochloride (Concurrent use is not recommended). Products include:
- Accupril Tablets ... 1893

Ramipril (Concurrent use is not recommended). Products include:
- Altace Capsules ... 1232

Rauwolfia Serpentina (Concurrent use is not recommended).
- No products indexed under this heading.

Rescinnamine (Concurrent use is not recommended).
- No products indexed under this heading.

Reserpine (Concurrent use is not recommended). Products include:
- Diupres Tablets ... 1650
- Hydropres Tablets ... 1675
- Ser-Ap-Es Tablets ... 849

Secobarbital Sodium (May increase drowsiness effect; consult your doctor). Products include:
- Seconal Sodium Pulvules ... 1474

Selegiline Hydrochloride (Concurrent use not recommended; consult your doctor). Products include:
- Eldepryl Tablets ... 2550

Sodium Nitroprusside (Concurrent use is not recommended).
- No products indexed under this heading.

Sotalol Hydrochloride (Concurrent use is not recommended). Products include:
- Betapace Tablets ... 641

Spirapril Hydrochloride (Concurrent use is not recommended).
- No products indexed under this heading.

Temazepam (May increase drowsiness effect; consult your doctor). Products include:
- Restoril Capsules ... 2284

Terazosin Hydrochloride (Concurrent use is not recommended). Products include:
- Hytrin Capsules ... 430

Thioridazine Hydrochloride (May increase drowsiness effect; consult your doctor). Products include:
- Mellaril ... 2269

Thiothixene (May increase drowsiness effect; consult your doctor). Products include:
- Navane Capsules and Concentrate 2201
- Navane Intramuscular ... 2202

Timolol Maleate (Concurrent use is not recommended). Products include:
- Blocadren Tablets ... 1614
- Timolide Tablets ... 1748
- Timoptic in Ocudose ... 1753
- Timoptic Sterile Ophthalmic Solution ... 1751
- Timoptic-XE ... 1755

Torsemide (Concurrent use is not recommended). Products include:
- Demadex Tablets and Injection ... 686

Tranylcypromine Sulfate (Concurrent use not recommended; consult your doctor). Products include:
- Parnate Tablets ... 2503

Triazolam (May increase drowsiness effect; consult your doctor). Products include:
- Halcion Tablets ... 2611

Trifluoperazine Hydrochloride (May increase drowsiness effect; consult your doctor). Products include:
- Stelazine ... 2514

Trimethaphan Camsylate (Concurrent use is not recommended). Products include:
- Arfonad Ampuls ... 2080

Verapamil Hydrochloride (Concurrent use is not recommended). Products include:
- Calan SR Caplets ... 2422
- Calan Tablets ... 2419
- Isoptin Injectable ... 1344
- Isoptin Oral Tablets ... 1346
- Isoptin SR Tablets ... 1348
- Verelan Capsules ... 1410

(▣ Described in PDR For Nonprescription Drugs) (◉ Described in PDR For Ophthalmology)

Verelan Capsules 2824

Zolpidem Tartrate (May increase drowsiness effect; consult your doctor). Products include:

Ambien Tablets 2416

Food Interactions

Alcohol (May increase drowsiness effect; consult your doctor).

ALKA-SELTZER PLUS COLD & COUGH MEDICINE

(Aspirin, Chlorpheniramine Maleate, Dextromethorphan Hydrobromide, Phenylpropanolamine Bitartrate) .... ▣ 708

May interact with hypnotics and sedatives, tranquilizers, oral anticoagulants, antihypertensives, monoamine oxidase inhibitors, and certain other agents. Compounds in these categories include:

Acebutolol Hydrochloride (Concurrent use is not recommended). Products include:

Sectral Capsules 2807

Alprazolam (May increase drowsiness effect). Products include:

Xanax Tablets 2649

Amlodipine Besylate (Concurrent use is not recommended). Products include:

Lotrel Capsules 840
Norvasc Tablets 1940

Antiarthritic Drugs, unspecified (Effects not specified).

Antidiabetic Drugs, unspecified (Effects not specified).

Atenolol (Concurrent use is not recommended). Products include:

Tenoretic Tablets 2845
Tenormin Tablets and I.V. Injection 2847

Benazepril Hydrochloride (Concurrent use is not recommended). Products include:

Lotensin Tablets 834
Lotensin HCT 837
Lotrel Capsules 840

Bendroflumethiazide (Concurrent use is not recommended).

No products indexed under this heading.

Betaxolol Hydrochloride (Concurrent use is not recommended). Products include:

Betoptic Ophthalmic Solution 469
Betoptic S Ophthalmic Suspension 471
Kerlone Tablets 2436

Bisoprolol Fumarate (Concurrent use is not recommended). Products include:

Zebeta Tablets 1413
Ziac 1415

Buspirone Hydrochloride (May increase drowsiness effect). Products include:

BuSpar 737

Captopril (Concurrent use is not recommended). Products include:

Capoten 739
Capozide 742

Carteolol Hydrochloride (Concurrent use is not recommended). Products include:

Cartrol Tablets 410
Ocupress Ophthalmic Solution, 1% Sterile .... ⊙ 309

Chlordiazepoxide (May increase drowsiness effect). Products include:

Libritabs Tablets 2177
Limbitrol 2180

Chlordiazepoxide Hydrochloride (May increase drowsiness effect). Products include:

Librax Capsules 2176
Librium Capsules 2178
Librium Injectable 2179

Chlorothiazide (Concurrent use is not recommended). Products include:

Aldoclor Tablets 1598
Diupres Tablets 1650
Diuril Oral 1653

Chlorothiazide Sodium (Concurrent use is not recommended). Products include:

Diuril Sodium Intravenous 1652

Chlorpromazine (May increase drowsiness effect). Products include:

Thorazine Suppositories 2523

Chlorpromazine Hydrochloride (May increase drowsiness effect). Products include:

Thorazine 2523

Chlorprothixene (May increase drowsiness effect).

No products indexed under this heading.

Chlorprothixene Hydrochloride (May increase drowsiness effect).

No products indexed under this heading.

Chlorthalidone (Concurrent use is not recommended). Products include:

Combipres Tablets 677
Tenoretic Tablets 2845
Thalitone 1245

Clonidine (Concurrent use is not recommended). Products include:

Catapres-TTS 675

Clonidine Hydrochloride (Concurrent use is not recommended). Products include:

Catapres Tablets 674
Combipres Tablets 677

Clorazepate Dipotassium (May increase drowsiness effect). Products include:

Tranxene 451

Deserpidine (Concurrent use is not recommended).

No products indexed under this heading.

Diazepam (May increase drowsiness effect). Products include:

Dizac 1809
Valium Injectable 2182
Valium Tablets 2183
Valrelease Capsules 2169

Diazoxide (Concurrent use is not recommended). Products include:

Hyperstat I.V. Injection 2363
Proglycem 580

Dicumarol (Concurrent use is not recommended).

No products indexed under this heading.

Diltiazem Hydrochloride (Concurrent use is not recommended). Products include:

Cardizem CD Capsules 1506
Cardizem SR Capsules 1510
Cardizem Injectable 1508
Cardizem Tablets 1512
Dilacor XR Extended-release Capsules 2018

Doxazosin Mesylate (Concurrent use is not recommended). Products include:

Cardura Tablets 2186

Droperidol (May increase drowsiness effect). Products include:

Inapsine Injection 1296

Enalapril Maleate (Concurrent use is not recommended). Products include:

Vaseretic Tablets 1765
Vasotec Tablets 1771

Enalaprilat (Concurrent use is not recommended). Products include:

Vasotec I.V. 1768

Esmolol Hydrochloride (Concurrent use is not recommended). Products include:

Brevibloc Injection 1808

Estazolam (May increase drowsiness effect). Products include:

ProSom Tablets 449

Ethchlorvynol (May increase drowsiness effect). Products include:

Placidyl Capsules 448

Ethinamate (May increase drowsiness effect).

No products indexed under this heading.

Felodipine (Concurrent use is not recommended). Products include:

Plendil Extended-Release Tablets 527

Fluphenazine Decanoate (May increase drowsiness effect). Products include:

Prolixin Decanoate 509

Fluphenazine Enanthate (May increase drowsiness effect). Products include:

Prolixin Enanthate 509

Fluphenazine Hydrochloride (May increase drowsiness effect). Products include:

Prolixin 509

Flurazepam Hydrochloride (May increase drowsiness effect). Products include:

Dalmane Capsules 2173

Fosinopril Sodium (Concurrent use is not recommended). Products include:

Monopril Tablets 757

Furazolidone (Concurrent or sequential use is not recommended). Products include:

Furoxone 2046

Furosemide (Concurrent use is not recommended). Products include:

Lasix Injection, Oral Solution and Tablets 1240

Glutethimide (May increase drowsiness effect).

No products indexed under this heading.

Guanabenz Acetate (Concurrent use is not recommended).

No products indexed under this heading.

Guanethidine Monosulfate (Concurrent use is not recommended). Products include:

Esimil Tablets 822
Ismelin Tablets 827

Haloperidol (May increase drowsiness effect). Products include:

Haldol Injection, Tablets and Concentrate 1575

Haloperidol Decanoate (May increase drowsiness effect). Products include:

Haldol Decanoate 1577

Hydralazine Hydrochloride (Concurrent use is not recommended). Products include:

Apresazide Capsules 808
Apresoline Hydrochloride Tablets .. 809
Ser-Ap-Es Tablets 849

Hydrochlorothiazide (Concurrent use is not recommended). Products include:

Aldactazide 2413
Aldoril Tablets 1604
Apresazide Capsules 808
Capozide 742
Dyazide 2479
Esidrix Tablets 821
Esimil Tablets 822
HydroDIURIL Tablets 1674
Hydropres Tablets 1675
Hyzaar Tablets 1677
Inderide Tablets 2732
Inderide LA Long Acting Capsules .. 2734
Lopressor HCT Tablets 832
Lotensin HCT 837
Maxzide 1380
Moduretic Tablets 1705
Oretic Tablets 443
Prinzide Tablets 1737
Ser-Ap-Es Tablets 849
Timolide Tablets 1748
Vaseretic Tablets 1765
Zestoretic 2850
Ziac 1415

Hydroflumethiazide (Concurrent use is not recommended). Products include:

Diucardin Tablets 2718

Hydroxyzine Hydrochloride (May increase drowsiness effect). Products include:

Atarax Tablets & Syrup 2185
Marax Tablets & DF Syrup 2200
Vistaril Intramuscular Solution 2216

Indapamide (Concurrent use is not recommended). Products include:

Lozol Tablets 2022

Isocarboxazid (Concurrent or sequential use is not recommended).

No products indexed under this heading.

Isradipine (Concurrent use is not recommended). Products include:

DynaCirc Capsules 2256

Labetalol Hydrochloride (Concurrent use is not recommended). Products include:

Normodyne Injection 2377
Normodyne Tablets 2379
Trandate 1185

Levobunolol Hydrochloride (Concurrent use is not recommended). Products include:

Betagan .... ⊙ 233

Lisinopril (Concurrent use is not recommended). Products include:

Prinivil Tablets 1733
Prinzide Tablets 1737
Zestoretic 2850
Zestril Tablets 2854

Lorazepam (May increase drowsiness effect). Products include:

Ativan Injection 2698
Ativan Tablets 2700

Losartan Potassium (Concurrent use is not recommended). Products include:

Cozaar Tablets 1628
Hyzaar Tablets 1677

Loxapine Hydrochloride (May increase drowsiness effect). Products include:

Loxitane 1378

Loxapine Succinate (May increase drowsiness effect). Products include:

Loxitane Capsules 1378

Mecamylamine Hydrochloride (Concurrent use is not recommended). Products include:

Inversine Tablets 1686

Meprobamate (May increase drowsiness effect). Products include:

Miltown Tablets 2672
PMB 200 and PMB 400 2783

Mesoridazine Besylate (May increase drowsiness effect). Products include:

Serentil 684

Methyclothiazide (Concurrent use is not recommended). Products include:

Enduron Tablets 420

Methyldopa (Concurrent use is not recommended). Products include:

Aldoclor Tablets 1598
Aldomet Oral 1600
Aldoril Tablets 1604

Methyldopate Hydrochloride (Concurrent use is not recommended). Products include:

Aldomet Ester HCl Injection 1602

Metolazone (Concurrent use is not recommended). Products include:

Mykrox Tablets 993
Zaroxolyn Tablets 1000

IMPORTANT NOTE: Always consult each drug listing in the patient's regimen for possible interactions.

Alka-Seltzer Plus Cold & Cough **Interactions Index** 40

Metoprolol Succinate (Concurrent use is not recommended). Products include:
- Toprol-XL Tablets 565

Metoprolol Tartrate (Concurrent use is not recommended). Products include:
- Lopressor Ampuls 830
- Lopressor HCT Tablets 832
- Lopressor Tablets 830

Metyrosine (Concurrent use is not recommended). Products include:
- Demser Capsules 1649

Midazolam Hydrochloride (May increase drowsiness effect). Products include:
- Versed Injection 2170

Minoxidil (Concurrent use is not recommended). Products include:
- Loniten Tablets 2618
- Rogaine Topical Solution 2637

Moexipril Hydrochloride (Concurrent use is not recommended). Products include:
- Univasc Tablets 2410

Molindone Hydrochloride (May increase drowsiness effect). Products include:
- Moban Tablets and Concentrate 1048

Nadolol (Concurrent use is not recommended).
- No products indexed under this heading.

Nicardipine Hydrochloride (Concurrent use is not recommended). Products include:
- Cardene Capsules 2095
- Cardene I.V. 2709
- Cardene SR Capsules 2097

Nifedipine (Concurrent use is not recommended). Products include:
- Adalat Capsules (10 mg and 20 mg) 587
- Adalat CC 589
- Procardia Capsules 1971
- Procardia XL Extended Release Tablets 1972

Nisoldipine (Concurrent use is not recommended).
- No products indexed under this heading.

Nitroglycerin (Concurrent use is not recommended). Products include:
- Deponit NTG Transdermal Delivery System 2397
- Nitro-Bid IV 1523
- Nitro-Bid Ointment 1524
- Nitrodisc 2047
- Nitro-Dur (nitroglycerin) Transdermal Infusion System 1326
- Nitrolingual Spray 2027
- Nitrostat Tablets 1925
- Transderm-Nitro Transdermal Therapeutic System 859

Oxazepam (May increase drowsiness effect). Products include:
- Serax Capsules 2810
- Serax Tablets 2810

Penbutolol Sulfate (Concurrent use is not recommended). Products include:
- Levatol 2403

Perphenazine (May increase drowsiness effect). Products include:
- Etrafon 2355
- Triavil Tablets 1757
- Trilafon 2389

Phenelzine Sulfate (Concurrent or sequential use is not recommended). Products include:
- Nardil 1920

Phenoxybenzamine Hydrochloride (Concurrent use is not recommended). Products include:
- Dibenzyline Capsules 2476

Phentolamine Mesylate (Concurrent use is not recommended). Products include:
- Regitine 846

Pindolol (Concurrent use is not recommended). Products include:
- Visken Tablets 2299

Polythiazide (Concurrent use is not recommended). Products include:
- Minizide Capsules 1938

Prazepam (May increase drowsiness effect).
- No products indexed under this heading.

Prazosin Hydrochloride (Concurrent use is not recommended). Products include:
- Minipress Capsules 1937
- Minizide Capsules 1938

Prochlorperazine (May increase drowsiness effect). Products include:
- Compazine 2470

Promethazine Hydrochloride (May increase drowsiness effect). Products include:
- Mepergan Injection 2753
- Phenergan with Codeine 2777
- Phenergan with Dextromethorphan 2778
- Phenergan Injection 2773
- Phenergan Suppositories 2775
- Phenergan Syrup 2774
- Phenergan Tablets 2775
- Phenergan VC 2779
- Phenergan VC with Codeine 2781

Propofol (May increase drowsiness effect). Products include:
- Diprivan Injection 2833

Propranolol Hydrochloride (Concurrent use is not recommended). Products include:
- Inderal 2728
- Inderal LA Long Acting Capsules 2730
- Inderide Tablets 2732
- Inderide LA Long Acting Capsules 2734

Quazepam (May increase drowsiness effect). Products include:
- Doral Tablets 2664

Quinapril Hydrochloride (Concurrent use is not recommended). Products include:
- Accupril Tablets 1893

Ramipril (Concurrent use is not recommended). Products include:
- Altace Capsules 1232

Rauwolfia Serpentina (Concurrent use is not recommended).
- No products indexed under this heading.

Rescinnamine (Concurrent use is not recommended).
- No products indexed under this heading.

Reserpine (Concurrent use is not recommended). Products include:
- Diupres Tablets 1650
- Hydropres Tablets 1675
- Ser-Ap-Es Tablets 849

Secobarbital Sodium (May increase drowsiness effect). Products include:
- Seconal Sodium Pulvules 1474

Selegiline Hydrochloride (Concurrent or sequential use is not recommended). Products include:
- Eldepryl Tablets 2550

Sodium Nitroprusside (Concurrent use is not recommended).
- No products indexed under this heading.

Sotalol Hydrochloride (Concurrent use is not recommended). Products include:
- Betapace Tablets 641

Spirapril Hydrochloride (Concurrent use is not recommended).
- No products indexed under this heading.

Temazepam (May increase drowsiness effect). Products include:
- Restoril Capsules 2284

Terazosin Hydrochloride (Concurrent use is not recommended). Products include:
- Hytrin Capsules 430

Thioridazine Hydrochloride (May increase drowsiness effect). Products include:
- Mellaril 2269

Thiothixene (May increase drowsiness effect). Products include:
- Navane Capsules and Concentrate 2201
- Navane Intramuscular 2202

Timolol Maleate (Concurrent use is not recommended). Products include:
- Blocadren Tablets 1614
- Timolide Tablets 1748
- Timoptic in Ocudose 1753
- Timoptic Sterile Ophthalmic Solution 1751
- Timoptic-XE 1755

Torsemide (Concurrent use is not recommended). Products include:
- Demadex Tablets and Injection 686

Tranylcypromine Sulfate (Concurrent or sequential use is not recommended). Products include:
- Parnate Tablets 2503

Triazolam (May increase drowsiness effect). Products include:
- Halcion Tablets 2611

Trifluoperazine Hydrochloride (May increase drowsiness effect). Products include:
- Stelazine 2514

Trimethaphan Camsylate (Concurrent use is not recommended). Products include:
- Arfonad Ampuls 2080

Verapamil Hydrochloride (Concurrent use is not recommended). Products include:
- Calan SR Caplets 2422
- Calan Tablets 2419
- Isoptin Injectable 1344
- Isoptin Oral Tablets 1346
- Isoptin SR Tablets 1348
- Verelan Capsules 1410
- Verelan Capsules 2824

Warfarin Sodium (Concurrent use is not recommended). Products include:
- Coumadin 926

Zolpidem Tartrate (May increase drowsiness effect). Products include:
- Ambien Tablets 2416

Food Interactions

Alcohol (Increases drowsiness effect).

ALKA-SELTZER PLUS COLD & COUGH MEDICINE LIQUI-GELS

(Dextromethorphan Hydrobromide, Chlorpheniramine Maleate, Pseudoephedrine Hydrochloride, Acetaminophen) .... ▣ 705

May interact with hypnotics and sedatives, tranquilizers, monoamine oxidase inhibitors, antihypertensives, and certain other agents. Compounds in these categories include:

Acebutolol Hydrochloride (Concurrent use is not recommended). Products include:
- Sectral Capsules 2807

Alprazolam (May increase drowsiness effect; consult your doctor). Products include:
- Xanax Tablets 2649

Amlodipine Besylate (Concurrent use is not recommended). Products include:
- Lotrel Capsules 840
- Norvasc Tablets 1940

Atenolol (Concurrent use is not recommended). Products include:
- Tenoretic Tablets 2845
- Tenormin Tablets and I.V. Injection 2847

Benazepril Hydrochloride (Concurrent use is not recommended). Products include:
- Lotensin Tablets 834
- Lotensin HCT 837
- Lotrel Capsules 840

Bendroflumethiazide (Concurrent use is not recommended).
- No products indexed under this heading.

Betaxolol Hydrochloride (Concurrent use is not recommended). Products include:
- Betoptic Ophthalmic Solution 469
- Betoptic S Ophthalmic Suspension 471
- Kerlone Tablets 2436

Bisoprolol Fumarate (Concurrent use is not recommended). Products include:
- Zebeta Tablets 1413
- Ziac 1415

Buspirone Hydrochloride (May increase drowsiness effect; consult your doctor). Products include:
- BuSpar 737

Captopril (Concurrent use is not recommended). Products include:
- Capoten 739
- Capozide 742

Carteolol Hydrochloride (Concurrent use is not recommended). Products include:
- Cartrol Tablets 410
- Ocupress Ophthalmic Solution, 1% Sterile .... ⊙ 309

Chlordiazepoxide (May increase drowsiness effect; consult your doctor). Products include:
- Libritabs Tablets 2177
- Limbitrol 2180

Chlordiazepoxide Hydrochloride (May increase drowsiness effect; consult your doctor). Products include:
- Librax Capsules 2176
- Librium Capsules 2178
- Librium Injectable 2179

Chlorothiazide (Concurrent use is not recommended). Products include:
- Aldoclor Tablets 1598
- Diupres Tablets 1650
- Diuril Oral 1653

Chlorothiazide Sodium (Concurrent use is not recommended). Products include:
- Diuril Sodium Intravenous 1652

Chlorpromazine (May increase drowsiness effect; consult your doctor). Products include:
- Thorazine Suppositories 2523

Chlorpromazine Hydrochloride (May increase drowsiness effect; consult your doctor). Products include:
- Thorazine 2523

Chlorprothixene (May increase drowsiness effect; consult your doctor).
- No products indexed under this heading.

Chlorprothixene Hydrochloride (May increase drowsiness effect; consult your doctor).
- No products indexed under this heading.

Chlorthalidone (Concurrent use is not recommended). Products include:
- Combipres Tablets 677
- Tenoretic Tablets 2845
- Thalitone 1245

Clonidine (Concurrent use is not recommended). Products include:
- Catapres-TTS 675

Clonidine Hydrochloride (Concurrent use is not recommended). Products include:
- Catapres Tablets 674

(▣ Described in PDR For Nonprescription Drugs) (⊙ Described in PDR For Ophthalmology)

Combipres Tablets 677

Clorazepate Dipotassium (May increase drowsiness effect; consult your doctor). Products include:
- Tranxene 451

Deserpidine (Concurrent use is not recommended).
- No products indexed under this heading.

Diazepam (May increase drowsiness effect; consult your doctor). Products include:
- Dizac 1809
- Valium Injectable 2182
- Valium Tablets 2183
- Valrelease Capsules 2169

Diazoxide (Concurrent use is not recommended). Products include:
- Hyperstat I.V. Injection 2363
- Proglycem 580

Diltiazem Hydrochloride (Concurrent use is not recommended). Products include:
- Cardizem CD Capsules 1506
- Cardizem SR Capsules 1510
- Cardizem Injectable 1508
- Cardizem Tablets 1512
- Dilacor XR Extended-release Capsules 2018

Doxazosin Mesylate (Concurrent use is not recommended). Products include:
- Cardura Tablets 2186

Droperidol (May increase drowsiness effect; consult your doctor). Products include:
- Inapsine Injection 1296

Enalapril Maleate (Concurrent use is not recommended). Products include:
- Vaseretic Tablets 1765
- Vasotec Tablets 1771

Enalaprilat (Concurrent use is not recommended). Products include:
- Vasotec I.V. 1768

Esmolol Hydrochloride (Concurrent use is not recommended). Products include:
- Brevibloc Injection 1808

Estazolam (May increase drowsiness effect; consult your doctor). Products include:
- ProSom Tablets 449

Ethchlorvynol (May increase drowsiness effect; consult your doctor). Products include:
- Placidyl Capsules 448

Ethinamate (May increase drowsiness effect; consult your doctor).
- No products indexed under this heading.

Felodipine (Concurrent use is not recommended). Products include:
- Plendil Extended-Release Tablets 527

Fluphenazine Decanoate (May increase drowsiness effect; consult your doctor). Products include:
- Prolixin Decanoate 509

Fluphenazine Enanthate (May increase drowsiness effect; consult your doctor). Products include:
- Prolixin Enanthate 509

Fluphenazine Hydrochloride (May increase drowsiness effect; consult your doctor). Products include:
- Prolixin 509

Flurazepam Hydrochloride (May increase drowsiness effect; consult your doctor). Products include:
- Dalmane Capsules 2173

Fosinopril Sodium (Concurrent use is not recommended). Products include:
- Monopril Tablets 757

Furazolidone (Concurrent use not recommended; consult your doctor). Products include:
- Furoxone 2046

Furosemide (Concurrent use is not recommended). Products include:
- Lasix Injection, Oral Solution and Tablets 1240

Glutethimide (May increase drowsiness effect; consult your doctor).
- No products indexed under this heading.

Guanabenz Acetate (Concurrent use is not recommended).
- No products indexed under this heading.

Guanethidine Monosulfate (Concurrent use is not recommended). Products include:
- Esimil Tablets 822
- Ismelin Tablets 827

Haloperidol (May increase drowsiness effect; consult your doctor). Products include:
- Haldol Injection, Tablets and Concentrate 1575

Haloperidol Decanoate (May increase drowsiness effect; consult your doctor). Products include:
- Haldol Decanoate 1577

Hydralazine Hydrochloride (Concurrent use is not recommended). Products include:
- Apresazide Capsules 808
- Apresoline Hydrochloride Tablets 809
- Ser-Ap-Es Tablets 849

Hydrochlorothiazide (Concurrent use is not recommended). Products include:
- Aldactazide 2413
- Aldoril Tablets 1604
- Apresazide Capsules 808
- Capozide 742
- Dyazide 2479
- Esidrix Tablets 821
- Esimil Tablets 822
- HydroDIURIL Tablets 1674
- Hydropres Tablets 1675
- Hyzaar Tablets 1677
- Inderide Tablets 2732
- Inderide LA Long Acting Capsules 2734
- Lopressor HCT Tablets 832
- Lotensin HCT 837
- Maxzide 1380
- Moduretic Tablets 1705
- Oretic Tablets 443
- Prinzide Tablets 1737
- Ser-Ap-Es Tablets 849
- Timolide Tablets 1748
- Vaseretic Tablets 1765
- Zestoretic 2850
- Ziac 1415

Hydroflumethiazide (Concurrent use is not recommended). Products include:
- Diucardin Tablets 2718

Hydroxyzine Hydrochloride (May increase drowsiness effect; consult your doctor). Products include:
- Atarax Tablets & Syrup 2185
- Marax Tablets & DF Syrup 2200
- Vistaril Intramuscular Solution 2216

Indapamide (Concurrent use is not recommended). Products include:
- Lozol Tablets 2022

Isocarboxazid (Concurrent use not recommended; consult your doctor).
- No products indexed under this heading.

Isradipine (Concurrent use is not recommended). Products include:
- DynaCirc Capsules 2256

Labetalol Hydrochloride (Concurrent use is not recommended). Products include:
- Normodyne Injection 2377
- Normodyne Tablets 2379
- Trandate 1185

Levobunolol Hydrochloride (Concurrent use is not recommended). Products include:
- Betagan .... ◉ 233

Lisinopril (Concurrent use is not recommended). Products include:
- Prinivil Tablets 1733
- Prinzide Tablets 1737
- Zestoretic 2850
- Zestril Tablets 2854

Lorazepam (May increase drowsiness effect; consult your doctor). Products include:
- Ativan Injection 2698
- Ativan Tablets 2700

Losartan Potassium (Concurrent use is not recommended). Products include:
- Cozaar Tablets 1628
- Hyzaar Tablets 1677

Loxapine Hydrochloride (May increase drowsiness effect; consult your doctor). Products include:
- Loxitane 1378

Loxapine Succinate (May increase drowsiness effect; consult your doctor). Products include:
- Loxitane Capsules 1378

Mecamylamine Hydrochloride (Concurrent use is not recommended). Products include:
- Inversine Tablets 1686

Meprobamate (May increase drowsiness effect; consult your doctor). Products include:
- Miltown Tablets 2672
- PMB 200 and PMB 400 2783

Mesoridazine Besylate (May increase drowsiness effect; consult your doctor). Products include:
- Serentil 684

Methyclothiazide (Concurrent use is not recommended). Products include:
- Enduron Tablets 420

Methyldopa (Concurrent use is not recommended). Products include:
- Aldoclor Tablets 1598
- Aldomet Oral 1600
- Aldoril Tablets 1604

Methyldopate Hydrochloride (Concurrent use is not recommended). Products include:
- Aldomet Ester HCl Injection 1602

Metipranolol Hydrochloride (Concurrent use is not recommended). Products include:
- OptiPranolol (Metipranolol 0.3%) Sterile Ophthalmic Solution .... ◉ 258

Metolazone (Concurrent use is not recommended). Products include:
- Mykrox Tablets 993
- Zaroxolyn Tablets 1000

Metoprolol Succinate (Concurrent use is not recommended). Products include:
- Toprol-XL Tablets 565

Metoprolol Tartrate (Concurrent use is not recommended). Products include:
- Lopressor Ampuls 830
- Lopressor HCT Tablets 832
- Lopressor Tablets 830

Metyrosine (Concurrent use is not recommended). Products include:
- Demser Capsules 1649

Midazolam Hydrochloride (May increase drowsiness effect; consult your doctor). Products include:
- Versed Injection 2170

Minoxidil (Concurrent use is not recommended). Products include:
- Loniten Tablets 2618
- Rogaine Topical Solution 2637

Moexipril Hydrochloride (Concurrent use is not recommended). Products include:
- Univasc Tablets 2410

Molindone Hydrochloride (May increase drowsiness effect; consult your doctor). Products include:
- Moban Tablets and Concentrate 1048

Nadolol (Concurrent use is not recommended).
- No products indexed under this heading.

Nicardipine Hydrochloride (Concurrent use is not recommended). Products include:
- Cardene Capsules 2095
- Cardene I.V. 2709
- Cardene SR Capsules 2097

Nifedipine (Concurrent use is not recommended). Products include:
- Adalat Capsules (10 mg and 20 mg) 587
- Adalat CC 589
- Procardia Capsules 1971
- Procardia XL Extended Release Tablets 1972

Nisoldipine (Concurrent use is not recommended).
- No products indexed under this heading.

Nitroglycerin (Concurrent use is not recommended). Products include:
- Deponit NTG Transdermal Delivery System 2397
- Nitro-Bid IV 1523
- Nitro-Bid Ointment 1524
- Nitrodisc 2047
- Nitro-Dur (nitroglycerin) Transdermal Infusion System 1326
- Nitrolingual Spray 2027
- Nitrostat Tablets 1925
- Transderm-Nitro Transdermal Therapeutic System 859

Oxazepam (May increase drowsiness effect; consult your doctor). Products include:
- Serax Capsules 2810
- Serax Tablets 2810

Penbutolol Sulfate (Concurrent use is not recommended). Products include:
- Levatol 2403

Perphenazine (May increase drowsiness effect; consult your doctor). Products include:
- Etrafon 2355
- Triavil Tablets 1757
- Trilafon 2389

Phenelzine Sulfate (Concurrent use not recommended; consult your doctor). Products include:
- Nardil 1920

Phenoxybenzamine Hydrochloride (Concurrent use is not recommended). Products include:
- Dibenzyline Capsules 2476

Phentolamine Mesylate (Concurrent use is not recommended). Products include:
- Regitine 846

Pindolol (Concurrent use is not recommended). Products include:
- Visken Tablets 2299

Polythiazide (Concurrent use is not recommended). Products include:
- Minizide Capsules 1938

Prazepam (May increase drowsiness effect; consult your doctor).
- No products indexed under this heading.

Prazosin Hydrochloride (Concurrent use is not recommended). Products include:
- Minipress Capsules 1937
- Minizide Capsules 1938

Prochlorperazine (May increase drowsiness effect; consult your doctor). Products include:
- Compazine 2470

IMPORTANT NOTE: Always consult each drug listing in the patient's regimen for possible interactions.

Promethazine Hydrochloride (May increase drowsiness effect; consult your doctor). Products include:
- Mepergan Injection 2753
- Phenergan with Codeine 2777
- Phenergan with Dextromethorphan 2778
- Phenergan Injection 2773
- Phenergan Suppositories 2775
- Phenergan Syrup 2774
- Phenergan Tablets 2775
- Phenergan VC 2779
- Phenergan VC with Codeine 2781

Propofol (May increase drowsiness effect; consult your doctor). Products include:
- Diprivan Injection 2833

Propranolol Hydrochloride (Concurrent use is not recommended). Products include:
- Inderal 2728
- Inderal LA Long Acting Capsules 2730
- Inderide Tablets 2732
- Inderide LA Long Acting Capsules .. 2734

Quazepam (May increase drowsiness effect; consult your doctor). Products include:
- Doral Tablets 2664

Quinapril Hydrochloride (Concurrent use is not recommended). Products include:
- Accupril Tablets 1893

Ramipril (Concurrent use is not recommended). Products include:
- Altace Capsules 1232

Rauwolfia Serpentina (Concurrent use is not recommended).
- No products indexed under this heading.

Rescinnamine (Concurrent use is not recommended).
- No products indexed under this heading.

Reserpine (Concurrent use is not recommended). Products include:
- Diupres Tablets 1650
- Hydropres Tablets 1675
- Ser-Ap-Es Tablets 849

Secobarbital Sodium (May increase drowsiness effect; consult your doctor). Products include:
- Seconal Sodium Pulvules 1474

Selegiline Hydrochloride (Concurrent use not recommended; consult your doctor). Products include:
- Eldepryl Tablets 2550

Sodium Nitroprusside (Concurrent use is not recommended).
- No products indexed under this heading.

Sotalol Hydrochloride (Concurrent use is not recommended). Products include:
- Betapace Tablets 641

Spirapril Hydrochloride (Concurrent use is not recommended).
- No products indexed under this heading.

Temazepam (May increase drowsiness effect; consult your doctor). Products include:
- Restoril Capsules 2284

Terazosin Hydrochloride (Concurrent use is not recommended). Products include:
- Hytrin Capsules 430

Thioridazine Hydrochloride (May increase drowsiness effect; consult your doctor). Products include:
- Mellaril 2269

Thiothixene (May increase drowsiness effect; consult your doctor). Products include:
- Navane Capsules and Concentrate 2201
- Navane Intramuscular 2202

Timolol Maleate (Concurrent use is not recommended). Products include:
- Blocadren Tablets 1614
- Timolide Tablets 1748
- Timoptic in Ocudose 1753
- Timoptic Sterile Ophthalmic Solution 1751
- Timoptic-XE 1755

Torsemide (Concurrent use is not recommended). Products include:
- Demadex Tablets and Injection 686

Tranylcypromine Sulfate (Concurrent use not recommended; consult your doctor). Products include:
- Parnate Tablets 2503

Triazolam (May increase drowsiness effect; consult your doctor). Products include:
- Halcion Tablets 2611

Trifluoperazine Hydrochloride (May increase drowsiness effect; consult your doctor). Products include:
- Stelazine 2514

Trimethaphan Camsylate (Concurrent use is not recommended). Products include:
- Arfonad Ampuls 2080

Verapamil Hydrochloride (Concurrent use is not recommended). Products include:
- Calan SR Caplets 2422
- Calan Tablets 2419
- Isoptin Injectable 1344
- Isoptin Oral Tablets 1346
- Isoptin SR Tablets 1348
- Verelan Capsules 1410
- Verelan Capsules 2824

Zolpidem Tartrate (May increase drowsiness effect; consult your doctor). Products include:
- Ambien Tablets 2416

Food Interactions

Alcohol (May increase drowsiness effect; consult your doctor).

ALKA-SELTZER PLUS NIGHT-TIME COLD MEDICINE

(Aspirin, Phenylpropanolamine Bitartrate, Doxylamine Succinate, Dextromethorphan Hydrobromide) ▣ 707

May interact with hypnotics and sedatives, tranquilizers, oral anticoagulants, monoamine oxidase inhibitors, antihypertensives, and certain other agents. Compounds in these categories include:

Acebutolol Hydrochloride (Concurrent use is not recommended). Products include:
- Sectral Capsules 2807

Alprazolam (May increase drowsiness effect). Products include:
- Xanax Tablets 2649

Amlodipine Besylate (Concurrent use is not recommended). Products include:
- Lotrel Capsules 840
- Norvasc Tablets 1940

Antiarthritic Drugs, unspecified (Effect not specified).

Antidiabetic Drugs, unspecified (Effect not specified).

Antigout Drugs, unspecified (Effect not specified).

Atenolol (Concurrent use is not recommended). Products include:
- Tenoretic Tablets 2845
- Tenormin Tablets and I.V. Injection 2847

Benazepril Hydrochloride (Concurrent use is not recommended). Products include:
- Lotensin Tablets 834
- Lotensin HCT 837
- Lotrel Capsules 840

Bendroflumethiazide (Concurrent use is not recommended).
- No products indexed under this heading.

Betaxolol Hydrochloride (Concurrent use is not recommended). Products include:
- Betoptic Ophthalmic Solution 469
- Betoptic S Ophthalmic Suspension 471
- Kerlone Tablets 2436

Bisoprolol Fumarate (Concurrent use is not recommended). Products include:
- Zebeta Tablets 1413
- Ziac 1415

Buspirone Hydrochloride (May increase drowsiness effect). Products include:
- BuSpar 737

Captopril (Concurrent use is not recommended). Products include:
- Capoten 739
- Capozide 742

Carteolol Hydrochloride (Concurrent use is not recommended). Products include:
- Cartrol Tablets 410
- Ocupress Ophthalmic Solution, 1% Sterile .... ⊙ 309

Chlordiazepoxide (May increase drowsiness effect). Products include:
- Libritabs Tablets 2177
- Limbitrol 2180

Chlordiazepoxide Hydrochloride (May increase drowsiness effect). Products include:
- Librax Capsules 2176
- Librium Capsules 2178
- Librium Injectable 2179

Chlorothiazide (Concurrent use is not recommended). Products include:
- Aldoclor Tablets 1598
- Diupres Tablets 1650
- Diuril Oral 1653

Chlorothiazide Sodium (Concurrent use is not recommended). Products include:
- Diuril Sodium Intravenous 1652

Chlorpromazine (May increase drowsiness effect). Products include:
- Thorazine Suppositories 2523

Chlorpromazine Hydrochloride (May increase drowsiness effect). Products include:
- Thorazine 2523

Chlorprothixene (May increase drowsiness effect).
- No products indexed under this heading.

Chlorprothixene Hydrochloride (May increase drowsiness effect).
- No products indexed under this heading.

Chlorthalidone (Concurrent use is not recommended). Products include:
- Combipres Tablets 677
- Tenoretic Tablets 2845
- Thalitone 1245

Clonidine (Concurrent use is not recommended). Products include:
- Catapres-TTS 675

Clonidine Hydrochloride (Concurrent use is not recommended). Products include:
- Catapres Tablets 674
- Combipres Tablets 677

Clorazepate Dipotassium (May increase drowsiness effect). Products include:
- Tranxene 451

Deserpidine (Concurrent use is not recommended).
- No products indexed under this heading.

Diazepam (May increase drowsiness effect). Products include:
- Dizac 1809
- Valium Injectable 2182
- Valium Tablets 2183
- Valrelease Capsules 2169

Diazoxide (Concurrent use is not recommended). Products include:
- Hyperstat I.V. Injection 2363
- Proglycem 580

Dicumarol (Effect not specified).
- No products indexed under this heading.

Diltiazem Hydrochloride (Concurrent use is not recommended). Products include:
- Cardizem CD Capsules 1506
- Cardizem SR Capsules 1510
- Cardizem Injectable 1508
- Cardizem Tablets 1512
- Dilacor XR Extended-release Capsules 2018

Doxazosin Mesylate (Concurrent use is not recommended). Products include:
- Cardura Tablets 2186

Droperidol (May increase drowsiness effect). Products include:
- Inapsine Injection 1296

Enalapril Maleate (Concurrent use is not recommended). Products include:
- Vaseretic Tablets 1765
- Vasotec Tablets 1771

Enalaprilat (Concurrent use is not recommended). Products include:
- Vasotec I.V. 1768

Esmolol Hydrochloride (Concurrent use is not recommended). Products include:
- Brevibloc Injection 1808

Estazolam (May increase the drowsiness effect). Products include:
- ProSom Tablets 449

Ethchlorvynol (May increase the drowsiness effect). Products include:
- Placidyl Capsules 448

Ethinamate (May increase the drowsiness effect).
- No products indexed under this heading.

Felodipine (Concurrent use is not recommended). Products include:
- Plendil Extended-Release Tablets 527

Fluphenazine Decanoate (May increase drowsiness effect). Products include:
- Prolixin Decanoate 509

Fluphenazine Enanthate (May increase drowsiness effect). Products include:
- Prolixin Enanthate 509

Fluphenazine Hydrochloride (May increase drowsiness effect). Products include:
- Prolixin 509

Flurazepam Hydrochloride (May increase the drowsiness effect). Products include:
- Dalmane Capsules 2173

Fosinopril Sodium (Concurrent use is not recommended). Products include:
- Monopril Tablets 757

Furazolidone (Concurrent and/or sequential use is not recommended). Products include:
- Furoxone 2046

Furosemide (Concurrent use is not recommended). Products include:
- Lasix Injection, Oral Solution and Tablets 1240

Glutethimide (May increase the drowsiness effect).
- No products indexed under this heading.

Guanabenz Acetate (Concurrent use is not recommended).
- No products indexed under this heading.

(▣ Described in PDR For Nonprescription Drugs) (⊙ Described in PDR For Ophthalmology)

43 **Interactions Index** **Alka-Seltzer Plus Night-Time**

Guanethidine Monosulfate (Concurrent use is not recommended). Products include:
- Esimil Tablets ... 822
- Ismelin Tablets ... 827

Haloperidol (May increase drowsiness effect). Products include:
- Haldol Injection, Tablets and Concentrate ... 1575

Haloperidol Decanoate (May increase drowsiness effect). Products include:
- Haldol Decanoate ... 1577

Hydralazine Hydrochloride (Concurrent use is not recommended). Products include:
- Apresazide Capsules ... 808
- Apresoline Hydrochloride Tablets ... 809
- Ser-Ap-Es Tablets ... 849

Hydrochlorothiazide (Concurrent use is not recommended). Products include:
- Aldactazide ... 2413
- Aldoril Tablets ... 1604
- Apresazide Capsules ... 808
- Capozide ... 742
- Dyazide ... 2479
- Esidrix Tablets ... 821
- Esimil Tablets ... 822
- HydroDIURIL Tablets ... 1674
- Hydropres Tablets ... 1675
- Hyzaar Tablets ... 1677
- Inderide Tablets ... 2732
- Inderide LA Long Acting Capsules ... 2734
- Lopressor HCT Tablets ... 832
- Lotensin HCT ... 837
- Maxzide ... 1380
- Moduretic Tablets ... 1705
- Oretic Tablets ... 443
- Prinzide Tablets ... 1737
- Ser-Ap-Es Tablets ... 849
- Timolide Tablets ... 1748
- Vaseretic Tablets ... 1765
- Zestoretic ... 2850
- Ziac ... 1415

Hydroflumethiazide (Concurrent use is not recommended). Products include:
- Diucardin Tablets ... 2718

Hydroxyzine Hydrochloride (May increase drowsiness effect). Products include:
- Atarax Tablets & Syrup ... 2185
- Marax Tablets & DF Syrup ... 2200
- Vistaril Intramuscular Solution ... 2216

Indapamide (Concurrent use is not recommended). Products include:
- Lozol Tablets ... 2022

Isocarboxazid (Concurrent and/or sequential use is not recommended).
- No products indexed under this heading.

Isradipine (Concurrent use is not recommended). Products include:
- DynaCirc Capsules ... 2256

Labetalol Hydrochloride (Concurrent use is not recommended). Products include:
- Normodyne Injection ... 2377
- Normodyne Tablets ... 2379
- Trandate ... 1185

Levobunolol Hydrochloride (Concurrent use is not recommended). Products include:
- Betagan ... ◉ 233

Lisinopril (Concurrent use is not recommended). Products include:
- Prinivil Tablets ... 1733
- Prinzide Tablets ... 1737
- Zestoretic ... 2850
- Zestril Tablets ... 2854

Lorazepam (May increase drowsiness effect). Products include:
- Ativan Injection ... 2698
- Ativan Tablets ... 2700

Losartan Potassium (Concurrent use is not recommended). Products include:
- Cozaar Tablets ... 1628
- Hyzaar Tablets ... 1677

Loxapine Hydrochloride (May increase drowsiness effect). Products include:
- Loxitane ... 1378

Loxapine Succinate (May increase drowsiness effect). Products include:
- Loxitane Capsules ... 1378

Mecamylamine Hydrochloride (Concurrent use is not recommended). Products include:
- Inversine Tablets ... 1686

Meprobamate (May increase drowsiness effect). Products include:
- Miltown Tablets ... 2672
- PMB 200 and PMB 400 ... 2783

Mesoridazine Besylate (May increase drowsiness effect). Products include:
- Serentil ... 684

Methyclothiazide (Concurrent use is not recommended). Products include:
- Enduron Tablets ... 420

Methyldopa (Concurrent use is not recommended). Products include:
- Aldoclor Tablets ... 1598
- Aldomet Oral ... 1600
- Aldoril Tablets ... 1604

Methyldopate Hydrochloride (Concurrent use is not recommended). Products include:
- Aldomet Ester HCl Injection ... 1602

Metipranolol Hydrochloride (Concurrent use is not recommended). Products include:
- OptiPranolol (Metipranolol 0.3%) Sterile Ophthalmic Solution ... ◉ 258

Metolazone (Concurrent use is not recommended). Products include:
- Mykrox Tablets ... 993
- Zaroxolyn Tablets ... 1000

Metoprolol Succinate (Concurrent use is not recommended). Products include:
- Toprol-XL Tablets ... 565

Metoprolol Tartrate (Concurrent use is not recommended). Products include:
- Lopressor Ampuls ... 830
- Lopressor HCT Tablets ... 832
- Lopressor Tablets ... 830

Metyrosine (Concurrent use is not recommended). Products include:
- Demser Capsules ... 1649

Midazolam Hydrochloride (May increase the drowsiness effect). Products include:
- Versed Injection ... 2170

Minoxidil (Concurrent use is not recommended). Products include:
- Loniten Tablets ... 2618
- Rogaine Topical Solution ... 2637

Moexipril Hydrochloride (Concurrent use is not recommended). Products include:
- Univasc Tablets ... 2410

Molindone Hydrochloride (May increase drowsiness effect). Products include:
- Moban Tablets and Concentrate ... 1048

Nadolol (Concurrent use is not recommended).
- No products indexed under this heading.

Nicardipine Hydrochloride (Concurrent use is not recommended). Products include:
- Cardene Capsules ... 2095
- Cardene I.V. ... 2709
- Cardene SR Capsules ... 2097

Nifedipine (Concurrent use is not recommended). Products include:
- Adalat Capsules (10 mg and 20 mg) ... 587
- Adalat CC ... 589
- Procardia Capsules ... 1971
- Procardia XL Extended Release Tablets ... 1972

Nisoldipine (Concurrent use is not recommended).
- No products indexed under this heading.

Nitroglycerin (Concurrent use is not recommended). Products include:
- Deponit NTG Transdermal Delivery System ... 2397
- Nitro-Bid IV ... 1523
- Nitro-Bid Ointment ... 1524
- Nitrodisc ... 2047
- Nitro-Dur (nitroglycerin) Transdermal Infusion System ... 1326
- Nitrolingual Spray ... 2027
- Nitrostat Tablets ... 1925
- Transderm-Nitro Transdermal Therapeutic System ... 859

Oxazepam (May increase drowsiness effect). Products include:
- Serax Capsules ... 2810
- Serax Tablets ... 2810

Penbutolol Sulfate (Concurrent use is not recommended). Products include:
- Levatol ... 2403

Perphenazine (May increase drowsiness effect). Products include:
- Etrafon ... 2355
- Triavil Tablets ... 1757
- Trilafon ... 2389

Phenelzine Sulfate (Concurrent and/or sequential use is not recommended). Products include:
- Nardil ... 1920

Phenoxybenzamine Hydrochloride (Concurrent use is not recommended). Products include:
- Dibenzyline Capsules ... 2476

Phentolamine Mesylate (Concurrent use is not recommended). Products include:
- Regitine ... 846

Pindolol (Concurrent use is not recommended). Products include:
- Visken Tablets ... 2299

Polythiazide (Concurrent use is not recommended). Products include:
- Minizide Capsules ... 1938

Prazepam (May increase drowsiness effect).
- No products indexed under this heading.

Prazosin Hydrochloride (Concurrent use is not recommended). Products include:
- Minipress Capsules ... 1937
- Minizide Capsules ... 1938

Prochlorperazine (May increase drowsiness effect). Products include:
- Compazine ... 2470

Promethazine Hydrochloride (May increase drowsiness effect). Products include:
- Mepergan Injection ... 2753
- Phenergan with Codeine ... 2777
- Phenergan with Dextromethorphan ... 2778
- Phenergan Injection ... 2773
- Phenergan Suppositories ... 2775
- Phenergan Syrup ... 2774
- Phenergan Tablets ... 2775
- Phenergan VC ... 2779
- Phenergan VC with Codeine ... 2781

Propofol (May increase the drowsiness effect). Products include:
- Diprivan Injection ... 2833

Propranolol Hydrochloride (Concurrent use is not recommended). Products include:
- Inderal ... 2728
- Inderal LA Long Acting Capsules ... 2730
- Inderide Tablets ... 2732
- Inderide LA Long Acting Capsules ... 2734

Quazepam (May increase the drowsiness effect). Products include:
- Doral Tablets ... 2664

Quinapril Hydrochloride (Concurrent use is not recommended). Products include:
- Accupril Tablets ... 1893

Ramipril (Concurrent use is not recommended). Products include:
- Altace Capsules ... 1232

Rauwolfia Serpentina (Concurrent use is not recommended).
- No products indexed under this heading.

Rescinnamine (Concurrent use is not recommended).
- No products indexed under this heading.

Reserpine (Concurrent use is not recommended). Products include:
- Diupres Tablets ... 1650
- Hydropres Tablets ... 1675
- Ser-Ap-Es Tablets ... 849

Secobarbital Sodium (May increase the drowsiness effect). Products include:
- Seconal Sodium Pulvules ... 1474

Selegiline Hydrochloride (Concurrent and/or sequential use is not recommended). Products include:
- Eldepryl Tablets ... 2550

Sodium Nitroprusside (Concurrent use is not recommended).
- No products indexed under this heading.

Sotalol Hydrochloride (Concurrent use is not recommended). Products include:
- Betapace Tablets ... 641

Spirapril Hydrochloride (Concurrent use is not recommended).
- No products indexed under this heading.

Temazepam (May increase the drowsiness effect). Products include:
- Restoril Capsules ... 2284

Terazosin Hydrochloride (Concurrent use is not recommended). Products include:
- Hytrin Capsules ... 430

Thioridazine Hydrochloride (May increase drowsiness effect). Products include:
- Mellaril ... 2269

Thiothixene (May increase drowsiness effect). Products include:
- Navane Capsules and Concentrate ... 2201
- Navane Intramuscular ... 2202

Timolol Maleate (Concurrent use is not recommended). Products include:
- Blocadren Tablets ... 1614
- Timolide Tablets ... 1748
- Timoptic in Ocudose ... 1753
- Timoptic Sterile Ophthalmic Solution ... 1751
- Timoptic-XE ... 1755

Torsemide (Concurrent use is not recommended). Products include:
- Demadex Tablets and Injection ... 686

Tranylcypromine Sulfate (Concurrent and/or sequential use is not recommended). Products include:
- Parnate Tablets ... 2503

Triazolam (May increase the drowsiness effect). Products include:
- Halcion Tablets ... 2611

Trifluoperazine Hydrochloride (May increase drowsiness effect). Products include:
- Stelazine ... 2514

Trimethaphan Camsylate (Concurrent use is not recommended). Products include:
- Arfonad Ampuls ... 2080

Verapamil Hydrochloride (Concurrent use is not recommended). Products include:
- Calan SR Caplets ... 2422
- Calan Tablets ... 2419
- Isoptin Injectable ... 1344

IMPORTANT NOTE: Always consult each drug listing in the patient's regimen for possible interactions.

Isoptin Oral Tablets 1346
Isoptin SR Tablets 1348
Verelan Capsules 1410
Verelan Capsules 2824

Warfarin Sodium (Effect not specified). Products include:
Coumadin 926

Zolpidem Tartrate (May increase the drowsiness effect). Products include:
Ambien Tablets 2416

Food Interactions

Alcohol (May increase the drowsiness effect; avoid concurrent use).

ALKA-SELTZER PLUS NIGHT-TIME COLD MEDICINE LIQUI-GELS

(Dextromethorphan Hydrobromide, Doxylamine Succinate, Pseudoephedrine Hydrochloride, Acetaminophen) ▣ 706

May interact with hypnotics and sedatives, tranquilizers, monoamine oxidase inhibitors, antihypertensives, and certain other agents. Compounds in these categories include:

Acebutolol Hydrochloride (Concurrent use is not recommended). Products include:
Sectral Capsules 2807

Alprazolam (May increase drowsiness effect; consult your doctor). Products include:
Xanax Tablets 2649

Amlodipine Besylate (Concurrent use is not recommended). Products include:
Lotrel Capsules 840
Norvasc Tablets 1940

Atenolol (Concurrent use is not recommended). Products include:
Tenoretic Tablets 2845
Tenormin Tablets and I.V. Injection 2847

Benazepril Hydrochloride (Concurrent use is not recommended). Products include:
Lotensin Tablets 834
Lotensin HCT 837
Lotrel Capsules 840

Bendroflumethiazide (Concurrent use is not recommended).
No products indexed under this heading.

Betaxolol Hydrochloride (Concurrent use is not recommended). Products include:
Betoptic Ophthalmic Solution 469
Betoptic S Ophthalmic Suspension 471
Kerlone Tablets 2436

Bisoprolol Fumarate (Concurrent use is not recommended). Products include:
Zebeta Tablets 1413
Ziac 1415

Buspirone Hydrochloride (May increase drowsiness effect; consult your doctor). Products include:
BuSpar 737

Captopril (Concurrent use is not recommended). Products include:
Capoten 739
Capozide 742

Carteolol Hydrochloride (Concurrent use is not recommended). Products include:
Cartrol Tablets 410
Ocupress Ophthalmic Solution, 1% Sterile ◉ 309

Chlordiazepoxide (May increase drowsiness effect; consult your doctor). Products include:
Libritabs Tablets 2177
Limbitrol 2180

Chlordiazepoxide Hydrochloride (May increase drowsiness effect; consult your doctor). Products include:
Librax Capsules 2176
Librium Capsules 2178
Librium Injectable 2179

Chlorothiazide (Concurrent use is not recommended). Products include:
Aldoclor Tablets 1598
Diupres Tablets 1650
Diuril Oral 1653

Chlorothiazide Sodium (Concurrent use is not recommended). Products include:
Diuril Sodium Intravenous 1652

Chlorpromazine (May increase drowsiness effect; consult your doctor). Products include:
Thorazine Suppositories 2523

Chlorpromazine Hydrochloride (May increase drowsiness effect; consult your doctor). Products include:
Thorazine 2523

Chlorprothixene (May increase drowsiness effect; consult your doctor).
No products indexed under this heading.

Chlorprothixene Hydrochloride (May increase drowsiness effect; consult your doctor).
No products indexed under this heading.

Chlorthalidone (Concurrent use is not recommended). Products include:
Combipres Tablets 677
Tenoretic Tablets 2845
Thalitone 1245

Clonidine (Concurrent use is not recommended). Products include:
Catapres-TTS 675

Clonidine Hydrochloride (Concurrent use is not recommended). Products include:
Catapres Tablets 674
Combipres Tablets 677

Clorazepate Dipotassium (May increase drowsiness effect; consult your doctor). Products include:
Tranxene 451

Deserpidine (Concurrent use is not recommended).
No products indexed under this heading.

Diazepam (May increase drowsiness effect; consult your doctor). Products include:
Dizac 1809
Valium Injectable 2182
Valium Tablets 2183
Valrelease Capsules 2169

Diazoxide (Concurrent use is not recommended). Products include:
Hyperstat I.V. Injection 2363
Proglycem 580

Diltiazem Hydrochloride (Concurrent use is not recommended). Products include:
Cardizem CD Capsules 1506
Cardizem SR Capsules 1510
Cardizem Injectable 1508
Cardizem Tablets 1512
Dilacor XR Extended-release Capsules 2018

Doxazosin Mesylate (Concurrent use is not recommended). Products include:
Cardura Tablets 2186

Droperidol (May increase drowsiness effect; consult your doctor). Products include:
Inapsine Injection 1296

Enalapril Maleate (Concurrent use is not recommended). Products include:
Vaseretic Tablets 1765
Vasotec Tablets 1771

Enalaprilat (Concurrent use is not recommended). Products include:
Vasotec I.V. 1768

Esmolol Hydrochloride (Concurrent use is not recommended). Products include:
Brevibloc Injection 1808

Estazolam (May increase drowsiness effect; consult your doctor). Products include:
ProSom Tablets 449

Ethchlorvynol (May increase drowsiness effect; consult your doctor). Products include:
Placidyl Capsules 448

Ethinamate (May increase drowsiness effect; consult your doctor).
No products indexed under this heading.

Felodipine (Concurrent use is not recommended). Products include:
Plendil Extended-Release Tablets 527

Fluphenazine Decanoate (May increase drowsiness effect; consult your doctor). Products include:
Prolixin Decanoate 509

Fluphenazine Enanthate (May increase drowsiness effect; consult your doctor). Products include:
Prolixin Enanthate 509

Fluphenazine Hydrochloride (May increase drowsiness effect; consult your doctor). Products include:
Prolixin 509

Flurazepam Hydrochloride (May increase drowsiness effect; consult your doctor). Products include:
Dalmane Capsules 2173

Fosinopril Sodium (Concurrent use is not recommended). Products include:
Monopril Tablets 757

Furazolidone (Concurrent use not recommended; consult your doctor). Products include:
Furoxone 2046

Furosemide (Concurrent use is not recommended). Products include:
Lasix Injection, Oral Solution and Tablets 1240

Glutethimide (May increase drowsiness effect; consult your doctor).
No products indexed under this heading.

Guanabenz Acetate (Concurrent use is not recommended).
No products indexed under this heading.

Guanethidine Monosulfate (Concurrent use is not recommended). Products include:
Esimil Tablets 822
Ismelin Tablets 827

Haloperidol (May increase drowsiness effect; consult your doctor). Products include:
Haldol Injection, Tablets and Concentrate 1575

Haloperidol Decanoate (May increase drowsiness effect; consult your doctor). Products include:
Haldol Decanoate 1577

Hydralazine Hydrochloride (Concurrent use is not recommended). Products include:
Apresazide Capsules 808
Apresoline Hydrochloride Tablets 809
Ser-Ap-Es Tablets 849

Hydrochlorothiazide (Concurrent use is not recommended). Products include:
Aldactazide 2413
Aldoril Tablets 1604
Apresazide Capsules 808
Capozide 742
Dyazide 2479
Esidrix Tablets 821
Esimil Tablets 822
HydroDIURIL Tablets 1674
Hydropres Tablets 1675
Hyzaar Tablets 1677
Inderide Tablets 2732
Inderide LA Long Acting Capsules 2734
Lopressor HCT Tablets 832
Lotensin HCT 837
Maxzide 1380
Moduretic Tablets 1705
Oretic Tablets 443
Prinzide Tablets 1737
Ser-Ap-Es Tablets 849
Timolide Tablets 1748
Vaseretic Tablets 1765
Zestoretic 2850
Ziac 1415

Hydroflumethiazide (Concurrent use is not recommended). Products include:
Diucardin Tablets 2718

Hydroxyzine Hydrochloride (May increase drowsiness effect; consult your doctor). Products include:
Atarax Tablets & Syrup 2185
Marax Tablets & DF Syrup 2200
Vistaril Intramuscular Solution 2216

Indapamide (Concurrent use is not recommended). Products include:
Lozol Tablets 2022

Isocarboxazid (Concurrent use not recommended; consult your doctor).
No products indexed under this heading.

Isradipine (Concurrent use is not recommended). Products include:
DynaCirc Capsules 2256

Labetalol Hydrochloride (Concurrent use is not recommended). Products include:
Normodyne Injection 2377
Normodyne Tablets 2379
Trandate 1185

Levobunolol Hydrochloride (Concurrent use is not recommended). Products include:
Betagan ◉ 233

Lisinopril (Concurrent use is not recommended). Products include:
Prinivil Tablets 1733
Prinzide Tablets 1737
Zestoretic 2850
Zestril Tablets 2854

Lorazepam (May increase drowsiness effect; consult your doctor). Products include:
Ativan Injection 2698
Ativan Tablets 2700

Losartan Potassium (Concurrent use is not recommended). Products include:
Cozaar Tablets 1628
Hyzaar Tablets 1677

Loxapine Hydrochloride (May increase drowsiness effect; consult your doctor). Products include:
Loxitane 1378

Loxapine Succinate (May increase drowsiness effect; consult your doctor). Products include:
Loxitane Capsules 1378

Mecamylamine Hydrochloride (Concurrent use is not recommended). Products include:
Inversine Tablets 1686

Meprobamate (May increase drowsiness effect; consult your doctor). Products include:
Miltown Tablets 2672
PMB 200 and PMB 400 2783

(▣ Described in PDR For Nonprescription Drugs) (◉ Described in PDR For Ophthalmology)

Interactions Index

Alka Seltzer Plus Sinus

Mesoridazine Besylate (May increase drowsiness effect; consult your doctor). Products include:

Serentil 684

Methyclothiazide (Concurrent use is not recommended). Products include:

Enduron Tablets... 420

Methyldopa (Concurrent use is not recommended). Products include:

Aldoclor Tablets 1598
Aldomet Oral 1600
Aldoril Tablets.. 1604

Methyldopate Hydrochloride (Concurrent use is not recommended). Products include:

Aldomet Ester HCl Injection 1602

Metipranolol Hydrochloride (Concurrent use is not recommended). Products include:

OptiPranolol (Metipranolol 0.3%) Sterile Ophthalmic Solution......... ◎ 258

Metolazone (Concurrent use is not recommended). Products include:

Mykrox Tablets 993
Zaroxolyn Tablets 1000

Metoprolol Succinate (Concurrent use is not recommended). Products include:

Toprol-XL Tablets 565

Metoprolol Tartrate (Concurrent use is not recommended). Products include:

Lopressor Ampuls 830
Lopressor HCT Tablets 832
Lopressor Tablets 830

Metyrosine (Concurrent use is not recommended). Products include:

Demser Capsules 1649

Midazolam Hydrochloride (May increase drowsiness effect; consult your doctor). Products include:

Versed Injection 2170

Minoxidil (Concurrent use is not recommended). Products include:

Loniten Tablets.. 2618
Rogaine Topical Solution 2637

Moexipril Hydrochloride (Concurrent use is not recommended). Products include:

Univasc Tablets 2410

Molindone Hydrochloride (May increase drowsiness effect; consult your doctor). Products include:

Moban Tablets and Concentrate...... 1048

Nadolol (Concurrent use is not recommended).

No products indexed under this heading.

Nicardipine Hydrochloride (Concurrent use is not recommended). Products include:

Cardene Capsules 2095
Cardene I.V. 2709
Cardene SR Capsules................................. 2097

Nifedipine (Concurrent use is not recommended). Products include:

Adalat Capsules (10 mg and 20 mg) 587
Adalat CC 589
Procardia Capsules 1971
Procardia XL Extended Release Tablets 1972

Nisoldipine (Concurrent use is not recommended).

No products indexed under this heading.

Nitroglycerin (Concurrent use is not recommended). Products include:

Deponit NTG Transdermal Delivery System 2397
Nitro-Bid IV.. 1523
Nitro-Bid Ointment 1524
Nitrodisc 2047
Nitro-Dur (nitroglycerin) Transdermal Infusion System 1326
Nitrolingual Spray 2027
Nitrostat Tablets 1925

Transderm-Nitro Transdermal Therapeutic System 859

Oxazepam (May increase drowsiness effect; consult your doctor). Products include:

Serax Capsules 2810
Serax Tablets.. 2810

Penbutolol Sulfate (Concurrent use is not recommended). Products include:

Levatol 2403

Perphenazine (May increase drowsiness effect; consult your doctor). Products include:

Etrafon 2355
Triavil Tablets 1757
Trilafon.. 2389

Phenelzine Sulfate (Concurrent use not recommended; consult your doctor). Products include:

Nardil 1920

Phenoxybenzamine Hydrochloride (Concurrent use is not recommended). Products include:

Dibenzyline Capsules 2476

Phentolamine Mesylate (Concurrent use is not recommended). Products include:

Regitine 846

Pindolol (Concurrent use is not recommended). Products include:

Visken Tablets.. 2299

Polythiazide (Concurrent use is not recommended). Products include:

Minizide Capsules 1938

Prazepam (May increase drowsiness effect; consult your doctor).

No products indexed under this heading.

Prazosin Hydrochloride (Concurrent use is not recommended). Products include:

Minipress Capsules..................................... 1937
Minizide Capsules 1938

Prochlorperazine (May increase drowsiness effect; consult your doctor). Products include:

Compazine 2470

Promethazine Hydrochloride (May increase drowsiness effect; consult your doctor). Products include:

Mepergan Injection 2753
Phenergan with Codeine........................... 2777
Phenergan with Dextromethorphan 2778
Phenergan Injection 2773
Phenergan Suppositories 2775
Phenergan Syrup 2774
Phenergan Tablets 2775
Phenergan VC 2779
Phenergan VC with Codeine.................... 2781

Propofol (May increase drowsiness effect; consult your doctor). Products include:

Diprivan Injection....................................... 2833

Propranolol Hydrochloride (Concurrent use is not recommended). Products include:

Inderal 2728
Inderal LA Long Acting Capsules 2730
Inderide Tablets... 2732
Inderide LA Long Acting Capsules .. 2734

Quazepam (May increase drowsiness effect; consult your doctor). Products include:

Doral Tablets 2664

Quinapril Hydrochloride (Concurrent use is not recommended). Products include:

Accupril Tablets 1893

Ramipril (Concurrent use is not recommended). Products include:

Altace Capsules 1232

Rauwolfia Serpentina (Concurrent use is not recommended).

No products indexed under this heading.

Rescinnamine (Concurrent use is not recommended).

No products indexed under this heading.

Reserpine (Concurrent use is not recommended). Products include:

Diupres Tablets 1650
Hydropres Tablets....................................... 1675
Ser-Ap-Es Tablets 849

Secobarbital Sodium (May increase drowsiness effect; consult your doctor). Products include:

Seconal Sodium Pulvules 1474

Selegiline Hydrochloride (Concurrent use not recommended; consult your doctor). Products include:

Eldepryl Tablets 2550

Sodium Nitroprusside (Concurrent use is not recommended).

No products indexed under this heading.

Sotalol Hydrochloride (Concurrent use is not recommended). Products include:

Betapace Tablets 641

Spirapril Hydrochloride (Concurrent use is not recommended).

No products indexed under this heading.

Temazepam (May increase drowsiness effect; consult your doctor). Products include:

Restoril Capsules 2284

Terazosin Hydrochloride (Concurrent use is not recommended). Products include:

Hytrin Capsules 430

Thioridazine Hydrochloride (May increase drowsiness effect; consult your doctor). Products include:

Mellaril 2269

Thiothixene (May increase drowsiness effect; consult your doctor). Products include:

Navane Capsules and Concentrate 2201
Navane Intramuscular 2202

Timolol Maleate (Concurrent use is not recommended). Products include:

Blocadren Tablets 1614
Timolide Tablets.. 1748
Timoptic in Ocudose 1753
Timoptic Sterile Ophthalmic Solution.. 1751
Timoptic-XE 1755

Torsemide (Concurrent use is not recommended). Products include:

Demadex Tablets and Injection 686

Tranylcypromine Sulfate (Concurrent use not recommended; consult your doctor). Products include:

Parnate Tablets 2503

Triazolam (May increase drowsiness effect; consult your doctor). Products include:

Halcion Tablets.. 2611

Trifluoperazine Hydrochloride (May increase drowsiness effect; consult your doctor). Products include:

Stelazine 2514

Trimethaphan Camsylate (Concurrent use is not recommended). Products include:

Arfonad Ampuls 2080

Verapamil Hydrochloride (Concurrent use is not recommended). Products include:

Calan SR Caplets 2422
Calan Tablets.. 2419
Isoptin Injectable 1344
Isoptin Oral Tablets 1346
Isoptin SR Tablets 1348
Verelan Capsules... 1410
Verelan Capsules... 2824

Zolpidem Tartrate (May increase drowsiness effect; consult your doctor). Products include:

Ambien Tablets.. 2416

Food Interactions

Alcohol (May increase drowsiness effect; consult your doctor).

ALKA SELTZER PLUS SINUS MEDICINE

(Phenylpropanolamine Bitartrate, Aspirin, Brompheniramine Maleate) ®◎ 707

May interact with hypnotics and sedatives, tranquilizers, oral anticoagulants, monoamine oxidase inhibitors, antihypertensives, and certain other agents. Compounds in these categories include:

Acebutolol Hydrochloride (Effect not specified). Products include:

Sectral Capsules 2807

Alprazolam (May increase the drowsiness effect). Products include:

Xanax Tablets 2649

Amlodipine Besylate (Effect not specified). Products include:

Lotrel Capsules.. 840
Norvasc Tablets 1940

Antiarthritic Drugs, unspecified (Effect not specified).

Antidiabetic Drugs, unspecified (Effect not specified).

Antigout Drugs, unspecified (Effect not specified).

Atenolol (Effect not specified). Products include:

Tenoretic Tablets... 2845
Tenormin Tablets and I.V. Injection 2847

Benazepril Hydrochloride (Effect not specified). Products include:

Lotensin Tablets... 834
Lotensin HCT... 837
Lotrel Capsules.. 840

Bendroflumethiazide (Effect not specified).

No products indexed under this heading.

Betaxolol Hydrochloride (Effect not specified). Products include:

Betoptic Ophthalmic Solution........... 469
Betoptic S Ophthalmic Suspension 471
Kerlone Tablets.. 2436

Bisoprolol Fumarate (Effect not specified). Products include:

Zebeta Tablets 1413
Ziac 1415

Buspirone Hydrochloride (May increase the drowsiness effect). Products include:

BuSpar 737

Captopril (Effect not specified). Products include:

Capoten 739
Capozide 742

Carteolol Hydrochloride (Effect not specified). Products include:

Cartrol Tablets 410
Ocupress Ophthalmic Solution, 1% Sterile.. ◎ 309

Chlordiazepoxide (May increase the drowsiness effect). Products include:

Libritabs Tablets 2177
Limbitrol 2180

Chlordiazepoxide Hydrochloride (May increase the drowsiness effect). Products include:

Librax Capsules 2176
Librium Capsules... 2178
Librium Injectable 2179

Chlorothiazide (Effect not specified). Products include:

Aldoclor Tablets 1598
Diupres Tablets 1650
Diuril Oral 1653

IMPORTANT NOTE: Always consult each drug listing in the patient's regimen for possible interactions.

Alka Seltzer Plus Sinus — Interactions Index — 46

Chlorothiazide Sodium (Effect not specified). Products include:
- Diuril Sodium Intravenous ... 1652

Chlorpromazine (May increase the drowsiness effect). Products include:
- Thorazine Suppositories ... 2523

Chlorpromazine Hydrochloride (May increase the drowsiness effect). Products include:
- Thorazine ... 2523

Chlorprothixene (May increase the drowsiness effect).
- No products indexed under this heading.

Chlorprothixene Hydrochloride (May increase the drowsiness effect).
- No products indexed under this heading.

Chlorthalidone (Effect not specified). Products include:
- Combipres Tablets ... 677
- Tenoretic Tablets ... 2845
- Thalitone ... 1245

Clonidine (Effect not specified). Products include:
- Catapres-TTS ... 675

Clonidine Hydrochloride (Effect not specified). Products include:
- Catapres Tablets ... 674
- Combipres Tablets ... 677

Clorazepate Dipotassium (May increase the drowsiness effect). Products include:
- Tranxene ... 451

Deserpidine (Effect not specified).
- No products indexed under this heading.

Diazepam (May increase the drowsiness effect). Products include:
- Dizac ... 1809
- Valium Injectable ... 2182
- Valium Tablets ... 2183
- Valrelease Capsules ... 2169

Diazoxide (Effect not specified). Products include:
- Hyperstat I.V. Injection ... 2363
- Proglycem ... 580

Dicumarol (Effect not specified).
- No products indexed under this heading.

Diltiazem Hydrochloride (Effect not specified). Products include:
- Cardizem CD Capsules ... 1506
- Cardizem SR Capsules ... 1510
- Cardizem Injectable ... 1508
- Cardizem Tablets ... 1512
- Dilacor XR Extended-release Capsules ... 2018

Doxazosin Mesylate (Effect not specified). Products include:
- Cardura Tablets ... 2186

Droperidol (May increase the drowsiness effect). Products include:
- Inapsine Injection ... 1296

Enalapril Maleate (Effect not specified). Products include:
- Vaseretic Tablets ... 1765
- Vasotec Tablets ... 1771

Enalaprilat (Effect not specified). Products include:
- Vasotec I.V. ... 1768

Esmolol Hydrochloride (Effect not specified). Products include:
- Brevibloc Injection ... 1808

Estazolam (May increase the drowsiness effect). Products include:
- ProSom Tablets ... 449

Ethchlorvynol (May increase the drowsiness effect). Products include:
- Placidyl Capsules ... 448

Ethinamate (May increase the drowsiness effect).
- No products indexed under this heading.

Felodipine (Effect not specified). Products include:
- Plendil Extended-Release Tablets ... 527

Fluphenazine Decanoate (May increase the drowsiness effect). Products include:
- Prolixin Decanoate ... 509

Fluphenazine Enanthate (May increase the drowsiness effect). Products include:
- Prolixin Enanthate ... 509

Fluphenazine Hydrochloride (May increase the drowsiness effect). Products include:
- Prolixin ... 509

Flurazepam Hydrochloride (May increase the drowsiness effect). Products include:
- Dalmane Capsules ... 2173

Fosinopril Sodium (Effect not specified). Products include:
- Monopril Tablets ... 757

Furazolidone (Concurrent and/or sequential use is not recommended). Products include:
- Furoxone ... 2046

Furosemide (Effect not specified). Products include:
- Lasix Injection, Oral Solution and Tablets ... 1240

Glutethimide (May increase the drowsiness effect).
- No products indexed under this heading.

Guanabenz Acetate (Effect not specified).
- No products indexed under this heading.

Guanethidine Monosulfate (Effect not specified). Products include:
- Esimil Tablets ... 822
- Ismelin Tablets ... 827

Haloperidol (May increase the drowsiness effect). Products include:
- Haldol Injection, Tablets and Concentrate ... 1575

Haloperidol Decanoate (May increase the drowsiness effect). Products include:
- Haldol Decanoate ... 1577

Hydralazine Hydrochloride (Effect not specified). Products include:
- Apresazide Capsules ... 808
- Apresoline Hydrochloride Tablets ... 809
- Ser-Ap-Es Tablets ... 849

Hydrochlorothiazide (Effect not specified). Products include:
- Aldactazide ... 2413
- Aldoril Tablets ... 1604
- Apresazide Capsules ... 808
- Capozide ... 742
- Dyazide ... 2479
- Esidrix Tablets ... 821
- Esimil Tablets ... 822
- HydroDIURIL Tablets ... 1674
- Hydropres Tablets ... 1675
- Hyzaar Tablets ... 1677
- Inderide Tablets ... 2732
- Inderide LA Long Acting Capsules ... 2734
- Lopressor HCT Tablets ... 832
- Lotensin HCT ... 837
- Maxzide ... 1380
- Moduretic Tablets ... 1705
- Oretic Tablets ... 443
- Prinzide Tablets ... 1737
- Ser-Ap-Es Tablets ... 849
- Timolide Tablets ... 1748
- Vaseretic Tablets ... 1765
- Zestoretic ... 2850
- Ziac ... 1415

Hydroflumethiazide (Effect not specified). Products include:
- Diucardin Tablets ... 2718

Hydroxyzine Hydrochloride (May increase the drowsiness effect). Products include:
- Atarax Tablets & Syrup ... 2185
- Marax Tablets & DF Syrup ... 2200
- Vistaril Intramuscular Solution ... 2216

Indapamide (Effect not specified). Products include:
- Lozol Tablets ... 2022

Isocarboxazid (Concurrent and/or sequential use is not recommended).
- No products indexed under this heading.

Isradipine (Effect not specified). Products include:
- DynaCirc Capsules ... 2256

Labetalol Hydrochloride (Effect not specified). Products include:
- Normodyne Injection ... 2377
- Normodyne Tablets ... 2379
- Trandate ... 1185

Levobunolol Hydrochloride (May increase the drowsiness effect). Products include:
- Betagan ... ⊙ 233

Lisinopril (Effect not specified). Products include:
- Prinivil Tablets ... 1733
- Prinzide Tablets ... 1737
- Zestoretic ... 2850
- Zestril Tablets ... 2854

Lorazepam (May increase the drowsiness effect). Products include:
- Ativan Injection ... 2698
- Ativan Tablets ... 2700

Losartan Potassium (Effect not specified). Products include:
- Cozaar Tablets ... 1628
- Hyzaar Tablets ... 1677

Loxapine Hydrochloride (May increase the drowsiness effect). Products include:
- Loxitane ... 1378

Loxapine Succinate (May increase the drowsiness effect). Products include:
- Loxitane Capsules ... 1378

Mecamylamine Hydrochloride (Effect not specified). Products include:
- Inversine Tablets ... 1686

Meprobamate (May increase the drowsiness effect). Products include:
- Miltown Tablets ... 2672
- PMB 200 and PMB 400 ... 2783

Mesoridazine Besylate (May increase the drowsiness effect). Products include:
- Serentil ... 684

Methyclothiazide (Effect not specified). Products include:
- Enduron Tablets ... 420

Methyldopa (Effect not specified). Products include:
- Aldoclor Tablets ... 1598
- Aldomet Oral ... 1600
- Aldoril Tablets ... 1604

Methyldopate Hydrochloride (Effect not specified). Products include:
- Aldomet Ester HCl Injection ... 1602

Metipranolol Hydrochloride (Effect not specified). Products include:
- OptiPranolol (Metipranolol 0.3%) Sterile Ophthalmic Solution ... ⊙ 258

Metolazone (Effect not specified). Products include:
- Mykrox Tablets ... 993
- Zaroxolyn Tablets ... 1000

Metoprolol Succinate (Effect not specified). Products include:
- Toprol-XL Tablets ... 565

Metoprolol Tartrate (Effect not specified). Products include:
- Lopressor Ampuls ... 830
- Lopressor HCT Tablets ... 832
- Lopressor Tablets ... 830

Metyrosine (Effect not specified). Products include:
- Demser Capsules ... 1649

Midazolam Hydrochloride (May increase the drowsiness effect). Products include:
- Versed Injection ... 2170

Minoxidil (Effect not specified). Products include:
- Loniten Tablets ... 2618
- Rogaine Topical Solution ... 2637

Moexipril Hydrochloride (Effect not specified). Products include:
- Univasc Tablets ... 2410

Molindone Hydrochloride (May increase the drowsiness effect). Products include:
- Moban Tablets and Concentrate ... 1048

Nadolol (Effect not specified).
- No products indexed under this heading.

Nicardipine Hydrochloride (Effect not specified). Products include:
- Cardene Capsules ... 2095
- Cardene I.V. ... 2709
- Cardene SR Capsules ... 2097

Nifedipine (Effect not specified). Products include:
- Adalat Capsules (10 mg and 20 mg) ... 587
- Adalat CC ... 589
- Procardia Capsules ... 1971
- Procardia XL Extended Release Tablets ... 1972

Nisoldipine (Effect not specified).
- No products indexed under this heading.

Nitroglycerin (Effect not specified). Products include:
- Deponit NTG Transdermal Delivery System ... 2397
- Nitro-Bid IV ... 1523
- Nitro-Bid Ointment ... 1524
- Nitrodisc ... 2047
- Nitro-Dur (nitroglycerin) Transdermal Infusion System ... 1326
- Nitrolingual Spray ... 2027
- Nitrostat Tablets ... 1925
- Transderm-Nitro Transdermal Therapeutic System ... 859

Oxazepam (May increase the drowsiness effect). Products include:
- Serax Capsules ... 2810
- Serax Tablets ... 2810

Penbutolol Sulfate (Effect not specified). Products include:
- Levatol ... 2403

Perphenazine (May increase the drowsiness effect). Products include:
- Etrafon ... 2355
- Triavil Tablets ... 1757
- Trilafon ... 2389

Phenelzine Sulfate (Concurrent and/or sequential use is not recommended). Products include:
- Nardil ... 1920

Phenoxybenzamine Hydrochloride (Effect not specified). Products include:
- Dibenzyline Capsules ... 2476

Phentolamine Mesylate (Effect not specified). Products include:
- Regitine ... 846

Pindolol (Effect not specified). Products include:
- Visken Tablets ... 2299

Polythiazide (Effect not specified). Products include:
- Minizide Capsules ... 1938

Prazepam (May increase the drowsiness effect).
- No products indexed under this heading.

Prazosin Hydrochloride (Effect not specified). Products include:
- Minipress Capsules ... 1937
- Minizide Capsules ... 1938

Prochlorperazine (May increase the drowsiness effect). Products include:
- Compazine ... 2470

(▣ Described in PDR For Nonprescription Drugs) (⊙ Described in PDR For Ophthalmology)

Promethazine Hydrochloride (May increase the drowsiness effect). Products include:
Mepergan Injection ... 2753
Phenergan with Codeine ... 2777
Phenergan with Dextromethorphan 2778
Phenergan Injection ... 2773
Phenergan Suppositories ... 2775
Phenergan Syrup ... 2774
Phenergan Tablets ... 2775
Phenergan VC ... 2779
Phenergan VC with Codeine ... 2781

Propofol (May increase the drowsiness effect). Products include:
Diprivan Injection ... 2833

Propranolol Hydrochloride (Effect not specified). Products include:
Inderal ... 2728
Inderal LA Long Acting Capsules ... 2730
Inderide Tablets ... 2732
Inderide LA Long Acting Capsules .. 2734

Quazepam (May increase the drowsiness effect). Products include:
Doral Tablets ... 2664

Quinapril Hydrochloride (Effect not specified). Products include:
Accupril Tablets ... 1893

Ramipril (Effect not specified). Products include:
Altace Capsules ... 1232

Rauwolfia Serpentina (Effect not specified).
No products indexed under this heading.

Rescinnamine (Effect not specified).
No products indexed under this heading.

Reserpine (Effect not specified). Products include:
Diupres Tablets ... 1650
Hydropres Tablets ... 1675
Ser-Ap-Es Tablets ... 849

Secobarbital Sodium (May increase the drowsiness effect). Products include:
Seconal Sodium Pulvules ... 1474

Selegiline Hydrochloride (Concurrent and/or sequential use is not recommended). Products include:
Eldepryl Tablets ... 2550

Sodium Nitroprusside (Effect not specified).
No products indexed under this heading.

Sotalol Hydrochloride (Effect not specified). Products include:
Betapace Tablets ... 641

Spirapril Hydrochloride (Effect not specified).
No products indexed under this heading.

Temazepam (May increase the drowsiness effect). Products include:
Restoril Capsules ... 2284

Terazosin Hydrochloride (Effect not specified). Products include:
Hytrin Capsules ... 430

Thioridazine Hydrochloride (May increase the drowsiness effect). Products include:
Mellaril ... 2269

Thiothixene (May increase the drowsiness effect). Products include:
Navane Capsules and Concentrate 2201
Navane Intramuscular ... 2202

Timolol Maleate (Effect not specified). Products include:
Blocadren Tablets ... 1614
Timolide Tablets ... 1748
Timoptic in Ocudose ... 1753
Timoptic Sterile Ophthalmic Solution ... 1751
Timoptic-XE ... 1755

Torsemide (Effect not specified). Products include:
Demadex Tablets and Injection ... 686

Tranylcypromine Sulfate (Concurrent and/or sequential use is not recommended). Products include:
Parnate Tablets ... 2503

Triazolam (May increase the drowsiness effect). Products include:
Halcion Tablets ... 2611

Trifluoperazine Hydrochloride (May increase the drowsiness effect). Products include:
Stelazine ... 2514

Trimethaphan Camsylate (Effect not specified). Products include:
Arfonad Ampuls ... 2080

Verapamil Hydrochloride (Effect not specified). Products include:
Calan SR Caplets ... 2422
Calan Tablets ... 2419
Isoptin Injectable ... 1344
Isoptin Oral Tablets ... 1346
Isoptin SR Tablets ... 1348
Verelan Capsules ... 1410
Verelan Capsules ... 2824

Warfarin Sodium (Effect not specified). Products include:
Coumadin ... 926

Zolpidem Tartrate (May increase the drowsiness effect). Products include:
Ambien Tablets ... 2416

Food Interactions

Alcohol (May increase the drowsiness effect; avoid concurrent use).

ALKERAN FOR INJECTION

(Melphalan Hydrochloride) ... 1070
May interact with:

Carmustine (BCNU) (Reduced threshold for BCNU lung toxicity). Products include:
BiCNU ... 691

Cisplatin (Affects melphalan kinetics by inducing renal dysfunction and subsequently altering melphalan clearance). Products include:
Platinol ... 708
Platinol-AQ Injection ... 710

Cyclosporine (Potential for severe renal failure). Products include:
Neoral ... 2276
Sandimmune ... 2286

Nalidixic Acid (Increased incidence of severe hemorrhagic necrotic enterocolitis). Products include:
NegGram ... 2323

ALKERAN TABLETS

(Melphalan) ... 1071
None cited in PDR database.

ALLEREST CHILDREN'S CHEWABLE TABLETS

(Chlorpheniramine Maleate, Phenylpropanolamine Hydrochloride) ... ▣ 627
See **Allerest Maximum Strength Tablets**

ALLEREST HEADACHE STRENGTH TABLETS

(Acetaminophen, Chlorpheniramine Maleate, Pseudoephedrine Hydrochloride) ... ▣ 627
See **Allerest Maximum Strength Tablets**

ALLEREST MAXIMUM STRENGTH TABLETS

(Chlorpheniramine Maleate, Pseudoephedrine Hydrochloride) ... ▣ 627
May interact with monoamine oxidase inhibitors, central nervous system depressants, and certain other agents. Compounds in these categories include:

Alfentanil Hydrochloride (Concurrent use produces additive effects). Products include:
Alfenta Injection ... 1286

Alprazolam (Concurrent use produces additive effects). Products include:
Xanax Tablets ... 2649

Aprobarbital (Concurrent use produces additive effects).
No products indexed under this heading.

Buprenorphine (Concurrent use produces additive effects). Products include:
Buprenex Injectable ... 2006

Buspirone Hydrochloride (Concurrent use produces additive effects). Products include:
BuSpar ... 737

Butabarbital (Concurrent use produces additive effects).
No products indexed under this heading.

Butalbital (Concurrent use produces additive effects). Products include:
Esgic-plus Tablets ... 1013
Fioricet Tablets ... 2258
Fioricet with Codeine Capsules ... 2260
Fiorinal Capsules ... 2261
Fiorinal with Codeine Capsules ... 2262
Fiorinal Tablets ... 2261
Phrenilin ... 785
Sedapap Tablets 50 mg/650 mg . 1543

Chlordiazepoxide (Concurrent use produces additive effects). Products include:
Libritabs Tablets ... 2177
Limbitrol ... 2180

Chlordiazepoxide Hydrochloride (Concurrent use produces additive effects). Products include:
Librax Capsules ... 2176
Librium Capsules ... 2178
Librium Injectable ... 2179

Chlorpromazine (Concurrent use produces additive effects). Products include:
Thorazine Suppositories ... 2523

Chlorprothixene (Concurrent use produces additive effects).
No products indexed under this heading.

Chlorprothixene Hydrochloride (Concurrent use produces additive effects).
No products indexed under this heading.

Clorazepate Dipotassium (Concurrent use produces additive effects). Products include:
Tranxene ... 451

Clozapine (Concurrent use produces additive effects). Products include:
Clozaril Tablets ... 2252

Codeine Phosphate (Concurrent use produces additive effects). Products include:
Actifed with Codeine Cough Syrup.. 1067
Brontex ... 1981
Deconsal C Expectorant Syrup ... 456
Deconsal Pediatric Syrup ... 457
Dimetane-DC Cough Syrup ... 2059
Empirin with Codeine Tablets ... 1093
Fioricet with Codeine Capsules ... 2260
Fiorinal with Codeine Capsules ... 2262
Isoclor Expectorant ... 990
Novahistine DH ... 2462
Novahistine Expectorant ... 2463
Nucofed ... 2051
Phenergan with Codeine ... 2777
Phenergan VC with Codeine ... 2781
Robitussin A-C Syrup ... 2073
Robitussin-DAC Syrup ... 2074
Ryna ... ▣ 841
Soma Compound w/Codeine Tablets ... 2676
Tussi-Organidin NR Liquid and S NR Liquid ... 2677
Tylenol with Codeine ... 1583

Desflurane (Concurrent use produces additive effects). Products include:
Suprane ... 1813

Dezocine (Concurrent use produces additive effects). Products include:
Dalgan Injection ... 538

Diazepam (Concurrent use produces additive effects). Products include:
Dizac ... 1809
Valium Injectable ... 2182
Valium Tablets ... 2183
Valrelease Capsules ... 2169

Droperidol (Concurrent use produces additive effects). Products include:
Inapsine Injection ... 1296

Enflurane (Concurrent use produces additive effects).
No products indexed under this heading.

Estazolam (Concurrent use produces additive effects). Products include:
ProSom Tablets ... 449

Ethchlorvynol (Concurrent use produces additive effects). Products include:
Placidyl Capsules ... 448

Ethinamate (Concurrent use produces additive effects).
No products indexed under this heading.

Fentanyl (Concurrent use produces additive effects). Products include:
Duragesic Transdermal System ... 1288

Fentanyl Citrate (Concurrent use produces additive effects). Products include:
Sublimaze Injection ... 1307

Fluphenazine Decanoate (Concurrent use produces additive effects). Products include:
Prolixin Decanoate ... 509

Fluphenazine Enanthate (Concurrent use produces additive effects). Products include:
Prolixin Enanthate ... 509

Fluphenazine Hydrochloride (Concurrent use produces additive effects). Products include:
Prolixin ... 509

Flurazepam Hydrochloride (Concurrent use produces additive effects). Products include:
Dalmane Capsules ... 2173

Furazolidone (Concurrent use is not recommended). Products include:
Furoxone ... 2046

Glutethimide (Concurrent use produces additive effects).
No products indexed under this heading.

Haloperidol (Concurrent use produces additive effects). Products include:
Haldol Injection, Tablets and Concentrate ... 1575

Haloperidol Decanoate (Concurrent use produces additive effects). Products include:
Haldol Decanoate ... 1577

Hydrocodone Bitartrate (Concurrent use produces additive effects). Products include:
Anexsia 5/500 Elixir ... 1781
Anexia Tablets ... 1782
Codiclear DH Syrup ... 791
Deconamine CX Cough and Cold Liquid and Tablets ... 1319
Duratuss HD Elixir ... 2565

IMPORTANT NOTE: Always consult each drug listing in the patient's regimen for possible interactions.

Allerest Maximum

Hycodan Tablets and Syrup 930
Hycomine Compound Tablets 932
Hycomine 931
Hycotuss Expectorant Syrup 933
Hydrocet Capsules 782
Lorcet 10/650.. 1018
Lortab 2566
Tussend 1783
Tussend Expectorant 1785
Vicodin Tablets...................................... 1356
Vicodin ES Tablets 1357
Vicodin Tuss Expectorant 1358
Zydone Capsules 949

Hydrocodone Polistirex (Concurrent use produces additive effects). Products include:

Tussionex Pennkinetic Extended-Release Suspension 998

Hydroxyzine Hydrochloride (Concurrent use produces additive effects). Products include:

Atarax Tablets & Syrup........................ 2185
Marax Tablets & DF Syrup.................. 2200
Vistaril Intramuscular Solution......... 2216

Isocarboxazid (Concurrent use is not recommended).

No products indexed under this heading.

Isoflurane (Concurrent use produces additive effects).

No products indexed under this heading.

Ketamine Hydrochloride (Concurrent use produces additive effects).

No products indexed under this heading.

Levomethadyl Acetate Hydrochloride (Concurrent use produces additive effects). Products include:

Orlaam 2239

Levorphanol Tartrate (Concurrent use produces additive effects). Products include:

Levo-Dromoran...................................... 2129

Lorazepam (Concurrent use produces additive effects). Products include:

Ativan Injection..................................... 2698
Ativan Tablets 2700

Loxapine Hydrochloride (Concurrent use produces additive effects). Products include:

Loxitane 1378

Loxapine Succinate (Concurrent use produces additive effects). Products include:

Loxitane Capsules 1378

Meperidine Hydrochloride (Concurrent use produces additive effects). Products include:

Demerol 2308
Mepergan Injection 2753

Mephobarbital (Concurrent use produces additive effects). Products include:

Mebaral Tablets 2322

Meprobamate (Concurrent use produces additive effects). Products include:

Miltown Tablets 2672
PMB 200 and PMB 400 2783

Mesoridazine Besylate (Concurrent use produces additive effects). Products include:

Serentil.. 684

Methadone Hydrochloride (Concurrent use produces additive effects). Products include:

Methadone Hydrochloride Oral Concentrate 2233
Methadone Hydrochloride Oral Solution & Tablets............................... 2235

Methohexital Sodium (Concurrent use produces additive effects). Products include:

Brevital Sodium Vials........................... 1429

Methotrimeprazine (Concurrent use produces additive effects). Products include:

Levoprome 1274

Methoxyflurane (Concurrent use produces additive effects).

No products indexed under this heading.

Midazolam Hydrochloride (Concurrent use produces additive effects). Products include:

Versed Injection 2170

Molindone Hydrochloride (Concurrent use produces additive effects). Products include:

Moban Tablets and Concentrate 1048

Morphine Sulfate (Concurrent use produces additive effects). Products include:

Astramorph/PF Injection, USP (Preservative-Free) 535
Duramorph 962
Infumorph 200 and Infumorph 500 Sterile Solutions......................... 965
MS Contin Tablets................................ 1994
MSIR 1997
Oramorph SR (Morphine Sulfate Sustained Release Tablets) 2236
RMS Suppositories 2657
Roxanol 2243

Opium Alkaloids (Concurrent use produces additive effects).

No products indexed under this heading.

Oxazepam (Concurrent use produces additive effects). Products include:

Serax Capsules 2810
Serax Tablets... 2810

Oxycodone Hydrochloride (Concurrent use produces additive effects). Products include:

Percocet Tablets 938
Percodan Tablets.................................. 939
Percodan-Demi Tablets....................... 940
Roxicodone Tablets, Oral Solution & Intensol (Oxycodone) 2244
Tylox Capsules 1584

Pentobarbital Sodium (Concurrent use produces additive effects). Products include:

Nembutal Sodium Capsules 436
Nembutal Sodium Solution 438
Nembutal Sodium Suppositories...... 440

Perphenazine (Concurrent use produces additive effects). Products include:

Etrafon 2355
Triavil Tablets 1757
Trilafon... 2389

Phenelzine Sulfate (Concurrent use is not recommended). Products include:

Nardil 1920

Phenobarbital (Concurrent use produces additive effects). Products include:

Arco-Lase Plus Tablets 512
Bellergal-S Tablets 2250
Donnatal 2060
Donnatal Extentabs.............................. 2061
Donnatal Tablets 2060
Phenobarbital Elixir and Tablets 1469
Quadrinal Tablets 1350

Prazepam (Concurrent use produces additive effects).

No products indexed under this heading.

Prochlorperazine (Concurrent use produces additive effects). Products include:

Compazine 2470

Promethazine Hydrochloride (Concurrent use produces additive effects). Products include:

Mepergan Injection 2753
Phenergan with Codeine.................... 2777
Phenergan with Dextromethorphan 2778
Phenergan Injection 2773
Phenergan Suppositories 2775
Phenergan Syrup 2774

Phenergan Tablets 2775
Phenergan VC 2779
Phenergan VC with Codeine 2781

Propofol (Concurrent use produces additive effects). Products include:

Diprivan Injection.................................. 2833

Propoxyphene Hydrochloride (Concurrent use produces additive effects). Products include:

Darvon 1435
Wygesic Tablets 2827

Propoxyphene Napsylate (Concurrent use produces additive effects). Products include:

Darvon-N/Darvocet-N 1433

Quazepam (Concurrent use produces additive effects). Products include:

Doral Tablets 2664

Risperidone (Concurrent use produces additive effects). Products include:

Risperdal 1301

Secobarbital Sodium (Concurrent use produces additive effects). Products include:

Seconal Sodium Pulvules 1474

Selegiline Hydrochloride (Concurrent use is not recommended). Products include:

Eldepryl Tablets 2550

Sufentanil Citrate (Concurrent use produces additive effects). Products include:

Sufenta Injection 1309

Temazepam (Concurrent use produces additive effects). Products include:

Restoril Capsules 2284

Thiamylal Sodium (Concurrent use produces additive effects).

No products indexed under this heading.

Thioridazine Hydrochloride (Concurrent use produces additive effects). Products include:

Mellaril 2269

Thiothixene (Concurrent use produces additive effects). Products include:

Navane Capsules and Concentrate 2201
Navane Intramuscular 2202

Tranylcypromine Sulfate (Concurrent use is not recommended). Products include:

Parnate Tablets 2503

Triazolam (Concurrent use produces additive effects). Products include:

Halcion Tablets...................................... 2611

Trifluoperazine Hydrochloride (Concurrent use produces additive effects). Products include:

Stelazine 2514

Zolpidem Tartrate (Concurrent use produces additive effects). Products include:

Ambien Tablets...................................... 2416

Food Interactions

Alcohol (Concurrent use produces additive effects).

ALLEREST NO DROWSINESS TABLETS

(Acetaminophen, Pseudoephedrine Hydrochloride)... ⊞ 627

See **Allerest Maximum Strength Tablets**

ALLEREST SINUS PAIN FORMULA

(Acetaminophen, Chlorpheniramine Maleate, Pseudoephedrine Hydrochloride)... ⊞ 627

See **Allerest Maximum Strength Tablets**

ALLEREST 12 HOUR CAPLETS

(Chlorpheniramine Maleate, Phenylpropanolamine Hydrochloride)... ⊞ 627

See **Allerest Maximum Strength Tablets**

ALL-FLEX ARCING SPRING DIAPHRAGM (SEE ALSO ORTHO DIAPHRAGM KITS)

(Diaphragm) 1865
None cited in PDR database.

ALOMIDE

(Lodoxamide Tromethamine).............. 469
None cited in PDR database.

ALPHA KERI MOISTURE RICH BODY OIL

(Lanolin Oil) .... ⊞ 613
None cited in PDR database.

ALTACE CAPSULES

(Ramipril) 1232
May interact with potassium sparing diuretics, diuretics, potassium preparations, lithium preparations, and certain other agents. Compounds in these categories include:

Amiloride Hydrochloride (May result in excessive reduction of blood pressure after initiation of therapy; increased risk of hyperkalemia). Products include:

Midamor Tablets 1703
Moduretic Tablets 1705

Bendroflumethiazide (May result in excessive reduction of blood pressure after initiation of therapy).

No products indexed under this heading.

Bumetanide (May result in excessive reduction of blood pressure after initiation of therapy). Products include:

Bumex 2093

Chlorothiazide (May result in excessive reduction of blood pressure after initiation of therapy). Products include:

Aldoclor Tablets 1598
Diupres Tablets 1650
Diuril Oral 1653

Chlorothiazide Sodium (May result in excessive reduction of blood pressure after initiation of therapy). Products include:

Diuril Sodium Intravenous 1652

Chlorthalidone (May result in excessive reduction of blood pressure after initiation of therapy). Products include:

Combipres Tablets 677
Tenoretic Tablets................................... 2845
Thalitone 1245

Ethacrynic Acid (May result in excessive reduction of blood pressure after initiation of therapy). Products include:

Edecrin Tablets...................................... 1657

Furosemide (May result in excessive reduction of blood pressure after initiation of therapy). Products include:

Lasix Injection, Oral Solution and Tablets 1240

Hydrochlorothiazide (May result in excessive reduction of blood pressure after initiation of therapy). Products include:

Aldactazide... 2413
Aldoril Tablets.. 1604
Apresazide Capsules 808
Capozide 742
Dyazide 2479
Esidrix Tablets 821
Esimil Tablets 822
HydroDIURIL Tablets 1674

(⊞ Described in PDR For Nonprescription Drugs) (◉ Described in PDR For Ophthalmology)

49 **Interactions Index** **Alupent**

Hydropres Tablets ... 1675
Hyzaar Tablets ... 1677
Inderide Tablets ... 2732
Inderide LA Long Acting Capsules .. 2734
Lopressor HCT Tablets ... 832
Lotensin HCT ... 837
Maxzide ... 1380
Moduretic Tablets ... 1705
Oretic Tablets ... 443
Prinzide Tablets ... 1737
Ser-Ap-Es Tablets ... 849
Timolide Tablets ... 1748
Vaseretic Tablets ... 1765
Zestoretic ... 2850
Ziac ... 1415

Hydroflumethiazide (May result in excessive reduction of blood pressure after initiation of therapy). Products include:
Diucardin Tablets ... 2718

Indapamide (May result in excessive reduction of blood pressure after initiation of therapy). Products include:
Lozol Tablets ... 2022

Lithium Carbonate (Increased serum lithium levels and symptoms of lithium toxicity). Products include:
Eskalith ... 2485
Lithium Carbonate Capsules & Tablets ... 2230
Lithonate/Lithotabs/Lithobid ... 2543

Lithium Citrate (Increased serum lithium levels and symptoms of lithium toxicity).
No products indexed under this heading.

Methyclothiazide (May result in excessive reduction of blood pressure after initiation of therapy). Products include:
Enduron Tablets ... 420

Metolazone (May result in excessive reduction of blood pressure after initiation of therapy). Products include:
Mykrox Tablets ... 993
Zaroxolyn Tablets ... 1000

Polythiazide (May result in excessive reduction of blood pressure after initiation of therapy). Products include:
Minizide Capsules ... 1938

Potassium Acid Phosphate (Increased risk of hyperkalemia). Products include:
K-Phos Original Formula 'Sodium Free' Tablets ... 639

Potassium Bicarbonate (Increased risk of hyperkalemia). Products include:
Alka-Seltzer Gold Effervescent Antacid ... 703

Potassium Chloride (Increased risk of hyperkalemia). Products include:
Chlor-3 Condiment ... 1004
K-Dur Microburst Release System (potassium chloride, USP) E.R. Tablets ... 1325
K-Lor Powder Packets ... 434
K-Norm Extended-Release Capsules ... 991
K-Tab Filmtab ... 434
Kolyum Liquid ... 992
Micro-K ... 2063
Micro-K LS Packets ... 2064
NuLYTELY ... 689
Cherry Flavor NuLYTELY ... 689
Rum-K Syrup ... 1005
Slow-K Extended-Release Tablets ... 851

Potassium Citrate (Increased risk of hyperkalemia). Products include:
Polycitra Syrup ... 578
Polycitra-K Crystals ... 579
Polycitra-K Oral Solution ... 579
Polycitra-LC ... 578

Potassium Gluconate (Increased risk of hyperkalemia). Products include:
Kolyum Liquid ... 992

Potassium Phosphate, Dibasic (Increased risk of hyperkalemia).
No products indexed under this heading.

Potassium Phosphate, Monobasic (Increased risk of hyperkalemia). Products include:
K-Phos Neutral Tablets ... 639
K-Phos Original Formula 'Sodium Free' Tablets ... 639

Spironolactone (May result in excessive reduction of blood pressure after initiation of therapy; increased risk of hyperkalemia). Products include:
Aldactazide ... 2413
Aldactone ... 2414

Torsemide (May result in excessive reduction of blood pressure after initiation of therapy). Products include:
Demadex Tablets and Injection ... 686

Triamterene (May result in excessive reduction of blood pressure after initiation of therapy; increased risk of hyperkalemia). Products include:
Dyazide ... 2479
Dyrenium Capsules ... 2481
Maxzide ... 1380

Food Interactions

Food, unspecified (The rate of absorption is reduced, not the extent of absorption).

Salt substitutes, potassium-containing (Increases risk of hyperkalemia).

ALTERNAGEL LIQUID
(Aluminum Hydroxide) ... 1316
May interact with tetracyclines. Compounds in this category include:

Demeclocycline Hydrochloride (Should not be taken concurrently). Products include:
Declomycin Tablets ... 1371

Doxycycline Calcium (Should not be taken concurrently). Products include:
Vibramycin Calcium Oral Suspension Syrup ... 1941

Doxycycline Hyclate (Should not be taken concurrently). Products include:
Doryx Capsules ... 1913
Vibramycin Hyclate Capsules ... 1941
Vibramycin Hyclate Intravenous ... 2215
Vibra-Tabs Film Coated Tablets ... 1941

Doxycycline Monohydrate (Should not be taken concurrently). Products include:
Monodox Capsules ... 1805
Vibramycin Monohydrate for Oral Suspension ... 1941

Methacycline Hydrochloride (Should not be taken concurrently).
No products indexed under this heading.

Minocycline Hydrochloride (Should not be taken concurrently). Products include:
Dynacin Capsules ... 1590
Minocin Intravenous ... 1382
Minocin Oral Suspension ... 1385
Minocin Pellet-Filled Capsules ... 1383

Oxytetracycline (Should not be taken concurrently). Products include:
Terramycin Intramuscular Solution 2210

Oxytetracycline Hydrochloride (Should not be taken concurrently). Products include:
TERAK Ointment ... ◉ 209
Terra-Cortril Ophthalmic Suspension ... 2210
Terramycin with Polymyxin B Sulfate Ophthalmic Ointment ... 2211
Urobiotic-250 Capsules ... 2214

Tetracycline Hydrochloride (Should not be taken concurrently). Products include:
Achromycin V Capsules ... 1367

ALUDROX ORAL SUSPENSION
(Aluminum Hydroxide Gel, Magnesium Hydroxide) ... 2695
May interact with tetracyclines. Compounds in this category include:

Demeclocycline Hydrochloride (Avoid concurrent administration). Products include:
Declomycin Tablets ... 1371

Doxycycline Calcium (Avoid concurrent administration). Products include:
Vibramycin Calcium Oral Suspension Syrup ... 1941

Doxycycline Hyclate (Avoid concurrent administration). Products include:
Doryx Capsules ... 1913
Vibramycin Hyclate Capsules ... 1941
Vibramycin Hyclate Intravenous ... 2215
Vibra-Tabs Film Coated Tablets ... 1941

Doxycycline Monohydrate (Avoid concurrent administration). Products include:
Monodox Capsules ... 1805
Vibramycin Monohydrate for Oral Suspension ... 1941

Methacycline Hydrochloride (Avoid concurrent administration).
No products indexed under this heading.

Minocycline Hydrochloride (Avoid concurrent administration). Products include:
Dynacin Capsules ... 1590
Minocin Intravenous ... 1382
Minocin Oral Suspension ... 1385
Minocin Pellet-Filled Capsules ... 1383

Oxytetracycline (Avoid concurrent administration). Products include:
Terramycin Intramuscular Solution 2210

Oxytetracycline Hydrochloride (Avoid concurrent administration). Products include:
TERAK Ointment ... ◉ 209
Terra-Cortril Ophthalmic Suspension ... 2210
Terramycin with Polymyxin B Sulfate Ophthalmic Ointment ... 2211
Urobiotic-250 Capsules ... 2214

Tetracycline Hydrochloride (Avoid concurrent administration). Products include:
Achromycin V Capsules ... 1367

ALUPENT INHALATION AEROSOL
(Metaproterenol Sulfate) ... 669
See **Alupent Inhalation Solution**

ALUPENT INHALATION SOLUTION
(Metaproterenol Sulfate) ... 669
May interact with monoamine oxidase inhibitors, tricyclic antidepressants, and sympathomimetic aerosol bronchodilators. Compounds in these categories include:

Albuterol (Possible potentiation of adrenergic effects with beta adrenergic aerosol bronchodilators). Products include:
Proventil Inhalation Aerosol ... 2382
Ventolin Inhalation Aerosol and Refill ... 1197

Amitriptyline Hydrochloride (The action of beta adrenergic agonists on the vascular system may be potentiated). Products include:
Elavil ... 2838
Endep Tablets ... 2174
Etrafon ... 2355
Limbitrol ... 2180
Triavil Tablets ... 1757

Amoxapine (The action of beta adrenergic agonists on the vascular system may be potentiated). Products include:
Asendin Tablets ... 1369

Bitolterol Mesylate (Possible potentiation of adrenergic effects with beta adrenergic aerosol bronchodilators). Products include:
Tornalate Solution for Inhalation, 0.2% ... 956
Tornalate Metered Dose Inhaler ... 957

Clomipramine Hydrochloride (The action of beta adrenergic agonists on the vascular system may be potentiated). Products include:
Anafranil Capsules ... 803

Desipramine Hydrochloride (The action of beta adrenergic agonists on the vascular system may be potentiated). Products include:
Norpramin Tablets ... 1526

Doxepin Hydrochloride (The action of beta adrenergic agonists on the vascular system may be potentiated). Products include:
Sinequan ... 2205
Zonalon Cream ... 1055

Furazolidone (The action of beta adrenergic agonists on the vascular system may be potentiated). Products include:
Furoxone ... 2046

Imipramine Hydrochloride (The action of beta adrenergic agonists on the vascular system may be potentiated). Products include:
Tofranil Ampuls ... 854
Tofranil Tablets ... 856

Imipramine Pamoate (The action of beta adrenergic agonists on the vascular system may be potentiated). Products include:
Tofranil-PM Capsules ... 857

Isocarboxazid (The action of beta adrenergic agonists on the vascular system may be potentiated).
No products indexed under this heading.

Isoetharine (Possible potentiation of adrenergic effects with beta adrenergic aerosol bronchodilators). Products include:
Bronkometer Aerosol ... 2302
Bronkosol Solution ... 2302
Isoetharine Inhalation Solution, USP, Arm-a-Med ... 551

Isoproterenol Hydrochloride (Possible potentiation of adrenergic effects with beta adrenergic aerosol bronchodilators). Products include:
Isuprel Hydrochloride Injection 1:5000 ... 2311
Isuprel Hydrochloride Solution 1:200 & 1:100 ... 2313
Isuprel Mistometer ... 2312

Maprotiline Hydrochloride (The action of beta adrenergic agonists on the vascular system may be potentiated). Products include:
Ludiomil Tablets ... 843

Nortriptyline Hydrochloride (The action of beta adrenergic agonists on the vascular system may be potentiated). Products include:
Pamelor ... 2280

Phenelzine Sulfate (The action of beta adrenergic agonists on the vascular system may be potentiated). Products include:
Nardil ... 1920

Pirbuterol Acetate (Possible potentiation of adrenergic effects with beta adrenergic aerosol bronchodilators). Products include:
Maxair Autohaler ... 1492
Maxair Inhaler ... 1494

IMPORTANT NOTE: Always consult each drug listing in the patient's regimen for possible interactions.

Alupent

Interactions Index

Protriptyline Hydrochloride (The action of beta adrenergic agonists on the vascular system may be potentiated). Products include:

Vivactil Tablets 1774

Salmeterol Xinafoate (Possible potentiation of adrenergic effects with beta adrenergic aerosol bronchodilators). Products include:

Serevent Inhalation Aerosol................. 1176

Selegiline Hydrochloride (The action of beta adrenergic agonists on the vascular system may be potentiated). Products include:

Eldepryl Tablets 2550

Terbutaline Sulfate (Possible potentiation of adrenergic effects with beta adrenergic aerosol bronchodilators). Products include:

Brethaire Inhaler 813
Brethine Ampuls 815
Brethine Tablets....................................... 814
Bricanyl Subcutaneous Injection 1502
Bricanyl Tablets 1503

Tranylcypromine Sulfate (The action of beta adrenergic agonists on the vascular system may be potentiated). Products include:

Parnate Tablets 2503

Trimipramine Maleate (The action of beta adrenergic agonists on the vascular system may be potentiated). Products include:

Surmontil Capsules................................. 2811

ALUPENT SYRUP

(Metaproterenol Sulfate)........................ 669
See Alupent Inhalation Solution

ALUPENT TABLETS

(Metaproterenol Sulfate)........................ 669
See Alupent Inhalation Solution

AMBIEN TABLETS

(Zolpidem Tartrate).................................2416
May interact with central nervous system depressants and certain other agents. Compounds in these categories include:

Alfentanil Hydrochloride (Potential for enhanced CNS depressant effects of zolpidem). Products include:

Alfenta Injection 1286

Alprazolam (Potential for enhanced CNS depressant effects of zolpidem). Products include:

Xanax Tablets 2649

Aprobarbital (Potential for enhanced CNS depressant effects of zolpidem).

No products indexed under this heading.

Buprenorphine (Potential for enhanced CNS depressant effects of zolpidem). Products include:

Buprenex Injectable 2006

Buspirone Hydrochloride (Potential for enhanced CNS depressant effects of zolpidem). Products include:

BuSpar 737

Butabarbital (Potential for enhanced CNS depressant effects of zolpidem).

No products indexed under this heading.

Butalbital (Potential for enhanced CNS depressant effects of zolpidem). Products include:

Esgic-plus Tablets 1013
Fioricet Tablets... 2258
Fioricet with Codeine Capsules 2260
Fiorinal Capsules 2261
Fiorinal with Codeine Capsules 2262
Fiorinal Tablets... 2261
Phrenilin 785

Sedapap Tablets 50 mg/650 mg .. 1543

Chlordiazepoxide (Potential for enhanced CNS depressant effects of zolpidem). Products include:

Libritabs Tablets 2177
Limbitrol 2180

Chlordiazepoxide Hydrochloride (Potential for enhanced CNS depressant effects of zolpidem). Products include:

Librax Capsules 2176
Librium Capsules...................................... 2178
Librium Injectable 2179

Chlorpromazine (Additive effect of decreased alertness and psychomotor performance; potential for enhanced CNS depressant effects of zolpidem). Products include:

Thorazine Suppositories........................ 2523

Chlorpromazine Hydrochloride (Additive effect of decreased alertness and psychomotor performance; potential for enhanced CNS depressant effects of zolpidem). Products include:

Thorazine 2523

Chlorprothixene (Potential for enhanced CNS depressant effects of zolpidem).

No products indexed under this heading.

Chlorprothixene Hydrochloride (Potential for enhanced CNS depressant effects of zolpidem).

No products indexed under this heading.

Clorazepate Dipotassium (Potential for enhanced CNS depressant effects of zolpidem). Products include:

Tranxene 451

Clozapine (Potential for enhanced CNS depressant effects of zolpidem). Products include:

Clozaril Tablets.. 2252

Codeine Phosphate (Potential for enhanced CNS depressant effects of zolpidem). Products include:

Actifed with Codeine Cough Syrup.. 1067
Brontex 1981
Deconsal C Expectorant Syrup 456
Deconsal Pediatric Syrup 457
Dimetane-DC Cough Syrup 2059
Empirin with Codeine Tablets............ 1093
Fioricet with Codeine Capsules 2260
Fiorinal with Codeine Capsules 2262
Isoclor Expectorant.................................. 990
Novahistine DH... 2462
Novahistine Expectorant....................... 2463
Nucofed 2051
Phenergan with Codeine 2777
Phenergan VC with Codeine 2781
Robitussin A-C Syrup.............................. 2073
Robitussin-DAC Syrup 2074
Ryna .... ◻ 841
Soma Compound w/Codeine Tablets 2676
Tussi-Organidin NR Liquid and S NR Liquid 2677
Tylenol with Codeine 1583

Desflurane (Potential for enhanced CNS depressant effects of zolpidem). Products include:

Suprane 1813

Dezocine (Potential for enhanced CNS depressant effects of zolpidem). Products include:

Dalgan Injection 538

Diazepam (Potential for enhanced CNS depressant effects of zolpidem). Products include:

Dizac 1809
Valium Injectable 2182
Valium Tablets 2183
Valrelease Capsules 2169

Droperidol (Potential for enhanced CNS depressant effects of zolpidem). Products include:

Inapsine Injection..................................... 1296

Enflurane (Potential for enhanced CNS depressant effects of zolpidem).

No products indexed under this heading.

Estazolam (Potential for enhanced CNS depressant effects of zolpidem). Products include:

ProSom Tablets 449

Ethchlorvynol (Potential for enhanced CNS depressant effects of zolpidem). Products include:

Placidyl Capsules...................................... 448

Ethinamate (Potential for enhanced CNS depressant effects of zolpidem).

No products indexed under this heading.

Fentanyl (Potential for enhanced CNS depressant effects of zolpidem). Products include:

Duragesic Transdermal System......... 1288

Fentanyl Citrate (Potential for enhanced CNS depressant effects of zolpidem). Products include:

Sublimaze Injection................................. 1307

Flumazenil (Flumazenil reverses sedative/hypnotic effects of Zolpidem). Products include:

Romazicon 2147

Fluphenazine Decanoate (Potential for enhanced CNS depressant effects of zolpidem). Products include:

Prolixin Decanoate 509

Fluphenazine Enanthate (Potential for enhanced CNS depressant effects of zolpidem). Products include:

Prolixin Enanthate 509

Fluphenazine Hydrochloride (Potential for enhanced CNS depressant effects of zolpidem). Products include:

Prolixin 509

Flurazepam Hydrochloride (Potential for enhanced CNS depressant effects of zolpidem). Products include:

Dalmane Capsules.................................... 2173

Glutethimide (Potential for enhanced CNS depressant effects of zolpidem).

No products indexed under this heading.

Haloperidol (Potential for enhanced CNS depressant effects of zolpidem). Products include:

Haldol Injection, Tablets and Concentrate 1575

Haloperidol Decanoate (Potential for enhanced CNS depressant effects of zolpidem). Products include:

Haldol Decanoate...................................... 1577

Hydrocodone Bitartrate (Potential for enhanced CNS depressant effects of zolpidem). Products include:

Anexsia 5/500 Elixir 1781
Anexia Tablets.. 1782
Codiclear DH Syrup 791
Deconamine CX Cough and Cold Liquid and Tablets................................ 1319
Duratuss HD Elixir.................................... 2565
Hycodan Tablets and Syrup 930
Hycomine Compound Tablets 932
Hycomine 931
Hycotuss Expectorant Syrup 933
Hydrocet Capsules 782
Lorcet 10/650... 1018
Lortab 2566
Tussend 1783
Tussend Expectorant 1785
Vicodin Tablets... 1356
Vicodin ES Tablets 1357
Vicodin Tuss Expectorant 1358
Zydone Capsules 949

Hydrocodone Polistirex (Potential for enhanced CNS depressant effects of zolpidem). Products include:

Tussionex Pennkinetic Extended-Release Suspension 998

Hydroxyzine Hydrochloride (Potential for enhanced CNS depressant effects of zolpidem). Products include:

Atarax Tablets & Syrup.......................... 2185
Marax Tablets & DF Syrup.................... 2200
Vistaril Intramuscular Solution.......... 2216

Imipramine Hydrochloride (Coadministration produces 20% decrease in peak levels of imipramine with an additive effect of decreased alertness). Products include:

Tofranil Ampuls 854
Tofranil Tablets 856

Imipramine Pamoate (Coadministration produces 20% decrease in peak levels of imipramine with an additive effect of decreased alertness). Products include:

Tofranil-PM Capsules............................... 857

Isoflurane (Potential for enhanced CNS depressant effects of zolpidem).

No products indexed under this heading.

Ketamine Hydrochloride (Potential for enhanced CNS depressant effects of zolpidem).

No products indexed under this heading.

Levomethadyl Acetate Hydrochloride (Potential for enhanced CNS depressant effects of zolpidem). Products include:

Orlaam 2239

Levorphanol Tartrate (Potential for enhanced CNS depressant effects of zolpidem). Products include:

Levo-Dromoran 2129

Lorazepam (Potential for enhanced CNS depressant effects of zolpidem). Products include:

Ativan Injection.. 2698
Ativan Tablets 2700

Loxapine Hydrochloride (Potential for enhanced CNS depressant effects of zolpidem). Products include:

Loxitane 1378

Loxapine Succinate (Potential for enhanced CNS depressant effects of zolpidem). Products include:

Loxitane Capsules 1378

Meperidine Hydrochloride (Potential for enhanced CNS depressant effects of zolpidem). Products include:

Demerol 2308
Mepergan Injection 2753

Mephobarbital (Potential for enhanced CNS depressant effects of zolpidem). Products include:

Mebaral Tablets 2322

Meprobamate (Potential for enhanced CNS depressant effects of zolpidem). Products include:

Miltown Tablets 2672
PMB 200 and PMB 400 2783

Mesoridazine Besylate (Potential for enhanced CNS depressant effects of zolpidem). Products include:

Serentil 684

Methadone Hydrochloride (Potential for enhanced CNS depressant effects of zolpidem). Products include:

Methadone Hydrochloride Oral Concentrate 2233
Methadone Hydrochloride Oral Solution & Tablets................................ 2235

(◻ Described in PDR For Nonprescription Drugs) (◉ Described in PDR For Ophthalmology)

Methohexital Sodium (Potential for enhanced CNS depressant effects of zolpidem). Products include:

Brevital Sodium Vials 1429

Methotrimeprazine (Potential for enhanced CNS depressant effects of zolpidem). Products include:

Levoprome 1274

Methoxyflurane (Potential for enhanced CNS depressant effects of zolpidem).

No products indexed under this heading.

Midazolam Hydrochloride (Potential for enhanced CNS depressant effects of zolpidem). Products include:

Versed Injection 2170

Molindone Hydrochloride (Potential for enhanced CNS depressant effects of zolpidem). Products include:

Moban Tablets and Concentrate 1048

Morphine Sulfate (Potential for enhanced CNS depressant effects of zolpidem). Products include:

Astramorph/PF Injection, USP (Preservative-Free) 535
Duramorph 962
Infumorph 200 and Infumorph 500 Sterile Solutions 965
MS Contin Tablets 1994
MSIR 1997
Oramorph SR (Morphine Sulfate Sustained Release Tablets) 2236
RMS Suppositories 2657
Roxanol 2243

Opium Alkaloids (Potential for enhanced CNS depressant effects of zolpidem).

No products indexed under this heading.

Oxazepam (Potential for enhanced CNS depressant effects of zolpidem). Products include:

Serax Capsules 2810
Serax Tablets 2810

Oxycodone Hydrochloride (Potential for enhanced CNS depressant effects of zolpidem). Products include:

Percocet Tablets 938
Percodan Tablets 939
Percodan-Demi Tablets 940
Roxicodone Tablets, Oral Solution & Intensol (Oxycodone) 2244
Tylox Capsules 1584

Pentobarbital Sodium (Potential for enhanced CNS depressant effects of zolpidem). Products include:

Nembutal Sodium Capsules 436
Nembutal Sodium Solution 438
Nembutal Sodium Suppositories 440

Perphenazine (Potential for enhanced CNS depressant effects of zolpidem). Products include:

Etrafon 2355
Triavil Tablets 1757
Trilafon 2389

Phenobarbital (Potential for enhanced CNS depressant effects of zolpidem). Products include:

Arco-Lase Plus Tablets 512
Bellergal-S Tablets 2250
Donnatal 2060
Donnatal Extentabs 2061
Donnatal Tablets 2060
Phenobarbital Elixir and Tablets 1469
Quadrinal Tablets 1350

Prazepam (Potential for enhanced CNS depressant effects of zolpidem).

No products indexed under this heading.

Prochlorperazine (Potential for enhanced CNS depressant effects of zolpidem). Products include:

Compazine 2470

Promethazine Hydrochloride (Potential for enhanced CNS depressant effects of zolpidem). Products include:

Mepergan Injection 2753
Phenergan with Codeine 2777
Phenergan with Dextromethorphan 2778
Phenergan Injection 2773
Phenergan Suppositories 2775
Phenergan Syrup 2774
Phenergan Tablets 2775
Phenergan VC 2779
Phenergan VC with Codeine 2781

Propofol (Potential for enhanced CNS depressant effects of zolpidem). Products include:

Diprivan Injection 2833

Propoxyphene Hydrochloride (Potential for enhanced CNS depressant effects of zolpidem). Products include:

Darvon 1435
Wygesic Tablets 2827

Propoxyphene Napsylate (Potential for enhanced CNS depressant effects of zolpidem). Products include:

Darvon-N/Darvocet-N 1433

Quazepam (Potential for enhanced CNS depressant effects of zolpidem). Products include:

Doral Tablets 2664

Risperidone (Potential for enhanced CNS depressant effects of zolpidem). Products include:

Risperdal 1301

Secobarbital Sodium (Potential for enhanced CNS depressant effects of zolpidem). Products include:

Seconal Sodium Pulvules 1474

Sufentanil Citrate (Potential for enhanced CNS depressant effects of zolpidem). Products include:

Sufenta Injection 1309

Temazepam (Potential for enhanced CNS depressant effects of zolpidem). Products include:

Restoril Capsules 2284

Thiamylal Sodium (Potential for enhanced CNS depressant effects of zolpidem).

No products indexed under this heading.

Thioridazine Hydrochloride (Potential for enhanced CNS depressant effects of zolpidem). Products include:

Mellaril 2269

Thiothixene (Potential for enhanced CNS depressant effects of zolpidem). Products include:

Navane Capsules and Concentrate 2201
Navane Intramuscular 2202

Triazolam (Potential for enhanced CNS depressant effects of zolpidem). Products include:

Halcion Tablets 2611

Trifluoperazine Hydrochloride (Potential for enhanced CNS depressant effects of zolpidem). Products include:

Stelazine 2514

Food Interactions

Alcohol (Coadministration produces additive effects on psychomotor performance).

Meal, unspecified (Mean AUC and C_{max} decreased by 15% and 25% respectively, while T_{max} was prolonged by 60%; for faster sleep onset, Ambien should not be administered with or immediately after meal).

AMEN TABLETS

(Medroxyprogesterone Acetate) .... 780 May interact with estrogens and certain other agents. Compounds in these categories include:

Aminoglutethimide (Concomitant administration may depress the bioavailability of Amen). Products include:

Cytadren Tablets 819

Chlorotrianisene (Potential for adverse effects on carbohydrate and lipid metabolism).

No products indexed under this heading.

Dienestrol (Potential for adverse effects on carbohydrate and lipid metabolism). Products include:

Ortho Dienestrol Cream 1866

Diethylstilbestrol (Potential for adverse effects on carbohydrate and lipid metabolism). Products include:

Diethylstilbestrol Tablets 1437

Estradiol (Potential for adverse effects on carbohydrate and lipid metabolism). Products include:

Climara Transdermal System 645
Estrace Cream and Tablets 749
Estraderm Transdermal System 824

Estrogens, Conjugated (Potential for adverse effects on carbohydrate and lipid metabolism). Products include:

PMB 200 and PMB 400 2783
Premarin Intravenous 2787
Premarin with Methyltestosterone .. 2794
Premarin Tablets 2789
Premarin Vaginal Cream 2791
Premphase 2797
Prempro 2801

Estrogens, Esterified (Potential for adverse effects on carbohydrate and lipid metabolism). Products include:

ESTRATAB Tablets (0.3, 0.625, 1.25, 2.5 mg) 2536
Estratest 2539
Menest Tablets 2494

Estropipate (Potential for adverse effects on carbohydrate and lipid metabolism). Products include:

Ogen Tablets 2627
Ogen Vaginal Cream 2630
Ortho-Est 1869

Ethinyl Estradiol (Potential for adverse effects on carbohydrate and lipid metabolism). Products include:

Brevicon 2088
Demulen 2428
Desogen Tablets 1817
Levlen/Tri-Levlen 651
Lo/Ovral Tablets 2746
Lo/Ovral-28 Tablets 2751
Modicon 1872
Nordette-21 Tablets 2755
Nordette-28 Tablets 2758
Norinyl 2088
Ortho-Cept 1851
Ortho-Cyclen/Ortho-Tri-Cyclen 1858
Ortho-Novum 1872
Ortho-Cyclen/Ortho Tri-Cyclen 1858
Ovcon 760
Ovral Tablets 2770
Ovral-28 Tablets 2770
Levlen/Tri-Levlen 651
Tri-Norinyl 2164
Triphasil-21 Tablets 2814
Triphasil-28 Tablets 2819

Polyestradiol Phosphate (Potential for adverse effects on carbohydrate and lipid metabolism).

No products indexed under this heading.

Quinestrol (Potential for adverse effects on carbohydrate and lipid metabolism).

No products indexed under this heading.

AMERICAINE ANESTHETIC LUBRICANT

(Benzocaine) .... 983 None cited in PDR database.

AMERICAINE HEMORRHOIDAL OINTMENT

(Benzocaine) .... ⊕ 629 None cited in PDR database.

AMERICAINE OTIC TOPICAL ANESTHETIC EAR DROPS

(Benzocaine) .... 983 None cited in PDR database.

AMERICAINE TOPICAL ANESTHETIC FIRST AID OINTMENT

(Benzocaine) .... ⊕ 629 None cited in PDR database.

AMERICAINE TOPICAL ANESTHETIC SPRAY

(Benzocaine) .... ⊕ 629 None cited in PDR database.

AMICAR SYRUP, TABLETS, AND INJECTION

(Aminocaproic Acid) .... 1267 None cited in PDR database.

AMIKACIN SULFATE INJECTION, USP

(Amikacin Sulfate) .... 960 May interact with aminoglycosides, anesthetics, cephalosporins, neuromuscular blocking agents, penicillins, and certain other agents. Compounds in these categories include:

Alfentanil Hydrochloride (Increased potential for neuromuscular blockade and respiratory paralysis). Products include:

Alfenta Injection 1286

Amoxicillin Trihydrate (Potential for mutual inactivation and a reduction in serum half-life may occur). Products include:

Amoxil 2464
Augmentin 2468

Amphotericin B (Concurrent and/or sequential use may increase the potential for increased toxicity). Products include:

Fungizone Intravenous 506

Ampicillin Sodium (Potential for mutual inactivation and a reduction in serum half-life may occur). Products include:

Unasyn 2212

Atracurium Besylate (Increased potential for neuromuscular blockade and respiratory paralysis). Products include:

Tracrium Injection 1183

Azlocillin Sodium (Potential for mutual inactivation and a reduction in serum half-life may occur).

No products indexed under this heading.

Bacampicillin Hydrochloride (Potential for mutual inactivation and a reduction in serum half-life may occur). Products include:

Spectrobid Tablets 2206

Bacitracin Zinc (Concurrent and/or sequential use may increase the potential for increased toxicity). Products include:

AK-Spore Ointment .... © 204
Bactine First Aid Antibiotic Plus Anesthetic Ointment .... ⊕ 708
Betadine Brand First Aid Antibiotics & Moisturizer Ointment 1991
Campho-Phenique Maximum Strength First Aid Antibiotic Plus Pain Reliever Ointment .... ⊕ 719
Cortisporin Ointment 1085
Cortisporin Ophthalmic Ointment Sterile 1085
Neosporin Ointment .... ⊕ 857

IMPORTANT NOTE: Always consult each drug listing in the patient's regimen for possible interactions.

Amikacin

Neosporin Plus Maximum Strength Ointment .... ◼ 858
Neosporin Ophthalmic Ointment Sterile 1148
Polysporin Ointment............................ ◼ 858
Polysporin Ophthalmic Ointment Sterile 1154
Polysporin Powder .... ◼ 859

Carbenicillin Indanyl Sodium (Potential for mutual inactivation and a reduction in serum half-life may occur). Products include:

Geocillin Tablets.. 2199

Cefaclor (Potential for increased nephrotoxicity and concomitant cephalosporins may spuriously elevate creatinine determinations). Products include:

Ceclor Pulvules & Suspension 1431

Cefadroxil Monohydrate (Potential for increased nephrotoxicity and concomitant cephalosporins may spuriously elevate creatinine determinations). Products include:

Duricef 748

Cefamandole Nafate (Potential for increased nephrotoxicity and concomitant cephalosporins may spuriously elevate creatinine determinations). Products include:

Mandol Vials, Faspak & ADD-Vantage 1461

Cefazolin Sodium (Potential for increased nephrotoxicity and concomitant cephalosporins may spuriously elevate creatinine determinations). Products include:

Ancef Injection 2465
Kefzol Vials, Faspak & ADD-Vantage 1456

Cefixime (Potential for increased nephrotoxicity and concomitant cephalosporins may spuriously elevate creatinine determinations). Products include:

Suprax 1399

Cefmetazole Sodium (Potential for increased nephrotoxicity and concomitant cephalosporins may spuriously elevate creatinine determinations). Products include:

Zefazone 2654

Cefonicid Sodium (Potential for increased nephrotoxicity and concomitant cephalosporins may spuriously elevate creatinine determinations). Products include:

Monocid Injection 2497

Cefoperazone Sodium (Potential for increased nephrotoxicity and concomitant cephalosporins may spuriously elevate creatinine determinations). Products include:

Cefobid Intravenous/Intramuscular 2189
Cefobid Pharmacy Bulk Package - Not for Direct Infusion....................... 2192

Ceforanide (Potential for increased nephrotoxicity and concomitant cephalosporins may spuriously elevate creatinine determinations).

No products indexed under this heading.

Cefotaxime Sodium (Potential for increased nephrotoxicity and concomitant cephalosporins may spuriously elevate creatinine determinations). Products include:

Claforan Sterile and Injection 1235

Cefotetan (Potential for increased nephrotoxicity and concomitant cephalosporins may spuriously elevate creatinine determinations). Products include:

Cefotan.. 2829

Cefoxitin Sodium (Potential for increased nephrotoxicity and concomitant cephalosporins may spuriously elevate creatinine determinations). Products include:

Mefoxin 1691
Mefoxin Premixed Intravenous Solution 1694

Cefpodoxime Proxetil (Potential for increased nephrotoxicity and concomitant cephalosporins may spuriously elevate creatinine determinations). Products include:

Vantin for Oral Suspension and Vantin Tablets 2646

Cefprozil (Potential for increased nephrotoxicity and concomitant cephalosporins may spuriously elevate creatinine determinations). Products include:

Cefzil Tablets and Oral Suspension 746

Ceftazidime (Potential for increased nephrotoxicity and concomitant cephalosporins may spuriously elevate creatinine determinations). Products include:

Ceptaz 1081
Fortaz 1100
Tazicef for Injection 2519
Tazidime Vials, Faspak & ADD-Vantage 1478

Ceftizoxime Sodium (Potential for increased nephrotoxicity and concomitant cephalosporins may spuriously elevate creatinine determinations). Products include:

Cefizox for Intramuscular or Intravenous Use 1034

Ceftriaxone Sodium (Potential for increased nephrotoxicity and concomitant cephalosporins may spuriously elevate creatinine determinations). Products include:

Rocephin Injectable Vials, ADD-Vantage, Galaxy Container............... 2142

Cefuroxime Axetil (Potential for increased nephrotoxicity and concomitant cephalosporins may spuriously elevate creatinine determinations). Products include:

Ceftin 1078

Cefuroxime Sodium (Potential for increased nephrotoxicity and concomitant cephalosporins may spuriously elevate creatinine determinations). Products include:

Kefurox Vials, Faspak & ADD-Vantage 1454
Zinacef 1211

Cephalexin (Potential for increased nephrotoxicity and concomitant cephalosporins may spuriously elevate creatinine determinations). Products include:

Keflex Pulvules & Oral Suspension 914

Cephaloridine (Concurrent and/or sequential use may increase the potential for increased toxicity).

Cephalothin Sodium (Potential for increased nephrotoxicity and concomitant cephalosporins may spuriously elevate creatinine determinations).

Cephapirin Sodium (Potential for increased nephrotoxicity and concomitant cephalosporins may spuriously elevate creatinine determinations).

No products indexed under this heading.

Cephradine (Potential for increased nephrotoxicity and concomitant cephalosporins may spuriously elevate creatinine determinations).

No products indexed under this heading.

Cisplatin (Concurrent and/or sequential use may increase the potential for increased toxicity). Products include:

Platinol 708
Platinol-AQ Injection............................... 710

Colistin Sulfate (Concurrent and/or sequential use may increase the potential for increased toxicity). Products include:

Coly-Mycin S Otic w/Neomycin & Hydrocortisone 1906

Dicloxacillin Sodium (Potential for mutual inactivation and a reduction in serum half-life may occur).

No products indexed under this heading.

Doxacurium Chloride (Increased potential for neuromuscular blockade and respiratory paralysis). Products include:

Nuromax Injection................................... 1149

Enflurane (Increased potential for neuromuscular blockade and respiratory paralysis).

No products indexed under this heading.

Ethacrynic Acid (Potential for increased ototoxicity; concurrent use should be avoided). Products include:

Edecrin Tablets.. 1657

Fentanyl Citrate (Increased potential for neuromuscular blockade and respiratory paralysis). Products include:

Sublimaze Injection................................. 1307

Furosemide (Potential for increased ototoxicity; concurrent use should be avoided). Products include:

Lasix Injection, Oral Solution and Tablets 1240

Gentamicin Sulfate (Concurrent and/or sequential use may increase the potential for increased toxicity). Products include:

Garamycin Injectable 2360
Genoptic Sterile Ophthalmic Solution.. ◉ 243
Genoptic Sterile Ophthalmic Ointment .... ◉ 243
Gentacidin Ointment .... ◉ 264
Gentacidin Solution................................ ◉ 264
Gentak .... ◉ 208
Pred-G Liquifilm Sterile Ophthalmic Suspension .... ◉ 251
Pred-G S.O.P. Sterile Ophthalmic Ointment .... ◉ 252

Halothane (Increased potential for neuromuscular blockade and respiratory paralysis). Products include:

Fluothane 2724

Isoflurane (Increased potential for neuromuscular blockade and respiratory paralysis).

No products indexed under this heading.

Kanamycin Sulfate (Concurrent and/or sequential use may increase the potential for increased toxicity).

No products indexed under this heading.

Ketamine Hydrochloride (Increased potential for neuromuscular blockade and respiratory paralysis).

No products indexed under this heading.

Lithium Carbonate (Increased potential for neuromuscular blockade and respiratory paralysis). Products include:

Eskalith 2485
Lithium Carbonate Capsules & Tablets 2230
Lithonate/Lithotabs/Lithobid.............. 2543

Lithium Citrate (Increased potential for neuromuscular blockade and respiratory paralysis).

No products indexed under this heading.

Loracarbef (Potential for increased nephrotoxicity and concomitant cephalosporins may spuriously elevate creatinine determinations). Products include:

Lorabid Suspension and Pulvules.... 1459

Methohexital Sodium (Increased potential for neuromuscular blockade and respiratory paralysis). Products include:

Brevital Sodium Vials............................. 1429

Metocurine Iodide (Increased potential for neuromuscular blockade and respiratory paralysis). Products include:

Metubine Iodide Vials............................ 916

Mezlocillin Sodium (Potential for mutual inactivation and a reduction in serum half-life may occur). Products include:

Mezlin 601
Mezlin Pharmacy Bulk Package......... 604

Midazolam Hydrochloride (Increased potential for neuromuscular blockade and respiratory paralysis). Products include:

Versed Injection 2170

Mivacurium Chloride (Increased potential for neuromuscular blockade and respiratory paralysis). Products include:

Mivacron 1138

Nafcillin Sodium (Potential for mutual inactivation and a reduction in serum half-life may occur).

No products indexed under this heading.

Pancuronium Bromide Injection (Increased potential for neuromuscular blockade and respiratory paralysis).

No products indexed under this heading.

Paromomycin Sulfate (Concurrent and/or sequential use may increase the potential for increased toxicity).

No products indexed under this heading.

Penicillin G Benzathine (Potential for mutual inactivation and a reduction in serum half-life may occur). Products include:

Bicillin C-R Injection 2704
Bicillin C-R 900/300 Injection 2706
Bicillin L-A Injection 2707

Penicillin G Potassium (Potential for mutual inactivation and a reduction in serum half-life may occur). Products include:

Pfizerpen for Injection........................... 2203

Penicillin G Procaine (Potential for mutual inactivation and a reduction in serum half-life may occur). Products include:

Bicillin C-R Injection 2704
Bicillin C-R 900/300 Injection 2706

Penicillin G Sodium (Potential for mutual inactivation and a reduction in serum half-life may occur).

No products indexed under this heading.

Penicillin V Potassium (Potential for mutual inactivation and a reduction in serum half-life may occur). Products include:

Pen•Vee K... 2772

Polymyxin B Sulfate (Concurrent and/or sequential use may increase the potential for increased toxicity). Products include:

AK-Spore .... ◉ 204
AK-Trol Ointment & Suspension .... ◉ 205

(◼ Described in PDR For Nonprescription Drugs)

(◉ Described in PDR For Ophthalmology)

53 **Interactions Index** **Amikin**

Bactine First Aid Antibiotic Plus Anesthetic Ointment ⊡ 708
Betadine Brand First Aid Antibiotics & Moisturizer Ointment 1991
Campho-Phenique Maximum Strength First Aid Antibiotic Plus Pain Reliever Ointment ⊡ 719
Cortisporin Cream 1084
Cortisporin Ointment 1085
Cortisporin Ophthalmic Ointment Sterile 1085
Cortisporin Ophthalmic Suspension Sterile 1086
Cortisporin Otic Solution Sterile 1087
Cortisporin Otic Suspension Sterile 1088
Dexacidin Ointment ◉ 263
Maxitrol Ophthalmic Ointment and Suspension ◉ 224
Mycitracin ⊡ 839
Neosporin G.U. Irrigant Sterile 1148
Neosporin Ointment ⊡ 857
Neosporin Plus Maximum Strength Cream ⊡ 858
Neosporin Plus Maximum Strength Ointment ⊡ 858
Neosporin Ophthalmic Ointment Sterile 1148
Neosporin Ophthalmic Solution Sterile 1149
Ophthocort ◉ 311
PediOtic Suspension Sterile 1153
Polymyxin B Sulfate, Aerosporin Brand Sterile Powder 1154
Poly-Pred Liquifilm ◉ 248
Polysporin Ointment ⊡ 858
Polysporin Ophthalmic Ointment Sterile 1154
Polysporin Powder ⊡ 859
Polytrim Ophthalmic Solution Sterile 482
TERAK Ointment ◉ 209
Terramycin with Polymyxin B Sulfate Ophthalmic Ointment 2211

Propofol (Increased potential for neuromuscular blockade and respiratory paralysis). Products include:
Diprivan Injection 2833

Rocuronium Bromide (Increased potential for neuromuscular blockade and respiratory paralysis). Products include:
Zemuron 1830

Streptomycin Sulfate (Concurrent and/or sequential use may increase the potential for increased toxicity). Products include:
Streptomycin Sulfate Injection 2208

Succinylcholine Chloride (Increased potential for neuromuscular blockade and respiratory paralysis). Products include:
Anectine 1073

Sufentanil Citrate (Increased potential for neuromuscular blockade and respiratory paralysis). Products include:
Sufenta Injection 1309

Thiamylal Sodium (Increased potential for neuromuscular blockade and respiratory paralysis).
No products indexed under this heading.

Ticarcillin Disodium (Potential for mutual inactivation and a reduction in serum half-life may occur). Products include:
Ticar for Injection 2526
Timentin for Injection 2528

Tobramycin (Concurrent and/or sequential use may increase the potential for increased toxicity). Products include:
AKTOB ◉ 206
TobraDex Ophthalmic Suspension and Ointment 473
Tobrex Ophthalmic Ointment and Solution ◉ 229

Tobramycin Sulfate (Concurrent and/or sequential use may increase the potential for increased toxicity). Products include:
Nebcin Vials, Hyporets & ADD-Vantage 1464
Tobramycin Sulfate Injection 968

Tubocurarine Chloride (Increased potential for neuromuscular blockade and respiratory paralysis).
No products indexed under this heading.

Vancomycin Hydrochloride (Concurrent and/or sequential use may increase the potential for increased toxicity). Products include:
Vancocin HCl, Oral Solution & Pulvules 1483
Vancocin HCl, Vials & ADD-Vantage 1481

Vecuronium Bromide (Increased potential for neuromuscular blockade and respiratory paralysis). Products include:
Norcuron 1826

Viomycin (Concurrent and/or sequential use may increase the potential for increased toxicity).

AMIKIN INJECTABLE
(Amikacin Sulfate) 501
May interact with aminoglycosides, cephalosporins, penicillins, neuromuscular blocking agents, anesthetics, and certain other agents. Compounds in these categories include:

Alfentanil Hydrochloride (Increased potential for neuromuscular blockade and respiratory paralysis). Products include:
Alfenta Injection 1286

Amoxicillin Trihydrate (Potential for mutual inactivation and a reduction in serum half-life may occur). Products include:
Amoxil 2464
Augmentin 2468

Amphotericin B (Concurrent and/or sequential use may increase the potential for increased toxicity). Products include:
Fungizone Intravenous 506

Ampicillin Sodium (Potential for mutual inactivation and a reduction in serum half-life may occur). Products include:
Unasyn 2212

Atracurium Besylate (Increased potential for neuromuscular blockade and respiratory paralysis). Products include:
Tracrium Injection 1183

Azlocillin Sodium (Potential for mutual inactivation and a reduction in serum half-life may occur).
No products indexed under this heading.

Bacampicillin Hydrochloride (Potential for mutual inactivation and a reduction in serum half-life may occur). Products include:
Spectrobid Tablets 2206

Bacitracin Zinc (Concurrent and/or sequential use may increase the potential for increased toxicity). Products include:
AK-Spore Ointment ◉ 204
Bactine First Aid Antibiotic Plus Anesthetic Ointment ⊡ 708
Betadine Brand First Aid Antibiotics & Moisturizer Ointment 1991
Campho-Phenique Maximum Strength First Aid Antibiotic Plus Pain Reliever Ointment ⊡ 719
Cortisporin Ointment 1085
Cortisporin Ophthalmic Ointment Sterile 1085
Neosporin Ointment ⊡ 857
Neosporin Plus Maximum Strength Ointment ⊡ 858
Neosporin Ophthalmic Ointment Sterile 1148
Polysporin Ointment ⊡ 858
Polysporin Ophthalmic Ointment Sterile 1154
Polysporin Powder ⊡ 859

Carbenicillin Indanyl Sodium (Potential for mutual inactivation and a reduction in serum half-life may occur). Products include:
Geocillin Tablets 2199

Cefaclor (Potential for increased nephrotoxicity and concomitant cephalosporins may spuriously elevate creatinine determinations). Products include:
Ceclor Pulvules & Suspension 1431

Cefadroxil Monohydrate (Potential for increased nephrotoxicity and concomitant cephalosporins may spuriously elevate creatinine determinations). Products include:
Duricef 748

Cefamandole Nafate (Potential for increased nephrotoxicity and concomitant cephalosporins may spuriously elevate creatinine determinations). Products include:
Mandol Vials, Faspak & ADD-Vantage 1461

Cefazolin Sodium (Potential for increased nephrotoxicity and concomitant cephalosporins may spuriously elevate creatinine determinations). Products include:
Ancef Injection 2465
Kefzol Vials, Faspak & ADD-Vantage 1456

Cefixime (Potential for increased nephrotoxicity and concomitant cephalosporins may spuriously elevate creatinine determinations). Products include:
Suprax 1399

Cefmetazole Sodium (Potential for increased nephrotoxicity and concomitant cephalosporins may spuriously elevate creatinine determinations). Products include:
Zefazone 2654

Cefonicid Sodium (Potential for increased nephrotoxicity and concomitant cephalosporins may spuriously elevate creatinine determinations). Products include:
Monocid Injection 2497

Cefoperazone Sodium (Potential for increased nephrotoxicity and concomitant cephalosporins may spuriously elevate creatinine determinations). Products include:
Cefobid Intravenous/Intramuscular 2189
Cefobid Pharmacy Bulk Package - Not for Direct Infusion 2192

Ceforanide (Potential for increased nephrotoxicity and concomitant cephalosporins may spuriously elevate creatinine determinations).
No products indexed under this heading.

Cefotaxime Sodium (Potential for increased nephrotoxicity and concomitant cephalosporins may spuriously elevate creatinine determinations). Products include:
Claforan Sterile and Injection 1235

Cefotetan (Potential for increased nephrotoxicity and concomitant cephalosporins may spuriously elevate creatinine determinations). Products include:
Cefotan 2829

Cefoxitin Sodium (Potential for increased nephrotoxicity and concomitant cephalosporins may spuriously elevate creatinine determinations). Products include:
Mefoxin 1691
Mefoxin Premixed Intravenous Solution 1694

Cefpodoxime Proxetil (Potential for increased nephrotoxicity and concomitant cephalosporins may spuriously elevate creatinine determinations). Products include:
Vantin for Oral Suspension and Vantin Tablets 2646

Cefprozil (Potential for increased nephrotoxicity and concomitant cephalosporins may spuriously elevate creatinine determinations). Products include:
Cefzil Tablets and Oral Suspension 746

Ceftazidime (Potential for increased nephrotoxicity and concomitant cephalosporins may spuriously elevate creatinine determinations). Products include:
Ceptaz 1081
Fortaz 1100
Tazicef for Injection 2519
Tazidime Vials, Faspak & ADD-Vantage 1478

Ceftizoxime Sodium (Potential for increased nephrotoxicity and concomitant cephalosporins may spuriously elevate creatinine determinations). Products include:
Cefizox for Intramuscular or Intravenous Use 1034

Ceftriaxone Sodium (Potential for increased nephrotoxicity and concomitant cephalosporins may spuriously elevate creatinine determinations). Products include:
Rocephin Injectable Vials, ADD-Vantage, Galaxy Container 2142

Cefuroxime Axetil (Potential for increased nephrotoxicity and concomitant cephalosporins may spuriously elevate creatinine determinations). Products include:
Ceftin 1078

Cefuroxime Sodium (Potential for increased nephrotoxicity and concomitant cephalosporins may spuriously elevate creatinine determinations). Products include:
Kefurox Vials, Faspak & ADD-Vantage 1454
Zinacef 1211

Cephalexin (Potential for increased nephrotoxicity and concomitant cephalosporins may spuriously elevate creatinine determinations). Products include:
Keflex Pulvules & Oral Suspension 914

Cephaloridine (Concurrent and/or sequential use may increase the potential for increased toxicity).

Cephalothin Sodium (Potential for increased nephrotoxicity and concomitant cephalosporins may spuriously elevate creatinine determinations).

Cephapirin Sodium (Potential for increased nephrotoxicity and concomitant cephalosporins may spuriously elevate creatinine determinations).
No products indexed under this heading.

Cephradine (Potential for increased nephrotoxicity and concomitant cephalosporins may spuriously elevate creatinine determinations).
No products indexed under this heading.

Cisplatin (Concurrent and/or sequential use may increase the potential for increased toxicity). Products include:
Platinol 708
Platinol-AQ Injection 710

IMPORTANT NOTE: Always consult each drug listing in the patient's regimen for possible interactions.

Amikin **Interactions Index** 54

Colistin Sulfate (Concurrent and/or sequential use may increase the potential for increased toxicity). Products include:
- Coly-Mycin S Otic w/Neomycin & Hydrocortisone ... 1906

Dicloxacillin Sodium (Potential for mutual inactivation and a reduction in serum half-life may occur).
- No products indexed under this heading.

Doxacurium Chloride (Increased potential for neuromuscular blockade and respiratory paralysis). Products include:
- Nuromax Injection ... 1149

Enflurane (Increased potential for neuromuscular blockade and respiratory paralysis).
- No products indexed under this heading.

Ethacrynic Acid (Potential for increased ototoxicity; concurrent use should be avoided). Products include:
- Edecrin Tablets ... 1657

Fentanyl Citrate (Increased potential for neuromuscular blockade and respiratory paralysis). Products include:
- Sublimaze Injection ... 1307

Furosemide (Potential for increased ototoxicity; concurrent use should be avoided). Products include:
- Lasix Injection, Oral Solution and Tablets ... 1240

Gentamicin Sulfate (Concurrent and/or sequential use may increase the potential for increased toxicity). Products include:
- Garamycin Injectable ... 2360
- Genoptic Sterile Ophthalmic Solution ... ◉ 243
- Genoptic Sterile Ophthalmic Ointment ... ◉ 243
- Gentacidin Ointment ... ◉ 264
- Gentacidin Solution ... ◉ 264
- Gentak ... ◉ 208
- Pred-G Liquifilm Sterile Ophthalmic Suspension ... ◉ 251
- Pred-G S.O.P. Sterile Ophthalmic Ointment ... ◉ 252

Halothane (Increased potential for neuromuscular blockade and respiratory paralysis). Products include:
- Fluothane ... 2724

Isoflurane (Increased potential for neuromuscular blockade and respiratory paralysis).
- No products indexed under this heading.

Kanamycin Sulfate (Concurrent and/or sequential use may increase the potential for increased toxicity).
- No products indexed under this heading.

Ketamine Hydrochloride (Increased potential for neuromuscular blockade and respiratory paralysis).
- No products indexed under this heading.

Lithium Carbonate (Increased potential for neuromuscular blockade and respiratory paralysis). Products include:
- Eskalith ... 2485
- Lithium Carbonate Capsules & Tablets ... 2230
- Lithonate/Lithotabs/Lithobid ... 2543

Lithium Citrate (Increased potential for neuromuscular blockade and respiratory paralysis).
- No products indexed under this heading.

Loracarbef (Potential for increased nephrotoxicity and concomitant cephalosporins may spuriously elevate creatinine determinations). Products include:
- Lorabid Suspension and Pulvules ... 1459

Methohexital Sodium (Increased potential for neuromuscular blockade and respiratory paralysis). Products include:
- Brevital Sodium Vials ... 1429

Metocurine Iodide (Increased potential for neuromuscular blockade and respiratory paralysis). Products include:
- Metubine Iodide Vials ... 916

Mezlocillin Sodium (Potential for mutual inactivation and a reduction in serum half-life may occur). Products include:
- Mezlin ... 601
- Mezlin Pharmacy Bulk Package ... 604

Midazolam Hydrochloride (Increased potential for neuromuscular blockade and respiratory paralysis). Products include:
- Versed Injection ... 2170

Mivacurium Chloride (Increased potential for neuromuscular blockade and respiratory paralysis). Products include:
- Mivacron ... 1138

Nafcillin Sodium (Potential for mutual inactivation and a reduction in serum half-life may occur).
- No products indexed under this heading.

Pancuronium Bromide Injection (Increased potential for neuromuscular blockade and respiratory paralysis).
- No products indexed under this heading.

Paromomycin Sulfate (Concurrent and/or sequential use may increase the potential for increased toxicity).
- No products indexed under this heading.

Penicillin G Benzathine (Potential for mutual inactivation and a reduction in serum half-life may occur). Products include:
- Bicillin C-R Injection ... 2704
- Bicillin C-R 900/300 Injection ... 2706
- Bicillin L-A Injection ... 2707

Penicillin G Potassium (Potential for mutual inactivation and a reduction in serum half-life may occur). Products include:
- Pfizerpen for Injection ... 2203

Penicillin G Procaine (Potential for mutual inactivation and a reduction in serum half-life may occur). Products include:
- Bicillin C-R Injection ... 2704
- Bicillin C-R 900/300 Injection ... 2706

Penicillin G Sodium (Potential for mutual inactivation and a reduction in serum half-life may occur).
- No products indexed under this heading.

Penicillin V Potassium (Potential for mutual inactivation and a reduction in serum half-life may occur). Products include:
- Pen•Vee K ... 2772

Polymyxin B Sulfate (Concurrent and/or sequential use may increase the potential for increased toxicity). Products include:
- AK-Spore ... ◉ 204
- AK-Trol Ointment & Suspension ... ◉ 205
- Bactine First Aid Antibiotic Plus Anesthetic Ointment ... ▣ 708
- Betadine Brand First Aid Antibiotics & Moisturizer Ointment ... 1991
- Campho-Phenique Maximum Strength First Aid Antibiotic Plus Pain Reliever Ointment ... ▣ 719
- Cortisporin Cream ... 1084
- Cortisporin Ointment ... 1085
- Cortisporin Ophthalmic Ointment Sterile ... 1085
- Cortisporin Ophthalmic Suspension Sterile ... 1086
- Cortisporin Otic Solution Sterile ... 1087
- Cortisporin Otic Suspension Sterile ... 1088
- Dexacidin Ointment ... ◉ 263
- Maxitrol Ophthalmic Ointment and Suspension ... ◉ 224
- Mycitracin ... ▣ 839
- Neosporin G.U. Irrigant Sterile ... 1148
- Neosporin Ointment ... ▣ 857
- Neosporin Plus Maximum Strength Cream ... ▣ 858
- Neosporin Plus Maximum Strength Ointment ... ▣ 858
- Neosporin Ophthalmic Ointment Sterile ... 1148
- Neosporin Ophthalmic Solution Sterile ... 1149
- Ophthocort ... ◉ 311
- PediOtic Suspension Sterile ... 1153
- Polymyxin B Sulfate, Aerosporin Brand Sterile Powder ... 1154
- Poly-Pred Liquifilm ... ◉ 248
- Polysporin Ointment ... ▣ 858
- Polysporin Ophthalmic Ointment Sterile ... 1154
- Polysporin Powder ... ▣ 859
- Polytrim Ophthalmic Solution Sterile ... 482
- TERAK Ointment ... ◉ 209
- Terramycin with Polymyxin B Sulfate Ophthalmic Ointment ... 2211

Propofol (Increased potential for neuromuscular blockade and respiratory paralysis). Products include:
- Diprivan Injection ... 2833

Rocuronium Bromide (Increased potential for neuromuscular blockade and respiratory paralysis). Products include:
- Zemuron ... 1830

Streptomycin Sulfate (Concurrent and/or sequential use may increase the potential for increased toxicity). Products include:
- Streptomycin Sulfate Injection ... 2208

Succinylcholine Chloride (Increased potential for neuromuscular blockade and respiratory paralysis). Products include:
- Anectine ... 1073

Sufentanil Citrate (Increased potential for neuromuscular blockade and respiratory paralysis). Products include:
- Sufenta Injection ... 1309

Thiamylal Sodium (Increased potential for neuromuscular blockade and respiratory paralysis).
- No products indexed under this heading.

Ticarcillin Disodium (Potential for mutual inactivation and a reduction in serum half-life may occur). Products include:
- Ticar for Injection ... 2526
- Timentin for Injection ... 2528

Tobramycin (Concurrent and/or sequential use may increase the potential for increased toxicity). Products include:
- AKTOB ... ◉ 206
- TobraDex Ophthalmic Suspension and Ointment ... 473
- Tobrex Ophthalmic Ointment and Solution ... ◉ 229

Tobramycin Sulfate (Concurrent and/or sequential use may increase the potential for increased toxicity). Products include:
- Nebcin Vials, Hyporets & ADD-Vantage ... 1464
- Tobramycin Sulfate Injection ... 968

Tubocurarine Chloride (Increased potential for neuromuscular blockade and respiratory paralysis).
- No products indexed under this heading.

Vancomycin Hydrochloride (Concurrent and/or sequential use may increase the potential for increased toxicity). Products include:
- Vancocin HCl, Oral Solution & Pulvules ... 1483
- Vancocin HCl, Vials & ADD-Vantage ... 1481

Vecuronium Bromide (Increased potential for neuromuscular blockade and respiratory paralysis). Products include:
- Norcuron ... 1826

Viomycin (Concurrent and/or sequential use may increase the potential for increased toxicity).

AMIN-AID INSTANT DRINK
(Nutritional Supplement) ... 2004
None cited in PDR database.

AMINO-CERV
(Urea, Benzalkonium Chloride, L-Cystine, Sodium Propionate, Methionine, Inositol) ... 1779
None cited in PDR database.

AMINOHIPPURATE SODIUM INJECTION
(Aminohippurate Sodium) ... 1606
May interact with sulfonamides and certain other agents. Compounds in these categories include:

Bendroflumethiazide (Renal clearance measurements impaired).
- No products indexed under this heading.

Chlorothiazide (Renal clearance measurements impaired). Products include:
- Aldoclor Tablets ... 1598
- Diupres Tablets ... 1650
- Diuril Oral ... 1653

Chlorothiazide Sodium (Renal clearance measurements impaired). Products include:
- Diuril Sodium Intravenous ... 1652

Chlorpropamide (Renal clearance measurements impaired). Products include:
- Diabinese Tablets ... 1935

Glipizide (Renal clearance measurements impaired). Products include:
- Glucotrol Tablets ... 1967
- Glucotrol XL Extended Release Tablets ... 1968

Glyburide (Renal clearance measurements impaired). Products include:
- DiaBeta Tablets ... 1239
- Glynase PresTab Tablets ... 2609
- Micronase Tablets ... 2623

Hydrochlorothiazide (Renal clearance measurements impaired). Products include:
- Aldactazide ... 2413
- Aldoril Tablets ... 1604
- Apresazide Capsules ... 808
- Capozide ... 742
- Dyazide ... 2479
- Esidrix Tablets ... 821
- Esimil Tablets ... 822
- HydroDIURIL Tablets ... 1674
- Hydropres Tablets ... 1675
- Hyzaar Tablets ... 1677
- Inderide Tablets ... 2732
- Inderide LA Long Acting Capsules ... 2734
- Lopressor HCT Tablets ... 832
- Lotensin HCT ... 837
- Maxzide ... 1380
- Moduretic Tablets ... 1705
- Oretic Tablets ... 443
- Prinzide Tablets ... 1737
- Ser-Ap-Es Tablets ... 849
- Timolide Tablets ... 1748

(▣ Described in PDR For Nonprescription Drugs) (◉ Described in PDR For Ophthalmology)

55 **Interactions Index** **Anafranil**

Vaseretic Tablets 1765
Zestoretic 2850
Ziac 1415

Hydroflumethiazide (Renal clearance measurements impaired). Products include:
Diucardin Tablets 2718

Methyclothiazide (Renal clearance measurements impaired). Products include:
Enduron Tablets 420

Polythiazide (Renal clearance measurements impaired). Products include:
Minizide Capsules 1938

Probenecid (Tubular secretion of PAH depressed). Products include:
Benemid Tablets 1611
ColBENEMID Tablets 1622

Procaine Hydrochloride (Renal clearance measurements impaired). Products include:
Novocain Hydrochloride for Spinal Anesthesia 2326

Sulfamethizole (Renal clearance measurements impaired). Products include:
Urobiotic-250 Capsules 2214

Sulfamethoxazole (Renal clearance measurements impaired). Products include:
Azo Gantanol Tablets 2080
Bactrim DS Tablets 2084
Bactrim I.V. Infusion 2082
Bactrim 2084
Gantanol Tablets 2119
Septra 1174
Septra I.V. Infusion 1169
Septra I.V. Infusion ADD-Vantage Vials 1171
Septra 1174

Sulfasalazine (Renal clearance measurements impaired). Products include:
Azulfidine 1949

Sulfinpyrazone (Renal clearance measurements impaired). Products include:
Anturane 807

Sulfisoxazole (Renal clearance measurements impaired). Products include:
Azo Gantrisin Tablets 2081
Gantrisin Tablets 2120

Sulfisoxazole Diolamine (Renal clearance measurements impaired).
No products indexed under this heading.

Tolazamide (Renal clearance measurements impaired).
No products indexed under this heading.

Tolbutamide (Renal clearance measurements impaired).
No products indexed under this heading.

AMINOPLEX CAPSULES
(Amino Acid Preparations) 2564
None cited in PDR database.

AMINOTATE CAPSULES
(Amino Acid Preparations) 2565
None cited in PDR database.

AMOXIL CAPSULES AND CHEWABLE TABLETS
(Amoxicillin Trihydrate) 2464
May interact with:

Probenecid (Concurrent administration delays excretion of amoxicillin). Products include:
Benemid Tablets 1611
ColBENEMID Tablets 1622

AMOXIL PEDIATRIC DROPS, POWDER FOR ORAL SUSPENSION
(Amoxicillin Trihydrate) 2464
See **Amoxil Capsules and Chewable Tablets**

AMPHOJEL SUSPENSION
(Aluminum Hydroxide Gel) 2695
May interact with tetracyclines. Compounds in this category include:

Demeclocycline Hydrochloride (Concurrent administration should be avoided). Products include:
Declomycin Tablets 1371

Doxycycline Calcium (Concurrent administration should be avoided). Products include:
Vibramycin Calcium Oral Suspension Syrup 1941

Doxycycline Hyclate (Concurrent administration should be avoided). Products include:
Doryx Capsules 1913
Vibramycin Hyclate Capsules 1941
Vibramycin Hyclate Intravenous 2215
Vibra-Tabs Film Coated Tablets 1941

Doxycycline Monohydrate (Concurrent administration should be avoided). Products include:
Monodox Capsules 1805
Vibramycin Monohydrate for Oral Suspension 1941

Methacycline Hydrochloride (Concurrent administration should be avoided).
No products indexed under this heading.

Minocycline Hydrochloride (Concurrent administration should be avoided). Products include:
Dynacin Capsules 1590
Minocin Intravenous 1382
Minocin Oral Suspension 1385
Minocin Pellet-Filled Capsules 1383

Oxytetracycline (Concurrent administration should be avoided). Products include:
Terramycin Intramuscular Solution 2210

Oxytetracycline Hydrochloride (Concurrent administration should be avoided). Products include:
TERAK Ointment ..... ◎ 209
Terra-Cortril Ophthalmic Suspension 2210
Terramycin with Polymyxin B Sulfate Ophthalmic Ointment 2211
Urobiotic-250 Capsules 2214

Prescription Drugs, unspecified (Effect resulting from coadministration not specified).

Tetracycline Hydrochloride (Concurrent administration should be avoided). Products include:
Achromycin V Capsules 1367

AMPHOJEL SUSPENSION WITHOUT FLAVOR
(Aluminum Hydroxide Gel) 2695
See **Amphojel Suspension**

AMPHOJEL TABLETS
(Aluminum Hydroxide Gel) 2695
See **Amphojel Suspension**

ANAFRANIL CAPSULES
(Clomipramine Hydrochloride) 803
May interact with sympathomimetics, anticholinergics, central nervous system depressants, monoamine oxidase inhibitors, barbiturates, and certain other agents. Compounds in these categories include:

Albuterol (Effect not specified; close supervision and careful adjustment of dosage are required). Products include:
Proventil Inhalation Aerosol 2382
Ventolin Inhalation Aerosol and Refill 1197

Albuterol Sulfate (Effect not specified; close supervision and careful adjustment of dosage are required). Products include:
Airet Solution for Inhalation 452
Proventil Inhalation Solution 0.083% 2384
Proventil Repetabs Tablets 2386
Proventil Solution for Inhalation 0.5% 2383
Proventil Syrup 2385
Proventil Tablets 2386
Ventolin Inhalation Solution 1198
Ventolin Nebules Inhalation Solution 1199
Ventolin Rotacaps for Inhalation 1200
Ventolin Syrup 1202
Ventolin Tablets 1203
Volmax Extended-Release Tablets .. 1788

Alfentanil Hydrochloride (Anafranil may exaggerate patients' response to CNS depressants). Products include:
Alfenta Injection 1286

Alprazolam (Anafranil may exaggerate patients' response to CNS depressants). Products include:
Xanax Tablets 2649

Aprobarbital (Anafranil may exaggerate patients' response to CNS depressants; decreases plasma levels of clomipramine).
No products indexed under this heading.

Atropine Sulfate (Effect not specified; close supervision and careful adjustment of dosage are required). Products include:
Arco-Lase Plus Tablets 512
Atrohist Plus Tablets 454
Atropine Sulfate Sterile Ophthalmic Solution ..... ◎ 233
Donnatal 2060
Donnatal Extentabs 2061
Donnatal Tablets 2060
Lomotil 2439
Motofen Tablets 784
Urised Tablets 1964

Belladonna Alkaloids (Effect not specified; close supervision and careful adjustment of dosage are required). Products include:
Bellergal-S Tablets 2250
Hyland's Bed Wetting Tablets ..... ▣ 828
Hyland's EnurAid Tablets ..... ▣ 829
Hyland's Teething Tablets ..... ▣ 830

Benztropine Mesylate (Effect not specified; close supervision and careful adjustment of dosage are required). Products include:
Cogentin 1621

Biperiden Hydrochloride (Effect not specified; close supervision and careful adjustment of dosage are required). Products include:
Akineton 1333

Buprenorphine (Anafranil may exaggerate patients' response to CNS depressants). Products include:
Buprenex Injectable 2006

Buspirone Hydrochloride (Anafranil may exaggerate patients' response to CNS depressants). Products include:
BuSpar 737

Butabarbital (Anafranil may exaggerate patients' response to CNS depressants; decreases plasma levels of clomipramine).
No products indexed under this heading.

Butalbital (Anafranil may exaggerate patients' response to CNS depressants; decreases plasma levels of clomipramine). Products include:
Esgic-plus Tablets 1013
Fioricet Tablets 2258
Fioricet with Codeine Capsules 2260
Fiorinal Capsules 2261
Fiorinal with Codeine Capsules 2262
Fiorinal Tablets 2261

Phrenilin 785
Sedapap Tablets 50 mg/650 mg .. 1543

Chlordiazepoxide (Anafranil may exaggerate patients' response to CNS depressants). Products include:
Libritabs Tablets 2177
Limbitrol 2180

Chlordiazepoxide Hydrochloride (Anafranil may exaggerate patients' response to CNS depressants). Products include:
Librax Capsules 2176
Librium Capsules 2178
Librium Injectable 2179

Chlorpromazine (Anafranil may exaggerate patients' response to CNS depressants). Products include:
Thorazine Suppositories 2523

Chlorprothixene (Anafranil may exaggerate patients' response to CNS depressants).
No products indexed under this heading.

Chlorprothixene Hydrochloride (Anafranil may exaggerate patients' response to CNS depressants).
No products indexed under this heading.

Cimetidine (May increase plasma concentration of clomipramine). Products include:
Tagamet Tablets 2516

Cimetidine Hydrochloride (May increase plasma concentration of clomipramine). Products include:
Tagamet 2516

Clidinium Bromide (Effect not specified; close supervision and careful adjustment of dosage are required). Products include:
Librax Capsules 2176
Quarzan Capsules 2181

Clonidine (Pharmacological effects of clonidine blocked). Products include:
Catapres-TTS 675

Clonidine Hydrochloride (Pharmacological effects of clonidine blocked). Products include:
Catapres Tablets 674
Combipres Tablets 677

Clorazepate Dipotassium (Anafranil may exaggerate patients' response to CNS depressants). Products include:
Tranxene 451

Clozapine (Anafranil may exaggerate patients' response to CNS depressants). Products include:
Clozaril Tablets 2252

Codeine Phosphate (Anafranil may exaggerate patients' response to CNS depressants). Products include:
Actifed with Codeine Cough Syrup.. 1067
Brontex 1981
Deconsal C Expectorant Syrup 456
Deconsal Pediatric Syrup 457
Dimetane-DC Cough Syrup 2059
Empirin with Codeine Tablets 1093
Fioricet with Codeine Capsules 2260
Fiorinal with Codeine Capsules 2262
Isoclor Expectorant 990
Novahistine DH 2462
Novahistine Expectorant 2463
Nucofed 2051
Phenergan with Codeine 2777
Phenergan VC with Codeine 2781
Robitussin A-C Syrup 2073
Robitussin-DAC Syrup 2074
Ryna ..... ▣ 841
Soma Compound w/Codeine Tablets 2676
Tussi-Organidin NR Liquid and S NR Liquid 2677
Tylenol with Codeine 1583

Desflurane (Anafranil may exaggerate patients' response to CNS depressants). Products include:
Suprane 1813

IMPORTANT NOTE: Always consult each drug listing in the patient's regimen for possible interactions.

Anafranil

Dezocine (Anafranil may exaggerate patients' response to CNS depressants). Products include:

Dalgan Injection 538

Diazepam (Anafranil may exaggerate patients' response to CNS depressants). Products include:

Dizac 1809
Valium Injectable 2182
Valium Tablets 2183
Valrelease Capsules 2169

Dicyclomine Hydrochloride (Effect not specified; close supervision and careful adjustment of dosage are required). Products include:

Bentyl 1501

Digoxin (Potential for adverse effects due to displacement of either drug from protein binding site). Products include:

Lanoxicaps 1117
Lanoxin Elixir Pediatric 1120
Lanoxin Injection 1123
Lanoxin Injection Pediatric................... 1126
Lanoxin Tablets 1128

Dobutamine Hydrochloride (Effect not specified; close supervision and careful adjustment of dosage are required). Products include:

Dobutrex Solution Vials......................... 1439

Dopamine Hydrochloride (Effect not specified; close supervision and careful adjustment of dosage are required).

No products indexed under this heading.

Droperidol (Anafranil may exaggerate patients' response to CNS depressants). Products include:

Inapsine Injection..................................... 1296

Enflurane (Anafranil may exaggerate patients' response to CNS depressants).

No products indexed under this heading.

Ephedrine Hydrochloride (Effect not specified; close supervision and careful adjustment of dosage are required). Products include:

Primatene Dual Action Formula...... ⊞ 872
Primatene Tablets .... ⊞ 873
Quadrinal Tablets 1350

Ephedrine Sulfate (Effect not specified; close supervision and careful adjustment of dosage are required). Products include:

Bronkaid Caplets .... ⊞ 717
Marax Tablets & DF Syrup................... 2200

Ephedrine Tannate (Effect not specified; close supervision and careful adjustment of dosage are required). Products include:

Rynatuss 2673

Epinephrine (Effect not specified; close supervision and careful adjustment of dosage are required). Products include:

Bronkaid Mist .... ⊞ 717
EPIFRIN .... ⊙ 239
EpiPen 790
Marcaine Hydrochloride with Epinephrine 1:200,000 2316
Primatene Mist .... ⊞ 873
Sensorcaine with Epinephrine Injection 559
Sus-Phrine Injection 1019
Xylocaine with Epinephrine Injections.. 567

Epinephrine Bitartrate (Effect not specified; close supervision and careful adjustment of dosage are required). Products include:

Bronkaid Mist Suspension .... ⊞ 718
Sensorcaine-MPF with Epinephrine Injection 559

Epinephrine Hydrochloride (Effect not specified; close supervision and careful adjustment of dosage are required). Products include:

Ana-Kit Anaphylaxis Emergency Treatment Kit 617

Estazolam (Anafranil may exaggerate patients' response to CNS depressants). Products include:

ProSom Tablets 449

Ethchlorvynol (Anafranil may exaggerate patients' response to CNS depressants). Products include:

Placidyl Capsules..................................... 448

Ethinamate (Anafranil may exaggerate patients' response to CNS depressants).

No products indexed under this heading.

Fentanyl (Anafranil may exaggerate patients' response to CNS depressants). Products include:

Duragesic Transdermal System........ 1288

Fentanyl Citrate (Anafranil may exaggerate patients' response to CNS depressants). Products include:

Sublimaze Injection................................. 1307

Fluoxetine Hydrochloride (May increase plasma concentration of clomipramine). Products include:

Prozac Pulvules & Liquid, Oral Solution 919

Fluphenazine Decanoate (Anafranil may exaggerate patients' response to CNS depressants). Products include:

Prolixin Decanoate 509

Fluphenazine Enanthate (Anafranil may exaggerate patients' response to CNS depressants). Products include:

Prolixin Enanthate 509

Fluphenazine Hydrochloride (Anafranil may exaggerate patients' response to CNS depressants). Products include:

Prolixin 509

Flurazepam Hydrochloride (Anafranil may exaggerate patients' response to CNS depressants). Products include:

Dalmane Capsules.................................... 2173

Furazolidone (Concurrent therapy is contraindicated, or should not be used within 14 days before or after treatment with MAOI). Products include:

Furoxone 2046

Glutethimide (Anafranil may exaggerate patients' response to CNS depressants).

No products indexed under this heading.

Glycopyrrolate (Effect not specified; close supervision and careful adjustment of dosage are required). Products include:

Robinul Forte Tablets.............................. 2072
Robinul Injectable 2072
Robinul Tablets.. 2072

Guanethidine Monosulfate (Pharmacological effects of guanethidine blocked). Products include:

Esimil Tablets 822
Ismelin Tablets 827

Haloperidol (Increases plasma concentration of clomipramine). Products include:

Haldol Injection, Tablets and Concentrate 1575

Haloperidol Decanoate (Increases plasma concentration of clomipramine). Products include:

Haldol Decanoate..................................... 1577

Hydrocodone Bitartrate (Anafranil may exaggerate patients' response to CNS depressants). Products include:

Anexsia 5/500 Elixir 1781
Anexia Tablets... 1782
Codiclear DH Syrup 791
Deconamine CX Cough and Cold Liquid and Tablets.................................. 1319
Duratuss HD Elixir................................... 2565
Hycodan Tablets and Syrup 930
Hycomine Compound Tablets 932
Hycomine 931
Hycotuss Expectorant Syrup 933
Hydrocet Capsules 782
Lorcet 10/650... 1018
Lortab 2566
Tussend 1783
Tussend Expectorant 1785
Vicodin Tablets.. 1356
Vicodin ES Tablets................................... 1357
Vicodin Tuss Expectorant 1358
Zydone Capsules 949

Hydrocodone Polistirex (Anafranil may exaggerate patients' response to CNS depressants). Products include:

Tussionex Pennkinetic Extended-Release Suspension 998

Hydroxyzine Hydrochloride (Anafranil may exaggerate patients' response to CNS depressants). Products include:

Atarax Tablets & Syrup.......................... 2185
Marax Tablets & DF Syrup................... 2200
Vistaril Intramuscular Solution.......... 2216

Hyoscyamine (Effect not specified; close supervision and careful adjustment of dosage are required). Products include:

Cystospaz Tablets 1963
Urised Tablets.. 1964

Hyoscyamine Sulfate (Effect not specified; close supervision and careful adjustment of dosage are required). Products include:

Arco-Lase Plus Tablets 512
Atrohist Plus Tablets 454
Cystospaz-M Capsules 1963
Donnatal 2060
Donnatal Extentabs................................. 2061
Donnatal Tablets 2060
Kutrase Capsules...................................... 2402
Levsin/Levsinex/Levbid 2405

Ipratropium Bromide (Effect not specified; close supervision and careful adjustment of dosage are required). Products include:

Atrovent Inhalation Aerosol................ 671
Atrovent Inhalation Solution 673

Isocarboxazid (Concurrent therapy is contraindicated, or should not be used within 14 days before or after treatment with MAOI).

No products indexed under this heading.

Isoflurane (Anafranil may exaggerate patients' response to CNS depressants).

No products indexed under this heading.

Isoproterenol Hydrochloride (Effect not specified; close supervision and careful adjustment of dosage are required). Products include:

Isuprel Hydrochloride Injection 1:5000 2311
Isuprel Hydrochloride Solution 1:200 & 1:100 2313
Isuprel Mistometer 2312

Isoproterenol Sulfate (Effect not specified; close supervision and careful adjustment of dosage are required). Products include:

Norisodrine with Calcium Iodide Syrup... 442

Ketamine Hydrochloride (Anafranil may exaggerate patients' response to CNS depressants).

No products indexed under this heading.

Levomethadyl Acetate Hydrochloride (Anafranil may exaggerate patients' response to CNS depressants). Products include:

Orlaam 2239

Levorphanol Tartrate (Anafranil may exaggerate patients' response to CNS depressants). Products include:

Levo-Dromoran.. 2129

Lorazepam (Anafranil may exaggerate patients' response to CNS depressants). Products include:

Ativan Injection... 2698
Ativan Tablets 2700

Loxapine Hydrochloride (Anafranil may exaggerate patients' response to CNS depressants). Products include:

Loxitane 1378

Loxapine Succinate (Anafranil may exaggerate patients' response to CNS depressants). Products include:

Loxitane Capsules 1378

Mepenzolate Bromide (Effect not specified; close supervision and careful adjustment of dosage are required).

No products indexed under this heading.

Meperidine Hydrochloride (Anafranil may exaggerate patients' response to CNS depressants). Products include:

Demerol 2308
Mepergan Injection 2753

Mephobarbital (Anafranil may exaggerate patients' response to CNS depressants; decreases plasma levels of clomipramine). Products include:

Mebaral Tablets 2322

Meprobamate (Anafranil may exaggerate patients' response to CNS depressants). Products include:

Miltown Tablets 2672
PMB 200 and PMB 400 2783

Mesoridazine Besylate (Anafranil may exaggerate patients' response to CNS depressants). Products include:

Serentil.. 684

Metaproterenol Sulfate (Effect not specified; close supervision and careful adjustment of dosage are required). Products include:

Alupent.. 669
Metaproterenol Sulfate Inhalation Solution, USP, Arm-a-Med 552

Metaraminol Bitartrate (Effect not specified; close supervision and careful adjustment of dosage are required). Products include:

Aramine Injection..................................... 1609

Methadone Hydrochloride (Anafranil may exaggerate patients' response to CNS depressants). Products include:

Methadone Hydrochloride Oral Concentrate 2233
Methadone Hydrochloride Oral Solution & Tablets................................ 2235

Methohexital Sodium (Anafranil may exaggerate patients' response to CNS depressants). Products include:

Brevital Sodium Vials............................. 1429

Methotrimeprazine (Anafranil may exaggerate patients' response to CNS depressants). Products include:

Levoprome 1274

Methoxamine Hydrochloride (Effect not specified; close supervision and careful adjustment of dosage are required). Products include:

Vasoxyl Injection 1196

(⊞ Described in PDR For Nonprescription Drugs) (⊙ Described in PDR For Ophthalmology)

Interactions Index — Anafranil

Methoxyflurane (Anafranil may exaggerate patients' response to CNS depressants).

No products indexed under this heading.

Methylphenidate Hydrochloride (May increase plasma concentration of clomipramine). Products include:

Ritalin 848

Midazolam Hydrochloride (Anafranil may exaggerate patients' response to CNS depressants). Products include:

Versed Injection 2170

Molindone Hydrochloride (Anafranil may exaggerate patients' response to CNS depressants). Products include:

Moban Tablets and Concentrate...... 1048

Morphine Sulfate (Anafranil may exaggerate patients' response to CNS depressants). Products include:

Astramorph/PF Injection, USP (Preservative-Free) 535
Duramorph 962
Infumorph 200 and Infumorph 500 Sterile Solutions 965
MS Contin Tablets 1994
MSIR 1997
Oramorph SR (Morphine Sulfate Sustained Release Tablets) 2236
RMS Suppositories 2657
Roxanol 2243

Norepinephrine Bitartrate (Effect not specified; close supervision and careful adjustment of dosage are required). Products include:

Levophed Bitartrate Injection 2315

Opium Alkaloids (Anafranil may exaggerate patients' response to CNS depressants).

No products indexed under this heading.

Oxazepam (Anafranil may exaggerate patients' response to CNS depressants). Products include:

Serax Capsules 2810
Serax Tablets 2810

Oxybutynin Chloride (Effect not specified; close supervision and careful adjustment of dosage are required). Products include:

Ditropan 1516

Oxycodone Hydrochloride (Anafranil may exaggerate patients' response to CNS depressants). Products include:

Percocet Tablets 938
Percodan Tablets 939
Percodan-Demi Tablets 940
Roxicodone Tablets, Oral Solution & Intensol (Oxycodone) 2244
Tylox Capsules 1584

Pentobarbital Sodium (Anafranil may exaggerate patients' response to CNS depressants; decreases plasma levels of clomipramine). Products include:

Nembutal Sodium Capsules 436
Nembutal Sodium Solution 438
Nembutal Sodium Suppositories...... 440

Perphenazine (Anafranil may exaggerate patients' response to CNS depressants). Products include:

Etrafon 2355
Triavil Tablets 1757
Trilafon 2389

Phenelzine Sulfate (Concurrent therapy is contraindicated, or should not be used within 14 days before or after treatment with MAOI). Products include:

Nardil 1920

Phenobarbital (Anafranil may exaggerate patients' response to CNS depressants; decreases plasma levels of clomipramine). Products include:

Arco-Lase Plus Tablets 512
Bellergal-S Tablets 2250
Donnatal 2060
Donnatal Extentabs 2061
Donnatal Tablets 2060
Phenobarbital Elixir and Tablets 1469
Quadrinal Tablets 1350

Phenylephrine Bitartrate (Effect not specified; close supervision and careful adjustment of dosage are required).

No products indexed under this heading.

Phenylephrine Hydrochloride (Effect not specified; close supervision and careful adjustment of dosage are required). Products include:

Atrohist Plus Tablets 454
Cerose DM .... ⓔ 878
Comhist 2038
D.A. Chewable Tablets 951
Deconsal Pediatric Capsules 454
Dura-Vent/DA Tablets 953
Entex Capsules 1986
Entex Liquid 1986
Extendryl 1005
4-Way Fast Acting Nasal Spray (regular & mentholated) .... ⓔ 621
Hemorid For Women .... ⓔ 834
Hycomine Compound Tablets 932
Neo-Synephrine Hydrochloride 1% Carpuject 2324
Neo-Synephrine Hydrochloride 1% Injection 2324
Neo-Synephrine Hydrochloride (Ophthalmic) 2325
Neo-Synephrine .... ⓔ 726
Nöstril .... ⓔ 644
Novahistine Elixir .... ⓔ 823
Phenergan VC 2779
Phenergan VC with Codeine 2781
Preparation H .... ⓔ 871
Tympagesic Ear Drops 2342
Vasosulf .... © 271
Vicks Sinex Nasal Spray and Ultra Fine Mist .... ⓔ 765

Phenylephrine Tannate (Effect not specified; close supervision and careful adjustment of dosage are required). Products include:

Atrohist Pediatric Suspension 454
Ricobid-D Pediatric Suspension....... 2038
Ricobid Tablets and Pediatric Suspension 2038
Rynatan 2673
Rynatuss 2673

Phenylpropanolamine Hydrochloride (Effect not specified; close supervision and careful adjustment of dosage are required). Products include:

Acutrim .... ⓔ 628
Allerest Children's Chewable Tablets .... ⓔ 627
Allerest 12 Hour Caplets .... ⓔ 627
Atrohist Plus Tablets 454
BC Cold Powder Multi-Symptom Formula (Cold-Sinus-Allergy) ...... ⓔ 609
BC Cold Powder Non-Drowsy Formula (Cold-Sinus) .... ⓔ 609
Cheracol Plus Head Cold/Cough Formula .... ⓔ 769
Comtrex Multi-Symptom Non-Drowsy Liqui-gels .... ⓔ 618
Contac Continuous Action Nasal Decongestant/Antihistamine 12 Hour Capsules .... ⓔ 813
Contac Maximum Strength Continuous Action Decongestant/ Antihistamine 12 Hour Caplets.. ⓔ 813
Contac Severe Cold and Flu Formula Caplets .... ⓔ 814
Coricidin 'D' Decongestant Tablets .... ⓔ 800
Dexatrim .... ⓔ 832
Dexatrim Plus Vitamins Caplets .... ⓔ 832
Dimetane-DC Cough Syrup 2059
Dimetapp Elixir .... ⓔ 773
Dimetapp Extentabs .... ⓔ 774
Dimetapp Tablets/Liqui-Gels .... ⓔ 775
Dimetapp Cold & Allergy Chewable Tablets .... ⓔ 773
Dimetapp DM Elixir .... ⓔ 774
Dura-Vent Tablets 952
Entex Capsules 1986
Entex LA Tablets 1987
Entex Liquid 1986
Exgest LA Tablets 782

Hycomine 931
Isoclor Timesule Capsules .... ⓔ 637
Nolamine Timed-Release Tablets 785
Ornade Spansule Capsules 2502
Propagest Tablets 786
Pyrroxate Caplets .... ⓔ 772
Robitussin-CF .... ⓔ 777
Sinulin Tablets 787
Tavist-D 12 Hour Relief Tablets .... ⓔ 787
Teldrin 12 Hour Antihistamine/ Nasal Decongestant Allergy Relief Capsules .... ⓔ 826
Triaminic Allergy Tablets .... ⓔ 789
Triaminic Cold Tablets .... ⓔ 790
Triaminic Expectorant .... ⓔ 790
Triaminic Syrup .... ⓔ 792
Triaminic-12 Tablets .... ⓔ 792
Triaminic-DM Syrup .... ⓔ 792
Triaminicin Tablets .... ⓔ 793
Triaminicol Multi-Symptom Cold Tablets .... ⓔ 793
Triaminicol Multi-Symptom Relief ⓔ 794
Vicks DayQuil Allergy Relief 12-Hour Extended Release Tablets.. ⓔ 760
Vicks DayQuil Allergy Relief 4-Hour Tablets .... ⓔ 760
Vicks DayQuil SINUS Pressure & CONGESTION Relief .... ⓔ 761

Phenytoin (Decreases plasma levels of clomipramine). Products include:

Dilantin Infatabs 1908
Dilantin-125 Suspension 1911

Phenytoin Sodium (Decreases plasma levels of clomipramine). Products include:

Dilantin Kapseals 1906
Dilantin Parenteral 1910

Pirbuterol Acetate (Effect not specified; close supervision and careful adjustment of dosage are required). Products include:

Maxair Autohaler 1492
Maxair Inhaler 1494

Prazepam (Anafranil may exaggerate patients' response to CNS depressants).

No products indexed under this heading.

Prochlorperazine (Anafranil may exaggerate patients' response to CNS depressants). Products include:

Compazine 2470

Procyclidine Hydrochloride (Effect not specified; close supervision and careful adjustment of dosage are required). Products include:

Kemadrin Tablets 1112

Promethazine Hydrochloride (Anafranil may exaggerate patients' response to CNS depressants). Products include:

Mepergan Injection 2753
Phenergan with Codeine 2777
Phenergan with Dextromethorphan 2778
Phenergan Injection 2773
Phenergan Suppositories 2775
Phenergan Syrup 2774
Phenergan Tablets 2775
Phenergan VC 2779
Phenergan VC with Codeine 2781

Propantheline Bromide (Effect not specified; close supervision and careful adjustment of dosage are required). Products include:

Pro-Banthine Tablets 2052

Propofol (Anafranil may exaggerate patients' response to CNS depressants). Products include:

Diprivan Injection 2833

Propoxyphene Hydrochloride (Anafranil may exaggerate patients' response to CNS depressants). Products include:

Darvon 1435
Wygesic Tablets 2827

Propoxyphene Napsylate (Anafranil may exaggerate patients' response to CNS depressants). Products include:

Darvon-N/Darvocet-N 1433

Pseudoephedrine Hydrochloride (Effect not specified; close supervision and careful adjustment of dosage are required). Products include:

Actifed Allergy Daytime/Nighttime Caplets .... ⓔ 844
Actifed Plus Caplets .... ⓔ 845
Actifed Plus Tablets .... ⓔ 845
Actifed with Codeine Cough Syrup.. 1067
Actifed Sinus Daytime/Nighttime Tablets and Caplets .... ⓔ 846
Actifed Syrup .... ⓔ 846
Actifed Tablets .... ⓔ 844
Advil Cold and Sinus Caplets and Tablets (formerly CoAdvil) .... ⓔ 870
Alka-Seltzer Plus Cold Medicine Liqui-Gels .... ⓔ 706
Alka-Seltzer Plus Cold & Cough Medicine Liqui-Gels .... ⓔ 705
Alka-Seltzer Plus Night-Time Cold Medicine Liqui-Gels .... ⓔ 706
Allerest Headache Strength Tablets .... ⓔ 627
Allerest Maximum Strength Tablets .... ⓔ 627
Allerest No Drowsiness Tablets ...... ⓔ 627
Allerest Sinus Pain Formula .... ⓔ 627
Anatuss LA Tablets 1542
Atrohist Pediatric Capsules 453
Bayer Select Sinus Pain Relief Formula .... ⓔ 717
Benadryl Allergy Decongestant Liquid Medication .... ⓔ 848
Benadryl Allergy Decongestant Tablets .... ⓔ 848
Benadryl Allergy Sinus Headache Formula Caplets .... ⓔ 849
Benylin Multisymptom .... ⓔ 852
Bromfed Capsules (Extended-Release) 1785
Bromfed Syrup .... ⓔ 733
Bromfed Tablets 1785
Bromfed-DM Cough Syrup 1786
Bromfed-PD Capsules (Extended-Release) 1785
Children's Vicks DayQuil Allergy Relief .... ⓔ 757
Children's Vicks NyQuil Cold/ Cough Relief .... ⓔ 758
Comtrex Multi-Symptom Cold Reliever Tablets/Caplets/Liqui-Gels/Liquid .... ⓔ 615
Allergy-Sinus Comtrex Multi-Symptom Allergy-Sinus Formula Tablets .... ⓔ 617
Comtrex Multi-Symptom Non-Drowsy Caplets .... ⓔ 618
Congess 1004
Contac Day Allergy/Sinus Caplets ⓔ 812
Contac Day & Night .... ⓔ 812
Contac Night Allergy/Sinus Caplets .... ⓔ 812
Contac Severe Cold & Flu Non-Drowsy .... ⓔ 815
Deconamine Chewable Tablets 1320
Deconamine CX Cough and Cold Liquid and Tablets 1319
Deconamine 1320
Deconsal C Expectorant Syrup 456
Deconsal Pediatric Syrup 457
Deconsal II Tablets 454
Dimetane-DX Cough Syrup 2059
Dimetapp Sinus Caplets .... ⓔ 775
Dorcol Children's Cough Syrup ...... ⓔ 785
Drixoral Cough + Congestion Liquid Caps .... ⓔ 802
Dura-Tap/PD Capsules 2867
Duratuss Tablets 2565
Duratuss HD Elixir 2565
Efidac/24 .... ⓔ 635
Entex PSE Tablets 1987
Fedahist Gyrocaps 2401
Fedahist Timecaps 2401
Guaifed 1787
Guaifed Syrup .... ⓔ 734
Guaimax-D Tablets 792
Guaitab Tablets .... ⓔ 734
Isoclor Expectorant 990
Kronofed-A 977
Motrin IB Sinus .... ⓔ 838
Novahistine DH 2462
Novahistine DMX .... ⓔ 822
Novahistine Expectorant 2463
Nucofed 2051
PediaCare Cold Allergy Chewable Tablets .... ⓔ 677
PediaCare Cough-Cold Chewable Tablets 1553
PediaCare 1553

IMPORTANT NOTE: Always consult each drug listing in the patient's regimen for possible interactions.

Anafranil Interactions Index 58

PediaCare Infants' Decongestant Drops ■ 677
PediCare Infant's Drops Decongestant Plus Cough 1553
PediaCare NightRest Cough-Cold Liquid 1553
Pediatric Vicks 44d Dry Hacking Cough & Head Congestion ■ 763
Pediatric Vicks 44m Cough & Cold Relief ■ 764
Robitussin Cold & Cough Liqui-Gels ■ 776
Robitussin Maximum Strength Cough & Cold ■ 778
Robitussin Pediatric Cough & Cold Formula ■ 779
Robitussin Severe Congestion Liqui-Gels ■ 776
Robitussin-DAC Syrup 2074
Robitussin-PE ■ 778
Rondec Oral Drops 953
Rondec Syrup 953
Rondec Tablet 953
Rondec-DM Oral Drops 954
Rondec-DM Syrup 954
Rondec-TR Tablet 953
Ryna ■ 841
Seldane-D Extended-Release Tablets 1538
Semprex-D Capsules 463
Semprex-D Capsules 1167
Sinarest Tablets ■ 648
Sinarest Extra Strength Tablets ■ 648
Sinarest No Drowsiness Tablets ■ 648
Sine-Aid IB Caplets 1554
Sine-Aid Maximum Strength Sinus Medication Gelcaps, Caplets and Tablets 1554
Sine-Off No Drowsiness Formula Caplets ■ 824
Sine-Off Sinus Medicine ■ 825
Singlet Tablets ■ 825
Sinutab Non-Drying Liquid Caps ■ 859
Sinutab Sinus Allergy Medication, Maximum Strength Tablets and Caplets ■ 860
Sinutab Sinus Medication, Maximum Strength Without Drowsiness Formula, Tablets & Caplets ■ 860
Sinutab Sinus Medication, Regular Strength Without Drowsiness Formula ■ 859
Sudafed Children's Liquid ■ 861
Sudafed Cold and Cough Liquidcaps ■ 862
Sudafed Cough Syrup ■ 862
Sudafed Plus Liquid ■ 862
Sudafed Plus Tablets ■ 863
Sudafed Severe Cold Formula Caplets ■ 863
Sudafed Severe Cold Formula Tablets ■ 864
Sudafed Sinus Caplets ■ 864
Sudafed Sinus Tablets ■ 864
Sudafed Tablets, 30 mg ■ 861
Sudafed Tablets, 60 mg ■ 861
Sudafed 12 Hour Caplets ■ 861
Syn-Rx Tablets 465
Syn-Rx DM Tablets 466
TheraFlu ■ 787
TheraFlu Maximum Strength Nighttime Flu, Cold & Cough Medicine ■ 788
TheraFlu Maximum Strength Non-Drowsy Formula Flu, Cold & Cough Medicine ■ 788
Thera Flu Maximum Strength, Non-Drowsy Formula Flu, Cold and Cough Caplets ■ 789
Triaminic AM Cough and Decongestant Formula ■ 789
Triaminic AM Decongestant Formula ■ 790
Triaminic Nite Light ■ 791
Triaminic Sore Throat Formula ■ 791
Tussend 1783
Tussend Expectorant 1785
Children's TYLENOL Cold Multi-Symptom Liquid Formula and Chewable Tablets 1561
Children's TYLENOL Cold Plus Cough Multi Symptom Tablets and Liquid ■ 681
Infants' TYLENOL Cold Decongestant & Fever-Reducer Drops 1556
TYLENOL Maximum Strength Allergy Sinus Medication Gelcaps and Caplets 1563
TYLENOL Maximum Strength Allergy Sinus NightTime Medication Caplets 1555
TYLENOL Flu Maximum Strength Gelcaps 1565
TYLENOL Flu NightTime, Maximum Strength, Gelcaps 1566
TYLENOL Maximum Strength Flu NightTime Hot Medication Packets 1562
TYLENOL, Maximum Strength, Sinus Medication Geltabs, Gelcaps, Caplets and Tablets 1566
TYLENOL Cold Multi-Symptom Formula Medication Tablets and Caplets 1561
TYLENOL Cold Medication No Drowsiness Formula Gelcaps and Caplets 1562
TYLENOL Cold Multi-Symptom Hot Medication Liquid Packets 1557
TYLENOL Cough Multi-Symptom Medication with Decongestant 1565
Ursinus Inlay-Tabs ■ 794
Vicks 44 LiquiCaps Cough, Cold & Flu Relief ■ 755
Vicks 44 LiquiCaps Non-Drowsy Cough & Cold Relief ■ 756
Vicks 44D Dry Hacking Cough & Head Congestion ■ 755
Vicks 44M Cough, Cold & Flu Relief ■ 756
Vicks DayQuil ■ 761
Vicks DayQuil SINUS Pressure & PAIN Relief with IBUPROFEN ■ 762
Vicks Nyquil Hot Therapy ■ 762
Vicks NyQuil LiquiCaps Multi-Symptom Cold/Flu Relief ■ 763
Vicks NyQuil Multi-Symptom Cold/Flu Relief - (Original & Cherry Flavor) ■ 763

Pseudoephedrine Sulfate (Effect not specified; close supervision and careful adjustment of dosage are required). Products include:
Cheracol Sinus ■ 768
Chlor-Trimeton Allergy Decongestant Tablets ■ 799
Claritin-D 2350
Drixoral Cold and Allergy Sustained-Action Tablets ■ 802
Drixoral Cold and Flu Extended-Release Tablets ■ 803
Drixoral Non-Drowsy Formula Extended-Release Tablets ■ 803
Drixoral Allergy/Sinus Extended Release Tablets ■ 804
Trinalin Repetabs Tablets 1330

Quazepam (Anafranil may exaggerate patients' response to CNS depressants). Products include:
Doral Tablets 2664

Risperidone (Anafranil may exaggerate patients' response to CNS depressants). Products include:
Risperdal 1301

Salmeterol Xinafoate (Effect not specified; close supervision and careful adjustment of dosage are required). Products include:
Serevent Inhalation Aerosol 1176

Scopolamine (Effect not specified; close supervision and careful adjustment of dosage are required). Products include:
Transderm Scōp Transdermal Therapeutic System 869

Scopolamine Hydrobromide (Effect not specified; close supervision and careful adjustment of dosage are required). Products include:
Atrohist Plus Tablets 454
Donnatal 2060
Donnatal Extentabs 2061
Donnatal Tablets 2060

Secobarbital Sodium (Anafranil may exaggerate patients' response to CNS depressants; decreases plasma levels of clomipramine). Products include:
Seconal Sodium Pulvules 1474

Selegiline Hydrochloride (Concurrent therapy is contraindicated, or should not be used within 14 days before or after treatment with MAOI). Products include:
Eldepryl Tablets 2550

Sufentanil Citrate (Anafranil may exaggerate patients' response to CNS depressants). Products include:
Sufenta Injection 1309

Temazepam (Anafranil may exaggerate patients' response to CNS depressants). Products include:
Restoril Capsules 2284

Terbutaline Sulfate (Effect not specified; close supervision and careful adjustment of dosage are required). Products include:
Brethaire Inhaler 813
Brethine Ampuls 815
Brethine Tablets 814
Bricanyl Subcutaneous Injection 1502
Bricanyl Tablets 1503

Thiamylal Sodium (Anafranil may exaggerate patients' response to CNS depressants; decreases plasma levels of clomipramine).
No products indexed under this heading.

Thioridazine Hydrochloride (Anafranil may exaggerate patients' response to CNS depressants). Products include:
Mellaril 2269

Thiothixene (Anafranil may exaggerate patients' response to CNS depressants). Products include:
Navane Capsules and Concentrate 2201
Navane Intramuscular 2202

Tranylcypromine Sulfate (Concurrent therapy is contraindicated, or should not be used within 14 days before or after treatment with MAOI). Products include:
Parnate Tablets 2503

Triazolam (Anafranil may exaggerate patients' response to CNS depressants). Products include:
Halcion Tablets 2611

Tridihexethyl Chloride (Effect not specified; close supervision and careful adjustment of dosage are required).
No products indexed under this heading.

Trifluoperazine Hydrochloride (Anafranil may exaggerate patients' response to CNS depressants). Products include:
Stelazine 2514

Trihexyphenidyl Hydrochloride (Effect not specified; close supervision and careful adjustment of dosage are required). Products include:
Artane 1368

Warfarin Sodium (Potential for adverse effects due to displacement of either drug from protein binding site). Products include:
Coumadin 926

Zolpidem Tartrate (Anafranil may exaggerate patients' response to CNS depressants). Products include:
Ambien Tablets 2416

Food Interactions

Alcohol (Anafranil may exaggerate patients' response to alcohol).

ANA-KIT ANAPHYLAXIS EMERGENCY TREATMENT KIT

(Epinephrine Hydrochloride, Chlorpheniramine Maleate) 617
May interact with tricyclic antidepressants, sympathomimetics, cardiac glycosides, beta blockers, ergot-containing drugs, phenothiazines, insulin, oral hypoglycemic agents, and certain other agents. Compounds in these categories include:

Acarbose (Diabetics may require an increased dose of oral hypoglycemic drugs).
No products indexed under this heading.

Acebutolol Hydrochloride (Antagonizes the cardiostimulating and bronchodilating effects of epinephrine). Products include:
Sectral Capsules 2807

Albuterol (Additive effects may be detrimental to the patient). Products include:
Proventil Inhalation Aerosol 2382
Ventolin Inhalation Aerosol and Refill 1197

Albuterol Sulfate (Additive effects may be detrimental to the patient). Products include:
Airet Solution for Inhalation 452
Proventil Inhalation Solution 0.083% 2384
Proventil Repetabs Tablets 2386
Proventil Solution for Inhalation 0.5% 2383
Proventil Syrup 2385
Proventil Tablets 2386
Ventolin Inhalation Solution 1198
Ventolin Nebules Inhalation Solution 1199
Ventolin Rotacaps for Inhalation 1200
Ventolin Syrup 1202
Ventolin Tablets 1203
Volmax Extended-Release Tablets 1788

Amitriptyline Hydrochloride (Potentiation of epinephrine). Products include:
Elavil 2838
Endep Tablets 2174
Etrafon 2355
Limbitrol 2180
Triavil Tablets 1757

Amoxapine (Potentiation of epinephrine). Products include:
Asendin Tablets 1369

Atenolol (Antagonizes the cardiostimulating and bronchodilating effects of epinephrine). Products include:
Tenoretic Tablets 2845
Tenormin Tablets and I.V. Injection 2847

Betaxolol Hydrochloride (Antagonizes the cardiostimulating and bronchodilating effects of epinephrine). Products include:
Betoptic Ophthalmic Solution 469
Betoptic S Ophthalmic Suspension 471
Kerlone Tablets 2436

Bisoprolol Fumarate (Antagonizes the cardiostimulating and bronchodilating effects of epinephrine). Products include:
Zebeta Tablets 1413
Ziac 1415

Carteolol Hydrochloride (Antagonizes the cardiostimulating and bronchodilating effects of epinephrine). Products include:
Cartrol Tablets 410
Ocupress Ophthalmic Solution, 1% Sterile ⊙ 309

Chlorpheniramine Polistirex (Potentiation of epinephrine). Products include:
Tussionex Pennkinetic Extended-Release Suspension 998

Chlorpheniramine Tannate (Potentiation of epinephrine). Products include:
Atrohist Pediatric Suspension 454
Ricobid Tablets and Pediatric Suspension 2038
Rynatan 2673
Rynatuss 2673

Chlorpromazine (May reverse the pressor effects of epinephrine). Products include:
Thorazine Suppositories 2523

(■ Described in PDR For Nonprescription Drugs) (⊙ Described in PDR For Ophthalmology)

Chlorpromazine Hydrochloride (May reverse the presser effects of epinephrine). Products include:
- Thorazine 2523

Chlorpropamide (Diabetics may require an increased dose of oral hypoglycemic drugs). Products include:
- Diabinese Tablets 1935

Clomipramine Hydrochloride (Potentiation of epinephrine). Products include:
- Anafranil Capsules 803

Desipramine Hydrochloride (Potentiation of epinephrine). Products include:
- Norpramin Tablets 1526

Deslanoside (Cardiac glycosides may sensitize the myocardium to beta-adrenergic stimulation and cardiac arrhythmias more likely).
- No products indexed under this heading.

Dexchlorpheniramine Maleate (Potentiation of epinephrine).
- No products indexed under this heading.

Digitoxin (Cardiac glycosides may sensitize the myocardium to beta-adrenergic stimulation and cardiac arrhythmias more likely). Products include:
- Crystodigin Tablets 1433

Digoxin (Cardiac glycosides may sensitize the myocardium to beta-adrenergic stimulation and cardiac arrhythmias more likely). Products include:
- Lanoxicaps 1117
- Lanoxin Elixir Pediatric 1120
- Lanoxin Injection 1123
- Lanoxin Injection Pediatric 1126
- Lanoxin Tablets 1128

Dihydroergotamine Mesylate (May reverse the pressor effects of epinephrine). Products include:
- D.H.E. 45 Injection 2255

Diphenhydramine Citrate (Potentiation of epinephrine). Products include:
- Excedrin P.M. Analgesic/Sleeping Aid Tablets, Caplets, Liquigels 733

Diphenhydramine Hydrochloride (Potentiation of epinephrine). Products include:
- Actifed Allergy Daytime/Nighttime Caplets .... ▣ 844
- Actifed Sinus Daytime/Nighttime Tablets and Caplets .... ▣ 846
- Arthritis Foundation NightTime Caplets .... ▣ 674
- Extra Strength Bayer PM Aspirin .. ▣ 713
- Bayer Select Night Time Pain Relief Formula .... ▣ 716
- Benadryl Allergy Decongestant Liquid Medication .... ▣ 848
- Benadryl Allergy Decongestant Tablets .... ▣ 848
- Benadryl Allergy Liquid Medication .... ▣ 849
- Benadryl Allergy .... ▣ 848
- Benadryl Allergy Sinus Headache Formula Caplets .... ▣ 849
- Benadryl Capsules 1898
- Benadryl Dye-Free Allergy Liqui-gel Softgels .... ▣ 850
- Benadryl Dye-Free Allergy Liquid Medication .... ▣ 850
- Benadryl Itch Relief Cream, Children's Formula and Maximum Strength 2% .... ▣ 851
- Benadryl Itch Relief Spray, Children's Formula and Maximum Strength 2% .... ▣ 851
- Benadryl Itch Relief Stick Maximum Strength 2% .... ▣ 850
- Benadryl Itch Stopping Gel, Children's Formula and Maximum Strength 2% .... ▣ 851
- Benadryl Kapseals 1898
- Benadryl Injection 1898
- Contac Day & Night Cold/Flu Night Caplets .... ▣ 812
- Contac Night Allergy/Sinus Caplets .... ▣ 812
- Extra Strength Doan's P.M. .... ▣ 633
- Legatrin PM .... ▣ 651
- Miles Nervine Nighttime Sleep-Aid ▣ 723
- Nytol QuickCaps Caplets .... ▣ 610
- Sleepinal Night-time Sleep Aid Capsules and Softgels .... ▣ 834
- TYLENOL Maximum Strength Allergy Sinus NightTime Medication Caplets 1555
- TYLENOL Flu NightTime, Maximum Strength, Gelcaps 1566
- TYLENOL Maximum Strength Flu NightTime Hot Medication Packets 1562
- TYLENOL PM, Extra Strength Pain Reliever/Sleep Aid Caplets, Geltabs, Gelcaps 1560
- TYLENOL Severe Allergy Medication Caplets 1564
- Maximum Strength Unisom Sleepgels 1934
- Unisom With Pain Relief-Nighttime Sleep Aid and Pain Reliever 1934

Dobutamine Hydrochloride (Additive effects may be detrimental to the patient). Products include:
- Dobutrex Solution Vials 1439

Dopamine Hydrochloride (Additive effects may be detrimental to the patient).
- No products indexed under this heading.

Doxepin Hydrochloride (Potentiation of epinephrine). Products include:
- Sinequan 2205
- Zonalon Cream 1055

Ephedrine Hydrochloride (Additive effects may be detrimental to the patient). Products include:
- Primatene Dual Action Formula .... ▣ 872
- Primatene Tablets .... ▣ 873
- Quadrinal Tablets 1350

Ephedrine Sulfate (Additive effects may be detrimental to the patient). Products include:
- Bronkaid Caplets .... ▣ 717
- Marax Tablets & DF Syrup 2200

Ephedrine Tannate (Additive effects may be detrimental to the patient). Products include:
- Rynatuss 2673

Epinephrine (Additive effects may be detrimental to the patient). Products include:
- Bronkaid Mist .... ▣ 717
- EPIFRIN .... ◉ 239
- EpiPen 790
- Marcaine Hydrochloride with Epinephrine 1:200,000 2316
- Primatene Mist .... ▣ 873
- Sensorcaine with Epinephrine Injection 559
- Sus-Phrine Injection 1019
- Xylocaine with Epinephrine Injections 567

Epinephrine Bitartrate (Additive effects may be detrimental to the patient). Products include:
- Bronkaid Mist Suspension .... ▣ 718
- Sensorcaine-MPF with Epinephrine Injection 559

Ergotamine Tartrate (May reverse the pressor effects of epinephrine). Products include:
- Bellergal-S Tablets 2250
- Cafergot 2251
- Ergomar 1486
- Wigraine Tablets & Suppositories .. 1829

Esmolol Hydrochloride (Antagonizes the cardiostimulating and bronchodilating effects of epinephrine). Products include:
- Brevibloc Injection 1808

Fluphenazine Decanoate (May reverse the pressor effects of epinephrine). Products include:
- Prolixin Decanoate 509

Fluphenazine Enanthate (May reverse the pressor effects of epinephrine). Products include:
- Prolixin Enanthate 509

Fluphenazine Hydrochloride (May reverse the pressor effects of epinephrine). Products include:
- Prolixin 509

Glipizide (Diabetics may require an increased dose of oral hypoglycemic drugs). Products include:
- Glucotrol Tablets 1967
- Glucotrol XL Extended Release Tablets 1968

Glyburide (Diabetics may require an increased dose of oral hypoglycemic drugs). Products include:
- DiaBeta Tablets 1239
- Glynase PresTab Tablets 2609
- Micronase Tablets 2623

Imipramine Hydrochloride (Potentiation of epinephrine). Products include:
- Tofranil Ampuls 854
- Tofranil Tablets 856

Imipramine Pamoate (Potentiation of epinephrine). Products include:
- Tofranil-PM Capsules 857

Insulin, Human (Diabetics may require an increased dose of insulin).
- No products indexed under this heading.

Insulin, Human Isophane Suspension (Diabetics may require an increased dose of insulin). Products include:
- Novolin N Human Insulin 10 ml Vials 1795

Insulin, Human NPH (Diabetics may require an increased dose of insulin). Products include:
- Humulin N, 100 Units 1448
- Novolin N PenFill Cartridges Durable Insulin Delivery System 1798
- Novolin N Prefilled Syringe Disposable Insulin Delivery System 1798

Insulin, Human Regular (Diabetics may require an increased dose of insulin). Products include:
- Humulin R, 100 Units 1449
- Novolin R Human Insulin 10 ml Vials 1795
- Novolin R PenFill Cartridges Durable Insulin Delivery System 1798
- Novolin R Prefilled Syringe Disposable Insulin Delivery System 1798
- Velosulin BR Human Insulin 10 ml Vials 1795

Insulin, Human, Zinc Suspension (Diabetics may require an increased dose of insulin). Products include:
- Humulin L, 100 Units 1446
- Humulin U, 100 Units 1450
- Novolin L Human Insulin 10 ml Vials 1795

Insulin, NPH (Diabetics may require an increased dose of insulin). Products include:
- NPH, 100 Units 1450
- Pork NPH, 100 Units 1452
- Purified Pork NPH Isophane Insulin 1801

Insulin, Regular (Diabetics may require an increased dose of insulin). Products include:
- Regular, 100 Units 1450
- Pork Regular, 100 Units 1452
- Pork Regular (Concentrated), 500 Units 1453
- Purified Pork Regular Insulin 1801

Insulin, Zinc Crystals (Diabetics may require an increased dose of insulin). Products include:
- NPH, 100 Units 1450

Insulin, Zinc Suspension (Diabetics may require an increased dose of insulin). Products include:
- Iletin I 1450
- Lente, 100 Units 1450
- Iletin II 1452
- Pork Lente, 100 Units 1452
- Purified Pork Lente Insulin 1801

Isoproterenol Hydrochloride (Additive effects may be detrimental to the patient). Products include:
- Isuprel Hydrochloride Injection 1:5000 2311
- Isuprel Hydrochloride Solution 1:200 & 1:100 2313
- Isuprel Mistometer 2312

Isoproterenol Sulfate (Additive effects may be detrimental to the patient). Products include:
- Norisodrine with Calcium Iodide Syrup 442

Labetalol Hydrochloride (Antagonizes the cardiostimulating and bronchodilating effects of epinephrine). Products include:
- Normodyne Injection 2377
- Normodyne Tablets 2379
- Trandate 1185

Levobunolol Hydrochloride (Antagonizes the cardiostimulating and bronchodilating effects of epinephrine). Products include:
- Betagan .... ◉ 233

Maprotiline Hydrochloride (Potentiation of epinephrine). Products include:
- Ludiomil Tablets 843

Mercurial Diuretics (Mercurial diuretics may sensitize the myocardium to beta-adrenergic stimulation and cardiac arrhythmias more likely).

Mesoridazine Besylate (May reverse the pressor effects of epinephrine). Products include:
- Serentil 684

Metaproterenol Sulfate (Additive effects may be detrimental to the patient). Products include:
- Alupent 669
- Metaproterenol Sulfate Inhalation Solution, USP, Arm-a-Med 552

Metaraminol Bitartrate (Additive effects may be detrimental to the patient). Products include:
- Aramine Injection 1609

Metformin Hydrochloride (Diabetics may require an increased dose of oral hypoglycemic drugs). Products include:
- Glucophage 752

Methotrimeprazine (May reverse the pressor effects of epinephrine). Products include:
- Levoprome 1274

Methoxamine Hydrochloride (Additive effects may be detrimental to the patient). Products include:
- Vasoxyl Injection 1196

Methylergonovine Maleate (May reverse the pressor effects of epinephrine). Products include:
- Methergine 2272

Methysergide Maleate (May reverse the pressor effects of epinephrine). Products include:
- Sansert Tablets 2295

Metipranolol Hydrochloride (Antagonizes the cardiostimulating and bronchodilating effects of epinephrine). Products include:
- OptiPranolol (Metipranolol 0.3%) Sterile Ophthalmic Solution .... ◉ 258

Metoprolol Succinate (Antagonizes the cardiostimulating and bronchodilating effects of epinephrine). Products include:
- Toprol-XL Tablets 565

Metoprolol Tartrate (Antagonizes the cardiostimulating and bronchodilating effects of epinephrine). Products include:
- Lopressor Ampuls 830
- Lopressor HCT Tablets 832

IMPORTANT NOTE: Always consult each drug listing in the patient's regimen for possible interactions.

Ana-Kit Interactions Index 60

Lopressor Tablets 830

Nadolol (Antagonizes the cardiostimulating and bronchodilating effects of epinephrine).

No products indexed under this heading.

Norepinephrine Bitartrate (Additive effects may be detrimental to the patient). Products include:

Levophed Bitartrate Injection 2315

Nortriptyline Hydrochloride (Potentiation of epinephrine). Products include:

Pamelor 2280

Penbutolol Sulfate (Antagonizes the cardiostimulating and bronchodilating effects of epinephrine). Products include:

Levatol 2403

Perphenazine (May reverse the pressor effects of epinephrine). Products include:

Etrafon 2355
Triavil Tablets 1757
Trilafon 2389

Phentolamine Mesylate (Antagonizes the vasoconstrictive and hypertensive effects of epinephrine). Products include:

Regitine 846

Phenylephrine Bitartrate (Additive effects may be detrimental to the patient).

No products indexed under this heading.

Phenylephrine Hydrochloride (Additive effects may be detrimental to the patient). Products include:

Atrohist Plus Tablets 454
Cerose DM .... ▣ 878
Comhist 2038
D.A. Chewable Tablets 951
Deconsal Pediatric Capsules 454
Dura-Vent/DA Tablets 953
Entex Capsules 1986
Entex Liquid 1986
Extendryl 1005
4-Way Fast Acting Nasal Spray (regular & mentholated) .... ▣ 621
Hemorid For Women .... ▣ 834
Hycomine Compound Tablets 932
Neo-Synephrine Hydrochloride 1% Carpuject 2324
Neo-Synephrine Hydrochloride 1% Injection 2324
Neo-Synephrine Hydrochloride (Ophthalmic) 2325
Neo-Synephrine .... ▣ 726
Nōstril .... ▣ 644
Novahistine Elixir .... ▣ 823
Phenergan VC 2779
Phenergan VC with Codeine 2781
Preparation H .... ▣ 871
Tympagesic Ear Drops 2342
Vasosulf .... ⊙ 271
Vicks Sinex Nasal Spray and Ultra Fine Mist .... ▣ 765

Phenylephrine Tannate (Additive effects may be detrimental to the patient). Products include:

Atrohist Pediatric Suspension 454
Ricobid-D Pediatric Suspension 2038
Ricobid Tablets and Pediatric Suspension 2038
Rynatan 2673
Rynatuss 2673

Phenylpropanolamine Hydrochloride (Additive effects may be detrimental to the patient). Products include:

Acutrim .... ▣ 628
Allerest Children's Chewable Tablets .... ▣ 627
Allerest 12 Hour Caplets .... ▣ 627
Atrohist Plus Tablets 454
BC Cold Powder Multi-Symptom Formula (Cold-Sinus-Allergy) .... ▣ 609
BC Cold Powder Non-Drowsy Formula (Cold-Sinus) .... ▣ 609
Cheracol Plus Head Cold/Cough Formula .... ▣ 769
Comtrex Multi-Symptom Non-Drowsy Liqui-gels .... ▣ 618
Contac Continuous Action Nasal Decongestant/Antihistamine 12 Hour Capsules .... ▣ 813
Contac Maximum Strength Continuous Action Decongestant/Antihistamine 12 Hour Caplets .... ▣ 813
Contac Severe Cold and Flu Formula Caplets .... ▣ 814
Coricidin 'D' Decongestant Tablets .... ▣ 800
Dexatrim .... ▣ 832
Dexatrim Plus Vitamins Caplets .... ▣ 832
Dimetane-DC Cough Syrup 2059
Dimetapp Elixir .... ▣ 773
Dimetapp Extentabs .... ▣ 774
Dimetapp Tablets/Liqui-Gels .... ▣ 775
Dimetapp Cold & Allergy Chewable Tablets .... ▣ 773
Dimetapp DM Elixir .... ▣ 774
Dura-Vent Tablets 952
Entex Capsules 1986
Entex LA Tablets 1987
Entex Liquid 1986
Exgest LA Tablets 782
Hycomine 931
Isoclor Timesule Capsules .... ▣ 637
Nolamine Timed-Release Tablets 785
Ornade Spansule Capsules 2502
Propagest Tablets 786
Pyrroxate Caplets .... ▣ 772
Robitussin-CF .... ▣ 777
Sinulin Tablets 787
Tavist-D 12 Hour Relief Tablets .... ▣ 787
Teldrin 12 Hour Antihistamine/Nasal Decongestant Allergy Relief Capsules .... ▣ 826
Triaminic Allergy Tablets .... ▣ 789
Triaminic Cold Tablets .... ▣ 790
Triaminic Expectorant .... ▣ 790
Triaminic Syrup .... ▣ 792
Triaminic-12 Tablets .... ▣ 792
Triaminic-DM Syrup .... ▣ 792
Triaminicin Tablets .... ▣ 793
Triaminicol Multi-Symptom Cold Tablets .... ▣ 793
Triaminicol Multi-Symptom Relief .... ▣ 794
Vicks DayQuil Allergy Relief 12-Hour Extended Release Tablets .... ▣ 760
Vicks DayQuil Allergy Relief 4-Hour Tablets .... ▣ 760
Vicks DayQuil SINUS Pressure & CONGESTION Relief .... ▣ 761

Pindolol (Antagonizes the cardiostimulating and bronchodilating effects of epinephrine). Products include:

Visken Tablets 2299

Pirbuterol Acetate (Additive effects may be detrimental to the patient). Products include:

Maxair Autohaler 1492
Maxair Inhaler 1494

Prochlorperazine (May reverse the pressor effects of epinephrine). Products include:

Compazine 2470

Promethazine Hydrochloride (May reverse the pressor effects of epinephrine). Products include:

Mepergan Injection 2753
Phenergan with Codeine 2777
Phenergan with Dextromethorphan 2778
Phenergan Injection 2773
Phenergan Suppositories 2775
Phenergan Syrup 2774
Phenergan Tablets 2775
Phenergan VC 2779
Phenergan VC with Codeine 2781

Propranolol Hydrochloride (Antagonizes the cardiostimulating and bronchodilating effects of epinephrine). Products include:

Inderal 2728
Inderal LA Long Acting Capsules 2730
Inderide Tablets 2732
Inderide LA Long Acting Capsules 2734

Protriptyline Hydrochloride (Potentiation of epinephrine). Products include:

Vivactil Tablets 1774

Pseudoephedrine Hydrochloride (Additive effects may be detrimental to the patient). Products include:

Actifed Allergy Daytime/Nighttime Caplets .... ▣ 844
Actifed Plus Caplets .... ▣ 845
Actifed Plus Tablets .... ▣ 845
Actifed with Codeine Cough Syrup 1067
Actifed Sinus Daytime/Nighttime Tablets and Caplets .... ▣ 846
Actifed Syrup .... ▣ 846
Actifed Tablets .... ▣ 844
Advil Cold and Sinus Caplets and Tablets (formerly CoAdvil) .... ▣ 870
Alka-Seltzer Plus Cold Medicine Liqui-Gels .... ▣ 706
Alka-Seltzer Plus Cold & Cough Medicine Liqui-Gels .... ▣ 705
Alka-Seltzer Plus Night-Time Cold Medicine Liqui-Gels .... ▣ 706
Allerest Headache Strength Tablets .... ▣ 627
Allerest Maximum Strength Tablets .... ▣ 627
Allerest No Drowsiness Tablets .... ▣ 627
Allerest Sinus Pain Formula .... ▣ 627
Anatuss LA Tablets 1542
Atrohist Pediatric Capsules 453
Bayer Select Sinus Pain Relief Formula .... ▣ 717
Benadryl Allergy Decongestant Liquid Medication .... ▣ 848
Benadryl Allergy Decongestant Tablets .... ▣ 848
Benadryl Allergy Sinus Headache Formula Caplets .... ▣ 849
Benylin Multisymptom .... ▣ 852
Bromfed Capsules (Extended-Release) 1785
Bromfed Syrup .... ▣ 733
Bromfed Tablets 1785
Bromfed-DM Cough Syrup 1786
Bromfed-PD Capsules (Extended-Release) 1785
Children's Vicks DayQuil Allergy Relief .... ▣ 757
Children's Vicks NyQuil Cold/Cough Relief .... ▣ 758
Comtrex Multi-Symptom Cold Reliever Tablets/Caplets/Liqui-Gels/Liquid .... ▣ 615
Allergy-Sinus Comtrex Multi-Symptom Allergy-Sinus Formula Tablets .... ▣ 617
Comtrex Multi-Symptom Non-Drowsy Caplets .... ▣ 618
Congess 1004
Contac Day Allergy/Sinus Caplets .... ▣ 812
Contac Day & Night .... ▣ 812
Contac Night Allergy/Sinus Caplets .... ▣ 812
Contac Severe Cold & Flu Non-Drowsy .... ▣ 815
Deconamine Chewable Tablets 1320
Deconamine CX Cough and Cold Liquid and Tablets 1319
Deconamine 1320
Deconsal C Expectorant Syrup 456
Deconsal Pediatric Syrup 457
Deconsal II Tablets 454
Dimetane-DX Cough Syrup 2059
Dimetapp Sinus Caplets .... ▣ 775
Dorcol Children's Cough Syrup .... ▣ 785
Drixoral Cough + Congestion Liquid Caps .... ▣ 802
Dura-Tap/PD Capsules 2867
Duratuss Tablets 2565
Duratuss HD Elixir 2565
Efidac/24 .... ▣ 635
Entex PSE Tablets 1987
Fedahist Gyrocaps 2401
Fedahist Timecaps 2401
Guaifed 1787
Guaifed Syrup .... ▣ 734
Guaimax-D Tablets 792
Guaitab Tablets .... ▣ 734
Isoclor Expectorant 990
Kronofed-A 977
Motrin IB Sinus .... ▣ 838
Novahistine DH 2462
Novahistine DMX .... ▣ 822
Novahistine Expectorant 2463
Nucofed 2051
PediaCare Cold Allergy Chewable Tablets .... ▣ 677
PediaCare Cough-Cold Chewable Tablets 1553
PediaCare 1553
PediaCare Infants' Decongestant Drops .... ▣ 677
PediCare Infant's Drops Decongestant Plus Cough 1553
PediaCare NightRest Cough-Cold Liquid 1553
Pediatric Vicks 44d Dry Hacking Cough & Head Congestion .... ▣ 763
Pediatric Vicks 44m Cough & Cold Relief .... ▣ 764
Robitussin Cold & Cough Liqui-Gels .... ▣ 776
Robitussin Maximum Strength Cough & Cold .... ▣ 778
Robitussin Pediatric Cough & Cold Formula .... ▣ 779
Robitussin Severe Congestion Liqui-Gels .... ▣ 776
Robitussin-DAC Syrup 2074
Robitussin-PE .... ▣ 778
Rondec Oral Drops 953
Rondec Syrup 953
Rondec Tablet 953
Rondec-DM Oral Drops 954
Rondec-DM Syrup 954
Rondec-TR Tablet 953
Ryna .... ▣ 841
Seldane-D Extended-Release Tablets 1538
Semprex-D Capsules 463
Semprex-D Capsules 1167
Sinarest Tablets .... ▣ 648
Sinarest Extra Strength Tablets .... ▣ 648
Sinarest No Drowsiness Tablets .... ▣ 648
Sine-Aid IB Caplets 1554
Sine-Aid Maximum Strength Sinus Medication Gelcaps, Caplets and Tablets 1554
Sine-Off No Drowsiness Formula Caplets .... ▣ 824
Sine-Off Sinus Medicine .... ▣ 825
Singlet Tablets .... ▣ 825
Sinutab Non-Drying Liquid Caps .... ▣ 859
Sinutab Sinus Allergy Medication, Maximum Strength Tablets and Caplets .... ▣ 860
Sinutab Sinus Medication, Maximum Strength Without Drowsiness Formula, Tablets & Caplets .... ▣ 860
Sinutab Sinus Medication, Regular Strength Without Drowsiness Formula .... ▣ 859
Sudafed Children's Liquid .... ▣ 861
Sudafed Cold and Cough Liquidcaps .... ▣ 862
Sudafed Cough Syrup .... ▣ 862
Sudafed Plus Liquid .... ▣ 862
Sudafed Plus Tablets .... ▣ 863
Sudafed Severe Cold Formula Caplets .... ▣ 863
Sudafed Severe Cold Formula Tablets .... ▣ 864
Sudafed Sinus Caplets .... ▣ 864
Sudafed Sinus Tablets .... ▣ 864
Sudafed Tablets, 30 mg .... ▣ 861
Sudafed Tablets, 60 mg .... ▣ 861
Sudafed 12 Hour Caplets .... ▣ 861
Syn-Rx Tablets 465
Syn-Rx DM Tablets 466
TheraFlu .... ▣ 787
TheraFlu Maximum Strength Nighttime Flu, Cold & Cough Medicine .... ▣ 788
TheraFlu Maximum Strength Non-Drowsy Formula Flu, Cold & Cough Medicine .... ▣ 788
Thera Flu Maximum Strength, Non-Drowsy Formula Flu, Cold and Cough Caplets .... ▣ 789
Triaminic AM Cough and Decongestant Formula .... ▣ 789
Triaminic AM Decongestant Formula .... ▣ 790
Triaminic Nite Light .... ▣ 791
Triaminic Sore Throat Formula .... ▣ 791
Tussend 1783
Tussend Expectorant 1785
Children's TYLENOL Cold Multi-Symptom Liquid Formula and Chewable Tablets 1561
Children's TYLENOL Cold Plus Cough Multi Symptom Tablets and Liquid .... ▣ 681
Infants' TYLENOL Cold Decongestant & Fever-Reducer Drops 1556
TYLENOL Maximum Strength Allergy Sinus Medication Gelcaps and Caplets 1563
TYLENOL Maximum Strength Allergy Sinus NightTime Medication Caplets 1555
TYLENOL Flu Maximum Strength Gelcaps 1565
TYLENOL Flu NightTime, Maximum Strength, Gelcaps 1566
TYLENOL Maximum Strength Flu NightTime Hot Medication Packets 1562

(▣ Described in PDR For Nonprescription Drugs) (⊙ Described in PDR For Ophthalmology)

TYLENOL, Maximum Strength, Sinus Medication Geltabs, Gelcaps, Caplets and Tablets 1566
TYLENOL Cold Multi-Symptom Formula Medication Tablets and Caplets 1561
TYLENOL Cold Medication No Drowsiness Formula Gelcaps and Caplets 1562
TYLENOL Cold Multi-Symptom Hot Medication Liquid Packets 1557
TYLENOL Cough Multi-Symptom Medication with Decongestant 1565
Ursinus Inlay-Tabs .... ■ 794
Vicks 44 LiquiCaps Cough, Cold & Flu Relief .... ■ 755
Vicks 44 LiquiCaps Non-Drowsy Cough & Cold Relief .... ■ 756
Vicks 44D Dry Hacking Cough & Head Congestion .... ■ 755
Vicks 44M Cough, Cold & Flu Relief .... ■ 756
Vicks DayQuil .... ■ 761
Vicks DayQuil SINUS Pressure & PAIN Relief with IBUPROFEN .... ■ 762
Vicks Nyquil Hot Therapy .... ■ 762
Vicks NyQuil LiquiCaps Multi-Symptom Cold/Flu Relief .... ■ 763
Vicks NyQuil Multi-Symptom Cold/Flu Relief - (Original & Cherry Flavor) .... ■ 763

Pseudoephedrine Sulfate (Additive effects may be detrimental to the patient). Products include:
Cheracol Sinus .... ■ 768
Chlor-Trimeton Allergy Decongestant Tablets .... ■ 799
Claritin-D 2350
Drixoral Cold and Allergy Sustained-Action Tablets .... ■ 802
Drixoral Cold and Flu Extended-Release Tablets .... ■ 803
Drixoral Non-Drowsy Formula Extended-Release Tablets .... ■ 803
Drixoral Allergy/Sinus Extended Release Tablets .... ■ 804
Trinalin Repetabs Tablets 1330

Salmeterol Xinafoate (Additive effects may be detrimental to the patient). Products include:
Serevent Inhalation Aerosol 1176

Sodium Levothyroxine (Potentiation of epinephrine).
No products indexed under this heading.

Sotalol Hydrochloride (Antagonizes the cardiostimulating and bronchodilating effects of epinephrine). Products include:
Betapace Tablets 641

Terbutaline Sulfate (Additive effects may be detrimental to the patient). Products include:
Brethaire Inhaler 813
Brethine Ampuls 815
Brethine Tablets 814
Bricanyl Subcutaneous Injection 1502
Bricanyl Tablets 1503

Thioridazine Hydrochloride (May reverse the pressor effects of epinephrine). Products include:
Mellaril 2269

Timolol Hemihydrate (Antagonizes the cardiostimulating and bronchodilating effects of epinephrine). Products include:
Betimol 0.25%, 0.5% .... ◎ 261

Timolol Maleate (Antagonizes the cardiostimulating and bronchodilating effects of epinephrine). Products include:
Blocadren Tablets 1614
Timolide Tablets 1748
Timoptic in Ocudose 1753
Timoptic Sterile Ophthalmic Solution 1751
Timoptic-XE 1755

Tolazamide (Diabetics may require an increased dose of oral hypoglycemic drugs).
No products indexed under this heading.

Tolbutamide (Diabetics may require an increased dose of oral hypoglycemic drugs).
No products indexed under this heading.

Trifluoperazine Hydrochloride (May reverse the pressor effects of epinephrine). Products include:
Stelazine 2514

Trimeprazine Tartrate (Potentiation of epinephrine). Products include:
Temaril Tablets, Syrup and Spansule Extended-Release Capsules 483

Trimipramine Maleate (Potentiation of epinephrine). Products include:
Surmontil Capsules 2811

Tripelennamine Hydrochloride (Potentiation of epinephrine). Products include:
PBZ Tablets 845
PBZ-SR Tablets 844

ANALPRAM-HC RECTAL CREAM 1% AND 2.5%

(Hydrocortisone Acetate, Pramoxine Hydrochloride) 977
None cited in PDR database.

ANAPROX TABLETS

(Naproxen Sodium) 2117
See **EC-Naprosyn Delayed-Release Tablets**

ANAPROX DS TABLETS

(Naproxen Sodium) 2117
See **EC-Naprosyn Delayed-Release Tablets**

ANATUSS LA TABLETS

(Guaifenesin, Pseudoephedrine Hydrochloride) 1542
May interact with veratrum alkaloids, monoamine oxidase inhibitors, beta blockers, catecholamine depleting drugs, and certain other agents. Compounds in these categories include:

Acebutolol Hydrochloride (Potentiates the effects of sympathomimetics). Products include:
Sectral Capsules 2807

Atenolol (Potentiates the effects of sympathomimetics). Products include:
Tenoretic Tablets 2845
Tenormin Tablets and I.V. Injection 2847

Betaxolol Hydrochloride (Potentiates the effects of sympathomimetics). Products include:
Betoptic Ophthalmic Solution 469
Betoptic S Ophthalmic Suspension 471
Kerlone Tablets 2436

Bisoprolol Fumarate (Potentiates the effects of sympathomimetics). Products include:
Zebeta Tablets 1413
Ziac 1415

Carteolol Hydrochloride (Potentiates the effects of sympathomimetics). Products include:
Cartrol Tablets 410
Ocupress Ophthalmic Solution, 1% Sterile .... ◎ 309

Cryptenamine Preparations (Reduced antihypertensive effect).

Deserpidine (Reduced antihypertensive effect).
No products indexed under this heading.

Esmolol Hydrochloride (Potentiates the effects of sympathomimetics). Products include:
Brevibloc Injection 1808

Furazolidone (Potentiates the effects of sympathomimetics; concurrent use is contraindicated). Products include:
Furoxone 2046

Guanethidine Monosulfate (Reduced antihypertensive effect). Products include:
Esimil Tablets 822
Ismelin Tablets 827

Isocarboxazid (Potentiates the effects of sympathomimetics; concurrent use is contraindicated).
No products indexed under this heading.

Labetalol Hydrochloride (Potentiates the effects of sympathomimetics). Products include:
Normodyne Injection 2377
Normodyne Tablets 2379
Trandate 1185

Levobunolol Hydrochloride (Potentiates the effects of sympathomimetics). Products include:
Betagan .... ◎ 233

Mecamylamine Hydrochloride (Reduced antihypertensive effect). Products include:
Inversine Tablets 1686

Methyldopa (Reduced antihypertensive effect). Products include:
Aldoclor Tablets 1598
Aldomet Oral 1600
Aldoril Tablets 1604

Methyldopate Hydrochloride (Reduced antihypertensive effect). Products include:
Aldomet Ester HCl Injection 1602

Metipranolol Hydrochloride (Potentiates the effects of sympathomimetics). Products include:
OptiPranolol (Metipranolol 0.3%) Sterile Ophthalmic Solution .... ◎ 258

Metoprolol Succinate (Potentiates the effects of sympathomimetics). Products include:
Toprol-XL Tablets 565

Metoprolol Tartrate (Potentiates the effects of sympathomimetics). Products include:
Lopressor Ampuls 830
Lopressor HCT Tablets 832
Lopressor Tablets 830

Nadolol (Potentiates the effects of sympathomimetics).
No products indexed under this heading.

Penbutolol Sulfate (Potentiates the effects of sympathomimetics). Products include:
Levatol 2403

Phenelzine Sulfate (Potentiates the effects of sympathomimetics; concurrent use is contraindicated). Products include:
Nardil 1920

Pindolol (Potentiates the effects of sympathomimetics). Products include:
Visken Tablets 2299

Propranolol Hydrochloride (Potentiates the effects of sympathomimetics). Products include:
Inderal 2728
Inderal LA Long Acting Capsules 2730
Inderide Tablets 2732
Inderide LA Long Acting Capsules .. 2734

Rauwolfia Serpentina (Reduced antihypertensive effect).
No products indexed under this heading.

Rescinnamine (Reduced antihypertensive effect).
No products indexed under this heading.

Reserpine (Reduced antihypertensive effect). Products include:
Diupres Tablets 1650
Hydropres Tablets 1675
Ser-Ap-Es Tablets 849

Selegiline Hydrochloride (Potentiates the effects of sympathomimetics; concurrent use is contraindicated). Products include:
Eldepryl Tablets 2550

Sotalol Hydrochloride (Potentiates the effects of sympathomimetics). Products include:
Betapace Tablets 641

Timolol Hemihydrate (Potentiates the effects of sympathomimetics). Products include:
Betimol 0.25%, 0.5% .... ◎ 261

Timolol Maleate (Potentiates the effects of sympathomimetics). Products include:
Blocadren Tablets 1614
Timolide Tablets 1748
Timoptic in Ocudose 1753
Timoptic Sterile Ophthalmic Solution 1751
Timoptic-XE 1755

Tranylcypromine Sulfate (Potentiates the effects of sympathomimetics; concurrent use is contraindicated). Products include:
Parnate Tablets 2503

ANCEF INJECTION

(Cefazolin Sodium) 2465
May interact with:

Probenecid (Increased and prolonged cephalosporin blood levels). Products include:
Benemid Tablets 1611
ColBENEMID Tablets 1622

ANCOBON CAPSULES

(Flucytosine) 2079
May interact with:

Amphotericin B (Antifungal synergism). Products include:
Fungizone Intravenous 506

Cytosine Arabinoside (Inactivation of Ancobon's antifungal activity).

Drugs That Impair Glomerular Filtration (Biological half-life of Ancobon may be prolonged).

ANDROID CAPSULES, 10 MG

(Methyltestosterone) 1250
May interact with oral anticoagulants, insulin, and certain other agents. Compounds in these categories include:

Dicumarol (Decreased anticoagulant requirements).
No products indexed under this heading.

Insulin, Human (In diabetic patients the metabolic effects of androgens may decrease blood glucose and insulin requirements).
No products indexed under this heading.

Insulin, Human Isophane Suspension (In diabetic patients the metabolic effects of androgens may decrease blood glucose and insulin requirements). Products include:
Novolin N Human Insulin 10 ml Vials 1795

Insulin, Human NPH (In diabetic patients the metabolic effects of androgens may decrease blood glucose and insulin requirements). Products include:
Humulin N, 100 Units 1448
Novolin N PenFill Cartridges Durable Insulin Delivery System 1798
Novolin N Prefilled Syringe Disposable Insulin Delivery System 1798

IMPORTANT NOTE: Always consult each drug listing in the patient's regimen for possible interactions.

Insulin, Human Regular (In diabetic patients the metabolic effects of androgens may decrease blood glucose and insulin requirements). Products include:

Humulin R, 100 Units 1449
Novolin R Human Insulin 10 ml Vials 1795
Novolin R PenFill Cartridges Durable Insulin Delivery System 1798
Novolin R Prefilled Syringe Disposable Insulin Delivery System 1798
Velosulin BR Human Insulin 10 ml Vials 1795

Insulin, Human, Zinc Suspension (In diabetic patients the metabolic effects of androgens may decrease blood glucose and insulin requirements). Products include:

Humulin L, 100 Units 1446
Humulin U, 100 Units 1450
Novolin L Human Insulin 10 ml Vials 1795

Insulin, NPH (In diabetic patients the metabolic effects of androgens may decrease blood glucose and insulin requirements). Products include:

NPH, 100 Units 1450
Pork NPH, 100 Units 1452
Purified Pork NPH Isophane Insulin 1801

Insulin, Regular (In diabetic patients the metabolic effects of androgens may decrease blood glucose and insulin requirements). Products include:

Regular, 100 Units 1450
Pork Regular, 100 Units 1452
Pork Regular (Concentrated), 500 Units 1453
Purified Pork Regular Insulin 1801

Insulin, Zinc Crystals (In diabetic patients the metabolic effects of androgens may decrease blood glucose and insulin requirements). Products include:

NPH, 100 Units 1450

Insulin, Zinc Suspension (In diabetic patients the metabolic effects of androgens may decrease blood glucose and insulin requirements). Products include:

Iletin I 1450
Lente, 100 Units 1450
Iletin II 1452
Pork Lente, 100 Units 1452
Purified Pork Lente Insulin 1801

Oxyphenbutazone (Concurrent use may result in elevated serum levels of oxyphenbutazone).

Warfarin Sodium (Decreased anticoagulant requirements). Products include:

Coumadin 926

ANDROID-10 TABLETS

(Methyltestosterone) 1251

May interact with oral anticoagulants, insulin, and certain other agents. Compounds in these categories include:

Dicumarol (Decreased anticoagulant requirements).

No products indexed under this heading.

Insulin, Human (Concurrent use may decrease blood glucose and insulin requirements).

No products indexed under this heading.

Insulin, Human Isophane Suspension (Concurrent use may decrease blood glucose and insulin requirements). Products include:

Novolin N Human Insulin 10 ml Vials 1795

Insulin, Human NPH (Concurrent use may decrease blood glucose and insulin requirements). Products include:

Humulin N, 100 Units 1448
Novolin N PenFill Cartridges Durable Insulin Delivery System 1798
Novolin N Prefilled Syringe Disposable Insulin Delivery System 1798

Insulin, Human Regular (Concurrent use may decrease blood glucose and insulin requirements). Products include:

Humulin R, 100 Units 1449
Novolin R Human Insulin 10 ml Vials 1795
Novolin R PenFill Cartridges Durable Insulin Delivery System 1798
Novolin R Prefilled Syringe Disposable Insulin Delivery System 1798
Velosulin BR Human Insulin 10 ml Vials 1795

Insulin, Human, Zinc Suspension (Concurrent use may decrease blood glucose and insulin requirements). Products include:

Humulin L, 100 Units 1446
Humulin U, 100 Units 1450
Novolin L Human Insulin 10 ml Vials 1795

Insulin, NPH (Concurrent use may decrease blood glucose and insulin requirements). Products include:

NPH, 100 Units 1450
Pork NPH, 100 Units 1452
Purified Pork NPH Isophane Insulin 1801

Insulin, Regular (Concurrent use may decrease blood glucose and insulin requirements). Products include:

Regular, 100 Units 1450
Pork Regular, 100 Units 1452
Pork Regular (Concentrated), 500 Units 1453
Purified Pork Regular Insulin 1801

Insulin, Zinc Crystals (Concurrent use may decrease blood glucose and insulin requirements). Products include:

NPH, 100 Units 1450

Insulin, Zinc Suspension (Concurrent use may decrease blood glucose and insulin requirements). Products include:

Iletin I 1450
Lente, 100 Units 1450
Iletin II 1452
Pork Lente, 100 Units 1452
Purified Pork Lente Insulin 1801

Oxyphenbutazone (Elevated serum levels of oxyphenbutazone).

Warfarin Sodium (Decreased anticoagulant requirements). Products include:

Coumadin 926

ANDROID-25 TABLETS

(Methyltestosterone) 1251

See **Android-10 Tablets**

ANECTINE INJECTION

(Succinylcholine Chloride) 1073

See **Anectine Sterile Powder Flo-Pack**

ANECTINE STERILE POWDER FLO-PACK

(Succinylcholine Chloride) 1073

May interact with beta blockers, monoamine oxidase inhibitors, oral contraceptives, glucocorticoids, neuromuscular blocking agents, and certain other agents. Compounds in these categories include:

Acebutolol Hydrochloride (Enhances neuromuscular blocking action). Products include:

Sectral Capsules 2807

Antibiotics, non-penicillin, unspecified (Enhances neuromuscular blocking action).

Anticancer Drugs, unspecified (Prolong respiratory depression).

Aprotinin (Enhances neuromuscular blocking action). Products include:

Trasylol 613

Atenolol (Enhances neuromuscular blocking action). Products include:

Tenoretic Tablets 2845
Tenormin Tablets and I.V. Injection 2847

Atracurium Besylate (Possible synergistic or antagonistic effect if co-administered during the same procedure). Products include:

Tracrium Injection 1183

Betamethasone Acetate (Chronic use of glucocorticoids enhances neuromuscular blocking effect by reducing plasma cholinesterase activity). Products include:

Celestone Soluspan Suspension 2347

Betamethasone Sodium Phosphate (Chronic use of glucocorticoids enhances neuromuscular blocking effect by reducing plasma cholinesterase activity). Products include:

Celestone Soluspan Suspension 2347

Betaxolol Hydrochloride (Enhances neuromuscular blocking action). Products include:

Betoptic Ophthalmic Solution 469
Betoptic S Ophthalmic Suspension 471
Kerlone Tablets 2436

Bisoprolol Fumarate (Enhances neuromuscular blocking action). Products include:

Zebeta Tablets 1413
Ziac 1415

Carteolol Hydrochloride (Enhances neuromuscular blocking action). Products include:

Cartrol Tablets 410
Ocupress Ophthalmic Solution, 1% Sterile .... ◉ 309

Chloroquine Hydrochloride (Enhances neuromuscular blocking action). Products include:

Aralen Hydrochloride Injection 2301

Chloroquine Phosphate (Enhances neuromuscular blocking action). Products include:

Aralen Phosphate Tablets 2301

Cortisone Acetate (Chronic use of glucocorticoids enhances neuromuscular blocking effect by reducing plasma cholinesterase activity). Products include:

Cortone Acetate Sterile Suspension 1623
Cortone Acetate Tablets 1624

Desflurane (Enhances neuromuscular blocking action). Products include:

Suprane 1813

Desogestrel (Chronic use of oral contraceptives enhances neuromuscular blocking effect by reducing plasma cholinesterase activity). Products include:

Desogen Tablets 1817
Ortho-Cept 1851

Dexamethasone (Chronic use of glucocorticoids enhances neuromuscular blocking effect by reducing plasma cholinesterase activity). Products include:

AK-Trol Ointment & Suspension .... ◉ 205
Decadron Elixir 1633
Decadron Tablets 1635
Decaspray Topical Aerosol 1648
Dexacidin Ointment .... ◉ 263
Maxitrol Ophthalmic Ointment and Suspension .... ◉ 224
TobraDex Ophthalmic Suspension and Ointment 473

Dexamethasone Acetate (Chronic use of glucocorticoids enhances neuromuscular blocking effect by reducing plasma cholinesterase activity). Products include:

Dalalone D.P. Injectable 1011
Decadron-LA Sterile Suspension 1646

Dexamethasone Sodium Phosphate (Chronic use of glucocorticoids enhances neuromuscular blocking effect by reducing plasma cholinesterase activity). Products include:

Decadron Phosphate Injection 1637
Decadron Phosphate Respihaler 1642
Decadron Phosphate Sterile Ophthalmic Ointment 1641
Decadron Phosphate Sterile Ophthalmic Solution 1642
Decadron Phosphate Topical Cream 1644
Decadron Phosphate Turbinaire 1645
Decadron Phosphate with Xylocaine Injection, Sterile 1639
Dexacort Phosphate in Respihaler .. 458
Dexacort Phosphate in Turbinaire .. 459
NeoDecadron Sterile Ophthalmic Ointment 1712
NeoDecadron Sterile Ophthalmic Solution 1713
NeoDecadron Topical Cream 1714

Diethyl Ether (Enhances neuromuscular blocking action).

Doxacurium Chloride (Possible synergistic or antagonistic effect if co-administered during the same procedure). Products include:

Nuromax Injection 1149

Echothiophate Iodide (Prolongs respiratory depression). Products include:

Phospholine Iodide .... ◉ 326

Esmolol Hydrochloride (Enhances neuromuscular blocking action). Products include:

Brevibloc Injection 1808

Ethinyl Estradiol (Chronic use of oral contraceptives enhances neuromuscular blocking effect by reducing plasma cholinesterase activity). Products include:

Brevicon 2088
Demulen 2428
Desogen Tablets 1817
Levlen/Tri-Levlen 651
Lo/Ovral Tablets 2746
Lo/Ovral-28 Tablets 2751
Modicon 1872
Nordette-21 Tablets 2755
Nordette-28 Tablets 2758
Norinyl 2088
Ortho-Cept 1851
Ortho-Cyclen/Ortho-Tri-Cyclen 1858
Ortho-Novum 1872
Ortho-Cyclen/Ortho Tri-Cyclen 1858
Ovcon 760
Ovral Tablets 2770
Ovral-28 Tablets 2770
Levlen/Tri-Levlen 651
Tri-Norinyl 2164
Triphasil-21 Tablets 2814
Triphasil-28 Tablets 2819

Ethynodiol Diacetate (Chronic use of oral contraceptives enhances neuromuscular blocking effect by reducing plasma cholinesterase activity). Products include:

Demulen 2428

Fludrocortisone Acetate (Chronic use of glucocorticoids enhances neuromuscular blocking effect by reducing plasma cholinesterase activity). Products include:

Florinef Acetate Tablets 505

Furazolidone (Chronic use of certain unspecified MAO inhibitors enhances neuromuscular blocking effect by reducing plasma cholinesterase activity). Products include:

Furoxone 2046

(▭ Described in PDR For Nonprescription Drugs) (◉ Described in PDR For Ophthalmology)

Interactions Index

Hydrocortisone (Chronic use of glucocorticoids enhances neuromuscular blocking effect by reducing plasma cholinesterase activity). Products include:

Anusol-HC Cream 2.5%........................ 1896
Aquanil HC Lotion................................. 1931
Bactine Hydrocortisone Anti-Itch Cream.. ⊕ 709
Caldecort Anti-Itch Hydrocortisone Spray.. ⊕ 631
Cortaid.. ⊕ 836
CORTENEMA.. 2535
Cortisporin Ointment.............................. 1085
Cortisporin Ophthalmic Ointment Sterile.. 1085
Cortisporin Ophthalmic Suspension Sterile.. 1086
Cortisporin Otic Solution Sterile...... 1087
Cortisporin Otic Suspension Sterile 1088
Cortizone-5... ⊕ 831
Cortizone-10.. ⊕ 831
Hydrocortone Tablets............................. 1672
Hytone.. 907
Massengill Medicated Soft Cloth Towelettes... 2458
PediOtic Suspension Sterile.............. 1153
Preparation H Hydrocortisone 1% Cream.. ⊕ 872
ProctoCream-HC 2.5%.......................... 2408
VoSoL HC Otic Solution........................ 2678

Hydrocortisone Acetate

(Chronic use of glucocorticoids enhances neuromuscular blocking effect by reducing plasma cholinesterase activity). Products include:

Analpram-HC Rectal Cream 1% and 2.5%.. 977
Anusol HC-1 Anti-Itch Hydrocortisone Ointment.. ⊕ 847
Anusol-HC Suppositories..................... 1897
Caldecort... ⊕ 631
Carmol HC... 924
Coly-Mycin S Otic w/Neomycin & Hydrocortisone...................................... 1906
Cortaid.. ⊕ 836
Cortifoam... 2396
Cortisporin Cream................................... 1084
Epifoam.. 2399
Hydrocortone Acetate Sterile Suspension.. 1669
Mantadil Cream....................................... 1135
Nupercainal Hydrocortisone 1% Cream.. ⊕ 645
Ophthocort.. © 311
Pramosone Cream, Lotion & Ointment.. 978
ProctoCream-HC..................................... 2408
ProctoFoam-HC...................................... 2409
Terra-Cortril Ophthalmic Suspension.. 2210

Hydrocortisone Sodium Phosphate

(Chronic use of glucocorticoids enhances neuromuscular blocking effect by reducing plasma cholinesterase activity). Products include:

Hydrocortone Phosphate Injection, Sterile.. 1670

Hydrocortisone Sodium Succinate

(Chronic use of glucocorticoids enhances neuromuscular blocking effect by reducing plasma cholinesterase activity). Products include:

Solu-Cortef Sterile Powder.................. 2641

Isocarboxazid (Chronic use of certain unspecified MAO inhibitors enhances neuromuscular blocking effect by reducing plasma cholinesterase activity).

No products indexed under this heading.

Isoflurane (Enhances neuromuscular blocking action).

No products indexed under this heading.

Labetalol Hydrochloride (Enhances neuromuscular blocking action). Products include:

Normodyne Injection.............................. 2377
Normodyne Tablets................................. 2379
Trandate... 1185

Levobunolol Hydrochloride (Enhances neuromuscular blocking action). Products include:

Betagan.. © 233

Levonorgestrel (Chronic use of oral contraceptives enhances neuromuscular blocking effect by reducing plasma cholinesterase activity). Products include:

Levlen/Tri-Levlen.................................... 651
Nordette-21 Tablets................................ 2755
Nordette-28 Tablets................................ 2758
Norplant System...................................... 2759
Levlen/Tri-Levlen.................................... 651
Triphasil-21 Tablets................................ 2814
Triphasil-28 Tablets................................ 2819

Lidocaine Hydrochloride (Enhances neuromuscular blocking action). Products include:

Bactine Antiseptic/Anesthetic First Aid Liquid...................................... ⊕ 708
Campho-Phenique Maximum Strength First Aid Antibiotic Plus Pain Reliever Ointment......... ⊕ 719
Decadron Phosphate with Xylocaine Injection, Sterile...................... 1639
Xylocaine Injections............................... 567

Lithium Carbonate (Enhances neuromuscular blocking action). Products include:

Eskalith.. 2485
Lithium Carbonate Capsules & Tablets.. 2230
Lithonate/Lithotabs/Lithobid.............. 2543

Magnesium Sulfate Injection (Enhances neuromuscular blocking action).

Mestranol (Chronic use of oral contraceptives enhances neuromuscular blocking effect by reducing plasma cholinesterase activity). Products include:

Norinyl.. 2088
Ortho-Novum... 1872

Methylprednisolone Acetate (Chronic use of glucocorticoids enhances neuromuscular blocking effect by reducing plasma cholinesterase activity). Products include:

Depo-Medrol Single-Dose Vial......... 2600
Depo-Medrol Sterile Aqueous Suspension.. 2597

Methylprednisolone Sodium Succinate (Chronic use of glucocorticoids enhances neuromuscular blocking effect by reducing plasma cholinesterase activity). Products include:

Solu-Medrol Sterile Powder................ 2643

Metipranolol Hydrochloride (Enhances neuromuscular blocking action). Products include:

OptiPranolol (Metipranolol 0.3%) Sterile Ophthalmic Solution.......... © 258

Metoclopramide Hydrochloride (Enhances neuromuscular blocking action). Products include:

Reglan... 2068

Metocurine Iodide (Possible synergistic or antagonistic effect if co-administered during the same procedure). Products include:

Metubine Iodide Vials............................ 916

Metoprolol Succinate (Enhances neuromuscular blocking action). Products include:

Toprol-XL Tablets.................................... 565

Metoprolol Tartrate (Enhances neuromuscular blocking action). Products include:

Lopressor Ampuls.................................... 830
Lopressor HCT Tablets.......................... 832
Lopressor Tablets.................................... 830

Mivacurium Chloride (Possible synergistic or antagonistic effect if co-administered during the same procedure). Products include:

Mivacron.. 1138

Nadolol (Enhances neuromuscular blocking action).

No products indexed under this heading.

Norethindrone (Chronic use of oral contraceptives enhances neuromuscular blocking effect by reducing plasma cholinesterase activity). Products include:

Brevicon.. 2088
Micronor Tablets...................................... 1872
Modicon.. 1872
Norinyl.. 2088
Nor-Q D Tablets....................................... 2135
Ortho-Novum... 1872
Ovcon... 760
Tri-Norinyl.. 2164

Norethynodrel (Chronic use of oral contraceptives enhances neuromuscular blocking effect by reducing plasma cholinesterase activity).

No products indexed under this heading.

Norgestimate (Chronic use of oral contraceptives enhances neuromuscular blocking effect by reducing plasma cholinesterase activity). Products include:

Ortho-Cyclen/Ortho-Tri-Cyclen........ 1858
Ortho-Cyclen/Ortho Tri-Cyclen........ 1858

Norgestrel (Chronic use of oral contraceptives enhances neuromuscular blocking effect by reducing plasma cholinesterase activity). Products include:

Lo/Ovral Tablets...................................... 2746
Lo/Ovral-28 Tablets................................ 2751
Ovral Tablets... 2770
Ovral-28 Tablets...................................... 2770
Ovrette Tablets... 2771

Oxytocin (Enhances neuromuscular blocking action). Products include:

Oxytocin Injection................................... 2771
Syntocinon Injection............................... 2296

Oxytocin (Nasal Spray) (Enhances neuromuscular blocking action).

Pancuronium Bromide Injection (Possible synergistic or antagonistic effect if co-administered during the same procedure).

No products indexed under this heading.

Penbutolol Sulfate (Enhances neuromuscular blocking action). Products include:

Levatol.. 2403

Phenelzine Sulfate (Chronic use of certain unspecified MAO inhibitors enhances neuromuscular blocking effect by reducing plasma cholinesterase activity). Products include:

Nardil.. 1920

Pindolol (Enhances neuromuscular blocking action). Products include:

Visken Tablets... 2299

Prednisolone Acetate (Chronic use of glucocorticoids enhances neuromuscular blocking effect by reducing plasma cholinesterase activity). Products include:

AK-CIDE.. © 202
AK-CIDE Ointment................................. © 202
Blephamide Liquifilm Sterile Ophthalmic Suspension.............................. 476
Blephamide Ointment............................ © 237
Econopred & Econopred Plus Ophthalmic Suspensions.................. © 217
Poly-Pred Liquifilm................................. © 248
Pred Forte.. © 250
Pred Mild.. © 253
Pred-G Liquifilm Sterile Ophthalmic Suspension.................................. © 251
Pred-G S.O.P. Sterile Ophthalmic Ointment.. © 252
Vasocidin Ointment................................. © 268

Prednisolone Sodium Phosphate (Chronic use of glucocorticoids enhances neuromuscular blocking effect by reducing plasma cholinesterase activity). Products include:

AK-Pred.. © 204
Hydeltrasol Injection, Sterile............... 1665
Inflamase.. © 265
Pediapred Oral Liquid............................ 995
Vasocidin Ophthalmic Solution....... © 270

Prednisolone Tebutate (Chronic use of glucocorticoids enhances neuromuscular blocking effect by reducing plasma cholinesterase activity). Products include:

Hydeltra-T.B.A. Sterile Suspension 1667

Prednisone (Chronic use of glucocorticoids enhances neuromuscular blocking effect by reducing plasma cholinesterase activity). Products include:

Deltasone Tablets.................................... 2595

Procainamide Hydrochloride (Enhances neuromuscular blocking action). Products include:

Procan SR Tablets.................................... 1926

Promazine Hydrochloride (Enhances neuromuscular blocking action).

No products indexed under this heading.

Propranolol Hydrochloride (Enhances neuromuscular blocking action). Products include:

Inderal.. 2728
Inderal LA Long Acting Capsules..... 2730
Inderide Tablets....................................... 2732
Inderide LA Long Acting Capsules.. 2734

Quinidine Gluconate (Enhances neuromuscular blocking action). Products include:

Quinaglute Dura-Tabs Tablets........... 649

Quinidine Polygalacturonate (Enhances neuromuscular blocking action).

No products indexed under this heading.

Quinidine Sulfate (Enhances neuromuscular blocking action). Products include:

Quinidex Extentabs................................. 2067

Quinine (Enhances neuromuscular blocking action).

Rocuronium Bromide (Possible synergistic or antagonistic effect if co-administered during the same procedure). Products include:

Zemuron... 1830

Selegiline Hydrochloride (Chronic use of certain unspecified MAO inhibitors enhances neuromuscular blocking effect by reducing plasma cholinesterase activity). Products include:

Eldepryl Tablets....................................... 2550

Sotalol Hydrochloride (Enhances neuromuscular blocking action). Products include:

Betapace Tablets...................................... 641

Terbutaline Sulfate (Enhances neuromuscular blocking action). Products include:

Brethaire Inhaler..................................... 813
Brethine Ampuls...................................... 815
Brethine Tablets....................................... 814
Bricanyl Subcutaneous Injection...... 1502
Bricanyl Tablets....................................... 1503

Timolol Hemihydrate (Enhances neuromuscular blocking action). Products include:

Betimol 0.25%, 0.5%............................ © 261

Timolol Maleate (Enhances neuromuscular blocking action). Products include:

Blocadren Tablets.................................... 1614
Timolide Tablets....................................... 1748
Timoptic in Ocudose.............................. 1753

IMPORTANT NOTE: Always consult each drug listing in the patient's regimen for possible interactions.

Anectine — Interactions Index — 64

Timoptic Sterile Ophthalmic Solution.... 1751
Timoptic-XE 1755

Tranylcypromine Sulfate (Chronic use of certain unspecified MAO inhibitors enhances neuromuscular blocking effect by reducing plasma cholinesterase activity). Products include:
Parnate Tablets 2503

Triamcinolone (Chronic use of glucocorticoids enhances neuromuscular blocking effect by reducing plasma cholinesterase activity). Products include:
Aristocort Tablets 1022

Triamcinolone Acetonide (Chronic use of glucocorticoids enhances neuromuscular blocking effect by reducing plasma cholinesterase activity). Products include:
Aristocort A 0.025% Cream 1027
Aristocort A 0.5% Cream 1031
Aristocort A 0.1% Cream 1029
Aristocort A 0.1% Ointment 1030
Azmacort Oral Inhaler 2011
Nasacort Nasal Inhaler 2024

Triamcinolone Diacetate (Chronic use of glucocorticoids enhances neuromuscular blocking effect by reducing plasma cholinesterase activity). Products include:
Aristocort Suspension (Forte Parenteral) 1027
Aristocort Suspension (Intralesional) 1025

Triamcinolone Hexacetonide (Chronic use of glucocorticoids enhances neuromuscular blocking effect by reducing plasma cholinesterase activity). Products include:
Aristospan Suspension (Intra-articular) 1033
Aristospan Suspension (Intralesional) 1032

Trimethaphan Camsylate (Enhances neuromuscular blocking action). Products include:
Arfonad Ampuls 2080

Vecuronium Bromide (Possible synergistic or antagonistic effect if co-administered during the same procedure). Products include:
Norcuron 1826

ANEXSIA 5/500 ELIXIR
(Acetaminophen, Hydrocodone Bitartrate) 1781
May interact with antipsychotic agents, narcotic analgesics, antihistamines, tranquilizers, central nervous system depressants, monoamine oxidase inhibitors, tricyclic antidepressants, anticholinergics, and certain other agents. Compounds in these categories include:

Acrivastine (Exhibits an additive CNS depression). Products include:
Semprex-D Capsules 463
Semprex-D Capsules 1167

Alfentanil Hydrochloride (Exhibits an additive CNS depression). Products include:
Alfenta Injection 1286

Alprazolam (Exhibits an additive CNS depression). Products include:
Xanax Tablets 2649

Amitriptyline Hydrochloride (Increased effect of either antidepressant or hydrocodone). Products include:
Elavil 2838
Endep Tablets 2174
Etrafon 2355
Limbitrol 2180
Triavil Tablets 1757

Amoxapine (Increased effect of either antidepressant or hydrocodone). Products include:
Asendin Tablets 1369

Aprobarbital (Exhibits an additive CNS depression).
No products indexed under this heading.

Astemizole (Exhibits an additive CNS depression). Products include:
Hismanal Tablets 1293

Atropine Sulfate (Potential for paralytic ileus). Products include:
Arco-Lase Plus Tablets 512
Atrohist Plus Tablets 454
Atropine Sulfate Sterile Ophthalmic Solution .... ◉ 233
Donnatal 2060
Donnatal Extentabs 2061
Donnatal Tablets 2060
Lomotil 2439
Motofen Tablets 784
Urised Tablets 1964

Azatadine Maleate (Exhibits an additive CNS depression). Products include:
Trinalin Repetabs Tablets 1330

Belladonna Alkaloids (Potential for paralytic ileus). Products include:
Bellergal-S Tablets 2250
Hyland's Bed Wetting Tablets .... ■ 828
Hyland's EnurAid Tablets .... ■ 829
Hyland's Teething Tablets .... ■ 830

Benztropine Mesylate (Potential for paralytic ileus). Products include:
Cogentin 1621

Biperiden Hydrochloride (Potential for paralytic ileus). Products include:
Akineton 1333

Bromodiphenhydramine Hydrochloride (Exhibits an additive CNS depression).
No products indexed under this heading.

Brompheniramine Maleate (Exhibits an additive CNS depression). Products include:
Alka Seltzer Plus Sinus Medicine .. ■ 707
Bromfed Capsules (Extended-Release) 1785
Bromfed Syrup .... ■ 733
Bromfed Tablets 1785
Bromfed-DM Cough Syrup 1786
Bromfed-PD Capsules (Extended-Release) 1785
Dimetane-DC Cough Syrup 2059
Dimetane-DX Cough Syrup 2059
Dimetapp Elixir .... ■ 773
Dimetapp Extentabs .... ■ 774
Dimetapp Tablets/Liqui-Gels .... ■ 775
Dimetapp Cold & Allergy Chewable Tablets .... ■ 773
Dimetapp DM Elixir .... ■ 774
Vicks DayQuil Allergy Relief 12-Hour Extended Release Tablets .... ■ 760
Vicks DayQuil Allergy Relief 4-Hour Tablets .... ■ 760

Buprenorphine (Exhibits an additive CNS depression). Products include:
Buprenex Injectable 2006

Buspirone Hydrochloride (Exhibits an additive CNS depression). Products include:
BuSpar 737

Butabarbital (Exhibits an additive CNS depression).
No products indexed under this heading.

Butalbital (Exhibits an additive CNS depression). Products include:
Esgic-plus Tablets 1013
Fioricet Tablets 2258
Fioricet with Codeine Capsules 2260
Fiorinal Capsules 2261
Fiorinal with Codeine Capsules 2262
Fiorinal Tablets 2261
Phrenilin 785
Sedapap Tablets 50 mg/650 mg .. 1543

Chlordiazepoxide (Exhibits an additive CNS depression). Products include:
Libritabs Tablets 2177
Limbitrol 2180

Chlordiazepoxide Hydrochloride (Exhibits an additive CNS depression). Products include:
Librax Capsules 2176
Librium Capsules 2178
Librium Injectable 2179

Chlorpheniramine Maleate (Exhibits an additive CNS depression). Products include:
Alka-Seltzer Plus Cold Medicine .... ■ 705
Alka-Seltzer Plus Cold Medicine Liqui-Gels .... ■ 706
Alka-Seltzer Plus Cold & Cough Medicine .... ■ 708
Alka-Seltzer Plus Cold & Cough Medicine Liqui-Gels .... ■ 705
Allerest Children's Chewable Tablets .... ■ 627
Allerest Headache Strength Tablets .... ■ 627
Allerest Maximum Strength Tablets .... ■ 627
Allerest Sinus Pain Formula .... ■ 627
Allerest 12 Hour Caplets .... ■ 627
Ana-Kit Anaphylaxis Emergency Treatment Kit 617
Atrohist Pediatric Capsules 453
Atrohist Plus Tablets 454
BC Cold Powder Multi-Symptom Formula (Cold-Sinus-Allergy) .... ■ 609
Cerose DM .... ■ 878
Cheracol Plus Head Cold/Cough Formula .... ■ 769
Children's Vicks DayQuil Allergy Relief .... ■ 757
Children's Vicks NyQuil Cold/Cough Relief .... ■ 758
Chlor-Trimeton Allergy Decongestant Tablets .... ■ 799
Chlor-Trimeton Allergy Tablets .... ■ 798
Comhist 2038
Comtrex Multi-Symptom Cold Reliever Tablets/Caplets/Liqui-Gels/Liquid .... ■ 615
Allergy-Sinus Comtrex Multi-Symptom Allergy-Sinus Formula Tablets .... ■ 617
Contac Continuous Action Nasal Decongestant/Antihistamine 12 Hour Capsules .... ■ 813
Contac Maximum Strength Continuous Action Decongestant/Antihistamine 12 Hour Caplets .... ■ 813
Contac Severe Cold and Flu Formula Caplets .... ■ 814
Coricidin 'D' Decongestant Tablets .... ■ 800
Coricidin Tablets .... ■ 800
D.A. Chewable Tablets 951
Deconamine 1320
Dura-Tap/PD Capsules 2867
Dura-Vent/DA Tablets 953
Extendryl 1005
Fedahist Gyrocaps 2401
Fedahist Timecaps 2401
Hycomine Compound Tablets 932
Isoclor Timesule Capsules .... ■ 637
Kronofed-A 977
Nolamine Timed-Release Tablets 785
Novahistine DH 2462
Novahistine Elixir .... ■ 823
Ornade Spansule Capsules 2502
PediaCare Cold Allergy Chewable Tablets .... ■ 677
PediaCare Cough-Cold Chewable Tablets 1553
PediaCare Cough-Cold Liquid 1553
PediaCare NightRest Cough-Cold Liquid 1553
Pediatric Vicks 44m Cough & Cold Relief .... ■ 764
Pyrroxate Caplets .... ■ 772
Ryna .... ■ 841
Sinarest Tablets .... ■ 648
Sinarest Extra Strength Tablets .... ■ 648
Sine-Off Sinus Medicine .... ■ 825
Singlet Tablets .... ■ 825
Sinulin Tablets 787
Sinutab Sinus Allergy Medication, Maximum Strength Tablets and Caplets .... ■ 860
Sudafed Plus Liquid .... ■ 862
Sudafed Plus Tablets .... ■ 863
Teldrin 12 Hour Antihistamine/Nasal Decongestant Allergy Relief Capsules .... ■ 826
TheraFlu .... ■ 787
TheraFlu Maximum Strength Nighttime Flu, Cold & Cough Medicine .... ■ 788
Triaminic Allergy Tablets .... ■ 789
Triaminic Cold Tablets .... ■ 790
Triaminic Nite Light .... ■ 791
Triaminic Syrup .... ■ 792
Triaminic-12 Tablets .... ■ 792
Triaminicin Tablets .... ■ 793
Triaminicol Multi-Symptom Cold Tablets .... ■ 793
Triaminicol Multi-Symptom Relief .... ■ 794
Tussend 1783
Children's TYLENOL Cold Multi-Symptom Liquid Formula and Chewable Tablets 1561
Children's TYLENOL Cold Plus Cough Multi Symptom Tablets and Liquid .... ■ 681
TYLENOL Maximum Strength Allergy Sinus Medication Gelcaps and Caplets 1563
TYLENOL Cold Multi-Symptom Formula Medication Tablets and Caplets 1561
TYLENOL Cold Multi-Symptom Hot Medication Liquid Packets 1557
Vicks 44 LiquiCaps Cough, Cold & Flu Relief .... ■ 755
Vicks 44M Cough, Cold & Flu Relief .... ■ 756

Chlorpheniramine Polistirex (Exhibits an additive CNS depression). Products include:
Tussionex Pennkinetic Extended-Release Suspension 998

Chlorpheniramine Tannate (Exhibits an additive CNS depression). Products include:
Atrohist Pediatric Suspension 454
Ricobid Tablets and Pediatric Suspension 2038
Rynatan 2673
Rynatuss 2673

Chlorpromazine (Exhibits an additive CNS depression). Products include:
Thorazine Suppositories 2523

Chlorpromazine Hydrochloride (Exhibits an additive CNS depression). Products include:
Thorazine 2523

Chlorprothixene (Exhibits an additive CNS depression).
No products indexed under this heading.

Chlorprothixene Hydrochloride (Exhibits an additive CNS depression).
No products indexed under this heading.

Clemastine Fumarate (Exhibits an additive CNS depression). Products include:
Tavist Syrup 2297
Tavist Tablets 2298
Tavist-1 12 Hour Relief Tablets .... ■ 787
Tavist-D 12 Hour Relief Tablets .... ■ 787

Clidinium Bromide (Potential for paralytic ileus). Products include:
Librax Capsules 2176
Quarzan Capsules 2181

Clomipramine Hydrochloride (Increased effect of either antidepressant or hydrocodone). Products include:
Anafranil Capsules 803

Clorazepate Dipotassium (Exhibits an additive CNS depression). Products include:
Tranxene 451

Clozapine (Exhibits an additive CNS depression). Products include:
Clozaril Tablets 2252

Codeine Phosphate (Exhibits an additive CNS depression). Products include:
Actifed with Codeine Cough Syrup.. 1067
Brontex 1981
Deconsal C Expectorant Syrup 456
Deconsal Pediatric Syrup 457
Dimetane-DC Cough Syrup 2059
Empirin with Codeine Tablets 1093
Fioricet with Codeine Capsules 2260
Fiorinal with Codeine Capsules 2262
Isoclor Expectorant 990
Novahistine DH 2462

(■ Described in PDR For Nonprescription Drugs) (◉ Described in PDR For Ophthalmology)

Novahistine Expectorant 2463
Nucofed 2051
Phenergan with Codeine 2777
Phenergan VC with Codeine 2781
Robitussin A-C Syrup 2073
Robitussin-DAC Syrup 2074
Ryna 841
Soma Compound w/Codeine Tablets 2676
Tussi-Organidin NR Liquid and S NR Liquid 2677
Tylenol with Codeine 1583

Cyproheptadine Hydrochloride (Exhibits an additive CNS depression). Products include:
Periactin 1724

Desflurane (Exhibits an additive CNS depression). Products include:
Suprane 1813

Desipramine Hydrochloride (Increased effect of either antidepressant or hydrocodone). Products include:
Norpramin Tablets 1526

Dexchlorpheniramine Maleate (Exhibits an additive CNS depression).
No products indexed under this heading.

Dezocine (Exhibits an additive CNS depression). Products include:
Dalgan Injection 538

Diazepam (Exhibits an additive CNS depression). Products include:
Dizac 1809
Valium Injectable 2182
Valium Tablets 2183
Valrelease Capsules 2169

Dicyclomine Hydrochloride (Potential for paralytic ileus). Products include:
Bentyl 1501

Diphenhydramine Citrate (Exhibits an additive CNS depression). Products include:
Excedrin P.M. Analgesic/Sleeping Aid Tablets, Caplets, Liquigels 733

Diphenhydramine Hydrochloride (Exhibits an additive CNS depression). Products include:
Actifed Allergy Daytime/Nighttime Caplets 844
Actifed Sinus Daytime/Nighttime Tablets and Caplets 846
Arthritis Foundation NightTime Caplets 674
Extra Strength Bayer PM Aspirin 713
Bayer Select Night Time Pain Relief Formula 716
Benadryl Allergy Decongestant Liquid Medication 848
Benadryl Allergy Decongestant Tablets 848
Benadryl Allergy Liquid Medication 849
Benadryl Allergy 848
Benadryl Allergy Sinus Headache Formula Caplets 849
Benadryl Capsules 1898
Benadryl Dye-Free Allergy Liquigel Softgels 850
Benadryl Dye-Free Allergy Liquid Medication 850
Benadryl Itch Relief Cream, Children's Formula and Maximum Strength 2% 851
Benadryl Itch Relief Spray, Children's Formula and Maximum Strength 2% 851
Benadryl Itch Relief Stick Maximum Strength 2% 850
Benadryl Itch Stopping Gel, Children's Formula and Maximum Strength 2% 851
Benadryl Kapseals 1898
Benadryl Injection 1898
Contac Day & Night Cold/Flu Night Caplets 812
Contac Night Allergy/Sinus Caplets 812
Extra Strength Doan's P.M. 633
Legatrin PM 651
Miles Nervine Nighttime Sleep-Aid 723
Nytol QuickCaps Caplets 610
Sleepinal Night-time Sleep Aid Capsules and Softgels 834
TYLENOL Maximum Strength Allergy Sinus NightTime Medication Caplets 1555
TYLENOL Flu NightTime, Maximum Strength, Gelcaps 1566
TYLENOL Maximum Strength Flu NightTime Hot Medication Packets 1562
TYLENOL PM, Extra Strength Pain Reliever/Sleep Aid Caplets, Geltabs, Gelcaps 1560
TYLENOL Severe Allergy Medication Caplets 1564
Maximum Strength Unisom Sleepgels 1934
Unisom With Pain Relief-Nighttime Sleep Aid and Pain Reliever 1934

Diphenylpyraline Hydrochloride (Exhibits an additive CNS depression).
No products indexed under this heading.

Doxepin Hydrochloride (Increased effect of either antidepressant or hydrocodone). Products include:
Sinequan 2205
Zonalon Cream 1055

Droperidol (Exhibits an additive CNS depression). Products include:
Inapsine Injection 1296

Enflurane (Exhibits an additive CNS depression).
No products indexed under this heading.

Estazolam (Exhibits an additive CNS depression). Products include:
ProSom Tablets 449

Ethchlorvynol (Exhibits an additive CNS depression). Products include:
Placidyl Capsules 448

Ethinamate (Exhibits an additive CNS depression).
No products indexed under this heading.

Fentanyl (Exhibits an additive CNS depression). Products include:
Duragesic Transdermal System 1288

Fentanyl Citrate (Exhibits an additive CNS depression). Products include:
Sublimaze Injection 1307

Fluphenazine Decanoate (Exhibits an additive CNS depression). Products include:
Prolixin Decanoate 509

Fluphenazine Enanthate (Exhibits an additive CNS depression). Products include:
Prolixin Enanthate 509

Fluphenazine Hydrochloride (Exhibits an additive CNS depression). Products include:
Prolixin 509

Flurazepam Hydrochloride (Exhibits an additive CNS depression). Products include:
Dalmane Capsules 2173

Furazolidone (Increased effect of either MAO inhibitor or hydrocodone). Products include:
Furoxone 2046

Glutethimide (Exhibits an additive CNS depression).
No products indexed under this heading.

Glycopyrrolate (Potential for paralytic ileus). Products include:
Robinul Forte Tablets 2072
Robinul Injectable 2072
Robinul Tablets 2072

Haloperidol (Exhibits an additive CNS depression). Products include:
Haldol Injection, Tablets and Concentrate 1575

Haloperidol Decanoate (Exhibits an additive CNS depression). Products include:
Haldol Decanoate 1577

Hydrocodone Polistirex (Exhibits an additive CNS depression). Products include:
Tussionex Pennkinetic Extended-Release Suspension 998

Hydroxyzine Hydrochloride (Exhibits an additive CNS depression). Products include:
Atarax Tablets & Syrup 2185
Marax Tablets & DF Syrup 2200
Vistaril Intramuscular Solution 2216

Hyoscyamine (Potential for paralytic ileus). Products include:
Cystospaz Tablets 1963
Urised Tablets 1964

Hyoscyamine Sulfate (Potential for paralytic ileus). Products include:
Arco-Lase Plus Tablets 512
Atrohist Plus Tablets 454
Cystospaz-M Capsules 1963
Donnatal 2060
Donnatal Extentabs 2061
Donnatal Tablets 2060
Kutrase Capsules 2402
Levsin/Levsinex/Levbid 2405

Imipramine Hydrochloride (Increased effect of either antidepressant or hydrocodone). Products include:
Tofranil Ampuls 854
Tofranil Tablets 856

Imipramine Pamoate (Increased effect of either antidepressant or hydrocodone). Products include:
Tofranil-PM Capsules 857

Ipratropium Bromide (Potential for paralytic ileus). Products include:
Atrovent Inhalation Aerosol 671
Atrovent Inhalation Solution 673

Isocarboxazid (Increased effect of either MAO inhibitor or hydrocodone).
No products indexed under this heading.

Isoflurane (Exhibits an additive CNS depression).
No products indexed under this heading.

Ketamine Hydrochloride (Exhibits an additive CNS depression).
No products indexed under this heading.

Levomethadyl Acetate Hydrochloride (Exhibits an additive CNS depression). Products include:
Orlamm 2239

Levorphanol Tartrate (Exhibits an additive CNS depression). Products include:
Levo-Dromoran 2129

Lithium Carbonate (Exhibits an additive CNS depression). Products include:
Eskalith 2485
Lithium Carbonate Capsules & Tablets 2230
Lithonate/Lithotabs/Lithobid 2543

Lithium Citrate (Exhibits an additive CNS depression).
No products indexed under this heading.

Loratadine (Exhibits an additive CNS depression). Products include:
Claritin 2349
Claritin-D 2350

Lorazepam (Exhibits an additive CNS depression). Products include:
Ativan Injection 2698
Ativan Tablets 2700

Loxapine Hydrochloride (Exhibits an additive CNS depression). Products include:
Loxitane 1378

Loxapine Succinate (Exhibits an additive CNS depression). Products include:
Loxitane Capsules 1378

Maprotiline Hydrochloride (Increased effect of either antidepressant or hydrocodone). Products include:
Ludiomil Tablets 843

Mepenzolate Bromide (Potential for paralytic ileus).
No products indexed under this heading.

Meperidine Hydrochloride (Exhibits an additive CNS depression). Products include:
Demerol 2308
Mepergan Injection 2753

Mephobarbital (Exhibits an additive CNS depression). Products include:
Mebaral Tablets 2322

Meprobamate (Exhibits an additive CNS depression). Products include:
Miltown Tablets 2672
PMB 200 and PMB 400 2783

Mesoridazine (Exhibits an additive CNS depression).

Mesoridazine Besylate (Exhibits an additive CNS depression). Products include:
Serentil 684

Methadone Hydrochloride (Exhibits an additive CNS depression). Products include:
Methadone Hydrochloride Oral Concentrate 2233
Methadone Hydrochloride Oral Solution & Tablets 2235

Methdilazine Hydrochloride (Exhibits an additive CNS depression).
No products indexed under this heading.

Methohexital Sodium (Exhibits an additive CNS depression). Products include:
Brevital Sodium Vials 1429

Methotrimeprazine (Exhibits an additive CNS depression). Products include:
Levoprome 1274

Methoxyflurane (Exhibits an additive CNS depression).
No products indexed under this heading.

Midazolam Hydrochloride (Exhibits an additive CNS depression). Products include:
Versed Injection 2170

Molindone Hydrochloride (Exhibits an additive CNS depression). Products include:
Moban Tablets and Concentrate 1048

Morphine Sulfate (Exhibits an additive CNS depression). Products include:
Astramorph/PF Injection, USP (Preservative-Free) 535
Duramorph 962
Infumorph 200 and Infumorph 500 Sterile Solutions 965
MS Contin Tablets 1994
MSIR 1997
Oramorph SR (Morphine Sulfate Sustained Release Tablets) 2236
RMS Suppositories 2657
Roxanol 2243

Nortriptyline Hydrochloride (Increased effect of either antidepressant or hydrocodone). Products include:
Pamelor 2280

Opium Alkaloids (Exhibits an additive CNS depression).
No products indexed under this heading.

Oxazepam (Exhibits an additive CNS depression). Products include:
Serax Capsules 2810
Serax Tablets 2810

IMPORTANT NOTE: Always consult each drug listing in the patient's regimen for possible interactions.

Anexsia Elixir

Interactions Index

Oxybutynin Chloride (Potential for paralytic ileus). Products include:

Ditropan 1516

Oxycodone Hydrochloride (Exhibits an additive CNS depression). Products include:

Percocet Tablets 938
Percodan Tablets.................................... 939
Percodan-Demi Tablets.......................... 940
Roxicodone Tablets, Oral Solution & Intensol (Oxycodone) 2244
Tylox Capsules 1584

Pentobarbital Sodium (Exhibits an additive CNS depression). Products include:

Nembutal Sodium Capsules 436
Nembutal Sodium Solution 438
Nembutal Sodium Suppositories...... 440

Perphenazine (Exhibits an additive CNS depression). Products include:

Etrafon 2355
Triavil Tablets 1757
Trilafon... 2389

Phenelzine Sulfate (Increased effect of either MAO inhibitor or hydrocodone). Products include:

Nardil 1920

Phenobarbital (Exhibits an additive CNS depression). Products include:

Arco-Lase Plus Tablets 512
Bellergal-S Tablets 2250
Donnatal 2060
Donnatal Extentabs............................... 2061
Donnatal Tablets 2060
Phenobarbital Elixir and Tablets 1469
Quadrinal Tablets 1350

Pimozide (Exhibits an additive CNS depression). Products include:

Orap Tablets 1050

Prazepam (Exhibits an additive CNS depression).

No products indexed under this heading.

Prochlorperazine (Exhibits an additive CNS depression). Products include:

Compazine 2470

Procyclidine Hydrochloride (Potential for paralytic ileus). Products include:

Kemadrin Tablets 1112

Promethazine Hydrochloride (Exhibits an additive CNS depression). Products include:

Mepergan Injection 2753
Phenergan with Codeine 2777
Phenergan with Dextromethorphan 2778
Phenergan Injection 2773
Phenergan Suppositories 2775
Phenergan Syrup 2774
Phenergan Tablets 2775
Phenergan VC 2779
Phenergan VC with Codeine 2781

Propantheline Bromide (Potential for paralytic ileus). Products include:

Pro-Banthine Tablets 2052

Propofol (Exhibits an additive CNS depression). Products include:

Diprivan Injection................................... 2833

Propoxyphene Hydrochloride (Exhibits an additive CNS depression). Products include:

Darvon 1435
Wygesic Tablets 2827

Propoxyphene Napsylate (Exhibits an additive CNS depression). Products include:

Darvon-N/Darvocet-N 1433

Protriptyline Hydrochloride (Increased effect of either antidepressant or hydrocodone). Products include:

Vivactil Tablets 1774

Pyrilamine Maleate (Exhibits an additive CNS depression). Products include:

4-Way Fast Acting Nasal Spray (regular & mentholated) .... 𝍍 621
Maximum Strength Multi-Symptom Formula Midol .... 𝍍 722
PMS Multi-Symptom Formula Midol .... 𝍍 723

Pyrilamine Tannate (Exhibits an additive CNS depression). Products include:

Atrohist Pediatric Suspension 454
Rynatan 2673

Quazepam (Exhibits an additive CNS depression). Products include:

Doral Tablets 2664

Risperidone (Exhibits an additive CNS depression). Products include:

Risperdal 1301

Scopolamine (Potential for paralytic ileus). Products include:

Transderm Scōp Transdermal Therapeutic System 869

Scopolamine Hydrobromide (Potential for paralytic ileus). Products include:

Atrohist Plus Tablets 454
Donnatal 2060
Donnatal Extentabs................................ 2061
Donnatal Tablets 2060

Secobarbital Sodium (Exhibits an additive CNS depression). Products include:

Seconal Sodium Pulvules 1474

Selegiline Hydrochloride (Increased effect of either MAO inhibitor or hydrocodone). Products include:

Eldepryl Tablets 2550

Sufentanil Citrate (Exhibits an additive CNS depression). Products include:

Sufenta Injection 1309

Temazepam (Exhibits an additive CNS depression). Products include:

Restoril Capsules 2284

Terfenadine (Exhibits an additive CNS depression). Products include:

Seldane Tablets 1536
Seldane-D Extended-Release Tablets 1538

Thiamylal Sodium (Exhibits an additive CNS depression).

No products indexed under this heading.

Thioridazine Hydrochloride (Exhibits an additive CNS depression). Products include:

Mellaril 2269

Thiothixene (Exhibits an additive CNS depression). Products include:

Navane Capsules and Concentrate 2201
Navane Intramuscular.......................... 2202

Tranylcypromine Sulfate (Increased effect of either MAO inhibitor or hydrocodone). Products include:

Parnate Tablets 2503

Triazolam (Exhibits an additive CNS depression). Products include:

Halcion Tablets....................................... 2611

Tridihexethyl Chloride (Potential for paralytic ileus).

No products indexed under this heading.

Trifluoperazine Hydrochloride (Exhibits an additive CNS depression). Products include:

Stelazine 2514

Trihexyphenidyl Hydrochloride (Potential for paralytic ileus). Products include:

Artane.. 1368

Trimeprazine Tartrate (Exhibits an additive CNS depression). Products include:

Temaril Tablets, Syrup and Spansule Extended-Release Capsules.. 483

Trimipramine Maleate (Increased effect of either antidepressant or hydrocodone). Products include:

Surmontil Capsules................................ 2811

Tripelennamine Hydrochloride (Exhibits an additive CNS depression). Products include:

PBZ Tablets 845
PBZ-SR Tablets....................................... 844

Triprolidine Hydrochloride (Exhibits an additive CNS depression). Products include:

Actifed Plus Caplets .... 𝍍 845
Actifed Plus Tablets .... 𝍍 845
Actifed with Codeine Cough Syrup.. 1067
Actifed Syrup... 𝍍 846
Actifed Tablets .... 𝍍 844

Zolpidem Tartrate (Exhibits an additive CNS depression). Products include:

Ambien Tablets.. 2416

Food Interactions

Alcohol (Exhibits an additive CNS depression).

ANEXSIA 5/500 TABLETS

(Acetaminophen, Hydrocodone Bitartrate) 1782

May interact with narcotic analgesics, antihistamines, tranquilizers, antipsychotic agents, central nervous system depressants, monoamine oxidase inhibitors, tricyclic antidepressants, and certain other agents. Compounds in these categories include:

Acrivastine (Exhibits an additive CNS depression). Products include:

Semprex-D Capsules 463
Semprex-D Capsules 1167

Alfentanil Hydrochloride (Exhibits an additive CNS depression). Products include:

Alfenta Injection 1286

Alprazolam (Exhibits an additive CNS depression). Products include:

Xanax Tablets 2649

Amitriptyline Hydrochloride (Increased effect of either antidepressant or hydrocodone). Products include:

Elavil 2838
Endep Tablets 2174
Etrafon 2355
Limbitrol 2180
Triavil Tablets 1757

Amoxapine (Increased effect of either antidepressant or hydrocodone). Products include:

Asendin Tablets 1369

Aprobarbital (Exhibits an additive CNS depression).

No products indexed under this heading.

Astemizole (Exhibits an additive CNS depression). Products include:

Hismanal Tablets 1293

Azatadine Maleate (Exhibits an additive CNS depression). Products include:

Trinalin Repetabs Tablets 1330

Bromodiphenhydramine Hydrochloride (Exhibits an additive CNS depression).

No products indexed under this heading.

Brompheniramine Maleate (Exhibits an additive CNS depression). Products include:

Alka Seltzer Plus Sinus Medicine ..𝍍 707
Bromfed Capsules (Extended-Release) 1785
Bromfed Syrup .... 𝍍 733
Bromfed Tablets 1785
Bromfed-DM Cough Syrup.................. 1786
Bromfed-PD Capsules (Extended-Release).. 1785
Dimetane-DC Cough Syrup 2059

Dimetane-DX Cough Syrup 2059
Dimetapp Elixir .... 𝍍 773
Dimetapp Extentabs............................... 𝍍 774
Dimetapp Tablets/Liqui-Gels .... 𝍍 775
Dimetapp Cold & Allergy Chewable Tablets .... 𝍍 773
Dimetapp DM Elixir............................... 𝍍 774
Vicks DayQuil Allergy Relief 12-Hour Extended Release Tablets..𝍍 760
Vicks DayQuil Allergy Relief 4-Hour Tablets .... 𝍍 760

Buprenorphine (Exhibits an additive CNS depression). Products include:

Buprenex Injectable 2006

Buspirone Hydrochloride (Exhibits an additive CNS depression). Products include:

BuSpar 737

Butabarbital (Exhibits an additive CNS depression).

No products indexed under this heading.

Butalbital (Exhibits an additive CNS depression). Products include:

Esgic-plus Tablets 1013
Fioricet Tablets 2258
Fioricet with Codeine Capsules 2260
Fiorinal Capsules 2261
Fiorinal with Codeine Capsules 2262
Fiorinal Tablets 2261
Phrenilin 785
Sedapap Tablets 50 mg/650 mg .. 1543

Chlordiazepoxide (Exhibits an additive CNS depression). Products include:

Libritabs Tablets 2177
Limbitrol 2180

Chlordiazepoxide Hydrochloride (Exhibits an additive CNS depression). Products include:

Librax Capsules 2176
Librium Capsules.................................... 2178
Librium Injectable 2179

Chlorpheniramine Maleate (Exhibits an additive CNS depression). Products include:

Alka-Seltzer Plus Cold Medicine .... 𝍍 705
Alka-Seltzer Plus Cold Medicine Liqui-Gels .... 𝍍 706
Alka-Seltzer Plus Cold & Cough Medicine .... 𝍍 708
Alka-Seltzer Plus Cold & Cough Medicine Liqui-Gels.......................... 𝍍 705
Allerest Children's Chewable Tablets .... 𝍍 627
Allerest Headache Strength Tablets .... 𝍍 627
Allerest Maximum Strength Tablets .... 𝍍 627
Allerest Sinus Pain Formula .... 𝍍 627
Allerest 12 Hour Caplets .... 𝍍 627
Ana-Kit Anaphylaxis Emergency Treatment Kit 617
Atrohist Pediatric Capsules................. 453
Atrohist Plus Tablets 454
BC Cold Powder Multi-Symptom Formula (Cold-Sinus-Allergy) ...... 𝍍 609
Cerose DM .... 𝍍 878
Cheracol Plus Head Cold/Cough Formula .... 𝍍 769
Children's Vicks DayQuil Allergy Relief .... 𝍍 757
Children's Vicks NyQuil Cold/Cough Relief.. 𝍍 758
Chlor-Trimeton Allergy Decongestant Tablets .... 𝍍 799
Chlor-Trimeton Allergy Tablets ...... 𝍍 798
Comhist 2038
Comtrex Multi-Symptom Cold Reliever Tablets/Caplets/Liqui-Gels/Liquid... 𝍍 615
Allergy-Sinus Comtrex Multi-Symptom Allergy-Sinus Formula Tablets .... 𝍍 617
Contac Continuous Action Nasal Decongestant/Antihistamine 12 Hour Capsules.. 𝍍 813
Contac Maximum Strength Continuous Action Decongestant/Antihistamine 12 Hour Caplets..𝍍 813
Contac Severe Cold and Flu Formula Caplets .... 𝍍 814
Coricidin 'D' Decongestant Tablets .... 𝍍 800
Coricidin Tablets .... 𝍍 800
D.A. Chewable Tablets........................... 951

(𝍍 Described in PDR For Nonprescription Drugs) (◆ Described in PDR For Ophthalmology)

Interactions Index

Anexsia Tablets

Deconamine 1320
Dura-Tap/PD Capsules 2867
Dura-Vent/DA Tablets 953
Extendryl 1005
Fedahist Gyrocaps................................... 2401
Fedahist Timecaps 2401
Hycomine Compound Tablets 932
Isoclor Timesule Capsules .... ⊞ 637
Kronofed-A 977
Nolamine Timed-Release Tablets 785
Novahistine DH....................................... 2462
Novahistine Elixir .... ⊞ 823
Ornade Spansule Capsules 2502
PediaCare Cold Allergy Chewable Tablets .... ⊞ 677
PediaCare Cough-Cold Chewable Tablets 1553
PediaCare Cough-Cold Liquid............ 1553
PediaCare NightRest Cough-Cold Liquid 1553
Pediatric Vicks 44m Cough & Cold Relief .... ⊞ 764
Pyrroxate Caplets .... ⊞ 772
Ryna .... ⊞ 841
Sinarest Tablets .... ⊞ 648
Sinarest Extra Strength Tablets...... ⊞ 648
Sine-Off Sinus Medicine .... ⊞ 825
Singlet Tablets .... ⊞ 825
Sinulin Tablets 787
Sinutab Sinus Allergy Medication, Maximum Strength Tablets and Caplets .... ⊞ 860
Sudafed Plus Liquid .... ⊞ 862
Sudafed Plus Tablets .... ⊞ 863
Teldrin 12 Hour Antihistamine/ Nasal Decongestant Allergy Relief Capsules .... ⊞ 826
TheraFlu.. ⊞ 787
TheraFlu Maximum Strength Nighttime Flu, Cold & Cough Medicine .... ⊞ 788
Triaminic Allergy Tablets .... ⊞ 789
Triaminic Cold Tablets .... ⊞ 790
Triaminic Nite Light .... ⊞ 791
Triaminic Syrup .... ⊞ 792
Triaminic-12 Tablets .... ⊞ 792
Triaminicin Tablets .... ⊞ 793
Triaminicol Multi-Symptom Cold Tablets .... ⊞ 793
Triaminicol Multi-Symptom Relief ⊞ 794
Tussend 1783
Children's TYLENOL Cold Multi-Symptom Liquid Formula and Chewable Tablets.................................. 1561
Children's TYLENOL Cold Plus Cough Multi Symptom Tablets and Liquid .... ⊞ 681
TYLENOL Maximum Strength Allergy Sinus Medication Gelcaps and Caplets 1563
TYLENOL Cold Multi-Symptom Formula Medication Tablets and Caplets.. 1561
TYLENOL Cold Multi-Symptom Hot Medication Liquid Packets.............. 1557
Vicks 44 LiquiCaps Cough, Cold & Flu Relief .... ⊞ 755
Vicks 44M Cough, Cold & Flu Relief .... ⊞ 756

Chlorpheniramine Polistirex (Exhibits an additive CNS depression). Products include:

Tussionex Pennkinetic Extended-Release Suspension 998

Chlorpheniramine Tannate (Exhibits an additive CNS depression). Products include:

Atrohist Pediatric Suspension 454
Ricobid Tablets and Pediatric Suspension.. 2038
Rynatan 2673
Rynatuss 2673

Chlorpromazine (Exhibits an additive CNS depression). Products include:

Thorazine Suppositories 2523

Chlorpromazine Hydrochloride (Exhibits an additive CNS depression). Products include:

Thorazine 2523

Chlorprothixene (Exhibits an additive CNS depression).

No products indexed under this heading.

Chlorprothixene Hydrochloride (Exhibits an additive CNS depression).

No products indexed under this heading.

Clemastine Fumarate (Exhibits an additive CNS depression). Products include:

Tavist Syrup... 2297
Tavist Tablets 2298
Tavist-1 12 Hour Relief Tablets .... ⊞ 787
Tavist-D 12 Hour Relief Tablets .... ⊞ 787

Clomipramine Hydrochloride (Increased effect of either antidepressant or hydrocodone). Products include:

Anafranil Capsules 803

Clorazepate Dipotassium (Exhibits an additive CNS depression). Products include:

Tranxene 451

Clozapine (Exhibits an additive CNS depression). Products include:

Clozaril Tablets....................................... 2252

Codeine Phosphate (Exhibits an additive CNS depression). Products include:

Actifed with Codeine Cough Syrup.. 1067
Brontex 1981
Deconsal C Expectorant Syrup 456
Deconsal Pediatric Syrup 457
Dimetane-DC Cough Syrup 2059
Empirin with Codeine Tablets............ 1093
Fioricet with Codeine Capsules 2260
Fiorinal with Codeine Capsules 2262
Isoclor Expectorant................................ 990
Novahistine DH....................................... 2462
Novahistine Expectorant...................... 2463
Nucofed 2051
Phenergan with Codeine...................... 2777
Phenergan VC with Codeine 2781
Robitussin A-C Syrup............................. 2073
Robitussin-DAC Syrup 2074
Ryna .... ⊞ 841
Soma Compound w/Codeine Tablets 2676
Tussi-Organidin NR Liquid and S NR Liquid 2677
Tylenol with Codeine 1583

Cyproheptadine Hydrochloride (Exhibits an additive CNS depression). Products include:

Periactin 1724

Desflurane (Exhibits an additive CNS depression). Products include:

Suprane 1813

Desipramine Hydrochloride (Increased effect of either antidepressant or hydrocodone). Products include:

Norpramin Tablets 1526

Dexchlorpheniramine Maleate (Exhibits an additive CNS depression).

No products indexed under this heading.

Dezocine (Exhibits an additive CNS depression). Products include:

Dalgan Injection 538

Diazepam (Exhibits an additive CNS depression). Products include:

Dizac... 1809
Valium Injectable 2182
Valium Tablets 2183
Valrelease Capsules 2169

Diphenhydramine Citrate (Exhibits an additive CNS depression). Products include:

Excedrin P.M. Analgesic/Sleeping Aid Tablets, Caplets, Liquigels...... 733

Diphenhydramine Hydrochloride (Exhibits an additive CNS depression). Products include:

Actifed Allergy Daytime/Nighttime Caplets.. ⊞ 844
Actifed Sinus Daytime/Nighttime Tablets and Caplets .... ⊞ 846
Arthritis Foundation NightTime Caplets.. ⊞ 674
Extra Strength Bayer PM Aspirin .. ⊞ 713
Bayer Select Night Time Pain Relief Formula .... ⊞ 716

Benadryl Allergy Decongestant Liquid Medication .... ⊞ 848
Benadryl Allergy Decongestant Tablets .... ⊞ 848
Benadryl Allergy Liquid Medication... ⊞ 849
Benadryl Allergy .... ⊞ 848
Benadryl Allergy Sinus Headache Formula Caplets................................ ⊞ 849
Benadryl Capsules.................................. 1898
Benadryl Dye-Free Allergy Liquigel Softgels .... ⊞ 850
Benadryl Dye-Free Allergy Liquid Medication .... ⊞ 850
Benadryl Itch Relief Cream, Children's Formula and Maximum Strength 2% .... ⊞ 851
Benadryl Itch Relief Spray, Children's Formula and Maximum Strength 2% .... ⊞ 851
Benadryl Itch Relief Stick Maximum Strength 2% .... ⊞ 850
Benadryl Itch Stopping Gel, Children's Formula and Maximum Strength 2% .... ⊞ 851
Benadryl Kapseals 1898
Benadryl Injection 1898
Contac Day & Night Cold/Flu Night Caplets.. ⊞ 812
Contac Night Allergy/Sinus Caplets .... ⊞ 812
Extra Strength Doan's P.M................... ⊞ 633
Legatrin PM .... ⊞ 651
Miles Nervine Nighttime Sleep-Aid ⊞ 723
Nytol QuickCaps Caplets .... ⊞ 610
Sleepinal Night-time Sleep Aid Capsules and Softgels .... ⊞ 834
TYLENOL Maximum Strength Allergy Sinus NightTime Medication Caplets 1555
TYLENOL Flu NightTime, Maximum Strength, Gelcaps 1566
TYLENOL Maximum Strength Flu NightTime Hot Medication Packets 1562
TYLENOL PM, Extra Strength Pain Reliever/Sleep Aid Caplets, Geltabs, Gelcaps 1560
TYLENOL Severe Allergy Medication Caplets 1564
Maximum Strength Unisom Sleepgels 1934
Unisom With Pain Relief-Nighttime Sleep Aid and Pain Reliever.............. 1934

Diphenylpyraline Hydrochloride (Exhibits an additive CNS depression).

No products indexed under this heading.

Doxepin Hydrochloride (Increased effect of either antidepressant or hydrocodone). Products include:

Sinequan 2205
Zonalon Cream 1055

Droperidol (Exhibits an additive CNS depression). Products include:

Inapsine Injection................................... 1296

Enflurane (Exhibits an additive CNS depression).

No products indexed under this heading.

Estazolam (Exhibits an additive CNS depression). Products include:

ProSom Tablets 449

Ethchlorvynol (Exhibits an additive CNS depression). Products include:

Placidyl Capsules.................................... 448

Ethinamate (Exhibits an additive CNS depression).

No products indexed under this heading.

Fentanyl (Exhibits an additive CNS depression). Products include:

Duragesic Transdermal System........ 1288

Fentanyl Citrate (Exhibits an additive CNS depression). Products include:

Sublimaze Injection................................ 1307

Fluphenazine Decanoate (Exhibits an additive CNS depression). Products include:

Prolixin Decanoate 509

Fluphenazine Enanthate (Exhibits an additive CNS depression). Products include:

Prolixin Enanthate 509

Fluphenazine Hydrochloride (Exhibits an additive CNS depression). Products include:

Prolixin 509

Flurazepam Hydrochloride (Exhibits an additive CNS depression). Products include:

Dalmane Capsules................................... 2173

Furazolidone (Increased effect of either MAO inhibitor or hydrocodone). Products include:

Furoxone 2046

Glutethimide (Exhibits an additive CNS depression).

No products indexed under this heading.

Haloperidol (Exhibits an additive CNS depression). Products include:

Haldol Injection, Tablets and Concentrate 1575

Haloperidol Decanoate (Exhibits an additive CNS depression). Products include:

Haldol Decanoate.................................... 1577

Hydrocodone Polistirex (Exhibits an additive CNS depression). Products include:

Tussionex Pennkinetic Extended-Release Suspension 998

Hydroxyzine Hydrochloride (Exhibits an additive CNS depression). Products include:

Atarax Tablets & Syrup......................... 2185
Marax Tablets & DF Syrup................... 2200
Vistaril Intramuscular Solution......... 2216

Imipramine Hydrochloride (Increased effect of either antidepressant or hydrocodone). Products include:

Tofranil Ampuls 854
Tofranil Tablets 856

Imipramine Pamoate (Increased effect of either antidepressant or hydrocodone). Products include:

Tofranil-PM Capsules............................ 857

Isocarboxazid (Increased effect of either MAO inhibitor or hydrocodone).

No products indexed under this heading.

Isoflurane (Exhibits an additive CNS depression).

No products indexed under this heading.

Ketamine Hydrochloride (Exhibits an additive CNS depression).

No products indexed under this heading.

Levomethadyl Acetate Hydrochloride (Exhibits an additive CNS depression). Products include:

Orlaam 2239

Levorphanol Tartrate (Exhibits an additive CNS depression). Products include:

Levo-Dromoran.. 2129

Lithium Carbonate (Exhibits an additive CNS depression). Products include:

Eskalith 2485
Lithium Carbonate Capsules & Tablets 2230
Lithonate/Lithotabs/Lithobid 2543

Lithium Citrate (Exhibits an additive CNS depression).

No products indexed under this heading.

Loratadine (Exhibits an additive CNS depression). Products include:

Claritin 2349
Claritin-D 2350

Lorazepam (Exhibits an additive CNS depression). Products include:

Ativan Injection....................................... 2698

IMPORTANT NOTE: Always consult each drug listing in the patient's regimen for possible interactions.

Anexsia Tablets — Interactions Index — 68

Ativan Tablets 2700

Loxapine Hydrochloride (Exhibits an additive CNS depression). Products include:
- Loxitane 1378

Loxapine Succinate (Exhibits an additive CNS depression). Products include:
- Loxitane Capsules 1378

Maprotiline Hydrochloride (Increased effect of either antidepressant or hydrocodone). Products include:
- Ludiomil Tablets 843

Meperidine Hydrochloride (Exhibits an additive CNS depression). Products include:
- Demerol 2308
- Mepergan Injection 2753

Mephobarbital (Exhibits an additive CNS depression). Products include:
- Mebaral Tablets 2322

Meprobamate (Exhibits an additive CNS depression). Products include:
- Miltown Tablets 2672
- PMB 200 and PMB 400 2783

Mesoridazine (Exhibits an additive CNS depression).

Mesoridazine Besylate (Exhibits an additive CNS depression). Products include:
- Serentil 684

Methadone Hydrochloride (Exhibits an additive CNS depression). Products include:
- Methadone Hydrochloride Oral Concentrate 2233
- Methadone Hydrochloride Oral Solution & Tablets 2235

Methdilazine Hydrochloride (Exhibits an additive CNS depression).
- No products indexed under this heading.

Methohexital Sodium (Exhibits an additive CNS depression). Products include:
- Brevital Sodium Vials 1429

Methotrimeprazine (Exhibits an additive CNS depression). Products include:
- Levoprome 1274

Methoxyflurane (Exhibits an additive CNS depression).
- No products indexed under this heading.

Midazolam Hydrochloride (Exhibits an additive CNS depression). Products include:
- Versed Injection 2170

Molindone Hydrochloride (Exhibits an additive CNS depression). Products include:
- Moban Tablets and Concentrate 1048

Morphine Sulfate (Exhibits an additive CNS depression). Products include:
- Astramorph/PF Injection, USP (Preservative-Free) 535
- Duramorph 962
- Infumorph 200 and Infumorph 500 Sterile Solutions 965
- MS Contin Tablets 1994
- MSIR 1997
- Oramorph SR (Morphine Sulfate Sustained Release Tablets) 2236
- RMS Suppositories 2657
- Roxanol 2243

Nortriptyline Hydrochloride (Increased effect of either antidepressant or hydrocodone). Products include:
- Pamelor 2280

Opium Alkaloids (Exhibits an additive CNS depression).
- No products indexed under this heading.

Oxazepam (Exhibits an additive CNS depression). Products include:
- Serax Capsules 2810
- Serax Tablets 2810

Oxycodone Hydrochloride (Exhibits an additive CNS depression). Products include:
- Percocet Tablets 938
- Percodan Tablets 939
- Percodan-Demi Tablets 940
- Roxicodone Tablets, Oral Solution & Intensol (Oxycodone) 2244
- Tylox Capsules 1584

Pentobarbital Sodium (Exhibits an additive CNS depression). Products include:
- Nembutal Sodium Capsules 436
- Nembutal Sodium Solution 438
- Nembutal Sodium Suppositories 440

Perphenazine (Exhibits an additive CNS depression). Products include:
- Etrafon 2355
- Triavil Tablets 1757
- Trilafon 2389

Phenelzine Sulfate (Increased effect of either MAO inhibitor or hydrocodone). Products include:
- Nardil 1920

Phenobarbital (Exhibits an additive CNS depression). Products include:
- Arco-Lase Plus Tablets 512
- Bellergal-S Tablets 2250
- Donnatal 2060
- Donnatal Extentabs 2061
- Donnatal Tablets 2060
- Phenobarbital Elixir and Tablets 1469
- Quadrinal Tablets 1350

Pimozide (Exhibits an additive CNS depression). Products include:
- Orap Tablets 1050

Prazepam (Exhibits an additive CNS depression).
- No products indexed under this heading.

Prochlorperazine (Exhibits an additive CNS depression). Products include:
- Compazine 2470

Promethazine Hydrochloride (Exhibits an additive CNS depression). Products include:
- Mepergan Injection 2753
- Phenergan with Codeine 2777
- Phenergan with Dextromethorphan 2778
- Phenergan Injection 2773
- Phenergan Suppositories 2775
- Phenergan Syrup 2774
- Phenergan Tablets 2775
- Phenergan VC 2779
- Phenergan VC with Codeine 2781

Propofol (Exhibits an additive CNS depression). Products include:
- Diprivan Injection 2833

Propoxyphene Hydrochloride (Exhibits an additive CNS depression). Products include:
- Darvon 1435
- Wygesic Tablets 2827

Propoxyphene Napsylate (Exhibits an additive CNS depression). Products include:
- Darvon-N/Darvocet-N 1433

Protriptyline Hydrochloride (Increased effect of either antidepressant or hydrocodone). Products include:
- Vivactil Tablets 1774

Pyrilamine Maleate (Exhibits an additive CNS depression). Products include:
- 4-Way Fast Acting Nasal Spray (regular & mentholated) .... ▣ 621
- Maximum Strength Multi-Symptom Formula Midol .... ▣ 722
- PMS Multi-Symptom Formula Midol .... ▣ 723

Pyrilamine Tannate (Exhibits an additive CNS depression). Products include:
- Atrohist Pediatric Suspension 454
- Rynatan 2673

Quazepam (Exhibits an additive CNS depression). Products include:
- Doral Tablets 2664

Risperidone (Exhibits an additive CNS depression). Products include:
- Risperdal 1301

Secobarbital Sodium (Exhibits an additive CNS depression). Products include:
- Seconal Sodium Pulvules 1474

Selegiline Hydrochloride (Increased effect of either MAO inhibitor or hydrocodone). Products include:
- Eldepryl Tablets 2550

Sufentanil Citrate (Exhibits an additive CNS depression). Products include:
- Sufenta Injection 1309

Temazepam (Exhibits an additive CNS depression). Products include:
- Restoril Capsules 2284

Terfenadine (Exhibits an additive CNS depression). Products include:
- Seldane Tablets 1536
- Seldane-D Extended-Release Tablets 1538

Thiamylal Sodium (Exhibits an additive CNS depression).
- No products indexed under this heading.

Thioridazine Hydrochloride (Exhibits an additive CNS depression). Products include:
- Mellaril 2269

Thiothixene (Exhibits an additive CNS depression). Products include:
- Navane Capsules and Concentrate 2201
- Navane Intramuscular 2202

Tranylcypromine Sulfate (Increased effect of either MAO inhibitor or hydrocodone). Products include:
- Parnate Tablets 2503

Triazolam (Exhibits an additive CNS depression). Products include:
- Halcion Tablets 2611

Trifluoperazine Hydrochloride (Exhibits an additive CNS depression). Products include:
- Stelazine 2514

Trimeprazine Tartrate (Exhibits an additive CNS depression). Products include:
- Temaril Tablets, Syrup and Spansule Extended-Release Capsules 483

Trimipramine Maleate (Increased effect of either antidepressant or hydrocodone). Products include:
- Surmontil Capsules 2811

Tripelennamine Hydrochloride (Exhibits an additive CNS depression). Products include:
- PBZ Tablets 845
- PBZ-SR Tablets 844

Triprolidine Hydrochloride (Exhibits an additive CNS depression). Products include:
- Actifed Plus Caplets .... ▣ 845
- Actifed Plus Tablets .... ▣ 845
- Actifed with Codeine Cough Syrup 1067
- Actifed Syrup .... ▣ 846
- Actifed Tablets .... ▣ 844

Zolpidem Tartrate (Exhibits an additive CNS depression). Products include:
- Ambien Tablets 2416

Food Interactions

Alcohol (Exhibits an additive CNS depression).

ANEXSIA 7.5/650 TABLETS
(Acetaminophen, Hydrocodone Bitartrate) 1782
- See **Anexsia 5/500 Tablets**

ANSAID TABLETS
(Flurbiprofen) 2579

May interact with antacids, oral hypoglycemic agents, diuretics, beta blockers, anticoagulants, and certain other agents. Compounds in these categories include:

Acarbose (Slight reduction in blood sugar concentrations).
- No products indexed under this heading.

Acebutolol Hydrochloride (Potential interference with hypotensive effect). Products include:
- Sectral Capsules 2807

Aluminum Carbonate Gel (Possible reduction in rate of absorption in geriatric subjects). Products include:
- Basaljel 2703

Aluminum Hydroxide (Possible reduction in rate of absorption in geriatric subjects). Products include:
- ALternaGEL Liquid 1316
- Maximum Strength Ascriptin .... ▣ 630
- Cama Arthritis Pain Reliever .... ▣ 785
- Gaviscon Extra Strength Relief Formula Antacid Tablets .... ▣ 819
- Gaviscon Extra Strength Relief Formula Liquid Antacid .... ▣ 819
- Gaviscon Liquid Antacid .... ▣ 820
- Gelusil Liquid & Tablets .... ▣ 855
- Maalox Heartburn Relief Suspension .... ▣ 642
- Maalox Heartburn Relief Tablets .... ▣ 641
- Maalox Magnesia and Alumina Oral Suspension .... ▣ 642
- Maalox Plus Tablets .... ▣ 643
- Extra Strength Maalox Antacid Plus Antigas Liquid and Tablets .... ▣ 638
- Tempo Soft Antacid .... ▣ 835

Aluminum Hydroxide Gel (Possible reduction in rate of absorption in geriatric subjects). Products include:
- ALternaGEL Liquid .... ▣ 659
- Aludrox Oral Suspension 2695
- Amphojel Suspension 2695
- Amphojel Suspension without Flavor 2695
- Amphojel Tablets 2695
- Arthritis Pain Ascriptin .... ▣ 631
- Regular Strength Ascriptin Tablets .... ▣ 629
- Gaviscon Antacid Tablets .... ▣ 819
- Gaviscon-2 Antacid Tablets .... ▣ 820
- Mylanta Liquid 1317
- Mylanta Tablets .... ▣ 660
- Mylanta Double Strength Liquid 1317
- Mylanta Double Strength Tablets .... ▣ 660
- Nephrox Suspension .... ▣ 655

Amiloride Hydrochloride (Flurbiprofen may interfere with diuretic effect). Products include:
- Midamor Tablets 1703
- Moduretic Tablets 1705

Aspirin (Lowers serum flurbiprofen concentrations by 50%). Products include:
- Alka-Seltzer Effervescent Antacid and Pain Reliever .... ▣ 701
- Alka-Seltzer Extra Strength Effervescent Antacid and Pain Reliever .... ▣ 703
- Alka-Seltzer Lemon Lime Effervescent Antacid and Pain Reliever .... ▣ 703
- Alka-Seltzer Plus Cold Medicine .... ▣ 705
- Alka-Seltzer Plus Cold & Cough Medicine .... ▣ 708
- Alka-Seltzer Plus Night-Time Cold Medicine .... ▣ 707
- Alka Seltzer Plus Sinus Medicine .... ▣ 707
- Arthritis Foundation Safety Coated Aspirin Tablets .... ▣ 675
- Arthritis Pain Ascriptin .... ▣ 631
- Maximum Strength Ascriptin .... ▣ 630
- Regular Strength Ascriptin Tablets .... ▣ 629
- Arthritis Strength BC Powder .... ▣ 609

(▣ Described in PDR For Nonprescription Drugs) (⊙ Described in PDR For Ophthalmology)

69 **Interactions Index** **Ansaid**

BC Cold Powder Multi-Symptom Formula (Cold-Sinus-Allergy) ⊡ 609
BC Cold Powder Non-Drowsy Formula (Cold-Sinus) ⊡ 609
BC Powder ⊡ 609
Bayer Children's Chewable Aspirin ⊡ 711
Genuine Bayer Aspirin Tablets & Caplets ⊡ 713
Extra Strength Bayer Arthritis Pain Regimen Formula ⊡ 711
Extra Strength Bayer Aspirin Caplets & Tablets ⊡ 712
Extended-Release Bayer 8-Hour Aspirin ⊡ 712
Extra Strength Bayer Plus Aspirin Caplets ⊡ 713
Extra Strength Bayer PM Aspirin .. ⊡ 713
Bayer Enteric Aspirin ⊡ 709
Bufferin Analgesic Tablets and Caplets ⊡ 613
Arthritis Strength Bufferin Analgesic Caplets ⊡ 614
Extra Strength Bufferin Analgesic Tablets ⊡ 615
Cama Arthritis Pain Reliever ⊡ 785
Darvon Compound-65 Pulvules 1435
Easprin 1914
Ecotrin 2455
Ecotrin Enteric Coated Aspirin Maximum Strength Tablets and Caplets ⊡ 816
Ecotrin Enteric Coated Aspirin Regular Strength Tablets 2455
Empirin Aspirin Tablets ⊡ 854
Empirin with Codeine Tablets 1093
Excedrin Extra-Strength Analgesic Tablets & Caplets 732
Fiorinal Capsules 2261
Fiorinal with Codeine Capsules 2262
Fiorinal Tablets 2261
Halfprin 1362
Healthprin Aspirin 2455
Norgesic 1496
Percodan Tablets 939
Percodan-Demi Tablets 940
Robaxisal Tablets 2071
Soma Compound w/Codeine Tablets 2676
Soma Compound Tablets 2675
St. Joseph Adult Chewable Aspirin (81 mg.) ⊡ 808
Talwin Compound 2335
Ursinus Inlay-Tabs ⊡ 794
Vanquish Analgesic Caplets ⊡ 731

Atenolol (Potential interference with hypotensive effect). Products include:
Tenoretic Tablets 2845
Tenormin Tablets and I.V. Injection 2847

Bendroflumethiazide (Flurbiprofen may interfere with diuretic effect).
No products indexed under this heading.

Betaxolol Hydrochloride (Potential interference with hypotensive effect). Products include:
Betoptic Ophthalmic Solution 469
Betoptic S Ophthalmic Suspension 471
Kerlone Tablets 2436

Bisoprolol Fumarate (Potential interference with hypotensive effect). Products include:
Zebeta Tablets 1413
Ziac 1415

Bumetanide (Flurbiprofen may interfere with diuretic effect). Products include:
Bumex 2093

Carteolol Hydrochloride (Potential interference with hypotensive effect). Products include:
Cartrol Tablets 410
Ocupress Ophthalmic Solution, 1% Sterile ⊙ 309

Chlorothiazide (Flurbiprofen may interfere with diuretic effect). Products include:
Aldoclor Tablets 1598
Diupres Tablets 1650
Diuril Oral 1653

Chlorothiazide Sodium (Flurbiprofen may interfere with diuretic effect). Products include:
Diuril Sodium Intravenous 1652

Chlorpropamide (Slight reduction in blood sugar concentrations). Products include:
Diabinese Tablets 1935

Chlorthalidone (Flurbiprofen may interfere with diuretic effect). Products include:
Combipres Tablets 677
Tenoretic Tablets 2845
Thalitone 1245

Cimetidine (Small increase in the AUC of flurbiprofen). Products include:
Tagamet Tablets 2516

Cimetidine Hydrochloride (Small increase in the AUC of flurbiprofen). Products include:
Tagamet 2516

Dalteparin Sodium (Possible serious clinical bleeding). Products include:
Fragmin 1954

Dicumarol (Possible serious clinical bleeding).
No products indexed under this heading.

Dihydroxyaluminum Sodium Carbonate (Possible reduction in rate of absorption in geriatric subjects).
No products indexed under this heading.

Enoxaparin (Possible serious clinical bleeding). Products include:
Lovenox Injection 2020

Esmolol Hydrochloride (Potential interference with hypotensive effect). Products include:
Brevibloc Injection 1808

Ethacrynic Acid (Flurbiprofen may interfere with diuretic effect). Products include:
Edecrin Tablets 1657

Furosemide (Flurbiprofen may interfere with diuretic effect). Products include:
Lasix Injection, Oral Solution and Tablets 1240

Glipizide (Slight reduction in blood sugar concentrations). Products include:
Glucotrol Tablets 1967
Glucotrol XL Extended Release Tablets 1968

Glyburide (Slight reduction in blood sugar concentrations). Products include:
DiaBeta Tablets 1239
Glynase PresTab Tablets 2609
Micronase Tablets 2623

Heparin Calcium (Possible serious clinical bleeding).
No products indexed under this heading.

Heparin Sodium (Possible serious clinical bleeding). Products include:
Heparin Lock Flush Solution 2725
Heparin Sodium Injection 2726
Heparin Sodium Injection, USP, Sterile Solution 2615
Heparin Sodium Vials 1441

Hydrochlorothiazide (Flurbiprofen may interfere with diuretic effect). Products include:
Aldactazide 2413
Aldoril Tablets 1604
Apresazide Capsules 808
Capozide 742
Dyazide 2479
Esidrix Tablets 821
Esimil Tablets 822
HydroDIURIL Tablets 1674
Hydropres Tablets 1675
Hyzaar Tablets 1677
Inderide Tablets 2732
Inderide LA Long Acting Capsules .. 2734
Lopressor HCT Tablets 832
Lotensin HCT 837
Maxzide 1380
Moduretic Tablets 1705
Oretic Tablets 443
Prinzide Tablets 1737
Ser-Ap-Es Tablets 849
Timolide Tablets 1748
Vaseretic Tablets 1765
Zestoretic 2850
Ziac 1415

Hydroflumethiazide (Flurbiprofen may interfere with diuretic effect). Products include:
Diucardin Tablets 2718

Indapamide (Flurbiprofen may interfere with diuretic effect). Products include:
Lozol Tablets 2022

Labetalol Hydrochloride (Potential interference with hypotensive effect). Products include:
Normodyne Injection 2377
Normodyne Tablets 2379
Trandate 1185

Levobunolol Hydrochloride (Potential interference with hypotensive effect). Products include:
Betagan ⊙ 233

Magaldrate (Possible reduction in rate of absorption in geriatric subjects).
No products indexed under this heading.

Magnesium Hydroxide (Possible reduction in rate of absorption in geriatric subjects). Products include:
Aludrox Oral Suspension 2695
Arthritis Pain Ascriptin ⊡ 631
Maximum Strength Ascriptin ⊡ 630
Regular Strength Ascriptin Tablets ⊡ 629
Di-Gel Antacid/Anti-Gas ⊡ 801
Gelusil Liquid & Tablets ⊡ 855
Maalox Magnesia and Alumina Oral Suspension ⊡ 642
Maalox Plus Tablets ⊡ 643
Extra Strength Maalox Antacid Plus Antigas Liquid and Tablets ⊡ 638
Mylanta Calcium Carbonate and Magnesium Hydroxide Tablets 1318
Mylanta Liquid 1317
Mylanta Tablets ⊡ 660
Mylanta Double Strength Liquid 1317
Mylanta Double Strength Tablets .. ⊡ 660
Phillips' Milk of Magnesia Liquid ⊡ 729
Rolaids Tablets ⊡ 843
Tempo Soft Antacid ⊡ 835

Magnesium Oxide (Possible reduction in rate of absorption in geriatric subjects). Products include:
Beelith Tablets 639
Bufferin Analgesic Tablets and Caplets ⊡ 613
Caltrate PLUS ⊡ 665
Cama Arthritis Pain Reliever ⊡ 785
Mag-Ox 400 668
Uro-Mag 668

Metformin Hydrochloride (Slight reduction in blood sugar concentrations). Products include:
Glucophage 752

Methyclothiazide (Flurbiprofen may interfere with diuretic effect). Products include:
Enduron Tablets 420

Metipranolol Hydrochloride (Potential interference with hypotensive effect). Products include:
OptiPranolol (Metipranolol 0.3%) Sterile Ophthalmic Solution ⊙ 258

Metolazone (Flurbiprofen may interfere with diuretic effect). Products include:
Mykrox Tablets 993
Zaroxolyn Tablets 1000

Metoprolol Succinate (Potential interference with hypotensive effect). Products include:
Toprol-XL Tablets 565

Metoprolol Tartrate (Potential interference with hypotensive effect). Products include:
Lopressor Ampuls 830
Lopressor HCT Tablets 832
Lopressor Tablets 830

Nadolol (Potential interference with hypotensive effect).
No products indexed under this heading.

Penbutolol Sulfate (Potential interference with hypotensive effect). Products include:
Levatol 2403

Pindolol (Potential interference with hypotensive effect). Products include:
Visken Tablets 2299

Polythiazide (Flurbiprofen may interfere with diuretic effect). Products include:
Minizide Capsules 1938

Propranolol Hydrochloride (Potential interference with hypotensive effect). Products include:
Inderal 2728
Inderal LA Long Acting Capsules 2730
Inderide Tablets 2732
Inderide LA Long Acting Capsules .. 2734

Ranitidine Hydrochloride (Small increase in the AUC of flurbiprofen). Products include:
Zantac 1209
Zantac Injection 1207
Zantac Syrup 1209

Sodium Bicarbonate (Possible reduction in rate of absorption in geriatric subjects). Products include:
Alka-Seltzer Effervescent Antacid and Pain Reliever ⊡ 701
Alka-Seltzer Extra Strength Effervescent Antacid and Pain Reliever ⊡ 703
Alka-Seltzer Gold Effervescent Antacid ⊡ 703
Alka-Seltzer Lemon Lime Effervescent Antacid and Pain Reliever ⊡ 703
Arm & Hammer Pure Baking Soda ⊡ 627
Ceo-Two Rectal Suppositories 666
Citrocarbonate Antacid ⊡ 770
Massengill Disposable Douches ⊡ 820
Massengill Liquid Concentrate ⊡ 820
NuLYTELY 689
Cherry Flavor NuLYTELY 689

Sotalol Hydrochloride (Potential interference with hypotensive effect). Products include:
Betapace Tablets 641

Spironolactone (Flurbiprofen may interfere with diuretic effect). Products include:
Aldactazide 2413
Aldactone 2414

Timolol Hemihydrate (Potential interference with hypotensive effect). Products include:
Betimol 0.25%, 0.5% ⊙ 261

Timolol Maleate (Potential interference with hypotensive effect). Products include:
Blocadren Tablets 1614
Timolide Tablets 1748
Timoptic in Ocudose 1753
Timoptic Sterile Ophthalmic Solution 1751
Timoptic-XE 1755

Tolazamide (Slight reduction in blood sugar concentrations).
No products indexed under this heading.

Tolbutamide (Slight reduction in blood sugar concentrations).
No products indexed under this heading.

Torsemide (Flurbiprofen may interfere with diuretic effect). Products include:
Demadex Tablets and Injection 686

Triamterene (Flurbiprofen may interfere with diuretic effect). Products include:
Dyazide 2479
Dyrenium Capsules 2481
Maxzide 1380

IMPORTANT NOTE: Always consult each drug listing in the patient's regimen for possible interactions.

Warfarin Sodium (Possible serious clinical bleeding). Products include:

Coumadin 926

Food Interactions

Food, unspecified (Alters the rate of absorption but does not affect the extent of drug availability).

ANTABUSE TABLETS

(Disulfiram) 2695

May interact with oral anticoagulants and certain other agents. Compounds in these categories include:

Dicumarol (Prolonged prothrombin time).

No products indexed under this heading.

Isoniazid (Potential for the appearance of unsteady gait or marked changes in mental status). Products include:

Nydrazid Injection 508
Rifamate Capsules 1530
Rifater 1532

Metronidazole (Psychotic reactions due to combined toxicity). Products include:

Flagyl 375 Capsules 2434
Flagyl I.V. RTU 2247
MetroGel 1047
MetroGel-Vaginal 902
Protostat Tablets 1883

Metronidazole Hydrochloride (Psychotic reactions due to combined toxicity). Products include:

Flagyl I.V. 2247

Paraldehyde (Contraindicated).

Phenytoin (Phenytoin intoxication). Products include:

Dilantin Infatabs 1908
Dilantin-125 Suspension 1911

Phenytoin Sodium (Phenytoin intoxication). Products include:

Dilantin Kapseals 1906
Dilantin Parenteral 1910

Warfarin Sodium (Prolonged prothrombin time). Products include:

Coumadin 926

Food Interactions

Alcohol (Antabuse plus alcohol, even small amounts, produces flushing, throbbing in head and neck, respiratory difficulty, headache and other serious reactions including convulsions and death; concurrent use is contraindicated).

ANTILIRIUM INJECTABLE

(Physostigmine Salicylate) 1009

May interact with:

Atropine Sulfate (Atropine antagonizes the action of Physostigmine). Products include:

Arco-Lase Plus Tablets 512
Atrohist Plus Tablets 454
Atropine Sulfate Sterile Ophthalmic Solution .... ⊙ 233
Donnatal 2060
Donnatal Extentabs 2061
Donnatal Tablets 2060
Lomotil 2439
Motofen Tablets 784
Urised Tablets 1964

Decamethonium (Concurrent administration contraindicated).

Succinylcholine Chloride (Concurrent administration contraindicated). Products include:

Anectine 1073

ANTIOX CAPSULES

(Beta Carotene, Vitamin C, Vitamin E) 1543

None cited in PDR database.

ANTIVENIN (BLACK WIDOW SPIDER)

(Black Widow Spider Antivenin (Equine)) 1607

None cited in PDR database.

ANTIVENIN (CROTALIDAE) POLYVALENT

(Antivenin (Crotalidae) Polyvalent) 2696

May interact with beta blockers. Compounds in this category include:

Acebutolol Hydrochloride (Potential for increased severity of acute and prolonged anaphylaxis). Products include:

Sectral Capsules 2807

Atenolol (Potential for increased severity of acute and prolonged anaphylaxis). Products include:

Tenoretic Tablets 2845
Tenormin Tablets and I.V. Injection 2847

Betaxolol Hydrochloride (Potential for increased severity of acute and prolonged anaphylaxis). Products include:

Betoptic Ophthalmic Solution 469
Betoptic S Ophthalmic Suspension 471
Kerlone Tablets 2436

Bisoprolol Fumarate (Potential for increased severity of acute and prolonged anaphylaxis). Products include:

Zebeta Tablets 1413
Ziac 1415

Carteolol Hydrochloride (Potential for increased severity of acute and prolonged anaphylaxis). Products include:

Cartrol Tablets 410
Ocupress Ophthalmic Solution, 1% Sterile .... ⊙ 309

Esmolol Hydrochloride (Potential for increased severity of acute and prolonged anaphylaxis). Products include:

Brevibloc Injection 1808

Labetalol Hydrochloride (Potential for increased severity of acute and prolonged anaphylaxis). Products include:

Normodyne Injection 2377
Normodyne Tablets 2379
Trandate 1185

Levobunolol Hydrochloride (Potential for increased severity of acute and prolonged anaphylaxis). Products include:

Betagan .... ⊙ 233

Metipranolol Hydrochloride (Potential for increased severity of acute and prolonged anaphylaxis). Products include:

OptiPranolol (Metipranolol 0.3%) Sterile Ophthalmic Solution .... ⊙ 258

Metoprolol Succinate (Potential for increased severity of acute and prolonged anaphylaxis). Products include:

Toprol-XL Tablets 565

Metoprolol Tartrate (Potential for increased severity of acute and prolonged anaphylaxis). Products include:

Lopressor Ampuls 830
Lopressor HCT Tablets 832
Lopressor Tablets 830

Nadolol (Potential for increased severity of acute and prolonged anaphylaxis).

No products indexed under this heading.

Penbutolol Sulfate (Potential for increased severity of acute and prolonged anaphylaxis). Products include:

Levatol 2403

Pindolol (Potential for increased severity of acute and prolonged anaphylaxis). Products include:

Visken Tablets 2299

Propranolol Hydrochloride (Potential for increased severity of acute and prolonged anaphylaxis). Products include:

Inderal 2728
Inderal LA Long Acting Capsules 2730
Inderide Tablets 2732
Inderide LA Long Acting Capsules 2734

Sotalol Hydrochloride (Potential for increased severity of acute and prolonged anaphylaxis). Products include:

Betapace Tablets 641

Timolol Hemihydrate (Potential for increased severity of acute and prolonged anaphylaxis). Products include:

Betimol 0.25%, 0.5% .... ⊙ 261

Timolol Maleate (Potential for increased severity of acute and prolonged anaphylaxis). Products include:

Blocadren Tablets 1614
Timolide Tablets 1748
Timoptic in Ocudose 1753
Timoptic Sterile Ophthalmic Solution 1751
Timoptic-XE 1755

ANTIVERT, ANTIVERT/25 TABLETS, & ANTIVERT/50 TABLETS

(Meclizine Hydrochloride) 2185

Food Interactions

Alcohol (Concurrent use should be avoided).

ANTURANE CAPSULES

(Sulfinpyrazone) 807

May interact with oral anticoagulants, salicylates, sulfonylureas, insulin, and certain other agents. Compounds in these categories include:

Aspirin (Uricosuric action antagonized). Products include:

Alka-Seltzer Effervescent Antacid and Pain Reliever .... ▣ 701
Alka-Seltzer Extra Strength Effervescent Antacid and Pain Reliever .... ▣ 703
Alka-Seltzer Lemon Lime Effervescent Antacid and Pain Reliever .... ▣ 703
Alka-Seltzer Plus Cold Medicine .... ▣ 705
Alka-Seltzer Plus Cold & Cough Medicine .... ▣ 708
Alka-Seltzer Plus Night-Time Cold Medicine .... ▣ 707
Alka Seltzer Plus Sinus Medicine .... ▣ 707
Arthritis Foundation Safety Coated Aspirin Tablets .... ▣ 675
Arthritis Pain Ascriptin .... ▣ 631
Maximum Strength Ascriptin .... ▣ 630
Regular Strength Ascriptin Tablets .... ▣ 629
Arthritis Strength BC Powder .... ▣ 609
BC Cold Powder Multi-Symptom Formula (Cold-Sinus-Allergy) .... ▣ 609
BC Cold Powder Non-Drowsy Formula (Cold-Sinus) .... ▣ 609
BC Powder .... ▣ 609
Bayer Children's Chewable Aspirin .... ▣ 711
Genuine Bayer Aspirin Tablets & Caplets .... ▣ 713
Extra Strength Bayer Arthritis Pain Regimen Formula .... ▣ 711
Extra Strength Bayer Aspirin Caplets & Tablets .... ▣ 712
Extended-Release Bayer 8-Hour Aspirin .... ▣ 712
Extra Strength Bayer Plus Aspirin Caplets .... ▣ 713
Extra Strength Bayer PM Aspirin .... ▣ 713
Bayer Enteric Aspirin .... ▣ 709
Bufferin Analgesic Tablets and Caplets .... ▣ 613
Arthritis Strength Bufferin Analgesic Caplets .... ▣ 614
Extra Strength Bufferin Analgesic Tablets .... ▣ 615
Cama Arthritis Pain Reliever .... ▣ 785
Darvon Compound-65 Pulvules 1435
Easprin 1914
Ecotrin 2455
Ecotrin Enteric Coated Aspirin Maximum Strength Tablets and Caplets .... ▣ 816
Ecotrin Enteric Coated Aspirin Regular Strength Tablets 2455
Empirin Aspirin Tablets .... ▣ 854
Empirin with Codeine Tablets 1093
Excedrin Extra-Strength Analgesic Tablets & Caplets 732
Fiorinal Capsules 2261
Fiorinal with Codeine Capsules 2262
Fiorinal Tablets 2261
Halfprin 1362
Healthprin Aspirin 2455
Norgesic 1496
Percodan Tablets 939
Percodan-Demi Tablets 940
Robaxisal Tablets 2071
Soma Compound w/Codeine Tablets 2676
Soma Compound Tablets 2675
St. Joseph Adult Chewable Aspirin (81 mg.) .... ▣ 808
Talwin Compound 2335
Ursinus Inlay-Tabs .... ▣ 794
Vanquish Analgesic Caplets .... ▣ 731

Chlorpropamide (Potentiated). Products include:

Diabinese Tablets 1935

Choline Magnesium Trisalicylate (Uricosuric action antagonized). Products include:

Trilisate 2000

Dicumarol (Action of coumarin-type anticoagulants may be accentuated).

No products indexed under this heading.

Diflunisal (Uricosuric action antagonized). Products include:

Dolobid Tablets 1654

Glipizide (Potentiated). Products include:

Glucotrol Tablets 1967
Glucotrol XL Extended Release Tablets 1968

Glyburide (Potentiated). Products include:

DiaBeta Tablets 1239
Glynase PresTab Tablets 2609
Micronase Tablets 2623

Insulin, Human (Potentiated).

No products indexed under this heading.

Insulin, Human Isophane Suspension (Potentiated). Products include:

Novolin N Human Insulin 10 ml Vials 1795

Insulin, Human NPH (Potentiated). Products include:

Humulin N, 100 Units 1448
Novolin N PenFill Cartridges Durable Insulin Delivery System 1798
Novolin N Prefilled Syringe Disposable Insulin Delivery System 1798

Insulin, Human Regular (Potentiated). Products include:

Humulin R, 100 Units 1449
Novolin R Human Insulin 10 ml Vials 1795
Novolin R PenFill Cartridges Durable Insulin Delivery System 1798
Novolin R Prefilled Syringe Disposable Insulin Delivery System 1798
Velosulin BR Human Insulin 10 ml Vials 1795

Insulin, Human, Zinc Suspension (Potentiated). Products include:

Humulin L, 100 Units 1446
Humulin U, 100 Units 1450
Novolin L Human Insulin 10 ml Vials 1795

Insulin, NPH (Potentiated). Products include:

NPH, 100 Units 1450
Pork NPH, 100 Units 1452

(▣ Described in PDR For Nonprescription Drugs)
(⊙ Described in PDR For Ophthalmology)

71 Interactions Index Apresazide

Purified Pork NPH Isophane Insulin 1801

Insulin, Regular (Potentiated). Products include:
- Regular, 100 Units 1450
- Pork Regular, 100 Units 1452
- Pork Regular (Concentrated), 500 Units 1453
- Purified Pork Regular Insulin 1801

Insulin, Zinc Crystals (Potentiated). Products include:
- NPH, 100 Units 1450

Insulin, Zinc Suspension (Potentiated). Products include:
- Iletin I 1450
- Lente, 100 Units 1450
- Iletin II 1452
- Pork Lente, 100 Units 1452
- Purified Pork Lente Insulin 1801

Magnesium Salicylate (Uricosuric action antagonized). Products include:
- Backache Caplets .... ▣ 613
- Bayer Select Backache Pain Relief Formula .... ▣ 715
- Doan's Extra-Strength Analgesic .... ▣ 633
- Extra Strength Doan's P.M. .... ▣ 633
- Doan's Regular Strength Analgesic .... ▣ 634
- Mobigesic Tablets .... ▣ 602

Salsalate (Uricosuric action antagonized). Products include:
- Mono-Gesic Tablets 792
- Salflex Tablets 786

Sulfisoxazole (Potentiated). Products include:
- Azo Gantrisin Tablets 2081
- Gantrisin Tablets 2120

Tolazamide (Potentiated).
- No products indexed under this heading.

Tolbutamide (Potentiated).
- No products indexed under this heading.

Warfarin Sodium (Action of coumarin-type anticoagulants may be accentuated). Products include:
- Coumadin 926

ANTURANE TABLETS
(Sulfinpyrazone) 807
See **Anturane Capsules**

ANUSOL HEMORRHOIDAL SUPPOSITORIES
(Starch) .... ▣ 847
None cited in PDR database.

ANUSOL OINTMENT
(Pramoxine Hydrochloride, Zinc Oxide, Mineral Oil) .... ▣ 847
None cited in PDR database.

ANUSOL HC-1 ANTI-ITCH HYDROCORTISONE OINTMENT
(Hydrocortisone Acetate) .... ▣ 847
None cited in PDR database.

ANUSOL-HC CREAM 2.5%
(Hydrocortisone) 1896
None cited in PDR database.

ANUSOL-HC SUPPOSITORIES
(Hydrocortisone Acetate) 1897
None cited in PDR database.

APRESAZIDE CAPSULES
(Hydralazine Hydrochloride, Hydrochlorothiazide) 808
May interact with monoamine oxidase inhibitors, corticosteroids, antihypertensives, insulin, narcotic analgesics, barbiturates, cardiac glycosides, non-steroidal anti-inflammatory agents, and certain other agents. Compounds in these categories include:

Acebutolol Hydrochloride (Additive or potentiated action). Products include:
- Sectral Capsules 2807

ACTH (Hypokalemia).
- No products indexed under this heading.

Alfentanil Hydrochloride (May potentiate orthostatic hypotension). Products include:
- Alfenta Injection 1286

Amlodipine Besylate (Additive or potentiated action). Products include:
- Lotrel Capsules 840
- Norvasc Tablets 1940

Aprobarbital (May potentiate orthostatic hypotension).
- No products indexed under this heading.

Atenolol (Additive or potentiated action). Products include:
- Tenoretic Tablets 2845
- Tenormin Tablets and I.V. Injection 2847

Benazepril Hydrochloride (Additive or potentiated action). Products include:
- Lotensin Tablets 834
- Lotensin HCT 837
- Lotrel Capsules 840

Bendroflumethiazide (Additive or potentiated action).
- No products indexed under this heading.

Betamethasone Acetate (Concomitant use may result in hypokalemia). Products include:
- Celestone Soluspan Suspension 2347

Betamethasone Sodium Phosphate (Concomitant use may result in hypokalemia). Products include:
- Celestone Soluspan Suspension 2347

Betaxolol Hydrochloride (Additive or potentiated action). Products include:
- Betoptic Ophthalmic Solution 469
- Betoptic S Ophthalmic Suspension 471
- Kerlone Tablets 2436

Bisoprolol Fumarate (Additive or potentiated action). Products include:
- Zebeta Tablets 1413
- Ziac 1415

Buprenorphine (May potentiate orthostatic hypotension). Products include:
- Buprenex Injectable 2006

Butabarbital (May potentiate orthostatic hypotension).
- No products indexed under this heading.

Butalbital (May potentiate orthostatic hypotension). Products include:
- Esgic-plus Tablets 1013
- Fioricet Tablets 2258
- Fioricet with Codeine Capsules 2260
- Fiorinal Capsules 2261
- Fiorinal with Codeine Capsules 2262
- Fiorinal Tablets 2261
- Phrenilin 785
- Sedapap Tablets 50 mg/650 mg .. 1543

Captopril (Additive or potentiated action). Products include:
- Capoten 739
- Capozide 742

Carteolol Hydrochloride (Additive or potentiated action). Products include:
- Cartrol Tablets 410
- Ocupress Ophthalmic Solution, 1% Sterile .... ◉ 309

Chlorothiazide (Additive or potentiated action). Products include:
- Aldoclor Tablets 1598
- Diupres Tablets 1650
- Diuril Oral 1653

Chlorothiazide Sodium (Additive or potentiated action). Products include:
- Diuril Sodium Intravenous 1652

Chlorthalidone (Additive or potentiated action). Products include:
- Combipres Tablets 677
- Tenoretic Tablets 2845
- Thalitone 1245

Clonidine (Additive or potentiated action). Products include:
- Catapres-TTS 675

Clonidine Hydrochloride (Additive or potentiated action). Products include:
- Catapres Tablets 674
- Combipres Tablets 677

Codeine Phosphate (May potentiate orthostatic hypotension). Products include:
- Actifed with Codeine Cough Syrup .. 1067
- Brontex 1981
- Deconsal C Expectorant Syrup 456
- Deconsal Pediatric Syrup 457
- Dimetane-DC Cough Syrup 2059
- Empirin with Codeine Tablets 1093
- Fioricet with Codeine Capsules 2260
- Fiorinal with Codeine Capsules 2262
- Isoclor Expectorant 990
- Novahistine DH 2462
- Novahistine Expectorant 2463
- Nucofed 2051
- Phenergan with Codeine 2777
- Phenergan VC with Codeine 2781
- Robitussin A-C Syrup 2073
- Robitussin-DAC Syrup 2074
- Ryna .... ▣ 841
- Soma Compound w/Codeine Tablets 2676
- Tussi-Organidin NR Liquid and S NR Liquid 2677
- Tylenol with Codeine 1583

Cortisone Acetate (Concomitant use may result in hypokalemia). Products include:
- Cortone Acetate Sterile Suspension 1623
- Cortone Acetate Tablets 1624

Deserpidine (Additive or potentiated action).
- No products indexed under this heading.

Deslanoside (Hypokalemia can exaggerate cardiotoxicity of digitalis).
- No products indexed under this heading.

Dexamethasone (Concomitant use may result in hypokalemia). Products include:
- AK-Trol Ointment & Suspension .... ◉ 205
- Decadron Elixir 1633
- Decadron Tablets 1635
- Decaspray Topical Aerosol 1648
- Dexacidin Ointment .... ◉ 263
- Maxitrol Ophthalmic Ointment and Suspension .... ◉ 224
- TobraDex Ophthalmic Suspension and Ointment 473

Dexamethasone Acetate (Concomitant use may result in hypokalemia). Products include:
- Dalalone D.P. Injectable 1011
- Decadron-LA Sterile Suspension 1646

Dexamethasone Sodium Phosphate (Concomitant use may result in hypokalemia). Products include:
- Decadron Phosphate Injection 1637
- Decadron Phosphate Respihaler 1642
- Decadron Phosphate Sterile Ophthalmic Ointment 1641
- Decadron Phosphate Sterile Ophthalmic Solution 1642
- Decadron Phosphate Topical Cream 1644
- Decadron Phosphate Turbinaire 1645
- Decadron Phosphate with Xylocaine Injection, Sterile 1639
- Dexacort Phosphate in Respihaler .. 458
- Dexacort Phosphate in Turbinaire .. 459
- NeoDecadron Sterile Ophthalmic Ointment 1712
- NeoDecadron Sterile Ophthalmic Solution 1713
- NeoDecadron Topical Cream 1714

Dezocine (May potentiate orthostatic hypotension). Products include:
- Dalgan Injection 538

Diazoxide (Profound hypotensive episodes; additive or potentiated action). Products include:
- Hyperstat I.V. Injection 2363
- Proglycem 580

Diclofenac Potassium (Concurrent administration may reduce the diuretic, natriuretic and antihypertensive effects of thiazide diuretics). Products include:
- Cataflam 816

Diclofenac Sodium (Concurrent administration may reduce the diuretic, natriuretic and antihypertensive effects of thiazide diuretics). Products include:
- Voltaren Ophthalmic Sterile Ophthalmic Solution .... ◉ 272
- Voltaren Tablets 861

Digitoxin (Hypokalemia can exaggerate cardiotoxicity of digitalis). Products include:
- Crystodigin Tablets 1433

Digoxin (Hypokalemia can exaggerate cardiotoxicity of digitalis). Products include:
- Lanoxicaps 1117
- Lanoxin Elixir Pediatric 1120
- Lanoxin Injection 1123
- Lanoxin Injection Pediatric 1126
- Lanoxin Tablets 1128

Diltiazem Hydrochloride (Additive or potentiated action). Products include:
- Cardizem CD Capsules 1506
- Cardizem SR Capsules 1510
- Cardizem Injectable 1508
- Cardizem Tablets 1512
- Dilacor XR Extended-release Capsules 2018

Doxazosin Mesylate (Additive or potentiated action). Products include:
- Cardura Tablets 2186

Enalapril Maleate (Additive or potentiated action). Products include:
- Vaseretic Tablets 1765
- Vasotec Tablets 1771

Enalaprilat (Additive or potentiated action). Products include:
- Vasotec I.V. 1768

Epinephrine (Pressor responses may be reduced). Products include:
- Bronkaid Mist .... ▣ 717
- EPIFRIN .... ◉ 239
- EpiPen 790
- Marcaine Hydrochloride with Epinephrine 1:200,000 2316
- Primatene Mist .... ▣ 873
- Sensorcaine with Epinephrine Injection 559
- Sus-Phrine Injection 1019
- Xylocaine with Epinephrine Injections 567

Epinephrine Bitartrate (Pressor responses may be reduced). Products include:
- Bronkaid Mist Suspension .... ▣ 718
- Sensorcaine-MPF with Epinephrine Injection 559

Esmolol Hydrochloride (Additive or potentiated action). Products include:
- Brevibloc Injection 1808

Etodolac (Concurrent administration may reduce the diuretic, natriuretic and antihypertensive effects of thiazide diuretics). Products include:
- Lodine Capsules and Tablets 2743

Felodipine (Additive or potentiated action). Products include:
- Plendil Extended-Release Tablets 527

IMPORTANT NOTE: Always consult each drug listing in the patient's regimen for possible interactions.

Apresazide Interactions Index 72

Fenoprofen Calcium (Concurrent administration may reduce the diuretic, natriuretic and antihypertensive effects of thiazide diuretics). Products include:
Nalfon 200 Pulvules & Nalfon Tablets 917

Fentanyl (May potentiate orthostatic hypotension). Products include:
Duragesic Transdermal System 1288

Fentanyl Citrate (May potentiate orthostatic hypotension). Products include:
Sublimaze Injection 1307

Fludrocortisone Acetate (Concomitant use may result in hypokalemia). Products include:
Florinef Acetate Tablets 505

Flurbiprofen (Concurrent administration may reduce the diuretic, natriuretic and antihypertensive effects of thiazide diuretics). Products include:
Ansaid Tablets 2579

Fosinopril Sodium (Additive or potentiated action). Products include:
Monopril Tablets 757

Furazolidone (Concurrent use requires caution). Products include:
Furoxone 2046

Furosemide (Additive or potentiated action). Products include:
Lasix Injection, Oral Solution and Tablets 1240

Guanabenz Acetate (Additive or potentiated action).
No products indexed under this heading.

Guanethidine Monosulfate (Additive or potentiated action). Products include:
Esimil Tablets 822
Ismelin Tablets 827

Hydrocodone Bitartrate (May potentiate orthostatic hypotension). Products include:
Anexsia 5/500 Elixir 1781
Anexia Tablets 1782
Codiclear DH Syrup 791
Deconamine CX Cough and Cold Liquid and Tablets 1319
Duratuss HD Elixir 2565
Hycodan Tablets and Syrup 930
Hycomine Compound Tablets 932
Hycomine 931
Hycotuss Expectorant Syrup 933
Hydrocet Capsules 782
Lorcet 10/650 1018
Lortab 2566
Tussend 1783
Tussend Expectorant 1785
Vicodin Tablets 1356
Vicodin ES Tablets 1357
Vicodin Tuss Expectorant 1358
Zydone Capsules 949

Hydrocodone Polistirex (May potentiate orthostatic hypotension). Products include:
Tussionex Pennkinetic Extended-Release Suspension 998

Hydrocortisone (Concomitant use may result in hypokalemia). Products include:
Anusol-HC Cream 2.5% 1896
Aquanil HC Lotion 1931
Bactine Hydrocortisone Anti-Itch Cream ▣ 709
Caldecort Anti-Itch Hydrocortisone Spray ▣ 631
Cortaid ▣ 836
CORTENEMA 2535
Cortisporin Ointment 1085
Cortisporin Ophthalmic Ointment Sterile 1085
Cortisporin Ophthalmic Suspension Sterile 1086
Cortisporin Otic Solution Sterile 1087
Cortisporin Otic Suspension Sterile 1088
Cortizone-5 ▣ 831
Cortizone-10 ▣ 831
Hydrocortone Tablets 1672
Hytone 907
Massengill Medicated Soft Cloth Towelettes 2458
PediOtic Suspension Sterile 1153
Preparation H Hydrocortisone 1% Cream ▣ 872
ProctoCream-HC 2.5% 2408
VōSoL HC Otic Solution 2678

Hydrocortisone Acetate (Concomitant use may result in hypokalemia). Products include:
Analpram-HC Rectal Cream 1% and 2.5% 977
Anusol HC-1 Anti-Itch Hydrocortisone Ointment ▣ 847
Anusol-HC Suppositories 1897
Caldecort ▣ 631
Carmol HC 924
Coly-Mycin S Otic w/Neomycin & Hydrocortisone 1906
Cortaid ▣ 836
Cortifoam 2396
Cortisporin Cream 1084
Epifoam 2399
Hydrocortone Acetate Sterile Suspension 1669
Mantadil Cream 1135
Nupercainal Hydrocortisone 1% Cream ▣ 645
Ophthocort ⊙ 311
Pramosone Cream, Lotion & Ointment 978
ProctoCream-HC 2408
ProctoFoam-HC 2409
Terra-Cortril Ophthalmic Suspension 2210

Hydrocortisone Sodium Phosphate (Concomitant use may result in hypokalemia). Products include:
Hydrocortone Phosphate Injection, Sterile 1670

Hydrocortisone Sodium Succinate (Concomitant use may result in hypokalemia). Products include:
Solu-Cortef Sterile Powder 2641

Hydroflumethiazide (Additive or potentiated action). Products include:
Diucardin Tablets 2718

Ibuprofen (Concurrent administration may reduce the diuretic, natriuretic and antihypertensive effects of thiazide diuretics). Products include:
Advil Cold and Sinus Caplets and Tablets (formerly CoAdvil) ▣ 870
Advil Ibuprofen Tablets and Caplets ▣ 870
Children's Advil Suspension 2692
Arthritis Foundation Ibuprofen Tablets ▣ 674
Bayer Select Ibuprofen Pain Relief Formula ▣ 715
Cramp End Tablets ▣ 735
Dimetapp Sinus Caplets ▣ 775
Haltran Tablets ▣ 771
IBU Tablets 1342
Ibuprohm ▣ 735
Children's Motrin Ibuprofen Oral Suspension 1546
Motrin Tablets 2625
Motrin IB Caplets, Tablets, and Geltabs ▣ 838
Motrin IB Sinus ▣ 838
Motrin Ibuprofen Suspension, Oral Drops, Chewable Tablets, Caplets 1546
Nuprin Ibuprofen/Analgesic Tablets & Caplets ▣ 622
Sine-Aid IB Caplets 1554
Vicks DayQuil SINUS Pressure & PAIN Relief with IBUPROFEN ▣ 762

Indapamide (Additive or potentiated action). Products include:
Lozol Tablets 2022

Indomethacin (Concurrent administration may reduce the diuretic, natriuretic and antihypertensive effects of thiazide diuretics). Products include:
Indocin 1680

Indomethacin Sodium Trihydrate (Concurrent administration may reduce the diuretic, natriuretic and antihypertensive effects of thiazide diuretics). Products include:
Indocin I.V. 1684

Insulin, Human (Insulin requirements may be altered).
No products indexed under this heading.

Insulin, Human Isophane Suspension (Insulin requirements may be altered). Products include:
Novolin N Human Insulin 10 ml Vials 1795

Insulin, Human NPH (Insulin requirements may be altered). Products include:
Humulin N, 100 Units 1448
Novolin N PenFill Cartridges Durable Insulin Delivery System 1798
Novolin N Prefilled Syringe Disposable Insulin Delivery System 1798

Insulin, Human Regular (Insulin requirements may be altered). Products include:
Humulin R, 100 Units 1449
Novolin R Human Insulin 10 ml Vials 1795
Novolin R PenFill Cartridges Durable Insulin Delivery System 1798
Novolin R Prefilled Syringe Disposable Insulin Delivery System 1798
Velosulin BR Human Insulin 10 ml Vials 1795

Insulin, Human, Zinc Suspension (Insulin requirements may be altered). Products include:
Humulin L, 100 Units 1446
Humulin U, 100 Units 1450
Novolin L Human Insulin 10 ml Vials 1795

Insulin, NPH (Insulin requirements may be altered). Products include:
NPH, 100 Units 1450
Pork NPH, 100 Units 1452
Purified Pork NPH Isophane Insulin 1801

Insulin, Regular (Insulin requirements may be altered). Products include:
Regular, 100 Units 1450
Pork Regular, 100 Units 1452
Pork Regular (Concentrated), 500 Units 1453
Purified Pork Regular Insulin 1801

Insulin, Zinc Crystals (Insulin requirements may be altered). Products include:
NPH, 100 Units 1450

Insulin, Zinc Suspension (Insulin requirements may be altered). Products include:
Iletin I 1450
Lente, 100 Units 1450
Iletin II 1452
Pork Lente, 100 Units 1452
Purified Pork Lente Insulin 1801

Isocarboxazid (Concurrent use requires caution).
No products indexed under this heading.

Isradipine (Additive or potentiated action). Products include:
DynaCirc Capsules 2256

Ketoprofen (Concurrent administration may reduce the diuretic, natriuretic and antihypertensive effects of thiazide diuretics). Products include:
Orudis Capsules 2766
Oruvail Capsules 2766

Ketorolac Tromethamine (Concurrent administration may reduce the diuretic, natriuretic and antihypertensive effects of thiazide diuretics). Products include:
Acular 474
Acular ⊙ 277
Toradol 2159

Labetalol Hydrochloride (Additive or potentiated action). Products include:
Normodyne Injection 2377
Normodyne Tablets 2379
Trandate 1185

Levorphanol Tartrate (May potentiate orthostatic hypotension). Products include:
Levo-Dromoran 2129

Lisinopril (Additive or potentiated action). Products include:
Prinivil Tablets 1733
Prinzide Tablets 1737
Zestoretic 2850
Zestril Tablets 2854

Lithium Carbonate (Increased risk of lithium toxicity). Products include:
Eskalith 2485
Lithium Carbonate Capsules & Tablets 2230
Lithonate/Lithotabs/Lithobid 2543

Lithium Citrate (Increased risk of lithium toxicity).
No products indexed under this heading.

Losartan Potassium (Additive or potentiated action). Products include:
Cozaar Tablets 1628
Hyzaar Tablets 1677

Mecamylamine Hydrochloride (Additive or potentiated action). Products include:
Inversine Tablets 1686

Meclofenamate Sodium (Concurrent administration may reduce the diuretic, natriuretic and antihypertensive effects of thiazide diuretics).
No products indexed under this heading.

Mefenamic Acid (Concurrent administration may reduce the diuretic, natriuretic and antihypertensive effects of thiazide diuretics). Products include:
Ponstel 1925

Meperidine Hydrochloride (May potentiate orthostatic hypotension). Products include:
Demerol 2308
Mepergan Injection 2753

Mephobarbital (May potentiate orthostatic hypotension). Products include:
Mebaral Tablets 2322

Methadone Hydrochloride (May potentiate orthostatic hypotension). Products include:
Methadone Hydrochloride Oral Concentrate 2233
Methadone Hydrochloride Oral Solution & Tablets 2235

Methyclothiazide (Additive or potentiated action). Products include:
Enduron Tablets 420

Methyldopa (Additive or potentiated action; concomitant use may cause hemolytic anemia). Products include:
Aldoclor Tablets 1598
Aldomet Oral 1600
Aldoril Tablets 1604

Methyldopate Hydrochloride (Additive or potentiated action; concomitant use may cause hemolytic anemia). Products include:
Aldomet Ester HCl Injection 1602

Methylprednisolone (Concomitant use may result in hypokalemia). Products include:
Medrol 2621

Methylprednisolone Acetate (Concomitant use may result in hypokalemia). Products include:
Depo-Medrol Single-Dose Vial 2600

Depo-Medrol Sterile Aqueous Suspension 2597

Methylprednisolone Sodium Succinate (Concomitant use may result in hypokalemia). Products include:
Solu-Medrol Sterile Powder 2643

Metolazone (Additive or potentiated action). Products include:
Mykrox Tablets 993
Zaroxolyn Tablets 1000

Metoprolol Succinate (Additive or potentiated action). Products include:
Toprol-XL Tablets 565

Metoprolol Tartrate (Additive or potentiated action). Products include:
Lopressor Ampuls 830
Lopressor HCT Tablets 832
Lopressor Tablets 830

Metyrosine (Additive or potentiated action). Products include:
Demser Capsules 1649

Minoxidil (Additive or potentiated action). Products include:
Loniten Tablets 2618
Rogaine Topical Solution 2637

Moexipril Hydrochloride (Additive or potentiated action). Products include:
Univasc Tablets 2410

Morphine Sulfate (May potentiate orthostatic hypotension). Products include:
Astramorph/PF Injection, USP (Preservative-Free) 535
Duramorph 962
Infumorph 200 and Infumorph 500 Sterile Solutions 965
MS Contin Tablets 1994
MSIR 1997
Oramorph SR (Morphine Sulfate Sustained Release Tablets) 2236
RMS Suppositories 2657
Roxanol 2243

Nabumetone (Concurrent administration may reduce the diuretic, natriuretic and antihypertensive effects of thiazide diuretics). Products include:
Relafen Tablets 2510

Nadolol (Additive or potentiated action).
No products indexed under this heading.

Naproxen (Concurrent administration may reduce the diuretic, natriuretic and antihypertensive effects of thiazide diuretics). Products include:
Anaprox/Naprosyn 2117

Naproxen Sodium (Concurrent administration may reduce the diuretic, natriuretic and antihypertensive effects of thiazide diuretics). Products include:
Aleve 1975
Anaprox/Naprosyn 2117

Nicardipine Hydrochloride (Additive or potentiated action). Products include:
Cardene Capsules 2095
Cardene I.V. 2709
Cardene SR Capsules 2097

Nifedipine (Additive or potentiated action). Products include:
Adalat Capsules (10 mg and 20 mg) 587
Adalat CC 589
Procardia Capsules 1971
Procardia XL Extended Release Tablets 1972

Nisoldipine (Additive or potentiated action).
No products indexed under this heading.

Nitroglycerin (Additive or potentiated action). Products include:
Deponit NTG Transdermal Delivery System 2397
Nitro-Bid IV 1523
Nitro-Bid Ointment 1524
Nitrodisc 2047
Nitro-Dur (nitroglycerin) Transdermal Infusion System 1326
Nitrolingual Spray 2027
Nitrostat Tablets 1925
Transderm-Nitro Transdermal Therapeutic System 859

Norepinephrine Bitartrate (Decreased arterial response to norepinephrine). Products include:
Levophed Bitartrate Injection 2315

Opium Alkaloids (May potentiate orthostatic hypotension).
No products indexed under this heading.

Oxaprozin (Concurrent administration may reduce the diuretic, natriuretic and antihypertensive effects of thiazide diuretics). Products include:
Daypro Caplets 2426

Oxycodone Hydrochloride (May potentiate orthostatic hypotension). Products include:
Percocet Tablets 938
Percodan Tablets 939
Percodan-Demi Tablets 940
Roxicodone Tablets, Oral Solution & Intensol (Oxycodone) 2244
Tylox Capsules 1584

Pargyline Hydrochloride (Concurrent administration contraindicated).
No products indexed under this heading.

Penbutolol Sulfate (Additive or potentiated action). Products include:
Levatol 2403

Pentobarbital Sodium (May potentiate orthostatic hypotension). Products include:
Nembutal Sodium Capsules 436
Nembutal Sodium Solution 438
Nembutal Sodium Suppositories 440

Phenelzine Sulfate (Concurrent use requires caution). Products include:
Nardil 1920

Phenobarbital (May potentiate orthostatic hypotension). Products include:
Arco-Lase Plus Tablets 512
Bellergal-S Tablets 2250
Donnatal 2060
Donnatal Extentabs 2061
Donnatal Tablets 2060
Phenobarbital Elixir and Tablets 1469
Quadrinal Tablets 1350

Phenoxybenzamine Hydrochloride (Additive or potentiated action). Products include:
Dibenzyline Capsules 2476

Phentolamine Mesylate (Additive or potentiated action). Products include:
Regitine 846

Phenylbutazone (Concurrent administration may reduce the diuretic, natriuretic and antihypertensive effects of thiazide diuretics).
No products indexed under this heading.

Pindolol (Additive or potentiated action). Products include:
Visken Tablets 2299

Piroxicam (Concurrent administration may reduce the diuretic, natriuretic and antihypertensive effects of thiazide diuretics). Products include:
Feldene Capsules 1965

Polythiazide (Additive or potentiated action). Products include:
Minizide Capsules 1938

Prazosin Hydrochloride (Additive or potentiated action). Products include:
Minipress Capsules 1937
Minizide Capsules 1938

Prednisolone Acetate (Concomitant use may result in hypokalemia). Products include:
AK-CIDE .... ◉ 202
AK-CIDE Ointment .... ◉ 202
Blephamide Liquifilm Sterile Ophthalmic Suspension 476
Blephamide Ointment .... ◉ 237
Econopred & Econopred Plus Ophthalmic Suspensions .... ◉ 217
Poly-Pred Liquifilm .... ◉ 248
Pred Forte .... ◉ 250
Pred Mild .... ◉ 253
Pred-G Liquifilm Sterile Ophthalmic Suspension .... ◉ 251
Pred-G S.O.P. Sterile Ophthalmic Ointment .... ◉ 252
Vasocidin Ointment .... ◉ 268

Prednisolone Sodium Phosphate (Concomitant use may result in hypokalemia). Products include:
AK-Pred .... ◉ 204
Hydeltrasol Injection, Sterile 1665
Inflamase .... ◉ 265
Pediapred Oral Liquid 995
Vasocidin Ophthalmic Solution .... ◉ 270

Prednisolone Tebutate (Concomitant use may result in hypokalemia). Products include:
Hydeltra-T.B.A. Sterile Suspension 1667

Prednisone (Concomitant use may result in hypokalemia). Products include:
Deltasone Tablets 2595

Propoxyphene Hydrochloride (May potentiate orthostatic hypotension). Products include:
Darvon 1435
Wygesic Tablets 2827

Propoxyphene Napsylate (May potentiate orthostatic hypotension). Products include:
Darvon-N/Darvocet-N 1433

Propranolol Hydrochloride (Additive or potentiated action). Products include:
Inderal 2728
Inderal LA Long Acting Capsules 2730
Inderide Tablets 2732
Inderide LA Long Acting Capsules 2734

Quinapril Hydrochloride (Additive or potentiated action). Products include:
Accupril Tablets 1893

Ramipril (Additive or potentiated action). Products include:
Altace Capsules 1232

Rauwolfia Serpentina (Additive or potentiated action).
No products indexed under this heading.

Rescinnamine (Additive or potentiated action).
No products indexed under this heading.

Reserpine (Additive or potentiated action). Products include:
Diupres Tablets 1650
Hydropres Tablets 1675
Ser-Ap-Es Tablets 849

Secobarbital Sodium (May potentiate orthostatic hypotension). Products include:
Seconal Sodium Pulvules 1474

Selegiline Hydrochloride (Concurrent use requires caution). Products include:
Eldepryl Tablets 2550

Sodium Nitroprusside (Additive or potentiated action).
No products indexed under this heading.

Sotalol Hydrochloride (Additive or potentiated action). Products include:
Betapace Tablets 641

Spirapril Hydrochloride (Additive or potentiated action).
No products indexed under this heading.

Sufentanil Citrate (May potentiate orthostatic hypotension). Products include:
Sufenta Injection 1309

Sulindac (Concurrent administration may reduce the diuretic, natriuretic and antihypertensive effects of thiazide diuretics). Products include:
Clinoril Tablets 1618

Terazosin Hydrochloride (Additive or potentiated action). Products include:
Hytrin Capsules 430

Thiamylal Sodium (May potentiate orthostatic hypotension).
No products indexed under this heading.

Timolol Maleate (Additive or potentiated action). Products include:
Blocadren Tablets 1614
Timolide Tablets 1748
Timoptic in Ocudose 1753
Timoptic Sterile Ophthalmic Solution 1751
Timoptic-XE 1755

Tolmetin Sodium (Concurrent administration may reduce the diuretic, natriuretic and antihypertensive effects of thiazide diuretics). Products include:
Tolectin (200, 400 and 600 mg) 1581

Torsemide (Additive or potentiated action). Products include:
Demadex Tablets and Injection 686

Tranylcypromine Sulfate (Concurrent use requires caution). Products include:
Parnate Tablets 2503

Triamcinolone (Concomitant use may result in hypokalemia). Products include:
Aristocort Tablets 1022

Triamcinolone Acetonide (Concomitant use may result in hypokalemia). Products include:
Aristocort A 0.025% Cream 1027
Aristocort A 0.5% Cream 1031
Aristocort A 0.1% Cream 1029
Aristocort A 0.1% Ointment 1030
Azmacort Oral Inhaler 2011
Nasacort Nasal Inhaler 2024

Triamcinolone Diacetate (Concomitant use may result in hypokalemia). Products include:
Aristocort Suspension (Forte Parenteral) 1027
Aristocort Suspension (Intralesional) 1025

Triamcinolone Hexacetonide (Concomitant use may result in hypokalemia). Products include:
Aristospan Suspension (Intra-articular) 1033
Aristospan Suspension (Intralesional) 1032

Trimethaphan Camsylate (Additive or potentiated action). Products include:
Arfonad Ampuls 2080

Tubocurarine Chloride (Increased responsiveness to tubocurarine).
No products indexed under this heading.

Verapamil Hydrochloride (Additive or potentiated action). Products include:
Calan SR Caplets 2422
Calan Tablets 2419

IMPORTANT NOTE: Always consult each drug listing in the patient's regimen for possible interactions.

Isoptin Injectable 1344
Isoptin Oral Tablets 1346
Isoptin SR Tablets 1348
Verelan Capsules 1410
Verelan Capsules 2824

Food Interactions

Alcohol (May potentiate orthostatic hypotension).

Food, unspecified (Enhances gastrointestinal absorption of hydrochlorothiazide).

APRESOLINE HYDROCHLORIDE TABLETS

(Hydralazine Hydrochloride) 809

May interact with monoamine oxidase inhibitors and certain other agents. Compounds in these categories include:

Diazoxide (Profound hypotensive episodes). Products include:

Hyperstat I.V. Injection 2363
Proglycem 580

Epinephrine (Pressor responses to epinephrine may be reduced). Products include:

Bronkaid Mist .... ▣ 717
EPIFRIN .... ◉ 239
EpiPen 790
Marcaine Hydrochloride with Epinephrine 1:200,000 2316
Primatene Mist .... ▣ 873
Sensorcaine with Epinephrine Injection 559
Sus-Phrine Injection 1019
Xylocaine with Epinephrine Injections 567

Epinephrine Bitartrate (Pressor responses to epinephrine may be reduced). Products include:

Bronkaid Mist Suspension .... ▣ 718
Sensorcaine-MPF with Epinephrine Injection 559

Furazolidone (Concurrent administration contraindicated). Products include:

Furoxone 2046

Isocarboxazid (Concurrent administration contraindicated).

No products indexed under this heading.

Phenelzine Sulfate (Concurrent administration contraindicated). Products include:

Nardil 1920

Selegiline Hydrochloride (Concurrent administration contraindicated). Products include:

Eldepryl Tablets 2550

Tranylcypromine Sulfate (Concurrent administration contraindicated). Products include:

Parnate Tablets 2503

Food Interactions

Food, unspecified (Results in higher plasma levels).

AQUADERM CREAM

(Caprylic/Capric Triglyceride) .... ▣ 604
None cited in PDR database.

AQUADERM LOTION

(Caprylic/Capric Triglyceride) .... ▣ 604
None cited in PDR database.

AQUADERM SUNSCREEN/MOISTURIZER-SPF 15

(Octyl Methoxycinnamate, Oxybenzone) .... ▣ 604
None cited in PDR database.

AQUAMEPHYTON INJECTION

(Phytonadione) 1608

May interact with oral anticoagulants. Compounds in this category include:

Dicumarol (Temporary resistance to anticoagulants).

No products indexed under this heading.

Warfarin Sodium (Temporary resistance to anticoagulants). Products include:

Coumadin 926

AQUANIL LOTION

(Cetyl Alcohol, Glycerin) 1932
None cited in PDR database.

AQUANIL HC LOTION

(Hydrocortisone) 1931
None cited in PDR database.

AQUAPHOR HEALING OINTMENT

(Petrolatum, Mineral Oil) 640
None cited in PDR database.

AQUAPHOR HEALING OINTMENT, ORIGINAL FORMULA

(Mineral Oil, Petrolatum) 640
None cited in PDR database.

AQUASITE EYE DROPS

(Polyethylene Glycol, Dextran 70) .. ◉ 261
None cited in PDR database.

AQUASOL A VITAMIN A CAPSULES, USP

(Vitamin A) 534

May interact with oral contraceptives. Compounds in this category include:

Desogestrel (Potential for a significant increase in plasma vitamin A levels). Products include:

Desogen Tablets 1817
Ortho-Cept 1851

Ethinyl Estradiol (Potential for a significant increase in plasma vitamin A levels). Products include:

Brevicon 2088
Demulen 2428
Desogen Tablets 1817
Levlen/Tri-Levlen 651
Lo/Ovral Tablets 2746
Lo/Ovral-28 Tablets 2751
Modicon 1872
Nordette-21 Tablets 2755
Nordette-28 Tablets 2758
Norinyl 2088
Ortho-Cept 1851
Ortho-Cyclen/Ortho-Tri-Cyclen 1858
Ortho-Novum 1872
Ortho-Cyclen/Ortho Tri-Cyclen 1858
Ovcon 760
Ovral Tablets 2770
Ovral-28 Tablets 2770
Levlen/Tri-Levlen 651
Tri-Norinyl 2164
Triphasil-21 Tablets 2814
Triphasil-28 Tablets 2819

Ethynodiol Diacetate (Potential for a significant increase in plasma vitamin A levels). Products include:

Demulen 2428

Levonorgestrel (Potential for a significant increase in plasma vitamin A levels). Products include:

Levlen/Tri-Levlen 651
Nordette-21 Tablets 2755
Nordette-28 Tablets 2758
Norplant System 2759
Levlen/Tri-Levlen 651
Triphasil-21 Tablets 2814
Triphasil-28 Tablets 2819

Mestranol (Potential for a significant increase in plasma vitamin A levels). Products include:

Norinyl 2088
Ortho-Novum 1872

Norethindrone (Potential for a significant increase in plasma vitamin A levels). Products include:

Brevicon 2088
Micronor Tablets 1872
Modicon 1872
Norinyl 2088
Nor-Q D Tablets 2135
Ortho-Novum 1872
Ovcon 760
Tri-Norinyl 2164

Norethynodrel (Potential for a significant increase in plasma vitamin A levels).

No products indexed under this heading.

Norgestimate (Potential for a significant increase in plasma vitamin A levels). Products include:

Ortho-Cyclen/Ortho-Tri-Cyclen 1858
Ortho-Cyclen/Ortho Tri-Cyclen 1858

Norgestrel (Potential for a significant increase in plasma vitamin A levels). Products include:

Lo/Ovral Tablets 2746
Lo/Ovral-28 Tablets 2751
Ovral Tablets 2770
Ovral-28 Tablets 2770
Ovrette Tablets 2771

AQUASOL A PARENTERAL

(Vitamin A) 534

May interact with oral contraceptives. Compounds in this category include:

Desogestrel (Potential for a significant increase in plasma vitamin A levels). Products include:

Desogen Tablets 1817
Ortho-Cept 1851

Ethinyl Estradiol (Potential for a significant increase in plasma vitamin A levels). Products include:

Brevicon 2088
Demulen 2428
Desogen Tablets 1817
Levlen/Tri-Levlen 651
Lo/Ovral Tablets 2746
Lo/Ovral-28 Tablets 2751
Modicon 1872
Nordette-21 Tablets 2755
Nordette-28 Tablets 2758
Norinyl 2088
Ortho-Cept 1851
Ortho-Cyclen/Ortho-Tri-Cyclen 1858
Ortho-Novum 1872
Ortho-Cyclen/Ortho Tri-Cyclen 1858
Ovcon 760
Ovral Tablets 2770
Ovral-28 Tablets 2770
Levlen/Tri-Levlen 651
Tri-Norinyl 2164
Triphasil-21 Tablets 2814
Triphasil-28 Tablets 2819

Ethynodiol Diacetate (Potential for a significant increase in plasma vitamin A levels). Products include:

Demulen 2428

Levonorgestrel (Potential for a significant increase in plasma vitamin A levels). Products include:

Levlen/Tri-Levlen 651
Nordette-21 Tablets 2755
Nordette-28 Tablets 2758
Norplant System 2759
Levlen/Tri-Levlen 651
Triphasil-21 Tablets 2814
Triphasil-28 Tablets 2819

Mestranol (Potential for a significant increase in plasma vitamin A levels). Products include:

Norinyl 2088
Ortho-Novum 1872

Norethindrone (Potential for a significant increase in plasma vitamin A levels). Products include:

Brevicon 2088
Micronor Tablets 1872
Modicon 1872
Norinyl 2088
Nor-Q D Tablets 2135
Ortho-Novum 1872
Ovcon 760
Tri-Norinyl 2164

Norethynodrel (Potential for a significant increase in plasma vitamin A levels).

No products indexed under this heading.

Norgestimate (Potential for a significant increase in plasma vitamin A levels). Products include:

Ortho-Cyclen/Ortho-Tri-Cyclen 1858
Ortho-Cyclen/Ortho Tri-Cyclen 1858

Norgestrel (Potential for a significant increase in plasma vitamin A levels). Products include:

Lo/Ovral Tablets 2746
Lo/Ovral-28 Tablets 2751
Ovral Tablets 2770
Ovral-28 Tablets 2770
Ovrette Tablets 2771

ARALEN HYDROCHLORIDE INJECTION

(Chloroquine Hydrochloride) 2301

May interact with:

Hepatotoxic Drugs, unspecified (Concurrent use requires caution).

ARALEN PHOSPHATE TABLETS

(Chloroquine Phosphate) 2301

May interact with:

Hepatotoxic Drugs, unspecified (Caution should be exercised when used in conjunction with known hepatotoxic drugs).

ARAMINE INJECTION

(Metaraminol Bitartrate) 1609

May interact with cardiac glycosides, monoamine oxidase inhibitors, tricyclic antidepressants, and certain other agents. Compounds in these categories include:

Amitriptyline Hydrochloride (Potentiates pressor effect). Products include:

Elavil 2838
Endep Tablets 2174
Etrafon 2355
Limbitrol 2180
Triavil Tablets 1757

Amoxapine (Potentiates pressor effect). Products include:

Asendin Tablets 1369

Clomipramine Hydrochloride (Potentiates pressor effect). Products include:

Anafranil Capsules 803

Desipramine Hydrochloride (Potentiates pressor effect). Products include:

Norpramin Tablets 1526

Deslanoside (May cause ectopic arrhythmic reaction).

No products indexed under this heading.

Digitoxin (May cause ectopic arrhythmic reaction). Products include:

Crystodigin Tablets 1433

Digoxin (May cause ectopic arrhythmic reaction). Products include:

Lanoxicaps 1117
Lanoxin Elixir Pediatric 1120
Lanoxin Injection 1123
Lanoxin Injection Pediatric 1126
Lanoxin Tablets 1128

Doxepin Hydrochloride (Potentiates pressor effect). Products include:

Sinequan 2205
Zonalon Cream 1055

Furazolidone (Potentiates pressor effect). Products include:

Furoxone 2046

Halothane (Concurrent use should be avoided). Products include:

Fluothane 2724

Imipramine Hydrochloride (Potentiates pressor effect). Products include:
Tofranil Ampuls 854
Tofranil Tablets 856

Imipramine Pamoate (Potentiates pressor effect). Products include:
Tofranil-PM Capsules 857

Isocarboxazid (Potentiates pressor effect).
No products indexed under this heading.

Maprotiline Hydrochloride (Potentiates pressor effect). Products include:
Ludiomil Tablets 843

Nortriptyline Hydrochloride (Potentiates pressor effect). Products include:
Pamelor 2280

Phenelzine Sulfate (Potentiates pressor effect). Products include:
Nardil 1920

Protriptyline Hydrochloride (Potentiates pressor effect). Products include:
Vivactil Tablets 1774

Selegiline Hydrochloride (Potentiates pressor effect). Products include:
Eldepryl Tablets 2550

Tranylcypromine Sulfate (Potentiates pressor effect). Products include:
Parnate Tablets 2503

Trimipramine Maleate (Potentiates pressor effect). Products include:
Surmontil Capsules 2811

ARCO-LASE PLUS TABLETS
(Enzymes, Digestive) 512
None cited in PDR database.

ARCO-LASE TABLETS
(Enzymes, Digestive) 512
None cited in PDR database.

AREDIA FOR INJECTION
(Pamidronate Disodium) 810
None cited in PDR database.

ARFONAD AMPULS
(Trimethaphan Camsylate) 2080
May interact with antihypertensives, diuretics, nondepolarizing neuromuscular blocking agents, and certain other agents. Compounds in these categories include:

Acebutolol Hydrochloride (Additive hypotensive effect). Products include:
Sectral Capsules 2807

Amiloride Hydrochloride (Enhances ganglionic blocking effects). Products include:
Midamor Tablets 1703
Moduretic Tablets 1705

Amlodipine Besylate (Additive hypotensive effect). Products include:
Lotrel Capsules 840
Norvasc Tablets 1940

Atenolol (Additive hypotensive effect). Products include:
Tenoretic Tablets 2845
Tenormin Tablets and I.V. Injection 2847

Atracurium Besylate (Prolonged effects of neuromuscular blocking agents). Products include:
Tracrium Injection 1183

Benazepril Hydrochloride (Additive hypotensive effect). Products include:
Lotensin Tablets 834
Lotensin HCT 837
Lotrel Capsules 840

Bendroflumethiazide (Enhances ganglionic blocking effects; additive hypotensive effect).
No products indexed under this heading.

Betaxolol Hydrochloride (Additive hypotensive effect). Products include:
Betoptic Ophthalmic Solution 469
Betoptic S Ophthalmic Suspension 471
Kerlone Tablets 2436

Bisoprolol Fumarate (Additive hypotensive effect). Products include:
Zebeta Tablets 1413
Ziac 1415

Bumetanide (Enhances ganglionic blocking effects). Products include:
Bumex 2093

Bupivacaine Hydrochloride (Additive hypotensive effect). Products include:
Marcaine Hydrochloride with Epinephrine 1:200,000 2316
Marcaine Hydrochloride Injection 2316
Marcaine Spinal 2319
Sensorcaine 559

Captopril (Additive hypotensive effect). Products include:
Capoten 739
Capozide 742

Carteolol Hydrochloride (Additive hypotensive effect). Products include:
Cartrol Tablets 410
Ocupress Ophthalmic Solution, 1% Sterile .... ◉ 309

Chlorothiazide (Enhances ganglionic blocking effects; additive hypotensive effect). Products include:
Aldoclor Tablets 1598
Diupres Tablets 1650
Diuril Oral 1653

Chlorothiazide Sodium (Enhances ganglionic blocking effects; additive hypotensive effect). Products include:
Diuril Sodium Intravenous 1652

Chlorthalidone (Additive hypotensive effect; enhances ganglionic blocking effects). Products include:
Combipres Tablets 677
Tenoretic Tablets 2845
Thalitone 1245

Clonidine (Additive hypotensive effect). Products include:
Catapres-TTS 675

Clonidine Hydrochloride (Additive hypotensive effect). Products include:
Catapres Tablets 674
Combipres Tablets 677

Deserpidine (Additive hypotensive effect).
No products indexed under this heading.

Diazoxide (Additive hypotensive effect). Products include:
Hyperstat I.V. Injection 2363
Proglycem 580

Diltiazem Hydrochloride (Additive hypotensive effect). Products include:
Cardizem CD Capsules 1506
Cardizem SR Capsules 1510
Cardizem Injectable 1508
Cardizem Tablets 1512
Dilacor XR Extended-release Capsules 2018

Doxazosin Mesylate (Additive hypotensive effect). Products include:
Cardura Tablets 2186

Enalapril Maleate (Additive hypotensive effect). Products include:
Vaseretic Tablets 1765
Vasotec Tablets 1771

Enalaprilat (Additive hypotensive effect). Products include:
Vasotec I.V. 1768

Esmolol Hydrochloride (Additive hypotensive effect). Products include:
Brevibloc Injection 1808

Ethacrynic Acid (Enhances ganglionic blocking effects). Products include:
Edecrin Tablets 1657

Felodipine (Additive hypotensive effect). Products include:
Plendil Extended-Release Tablets 527

Fosinopril Sodium (Additive hypotensive effect). Products include:
Monopril Tablets 757

Furosemide (Enhances ganglionic blocking effects; additive hypotensive effect). Products include:
Lasix Injection, Oral Solution and Tablets 1240

Guanabenz Acetate (Additive hypotensive effect).
No products indexed under this heading.

Guanethidine Monosulfate (Additive hypotensive effect). Products include:
Esimil Tablets 822
Ismelin Tablets 827

Hydralazine Hydrochloride (Additive hypotensive effect). Products include:
Apresazide Capsules 808
Apresoline Hydrochloride Tablets .. 809
Ser-Ap-Es Tablets 849

Hydrochlorothiazide (Enhances ganglionic blocking effects; additive hypotensive effect). Products include:
Aldactazide 2413
Aldoril Tablets 1604
Apresazide Capsules 808
Capozide 742
Dyazide 2479
Esidrix Tablets 821
Esimil Tablets 822
HydroDIURIL Tablets 1674
Hydropres Tablets 1675
Hyzaar Tablets 1677
Inderide Tablets 2732
Inderide LA Long Acting Capsules .. 2734
Lopressor HCT Tablets 832
Lotensin HCT 837
Maxzide 1380
Moduretic Tablets 1705
Oretic Tablets 443
Prinzide Tablets 1737
Ser-Ap-Es Tablets 849
Timolide Tablets 1748
Vaseretic Tablets 1765
Zestoretic 2850
Ziac 1415

Hydroflumethiazide (Enhances ganglionic blocking effects; additive hypotensive effect). Products include:
Diucardin Tablets 2718

Indapamide (Enhances ganglionic blocking effects; additive hypotensive effect). Products include:
Lozol Tablets 2022

Isradipine (Additive hypotensive effect). Products include:
DynaCirc Capsules 2256

Labetalol Hydrochloride (Additive hypotensive effect). Products include:
Normodyne Injection 2377
Normodyne Tablets 2379
Trandate 1185

Lisinopril (Additive hypotensive effect). Products include:
Prinivil Tablets 1733
Prinzide Tablets 1737
Zestoretic 2850
Zestril Tablets 2854

Losartan Potassium (Additive hypotensive effect). Products include:
Cozaar Tablets 1628
Hyzaar Tablets 1677

Mecamylamine Hydrochloride (Additive hypotensive effect). Products include:
Inversine Tablets 1686

Methyclothiazide (Enhances ganglionic blocking effects; additive hypotensive effect). Products include:
Enduron Tablets 420

Methyldopa (Additive hypotensive effect). Products include:
Aldoclor Tablets 1598
Aldomet Oral 1600
Aldoril Tablets 1604

Methyldopate Hydrochloride (Additive hypotensive effect). Products include:
Aldomet Ester HCl Injection 1602

Metocurine Iodide (Prolonged effects of neuromuscular blocking agents). Products include:
Metubine Iodide Vials 916

Metolazone (Enhances ganglionic blocking effects; additive hypotensive effect). Products include:
Mykrox Tablets 993
Zaroxolyn Tablets 1000

Metoprolol Succinate (Additive hypotensive effect). Products include:
Toprol-XL Tablets 565

Metoprolol Tartrate (Additive hypotensive effect). Products include:
Lopressor Ampuls 830
Lopressor HCT Tablets 832
Lopressor Tablets 830

Metyrosine (Additive hypotensive effect). Products include:
Demser Capsules 1649

Minoxidil (Additive hypotensive effect). Products include:
Loniten Tablets 2618
Rogaine Topical Solution 2637

Mivacurium Chloride (Prolonged effects of neuromuscular blocking agents). Products include:
Mivacron 1138

Moexipril Hydrochloride (Additive hypotensive effect). Products include:
Univasc Tablets 2410

Nadolol (Additive hypotensive effect).
No products indexed under this heading.

Nicardipine Hydrochloride (Additive hypotensive effect). Products include:
Cardene Capsules 2095
Cardene I.V. 2709
Cardene SR Capsules 2097

Nifedipine (Additive hypotensive effect). Products include:
Adalat Capsules (10 mg and 20 mg) 587
Adalat CC 589
Procardia Capsules 1971
Procardia XL Extended Release Tablets 1972

Nisoldipine (Additive hypotensive effect).
No products indexed under this heading.

Nitroglycerin (Additive hypotensive effect). Products include:
Deponit NTG Transdermal Delivery System 2397
Nitro-Bid IV 1523
Nitro-Bid Ointment 1524
Nitrodisc 2047
Nitro-Dur (nitroglycerin) Transdermal Infusion System 1326
Nitrolingual Spray 2027
Nitrostat Tablets 1925

IMPORTANT NOTE: Always consult each drug listing in the patient's regimen for possible interactions.

Arfonad Interactions Index 76

Transderm-Nitro Transdermal Therapeutic System 859

Pancuronium Bromide Injection (Prolonged effects of neuromuscular blocking agents).
No products indexed under this heading.

Penbutolol Sulfate (Additive hypotensive effect). Products include:
Levatol 2403

Phenoxybenzamine Hydrochloride (Additive hypotensive effect). Products include:
Dibenzyline Capsules 2476

Phentolamine Mesylate (Additive hypotensive effect). Products include:
Regitine 846

Pindolol (Additive hypotensive effect). Products include:
Visken Tablets 2299

Polythiazide (Enhances ganglionic blocking effects; additive hypotensive effect). Products include:
Minizide Capsules 1938

Prazosin Hydrochloride (Additive hypotensive effect). Products include:
Minipress Capsules 1937
Minizide Capsules 1938

Procainamide Hydrochloride (Additive hypotensive effect). Products include:
Procan SR Tablets 1926

Procaine Hydrochloride (Additive hypotensive effect). Products include:
Novocain Hydrochloride for Spinal Anesthesia 2326

Propranolol Hydrochloride (Additive hypotensive effect). Products include:
Inderal 2728
Inderal LA Long Acting Capsules 2730
Inderide Tablets 2732
Inderide LA Long Acting Capsules 2734

Quinapril Hydrochloride (Additive hypotensive effect). Products include:
Accupril Tablets 1893

Ramipril (Additive hypotensive effect). Products include:
Altace Capsules 1232

Rauwolfia Serpentina (Additive hypotensive effect).
No products indexed under this heading.

Rescinnamine (Additive hypotensive effect).
No products indexed under this heading.

Reserpine (Additive hypotensive effect). Products include:
Diupres Tablets 1650
Hydropres Tablets 1675
Ser-Ap-Es Tablets 849

Rocuronium Bromide (Prolonged effects of neuromuscular blocking agents). Products include:
Zemuron 1830

Sodium Nitroprusside (Additive hypotensive effect).
No products indexed under this heading.

Sotalol Hydrochloride (Additive hypotensive effect). Products include:
Betapace Tablets 641

Spirapril Hydrochloride (Additive hypotensive effect).
No products indexed under this heading.

Spironolactone (Enhances ganglionic blocking effects). Products include:
Aldactazide 2413
Aldactone 2414

Terazosin Hydrochloride (Additive hypotensive effect). Products include:
Hytrin Capsules 430

Tetracaine Hydrochloride (Additive hypotensive effect). Products include:
Cetacaine Topical Anesthetic 794
Pontocaine Hydrochloride for Spinal Anesthesia 2330

Timolol Maleate (Additive hypotensive effect). Products include:
Blocadren Tablets 1614
Timolide Tablets 1748
Timoptic in Ocudose 1753
Timoptic Sterile Ophthalmic Solution 1751
Timoptic-XE 1755

Torsemide (Additive hypotensive effect). Products include:
Demadex Tablets and Injection 686

Triamterene (Enhances ganglionic blocking effects). Products include:
Dyazide 2479
Dyrenium Capsules 2481
Maxzide 1380

Vecuronium Bromide (Prolonged effects of neuromuscular blocking agents). Products include:
Norcuron 1826

Verapamil Hydrochloride (Additive hypotensive effect). Products include:
Calan SR Caplets 2422
Calan Tablets 2419
Isoptin Injectable 1344
Isoptin Oral Tablets 1346
Isoptin SR Tablets 1348
Verelan Capsules 1410
Verelan Capsules 2824

ARISTOCORT SUSPENSION (FORTE PARENTERAL)

(Triamcinolone Diacetate) 1027
May interact with oral hypoglycemic agents. Compounds in this category include:

Acarbose (Increased requirements for oral hypoglycemic agents in diabetes).
No products indexed under this heading.

Aspirin (Aspirin should be used cautiously in conjunction with corticosteroids in hypoprothrombinemia). Products include:
Alka-Seltzer Effervescent Antacid and Pain Reliever .... ▣ 701
Alka-Seltzer Extra Strength Effervescent Antacid and Pain Reliever .... ▣ 703
Alka-Seltzer Lemon Lime Effervescent Antacid and Pain Reliever .... ▣ 703
Alka-Seltzer Plus Cold Medicine .... ▣ 705
Alka-Seltzer Plus Cold & Cough Medicine .... ▣ 708
Alka-Seltzer Plus Night-Time Cold Medicine .... ▣ 707
Alka Seltzer Plus Sinus Medicine .... ▣ 707
Arthritis Foundation Safety Coated Aspirin Tablets .... ▣ 675
Arthritis Pain Ascriptin .... ▣ 631
Maximum Strength Ascriptin .... ▣ 630
Regular Strength Ascriptin Tablets .... ▣ 629
Arthritis Strength BC Powder .... ▣ 609
BC Cold Powder Multi-Symptom Formula (Cold-Sinus-Allergy) .... ▣ 609
BC Cold Powder Non-Drowsy Formula (Cold-Sinus) .... ▣ 609
BC Powder .... ▣ 609
Bayer Children's Chewable Aspirin .... ▣ 711
Genuine Bayer Aspirin Tablets & Caplets .... ▣ 713
Extra Strength Bayer Arthritis Pain Regimen Formula .... ▣ 711
Extra Strength Bayer Aspirin Caplets & Tablets .... ▣ 712
Extended-Release Bayer 8-Hour Aspirin .... ▣ 712
Extra Strength Bayer Plus Aspirin Caplets .... ▣ 713
Extra Strength Bayer PM Aspirin .... ▣ 713
Bayer Enteric Aspirin .... ▣ 709
Bufferin Analgesic Tablets and Caplets .... ▣ 613
Arthritis Strength Bufferin Analgesic Caplets .... ▣ 614
Extra Strength Bufferin Analgesic Tablets .... ▣ 615
Cama Arthritis Pain Reliever .... ▣ 785
Darvon Compound-65 Pulvules 1435
Easprin 1914
Ecotrin 2455
Ecotrin Enteric Coated Aspirin Maximum Strength Tablets and Caplets .... ▣ 816
Ecotrin Enteric Coated Aspirin Regular Strength Tablets 2455
Empirin Aspirin Tablets .... ▣ 854
Empirin with Codeine Tablets 1093
Excedrin Extra-Strength Analgesic Tablets & Caplets 732
Fiorinal Capsules 2261
Fiorinal with Codeine Capsules 2262
Fiorinal Tablets 2261
Halfprin 1362
Healthprin Aspirin 2455
Norgesic 1496
Percodan Tablets 939
Percodan-Demi Tablets 940
Robaxisal Tablets 2071
Soma Compound w/Codeine Tablets 2676
Soma Compound Tablets 2675
St. Joseph Adult Chewable Aspirin (81 mg.) .... ▣ 808
Talwin Compound 2335
Ursinus Inlay-Tabs .... ▣ 794
Vanquish Analgesic Caplets .... ▣ 731

Chlorpropamide (Increased requirements for oral hypoglycemic agents in diabetes). Products include:
Diabinese Tablets 1935

Glipizide (Increased requirements for oral hypoglycemic agents in diabetes). Products include:
Glucotrol Tablets 1967
Glucotrol XL Extended Release Tablets 1968

Glyburide (Increased requirements for oral hypoglycemic agents in diabetes). Products include:
DiaBeta Tablets 1239
Glynase PresTab Tablets 2609
Micronase Tablets 2623

Immunization (Potential for neurological complications and lack of antibody response, especially, in patients on high dose of corticosteroids).

Insulin, Human (Increased requirements for insulin in diabetes).
No products indexed under this heading.

Insulin, Human Isophane Suspension (Increased requirements for insulin in diabetes). Products include:
Novolin N Human Insulin 10 ml Vials 1795

Insulin, Human NPH (Increased requirements for insulin in diabetes). Products include:
Humulin N, 100 Units 1448
Novolin N PenFill Cartridges Durable Insulin Delivery System 1798
Novolin N Prefilled Syringe Disposable Insulin Delivery System 1798

Insulin, Human Regular (Increased requirements for insulin in diabetes). Products include:
Humulin R, 100 Units 1449
Novolin R Human Insulin 10 ml Vials 1795
Novolin R PenFill Cartridges Durable Insulin Delivery System 1798
Novolin R Prefilled Syringe Disposable Insulin Delivery System 1798
Velosulin BR Human Insulin 10 ml Vials 1795

Insulin, Human, Zinc Suspension (Increased requirements for insulin in diabetes). Products include:
Humulin L, 100 Units 1446
Humulin U, 100 Units 1450
Novolin L Human Insulin 10 ml Vials 1795

Insulin, NPH (Increased requirements for insulin in diabetes). Products include:
NPH, 100 Units 1450
Pork NPH, 100 Units 1452
Purified Pork NPH Isophane Insulin 1801

Insulin, Regular (Increased requirements for insulin in diabetes). Products include:
Regular, 100 Units 1450
Pork Regular, 100 Units 1452
Pork Regular (Concentrated), 500 Units 1453
Purified Pork Regular Insulin 1801

Insulin, Zinc Crystals (Increased requirements for insulin in diabetes). Products include:
NPH, 100 Units 1450

Insulin, Zinc Suspension (Increased requirements for insulin in diabetes). Products include:
Iletin I 1450
Lente, 100 Units 1450
Iletin II 1452
Pork Lente, 100 Units 1452
Purified Pork Lente Insulin 1801

Metformin Hydrochloride (Increased requirements for oral hypoglycemic agents in diabetes). Products include:
Glucophage 752

Smallpox Vaccine (Potential for neurological complications and lack of antibody response, especially, in patients on high dose of corticosteroids).

Tolazamide (Increased requirements for oral hypoglycemic agents in diabetes).
No products indexed under this heading.

Tolbutamide (Increased requirements for oral hypoglycemic agents in diabetes).
No products indexed under this heading.

ARISTOCORT SUSPENSION (INTRALESIONAL)

(Triamcinolone Diacetate) 1025
May interact with oral hypoglycemic agents, insulin, and certain other agents. Compounds in these categories include:

Acarbose (Increased requirements for oral hypoglycemic agents in diabetes).
No products indexed under this heading.

Aspirin (Aspirin should be used cautiously in conjunction with corticosteroid in hypoprothrombinemia). Products include:
Alka-Seltzer Effervescent Antacid and Pain Reliever .... ▣ 701
Alka-Seltzer Extra Strength Effervescent Antacid and Pain Reliever .... ▣ 703
Alka-Seltzer Lemon Lime Effervescent Antacid and Pain Reliever .... ▣ 703
Alka-Seltzer Plus Cold Medicine .... ▣ 705
Alka-Seltzer Plus Cold & Cough Medicine .... ▣ 708
Alka-Seltzer Plus Night-Time Cold Medicine .... ▣ 707
Alka Seltzer Plus Sinus Medicine .... ▣ 707
Arthritis Foundation Safety Coated Aspirin Tablets .... ▣ 675
Arthritis Pain Ascriptin .... ▣ 631
Maximum Strength Ascriptin .... ▣ 630

(▣ Described in PDR For Nonprescription Drugs) (◉ Described in PDR For Ophthalmology)

Interactions Index

Aristospan Suspension 20 mg/mL

Regular Strength Ascriptin Tablets .... ✦D 629
Arthritis Strength BC Powder .... ✦D 609
BC Cold Powder Multi-Symptom Formula (Cold-Sinus-Allergy) ...... ✦D 609
BC Cold Powder Non-Drowsy Formula (Cold-Sinus) .... ✦D 609
BC Powder .... ✦D 609
Bayer Children's Chewable Aspirin .... ✦D 711
Genuine Bayer Aspirin Tablets & Caplets .... ✦D 713
Extra Strength Bayer Arthritis Pain Regimen Formula .... ✦D 711
Extra Strength Bayer Aspirin Caplets & Tablets .... ✦D 712
Extended-Release Bayer 8-Hour Aspirin .... ✦D 712
Extra Strength Bayer Plus Aspirin Caplets .... ✦D 713
Extra Strength Bayer PM Aspirin .. ✦D 713
Bayer Enteric Aspirin .... ✦D 709
Bufferin Analgesic Tablets and Caplets .... ✦D 613
Arthritis Strength Bufferin Analgesic Caplets .... ✦D 614
Extra Strength Bufferin Analgesic Tablets .... ✦D 615
Cama Arthritis Pain Reliever............. ✦D 785
Darvon Compound-65 Pulvules 1435
Easprin 1914
Ecotrin 2455
Ecotrin Enteric Coated Aspirin Maximum Strength Tablets and Caplets .... ✦D 816
Ecotrin Enteric Coated Aspirin Regular Strength Tablets 2455
Empirin Aspirin Tablets .... ✦D 854
Empirin with Codeine Tablets............ 1093
Excedrin Extra-Strength Analgesic Tablets & Caplets 732
Fiorinal Capsules 2261
Fiorinal with Codeine Capsules 2262
Fiorinal Tablets 2261
Halfprin 1362
Healthprin Aspirin 2455
Norgesic... 1496
Percodan Tablets 939
Percodan-Demi Tablets......................... 940
Robaxisal Tablets..................................... 2071
Soma Compound w/Codeine Tablets 2676
Soma Compound Tablets..................... 2675
St. Joseph Adult Chewable Aspirin (81 mg.) .... ✦D 808
Talwin Compound 2335
Ursinus Inlay-Tabs.................................. ✦D 794
Vanquish Analgesic Caplets .... ✦D 731

Chlorpropamide (Increased requirements for oral hypoglycemic agents in diabetes). Products include:

Diabinese Tablets 1935

Glipizide (Increased requirements for oral hypoglycemic agents in diabetes). Products include:

Glucotrol Tablets 1967
Glucotrol XL Extended Release Tablets 1968

Glyburide (Increased requirements for oral hypoglycemic agents in diabetes). Products include:

DiaBeta Tablets 1239
Glynase PresTab Tablets 2609
Micronase Tablets 2623

Insulin, Human (Increased requirements for insulin in diabetes).

No products indexed under this heading.

Insulin, Human Isophane Suspension (Increased requirements for insulin in diabetes). Products include:

Novolin N Human Insulin 10 ml Vials.. 1795

Insulin, Human NPH (Increased requirements for insulin in diabetes). Products include:

Humulin N, 100 Units 1448
Novolin N PenFill Cartridges Durable Insulin Delivery System 1798
Novolin N Prefilled Syringe Disposable Insulin Delivery System 1798

Insulin, Human Regular (Increased requirements for insulin in diabetes). Products include:

Humulin R, 100 Units 1449
Novolin R Human Insulin 10 ml Vials.. 1795
Novolin R PenFill Cartridges Durable Insulin Delivery System 1798
Novolin R Prefilled Syringe Disposable Insulin Delivery System 1798
Velosulin BR Human Insulin 10 ml Vials.. 1795

Insulin, Human, Zinc Suspension (Increased requirements for insulin in diabetes). Products include:

Humulin L, 100 Units 1446
Humulin U, 100 Units 1450
Novolin L Human Insulin 10 ml Vials.. 1795

Insulin, NPH (Increased requirements for insulin in diabetes). Products include:

NPH, 100 Units 1450
Pork NPH, 100 Units............................. 1452
Purified Pork NPH Isophane Insulin 1801

Insulin, Regular (Increased requirements for insulin in diabetes). Products include:

Regular, 100 Units 1450
Pork Regular, 100 Units 1452
Pork Regular (Concentrated), 500 Units 1453
Purified Pork Regular Insulin 1801

Insulin, Zinc Crystals (Increased requirements for insulin in diabetes). Products include:

NPH, 100 Units 1450

Insulin, Zinc Suspension (Increased requirements for insulin in diabetes). Products include:

Iletin I 1450
Lente, 100 Units 1450
Iletin II 1452
Pork Lente, 100 Units........................... 1452
Purified Pork Lente Insulin 1801

Metformin Hydrochloride (Increased requirements for oral hypoglycemic agents in diabetes). Products include:

Glucophage 752

Tolazamide (Increased requirements for oral hypoglycemic agents in diabetes).

No products indexed under this heading.

Tolbutamide (Increased requirements for oral hypoglycemic agents in diabetes).

No products indexed under this heading.

Vaccines (Live) (Administration of live or live attenuated vaccines is contraindicated).

ARISTOCORT TABLETS

(Triamcinolone) 1022
May interact with:

Aspirin (Aspirin should be used cautiously in conjunction with corticosteroids in hypoprothrombinemia). Products include:

Alka-Seltzer Effervescent Antacid and Pain Reliever................................ ✦D 701
Alka-Seltzer Extra Strength Effervescent Antacid and Pain Reliever .... ✦D 703
Alka-Seltzer Lemon Lime Effervescent Antacid and Pain Reliever .... ✦D 703
Alka-Seltzer Plus Cold Medicine .... ✦D 705
Alka-Seltzer Plus Cold & Cough Medicine .... ✦D 708
Alka-Seltzer Plus Night-Time Cold Medicine .... ✦D 707
Alka Seltzer Plus Sinus Medicine .. ✦D 707
Arthritis Foundation Safety Coated Aspirin Tablets .... ✦D 675
Arthritis Pain Ascriptin .... ✦D 631
Maximum Strength Ascriptin .... ✦D 630

Regular Strength Ascriptin Tablets .... ✦D 629
Arthritis Strength BC Powder .... ✦D 609
BC Cold Powder Multi-Symptom Formula (Cold-Sinus-Allergy) ...... ✦D 609
BC Cold Powder Non-Drowsy Formula (Cold-Sinus) .... ✦D 609
BC Powder .... ✦D 609
Bayer Children's Chewable Aspirin .... ✦D 711
Genuine Bayer Aspirin Tablets & Caplets .... ✦D 713
Extra Strength Bayer Arthritis Pain Regimen Formula .... ✦D 711
Extra Strength Bayer Aspirin Caplets & Tablets .... ✦D 712
Extended-Release Bayer 8-Hour Aspirin .... ✦D 712
Extra Strength Bayer Plus Aspirin Caplets .... ✦D 713
Extra Strength Bayer PM Aspirin .. ✦D 713
Bayer Enteric Aspirin .... ✦D 709
Bufferin Analgesic Tablets and Caplets .... ✦D 613
Arthritis Strength Bufferin Analgesic Caplets .... ✦D 614
Extra Strength Bufferin Analgesic Tablets .... ✦D 615
Cama Arthritis Pain Reliever............. ✦D 785
Darvon Compound-65 Pulvules 1435
Easprin 1914
Ecotrin 2455
Ecotrin Enteric Coated Aspirin Maximum Strength Tablets and Caplets .... ✦D 816
Ecotrin Enteric Coated Aspirin Regular Strength Tablets 2455
Empirin Aspirin Tablets .... ✦D 854
Empirin with Codeine Tablets............ 1093
Excedrin Extra-Strength Analgesic Tablets & Caplets 732
Fiorinal Capsules 2261
Fiorinal with Codeine Capsules 2262
Fiorinal Tablets 2261
Halfprin 1362
Healthprin Aspirin 2455
Norgesic... 1496
Percodan Tablets 939
Percodan-Demi Tablets......................... 940
Robaxisal Tablets..................................... 2071
Soma Compound w/Codeine Tablets 2676
Soma Compound Tablets..................... 2675
St. Joseph Adult Chewable Aspirin (81 mg.) .... ✦D 808
Talwin Compound 2335
Ursinus Inlay-Tabs.................................. ✦D 794
Vanquish Analgesic Caplets .... ✦D 731

Immunization (Possible neurological complications and lack of antibody response, especially in patients on high dose of corticosteroids).

Smallpox Vaccine (Patients on corticosteroid therapy should not be vaccinated).

ARISTOCORT A 0.025% CREAM

(Triamcinolone Acetonide) 1027
None cited in PDR database.

ARISTOCORT A 0.5% CREAM

(Triamcinolone Acetonide) 1031
None cited in PDR database.

ARISTOCORT A 0.1% CREAM

(Triamcinolone Acetonide) 1029
None cited in PDR database.

ARISTOCORT A 0.1% OINTMENT

(Triamcinolone Acetonide) 1030
None cited in PDR database.

ARISTOSPAN SUSPENSION (INTRA-ARTICULAR)

(Triamcinolone Hexacetonide) 1033
May interact with oral hypoglycemic agents, insulin, and certain other agents. Compounds in these categories include:

Acarbose (Increased requirements for oral hypoglycemic agents in diabetes).

No products indexed under this heading.

Aspirin (Aspirin should be used cautiously in conjunction with corticosteroids in hypoprothrombinemia). Products include:

Alka-Seltzer Effervescent Antacid and Pain Reliever................................ ✦D 701
Alka-Seltzer Extra Strength Effervescent Antacid and Pain Reliever .... ✦D 703
Alka-Seltzer Lemon Lime Effervescent Antacid and Pain Reliever .... ✦D 703
Alka-Seltzer Plus Cold Medicine .... ✦D 705
Alka-Seltzer Plus Cold & Cough Medicine .... ✦D 708
Alka-Seltzer Plus Night-Time Cold Medicine .... ✦D 707
Alka Seltzer Plus Sinus Medicine .. ✦D 707
Arthritis Foundation Safety Coated Aspirin Tablets .... ✦D 675
Arthritis Pain Ascriptin .... ✦D 631
Maximum Strength Ascriptin .... ✦D 630
Regular Strength Ascriptin Tablets .... ✦D 629
Arthritis Strength BC Powder........... ✦D 609
BC Cold Powder Multi-Symptom Formula (Cold-Sinus-Allergy) ...... ✦D 609
BC Cold Powder Non-Drowsy Formula (Cold-Sinus) .... ✦D 609
BC Powder .... ✦D 609
Bayer Children's Chewable Aspirin .... ✦D 711
Genuine Bayer Aspirin Tablets & Caplets .... ✦D 713
Extra Strength Bayer Arthritis Pain Regimen Formula .... ✦D 711
Extra Strength Bayer Aspirin Caplets & Tablets .... ✦D 712
Extended-Release Bayer 8-Hour Aspirin .... ✦D 712
Extra Strength Bayer Plus Aspirin Caplets .... ✦D 713
Extra Strength Bayer PM Aspirin .. ✦D 713
Bayer Enteric Aspirin .... ✦D 709
Bufferin Analgesic Tablets and Caplets .... ✦D 613
Arthritis Strength Bufferin Analgesic Caplets .... ✦D 614
Extra Strength Bufferin Analgesic Tablets .... ✦D 615
Cama Arthritis Pain Reliever............. ✦D 785
Darvon Compound-65 Pulvules 1435
Easprin 1914
Ecotrin 2455
Ecotrin Enteric Coated Aspirin Maximum Strength Tablets and Caplets .... ✦D 816
Ecotrin Enteric Coated Aspirin Regular Strength Tablets 2455
Empirin Aspirin Tablets .... ✦D 854
Empirin with Codeine Tablets............ 1093
Excedrin Extra-Strength Analgesic Tablets & Caplets 732
Fiorinal Capsules 2261
Fiorinal with Codeine Capsules 2262
Fiorinal Tablets 2261
Halfprin 1362
Healthprin Aspirin 2455
Norgesic... 1496
Percodan Tablets 939
Percodan-Demi Tablets......................... 940
Robaxisal Tablets..................................... 2071
Soma Compound w/Codeine Tablets 2676
Soma Compound Tablets..................... 2675
St. Joseph Adult Chewable Aspirin (81 mg.) .... ✦D 808
Talwin Compound 2335
Ursinus Inlay-Tabs.................................. ✦D 794
Vanquish Analgesic Caplets .... ✦D 731

Chlorpropamide (Increased requirements for oral hypoglycemic agents in diabetes). Products include:

Diabinese Tablets 1935

Glipizide (Increased requirements for oral hypoglycemic agents in diabetes). Products include:

Glucotrol Tablets 1967
Glucotrol XL Extended Release Tablets 1968

IMPORTANT NOTE: Always consult each drug listing in the patient's regimen for possible interactions.

Aristospan Suspension 20 mg/mL Interactions Index

Glyburide (Increased requirements for oral hypoglycemic agents in diabetes). Products include:

DiaBeta Tablets 1239
Glynase PresTab Tablets 2609
Micronase Tablets 2623

Immunization (Potential for neurological complications and lack of antibody response, especially, in patients on high dose of corticosteroids).

Insulin, Human (Increased requirements for insulin in diabetes).

No products indexed under this heading.

Insulin, Human Isophane Suspension (Increased requirements for insulin in diabetes). Products include:

Novolin N Human Insulin 10 ml Vials 1795

Insulin, Human NPH (Increased requirements for insulin in diabetes). Products include:

Humulin N, 100 Units 1448
Novolin N PenFill Cartridges Durable Insulin Delivery System 1798
Novolin N Prefilled Syringe Disposable Insulin Delivery System 1798

Insulin, Human Regular (Increased requirements for insulin in diabetes). Products include:

Humulin R, 100 Units 1449
Novolin R Human Insulin 10 ml Vials 1795
Novolin R PenFill Cartridges Durable Insulin Delivery System 1798
Novolin R Prefilled Syringe Disposable Insulin Delivery System 1798
Velosulin BR Human Insulin 10 ml Vials 1795

Insulin, Human, Zinc Suspension (Increased requirements for insulin in diabetes). Products include:

Humulin L, 100 Units 1446
Humulin U, 100 Units 1450
Novolin L Human Insulin 10 ml Vials 1795

Insulin, NPH (Increased requirements for insulin in diabetes). Products include:

NPH, 100 Units 1450
Pork NPH, 100 Units 1452
Purified Pork NPH Isophane Insulin 1801

Insulin, Regular (Increased requirements for insulin in diabetes). Products include:

Regular, 100 Units 1450
Pork Regular, 100 Units 1452
Pork Regular (Concentrated), 500 Units 1453
Purified Pork Regular Insulin 1801

Insulin, Zinc Crystals (Increased requirements for insulin in diabetes). Products include:

NPH, 100 Units 1450

Insulin, Zinc Suspension (Increased requirements for insulin in diabetes). Products include:

Iletin I 1450
Lente, 100 Units 1450
Iletin II 1452
Pork Lente, 100 Units 1452
Purified Pork Lente Insulin 1801

Metformin Hydrochloride (Increased requirements for oral hypoglycemic agents in diabetes). Products include:

Glucophage 752

Smallpox Vaccine (Potential for neurological complications and lack of antibody response, especially, in patients on high dose of corticosteroids).

Tolazamide (Increased requirements for oral hypoglycemic agents in diabetes).

No products indexed under this heading.

Tolbutamide (Increased requirements for oral hypoglycemic agents in diabetes).

No products indexed under this heading.

ARISTOSPAN SUSPENSION (INTRALESIONAL)

(Triamcinolone Hexacetonide) 1032

May interact with oral hypoglycemic agents, insulin, and certain other agents. Compounds in these categories include:

Acarbose (Increased requirements for oral hypoglycemia agents in diabetes).

No products indexed under this heading.

Aspirin (Aspirin should be used cautiously in conjunction with corticosteroids in hypoprothrombinemia). Products include:

Alka-Seltzer Effervescent Antacid and Pain Reliever .... ᵃᴰ 701
Alka-Seltzer Extra Strength Effervescent Antacid and Pain Reliever .... ᵃᴰ 703
Alka-Seltzer Lemon Lime Effervescent Antacid and Pain Reliever .... ᵃᴰ 703
Alka-Seltzer Plus Cold Medicine .... ᵃᴰ 705
Alka-Seltzer Plus Cold & Cough Medicine .... ᵃᴰ 708
Alka-Seltzer Plus Night-Time Cold Medicine .... ᵃᴰ 707
Alka Seltzer Plus Sinus Medicine .. ᵃᴰ 707
Arthritis Foundation Safety Coated Aspirin Tablets .... ᵃᴰ 675
Arthritis Pain Ascriptin .... ᵃᴰ 631
Maximum Strength Ascriptin .... ᵃᴰ 630
Regular Strength Ascriptin Tablets .... ᵃᴰ 629
Arthritis Strength BC Powder .... ᵃᴰ 609
BC Cold Powder Multi-Symptom Formula (Cold-Sinus-Allergy) ...... ᵃᴰ 609
BC Cold Powder Non-Drowsy Formula (Cold-Sinus) .... ᵃᴰ 609
BC Powder .... ᵃᴰ 609
Bayer Children's Chewable Aspirin .... ᵃᴰ 711
Genuine Bayer Aspirin Tablets & Caplets .... ᵃᴰ 713
Extra Strength Bayer Arthritis Pain Regimen Formula .... ᵃᴰ 711
Extra Strength Bayer Aspirin Caplets & Tablets .... ᵃᴰ 712
Extended-Release Bayer 8-Hour Aspirin .... ᵃᴰ 712
Extra Strength Bayer Plus Aspirin Caplets .... ᵃᴰ 713
Extra Strength Bayer PM Aspirin .. ᵃᴰ 713
Bayer Enteric Aspirin .... ᵃᴰ 709
Bufferin Analgesic Tablets and Caplets .... ᵃᴰ 613
Arthritis Strength Bufferin Analgesic Caplets .... ᵃᴰ 614
Extra Strength Bufferin Analgesic Tablets .... ᵃᴰ 615
Cama Arthritis Pain Reliever .... ᵃᴰ 785
Darvon Compound-65 Pulvules 1435
Easprin 1914
Ecotrin 2455
Ecotrin Enteric Coated Aspirin Maximum Strength Tablets and Caplets .... ᵃᴰ 816
Ecotrin Enteric Coated Aspirin Regular Strength Tablets 2455
Empirin Aspirin Tablets .... ᵃᴰ 854
Empirin with Codeine Tablets 1093
Excedrin Extra-Strength Analgesic Tablets & Caplets 732
Fiorinal Capsules 2261
Fiorinal with Codeine Capsules 2262
Fiorinal Tablets 2261
Halfprin 1362
Healthprin Aspirin 2455
Norgesic 1496
Percodan Tablets 939
Percodan-Demi Tablets 940
Robaxisal Tablets 2071
Soma Compound w/Codeine Tablets 2676
Soma Compound Tablets 2675
St. Joseph Adult Chewable Aspirin (81 mg.) .... ᵃᴰ 808

Talwin Compound 2335
Ursinus Inlay-Tabs .... ᵃᴰ 794
Vanquish Analgesic Caplets .... ᵃᴰ 731

Chlorpropamide (Increased requirements for oral hypoglycemia agents in diabetes). Products include:

Diabinese Tablets 1935

Glipizide (Increased requirements for oral hypoglycemia agents in diabetes). Products include:

Glucotrol Tablets 1967
Glucotrol XL Extended Release Tablets 1968

Glyburide (Increased requirements for oral hypoglycemia agents in diabetes). Products include:

DiaBeta Tablets 1239
Glynase PresTab Tablets 2609
Micronase Tablets 2623

Insulin, Human (Increased requirements for insulin in diabetes).

No products indexed under this heading.

Insulin, Human Isophane Suspension (Increased requirements for insulin in diabetes). Products include:

Novolin N Human Insulin 10 ml Vials 1795

Insulin, Human NPH (Increased requirements for insulin in diabetes). Products include:

Humulin N, 100 Units 1448
Novolin N PenFill Cartridges Durable Insulin Delivery System 1798
Novolin N Prefilled Syringe Disposable Insulin Delivery System 1798

Insulin, Human Regular (Increased requirements for insulin in diabetes). Products include:

Humulin R, 100 Units 1449
Novolin R Human Insulin 10 ml Vials 1795
Novolin R PenFill Cartridges Durable Insulin Delivery System 1798
Novolin R Prefilled Syringe Disposable Insulin Delivery System 1798
Velosulin BR Human Insulin 10 ml Vials 1795

Insulin, Human, Zinc Suspension (Increased requirements for insulin in diabetes). Products include:

Humulin L, 100 Units 1446
Humulin U, 100 Units 1450
Novolin L Human Insulin 10 ml Vials 1795

Insulin, NPH (Increased requirements for insulin in diabetes). Products include:

NPH, 100 Units 1450
Pork NPH, 100 Units 1452
Purified Pork NPH Isophane Insulin 1801

Insulin, Regular (Increased requirements for insulin in diabetes). Products include:

Regular, 100 Units 1450
Pork Regular, 100 Units 1452
Pork Regular (Concentrated), 500 Units 1453
Purified Pork Regular Insulin 1801

Insulin, Zinc Crystals (Increased requirements for insulin in diabetes). Products include:

NPH, 100 Units 1450

Insulin, Zinc Suspension (Increased requirements for insulin in diabetes). Products include:

Iletin I 1450
Lente, 100 Units 1450
Iletin II 1452
Pork Lente, 100 Units 1452
Purified Pork Lente Insulin 1801

Metformin Hydrochloride (Increased requirements for oral hypoglycemia agents in diabetes). Products include:

Glucophage 752

Tolazamide (Increased requirements for oral hypoglycemia agents in diabetes).

No products indexed under this heading.

Tolbutamide (Increased requirements for oral hypoglycemia agents in diabetes).

No products indexed under this heading.

ARM & HAMMER PURE BAKING SODA

(Sodium Bicarbonate) .... ᵃᴰ 627

None cited in PDR database.

ARTANE ELIXIR

(Trihexyphenidyl Hydrochloride) 1368

May interact with:

Levodopa (The usual dose of each may need to be reduced when used concomitantly). Products include:

Atamet 572
Larodopa Tablets 2129
Sinemet Tablets 943
Sinemet CR Tablets 944

ARTANE TABLETS

(Trihexyphenidyl Hydrochloride) 1368

See Artane Elixir

ARTHRICARE ODOR FREE RUB

(Capsaicin, Menthol, Methyl Nicotinate) .... ᵃᴰ 651

None cited in PDR database.

ARTHRICARE TRIPLE MEDICATED RUB

(Menthol, Methyl Nicotinate, Methyl Salicylate) .... ᵃᴰ 651

None cited in PDR database.

ARTHRITIS FOUNDATION ASPIRIN FREE CAPLETS

(Acetaminophen) .... ᵃᴰ 673

Food Interactions

Alcohol (Patients consuming 3 or more drinks per day on a regular basis should consult their physician for advice on when and how they should take acetaminophen-containing products).

ARTHRITIS FOUNDATION IBUPROFEN TABLETS

(Ibuprofen) .... ᵃᴰ 674

May interact with:

Prescription Drugs, unspecified (Consult your doctor).

ARTHRITIS FOUNDATION NIGHTTIME CAPLETS

(Acetaminophen, Diphenhydramine Hydrochloride) .... ᵃᴰ 674

May interact with hypnotics and sedatives, tranquilizers, and certain other agents. Compounds in these categories include:

Alprazolam (Concomitant use not recommended; consult your doctor). Products include:

Xanax Tablets 2649

Buspirone Hydrochloride (Concomitant use not recommended; consult your doctor). Products include:

BuSpar 737

Chlordiazepoxide (Concomitant use not recommended; consult your doctor). Products include:

Libritabs Tablets 2177
Limbitrol 2180

(ᵃᴰ Described in PDR For Nonprescription Drugs) (◉ Described in PDR For Ophthalmology)

Interactions Index — Ascriptin Maximum Strength

Chlordiazepoxide Hydrochloride (Concomitant use not recommended; consult your doctor). Products include:

Librax Capsules 2176
Librium Capsules 2178
Librium Injectable 2179

Chlorpromazine (Concomitant use not recommended; consult your doctor). Products include:

Thorazine Suppositories 2523

Chlorpromazine Hydrochloride (Concomitant use not recommended; consult your doctor). Products include:

Thorazine 2523

Chlorprothixene (Concomitant use not recommended; consult your doctor).

No products indexed under this heading.

Chlorprothixene Hydrochloride (Concomitant use not recommended; consult your doctor).

No products indexed under this heading.

Clorazepate Dipotassium (Concomitant use not recommended; consult your doctor). Products include:

Tranxene 451

Diazepam (Concomitant use not recommended; consult your doctor). Products include:

Dizac 1809
Valium Injectable 2182
Valium Tablets 2183
Valrelease Capsules 2169

Droperidol (Concomitant use not recommended; consult your doctor). Products include:

Inapsine Injection 1296

Estazolam (Concomitant use not recommended; consult your doctor). Products include:

ProSom Tablets 449

Ethchlorvynol (Concomitant use not recommended; consult your doctor). Products include:

Placidyl Capsules 448

Ethinamate (Concomitant use not recommended; consult your doctor).

No products indexed under this heading.

Fluphenazine Decanoate (Concomitant use not recommended; consult your doctor). Products include:

Prolixin Decanoate 509

Fluphenazine Enanthate (Concomitant use not recommended; consult your doctor). Products include:

Prolixin Enanthate 509

Fluphenazine Hydrochloride (Concomitant use not recommended; consult your doctor). Products include:

Prolixin 509

Flurazepam Hydrochloride (Concomitant use not recommended; consult your doctor). Products include:

Dalmane Capsules 2173

Glutethimide (Concomitant use not recommended; consult your doctor).

No products indexed under this heading.

Haloperidol (Concomitant use not recommended; consult your doctor). Products include:

Haldol Injection, Tablets and Concentrate 1575

Haloperidol Decanoate (Concomitant use not recommended; consult your doctor). Products include:

Haldol Decanoate 1577

Hydroxyzine Hydrochloride (Concomitant use not recommended; consult your doctor). Products include:

Atarax Tablets & Syrup 2185
Marax Tablets & DF Syrup 2200
Vistaril Intramuscular Solution 2216

Lorazepam (Concomitant use not recommended; consult your doctor). Products include:

Ativan Injection 2698
Ativan Tablets 2700

Loxapine Hydrochloride (Concomitant use not recommended; consult your doctor). Products include:

Loxitane 1378

Loxapine Succinate (Concomitant use not recommended; consult your doctor). Products include:

Loxitane Capsules 1378

Meprobamate (Concomitant use not recommended; consult your doctor). Products include:

Miltown Tablets 2672
PMB 200 and PMB 400 2783

Mesoridazine Besylate (Concomitant use not recommended; consult your doctor). Products include:

Serentil 684

Midazolam Hydrochloride (Concomitant use not recommended; consult your doctor). Products include:

Versed Injection 2170

Molindone Hydrochloride (Concomitant use not recommended; consult your doctor). Products include:

Moban Tablets and Concentrate 1048

Oxazepam (Concomitant use not recommended; consult your doctor). Products include:

Serax Capsules 2810
Serax Tablets 2810

Perphenazine (Concomitant use not recommended; consult your doctor). Products include:

Etrafon 2355
Triavil Tablets 1757
Trilafon 2389

Prazepam (Concomitant use not recommended; consult your doctor).

No products indexed under this heading.

Prochlorperazine (Concomitant use not recommended; consult your doctor). Products include:

Compazine 2470

Promethazine Hydrochloride (Concomitant use not recommended; consult your doctor). Products include:

Mepergan Injection 2753
Phenergan with Codeine 2777
Phenergan with Dextromethorphan 2778
Phenergan Injection 2773
Phenergan Suppositories 2775
Phenergan Syrup 2774
Phenergan Tablets 2775
Phenergan VC 2779
Phenergan VC with Codeine 2781

Propofol (Concomitant use not recommended; consult your doctor). Products include:

Diprivan Injection 2833

Quazepam (Concomitant use not recommended; consult your doctor). Products include:

Doral Tablets 2664

Secobarbital Sodium (Concomitant use not recommended; consult your doctor). Products include:

Seconal Sodium Pulvules 1474

Temazepam (Concomitant use not recommended; consult your doctor). Products include:

Restoril Capsules 2284

Thioridazine Hydrochloride (Concomitant use not recommended; consult your doctor). Products include:

Mellaril 2269

Thiothixene (Concomitant use not recommended; consult your doctor). Products include:

Navane Capsules and Concentrate 2201
Navane Intramuscular 2202

Triazolam (Concomitant use not recommended; consult your doctor). Products include:

Halcion Tablets 2611

Trifluoperazine Hydrochloride (Concomitant use not recommended; consult your doctor). Products include:

Stelazine 2514

Zolpidem Tartrate (Concomitant use not recommended; consult your doctor). Products include:

Ambien Tablets 2416

Food Interactions

Alcohol (Patients consuming 3 or more alcohol-containing drinks per day should consult their physician for advice on when and how they should take acetaminophen-containing products).

ARTHRITIS FOUNDATION SAFETY COATED ASPIRIN TABLETS

(Aspirin) .... ⒷⒹ 675

May interact with oral anticoagulants and certain other agents. Compounds in these categories include:

Antiarthritic Drugs, unspecified (Concurrent use not recommended).

Antidiabetic Drugs, unspecified (Concurrent use not recommended).

Antigout Drugs, unspecified (Concurrent use not recommended).

Dicumarol (Effect not specified).

No products indexed under this heading.

Warfarin Sodium (Effect not specified). Products include:

Coumadin 926

ASACOL DELAYED-RELEASE TABLETS

(Mesalamine) 1979

None cited in PDR database.

ARTHRITIS PAIN ASCRIPTIN

(Aspirin Buffered, Calcium Carbonate) .... ⒷⒹ 631

May interact with oral anticoagulants, tetracyclines, and certain other agents. Compounds in these categories include:

Antiarthritic Drugs, unspecified (Concurrent use is not recommended; consult your doctor).

Antidiabetic Drugs, unspecified (Concurrent use is not recommended; consult your doctor).

Antigout Drugs, unspecified (Concurrent use is not recommended; consult your doctor).

Demeclocycline Hydrochloride (Concurrent use is not recommended; consult your doctor). Products include:

Declomycin Tablets 1371

Dicumarol (Concurrent use is not recommended; consult your doctor).

No products indexed under this heading.

Doxycycline Calcium (Concurrent use is not recommended; consult your doctor). Products include:

Vibramycin Calcium Oral Suspension Syrup 1941

Doxycycline Hyclate (Concurrent use is not recommended; consult your doctor). Products include:

Doryx Capsules 1913
Vibramycin Hyclate Capsules 1941
Vibramycin Hyclate Intravenous 2215
Vibra-Tabs Film Coated Tablets 1941

Doxycycline Monohydrate (Concurrent use is not recommended; consult your doctor). Products include:

Monodox Capsules 1805
Vibramycin Monohydrate for Oral Suspension 1941

Methacycline Hydrochloride (Concurrent use is not recommended; consult your doctor).

No products indexed under this heading.

Minocycline Hydrochloride (Concurrent use is not recommended; consult your doctor). Products include:

Dynacin Capsules 1590
Minocin Intravenous 1382
Minocin Oral Suspension 1385
Minocin Pellet-Filled Capsules 1383

Oxytetracycline Hydrochloride (Concurrent use is not recommended; consult your doctor). Products include:

TERAK Ointment .... © 209
Terra-Cortril Ophthalmic Suspension 2210
Terramycin with Polymyxin B Sulfate Ophthalmic Ointment 2211
Urobiotic-250 Capsules 2214

Tetracycline Hydrochloride (Concurrent use is not recommended; consult your doctor). Products include:

Achromycin V Capsules 1367

Warfarin Sodium (Concurrent use is not recommended; consult your doctor). Products include:

Coumadin 926

MAXIMUM STRENGTH ASCRIPTIN

(Aspirin Buffered, Calcium Carbonate) .... ⒷⒹ 630

May interact with tetracyclines, oral anticoagulants, and certain other agents. Compounds in these categories include:

Antiarthritic Drugs, unspecified (Concurrent use not advisable; consult your doctor).

Antidiabetic Drugs, unspecified (Concurrent use not advisable; consult your doctor).

Antigout Drugs, unspecified (Concurrent use not advisable; consult your doctor).

Demeclocycline Hydrochloride (Concurrent use not advisable; consult your doctor). Products include:

Declomycin Tablets 1371

Dicumarol (Concurrent use not recommended; consult your doctor).

No products indexed under this heading.

Doxycycline Calcium (Concurrent use not advisable; consult your doctor). Products include:

Vibramycin Calcium Oral Suspension Syrup 1941

IMPORTANT NOTE: Always consult each drug listing in the patient's regimen for possible interactions.

Ascriptin Maximum Strength — Interactions Index — 80

Doxycycline Hyclate (Concurrent use not advisable; consult your doctor). Products include:
- Doryx Capsules 1913
- Vibramycin Hyclate Capsules 1941
- Vibramycin Hyclate Intravenous 2215
- Vibra-Tabs Film Coated Tablets 1941

Doxycycline Monohydrate (Concurrent use not advisable; consult your doctor). Products include:
- Monodox Capsules 1805
- Vibramycin Monohydrate for Oral Suspension 1941

Methacycline Hydrochloride (Concurrent use not advisable; consult your doctor).
- No products indexed under this heading.

Minocycline Hydrochloride (Concurrent use not advisable; consult your doctor). Products include:
- Dynacin Capsules 1590
- Minocin Intravenous 1382
- Minocin Oral Suspension 1385
- Minocin Pellet-Filled Capsules 1383

Oxytetracycline Hydrochloride (Concurrent use not advisable; consult your doctor). Products include:
- TERAK Ointment .... ⊚ 209
- Terra-Cortril Ophthalmic Suspension 2210
- Terramycin with Polymyxin B Sulfate Ophthalmic Ointment 2211
- Urobiotic-250 Capsules 2214

Tetracycline Hydrochloride (Concurrent use not advisable; consult your doctor). Products include:
- Achromycin V Capsules 1367

Warfarin Sodium (Concurrent use not recommended; consult your doctor). Products include:
- Coumadin 926

REGULAR STRENGTH ASCRIPTIN TABLETS

(Aspirin Buffered, Calcium Carbonate) .... ▣ 629

May interact with oral anticoagulants, tetracyclines, and certain other agents. Compounds in these categories include:

Antiarthritic Drugs, unspecified (Concurrent use is not recommended; consult your doctor).

Antidiabetic Drugs, unspecified (Concurrent use is not recommended; consult your doctor).

Antigout Drugs, unspecified (Concurrent use is not recommended; consult your doctor).

Demeclocycline Hydrochloride (Concurrent use is not recommended; consult your doctor). Products include:
- Declomycin Tablets 1371

Dicumarol (Concurrent use is not recommended; consult your doctor).
- No products indexed under this heading.

Doxycycline Calcium (Concurrent use is not recommended; consult your doctor). Products include:
- Vibramycin Calcium Oral Suspension Syrup 1941

Doxycycline Hyclate (Concurrent use is not recommended; consult your doctor). Products include:
- Doryx Capsules 1913
- Vibramycin Hyclate Capsules 1941
- Vibramycin Hyclate Intravenous 2215
- Vibra-Tabs Film Coated Tablets 1941

Doxycycline Monohydrate (Concurrent use is not recommended; consult your doctor). Products include:
- Monodox Capsules 1805
- Vibramycin Monohydrate for Oral Suspension 1941

Methacycline Hydrochloride (Concurrent use is not recommended; consult your doctor).
- No products indexed under this heading.

Minocycline Hydrochloride (Concurrent use is not recommended; consult your doctor). Products include:
- Dynacin Capsules 1590
- Minocin Intravenous 1382
- Minocin Oral Suspension 1385
- Minocin Pellet-Filled Capsules 1383

Oxytetracycline Hydrochloride (Concurrent use is not recommended; consult your doctor). Products include:
- TERAK Ointment .... ⊚ 209
- Terra-Cortril Ophthalmic Suspension 2210
- Terramycin with Polymyxin B Sulfate Ophthalmic Ointment 2211
- Urobiotic-250 Capsules 2214

Tetracycline Hydrochloride (Concurrent use is not recommended; consult your doctor). Products include:
- Achromycin V Capsules 1367

Warfarin Sodium (Concurrent use is not recommended; consult your doctor). Products include:
- Coumadin 926

ASENDIN TABLETS

(Amoxapine) 1369

May interact with monoamine oxidase inhibitors, anticholinergics, barbiturates, central nervous system depressants, selective serotonin reuptake inhibitors, antidepressant drugs, phenothiazines, and certain other agents. Compounds in these categories include:

Alfentanil Hydrochloride (Enhanced response to central nervous system depressants). Products include:
- Alfenta Injection 1286

Alprazolam (Enhanced response to central nervous system depressants). Products include:
- Xanax Tablets 2649

Amitriptyline Hydrochloride (Concomitant use of amoxapine with other drugs that inhibit cytochrome $P_{450}IID_6$ may require lower than usual doses prescribed for either drug). Products include:
- Elavil 2838
- Endep Tablets 2174
- Etrafon 2355
- Limbitrol 2180
- Triavil Tablets 1757

Aprobarbital (Enhanced response to barbiturates and central nervous system depressants).
- No products indexed under this heading.

Atropine Sulfate (Paralytic ileus may occur). Products include:
- Arco-Lase Plus Tablets 512
- Atrohist Plus Tablets 454
- Atropine Sulfate Sterile Ophthalmic Solution .... ⊚ 233
- Donnatal 2060
- Donnatal Extentabs 2061
- Donnatal Tablets 2060
- Lomotil 2439
- Motofen Tablets 784
- Urised Tablets 1964

Belladonna Alkaloids (Paralytic ileus may occur). Products include:
- Bellergal-S Tablets 2250
- Hyland's Bed Wetting Tablets .... ▣ 828
- Hyland's EnurAid Tablets .... ▣ 829
- Hyland's Teething Tablets .... ▣ 830

Benztropine Mesylate (Paralytic ileus may occur). Products include:
- Cogentin 1621

Biperiden Hydrochloride (Paralytic ileus may occur). Products include:
- Akineton 1333

Buprenorphine (Enhanced response to central nervous system depressants). Products include:
- Buprenex Injectable 2006

Bupropion Hydrochloride (Concomitant use of amoxapine with other drugs that inhibit cytochrome $P_{450}IID_6$ may require lower than usual doses prescribed for either drug). Products include:
- Wellbutrin Tablets 1204

Buspirone Hydrochloride (Enhanced response to central nervous system depressants). Products include:
- BuSpar 737

Butabarbital (Enhanced response to barbiturates and central nervous system depressants).
- No products indexed under this heading.

Butalbital (Enhanced response to barbiturates and central nervous system depressants). Products include:
- Esgic-plus Tablets 1013
- Fioricet Tablets 2258
- Fioricet with Codeine Capsules 2260
- Fiorinal Capsules 2261
- Fiorinal with Codeine Capsules 2262
- Fiorinal Tablets 2261
- Phrenilin 785
- Sedapap Tablets 50 mg/650 mg 1543

Chlordiazepoxide (Enhanced response to central nervous system depressants). Products include:
- Libritabs Tablets 2177
- Limbitrol 2180

Chlordiazepoxide Hydrochloride (Enhanced response to central nervous system depressants). Products include:
- Librax Capsules 2176
- Librium Capsules 2178
- Librium Injectable 2179

Chlorpromazine (Concomitant use of amoxapine with other drugs that inhibit cytochrome $P_{450}IID_6$ may require lower than usual doses prescribed for either drug; enhanced response to central nervous system depressants). Products include:
- Thorazine Suppositories 2523

Chlorpromazine Hydrochloride (Concomitant use of amoxapine with other drugs that inhibit cytochrome $P_{450}IID_6$ may require lower than usual doses prescribed for either drug). Products include:
- Thorazine 2523

Chlorprothixene (Enhanced response to central nervous system depressants).
- No products indexed under this heading.

Chlorprothixene Hydrochloride (Enhanced response to central nervous system depressants).
- No products indexed under this heading.

Cimetidine (Significant increase in serum levels of several tricyclic antidepressants; not documented with Asendin; concomitant use of amoxapine with other drugs that inhibit cytochrome $P_{450}IID_6$ may require lower than usual doses prescribed for either drug). Products include:
- Tagamet Tablets 2516

Cimetidine Hydrochloride (Significant increase in serum levels of several tricyclic antidepressants; not documented with Asendin; concomitant use of amoxapine with other drugs that inhibit cytochrome $P_{450}IID_6$ may require lower than usual doses prescribed for either drug). Products include:
- Tagamet 2516

Clidinium Bromide (Paralytic ileus may occur; enhanced response to central nervous system depressants). Products include:
- Librax Capsules 2176
- Quarzan Capsules 2181

Clorazepate Dipotassium (Enhanced response to central nervous system depressants). Products include:
- Tranxene 451

Clozapine (Enhanced response to central nervous system depressants). Products include:
- Clozaril Tablets 2252

Codeine Phosphate (Enhanced response to central nervous system depressants). Products include:
- Actifed with Codeine Cough Syrup 1067
- Brontex 1981
- Deconsal C Expectorant Syrup 456
- Deconsal Pediatric Syrup 457
- Dimetane-DC Cough Syrup 2059
- Empirin with Codeine Tablets 1093
- Fioricet with Codeine Capsules 2260
- Fiorinal with Codeine Capsules 2262
- Isoclor Expectorant 990
- Novahistine DH 2462
- Novahistine Expectorant 2463
- Nucofed 2051
- Phenergan with Codeine 2777
- Phenergan VC with Codeine 2781
- Robitussin A-C Syrup 2073
- Robitussin-DAC Syrup 2074
- Ryna .... ▣ 841
- Soma Compound w/Codeine Tablets 2676
- Tussi-Organidin NR Liquid and S NR Liquid 2677
- Tylenol with Codeine 1583

Desflurane (Enhanced response to central nervous system depressants). Products include:
- Suprane 1813

Desipramine Hydrochloride (Concomitant use of amoxapine with other drugs that inhibit cytochrome $P_{450}IID_6$ may require lower than usual doses prescribed for either drug). Products include:
- Norpramin Tablets 1526

Dezocine (Enhanced response to central nervous system depressants). Products include:
- Dalgan Injection 538

Diazepam (Enhanced response to central nervous system depressants). Products include:
- Dizac 1809
- Valium Injectable 2182
- Valium Tablets 2183
- Valrelease Capsules 2169

Dicyclomine Hydrochloride (Paralytic ileus may occur). Products include:
- Bentyl 1501

Doxepin Hydrochloride (Concomitant use of amoxapine with other drugs that inhibit cytochrome $P_{450}IID_6$ may require lower than usual doses prescribed for either drug). Products include:
- Sinequan 2205
- Zonalon Cream 1055

Droperidol (Enhanced response to central nervous system depressants). Products include:
- Inapsine Injection 1296

(▣ Described in PDR For Nonprescription Drugs) (⊚ Described in PDR For Ophthalmology)

81 **Interactions Index** **Asendin Tablets**

Enflurane (Enhanced response to central nervous system depressants).
No products indexed under this heading.

Estazolam (Enhanced response to central nervous system depressants). Products include:
ProSom Tablets 449

Ethchlorvynol (Enhanced response to central nervous system depressants). Products include:
Placidyl Capsules 448

Ethinamate (Enhanced response to central nervous system depressants).
No products indexed under this heading.

Ethopropazine Hydrochloride (Paralytic ileus may occur).

Fentanyl (Enhanced response to central nervous system depressants). Products include:
Duragesic Transdermal System 1288

Fentanyl Citrate (Enhanced response to central nervous system depressants). Products include:
Sublimaze Injection 1307

Flecainide Acetate (Concomitant use of amoxapine with other drugs that inhibit cytochrome $P_{450}IID_6$ may require lower than usual doses prescribed for either drug). Products include:
Tambocor Tablets 1497

Fluoxetine Hydrochloride (Concomitant use of amoxapine with other drugs that inhibit cytochrome $P_{450}IID_6$ may require lower than usual doses prescribed for either drug; sufficient time must elapse before initiating Asendin treatment in a patient being withdrawn from fluoxetine due to its long half-life). Products include:
Prozac Pulvules & Liquid, Oral Solution 919

Fluphenazine Decanoate (Concomitant use of amoxapine with other drugs that inhibit cytochrome $P_{450}IID_6$ may require lower than usual doses prescribed for either drug; enhanced response to central nervous system depressants). Products include:
Prolixin Decanoate 509

Fluphenazine Enanthate (Concomitant use of amoxapine with other drugs that inhibit cytochrome $P_{450}IID_6$ may require lower than usual doses prescribed for either drug; enhanced response to central nervous system depressants). Products include:
Prolixin Enanthate 509

Fluphenazine Hydrochloride (Concomitant use of amoxapine with other drugs that inhibit cytochrome $P_{450}IID_6$ may require lower than usual doses prescribed for either drug; enhanced response to central nervous system depressants). Products include:
Prolixin 509

Flurazepam Hydrochloride (Enhanced response to central nervous system depressants). Products include:
Dalmane Capsules 2173

Fluvoxamine Maleate (Concomitant use of amoxapine with other drugs that inhibit cytochrome $P_{450}IID_6$ may require lower than usual doses prescribed for either drug; sufficient time must elapse before initiating Asendin treatment in a patient being withdrawn from fluoxetine due to its long half-life). Products include:
Luvox Tablets 2544

Furazolidone (Concurrent and/or sequential use may result in hyperpyretic crises, severe convulsions, and fatalities; coadministration is contraindicated). Products include:
Furoxone 2046

Glutethimide (Enhanced response to central nervous system depressants).
No products indexed under this heading.

Glycopyrrolate (Paralytic ileus may occur). Products include:
Robinul Forte Tablets 2072
Robinul Injectable 2072
Robinul Tablets 2072

Haloperidol (Enhanced response to central nervous system depressants). Products include:
Haldol Injection, Tablets and Concentrate 1575

Haloperidol Decanoate (Enhanced response to central nervous system depressants). Products include:
Haldol Decanoate 1577

Hydrocodone Bitartrate (Enhanced response to central nervous system depressants). Products include:
Anexsia 5/500 Elixir 1781
Anexia Tablets 1782
Codiclear DH Syrup 791
Deconamine CX Cough and Cold Liquid and Tablets 1319
Duratuss HD Elixir 2565
Hycodan Tablets and Syrup 930
Hycomine Compound Tablets 932
Hycomine 931
Hycotuss Expectorant Syrup 933
Hydrocet Capsules 782
Lorcet 10/650 1018
Lortab 2566
Tussend 1783
Tussend Expectorant 1785
Vicodin Tablets 1356
Vicodin ES Tablets 1357
Vicodin Tuss Expectorant 1358
Zydone Capsules 949

Hydrocodone Polistirex (Enhanced response to central nervous system depressants). Products include:
Tussionex Pennkinetic Extended-Release Suspension 998

Hydroxyzine Hydrochloride (Enhanced response to central nervous system depressants). Products include:
Atarax Tablets & Syrup 2185
Marax Tablets & DF Syrup 2200
Vistaril Intramuscular Solution 2216

Hyoscyamine (Paralytic ileus may occur). Products include:
Cystospaz Tablets 1963
Urised Tablets 1964

Hyoscyamine Sulfate (Paralytic ileus may occur). Products include:
Arco-Lase Plus Tablets 512
Atrohist Plus Tablets 454
Cystospaz-M Capsules 1963
Donnatal 2060
Donnatal Extentabs 2061
Donnatal Tablets 2060
Kutrase Capsules 2402
Levsin/Levsinex/Levbid 2405

Imipramine Hydrochloride (Concomitant use of amoxapine with other drugs that inhibit cytochrome $P_{450}IID_6$ may require lower than usual doses prescribed for either drug). Products include:
Tofranil Ampuls 854
Tofranil Tablets 856

Imipramine Pamoate (Concomitant use of amoxapine with other drugs that inhibit cytochrome $P_{450}IID_6$ may require lower than usual doses prescribed for either drug). Products include:
Tofranil-PM Capsules 857

Ipratropium Bromide (Paralytic ileus may occur). Products include:
Atrovent Inhalation Aerosol 671
Atrovent Inhalation Solution 673

Isocarboxazid (Concurrent and/or sequential use may result in hyperpyretic crises, severe convulsions, and fatalities; coadministration is contraindicated).
No products indexed under this heading.

Isoflurane (Enhanced response to central nervous system depressants).
No products indexed under this heading.

Ketamine Hydrochloride (Enhanced response to central nervous system depressants).
No products indexed under this heading.

Levomethadyl Acetate Hydrochloride (Enhanced response to central nervous system depressants). Products include:
Orlamm 2239

Levorphanol Tartrate (Enhanced response to central nervous system depressants). Products include:
Levo-Dromoran 2129

Lorazepam (Enhanced response to central nervous system depressants). Products include:
Ativan Injection 2698
Ativan Tablets 2700

Loxapine Hydrochloride (Enhanced response to central nervous system depressants). Products include:
Loxitane 1378

Loxapine Succinate (Enhanced response to central nervous system depressants). Products include:
Loxitane Capsules 1378

Maprotiline Hydrochloride (Concomitant use of amoxapine with other drugs that inhibit cytochrome $P_{450}IID_6$ may require lower than usual doses prescribed for either drug). Products include:
Ludiomil Tablets 843

Mepenzolate Bromide (Paralytic ileus may occur).
No products indexed under this heading.

Meperidine Hydrochloride (Enhanced response to central nervous system depressants). Products include:
Demerol 2308
Mepergan Injection 2753

Mephobarbital (Enhanced response to barbiturates and central nervous system depressants). Products include:
Mebaral Tablets 2322

Meprobamate (Enhanced response to central nervous system depressants). Products include:
Miltown Tablets 2672
PMB 200 and PMB 400 2783

Mesoridazine Besylate (Concomitant use of amoxapine with other drugs that inhibit cytochrome $P_{450}IID_6$ may require lower than usual doses prescribed for either drug; enhanced response to central nervous system depressants). Products include:
Serentil 684

Methadone Hydrochloride (Enhanced response to central nervous system depressants). Products include:
Methadone Hydrochloride Oral Concentrate 2233
Methadone Hydrochloride Oral Solution & Tablets 2235

Methohexital Sodium (Enhanced response to central nervous system depressants). Products include:
Brevital Sodium Vials 1429

Methotrimeprazine (Concomitant use of amoxapine with other drugs that inhibit cytochrome $P_{450}IID_6$ may require lower than usual doses prescribed for either drug; enhanced response to central nervous system depressants). Products include:
Levoprome 1274

Methoxyflurane (Enhanced response to central nervous system depressants).
No products indexed under this heading.

Midazolam Hydrochloride (Enhanced response to central nervous system depressants). Products include:
Versed Injection 2170

Molindone Hydrochloride (Enhanced response to central nervous system depressants). Products include:
Moban Tablets and Concentrate 1048

Morphine Sulfate (Enhanced response to central nervous system depressants). Products include:
Astramorph/PF Injection, USP (Preservative-Free) 535
Duramorph 962
Infumorph 200 and Infumorph 500 Sterile Solutions 965
MS Contin Tablets 1994
MSIR 1997
Oramorph SR (Morphine Sulfate Sustained Release Tablets) 2236
RMS Suppositories 2657
Roxanol 2243

Nefazodone Hydrochloride (Concomitant use of amoxapine with other drugs that inhibit cytochrome $P_{450}IID_6$ may require lower than usual doses prescribed for either drug). Products include:
Serzone Tablets 771

Nortriptyline Hydrochloride (Concomitant use of amoxapine with other drugs that inhibit cytochrome $P_{450}IID_6$ may require lower than usual doses prescribed for either drug). Products include:
Pamelor 2280

Opium Alkaloids (Enhanced response to central nervous system depressants).
No products indexed under this heading.

Oxazepam (Enhanced response to central nervous system depressants). Products include:
Serax Capsules 2810
Serax Tablets 2810

Oxybutynin Chloride (Paralytic ileus may occur). Products include:
Ditropan 1516

IMPORTANT NOTE: Always consult each drug listing in the patient's regimen for possible interactions.

Oxycodone Hydrochloride (Enhanced response to central nervous system depressants). Products include:

Percocet Tablets ... 938
Percodan Tablets ... 939
Percodan-Demi Tablets ... 940
Roxicodone Tablets, Oral Solution & Intensol (Oxycodone) ... 2244
Tylox Capsules ... 1584

Oxyphenonium Bromide (Paralytic ileus may occur).

Paroxetine Hydrochloride (Concomitant use of amoxapine with other drugs that inhibit cytochrome $P_{450}IID_6$ may require lower than usual doses prescribed for either drug). Products include:

Paxil Tablets ... 2505

Pentobarbital Sodium (Enhanced response to barbiturates and central nervous system depressants). Products include:

Nembutal Sodium Capsules ... 436
Nembutal Sodium Solution ... 438
Nembutal Sodium Suppositories ... 440

Perphenazine (Concomitant use of amoxapine with other drugs that inhibit cytochrome $P_{450}IID_6$ may require lower than usual doses prescribed for either drug; enhanced response to central nervous system depressants). Products include:

Etrafon ... 2355
Triavil Tablets ... 1757
Trilafon ... 2389

Phenelzine Sulfate (Concurrent and/or sequential use may result in hyperpyretic crises, severe convulsions, and fatalities; coadministration is contraindicated). Products include:

Nardil ... 1920

Phenobarbital (Enhanced response to barbiturates and central nervous system depressants). Products include:

Arco-Lase Plus Tablets ... 512
Bellergal-S Tablets ... 2250
Donnatal ... 2060
Donnatal Extentabs ... 2061
Donnatal Tablets ... 2060
Phenobarbital Elixir and Tablets ... 1469
Quadrinal Tablets ... 1350

Prazepam (Enhanced response to central nervous system depressants).

No products indexed under this heading.

Prochlorperazine (Concomitant use of amoxapine with other drugs that inhibit cytochrome $P_{450}IID_6$ may require lower than usual doses prescribed for either drug; enhanced response to central nervous system depressants). Products include:

Compazine ... 2470

Procyclidine Hydrochloride (Paralytic ileus may occur). Products include:

Kemadrin Tablets ... 1112

Promethazine Hydrochloride (Concomitant use of amoxapine with other drugs that inhibit cytochrome $P_{450}IID_6$ may require lower than usual doses prescribed for either drug; enhanced response to central nervous system depressants). Products include:

Mepergan Injection ... 2753
Phenergan with Codeine ... 2777
Phenergan with Dextromethorphan 2778
Phenergan Injection ... 2773
Phenergan Suppositories ... 2775
Phenergan Syrup ... 2774
Phenergan Tablets ... 2775
Phenergan VC ... 2779
Phenergan VC with Codeine ... 2781

Propafenone Hydrochloride (Concomitant use of amoxapine with other drugs that inhibit cytochrome $P_{450}IID_6$ may require lower than usual doses prescribed for either drug). Products include:

Rythmol Tablets–150mg, 225mg, 300mg ... 1352

Propantheline Bromide (Paralytic ileus may occur). Products include:

Pro-Banthīne Tablets ... 2052

Propofol (Enhanced response to central nervous system depressants). Products include:

Diprivan Injection ... 2833

Propoxyphene Hydrochloride (Enhanced response to central nervous system depressants). Products include:

Darvon ... 1435
Wygesic Tablets ... 2827

Propoxyphene Napsylate (Enhanced response to central nervous system depressants). Products include:

Darvon-N/Darvocet-N ... 1433

Protriptyline Hydrochloride (Concomitant use of amoxapine with other drugs that inhibit cytochrome $P_{450}IID_6$ may require lower than usual doses prescribed for either drug). Products include:

Vivactil Tablets ... 1774

Quazepam (Enhanced response to central nervous system depressants). Products include:

Doral Tablets ... 2664

Quinidine Gluconate (Concomitant use of amoxapine with other drugs that inhibit cytochrome $P_{450}IID_6$ may require lower than usual doses prescribed for either drug). Products include:

Quinaglute Dura-Tabs Tablets ... 649

Quinidine Polygalacturonate (Concomitant use of amoxapine with other drugs that inhibit cytochrome $P_{450}IID_6$ may require lower than usual doses prescribed for either drug).

No products indexed under this heading.

Quinidine Sulfate (Concomitant use of amoxapine with other drugs that inhibit cytochrome $P_{450}IID_6$ may require lower than usual doses prescribed for either drug). Products include:

Quinidex Extentabs ... 2067

Risperidone (Enhanced response to central nervous system depressants). Products include:

Risperdal ... 1301

Scopolamine (Paralytic ileus may occur). Products include:

Transderm Scōp Transdermal Therapeutic System ... 869

Scopolamine Hydrobromide (Paralytic ileus may occur). Products include:

Atrohist Plus Tablets ... 454
Donnatal ... 2060
Donnatal Extentabs ... 2061
Donnatal Tablets ... 2060

Secobarbital Sodium (Enhanced response to barbiturates and central nervous system depressants). Products include:

Seconal Sodium Pulvules ... 1474

Selegiline Hydrochloride (Concurrent and/or sequential use may result in hyperpyretic crises, severe convulsions, and fatalities; coadministration is contraindicated). Products include:

Eldepryl Tablets ... 2550

Sertraline Hydrochloride (Concomitant use of amoxapine with other drugs that inhibit cytochrome $P_{450}IID_6$ may require lower than usual doses prescribed for either drug). Products include:

Zoloft Tablets ... 2217

Sufentanil Citrate (Enhanced response to central nervous system depressants). Products include:

Sufenta Injection ... 1309

Temazepam (Enhanced response to central nervous system depressants). Products include:

Restoril Capsules ... 2284

Thiamylal Sodium (Enhanced response to barbiturates and central nervous system depressants).

No products indexed under this heading.

Thioridazine Hydrochloride (Concomitant use of amoxapine with other drugs that inhibit cytochrome $P_{450}IID_6$ may require lower than usual doses prescribed for either drug; enhanced response to central nervous system depressants). Products include:

Mellaril ... 2269

Thiothixene (Enhanced response to central nervous system depressants). Products include:

Navane Capsules and Concentrate 2201
Navane Intramuscular ... 2202

Tranylcypromine Sulfate (Concurrent and/or sequential use may result in hyperpyretic crises, severe convulsions, and fatalities; coadministration is contraindicated). Products include:

Parnate Tablets ... 2503

Trazodone Hydrochloride (Concomittant use of amoxapine with other drugs that inhibit cytochrome $P_{450}IID_6$ may require lower than usual doses prescribed for either drug). Products include:

Desyrel and Desyrel Dividose ... 503

Triazolam (Enhanced response to central nervous system depressants). Products include:

Halcion Tablets ... 2611

Tridihexethyl Chloride (Paralytic ileus may occur).

No products indexed under this heading.

Trifluoperazine Hydrochloride (Concomitant use of amoxapine with other drugs that inhibit cytochrome $P_{450}IID_6$ may require lower than usual doses prescribed for either drug; enhanced response to central nervous system depressants). Products include:

Stelazine ... 2514

Trihexyphenidyl Hydrochloride (Paralytic ileus may occur). Products include:

Artane ... 1368

Trimipramine Maleate (Concomitant use of amoxapine with other drugs that inhibit cytochrome $P_{450}IID_6$ may require lower than usual doses prescribed for either drug). Products include:

Surmontil Capsules ... 2811

Venlafaxine Hydrochloride (Concomitant use of amoxapine with other drugs that inhibit cytochrome $P_{450}IID_6$ may require lower than usual doses prescribed for either drug). Products include:

Effexor ... 2719

Zolpidem Tartrate (Enhanced response to central nervous system depressants). Products include:

Ambien Tablets ... 2416

Food Interactions

Alcohol (Enhanced response to alcohol).

ASPERCREME CREME, LOTION ANALGESIC RUB

(Trolamine Salicylate) ... ▣ 830
None cited in PDR database.

ASTRAMORPH/PF INJECTION, USP (PRESERVATIVE-FREE)

(Morphine Sulfate) ... 535
May interact with central nervous system depressants, psychotropics, antihistamines, antipsychotic agents, and certain other agents. Compounds in these categories include:

Acrivastine (Potentiation of depressant effects of morphine). Products include:

Semprex-D Capsules ... 463
Semprex-D Capsules ... 1167

Alfentanil Hydrochloride (Potentiation of depressant effects of morphine). Products include:

Alfenta Injection ... 1286

Alprazolam (Potentiation of depressant effects of morphine). Products include:

Xanax Tablets ... 2649

Amitriptyline Hydrochloride (Potentiation of depressant effects of morphine). Products include:

Elavil ... 2838
Endep Tablets ... 2174
Etrafon ... 2355
Limbitrol ... 2180
Triavil Tablets ... 1757

Amoxapine (Potentiation of depressant effects of morphine). Products include:

Asendin Tablets ... 1369

Aprobarbital (Potentiation of depressant effects of morphine).

No products indexed under this heading.

Astemizole (Potentiation of depressant effects of morphine). Products include:

Hismanal Tablets ... 1293

Azatadine Maleate (Potentiation of depressant effects of morphine). Products include:

Trinalin Repetabs Tablets ... 1330

Bromodiphenhydramine Hydrochloride (Potentiation of depressant effects of morphine).

No products indexed under this heading.

Brompheniramine Maleate (Potentiation of depressant effects of morphine). Products include:

Alka Seltzer Plus Sinus Medicine .. ▣ 707
Bromfed Capsules (Extended-Release) ... 1785
Bromfed Syrup ... ▣ 733
Bromfed Tablets ... 1785
Bromfed-DM Cough Syrup ... 1786
Bromfed-PD Capsules (Extended-Release) ... 1785
Dimetane-DC Cough Syrup ... 2059
Dimetane-DX Cough Syrup ... 2059
Dimetapp Elixir ... ▣ 773
Dimetapp Extentabs ... ▣ 774
Dimetapp Tablets/Liqui-Gels ... ▣ 775
Dimetapp Cold & Allergy Chewable Tablets ... ▣ 773
Dimetapp DM Elixir ... ▣ 774
Vicks DayQuil Allergy Relief 12-Hour Extended Release Tablets .. ▣ 760
Vicks DayQuil Allergy Relief 4-Hour Tablets ... ▣ 760

Buprenorphine (Potentiation of depressant effects of morphine). Products include:

Buprenex Injectable ... 2006

Buspirone Hydrochloride (Potentiation of depressant effects of morphine). Products include:

BuSpar ... 737

(▣ Described in PDR For Nonprescription Drugs) (⊙ Described in PDR For Ophthalmology)

Interactions Index — Astramorph PF

Butabarbital (Potentiation of depressant effects of morphine).

No products indexed under this heading.

Butalbital (Potentiation of depressant effects of morphine). Products include:

Esgic-plus Tablets 1013
Fioricet Tablets 2258
Fioricet with Codeine Capsules 2260
Fiorinal Capsules 2261
Fiorinal with Codeine Capsules 2262
Fiorinal Tablets 2261
Phrenilin 785
Sedapap Tablets 50 mg/650 mg .. 1543

Chlordiazepoxide (Potentiation of depressant effects of morphine). Products include:

Libritabs Tablets 2177
Limbitrol 2180

Chlordiazepoxide Hydrochloride (Potentiation of depressant effects of morphine). Products include:

Librax Capsules 2176
Librium Capsules 2178
Librium Injectable 2179

Chlorpheniramine Maleate (Potentiation of depressant effects of morphine). Products include:

Alka-Seltzer Plus Cold Medicine .... ⊞ 705
Alka-Seltzer Plus Cold Medicine Liqui-Gels .... ⊞ 706
Alka-Seltzer Plus Cold & Cough Medicine .... ⊞ 708
Alka-Seltzer Plus Cold & Cough Medicine Liqui-Gels .... ⊞ 705
Allerest Children's Chewable Tablets .... ⊞ 627
Allerest Headache Strength Tablets .... ⊞ 627
Allerest Maximum Strength Tablets .... ⊞ 627
Allerest Sinus Pain Formula .... ⊞ 627
Allerest 12 Hour Caplets .... ⊞ 627
Ana-Kit Anaphylaxis Emergency Treatment Kit 617
Atrohist Pediatric Capsules 453
Atrohist Plus Tablets 454
BC Cold Powder Multi-Symptom Formula (Cold-Sinus-Allergy) ...... ⊞ 609
Cerose DM .... ⊞ 878
Cheracol Plus Head Cold/Cough Formula .... ⊞ 769
Children's Vicks DayQuil Allergy Relief .... ⊞ 757
Children's Vicks NyQuil Cold/ Cough Relief .... ⊞ 758
Chlor-Trimeton Allergy Decongestant Tablets .... ⊞ 799
Chlor-Trimeton Allergy Tablets ...... ⊞ 798
Comhist 2038
Comtrex Multi-Symptom Cold Reliever Tablets/Caplets/Liqui-Gels/Liquid .... ⊞ 615
Allergy-Sinus Comtrex Multi-Symptom Allergy-Sinus Formula Tablets .... ⊞ 617
Contac Continuous Action Nasal Decongestant/Antihistamine 12 Hour Capsules .... ⊞ 813
Contac Maximum Strength Continuous Action Decongestant/ Antihistamine 12 Hour Caplets .. ⊞ 813
Contac Severe Cold and Flu Formula Caplets .... ⊞ 814
Coricidin 'D' Decongestant Tablets .... ⊞ 800
Coricidin Tablets .... ⊞ 800
D.A. Chewable Tablets 951
Deconamine 1320
Dura-Tap/PD Capsules 2867
Dura-Vent/DA Tablets 953
Extendryl 1005
Fedahist Gyrocaps 2401
Fedahist Timecaps 2401
Hycomine Compound Tablets 932
Isoclor Timesule Capsules .... ⊞ 637
Kronofed-A 977
Nolamine Timed-Release Tablets 785
Novahistine DH 2462
Novahistine Elixir .... ⊞ 823
Ornade Spansule Capsules 2502
PediaCare Cold Allergy Chewable Tablets .... ⊞ 677
PediaCare Cough-Cold Chewable Tablets 1553
PediaCare Cough-Cold Liquid 1553
PediaCare NightRest Cough-Cold Liquid 1553
Pediatric Vicks 44m Cough & Cold Relief .... ⊞ 764
Pyrroxate Caplets .... ⊞ 772
Ryna .... ⊞ 841
Sinarest Tablets .... ⊞ 648
Sinarest Extra Strength Tablets ...... ⊞ 648
Sine-Off Sinus Medicine .... ⊞ 825
Singlet Tablets .... ⊞ 825
Sinulin Tablets 787
Sinutab Sinus Allergy Medication, Maximum Strength Tablets and Caplets .... ⊞ 860
Sudafed Plus Liquid .... ⊞ 862
Sudafed Plus Tablets .... ⊞ 863
Teldrin 12 Hour Antihistamine/ Nasal Decongestant Allergy Relief Capsules .... ⊞ 826
TheraFlu .... ⊞ 787
TheraFlu Maximum Strength Nighttime Flu, Cold & Cough Medicine .... ⊞ 788
Triaminic Allergy Tablets .... ⊞ 789
Triaminic Cold Tablets .... ⊞ 790
Triaminic Nite Light .... ⊞ 791
Triaminic Syrup .... ⊞ 792
Triaminic-12 Tablets .... ⊞ 792
Triaminicin Tablets .... ⊞ 793
Triaminicol Multi-Symptom Cold Tablets .... ⊞ 793
Triaminicol Multi-Symptom Relief ⊞ 794
Tussend 1783
Children's TYLENOL Cold Multi-Symptom Liquid Formula and Chewable Tablets 1561
Children's TYLENOL Cold Plus Cough Multi Symptom Tablets and Liquid .... ⊞ 681
TYLENOL Maximum Strength Allergy Sinus Medication Gelcaps and Caplets 1563
TYLENOL Cold Multi-Symptom Formula Medication Tablets and Caplets 1561
TYLENOL Cold Multi-Symptom Hot Medication Liquid Packets 1557
Vicks 44 LiquiCaps Cough, Cold & Flu Relief .... ⊞ 755
Vicks 44M Cough, Cold & Flu Relief .... ⊞ 756

Chlorpheniramine Polistirex (Potentiation of depressant effects of morphine). Products include:

Tussionex Pennkinetic Extended-Release Suspension 998

Chlorpheniramine Tannate (Potentiation of depressant effects of morphine). Products include:

Atrohist Pediatric Suspension 454
Ricobid Tablets and Pediatric Suspension 2038
Rynatan 2673
Rynatuss 2673

Chlorpromazine (Potentiation of depressant effects of morphine; increased risk of respiratory depression). Products include:

Thorazine Suppositories 2523

Chlorprothixene (Potentiation of depressant effects of morphine; increased risk of respiratory depression).

No products indexed under this heading.

Chlorprothixene Hydrochloride (Potentiation of depressant effects of morphine; increased risk of respiratory depression).

No products indexed under this heading.

Clemastine Fumarate (Potentiation of depressant effects of morphine). Products include:

Tavist Syrup 2297
Tavist Tablets 2298
Tavist-1 12 Hour Relief Tablets .... ⊞ 787
Tavist-D 12 Hour Relief Tablets .... ⊞ 787

Clorazepate Dipotassium (Potentiation of depressant effects of morphine). Products include:

Tranxene 451

Clozapine (Potentiation of depressant effects of morphine; increased risk of respiratory depression). Products include:

Clozaril Tablets 2252

Codeine Phosphate (Potentiation of depressant effects of morphine). Products include:

Actifed with Codeine Cough Syrup .. 1067
Brontex 1981
Deconsal C Expectorant Syrup 456
Deconsal Pediatric Syrup 457
Dimetane-DC Cough Syrup 2059
Empirin with Codeine Tablets 1093
Fioricet with Codeine Capsules 2260
Fiorinal with Codeine Capsules 2262
Isoclor Expectorant 990
Novahistine DH 2462
Novahistine Expectorant 2463
Nucofed 2051
Phenergan with Codeine 2777
Phenergan VC with Codeine 2781
Robitussin A-C Syrup 2073
Robitussin-DAC Syrup 2074
Ryna .... ⊞ 841
Soma Compound w/Codeine Tablets 2676
Tussi-Organidin NR Liquid and S NR Liquid 2677
Tylenol with Codeine 1583

Cyproheptadine Hydrochloride (Potentiation of depressant effects of morphine). Products include:

Periactin 1724

Desflurane (Potentiation of depressant effects of morphine). Products include:

Suprane 1813

Desipramine Hydrochloride (Potentiation of depressant effects of morphine). Products include:

Norpramin Tablets 1526

Dexchlorpheniramine Maleate (Potentiation of depressant effects of morphine).

No products indexed under this heading.

Dezocine (Potentiation of depressant effects of morphine). Products include:

Dalgan Injection 538

Diazepam (Potentiation of depressant effects of morphine). Products include:

Dizac 1809
Valium Injectable 2182
Valium Tablets 2183
Valrelease Capsules 2169

Diethylpropion Hydrochloride (Potentiation of depressant effects of morphine).

No products indexed under this heading.

Diphenhydramine Citrate (Potentiation of depressant effects of morphine). Products include:

Excedrin P.M. Analgesic/Sleeping Aid Tablets, Caplets, Liquigels 733

Diphenhydramine Hydrochloride (Potentiation of depressant effects of morphine). Products include:

Actifed Allergy Daytime/Nighttime Caplets .... ⊞ 844
Actifed Sinus Daytime/Nighttime Tablets and Caplets .... ⊞ 846
Arthritis Foundation NightTime Caplets .... ⊞ 674
Extra Strength Bayer PM Aspirin .. ⊞ 713
Bayer Select Night Time Pain Relief Formula .... ⊞ 716
Benadryl Allergy Decongestant Liquid Medication .... ⊞ 848
Benadryl Allergy Decongestant Tablets .... ⊞ 848
Benadryl Allergy Liquid Medication .... ⊞ 849
Benadryl Allergy .... ⊞ 848
Benadryl Allergy Sinus Headache Formula Caplets .... ⊞ 849
Benadryl Capsules 1898
Benadryl Dye-Free Allergy Liquigel Softgels .... ⊞ 850
Benadryl Dye-Free Allergy Liquid Medication .... ⊞ 850
Benadryl Itch Relief Cream, Children's Formula and Maximum Strength 2% .... ⊞ 851
Benadryl Itch Relief Spray, Children's Formula and Maximum Strength 2% .... ⊞ 851
Benadryl Itch Relief Stick Maximum Strength 2% .... ⊞ 850
Benadryl Itch Stopping Gel, Children's Formula and Maximum Strength 2% .... ⊞ 851
Benadryl Kapseals 1898
Benadryl Injection 1898
Contac Day & Night Cold/Flu Night Caplets .... ⊞ 812
Contac Night Allergy/Sinus Caplets .... ⊞ 812
Extra Strength Doan's P.M. .... ⊞ 633
Legatrin PM .... ⊞ 651
Miles Nervine Nighttime Sleep-Aid ⊞ 723
Nytol QuickCaps Caplets .... ⊞ 610
Sleepinal Night-time Sleep Aid Capsules and Softgels .... ⊞ 834
TYLENOL Maximum Strength Allergy Sinus NightTime Medication Caplets 1555
TYLENOL Flu NightTime, Maximum Strength, Gelcaps 1566
TYLENOL Maximum Strength Flu NightTime Hot Medication Packets 1562
TYLENOL PM, Extra Strength Pain Reliever/Sleep Aid Caplets, Geltabs, Gelcaps 1560
TYLENOL Severe Allergy Medication Caplets 1564
Maximum Strength Unisom Sleepgels 1934
Unisom With Pain Relief-Nighttime Sleep Aid and Pain Reliever 1934

Diphenylpyraline Hydrochloride (Potentiation of depressant effects of morphine).

No products indexed under this heading.

Doxepin Hydrochloride (Potentiation of depressant effects of morphine). Products include:

Sinequan 2205
Zonalon Cream 1055

Droperidol (Potentiation of depressant effects of morphine). Products include:

Inapsine Injection 1296

Enflurane (Potentiation of depressant effects of morphine).

No products indexed under this heading.

Estazolam (Potentiation of depressant effects of morphine). Products include:

ProSom Tablets 449

Ethchlorvynol (Potentiation of depressant effects of morphine). Products include:

Placidyl Capsules 448

Ethinamate (Potentiation of depressant effects of morphine).

No products indexed under this heading.

Fentanyl (Potentiation of depressant effects of morphine). Products include:

Duragesic Transdermal System 1288

Fentanyl Citrate (Potentiation of depressant effects of morphine). Products include:

Sublimaze Injection 1307

Fluphenazine Decanoate (Potentiation of depressant effects of morphine; increased risk of respiratory depression). Products include:

Prolixin Decanoate 509

Fluphenazine Enanthate (Potentiation of depressant effects of morphine; increased risk of respiratory depression). Products include:

Prolixin Enanthate 509

IMPORTANT NOTE: Always consult each drug listing in the patient's regimen for possible interactions.

Astramorph PF — Interactions Index — 84

Fluphenazine Hydrochloride (Potentiation of depressant effects of morphine; increased risk of respiratory depression). Products include:
- Prolixin ... 509

Flurazepam Hydrochloride (Potentiation of depressant effects of morphine). Products include:
- Dalmane Capsules ... 2173

Glutethimide (Potentiation of depressant effects of morphine).
- No products indexed under this heading.

Haloperidol (Potentiation of depressant effects of morphine). Products include:
- Haldol Injection, Tablets and Concentrate ... 1575

Haloperidol Decanoate (Potentiation of depressant effects of morphine; increased risk of respiratory depression). Products include:
- Haldol Decanoate ... 1577

Hydrocodone Bitartrate (Potentiation of depressant effects of morphine). Products include:
- Anexsia 5/500 Elixir ... 1781
- Anexia Tablets ... 1782
- Codiclear DH Syrup ... 791
- Deconamine CX Cough and Cold Liquid and Tablets ... 1319
- Duratuss HD Elixir ... 2565
- Hycodan Tablets and Syrup ... 930
- Hycomine Compound Tablets ... 932
- Hycomine ... 931
- Hycotuss Expectorant Syrup ... 933
- Hydrocet Capsules ... 782
- Lorcet 10/650 ... 1018
- Lortab ... 2566
- Tussend ... 1783
- Tussend Expectorant ... 1785
- Vicodin Tablets ... 1356
- Vicodin ES Tablets ... 1357
- Vicodin Tuss Expectorant ... 1358
- Zydone Capsules ... 949

Hydrocodone Polistirex (Potentiation of depressant effects of morphine). Products include:
- Tussionex Pennkinetic Extended-Release Suspension ... 998

Hydroxyzine Hydrochloride (Potentiation of depressant effects of morphine). Products include:
- Atarax Tablets & Syrup ... 2185
- Marax Tablets & DF Syrup ... 2200
- Vistaril Intramuscular Solution ... 2216

Imipramine Hydrochloride (Potentiation of depressant effects of morphine). Products include:
- Tofranil Ampuls ... 854
- Tofranil Tablets ... 856

Imipramine Pamoate (Potentiation of depressant effects of morphine). Products include:
- Tofranil-PM Capsules ... 857

Isocarboxazid (Potentiation of depressant effects of morphine).
- No products indexed under this heading.

Isoflurane (Potentiation of depressant effects of morphine).
- No products indexed under this heading.

Ketamine Hydrochloride (Potentiation of depressant effects of morphine).
- No products indexed under this heading.

Levomethadyl Acetate Hydrochloride (Potentiation of depressant effects of morphine). Products include:
- Orlamm ... 2239

Levorphanol Tartrate (Potentiation of depressant effects of morphine). Products include:
- Levo-Dromoran ... 2129

Lithium Carbonate (Potentiation of depressant effects of morphine; increased risk of respiratory depression). Products include:
- Eskalith ... 2485
- Lithium Carbonate Capsules & Tablets ... 2230
- Lithonate/Lithotabs/Lithobid ... 2543

Lithium Citrate (Potentiation of depressant effects of morphine; increased risk of respiratory depression).
- No products indexed under this heading.

Loratadine (Potentiation of depressant effects of morphine). Products include:
- Claritin ... 2349
- Claritin-D ... 2350

Lorazepam (Potentiation of depressant effects of morphine). Products include:
- Ativan Injection ... 2698
- Ativan Tablets ... 2700

Loxapine Hydrochloride (Potentiation of depressant effects of morphine; increased risk of respiratory depression). Products include:
- Loxitane ... 1378

Loxapine Succinate (Potentiation of depressant effects of morphine). Products include:
- Loxitane Capsules ... 1378

Maprotiline Hydrochloride (Potentiation of depressant effects of morphine). Products include:
- Ludiomil Tablets ... 843

Meperidine Hydrochloride (Potentiation of depressant effects of morphine). Products include:
- Demerol ... 2308
- Mepergan Injection ... 2753

Mephobarbital (Potentiation of depressant effects of morphine). Products include:
- Mebaral Tablets ... 2322

Meprobamate (Potentiation of depressant effects of morphine). Products include:
- Miltown Tablets ... 2672
- PMB 200 and PMB 400 ... 2783

Mesoridazine Besylate (Potentiation of depressant effects of morphine; increased risk of respiratory depression). Products include:
- Serentil ... 684

Methadone Hydrochloride (Potentiation of depressant effects of morphine). Products include:
- Methadone Hydrochloride Oral Concentrate ... 2233
- Methadone Hydrochloride Oral Solution & Tablets ... 2235

Methdilazine Hydrochloride (Potentiation of depressant effects of morphine).
- No products indexed under this heading.

Methohexital Sodium (Potentiation of depressant effects of morphine). Products include:
- Brevital Sodium Vials ... 1429

Methotrimeprazine (Potentiation of depressant effects of morphine). Products include:
- Levoprome ... 1274

Methoxyflurane (Potentiation of depressant effects of morphine).
- No products indexed under this heading.

Midazolam Hydrochloride (Potentiation of depressant effects of morphine). Products include:
- Versed Injection ... 2170

Molindone Hydrochloride (Potentiation of depressant effects of morphine; increased risk of respiratory depression with neuroleptics). Products include:
- Moban Tablets and Concentrate ... 1048

Nortriptyline Hydrochloride (Potentiation of depressant effects of morphine). Products include:
- Pamelor ... 2280

Opium Alkaloids (Potentiation of depressant effects of morphine).
- No products indexed under this heading.

Oxazepam (Potentiation of depressant effects of morphine). Products include:
- Serax Capsules ... 2810
- Serax Tablets ... 2810

Oxycodone Hydrochloride (Potentiation of depressant effects of morphine). Products include:
- Percocet Tablets ... 938
- Percodan Tablets ... 939
- Percodan-Demi Tablets ... 940
- Roxicodone Tablets, Oral Solution & Intensol (Oxycodone) ... 2244
- Tylox Capsules ... 1584

Pentobarbital Sodium (Potentiation of depressant effects of morphine). Products include:
- Nembutal Sodium Capsules ... 436
- Nembutal Sodium Solution ... 438
- Nembutal Sodium Suppositories ... 440

Perphenazine (Potentiation of depressant effects of morphine). Products include:
- Etrafon ... 2355
- Triavil Tablets ... 1757
- Trilafon ... 2389

Phenelzine Sulfate (Potentiation of depressant effects of morphine). Products include:
- Nardil ... 1920

Phenobarbital (Potentiation of depressant effects of morphine). Products include:
- Arco-Lase Plus Tablets ... 512
- Bellergal-S Tablets ... 2250
- Donnatal ... 2060
- Donnatal Extentabs ... 2061
- Donnatal Tablets ... 2060
- Phenobarbital Elixir and Tablets ... 1469
- Quadrinal Tablets ... 1350

Pimozide (Potentiation of depressant effects of morphine; increased risk of respiratory depression). Products include:
- Orap Tablets ... 1050

Prazepam (Potentiation of depressant effects of morphine).
- No products indexed under this heading.

Prochlorperazine (Potentiation of depressant effects of morphine; increased risk of respiratory depression). Products include:
- Compazine ... 2470

Promethazine Hydrochloride (Potentiation of depressant effects of morphine; increased risk of respiratory depression). Products include:
- Mepergan Injection ... 2753
- Phenergan with Codeine ... 2777
- Phenergan with Dextromethorphan 2778
- Phenergan Injection ... 2773
- Phenergan Suppositories ... 2775
- Phenergan Syrup ... 2774
- Phenergan Tablets ... 2775
- Phenergan VC ... 2779
- Phenergan VC with Codeine ... 2781

Propofol (Potentiation of depressant effects of morphine). Products include:
- Diprivan Injection ... 2833

Propoxyphene Hydrochloride (Potentiation of depressant effects of morphine). Products include:
- Darvon ... 1435
- Wygesic Tablets ... 2827

Propoxyphene Napsylate (Potentiation of depressant effects of morphine). Products include:
- Darvon-N/Darvocet-N ... 1433

Protriptyline Hydrochloride (Potentiation of depressant effects of morphine). Products include:
- Vivactil Tablets ... 1774

Pyrilamine Maleate (Potentiation of depressant effects of morphine). Products include:
- 4-Way Fast Acting Nasal Spray (regular & mentholated) ... ▣ 621
- Maximum Strength Multi-Symptom Formula Midol ... ▣ 722
- PMS Multi-Symptom Formula Midol ... ▣ 723

Pyrilamine Tannate (Potentiation of depressant effects of morphine). Products include:
- Atrohist Pediatric Suspension ... 454
- Rynatan ... 2673

Quazepam (Potentiation of depressant effects of morphine). Products include:
- Doral Tablets ... 2664

Risperidone (Potentiation of depressant effects of morphine). Products include:
- Risperdal ... 1301

Secobarbital Sodium (Potentiation of depressant effects of morphine). Products include:
- Seconal Sodium Pulvules ... 1474

Sufentanil Citrate (Potentiation of depressant effects of morphine). Products include:
- Sufenta Injection ... 1309

Temazepam (Potentiation of depressant effects of morphine). Products include:
- Restoril Capsules ... 2284

Terfenadine (Potentiation of depressant effects of morphine). Products include:
- Seldane Tablets ... 1536
- Seldane-D Extended-Release Tablets ... 1538

Thiamylal Sodium (Potentiation of depressant effects of morphine).
- No products indexed under this heading.

Thioridazine Hydrochloride (Potentiation of depressant effects of morphine; increased risk of respiratory depression). Products include:
- Mellaril ... 2269

Thiothixene (Potentiation of depressant effects of morphine; increased risk of respiratory depression). Products include:
- Navane Capsules and Concentrate 2201
- Navane Intramuscular ... 2202

Tranylcypromine Sulfate (Potentiation of depressant effects of morphine). Products include:
- Parnate Tablets ... 2503

Triazolam (Potentiation of depressant effects of morphine). Products include:
- Halcion Tablets ... 2611

Trifluoperazine Hydrochloride (Potentiation of depressant effects of morphine; increased risk of respiratory depression). Products include:
- Stelazine ... 2514

Trimeprazine Tartrate (Potentiation of depressant effects of morphine). Products include:
- Temaril Tablets, Syrup and Spansule Extended-Release Capsules .. 483

Trimipramine Maleate (Potentiation of depressant effects of morphine). Products include:
- Surmontil Capsules ... 2811

(▣ Described in PDR For Nonprescription Drugs) (◉ Described in PDR For Ophthalmology)

Interactions Index

Tripelennamine Hydrochloride (Potentiation of depressant effects of morphine). Products include:

PBZ Tablets 845
PBZ-SR Tablets................................... 844

Triprolidine Hydrochloride (Potentiation of depressant effects of morphine). Products include:

Actifed Plus Caplets .... ◻️ 845
Actifed Plus Tablets .... ◻️ 845
Actifed with Codeine Cough Syrup.. 1067
Actifed Syrup....................................... ◻️ 846
Actifed Tablets .... ◻️ 844

Zolpidem Tartrate (Potentiation of depressant effects of morphine). Products include:

Ambien Tablets.................................... 2416

Food Interactions

Alcohol (Potentiation of depressant effects of morphine).

ATAMET

(Carbidopa, Levodopa) 572

May interact with monoamine oxidase inhibitors, antihypertensives, tricyclic antidepressants, phenothiazines, and butyrophenones. Compounds in these categories include:

Acebutolol Hydrochloride (Potential for symptomatic postural hypotension). Products include:

Sectral Capsules 2807

Amitriptyline Hydrochloride (Potential for rare adverse reactions, including hypertension and dyskinesia). Products include:

Elavil 2838
Endep Tablets 2174
Etrafon 2355
Limbitrol 2180
Triavil Tablets 1757

Amlodipine Besylate (Potential for symptomatic postural hypotension). Products include:

Lotrel Capsules 840
Norvasc Tablets 1940

Amoxapine (Potential for rare adverse reactions, including hypertension and dyskinesia). Products include:

Asendin Tablets 1369

Atenolol (Potential for symptomatic postural hypotension). Products include:

Tenoretic Tablets 2845
Tenormin Tablets and I.V. Injection 2847

Benazepril Hydrochloride (Potential for symptomatic postural hypotension). Products include:

Lotensin Tablets 834
Lotensin HCT...................................... 837
Lotrel Capsules 840

Bendroflumethiazide (Potential for symptomatic postural hypotension).

No products indexed under this heading.

Betaxolol Hydrochloride (Potential for symptomatic postural hypotension). Products include:

Betoptic Ophthalmic Solution............ 469
Betoptic S Ophthalmic Suspension 471
Kerlone Tablets................................... 2436

Bisoprolol Fumarate (Potential for symptomatic postural hypotension). Products include:

Zebeta Tablets 1413
Ziac 1415

Captopril (Potential for symptomatic postural hypotension). Products include:

Capoten 739
Capozide 742

Carteolol Hydrochloride (Potential for symptomatic postural hypotension). Products include:

Cartrol Tablets 410
Ocupress Ophthalmic Solution, 1% Sterile.. ◎ 309

Chlorothiazide (Potential for symptomatic postural hypotension). Products include:

Aldoclor Tablets 1598
Diupres Tablets 1650
Diuril Oral 1653

Chlorothiazide Sodium (Potential for symptomatic postural hypotension). Products include:

Diuril Sodium Intravenous 1652

Chlorpromazine (Reduces therapeutic effect of levodopa). Products include:

Thorazine Suppositories 2523

Chlorpromazine Hydrochloride (Reduces therapeutic effect of levodopa). Products include:

Thorazine 2523

Chlorthalidone (Potential for symptomatic postural hypotension). Products include:

Combipres Tablets 677
Tenoretic Tablets 2845
Thalitone 1245

Clomipramine Hydrochloride (Potential for rare adverse reactions, including hypertension and dyskinesia). Products include:

Anafranil Capsules 803

Clonidine (Potential for symptomatic postural hypotension). Products include:

Catapres-TTS...................................... 675

Clonidine Hydrochloride (Potential for symptomatic postural hypotension). Products include:

Catapres Tablets 674
Combipres Tablets 677

Deserpidine (Potential for symptomatic postural hypotension).

No products indexed under this heading.

Desipramine Hydrochloride (Potential for rare adverse reactions, including hypertension and dyskinesia). Products include:

Norpramin Tablets 1526

Diazoxide (Potential for symptomatic postural hypotension). Products include:

Hyperstat I.V. Injection 2363
Proglycem... 580

Diltiazem Hydrochloride (Potential for symptomatic postural hypotension). Products include:

Cardizem CD Capsules 1506
Cardizem SR Capsules 1510
Cardizem Injectable 1508
Cardizem Tablets................................. 1512
Dilacor XR Extended-release Capsules 2018

Doxazosin Mesylate (Potential for symptomatic postural hypotension). Products include:

Cardura Tablets 2186

Doxepin Hydrochloride (Potential for rare adverse reactions, including hypertension and dyskinesia). Products include:

Sinequan 2205
Zonalon Cream 1055

Enalapril Maleate (Potential for symptomatic postural hypotension). Products include:

Vaseretic Tablets 1765
Vasotec Tablets 1771

Enalaprilat (Potential for symptomatic postural hypotension). Products include:

Vasotec I.V.. 1768

Esmolol Hydrochloride (Potential for symptomatic postural hypotension). Products include:

Brevibloc Injection............................... 1808

Felodipine (Potential for symptomatic postural hypotension). Products include:

Plendil Extended-Release Tablets..... 527

Fluphenazine Decanoate (Reduces therapeutic effect of levodopa). Products include:

Prolixin Decanoate 509

Fluphenazine Enanthate (Reduces therapeutic effect of levodopa). Products include:

Prolixin Enanthate 509

Fluphenazine Hydrochloride (Reduces therapeutic effect of levodopa). Products include:

Prolixin 509

Fosinopril Sodium (Potential for symptomatic postural hypotension). Products include:

Monopril Tablets 757

Furazolidone (Concurrent use is contraindicated). Products include:

Furoxone 2046

Furosemide (Potential for symptomatic postural hypotension). Products include:

Lasix Injection, Oral Solution and Tablets 1240

Guanabenz Acetate (Potential for symptomatic postural hypotension).

No products indexed under this heading.

Guanethidine Monosulfate (Potential for symptomatic postural hypotension). Products include:

Esimil Tablets 822
Ismelin Tablets 827

Haloperidol (Reduces therapeutic effect of levodopa). Products include:

Haldol Injection, Tablets and Concentrate 1575

Haloperidol Decanoate (Reduces therapeutic effect of levodopa). Products include:

Haldol Decanoate................................. 1577

Hydralazine Hydrochloride (Potential for symptomatic postural hypotension). Products include:

Apresazide Capsules 808
Apresoline Hydrochloride Tablets .. 809
Ser-Ap-Es Tablets 849

Hydrochlorothiazide (Potential for symptomatic postural hypotension). Products include:

Aldactazide.. 2413
Aldoril Tablets..................................... 1604
Apresazide Capsules 808
Capozide 742
Dyazide 2479
Esidrix Tablets 821
Esimil Tablets 822
HydroDIURIL Tablets 1674
Hydropres Tablets................................ 1675
Hyzaar Tablets 1677
Inderide Tablets 2732
Inderide LA Long Acting Capsules.. 2734
Lopressor HCT Tablets 832
Lotensin HCT...................................... 837
Maxzide 1380
Moduretic Tablets 1705
Oretic Tablets 443
Prinzide Tablets................................... 1737
Ser-Ap-Es Tablets 849
Timolide Tablets................................... 1748
Vaseretic Tablets 1765
Zestoretic 2850
Ziac 1415

Hydroflumethiazide (Potential for symptomatic postural hypotension). Products include:

Diucardin Tablets................................. 2718

Imipramine Hydrochloride (Potential for rare adverse reactions, including hypertension and dyskinesia). Products include:

Tofranil Ampuls 854
Tofranil Tablets 856

Imipramine Pamoate (Potential for rare adverse reactions, including hypertension and dyskinesia). Products include:

Tofranil-PM Capsules.......................... 857

Indapamide (Potential for symptomatic postural hypotension). Products include:

Lozol Tablets 2022

Isocarboxazid (Concurrent use is contraindicated).

No products indexed under this heading.

Isradipine (Potential for symptomatic postural hypotension). Products include:

DynaCirc Capsules 2256

Labetalol Hydrochloride (Potential for symptomatic postural hypotension). Products include:

Normodyne Injection 2377
Normodyne Tablets 2379
Trandate 1185

Lisinopril (Potential for symptomatic postural hypotension). Products include:

Prinivil Tablets 1733
Prinzide Tablets 1737
Zestoretic 2850
Zestril Tablets 2854

Losartan Potassium (Potential for symptomatic postural hypotension). Products include:

Cozaar Tablets 1628
Hyzaar Tablets 1677

Maprotiline Hydrochloride (Potential for rare adverse reactions, including hypertension and dyskinesia). Products include:

Ludiomil Tablets.................................. 843

Mecamylamine Hydrochloride (Potential for symptomatic postural hypotension). Products include:

Inversine Tablets 1686

Mesoridazine Besylate (Reduces therapeutic effect of levodopa). Products include:

Serentil... 684

Methotrimeprazine (Reduces therapeutic effect of levodopa). Products include:

Levoprome 1274

Methyclothiazide (Potential for symptomatic postural hypotension). Products include:

Enduron Tablets................................... 420

Methyldopa (Potential for symptomatic postural hypotension). Products include:

Aldoclor Tablets 1598
Aldomet Oral 1600
Aldoril Tablets..................................... 1604

Methyldopate Hydrochloride (Potential for symptomatic postural hypotension). Products include:

Aldomet Ester HCl Injection 1602

Metolazone (Potential for symptomatic postural hypotension). Products include:

Mykrox Tablets 993
Zaroxolyn Tablets 1000

Metoprolol Succinate (Potential for symptomatic postural hypotension). Products include:

Toprol-XL Tablets 565

Metoprolol Tartrate (Potential for symptomatic postural hypotension). Products include:

Lopressor Ampuls 830
Lopressor HCT Tablets 832
Lopressor Tablets 830

Metyrosine (Potential for symptomatic postural hypotension). Products include:

Demser Capsules 1649

Minoxidil (Potential for symptomatic postural hypotension). Products include:

Loniten Tablets 2618
Rogaine Topical Solution 2637

IMPORTANT NOTE: Always consult each drug listing in the patient's regimen for possible interactions.

Moexipril Hydrochloride (Potential for symptomatic postural hypotension). Products include:
- Univasc Tablets 2410

Nadolol (Potential for symptomatic postural hypotension).
- No products indexed under this heading.

Nicardipine Hydrochloride (Potential for symptomatic postural hypotension). Products include:
- Cardene Capsules 2095
- Cardene I.V. 2709
- Cardene SR Capsules 2097

Nifedipine (Potential for symptomatic postural hypotension). Products include:
- Adalat Capsules (10 mg and 20 mg) 587
- Adalat CC 589
- Procardia Capsules 1971
- Procardia XL Extended Release Tablets 1972

Nisoldipine (Potential for symptomatic postural hypotension).
- No products indexed under this heading.

Nitroglycerin (Potential for symptomatic postural hypotension). Products include:
- Deponit NTG Transdermal Delivery System 2397
- Nitro-Bid IV 1523
- Nitro-Bid Ointment 1524
- Nitrodisc 2047
- Nitro-Dur (nitroglycerin) Transdermal Infusion System 1326
- Nitrolingual Spray 2027
- Nitrostat Tablets 1925
- Transderm-Nitro Transdermal Therapeutic System 859

Nortriptyline Hydrochloride (Potential for rare adverse reactions, including hypertension and dyskinesia). Products include:
- Pamelor 2280

Papaverine Hydrochloride (Beneficial effects of levodopa reversed in Parkinson's disease). Products include:
- Papaverine Hydrochloride Vials and Ampoules 1468

Penbutolol Sulfate (Potential for symptomatic postural hypotension). Products include:
- Levatol 2403

Perphenazine (Reduces therapeutic effect of levodopa). Products include:
- Etrafon 2355
- Triavil Tablets 1757
- Trilafon 2389

Phenelzine Sulfate (Concurrent use is contraindicated). Products include:
- Nardil 1920

Phenoxybenzamine Hydrochloride (Potential for symptomatic postural hypotension). Products include:
- Dibenzyline Capsules 2476

Phentolamine Mesylate (Potential for symptomatic postural hypotension). Products include:
- Regitine 846

Phenytoin (Beneficial effects of levodopa reversed in Parkinson's disease). Products include:
- Dilantin Infatabs 1908
- Dilantin-125 Suspension 1911

Phenytoin Sodium (Beneficial effects of levodopa reversed in Parkinson's disease). Products include:
- Dilantin Kapseals 1906
- Dilantin Parenteral 1910

Pindolol (Potential for symptomatic postural hypotension). Products include:
- Visken Tablets 2299

Polythiazide (Potential for symptomatic postural hypotension). Products include:
- Minizide Capsules 1938

Prazosin Hydrochloride (Potential for symptomatic postural hypotension). Products include:
- Minipress Capsules 1937
- Minizide Capsules 1938

Prochlorperazine (Reduces therapeutic effect of levodopa). Products include:
- Compazine 2470

Promethazine Hydrochloride (Reduces therapeutic effect of levodopa). Products include:
- Mepergan Injection 2753
- Phenergan with Codeine 2777
- Phenergan with Dextromethorphan 2778
- Phenergan Injection 2773
- Phenergan Suppositories 2775
- Phenergan Syrup 2774
- Phenergan Tablets 2775
- Phenergan VC 2779
- Phenergan VC with Codeine 2781

Propranolol Hydrochloride (Potential for symptomatic postural hypotension). Products include:
- Inderal 2728
- Inderal LA Long Acting Capsules 2730
- Inderide Tablets 2732
- Inderide LA Long Acting Capsules 2734

Protriptyline Hydrochloride (Potential for rare adverse reactions, including hypertension and dyskinesia). Products include:
- Vivactil Tablets 1774

Quinapril Hydrochloride (Potential for symptomatic postural hypotension). Products include:
- Accupril Tablets 1893

Ramipril (Potential for symptomatic postural hypotension). Products include:
- Altace Capsules 1232

Rauwolfia Serpentina (Potential for symptomatic postural hypotension).
- No products indexed under this heading.

Rescinnamine (Potential for symptomatic postural hypotension).
- No products indexed under this heading.

Reserpine (Potential for symptomatic postural hypotension). Products include:
- Diupres Tablets 1650
- Hydropres Tablets 1675
- Ser-Ap-Es Tablets 849

Sodium Nitroprusside (Potential for symptomatic postural hypotension).
- No products indexed under this heading.

Sotalol Hydrochloride (Potential for symptomatic postural hypotension). Products include:
- Betapace Tablets 641

Spirapril Hydrochloride (Potential for symptomatic postural hypotension).
- No products indexed under this heading.

Terazosin Hydrochloride (Potential for symptomatic postural hypotension). Products include:
- Hytrin Capsules 430

Thioridazine Hydrochloride (Reduces therapeutic effect of levodopa). Products include:
- Mellaril 2269

Timolol Maleate (Potential for symptomatic postural hypotension). Products include:
- Blocadren Tablets 1614
- Timolide Tablets 1748
- Timoptic in Ocudose 1753
- Timoptic Sterile Ophthalmic Solution 1751
- Timoptic-XE 1755

Torsemide (Potential for symptomatic postural hypotension). Products include:
- Demadex Tablets and Injection 686

Tranylcypromine Sulfate (Concurrent use is contraindicated). Products include:
- Parnate Tablets 2503

Trifluoperazine Hydrochloride (Reduces therapeutic effect of levodopa). Products include:
- Stelazine 2514

Trimethaphan Camsylate (Potential for symptomatic postural hypotension). Products include:
- Arfonad Ampuls 2080

Trimipramine Maleate (Potential for rare adverse reactions, including hypertension and dyskinesia). Products include:
- Surmontil Capsules 2811

Verapamil Hydrochloride (Potential for symptomatic postural hypotension). Products include:
- Calan SR Caplets 2422
- Calan Tablets 2419
- Isoptin Injectable 1344
- Isoptin Oral Tablets 1346
- Isoptin SR Tablets 1348
- Verelan Capsules 1410
- Verelan Capsules 2824

Food Interactions

Diet high in protein (Levodopa competes with certain amino acids, the absorption of levodopa may be impaired in some patients on a high protein diet).

ATARAX TABLETS & SYRUP

(Hydroxyzine Hydrochloride) 2185

May interact with narcotic analgesics, barbiturates, central nervous system depressants, and certain other agents. Compounds in these categories include:

Alfentanil Hydrochloride (The potentiating action of hydroxyzine must be considered when it is used concurrently). Products include:
- Alfenta Injection 1286

Alprazolam (The potentiating action of hydroxyzine must be considered when it is used concurrently). Products include:
- Xanax Tablets 2649

Aprobarbital (The potentiating action of hydroxyzine must be considered when it is used concurrently).
- No products indexed under this heading.

Buprenorphine (The potentiating action of hydroxyzine must be considered when it is used concurrently). Products include:
- Buprenex Injectable 2006

Buspirone Hydrochloride (The potentiating action of hydroxyzine must be considered when it is used concurrently). Products include:
- BuSpar 737

Butabarbital (The potentiating action of hydroxyzine must be considered when it is used concurrently).
- No products indexed under this heading.

Butalbital (The potentiating action of hydroxyzine must be considered when it is used concurrently). Products include:
- Esgic-plus Tablets 1013
- Fioricet Tablets 2258
- Fioricet with Codeine Capsules 2260
- Fiorinal Capsules 2261
- Fiorinal with Codeine Capsules 2262
- Fiorinal Tablets 2261
- Phrenilin 785
- Sedapap Tablets 50 mg/650 mg 1543

Chlordiazepoxide (The potentiating action of hydroxyzine must be considered when it is used concurrently). Products include:
- Libritabs Tablets 2177
- Limbitrol 2180

Chlordiazepoxide Hydrochloride (The potentiating action of hydroxyzine must be considered when it is used concurrently). Products include:
- Librax Capsules 2176
- Librium Capsules 2178
- Librium Injectable 2179

Chlorpromazine (The potentiating action of hydroxyzine must be considered when it is used concurrently). Products include:
- Thorazine Suppositories 2523

Chlorpromazine Hydrochloride (The potentiating action of hydroxyzine must be considered when it is used concurrently). Products include:
- Thorazine 2523

Chlorprothixene (The potentiating action of hydroxyzine must be considered when it is used concurrently).
- No products indexed under this heading.

Chlorprothixene Hydrochloride (The potentiating action of hydroxyzine must be considered when it is used concurrently).
- No products indexed under this heading.

Clorazepate Dipotassium (The potentiating action of hydroxyzine must be considered when it is used concurrently). Products include:
- Tranxene 451

Clozapine (The potentiating action of hydroxyzine must be considered when it is used concurrently). Products include:
- Clozaril Tablets 2252

Codeine Phosphate (The potentiating action of hydroxyzine must be considered when it is used concurrently). Products include:
- Actifed with Codeine Cough Syrup 1067
- Brontex 1981
- Deconsal C Expectorant Syrup 456
- Deconsal Pediatric Syrup 457
- Dimetane-DC Cough Syrup 2059
- Empirin with Codeine Tablets 1093
- Fioricet with Codeine Capsules 2260
- Fiorinal with Codeine Capsules 2262
- Isoclor Expectorant 990
- Novahistine DH 2462
- Novahistine Expectorant 2463
- Nucofed 2051
- Phenergan with Codeine 2777
- Phenergan VC with Codeine 2781
- Robitussin A-C Syrup 2073
- Robitussin-DAC Syrup 2074
- Ryna ◘ 841
- Soma Compound w/Codeine Tablets 2676
- Tussi-Organidin NR Liquid and S NR Liquid 2677
- Tylenol with Codeine 1583

Desflurane (The potentiating action of hydroxyzine must be considered when it is used concurrently). Products include:
- Suprane 1813

Dezocine (The potentiating action of hydroxyzine must be considered when it is used concurrently). Products include:
- Dalgan Injection 538

Diazepam (The potentiating action of hydroxyzine must be considered when it is used concurrently). Products include:
- Dizac 1809
- Valium Injectable 2182

(◘ Described in PDR For Nonprescription Drugs) (◉ Described in PDR For Ophthalmology)

87 **Interactions Index** **Atarax**

Valium Tablets 2183
Valrelease Capsules 2169

Droperidol (The potentiating action of hydroxyzine must be considered when it is used concurrently). Products include:
Inapsine Injection 1296

Enflurane (The potentiating action of hydroxyzine must be considered when it is used concurrently).
No products indexed under this heading.

Estazolam (The potentiating action of hydroxyzine must be considered when it is used concurrently). Products include:
ProSom Tablets 449

Ethchlorvynol (The potentiating action of hydroxyzine must be considered when it is used concurrently). Products include:
Placidyl Capsules 448

Ethinamate (The potentiating action of hydroxyzine must be considered when it is used concurrently).
No products indexed under this heading.

Fentanyl (The potentiating action of hydroxyzine must be considered when it is used concurrently). Products include:
Duragesic Transdermal System 1288

Fentanyl Citrate (The potentiating action of hydroxyzine must be considered when it is used concurrently). Products include:
Sublimaze Injection 1307

Fluphenazine Decanoate (The potentiating action of hydroxyzine must be considered when it is used concurrently). Products include:
Prolixin Decanoate 509

Fluphenazine Enanthate (The potentiating action of hydroxyzine must be considered when it is used concurrently). Products include:
Prolixin Enanthate 509

Fluphenazine Hydrochloride (The potentiating action of hydroxyzine must be considered when it is used concurrently). Products include:
Prolixin 509

Flurazepam Hydrochloride (The potentiating action of hydroxyzine must be considered when it is used concurrently). Products include:
Dalmane Capsules 2173

Glutethimide (The potentiating action of hydroxyzine must be considered when it is used concurrently).
No products indexed under this heading.

Haloperidol (The potentiating action of hydroxyzine must be considered when it is used concurrently). Products include:
Haldol Injection, Tablets and Concentrate 1575

Haloperidol Decanoate (The potentiating action of hydroxyzine must be considered when it is used concurrently). Products include:
Haldol Decanoate 1577

Hydrocodone Bitartrate (The potentiating action of hydroxyzine must be considered when it is used concurrently). Products include:
Anexsia 5/500 Elixir 1781
Anexia Tablets 1782
Codiclear DH Syrup 791
Deconamine CX Cough and Cold Liquid and Tablets 1319
Duratuss HD Elixir 2565
Hycodan Tablets and Syrup 930
Hycomine Compound Tablets 932
Hycomine 931
Hycotuss Expectorant Syrup 933
Hydrocet Capsules 782
Lorcet 10/650 1018
Lortab 2566
Tussend 1783
Tussend Expectorant 1785
Vicodin Tablets 1356
Vicodin ES Tablets 1357
Vicodin Tuss Expectorant 1358
Zydone Capsules 949

Hydrocodone Polistirex (The potentiating action of hydroxyzine must be considered when it is used concurrently). Products include:
Tussionex Pennkinetic Extended-Release Suspension 998

Isoflurane (The potentiating action of hydroxyzine must be considered when it is used concurrently).
No products indexed under this heading.

Ketamine Hydrochloride (The potentiating action of hydroxyzine must be considered when it is used concurrently).
No products indexed under this heading.

Levomethadyl Acetate Hydrochloride (The potentiating action of hydroxyzine must be considered when it is used concurrently). Products include:
Orlamm 2239

Levorphanol Tartrate (The potentiating action of hydroxyzine must be considered when it is used concurrently). Products include:
Levo-Dromoran 2129

Lorazepam (The potentiating action of hydroxyzine must be considered when it is used concurrently). Products include:
Ativan Injection 2698
Ativan Tablets 2700

Loxapine Hydrochloride (The potentiating action of hydroxyzine must be considered when it is used concurrently). Products include:
Loxitane 1378

Loxapine Succinate (The potentiating action of hydroxyzine must be considered when it is used concurrently). Products include:
Loxitane Capsules 1378

Meperidine Hydrochloride (The potentiating action of hydroxyzine must be considered when it is used concurrently). Products include:
Demerol 2308
Mepergan Injection 2753

Mephobarbital (The potentiating action of hydroxyzine must be considered when it is used concurrently). Products include:
Mebaral Tablets 2322

Meprobamate (The potentiating action of hydroxyzine must be considered when it is used concurrently). Products include:
Miltown Tablets 2672
PMB 200 and PMB 400 2783

Mesoridazine (The potentiating action of hydroxyzine must be considered when it is used concurrently).

Methadone Hydrochloride (The potentiating action of hydroxyzine must be considered when it is used concurrently). Products include:
Methadone Hydrochloride Oral Concentrate 2233
Methadone Hydrochloride Oral Solution & Tablets 2235

Methohexital Sodium (The potentiating action of hydroxyzine must be considered when it is used concurrently). Products include:
Brevital Sodium Vials 1429

Methotrimeprazine (The potentiating action of hydroxyzine must be considered when it is used concurrently). Products include:
Levoprome 1274

Methoxyflurane (The potentiating action of hydroxyzine must be considered when it is used concurrently).
No products indexed under this heading.

Midazolam Hydrochloride (The potentiating action of hydroxyzine must be considered when it is used concurrently). Products include:
Versed Injection 2170

Molindone Hydrochloride (The potentiating action of hydroxyzine must be considered when it is used concurrently). Products include:
Moban Tablets and Concentrate 1048

Morphine Sulfate (The potentiating action of hydroxyzine must be considered when it is used concurrently). Products include:
Astramorph/PF Injection, USP (Preservative-Free) 535
Duramorph 962
Infumorph 200 and Infumorph 500 Sterile Solutions 965
MS Contin Tablets 1994
MSIR 1997
Oramorph SR (Morphine Sulfate Sustained Release Tablets) 2236
RMS Suppositories 2657
Roxanol 2243

Non-narcotic Analgesics, unspecified (Potentiated action of non-narcotic analgesics).

Opium Alkaloids (The potentiating action of hydroxyzine must be considered when it is used concurrently).
No products indexed under this heading.

Oxazepam (The potentiating action of hydroxyzine must be considered when it is used concurrently). Products include:
Serax Capsules 2810
Serax Tablets 2810

Oxycodone Hydrochloride (The potentiating action of hydroxyzine must be considered when it is used concurrently). Products include:
Percocet Tablets 938
Percodan Tablets 939
Percodan-Demi Tablets 940
Roxicodone Tablets, Oral Solution & Intensol (Oxycodone) 2244
Tylox Capsules 1584

Pentobarbital Sodium (The potentiating action of hydroxyzine must be considered when it is used concurrently). Products include:
Nembutal Sodium Capsules 436
Nembutal Sodium Solution 438
Nembutal Sodium Suppositories 440

Perphenazine (The potentiating action of hydroxyzine must be considered when it is used concurrently). Products include:
Etrafon 2355
Triavil Tablets 1757
Trilafon 2389

Phenobarbital (The potentiating action of hydroxyzine must be considered when it is used concurrently). Products include:
Arco-Lase Plus Tablets 512
Bellergal-S Tablets 2250
Donnatal 2060
Donnatal Extentabs 2061
Donnatal Tablets 2060
Phenobarbital Elixir and Tablets 1469
Quadrinal Tablets 1350

Prazepam (The potentiating action of hydroxyzine must be considered when it is used concurrently).
No products indexed under this heading.

Prochlorperazine (The potentiating action of hydroxyzine must be considered when it is used concurrently). Products include:
Compazine 2470

Promethazine Hydrochloride (The potentiating action of hydroxyzine must be considered when it is used concurrently). Products include:
Mepergan Injection 2753
Phenergan with Codeine 2777
Phenergan with Dextromethorphan 2778
Phenergan Injection 2773
Phenergan Suppositories 2775
Phenergan Syrup 2774
Phenergan Tablets 2775
Phenergan VC 2779
Phenergan VC with Codeine 2781

Propofol (The potentiating action of hydroxyzine must be considered when it is used concurrently). Products include:
Diprivan Injection 2833

Propoxyphene Hydrochloride (The potentiating action of hydroxyzine must be considered when it is used concurrently). Products include:
Darvon 1435
Wygesic Tablets 2827

Propoxyphene Napsylate (The potentiating action of hydroxyzine must be considered when it is used concurrently). Products include:
Darvon-N/Darvocet-N 1433

Quazepam (The potentiating action of hydroxyzine must be considered when it is used concurrently). Products include:
Doral Tablets 2664

Risperidone (The potentiating action of hydroxyzine must be considered when it is used concurrently). Products include:
Risperdal 1301

Secobarbital Sodium (The potentiating action of hydroxyzine must be considered when it is used concurrently). Products include:
Seconal Sodium Pulvules 1474

Sufentanil Citrate (The potentiating action of hydroxyzine must be considered when it is used concurrently). Products include:
Sufenta Injection 1309

Temazepam (The potentiating action of hydroxyzine must be considered when it is used concurrently). Products include:
Restoril Capsules 2284

Thiamylal Sodium (The potentiating action of hydroxyzine must be considered when it is used concurrently).
No products indexed under this heading.

Thioridazine Hydrochloride (The potentiating action of hydroxyzine must be considered when it is used concurrently). Products include:
Mellaril 2269

Thiothixene (The potentiating action of hydroxyzine must be considered when it is used concurrently). Products include:
Navane Capsules and Concentrate 2201
Navane Intramuscular 2202

Triazolam (The potentiating action of hydroxyzine must be considered when it is used concurrently). Products include:
Halcion Tablets 2611

IMPORTANT NOTE: Always consult each drug listing in the patient's regimen for possible interactions.

Trifluoperazine Hydrochloride (The potentiating action of hydroxyzine must be considered when it is used concurrently). Products include:
- Stelazine 2514

Zolpidem Tartrate (The potentiating action of hydroxyzine must be considered when it is used concurrently). Products include:
- Ambien Tablets 2416

Food Interactions

Alcohol (Increased effect of alcohol).

ATGAM STERILE SOLUTION

(Lymphocyte Immune Globulin Anti-Thymocyte Globulin (Equine)) 2581

May interact with corticosteroids, immunosuppressive agents, and certain other agents. Compounds in these categories include:

Azathioprine (When the dose of corticosteroids is reduced, some previously masked reactions to Atgam may appear). Products include:
- Imuran 1110

Betamethasone Acetate (When the dose of corticosteroids is reduced, some previously masked reactions to Atgam may appear). Products include:
- Celestone Soluspan Suspension 2347

Betamethasone Sodium Phosphate (When the dose of corticosteroids is reduced, some previously masked reactions to Atgam may appear). Products include:
- Celestone Soluspan Suspension 2347

Cortisone Acetate (When the dose of corticosteroids is reduced, some previously masked reactions to Atgam may appear). Products include:
- Cortone Acetate Sterile Suspension 1623
- Cortone Acetate Tablets 1624

Cyclosporine (When the dose of corticosteroids is reduced, some previously masked reactions to Atgam may appear). Products include:
- Neoral 2276
- Sandimmune 2286

Dexamethasone (When the dose of corticosteroids is reduced, some previously masked reactions to Atgam may appear). Products include:
- AK-Trol Ointment & Suspension ..... ◉ 205
- Decadron Elixir 1633
- Decadron Tablets 1635
- Decaspray Topical Aerosol 1648
- Dexacidin Ointment ..... ◉ 263
- Maxitrol Ophthalmic Ointment and Suspension ..... ◉ 224
- TobraDex Ophthalmic Suspension and Ointment 473

Dexamethasone Acetate (When the dose of corticosteroids is reduced, some previously masked reactions to Atgam may appear). Products include:
- Dalalone D.P. Injectable 1011
- Decadron-LA Sterile Suspension 1646

Dexamethasone Sodium Phosphate (When the dose of corticosteroids is reduced, some previously masked reactions to Atgam may appear). Products include:
- Decadron Phosphate Injection 1637
- Decadron Phosphate Respihaler 1642
- Decadron Phosphate Sterile Ophthalmic Ointment 1641
- Decadron Phosphate Sterile Ophthalmic Solution 1642
- Decadron Phosphate Topical Cream 1644
- Decadron Phosphate Turbinaire 1645
- Decadron Phosphate with Xylocaine Injection, Sterile 1639
- Dexacort Phosphate in Respihaler 458
- Dexacort Phosphate in Turbinaire 459
- NeoDecadron Sterile Ophthalmic Ointment 1712
- NeoDecadron Sterile Ophthalmic Solution 1713
- NeoDecadron Topical Cream 1714

Fludrocortisone Acetate (When the dose of corticosteroids is reduced, some previously masked reactions to Atgam may appear). Products include:
- Florinef Acetate Tablets 505

Hydrocortisone (When the dose of corticosteroids is reduced, some previously masked reactions to Atgam may appear). Products include:
- Anusol-HC Cream 2.5% 1896
- Aquanil HC Lotion 1931
- Bactine Hydrocortisone Anti-Itch Cream ..... ▣ 709
- Caldecort Anti-Itch Hydrocortisone Spray ..... ▣ 631
- Cortaid ..... ▣ 836
- CORTENEMA 2535
- Cortisporin Ointment 1085
- Cortisporin Ophthalmic Ointment Sterile 1085
- Cortisporin Ophthalmic Suspension Sterile 1086
- Cortisporin Otic Solution Sterile 1087
- Cortisporin Otic Suspension Sterile 1088
- Cortizone-5 ..... ▣ 831
- Cortizone-10 ..... ▣ 831
- Hydrocortone Tablets 1672
- Hytone 907
- Massengill Medicated Soft Cloth Towelettes 2458
- PediOtic Suspension Sterile 1153
- Preparation H Hydrocortisone 1% Cream ..... ▣ 872
- ProctoCream-HC 2.5% 2408
- VōSoL HC Otic Solution 2678

Hydrocortisone Acetate (When the dose of corticosteroids is reduced, some previously masked reactions to Atgam may appear). Products include:
- Analpram-HC Rectal Cream 1% and 2.5% 977
- Anusol HC-1 Anti-Itch Hydrocortisone Ointment ..... ▣ 847
- Anusol-HC Suppositories 1897
- Caldecort ..... ▣ 631
- Carmol HC 924
- Coly-Mycin S Otic w/Neomycin & Hydrocortisone 1906
- Cortaid ..... ▣ 836
- Cortifoam 2396
- Cortisporin Cream 1084
- Epifoam 2399
- Hydrocortone Acetate Sterile Suspension 1669
- Mantadil Cream 1135
- Nupercainal Hydrocortisone 1% Cream ..... ▣ 645
- Ophthocort ..... ◉ 311
- Pramosone Cream, Lotion & Ointment 978
- ProctoCream-HC 2408
- ProctoFoam-HC 2409
- Terra-Cortril Ophthalmic Suspension 2210

Hydrocortisone Sodium Phosphate (When the dose of corticosteroids is reduced, some previously masked reactions to Atgam may appear). Products include:
- Hydrocortone Phosphate Injection, Sterile 1670

Hydrocortisone Sodium Succinate (When the dose of corticosteroids is reduced, some previously masked reactions to Atgam may appear). Products include:
- Solu-Cortef Sterile Powder 2641

Immune Globulin (Human) (When the dose of corticosteroids is reduced, some previously masked reactions to Atgam may appear).
- No products indexed under this heading.

Immune Globulin Intravenous (Human) (When the dose of corticosteroids is reduced, some previously masked reactions to Atgam may appear).

Methylprednisolone Acetate (When the dose of corticosteroids is reduced, some previously masked reactions to Atgam may appear). Products include:
- Depo-Medrol Single-Dose Vial 2600
- Depo-Medrol Sterile Aqueous Suspension 2597

Methylprednisolone Sodium Succinate (When the dose of corticosteroids is reduced, some previously masked reactions to Atgam may appear). Products include:
- Solu-Medrol Sterile Powder 2643

Muromonab-CD3 (When the dose of corticosteroids is reduced, some previously masked reactions to Atgam may appear). Products include:
- Orthoclone OKT3 Sterile Solution 1837

Mycophenolate Mofetil (When the dose of corticosteroids is reduced, some previously masked reactions to Atgam may appear). Products include:
- CellCept Capsules 2099

Prednisolone Acetate (When the dose of corticosteroids is reduced, some previously masked reactions to Atgam may appear). Products include:
- AK-CIDE ..... ◉ 202
- AK-CIDE Ointment ..... ◉ 202
- Blephamide Liquifilm Sterile Ophthalmic Suspension 476
- Blephamide Ointment ..... ◉ 237
- Econopred & Econopred Plus Ophthalmic Suspensions ..... ◉ 217
- Poly-Pred Liquifilm ..... ◉ 248
- Pred Forte ..... ◉ 250
- Pred Mild ..... ◉ 253
- Pred-G Liquifilm Sterile Ophthalmic Suspension ..... ◉ 251
- Pred-G S.O.P. Sterile Ophthalmic Ointment ..... ◉ 252
- Vasocidin Ointment ..... ◉ 268

Prednisolone Sodium Phosphate (When the dose of corticosteroids is reduced, some previously masked reactions to Atgam may appear). Products include:
- AK-Pred ..... ◉ 204
- Hydeltrasol Injection, Sterile 1665
- Inflamase ..... ◉ 265
- Pediapred Oral Liquid 995
- Vasocidin Ophthalmic Solution ..... ◉ 270

Prednisolone Tebutate (When the dose of corticosteroids is reduced, some previously masked reactions to Atgam may appear). Products include:
- Hydeltra-T.B.A. Sterile Suspension 1667

Prednisone (When the dose of corticosteroids is reduced, some previously masked reactions to Atgam may appear). Products include:
- Deltasone Tablets 2595

Tacrolimus (When the dose of corticosteroids is reduced, some previously masked reactions to Atgam may appear). Products include:
- Prograf 1042

Triamcinolone (When the dose of corticosteroids is reduced, some previously masked reactions to Atgam may appear). Products include:
- Aristocort Tablets 1022

Triamcinolone Acetonide (When the dose of corticosteroids is reduced, some previously masked reactions to Atgam may appear). Products include:
- Aristocort A 0.025% Cream 1027
- Aristocort A 0.5% Cream 1031
- Aristocort A 0.1% Cream 1029
- Aristocort A 0.1% Ointment 1030
- Azmacort Oral Inhaler 2011
- Nasacort Nasal Inhaler 2024

Triamcinolone Diacetate (When the dose of corticosteroids is reduced, some previously masked reactions to Atgam may appear). Products include:
- Aristocort Suspension (Forte Parenteral) 1027
- Aristocort Suspension (Intralesional) 1025

Triamcinolone Hexacetonide (When the dose of corticosteroids is reduced, some previously masked reactions to Atgam may appear). Products include:
- Aristospan Suspension (Intra-articular) 1033
- Aristospan Suspension (Intralesional) 1032

ATIVAN INJECTION

(Lorazepam) 2698

May interact with phenothiazines, barbiturates, monoamine oxidase inhibitors, narcotic analgesics, central nervous system depressants, and certain other agents. Compounds in these categories include:

Alfentanil Hydrochloride (Additive CNS depressant effects). Products include:
- Alfenta Injection 1286

Alprazolam (Additive CNS depressant effects). Products include:
- Xanax Tablets 2649

Aprobarbital (Additive CNS depressant effects).
- No products indexed under this heading.

Buprenorphine (Additive CNS depressant effects). Products include:
- Buprenex Injectable 2006

Buspirone Hydrochloride (Additive CNS depressant effects). Products include:
- BuSpar 737

Butabarbital (Additive CNS depressant effects).
- No products indexed under this heading.

Butalbital (Additive CNS depressant effects). Products include:
- Esgic-plus Tablets 1013
- Fioricet Tablets 2258
- Fioricet with Codeine Capsules 2260
- Fiorinal Capsules 2261
- Fiorinal with Codeine Capsules 2262
- Fiorinal Tablets 2261
- Phrenilin 785
- Sedapap Tablets 50 mg/650 mg 1543

Chlordiazepoxide (Additive CNS depressant effects). Products include:
- Libritabs Tablets 2177
- Limbitrol 2180

Chlordiazepoxide Hydrochloride (Additive CNS depressant effects). Products include:
- Librax Capsules 2176
- Librium Capsules 2178
- Librium Injectable 2179

Chlorpromazine (Additive CNS depressant effects). Products include:
- Thorazine Suppositories 2523

Chlorprothixene (Additive CNS depressant effects).
- No products indexed under this heading.

Chlorprothixene Hydrochloride (Additive CNS depressant effects).
- No products indexed under this heading.

Clorazepate Dipotassium (Additive CNS depressant effects). Products include:
- Tranxene 451

Clozapine (Additive CNS depressant effects). Products include:
- Clozaril Tablets 2252

Codeine Phosphate (Additive CNS depressant effects). Products include:
- Actifed with Codeine Cough Syrup 1067
- Brontex 1981
- Deconsal C Expectorant Syrup 456
- Deconsal Pediatric Syrup 457
- Dimetane-DC Cough Syrup 2059
- Empirin with Codeine Tablets 1093
- Fioricet with Codeine Capsules 2260
- Fiorinal with Codeine Capsules 2262
- Isoclor Expectorant 990
- Novahistine DH 2462
- Novahistine Expectorant 2463
- Nucofed 2051
- Phenergan with Codeine 2777
- Phenergan VC with Codeine 2781
- Robitussin A-C Syrup 2073
- Robitussin-DAC Syrup 2074
- Ryna 841
- Soma Compound w/Codeine Tablets 2676
- Tussi-Organidin NR Liquid and S NR Liquid 2677
- Tylenol with Codeine 1583

Desflurane (Additive CNS depressant effects). Products include:
- Suprane 1813

Dezocine (Additive CNS depressant effects). Products include:
- Dalgan Injection 538

Diazepam (Additive CNS depressant effects). Products include:
- Dizac 1809
- Valium Injectable 2182
- Valium Tablets 2183
- Valrelease Capsules 2169

Droperidol (Additive CNS depressant effects). Products include:
- Inapsine Injection 1296

Enflurane (Additive CNS depressant effects).
- No products indexed under this heading.

Estazolam (Additive CNS depressant effects). Products include:
- ProSom Tablets 449

Ethchlorvynol (Additive CNS depressant effects). Products include:
- Placidyl Capsules 448

Ethinamate (Additive CNS depressant effects).
- No products indexed under this heading.

Fentanyl (Additive CNS depressant effects). Products include:
- Duragesic Transdermal System 1288

Fentanyl Citrate (Additive CNS depressant effects). Products include:
- Sublimaze Injection 1307

Fluphenazine Decanoate (Additive CNS depressant effects). Products include:
- Prolixin Decanoate 509

Fluphenazine Enanthate (Additive CNS depressant effects). Products include:
- Prolixin Enanthate 509

Fluphenazine Hydrochloride (Additive CNS depressant effects). Products include:
- Prolixin 509

Flurazepam Hydrochloride (Additive CNS depressant effects). Products include:
- Dalmane Capsules 2173

Furazolidone (Additive CNS depressant effects). Products include:
- Furoxone 2046

Glutethimide (Additive CNS depressant effects).
- No products indexed under this heading.

Haloperidol (Additive CNS depressant effects). Products include:
- Haldol Injection, Tablets and Concentrate 1575

Haloperidol Decanoate (Additive CNS depressant effects). Products include:
- Haldol Decanoate 1577

Hydrocodone Bitartrate (Additive CNS depressant effects). Products include:
- Anexsia 5/500 Elixir 1781
- Anexia Tablets 1782
- Codiclear DH Syrup 791
- Deconamine CX Cough and Cold Liquid and Tablets 1319
- Duratuss HD Elixir 2565
- Hycodan Tablets and Syrup 930
- Hycomine Compound Tablets 932
- Hycomine 931
- Hycotuss Expectorant Syrup 933
- Hydrocet Capsules 782
- Lorcet 10/650 1018
- Lortab 2566
- Tussend 1783
- Tussend Expectorant 1785
- Vicodin Tablets 1356
- Vicodin ES Tablets 1357
- Vicodin Tuss Expectorant 1358
- Zydone Capsules 949

Hydrocodone Polistirex (Additive CNS depressant effects). Products include:
- Tussionex Pennkinetic Extended-Release Suspension 998

Hydroxyzine Hydrochloride (Additive CNS depressant effects). Products include:
- Atarax Tablets & Syrup 2185
- Marax Tablets & DF Syrup 2200
- Vistaril Intramuscular Solution 2216

Isocarboxazid (Additive CNS depressant effects).
- No products indexed under this heading.

Isoflurane (Additive CNS depressant effects).
- No products indexed under this heading.

Ketamine Hydrochloride (Additive CNS depressant effects).
- No products indexed under this heading.

Levomethadyl Acetate Hydrochloride (Additive CNS depressant effects). Products include:
- Orlamm 2239

Levorphanol Tartrate (Additive CNS depressant effects). Products include:
- Levo-Dromoran 2129

Loxapine Hydrochloride (Additive CNS depressant effects). Products include:
- Loxitane 1378

Loxapine Succinate (Additive CNS depressant effects). Products include:
- Loxitane Capsules 1378

Meperidine Hydrochloride (Additive CNS depressant effects). Products include:
- Demerol 2308
- Mepergan Injection 2753

Mephobarbital (Additive CNS depressant effects). Products include:
- Mebaral Tablets 2322

Meprobamate (Additive CNS depressant effects). Products include:
- Miltown Tablets 2672
- PMB 200 and PMB 400 2783

Mesoridazine Besylate (Additive CNS depressant effects). Products include:
- Serentil 684

Methadone Hydrochloride (Additive CNS depressant effects). Products include:
- Methadone Hydrochloride Oral Concentrate 2233
- Methadone Hydrochloride Oral Solution & Tablets 2235

Methohexital Sodium (Additive CNS depressant effects). Products include:
- Brevital Sodium Vials 1429

Methotrimeprazine (Additive CNS depressant effects). Products include:
- Levoprome 1274

Methoxyflurane (Additive CNS depressant effects).
- No products indexed under this heading.

Midazolam Hydrochloride (Additive CNS depressant effects). Products include:
- Versed Injection 2170

Molindone Hydrochloride (Additive CNS depressant effects). Products include:
- Moban Tablets and Concentrate 1048

Morphine Sulfate (Additive CNS depressant effects). Products include:
- Astramorph/PF Injection, USP (Preservative-Free) 535
- Duramorph 962
- Infumorph 200 and Infumorph 500 Sterile Solutions 965
- MS Contin Tablets 1994
- MSIR 1997
- Oramorph SR (Morphine Sulfate Sustained Release Tablets) 2236
- RMS Suppositories 2657
- Roxanol 2243

Opium Alkaloids (Additive CNS depressant effects).
- No products indexed under this heading.

Oxazepam (Additive CNS depressant effects). Products include:
- Serax Capsules 2810
- Serax Tablets 2810

Oxycodone Hydrochloride (Additive CNS depressant effects). Products include:
- Percocet Tablets 938
- Percodan Tablets 939
- Percodan-Demi Tablets 940
- Roxicodone Tablets, Oral Solution & Intensol (Oxycodone) 2244
- Tylox Capsules 1584

Pentobarbital Sodium (Additive CNS depressant effects). Products include:
- Nembutal Sodium Capsules 436
- Nembutal Sodium Solution 438
- Nembutal Sodium Suppositories 440

Perphenazine (Additive CNS depressant effects). Products include:
- Etrafon 2355
- Triavil Tablets 1757
- Trilafon 2389

Phenelzine Sulfate (Additive CNS depressant effects). Products include:
- Nardil 1920

Phenobarbital (Additive CNS depressant effects). Products include:
- Arco-Lase Plus Tablets 512
- Bellergal-S Tablets 2250
- Donnatal 2060
- Donnatal Extentabs 2061
- Donnatal Tablets 2060
- Phenobarbital Elixir and Tablets 1469
- Quadrinal Tablets 1350

Prazepam (Additive CNS depressant effects).
- No products indexed under this heading.

Prochlorperazine (Additive CNS depressant effects). Products include:
- Compazine 2470

Promethazine Hydrochloride (Additive CNS depressant effects). Products include:
- Mepergan Injection 2753
- Phenergan with Codeine 2777
- Phenergan with Dextromethorphan 2778
- Phenergan Injection 2773
- Phenergan Suppositories 2775
- Phenergan Syrup 2774
- Phenergan Tablets 2775
- Phenergan VC 2779
- Phenergan VC with Codeine 2781

Propofol (Additive CNS depressant effects). Products include:
- Diprivan Injection 2833

Propoxyphene Hydrochloride (Additive CNS depressant effects). Products include:
- Darvon 1435
- Wygesic Tablets 2827

Propoxyphene Napsylate (Additive CNS depressant effects). Products include:
- Darvon-N/Darvocet-N 1433

Quazepam (Additive CNS depressant effects). Products include:
- Doral Tablets 2664

Risperidone (Additive CNS depressant effects). Products include:
- Risperdal 1301

Scopolamine (Increased incidence of sedation, hallucinations, and irrational behavior). Products include:
- Transderm Scōp Transdermal Therapeutic System 869

Scopolamine Hydrobromide (Increased incidence of sedation, hallucinations, and irrational behavior). Products include:
- Atrohist Plus Tablets 454
- Donnatal 2060
- Donnatal Extentabs 2061
- Donnatal Tablets 2060

Secobarbital Sodium (Additive CNS depressant effects). Products include:
- Seconal Sodium Pulvules 1474

Selegiline Hydrochloride (Additive CNS depressant effects). Products include:
- Eldepryl Tablets 2550

Sufentanil Citrate (Additive CNS depressant effects). Products include:
- Sufenta Injection 1309

Temazepam (Additive CNS depressant effects). Products include:
- Restoril Capsules 2284

Thiamylal Sodium (Additive CNS depressant effects).
- No products indexed under this heading.

Thioridazine Hydrochloride (Additive CNS depressant effects). Products include:
- Mellaril 2269

Thiothixene (Additive CNS depressant effects). Products include:
- Navane Capsules and Concentrate 2201
- Navane Intramuscular 2202

Tranylcypromine Sulfate (Additive CNS depressant effects). Products include:
- Parnate Tablets 2503

Triazolam (Additive CNS depressant effects). Products include:
- Halcion Tablets 2611

Trifluoperazine Hydrochloride (Additive CNS depressant effects). Products include:
- Stelazine 2514

Zolpidem Tartrate (Additive CNS depressant effects). Products include:
- Ambien Tablets 2416

Food Interactions

Alcohol (Additive CNS depressant effects).

IMPORTANT NOTE: Always consult each drug listing in the patient's regimen for possible interactions.

Ativan Tablets Interactions Index 90

ATIVAN TABLETS
(Lorazepam) 2700
May interact with barbiturates and certain other agents. Compounds in these categories include:

Aprobarbital (Depressant effect).
No products indexed under this heading.

Butabarbital (Depressant effect).
No products indexed under this heading.

Butalbital (Depressant effect). Products include:
- Esgic-plus Tablets 1013
- Fioricet Tablets 2258
- Fioricet with Codeine Capsules 2260
- Fiorinal Capsules 2261
- Fiorinal with Codeine Capsules 2262
- Fiorinal Tablets 2261
- Phrenilin 785
- Sedapap Tablets 50 mg/650 mg .. 1543

Mephobarbital (Depressant effect). Products include:
- Mebaral Tablets 2322

Pentobarbital Sodium (Depressant effect). Products include:
- Nembutal Sodium Capsules 436
- Nembutal Sodium Solution 438
- Nembutal Sodium Suppositories 440

Phenobarbital (Depressant effect). Products include:
- Arco-Lase Plus Tablets 512
- Bellergal-S Tablets 2250
- Donnatal 2060
- Donnatal Extentabs 2061
- Donnatal Tablets 2060
- Phenobarbital Elixir and Tablets 1469
- Quadrinal Tablets 1350

Secobarbital Sodium (Depressant effect). Products include:
- Seconal Sodium Pulvules 1474

Thiamylal Sodium (Depressant effect).
No products indexed under this heading.

Food Interactions

Alcohol (Depressant effect).

ATRAC-TAIN, MOISTURIZING CREAM
(Urea, Lactic Acid) 2554
None cited in PDR database.

ATRETOL TABLETS
(Carbamazepine) 573
May interact with calcium channel blockers, monoamine oxidase inhibitors, lithium preparations, anticonvulsants, oral contraceptives, xanthine bronchodilators, and certain other agents. Compounds in these categories include:

Aminophylline (Half-life of theophyllin is shortened when concurrently administered).
No products indexed under this heading.

Amlodipine Besylate (Concomitant administration has been reported to result in elevated plasma levels of carbamazepine resulting in toxicity is some cases). Products include:
- Lotrel Capsules 840
- Norvasc Tablets 1940

Bepridil Hydrochloride (Concomitant administration has been reported to result in elevated plasma levels of carbamazepine resulting in toxicity is some cases). Products include:
- Vascor (200, 300 and 400 mg) Tablets 1587

Cimetidine (Concomitant administration has been reported to result in elevated plasma levels of carbamazepine resulting in toxicity is some cases). Products include:
- Tagamet Tablets 2516

Cimetidine Hydrochloride (Concomitant administration has been reported to result in elevated plasma levels of carbamazepine resulting in toxicity is some cases). Products include:
- Tagamet 2516

Desogestrel (Potential for breakthrough bleeding in patients receiving concomitant oral contraceptives; reliability may be adversely affected). Products include:
- Desogen Tablets 1817
- Ortho-Cept 1851

Diltiazem Hydrochloride (Concomitant administration has been reported to result in elevated plasma levels of carbamazepine resulting in toxicity is some cases). Products include:
- Cardizem CD Capsules 1506
- Cardizem SR Capsules 1510
- Cardizem Injectable 1508
- Cardizem Tablets 1512
- Dilacor XR Extended-release Capsules 2018

Divalproex Sodium (Potential for an increase in the ratio of active 10,11-epoxide metabolite to parent compound; valproic acid serum levels may be reduced when divalproex is administered with carbamazepine; combination therapy with other anticonvulsant has resulted in alteration of thyroid function). Products include:
- Depakote Tablets 415

Doxycycline Calcium (Half-life of doxycyclline is shortened when concurrently administered). Products include:
- Vibramycin Calcium Oral Suspension Syrup 1941

Doxycycline Hyclate (Half-life of doxycyclline is shortened when concurrently administered). Products include:
- Doryx Capsules 1913
- Vibramycin Hyclate Capsules 1941
- Vibramycin Hyclate Intravenous 2215
- Vibra-Tabs Film Coated Tablets 1941

Doxycycline Monohydrate (Half-life of doxycyclline is shortened when concurrently administered). Products include:
- Monodox Capsules 1805
- Vibramycin Monohydrate for Oral Suspension 1941

Dyphylline (Half-life of theophyllin is shortened when concurrently administered). Products include:
- Lufyllin & Lufyllin-400 Tablets 2670
- Lufyllin-GG Elixir & Tablets 2671

Erythromycin (Concomitant administration has been reported to result in elevated plasma levels of carbamazepine resulting in toxicity is some cases). Products include:
- A/T/S 2% Acne Topical Gel and Solution 1234
- Benzamycin Topical Gel 905
- E-Mycin Tablets 1341
- Emgel 2% Topical Gel 1093
- ERYC 1915
- Erycette (erythromycin 2%) Topical Solution 1888
- Ery-Tab Tablets 422
- Erythromycin Base Filmtab 426
- Erythromycin Delayed-Release Capsules, USP 427
- Ilotycin Ophthalmic Ointment 912
- PCE Dispertab Tablets 444
- T-Stat 2.0% Topical Solution and Pads 2688
- Theramycin Z Topical Solution 2% 1592

Erythromycin Estolate (Concomitant administration has been reported to result in elevated plasma levels of carbamazepine resulting in toxicity is some cases). Products include:
- Ilosone 911

Erythromycin Ethylsuccinate (Concomitant administration has been reported to result in elevated plasma levels of carbamazepine resulting in toxicity is some cases). Products include:
- E.E.S. 424
- EryPed 421

Erythromycin Gluceptate (Concomitant administration has been reported to result in elevated plasma levels of carbamazepine resulting in toxicity is some cases). Products include:
- Ilotycin Gluceptate, IV, Vials 913

Erythromycin Stearate (Concomitant administration has been reported to result in elevated plasma levels of carbamazepine resulting in toxicity is some cases). Products include:
- Erythrocin Stearate Filmtab 425

Ethinyl Estradiol (Potential for breakthrough bleeding in patients receiving concomitant oral contraceptives; reliability may be adversely affected). Products include:
- Brevicon 2088
- Demulen 2428
- Desogen Tablets 1817
- Levlen/Tri-Levlen 651
- Lo/Ovral Tablets 2746
- Lo/Ovral-28 Tablets 2751
- Modicon 1872
- Nordette-21 Tablets 2755
- Nordette-28 Tablets 2758
- Norinyl 2088
- Ortho-Cept 1851
- Ortho-Cyclen/Ortho-Tri-Cyclen 1858
- Ortho-Novum 1872
- Ortho-Cyclen/Ortho Tri-Cyclen 1858
- Ovcon 760
- Ovral Tablets 2770
- Ovral-28 Tablets 2770
- Levlen/Tri-Levlen 651
- Tri-Norinyl 2164
- Triphasil-21 Tablets 2814
- Triphasil-28 Tablets 2819

Ethosuximide (Combination therapy with other anticonvulsant has resulted in alteration of thyroid function). Products include:
- Zarontin Capsules 1928
- Zarontin Syrup 1929

Ethotoin (Combination therapy with other anticonvulsant has resulted in alteration of thyroid function). Products include:
- Peganone Tablets 446

Ethynodiol Diacetate (Potential for breakthrough bleeding in patients receiving concomitant oral contraceptives; reliability may be adversely affected). Products include:
- Demulen 2428

Felbamate (Combination therapy with other anticonvulsant has resulted in alteration of thyroid function). Products include:
- Felbatol 2666

Felodipine (Concomitant administration has been reported to result in elevated plasma levels of carbamazepine resulting in toxicity is some cases). Products include:
- Plendil Extended-Release Tablets 527

Furazolidone (On theoretical grounds concurrent and/or sequential use is contraindicated). Products include:
- Furoxone 2046

Haloperidol (Haloperidol serum levels may be reduced when it is administered with carbamazepine). Products include:
- Haldol Injection, Tablets and Concentrate 1575

Haloperidol Decanoate (Haloperidol serum levels may be reduced when it is administered with carbamazepine). Products include:
- Haldol Decanoate 1577

Isocarboxazid (On theoretical grounds concurrent and/or sequential use is contraindicated).
No products indexed under this heading.

Isoniazid (Concomitant administration has been reported to result in elevated plasma levels of carbamazepine resulting in toxicity in some cases). Products include:
- Nydrazid Injection 508
- Rifamate Capsules 1530
- Rifater 1532

Isradipine (Concomitant administration has been reported to result in elevated plasma levels of carbamazepine resulting in toxicity is some cases). Products include:
- DynaCirc Capsules 2256

Lamotrigine (Combination therapy with other anticonvulsant has resulted in alteration of thyroid function). Products include:
- Lamictal Tablets 1112

Levonorgestrel (Potential for breakthrough bleeding in patients receiving concomitant oral contraceptives; reliability may be adversely affected). Products include:
- Levlen/Tri-Levlen 651
- Nordette-21 Tablets 2755
- Nordette-28 Tablets 2758
- Norplant System 2759
- Levlen/Tri-Levlen 651
- Triphasil-21 Tablets 2814
- Triphasil-28 Tablets 2819

Lithium Carbonate (Concomitant administration may increase the risk of neurotoxic side effects). Products include:
- Eskalith 2485
- Lithium Carbonate Capsules & Tablets 2230
- Lithonate/Lithotabs/Lithobid 2543

Lithium Citrate (Concomitant administration may increase the risk of neurotoxic side effects).
No products indexed under this heading.

Mephenytoin (Combination therapy with other anticonvulsant has resulted in alteration of thyroid function). Products include:
- Mesantoin Tablets 2272

Mestranol (Potential for breakthrough bleeding in patients receiving concomitant oral contraceptives; reliability may be adversely affected). Products include:
- Norinyl 2088
- Ortho-Novum 1872

Methsuximide (Combination therapy with other anticonvulsant has resulted in alteration of thyroid function). Products include:
- Celontin Kapseals 1899

Nicardipine Hydrochloride (Concomitant administration has been reported to result in elevated plasma levels of carbamazepine resulting in toxicity is some cases). Products include:
- Cardene Capsules 2095
- Cardene I.V. 2709
- Cardene SR Capsules 2097

(▣ Described in PDR For Nonprescription Drugs) (◉ Described in PDR For Ophthalmology)

Nifedipine (Concomitant administration has been reported to result in elevated plasma levels of carbamazepine resulting in toxicity is some cases). Products include:

Adalat Capsules (10 mg and 20 mg) **587**
Adalat CC **589**
Procardia Capsules **1971**
Procardia XL Extended Release Tablets **1972**

Nimodipine (Concomitant administration has been reported to result in elevated plasma levels of carbamazepine resulting in toxicity is some cases). Products include:

Nimotop Capsules **610**

Nisoldipine (Concomitant administration has been reported to result in elevated plasma levels of carbamazepine resulting in toxicity is some cases).

No products indexed under this heading.

Norethindrone (Potential for breakthrough bleeding in patients receiving concomitant oral contraceptives; reliability may be adversely affected). Products include:

Brevicon **2088**
Micronor Tablets **1872**
Modicon **1872**
Norinyl **2088**
Nor-Q D Tablets **2135**
Ortho-Novum **1872**
Ovcon **760**
Tri-Norinyl **2164**

Norethynodrel (Potential for breakthrough bleeding in patients receiving concomitant oral contraceptives; reliability may be adversely affected).

No products indexed under this heading.

Norgestimate (Potential for breakthrough bleeding in patients receiving concomitant oral contraceptives; reliability may be adversely affected). Products include:

Ortho-Cyclen/Ortho-Tri-Cyclen **1858**
Ortho-Cyclen/Ortho Tri-Cyclen **1858**

Norgestrel (Potential for breakthrough bleeding in patients receiving concomitant oral contraceptives; reliability may be adversely affected). Products include:

Lo/Ovral Tablets **2746**
Lo/Ovral-28 Tablets **2751**
Ovral Tablets **2770**
Ovral-28 Tablets **2770**
Ovrette Tablets **2771**

Paramethadione (Combination therapy with other anticonvulsant has resulted in alteration of thyroid function).

No products indexed under this heading.

Phenacemide (Combination therapy with other anticonvulsant has resulted in alteration of thyroid function). Products include:

Phenurone Tablets **447**

Phenelzine Sulfate (On theoretical grounds concurrent and/or sequential use is contraindicated). Products include:

Nardil **1920**

Phenobarbital (Simultaneous administration produces a marked lowering of serum levels of carbamazepine; combination therapy with other anticonvulsant has resulted in alteration of thyroid function). Products include:

Arco-Lase Plus Tablets **512**
Bellergal-S Tablets **2250**
Donnatal **2060**
Donnatal Extentabs **2061**
Donnatal Tablets **2060**
Phenobarbital Elixir and Tablets **1469**

Quadrinal Tablets **1350**

Phensuximide (Combination therapy with other anticonvulsant has resulted in alteration of thyroid function). Products include:

Milontin Kapseals **1920**

Phenytoin (Simultaneous administration produces a marked lowering of serum levels of carbamazepine; half-life of phenytoin is shortened when concurrently administered; combination therapy with other anticonvulsant has resulted in alteration of thyroid function). Products include:

Dilantin Infatabs **1908**
Dilantin-125 Suspension **1911**

Phenytoin Sodium (Simultaneous administration produces a marked lowering of serum levels of carbamazepine; half-life of phenytoin is shortened when concurrently administered; combination therapy with other anticonvulsant has resulted in alteration of thyroid function). Products include:

Dilantin Kapseals **1906**
Dilantin Parenteral **1910**

Primidone (Simultaneous administration produces a marked lowering of serum levels of carbamazepine; combination therapy with other anticonvulsant has resulted in alteration of thyroid function). Products include:

Mysoline **2754**

Propoxyphene Hydrochloride (Concomitant administration has been reported to result in elevated plasma levels of carbamazepine resulting in toxicity is some cases). Products include:

Darvon **1435**
Wygesic Tablets **2827**

Propoxyphene Napsylate (Concomitant administration has been reported to result in elevated plasma levels of carbamazepine resulting in toxicity is some cases). Products include:

Darvon-N/Darvocet-N **1433**

Selegiline Hydrochloride (On theoretical grounds concurrent and/ or sequential use is contraindicated). Products include:

Eldepryl Tablets **2550**

Theophylline (Half-life of theophyllin is shortened when concurrently administered). Products include:

Marax Tablets & DF Syrup **2200**
Quibron **2053**

Theophylline Anhydrous (Half-life of theophyllin is shortened when concurrently administered). Products include:

Aerolate **1004**
Primatene Dual Action Formula ...... ᴹᴰ **872**
Primatene Tablets .... ᴹᴰ **873**
Respbid Tablets **682**
Slo-bid Gyrocaps **2033**
Theo-24 Extended Release Capsules **2568**
Theo-Dur Extended-Release Tablets **1327**
Theo-X Extended-Release Tablets .. **788**
Uni-Dur Extended-Release Tablets.. **1331**
Uniphyl 400 mg Tablets **2001**

Theophylline Calcium Salicylate (Half-life of theophyllin is shortened when concurrently administered). Products include:

Quadrinal Tablets **1350**

Theophylline Sodium Glycinate (Half-life of theophyllin is shortened when concurrently administered).

No products indexed under this heading.

Tranylcypromine Sulfate (On theoretical grounds concurrent and/ or sequential use is contraindicated). Products include:

Parnate Tablets **2503**

Trimethadione (Combination therapy with other anticonvulsant has resulted in alteration of thyroid function).

No products indexed under this heading.

Valproic Acid (Potential for an increase in the ratio of active 10,11-epoxide metabolite to parent compound; valproic acid serum levels may be reduced when valproic acid is administered with carbamazepine; combination therapy with other anticonvulsant has resulted in alteration of thyroid function). Products include:

Depakene **413**

Verapamil Hydrochloride (Concomitant administration has been reported to result in elevated plasma levels of carbamazepine resulting in toxicity is some cases). Products include:

Calan SR Caplets **2422**
Calan Tablets **2419**
Isoptin Injectable **1344**
Isoptin Oral Tablets **1346**
Isoptin SR Tablets **1348**
Verelan Capsules **1410**
Verelan Capsules **2824**

Warfarin Sodium (Half-life of warfarin is shortened when concurrently administered). Products include:

Coumadin **926**

ATROHIST PEDIATRIC CAPSULES

(Chlorpheniramine Maleate, Pseudoephedrine Hydrochloride) **453**
May interact with monoamine oxidase inhibitors, beta blockers, veratrum alkaloids, central nervous system depressants, and certain other agents. Compounds in these categories include:

Acebutolol Hydrochloride (Increases the effects of sympathomimetics). Products include:

Sectral Capsules **2807**

Alfentanil Hydrochloride (Potential for additive effects). Products include:

Alfenta Injection **1286**

Alprazolam (Potential for additive effects). Products include:

Xanax Tablets **2649**

Aprobarbital (Potential for additive effects).

No products indexed under this heading.

Atenolol (Increases the effects of sympathomimetics). Products include:

Tenoretic Tablets **2845**
Tenormin Tablets and I.V. Injection **2847**

Betaxolol Hydrochloride (Increases the effects of sympathomimetics). Products include:

Betoptic Ophthalmic Solution **469**
Betoptic S Ophthalmic Suspension **471**
Kerlone Tablets **2436**

Bisoprolol Fumarate (Increases the effects of sympathomimetics). Products include:

Zebeta Tablets **1413**
Ziac **1415**

Buprenorphine (Potential for additive effects). Products include:

Buprenex Injectable **2006**

Buspirone Hydrochloride (Potential for additive effects). Products include:

BuSpar **737**

Butabarbital (Potential for additive effects).

No products indexed under this heading.

Butalbital (Potential for additive effects). Products include:

Esgic-plus Tablets **1013**
Fioricet Tablets **2258**
Fioricet with Codeine Capsules **2260**
Fiorinal Capsules **2261**
Fiorinal with Codeine Capsules **2262**
Fiorinal Tablets **2261**
Phrenilin **785**
Sedapap Tablets 50 mg/650 mg .. **1543**

Carteolol Hydrochloride (Increases the effects of sympathomimetics). Products include:

Cartrol Tablets **410**
Ocupress Ophthalmic Solution, 1% Sterile .... ⓒ **309**

Chlordiazepoxide (Potential for additive effects). Products include:

Libritabs Tablets **2177**
Limbitrol **2180**

Chlordiazepoxide Hydrochloride (Potential for additive effects). Products include:

Librax Capsules **2176**
Librium Capsules **2178**
Librium Injectable **2179**

Chlorpromazine (Potential for additive effects). Products include:

Thorazine Suppositories **2523**

Chlorpromazine Hydrochloride (Potential for additive effects). Products include:

Thorazine **2523**

Chlorprothixene (Potential for additive effects).

No products indexed under this heading.

Chlorprothixene Hydrochloride (Potential for additive effects).

No products indexed under this heading.

Clorazepate Dipotassium (Potential for additive effects). Products include:

Tranxene **451**

Clozapine (Potential for additive effects). Products include:

Clozaril Tablets **2252**

Codeine Phosphate (Potential for additive effects). Products include:

Actifed with Codeine Cough Syrup.. **1067**
Brontex **1981**
Deconsal C Expectorant Syrup **456**
Deconsal Pediatric Syrup **457**
Dimetane-DC Cough Syrup **2059**
Empirin with Codeine Tablets **1093**
Fioricet with Codeine Capsules **2260**
Fiorinal with Codeine Capsules **2262**
Isoclor Expectorant **990**
Novahistine DH **2462**
Novahistine Expectorant **2463**
Nucofed **2051**
Phenergan with Codeine **2777**
Phenergan VC with Codeine **2781**
Robitussin A-C Syrup **2073**
Robitussin-DAC Syrup **2074**
Ryna .... ᴹᴰ **841**
Soma Compound w/Codeine Tablets **2676**
Tussi-Organidin NR Liquid and S NR Liquid **2677**
Tylenol with Codeine **1583**

Cryptenamine Preparations (Reduced antihypertensive effects).

Desflurane (Potential for additive effects). Products include:

Suprane **1813**

Dezocine (Potential for additive effects). Products include:

Dalgan Injection **538**

Diazepam (Potential for additive effects). Products include:

Dizac **1809**

IMPORTANT NOTE: Always consult each drug listing in the patient's regimen for possible interactions.

Atrohist **Interactions Index** **92**

Valium Injectable 2182
Valium Tablets 2183
Valrelease Capsules 2169

Droperidol (Potential for additive effects). Products include:
Inapsine Injection 1296

Enflurane (Potential for additive effects).
No products indexed under this heading.

Esmolol Hydrochloride (Increases the effects of sympathomimetics). Products include:
Brevibloc Injection 1808

Estazolam (Potential for additive effects). Products include:
ProSom Tablets 449

Ethchlorvynol (Potential for additive effects). Products include:
Placidyl Capsules 448

Ethinamate (Potential for additive effects).
No products indexed under this heading.

Fentanyl (Potential for additive effects). Products include:
Duragesic Transdermal System 1288

Fentanyl Citrate (Potential for additive effects). Products include:
Sublimaze Injection 1307

Fluphenazine Decanoate (Potential for additive effects). Products include:
Prolixin Decanoate 509

Fluphenazine Enanthate (Potential for additive effects). Products include:
Prolixin Enanthate 509

Fluphenazine Hydrochloride (Potential for additive effects). Products include:
Prolixin 509

Flurazepam Hydrochloride (Potential for additive effects). Products include:
Dalmane Capsules 2173

Furazolidone (Increases the effects of sympathomimetics; concurrent and/or sequential use is contraindicated). Products include:
Furoxone 2046

Glutethimide (Potential for additive effects).
No products indexed under this heading.

Haloperidol (Potential for additive effects). Products include:
Haldol Injection, Tablets and Concentrate 1575

Haloperidol Decanoate (Potential for additive effects). Products include:
Haldol Decanoate 1577

Hydrocodone Bitartrate (Potential for additive effects). Products include:
Anexsia 5/500 Elixir 1781
Anexia Tablets 1782
Codiclear DH Syrup 791
Deconamine CX Cough and Cold Liquid and Tablets 1319
Duratuss HD Elixir 2565
Hycodan Tablets and Syrup 930
Hycomine Compound Tablets 932
Hycomine 931
Hycotuss Expectorant Syrup 933
Hydrocet Capsules 782
Lorcet 10/650 1018
Lortab 2566
Tussend 1783
Tussend Expectorant 1785
Vicodin Tablets 1356
Vicodin ES Tablets 1357
Vicodin Tuss Expectorant 1358
Zydone Capsules 949

Hydrocodone Polistirex (Potential for additive effects). Products include:
Tussionex Pennkinetic Extended-Release Suspension 998

Hydroxyzine Hydrochloride (Potential for additive effects). Products include:
Atarax Tablets & Syrup 2185
Marax Tablets & DF Syrup 2200
Vistaril Intramuscular Solution 2216

Isocarboxazid (Increases the effects of sympathomimetics; concurrent and/or sequential use is contraindicated).
No products indexed under this heading.

Isoflurane (Potential for additive effects).
No products indexed under this heading.

Ketamine Hydrochloride (Potential for additive effects).
No products indexed under this heading.

Labetalol Hydrochloride (Increases the effects of sympathomimetics). Products include:
Normodyne Injection 2377
Normodyne Tablets 2379
Trandate 1185

Levobunolol Hydrochloride (Increases the effects of sympathomimetics). Products include:
Betagan .... ◉ 233

Levomethadyl Acetate Hydrochloride (Potential for additive effects). Products include:
Orlamm 2239

Levorphanol Tartrate (Potential for additive effects). Products include:
Levo-Dromoran 2129

Lorazepam (Potential for additive effects). Products include:
Ativan Injection 2698
Ativan Tablets 2700

Loxapine Hydrochloride (Potential for additive effects). Products include:
Loxitane 1378

Loxapine Succinate (Potential for additive effects). Products include:
Loxitane Capsules 1378

Mecamylamine Hydrochloride (Reduced antihypertensive effects). Products include:
Inversine Tablets 1686

Meperidine Hydrochloride (Potential for additive effects). Products include:
Demerol 2308
Mepergan Injection 2753

Mephobarbital (Potential for additive effects). Products include:
Mebaral Tablets 2322

Meprobamate (Potential for additive effects). Products include:
Miltown Tablets 2672
PMB 200 and PMB 400 2783

Mesoridazine (Potential for additive effects).

Methadone Hydrochloride (Potential for additive effects). Products include:
Methadone Hydrochloride Oral Concentrate 2233
Methadone Hydrochloride Oral Solution & Tablets 2235

Methohexital Sodium (Potential for additive effects). Products include:
Brevital Sodium Vials 1429

Methotrimeprazine (Potential for additive effects). Products include:
Levoprome 1274

Methoxyflurane (Potential for additive effects).
No products indexed under this heading.

Methyldopa (Reduced antihypertensive effects). Products include:
Aldoclor Tablets 1598
Aldomet Oral 1600
Aldoril Tablets 1604

Methyldopate Hydrochloride (Reduced antihypertensive effects). Products include:
Aldomet Ester HCl Injection 1602

Metipranolol Hydrochloride (Increases the effects of sympathomimetics). Products include:
OptiPranolol (Metipranolol 0.3%) Sterile Ophthalmic Solution .... ◉ 258

Metoprolol Succinate (Increases the effects of sympathomimetics). Products include:
Toprol-XL Tablets 565

Metoprolol Tartrate (Increases the effects of sympathomimetics). Products include:
Lopressor Ampuls 830
Lopressor HCT Tablets 832
Lopressor Tablets 830

Midazolam Hydrochloride (Potential for additive effects). Products include:
Versed Injection 2170

Molindone Hydrochloride (Potential for additive effects). Products include:
Moban Tablets and Concentrate 1048

Morphine Sulfate (Potential for additive effects). Products include:
Astramorph/PF Injection, USP (Preservative-Free) 535
Duramorph 962
Infumorph 200 and Infumorph 500 Sterile Solutions 965
MS Contin Tablets 1994
MSIR 1997
Oramorph SR (Morphine Sulfate Sustained Release Tablets) 2236
RMS Suppositories 2657
Roxanol 2243

Nadolol (Increases the effects of sympathomimetics).
No products indexed under this heading.

Opium Alkaloids (Potential for additive effects).
No products indexed under this heading.

Oxazepam (Potential for additive effects). Products include:
Serax Capsules 2810
Serax Tablets 2810

Oxycodone Hydrochloride (Potential for additive effects). Products include:
Percocet Tablets 938
Percodan Tablets 939
Percodan-Demi Tablets 940
Roxicodone Tablets, Oral Solution & Intensol (Oxycodone) 2244
Tylox Capsules 1584

Penbutolol Sulfate (Increases the effects of sympathomimetics). Products include:
Levatol 2403

Pentobarbital Sodium (Potential for additive effects). Products include:
Nembutal Sodium Capsules 436
Nembutal Sodium Solution 438
Nembutal Sodium Suppositories 440

Perphenazine (Potential for additive effects). Products include:
Etrafon 2355
Triavil Tablets 1757
Trilafon 2389

Phenelzine Sulfate (Increases the effects of sympathomimetics; concurrent and/or sequential use is contraindicated). Products include:
Nardil 1920

Phenobarbital (Potential for additive effects). Products include:
Arco-Lase Plus Tablets 512
Bellergal-S Tablets 2250
Donnatal 2060
Donnatal Extentabs 2061
Donnatal Tablets 2060
Phenobarbital Elixir and Tablets 1469
Quadrinal Tablets 1350

Pindolol (Increases the effects of sympathomimetics). Products include:
Visken Tablets 2299

Prazepam (Potential for additive effects).
No products indexed under this heading.

Prochlorperazine (Potential for additive effects). Products include:
Compazine 2470

Promethazine Hydrochloride (Potential for additive effects). Products include:
Mepergan Injection 2753
Phenergan with Codeine 2777
Phenergan with Dextromethorphan 2778
Phenergan Injection 2773
Phenergan Suppositories 2775
Phenergan Syrup 2774
Phenergan Tablets 2775
Phenergan VC 2779
Phenergan VC with Codeine 2781

Propofol (Potential for additive effects). Products include:
Diprivan Injection 2833

Propoxyphene Hydrochloride (Potential for additive effects). Products include:
Darvon 1435
Wygesic Tablets 2827

Propoxyphene Napsylate (Potential for additive effects). Products include:
Darvon-N/Darvocet-N 1433

Propranolol Hydrochloride (Increases the effects of sympathomimetics). Products include:
Inderal 2728
Inderal LA Long Acting Capsules 2730
Inderide Tablets 2732
Inderide LA Long Acting Capsules 2734

Quazepam (Potential for additive effects). Products include:
Doral Tablets 2664

Reserpine (Reduced antihypertensive effects). Products include:
Diupres Tablets 1650
Hydropres Tablets 1675
Ser-Ap-Es Tablets 849

Risperidone (Potential for additive effects). Products include:
Risperdal 1301

Secobarbital Sodium (Potential for additive effects). Products include:
Seconal Sodium Pulvules 1474

Selegiline Hydrochloride (Increases the effects of sympathomimetics; concurrent and/or sequential use is contraindicated). Products include:
Eldepryl Tablets 2550

Sotalol Hydrochloride (Increases the effects of sympathomimetics). Products include:
Betapace Tablets 641

Sufentanil Citrate (Potential for additive effects). Products include:
Sufenta Injection 1309

Temazepam (Potential for additive effects). Products include:
Restoril Capsules 2284

Thiamylal Sodium (Potential for additive effects).
No products indexed under this heading.

Thioridazine Hydrochloride (Potential for additive effects). Products include:
Mellaril 2269

Thiothixene (Potential for additive effects). Products include:
Navane Capsules and Concentrate 2201
Navane Intramuscular 2202

(▭ Described in PDR For Nonprescription Drugs) (◉ Described in PDR For Ophthalmology)

Interactions Index — Atrohist Pediatric

Timolol Hemihydrate (Increases the effects of sympathomimetics). Products include:

Betimol 0.25%, 0.5% .... ◉ 261

Timolol Maleate (Increases the effects of sympathomimetics). Products include:

Blocadren Tablets 1614
Timolide Tablets.................................... 1748
Timoptic in Ocudose 1753
Timoptic Sterile Ophthalmic Solution.. 1751
Timoptic-XE 1755

Tranylcypromine Sulfate (Increases the effects of sympathomimetics; concurrent and/or sequential use is contraindicated). Products include:

Parnate Tablets 2503

Triazolam (Potential for additive effects). Products include:

Halcion Tablets...................................... 2611

Trifluoperazine Hydrochloride (Potential for additive effects). Products include:

Stelazine 2514

Zolpidem Tartrate (Potential for additive effects). Products include:

Ambien Tablets...................................... 2416

Food Interactions

Alcohol (Potential for additive effects).

ATROHIST PEDIATRIC SUSPENSION

(Chlorpheniramine Tannate, Phenylephrine Tannate, Pyrilamine Tannate) 454

May interact with monoamine oxidase inhibitors, central nervous system depressants, tranquilizers, hypnotics and sedatives, and certain other agents. Compounds in these categories include:

Alfentanil Hydrochloride (Potential for additive central nervous system effects). Products include:

Alfenta Injection 1286

Alprazolam (Potential for additive central nervous system effects). Products include:

Xanax Tablets 2649

Aprobarbital (Potential for additive central nervous system effects).

No products indexed under this heading.

Buprenorphine (Potential for additive central nervous system effects). Products include:

Buprenex Injectable 2006

Buspirone Hydrochloride (Potential for additive central nervous system effects). Products include:

BuSpar 737

Butabarbital (Potential for additive central nervous system effects).

No products indexed under this heading.

Butalbital (Potential for additive central nervous system effects). Products include:

Esgic-plus Tablets 1013
Fioricet Tablets...................................... 2258
Fioricet with Codeine Capsules 2260
Fiorinal Capsules 2261
Fiorinal with Codeine Capsules 2262
Fiorinal Tablets 2261
Phrenilin 785
Sedapap Tablets 50 mg/650 mg .. 1543

Chlordiazepoxide (Potential for additive central nervous system effects). Products include:

Libritabs Tablets 2177
Limbitrol 2180

Chlordiazepoxide Hydrochloride (Potential for additive central nervous system effects). Products include:

Librax Capsules 2176

Librium Capsules................................... 2178
Librium Injectable 2179

Chlorpromazine (Potential for additive central nervous system effects). Products include:

Thorazine Suppositories....................... 2523

Chlorpromazine Hydrochloride (Potential for additive central nervous system effects). Products include:

Thorazine 2523

Chlorprothixene (Potential for additive central nervous system effects).

No products indexed under this heading.

Chlorprothixene Hydrochloride (Potential for additive central nervous system effects).

No products indexed under this heading.

Clorazepate Dipotassium (Potential for additive central nervous system effects). Products include:

Tranxene 451

Clozapine (Potential for additive central nervous system effects). Products include:

Clozaril Tablets..................................... 2252

Codeine Phosphate (Potential for additive central nervous system effects). Products include:

Actifed with Codeine Cough Syrup.. 1067
Brontex 1981
Deconsal C Expectorant Syrup 456
Deconsal Pediatric Syrup..................... 457
Dimetane-DC Cough Syrup 2059
Empirin with Codeine Tablets.............. 1093
Fioricet with Codeine Capsules 2260
Fiorinal with Codeine Capsules 2262
Isoclor Expectorant................................ 990
Novahistine DH..................................... 2462
Novahistine Expectorant...................... 2463
Nucofed 2051
Phenergan with Codeine...................... 2777
Phenergan VC with Codeine 2781
Robitussin A-C Syrup............................ 2073
Robitussin-DAC Syrup 2074
Ryna .... ◉◻ 841
Soma Compound w/Codeine Tablets 2676
Tussi-Organidin NR Liquid and S NR Liquid 2677
Tylenol with Codeine 1583

Desflurane (Potential for additive central nervous system effects). Products include:

Suprane 1813

Dezocine (Potential for additive central nervous system effects). Products include:

Dalgan Injection 538

Diazepam (Potential for additive central nervous system effects). Products include:

Dizac 1809
Valium Injectable 2182
Valium Tablets 2183
Valrelease Capsules 2169

Droperidol (Potential for additive central nervous system effects). Products include:

Inapsine Injection.................................. 1296

Enflurane (Potential for additive central nervous system effects).

No products indexed under this heading.

Estazolam (Potential for additive central nervous system effects). Products include:

ProSom Tablets 449

Ethchlorvynol (Potential for additive central nervous system effects). Products include:

Placidyl Capsules.................................. 448

Ethinamate (Potential for additive central nervous system effects).

No products indexed under this heading.

Fentanyl (Potential for additive central nervous system effects). Products include:

Duragesic Transdermal System......... 1288

Fentanyl Citrate (Potential for additive central nervous system effects). Products include:

Sublimaze Injection............................... 1307

Fluphenazine Decanoate (Potential for additive central nervous system effects). Products include:

Prolixin Decanoate 509

Fluphenazine Enanthate (Potential for additive central nervous system effects). Products include:

Prolixin Enanthate 509

Fluphenazine Hydrochloride (Potential for additive central nervous system effects). Products include:

Prolixin 509

Flurazepam Hydrochloride (Potential for additive central nervous system effects). Products include:

Dalmane Capsules................................. 2173

Furazolidone (Prolongs and intensifies the anticholingeric effects of antihistamines and the overall effects of sympathomimetics; concurrent and/or sequential treatment should not be undertaken). Products include:

Furoxone 2046

Glutethimide (Potential for additive central nervous system effects).

No products indexed under this heading.

Haloperidol (Potential for additive central nervous system effects). Products include:

Haldol Injection, Tablets and Concentrate 1575

Haloperidol Decanoate (Potential for additive central nervous system effects). Products include:

Haldol Decanoate.................................. 1577

Hydrocodone Bitartrate (Potential for additive central nervous system effects). Products include:

Anexsia 5/500 Elixir 1781
Anexia Tablets....................................... 1782
Codiclear DH Syrup 791
Deconamine CX Cough and Cold Liquid and Tablets................................ 1319
Duratuss HD Elixir................................. 2565
Hycodan Tablets and Syrup 930
Hycomine Compound Tablets 932
Hycomine 931
Hycotuss Expectorant Syrup 933
Hydrocet Capsules 782
Lorcet 10/650.. 1018
Lortab 2566
Tussend 1783
Tussend Expectorant 1785
Vicodin Tablets 1356
Vicodin ES Tablets 1357
Vicodin Tuss Expectorant 1358
Zydone Capsules 949

Hydrocodone Polistirex (Potential for additive central nervous system effects). Products include:

Tussionex Pennkinetic Extended-Release Suspension 998

Hydroxyzine Hydrochloride (Potential for additive central nervous system effects). Products include:

Atarax Tablets & Syrup......................... 2185
Marax Tablets & DF Syrup.................... 2200
Vistaril Intramuscular Solution........... 2216

Isocarboxazid (Prolongs and intensifies the anticholingeric effects of antihistamines and the overall effects of sympathomimetics; concurrent and/or sequential treatment should not be undertaken).

No products indexed under this heading.

Isoflurane (Potential for additive central nervous system effects).

No products indexed under this heading.

Ketamine Hydrochloride (Potential for additive central nervous system effects).

No products indexed under this heading.

Levomethadyl Acetate Hydrochloride (Potential for additive central nervous system effects). Products include:

Orlaam 2239

Levorphanol Tartrate (Potential for additive central nervous system effects). Products include:

Levo-Dromoran...................................... 2129

Lorazepam (Potential for additive central nervous system effects). Products include:

Ativan Injection..................................... 2698
Ativan Tablets 2700

Loxapine Hydrochloride (Potential for additive central nervous system effects). Products include:

Loxitane 1378

Loxapine Succinate (Potential for additive central nervous system effects). Products include:

Loxitane Capsules 1378

Meperidine Hydrochloride (Potential for additive central nervous system effects). Products include:

Demerol 2308
Mepergan Injection 2753

Mephobarbital (Potential for additive central nervous system effects). Products include:

Mebaral Tablets 2322

Meprobamate (Potential for additive central nervous system effects). Products include:

Miltown Tablets 2672
PMB 200 and PMB 400 2783

Mesoridazine (Potential for additive central nervous system effects).

Mesoridazine Besylate (Potential for additive central nervous system effects). Products include:

Serentil... 684

Methadone Hydrochloride (Potential for additive central nervous system effects). Products include:

Methadone Hydrochloride Oral Concentrate 2233
Methadone Hydrochloride Oral Solution & Tablets................................ 2235

Methohexital Sodium (Potential for additive central nervous system effects). Products include:

Brevital Sodium Vials............................ 1429

Methotrimeprazine (Potential for additive central nervous system effects). Products include:

Levoprome 1274

Methoxyflurane (Potential for additive central nervous system effects).

No products indexed under this heading.

Midazolam Hydrochloride (Potential for additive central nervous system effects). Products include:

Versed Injection 2170

Molindone Hydrochloride (Potential for additive central nervous system effects). Products include:

Moban Tablets and Concentrate 1048

Morphine Sulfate (Potential for additive central nervous system effects). Products include:

Astramorph/PF Injection, USP (Preservative-Free) 535
Duramorph 962
Infumorph 200 and Infumorph 500 Sterile Solutions........................ 965
MS Contin Tablets.................................. 1994

IMPORTANT NOTE: Always consult each drug listing in the patient's regimen for possible interactions.

Atrohist Pediatric — Interactions Index — 94

MSIR ... 1997
Oramorph SR (Morphine Sulfate Sustained Release Tablets) ... 2236
RMS Suppositories ... 2657
Roxanol ... 2243

Opium Alkaloids (Potential for additive central nervous system effects).
No products indexed under this heading.

Oxazepam (Potential for additive central nervous system effects). Products include:
Serax Capsules ... 2810
Serax Tablets ... 2810

Oxycodone Hydrochloride (Potential for additive central nervous system effects). Products include:
Percocet Tablets ... 938
Percodan Tablets ... 939
Percodan-Demi Tablets ... 940
Roxicodone Tablets, Oral Solution & Intensol (Oxycodone) ... 2244
Tylox Capsules ... 1584

Pentobarbital Sodium (Potential for additive central nervous system effects). Products include:
Nembutal Sodium Capsules ... 436
Nembutal Sodium Solution ... 438
Nembutal Sodium Suppositories ... 440

Perphenazine (Potential for additive central nervous system effects). Products include:
Etrafon ... 2355
Triavil Tablets ... 1757
Trilafon ... 2389

Phenelzine Sulfate (Prolongs and intensifies the anticholinergic effects of antihistamines and the overall effects of sympathomimetics; concurrent and/or sequential treatment should not be undertaken). Products include:
Nardil ... 1920

Phenobarbital (Potential for additive central nervous system effects). Products include:
Arco-Lase Plus Tablets ... 512
Bellergal-S Tablets ... 2250
Donnatal ... 2060
Donnatal Extentabs ... 2061
Donnatal Tablets ... 2060
Phenobarbital Elixir and Tablets ... 1469
Quadrinal Tablets ... 1350

Prazepam (Potential for additive central nervous system effects).
No products indexed under this heading.

Prochlorperazine (Potential for additive central nervous system effects). Products include:
Compazine ... 2470

Promethazine Hydrochloride (Potential for additive central nervous system effects). Products include:
Mepergan Injection ... 2753
Phenergan with Codeine ... 2777
Phenergan with Dextromethorphan 2778
Phenergan Injection ... 2773
Phenergan Suppositories ... 2775
Phenergan Syrup ... 2774
Phenergan Tablets ... 2775
Phenergan VC ... 2779
Phenergan VC with Codeine ... 2781

Propofol (Potential for additive central nervous system effects). Products include:
Diprivan Injection ... 2833

Propoxyphene Hydrochloride (Potential for additive central nervous system effects). Products include:
Darvon ... 1435
Wygesic Tablets ... 2827

Propoxyphene Napsylate (Potential for additive central nervous system effects). Products include:
Darvon-N/Darvocet-N ... 1433

Quazepam (Potential for additive central nervous system effects). Products include:
Doral Tablets ... 2664

Risperidone (Potential for additive central nervous system effects). Products include:
Risperdal ... 1301

Secobarbital Sodium (Potential for additive central nervous system effects). Products include:
Seconal Sodium Pulvules ... 1474

Selegiline Hydrochloride (Prolongs and intensifies the anticholinergic effects of antihistamines and the overall effects of sympathomimetics; concurrent and/or sequential treatment should not be undertaken). Products include:
Eldepryl Tablets ... 2550

Sufentanil Citrate (Potential for additive central nervous system effects). Products include:
Sufenta Injection ... 1309

Temazepam (Potential for additive central nervous system effects). Products include:
Restoril Capsules ... 2284

Thiamylal Sodium (Potential for additive central nervous system effects).
No products indexed under this heading.

Thioridazine Hydrochloride (Potential for additive central nervous system effects). Products include:
Mellaril ... 2269

Thiothixene (Potential for additive central nervous system effects). Products include:
Navane Capsules and Concentrate 2201
Navane Intramuscular ... 2202

Tranylcypromine Sulfate (Prolongs and intensifies the anticholinergic effects of antihistamines and the overall effects of sympathomimetics; concurrent and/or sequential treatment should not be undertaken). Products include:
Parnate Tablets ... 2503

Triazolam (Potential for additive central nervous system effects). Products include:
Halcion Tablets ... 2611

Trifluoperazine Hydrochloride (Potential for additive central nervous system effects). Products include:
Stelazine ... 2514

Zolpidem Tartrate (Potential for additive central nervous system effects). Products include:
Ambien Tablets ... 2416

Food Interactions

Alcohol (Potential for additive central nervous system effects).

ATROHIST PLUS TABLETS

(Chlorpheniramine Maleate, Phenylpropanolamine Hydrochloride, Phenylephrine Hydrochloride, Hyoscyamine Sulfate, Atropine Sulfate, Scopolamine Hydrobromide) 454

May interact with monoamine oxidase inhibitors, hypnotics and sedatives, tranquilizers, and certain other agents. Compounds in these categories include:

Alprazolam (Possible additive drowsiness effects). Products include:
Xanax Tablets ... 2649

Buspirone Hydrochloride (Possible additive drowsiness effects). Products include:
BuSpar ... 737

Chlordiazepoxide (Possible additive drowsiness effects). Products include:
Libritabs Tablets ... 2177
Limbitrol ... 2180

Chlordiazepoxide Hydrochloride (Possible additive drowsiness effects). Products include:
Librax Capsules ... 2176
Librium Capsules ... 2178
Librium Injectable ... 2179

Chlorpromazine (Possible additive drowsiness effects). Products include:
Thorazine Suppositories ... 2523

Chlorpromazine Hydrochloride (Possible additive drowsiness effects). Products include:
Thorazine ... 2523

Chlorprothixene (Possible additive drowsiness effects).
No products indexed under this heading.

Chlorprothixene Hydrochloride (Possible additive drowsiness effects).
No products indexed under this heading.

Clorazepate Dipotassium (Possible additive drowsiness effects). Products include:
Tranxene ... 451

Diazepam (Possible additive drowsiness effects). Products include:
Dizac ... 1809
Valium Injectable ... 2182
Valium Tablets ... 2183
Valrelease Capsules ... 2169

Droperidol (Possible additive drowsiness effects). Products include:
Inapsine Injection ... 1296

Estazolam (Possible additive drowsiness effects). Products include:
ProSom Tablets ... 449

Ethchlorvynol (Possible additive drowsiness effects). Products include:
Placidyl Capsules ... 448

Ethinamate (Possible additive drowsiness effects).
No products indexed under this heading.

Fluphenazine Decanoate (Possible additive drowsiness effects). Products include:
Prolixin Decanoate ... 509

Fluphenazine Enanthate (Possible additive drowsiness effects). Products include:
Prolixin Enanthate ... 509

Fluphenazine Hydrochloride (Possible additive drowsiness effects). Products include:
Prolixin ... 509

Flurazepam Hydrochloride (Possible additive drowsiness effects). Products include:
Dalmane Capsules ... 2173

Furazolidone (Concurrent and/or sequential therapy should not be undertaken). Products include:
Furoxone ... 2046

Glutethimide (Possible additive drowsiness effects).
No products indexed under this heading.

Haloperidol (Possible additive drowsiness effects). Products include:
Haldol Injection, Tablets and Concentrate ... 1575

Haloperidol Decanoate (Possible additive drowsiness effects). Products include:
Haldol Decanoate ... 1577

Hydroxyzine Hydrochloride (Possible additive drowsiness effects). Products include:
Atarax Tablets & Syrup ... 2185
Marax Tablets & DF Syrup ... 2200
Vistaril Intramuscular Solution ... 2216

Isocarboxazid (Concurrent and/or sequential therapy should not be undertaken).
No products indexed under this heading.

Lorazepam (Possible additive drowsiness effects). Products include:
Ativan Injection ... 2698
Ativan Tablets ... 2700

Loxapine Hydrochloride (Possible additive drowsiness effects). Products include:
Loxitane ... 1378

Loxapine Succinate (Possible additive drowsiness effects). Products include:
Loxitane Capsules ... 1378

Meprobamate (Possible additive drowsiness effects). Products include:
Miltown Tablets ... 2672
PMB 200 and PMB 400 ... 2783

Mesoridazine Besylate (Possible additive drowsiness effects). Products include:
Serentil ... 684

Midazolam Hydrochloride (Possible additive drowsiness effects). Products include:
Versed Injection ... 2170

Molindone Hydrochloride (Possible additive drowsiness effects). Products include:
Moban Tablets and Concentrate ... 1048

Oxazepam (Possible additive drowsiness effects). Products include:
Serax Capsules ... 2810
Serax Tablets ... 2810

Perphenazine (Possible additive drowsiness effects). Products include:
Etrafon ... 2355
Triavil Tablets ... 1757
Trilafon ... 2389

Phenelzine Sulfate (Concurrent and/or sequential therapy should not be undertaken). Products include:
Nardil ... 1920

Prazepam (Possible additive drowsiness effects).
No products indexed under this heading.

Prochlorperazine (Possible additive drowsiness effects). Products include:
Compazine ... 2470

Promethazine Hydrochloride (Possible additive drowsiness effects). Products include:
Mepergan Injection ... 2753
Phenergan with Codeine ... 2777
Phenergan with Dextromethorphan 2778
Phenergan Injection ... 2773
Phenergan Suppositories ... 2775
Phenergan Syrup ... 2774
Phenergan Tablets ... 2775
Phenergan VC ... 2779
Phenergan VC with Codeine ... 2781

Propofol (Possible additive drowsiness effects). Products include:
Diprivan Injection ... 2833

Quazepam (Possible additive drowsiness effects). Products include:
Doral Tablets ... 2664

Secobarbital Sodium (Possible additive drowsiness effects). Products include:
Seconal Sodium Pulvules ... 1474

Selegiline Hydrochloride (Concurrent and/or sequential therapy should not be undertaken). Products include:
- Eldepryl Tablets 2550

Temazepam (Possible additive drowsiness effects). Products include:
- Restoril Capsules 2284

Thioridazine Hydrochloride (Possible additive drowsiness effects). Products include:
- Mellaril 2269

Thiothixene (Possible additive drowsiness effects). Products include:
- Navane Capsules and Concentrate 2201
- Navane Intramuscular 2202

Tranylcypromine Sulfate (Concurrent and/or sequential therapy should not be undertaken). Products include:
- Parnate Tablets 2503

Triazolam (Possible additive drowsiness effects). Products include:
- Halcion Tablets 2611

Trifluoperazine Hydrochloride (Possible additive drowsiness effects). Products include:
- Stelazine 2514

Zolpidem Tartrate (Possible additive drowsiness effects). Products include:
- Ambien Tablets 2416

Food Interactions

Alcohol (Possible additive drowsiness effects).

ATROMID-S CAPSULES

(Clofibrate) 2701
May interact with anticoagulants and certain other agents. Compounds in these categories include:

Dalteparin Sodium (To prevent bleeding complications, anticoagulant dosage should be reduced generally by one-half). Products include:
- Fragmin 1954

Dicumarol (To prevent bleeding complications, anticoagulant dosage should be reduced generally by one-half).
- No products indexed under this heading.

Enoxaparin (To prevent bleeding complications, anticoagulant dosage should be reduced generally by one-half). Products include:
- Lovenox Injection 2020

Heparin Calcium (To prevent bleeding complications, anticoagulant dosage should be reduced generally by one-half).
- No products indexed under this heading.

Heparin Sodium (To prevent bleeding complications, anticoagulant dosage should be reduced generally by one-half). Products include:
- Heparin Lock Flush Solution 2725
- Heparin Sodium Injection 2726
- Heparin Sodium Injection, USP, Sterile Solution 2615
- Heparin Sodium Vials 1441

Lovastatin (Potential for fulminant rhabdomyolysis, myopathy, and acute renal failure). Products include:
- Mevacor Tablets 1699

Phenytoin (Atromid-S may displace phenytoin from its binding site). Products include:
- Dilantin Infatabs 1908
- Dilantin-125 Suspension 1911

Phenytoin Sodium (Atromid-S may displace phenytoin from its binding site). Products include:
- Dilantin Kapseals 1906
- Dilantin Parenteral 1910

Tolbutamide (Increased hypoglycemic effect; Atromid-S may displace tolbutamide from its binding site).
- No products indexed under this heading.

Warfarin Sodium (To prevent bleeding complications, anticoagulant dosage should be reduced generally by one-half). Products include:
- Coumadin 926

ATROPINE SULFATE STERILE OPHTHALMIC SOLUTION

(Atropine Sulfate) .... ⊙ 233
None cited in PDR database.

ATROVENT INHALATION AEROSOL

(Ipratropium Bromide) 671
None cited in PDR database.

ATROVENT INHALATION SOLUTION

(Ipratropium Bromide) 673
None cited in PDR database.

ATTENUVAX

(Measles Virus Vaccine Live) 1610
May interact with immunosuppressive agents. Compounds in this category include:

Azathioprine (Concurrent use in individuals on immunosuppressive therapy is contraindicated). Products include:
- Imuran 1110

Cyclosporine (Concurrent use in individuals on immunosuppressive therapy is contraindicated). Products include:
- Neoral 2276
- Sandimmune 2286

Immune Globulin (Human) (Concurrent use in individuals on immunosuppressive therapy is contraindicated).
- No products indexed under this heading.

Muromonab-CD3 (Concurrent use in individuals on immunosuppressive therapy is contraindicated). Products include:
- Orthoclone OKT3 Sterile Solution .. 1837

Mycophenolate Mofetil (Concurrent use in individuals on immunosuppressive therapy is contraindicated). Products include:
- CellCept Capsules 2099

Tacrolimus (Concurrent use in individuals on immunosuppressive therapy is contraindicated). Products include:
- Prograf 1042

AUGMENTIN POWDER FOR ORAL SUSPENSION

(Amoxicillin Trihydrate, Clavulanate Potassium) 2468
See **Augmentin Tablets and Chewable Tablets**

AUGMENTIN TABLETS AND CHEWABLE TABLETS

(Amoxicillin Trihydrate, Clavulanate Potassium) 2468
May interact with:

Allopurinol (Substantially increased incidence of rashes has been reported with ampicillin; no data with Augmentin). Products include:
- Zyloprim Tablets 1226

Disulfiram (Co-administration should be avoided). Products include:
- Antabuse Tablets 2695

Probenecid (Delays amoxicillin excretion). Products include:
- Benemid Tablets 1611
- ColBENEMID Tablets 1622

AURALGAN OTIC SOLUTION

(Antipyrine, Benzocaine, Glycerin) 2703
None cited in PDR database.

AXID PULVULES

(Nizatidine) 1427
May interact with:

Aspirin (Increased serum salicylate levels when nizatidine is given concurrently with very high doses (3,900 mg) of aspirin). Products include:
- Alka-Seltzer Effervescent Antacid and Pain Reliever .... ▣ 701
- Alka-Seltzer Extra Strength Effervescent Antacid and Pain Reliever .... ▣ 703
- Alka-Seltzer Lemon Lime Effervescent Antacid and Pain Reliever .... ▣ 703
- Alka-Seltzer Plus Cold Medicine .... ▣ 705
- Alka-Seltzer Plus Cold & Cough Medicine .... ▣ 708
- Alka-Seltzer Plus Night-Time Cold Medicine .... ▣ 707
- Alka Seltzer Plus Sinus Medicine .. ▣ 707
- Arthritis Foundation Safety Coated Aspirin Tablets .... ▣ 675
- Arthritis Pain Ascriptin .... ▣ 631
- Maximum Strength Ascriptin .... ▣ 630
- Regular Strength Ascriptin Tablets .... ▣ 629
- Arthritis Strength BC Powder .... ▣ 609
- BC Cold Powder Multi-Symptom Formula (Cold-Sinus-Allergy) .... ▣ 609
- BC Cold Powder Non-Drowsy Formula (Cold-Sinus) .... ▣ 609
- BC Powder .... ▣ 609
- Bayer Children's Chewable Aspirin .... ▣ 711
- Genuine Bayer Aspirin Tablets & Caplets .... ▣ 713
- Extra Strength Bayer Arthritis Pain Regimen Formula .... ▣ 711
- Extra Strength Bayer Aspirin Caplets & Tablets .... ▣ 712
- Extended-Release Bayer 8-Hour Aspirin .... ▣ 712
- Extra Strength Bayer Plus Aspirin Caplets .... ▣ 713
- Extra Strength Bayer PM Aspirin .. ▣ 713
- Bayer Enteric Aspirin .... ▣ 709
- Bufferin Analgesic Tablets and Caplets .... ▣ 613
- Arthritis Strength Bufferin Analgesic Caplets .... ▣ 614
- Extra Strength Bufferin Analgesic Tablets .... ▣ 615
- Cama Arthritis Pain Reliever .... ▣ 785
- Darvon Compound-65 Pulvules 1435
- Easprin 1914
- Ecotrin 2455
- Ecotrin Enteric Coated Aspirin Maximum Strength Tablets and Caplets .... ▣ 816
- Ecotrin Enteric Coated Aspirin Regular Strength Tablets 2455
- Empirin Aspirin Tablets .... ▣ 854
- Empirin with Codeine Tablets 1093
- Excedrin Extra-Strength Analgesic Tablets & Caplets 732
- Fiorinal Capsules 2261
- Fiorinal with Codeine Capsules 2262
- Fiorinal Tablets 2261
- Halfprin 1362
- Healthprin Aspirin 2455
- Norgesic 1496
- Percodan Tablets 939
- Percodan-Demi Tablets 940
- Robaxisal Tablets 2071
- Soma Compound w/Codeine Tablets 2676
- Soma Compound Tablets 2675
- St. Joseph Adult Chewable Aspirin (81 mg.) .... ▣ 808
- Talwin Compound 2335
- Ursinus Inlay-Tabs .... ▣ 794
- Vanquish Analgesic Caplets .... ▣ 731

AYGESTIN TABLETS

(Norethindrone Acetate) 974
None cited in PDR database.

AYR SALINE NASAL DROPS

(Sodium Chloride) .... ▣ 602
None cited in PDR database.

AYR SALINE NASAL MIST

(Sodium Chloride) .... ▣ 602
None cited in PDR database.

AZACTAM FOR INJECTION

(Aztreonam) 734
May interact with aminoglycosides and certain other agents. Compounds in these categories include:

Amikacin Sulfate (Renal function should be monitored if used concurrently or if higher dosages of aminoglycosides are used). Products include:
- Amikacin Sulfate Injection, USP 960
- Amikin Injectable 501

Cefoxitin Sodium (Beta-lactamase inducing antibiotics may antagonize aztreonam). Products include:
- Mefoxin 1691
- Mefoxin Premixed Intravenous Solution 1694

Gentamicin Sulfate (Renal function should be monitored if used concurrently or if higher dosages of aminoglycosides are used). Products include:
- Garamycin Injectable 2360
- Genoptic Sterile Ophthalmic Solution .... ⊙ 243
- Genoptic Sterile Ophthalmic Ointment .... ⊙ 243
- Gentacidin Ointment .... ⊙ 264
- Gentacidin Solution .... ⊙ 264
- Gentak .... ⊙ 208
- Pred-G Liquifilm Sterile Ophthalmic Suspension .... ⊙ 251
- Pred-G S.O.P. Sterile Ophthalmic Ointment .... ⊙ 252

Kanamycin Sulfate (Renal function should be monitored if used concurrently or if higher dosages of aminoglycosides are used).
- No products indexed under this heading.

Streptomycin Sulfate (Renal function should be monitored if used concurrently or if higher dosages of aminoglycosides are used). Products include:
- Streptomycin Sulfate Injection 2208

Tobramycin (Renal function should be monitored if used concurrently or if higher dosages of aminoglycosides are used). Products include:
- AKTOB .... ⊙ 206
- TobraDex Ophthalmic Suspension and Ointment 473
- Tobrex Ophthalmic Ointment and Solution .... ⊙ 229

Tobramycin Sulfate (Renal function should be monitored if used concurrently or if higher dosages of aminoglycosides are used). Products include:
- Nebcin Vials, Hyporets & ADD-Vantage 1464

IMPORTANT NOTE: Always consult each drug listing in the patient's regimen for possible interactions.

Azactam

Tobramycin Sulfate Injection 968

AZEC

(Vitamin A, Vitamin C, Vitamin E) 667
None cited in PDR database.

AZMACORT ORAL INHALER

(Triamcinolone Acetonide) 2011
May interact with:

Prednisone (Potential for increased likelihood of HPA suppression). Products include:

Deltasone Tablets 2595

AZO GANTANOL TABLETS

(Sulfamethoxazole, Phenazopyridine Hydrochloride) 2080
None cited in PDR database.

AZO GANTRISIN TABLETS

(Sulfisoxazole, Phenazopyridine Hydrochloride) 2081
May interact with oral anticoagulants, sulfonylureas, and certain other agents. Compounds in these categories include:

Chlorpropamide (Blood sugar-lowering activity of sulfonylureas potentiated). Products include:

Diabinese Tablets 1935

Dicumarol (Sulfisoxazole prolongs the prothrombin time).

No products indexed under this heading.

Glipizide (Blood sugar-lowering activity of sulfonylureas potentiated). Products include:

Glucotrol Tablets 1967
Glucotrol XL Extended Release Tablets 1968

Glyburide (Blood sugar-lowering activity of sulfonylureas potentiated). Products include:

DiaBeta Tablets 1239
Glynase PresTab Tablets 2609
Micronase Tablets 2623

Methotrexate Sodium (Displacement from protein binding sites). Products include:

Methotrexate Sodium Tablets, Injection, for Injection and LPF Injection 1275

Sodium Thiopental (Sulfisoxazole competes with thiopental for plasma protein binding).

No products indexed under this heading.

Tolazamide (Blood sugar-lowering activity of sulfonylureas potentiated).

No products indexed under this heading.

Tolbutamide (Blood sugar-lowering activity of sulfonylureas potentiated).

No products indexed under this heading.

Warfarin Sodium (Sulfisoxazole prolongs the prothrombin time). Products include:

Coumadin 926

AZULFIDINE EN-TABS

(Sulfasalazine) 1949
See Azulfidine Tablets

AZULFIDINE TABLETS

(Sulfasalazine) 1949
May interact with:

Digoxin (Reduced absorption of digoxin). Products include:

Lanoxicaps 1117
Lanoxin Elixir Pediatric 1120
Lanoxin Injection 1123
Lanoxin Injection Pediatric.................. 1126
Lanoxin Tablets 1128

Folic Acid (Reduced absorption of folic acid). Products include:

Cefol Filmtab.. 412
Fero-Folic-500 Filmtab 429
Iberet-Folic-500 Filmtab...................... 429
Materna Tablets 1379
Mega-B 512
Megadose 512
Nephro-Fer Rx Tablets.......................... 2005
Nephro-Vite + Fe Tablets 2006
Nephro-Vite Rx Tablets 2006
Niferex-150 Forte Capsules 794
Niferex Forte Elixir 794
Sigtab Tablets .... ⊞ 772
Slow Fe with Folic Acid 869
Stuart Prenatal Tablets .... ⊞ 881
The Stuart Formula Tablets................ ⊞ 663
Trinsicon Capsules 2570
Zymacap Capsules .... ⊞ 772

ARTHRITIS STRENGTH BC POWDER

(Aspirin, Salicylamide, Caffeine) ...... ⊞ 609
See BC Cold Powder Multi-Symptom Formula (Cold-Sinus-Allergy)

BC COLD POWDER MULTI-SYMPTOM FORMULA (COLD-SINUS-ALLERGY)

(Aspirin, Phenylpropanolamine Hydrochloride, Chlorpheniramine Maleate) .... ⊞ 609
May interact with monoamine oxidase inhibitors and certain other agents. Compounds in these categories include:

Furazolidone (Concurrent use not recommended; consult your doctor). Products include:

Furoxone 2046

Isocarboxazid (Concurrent use not recommended; consult your doctor).

No products indexed under this heading.

Phenelzine Sulfate (Concurrent use not recommended; consult your doctor). Products include:

Nardil 1920

Selegiline Hydrochloride (Concurrent use not recommended; consult your doctor). Products include:

Eldepryl Tablets 2550

Tranylcypromine Sulfate (Concurrent use not recommended; consult your doctor). Products include:

Parnate Tablets 2503

Food Interactions

Alcohol (Concurrent use not recommended; consult your doctor).

BC COLD POWDER NON-DROWSY FORMULA (COLD-SINUS)

(Aspirin, Phenylpropanolamine Hydrochloride)....................................... ⊞ 609
See BC Cold Powder Multi-Symptom Formula (Cold-Sinus-Allergy)

BC POWDER

(Aspirin, Salicylamide, Caffeine) ...... ⊞ 609
See BC Cold Powder Multi-Symptom Formula (Cold-Sinus-Allergy)

BCG VACCINE, USP (TICE)

(BCG Vaccine) 1814
May interact with immunosuppressive agents and certain other agents. Compounds in these categories include:

Antimicrobial therapy, unspecified (May interfere with the effectiveness of TICE BCG therapy).

Azathioprine (May interfere with development of immune response). Products include:

Imuran 1110

Cyclosporine (May interfere with development of immune response). Products include:

Neoral 2276
Sandimmune 2286

Immune Globulin (Human) (May interfere with development of immune response).

No products indexed under this heading.

Muromonab-CD3 (May interfere with development of immune response). Products include:

Orthoclone OKT3 Sterile Solution .. 1837

Mycophenolate Mofetil (May interfere with development of immune response). Products include:

CellCept Capsules 2099

Tacrolimus (May interfere with development of immune response). Products include:

Prograf 1042

BSS (15 ML & 30 ML) STERILE IRRIGATION SOLUTION

(Balanced Salt Solution)...................... ◉ 214
None cited in PDR database.

BSS (250 ML) STERILE IRRIGATION SOLUTION

(Balanced Salt Solution)...................... ◉ 214
None cited in PDR database.

BSS (500 ML) STERILE IRRIGATION SOLUTION

(Balanced Salt Solution)...................... ◉ 214
None cited in PDR database.

BSS PLUS (500 ML) STERILE IRRIGATION SOLUTION

(Balanced Salt Solution)...................... ◉ 215
None cited in PDR database.

BACKACHE CAPLETS

(Magnesium Salicylate) .... ⊞ 613
May interact with oral anticoagulants and certain other agents. Compounds in these categories include:

Antiarthritic Drugs, unspecified (Concurrent use is not recommended).

Antidiabetic Drugs, unspecified (Concurrent use is not recommended).

Antigout Drugs, unspecified (Concurrent use is not recommended).

Dicumarol (Concurrent use is not recommended).

No products indexed under this heading.

Warfarin Sodium (Concurrent use is not recommended). Products include:

Coumadin 926

BACTINE ANTISEPTIC/ANESTHETIC FIRST AID LIQUID

(Benzalkonium Chloride, Lidocaine Hydrochloride)....................................... ⊞ 708
None cited in PDR database.

BACTINE FIRST AID ANTIBIOTIC PLUS ANESTHETIC OINTMENT

(Bacitracin Zinc, Neomycin Sulfate, Polymyxin B Sulfate, Lidocaine) ...... ⊞ 708
None cited in PDR database.

BACTINE HYDROCORTISONE ANTI-ITCH CREAM

(Hydrocortisone) .... ⊞ 709
None cited in PDR database.

BACTRIM DS TABLETS

(Trimethoprim, Sulfamethoxazole) 2084
May interact with thiazides, oral anticoagulants, and certain other agents. Compounds in these categories include:

Bendroflumethiazide (Increased incidence of thrombocytopenia with purpura in elderly).

No products indexed under this heading.

Chlorothiazide (Increased incidence of thrombocytopenia with purpura in elderly). Products include:

Aldoclor Tablets 1598
Diupres Tablets 1650
Diuril Oral 1653

Chlorothiazide Sodium (Increased incidence of thrombocytopenia with purpura in elderly). Products include:

Diuril Sodium Intravenous 1652

Dicumarol (Prolonged prothrombin time).

No products indexed under this heading.

Hydrochlorothiazide (Increased incidence of thrombocytopenia with purpura in elderly). Products include:

Aldactazide.. 2413
Aldoril Tablets... 1604
Apresazide Capsules 808
Capozide 742
Dyazide 2479
Esidrix Tablets 821
Esimil Tablets 822
HydroDIURIL Tablets 1674
Hydropres Tablets.................................. 1675
Hyzaar Tablets 1677
Inderide Tablets 2732
Inderide LA Long Acting Capsules .. 2734
Lopressor HCT Tablets 832
Lotensin HCT.. 837
Maxzide 1380
Moduretic Tablets 1705
Oretic Tablets 443
Prinzide Tablets 1737
Ser-Ap-Es Tablets 849
Timolide Tablets..................................... 1748
Vaseretic Tablets 1765
Zestoretic 2850
Ziac 1415

Hydroflumethiazide (Increased incidence of thrombocytopenia with purpura in elderly). Products include:

Diucardin Tablets................................... 2718

Methotrexate Sodium (Increased free methotrexate concentrations). Products include:

Methotrexate Sodium Tablets, Injection, for Injection and LPF Injection 1275

Methyclothiazide (Increased incidence of thrombocytopenia with purpura in elderly). Products include:

Enduron Tablets..................................... 420

Phenytoin (Decreased hepatic metabolism of phenytoin). Products include:

Dilantin Infatabs 1908
Dilantin-125 Suspension 1911

Phenytoin Sodium (Decreased hepatic metabolism of phenytoin). Products include:

Dilantin Kapseals 1906
Dilantin Parenteral 1910

Polythiazide (Increased incidence of thrombocytopenia with purpura in elderly). Products include:

Minizide Capsules 1938

(⊞ Described in PDR For Nonprescription Drugs) (◉ Described in PDR For Ophthalmology)

Warfarin Sodium (Prolonged prothrombin time). Products include:

Coumadin 926

BACTRIM I.V. INFUSION

(Trimethoprim, Sulfamethoxazole) ....2082 May interact with thiazides, oral anticoagulants, and certain other agents. Compounds in these categories include:

Bendroflumethiazide (Increased incidence of thrombocytopenia with purpura in elderly).

No products indexed under this heading.

Chlorothiazide (Increased incidence of thrombocytopenia with purpura in elderly). Products include:

Aldoclor Tablets	1598
Diupres Tablets	1650
Diuril Oral	1653

Chlorothiazide Sodium (Increased incidence of thrombocytopenia with purpura in elderly). Products include:

Diuril Sodium Intravenous 1652

Dicumarol (Prolonged prothrombin time).

No products indexed under this heading.

Hydrochlorothiazide (Increased incidence of thrombocytopenia with purpura in elderly). Products include:

Aldactazide	2413
Aldoril Tablets	1604
Apresazide Capsules	808
Capozide	742
Dyazide	2479
Esidrix Tablets	821
Esimil Tablets	822
HydroDIURIL Tablets	1674
Hydropres Tablets	1675
Hyzaar Tablets	1677
Inderide Tablets	2732
Inderide LA Long Acting Capsules	2734
Lopressor HCT Tablets	832
Lotensin HCT	837
Maxzide	1380
Moduretic Tablets	1705
Oretic Tablets	443
Prinzide Tablets	1737
Ser-Ap-Es Tablets	849
Timolide Tablets	1748
Vaseretic Tablets	1765
Zestoretic	2850
Ziac	1415

Hydroflumethiazide (Increased incidence of thrombocytopenia with purpura in elderly). Products include:

Diucardin Tablets................................... 2718

Methotrexate Sodium (Increased free methotrexate concentrations). Products include:

Methotrexate Sodium Tablets, Injection, for Injection and LPF Injection 1275

Methyclothiazide (Increased incidence of thrombocytopenia with purpura in elderly). Products include:

Enduron Tablets...................................... 420

Phenytoin (Decreased hepatic metabolism of phenytoin). Products include:

Dilantin Infatabs	1908
Dilantin-125 Suspension	1911

Phenytoin Sodium (Decreased hepatic metabolism of phenytoin). Products include:

Dilantin Kapseals	1906
Dilantin Parenteral	1910

Polythiazide (Increased incidence of thrombocytopenia with purpura in elderly). Products include:

Minizide Capsules 1938

Warfarin Sodium (Prolonged prothrombin time). Products include:

Coumadin 926

BACTRIM PEDIATRIC SUSPENSION

(Trimethoprim, Sulfamethoxazole) ....2084 See Bactrim DS Tablets

BACTRIM TABLETS

(Trimethoprim, Sulfamethoxazole) ....2084 See Bactrim DS Tablets

BACTROBAN OINTMENT

(Mupirocin) ....2470 None cited in PDR database.

BALMEX OINTMENT

(Zinc Oxide) ....ⓢⓓ 609 None cited in PDR database.

BARRI-CARE ANTIMICROBIAL BARRIER OINTMENT

(Chloroxylenol) ....ⓢⓓ 624 None cited in PDR database.

BASALJEL CAPSULES

(Aluminum Carbonate Gel).................2703 May interact with tetracyclines. Compounds in this category include:

Demeclocycline Hydrochloride (Concurrent oral administration should be avoided). Products include:

Declomycin Tablets................................. 1371

Doxycycline Calcium (Concurrent oral administration should be avoided). Products include:

Vibramycin Calcium Oral Suspension Syrup 1941

Doxycycline Hyclate (Concurrent oral administration should be avoided). Products include:

Doryx Capsules	1913
Vibramycin Hyclate Capsules	1941
Vibramycin Hyclate Intravenous	2215
Vibra-Tabs Film Coated Tablets	1941

Doxycycline Monohydrate (Concurrent oral administration should be avoided). Products include:

Monodox Capsules	1805
Vibramycin Monohydrate for Oral Suspension	1941

Methacycline Hydrochloride (Concurrent oral administration should be avoided).

No products indexed under this heading.

Minocycline Hydrochloride (Concurrent oral administration should be avoided). Products include:

Dynacin Capsules	1590
Minocin Intravenous	1382
Minocin Oral Suspension	1385
Minocin Pellet-Filled Capsules	1383

Oxytetracycline (Concurrent oral administration should be avoided). Products include:

Terramycin Intramuscular Solution 2210

Oxytetracycline Hydrochloride (Concurrent oral administration should be avoided). Products include:

TERAK Ointment	ⓒ 209
Terra-Cortril Ophthalmic Suspension	2210
Terramycin with Polymyxin B Sulfate Ophthalmic Ointment	2211
Urobiotic-250 Capsules	2214

Tetracycline Hydrochloride (Concurrent oral administration should be avoided). Products include:

Achromycin V Capsules 1367

BASALJEL SUSPENSION

(Aluminum Carbonate Gel).................2703 See Basaljel Capsules

BASALJEL TABLETS

(Aluminum Carbonate Gel).................2703 See Basaljel Capsules

BAYER CHILDREN'S CHEWABLE ASPIRIN

(Aspirin) ....ⓢⓓ 711 May interact with oral anticoagulants and certain other agents. Compounds in these categories include:

Antiarthritic Drugs, unspecified (Effect not specified).

Antidiabetic Drugs, unspecified (Effect not specified).

Antigout Drugs, unspecified (Effect not specified).

Dicumarol (Effect not specified).

No products indexed under this heading.

Warfarin Sodium (Effect not specified). Products include:

Coumadin 926

GENUINE BAYER ASPIRIN TABLETS & CAPLETS

(Aspirin) ....ⓢⓓ 713 May interact with oral anticoagulants and certain other agents. Compounds in these categories include:

Aluminum Carbonate Gel (Concurrent administration of nonabsorbable antacids may alter the rate of absorption of aspirin, thereby resulting in a decreased acetylsalicylic acid/salicylate ratio in plasma). Products include:

Basaljel... 2703

Aluminum Hydroxide (Concurrent administration of nonabsorbable antacids may alter the rate of absorption of aspirin, thereby resulting in a decreased acetylsalicylic acid/salicylate ratio in plasma). Products include:

ALternaGEL Liquid	1316
Maximum Strength Ascriptin	ⓢⓓ 630
Cama Arthritis Pain Reliever	ⓢⓓ 785
Gaviscon Extra Strength Relief Formula Antacid Tablets	ⓢⓓ 819
Gaviscon Extra Strength Relief Formula Liquid Antacid	ⓢⓓ 819
Gaviscon Liquid Antacid	ⓢⓓ 820
Gelusil Liquid & Tablets	ⓢⓓ 855
Maalox Heartburn Relief Suspension	ⓢⓓ 642
Maalox Heartburn Relief Tablets	ⓢⓓ 641
Maalox Magnesia and Alumina Oral Suspension	ⓢⓓ 642
Maalox Plus Tablets	ⓢⓓ 643
Extra Strength Maalox Antacid Plus Antigas Liquid and Tablets	ⓢⓓ 638
Tempo Soft Antacid	ⓢⓓ 835

Aluminum Hydroxide Gel (Concurrent administration of nonabsorbable antacids may alter the rate of absorption of aspirin, thereby resulting in a decreased acetylsalicylic acid/salicylate ratio in plasma). Products include:

ALternaGEL Liquid	ⓢⓓ 659
Aludrox Oral Suspension	2695
Amphojel Suspension	2695
Amphojel Suspension without Flavor	2695
Amphojel Tablets	2695
Arthritis Pain Ascriptin	ⓢⓓ 631
Regular Strength Ascriptin Tablets	ⓢⓓ 629
Gaviscon Antacid Tablets	ⓢⓓ 819
Gaviscon-2 Antacid Tablets	ⓢⓓ 820
Mylanta Liquid	1317
Mylanta Tablets	ⓢⓓ 660
Mylanta Double Strength Liquid	1317
Mylanta Double Strength Tablets	ⓢⓓ 660
Nephrox Suspension	ⓢⓓ 655

Antiarthritic Drugs, unspecified (Effect not specified).

Antidiabetic Drugs, unspecified (Effect not specified).

Antigout Drugs, unspecified (Effect not specified).

Dicumarol (Effect not specified).

No products indexed under this heading.

Magnesium Hydroxide (Concurrent administration of nonabsorbable antacids may alter the rate of absorption of aspirin, thereby resulting in a decreased acetylsalicylic acid/salicylate ratio in plasma). Products include:

Aludrox Oral Suspension	2695
Arthritis Pain Ascriptin	ⓢⓓ 631
Maximum Strength Ascriptin	ⓢⓓ 630
Regular Strength Ascriptin Tablets	ⓢⓓ 629
Di-Gel Antacid/Anti-Gas	ⓢⓓ 801
Gelusil Liquid & Tablets	ⓢⓓ 855
Maalox Magnesia and Alumina Oral Suspension	ⓢⓓ 642
Maalox Plus Tablets	ⓢⓓ 643
Extra Strength Maalox Antacid Plus Antigas Liquid and Tablets	ⓢⓓ 638
Mylanta Calcium Carbonate and Magnesium Hydroxide Tablets	1318
Mylanta Liquid	1317
Mylanta Tablets	ⓢⓓ 660
Mylanta Double Strength Liquid	1317
Mylanta Double Strength Tablets	ⓢⓓ 660
Phillips' Milk of Magnesia Liquid	ⓢⓓ 729
Rolaids Tablets	ⓢⓓ 843
Tempo Soft Antacid	ⓢⓓ 835

Magnesium Oxide (Concurrent administration of nonabsorbable antacids may alter the rate of absorption of aspirin, thereby resulting in a decreased acetylsalicylic acid/salicylate ratio in plasma). Products include:

Beelith Tablets	639
Bufferin Analgesic Tablets and Caplets	ⓢⓓ 613
Caltrate PLUS	ⓢⓓ 665
Cama Arthritis Pain Reliever	ⓢⓓ 785
Mag-Ox 400	668
Uro-Mag	668

Sodium Bicarbonate (Concurrent administration of absorbable antacids at therapeutic doses may increase the clearance of salicylates in some individuals). Products include:

Alka-Seltzer Effervescent Antacid and Pain Reliever	ⓢⓓ 701
Alka-Seltzer Extra Strength Effervescent Antacid and Pain Reliever	ⓢⓓ 703
Alka-Seltzer Gold Effervescent Antacid	ⓢⓓ 703
Alka-Seltzer Lemon Lime Effervescent Antacid and Pain Reliever	ⓢⓓ 703
Arm & Hammer Pure Baking Soda	ⓢⓓ 627
Ceo-Two Rectal Suppositories	666
Citrocarbonate Antacid	ⓢⓓ 770
Massengill Disposable Douches	ⓢⓓ 820
Massengill Liquid Concentrate	ⓢⓓ 820
NuLYTELY	689
Cherry Flavor NuLYTELY	689

Warfarin Sodium (Effect not specified). Products include:

Coumadin 926

EXTRA STRENGTH BAYER ARTHRITIS PAIN REGIMEN FORMULA

(Aspirin, Enteric Coated) ....ⓢⓓ 711 May interact with oral anticoagulants and certain other agents. Compounds in these categories include:

Antiarthritic Drugs, unspecified (Concurrent use not recommended; consult your doctor).

Antidiabetic Drugs, unspecified (Concurrent use not recommended; consult your doctor).

Antigout Drugs, unspecified (Concurrent use not recommended; consult your doctor).

Dicumarol (Concurrent use not recommended; consult your doctor).

No products indexed under this heading.

IMPORTANT NOTE: Always consult each drug listing in the patient's regimen for possible interactions.

Bayer Arthritis Extra | Interactions Index | 98

Warfarin Sodium (Concurrent use not recommended; consult your doctor). Products include:
Coumadin 926

EXTRA STRENGTH BAYER ASPIRIN CAPLETS & TABLETS
(Aspirin) .... ▣ 712
May interact with oral anticoagulants and certain other agents. Compounds in these categories include:
Antiarthritic Drugs, unspecified (Effect not specified).
Antidiabetic Drugs, unspecified (Effect not specified).
Antigout Drugs, unspecified (Effect not specified).
Dicumarol (Effect not specified).
No products indexed under this heading.
Warfarin Sodium (Effect not specified). Products include:
Coumadin 926

EXTENDED-RELEASE BAYER 8-HOUR ASPIRIN
(Aspirin) .... ▣ 712
May interact with oral anticoagulants and certain other agents. Compounds in these categories include:
Antiarthritic Drugs, unspecified (Effect not specified).
Antidiabetic Drugs, unspecified (Effect not specified).
Antigout Drugs, unspecified (Effect not specified).
Dicumarol (Effect not specified).
No products indexed under this heading.
Warfarin Sodium (Effect not specified). Products include:
Coumadin 926

EXTRA STRENGTH BAYER PLUS ASPIRIN CAPLETS
(Aspirin, Calcium Carbonate) .... ▣ 713
May interact with oral anticoagulants and certain other agents. Compounds in these categories include:
Antiarthritic Drugs, unspecified (Concurrent use is not recommended unless directed by a doctor).
Antidiabetic Drugs, unspecified (Concurrent use is not recommended unless directed by a doctor).
Antigout Drugs, unspecified (Concurrent use is not recommended unless directed by a doctor).
Dicumarol (Concurrent use is not recommended unless directed by a doctor).
No products indexed under this heading.
Warfarin Sodium (Concurrent use is not recommended unless directed by a doctor). Products include:
Coumadin 926

EXTRA STRENGTH BAYER PM ASPIRIN
(Aspirin, Diphenhydramine Hydrochloride) .... ▣ 713
May interact with oral anticoagulants, hypnotics and sedatives, tranquilizers, and certain other agents. Compounds in these categories include:
Alprazolam (Concurrent use not recommended). Products include:
Xanax Tablets 2649
Antiarthritic Drugs, unspecified (Concurrent use not recommended; consult your doctor).
Antidiabetic Drugs, unspecified (Concurrent use not recommended; consult your doctor).
Antigout Drugs, unspecified (Concurrent use not recommended; consult your doctor).
Buspirone Hydrochloride (Concurrent use not recommended). Products include:
BuSpar 737
Chlordiazepoxide (Concurrent use not recommended). Products include:
Libritabs Tablets 2177
Limbitrol 2180
Chlordiazepoxide Hydrochloride (Concurrent use not recommended). Products include:
Librax Capsules 2176
Librium Capsules 2178
Librium Injectable 2179
Chlorpromazine (Concurrent use not recommended). Products include:
Thorazine Suppositories 2523
Chlorpromazine Hydrochloride (Concurrent use not recommended). Products include:
Thorazine 2523
Chlorprothixene (Concurrent use not recommended).
No products indexed under this heading.
Chlorprothixene Hydrochloride (Concurrent use not recommended).
No products indexed under this heading.
Clorazepate Dipotassium (Concurrent use not recommended). Products include:
Tranxene 451
Diazepam (Concurrent use not recommended). Products include:
Dizac 1809
Valium Injectable 2182
Valium Tablets 2183
Valrelease Capsules 2169
Dicumarol (Concurrent use not recommended; consult your doctor).
No products indexed under this heading.
Droperidol (Concurrent use not recommended). Products include:
Inapsine Injection 1296
Estazolam (Concurrent use not recommended). Products include:
ProSom Tablets 449
Ethchlorvynol (Concurrent use not recommended). Products include:
Placidyl Capsules 448
Ethinamate (Concurrent use not recommended).
No products indexed under this heading.
Fluphenazine Decanoate (Concurrent use not recommended). Products include:
Prolixin Decanoate 509
Fluphenazine Enanthate (Concurrent use not recommended). Products include:
Prolixin Enanthate 509
Fluphenazine Hydrochloride (Concurrent use not recommended). Products include:
Prolixin 509
Flurazepam Hydrochloride (Concurrent use not recommended). Products include:
Dalmane Capsules 2173
Glutethimide (Concurrent use not recommended).
No products indexed under this heading.
Haloperidol (Concurrent use not recommended). Products include:
Haldol Injection, Tablets and Concentrate 1575
Haloperidol Decanoate (Concurrent use not recommended). Products include:
Haldol Decanoate 1577
Hydroxyzine Hydrochloride (Concurrent use not recommended). Products include:
Atarax Tablets & Syrup 2185
Marax Tablets & DF Syrup 2200
Vistaril Intramuscular Solution 2216
Lorazepam (Concurrent use not recommended). Products include:
Ativan Injection 2698
Ativan Tablets 2700
Loxapine Hydrochloride (Concurrent use not recommended). Products include:
Loxitane 1378
Loxapine Succinate (Concurrent use not recommended). Products include:
Loxitane Capsules 1378
Meprobamate (Concurrent use not recommended). Products include:
Miltown Tablets 2672
PMB 200 and PMB 400 2783
Mesoridazine Besylate (Concurrent use not recommended). Products include:
Serentil 684
Midazolam Hydrochloride (Concurrent use not recommended). Products include:
Versed Injection 2170
Molindone Hydrochloride (Concurrent use not recommended). Products include:
Moban Tablets and Concentrate 1048
Oxazepam (Concurrent use not recommended). Products include:
Serax Capsules 2810
Serax Tablets 2810
Perphenazine (Concurrent use not recommended). Products include:
Etrafon 2355
Triavil Tablets 1757
Trilafon 2389
Prazepam (Concurrent use not recommended).
No products indexed under this heading.
Prochlorperazine (Concurrent use not recommended). Products include:
Compazine 2470
Promethazine Hydrochloride (Concurrent use not recommended). Products include:
Mepergan Injection 2753
Phenergan with Codeine 2777
Phenergan with Dextromethorphan 2778
Phenergan Injection 2773
Phenergan Suppositories 2775
Phenergan Syrup 2774
Phenergan Tablets 2775
Phenergan VC 2779
Phenergan VC with Codeine 2781
Propofol (Concurrent use not recommended). Products include:
Diprivan Injection 2833
Quazepam (Concurrent use not recommended). Products include:
Doral Tablets 2664
Secobarbital Sodium (Concurrent use not recommended). Products include:
Seconal Sodium Pulvules 1474
Temazepam (Concurrent use not recommended). Products include:
Restoril Capsules 2284
Thioridazine Hydrochloride (Concurrent use not recommended). Products include:
Mellaril 2269
Thiothixene (Concurrent use not recommended). Products include:
Navane Capsules and Concentrate 2201
Navane Intramuscular 2202
Triazolam (Concurrent use not recommended). Products include:
Halcion Tablets 2611
Trifluoperazine Hydrochloride (Concurrent use not recommended). Products include:
Stelazine 2514
Warfarin Sodium (Concurrent use not recommended; consult your doctor). Products include:
Coumadin 926
Zolpidem Tartrate (Concurrent use not recommended). Products include:
Ambien Tablets 2416

Food Interactions
Alcohol (Avoid concurrent use).

ASPIRIN REGIMEN BAYER ADULT LOW STRENGTH 81 MG TABLETS
(Aspirin, Enteric Coated) .... ▣ 709
See **Aspirin Regimen Bayer Regular Strength 325 mg Caplets**

ASPIRIN REGIMEN BAYER REGULAR STRENGTH 325 MG CAPLETS
(Aspirin, Enteric Coated) .... ▣ 709
May interact with oral anticoagulants, antigout agents, antacids containing aluminium, calcium and magnesium, and certain other agents. Compounds in these categories include:
Allopurinol (Effect not specified). Products include:
Zyloprim Tablets 1226
Aluminum Carbonate Gel (Concurrent use of absorbable antacids at therapeutic doses may increase the clearance of salicylates in some individuals). Products include:
Basaljel 2703
Aluminum Hydroxide (Concurrent use of absorbable antacids at therapeutic doses may increase the clearance of salicylates in some individuals). Products include:
ALternaGEL Liquid 1316
Maximum Strength Ascriptin .... ▣ 630
Cama Arthritis Pain Reliever .... ▣ 785
Gaviscon Extra Strength Relief Formula Antacid Tablets .... ▣ 819
Gaviscon Extra Strength Relief Formula Liquid Antacid .... ▣ 819
Gaviscon Liquid Antacid .... ▣ 820
Gelusil Liquid & Tablets .... ▣ 855
Maalox Heartburn Relief Suspension .... ▣ 642
Maalox Heartburn Relief Tablets .... ▣ 641
Maalox Magnesia and Alumina Oral Suspension .... ▣ 642
Maalox Plus Tablets .... ▣ 643
Extra Strength Maalox Antacid Plus Antigas Liquid and Tablets ▣ 638
Tempo Soft Antacid .... ▣ 835
Aluminum Hydroxide Gel (Concurrent use of absorbable antacids at therapeutic doses may increase the clearance of salicylates in some individuals). Products include:
ALternaGEL Liquid .... ▣ 659
Aludrox Oral Suspension 2695
Amphojel Suspension 2695
Amphojel Suspension without Flavor 2695
Amphojel Tablets 2695
Arthritis Pain Ascriptin .... ▣ 631
Regular Strength Ascriptin Tablets .... ▣ 629
Gaviscon Antacid Tablets .... ▣ 819
Gaviscon-2 Antacid Tablets .... ▣ 820
Mylanta Liquid 1317
Mylanta Tablets .... ▣ 660
Mylanta Double Strength Liquid 1317
Mylanta Double Strength Tablets .. ▣ 660

(▣ Described in PDR For Nonprescription Drugs) (◉ Described in PDR For Ophthalmology)

Nephrox Suspension ....ℬ 655

Antiarthritic Drugs, unspecified (Effect not specified).

Antidiabetic Drugs, unspecified (Effect not specified).

Dicumarol (Effect not specified).

No products indexed under this heading.

Dihydroxyaluminum Sodium Carbonate (Concurrent use of absorbable antacids at therapeutic doses may increase the clearance of salicylates in some individuals).

No products indexed under this heading.

Magaldrate (Concurrent use of absorbable antacids at therapeutic doses may increase the clearance of salicylates in some individuals).

No products indexed under this heading.

Magnesium Hydroxide (Concurrent use of absorbable antacids at therapeutic doses may increase the clearance of salicylates in some individuals). Products include:

Aludrox Oral Suspension 2695
Arthritis Pain Ascriptin ....ℬ 631
Maximum Strength Ascriptin ....ℬ 630
Regular Strength Ascriptin Tablets ....ℬ 629
Di-Gel Antacid/Anti-Gas ....ℬ 801
Gelusil Liquid & Tablets ....ℬ 855
Maalox Magnesia and Alumina Oral Suspension ....ℬ 642
Maalox Plus Tablets ....ℬ 643
Extra Strength Maalox Antacid Plus Antigas Liquid and Tablets ℬ 638
Mylanta Calcium Carbonate and Magnesium Hydroxide Tablets...... 1318
Mylanta Liquid 1317
Mylanta Tablets ....ℬ 660
Mylanta Double Strength Liquid 1317
Mylanta Double Strength Tablets ..ℬ 660
Phillips' Milk of Magnesia Liquid....ℬ 729
Rolaids Tablets ....ℬ 843
Tempo Soft Antacid ....ℬ 835

Magnesium Oxide (Concurrent use of absorbable antacids at therapeutic doses may increase the clearance of salicylates in some individuals). Products include:

Beelith Tablets 639
Bufferin Analgesic Tablets and Caplets ....ℬ 613
Caltrate PLUS ....ℬ 665
Cama Arthritis Pain Reliever.............ℬ 785
Mag-Ox 400 668
Uro-Mag... 668

Probenecid (Effect not specified). Products include:

Benemid Tablets 1611
ColBENEMID Tablets 1622

Sodium Bicarbonate (Concurrent use of nonabsorbable antacids may alter the rate of absorption of aspirin resulting in a decreased acetylsalicylic acid/salicylate ratio in plasma). Products include:

Alka-Seltzer Effervescent Antacid and Pain Reliever ....ℬ 701
Alka-Seltzer Extra Strength Effervescent Antacid and Pain Reliever ....ℬ 703
Alka-Seltzer Gold Effervescent Antacid...ℬ 703
Alka-Seltzer Lemon Lime Effervescent Antacid and Pain Reliever ....ℬ 703
Arm & Hammer Pure Baking Soda ....ℬ 627
Ceo-Two Rectal Suppositories 666
Citrocarbonate Antacid ....ℬ 770
Massengill Disposable Douches......ℬ 820
Massengill Liquid Concentrate.........ℬ 820
NuLYTELY.. 689
Cherry Flavor NuLYTELY 689

Sulfinpyrazone (Effect not specified). Products include:

Anturane 807

Warfarin Sodium (Effect not specified). Products include:

Coumadin 926

BAYER SELECT BACKACHE PAIN RELIEF FORMULA

(Magnesium Salicylate) ....ℬ 715

May interact with oral anticoagulants and certain other agents. Compounds in these categories include:

Antiarthritic Drugs, unspecified (Effect not specified).

Antidiabetic Drugs, unspecified (Effect not specified).

Antigout Drugs, unspecified (Effect not specified).

Dicumarol (Effect not specified).

No products indexed under this heading.

Warfarin Sodium (Effect not specified). Products include:

Coumadin 926

BAYER SELECT HEADACHE PAIN RELIEF FORMULA

(Acetaminophen, Caffeine) ....ℬ 716

Food Interactions

Beverages, caffeine-containing (Concurrent use may cause nervousness, irritability, and occasionally rapid heart beat).

Food, caffeine containing (Concurrent use may cause nervousness, irritability, and occasionally rapid heart beat).

BAYER SELECT IBUPROFEN PAIN RELIEF FORMULA

(Ibuprofen)..ℬ 715

May interact with aspirin and acetaminophen containing products and certain other agents. Compounds in these categories include:

Acetaminophen (Concurrent use is not recommended except under a doctor's direction). Products include:

Actifed Plus Caplets ....ℬ 845
Actifed Plus Tablets ....ℬ 845
Actifed Sinus Daytime/Nighttime Tablets and Caplets ....ℬ 846
Alka-Seltzer Plus Cold Medicine Liqui-Gels ....ℬ 706
Alka-Seltzer Plus Cold & Cough Medicine Liqui-Gels..........................ℬ 705
Alka-Seltzer Plus Night-Time Cold Medicine Liqui-Gels..........................ℬ 706
Allerest Headache Strength Tablets ....ℬ 627
Allerest No Drowsiness Tablets ......ℬ 627
Allerest Sinus Pain Formula ....ℬ 627
Anexsia 5/500 Elixir 1781
Anexia Tablets.. 1782
Arthritis Foundation Aspirin Free Caplets ....ℬ 673
Arthritis Foundation NightTime Caplets ....ℬ 674
Bayer Select Headache Pain Relief Formula ....ℬ 716
Bayer Select Menstrual Multi-Symptom Formula...........................ℬ 716
Bayer Select Night Time Pain Relief Formula.....................................ℬ 716
Bayer Select Sinus Pain Relief Formula ....ℬ 717
Benadryl Allergy Sinus Headache Formula Caplets................................ℬ 849
Comtrex Multi-Symptom Cold Reliever Tablets/Caplets/Liqui-Gels/Liquid..ℬ 615
Allergy-Sinus Comtrex Multi-Symptom Allergy-Sinus Formula Tablets ....ℬ 617
Comtrex Non-Drowsy..........................ℬ 618
Contac Day Allergy/Sinus Caplets ℬ 812
Contac Day & Night ....ℬ 812
Contac Night Allergy/Sinus Caplets ....ℬ 812
Contac Severe Cold and Flu Formula Caplets ....ℬ 814
Contac Severe Cold & Flu Non-Drowsy ....ℬ 815
Coricidin 'D' Decongestant Tablets ....ℬ 800
Coricidin Tablets ....ℬ 800

DHCplus Capsules................................. 1993
Darvon-N/Darvocet-N 1433
Drixoral Cold and Flu Extended-Release Tablets.....................................ℬ 803
Drixoral Cough + Sore Throat Liquid Caps ....ℬ 802
Drixoral Allergy/Sinus Extended Release Tablets.....................................ℬ 804
Esgic-plus Tablets 1013
Aspirin Free Excedrin Analgesic Caplets and Geltabs 732
Excedrin Extra-Strength Analgesic Tablets & Caplets 732
Excedrin P.M. Analgesic/Sleeping Aid Tablets, Caplets, Liquigels 733
Fioricet Tablets...................................... 2258
Fioricet with Codeine Capsules 2260
Hycomine Compound Tablets 932
Hydrocet Capsules 782
Legatrin PM ....ℬ 651
Lorcet 10/650... 1018
Lortab 2566
Lurline PMS Tablets 982
Maximum Strength Multi-Symptom Formula Midol ....ℬ 722
PMS Multi-Symptom Formula Midol ....ℬ 723
Teen Multi-Symptom Formula Midol ....ℬ 722
Midrin Capsules 783
Migralam Capsules 2038
Panodol Tablets and Caplets ....ℬ 824
Children's Panadol Chewable Tablets, Liquid, Infant's Drops ....ℬ 824
Percocet Tablets 938
Percogesic Analgesic Tablets ....ℬ 754
Phrenilin 785
Pyrroxate Caplets ....ℬ 772
Sedapap Tablets 50 mg/650 mg .. 1543
Sinarest Tablets ....ℬ 648
Sinarest Extra Strength Tablets......ℬ 648
Sinarest No Drowsiness Tablets ....ℬ 648
Sine-Aid Maximum Strength Sinus Medication Gelcaps, Caplets and Tablets 1554
Sine-Off No Drowsiness Formula Caplets ....ℬ 824
Sine-Off Sinus Medicine ....ℬ 825
Singlet Tablets ....ℬ 825
Sinulin Tablets 787
Sinutab Sinus Allergy Medication, Maximum Strength Tablets and Caplets ....ℬ 860
Sinutab Sinus Medication, Maximum Strength Without Drowsiness Formula, Tablets & Caplets ....ℬ 860
Sinutab Sinus Medication, Regular Strength Without Drowsiness Formula ....ℬ 859
Sudafed Cold and Cough Liquidcaps ....ℬ 862
Sudafed Severe Cold Formula Caplets ....ℬ 863
Sudafed Severe Cold Formula Tablets ....ℬ 864
Sudafed Sinus Caplets........................ℬ 864
Sudafed Sinus Tablets........................ℬ 864
Talacen.. 2333
TheraFlu...ℬ 787
TheraFlu Maximum Strength Nighttime Flu, Cold & Cough Medicine ....ℬ 788
TheraFlu Maximum Strength Non-Drowsy Formula Flu, Cold & Cough Medicine ....ℬ 788
Thera Flu Maximum Strength, Non-Drowsy Formula Flu, Cold and Cough Caplets ....ℬ 789
Triaminic Sore Throat Formula ......ℬ 791
Triaminicin Tablets ....ℬ 793
Children's TYLENOL acetaminophen Chewable Tablets, Elixir, Suspension Liquid............................. 1555
Children's TYLENOL Cold Multi-Symptom Liquid Formula and Chewable Tablets.................................. 1561
Children's TYLENOL Cold Plus Cough Multi Symptom Tablets and Liquid...ℬ 681
Infants' TYLENOL acetaminophen Drops and Suspension Drops........ 1555
Infants' TYLENOL Cold Decongestant & Fever-Reducer Drops.......... 1556
TYLENOL Extended Relief Caplets.. 1558
TYLENOL, Extra Strength, Acetaminophen Adult Liquid Pain Reliever 1560
TYLENOL, Extra Strength, acetaminophen Gelcaps, Geltabs, Caplets, Tablets 1559

TYLENOL, Extra Strength, Headache Plus Pain Reliever with Antacid Caplets 1559
TYLENOL, Junior Strength, acetaminophen Coated Caplets, Grape and Fruit Chewable Tablets 1557
TYLENOL Maximum Strength Allergy Sinus Medication Gelcaps and Caplets 1563
TYLENOL Maximum Strength Allergy Sinus NightTime Medication Caplets 1555
TYLENOL Flu Maximum Strength Gelcaps 1565
TYLENOL Flu NightTime, Maximum Strength, Gelcaps 1566
TYLENOL Maximum Strength Flu NightTime Hot Medication Packets 1562
TYLENOL, Maximum Strength, Sinus Medication Geltabs, Gelcaps, Caplets and Tablets 1566
TYLENOL Cold Multi-Symptom Formula Medication Tablets and Caplets 1561
TYLENOL Cold Medication No Drowsiness Formula Gelcaps and Caplets 1562
TYLENOL Cold Multi-Symptom Hot Medication Liquid Packets.............. 1557
TYLENOL Cough Multi-Symptom Medication 1564
TYLENOL Cough Multi-Symptom Medication with Decongestant...... 1565
TYLENOL, Regular Strength, acetaminophen Caplets and Tablets .. 1558
TYLENOL PM, Extra Strength Pain Reliever/Sleep Aid Caplets, Geltabs, Gelcaps 1560
TYLENOL Severe Allergy Medication Caplets 1564
Tylenol with Codeine 1583
Tylox Capsules 1584
Unisom With Pain Relief-Nighttime Sleep Aid and Pain Reliever............ 1934
Vanquish Analgesic Caplets ....ℬ 731
Vicks 44 LiquiCaps Cough, Cold & Flu Relief ....ℬ 755
Vicks 44M Cough, Cold & Flu Relief..ℬ 756
Vicks DayQuil ....ℬ 761
Vicks Nyquil Hot Therapy...................ℬ 762
Vicks NyQuil LiquiCaps Multi-Symptom Cold/Flu Relief ....ℬ 763
Vicks NyQuil Multi-Symptom Cold/Flu Relief - (Original & Cherry Flavor)....................................ℬ 763
Vicodin Tablets....................................... 1356
Vicodin ES Tablets 1357
Wygesic Tablets 2827
Zydone Capsules 949

Aspirin (Concurrent use is not recommended except under a doctor's direction). Products include:

Alka-Seltzer Effervescent Antacid and Pain Reliever ....ℬ 701
Alka-Seltzer Extra Strength Effervescent Antacid and Pain Reliever ....ℬ 703
Alka-Seltzer Lemon Lime Effervescent Antacid and Pain Reliever ....ℬ 703
Alka-Seltzer Plus Cold Medicine ....ℬ 705
Alka-Seltzer Plus Cold & Cough Medicine ....ℬ 708
Alka-Seltzer Plus Night-Time Cold Medicine ....ℬ 707
Alka Seltzer Plus Sinus Medicine ..ℬ 707
Arthritis Foundation Safety Coated Aspirin Tablets ....ℬ 675
Arthritis Pain Ascriptin ....ℬ 631
Maximum Strength Ascriptin ....ℬ 630
Regular Strength Ascriptin Tablets ....ℬ 629
Arthritis Strength BC Powder..........ℬ 609
BC Cold Powder Multi-Symptom Formula (Cold-Sinus-Allergy) ......ℬ 609
BC Cold Powder Non-Drowsy Formula (Cold-Sinus) ....ℬ 609
BC Powder ....ℬ 609
Bayer Children's Chewable Aspirin ....ℬ 711
Genuine Bayer Aspirin Tablets & Caplets ....ℬ 713
Extra Strength Bayer Arthritis Pain Regimen Formula ....ℬ 711
Extra Strength Bayer Aspirin Caplets & Tablets ....ℬ 712
Extended-Release Bayer 8-Hour Aspirin ....ℬ 712

IMPORTANT NOTE: Always consult each drug listing in the patient's regimen for possible interactions.

Bayer Select Ibuprofen — Interactions Index — 100

Extra Strength Bayer Plus Aspirin Caplets ▣ 713
Extra Strength Bayer PM Aspirin .. ▣ 713
Bayer Enteric Aspirin ▣ 709
Bufferin Analgesic Tablets and Caplets ▣ 613
Arthritis Strength Bufferin Analgesic Caplets ▣ 614
Extra Strength Bufferin Analgesic Tablets ▣ 615
Cama Arthritis Pain Reliever ▣ 785
Darvon Compound-65 Pulvules 1435
Easprin 1914
Ecotrin 2455
Ecotrin Enteric Coated Aspirin Maximum Strength Tablets and Caplets ▣ 816
Ecotrin Enteric Coated Aspirin Regular Strength Tablets 2455
Empirin Aspirin Tablets ▣ 854
Empirin with Codeine Tablets 1093
Excedrin Extra-Strength Analgesic Tablets & Caplets 732
Fiorinal Capsules 2261
Fiorinal with Codeine Capsules 2262
Fiorinal Tablets 2261
Halfprin 1362
Healthprin Aspirin 2455
Norgesic 1496
Percodan Tablets 939
Percodan-Demi Tablets 940
Robaxisal Tablets 2071
Soma Compound w/Codeine Tablets 2676
Soma Compound Tablets 2675
St. Joseph Adult Chewable Aspirin (81 mg.) ▣ 808
Talwin Compound 2335
Ursinus Inlay-Tabs ▣ 794
Vanquish Analgesic Caplets ▣ 731

BAYER SELECT MENSTRUAL MULTI-SYMPTOM FORMULA
(Acetaminophen, Pamabrom) ▣ 716
None cited in PDR database.

BAYER SELECT NIGHT TIME PAIN RELIEF FORMULA
(Acetaminophen, Diphenhydramine Hydrochloride) ▣ 716
May interact with hypnotics and sedatives, tranquilizers, and certain other agents. Compounds in these categories include:

Alprazolam (Effect not specified). Products include:
Xanax Tablets 2649
Buspirone Hydrochloride (Effect not specified). Products include:
BuSpar 737
Chlordiazepoxide (Effect not specified). Products include:
Libritabs Tablets 2177
Limbitrol 2180
Chlordiazepoxide Hydrochloride (Effect not specified). Products include:
Librax Capsules 2176
Librium Capsules 2178
Librium Injectable 2179
Chlorpromazine (Effect not specified). Products include:
Thorazine Suppositories 2523
Chlorpromazine Hydrochloride (Effect not specified). Products include:
Thorazine 2523
Chlorprothixene (Effect not specified).
No products indexed under this heading.
Chlorprothixene Hydrochloride (Effect not specified).
No products indexed under this heading.
Clorazepate Dipotassium (Effect not specified). Products include:
Tranxene 451
Diazepam (Effect not specified). Products include:
Dizac 1809
Valium Injectable 2182
Valium Tablets 2183
Valrelease Capsules 2169
Droperidol (Effect not specified). Products include:
Inapsine Injection 1296
Estazolam (Effect not specified). Products include:
ProSom Tablets 449
Ethchlorvynol (Effect not specified). Products include:
Placidyl Capsules 448
Ethinamate (Effect not specified).
No products indexed under this heading.
Fluphenazine Decanoate (Effect not specified). Products include:
Prolixin Decanoate 509
Fluphenazine Enanthate (Effect not specified). Products include:
Prolixin Enanthate 509
Fluphenazine Hydrochloride (Effect not specified). Products include:
Prolixin 509
Flurazepam Hydrochloride (Effect not specified). Products include:
Dalmane Capsules 2173
Glutethimide (Effect not specified).
No products indexed under this heading.
Haloperidol (Effect not specified). Products include:
Haldol Injection, Tablets and Concentrate 1575
Haloperidol Decanoate (Effect not specified). Products include:
Haldol Decanoate 1577
Hydroxyzine Hydrochloride (Effect not specified). Products include:
Atarax Tablets & Syrup 2185
Marax Tablets & DF Syrup 2200
Vistaril Intramuscular Solution 2216
Lorazepam (Effect not specified). Products include:
Ativan Injection 2698
Ativan Tablets 2700
Loxapine Hydrochloride (Effect not specified). Products include:
Loxitane 1378
Loxapine Succinate (Effect not specified). Products include:
Loxitane Capsules 1378
Meprobamate (Effect not specified). Products include:
Miltown Tablets 2672
PMB 200 and PMB 400 2783
Mesoridazine Besylate (Effect not specified). Products include:
Serentil 684
Midazolam Hydrochloride (Effect not specified). Products include:
Versed Injection 2170
Molindone Hydrochloride (Effect not specified). Products include:
Moban Tablets and Concentrate 1048
Oxazepam (Effect not specified). Products include:
Serax Capsules 2810
Serax Tablets 2810
Perphenazine (Effect not specified). Products include:
Etrafon 2355
Triavil Tablets 1757
Trilafon 2389
Prazepam (Effect not specified).
No products indexed under this heading.
Prochlorperazine (Effect not specified). Products include:
Compazine 2470
Promethazine Hydrochloride (Effect not specified). Products include:
Mepergan Injection 2753
Phenergan with Codeine 2777
Phenergan with Dextromethorphan 2778
Phenergan Injection 2773
Phenergan Suppositories 2775
Phenergan Syrup 2774
Phenergan Tablets 2775
Phenergan VC 2779
Phenergan VC with Codeine 2781
Propofol (Effect not specified). Products include:
Diprivan Injection 2833
Quazepam (Effect not specified). Products include:
Doral Tablets 2664
Secobarbital Sodium (Effect not specified). Products include:
Seconal Sodium Pulvules 1474
Temazepam (Effect not specified). Products include:
Restoril Capsules 2284
Thioridazine Hydrochloride (Effect not specified). Products include:
Mellaril 2269
Thiothixene (Effect not specified). Products include:
Navane Capsules and Concentrate 2201
Navane Intramuscular 2202
Triazolam (Effect not specified). Products include:
Halcion Tablets 2611
Trifluoperazine Hydrochloride (Effect not specified). Products include:
Stelazine 2514
Zolpidem Tartrate (Effect not specified). Products include:
Ambien Tablets 2416

Food Interactions
Alcohol (Avoid concurrent use).

BAYER SELECT SINUS PAIN RELIEF FORMULA
(Acetaminophen, Pseudoephedrine Hydrochloride) ▣ 717
May interact with monoamine oxidase inhibitors. Compounds in this category include:

Furazolidone (Concurrent and/or sequential use not recommended). Products include:
Furoxone 2046
Isocarboxazid (Concurrent and/or sequential use not recommended).
No products indexed under this heading.
Phenelzine Sulfate (Concurrent and/or sequential use not recommended). Products include:
Nardil 1920
Selegiline Hydrochloride (Concurrent and/or sequential use not recommended). Products include:
Eldepryl Tablets 2550
Tranylcypromine Sulfate (Concurrent and/or sequential use not recommended). Products include:
Parnate Tablets 2503

BECLOVENT INHALATION AEROSOL AND REFILL
(Beclomethasone Dipropionate) 1075
None cited in PDR database.

BECONASE AQ NASAL SPRAY
(Beclomethasone Dipropionate) 1076
None cited in PDR database.

BECONASE INHALATION AEROSOL AND REFILL
(Beclomethasone Dipropionate) 1076
None cited in PDR database.

BEELITH TABLETS
(Magnesium Oxide, Vitamin B_6) 639
May interact with:

Prescription Drugs, unspecified (Concurrent use should be avoided).

BELLERGAL-S TABLETS
(Phenobarbital, Ergotamine Tartrate, Belladonna Alkaloids) 2250
May interact with oral anticoagulants, tricyclic antidepressants, phenothiazines, narcotic analgesics, beta blockers, estrogens, central nervous system depressants, and certain other agents. Compounds in these categories include:

Acebutolol Hydrochloride (A possible interaction may result in excessive vasoconstriction). Products include:
Sectral Capsules 2807
Alfentanil Hydrochloride (Combined use may result in a potentiation of the depressant action). Products include:
Alfenta Injection 1286
Alprazolam (Combined use may result in a potentiation of the depressant action). Products include:
Xanax Tablets 2649
Amitriptyline Hydrochloride (Combined use may result in a potentiation of the depressant action; additive anticholinergic effect). Products include:
Elavil 2838
Endep Tablets 2174
Etrafon 2355
Limbitrol 2180
Triavil Tablets 1757
Amoxapine (Combined use may result in a potentiation of the depressant action; additive anticholinergic effect). Products include:
Asendin Tablets 1369
Aprobarbital (Combined use may result in a potentiation of the depressant action).
No products indexed under this heading.
Atenolol (A possible interaction may result in excessive vasoconstriction). Products include:
Tenoretic Tablets 2845
Tenormin Tablets and I.V. Injection 2847
Betaxolol Hydrochloride (A possible interaction may result in excessive vasoconstriction). Products include:
Betoptic Ophthalmic Solution 469
Betoptic S Ophthalmic Suspension 471
Kerlone Tablets 2436
Bisoprolol Fumarate (A possible interaction may result in excessive vasoconstriction). Products include:
Zebeta Tablets 1413
Ziac 1415
Buprenorphine (Combined use may result in a potentiation of the depressant action). Products include:
Buprenex Injectable 2006
Buspirone Hydrochloride (Combined use may result in a potentiation of the depressant action). Products include:
BuSpar 737
Butabarbital (Combined use may result in a potentiation of the depressant action).
No products indexed under this heading.
Butalbital (Combined use may result in a potentiation of the depressant action). Products include:
Esgic-plus Tablets 1013
Fioricet Tablets 2258

(▣ Described in PDR For Nonprescription Drugs) (◉ Described in PDR For Ophthalmology)

101 Interactions Index Bellergal-S

Fioricet with Codeine Capsules 2260
Fiorinal Capsules 2261
Fiorinal with Codeine Capsules 2262
Fiorinal Tablets 2261
Phrenilin 785
Sedapap Tablets 50 mg/650 mg .. 1543

Carteolol Hydrochloride (A possible interaction may result in excessive vasoconstriction). Products include:
Cartrol Tablets 410
Ocupress Ophthalmic Solution, 1% Sterile........ ◉ 309

Chlordiazepoxide (Combined use may result in a potentiation of the depressant action). Products include:
Libritabs Tablets 2177
Limbitrol 2180

Chlordiazepoxide Hydrochloride (Combined use may result in a potentiation of the depressant action). Products include:
Librax Capsules 2176
Librium Capsules 2178
Librium Injectable 2179

Chlorotrianisene (Potential for increased metabolism rate).
No products indexed under this heading.

Chlorpromazine (Combined use may result in a potentiation of the depressant action). Products include:
Thorazine Suppositories 2523

Chlorpromazine Hydrochloride (Combined use may result in a potentiation of the depressant action). Products include:
Thorazine 2523

Chlorprothixene (Combined use may result in a potentiation of the depressant action).
No products indexed under this heading.

Chlorprothixene Hydrochloride (Combined use may result in a potentiation of the depressant action).
No products indexed under this heading.

Clomipramine Hydrochloride (Combined use may result in a potentiation of the depressant action; additive anticholinergic effect). Products include:
Anafranil Capsules 803

Clorazepate Dipotassium (Combined use may result in a potentiation of the depressant action). Products include:
Tranxene 451

Clozapine (Combined use may result in a potentiation of the depressant action). Products include:
Clozaril Tablets 2252

Codeine Phosphate (Combined use may result in a potentiation of the depressant action). Products include:
Actifed with Codeine Cough Syrup.. 1067
Brontex 1981
Deconsal C Expectorant Syrup 456
Deconsal Pediatric Syrup 457
Dimetane-DC Cough Syrup 2059
Empirin with Codeine Tablets........ 1093
Fioricet with Codeine Capsules 2260
Fiorinal with Codeine Capsules 2262
Isoclor Expectorant........ 990
Novahistine DH........ 2462
Novahistine Expectorant........ 2463
Nucofed 2051
Phenergan with Codeine........ 2777
Phenergan VC with Codeine 2781
Robitussin A-C Syrup........ 2073
Robitussin-DAC Syrup........ 2074
Ryna .... ▣ 841
Soma Compound w/Codeine Tablets........ 2676
Tussi-Organidin NR Liquid and S NR Liquid 2677
Tylenol with Codeine 1583

Desflurane (Combined use may result in a potentiation of the depressant action). Products include:
Suprane 1813

Desipramine Hydrochloride (Combined use may result in a potentiation of the depressant action; additive anticholinergic effect). Products include:
Norpramin Tablets 1526

Dezocine (Combined use may result in a potentiation of the depressant action). Products include:
Dalgan Injection 538

Diazepam (Combined use may result in a potentiation of the depressant action). Products include:
Dizac 1809
Valium Injectable 2182
Valium Tablets 2183
Valrelease Capsules 2169

Dicumarol (Phenobarbital may lower the plasma levels of oral anticoagulant and may cause a decrease in anticoagulant activity).
No products indexed under this heading.

Dienestrol (Potential for increased metabolism rate). Products include:
Ortho Dienestrol Cream 1866

Diethylstilbestrol (Potential for increased metabolism rate). Products include:
Diethylstilbestrol Tablets 1437

Divalproex Sodium (May increase barbiturate metabolism). Products include:
Depakote Tablets........ 415

Doxepin Hydrochloride (Combined use may result in a potentiation of the depressant action; additive anticholinergic effect). Products include:
Sinequan 2205
Zonalon Cream 1055

Doxycycline Calcium (Potential for increased metabolism rate). Products include:
Vibramycin Calcium Oral Suspension Syrup........ 1941

Doxycycline Hyclate (Potential for increased metabolism rate). Products include:
Doryx Capsules........ 1913
Vibramycin Hyclate Capsules........ 1941
Vibramycin Hyclate Intravenous 2215
Vibra-Tabs Film Coated Tablets 1941

Doxycycline Monohydrate (Potential for increased metabolism rate). Products include:
Monodox Capsules 1805
Vibramycin Monohydrate for Oral Suspension........ 1941

Droperidol (Combined use may result in a potentiation of the depressant action). Products include:
Inapsine Injection........ 1296

Enflurane (Combined use may result in a potentiation of the depressant action).
No products indexed under this heading.

Esmolol Hydrochloride (A possible interaction may result in excessive vasoconstriction). Products include:
Brevibloc Injection........ 1808

Estazolam (Combined use may result in a potentiation of the depressant action). Products include:
ProSom Tablets 449

Estradiol (Potential for increased metabolism rate). Products include:
Climara Transdermal System........ 645
Estrace Cream and Tablets........ 749
Estraderm Transdermal System 824

Estrogens, Conjugated (Potential for increased metabolism rate). Products include:
PMB 200 and PMB 400 2783
Premarin Intravenous 2787
Premarin with Methyltestosterone .. 2794
Premarin Tablets 2789
Premarin Vaginal Cream........ 2791
Premphase 2797
Prempro........ 2801

Estrogens, Esterified (Potential for increased metabolism rate). Products include:
ESTRATAB Tablets (0.3, 0.625, 1.25, 2.5 mg)........ 2536
Estratest 2539
Menest Tablets 2494

Estropipate (Potential for increased metabolism rate). Products include:
Ogen Tablets 2627
Ogen Vaginal Cream........ 2630
Ortho-Est........ 1869

Ethchlorvynol (Combined use may result in a potentiation of the depressant action). Products include:
Placidyl Capsules 448

Ethinamate (Combined use may result in a potentiation of the depressant action).
No products indexed under this heading.

Ethinyl Estradiol (Potential for increased metabolism rate). Products include:
Brevicon........ 2088
Demulen 2428
Desogen Tablets........ 1817
Levlen/Tri-Levlen........ 651
Lo/Ovral Tablets 2746
Lo/Ovral-28 Tablets........ 2751
Modicon 1872
Nordette-21 Tablets........ 2755
Nordette-28 Tablets........ 2758
Norinyl 2088
Ortho-Cept 1851
Ortho-Cyclen/Ortho-Tri-Cyclen 1858
Ortho-Novum........ 1872
Ortho-Cyclen/Ortho Tri-Cyclen 1858
Ovcon 760
Ovral Tablets 2770
Ovral-28 Tablets 2770
Levlen/Tri-Levlen........ 651
Tri-Norinyl........ 2164
Triphasil-21 Tablets........ 2814
Triphasil-28 Tablets........ 2819

Fentanyl (Combined use may result in a potentiation of the depressant action). Products include:
Duragesic Transdermal System........ 1288

Fentanyl Citrate (Combined use may result in a potentiation of the depressant action). Products include:
Sublimaze Injection........ 1307

Fluphenazine Decanoate (Combined use may result in a potentiation of the depressant action). Products include:
Prolixin Decanoate 509

Fluphenazine Enanthate (Combined use may result in a potentiation of the depressant action). Products include:
Prolixin Enanthate 509

Fluphenazine Hydrochloride (Combined use may result in a potentiation of the depressant action). Products include:
Prolixin 509

Flurazepam Hydrochloride (Combined use may result in a potentiation of the depressant action). Products include:
Dalmane Capsules........ 2173

Glutethimide (Combined use may result in a potentiation of the depressant action).
No products indexed under this heading.

Griseofulvin (Potential for increased metabolism rate). Products include:
Fulvicin P/G Tablets 2359
Fulvicin P/G 165 & 330 Tablets 2359
Grifulvin V (griseofulvin tablets) Microsize (griseofulvin oral suspension) Microsize 1888
Gris-PEG Tablets, 125 mg & 250 mg 479

Haloperidol (Combined use may result in a potentiation of the depressant action). Products include:
Haldol Injection, Tablets and Concentrate 1575

Haloperidol Decanoate (Combined use may result in a potentiation of the depressant action). Products include:
Haldol Decanoate........ 1577

Hydrocodone Bitartrate (Combined use may result in a potentiation of the depressant action). Products include:
Anexsia 5/500 Elixir 1781
Anexia Tablets........ 1782
Codiclear DH Syrup 791
Deconamine CX Cough and Cold Liquid and Tablets........ 1319
Duratuss HD Elixir........ 2565
Hycodan Tablets and Syrup 930
Hycomine Compound Tablets 932
Hycomine 931
Hycotuss Expectorant Syrup 933
Hydrocet Capsules 782
Lorcet 10/650........ 1018
Lortab 2566
Tussend 1783
Tussend Expectorant 1785
Vicodin Tablets 1356
Vicodin ES Tablets 1357
Vicodin Tuss Expectorant 1358
Zydone Capsules 949

Hydrocodone Polistirex (Combined use may result in a potentiation of the depressant action). Products include:
Tussionex Pennkinetic Extended-Release Suspension 998

Hydroxyzine Hydrochloride (Combined use may result in a potentiation of the depressant action). Products include:
Atarax Tablets & Syrup........ 2185
Marax Tablets & DF Syrup........ 2200
Vistaril Intramuscular Solution........ 2216

Imipramine Hydrochloride (Combined use may result in a potentiation of the depressant action; additive anticholinergic effect). Products include:
Tofranil Ampuls 854
Tofranil Tablets 856

Imipramine Pamoate (Combined use may result in a potentiation of the depressant action; additive anticholinergic effect). Products include:
Tofranil-PM Capsules........ 857

Isoflurane (Combined use may result in a potentiation of the depressant action).
No products indexed under this heading.

Ketamine Hydrochloride (Combined use may result in a potentiation of the depressant action).
No products indexed under this heading.

Labetalol Hydrochloride (A possible interaction may result in excessive vasoconstriction). Products include:
Normodyne Injection 2377
Normodyne Tablets 2379
Trandate 1185

Levobunolol Hydrochloride (A possible interaction may result in excessive vasoconstriction). Products include:
Betagan .... ◉ 233

IMPORTANT NOTE: Always consult each drug listing in the patient's regimen for possible interactions.

Levomethadyl Acetate Hydrochloride (Combined use may result in a potentiation of the depressant action). Products include:

Orlamm ... 2239

Levorphanol Tartrate (Combined use may result in a potentiation of the depressant action). Products include:

Levo-Dromoran ... 2129

Lorazepam (Combined use may result in a potentiation of the depressant action). Products include:

Ativan Injection ... 2698
Ativan Tablets ... 2700

Loxapine Hydrochloride (Combined use may result in a potentiation of the depressant action). Products include:

Loxitane ... 1378

Loxapine Succinate (Combined use may result in a potentiation of the depressant action). Products include:

Loxitane Capsules ... 1378

Maprotiline Hydrochloride (Combined use may result in a potentiation of the depressant action; additive anticholinergic effect). Products include:

Ludiomil Tablets ... 843

Meperidine Hydrochloride (Combined use may result in a potentiation of the depressant action). Products include:

Demerol ... 2308
Mepergan Injection ... 2753

Mephobarbital (Combined use may result in a potentiation of the depressant action). Products include:

Mebaral Tablets ... 2322

Meprobamate (Combined use may result in a potentiation of the depressant action). Products include:

Miltown Tablets ... 2672
PMB 200 and PMB 400 ... 2783

Mesoridazine Besylate (Combined use may result in a potentiation of the depressant action). Products include:

Serentil ... 684

Methadone Hydrochloride (Combined use may result in a potentiation of the depressant action). Products include:

Methadone Hydrochloride Oral Concentrate ... 2233
Methadone Hydrochloride Oral Solution & Tablets ... 2235

Methohexital Sodium (Combined use may result in a potentiation of the depressant action). Products include:

Brevital Sodium Vials ... 1429

Methotrimeprazine (Combined use may result in a potentiation of the depressant action). Products include:

Levoprome ... 1274

Methoxyflurane (Combined use may result in a potentiation of the depressant action).

No products indexed under this heading.

Metipranolol Hydrochloride (A possible interaction may result in excessive vasoconstriction). Products include:

OptiPranolol (Metipranolol 0.3%) Sterile Ophthalmic Solution ... ⊙ 258

Metoprolol Succinate (A possible interaction may result in excessive vasoconstriction). Products include:

Toprol-XL Tablets ... 565

Metoprolol Tartrate (A possible interaction may result in excessive vasoconstriction). Products include:

Lopressor Ampuls ... 830
Lopressor HCT Tablets ... 832
Lopressor Tablets ... 830

Midazolam Hydrochloride (Combined use may result in a potentiation of the depressant action). Products include:

Versed Injection ... 2170

Molindone Hydrochloride (Combined use may result in a potentiation of the depressant action). Products include:

Moban Tablets and Concentrate ... 1048

Morphine Sulfate (Combined use may result in a potentiation of the depressant action). Products include:

Astramorph/PF Injection, USP (Preservative-Free) ... 535
Duramorph ... 962
Infumorph 200 and Infumorph 500 Sterile Solutions ... 965
MS Contin Tablets ... 1994
MSIR ... 1997
Oramorph SR (Morphine Sulfate Sustained Release Tablets) ... 2236
RMS Suppositories ... 2657
Roxanol ... 2243

Nadolol (A possible interaction may result in excessive vasoconstriction).

No products indexed under this heading.

Nortriptyline Hydrochloride (Combined use may result in a potentiation of the depressant action; additive anticholinergic effect). Products include:

Pamelor ... 2280

Opium Alkaloids (Combined use may result in a potentiation of the depressant action).

No products indexed under this heading.

Oxazepam (Combined use may result in a potentiation of the depressant action). Products include:

Serax Capsules ... 2810
Serax Tablets ... 2810

Oxycodone Hydrochloride (Combined use may result in a potentiation of the depressant action). Products include:

Percocet Tablets ... 938
Percodan Tablets ... 939
Percodan-Demi Tablets ... 940
Roxicodone Tablets, Oral Solution & Intensol (Oxycodone) ... 2244
Tylox Capsules ... 1584

Penbutolol Sulfate (A possible interaction may result in excessive vasoconstriction). Products include:

Levatol ... 2403

Pentobarbital Sodium (Combined use may result in a potentiation of the depressant action). Products include:

Nembutal Sodium Capsules ... 436
Nembutal Sodium Solution ... 438
Nembutal Sodium Suppositories ... 440

Perphenazine (Combined use may result in a potentiation of the depressant action). Products include:

Etrafon ... 2355
Triavil Tablets ... 1757
Trilafon ... 2389

Phenytoin (Variable effect on phenytoin metabolism with possible accelerating effect). Products include:

Dilantin Infatabs ... 1908
Dilantin-125 Suspension ... 1911

Phenytoin Sodium (Variable effect on phenytoin metabolism with possible accelerating effect). Products include:

Dilantin Kapseals ... 1906
Dilantin Parenteral ... 1910

Pindolol (A possible interaction may result in excessive vasoconstriction). Products include:

Visken Tablets ... 2299

Polyestradiol Phosphate (Potential for increased metabolism rate).

No products indexed under this heading.

Prazepam (Combined use may result in a potentiation of the depressant action).

No products indexed under this heading.

Prochlorperazine (Combined use may result in a potentiation of the depressant action). Products include:

Compazine ... 2470

Promethazine Hydrochloride (Combined use may result in a potentiation of the depressant action). Products include:

Mepergan Injection ... 2753
Phenergan with Codeine ... 2777
Phenergan with Dextromethorphan 2778
Phenergan Injection ... 2773
Phenergan Suppositories ... 2775
Phenergan Syrup ... 2774
Phenergan Tablets ... 2775
Phenergan VC ... 2779
Phenergan VC with Codeine ... 2781

Propofol (Combined use may result in a potentiation of the depressant action). Products include:

Diprivan Injection ... 2833

Propoxyphene Hydrochloride (Combined use may result in a potentiation of the depressant action). Products include:

Darvon ... 1435
Wygesic Tablets ... 2827

Propoxyphene Napsylate (Combined use may result in a potentiation of the depressant action). Products include:

Darvon-N/Darvocet-N ... 1433

Propranolol Hydrochloride (A possible interaction may result in excessive vasoconstriction). Products include:

Inderal ... 2728
Inderal LA Long Acting Capsules ... 2730
Inderide Tablets ... 2732
Inderide LA Long Acting Capsules .. 2734

Protriptyline Hydrochloride (Combined use may result in a potentiation of the depressant action; additive anticholinergic effect). Products include:

Vivactil Tablets ... 1774

Quazepam (Combined use may result in a potentiation of the depressant action). Products include:

Doral Tablets ... 2664

Quinestrol (Potential for increased metabolism rate).

No products indexed under this heading.

Quinidine Gluconate (Potential for increased metabolism rate). Products include:

Quinaglute Dura-Tabs Tablets ... 649

Quinidine Polygalacturonate (Potential for increased metabolism rate).

No products indexed under this heading.

Quinidine Sulfate (Potential for increased metabolism rate). Products include:

Quinidex Extentabs ... 2067

Risperidone (Combined use may result in a potentiation of the depressant action). Products include:

Risperdal ... 1301

Secobarbital Sodium (Combined use may result in a potentiation of the depressant action). Products include:

Seconal Sodium Pulvules ... 1474

Sotalol Hydrochloride (A possible interaction may result in excessive vasoconstriction). Products include:

Betapace Tablets ... 641

Sufentanil Citrate (Combined use may result in a potentiation of the depressant action). Products include:

Sufenta Injection ... 1309

Temazepam (Combined use may result in a potentiation of the depressant action). Products include:

Restoril Capsules ... 2284

Thiamylal Sodium (Combined use may result in a potentiation of the depressant action).

No products indexed under this heading.

Thioridazine Hydrochloride (Combined use may result in a potentiation of the depressant action). Products include:

Mellaril ... 2269

Thiothixene (Combined use may result in a potentiation of the depressant action). Products include:

Navane Capsules and Concentrate 2201
Navane Intramuscular ... 2202

Timolol Hemihydrate (A possible interaction may result in excessive vasoconstriction). Products include:

Betimol 0.25%, 0.5% ... ⊙ 261

Timolol Maleate (A possible interaction may result in excessive vasoconstriction). Products include:

Blocadren Tablets ... 1614
Timolide Tablets ... 1748
Timoptic in Ocudose ... 1753
Timoptic Sterile Ophthalmic Solution ... 1751
Timoptic-XE ... 1755

Triazolam (Combined use may result in a potentiation of the depressant action). Products include:

Halcion Tablets ... 2611

Trifluoperazine Hydrochloride (Combined use may result in a potentiation of the depressant action). Products include:

Stelazine ... 2514

Trimipramine Maleate (Combined use may result in a potentiation of the depressant action; additive anticholinergic effect). Products include:

Surmontil Capsules ... 2811

Valproic Acid (May increase barbiturate metabolism). Products include:

Depakene ... 413

Warfarin Sodium (Phenobarbital may lower the plasma levels of oral anticoagulant and may cause a decrease in anticoagulant activity). Products include:

Coumadin ... 926

Zolpidem Tartrate (Combined use may result in a potentiation of the depressant action). Products include:

Ambien Tablets ... 2416

Food Interactions

Alcohol (Combined use may result in a potentiation of the depressant action).

BENADRYL ALLERGY DECONGESTANT LIQUID MEDICATION

(Diphenhydramine Hydrochloride, Pseudoephedrine Hydrochloride) ... ▣ 848
May interact with hypnotics and

sedatives, tranquilizers, monoamine oxidase inhibitors, and certain other agents. Compounds in these categories include:

Alprazolam (May increase drowsiness effect; consult your physician). Products include:

Xanax Tablets 2649

Buspirone Hydrochloride (May increase drowsiness effect; consult your physician). Products include:

BuSpar 737

Chlordiazepoxide (May increase drowsiness effect; consult your physician). Products include:

Libritabs Tablets 2177
Limbitrol 2180

Chlordiazepoxide Hydrochloride (May increase drowsiness effect; consult your physician). Products include:

Librax Capsules 2176
Librium Capsules 2178
Librium Injectable 2179

Chlorpromazine (May increase drowsiness effect; consult your physician). Products include:

Thorazine Suppositories 2523

Chlorpromazine Hydrochloride (May increase drowsiness effect; consult your physician). Products include:

Thorazine 2523

Chlorprothixene (May increase drowsiness effect; consult your physician).

No products indexed under this heading.

Chlorprothixene Hydrochloride (May increase drowsiness effect; consult your physician).

No products indexed under this heading.

Clorazepate Dipotassium (May increase drowsiness effect; consult your physician). Products include:

Tranxene 451

Diazepam (May increase drowsiness effect; consult your physician). Products include:

Dizac 1809
Valium Injectable 2182
Valium Tablets 2183
Valrelease Capsules 2169

Droperidol (May increase drowsiness effect; consult your physician). Products include:

Inapsine Injection 1296

Estazolam (May increase drowsiness effect; consult your physician). Products include:

ProSom Tablets 449

Ethchlorvynol (May increase drowsiness effect; consult your physician). Products include:

Placidyl Capsules 448

Ethinamate (May increase drowsiness effect; consult your physician).

No products indexed under this heading.

Fluphenazine Decanoate (May increase drowsiness effect; consult your physician). Products include:

Prolixin Decanoate 509

Fluphenazine Enanthate (May increase drowsiness effect; consult your physician). Products include:

Prolixin Enanthate 509

Fluphenazine Hydrochloride (May increase drowsiness effect; consult your physician). Products include:

Prolixin 509

Flurazepam Hydrochloride (May increase drowsiness effect; consult your physician). Products include:

Dalmane Capsules 2173

Furazolidone (Concurrent and/or sequential use is not recommended). Products include:

Furoxone 2046

Glutethimide (May increase drowsiness effect; consult your physician).

No products indexed under this heading.

Haloperidol (May increase drowsiness effect; consult your physician). Products include:

Haldol Injection, Tablets and Concentrate 1575

Haloperidol Decanoate (May increase drowsiness effect; consult your physician). Products include:

Haldol Decanoate 1577

Hydroxyzine Hydrochloride (May increase drowsiness effect; consult your physician). Products include:

Atarax Tablets & Syrup 2185
Marax Tablets & DF Syrup 2200
Vistaril Intramuscular Solution 2216

Isocarboxazid (Concurrent and/or sequential use is not recommended).

No products indexed under this heading.

Lorazepam (May increase drowsiness effect; consult your physician). Products include:

Ativan Injection 2698
Ativan Tablets 2700

Loxapine Hydrochloride (May increase drowsiness effect; consult your physician). Products include:

Loxitane 1378

Loxapine Succinate (May increase drowsiness effect; consult your physician). Products include:

Loxitane Capsules 1378

Meprobamate (May increase drowsiness effect; consult your physician). Products include:

Miltown Tablets 2672
PMB 200 and PMB 400 2783

Mesoridazine Besylate (May increase drowsiness effect; consult your physician). Products include:

Serentil 684

Midazolam Hydrochloride (May increase drowsiness effect; consult your physician). Products include:

Versed Injection 2170

Molindone Hydrochloride (May increase drowsiness effect; consult your physician). Products include:

Moban Tablets and Concentrate 1048

Oxazepam (May increase drowsiness effect; consult your physician). Products include:

Serax Capsules 2810
Serax Tablets 2810

Perphenazine (May increase drowsiness effect; consult your physician). Products include:

Etrafon 2355
Triavil Tablets 1757
Trilafon 2389

Phenelzine Sulfate (Concurrent and/or sequential use is not recommended). Products include:

Nardil 1920

Prazepam (May increase drowsiness effect; consult your physician).

No products indexed under this heading.

Prochlorperazine (May increase drowsiness effect; consult your physician). Products include:

Compazine 2470

Promethazine Hydrochloride (May increase drowsiness effect; consult your physician). Products include:

Mepergan Injection 2753

Phenergan with Codeine 2777
Phenergan with Dextromethorphan 2778
Phenergan Injection 2773
Phenergan Suppositories 2775
Phenergan Syrup 2774
Phenergan Tablets 2775
Phenergan VC 2779
Phenergan VC with Codeine 2781

Propofol (May increase drowsiness effect; consult your physician). Products include:

Diprivan Injection 2833

Quazepam (May increase drowsiness effect; consult your physician). Products include:

Doral Tablets 2664

Secobarbital Sodium (May increase drowsiness effect; consult your physician). Products include:

Seconal Sodium Pulvules 1474

Selegiline Hydrochloride (Concurrent and/or sequential use is not recommended). Products include:

Eldepryl Tablets 2550

Temazepam (May increase drowsiness effect; consult your physician). Products include:

Restoril Capsules 2284

Thioridazine Hydrochloride (May increase drowsiness effect; consult your physician). Products include:

Mellaril 2269

Thiothixene (May increase drowsiness effect; consult your physician). Products include:

Navane Capsules and Concentrate 2201
Navane Intramuscular 2202

Tranylcypromine Sulfate (Concurrent and/or sequential use is not recommended). Products include:

Parnate Tablets 2503

Triazolam (May increase drowsiness effect; consult your physician). Products include:

Halcion Tablets 2611

Trifluoperazine Hydrochloride (May increase drowsiness effect; consult your physician). Products include:

Stelazine 2514

Zolpidem Tartrate (May increase drowsiness effect; consult your physician). Products include:

Ambien Tablets 2416

Food Interactions

Alcohol (May increase drowsiness effect; avoid concurrent use).

BENADRYL ALLERGY DECONGESTANT TABLETS

(Diphenhydramine Hydrochloride, Pseudoephedrine Hydrochloride) ....⊞ 848

May interact with hypnotics and sedatives, tranquilizers, monoamine oxidase inhibitors, and certain other agents. Compounds in these categories include:

Alprazolam (May increase the drowsiness effect). Products include:

Xanax Tablets 2649

Buspirone Hydrochloride (May increase the drowsiness effect). Products include:

BuSpar 737

Chlordiazepoxide (May increase the drowsiness effect). Products include:

Libritabs Tablets 2177
Limbitrol 2180

Chlordiazepoxide Hydrochloride (May increase the drowsiness effect). Products include:

Librax Capsules 2176
Librium Capsules 2178
Librium Injectable 2179

Chlorpromazine (May increase the drowsiness effect). Products include:

Thorazine Suppositories 2523

Chlorpromazine Hydrochloride (May increase the drowsiness effect). Products include:

Thorazine 2523

Chlorprothixene (May increase the drowsiness effect).

No products indexed under this heading.

Chlorprothixene Hydrochloride (May increase the drowsiness effect).

No products indexed under this heading.

Clorazepate Dipotassium (May increase the drowsiness effect). Products include:

Tranxene 451

Diazepam (May increase the drowsiness effect). Products include:

Dizac 1809
Valium Injectable 2182
Valium Tablets 2183
Valrelease Capsules 2169

Droperidol (May increase the drowsiness effect). Products include:

Inapsine Injection 1296

Estazolam (May increase the drowsiness effect). Products include:

ProSom Tablets 449

Ethchlorvynol (May increase the drowsiness effect). Products include:

Placidyl Capsules 448

Ethinamate (May increase the drowsiness effect).

No products indexed under this heading.

Fluphenazine Decanoate (May increase the drowsiness effect). Products include:

Prolixin Decanoate 509

Fluphenazine Enanthate (May increase the drowsiness effect). Products include:

Prolixin Enanthate 509

Fluphenazine Hydrochloride (May increase the drowsiness effect). Products include:

Prolixin 509

Flurazepam Hydrochloride (May increase the drowsiness effect). Products include:

Dalmane Capsules 2173

Furazolidone (Concurrent and/or sequential use is not recommended). Products include:

Furoxone 2046

Glutethimide (May increase the drowsiness effect).

No products indexed under this heading.

Haloperidol (May increase the drowsiness effect). Products include:

Haldol Injection, Tablets and Concentrate 1575

Haloperidol Decanoate (May increase the drowsiness effect). Products include:

Haldol Decanoate 1577

Hydroxyzine Hydrochloride (May increase the drowsiness effect). Products include:

Atarax Tablets & Syrup 2185
Marax Tablets & DF Syrup 2200
Vistaril Intramuscular Solution 2216

Isocarboxazid (Concurrent and/or sequential use is not recommended).

No products indexed under this heading.

Lorazepam (May increase the drowsiness effect). Products include:

Ativan Injection 2698
Ativan Tablets 2700

IMPORTANT NOTE: Always consult each drug listing in the patient's regimen for possible interactions.

Loxapine Hydrochloride (May increase the drowsiness effect). Products include:
- Loxitane ... 1378

Loxapine Succinate (May increase the drowsiness effect). Products include:
- Loxitane Capsules ... 1378

Meprobamate (May increase the drowsiness effect). Products include:
- Miltown Tablets ... 2672
- PMB 200 and PMB 400 ... 2783

Mesoridazine Besylate (May increase the drowsiness effect). Products include:
- Serentil ... 684

Midazolam Hydrochloride (May increase the drowsiness effect). Products include:
- Versed Injection ... 2170

Molindone Hydrochloride (May increase the drowsiness effect). Products include:
- Moban Tablets and Concentrate ... 1048

Oxazepam (May increase the drowsiness effect). Products include:
- Serax Capsules ... 2810
- Serax Tablets ... 2810

Perphenazine (May increase the drowsiness effect). Products include:
- Etrafon ... 2355
- Triavil Tablets ... 1757
- Trilafon ... 2389

Phenelzine Sulfate (Concurrent and/or sequential use is not recommended). Products include:
- Nardil ... 1920

Prazepam (May increase the drowsiness effect).
- No products indexed under this heading.

Prochlorperazine (May increase the drowsiness effect). Products include:
- Compazine ... 2470

Promethazine Hydrochloride (May increase the drowsiness effect). Products include:
- Mepergan Injection ... 2753
- Phenergan with Codeine ... 2777
- Phenergan with Dextromethorphan 2778
- Phenergan Injection ... 2773
- Phenergan Suppositories ... 2775
- Phenergan Syrup ... 2774
- Phenergan Tablets ... 2775
- Phenergan VC ... 2779
- Phenergan VC with Codeine ... 2781

Propofol (May increase the drowsiness effect). Products include:
- Diprivan Injection ... 2833

Quazepam (May increase the drowsiness effect). Products include:
- Doral Tablets ... 2664

Secobarbital Sodium (May increase the drowsiness effect). Products include:
- Seconal Sodium Pulvules ... 1474

Selegiline Hydrochloride (Concurrent and/or sequential use is not recommended). Products include:
- Eldepryl Tablets ... 2550

Temazepam (May increase the drowsiness effect). Products include:
- Restoril Capsules ... 2284

Thioridazine Hydrochloride (May increase the drowsiness effect). Products include:
- Mellaril ... 2269

Thiothixene (May increase the drowsiness effect). Products include:
- Navane Capsules and Concentrate 2201
- Navane Intramuscular ... 2202

Tranylcypromine Sulfate (Concurrent and/or sequential use is not recommended). Products include:
- Parnate Tablets ... 2503

Triazolam (May increase the drowsiness effect). Products include:
- Halcion Tablets ... 2611

Trifluoperazine Hydrochloride (May increase the drowsiness effect). Products include:
- Stelazine ... 2514

Zolpidem Tartrate (Increases the drowsiness effect). Products include:
- Ambien Tablets ... 2416

Food Interactions

Alcohol (Increases the drowsiness effect; avoid concomitant use).

BENADRYL ALLERGY LIQUID MEDICATION

(Diphenhydramine Hydrochloride) .. ▣ 849

May interact with hypnotics and sedatives, tranquilizers, and certain other agents. Compounds in these categories include:

Alprazolam (May increase drowsiness effect; consult your physician). Products include:
- Xanax Tablets ... 2649

Buspirone Hydrochloride (May increase drowsiness effect; consult your physician). Products include:
- BuSpar ... 737

Chlordiazepoxide (May increase drowsiness effect; consult your physician). Products include:
- Libritabs Tablets ... 2177
- Limbitrol ... 2180

Chlordiazepoxide Hydrochloride (May increase drowsiness effect; consult your physician). Products include:
- Librax Capsules ... 2176
- Librium Capsules ... 2178
- Librium Injectable ... 2179

Chlorpromazine (May increase drowsiness effect; consult your physician). Products include:
- Thorazine Suppositories ... 2523

Chlorpromazine Hydrochloride (May increase drowsiness effect; consult your physician). Products include:
- Thorazine ... 2523

Chlorprothixene (May increase drowsiness effect; consult your physician).
- No products indexed under this heading.

Chlorprothixene Hydrochloride (May increase drowsiness effect; consult your physician).
- No products indexed under this heading.

Clorazepate Dipotassium (May increase drowsiness effect; consult your physician). Products include:
- Tranxene ... 451

Diazepam (May increase drowsiness effect; consult your physician). Products include:
- Dizac ... 1809
- Valium Injectable ... 2182
- Valium Tablets ... 2183
- Valrelease Capsules ... 2169

Droperidol (May increase drowsiness effect; consult your physician). Products include:
- Inapsine Injection ... 1296

Estazolam (May increase drowsiness effect; consult your physician). Products include:
- ProSom Tablets ... 449

Ethchlorvynol (May increase drowsiness effect; consult your physician). Products include:
- Placidyl Capsules ... 448

Ethinamate (May increase drowsiness effect; consult your physician).
- No products indexed under this heading.

Fluphenazine Decanoate (May increase drowsiness effect; consult your physician). Products include:
- Prolixin Decanoate ... 509

Fluphenazine Enanthate (May increase drowsiness effect; consult your physician). Products include:
- Prolixin Enanthate ... 509

Fluphenazine Hydrochloride (May increase drowsiness effect; consult your physician). Products include:
- Prolixin ... 509

Flurazepam Hydrochloride (May increase drowsiness effect; consult your physician). Products include:
- Dalmane Capsules ... 2173

Glutethimide (May increase drowsiness effect; consult your physician).
- No products indexed under this heading.

Haloperidol (May increase drowsiness effect; consult your physician). Products include:
- Haldol Injection, Tablets and Concentrate ... 1575

Haloperidol Decanoate (May increase drowsiness effect; consult your physician). Products include:
- Haldol Decanoate ... 1577

Hydroxyzine Hydrochloride (May increase drowsiness effect; consult your physician). Products include:
- Atarax Tablets & Syrup ... 2185
- Marax Tablets & DF Syrup ... 2200
- Vistaril Intramuscular Solution ... 2216

Lorazepam (May increase drowsiness effect; consult your physician). Products include:
- Ativan Injection ... 2698
- Ativan Tablets ... 2700

Loxapine Hydrochloride (May increase drowsiness effect; consult your physician). Products include:
- Loxitane ... 1378

Loxapine Succinate (May increase drowsiness effect; consult your physician). Products include:
- Loxitane Capsules ... 1378

Meprobamate (May increase drowsiness effect; consult your physician). Products include:
- Miltown Tablets ... 2672
- PMB 200 and PMB 400 ... 2783

Mesoridazine Besylate (May increase drowsiness effect; consult your physician). Products include:
- Serentil ... 684

Midazolam Hydrochloride (May increase drowsiness effect; consult your physician). Products include:
- Versed Injection ... 2170

Molindone Hydrochloride (May increase drowsiness effect; consult your physician). Products include:
- Moban Tablets and Concentrate ... 1048

Oxazepam (May increase drowsiness effect; consult your physician). Products include:
- Serax Capsules ... 2810
- Serax Tablets ... 2810

Perphenazine (May increase drowsiness effect; consult your physician). Products include:
- Etrafon ... 2355
- Triavil Tablets ... 1757
- Trilafon ... 2389

Prazepam (May increase drowsiness effect; consult your physician).
- No products indexed under this heading.

Prochlorperazine (May increase drowsiness effect; consult your physician). Products include:
- Compazine ... 2470

Promethazine Hydrochloride (May increase drowsiness effect; consult your physician). Products include:
- Mepergan Injection ... 2753
- Phenergan with Codeine ... 2777
- Phenergan with Dextromethorphan 2778
- Phenergan Injection ... 2773
- Phenergan Suppositories ... 2775
- Phenergan Syrup ... 2774
- Phenergan Tablets ... 2775
- Phenergan VC ... 2779
- Phenergan VC with Codeine ... 2781

Propofol (May increase drowsiness effect; consult your physician). Products include:
- Diprivan Injection ... 2833

Quazepam (May increase drowsiness effect; consult your physician). Products include:
- Doral Tablets ... 2664

Secobarbital Sodium (May increase drowsiness effect; consult your physician). Products include:
- Seconal Sodium Pulvules ... 1474

Temazepam (May increase drowsiness effect; consult your physician). Products include:
- Restoril Capsules ... 2284

Thioridazine Hydrochloride (May increase drowsiness effect; consult your physician). Products include:
- Mellaril ... 2269

Thiothixene (May increase drowsiness effect; consult your physician). Products include:
- Navane Capsules and Concentrate 2201
- Navane Intramuscular ... 2202

Triazolam (May increase drowsiness effect; consult your physician). Products include:
- Halcion Tablets ... 2611

Trifluoperazine Hydrochloride (May increase drowsiness effect; consult your physician). Products include:
- Stelazine ... 2514

Zolpidem Tartrate (May increase drowsiness effect; consult your physician). Products include:
- Ambien Tablets ... 2416

Food Interactions

Alcohol (Increases drowsiness effect).

BENADRYL ALLERGY KAPSEALS

(Diphenhydramine Hydrochloride) .. ▣ 848

May interact with hypnotics and sedatives, tranquilizers, and certain other agents. Compounds in these categories include:

Alprazolam (May increase drowsiness effect). Products include:
- Xanax Tablets ... 2649

Buspirone Hydrochloride (May increase drowsiness effect). Products include:
- BuSpar ... 737

Chlordiazepoxide (May increase drowsiness effect). Products include:
- Libritabs Tablets ... 2177
- Limbitrol ... 2180

Chlordiazepoxide Hydrochloride (May increase drowsiness effect). Products include:
- Librax Capsules ... 2176
- Librium Capsules ... 2178
- Librium Injectable ... 2179

Chlorpromazine (May increase drowsiness effect). Products include:
- Thorazine Suppositories ... 2523

Chlorpromazine Hydrochloride (May increase drowsiness effect). Products include:
- Thorazine ... 2523

Chlorprothixene (May increase drowsiness effect).
No products indexed under this heading.

Chlorprothixene Hydrochloride (May increase drowsiness effect).
No products indexed under this heading.

Clorazepate Dipotassium (May increase drowsiness effect). Products include:
Tranxene ... 451

Diazepam (May increase drowsiness effect). Products include:
Dizac ... 1809
Valium Injectable ... 2182
Valium Tablets ... 2183
Valrelease Capsules ... 2169

Droperidol (May increase drowsiness effect). Products include:
Inapsine Injection ... 1296

Estazolam (May increase drowsiness effect). Products include:
ProSom Tablets ... 449

Ethchlorvynol (May increase drowsiness effect). Products include:
Placidyl Capsules ... 448

Ethinamate (May increase drowsiness effect).
No products indexed under this heading.

Fluphenazine Decanoate (May increase drowsiness effect). Products include:
Prolixin Decanoate ... 509

Fluphenazine Enanthate (May increase drowsiness effect). Products include:
Prolixin Enanthate ... 509

Fluphenazine Hydrochloride (May increase drowsiness effect). Products include:
Prolixin ... 509

Flurazepam Hydrochloride (May increase drowsiness effect). Products include:
Dalmane Capsules ... 2173

Glutethimide (May increase drowsiness effect).
No products indexed under this heading.

Haloperidol (May increase drowsiness effect). Products include:
Haldol Injection, Tablets and Concentrate ... 1575

Haloperidol Decanoate (May increase drowsiness effect). Products include:
Haldol Decanoate ... 1577

Hydroxyzine Hydrochloride (May increase drowsiness effect). Products include:
Atarax Tablets & Syrup ... 2185
Marax Tablets & DF Syrup ... 2200
Vistaril Intramuscular Solution ... 2216

Lorazepam (May increase drowsiness effect). Products include:
Ativan Injection ... 2698
Ativan Tablets ... 2700

Loxapine Hydrochloride (May increase drowsiness effect). Products include:
Loxitane ... 1378

Loxapine Succinate (May increase drowsiness effect). Products include:
Loxitane Capsules ... 1378

Meprobamate (May increase drowsiness effect). Products include:
Miltown Tablets ... 2672
PMB 200 and PMB 400 ... 2783

Mesoridazine Besylate (May increase drowsiness effect). Products include:
Serentil ... 684

Midazolam Hydrochloride (May increase drowsiness effect). Products include:
Versed Injection ... 2170

Molindone Hydrochloride (May increase drowsiness effect). Products include:
Moban Tablets and Concentrate ... 1048

Oxazepam (May increase drowsiness effect). Products include:
Serax Capsules ... 2810
Serax Tablets ... 2810

Perphenazine (May increase drowsiness effect). Products include:
Etrafon ... 2355
Triavil Tablets ... 1757
Trilafon ... 2389

Prazepam (May increase drowsiness effect).
No products indexed under this heading.

Prochlorperazine (May increase drowsiness effect). Products include:
Compazine ... 2470

Promethazine Hydrochloride (May increase drowsiness effect). Products include:
Mepergan Injection ... 2753
Phenergan with Codeine ... 2777
Phenergan with Dextromethorphan 2778
Phenergan Injection ... 2773
Phenergan Suppositories ... 2775
Phenergan Syrup ... 2774
Phenergan Tablets ... 2775
Phenergan VC ... 2779
Phenergan VC with Codeine ... 2781

Propofol (May increase drowsiness effect). Products include:
Diprivan Injection ... 2833

Quazepam (May increase drowsiness effect). Products include:
Doral Tablets ... 2664

Secobarbital Sodium (May increase drowsiness effect). Products include:
Seconal Sodium Pulvules ... 1474

Temazepam (May increase drowsiness effect). Products include:
Restoril Capsules ... 2284

Thioridazine Hydrochloride (May increase drowsiness effect). Products include:
Mellaril ... 2269

Thiothixene (May increase drowsiness effect). Products include:
Navane Capsules and Concentrate 2201
Navane Intramuscular ... 2202

Triazolam (May increase drowsiness effect). Products include:
Halcion Tablets ... 2611

Trifluoperazine Hydrochloride (May increase drowsiness effect). Products include:
Stelazine ... 2514

Zolpidem Tartrate (May increase drowsiness effect). Products include:
Ambien Tablets ... 2416

Food Interactions

Alcohol (May increase drowsiness effect).

BENADRYL ALLERGY TABLETS
(Diphenhydramine Hydrochloride) .. ▣ 848
See **Benadryl Allergy Kapseals**

BENADRYL ALLERGY SINUS HEADACHE FORMULA CAPLETS
(Diphenhydramine Hydrochloride, Pseudoephedrine Hydrochloride, Acetaminophen) ... ▣ 849
May interact with hypnotics and sedatives, tranquilizers, monoamine oxidase inhibitors, and certain other agents. Compounds in these categories include:

Alprazolam (May increase drowsiness effect). Products include:
Xanax Tablets ... 2649

Buspirone Hydrochloride (May increase drowsiness effect). Products include:
BuSpar ... 737

Chlordiazepoxide (May increase drowsiness effect). Products include:
Libritabs Tablets ... 2177
Limbitrol ... 2180

Chlordiazepoxide Hydrochloride (May increase drowsiness effect). Products include:
Librax Capsules ... 2176
Librium Capsules ... 2178
Librium Injectable ... 2179

Chlorpromazine (May increase drowsiness effect). Products include:
Thorazine Suppositories ... 2523

Chlorpromazine Hydrochloride (May increase drowsiness effect). Products include:
Thorazine ... 2523

Chlorprothixene (May increase drowsiness effect).
No products indexed under this heading.

Chlorprothixene Hydrochloride (May increase drowsiness effect).
No products indexed under this heading.

Clorazepate Dipotassium (May increase drowsiness effect). Products include:
Tranxene ... 451

Diazepam (May increase drowsiness effect). Products include:
Dizac ... 1809
Valium Injectable ... 2182
Valium Tablets ... 2183
Valrelease Capsules ... 2169

Droperidol (May increase drowsiness effect). Products include:
Inapsine Injection ... 1296

Estazolam (May increase drowsiness effect). Products include:
ProSom Tablets ... 449

Ethchlorvynol (May increase drowsiness effect). Products include:
Placidyl Capsules ... 448

Ethinamate (May increase drowsiness effect).
No products indexed under this heading.

Fluphenazine Decanoate (May increase drowsiness effect). Products include:
Prolixin Decanoate ... 509

Fluphenazine Enanthate (May increase drowsiness effect). Products include:
Prolixin Enanthate ... 509

Fluphenazine Hydrochloride (May increase drowsiness effect). Products include:
Prolixin ... 509

Flurazepam Hydrochloride (May increase drowsiness effect). Products include:
Dalmane Capsules ... 2173

Furazolidone (Concurrent and/or sequential use is not recommended). Products include:
Furoxone ... 2046

Glutethimide (May increase drowsiness effect).
No products indexed under this heading.

Haloperidol (May increase drowsiness effect). Products include:
Haldol Injection, Tablets and Concentrate ... 1575

Haloperidol Decanoate (May increase drowsiness effect). Products include:
Haldol Decanoate ... 1577

Hydroxyzine Hydrochloride (May increase drowsiness effect). Products include:
Atarax Tablets & Syrup ... 2185
Marax Tablets & DF Syrup ... 2200
Vistaril Intramuscular Solution ... 2216

Isocarboxazid (Concurrent and/or sequential use is not recommended).
No products indexed under this heading.

Lorazepam (May increase drowsiness effect). Products include:
Ativan Injection ... 2698
Ativan Tablets ... 2700

Loxapine Hydrochloride (May increase drowsiness effect). Products include:
Loxitane ... 1378

Loxapine Succinate (May increase drowsiness effect). Products include:
Loxitane Capsules ... 1378

Meprobamate (May increase drowsiness effect). Products include:
Miltown Tablets ... 2672
PMB 200 and PMB 400 ... 2783

Mesoridazine Besylate (May increase drowsiness effect). Products include:
Serentil ... 684

Midazolam Hydrochloride (May increase drowsiness effect). Products include:
Versed Injection ... 2170

Molindone Hydrochloride (May increase drowsiness effect). Products include:
Moban Tablets and Concentrate ... 1048

Oxazepam (May increase drowsiness effect). Products include:
Serax Capsules ... 2810
Serax Tablets ... 2810

Perphenazine (May increase drowsiness effect). Products include:
Etrafon ... 2355
Triavil Tablets ... 1757
Trilafon ... 2389

Phenelzine Sulfate (Concurrent and/or sequential use is not recommended). Products include:
Nardil ... 1920

Prazepam (May increase drowsiness effect).
No products indexed under this heading.

Prochlorperazine (May increase drowsiness effect). Products include:
Compazine ... 2470

Promethazine Hydrochloride (May increase drowsiness effect). Products include:
Mepergan Injection ... 2753
Phenergan with Codeine ... 2777
Phenergan with Dextromethorphan 2778
Phenergan Injection ... 2773
Phenergan Suppositories ... 2775
Phenergan Syrup ... 2774
Phenergan Tablets ... 2775
Phenergan VC ... 2779
Phenergan VC with Codeine ... 2781

Propofol (May increase drowsiness effect). Products include:
Diprivan Injection ... 2833

Quazepam (May increase drowsiness effect). Products include:
Doral Tablets ... 2664

Secobarbital Sodium (May increase drowsiness effect). Products include:
Seconal Sodium Pulvules ... 1474

Selegiline Hydrochloride (Concurrent and/or sequential use is not recommended). Products include:
Eldepryl Tablets ... 2550

IMPORTANT NOTE: Always consult each drug listing in the patient's regimen for possible interactions.

Temazepam (May increase drowsiness effect). Products include:
Restoril Capsules ... 2284

Thioridazine Hydrochloride (May increase drowsiness effect). Products include:
Mellaril ... 2269

Thiothixene (May increase drowsiness effect). Products include:
Navane Capsules and Concentrate 2201
Navane Intramuscular ... 2202

Tranylcypromine Sulfate (Concurrent and/or sequential use is not recommended). Products include:
Parnate Tablets ... 2503

Triazolam (May increase drowsiness effect). Products include:
Halcion Tablets ... 2611

Trifluoperazine Hydrochloride (May increase drowsiness effect). Products include:
Stelazine ... 2514

Zolpidem Tartrate (May increase drowsiness effect). Products include:
Ambien Tablets ... 2416

Food Interactions

Alcohol (May increase drowsiness effect).

BENADRYL CAPSULES

(Diphenhydramine Hydrochloride) ... 1898

May interact with central nervous system depressants, monoamine oxidase inhibitors, and certain other agents. Compounds in these categories include:

Alfentanil Hydrochloride (Additive effects). Products include:
Alfenta Injection ... 1286

Alprazolam (Additive effects). Products include:
Xanax Tablets ... 2649

Aprobarbital (Additive effects).
No products indexed under this heading.

Buprenorphine (Additive effects). Products include:
Buprenex Injectable ... 2006

Buspirone Hydrochloride (Additive effects). Products include:
BuSpar ... 737

Butabarbital (Additive effects).
No products indexed under this heading.

Butalbital (Additive effects). Products include:
Esgic-plus Tablets ... 1013
Fioricet Tablets ... 2258
Fioricet with Codeine Capsules ... 2260
Fiorinal Capsules ... 2261
Fiorinal with Codeine Capsules ... 2262
Fiorinal Tablets ... 2261
Phrenilin ... 785
Sedapap Tablets 50 mg/650 mg .. 1543

Chlordiazepoxide (Additive effects). Products include:
Libritabs Tablets ... 2177
Limbitrol ... 2180

Chlordiazepoxide Hydrochloride (Additive effects). Products include:
Librax Capsules ... 2176
Librium Capsules ... 2178
Librium Injectable ... 2179

Chlorpromazine (Additive effects). Products include:
Thorazine Suppositories ... 2523

Chlorprothixene (Additive effects).
No products indexed under this heading.

Chlorprothixene Hydrochloride (Additive effects).
No products indexed under this heading.

Chlorprothixene Lactate (Additive effects).
No products indexed under this heading.

Clorazepate Dipotassium (Additive effects). Products include:
Tranxene ... 451

Clozapine (Additive effects). Products include:
Clozaril Tablets ... 2252

Codeine Phosphate (Additive effects). Products include:
Actifed with Codeine Cough Syrup.. 1067
Brontex ... 1981
Deconsal C Expectorant Syrup ... 456
Deconsal Pediatric Syrup ... 457
Dimetane-DC Cough Syrup ... 2059
Empirin with Codeine Tablets ... 1093
Fioricet with Codeine Capsules ... 2260
Fiorinal with Codeine Capsules ... 2262
Isoclor Expectorant ... 990
Novahistine DH ... 2462
Novahistine Expectorant ... 2463
Nucofed ... 2051
Phenergan with Codeine ... 2777
Phenergan VC with Codeine ... 2781
Robitussin A-C Syrup ... 2073
Robitussin-DAC Syrup ... 2074
Ryna ... ▣ 841
Soma Compound w/Codeine Tablets ... 2676
Tussi-Organidin NR Liquid and S NR Liquid ... 2677
Tylenol with Codeine ... 1583

Desflurane (Additive effects). Products include:
Suprane ... 1813

Dezocine (Additive effects). Products include:
Dalgan Injection ... 538

Diazepam (Additive effects). Products include:
Dizac ... 1809
Valium Injectable ... 2182
Valium Tablets ... 2183
Valrelease Capsules ... 2169

Droperidol (Additive effects). Products include:
Inapsine Injection ... 1296

Enflurane (Additive effects).
No products indexed under this heading.

Estazolam (Additive effects). Products include:
ProSom Tablets ... 449

Ethchlorvynol (Additive effects). Products include:
Placidyl Capsules ... 448

Ethinamate (Additive effects).
No products indexed under this heading.

Fentanyl (Additive effects). Products include:
Duragesic Transdermal System ... 1288

Fentanyl Citrate (Additive effects). Products include:
Sublimaze Injection ... 1307

Fluphenazine Decanoate (Additive effects). Products include:
Prolixin Decanoate ... 509

Fluphenazine Enanthate (Additive effects). Products include:
Prolixin Enanthate ... 509

Fluphenazine Hydrochloride (Additive effects). Products include:
Prolixin ... 509

Flurazepam Hydrochloride (Additive effects). Products include:
Dalmane Capsules ... 2173

Furazolidone (Anticholinergic effects of antihistamines prolonged and intensified). Products include:
Furoxone ... 2046

Glutethimide (Additive effects).
No products indexed under this heading.

Haloperidol (Additive effects). Products include:
Haldol Injection, Tablets and Concentrate ... 1575

Haloperidol Decanoate (Additive effects). Products include:
Haldol Decanoate ... 1577

Hydrocodone Bitartrate (Additive effects). Products include:
Anexsia 5/500 Elixir ... 1781
Anexia Tablets ... 1782
Codiclear DH Syrup ... 791
Deconamine CX Cough and Cold Liquid and Tablets ... 1319
Duratuss HD Elixir ... 2565
Hycodan Tablets and Syrup ... 930
Hycomine Compound Tablets ... 932
Hycomine ... 931
Hycotuss Expectorant Syrup ... 933
Hydrocet Capsules ... 782
Lorcet 10/650 ... 1018
Lortab ... 2566
Tussend ... 1783
Tussend Expectorant ... 1785
Vicodin Tablets ... 1356
Vicodin ES Tablets ... 1357
Vicodin Tuss Expectorant ... 1358
Zydone Capsules ... 949

Hydrocodone Polistirex (Additive effects). Products include:
Tussionex Pennkinetic Extended-Release Suspension ... 998

Hydroxyzine Hydrochloride (Additive effects). Products include:
Atarax Tablets & Syrup ... 2185
Marax Tablets & DF Syrup ... 2200
Vistaril Intramuscular Solution ... 2216

Isocarboxazid (Anticholinergic effects of antihistamines prolonged and intensified).
No products indexed under this heading.

Isoflurane (Additive effects).
No products indexed under this heading.

Ketamine Hydrochloride (Additive effects).
No products indexed under this heading.

Levomethadyl Acetate Hydrochloride (Additive effects). Products include:
Orlamm ... 2239

Levorphanol Tartrate (Additive effects). Products include:
Levo-Dromoran ... 2129

Lorazepam (Additive effects). Products include:
Ativan Injection ... 2698
Ativan Tablets ... 2700

Loxapine Hydrochloride (Additive effects). Products include:
Loxitane ... 1378

Loxapine Succinate (Additive effects). Products include:
Loxitane Capsules ... 1378

Meperidine Hydrochloride (Additive effects). Products include:
Demerol ... 2308
Mepergan Injection ... 2753

Mephobarbital (Additive effects). Products include:
Mebaral Tablets ... 2322

Meprobamate (Additive effects). Products include:
Miltown Tablets ... 2672
PMB 200 and PMB 400 ... 2783

Mesoridazine Besylate (Additive effects). Products include:
Serentil ... 684

Methadone Hydrochloride (Additive effects). Products include:
Methadone Hydrochloride Oral Concentrate ... 2233
Methadone Hydrochloride Oral Solution & Tablets ... 2235

Methohexital Sodium (Additive effects). Products include:
Brevital Sodium Vials ... 1429

Methotrimeprazine (Additive effects). Products include:
Levoprome ... 1274

Methoxyflurane (Additive effects).
No products indexed under this heading.

Midazolam Hydrochloride (Additive effects). Products include:
Versed Injection ... 2170

Molindone Hydrochloride (Additive effects). Products include:
Moban Tablets and Concentrate ... 1048

Morphine Sulfate (Additive effects). Products include:
Astramorph/PF Injection, USP (Preservative-Free) ... 535
Duramorph ... 962
Infumorph 200 and Infumorph 500 Sterile Solutions ... 965
MS Contin Tablets ... 1994
MSIR ... 1997
Oramorph SR (Morphine Sulfate Sustained Release Tablets) ... 2236
RMS Suppositories ... 2657
Roxanol ... 2243

Opium Alkaloids (Additive effects).
No products indexed under this heading.

Oxazepam (Additive effects). Products include:
Serax Capsules ... 2810
Serax Tablets ... 2810

Oxycodone Hydrochloride (Additive effects). Products include:
Percocet Tablets ... 938
Percodan Tablets ... 939
Percodan-Demi Tablets ... 940
Roxicodone Tablets, Oral Solution & Intensol (Oxycodone) ... 2244
Tylox Capsules ... 1584

Pentobarbital Sodium (Additive effects). Products include:
Nembutal Sodium Capsules ... 436
Nembutal Sodium Solution ... 438
Nembutal Sodium Suppositories ... 440

Perphenazine (Additive effects). Products include:
Etrafon ... 2355
Triavil Tablets ... 1757
Trilafon ... 2389

Phenelzine Sulfate (Anticholinergic effects of antihistamines prolonged and intensified). Products include:
Nardil ... 1920

Phenobarbital (Additive effects). Products include:
Arco-Lase Plus Tablets ... 512
Bellergal-S Tablets ... 2250
Donnatal ... 2060
Donnatal Extentabs ... 2061
Donnatal Tablets ... 2060
Phenobarbital Elixir and Tablets ... 1469
Quadrinal Tablets ... 1350

Prazepam (Additive effects).
No products indexed under this heading.

Prochlorperazine (Additive effects). Products include:
Compazine ... 2470

Promethazine Hydrochloride (Additive effects). Products include:
Mepergan Injection ... 2753
Phenergan with Codeine ... 2777
Phenergan with Dextromethorphan 2778
Phenergan Injection ... 2773
Phenergan Suppositories ... 2775
Phenergan Syrup ... 2774
Phenergan Tablets ... 2775
Phenergan VC ... 2779
Phenergan VC with Codeine ... 2781

Propofol (Additive effects). Products include:
Diprivan Injection ... 2833

Propoxyphene Hydrochloride (Additive effects). Products include:
Darvon ... 1435
Wygesic Tablets ... 2827

Propoxyphene Napsylate (Additive effects). Products include:
Darvon-N/Darvocet-N ... 1433

Quazepam (Additive effects). Products include:
Doral Tablets ... 2664
Risperidone (Additive effects). Products include:
Risperdal ... 1301
Secobarbital Sodium (Additive effects). Products include:
Seconal Sodium Pulvules ... 1474
Selegiline Hydrochloride (Anticholinergic effects of antihistamines prolonged and intensified). Products include:
Eldepryl Tablets ... 2550
Sufentanil Citrate (Additive effects). Products include:
Sufenta Injection ... 1309
Temazepam (Additive effects). Products include:
Restoril Capsules ... 2284
Thiamylal Sodium (Additive effects).
No products indexed under this heading.
Thioridazine Hydrochloride (Additive effects). Products include:
Mellaril ... 2269
Thiothixene (Additive effects). Products include:
Navane Capsules and Concentrate 2201
Navane Intramuscular ... 2202
Tranylcypromine Sulfate (Anticholinergic effects of antihistamines prolonged and intensified). Products include:
Parnate Tablets ... 2503
Triazolam (Additive effects). Products include:
Halcion Tablets ... 2611
Trifluoperazine Hydrochloride (Additive effects). Products include:
Stelazine ... 2514
Zolpidem Tartrate (Additive effects). Products include:
Ambien Tablets ... 2416

Food Interactions

Alcohol (Additive effects).

BENADRYL DYE-FREE ALLERGY LIQUI-GEL SOFTGELS

(Diphenhydramine Hydrochloride) .. 850
May interact with hypnotics and sedatives, tranquilizers, and certain other agents. Compounds in these categories include:

Alprazolam (May increase the drowsiness effect). Products include:
Xanax Tablets ... 2649
Buspirone Hydrochloride (May increase the drowsiness effect). Products include:
BuSpar ... 737
Chlordiazepoxide (May increase the drowsiness effect). Products include:
Libritabs Tablets ... 2177
Limbitrol ... 2180
Chlordiazepoxide Hydrochloride (May increase the drowsiness effect). Products include:
Librax Capsules ... 2176
Librium Capsules ... 2178
Librium Injectable ... 2179
Chlorpromazine (May increase the drowsiness effect). Products include:
Thorazine Suppositories ... 2523
Chlorpromazine Hydrochloride (May increase the drowsiness effect). Products include:
Thorazine ... 2523
Chlorprothixene (May increase the drowsiness effect).
No products indexed under this heading.
Chlorprothixene Hydrochloride (May increase the drowsiness effect).
No products indexed under this heading.
Clorazepate Dipotassium (May increase the drowsiness effect). Products include:
Tranxene ... 451
Diazepam (May increase the drowsiness effect). Products include:
Dizac ... 1809
Valium Injectable ... 2182
Valium Tablets ... 2183
Valrelease Capsules ... 2169
Droperidol (May increase the drowsiness effect). Products include:
Inapsine Injection ... 1296
Estazolam (May increase the drowsiness effect). Products include:
ProSom Tablets ... 449
Ethchlorvynol (May increase the drowsiness effect). Products include:
Placidyl Capsules ... 448
Ethinamate (May increase the drowsiness effect).
No products indexed under this heading.
Fluphenazine Decanoate (May increase the drowsiness effect). Products include:
Prolixin Decanoate ... 509
Fluphenazine Enanthate (May increase the drowsiness effect). Products include:
Prolixin Enanthate ... 509
Fluphenazine Hydrochloride (May increase the drowsiness effect). Products include:
Prolixin ... 509
Flurazepam Hydrochloride (May increase the drowsiness effect). Products include:
Dalmane Capsules ... 2173
Glutethimide (May increase the drowsiness effect).
No products indexed under this heading.
Haloperidol (May increase the drowsiness effect). Products include:
Haldol Injection, Tablets and Concentrate ... 1575
Haloperidol Decanoate (May increase the drowsiness effect). Products include:
Haldol Decanoate ... 1577
Hydroxyzine Hydrochloride (May increase the drowsiness effect). Products include:
Atarax Tablets & Syrup ... 2185
Marax Tablets & DF Syrup ... 2200
Vistaril Intramuscular Solution ... 2216
Lorazepam (May increase the drowsiness effect). Products include:
Ativan Injection ... 2698
Ativan Tablets ... 2700
Loxapine Hydrochloride (May increase the drowsiness effect). Products include:
Loxitane ... 1378
Loxapine Succinate (May increase the drowsiness effect). Products include:
Loxitane Capsules ... 1378
Meprobamate (May increase the drowsiness effect). Products include:
Miltown Tablets ... 2672
PMB 200 and PMB 400 ... 2783
Mesoridazine Besylate (May increase the drowsiness effect). Products include:
Serentil ... 684
Midazolam Hydrochloride (May increase the drowsiness effect). Products include:
Versed Injection ... 2170
Molindone Hydrochloride (May increase the drowsiness effect). Products include:
Moban Tablets and Concentrate ... 1048
Oxazepam (May increase the drowsiness effect). Products include:
Serax Capsules ... 2810
Serax Tablets ... 2810
Perphenazine (May increase the drowsiness effect). Products include:
Etrafon ... 2355
Triavil Tablets ... 1757
Trilafon ... 2389
Prazepam (May increase the drowsiness effect).
No products indexed under this heading.
Prochlorperazine (May increase the drowsiness effect). Products include:
Compazine ... 2470
Promethazine Hydrochloride (May increase the drowsiness effect). Products include:
Mepergan Injection ... 2753
Phenergan with Codeine ... 2777
Phenergan with Dextromethorphan 2778
Phenergan Injection ... 2773
Phenergan Suppositories ... 2775
Phenergan Syrup ... 2774
Phenergan Tablets ... 2775
Phenergan VC ... 2779
Phenergan VC with Codeine ... 2781
Propofol (May increase the drowsiness effect). Products include:
Diprivan Injection ... 2833
Quazepam (May increase the drowsiness effect). Products include:
Doral Tablets ... 2664
Secobarbital Sodium (May increase the drowsiness effect). Products include:
Seconal Sodium Pulvules ... 1474
Temazepam (May increase the drowsiness effect). Products include:
Restoril Capsules ... 2284
Thioridazine Hydrochloride (May increase the drowsiness effect). Products include:
Mellaril ... 2269
Thiothixene (May increase the drowsiness effect). Products include:
Navane Capsules and Concentrate 2201
Navane Intramuscular ... 2202
Triazolam (May increase the drowsiness effect). Products include:
Halcion Tablets ... 2611
Trifluoperazine Hydrochloride (May increase the drowsiness effect). Products include:
Stelazine ... 2514
Zolpidem Tartrate (May increase the drowsiness effect). Products include:
Ambien Tablets ... 2416

Food Interactions

Alcohol (May increase the drowsiness effect).

BENADRYL DYE-FREE ALLERGY LIQUID MEDICATION

(Diphenhydramine Hydrochloride) .. 850
May interact with hypnotics and sedatives, tranquilizers, and certain other agents. Compounds in these categories include:

Alprazolam (May increase the drowsiness effect). Products include:
Xanax Tablets ... 2649
Buspirone Hydrochloride (May increase the drowsiness effect). Products include:
BuSpar ... 737
Chlordiazepoxide (May increase the drowsiness effect). Products include:
Libritabs Tablets ... 2177
Limbitrol ... 2180
Chlordiazepoxide Hydrochloride (May increase the drowsiness effect). Products include:
Librax Capsules ... 2176
Librium Capsules ... 2178
Librium Injectable ... 2179
Chlorpromazine (May increase the drowsiness effect). Products include:
Thorazine Suppositories ... 2523
Chlorpromazine Hydrochloride (May increase the drowsiness effect). Products include:
Thorazine ... 2523
Chlorprothixene (May increase the drowsiness effect).
No products indexed under this heading.
Chlorprothixene Hydrochloride (May increase the drowsiness effect).
No products indexed under this heading.
Clorazepate Dipotassium (May increase the drowsiness effect). Products include:
Tranxene ... 451
Diazepam (May increase the drowsiness effect). Products include:
Dizac ... 1809
Valium Injectable ... 2182
Valium Tablets ... 2183
Valrelease Capsules ... 2169
Droperidol (May increase the drowsiness effect). Products include:
Inapsine Injection ... 1296
Estazolam (May increase the drowsiness effect). Products include:
ProSom Tablets ... 449
Ethchlorvynol (May increase the drowsiness effect). Products include:
Placidyl Capsules ... 448
Ethinamate (May increase the drowsiness effect).
No products indexed under this heading.
Fluphenazine Decanoate (May increase the drowsiness effect). Products include:
Prolixin Decanoate ... 509
Fluphenazine Enanthate (May increase the drowsiness effect). Products include:
Prolixin Enanthate ... 509
Fluphenazine Hydrochloride (May increase the drowsiness effect). Products include:
Prolixin ... 509
Flurazepam Hydrochloride (May increase the drowsiness effect). Products include:
Dalmane Capsules ... 2173
Glutethimide (May increase the drowsiness effect).
No products indexed under this heading.
Haloperidol (May increase the drowsiness effect). Products include:
Haldol Injection, Tablets and Concentrate ... 1575
Haloperidol Decanoate (May increase the drowsiness effect). Products include:
Haldol Decanoate ... 1577
Hydroxyzine Hydrochloride (May increase the drowsiness effect). Products include:
Atarax Tablets & Syrup ... 2185
Marax Tablets & DF Syrup ... 2200
Vistaril Intramuscular Solution ... 2216
Lorazepam (May increase the drowsiness effect). Products include:
Ativan Injection ... 2698

IMPORTANT NOTE: Always consult each drug listing in the patient's regimen for possible interactions.

Ativan Tablets 2700

Loxapine Hydrochloride (May increase the drowsiness effect). Products include:

Loxitane 1378

Loxapine Succinate (May increase the drowsiness effect). Products include:

Loxitane Capsules 1378

Meprobamate (May increase the drowsiness effect). Products include:

Miltown Tablets 2672
PMB 200 and PMB 400 2783

Mesoridazine Besylate (May increase the drowsiness effect). Products include:

Serentil 684

Midazolam Hydrochloride (May increase the drowsiness effect). Products include:

Versed Injection 2170

Molindone Hydrochloride (May increase the drowsiness effect). Products include:

Moban Tablets and Concentrate 1048

Oxazepam (May increase the drowsiness effect). Products include:

Serax Capsules 2810
Serax Tablets 2810

Perphenazine (May increase the drowsiness effect). Products include:

Etrafon 2355
Triavil Tablets 1757
Trilafon 2389

Prazepam (May increase the drowsiness effect).

No products indexed under this heading.

Prochlorperazine (May increase the drowsiness effect). Products include:

Compazine 2470

Promethazine Hydrochloride (May increase the drowsiness effect). Products include:

Mepergan Injection 2753
Phenergan with Codeine 2777
Phenergan with Dextromethorphan 2778
Phenergan Injection 2773
Phenergan Suppositories 2775
Phenergan Syrup 2774
Phenergan Tablets 2775
Phenergan VC 2779
Phenergan VC with Codeine 2781

Propofol (May increase the drowsiness effect). Products include:

Diprivan Injection 2833

Quazepam (May increase the drowsiness effect). Products include:

Doral Tablets 2664

Secobarbital Sodium (May increase the drowsiness effect). Products include:

Seconal Sodium Pulvules 1474

Temazepam (May increase the drowsiness effect). Products include:

Restoril Capsules 2284

Thioridazine Hydrochloride (May increase the drowsiness effect). Products include:

Mellaril 2269

Thiothixene (May increase the drowsiness effect). Products include:

Navane Capsules and Concentrate 2201
Navane Intramuscular 2202

Triazolam (May increase the drowsiness effect). Products include:

Halcion Tablets 2611

Trifluoperazine Hydrochloride (May increase the drowsiness effect). Products include:

Stelazine 2514

Zolpidem Tartrate (May increase the drowsiness effect). Products include:

Ambien Tablets 2416

Food Interactions

Alcohol (May increase the drowsiness effect).

BENADRYL ITCH RELIEF CREAM, CHILDREN'S FORMULA AND MAXIMUM STRENGTH 2%

(Diphenhydramine Hydrochloride, Zinc Acetate) .... ▣ 851
May interact with:

Diphenhydramine (Concurrent use is not recommended).

No products indexed under this heading.

BENADRYL ITCH RELIEF SPRAY, CHILDREN'S FORMULA AND MAXIMUM STRENGTH 2%

(Diphenhydramine Hydrochloride, Zinc Acetate) .... ▣ 851
None cited in PDR database.

BENADRYL ITCH RELIEF STICK MAXIMUM STRENGTH 2%

(Diphenhydramine Hydrochloride, Zinc Acetate) .... ▣ 850
None cited in PDR database.

BENADRYL ITCH STOPPING GEL, CHILDREN'S FORMULA AND MAXIMUM STRENGTH 2%

(Diphenhydramine Hydrochloride, Zinc Acetate) .... ▣ 851
None cited in PDR database.

BENADRYL KAPSEALS

(Diphenhydramine Hydrochloride) 1898
See **Benadryl Capsules**

BENADRYL PARENTERAL

(Diphenhydramine Hydrochloride) 1898
May interact with central nervous system depressants, monoamine oxidase inhibitors, and certain other agents. Compounds in these categories include:

Alfentanil Hydrochloride (Additive effects). Products include:

Alfenta Injection 1286

Alprazolam (Additive effects). Products include:

Xanax Tablets 2649

Aprobarbital (Additive effects).

No products indexed under this heading.

Buprenorphine (Additive effects). Products include:

Buprenex Injectable 2006

Buspirone Hydrochloride (Additive effects). Products include:

BuSpar 737

Butabarbital (Additive effects).

No products indexed under this heading.

Butalbital (Additive effects). Products include:

Esgic-plus Tablets 1013
Fioricet Tablets 2258
Fioricet with Codeine Capsules 2260
Fiorinal Capsules 2261
Fiorinal with Codeine Capsules 2262
Fiorinal Tablets 2261
Phrenilin 785
Sedapap Tablets 50 mg/650 mg .. 1543

Chlordiazepoxide (Additive effects). Products include:

Libritabs Tablets 2177
Limbitrol 2180

Chlordiazepoxide Hydrochloride (Additive effects). Products include:

Librax Capsules 2176
Librium Capsules 2178
Librium Injectable 2179

Chlorpromazine (Additive effects). Products include:

Thorazine Suppositories 2523

Chlorprothixene (Additive effects).

No products indexed under this heading.

Chlorprothixene Hydrochloride (Additive effects).

No products indexed under this heading.

Clorazepate Dipotassium (Additive effects). Products include:

Tranxene 451

Clozapine (Additive effects). Products include:

Clozaril Tablets 2252

Codeine Phosphate (Additive effects). Products include:

Actifed with Codeine Cough Syrup.. 1067
Brontex 1981
Deconsal C Expectorant Syrup 456
Deconsal Pediatric Syrup 457
Dimetane-DC Cough Syrup 2059
Empirin with Codeine Tablets........ 1093
Fioricet with Codeine Capsules 2260
Fiorinal with Codeine Capsules 2262
Isoclor Expectorant 990
Novahistine DH 2462
Novahistine Expectorant 2463
Nucofed 2051
Phenergan with Codeine 2777
Phenergan VC with Codeine 2781
Robitussin A-C Syrup 2073
Robitussin-DAC Syrup 2074
Ryna .... ▣ 841
Soma Compound w/Codeine Tablets 2676
Tussi-Organidin NR Liquid and S NR Liquid 2677
Tylenol with Codeine 1583

Desflurane (Additive effects). Products include:

Suprane 1813

Dezocine (Additive effects). Products include:

Dalgan Injection 538

Diazepam (Additive effects). Products include:

Dizac 1809
Valium Injectable 2182
Valium Tablets 2183
Valrelease Capsules 2169

Droperidol (Additive effects). Products include:

Inapsine Injection 1296

Enflurane (Additive effects).

No products indexed under this heading.

Estazolam (Additive effects). Products include:

ProSom Tablets 449

Ethchlorvynol (Additive effects). Products include:

Placidyl Capsules 448

Ethinamate (Additive effects).

No products indexed under this heading.

Fentanyl (Additive effects). Products include:

Duragesic Transdermal System........ 1288

Fentanyl Citrate (Additive effects). Products include:

Sublimaze Injection 1307

Fluphenazine Decanoate (Additive effects). Products include:

Prolixin Decanoate 509

Fluphenazine Enanthate (Additive effects). Products include:

Prolixin Enanthate 509

Fluphenazine Hydrochloride (Additive effects). Products include:

Prolixin 509

Flurazepam Hydrochloride (Additive effects). Products include:

Dalmane Capsules 2173

Furazolidone (Anticholinergic effects of antihistamines prolonged and intensified). Products include:

Furoxone 2046

Glutethimide (Additive effects).

No products indexed under this heading.

Haloperidol (Additive effects). Products include:

Haldol Injection, Tablets and Concentrate 1575

Haloperidol Decanoate (Additive effects). Products include:

Haldol Decanoate 1577

Hydrocodone Bitartrate (Additive effects). Products include:

Anexsia 5/500 Elixir 1781
Anexia Tablets 1782
Codiclear DH Syrup 791
Deconamine CX Cough and Cold Liquid and Tablets 1319
Duratuss HD Elixir 2565
Hycodan Tablets and Syrup 930
Hycomine Compound Tablets 932
Hycomine 931
Hycotuss Expectorant Syrup 933
Hydrocet Capsules 782
Lorcet 10/650 1018
Lortab 2566
Tussend 1783
Tussend Expectorant 1785
Vicodin Tablets 1356
Vicodin ES Tablets 1357
Vicodin Tuss Expectorant 1358
Zydone Capsules 949

Hydrocodone Polistirex (Additive effects). Products include:

Tussionex Pennkinetic Extended-Release Suspension 998

Hydroxyzine Hydrochloride (Additive effects). Products include:

Atarax Tablets & Syrup 2185
Marax Tablets & DF Syrup 2200
Vistaril Intramuscular Solution 2216

Isocarboxazid (Anticholinergic effects of antihistamines prolonged and intensified).

No products indexed under this heading.

Isoflurane (Additive effects).

No products indexed under this heading.

Ketamine Hydrochloride (Additive effects).

No products indexed under this heading.

Levomethadyl Acetate Hydrochloride (Additive effects). Products include:

Orlamm 2239

Levorphanol Tartrate (Additive effects). Products include:

Levo-Dromoran 2129

Lorazepam (Additive effects). Products include:

Ativan Injection 2698
Ativan Tablets 2700

Loxapine Hydrochloride (Additive effects). Products include:

Loxitane 1378

Loxapine Succinate (Additive effects). Products include:

Loxitane Capsules 1378

Meperidine Hydrochloride (Additive effects). Products include:

Demerol 2308
Mepergan Injection 2753

Mephobarbital (Additive effects). Products include:

Mebaral Tablets 2322

Meprobamate (Additive effects). Products include:

Miltown Tablets 2672
PMB 200 and PMB 400 2783

Mesoridazine Besylate (Additive effects). Products include:

Serentil 684

(▣ Described in PDR For Nonprescription Drugs) (◉ Described in PDR For Ophthalmology)

109 Interactions Index Benemid

Methadone Hydrochloride (Additive effects). Products include:
Methadone Hydrochloride Oral Concentrate 2233
Methadone Hydrochloride Oral Solution & Tablets 2235

Methohexital Sodium (Additive effects). Products include:
Brevital Sodium Vials 1429

Methotrimeprazine (Additive effects). Products include:
Levoprome 1274

Methoxyflurane (Additive effects).
No products indexed under this heading.

Midazolam Hydrochloride (Additive effects). Products include:
Versed Injection 2170

Molindone Hydrochloride (Additive effects). Products include:
Moban Tablets and Concentrate 1048

Morphine Sulfate (Additive effects). Products include:
Astramorph/PF Injection, USP (Preservative-Free) 535
Duramorph 962
Infumorph 200 and Infumorph 500 Sterile Solutions 965
MS Contin Tablets 1994
MSIR 1997
Oramorph SR (Morphine Sulfate Sustained Release Tablets) 2236
RMS Suppositories 2657
Roxanol 2243

Opium Alkaloids (Additive effects).
No products indexed under this heading.

Oxazepam (Additive effects). Products include:
Serax Capsules 2810
Serax Tablets 2810

Oxycodone Hydrochloride (Additive effects). Products include:
Percocet Tablets 938
Percodan Tablets 939
Percodan-Demi Tablets 940
Roxicodone Tablets, Oral Solution & Intensol (Oxycodone) 2244
Tylox Capsules 1584

Pentobarbital Sodium (Additive effects). Products include:
Nembutal Sodium Capsules 436
Nembutal Sodium Solution 438
Nembutal Sodium Suppositories 440

Perphenazine (Additive effects). Products include:
Etrafon 2355
Triavil Tablets 1757
Trilafon 2389

Phenelzine Sulfate (Anticholinergic effects of antihistamines prolonged and intensified). Products include:
Nardil 1920

Phenobarbital (Additive effects). Products include:
Arco-Lase Plus Tablets 512
Bellergal-S Tablets 2250
Donnatal 2060
Donnatal Extentabs 2061
Donnatal Tablets 2060
Phenobarbital Elixir and Tablets 1469
Quadrinal Tablets 1350

Prazepam (Additive effects).
No products indexed under this heading.

Prochlorperazine (Additive effects). Products include:
Compazine 2470

Promethazine Hydrochloride (Additive effects). Products include:
Mepergan Injection 2753
Phenergan with Codeine 2777
Phenergan with Dextromethorphan 2778
Phenergan Injection 2773
Phenergan Suppositories 2775
Phenergan Syrup 2774
Phenergan Tablets 2775
Phenergan VC 2779
Phenergan VC with Codeine 2781

Propofol (Additive effects). Products include:
Diprivan Injection 2833

Propoxyphene Hydrochloride (Additive effects). Products include:
Darvon 1435
Wygesic Tablets 2827

Propoxyphene Napsylate (Additive effects). Products include:
Darvon-N/Darvocet-N 1433

Quazepam (Additive effects). Products include:
Doral Tablets 2664

Risperidone (Additive effects). Products include:
Risperdal 1301

Secobarbital Sodium (Additive effects). Products include:
Seconal Sodium Pulvules 1474

Selegiline Hydrochloride (Anticholinergic effects of antihistamines prolonged and intensified). Products include:
Eldepryl Tablets 2550

Sufentanil Citrate (Additive effects). Products include:
Sufenta Injection 1309

Temazepam (Additive effects). Products include:
Restoril Capsules 2284

Thiamylal Sodium (Additive effects).
No products indexed under this heading.

Thioridazine Hydrochloride (Additive effects). Products include:
Mellaril 2269

Thiothixene (Additive effects). Products include:
Navane Capsules and Concentrate 2201
Navane Intramuscular 2202

Tranylcypromine Sulfate (Anticholinergic effects of antihistamines prolonged and intensified). Products include:
Parnate Tablets 2503

Triazolam (Additive effects). Products include:
Halcion Tablets 2611

Trifluoperazine Hydrochloride (Additive effects). Products include:
Stelazine 2514

Zolpidem Tartrate (Additive effects). Products include:
Ambien Tablets 2416

Food Interactions

Alcohol (Additive effects).

BENADRYL STERI-VIALS, AMPOULES, AND STERI-DOSE SYRINGE
(Diphenhydramine Hydrochloride) 1898
See **Benadryl Parenteral**

BENEMID TABLETS
(Probenecid) 1611
May interact with sulfonylureas, salicylates, penicillins, sulfonamides, and certain other agents. Compounds in these categories include:

Acetaminophen (Increased peak plasma concentrations of acetaminophen). Products include:
Actifed Plus Caplets 845
Actifed Plus Tablets 845
Actifed Sinus Daytime/Nighttime Tablets and Caplets 846
Alka-Seltzer Plus Cold Medicine Liqui-Gels 706
Alka-Seltzer Plus Cold & Cough Medicine Liqui-Gels 705
Alka-Seltzer Plus Night-Time Cold Medicine Liqui-Gels 706
Allerest Headache Strength Tablets 627
Allerest No Drowsiness Tablets 627
Allerest Sinus Pain Formula 627
Anexsia 5/500 Elixir 1781
Anexia Tablets 1782
Arthritis Foundation Aspirin Free Caplets 673
Arthritis Foundation NightTime Caplets 674
Bayer Select Headache Pain Relief Formula 716
Bayer Select Menstrual Multi-Symptom Formula 716
Bayer Select Night Time Pain Relief Formula 716
Bayer Select Sinus Pain Relief Formula 717
Benadryl Allergy Sinus Headache Formula Caplets 849
Comtrex Multi-Symptom Cold Reliever Tablets/Caplets/Liqui-Gels/Liquid 615
Allergy-Sinus Comtrex Multi-Symptom Allergy-Sinus Formula Tablets 617
Comtrex Non-Drowsy 618
Contac Day Allergy/Sinus Caplets 812
Contac Day & Night 812
Contac Night Allergy/Sinus Caplets 812
Contac Severe Cold and Flu Formula Caplets 814
Contac Severe Cold & Flu Non-Drowsy 815
Coricidin 'D' Decongestant Tablets 800
Coricidin Tablets 800
DHCplus Capsules 1993
Darvon-N/Darvocet-N 1433
Drixoral Cold and Flu Extended-Release Tablets 803
Drixoral Cough + Sore Throat Liquid Caps 802
Drixoral Allergy/Sinus Extended Release Tablets 804
Esgic-plus Tablets 1013
Aspirin Free Excedrin Analgesic Caplets and Geltabs 732
Excedrin Extra-Strength Analgesic Tablets & Caplets 732
Excedrin P.M. Analgesic/Sleeping Aid Tablets, Caplets, Liquigels 733
Fioricet Tablets 2258
Fioricet with Codeine Capsules 2260
Hycomine Compound Tablets 932
Hydrocet Capsules 782
Legatrin PM 651
Lorcet 10/650 1018
Lortab 2566
Lurline PMS Tablets 982
Maximum Strength Multi-Symptom Formula Midol 722
PMS Multi-Symptom Formula Midol 723
Teen Multi-Symptom Formula Midol 722
Midrin Capsules 783
Migralam Capsules 2038
Panodol Tablets and Caplets 824
Children's Panadol Chewable Tablets, Liquid, Infant's Drops 824
Percocet Tablets 938
Percogesic Analgesic Tablets 754
Phrenilin 785
Pyrroxate Caplets 772
Sedapap Tablets 50 mg/650 mg 1543
Sinarest Tablets 648
Sinarest Extra Strength Tablets 648
Sinarest No Drowsiness Tablets 648
Sine-Aid Maximum Strength Sinus Medication Gelcaps, Caplets and Tablets 1554
Sine-Off No Drowsiness Formula Caplets 824
Sine-Off Sinus Medicine 825
Singlet Tablets 825
Sinulin Tablets 787
Sinutab Sinus Allergy Medication, Maximum Strength Tablets and Caplets 860
Sinutab Sinus Medication, Maximum Strength Without Drowsiness Formula, Tablets & Caplets 860
Sinutab Sinus Medication, Regular Strength Without Drowsiness Formula 859
Sudafed Cold and Cough Liquidcaps 862
Sudafed Severe Cold Formula Caplets 863
Sudafed Severe Cold Formula Tablets 864
Sudafed Sinus Caplets 864
Sudafed Sinus Tablets 864
Talacen 2333
TheraFlu 787
TheraFlu Maximum Strength Nighttime Flu, Cold & Cough Medicine 788
TheraFlu Maximum Strength Non-Drowsy Formula Flu, Cold & Cough Medicine 788
Thera Flu Maximum Strength, Non-Drowsy Formula Flu, Cold and Cough Caplets 789
Triaminic Sore Throat Formula 791
Triaminicin Tablets 793
Children's TYLENOL acetaminophen Chewable Tablets, Elixir, Suspension Liquid 1555
Children's TYLENOL Cold Multi-Symptom Liquid Formula and Chewable Tablets 1561
Children's TYLENOL Cold Plus Cough Multi Symptom Tablets and Liquid 681
Infants' TYLENOL acetaminophen Drops and Suspension Drops 1555
Infants' TYLENOL Cold Decongestant & Fever-Reducer Drops 1556
TYLENOL Extended Relief Caplets 1558
TYLENOL, Extra Strength, Acetaminophen Adult Liquid Pain Reliever 1560
TYLENOL, Extra Strength, acetaminophen Gelcaps, Geltabs, Caplets, Tablets 1559
TYLENOL, Extra Strength, Headache Plus Pain Reliever with Antacid Caplets 1559
TYLENOL, Junior Strength, acetaminophen Coated Caplets, Grape and Fruit Chewable Tablets 1557
TYLENOL Maximum Strength Allergy Sinus Medication Gelcaps and Caplets 1563
TYLENOL Maximum Strength Allergy Sinus NightTime Medication Caplets 1555
TYLENOL Flu Maximum Strength Gelcaps 1565
TYLENOL Flu NightTime, Maximum Strength, Gelcaps 1566
TYLENOL Maximum Strength Flu NightTime Hot Medication Packets 1562
TYLENOL, Maximum Strength, Sinus Medication Geltabs, Gelcaps, Caplets and Tablets 1566
TYLENOL Cold Multi-Symptom Formula Medication Tablets and Caplets 1561
TYLENOL Cold Medication No Drowsiness Formula Gelcaps and Caplets 1562
TYLENOL Cold Multi-Symptom Hot Medication Liquid Packets 1557
TYLENOL Cough Multi-Symptom Medication 1564
TYLENOL Cough Multi-Symptom Medication with Decongestant 1565
TYLENOL, Regular Strength, acetaminophen Caplets and Tablets 1558
TYLENOL PM, Extra Strength Pain Reliever/Sleep Aid Caplets, Geltabs, Gelcaps 1560
TYLENOL Severe Allergy Medication Caplets 1564
Tylenol with Codeine 1583
Tylox Capsules 1584
Unisom With Pain Relief-Nighttime Sleep Aid and Pain Reliever 1934
Vanquish Analgesic Caplets 731
Vicks 44 LiquiCaps Cough, Cold & Flu Relief 755
Vicks 44M Cough, Cold & Flu Relief 756
Vicks DayQuil 761
Vicks Nyquil Hot Therapy 762
Vicks NyQuil LiquiCaps Multi-Symptom Cold/Flu Relief 763
Vicks NyQuil Multi-Symptom Cold/Flu Relief - (Original & Cherry Flavor) 763
Vicodin Tablets 1356
Vicodin ES Tablets 1357
Wygesic Tablets 2827
Zydone Capsules 949

Aminophylline (Falsely high theophylline readings in an in vitro study).
No products indexed under this heading.

IMPORTANT NOTE: Always consult each drug listing in the patient's regimen for possible interactions.

Benemid Interactions Index 110

Amoxicillin Trihydrate (May result in high plasma levels of amoxicillin). Products include:
- Amoxil 2464
- Augmentin 2468

Ampicillin (May result in high plasma levels of ampicillin). Products include:
- Omnipen Capsules 2764
- Omnipen for Oral Suspension 2765

Ampicillin Sodium (May result in high plasma levels of ampicillin). Products include:
- Unasyn 2212

Aspirin (Uricosuric action of probenecid antagonized). Products include:
- Alka-Seltzer Effervescent Antacid and Pain Reliever .... ▣ 701
- Alka-Seltzer Extra Strength Effervescent Antacid and Pain Reliever .... ▣ 703
- Alka-Seltzer Lemon Lime Effervescent Antacid and Pain Reliever .... ▣ 703
- Alka-Seltzer Plus Cold Medicine .... ▣ 705
- Alka-Seltzer Plus Cold & Cough Medicine .... ▣ 708
- Alka-Seltzer Plus Night-Time Cold Medicine .... ▣ 707
- Alka Seltzer Plus Sinus Medicine .... ▣ 707
- Arthritis Foundation Safety Coated Aspirin Tablets .... ▣ 675
- Arthritis Pain Ascriptin .... ▣ 631
- Maximum Strength Ascriptin .... ▣ 630
- Regular Strength Ascriptin Tablets .... ▣ 629
- Arthritis Strength BC Powder .... ▣ 609
- BC Cold Powder Multi-Symptom Formula (Cold-Sinus-Allergy) .... ▣ 609
- BC Cold Powder Non-Drowsy Formula (Cold-Sinus) .... ▣ 609
- BC Powder .... ▣ 609
- Bayer Children's Chewable Aspirin .... ▣ 711
- Genuine Bayer Aspirin Tablets & Caplets .... ▣ 713
- Extra Strength Bayer Arthritis Pain Regimen Formula .... ▣ 711
- Extra Strength Bayer Aspirin Caplets & Tablets .... ▣ 712
- Extended-Release Bayer 8-Hour Aspirin .... ▣ 712
- Extra Strength Bayer Plus Aspirin Caplets .... ▣ 713
- Extra Strength Bayer PM Aspirin .... ▣ 713
- Bayer Enteric Aspirin .... ▣ 709
- Bufferin Analgesic Tablets and Caplets .... ▣ 613
- Arthritis Strength Bufferin Analgesic Caplets .... ▣ 614
- Extra Strength Bufferin Analgesic Tablets .... ▣ 615
- Cama Arthritis Pain Reliever .... ▣ 785
- Darvon Compound-65 Pulvules 1435
- Easprin 1914
- Ecotrin 2455
- Ecotrin Enteric Coated Aspirin Maximum Strength Tablets and Caplets .... ▣ 816
- Ecotrin Enteric Coated Aspirin Regular Strength Tablets 2455
- Empirin Aspirin Tablets .... ▣ 854
- Empirin with Codeine Tablets 1093
- Excedrin Extra-Strength Analgesic Tablets & Caplets 732
- Fiorinal Capsules 2261
- Fiorinal with Codeine Capsules 2262
- Fiorinal Tablets 2261
- Halfprin 1362
- Healthprin Aspirin 2455
- Norgesic 1496
- Percodan Tablets 939
- Percodan-Demi Tablets 940
- Robaxisal Tablets 2071
- Soma Compound w/Codeine Tablets 2676
- Soma Compound Tablets 2675
- St. Joseph Adult Chewable Aspirin (81 mg.) .... ▣ 808
- Talwin Compound 2335
- Ursinus Inlay-Tabs .... ▣ 794
- Vanquish Analgesic Caplets .... ▣ 731

Azlocillin Sodium (May result in high plasma levels of azlocillin).
- No products indexed under this heading.

Bacampicillin Hydrochloride (May result in high plasma levels of bacampicillin). Products include:
- Spectrobid Tablets 2206

Bendroflumethiazide (Significant increase in total sulfonamide plasma levels).
- No products indexed under this heading.

Carbenicillin Disodium (May result in high plasma levels of carbenicillin).
- No products indexed under this heading.

Carbenicillin Indanyl Sodium (May result in high plasma levels of carbenicillin). Products include:
- Geocillin Tablets 2199

Chlorothiazide (Significant increase in total sulfonamide plasma levels). Products include:
- Aldoclor Tablets 1598
- Diupres Tablets 1650
- Diuril Oral 1653

Chlorothiazide Sodium (Significant increase in total sulfonamide plasma levels). Products include:
- Diuril Sodium Intravenous 1652

Chlorpropamide (Significant increase in total sulfonamide plasma levels; increased risk of hypoglycemia). Products include:
- Diabinese Tablets 1935

Choline Magnesium Trisalicylate (Uricosuric action of probenecid antagonized). Products include:
- Trilisate 2000

Dicloxacillin Sodium (May result in high plasma levels of amoxicillin).
- No products indexed under this heading.

Diflunisal (Uricosuric action of probenecid antagonized). Products include:
- Dolobid Tablets 1654

Dyphylline (Falsely high theophylline readings in an in vitro study). Products include:
- Lufyllin & Lufyllin-400 Tablets 2670
- Lufyllin-GG Elixir & Tablets 2671

Glipizide (Significant increase in total sulfonamide plasma levels; increased risk of hypoglycemia). Products include:
- Glucotrol Tablets 1967
- Glucotrol XL Extended Release Tablets 1968

Glyburide (Significant increase in total sulfonamide plasma levels; increased risk of hypoglycemia). Products include:
- DiaBeta Tablets 1239
- Glynase PresTab Tablets 2609
- Micronase Tablets 2623

Hydrochlorothiazide (Significant increase in total sulfonamide plasma levels). Products include:
- Aldactazide 2413
- Aldoril Tablets 1604
- Apresazide Capsules 808
- Capozide 742
- Dyazide 2479
- Esidrix Tablets 821
- Esimil Tablets 822
- HydroDIURIL Tablets 1674
- Hydropres Tablets 1675
- Hyzaar Tablets 1677
- Inderide Tablets 2732
- Inderide LA Long Acting Capsules 2734
- Lopressor HCT Tablets 832
- Lotensin HCT 837
- Maxzide 1380
- Moduretic Tablets 1705
- Oretic Tablets 443
- Prinzide Tablets 1737
- Ser-Ap-Es Tablets 849
- Timolide Tablets 1748
- Vaseretic Tablets 1765
- Zestoretic 2850
- Ziac 1415

Hydroflumethiazide (Significant increase in total sulfonamide plasma levels). Products include:
- Diucardin Tablets 2718

Indomethacin (Increased plasma levels of indomethacin). Products include:
- Indocin 1680

Indomethacin Sodium Trihydrate (Increased plasma levels of indomethacin). Products include:
- Indocin I.V. 1684

Ketamine Hydrochloride (Anesthesia prolonged).
- No products indexed under this heading.

Ketoprofen (Increased peak plasma levels of ketoprofen). Products include:
- Orudis Capsules 2766
- Oruvail Capsules 2766

Lorazepam (Increased peak plasma levels of lorazepam). Products include:
- Ativan Injection 2698
- Ativan Tablets 2700

Magnesium Salicylate (Uricosuric action of probenecid antagonized). Products include:
- Backache Caplets .... ▣ 613
- Bayer Select Backache Pain Relief Formula .... ▣ 715
- Doan's Extra-Strength Analgesic .... ▣ 633
- Extra Strength Doan's P.M. .... ▣ 633
- Doan's Regular Strength Analgesic .... ▣ 634
- Mobigesic Tablets .... ▣ 602

Meclofenamate Sodium (Increased peak plasma concentrations of meclofenamate).
- No products indexed under this heading.

Methotrexate Sodium (Methotrexate toxicity). Products include:
- Methotrexate Sodium Tablets, Injection, for Injection and LPF Injection 1275

Methyclothiazide (Significant increase in total sulfonamide plasma levels). Products include:
- Enduron Tablets 420

Mezlocillin Sodium (May result in high plasma levels of mezlocillin). Products include:
- Mezlin 601
- Mezlin Pharmacy Bulk Package 604

Nafcillin Sodium (May result in high plasma levels of nafcillin).
- No products indexed under this heading.

Naproxen (Increased peak plasma concentrations of naproxen). Products include:
- Anaprox/Naprosyn 2117

Naproxen Sodium (Increased peak plasma concentrations of naproxen). Products include:
- Aleve 1975
- Anaprox/Naprosyn 2117

Penicillin G Benzathine (May result in high plasma levels of penicillin). Products include:
- Bicillin C-R Injection 2704
- Bicillin C-R 900/300 Injection 2706
- Bicillin L-A Injection 2707

Penicillin G Potassium (May result in high plasma levels of penicillin). Products include:
- Pfizerpen for Injection 2203

Penicillin G Procaine (May result in high plasma levels of penicillin). Products include:
- Bicillin C-R Injection 2704
- Bicillin C-R 900/300 Injection 2706

Penicillin V Potassium (May result in high plasma levels of penicillin). Products include:
- Pen•Vee K 2772

Polythiazide (Significant increase in total sulfonamide plasma levels). Products include:
- Minizide Capsules 1938

Pyrazinamide (Uricosuric action of probenecid antagonized). Products include:
- Pyrazinamide Tablets 1398
- Rifater 1532

Rifampin (Increased peak plasma concentrations of rifampin). Products include:
- Rifadin 1528
- Rifamate Capsules 1530
- Rifater 1532
- Rimactane Capsules 847

Salsalate (Uricosuric action of probenecid antagonized). Products include:
- Mono-Gesic Tablets 792
- Salflex Tablets 786

Sulfamethizole (Significant increase in total sulfonamide plasma levels). Products include:
- Urobiotic-250 Capsules 2214

Sulfamethoxazole (Significant increase in total sulfonamide plasma levels). Products include:
- Azo Gantanol Tablets 2080
- Bactrim DS Tablets 2084
- Bactrim I.V. Infusion 2082
- Bactrim 2084
- Gantanol Tablets 2119
- Septra 1174
- Septra I.V. Infusion 1169
- Septra I.V. Infusion ADD-Vantage Vials 1171
- Septra 1174

Sulfasalazine (Significant increase in total sulfonamide plasma levels). Products include:
- Azulfidine 1949

Sulfinpyrazone (Significant increase in total sulfonamide plasma levels). Products include:
- Anturane 807

Sulfisoxazole (Significant increase in total sulfonamide plasma levels). Products include:
- Azo Gantrisin Tablets 2081
- Gantrisin Tablets 2120

Sulfisoxazole Diolamine (Significant increase in total sulfonamide plasma levels).
- No products indexed under this heading.

Sulindac (Modest reduction in uricosuric action of probenecid). Products include:
- Clinoril Tablets 1618

Theophylline (Falsely high theophylline readings in an in vitro study). Products include:
- Marax Tablets & DF Syrup 2200
- Quibron 2053

Theophylline Anhydrous (Falsely high theophylline readings in an in vitro study). Products include:
- Aerolate 1004
- Primatene Dual Action Formula .... ▣ 872
- Primatene Tablets .... ▣ 873
- Respbid Tablets 682
- Slo-bid Gyrocaps 2033
- Theo-24 Extended Release Capsules 2568
- Theo-Dur Extended-Release Tablets 1327
- Theo-X Extended-Release Tablets 788
- Uni-Dur Extended-Release Tablets 1331
- Uniphyl 400 mg Tablets 2001

Theophylline Calcium Salicylate (Falsely high theophylline readings in an in vitro study). Products include:
- Quadrinal Tablets 1350

Theophylline Sodium Glycinate (Falsely high theophylline readings in an in vitro study).
- No products indexed under this heading.

(▣ Described in PDR For Nonprescription Drugs) (⊙ Described in PDR For Ophthalmology)

Ticarcillin Disodium (May result in high plasma levels of ticarcillin). Products include:
- Ticar for Injection 2526
- Timentin for Injection 2528

Tolazamide (Significant increase in total sulfonamide plasma levels; increased risk of hypoglycemia).
- No products indexed under this heading.

Tolbutamide (Significant increase in total sulfonamide plasma levels; increased risk of hypoglycemia).
- No products indexed under this heading.

BENGAY EXTERNAL ANALGESIC PRODUCTS
(Menthol, Methyl Salicylate) .... ◘ 741
None cited in PDR database.

BENOQUIN CREAM 20%
(Monobenzone) 2868
None cited in PDR database.

BENTYL 10 MG CAPSULES
(Dicyclomine Hydrochloride) 1501
May interact with antacids, agents used to treat achlorhydria and/or to test gastric secretion, nitrates and nitrites, monoamine oxidase inhibitors, phenothiazines, antihistamines, narcotic analgesics, tricyclic antidepressants, benzodiazepines, corticosteroids, sympathomimetics, type 1 antiarrhythmic drugs, antiglaucoma agents, anticholinergics, and certain other agents. Compounds in these categories include:

Acetazolamide (Effects of antiglaucoma agents antagonized). Products include:
- Diamox Sequels (Sustained Release) 1373
- Diamox Sequels (Sustained Release) .... ◉ 319
- Diamox Tablets 1372
- Diamox Tablets .... ◉ 317

Acetylcholine Chloride (Effects of antiglaucoma agents antagonized). Products include:
- Miochol-E with Iocare Steri-Tags and Miochol-E System Pak .... ◉ 273

Acrivastine (Increases certain actions or side effects). Products include:
- Semprex-D Capsules 463
- Semprex-D Capsules 1167

Albuterol (Increases certain actions or side effects). Products include:
- Proventil Inhalation Aerosol 2382
- Ventolin Inhalation Aerosol and Refill 1197

Albuterol Sulfate (Increases certain actions or side effects). Products include:
- Airet Solution for Inhalation 452
- Proventil Inhalation Solution 0.083% 2384
- Proventil Repetabs Tablets 2386
- Proventil Solution for Inhalation 0.5% 2383
- Proventil Syrup 2385
- Proventil Tablets 2386
- Ventolin Inhalation Solution 1198
- Ventolin Nebules Inhalation Solution 1199
- Ventolin Rotacaps for Inhalation 1200
- Ventolin Syrup 1202
- Ventolin Tablets 1203
- Volmax Extended-Release Tablets .. 1788

Alfentanil Hydrochloride (Increases certain actions or side effects). Products include:
- Alfenta Injection 1286

Alprazolam (Increases certain actions or side effects). Products include:
- Xanax Tablets 2649

Aluminum Carbonate Gel (Interferes with the absorption). Products include:
- Basaljel 2703

Aluminum Hydroxide (Interferes with the absorption). Products include:
- ALternaGEL Liquid 1316
- Maximum Strength Ascriptin .... ◘ 630
- Cama Arthritis Pain Reliever .... ◘ 785
- Gaviscon Extra Strength Relief Formula Antacid Tablets .... ◘ 819
- Gaviscon Extra Strength Relief Formula Liquid Antacid .... ◘ 819
- Gaviscon Liquid Antacid .... ◘ 820
- Gelusil Liquid & Tablets .... ◘ 855
- Maalox Heartburn Relief Suspension .... ◘ 642
- Maalox Heartburn Relief Tablets .... ◘ 641
- Maalox Magnesia and Alumina Oral Suspension .... ◘ 642
- Maalox Plus Tablets .... ◘ 643
- Extra Strength Maalox Antacid Plus Antigas Liquid and Tablets ◘ 638
- Tempo Soft Antacid .... ◘ 835

Aluminum Hydroxide Gel (Interferes with the absorption). Products include:
- ALternaGEL Liquid .... ◘ 659
- Aludrox Oral Suspension 2695
- Amphojel Suspension 2695
- Amphojel Suspension without Flavor 2695
- Amphojel Tablets 2695
- Arthritis Pain Ascriptin .... ◘ 631
- Regular Strength Ascriptin Tablets .... ◘ 629
- Gaviscon Antacid Tablets .... ◘ 819
- Gaviscon-2 Antacid Tablets .... ◘ 820
- Mylanta Liquid 1317
- Mylanta Tablets .... ◘ 660
- Mylanta Double Strength Liquid 1317
- Mylanta Double Strength Tablets .. ◘ 660
- Nephrox Suspension .... ◘ 655

Amantadine Hydrochloride (Increases certain actions or side effects). Products include:
- Symmetrel Capsules and Syrup 946

Amitriptyline Hydrochloride (Increases certain actions or side effects). Products include:
- Elavil 2838
- Endep Tablets 2174
- Etrafon 2355
- Limbitrol 2180
- Triavil Tablets 1757

Amoxapine (Increases certain actions or side effects). Products include:
- Asendin Tablets 1369

Amyl Nitrite (Increases certain actions and side effects).
- No products indexed under this heading.

Astemizole (Increases certain actions or side effects). Products include:
- Hismanal Tablets 1293

Atropine Sulfate (Increases certain actions or side effects). Products include:
- Arco-Lase Plus Tablets 512
- Atrohist Plus Tablets 454
- Atropine Sulfate Sterile Ophthalmic Solution .... ◉ 233
- Donnatal 2060
- Donnatal Extentabs 2061
- Donnatal Tablets 2060
- Lomotil 2439
- Motofen Tablets 784
- Urised Tablets 1964

Azatadine Maleate (Increases certain actions or side effects). Products include:
- Trinalin Repetabs Tablets 1330

Belladonna Alkaloids (Increases certain actions or side effects). Products include:
- Bellergal-S Tablets 2250
- Hyland's Bed Wetting Tablets .... ◘ 828
- Hyland's EnurAid Tablets .... ◘ 829
- Hyland's Teething Tablets .... ◘ 830

Benztropine Mesylate (Increases certain actions or side effects). Products include:
- Cogentin 1621

Betamethasone Acetate (Concurrent use in the presence of increased intraocular pressure may be hazardous). Products include:
- Celestone Soluspan Suspension 2347

Betamethasone Sodium Phosphate (Concurrent use in the presence of increased intraocular pressure may be hazardous). Products include:
- Celestone Soluspan Suspension 2347

Betaxolol Hydrochloride (Effects of antiglaucoma agents antagonized). Products include:
- Betoptic Ophthalmic Solution 469
- Betoptic S Ophthalmic Suspension 471
- Kerlone Tablets 2436

Biperiden Hydrochloride (Increases certain actions or side effects). Products include:
- Akineton 1333

Bromodiphenhydramine Hydrochloride (Increases certain actions or side effects).
- No products indexed under this heading.

Brompheniramine Maleate (Increases certain actions or side effects). Products include:
- Alka Seltzer Plus Sinus Medicine .. ◘ 707
- Bromfed Capsules (Extended-Release) 1785
- Bromfed Syrup .... ◘ 733
- Bromfed Tablets 1785
- Bromfed-DM Cough Syrup 1786
- Bromfed-PD Capsules (Extended-Release) 1785
- Dimetane-DC Cough Syrup 2059
- Dimetane-DX Cough Syrup 2059
- Dimetapp Elixir .... ◘ 773
- Dimetapp Extentabs .... ◘ 774
- Dimetapp Tablets/Liqui-Gels .... ◘ 775
- Dimetapp Cold & Allergy Chewable Tablets .... ◘ 773
- Dimetapp DM Elixir .... ◘ 774
- Vicks DayQuil Allergy Relief 12-Hour Extended Release Tablets .. ◘ 760
- Vicks DayQuil Allergy Relief 4-Hour Tablets .... ◘ 760

Buprenorphine (Increases certain actions or side effects). Products include:
- Buprenex Injectable 2006

Carbachol (Effects of antiglaucoma agents antagonized). Products include:
- Isopto Carbachol Ophthalmic Solution .... ◉ 223
- MIOSTAT Intraocular Solution .... ◉ 224

Chlordiazepoxide (Increases certain actions or side effects). Products include:
- Libritabs Tablets 2177
- Limbitrol 2180

Chlordiazepoxide Hydrochloride (Increases certain actions or side effects). Products include:
- Librax Capsules 2176
- Librium Capsules 2178
- Librium Injectable 2179

Chlorpheniramine Maleate (Increases certain actions or side effects). Products include:
- Alka-Seltzer Plus Cold Medicine .... ◘ 705
- Alka-Seltzer Plus Cold Medicine Liqui-Gels .... ◘ 706
- Alka-Seltzer Plus Cold & Cough Medicine .... ◘ 708
- Alka-Seltzer Plus Cold & Cough Medicine Liqui-Gels .... ◘ 705
- Allerest Children's Chewable Tablets .... ◘ 627
- Allerest Headache Strength Tablets .... ◘ 627
- Allerest Maximum Strength Tablets .... ◘ 627
- Allerest Sinus Pain Formula .... ◘ 627
- Allerest 12 Hour Caplets .... ◘ 627
- Ana-Kit Anaphylaxis Emergency Treatment Kit 617
- Atrohist Pediatric Capsules 453
- Atrohist Plus Tablets 454
- BC Cold Powder Multi-Symptom Formula (Cold-Sinus-Allergy) ...... ◘ 609
- Cerose DM .... ◘ 878
- Cheracol Plus Head Cold/Cough Formula .... ◘ 769
- Children's Vicks DayQuil Allergy Relief .... ◘ 757
- Children's Vicks NyQuil Cold/Cough Relief .... ◘ 758
- Chlor-Trimeton Allergy Decongestant Tablets .... ◘ 799
- Chlor-Trimeton Allergy Tablets ...... ◘ 798
- Comhist 2038
- Comtrex Multi-Symptom Cold Reliever Tablets/Caplets/Liqui-Gels/Liquid .... ◘ 615
- Allergy-Sinus Comtrex Multi-Symptom Allergy-Sinus Formula Tablets .... ◘ 617
- Contac Continuous Action Nasal Decongestant/Antihistamine 12 Hour Capsules .... ◘ 813
- Contac Maximum Strength Continuous Action Decongestant/Antihistamine 12 Hour Caplets .. ◘ 813
- Contac Severe Cold and Flu Formula Caplets .... ◘ 814
- Coricidin 'D' Decongestant Tablets .... ◘ 800
- Coricidin Tablets .... ◘ 800
- D.A. Chewable Tablets 951
- Deconamine 1320
- Dura-Tap/PD Capsules 2867
- Dura-Vent/DA Tablets 953
- Extendryl 1005
- Fedahist Gyrocaps 2401
- Fedahist Timecaps 2401
- Hycomine Compound Tablets 932
- Isoclor Timesule Capsules .... ◘ 637
- Kronofed-A 977
- Nolamine Timed-Release Tablets 785
- Novahistine DH 2462
- Novahistine Elixir .... ◘ 823
- Ornade Spansule Capsules 2502
- PediaCare Cold Allergy Chewable Tablets .... ◘ 677
- PediaCare Cough-Cold Chewable Tablets 1553
- PediaCare Cough-Cold Liquid 1553
- PediaCare NightRest Cough-Cold Liquid 1553
- Pediatric Vicks 44m Cough & Cold Relief .... ◘ 764
- Pyrroxate Caplets .... ◘ 772
- Ryna .... ◘ 841
- Sinarest Tablets .... ◘ 648
- Sinarest Extra Strength Tablets ...... ◘ 648
- Sine-Off Sinus Medicine .... ◘ 825
- Singlet Tablets .... ◘ 825
- Sinulin Tablets 787
- Sinutab Sinus Allergy Medication, Maximum Strength Tablets and Caplets .... ◘ 860
- Sudafed Plus Liquid .... ◘ 862
- Sudafed Plus Tablets .... ◘ 863
- Teldrin 12 Hour Antihistamine/Nasal Decongestant Allergy Relief Capsules .... ◘ 826
- TheraFlu .... ◘ 787
- TheraFlu Maximum Strength Nighttime Flu, Cold & Cough Medicine .... ◘ 788
- Triaminic Allergy Tablets .... ◘ 789
- Triaminic Cold Tablets .... ◘ 790
- Triaminic Nite Light .... ◘ 791
- Triaminic Syrup .... ◘ 792
- Triaminic-12 Tablets .... ◘ 792
- Triaminicin Tablets .... ◘ 793
- Triaminicol Multi-Symptom Cold Tablets .... ◘ 793
- Triaminicol Multi-Symptom Relief ◘ 794
- Tussend 1783
- Children's TYLENOL Cold Multi-Symptom Liquid Formula and Chewable Tablets 1561
- Children's TYLENOL Cold Plus Cough Multi Symptom Tablets and Liquid .... ◘ 681
- TYLENOL Maximum Strength Allergy Sinus Medication Gelcaps and Caplets 1563
- TYLENOL Cold Multi-Symptom Formula Medication Tablets and Caplets 1561
- TYLENOL Cold Multi-Symptom Hot Medication Liquid Packets 1557

IMPORTANT NOTE: Always consult each drug listing in the patient's regimen for possible interactions.

Bentyl — **Interactions Index** — **112**

Vicks 44 LiquiCaps Cough, Cold & Flu Relief ▣ 755
Vicks 44M Cough, Cold & Flu Relief ▣ 756

Chlorpheniramine Polistirex (Increases certain actions or side effects). Products include:
Tussionex Pennkinetic Extended-Release Suspension 998

Chlorpheniramine Tannate (Increases certain actions or side effects). Products include:
Atrohist Pediatric Suspension 454
Ricobid Tablets and Pediatric Suspension 2038
Rynatan 2673
Rynatuss 2673

Chlorpromazine (Increases certain actions or side effects). Products include:
Thorazine Suppositories 2523

Chlorpromazine Hydrochloride (Increases certain actions or side effects). Products include:
Thorazine 2523

Clemastine Fumarate (Increases certain actions or side effects). Products include:
Tavist Syrup 2297
Tavist Tablets 2298
Tavist-1 12 Hour Relief Tablets ▣ 787
Tavist-D 12 Hour Relief Tablets ▣ 787

Clidinium Bromide (Increases certain actions or side effects). Products include:
Librax Capsules 2176
Quarzan Capsules 2181

Clomipramine Hydrochloride (Increases certain actions or side effects). Products include:
Anafranil Capsules 803

Clorazepate Dipotassium (Increases certain actions or side effects). Products include:
Tranxene 451

Codeine Phosphate (Increases certain actions or side effects). Products include:
Actifed with Codeine Cough Syrup 1067
Brontex 1981
Deconsal C Expectorant Syrup 456
Deconsal Pediatric Syrup 457
Dimetane-DC Cough Syrup 2059
Empirin with Codeine Tablets 1093
Fioricet with Codeine Capsules 2260
Fiorinal with Codeine Capsules 2262
Isoclor Expectorant 990
Novahistine DH 2462
Novahistine Expectorant 2463
Nucofed 2051
Phenergan with Codeine 2777
Phenergan VC with Codeine 2781
Robitussin A-C Syrup 2073
Robitussin-DAC Syrup 2074
Ryna ▣ 841
Soma Compound w/Codeine Tablets 2676
Tussi-Organidin NR Liquid and S NR Liquid 2677
Tylenol with Codeine 1583

Cortisone Acetate (Concurrent use in the presence of increased intraocular pressure may be hazardous). Products include:
Cortone Acetate Sterile Suspension 1623
Cortone Acetate Tablets 1624

Cyproheptadine Hydrochloride (Increases certain actions or side effects). Products include:
Periactin 1724

Demecarium Bromide (Effects of antiglaucoma agents antagonized). Products include:
Humorsol Sterile Ophthalmic Solution 1664

Desipramine Hydrochloride (Increases certain actions or side effects). Products include:
Norpramin Tablets 1526

Dexamethasone (Concurrent use in the presence of increased intraocular pressure may be hazardous). Products include:
AK-Trol Ointment & Suspension ◉ 205
Decadron Elixir 1633
Decadron Tablets 1635
Decaspray Topical Aerosol 1648
Dexacidin Ointment ◉ 263
Maxitrol Ophthalmic Ointment and Suspension ◉ 224
TobraDex Ophthalmic Suspension and Ointment 473

Dexamethasone Acetate (Concurrent use in the presence of increased intraocular pressure may be hazardous). Products include:
Dalalone D.P. Injectable 1011
Decadron-LA Sterile Suspension 1646

Dexamethasone Sodium Phosphate (Concurrent use in the presence of increased intraocular pressure may be hazardous). Products include:
Decadron Phosphate Injection 1637
Decadron Phosphate Respihaler 1642
Decadron Phosphate Sterile Ophthalmic Ointment 1641
Decadron Phosphate Sterile Ophthalmic Solution 1642
Decadron Phosphate Topical Cream 1644
Decadron Phosphate Turbinaire 1645
Decadron Phosphate with Xylocaine Injection, Sterile 1639
Dexacort Phosphate in Respihaler 458
Dexacort Phosphate in Turbinaire 459
NeoDecadron Sterile Ophthalmic Ointment 1712
NeoDecadron Sterile Ophthalmic Solution 1713
NeoDecadron Topical Cream 1714

Dexchlorpheniramine Maleate (Increases certain actions or side effects).
No products indexed under this heading.

Dezocine (Increases certain actions or side effects). Products include:
Dalgan Injection 538

Diazepam (Increases certain actions or side effects). Products include:
Dizac 1809
Valium Injectable 2182
Valium Tablets 2183
Valrelease Capsules 2169

Dichlorphenamide (Effects of antiglaucoma agents antagonized). Products include:
Daranide Tablets 1633

Digoxin (Increased serum digoxin levels). Products include:
Lanoxicaps 1117
Lanoxin Elixir Pediatric 1120
Lanoxin Injection 1123
Lanoxin Injection Pediatric 1126
Lanoxin Tablets 1128

Dihydroxyaluminum Sodium Carbonate (Interferes with the absorption).
No products indexed under this heading.

Diphenhydramine Citrate (Increases certain actions or side effects). Products include:
Excedrin P.M. Analgesic/Sleeping Aid Tablets, Caplets, Liquigels 733

Diphenhydramine Hydrochloride (Increases certain actions or side effects). Products include:
Actifed Allergy Daytime/Nighttime Caplets ▣ 844
Actifed Sinus Daytime/Nighttime Tablets and Caplets ▣ 846
Arthritis Foundation NightTime Caplets ▣ 674
Extra Strength Bayer PM Aspirin ▣ 713
Bayer Select Night Time Pain Relief Formula ▣ 716
Benadryl Allergy Decongestant Liquid Medication ▣ 848
Benadryl Allergy Decongestant Tablets ▣ 848
Benadryl Allergy Liquid Medication ▣ 849
Benadryl Allergy ▣ 848
Benadryl Allergy Sinus Headache Formula Caplets ▣ 849
Benadryl Capsules 1898
Benadryl Dye-Free Allergy Liquigel Softgels ▣ 850
Benadryl Dye-Free Allergy Liquid Medication ▣ 850
Benadryl Itch Relief Cream, Children's Formula and Maximum Strength 2% ▣ 851
Benadryl Itch Relief Spray, Children's Formula and Maximum Strength 2% ▣ 851
Benadryl Itch Relief Stick Maximum Strength 2% ▣ 850
Benadryl Itch Stopping Gel, Children's Formula and Maximum Strength 2% ▣ 851
Benadryl Kapseals 1898
Benadryl Injection 1898
Contac Day & Night Cold/Flu Night Caplets ▣ 812
Contac Night Allergy/Sinus Caplets ▣ 812
Extra Strength Doan's P.M. ▣ 633
Legatrin PM ▣ 651
Miles Nervine Nighttime Sleep-Aid ▣ 723
Nytol QuickCaps Caplets ▣ 610
Sleepinal Night-time Sleep Aid Capsules and Softgels ▣ 834
TYLENOL Maximum Strength Allergy Sinus NightTime Medication Caplets 1555
TYLENOL Flu NightTime, Maximum Strength, Gelcaps 1566
TYLENOL Maximum Strength Flu NightTime Hot Medication Packets 1562
TYLENOL PM, Extra Strength Pain Reliever/Sleep Aid Caplets, Geltabs, Gelcaps 1560
TYLENOL Severe Allergy Medication Caplets 1564
Maximum Strength Unisom Sleepgels 1934
Unisom With Pain Relief-Nighttime Sleep Aid and Pain Reliever 1934

Dipivefrin Hydrochloride (Effects of antiglaucoma agents antagonized). Products include:
PROPINE with C CAP Compliance Cap ◉ 253

Disopyramide Phosphate (Increases certain actions or side effects). Products include:
Norpace 2444

Dobutamine Hydrochloride (Increases certain actions or side effects). Products include:
Dobutrex Solution Vials 1439

Dopamine Hydrochloride (Increases certain actions or side effects).
No products indexed under this heading.

Doxepin Hydrochloride (Increases certain actions or side effects). Products include:
Sinequan 2205
Zonalon Cream 1055

Echothiophate Iodide (Effects of antiglaucoma agents antagonized). Products include:
Phospholine Iodide ◉ 326

Ephedrine Hydrochloride (Effects of antiglaucoma agents antagonized). Products include:
Primatene Dual Action Formula ▣ 872
Primatene Tablets ▣ 873
Quadrinal Tablets 1350

Ephedrine Sulfate (Increases certain actions or side effects). Products include:
Bronkaid Caplets ▣ 717
Marax Tablets & DF Syrup 2200

Ephedrine Tannate (Increases certain actions or side effects). Products include:
Rynatuss 2673

Epinephrine (Increases certain actions or side effects). Products include:
Bronkaid Mist ▣ 717
EPIFRIN ◉ 239
EpiPen 790
Marcaine Hydrochloride with Epinephrine 1:200,000 2316
Primatene Mist ▣ 873
Sensorcaine with Epinephrine Injection 559
Sus-Phrine Injection 1019
Xylocaine with Epinephrine Injections 567

Epinephrine Bitartrate (Effects of antiglaucoma agents antagonized). Products include:
Bronkaid Mist Suspension ▣ 718
Sensorcaine-MPF with Epinephrine Injection 559

Epinephrine Hydrochloride (Increases certain actions or side effects; effects of antiglaucoma agents antagonized). Products include:
Ana-Kit Anaphylaxis Emergency Treatment Kit 617

Epinephryl Borate (Effects of antiglaucoma agents antagonized).
No products indexed under this heading.

Erythrityl Tetranitrate (Increases certain actions and side effects).
No products indexed under this heading.

Estazolam (Increases certain actions or side effects). Products include:
ProSom Tablets 449

Fentanyl (Increases certain actions or side effects). Products include:
Duragesic Transdermal System 1288

Fentanyl Citrate (Increases certain actions or side effects). Products include:
Sublimaze Injection 1307

Fludrocortisone Acetate (Concurrent use in the presence of increased intraocular pressure may be hazardous). Products include:
Florinef Acetate Tablets 505

Fluphenazine Decanoate (Increases certain actions or side effects). Products include:
Prolixin Decanoate 509

Fluphenazine Enanthate (Increases certain actions or side effects). Products include:
Prolixin Enanthate 509

Fluphenazine Hydrochloride (Increases certain actions or side effects). Products include:
Prolixin 509

Flurazepam Hydrochloride (Increases certain actions or side effects). Products include:
Dalmane Capsules 2173

Furazolidone (Increases certain actions or side effects). Products include:
Furoxone 2046

Glutamic Acid Hydrochloride (Antagonizes the inhibiting effects on gastric hydrochloric acid).
No products indexed under this heading.

Glycopyrrolate (Increases certain actions or side effects). Products include:
Robinul Forte Tablets 2072
Robinul Injectable 2072
Robinul Tablets 2072

Halazepam (Increases certain actions or side effects).
No products indexed under this heading.

(▣ Described in PDR For Nonprescription Drugs) (◉ Described in PDR For Ophthalmology)

Hydrocodone Bitartrate (Increases certain actions or side effects). Products include:

Anexsia 5/500 Elixir 1781
Anexia Tablets.. 1782
Codiclear DH Syrup 791
Deconamine CX Cough and Cold Liquid and Tablets................................ 1319
Duratuss HD Elixir.................................. 2565
Hycodan Tablets and Syrup 930
Hycomine Compound Tablets 932
Hycomine 931
Hycotuss Expectorant Syrup 933
Hydrocet Capsules 782
Lorcet 10/650... 1018
Lortab 2566
Tussend 1783
Tussend Expectorant 1785
Vicodin Tablets 1356
Vicodin ES Tablets 1357
Vicodin Tuss Expectorant 1358
Zydone Capsules 949

Hydrocodone Polistirex (Increases certain actions or side effects). Products include:

Tussionex Pennkinetic Extended-Release Suspension 998

Hydrocortisone (Concurrent use in the presence of increased intraocular pressure may be hazardous). Products include:

Anusol-HC Cream 2.5% 1896
Aquanil HC Lotion 1931
Bactine Hydrocortisone Anti-Itch Cream .... ⊞ 709
Caldecort Anti-Itch Hydrocortisone Spray .... ⊞ 631
Cortaid .... ⊞ 836
CORTENEMA... 2535
Cortisporin Ointment 1085
Cortisporin Ophthalmic Ointment Sterile 1085
Cortisporin Ophthalmic Suspension Sterile 1086
Cortisporin Otic Solution Sterile 1087
Cortisporin Otic Suspension Sterile 1088
Cortizone-5 .... ⊞ 831
Cortizone-10 .... ⊞ 831
Hydrocortone Tablets 1672
Hytone 907
Massengill Medicated Soft Cloth Towelettes.. 2458
PediOtic Suspension Sterile 1153
Preparation H Hydrocortisone 1% Cream .... ⊞ 872
ProctoCream-HC 2.5% 2408
VōSoL HC Otic Solution....................... 2678

Hydrocortisone Acetate (Concurrent use in the presence of increased intraocular pressure may be hazardous). Products include:

Analpram-HC Rectal Cream 1% and 2.5% 977
Anusol HC-1 Anti-Itch Hydrocortisone Ointment.................................... ⊞ 847
Anusol-HC Suppositories 1897
Caldecort.. ⊞ 631
Carmol HC 924
Coly-Mycin S Otic w/Neomycin & Hydrocortisone 1906
Cortaid .... ⊞ 836
Cortifoam 2396
Cortisporin Cream................................. 1084
Epifoam 2399
Hydrocortone Acetate Sterile Suspension.. 1669
Mantadil Cream 1135
Nupercainal Hydrocortisone 1% Cream .... ⊞ 645
Ophthocort .... ◎ 311
Pramosone Cream, Lotion & Ointment 978
ProctoCream-HC 2408
ProctoFoam-HC 2409
Terra-Cortril Ophthalmic Suspension 2210

Hydrocortisone Sodium Phosphate (Concurrent use in the presence of increased intraocular pressure may be hazardous). Products include:

Hydrocortone Phosphate Injection, Sterile 1670

Hydrocortisone Sodium Succinate (Concurrent use in the presence of increased intraocular pressure may be hazardous). Products include:

Solu-Cortef Sterile Powder................. 2641

Hyoscyamine (Increases certain actions or side effects). Products include:

Cystospaz Tablets 1963
Urised Tablets... 1964

Hyoscyamine Sulfate (Increases certain actions or side effects). Products include:

Arco-Lase Plus Tablets 512
Atrohist Plus Tablets 454
Cystospaz-M Capsules 1963
Donnatal 2060
Donnatal Extentabs............................... 2061
Donnatal Tablets 2060
Kutrase Capsules................................... 2402
Levsin/Levsinex/Levbid 2405

Imipramine Hydrochloride (Increases certain actions or side effects). Products include:

Tofranil Ampuls 854
Tofranil Tablets 856

Imipramine Pamoate (Increases certain actions or side effects). Products include:

Tofranil-PM Capsules........................... 857

Ipratropium Bromide (Increases certain actions or side effects). Products include:

Atrovent Inhalation Aerosol............... 671
Atrovent Inhalation Solution 673

Isocarboxazid (Increases certain actions or side effects).

No products indexed under this heading.

Isoflurophate (Effects of antiglaucoma agents antagonized). Products include:

Floropryl Sterile Ophthalmic Ointment 1662

Isoproterenol Hydrochloride (Increases certain actions or side effects). Products include:

Isuprel Hydrochloride Injection 1:5000 2311
Isuprel Hydrochloride Solution 1:200 & 1:100 2313
Isuprel Mistometer 2312

Isoproterenol Sulfate (Increases certain actions or side effects). Products include:

Norisodrine with Calcium Iodide Syrup... 442

Isosorbide Dinitrate (Increases certain actions and side effects). Products include:

Dilatrate-SR 2398
Isordil Sublingual Tablets 2739
Isordil Tembids....................................... 2741
Isordil Titradose Tablets...................... 2742
Sorbitrate 2843

Isosorbide Mononitrate (Increases certain actions and side effects). Products include:

Imdur 1323
Ismo Tablets 2738
Monoket.. 2406

Levobunolol Hydrochloride (Effects of antiglaucoma agents antagonized). Products include:

Betagan .... ◎ 233

Levorphanol Tartrate (Increases certain actions or side effects). Products include:

Levo-Dromoran 2129

Loratadine (Increases certain actions or side effects). Products include:

Claritin 2349
Claritin-D 2350

Lorazepam (Increases certain actions or side effects). Products include:

Ativan Injection 2698

Ativan Tablets 2700

Magaldrate (Interferes with the absorption).

No products indexed under this heading.

Magnesium Hydroxide (Interferes with the absorption). Products include:

Aludrox Oral Suspension 2695
Arthritis Pain Ascriptin .... ⊞ 631
Maximum Strength Ascriptin .... ⊞ 630
Regular Strength Ascriptin Tablets .... ⊞ 629
Di-Gel Antacid/Anti-Gas .... ⊞ 801
Gelusil Liquid & Tablets .... ⊞ 855
Maalox Magnesia and Alumina Oral Suspension .... ⊞ 642
Maalox Plus Tablets .... ⊞ 643
Extra Strength Maalox Antacid Plus Antigas Liquid and Tablets ⊞ 638
Mylanta Calcium Carbonate and Magnesium Hydroxide Tablets...... 1318
Mylanta Liquid 1317
Mylanta Tablets .... ⊞ 660
Mylanta Double Strength Liquid 1317
Mylanta Double Strength Tablets.. ⊞ 660
Phillips' Milk of Magnesia Liquid.... ⊞ 729
Rolaids Tablets .... ⊞ 843
Tempo Soft Antacid .... ⊞ 835

Magnesium Oxide (Interferes with the absorption). Products include:

Beelith Tablets 639
Bufferin Analgesic Tablets and Caplets .... ⊞ 613
Caltrate PLUS .... ⊞ 665
Cama Arthritis Pain Reliever.............. ⊞ 785
Mag-Ox 400 668
Uro-Mag.. 668

Maprotiline Hydrochloride (Increases certain actions or side effects). Products include:

Ludiomil Tablets.................................... 843

Mepenzolate Bromide (Increases certain actions or side effects).

No products indexed under this heading.

Meperidine Hydrochloride (Increases certain actions or side effects). Products include:

Demerol 2308
Mepergan Injection 2753

Mesoridazine Besylate (Increases certain actions or side effects). Products include:

Serentil 684

Metaproterenol Sulfate (Increases certain actions or side effects). Products include:

Alupent.. 669
Metaproterenol Sulfate Inhalation Solution, USP, Arm-a-Med 552

Metaraminol Bitartrate (Increases certain actions or side effects). Products include:

Aramine Injection.................................. 1609

Methadone Hydrochloride (Increases certain actions or side effects). Products include:

Methadone Hydrochloride Oral Concentrate 2233
Methadone Hydrochloride Oral Solution & Tablets.............................. 2235

Methazolamide (Effects of antiglaucoma agents antagonized). Products include:

Glauctabs .... ◎ 208
MZM .... ◎ 267
Neptazane Tablets 1388
Neptazane Tablets .... ◎ 320

Methdilazine Hydrochloride (Increases certain actions or side effects).

No products indexed under this heading.

Methotrimeprazine (Increases certain actions or side effects). Products include:

Levoprome 1274

Methoxamine Hydrochloride (Increases certain actions or side effects). Products include:

Vasoxyl Injection 1196

Methylprednisolone Acetate (Concurrent use in the presence of increased intraocular pressure may be hazardous). Products include:

Depo-Medrol Single-Dose Vial 2600
Depo-Medrol Sterile Aqueous Suspension.. 2597

Methylprednisolone Sodium Succinate (Concurrent use in the presence of increased intraocular pressure may be hazardous). Products include:

Solu-Medrol Sterile Powder............... 2643

Metoclopramide Hydrochloride (Gastrointestinal motility effects of metoclopramide may be antagonized). Products include:

Reglan.. 2068

Midazolam Hydrochloride (Increases certain actions or side effects). Products include:

Versed Injection 2170

Moricizine Hydrochloride (Increases certain actions or side effects). Products include:

Ethmozine Tablets................................. 2041

Morphine Sulfate (Increases certain actions or side effects). Products include:

Astramorph/PF Injection, USP (Preservative-Free) 535
Duramorph 962
Infumorph 200 and Infumorph 500 Sterile Solutions.......................... 965
MS Contin Tablets.................................. 1994
MSIR 1997
Oramorph SR (Morphine Sulfate Sustained Release Tablets)............. 2236
RMS Suppositories 2657
Roxanol 2243

Nitroglycerin (Increases certain actions and side effects). Products include:

Deponit NTG Transdermal Delivery System 2397
Nitro-Bid IV.. 1523
Nitro-Bid Ointment 1524
Nitrodisc 2047
Nitro-Dur (nitroglycerin) Transdermal Infusion System 1326
Nitrolingual Spray 2027
Nitrostat Tablets 1925
Transderm-Nitro Transdermal Therapeutic System 859

Norepinephrine Bitartrate (Increases certain actions or side effects). Products include:

Levophed Bitartrate Injection 2315

Nortriptyline Hydrochloride (Increases certain actions or side effects). Products include:

Pamelor 2280

Opium Alkaloids (Increases certain actions or side effects).

No products indexed under this heading.

Oxazepam (Increases certain actions or side effects). Products include:

Serax Capsules 2810
Serax Tablets... 2810

Oxybutynin Chloride (Increases certain actions or side effects). Products include:

Ditropan... 1516

Oxycodone Hydrochloride (Increases certain actions or side effects). Products include:

Percocet Tablets 938
Percodan Tablets................................... 939
Percodan-Demi Tablets........................ 940
Roxicodone Tablets, Oral Solution & Intensol (Oxycodone) 2244
Tylox Capsules 1584

IMPORTANT NOTE: Always consult each drug listing in the patient's regimen for possible interactions.

Bentyl
Interactions Index
114

Pentaerythritol Tetranitrate (Increases certain actions and side effects).
No products indexed under this heading.

Pentagastrin (Antagonizes the inhibiting effects on gastric hydrochloric acid). Products include:
Peptavlon 2878

Perphenazine (Increases certain actions or side effects). Products include:
Etrafon 2355
Triavil Tablets 1757
Trilafon 2389

Phenelzine Sulfate (Increases certain actions or side effects). Products include:
Nardil 1920

Phenylephrine Bitartrate (Increases certain actions or side effects).
No products indexed under this heading.

Phenylephrine Hydrochloride (Increases certain actions or side effects). Products include:
Atrohist Plus Tablets 454
Cerose DM ▣ 878
Comhist 2038
D.A. Chewable Tablets 951
Deconsal Pediatric Capsules 454
Dura-Vent/DA Tablets 953
Entex Capsules 1986
Entex Liquid 1986
Extendryl 1005
4-Way Fast Acting Nasal Spray (regular & mentholated) ▣ 621
Hemorid For Women ▣ 834
Hycomine Compound Tablets 932
Neo-Synephrine Hydrochloride 1% Carpuject 2324
Neo-Synephrine Hydrochloride 1% Injection 2324
Neo-Synephrine Hydrochloride (Ophthalmic) 2325
Neo-Synephrine ▣ 726
Nōstril ▣ 644
Novahistine Elixir ▣ 823
Phenergan VC 2779
Phenergan VC with Codeine 2781
Preparation H ▣ 871
Tympagesic Ear Drops 2342
Vasosulf ◉ 271
Vicks Sinex Nasal Spray and Ultra Fine Mist ▣ 765

Phenylephrine Tannate (Increases certain actions or side effects). Products include:
Atrohist Pediatric Suspension 454
Ricobid-D Pediatric Suspension 2038
Ricobid Tablets and Pediatric Suspension 2038
Rynatan 2673
Rynatuss 2673

Phenylpropanolamine Hydrochloride (Increases certain actions or side effects). Products include:
Acutrim ▣ 628
Allerest Children's Chewable Tablets ▣ 627
Allerest 12 Hour Caplets ▣ 627
Atrohist Plus Tablets 454
BC Cold Powder Multi-Symptom Formula (Cold-Sinus-Allergy) ▣ 609
BC Cold Powder Non-Drowsy Formula (Cold-Sinus) ▣ 609
Cheracol Plus Head Cold/Cough Formula ▣ 769
Comtrex Multi-Symptom Non-Drowsy Liqui-gels ▣ 618
Contac Continuous Action Nasal Decongestant/Antihistamine 12 Hour Capsules ▣ 813
Contac Maximum Strength Continuous Action Decongestant/Antihistamine 12 Hour Caplets ▣ 813
Contac Severe Cold and Flu Formula Caplets ▣ 814
Coricidin 'D' Decongestant Tablets ▣ 800
Dexatrim ▣ 832
Dexatrim Plus Vitamins Caplets ▣ 832
Dimetane-DC Cough Syrup 2059
Dimetapp Elixir ▣ 773
Dimetapp Extentabs ▣ 774
Dimetapp Tablets/Liqui-Gels ▣ 775
Dimetapp Cold & Allergy Chewable Tablets ▣ 773
Dimetapp DM Elixir ▣ 774
Dura-Vent Tablets 952
Entex Capsules 1986
Entex LA Tablets 1987
Entex Liquid 1986
Exgest LA Tablets 782
Hycomine 931
Isoclor Timesule Capsules ▣ 637
Nolamine Timed-Release Tablets 785
Ornade Spansule Capsules 2502
Propagest Tablets 786
Pyrroxate Caplets ▣ 772
Robitussin-CF ▣ 777
Sinulin Tablets 787
Tavist-D 12 Hour Relief Tablets ▣ 787
Teldrin 12 Hour Antihistamine/Nasal Decongestant Allergy Relief Capsules ▣ 826
Triaminic Allergy Tablets ▣ 789
Triaminic Cold Tablets ▣ 790
Triaminic Expectorant ▣ 790
Triaminic Syrup ▣ 792
Triaminic-12 Tablets ▣ 792
Triaminic-DM Syrup ▣ 792
Triaminicin Tablets ▣ 793
Triaminicol Multi-Symptom Cold Tablets ▣ 793
Triaminicol Multi-Symptom Relief ▣ 794
Vicks DayQuil Allergy Relief 12-Hour Extended Release Tablets ▣ 760
Vicks DayQuil Allergy Relief 4-Hour Tablets ▣ 760
Vicks DayQuil SINUS Pressure & CONGESTION Relief ▣ 761

Pilocarpine (Effects of antiglaucoma agents antagonized). Products include:
Ocusert Pilo-20 and Pilo-40 Ocular Therapeutic Systems ◉ 254

Pilocarpine Hydrochloride (Effects of antiglaucoma agents antagonized). Products include:
Isopto Carpine Ophthalmic Solution ◉ 223
Pilocar ◉ 268
Pilopine HS Ophthalmic Gel ◉ 226
Salagen Tablets 1489

Pirbuterol Acetate (Increases certain actions or side effects). Products include:
Maxair Autohaler 1492
Maxair Inhaler 1494

Prazepam (Increases certain actions or side effects).
No products indexed under this heading.

Prednisolone Acetate (Concurrent use in the presence of increased intraocular pressure may be hazardous). Products include:
AK-CIDE ◉ 202
AK-CIDE Ointment ◉ 202
Blephamide Liquifilm Sterile Ophthalmic Suspension 476
Blephamide Ointment ◉ 237
Econopred & Econopred Plus Ophthalmic Suspensions ◉ 217
Poly-Pred Liquifilm ◉ 248
Pred Forte ◉ 250
Pred Mild ◉ 253
Pred-G Liquifilm Sterile Ophthalmic Suspension ◉ 251
Pred-G S.O.P. Sterile Ophthalmic Ointment ◉ 252
Vasocidin Ointment ◉ 268

Prednisolone Sodium Phosphate (Concurrent use in the presence of increased intraocular pressure may be hazardous). Products include:
AK-Pred ◉ 204
Hydeltrasol Injection, Sterile 1665
Inflamase ◉ 265
Pediapred Oral Liquid 995
Vasocidin Ophthalmic Solution ◉ 270

Prednisolone Tebutate (Concurrent use in the presence of increased intraocular pressure may be hazardous). Products include:
Hydeltra-T.B.A. Sterile Suspension 1667

Prednisone (Concurrent use in the presence of increased intraocular pressure may be hazardous). Products include:
Deltasone Tablets 2595

Procainamide Hydrochloride (Increases certain actions or side effects). Products include:
Procan SR Tablets 1926

Prochlorperazine (Increases certain actions or side effects). Products include:
Compazine 2470

Procyclidine Hydrochloride (Increases certain actions or side effects). Products include:
Kemadrin Tablets 1112

Promethazine Hydrochloride (Increases certain actions or side effects). Products include:
Mepergan Injection 2753
Phenergan with Codeine 2777
Phenergan with Dextromethorphan 2778
Phenergan Injection 2773
Phenergan Suppositories 2775
Phenergan Syrup 2774
Phenergan Tablets 2775
Phenergan VC 2779
Phenergan VC with Codeine 2781

Propafenone Hydrochloride (Increases certain actions or side effects). Products include:
Rythmol Tablets–150mg, 225mg, 300mg 1352

Propantheline Bromide (Increases certain actions or side effects). Products include:
Pro-Banthīne Tablets 2052

Propoxyphene Hydrochloride (Increases certain actions or side effects). Products include:
Darvon 1435
Wygesic Tablets 2827

Propoxyphene Napsylate (Increases certain actions or side effects). Products include:
Darvon-N/Darvocet-N 1433

Protriptyline Hydrochloride (Increases certain actions or side effects). Products include:
Vivactil Tablets 1774

Pseudoephedrine Hydrochloride (Increases certain actions or side effects). Products include:
Actifed Allergy Daytime/Nighttime Caplets ▣ 844
Actifed Plus Caplets ▣ 845
Actifed Plus Tablets ▣ 845
Actifed with Codeine Cough Syrup 1067
Actifed Sinus Daytime/Nighttime Tablets and Caplets ▣ 846
Actifed Syrup ▣ 846
Actifed Tablets ▣ 844
Advil Cold and Sinus Caplets and Tablets (formerly CoAdvil) ▣ 870
Alka-Seltzer Plus Cold Medicine Liqui-Gels ▣ 706
Alka-Seltzer Plus Cold & Cough Medicine Liqui-Gels ▣ 705
Alka-Seltzer Plus Night-Time Cold Medicine Liqui-Gels ▣ 706
Allerest Headache Strength Tablets ▣ 627
Allerest Maximum Strength Tablets ▣ 627
Allerest No Drowsiness Tablets ▣ 627
Allerest Sinus Pain Formula ▣ 627
Anatuss LA Tablets 1542
Atrohist Pediatric Capsules 453
Bayer Select Sinus Pain Relief Formula ▣ 717
Benadryl Allergy Decongestant Liquid Medication ▣ 848
Benadryl Allergy Decongestant Tablets ▣ 848
Benadryl Allergy Sinus Headache Formula Caplets ▣ 849
Benylin Multisymptom ▣ 852
Bromfed Capsules (Extended-Release) 1785
Bromfed Syrup ▣ 733
Bromfed Tablets 1785
Bromfed-DM Cough Syrup 1786
Bromfed-PD Capsules (Extended-Release) 1785
Children's Vicks DayQuil Allergy Relief ▣ 757
Children's Vicks NyQuil Cold/Cough Relief ▣ 758
Comtrex Multi-Symptom Cold Reliever Tablets/Caplets/Liqui-Gels/Liquid ▣ 615
Allergy-Sinus Comtrex Multi-Symptom Allergy-Sinus Formula Tablets ▣ 617
Comtrex Multi-Symptom Non-Drowsy Caplets ▣ 618
Congess 1004
Contac Day Allergy/Sinus Caplets ▣ 812
Contac Day & Night ▣ 812
Contac Night Allergy/Sinus Caplets ▣ 812
Contac Severe Cold & Flu Non-Drowsy ▣ 815
Deconamine Chewable Tablets 1320
Deconamine CX Cough and Cold Liquid and Tablets 1319
Deconamine 1320
Deconsal C Expectorant Syrup 456
Deconsal Pediatric Syrup 457
Deconsal II Tablets 454
Dimetane-DX Cough Syrup 2059
Dimetapp Sinus Caplets ▣ 775
Dorcol Children's Cough Syrup ▣ 785
Drixoral Cough + Congestion Liquid Caps ▣ 802
Dura-Tap/PD Capsules 2867
Duratuss Tablets 2565
Duratuss HD Elixir 2565
Efidac/24 ▣ 635
Entex PSE Tablets 1987
Fedahist Gyrocaps 2401
Fedahist Timecaps 2401
Guaifed 1787
Guaifed Syrup ▣ 734
Guaimax-D Tablets 792
Guaitab Tablets ▣ 734
Isoclor Expectorant 990
Kronofed-A 977
Motrin IB Sinus ▣ 838
Novahistine DH 2462
Novahistine DMX ▣ 822
Novahistine Expectorant 2463
Nucofed 2051
PediaCare Cold Allergy Chewable Tablets ▣ 677
PediaCare Cough-Cold Chewable Tablets 1553
PediaCare 1553
PediaCare Infants' Decongestant Drops ▣ 677
PediCare Infant's Drops Decongestant Plus Cough 1553
PediaCare NightRest Cough-Cold Liquid 1553
Pediatric Vicks 44d Dry Hacking Cough & Head Congestion ▣ 763
Pediatric Vicks 44m Cough & Cold Relief ▣ 764
Robitussin Cold & Cough Liqui-Gels ▣ 776
Robitussin Maximum Strength Cough & Cold ▣ 778
Robitussin Pediatric Cough & Cold Formula ▣ 779
Robitussin Severe Congestion Liqui-Gels ▣ 776
Robitussin-DAC Syrup 2074
Robitussin-PE ▣ 778
Rondec Oral Drops 953
Rondec Syrup 953
Rondec Tablet 953
Rondec-DM Oral Drops 954
Rondec-DM Syrup 954
Rondec-TR Tablet 953
Ryna ▣ 841
Seldane-D Extended-Release Tablets 1538
Semprex-D Capsules 463
Semprex-D Capsules 1167
Sinarest Tablets ▣ 648
Sinarest Extra Strength Tablets ▣ 648
Sinarest No Drowsiness Tablets ▣ 648
Sine-Aid IB Caplets 1554
Sine-Aid Maximum Strength Sinus Medication Gelcaps, Caplets and Tablets 1554
Sine-Off No Drowsiness Formula Caplets ▣ 824
Sine-Off Sinus Medicine ▣ 825
Singlet Tablets ▣ 825
Sinutab Non-Drying Liquid Caps ▣ 859

(▣ Described in PDR For Nonprescription Drugs)
(◉ Described in PDR For Ophthalmology)

115 Interactions Index Benylin Multisymptom

Sinutab Sinus Allergy Medication, Maximum Strength Tablets and Caplets ... 860
Sinutab Sinus Medication, Maximum Strength Without Drowsiness Formula, Tablets & Caplets ... 860
Sinutab Sinus Medication, Regular Strength Without Drowsiness Formula ... 859
Sudafed Children's Liquid ... 861
Sudafed Cold and Cough Liquidcaps ... 862
Sudafed Cough Syrup ... 862
Sudafed Plus Liquid ... 862
Sudafed Plus Tablets ... 863
Sudafed Severe Cold Formula Caplets ... 863
Sudafed Severe Cold Formula Tablets ... 864
Sudafed Sinus Caplets ... 864
Sudafed Sinus Tablets ... 864
Sudafed Tablets, 30 mg ... 861
Sudafed Tablets, 60 mg ... 861
Sudafed 12 Hour Caplets ... 861
Syn-Rx Tablets ... 465
Syn-Rx DM Tablets ... 466
TheraFlu ... 787
TheraFlu Maximum Strength Nighttime Flu, Cold & Cough Medicine ... 788
TheraFlu Maximum Strength Non-Drowsy Formula Flu, Cold & Cough Medicine ... 788
Thera Flu Maximum Strength, Non-Drowsy Formula Flu, Cold and Cough Caplets ... 789
Triaminic AM Cough and Decongestant Formula ... 789
Triaminic AM Decongestant Formula ... 790
Triaminic Nite Light ... 791
Triaminic Sore Throat Formula ... 791
Tussend ... 1783
Tussend Expectorant ... 1785
Children's TYLENOL Cold Multi-Symptom Liquid Formula and Chewable Tablets ... 1561
Children's TYLENOL Cold Plus Cough Multi Symptom Tablets and Liquid ... 681
Infants' TYLENOL Cold Decongestant & Fever-Reducer Drops ... 1556
TYLENOL Maximum Strength Allergy Sinus Medication Gelcaps and Caplets ... 1563
TYLENOL Maximum Strength Allergy Sinus NightTime Medication Caplets ... 1555
TYLENOL Flu Maximum Strength Gelcaps ... 1565
TYLENOL Flu NightTime, Maximum Strength, Gelcaps ... 1566
TYLENOL Maximum Strength Flu NightTime Hot Medication Packets ... 1562
TYLENOL, Maximum Strength, Sinus Medication Geltabs, Gelcaps, Caplets and Tablets ... 1566
TYLENOL Cold Multi-Symptom Formula Medication Tablets and Caplets ... 1561
TYLENOL Cold Medication No Drowsiness Formula Gelcaps and Caplets ... 1562
TYLENOL Cold Multi-Symptom Hot Medication Liquid Packets ... 1557
TYLENOL Cough Multi-Symptom Medication with Decongestant ... 1565
Ursinus Inlay-Tabs ... 794
Vicks 44 LiquiCaps Cough, Cold & Flu Relief ... 755
Vicks 44 LiquiCaps Non-Drowsy Cough & Cold Relief ... 756
Vicks 44D Dry Hacking Cough & Head Congestion ... 755
Vicks 44M Cough, Cold & Flu Relief ... 756
Vicks DayQuil ... 761
Vicks DayQuil SINUS Pressure & PAIN Relief with IBUPROFEN ... 762
Vicks Nyquil Hot Therapy ... 762
Vicks NyQuil LiquiCaps Multi-Symptom Cold/Flu Relief ... 763
Vicks NyQuil Multi-Symptom Cold/Flu Relief - (Original & Cherry Flavor) ... 763

Pseudoephedrine Sulfate (Increases certain actions or side effects). Products include:
Cheracol Sinus ... 768
Chlor-Trimeton Allergy Decongestant Tablets ... 799
Claritin-D ... 2350
Drixoral Cold and Allergy Sustained-Action Tablets ... 802
Drixoral Cold and Flu Extended-Release Tablets ... 803
Drixoral Non-Drowsy Formula Extended-Release Tablets ... 803
Drixoral Allergy/Sinus Extended Release Tablets ... 804
Trinalin Repetabs Tablets ... 1330

Pyrilamine Maleate (Increases certain actions or side effects). Products include:
4-Way Fast Acting Nasal Spray (regular & mentholated) ... 621
Maximum Strength Multi-Symptom Formula Midol ... 722
PMS Multi-Symptom Formula Midol ... 723

Pyrilamine Tannate (Increases certain actions or side effects). Products include:
Atrohist Pediatric Suspension ... 454
Rynatan ... 2673

Quazepam (Increases certain actions or side effects). Products include:
Doral Tablets ... 2664

Quinidine Gluconate (Increases certain actions or side effects). Products include:
Quinaglute Dura-Tabs Tablets ... 649

Quinidine Polygalacturonate (Increases certain actions or side effects).
No products indexed under this heading.

Quinidine Sulfate (Increases certain actions or side effects). Products include:
Quinidex Extentabs ... 2067

Salmeterol Xinafoate (Increases certain actions or side effects). Products include:
Serevent Inhalation Aerosol ... 1176

Scopolamine (Increases certain actions or side effects). Products include:
Transderm Scōp Transdermal Therapeutic System ... 869

Scopolamine Hydrobromide (Increases certain actions or side effects). Products include:
Atrohist Plus Tablets ... 454
Donnatal ... 2060
Donnatal Extentabs ... 2061
Donnatal Tablets ... 2060

Selegiline Hydrochloride (Increases certain actions or side effects). Products include:
Eldepryl Tablets ... 2550

Sodium Bicarbonate (Interferes with the absorption). Products include:
Alka-Seltzer Effervescent Antacid and Pain Reliever ... 701
Alka-Seltzer Extra Strength Effervescent Antacid and Pain Reliever ... 703
Alka-Seltzer Gold Effervescent Antacid ... 703
Alka-Seltzer Lemon Lime Effervescent Antacid and Pain Reliever ... 703
Arm & Hammer Pure Baking Soda ... 627
Ceo-Two Rectal Suppositories ... 666
Citrocarbonate Antacid ... 770
Massengill Disposable Douches ... 820
Massengill Liquid Concentrate ... 820
NuLYTELY ... 689
Cherry Flavor NuLYTELY ... 689

Sufentanil Citrate (Increases certain actions or side effects). Products include:
Sufenta Injection ... 1309

Temazepam (Increases certain actions or side effects). Products include:
Restoril Capsules ... 2284

Terbutaline Sulfate (Increases certain actions or side effects). Products include:
Brethaire Inhaler ... 813
Brethine Ampuls ... 815
Brethine Tablets ... 814
Bricanyl Subcutaneous Injection ... 1502
Bricanyl Tablets ... 1503

Terfenadine (Increases certain actions or side effects). Products include:
Seldane Tablets ... 1536
Seldane-D Extended-Release Tablets ... 1538

Thioridazine Hydrochloride (Increases certain actions or side effects). Products include:
Mellaril ... 2269

Timolol Maleate (Effects of anti-glaucoma agents antagonized). Products include:
Blocadren Tablets ... 1614
Timolide Tablets ... 1748
Timoptic in Ocudose ... 1753
Timoptic Sterile Ophthalmic Solution ... 1751
Timoptic-XE ... 1755

Tranylcypromine Sulfate (Increases certain actions or side effects). Products include:
Parnate Tablets ... 2503

Triamcinolone (Concurrent use in the presence of increased intraocular pressure may be hazardous). Products include:
Aristocort Tablets ... 1022

Triamcinolone Acetonide (Concurrent use in the presence of increased intraocular pressure may be hazardous). Products include:
Aristocort A 0.025% Cream ... 1027
Aristocort A 0.5% Cream ... 1031
Aristocort A 0.1% Cream ... 1029
Aristocort A 0.1% Ointment ... 1030
Azmacort Oral Inhaler ... 2011
Nasacort Nasal Inhaler ... 2024

Triamcinolone Diacetate (Concurrent use in the presence of increased intraocular pressure may be hazardous). Products include:
Aristocort Suspension (Forte Parenteral) ... 1027
Aristocort Suspension (Intralesional) ... 1025

Triamcinolone Hexacetonide (Concurrent use in the presence of increased intraocular pressure may be hazardous). Products include:
Aristospan Suspension (Intra-articular) ... 1033
Aristospan Suspension (Intralesional) ... 1032

Triazolam (Increases certain actions or side effects). Products include:
Halcion Tablets ... 2611

Tridihexethyl Chloride (Increases certain actions or side effects).
No products indexed under this heading.

Trifluoperazine Hydrochloride (Increases certain actions or side effects). Products include:
Stelazine ... 2514

Trihexyphenidyl Hydrochloride (Increases certain actions or side effects). Products include:
Artane ... 1368

Trimeprazine Tartrate (Increases certain actions or side effects). Products include:
Temaril Tablets, Syrup and Spansule Extended-Release Capsules ... 483

Trimipramine Maleate (Increases certain actions or side effects). Products include:
Surmontil Capsules ... 2811

Tripelennamine Hydrochloride (Increases certain actions or side effects). Products include:
PBZ Tablets ... 845
PBZ-SR Tablets ... 844

Triprolidine Hydrochloride (Increases certain actions or side effects). Products include:
Actifed Plus Caplets ... 845
Actifed Plus Tablets ... 845
Actifed with Codeine Cough Syrup ... 1067
Actifed Syrup ... 846
Actifed Tablets ... 844

BENTYL INJECTION
(Dicyclomine Hydrochloride) ... 1501
See **Bentyl 10 mg Capsules**

BENTYL SYRUP
(Dicyclomine Hydrochloride) ... 1501
See **Bentyl 10 mg Capsules**

BENTYL 20 MG TABLETS
(Dicyclomine Hydrochloride) ... 1501
See **Bentyl 10 mg Capsules**

BENYLIN ADULT FORMULA COUGH SUPPRESSANT
(Dextromethorphan Hydrobromide) ... 852
May interact with monoamine oxidase inhibitors. Compounds in this category include:

Furazolidone (Concurrent and/or sequential use should be avoided). Products include:
Furoxone ... 2046

Isocarboxazid (Concurrent and/or sequential use should be avoided).
No products indexed under this heading.

Phenelzine Sulfate (Concurrent and/or sequential use should be avoided). Products include:
Nardil ... 1920

Selegiline Hydrochloride (Concurrent and/or sequential use should be avoided). Products include:
Eldepryl Tablets ... 2550

Tranylcypromine Sulfate (Concurrent and/or sequential use should be avoided). Products include:
Parnate Tablets ... 2503

BENYLIN EXPECTORANT
(Dextromethorphan Hydrobromide, Guaifenesin) ... 852
May interact with monoamine oxidase inhibitors. Compounds in this category include:

Furazolidone (Concurrent and/or sequential use is not recommended). Products include:
Furoxone ... 2046

Isocarboxazid (Concurrent and/or sequential use is not recommended).
No products indexed under this heading.

Phenelzine Sulfate (Concurrent and/or sequential use is not recommended). Products include:
Nardil ... 1920

Selegiline Hydrochloride (Concurrent and/or sequential use is not recommended). Products include:
Eldepryl Tablets ... 2550

Tranylcypromine Sulfate (Concurrent and/or sequential use is not recommended.). Products include:
Parnate Tablets ... 2503

BENYLIN MULTISYMPTOM
(Dextromethorphan Hydrobromide, Pseudoephedrine Hydrochloride, Guaifenesin) ... 852
May interact with monoamine oxi-

IMPORTANT NOTE: Always consult each drug listing in the patient's regimen for possible interactions.

Benylin Multisymptom

dase inhibitors. Compounds in this category include:

Furazolidone (Concurrent and/or sequential use is not recommended). Products include:

Furoxone 2046

Isocarboxazid (Concurrent and/or sequential use is not recommended). No products indexed under this heading.

Phenelzine Sulfate (Concurrent and/or sequential use is not recommended). Products include:

Nardil 1920

Selegiline Hydrochloride (Concurrent and/or sequential use is not recommended). Products include:

Eldepryl Tablets 2550

Tranylcypromine Sulfate (Concurrent and/or sequential use is not recommended). Products include:

Parnate Tablets 2503

BENYLIN PEDIATRIC COUGH SUPPRESSANT

(Dextromethorphan Hydrobromide) .... ⊞ 853

May interact with monoamine oxidase inhibitors. Compounds in this category include:

Furazolidone (Concurrent and/or sequential use should be avoided). Products include:

Furoxone 2046

Isocarboxazid (Concurrent and/or sequential use should be avoided). No products indexed under this heading.

Phenelzine Sulfate (Concurrent and/or sequential use should be avoided). Products include:

Nardil 1920

Selegiline Hydrochloride (Concurrent and/or sequential use should be avoided). Products include:

Eldepryl Tablets 2550

Tranylcypromine Sulfate (Concurrent and/or sequential use should be avoided). Products include:

Parnate Tablets 2503

BENZAC 5 & 10 GEL

(Benzoyl Peroxide) .... 1045 None cited in PDR database.

BENZAC AC 2½%, 5%, AND 10% WATER-BASE GEL

(Benzoyl Peroxide) .... 1045 None cited in PDR database.

BENZAC AC WASH 2½%, 5%, 10% WATER-BASE CLEANSER

(Benzoyl Peroxide) .... 1045 None cited in PDR database.

BENZAC W WASH 5 & 10 WATER-BASE CLEANSER

(Benzoyl Peroxide) .... 1045 None cited in PDR database.

BENZAC W 2½, 5 & 10 WATER-BASE GEL

(Benzoyl Peroxide) .... 1045 None cited in PDR database.

BENZAMYCIN TOPICAL GEL

(Erythromycin, Benzoyl Peroxide) ...... 905 May interact with:

Clindamycin Palmitate Hydrochloride (Erythromycin antagonist). No products indexed under this heading.

Clindamycin Phosphate (Erythromycin antagonist). Products include:

Cleocin Phosphate Injection 2586
Cleocin T Topical 2590
Cleocin Vaginal Cream......................... 2589

BENZASHAVE MEDICATED SHAVE CREAM 5% AND 10%

(Benzoyl Peroxide) .... 1590 None cited in PDR database.

BEROCCA PLUS TABLETS

(Vitamins with Minerals) .... 2087 May interact with:

Levodopa (Decreased efficacy). Products include:

Atamet 572
Larodopa Tablets 2129
Sinemet Tablets 943
Sinemet CR Tablets 944

BEROCCA TABLETS

(Vitamin B Complex With Vitamin C) 2087 May interact with:

Levodopa (Decreased efficacy). Products include:

Atamet 572
Larodopa Tablets 2129
Sinemet Tablets 943
Sinemet CR Tablets 944

BETADINE BRAND FIRST AID ANTIBIOTICS & MOISTURIZER OINTMENT

(Polymyxin B Sulfate, Bacitracin Zinc) .... 1991 None cited in PDR database.

BETADINE DISPOSABLE MEDICATED DOUCHE

(Povidone Iodine) .... 1992 None cited in PDR database.

BETADINE FIRST AID CREAM

(Povidone Iodine) .... 1991 None cited in PDR database.

BETADINE MEDICATED DOUCHE

(Povidone Iodine) .... 1992 None cited in PDR database.

BETADINE MEDICATED GEL

(Povidone Iodine) .... 1992 None cited in PDR database.

BETADINE MEDICATED VAGINAL SUPPOSITORIES

(Povidone Iodine) .... 1992 None cited in PDR database.

BETADINE OINTMENT

(Povidone Iodine) .... 1992 None cited in PDR database.

BETADINE PRE-MIXED MEDICATED DISPOSABLE DOUCHE

(Povidone Iodine) .... 1992 None cited in PDR database.

BETADINE SKIN CLEANSER

(Povidone Iodine) .... 1992 None cited in PDR database.

BETADINE SOLUTION

(Povidone Iodine) .... 1992 None cited in PDR database.

BETADINE 5% STERILE OPHTHALMIC PREP SOLUTION

(Povidone Iodine) .... ⊙ 274 None cited in PDR database.

BETADINE SURGICAL SCRUB

(Povidone Iodine) .... 1992 None cited in PDR database.

BETAGAN LIQUIFILM

(Levobunolol Hydrochloride) .... ⊙ 233

See BETAGAN Liquifilm with C CAP Compliance Cap

BETAGAN LIQUIFILM WITH C CAP COMPLIANCE CAP

(Levobunolol Hydrochloride) .... ⊙ 233

May interact with beta blockers, catecholamine depleting drugs, oral hypoglycemic agents, insulin, phenothiazines, sympathomimetic bronchodilators, calcium channel blockers, cardiac glycosides, and certain other agents. Compounds in these categories include:

Acebutolol Hydrochloride (Additive effects on systemic beta-blockade from concomitant therapy with orally administered beta-blockers). Products include:

Sectral Capsules 2807

Albuterol (Betagan may block bronchodilation produced by $beta_2$adrenergic agonists). Products include:

Proventil Inhalation Aerosol 2382
Ventolin Inhalation Aerosol and Refill 1197

Albuterol Sulfate (Betagan may block bronchodilation produced by $beta_2$adrenergic agonists). Products include:

Airet Solution for Inhalation 452
Proventil Inhalation Solution 0.083% 2384
Proventil Repetabs Tablets 2386
Proventil Solution for Inhalation 0.5% 2383
Proventil Syrup 2385
Proventil Tablets 2386
Ventolin Inhalation Solution 1198
Ventolin Nebules Inhalation Solution 1199
Ventolin Rotacaps for Inhalation 1200
Ventolin Syrup 1202
Ventolin Tablets 1203
Volmax Extended-Release Tablets .. 1788

Amlodipine Besylate (Concurrent use with either oral or intravenous calcium antagonists may produce AV conduction disturbances, LVF and hypotension). Products include:

Lotrel Capsules 840
Norvasc Tablets 1940

Atenolol (Additive effects on systemic beta-blockade from concomitant therapy with orally administered beta-blockers). Products include:

Tenoretic Tablets 2845
Tenormin Tablets and I.V. Injection 2847

Bepridil Hydrochloride (Concurrent use with either oral or intravenous calcium antagonists may produce AV conduction disturbances, LVF and hypotension). Products include:

Vascor (200, 300 and 400 mg) Tablets 1587

Betaxolol Hydrochloride (Additive effects on systemic beta-blockade from concomitant therapy with orally administered beta-blockers). Products include:

Betoptic Ophthalmic Solution 469
Betoptic S Ophthalmic Suspension 471

Kerlone Tablets 2436

Bisoprolol Fumarate (Additive effects on systemic beta-blockade from concomitant therapy with orally administered beta-blockers). Products include:

Zebeta Tablets 1413
Ziac 1415

Bitolterol Mesylate (Betagan may block bronchodilation produced by $beta_2$adrenergic agonists). Products include:

Tornalate Solution for Inhalation, 0.2% 956
Tornalate Metered Dose Inhaler 957

Chlorpromazine (Possible additive hypotensive effects). Products include:

Thorazine Suppositories 2523

Chlorpropamide (Beta-blockers may mask the signs and symptoms of acute hypoglycemia). Products include:

Diabinese Tablets 1935

Deserpidine (Possible additive effects and production of hypotension and/or bradycardia).

No products indexed under this heading.

Deslanoside (Concomitant use with digitalis and calcium antagonists may result in additive effects on prolonging AV conduction time).

No products indexed under this heading.

Digitoxin (Concomitant use with digitalis and calcium antagonists may result in additive effects on prolonging AV conduction time). Products include:

Crystodigin Tablets 1433

Digoxin (Concomitant use with digitalis and calcium antagonists may result in additive effects on prolonging AV conduction time). Products include:

Lanoxicaps 1117
Lanoxin Elixir Pediatric 1120
Lanoxin Injection 1123
Lanoxin Injection Pediatric 1126
Lanoxin Tablets 1128

Diltiazem Hydrochloride (Concurrent use with either oral or intravenous calcium antagonists may produce AV conduction disturbances, LVF and hypotension). Products include:

Cardizem CD Capsules 1506
Cardizem SR Capsules 1510
Cardizem Injectable 1508
Cardizem Tablets 1512
Dilacor XR Extended-release Capsules 2018

Epinephrine (Mydriasis may result from concomitant ocular therapy). Products include:

Bronkaid Mist .... ⊞ 717
EPIFRIN .... ⊙ 239
EpiPen 790
Marcaine Hydrochloride with Epinephrine 1:200,000 2316
Primatene Mist .... ⊞ 873
Sensorcaine with Epinephrine Injection 559
Sus-Phrine Injection 1019
Xylocaine with Epinephrine Injections 567

Epinephrine Bitartrate (Mydriasis may result from concomitant ocular therapy). Products include:

Bronkaid Mist Suspension .... ⊞ 718
Sensorcaine-MPF with Epinephrine Injection 559

Epinephrine Hydrochloride (Mydriasis may result from concomitant ocular therapy). Products include:

Ana-Kit Anaphylaxis Emergency Treatment Kit 617

(⊞ Described in PDR For Nonprescription Drugs)

(⊙ Described in PDR For Ophthalmology)

117 Interactions Index Betapace

Esmolol Hydrochloride (Additive effects on systemic beta-blockade from concomitant therapy with orally administered beta-blockers). Products include:
- Brevibloc Injection ... 1808

Felodipine (Concurrent use with either oral or intravenous calcium antagonists may produce AV conduction disturbances, LVF and hypotension). Products include:
- Plendil Extended-Release Tablets ... 527

Fluphenazine Decanoate (Possible additive hypotensive effects). Products include:
- Prolixin Decanoate ... 509

Fluphenazine Enanthate (Possible additive hypotensive effects). Products include:
- Prolixin Enanthate ... 509

Fluphenazine Hydrochloride (Possible additive hypotensive effects). Products include:
- Prolixin ... 509

Glipizide (Beta-blockers may mask the signs and symptoms of acute hypoglycemia). Products include:
- Glucotrol Tablets ... 1967
- Glucotrol XL Extended Release Tablets ... 1968

Glyburide (Beta-blockers may mask the signs and symptoms of acute hypoglycemia). Products include:
- DiaBeta Tablets ... 1239
- Glynase PresTab Tablets ... 2609
- Micronase Tablets ... 2623

Guanethidine Monosulfate (Possible additive effects and production of hypotension and/or bradycardia). Products include:
- Esimil Tablets ... 822
- Ismelin Tablets ... 827

Insulin, Human (Beta-blockers may mask the signs and symptoms of acute hypoglycemia).
- No products indexed under this heading.

Insulin, Human Isophane Suspension (Beta-blockers may mask the signs and symptoms of acute hypoglycemia). Products include:
- Novolin N Human Insulin 10 ml Vials ... 1795

Insulin, Human NPH (Beta-blockers may mask the signs and symptoms of acute hypoglycemia). Products include:
- Humulin N, 100 Units ... 1448
- Novolin N PenFill Cartridges Durable Insulin Delivery System ... 1798
- Novolin N Prefilled Syringe Disposable Insulin Delivery System ... 1798

Insulin, Human Regular (Beta-blockers may mask the signs and symptoms of acute hypoglycemia). Products include:
- Humulin R, 100 Units ... 1449
- Novolin R Human Insulin 10 ml Vials ... 1795
- Novolin R PenFill Cartridges Durable Insulin Delivery System ... 1798
- Novolin R Prefilled Syringe Disposable Insulin Delivery System ... 1798
- Velosulin BR Human Insulin 10 ml Vials ... 1795

Insulin, Human, Zinc Suspension (Beta-blockers may mask the signs and symptoms of acute hypoglycemia). Products include:
- Humulin L, 100 Units ... 1446
- Humulin U, 100 Units ... 1450
- Novolin L Human Insulin 10 ml Vials ... 1795

Insulin, NPH (Beta-blockers may mask the signs and symptoms of acute hypoglycemia). Products include:
- NPH, 100 Units ... 1450
- Pork NPH, 100 Units ... 1452
- Purified Pork NPH Isophane Insulin ... 1801

Insulin, Regular (Beta-blockers may mask the signs and symptoms of acute hypoglycemia). Products include:
- Regular, 100 Units ... 1450
- Pork Regular, 100 Units ... 1452
- Pork Regular (Concentrated), 500 Units ... 1453
- Purified Pork Regular Insulin ... 1801

Insulin, Zinc Crystals (Beta-blockers may mask the signs and symptoms of acute hypoglycemia). Products include:
- NPH, 100 Units ... 1450

Insulin, Zinc Suspension (Beta-blockers may mask the signs and symptoms of acute hypoglycemia). Products include:
- Iletin I ... 1450
- Lente, 100 Units ... 1450
- Iletin II ... 1452
- Pork Lente, 100 Units ... 1452
- Purified Pork Lente Insulin ... 1801

Isoproterenol Hydrochloride (Betagan may block bronchodilation produced by $beta_2$adrenergic agonists). Products include:
- Isuprel Hydrochloride Injection 1:5000 ... 2311
- Isuprel Hydrochloride Solution 1:200 & 1:100 ... 2313
- Isuprel Mistometer ... 2312

Isoproterenol Sulfate (Betagan may block bronchodilation produced by $beta_2$adrenergic agonists). Products include:
- Norisodrine with Calcium Iodide Syrup ... 442

Isradipine (Concurrent use with either oral or intravenous calcium antagonists may produce AV conduction disturbances, LVF and hypotension). Products include:
- DynaCirc Capsules ... 2256

Labetalol Hydrochloride (Additive effects on systemic beta-blockade from concomitant therapy with orally administered beta-blockers). Products include:
- Normodyne Injection ... 2377
- Normodyne Tablets ... 2379
- Trandate ... 1185

Mesoridazine Besylate (Possible additive hypotensive effects). Products include:
- Serentil ... 684

Metaproterenol Sulfate (Betagan may block bronchodilation produced by $beta_2$adrenergic agonists). Products include:
- Alupent ... 669
- Metaproterenol Sulfate Inhalation Solution, USP, Arm-a-Med ... 552

Methotrimeprazine (Possible additive hypotensive effects). Products include:
- Levoprome ... 1274

Metipranolol Hydrochloride (Additive effects on systemic beta-blockade from concomitant therapy with orally administered beta-blockers). Products include:
- OptiPranolol (Metipranolol 0.3%) Sterile Ophthalmic Solution ... ◉ 258

Metoprolol Succinate (Additive effects on systemic beta-blockade from concomitant therapy with orally administered beta-blockers). Products include:
- Toprol-XL Tablets ... 565

Metoprolol Tartrate (Additive effects on systemic beta-blockade from concomitant therapy with orally administered beta-blockers). Products include:
- Lopressor Ampuls ... 830
- Lopressor HCT Tablets ... 832
- Lopressor Tablets ... 830

Nadolol (Additive effects on systemic beta-blockade from concomitant therapy with orally administered beta-blockers).
- No products indexed under this heading.

Nicardipine Hydrochloride (Concurrent use with either oral or intravenous calcium antagonists may produce AV conduction disturbances, LVF and hypotension). Products include:
- Cardene Capsules ... 2095
- Cardene I.V. ... 2709
- Cardene SR Capsules ... 2097

Nifedipine (Concurrent use with either oral or intravenous calcium antagonists may produce AV conduction disturbances, LVF and hypotension). Products include:
- Adalat Capsules (10 mg and 20 mg) ... 587
- Adalat CC ... 589
- Procardia Capsules ... 1971
- Procardia XL Extended Release Tablets ... 1972

Nimodipine (Concurrent use with either oral or intravenous calcium antagonists may produce AV conduction disturbances, LVF and hypotension). Products include:
- Nimotop Capsules ... 610

Nisoldipine (Concurrent use with either oral or intravenous calcium antagonists may produce AV conduction disturbances, LVF and hypotension).
- No products indexed under this heading.

Perphenazine (Possible additive hypotensive effects). Products include:
- Etrafon ... 2355
- Triavil Tablets ... 1757
- Trilafon ... 2389

Pindolol (Additive effects on systemic beta-blockade from concomitant therapy with orally administered beta-blockers). Products include:
- Visken Tablets ... 2299

Pirbuterol Acetate (Betagan may block bronchodilation produced by $beta_2$adrenergic agonists). Products include:
- Maxair Autohaler ... 1492
- Maxair Inhaler ... 1494

Prochlorperazine (Possible additive hypotensive effects). Products include:
- Compazine ... 2470

Promethazine Hydrochloride (Possible additive hypotensive effects). Products include:
- Mepergan Injection ... 2753
- Phenergan with Codeine ... 2777
- Phenergan with Dextromethorphan ... 2778
- Phenergan Injection ... 2773
- Phenergan Suppositories ... 2775
- Phenergan Syrup ... 2774
- Phenergan Tablets ... 2775
- Phenergan VC ... 2779
- Phenergan VC with Codeine ... 2781

Propranolol Hydrochloride (Additive effects on systemic beta-blockade from concomitant therapy with orally administered beta-blockers). Products include:
- Inderal ... 2728
- Inderal LA Long Acting Capsules ... 2730
- Inderide Tablets ... 2732
- Inderide LA Long Acting Capsules ... 2734

Rauwolfia Serpentina (Possible additive effects and production of hypotension and/or bradycardia).
- No products indexed under this heading.

Rescinnamine (Possible additive effects and production of hypotension and/or bradycardia).
- No products indexed under this heading.

Reserpine (Possible additive effects and production of hypotension and/or bradycardia). Products include:
- Diupres Tablets ... 1650
- Hydropres Tablets ... 1675
- Ser-Ap-Es Tablets ... 849

Salmeterol Xinafoate (Betagan may block bronchodilation produced by $beta_2$adrenergic agonists). Products include:
- Serevent Inhalation Aerosol ... 1176

Sotalol Hydrochloride (Additive effects on systemic beta-blockade from concomitant therapy with orally administered beta-blockers). Products include:
- Betapace Tablets ... 641

Terbutaline Sulfate (Betagan may block bronchodilation produced by $beta_2$adrenergic agonists). Products include:
- Brethaire Inhaler ... 813
- Brethine Ampuls ... 815
- Brethine Tablets ... 814
- Bricanyl Subcutaneous Injection ... 1502
- Bricanyl Tablets ... 1503

Thioridazine Hydrochloride (Possible additive hypotensive effects). Products include:
- Mellaril ... 2269

Timolol Hemihydrate (Additive effects on systemic beta-blockade from concomitant therapy with orally administered beta-blockers). Products include:
- Betimol 0.25%, 0.5% ... ◉ 261

Timolol Maleate (Additive effects on systemic beta-blockade from concomitant therapy with orally administered beta-blockers). Products include:
- Blocadren Tablets ... 1614
- Timolide Tablets ... 1748
- Timoptic in Ocudose ... 1753
- Timoptic Sterile Ophthalmic Solution ... 1751
- Timoptic-XE ... 1755

Tolazamide (Beta-blockers may mask the signs and symptoms of acute hypoglycemia).
- No products indexed under this heading.

Tolbutamide (Beta-blockers may mask the signs and symptoms of acute hypoglycemia).
- No products indexed under this heading.

Trifluoperazine Hydrochloride (Possible additive hypotensive effects). Products include:
- Stelazine ... 2514

Verapamil Hydrochloride (Concurrent use with either oral or intravenous calcium antagonists may produce AV conduction disturbances, LVF and hypotension). Products include:
- Calan SR Caplets ... 2422
- Calan Tablets ... 2419
- Isoptin Injectable ... 1344
- Isoptin Oral Tablets ... 1346
- Isoptin SR Tablets ... 1348
- Verelan Capsules ... 1410
- Verelan Capsules ... 2824

BETAPACE TABLETS

(Sotalol Hydrochloride) ... 641

May interact with drugs that prolong the qt interval, cardiac glycosides, calcium channel blockers, catecholamine depleting drugs, insulin, oral hypoglycemic agents, $beta_2$ agonists, antiarrhythmics, and certain other

IMPORTANT NOTE: Always consult each drug listing in the patient's regimen for possible interactions.

agents. Compounds in these categories include:

Acarbose (Potential for hyperglycemia; symptoms of hypoglycemia may be masked; dosage of antidiabetic drugs may require adjustment).
- No products indexed under this heading.

Acebutolol Hydrochloride (Potential for prolonged refractoriness; concomitant therapy is not recommended). Products include:
- Sectral Capsules 2807

Adenosine (Potential for prolonged refractoriness; concomitant therapy is not recommended). Products include:
- Adenocard Injection 1021
- Adenoscan 1024

Albuterol (Beta-agonist may have to be administered in increased dosage when used concomitantly). Products include:
- Proventil Inhalation Aerosol 2382
- Ventolin Inhalation Aerosol and Refill 1197

Albuterol Sulfate (Beta-agonist may have to be administered in increased dosage when used concomitantly). Products include:
- Airet Solution for Inhalation 452
- Proventil Inhalation Solution 0.083% 2384
- Proventil Repetabs Tablets 2386
- Proventil Solution for Inhalation 0.5% 2383
- Proventil Syrup 2385
- Proventil Tablets 2386
- Ventolin Inhalation Solution 1198
- Ventolin Nebules Inhalation Solution 1199
- Ventolin Rotacaps for Inhalation 1200
- Ventolin Syrup 1202
- Ventolin Tablets 1203
- Volmax Extended-Release Tablets .. 1788

Amiodarone Hydrochloride (Potential for prolonged refractoriness; concomitant therapy is not recommended; caution is advised if used concurrently due to sotalol's effect on cardiac repolarization (QT*c* prolongation) torsade de pointes, a polymorphic ventricular tachycardia with prolonged QT interval). Products include:
- Cordarone Intravenous 2715
- Cordarone Tablets 2712

Amitriptyline Hydrochloride (Caution is advised if used concurrently due to sotalol's effect on cardiac repolarization (QT*c* prolongation) torsade de pointes, a polymorphic ventricular tachycardia with prolonged QT interval). Products include:
- Elavil 2838
- Endep Tablets 2174
- Etrafon 2355
- Limbitrol 2180
- Triavil Tablets 1757

Amlodipine Besylate (Possible additive effects on AV conduction or ventricular conduction; co-administration may result in hypotension). Products include:
- Lotrel Capsules 840
- Norvasc Tablets 1940

Amoxapine (Caution is advised if used concurrently due to sotalol's effect on cardiac repolarization (QT*c* prolongation) torsade de pointes, a polymorphic ventricular tachycardia with prolonged QT interval). Products include:
- Asendin Tablets 1369

Astemizole (Caution is advised if used concurrently due to sotalol's effect on cardiac repolarization (QT*c* prolongation) torsade de pointes, a polymorphic ventricular tachycardia with prolonged QT interval). Products include:
- Hismanal Tablets 1293

Bepridil Hydrochloride (Possible additive effects on AV conduction or ventricular conduction; co-administration may result in hypotension). Products include:
- Vascor (200, 300 and 400 mg) Tablets 1587

Bitolterol Mesylate (Beta-agonist may have to be administered in increased dosage when used concomitantly). Products include:
- Tornalate Solution for Inhalation, 0.2% 956
- Tornalate Metered Dose Inhaler 957

Bretylium Tosylate (Potential for prolonged refractoriness; concomitant therapy is not recommended; caution is advised if used concurrently due to sotalol's effect on cardiac repolarization (QT*c* prolongation) torsade de pointes, a polymorphic ventricular tachycardia with prolonged QT interval).
- No products indexed under this heading.

Chlorpromazine (Caution is advised if used concurrently due to sotalol's effect on cardiac repolarization (QT*c* prolongation) torsade de pointes, a polymorphic ventricular tachycardia with prolonged QT interval). Products include:
- Thorazine Suppositories 2523

Chlorpromazine Hydrochloride (Caution is advised if used concurrently due to sotalol's effect on cardiac repolarization (QT*c* prolongation) torsade de pointes, a polymorphic ventricular tachycardia with prolonged QT interval). Products include:
- Thorazine 2523

Chlorpropamide (Potential for hyperglycemia; symptoms of hypoglycemia may be masked; dosage of antidiabetic drugs may require adjustment). Products include:
- Diabinese Tablets 1935

Clomipramine Hydrochloride (Caution is advised if used concurrently due to sotalol's effect on cardiac repolarization (QT*c* prolongation) torsade de pointes, a polymorphic ventricular tachycardia with prolonged QT interval). Products include:
- Anafranil Capsules 803

Clonidine (Beta-blocking drugs may potentiate the rebound hypertension sometimes observed after discontinuation of clonidine). Products include:
- Catapres-TTS 675

Clonidine Hydrochloride (Beta-blocking drugs may potentiate the rebound hypertension sometimes observed after discontinuation of clonidine). Products include:
- Catapres Tablets 674
- Combipres Tablets 677

Deserpidine (Produces an excessive reduction of resting sympathetic nervous tone).
- No products indexed under this heading.

Desipramine Hydrochloride (Caution is advised if used concurrently due to sotalol's effect on cardiac repolarization (QT*c* prolongation) torsade de pointes, a polymorphic ventricular tachycardia with prolonged QT interval). Products include:
- Norpramin Tablets 1526

Deslanoside (Potential for proarrhythmic events when co-administered).
- No products indexed under this heading.

Digitoxin (Potential for proarrhythmic events when co-administered). Products include:
- Crystodigin Tablets 1433

Digoxin (Potential for proarrhythmic events when co-administered). Products include:
- Lanoxicaps 1117
- Lanoxin Elixir Pediatric 1120
- Lanoxin Injection 1123
- Lanoxin Injection Pediatric 1126
- Lanoxin Tablets 1128

Diltiazem Hydrochloride (Possible additive effects on AV conduction or ventricular conduction; co-administration may result in hypotension). Products include:
- Cardizem CD Capsules 1506
- Cardizem SR Capsules 1510
- Cardizem Injectable 1508
- Cardizem Tablets 1512
- Dilacor XR Extended-release Capsules 2018

Disopyramide Phosphate (Potential for prolonged refractoriness; concomitant therapy is not recommended; caution is advised if used concurrently due to sotalol's effect on cardiac repolarization (QT*c* prolongation) torsade de pointes, a polymorphic ventricular tachycardia with prolonged QT interval). Products include:
- Norpace 2444

Doxepin Hydrochloride (Caution is advised if used concurrently due to sotalol's effect on cardiac repolarization (QT*c* prolongation) torsade de pointes, a polymorphic ventricular tachycardia with prolonged QT interval). Products include:
- Sinequan 2205
- Zonalon Cream 1055

Ephedrine Hydrochloride (Beta-agonist may have to be administered in increased dosage when used concomitantly). Products include:
- Primatene Dual Action Formula .... ▣ 872
- Primatene Tablets .... ▣ 873
- Quadrinal Tablets 1350

Ephedrine Sulfate (Beta-agonist may have to be administered in increased dosage when used concomitantly). Products include:
- Bronkaid Caplets .... ▣ 717
- Marax Tablets & DF Syrup 2200

Ephedrine Tannate (Beta-agonist may have to be administered in increased dosage when used concomitantly). Products include:
- Rynatuss 2673

Epinephrine (Beta-agonist may have to be administered in increased dosage when used concomitantly). Products include:
- Bronkaid Mist .... ▣ 717
- EPIFRIN .... ◉ 239
- EpiPen 790
- Marcaine Hydrochloride with Epinephrine 1:200,000 2316
- Primatene Mist .... ▣ 873
- Sensorcaine with Epinephrine Injection 559
- Sus-Phrine Injection 1019
- Xylocaine with Epinephrine Injections 567

Epinephrine Hydrochloride (Beta-agonist may have to be administered in increased dosage when used concomitantly; potential for unresponsiveness to the usual dose of epinephrine to treat allergic reaction). Products include:
- Ana-Kit Anaphylaxis Emergency Treatment Kit 617

Ethylnorepinephrine Hydrochloride (Beta-agonist may have to be administered in increased dosage when used concomitantly).
- No products indexed under this heading.

Felodipine (Possible additive effects on AV conduction or ventricular conduction; co-administration may result in hypotension). Products include:
- Plendil Extended-Release Tablets 527

Flecainide Acetate (Potential for prolonged refractoriness; concomitant therapy is not recommended; caution is advised if used concurrently due to sotalol's effect on cardiac repolarization (QT*c* prolongation) torsade de pointes, a polymorphic ventricular tachycardia with prolonged QT interval). Products include:
- Tambocor Tablets 1497

Fluphenazine Decanoate (Caution is advised if used concurrently due to sotalol's effect on cardiac repolarization (QT*c* prolongation) torsade de pointes, a polymorphic ventricular tachycardia with prolonged QT interval). Products include:
- Prolixin Decanoate 509

Fluphenazine Enanthate (Caution is advised if used concurrently due to sotalol's effect on cardiac repolarization (QT*c* prolongation) torsade de pointes, a polymorphic ventricular tachycardia with prolonged QT interval). Products include:
- Prolixin Enanthate 509

Fluphenazine Hydrochloride (Caution is advised if used concurrently due to sotalol's effect on cardiac repolarization (QT*c* prolongation) torsade de pointes, a polymorphic ventricular tachycardia with prolonged QT interval). Products include:
- Prolixin 509

Glipizide (Potential for hyperglycemia; symptoms of hypoglycemia may be masked; dosage of antidiabetic drugs may require adjustment). Products include:
- Glucotrol Tablets 1967
- Glucotrol XL Extended Release Tablets 1968

Glyburide (Potential for hyperglycemia; symptoms of hypoglycemia may be masked; dosage of antidiabetic drugs may require adjustment). Products include:
- DiaBeta Tablets 1239
- Glynase PresTab Tablets 2609
- Micronase Tablets 2623

Guanethidine Monosulfate (Produces an excessive reduction of resting sympathetic nervous tone). Products include:
- Esimil Tablets 822
- Ismelin Tablets 827

(▣ Described in PDR For Nonprescription Drugs) (◉ Described in PDR For Ophthalmology)

Interactions Index

Imipramine Hydrochloride
(Caution is advised if used concurrently due to sotalol's effect on cardiac repolarization (QTc prolongation) torsade de pointes, a polymorphic ventricular tachycardia with prolonged QT interval). Products include:

Tofranil Ampuls 854
Tofranil Tablets 856

Imipramine Pamoate
(Caution is advised if used concurrently due to sotalol's effect on cardiac repolarization (QTc prolongation) torsade de pointes, a polymorphic ventricular tachycardia with prolonged QT interval). Products include:

Tofranil-PM Capsules 857

Insulin, Human
(Potential for hyperglycemia; symptoms of hypoglycemia may be masked; dosage of insulin may require adjustment).

No products indexed under this heading.

Insulin, Human Isophane Suspension
(Potential for hyperglycemia; symptoms of hypoglycemia may be masked; dosage of insulin may require adjustment). Products include:

Novolin N Human Insulin 10 ml Vials 1795

Insulin, Human NPH
(Potential for hyperglycemia; symptoms of hypoglycemia may be masked; dosage of insulin may require adjustment). Products include:

Humulin N, 100 Units 1448
Novolin N PenFill Cartridges Durable Insulin Delivery System 1798
Novolin N Prefilled Syringe Disposable Insulin Delivery System 1798

Insulin, Human Regular
(Potential for hyperglycemia; symptoms of hypoglycemia may be masked; dosage of insulin may require adjustment). Products include:

Humulin R, 100 Units 1449
Novolin R Human Insulin 10 ml Vials 1795
Novolin R PenFill Cartridges Durable Insulin Delivery System 1798
Novolin R Prefilled Syringe Disposable Insulin Delivery System 1798
Velosulin BR Human Insulin 10 ml Vials 1795

Insulin, Human, Zinc Suspension
(Potential for hyperglycemia; symptoms of hypoglycemia may be masked; dosage of insulin may require adjustment). Products include:

Humulin L, 100 Units 1446
Humulin U, 100 Units 1450
Novolin L Human Insulin 10 ml Vials 1795

Insulin, NPH
(Potential for hyperglycemia; symptoms of hypoglycemia may be masked; dosage of insulin may require adjustment). Products include:

NPH, 100 Units 1450
Pork NPH, 100 Units 1452
Purified Pork NPH Isophane Insulin 1801

Insulin, Regular
(Potential for hyperglycemia; symptoms of hypoglycemia may be masked; dosage of insulin may require adjustment). Products include:

Regular, 100 Units 1450
Pork Regular, 100 Units 1452
Pork Regular (Concentrated), 500 Units 1453
Purified Pork Regular Insulin 1801

Insulin, Zinc Crystals
(Potential for hyperglycemia; symptoms of hypoglycemia may be masked; dosage of insulin may require adjustment). Products include:

NPH, 100 Units 1450

Insulin, Zinc Suspension
(Potential for hyperglycemia; symptoms of hypoglycemia may be masked; dosage of insulin may require adjustment). Products include:

Iletin I 1450
Lente, 100 Units 1450
Iletin II 1452
Pork Lente, 100 Units 1452
Purified Pork Lente Insulin 1801

Isoetharine
(Beta-agonist may have to be administered in increased dosage when used concomitantly). Products include:

Bronkometer Aerosol 2302
Bronkosol Solution 2302
Isoetharine Inhalation Solution, USP, Arm-a-Med 551

Isoproterenol Hydrochloride
(Beta-agonist may have to be administered in increased dosage when used concomitantly). Products include:

Isuprel Hydrochloride Injection 1:5000 2311
Isuprel Hydrochloride Solution 1:200 & 1:100 2313
Isuprel Mistometer 2312

Isoproterenol Sulfate
(Beta-agonist may have to be administered in increased dosage when used concomitantly). Products include:

Norisodrine with Calcium Iodide Syrup 442

Isradipine
(Possible additive effects on AV conduction or ventricular conduction; co-administration may result in hypotension). Products include:

DynaCirc Capsules 2256

Lidocaine Hydrochloride
(Potential for prolonged refractoriness; concomitant therapy is not recommended; caution is advised if used concurrently due to sotalol's effect on cardiac repolarization (QTc prolongation) torsade de pointes, a polymorphic ventricular tachycardia with prolonged QT interval). Products include:

Bactine Antiseptic/Anesthetic First Aid Liquid .... ᴮᴰ 708
Campho-Phenique Maximum Strength First Aid Antibiotic Plus Pain Reliever Ointment .... ᴮᴰ 719
Decadron Phosphate with Xylocaine Injection, Sterile 1639
Xylocaine Injections 567

Maprotiline Hydrochloride
(Caution is advised if used concurrently due to sotalol's effect on cardiac repolarization (QTc prolongation) torsade de pointes, a polymorphic ventricular tachycardia with prolonged QT interval). Products include:

Ludiomil Tablets 843

Mesoridazine
(Caution is advised if used concurrently due to sotalol's effect on cardiac repolarization (QTc prolongation) torsade de pointes, a polymorphic ventricular tachycardia with prolonged QT interval).

Metaproterenol Sulfate
(Beta-agonist may have to be administered in increased dosage when used concomitantly). Products include:

Alupent 669
Metaproterenol Sulfate Inhalation Solution, USP, Arm-a-Med 552

Metformin Hydrochloride
(Potential for hyperglycemia; symptoms of hypoglycemia may be masked; dosage of antidiabetic drugs may require adjustment). Products include:

Glucophage 752

Mexiletine Hydrochloride
(Potential for prolonged refractoriness; concomitant therapy is not recommended; caution is advised if used concurrently due to sotalol's effect on cardiac repolarization (QTc prolongation) torsade de pointes, a polymorphic ventricular tachycardia with prolonged QT interval). Products include:

Mexitil Capsules 678

Moricizine Hydrochloride
(Potential for prolonged refractoriness; concomitant therapy is not recommended). Products include:

Ethmozine Tablets 2041

Nicardipine Hydrochloride
(Possible additive effects on AV conduction or ventricular conduction; co-administration may result in hypotension). Products include:

Cardene Capsules 2095
Cardene I.V. 2709
Cardene SR Capsules 2097

Nifedipine
(Possible additive effects on AV conduction or ventricular conduction; co-administration may result in hypotension). Products include:

Adalat Capsules (10 mg and 20 mg) 587
Adalat CC 589
Procardia Capsules 1971
Procardia XL Extended Release Tablets 1972

Nimodipine
(Possible additive effects on AV conduction or ventricular conduction; co-administration may result in hypotension). Products include:

Nimotop Capsules 610

Nisoldipine
(Possible additive effects on AV conduction or ventricular conduction; co-administration may result in hypotension).

No products indexed under this heading.

Nortriptyline Hydrochloride
(Caution is advised if used concurrently due to sotalol's effect on cardiac repolarization (QTc prolongation) torsade de pointes, a polymorphic ventricular tachycardia with prolonged QT interval). Products include:

Pamelor 2280

Perphenazine
(Caution is advised if used concurrently due to sotalol's effect on cardiac repolarization (QTc prolongation) torsade de pointes, a polymorphic ventricular tachycardia with prolonged QT interval). Products include:

Etrafon 2355
Triavil Tablets 1757
Trilafon 2389

Pirbuterol Acetate
(Beta-agonist may have to be administered in increased dosage when used concomitantly). Products include:

Maxair Autohaler 1492
Maxair Inhaler 1494

Procainamide Hydrochloride
(Potential for prolonged refractoriness; concomitant therapy is not recommended; caution is advised if used concurrently due to sotalol's effect on cardiac repolarization (QTc prolongation) torsade de pointes, a polymorphic ventricular tachycardia with prolonged QT interval). Products include:

Procan SR Tablets 1926

Prochlorperazine
(Caution is advised if used concurrently due to sotalol's effect on cardiac repolarization (QTc prolongation) torsade de pointes, a polymorphic ventricular tachycardia with prolonged QT interval). Products include:

Compazine 2470

Promethazine Hydrochloride
(Caution is advised if used concurrently due to sotalol's effect on cardiac repolarization (QTc prolongation) torsade de pointes, a polymorphic ventricular tachycardia with prolonged QT interval). Products include:

Mepergan Injection 2753
Phenergan with Codeine 2777
Phenergan with Dextromethorphan 2778
Phenergan Injection 2773
Phenergan Suppositories 2775
Phenergan Syrup 2774
Phenergan Tablets 2775
Phenergan VC 2779
Phenergan VC with Codeine 2781

Propafenone Hydrochloride
(Potential for prolonged refractoriness; concomitant therapy is not recommended; caution is advised if used concurrently due to sotalol's effect on cardiac repolarization (QTc prolongation) torsade de pointes, a polymorphic ventricular tachycardia with prolonged QT interval). Products include:

Rythmol Tablets–150mg, 225mg, 300mg 1352

Propranolol Hydrochloride
(Potential for prolonged refractoriness; concomitant therapy is not recommended). Products include:

Inderal 2728
Inderal LA Long Acting Capsules 2730
Inderide Tablets 2732
Inderide LA Long Acting Capsules .. 2734

Protriptyline Hydrochloride
(Caution is advised if used concurrently due to sotalol's effect on cardiac repolarization (QTc prolongation) torsade de pointes, a polymorphic ventricular tachycardia with prolonged QT interval). Products include:

Vivactil Tablets 1774

Quinidine Gluconate
(Potential for prolonged refractoriness; concomitant therapy is not recommended; caution is advised if used concurrently due to sotalol's effect on cardiac repolarization (QTc prolongation) torsade de pointes, a polymorphic ventricular tachycardia with prolonged QT interval). Products include:

Quinaglute Dura-Tabs Tablets 649

Quinidine Polygalacturonate
(Potential for prolonged refractoriness; concomitant therapy is not recommended; caution is advised if used concurrently due to sotalol's effect on cardiac repolarization (QTc prolongation) torsade de pointes, a polymorphic ventricular tachycardia with prolonged QT interval).

No products indexed under this heading.

Quinidine Sulfate
(Potential for prolonged refractoriness; concomitant therapy is not recommended; caution is advised if used concurrently due to sotalol's effect on cardiac repolarization (QTc prolongation) torsade de pointes, a polymorphic ventricular tachycardia with prolonged QT interval). Products include:

Quinidex Extentabs 2067

IMPORTANT NOTE: Always consult each drug listing in the patient's regimen for possible interactions.

Rauwolfia Serpentina (Produces an excessive reduction of resting sympathetic nervous tone).
No products indexed under this heading.

Rescinnamine (Produces an excessive reduction of resting sympathetic nervous tone).
No products indexed under this heading.

Reserpine (Produces an excessive reduction of resting sympathetic nervous tone). Products include:
- Diupres Tablets 1650
- Hydropres Tablets 1675
- Ser-Ap-Es Tablets 849

Salmeterol Xinafoate (Beta-agonist may have to be administered in increased dosage when used concomitantly). Products include:
- Serevent Inhalation Aerosol 1176

Terbutaline Sulfate (Beta-agonist may have to be administered in increased dosage when used concomitantly). Products include:
- Brethaire Inhaler 813
- Brethine Ampuls 815
- Brethine Tablets 814
- Bricanyl Subcutaneous Injection 1502
- Bricanyl Tablets 1503

Terfenadine (Caution is advised if used concurrently due to sotalol's effect on cardiac repolarization (QT*c* prolongation) torsade de pointes, a polymorphic ventricular tachycardia with prolonged QT interval). Products include:
- Seldane Tablets 1536
- Seldane-D Extended-Release Tablets 1538

Thioridazine Hydrochloride (Caution is advised if used concurrently due to sotalol's effect on cardiac repolarization (QT*c* prolongation) torsade de pointes, a polymorphic ventricular tachycardia with prolonged QT interval). Products include:
- Mellaril 2269

Tocainide Hydrochloride (Potential for prolonged refractoriness; concomitant therapy is not recommended; caution is advised if used concurrently due to sotalol's effect on cardiac repolarization (QT*c* prolongation) torsade de pointes, a polymorphic ventricular tachycardia with prolonged QT interval). Products include:
- Tonocard Tablets 531

Tolazamide (Potential for hyperglycemia; symptoms of hypoglycemia may be masked; dosage of antidiabetic drugs may require adjustment).
No products indexed under this heading.

Tolbutamide (Potential for hyperglycemia; symptoms of hypoglycemia may be masked; dosage of antidiabetic drugs may require adjustment).
No products indexed under this heading.

Trifluoperazine Hydrochloride (Caution is advised if used concurrently due to sotalol's effect on cardiac repolarization (QT*c* prolongation) torsade de pointes, a polymorphic ventricular tachycardia with prolonged QT interval). Products include:
- Stelazine 2514

Trimipramine Maleate (Caution is advised if used concurrently due to sotalol's effect on cardiac repolarization (QT*c* prolongation) torsade de pointes, a polymorphic ventricular tachycardia with prolonged QT interval). Products include:
- Surmontil Capsules 2811

Verapamil Hydrochloride (Potential for prolonged refractoriness; concomitant therapy is not recommended; possible additive effects on AV conduction or ventricular conduction; co-administration may result in hypotension). Products include:
- Calan SR Caplets 2422
- Calan Tablets 2419
- Isoptin Injectable 1344
- Isoptin Oral Tablets 1346
- Isoptin SR Tablets 1348
- Verelan Capsules 1410
- Verelan Capsules 2824

Food Interactions

Meal, unspecified (Reduces oral absorption by 20%).

BETASEPT SURGICAL SCRUB

(Chlorhexidine Gluconate) 1993
None cited in PDR database.

BETASERON FOR SC INJECTION

(Interferon Beta-1b) 658
None cited in PDR database.

BETIMOL 0.25%, 0.5%

(Timolol Hemihydrate) ..... ◎ 261
May interact with beta blockers, catecholamine depleting drugs, calcium channel blockers, cardiac glycosides, and certain other agents. Compounds in these categories include:

Acebutolol Hydrochloride (Concurrent use with systemic beta blockers may result in additive effect either on the intraocular pressure or the known systemic effect of beta blockade). Products include:
- Sectral Capsules 2807

Amlodipine Besylate (Possible atrioventricular conduction disturbances, left ventricular failure, and hypotension). Products include:
- Lotrel Capsules 840
- Norvasc Tablets 1940

Atenolol (Concurrent use with systemic beta blockers may result in additive effect either on the intraocular pressure or the known systemic effect of beta blockade). Products include:
- Tenoretic Tablets 2845
- Tenormin Tablets and I.V. Injection 2847

Bepridil Hydrochloride (Possible atrioventricular conduction disturbances, left ventricular failure, and hypotension). Products include:
- Vascor (200, 300 and 400 mg) Tablets 1587

Betaxolol Hydrochloride (Concurrent use with systemic beta blockers may result in additive effect either on the intraocular pressure or the known systemic effect of beta blockade). Products include:
- Betoptic Ophthalmic Solution 469
- Betoptic S Ophthalmic Suspension 471
- Kerlone Tablets 2436

Bisoprolol Fumarate (Concurrent use with systemic beta blockers may result in additive effect either on the intraocular pressure or the known systemic effect of beta blockade). Products include:
- Zebeta Tablets 1413
- Ziac 1415

Carteolol Hydrochloride (Concurrent use with systemic beta blockers may result in additive effect either on the intraocular pressure or the known systemic effect of beta blockade). Products include:
- Cartrol Tablets 410
- Ocupress Ophthalmic Solution, 1% Sterile ..... ◎ 309

Deserpidine (Possible additive effects and the production of hypotension and/or marked bradycardia).
No products indexed under this heading.

Deslanoside (Concomitant use of beta blockers with digitalis and calcium antagonists may have additive effects in prolonging atrioventricular conduction time).
No products indexed under this heading.

Digitoxin (Concomitant use of beta blockers with digitalis and calcium antagonists may have additive effects in prolonging atrioventricular conduction time). Products include:
- Crystodigin Tablets 1433

Digoxin (Concomitant use of beta blockers with digitalis and calcium antagonists may have additive effects in prolonging atrioventricular conduction time). Products include:
- Lanoxicaps 1117
- Lanoxin Elixir Pediatric 1120
- Lanoxin Injection 1123
- Lanoxin Injection Pediatric 1126
- Lanoxin Tablets 1128

Diltiazem Hydrochloride (Possible atrioventricular conduction disturbances, left ventricular failure, and hypotension). Products include:
- Cardizem CD Capsules 1506
- Cardizem SR Capsules 1510
- Cardizem Injectable 1508
- Cardizem Tablets 1512
- Dilacor XR Extended-release Capsules 2018

Epinephrine (Patients with a history of atopy or anaphylactic reactions to a variety of allergens may be unresponsive to the usual dose of injectable epinephrine used to treat allergic reactions). Products include:
- Bronkaid Mist ..... ▣ 717
- EPIFRIN ..... ◎ 239
- EpiPen 790
- Marcaine Hydrochloride with Epinephrine 1:200,000 2316
- Primatene Mist ..... ▣ 873
- Sensorcaine with Epinephrine Injection 559
- Sus-Phrine Injection 1019
- Xylocaine with Epinephrine Injections 567

Epinephrine Bitartrate (Patients with a history of atopy or anaphylactic reactions to a variety of allergens may be unresponsive to the usual dose of injectable epinephrine used to treat allergic reactions). Products include:
- Bronkaid Mist Suspension ..... ▣ 718
- Sensorcaine-MPF with Epinephrine Injection 559

Esmolol Hydrochloride (Concurrent use with systemic beta blockers may result in additive effect either on the intraocular pressure or the known systemic effect of beta blockade). Products include:
- Brevibloc Injection 1808

Felodipine (Possible atrioventricular conduction disturbances, left ventricular failure, and hypotension). Products include:
- Plendil Extended-Release Tablets 527

Guanethidine Monosulfate (Possible additive effects and the production of hypotension and/or marked bradycardia). Products include:
- Esimil Tablets 822
- Ismelin Tablets 827

Isradipine (Possible atrioventricular conduction disturbances, left ventricular failure, and hypotension). Products include:
- DynaCirc Capsules 2256

Labetalol Hydrochloride (Concurrent use with systemic beta blockers may result in additive effect either on the intraocular pressure or the known systemic effect of beta blockade). Products include:
- Normodyne Injection 2377
- Normodyne Tablets 2379
- Trandate 1185

Levobunolol Hydrochloride (Concurrent use with systemic beta blockers may result in additive effect either on the intraocular pressure or the known systemic effect of beta blockade). Products include:
- Betagan ..... ◎ 233

Metipranolol Hydrochloride (Concurrent use with systemic beta blockers may result in additive effect either on the intraocular pressure or the known systemic effect of beta blockade). Products include:
- OptiPranolol (Metipranolol 0.3%) Sterile Ophthalmic Solution ..... ◎ 258

Metoprolol Succinate (Concurrent use with systemic beta blockers may result in additive effect either on the intraocular pressure or the known systemic effect of beta blockade). Products include:
- Toprol-XL Tablets 565

Metoprolol Tartrate (Concurrent use with systemic beta blockers may result in additive effect either on the intraocular pressure or the known systemic effect of beta blockade). Products include:
- Lopressor Ampuls 830
- Lopressor HCT Tablets 832
- Lopressor Tablets 830

Nadolol (Concurrent use with systemic beta blockers may result in additive effect either on the intraocular pressure or the known systemic effect of beta blockade).
No products indexed under this heading.

Nicardipine Hydrochloride (Possible atrioventricular conduction disturbances, left ventricular failure, and hypotension). Products include:
- Cardene Capsules 2095
- Cardene I.V. 2709
- Cardene SR Capsules 2097

Nifedipine (Possible atrioventricular conduction disturbances, left ventricular failure, and hypotension). Products include:
- Adalat Capsules (10 mg and 20 mg) 587
- Adalat CC 589
- Procardia Capsules 1971
- Procardia XL Extended Release Tablets 1972

Nimodipine (Possible atrioventricular conduction disturbances, left ventricular failure, and hypotension). Products include:
- Nimotop Capsules 610

Nisoldipine (Possible atrioventricular conduction disturbances, left ventricular failure, and hypotension).
No products indexed under this heading.

(▣ Described in PDR For Nonprescription Drugs) (◎ Described in PDR For Ophthalmology)

Penbutolol Sulfate (Concurrent use with systemic beta blockers may result in additive effect either on the intraocular pressure or the known systemic effect of beta blockade). Products include:

Levatol 2403

Pindolol (Concurrent use with systemic beta blockers may result in additive effect either on the intraocular pressure or the known systemic effect of beta blockade). Products include:

Visken Tablets 2299

Propranolol Hydrochloride (Concurrent use with systemic beta blockers may result in additive effect either on the intraocular pressure or the known systemic effect of beta blockade). Products include:

Inderal 2728
Inderal LA Long Acting Capsules 2730
Inderide Tablets 2732
Inderide LA Long Acting Capsules 2734

Rauwolfia Serpentina (Possible additive effects and the production of hypotension and/or marked bradycardia).

No products indexed under this heading.

Rescinnamine (Possible additive effects and the production of hypotension and/or marked bradycardia).

No products indexed under this heading.

Reserpine (Possible additive effects and the production of hypotension and/or marked bradycardia). Products include:

Diupres Tablets 1650
Hydropres Tablets 1675
Ser-Ap-Es Tablets 849

Sotalol Hydrochloride (Concurrent use with systemic beta blockers may result in additive effect either on the intraocular pressure or the known systemic effect of beta blockade). Products include:

Betapace Tablets 641

Timolol Maleate (Concurrent use with systemic beta blockers may result in additive effect either on the intraocular pressure or the known systemic effect of beta blockade). Products include:

Blocadren Tablets 1614
Timolide Tablets 1748
Timoptic in Ocudose 1753
Timoptic Sterile Ophthalmic Solution 1751
Timoptic-XE 1755

Verapamil Hydrochloride (Possible atrioventricular conduction disturbances, left ventricular failure, and hypotension). Products include:

Calan SR Caplets 2422
Calan Tablets 2419
Isoptin Injectable 1344
Isoptin Oral Tablets 1346
Isoptin SR Tablets 1348
Verelan Capsules 1410
Verelan Capsules 2824

BETOPTIC OPHTHALMIC SOLUTION

(Betaxolol Hydrochloride) 469

May interact with beta blockers, general anesthetics, catecholamine depleting drugs, adrenergic augmenting psychotropics, and certain other agents. Compounds in these categories include:

Acebutolol Hydrochloride (Potential additive effects either on the intraocular pressure or on the known systemic effects of beta blockade). Products include:

Sectral Capsules 2807

Atenolol (Potential additive effects either on the intraocular pressure or on the known systemic effects of beta blockade). Products include:

Tenoretic Tablets 2845
Tenormin Tablets and I.V. Injection 2847

Bisoprolol Fumarate (Potential additive effects either on the intraocular pressure or on the known systemic effects of beta blockade). Products include:

Zebeta Tablets 1413
Ziac 1415

Carteolol Hydrochloride (Potential additive effects either on the intraocular pressure or on the known systemic effects of beta blockade). Products include:

Cartrol Tablets 410
Ocupress Ophthalmic Solution, 1% Sterile .... ◉ 309

Deserpidine (Possible additive effects and the production of hypotension and/or bradycardia).

No products indexed under this heading.

Enflurane (Impairment of heart's ability to respond to beta-adrenergically mediated sympathetic reflex stimuli).

No products indexed under this heading.

Esmolol Hydrochloride (Potential additive effects either on the intraocular pressure or on the known systemic effects of beta blockade). Products include:

Brevibloc Injection 1808

Guanethidine Monosulfate (Possible additive effects and the production of hypotension and/or bradycardia). Products include:

Esimil Tablets 822
Ismelin Tablets 827

Isocarboxazid (Exercise caution when used concomitantly).

No products indexed under this heading.

Isoflurane (Impairment of heart's ability to respond to beta-adrenergically mediated sympathetic reflex stimuli).

No products indexed under this heading.

Ketamine Hydrochloride (Impairment of heart's ability to respond to beta-adrenergically mediated sympathetic reflex stimuli).

No products indexed under this heading.

Labetalol Hydrochloride (Potential additive effects either on the intraocular pressure or on the known systemic effects of beta blockade). Products include:

Normodyne Injection 2377
Normodyne Tablets 2379
Trandate 1185

Levobunolol Hydrochloride (Potential additive effects either on the intraocular pressure or on the known systemic effects of beta blockade). Products include:

Betagan .... ◉ 233

Methohexital Sodium (Impairment of heart's ability to respond to beta-adrenergically mediated sympathetic reflex stimuli). Products include:

Brevital Sodium Vials 1429

Methoxyflurane (Impairment of heart's ability to respond to beta-adrenergically mediated sympathetic reflex stimuli).

No products indexed under this heading.

Metipranolol Hydrochloride (Potential additive effects either on the intraocular pressure or on the known systemic effects of beta blockade). Products include:

OptiPranolol (Metipranolol 0.3%) Sterile Ophthalmic Solution .... ◉ 258

Metoprolol Succinate (Potential additive effects either on the intraocular pressure or on the known systemic effects of beta blockade). Products include:

Toprol-XL Tablets 565

Metoprolol Tartrate (Potential additive effects either on the intraocular pressure or on the known systemic effects of beta blockade). Products include:

Lopressor Ampuls 830
Lopressor HCT Tablets 832
Lopressor Tablets 830

Nadolol (Potential additive effects either on the intraocular pressure or on the known systemic effects of beta blockade).

No products indexed under this heading.

Pargyline Hydrochloride (Exercise caution when used concomitantly).

No products indexed under this heading.

Penbutolol Sulfate (Potential additive effects either on the intraocular pressure or on the known systemic effects of beta blockade). Products include:

Levatol 2403

Phenelzine Sulfate (Exercise caution when used concomitantly). Products include:

Nardil 1920

Pindolol (Potential additive effects either on the intraocular pressure or on the known systemic effects of beta blockade). Products include:

Visken Tablets 2299

Propofol (Impairment of heart's ability to respond to beta-adrenergically mediated sympathetic reflex stimuli). Products include:

Diprivan Injection 2833

Propranolol Hydrochloride (Potential additive effects either on the intraocular pressure or on the known systemic effects of beta blockade). Products include:

Inderal 2728
Inderal LA Long Acting Capsules 2730
Inderide Tablets 2732
Inderide LA Long Acting Capsules 2734

Rauwolfia Serpentina (Possible additive effects and the production of hypotension and/or bradycardia).

No products indexed under this heading.

Rescinnamine (Possible additive effects and the production of hypotension and/or bradycardia).

No products indexed under this heading.

Reserpine (Possible additive effects and the production of hypotension and/or bradycardia). Products include:

Diupres Tablets 1650
Hydropres Tablets 1675
Ser-Ap-Es Tablets 849

Sotalol Hydrochloride (Potential additive effects either on the intraocular pressure or on the known systemic effects of beta blockade). Products include:

Betapace Tablets 641

Timolol Hemihydrate (Potential additive effects either on the intraocular pressure or on the known systemic effects of beta blockade). Products include:

Betimol 0.25%, 0.5% .... ◉ 261

Timolol Maleate (Potential additive effects either on the intraocular pressure or on the known systemic effects of beta blockade). Products include:

Blocadren Tablets 1614
Timolide Tablets 1748
Timoptic in Ocudose 1753
Timoptic Sterile Ophthalmic Solution 1751
Timoptic-XE 1755

Tranylcypromine Sulfate (Exercise caution when used concomitantly). Products include:

Parnate Tablets 2503

BETOPTIC S OPHTHALMIC SUSPENSION

(Betaxolol Hydrochloride) 471

May interact with catecholamine depleting drugs, adrenergic augmenting psychotropics, beta blockers, and general anesthetics. Compounds in these categories include:

Acebutolol Hydrochloride (Potential for additive effects). Products include:

Sectral Capsules 2807

Atenolol (Potential for additive effects). Products include:

Tenoretic Tablets 2845
Tenormin Tablets and I.V. Injection 2847

Bisoprolol Fumarate (Potential for additive effects). Products include:

Zebeta Tablets 1413
Ziac 1415

Carteolol Hydrochloride (Potential for additive effects). Products include:

Cartrol Tablets 410
Ocupress Ophthalmic Solution, 1% Sterile .... ◉ 309

Deserpidine (Potential for additive effects and production of hypotension and/or bradycardia).

No products indexed under this heading.

Enflurane (Impairment of heart's ability to respond to beta-adrenergically mediated sympathetic reflex stimuli).

No products indexed under this heading.

Esmolol Hydrochloride (Potential for additive effects). Products include:

Brevibloc Injection 1808

Guanethidine Monosulfate (Potential for additive effects and production of hypotension and/or bradycardia). Products include:

Esimil Tablets 822
Ismelin Tablets 827

Isocarboxazid (Exercise caution when used concomitantly).

No products indexed under this heading.

Isoflurane (Impairment of heart's ability to respond to beta-adrenergically mediated sympathetic reflex stimuli).

No products indexed under this heading.

Ketamine Hydrochloride (Impairment of heart's ability to respond to beta-adrenergically mediated sympathetic reflux stimuli).

No products indexed under this heading.

IMPORTANT NOTE: Always consult each drug listing in the patient's regimen for possible interactions.

Labetalol Hydrochloride (Potential for additive effects). Products include:
- Normodyne Injection ... 2377
- Normodyne Tablets ... 2379
- Trandate ... 1185

Levobunolol Hydrochloride (Potential for additive effects). Products include:
- Betagan ... ◉ 233

Methohexital Sodium (Impairment of heart's ability to respond to beta-adrenergically mediated sympathetic reflex stimuli). Products include:
- Brevital Sodium Vials ... 1429

Methoxyflurane (Impairment of heart's ability to respond to beta-adrenergically mediated sympathetic reflex stimuli).
- No products indexed under this heading.

Metipranolol Hydrochloride (Potential for additive effects). Products include:
- OptiPranolol (Metipranolol 0.3%) Sterile Ophthalmic Solution ... ◉ 258

Metoprolol Succinate (Potential for additive effects). Products include:
- Toprol-XL Tablets ... 565

Metoprolol Tartrate (Potential for additive effects). Products include:
- Lopressor Ampuls ... 830
- Lopressor HCT Tablets ... 832
- Lopressor Tablets ... 830

Nadolol (Potential for additive effects).
- No products indexed under this heading.

Pargyline Hydrochloride (Exercise caution when used concomitantly).
- No products indexed under this heading.

Penbutolol Sulfate (Potential for additive effects). Products include:
- Levatol ... 2403

Phenelzine Sulfate (Exercise caution when used concomitantly). Products include:
- Nardil ... 1920

Pindolol (Potential for additive effects). Products include:
- Visken Tablets ... 2299

Propofol (Impairment of heart's ability to respond to beta-adrenergically mediated sympathetic reflex stimuli). Products include:
- Diprivan Injection ... 2833

Propranolol Hydrochloride (Potential for additive effects). Products include:
- Inderal ... 2728
- Inderal LA Long Acting Capsules ... 2730
- Inderide Tablets ... 2732
- Inderide LA Long Acting Capsules .. 2734

Reserpine (Potential for additive effects and production of hypotension and/or bradycardia). Products include:
- Diupres Tablets ... 1650
- Hydropres Tablets ... 1675
- Ser-Ap-Es Tablets ... 849

Sotalol Hydrochloride (Potential for additive effects). Products include:
- Betapace Tablets ... 641

Timolol Hemihydrate (Potential for additive effects). Products include:
- Betimol 0.25%, 0.5% ... ◉ 261

Timolol Maleate (Potential for additive effects). Products include:
- Blocadren Tablets ... 1614
- Timolide Tablets ... 1748
- Timoptic in Ocudose ... 1753
- Timoptic Sterile Ophthalmic Solution ... 1751
- Timoptic-XE ... 1755

Tranylcypromine Sulfate (Exercise caution when used concomitantly). Products include:
- Parnate Tablets ... 2503

BIAVAX II
(Rubella & Mumps Virus Vaccine Live) ... 1613
May interact with:

Azathioprine (Contraindication). Products include:
- Imuran ... 1110

Cyclosporine (Contraindication). Products include:
- Neoral ... 2276
- Sandimmune ... 2286

Immune Globulin (Human) (Contraindication).
- No products indexed under this heading.

Immune Globulin Intravenous (Human) (Contraindication).

Muromonab-CD3 (Contraindication). Products include:
- Orthoclone OKT3 Sterile Solution .. 1837

BIAXIN GRANULES
(Clarithromycin) ... 405
See **Biaxin Tablets**

BIAXIN TABLETS
(Clarithromycin) ... 405
May interact with xanthine bronchodilators, oral anticoagulants, and certain other agents. Compounds in these categories include:

Aminophylline (Potential for increased serum theophylline concentration).
- No products indexed under this heading.

Carbamazepine (Potential for increased serum concentration of carbamazepine). Products include:
- Atretol Tablets ... 573
- Tegretol Chewable Tablets ... 852
- Tegretol Suspension ... 852
- Tegretol Tablets ... 852

Cyclosporine (Potential exists for elevated serum levels due to structural relationship with erythromycin group). Products include:
- Neoral ... 2276
- Sandimmune ... 2286

Dicumarol (Potential exists for increased anticoagulant effects due to structural relationship with erythromycin group).
- No products indexed under this heading.

Digoxin (Potential exists for elevated digoxin levels due to structural relationship with erythromycin group). Products include:
- Lanoxicaps ... 1117
- Lanoxin Elixir Pediatric ... 1120
- Lanoxin Injection ... 1123
- Lanoxin Injection Pediatric ... 1126
- Lanoxin Tablets ... 1128

Dihydroergotamine Mesylate (Concurrent use is associated with acute ergot toxicity characterized by severe peripheral vasospasm and dysesthesia). Products include:
- D.H.E. 45 Injection ... 2255

Dyphylline (Potential for increased serum theophylline concentration). Products include:
- Lufyllin & Lufyllin-400 Tablets ... 2670
- Lufyllin-GG Elixir & Tablets ... 2671

Ergotamine Tartrate (Concurrent use is associated with acute ergot toxicity characterized by severe peripheral vasospasm and dysesthesia). Products include:
- Bellergal-S Tablets ... 2250
- Cafergot ... 2251
- Ergomar ... 1486
- Wigraine Tablets & Suppositories .. 1829

Hexobarbital (Potential exists for elevated serum levels due to structural relationship with erythromycin group).

Phenytoin (Potential exists for elevated serum levels due to structural relationship with erythromycin group). Products include:
- Dilantin Infatabs ... 1908
- Dilantin-125 Suspension ... 1911

Phenytoin Sodium (Potential exists for elevated serum levels due to structural relationship with erythromycin group). Products include:
- Dilantin Kapseals ... 1906
- Dilantin Parenteral ... 1910

Terfenadine (When coadministered plasma concentration of active acid metabolite of terfenadine were three-fold higher, on average, than the values observed when terfenadine was administered alone). Products include:
- Seldane Tablets ... 1536
- Seldane-D Extended-Release Tablets ... 1538

Theophylline (Potential for increased serum theophylline concentration). Products include:
- Marax Tablets & DF Syrup ... 2200
- Quibron ... 2053

Theophylline Anhydrous (Potential for increased serum theophylline concentration). Products include:
- Aerolate ... 1004
- Primatene Dual Action Formula ... ▣ 872
- Primatene Tablets ... ▣ 873
- Respbid Tablets ... 682
- Slo-bid Gyrocaps ... 2033
- Theo-24 Extended Release Capsules ... 2568
- Theo-Dur Extended-Release Tablets ... 1327
- Theo-X Extended-Release Tablets .. 788
- Uni-Dur Extended-Release Tablets .. 1331
- Uniphyl 400 mg Tablets ... 2001

Theophylline Calcium Salicylate (Potential for increased serum theophylline concentration). Products include:
- Quadrinal Tablets ... 1350

Theophylline Sodium Glycinate (Potential for increased serum theophylline concentration).
- No products indexed under this heading.

Triazolam (Potential exists for decreased clearance of triazolam and thus increase pharmacologic effect of triazolam due to structural relationship with erythromycin group). Products include:
- Halcion Tablets ... 2611

Warfarin Sodium (Potential exists for increased anticoagulant effects due to structural relationship with erythromycin group). Products include:
- Coumadin ... 926

Zidovudine (Potential for decreased steady-state zidovudine concentration). Products include:
- Retrovir Capsules ... 1158
- Retrovir I.V. Infusion ... 1163
- Retrovir Syrup ... 1158

BICHLORACETIC ACID KAHLENBERG
(Dichloroacetic Acid) ... 1229
None cited in PDR database.

BICILLIN C-R INJECTION
(Penicillin G Procaine, Penicillin G Benzathine) ... 2704
May interact with tetracyclines and certain other agents. Compounds in these categories include:

Demeclocycline Hydrochloride (May antagonize the bactericidal effect of penicillin). Products include:
- Declomycin Tablets ... 1371

Doxycycline Calcium (May antagonize the bactericidal effect of penicillin). Products include:
- Vibramycin Calcium Oral Suspension Syrup ... 1941

Doxycycline Hyclate (May antagonize the bactericidal effect of penicillin). Products include:
- Doryx Capsules ... 1913
- Vibramycin Hyclate Capsules ... 1941
- Vibramycin Hyclate Intravenous ... 2215
- Vibra-Tabs Film Coated Tablets ... 1941

Doxycycline Monohydrate (May antagonize the bactericidal effect of penicillin). Products include:
- Monodox Capsules ... 1805
- Vibramycin Monohydrate for Oral Suspension ... 1941

Methacycline Hydrochloride (May antagonize the bactericidal effect of penicillin).
- No products indexed under this heading.

Minocycline Hydrochloride (May antagonize the bactericidal effect of penicillin). Products include:
- Dynacin Capsules ... 1590
- Minocin Intravenous ... 1382
- Minocin Oral Suspension ... 1385
- Minocin Pellet-Filled Capsules ... 1383

Oxytetracycline Hydrochloride (May antagonize the bactericidal effect of penicillin). Products include:
- TERAK Ointment ... ◉ 209
- Terra-Cortril Ophthalmic Suspension ... 2210
- Terramycin with Polymyxin B Sulfate Ophthalmic Ointment ... 2211
- Urobiotic-250 Capsules ... 2214

Probenecid (Increases serum penicillin levels). Products include:
- Benemid Tablets ... 1611
- ColBENEMID Tablets ... 1622

Tetracycline Hydrochloride (May antagonize the bactericidal effect of penicillin). Products include:
- Achromycin V Capsules ... 1367

BICILLIN C-R 900/300 INJECTION
(Penicillin G Procaine, Penicillin G Benzathine) ... 2706
May interact with tetracyclines and certain other agents. Compounds in these categories include:

Demeclocycline Hydrochloride (May antagonize the bactericidal effect of penicillin). Products include:
- Declomycin Tablets ... 1371

Doxycycline Calcium (May antagonize the bactericidal effect of penicillin). Products include:
- Vibramycin Calcium Oral Suspension Syrup ... 1941

Doxycycline Hyclate (May antagonize the bactericidal effect of penicillin). Products include:
- Doryx Capsules ... 1913
- Vibramycin Hyclate Capsules ... 1941
- Vibramycin Hyclate Intravenous ... 2215
- Vibra-Tabs Film Coated Tablets ... 1941

Doxycycline Monohydrate (May antagonize the bactericidal effect of penicillin). Products include:
- Monodox Capsules ... 1805

Vibramycin Monohydrate for Oral Suspension 1941

Methacycline Hydrochloride (May antagonize the bactericidal effect of penicillin).

No products indexed under this heading.

Minocycline Hydrochloride (May antagonize the bactericidal effect of penicillin). Products include:

Dynacin Capsules 1590
Minocin Intravenous 1382
Minocin Oral Suspension 1385
Minocin Pellet-Filled Capsules 1383

Oxytetracycline Hydrochloride (May antagonize the bactericidal effect of penicillin). Products include:

TERAK Ointment .... ◉ 209
Terra-Cortril Ophthalmic Suspension 2210
Terramycin with Polymyxin B Sulfate Ophthalmic Ointment 2211
Urobiotic-250 Capsules 2214

Probenecid (Concurrent administration increases and prolongs serum penicillin levels). Products include:

Benemid Tablets 1611
ColBENEMID Tablets 1622

Tetracycline Hydrochloride (May antagonize the bactericidal effect of penicillin). Products include:

Achromycin V Capsules 1367

BICILLIN L-A INJECTION

(Penicillin G Benzathine)........................2707
May interact with tetracyclines and certain other agents. Compounds in these categories include:

Demeclocycline Hydrochloride (May antagonize the bactericidal effect of penicillin). Products include:

Declomycin Tablets............................... 1371

Doxycycline Calcium (May antagonize the bactericidal effect of penicillin). Products include:

Vibramycin Calcium Oral Suspension Syrup 1941

Doxycycline Hyclate (May antagonize the bactericidal effect of penicillin). Products include:

Doryx Capsules...................................... 1913
Vibramycin Hyclate Capsules 1941
Vibramycin Hyclate Intravenous 2215
Vibra-Tabs Film Coated Tablets 1941

Doxycycline Monohydrate (May antagonize the bactericidal effect of penicillin). Products include:

Monodox Capsules 1805
Vibramycin Monohydrate for Oral Suspension 1941

Methacycline Hydrochloride (May antagonize the bactericidal effect of penicillin).

No products indexed under this heading.

Minocycline Hydrochloride (May antagonize the bactericidal effect of penicillin). Products include:

Dynacin Capsules 1590
Minocin Intravenous 1382
Minocin Oral Suspension 1385
Minocin Pellet-Filled Capsules 1383

Oxytetracycline Hydrochloride (May antagonize the bactericidal effect of penicillin). Products include:

TERAK Ointment .... ◉ 209
Terra-Cortril Ophthalmic Suspension 2210
Terramycin with Polymyxin B Sulfate Ophthalmic Ointment 2211
Urobiotic-250 Capsules 2214

Probenecid (Increases serum penicillin levels). Products include:

Benemid Tablets 1611
ColBENEMID Tablets 1622

Tetracycline Hydrochloride (May antagonize the bactericidal effect of penicillin). Products include:

Achromycin V Capsules 1367

BICITRA

(Sodium Citrate, Citric Acid) 578
May interact with:

Aluminum Carbonate Gel (Avoid concomitant use of aluminum-based antacids). Products include:

Basaljel... 2703

Aluminum Hydroxide (Avoid concomitant use of aluminum-based antacids). Products include:

ALternaGEL Liquid 1316
Maximum Strength Ascriptin .... ⊕ 630
Cama Arthritis Pain Reliever............ ⊕ 785
Gaviscon Extra Strength Relief Formula Antacid Tablets.................. ⊕ 819
Gaviscon Extra Strength Relief Formula Liquid Antacid................... ⊕ 819
Gaviscon Liquid Antacid .... ⊕ 820
Gelusil Liquid & Tablets .... ⊕ 855
Maalox Heartburn Relief Suspension .... ⊕ 642
Maalox Heartburn Relief Tablets.... ⊕ 641
Maalox Magnesia and Alumina Oral Suspension .... ⊕ 642
Maalox Plus Tablets .... ⊕ 643
Extra Strength Maalox Antacid Plus Antigas Liquid and Tablets ⊕ 638
Tempo Soft Antacid .... ⊕ 835

Aluminum Hydroxide Gel (Avoid concomitant use of aluminum-based antacids). Products include:

ALternaGEL Liquid .... ⊕ 659
Aludrox Oral Suspension 2695
Amphojel Suspension 2695
Amphojel Suspension without Flavor 2695
Amphojel Tablets................................... 2695
Arthritis Pain Ascriptin .... ⊕ 631
Regular Strength Ascriptin Tablets .... ⊕ 629
Gaviscon Antacid Tablets.................... ⊕ 819
Gaviscon-2 Antacid Tablets .... ⊕ 820
Mylanta Liquid 1317
Mylanta Tablets .... ⊕ 660
Mylanta Double Strength Liquid 1317
Mylanta Double Strength Tablets .. ⊕ 660
Nephrox Suspension .... ⊕ 655

BICNU

(Carmustine (BCNU)) 691
None cited in PDR database.

BICOZENE CREME

(Benzocaine, Resorcinol) .... ⊕ 785
None cited in PDR database.

BILTRICIDE TABLETS

(Praziquantel)... 591
None cited in PDR database.

BIOCLATE, ANTIHEMOPHILIC FACTOR (RECOMBINANT)

(Antihemophilic Factor (Recombinant)) 513
None cited in PDR database.

BIO-COMPLEX 5000 GENTLE FOAMING CLEANSER

(Aloe Vera) .... ⊕ 865
None cited in PDR database.

BIO-COMPLEX 5000 REVITALIZING CONDITIONER

(Cleanser).. ⊕ 865
None cited in PDR database.

BIO-COMPLEX 5000 REVITALIZING SHAMPOO

(Cleanser).. ⊕ 865
None cited in PDR database.

BIOLEAN

(Nutritional Supplement) .... ⊕ 866
May interact with anorexiants and antidepressant drugs. Compounds in these categories include:

Amitriptyline Hydrochloride (Concurrent use is not recommended). Products include:

Elavil 2838
Endep Tablets 2174
Etrafon 2355
Limbitrol 2180
Triavil Tablets 1757

Amoxapine (Concurrent use is not recommended). Products include:

Asendin Tablets 1369

Amphetamine Resins (Concurrent use is not recommended). Products include:

Biphetamine Capsules 983

Benzphetamine Hydrochloride (Concurrent use is not recommended). Products include:

Didrex Tablets... 2607

Bupropion Hydrochloride (Concurrent use is not recommended). Products include:

Wellbutrin Tablets 1204

Desipramine Hydrochloride (Concurrent use is not recommended). Products include:

Norpramin Tablets 1526

Dextroamphetamine Sulfate (Concurrent use is not recommended). Products include:

Dexedrine 2474
DextroStat Dextroamphetamine Tablets 2036

Diethylpropion Hydrochloride (Concurrent use is not recommended).

No products indexed under this heading.

Doxepin Hydrochloride (Concurrent use is not recommended). Products include:

Sinequan 2205
Zonalon Cream 1055

Fenfluramine Hydrochloride (Concurrent use is not recommended). Products include:

Pondimin Tablets 2066

Fluoxetine Hydrochloride (Concurrent use is not recommended). Products include:

Prozac Pulvules & Liquid, Oral Solution 919

Imipramine Hydrochloride (Concurrent use is not recommended). Products include:

Tofranil Ampuls 854
Tofranil Tablets 856

Imipramine Pamoate (Concurrent use is not recommended). Products include:

Tofranil-PM Capsules............................ 857

Isocarboxazid (Concurrent use is not recommended).

No products indexed under this heading.

Maprotiline Hydrochloride (Concurrent use is not recommended). Products include:

Ludiomil Tablets..................................... 843

Mazindol (Concurrent use is not recommended). Products include:

Sanorex Tablets 2294

Methamphetamine Hydrochloride (Concurrent use is not recommended). Products include:

Desoxyn Gradumet Tablets 419

Nefazodone Hydrochloride (Concurrent use is not recommended). Products include:

Serzone Tablets 771

Nortriptyline Hydrochloride (Concurrent use is not recommended). Products include:

Pamelor 2280

Paroxetine Hydrochloride (Concurrent use is not recommended). Products include:

Paxil Tablets 2505

Phendimetrazine Tartrate (Concurrent use is not recommended). Products include:

Bontril Slow-Release Capsules 781
Prelu-2 Timed Release Capsules....... 681

Phenelzine Sulfate (Concurrent use is not recommended). Products include:

Nardil 1920

Phenmetrazine Hydrochloride (Concurrent use is not recommended).

No products indexed under this heading.

Protriptyline Hydrochloride (Concurrent use is not recommended). Products include:

Vivactil Tablets 1774

Sertraline Hydrochloride (Concurrent use is not recommended). Products include:

Zoloft Tablets 2217

Tranylcypromine Sulfate (Concurrent use is not recommended). Products include:

Parnate Tablets 2503

Trazodone Hydrochloride (Concurrent use is not recommended). Products include:

Desyrel and Desyrel Dividose 503

Trimipramine Maleate (Concurrent use is not recommended). Products include:

Surmontil Capsules................................ 2811

Venlafaxine Hydrochloride (Concurrent use is not recommended). Products include:

Effexor 2719

BIOLEAN ACCELERATOR

(Nutritional Supplement) .... ⊕ 866
May interact with antidepressant drugs and anorexiants. Compounds in these categories include:

Amitriptyline Hydrochloride (Effect of concurrent use is not specified). Products include:

Elavil 2838
Endep Tablets 2174
Etrafon 2355
Limbitrol 2180
Triavil Tablets 1757

Amoxapine (Effect of concurrent use is not specified). Products include:

Asendin Tablets 1369

Amphetamine Resins (Effect of concurrent use is not specified). Products include:

Biphetamine Capsules 983

Benzphetamine Hydrochloride (Effect of concurrent use is not specified). Products include:

Didrex Tablets... 2607

Bupropion Hydrochloride (Effect of concurrent use is not specified). Products include:

Wellbutrin Tablets 1204

Desipramine Hydrochloride (Effect of concurrent use is not specified). Products include:

Norpramin Tablets 1526

Dextroamphetamine Sulfate (Effect of concurrent use is not specified). Products include:

Dexedrine 2474
DextroStat Dextroamphetamine Tablets 2036

Diethylpropion Hydrochloride (Effect of concurrent use is not specified).

No products indexed under this heading.

IMPORTANT NOTE: Always consult each drug listing in the patient's regimen for possible interactions.

Doxepin Hydrochloride (Effect of concurrent use is not specified). Products include:
- Sinequan ... 2205
- Zonalon Cream ... 1055

Fenfluramine Hydrochloride (Effect of concurrent use is not specified). Products include:
- Pondimin Tablets ... 2066

Fluoxetine Hydrochloride (Effect of concurrent use is not specified). Products include:
- Prozac Pulvules & Liquid, Oral Solution ... 919

Imipramine Hydrochloride (Effect of concurrent use is not specified). Products include:
- Tofranil Ampuls ... 854
- Tofranil Tablets ... 856

Imipramine Pamoate (Effect of concurrent use is not specified). Products include:
- Tofranil-PM Capsules ... 857

Isocarboxazid (Effect of concurrent use is not specified).
- No products indexed under this heading.

Maprotiline Hydrochloride (Effect of concurrent use is not specified). Products include:
- Ludiomil Tablets ... 843

Mazindol (Effect of concurrent use is not specified). Products include:
- Sanorex Tablets ... 2294

Methamphetamine Hydrochloride (Effect of concurrent use is not specified). Products include:
- Desoxyn Gradumet Tablets ... 419

Nefazodone Hydrochloride (Effect of concurrent use is not specified). Products include:
- Serzone Tablets ... 771

Nortriptyline Hydrochloride (Effect of concurrent use is not specified). Products include:
- Pamelor ... 2280

Paroxetine Hydrochloride (Effect of concurrent use is not specified). Products include:
- Paxil Tablets ... 2505

Phendimetrazine Tartrate (Effect of concurrent use is not specified). Products include:
- Bontril Slow-Release Capsules ... 781
- Prelu-2 Timed Release Capsules ... 681

Phenelzine Sulfate (Effect of concurrent use is not specified). Products include:
- Nardil ... 1920

Phenmetrazine Hydrochloride (Effect of concurrent use is not specified).
- No products indexed under this heading.

Protriptyline Hydrochloride (Effect of concurrent use is not specified). Products include:
- Vivactil Tablets ... 1774

Sertraline Hydrochloride (Effect of concurrent use is not specified). Products include:
- Zoloft Tablets ... 2217

Tranylcypromine Sulfate (Effect of concurrent use is not specified). Products include:
- Parnate Tablets ... 2503

Trazodone Hydrochloride (Effect of concurrent use is not specified). Products include:
- Desyrel and Desyrel Dividose ... 503

Trimipramine Maleate (Effect of concurrent use is not specified). Products include:
- Surmontil Capsules ... 2811

Venlafaxine Hydrochloride (Effect of concurrent use is not specified). Products include:
- Effexor ... 2719

BIOLEAN LIPOTRIM
(Nutritional Supplement) ... ▣ 866
None cited in PDR database.

BIOLEAN MEAL
(Nutritional Beverage) ... ▣ 867
None cited in PDR database.

BION TEARS
(Lubricant) ... ◉ 213
None cited in PDR database.

BIPHETAMINE CAPSULES
(Amphetamine Resins) ... 983
May interact with monoamine oxidase inhibitors, insulin, and certain other agents. Compounds in these categories include:

Furazolidone (Hypertensive crisis may result; concurrent use is contraindicated). Products include:
- Furoxone ... 2046

Guanethidine Monosulfate (Decreased hypotensive effect of guanethidine). Products include:
- Esimil Tablets ... 822
- Ismelin Tablets ... 827

Insulin, Human (Insulin requirements in diabetic patients may be altered).
- No products indexed under this heading.

Insulin, Human Isophane Suspension (Insulin requirements in diabetic patients may be altered). Products include:
- Novolin N Human Insulin 10 ml Vials ... 1795

Insulin, Human NPH (Insulin requirements in diabetic patients may be altered). Products include:
- Humulin N, 100 Units ... 1448
- Novolin N PenFill Cartridges Durable Insulin Delivery System ... 1798
- Novolin N Prefilled Syringe Disposable Insulin Delivery System ... 1798

Insulin, Human Regular (Insulin requirements in diabetic patients may be altered). Products include:
- Humulin R, 100 Units ... 1449
- Novolin R Human Insulin 10 ml Vials ... 1795
- Novolin R PenFill Cartridges Durable Insulin Delivery System ... 1798
- Novolin R Prefilled Syringe Disposable Insulin Delivery System ... 1798
- Velosulin BR Human Insulin 10 ml Vials ... 1795

Insulin, Human, Zinc Suspension (Insulin requirements in diabetic patients may be altered). Products include:
- Humulin L, 100 Units ... 1446
- Humulin U, 100 Units ... 1450
- Novolin L Human Insulin 10 ml Vials ... 1795

Insulin, NPH (Insulin requirements in diabetic patients may be altered). Products include:
- NPH, 100 Units ... 1450
- Pork NPH, 100 Units ... 1452
- Purified Pork NPH Isophane Insulin ... 1801

Insulin, Regular (Insulin requirements in diabetic patients may be altered). Products include:
- Regular, 100 Units ... 1450
- Pork Regular, 100 Units ... 1452
- Pork Regular (Concentrated), 500 Units ... 1453
- Purified Pork Regular Insulin ... 1801

Insulin, Zinc Crystals (Insulin requirements in diabetic patients may be altered). Products include:
- NPH, 100 Units ... 1450

Insulin, Zinc Suspension (Insulin requirements in diabetic patients may be altered). Products include:
- Iletin I ... 1450
- Lente, 100 Units ... 1450
- Iletin II ... 1452
- Pork Lente, 100 Units ... 1452
- Purified Pork Lente Insulin ... 1801

Isocarboxazid (Hypertensive crisis may result; concurrent use is contraindicated).
- No products indexed under this heading.

Phenelzine Sulfate (Hypertensive crisis may result; concurrent use is contraindicated). Products include:
- Nardil ... 1920

Selegiline Hydrochloride (Hypertensive crisis may result; concurrent use is contraindicated). Products include:
- Eldepryl Tablets ... 2550

Tranylcypromine Sulfate (Hypertensive crisis may result; concurrent use is contraindicated). Products include:
- Parnate Tablets ... 2503

BLENOXANE
(Bleomycin Sulfate) ... 692
None cited in PDR database.

BLEPH-10 OPHTHALMIC OINTMENT 10%
(Sulfacetamide Sodium) ... 475
May interact with silver preparations. Compounds in this category include:

Silver Nitrate (Incompatible).
- No products indexed under this heading.

BLEPH-10 OPHTHALMIC SOLUTION 10%
(Sulfacetamide Sodium) ... 475
May interact with silver preparations. Compounds in this category include:

Silver Nitrate (Incompatible).
- No products indexed under this heading.

BLEPHAMIDE LIQUIFILM STERILE OPHTHALMIC SUSPENSION
(Prednisolone Acetate, Sulfacetamide Sodium) ... 476
None cited in PDR database.

BLEPHAMIDE OINTMENT
(Sulfacetamide Sodium, Prednisolone Acetate) ... ◉ 237
May interact with silver preparations and para-aminobenzoic acid based local anesthetics. Compounds in these categories include:

Procaine Hydrochloride (May antagonize the action of sulfonamide). Products include:
- Novocain Hydrochloride for Spinal Anesthesia ... 2326

Silver Nitrate (Blephamide ointment is incompatible with silver preparations).
- No products indexed under this heading.

Tetracaine Hydrochloride (May antagonize the action of sulfonamide). Products include:
- Cetacaine Topical Anesthetic ... 794
- Pontocaine Hydrochloride for Spinal Anesthesia ... 2330

BLOCADREN TABLETS
(Timolol Maleate) ... 1614
May interact with cardiac glycosides, insulin, oral hypoglycemic agents, catecholamine depleting drugs, calcium channel blockers, non-steroidal anti-inflammatory agents, and certain other agents. Compounds in these categories include:

Acarbose (Beta blockers may mask the signs and symptoms of acute hypoglycemia).
- No products indexed under this heading.

Amlodipine Besylate (AV conduction disturbances; left ventricular failure). Products include:
- Lotrel Capsules ... 840
- Norvasc Tablets ... 1940

Bepridil Hydrochloride (AV conduction disturbances; left ventricular failure). Products include:
- Vascor (200, 300 and 400 mg) Tablets ... 1587

Chlorpropamide (Beta blockers may mask the signs and symptoms of acute hypoglycemia). Products include:
- Diabinese Tablets ... 1935

Diclofenac Potassium (Blunting of the antihypertensive effect). Products include:
- Cataflam ... 816

Diclofenac Sodium (Blunting of the antihypertensive effect). Products include:
- Voltaren Ophthalmic Sterile Ophthalmic Solution ... ◉ 272
- Voltaren Tablets ... 861

Digitoxin (Additive effects in prolonging AV conduction time). Products include:
- Crystodigin Tablets ... 1433

Digoxin (Additive effects in prolonging AV conduction time). Products include:
- Lanoxicaps ... 1117
- Lanoxin Elixir Pediatric ... 1120
- Lanoxin Injection ... 1123
- Lanoxin Injection Pediatric ... 1126
- Lanoxin Tablets ... 1128

Diltiazem Hydrochloride (AV conduction disturbances; left ventricular failure). Products include:
- Cardizem CD Capsules ... 1506
- Cardizem SR Capsules ... 1510
- Cardizem Injectable ... 1508
- Cardizem Tablets ... 1512
- Dilacor XR Extended-release Capsules ... 2018

Epinephrine (Patients with a history of atopy or severe anaphylactic reaction to variety of allergens may be unresponsive to the usual dose of epinephrine to treat anaphylactic reactions). Products include:
- Bronkaid Mist ... ▣ 717
- EPIFRIN ... ◉ 239
- EpiPen ... 790
- Marcaine Hydrochloride with Epinephrine 1:200,000 ... 2316
- Primatene Mist ... ▣ 873
- Sensorcaine with Epinephrine Injection ... 559
- Sus-Phrine Injection ... 1019
- Xylocaine with Epinephrine Injections ... 567

Epinephrine Hydrochloride (Patients with a history of atopy or severe anaphylactic reaction to variety of allergens may be unresponsive to the usual dose of epinephrine to treat anaphylactic reactions). Products include:
- Ana-Kit Anaphylaxis Emergency Treatment Kit ... 617

Etodolac (Blunting of the antihypertensive effect). Products include:
- Lodine Capsules and Tablets ... 2743

Felodipine (AV conduction disturbances; left ventricular failure). Products include:
- Plendil Extended-Release Tablets ... 527

(▣ Described in PDR For Nonprescription Drugs) (◉ Described in PDR For Ophthalmology)

125 **Interactions Index** **Bonine Tablets**

Fenoprofen Calcium (Blunting of the antihypertensive effect). Products include:
- Nalfon 200 Pulvules & Nalfon Tablets ... 917

Flurbiprofen (Blunting of the antihypertensive effect). Products include:
- Ansaid Tablets ... 2579

Glipizide (Beta blockers may mask the signs and symptoms of acute hypoglycemia). Products include:
- Glucotrol Tablets ... 1967
- Glucotrol XL Extended Release Tablets ... 1968

Glyburide (Beta blockers may mask the signs and symptoms of acute hypoglycemia). Products include:
- DiaBeta Tablets ... 1239
- Glynase PresTab Tablets ... 2609
- Micronase Tablets ... 2623

Guanethidine Monosulfate (Additive effects; hypotension and/or bradycardia). Products include:
- Esimil Tablets ... 822
- Ismelin Tablets ... 827

Ibuprofen (Blunting of the antihypertensive effect). Products include:
- Advil Cold and Sinus Caplets and Tablets (formerly CoAdvil) ... ▣ 870
- Advil Ibuprofen Tablets and Caplets ... ▣ 870
- Children's Advil Suspension ... 2692
- Arthritis Foundation Ibuprofen Tablets ... ▣ 674
- Bayer Select Ibuprofen Pain Relief Formula ... ▣ 715
- Cramp End Tablets ... ▣ 735
- Dimetapp Sinus Caplets ... ▣ 775
- Haltran Tablets ... ▣ 771
- IBU Tablets ... 1342
- Ibuprohm ... ▣ 735
- Children's Motrin Ibuprofen Oral Suspension ... 1546
- Motrin Tablets ... 2625
- Motrin IB Caplets, Tablets, and Geltabs ... ▣ 838
- Motrin IB Sinus ... ▣ 838
- Motrin Ibuprofen Suspension, Oral Drops, Chewable Tablets, Caplets ... 1546
- Nuprin Ibuprofen/Analgesic Tablets & Caplets ... ▣ 622
- Sine-Aid IB Caplets ... 1554
- Vicks DayQuil SINUS Pressure & PAIN Relief with IBUPROFEN ... ▣ 762

Indomethacin (Blunting of the antihypertensive effect). Products include:
- Indocin ... 1680

Indomethacin Sodium Trihydrate (Blunting of the antihypertensive effect). Products include:
- Indocin I.V. ... 1684

Insulin, Human Isophane Suspension (Beta blockers may mask the signs and symptoms of acute hypoglycemia). Products include:
- Novolin N Human Insulin 10 ml Vials ... 1795

Insulin, Human NPH (Beta blockers may mask the signs and symptoms of acute hypoglycemia). Products include:
- Humulin N, 100 Units ... 1448
- Novolin N PenFill Cartridges Durable Insulin Delivery System ... 1798
- Novolin N Prefilled Syringe Disposable Insulin Delivery System ... 1798

Insulin, Human Regular (Beta blockers may mask the signs and symptoms of acute hypoglycemia). Products include:
- Humulin R, 100 Units ... 1449
- Novolin R Human Insulin 10 ml Vials ... 1795
- Novolin R PenFill Cartridges Durable Insulin Delivery System ... 1798
- Novolin R Prefilled Syringe Disposable Insulin Delivery System ... 1798
- Velosulin BR Human Insulin 10 ml Vials ... 1795

Insulin, Human, Zinc Suspension (Beta blockers may mask the signs and symptoms of acute hypoglycemia). Products include:
- Humulin L, 100 Units ... 1446
- Humulin U, 100 Units ... 1450
- Novolin L Human Insulin 10 ml Vials ... 1795

Insulin, NPH (Beta blockers may mask the signs and symptoms of acute hypoglycemia). Products include:
- NPH, 100 Units ... 1450
- Pork NPH, 100 Units ... 1452
- Purified Pork NPH Isophane Insulin ... 1801

Insulin, Regular (Beta blockers may mask the signs and symptoms of acute hypoglycemia). Products include:
- Regular, 100 Units ... 1450
- Pork Regular, 100 Units ... 1452
- Pork Regular (Concentrated), 500 Units ... 1453
- Purified Pork Regular Insulin ... 1801

Insulin, Zinc Crystals (Beta blockers may mask the signs and symptoms of acute hypoglycemia). Products include:
- NPH, 100 Units ... 1450

Insulin, Zinc Suspension (Beta blockers may mask the signs and symptoms of acute hypoglycemia). Products include:
- Iletin I ... 1450
- Lente, 100 Units ... 1450
- Iletin II ... 1452
- Pork Lente, 100 Units ... 1452
- Purified Pork Lente Insulin ... 1801

Isradipine (AV conduction disturbances; left ventricular failure). Products include:
- DynaCirc Capsules ... 2256

Ketoprofen (Blunting of the antihypertensive effect). Products include:
- Orudis Capsules ... 2766
- Oruvail Capsules ... 2766

Ketorolac Tromethamine (Blunting of the antihypertensive effect). Products include:
- Acular ... 474
- Acular ... ◉ 277
- Toradol ... 2159

Meclofenamate Sodium (Blunting of the antihypertensive effect).
- No products indexed under this heading.

Mefenamic Acid (Blunting of the antihypertensive effect). Products include:
- Ponstel ... 1925

Metformin Hydrochloride (Beta blockers may mask the signs and symptoms of acute hypoglycemia). Products include:
- Glucophage ... 752

Nabumetone (Blunting of the antihypertensive effect). Products include:
- Relafen Tablets ... 2510

Naproxen (Blunting of the antihypertensive effect). Products include:
- Anaprox/Naprosyn ... 2117

Naproxen Sodium (Blunting of the antihypertensive effect). Products include:
- Aleve ... 1975
- Anaprox/Naprosyn ... 2117

Nicardipine Hydrochloride (AV conduction disturbances; left ventricular failure). Products include:
- Cardene Capsules ... 2095
- Cardene I.V. ... 2709
- Cardene SR Capsules ... 2097

Nifedipine (Hypotension). Products include:
- Adalat Capsules (10 mg and 20 mg) ... 587
- Adalat CC ... 589
- Procardia Capsules ... 1971
- Procardia XL Extended Release Tablets ... 1972

Nimodipine (AV conduction disturbances; left ventricular failure). Products include:
- Nimotop Capsules ... 610

Nisoldipine (AV conduction disturbances; left ventricular failure).
- No products indexed under this heading.

Oxaprozin (Blunting of the antihypertensive effect). Products include:
- Daypro Caplets ... 2426

Phenylbutazone (Blunting of the antihypertensive effect).
- No products indexed under this heading.

Piroxicam (Blunting of the antihypertensive effect). Products include:
- Feldene Capsules ... 1965

Reserpine (Additive effects; hypotension and/or bradycardia). Products include:
- Diupres Tablets ... 1650
- Hydropres Tablets ... 1675
- Ser-Ap-Es Tablets ... 849

Sulindac (Blunting of the antihypertensive effect). Products include:
- Clinoril Tablets ... 1618

Tolazamide (Beta blockers may mask the signs and symptoms of acute hypoglycemia).
- No products indexed under this heading.

Tolbutamide (Beta blockers may mask the signs and symptoms of acute hypoglycemia).
- No products indexed under this heading.

Tolmetin Sodium (Blunting of the antihypertensive effect). Products include:
- Tolectin (200, 400 and 600 mg) .. 1581

Verapamil Hydrochloride (AV conduction disturbances; left ventricular failure). Products include:
- Calan SR Caplets ... 2422
- Calan Tablets ... 2419
- Isoptin Injectable ... 1344
- Isoptin Oral Tablets ... 1346
- Isoptin SR Tablets ... 1348
- Verelan Capsules ... 1410
- Verelan Capsules ... 2824

BONAMIL INFANT FORMULA WITH IRON, POWDER, READY-TO-FEED AND CONCENTRATED LIQUIDS

(Infant Formula, Ferrous Sulfate) 2709

None cited in PDR database.

BONINE TABLETS

(Meclizine Hydrochloride)...................1933

May interact with hypnotics and sedatives, tranquilizers, and certain other agents. Compounds in these categories include:

Alprazolam (May increase drowsiness effect). Products include:
- Xanax Tablets ... 2649

Buspirone Hydrochloride (May increase drowsiness effect). Products include:
- BuSpar ... 737

Chlordiazepoxide (May increase drowsiness effect). Products include:
- Libritabs Tablets ... 2177
- Limbitrol ... 2180

Chlordiazepoxide Hydrochloride (May increase drowsiness effect). Products include:
- Librax Capsules ... 2176
- Librium Capsules ... 2178
- Librium Injectable ... 2179

Chlorpromazine (May increase drowsiness effect). Products include:
- Thorazine Suppositories ... 2523

Chlorprothixene (May increase drowsiness effect).
- No products indexed under this heading.

Chlorprothixene Hydrochloride (May increase drowsiness effect).
- No products indexed under this heading.

Clorazepate Dipotassium (May increase drowsiness effect). Products include:
- Tranxene ... 451

Diazepam (May increase drowsiness effect). Products include:
- Dizac ... 1809
- Valium Injectable ... 2182
- Valium Tablets ... 2183
- Valrelease Capsules ... 2169

Droperidol (May increase drowsiness effect). Products include:
- Inapsine Injection ... 1296

Estazolam (May increase drowsiness effect). Products include:
- ProSom Tablets ... 449

Ethchlorvynol (May increase drowsiness effect). Products include:
- Placidyl Capsules ... 448

Ethinamate (May increase drowsiness effect).
- No products indexed under this heading.

Fluphenazine Decanoate (May increase drowsiness effect). Products include:
- Prolixin Decanoate ... 509

Fluphenazine Enanthate (May increase drowsiness effect). Products include:
- Prolixin Enanthate ... 509

Fluphenazine Hydrochloride (May increase drowsiness effect). Products include:
- Prolixin ... 509

Flurazepam Hydrochloride (May increase drowsiness effect). Products include:
- Dalmane Capsules ... 2173

Glutethimide (May increase drowsiness effect).
- No products indexed under this heading.

Haloperidol (May increase drowsiness effect). Products include:
- Haldol Injection, Tablets and Concentrate ... 1575

Haloperidol Decanoate (May increase drowsiness effect). Products include:
- Haldol Decanoate ... 1577

Hydroxyzine Hydrochloride (May increase drowsiness effect). Products include:
- Atarax Tablets & Syrup ... 2185
- Marax Tablets & DF Syrup ... 2200
- Vistaril Intramuscular Solution ... 2216

Lorazepam (May increase drowsiness effect). Products include:
- Ativan Injection ... 2698
- Ativan Tablets ... 2700

Loxapine Hydrochloride (May increase drowsiness effect). Products include:
- Loxitane ... 1378

Loxapine Succinate (May increase drowsiness effect). Products include:
- Loxitane Capsules ... 1378

Meprobamate (May increase drowsiness effect). Products include:
- Miltown Tablets ... 2672
- PMB 200 and PMB 400 ... 2783

Mesoridazine Besylate (May increas drowsiness effect). Products include:
- Serentil ... 684

IMPORTANT NOTE: Always consult each drug listing in the patient's regimen for possible interactions.

Bonine Tablets | Interactions Index | 126

Midazolam Hydrochloride (May increase drowsiness effect). Products include:

Versed Injection 2170

Molindone Hydrochloride (May increase drowsiness effect). Products include:

Moban Tablets and Concentrate 1048

Oxazepam (May increase drowsiness effect). Products include:

Serax Capsules 2810
Serax Tablets 2810

Perphenazine (May increase drowsiness effect). Products include:

Etrafon 2355
Triavil Tablets 1757
Trilafon 2389

Prazepam (May increase drowsiness effect).

No products indexed under this heading.

Prochlorperazine (May increase drowsiness effect). Products include:

Compazine 2470

Promethazine Hydrochloride (May increase drowsiness effect). Products include:

Mepergan Injection 2753
Phenergan with Codeine 2777
Phenergan with Dextromethorphan 2778
Phenergan Injection 2773
Phenergan Suppositories 2775
Phenergan Syrup 2774
Phenergan Tablets 2775
Phenergan VC 2779
Phenergan VC with Codeine 2781

Propofol (May increase drowsiness effect). Products include:

Diprivan Injection 2833

Quazepam (May increase drowsiness effect). Products include:

Doral Tablets 2664

Secobarbital Sodium (May increase drowsiness effect). Products include:

Seconal Sodium Pulvules 1474

Temazepam (May increase drowsiness effect). Products include:

Restoril Capsules 2284

Thioridazine Hydrochloride (May increase drowsiness effect). Products include:

Mellaril 2269

Thiothixene (May increase drowsiness effect). Products include:

Navane Capsules and Concentrate 2201
Navane Intramuscular 2202

Triazolam (May increase drowsiness effect). Products include:

Halcion Tablets 2611

Trifluoperazine Hydrochloride (May increase drowsiness effect). Products include:

Stelazine 2514

Zolpidem Tartrate (May increase drowsiness effect). Products include:

Ambien Tablets 2416

Food Interactions

Alcohol (May increase drowsiness effect).

BONTRIL SLOW-RELEASE CAPSULES
(Phendimetrazine Tartrate) 781
May interact with monoamine oxidase inhibitors, insulin, and certain other agents. Compounds in these categories include:

Furazolidone (Potential for hypertensive crisis). Products include:

Furoxone 2046

Guanethidine Monosulfate (Hypotensive effect of guanethidine may be decreased). Products include:

Esimil Tablets 822
Ismelin Tablets 827

Insulin, Human (Insulin requirement may be altered).

No products indexed under this heading.

Insulin, Human Isophane Suspension (Insulin requirement may be altered). Products include:

Novolin N Human Insulin 10 ml Vials 1795

Insulin, Human NPH (Insulin requirement may be altered). Products include:

Humulin N, 100 Units 1448
Novolin N PenFill Cartridges Durable Insulin Delivery System 1798
Novolin N Prefilled Syringe Disposable Insulin Delivery System 1798

Insulin, Human Regular (Insulin requirement may be altered). Products include:

Humulin R, 100 Units 1449
Novolin R Human Insulin 10 ml Vials 1795
Novolin R PenFill Cartridges Durable Insulin Delivery System 1798
Novolin R Prefilled Syringe Disposable Insulin Delivery System 1798
Velosulin BR Human Insulin 10 ml Vials 1795

Insulin, Human, Zinc Suspension (Insulin requirement may be altered). Products include:

Humulin L, 100 Units 1446
Humulin U, 100 Units 1450
Novolin L Human Insulin 10 ml Vials 1795

Insulin, NPH (Insulin requirement may be altered). Products include:

NPH, 100 Units 1450
Pork NPH, 100 Units 1452
Purified Pork NPH Isophane Insulin 1801

Insulin, Regular (Insulin requirement may be altered). Products include:

Regular, 100 Units 1450
Pork Regular, 100 Units 1452
Pork Regular (Concentrated), 500 Units 1453
Purified Pork Regular Insulin 1801

Insulin, Zinc Crystals (Insulin requirement may be altered). Products include:

NPH, 100 Units 1450

Insulin, Zinc Suspension (Insulin requirement may be altered). Products include:

Iletin I 1450
Lente, 100 Units 1450
Iletin II 1452
Pork Lente, 100 Units 1452
Purified Pork Lente Insulin 1801

Isocarboxazid (Potential for hypertensive crisis).

No products indexed under this heading.

Phenelzine Sulfate (Potential for hypertensive crisis). Products include:

Nardil 1920

Selegiline Hydrochloride (Potential for hypertensive crisis). Products include:

Eldepryl Tablets 2550

Tranylcypromine Sulfate (Potential for hypertensive crisis). Products include:

Parnate Tablets 2503

BOROFAX SKIN PROTECTANT OINTMENT
(Zinc Oxide, Petrolatum, White) .... ▣ 853
None cited in PDR database.

BOTOX (BOTULINUM TOXIN TYPE A) PURIFIED NEUROTOXIN COMPLEX
(Botulinum Toxin Type A) 477
None cited in PDR database.

BRETHAIRE INHALER
(Terbutaline Sulfate) 813
May interact with monoamine oxidase inhibitors, tricyclic antidepressants, beta blockers, sympathomimetic aerosol bronchodilators, and certain other agents. Compounds in these categories include:

Acebutolol Hydrochloride (Beta receptor blocking agents and terbutaline sulfate inhibit each other). Products include:

Sectral Capsules 2807

Albuterol (Concomitant therapy with other sympathomimetic aerosol bronchodilators should be avoided). Products include:

Proventil Inhalation Aerosol 2382
Ventolin Inhalation Aerosol and Refill 1197

Amitriptyline Hydrochloride (May potentiate action of terbutaline sulfate on vascular system). Products include:

Elavil 2838
Endep Tablets 2174
Etrafon 2355
Limbitrol 2180
Triavil Tablets 1757

Amoxapine (May potentiate action of terbutaline sulfate on vascular system). Products include:

Asendin Tablets 1369

Atenolol (Beta receptor blocking agents and terbutaline sulfate inhibit each other). Products include:

Tenoretic Tablets 2845
Tenormin Tablets and I.V. Injection 2847

Betaxolol Hydrochloride (Beta receptor blocking agents and terbutaline sulfate inhibit each other). Products include:

Betoptic Ophthalmic Solution 469
Betoptic S Ophthalmic Suspension 471
Kerlone Tablets 2436

Bisoprolol Fumarate (Beta receptor blocking agents and terbutaline sulfate inhibit each other). Products include:

Zebeta Tablets 1413
Ziac 1415

Bitolterol Mesylate (Concomitant therapy with other sympathomimetic aerosol bronchodilators should be avoided). Products include:

Tornalate Solution for Inhalation, 0.2% 956
Tornalate Metered Dose Inhaler 957

Carteolol Hydrochloride (Beta receptor blocking agents and terbutaline sulfate inhibit each other). Products include:

Cartrol Tablets 410
Ocupress Ophthalmic Solution, 1% Sterile .... ◉ 309

Clomipramine Hydrochloride (May potentiate action of terbutaline sulfate on vascular system). Products include:

Anafranil Capsules 803

Desipramine Hydrochloride (May potentiate action of terbutaline sulfate on vascular system). Products include:

Norpramin Tablets 1526

Doxepin Hydrochloride (May potentiate action of terbutaline sulfate on vascular system). Products include:

Sinequan 2205
Zonalon Cream 1055

Epinephrine (Concomitant administration is not advised). Products include:

Bronkaid Mist .... ▣ 717
EPIFRIN .... ◉ 239
EpiPen 790
Marcaine Hydrochloride with Epinephrine 1:200,000 2316
Primatene Mist .... ▣ 873
Sensorcaine with Epinephrine Injection 559
Sus-Phrine Injection 1019
Xylocaine with Epinephrine Injections 567

Epinephrine Bitartrate (Concomitant administration is not advised). Products include:

Bronkaid Mist Suspension .... ▣ 718
Sensorcaine-MPF with Epinephrine Injection 559

Epinephrine Hydrochloride (Concomitant administration is not advised). Products include:

Ana-Kit Anaphylaxis Emergency Treatment Kit 617

Esmolol Hydrochloride (Beta receptors blocking agents and terbutaline sulfate inhibit each other). Products include:

Brevibloc Injection 1808

Furazolidone (May potentiate action of terbutaline sulfate on vascular system). Products include:

Furoxone 2046

Imipramine Hydrochloride (May potentiate action of terbutaline sulfate on vascular system). Products include:

Tofranil Ampuls 854
Tofranil Tablets 856

Imipramine Pamoate (May potentiate action of terbutaline sulfate on vascular system). Products include:

Tofranil-PM Capsules 857

Isocarboxazid (May potentiate action of terbutaline sulfate on vascular system).

No products indexed under this heading.

Isoetharine (Concomitant therapy with other sympathomimetic aerosol bronchodilators should be avoided). Products include:

Bronkometer Aerosol 2302
Bronkosol Solution 2302
Isoetharine Inhalation Solution, USP, Arm-a-Med 551

Isoproterenol Hydrochloride (Concomitant therapy with other sympathomimetic aerosol bronchodilators should be avoided). Products include:

Isuprel Hydrochloride Injection 1:5000 2311
Isuprel Hydrochloride Solution 1:200 & 1:100 2313
Isuprel Mistometer 2312

Isoproterenol Sulfate (Concomitant administration is not advised). Products include:

Norisodrine with Calcium Iodide Syrup 442

Labetalol Hydrochloride (Beta receptor blocking agents and terbutaline sulfate inhibit each other). Products include:

Normodyne Injection 2377
Normodyne Tablets 2379
Trandate 1185

Levobunolol Hydrochloride (Beta receptor blocking agents and terbutaline sulfate inhibit each other). Products include:

Betagan .... ◉ 233

Maprotiline Hydrochloride (May potentiate action of terbutaline sulfate on vascular system). Products include:

Ludiomil Tablets 843

Metaproterenol Sulfate (Concomitant therapy with other sympathomimetic aerosol bronchodilators should be avoided). Products include:

Alupent 669
Metaproterenol Sulfate Inhalation Solution, USP, Arm-a-Med 552

(▣ Described in PDR For Nonprescription Drugs) (◉ Described in PDR For Ophthalmology)

Interactions Index — Brethine

Metipranolol Hydrochloride (Beta receptor blocking agents and terbutaline sulfate inhibit each other). Products include:

OptiPranolol (Metipranolol 0.3%) Sterile Ophthalmic Solution.......... © 258

Metoprolol Succinate (Beta receptor blocking agents and terbutaline sulfate inhibit each other). Products include:

Toprol-XL Tablets 565

Metoprolol Tartrate (Beta receptor blocking agents and terbutaline sulfate inhibit each other). Products include:

Lopressor Ampuls 830
Lopressor HCT Tablets 832
Lopressor Tablets 830

Nadolol (Beta receptor blocking agents and terbutaline sulfate inhibit each other).

No products indexed under this heading.

Nortriptyline Hydrochloride (May potentiate action of terbutaline sulfate on vascular system). Products include:

Pamelor 2280

Penbutolol Sulfate (Beta receptor blocking agents and terbutaline sulfate inhibit each other). Products include:

Levatol 2403

Phenelzine Sulfate (May potentiate action of terbutaline sulfate on vascular system). Products include:

Nardil 1920

Pindolol (Beta receptor blocking agents and terbutaline sulfate inhibit each other). Products include:

Visken Tablets... 2299

Pirbuterol Acetate (Concomitant therapy with other sympathomimetic aerosol bronchodilators should be avoided). Products include:

Maxair Autohaler 1492
Maxair Inhaler 1494

Propranolol Hydrochloride (Beta receptor blocking agents and terbutaline sulfate inhibit each other). Products include:

Inderal 2728
Inderal LA Long Acting Capsules 2730
Inderide Tablets 2732
Inderide LA Long Acting Capsules .. 2734

Protriptyline Hydrochloride (May potentiate action of terbutaline sulfate on vascular system). Products include:

Vivactil Tablets 1774

Salmeterol Xinafoate (Concomitant therapy with other sympathomimetic aerosol bronchodilators should be avoided). Products include:

Serevent Inhalation Aerosol................ 1176

Selegiline Hydrochloride (May potentiate action of terbutaline sulfate on vascular system). Products include:

Eldepryl Tablets 2550

Sotalol Hydrochloride (Beta receptor blocking agents and terbutaline sulfate inhibit each other). Products include:

Betapace Tablets 641

Timolol Hemihydrate (Beta receptor blocking agents and terbutaline sulfate inhibit each other). Products include:

Betimol 0.25%, 0.5% .... © 261

Timolol Maleate (Beta receptor blocking agents and terbutaline sulfate inhibit each other). Products include:

Blocadren Tablets 1614
Timolide Tablets..................................... 1748
Timoptic in Ocudose 1753

Timoptic Sterile Ophthalmic Solution... 1751
Timoptic-XE 1755

Tranylcypromine Sulfate (May potentiate action of terbutaline sulfate on vascular system). Products include:

Parnate Tablets 2503

Trimipramine Maleate (May potentiate action of terbutaline sulfate on vascular system). Products include:

Surmontil Capsules............................... 2811

BRETHINE AMPULS

(Terbutaline Sulfate) 815
May interact with sympathomimetics, monoamine oxidase inhibitors, and tricyclic antidepressants. Compounds in these categories include:

Albuterol (Combined effect on cardiovascular system may be deleterious). Products include:

Proventil Inhalation Aerosol 2382
Ventolin Inhalation Aerosol and Refill 1197

Albuterol Sulfate (Combined effect on cardiovascular system may be deleterious). Products include:

Airet Solution for Inhalation 452
Proventil Inhalation Solution 0.083% 2384
Proventil Repetabs Tablets 2386
Proventil Solution for Inhalation 0.5% 2383
Proventil Syrup 2385
Proventil Tablets 2386
Ventolin Inhalation Solution................ 1198
Ventolin Nebules Inhalation Solution... 1199
Ventolin Rotacaps for Inhalation 1200
Ventolin Syrup.. 1202
Ventolin Tablets 1203
Volmax Extended-Release Tablets .. 1788

Amitriptyline Hydrochloride (The action of beta-adrenergic agonists on the vascular system may be potentiated). Products include:

Elavil 2838
Endep Tablets 2174
Etrafon.. 2355
Limbitrol 2180
Triavil Tablets 1757

Amoxapine (The action of beta-adrenergic agonists on the vascular system may be potentiated). Products include:

Asendin Tablets 1369

Clomipramine Hydrochloride (The action of beta-adrenergic agonists on the vascular system may be potentiated). Products include:

Anafranil Capsules 803

Desipramine Hydrochloride (The action of beta-adrenergic agonists on the vascular system may be potentiated). Products include:

Norpramin Tablets 1526

Dobutamine Hydrochloride (Combined effect on cardiovascular system may be deleterious). Products include:

Dobutrex Solution Vials....................... 1439

Dopamine Hydrochloride (Combined effect on cardiovascular system may be deleterious).

No products indexed under this heading.

Doxepin Hydrochloride (The action of beta-adrenergic agonists on the vascular system may be potentiated). Products include:

Sinequan 2205
Zonalon Cream 1055

Ephedrine Hydrochloride (Combined effect on cardiovascular system may be deleterious). Products include:

Primatene Dual Action Formula...... ⊞ 872
Primatene Tablets .... ⊞ 873

Quadrinal Tablets 1350

Ephedrine Sulfate (Combined effect on cardiovascular system may be deleterious). Products include:

Bronkaid Caplets .... ⊞ 717
Marax Tablets & DF Syrup.................. 2200

Ephedrine Tannate (Combined effect on cardiovascular system may be deleterious). Products include:

Rynatuss 2673

Epinephrine (Combined effect on cardiovascular system may be deleterious). Products include:

Bronkaid Mist .... ⊞ 717
EPIFRIN .... © 239
EpiPen 790
Marcaine Hydrochloride with Epinephrine 1:200,000 2316
Primatene Mist .... ⊞ 873
Sensorcaine with Epinephrine Injection.. 559
Sus-Phrine Injection 1019
Xylocaine with Epinephrine Injections.. 567

Epinephrine Bitartrate (Combined effect on cardiovascular system may be deleterious). Products include:

Bronkaid Mist Suspension .... ⊞ 718
Sensorcaine-MPF with Epinephrine Injection 559

Epinephrine Hydrochloride (Combined effect on cardiovascular system may be deleterious). Products include:

Ana-Kit Anaphylaxis Emergency Treatment Kit 617

Furazolidone (The action of beta-adrenergic agonists on the vascular system may be potentiated). Products include:

Furoxone 2046

Imipramine Hydrochloride (The action of beta-adrenergic agonists on the vascular system may be potentiated). Products include:

Tofranil Ampuls 854
Tofranil Tablets 856

Imipramine Pamoate (The action of beta-adrenergic agonists on the vascular system may be potentiated). Products include:

Tofranil-PM Capsules........................... 857

Isocarboxazid (The action of beta-adrenergic agonists on the vascular system may be potentiated).

No products indexed under this heading.

Isoproterenol Hydrochloride (Combined effect on cardiovascular system may be deleterious). Products include:

Isuprel Hydrochloride Injection 1:5000 2311
Isuprel Hydrochloride Solution 1:200 & 1:100 2313
Isuprel Mistometer 2312

Isoproterenol Sulfate (Combined effect on cardiovascular system may be deleterious). Products include:

Norisodrine with Calcium Iodide Syrup... 442

Maprotiline Hydrochloride (The action of beta-adrenergic agonists on the vascular system may be potentiated). Products include:

Ludiomil Tablets.................................... 843

Metaproterenol Sulfate (Combined effect on cardiovascular system may be deleterious). Products include:

Alupent... 669
Metaproterenol Sulfate Inhalation Solution, USP, Arm-a-Med 552

Metaraminol Bitartrate (Combined effect on cardiovascular system may be deleterious). Products include:

Aramine Injection.................................. 1609

Norepinephrine Bitartrate (Combined effect on cardiovascular system may be deleterious). Products include:

Levophed Bitartrate Injection 2315

Nortriptyline Hydrochloride (The action of beta-adrenergic agonists on the vascular system may be potentiated). Products include:

Pamelor 2280

Phenelzine Sulfate (The action of beta-adrenergic agonists on the vascular system may be potentiated). Products include:

Nardil 1920

Phenylephrine Bitartrate (Combined effect on cardiovascular system may be deleterious).

No products indexed under this heading.

Phenylephrine Hydrochloride (Combined effect on cardiovascular system may be deleterious). Products include:

Atrohist Plus Tablets 454
Cerose DM .... ⊞ 878
Comhist 2038
D.A. Chewable Tablets......................... 951
Deconsal Pediatric Capsules.............. 454
Dura-Vent/DA Tablets 953
Entex Capsules 1986
Entex Liquid 1986
Extendryl 1005
4-Way Fast Acting Nasal Spray (regular & mentholated) .... ⊞ 621
Hemorid For Women .... ⊞ 834
Hycomine Compound Tablets 932
Neo-Synephrine Hydrochloride 1% Carpuject... 2324
Neo-Synephrine Hydrochloride 1% Injection 2324
Neo-Synephrine Hydrochloride (Ophthalmic) 2325
Neo-Synephrine .... ⊞ 726
Nōstril .... ⊞ 644
Novahistine Elixir .... ⊞ 823
Phenergan VC 2779
Phenergan VC with Codeine 2781
Preparation H .... ⊞ 871
Tympagesic Ear Drops 2342
Vasosulf .... © 271
Vicks Sinex Nasal Spray and Ultra Fine Mist .... ⊞ 765

Phenylephrine Tannate (Combined effect on cardiovascular system may be deleterious). Products include:

Atrohist Pediatric Suspension 454
Ricobid-D Pediatric Suspension........ 2038
Ricobid Tablets and Pediatric Suspension.. 2038
Rynatan 2673
Rynatuss 2673

Phenylpropanolamine Hydrochloride (Combined effect on cardiovascular system may be deleterious). Products include:

Acutrim .... ⊞ 628
Allerest Children's Chewable Tablets .... ⊞ 627
Allerest 12 Hour Caplets .... ⊞ 627
Atrohist Plus Tablets 454
BC Cold Powder Multi-Symptom Formula (Cold-Sinus-Allergy) ...... ⊞ 609
BC Cold Powder Non-Drowsy Formula (Cold-Sinus) .... ⊞ 609
Cheracol Plus Head Cold/Cough Formula .... ⊞ 769
Comtrex Multi-Symptom Non-Drowsy Liqui-gels............................... ⊞ 618
Contac Continuous Action Nasal Decongestant/Antihistamine 12 Hour Capsules..................................... ⊞ 813
Contac Maximum Strength Continuous Action Decongestant/ Antihistamine 12 Hour Caplets.. ⊞ 813
Contac Severe Cold and Flu Formula Caplets .... ⊞ 814
Coricidin 'D' Decongestant Tablets .... ⊞ 800
Dexatrim .... ⊞ 832
Dexatrim Plus Vitamins Caplets .... ⊞ 832
Dimetane-DC Cough Syrup 2059
Dimetapp Elixir .... ⊞ 773
Dimetapp Extentabs .... ⊞ 774
Dimetapp Tablets/Liqui-Gels .... ⊞ 775

IMPORTANT NOTE: Always consult each drug listing in the patient's regimen for possible interactions.

Brethine Interactions Index 128

Dimetapp Cold & Allergy Chewable Tablets ■ 773
Dimetapp DM Elixir ■ 774
Dura-Vent Tablets 952
Entex Capsules 1986
Entex LA Tablets 1987
Entex Liquid 1986
Exgest LA Tablets 782
Hycomine 931
Isoclor Timesule Capsules ■ 637
Nolamine Timed-Release Tablets 785
Ornade Spansule Capsules 2502
Propagest Tablets 786
Pyrroxate Caplets ■ 772
Robitussin-CF ■ 777
Sinulin Tablets 787
Tavist-D 12 Hour Relief Tablets ■ 787
Teldrin 12 Hour Antihistamine/Nasal Decongestant Allergy Relief Capsules ■ 826
Triaminic Allergy Tablets ■ 789
Triaminic Cold Tablets ■ 790
Triaminic Expectorant ■ 790
Triaminic Syrup ■ 792
Triaminic-12 Tablets ■ 792
Triaminic-DM Syrup ■ 792
Triaminicin Tablets ■ 793
Triaminicol Multi-Symptom Cold Tablets ■ 793
Triaminicol Multi-Symptom Relief ■ 794
Vicks DayQuil Allergy Relief 12-Hour Extended Release Tablets ■ 760
Vicks DayQuil Allergy Relief 4-Hour Tablets ■ 760
Vicks DayQuil SINUS Pressure & CONGESTION Relief ■ 761

Pirbuterol Acetate (Combined effect on cardiovascular system may be deleterious). Products include:
Maxair Autohaler 1492
Maxair Inhaler 1494

Protriptyline Hydrochloride (The action of beta-adrenergic agonists on the vascular system may be potentiated). Products include:
Vivactil Tablets 1774

Pseudoephedrine Hydrochloride (Combined effect on cardiovascular system may be deleterious). Products include:
Actifed Allergy Daytime/Nighttime Caplets ■ 844
Actifed Plus Caplets ■ 845
Actifed Plus Tablets ■ 845
Actifed with Codeine Cough Syrup 1067
Actifed Sinus Daytime/Nighttime Tablets and Caplets ■ 846
Actifed Syrup ■ 846
Actifed Tablets ■ 844
Advil Cold and Sinus Caplets and Tablets (formerly CoAdvil) ■ 870
Alka-Seltzer Plus Cold Medicine Liqui-Gels ■ 706
Alka-Seltzer Plus Cold & Cough Medicine Liqui-Gels ■ 705
Alka-Seltzer Plus Night-Time Cold Medicine Liqui-Gels ■ 706
Allerest Headache Strength Tablets ■ 627
Allerest Maximum Strength Tablets ■ 627
Allerest No Drowsiness Tablets ■ 627
Allerest Sinus Pain Formula ■ 627
Anatuss LA Tablets 1542
Atrohist Pediatric Capsules 453
Bayer Select Sinus Pain Relief Formula ■ 717
Benadryl Allergy Decongestant Liquid Medication ■ 848
Benadryl Allergy Decongestant Tablets ■ 848
Benadryl Allergy Sinus Headache Formula Caplets ■ 849
Benylin Multisymptom ■ 852
Bromfed Capsules (Extended-Release) 1785
Bromfed Syrup ■ 733
Bromfed Tablets 1785
Bromfed-DM Cough Syrup 1786
Bromfed-PD Capsules (Extended-Release) 1785
Children's Vicks DayQuil Allergy Relief ■ 757
Children's Vicks NyQuil Cold/Cough Relief ■ 758
Comtrex Multi-Symptom Cold Reliever Tablets/Caplets/Liqui-Gels/Liquid ■ 615
Allergy-Sinus Comtrex Multi-Symptom Allergy-Sinus Formula Tablets ■ 617
Comtrex Multi-Symptom Non-Drowsy Caplets ■ 618
Congess 1004
Contac Day Allergy/Sinus Caplets ■ 812
Contac Day & Night ■ 812
Contac Night Allergy/Sinus Caplets ■ 812
Contac Severe Cold & Flu Non-Drowsy ■ 815
Deconamine Chewable Tablets 1320
Deconamine CX Cough and Cold Liquid and Tablets 1319
Deconamine 1320
Deconsal C Expectorant Syrup 456
Deconsal Pediatric Syrup 457
Deconsal II Tablets 454
Dimetane-DX Cough Syrup 2059
Dimetapp Sinus Caplets ■ 775
Dorcol Children's Cough Syrup ■ 785
Drixoral Cough + Congestion Liquid Caps ■ 802
Dura-Tap/PD Capsules 2867
Duratuss Tablets 2565
Duratuss HD Elixir 2565
Efidac/24 ■ 635
Entex PSE Tablets 1987
Fedahist Gyrocaps 2401
Fedahist Timecaps 2401
Guaifed 1787
Guaifed Syrup ■ 734
Guaimax-D Tablets 792
Guaitab Tablets ■ 734
Isoclor Expectorant 990
Kronofed-A 977
Motrin IB Sinus ■ 838
Novahistine DH 2462
Novahistine DMX ■ 822
Novahistine Expectorant 2463
Nucofed 2051
PediaCare Cold Allergy Chewable Tablets ■ 677
PediaCare Cough-Cold Chewable Tablets 1553
PediaCare 1553
PediaCare Infants' Decongestant Drops ■ 677
PediCare Infant's Drops Decongestant Plus Cough 1553
PediaCare NightRest Cough-Cold Liquid 1553
Pediatric Vicks 44d Dry Hacking Cough & Head Congestion ■ 763
Pediatric Vicks 44m Cough & Cold Relief ■ 764
Robitussin Cold & Cough Liqui-Gels ■ 776
Robitussin Maximum Strength Cough & Cold ■ 778
Robitussin Pediatric Cough & Cold Formula ■ 779
Robitussin Severe Congestion Liqui-Gels ■ 776
Robitussin-DAC Syrup 2074
Robitussin-PE ■ 778
Rondec Oral Drops 953
Rondec Syrup 953
Rondec Tablet 953
Rondec-DM Oral Drops 954
Rondec-DM Syrup 954
Rondec-TR Tablet 953
Ryna ■ 841
Seldane-D Extended-Release Tablets 1538
Semprex-D Capsules 463
Semprex-D Capsules 1167
Sinarest Tablets ■ 648
Sinarest Extra Strength Tablets ■ 648
Sinarest No Drowsiness Tablets ■ 648
Sine-Aid IB Caplets 1554
Sine-Aid Maximum Strength Sinus Medication Gelcaps, Caplets and Tablets 1554
Sine-Off No Drowsiness Formula Caplets ■ 824
Sine-Off Sinus Medicine ■ 825
Singlet Tablets ■ 825
Sinutab Non-Drying Liquid Caps ■ 859
Sinutab Sinus Allergy Medication, Maximum Strength Tablets and Caplets ■ 860
Sinutab Sinus Medication, Maximum Strength Without Drowsiness Formula, Tablets & Caplets ■ 860
Sinutab Sinus Medication, Regular Strength Without Drowsiness Formula ■ 859
Sudafed Children's Liquid ■ 861
Sudafed Cold and Cough Liquidcaps ■ 862
Sudafed Cough Syrup ■ 862
Sudafed Plus Liquid ■ 862
Sudafed Plus Tablets ■ 863
Sudafed Severe Cold Formula Caplets ■ 863
Sudafed Severe Cold Formula Tablets ■ 864
Sudafed Sinus Caplets ■ 864
Sudafed Sinus Tablets ■ 864
Sudafed Tablets, 30 mg ■ 861
Sudafed Tablets, 60 mg ■ 861
Sudafed 12 Hour Caplets ■ 861
Syn-Rx Tablets 465
Syn-Rx DM Tablets 466
TheraFlu ■ 787
TheraFlu Maximum Strength Nighttime Flu, Cold & Cough Medicine ■ 788
TheraFlu Maximum Strength Non-Drowsy Formula Flu, Cold & Cough Medicine ■ 788
Thera Flu Maximum Strength, Non-Drowsy Formula Flu, Cold and Cough Caplets ■ 789
Triaminic AM Cough and Decongestant Formula ■ 789
Triaminic AM Decongestant Formula ■ 790
Triaminic Nite Light ■ 791
Triaminic Sore Throat Formula ■ 791
Tussend 1783
Tussend Expectorant 1785
Children's TYLENOL Cold Multi-Symptom Liquid Formula and Chewable Tablets 1561
Children's TYLENOL Cold Plus Cough Multi Symptom Tablets and Liquid ■ 681
Infants' TYLENOL Cold Decongestant & Fever-Reducer Drops 1556
TYLENOL Maximum Strength Allergy Sinus Medication Gelcaps and Caplets 1563
TYLENOL Maximum Strength Allergy Sinus NightTime Medication Caplets 1555
TYLENOL Flu Maximum Strength Gelcaps 1565
TYLENOL Flu NightTime, Maximum Strength, Gelcaps 1566
TYLENOL Maximum Strength Flu NightTime Hot Medication Packets 1562
TYLENOL, Maximum Strength, Sinus Medication Geltabs, Gelcaps, Caplets and Tablets 1566
TYLENOL Cold Multi-Symptom Formula Medication Tablets and Caplets 1561
TYLENOL Cold Medication No Drowsiness Formula Gelcaps and Caplets 1562
TYLENOL Cold Multi-Symptom Hot Medication Liquid Packets 1557
TYLENOL Cough Multi-Symptom Medication with Decongestant 1565
Ursinus Inlay-Tabs ■ 794
Vicks 44 LiquiCaps Cough, Cold & Flu Relief ■ 755
Vicks 44 LiquiCaps Non-Drowsy Cough & Cold Relief ■ 756
Vicks 44D Dry Hacking Cough & Head Congestion ■ 755
Vicks 44M Cough, Cold & Flu Relief ■ 756
Vicks DayQuil ■ 761
Vicks DayQuil SINUS Pressure & PAIN Relief with IBUPROFEN ■ 762
Vicks Nyquil Hot Therapy ■ 762
Vicks NyQuil LiquiCaps Multi-Symptom Cold/Flu Relief ■ 763
Vicks NyQuil Multi-Symptom Cold/Flu Relief - (Original & Cherry Flavor) ■ 763

Pseudoephedrine Sulfate (Combined effect on cardiovascular system may be deleterious). Products include:
Cheracol Sinus ■ 768
Chlor-Trimeton Allergy Decongestant Tablets ■ 799
Claritin-D 2350
Drixoral Cold and Allergy Sustained-Action Tablets ■ 802
Drixoral Cold and Flu Extended-Release Tablets ■ 803
Drixoral Non-Drowsy Formula Extended-Release Tablets ■ 803
Drixoral Allergy/Sinus Extended Release Tablets ■ 804
Trinalin Repetabs Tablets 1330

Salmeterol Xinafoate (Combined effect on cardiovascular system may be deleterious). Products include:
Serevent Inhalation Aerosol 1176

Selegiline Hydrochloride (The action of beta-adrenergic agonists on the vascular system may be potentiated). Products include:
Eldepryl Tablets 2550

Tranylcypromine Sulfate (The action of beta-adrenergic agonists on the vascular system may be potentiated). Products include:
Parnate Tablets 2503

Trimipramine Maleate (The action of beta-adrenergic agonists on the vascular system may be potentiated). Products include:
Surmontil Capsules 2811

BRETHINE TABLETS
(Terbutaline Sulfate) 814
May interact with sympathomimetics. Compounds in this category include:

Albuterol (Concomitant use not recommended; combined effect on the cardiovascular system may be deleterious). Products include:
Proventil Inhalation Aerosol 2382
Ventolin Inhalation Aerosol and Refill 1197

Albuterol Sulfate (Concomitant use not recommended; combined effect on the cardiovascular system may be deleterious). Products include:
Airet Solution for Inhalation 452
Proventil Inhalation Solution 0.083% 2384
Proventil Repetabs Tablets 2386
Proventil Solution for Inhalation 0.5% 2383
Proventil Syrup 2385
Proventil Tablets 2386
Ventolin Inhalation Solution 1198
Ventolin Nebules Inhalation Solution 1199
Ventolin Rotacaps for Inhalation 1200
Ventolin Syrup 1202
Ventolin Tablets 1203
Volmax Extended-Release Tablets 1788

Dobutamine Hydrochloride (Concomitant use not recommended; combined effect on the cardiovascular system may be deleterious). Products include:
Dobutrex Solution Vials 1439

Dopamine Hydrochloride (Concomitant use not recommended; combined effect on the cardiovascular system may be deleterious).
No products indexed under this heading.

Ephedrine Hydrochloride (Concomitant use not recommended; combined effect on the cardiovascular system may be deleterious). Products include:
Primatene Dual Action Formula ■ 872
Primatene Tablets ■ 873
Quadrinal Tablets 1350

Ephedrine Sulfate (Concomitant use not recommended; combined effect on the cardiovascular system may be deleterious). Products include:
Bronkaid Caplets ■ 717
Marax Tablets & DF Syrup 2200

Ephedrine Tannate (Concomitant use not recommended; combined effect on the cardiovascular system may be deleterious). Products include:
Rynatuss 2673

(■ Described in PDR For Nonprescription Drugs) (◉ Described in PDR For Ophthalmology)

129 **Interactions Index** **Brethine Tablets**

Epinephrine (Concomitant use not recommended; combined effect on the cardiovascular system may be deleterious). Products include:
- Bronkaid Mist ▣ 717
- EPIFRIN ◉ 239
- EpiPen 790
- Marcaine Hydrochloride with Epinephrine 1:200,000 2316
- Primatene Mist ▣ 873
- Sensorcaine with Epinephrine Injection 559
- Sus-Phrine Injection 1019
- Xylocaine with Epinephrine Injections 567

Epinephrine Bitartrate (Concomitant use not recommended; combined effect on the cardiovascular system may be deleterious). Products include:
- Bronkaid Mist Suspension ▣ 718
- Sensorcaine-MPF with Epinephrine Injection 559

Epinephrine Hydrochloride (Concomitant use not recommended; combined effect on the cardiovascular system may be deleterious). Products include:
- Ana-Kit Anaphylaxis Emergency Treatment Kit 617

Isoproterenol Hydrochloride (Concomitant use not recommended; combined effect on the cardiovascular system may be deleterious). Products include:
- Isuprel Hydrochloride Injection 1:5000 2311
- Isuprel Hydrochloride Solution 1:200 & 1:100 2313
- Isuprel Mistometer 2312

Isoproterenol Sulfate (Concomitant use not recommended; combined effect on the cardiovascular system may be deleterious). Products include:
- Norisodrine with Calcium Iodide Syrup 442

Metaproterenol Sulfate (Concomitant use not recommended; combined effect on the cardiovascular system may be deleterious). Products include:
- Alupent 669
- Metaproterenol Sulfate Inhalation Solution, USP, Arm-a-Med 552

Metaraminol Bitartrate (Concomitant use not recommended; combined effect on the cardiovascular system may be deleterious). Products include:
- Aramine Injection 1609

Methoxamine Hydrochloride (Concomitant use not recommended; combined effect on the cardiovascular system may be deleterious). Products include:
- Vasoxyl Injection 1196

Norepinephrine Bitartrate (Concomitant use not recommended; combined effect on the cardiovascular system may be deleterious). Products include:
- Levophed Bitartrate Injection 2315

Phenylephrine Bitartrate (Concomitant use not recommended; combined effect on the cardiovascular system may be deleterious).
- No products indexed under this heading.

Phenylephrine Hydrochloride (Concomitant use not recommended; combined effect on the cardiovascular system may be deleterious). Products include:
- Atrohist Plus Tablets 454
- Cerose DM ▣ 878
- Comhist 2038
- D.A. Chewable Tablets 951
- Deconsal Pediatric Capsules 454
- Dura-Vent/DA Tablets 953
- Entex Capsules 1986
- Entex Liquid 1986
- Extendryl 1005
- 4-Way Fast Acting Nasal Spray (regular & mentholated) ▣ 621
- Hemorid For Women ▣ 834
- Hycomine Compound Tablets 932
- Neo-Synephrine Hydrochloride 1% Carpuject 2324
- Neo-Synephrine Hydrochloride 1% Injection 2324
- Neo-Synephrine Hydrochloride (Ophthalmic) 2325
- Neo-Synephrine ▣ 726
- Nōstril ▣ 644
- Novahistine Elixir ▣ 823
- Phenergan VC 2779
- Phenergan VC with Codeine 2781
- Preparation H ▣ 871
- Tympagesic Ear Drops 2342
- Vasosulf ◉ 271
- Vicks Sinex Nasal Spray and Ultra Fine Mist ▣ 765

Phenylephrine Tannate (Concomitant use not recommended; combined effect on the cardiovascular system may be deleterious). Products include:
- Atrohist Pediatric Suspension 454
- Ricobid-D Pediatric Suspension 2038
- Ricobid Tablets and Pediatric Suspension 2038
- Rynatan 2673
- Rynatuss 2673

Phenylpropanolamine Hydrochloride (Concomitant use not recommended; combined effect on the cardiovascular system may be deleterious). Products include:
- Acutrim ▣ 628
- Allerest Children's Chewable Tablets ▣ 627
- Allerest 12 Hour Caplets ▣ 627
- Atrohist Plus Tablets 454
- BC Cold Powder Multi-Symptom Formula (Cold-Sinus-Allergy) ▣ 609
- BC Cold Powder Non-Drowsy Formula (Cold-Sinus) ▣ 609
- Cheracol Plus Head Cold/Cough Formula ▣ 769
- Comtrex Multi-Symptom Non-Drowsy Liqui-gels ▣ 618
- Contac Continuous Action Nasal Decongestant/Antihistamine 12 Hour Capsules ▣ 813
- Contac Maximum Strength Continuous Action Decongestant/Antihistamine 12 Hour Caplets ▣ 813
- Contac Severe Cold and Flu Formula Caplets ▣ 814
- Coricidin 'D' Decongestant Tablets ▣ 800
- Dexatrim ▣ 832
- Dexatrim Plus Vitamins Caplets ▣ 832
- Dimetane-DC Cough Syrup 2059
- Dimetapp Elixir ▣ 773
- Dimetapp Extentabs ▣ 774
- Dimetapp Tablets/Liqui-Gels ▣ 775
- Dimetapp Cold & Allergy Chewable Tablets ▣ 773
- Dimetapp DM Elixir ▣ 774
- Dura-Vent Tablets 952
- Entex Capsules 1986
- Entex LA Tablets 1987
- Entex Liquid 1986
- Exgest LA Tablets 782
- Hycomine 931
- Isoclor Timesule Capsules ▣ 637
- Nolamine Timed-Release Tablets 785
- Ornade Spansule Capsules 2502
- Propagest Tablets 786
- Pyrroxate Caplets ▣ 772
- Robitussin-CF ▣ 777
- Sinulin Tablets 787
- Tavist-D 12 Hour Relief Tablets ▣ 787
- Teldrin 12 Hour Antihistamine/Nasal Decongestant Allergy Relief Capsules ▣ 826
- Triaminic Allergy Tablets ▣ 789
- Triaminic Cold Tablets ▣ 790
- Triaminic Expectorant ▣ 790
- Triaminic Syrup ▣ 792
- Triaminic-12 Tablets ▣ 792
- Triaminic-DM Syrup ▣ 792
- Triaminicin Tablets ▣ 793
- Triaminicol Multi-Symptom Cold Tablets ▣ 793
- Triaminicol Multi-Symptom Relief ▣ 794
- Vicks DayQuil Allergy Relief 12-Hour Extended Release Tablets ▣ 760
- Vicks DayQuil Allergy Relief 4-Hour Tablets ▣ 760
- Vicks DayQuil SINUS Pressure & CONGESTION Relief ▣ 761

Pirbuterol Acetate (Concomitant use not recommended; combined effect on the cardiovascular system may be deleterious). Products include:
- Maxair Autohaler 1492
- Maxair Inhaler 1494

Pseudoephedrine Hydrochloride (Concomitant use not recommended; combined effect on the cardiovascular system may be deleterious). Products include:
- Actifed Allergy Daytime/Nighttime Caplets ▣ 844
- Actifed Plus Caplets ▣ 845
- Actifed Plus Tablets ▣ 845
- Actifed with Codeine Cough Syrup 1067
- Actifed Sinus Daytime/Nighttime Tablets and Caplets ▣ 846
- Actifed Syrup ▣ 846
- Actifed Tablets ▣ 844
- Advil Cold and Sinus Caplets and Tablets (formerly CoAdvil) ▣ 870
- Alka-Seltzer Plus Cold Medicine Liqui-Gels ▣ 706
- Alka-Seltzer Plus Cold & Cough Medicine Liqui-Gels ▣ 705
- Alka-Seltzer Plus Night-Time Cold Medicine Liqui-Gels ▣ 706
- Allerest Headache Strength Tablets ▣ 627
- Allerest Maximum Strength Tablets ▣ 627
- Allerest No Drowsiness Tablets ▣ 627
- Allerest Sinus Pain Formula ▣ 627
- Anatuss LA Tablets 1542
- Atrohist Pediatric Capsules 453
- Bayer Select Sinus Pain Relief Formula ▣ 717
- Benadryl Allergy Decongestant Liquid Medication ▣ 848
- Benadryl Allergy Decongestant Tablets ▣ 848
- Benadryl Allergy Sinus Headache Formula Caplets ▣ 849
- Benylin Multisymptom ▣ 852
- Bromfed Capsules (Extended-Release) 1785
- Bromfed Syrup ▣ 733
- Bromfed Tablets 1785
- Bromfed-DM Cough Syrup 1786
- Bromfed-PD Capsules (Extended-Release) 1785
- Children's Vicks DayQuil Allergy Relief ▣ 757
- Children's Vicks NyQuil Cold/Cough Relief ▣ 758
- Comtrex Multi-Symptom Cold Reliever Tablets/Caplets/Liqui-Gels/Liquid ▣ 615
- Allergy-Sinus Comtrex Multi-Symptom Allergy-Sinus Formula Tablets ▣ 617
- Comtrex Multi-Symptom Non-Drowsy Caplets ▣ 618
- Congess 1004
- Contac Day Allergy/Sinus Caplets ▣ 812
- Contac Day & Night ▣ 812
- Contac Night Allergy/Sinus Caplets ▣ 812
- Contac Severe Cold & Flu Non-Drowsy ▣ 815
- Deconamine Chewable Tablets 1320
- Deconamine CX Cough and Cold Liquid and Tablets 1319
- Deconamine 1320
- Deconsal C Expectorant Syrup 456
- Deconsal Pediatric Syrup 457
- Deconsal II Tablets 454
- Dimetane-DX Cough Syrup 2059
- Dimetapp Sinus Caplets ▣ 775
- Dorcol Children's Cough Syrup ▣ 785
- Drixoral Cough + Congestion Liquid Caps ▣ 802
- Dura-Tap/PD Capsules 2867
- Duratuss Tablets 2565
- Duratuss HD Elixir 2565
- Efidac/24 ▣ 635
- Entex PSE Tablets 1987
- Fedahist Gyrocaps 2401
- Fedahist Timecaps 2401
- Guaifed 1787
- Guaifed Syrup ▣ 734
- Guaimax-D Tablets 792
- Guaitab Tablets ▣ 734
- Isoclor Expectorant 990
- Kronofed-A 977
- Motrin IB Sinus ▣ 838
- Novahistine DH 2462
- Novahistine DMX ▣ 822
- Novahistine Expectorant 2463
- Nucofed 2051
- PediaCare Cold Allergy Chewable Tablets ▣ 677
- PediaCare Cough-Cold Chewable Tablets 1553
- PediaCare 1553
- PediaCare Infants' Decongestant Drops ▣ 677
- PediCare Infant's Drops Decongestant Plus Cough 1553
- PediaCare NightRest Cough-Cold Liquid 1553
- Pediatric Vicks 44d Dry Hacking Cough & Head Congestion ▣ 763
- Pediatric Vicks 44m Cough & Cold Relief ▣ 764
- Robitussin Cold & Cough Liqui-Gels ▣ 776
- Robitussin Maximum Strength Cough & Cold ▣ 778
- Robitussin Pediatric Cough & Cold Formula ▣ 779
- Robitussin Severe Congestion Liqui-Gels ▣ 776
- Robitussin-DAC Syrup 2074
- Robitussin-PE ▣ 778
- Rondec Oral Drops 953
- Rondec Syrup 953
- Rondec Tablet 953
- Rondec-DM Oral Drops 954
- Rondec-DM Syrup 954
- Rondec-TR Tablet 953
- Ryna ▣ 841
- Seldane-D Extended-Release Tablets 1538
- Semprex-D Capsules 463
- Semprex-D Capsules 1167
- Sinarest Tablets ▣ 648
- Sinarest Extra Strength Tablets ▣ 648
- Sinarest No Drowsiness Tablets ▣ 648
- Sine-Aid IB Caplets 1554
- Sine-Aid Maximum Strength Sinus Medication Gelcaps, Caplets and Tablets 1554
- Sine-Off No Drowsiness Formula Caplets ▣ 824
- Sine-Off Sinus Medicine ▣ 825
- Singlet Tablets ▣ 825
- Sinutab Non-Drying Liquid Caps ▣ 859
- Sinutab Sinus Allergy Medication, Maximum Strength Tablets and Caplets ▣ 860
- Sinutab Sinus Medication, Maximum Strength Without Drowsiness Formula, Tablets & Caplets ▣ 860
- Sinutab Sinus Medication, Regular Strength Without Drowsiness Formula ▣ 859
- Sudafed Children's Liquid ▣ 861
- Sudafed Cold and Cough Liquidcaps ▣ 862
- Sudafed Cough Syrup ▣ 862
- Sudafed Plus Liquid ▣ 862
- Sudafed Plus Tablets ▣ 863
- Sudafed Severe Cold Formula Caplets ▣ 863
- Sudafed Severe Cold Formula Tablets ▣ 864
- Sudafed Sinus Caplets ▣ 864
- Sudafed Sinus Tablets ▣ 864
- Sudafed Tablets, 30 mg ▣ 861
- Sudafed Tablets, 60 mg ▣ 861
- Sudafed 12 Hour Caplets ▣ 861
- Syn-Rx Tablets 465
- Syn-Rx DM Tablets 466
- TheraFlu ▣ 787
- TheraFlu Maximum Strength Nighttime Flu, Cold & Cough Medicine ▣ 788
- TheraFlu Maximum Strength Non-Drowsy Formula Flu, Cold & Cough Medicine ▣ 788
- Thera Flu Maximum Strength, Non-Drowsy Formula Flu, Cold and Cough Caplets ▣ 789
- Triaminic AM Cough and Decongestant Formula ▣ 789
- Triaminic AM Decongestant Formula ▣ 790
- Triaminic Nite Light ▣ 791
- Triaminic Sore Throat Formula ▣ 791
- Tussend 1783
- Tussend Expectorant 1785

IMPORTANT NOTE: Always consult each drug listing in the patient's regimen for possible interactions.

Children's TYLENOL Cold Multi-Symptom Liquid Formula and Chewable Tablets 1561
Children's TYLENOL Cold Plus Cough Multi Symptom Tablets and Liquid .... ▣ 681
Infants' TYLENOL Cold Decongestant & Fever-Reducer Drops 1556
TYLENOL Maximum Strength Allergy Sinus Medication Gelcaps and Caplets 1563
TYLENOL Maximum Strength Allergy Sinus NightTime Medication Caplets 1555
TYLENOL Flu Maximum Strength Gelcaps 1565
TYLENOL Flu NightTime, Maximum Strength, Gelcaps 1566
TYLENOL Maximum Strength Flu NightTime Hot Medication Packets 1562
TYLENOL, Maximum Strength, Sinus Medication Geltabs, Gelcaps, Caplets and Tablets 1566
TYLENOL Cold Multi-Symptom Formula Medication Tablets and Caplets 1561
TYLENOL Cold Medication No Drowsiness Formula Gelcaps and Caplets 1562
TYLENOL Cold Multi-Symptom Hot Medication Liquid Packets 1557
TYLENOL Cough Multi-Symptom Medication with Decongestant 1565
Ursinus Inlay-Tabs .... ▣ 794
Vicks 44 LiquiCaps Cough, Cold & Flu Relief .... ▣ 755
Vicks 44 LiquiCaps Non-Drowsy Cough & Cold Relief .... ▣ 756
Vicks 44D Dry Hacking Cough & Head Congestion .... ▣ 755
Vicks 44M Cough, Cold & Flu Relief .... ▣ 756
Vicks DayQuil .... ▣ 761
Vicks DayQuil SINUS Pressure & PAIN Relief with IBUPROFEN .... ▣ 762
Vicks Nyquil Hot Therapy .... ▣ 762
Vicks NyQuil LiquiCaps Multi-Symptom Cold/Flu Relief .... ▣ 763
Vicks NyQuil Multi-Symptom Cold/Flu Relief - (Original & Cherry Flavor) .... ▣ 763

Pseudoephedrine Sulfate (Concomitant use not recommended; combined effect on the cardiovascular system may be deleterious). Products include:
Cheracol Sinus .... ▣ 768
Chlor-Trimeton Allergy Decongestant Tablets .... ▣ 799
Claritin-D 2350
Drixoral Cold and Allergy Sustained-Action Tablets .... ▣ 802
Drixoral Cold and Flu Extended-Release Tablets .... ▣ 803
Drixoral Non-Drowsy Formula Extended-Release Tablets .... ▣ 803
Drixoral Allergy/Sinus Extended Release Tablets .... ▣ 804
Trinalin Repetabs Tablets 1330

Salmeterol Xinafoate (Concomitant use not recommended; combined effect on the cardiovascular system may be deleterious). Products include:
Serevent Inhalation Aerosol 1176

BREVIBLOC INJECTION
(Esmolol Hydrochloride) 1808
May interact with catecholamine depleting drugs and certain other agents. Compounds in these categories include:

Deserpidine (Potential for additive effect; hypotension or marked bradycardia which may result in vertigo, syncope, or postural hypotension).
No products indexed under this heading.

Digoxin (Increased digoxin levels by 10-20% when concomitantly administered by intravenous route). Products include:
Lanoxicaps 1117
Lanoxin Elixir Pediatric 1120
Lanoxin Injection 1123
Lanoxin Injection Pediatric 1126
Lanoxin Tablets 1128

Dopamine Hydrochloride (Concurrent use is not recommended to control supraventricular tachycardia because of the danger of blocking cardiac contractility when systemic vascular resistance is high).
No products indexed under this heading.

Epinephrine Hydrochloride (Concurrent use is not recommended to control supraventricular tachycardia because of the danger of blocking cardiac contractility when systemic vascular resistance is high; potential for unresponsiveness to the usual dose of epinephrine to treat allergic reaction). Products include:
Ana-Kit Anaphylaxis Emergency Treatment Kit 617

Guanethidine Monosulfate (Potential for additive effect; hypotension or marked bradycardia which may result in vertigo, syncope, or postural hypotension). Products include:
Esimil Tablets 822
Ismelin Tablets 827

Morphine Sulfate (Intravenous morphine increases Brevibloc steady-state blood levels by 46%). Products include:
Astramorph/PF Injection, USP (Preservative-Free) 535
Duramorph 962
Infumorph 200 and Infumorph 500 Sterile Solutions 965
MS Contin Tablets 1994
MSIR 1997
Oramorph SR (Morphine Sulfate Sustained Release Tablets) 2236
RMS Suppositories 2657
Roxanol 2243

Norepinephrine Hydrochloride (Concurrent use is not recommended to control supraventricular tachycardia because of the danger of blocking cardiac contractility when systemic vascular resistance is high).

Rauwolfia Serpentina (Potential for additive effect; hypotension or marked bradycardia which may result in vertigo, syncope, or postural hypotension).
No products indexed under this heading.

Rescinnamine (Potential for additive effect; hypotension or marked bradycardia which may result in vertigo, syncope, or postural hypotension).
No products indexed under this heading.

Reserpine (Potential for additive effect; hypotension or marked bradycardia which may result in vertigo, syncope, or postural hypotension). Products include:
Diupres Tablets 1650
Hydropres Tablets 1675
Ser-Ap-Es Tablets 849

Succinylcholine Chloride (Prolonged neuromuscular blockade from 5 minutes to eight minutes). Products include:
Anectine 1073

Verapamil Hydrochloride (Potential for fatal cardiac arrests in patients with depressed myocardial function). Products include:
Calan SR Caplets 2422
Calan Tablets 2419
Isoptin Injectable 1344
Isoptin Oral Tablets 1346
Isoptin SR Tablets 1348
Verelan Capsules 1410
Verelan Capsules 2824

Warfarin Sodium (Brevibloc concentrations were equivocally higher when given with Warfarin). Products include:
Coumadin 926

BREVICON 21-DAY TABLETS
(Norethindrone, Ethinyl Estradiol) 2088
May interact with barbiturates, tetracyclines, and certain other agents. Compounds in these categories include:

Ampicillin Sodium (Possibility of reduced efficacy, increased incidence of breakthrough bleeding, and menstrual irregularities). Products include:
Unasyn 2212

Aprobarbital (Reduced efficacy; increased incidence of breakthrough bleeding; menstrual irregularities).
No products indexed under this heading.

Butabarbital (Reduced efficacy; increased incidence of breakthrough bleeding; menstrual irregularities).
No products indexed under this heading.

Butalbital (Reduced efficacy; increased incidence of breakthrough bleeding; menstrual irregularities). Products include:
Esgic-plus Tablets 1013
Fioricet Tablets 2258
Fioricet with Codeine Capsules 2260
Fiorinal Capsules 2261
Fiorinal with Codeine Capsules 2262
Fiorinal Tablets 2261
Phrenilin 785
Sedapap Tablets 50 mg/650 mg 1543

Demeclocycline Hydrochloride (Possibility of reduced efficacy, increased incidence of breakthrough bleeding, and menstrual irregularities). Products include:
Declomycin Tablets 1371

Doxycycline Calcium (Possibility of reduced efficacy, increased incidence of breakthrough bleeding, and menstrual irregularities). Products include:
Vibramycin Calcium Oral Suspension Syrup 1941

Doxycycline Hyclate (Possibility of reduced efficacy, increased incidence of breakthrough bleeding, and menstrual irregularities). Products include:
Doryx Capsules 1913
Vibramycin Hyclate Capsules 1941
Vibramycin Hyclate Intravenous 2215
Vibra-Tabs Film Coated Tablets 1941

Doxycycline Monohydrate (Possibility of reduced efficacy, increased incidence of breakthrough bleeding, and menstrual irregularities). Products include:
Monodox Capsules 1805
Vibramycin Monohydrate for Oral Suspension 1941

Griseofulvin (Possibility of reduced efficacy, increased incidence of breakthrough bleeding, and menstrual irregularities). Products include:
Fulvicin P/G Tablets 2359
Fulvicin P/G 165 & 330 Tablets 2359
Grifulvin V (griseofulvin tablets) Microsize (griseofulvin oral suspension) Microsize 1888
Gris-PEG Tablets, 125 mg & 250 mg 479

Mephobarbital (Reduced efficacy; increased incidence of breakthrough bleeding; menstrual irregularities). Products include:
Mebaral Tablets 2322

Methacycline Hydrochloride (Possibility of reduced efficacy, increased incidence of breakthrough bleeding, and menstrual irregularities).
No products indexed under this heading.

Minocycline Hydrochloride (Possibility of reduced efficacy, increased incidence of breakthrough bleeding, and menstrual irregularities). Products include:
Dynacin Capsules 1590
Minocin Intravenous 1382
Minocin Oral Suspension 1385
Minocin Pellet-Filled Capsules 1383

Oxytetracycline Hydrochloride (Possibility of reduced efficacy, increased incidence of breakthrough bleeding, and menstrual irregularities). Products include:
TERAK Ointment .... ◉ 209
Terra-Cortril Ophthalmic Suspension 2210
Terramycin with Polymyxin B Sulfate Ophthalmic Ointment 2211
Urobiotic-250 Capsules 2214

Pentobarbital Sodium (Reduced efficacy; increased incidence of breakthrough bleeding; menstrual irregularities). Products include:
Nembutal Sodium Capsules 436
Nembutal Sodium Solution 438
Nembutal Sodium Suppositories 440

Phenobarbital (Reduced efficacy; increased incidence of breakthrough bleeding; menstrual irregularities). Products include:
Arco-Lase Plus Tablets 512
Bellergal-S Tablets 2250
Donnatal 2060
Donnatal Extentabs 2061
Donnatal Tablets 2060
Phenobarbital Elixir and Tablets 1469
Quadrinal Tablets 1350

Phenylbutazone (Reduced efficacy; increased incidence of breakthrough bleeding; menstrual irregularities).
No products indexed under this heading.

Phenytoin Sodium (Reduced efficacy; increased incidence of breakthrough bleeding; menstrual irregularities). Products include:
Dilantin Kapseals 1906
Dilantin Parenteral 1910

Rifampin (Reduced efficacy; increased incidence of breakthrough bleeding; menstrual irregularities). Products include:
Rifadin 1528
Rifamate Capsules 1530
Rifater 1532
Rimactane Capsules 847

Secobarbital Sodium (Reduced efficacy; increased incidence of breakthrough bleeding; menstrual irregularities). Products include:
Seconal Sodium Pulvules 1474

Tetracycline Hydrochloride (Possibility of reduced efficacy, increased incidence of breakthrough bleeding, and menstrual irregularities). Products include:
Achromycin V Capsules 1367

Thiamylal Sodium (Reduced efficacy; increased incidence of breakthrough bleeding; menstrual irregularities).
No products indexed under this heading.

BREVICON 28-DAY TABLETS
(Norethindrone, Ethinyl Estradiol) 2088
See **Brevicon 21-Day Tablets**

BREVITAL SODIUM VIALS
(Methohexital Sodium) 1429
May interact with central nervous

(▣ Described in PDR For Nonprescription Drugs) (◉ Described in PDR For Ophthalmology)

system depressants, oral anticoagulants, corticosteroids, and certain other agents. Compounds in these categories include:

Alfentanil Hydrochloride (Additive effect). Products include:
Alfenta Injection 1286

Alprazolam (Additive effect). Products include:
Xanax Tablets 2649

Aprobarbital (Additive effect).
No products indexed under this heading.

Betamethasone Acetate (Barbiturates may influence the absorption and elimination of concomitantly used corticosteroids). Products include:
Celestone Soluspan Suspension 2347

Betamethasone Sodium Phosphate (Barbiturates may influence the absorption and elimination of concomitantly used corticosteroids). Products include:
Celestone Soluspan Suspension 2347

Buprenorphine (Additive effect). Products include:
Buprenex Injectable 2006

Buspirone Hydrochloride (Additive effect). Products include:
BuSpar 737

Butabarbital (Additive effect).
No products indexed under this heading.

Butalbital (Additive effect). Products include:
Esgic-plus Tablets 1013
Fioricet Tablets 2258
Fioricet with Codeine Capsules 2260
Fiorinal Capsules 2261
Fiorinal with Codeine Capsules 2262
Fiorinal Tablets 2261
Phrenilin 785
Sedapap Tablets 50 mg/650 mg 1543

Chlordiazepoxide (Additive effect). Products include:
Libritabs Tablets 2177
Limbitrol 2180

Chlordiazepoxide Hydrochloride (Additive effect). Products include:
Librax Capsules 2176
Librium Capsules 2178
Librium Injectable 2179

Chlorpromazine (Additive effect). Products include:
Thorazine Suppositories 2523

Chlorprothixene (Additive effect).
No products indexed under this heading.

Chlorprothixene Hydrochloride (Additive effect).
No products indexed under this heading.

Clorazepate Dipotassium (Additive effect). Products include:
Tranxene 451

Clozapine (Additive effect). Products include:
Clozaril Tablets 2252

Codeine Phosphate (Additive effect). Products include:
Actifed with Codeine Cough Syrup 1067
Brontex 1981
Deconsal C Expectorant Syrup 456
Deconsal Pediatric Syrup 457
Dimetane-DC Cough Syrup 2059
Empirin with Codeine Tablets 1093
Fioricet with Codeine Capsules 2260
Fiorinal with Codeine Capsules 2262
Isoclor Expectorant 990
Novahistine DH 2462
Novahistine Expectorant 2463
Nucofed 2051
Phenergan with Codeine 2777
Phenergan VC with Codeine 2781
Robitussin A-C Syrup 2073
Robitussin-DAC Syrup 2074
Ryna .... ▣ 841
Soma Compound w/Codeine Tablets 2676
Tussi-Organidin NR Liquid and S NR Liquid 2677
Tylenol with Codeine 1583

Cortisone Acetate (Barbiturates may influence the absorption and elimination of concomitantly used corticosteroids). Products include:
Cortone Acetate Sterile Suspension 1623
Cortone Acetate Tablets 1624

Desflurane (Additive effect). Products include:
Suprane 1813

Dexamethasone (Barbiturates may influence the absorption and elimination of concomitantly used corticosteroids). Products include:
AK-Trol Ointment & Suspension .... ◉ 205
Decadron Elixir 1633
Decadron Tablets 1635
Decaspray Topical Aerosol 1648
Dexacidin Ointment .... ◉ 263
Maxitrol Ophthalmic Ointment and Suspension .... ◉ 224
TobraDex Ophthalmic Suspension and Ointment 473

Dexamethasone Acetate (Barbiturates may influence the absorption and elimination of concomitantly used corticosteroids). Products include:
Dalalone D.P. Injectable 1011
Decadron-LA Sterile Suspension 1646

Dexamethasone Sodium Phosphate (Barbiturates may influence the absorption and elimination of concomitantly used corticosteroids). Products include:
Decadron Phosphate Injection 1637
Decadron Phosphate Respihaler 1642
Decadron Phosphate Sterile Ophthalmic Ointment 1641
Decadron Phosphate Sterile Ophthalmic Solution 1642
Decadron Phosphate Topical Cream 1644
Decadron Phosphate Turbinaire 1645
Decadron Phosphate with Xylocaine Injection, Sterile 1639
Dexacort Phosphate in Respihaler 458
Dexacort Phosphate in Turbinaire 459
NeoDecadron Sterile Ophthalmic Ointment 1712
NeoDecadron Sterile Ophthalmic Solution 1713
NeoDecadron Topical Cream 1714

Dezocine (Additive effect). Products include:
Dalgan Injection 538

Diazepam (Additive effect). Products include:
Dizac 1809
Valium Injectable 2182
Valium Tablets 2183
Valrelease Capsules 2169

Dicumarol (Barbiturates may influence the absorption and elimination of concomitantly used anticoagulants).
No products indexed under this heading.

Droperidol (Additive effect). Products include:
Inapsine Injection 1296

Enflurane (Additive effect).
No products indexed under this heading.

Estazolam (Additive effect). Products include:
ProSom Tablets 449

Ethchlorvynol (Additive effect). Products include:
Placidyl Capsules 448

Ethinamate (Additive effect).
No products indexed under this heading.

Fentanyl (Additive effect). Products include:
Duragesic Transdermal System 1288

Fentanyl Citrate (Additive effect). Products include:
Sublimaze Injection 1307

Fludrocortisone Acetate (Barbiturates may influence the absorption and elimination of concomitantly used corticosteroids). Products include:
Florinef Acetate Tablets 505

Fluphenazine Decanoate (Additive effect). Products include:
Prolixin Decanoate 509

Fluphenazine Enanthate (Additive effect). Products include:
Prolixin Enanthate 509

Fluphenazine Hydrochloride (Additive effect). Products include:
Prolixin 509

Flurazepam Hydrochloride (Additive effect). Products include:
Dalmane Capsules 2173

Glutethimide (Additive effect).
No products indexed under this heading.

Haloperidol (Additive effect). Products include:
Haldol Injection, Tablets and Concentrate 1575

Haloperidol Decanoate (Additive effect). Products include:
Haldol Decanoate 1577

Halothane (Barbiturates may influence the absorption and elimination of concomitantly used halothane). Products include:
Fluothane 2724

Hydrocodone Bitartrate (Additive effect). Products include:
Anexsia 5/500 Elixir 1781
Anexia Tablets 1782
Codiclear DH Syrup 791
Deconamine CX Cough and Cold Liquid and Tablets 1319
Duratuss HD Elixir 2565
Hycodan Tablets and Syrup 930
Hycomine Compound Tablets 932
Hycomine 931
Hycotuss Expectorant Syrup 933
Hydrocet Capsules 782
Lorcet 10/650 1018
Lortab 2566
Tussend 1783
Tussend Expectorant 1785
Vicodin Tablets 1356
Vicodin ES Tablets 1357
Vicodin Tuss Expectorant 1358
Zydone Capsules 949

Hydrocodone Polistirex (Additive effect). Products include:
Tussionex Pennkinetic Extended-Release Suspension 998

Hydrocortisone (Barbiturates may influence the absorption and elimination of concomitantly used corticosteroids). Products include:
Anusol-HC Cream 2.5% 1896
Aquanil HC Lotion 1931
Bactine Hydrocortisone Anti-Itch Cream .... ▣ 709
Caldecort Anti-Itch Hydrocortisone Spray .... ▣ 631
Cortaid .... ▣ 836
CORTENEMA 2535
Cortisporin Ointment 1085
Cortisporin Ophthalmic Ointment Sterile 1085
Cortisporin Ophthalmic Suspension Sterile 1086
Cortisporin Otic Solution Sterile 1087
Cortisporin Otic Suspension Sterile 1088
Cortizone-5 .... ▣ 831
Cortizone-10 .... ▣ 831
Hydrocortone Tablets 1672
Hytone 907
Massengill Medicated Soft Cloth Towelettes 2458
PediOtic Suspension Sterile 1153
Preparation H Hydrocortisone 1% Cream .... ▣ 872
ProctoCream-HC 2.5% 2408
VōSoL HC Otic Solution 2678

Hydrocortisone Acetate (Barbiturates may influence the absorption and elimination of concomitantly used corticosteroids). Products include:
Analpram-HC Rectal Cream 1% and 2.5% 977
Anusol HC-1 Anti-Itch Hydrocortisone Ointment .... ▣ 847
Anusol-HC Suppositories 1897
Caldecort .... ▣ 631
Carmol HC 924
Coly-Mycin S Otic w/Neomycin & Hydrocortisone 1906
Cortaid .... ▣ 836
Cortifoam 2396
Cortisporin Cream 1084
Epifoam 2399
Hydrocortone Acetate Sterile Suspension 1669
Mantadil Cream 1135
Nupercainal Hydrocortisone 1% Cream .... ▣ 645
Ophthocort .... ◉ 311
Pramosone Cream, Lotion & Ointment 978
ProctoCream-HC 2408
ProctoFoam-HC 2409
Terra-Cortril Ophthalmic Suspension 2210

Hydrocortisone Sodium Phosphate (Barbiturates may influence the absorption and elimination of concomitantly used corticosteroids). Products include:
Hydrocortone Phosphate Injection, Sterile 1670

Hydrocortisone Sodium Succinate (Barbiturates may influence the absorption and elimination of concomitantly used corticosteroids). Products include:
Solu-Cortef Sterile Powder 2641

Hydroxyzine Hydrochloride (Additive effect). Products include:
Atarax Tablets & Syrup 2185
Marax Tablets & DF Syrup 2200
Vistaril Intramuscular Solution 2216

Isoflurane (Additive effect).
No products indexed under this heading.

Ketamine Hydrochloride (Additive effect).
No products indexed under this heading.

Levomethadyl Acetate Hydrochloride (Additive effect). Products include:
Orlamm 2239

Levorphanol Tartrate (Additive effect). Products include:
Levo-Dromoran 2129

Lorazepam (Additive effect). Products include:
Ativan Injection 2698
Ativan Tablets 2700

Loxapine Hydrochloride (Additive effect). Products include:
Loxitane 1378

Loxapine Succinate (Additive effect). Products include:
Loxitane Capsules 1378

Meperidine Hydrochloride (Additive effect). Products include:
Demerol 2308
Mepergan Injection 2753

Mephobarbital (Additive effect). Products include:
Mebaral Tablets 2322

Meprobamate (Additive effect). Products include:
Miltown Tablets 2672
PMB 200 and PMB 400 2783

Mesoridazine Besylate (Additive effect). Products include:
Serentil 684

Methadone Hydrochloride (Additive effect). Products include:
Methadone Hydrochloride Oral Concentrate 2233

IMPORTANT NOTE: Always consult each drug listing in the patient's regimen for possible interactions.

Methadone Hydrochloride Oral Solution & Tablets 2235

Methotrimeprazine (Additive effect). Products include:

Levoprome 1274

Methoxyflurane (Additive effect).

No products indexed under this heading.

Methylprednisolone Acetate (Barbiturates may influence the absorption and elimination of concomitantly used corticosteroids). Products include:

Depo-Medrol Single-Dose Vial 2600
Depo-Medrol Sterile Aqueous Suspension 2597

Methylprednisolone Sodium Succinate (Barbiturates may influence the absorption and elimination of concomitantly used corticosteroids). Products include:

Solu-Medrol Sterile Powder 2643

Midazolam Hydrochloride (Additive effect). Products include:

Versed Injection 2170

Molindone Hydrochloride (Additive effect). Products include:

Moban Tablets and Concentrate 1048

Morphine Sulfate (Additive effect). Products include:

Astramorph/PF Injection, USP (Preservative-Free) 535
Duramorph 962
Infumorph 200 and Infumorph 500 Sterile Solutions 965
MS Contin Tablets 1994
MSIR 1997
Oramorph SR (Morphine Sulfate Sustained Release Tablets) 2236
RMS Suppositories 2657
Roxanol 2243

Opium Alkaloids (Additive effect).

No products indexed under this heading.

Oxazepam (Additive effect). Products include:

Serax Capsules 2810
Serax Tablets 2810

Oxycodone Hydrochloride (Additive effect). Products include:

Percocet Tablets 938
Percodan Tablets 939
Percodan-Demi Tablets 940
Roxicodone Tablets, Oral Solution & Intensol (Oxycodone) 2244
Tylox Capsules 1584

Pentobarbital Sodium (Additive effect). Products include:

Nembutal Sodium Capsules 436
Nembutal Sodium Solution 438
Nembutal Sodium Suppositories 440

Perphenazine (Additive effect). Products include:

Etrafon 2355
Triavil Tablets 1757
Trilafon 2389

Phenobarbital (Additive effect). Products include:

Arco-Lase Plus Tablets 512
Bellergal-S Tablets 2250
Donnatal 2060
Donnatal Extentabs 2061
Donnatal Tablets 2060
Phenobarbital Elixir and Tablets 1469
Quadrinal Tablets 1350

Phenytoin (Barbiturates may influence the absorption and elimination of concomitantly used diphenylhydantoin). Products include:

Dilantin Infatabs 1908
Dilantin-125 Suspension 1911

Phenytoin Sodium (Barbiturates may influence the absorption and elimination of concomitantly used diphenylhydantoin). Products include:

Dilantin Kapseals 1906
Dilantin Parenteral 1910

Prazepam (Additive effect).

No products indexed under this heading.

Prednisolone Acetate (Barbiturates may influence the absorption and elimination of concomitantly used corticosteroids). Products include:

AK-CIDE .... ◉ 202
AK-CIDE Ointment .... ◉ 202
Blephamide Liquifilm Sterile Ophthalmic Suspension 476
Blephamide Ointment .... ◉ 237
Econopred & Econopred Plus Ophthalmic Suspensions .... ◉ 217
Poly-Pred Liquifilm .... ◉ 248
Pred Forte .... ◉ 250
Pred Mild .... ◉ 253
Pred-G Liquifilm Sterile Ophthalmic Suspension .... ◉ 251
Pred-G S.O.P. Sterile Ophthalmic Ointment .... ◉ 252
Vasocidin Ointment .... ◉ 268

Prednisolone Sodium Phosphate (Barbiturates may influence the absorption and elimination of concomitantly used corticosteroids). Products include:

AK-Pred .... ◉ 204
Hydeltrasol Injection, Sterile 1665
Inflamase .... ◉ 265
Pediapred Oral Liquid 995
Vasocidin Ophthalmic Solution .... ◉ 270

Prednisolone Tebutate (Barbiturates may influence the absorption and elimination of concomitantly used corticosteroids). Products include:

Hydeltra-T.B.A. Sterile Suspension 1667

Prednisone (Barbiturates may influence the absorption and elimination of concomitantly used corticosteroids). Products include:

Deltasone Tablets 2595

Prochlorperazine (Additive effect). Products include:

Compazine 2470

Promethazine Hydrochloride (Additive effect). Products include:

Mepergan Injection 2753
Phenergan with Codeine 2777
Phenergan with Dextromethorphan 2778
Phenergan Injection 2773
Phenergan Suppositories 2775
Phenergan Syrup 2774
Phenergan Tablets 2775
Phenergan VC 2779
Phenergan VC with Codeine 2781

Propofol (Additive effect). Products include:

Diprivan Injection 2833

Propoxyphene Hydrochloride (Additive effect). Products include:

Darvon 1435
Wygesic Tablets 2827

Propoxyphene Napsylate (Additive effect). Products include:

Darvon-N/Darvocet-N 1433

Propylene glycol-containing solutions (Barbiturates may influence the absorption and elimination of concomitantly used propylene glycol-containing solutions).

Quazepam (Additive effect). Products include:

Doral Tablets 2664

Risperidone (Additive effect). Products include:

Risperdal 1301

Secobarbital Sodium (Additive effect). Products include:

Seconal Sodium Pulvules 1474

Sufentanil Citrate (Additive effect). Products include:

Sufenta Injection 1309

Temazepam (Additive effect). Products include:

Restoril Capsules 2284

Thiamylal Sodium (Additive effect).

No products indexed under this heading.

Thioridazine Hydrochloride (Additive effect). Products include:

Mellaril 2269

Thiothixene (Additive effect). Products include:

Navane Capsules and Concentrate 2201
Navane Intramuscular 2202

Triamcinolone (Barbiturates may influence the absorption and elimination of concomitantly used corticosteroids). Products include:

Aristocort Tablets 1022

Triamcinolone Acetonide (Barbiturates may influence the absorption and elimination of concomitantly used corticosteroids). Products include:

Aristocort A 0.025% Cream 1027
Aristocort A 0.5% Cream 1031
Aristocort A 0.1% Cream 1029
Aristocort A 0.1% Ointment 1030
Azmacort Oral Inhaler 2011
Nasacort Nasal Inhaler 2024

Triamcinolone Diacetate (Barbiturates may influence the absorption and elimination of concomitantly used corticosteroids). Products include:

Aristocort Suspension (Forte Parenteral) 1027
Aristocort Suspension (Intralesional) 1025

Triamcinolone Hexacetonide (Barbiturates may influence the absorption and elimination of concomitantly used corticosteroids). Products include:

Aristospan Suspension (Intra-articular) 1033
Aristospan Suspension (Intralesional) 1032

Triazolam (Additive effect). Products include:

Halcion Tablets 2611

Trifluoperazine Hydrochloride (Additive effect). Products include:

Stelazine 2514

Warfarin Sodium (Barbiturates may influence the absorption and elimination of concomitantly used anticoagulants). Products include:

Coumadin 926

Zolpidem Tartrate (Additive effect). Products include:

Ambien Tablets 2416

Food Interactions

Alcohol (Additive effect).

BREVOXYL GEL

(Benzoyl Peroxide) 2552
None cited in PDR database.

BREVOXYL CLEANSING LOTION

(Benzoyl Peroxide) 2553
None cited in PDR database.

BRICANYL SUBCUTANEOUS INJECTION

(Terbutaline Sulfate) 1502
May interact with sympathomimetic bronchodilators, monoamine oxidase inhibitors, tricyclic antidepressants, and beta blockers. Compounds in these categories include:

Acebutolol Hydrochloride (Blocked pulmonary effects; may produce severe asthma attacks in asthmatic patients). Products include:

Sectral Capsules 2807

Albuterol (Deleterious cardiovascular effects). Products include:

Proventil Inhalation Aerosol 2382
Ventolin Inhalation Aerosol and Refill 1197

Albuterol Sulfate (Deleterious cardiovascular effects). Products include:

Airet Solution for Inhalation 452
Proventil Inhalation Solution 0.083% 2384
Proventil Repetabs Tablets 2386
Proventil Solution for Inhalation 0.5% 2383
Proventil Syrup 2385
Proventil Tablets 2386
Ventolin Inhalation Solution 1198
Ventolin Nebules Inhalation Solution 1199
Ventolin Rotacaps for Inhalation 1200
Ventolin Syrup 1202
Ventolin Tablets 1203
Volmax Extended-Release Tablets .. 1788

Amitriptyline Hydrochloride (Potentiates terbutaline's vascular effects). Products include:

Elavil 2838
Endep Tablets 2174
Etrafon 2355
Limbitrol 2180
Triavil Tablets 1757

Amoxapine (Potentiates terbutaline's vascular effects). Products include:

Asendin Tablets 1369

Atenolol (Blocked pulmonary effects; may produce severe asthma attacks in asthmatic patients). Products include:

Tenoretic Tablets 2845
Tenormin Tablets and I.V. Injection 2847

Betaxolol Hydrochloride (Blocked pulmonary effects; may produce severe asthma attacks in asthmatic patients). Products include:

Betoptic Ophthalmic Solution 469
Betoptic S Ophthalmic Suspension 471
Kerlone Tablets 2436

Bisoprolol Fumarate (Blocked pulmonary effects; may produce severe asthma attacks in asthmatic patients). Products include:

Zebeta Tablets 1413
Ziac 1415

Bitolterol Mesylate (Deleterious cardiovascular effects). Products include:

Tornalate Solution for Inhalation, 0.2% 956
Tornalate Metered Dose Inhaler 957

Carteolol Hydrochloride (Blocked pulmonary effects; may produce severe asthma attacks in asthmatic patients). Products include:

Cartrol Tablets 410
Ocupress Ophthalmic Solution, 1% Sterile .... ◉ 309

Clomipramine Hydrochloride (Potentiates terbutaline's vascular effects). Products include:

Anafranil Capsules 803

Desipramine Hydrochloride (Potentiates terbutaline's vascular effects). Products include:

Norpramin Tablets 1526

Doxepin Hydrochloride (Potentiates terbutaline's vascular effects). Products include:

Sinequan 2205
Zonalon Cream 1055

Ephedrine Hydrochloride (Deleterious cardiovascular effects). Products include:

Primatene Dual Action Formula .... ▣ 872
Primatene Tablets .... ▣ 873
Quadrinal Tablets 1350

Ephedrine Sulfate (Deleterious cardiovascular effects). Products include:

Bronkaid Caplets .... ▣ 717
Marax Tablets & DF Syrup 2200

(▣ Described in PDR For Nonprescription Drugs) (◉ Described in PDR For Ophthalmology)

133 **Interactions Index** **Bricanyl Tablets**

Ephedrine Tannate (Deleterious cardiovascular effects). Products include:
- Rynatuss 2673

Epinephrine (Deleterious cardiovascular effects). Products include:
- Bronkaid Mist .... 📖 717
- EPIFRIN .... ⊙ 239
- EpiPen 790
- Marcaine Hydrochloride with Epinephrine 1:200,000 2316
- Primatene Mist .... 📖 873
- Sensorcaine with Epinephrine Injection 559
- Sus-Phrine Injection 1019
- Xylocaine with Epinephrine Injections 567

Epinephrine Hydrochloride (Deleterious cardiovascular effects). Products include:
- Ana-Kit Anaphylaxis Emergency Treatment Kit 617

Esmolol Hydrochloride (Blocked pulmonary effects; may produce severe asthma attacks in asthmatic patients). Products include:
- Brevibloc Injection 1808

Ethylnorepinephrine Hydrochloride (Deleterious cardiovascular effects).
- No products indexed under this heading.

Furazolidone (Potentiates terbutaline's vascular effects). Products include:
- Furoxone 2046

Imipramine Hydrochloride (Potentiates terbutaline's vascular effects). Products include:
- Tofranil Ampuls 854
- Tofranil Tablets 856

Imipramine Pamoate (Potentiates terbutaline's vascular effects). Products include:
- Tofranil-PM Capsules 857

Isocarboxazid (Potentiates terbutaline's vascular effects).
- No products indexed under this heading.

Isoetharine (Deleterious cardiovascular effects). Products include:
- Bronkometer Aerosol 2302
- Bronkosol Solution 2302
- Isoetharine Inhalation Solution, USP, Arm-a-Med 551

Isoproterenol Hydrochloride (Deleterious cardiovascular effects). Products include:
- Isuprel Hydrochloride Injection 1:5000 2311
- Isuprel Hydrochloride Solution 1:200 & 1:100 2313
- Isuprel Mistometer 2312

Isoproterenol Sulfate (Deleterious cardiovascular effects). Products include:
- Norisodrine with Calcium Iodide Syrup 442

Labetalol Hydrochloride (Blocked pulmonary effects; may produce severe asthma attacks in asthmatic patients). Products include:
- Normodyne Injection 2377
- Normodyne Tablets 2379
- Trandate 1185

Levobunolol Hydrochloride (Blocked pulmonary effects; may produce severe asthma attacks in asthmatic patients). Products include:
- Betagan .... ⊙ 233

Maprotiline Hydrochloride (Potentiates terbutaline's vascular effects). Products include:
- Ludiomil Tablets 843

Metaproterenol Sulfate (Deleterious cardiovascular effects). Products include:
- Alupent 669
- Metaproterenol Sulfate Inhalation Solution, USP, Arm-a-Med 552

Metipranolol Hydrochloride (Blocked pulmonary effects; may produce severe asthma attacks in asthmatic patients). Products include:
- OptiPranolol (Metipranolol 0.3%) Sterile Ophthalmic Solution .... ⊙ 258

Metoprolol Succinate (Blocked pulmonary effects; may produce severe asthma attacks in asthmatic patients). Products include:
- Toprol-XL Tablets 565

Metoprolol Tartrate (Blocked pulmonary effects; may produce severe asthma attacks in asthmatic patients). Products include:
- Lopressor Ampuls 830
- Lopressor HCT Tablets 832
- Lopressor Tablets 830

Nadolol (Blocked pulmonary effects; may produce severe asthma attacks in asthmatic patients).
- No products indexed under this heading.

Nortriptyline Hydrochloride (Potentiates terbutaline's vascular effects). Products include:
- Pamelor 2280

Penbutolol Sulfate (Blocked pulmonary effects; may produce severe asthma attacks in asthmatic patients). Products include:
- Levatol 2403

Phenelzine Sulfate (Potentiates terbutaline's vascular effects). Products include:
- Nardil 1920

Pindolol (Blocked pulmonary effects; may produce severe asthma attacks in asthmatic patients). Products include:
- Visken Tablets 2299

Pirbuterol Acetate (Deleterious cardiovascular effects). Products include:
- Maxair Autohaler 1492
- Maxair Inhaler 1494

Propranolol Hydrochloride (Blocked pulmonary effects; may produce severe asthma attacks in asthmatic patients). Products include:
- Inderal 2728
- Inderal LA Long Acting Capsules 2730
- Inderide Tablets 2732
- Inderide LA Long Acting Capsules 2734

Protriptyline Hydrochloride (Potentiates terbutaline's vascular effects). Products include:
- Vivactil Tablets 1774

Salmeterol Xinafoate (Deleterious cardiovascular effects). Products include:
- Serevent Inhalation Aerosol 1176

Selegiline Hydrochloride (Potentiates terbutaline's vascular effects). Products include:
- Eldepryl Tablets 2550

Sotalol Hydrochloride (Blocked pulmonary effects; may produce severe asthma attacks in asthmatic patients). Products include:
- Betapace Tablets 641

Timolol Hemihydrate (Blocked pulmonary effects; may produce severe asthma attacks in asthmatic patients). Products include:
- Betimol 0.25%, 0.5% .... ⊙ 261

Timolol Maleate (Blocked pulmonary effects; may produce severe asthma attacks in asthmatic patients). Products include:
- Blocadren Tablets 1614
- Timolide Tablets 1748
- Timoptic in Ocudose 1753
- Timoptic Sterile Ophthalmic Solution 1751
- Timoptic-XE 1755

Tranylcypromine Sulfate (Potentiates terbutaline's vascular effects). Products include:
- Parnate Tablets 2503

Trimipramine Maleate (Potentiates terbutaline's vascular effects). Products include:
- Surmontil Capsules 2811

BRICANYL TABLETS
(Terbutaline Sulfate) 1503
May interact with sympathomimetic bronchodilators, monoamine oxidase inhibitors, tricyclic antidepressants, and beta blockers. Compounds in these categories include:

Acebutolol Hydrochloride (Blocked pulmonary effects; may produce severe asthma attacks in asthmatic patients). Products include:
- Sectral Capsules 2807

Albuterol (Deleterious cardiovascular effects). Products include:
- Proventil Inhalation Aerosol 2382
- Ventolin Inhalation Aerosol and Refill 1197

Albuterol Sulfate (Deleterious cardiovascular effects). Products include:
- Airet Solution for Inhalation 452
- Proventil Inhalation Solution 0.083% 2384
- Proventil Repetabs Tablets 2386
- Proventil Solution for Inhalation 0.5% 2383
- Proventil Syrup 2385
- Proventil Tablets 2386
- Ventolin Inhalation Solution 1198
- Ventolin Nebules Inhalation Solution 1199
- Ventolin Rotacaps for Inhalation 1200
- Ventolin Syrup 1202
- Ventolin Tablets 1203
- Volmax Extended-Release Tablets 1788

Amitriptyline Hydrochloride (Potentiates terbutaline's vascular effects). Products include:
- Elavil 2838
- Endep Tablets 2174
- Etrafon 2355
- Limbitrol 2180
- Triavil Tablets 1757

Amoxapine (Potentiates terbutaline's vascular effects). Products include:
- Asendin Tablets 1369

Atenolol (Blocked pulmonary effects; may produce severe asthma attacks in asthmatic patients). Products include:
- Tenoretic Tablets 2845
- Tenormin Tablets and I.V. Injection 2847

Betaxolol Hydrochloride (Blocked pulmonary effects; may produce severe asthma attacks in asthmatic patients). Products include:
- Betoptic Ophthalmic Solution 469
- Betoptic S Ophthalmic Suspension 471
- Kerlone Tablets 2436

Bisoprolol Fumarate (Blocked pulmonary effects; may produce severe asthma attacks in asthmatic patients). Products include:
- Zebeta Tablets 1413
- Ziac 1415

Bitolterol Mesylate (Deleterious cardiovascular effects). Products include:
- Tornalate Solution for Inhalation, 0.2% 956
- Tornalate Metered Dose Inhaler 957

Carteolol Hydrochloride (Blocked pulmonary effects; may produce severe asthma attacks in asthmatic patients). Products include:
- Cartrol Tablets 410
- Ocupress Ophthalmic Solution, 1% Sterile .... ⊙ 309

Clomipramine Hydrochloride (Potentiates terbutaline's vascular effects). Products include:
- Anafranil Capsules 803

Desipramine Hydrochloride (Potentiates terbutaline's vascular effects). Products include:
- Norpramin Tablets 1526

Doxepin Hydrochloride (Potentiates terbutaline's vascular effects). Products include:
- Sinequan 2205
- Zonalon Cream 1055

Ephedrine Hydrochloride (Deleterious cardiovascular effects). Products include:
- Primatene Dual Action Formula .... 📖 872
- Primatene Tablets .... 📖 873
- Quadrinal Tablets 1350

Ephedrine Sulfate (Deleterious cardiovascular effects). Products include:
- Bronkaid Caplets .... 📖 717
- Marax Tablets & DF Syrup 2200

Ephedrine Tannate (Deleterious cardiovascular effects). Products include:
- Rynatuss 2673

Epinephrine (Deleterious cardiovascular effects). Products include:
- Bronkaid Mist .... 📖 717
- EPIFRIN .... ⊙ 239
- EpiPen 790
- Marcaine Hydrochloride with Epinephrine 1:200,000 2316
- Primatene Mist .... 📖 873
- Sensorcaine with Epinephrine Injection 559
- Sus-Phrine Injection 1019
- Xylocaine with Epinephrine Injections 567

Epinephrine Hydrochloride (Deleterious cardiovascular effects). Products include:
- Ana-Kit Anaphylaxis Emergency Treatment Kit 617

Esmolol Hydrochloride (Blocked pulmonary effects; may produce severe asthma attacks in asthmatic patients). Products include:
- Brevibloc Injection 1808

Ethylnorepinephrine Hydrochloride (Deleterious cardiovascular effects).
- No products indexed under this heading.

Furazolidone (Potentiates terbutaline's vascular effects). Products include:
- Furoxone 2046

Imipramine Hydrochloride (Potentiates terbutaline's vascular effects). Products include:
- Tofranil Ampuls 854
- Tofranil Tablets 856

Imipramine Pamoate (Potentiates terbutaline's vascular effects). Products include:
- Tofranil-PM Capsules 857

Isocarboxazid (Potentiates terbutaline's vascular effects).
- No products indexed under this heading.

Isoetharine (Deleterious cardiovascular effects). Products include:
- Bronkometer Aerosol 2302
- Bronkosol Solution 2302
- Isoetharine Inhalation Solution, USP, Arm-a-Med 551

Isoproterenol Hydrochloride (Deleterious cardiovascular effects). Products include:
- Isuprel Hydrochloride Injection 1:5000 2311
- Isuprel Hydrochloride Solution 1:200 & 1:100 2313
- Isuprel Mistometer 2312

IMPORTANT NOTE: Always consult each drug listing in the patient's regimen for possible interactions.

Bricanyl Tablets **Interactions Index** **134**

Isoproterenol Sulfate (Deleterious cardiovascular effects). Products include:
- Norisodrine with Calcium Iodide Syrup 442

Labetalol Hydrochloride (Blocked pulmonary effects; may produce severe asthma attacks in asthmatic patients). Products include:
- Normodyne Injection 2377
- Normodyne Tablets 2379
- Trandate 1185

Levobunolol Hydrochloride (Blocked pulmonary effects; may produce severe asthma attacks in asthmatic patients). Products include:
- Betagan .... ◉ 233

Maprotiline Hydrochloride (Potentiates terbutaline's vascular effects). Products include:
- Ludiomil Tablets 843

Metaproterenol Sulfate (Deleterious cardiovascular effects). Products include:
- Alupent 669
- Metaproterenol Sulfate Inhalation Solution, USP, Arm-a-Med 552

Metipranolol Hydrochloride (Blocked pulmonary effects; may produce severe asthma attacks in asthmatic patients). Products include:
- OptiPranolol (Metipranolol 0.3%) Sterile Ophthalmic Solution .... ◉ 258

Metoprolol Succinate (Blocked pulmonary effects; may produce severe asthma attacks in asthmatic patients). Products include:
- Toprol-XL Tablets 565

Metoprolol Tartrate (Blocked pulmonary effects; may produce severe asthma attacks in asthmatic patients). Products include:
- Lopressor Ampuls 830
- Lopressor HCT Tablets 832
- Lopressor Tablets 830

Nadolol (Blocked pulmonary effects; may produce severe asthma attacks in asthmatic patients).
- No products indexed under this heading.

Nortriptyline Hydrochloride (Potentiates terbutaline's vascular effects). Products include:
- Pamelor 2280

Penbutolol Sulfate (Blocked pulmonary effects; may produce severe asthma attacks in asthmatic patients). Products include:
- Levatol 2403

Phenelzine Sulfate (Potentiates terbutaline's vascular effects). Products include:
- Nardil 1920

Pindolol (Blocked pulmonary effects; may produce severe asthma attacks in asthmatic patients). Products include:
- Visken Tablets 2299

Pirbuterol Acetate (Deleterious cardiovascular effects). Products include:
- Maxair Autohaler 1492
- Maxair Inhaler 1494

Propranolol Hydrochloride (Blocked pulmonary effects; may produce severe asthma attacks in asthmatic patients). Products include:
- Inderal 2728
- Inderal LA Long Acting Capsules 2730
- Inderide Tablets 2732
- Inderide LA Long Acting Capsules 2734

Protriptyline Hydrochloride (Potentiates terbutaline's vascular effects). Products include:
- Vivactil Tablets 1774

Salmeterol Xinafoate (Deleterious cardiovascular effects). Products include:
- Serevent Inhalation Aerosol 1176

Selegiline Hydrochloride (Potentiates terbutaline's vascular effects). Products include:
- Eldepryl Tablets 2550

Sotalol Hydrochloride (Blocked pulmonary effects; may produce severe asthma attacks in asthmatic patients). Products include:
- Betapace Tablets 641

Timolol Hemihydrate (Blocked pulmonary effects; may produce severe asthma attacks in asthmatic patients). Products include:
- Betimol 0.25%, 0.5% .... ◉ 261

Timolol Maleate (Blocked pulmonary effects; may produce severe asthma attacks in asthmatic patients). Products include:
- Blocadren Tablets 1614
- Timolide Tablets 1748
- Timoptic in Ocudose 1753
- Timoptic Sterile Ophthalmic Solution 1751
- Timoptic-XE 1755

Tranylcypromine Sulfate (Potentiates terbutaline's vascular effects). Products include:
- Parnate Tablets 2503

Trimipramine Maleate (Potentiates terbutaline's vascular effects). Products include:
- Surmontil Capsules 2811

BROMASE

(Proteolytic Enzymes) **667**

May interact with oral anticoagulants. Compounds in this category include:

Dicumarol (Concomitant use not recommended).
- No products indexed under this heading.

Warfarin Sodium (Concomitant use not recommended). Products include:
- Coumadin 926

BROMFED CAPSULES (EXTENDED-RELEASE)

(Brompheniramine Maleate, Pseudoephedrine Hydrochloride) **1785**

May interact with central nervous system depressants, monoamine oxidase inhibitors, beta blockers, veratrum alkaloids, and certain other agents. Compounds in these categories include:

Acebutolol Hydrochloride (Increased sympathomimetic effect). Products include:
- Sectral Capsules 2807

Alfentanil Hydrochloride (Additive effects). Products include:
- Alfenta Injection 1286

Alprazolam (Additive effects). Products include:
- Xanax Tablets 2649

Aprobarbital (Additive effects).
- No products indexed under this heading.

Atenolol (Increased sympathomimetic effect). Products include:
- Tenoretic Tablets 2845
- Tenormin Tablets and I.V. Injection 2847

Betaxolol Hydrochloride (Increased sympathomimetic effect). Products include:
- Betoptic Ophthalmic Solution 469
- Betoptic S Ophthalmic Suspension 471
- Kerlone Tablets 2436

Bisoprolol Fumarate (Increased sympathomimetic effect). Products include:
- Zebeta Tablets 1413
- Ziac 1415

Buprenorphine (Additive effects). Products include:
- Buprenex Injectable 2006

Buspirone Hydrochloride (Additive effects). Products include:
- BuSpar 737

Butabarbital (Additive effects).
- No products indexed under this heading.

Butalbital (Additive effects). Products include:
- Esgic-plus Tablets 1013
- Fioricet Tablets 2258
- Fioricet with Codeine Capsules 2260
- Fiorinal Capsules 2261
- Fiorinal with Codeine Capsules 2262
- Fiorinal Tablets 2261
- Phrenilin 785
- Sedapap Tablets 50 mg/650 mg 1543

Carteolol Hydrochloride (Increased sympathomimetic effect). Products include:
- Cartrol Tablets 410
- Ocupress Ophthalmic Solution, 1% Sterile .... ◉ 309

Chlordiazepoxide (Additive effects). Products include:
- Libritabs Tablets 2177
- Limbitrol 2180

Chlordiazepoxide Hydrochloride (Additive effects). Products include:
- Librax Capsules 2176
- Librium Capsules 2178
- Librium Injectable 2179

Chlorpromazine (Additive effects). Products include:
- Thorazine Suppositories 2523

Chlorprothixene (Additive effects).
- No products indexed under this heading.

Chlorprothixene Hydrochloride (Additive effects).
- No products indexed under this heading.

Clorazepate Dipotassium (Additive effects). Products include:
- Tranxene 451

Clozapine (Additive effects). Products include:
- Clozaril Tablets 2252

Codeine Phosphate (Additive effects). Products include:
- Actifed with Codeine Cough Syrup 1067
- Brontex 1981
- Deconsal C Expectorant Syrup 456
- Deconsal Pediatric Syrup 457
- Dimetane-DC Cough Syrup 2059
- Empirin with Codeine Tablets 1093
- Fioricet with Codeine Capsules 2260
- Fiorinal with Codeine Capsules 2262
- Isoclor Expectorant 990
- Novahistine DH 2462
- Novahistine Expectorant 2463
- Nucofed 2051
- Phenergan with Codeine 2777
- Phenergan VC with Codeine 2781
- Robitussin A-C Syrup 2073
- Robitussin-DAC Syrup 2074
- Ryna .... ▣ 841
- Soma Compound w/Codeine Tablets 2676
- Tussi-Organidin NR Liquid and S NR Liquid 2677
- Tylenol with Codeine 1583

Cryptenamine Preparations (Reduced antihypertensive effects).

Desflurane (Additive effects). Products include:
- Suprane 1813

Dezocine (Additive effects). Products include:
- Dalgan Injection 538

Diazepam (Additive effects). Products include:
- Dizac 1809
- Valium Injectable 2182
- Valium Tablets 2183
- Valrelease Capsules 2169

Droperidol (Additive effects). Products include:
- Inapsine Injection 1296

Enflurane (Additive effects).
- No products indexed under this heading.

Esmolol Hydrochloride (Increased sympathomimetic effect). Products include:
- Brevibloc Injection 1808

Estazolam (Additive effects). Products include:
- ProSom Tablets 449

Ethchlorvynol (Additive effects). Products include:
- Placidyl Capsules 448

Ethinamate (Additive effects).
- No products indexed under this heading.

Fentanyl (Additive effects). Products include:
- Duragesic Transdermal System 1288

Fentanyl Citrate (Additive effects). Products include:
- Sublimaze Injection 1307

Fluphenazine Decanoate (Additive effects). Products include:
- Prolixin Decanoate 509

Fluphenazine Enanthate (Additive effects). Products include:
- Prolixin Enanthate 509

Fluphenazine Hydrochloride (Additive effects). Products include:
- Prolixin 509

Flurazepam Hydrochloride (Additive effects). Products include:
- Dalmane Capsules 2173

Furazolidone (Increased sympathomimetic effect; concurrent therapy is contraindicated). Products include:
- Furoxone 2046

Glutethimide (Additive effects).
- No products indexed under this heading.

Haloperidol (Additive effects). Products include:
- Haldol Injection, Tablets and Concentrate 1575

Haloperidol Decanoate (Additive effects). Products include:
- Haldol Decanoate 1577

Hydrocodone Bitartrate (Additive effects). Products include:
- Anexsia 5/500 Elixir 1781
- Anexia Tablets 1782
- Codiclear DH Syrup 791
- Deconamine CX Cough and Cold Liquid and Tablets 1319
- Duratuss HD Elixir 2565
- Hycodan Tablets and Syrup 930
- Hycomine Compound Tablets 932
- Hycomine 931
- Hycotuss Expectorant Syrup 933
- Hydrocet Capsules 782
- Lorcet 10/650 1018
- Lortab 2566
- Tussend 1783
- Tussend Expectorant 1785
- Vicodin Tablets 1356
- Vicodin ES Tablets 1357
- Vicodin Tuss Expectorant 1358
- Zydone Capsules 949

Hydrocodone Polistirex (Additive effects). Products include:
- Tussionex Pennkinetic Extended-Release Suspension 998

Hydroxyzine Hydrochloride (Additive effects). Products include:
- Atarax Tablets & Syrup 2185
- Marax Tablets & DF Syrup 2200
- Vistaril Intramuscular Solution 2216

Isocarboxazid (Increased sympathomimetic effect; concurrent therapy is contraindicated).
- No products indexed under this heading.

Isoflurane (Additive effects).
- No products indexed under this heading.

(▣ Described in PDR For Nonprescription Drugs) (◉ Described in PDR For Ophthalmology)

135 **Interactions Index** **Bromfed-DM Cough**

Ketamine Hydrochloride (Additive effects).
No products indexed under this heading.

Labetalol Hydrochloride (Increased sympathomimetic effect). Products include:
Normodyne Injection ... 2377
Normodyne Tablets ... 2379
Trandate ... 1185

Levobunolol Hydrochloride (Increased sympathomimetic effect). Products include:
Betagan ... ◉ 233

Levomethadyl Acetate Hydrochloride (Additive effects). Products include:
Orlamm ... 2239

Levorphanol Tartrate (Additive effects). Products include:
Levo-Dromoran ... 2129

Lorazepam (Additive effects). Products include:
Ativan Injection ... 2698
Ativan Tablets ... 2700

Loxapine Hydrochloride (Additive effects). Products include:
Loxitane ... 1378

Loxapine Succinate (Additive effects). Products include:
Loxitane Capsules ... 1378

Mecamylamine Hydrochloride (Reduced antihypertensive effects). Products include:
Inversine Tablets ... 1686

Meperidine Hydrochloride (Additive effects). Products include:
Demerol ... 2308
Mepergan Injection ... 2753

Mephobarbital (Additive effects). Products include:
Mebaral Tablets ... 2322

Meprobamate (Additive effects). Products include:
Miltown Tablets ... 2672
PMB 200 and PMB 400 ... 2783

Mesoridazine Besylate (Additive effects). Products include:
Serentil ... 684

Methadone Hydrochloride (Additive effects). Products include:
Methadone Hydrochloride Oral Concentrate ... 2233
Methadone Hydrochloride Oral Solution & Tablets ... 2235

Methohexital Sodium (Additive effects). Products include:
Brevital Sodium Vials ... 1429

Methotrimeprazine (Additive effects). Products include:
Levoprome ... 1274

Methoxyflurane (Additive effects).
No products indexed under this heading.

Methyldopa (Reduced antihypertensive effects). Products include:
Aldoclor Tablets ... 1598
Aldomet Oral ... 1600
Aldoril Tablets ... 1604

Methyldopate Hydrochloride (Reduced antihypertensive effects). Products include:
Aldomet Ester HCl Injection ... 1602

Metipranolol Hydrochloride (Increased sympathomimetic effect). Products include:
OptiPranolol (Metipranolol 0.3%) Sterile Ophthalmic Solution ... ◉ 258

Metoprolol Succinate (Increased sympathomimetic effect). Products include:
Toprol-XL Tablets ... 565

Metoprolol Tartrate (Increased sympathomimetic effect). Products include:
Lopressor Ampuls ... 830
Lopressor HCT Tablets ... 832
Lopressor Tablets ... 830

Midazolam Hydrochloride (Additive effects). Products include:
Versed Injection ... 2170

Molindone Hydrochloride (Additive effects). Products include:
Moban Tablets and Concentrate ... 1048

Morphine Sulfate (Additive effects). Products include:
Astramorph/PF Injection, USP (Preservative-Free) ... 535
Duramorph ... 962
Infumorph 200 and Infumorph 500 Sterile Solutions ... 965
MS Contin Tablets ... 1994
MSIR ... 1997
Oramorph SR (Morphine Sulfate Sustained Release Tablets) ... 2236
RMS Suppositories ... 2657
Roxanol ... 2243

Nadolol (Increased sympathomimetic effect).
No products indexed under this heading.

Opium Alkaloids (Additive effects).
No products indexed under this heading.

Oxazepam (Additive effects). Products include:
Serax Capsules ... 2810
Serax Tablets ... 2810

Oxycodone Hydrochloride (Additive effects). Products include:
Percocet Tablets ... 938
Percodan Tablets ... 939
Percodan-Demi Tablets ... 940
Roxicodone Tablets, Oral Solution & Intensol (Oxycodone) ... 2244
Tylox Capsules ... 1584

Penbutolol Sulfate (Increased sympathomimetic effect). Products include:
Levatol ... 2403

Pentobarbital Sodium (Additive effects). Products include:
Nembutal Sodium Capsules ... 436
Nembutal Sodium Solution ... 438
Nembutal Sodium Suppositories ... 440

Perphenazine (Additive effects). Products include:
Etrafon ... 2355
Triavil Tablets ... 1757
Trilafon ... 2389

Phenelzine Sulfate (Increased sympathomimetic effect; concurrent therapy is contraindicated). Products include:
Nardil ... 1920

Phenobarbital (Additive effects). Products include:
Arco-Lase Plus Tablets ... 512
Bellergal-S Tablets ... 2250
Donnatal ... 2060
Donnatal Extentabs ... 2061
Donnatal Tablets ... 2060
Phenobarbital Elixir and Tablets ... 1469
Quadrinal Tablets ... 1350

Pindolol (Increased sympathomimetic effect). Products include:
Visken Tablets ... 2299

Prazepam (Additive effects).
No products indexed under this heading.

Prochlorperazine (Additive effects). Products include:
Compazine ... 2470

Promethazine Hydrochloride (Additive effects). Products include:
Mepergan Injection ... 2753
Phenergan with Codeine ... 2777
Phenergan with Dextromethorphan 2778
Phenergan Injection ... 2773
Phenergan Suppositories ... 2775
Phenergan Syrup ... 2774
Phenergan Tablets ... 2775
Phenergan VC ... 2779
Phenergan VC with Codeine ... 2781

Propofol (Additive effects). Products include:
Diprivan Injection ... 2833

Propoxyphene Hydrochloride (Additive effects). Products include:
Darvon ... 1435
Wygesic Tablets ... 2827

Propoxyphene Napsylate (Additive effects). Products include:
Darvon-N/Darvocet-N ... 1433

Propranolol Hydrochloride (Increased sympathomimetic effect). Products include:
Inderal ... 2728
Inderal LA Long Acting Capsules ... 2730
Inderide Tablets ... 2732
Inderide LA Long Acting Capsules .. 2734

Quazepam (Additive effects). Products include:
Doral Tablets ... 2664

Reserpine (Reduced antihypertensive effects). Products include:
Diupres Tablets ... 1650
Hydropres Tablets ... 1675
Ser-Ap-Es Tablets ... 849

Risperidone (Additive effects). Products include:
Risperdal ... 1301

Secobarbital Sodium (Additive effects). Products include:
Seconal Sodium Pulvules ... 1474

Selegiline Hydrochloride (Increased sympathomimetic effect; concurrent therapy is contraindicated). Products include:
Eldepryl Tablets ... 2550

Sotalol Hydrochloride (Increased sympathomimetic effect). Products include:
Betapace Tablets ... 641

Sufentanil Citrate (Additive effects). Products include:
Sufenta Injection ... 1309

Temazepam (Additive effects). Products include:
Restoril Capsules ... 2284

Thiamylal Sodium (Additive effects).
No products indexed under this heading.

Thioridazine Hydrochloride (Additive effects). Products include:
Mellaril ... 2269

Thiothixene (Additive effects). Products include:
Navane Capsules and Concentrate 2201
Navane Intramuscular ... 2202

Timolol Hemihydrate (Increased sympathomimetic effect). Products include:
Betimol 0.25%, 0.5% ... ◉ 261

Timolol Maleate (Increased sympathomimetic effect). Products include:
Blocadren Tablets ... 1614
Timolide Tablets ... 1748
Timoptic in Ocudose ... 1753
Timoptic Sterile Ophthalmic Solution ... 1751
Timoptic-XE ... 1755

Tranylcypromine Sulfate (Increased sympathomimetic effect; concurrent therapy is contraindicated). Products include:
Parnate Tablets ... 2503

Triazolam (Additive effects). Products include:
Halcion Tablets ... 2611

Trifluoperazine Hydrochloride (Additive effects). Products include:
Stelazine ... 2514

Zolpidem Tartrate (Additive effects). Products include:
Ambien Tablets ... 2416

Food Interactions

Alcohol (Additive effects).

BROMFED SYRUP
(Brompheniramine Maleate, Pseudoephedrine Hydrochloride) ... 733
May interact with monoamine oxidase inhibitors. Compounds in this category include:

Furazolidone (Effect not specified). Products include:
Furoxone ... 2046

Isocarboxazid (Effect not specified).
No products indexed under this heading.

Pargyline Hydrochloride (Effect not specified).
No products indexed under this heading.

Phenelzine Sulfate (Effect not specified). Products include:
Nardil ... 1920

Selegiline Hydrochloride (Effect not specified). Products include:
Eldepryl Tablets ... 2550

Tranylcypromine Sulfate (Effect not specified). Products include:
Parnate Tablets ... 2503

Food Interactions

Alcohol (Effect not specified).

BROMFED TABLETS
(Brompheniramine Maleate, Pseudoephedrine Hydrochloride) ... 1785
See **Bromfed Capsules (Extended-Release)**

BROMFED-DM COUGH SYRUP
(Brompheniramine Maleate, Pseudoephedrine Hydrochloride, Dextromethorphan Hydrobromide) ... 1786
May interact with central nervous system depressants, tranquilizers, hypnotics and sedatives, monoamine oxidase inhibitors, antihypertensives, and certain other agents. Compounds in these categories include:

Acebutolol Hydrochloride (Sympathomimetic, pseudoephedrine, may reduce the effects of antihypertensives). Products include:
Sectral Capsules ... 2807

Alfentanil Hydrochloride (Potential for additive effects). Products include:
Alfenta Injection ... 1286

Alprazolam (Potential for additive effects). Products include:
Xanax Tablets ... 2649

Amlodipine Besylate (Sympathomimetic, pseudoephedrine, may reduce the effects of antihypertensives). Products include:
Lotrel Capsules ... 840
Norvasc Tablets ... 1940

Aprobarbital (Potential for additive effects).
No products indexed under this heading.

Atenolol (Sympathomimetic, pseudoephedrine, may reduce the effects of antihypertensives). Products include:
Tenoretic Tablets ... 2845
Tenormin Tablets and I.V. Injection 2847

Benazepril Hydrochloride (Sympathomimetic, pseudoephedrine, may reduce the effects of antihypertensives). Products include:
Lotensin Tablets ... 834
Lotensin HCT ... 837
Lotrel Capsules ... 840

Bendroflumethiazide (Sympathomimetic, pseudoephedrine, may reduce the effects of antihypertensives).
No products indexed under this heading.

IMPORTANT NOTE: Always consult each drug listing in the patient's regimen for possible interactions.

Bromfed-DM Cough **Interactions Index** **136**

Betaxolol Hydrochloride (Sympathomimetic, pseudoephedrine, may reduce the effects of antihypertensives). Products include:
- Betoptic Ophthalmic Solution 469
- Betoptic S Ophthalmic Suspension 471
- Kerlone Tablets 2436

Bisoprolol Fumarate (Sympathomimetic, pseudoephedrine, may reduce the effects of antihypertensives). Products include:
- Zebeta Tablets 1413
- Ziac 1415

Buprenorphine (Potential for additive effects). Products include:
- Buprenex Injectable 2006

Buspirone Hydrochloride (Potential for additive effects). Products include:
- BuSpar 737

Butabarbital (Potential for additive effects).
- No products indexed under this heading.

Butalbital (Potential for additive effects). Products include:
- Esgic-plus Tablets 1013
- Fioricet Tablets 2258
- Fioricet with Codeine Capsules 2260
- Fiorinal Capsules 2261
- Fiorinal with Codeine Capsules 2262
- Fiorinal Tablets 2261
- Phrenilin 785
- Sedapap Tablets 50 mg/650 mg .. 1543

Captopril (Sympathomimetic, pseudoephedrine, may reduce the effects of antihypertensives). Products include:
- Capoten 739
- Capozide 742

Carteolol Hydrochloride (Sympathomimetic, pseudoephedrine, may reduce the effects of antihypertensives). Products include:
- Cartrol Tablets 410
- Ocupress Ophthalmic Solution, 1% Sterile .... ⊚ 309

Chlordiazepoxide (Potential for additive effects). Products include:
- Libritabs Tablets 2177
- Limbitrol 2180

Chlordiazepoxide Hydrochloride (Potential for additive effects). Products include:
- Librax Capsules 2176
- Librium Capsules 2178
- Librium Injectable 2179

Chlorothiazide (Sympathomimetic, pseudoephedrine, may reduce the effects of antihypertensives). Products include:
- Aldoclor Tablets 1598
- Diupres Tablets 1650
- Diuril Oral 1653

Chlorothiazide Sodium (Sympathomimetic, pseudoephedrine, may reduce the effects of antihypertensives). Products include:
- Diuril Sodium Intravenous 1652

Chlorpromazine (Potential for additive effects). Products include:
- Thorazine Suppositories 2523

Chlorpromazine Hydrochloride (Potential for additive effects). Products include:
- Thorazine 2523

Chlorprothixene (Potential for additive effects).
- No products indexed under this heading.

Chlorprothixene Hydrochloride (Potential for additive effects).
- No products indexed under this heading.

Chlorthalidone (Sympathomimetic, pseudoephedrine, may reduce the effects of antihypertensives). Products include:
- Combipres Tablets 677
- Tenoretic Tablets 2845
- Thalitone 1245

Clonidine (Sympathomimetic, pseudoephedrine, may reduce the effects of antihypertensives). Products include:
- Catapres-TTS 675

Clonidine Hydrochloride (Sympathomimetic, pseudoephedrine, may reduce the effects of antihypertensives). Products include:
- Catapres Tablets 674
- Combipres Tablets 677

Clorazepate Dipotassium (Potential for additive effects). Products include:
- Tranxene 451

Clozapine (Potential for additive effects). Products include:
- Clozaril Tablets 2252

Codeine Phosphate (Potential for additive effects). Products include:
- Actifed with Codeine Cough Syrup.. 1067
- Brontex 1981
- Deconsal C Expectorant Syrup 456
- Deconsal Pediatric Syrup 457
- Dimetane-DC Cough Syrup 2059
- Empirin with Codeine Tablets 1093
- Fioricet with Codeine Capsules 2260
- Fiorinal with Codeine Capsules 2262
- Isoclor Expectorant 990
- Novahistine DH 2462
- Novahistine Expectorant 2463
- Nucofed 2051
- Phenergan with Codeine 2777
- Phenergan VC with Codeine 2781
- Robitussin A-C Syrup 2073
- Robitussin-DAC Syrup 2074
- Ryna .... ■ 841
- Soma Compound w/Codeine Tablets 2676
- Tussi-Organidin NR Liquid and S NR Liquid 2677
- Tylenol with Codeine 1583

Deserpidine (Sympathomimetic, pseudoephedrine, may reduce the effects of antihypertensives).
- No products indexed under this heading.

Desflurane (Potential for additive effects). Products include:
- Suprane 1813

Dezocine (Potential for additive effects). Products include:
- Dalgan Injection 538

Diazepam (Potential for additive effects). Products include:
- Dizac 1809
- Valium Injectable 2182
- Valium Tablets 2183
- Valrelease Capsules 2169

Diazoxide (Sympathomimetic, pseudoephedrine, may reduce the effects of antihypertensives). Products include:
- Hyperstat I.V. Injection 2363
- Proglycem 580

Diltiazem Hydrochloride (Sympathomimetic, pseudoephedrine, may reduce the effects of antihypertensives). Products include:
- Cardizem CD Capsules 1506
- Cardizem SR Capsules 1510
- Cardizem Injectable 1508
- Cardizem Tablets 1512
- Dilacor XR Extended-release Capsules 2018

Doxazosin Mesylate (Sympathomimetic, pseudoephedrine, may reduce the effects of antihypertensives). Products include:
- Cardura Tablets 2186

Droperidol (Potential for additive effects). Products include:
- Inapsine Injection 1296

Enalapril Maleate (Sympathomimetic, pseudoephedrine, may reduce the effects of antihypertensives). Products include:
- Vaseretic Tablets 1765
- Vasotec Tablets 1771

Enalaprilat (Sympathomimetic, pseudoephedrine, may reduce the effects of antihypertensives). Products include:
- Vasotec I.V. 1768

Enflurane (Potential for additive effects).
- No products indexed under this heading.

Esmolol Hydrochloride (Sympathomimetic, pseudoephedrine, may reduce the effects of antihypertensives). Products include:
- Brevibloc Injection 1808

Estazolam (Potential for additive effects). Products include:
- ProSom Tablets 449

Ethchlorvynol (Potential for additive effects). Products include:
- Placidyl Capsules 448

Ethinamate (Potential for additive effects).
- No products indexed under this heading.

Felodipine (Sympathomimetic, pseudoephedrine, may reduce the effects of antihypertensives). Products include:
- Plendil Extended-Release Tablets 527

Fentanyl (Potential for additive effects). Products include:
- Duragesic Transdermal System 1288

Fentanyl Citrate (Potential for additive effects). Products include:
- Sublimaze Injection 1307

Fluphenazine Decanoate (Potential for additive effects). Products include:
- Prolixin Decanoate 509

Fluphenazine Enanthate (Potential for additive effects). Products include:
- Prolixin Enanthate 509

Fluphenazine Hydrochloride (Potential for additive effects). Products include:
- Prolixin 509

Flurazepam Hydrochloride (Potential for additive effects). Products include:
- Dalmane Capsules 2173

Fosinopril Sodium (Sympathomimetic, pseudoephedrine, may reduce the effects of antihypertensives). Products include:
- Monopril Tablets 757

Furazolidone (Prolongs and intensifies the anticholinergic effects; enhances pseudoephedrine effects; concurrent use is contraindicated). Products include:
- Furoxone 2046

Furosemide (Sympathomimetic, pseudoephedrine, may reduce the effects of antihypertensives). Products include:
- Lasix Injection, Oral Solution and Tablets 1240

Glutethimide (Potential for additive effects).
- No products indexed under this heading.

Guanabenz Acetate (Sympathomimetic, pseudoephedrine, may reduce the effects of antihypertensives).
- No products indexed under this heading.

Guanethidine Monosulfate (Sympathomimetic, pseudoephedrine, may reduce the effects of antihypertensives). Products include:
- Esimil Tablets 822
- Ismelin Tablets 827

Haloperidol (Potential for additive effects). Products include:
- Haldol Injection, Tablets and Concentrate 1575

Haloperidol Decanoate (Potential for additive effects). Products include:
- Haldol Decanoate 1577

Hydralazine Hydrochloride (Sympathomimetic, pseudoephedrine, may reduce the effects of antihypertensives). Products include:
- Apresazide Capsules 808
- Apresoline Hydrochloride Tablets .. 809
- Ser-Ap-Es Tablets 849

Hydrochlorothiazide (Sympathomimetic, pseudoephedrine, may reduce the effects of antihypertensives). Products include:
- Aldactazide 2413
- Aldoril Tablets 1604
- Apresazide Capsules 808
- Capozide 742
- Dyazide 2479
- Esidrix Tablets 821
- Esimil Tablets 822
- HydroDIURIL Tablets 1674
- Hydropres Tablets 1675
- Hyzaar Tablets 1677
- Inderide Tablets 2732
- Inderide LA Long Acting Capsules .. 2734
- Lopressor HCT Tablets 832
- Lotensin HCT 837
- Maxzide 1380
- Moduretic Tablets 1705
- Oretic Tablets 443
- Prinzide Tablets 1737
- Ser-Ap-Es Tablets 849
- Timolide Tablets 1748
- Vaseretic Tablets 1765
- Zestoretic 2850
- Ziac 1415

Hydrocodone Bitartrate (Potential for additive effects). Products include:
- Anexsia 5/500 Elixir 1781
- Anexia Tablets 1782
- Codiclear DH Syrup 791
- Deconamine CX Cough and Cold Liquid and Tablets 1319
- Duratuss HD Elixir 2565
- Hycodan Tablets and Syrup 930
- Hycomine Compound Tablets 932
- Hycomine 931
- Hycotuss Expectorant Syrup 933
- Hydrocet Capsules 782
- Lorcet 10/650 1018
- Lortab 2566
- Tussend 1783
- Tussend Expectorant 1785
- Vicodin Tablets 1356
- Vicodin ES Tablets 1357
- Vicodin Tuss Expectorant 1358
- Zydone Capsules 949

Hydrocodone Polistirex (Potential for additive effects). Products include:
- Tussionex Pennkinetic Extended-Release Suspension 998

Hydroflumethiazide (Sympathomimetic, pseudoephedrine, may reduce the effects of antihypertensives). Products include:
- Diucardin Tablets 2718

Hydroxyzine Hydrochloride (Potential for additive effects). Products include:
- Atarax Tablets & Syrup 2185
- Marax Tablets & DF Syrup 2200
- Vistaril Intramuscular Solution 2216

Indapamide (Sympathomimetic, pseudoephedrine, may reduce the effects of antihypertensives). Products include:
- Lozol Tablets 2022

Isocarboxazid (Prolongs and intensifies the anticholinergic effects; enhances pseudoephedrine effects; concurrent use is contraindicated).
- No products indexed under this heading.

137 **Interactions Index** **Bromfed-DM Cough**

Isoflurane (Potential for additive effects).
No products indexed under this heading.

Isradipine (Sympathomimetic, pseudoephedrine, may reduce the effects of antihypertensives). Products include:
DynaCirc Capsules ... 2256

Ketamine Hydrochloride (Potential for additive effects).
No products indexed under this heading.

Labetalol Hydrochloride (Sympathomimetic, pseudoephedrine, may reduce the effects of antihypertensives). Products include:
Normodyne Injection ... 2377
Normodyne Tablets ... 2379
Trandate ... 1185

Levobunolol Hydrochloride (Sympathomimetic, pseudoephedrine, may reduce the effects of antihypertensives). Products include:
Betagan ... ◉ 233

Levomethadyl Acetate Hydrochloride (Potential for additive effects). Products include:
Orlamm ... 2239

Levorphanol Tartrate (Potential for additive effects). Products include:
Levo-Dromoran ... 2129

Lisinopril (Sympathomimetic, pseudoephedrine, may reduce the effects of antihypertensives). Products include:
Prinivil Tablets ... 1733
Prinzide Tablets ... 1737
Zestoretic ... 2850
Zestril Tablets ... 2854

Lorazepam (Potential for additive effects). Products include:
Ativan Injection ... 2698
Ativan Tablets ... 2700

Losartan Potassium (Sympathomimetic, pseudoephedrine, may reduce the effects of antihypertensives). Products include:
Cozaar Tablets ... 1628
Hyzaar Tablets ... 1677

Loxapine Hydrochloride (Potential for additive effects). Products include:
Loxitane ... 1378

Loxapine Succinate (Potential for additive effects). Products include:
Loxitane Capsules ... 1378

Mecamylamine Hydrochloride (Sympathomimetic, pseudoephedrine, may reduce the effects of antihypertensives). Products include:
Inversine Tablets ... 1686

Meperidine Hydrochloride (Potential for additive effects). Products include:
Demerol ... 2308
Mepergan Injection ... 2753

Mephobarbital (Potential for additive effects). Products include:
Mebaral Tablets ... 2322

Meprobamate (Potential for additive effects). Products include:
Miltown Tablets ... 2672
PMB 200 and PMB 400 ... 2783

Mesoridazine Besylate (Potential for additive effects). Products include:
Serentil ... 684

Methadone Hydrochloride (Potential for additive effects). Products include:
Methadone Hydrochloride Oral Concentrate ... 2233
Methadone Hydrochloride Oral Solution & Tablets ... 2235

Methohexital Sodium (Potential for additive effects). Products include:
Brevital Sodium Vials ... 1429

Methotrimeprazine (Potential for additive effects). Products include:
Levoprome ... 1274

Methoxyflurane (Potential for additive effects).
No products indexed under this heading.

Methyclothiazide (Sympathomimetic, pseudoephedrine, may reduce the effects of antihypertensives). Products include:
Enduron Tablets ... 420

Methyldopa (Sympathomimetic, pseudoephedrine, may reduce the effects of antihypertensives). Products include:
Aldoclor Tablets ... 1598
Aldomet Oral ... 1600
Aldoril Tablets ... 1604

Methyldopate Hydrochloride (Sympathomimetic, pseudoephedrine, may reduce the effects of antihypertensives). Products include:
Aldomet Ester HCl Injection ... 1602

Metipranolol Hydrochloride (Sympathomimetic, pseudoephedrine, may reduce the effects of antihypertensives). Products include:
OptiPranolol (Metipranolol 0.3%) Sterile Ophthalmic Solution ... ◉ 258

Metolazone (Sympathomimetic, pseudoephedrine, may reduce the effects of antihypertensives). Products include:
Mykrox Tablets ... 993
Zaroxolyn Tablets ... 1000

Metoprolol Succinate (Sympathomimetic, pseudoephedrine, may reduce the effects of antihypertensives). Products include:
Toprol-XL Tablets ... 565

Metoprolol Tartrate (Sympathomimetic, pseudoephedrine, may reduce the effects of antihypertensives). Products include:
Lopressor Ampuls ... 830
Lopressor HCT Tablets ... 832
Lopressor Tablets ... 830

Metyrosine (Sympathomimetic, pseudoephedrine, may reduce the effects of antihypertensives). Products include:
Demser Capsules ... 1649

Midazolam Hydrochloride (Potential for additive effects). Products include:
Versed Injection ... 2170

Minoxidil (Sympathomimetic, pseudoephedrine, may reduce the effects of antihypertensives). Products include:
Loniten Tablets ... 2618
Rogaine Topical Solution ... 2637

Moexipril Hydrochloride (Sympathomimetic, pseudoephedrine, may reduce the effects of antihypertensives). Products include:
Univasc Tablets ... 2410

Molindone Hydrochloride (Potential for additive effects). Products include:
Moban Tablets and Concentrate ... 1048

Morphine Sulfate (Potential for additive effects). Products include:
Astramorph/PF Injection, USP (Preservative-Free) ... 535
Duramorph ... 962
Infumorph 200 and Infumorph 500 Sterile Solutions ... 965
MS Contin Tablets ... 1994
MSIR ... 1997
Oramorph SR (Morphine Sulfate Sustained Release Tablets) ... 2236
RMS Suppositories ... 2657
Roxanol ... 2243

Nadolol (Sympathomimetic, pseudoephedrine, may reduce the effects of antihypertensives).
No products indexed under this heading.

Nicardipine Hydrochloride (Sympathomimetic, pseudoephedrine, may reduce the effects of antihypertensives). Products include:
Cardene Capsules ... 2095
Cardene I.V. ... 2709
Cardene SR Capsules ... 2097

Nifedipine (Sympathomimetic, pseudoephedrine, may reduce the effects of antihypertensives). Products include:
Adalat Capsules (10 mg and 20 mg) ... 587
Adalat CC ... 589
Procardia Capsules ... 1971
Procardia XL Extended Release Tablets ... 1972

Nisoldipine (Sympathomimetic, pseudoephedrine, may reduce the effects of antihypertensives).
No products indexed under this heading.

Nitroglycerin (Sympathomimetic, pseudoephedrine, may reduce the effects of antihypertensives). Products include:
Deponit NTG Transdermal Delivery System ... 2397
Nitro-Bid IV ... 1523
Nitro-Bid Ointment ... 1524
Nitrodisc ... 2047
Nitro-Dur (nitroglycerin) Transdermal Infusion System ... 1326
Nitrolingual Spray ... 2027
Nitrostat Tablets ... 1925
Transderm-Nitro Transdermal Therapeutic System ... 859

Opium Alkaloids (Potential for additive effects).
No products indexed under this heading.

Oxazepam (Potential for additive effects). Products include:
Serax Capsules ... 2810
Serax Tablets ... 2810

Oxycodone Hydrochloride (Potential for additive effects). Products include:
Percocet Tablets ... 938
Percodan Tablets ... 939
Percodan-Demi Tablets ... 940
Roxicodone Tablets, Oral Solution & Intensol (Oxycodone) ... 2244
Tylox Capsules ... 1584

Penbutolol Sulfate (Sympathomimetic, pseudoephedrine, may reduce the effects of antihypertensives). Products include:
Levatol ... 2403

Pentobarbital Sodium (Potential for additive effects). Products include:
Nembutal Sodium Capsules ... 436
Nembutal Sodium Solution ... 438
Nembutal Sodium Suppositories ... 440

Perphenazine (Potential for additive effects). Products include:
Etrafon ... 2355
Triavil Tablets ... 1757
Trilafon ... 2389

Phenelzine Sulfate (Prolongs and intensifies the anticholinergic effects; enhances pseudoephedrine effects; concurrent use is contraindicated). Products include:
Nardil ... 1920

Phenobarbital (Potential for additive effects). Products include:
Arco-Lase Plus Tablets ... 512
Bellergal-S Tablets ... 2250
Donnatal ... 2060
Donnatal Extentabs ... 2061
Donnatal Tablets ... 2060
Phenobarbital Elixir and Tablets ... 1469
Quadrinal Tablets ... 1350

Phenoxybenzamine Hydrochloride (Sympathomimetic, pseudoephedrine, may reduce the effects of antihypertensives). Products include:
Dibenzyline Capsules ... 2476

Phentolamine Mesylate (Sympathomimetic, pseudoephedrine, may reduce the effects of antihypertensives). Products include:
Regitine ... 846

Pindolol (Sympathomimetic, pseudoephedrine, may reduce the effects of antihypertensives). Products include:
Visken Tablets ... 2299

Polythiazide (Sympathomimetic, pseudoephedrine, may reduce the effects of antihypertensives). Products include:
Minizide Capsules ... 1938

Prazepam (Potential for additive effects).
No products indexed under this heading.

Prazosin Hydrochloride (Sympathomimetic, pseudoephedrine, may reduce the effects of antihypertensives). Products include:
Minipress Capsules ... 1937
Minizide Capsules ... 1938

Prochlorperazine (Potential for additive effects). Products include:
Compazine ... 2470

Promethazine Hydrochloride (Potential for additive effects). Products include:
Mepergan Injection ... 2753
Phenergan with Codeine ... 2777
Phenergan with Dextromethorphan 2778
Phenergan Injection ... 2773
Phenergan Suppositories ... 2775
Phenergan Syrup ... 2774
Phenergan Tablets ... 2775
Phenergan VC ... 2779
Phenergan VC with Codeine ... 2781

Propofol (Potential for additive effects). Products include:
Diprivan Injection ... 2833

Propoxyphene Hydrochloride (Potential for additive effects). Products include:
Darvon ... 1435
Wygesic Tablets ... 2827

Propoxyphene Napsylate (Potential for additive effects). Products include:
Darvon-N/Darvocet-N ... 1433

Propranolol Hydrochloride (Sympathomimetic, pseudoephedrine, may reduce the effects of antihypertensives). Products include:
Inderal ... 2728
Inderal LA Long Acting Capsules ... 2730
Inderide Tablets ... 2732
Inderide LA Long Acting Capsules .. 2734

Quazepam (Potential for additive effects). Products include:
Doral Tablets ... 2664

Quinapril Hydrochloride (Sympathomimetic, pseudoephedrine, may reduce the effects of antihypertensives). Products include:
Accupril Tablets ... 1893

Ramipril (Sympathomimetic, pseudoephedrine, may reduce the effects of antihypertensives). Products include:
Altace Capsules ... 1232

Rauwolfia Serpentina (Sympathomimetic, pseudoephedrine, may reduce the effects of antihypertensives).
No products indexed under this heading.

Rescinnamine (Sympathomimetic, pseudoephedrine, may reduce the effects of antihypertensives).
No products indexed under this heading.

IMPORTANT NOTE: Always consult each drug listing in the patient's regimen for possible interactions.

Bromfed - DM Cough **Interactions Index** **138**

Reserpine (Sympathomimetic, pseudoephedrine, may reduce the effects of antihypertensives). Products include:
Diupres Tablets 1650
Hydropres Tablets 1675
Ser-Ap-Es Tablets 849

Risperidone (Potential for additive effects). Products include:
Risperdal 1301

Secobarbital Sodium (Potential for additive effects). Products include:
Seconal Sodium Pulvules 1474

Selegiline Hydrochloride (Prolongs and intensifies the anticholinergic effects; enhances pseudoephedrine effects; concurrent use is contraindicated). Products include:
Eldepryl Tablets 2550

Sodium Nitroprusside (Sympathomimetic, pseudoephedrine, may reduce the effects of antihypertensives).
No products indexed under this heading.

Sotalol Hydrochloride (Sympathomimetic, pseudoephedrine, may reduce the effects of antihypertensives). Products include:
Betapace Tablets 641

Spirapril Hydrochloride (Sympathomimetic, pseudoephedrine, may reduce the effects of antihypertensives).
No products indexed under this heading.

Sufentanil Citrate (Potential for additive effects). Products include:
Sufenta Injection 1309

Temazepam (Potential for additive effects). Products include:
Restoril Capsules 2284

Terazosin Hydrochloride (Sympathomimetic, pseudoephedrine, may reduce the effects of antihypertensives). Products include:
Hytrin Capsules 430

Thiamylal Sodium (Potential for additive effects).
No products indexed under this heading.

Thioridazine Hydrochloride (Potential for additive effects). Products include:
Mellaril 2269

Thiothixene (Potential for additive effects). Products include:
Navane Capsules and Concentrate 2201
Navane Intramuscular 2202

Timolol Maleate (Sympathomimetic, pseudoephedrine, may reduce the effects of antihypertensives). Products include:
Blocadren Tablets 1614
Timolide Tablets 1748
Timoptic in Ocudose 1753
Timoptic Sterile Ophthalmic Solution 1751
Timoptic-XE 1755

Torsemide (Sympathomimetic, pseudoephedrine, may reduce the effects of antihypertensives). Products include:
Demadex Tablets and Injection 686

Tranylcypromine Sulfate (Prolongs and intensifies the anticholinergic effects; enhances pseudoephedrine effects; concurrent use is contraindicated). Products include:
Parnate Tablets 2503

Triazolam (Potential for additive effects). Products include:
Halcion Tablets 2611

Trifluoperazine Hydrochloride (Potential for additive effects). Products include:
Stelazine 2514

Trimethaphan Camsylate (Sympathomimetic, pseudoephedrine, may reduce the effects of antihypertensives). Products include:
Arfonad Ampuls 2080

Verapamil Hydrochloride (Sympathomimetic, pseudoephedrine, may reduce the effects of antihypertensives). Products include:
Calan SR Caplets 2422
Calan Tablets 2419
Isoptin Injectable 1344
Isoptin Oral Tablets 1346
Isoptin SR Tablets 1348
Verelan Capsules 1410
Verelan Capsules 2824

Zolpidem Tartrate (Potential for additive effects). Products include:
Ambien Tablets 2416

Food Interactions

Alcohol (Potential for additive effects).

BROMFED-PD CAPSULES (EXTENDED-RELEASE)

(Brompheniramine Maleate, Pseudoephedrine Hydrochloride) 1785
See **Bromfed Capsules (Extended-Release)**

BRONKAID MIST

(Epinephrine) ..... ⊞ 717
May interact with antihypertensives, antidepressant drugs, and monoamine oxidase inhibitors. Compounds in these categories include:

Acebutolol Hydrochloride (Concurrent use is not recommended without physician's consultation). Products include:
Sectral Capsules 2807

Amitriptyline Hydrochloride (Concurrent use is not recommended without physician's consultation). Products include:
Elavil 2838
Endep Tablets 2174
Etrafon 2355
Limbitrol 2180
Triavil Tablets 1757

Amlodipine Besylate (Concurrent use is not recommended without physician's consultation). Products include:
Lotrel Capsules 840
Norvasc Tablets 1940

Amoxapine (Concurrent use is not recommended without physician's consultation). Products include:
Asendin Tablets 1369

Atenolol (Concurrent use is not recommended without physician's consultation). Products include:
Tenoretic Tablets 2845
Tenormin Tablets and I.V. Injection 2847

Benazepril Hydrochloride (Concurrent use is not recommended without physician's consultation). Products include:
Lotensin Tablets 834
Lotensin HCT 837
Lotrel Capsules 840

Bendroflumethiazide (Concurrent use is not recommended without physician's consultation).
No products indexed under this heading.

Betaxolol Hydrochloride (Concurrent use is not recommended without physician's consultation). Products include:
Betoptic Ophthalmic Solution 469
Betoptic S Ophthalmic Suspension 471
Kerlone Tablets 2436

Bisoprolol Fumarate (Concurrent use is not recommended without physician's consultation). Products include:
Zebeta Tablets 1413
Ziac 1415

Bupropion Hydrochloride (Concurrent use is not recommended without physician's consultation). Products include:
Wellbutrin Tablets 1204

Captopril (Concurrent use is not recommended without physician's consultation). Products include:
Capoten 739
Capozide 742

Carteolol Hydrochloride (Concurrent use is not recommended without physician's consultation). Products include:
Cartrol Tablets 410
Ocupress Ophthalmic Solution, 1% Sterile ..... ◉ 309

Chlorothiazide (Concurrent use is not recommended without physician's consultation). Products include:
Aldoclor Tablets 1598
Diupres Tablets 1650
Diuril Oral 1653

Chlorothiazide Sodium (Concurrent use is not recommended without physician's consultation). Products include:
Diuril Sodium Intravenous 1652

Chlorthalidone (Concurrent use is not recommended without physician's consultation). Products include:
Combipres Tablets 677
Tenoretic Tablets 2845
Thalitone 1245

Clonidine (Concurrent use is not recommended without physician's consultation). Products include:
Catapres-TTS 675

Clonidine Hydrochloride (Concurrent use is not recommended without physician's consultation). Products include:
Catapres Tablets 674
Combipres Tablets 677

Deserpidine (Concurrent use is not recommended without physician's consultation).
No products indexed under this heading.

Desipramine Hydrochloride (Concurrent use is not recommended without physician's consultation). Products include:
Norpramin Tablets 1526

Diazoxide (Concurrent use is not recommended without physician's consultation). Products include:
Hyperstat I.V. Injection 2363
Proglycem 580

Diltiazem Hydrochloride (Concurrent use is not recommended without physician's consultation). Products include:
Cardizem CD Capsules 1506
Cardizem SR Capsules 1510
Cardizem Injectable 1508
Cardizem Tablets 1512
Dilacor XR Extended-release Capsules 2018

Doxazosin Mesylate (Concurrent use is not recommended without physician's consultation). Products include:
Cardura Tablets 2186

Doxepin Hydrochloride (Concurrent use is not recommended without physician's consultation). Products include:
Sinequan 2205
Zonalon Cream 1055

Enalapril Maleate (Concurrent use is not recommended without physician's consultation). Products include:
Vaseretic Tablets 1765
Vasotec Tablets 1771

Enalaprilat (Concurrent use is not recommended without physician's consultation). Products include:
Vasotec I.V. 1768

Esmolol Hydrochloride (Concurrent use is not recommended without physician's consultation). Products include:
Brevibloc Injection 1808

Felodipine (Concurrent use is not recommended without physician's consultation). Products include:
Plendil Extended-Release Tablets 527

Fluoxetine Hydrochloride (Concurrent use is not recommended without physician's consultation). Products include:
Prozac Pulvules & Liquid, Oral Solution 919

Fosinopril Sodium (Concurrent use is not recommended without physician's consultation). Products include:
Monopril Tablets 757

Furazolidone (Concurrent use is not recommended without physician's consultation). Products include:
Furoxone 2046

Furosemide (Concurrent use is not recommended without physician's consultation). Products include:
Lasix Injection, Oral Solution and Tablets 1240

Guanabenz Acetate (Concurrent use is not recommended without physician's consultation).
No products indexed under this heading.

Guanethidine Monosulfate (Concurrent use is not recommended without physician's consultation). Products include:
Esimil Tablets 822
Ismelin Tablets 827

Hydralazine Hydrochloride (Concurrent use is not recommended without physician's consultation). Products include:
Apresazide Capsules 808
Apresoline Hydrochloride Tablets 809
Ser-Ap-Es Tablets 849

Hydrochlorothiazide (Concurrent use is not recommended without physician's consultation). Products include:
Aldactazide 2413
Aldoril Tablets 1604
Apresazide Capsules 808
Capozide 742
Dyazide 2479
Esidrix Tablets 821
Esimil Tablets 822
HydroDIURIL Tablets 1674
Hydropres Tablets 1675
Hyzaar Tablets 1677
Inderide Tablets 2732
Inderide LA Long Acting Capsules 2734
Lopressor HCT Tablets 832
Lotensin HCT 837
Maxzide 1380
Moduretic Tablets 1705
Oretic Tablets 443
Prinzide Tablets 1737
Ser-Ap-Es Tablets 849
Timolide Tablets 1748
Vaseretic Tablets 1765
Zestoretic 2850
Ziac 1415

Hydroflumethiazide (Concurrent use is not recommended without physician's consultation). Products include:
Diucardin Tablets 2718

Imipramine Hydrochloride (Concurrent use is not recommended without physician's consultation). Products include:
Tofranil Ampuls 854
Tofranil Tablets 856

(⊞ Described in PDR For Nonprescription Drugs) (◉ Described in PDR For Ophthalmology)

Imipramine Pamoate (Concurrent use is not recommended without physician's consultation). Products include:
Tofranil-PM Capsules ... 857
Indapamide (Concurrent use is not recommended without physician's consultation). Products include:
Lozol Tablets ... 2022
Isocarboxazid (Concurrent use is not recommended without physician's consultation).
No products indexed under this heading.
Isradipine (Concurrent use is not recommended without physician's consultation). Products include:
DynaCirc Capsules ... 2256
Labetalol Hydrochloride (Concurrent use is not recommended without physician's consultation). Products include:
Normodyne Injection ... 2377
Normodyne Tablets ... 2379
Trandate ... 1185
Lisinopril (Concurrent use is not recommended without physician's consultation). Products include:
Prinivil Tablets ... 1733
Prinzide Tablets ... 1737
Zestoretic ... 2850
Zestril Tablets ... 2854
Losartan Potassium (Concurrent use is not recommended without physician's consultation). Products include:
Cozaar Tablets ... 1628
Hyzaar Tablets ... 1677
Maprotiline Hydrochloride (Concurrent use is not recommended without physician's consultation). Products include:
Ludiomil Tablets ... 843
Mecamylamine Hydrochloride (Concurrent use is not recommended without physician's consultation). Products include:
Inversine Tablets ... 1686
Methyclothiazide (Concurrent use is not recommended without physician's consultation). Products include:
Enduron Tablets ... 420
Methyldopa (Concurrent use is not recommended without physician's consultation). Products include:
Aldoclor Tablets ... 1598
Aldomet Oral ... 1600
Aldoril Tablets ... 1604
Methyldopate Hydrochloride (Concurrent use is not recommended without physician's consultation). Products include:
Aldomet Ester HCl Injection ... 1602
Metolazone (Concurrent use is not recommended without physician's consultation). Products include:
Mykrox Tablets ... 993
Zaroxolyn Tablets ... 1000
Metoprolol Succinate (Concurrent use is not recommended without physician's consultation). Products include:
Toprol-XL Tablets ... 565
Metoprolol Tartrate (Concurrent use is not recommended without physician's consultation). Products include:
Lopressor Ampuls ... 830
Lopressor HCT Tablets ... 832
Lopressor Tablets ... 830
Metyrosine (Concurrent use is not recommended without physician's consultation). Products include:
Demser Capsules ... 1649
Minoxidil (Concurrent use is not recommended without physician's consultation). Products include:
Loniten Tablets ... 2618
Rogaine Topical Solution ... 2637
Moexipril Hydrochloride (Concurrent use is not recommended without physician's consultation). Products include:
Univasc Tablets ... 2410
Nadolol (Concurrent use is not recommended without physician's consultation).
No products indexed under this heading.
Nefazodone Hydrochloride (Concurrent use is not recommended without physician's consultation). Products include:
Serzone Tablets ... 771
Nicardipine Hydrochloride (Concurrent use is not recommended without physician's consultation). Products include:
Cardene Capsules ... 2095
Cardene I.V. ... 2709
Cardene SR Capsules ... 2097
Nifedipine (Concurrent use is not recommended without physician's consultation). Products include:
Adalat Capsules (10 mg and 20 mg) ... 587
Adalat CC ... 589
Procardia Capsules ... 1971
Procardia XL Extended Release Tablets ... 1972
Nisoldipine (Concurrent use is not recommended without physician's consultation).
No products indexed under this heading.
Nitroglycerin (Concurrent use is not recommended without physician's consultation). Products include:
Deponit NTG Transdermal Delivery System ... 2397
Nitro-Bid IV ... 1523
Nitro-Bid Ointment ... 1524
Nitrodisc ... 2047
Nitro-Dur (nitroglycerin) Transdermal Infusion System ... 1326
Nitrolingual Spray ... 2027
Nitrostat Tablets ... 1925
Transderm-Nitro Transdermal Therapeutic System ... 859
Nortriptyline Hydrochloride (Concurrent use is not recommended without physician's consultation). Products include:
Pamelor ... 2280
Paroxetine Hydrochloride (Concurrent use is not recommended without physician's consultation). Products include:
Paxil Tablets ... 2505
Penbutolol Sulfate (Concurrent use is not recommended without physician's consultation). Products include:
Levatol ... 2403
Phenelzine Sulfate (Concurrent use is not recommended without physician's consultation). Products include:
Nardil ... 1920
Phenoxybenzamine Hydrochloride (Concurrent use is not recommended without physician's consultation). Products include:
Dibenzyline Capsules ... 2476
Phentolamine Mesylate (Concurrent use is not recommended without physician's consultation). Products include:
Regitine ... 846
Pindolol (Concurrent use is not recommended without physician's consultation). Products include:
Visken Tablets ... 2299
Polythiazide (Concurrent use is not recommended without physician's consultation). Products include:
Minizide Capsules ... 1938
Prazosin Hydrochloride (Concurrent use is not recommended without physician's consultation). Products include:
Minipress Capsules ... 1937
Minizide Capsules ... 1938
Propranolol Hydrochloride (Concurrent use is not recommended without physician's consultation). Products include:
Inderal ... 2728
Inderal LA Long Acting Capsules ... 2730
Inderide Tablets ... 2732
Inderide LA Long Acting Capsules .. 2734
Protriptyline Hydrochloride (Concurrent use is not recommended without physician's consultation). Products include:
Vivactil Tablets ... 1774
Quinapril Hydrochloride (Concurrent use is not recommended without physician's consultation). Products include:
Accupril Tablets ... 1893
Ramipril (Concurrent use is not recommended without physician's consultation). Products include:
Altace Capsules ... 1232
Rauwolfia Serpentina (Concurrent use is not recommended without physician's consultation).
No products indexed under this heading.
Rescinnamine (Concurrent use is not recommended without physician's consultation).
No products indexed under this heading.
Reserpine (Concurrent use is not recommended without physician's consultation). Products include:
Diupres Tablets ... 1650
Hydropres Tablets ... 1675
Ser-Ap-Es Tablets ... 849
Selegiline Hydrochloride (Concurrent use is not recommended without physician's consultation). Products include:
Eldepryl Tablets ... 2550
Sertraline Hydrochloride (Concurrent use is not recommended without physician's consultation). Products include:
Zoloft Tablets ... 2217
Sodium Nitroprusside (Concurrent use is not recommended without physician's consultation).
No products indexed under this heading.
Sotalol Hydrochloride (Concurrent use is not recommended without physician's consultation). Products include:
Betapace Tablets ... 641
Spirapril Hydrochloride (Concurrent use is not recommended without physician's consultation).
No products indexed under this heading.
Terazosin Hydrochloride (Concurrent use is not recommended without physician's consultation). Products include:
Hytrin Capsules ... 430
Timolol Maleate (Concurrent use is not recommended without physician's consultation). Products include:
Blocadren Tablets ... 1614
Timolide Tablets ... 1748
Timoptic in Ocudose ... 1753
Timoptic Sterile Ophthalmic Solution ... 1751
Timoptic-XE ... 1755
Torsemide (Concurrent use is not recommended without physician's consultation). Products include:
Demadex Tablets and Injection ... 686
Tranylcypromine Sulfate (Concurrent use is not recommended without physician's consultation). Products include:
Parnate Tablets ... 2503
Trazodone Hydrochloride (Concurrent use is not recommended without physician's consultation). Products include:
Desyrel and Desyrel Dividose ... 503
Trimethaphan Camsylate (Concurrent use is not recommended without physician's consultation). Products include:
Arfonad Ampuls ... 2080
Trimipramine Maleate (Concurrent use is not recommended without physician's consultation). Products include:
Surmontil Capsules ... 2811
Venlafaxine Hydrochloride (Concurrent use is not recommended without physician's consultation). Products include:
Effexor ... 2719
Verapamil Hydrochloride (Concurrent use is not recommended without physician's consultation). Products include:
Calan SR Caplets ... 2422
Calan Tablets ... 2419
Isoptin Injectable ... 1344
Isoptin Oral Tablets ... 1346
Isoptin SR Tablets ... 1348
Verelan Capsules ... 1410
Verelan Capsules ... 2824

BRONKAID MIST SUSPENSION

(Epinephrine Bitartrate) ... 718
May interact with antihypertensives, antidepressant drugs, and monoamine oxidase inhibitors. Compounds in these categories include:
Acebutolol Hydrochloride (Concurrent use is not recommended without physician's consultation). Products include:
Sectral Capsules ... 2807
Amitriptyline Hydrochloride (Concurrent use is not recommended without physician's consultation). Products include:
Elavil ... 2838
Endep Tablets ... 2174
Etrafon ... 2355
Limbitrol ... 2180
Triavil Tablets ... 1757
Amlodipine Besylate (Concurrent use is not recommended without physician's consultation). Products include:
Lotrel Capsules ... 840
Norvasc Tablets ... 1940
Amoxapine (Concurrent use is not recommended without physician's consultation). Products include:
Asendin Tablets ... 1369
Atenolol (Concurrent use is not recommended without physician's consultation). Products include:
Tenoretic Tablets ... 2845
Tenormin Tablets and I.V. Injection 2847
Benazepril Hydrochloride (Concurrent use is not recommended without physician's consultation). Products include:
Lotensin Tablets ... 834
Lotensin HCT ... 837
Lotrel Capsules ... 840
Bendroflumethiazide (Concurrent use is not recommended without physician's consultation).
No products indexed under this heading.

IMPORTANT NOTE: Always consult each drug listing in the patient's regimen for possible interactions.

Bronkaid Mist Suspension Interactions Index 140

Betaxolol Hydrochloride (Concurrent use is not recommended without physician's consultation). Products include:
Betoptic Ophthalmic Solution 469
Betoptic S Ophthalmic Suspension 471
Kerlone Tablets 2436

Bisoprolol Fumarate (Concurrent use is not recommended without physician's consultation). Products include:
Zebeta Tablets 1413
Ziac 1415

Bupropion Hydrochloride (Concurrent use is not recommended without physician's consultation). Products include:
Wellbutrin Tablets 1204

Captopril (Concurrent use is not recommended without physician's consultation). Products include:
Capoten 739
Capozide 742

Carteolol Hydrochloride (Concurrent use is not recommended without physician's consultation). Products include:
Cartrol Tablets 410
Ocupress Ophthalmic Solution, 1% Sterile ⊚ 309

Chlorothiazide (Concurrent use is not recommended without physician's consultation). Products include:
Aldoclor Tablets 1598
Diupres Tablets 1650
Diuril Oral 1653

Chlorothiazide Sodium (Concurrent use is not recommended without physician's consultation). Products include:
Diuril Sodium Intravenous 1652

Chlorthalidone (Concurrent use is not recommended without physician's consultation). Products include:
Combipres Tablets 677
Tenoretic Tablets 2845
Thalitone 1245

Clonidine (Concurrent use is not recommended without physician's consultation). Products include:
Catapres-TTS 675

Clonidine Hydrochloride (Concurrent use is not recommended without physician's consultation). Products include:
Catapres Tablets 674
Combipres Tablets 677

Deserpidine (Concurrent use is not recommended without physician's consultation).
No products indexed under this heading.

Desipramine Hydrochloride (Concurrent use is not recommended without physician's consultation). Products include:
Norpramin Tablets 1526

Diazoxide (Concurrent use is not recommended without physician's consultation). Products include:
Hyperstat I.V. Injection 2363
Proglycem 580

Diltiazem Hydrochloride (Concurrent use is not recommended without physician's consultation). Products include:
Cardizem CD Capsules 1506
Cardizem SR Capsules 1510
Cardizem Injectable 1508
Cardizem Tablets 1512
Dilacor XR Extended-release Capsules 2018

Doxazosin Mesylate (Concurrent use is not recommended without physician's consultation). Products include:
Cardura Tablets 2186

Doxepin Hydrochloride (Concurrent use is not recommended without physician's consultation). Products include:
Sinequan 2205
Zonalon Cream 1055

Enalapril Maleate (Concurrent use is not recommended without physician's consultation). Products include:
Vaseretic Tablets 1765
Vasotec Tablets 1771

Enalaprilat (Concurrent use is not recommended without physician's consultation). Products include:
Vasotec I.V. 1768

Esmolol Hydrochloride (Concurrent use is not recommended without physician's consultation). Products include:
Brevibloc Injection 1808

Felodipine (Concurrent use is not recommended without physician's consultation). Products include:
Plendil Extended-Release Tablets 527

Fluoxetine Hydrochloride (Concurrent use is not recommended without physician's consultation). Products include:
Prozac Pulvules & Liquid, Oral Solution 919

Fosinopril Sodium (Concurrent use is not recommended without physician's consultation). Products include:
Monopril Tablets 757

Furazolidone (Concurrent use is not recommended without physician's consultation). Products include:
Furoxone 2046

Furosemide (Concurrent use is not recommended without physician's consultation). Products include:
Lasix Injection, Oral Solution and Tablets 1240

Guanabenz Acetate (Concurrent use is not recommended without physician's consultation).
No products indexed under this heading.

Guanethidine Monosulfate (Concurrent use is not recommended without physician's consultation). Products include:
Esimil Tablets 822
Ismelin Tablets 827

Hydralazine Hydrochloride (Concurrent use is not recommended without physician's consultation). Products include:
Apresazide Capsules 808
Apresoline Hydrochloride Tablets 809
Ser-Ap-Es Tablets 849

Hydrochlorothiazide (Concurrent use is not recommended without physician's consultation). Products include:
Aldactazide 2413
Aldoril Tablets 1604
Apresazide Capsules 808
Capozide 742
Dyazide 2479
Esidrix Tablets 821
Esimil Tablets 822
HydroDIURIL Tablets 1674
Hydropres Tablets 1675
Hyzaar Tablets 1677
Inderide Tablets 2732
Inderide LA Long Acting Capsules 2734
Lopressor HCT Tablets 837
Lotensin HCT 837
Maxzide 1380
Moduretic Tablets 1705
Oretic Tablets 443
Prinzide Tablets 1737
Ser-Ap-Es Tablets 849
Timolide Tablets 1748
Vaseretic Tablets 1765
Zestoretic 2850
Ziac 1415

Hydroflumethiazide (Concurrent use is not recommended without physician's consultation). Products include:
Diucardin Tablets 2718

Imipramine Hydrochloride (Concurrent use is not recommended without physician's consultation). Products include:
Tofranil Ampuls 854
Tofranil Tablets 856

Imipramine Pamoate (Concurrent use is not recommended without physician's consultation). Products include:
Tofranil-PM Capsules 857

Indapamide (Concurrent use is not recommended without physician's consultation). Products include:
Lozol Tablets 2022

Isocarboxazid (Concurrent use is not recommended without physician's consultation).
No products indexed under this heading.

Isradipine (Concurrent use is not recommended without physician's consultation). Products include:
DynaCirc Capsules 2256

Labetalol Hydrochloride (Concurrent use is not recommended without physician's consultation). Products include:
Normodyne Injection 2377
Normodyne Tablets 2379
Trandate 1185

Lisinopril (Concurrent use is not recommended without physician's consultation). Products include:
Prinivil Tablets 1733
Prinzide Tablets 1737
Zestoretic 2850
Zestril Tablets 2854

Losartan Potassium (Concurrent use is not recommended without physician's consultation). Products include:
Cozaar Tablets 1628
Hyzaar Tablets 1677

Maprotiline Hydrochloride (Concurrent use is not recommended without physician's consultation). Products include:
Ludiomil Tablets 843

Mecamylamine Hydrochloride (Concurrent use is not recommended without physician's consultation). Products include:
Inversine Tablets 1686

Methyclothiazide (Concurrent use is not recommended without physician's consultation). Products include:
Enduron Tablets 420

Methyldopa (Concurrent use is not recommended without physician's consultation). Products include:
Aldoclor Tablets 1598
Aldomet Oral 1600
Aldoril Tablets 1604

Methyldopate Hydrochloride (Concurrent use is not recommended without physician's consultation). Products include:
Aldomet Ester HCl Injection 1602

Metolazone (Concurrent use is not recommended without physician's consultation). Products include:
Mykrox Tablets 993
Zaroxolyn Tablets 1000

Metoprolol Succinate (Concurrent use is not recommended without physician's consultation). Products include:
Toprol-XL Tablets 565

Metoprolol Tartrate (Concurrent use is not recommended without physician's consultation). Products include:
Lopressor Ampuls 830
Lopressor HCT Tablets 832
Lopressor Tablets 830

Metyrosine (Concurrent use is not recommended without physician's consultation). Products include:
Demser Capsules 1649

Minoxidil (Concurrent use is not recommended without physician's consultation). Products include:
Loniten Tablets 2618
Rogaine Topical Solution 2637

Moexipril Hydrochloride (Concurrent use is not recommended without physician's consultation). Products include:
Univasc Tablets 2410

Nadolol (Concurrent use is not recommended without physician's consultation).
No products indexed under this heading.

Nefazodone Hydrochloride (Concurrent use is not recommended without physician's consultation). Products include:
Serzone Tablets 771

Nicardipine Hydrochloride (Concurrent use is not recommended without physician's consultation). Products include:
Cardene Capsules 2095
Cardene I.V. 2709
Cardene SR Capsules 2097

Nifedipine (Concurrent use is not recommended without physician's consultation). Products include:
Adalat Capsules (10 mg and 20 mg) 587
Adalat CC 589
Procardia Capsules 1971
Procardia XL Extended Release Tablets 1972

Nisoldipine (Concurrent use is not recommended without physician's consultation).
No products indexed under this heading.

Nitroglycerin (Concurrent use is not recommended without physician's consultation). Products include:
Deponit NTG Transdermal Delivery System 2397
Nitro-Bid IV 1523
Nitro-Bid Ointment 1524
Nitrodisc 2047
Nitro-Dur (nitroglycerin) Transdermal Infusion System 1326
Nitrolingual Spray 2027
Nitrostat Tablets 1925
Transderm-Nitro Transdermal Therapeutic System 859

Nortriptyline Hydrochloride (Concurrent use is not recommended without physician's consultation). Products include:
Pamelor 2280

Paroxetine Hydrochloride (Concurrent use is not recommended without physician's consultation). Products include:
Paxil Tablets 2505

Penbutolol Sulfate (Concurrent use is not recommended without physician's consultation). Products include:
Levatol 2403

Phenelzine Sulfate (Concurrent use is not recommended without physician's consultation). Products include:
Nardil 1920

(▭ Described in PDR For Nonprescription Drugs) (⊚ Described in PDR For Ophthalmology)

141 Interactions Index Bronkaid Caplets

Phenoxybenzamine Hydrochloride (Concurrent use is not recommended without physician's consultation). Products include:
Dibenzyline Capsules ... 2476

Phentolamine Mesylate (Concurrent use is not recommended without physician's consultation). Products include:
Regitine ... 846

Pindolol (Concurrent use is not recommended without physician's consultation). Products include:
Visken Tablets ... 2299

Polythiazide (Concurrent use is not recommended without physician's consultation). Products include:
Minizide Capsules ... 1938

Prazosin Hydrochloride (Concurrent use is not recommended without physician's consultation). Products include:
Minipress Capsules ... 1937
Minizide Capsules ... 1938

Propranolol Hydrochloride (Concurrent use is not recommended without physician's consultation). Products include:
Inderal ... 2728
Inderal LA Long Acting Capsules ... 2730
Inderide Tablets ... 2732
Inderide LA Long Acting Capsules ... 2734

Protriptyline Hydrochloride (Concurrent use is not recommended without physician's consultation). Products include:
Vivactil Tablets ... 1774

Quinapril Hydrochloride (Concurrent use is not recommended without physician's consultation). Products include:
Accupril Tablets ... 1893

Ramipril (Concurrent use is not recommended without physician's consultation). Products include:
Altace Capsules ... 1232

Rauwolfia Serpentina (Concurrent use is not recommended without physician's consultation).
No products indexed under this heading.

Rescinnamine (Concurrent use is not recommended without physician's consultation).
No products indexed under this heading.

Reserpine (Concurrent use is not recommended without physician's consultation). Products include:
Diupres Tablets ... 1650
Hydropres Tablets ... 1675
Ser-Ap-Es Tablets ... 849

Selegiline Hydrochloride (Concurrent use is not recommended without physician's consultation). Products include:
Eldepryl Tablets ... 2550

Sertraline Hydrochloride (Concurrent use is not recommended without physician's consultation). Products include:
Zoloft Tablets ... 2217

Sodium Nitroprusside (Concurrent use is not recommended without physician's consultation).
No products indexed under this heading.

Sotalol Hydrochloride (Concurrent use is not recommended without physician's consultation). Products include:
Betapace Tablets ... 641

Spirapril Hydrochloride (Concurrent use is not recommended without physician's consultation).
No products indexed under this heading.

Terazosin Hydrochloride (Concurrent use is not recommended without physician's consultation). Products include:
Hytrin Capsules ... 430

Timolol Maleate (Concurrent use is not recommended without physician's consultation). Products include:
Blocadren Tablets ... 1614
Timolide Tablets ... 1748
Timoptic in Ocudose ... 1753
Timoptic Sterile Ophthalmic Solution ... 1751
Timoptic-XE ... 1755

Torsemide (Concurrent use is not recommended without physician's consultation). Products include:
Demadex Tablets and Injection ... 686

Tranylcypromine Sulfate (Concurrent use is not recommended without physician's consultation). Products include:
Parnate Tablets ... 2503

Trazodone Hydrochloride (Concurrent use is not recommended without physician's consultation). Products include:
Desyrel and Desyrel Dividose ... 503

Trimethaphan Camsylate (Concurrent use is not recommended without physician's consultation). Products include:
Arfonad Ampuls ... 2080

Trimipramine Maleate (Concurrent use is not recommended without physician's consultation). Products include:
Surmontil Capsules ... 2811

Venlafaxine Hydrochloride (Concurrent use is not recommended without physician's consultation). Products include:
Effexor ... 2719

Verapamil Hydrochloride (Concurrent use is not recommended without physician's consultation). Products include:
Calan SR Caplets ... 2422
Calan Tablets ... 2419
Isoptin Injectable ... 1344
Isoptin Oral Tablets ... 1346
Isoptin SR Tablets ... 1348
Verelan Capsules ... 1410
Verelan Capsules ... 2824

BRONKAID CAPLETS
(Ephedrine Sulfate, Guaifenesin) ... 717
May interact with antihypertensives, antidepressant drugs, and monoamine oxidase inhibitors. Compounds in these categories include:

Acebutolol Hydrochloride (Concurrent use is not recommended). Products include:
Sectral Capsules ... 2807

Amitriptyline Hydrochloride (Concurrent use is not recommended). Products include:
Elavil ... 2838
Endep Tablets ... 2174
Etrafon ... 2355
Limbitrol ... 2180
Triavil Tablets ... 1757

Amlodipine Besylate (Concurrent use is not recommended). Products include:
Lotrel Capsules ... 840
Norvasc Tablets ... 1940

Amoxapine (Concurrent use is not recommended). Products include:
Asendin Tablets ... 1369

Atenolol (Concurrent use is not recommended). Products include:
Tenoretic Tablets ... 2845
Tenormin Tablets and I.V. Injection ... 2847

Benazepril Hydrochloride (Concurrent use is not recommended). Products include:
Lotensin Tablets ... 834
Lotensin HCT ... 837
Lotrel Capsules ... 840

Bendroflumethiazide (Concurrent use is not recommended).
No products indexed under this heading.

Betaxolol Hydrochloride (Concurrent use is not recommended). Products include:
Betoptic Ophthalmic Solution ... 469
Betoptic S Ophthalmic Suspension ... 471
Kerlone Tablets ... 2436

Bisoprolol Fumarate (Concurrent use is not recommended). Products include:
Zebeta Tablets ... 1413
Ziac ... 1415

Bupropion Hydrochloride (Concurrent use is not recommended). Products include:
Wellbutrin Tablets ... 1204

Captopril (Concurrent use is not recommended). Products include:
Capoten ... 739
Capozide ... 742

Carteolol Hydrochloride (Concurrent use is not recommended). Products include:
Cartrol Tablets ... 410
Ocupress Ophthalmic Solution, 1% Sterile ... ◉ 309

Chlorothiazide (Concurrent use is not recommended). Products include:
Aldoclor Tablets ... 1598
Diupres Tablets ... 1650
Diuril Oral ... 1653

Chlorothiazide Sodium (Concurrent use is not recommended). Products include:
Diuril Sodium Intravenous ... 1652

Chlorthalidone (Concurrent use is not recommended). Products include:
Combipres Tablets ... 677
Tenoretic Tablets ... 2845
Thalitone ... 1245

Clonidine (Concurrent use is not recommended). Products include:
Catapres-TTS ... 675

Clonidine Hydrochloride (Concurrent use is not recommended). Products include:
Catapres Tablets ... 674
Combipres Tablets ... 677

Deserpidine (Concurrent use is not recommended).
No products indexed under this heading.

Desipramine Hydrochloride (Concurrent use is not recommended). Products include:
Norpramin Tablets ... 1526

Diazoxide (Concurrent use is not recommended). Products include:
Hyperstat I.V. Injection ... 2363
Proglycem ... 580

Diltiazem Hydrochloride (Concurrent use is not recommended). Products include:
Cardizem CD Capsules ... 1506
Cardizem SR Capsules ... 1510
Cardizem Injectable ... 1508
Cardizem Tablets ... 1512
Dilacor XR Extended-release Capsules ... 2018

Doxazosin Mesylate (Concurrent use is not recommended). Products include:
Cardura Tablets ... 2186

Doxepin Hydrochloride (Concurrent use is not recommended). Products include:
Sinequan ... 2205

Zonalon Cream ... 1055

Enalapril Maleate (Concurrent use is not recommended). Products include:
Vaseretic Tablets ... 1765
Vasotec Tablets ... 1771

Enalaprilat (Concurrent use is not recommended). Products include:
Vasotec I.V. ... 1768

Esmolol Hydrochloride (Concurrent use is not recommended). Products include:
Brevibloc Injection ... 1808

Felodipine (Concurrent use is not recommended). Products include:
Plendil Extended-Release Tablets ... 527

Fluoxetine Hydrochloride (Concurrent use is not recommended). Products include:
Prozac Pulvules & Liquid, Oral Solution ... 919

Fosinopril Sodium (Concurrent use is not recommended). Products include:
Monopril Tablets ... 757

Furazolidone (Concurrent use is not recommended). Products include:
Furoxone ... 2046

Furosemide (Concurrent use is not recommended). Products include:
Lasix Injection, Oral Solution and Tablets ... 1240

Guanabenz Acetate (Concurrent use is not recommended).
No products indexed under this heading.

Guanethidine Monosulfate (Concurrent use is not recommended). Products include:
Esimil Tablets ... 822
Ismelin Tablets ... 827

Hydralazine Hydrochloride (Concurrent use is not recommended). Products include:
Apresazide Capsules ... 808
Apresoline Hydrochloride Tablets ... 809
Ser-Ap-Es Tablets ... 849

Hydrochlorothiazide (Concurrent use is not recommended). Products include:
Aldactazide ... 2413
Aldoril Tablets ... 1604
Apresazide Capsules ... 808
Capozide ... 742
Dyazide ... 2479
Esidrix Tablets ... 821
Esimil Tablets ... 822
HydroDIURIL Tablets ... 1674
Hydropres Tablets ... 1675
Hyzaar Tablets ... 1677
Inderide Tablets ... 2732
Inderide LA Long Acting Capsules ... 2734
Lopressor HCT Tablets ... 832
Lotensin HCT ... 837
Maxzide ... 1380
Moduretic Tablets ... 1705
Oretic Tablets ... 443
Prinzide Tablets ... 1737
Ser-Ap-Es Tablets ... 849
Timolide Tablets ... 1748
Vaseretic Tablets ... 1765
Zestoretic ... 2850
Ziac ... 1415

Hydroflumethiazide (Concurrent use is not recommended). Products include:
Diucardin Tablets ... 2718

Imipramine Hydrochloride (Concurrent use is not recommended). Products include:
Tofranil Ampuls ... 854
Tofranil Tablets ... 856

Imipramine Pamoate (Concurrent use is not recommended). Products include:
Tofranil-PM Capsules ... 857

Indapamide (Concurrent use is not recommended). Products include:
Lozol Tablets ... 2022

IMPORTANT NOTE: Always consult each drug listing in the patient's regimen for possible interactions.

Bronkaid Caplets — **Interactions Index** — **142**

Isocarboxazid (Concurrent use is not recommended).
- No products indexed under this heading.

Isradipine (Concurrent use is not recommended). Products include:
- DynaCirc Capsules ... 2256

Labetalol Hydrochloride (Concurrent use is not recommended). Products include:
- Normodyne Injection ... 2377
- Normodyne Tablets ... 2379
- Trandate ... 1185

Lisinopril (Concurrent use is not recommended). Products include:
- Prinivil Tablets ... 1733
- Prinzide Tablets ... 1737
- Zestoretic ... 2850
- Zestril Tablets ... 2854

Losartan Potassium (Concurrent use is not recommended). Products include:
- Cozaar Tablets ... 1628
- Hyzaar Tablets ... 1677

Maprotiline Hydrochloride (Concurrent use is not recommended). Products include:
- Ludiomil Tablets ... 843

Mecamylamine Hydrochloride (Concurrent use is not recommended). Products include:
- Inversine Tablets ... 1686

Methyclothiazide (Concurrent use is not recommended). Products include:
- Enduron Tablets ... 420

Methyldopa (Concurrent use is not recommended). Products include:
- Aldoclor Tablets ... 1598
- Aldomet Oral ... 1600
- Aldoril Tablets ... 1604

Methyldopate Hydrochloride (Concurrent use is not recommended). Products include:
- Aldomet Ester HCl Injection ... 1602

Metolazone (Concurrent use is not recommended). Products include:
- Mykrox Tablets ... 993
- Zaroxolyn Tablets ... 1000

Metoprolol Succinate (Concurrent use is not recommended). Products include:
- Toprol-XL Tablets ... 565

Metoprolol Tartrate (Concurrent use is not recommended). Products include:
- Lopressor Ampuls ... 830
- Lopressor HCT Tablets ... 832
- Lopressor Tablets ... 830

Metyrosine (Concurrent use is not recommended). Products include:
- Demser Capsules ... 1649

Minoxidil (Concurrent use is not recommended). Products include:
- Loniten Tablets ... 2618
- Rogaine Topical Solution ... 2637

Moexipril Hydrochloride (Concurrent use is not recommended). Products include:
- Univasc Tablets ... 2410

Nadolol (Concurrent use is not recommended).
- No products indexed under this heading.

Nefazodone Hydrochloride (Concurrent use is not recommended). Products include:
- Serzone Tablets ... 771

Nicardipine Hydrochloride (Concurrent use is not recommended). Products include:
- Cardene Capsules ... 2095
- Cardene I.V. ... 2709
- Cardene SR Capsules ... 2097

Nifedipine (Concurrent use is not recommended). Products include:
- Adalat Capsules (10 mg and 20 mg) ... 587
- Adalat CC ... 589
- Procardia Capsules ... 1971
- Procardia XL Extended Release Tablets ... 1972

Nisoldipine (Concurrent use is not recommended).
- No products indexed under this heading.

Nitroglycerin (Concurrent use is not recommended). Products include:
- Deponit NTG Transdermal Delivery System ... 2397
- Nitro-Bid IV ... 1523
- Nitro-Bid Ointment ... 1524
- Nitrodisc ... 2047
- Nitro-Dur (nitroglycerin) Transdermal Infusion System ... 1326
- Nitrolingual Spray ... 2027
- Nitrostat Tablets ... 1925
- Transderm-Nitro Transdermal Therapeutic System ... 859

Nortriptyline Hydrochloride (Concurrent use is not recommended). Products include:
- Pamelor ... 2280

Paroxetine Hydrochloride (Concurrent use is not recommended). Products include:
- Paxil Tablets ... 2505

Penbutolol Sulfate (Concurrent use is not recommended). Products include:
- Levatol ... 2403

Phenelzine Sulfate (Concurrent use is not recommended). Products include:
- Nardil ... 1920

Phenoxybenzamine Hydrochloride (Concurrent use is not recommended). Products include:
- Dibenzyline Capsules ... 2476

Phentolamine Mesylate (Concurrent use is not recommended). Products include:
- Regitine ... 846

Pindolol (Concurrent use is not recommended). Products include:
- Visken Tablets ... 2299

Polythiazide (Concurrent use is not recommended). Products include:
- Minizide Capsules ... 1938

Prazosin Hydrochloride (Concurrent use is not recommended). Products include:
- Minipress Capsules ... 1937
- Minizide Capsules ... 1938

Propranolol Hydrochloride (Concurrent use is not recommended). Products include:
- Inderal ... 2728
- Inderal LA Long Acting Capsules ... 2730
- Inderide Tablets ... 2732
- Inderide LA Long Acting Capsules .. 2734

Protriptyline Hydrochloride (Concurrent use is not recommended). Products include:
- Vivactil Tablets ... 1774

Quinapril Hydrochloride (Concurrent use is not recommended). Products include:
- Accupril Tablets ... 1893

Ramipril (Concurrent use is not recommended). Products include:
- Altace Capsules ... 1232

Rauwolfia Serpentina (Concurrent use is not recommended).
- No products indexed under this heading.

Rescinnamine (Concurrent use is not recommended).
- No products indexed under this heading.

Reserpine (Concurrent use is not recommended). Products include:
- Diupres Tablets ... 1650
- Hydropres Tablets ... 1675
- Ser-Ap-Es Tablets ... 849

Selegiline Hydrochloride (Concurrent use is not recommended). Products include:
- Eldepryl Tablets ... 2550

Sertraline Hydrochloride (Concurrent use is not recommended). Products include:
- Zoloft Tablets ... 2217

Sodium Nitroprusside (Concurrent use is not recommended).
- No products indexed under this heading.

Sotalol Hydrochloride (Concurrent use is not recommended). Products include:
- Betapace Tablets ... 641

Spirapril Hydrochloride (Concurrent use is not recommended).
- No products indexed under this heading.

Terazosin Hydrochloride (Concurrent use is not recommended). Products include:
- Hytrin Capsules ... 430

Timolol Maleate (Concurrent use is not recommended). Products include:
- Blocadren Tablets ... 1614
- Timolide Tablets ... 1748
- Timoptic in Ocudose ... 1753
- Timoptic Sterile Ophthalmic Solution ... 1751
- Timoptic-XE ... 1755

Torsemide (Concurrent use is not recommended). Products include:
- Demadex Tablets and Injection ... 686

Tranylcypromine Sulfate (Concurrent use is not recommended). Products include:
- Parnate Tablets ... 2503

Trazodone Hydrochloride (Concurrent use is not recommended). Products include:
- Desyrel and Desyrel Dividose ... 503

Trimethaphan Camsylate (Concurrent use is not recommended). Products include:
- Arfonad Ampuls ... 2080

Trimipramine Maleate (Concurrent use is not recommended). Products include:
- Surmontil Capsules ... 2811

Venlafaxine Hydrochloride (Concurrent use is not recommended). Products include:
- Effexor ... 2719

Verapamil Hydrochloride (Concurrent use is not recommended). Products include:
- Calan SR Caplets ... 2422
- Calan Tablets ... 2419
- Isoptin Injectable ... 1344
- Isoptin Oral Tablets ... 1346
- Isoptin SR Tablets ... 1348
- Verelan Capsules ... 1410
- Verelan Capsules ... 2824

BRONKOMETER AEROSOL

(Isoetharine) ... 2302
See **Bronkosol Solution**

BRONKOSOL SOLUTION

(Isoetharine) ... 2302
May interact with sympathomimetics. Compounds in this category include:

Albuterol (May cause excessive tachycardia due to direct cardiac stimulation). Products include:
- Proventil Inhalation Aerosol ... 2382
- Ventolin Inhalation Aerosol and Refill ... 1197

Albuterol Sulfate (May cause excessive tachycardia due to direct cardiac stimulation). Products include:
- Airet Solution for Inhalation ... 452
- Proventil Inhalation Solution 0.083% ... 2384
- Proventil Repetabs Tablets ... 2386
- Proventil Solution for Inhalation 0.5% ... 2383
- Proventil Syrup ... 2385
- Proventil Tablets ... 2386
- Ventolin Inhalation Solution ... 1198
- Ventolin Nebules Inhalation Solution ... 1199
- Ventolin Rotacaps for Inhalation ... 1200
- Ventolin Syrup ... 1202
- Ventolin Tablets ... 1203
- Volmax Extended-Release Tablets .. 1788

Dobutamine Hydrochloride (May cause excessive tachycardia due to direct cardiac stimulation). Products include:
- Dobutrex Solution Vials ... 1439

Dopamine Hydrochloride (May cause excessive tachycardia due to direct cardiac stimulation).
- No products indexed under this heading.

Ephedrine Hydrochloride (May cause excessive tachycardia due to direct cardiac stimulation). Products include:
- Primatene Dual Action Formula ... ▣ 872
- Primatene Tablets ... ▣ 873
- Quadrinal Tablets ... 1350

Ephedrine Sulfate (May cause excessive tachycardia due to direct cardiac stimulation). Products include:
- Bronkaid Caplets ... ▣ 717
- Marax Tablets & DF Syrup ... 2200

Ephedrine Tannate (May cause excessive tachycardia due to direct cardiac stimulation). Products include:
- Rynatuss ... 2673

Epinephrine (May cause excessive tachycardia due to direct cardiac stimulation). Products include:
- Bronkaid Mist ... ▣ 717
- EPIFRIN ... ◉ 239
- EpiPen ... 790
- Marcaine Hydrochloride with Epinephrine 1:200,000 ... 2316
- Primatene Mist ... ▣ 873
- Sensorcaine with Epinephrine Injection ... 559
- Sus-Phrine Injection ... 1019
- Xylocaine with Epinephrine Injections ... 567

Epinephrine Bitartrate (May cause excessive tachycardia due to direct cardiac stimulation). Products include:
- Bronkaid Mist Suspension ... ▣ 718
- Sensorcaine-MPF with Epinephrine Injection ... 559

Epinephrine Hydrochloride (May cause excessive tachycardia due to direct cardiac stimulation). Products include:
- Ana-Kit Anaphylaxis Emergency Treatment Kit ... 617

Isoproterenol Hydrochloride (May cause excessive tachycardia due to direct cardiac stimulation). Products include:
- Isuprel Hydrochloride Injection 1:5000 ... 2311
- Isuprel Hydrochloride Solution 1:200 & 1:100 ... 2313
- Isuprel Mistometer ... 2312

Isoproterenol Sulfate (May cause excessive tachycardia due to direct cardiac stimulation). Products include:
- Norisodrine with Calcium Iodide Syrup ... 442

Metaproterenol Sulfate (May cause excessive tachycardia due to direct cardiac stimulation). Products include:
- Alupent ... 669
- Metaproterenol Sulfate Inhalation Solution, USP, Arm-a-Med ... 552

Interactions Index

Bronkosol

Metaraminol Bitartrate (May cause excessive tachycardia due to direct cardiac stimulation). Products include:

Aramine Injection................................. 1609

Methoxamine Hydrochloride (May cause excessive tachycardia due to direct cardiac stimulation). Products include:

Vasoxyl Injection 1196

Norepinephrine Bitartrate (May cause excessive tachycardia due to direct cardiac stimulation). Products include:

Levophed Bitartrate Injection 2315

Phenylephrine Bitartrate (May cause excessive tachycardia due to direct cardiac stimulation).

No products indexed under this heading.

Phenylephrine Hydrochloride (May cause excessive tachycardia due to direct cardiac stimulation). Products include:

Atrohist Plus Tablets 454
Cerose DM .... ⊞ 878
Comhist 2038
D.A. Chewable Tablets......................... 951
Deconsal Pediatric Capsules............... 454
Dura-Vent/DA Tablets 953
Entex Capsules 1986
Entex Liquid 1986
Extendryl 1005
4-Way Fast Acting Nasal Spray (regular & mentholated) .... ⊞ 621
Hemorid For Women .... ⊞ 834
Hycomine Compound Tablets 932
Neo-Synephrine Hydrochloride 1%
Carpuject... 2324
Neo-Synephrine Hydrochloride 1%
Injection 2324
Neo-Synephrine Hydrochloride (Ophthalmic) 2325
Neo-Synephrine .... ⊞ 726
Nöstril... ⊞ 644
Novahistine Elixir .... ⊞ 823
Phenergan VC 2779
Phenergan VC with Codeine 2781
Preparation H .... ⊞ 871
Tympagesic Ear Drops 2342
Vasosulf .... © 271
Vicks Sinex Nasal Spray and Ultra
Fine Mist .... ⊞ 765

Phenylephrine Tannate (May cause excessive tachycardia due to direct cardiac stimulation). Products include:

Atrohist Pediatric Suspension 454
Ricobid-D Pediatric Suspension........ 2038
Ricobid Tablets and Pediatric Suspension... 2038
Rynatan 2673
Rynatuss 2673

Phenylpropanolamine Hydrochloride (May cause excessive tachycardia due to direct cardiac stimulation). Products include:

Acutrim .... ⊞ 628
Allerest Children's Chewable Tablets .... ⊞ 627
Allerest 12 Hour Caplets .... ⊞ 627
Atrohist Plus Tablets 454
BC Cold Powder Multi-Symptom
Formula (Cold-Sinus-Allergy) ...... ⊞ 609
BC Cold Powder Non-Drowsy
Formula (Cold-Sinus)...................... ⊞ 609
Cheracol Plus Head Cold/Cough
Formula .... ⊞ 769
Comtrex Multi-Symptom Non-Drowsy Liqui-gels............................... ⊞ 618
Contac Continuous Action Nasal
Decongestant/Antihistamine 12
Hour Capsules.................................... ⊞ 813
Contac Maximum Strength Continuous Action Decongestant/
Antihistamine 12 Hour Caplets.. ⊞ 813
Contac Severe Cold and Flu Formula Caplets .... ⊞ 814
Coricidin 'D' Decongestant Tablets .... ⊞ 800
Dexatrim .... ⊞ 832
Dexatrim Plus Vitamins Caplets .... ⊞ 832
Dimetane-DC Cough Syrup 2059
Dimetapp Elixir .... ⊞ 773
Dimetapp Extentabs .... ⊞ 774

Dimetapp Tablets/Liqui-Gels .... ⊞ 775
Dimetapp Cold & Allergy Chewable Tablets .... ⊞ 773
Dimetapp DM Elixir .... ⊞ 774
Dura-Vent Tablets 952
Entex Capsules 1986
Entex LA Tablets 1987
Entex Liquid 1986
Exgest LA Tablets 782
Hycomine 931
Isoclor Timesule Capsules .... ⊞ 637
Nolamine Timed-Release Tablets 785
Ornade Spansule Capsules 2502
Propagest Tablets 786
Pyrroxate Caplets .... ⊞ 772
Robitussin-CF .... ⊞ 777
Sinulin Tablets 787
Tavist-D 12 Hour Relief Tablets .... ⊞ 787
Teldrin 12 Hour Antihistamine/
Nasal Decongestant Allergy
Relief Capsules .... ⊞ 826
Triaminic Allergy Tablets .... ⊞ 789
Triaminic Cold Tablets .... ⊞ 790
Triaminic Expectorant .... ⊞ 790
Triaminic Syrup .... ⊞ 792
Triaminic-12 Tablets .... ⊞ 792
Triaminic-DM Syrup .... ⊞ 792
Triaminicin Tablets .... ⊞ 793
Triaminicol Multi-Symptom Cold
Tablets .... ⊞ 793
Triaminicol Multi-Symptom Relief ⊞ 794
Vicks DayQuil Allergy Relief 12-
Hour Extended Release Tablets.. ⊞ 760
Vicks DayQuil Allergy Relief 4-
Hour Tablets .... ⊞ 760
Vicks DayQuil SINUS Pressure &
CONGESTION Relief......................... ⊞ 761

Pirbuterol Acetate (May cause excessive tachycardia due to direct cardiac stimulation). Products include:

Maxair Autohaler 1492
Maxair Inhaler 1494

Pseudoephedrine Hydrochloride (May cause excessive tachycardia due to direct cardiac stimulation). Products include:

Actifed Allergy Daytime/Nighttime Caplets.. ⊞ 844
Actifed Plus Caplets .... ⊞ 845
Actifed Plus Tablets .... ⊞ 845
Actifed with Codeine Cough Syrup.. 1067
Actifed Sinus Daytime/Nighttime
Tablets and Caplets .... ⊞ 846
Actifed Syrup... ⊞ 846
Actifed Tablets .... ⊞ 844
Advil Cold and Sinus Caplets and
Tablets (formerly CoAdvil) .... ⊞ 870
Alka-Seltzer Plus Cold Medicine
Liqui-Gels .... ⊞ 706
Alka-Seltzer Plus Cold & Cough
Medicine Liqui-Gels.......................... ⊞ 705
Alka-Seltzer Plus Night-Time Cold
Medicine Liqui-Gels........................ ⊞ 706
Allerest Headache Strength Tablets .... ⊞ 627
Allerest Maximum Strength Tablets .... ⊞ 627
Allerest No Drowsiness Tablets........ ⊞ 627
Allerest Sinus Pain Formula .... ⊞ 627
Anatuss LA Tablets............................... 1542
Atrohist Pediatric Capsules................ 453
Bayer Select Sinus Pain Relief
Formula .... ⊞ 717
Benadryl Allergy Decongestant
Liquid Medication .... ⊞ 848
Benadryl Allergy Decongestant
Tablets .... ⊞ 848
Benadryl Allergy Sinus Headache
Formula Caplets .... ⊞ 849
Benylin Multisymptom .... ⊞ 852
Bromfed Capsules (Extended-Release) 1785
Bromfed Syrup .... ⊞ 733
Bromfed Tablets 1785
Bromfed-DM Cough Syrup................. 1786
Bromfed-PD Capsules (Extended-Release).. 1785
Children's Vicks DayQuil Allergy
Relief.. ⊞ 757
Children's Vicks NyQuil Cold/
Cough Relief.. ⊞ 758
Comtrex Multi-Symptom Cold
Reliever Tablets/Caplets/Liqui-Gels/Liquid.. ⊞ 615
Allergy-Sinus Comtrex Multi-Symptom Allergy-Sinus Formula
Tablets .... ⊞ 617

Comtrex Multi-Symptom Non-Drowsy Caplets.................................... ⊞ 618
Congess 1004
Contac Day Allergy/Sinus Caplets ⊞ 812
Contac Day & Night .... ⊞ 812
Contac Night Allergy/Sinus Caplets .... ⊞ 812
Contac Severe Cold & Flu Non-Drowsy .... ⊞ 815
Deconamine Chewable Tablets 1320
Deconamine CX Cough and Cold
Liquid and Tablets.............................. 1319
Deconamine 1320
Deconsal C Expectorant Syrup 456
Deconsal Pediatric Syrup 457
Deconsal II Tablets 454
Dimetane-DX Cough Syrup 2059
Dimetapp Sinus Caplets .... ⊞ 775
Dorcol Children's Cough Syrup...... ⊞ 785
Drixoral Cough + Congestion
Liquid Caps .... ⊞ 802
Dura-Tap/PD Capsules 2867
Duratuss Tablets 2565
Duratuss HD Elixir................................ 2565
Efidac/24 .... ⊞ 635
Entex PSE Tablets 1987
Fedahist Gyrocaps................................ 2401
Fedahist Timecaps 2401
Guaifed.. 1787
Guaifed Syrup .... ⊞ 734
Guaimax-D Tablets 792
Guaitab Tablets .... ⊞ 734
Isoclor Expectorant 990
Kronofed-A 977
Motrin IB Sinus..................................... ⊞ 838
Novahistine DH..................................... 2462
Novahistine DMX .... ⊞ 822
Novahistine Expectorant..................... 2463
Nucofed 2051
PediaCare Cold Allergy Chewable
Tablets .... ⊞ 677
PediaCare Cough-Cold Chewable
Tablets 1553
PediaCare 1553
PediaCare Infants' Decongestant
Drops .... ⊞ 677
PediCare Infant's Drops Decongestant Plus Cough 1553
PediaCare NightRest Cough-Cold
Liquid 1553
Pediatric Vicks 44d Dry Hacking
Cough & Head Congestion............ ⊞ 763
Pediatric Vicks 44m Cough &
Cold Relief .... ⊞ 764
Robitussin Cold & Cough Liqui-Gels .... ⊞ 776
Robitussin Maximum Strength
Cough & Cold .... ⊞ 778
Robitussin Pediatric Cough &
Cold Formula....................................... ⊞ 779
Robitussin Severe Congestion
Liqui-Gels .... ⊞ 776
Robitussin-DAC Syrup 2074
Robitussin-PE .... ⊞ 778
Rondec Oral Drops 953
Rondec Syrup 953
Rondec Tablet 953
Rondec-DM Oral Drops 954
Rondec-DM Syrup 954
Rondec-TR Tablet 953
Ryna .... ⊞ 841
Seldane-D Extended-Release Tablets 1538
Semprex-D Capsules 463
Semprex-D Capsules 1167
Sinarest Tablets .... ⊞ 648
Sinarest Extra Strength Tablets....... ⊞ 648
Sinarest No Drowsiness Tablets .... ⊞ 648
Sine-Aid IB Caplets 1554
Sine-Aid Maximum Strength Sinus
Medication Gelcaps, Caplets and
Tablets 1554
Sine-Off No Drowsiness Formula
Caplets .... ⊞ 824
Sine-Off Sinus Medicine .... ⊞ 825
Singlet Tablets .... ⊞ 825
Sinutab Non-Drying Liquid Caps .... ⊞ 859
Sinutab Sinus Allergy Medication,
Maximum Strength Tablets and
Caplets .... ⊞ 860
Sinutab Sinus Medication, Maximum Strength Without Drowsiness Formula, Tablets & Caplets .... ⊞ 860
Sinutab Sinus Medication, Regular
Strength Without Drowsiness
Formula .... ⊞ 859
Sudafed Children's Liquid .... ⊞ 861
Sudafed Cold and Cough Liquidcaps .... ⊞ 862
Sudafed Cough Syrup .... ⊞ 862

Sudafed Plus Liquid .... ⊞ 862
Sudafed Plus Tablets............................ ⊞ 863
Sudafed Severe Cold Formula
Caplets .... ⊞ 863
Sudafed Severe Cold Formula
Tablets .... ⊞ 864
Sudafed Sinus Caplets......................... ⊞ 864
Sudafed Sinus Tablets.......................... ⊞ 864
Sudafed Tablets, 30 mg....................... ⊞ 861
Sudafed Tablets, 60 mg....................... ⊞ 861
Sudafed 12 Hour Caplets .... ⊞ 861
Syn-Rx Tablets 465
Syn-Rx DM Tablets 466
TheraFlu.. ⊞ 787
TheraFlu Maximum Strength
Nighttime Flu, Cold & Cough
Medicine .... ⊞ 788
TheraFlu Maximum Strength Non-Drowsy Formula Flu, Cold &
Cough Medicine .... ⊞ 788
Thera Flu Maximum Strength,
Non-Drowsy Formula Flu, Cold
and Cough Caplets .... ⊞ 789
Triaminic AM Cough and Decongestant Formula .... ⊞ 789
Triaminic AM Decongestant Formula .... ⊞ 790
Triaminic Nite Light .... ⊞ 791
Triaminic Sore Throat Formula ...... ⊞ 791
Tussend 1783
Tussend Expectorant 1785
Children's TYLENOL Cold Multi-Symptom Liquid Formula and
Chewable Tablets................................ 1561
Children's TYLENOL Cold Plus
Cough Multi Symptom Tablets
and Liquid... ⊞ 681
Infants' TYLENOL Cold Decongestant & Fever-Reducer Drops 1556
TYLENOL Maximum Strength Allergy Sinus Medication Gelcaps
and Caplets 1563
TYLENOL Maximum Strength Allergy Sinus NightTime Medication Caplets 1555
TYLENOL Flu Maximum Strength
Gelcaps 1565
TYLENOL Flu NightTime, Maximum Strength, Gelcaps 1566
TYLENOL Maximum Strength Flu
NightTime Hot Medication Packets 1562
TYLENOL, Maximum Strength,
Sinus Medication Geltabs, Gelcaps, Caplets and Tablets 1566
TYLENOL Cold Multi-Symptom
Formula Medication Tablets and
Caplets 1561
TYLENOL Cold Medication No
Drowsiness Formula Gelcaps and
Caplets 1562
TYLENOL Cold Multi-Symptom Hot
Medication Liquid Packets............... 1557
TYLENOL Cough Multi-Symptom
Medication with Decongestant 1565
Ursinus Inlay-Tabs................................ ⊞ 794
Vicks 44 LiquiCaps Cough, Cold
& Flu Relief.. ⊞ 755
Vicks 44 LiquiCaps Non-Drowsy
Cough & Cold Relief .... ⊞ 756
Vicks 44D Dry Hacking Cough &
Head Congestion................................ ⊞ 755
Vicks 44M Cough, Cold & Flu
Relief .... ⊞ 756
Vicks DayQuil .... ⊞ 761
Vicks DayQuil SINUS Pressure &
PAIN Relief with IBUPROFEN ...... ⊞ 762
Vicks Nyquil Hot Therapy.................... ⊞ 762
Vicks NyQuil LiquiCaps Multi-Symptom Cold/Flu Relief .... ⊞ 763
Vicks NyQuil Multi-Symptom
Cold/Flu Relief - (Original &
Cherry Flavor)..................................... ⊞ 763

Pseudoephedrine Sulfate (May cause excessive tachycardia due to direct cardiac stimulation). Products include:

Cheracol Sinus .... ⊞ 768
Chlor-Trimeton Allergy Decongestant Tablets .... ⊞ 799
Claritin-D 2350
Drixoral Cold and Allergy Sustained-Action Tablets .... ⊞ 802
Drixoral Cold and Flu Extended-Release Tablets..................................... ⊞ 803
Drixoral Non-Drowsy Formula
Extended-Release Tablets .... ⊞ 803
Drixoral Allergy/Sinus Extended
Release Tablets................................... ⊞ 804
Trinalin Repetabs Tablets 1330

IMPORTANT NOTE: Always consult each drug listing in the patient's regimen for possible interactions.

Bronkosol Interactions Index 144

Salmeterol Xinafoate (May cause excessive tachycardia due to direct cardiac stimulation). Products include:
- Serevent Inhalation Aerosol ... 1176

Terbutaline Sulfate (May cause excessive tachycardia due to direct cardiac stimulation). Products include:
- Brethaire Inhaler ... 813
- Brethine Ampuls ... 815
- Brethine Tablets ... 814
- Bricanyl Subcutaneous Injection ... 1502
- Bricanyl Tablets ... 1503

BRONTEX
(Codeine Phosphate, Guaifenesin) ... 1981
May interact with central nervous system depressants, hypnotics and sedatives, tranquilizers, antidepressant drugs, narcotic analgesics, and certain other agents. Compounds in these categories include:

Alfentanil Hydrochloride (Potential for greater sedation). Products include:
- Alfenta Injection ... 1286

Alprazolam (Potential for greater sedation). Products include:
- Xanax Tablets ... 2649

Amitriptyline Hydrochloride (Potential for greater sedation). Products include:
- Elavil ... 2838
- Endep Tablets ... 2174
- Etrafon ... 2355
- Limbitrol ... 2180
- Triavil Tablets ... 1757

Amoxapine (Potential for greater sedation). Products include:
- Asendin Tablets ... 1369

Aprobarbital (Potential for greater sedation).
- No products indexed under this heading.

Buprenorphine (Potential for greater sedation). Products include:
- Buprenex Injectable ... 2006

Bupropion Hydrochloride (Potential for greater sedation). Products include:
- Wellbutrin Tablets ... 1204

Buspirone Hydrochloride (Potential for greater sedation). Products include:
- BuSpar ... 737

Butabarbital (Potential for greater sedation).
- No products indexed under this heading.

Butalbital (Potential for greater sedation). Products include:
- Esgic-plus Tablets ... 1013
- Fioricet Tablets ... 2258
- Fioricet with Codeine Capsules ... 2260
- Fiorinal Capsules ... 2261
- Fiorinal with Codeine Capsules ... 2262
- Fiorinal Tablets ... 2261
- Phrenilin ... 785
- Sedapap Tablets 50 mg/650 mg .. 1543

Chlordiazepoxide (Potential for greater sedation). Products include:
- Libritabs Tablets ... 2177
- Limbitrol ... 2180

Chlordiazepoxide Hydrochloride (Potential for greater sedation). Products include:
- Librax Capsules ... 2176
- Librium Capsules ... 2178
- Librium Injectable ... 2179

Chlorpromazine (Potential for greater sedation). Products include:
- Thorazine Suppositories ... 2523

Chlorpromazine Hydrochloride (Potential for greater sedation). Products include:
- Thorazine ... 2523

Chlorprothixene (Potential for greater sedation).
- No products indexed under this heading.

Chlorprothixene Hydrochloride (Potential for greater sedation).
- No products indexed under this heading.

Clorazepate Dipotassium (Potential for greater sedation). Products include:
- Tranxene ... 451

Clozapine (Potential for greater sedation). Products include:
- Clozaril Tablets ... 2252

Desflurane (Potential for greater sedation). Products include:
- Suprane ... 1813

Desipramine Hydrochloride (Potential for greater sedation). Products include:
- Norpramin Tablets ... 1526

Dezocine (Potential for greater sedation). Products include:
- Dalgan Injection ... 538

Diazepam (Potential for greater sedation). Products include:
- Dizac ... 1809
- Valium Injectable ... 2182
- Valium Tablets ... 2183
- Valrelease Capsules ... 2169

Doxepin Hydrochloride (Potential for greater sedation). Products include:
- Sinequan ... 2205
- Zonalon Cream ... 1055

Droperidol (Potential for greater sedation). Products include:
- Inapsine Injection ... 1296

Enflurane (Potential for greater sedation).
- No products indexed under this heading.

Estazolam (Potential for greater sedation). Products include:
- ProSom Tablets ... 449

Ethchlorvynol (Potential for greater sedation). Products include:
- Placidyl Capsules ... 448

Ethinamate (Potential for greater sedation).
- No products indexed under this heading.

Fentanyl (Potential for greater sedation). Products include:
- Duragesic Transdermal System ... 1288

Fentanyl Citrate (Potential for greater sedation). Products include:
- Sublimaze Injection ... 1307

Fluoxetine Hydrochloride (Potential for greater sedation). Products include:
- Prozac Pulvules & Liquid, Oral Solution ... 919

Fluphenazine Decanoate (Potential for greater sedation). Products include:
- Prolixin Decanoate ... 509

Fluphenazine Enanthate (Potential for greater sedation). Products include:
- Prolixin Enanthate ... 509

Fluphenazine Hydrochloride (Potential for greater sedation). Products include:
- Prolixin ... 509

Flurazepam Hydrochloride (Potential for greater sedation). Products include:
- Dalmane Capsules ... 2173

Glutethimide (Potential for greater sedation).
- No products indexed under this heading.

Haloperidol (Potential for greater sedation). Products include:
- Haldol Injection, Tablets and Concentrate ... 1575

Haloperidol Decanoate (Potential for greater sedation). Products include:
- Haldol Decanoate ... 1577

Hydrocodone Bitartrate (Potential for greater sedation). Products include:
- Anexsia 5/500 Elixir ... 1781
- Anexia Tablets ... 1782
- Codiclear DH Syrup ... 791
- Deconamine CX Cough and Cold Liquid and Tablets ... 1319
- Duratuss HD Elixir ... 2565
- Hycodan Tablets and Syrup ... 930
- Hycomine Compound Tablets ... 932
- Hycomine ... 931
- Hycotuss Expectorant Syrup ... 933
- Hydrocet Capsules ... 782
- Lorcet 10/650 ... 1018
- Lortab ... 2566
- Tussend ... 1783
- Tussend Expectorant ... 1785
- Vicodin Tablets ... 1356
- Vicodin ES Tablets ... 1357
- Vicodin Tuss Expectorant ... 1358
- Zydone Capsules ... 949

Hydrocodone Polistirex (Potential for greater sedation). Products include:
- Tussionex Pennkinetic Extended-Release Suspension ... 998

Hydroxyzine Hydrochloride (Potential for greater sedation). Products include:
- Atarax Tablets & Syrup ... 2185
- Marax Tablets & DF Syrup ... 2200
- Vistaril Intramuscular Solution ... 2216

Imipramine Hydrochloride (Potential for greater sedation). Products include:
- Tofranil Ampuls ... 854
- Tofranil Tablets ... 856

Imipramine Pamoate (Potential for greater sedation). Products include:
- Tofranil-PM Capsules ... 857

Isocarboxazid (Potential for greater sedation).
- No products indexed under this heading.

Isoflurane (Potential for greater sedation).
- No products indexed under this heading.

Ketamine Hydrochloride (Potential for greater sedation).
- No products indexed under this heading.

Levomethadyl Acetate Hydrochloride (Potential for greater sedation). Products include:
- Orlamm ... 2239

Levorphanol Tartrate (Potential for greater sedation). Products include:
- Levo-Dromoran ... 2129

Lorazepam (Potential for greater sedation). Products include:
- Ativan Injection ... 2698
- Ativan Tablets ... 2700

Loxapine Hydrochloride (Potential for greater sedation). Products include:
- Loxitane ... 1378

Loxapine Succinate (Potential for greater sedation). Products include:
- Loxitane Capsules ... 1378

Maprotiline Hydrochloride (Potential for greater sedation). Products include:
- Ludiomil Tablets ... 843

Meperidine Hydrochloride (Potential for greater sedation). Products include:
- Demerol ... 2308
- Mepergan Injection ... 2753

Mephobarbital (Potential for greater sedation). Products include:
- Mebaral Tablets ... 2322

Meprobamate (Potential for greater sedation). Products include:
- Miltown Tablets ... 2672
- PMB 200 and PMB 400 ... 2783

Mesoridazine Besylate (Potential for greater sedation). Products include:
- Serentil ... 684

Methadone Hydrochloride (Potential for greater sedation). Products include:
- Methadone Hydrochloride Oral Concentrate ... 2233
- Methadone Hydrochloride Oral Solution & Tablets ... 2235

Methohexital Sodium (Potential for greater sedation). Products include:
- Brevital Sodium Vials ... 1429

Methotrimeprazine (Potential for greater sedation). Products include:
- Levoprome ... 1274

Methoxyflurane (Potential for greater sedation).
- No products indexed under this heading.

Midazolam Hydrochloride (Potential for greater sedation). Products include:
- Versed Injection ... 2170

Molindone Hydrochloride (Potential for greater sedation). Products include:
- Moban Tablets and Concentrate ... 1048

Morphine Sulfate (Potential for greater sedation). Products include:
- Astramorph/PF Injection, USP (Preservative-Free) ... 535
- Duramorph ... 962
- Infumorph 200 and Infumorph 500 Sterile Solutions ... 965
- MS Contin Tablets ... 1994
- MSIR ... 1997
- Oramorph SR (Morphine Sulfate Sustained Release Tablets) ... 2236
- RMS Suppositories ... 2657
- Roxanol ... 2243

Nefazodone Hydrochloride (Potential for greater sedation). Products include:
- Serzone Tablets ... 771

Nortriptyline Hydrochloride (Potential for greater sedation). Products include:
- Pamelor ... 2280

Opium Alkaloids (Potential for greater sedation).
- No products indexed under this heading.

Oxazepam (Potential for greater sedation). Products include:
- Serax Capsules ... 2810
- Serax Tablets ... 2810

Oxycodone Hydrochloride (Potential for greater sedation). Products include:
- Percocet Tablets ... 938
- Percodan Tablets ... 939
- Percodan-Demi Tablets ... 940
- Roxicodone Tablets, Oral Solution & Intensol (Oxycodone) ... 2244
- Tylox Capsules ... 1584

Paroxetine Hydrochloride (Potential for greater sedation). Products include:
- Paxil Tablets ... 2505

Pentobarbital Sodium (Potential for greater sedation). Products include:
- Nembutal Sodium Capsules ... 436
- Nembutal Sodium Solution ... 438
- Nembutal Sodium Suppositories ... 440

Perphenazine (Potential for greater sedation). Products include:
- Etrafon ... 2355
- Triavil Tablets ... 1757
- Trilafon ... 2389

(▣ Described in PDR For Nonprescription Drugs) (◉ Described in PDR For Ophthalmology)

Phenelzine Sulfate (Potential for greater sedation). Products include:

Nardil 1920

Phenobarbital (Potential for greater sedation). Products include:

Arco-Lase Plus Tablets 512
Bellergal-S Tablets 2250
Donnatal 2060
Donnatal Extentabs.............................. 2061
Donnatal Tablets 2060
Phenobarbital Elixir and Tablets 1469
Quadrinal Tablets 1350

Prazepam (Potential for greater sedation).

No products indexed under this heading.

Prochlorperazine (Potential for greater sedation). Products include:

Compazine 2470

Promethazine Hydrochloride (Potential for greater sedation). Products include:

Mepergan Injection 2753
Phenergan with Codeine 2777
Phenergan with Dextromethorphan 2778
Phenergan Injection 2773
Phenergan Suppositories 2775
Phenergan Syrup 2774
Phenergan Tablets 2775
Phenergan VC 2779
Phenergan VC with Codeine 2781

Propofol (Potential for greater sedation). Products include:

Diprivan Injection................................. 2833

Propoxyphene Hydrochloride (Potential for greater sedation). Products include:

Darvon 1435
Wygesic Tablets 2827

Propoxyphene Napsylate (Potential for greater sedation). Products include:

Darvon-N/Darvocet-N 1433

Protriptyline Hydrochloride (Potential for greater sedation). Products include:

Vivactil Tablets 1774

Quazepam (Potential for greater sedation). Products include:

Doral Tablets 2664

Risperidone (Potential for greater sedation). Products include:

Risperdal 1301

Secobarbital Sodium (Potential for greater sedation). Products include:

Seconal Sodium Pulvules 1474

Sertraline Hydrochloride (Potential for greater sedation). Products include:

Zoloft Tablets 2217

Sufentanil Citrate (Potential for greater sedation). Products include:

Sufenta Injection 1309

Temazepam (Potential for greater sedation). Products include:

Restoril Capsules 2284

Thiamylal Sodium (Potential for greater sedation).

No products indexed under this heading.

Thioridazine Hydrochloride (Potential for greater sedation). Products include:

Mellaril 2269

Thiothixene (Potential for greater sedation). Products include:

Navane Capsules and Concentrate 2201
Navane Intramuscular 2202

Tranylcypromine Sulfate (Potential for greater sedation). Products include:

Parnate Tablets 2503

Trazodone Hydrochloride (Potential for greater sedation). Products include:

Desyrel and Desyrel Dividose 503

Triazolam (Potential for greater sedation). Products include:

Halcion Tablets..................................... 2611

Trifluoperazine Hydrochloride (Potential for greater sedation). Products include:

Stelazine 2514

Trimipramine Maleate (Potential for greater sedation). Products include:

Surmontil Capsules.............................. 2811

Venlafaxine Hydrochloride (Potential for greater sedation). Products include:

Effexor 2719

Zolpidem Tartrate (Potential for greater sedation). Products include:

Ambien Tablets..................................... 2416

Food Interactions

Alcohol (Potential for greater sedation).

BUCKLEY'S MIXTURE

(Dextromethorphan Hydrobromide) .... ℞ 624

May interact with monoamine oxidase inhibitors. Compounds in this category include:

Furazolidone (Concurrent use not recommended; consult your doctor). Products include:

Furoxone 2046

Isocarboxazid (Concurrent use not recommended; consult your doctor).

No products indexed under this heading.

Phenelzine Sulfate (Concurrent use not recommended; consult your doctor). Products include:

Nardil 1920

Selegiline Hydrochloride (Concurrent use not recommended; consult your doctor). Products include:

Eldepryl Tablets 2550

Tranylcypromine Sulfate (Concurrent use not recommended; consult your doctor). Products include:

Parnate Tablets 2503

BUFFERIN ANALGESIC TABLETS AND CAPLETS

(Aspirin) .... ℞ 613

May interact with:

Aluminum Carbonate Gel (Concurrent administration of nonabsorbable antacids may alter the rate of absorption of aspirin). Products include:

Basaljel... 2703

Aluminum Hydroxide (Concurrent administration of nonabsorbable antacids may alter the rate of absorption of aspirin). Products include:

ALternaGEL Liquid 1316
Maximum Strength Ascriptin .... ℞ 630
Cama Arthritis Pain Reliever............ ℞ 785
Gaviscon Extra Strength Relief Formula Antacid Tablets................. ℞ 819
Gaviscon Extra Strength Relief Formula Liquid Antacid .... ℞ 819
Gaviscon Liquid Antacid .... ℞ 820
Gelusil Liquid & Tablets .... ℞ 855
Maalox Heartburn Relief Suspension .... ℞ 642
Maalox Heartburn Relief Tablets.... ℞ 641
Maalox Magnesia and Alumina Oral Suspension .... ℞ 642
Maalox Plus Tablets .... ℞ 643
Extra Strength Maalox Antacid Plus Antigas Liquid and Tablets ℞ 638
Tempo Soft Antacid .... ℞ 835

Aluminum Hydroxide Gel (Concurrent administration of nonabsorbable antacids may alter the rate of absorption of aspirin). Products include:

ALternaGEL Liquid .... ℞ 659

Aludrox Oral Suspension 2695
Amphojel Suspension 2695
Amphojel Suspension without Flavor 2695
Amphojel Tablets.................................. 2695
Arthritis Pain Ascriptin .... ℞ 631
Regular Strength Ascriptin Tablets .... ℞ 629
Gaviscon Antacid Tablets.................... ℞ 819
Gaviscon-2 Antacid Tablets .... ℞ 820
Mylanta Liquid 1317
Mylanta Tablets .... ℞ 660
Mylanta Double Strength Liquid 1317
Mylanta Double Strength Tablets .. ℞ 660
Nephrox Suspension .... ℞ 655

Antiarthritic Drugs, unspecified (Effect not specified).

Anticoagulant Drugs, unspecified (Effect not specified).

Antidiabetic Drugs, unspecified (Effect not specified).

Antigout Drugs, unspecified (Effect not specified).

Magnesium Hydroxide (Concurrent administration of nonabsorbable antacids may alter the rate of absorption of aspirin). Products include:

Aludrox Oral Suspension 2695
Arthritis Pain Ascriptin .... ℞ 631
Maximum Strength Ascriptin .... ℞ 630
Regular Strength Ascriptin Tablets .... ℞ 629
Di-Gel Antacid/Anti-Gas .... ℞ 801
Gelusil Liquid & Tablets .... ℞ 855
Maalox Magnesia and Alumina Oral Suspension .... ℞ 642
Maalox Plus Tablets .... ℞ 643
Extra Strength Maalox Antacid Plus Antigas Liquid and Tablets ℞ 638
Mylanta Calcium Carbonate and Magnesium Hydroxide Tablets...... 1318
Mylanta Liquid 1317
Mylanta Tablets .... ℞ 660
Mylanta Double Strength Liquid 1317
Mylanta Double Strength Tablets.. ℞ 660
Phillips' Milk of Magnesia Liquid.... ℞ 729
Rolaids Tablets..................................... ℞ 843
Tempo Soft Antacid .... ℞ 835

Magnesium Oxide (Concurrent administration of nonabsorbable antacids may alter the rate of absorption of aspirin). Products include:

Beelith Tablets 639
Bufferin Analgesic Tablets and Caplets .... ℞ 613
Caltrate PLUS .... ℞ 665
Cama Arthritis Pain Reliever............ ℞ 785
Mag-Ox 400 668
Uro-Mag.. 668

Sodium Bicarbonate (Concurrent administration with absorbable antacids may increase the clearance of salicylates). Products include:

Alka-Seltzer Effervescent Antacid and Pain Reliever.............................. ℞ 701
Alka-Seltzer Extra Strength Effervescent Antacid and Pain Reliever .... ℞ 703
Alka-Seltzer Gold Effervescent Antacid... ℞ 703
Alka-Seltzer Lemon Lime Effervescent Antacid and Pain Reliever .... ℞ 703
Arm & Hammer Pure Baking Soda .... ℞ 627
Ceo-Two Rectal Suppositories 666
Citrocarbonate Antacid .... ℞ 770
Massengill Disposable Douches...... ℞ 820
Massengill Liquid Concentrate .... ℞ 820
NuLYTELY... 689
Cherry Flavor NuLYTELY 689

ARTHRITIS STRENGTH BUFFERIN ANALGESIC CAPLETS

(Aspirin) .... ℞ 614

May interact with:

Antiarthritic Drugs, unspecified (Effect not specified).

Anticoagulant Drugs, unspecified (Effect not specified).

Antidiabetic Drugs, unspecified (Effect not specified).

Antigout Drugs, unspecified (Effect not specified).

EXTRA STRENGTH BUFFERIN ANALGESIC TABLETS

(Aspirin) .... ℞ 615

May interact with:

Antiarthritic Drugs, unspecified (Effect not specified).

Anticoagulant Drugs, unspecified (Effect not specified).

Antidiabetic Drugs, unspecified (Effect not specified).

Antigout Drugs, unspecified (Effect not specified).

BUGS BUNNY COMPLETE CHILDREN'S CHEWABLE VITAMINS + MINERALS WITH IRON AND CALCIUM (SUGAR FREE)

(Vitamins with Minerals) .... ℞ 721

None cited in PDR database.

BUGS BUNNY WITH EXTRA C CHILDREN'S CHEWABLE VITAMINS (SUGAR FREE)

(Vitamins with Minerals) .... ℞ 722

None cited in PDR database.

BUGS BUNNY PLUS IRON CHILDREN'S CHEWABLE VITAMINS (SUGAR FREE)

(Vitamins with Iron) .... ℞ 718

None cited in PDR database.

BUMEX INJECTION

(Bumetanide) 2093

May interact with aminoglycosides, lithium preparations, antihypertensives, and certain other agents. Compounds in these categories include:

Acebutolol Hydrochloride (Antihypertensive effect potentiated). Products include:

Sectral Capsules 2807

Amikacin Sulfate (Potential for ototoxicity and/or nephrotoxicity). Products include:

Amikacin Sulfate Injection, USP 960
Amikin Injectable 501

Amlodipine Besylate (Antihypertensive effect potentiated). Products include:

Lotrel Capsules.................................... 840
Norvasc Tablets 1940

Atenolol (Antihypertensive effect potentiated). Products include:

Tenoretic Tablets.................................. 2845
Tenormin Tablets and I.V. Injection 2847

Benazepril Hydrochloride (Antihypertensive effect potentiated). Products include:

Lotensin Tablets................................... 834
Lotensin HCT....................................... 837
Lotrel Capsules.................................... 840

Bendroflumethiazide (Antihypertensive effect potentiated).

No products indexed under this heading.

Betaxolol Hydrochloride (Antihypertensive effect potentiated). Products include:

Betoptic Ophthalmic Solution............ 469
Betoptic S Ophthalmic Suspension 471
Kerlone Tablets.................................... 2436

Bisoprolol Fumarate (Antihypertensive effect potentiated). Products include:

Zebeta Tablets 1413
Ziac 1415

IMPORTANT NOTE: Always consult each drug listing in the patient's regimen for possible interactions.

Bumex Interactions Index 146

Captopril (Antihypertensive effect potentiated). Products include:
Capoten ... 739
Capozide ... 742
Carteolol Hydrochloride (Antihypertensive effect potentiated). Products include:
Cartrol Tablets ... 410
Ocupress Ophthalmic Solution, 1% Sterile ... ◉ 309
Chlorothiazide (Antihypertensive effect potentiated). Products include:
Aldoclor Tablets ... 1598
Diupres Tablets ... 1650
Diuril Oral ... 1653
Chlorothiazide Sodium (Antihypertensive effect potentiated). Products include:
Diuril Sodium Intravenous ... 1652
Chlorthalidone (Antihypertensive effect potentiated). Products include:
Combipres Tablets ... 677
Tenoretic Tablets ... 2845
Thalitone ... 1245
Clonidine (Antihypertensive effect potentiated). Products include:
Catapres-TTS ... 675
Clonidine Hydrochloride (Antihypertensive effect potentiated). Products include:
Catapres Tablets ... 674
Combipres Tablets ... 677
Deserpidine (Antihypertensive effect potentiated).
No products indexed under this heading.
Diazoxide (Antihypertensive effect potentiated). Products include:
Hyperstat I.V. Injection ... 2363
Proglycem ... 580
Diltiazem Hydrochloride (Antihypertensive effect potentiated). Products include:
Cardizem CD Capsules ... 1506
Cardizem SR Capsules ... 1510
Cardizem Injectable ... 1508
Cardizem Tablets ... 1512
Dilacor XR Extended-release Capsules ... 2018
Doxazosin Mesylate (Antihypertensive effect potentiated). Products include:
Cardura Tablets ... 2186
Enalapril Maleate (Antihypertensive effect potentiated). Products include:
Vaseretic Tablets ... 1765
Vasotec Tablets ... 1771
Enalaprilat (Antihypertensive effect potentiated). Products include:
Vasotec I.V. ... 1768
Esmolol Hydrochloride (Antihypertensive effect potentiated). Products include:
Brevibloc Injection ... 1808
Felodipine (Antihypertensive effect potentiated). Products include:
Plendil Extended-Release Tablets ... 527
Fosinopril Sodium (Antihypertensive effect potentiated). Products include:
Monopril Tablets ... 757
Furosemide (Antihypertensive effect potentiated). Products include:
Lasix Injection, Oral Solution and Tablets ... 1240
Gentamicin Sulfate (Potential for ototoxicity and/or nephrotoxicity). Products include:
Garamycin Injectable ... 2360
Genoptic Sterile Ophthalmic Solution ... ◉ 243
Genoptic Sterile Ophthalmic Ointment ... ◉ 243
Gentacidin Ointment ... ◉ 264
Gentacidin Solution ... ◉ 264
Gentak ... ◉ 208
Pred-G Liquifilm Sterile Ophthalmic Suspension ... ◉ 251
Pred-G S.O.P. Sterile Ophthalmic Ointment ... ◉ 252
Guanabenz Acetate (Antihypertensive effect potentiated).
No products indexed under this heading.
Guanethidine Monosulfate (Antihypertensive effect potentiated). Products include:
Esimil Tablets ... 822
Ismelin Tablets ... 827
Hydralazine Hydrochloride (Antihypertensive effect potentiated). Products include:
Apresazide Capsules ... 808
Apresoline Hydrochloride Tablets ... 809
Ser-Ap-Es Tablets ... 849
Hydrochlorothiazide (Antihypertensive effect potentiated). Products include:
Aldactazide ... 2413
Aldoril Tablets ... 1604
Apresazide Capsules ... 808
Capozide ... 742
Dyazide ... 2479
Esidrix Tablets ... 821
Esimil Tablets ... 822
HydroDIURIL Tablets ... 1674
Hydropres Tablets ... 1675
Hyzaar Tablets ... 1677
Inderide Tablets ... 2732
Inderide LA Long Acting Capsules ... 2734
Lopressor HCT Tablets ... 832
Lotensin HCT ... 837
Maxzide ... 1380
Moduretic Tablets ... 1705
Oretic Tablets ... 443
Prinzide Tablets ... 1737
Ser-Ap-Es Tablets ... 849
Timolide Tablets ... 1748
Vaseretic Tablets ... 1765
Zestoretic ... 2850
Ziac ... 1415
Hydroflumethiazide (Antihypertensive effect potentiated). Products include:
Diucardin Tablets ... 2718
Indapamide (Antihypertensive effect potentiated). Products include:
Lozol Tablets ... 2022
Indomethacin (Decreased plasma renin activity). Products include:
Indocin ... 1680
Indomethacin Sodium Trihydrate (Decreased plasma renin activity). Products include:
Indocin I.V. ... 1684
Isradipine (Antihypertensive effect potentiated). Products include:
DynaCirc Capsules ... 2256
Kanamycin Sulfate (Potential for ototoxicity and/or nephrotoxicity).
No products indexed under this heading.
Labetalol Hydrochloride (Antihypertensive effect potentiated). Products include:
Normodyne Injection ... 2377
Normodyne Tablets ... 2379
Trandate ... 1185
Lisinopril (Antihypertensive effect potentiated). Products include:
Prinivil Tablets ... 1733
Prinzide Tablets ... 1737
Zestoretic ... 2850
Zestril Tablets ... 2854
Lithium Carbonate (Reduced renal clearance and added high risk of lithium toxicity). Products include:
Eskalith ... 2485
Lithium Carbonate Capsules & Tablets ... 2230
Lithonate/Lithotabs/Lithobid ... 2543
Lithium Citrate (Reduced renal clearance and added high risk of lithium toxicity).
No products indexed under this heading.
Losartan Potassium (Antihypertensive effect potentiated). Products include:
Cozaar Tablets ... 1628
Hyzaar Tablets ... 1677
Mecamylamine Hydrochloride (Antihypertensive effect potentiated). Products include:
Inversine Tablets ... 1686
Methyclothiazide (Antihypertensive effect potentiated). Products include:
Enduron Tablets ... 420
Methyldopa (Antihypertensive effect potentiated). Products include:
Aldoclor Tablets ... 1598
Aldomet Oral ... 1600
Aldoril Tablets ... 1604
Methyldopate Hydrochloride (Antihypertensive effect potentiated). Products include:
Aldomet Ester HCl Injection ... 1602
Metolazone (Antihypertensive effect potentiated). Products include:
Mykrox Tablets ... 993
Zaroxolyn Tablets ... 1000
Metoprolol Succinate (Antihypertensive effect potentiated). Products include:
Toprol-XL Tablets ... 565
Metoprolol Tartrate (Antihypertensive effect potentiated). Products include:
Lopressor Ampuls ... 830
Lopressor HCT Tablets ... 832
Lopressor Tablets ... 830
Metyrosine (Antihypertensive effect potentiated). Products include:
Demser Capsules ... 1649
Minoxidil (Antihypertensive effect potentiated). Products include:
Loniten Tablets ... 2618
Rogaine Topical Solution ... 2637
Moexipril Hydrochloride (Antihypertensive effect potentiated). Products include:
Univasc Tablets ... 2410
Nadolol (Antihypertensive effect potentiated).
No products indexed under this heading.
Nicardipine Hydrochloride (Antihypertensive effect potentiated). Products include:
Cardene Capsules ... 2095
Cardene I.V. ... 2709
Cardene SR Capsules ... 2097
Nifedipine (Antihypertensive effect potentiated). Products include:
Adalat Capsules (10 mg and 20 mg) ... 587
Adalat CC ... 589
Procardia Capsules ... 1971
Procardia XL Extended Release Tablets ... 1972
Nisoldipine (Antihypertensive effect potentiated).
No products indexed under this heading.
Nitroglycerin (Antihypertensive effect potentiated). Products include:
Deponit NTG Transdermal Delivery System ... 2397
Nitro-Bid IV ... 1523
Nitro-Bid Ointment ... 1524
Nitrodisc ... 2047
Nitro-Dur (nitroglycerin) Transdermal Infusion System ... 1326
Nitrolingual Spray ... 2027
Nitrostat Tablets ... 1925
Transderm-Nitro Transdermal Therapeutic System ... 859
Penbutolol Sulfate (Antihypertensive effect potentiated). Products include:
Levatol ... 2403
Phenoxybenzamine Hydrochloride (Antihypertensive effect potentiated). Products include:
Dibenzyline Capsules ... 2476
Phentolamine Mesylate (Antihypertensive effect potentiated). Products include:
Regitine ... 846
Pindolol (Antihypertensive effect potentiated). Products include:
Visken Tablets ... 2299
Polythiazide (Antihypertensive effect potentiated). Products include:
Minizide Capsules ... 1938
Prazosin Hydrochloride (Antihypertensive effect potentiated). Products include:
Minipress Capsules ... 1937
Minizide Capsules ... 1938
Probenecid (Decreases natriuresis and hyperreninemia; concurrent use should be avoided). Products include:
Benemid Tablets ... 1611
ColBENEMID Tablets ... 1622
Propranolol Hydrochloride (Antihypertensive effect potentiated). Products include:
Inderal ... 2728
Inderal LA Long Acting Capsules ... 2730
Inderide Tablets ... 2732
Inderide LA Long Acting Capsules ... 2734
Quinapril Hydrochloride (Antihypertensive effect potentiated). Products include:
Accupril Tablets ... 1893
Ramipril (Antihypertensive effect potentiated). Products include:
Altace Capsules ... 1232
Rauwolfia Serpentina (Antihypertensive effect potentiated).
No products indexed under this heading.
Rescinnamine (Antihypertensive effect potentiated).
No products indexed under this heading.
Reserpine (Antihypertensive effect potentiated). Products include:
Diupres Tablets ... 1650
Hydropres Tablets ... 1675
Ser-Ap-Es Tablets ... 849
Sodium Nitroprusside (Antihypertensive effect potentiated).
No products indexed under this heading.
Sotalol Hydrochloride (Antihypertensive effect potentiated). Products include:
Betapace Tablets ... 641
Spirapril Hydrochloride (Antihypertensive effect potentiated).
No products indexed under this heading.
Streptomycin Sulfate (Potential for ototoxicity and/or nephrotoxicity). Products include:
Streptomycin Sulfate Injection ... 2208
Terazosin Hydrochloride (Antihypertensive effect potentiated). Products include:
Hytrin Capsules ... 430
Timolol Maleate (Antihypertensive effect potentiated). Products include:
Blocadren Tablets ... 1614
Timolide Tablets ... 1748
Timoptic in Ocudose ... 1753
Timoptic Sterile Ophthalmic Solution ... 1751
Timoptic-XE ... 1755
Tobramycin (Potential for ototoxicity and/or nephrotoxicity). Products include:
AKTOB ... ◉ 206
TobraDex Ophthalmic Suspension and Ointment ... 473

(▣ Described in PDR For Nonprescription Drugs) (◉ Described in PDR For Ophthalmology)

Tobrex Ophthalmic Ointment and Solution ⓒ 229

Tobramycin Sulfate (Potential for ototoxicity and/or nephrotoxicity). Products include:

Nebcin Vials, Hyporets & ADD-Vantage 1464
Tobramycin Sulfate Injection 968

Torsemide (Antihypertensive effect potentiated). Products include:

Demadex Tablets and Injection 686

Trimethaphan Camsylate (Antihypertensive effect potentiated). Products include:

Arfonad Ampuls 2080

Verapamil Hydrochloride (Antihypertensive effect potentiated). Products include:

Calan SR Caplets 2422
Calan Tablets 2419
Isoptin Injectable 1344
Isoptin Oral Tablets 1346
Isoptin SR Tablets 1348
Verelan Capsules 1410
Verelan Capsules 2824

BUMEX TABLETS

(Bumetanide) 2093
See Bumex Injection

BUPRENEX INJECTABLE

(Buprenorphine) 2006
May interact with central nervous system depressants, narcotic analgesics, general anesthetics, antihistamines, benzodiazepines, monoamine oxidase inhibitors, phenothiazines, hypnotics and sedatives, tranquilizers, and certain other agents. Compounds in these categories include:

Acrivastine (Increased CNS depression). Products include:

Semprex-D Capsules 463
Semprex-D Capsules 1167

Alfentanil Hydrochloride (Increased CNS depression). Products include:

Alfenta Injection 1286

Alprazolam (Increased CNS depression). Products include:

Xanax Tablets 2649

Aprobarbital (Increased CNS depression).

No products indexed under this heading.

Astemizole (Increased CNS depression). Products include:

Hismanal Tablets 1293

Azatadine Maleate (Increased CNS depression). Products include:

Trinalin Repetabs Tablets 1330

Bromodiphenhydramine Hydrochloride (Increased CNS depression).

No products indexed under this heading.

Brompheniramine Maleate (Increased CNS depression). Products include:

Alka Seltzer Plus Sinus Medicine ⊞ 707
Bromfed Capsules (Extended-Release) 1785
Bromfed Syrup ⊞ 733
Bromfed Tablets 1785
Bromfed-DM Cough Syrup 1786
Bromfed-PD Capsules (Extended-Release) 1785
Dimetane-DC Cough Syrup 2059
Dimetane-DX Cough Syrup 2059
Dimetapp Elixir ⊞ 773
Dimetapp Extentabs ⊞ 774
Dimetapp Tablets/Liqui-Gels ⊞ 775
Dimetapp Cold & Allergy Chewable Tablets ⊞ 773
Dimetapp DM Elixir ⊞ 774
Vicks DayQuil Allergy Relief 12-Hour Extended Release Tablets.. ⊞ 760
Vicks DayQuil Allergy Relief 4-Hour Tablets ⊞ 760

Buspirone Hydrochloride (Increased CNS depression). Products include:

BuSpar 737

Butabarbital (Increased CNS depression).

No products indexed under this heading.

Butalbital (Increased CNS depression). Products include:

Esgic-plus Tablets 1013
Fioricet Tablets 2258
Fioricet with Codeine Capsules 2260
Fiorinal Capsules 2261
Fiorinal with Codeine Capsules 2262
Fiorinal Tablets 2261
Phrenilin 785
Sedapap Tablets 50 mg/650 mg .. 1543

Chlordiazepoxide (Increased CNS depression). Products include:

Libritabs Tablets 2177
Limbitrol 2180

Chlordiazepoxide Hydrochloride (Increased CNS depression). Products include:

Librax Capsules 2176
Librium Capsules 2178
Librium Injectable 2179

Chlorpheniramine Maleate (Increased CNS depression). Products include:

Alka-Seltzer Plus Cold Medicine .... ⊞ 705
Alka-Seltzer Plus Cold Medicine Liqui-Gels ⊞ 706
Alka-Seltzer Plus Cold & Cough Medicine ⊞ 708
Alka-Seltzer Plus Cold & Cough Medicine Liqui-Gels ⊞ 705
Allerest Children's Chewable Tablets ⊞ 627
Allerest Headache Strength Tablets ⊞ 627
Allerest Maximum Strength Tablets ⊞ 627
Allerest Sinus Pain Formula ⊞ 627
Allerest 12 Hour Caplets ⊞ 627
Ana-Kit Anaphylaxis Emergency Treatment Kit 617
Atrohist Pediatric Capsules 453
Atrohist Plus Tablets 454
BC Cold Powder Multi-Symptom Formula (Cold-Sinus-Allergy) ⊞ 609
Cerose DM ⊞ 878
Cheracol Plus Head Cold/Cough Formula ⊞ 769
Children's Vicks DayQuil Allergy Relief ⊞ 757
Children's Vicks NyQuil Cold/Cough Relief ⊞ 758
Chlor-Trimeton Allergy Decongestant Tablets ⊞ 799
Chlor-Trimeton Allergy Tablets ⊞ 798
Comhist 2038
Comtrex Multi-Symptom Cold Reliever Tablets/Caplets/Liqui-Gels/Liquid ⊞ 615
Allergy-Sinus Comtrex Multi-Symptom Allergy-Sinus Formula Tablets ⊞ 617
Contac Continuous Action Nasal Decongestant/Antihistamine 12 Hour Capsules ⊞ 813
Contac Maximum Strength Continuous Action Decongestant/Antihistamine 12 Hour Caplets.. ⊞ 813
Contac Severe Cold and Flu Formula Caplets ⊞ 814
Coricidin 'D' Decongestant Tablets ⊞ 800
Coricidin Tablets ⊞ 800
D.A. Chewable Tablets 951
Deconamine 1320
Dura-Tap/PD Capsules 2867
Dura-Vent/DA Tablets 953
Extendryl 1005
Fedahist Gyrocaps 2401
Fedahist Timecaps 2401
Hycomine Compound Tablets 932
Isoclor Timesule Capsules ⊞ 637
Kronofed-A 977
Nolamine Timed-Release Tablets 785
Novahistine DH 2462
Novahistine Elixir ⊞ 823
Ornade Spansule Capsules 2502
PediaCare Cold Allergy Chewable Tablets ⊞ 677
PediaCare Cough-Cold Chewable Tablets 1553

PediaCare Cough-Cold Liquid 1553
PediaCare NightRest Cough-Cold Liquid 1553
Pediatric Vicks 44m Cough & Cold Relief ⊞ 764
Pyrroxate Caplets ⊞ 772
Ryna ⊞ 841
Sinarest Tablets ⊞ 648
Sinarest Extra Strength Tablets ⊞ 648
Sine-Off Sinus Medicine ⊞ 825
Singlet Tablets ⊞ 825
Sinutin Tablets 787
Sinutab Sinus Allergy Medication, Maximum Strength Tablets and Caplets ⊞ 860
Sudafed Plus Liquid ⊞ 862
Sudafed Plus Tablets ⊞ 863
Teldrin 12 Hour Antihistamine/Nasal Decongestant Allergy Relief Capsules ⊞ 826
TheraFlu ⊞ 787
TheraFlu Maximum Strength Nighttime Flu, Cold & Cough Medicine ⊞ 788
Triaminic Allergy Tablets ⊞ 789
Triaminic Cold Tablets ⊞ 790
Triaminic Nite Light ⊞ 791
Triaminic Syrup ⊞ 792
Triaminic-12 Tablets ⊞ 792
Triaminicin Tablets ⊞ 793
Triaminicol Multi-Symptom Cold Tablets ⊞ 793
Triaminicol Multi-Symptom Relief ⊞ 794
Tussend 1783
Children's TYLENOL Cold Multi-Symptom Liquid Formula and Chewable Tablets 1561
Children's TYLENOL Cold Plus Cough Multi Symptom Tablets and Liquid ⊞ 681
TYLENOL Maximum Strength Allergy Sinus Medication Gelcaps and Caplets 1563
TYLENOL Cold Multi-Symptom Formula Medication Tablets and Caplets 1561
TYLENOL Cold Multi-Symptom Hot Medication Liquid Packets 1557
Vicks 44 LiquiCaps Cough, Cold & Flu Relief ⊞ 755
Vicks 44M Cough, Cold & Flu Relief ⊞ 756

Chlorpheniramine Polistirex (Increased CNS depression). Products include:

Tussionex Pennkinetic Extended-Release Suspension 998

Chlorpheniramine Tannate (Increased CNS depression). Products include:

Atrohist Pediatric Suspension 454
Ricobid Tablets and Pediatric Suspension 2038
Rynatan 2673
Rynatuss 2673

Chlorpromazine (Increased CNS depression). Products include:

Thorazine Suppositories 2523

Chlorprothixene (Increased CNS depression).

No products indexed under this heading.

Chlorprothixene Hydrochloride (Increased CNS depression).

No products indexed under this heading.

Clemastine Fumarate (Increased CNS depression). Products include:

Tavist Syrup 2297
Tavist Tablets 2298
Tavist-1 12 Hour Relief Tablets ⊞ 787
Tavist-D 12 Hour Relief Tablets ⊞ 787

Clorazepate Dipotassium (Increased CNS depression). Products include:

Tranxene 451

Clozapine (Increased CNS depression). Products include:

Clozaril Tablets 2252

Codeine Phosphate (Increased CNS depression). Products include:

Actifed with Codeine Cough Syrup.. 1067
Brontex 1981
Deconsal C Expectorant Syrup 456
Deconsal Pediatric Syrup 457
Dimetane-DC Cough Syrup 2059

Empirin with Codeine Tablets 1093
Fioricet with Codeine Capsules 2260
Fiorinal with Codeine Capsules 2262
Isoclor Expectorant 990
Novahistine DH 2462
Novahistine Expectorant 2463
Nucofed 2051
Phenergan with Codeine 2777
Phenergan VC with Codeine 2781
Robitussin A-C Syrup 2073
Robitussin-DAC Syrup 2074
Ryna ⊞ 841
Soma Compound w/Codeine Tablets 2676
Tussi-Organidin NR Liquid and S NR Liquid 2677
Tylenol with Codeine 1583

Cyproheptadine Hydrochloride (Increased CNS depression). Products include:

Periactin 1724

Desflurane (Increased CNS depression). Products include:

Suprane 1813

Dexchlorpheniramine Maleate (Increased CNS depression).

No products indexed under this heading.

Dezocine (Increased CNS depression). Products include:

Dalgan Injection 538

Diazepam (Concurrent use has resulted in respiratory and cardiovascular collapse; increased CNS depression). Products include:

Dizac 1809
Valium Injectable 2182
Valium Tablets 2183
Valrelease Capsules 2169

Diphenhydramine Citrate (Increased CNS depression). Products include:

Excedrin P.M. Analgesic/Sleeping Aid Tablets, Caplets, Liquigels 733

Diphenhydramine Hydrochloride (Increased CNS depression). Products include:

Actifed Allergy Daytime/Nighttime Caplets ⊞ 844
Actifed Sinus Daytime/Nighttime Tablets and Caplets ⊞ 846
Arthritis Foundation NightTime Caplets ⊞ 674
Extra Strength Bayer PM Aspirin .. ⊞ 713
Bayer Select Night Time Pain Relief Formula ⊞ 716
Benadryl Allergy Decongestant Liquid Medication ⊞ 848
Benadryl Allergy Decongestant Tablets ⊞ 848
Benadryl Allergy Liquid Medication ⊞ 849
Benadryl Allergy ⊞ 848
Benadryl Allergy Sinus Headache Formula Caplets ⊞ 849
Benadryl Capsules 1898
Benadryl Dye-Free Allergy Liquigel Softgels ⊞ 850
Benadryl Dye-Free Allergy Liquid Medication ⊞ 850
Benadryl Itch Relief Cream, Children's Formula and Maximum Strength 2% ⊞ 851
Benadryl Itch Relief Spray, Children's Formula and Maximum Strength 2% ⊞ 851
Benadryl Itch Relief Stick Maximum Strength 2% ⊞ 850
Benadryl Itch Stopping Gel, Children's Formula and Maximum Strength 2% ⊞ 851
Benadryl Kapseals 1898
Benadryl Injection 1898
Contac Day & Night Cold/Flu Night Caplets ⊞ 812
Contac Night Allergy/Sinus Caplets ⊞ 812
Extra Strength Doan's P.M. ⊞ 633
Legatrin PM ⊞ 651
Miles Nervine Nighttime Sleep-Aid ⊞ 723
Nytol QuickCaps Caplets ⊞ 610
Sleepinal Night-time Sleep Aid Capsules and Softgels ⊞ 834
TYLENOL Maximum Strength Allergy Sinus NightTime Medication Caplets 1555

IMPORTANT NOTE: Always consult each drug listing in the patient's regimen for possible interactions.

Buprenex **Interactions Index** **148**

TYLENOL Flu NightTime, Maximum Strength, Gelcaps 1566
TYLENOL Maximum Strength Flu NightTime Hot Medication Packets 1562
TYLENOL PM, Extra Strength Pain Reliever/Sleep Aid Caplets, Geltabs, Gelcaps 1560
TYLENOL Severe Allergy Medication Caplets 1564
Maximum Strength Unisom Sleepgels 1934
Unisom With Pain Relief-Nighttime Sleep Aid and Pain Reliever 1934

Diphenylpyraline Hydrochloride (Increased CNS depression).
No products indexed under this heading.

Droperidol (Increased CNS depression). Products include:
Inapsine Injection 1296

Enflurane (Increased CNS depression).
No products indexed under this heading.

Estazolam (Increased CNS depression). Products include:
ProSom Tablets 449

Ethchlorvynol (Increased CNS depression). Products include:
Placidyl Capsules 448

Ethinamate (Increased CNS depression).
No products indexed under this heading.

Fentanyl (Increased CNS depression). Products include:
Duragesic Transdermal System 1288

Fentanyl Citrate (Increased CNS depression). Products include:
Sublimaze Injection 1307

Fluphenazine Decanoate (Increased CNS depression). Products include:
Prolixin Decanoate 509

Fluphenazine Enanthate (Increased CNS depression). Products include:
Prolixin Enanthate 509

Fluphenazine Hydrochloride (Increased CNS depression). Products include:
Prolixin 509

Flurazepam Hydrochloride (Increased CNS depression). Products include:
Dalmane Capsules 2173

Furazolidone (Effect unspecified; caution should be exercised). Products include:
Furoxone 2046

Glutethimide (Increased CNS depression).
No products indexed under this heading.

Halazepam (Increased CNS depression).
No products indexed under this heading.

Haloperidol (Increased CNS depression). Products include:
Haldol Injection, Tablets and Concentrate 1575

Haloperidol Decanoate (Increased CNS depression). Products include:
Haldol Decanoate 1577

Hydrocodone Bitartrate (Increased CNS depression). Products include:
Anexsia 5/500 Elixir 1781
Anexia Tablets 1782
Codiclear DH Syrup 791
Deconamine CX Cough and Cold Liquid and Tablets 1319
Duratuss HD Elixir 2565
Hycodan Tablets and Syrup 930
Hycomine Compound Tablets 932
Hycomine 931
Hycotuss Expectorant Syrup 933
Hydrocet Capsules 782
Lorcet 10/650 1018
Lortab 2566
Tussend 1783
Tussend Expectorant 1785
Vicodin Tablets 1356
Vicodin ES Tablets 1357
Vicodin Tuss Expectorant 1358
Zydone Capsules 949

Hydrocodone Polistirex (Increased CNS depression). Products include:
Tussionex Pennkinetic Extended-Release Suspension 998

Hydroxyzine Hydrochloride (Increased CNS depression). Products include:
Atarax Tablets & Syrup 2185
Marax Tablets & DF Syrup 2200
Vistaril Intramuscular Solution 2216

Isocarboxazid (Effect unspecified; caution should be exercised).
No products indexed under this heading.

Isoflurane (Increased CNS depression).
No products indexed under this heading.

Ketamine Hydrochloride (Increased CNS depression).
No products indexed under this heading.

Levomethadyl Acetate Hydrochloride (Increased CNS depression). Products include:
Orlamm 2239

Levorphanol Tartrate (Increased CNS depression). Products include:
Levo-Dromoran 2129

Loratadine (Increased CNS depression). Products include:
Claritin 2349
Claritin-D 2350

Lorazepam (Increased CNS depression). Products include:
Ativan Injection 2698
Ativan Tablets 2700

Loxapine Hydrochloride (Increased CNS depression). Products include:
Loxitane 1378

Loxapine Succinate (Increased CNS depression). Products include:
Loxitane Capsules 1378

Meperidine Hydrochloride (Increased CNS depression). Products include:
Demerol 2308
Mepergan Injection 2753

Mephobarbital (Increased CNS depression). Products include:
Mebaral Tablets 2322

Meprobamate (Increased CNS depression). Products include:
Miltown Tablets 2672
PMB 200 and PMB 400 2783

Mesoridazine Besylate (Increased CNS depression). Products include:
Serentil 684

Methadone Hydrochloride (Increased CNS depression). Products include:
Methadone Hydrochloride Oral Concentrate 2233
Methadone Hydrochloride Oral Solution & Tablets 2235

Methdilazine Hydrochloride (Increased CNS depression).
No products indexed under this heading.

Methohexital Sodium (Increased CNS depression). Products include:
Brevital Sodium Vials 1429

Methotrimeprazine (Increased CNS depression). Products include:
Levoprome 1274

Methoxyflurane (Increased CNS depression).
No products indexed under this heading.

Midazolam Hydrochloride (Increased CNS depression). Products include:
Versed Injection 2170

Molindone Hydrochloride (Increased CNS depression). Products include:
Moban Tablets and Concentrate 1048

Morphine Sulfate (Increased CNS depression). Products include:
Astramorph/PF Injection, USP (Preservative-Free) 535
Duramorph 962
Infumorph 200 and Infumorph 500 Sterile Solutions 965
MS Contin Tablets 1994
MSIR 1997
Oramorph SR (Morphine Sulfate Sustained Release Tablets) 2236
RMS Suppositories 2657
Roxanol 2243

Opium Alkaloids (Increased CNS depression).
No products indexed under this heading.

Oxazepam (Increased CNS depression). Products include:
Serax Capsules 2810
Serax Tablets 2810

Oxycodone Hydrochloride (Increased CNS depression). Products include:
Percocet Tablets 938
Percodan Tablets 939
Percodan-Demi Tablets 940
Roxicodone Tablets, Oral Solution & Intensol (Oxycodone) 2244
Tylox Capsules 1584

Pentobarbital Sodium (Increased CNS depression). Products include:
Nembutal Sodium Capsules 436
Nembutal Sodium Solution 438
Nembutal Sodium Suppositories 440

Perphenazine (Increased CNS depression). Products include:
Etrafon 2355
Triavil Tablets 1757
Trilafon 2389

Phenelzine Sulfate (Effect unspecified; caution should be exercised). Products include:
Nardil 1920

Phenobarbital (Increased CNS depression). Products include:
Arco-Lase Plus Tablets 512
Bellergal-S Tablets 2250
Donnatal 2060
Donnatal Extentabs 2061
Donnatal Tablets 2060
Phenobarbital Elixir and Tablets 1469
Quadrinal Tablets 1350

Phenprocoumon (Potential for purpura).

Prazepam (Increased CNS depression).
No products indexed under this heading.

Prochlorperazine (Increased CNS depression). Products include:
Compazine 2470

Promethazine Hydrochloride (Increased CNS depression). Products include:
Mepergan Injection 2753
Phenergan with Codeine 2777
Phenergan with Dextromethorphan 2778
Phenergan Injection 2773
Phenergan Suppositories 2775
Phenergan Syrup 2774
Phenergan Tablets 2775
Phenergan VC 2779
Phenergan VC with Codeine 2781

Propofol (Increased CNS depression). Products include:
Diprivan Injection 2833

Propoxyphene Hydrochloride (Increased CNS depression). Products include:
Darvon 1435
Wygesic Tablets 2827

Propoxyphene Napsylate (Increased CNS depression). Products include:
Darvon-N/Darvocet-N 1433

Pyrilamine Maleate (Increased CNS depression). Products include:
4-Way Fast Acting Nasal Spray (regular & mentholated) .... ■ 621
Maximum Strength Multi-Symptom Formula Midol .... ■ 722
PMS Multi-Symptom Formula Midol .... ■ 723

Pyrilamine Tannate (Increased CNS depression). Products include:
Atrohist Pediatric Suspension 454
Rynatan 2673

Quazepam (Increased CNS depression). Products include:
Doral Tablets 2664

Risperidone (Increased CNS depression). Products include:
Risperdal 1301

Secobarbital Sodium (Increased CNS depression). Products include:
Seconal Sodium Pulvules 1474

Selegiline Hydrochloride (Effect unspecified; caution should be exercised). Products include:
Eldepryl Tablets 2550

Sufentanil Citrate (Increased CNS depression). Products include:
Sufenta Injection 1309

Temazepam (Increased CNS depression). Products include:
Restoril Capsules 2284

Terfenadine (Increased CNS depression). Products include:
Seldane Tablets 1536
Seldane-D Extended-Release Tablets 1538

Thiamylal Sodium (Increased CNS depression).
No products indexed under this heading.

Thioridazine Hydrochloride (Increased CNS depression). Products include:
Mellaril 2269

Thiothixene (Increased CNS depression). Products include:
Navane Capsules and Concentrate 2201
Navane Intramuscular 2202

Tranylcypromine Sulfate (Effect unspecified; caution should be exercised). Products include:
Parnate Tablets 2503

Triazolam (Increased CNS depression). Products include:
Halcion Tablets 2611

Trifluoperazine Hydrochloride (Increased CNS depression). Products include:
Stelazine 2514

Trimeprazine Tartrate (Increased CNS depression). Products include:
Temaril Tablets, Syrup and Spansule Extended-Release Capsules.. 483

Tripelennamine Hydrochloride (Increased CNS depression). Products include:
PBZ Tablets 845
PBZ-SR Tablets 844

Triprolidine Hydrochloride (Increased CNS depression). Products include:
Actifed Plus Caplets .... ■ 845
Actifed Plus Tablets .... ■ 845
Actifed with Codeine Cough Syrup.. 1067
Actifed Syrup .... ■ 846
Actifed Tablets .... ■ 844

Zolpidem Tartrate (Increased CNS depression). Products include:
Ambien Tablets 2416

(■ Described in PDR For Nonprescription Drugs) (⊙ Described in PDR For Ophthalmology)

Food Interactions

Alcohol (Increased CNS depression).

BUSPAR

(Buspirone Hydrochloride) 737

May interact with monoamine oxidase inhibitors and certain other agents. Compounds in these categories include:

Digoxin (*In vitro* buspirone may displace less firmly bound drugs like digoxin; the clinical significance is unknown). Products include:

Lanoxicaps 1117
Lanoxin Elixir Pediatric 1120
Lanoxin Injection 1123
Lanoxin Injection Pediatric................... 1126
Lanoxin Tablets 1128

Furazolidone (Co-administration may pose a hazard due to potential for elevated blood pressure; concomitant administration is not recommended). Products include:

Furoxone 2046

Haloperidol (Increased serum haloperidol concentrations). Products include:

Haldol Injection, Tablets and Concentrate 1575

Haloperidol Decanoate (Increased serum haloperidol concentrations). Products include:

Haldol Decanoate.................................... 1577

Isocarboxazid (Co-administration may pose a hazard due to potential for elevated blood pressure; concomitant administration is not recommended).

No products indexed under this heading.

Phenelzine Sulfate (Co-administration may pose a hazard due to potential for elevated blood pressure; concomitant administration is not recommended). Products include:

Nardil 1920

Psychotropic drugs, unspecified (Concomitant use of BuSpar with other CNS-active drugs should be approached with caution).

Selegiline Hydrochloride (Co-administration may pose a hazard due to potential for elevated blood pressure; concomitant administration is not recommended). Products include:

Eldepryl Tablets 2550

Tranylcypromine Sulfate (Co-administration may pose a hazard due to potential for elevated blood pressure; concomitant administration is not recommended). Products include:

Parnate Tablets 2503

Trazodone Hydrochloride (Possible SGPT elevation). Products include:

Desyrel and Desyrel Dividose 503

Warfarin Sodium (Single report of prolonged prothrombin time in a patient on other tightly protein bound drugs). Products include:

Coumadin 926

Food Interactions

Alcohol (Concomitant use should be avoided).

Food, unspecified (Food may decrease presystemic clearance of buspirone).

BUTISOL SODIUM ELIXIR & TABLETS

(Butabarbital Sodium)...........................2660

May interact with oral anticoagulants, anticoagulants, corticosteroids, central nervous system depressants, monoamine oxidase inhibitors, hypnotics and sedatives, tranquilizers, antihistamines, estrogens, oral contraceptives, and certain other agents. Compounds in these categories include:

Acrivastine (Additive CNS depressant effects). Products include:

Semprex-D Capsules 463
Semprex-D Capsules 1167

Alfentanil Hydrochloride (Additive CNS depressant effects). Products include:

Alfenta Injection 1286

Alprazolam (Additive CNS depressant effects). Products include:

Xanax Tablets 2649

Aprobarbital (Additive CNS depressant effects).

No products indexed under this heading.

Astemizole (Additive CNS depressant effects). Products include:

Hismanal Tablets 1293

Azatadine Maleate (Additive CNS depressant effects). Products include:

Trinalin Repetabs Tablets 1330

Betamethasone Acetate (Enhanced metabolism of corticosteroids; dosage adjustment may be necessary). Products include:

Celestone Soluspan Suspension 2347

Betamethasone Sodium Phosphate (Enhanced metabolism of corticosteroids; dosage adjustment may be necessary). Products include:

Celestone Soluspan Suspension 2347

Bromodiphenhydramine Hydrochloride (Additive CNS depressant effects).

No products indexed under this heading.

Brompheniramine Maleate (Additive CNS depressant effects). Products include:

Alka Seltzer Plus Sinus Medicine .. ᴿᴰ 707
Bromfed Capsules (Extended-Release) 1785
Bromfed Syrup .... ᴿᴰ 733
Bromfed Tablets 1785
Bromfed-DM Cough Syrup.................... 1786
Bromfed-PD Capsules (Extended-Release)... 1785
Dimetane-DC Cough Syrup 2059
Dimetane-DX Cough Syrup 2059
Dimetapp Elixir .... ᴿᴰ 773
Dimetapp Extentabs................................ ᴿᴰ 774
Dimetapp Tablets/Liqui-Gels .... ᴿᴰ 775
Dimetapp Cold & Allergy Chewable Tablets .... ᴿᴰ 773
Dimetapp DM Elixir .... ᴿᴰ 774
Vicks DayQuil Allergy Relief 12-Hour Extended Release Tablets.. ᴿᴰ 760
Vicks DayQuil Allergy Relief 4-Hour Tablets .... ᴿᴰ 760

Buprenorphine (Additive CNS depressant effects). Products include:

Buprenex Injectable 2006

Buspirone Hydrochloride (Additive CNS depressant effects). Products include:

BuSpar 737

Butabarbital (Additive CNS depressant effects).

No products indexed under this heading.

Butalbital (Additive CNS depressant effects). Products include:

Esgic-plus Tablets 1013
Fioricet Tablets.. 2258
Fioricet with Codeine Capsules 2260
Fiorinal Capsules 2261
Fiorinal with Codeine Capsules 2262
Fiorinal Tablets.. 2261
Phrenilin 785
Sedapap Tablets 50 mg/650 mg .. 1543

Chlordiazepoxide (Additive CNS depressant effects). Products include:

Libritabs Tablets 2177
Limbitrol 2180

Chlordiazepoxide Hydrochloride (Additive CNS depressant effects). Products include:

Librax Capsules 2176
Librium Capsules..................................... 2178
Librium Injectable 2179

Chlorotrianisene (Increased metabolism of estradiol).

No products indexed under this heading.

Chlorpheniramine Maleate (Additive CNS depressant effects). Products include:

Alka-Seltzer Plus Cold Medicine .... ᴿᴰ 705
Alka-Seltzer Plus Cold Medicine Liqui-Gels .... ᴿᴰ 706
Alka-Seltzer Plus Cold & Cough Medicine .... ᴿᴰ 708
Alka-Seltzer Plus Cold & Cough Medicine Liqui-Gels........................... ᴿᴰ 705
Allerest Children's Chewable Tablets .... ᴿᴰ 627
Allerest Headache Strength Tablets .... ᴿᴰ 627
Allerest Maximum Strength Tablets .... ᴿᴰ 627
Allerest Sinus Pain Formula .... ᴿᴰ 627
Allerest 12 Hour Caplets .... ᴿᴰ 627
Ana-Kit Anaphylaxis Emergency Treatment Kit 617
Atrohist Pediatric Capsules................... 453
Atrohist Plus Tablets 454
BC Cold Powder Multi-Symptom Formula (Cold-Sinus-Allergy) ...... ᴿᴰ 609
Cerose DM .... ᴿᴰ 878
Cheracol Plus Head Cold/Cough Formula .... ᴿᴰ 769
Children's Vicks DayQuil Allergy Relief.. ᴿᴰ 757
Children's Vicks NyQuil Cold/Cough Relief... ᴿᴰ 758
Chlor-Trimeton Allergy Decongestant Tablets .... ᴿᴰ 799
Chlor-Trimeton Allergy Tablets ...... ᴿᴰ 798
Comhist 2038
Comtrex Multi-Symptom Cold Reliever Tablets/Caplets/Liqui-Gels/Liquid.. ᴿᴰ 615
Allergy-Sinus Comtrex Multi-Symptom Allergy-Sinus Formula Tablets .... ᴿᴰ 617
Contac Continuous Action Nasal Decongestant/Antihistamine 12 Hour Capsules...................................... ᴿᴰ 813
Contac Maximum Strength Continuous Action Decongestant/Antihistamine 12 Hour Caplets.. ᴿᴰ 813
Contac Severe Cold and Flu Formula Caplets .... ᴿᴰ 814
Coricidin 'D' Decongestant Tablets .... ᴿᴰ 800
Coricidin Tablets .... ᴿᴰ 800
D.A. Chewable Tablets............................ 951
Deconamine 1320
Dura-Tap/PD Capsules 2867
Dura-Vent/DA Tablets 953
Extendryl 1005
Fedahist Gyrocaps................................... 2401
Fedahist Timecaps 2401
Hycomine Compound Tablets 932
Isoclor Timesule Capsules .... ᴿᴰ 637
Kronofed-A 977
Nolamine Timed-Release Tablets 785
Novahistine DH.. 2462
Novahistine Elixir .... ᴿᴰ 823
Ornade Spansule Capsules 2502
PediaCare Cold Allergy Chewable Tablets .... ᴿᴰ 677
PediaCare Cough-Cold Chewable Tablets 1553
PediaCare Cough-Cold Liquid.............. 1553
PediaCare NightRest Cough-Cold Liquid 1553
Pediatric Vicks 44m Cough & Cold Relief .... ᴿᴰ 764
Pyrroxate Caplets .... ᴿᴰ 772
Ryna .... ᴿᴰ 841
Sinarest Tablets .... ᴿᴰ 648
Sinarest Extra Strength Tablets....... ᴿᴰ 648
Sine-Off Sinus Medicine .... ᴿᴰ 825
Singlet Tablets .... ᴿᴰ 825
Sinutab Sinus Allergy Medication, Maximum Strength Tablets and Caplets .... ᴿᴰ 860
Sudafed Plus Liquid .... ᴿᴰ 862
Sudafed Plus Tablets .... ᴿᴰ 863
Teldrin 12 Hour Antihistamine/Nasal Decongestant Allergy Relief Capsules .... ᴿᴰ 826
TheraFlu.. ᴿᴰ 787
TheraFlu Maximum Strength Nighttime Flu, Cold & Cough Medicine .... ᴿᴰ 788
Triaminic Allergy Tablets .... ᴿᴰ 789
Triaminic Cold Tablets .... ᴿᴰ 790
Triaminic Nite Light .... ᴿᴰ 791
Triaminic Syrup .... ᴿᴰ 792
Triaminic-12 Tablets .... ᴿᴰ 792
Triaminicin Tablets.................................. ᴿᴰ 793
Triaminicol Multi-Symptom Cold Tablets .... ᴿᴰ 793
Triaminicol Multi-Symptom Relief ᴿᴰ 794
Tussend 1783
Children's TYLENOL Cold Multi-Symptom Liquid Formula and Chewable Tablets................................... 1561
Children's TYLENOL Cold Plus Cough Multi Symptom Tablets and Liquid .... ᴿᴰ 681
TYLENOL Maximum Strength Allergy Sinus Medication Gelcaps and Caplets 1563
TYLENOL Cold Multi-Symptom Formula Medication Tablets and Caplets 1561
TYLENOL Cold Multi-Symptom Hot Medication Liquid Packets.............. 1557
Vicks 44 LiquiCaps Cough, Cold & Flu Relief... ᴿᴰ 755
Vicks 44M Cough, Cold & Flu Relief... ᴿᴰ 756

Chlorpheniramine Polistirex (Additive CNS depressant effects). Products include:

Tussionex Pennkinetic Extended-Release Suspension 998

Chlorpheniramine Tannate (Additive CNS depressant effects). Products include:

Atrohist Pediatric Suspension 454
Ricobid Tablets and Pediatric Suspension.. 2038
Rynatan 2673
Rynatuss 2673

Chlorpromazine (Additive CNS depressant effects). Products include:

Thorazine Suppositories......................... 2523

Chlorpromazine Hydrochloride (Additive CNS depressant effects). Products include:

Thorazine 2523

Chlorprothixene (Additive CNS depressant effects).

No products indexed under this heading.

Chlorprothixene Hydrochloride (Additive CNS depressant effects).

No products indexed under this heading.

Clemastine Fumarate (Additive CNS depressant effects). Products include:

Tavist Syrup.. 2297
Tavist Tablets 2298
Tavist-1 12 Hour Relief Tablets .... ᴿᴰ 787
Tavist-D 12 Hour Relief Tablets .... ᴿᴰ 787

Clorazepate Dipotassium (Additive CNS depressant effects). Products include:

Tranxene 451

Clozapine (Additive CNS depressant effects). Products include:

Clozaril Tablets.. 2252

Codeine Phosphate (Additive CNS depressant effects). Products include:

Actifed with Codeine Cough Syrup.. 1067
Brontex 1981
Deconsal C Expectorant Syrup 456
Deconsal Pediatric Syrup 457
Dimetane-DC Cough Syrup 2059
Empirin with Codeine Tablets.............. 1093
Fioricet with Codeine Capsules 2260
Fiorinal with Codeine Capsules 2262
Isoclor Expectorant................................. 990

Sinulin Tablets 787

IMPORTANT NOTE: Always consult each drug listing in the patient's regimen for possible interactions.

Butisol Sodium **Interactions Index** **150**

Novahistine DH 2462
Novahistine Expectorant 2463
Nucofed 2051
Phenergan with Codeine 2777
Phenergan VC with Codeine 2781
Robitussin A-C Syrup 2073
Robitussin-DAC Syrup 2074
Ryna ..... ⊡ 841
Soma Compound w/Codeine Tablets 2676
Tussi-Organidin NR Liquid and S NR Liquid 2677
Tylenol with Codeine 1583

Cortisone Acetate (Enhanced metabolism of corticosteroids; dosage adjustment may be necessary). Products include:
Cortone Acetate Sterile Suspension 1623
Cortone Acetate Tablets 1624

Cyproheptadine Hydrochloride (Additive CNS depressant effects). Products include:
Periactin 1724

Dalteparin Sodium (Decreased anticoagulant response). Products include:
Fragmin 1954

Desflurane (Additive CNS depressant effects). Products include:
Suprane 1813

Desogestrel (Increased metabolism of estradiol). Products include:
Desogen Tablets 1817
Ortho-Cept 1851

Dexamethasone (Enhanced metabolism of corticosteroids; dosage adjustment may be necessary). Products include:
AK-Trol Ointment & Suspension ..... ⊙ 205
Decadron Elixir 1633
Decadron Tablets 1635
Decaspray Topical Aerosol 1648
Dexacidin Ointment ..... ⊙ 263
Maxitrol Ophthalmic Ointment and Suspension ..... ⊙ 224
TobraDex Ophthalmic Suspension and Ointment 473

Dexamethasone Acetate (Enhanced metabolism of corticosteroids; dosage adjustment may be necessary). Products include:
Dalalone D.P. Injectable 1011
Decadron-LA Sterile Suspension 1646

Dexamethasone Sodium Phosphate (Enhanced metabolism of corticosteroids; dosage adjustment may be necessary). Products include:
Decadron Phosphate Injection 1637
Decadron Phosphate Respihaler 1642
Decadron Phosphate Sterile Ophthalmic Ointment 1641
Decadron Phosphate Sterile Ophthalmic Solution 1642
Decadron Phosphate Topical Cream 1644
Decadron Phosphate Turbinaire 1645
Decadron Phosphate with Xylocaine Injection, Sterile 1639
Dexacort Phosphate in Respihaler 458
Dexacort Phosphate in Turbinaire 459
NeoDecadron Sterile Ophthalmic Ointment 1712
NeoDecadron Sterile Ophthalmic Solution 1713
NeoDecadron Topical Cream 1714

Dexchlorpheniramine Maleate (Additive CNS depressant effects).
No products indexed under this heading.

Dezocine (Additive CNS depressant effects). Products include:
Dalgan Injection 538

Diazepam (Additive CNS depressant effects). Products include:
Dizac 1809
Valium Injectable 2182
Valium Tablets 2183
Valrelease Capsules 2169

Dicumarol (Decreased anticoagulant response).
No products indexed under this heading.

Dienestrol (Increased metabolism of estradiol). Products include:
Ortho Dienestrol Cream 1866

Diethylstilbestrol (Increased metabolism of estradiol). Products include:
Diethylstilbestrol Tablets 1437

Diphenhydramine Citrate (Additive CNS depressant effects). Products include:
Excedrin P.M. Analgesic/Sleeping Aid Tablets, Caplets, Liquigels 733

Diphenhydramine Hydrochloride (Additive CNS depressant effects). Products include:
Actifed Allergy Daytime/Nighttime Caplets ..... ⊡ 844
Actifed Sinus Daytime/Nighttime Tablets and Caplets ..... ⊡ 846
Arthritis Foundation NightTime Caplets ..... ⊡ 674
Extra Strength Bayer PM Aspirin ..... ⊡ 713
Bayer Select Night Time Pain Relief Formula ..... ⊡ 716
Benadryl Allergy Decongestant Liquid Medication ..... ⊡ 848
Benadryl Allergy Decongestant Tablets ..... ⊡ 848
Benadryl Allergy Liquid Medication ..... ⊡ 849
Benadryl Allergy ..... ⊡ 848
Benadryl Allergy Sinus Headache Formula Caplets ..... ⊡ 849
Benadryl Capsules 1898
Benadryl Dye-Free Allergy Liqui-gel Softgels ..... ⊡ 850
Benadryl Dye-Free Allergy Liquid Medication ..... ⊡ 850
Benadryl Itch Relief Cream, Children's Formula and Maximum Strength 2% ..... ⊡ 851
Benadryl Itch Relief Spray, Children's Formula and Maximum Strength 2% ..... ⊡ 851
Benadryl Itch Relief Stick Maximum Strength 2% ..... ⊡ 850
Benadryl Itch Stopping Gel, Children's Formula and Maximum Strength 2% ..... ⊡ 851
Benadryl Kapseals 1898
Benadryl Injection 1898
Contac Day & Night Cold/Flu Night Caplets ..... ⊡ 812
Contac Night Allergy/Sinus Caplets ..... ⊡ 812
Extra Strength Doan's P.M. ..... ⊡ 633
Legatrin PM ..... ⊡ 651
Miles Nervine Nighttime Sleep-Aid ..... ⊡ 723
Nytol QuickCaps Caplets ..... ⊡ 610
Sleepinal Night-time Sleep Aid Capsules and Softgels ..... ⊡ 834
TYLENOL Maximum Strength Allergy Sinus NightTime Medication Caplets 1555
TYLENOL Flu NightTime, Maximum Strength, Gelcaps 1566
TYLENOL Maximum Strength Flu NightTime Hot Medication Packets 1562
TYLENOL PM, Extra Strength Pain Reliever/Sleep Aid Caplets, Geltabs, Gelcaps 1560
TYLENOL Severe Allergy Medication Caplets 1564
Maximum Strength Unisom Sleepgels 1934
Unisom With Pain Relief-Nighttime Sleep Aid and Pain Reliever 1934

Diphenylpyraline Hydrochloride (Additive CNS depressant effects).
No products indexed under this heading.

Doxycycline Calcium (Phenobarbital has been shown to shorten the half-life of doxycycline). Products include:
Vibramycin Calcium Oral Suspension Syrup 1941

Doxycycline Hyclate (Phenobarbital has been shown to shorten the half-life of doxycycline). Products include:
Doryx Capsules 1913
Vibramycin Hyclate Capsules 1941
Vibramycin Hyclate Intravenous 2215
Vibra-Tabs Film Coated Tablets 1941

Doxycycline Monohydrate (Phenobarbital has been shown to shorten the half-life of doxycycline). Products include:
Monodox Capsules 1805
Vibramycin Monohydrate for Oral Suspension 1941

Droperidol (Additive CNS depressant effects). Products include:
Inapsine Injection 1296

Enflurane (Additive CNS depressant effects).
No products indexed under this heading.

Enoxaparin (Decreased anticoagulant response). Products include:
Lovenox Injection 2020

Estazolam (Additive CNS depressant effects). Products include:
ProSom Tablets 449

Estradiol (Increased metabolism of estradiol). Products include:
Climara Transdermal System 645
Estrace Cream and Tablets 749
Estraderm Transdermal System 824

Estrogens, Conjugated (Increased metabolism of estradiol). Products include:
PMB 200 and PMB 400 2783
Premarin Intravenous 2787
Premarin with Methyltestosterone 2794
Premarin Tablets 2789
Premarin Vaginal Cream 2791
Premphase 2797
Prempro 2801

Estrogens, Esterified (Increased metabolism of estradiol). Products include:
ESTRATAB Tablets (0.3, 0.625, 1.25, 2.5 mg) 2536
Estratest 2539
Menest Tablets 2494

Estropipate (Increased metabolism of estradiol). Products include:
Ogen Tablets 2627
Ogen Vaginal Cream 2630
Ortho-Est 1869

Ethchlorvynol (Additive CNS depressant effects). Products include:
Placidyl Capsules 448

Ethinamate (Additive CNS depressant effects).
No products indexed under this heading.

Ethinyl Estradiol (Increased metabolism of estradiol). Products include:
Brevicon 2088
Demulen 2428
Desogen Tablets 1817
Levlen/Tri-Levlen 651
Lo/Ovral Tablets 2746
Lo/Ovral-28 Tablets 2751
Modicon 1872
Nordette-21 Tablets 2755
Nordette-28 Tablets 2758
Norinyl 2088
Ortho-Cept 1851
Ortho-Cyclen/Ortho-Tri-Cyclen 1858
Ortho-Novum 1872
Ortho-Cyclen/Ortho Tri-Cyclen 1858
Ovcon 760
Ovral Tablets 2770
Ovral-28 Tablets 2770
Levlen/Tri-Levlen 651
Tri-Norinyl 2164
Triphasil-21 Tablets 2814
Triphasil-28 Tablets 2819

Ethynodiol Diacetate (Increased metabolism of estradiol). Products include:
Demulen 2428

Fentanyl (Additive CNS depressant effects). Products include:
Duragesic Transdermal System 1288

Fentanyl Citrate (Additive CNS depressant effects). Products include:
Sublimaze Injection 1307

Fludrocortisone Acetate (Enhanced metabolism of corticosteroids; dosage adjustment may be necessary). Products include:
Florinef Acetate Tablets 505

Fluphenazine Decanoate (Additive CNS depressant effects). Products include:
Prolixin Decanoate 509

Fluphenazine Enanthate (Additive CNS depressant effects). Products include:
Prolixin Enanthate 509

Fluphenazine Hydrochloride (Additive CNS depressant effects). Products include:
Prolixin 509

Flurazepam Hydrochloride (Additive CNS depressant effects). Products include:
Dalmane Capsules 2173

Furazolidone (Prolonged barbiturate effects). Products include:
Furoxone 2046

Glutethimide (Additive CNS depressant effects).
No products indexed under this heading.

Griseofulvin (Decreased griseofulvin blood levels). Products include:
Fulvicin P/G Tablets 2359
Fulvicin P/G 165 & 330 Tablets 2359
Grifulvin V (griseofulvin tablets) Microsize (griseofulvin oral suspension) Microsize 1888
Gris-PEG Tablets, 125 mg & 250 mg 479

Haloperidol (Additive CNS depressant effects). Products include:
Haldol Injection, Tablets and Concentrate 1575

Haloperidol Decanoate (Additive CNS depressant effects). Products include:
Haldol Decanoate 1577

Heparin Calcium (Decreased anticoagulant response).
No products indexed under this heading.

Heparin Sodium (Decreased anticoagulant response). Products include:
Heparin Lock Flush Solution 2725
Heparin Sodium Injection 2726
Heparin Sodium Injection, USP, Sterile Solution 2615
Heparin Sodium Vials 1441

Hydrocodone Bitartrate (Additive CNS depressant effects). Products include:
Anexsia 5/500 Elixir 1781
Anexia Tablets 1782
Codiclear DH Syrup 791
Deconamine CX Cough and Cold Liquid and Tablets 1319
Duratuss HD Elixir 2565
Hycodan Tablets and Syrup 930
Hycomine Compound Tablets 932
Hycomine 931
Hycotuss Expectorant Syrup 933
Hydrocet Capsules 782
Lorcet 10/650 1018
Lortab 2566
Tussend 1783
Tussend Expectorant 1785
Vicodin Tablets 1356
Vicodin ES Tablets 1357
Vicodin Tuss Expectorant 1358
Zydone Capsules 949

Hydrocodone Polistirex (Additive CNS depressant effects). Products include:
Tussionex Pennkinetic Extended-Release Suspension 998

(⊡ Described in PDR For Nonprescription Drugs) (⊙ Described in PDR For Ophthalmology)

Interactions Index — Butisol Sodium

Hydrocortisone (Enhanced metabolism of corticosteroids; dosage adjustment may be necessary). Products include:

Anusol-HC Cream 2.5% 1896
Aquanil HC Lotion 1931
Bactine Hydrocortisone Anti-Itch Cream .... ⊕ 709
Caldecort Anti-Itch Hydrocortisone Spray .... ⊕ 631
Cortaid .... ⊕ 836
CORTENEMA 2535
Cortisporin Ointment 1085
Cortisporin Ophthalmic Ointment Sterile 1085
Cortisporin Ophthalmic Suspension Sterile 1086
Cortisporin Otic Solution Sterile 1087
Cortisporin Otic Suspension Sterile 1088
Cortizone-5 .... ⊕ 831
Cortizone-10 .... ⊕ 831
Hydrocortone Tablets 1672
Hytone 907
Massengill Medicated Soft Cloth Towelettes 2458
PediOtic Suspension Sterile 1153
Preparation H Hydrocortisone 1% Cream .... ⊕ 872
ProctoCream-HC 2.5% 2408
VōSoL HC Otic Solution 2678

Hydrocortisone Acetate (Enhanced metabolism of corticosteroids; dosage adjustment may be necessary). Products include:

Analpram-HC Rectal Cream 1% and 2.5% 977
Anusol HC-1 Anti-Itch Hydrocortisone Ointment .... ⊕ 847
Anusol-HC Suppositories 1897
Caldecort .... ⊕ 631
Carmol HC 924
Coly-Mycin S Otic w/Neomycin & Hydrocortisone 1906
Cortaid .... ⊕ 836
Cortifoam 2396
Cortisporin Cream 1084
Epifoam 2399
Hydrocortone Acetate Sterile Suspension 1669
Mantadil Cream 1135
Nupercainal Hydrocortisone 1% Cream .... ⊕ 645
Ophthocort .... ⊙ 311
Pramosone Cream, Lotion & Ointment 978
ProctoCream-HC 2408
ProctoFoam-HC 2409
Terra-Cortril Ophthalmic Suspension 2210

Hydrocortisone Sodium Phosphate (Enhanced metabolism of corticosteroids; dosage adjustment may be necessary). Products include:

Hydrocortone Phosphate Injection, Sterile 1670

Hydrocortisone Sodium Succinate (Enhanced metabolism of corticosteroids; dosage adjustment may be necessary). Products include:

Solu-Cortef Sterile Powder 2641

Hydroxyzine Hydrochloride (Additive CNS depressant effects). Products include:

Atarax Tablets & Syrup 2185
Marax Tablets & DF Syrup 2200
Vistaril Intramuscular Solution 2216

Isocarboxazid (Prolonged barbiturate effects).

No products indexed under this heading.

Isoflurane (Additive CNS depressant effects).

No products indexed under this heading.

Ketamine Hydrochloride (Additive CNS depressant effects).

No products indexed under this heading.

Levomethadyl Acetate Hydrochloride (Additive CNS depressant effects). Products include:

Orlamm 2239

Levonorgestrel (Increased metabolism of estradiol). Products include:

Levlen/Tri-Levlen 651
Nordette-21 Tablets 2755
Nordette-28 Tablets 2758
Norplant System 2759
Levlen/Tri-Levlen 651
Triphasil-21 Tablets 2814
Triphasil-28 Tablets 2819

Levorphanol Tartrate (Additive CNS depressant effects). Products include:

Levo-Dromoran 2129

Loratadine (Additive CNS depressant effects). Products include:

Claritin 2349
Claritin-D 2350

Lorazepam (Additive CNS depressant effects). Products include:

Ativan Injection 2698
Ativan Tablets 2700

Loxapine Hydrochloride (Additive CNS depressant effects). Products include:

Loxitane 1378

Loxapine Succinate (Additive CNS depressant effects). Products include:

Loxitane Capsules 1378

Meperidine Hydrochloride (Additive CNS depressant effects). Products include:

Demerol 2308
Mepergan Injection 2753

Mephobarbital (Additive CNS depressant effects). Products include:

Mebaral Tablets 2322

Meprobamate (Additive CNS depressant effects). Products include:

Miltown Tablets 2672
PMB 200 and PMB 400 2783

Mesoridazine Besylate (Additive CNS depressant effects). Products include:

Serentil 684

Mestranol (Increased metabolism of estradiol). Products include:

Norinyl 2088
Ortho-Novum 1872

Methadone Hydrochloride (Additive CNS depressant effects). Products include:

Methadone Hydrochloride Oral Concentrate 2233
Methadone Hydrochloride Oral Solution & Tablets 2235

Methdilazine Hydrochloride (Additive CNS depressant effects).

No products indexed under this heading.

Methohexital Sodium (Additive CNS depressant effects). Products include:

Brevital Sodium Vials 1429

Methotrimeprazine (Additive CNS depressant effects). Products include:

Levoprome 1274

Methoxyflurane (Additive CNS depressant effects).

No products indexed under this heading.

Methylprednisolone (Enhanced metabolism of corticosteroids; dosage adjustment may be necessary). Products include:

Medrol 2621

Methylprednisolone Acetate (Enhanced metabolism of corticosteroids; dosage adjustment may be necessary). Products include:

Depo-Medrol Single-Dose Vial 2600
Depo-Medrol Sterile Aqueous Suspension 2597

Methylprednisolone Sodium Succinate (Enhanced metabolism of corticosteroids; dosage adjustment may be necessary). Products include:

Solu-Medrol Sterile Powder 2643

Midazolam Hydrochloride (Additive CNS depressant effects). Products include:

Versed Injection 2170

Molindone Hydrochloride (Additive CNS depressant effects). Products include:

Moban Tablets and Concentrate 1048

Morphine Sulfate (Additive CNS depressant effects). Products include:

Astramorph/PF Injection, USP (Preservative-Free) 535
Duramorph 962
Infumorph 200 and Infumorph 500 Sterile Solutions 965
MS Contin Tablets 1994
MSIR 1997
Oramorph SR (Morphine Sulfate Sustained Release Tablets) 2236
RMS Suppositories 2657
Roxanol 2243

Norethindrone (Increased metabolism of estradiol). Products include:

Brevicon 2088
Micronor Tablets 1872
Modicon 1872
Norinyl 2088
Nor-Q D Tablets 2135
Ortho-Novum 1872
Ovcon 760
Tri-Norinyl 2164

Norethynodrel (Increased metabolism of estradiol).

No products indexed under this heading.

Norgestimate (Increased metabolism of estradiol). Products include:

Ortho-Cyclen/Ortho-Tri-Cyclen 1858
Ortho-Cyclen/Ortho Tri-Cyclen 1858

Norgestrel (Increased metabolism of estradiol). Products include:

Lo/Ovral Tablets 2746
Lo/Ovral-28 Tablets 2751
Ovral Tablets 2770
Ovral-28 Tablets 2770
Ovrette Tablets 2771

Opium Alkaloids (Additive CNS depressant effects).

No products indexed under this heading.

Oxazepam (Additive CNS depressant effects). Products include:

Serax Capsules 2810
Serax Tablets 2810

Oxycodone Hydrochloride (Additive CNS depressant effects). Products include:

Percocet Tablets 938
Percodan Tablets 939
Percodan-Demi Tablets 940
Roxicodone Tablets, Oral Solution & Intensol (Oxycodone) 2244
Tylox Capsules 1584

Pentobarbital Sodium (Additive CNS depressant effects). Products include:

Nembutal Sodium Capsules 436
Nembutal Sodium Solution 438
Nembutal Sodium Suppositories 440

Perphenazine (Additive CNS depressant effects). Products include:

Etrafon 2355
Triavil Tablets 1757
Trilafon 2389

Phenelzine Sulfate (Prolonged barbiturate effects). Products include:

Nardil 1920

Phenobarbital (Additive CNS depressant effects). Products include:

Arco-Lase Plus Tablets 512
Bellergal-S Tablets 2250
Donnatal 2060
Donnatal Extentabs 2061

Donnatal Tablets 2060
Phenobarbital Elixir and Tablets 1469
Quadrinal Tablets 1350

Phenprocoumon (Decreased anticoagulant effect).

Phenytoin (Variable effect on phenytoin metabolism). Products include:

Dilantin Infatabs 1908
Dilantin-125 Suspension 1911

Phenytoin Sodium (Variable effect on phenytoin metabolism). Products include:

Dilantin Kapseals 1906
Dilantin Parenteral 1910

Polyestradiol Phosphate (Increased metabolism of estradiol).

No products indexed under this heading.

Prazepam (Additive CNS depressant effects).

No products indexed under this heading.

Prednisolone Acetate (Enhanced metabolism of corticosteroids; dosage adjustment may be necessary). Products include:

AK-CIDE .... ⊙ 202
AK-CIDE Ointment .... ⊙ 202
Blephamide Liquifilm Sterile Ophthalmic Suspension 476
Blephamide Ointment .... ⊙ 237
Econopred & Econopred Plus Ophthalmic Suspensions .... ⊙ 217
Poly-Pred Liquifilm .... ⊙ 248
Pred Forte .... ⊙ 250
Pred Mild .... ⊙ 253
Pred-G Liquifilm Sterile Ophthalmic Suspension .... ⊙ 251
Pred-G S.O.P. Sterile Ophthalmic Ointment .... ⊙ 252
Vasocidin Ointment .... ⊙ 268

Prednisolone Sodium Phosphate (Enhanced metabolism of corticosteroids; dosage adjustment may be necessary). Products include:

AK-Pred .... ⊙ 204
Hydeltrasol Injection, Sterile 1665
Inflamase .... ⊙ 265
Pediapred Oral Liquid 995
Vasocidin Ophthalmic Solution .... ⊙ 270

Prednisolone Tebutate (Enhanced metabolism of corticosteroids; dosage adjustment may be necessary). Products include:

Hydeltra-T.B.A. Sterile Suspension 1667

Prednisone (Enhanced metabolism of corticosteroids; dosage adjustment may be necessary). Products include:

Deltasone Tablets 2595

Prochlorperazine (Additive CNS depressant effects). Products include:

Compazine 2470

Promethazine Hydrochloride (Additive CNS depressant effects). Products include:

Mepergan Injection 2753
Phenergan with Codeine 2777
Phenergan with Dextromethorphan 2778
Phenergan Injection 2773
Phenergan Suppositories 2775
Phenergan Syrup 2774
Phenergan Tablets 2775
Phenergan VC 2779
Phenergan VC with Codeine 2781

Propofol (Additive CNS depressant effects). Products include:

Diprivan Injection 2833

Propoxyphene Hydrochloride (Additive CNS depressant effects). Products include:

Darvon 1435
Wygesic Tablets 2827

Propoxyphene Napsylate (Additive CNS depressant effects). Products include:

Darvon-N/Darvocet-N 1433

IMPORTANT NOTE: Always consult each drug listing in the patient's regimen for possible interactions.

Pyrilamine Maleate (Additive CNS depressant effects). Products include:
- 4-Way Fast Acting Nasal Spray (regular & mentholated) .... ▣ 621
- Maximum Strength Multi-Symptom Formula Midol .... ▣ 722
- PMS Multi-Symptom Formula Midol .... ▣ 723

Pyrilamine Tannate (Additive CNS depressant effects). Products include:
- Atrohist Pediatric Suspension 454
- Rynatan 2673

Quazepam (Additive CNS depressant effects). Products include:
- Doral Tablets 2664

Quinestrol (Increased metabolism of estradiol).
- No products indexed under this heading.

Risperidone (Additive CNS depressant effects). Products include:
- Risperdal 1301

Secobarbital Sodium (Additive CNS depressant effects). Products include:
- Seconal Sodium Pulvules 1474

Selegiline Hydrochloride (Prolonged barbiturate effects). Products include:
- Eldepryl Tablets 2550

Sodium Valproate (Decreased barbiturate metabolism).

Sufentanil Citrate (Additive CNS depressant effects). Products include:
- Sufenta Injection 1309

Temazepam (Additive CNS depressant effects). Products include:
- Restoril Capsules 2284

Terfenadine (Additive CNS depressant effects). Products include:
- Seldane Tablets 1536
- Seldane-D Extended-Release Tablets 1538

Thiamylal Sodium (Additive CNS depressant effects).
- No products indexed under this heading.

Thioridazine Hydrochloride (Additive CNS depressant effects). Products include:
- Mellaril 2269

Thiothixene (Additive CNS depressant effects). Products include:
- Navane Capsules and Concentrate 2201
- Navane Intramuscular 2202

Tranylcypromine Sulfate (Prolonged barbiturate effects). Products include:
- Parnate Tablets 2503

Triamcinolone (Enhanced metabolism of corticosteroids; dosage adjustment may be necessary). Products include:
- Aristocort Tablets 1022

Triamcinolone Acetonide (Enhanced metabolism of corticosteroids; dosage adjustment may be necessary). Products include:
- Aristocort A 0.025% Cream 1027
- Aristocort A 0.5% Cream 1031
- Aristocort A 0.1% Cream 1029
- Aristocort A 0.1% Ointment 1030
- Azmacort Oral Inhaler 2011
- Nasacort Nasal Inhaler 2024

Triamcinolone Diacetate (Enhanced metabolism of corticosteroids; dosage adjustment may be necessary). Products include:
- Aristocort Suspension (Forte Parenteral) 1027
- Aristocort Suspension (Intralesional) 1025

Triamcinolone Hexacetonide (Enhanced metabolism of corticosteroids; dosage adjustment may be necessary). Products include:
- Aristospan Suspension (Intra-articular) 1033
- Aristospan Suspension (Intralesional) 1032

Triazolam (Additive CNS depressant effects). Products include:
- Halcion Tablets 2611

Trifluoperazine Hydrochloride (Additive CNS depressant effects). Products include:
- Stelazine 2514

Trimeprazine Tartrate (Additive CNS depressant effects). Products include:
- Temaril Tablets, Syrup and Spansule Extended-Release Capsules .. 483

Tripelennamine Hydrochloride (Additive CNS depressant effects). Products include:
- PBZ Tablets 845
- PBZ-SR Tablets 844

Triprolidine Hydrochloride (Additive CNS depressant effects). Products include:
- Actifed Plus Caplets .... ▣ 845
- Actifed Plus Tablets .... ▣ 845
- Actifed with Codeine Cough Syrup .. 1067
- Actifed Syrup .... ▣ 846
- Actifed Tablets .... ▣ 844

Valproic Acid (Decreased barbiturate metabolism). Products include:
- Depakene 413

Warfarin Sodium (Decreased anticoagulant response). Products include:
- Coumadin 926

Zolpidem Tartrate (Additive CNS depressant effects). Products include:
- Ambien Tablets 2416

Food Interactions

Alcohol (Additive CNS depressant effects).

CAFERGOT SUPPOSITORIES

(Ergotamine Tartrate, Caffeine) 2251
See **Cafergot Tablets**

CAFERGOT TABLETS

(Ergotamine Tartrate, Caffeine) 2251
May interact with vasopressors, macrolide antibiotics, and certain other agents. Compounds in these categories include:

Azithromycin (Elevates blood levels; potential for vasospastic reactions). Products include:
- Zithromax 1944

Clarithromycin (Elevates blood levels; potential for vasospastic reactions). Products include:
- Biaxin 405

Dopamine Hydrochloride (Potential for extreme hypertension; concurrent administration should be avoided).
- No products indexed under this heading.

Epinephrine Bitartrate (Potential for extreme hypertension; concurrent administration should be avoided). Products include:
- Bronkaid Mist Suspension .... ▣ 718
- Sensorcaine-MPF with Epinephrine Injection 559

Epinephrine Hydrochloride (Potential for extreme hypertension; concurrent administration should be avoided). Products include:
- Ana-Kit Anaphylaxis Emergency Treatment Kit 617

Erythromycin (Elevates blood levels; potential for vasospastic reactions). Products include:
- A/T/S 2% Acne Topical Gel and Solution 1234
- Benzamycin Topical Gel 905
- E-Mycin Tablets 1341
- Emgel 2% Topical Gel 1093
- ERYC 1915
- Erycette (erythromycin 2%) Topical Solution 1888
- Ery-Tab Tablets 422
- Erythromycin Base Filmtab 426
- Erythromycin Delayed-Release Capsules, USP 427
- Ilotycin Ophthalmic Ointment 912
- PCE Dispertab Tablets 444
- T-Stat 2.0% Topical Solution and Pads 2688
- Theramycin Z Topical Solution 2% 1592

Erythromycin Estolate (Elevates blood levels; potential for vasospastic reactions). Products include:
- Ilosone 911

Erythromycin Ethylsuccinate (Elevates blood levels; potential for vasospastic reactions). Products include:
- E.E.S. 424
- EryPed 421

Erythromycin Gluceptate (Elevates blood levels; potential for vasospastic reactions). Products include:
- Ilotycin Gluceptate, IV, Vials 913

Erythromycin Stearate (Elevates blood levels; potential for vasospastic reactions). Products include:
- Erythrocin Stearate Filmtab 425

Metaraminol Bitartrate (Potential for extreme hypertension; concurrent administration should be avoided). Products include:
- Aramine Injection 1609

Methoxamine Hydrochloride (Potential for extreme hypertension; concurrent administration should be avoided). Products include:
- Vasoxyl Injection 1196

Nicotine (Provokes vasoconstriction in some patients; predisposing to a greater ischemic response). Products include:
- Habitrol Nicotine Transdermal System 865
- Nicoderm (nicotine transdermal system) 1518
- Nicotrol Nicotine Transdermal System 1550
- Prostep (nicotine transdermal system) 1394

Nicotine Polacrilex (Provokes vasoconstriction in some patients; predisposing to a greater ischemic response). Products include:
- Nicorette 2458

Norepinephrine Bitartrate (Potential for extreme hypertension; concurrent administration should be avoided). Products include:
- Levophed Bitartrate Injection 2315

Phenylephrine Hydrochloride (Potential for extreme hypertension; concurrent administration should be avoided). Products include:
- Atrohist Plus Tablets 454
- Cerose DM .... ▣ 878
- Comhist 2038
- D.A. Chewable Tablets 951
- Deconsal Pediatric Capsules 454
- Dura-Vent/DA Tablets 953
- Entex Capsules 1986
- Entex Liquid 1986
- Extendryl 1005
- 4-Way Fast Acting Nasal Spray (regular & mentholated) .... ▣ 621
- Hemorid For Women .... ▣ 834
- Hycomine Compound Tablets 932
- Neo-Synephrine Hydrochloride 1% Carpuject 2324
- Neo-Synephrine Hydrochloride 1% Injection 2324
- Neo-Synephrine Hydrochloride (Ophthalmic) 2325
- Neo-Synephrine .... ▣ 726
- Nōstril .... ▣ 644
- Novahistine Elixir .... ▣ 823
- Phenergan VC 2779
- Phenergan VC with Codeine 2781
- Preparation H .... ▣ 871
- Tympagesic Ear Drops 2342
- Vasosulf .... ⊙ 271
- Vicks Sinex Nasal Spray and Ultra Fine Mist .... ▣ 765

Propranolol Hydrochloride (Potentiates vasoconstrictive action). Products include:
- Inderal 2728
- Inderal LA Long Acting Capsules 2730
- Inderide Tablets 2732
- Inderide LA Long Acting Capsules .. 2734

Troleandomycin (Elevates blood levels; potential for vasospastic reactions). Products include:
- Tao Capsules 2209

CALADRYL CLEAR LOTION

(Pramoxine Hydrochloride, Zinc Acetate) .... ▣ 853
None cited in PDR database.

CALADRYL CREAM FOR KIDS

(Calamine, Pramoxine Hydrochloride) .... ▣ 853
None cited in PDR database.

CALADRYL LOTION

(Calamine, Pramoxine Hydrochloride) .... ▣ 853
None cited in PDR database.

CALAN SR CAPLETS

(Verapamil Hydrochloride) 2422
May interact with beta blockers, lithium preparations, nondepolarizing neuromuscular blocking agents, inhalant anesthetics, alpha adrenergic blockers, cardiac glycosides, diuretics, ACE inhibitors, vasodilators, and certain other agents. Compounds in these categories include:

Acebutolol Hydrochloride (Additive effect on lowering blood pressure; additive negative effects on heart rate, atrioventricular conduction, and/or cardiac contractility). Products include:
- Sectral Capsules 2807

Amiloride Hydrochloride (Additive effect on lowering blood pressure). Products include:
- Midamor Tablets 1703
- Moduretic Tablets 1705

Aminophylline (Verapamil may inhibit the clearance and increase the plasma levels of theophylline).
- No products indexed under this heading.

Atenolol (Additive effect on lowering blood pressure; additive negative effects on heart rate, atrioventricular conduction, and/or cardiac contractility; variable effect in atenolol clearance). Products include:
- Tenoretic Tablets 2845
- Tenormin Tablets and I.V. Injection 2847

Atracurium Besylate (Activity of neuromuscular blocking agents potentiated). Products include:
- Tracrium Injection 1183

Benazepril Hydrochloride (Additive effect on lowering blood pressure). Products include:
- Lotensin Tablets 834
- Lotensin HCT 837
- Lotrel Capsules 840

Bendroflumethiazide (Additive effect on lowering blood pressure).
- No products indexed under this heading.

(▣ Described in PDR For Nonprescription Drugs) (⊙ Described in PDR For Ophthalmology)

153 **Interactions Index** **Calan SR Caplets**

Betaxolol Hydrochloride (Additive effect on lowering blood pressure; additive negative effects on heart rate, atrioventricular conduction, and/or cardiac contractility). Products include:
Betoptic Ophthalmic Solution ... 469
Betoptic S Ophthalmic Suspension 471
Kerlone Tablets ... 2436

Bisoprolol Fumarate (Additive effect on lowering blood pressure; additive negative effects on heart rate, atrioventricular conduction, and/or cardiac contractility). Products include:
Zebeta Tablets ... 1413
Ziac ... 1415

Bumetanide (Additive effect on lowering blood pressure). Products include:
Bumex ... 2093

Captopril (Additive effect on lowering blood pressure). Products include:
Capoten ... 739
Capozide ... 742

Carbamazepine (Increased concentrations of carbamazepine). Products include:
Atretol Tablets ... 573
Tegretol Chewable Tablets ... 852
Tegretol Suspension ... 852
Tegretol Tablets ... 852

Carteolol Hydrochloride (Additive effect on lowering blood pressure; additive negative effects on heart rate, atrioventricular conduction, and/or cardiac contractility). Products include:
Cartrol Tablets ... 410
Ocupress Ophthalmic Solution, 1% Sterile ... ⊚ 309

Chlorothiazide (Additive effect on lowering blood pressure). Products include:
Aldoclor Tablets ... 1598
Diupres Tablets ... 1650
Diuril Oral ... 1653

Chlorothiazide Sodium (Additive effect on lowering blood pressure). Products include:
Diuril Sodium Intravenous ... 1652

Chlorthalidone (Additive effect on lowering blood pressure). Products include:
Combipres Tablets ... 677
Tenoretic Tablets ... 2845
Thalitone ... 1245

Cimetidine (Possible reduction in verapamil clearance). Products include:
Tagamet Tablets ... 2516

Cimetidine Hydrochloride (Possible reduction in verapamil clearance). Products include:
Tagamet ... 2516

Clonidine (Additive effect on lowering blood pressure). Products include:
Catapres-TTS ... 675

Clonidine Hydrochloride (Additive effect on lowering blood pressure). Products include:
Catapres Tablets ... 674
Combipres Tablets ... 677

Cyclosporine (Possible increase in serum levels of cyclosporine). Products include:
Neoral ... 2276
Sandimmune ... 2286

Desflurane (Excessive cardiovascular depression). Products include:
Suprane ... 1813

Deslanoside (Chronic verapamil treatment can increase serum digoxin levels and this can result in digitalis toxicity).
No products indexed under this heading.

Diazoxide (Additive effect on lowering blood pressure). Products include:
Hyperstat I.V. Injection ... 2363
Proglycem ... 580

Digitoxin (Chronic verapamil treatment can increase serum digoxin levels and this can result in digitalis toxicity). Products include:
Crystodigin Tablets ... 1433

Digoxin (Chronic verapamil treatment can increase serum digoxin levels and this can result in digitalis toxicity). Products include:
Lanoxicaps ... 1117
Lanoxin Elixir Pediatric ... 1120
Lanoxin Injection ... 1123
Lanoxin Injection Pediatric ... 1126
Lanoxin Tablets ... 1128

Disopyramide Phosphate (Do not administer concomitantly). Products include:
Norpace ... 2444

Doxazosin Mesylate (May result in a reduction in blood pressure that is excessive in some patients). Products include:
Cardura Tablets ... 2186

Dyphylline (Verapamil may inhibit the clearance and increase the plasma levels of theophylline). Products include:
Lufyllin & Lufyllin-400 Tablets ... 2670
Lufyllin-GG Elixir & Tablets ... 2671

Enalapril Maleate (Additive effect on lowering blood pressure). Products include:
Vaseretic Tablets ... 1765
Vasotec Tablets ... 1771

Enalaprilat (Additive effect on lowering blood pressure). Products include:
Vasotec I.V. ... 1768

Enflurane (Excessive cardiovascular depression).
No products indexed under this heading.

Esmolol Hydrochloride (Additive effect on lowering blood pressure; additive negative effects on heart rate, atrioventricular conduction, and/or cardiac contractility). Products include:
Brevibloc Injection ... 1808

Ethacrynic Acid (Additive effect on lowering blood pressure). Products include:
Edecrin Tablets ... 1657

Flecainide Acetate (Possible additive effects on myocardial contractility, AV conduction, and repolarization). Products include:
Tambocor Tablets ... 1497

Fosinopril Sodium (Additive effect on lowering blood pressure). Products include:
Monopril Tablets ... 757

Furosemide (Additive effect on lowering blood pressure). Products include:
Lasix Injection, Oral Solution and Tablets ... 1240

Guanabenz Acetate (Additive effect on lowering blood pressure).
No products indexed under this heading.

Guanadrel Sulfate (Additive effect on lowering blood pressure). Products include:
Hylorel Tablets ... 985

Guanethidine Monosulfate (Additive effect on lowering blood pressure). Products include:
Esimil Tablets ... 822
Ismelin Tablets ... 827

Halothane (Excessive cardiovascular depression). Products include:
Fluothane ... 2724

Hydralazine Hydrochloride (Additive effect on lowering blood pressure). Products include:
Apresazide Capsules ... 808
Apresoline Hydrochloride Tablets .. 809
Ser-Ap-Es Tablets ... 849

Hydrochlorothiazide (Additive effect on lowering blood pressure). Products include:
Aldactazide ... 2413
Aldoril Tablets ... 1604
Apresazide Capsules ... 808
Capozide ... 742
Dyazide ... 2479
Esidrix Tablets ... 821
Esimil Tablets ... 822
HydroDIURIL Tablets ... 1674
Hydropres Tablets ... 1675
Hyzaar Tablets ... 1677
Inderide Tablets ... 2732
Inderide LA Long Acting Capsules .. 2734
Lopressor HCT Tablets ... 832
Lotensin HCT ... 837
Maxzide ... 1380
Moduretic Tablets ... 1705
Oretic Tablets ... 443
Prinzide Tablets ... 1737
Ser-Ap-Es Tablets ... 849
Timolide Tablets ... 1748
Vaseretic Tablets ... 1765
Zestoretic ... 2850
Ziac ... 1415

Hydroflumethiazide (Additive effect on lowering blood pressure). Products include:
Diucardin Tablets ... 2718

Indapamide (Additive effect on lowering blood pressure). Products include:
Lozol Tablets ... 2022

Isoflurane (Excessive cardiovascular depression).
No products indexed under this heading.

Labetalol Hydrochloride (Additive effect on lowering blood pressure; additive negative effects on heart rate, atrioventricular conduction, and/or cardiac contractility). Products include:
Normodyne Injection ... 2377
Normodyne Tablets ... 2379
Trandate ... 1185

Levobunolol Hydrochloride (Additive effect on lowering blood pressure; additive negative effects on heart rate, atrioventricular conduction, and/or cardiac contractility). Products include:
Betagan ... ⊚ 233

Lisinopril (Additive effect on lowering blood pressure). Products include:
Prinivil Tablets ... 1733
Prinzide Tablets ... 1737
Zestoretic ... 2850
Zestril Tablets ... 2854

Lithium Carbonate (Possible lowering of serum lithium levels; possible increased sensitivity to effects of lithium). Products include:
Eskalith ... 2485
Lithium Carbonate Capsules & Tablets ... 2230
Lithonate/Lithotabs/Lithobid ... 2543

Lithium Citrate (Possible lowering of serum lithium levels; possible increased sensitivity to effects of lithium).
No products indexed under this heading.

Mecamylamine Hydrochloride (Additive effect on lowering blood pressure). Products include:
Inversine Tablets ... 1686

Methoxyflurane (Excessive cardiovascular depression).
No products indexed under this heading.

Methyclothiazide (Additive effect on lowering blood pressure). Products include:
Enduron Tablets ... 420

Methyldopa (Additive effect on lowering blood pressure). Products include:
Aldoclor Tablets ... 1598
Aldomet Oral ... 1600
Aldoril Tablets ... 1604

Methyldopate Hydrochloride (Additive effect on lowering blood pressure). Products include:
Aldomet Ester HCl Injection ... 1602

Metipranolol Hydrochloride (Additive effect on lowering blood pressure; additive negative effects on heart rate, atrioventricular conduction, and/or cardiac contractility). Products include:
OptiPranolol (Metipranolol 0.3%) Sterile Ophthalmic Solution ... ⊚ 258

Metocurine Iodide (Activity of neuromuscular blocking agents potentiated). Products include:
Metubine Iodide Vials ... 916

Metolazone (Additive effect on lowering blood pressure). Products include:
Mykrox Tablets ... 993
Zaroxolyn Tablets ... 1000

Metoprolol Succinate (Additive effect on lowering blood pressure; additive negative effects on heart rate, atrioventricular conduction, and/or cardiac contractility). Products include:
Toprol-XL Tablets ... 565

Metoprolol Tartrate (Additive effect on lowering blood pressure; additive negative effects on heart rate, atrioventricular conduction, and/or cardiac contractility; decrease in metoprolol clearance). Products include:
Lopressor Ampuls ... 830
Lopressor HCT Tablets ... 832
Lopressor Tablets ... 830

Metyrosine (Additive effect on lowering blood pressure). Products include:
Demser Capsules ... 1649

Minoxidil (Additive effect on lowering blood pressure). Products include:
Loniten Tablets ... 2618
Rogaine Topical Solution ... 2637

Mivacurium Chloride (Activity of neuromuscular blocking agents potentiated). Products include:
Mivacron ... 1138

Moexipril Hydrochloride (Additive effect on lowering blood pressure). Products include:
Univasc Tablets ... 2410

Nadolol (Additive effect on lowering blood pressure; additive negative effects on heart rate, atrioventricular conduction, and/or cardiac contractility).
No products indexed under this heading.

Pancuronium Bromide Injection (Activity of neuromuscular blocking agents potentiated).
No products indexed under this heading.

Penbutolol Sulfate (Additive effect on lowering blood pressure; additive negative effects on heart rate, atrioventricular conduction, and/or cardiac contractility). Products include:
Levatol ... 2403

Phenobarbital (Verapamil clearance may be increased). Products include:
Arco-Lase Plus Tablets ... 512

IMPORTANT NOTE: Always consult each drug listing in the patient's regimen for possible interactions.

Bellergal-S Tablets 2250
Donnatal 2060
Donnatal Extentabs 2061
Donnatal Tablets 2060
Phenobarbital Elixir and Tablets 1469
Quadrinal Tablets 1350

Phenoxybenzamine Hydrochloride (Additive effect on lowering blood pressure). Products include:
Dibenzyline Capsules 2476

Phentolamine Mesylate (Additive effect on lowering blood pressure). Products include:
Regitine 846

Pindolol (Additive effect on lowering blood pressure; additive negative effects on heart rate, atrioventricular conduction, and/or cardiac contractility). Products include:
Visken Tablets 2299

Polythiazide (Additive effect on lowering blood pressure). Products include:
Minizide Capsules 1938

Prazosin Hydrochloride (May result in a reduction in blood pressure that is excessive in some patients). Products include:
Minipress Capsules 1937
Minizide Capsules 1938

Propranolol Hydrochloride (Additive effect on lowering blood pressure; additive negative effects on heart rate, atrioventricular conduction, and/or cardiac contractility; decrease in propranolol clearance). Products include:
Inderal 2728
Inderal LA Long Acting Capsules 2730
Inderide Tablets 2732
Inderide LA Long Acting Capsules 2734

Quinapril Hydrochloride (Additive effect on lowering blood pressure). Products include:
Accupril Tablets 1893

Quinidine Gluconate (Hypotension in patients with hypertrophic cardiomyopathy). Products include:
Quinaglute Dura-Tabs Tablets 649

Quinidine Polygalacturonate (Hypotension in patients with hypertrophic cardiomyopathy).
No products indexed under this heading.

Quinidine Sulfate (Hypotension in patients with hypertrophic cardiomyopathy). Products include:
Quinidex Extentabs 2067

Ramipril (Additive effect on lowering blood pressure). Products include:
Altace Capsules 1232

Rifampin (Reduced oral verapamil bioavailability). Products include:
Rifadin 1528
Rifamate Capsules 1530
Rifater 1532
Rimactane Capsules 847

Rocuronium Bromide (Activity of neuromuscular blocking agents potentiated). Products include:
Zemuron 1830

Sotalol Hydrochloride (Additive effect on lowering blood pressure; additive negative effects on heart rate, atrioventricular conduction, and/or cardiac contractility). Products include:
Betapace Tablets 641

Spirapril Hydrochloride (Additive effect on lowering blood pressure).
No products indexed under this heading.

Spironolactone (Additive effect on lowering blood pressure). Products include:
Aldactazide 2413
Aldactone 2414

Succinylcholine Chloride (Potentiation of neuromuscular blockers). Products include:
Anectine 1073

Terazosin Hydrochloride (May result in a reduction in blood pressure that is excessive in some patients). Products include:
Hytrin Capsules 430

Theophylline (Verapamil may inhibit the clearance and increase the plasma levels of theophylline). Products include:
Marax Tablets & DF Syrup 2200
Quibron 2053

Theophylline Anhydrous (Verapamil may inhibit the clearance and increase the plasma levels of theophylline). Products include:
Aerolate 1004
Primatene Dual Action Formula .... ▣ 872
Primatene Tablets .... ▣ 873
Respbid Tablets 682
Slo-bid Gyrocaps 2033
Theo-24 Extended Release Capsules 2568
Theo-Dur Extended-Release Tablets 1327
Theo-X Extended-Release Tablets 788
Uni-Dur Extended-Release Tablets 1331
Uniphyl 400 mg Tablets 2001

Theophylline Calcium Salicylate (Verapamil may inhibit the clearance and increase the plasma levels of theophylline). Products include:
Quadrinal Tablets 1350

Theophylline Sodium Glycinate (Verapamil may inhibit the clearance and increase the plasma levels of theophylline).
No products indexed under this heading.

Timolol Hemihydrate (Additive effect on lowering blood pressure; additive negative effects on heart rate, atrioventricular conduction, and/or cardiac contractility). Products include:
Betimol 0.25%, 0.5% .... ◉ 261

Timolol Maleate (Additive effect on lowering blood pressure; additive negative effects on heart rate, atrioventricular conduction, and/or cardiac contractility). Products include:
Blocadren Tablets 1614
Timolide Tablets 1748
Timoptic in Ocudose 1753
Timoptic Sterile Ophthalmic Solution 1751
Timoptic-XE 1755

Torsemide (Additive effect on lowering blood pressure). Products include:
Demadex Tablets and Injection 686

Triamterene (Additive effect on lowering blood pressure). Products include:
Dyazide 2479
Dyrenium Capsules 2481
Maxzide 1380

Vecuronium Bromide (Activity of neuromuscular blocking agents potentiated). Products include:
Norcuron 1826

Food Interactions

Food, unspecified (Produces decreased bioavailability (AUC) but a narrower peak-to-trough ratio).

CALAN TABLETS

(Verapamil Hydrochloride) 2419
May interact with beta blockers, cardiac glycosides, lithium preparations, diuretics, ACE inhibitors, vasodilators, nondepolarizing neuromuscular blocking agents, inhalant anesthetics, and certain other agents. Compounds in these categories include:

Acebutolol Hydrochloride (Additive negative effects on heart rate, AV conduction and/or cardiac contractility; additive hypotensive effect). Products include:
Sectral Capsules 2807

Amiloride Hydrochloride (Additive effect on lowering blood pressure). Products include:
Midamor Tablets 1703
Moduretic Tablets 1705

Aminophylline (Verapamil may inhibit the clearance and increase the plasma levels of theophylline).
No products indexed under this heading.

Atenolol (Additive negative effects on heart rate, AV conduction and/or cardiac contractility; additive hypotensive effect; variable effect in atenolol clearance). Products include:
Tenoretic Tablets 2845
Tenormin Tablets and I.V. Injection 2847

Atracurium Besylate (Activity of neuromuscular blocking agents potentiated). Products include:
Tracrium Injection 1183

Benazepril Hydrochloride (Additive effect on lowering blood pressure). Products include:
Lotensin Tablets 834
Lotensin HCT 837
Lotrel Capsules 840

Bendroflumethiazide (Additive effect on lowering blood pressure).
No products indexed under this heading.

Betaxolol Hydrochloride (Additive negative effects on heart rate, AV conduction and/or cardiac contractility; additive hypotensive effect). Products include:
Betoptic Ophthalmic Solution 469
Betoptic S Ophthalmic Suspension 471
Kerlone Tablets 2436

Bisoprolol Fumarate (Additive negative effects on heart rate, AV conduction and/or cardiac contractility; additive hypotensive effect). Products include:
Zebeta Tablets 1413
Ziac 1415

Bumetanide (Additive effect on lowering blood pressure). Products include:
Bumex 2093

Captopril (Additive effect on lowering blood pressure). Products include:
Capoten 739
Capozide 742

Carbamazepine (Increased carbamazepine concentrations). Products include:
Atretol Tablets 573
Tegretol Chewable Tablets 852
Tegretol Suspension 852
Tegretol Tablets 852

Carteolol Hydrochloride (Additive negative effects on heart rate, AV conduction, and/or cardiac contractility; additive hypotensive effect). Products include:
Cartrol Tablets 410
Ocupress Ophthalmic Solution, 1% Sterile .... ◉ 309

Chlorothiazide (Additive effect on lowering blood pressure). Products include:
Aldoclor Tablets 1598
Diupres Tablets 1650
Diuril Oral 1653

Chlorothiazide Sodium (Additive effect on lowering blood pressure). Products include:
Diuril Sodium Intravenous 1652

Chlorthalidone (Additive effect on lowering blood pressure). Products include:
Combipres Tablets 677
Tenoretic Tablets 2845
Thalitone 1245

Cimetidine (Possible reduction in verapamil clearance). Products include:
Tagamet Tablets 2516

Cimetidine Hydrochloride (Possible reduction in verapamil clearance). Products include:
Tagamet 2516

Clonidine (Additive effect on lowering blood pressure). Products include:
Catapres-TTS 675

Clonidine Hydrochloride (Additive effect on lowering blood pressure). Products include:
Catapres Tablets 674
Combipres Tablets 677

Cyclosporine (Possible increase in serum levels of cyclosporine). Products include:
Neoral 2276
Sandimmune 2286

Desflurane (Excessive cardiovascular depression). Products include:
Suprane 1813

Deslanoside (Chronic verapamil treatment can increase serum digoxin levels and this can result in digitalis toxicity).
No products indexed under this heading.

Diazoxide (Additive effect on lowering blood pressure). Products include:
Hyperstat I.V. Injection 2363
Proglycem 580

Digitoxin (Chronic verapamil treatment can increase serum digoxin levels and this can result in digitalis toxicity). Products include:
Crystodigin Tablets 1433

Digoxin (Chronic verapamil treatment can increase serum digoxin levels and this can result in digitalis toxicity). Products include:
Lanoxicaps 1117
Lanoxin Elixir Pediatric 1120
Lanoxin Injection 1123
Lanoxin Injection Pediatric 1126
Lanoxin Tablets 1128

Disopyramide Phosphate (Do not administer concomitantly). Products include:
Norpace 2444

Dyphylline (Verapamil may inhibit the clearance and increase the plasma levels of theophylline). Products include:
Lufyllin & Lufyllin-400 Tablets 2670
Lufyllin-GG Elixir & Tablets 2671

Enalapril Maleate (Additive effect on lowering blood pressure). Products include:
Vaseretic Tablets 1765
Vasotec Tablets 1771

Enalaprilat (Additive effect on lowering blood pressure). Products include:
Vasotec I.V. 1768

Enflurane (Excessive cardiovascular depression).
No products indexed under this heading.

(▣ Described in PDR For Nonprescription Drugs) (◉ Described in PDR For Ophthalmology)

155 Interactions Index Calan Tablets

Esmolol Hydrochloride (Additive negative effects on heart rate, AV conduction and/or cardiac contractility; additive hypotensive effect). Products include:
- Brevibloc Injection ... 1808

Ethacrynic Acid (Additive effect on lowering blood pressure). Products include:
- Edecrin Tablets ... 1657

Flecainide Acetate (Possible additive negative inotropic effect and prolongation of AV conduction). Products include:
- Tambocor Tablets ... 1497

Fosinopril Sodium (Additive effect on lowering blood pressure). Products include:
- Monopril Tablets ... 757

Furosemide (Additive effect on lowering blood pressure). Products include:
- Lasix Injection, Oral Solution and Tablets ... 1240

Guanabenz Acetate (Additive effect on lowering blood pressure).
- No products indexed under this heading.

Guanadrel Sulfate (Additive effect on lowering blood pressure). Products include:
- Hylorel Tablets ... 985

Guanethidine Monosulfate (Additive effect on lowering blood pressure). Products include:
- Esimil Tablets ... 822
- Ismelin Tablets ... 827

Halothane (Excessive cardiovascular depression). Products include:
- Fluothane ... 2724

Hydralazine Hydrochloride (Additive effect on lowering blood pressure). Products include:
- Apresazide Capsules ... 808
- Apresoline Hydrochloride Tablets ... 809
- Ser-Ap-Es Tablets ... 849

Hydrochlorothiazide (Additive effect on lowering blood pressure). Products include:
- Aldactazide ... 2413
- Aldoril Tablets ... 1604
- Apresazide Capsules ... 808
- Capozide ... 742
- Dyazide ... 2479
- Esidrix Tablets ... 821
- Esimil Tablets ... 822
- HydroDIURIL Tablets ... 1674
- Hydropres Tablets ... 1675
- Hyzaar Tablets ... 1677
- Inderide Tablets ... 2732
- Inderide LA Long Acting Capsules ... 2734
- Lopressor HCT Tablets ... 832
- Lotensin HCT ... 837
- Maxzide ... 1380
- Moduretic Tablets ... 1705
- Oretic Tablets ... 443
- Prinzide Tablets ... 1737
- Ser-Ap-Es Tablets ... 849
- Timolide Tablets ... 1748
- Vaseretic Tablets ... 1765
- Zestoretic ... 2850
- Ziac ... 1415

Hydroflumethiazide (Additive effect on lowering blood pressure). Products include:
- Diucardin Tablets ... 2718

Indapamide (Additive effect on lowering blood pressure). Products include:
- Lozol Tablets ... 2022

Isoflurane (Excessive cardiovascular depression).
- No products indexed under this heading.

Labetalol Hydrochloride (Additive negative effects on heart rate, AV conduction and/or cardiac contractility; additive hypotensive effect). Products include:
- Normodyne Injection ... 2377
- Normodyne Tablets ... 2379
- Trandate ... 1185

Levobunolol Hydrochloride (Additive negative effects on heart rate, AV conduction and/or cardiac contractility; additive hypotensive effect). Products include:
- Betagan ... ◉ 233

Lisinopril (Additive effect on lowering blood pressure). Products include:
- Prinivil Tablets ... 1733
- Prinzide Tablets ... 1737
- Zestoretic ... 2850
- Zestril Tablets ... 2854

Lithium Carbonate (May result in lowering of serum lithium levels and increased sensitivity to the effects of lithium). Products include:
- Eskalith ... 2485
- Lithium Carbonate Capsules & Tablets ... 2230
- Lithonate/Lithotabs/Lithobid ... 2543

Lithium Citrate (May result in lowering of serum lithium levels and increased sensitivity to the effects of lithium).
- No products indexed under this heading.

Mecamylamine Hydrochloride (Additive effect on lowering blood pressure). Products include:
- Inversine Tablets ... 1686

Methoxyflurane (Excessive cardiovascular depression).
- No products indexed under this heading.

Methyclothiazide (Additive effect on lowering blood pressure). Products include:
- Enduron Tablets ... 420

Methyldopa (Additive effect on lowering blood pressure). Products include:
- Aldoclor Tablets ... 1598
- Aldomet Oral ... 1600
- Aldoril Tablets ... 1604

Methyldopate Hydrochloride (Additive effect on lowering blood pressure). Products include:
- Aldomet Ester HCl Injection ... 1602

Metipranolol Hydrochloride (Additive negative effects on heart rate, AV conduction and/or cardiac contractility; additive hypotensive effect). Products include:
- OptiPranolol (Metipranolol 0.3%) Sterile Ophthalmic Solution ... ◉ 258

Metocurine Iodide (Activity of neuromuscular blocking agents potentiated). Products include:
- Metubine Iodide Vials ... 916

Metolazone (Additive effect on lowering blood pressure). Products include:
- Mykrox Tablets ... 993
- Zaroxolyn Tablets ... 1000

Metoprolol Succinate (Additive negative effects on heart rate, AV conduction and/or cardiac contractility; additive hypotensive effect). Products include:
- Toprol-XL Tablets ... 565

Metoprolol Tartrate (Additive negative effects on heart rate, AV conduction and/or cardiac contractility; additive hypotensive effect; decrease in metoprolol clearance). Products include:
- Lopressor Ampuls ... 830
- Lopressor HCT Tablets ... 832
- Lopressor Tablets ... 830

Metyrosine (Additive effect on lowering blood pressure). Products include:
- Demser Capsules ... 1649

Minoxidil (Additive effect on lowering blood pressure). Products include:
- Loniten Tablets ... 2618
- Rogaine Topical Solution ... 2637

Mivacurium Chloride (Activity of neuromuscular blocking agents potentiated). Products include:
- Mivacron ... 1138

Moexipril Hydrochloride (Additive effect on lowering blood pressure). Products include:
- Univasc Tablets ... 2410

Nadolol (Additive negative effects on heart rate, AV conduction and/or cardiac contractility; additive hypotensive effect).
- No products indexed under this heading.

Pancuronium Bromide Injection (Activity of neuromuscular blocking agents potentiated).
- No products indexed under this heading.

Pargyline Hydrochloride (Additive effect on lowering blood pressure).
- No products indexed under this heading.

Penbutolol Sulfate (Additive negative effects on heart rate, AV conduction, and/or cardiac contractility; additive hypotensive effect). Products include:
- Levatol ... 2403

Phenobarbital (Verapamil clearance may be increased). Products include:
- Arco-Lase Plus Tablets ... 512
- Bellergal-S Tablets ... 2250
- Donnatal ... 2060
- Donnatal Extentabs ... 2061
- Donnatal Tablets ... 2060
- Phenobarbital Elixir and Tablets ... 1469
- Quadrinal Tablets ... 1350

Phenoxybenzamine Hydrochloride (Additive effect on lowering blood pressure). Products include:
- Dibenzyline Capsules ... 2476

Phentolamine Mesylate (Additive effect on lowering blood pressure). Products include:
- Regitine ... 846

Pindolol (Additive negative effects on heart rate, AV conduction and/or cardiac contractility; additive hypotensive effect). Products include:
- Visken Tablets ... 2299

Polythiazide (Additive effect on lowering blood pressure). Products include:
- Minizide Capsules ... 1938

Prazosin Hydrochloride (May result in a reduction in blood pressure that is excessive in some patients). Products include:
- Minipress Capsules ... 1937
- Minizide Capsules ... 1938

Propranolol Hydrochloride (Additive negative effects on heart rate, AV conduction and/or cardiac contractility; additive hypotensive effect; decrease in propranolol clearance). Products include:
- Inderal ... 2728
- Inderal LA Long Acting Capsules ... 2730
- Inderide Tablets ... 2732
- Inderide LA Long Acting Capsules ... 2734

Quinapril Hydrochloride (Additive effect on lowering blood pressure). Products include:
- Accupril Tablets ... 1893

Quinidine Gluconate (Hypotension in patients with hypertrophic cardiomyopathy; increased quinidine levels). Products include:
- Quinaglute Dura-Tabs Tablets ... 649

Quinidine Polygalacturonate (Hypotension in patients with hypertrophic cardiomyopathy; increased quinidine levels).
- No products indexed under this heading.

Quinidine Sulfate (Hypotension in patients with hypertrophic cardiomyopathy; increased quinidine levels). Products include:
- Quinidex Extentabs ... 2067

Ramipril (Additive effect on lowering blood pressure). Products include:
- Altace Capsules ... 1232

Rifampin (Bioavailability of oral verapamil may be markedly reduced). Products include:
- Rifadin ... 1528
- Rifamate Capsules ... 1530
- Rifater ... 1532
- Rimactane Capsules ... 847

Rocuronium Bromide (Activity of neuromuscular blocking agents potentiated). Products include:
- Zemuron ... 1830

Sotalol Hydrochloride (Additive negative effects on heart rate, AV conduction and/or cardiac contractility; additive hypotensive effect). Products include:
- Betapace Tablets ... 641

Spirapril Hydrochloride (Additive effect on lowering blood pressure).
- No products indexed under this heading.

Spironolactone (Additive effect on lowering blood pressure). Products include:
- Aldactazide ... 2413
- Aldactone ... 2414

Succinylcholine Chloride (Potentiation of neuromuscular blockers). Products include:
- Anectine ... 1073

Terazosin Hydrochloride (May result in a reduction in blood pressure that is excessive in some patients). Products include:
- Hytrin Capsules ... 430

Theophylline (Verapamil may inhibit the clearance and increase the plasma levels of theophylline). Products include:
- Marax Tablets & DF Syrup ... 2200
- Quibron ... 2053

Theophylline Anhydrous (Verapamil may inhibit the clearance and increase the plasma levels of theophylline). Products include:
- Aerolate ... 1004
- Primatene Dual Action Formula ... ▣ 872
- Primatene Tablets ... ▣ 873
- Respbid Tablets ... 682
- Slo-bid Gyrocaps ... 2033
- Theo-24 Extended Release Capsules ... 2568
- Theo-Dur Extended-Release Tablets ... 1327
- Theo-X Extended-Release Tablets ... 788
- Uni-Dur Extended-Release Tablets ... 1331
- Uniphyl 400 mg Tablets ... 2001

Theophylline Calcium Salicylate (Verapamil may inhibit the clearance and increase the plasma levels of theophylline). Products include:
- Quadrinal Tablets ... 1350

Theophylline Sodium Glycinate (Verapamil may inhibit the clearance and increase the plasma levels of theophylline).
- No products indexed under this heading.

Timolol Hemihydrate (Additive negative effects on heart rate, AV conduction and/or cardiac contractility; additive hypotensive effect). Products include:
- Betimol 0.25%, 0.5% ... ◉ 261

IMPORTANT NOTE: Always consult each drug listing in the patient's regimen for possible interactions.

Timolol Maleate (Additive negative effects on heart rate, AV conduction and/or cardiac contractility; additive hypotensive effect). Products include:
- Blocadren Tablets 1614
- Timolide Tablets 1748
- Timoptic in Ocudose 1753
- Timoptic Sterile Ophthalmic Solution 1751
- Timoptic-XE 1755

Torsemide (Additive effect on lowering blood pressure). Products include:
- Demadex Tablets and Injection 686

Triamterene (Additive effect on lowering blood pressure). Products include:
- Dyazide 2479
- Dyrenium Capsules 2481
- Maxzide 1380

Vecuronium Bromide (Activity of neuromuscular blocking agents potentiated). Products include:
- Norcuron 1826

CALCI-CHEW TABLETS
(Calcium Carbonate) 2004
None cited in PDR database.

CALCIMAR INJECTION, SYNTHETIC
(Calcitonin, Synthetic) 2013
None cited in PDR database.

CALCI-MIX CAPSULES
(Calcium Carbonate) 2004
None cited in PDR database.

CALCIUM DISODIUM VERSENATE INJECTION
(Calcium Disodium Edetate) 1490
May interact with:

Insulin, Human, Zinc Suspension (Interference with the action of zinc insulin by chelating the zinc). Products include:
- Humulin L, 100 Units 1446
- Humulin U, 100 Units 1450
- Novolin L Human Insulin 10 ml Vials 1795

Insulin, Zinc Crystals (Interference with the action of zinc insulin by chelating the zinc). Products include:
- NPH, 100 Units 1450

Insulin, Zinc Suspension (Interference with the action of zinc insulin by chelating the zinc). Products include:
- Iletin I 1450
- Lente, 100 Units 1450
- Iletin II 1452
- Pork Lente, 100 Units 1452
- Purified Pork Lente Insulin 1801

Steroids, unspecified (Enhances renal toxicity of edetate calcium disodium in animals).
No products indexed under this heading.

CALDECORT ANTI-ITCH HYDROCORTISONE CREAM
(Hydrocortisone Acetate) .... ▣ 631
None cited in PDR database.

CALDECORT ANTI-ITCH HYDROCORTISONE SPRAY
(Hydrocortisone) .... ▣ 631
None cited in PDR database.

CALDECORT LIGHT CREAM
(Hydrocortisone Acetate) .... ▣ 631
None cited in PDR database.

CALDESENE MEDICATED OINTMENT
(Petrolatum, Zinc Oxide) .... ▣ 632
None cited in PDR database.

CALDESENE MEDICATED POWDER
(Calcium Undecylenate) .... ▣ 632
None cited in PDR database.

CALPHOSAN
(Calcium Glycerophosphate, Calcium Lactate) 1229
None cited in PDR database.

CALTRATE 600
(Calcium Carbonate) .... ▣ 665
None cited in PDR database.

CALTRATE PLUS
(Calcium Carbonate, Vitamin D) .... ▣ 665
None cited in PDR database.

CALTRATE 600 + D
(Calcium Carbonate, Vitamin D) .... ▣ 665
None cited in PDR database.

CAMA ARTHRITIS PAIN RELIEVER
(Aspirin, Aluminum Hydroxide, Magnesium Oxide) .... ▣ 785
May interact with oral hypoglycemic agents, oral anticoagulants, and antigout agents. Compounds in these categories include:

Acarbose (Do not use concomitantly).
No products indexed under this heading.

Allopurinol (Do not use concomitantly). Products include:
- Zyloprim Tablets 1226

Chlorpropamide (Do not use concomitantly). Products include:
- Diabinese Tablets 1935

Dicumarol (Do not use concomitantly).
No products indexed under this heading.

Glipizide (Do not use concomitantly). Products include:
- Glucotrol Tablets 1967
- Glucotrol XL Extended Release Tablets 1968

Glyburide (Do not use concomitantly). Products include:
- DiaBeta Tablets 1239
- Glynase PresTab Tablets 2609
- Micronase Tablets 2623

Metformin Hydrochloride (Do not use concomitantly). Products include:
- Glucophage 752

Probenecid (Do not use concomitantly). Products include:
- Benemid Tablets 1611
- ColBENEMID Tablets 1622

Sulfinpyrazone (Do not use concomitantly). Products include:
- Anturane 807

Tolazamide (Do not use concomitantly).
No products indexed under this heading.

Tolbutamide (Do not use concomitantly).
No products indexed under this heading.

Warfarin Sodium (Do not use concomitantly). Products include:
- Coumadin 926

CAMPHO-PHENIQUE ANTISEPTIC GEL
(Camphor, Phenol) .... ▣ 718
None cited in PDR database.

CAMPHO-PHENIQUE COLD SORE GEL
(Camphor, Phenol) .... ▣ 719
None cited in PDR database.

CAMPHO-PHENIQUE LIQUID
(Phenol, Camphor) .... ▣ 719
None cited in PDR database.

CAMPHO-PHENIQUE MAXIMUM STRENGTH FIRST AID ANTIBIOTIC PLUS PAIN RELIEVER OINTMENT
(Bacitracin Zinc, Lidocaine Hydrochloride, Neomycin Sulfate, Polymyxin B Sulfate) .... ▣ 719
None cited in PDR database.

CAPASTAT SULFATE VIALS
(Capreomycin Sulfate) 2868
May interact with aminoglycosides, antituberculosis drugs, and certain other agents. Compounds in these categories include:

Amikacin Sulfate (Additive ototoxicity and/or nephrotoxicity). Products include:
- Amikacin Sulfate Injection, USP 960
- Amikin Injectable 501

Aminosalicylic Acid (Potential for febrile reactions and abnormal liver function tests). Products include:
- PASER Granules 1285

p-Aminosalicylic Acid (Potential for febrile reactions and abnormal liver function tests).
No products indexed under this heading.

Colistin Sulfate (Additive ototoxicity and/or nephrotoxicity). Products include:
- Coly-Mycin S Otic w/Neomycin & Hydrocortisone 1906

Cycloserine (Potential for febrile reactions and abnormal liver function tests). Products include:
- Seromycin Pulvules 1476

Ethambutol Hydrochloride (Potential for febrile reactions and abnormal liver function tests). Products include:
- Myambutol Tablets 1386

Ether (Neuromuscular block enhanced).

Gentamicin Sulfate (Additive ototoxicity and/or nephrotoxicity). Products include:
- Garamycin Injectable 2360
- Genoptic Sterile Ophthalmic Solution .... ◉ 243
- Genoptic Sterile Ophthalmic Ointment .... ◉ 243
- Gentacidin Ointment .... ◉ 264
- Gentacidin Solution .... ◉ 264
- Gentak .... ◉ 208
- Pred-G Liquifilm Sterile Ophthalmic Suspension .... ◉ 251
- Pred-G S.O.P. Sterile Ophthalmic Ointment .... ◉ 252

Isoniazid (Potential for febrile reactions and abnormal liver function tests). Products include:
- Nydrazid Injection 508
- Rifamate Capsules 1530
- Rifater 1532

Kanamycin Sulfate (Additive ototoxicity and/or nephrotoxicity).
No products indexed under this heading.

Neomycin, oral (Additive ototoxicity and/or nephrotoxicity).

Paromomycin Sulfate (Additive ototoxicity and/or nephrotoxicity).
No products indexed under this heading.

Polymyxin B Sulfate (Additive ototoxicity and/or nephrotoxicity). Products include:
- AK-Spore .... ◉ 204
- AK-Trol Ointment & Suspension .... ◉ 205
- Bactine First Aid Antibiotic Plus Anesthetic Ointment .... ▣ 708
- Betadine Brand First Aid Antibiotics & Moisturizer Ointment 1991
- Campho-Phenique Maximum Strength First Aid Antibiotic Plus Pain Reliever Ointment .... ▣ 719
- Cortisporin Cream 1084
- Cortisporin Ointment 1085
- Cortisporin Ophthalmic Ointment Sterile 1085
- Cortisporin Ophthalmic Suspension Sterile 1086
- Cortisporin Otic Solution Sterile 1087
- Cortisporin Otic Suspension Sterile 1088
- Dexacidin Ointment .... ◉ 263
- Maxitrol Ophthalmic Ointment and Suspension .... ◉ 224
- Mycitracin .... ▣ 839
- Neosporin G.U. Irrigant Sterile 1148
- Neosporin Ointment .... ▣ 857
- Neosporin Plus Maximum Strength Cream .... ▣ 858
- Neosporin Plus Maximum Strength Ointment .... ▣ 858
- Neosporin Ophthalmic Ointment Sterile 1148
- Neosporin Ophthalmic Solution Sterile 1149
- Ophthocort .... ◉ 311
- PediOtic Suspension Sterile 1153
- Polymyxin B Sulfate, Aerosporin Brand Sterile Powder 1154
- Poly-Pred Liquifilm .... ◉ 248
- Polysporin Ointment .... ▣ 858
- Polysporin Ophthalmic Ointment Sterile 1154
- Polysporin Powder .... ▣ 859
- Polytrim Ophthalmic Solution Sterile 482
- TERAK Ointment .... ◉ 209
- Terramycin with Polymyxin B Sulfate Ophthalmic Ointment 2211

Pyrazinamide (Potential for febrile reactions and abnormal liver function tests). Products include:
- Pyrazinamide Tablets 1398
- Rifater 1532

Rifampin (Potential for febrile reactions and abnormal liver function tests). Products include:
- Rifadin 1528
- Rifamate Capsules 1530
- Rifater 1532
- Rimactane Capsules 847

Streptomycin Sulfate (Additive ototoxicity and/or nephrotoxicity). Products include:
- Streptomycin Sulfate Injection 2208

Tobramycin (Additive ototoxicity and/or nephrotoxicity). Products include:
- AKTOB .... ◉ 206
- TobraDex Ophthalmic Suspension and Ointment 473
- Tobrex Ophthalmic Ointment and Solution .... ◉ 229

Tobramycin Sulfate (Additive ototoxicity and/or nephrotoxicity). Products include:
- Nebcin Vials, Hyporets & ADD-Vantage 1464
- Tobramycin Sulfate Injection 968

Vancomycin Hydrochloride (Additive ototoxicity and/or nephrotoxicity). Products include:
- Vancocin HCl, Oral Solution & Pulvules 1483
- Vancocin HCl, Vials & ADD-Vantage 1481

Viomycin (Additive ototoxicity and/or nephrotoxicity).

CAPITROL SHAMPOO
(Chloroxine) 2683
None cited in PDR database.

CAPOTEN
(Captopril) 739

May interact with diuretics, thiazides, ganglionic blocking agents,

(▣ Described in PDR For Nonprescription Drugs) (◉ Described in PDR For Ophthalmology)

peripheral adrenergic blockers, potassium sparing diuretics, potassium preparations, non-steroidal anti-inflammatory agents, beta blockers, vasodilators, lithium preparations, nitrates and nitrites, agents causing renin release, inhibitors of endogenous prostaglandin synthesis, and certain other agents. Compounds in these categories include:

Acebutolol Hydrochloride (Less than additive antihypertensive effect). Products include:
- Sectral Capsules ... 2807

Amiloride Hydrochloride (Hypotension; increased serum potassium). Products include:
- Midamor Tablets ... 1703
- Moduretic Tablets ... 1705

Amyl Nitrite (Discontinue before starting captopril; if resumed administer at lower dosage).
- No products indexed under this heading.

Aspirin (Antihypertensive effects of captopril reduced). Products include:
- Alka-Seltzer Effervescent Antacid and Pain Reliever ... ▣ 701
- Alka-Seltzer Extra Strength Effervescent Antacid and Pain Reliever ... ▣ 703
- Alka-Seltzer Lemon Lime Effervescent Antacid and Pain Reliever ... ▣ 703
- Alka-Seltzer Plus Cold Medicine ... ▣ 705
- Alka-Seltzer Plus Cold & Cough Medicine ... ▣ 708
- Alka-Seltzer Plus Night-Time Cold Medicine ... ▣ 707
- Alka Seltzer Plus Sinus Medicine .. ▣ 707
- Arthritis Foundation Safety Coated Aspirin Tablets ... ▣ 675
- Arthritis Pain Ascriptin ... ▣ 631
- Maximum Strength Ascriptin ... ▣ 630
- Regular Strength Ascriptin Tablets ... ▣ 629
- Arthritis Strength BC Powder ... ▣ 609
- BC Cold Powder Multi-Symptom Formula (Cold-Sinus-Allergy) ... ▣ 609
- BC Cold Powder Non-Drowsy Formula (Cold-Sinus) ... ▣ 609
- BC Powder ... ▣ 609
- Bayer Children's Chewable Aspirin ... ▣ 711
- Genuine Bayer Aspirin Tablets & Caplets ... ▣ 713
- Extra Strength Bayer Arthritis Pain Regimen Formula ... ▣ 711
- Extra Strength Bayer Aspirin Caplets & Tablets ... ▣ 712
- Extended-Release Bayer 8-Hour Aspirin ... ▣ 712
- Extra Strength Bayer Plus Aspirin Caplets ... ▣ 713
- Extra Strength Bayer PM Aspirin .. ▣ 713
- Bayer Enteric Aspirin ... ▣ 709
- Bufferin Analgesic Tablets and Caplets ... ▣ 613
- Arthritis Strength Bufferin Analgesic Caplets ... ▣ 614
- Extra Strength Bufferin Analgesic Tablets ... ▣ 615
- Cama Arthritis Pain Reliever ... ▣ 785
- Darvon Compound-65 Pulvules ... 1435
- Easprin ... 1914
- Ecotrin ... 2455
- Ecotrin Enteric Coated Aspirin Maximum Strength Tablets and Caplets ... ▣ 816
- Ecotrin Enteric Coated Aspirin Regular Strength Tablets ... 2455
- Empirin Aspirin Tablets ... ▣ 854
- Empirin with Codeine Tablets ... 1093
- Excedrin Extra-Strength Analgesic Tablets & Caplets ... 732
- Fiorinal Capsules ... 2261
- Fiorinal with Codeine Capsules ... 2262
- Fiorinal Tablets ... 2261
- Halfprin ... 1362
- Healthprin Aspirin ... 2455
- Norgesic ... 1496
- Percodan Tablets ... 939
- Percodan-Demi Tablets ... 940
- Robaxisal Tablets ... 2071
- Soma Compound w/Codeine Tablets ... 2676
- Soma Compound Tablets ... 2675
- St. Joseph Adult Chewable Aspirin (81 mg.) ... ▣ 808
- Talwin Compound ... 2335
- Ursinus Inlay-Tabs ... ▣ 794
- Vanquish Analgesic Caplets ... ▣ 731

Atenolol (Less than additive antihypertensive effect). Products include:
- Tenoretic Tablets ... 2845
- Tenormin Tablets and I.V. Injection 2847

Bendroflumethiazide (Captopril's effect will be augmented).
- No products indexed under this heading.

Betaxolol Hydrochloride (Less than additive antihypertensive effect). Products include:
- Betoptic Ophthalmic Solution ... 469
- Betoptic S Ophthalmic Suspension 471
- Kerlone Tablets ... 2436

Bisoprolol Fumarate (Less than additive antihypertensive effect). Products include:
- Zebeta Tablets ... 1413
- Ziac ... 1415

Bumetanide (Captopril's effect will be augmented; hypotension). Products include:
- Bumex ... 2093

Carteolol Hydrochloride (Less than additive antihypertensive effect). Products include:
- Cartrol Tablets ... 410
- Ocupress Ophthalmic Solution, 1% Sterile ... ⊙ 309

Chlorothiazide (Captopril's effect will be augmented). Products include:
- Aldoclor Tablets ... 1598
- Diupres Tablets ... 1650
- Diuril Oral ... 1653

Chlorothiazide Sodium (Captopril's effect will be augmented). Products include:
- Diuril Sodium Intravenous ... 1652

Chlorthalidone (Captopril's effect will be augmented; hypotension; increased serum potassium). Products include:
- Combipres Tablets ... 677
- Tenoretic Tablets ... 2845
- Thalitone ... 1245

Deserpidine (Use with caution).
- No products indexed under this heading.

Diazoxide (Drugs having vasodilator activity should, if possible, be discontinued before starting Capoten). Products include:
- Hyperstat I.V. Injection ... 2363
- Proglycem ... 580

Diclofenac Potassium (Antihypertensive effects of captopril reduced). Products include:
- Cataflam ... 816

Diclofenac Sodium (Antihypertensive effects of captopril reduced). Products include:
- Voltaren Ophthalmic Sterile Ophthalmic Solution ... ⊙ 272
- Voltaren Tablets ... 861

Erythrityl Tetranitrate (Discontinue before starting captopril; if resumed administer at lower dosage).
- No products indexed under this heading.

Esmolol Hydrochloride (Less than additive antihypertensive effect). Products include:
- Brevibloc Injection ... 1808

Ethacrynic Acid (Captopril's effect will be augmented; hypotension). Products include:
- Edecrin Tablets ... 1657

Etodolac (Antihypertensive effects of captopril reduced). Products include:
- Lodine Capsules and Tablets ... 2743

Fenoprofen Calcium (Antihypertensive effects of captopril reduced). Products include:
- Nalfon 200 Pulvules & Nalfon Tablets ... 917

Flurbiprofen (Antihypertensive effects of captopril reduced). Products include:
- Ansaid Tablets ... 2579

Furosemide (Captopril's effect will be augmented; hypotension). Products include:
- Lasix Injection, Oral Solution and Tablets ... 1240

Guanethidine Monosulfate (Use with caution). Products include:
- Esimil Tablets ... 822
- Ismelin Tablets ... 827

Hydralazine Hydrochloride (Drugs having vasodilator activity should, if possible, be discontinued before starting Capoten). Products include:
- Apresazide Capsules ... 808
- Apresoline Hydrochloride Tablets .. 809
- Ser-Ap-Es Tablets ... 849

Hydrochlorothiazide (Captopril's effect will be augmented). Products include:
- Aldactazide ... 2413
- Aldoril Tablets ... 1604
- Apresazide Capsules ... 808
- Capozide ... 742
- Dyazide ... 2479
- Esidrix Tablets ... 821
- Esimil Tablets ... 822
- HydroDIURIL Tablets ... 1674
- Hydropres Tablets ... 1675
- Hyzaar Tablets ... 1677
- Inderide Tablets ... 2732
- Inderide LA Long Acting Capsules .. 2734
- Lopressor HCT Tablets ... 832
- Lotensin HCT ... 837
- Maxzide ... 1380
- Moduretic Tablets ... 1705
- Oretic Tablets ... 443
- Prinzide Tablets ... 1737
- Ser-Ap-Es Tablets ... 849
- Timolide Tablets ... 1748
- Vaseretic Tablets ... 1765
- Zestoretic ... 2850
- Ziac ... 1415

Hydroflumethiazide (Captopril's effect will be augmented). Products include:
- Diucardin Tablets ... 2718

Ibuprofen (Antihypertensive effects of captopril reduced). Products include:
- Advil Cold and Sinus Caplets and Tablets (formerly CoAdvil) ... ▣ 870
- Advil Ibuprofen Tablets and Caplets ... ▣ 870
- Children's Advil Suspension ... 2692
- Arthritis Foundation Ibuprofen Tablets ... ▣ 674
- Bayer Select Ibuprofen Pain Relief Formula ... ▣ 715
- Cramp End Tablets ... ▣ 735
- Dimetapp Sinus Caplets ... ▣ 775
- Haltran Tablets ... ▣ 771
- IBU Tablets ... 1342
- Ibuprohm ... ▣ 735
- Children's Motrin Ibuprofen Oral Suspension ... 1546
- Motrin Tablets ... 2625
- Motrin IB Caplets, Tablets, and Geltabs ... ▣ 838
- Motrin IB Sinus ... ▣ 838
- Motrin Ibuprofen Suspension, Oral Drops, Chewable Tablets, Caplets ... 1546
- Nuprin Ibuprofen/Analgesic Tablets & Caplets ... ▣ 622
- Sine-Aid IB Caplets ... 1554
- Vicks DayQuil SINUS Pressure & PAIN Relief with IBUPROFEN ... ▣ 762

Indapamide (Captopril's effect will be augmented; hypotension). Products include:
- Lozol Tablets ... 2022

Indomethacin (Antihypertensive effects of captopril reduced). Products include:
- Indocin ... 1680

Indomethacin Sodium Trihydrate (Antihypertensive effects of captopril reduced). Products include:
- Indocin I.V. ... 1684

Isosorbide Dinitrate (Discontinue before starting captopril; if resumed administer at lower dosage). Products include:
- Dilatrate-SR ... 2398
- Isordil Sublingual Tablets ... 2739
- Isordil Tembids ... 2741
- Isordil Titradose Tablets ... 2742
- Sorbitrate ... 2843

Isosorbide Mononitrate (Discontinue before starting captopril; if resumed administer at lower dosage). Products include:
- Imdur ... 1323
- Ismo Tablets ... 2738
- Monoket ... 2406

Ketoprofen (Antihypertensive effects of captopril reduced). Products include:
- Orudis Capsules ... 2766
- Oruvail Capsules ... 2766

Ketorolac Tromethamine (Antihypertensive effects of captopril reduced). Products include:
- Acular ... 474
- Acular ... ⊙ 277
- Toradol ... 2159

Labetalol Hydrochloride (Less than additive antihypertensive effect). Products include:
- Normodyne Injection ... 2377
- Normodyne Tablets ... 2379
- Trandate ... 1185

Levobunolol Hydrochloride (Less than additive antihypertensive effect). Products include:
- Betagan ... ⊙ 233

Lithium Carbonate (Increased serum lithium levels and symptoms of lithium toxicity). Products include:
- Eskalith ... 2485
- Lithium Carbonate Capsules & Tablets ... 2230
- Lithonate/Lithotabs/Lithobid ... 2543

Lithium Citrate (Increased serum lithium levels and symptoms of lithium toxicity).
- No products indexed under this heading.

Mecamylamine Hydrochloride (Use with caution). Products include:
- Inversine Tablets ... 1686

Meclofenamate Sodium (Antihypertensive effects of captopril reduced).
- No products indexed under this heading.

Mefenamic Acid (Antihypertensive effects of captopril reduced). Products include:
- Ponstel ... 1925

Methyclothiazide (Captopril's effect will be augmented). Products include:
- Enduron Tablets ... 420

Metipranolol Hydrochloride (Less than additive antihypertensive effect). Products include:
- OptiPranolol (Metipranolol 0.3%) Sterile Ophthalmic Solution ... ⊙ 258

Metolazone (Captopril's effect will be augmented; hypotension). Products include:
- Mykrox Tablets ... 993
- Zaroxolyn Tablets ... 1000

Metoprolol Succinate (Less than additive antihypertensive effect). Products include:
- Toprol-XL Tablets ... 565

IMPORTANT NOTE: Always consult each drug listing in the patient's regimen for possible interactions.

Capoten **Interactions Index** 158

Metoprolol Tartrate (Less than additive antihypertensive effect). Products include:
Lopressor Ampuls ... 830
Lopressor HCT Tablets ... 832
Lopressor Tablets ... 830

Minoxidil (Drugs having vasodilator activity should, if possible, be discontinued before starting Capoten). Products include:
Loniten Tablets ... 2618
Rogaine Topical Solution ... 2637

Nabumetone (Antihypertensive effects of captopril reduced). Products include:
Relafen Tablets ... 2510

Nadolol (Less than additive antihypertensive effect).
No products indexed under this heading.

Naproxen (Antihypertensive effects of captopril reduced). Products include:
Anaprox/Naprosyn ... 2117

Naproxen Sodium (Antihypertensive effects of captopril reduced). Products include:
Aleve ... 1975
Anaprox/Naprosyn ... 2117

Nitroglycerin (Discontinue before starting captopril; if resumed administer at lower dosage). Products include:
Deponit NTG Transdermal Delivery System ... 2397
Nitro-Bid IV ... 1523
Nitro-Bid Ointment ... 1524
Nitrodisc ... 2047
Nitro-Dur (nitroglycerin) Transdermal Infusion System ... 1326
Nitrolingual Spray ... 2027
Nitrostat Tablets ... 1925
Transderm-Nitro Transdermal Therapeutic System ... 859

Oxaprozin (Antihypertensive effects of captopril reduced). Products include:
Daypro Caplets ... 2426

Penbutolol Sulfate (Less than additive antihypertensive effect). Products include:
Levatol ... 2403

Pentaerythritol Tetranitrate (Discontinue before starting captopril; if resumed administer at lower dosage).
No products indexed under this heading.

Phenylbutazone (Antihypertensive effects of captopril reduced).
No products indexed under this heading.

Pindolol (Less than additive antihypertensive effect). Products include:
Visken Tablets ... 2299

Piroxicam (Antihypertensive effects of captopril reduced). Products include:
Feldene Capsules ... 1965

Polythiazide (Captopril's effect will be augmented). Products include:
Minizide Capsules ... 1938

Potassium Acid Phosphate (Potential for significant increase in serum potassium). Products include:
K-Phos Original Formula 'Sodium Free' Tablets ... 639

Potassium Bicarbonate (Potential for significant increase in serum potassium). Products include:
Alka-Seltzer Gold Effervescent Antacid ... ▣ 703

Potassium Chloride (Potential for significant increase in serum potassium). Products include:
Chlor-3 Condiment ... 1004
K-Dur Microburst Release System (potassium chloride, USP) E.R. Tablets ... 1325
K-Lor Powder Packets ... 434
K-Norm Extended-Release Capsules ... 991
K-Tab Filmtab ... 434
Kolyum Liquid ... 992
Micro-K ... 2063
Micro-K LS Packets ... 2064
NuLYTELY ... 689
Cherry Flavor NuLYTELY ... 689
Rum-K Syrup ... 1005
Slow-K Extended-Release Tablets ... 851

Potassium Citrate (Potential for significant increase in serum potassium). Products include:
Polycitra Syrup ... 578
Polycitra-K Crystals ... 579
Polycitra-K Oral Solution ... 579
Polycitra-LC ... 578

Potassium Gluconate (Potential for significant increase in serum potassium). Products include:
Kolyum Liquid ... 992

Potassium Phosphate, Dibasic (Potential for significant increase in serum potassium).
No products indexed under this heading.

Potassium Phosphate, Monobasic (Potential for significant increase in serum potassium). Products include:
K-Phos Neutral Tablets ... 639
K-Phos Original Formula 'Sodium Free' Tablets ... 639

Prazosin Hydrochloride (Use with caution). Products include:
Minipress Capsules ... 1937
Minizide Capsules ... 1938

Propranolol Hydrochloride (Less than additive antihypertensive effect). Products include:
Inderal ... 2728
Inderal LA Long Acting Capsules ... 2730
Inderide Tablets ... 2732
Inderide LA Long Acting Capsules ... 2734

Reserpine (Use with caution). Products include:
Diupres Tablets ... 1650
Hydropres Tablets ... 1675
Ser-Ap-Es Tablets ... 849

Sotalol Hydrochloride (Less than additive antihypertensive effect). Products include:
Betapace Tablets ... 641

Spironolactone (Captopril's effect will be augmented; hypotension; increased serum potassium). Products include:
Aldactazide ... 2413
Aldactone ... 2414

Sulindac (Antihypertensive effects of captopril reduced). Products include:
Clinoril Tablets ... 1618

Terazosin Hydrochloride (Use with caution). Products include:
Hytrin Capsules ... 430

Timolol Hemihydrate (Less than additive antihypertensive effect). Products include:
Betimol 0.25%, 0.5% ... ◉ 261

Timolol Maleate (Less than additive antihypertensive effect). Products include:
Blocadren Tablets ... 1614
Timolide Tablets ... 1748
Timoptic in Ocudose ... 1753
Timoptic Sterile Ophthalmic Solution ... 1751
Timoptic-XE ... 1755

Tolmetin Sodium (Antihypertensive effects of captopril reduced). Products include:
Tolectin (200, 400 and 600 mg) .. 1581

Torsemide (Captopril's effect will be augmented; hypotension). Products include:
Demadex Tablets and Injection ... 686

Triamterene (Captopril's effect will be augmented; hypotension; increased serum potassium). Products include:
Dyazide ... 2479
Dyrenium Capsules ... 2481
Maxzide ... 1380

Trimethaphan Camsylate (Use with caution). Products include:
Arfonad Ampuls ... 2080

Food Interactions

Food, unspecified (Reduces absorption by about 30% to 40%; should be given one hour before meals).

CAPOZIDE

(Captopril, Hydrochlorothiazide) ... 742
May interact with diuretics, thiazides, ganglionic blocking agents, peripheral adrenergic blockers, lithium preparations, potassium sparing diuretics, potassium preparations, oral anticoagulants, calcium preparations, cardiac glycosides, non-steroidal anti-inflammatory agents, barbiturates, agents causing renin release, inhibitors of endogenous prostaglandin synthesis, narcotic analgesics, antihypertensives, corticosteroids, preanesthetic medications, general anesthetics, nondepolarizing neuromuscular blocking agents, oral hypoglycemic agents, insulin, monoamine oxidase inhibitors, antigout agents, nitrates and nitrites, and certain other agents. Compounds in these categories include:

Acarbose (Thiazide-induced hyperglycemia may require dosage adjustment of antidiabetic drugs).
No products indexed under this heading.

Acebutolol Hydrochloride (Additive effect). Products include:
Sectral Capsules ... 2807

ACTH (Intensified electrolyte depletion, particularly hypokalemia).
No products indexed under this heading.

Alfentanil Hydrochloride (Potentiation of orthostatic hypotension). Products include:
Alfenta Injection ... 1286

Allopurinol (Dosage adjustment may be necessary since hydrochlorothiazide may have hyperuricemic effect). Products include:
Zyloprim Tablets ... 1226

Amiloride Hydrochloride (Precipitous reduction of blood pressure; elevated serum potassium; additive effect). Products include:
Midamor Tablets ... 1703
Moduretic Tablets ... 1705

Amlodipine Besylate (Additive effect; precipitous reduction of blood pressure). Products include:
Lotrel Capsules ... 840
Norvasc Tablets ... 1940

Amphotericin B (Intensified electrolyte depletion, particularly hypokalemia). Products include:
Fungizone Intravenous ... 506

Amyl Nitrite (Discontinue before starting captopril; if resumed administer at lower dosage).
No products indexed under this heading.

Aprobarbital (Potentiation of orthostatic hypotension).
No products indexed under this heading.

Aspirin (May reduce the antihypertensive effect of captopril). Products include:
Alka-Seltzer Effervescent Antacid and Pain Reliever ... ▣ 701
Alka-Seltzer Extra Strength Effervescent Antacid and Pain Reliever ... ▣ 703
Alka-Seltzer Lemon Lime Effervescent Antacid and Pain Reliever ... ▣ 703
Alka-Seltzer Plus Cold Medicine ... ▣ 705
Alka-Seltzer Plus Cold & Cough Medicine ... ▣ 708
Alka-Seltzer Plus Night-Time Cold Medicine ... ▣ 707
Alka Seltzer Plus Sinus Medicine .. ▣ 707
Arthritis Foundation Safety Coated Aspirin Tablets ... ▣ 675
Arthritis Pain Ascriptin ... ▣ 631
Maximum Strength Ascriptin ... ▣ 630
Regular Strength Ascriptin Tablets ... ▣ 629
Arthritis Strength BC Powder ... ▣ 609
BC Cold Powder Multi-Symptom Formula (Cold-Sinus-Allergy) ... ▣ 609
BC Cold Powder Non-Drowsy Formula (Cold-Sinus) ... ▣ 609
BC Powder ... ▣ 609
Bayer Children's Chewable Aspirin ... ▣ 711
Genuine Bayer Aspirin Tablets & Caplets ... ▣ 713
Extra Strength Bayer Arthritis Pain Regimen Formula ... ▣ 711
Extra Strength Bayer Aspirin Caplets & Tablets ... ▣ 712
Extended-Release Bayer 8-Hour Aspirin ... ▣ 712
Extra Strength Bayer Plus Aspirin Caplets ... ▣ 713
Extra Strength Bayer PM Aspirin .. ▣ 713
Bayer Enteric Aspirin ... ▣ 709
Bufferin Analgesic Tablets and Caplets ... ▣ 613
Arthritis Strength Bufferin Analgesic Caplets ... ▣ 614
Extra Strength Bufferin Analgesic Tablets ... ▣ 615
Cama Arthritis Pain Reliever ... ▣ 785
Darvon Compound-65 Pulvules ... 1435
Easprin ... 1914
Ecotrin ... 2455
Ecotrin Enteric Coated Aspirin Maximum Strength Tablets and Caplets ... ▣ 816
Ecotrin Enteric Coated Aspirin Regular Strength Tablets ... 2455
Empirin Aspirin Tablets ... ▣ 854
Empirin with Codeine Tablets ... 1093
Excedrin Extra-Strength Analgesic Tablets & Caplets ... 732
Fiorinal Capsules ... 2261
Fiorinal with Codeine Capsules ... 2262
Fiorinal Tablets ... 2261
Halfprin ... 1362
Healthprin Aspirin ... 2455
Norgesic ... 1496
Percodan Tablets ... 939
Percodan-Demi Tablets ... 940
Robaxisal Tablets ... 2071
Soma Compound w/Codeine Tablets ... 2676
Soma Compound Tablets ... 2675
St. Joseph Adult Chewable Aspirin (81 mg.) ... ▣ 808
Talwin Compound ... 2335
Ursinus Inlay-Tabs ... ▣ 794
Vanquish Analgesic Caplets ... ▣ 731

Atenolol (Additive effect). Products include:
Tenoretic Tablets ... 2845
Tenormin Tablets and I.V. Injection 2847

Atracurium Besylate (Increased response to relaxant). Products include:
Tracrium Injection ... 1183

Benazepril Hydrochloride (Additive effect; precipitous reduction of blood pressure). Products include:
Lotensin Tablets ... 834
Lotensin HCT ... 837
Lotrel Capsules ... 840

Bendroflumethiazide (Precipitous reduction of blood pressure; captopril's effect will be augmented).
No products indexed under this heading.

Betamethasone Acetate (Intensified electrolyte depletion, particularly hypokalemia). Products include:
Celestone Soluspan Suspension ... 2347

(▣ Described in PDR For Nonprescription Drugs) (◉ Described in PDR For Ophthalmology)

Betamethasone Sodium Phosphate (Intensified electrolyte depletion, particularly hypokalemia). Products include:

Celestone Soluspan Suspension 2347

Betaxolol Hydrochloride (Additive effect; precipitous reduction of blood pressure; elevated serum potassium). Products include:

Betoptic Ophthalmic Solution............ 469
Betoptic S Ophthalmic Suspension 471
Kerlone Tablets.. 2436

Bisoprolol Fumarate (Additive effect; precipitous reduction of blood pressure; elevated serum potassium). Products include:

Zebeta Tablets 1413
Ziac 1415

Bumetanide (Precipitous reduction of blood pressure). Products include:

Bumex 2093

Buprenorphine (Potentiation of orthostatic hypotension). Products include:

Buprenex Injectable 2006

Butabarbital (Potentiation of orthostatic hypotension).

No products indexed under this heading.

Butalbital (Potentiation of orthostatic hypotension). Products include:

Esgic-plus Tablets 1013
Fioricet Tablets.. 2258
Fioricet with Codeine Capsules 2260
Fiorinal Capsules 2261
Fiorinal with Codeine Capsules 2262
Fiorinal Tablets 2261
Phrenilin 785
Sedapap Tablets 50 mg/650 mg .. 1543

Calcium Carbonate (Potential for hypercalcemia). Products include:

Alka-Mints Chewable Antacid .... ⊞ 701
Arthritis Pain Ascriptin .... ⊞ 631
Maximum Strength Ascriptin .... ⊞ 630
Regular Strength Ascriptin Tablets .... ⊞ 629
Extra Strength Bayer Plus Aspirin Caplets .... ⊞ 713
Bufferin Analgesic Tablets and Caplets .... ⊞ 613
Calci-Chew Tablets 2004
Calci-Mix Capsules 2004
Caltrate 600 .... ⊞ 665
Caltrate PLUS .... ⊞ 665
Caltrate 600 + D .... ⊞ 665
Centrum Singles Calcium...................... ⊞ 669
Chooz Antacid Gum .... ⊞ 799
Di-Gel Antacid/Anti-Gas .... ⊞ 801
Gerimed Tablets.. 982
Maalox Antacid Caplets........................ ⊞ 638
Marblen .... ⊞ 655
Materna Tablets 1379
Mylanta Calcium Carbonate and Magnesium Hydroxide Tablets...... 1318
Mylanta Gelcaps Antacid .... ⊞ 662
Mylanta Soothing Lozenges................ 1319
Nephro-Calci Tablets 2004
Rolaids Tablets .... ⊞ 843
Rolaids (Calcium Rich/Sodium Free) Tablets .... ⊞ 843
Tempo Soft Antacid .... ⊞ 835
Titralac .... ⊞ 672
Titralac Plus.. ⊞ 672
Tums Antacid Tablets .... ⊞ 827
Tums Anti-gas/Antacid Formula Tablets, Assorted Fruit .... ⊞ 827
Tums E-X Antacid Tablets .... ⊞ 827
Tums 500 Calcium Supplement .... ⊞ 828
Tums ULTRA Antacid Tablets .... ⊞ 827
TYLENOL, Extra Strength, Headache Plus Pain Reliever with Antacid Caplets 1559

Calcium Chloride (Potential for hypercalcemia).

No products indexed under this heading.

Calcium Citrate (Potential for hypercalcemia). Products include:

Citracal.. 1779
Citracal Caplets + D 1780
Citracal Liquitab 1780

Calcium Glubionate (Potential for hypercalcemia).

No products indexed under this heading.

Carteolol Hydrochloride (Additive effect). Products include:

Cartrol Tablets 410
Ocupress Ophthalmic Solution, 1% Sterile.. ⊙ 309

Chlorothiazide (Precipitous reduction of blood pressure; captopril's effect will be augmented). Products include:

Aldoclor Tablets 1598
Diupres Tablets 1650
Diuril Oral 1653

Chlorothiazide Sodium (Precipitous reduction of blood pressure; captopril's effect will be augmented). Products include:

Diuril Sodium Intravenous 1652

Chlorpropamide (Thiazide-induced hyperglycemia may require dosage adjustment of antidiabetic drugs). Products include:

Diabinese Tablets 1935

Chlorthalidone (Additive effect; precipitous reduction of blood pressure). Products include:

Combipres Tablets 677
Tenoretic Tablets...................................... 2845
Thalitone 1245

Cholestyramine (Delays or decreases absorption of hydrochlorothiazide). Products include:

Questran Light 769
Questran Powder 770

Clonidine (Additive effect). Products include:

Catapres-TTS.. 675

Clonidine Hydrochloride (Additive effect). Products include:

Catapres Tablets 674
Combipres Tablets 677

Codeine Phosphate (Potentiation of orthostatic hypotension). Products include:

Actifed with Codeine Cough Syrup.. 1067
Brontex 1981
Deconsal C Expectorant Syrup 456
Deconsal Pediatric Syrup...................... 457
Dimetane-DC Cough Syrup 2059
Empirin with Codeine Tablets............ 1093
Fioricet with Codeine Capsules 2260
Fiorinal with Codeine Capsules 2262
Isoclor Expectorant................................. 990
Novahistine DH.. 2462
Novahistine Expectorant........................ 2463
Nucofed 2051
Phenergan with Codeine........................ 2777
Phenergan VC with Codeine 2781
Robitussin A-C Syrup.............................. 2073
Robitussin-DAC Syrup 2074
Ryna .... ⊞ 841
Soma Compound w/Codeine Tablets 2676
Tussi-Organidin NR Liquid and S NR Liquid 2677
Tylenol with Codeine 1583

Colestipol Hydrochloride (Delays or decreases absorption of hydrochlorothiazide). Products include:

Colestid Tablets 2591

Cortisone Acetate (Intensified electrolyte depletion, particularly hypokalemia). Products include:

Cortone Acetate Sterile Suspension 1623
Cortone Acetate Tablets........................ 1624

Deserpidine (Additive effect or potentiation; use with caution).

No products indexed under this heading.

Deslanoside (Enhanced possibility of digitalis toxicity).

No products indexed under this heading.

Dexamethasone (Intensified electrolyte depletion, particularly hypokalemia). Products include:

AK-Trol Ointment & Suspension .... ⊙ 205

Decadron Elixir 1633
Decadron Tablets...................................... 1635
Decaspray Topical Aerosol 1648
Dexacidin Ointment .... ⊙ 263
Maxitrol Ophthalmic Ointment and Suspension .... ⊙ 224
TobraDex Ophthalmic Suspension and Ointment.. 473

Dexamethasone Acetate (Intensified electrolyte depletion, particularly hypokalemia). Products include:

Dalalone D.P. Injectable 1011
Decadron-LA Sterile Suspension...... 1646

Dexamethasone Sodium Phosphate (Intensified electrolyte depletion, particularly hypokalemia). Products include:

Decadron Phosphate Injection 1637
Decadron Phosphate Respihaler 1642
Decadron Phosphate Sterile Ophthalmic Ointment.. 1641
Decadron Phosphate Sterile Ophthalmic Solution 1642
Decadron Phosphate Topical Cream.. 1644
Decadron Phosphate Turbinaire 1645
Decadron Phosphate with Xylocaine Injection, Sterile 1639
Dexacort Phosphate in Respihaler .. 458
Dexacort Phosphate in Turbinaire .. 459
NeoDecadron Sterile Ophthalmic Ointment 1712
NeoDecadron Sterile Ophthalmic Solution 1713
NeoDecadron Topical Cream 1714

Dezocine (Potentiation of orthostatic hypotension). Products include:

Dalgan Injection 538

Diazepam (Effects may be potentiated). Products include:

Dizac 1809
Valium Injectable 2182
Valium Tablets 2183
Valrelease Capsules 2169

Diazoxide (Enhanced hyperglycemic, hyperuricemic, and antihypertensive effect). Products include:

Hyperstat I.V. Injection 2363
Proglycem.. 580

Diclofenac Potassium (Antihypertensive effect of captopril may be reduced; reduces diuretic and natriuretic effects). Products include:

Cataflam 816

Diclofenac Sodium (Antihypertensive effect of captopril may be reduced; reduces diuretic and natriuretic effects). Products include:

Voltaren Ophthalmic Sterile Ophthalmic Solution .... ⊙ 272
Voltaren Tablets.. 861

Dicumarol (May decrease anticoagulant effect).

No products indexed under this heading.

Digitoxin (Enhanced possibility of digitalis toxicity). Products include:

Crystodigin Tablets.................................. 1433

Digoxin (Enhanced possibility of digitalis toxicity). Products include:

Lanoxicaps 1117
Lanoxin Elixir Pediatric 1120
Lanoxin Injection 1123
Lanoxin Injection Pediatric.................. 1126
Lanoxin Tablets 1128

Diltiazem Hydrochloride (Additive effect; precipitous reduction of blood pressure). Products include:

Cardizem CD Capsules 1506
Cardizem SR Capsules 1510
Cardizem Injectable 1508
Cardizem Tablets...................................... 1512
Dilacor XR Extended-release Capsules 2018

Dopamine Hydrochloride (Decreased response to pressor amines).

No products indexed under this heading.

Doxazosin Mesylate (Additive effect; precipitous reduction of blood pressure). Products include:

Cardura Tablets 2186

Droperidol (Effects may be potentiated). Products include:

Inapsine Injection...................................... 1296

Enalapril Maleate (Additive effect). Products include:

Vaseretic Tablets 1765
Vasotec Tablets 1771

Enalaprilat (Additive effect). Products include:

Vasotec I.V.. 1768

Enflurane (Effects may be potentiated).

No products indexed under this heading.

Epinephrine Hydrochloride (Decreased response to pressor amines). Products include:

Ana-Kit Anaphylaxis Emergency Treatment Kit 617

Erythrityl Tetranitrate (Discontinue before starting captopril; if resumed administer at lower dosage).

No products indexed under this heading.

Esmolol Hydrochloride (Additive effect). Products include:

Brevibloc Injection.................................... 1808

Ethacrynic Acid (Precipitous reduction of blood pressure; additive effect). Products include:

Edecrin Tablets.. 1657

Etodolac (Antihypertensive effect of captopril may be reduced; reduces diuretic and natriuretic effects). Products include:

Lodine Capsules and Tablets 2743

Felodipine (Additive effect; precipitous reduction of blood pressure). Products include:

Plendil Extended-Release Tablets.... 527

Fenoprofen Calcium (Antihypertensive effect of captopril may be reduced; reduces diuretic and natriuretic effects). Products include:

Nalfon 200 Pulvules & Nalfon Tablets 917

Fentanyl (Potentiation of orthostatic hypotension). Products include:

Duragesic Transdermal System........ 1288

Fentanyl Citrate (Effects may be potentiated; potentiation of orthostatic hypotension). Products include:

Sublimaze Injection.................................. 1307

Fludrocortisone Acetate (Intensified electrolyte depletion, particularly hypokalemia). Products include:

Florinef Acetate Tablets 505

Flurbiprofen (Antihypertensive effect of captopril may be reduced; reduces diuretic and natriuretic effects). Products include:

Ansaid Tablets 2579

Fosinopril Sodium (Additive effect; precipitous reduction of blood pressure). Products include:

Monopril Tablets 757

Furazolidone (Enhanced hypotensive effect; dosage adjustments of one or both agents may be necessary). Products include:

Furoxone 2046

Furosemide (Precipitous reduction of blood pressure; additive effect). Products include:

Lasix Injection, Oral Solution and Tablets 1240

Gallamine (Effects of gallamine may be potentiated).

IMPORTANT NOTE: Always consult each drug listing in the patient's regimen for possible interactions.

Capozide **Interactions Index** **160**

Glipizide (Thiazide-induced hyperglycemia may require dosage adjustment of antidiabetic drugs). Products include:

- Glucotrol Tablets 1967
- Glucotrol XL Extended Release Tablets 1968

Glyburide (Thiazide-induced hyperglycemia may require dosage adjustment of antidiabetic drugs). Products include:

- DiaBeta Tablets 1239
- Glynase PresTab Tablets 2609
- Micronase Tablets 2623

Guanabenz Acetate (Additive effect).

No products indexed under this heading.

Guanethidine Monosulfate (Additive effect or potentiation; use with caution). Products include:

- Esimil Tablets 822
- Ismelin Tablets 827

Hydralazine Hydrochloride (Additive effect). Products include:

- Apresazide Capsules 808
- Apresoline Hydrochloride Tablets .. 809
- Ser-Ap-Es Tablets 849

Hydrocodone Bitartrate (Potentiation of orthostatic hypotension). Products include:

- Anexsia 5/500 Elixir 1781
- Anexia Tablets 1782
- Codiclear DH Syrup 791
- Deconamine CX Cough and Cold Liquid and Tablets 1319
- Duratuss HD Elixir 2565
- Hycodan Tablets and Syrup 930
- Hycomine Compound Tablets 932
- Hycomine 931
- Hycotuss Expectorant Syrup 933
- Hydrocet Capsules 782
- Lorcet 10/650 1018
- Lortab 2566
- Tussend 1783
- Tussend Expectorant 1785
- Vicodin Tablets 1356
- Vicodin ES Tablets 1357
- Vicodin Tuss Expectorant 1358
- Zydone Capsules 949

Hydrocodone Polistirex (Potentiation of orthostatic hypotension). Products include:

- Tussionex Pennkinetic Extended-Release Suspension 998

Hydrocortisone (Intensified electrolyte depletion, particularly hypokalemia). Products include:

- Anusol-HC Cream 2.5% 1896
- Aquanil HC Lotion 1931
- Bactine Hydrocortisone Anti-Itch Cream .... ■ 709
- Caldecort Anti-Itch Hydrocortisone Spray .... ■ 631
- Cortaid .... ■ 836
- CORTENEMA 2535
- Cortisporin Ointment 1085
- Cortisporin Ophthalmic Ointment Sterile 1085
- Cortisporin Ophthalmic Suspension Sterile 1086
- Cortisporin Otic Solution Sterile 1087
- Cortisporin Otic Suspension Sterile 1088
- Cortizone-5 .... ■ 831
- Cortizone-10 .... ■ 831
- Hydrocortone Tablets 1672
- Hytone 907
- Massengill Medicated Soft Cloth Towelettes 2458
- PediOtic Suspension Sterile 1153
- Preparation H Hydrocortisone 1% Cream .... ■ 872
- ProctoCream-HC 2.5% 2408
- VōSoL HC Otic Solution 2678

Hydrocortisone Acetate (Intensified electrolyte depletion, particularly hypokalemia). Products include:

- Analpram-HC Rectal Cream 1% and 2.5% 977
- Anusol HC-1 Anti-Itch Hydrocortisone Ointment .... ■ 847
- Anusol-HC Suppositories 1897
- Caldecort .... ■ 631
- Carmol HC 924
- Coly-Mycin S Otic w/Neomycin & Hydrocortisone 1906
- Cortaid .... ■ 836
- Cortifoam 2396
- Cortisporin Cream 1084
- Epifoam 2399
- Hydrocortone Acetate Sterile Suspension 1669
- Mantadil Cream 1135
- Nupercainal Hydrocortisone 1% Cream .... ■ 645
- Ophthocort .... ⊙ 311
- Pramosone Cream, Lotion & Ointment 978
- ProctoCream-HC 2408
- ProctoFoam-HC 2409
- Terra-Cortril Ophthalmic Suspension 2210

Hydrocortisone Sodium Phosphate (Intensified electrolyte depletion, particularly hypokalemia). Products include:

- Hydrocortone Phosphate Injection, Sterile 1670

Hydrocortisone Sodium Succinate (Intensified electrolyte depletion, particularly hypokalemia). Products include:

- Solu-Cortef Sterile Powder 2641

Hydroflumethiazide (Precipitous reduction of blood pressure; captopril's effect will be augmented). Products include:

- Diucardin Tablets 2718

Hydroxyzine Hydrochloride (Effects may be potentiated). Products include:

- Atarax Tablets & Syrup 2185
- Marax Tablets & DF Syrup 2200
- Vistaril Intramuscular Solution 2216

Ibuprofen (Antihypertensive effect of captopril may be reduced; reduces diuretic and natriuretic effects). Products include:

- Advil Cold and Sinus Caplets and Tablets (formerly CoAdvil) .... ■ 870
- Advil Ibuprofen Tablets and Caplets .... ■ 870
- Children's Advil Suspension 2692
- Arthritis Foundation Ibuprofen Tablets .... ■ 674
- Bayer Select Ibuprofen Pain Relief Formula .... ■ 715
- Cramp End Tablets .... ■ 735
- Dimetapp Sinus Caplets .... ■ 775
- Haltran Tablets .... ■ 771
- IBU Tablets 1342
- Ibuprohm .... ■ 735
- Children's Motrin Ibuprofen Oral Suspension 1546
- Motrin Tablets 2625
- Motrin IB Caplets, Tablets, and Geltabs .... ■ 838
- Motrin IB Sinus .... ■ 838
- Motrin Ibuprofen Suspension, Oral Drops, Chewable Tablets, Caplets 1546
- Nuprin Ibuprofen/Analgesic Tablets & Caplets .... ■ 622
- Sine-Aid IB Caplets 1554
- Vicks DayQuil SINUS Pressure & PAIN Relief with IBUPROFEN .... ■ 762

Indapamide (Precipitous reduction of blood pressure; additive effect). Products include:

- Lozol Tablets 2022

Indomethacin (Antihypertensive effect of captopril may be reduced; reduces diuretic and natriuretic effects). Products include:

- Indocin 1680

Indomethacin Sodium Trihydrate (Antihypertensive effect of captopril may be reduced; reduces diuretic and natriuretic effects). Products include:

- Indocin I.V. 1684

Insulin, Human (Thiazide-induced hyperglycemia may require dosage adjustment of antidiabetic drugs).

No products indexed under this heading.

Insulin, Human Isophane Suspension (Thiazide-induced hyperglycemia may require dosage adjustment of antidiabetic drugs). Products include:

- Novolin N Human Insulin 10 ml Vials 1795

Insulin, Human NPH (Thiazide-induced hyperglycemia may require dosage adjustment of antidiabetic drugs). Products include:

- Humulin N, 100 Units 1448
- Novolin N PenFill Cartridges Durable Insulin Delivery System 1798
- Novolin N Prefilled Syringe Disposable Insulin Delivery System 1798

Insulin, Human Regular (Thiazide-induced hyperglycemia may require dosage adjustment of antidiabetic drugs). Products include:

- Humulin R, 100 Units 1449
- Novolin R Human Insulin 10 ml Vials 1795
- Novolin R PenFill Cartridges Durable Insulin Delivery System 1798
- Novolin R Prefilled Syringe Disposable Insulin Delivery System 1798
- Velosulin BR Human Insulin 10 ml Vials 1795

Insulin, Human, Zinc Suspension (Thiazide-induced hyperglycemia may require dosage adjustment of antidiabetic drugs). Products include:

- Humulin L, 100 Units 1446
- Humulin U, 100 Units 1450
- Novolin L Human Insulin 10 ml Vials 1795

Insulin, NPH (Thiazide-induced hyperglycemia may require dosage adjustment of antidiabetic drugs). Products include:

- NPH, 100 Units 1450
- Pork NPH, 100 Units 1452
- Purified Pork NPH Isophane Insulin 1801

Insulin, Regular (Thiazide-induced hyperglycemia may require dosage adjustment of antidiabetic drugs). Products include:

- Regular, 100 Units 1450
- Pork Regular, 100 Units 1452
- Pork Regular (Concentrated), 500 Units 1453
- Purified Pork Regular Insulin 1801

Insulin, Zinc Crystals (Thiazide-induced hyperglycemia may require dosage adjustment of antidiabetic drugs). Products include:

- NPH, 100 Units 1450

Insulin, Zinc Suspension (Thiazide-induced hyperglycemia may require dosage adjustment of antidiabetic drugs). Products include:

- Iletin I 1450
- Lente, 100 Units 1450
- Iletin II 1452
- Pork Lente, 100 Units 1452
- Purified Pork Lente Insulin 1801

Isocarboxazid (Enhanced hypotensive effect; dosage adjustments of one or both agents may be necessary).

No products indexed under this heading.

Isoflurane (Effects may be potentiated).

No products indexed under this heading.

Isosorbide Dinitrate (Discontinue before starting captopril; if resumed administer at lower dosage). Products include:

- Dilatrate-SR 2398
- Isordil Sublingual Tablets 2739
- Isordil Tembids 2741
- Isordil Titradose Tablets 2742
- Sorbitrate 2843

Isosorbide Mononitrate (Discontinue before starting captopril; if resumed administer at lower dosage). Products include:

- Imdur 1323
- Ismo Tablets 2738
- Monoket 2406

Isradipine (Additive effect; precipitous reduction of blood pressure). Products include:

- DynaCirc Capsules 2256

Ketamine Hydrochloride (Effects may be potentiated).

No products indexed under this heading.

Ketoprofen (Antihypertensive effect of captopril may be reduced; reduces diuretic and natriuretic effects). Products include:

- Orudis Capsules 2766
- Oruvail Capsules 2766

Ketorolac Tromethamine (Antihypertensive effect of captopril may be reduced; reduces diuretic and natriuretic effects). Products include:

- Acular 474
- Acular .... ⊙ 277
- Toradol 2159

Labetalol Hydrochloride (Additive effect). Products include:

- Normodyne Injection 2377
- Normodyne Tablets 2379
- Trandate 1185

Levobunolol Hydrochloride (Additive effect). Products include:

- Betagan .... ⊙ 233

Levorphanol Tartrate (Potentiation of orthostatic hypotension). Products include:

- Levo-Dromoran 2129

Lisinopril (Additive effect). Products include:

- Prinivil Tablets 1733
- Prinzide Tablets 1737
- Zestoretic 2850
- Zestril Tablets 2854

Lithium Carbonate (Increased serum lithium levels and symptoms of lithium toxicity). Products include:

- Eskalith 2485
- Lithium Carbonate Capsules & Tablets 2230
- Lithonate/Lithotabs/Lithobid 2543

Lithium Citrate (Increased serum lithium levels and symptoms of lithium toxicity).

No products indexed under this heading.

Lorazepam (Effects may be potentiated). Products include:

- Ativan Injection 2698
- Ativan Tablets 2700

Losartan Potassium (Additive effect; precipitous reduction of blood pressure; elevated serum potassium). Products include:

- Cozaar Tablets 1628
- Hyzaar Tablets 1677

Mecamylamine Hydrochloride (Additive effect or potentiation; use with caution). Products include:

- Inversine Tablets 1686

Meclofenamate Sodium (Antihypertensive effect of captopril may be reduced; reduces diuretic and natriuretic effects).

No products indexed under this heading.

Mefenamic Acid (Antihypertensive effect of captopril may be reduced; reduces diuretic and natriuretic effects). Products include:

- Ponstel 1925

Meperidine Hydrochloride (Effects may be potentiated; potentiation of orthostatic hypotension). Products include:

- Demerol 2308

(■ Described in PDR For Nonprescription Drugs) (⊙ Described in PDR For Ophthalmology)

161 **Interactions Index** **Capozide**

Mepergan Injection 2753

Mephobarbital (Potentiation of orthostatic hypotension). Products include:
Mebaral Tablets 2322

Metaraminol Bitartrate (Decreased response to pressor amines). Products include:
Aramine Injection 1609

Metformin Hydrochloride (Thiazide-induced hyperglycemia may require dosage adjustment of antidiabetic drugs). Products include:
Glucophage 752

Methadone Hydrochloride (Potentiation of orthostatic hypotension). Products include:
Methadone Hydrochloride Oral Concentrate 2233
Methadone Hydrochloride Oral Solution & Tablets 2235

Methenamine (Possible decreased effectiveness due to alkalinization of urine). Products include:
Urised Tablets 1964

Methohexital Sodium (Effects may be potentiated). Products include:
Brevital Sodium Vials 1429

Methoxamine Hydrochloride (Decreased response to pressor amines). Products include:
Vasoxyl Injection 1196

Methoxyflurane (Effects may be potentiated).
No products indexed under this heading.

Methyclothiazide (Precipitous reduction of blood pressure; captopril's effect will be augmented). Products include:
Enduron Tablets 420

Methyldopa (Additive effect). Products include:
Aldoclor Tablets 1598
Aldomet Oral 1600
Aldoril Tablets 1604

Methyldopate Hydrochloride (Additive effect). Products include:
Aldomet Ester HCl Injection 1602

Methylprednisolone Acetate (Intensified electrolyte depletion, particularly hypokalemia). Products include:
Depo-Medrol Single-Dose Vial 2600
Depo-Medrol Sterile Aqueous Suspension 2597

Methylprednisolone Sodium Succinate (Intensified electrolyte depletion, particularly hypokalemia). Products include:
Solu-Medrol Sterile Powder 2643

Metipranolol Hydrochloride (Additive effect). Products include:
OptiPranolol (Metipranolol 0.3%) Sterile Ophthalmic Solution .... ⊙ 258

Metocurine Iodide (Increased response to relaxant). Products include:
Metubine Iodide Vials 916

Metolazone (Precipitous reduction of blood pressure; additive effect). Products include:
Mykrox Tablets 993
Zaroxolyn Tablets 1000

Metoprolol Succinate (Additive effect; precipitous reduction of blood pressure). Products include:
Toprol-XL Tablets 565

Metoprolol Tartrate (Additive effect). Products include:
Lopressor Ampuls 830
Lopressor HCT Tablets 832
Lopressor Tablets 830

Metyrosine (Additive effect). Products include:
Demser Capsules 1649

Minoxidil (Additive effect). Products include:
Loniten Tablets 2618
Rogaine Topical Solution 2637

Mivacurium Chloride (Increased response to relaxant). Products include:
Mivacron 1138

Moexipril Hydrochloride (Additive effect; precipitous reduction of blood pressure; elevated serum potassium). Products include:
Univasc Tablets 2410

Morphine Sulfate (Effects may be potentiated; potentiation of orthostatic hypotension). Products include:
Astramorph/PF Injection, USP (Preservative-Free) 535
Duramorph 962
Infumorph 200 and Infumorph 500 Sterile Solutions 965
MS Contin Tablets 1994
MSIR 1997
Oramorph SR (Morphine Sulfate Sustained Release Tablets) 2236
RMS Suppositories 2657
Roxanol 2243

Nabumetone (Antihypertensive effect of captopril may be reduced; reduces diuretic and natriuretic effects). Products include:
Relafen Tablets 2510

Nadolol (Additive effect).
No products indexed under this heading.

Naproxen (Antihypertensive effect of captopril may be reduced; reduces diuretic and natriuretic effects). Products include:
Anaprox/Naprosyn 2117

Naproxen Sodium (Antihypertensive effect of captopril may be reduced; reduces diuretic and natriuretic effects). Products include:
Aleve 1975
Anaprox/Naprosyn 2117

Nicardipine Hydrochloride (Additive effect). Products include:
Cardene Capsules 2095
Cardene I.V. 2709
Cardene SR Capsules 2097

Nifedipine (Additive effect; precipitous reduction of blood pressure; elevated serum potassium). Products include:
Adalat Capsules (10 mg and 20 mg) 587
Adalat CC 589
Procardia Capsules 1971
Procardia XL Extended Release Tablets 1972

Nisoldipine (Additive effects).
No products indexed under this heading.

Nitroglycerin (Discontinue before starting captopril; if resumed administer at lower dosage; additive effects). Products include:
Deponit NTG Transdermal Delivery System 2397
Nitro-Bid IV 1523
Nitro-Bid Ointment 1524
Nitrodisc 2047
Nitro-Dur (nitroglycerin) Transdermal Infusion System 1326
Nitrolingual Spray 2027
Nitrostat Tablets 1925
Transderm-Nitro Transdermal Therapeutic System 859

Norepinephrine Bitartrate (Possible decreased response to pressor amines). Products include:
Levophed Bitartrate Injection 2315

Opium Alkaloids (Potentiation of orthostatic hypotension).
No products indexed under this heading.

Oxaprozin (Antihypertensive effect of captopril may be reduced; reduces diuretic and natriuretic effects). Products include:
Daypro Caplets 2426

Oxycodone Hydrochloride (Potentiation of orthostatic hypotension). Products include:
Percocet Tablets 938
Percodan Tablets 939
Percodan-Demi Tablets 940
Roxicodone Tablets, Oral Solution & Intensol (Oxycodone) 2244
Tylox Capsules 1584

Pancuronium Bromide Injection (Increased response to relaxant).
No products indexed under this heading.

Penbutolol Sulfate (Additive effect). Products include:
Levatol 2403

Pentaerythritol Tetranitrate (Discontinue before starting captopril; if resumed administer at lower dosage).
No products indexed under this heading.

Pentobarbital Sodium (Effects may be potentiated; potentiation of orthostatic hypotension). Products include:
Nembutal Sodium Capsules 436
Nembutal Sodium Solution 438
Nembutal Sodium Suppositories 440

Phenelzine Sulfate (Enhanced hypotensive effect; dosage adjusts of one or both agents may be necessary). Products include:
Nardil 1920

Phenobarbital (Potentiation of orthostatic hypotension). Products include:
Arco-Lase Plus Tablets 512
Bellergal-S Tablets 2250
Donnatal 2060
Donnatal Extentabs 2061
Donnatal Tablets 2060
Phenobarbital Elixir and Tablets 1469
Quadrinal Tablets 1350

Phenoxybenzamine Hydrochloride (Additive effect). Products include:
Dibenzyline Capsules 2476

Phentolamine Mesylate (Additive effect). Products include:
Regitine 846

Phenylbutazone (Antihypertensive effect of captopril may be reduced; reduces diuretic and natriuretic effects).
No products indexed under this heading.

Phenylephrine Hydrochloride (Decreased response to pressor amines). Products include:
Atrohist Plus Tablets 454
Cerose DM .... ▣ 878
Comhist 2038
D.A. Chewable Tablets 951
Deconsal Pediatric Capsules 454
Dura-Vent/DA Tablets 953
Entex Capsules 1986
Entex Liquid 1986
Extendryl 1005
4-Way Fast Acting Nasal Spray (regular & mentholated) .... ▣ 621
Hemorid For Women .... ▣ 834
Hycomine Compound Tablets 932
Neo-Synephrine Hydrochloride 1% Carpuject 2324
Neo-Synephrine Hydrochloride 1% Injection 2324
Neo-Synephrine Hydrochloride (Ophthalmic) 2325
Neo-Synephrine .... ▣ 726
Nōstril .... ▣ 644
Novahistine Elixir .... ▣ 823
Phenergan VC 2779
Phenergan VC with Codeine 2781
Preparation H .... ▣ 871
Tympagesic Ear Drops 2342

Vasosulf .... ⊙ 271
Vicks Sinex Nasal Spray and Ultra Fine Mist .... ▣ 765

Pindolol (Additive effect). Products include:
Visken Tablets 2299

Piroxicam (Antihypertensive effect of captopril may be reduced; reduces diuretic and natriuretic effects). Products include:
Feldene Capsules 1965

Polythiazide (Precipitous reduction of blood pressure; captopril's effect will be augmented). Products include:
Minizide Capsules 1938

Potassium Acid Phosphate (Potential for significant increase in serum potassium levels). Products include:
K-Phos Original Formula 'Sodium Free' Tablets 639

Potassium Bicarbonate (Potential for significant increase in serum potassium levels). Products include:
Alka-Seltzer Gold Effervescent Antacid .... ▣ 703

Potassium Chloride (Potential for significant increase in serum potassium levels). Products include:
Chlor-3 Condiment 1004
K-Dur Microburst Release System (potassium chloride, USP) E.R. Tablets 1325
K-Lor Powder Packets 434
K-Norm Extended-Release Capsules 991
K-Tab Filmtab 434
Kolyum Liquid 992
Micro-K 2063
Micro-K LS Packets 2064
NuLYTELY 689
Cherry Flavor NuLYTELY 689
Rum-K Syrup 1005
Slow-K Extended-Release Tablets 851

Potassium Citrate (Potential for significant increase in serum potassium levels). Products include:
Polycitra Syrup 578
Polycitra-K Crystals 579
Polycitra-K Oral Solution 579
Polycitra-LC 578

Potassium Gluconate (Potential for significant increase in serum potassium levels). Products include:
Kolyum Liquid 992

Potassium Phosphate, Dibasic (Potential for significant increase in serum potassium levels).
No products indexed under this heading.

Potassium Phosphate, Monobasic (Potential for significant increase in serum potassium levels). Products include:
K-Phos Neutral Tablets 639
K-Phos Original Formula 'Sodium Free' Tablets 639

Prazosin Hydrochloride (Additive effect or potentiation; use with caution). Products include:
Minipress Capsules 1937
Minizide Capsules 1938

Prednisolone Acetate (Intensified electrolyte depletion, particularly hypokalemia). Products include:
AK-CIDE .... ⊙ 202
AK-CIDE Ointment .... ⊙ 202
Blephamide Liquifilm Sterile Ophthalmic Suspension 476
Blephamide Ointment .... ⊙ 237
Econopred & Econopred Plus Ophthalmic Suspensions .... ⊙ 217
Poly-Pred Liquifilm .... ⊙ 248
Pred Forte .... ⊙ 250
Pred Mild .... ⊙ 253
Pred-G Liquifilm Sterile Ophthalmic Suspension .... ⊙ 251
Pred-G S.O.P. Sterile Ophthalmic Ointment .... ⊙ 252
Vasocidin Ointment .... ⊙ 268

IMPORTANT NOTE: Always consult each drug listing in the patient's regimen for possible interactions.

Capozide | Interactions Index | 162

Prednisolone Sodium Phosphate (Intensified electrolyte depletion, particularly hypokalemia). Products include:
- AK-Pred ◎ 204
- Hydeltrasol Injection, Sterile 1665
- Inflamase ◎ 265
- Pediapred Oral Liquid 995
- Vasocidin Ophthalmic Solution ◎ 270

Prednisolone Tebutate (Intensified electrolyte depletion, particularly hypokalemia). Products include:
- Hydeltra-T.B.A. Sterile Suspension 1667

Prednisone (Intensified electrolyte depletion, particularly hypokalemia). Products include:
- Deltasone Tablets 2595

Probenecid (Dosage adjustment may be necessary since hydrochlorothiazide may have hyperuricemic effect). Products include:
- Benemid Tablets 1611
- ColBENEMID Tablets 1622

Promethazine Hydrochloride (Effects may be potentiated). Products include:
- Mepergan Injection 2753
- Phenergan with Codeine 2777
- Phenergan with Dextromethorphan 2778
- Phenergan Injection 2773
- Phenergan Suppositories 2775
- Phenergan Syrup 2774
- Phenergan Tablets 2775
- Phenergan VC 2779
- Phenergan VC with Codeine 2781

Propofol (Effects may be potentiated). Products include:
- Diprivan Injection 2833

Propoxyphene Hydrochloride (Potentiation of orthostatic hypotension). Products include:
- Darvon 1435
- Wygesic Tablets 2827

Propoxyphene Napsylate (Potentiation of orthostatic hypotension). Products include:
- Darvon-N/Darvocet-N 1433

Propranolol Hydrochloride (Additive effect). Products include:
- Inderal 2728
- Inderal LA Long Acting Capsules 2730
- Inderide Tablets 2732
- Inderide LA Long Acting Capsules 2734

Quinapril Hydrochloride (Additive effect; precipitous reduction of blood pressure). Products include:
- Accupril Tablets 1893

Ramipril (Additive effect; precipitous reduction of blood pressure). Products include:
- Altace Capsules 1232

Rauwolfia Serpentina (Additive effect or potentiation; use with caution).
- No products indexed under this heading.

Rescinnamine (Additive effect or potentiation; use with caution).
- No products indexed under this heading.

Reserpine (Additive effect or potentiation; use with caution). Products include:
- Diupres Tablets 1650
- Hydropres Tablets 1675
- Ser-Ap-Es Tablets 849

Rocuronium Bromide (Increased response to relaxant). Products include:
- Zemuron 1830

Secobarbital Sodium (Effects may be potentiated; potentiation of orthostatic hypotension). Products include:
- Seconal Sodium Pulvules 1474

Selegiline Hydrochloride (Enhanced hypotensive effect; dosage adjustments of one or both agents may be necessary). Products include:
- Eldepryl Tablets 2550

Sodium Nitroprusside (Additive effect).
- No products indexed under this heading.

Sotalol Hydrochloride (Additive effect; precipitous reduction of blood pressure; elevated serum potassium). Products include:
- Betapace Tablets 641

Spirapril Hydrochloride (Additive effect).
- No products indexed under this heading.

Spironolactone (Precipitous reduction of blood pressure; elevated serum potassium; additive effect). Products include:
- Aldactazide 2413
- Aldactone 2414

Sufentanil Citrate (Potentiation of orthostatic hypotension). Products include:
- Sufenta Injection 1309

Sulfinpyrazone (Dosage adjustment may be necessary since hydrochlorothiazide may have hyperuricemic effect). Products include:
- Anturane 807

Sulindac (Antihypertensive effect of captopril may be reduced; reduces diuretic and natriuretic effects). Products include:
- Clinoril Tablets 1618

Terazosin Hydrochloride (Additive effect or potentiation; use with caution). Products include:
- Hytrin Capsules 430

Thiamylal Sodium (Potentiation of orthostatic hypotension).
- No products indexed under this heading.

Timolol Maleate (Additive effect). Products include:
- Blocadren Tablets 1614
- Timolide Tablets 1748
- Timoptic in Ocudose 1753
- Timoptic Sterile Ophthalmic Solution 1751
- Timoptic-XE 1755

Tolazamide (Thiazide-induced hyperglycemia may require dosage adjustment of antidiabetic drugs).
- No products indexed under this heading.

Tolbutamide (Thiazide-induced hyperglycemia may require dosage adjustment of antidiabetic drugs).
- No products indexed under this heading.

Tolmetin Sodium (Antihypertensive effect of captopril may be reduced; reduces diuretic and natriuretic effects). Products include:
- Tolectin (200, 400 and 600 mg) 1581

Torsemide (Additive effect; precipitous reduction of blood pressure). Products include:
- Demadex Tablets and Injection 686

Tranylcypromine Sulfate (Enhanced hypotensive effect; dosage adjustments of one or both agents may be necessary). Products include:
- Parnate Tablets 2503

Triamcinolone (Intensified electrolyte depletion, particularly hypokalemia). Products include:
- Aristocort Tablets 1022

Triamcinolone Acetonide (Intensified electrolyte depletion, particularly hypokalemia). Products include:
- Aristocort A 0.025% Cream 1027
- Aristocort A 0.5% Cream 1031
- Aristocort A 0.1% Cream 1029
- Aristocort A 0.1% Ointment 1030
- Azmacort Oral Inhaler 2011
- Nasacort Nasal Inhaler 2024

Triamcinolone Diacetate (Intensified electrolyte depletion, particularly hypokalemia). Products include:
- Aristocort Suspension (Forte Parenteral) 1027
- Aristocort Suspension (Intralesional) 1025

Triamcinolone Hexacetonide (Intensified electrolyte depletion, particularly hypokalemia). Products include:
- Aristospan Suspension (Intra-articular) 1033
- Aristospan Suspension (Intralesional) 1032

Triamterene (Precipitous reduction of blood pressure; elevated serum potassium; additive effect). Products include:
- Dyazide 2479
- Dyrenium Capsules 2481
- Maxzide 1380

Trimethaphan Camsylate (Additive effect or potentiation; use with caution). Products include:
- Arfonad Ampuls 2080

Tubocurarine Chloride (Effects of tubocurarine may be potentiated).
- No products indexed under this heading.

Vecuronium Bromide (Increased response to relaxant). Products include:
- Norcuron 1826

Verapamil Hydrochloride (Additive effect; precipitous reduction of blood pressure; elevated serum potassium). Products include:
- Calan SR Caplets 2422
- Calan Tablets 2419
- Isoptin Injectable 1344
- Isoptin Oral Tablets 1346
- Isoptin SR Tablets 1348
- Verelan Capsules 1410
- Verelan Capsules 2824

Warfarin Sodium (May decrease anticoagulant effect). Products include:
- Coumadin 926

Food Interactions

Alcohol (Potentation of orthostatic hypotension).

CAPSIN TOPICAL ANALGESIC LOTION 0.025% AND 0.075%

(Capsaicin) ▣ 655

None cited in PDR database.

CAPZASIN-P

(Capsaicin) ▣ 831

None cited in PDR database.

CARAFATE SUSPENSION

(Sucralfate) 1505

May interact with antacids, fluoroquinolone antibiotics, and certain other agents. Compounds in these categories include:

Aluminum Carbonate Gel (Simultaneous administration within one-half hour before or after sucralfate should be avoided; may increase the total body burden of aluminum). Products include:
- Basaljel 2703

Aluminum Hydroxide (Simultaneous administration within one-half hour before or after sucralfate should be avoided; may increase the total body burden of aluminum). Products include:
- ALternaGEL Liquid 1316
- Maximum Strength Ascriptin ▣ 630
- Cama Arthritis Pain Reliever ▣ 785
- Gaviscon Extra Strength Relief Formula Antacid Tablets ▣ 819
- Gaviscon Extra Strength Relief Formula Liquid Antacid ▣ 819
- Gaviscon Liquid Antacid ▣ 820
- Gelusil Liquid & Tablets ▣ 855
- Maalox Heartburn Relief Suspension ▣ 642
- Maalox Heartburn Relief Tablets ▣ 641
- Maalox Magnesia and Alumina Oral Suspension ▣ 642
- Maalox Plus Tablets ▣ 643
- Extra Strength Maalox Antacid Plus Antigas Liquid and Tablets ▣ 638
- Tempo Soft Antacid ▣ 835

Aluminum Hydroxide Gel (Simultaneous administration within one-half hour before or after sucralfate should be avoided; may increase the total body burden of aluminum). Products include:
- ALternaGEL Liquid ▣ 659
- Aludrox Oral Suspension 2695
- Amphojel Suspension 2695
- Amphojel Suspension without Flavor 2695
- Amphojel Tablets 2695
- Arthritis Pain Ascriptin ▣ 631
- Regular Strength Ascriptin Tablets ▣ 629
- Gaviscon Antacid Tablets ▣ 819
- Gaviscon-2 Antacid Tablets ▣ 820
- Mylanta Liquid 1317
- Mylanta Tablets ▣ 660
- Mylanta Double Strength Liquid 1317
- Mylanta Double Strength Tablets ▣ 660
- Nephrox Suspension ▣ 655

Aminophylline (Reduction in bioavailability of oral theophylline).
- No products indexed under this heading.

Cimetidine (Reduction in bioavailability of oral cimetidine). Products include:
- Tagamet Tablets 2516

Cimetidine Hydrochloride (Reduction in oral bioavailability of cimetidine). Products include:
- Tagamet 2516

Ciprofloxacin (Potential for reduced extent of absorption (bioavailability) with concomitant oral administration; dosing the concomitant medication 2 hours before sucralfate eliminates the interaction). Products include:
- Cipro I.V. 595
- Cipro I.V. Pharmacy Bulk Package 597

Ciprofloxacin Hydrochloride (Potential for reduced extent of absorption (bioavailability) with concomitant oral administration; dosing the concomitant medication 2 hours before sucralfate eliminates the interaction). Products include:
- Ciloxan Ophthalmic Solution 472
- Cipro Tablets 592

Digitoxin (Reduction in bioavailability of oral digitoxin). Products include:
- Crystodigin Tablets 1433

Digoxin (Reduction in bioavailability of oral digoxin). Products include:
- Lanoxicaps 1117
- Lanoxin Elixir Pediatric 1120
- Lanoxin Injection 1123
- Lanoxin Injection Pediatric 1126
- Lanoxin Tablets 1128

Dyphylline (Reduction in bioavailability of oral theophylline). Products include:
- Lufyllin & Lufyllin-400 Tablets 2670
- Lufyllin-GG Elixir & Tablets 2671

(▣ Described in PDR For Nonprescription Drugs) (◎ Described in PDR For Ophthalmology)

Interactions Index

Carafate

Enoxacin (Potential for reduced extent of absorption (bioavailability) with concomitant oral administration; dosing the concomitant medication 2 hours before sucralfate eliminates the interaction). Products include:

Penetrex Tablets 2031

Ketoconazole (Reduction in the extent of absorption (bioavailability) of oral ketoconazole). Products include:

Nizoral 2% Cream 1297
Nizoral 2% Shampoo........................... 1298
Nizoral Tablets 1298

Levothyroxine Sodium (Potential for reduced extent of absorption (bioavailability) with concomitant oral administration). Products include:

Levothroid Tablets 1016
Levoxyl Tablets.................................... 903
Synthroid.. 1359

Lomefloxacin Hydrochloride (Potential for reduced extent of absorption (bioavailability) with concomitant oral administration; dosing the concomitant medication 2 hours before sucralfate eliminates the interaction). Products include:

Maxaquin Tablets 2440

Magaldrate (Simultaneous administration within one-half hour before or after sucralfate should be avoided; may increase the total body burden of aluminum).

No products indexed under this heading.

Magnesium Hydroxide (Simultaneous administration within one-half hour before or after sucralfate should be avoided). Products include:

Aludrox Oral Suspension 2695
Arthritis Pain Ascriptin .... ◈ 631
Maximum Strength Ascriptin .... ◈ 630
Regular Strength Ascriptin Tablets .... ◈ 629
Di-Gel Antacid/Anti-Gas .... ◈ 801
Gelusil Liquid & Tablets .... ◈ 855
Maalox Magnesia and Alumina Oral Suspension .... ◈ 642
Maalox Plus Tablets .... ◈ 643
Extra Strength Maalox Antacid Plus Antigas Liquid and Tablets ◈ 638
Mylanta Calcium Carbonate and Magnesium Hydroxide Tablets..... 1318
Mylanta Liquid 1317
Mylanta Tablets .... ◈ 660
Mylanta Double Strength Liquid 1317
Mylanta Double Strength Tablets.. ◈ 660
Phillips' Milk of Magnesia Liquid... ◈ 729
Rolaids Tablets .... ◈ 843
Tempo Soft Antacid .... ◈ 835

Magnesium Oxide (Simultaneous administration within one-half hour before or after sucralfate should be avoided). Products include:

Beelith Tablets 639
Bufferin Analgesic Tablets and Caplets .... ◈ 613
Caltrate PLUS .... ◈ 665
Cama Arthritis Pain Reliever............... ◈ 785
Mag-Ox 400 668
Uro-Mag.. 668

Norfloxacin (Potential for reduced extent of absorption (bioavailability) with concomitant oral administration; dosing the concomitant medication 2 hours before sucralfate eliminates the interaction). Products include:

Chibroxin Sterile Ophthalmic Solution.. 1617
Noroxin Tablets 1715
Noroxin Tablets 2048

Ofloxacin (Potential for reduced extent of absorption (bioavailability) with concomitant oral administration; dosing the concomitant medication 2 hours before sucralfate eliminates the interaction). Products include:

Floxin I.V. 1571
Floxin Tablets (200 mg, 300 mg, 400 mg) 1567
Ocuflox... 481
Ocuflox... ◎ 246

Oxytetracycline (Reduction in bioavailability of oral oxytetracycline). Products include:

Terramycin Intramuscular Solution 2210

Oxytetracycline Hydrochloride (Reduction in bioavailability of oral oxytetracycline). Products include:

TERAK Ointment .... ◎ 209
Terra-Cortril Ophthalmic Suspension 2210
Terramycin with Polymyxin B Sulfate Ophthalmic Ointment 2211
Urobiotic-250 Capsules 2214

Phenytoin (Reduction in bioavailability of oral phenytoin). Products include:

Dilantin Infatabs 1908
Dilantin-125 Suspension 1911

Phenytoin Sodium (Reduction in bioavailability of oral phenytoin). Products include:

Dilantin Kapseals 1906
Dilantin Parenteral 1910

Quinidine Gluconate (Potential for reduced extent of absorption (bioavailability) with concomitant oral administration). Products include:

Quinaglute Dura-Tabs Tablets 649

Quinidine Polygalacturonate (Potential for reduced extent of absorption (bioavailability) with concomitant oral administration).

No products indexed under this heading.

Quinidine Sulfate (Potential for reduced extent of absorption (bioavailability) with concomitant oral administration). Products include:

Quinidex Extentabs 2067

Ranitidine Hydrochloride (Reduction in bioavailability of oral ranitidine). Products include:

Zantac.. 1209
Zantac Injection 1207
Zantac Syrup 1209

Temafloxacin Hydrochloride (Potential for reduced extent of absorption (bioavailability) with concomitant oral administration; dosing the concomitant medication 2 hours before sucralfate eliminates the interaction).

No products indexed under this heading.

Tetracycline Hydrochloride (Reduction in bioavailability of oral tetracycline). Products include:

Achromycin V Capsules 1367

Theophylline (Reduction in bioavailability of oral theophylline). Products include:

Marax Tablets & DF Syrup................... 2200
Quibron 2053

Theophylline Anhydrous (Reduction in bioavailability of oral theophylline). Products include:

Aerolate 1004
Primatene Dual Action Formula......◈ 872
Primatene Tablets ....◈ 873
Respbid Tablets 682
Slo-bid Gyrocaps 2033
Theo-24 Extended Release Capsules 2568
Theo-Dur Extended-Release Tablets 1327
Theo-X Extended-Release Tablets .. 788
Uni-Dur Extended-Release Tablets.. 1331
Uniphyl 400 mg Tablets....................... 2001

Theophylline Calcium Salicylate (Reduction in bioavailability of oral theophylline). Products include:

Quadrinal Tablets 1350

Theophylline Sodium Glycinate (Reduction in bioavailability of oral theophylline).

No products indexed under this heading.

Warfarin Sodium (Subtherapeutic prothrombin times with concomitant warfarin and sucralfate have been reported in spontaneous and published case reports; clinical studies have demonstrated no change in the prothrombin time with the addition of sucralfate to chronic warfarin therapy.). Products include:

Coumadin 926

CARAFATE TABLETS

(Sucralfate)... 1504

May interact with antacids, fluoroquinolone antibiotics, and certain other agents. Compounds in these categories include:

Aluminum Carbonate Gel (Simultaneous administration within one-half hour before or after sucralfate should be avoided; may increase the total body burden of aluminum). Products include:

Basaljel... 2703

Aluminum Hydroxide (Simultaneous administration within one-half hour before or after sucralfate should be avoided; may increase the total body burden of aluminum). Products include:

ALternaGEL Liquid 1316
Maximum Strength Ascriptin ....◈ 630
Cama Arthritis Pain Reliever..............◈ 785
Gaviscon Extra Strength Relief Formula Antacid Tablets...................◈ 819
Gaviscon Extra Strength Relief Formula Liquid Antacid.....................◈ 819
Gaviscon Liquid Antacid.....................◈ 820
Gelusil Liquid & Tablets ....◈ 855
Maalox Heartburn Relief Suspension ....◈ 642
Maalox Heartburn Relief Tablets....◈ 641
Maalox Magnesia and Alumina Oral Suspension..................................◈ 642
Maalox Plus Tablets ....◈ 643
Extra Strength Maalox Antacid Plus Antigas Liquid and Tablets ◈ 638
Tempo Soft Antacid ....◈ 835

Aluminum Hydroxide Gel (Simultaneous administration within one-half hour before or after sucralfate should be avoided; may increase the total body burden of aluminum). Products include:

ALternaGEL Liquid ....◈ 659
Aludrox Oral Suspension 2695
Amphojel Suspension 2695
Amphojel Suspension without Flavor 2695
Amphojel Tablets.................................. 2695
Arthritis Pain Ascriptin ....◈ 631
Regular Strength Ascriptin Tablets ....◈ 629
Gaviscon Antacid Tablets....................◈ 819
Gaviscon-2 Antacid Tablets ....◈ 820
Mylanta Liquid 1317
Mylanta Tablets ....◈ 660
Mylanta Double Strength Liquid 1317
Mylanta Double Strength Tablets ..◈ 660
Nephrox Suspension ....◈ 655

Aminophylline (Reduction in bioavailability of oral theophylline).

No products indexed under this heading.

Cimetidine (Reduction in bioavailability of oral cimetidine). Products include:

Tagamet Tablets 2516

Cimetidine Hydrochloride (Reduction in oral bioavailability of cimetidine). Products include:

Tagamet.. 2516

Ciprofloxacin (Potential for reduced extent of absorption (bioavailability) with concomitant oral administration; dosing the concomitant medication 2 hours before sucralfate eliminates the interaction). Products include:

Cipro I.V. 595
Cipro I.V. Pharmacy Bulk Package.. 597

Ciprofloxacin Hydrochloride (Potential for reduced extent of absorption (bioavailability) with concomitant oral administration; dosing the concomitant medication 2 hours before sucralfate eliminates the interaction). Products include:

Ciloxan Ophthalmic Solution............... 472
Cipro Tablets... 592

Digitoxin (Reduction in bioavailability of oral digitoxin). Products include:

Crystodigin Tablets............................... 1433

Digoxin (Reduction in bioavailability of oral digoxin). Products include:

Lanoxicaps 1117
Lanoxin Elixir Pediatric 1120
Lanoxin Injection 1123
Lanoxin Injection Pediatric.................. 1126
Lanoxin Tablets 1128

Dihydroxyaluminum Sodium Carbonate (Simultaneous administration within one-half hour before or after sucralfate should be avoided).

No products indexed under this heading.

Dyphylline (Reduction in bioavailability of oral theophylline). Products include:

Lufyllin & Lufyllin-400 Tablets 2670
Lufyllin-GG Elixir & Tablets 2671

Enoxacin (Potential for reduced extent of absorption (bioavailability) with concomitant oral administration; dosing the concomitant medication 2 hours before sucralfate eliminates the interaction). Products include:

Penetrex Tablets 2031

Ketoconazole (Reduction in the extent of absorption (bioavailability) of oral ketoconazole). Products include:

Nizoral 2% Cream 1297
Nizoral 2% Shampoo........................... 1298
Nizoral Tablets 1298

Levothyroxine Sodium (Potential for reduced extent of absorption (bioavailability) with concomitant oral administration). Products include:

Levothroid Tablets 1016
Levoxyl Tablets..................................... 903
Synthroid... 1359

Lomefloxacin Hydrochloride (Potential for reduced extent of absorption (bioavailability) with concomitant oral administration; dosing the concomitant medication 2 hours before sucralfate eliminates the interaction). Products include:

Maxaquin Tablets 2440

Magaldrate (Simultaneous administration within one-half hour before or after sucralfate should be avoided; may increase the total body burden of aluminum).

No products indexed under this heading.

Magnesium Hydroxide (Simultaneous administration within one-half hour before or after sucralfate should be avoided). Products include:

Aludrox Oral Suspension 2695
Arthritis Pain Ascriptin ....◈ 631
Maximum Strength Ascriptin ....◈ 630
Regular Strength Ascriptin Tablets ....◈ 629
Di-Gel Antacid/Anti-Gas ....◈ 801
Gelusil Liquid & Tablets ....◈ 855

IMPORTANT NOTE: Always consult each drug listing in the patient's regimen for possible interactions.

Maalox Magnesia and Alumina Oral Suspension ■ 642
Maalox Plus Tablets ■ 643
Extra Strength Maalox Antacid Plus Antigas Liquid and Tablets ■ 638
Mylanta Calcium Carbonate and Magnesium Hydroxide Tablets 1318
Mylanta Liquid 1317
Mylanta Tablets ■ 660
Mylanta Double Strength Liquid 1317
Mylanta Double Strength Tablets ■ 660
Phillips' Milk of Magnesia Liquid ■ 729
Rolaids Tablets ■ 843
Tempo Soft Antacid ■ 835

Magnesium Oxide (Simultaneous administration within one-half hour before or after sucralfate should be avoided). Products include:
Beelith Tablets 639
Bufferin Analgesic Tablets and Caplets ■ 613
Caltrate PLUS ■ 665
Cama Arthritis Pain Reliever ■ 785
Mag-Ox 400 668
Uro-Mag 668

Norfloxacin (Potential for reduced extent of absorption (bioavailability) with concomitant oral administration; dosing the concomitant medication 2 hours before sucralfate eliminates the interaction). Products include:
Chibroxin Sterile Ophthalmic Solution 1617
Noroxin Tablets 1715
Noroxin Tablets 2048

Ofloxacin (Potential for reduced extent of absorption (bioavailability) with concomitant oral administration; dosing the concomitant medication 2 hours before sucralfate eliminates the interaction). Products include:
Floxin I.V. 1571
Floxin Tablets (200 mg, 300 mg, 400 mg) 1567
Ocuflox 481
Ocuflox ◉ 246

Oxytetracycline (Reduction in bioavailability of oral oxytetracycline). Products include:
Terramycin Intramuscular Solution 2210

Oxytetracycline Hydrochloride (Reduction in bioavailability of oral oxytetracycline). Products include:
TERAK Ointment ◉ 209
Terra-Cortril Ophthalmic Suspension 2210
Terramycin with Polymyxin B Sulfate Ophthalmic Ointment 2211
Urobiotic-250 Capsules 2214

Phenytoin (Reduction in bioavailability of oral phenytoin). Products include:
Dilantin Infatabs 1908
Dilantin-125 Suspension 1911

Phenytoin Sodium (Reduction in bioavailability of oral phenytoin). Products include:
Dilantin Kapseals 1906
Dilantin Parenteral 1910

Quinidine Gluconate (Potential for reduced extent of absorption (bioavailability) with concomitant oral administration). Products include:
Quinaglute Dura-Tabs Tablets 649

Quinidine Polygalacturonate (Potential for reduced extent of absorption (bioavailability) with concomitant oral administration).
No products indexed under this heading.

Quinidine Sulfate (Potential for reduced extent of absorption (bioavailability) with concomitant oral administration). Products include:
Quinidex Extentabs 2067

Ranitidine Hydrochloride (Reduction in bioavailability of oral ranitidine). Products include:
Zantac 1209
Zantac Injection 1207
Zantac Syrup 1209

Temafloxacin Hydrochloride (Potential for reduced extent of absorption (bioavailability) with concomitant oral administration; dosing the concomitant medication 2 hours before sucralfate eliminates the interaction).
No products indexed under this heading.

Tetracycline Hydrochloride (Reduction in bioavailability of oral tetracycline). Products include:
Achromycin V Capsules 1367

Theophylline (Reduction in bioavailability of oral theophylline). Products include:
Marax Tablets & DF Syrup 2200
Quibron 2053

Theophylline Anhydrous (Reduction in bioavailability of oral theophylline). Products include:
Aerolate 1004
Primatene Dual Action Formula ■ 872
Primatene Tablets ■ 873
Respbid Tablets 682
Slo-bid Gyrocaps 2033
Theo-24 Extended Release Capsules 2568
Theo-Dur Extended-Release Tablets 1327
Theo-X Extended-Release Tablets 788
Uni-Dur Extended-Release Tablets 1331
Uniphyl 400 mg Tablets 2001

Theophylline Calcium Salicylate (Reduction in bioavailability of oral theophylline). Products include:
Quadrinal Tablets 1350

Theophylline Sodium Glycinate (Reduction in bioavailability of oral theophylline).
No products indexed under this heading.

Warfarin Sodium (Subtherapeutic prothrombin times with concomitant warfarin and sucralfate have been reported in spontaneous and published reports; clinical studies have demonstrated no changes in the prothrombin time with the addition of sucralfate to chronic warfarin therapy). Products include:
Coumadin 926

CARBOCAINE HYDROCHLORIDE INJECTION

(Mepivacaine Hydrochloride Injection) 2303
None cited in PDR database.

CARDENE CAPSULES

(Nicardipine Hydrochloride) 2095
May interact with cardiac glycosides and certain other agents. Compounds in these categories include:

Cimetidine (Increased Cardene plasma levels). Products include:
Tagamet Tablets 2516

Cimetidine Hydrochloride (Increased Cardene plasma levels). Products include:
Tagamet 2516

Cyclosporine (Concomitant administration results in elevated plasma cyclosporine levels). Products include:
Neoral 2276
Sandimmune 2286

Deslanoside (Potential for altered plasma deslanoside levels).
No products indexed under this heading.

Digitoxin (Potential for altered plasma digitoxin levels). Products include:
Crystodigin Tablets 1433

Digoxin (Potential for altered plasma digoxin levels). Products include:
Lanoxicaps 1117
Lanoxin Elixir Pediatric 1120
Lanoxin Injection 1123
Lanoxin Injection Pediatric 1126
Lanoxin Tablets 1128

Fentanyl Citrate (May require increased volume of circulating fluids if severe hypotension were to occur). Products include:
Sublimaze Injection 1307

CARDENE I.V.

(Nicardipine Hydrochloride) 2709
May interact with beta blockers and certain other agents. Compounds in these categories include:

Acebutolol Hydrochloride (In vitro and in some patients a negative inotropic effect has been observed with Cardene I.V., therefore, caution should be exercised when co-administered with beta blocker in patients with CHF or significant left ventricular dysfunction). Products include:
Sectral Capsules 2807

Atenolol (In vitro and in some patients a negative inotropic effect has been observed with Cardene I.V., therefore, caution should be exercised when co-administered with beta blocker in patients with CHF or significant left ventricular dysfunction). Products include:
Tenoretic Tablets 2845
Tenormin Tablets and I.V. Injection 2847

Betaxolol Hydrochloride (In vitro and in some patients a negative inotropic effect has been observed with Cardene I.V., therefore, caution should be exercised when co-administered with beta blocker in patients with CHF or significant left ventricular dysfunction). Products include:
Betoptic Ophthalmic Solution 469
Betoptic S Ophthalmic Suspension 471
Kerlone Tablets 2436

Bisoprolol Fumarate (In vitro and in some patients a negative inotropic effect has been observed with Cardene I.V., therefore, caution should be exercised when co-administered with beta blocker in patients with CHF or significant left ventricular dysfunction). Products include:
Zebeta Tablets 1413
Ziac 1415

Carteolol Hydrochloride (In vitro and in some patients a negative inotropic effect has been observed with Cardene I.V., therefore, caution should be exercised when co-administered with beta blocker in patients with CHF or significant left ventricular dysfunction). Products include:
Cartrol Tablets 410
Ocupress Ophthalmic Solution, 1% Sterile ◉ 309

Cimetidine (Co-administration of cimetidine with Cardene Capsules increases nicardipine plasma concentration). Products include:
Tagamet Tablets 2516

Cimetidine Hydrochloride (Co-administration of cimetidine with Cardene Capsules increases nicardipine plasma concentration). Products include:
Tagamet 2516

Cyclosporine (Co-administration of Cardene Capsules and cyclosporine results in elevated plasma cyclosporine levels). Products include:
Neoral 2276
Sandimmune 2286

Digoxin (No alteration in digoxin plasma levels, however, as a precaution, digoxin levels should be evaluated when concomitant therapy is initiated). Products include:
Lanoxicaps 1117
Lanoxin Elixir Pediatric 1120
Lanoxin Injection 1123
Lanoxin Injection Pediatric 1126
Lanoxin Tablets 1128

Esmolol Hydrochloride (In vitro and in some patients a negative inotropic effect has been observed with Cardene I.V., therefore, caution should be exercised when co-administered with beta blocker in patients with CHF or significant left ventricular dysfunction). Products include:
Brevibloc Injection 1808

Fentanyl (Potential for hypotension with fentanyl anesthesia when used with calcium channel blocker and beta blocker; such reaction has not been observed with Cardene I.V. during clinical trials). Products include:
Duragesic Transdermal System 1288

Fentanyl Citrate (Potential for hypotension with fentanyl anesthesia when used with calcium channel blocker and beta blocker; such reaction has not been observed with Cardene I.V. during clinical trials). Products include:
Sublimaze Injection 1307

Labetalol Hydrochloride (In vitro and in some patients a negative inotropic effect has been observed with Cardene I.V., therefore, caution should be exercised when co-administered with beta blocker in patients with CHF or significant left ventricular dysfunction). Products include:
Normodyne Injection 2377
Normodyne Tablets 2379
Trandate 1185

Levobunolol Hydrochloride (In vitro and in some patients a negative inotropic effect has been observed with Cardene I.V., therefore, caution should be exercised when co-administered with beta blocker in patients with CHF or significant left ventricular dysfunction). Products include:
Betagan ◉ 233

Metipranolol Hydrochloride (In vitro and in some patients a negative inotropic effect has been observed with Cardene I.V., therefore, caution should be exercised when co-administered with beta blocker in patients with CHF or significant left ventricular dysfunction). Products include:
OptiPranolol (Metipranolol 0.3%) Sterile Ophthalmic Solution ◉ 258

Metoprolol Succinate (In vitro and in some patients a negative inotropic effect has been observed with Cardene I.V., therefore, caution should be exercised when co-administered with beta blocker in patients with CHF or significant left ventricular dysfunction). Products include:
Toprol-XL Tablets 565

Metoprolol Tartrate (In vitro and in some patients a negative inotropic effect has been observed with Cardene I.V., therefore, caution should be exercised when co-administered with beta blocker in patients with CHF or significant left ventricular dysfunction). Products include:
Lopressor Ampuls 830
Lopressor HCT Tablets 832
Lopressor Tablets 830

(■ Described in PDR For Nonprescription Drugs) (◉ Described in PDR For Ophthalmology)

Nadolol (In vitro and in some patients a negative inotropic effect has been observed with Cardene I.V., therefore, caution should be exercised when co-administered with beta blocker in patients with CHF or significant left ventricular dysfunction).

No products indexed under this heading.

Penbutolol Sulfate (In vitro and in some patients a negative inotropic effect has been observed with Cardene I.V., therefore, caution should be exercised when co-administered with beta blocker in patients with CHF or significant left ventricular dysfunction). Products include:

Levatol 2403

Pindolol (In vitro and in some patients a negative inotropic effect has been observed with Cardene I.V., therefore, caution should be exercised when co-administered with beta blocker in patients with CHF or significant left ventricular dysfunction). Products include:

Visken Tablets 2299

Propranolol Hydrochloride (In vitro and in some patients a negative inotropic effect has been observed with Cardene I.V., therefore, caution should be exercised when co-administered with beta blocker in patients with CHF or significant left ventricular dysfunction). Products include:

Inderal 2728
Inderal LA Long Acting Capsules 2730
Inderide Tablets 2732
Inderide LA Long Acting Capsules 2734

Sotalol Hydrochloride (In vitro and in some patients a negative inotropic effect has been observed with Cardene I.V., therefore, caution should be exercised when co-administered with beta blocker in patients with CHF or significant left ventricular dysfunction). Products include:

Betapace Tablets 641

Timolol Hemihydrate (In vitro and in some patients a negative inotropic effect has been observed with Cardene I.V., therefore, caution should be exercised when co-administered with beta blocker in patients with CHF or significant left ventricular dysfunction). Products include:

Betimol 0.25%, 0.5% .... ◉ 261

Timolol Maleate (In vitro and in some patients a negative inotropic effect has been observed with Cardene I.V., therefore, caution should be exercised when co-administered with beta blocker in patients with CHF or significant left ventricular dysfunction). Products include:

Blocadren Tablets 1614
Timolide Tablets 1748
Timoptic in Ocudose 1753
Timoptic Sterile Ophthalmic Solution 1751
Timoptic-XE 1755

CARDENE SR CAPSULES

(Nicardipine Hydrochloride) 2097
May interact with:

Cimetidine (Increases plasma levels). Products include:

Tagamet Tablets 2516

Cimetidine Hydrochloride (Increases plasma levels). Products include:

Tagamet 2516

Cyclosporine (Elevated plasma cyclosporine levels). Products include:

Neoral 2276
Sandimmune 2286

Digoxin (Serum digoxin levels should be evaluated after concomitant therapy with Cardene is initiated because of the potential of increased digoxin serum concentrations). Products include:

Lanoxicaps 1117
Lanoxin Elixir Pediatric 1120
Lanoxin Injection 1123
Lanoxin Injection Pediatric 1126
Lanoxin Tablets 1128

Fentanyl (Potential for severe hypotension). Products include:

Duragesic Transdermal System 1288

Fentanyl Citrate (Potential for severe hypotension). Products include:

Sublimaze Injection 1307

Food Interactions

Diet, high-lipid (Results in lower C_{max} and AUC; higher trough levels).

CARDIZEM CD CAPSULES

(Diltiazem Hydrochloride) 1506
May interact with cardiac glycosides, anesthetics, beta blockers, and certain other agents. Compounds in these categories include:

Acebutolol Hydrochloride (Possible additive effects on cardiac conduction (prolonged AV conduction)). Products include:

Sectral Capsules 2807

Alfentanil Hydrochloride (Depression of cardiac contractility, conductivity, automaticity, and vasodilation associated with anesthetic may be potentiated). Products include:

Alfenta Injection 1286

Atenolol (Possible additive effects on cardiac conduction (prolonged AV conduction)). Products include:

Tenoretic Tablets 2845
Tenormin Tablets and I.V. Injection 2847

Betaxolol Hydrochloride (Possible additive effects on cardiac conduction (prolonged AV conduction)). Products include:

Betoptic Ophthalmic Solution 469
Betoptic S Ophthalmic Suspension 471
Kerlone Tablets 2436

Bisoprolol Fumarate (Possible additive effects on cardiac conduction (prolonged AV conduction)). Products include:

Zebeta Tablets 1413
Ziac 1415

Carbamazepine (Potential for elevated serum levels of carbamazepine (40% to 72% increase), resulting in toxicity in some cases). Products include:

Atretol Tablets 573
Tegretol Chewable Tablets 852
Tegretol Suspension 852
Tegretol Tablets 852

Carteolol Hydrochloride (Possible additive effects on cardiac conduction (prolonged AV conduction)). Products include:

Cartrol Tablets 410
Ocupress Ophthalmic Solution, 1% Sterile .... ◉ 309

Cimetidine (Potential for significant increase in peak plasma levels (58%) and AUC (53%); an adjustment in diltiazem dosage may be warranted). Products include:

Tagamet Tablets 2516

Cimetidine Hydrochloride (Potential for significant increase in peak plasma levels (58%) and AUC (53%); an adjustment in diltiazem dosage may be warranted). Products include:

Tagamet 2516

Cyclosporine (A pharmacokinetic interaction between diltiazem and cyclosporine has been observed in renal and cardiac transplant patients requiring a reduction of cyclosporine dose). Products include:

Neoral 2276
Sandimmune 2286

Deslanoside (Possible increase in digitalis levels; possible additive effects on cardiac conduction).

No products indexed under this heading.

Digitoxin (Possible increase in digitalis levels; possible additive effects on cardiac conduction). Products include:

Crystodigin Tablets 1433

Digoxin (Possible increase in digoxin levels; possible additive effects on cardiac conduction). Products include:

Lanoxicaps 1117
Lanoxin Elixir Pediatric 1120
Lanoxin Injection 1123
Lanoxin Injection Pediatric 1126
Lanoxin Tablets 1128

Drugs which undergo biotransformation by cytochrome P-450 mixed function oxidase (May result in competitive inhibition of metabolism).

Enflurane (Depression of cardiac contractility, conductivity, automaticity, and vasodilation associated with anesthetic may be potentiated).

No products indexed under this heading.

Esmolol Hydrochloride (Possible additive effects on cardiac conduction (prolonged AV conduction)). Products include:

Brevibloc Injection 1808

Fentanyl Citrate (Depression of cardiac contractility, conductivity, automaticity, and vasodilation associated with anesthetic may be potentiated). Products include:

Sublimaze Injection 1307

Halothane (Depression of cardiac contractility, conductivity, automaticity, and vasodilation associated with anesthetic may be potentiated). Products include:

Fluothane 2724

Isoflurane (Depression of cardiac contractility, conductivity, automaticity, and vasodilation associated with anesthetic may be potentiated).

No products indexed under this heading.

Ketamine Hydrochloride (Depression of cardiac contractility, conductivity, automaticity, and vasodilation associated with anesthetic may be potentiated).

No products indexed under this heading.

Labetalol Hydrochloride (Possible additive effects on cardiac conduction (prolonged AV conduction)). Products include:

Normodyne Injection 2377
Normodyne Tablets 2379
Trandate 1185

Levobunolol Hydrochloride (Possible additive effects on cardiac conduction (prolonged AV conduction)). Products include:

Betagan .... ◉ 233

Methohexital Sodium (Depression of cardiac contractility, conductivity, automaticity, and vasodilation associated with anesthetic may be potentiated). Products include:

Brevital Sodium Vials 1429

Metipranolol Hydrochloride (Possible additive effects on cardiac conduction (prolonged AV conduction)). Products include:

OptiPranolol (Metipranolol 0.3%) Sterile Ophthalmic Solution .... ◉ 258

Metoprolol Succinate (Possible additive effects on cardiac conduction (prolonged AV conduction)). Products include:

Toprol-XL Tablets 565

Metoprolol Tartrate (Possible additive effects on cardiac conduction (prolonged AV conduction)). Products include:

Lopressor Ampuls 830
Lopressor HCT Tablets 832
Lopressor Tablets 830

Midazolam Hydrochloride (Depression of cardiac contractility, conductivity, automaticity, and vasodilation associated with anesthetic may be potentiated). Products include:

Versed Injection 2170

Nadolol (Possible additive effects on cardiac conduction (prolonged AV conduction)).

No products indexed under this heading.

Penbutolol Sulfate (Possible additive effects on cardiac conduction (prolonged AV conduction)). Products include:

Levatol 2403

Pindolol (Possible additive effects on cardiac conduction (prolonged AV conduction)). Products include:

Visken Tablets 2299

Propofol (Depression of cardiac contractility, conductivity, automaticity, and vasodilation associated with anesthetic may be potentiated). Products include:

Diprivan Injection 2833

Propranolol Hydrochloride (Increased levels and bioavailability of propranolol; dosage of propranolol may need to be adjusted; possible additive effects on cardiac conduction (prolonged AV conduction)). Products include:

Inderal 2728
Inderal LA Long Acting Capsules 2730
Inderide Tablets 2732
Inderide LA Long Acting Capsules 2734

Ranitidine Hydrochloride (Produces smaller, nonsignificant increase in diltiazem plasma levels). Products include:

Zantac 1209
Zantac Injection 1207
Zantac Syrup 1209

Sotalol Hydrochloride (Possible additive effects on cardiac conduction (prolonged AV conduction)). Products include:

Betapace Tablets 641

Sufentanil Citrate (Depression of cardiac contractility, conductivity, automaticity, and vasodilation associated with anesthetic may be potentiated). Products include:

Sufenta Injection 1309

Thiamylal Sodium (Depression of cardiac contractility, conductivity, automaticity, and vasodilation associated with anesthetic may be potentiated).

No products indexed under this heading.

Timolol Hemihydrate (Possible additive effects on cardiac conduction (prolonged AV conduction)). Products include:

Betimol 0.25%, 0.5% .... ◉ 261

IMPORTANT NOTE: Always consult each drug listing in the patient's regimen for possible interactions.

Timolol Maleate (Possible additive effects on cardiac conduction (prolonged AV conduction)). Products include:

- Blocadren Tablets ... 1614
- Timolide Tablets ... 1748
- Timoptic in Ocudose ... 1753
- Timoptic Sterile Ophthalmic Solution ... 1751
- Timoptic-XE ... 1755

CARDIZEM SR CAPSULES

(Diltiazem Hydrochloride) ... 1510

May interact with beta blockers, cardiac glycosides, general anesthetics, drugs which undergo biotransformation by cytochrome p-450 mixed function oxidase, and certain other agents. Compounds in these categories include:

Acebutolol Hydrochloride (Concomitant administration may result in additive effects in prolonging AV conduction). Products include:

- Sectral Capsules ... 2807

Atenolol (Concomitant administration may result in additive effects in prolonging AV conduction). Products include:

- Tenoretic Tablets ... 2845
- Tenormin Tablets and I.V. Injection 2847

Betaxolol Hydrochloride (Concomitant administration may result in additive effects in prolonging AV conduction). Products include:

- Betoptic Ophthalmic Solution ... 469
- Betoptic S Ophthalmic Suspension 471
- Kerlone Tablets ... 2436

Bisoprolol Fumarate (Concomitant administration may result in additive effects in prolonging AV conduction). Products include:

- Zebeta Tablets ... 1413
- Ziac ... 1415

Carbamazepine (Potential for elevated serum levels of carbamazepine (40% to 72% increase), resulting in toxicity in some cases). Products include:

- Atretol Tablets ... 573
- Tegretol Chewable Tablets ... 852
- Tegretol Suspension ... 852
- Tegretol Tablets ... 852

Carteolol Hydrochloride (Concomitant administration may result in additive effects in prolonging AV conduction). Products include:

- Cartrol Tablets ... 410
- Ocupress Ophthalmic Solution, 1% Sterile ... ⊙ 309

Cimetidine (Increases peak diltiazem plasma levels (58%) and AUC (53%)). Products include:

- Tagamet Tablets ... 2516

Cimetidine Hydrochloride (Increases peak diltiazem plasma levels (58%) and AUC (53%)). Products include:

- Tagamet ... 2516

Cyclosporine (A pharmacokinetic interaction between diltiazem and cyclosporine has been observed in renal and cardiac transplant patients requiring a reduction of cyclosporine dose). Products include:

- Neoral ... 2276
- Sandimmune ... 2286

Deslanoside (Additive effects on cardiac conduction; variable effect on plasma digoxin).

No products indexed under this heading.

Digitoxin (Additive effects on cardiac conduction; variable effect on plasma digoxin). Products include:

- Crystodigin Tablets ... 1433

Digoxin (Additive effects on cardiac conduction; variable effect on plasma digoxin). Products include:

- Lanoxicaps ... 1117
- Lanoxin Elixir Pediatric ... 1120
- Lanoxin Injection ... 1123
- Lanoxin Injection Pediatric ... 1126
- Lanoxin Tablets ... 1128

Drugs which undergo biotransformation by cytochrome P-450 mixed function oxidase (Coadministration may result in the competitive inhibition of metabolism).

Enflurane (Depression of cardiac contractility, conductivity, automaticity, and vasodilation may be potentiated).

No products indexed under this heading.

Esmolol Hydrochloride (Concomitant administration may result in additive effects in prolonging AV conduction). Products include:

- Brevibloc Injection ... 1808

Isoflurane (Depression of cardiac contractility, conductivity, automaticity, and vasodilation may be potentiated).

No products indexed under this heading.

Ketamine Hydrochloride (Depression of cardiac contractility, conductivity, automaticity, and vasodilation may be potentiated).

No products indexed under this heading.

Labetalol Hydrochloride (Concomitant administration may result in additive effects in prolonging AV conduction). Products include:

- Normodyne Injection ... 2377
- Normodyne Tablets ... 2379
- Trandate ... 1185

Levobunolol Hydrochloride (Concomitant administration may result in additive effects in prolonging AV conduction). Products include:

- Betagan ... ⊙ 233

Methohexital Sodium (Depression of cardiac contractility, conductivity, automaticity, and vasodilation may be potentiated). Products include:

- Brevital Sodium Vials ... 1429

Methoxyflurane (Depression of cardiac contractility, conductivity, automaticity, and vasodilation may be potentiated).

No products indexed under this heading.

Metipranolol Hydrochloride (Concomitant administration may result in additive effects in prolonging AV conduction). Products include:

- OptiPranolol (Metipranolol 0.3%) Sterile Ophthalmic Solution ... ⊙ 258

Metoprolol Succinate (Concomitant administration may result in additive effects in prolonging AV conduction). Products include:

- Toprol-XL Tablets ... 565

Metoprolol Tartrate (Concomitant administration may result in additive effects in prolonging AV conduction). Products include:

- Lopressor Ampuls ... 830
- Lopressor HCT Tablets ... 832
- Lopressor Tablets ... 830

Nadolol (Concomitant administration may result in additive effects in prolonging AV conduction).

No products indexed under this heading.

Penbutolol Sulfate (Concomitant administration may result in additive effects in prolonging AV conduction). Products include:

- Levatol ... 2403

Pindolol (Concomitant administration may result in additive effects in prolonging AV conduction). Products include:

- Visken Tablets ... 2299

Propofol (Depression of cardiac contractility, conductivity, automaticity, and vasodilation may be potentiated). Products include:

- Diprivan Injection ... 2833

Propranolol Hydrochloride (Concomitant administration may result in additive effects in prolonging AV conduction; increased bioavailability of propranolol by 50%). Products include:

- Inderal ... 2728
- Inderal LA Long Acting Capsules ... 2730
- Inderide Tablets ... 2732
- Inderide LA Long Acting Capsules .. 2734

Ranitidine Hydrochloride (Produces smaller, nonsignificant increase in plasma levels). Products include:

- Zantac ... 1209
- Zantac Injection ... 1207
- Zantac Syrup ... 1209

Sotalol Hydrochloride (Concomitant administration may result in additive effects in prolonging AV conduction). Products include:

- Betapace Tablets ... 641

Timolol Hemihydrate (Concomitant administration may result in additive effects in prolonging AV conduction). Products include:

- Betimol 0.25%, 0.5% ... ⊙ 261

Timolol Maleate (Concomitant administration may result in additive effects in prolonging AV conduction). Products include:

- Blocadren Tablets ... 1614
- Timolide Tablets ... 1748
- Timoptic in Ocudose ... 1753
- Timoptic Sterile Ophthalmic Solution ... 1751
- Timoptic-XE ... 1755

CARDIZEM INJECTABLE

(Diltiazem Hydrochloride) ... 1508

May interact with beta blockers, intravenous beta-blockers, cardiac glycosides, anesthetics, agents known affect cardiac contractility and/or sa or av node conduction (selected), and certain other agents. Compounds in these categories include:

Acebutolol Hydrochloride (Potential for bradycardia, AV block, and/or depression of contractility in patients receiving chronic oral beta-blockers). Products include:

- Sectral Capsules ... 2807

Alfentanil Hydrochloride (Potential for additive effects; potential for the increased depression of cardiac contractility, conductivity and automaticity). Products include:

- Alfenta Injection ... 1286

Atenolol (Concurrent intravenous administration should not be undertaken together or in close proximity; potential for bradycardia, AV block, and/or depression of contractility in patients receiving chronic oral beta-blockers). Products include:

- Tenoretic Tablets ... 2845
- Tenormin Tablets and I.V. Injection 2847

Betaxolol Hydrochloride (Potential for bradycardia, AV block, and/or depression of contractility in patients receiving chronic oral beta-blockers). Products include:

- Betoptic Ophthalmic Solution ... 469
- Betoptic S Ophthalmic Suspension 471
- Kerlone Tablets ... 2436

Bisoprolol Fumarate (Potential for bradycardia, AV block, and/or depression of contractility in patients receiving chronic oral beta-blockers). Products include:

- Zebeta Tablets ... 1413
- Ziac ... 1415

Carbamazepine (Potential for elevated serum levels of carbamazepine (40% to 72% increase), resulting in toxicity in some cases). Products include:

- Atretol Tablets ... 573
- Tegretol Chewable Tablets ... 852
- Tegretol Suspension ... 852
- Tegretol Tablets ... 852

Carteolol Hydrochloride (Potential for bradycardia, AV block, and/or depression of contractility in patients receiving chronic oral beta-blockers). Products include:

- Cartrol Tablets ... 410
- Ocupress Ophthalmic Solution, 1% Sterile ... ⊙ 309

Cyclosporine (A pharmacokinetic interaction between diltiazem and cyclosporine has been observed in renal and cardiac transplant patients requiring a reduction of cyclosporine dose). Products include:

- Neoral ... 2276
- Sandimmune ... 2286

Deslanoside (Potential for additive effects; potential for excessive slowing of the heart rate and/or AV block).

No products indexed under this heading.

Digitoxin (Potential for additive effects; potential for excessive slowing of the heart rate and/or AV block). Products include:

- Crystodigin Tablets ... 1433

Digoxin (Potential for additive effects; potential for excessive slowing of the heart rate and/or AV block). Products include:

- Lanoxicaps ... 1117
- Lanoxin Elixir Pediatric ... 1120
- Lanoxin Injection ... 1123
- Lanoxin Injection Pediatric ... 1126
- Lanoxin Tablets ... 1128

Enflurane (Potential for additive effects; potential for the increased depression of cardiac contractility, conductivity and automaticity).

No products indexed under this heading.

Esmolol Hydrochloride (Concurrent intravenous administration should not be undertaken together or in close proximity; potential for bradycardia, AV block, and/or depression of contractility in patients receiving chronic oral beta-blockers). Products include:

- Brevibloc Injection ... 1808

Fentanyl Citrate (Potential for additive effects; potential for the increased depression of cardiac contractility, conductivity and automaticity). Products include:

- Sublimaze Injection ... 1307

Halothane (Potential for additive effects; potential for the increased depression of cardiac contractility, conductivity and automaticity). Products include:

- Fluothane ... 2724

(▣ Described in PDR For Nonprescription Drugs) (⊙ Described in PDR For Ophthalmology)

Isoflurane (Potential for additive effects; potential for the increased depression of cardiac contractility, conductivity and automaticity).

No products indexed under this heading.

Ketamine Hydrochloride (Potential for additive effects; potential for the increased depression of cardiac contractility, conductivity and automaticity).

No products indexed under this heading.

Labetalol Hydrochloride (Concurrent intravenous administration should not be undertaken together or in close proximity; potential for bradycardia, AV block, and/or depression of contractility in patients receiving chronic oral beta-blockers). Products include:

Normodyne Injection 2377
Normodyne Tablets 2379
Trandate 1185

Levobunolol Hydrochloride (Potential for bradycardia, AV block, and/or depression of contractility in patients receiving chronic oral beta-blockers). Products include:

Betagan .... ⊕ 233

Methohexital Sodium (Potential for additive effects; potential for the increased depression of cardiac contractility, conductivity and automaticity). Products include:

Brevital Sodium Vials 1429

Metipranolol Hydrochloride (Potential for bradycardia, AV block, and/or depression of contractility in patients receiving chronic oral beta-blockers). Products include:

OptiPranolol (Metipranolol 0.3%)
Sterile Ophthalmic Solution.......... ⊕ 258

Metoprolol Succinate (Potential for bradycardia, AV block, and/or depression of contractility in patients receiving chronic oral beta-blockers). Products include:

Toprol-XL Tablets 565

Metoprolol Tartrate (Concurrent intravenous administration should not be undertaken together or in close proximity; potential for bradycardia, AV block, and/or depression of contractility in patients receiving chronic oral beta-blockers). Products include:

Lopressor Ampuls 830
Lopressor HCT Tablets 832
Lopressor Tablets 830

Midazolam Hydrochloride (Potential for additive effects; potential for the increased depression of cardiac contractility, conductivity and automaticity). Products include:

Versed Injection 2170

Nadolol (Potential for bradycardia, AV block, and/or depression of contractility in patients receiving chronic oral beta-blockers).

No products indexed under this heading.

Penbutolol Sulfate (Potential for bradycardia, AV block, and/or depression of contractility in patients receiving chronic oral beta-blockers). Products include:

Levatol 2403

Pindolol (Potential for bradycardia, AV block, and/or depression of contractility in patients receiving chronic oral beta-blockers). Products include:

Visken Tablets... 2299

Propofol (Potential for additive effects; potential for the increased depression of cardiac contractility, conductivity and automaticity). Products include:

Diprivan Injection................................... 2833

Propranolol Hydrochloride (Concurrent intravenous administration should not be undertaken together or in close proximity; potential for bradycardia, AV block, and/or depression of contractility in patients receiving chronic oral beta-blockers). Products include:

Inderal 2728
Inderal LA Long Acting Capsules 2730
Inderide Tablets 2732
Inderide LA Long Acting Capsules .. 2734

Sotalol Hydrochloride (Potential for bradycardia, AV block, and/or depression of contractility in patients receiving chronic oral beta-blockers). Products include:

Betapace Tablets 641

Sufentanil Citrate (Potential for additive effects; potential for the increased depression of cardiac contractility, conductivity and automaticity). Products include:

Sufenta Injection 1309

Thiamylal Sodium (Potential for additive effects; potential for the increased depression of cardiac contractility, conductivity and automaticity).

No products indexed under this heading.

Timolol Hemihydrate (Potential for bradycardia, AV block, and/or depression of contractility in patients receiving chronic oral beta-blockers). Products include:

Betimol 0.25%, 0.5% .... ⊕ 261

Timolol Maleate (Potential for bradycardia, AV block, and/or depression of contractility in patients receiving chronic oral beta-blockers). Products include:

Blocadren Tablets 1614
Timolide Tablets..................................... 1748
Timoptic in Ocudose 1753
Timoptic Sterile Ophthalmic Solution.. 1751
Timoptic-XE 1755

CARDIZEM TABLETS

(Diltiazem Hydrochloride)....................1512

May interact with beta blockers, cardiac glycosides, anesthetics, and certain other agents. Compounds in these categories include:

Acebutolol Hydrochloride (Potential for additive effects on cardiac conduction). Products include:

Sectral Capsules 2807

Alfentanil Hydrochloride (Depression of cardiac contractility, conductivity, automaticity, and vasodilation associated with anesthetic may be potentiated). Products include:

Alfenta Injection 1286

Atenolol (Potential for additive effects on cardiac conduction). Products include:

Tenoretic Tablets.................................... 2845
Tenormin Tablets and I.V. Injection 2847

Betaxolol Hydrochloride (Potential for additive effects on cardiac conduction). Products include:

Betoptic Ophthalmic Solution............ 469
Betoptic S Ophthalmic Suspension 471
Kerlone Tablets....................................... 2436

Bisoprolol Fumarate (Potential for additive effects on cardiac conduction). Products include:

Zebeta Tablets 1413

Ziac 1415

Carbamazepine (Co-administration results in elevated serum levels of carbamazepine (40% to 72%) resulting in toxicity in some cases). Products include:

Atretol Tablets 573
Tegretol Chewable Tablets 852
Tegretol Suspension.............................. 852
Tegretol Tablets...................................... 852

Carteolol Hydrochloride (Potential for additive effects on cardiac conduction). Products include:

Cartrol Tablets 410
Ocupress Ophthalmic Solution,
1% Sterile... ⊕ 309

Cimetidine (May increase peak plasma levels and AUC when administered concurrently; an adjustment in the diltiazem dose may be warranted). Products include:

Tagamet Tablets 2516

Cimetidine Hydrochloride (May increase peak plasma levels and AUC when administered concurrently; an adjustment in the diltiazem dose may be warranted). Products include:

Tagamet... 2516

Cyclosporine (In renal and cardiac transplant recipients, a reduction of cyclosporine dose ranging from 15% to 48% may be necessary; monitor cyclosporine levels). Products include:

Neoral.. 2276
Sandimmune 2286

Deslanoside (Potential for additive effects on cardiac conduction; variable effect on plasma digoxin concentrations).

No products indexed under this heading.

Digitoxin (Potential for additive effects on cardiac conduction; variable effect on plasma digoxin concentrations). Products include:

Crystodigin Tablets................................ 1433

Digoxin (Potential for additive effects on cardiac conduction; variable effect on plasma digoxin concentrations). Products include:

Lanoxicaps 1117
Lanoxin Elixir Pediatric 1120
Lanoxin Injection 1123
Lanoxin Injection Pediatric.................. 1126
Lanoxin Tablets 1128

Drugs which undergo biotransformation by cytochrome P-450 mixed function oxidase (Co-administration may result in the competitive inhibition of metabolism).

Enflurane (Depression of cardiac contractility, conductivity, automaticity, and vasodilation associated with anesthetic may be potentiated).

No products indexed under this heading.

Esmolol Hydrochloride (Potential for additive effects on cardiac conduction). Products include:

Brevibloc Injection................................. 1808

Fentanyl Citrate (Depression of cardiac contractility, conductivity, automaticity, and vasodilation associated with anesthetic may be potentiated). Products include:

Sublimaze Injection................................ 1307

Halothane (Depression of cardiac contractility, conductivity, automaticity, and vasodilation associated with anesthetic may be potentiated). Products include:

Fluothane 2724

Isoflurane (Depression of cardiac contractility, conductivity, automaticity, and vasodilation associated with anesthetic may be potentiated).

No products indexed under this heading.

Ketamine Hydrochloride (Depression of cardiac contractility, conductivity, automaticity, and vasodilation associated with anesthetic may be potentiated).

No products indexed under this heading.

Labetalol Hydrochloride (Potential for additive effects on cardiac conduction). Products include:

Normodyne Injection 2377
Normodyne Tablets 2379
Trandate 1185

Levobunolol Hydrochloride (Potential for additive effects on cardiac conduction). Products include:

Betagan .... ⊕ 233

Methohexital Sodium (Depression of cardiac contractility, conductivity, automaticity, and vasodilation associated with anesthetic may be potentiated). Products include:

Brevital Sodium Vials............................. 1429

Metipranolol Hydrochloride (Potential for additive effects on cardiac conduction). Products include:

OptiPranolol (Metipranolol 0.3%)
Sterile Ophthalmic Solution.......... ⊕ 258

Metoprolol Succinate (Potential for additive effects on cardiac conduction). Products include:

Toprol-XL Tablets 565

Metoprolol Tartrate (Potential for additive effects on cardiac conduction). Products include:

Lopressor Ampuls 830
Lopressor HCT Tablets 832
Lopressor Tablets 830

Midazolam Hydrochloride (Depression of cardiac contractility, conductivity, automaticity, and vasodilation associated with anesthetic may be potentiated). Products include:

Versed Injection 2170

Nadolol (Potential for additive effects on cardiac conduction).

No products indexed under this heading.

Penbutolol Sulfate (Potential for additive effects on cardiac conduction). Products include:

Levatol 2403

Pindolol (Potential for additive effects on cardiac conduction). Products include:

Visken Tablets... 2299

Propofol (Depression of cardiac contractility, conductivity, automaticity, and vasodilation associated with anesthetic may be potentiated). Products include:

Diprivan Injection................................... 2833

Propranolol Hydrochloride (Potential for additive effects on cardiac conduction; increased propranolol levels, in vitro propranolol appears to be displaced from its binding sites by diltiazem). Products include:

Inderal 2728
Inderal LA Long Acting Capsules 2730
Inderide Tablets 2732
Inderide LA Long Acting Capsules .. 2734

Ranitidine Hydrochloride (Produces smaller increases in plasma levels). Products include:

Zantac.. 1209
Zantac Injection 1207
Zantac Syrup 1209

IMPORTANT NOTE: Always consult each drug listing in the patient's regimen for possible interactions.

Sotalol Hydrochloride (Potential for additive effects on cardiac conduction). Products include:
- Betapace Tablets 641

Sufentanil Citrate (Depression of cardiac contractility, conductivity, automaticity, and vasodilation associated with anesthetic may be potentiated). Products include:
- Sufenta Injection 1309

Thiamylal Sodium (Depression of cardiac contractility, conductivity, automaticity, and vasodilation associated with anesthetic may be potentiated).
- No products indexed under this heading.

Timolol Hemihydrate (Potential for additive effects on cardiac conduction). Products include:
- Betimol 0.25%, 0.5% .... ⊙ 261

Timolol Maleate (Potential for additive effects on cardiac conduction). Products include:
- Blocadren Tablets 1614
- Timolide Tablets 1748
- Timoptic in Ocudose 1753
- Timoptic Sterile Ophthalmic Solution 1751
- Timoptic-XE 1755

CARDURA TABLETS
(Doxazosin Mesylate) 2186
May interact with:

Cimetidine (Co-administration with oral cimetidine has resulted in a 10% increase in mean AUC of doxazosin and a slight but statistically insignificant increase in mean C_{max} and mean half-life of doxazosin). Products include:
- Tagamet Tablets 2516

Cimetidine Hydrochloride (Co-administration with oral cimetidine has resulted in a 10% increase in mean AUC of doxazosin and a slight but statistically insignificant increase in mean C_{max} and mean half-life of doxazosin). Products include:
- Tagamet 2516

Food Interactions

Food, unspecified (Reduction of 18% in mean maximum plasma concentration and 12% in the AUC occurred when Cardura was administered with food; neither of these differences were statistically or clinically significant).

CARE CREME ANTIMICROBIAL CREAM
(Chloroxylenol) .... ▣ 624
None cited in PDR database.

CARMOL HC
(Hydrocortisone Acetate) 924
None cited in PDR database.

L-CARNITINE 250MG AND 500MG TABLETS
(Levocarnitine) 2659
None cited in PDR database.

CARNITOR INJECTION
(Levocarnitine) 2452
None cited in PDR database.

CARNITOR TABLETS AND SOLUTION
(Levocarnitine) 2453
None cited in PDR database.

CARTILADE SHARK CARTILAGE CAPSULES, POWDER, AND CAPLETS
(Shark Cartilage) .... ▣ 626
None cited in PDR database.

CARTROL TABLETS
(Carteolol Hydrochloride) 410
May interact with calcium channel blockers, insulin, oral hypoglycemic agents, non-steroidal anti-inflammatory agents, sympathomimetic bronchodilators, catecholamine depleting drugs, and general anesthetics. Compounds in these categories include:

Acarbose (Concomitant administration may result in hypo- or hyperglycemia).
- No products indexed under this heading.

Albuterol (Diminished response to therapy with a beta-receptor agonist). Products include:
- Proventil Inhalation Aerosol 2382
- Ventolin Inhalation Aerosol and Refill 1197

Albuterol Sulfate (Diminished response to therapy with a beta-receptor agonist). Products include:
- Airet Solution for Inhalation 452
- Proventil Inhalation Solution 0.083% 2384
- Proventil Repetabs Tablets 2386
- Proventil Solution for Inhalation 0.5% 2383
- Proventil Syrup 2385
- Proventil Tablets 2386
- Ventolin Inhalation Solution 1198
- Ventolin Nebules Inhalation Solution 1199
- Ventolin Rotacaps for Inhalation 1200
- Ventolin Syrup 1202
- Ventolin Tablets 1203
- Volmax Extended-Release Tablets 1788

Amlodipine Besylate (Potential for hypotension, AV conduction disturbances and LVF in some patients). Products include:
- Lotrel Capsules 840
- Norvasc Tablets 1940

Bepridil Hydrochloride (Potential for hypotension, AV conduction disturbances and LVF in some patients). Products include:
- Vascor (200, 300 and 400 mg) Tablets 1587

Bitolterol Mesylate (Diminished response to therapy with a beta-receptor agonist). Products include:
- Tornalate Solution for Inhalation, 0.2% 956
- Tornalate Metered Dose Inhaler 957

Chlorpropamide (Concomitant administration may result in hypo- or hyperglycemia). Products include:
- Diabinese Tablets 1935

Deserpidine (Possible additive effect).
- No products indexed under this heading.

Diclofenac Potassium (Possible blunting of the antihypertensive effect). Products include:
- Cataflam 816

Diclofenac Sodium (Possible blunting of the antihypertensive effect). Products include:
- Voltaren Ophthalmic Sterile Ophthalmic Solution .... ⊙ 272
- Voltaren Tablets 861

Diltiazem Hydrochloride (Potential for hypotension, AV conduction disturbances and LVF in some patients). Products include:
- Cardizem CD Capsules 1506
- Cardizem SR Capsules 1510
- Cardizem Injectable 1508
- Cardizem Tablets 1512
- Dilacor XR Extended-release Capsules 2018

Enflurane (Possible exaggeration of hypotension).
- No products indexed under this heading.

Ephedrine Hydrochloride (Diminished response to therapy with a beta-receptor agonist). Products include:
- Primatene Dual Action Formula .... ▣ 872
- Primatene Tablets .... ▣ 873
- Quadrinal Tablets 1350

Ephedrine Sulfate (Diminished response to therapy with a beta-receptor agonist). Products include:
- Bronkaid Caplets .... ▣ 717
- Marax Tablets & DF Syrup 2200

Ephedrine Tannate (Diminished response to therapy with a beta-receptor agonist). Products include:
- Rynatuss 2673

Epinephrine (Diminished response to therapy with a beta-receptor agonist). Products include:
- Bronkaid Mist .... ▣ 717
- EPIFRIN .... ⊙ 239
- EpiPen 790
- Marcaine Hydrochloride with Epinephrine 1:200,000 2316
- Primatene Mist .... ▣ 873
- Sensorcaine with Epinephrine Injection 559
- Sus-Phrine Injection 1019
- Xylocaine with Epinephrine Injections 567

Epinephrine Hydrochloride (Diminished response to therapy with a beta-receptor agonist). Products include:
- Ana-Kit Anaphylaxis Emergency Treatment Kit 617

Ethylnorepinephrine Hydrochloride (Diminished response to therapy with a beta-receptor agonist).
- No products indexed under this heading.

Etodolac (Possible blunting of the antihypertensive effect). Products include:
- Lodine Capsules and Tablets 2743

Felodipine (Potential for hypotension, AV conduction disturbances and LVF in some patients). Products include:
- Plendil Extended-Release Tablets 527

Fenoprofen Calcium (Possible blunting of the antihypertensive effect). Products include:
- Nalfon 200 Pulvules & Nalfon Tablets 917

Flurbiprofen (Possible blunting of the antihypertensive effect). Products include:
- Ansaid Tablets 2579

Glipizide (Concomitant administration may result in hypo- or hyperglycemia). Products include:
- Glucotrol Tablets 1967
- Glucotrol XL Extended Release Tablets 1968

Glyburide (Concomitant administration may result in hypo- or hyperglycemia). Products include:
- DiaBeta Tablets 1239
- Glynase PresTab Tablets 2609
- Micronase Tablets 2623

Guanethidine Monosulfate (Possible additive effect). Products include:
- Esimil Tablets 822
- Ismelin Tablets 827

Ibuprofen (Possible blunting of the antihypertensive effect). Products include:
- Advil Cold and Sinus Caplets and Tablets (formerly CoAdvil) .... ▣ 870
- Advil Ibuprofen Tablets and Caplets .... ▣ 870
- Children's Advil Suspension 2692
- Arthritis Foundation Ibuprofen Tablets .... ▣ 674
- Bayer Select Ibuprofen Pain Relief Formula .... ▣ 715
- Cramp End Tablets .... ▣ 735
- Dimetapp Sinus Caplets .... ▣ 775
- Haltran Tablets .... ▣ 771
- IBU Tablets 1342
- Ibuprohm .... ▣ 735
- Children's Motrin Ibuprofen Oral Suspension 1546
- Motrin Tablets 2625
- Motrin IB Caplets, Tablets, and Geltabs .... ▣ 838
- Motrin IB Sinus .... ▣ 838
- Motrin Ibuprofen Suspension, Oral Drops, Chewable Tablets, Caplets 1546
- Nuprin Ibuprofen/Analgesic Tablets & Caplets .... ▣ 622
- Sine-Aid IB Caplets 1554
- Vicks DayQuil SINUS Pressure & PAIN Relief with IBUPROFEN .... ▣ 762

Indomethacin (Possible blunting of the antihypertensive effect). Products include:
- Indocin 1680

Indomethacin Sodium Trihydrate (Possible blunting of the antihypertensive effect). Products include:
- Indocin I.V. 1684

Insulin, Human (Concomitant administration may result in hypo- or hyperglycemia).
- No products indexed under this heading.

Insulin, Human Isophane Suspension (Concomitant administration may result in hypo- or hyperglycemia). Products include:
- Novolin N Human Insulin 10 ml Vials 1795

Insulin, Human NPH (Concomitant administration may result in hypo- or hyperglycemia). Products include:
- Humulin N, 100 Units 1448
- Novolin N PenFill Cartridges Durable Insulin Delivery System 1798
- Novolin N Prefilled Syringe Disposable Insulin Delivery System 1798

Insulin, Human Regular (Concomitant administration may result in hypo- or hyperglycemia). Products include:
- Humulin R, 100 Units 1449
- Novolin R Human Insulin 10 ml Vials 1795
- Novolin R PenFill Cartridges Durable Insulin Delivery System 1798
- Novolin R Prefilled Syringe Disposable Insulin Delivery System 1798
- Velosulin BR Human Insulin 10 ml Vials 1795

Insulin, Human, Zinc Suspension (Concomitant administration may result in hypo- or hyperglycemia). Products include:
- Humulin L, 100 Units 1446
- Humulin U, 100 Units 1450
- Novolin L Human Insulin 10 ml Vials 1795

Insulin, NPH (Concomitant administration may result in hypo- or hyperglycemia). Products include:
- NPH, 100 Units 1450
- Pork NPH, 100 Units 1452
- Purified Pork NPH Isophane Insulin 1801

Insulin, Regular (Concomitant administration may result in hypo- or hyperglycemia). Products include:
- Regular, 100 Units 1450
- Pork Regular, 100 Units 1452
- Pork Regular (Concentrated), 500 Units 1453
- Purified Pork Regular Insulin 1801

Insulin, Zinc Crystals (Concomitant administration may result in hypo- or hyperglycemia). Products include:
- NPH, 100 Units 1450

Insulin, Zinc Suspension (Concomitant administration may result in hypo- or hyperglycemia). Products include:
- Iletin I 1450
- Lente, 100 Units 1450

(▣ Described in PDR For Nonprescription Drugs) — (⊙ Described in PDR For Ophthalmology)

169 **Interactions Index** **Catapres**

Iletin II 1452
Pork Lente, 100 Units 1452
Purified Pork Lente Insulin 1801

Isoetharine (Diminished response to therapy with a beta-receptor agonist). Products include:
Bronkometer Aerosol 2302
Bronkosol Solution 2302
Isoetharine Inhalation Solution, USP, Arm-a-Med 551

Isoflurane (Possible exaggeration of hypotension).
No products indexed under this heading.

Isoproterenol Hydrochloride (Diminished response to therapy with a beta-receptor agonist). Products include:
Isuprel Hydrochloride Injection 1:5000 2311
Isuprel Hydrochloride Solution 1:200 & 1:100 2313
Isuprel Mistometer 2312

Isoproterenol Sulfate (Diminished response to therapy with a beta-receptor agonist). Products include:
Norisodrine with Calcium Iodide Syrup 442

Isradipine (Potential for hypotension, AV conduction disturbances and LVF in some patients). Products include:
DynaCirc Capsules 2256

Ketamine Hydrochloride (Possible exaggeration of hypotension).
No products indexed under this heading.

Ketoprofen (Possible blunting of the antihypertensive effect). Products include:
Orudis Capsules 2766
Oruvail Capsules 2766

Ketorolac Tromethamine (Possible blunting of the antihypertensive effect). Products include:
Acular 474
Acular .... ◉ 277
Toradol 2159

Meclofenamate Sodium (Possible blunting of the antihypertensive effect).
No products indexed under this heading.

Mefenamic Acid (Possible blunting of the antihypertensive effect). Products include:
Ponstel 1925

Metaproterenol Sulfate (Diminished response to therapy with a beta-receptor agonist). Products include:
Alupent 669
Metaproterenol Sulfate Inhalation Solution, USP, Arm-a-Med 552

Metformin Hydrochloride (Concomitant administration may result in hypo- or hyperglycemia). Products include:
Glucophage 752

Methohexital Sodium (Possible exaggeration of hypotension). Products include:
Brevital Sodium Vials 1429

Methoxyflurane (Possible exaggeration of hypotension).
No products indexed under this heading.

Nabumetone (Possible blunting of the antihypertensive effect). Products include:
Relafen Tablets 2510

Naproxen (Possible blunting of the antihypertensive effect). Products include:
Anaprox/Naprosyn 2117

Naproxen Sodium (Possible blunting of the antihypertensive effect). Products include:
Aleve 1975
Anaprox/Naprosyn 2117

Nicardipine Hydrochloride (Potential for hypotension, AV conduction disturbances and LVF in some patients). Products include:
Cardene Capsules 2095
Cardene I.V. 2709
Cardene SR Capsules 2097

Nifedipine (Potential for hypotension, AV conduction disturbances and LVF in some patients). Products include:
Adalat Capsules (10 mg and 20 mg) 587
Adalat CC 589
Procardia Capsules 1971
Procardia XL Extended Release Tablets 1972

Nimodipine (Potential for hypotension, AV conduction disturbances and LVF in some patients). Products include:
Nimotop Capsules 610

Nisoldipine (Potential for hypotension, AV conduction disturbances and LVF in some patients).
No products indexed under this heading.

Oxaprozin (Possible blunting of the antihypertensive effect). Products include:
Daypro Caplets 2426

Phenylbutazone (Possible blunting of the antihypertensive effect).
No products indexed under this heading.

Pirbuterol Acetate (Diminished response to therapy with a beta-receptor agonist). Products include:
Maxair Autohaler 1492
Maxair Inhaler 1494

Piroxicam (Possible blunting of the antihypertensive effect). Products include:
Feldene Capsules 1965

Propofol (Possible exaggeration of hypotension). Products include:
Diprivan Injection 2833

Rauwolfia Serpentina (Possible additive effect).
No products indexed under this heading.

Rescinnamine (Possible additive effect).
No products indexed under this heading.

Reserpine (Possible additive effect). Products include:
Diupres Tablets 1650
Hydropres Tablets 1675
Ser-Ap-Es Tablets 849

Salmeterol Xinafoate (Diminished response to therapy with a beta-receptor agonist). Products include:
Serevent Inhalation Aerosol 1176

Sulindac (Possible blunting of the antihypertensive effect). Products include:
Clinoril Tablets 1618

Terbutaline Sulfate (Diminished response to therapy with a beta-receptor agonist). Products include:
Brethaire Inhaler 813
Brethine Ampuls 815
Brethine Tablets 814
Bricanyl Subcutaneous Injection 1502
Bricanyl Tablets 1503

Tolazamide (Concomitant administration may result in hypo- or hyperglycemia).
No products indexed under this heading.

Tolbutamide (Concomitant administration may result in hypo- or hyperglycemia).
No products indexed under this heading.

Tolmetin Sodium (Possible blunting of the antihypertensive effect). Products include:
Tolectin (200, 400 and 600 mg) .. 1581

Verapamil Hydrochloride (Potential for hypotension, AV conduction disturbances and LVF in some patients). Products include:
Calan SR Caplets 2422
Calan Tablets 2419
Isoptin Injectable 1344
Isoptin Oral Tablets 1346
Isoptin SR Tablets 1348
Verelan Capsules 1410
Verelan Capsules 2824

CATAFLAM
(Diclofenac Potassium) 816
See **Voltaren Tablets**

CATAPRES TABLETS
(Clonidine Hydrochloride) 674
May interact with tricyclic antidepressants, barbiturates, hypnotics and sedatives, cardiac glycosides, beta blockers, and certain other agents. Compounds in these categories include:

Acebutolol Hydrochloride (Rapid rise in blood pressure following sudden cessation of Catapres). Products include:
Sectral Capsules 2807

Amitriptyline Hydrochloride (Enhanced manifestation of corneal lesions (in rats); reduced effect of clonidine). Products include:
Elavil 2838
Endep Tablets 2174
Etrafon 2355
Limbitrol 2180
Triavil Tablets 1757

Amoxapine (Reduced effect of clonidine). Products include:
Asendin Tablets 1369

Aprobarbital (Enhanced CNS-depressive effects).
No products indexed under this heading.

Atenolol (Rapid rise in blood pressure following sudden cessation of Catapres). Products include:
Tenoretic Tablets 2845
Tenormin Tablets and I.V. Injection 2847

Betaxolol Hydrochloride (Rapid rise in blood pressure following sudden cessation of Catapres). Products include:
Betoptic Ophthalmic Solution 469
Betoptic S Ophthalmic Suspension 471
Kerlone Tablets 2436

Bisoprolol Fumarate (Rapid rise in blood pressure following sudden cessation of Catapres). Products include:
Zebeta Tablets 1413
Ziac 1415

Butabarbital (Enhanced CNS-depressive effects).
No products indexed under this heading.

Butalbital (Enhanced CNS-depressive effects). Products include:
Esgic-plus Tablets 1013
Fioricet Tablets 2258
Fioricet with Codeine Capsules 2260
Fiorinal Capsules 2261
Fiorinal with Codeine Capsules 2262
Fiorinal Tablets 2261
Phrenilin 785
Sedapap Tablets 50 mg/650 mg .. 1543

Carteolol Hydrochloride (Rapid rise in blood pressure following sudden cessation of Catapres). Products include:
Cartrol Tablets 410
Ocupress Ophthalmic Solution, 1% Sterile .... ◉ 309

Clomipramine Hydrochloride (Enhanced manifestation of corneal lesions (in rats); reduced effect of clonidine). Products include:
Anafranil Capsules 803

Desipramine Hydrochloride (Reduced effect of clonidine). Products include:
Norpramin Tablets 1526

Deslanoside (Sinus bradycardia and atrioventricular block (rare)).
No products indexed under this heading.

Digitoxin (Sinus bradycardia and atrioventricular block (rare)). Products include:
Crystodigin Tablets 1433

Digoxin (Sinus bradycardia and atrioventricular block (rare)). Products include:
Lanoxicaps 1117
Lanoxin Elixir Pediatric 1120
Lanoxin Injection 1123
Lanoxin Injection Pediatric 1126
Lanoxin Tablets 1128

Doxepin Hydrochloride (Reduced effect of clonidine). Products include:
Sinequan 2205
Zonalon Cream 1055

Esmolol Hydrochloride (Rapid rise in blood pressure following sudden cessation of Catapres). Products include:
Brevibloc Injection 1808

Estazolam (Enhanced CNS-depressive effects). Products include:
ProSom Tablets 449

Ethchlorvynol (Enhanced CNS-depressive effects). Products include:
Placidyl Capsules 448

Ethinamate (Enhanced CNS-depressive effects).
No products indexed under this heading.

Flurazepam Hydrochloride (Enhanced CNS-depressive effects). Products include:
Dalmane Capsules 2173

Glutethimide (Enhanced CNS-depressive effects).
No products indexed under this heading.

Imipramine Hydrochloride (Reduced effect of clonidine). Products include:
Tofranil Ampuls 854
Tofranil Tablets 856

Imipramine Pamoate (Reduced effect of clonidine). Products include:
Tofranil-PM Capsules 857

Labetalol Hydrochloride (Rapid rise in blood pressure following sudden cessation of Catapres). Products include:
Normodyne Injection 2377
Normodyne Tablets 2379
Trandate 1185

Levobunolol Hydrochloride (Rapid rise in blood pressure following sudden cessation of Catapres). Products include:
Betagan .... ◉ 233

Lorazepam (Enhanced CNS-depressive effects). Products include:
Ativan Injection 2698
Ativan Tablets 2700

IMPORTANT NOTE: Always consult each drug listing in the patient's regimen for possible interactions.

Maprotiline Hydrochloride (Reduced effect of clonidine). Products include:
Ludiomil Tablets ... 843

Mephobarbital (Enhanced CNS-depressive effects). Products include:
Mebaral Tablets ... 2322

Methyltestosterone (Enhanced CNS-depressive effects). Products include:
Android Capsules, 10 mg ... 1250
Android ... 1251
Estratest ... 2539
Oreton Methyl ... 1255
Premarin with Methyltestosterone .. 2794
Testred Capsules ... 1262

Metipranolol Hydrochloride (Rapid rise in blood pressure following sudden cessation of Catapres). Products include:
OptiPranolol (Metipranolol 0.3%) Sterile Ophthalmic Solution ... ⊙ 258

Metoprolol Succinate (Rapid rise in blood pressure following sudden cessation of Catapres). Products include:
Toprol-XL Tablets ... 565

Metoprolol Tartrate (Rapid rise in blood pressure following sudden cessation of Catapres). Products include:
Lopressor Ampuls ... 830
Lopressor HCT Tablets ... 832
Lopressor Tablets ... 830

Midazolam Hydrochloride (Enhanced CNS-depressive effects). Products include:
Versed Injection ... 2170

Nadolol (Rapid rise in blood pressure following sudden cessation of Catapres).
No products indexed under this heading.

Nortriptyline Hydrochloride (Reduced effect of clonidine). Products include:
Pamelor ... 2280

Penbutolol Sulfate (Rapid rise in blood pressure following sudden cessation of Catapres). Products include:
Levatol ... 2403

Pentobarbital Sodium (Effect not specified). Products include:
Nembutal Sodium Capsules ... 436
Nembutal Sodium Solution ... 438
Nembutal Sodium Suppositories ... 440

Phenobarbital (Enhanced CNS-depressive effects). Products include:
Arco-Lase Plus Tablets ... 512
Bellergal-S Tablets ... 2250
Donnatal ... 2060
Donnatal Extentabs ... 2061
Donnatal Tablets ... 2060
Phenobarbital Elixir and Tablets ... 1469
Quadrinal Tablets ... 1350

Pindolol (Rapid rise in blood pressure following sudden cessation of Catapres). Products include:
Visken Tablets ... 2299

Propofol (Enhanced CNS-depressive effects). Products include:
Diprivan Injection ... 2833

Propranolol Hydrochloride (Rapid rise in blood pressure following sudden cessation of Catapres). Products include:
Inderal ... 2728
Inderal LA Long Acting Capsules ... 2730
Inderide Tablets ... 2732
Inderide LA Long Acting Capsules .. 2734

Protriptyline Hydrochloride (Reduced effect of clonidine). Products include:
Vivactil Tablets ... 1774

Quazepam (Enhanced CNS-depressive effects). Products include:
Doral Tablets ... 2664

Secobarbital Sodium (Enhanced CNS-depressive effects). Products include:
Seconal Sodium Pulvules ... 1474

Sotalol Hydrochloride (Rapid rise in blood pressure following sudden cessation of Catapres). Products include:
Betapace Tablets ... 641

Temazepam (Enhanced CNS-depressive effects). Products include:
Restoril Capsules ... 2284

Thiamylal Sodium (Enhanced CNS-depressive effects).
No products indexed under this heading.

Timolol Hemihydrate (Rapid rise in blood pressure following sudden cessation of Catapres). Products include:
Betimol 0.25%, 0.5% ... ⊙ 261

Timolol Maleate (Rapid rise in blood pressure following sudden cessation of Catapres). Products include:
Blocadren Tablets ... 1614
Timolide Tablets ... 1748
Timoptic in Ocudose ... 1753
Timoptic Sterile Ophthalmic Solution ... 1751
Timoptic-XE ... 1755

Triazolam (Enhanced CNS-depressive effects). Products include:
Halcion Tablets ... 2611

Trimipramine Maleate (Reduced effect of clonidine). Products include:
Surmontil Capsules ... 2811

Zolpidem Tartrate (Enhanced CNS-depressive effects). Products include:
Ambien Tablets ... 2416

Food Interactions

Alcohol (Enhanced CNS-depressive effects).

CATAPRES-TTS
(Clonidine) ... 675
May interact with tricyclic antidepressants, barbiturates, hypnotics and sedatives, and certain other agents. Compounds in these categories include:

Amitriptyline Hydrochloride (Enhanced manifestation of corneal lesions (in rats); reduced effect of clonidine). Products include:
Elavil ... 2838
Endep Tablets ... 2174
Etrafon ... 2355
Limbitrol ... 2180
Triavil Tablets ... 1757

Amoxapine (Reduced effect of clonidine). Products include:
Asendin Tablets ... 1369

Aprobarbital (Enhanced CNS-depressive effects).
No products indexed under this heading.

Butabarbital (Enhanced CNS-depressive effects).
No products indexed under this heading.

Butalbital (Enhanced CNS-depressive effects). Products include:
Esgic-plus Tablets ... 1013
Fioricet Tablets ... 2258
Fioricet with Codeine Capsules ... 2260
Fiorinal Capsules ... 2261
Fiorinal with Codeine Capsules ... 2262
Fiorinal Tablets ... 2261
Phrenilin ... 785
Sedapap Tablets 50 mg/650 mg .. 1543

Clomipramine Hydrochloride (Enhanced manifestation of corneal lesions (in rats); reduced effect of clonidine). Products include:
Anafranil Capsules ... 803

Desipramine Hydrochloride (Reduced effect of clonidine). Products include:
Norpramin Tablets ... 1526

Doxepin Hydrochloride (Reduced effect of clonidine). Products include:
Sinequan ... 2205
Zonalon Cream ... 1055

Estazolam (Enhanced CNS-depressive effects). Products include:
ProSom Tablets ... 449

Ethchlorvynol (Enhanced CNS-depressive effects). Products include:
Placidyl Capsules ... 448

Ethinamate (Enhanced CNS-depressive effects).
No products indexed under this heading.

Flurazepam Hydrochloride (Enhanced CNS-depressive effects). Products include:
Dalmane Capsules ... 2173

Glutethimide (Enhanced CNS-depressive effects).
No products indexed under this heading.

Imipramine Hydrochloride (Reduced effect of clonidine). Products include:
Tofranil Ampuls ... 854
Tofranil Tablets ... 856

Imipramine Pamoate (Reduced effect of clonidine). Products include:
Tofranil-PM Capsules ... 857

Lorazepam (Enhanced CNS-depressive effects). Products include:
Ativan Injection ... 2698
Ativan Tablets ... 2700

Maprotiline Hydrochloride (Reduced effect of clonidine). Products include:
Ludiomil Tablets ... 843

Mephobarbital (Enhanced CNS-depressive effects). Products include:
Mebaral Tablets ... 2322

Midazolam Hydrochloride (Enhanced CNS-depressive effects). Products include:
Versed Injection ... 2170

Nortriptyline Hydrochloride (Reduced effect of clonidine). Products include:
Pamelor ... 2280

Pentobarbital Sodium (Enhanced CNS-depressive effects). Products include:
Nembutal Sodium Capsules ... 436
Nembutal Sodium Solution ... 438
Nembutal Sodium Suppositories ... 440

Phenobarbital (Enhanced CNS-depressive effects). Products include:
Arco-Lase Plus Tablets ... 512
Bellergal-S Tablets ... 2250
Donnatal ... 2060
Donnatal Extentabs ... 2061
Donnatal Tablets ... 2060
Phenobarbital Elixir and Tablets ... 1469
Quadrinal Tablets ... 1350

Propofol (Enhanced CNS-depressive effects). Products include:
Diprivan Injection ... 2833

Protriptyline Hydrochloride (Reduced effect of clonidine). Products include:
Vivactil Tablets ... 1774

Quazepam (Enhanced CNS-depressive effects). Products include:
Doral Tablets ... 2664

Secobarbital Sodium (Enhanced CNS-depressive effects). Products include:
Seconal Sodium Pulvules ... 1474

Temazepam (Enhanced CNS-depressive effects). Products include:
Restoril Capsules ... 2284

Thiamylal Sodium (Enhanced CNS-depressive effects).
No products indexed under this heading.

Triazolam (Enhanced CNS-depressive effects). Products include:
Halcion Tablets ... 2611

Trimipramine Maleate (Reduced effect of clonidine). Products include:
Surmontil Capsules ... 2811

Zolpidem Tartrate (Enhanced CNS-depressive effects). Products include:
Ambien Tablets ... 2416

Food Interactions

Alcohol (Enhanced CNS-depressive effects).

CATEMINE ENTERIC TABLETS (TYROSINE)
(L-Tyrosine) ... 2565
None cited in PDR database.

CAVERJECT
(Alprostadil) ... 2583
May interact with anticoagulants. Compounds in this category include:

Dalteparin Sodium (Increased propensity for bleeding after intracavernosal injections). Products include:
Fragmin ... 1954

Dicumarol (Increased propensity for bleeding after intracavernosal injections).
No products indexed under this heading.

Enoxaparin (Increased propensity for bleeding after intracavernosal injections). Products include:
Lovenox Injection ... 2020

Heparin Calcium (Increased propensity for bleeding after intracavernosal injections).
No products indexed under this heading.

Heparin Sodium (Increased propensity for bleeding after intracavernosal injections). Products include:
Heparin Lock Flush Solution ... 2725
Heparin Sodium Injection ... 2726
Heparin Sodium Injection, USP, Sterile Solution ... 2615
Heparin Sodium Vials ... 1441

Warfarin Sodium (Increased propensity for bleeding after intracavernosal injections). Products include:
Coumadin ... 926

C-BUFF
(Vitamin C) ... 667
None cited in PDR database.

CECLOR PULVULES & SUSPENSION
(Cefaclor) ... 1431
May interact with:

Probenecid (Inhibits renal excretion of cefaclor). Products include:
Benemid Tablets ... 1611
ColBENEMID Tablets ... 1622

Warfarin Sodium (Rare reports of increased prothrombin time—with or without clinical bleeding—with concomitant use). Products include:
Coumadin ... 926

CEENU
(Lomustine (CCNU)) ... 693
None cited in PDR database.

CEFIZOX FOR INTRAMUSCULAR OR INTRAVENOUS USE
(Ceftizoxime Sodium) ... 1034
May interact with aminoglycosides. Compounds in this category include:

Amikacin Sulfate (Concomitant administration may result in possible nephrotoxicity). Products include:

Amikacin Sulfate Injection, USP 960
Amikin Injectable 501

Gentamicin Sulfate (Concomitant administration may result in possible nephrotoxicity). Products include:

Garamycin Injectable 2360
Genoptic Sterile Ophthalmic Solution .... ⊙ 243
Genoptic Sterile Ophthalmic Ointment .... ⊙ 243
Gentacidin Ointment .... ⊙ 264
Gentacidin Solution .... ⊙ 264
Gentak .... ⊙ 208
Pred-G Liquifilm Sterile Ophthalmic Suspension .... ⊙ 251
Pred-G S.O.P. Sterile Ophthalmic Ointment .... ⊙ 252

Kanamycin Sulfate (Concomitant administration may result in possible nephrotoxicity).

No products indexed under this heading.

Streptomycin Sulfate (Concomitant administration may result in possible nephrotoxicity). Products include:

Streptomycin Sulfate Injection 2208

Tobramycin (Concomitant administration may result in possible nephrotoxicity). Products include:

AKTOB .... ⊙ 206
TobraDex Ophthalmic Suspension and Ointment 473
Tobrex Ophthalmic Ointment and Solution .... ⊙ 229

Tobramycin Sulfate (Concomitant administration may result in possible nephrotoxicity). Products include:

Nebcin Vials, Hyporets & ADD-Vantage 1464
Tobramycin Sulfate Injection 968

CEFOBID INTRAVENOUS/INTRAMUSCULAR

(Cefoperazone Sodium) 2189
May interact with aminoglycosides and certain other agents. Compounds in these categories include:

Amikacin Sulfate (Nephrotoxicity). Products include:

Amikacin Sulfate Injection, USP 960
Amikin Injectable 501

Gentamicin Sulfate (Nephrotoxicity). Products include:

Garamycin Injectable 2360
Genoptic Sterile Ophthalmic Solution .... ⊙ 243
Genoptic Sterile Ophthalmic Ointment .... ⊙ 243
Gentacidin Ointment .... ⊙ 264
Gentacidin Solution .... ⊙ 264
Gentak .... ⊙ 208
Pred-G Liquifilm Sterile Ophthalmic Suspension .... ⊙ 251
Pred-G S.O.P. Sterile Ophthalmic Ointment .... ⊙ 252

Kanamycin Sulfate (Nephrotoxicity).

No products indexed under this heading.

Streptomycin Sulfate (Nephrotoxicity). Products include:

Streptomycin Sulfate Injection 2208

Tobramycin (Nephrotoxicity). Products include:

AKTOB .... ⊙ 206
TobraDex Ophthalmic Suspension and Ointment 473
Tobrex Ophthalmic Ointment and Solution .... ⊙ 229

Tobramycin Sulfate (Nephrotoxicity). Products include:

Nebcin Vials, Hyporets & ADD-Vantage 1464

Tobramycin Sulfate Injection 968

Food Interactions

Alcohol (When ingested within 72 hours, flushing, sweating, headache, and tachycardia have been reported).

CEFOBID PHARMACY BULK PACKAGE - NOT FOR DIRECT INFUSION

(Cefoperazone Sodium) 2192
May interact with aminoglycosides and certain other agents. Compounds in these categories include:

Amikacin Sulfate (Potential for nephrotoxicity). Products include:

Amikacin Sulfate Injection, USP 960
Amikin Injectable 501

Gentamicin Sulfate (Potential for nephrotoxicity). Products include:

Garamycin Injectable 2360
Genoptic Sterile Ophthalmic Solution .... ⊙ 243
Genoptic Sterile Ophthalmic Ointment .... ⊙ 243
Gentacidin Ointment .... ⊙ 264
Gentacidin Solution .... ⊙ 264
Gentak .... ⊙ 208
Pred-G Liquifilm Sterile Ophthalmic Suspension .... ⊙ 251
Pred-G S.O.P. Sterile Ophthalmic Ointment .... ⊙ 252

Kanamycin Sulfate (Potential for nephrotoxicity).

No products indexed under this heading.

Streptomycin Sulfate (Potential for nephrotoxicity). Products include:

Streptomycin Sulfate Injection 2208

Tobramycin (Potential for nephrotoxicity). Products include:

AKTOB .... ⊙ 206
TobraDex Ophthalmic Suspension and Ointment 473
Tobrex Ophthalmic Ointment and Solution .... ⊙ 229

Tobramycin Sulfate (Potential for nephrotoxicity). Products include:

Nebcin Vials, Hyporets & ADD-Vantage 1464
Tobramycin Sulfate Injection 968

Food Interactions

Alcohol (A disulfiram-like reaction characterized by flushing, sweating, headache, and tachycardia has been reported when alcohol was ingested within 72 hours after Cefobid administration).

CEFOL FILMTAB

(Vitamin B Complex With Vitamin C, Vitamin E, Folic Acid) 412
None cited in PDR database.

CEFOTAN

(Cefotetan) 2829
May interact with aminoglycosides and certain other agents. Compounds in these categories include:

Amikacin Sulfate (Cefotetan increases serum creatinine; concurrent use may lead to potentiation of nephrotoxicity). Products include:

Amikacin Sulfate Injection, USP 960
Amikin Injectable 501

Gentamicin Sulfate (Cefotetan increases serum creatinine; concurrent use may lead to potentiation of nephrotoxicity). Products include:

Garamycin Injectable 2360
Genoptic Sterile Ophthalmic Solution .... ⊙ 243
Genoptic Sterile Ophthalmic Ointment .... ⊙ 243
Gentacidin Ointment .... ⊙ 264
Gentacidin Solution .... ⊙ 264
Gentak .... ⊙ 208
Pred-G Liquifilm Sterile Ophthalmic Suspension .... ⊙ 251
Pred-G S.O.P. Sterile Ophthalmic Ointment .... ⊙ 252

Kanamycin Sulfate (Cefotetan increases serum creatinine; concurrent use may lead to potentiation of nephrotoxicity).

No products indexed under this heading.

Streptomycin Sulfate (Cefotetan increases serum creatinine; concurrent use may lead to potentiation of nephrotoxicity). Products include:

Streptomycin Sulfate Injection 2208

Tobramycin (Cefotetan increases serum creatinine; concurrent use may lead to potentiation of nephrotoxicity). Products include:

AKTOB .... ⊙ 206
TobraDex Ophthalmic Suspension and Ointment 473
Tobrex Ophthalmic Ointment and Solution .... ⊙ 229

Tobramycin Sulfate (Cefotetan increases serum creatinine; concurrent use may lead to potentiation of nephrotoxicity). Products include:

Nebcin Vials, Hyporets & ADD-Vantage 1464
Tobramycin Sulfate Injection 968

Food Interactions

Alcohol (When ingested within 72 hours after Cefotan administration may cause disulfiram-like reactions, including flushing, headache, sweating and tachycardia).

CEFOTAN INJECTION

(Cefotetan) 2829
See Cefotan

CEFTIN FOR ORAL SUSPENSION

(Cefuroxime Axetil) 1078
See Ceftin Tablets

CEFTIN TABLETS

(Cefuroxime Axetil) 1078
May interact with:

Amiloride Hydrochloride (Concurrent treatment with unspecified potent diuretics may adversely affect renal function; caution is advised). Products include:

Midamor Tablets 1703
Moduretic Tablets 1705

Bendroflumethiazide (Concurrent treatment with unspecified potent diuretics may adversely affect renal function; caution is advised).

No products indexed under this heading.

Bumetanide (Concurrent treatment with unspecified potent diuretics may adversely affect renal function; caution is advised). Products include:

Bumex 2093

Chlorothiazide (Concurrent treatment with unspecified potent diuretics may adversely affect renal function; caution is advised). Products include:

Aldoclor Tablets 1598
Diupres Tablets 1650
Diuril Oral 1653

Chlorothiazide Sodium (Concurrent treatment with unspecified potent diuretics may adversely affect renal function; caution is advised). Products include:

Diuril Sodium Intravenous 1652

Chlorthalidone (Concurrent treatment with unspecified potent diuretics may adversely affect renal function; caution is advised). Products include:

Combipres Tablets 677
Tenoretic Tablets 2845
Thalitone 1245

Ethacrynic Acid (Concurrent treatment with unspecified potent diuretics may adversely affect renal function; caution is advised). Products include:

Edecrin Tablets 1657

Furosemide (Concurrent treatment with unspecified potent diuretics may adversely affect renal function; caution is advised). Products include:

Lasix Injection, Oral Solution and Tablets 1240

Hydrochlorothiazide (Concurrent treatment with unspecified potent diuretics may adversely affect renal function; caution is advised). Products include:

Aldactazide 2413
Aldoril Tablets 1604
Apresazide Capsules 808
Capozide 742
Dyazide 2479
Esidrix Tablets 821
Esimil Tablets 822
HydroDIURIL Tablets 1674
Hydropres Tablets 1675
Hyzaar Tablets 1677
Inderide Tablets 2732
Inderide LA Long Acting Capsules .. 2734
Lopressor HCT Tablets 832
Lotensin HCT 837
Maxzide 1380
Moduretic Tablets 1705
Oretic Tablets 443
Prinzide Tablets 1737
Ser-Ap-Es Tablets 849
Timolide Tablets 1748
Vaseretic Tablets 1765
Zestoretic 2850
Ziac 1415

Hydroflumethiazide (Concurrent treatment with unspecified potent diuretics may adversely affect renal function; caution is advised). Products include:

Diucardin Tablets 2718

Indapamide (Concurrent treatment with unspecified potent diuretics may adversely affect renal function; caution is advised). Products include:

Lozol Tablets 2022

Methylclothiazide (Concurrent treatment with unspecified potent diuretics may adversely affect renal function; caution is advised). Products include:

Enduron Tablets 420

Metolazone (Concurrent treatment with unspecified potent diuretics may adversely affect renal function; caution is advised). Products include:

Mykrox Tablets 993
Zaroxolyn Tablets 1000

Polythiazide (Concurrent treatment with unspecified potent diuretics may adversely affect renal function; caution is advised). Products include:

Minizide Capsules 1938

Probenecid (Increases serum concentration of cefuroxime). Products include:

Benemid Tablets 1611
ColBENEMID Tablets 1622

Spironolactone (Concurrent treatment with unspecified potent diuretics may adversely affect renal function; caution is advised). Products include:

Aldactazide 2413
Aldactone 2414

Torsemide (Concurrent treatment with unspecified potent diuretics may adversely affect renal function; caution is advised). Products include:

Demadex Tablets and Injection 686

IMPORTANT NOTE: Always consult each drug listing in the patient's regimen for possible interactions.

Triamterene (Concurrent treatment with unspecified potent diuretics may adversely affect renal function; caution is advised). Products include:

Dyazide ... 2479
Dyrenium Capsules ... 2481
Maxzide ... 1380

Food Interactions

Food, unspecified (Absorption is greater when taken after food).

CEFZIL TABLETS AND ORAL SUSPENSION

(Cefprozil) ... 746
May interact with aminoglycosides and certain other agents. Compounds in these categories include:

Amikacin Sulfate (Potential for nephrotoxicity). Products include:

Amikacin Sulfate Injection, USP ... 960
Amikin Injectable ... 501

Gentamicin Sulfate (Potential for nephrotoxicity). Products include:

Garamycin Injectable ... 2360
Genoptic Sterile Ophthalmic Solution ... ⊙ 243
Genoptic Sterile Ophthalmic Ointment ... ⊙ 243
Gentacidin Ointment ... ⊙ 264
Gentacidin Solution ... ⊙ 264
Gentak ... ⊙ 208
Pred-G Liquifilm Sterile Ophthalmic Suspension ... ⊙ 251
Pred-G S.O.P. Sterile Ophthalmic Ointment ... ⊙ 252

Kanamycin Sulfate (Potential for nephrotoxicity).

No products indexed under this heading.

Probenecid (Doubles the AUC for cefprozil). Products include:

Benemid Tablets ... 1611
ColBENEMID Tablets ... 1622

Streptomycin Sulfate (Potential for nephrotoxicity). Products include:

Streptomycin Sulfate Injection ... 2208

Tobramycin (Potential for nephrotoxicity). Products include:

AKTOB ... ⊙ 206
TobraDex Ophthalmic Suspension and Ointment ... 473
Tobrex Ophthalmic Ointment and Solution ... ⊙ 229

Tobramycin Sulfate (Potential for nephrotoxicity). Products include:

Nebcin Vials, Hyporets & ADD-Vantage ... 1464
Tobramycin Sulfate Injection ... 968

CELESTIAL SEASONINGS SOOTHERS THROAT DROPS

(Menthol, Pectin) ... ■ 842
None cited in PDR database.

CELESTONE SOLUSPAN SUSPENSION

(Betamethasone Sodium Phosphate, Betamethasone Acetate) ... 2347
May interact with:

Aspirin (Concurrent use in hypoprothrombinemia may be undertaken with caution). Products include:

Alka-Seltzer Effervescent Antacid and Pain Reliever ... ■ 701
Alka-Seltzer Extra Strength Effervescent Antacid and Pain Reliever ... ■ 703
Alka-Seltzer Lemon Lime Effervescent Antacid and Pain Reliever ... ■ 703
Alka-Seltzer Plus Cold Medicine ... ■ 705
Alka-Seltzer Plus Cold & Cough Medicine ... ■ 708
Alka-Seltzer Plus Night-Time Cold Medicine ... ■ 707
Alka Seltzer Plus Sinus Medicine ... ■ 707
Arthritis Foundation Safety Coated Aspirin Tablets ... ■ 675
Arthritis Pain Ascriptin ... ■ 631
Maximum Strength Ascriptin ... ■ 630
Regular Strength Ascriptin Tablets ... ■ 629
Arthritis Strength BC Powder ... ■ 609
BC Cold Powder Multi-Symptom Formula (Cold-Sinus-Allergy) ... ■ 609
BC Cold Powder Non-Drowsy Formula (Cold-Sinus) ... ■ 609
BC Powder ... ■ 609
Bayer Children's Chewable Aspirin ... ■ 711
Genuine Bayer Aspirin Tablets & Caplets ... ■ 713
Extra Strength Bayer Arthritis Pain Regimen Formula ... ■ 711
Extra Strength Bayer Aspirin Caplets & Tablets ... ■ 712
Extended-Release Bayer 8-Hour Aspirin ... ■ 712
Extra Strength Bayer Plus Aspirin Caplets ... ■ 713
Extra Strength Bayer PM Aspirin ... ■ 713
Bayer Enteric Aspirin ... ■ 709
Bufferin Analgesic Tablets and Caplets ... ■ 613
Arthritis Strength Bufferin Analgesic Caplets ... ■ 614
Extra Strength Bufferin Analgesic Tablets ... ■ 615
Cama Arthritis Pain Reliever ... ■ 785
Darvon Compound-65 Pulvules ... 1435
Easprin ... 1914
Ecotrin ... 2455
Ecotrin Enteric Coated Aspirin Maximum Strength Tablets and Caplets ... ■ 816
Ecotrin Enteric Coated Aspirin Regular Strength Tablets ... 2455
Empirin Aspirin Tablets ... ■ 854
Empirin with Codeine Tablets ... 1093
Excedrin Extra-Strength Analgesic Tablets & Caplets ... 732
Fiorinal Capsules ... 2261
Fiorinal with Codeine Capsules ... 2262
Fiorinal Tablets ... 2261
Halfprin ... 1362
Healthprin Aspirin ... 2455
Norgesic ... 1496
Percodan Tablets ... 939
Percodan-Demi Tablets ... 940
Robaxisal Tablets ... 2071
Soma Compound w/Codeine Tablets ... 2676
Soma Compound Tablets ... 2675
St. Joseph Adult Chewable Aspirin (81 mg.) ... ■ 808
Talwin Compound ... 2335
Ursinus Inlay-Tabs ... ■ 794
Vanquish Analgesic Caplets ... ■ 731

Immunization (Neurological complications).

CELLCEPT CAPSULES

(Mycophenolate Mofetil) ... 2099
May interact with oral contraceptives and certain other agents. Compounds in these categories include:

Acyclovir (Potential for these two drugs to compete for tubular secretion further increasing the concentrations of both drugs; AUCs were increased 10.6% for phenolic glucuronide of mycophenolate mofetil and 21.9% for acyclovir). Products include:

Zovirax Capsules ... 1219
Zovirax Ointment 5% ... 1223
Zovirax ... 1219

Acyclovir Sodium (Potential for these two drugs to compete for tubular secretion further increasing the concentrations of both drugs; AUCs were increased 10.6% for phenolic glucuronide of mycophenolate mofetil and 21.9% for acyclovir). Products include:

Zovirax Sterile Powder ... 1223

Aluminum Hydroxide (Potential for decreased absorption when CellCept is administered with the antacids containing aluminum and magnesium hydroxide; avoid simultaneous administration). Products include:

ALternaGEL Liquid ... 1316
Maximum Strength Ascriptin ... ■ 630
Cama Arthritis Pain Reliever ... ■ 785
Gaviscon Extra Strength Relief Formula Antacid Tablets ... ■ 819
Gaviscon Extra Strength Relief Formula Liquid Antacid ... ■ 819
Gaviscon Liquid Antacid ... ■ 820
Gelusil Liquid & Tablets ... ■ 855
Maalox Heartburn Relief Suspension ... ■ 642
Maalox Heartburn Relief Tablets ... ■ 641
Maalox Magnesia and Alumina Oral Suspension ... ■ 642
Maalox Plus Tablets ... ■ 643
Extra Strength Maalox Antacid Plus Antigas Liquid and Tablets ... ■ 638
Tempo Soft Antacid ... ■ 835

Aluminum Hydroxide Gel (Potential for decreased absorption when CellCept is administered with the antacids containing aluminum and magnesium hydroxide; avoid simultaneous administration). Products include:

ALternaGEL Liquid ... ■ 659
Aludrox Oral Suspension ... 2695
Amphojel Suspension ... 2695
Amphojel Suspension without Flavor ... 2695
Amphojel Tablets ... 2695
Arthritis Pain Ascriptin ... ■ 631
Regular Strength Ascriptin Tablets ... ■ 629
Gaviscon Antacid Tablets ... ■ 819
Gaviscon-2 Antacid Tablets ... ■ 820
Mylanta Liquid ... 1317
Mylanta Tablets ... ■ 660
Mylanta Double Strength Liquid ... 1317
Mylanta Double Strength Tablets ... ■ 660
Nephrox Suspension ... ■ 655

Antibiotics, unspecified (Drugs that alter gastrointestinal flora may interact with mycophenolate mofetil by disrupting enterohepatic recirculation).

Azathioprine (Concomitant administration is not recommended because such co-administration has not been studied clinically). Products include:

Imuran ... 1110

Azathioprine Sodium (Concomitant administration is not recommended because such co-administration has not been studied clinically).

No products indexed under this heading.

Cholestyramine (Decreased AUC of mycophenolate mofetil by approximately 40%; concomitant use with agents that may interfere with enterohepatic circulation should be avoided). Products include:

Questran Light ... 769
Questran Powder ... 770

Desogestrel (Possibility of changes in the pharmacokinetics of the oral contraceptives under long term dosing conditions with CellCept which might adversely affect the efficacy of the oral contraceptive). Products include:

Desogen Tablets ... 1817
Ortho-Cept ... 1851

Ethinyl Estradiol (Possibility of changes in the pharmacokinetics of the oral contraceptives under long term dosing conditions with CellCept which might adversely affect the efficacy of the oral contraceptive). Products include:

Brevicon ... 2088
Demulen ... 2428
Desogen Tablets ... 1817
Levlen/Tri-Levlen ... 651
Lo/Ovral Tablets ... 2746
Lo/Ovral-28 Tablets ... 2751
Modicon ... 1872
Nordette-21 Tablets ... 2755
Nordette-28 Tablets ... 2758
Norinyl ... 2088
Ortho-Cept ... 1851
Ortho-Cyclen/Ortho-Tri-Cyclen ... 1858
Ortho-Novum ... 1872
Ortho-Cyclen/Ortho Tri-Cyclen ... 1858
Ovcon ... 760
Ovral Tablets ... 2770
Ovral-28 Tablets ... 2770
Levlen/Tri-Levlen ... 651
Tri-Norinyl ... 2164
Triphasil-21 Tablets ... 2814
Triphasil-28 Tablets ... 2819

Ethynodiol Diacetate (Possibility of changes in the pharmacokinetics of the oral contraceptives under long term dosing conditions with CellCept which might adversely affect the efficacy of the oral contraceptive). Products include:

Demulen ... 2428

Ganciclovir Sodium (Potential for these two drugs to compete for tubular secretion further increasing the concentrations of both drugs). Products include:

Cytovene-IV ... 2103

Levonorgestrel (Possibility of changes in the pharmacokinetics of the oral contraceptives under long term dosing conditions with CellCept which might adversely affect the efficacy of the oral contraceptive). Products include:

Levlen/Tri-Levlen ... 651
Nordette-21 Tablets ... 2755
Nordette-28 Tablets ... 2758
Norplant System ... 2759
Levlen/Tri-Levlen ... 651
Triphasil-21 Tablets ... 2814
Triphasil-28 Tablets ... 2819

Magnesium Hydroxide (Potential for decreased absorption when CellCept is administered with the antacids containing aluminum and magnesium hydroxide; avoid simultaneous administration). Products include:

Aludrox Oral Suspension ... 2695
Arthritis Pain Ascriptin ... ■ 631
Maximum Strength Ascriptin ... ■ 630
Regular Strength Ascriptin Tablets ... ■ 629
Di-Gel Antacid/Anti-Gas ... ■ 801
Gelusil Liquid & Tablets ... ■ 855
Maalox Magnesia and Alumina Oral Suspension ... ■ 642
Maalox Plus Tablets ... ■ 643
Extra Strength Maalox Antacid Plus Antigas Liquid and Tablets ... ■ 638
Mylanta Calcium Carbonate and Magnesium Hydroxide Tablets ... 1318
Mylanta Liquid ... 1317
Mylanta Tablets ... ■ 660
Mylanta Double Strength Liquid ... 1317
Mylanta Double Strength Tablets ... ■ 660
Phillips' Milk of Magnesia Liquid ... ■ 729
Rolaids Tablets ... ■ 843
Tempo Soft Antacid ... ■ 835

Mestranol (Possibility of changes in the pharmacokinetics of the oral contraceptives under long term dosing conditions with CellCept which might adversely affect the efficacy of the oral contraceptive). Products include:

Norinyl ... 2088
Ortho-Novum ... 1872

Norethindrone (Possibility of changes in the pharmacokinetics of the oral contraceptives under long term dosing conditions with CellCept which might adversely affect the efficacy of the oral contraceptive). Products include:

Brevicon ... 2088
Micronor Tablets ... 1872
Modicon ... 1872

Norinyl 2088
Nor-Q D Tablets 2135
Ortho-Novum.. 1872
Ovcon 760
Tri-Norinyl.. 2164

Norethynodrel (Possibility of changes in the pharmacokinetics of the oral contraceptives under long term dosing conditions with CellCept which might adversely affect the efficacy of the oral contraceptive).

No products indexed under this heading.

Norgestimate (Possibility of changes in the pharmacokinetics of the oral contraceptives under long term dosing conditions with CellCept which might adversely affect the efficacy of the oral contraceptive). Products include:

Ortho-Cyclen/Ortho-Tri-Cyclen 1858
Ortho-Cyclen/Ortho Tri-Cyclen 1858

Norgestrel (Possibility of changes in the pharmacokinetics of the oral contraceptives under long term dosing conditions with CellCept which might adversely affect the efficacy of the oral contraceptive). Products include:

Lo/Ovral Tablets 2746
Lo/Ovral-28 Tablets............................. 2751
Ovral Tablets 2770
Ovral-28 Tablets 2770
Ovrette Tablets.................................... 2771

Probenecid (Potential for increased plasma concentration of MPA). Products include:

Benemid Tablets 1611
ColBENEMID Tablets 1622

Food Interactions

Food, unspecified (Decreased Cmax of mycophenolate mofetil by 40% in the presence of food; no effect on the extent of absorption).

CELLUVISC LUBRICANT EYE DROPS

(Carboxymethylcellulose Sodium) .. ◎ 238
None cited in PDR database.

CELONTIN KAPSEALS

(Methsuximide) 1899
May interact with anticonvulsants. Compounds in this category include:

Carbamazepine (Effect not specified; periodic serum level determination may be necessary). Products include:

Atretol Tablets 573
Tegretol Chewable Tablets 852
Tegretol Suspension............................. 852
Tegretol Tablets 852

Divalproex Sodium (Effect not specified; periodic serum level determination may be necessary). Products include:

Depakote Tablets.................................. 415

Ethosuximide (Effect not specified; periodic serum level determination may be necessary). Products include:

Zarontin Capsules 1928
Zarontin Syrup 1929

Ethotoin (Effect not specified; periodic serum level determination may be necessary). Products include:

Peganone Tablets 446

Felbamate (Effect not specified; periodic serum level determination may be necessary). Products include:

Felbatol 2666

Lamotrigine (Effect not specified; periodic serum level determination may be necessary). Products include:

Lamictal Tablets................................... 1112

Mephenytoin (Effect not specified; periodic serum level determination may be necessary). Products include:

Mesantoin Tablets 2272

Paramethadione (Effect not specified; periodic serum level determination may be necessary).

No products indexed under this heading.

Phenacemide (Effect not specified; periodic serum level determination may be necessary). Products include:

Phenurone Tablets 447

Phenobarbital (Increased plasma concentration of phenobarbital). Products include:

Arco-Lase Plus Tablets 512
Bellergal-S Tablets 2250
Donnatal 2060
Donnatal Extentabs.............................. 2061
Donnatal Tablets 2060
Phenobarbital Elixir and Tablets 1469
Quadrinal Tablets 1350

Phensuximide (Effect not specified; periodic serum level determination may be necessary). Products include:

Milontin Kapseals................................. 1920

Phenytoin (Increased plasma concentration of phenytoin). Products include:

Dilantin Infatabs.................................. 1908
Dilantin-125 Suspension 1911

Phenytoin Sodium (Increased plasma concentration of phenytoin). Products include:

Dilantin Kapseals 1906
Dilantin Parenteral 1910

Primidone (Effect not specified; periodic serum level determination may be necessary). Products include:

Mysoline... 2754

Trimethadione (Effect not specified; periodic serum level determination may be necessary).

No products indexed under this heading.

Valproic Acid (Effect not specified; periodic serum level determination may be necessary). Products include:

Depakene 413

CENTRUM

(Vitamins with Minerals) ....ⓐⓓ 666
None cited in PDR database.

CENTRUM, JR. (CHILDREN'S CHEWABLE) + EXTRA C

(Vitamins with Minerals) ....ⓐⓓ 666
None cited in PDR database.

CENTRUM, JR. (CHILDREN'S CHEWABLE) + EXTRA CALCIUM

(Vitamins with Minerals) ....ⓐⓓ 667
None cited in PDR database.

CENTRUM, JR. (CHILDREN'S CHEWABLE) + IRON

(Vitamins with Minerals) ....ⓐⓓ 668
None cited in PDR database.

CENTRUM LIQUID

(Vitamins with Minerals) ....ⓐⓓ 666
None cited in PDR database.

CENTRUM SILVER

(Vitamins with Minerals) ....ⓐⓓ 668
None cited in PDR database.

CENTRUM SINGLES BETA CAROTENE

(Beta Carotene) ....ⓐⓓ 669
None cited in PDR database.

CENTRUM SINGLES CALCIUM

(Calcium Carbonate) ....ⓐⓓ 669
None cited in PDR database.

CENTRUM SINGLES VITAMIN C

(Vitamin C)...ⓐⓓ 669
None cited in PDR database.

CENTRUM SINGLES VITAMIN E

(Vitamin E) ....ⓐⓓ 669
None cited in PDR database.

CEO-TWO RECTAL SUPPOSITORIES

(Sodium Bicarbonate, Potassium Bitartrate) 666
None cited in PDR database.

CēPACOL ANESTHETIC LOZENGES

(Benzocaine, Cetylpyridinium Chloride)..ⓐⓓ 875
None cited in PDR database.

CēPACOL/CēPACOL MINT MOUTHWASH/GARGLE

(Cetylpyridinium Chloride)..................ⓐⓓ 875
None cited in PDR database.

CēPACOL DRY THROAT LOZENGES, CHERRY FLAVOR

(Menthol) ....ⓐⓓ 875
None cited in PDR database.

CēPACOL DRY THROAT LOZENGES, HONEY-LEMON FLAVOR

(Menthol) ....ⓐⓓ 875
None cited in PDR database.

CēPACOL DRY THROAT LOZENGES, MENTHOL-EUCALYPTUS FLAVOR

(Menthol) ....ⓐⓓ 875
None cited in PDR database.

CēPACOL DRY THROAT LOZENGES, ORIGINAL FLAVOR

(Benzyl Alcohol, Cetylpyridinium Chloride)..ⓐⓓ 875
None cited in PDR database.

CEPASTAT CHERRY FLAVOR SORE THROAT LOZENGES

(Menthol, Phenol) ....ⓐⓓ 810
None cited in PDR database.

CEPASTAT EXTRA STRENGTH SORE THROAT LOZENGES

(Phenol, Menthol) ....ⓐⓓ 810
None cited in PDR database.

CEPTAZ

(Ceftazidime) 1081
May interact with aminoglycosides and certain other agents. Compounds in these categories include:

Amikacin Sulfate (Potential for nephrotoxicity following concomitant administration). Products include:

Amikacin Sulfate Injection, USP 960
Amikin Injectable 501

Chloramphenicol (Possible antagonism in vivo). Products include:

Chloromycetin Ophthalmic Ointment, 1% .... ◎ 310
Chloromycetin Ophthalmic Solution... ◎ 310
Chloroptic S.O.P. .... ◎ 239
Chloroptic Sterile Ophthalmic Solution .... ◎ 239
Elase-Chloromycetin Ointment 1040
Ophthocort .... ◎ 311

Chloramphenicol Palmitate (Possible antagonism in vivo).

No products indexed under this heading.

Chloramphenicol Sodium Succinate (Possible antagonism in vivo). Products include:

Chloromycetin Sodium Succinate.... 1900

Furosemide (Potential for nephrotoxicity following concomitant administration). Products include:

Lasix Injection, Oral Solution and Tablets 1240

Gentamicin Sulfate (Potential for nephrotoxicity following concomitant administration). Products include:

Garamycin Injectable 2360
Genoptic Sterile Ophthalmic Solution... ◎ 243
Genoptic Sterile Ophthalmic Ointment .... ◎ 243
Gentacidin Ointment .... ◎ 264
Gentacidin Solution.............................. ◎ 264
Gentak .... ◎ 208
Pred-G Liquifilm Sterile Ophthalmic Suspension .... ◎ 251
Pred-G S.O.P. Sterile Ophthalmic Ointment .... ◎ 252

Kanamycin Sulfate (Potential for nephrotoxicity following concomitant administration).

No products indexed under this heading.

Streptomycin Sulfate (Potential for nephrotoxicity following concomitant administration). Products include:

Streptomycin Sulfate Injection.......... 2208

Tobramycin (Potential for nephrotoxicity following concomitant administration). Products include:

AKTOB .... ◎ 206
TobraDex Ophthalmic Suspension and Ointment.. 473
Tobrex Ophthalmic Ointment and Solution .... ◎ 229

Tobramycin Sulfate (Potential for nephrotoxicity following concomitant administration). Products include:

Nebcin Vials, Hyporets & ADD-Vantage 1464
Tobramycin Sulfate Injection 968

CEREDASE

(Alglucerase)...1065
None cited in PDR database.

CEREZYME

(Imiglucerase).......................................1066
None cited in PDR database.

CEROSE DM

(Chlorpheniramine Maleate, Dextromethorphan Hydrobromide, Phenylephrine Hydrochloride)..........ⓐⓓ 878
May interact with antihypertensives, antidepressant drugs, and certain other agents. Compounds in these categories include:

Acebutolol Hydrochloride (Effects not specified). Products include:

Sectral Capsules 2807

Amitriptyline Hydrochloride (Effects not specified). Products include:

Elavil 2838
Endep Tablets 2174
Etrafon 2355
Limbitrol 2180
Triavil Tablets 1757

IMPORTANT NOTE: Always consult each drug listing in the patient's regimen for possible interactions.

Cerose DM Interactions Index 174

Amlodipine Besylate (Effects not specified). Products include:
Lotrel Capsules 840
Norvasc Tablets 1940
Amoxapine (Effects not specified). Products include:
Asendin Tablets 1369
Atenolol (Effects not specified). Products include:
Tenoretic Tablets 2845
Tenormin Tablets and I.V. Injection 2847
Benazepril Hydrochloride (Effects not specified). Products include:
Lotensin Tablets 834
Lotensin HCT 837
Lotrel Capsules 840
Bendroflumethiazide (Effects not specified).
No products indexed under this heading.
Betaxolol Hydrochloride (Effects not specified). Products include:
Betoptic Ophthalmic Solution 469
Betoptic S Ophthalmic Suspension 471
Kerlone Tablets 2436
Bisoprolol Fumarate (Effects not specified). Products include:
Zebeta Tablets 1413
Ziac 1415
Bupropion Hydrochloride (Effects not specified). Products include:
Wellbutrin Tablets 1204
Captopril (Effects not specified). Products include:
Capoten 739
Capozide 742
Carteolol Hydrochloride (Effects not specified). Products include:
Cartrol Tablets 410
Ocupress Ophthalmic Solution, 1% Sterile .... ◉ 309
Chlorothiazide (Effects not specified). Products include:
Aldoclor Tablets 1598
Diupres Tablets 1650
Diuril Oral 1653
Chlorothiazide Sodium (Effects not specified). Products include:
Diuril Sodium Intravenous 1652
Chlorthalidone (Effects not specified). Products include:
Combipres Tablets 677
Tenoretic Tablets 2845
Thalitone 1245
Clonidine (Effects not specified). Products include:
Catapres-TTS 675
Clonidine Hydrochloride (Effects not specified). Products include:
Catapres Tablets 674
Combipres Tablets 677
Deserpidine (Effects not specified).
No products indexed under this heading.
Desipramine Hydrochloride (Effects not specified). Products include:
Norpramin Tablets 1526
Diazoxide (Effects not specified). Products include:
Hyperstat I.V. Injection 2363
Proglycem 580
Diltiazem Hydrochloride (Effects not specified). Products include:
Cardizem CD Capsules 1506
Cardizem SR Capsules 1510
Cardizem Injectable 1508
Cardizem Tablets 1512
Dilacor XR Extended-release Capsules 2018
Doxazosin Mesylate (Effects not specified). Products include:
Cardura Tablets 2186
Doxepin Hydrochloride (Effects not specified). Products include:
Sinequan 2205
Zonalon Cream 1055
Enalapril Maleate (Effects not specified). Products include:
Vaseretic Tablets 1765
Vasotec Tablets 1771
Enalaprilat (Effects not specified). Products include:
Vasotec I.V. 1768
Esmolol Hydrochloride (Effects not specified). Products include:
Brevibloc Injection 1808
Felodipine (Effects not specified). Products include:
Plendil Extended-Release Tablets 527
Fluoxetine Hydrochloride (Effects not specified). Products include:
Prozac Pulvules & Liquid, Oral Solution 919
Fosinopril Sodium (Effects not specified). Products include:
Monopril Tablets 757
Furosemide (Effects not specified). Products include:
Lasix Injection, Oral Solution and Tablets 1240
Guanabenz Acetate (Effects not specified).
No products indexed under this heading.
Guanethidine Monosulfate (Effects not specified). Products include:
Esimil Tablets 822
Ismelin Tablets 827
Hydralazine Hydrochloride (Effects not specified). Products include:
Apresazide Capsules 808
Apresoline Hydrochloride Tablets .. 809
Ser-Ap-Es Tablets 849
Hydrochlorothiazide (Effects not specified). Products include:
Aldactazide 2413
Aldoril Tablets 1604
Apresazide Capsules 808
Capozide 742
Dyazide 2479
Esidrix Tablets 821
Esimil Tablets 822
HydroDIURIL Tablets 1674
Hydropres Tablets 1675
Hyzaar Tablets 1677
Inderide Tablets 2732
Inderide LA Long Acting Capsules .. 2734
Lopressor HCT Tablets 832
Lotensin HCT 837
Maxzide 1380
Moduretic Tablets 1705
Oretic Tablets 443
Prinzide Tablets 1737
Ser-Ap-Es Tablets 849
Timolide Tablets 1748
Vaseretic Tablets 1765
Zestoretic 2850
Ziac 1415
Hydroflumethiazide (Effects not specified). Products include:
Diucardin Tablets 2718
Imipramine Hydrochloride (Effects not specified). Products include:
Tofranil Ampuls 854
Tofranil Tablets 856
Imipramine Pamoate (Effects not specified). Products include:
Tofranil-PM Capsules 857
Indapamide (Effects not specified). Products include:
Lozol Tablets 2022
Isocarboxazid (Effects not specified).
No products indexed under this heading.
Isradipine (Effects not specified). Products include:
DynaCirc Capsules 2256
Labetalol Hydrochloride (Effects not specified). Products include:
Normodyne Injection 2377
Normodyne Tablets 2379
Trandate 1185
Levobunolol Hydrochloride (Effects not specified). Products include:
Betagan .... ◉ 233
Lisinopril (Effects not specified). Products include:
Prinivil Tablets 1733
Prinzide Tablets 1737
Zestoretic 2850
Zestril Tablets 2854
Losartan Potassium (Effects not specified). Products include:
Cozaar Tablets 1628
Hyzaar Tablets 1677
Maprotiline Hydrochloride (Effects not specified). Products include:
Ludiomil Tablets 843
Mecamylamine Hydrochloride (Effects not specified). Products include:
Inversine Tablets 1686
Methyclothiazide (Effects not specified). Products include:
Enduron Tablets 420
Methyldopa (Effects not specified). Products include:
Aldoclor Tablets 1598
Aldomet Oral 1600
Aldoril Tablets 1604
Methyldopate Hydrochloride (Effects not specified). Products include:
Aldomet Ester HCl Injection 1602
Metipranolol Hydrochloride (Effects not specified). Products include:
OptiPranolol (Metipranolol 0.3%) Sterile Ophthalmic Solution .... ◉ 258
Metolazone (Effects not specified). Products include:
Mykrox Tablets 993
Zaroxolyn Tablets 1000
Metoprolol Succinate (Effects not specified). Products include:
Toprol-XL Tablets 565
Metoprolol Tartrate (Effects not specified). Products include:
Lopressor Ampuls 830
Lopressor HCT Tablets 832
Lopressor Tablets 830
Metyrosine (Effects not specified). Products include:
Demser Capsules 1649
Minoxidil (Effects not specified). Products include:
Loniten Tablets 2618
Rogaine Topical Solution 2637
Moexipril Hydrochloride (Effects not specified). Products include:
Univasc Tablets 2410
Nadolol (Effects not specified).
No products indexed under this heading.
Nefazodone Hydrochloride (Effects not specified). Products include:
Serzone Tablets 771
Nicardipine Hydrochloride (Effects not specified). Products include:
Cardene Capsules 2095
Cardene I.V. 2709
Cardene SR Capsules 2097
Nifedipine (Effects not specified). Products include:
Adalat Capsules (10 mg and 20 mg) 587
Adalat CC 589
Procardia Capsules 1971
Procardia XL Extended Release Tablets 1972
Nisoldipine (Effects not specified).
No products indexed under this heading.
Nitroglycerin (Effects not specified). Products include:
Deponit NTG Transdermal Delivery System 2397
Nitro-Bid IV 1523
Nitro-Bid Ointment 1524
Nitrodisc 2047
Nitro-Dur (nitroglycerin) Transdermal Infusion System 1326
Nitrolingual Spray 2027
Nitrostat Tablets 1925
Transderm-Nitro Transdermal Therapeutic System 859
Nortriptyline Hydrochloride (Effects not specified). Products include:
Pamelor 2280
Paroxetine Hydrochloride (Effects not specified). Products include:
Paxil Tablets 2505
Penbutolol Sulfate (Effects not specified). Products include:
Levatol 2403
Phenelzine Sulfate (Effects not specified). Products include:
Nardil 1920
Phenoxybenzamine Hydrochloride (Effects not specified). Products include:
Dibenzyline Capsules 2476
Phentolamine Mesylate (Effects not specified). Products include:
Regitine 846
Pindolol (Effects not specified). Products include:
Visken Tablets 2299
Polythiazide (Effects not specified). Products include:
Minizide Capsules 1938
Prazosin Hydrochloride (Effects not specified). Products include:
Minipress Capsules 1937
Minizide Capsules 1938
Propranolol Hydrochloride (Effects not specified). Products include:
Inderal 2728
Inderal LA Long Acting Capsules 2730
Inderide Tablets 2732
Inderide LA Long Acting Capsules .. 2734
Protriptyline Hydrochloride (Effects not specified). Products include:
Vivactil Tablets 1774
Quinapril Hydrochloride (Effects not specified). Products include:
Accupril Tablets 1893
Ramipril (Effects not specified). Products include:
Altace Capsules 1232
Rauwolfia Serpentina (Effects not specified).
No products indexed under this heading.
Rescinnamine (Effects not specified).
No products indexed under this heading.
Reserpine (Effects not specified). Products include:
Diupres Tablets 1650
Hydropres Tablets 1675
Ser-Ap-Es Tablets 849
Sertraline Hydrochloride (Effects not specified). Products include:
Zoloft Tablets 2217
Sodium Nitroprusside (Effects not specified).
No products indexed under this heading.
Sotalol Hydrochloride (Effects not specified). Products include:
Betapace Tablets 641

(▭ Described in PDR For Nonprescription Drugs) (◉ Described in PDR For Ophthalmology)

Spirapril Hydrochloride (Effects not specified).

No products indexed under this heading.

Terazosin Hydrochloride (Effects not specified). Products include:

Hytrin Capsules 430

Timolol Maleate (Effects not specified). Products include:

Blocadren Tablets 1614
Timolide Tablets....................................... 1748
Timoptic in Ocudose 1753
Timoptic Sterile Ophthalmic Solution... 1751
Timoptic-XE 1755

Torsemide (Effects not specified). Products include:

Demadex Tablets and Injection 686

Tranylcypromine Sulfate (Effects not specified). Products include:

Parnate Tablets 2503

Trazodone Hydrochloride (Effects not specified). Products include:

Desyrel and Desyrel Dividose 503

Trimethaphan Camsylate (Effects not specified). Products include:

Arfonad Ampuls 2080

Trimipramine Maleate (Effects not specified). Products include:

Surmontil Capsules................................. 2811

Venlafaxine Hydrochloride (Effects not specified). Products include:

Effexor 2719

Verapamil Hydrochloride (Effects not specified). Products include:

Calan SR Caplets 2422
Calan Tablets.. 2419
Isoptin Injectable 1344
Isoptin Oral Tablets 1346
Isoptin SR Tablets 1348
Verelan Capsules 1410
Verelan Capsules 2824

Food Interactions

Alcohol (May increase the drowsiness effect; avoid concurrent use).

CERUBIDINE

(Daunorubicin Hydrochloride) 795
May interact with:

Bone Marrow Depressants, unspecified (Therapy with Cerubidine should not be started in patients with pre-existing drug-induced myelosuppression).

CERUMENEX DROPS

(Triethanolamine Polypeptide Oleate-Condensate) 1993
None cited in PDR database.

CERVIDIL

(Dinoprostone) 1010
May interact with oxytocic drugs and certain other agents. Compounds in these categories include:

Ergonovine Maleate (Dinoprostone may augment the activity of oxytocic agents and concomitant use is not recommended; a dosing interval of at least 30 minutes is recommended for sequential use).

No products indexed under this heading.

Methylergonovine Maleate (Dinoprostone may augment the activity of oxytocic agents and concomitant use is not recommended; a dosing interval of at least 30 minutes is recommended for sequential use). Products include:

Methergine 2272

Oxytocin (Injection) (Dinoprostone may augment the activity of oxytocic agents and concomitant use is not recommended; a dosing interval of at least 30 minutes is recommended for sequential use).

CETACAINE TOPICAL ANESTHETIC

(Benzocaine, Tetracaine Hydrochloride, Butyl Aminobenzoate) 794
None cited in PDR database.

CETAPHIL GENTLE CLEANSING BAR

(Cleanser) 1046
None cited in PDR database.

CETAPHIL MOISTURIZING CREAM

(Moisturizing formula) 1046
None cited in PDR database.

CETAPHIL MOISTURIZING LOTION

(Moisturizing formula) 1046
None cited in PDR database.

CETAPHIL SKIN CLEANSER

(Cetyl Alcohol) 1046
None cited in PDR database.

CHARCOAID

(Charcoal, Activated) ....ⓢⓓ 768
None cited in PDR database.

CHARCOAID 2000

(Charcoal, Activated) ....ⓢⓓ 768
None cited in PDR database.

CHEMET (SUCCIMER) CAPSULES

(Succimer) 1545
May interact with:

Calcium Disodium Edetate (Concomitant administration is not recommended). Products include:

Calcium Disodium Versenate Injection... 1490

CHERACOL-D COUGH FORMULA

(Dextromethorphan Hydrobromide, Guaifenesin) ....ⓢⓓ 769
None cited in PDR database.

CHERACOL NASAL SPRAY PUMP

(Oxymetazoline Hydrochloride) ......ⓢⓓ 768
None cited in PDR database.

CHERACOL PLUS HEAD COLD/COUGH FORMULA

(Phenylpropanolamine Hydrochloride, Dextromethorphan Hydrobromide, Chlorpheniramine Maleate) ....ⓢⓓ 769
May interact with monoamine oxidase inhibitors. Compounds in this category include:

Furazolidone (Concurrent and/or sequential administration is not recommended). Products include:

Furoxone 2046

Isocarboxazid (Concurrent and/or sequential administration is not recommended).

No products indexed under this heading.

Phenelzine Sulfate (Concurrent and/or sequential administration is not recommended). Products include:

Nardil 1920

Selegiline Hydrochloride (Concurrent and/or sequential administration is not recommended). Products include:

Eldepryl Tablets 2550

Tranylcypromine Sulfate (Concurrent and/or sequential administration is not recommended). Products include:

Parnate Tablets 2503

CHERACOL SINUS

(Dexbrompheniramine Maleate, Pseudoephedrine Sulfate) ....ⓢⓓ 768
May interact with:

Antidepressant Medications, unspecified (Effect not specified).

Antihypertensive agents, unspecified (Effect not specified).

Food Interactions

Alcohol (May increase drowsiness effect).

CHERACOL SORE THROAT SPRAY

(Phenol) ....ⓢⓓ 769
None cited in PDR database.

CHIBROXIN STERILE OPHTHALMIC SOLUTION

(Norfloxacin)...1617
May interact with oral anticoagulants and certain other agents. Compounds in these categories include:

Aminophylline (Potential elevation of serum theophylline concentrations).

No products indexed under this heading.

Caffeine (Interferes with the metabolism of caffeine). Products include:

Arthritis Strength BC Powder..........ⓢⓓ 609
BC Powder ....ⓢⓓ 609
Bayer Select Headache Pain Relief Formula ....ⓢⓓ 716
Cafergot... 2251
DHCplus Capsules................................... 1993
Darvon Compound-65 Pulvules 1435
Esgic-plus Tablets 1013
Aspirin Free Excedrin Analgesic Caplets and Geltabs 732
Excedrin Extra-Strength Analgesic Tablets & Caplets 732
Fioricet Tablets... 2258
Fioricet with Codeine Capsules 2260
Fiorinal Capsules 2261
Fiorinal with Codeine Capsules 2262
Fiorinal Tablets... 2261
Maximum Strength Multi-Symptom Formula Midol ....ⓢⓓ 722
Migralam Capsules 2038
No Doz Maximum Strength Caplets...ⓢⓓ 622
Norgesic.. 1496
Vanquish Analgesic Caplets ....ⓢⓓ 731
Wigraine Tablets & Suppositories .. 1829

Cyclosporine (Elevated serum levels of cyclosporine). Products include:

Neoral... 2276
Sandimmune 2286

Dicumarol (Enhanced effects of anticoagulant).

No products indexed under this heading.

Dyphylline (Potential elevation of serum theophylline concentrations). Products include:

Lufyllin & Lufyllin-400 Tablets 2670
Lufyllin-GG Elixir & Tablets 2671

Theophylline (Potential elevation of serum theophylline concentrations). Products include:

Marax Tablets & DF Syrup................... 2200
Quibron 2053

Theophylline Anhydrous (Potential elevation of serum theophylline concentrations). Products include:

Aerolate 1004
Primatene Dual Action Formula......ⓢⓓ 872
Primatene Tablets ....ⓢⓓ 873
Respbid Tablets 682
Slo-bid Gyrocaps 2033
Theo-24 Extended Release Capsules 2568
Theo-Dur Extended-Release Tablets 1327
Theo-X Extended-Release Tablets .. 788
Uni-Dur Extended-Release Tablets.. 1331
Uniphyl 400 mg Tablets....................... 2001

Theophylline Calcium Salicylate (Potential elevation of serum theophylline concentrations). Products include:

Quadrinal Tablets 1350

Theophylline Sodium Glycinate (Potential elevation of serum theophylline concentrations).

No products indexed under this heading.

Warfarin Sodium (Enhanced effects of anticoagulant). Products include:

Coumadin 926

CHLOR-3 CONDIMENT

(Potassium Chloride)..............................1004
None cited in PDR database.

CHILDREN'S VICKS CHLORASEPTIC SORE THROAT LOZENGES

(Benzocaine) ....ⓢⓓ 757
None cited in PDR database.

CHILDREN'S VICKS CHLORASEPTIC SORE THROAT SPRAY

(Phenol) ....ⓢⓓ 757
None cited in PDR database.

CHILDREN'S VICKS DAYQUIL ALLERGY RELIEF

(Chlorpheniramine Maleate, Pseudoephedrine Hydrochloride) ....ⓢⓓ 757
May interact with tranquilizers, hypnotics and sedatives, monoamine oxidase inhibitors, and certain other agents. Compounds in these categories include:

Alprazolam (May increase drowsiness effect). Products include:

Xanax Tablets 2649

Buspirone Hydrochloride (May increase drowsiness effect). Products include:

BuSpar 737

Chlordiazepoxide (May increase drowsiness effect). Products include:

Libritabs Tablets 2177
Limbitrol 2180

Chlordiazepoxide Hydrochloride (May increase drowsiness effect). Products include:

Librax Capsules 2176
Librium Capsules..................................... 2178
Librium Injectable 2179

Chlorpromazine (May increase drowsiness effect). Products include:

Thorazine Suppositories 2523

Chlorpromazine Hydrochloride (May increase drowsiness effect). Products include:

Thorazine 2523

Chlorprothixene (May increase drowsiness effect).

No products indexed under this heading.

Chlorprothixene Hydrochloride (May increase drowsiness effect).

No products indexed under this heading.

IMPORTANT NOTE: Always consult each drug listing in the patient's regimen for possible interactions.

Children's Vicks DayQuil

Clorazepate Dipotassium (May increase drowsiness effect). Products include:

Tranxene 451

Diazepam (May increase drowsiness effect). Products include:

Dizac	1809
Valium Injectable	2182
Valium Tablets	2183
Valrelease Capsules	2169

Droperidol (May increase drowsiness effect). Products include:

Inapsine Injection 1296

Estazolam (May increase drowsiness effect). Products include:

ProSom Tablets 449

Ethchlorvynol (May increase drowsiness effect). Products include:

Placidyl Capsules 448

Ethinamate (May increase drowsiness effect).

No products indexed under this heading.

Fluphenazine Decanoate (May increase drowsiness effect). Products include:

Prolixin Decanoate 509

Fluphenazine Enanthate (May increase drowsiness effect). Products include:

Prolixin Enanthate 509

Fluphenazine Hydrochloride (May increase drowsiness effect). Products include:

Prolixin 509

Flurazepam Hydrochloride (May increase drowsiness effect). Products include:

Dalmane Capsules 2173

Furazolidone (Concurrent and/or sequential use is not recommended). Products include:

Furoxone 2046

Glutethimide (May increase drowsiness effect).

No products indexed under this heading.

Haloperidol (May increase drowsiness effect). Products include:

Haldol Injection, Tablets and Concentrate 1575

Haloperidol Decanoate (May increase drowsiness effect). Products include:

Haldol Decanoate 1577

Hydroxyzine Hydrochloride (May increase drowsiness effect). Products include:

Atarax Tablets & Syrup	2185
Marax Tablets & DF Syrup	2200
Vistaril Intramuscular Solution	2216

Isocarboxazid (Concurrent and/or sequential use is not recommended).

No products indexed under this heading.

Lorazepam (May increase drowsiness effect). Products include:

Ativan Injection	2698
Ativan Tablets	2700

Loxapine Hydrochloride (May increase drowsiness effect). Products include:

Loxitane 1378

Loxapine Succinate (May increase drowsiness effect). Products include:

Loxitane Capsules 1378

Meprobamate (May increase drowsiness effect). Products include:

Miltown Tablets	2672
PMB 200 and PMB 400	2783

Mesoridazine Besylate (May increase drowsiness effect). Products include:

Serentil 684

Midazolam Hydrochloride (May increase drowsiness effect). Products include:

Versed Injection 2170

Molindone Hydrochloride (May increase drowsiness effect). Products include:

Moban Tablets and Concentrate 1048

Oxazepam (May increase drowsiness effect). Products include:

Serax Capsules	2810
Serax Tablets	2810

Perphenazine (May increase drowsiness effect). Products include:

Etrafon	2355
Triavil Tablets	1757
Trilafon	2389

Phenelzine Sulfate (Concurrent and/or sequential use is not recommended). Products include:

Nardil 1920

Prazepam (May increase drowsiness effect).

No products indexed under this heading.

Prochlorperazine (May increase drowsiness effect). Products include:

Compazine 2470

Promethazine Hydrochloride (May increase drowsiness effect). Products include:

Mepergan Injection	2753
Phenergan with Codeine	2777
Phenergan with Dextromethorphan	2778
Phenergan Injection	2773
Phenergan Suppositories	2775
Phenergan Syrup	2774
Phenergan Tablets	2775
Phenergan VC	2779
Phenergan VC with Codeine	2781

Propofol (May increase drowsiness effect). Products include:

Diprivan Injection 2833

Quazepam (May increase drowsiness effect). Products include:

Doral Tablets 2664

Secobarbital Sodium (May increase drowsiness effect). Products include:

Seconal Sodium Pulvules 1474

Selegiline Hydrochloride (Concurrent and/or sequential use is not recommended). Products include:

Eldepryl Tablets 2550

Temazepam (May increase drowsiness effect). Products include:

Restoril Capsules 2284

Thioridazine Hydrochloride (May increase drowsiness effect). Products include:

Mellaril 2269

Thiothixene (May increase drowsiness effect). Products include:

Navane Capsules and Concentrate	2201
Navane Intramuscular	2202

Tranylcypromine Sulfate (Concurrent and/or sequential use is not recommended). Products include:

Parnate Tablets 2503

Triazolam (May increase drowsiness effect). Products include:

Halcion Tablets 2611

Trifluoperazine Hydrochloride (May increase drowsiness effect). Products include:

Stelazine 2514

Zolpidem Tartrate (May increase drowsiness effect). Products include:

Ambien Tablets 2416

Food Interactions

Alcohol (May increase drowsiness effect).

CHILDREN'S VICKS NYQUIL COLD/COUGH RELIEF

(Chlorpheniramine Maleate, Dextromethorphan Hydrobromide, Pseudoephedrine Hydrochloride) ....▣ 758

May interact with hypnotics and sedatives, tranquilizers, monoamine oxidase inhibitors, and certain other agents. Compounds in these categories include:

Alprazolam (May increase drowsiness effect). Products include:

Xanax Tablets 2649

Buspirone Hydrochloride (May increase drowsiness effect). Products include:

BuSpar 737

Chlordiazepoxide (May increase drowsiness effect). Products include:

Libritabs Tablets	2177
Limbitrol	2180

Chlordiazepoxide Hydrochloride (May increase drowsiness effect). Products include:

Librax Capsules	2176
Librium Capsules	2178
Librium Injectable	2179

Chlorpromazine (May increase drowsiness effect). Products include:

Thorazine Suppositories 2523

Chlorpromazine Hydrochloride (May increase drowsiness effect). Products include:

Thorazine 2523

Chlorprothixene (May increase drowsiness effect).

No products indexed under this heading.

Chlorprothixene Hydrochloride (May increase drowsiness effect).

No products indexed under this heading.

Clorazepate Dipotassium (May increase drowsiness effect). Products include:

Tranxene 451

Diazepam (May increase drowsiness effect). Products include:

Dizac	1809
Valium Injectable	2182
Valium Tablets	2183
Valrelease Capsules	2169

Droperidol (May increase drowsiness effect). Products include:

Inapsine Injection 1296

Estazolam (May increase drowsiness effect). Products include:

ProSom Tablets 449

Ethchlorvynol (May increase drowsiness effect). Products include:

Placidyl Capsules 448

Ethinamate (May increase drowsiness effect).

No products indexed under this heading.

Fluphenazine Decanoate (May increase drowsiness effect). Products include:

Prolixin Decanoate 509

Fluphenazine Enanthate (May increase drowsiness effect). Products include:

Prolixin Enanthate 509

Fluphenazine Hydrochloride (May increase drowsiness effect). Products include:

Prolixin 509

Flurazepam Hydrochloride (May increase drowsiness effect). Products include:

Dalmane Capsules 2173

Furazolidone (Concurrent and/or sequential use is not recommended). Products include:

Furoxone 2046

Glutethimide (May increase drowsiness effect).

No products indexed under this heading.

Haloperidol (May increase drowsiness effect). Products include:

Haldol Injection, Tablets and Concentrate 1575

Haloperidol Decanoate (May increase drowsiness effect). Products include:

Haldol Decanoate 1577

Hydroxyzine Hydrochloride (May increase drowsiness effect). Products include:

Atarax Tablets & Syrup	2185
Marax Tablets & DF Syrup	2200
Vistaril Intramuscular Solution	2216

Isocarboxazid (Concurrent and/or sequential use is not recommended).

No products indexed under this heading.

Lorazepam (May increase drowsiness effect). Products include:

Ativan Injection	2698
Ativan Tablets	2700

Loxapine Hydrochloride (May increase drowsiness effect). Products include:

Loxitane 1378

Loxapine Succinate (May increase drowsiness effect). Products include:

Loxitane Capsules 1378

Meprobamate (May increase drowsiness effect). Products include:

Miltown Tablets	2672
PMB 200 and PMB 400	2783

Mesoridazine Besylate (May increase drowsiness effect). Products include:

Serentil 684

Midazolam Hydrochloride (May increase drowsiness effect). Products include:

Versed Injection 2170

Molindone Hydrochloride (May increase drowsiness effect). Products include:

Moban Tablets and Concentrate 1048

Oxazepam (May increase drowsiness effect). Products include:

Serax Capsules	2810
Serax Tablets	2810

Perphenazine (May increase drowsiness effect). Products include:

Etrafon	2355
Triavil Tablets	1757
Trilafon	2389

Phenelzine Sulfate (Concurrent and/or sequential use is not recommended). Products include:

Nardil 1920

Prazepam (May increase drowsiness effect).

No products indexed under this heading.

Prochlorperazine (May increase drowsiness effect). Products include:

Compazine 2470

Promethazine Hydrochloride (May increase drowsiness effect). Products include:

Mepergan Injection	2753
Phenergan with Codeine	2777
Phenergan with Dextromethorphan	2778
Phenergan Injection	2773
Phenergan Suppositories	2775
Phenergan Syrup	2774
Phenergan Tablets	2775
Phenergan VC	2779
Phenergan VC with Codeine	2781

Propofol (May increase drowsiness effect). Products include:

Diprivan Injection 2833

Quazepam (May increase drowsiness effect). Products include:

Doral Tablets 2664

(▣ Described in PDR For Nonprescription Drugs) (◉ Described in PDR For Ophthalmology)

Secobarbital Sodium (May increase drowsiness effect). Products include:
- Seconal Sodium Pulvules 1474

Selegiline Hydrochloride (Concurrent and/or sequential use is not recommended). Products include:
- Eldepryl Tablets 2550

Temazepam (May increase drowsiness effect). Products include:
- Restoril Capsules 2284

Thioridazine Hydrochloride (May increase drowsiness effect). Products include:
- Mellaril 2269

Thiothixene (May increase drowsiness effect). Products include:
- Navane Capsules and Concentrate 2201
- Navane Intramuscular 2202

Tranylcypromine Sulfate (Concurrent and/or sequential use is not recommended). Products include:
- Parnate Tablets 2503

Triazolam (May increase drowsiness effect). Products include:
- Halcion Tablets 2611

Trifluoperazine Hydrochloride (May increase drowsiness effect). Products include:
- Stelazine 2514

Zolpidem Tartrate (May increase drowsiness effect). Products include:
- Ambien Tablets 2416

Food Interactions

Alcohol (May increase drowsiness effect).

CHLORESIUM OINTMENT
(Chlorophyllin Copper Complex) 2246
None cited in PDR database.

CHLORESIUM SOLUTION
(Chlorophyllin Copper Complex) 2246
None cited in PDR database.

CHLOROMYCETIN OPHTHALMIC OINTMENT, 1%
(Chloramphenicol) .... ◉ 310
None cited in PDR database.

CHLOROMYCETIN OPHTHALMIC SOLUTION
(Chloramphenicol) .... ◉ 310
None cited in PDR database.

CHLOROMYCETIN SODIUM SUCCINATE
(Chloramphenicol Sodium Succinate) 1900
May interact with:

Bone Marrow Depressants, unspecified (Concurrent therapy should be avoided).

CHLOROPTIC S.O.P.
(Chloramphenicol) .... ◉ 239
None cited in PDR database.

CHLOROPTIC STERILE OPHTHALMIC SOLUTION
(Chloramphenicol) .... ◉ 239
None cited in PDR database.

CHLOR-TRIMETON ALLERGY DECONGESTANT TABLETS
(Chlorpheniramine Maleate, Pseudoephedrine Sulfate) .... ▣ 799
May interact with monoamine oxidase inhibitors, hypnotics and sedatives, tranquilizers, and certain other agents. Compounds in these categories include:

Alprazolam (Increases the drowsiness effect). Products include:
- Xanax Tablets 2649

Buspirone Hydrochloride (Increases the drowsiness effect). Products include:
- BuSpar 737

Chlordiazepoxide (Increases the drowsiness effect). Products include:
- Libritabs Tablets 2177
- Limbitrol 2180

Chlordiazepoxide Hydrochloride (Increases the drowsiness effect). Products include:
- Librax Capsules 2176
- Librium Capsules 2178
- Librium Injectable 2179

Chlorpromazine (Increases the drowsiness effect). Products include:
- Thorazine Suppositories 2523

Chlorpromazine Hydrochloride (Increases the drowsiness effect). Products include:
- Thorazine 2523

Chlorprothixene (Increases the drowsiness effect).
- No products indexed under this heading.

Chlorprothixene Hydrochloride (Increases the drowsiness effect).
- No products indexed under this heading.

Clorazepate Dipotassium (Increases the drowsiness effect). Products include:
- Tranxene 451

Diazepam (Increases the drowsiness effect). Products include:
- Dizac 1809
- Valium Injectable 2182
- Valium Tablets 2183
- Valrelease Capsules 2169

Droperidol (Increases the drowsiness effect). Products include:
- Inapsine Injection 1296

Estazolam (Increases the drowsiness effect). Products include:
- ProSom Tablets 449

Ethchlorvynol (Increases the drowsiness effect). Products include:
- Placidyl Capsules 448

Ethinamate (Increases the drowsiness effect).
- No products indexed under this heading.

Fluphenazine Decanoate (Increases the drowsiness effect). Products include:
- Prolixin Decanoate 509

Fluphenazine Enanthate (Increases the drowsiness effect). Products include:
- Prolixin Enanthate 509

Fluphenazine Hydrochloride (Increases the drowsiness effect). Products include:
- Prolixin 509

Flurazepam Hydrochloride (Increases the drowsiness effect). Products include:
- Dalmane Capsules 2173

Furazolidone (Concurrent use is not recommended). Products include:
- Furoxone 2046

Glutethimide (Increases the drowsiness effect).
- No products indexed under this heading.

Haloperidol (Increases the drowsiness effect). Products include:
- Haldol Injection, Tablets and Concentrate 1575

Haloperidol Decanoate (Increases the drowsiness effect). Products include:
- Haldol Decanoate 1577

Hydroxyzine Hydrochloride (Increases the drowsiness effect). Products include:
- Atarax Tablets & Syrup 2185
- Marax Tablets & DF Syrup 2200
- Vistaril Intramuscular Solution 2216

Isocarboxazid (Concurrent use is not recommended).
- No products indexed under this heading.

Lorazepam (Increases the drowsiness effect). Products include:
- Ativan Injection 2698
- Ativan Tablets 2700

Loxapine Hydrochloride (Increases the drowsiness effect). Products include:
- Loxitane 1378

Loxapine Succinate (Increases the drowsiness effect). Products include:
- Loxitane Capsules 1378

Meprobamate (Increases the drowsiness effect). Products include:
- Miltown Tablets 2672
- PMB 200 and PMB 400 2783

Mesoridazine Besylate (Increases the drowsiness effect). Products include:
- Serentil 684

Midazolam Hydrochloride (Increases the drowsiness effect). Products include:
- Versed Injection 2170

Molindone Hydrochloride (Increases the drowsiness effect). Products include:
- Moban Tablets and Concentrate 1048

Oxazepam (Increases the drowsiness effect). Products include:
- Serax Capsules 2810
- Serax Tablets 2810

Perphenazine (Increases the drowsiness effect). Products include:
- Etrafon 2355
- Triavil Tablets 1757
- Trilafon 2389

Phenelzine Sulfate (Concurrent use is not recommended). Products include:
- Nardil 1920

Prazepam (Increases the drowsiness effect).
- No products indexed under this heading.

Prochlorperazine (Increases the drowsiness effect). Products include:
- Compazine 2470

Promethazine Hydrochloride (Increases the drowsiness effect). Products include:
- Mepergan Injection 2753
- Phenergan with Codeine 2777
- Phenergan with Dextromethorphan 2778
- Phenergan Injection 2773
- Phenergan Suppositories 2775
- Phenergan Syrup 2774
- Phenergan Tablets 2775
- Phenergan VC 2779
- Phenergan VC with Codeine 2781

Propofol (Increases the drowsiness effeet). Products include:
- Diprivan Injection 2833

Quazepam (Increases the drowsiness effect). Products include:
- Doral Tablets 2664

Secobarbital Sodium (Increases the drowsiness effect). Products include:
- Seconal Sodium Pulvules 1474

Selegiline Hydrochloride (Concurrent use is not recommended). Products include:
- Eldepryl Tablets 2550

Temazepam (Increases the drowsiness effect). Products include:
- Restoril Capsules 2284

Thioridazine Hydrochloride (Increases the drowsiness effect). Products include:
- Mellaril 2269

Thiothixene (Increases the drowsiness effect). Products include:
- Navane Capsules and Concentrate 2201
- Navane Intramuscular 2202

Tranylcypromine Sulfate (Concurrent use is not recommended). Products include:
- Parnate Tablets 2503

Triazolam (Increases the drowsiness effect). Products include:
- Halcion Tablets 2611

Trifluoperazine Hydrochloride (Increases the drowsiness effect). Products include:
- Stelazine 2514

Zolpidem Tartrate (Increases the drowsiness effect). Products include:
- Ambien Tablets 2416

Food Interactions

Alcohol (Increases the drowsiness effect).

CHLOR-TRIMETON ALLERGY TABLETS
(Chlorpheniramine Maleate) .... ▣ 798
May interact with hypnotics and sedatives, tranquilizers, and certain other agents. Compounds in these categories include:

Alprazolam (Do not use comcomitantly). Products include:
- Xanax Tablets 2649

Buspirone Hydrochloride (Do not use comcomitantly). Products include:
- BuSpar 737

Chlordiazepoxide (Do not use comcomitantly). Products include:
- Libritabs Tablets 2177
- Limbitrol 2180

Chlordiazepoxide Hydrochloride (Do not use comcomitantly). Products include:
- Librax Capsules 2176
- Librium Capsules 2178
- Librium Injectable 2179

Chlorpromazine (Do not use comcomitantly). Products include:
- Thorazine Suppositories 2523

Chlorpromazine Hydrochloride (Do not use comcomitantly). Products include:
- Thorazine 2523

Chlorprothixene (Do not use comcomitantly).
- No products indexed under this heading.

Chlorprothixene Hydrochloride (Do not use comcomitantly).
- No products indexed under this heading.

Clorazepate Dipotassium (Do not use comcomitantly). Products include:
- Tranxene 451

Diazepam (Do not use comcomitantly). Products include:
- Dizac 1809
- Valium Injectable 2182
- Valium Tablets 2183
- Valrelease Capsules 2169

Droperidol (Do not use comcomitantly). Products include:
- Inapsine Injection 1296

Estazolam (Do not use comcomitantly). Products include:
- ProSom Tablets 449

Ethchlorvynol (Do not use comcomitantly). Products include:
- Placidyl Capsules 448

IMPORTANT NOTE: Always consult each drug listing in the patient's regimen for possible interactions.

Ethinamate (Do not use comcomitantly).
No products indexed under this heading.

Fluphenazine Decanoate (Do not use comcomitantly). Products include:
Prolixin Decanoate 509

Fluphenazine Enanthate (Do not use comcomitantly). Products include:
Prolixin Enanthate 509

Fluphenazine Hydrochloride (Do not use comcomitantly). Products include:
Prolixin 509

Flurazepam Hydrochloride (Do not use comcomitantly). Products include:
Dalmane Capsules 2173

Glutethimide (Do not use comcomitantly).
No products indexed under this heading.

Haloperidol (Do not use comcomitantly). Products include:
Haldol Injection, Tablets and Concentrate 1575

Haloperidol Decanoate (Do not use comcomitantly). Products include:
Haldol Decanoate 1577

Hydroxyzine Hydrochloride (Do not use comcomitantly). Products include:
Atarax Tablets & Syrup 2185
Marax Tablets & DF Syrup 2200
Vistaril Intramuscular Solution 2216

Lorazepam (Do not use comcomitantly). Products include:
Ativan Injection 2698
Ativan Tablets 2700

Loxapine Hydrochloride (Do not use comcomitantly). Products include:
Loxitane 1378

Loxapine Succinate (Do not use comcomitantly). Products include:
Loxitane Capsules 1378

Meprobamate (Do not use comcomitantly). Products include:
Miltown Tablets 2672
PMB 200 and PMB 400 2783

Mesoridazine Besylate (Do not use comcomitantly). Products include:
Serentil 684

Midazolam Hydrochloride (Do not use comcomitantly). Products include:
Versed Injection 2170

Molindone Hydrochloride (Do not use comcomitantly). Products include:
Moban Tablets and Concentrate 1048

Oxazepam (Do not use comcomitantly). Products include:
Serax Capsules 2810
Serax Tablets 2810

Perphenazine (Do not use comcomitantly). Products include:
Etrafon 2355
Triavil Tablets 1757
Trilafon 2389

Prazepam (Do not use comcomitantly).
No products indexed under this heading.

Prochlorperazine (Do not use comcomitantly). Products include:
Compazine 2470

Promethazine Hydrochloride (Do not use comcomitantly). Products include:
Mepergan Injection 2753
Phenergan with Codeine 2777
Phenergan with Dextromethorphan 2778
Phenergan Injection 2773
Phenergan Suppositories 2775
Phenergan Syrup 2774
Phenergan Tablets 2775
Phenergan VC 2779
Phenergan VC with Codeine 2781

Propofol (Do not use comcomitantly). Products include:
Diprivan Injection 2833

Quazepam (Do not use comcomitantly). Products include:
Doral Tablets 2664

Secobarbital Sodium (Do not use comcomitantly). Products include:
Seconal Sodium Pulvules 1474

Temazepam (Do not use comcomitantly). Products include:
Restoril Capsules 2284

Thioridazine Hydrochloride (Do not use comcomitantly). Products include:
Mellaril 2269

Thiothixene (Do not use comcomitantly). Products include:
Navane Capsules and Concentrate 2201
Navane Intramuscular 2202

Triazolam (Do not use comcomitantly). Products include:
Halcion Tablets 2611

Trifluoperazine Hydrochloride (Do not use comcomitantly). Products include:
Stelazine 2514

Zolpidem Tartrate (Do not use comcomitantly). Products include:
Ambien Tablets 2416

Food Interactions

Alcohol (Do not use concomitantly).

CHOLERA VACCINE
(Cholera Vaccine) 2711
None cited in PDR database.

CHOOZ ANTACID GUM
(Calcium Carbonate) .... ◙ 799
None cited in PDR database.

CHROMAGEN CAPSULES
(Ferrous Fumarate, Vitamin C, Vitamin B_{12}) 2339
None cited in PDR database.

CILOXAN OPHTHALMIC SOLUTION
(Ciprofloxacin Hydrochloride) 472
May interact with xanthine bronchodilators, oral anticoagulants, and certain other agents. Compounds in these categories include:

Aminophylline (Systemic administration of quinolones elevates plasma concentrations of theophylline).
No products indexed under this heading.

Caffeine-containing medications (Interference with caffeine metabolism with systemic quinolones).

Cyclosporine (Concomitant administration with systemic quinolones may result in transient elevations in serum creatinine). Products include:
Neoral 2276
Sandimmune 2286

Dicumarol (Enhanced anticoagulant effect with systemic quinolones).
No products indexed under this heading.

Dyphylline (Systemic administration of quinolones elevates plasma concentrations of theophylline). Products include:
Lufyllin & Lufyllin-400 Tablets 2670
Lufyllin-GG Elixir & Tablets 2671

Theophylline (Systemic administration of quinolones elevates plasma concentrations of theophylline). Products include:
Marax Tablets & DF Syrup 2200
Quibron 2053

Theophylline Anhydrous (Systemic administration of quinolones elevates plasma concentrations of theophylline). Products include:
Aerolate 1004
Primatene Dual Action Formula .... ◙ 872
Primatene Tablets .... ◙ 873
Respbid Tablets 682
Slo-bid Gyrocaps 2033
Theo-24 Extended Release Capsules 2568
Theo-Dur Extended-Release Tablets 1327
Theo-X Extended-Release Tablets .. 788
Uni-Dur Extended-Release Tablets .. 1331
Uniphyl 400 mg Tablets 2001

Theophylline Calcium Salicylate (Systemic administration of quinolones elevates plasma concentrations of theophylline). Products include:
Quadrinal Tablets 1350

Theophylline Sodium Glycinate (Systemic administration of quinolones elevates plasma concentrations of theophylline).
No products indexed under this heading.

Warfarin Sodium (Enhanced anticoagulant effect with systemic quinolones). Products include:
Coumadin 926

CIPRO I.V.
(Ciprofloxacin) 595
May interact with oral anticoagulants and certain other agents. Compounds in these categories include:

Aminophylline (Potential for severe and fatal reactions including cardiac arrest, seizures, respiratory failure and status epilepticus; concurrent use should be avoided or serum levels of theophylline should be monitored carefully).
No products indexed under this heading.

Caffeine (Reduced clearance of caffeine and prolongation of its serum half-life). Products include:
Arthritis Strength BC Powder .... ◙ 609
BC Powder .... ◙ 609
Bayer Select Headache Pain Relief Formula .... ◙ 716
Cafergot 2251
DHCplus Capsules 1993
Darvon Compound-65 Pulvules 1435
Esgic-plus Tablets 1013
Aspirin Free Excedrin Analgesic Caplets and Geltabs 732
Excedrin Extra-Strength Analgesic Tablets & Caplets 732
Fioricet Tablets 2258
Fioricet with Codeine Capsules 2260
Fiorinal Capsules 2261
Fiorinal with Codeine Capsules 2262
Fiorinal Tablets 2261
Maximum Strength Multi-Symptom Formula Midol .... ◙ 722
Migralam Capsules 2038
No Doz Maximum Strength Caplets .... ◙ 622
Norgesic 1496
Vanquish Analgesic Caplets .... ◙ 731
Wigraine Tablets & Suppositories .. 1829

Cyclosporine (Potential for transient elevations in serum creatinine). Products include:
Neoral 2276
Sandimmune 2286

Dicumarol (Enhanced effects of anticoagulant).
No products indexed under this heading.

Dyphylline (Potential for severe and fatal reactions including cardiac arrest, seizures, respiratory failure and status epilepticus; concurrent use should be avoided or serum levels of theophylline should be monitored carefully). Products include:
Lufyllin & Lufyllin-400 Tablets 2670
Lufyllin-GG Elixir & Tablets 2671

Probenecid (Interferes with renal tubular secretion and produces an increase in the level of ciprofloxacin). Products include:
Benemid Tablets 1611
ColBENEMID Tablets 1622

Theophylline (Potential for severe and fatal reactions including cardiac arrest, seizures, respiratory failure and status epilepticus; concurrent use should be avoided or serum levels of theophylline should be monitored carefully). Products include:
Marax Tablets & DF Syrup 2200
Quibron 2053

Theophylline Anhydrous (Potential for severe and fatal reactions including cardiac arrest, seizures, respiratory failure and status epilepticus; concurrent use should be avoided or serum levels of theophylline should be monitored carefully). Products include:
Aerolate 1004
Primatene Dual Action Formula .... ◙ 872
Primatene Tablets .... ◙ 873
Respbid Tablets 682
Slo-bid Gyrocaps 2033
Theo-24 Extended Release Capsules 2568
Theo-Dur Extended-Release Tablets 1327
Theo-X Extended-Release Tablets .. 788
Uni-Dur Extended-Release Tablets .. 1331
Uniphyl 400 mg Tablets 2001

Theophylline Calcium Salicylate (Potential for severe and fatal reactions including cardiac arrest, seizures, respiratory failure and status epilepticus; concurrent use should be avoided or serum levels of theophylline should be monitored carefully). Products include:
Quadrinal Tablets 1350

Theophylline Sodium Glycinate (Potential for severe and fatal reactions including cardiac arrest, seizures, respiratory failure and status epilepticus; concurrent use should be avoided or serum levels of theophylline should be monitored carefully).
No products indexed under this heading.

Warfarin Sodium (Enhanced effects of anticoagulant). Products include:
Coumadin 926

CIPRO I.V. PHARMACY BULK PACKAGE
(Ciprofloxacin) 597
May interact with oral anticoagulants and certain other agents. Compounds in these categories include:

Aminophylline (Potential for severe and fatal reactions including cardiac arrest, seizures, respiratory failure and status epilepticus; concurrent use should be avoided or serum levels of theophylline should be monitored carefully).
No products indexed under this heading.

Caffeine (Reduced clearance of caffeine and a prolongation of serum half-life). Products include:
Arthritis Strength BC Powder .... ◙ 609
BC Powder .... ◙ 609
Bayer Select Headache Pain Relief Formula .... ◙ 716

(◙ Described in PDR For Nonprescription Drugs) (⊚ Described in PDR For Ophthalmology)

Interactions Index — Cipro

Cafergot 2251
DHCplus Capsules 1993
Darvon Compound-65 Pulvules 1435
Esgic-plus Tablets 1013
Aspirin Free Excedrin Analgesic Caplets and Geltabs 732
Excedrin Extra-Strength Analgesic Tablets & Caplets 732
Fioricet Tablets 2258
Fioricet with Codeine Capsules 2260
Fiorinal Capsules 2261
Fiorinal with Codeine Capsules 2262
Fiorinal Tablets 2261
Maximum Strength Multi-Symptom Formula Midol .... ⊞ 722
Migralam Capsules 2038
No Doz Maximum Strength Caplets .... ⊞ 622
Norgesic 1496
Vanquish Analgesic Caplets .... ⊞ 731
Wigraine Tablets & Suppositories .. 1829

Cyclosporine (Concomitant use may produce transient elevations in serum creatinine). Products include:

Neoral 2276
Sandimmune 2286

Dicumarol (Enhanced effects of oral anticoagulant).

No products indexed under this heading.

Dyphylline (Potential for severe and fatal reactions including cardiac arrest, seizures, respiratory failure and status epilepticus; concurrent use should be avoided or serum levels of theophylline should be monitored carefully). Products include:

Lufyllin & Lufyllin-400 Tablets 2670
Lufyllin-GG Elixir & Tablets 2671

Probenecid (Interferes with renal tubular secretion of ciprofloxacin). Products include:

Benemid Tablets 1611
ColBENEMID Tablets 1622

Theophylline (Potential for severe and fatal reactions including cardiac arrest, seizures, respiratory failure and status epilepticus; concurrent use should be avoided or serum levels of theophylline should be monitored carefully). Products include:

Marax Tablets & DF Syrup 2200
Quibron 2053

Theophylline Anhydrous (Potential for severe and fatal reactions including cardiac arrest, seizures, respiratory failure and status epilepticus; concurrent use should be avoided or serum levels of theophylline should be monitored carefully). Products include:

Aerolate 1004
Primatene Dual Action Formula ...... ⊞ 872
Primatene Tablets .... ⊞ 873
Respbid Tablets 682
Slo-bid Gyrocaps 2033
Theo-24 Extended Release Capsules 2568
Theo-Dur Extended-Release Tablets 1327
Theo-X Extended-Release Tablets .. 788
Uni-Dur Extended-Release Tablets .. 1331
Uniphyl 400 mg Tablets 2001

Theophylline Calcium Salicylate (Potential for severe and fatal reactions including cardiac arrest, seizures, respiratory failure and status epilepticus; concurrent use should be avoided or serum levels of theophylline should be monitored carefully). Products include:

Quadrinal Tablets 1350

Theophylline Sodium Glycinate (Potential for severe and fatal reactions including cardiac arrest, seizures, respiratory failure and status epilepticus; concurrent use should be avoided or serum levels of theophylline should be monitored carefully).

No products indexed under this heading.

Warfarin Sodium (Enhanced effects of oral anticoagulant). Products include:

Coumadin 926

CIPRO TABLETS

(Ciprofloxacin Hydrochloride) 592

May interact with xanthine bronchodilators, antacids containing aluminum, calcium and magnesium, oral anticoagulants, iron containing oral preparations, and certain other agents. Compounds in these categories include:

Aluminum Carbonate Gel (Concurrent administration of these antacids may substantially interfere with the oral absorption of ciprofloxacin; antacids may be administered either 2 hours after or 6 hours before ciprofloxacin dosing without a significant decrease in bioavailability). Products include:

Basaljel 2703

Aluminum Hydroxide (Concurrent administration of these antacids may substantially interfere with the oral absorption of ciprofloxacin; antacids may be administered either 2 hours after or 6 hours before ciprofloxacin dosing without a significant decrease in bioavailability). Products include:

ALternaGEL Liquid 1316
Maximum Strength Ascriptin .... ⊞ 630
Cama Arthritis Pain Reliever .... ⊞ 785
Gaviscon Extra Strength Relief Formula Antacid Tablets .... ⊞ 819
Gaviscon Extra Strength Relief Formula Liquid Antacid .... ⊞ 819
Gaviscon Liquid Antacid .... ⊞ 820
Gelusil Liquid & Tablets .... ⊞ 855
Maalox Heartburn Relief Suspension .... ⊞ 642
Maalox Heartburn Relief Tablets .... ⊞ 641
Maalox Magnesia and Alumina Oral Suspension .... ⊞ 642
Maalox Plus Tablets .... ⊞ 643
Extra Strength Maalox Antacid Plus Antigas Liquid and Tablets ⊞ 638
Tempo Soft Antacid .... ⊞ 835

Aluminum Hydroxide Gel (Concurrent administration of these antacids may substantially interfere with the oral absorption of ciprofloxacin; antacids may be administered either 2 hours after or 6 hours before ciprofloxacin dosing without a significant decrease in bioavailability). Products include:

ALternaGEL Liquid .... ⊞ 659
Aludrox Oral Suspension 2695
Amphojel Suspension 2695
Amphojel Suspension without Flavor 2695
Amphojel Tablets 2695
Arthritis Pain Ascriptin .... ⊞ 631
Regular Strength Ascriptin Tablets .... ⊞ 629
Gaviscon Antacid Tablets .... ⊞ 819
Gaviscon-2 Antacid Tablets .... ⊞ 820
Mylanta Liquid 1317
Mylanta Tablets .... ⊞ 660
Mylanta Double Strength Liquid 1317
Mylanta Double Strength Tablets .. ⊞ 660
Nephrox Suspension .... ⊞ 655

Aminophylline (Potential for severe and fatal reactions including cardiac arrest, seizures, respiratory failure and status epilepticus; concurrent use should be avoided or serum levels of theophylline should be monitored carefully).

No products indexed under this heading.

Caffeine (Reduced clearance of caffeine and a prolongation of its serum half-life). Products include:

Arthritis Strength BC Powder .... ⊞ 609
BC Powder .... ⊞ 609
Bayer Select Headache Pain Relief Formula .... ⊞ 716

Cafergot 2251
DHCplus Capsules 1993
Darvon Compound-65 Pulvules 1435
Esgic-plus Tablets 1013
Aspirin Free Excedrin Analgesic Caplets and Geltabs 732
Excedrin Extra-Strength Analgesic Tablets & Caplets 732
Fioricet Tablets 2258
Fioricet with Codeine Capsules 2260
Fiorinal Capsules 2261
Fiorinal with Codeine Capsules 2262
Fiorinal Tablets 2261
Maximum Strength Multi-Symptom Formula Midol .... ⊞ 722
Migralam Capsules 2038
No Doz Maximum Strength Caplets .... ⊞ 622
Norgesic 1496
Vanquish Analgesic Caplets .... ⊞ 731
Wigraine Tablets & Suppositories .. 1829

Cyclosporine (Transient elevations in serum creatinine). Products include:

Neoral 2276
Sandimmune 2286

Dicumarol (Enhanced effects of anticoagulant).

No products indexed under this heading.

Dihydroxyaluminum Sodium Carbonate (Concurrent administration of these antacids may substantially interfere with the oral absorption of ciprofloxacin; antacids may be administered either 2 hours after or 6 hours before ciprofloxacin dosing without a significant decrease in bioavailability).

No products indexed under this heading.

Dyphylline (Potential for severe and fatal reactions including cardiac arrest, seizures, respiratory failure and status epilepticus; concurrent use should be avoided or serum levels of theophylline should be monitored carefully). Products include:

Lufyllin & Lufyllin-400 Tablets 2670
Lufyllin-GG Elixir & Tablets 2671

Ferrous Fumarate (Concurrent administration of iron-containing products may substantially interfere with the oral absorption of ciprofloxacin). Products include:

Chromagen Capsules 2339
Ferro-Sequels .... ⊞ 669
Nephro-Fer Tablets 2004
Nephro-Fer Rx Tablets 2005
Nephro-Vite + Fe Tablets 2006
Sigtab-M Tablets .... ⊞ 772
Stresstabs + Iron .... ⊞ 671
The Stuart Formula Tablets .... ⊞ 663
Theragran-M Tablets with Beta Carotene .... ⊞ 623
Trinsicon Capsules 2570
Vitron-C Tablets .... ⊞ 650

Ferrous Gluconate (Concurrent administration of iron-containing products may substantially interfere with the oral absorption of ciprofloxacin). Products include:

Fergon Iron Supplement Tablets .... ⊞ 721
Megadose 512

Ferrous Sulfate (Concurrent administration of iron-containing products may substantially interfere with the oral absorption of ciprofloxacin). Products include:

Feosol Capsules 2456
Feosol Elixir 2456
Feosol Tablets 2457
Fero-Folic-500 Filmtab 429
Fero-Grad-500 Filmtab 429
Fero-Gradumet Filmtab 429
Iberet Tablets 433
Iberet-500 Liquid 433
Iberet-Folic-500 Filmtab 429
Iberet-Liquid 433
Irospan 982
Slow Fe Tablets 869
Slow Fe with Folic Acid 869

Glyburide (Co-administration, on rare occasions, has resulted in severe hypoglycemia). Products include:

DiaBeta Tablets 1239
Glynase PresTab Tablets 2609
Micronase Tablets 2623

Magaldrate (Concurrent administration of these antacids may substantially interfere with the oral absorption of ciprofloxacin; antacids may be administered either 2 hours after or 6 hours before ciprofloxacin dosing without a significant decrease in bioavailability).

No products indexed under this heading.

Magnesium Hydroxide (Concurrent administration of these antacids may substantially interfere with the oral absorption of ciprofloxacin; antacids may be administered either 2 hours after or 6 hours before ciprofloxacin dosing without a significant decrease in bioavailability). Products include:

Aludrox Oral Suspension 2695
Arthritis Pain Ascriptin .... ⊞ 631
Maximum Strength Ascriptin .... ⊞ 630
Regular Strength Ascriptin Tablets .... ⊞ 629
Di-Gel Antacid/Anti-Gas .... ⊞ 801
Gelusil Liquid & Tablets .... ⊞ 855
Maalox Magnesia and Alumina Oral Suspension .... ⊞ 642
Maalox Plus Tablets .... ⊞ 643
Extra Strength Maalox Antacid Plus Antigas Liquid and Tablets ⊞ 638
Mylanta Calcium Carbonate and Magnesium Hydroxide Tablets 1318
Mylanta Liquid 1317
Mylanta Tablets .... ⊞ 660
Mylanta Double Strength Liquid 1317
Mylanta Double Strength Tablets .. ⊞ 660
Phillips' Milk of Magnesia Liquid .... ⊞ 729
Rolaids Tablets .... ⊞ 843
Tempo Soft Antacid .... ⊞ 835

Magnesium Oxide (Concurrent administration of these antacids may substantially interfere with the oral absorption of ciprofloxacin; antacids may be administered either 2 hours after or 6 hours before ciprofloxacin dosing without a significant decrease in bioavailability). Products include:

Beelith Tablets 639
Bufferin Analgesic Tablets and Caplets .... ⊞ 613
Caltrate PLUS .... ⊞ 665
Cama Arthritis Pain Reliever .... ⊞ 785
Mag-Ox 400 668
Uro-Mag 668

Phenytoin (Potential for change in serum phenytoin levels). Products include:

Dilantin Infatabs 1908
Dilantin-125 Suspension 1911

Phenytoin Sodium (Potential for change in serum phenytoin levels). Products include:

Dilantin Kapseals 1906
Dilantin Parenteral 1910

Polysaccharide-Iron Complex (Concurrent administration of iron-containing products may substantially interfere with the oral absorption of ciprofloxacin). Products include:

Niferex-150 Capsules 793
Niferex Elixir 793
Niferex-150 Forte Capsules 794
Niferex Forte Elixir 794
Niferex 793
Niferex-PN Tablets 794
Nu-Iron 150 Capsules 1543
Nu-Iron Elixir 1543
Sunkist Children's Chewable Multivitamins - Plus Iron .... ⊞ 649

Probenecid (Interferes with renal tubular secretion of ciprofloxacin). Products include:

Benemid Tablets 1611
ColBENEMID Tablets 1622

IMPORTANT NOTE: Always consult each drug listing in the patient's regimen for possible interactions.

Cipro **Interactions Index** 180

Sucralfate (Substantially interferes with absorption of ciprofloxacin). Products include:
- Carafate Suspension 1505
- Carafate Tablets 1504

Theophylline (Potential for severe and fatal reactions including cardiac arrest, seizures, respiratory failure and status epilepticus; concurrent use should be avoided or serum levels of theophylline should be monitored carefully). Products include:
- Marax Tablets & DF Syrup 2200
- Quibron 2053

Theophylline Anhydrous (Potential for severe and fatal reactions including cardiac arrest, seizures, respiratory failure and status epilepticus; concurrent use should be avoided or serum levels of theophylline should be monitored carefully). Products include:
- Aerolate 1004
- Primatene Dual Action Formula .... ▣ 872
- Primatene Tablets .... ▣ 873
- Respbid Tablets 682
- Slo-bid Gyrocaps 2033
- Theo-24 Extended Release Capsules 2568
- Theo-Dur Extended-Release Tablets 1327
- Theo-X Extended-Release Tablets .. 788
- Uni-Dur Extended-Release Tablets .. 1331
- Uniphyl 400 mg Tablets 2001

Theophylline Calcium Salicylate (Potential for severe and fatal reactions including cardiac arrest, seizures, respiratory failure and status epilepticus; concurrent use should be avoided or serum levels of theophylline should be monitored carefully). Products include:
- Quadrinal Tablets 1350

Theophylline Sodium Glycinate (Potential for severe and fatal reactions including cardiac arrest, seizures, respiratory failure and status epilepticus; concurrent use should be avoided or serum levels of theophylline should be monitored carefully).
- No products indexed under this heading.

Warfarin Sodium (Enhanced effects of anticoagulant). Products include:
- Coumadin 926

Zinc Sulfate (Zinc-containing multivitamin preparations interfere with absorption of ciprofloxacin). Products include:
- Clear Eyes ACR Astringent/Lubricant Eye Redness Reliever Eye Drops .... ⊙ 316
- Visine Maximum Strength Allergy Relief .... ⊙ 313

Food Interactions

Food, unspecified (Delays the absorption of the drug resulting in peak concentrations that are closer to 2 hours after dosing).

CITRACAL
(Calcium Citrate) 1779
None cited in PDR database.

CITRACAL CAPLETS+ D
(Calcium Citrate, Vitamin D_3) 1780
None cited in PDR database.

CITRACAL LIQUITAB
(Calcium Citrate) 1780
None cited in PDR database.

CITROCARBONATE ANTACID
(Sodium Bicarbonate, Sodium Citrate) .... ▣ 770
None cited in PDR database.

CITRUCEL ORANGE FLAVOR
(Methylcellulose) .... ▣ 811
None cited in PDR database.

CITRUCEL SUGAR FREE ORANGE FLAVOR
(Methylcellulose) .... ▣ 811
None cited in PDR database.

CLAFORAN STERILE AND INJECTION
(Cefotaxime Sodium) 1235
May interact with aminoglycosides. Compounds in this category include:

Amikacin Sulfate (Increased nephrotoxicity). Products include:
- Amikacin Sulfate Injection, USP 960
- Amikin Injectable 501

Gentamicin Sulfate (Increased nephrotoxicity). Products include:
- Garamycin Injectable 2360
- Genoptic Sterile Ophthalmic Solution .... ⊙ 243
- Genoptic Sterile Ophthalmic Ointment .... ⊙ 243
- Gentacidin Ointment .... ⊙ 264
- Gentacidin Solution .... ⊙ 264
- Gentak .... ⊙ 208
- Pred-G Liquifilm Sterile Ophthalmic Suspension .... ⊙ 251
- Pred-G S.O.P. Sterile Ophthalmic Ointment .... ⊙ 252

Kanamycin Sulfate (Increased nephrotoxicity).
- No products indexed under this heading.

Streptomycin Sulfate (Increased nephrotoxicity). Products include:
- Streptomycin Sulfate Injection 2208

Tobramycin (Increased nephrotoxicity). Products include:
- AKTOB .... ⊙ 206
- TobraDex Ophthalmic Suspension and Ointment 473
- Tobrex Ophthalmic Ointment and Solution .... ⊙ 229

Tobramycin Sulfate (Increased nephrotoxicity). Products include:
- Nebcin Vials, Hyporets & ADD-Vantage 1464
- Tobramycin Sulfate Injection 968

CLARITIN
(Loratadine) 2349
May interact with drugs affecting hepatic drug metabolizing enzyme systems, xanthine bronchodilators, and certain other agents. Compounds in these categories include:

Aminophylline (The number of subjects who concomitantly received these drugs in the clinical trials is too small to rule out possible drug-drug interactions).
- No products indexed under this heading.

Carbamazepine (Coadministration should be undertaken with caution until definitive interaction studies are completed). Products include:
- Atretol Tablets 573
- Tegretol Chewable Tablets 852
- Tegretol Suspension 852
- Tegretol Tablets 852

Cimetidine (Increased plasma concentrations (AUC_{0-24} hours) of loratadine and/or decarboethoxyloratadine have been reported following co-administration; no clinically relevant changes in the safety profile of loratadine have been observed). Products include:
- Tagamet Tablets 2516

Cimetidine Hydrochloride (Increased plasma concentrations (AUC_{0-24} hours) of loratadine and/or decarboethoxyloratadine have been reported following co-administration; no clinically relevant changes in the safety profile of loratadine have been observed). Products include:
- Tagamet 2516

Dyphylline (The number of subjects who concomitantly received these drugs in the clinical trials is too small to rule out possible drug-drug interactions). Products include:
- Lufyllin & Lufyllin-400 Tablets 2670
- Lufyllin-GG Elixir & Tablets 2671

Erythromycin (Increased plasma concentrations (AUC_{0-24} hours) of loratadine and/or decarboethoxyloratadine have been reported following co-administration; no clinically relevant changes in the safety profile of loratadine have been observed). Products include:
- A/T/S 2% Acne Topical Gel and Solution 1234
- Benzamycin Topical Gel 905
- E-Mycin Tablets 1341
- Emgel 2% Topical Gel 1093
- ERYC 1915
- Erycette (erythromycin 2%) Topical Solution 1888
- Ery-Tab Tablets 422
- Erythromycin Base Filmtab 426
- Erythromycin Delayed-Release Capsules, USP 427
- Ilotycin Ophthalmic Ointment 912
- PCE Dispertab Tablets 444
- T-Stat 2.0% Topical Solution and Pads 2688
- Theramycin Z Topical Solution 2% 1592

Erythromycin Estolate (Increased plasma concentrations (AUC_{0-24} hours) of loratadine and/or decarboethoxyloratadine have been reported following co-administration; no clinically relevant changes in the safety profile of loratadine have been observed). Products include:
- Ilosone 911

Erythromycin Ethylsuccinate (Increased plasma concentrations (AUC_{0-24} hours) of loratadine and/or decarboethoxyloratadine have been reported following co-administration; no clinically relevant changes in the safety profile of loratadine have been observed). Products include:
- E.E.S. 424
- EryPed 421

Erythromycin Gluceptate (Increased plasma concentrations (AUC_{0-24} hours) of loratadine and/or decarboethoxyloratadine have been reported following co-administration; no clinically relevant changes in the safety profile of loratadine have been observed). Products include:
- Ilotycin Gluceptate, IV, Vials 913

Erythromycin Stearate (Increased plasma concentrations (AUC_{0-24} hours) of loratadine and/or decarboethoxyloratadine have been reported following co-administration; no clinically relevant changes in the safety profile of loratadine have been observed). Products include:
- Erythrocin Stearate Filmtab 425

Ketoconazole (Increased plasma concentrations (AUC_{0-24} hours) of loratadine and/or decarboethoxyloratadine have been reported following co-administration; no clinically relevant changes in the safety profile of loratadine have been observed). Products include:
- Nizoral 2% Cream 1297
- Nizoral 2% Shampoo 1298
- Nizoral Tablets 1298

Phenobarbital (Coadministration should be undertaken with caution until definitive interaction studies are completed). Products include:
- Arco-Lase Plus Tablets 512
- Bellergal-S Tablets 2250
- Donnatal 2060
- Donnatal Extentabs 2061
- Donnatal Tablets 2060
- Phenobarbital Elixir and Tablets 1469
- Quadrinal Tablets 1350

Phenytoin (Coadministration should be undertaken with caution until definitive interaction studies are completed). Products include:
- Dilantin Infatabs 1908
- Dilantin-125 Suspension 1911

Phenytoin Sodium (Coadministration should be undertaken with caution until definitive interaction studies are completed). Products include:
- Dilantin Kapseals 1906
- Dilantin Parenteral 1910

Ranitidine Hydrochloride (The number of subjects who concomitantly received these drugs in the clinical trials is too small to rule out possible drug-drug interactions). Products include:
- Zantac 1209
- Zantac Injection 1207
- Zantac Syrup 1209

Theophylline (The number of subjects who concomitantly received these drugs in the clinical trials is too small to rule out possible drug-drug interactions). Products include:
- Marax Tablets & DF Syrup 2200
- Quibron 2053

Theophylline Anhydrous (The number of subjects who concomitantly received these drugs in the clinical trials is too small to rule out possible drug-drug interactions). Products include:
- Aerolate 1004
- Primatene Dual Action Formula ...... ▣ 872
- Primatene Tablets .... ▣ 873
- Respbid Tablets 682
- Slo-bid Gyrocaps 2033
- Theo-24 Extended Release Capsules 2568
- Theo-Dur Extended-Release Tablets 1327
- Theo-X Extended-Release Tablets .. 788
- Uni-Dur Extended-Release Tablets .. 1331
- Uniphyl 400 mg Tablets 2001

Theophylline Calcium Salicylate (The number of subjects who concomitantly received these drugs in the clinical trials is too small to rule out possible drug-drug interactions). Products include:
- Quadrinal Tablets 1350

Theophylline Sodium Glycinate (The number of subjects who concomitantly received these drugs in the clinical trials is too small to rule out possible drug-drug interactions).
- No products indexed under this heading.

Food Interactions

Meal, unspecified (Food increases the AUC by approximately 73%, the time to peak plasma concentration is delayed by one-hour; Claritin should be administered on an empty stomach).

CLARITIN-D
(Loratadine, Pseudoephedrine Sulfate) 2350
May interact with monoamine oxidase inhibitors, beta blockers, veratrum alkaloids, and cardiac glyco-

(▣ Described in PDR For Nonprescription Drugs) (⊙ Described in PDR For Ophthalmology)

sides. Compounds in these categories include:

Acebutolol Hydrochloride (Antihypertensive effects may be reduced by sympathomimetics). Products include:

Sectral Capsules ... 2807

Atenolol (Antihypertensive effects may be reduced by sympathomimetics). Products include:

Tenoretic Tablets ... 2845
Tenormin Tablets and I.V. Injection 2847

Betaxolol Hydrochloride (Antihypertensive effects may be reduced by sympathomimetics). Products include:

Betoptic Ophthalmic Solution ... 469
Betoptic S Ophthalmic Suspension 471
Kerlone Tablets ... 2436

Bisoprolol Fumarate (Antihypertensive effects may be reduced by sympathomimetics). Products include:

Zebeta Tablets ... 1413
Ziac ... 1415

Carteolol Hydrochloride (Antihypertensive effects may be reduced by sympathomimetics). Products include:

Cartrol Tablets ... 410
Ocupress Ophthalmic Solution, 1% Sterile ... ⊙ 309

Cimetidine (Increased plasma concentrations (AUC_{0-24} hours) of loratadine and/or decarboethoxyloratadine have been reported following co-administration; no clinically relevant changes in the safety profile of loratadine have been observed). Products include:

Tagamet Tablets ... 2516

Cimetidine Hydrochloride (Increased plasma concentrations (AUC_{0-24} hours) of loratadine and/or decarboethoxyloratadine have been reported following co-administration; no clinically relevant changes in the safety profile of loratadine have been observed). Products include:

Tagamet ... 2516

Cryptenamine Preparations (Antihypertensive effects may be reduced by sympathomimetics).

Deslanoside (Increased ectopic pacemaker activity can occur when pseudoephedrine is used concomitantly with digitalis).

No products indexed under this heading.

Digitoxin (Increased ectopic pacemaker activity can occur when pseudoephedrine is used concomitantly with digitalis). Products include:

Crystodigin Tablets ... 1433

Digoxin (Increased ectopic pacemaker activity can occur when pseudoephedrine is used concomitantly with digitalis). Products include:

Lanoxicaps ... 1117
Lanoxin Elixir Pediatric ... 1120
Lanoxin Injection ... 1123
Lanoxin Injection Pediatric ... 1126
Lanoxin Tablets ... 1128

Erythromycin (Increased plasma concentrations (AUC_{0-24} hours) of loratadine and/or decarboethoxyloratadine have been reported following co-administration; plasma concentrations (AUC_{0-24} hours) of eryhromycin decreased 15% with co-administration; no clinically relevant changes in the safety profile of loratadine have been observed). Products include:

A/T/S 2% Acne Topical Gel and Solution ... 1234
Benzamycin Topical Gel ... 905
E-Mycin Tablets ... 1341
Emgel 2% Topical Gel ... 1093
ERYC ... 1915
Erycette (erythromycin 2%) Topical Solution ... 1888
Ery-Tab Tablets ... 422
Erythromycin Base Filmtab ... 426
Erythromycin Delayed-Release Capsules, USP ... 427
Ilotycin Ophthalmic Ointment ... 912
PCE Dispertab Tablets ... 444
T-Stat 2.0% Topical Solution and Pads ... 2688
Theramycin Z Topical Solution 2% 1592

Erythromycin Estolate (Increased plasma concentrations (AUC_{0-24} hours) of loratadine and/or decarboethoxyloratadine have been reported following co-administration; plasma concentrations (AUC_{0-24} hours) of eryhromycin decreased 15% with co-administration; no clinically relevant changes in the safety profile of loratadine have been observed). Products include:

Ilosone ... 911

Erythromycin Ethylsuccinate (Increased plasma concentrations (AUC_{0-24} hours) of loratadine and/or decarboethoxyloratadine have been reported following co-administration; plasma concentrations (AUC_{0-24} hours) of eryhromycin decreased 15% with co-administration; no clinically relevant changes in the safety profile of loratadine have been observed). Products include:

E.E.S. ... 424
EryPed ... 421

Erythromycin Gluceptate (Increased plasma concentrations (AUC_{0-24} hours) of loratadine and/or decarboethoxyloratadine have been reported following co-administration; plasma concentrations (AUC_{0-24} hours) of eryhromycin decreased 15% with co-administration; no clinically relevant changes in the safety profile of loratadine have been observed). Products include:

Ilotycin Gluceptate, IV, Vials ... 913

Erythromycin Stearate (Increased plasma concentrations (AUC_{0-24} hours) of loratadine and/or decarboethoxyloratadine have been reported following co-administration; plasma concentrations (AUC_{0-24} hours) of eryhromycin decreased 15% with co-administration; no clinically relevant changes in the safety profile of loratadine have been observed). Products include:

Erythrocin Stearate Filmtab ... 425

Esmolol Hydrochloride (Antihypertensive effects may be reduced by sympathomimetics). Products include:

Brevibloc Injection ... 1808

Furazolidone (Concurrent and/or sequential use is contraindicated). Products include:

Furoxone ... 2046

Isocarboxazid (Concurrent and/or sequential use is contraindicated).

No products indexed under this heading.

Ketoconazole (Increased plasma concentrations (AUC_{0-24} hours) of loratadine and/or decarboethoxyloratadine have been reported following co-administration; no clinically relevant changes in the safety profile of loratadine have been observed). Products include:

Nizoral 2% Cream ... 1297
Nizoral 2% Shampoo ... 1298
Nizoral Tablets ... 1298

Labetalol Hydrochloride (Antihypertensive effects may be reduced by sympathomimetics). Products include:

Normodyne Injection ... 2377
Normodyne Tablets ... 2379
Trandate ... 1185

Levobunolol Hydrochloride (Antihypertensive effects may be reduced by sympathomimetics). Products include:

Betagan ... ⊙ 233

Mecamylamine Hydrochloride (Antihypertensive effects may be reduced by sympathomimetics). Products include:

Inversine Tablets ... 1686

Methyldopa (Antihypertensive effects may be reduced by sympathomimetics). Products include:

Aldoclor Tablets ... 1598
Aldomet Oral ... 1600
Aldoril Tablets ... 1604

Methyldopate Hydrochloride (Antihypertensive effects may be reduced by sympathomimetics). Products include:

Aldomet Ester HCl Injection ... 1602

Metipranolol Hydrochloride (Antihypertensive effects may be reduced by sympathomimetics). Products include:

OptiPranolol (Metipranolol 0.3%) Sterile Ophthalmic Solution ... ⊙ 258

Metoprolol Succinate (Antihypertensive effects may be reduced by sympathomimetics). Products include:

Toprol-XL Tablets ... 565

Metoprolol Tartrate (Antihypertensive effects may be reduced by sympathomimetics). Products include:

Lopressor Ampuls ... 830
Lopressor HCT Tablets ... 832
Lopressor Tablets ... 830

Nadolol (Antihypertensive effects may be reduced by sympathomimetics).

No products indexed under this heading.

Penbutolol Sulfate (Antihypertensive effects may be reduced by sympathomimetics). Products include:

Levatol ... 2403

Phenelzine Sulfate (Concurrent and/or sequential use is contraindicated). Products include:

Nardil ... 1920

Pindolol (Antihypertensive effects may be reduced by sympathomimetics). Products include:

Visken Tablets ... 2299

Propranolol Hydrochloride (Antihypertensive effects may be reduced by sympathomimetics). Products include:

Inderal ... 2728
Inderal LA Long Acting Capsules ... 2730
Inderide Tablets ... 2732
Inderide LA Long Acting Capsules .. 2734

Selegiline Hydrochloride (Concurrent and/or sequential use is contraindicated). Products include:

Eldepryl Tablets ... 2550

Sotalol Hydrochloride (Antihypertensive effects may be reduced by sympathomimetics). Products include:

Betapace Tablets ... 641

Timolol Hemihydrate (Antihypertensive effects may be reduced by sympathomimetics). Products include:

Betimol 0.25%, 0.5% ... ⊙ 261

Timolol Maleate (Antihypertensive effects may be reduced by sympathomimetics). Products include:

Blocadren Tablets ... 1614
Timolide Tablets ... 1748
Timoptic in Ocudose ... 1753
Timoptic Sterile Ophthalmic Solution ... 1751
Timoptic-XE ... 1755

Tranylcypromine Sulfate (Concurrent and/or sequential use is contraindicated). Products include:

Parnate Tablets ... 2503

Food Interactions

Meal, unspecified (Food increases the AUC of loratadine by approximately 40% and of decarboethoxyloratadine by approximately 15%; the time of peak plasma concentration (T_{max}) of loratadine and decarboethoxyloratadine was delayed by 1 hour with meal).

CLEAR EYES ACR ASTRINGENT/LUBRICANT EYE REDNESS RELIEVER EYE DROPS

(Zinc Sulfate, Naphazoline Hydrochloride) ... ⊙ 316

None cited in PDR database.

CLEAR EYES LUBRICANT EYE REDNESS RELIEVER

(Glycerin, Naphazoline Hydrochloride) ... ⊙ 316

None cited in PDR database.

CLEOCIN PHOSPHATE IV SOLUTION

(Clindamycin Phosphate) ... 2586

See **Cleocin Phosphate Sterile Solution**

CLEOCIN PHOSPHATE STERILE SOLUTION

(Clindamycin Phosphate) ... 2586

May interact with neuromuscular blocking agents and certain other agents. Compounds in these categories include:

Atracurium Besylate (Enhanced action of neuromuscular blocking agents). Products include:

Tracrium Injection ... 1183

Diphenoxylate Hydrochloride (May prolong and/or worsen colitis). Products include:

Lomotil ... 2439

Doxacurium Chloride (Enhanced action of neuromuscular blocking agents). Products include:

Nuromax Injection ... 1149

Erythromycin (Should not be administered concurrently; in vivo antagonism). Products include:

A/T/S 2% Acne Topical Gel and Solution ... 1234
Benzamycin Topical Gel ... 905
E-Mycin Tablets ... 1341
Emgel 2% Topical Gel ... 1093
ERYC ... 1915
Erycette (erythromycin 2%) Topical Solution ... 1888
Ery-Tab Tablets ... 422
Erythromycin Base Filmtab ... 426
Erythromycin Delayed-Release Capsules, USP ... 427
Ilotycin Ophthalmic Ointment ... 912
PCE Dispertab Tablets ... 444
T-Stat 2.0% Topical Solution and Pads ... 2688
Theramycin Z Topical Solution 2% 1592

Erythromycin Estolate (Should not be administered concurrently; in vivo antagonism). Products include:

Ilosone ... 911

Erythromycin Ethylsuccinate (Should not be administered concurrently; in vivo antagonism). Products include:

E.E.S. ... 424
EryPed ... 421

Erythromycin Gluceptate (Should not be administered concurrently; in vivo antagonism). Products include:

Ilotycin Gluceptate, IV, Vials ... 913

IMPORTANT NOTE: Always consult each drug listing in the patient's regimen for possible interactions.

Cleocin Phosphate Injection Interactions Index 182

Erythromycin Stearate (Should not be administered concurrently; in vivo antagonism). Products include:

Erythrocin Stearate Filmtab 425

Metocurine Iodide (Enhanced action of neuromuscular blocking agents). Products include:

Metubine Iodide Vials 916

Mivacurium Chloride (Enhanced action of neuromuscular blocking agents). Products include:

Mivacron 1138

Pancuronium Bromide Injection (Enhanced action of neuromuscular blocking agents).

No products indexed under this heading.

Paregoric (May prolong and/or worsen colitis).

No products indexed under this heading.

Rocuronium Bromide (Enhanced action of neuromuscular blocking agents). Products include:

Zemuron 1830

Succinylcholine Chloride (Enhanced action of neuromuscular blocking agents). Products include:

Anectine 1073

Vecuronium Bromide (Enhanced action of neuromuscular blocking agents). Products include:

Norcuron 1826

CLEOCIN T TOPICAL GEL

(Clindamycin Phosphate) 2590

May interact with neuromuscular blocking agents. Compounds in this category include:

Atracurium Besylate (Clindamycin has neuromuscular blocking properties that may enhance the action of other neuromuscular blocking agents). Products include:

Tracrium Injection 1183

Doxacurium Chloride (Clindamycin has neuromuscular blocking properties that may enhance the action of other neuromuscular blocking agents). Products include:

Nuromax Injection 1149

Metocurine Iodide (Clindamycin has neuromuscular blocking properties that may enhance the action of other neuromuscular blocking agents). Products include:

Metubine Iodide Vials 916

Mivacurium Chloride (Clindamycin has neuromuscular blocking properties that may enhance the action of other neuromuscular blocking agents). Products include:

Mivacron 1138

Pancuronium Bromide Injection (Clindamycin has neuromuscular blocking properties that may enhance the action of other neuromuscular blocking agents).

No products indexed under this heading.

Rocuronium Bromide (Clindamycin has neuromuscular blocking properties that may enhance the action of other neuromuscular blocking agents). Products include:

Zemuron 1830

Succinylcholine Chloride (Clindamycin has neuromuscular blocking properties that may enhance the action of other neuromuscular blocking agents). Products include:

Anectine 1073

Vecuronium Bromide (Clindamycin has neuromuscular blocking properties that may enhance the action of other neuromuscular blocking agents). Products include:

Norcuron 1826

CLEOCIN T TOPICAL LOTION

(Clindamycin Phosphate) 2590

See **Cleocin T Topical Gel**

CLEOCIN T TOPICAL SOLUTION

(Clindamycin Phosphate) 2590

See **Cleocin T Topical Gel**

CLIMARA TRANSDERMAL SYSTEM

(Estradiol) 645

May interact with progestins. Compounds in this category include:

Desogestrel (Potential for adverse effects on carbohydrate and lipid metabolism). Products include:

Desogen Tablets 1817
Ortho-Cept 1851

Medroxyprogesterone Acetate (Potential for adverse effects on carbohydrate and lipid metabolism). Products include:

Amen Tablets 780
Cycrin Tablets 975
Depo-Provera Contraceptive Injection 2602
Depo-Provera Sterile Aqueous Suspension 2606
Premphase 2797
Prempro 2801
Provera Tablets 2636

Megestrol Acetate (Potential for adverse effects on carbohydrate and lipid metabolism). Products include:

Megace Oral Suspension 699
Megace Tablets 701

Norgestimate (Potential for adverse effects on carbohydrate and lipid metabolism). Products include:

Ortho-Cyclen/Ortho-Tri-Cyclen 1858
Ortho-Cyclen/Ortho Tri-Cyclen 1858

CLEOCIN VAGINAL CREAM

(Clindamycin Phosphate) 2589

May interact with neuromuscular blocking agents. Compounds in this category include:

Atracurium Besylate (Enhanced action of neuromuscular blocking agents; caution is advised when co-administered). Products include:

Tracrium Injection 1183

Doxacurium Chloride (Enhanced action of neuromuscular blocking agents; caution is advised when co-administered). Products include:

Nuromax Injection 1149

Metocurine Iodide (Enhanced action of neuromuscular blocking agents; caution is advised when co-administered). Products include:

Metubine Iodide Vials 916

Mivacurium Chloride (Enhanced action of neuromuscular blocking agents; caution is advised when co-administered). Products include:

Mivacron 1138

Pancuronium Bromide Injection (Enhanced action of neuromuscular blocking agents; caution is advised when co-administered).

No products indexed under this heading.

Rocuronium Bromide (Enhanced action of neuromuscular blocking agents; caution is advised when co-administered). Products include:

Zemuron 1830

Rubber or latex products (Use of such products within 72 hours following treatment with Cleocin Vaginal Cream is not recommended).

Succinylcholine Chloride (Enhanced action of neuromuscular blocking agents; caution is advised when co-administered). Products include:

Anectine 1073

Vecuronium Bromide (Enhanced action of neuromuscular blocking agents; caution is advised when co-administered). Products include:

Norcuron 1826

CLINICAL CARE DERMAL WOUND CLEANSER

(Benzethonium Chloride) .... ▣ 625

None cited in PDR database.

CLINORIL TABLETS

(Sulindac) 1618

May interact with oral anticoagulants, oral hypoglycemic agents, and certain other agents. Compounds in these categories include:

Acarbose (Special attention should be paid to patients taking higher doses than those recommended and to patients with renal or metabolic impairment).

No products indexed under this heading.

Aspirin (Increased gastrointestinal reactions). Products include:

Alka-Seltzer Effervescent Antacid and Pain Reliever .... ▣ 701
Alka-Seltzer Extra Strength Effervescent Antacid and Pain Reliever .... ▣ 703
Alka-Seltzer Lemon Lime Effervescent Antacid and Pain Reliever .... ▣ 703
Alka-Seltzer Plus Cold Medicine .... ▣ 705
Alka-Seltzer Plus Cold & Cough Medicine .... ▣ 708
Alka-Seltzer Plus Night-Time Cold Medicine .... ▣ 707
Alka Seltzer Plus Sinus Medicine .... ▣ 707
Arthritis Foundation Safety Coated Aspirin Tablets .... ▣ 675
Arthritis Pain Ascriptin .... ▣ 631
Maximum Strength Ascriptin .... ▣ 630
Regular Strength Ascriptin Tablets .... ▣ 629
Arthritis Strength BC Powder .... ▣ 609
BC Cold Powder Multi-Symptom Formula (Cold-Sinus-Allergy) .... ▣ 609
BC Cold Powder Non-Drowsy Formula (Cold-Sinus) .... ▣ 609
BC Powder .... ▣ 609
Bayer Children's Chewable Aspirin .... ▣ 711
Genuine Bayer Aspirin Tablets & Caplets .... ▣ 713
Extra Strength Bayer Arthritis Pain Regimen Formula .... ▣ 711
Extra Strength Bayer Aspirin Caplets & Tablets .... ▣ 712
Extended-Release Bayer 8-Hour Aspirin .... ▣ 712
Extra Strength Bayer Plus Aspirin Caplets .... ▣ 713
Extra Strength Bayer PM Aspirin .... ▣ 713
Bayer Enteric Aspirin .... ▣ 709
Bufferin Analgesic Tablets and Caplets .... ▣ 613
Arthritis Strength Bufferin Analgesic Caplets .... ▣ 614
Extra Strength Bufferin Analgesic Tablets .... ▣ 615
Cama Arthritis Pain Reliever .... ▣ 785
Darvon Compound-65 Pulvules 1435
Easprin 1914
Ecotrin 2455
Ecotrin Enteric Coated Aspirin Maximum Strength Tablets and Caplets .... ▣ 816
Ecotrin Enteric Coated Aspirin Regular Strength Tablets 2455
Empirin Aspirin Tablets .... ▣ 854
Empirin with Codeine Tablets 1093
Excedrin Extra-Strength Analgesic Tablets & Caplets 732
Fiorinal Capsules 2261
Fiorinal with Codeine Capsules 2262
Fiorinal Tablets 2261
Halfprin 1362
Healthprin Aspirin 2455
Norgesic 1496
Percodan Tablets 939
Percodan-Demi Tablets 940
Robaxisal Tablets 2071
Soma Compound w/Codeine Tablets 2676
Soma Compound Tablets 2675
St. Joseph Adult Chewable Aspirin (81 mg.) .... ▣ 808
Talwin Compound 2335
Ursinus Inlay-Tabs .... ▣ 794
Vanquish Analgesic Caplets .... ▣ 731

Aspirin, Enteric Coated (Increased gastrointestinal reactions). Products include:

Bayer Enteric Aspirin .... ▣ 709
Ecotrin 2455

Chlorpropamide (Special attention should be paid to patients taking higher doses than those recommended and to patients with renal or metabolic impairment). Products include:

Diabinese Tablets 1935

Cyclosporine (Increased cyclosporine-induced toxicity). Products include:

Neoral 2276
Sandimmune 2286

DMSO (Reduced efficacy of sulindac; peripheral neuropathy).

Dicumarol (Special attention should be paid to patients taking higher doses than those recommended and to patients with renal or metabolic impairment).

No products indexed under this heading.

Diflunisal (Decreased plasma levels of sulindac). Products include:

Dolobid Tablets 1654

Furosemide (Clinoril may blunt the renal response to I.V. furosemide). Products include:

Lasix Injection, Oral Solution and Tablets 1240

Glipizide (Special attention should be paid to patients taking higher doses than those recommended and to patients with renal or metabolic impairment). Products include:

Glucotrol Tablets 1967
Glucotrol XL Extended Release Tablets 1968

Glyburide (Special attention should be paid to patients taking higher doses than those recommended and to patients with renal or metabolic impairment). Products include:

DiaBeta Tablets 1239
Glynase PresTab Tablets 2609
Micronase Tablets 2623

Metformin Hydrochloride (Special attention should be paid to patients taking higher doses than those recommended and to patients with renal or metabolic impairment). Products include:

Glucophage 752

Methotrexate Sodium (Decreased tubular secretion of methotrexate and potentiation of its toxicity). Products include:

Methotrexate Sodium Tablets, Injection, for Injection and LPF Injection 1275

Probenecid (Increased plasma levels of sulindac; modest reduction in uricosuric action of probenecid). Products include:

Benemid Tablets 1611
ColBENEMID Tablets 1622

(▣ Described in PDR For Nonprescription Drugs) (◉ Described in PDR For Ophthalmology)

Tolazamide (Special attention should be paid to patients taking higher doses than those recommended and to patients with renal or metabolic impairment).
No products indexed under this heading.

Tolbutamide (Special attention should be paid to patients taking higher doses than those recommended and to patients with renal or metabolic impairment).
No products indexed under this heading.

Warfarin Sodium (Special attention should be paid to patients taking higher doses than those recommended and to patients with renal or metabolic impairment). Products include:
Coumadin 926

Food Interactions

Food, unspecified (The peak plasma concentrations of biologically active sulfide metabolite is delayed slightly in the presence of food).

CLOCREAM SKIN PROTECTANT CREAM

(Vitamin A & Vitamin D) .... ◙ 770
None cited in PDR database.

CLOMID

(Clomiphene Citrate) 1514
None cited in PDR database.

CLORPACTIN WCS-90

(Sodium Oxychlorosene) 1230
None cited in PDR database.

CLOZARIL TABLETS

(Clozapine) 2252
May interact with antihypertensives, belladona products, benzodiazepines, antidepressant drugs, phenothiazines, selective serotonin reuptake inhibitors, and certain other agents. Compounds in these categories include:

Acebutolol Hydrochloride (Hypotensive effects potentiated). Products include:
Sectral Capsules 2807

Alprazolam (Potential for profound collapse and respiratory depression). Products include:
Xanax Tablets 2649

Amitriptyline Hydrochloride (Concomitant use of clozapine with other drugs metabolized by cytochrome $P_{450}IID_6$ may require lower than usual doses prescribed for either drug). Products include:
Elavil 2838
Endep Tablets 2174
Etrafon 2355
Limbitrol 2180
Triavil Tablets 1757

Amlodipine Besylate (Hypotensive effects potentiated). Products include:
Lotrel Capsules 840
Norvasc Tablets 1940

Amoxapine (Concomitant use of clozapine with other drugs metabolized by cytochrome $P_{450}IID_6$ may require lower than usual doses prescribed for either drug). Products include:
Asendin Tablets 1369

Atenolol (Hypotensive effects potentiated). Products include:
Tenoretic Tablets 2845
Tenormin Tablets and I.V. Injection 2847

Atropine Sulfate (Anticholinergic effects potentiated). Products include:
Arco-Lase Plus Tablets 512
Atrohist Plus Tablets 454
Atropine Sulfate Sterile Ophthalmic Solution .... ⊙ 233
Donnatal 2060
Donnatal Extentabs 2061
Donnatal Tablets 2060
Lomotil 2439
Motofen Tablets 784
Urised Tablets 1964

Belladonna Alkaloids (Anticholinergic effects potentiated). Products include:
Bellergal-S Tablets 2250
Hyland's Bed Wetting Tablets .... ◙ 828
Hyland's EnurAid Tablets .... ◙ 829
Hyland's Teething Tablets .... ◙ 830

Benazepril Hydrochloride (Hypotensive effects potentiated). Products include:
Lotensin Tablets 834
Lotensin HCT 837
Lotrel Capsules 840

Bendroflumethiazide (Hypotensive effects potentiated).
No products indexed under this heading.

Betaxolol Hydrochloride (Hypotensive effects potentiated). Products include:
Betoptic Ophthalmic Solution 469
Betoptic S Ophthalmic Suspension 471
Kerlone Tablets 2436

Bisoprolol Fumarate (Hypotensive effects potentiated). Products include:
Zebeta Tablets 1413
Ziac 1415

Bone Marrow Depressants, unspecified (Increases the risk and/or severity of bone marrow suppression).

Bupropion Hydrochloride (Concomitant use of clozapine with other drugs metabolized by cytochrome $P_{450}IID_6$ may require lower than usual doses prescribed for either drug). Products include:
Wellbutrin Tablets 1204

Captopril (Hypotensive effects potentiated). Products include:
Capoten 739
Capozide 742

Carbamazepine (Concomitant use is not recommended; discontinuation of concomitant carbamazepine administration may result in increase in clozapine levels). Products include:
Atretol Tablets 573
Tegretol Chewable Tablets 852
Tegretol Suspension 852
Tegretol Tablets 852

Carteolol Hydrochloride (Hypotensive effects potentiated). Products include:
Cartrol Tablets 410
Ocupress Ophthalmic Solution, 1% Sterile .... ⊙ 309

Chlordiazepoxide (Potential for profound collapse and respiratory depression). Products include:
Libritabs Tablets 2177
Limbitrol 2180

Chlordiazepoxide Hydrochloride (Potential for profound collapse and respiratory depression). Products include:
Librax Capsules 2176
Librium Capsules 2178
Librium Injectable 2179

Chlorothiazide (Hypotensive effects potentiated). Products include:
Aldoclor Tablets 1598
Diupres Tablets 1650
Diuril Oral 1653

Chlorothiazide Sodium (Hypotensive effects potentiated). Products include:
Diuril Sodium Intravenous 1652

Chlorpromazine (Concomitant use of clozapine with other drugs metabolized by cytochrome $P_{450}IID_6$ may require lower than usual doses prescribed for either drug). Products include:
Thorazine Suppositories 2523

Chlorpromazine Hydrochloride (Concomitant use of clozapine with other drugs metabolized by cytochrome $P_{450}IID_6$ may require lower than usual doses prescribed for either drug). Products include:
Thorazine 2523

Chlorthalidone (Hypotensive effects potentiated). Products include:
Combipres Tablets 677
Tenoretic Tablets 2845
Thalitone 1245

Cimetidine (May increase plasma levels of clozapine, potentially resulting in adverse effects). Products include:
Tagamet Tablets 2516

Cimetidine Hydrochloride (May increase levels of clozapine potentially resulting in adverse effects). Products include:
Tagamet 2516

Clonidine (Hypotensive effects potentiated). Products include:
Catapres-TTS 675

Clonidine Hydrochloride (Hypotensive effects potentiated). Products include:
Catapres Tablets 674
Combipres Tablets 677

Clorazepate Dipotassium (Potential for profound collapse and respiratory depression). Products include:
Tranxene 451

CNS-Active Drugs, unspecified (Caution is advised).

Deserpidine (Hypotensive effects potentiated).
No products indexed under this heading.

Desipramine Hydrochloride (Concomitant use of clozapine with other drugs metabolized by cytochrome $P_{450}IID_6$ may require lower than usual doses prescribed for either drug). Products include:
Norpramin Tablets 1526

Diazepam (Potential for profound collapse and respiratory depression). Products include:
Dizac 1809
Valium Injectable 2182
Valium Tablets 2183
Valrelease Capsules 2169

Diazoxide (Hypotensive effects potentiated). Products include:
Hyperstat I.V. Injection 2363
Proglycem 580

Digitoxin (Potential for increased plasma levels and adverse effects). Products include:
Crystodigin Tablets 1433

Digoxin (Increase in plasma concentrations resulting in adverse effects). Products include:
Lanoxicaps 1117
Lanoxin Elixir Pediatric 1120
Lanoxin Injection 1123
Lanoxin Injection Pediatric 1126
Lanoxin Tablets 1128

Diltiazem Hydrochloride (Hypotensive effects potentiated). Products include:
Cardizem CD Capsules 1506
Cardizem SR Capsules 1510
Cardizem Injectable 1508
Cardizem Tablets 1512
Dilacor XR Extended-release Capsules 2018

Doxazosin Mesylate (Hypotensive effects potentiated). Products include:
Cardura Tablets 2186

Doxepin Hydrochloride (Concomitant use of clozapine with other drugs metabolized by cytochrome $P_{450}IID_6$ may require lower than usual doses prescribed for either drug). Products include:
Sinequan 2205
Zonalon Cream 1055

Enalapril Maleate (Hypotensive effects potentiated). Products include:
Vaseretic Tablets 1765
Vasotec Tablets 1771

Enalaprilat (Hypotensive effects potentiated). Products include:
Vasotec I.V. 1768

Encainide Hydrochloride (Concomitant use of clozapine with other drugs metabolized by cytochrome $P_{450}IID_6$ may require lower than usual doses).
No products indexed under this heading.

Epinephrine Hydrochloride (Possible reverse epinephrine effect). Products include:
Ana-Kit Anaphylaxis Emergency Treatment Kit 617

Esmolol Hydrochloride (Hypotensive effects potentiated). Products include:
Brevibloc Injection 1808

Estazolam (Potential for profound collapse and respiratory depression). Products include:
ProSom Tablets 449

Felodipine (Hypotensive effects potentiated). Products include:
Plendil Extended-Release Tablets 527

Flecainide Acetate (Concomitant use of clozapine with other drugs metabolized by cytochrome $P_{450}IID_6$ may require lower than usual doses prescribed for either drug). Products include:
Tambocor Tablets 1497

Fluoxetine Hydrochloride (Concomitant use of clozapine with other drugs metabolized by cytochrome $P_{450}IID_6$ may require lower than usual doses prescribed for either drug). Products include:
Prozac Pulvules & Liquid, Oral Solution 919

Fluphenazine Decanoate (Concomitant use of clozapine with other drugs metabolized by cytochrome $P_{450}IID_6$ may require lower than usual doses prescribed for either drug). Products include:
Prolixin Decanoate 509

Fluphenazine Enanthate (Concomitant use of clozapine with other drugs metabolized by cytochrome $P_{450}IID_6$ may require lower than usual doses prescribed for either drug). Products include:
Prolixin Enanthate 509

Fluphenazine Hydrochloride (Concomitant use of clozapine with other drugs metabolized by cytochrome $P_{450}IID_6$ may require lower than usual doses prescribed for either drug). Products include:
Prolixin 509

Flurazepam Hydrochloride (Potential for profound collapse and respiratory depression). Products include:
Dalmane Capsules 2173

IMPORTANT NOTE: Always consult each drug listing in the patient's regimen for possible interactions.

Fluvoxamine Maleate (Concomitant use of clozapine with other drugs metabolized by cytochrome $P_{450}IID_6$ may require lower than usual doses prescribed for either drug). Products include:
- Luvox Tablets 2544

Fosinopril Sodium (Hypotensive effects potentiated). Products include:
- Monopril Tablets 757

Furosemide (Hypotensive effects potentiated). Products include:
- Lasix Injection, Oral Solution and Tablets 1240

Guanabenz Acetate (Hypotensive effects potentiated).
- No products indexed under this heading.

Guanethidine Monosulfate (Hypotensive effects potentiated). Products include:
- Esimil Tablets 822
- Ismelin Tablets 827

Halazepam (Potential for profound collapse and respiratory depression).
- No products indexed under this heading.

Hydralazine Hydrochloride (Hypotensive effects potentiated). Products include:
- Apresazide Capsules 808
- Apresoline Hydrochloride Tablets .. 809
- Ser-Ap-Es Tablets 849

Hydrochlorothiazide (Hypotensive effects potentiated). Products include:
- Aldactazide 2413
- Aldoril Tablets 1604
- Apresazide Capsules 808
- Capozide 742
- Dyazide 2479
- Esidrix Tablets 821
- Esimil Tablets 822
- HydroDIURIL Tablets 1674
- Hydropres Tablets 1675
- Hyzaar Tablets 1677
- Inderide Tablets 2732
- Inderide LA Long Acting Capsules .. 2734
- Lopressor HCT Tablets 832
- Lotensin HCT 837
- Maxzide 1380
- Moduretic Tablets 1705
- Oretic Tablets 443
- Prinzide Tablets 1737
- Ser-Ap-Es Tablets 849
- Timolide Tablets 1748
- Vaseretic Tablets 1765
- Zestoretic 2850
- Ziac 1415

Hydroflumethiazide (Hypotensive effects potentiated). Products include:
- Diucardin Tablets 2718

Hyoscyamine (Anticholinergic effects potentiated). Products include:
- Cystospaz Tablets 1963
- Urised Tablets 1964

Hyoscyamine Sulfate (Anticholinergic effects potentiated). Products include:
- Arco-Lase Plus Tablets 512
- Atrohist Plus Tablets 454
- Cystospaz-M Capsules 1963
- Donnatal 2060
- Donnatal Extentabs 2061
- Donnatal Tablets 2060
- Kutrase Capsules 2402
- Levsin/Levsinex/Levbid 2405

Imipramine Hydrochloride (Concomitant use of clozapine with other drugs metabolized by cytochrome $P_{450}IID_6$ may require lower than usual doses prescribed for either drug). Products include:
- Tofranil Ampuls 854
- Tofranil Tablets 856

Imipramine Pamoate (Concomitant use of clozapine with other drugs metabolized by cytochrome $P_{450}IID_6$ may require lower than usual doses prescribed for either drug). Products include:
- Tofranil-PM Capsules 857

Indapamide (Hypotensive effects potentiated). Products include:
- Lozol Tablets 2022

Isocarboxazid (Concomitant use of clozapine with other drugs metabolized by cytochrome $P_{450}IID_6$ may require lower than usual doses prescribed for either drug).
- No products indexed under this heading.

Isradipine (Hypotensive effects potentiated). Products include:
- DynaCirc Capsules 2256

Labetalol Hydrochloride (Hypotensive effects potentiated). Products include:
- Normodyne Injection 2377
- Normodyne Tablets 2379
- Trandate 1185

Levobunolol Hydrochloride (Hypotensive effects potentiated). Products include:
- Betagan .... ⊙ 233

Lisinopril (Hypotensive effects potentiated). Products include:
- Prinivil Tablets 1733
- Prinzide Tablets 1737
- Zestoretic 2850
- Zestril Tablets 2854

Lorazepam (Potential for profound collapse and respiratory depression). Products include:
- Ativan Injection 2698
- Ativan Tablets 2700

Losartan Potassium (Hypotensive effects potentiated). Products include:
- Cozaar Tablets 1628
- Hyzaar Tablets 1677

Maprotiline Hydrochloride (Concomitant use of clozapine with other drugs metabolized by cytochrome $P_{450}IID_6$ may require lower than usual doses prescribed for either drug). Products include:
- Ludiomil Tablets 843

Mecamylamine Hydrochloride (Hypotensive effects potentiated). Products include:
- Inversine Tablets 1686

Mesoridazine Besylate (Concomitant use of clozapine with other drugs metabolized by cytochrome $P_{450}IID_6$ may require lower than usual doses prescribed for either drug). Products include:
- Serentil 684

Methotrimeprazine (Concomitant use of clozapine with other drugs metabolized by cytochrome $P_{450}IID_6$ may require lower than usual doses prescribed for either drug). Products include:
- Levoprome 1274

Methyclothiazide (Hypotensive effects potentiated). Products include:
- Enduron Tablets 420

Methyldopa (Hypotensive effects potentiated). Products include:
- Aldoclor Tablets 1598
- Aldomet Oral 1600
- Aldoril Tablets 1604

Methyldopate Hydrochloride (Hypotensive effects potentiated). Products include:
- Aldomet Ester HCl Injection 1602

Metipranolol Hydrochloride (Hypotensive effects potentiated). Products include:
- OptiPranolol (Metipranolol 0.3%) Sterile Ophthalmic Solution .... ⊙ 258

Metolazone (Hypotensive effects potentiated). Products include:
- Mykrox Tablets 993
- Zaroxolyn Tablets 1000

Metoprolol Succinate (Hypotensive effects potentiated). Products include:
- Toprol-XL Tablets 565

Metoprolol Tartrate (Hypotensive effects potentiated). Products include:
- Lopressor Ampuls 830
- Lopressor HCT Tablets 832
- Lopressor Tablets 830

Metyrosine (Hypotensive effects potentiated). Products include:
- Demser Capsules 1649

Midazolam Hydrochloride (Potential for profound collapse and respiratory depression). Products include:
- Versed Injection 2170

Minoxidil (Hypotensive effects potentiated). Products include:
- Loniten Tablets 2618
- Rogaine Topical Solution 2637

Moexipril Hydrochloride (Hypotensive effects potentiated). Products include:
- Univasc Tablets 2410

Nadolol (Hypotensive effects potentiated).
- No products indexed under this heading.

Nefazodone Hydrochloride (Concomitant use of clozapine with other drugs metabolized by cytochrome $P_{450}IID_6$ may require lower than usual doses prescribed for either drug). Products include:
- Serzone Tablets 771

Nicardipine Hydrochloride (Hypotensive effects potentiated). Products include:
- Cardene Capsules 2095
- Cardene I.V. 2709
- Cardene SR Capsules 2097

Nifedipine (Hypotensive effects potentiated). Products include:
- Adalat Capsules (10 mg and 20 mg) 587
- Adalat CC 589
- Procardia Capsules 1971
- Procardia XL Extended Release Tablets 1972

Nisoldipine (Hypotensive effects potentiated).
- No products indexed under this heading.

Nitroglycerin (Hypotensive effects potentiated). Products include:
- Deponit NTG Transdermal Delivery System 2397
- Nitro-Bid IV 1523
- Nitro-Bid Ointment 1524
- Nitrodisc 2047
- Nitro-Dur (nitroglycerin) Transdermal Infusion System 1326
- Nitrolingual Spray 2027
- Nitrostat Tablets 1925
- Transderm-Nitro Transdermal Therapeutic System 859

Norepinephrine Bitartrate (Possible reverse epinephrine effect). Products include:
- Levophed Bitartrate Injection 2315

Nortriptyline Hydrochloride (Concomitant use of clozapine with other drugs metabolized by cytochrome $P_{450}IID_6$ may require lower than usual doses prescribed for either drug). Products include:
- Pamelor 2280

Oxazepam (Potential for profound collapse and respiratory depression). Products include:
- Serax Capsules 2810
- Serax Tablets 2810

Paroxetine Hydrochloride (Concomitant use of clozapine with other drugs metabolized by cytochrome $P_{450}IID_6$ may require lower than usual doses prescribed for either drug). Products include:
- Paxil Tablets 2505

Penbutolol Sulfate (Hypotensive effects potentiated). Products include:
- Levatol 2403

Perphenazine (Concomitant use of clozapine with other drugs metabolized by cytochrome $P_{450}IID_6$ may require lower than usual doses prescribed for either drug). Products include:
- Etrafon 2355
- Triavil Tablets 1757
- Trilafon 2389

Phenelzine Sulfate (Concomitant use of clozapine with other drugs metabolized by cytochrome $P_{450}IID_6$ may require lower than usual doses prescribed for either drug). Products include:
- Nardil 1920

Phenoxybenzamine Hydrochloride (Hypotensive effects potentiated). Products include:
- Dibenzyline Capsules 2476

Phentolamine Mesylate (Hypotensive effects potentiated). Products include:
- Regitine 846

Phenytoin (May decrease clozapine plasma levels, a decrease in effectiveness of a previously effective clozapine dose). Products include:
- Dilantin Infatabs 1908
- Dilantin-125 Suspension 1911

Phenytoin Sodium (May decrease clozapine plasma levels, a decrease in effectiveness of a previously effective clozapine dose). Products include:
- Dilantin Kapseals 1906
- Dilantin Parenteral 1910

Pindolol (Hypotensive effects potentiated). Products include:
- Visken Tablets 2299

Polythiazide (Hypotensive effects potentiated). Products include:
- Minizide Capsules 1938

Prazepam (Potential for profound collapse and respiratory depression).
- No products indexed under this heading.

Prazosin Hydrochloride (Hypotensive effects potentiated). Products include:
- Minipress Capsules 1937
- Minizide Capsules 1938

Prochlorperazine (Concomitant use of clozapine with other drugs metabolized by cytochrome $P_{450}IID_6$ may require lower than usual doses prescribed for either drug). Products include:
- Compazine 2470

Promethazine Hydrochloride (Concomitant use of clozapine with other drugs metabolized by cytochrome $P_{450}IID_6$ may require lower than usual doses prescribed for either drug). Products include:
- Mepergan Injection 2753
- Phenergan with Codeine 2777
- Phenergan with Dextromethorphan 2778
- Phenergan Injection 2773
- Phenergan Suppositories 2775
- Phenergan Syrup 2774
- Phenergan Tablets 2775
- Phenergan VC 2779
- Phenergan VC with Codeine 2781

(▣ Described in PDR For Nonprescription Drugs) (⊙ Described in PDR For Ophthalmology)

Propafenone Hydrochloride (Concomitant use of clozapine with other drugs metabolized by cytochrome $P_{450}IID_6$ may require lower than usual doses prescribed for either drug). Products include:
- Rythmol Tablets–150mg, 225mg, 300mg 1352

Propranolol Hydrochloride (Hypotensive effects potentiated). Products include:
- Inderal 2728
- Inderal LA Long Acting Capsules 2730
- Inderide Tablets 2732
- Inderide LA Long Acting Capsules 2734

Protriptyline Hydrochloride (Concomitant use of clozapine with other drugs metabolized by cytochrome $P_{450}IID_6$ may require lower than usual doses prescribed for either drug). Products include:
- Vivactil Tablets 1774

Quazepam (Potential for profound collapse and respiratory depression). Products include:
- Doral Tablets 2664

Quinapril Hydrochloride (Hypotensive effects potentiated). Products include:
- Accupril Tablets 1893

Quinidine Gluconate (Concomitant use of clozapine with quinidine which inhibits cytochrome $P_{450}IID_6$ should be approached with caution). Products include:
- Quinaglute Dura-Tabs Tablets 649

Quinidine Polygalacturonate (Concomitant use of clozapine with quinidine which inhibits cytochrome $P_{450}IID_6$ should be approached with caution).
- No products indexed under this heading.

Quinidine Sulfate (Concomitant use of clozapine with quinidine which inhibits cytochrome $P_{450}IID_6$ should be approached with caution). Products include:
- Quinidex Extentabs 2067

Ramipril (Hypotensive effects potentiated). Products include:
- Altace Capsules 1232

Rauwolfia Serpentina (Hypotensive effects potentiated).
- No products indexed under this heading.

Rescinnamine (Hypotensive effects potentiated).
- No products indexed under this heading.

Reserpine (Hypotensive effects potentiated). Products include:
- Diupres Tablets 1650
- Hydropres Tablets 1675
- Ser-Ap-Es Tablets 849

Scopolamine (Anticholinergic effects potentiated). Products include:
- Transderm Scōp Transdermal Therapeutic System 869

Scopolamine Hydrobromide (Anticholinergic effects potentiated). Products include:
- Atrohist Plus Tablets 454
- Donnatal 2060
- Donnatal Extentabs 2061
- Donnatal Tablets 2060

Sertraline Hydrochloride (Concomitant use of clozapine with other drugs metabolized by cytochrome $P_{450}IID_6$ may require lower than usual doses prescribed for either drug). Products include:
- Zoloft Tablets 2217

Sodium Nitroprusside (Hypotensive effects potentiated).
- No products indexed under this heading.

Sotalol Hydrochloride (Hypotensive effects potentiated). Products include:
- Betapace Tablets 641

Spirapril Hydrochloride (Hypotensive effects potentiated).
- No products indexed under this heading.

Temazepam (Potential for profound collapse and respiratory depression). Products include:
- Restoril Capsules 2284

Terazosin Hydrochloride (Hypotensive effects potentiated). Products include:
- Hytrin Capsules 430

Thioridazine Hydrochloride (Concomitant use of clozapine with other drugs metabolized by cytochrome $P_{450}IID_6$ may require lower than usual doses prescribed for either drug). Products include:
- Mellaril 2269

Timolol Maleate (Hypotensive effects potentiated). Products include:
- Blocadren Tablets 1614
- Timolide Tablets 1748
- Timoptic in Ocudose 1753
- Timoptic Sterile Ophthalmic Solution 1751
- Timoptic-XE 1755

Torsemide (Hypotensive effects potentiated). Products include:
- Demadex Tablets and Injection 686

Tranylcypromine Sulfate (Concomitant use of clozapine with other drugs metabolized by cytochrome $P_{450}IID_6$ may require lower than usual doses prescribed for either drug). Products include:
- Parnate Tablets 2503

Trazodone Hydrochloride (Concomitant use of clozapine with other drugs metabolized by cytochrome $P_{450}IID_6$ may require lower than usual doses prescribed for either drug). Products include:
- Desyrel and Desyrel Dividose 503

Triazolam (Potential for profound collapse and respiratory depression). Products include:
- Halcion Tablets 2611

Trifluoperazine Hydrochloride (Concomitant use of clozapine with other drugs metabolized by cytochrome $P_{450}IID_6$ may require lower than usual doses prescribed for either drug). Products include:
- Stelazine 2514

Trimethaphan Camsylate (Hypotensive effects potentiated). Products include:
- Arfonad Ampuls 2080

Trimipramine Maleate (Concomitant use of clozapine with other drugs metabolized by cytochrome $P_{450}IID_6$ may require lower than usual doses prescribed for either drug). Products include:
- Surmontil Capsules 2811

Venlafaxine Hydrochloride (Concomitant use of clozapine with other drugs metabolized by cytochrome $P_{450}IID_6$ may require lower than usual doses prescribed for either drug). Products include:
- Effexor 2719

Verapamil Hydrochloride (Hypotensive effects potentiated). Products include:
- Calan SR Caplets 2422
- Calan Tablets 2419
- Isoptin Injectable 1344
- Isoptin Oral Tablets 1346
- Isoptin SR Tablets 1348
- Verelan Capsules 1410
- Verelan Capsules 2824

Warfarin Sodium (Potential for increased plasma levels and adverse effects). Products include:
- Coumadin 926

Food Interactions

Alcohol (Caution is advised with concomitant use).

COCAINE HYDROCHLORIDE TOPICAL SOLUTION

(Cocaine Hydrochloride) 537

None cited in PDR database.

CODICLEAR DH SYRUP

(Guaifenesin, Hydrocodone Bitartrate) 791

May interact with narcotic analgesics, hypnotics and sedatives, tranquilizers, central nervous system depressants, and certain other agents. Compounds in these categories include:

Alfentanil Hydrochloride (Additive CNS depression). Products include:
- Alfenta Injection 1286

Alprazolam (Additive CNS depression). Products include:
- Xanax Tablets 2649

Aprobarbital (Additive CNS depression).
- No products indexed under this heading.

Buprenorphine (Additive CNS depression). Products include:
- Buprenex Injectable 2006

Buspirone Hydrochloride (Additive CNS depression). Products include:
- BuSpar 737

Butabarbital (Additive CNS depression).
- No products indexed under this heading.

Butalbital (Additive CNS depression). Products include:
- Esgic-plus Tablets 1013
- Fioricet Tablets 2258
- Fioricet with Codeine Capsules 2260
- Fiorinal Capsules 2261
- Fiorinal with Codeine Capsules 2262
- Fiorinal Tablets 2261
- Phrenilin 785
- Sedapap Tablets 50 mg/650 mg 1543

Chlordiazepoxide (Additive CNS depression). Products include:
- Libritabs Tablets 2177
- Limbitrol 2180

Chlordiazepoxide Hydrochloride (Additive CNS depression). Products include:
- Librax Capsules 2176
- Librium Capsules 2178
- Librium Injectable 2179

Chlorpromazine (Additive CNS depression). Products include:
- Thorazine Suppositories 2523

Chlorprothixene (Additive CNS depression).
- No products indexed under this heading.

Chlorprothixene Hydrochloride (Additive CNS depression).
- No products indexed under this heading.

Chlorprothixene Lactate (Additive CNS depression).
- No products indexed under this heading.

Clorazepate Dipotassium (Additive CNS depression). Products include:
- Tranxene 451

Clozapine (Additive CNS depression). Products include:
- Clozaril Tablets 2252

Codeine Phosphate (Additive CNS depression). Products include:
- Actifed with Codeine Cough Syrup 1067
- Brontex 1981
- Deconsal C Expectorant Syrup 456
- Deconsal Pediatric Syrup 457
- Dimetane-DC Cough Syrup 2059
- Empirin with Codeine Tablets 1093
- Fioricet with Codeine Capsules 2260
- Fiorinal with Codeine Capsules 2262
- Isoclor Expectorant 990
- Novahistine DH 2462
- Novahistine Expectorant 2463
- Nucofed 2051
- Phenergan with Codeine 2777
- Phenergan VC with Codeine 2781
- Robitussin A-C Syrup 2073
- Robitussin-DAC Syrup 2074
- Ryna ..... ⓢⓓ 841
- Soma Compound w/Codeine Tablets 2676
- Tussi-Organidin NR Liquid and S NR Liquid 2677
- Tylenol with Codeine 1583

Desflurane (Additive CNS depression). Products include:
- Suprane 1813

Dezocine (Additive CNS depression). Products include:
- Dalgan Injection 538

Diazepam (Additive CNS depression). Products include:
- Dizac 1809
- Valium Injectable 2182
- Valium Tablets 2183
- Valrelease Capsules 2169

Droperidol (Additive CNS depression). Products include:
- Inapsine Injection 1296

Enflurane (Additive CNS depression).
- No products indexed under this heading.

Estazolam (Additive CNS depression). Products include:
- ProSom Tablets 449

Ethchlorvynol (Additive CNS depression). Products include:
- Placidyl Capsules 448

Ethinamate (Additive CNS depression).
- No products indexed under this heading.

Fentanyl (Additive CNS depression). Products include:
- Duragesic Transdermal System 1288

Fentanyl Citrate (Additive CNS depression). Products include:
- Sublimaze Injection 1307

Fluphenazine Decanoate (Additive CNS depression). Products include:
- Prolixin Decanoate 509

Fluphenazine Enanthate (Additive CNS depression). Products include:
- Prolixin Enanthate 509

Fluphenazine Hydrochloride (Additive CNS depression). Products include:
- Prolixin 509

Flurazepam Hydrochloride (Additive CNS depression). Products include:
- Dalmane Capsules 2173

Glutethimide (Additive CNS depression).
- No products indexed under this heading.

Haloperidol (Additive CNS depression). Products include:
- Haldol Injection, Tablets and Concentrate 1575

Haloperidol Decanoate (Additive CNS depression). Products include:
- Haldol Decanoate 1577

IMPORTANT NOTE: Always consult each drug listing in the patient's regimen for possible interactions.

Codiclear DH — Interactions Index — 186

Hydrocodone Polistirex (Additive CNS depression). Products include:
- Tussionex Pennkinetic Extended-Release Suspension ... 998

Hydroxyzine Hydrochloride (Additive CNS depression). Products include:
- Atarax Tablets & Syrup ... 2185
- Marax Tablets & DF Syrup ... 2200
- Vistaril Intramuscular Solution ... 2216

Isoflurane (Additive CNS depression).
- No products indexed under this heading.

Ketamine Hydrochloride (Additive CNS depression).
- No products indexed under this heading.

Levomethadyl Acetate Hydrochloride (Additive CNS depression). Products include:
- Orlamm ... 2239

Levorphanol Tartrate (Additive CNS depression). Products include:
- Levo-Dromoran ... 2129

Lorazepam (Additive CNS depression). Products include:
- Ativan Injection ... 2698
- Ativan Tablets ... 2700

Loxapine Hydrochloride (Additive CNS depression). Products include:
- Loxitane ... 1378

Loxapine Succinate (Additive CNS depression). Products include:
- Loxitane Capsules ... 1378

Meperidine Hydrochloride (Additive CNS depression). Products include:
- Demerol ... 2308
- Mepergan Injection ... 2753

Mephobarbital (Additive CNS depression). Products include:
- Mebaral Tablets ... 2322

Meprobamate (Additive CNS depression). Products include:
- Miltown Tablets ... 2672
- PMB 200 and PMB 400 ... 2783

Mesoridazine Besylate (Additive CNS depression). Products include:
- Serentil ... 684

Methadone Hydrochloride (Additive CNS depression). Products include:
- Methadone Hydrochloride Oral Concentrate ... 2233
- Methadone Hydrochloride Oral Solution & Tablets ... 2235

Methohexital Sodium (Additive CNS depression). Products include:
- Brevital Sodium Vials ... 1429

Methotrimeprazine (Additive CNS depression). Products include:
- Levoprome ... 1274

Methoxyflurane (Additive CNS depression).
- No products indexed under this heading.

Midazolam Hydrochloride (Additive CNS depression). Products include:
- Versed Injection ... 2170

Molindone Hydrochloride (Additive CNS depression). Products include:
- Moban Tablets and Concentrate ... 1048

Morphine Sulfate (Additive CNS depression). Products include:
- Astramorph/PF Injection, USP (Preservative-Free) ... 535
- Duramorph ... 962
- Infumorph 200 and Infumorph 500 Sterile Solutions ... 965
- MS Contin Tablets ... 1994
- MSIR ... 1997
- Oramorph SR (Morphine Sulfate Sustained Release Tablets) ... 2236
- RMS Suppositories ... 2657
- Roxanol ... 2243

Opium Alkaloids (Additive CNS depression).
- No products indexed under this heading.

Oxazepam (Additive CNS depression). Products include:
- Serax Capsules ... 2810
- Serax Tablets ... 2810

Oxycodone Hydrochloride (Additive CNS depression). Products include:
- Percocet Tablets ... 938
- Percodan Tablets ... 939
- Percodan-Demi Tablets ... 940
- Roxicodone Tablets, Oral Solution & Intensol (Oxycodone) ... 2244
- Tylox Capsules ... 1584

Pentobarbital Sodium (Additive CNS depression). Products include:
- Nembutal Sodium Capsules ... 436
- Nembutal Sodium Solution ... 438
- Nembutal Sodium Suppositories ... 440

Perphenazine (Additive CNS depression). Products include:
- Etrafon ... 2355
- Triavil Tablets ... 1757
- Trilafon ... 2389

Phenobarbital (Additive CNS depression). Products include:
- Arco-Lase Plus Tablets ... 512
- Bellergal-S Tablets ... 2250
- Donnatal ... 2060
- Donnatal Extentabs ... 2061
- Donnatal Tablets ... 2060
- Phenobarbital Elixir and Tablets ... 1469
- Quadrinal Tablets ... 1350

Prazepam (Additive CNS depression).
- No products indexed under this heading.

Prochlorperazine (Additive CNS depression). Products include:
- Compazine ... 2470

Promethazine Hydrochloride (Additive CNS depression). Products include:
- Mepergan Injection ... 2753
- Phenergan with Codeine ... 2777
- Phenergan with Dextromethorphan 2778
- Phenergan Injection ... 2773
- Phenergan Suppositories ... 2775
- Phenergan Syrup ... 2774
- Phenergan Tablets ... 2775
- Phenergan VC ... 2779
- Phenergan VC with Codeine ... 2781

Propofol (Additive CNS depression). Products include:
- Diprivan Injection ... 2833

Propoxyphene Hydrochloride (Additive CNS depression). Products include:
- Darvon ... 1435
- Wygesic Tablets ... 2827

Propoxyphene Napsylate (Additive CNS depression). Products include:
- Darvon-N/Darvocet-N ... 1433

Quazepam (Additive CNS depression). Products include:
- Doral Tablets ... 2664

Risperidone (Additive CNS depression). Products include:
- Risperdal ... 1301

Secobarbital Sodium (Additive CNS depression). Products include:
- Seconal Sodium Pulvules ... 1474

Sufentanil Citrate (Additive CNS depression). Products include:
- Sufenta Injection ... 1309

Temazepam (Additive CNS depression). Products include:
- Restoril Capsules ... 2284

Thiamylal Sodium (Additive CNS depression).
- No products indexed under this heading.

Thiothixene (Additive CNS depression). Products include:
- Navane Capsules and Concentrate 2201
- Navane Intramuscular ... 2202

Triazolam (Additive CNS depression). Products include:
- Halcion Tablets ... 2611

Trifluoperazine Hydrochloride (Additive CNS depression). Products include:
- Stelazine ... 2514

Zolpidem Tartrate (Additive CNS depression). Products include:
- Ambien Tablets ... 2416

Food Interactions

Alcohol (Additive CNS depression).

COENZYME Q10 200MG, 100MG & 60MG CHEWABLE WAFERS, AND 200MG, 60MG & 25MG TABLETS

(Coenzyme Q-10) ... 2659
None cited in PDR database.

COGENTIN INJECTION

(Benztropine Mesylate) ... 1621
May interact with phenothiazines, tricyclic antidepressants, belladona products, anticholinergics, butyrophenones, and dopamine antagonists. Compounds in these categories include:

Amitriptyline Hydrochloride (Potential for paralytic ileus, hyperthermia and heat stroke). Products include:
- Elavil ... 2838
- Endep Tablets ... 2174
- Etrafon ... 2355
- Limbitrol ... 2180
- Triavil Tablets ... 1757

Amoxapine (Potential for paralytic ileus, hyperthermia and heat stroke). Products include:
- Asendin Tablets ... 1369

Atropine Sulfate (Potential for paralytic ileus, hyperthermia and heat stroke). Products include:
- Arco-Lase Plus Tablets ... 512
- Atrohist Plus Tablets ... 454
- Atropine Sulfate Sterile Ophthalmic Solution ... ⊙ 233
- Donnatal ... 2060
- Donnatal Extentabs ... 2061
- Donnatal Tablets ... 2060
- Lomotil ... 2439
- Motofen Tablets ... 784
- Urised Tablets ... 1964

Belladonna Alkaloids (Potential for paralytic ileus, hyperthermia and heat stroke). Products include:
- Bellergal-S Tablets ... 2250
- Hyland's Bed Wetting Tablets ... ▣ 828
- Hyland's EnurAid Tablets ... ▣ 829
- Hyland's Teething Tablets ... ▣ 830

Biperiden Hydrochloride (Potential for paralytic ileus, hyperthermia and heat stroke). Products include:
- Akineton ... 1333

Chlorpromazine (Potential for paralytic ileus, hyperthermia and heat stroke). Products include:
- Thorazine Suppositories ... 2523

Clidinium Bromide (Potential for paralytic ileus, hyperthermia and heat stroke). Products include:
- Librax Capsules ... 2176
- Quarzan Capsules ... 2181

Clomipramine Hydrochloride (Potential for paralytic ileus, hyperthermia and heat stroke). Products include:
- Anafranil Capsules ... 803

Clozapine (Potential for paralytic ileus, hyperthermia and heat stroke). Products include:
- Clozaril Tablets ... 2252

Desipramine Hydrochloride (Potential for paralytic ileus, hyperthermia and heat stroke). Products include:
- Norpramin Tablets ... 1526

Dicyclomine Hydrochloride (Potential for paralytic ileus, hyperthermia and heat stroke). Products include:
- Bentyl ... 1501

Doxepin Hydrochloride (Potential for paralytic ileus, hyperthermia and heat stroke). Products include:
- Sinequan ... 2205
- Zonalon Cream ... 1055

Fluphenazine Decanoate (Potential for paralytic ileus, hyperthermia and heat stroke). Products include:
- Prolixin Decanoate ... 509

Fluphenazine Enanthate (Potential for paralytic ileus, hyperthermia and heat stroke). Products include:
- Prolixin Enanthate ... 509

Fluphenazine Hydrochloride (Potential for paralytic ileus, hyperthermia and heat stroke). Products include:
- Prolixin ... 509

Glycopyrrolate (Potential for paralytic ileus, hyperthermia and heat stroke). Products include:
- Robinul Forte Tablets ... 2072
- Robinul Injectable ... 2072
- Robinul Tablets ... 2072

Haloperidol (Potential for paralytic ileus, hyperthermia and heat stroke). Products include:
- Haldol Injection, Tablets and Concentrate ... 1575

Haloperidol Decanoate (Potential for paralytic ileus, hyperthermia and heat stroke). Products include:
- Haldol Decanoate ... 1577

Hyoscyamine (Potential for paralytic ileus, hyperthermia and heat stroke). Products include:
- Cystospaz Tablets ... 1963
- Urised Tablets ... 1964

Hyoscyamine Sulfate (Potential for paralytic ileus, hyperthermia and heat stroke). Products include:
- Arco-Lase Plus Tablets ... 512
- Atrohist Plus Tablets ... 454
- Cystospaz-M Capsules ... 1963
- Donnatal ... 2060
- Donnatal Extentabs ... 2061
- Donnatal Tablets ... 2060
- Kutrase Capsules ... 2402
- Levsin/Levsinex/Levbid ... 2405

Imipramine Hydrochloride (Potential for paralytic ileus, hyperthermia and heat stroke). Products include:
- Tofranil Ampuls ... 854
- Tofranil Tablets ... 856

Imipramine Pamoate (Potential for paralytic ileus, hyperthermia and heat stroke). Products include:
- Tofranil-PM Capsules ... 857

Ipratropium Bromide (Potential for paralytic ileus, hyperthermia and heat stroke). Products include:
- Atrovent Inhalation Aerosol ... 671
- Atrovent Inhalation Solution ... 673

Maprotiline Hydrochloride (Potential for paralytic ileus, hyperthermia and heat stroke). Products include:
- Ludiomil Tablets ... 843

Mepenzolate Bromide (Potential for paralytic ileus, hyperthermia and heat stroke).
- No products indexed under this heading.

Mesoridazine Besylate (Potential for paralytic ileus, hyperthermia and heat stroke). Products include:
- Serentil ... 684

(▣ Described in PDR For Nonprescription Drugs) (⊙ Described in PDR For Ophthalmology)

187 **Interactions Index** **Cognex**

Methotrimeprazine (Potential for paralytic ileus, hyperthermia and heat stroke). Products include:

- Levoprome 1274

Metoclopramide Hydrochloride (Potential for paralytic ileus, hyperthermia and heat stroke). Products include:

- Reglan 2068

Nortriptyline Hydrochloride (Potential for paralytic ileus, hyperthermia and heat stroke). Products include:

- Pamelor 2280

Oxybutynin Chloride (Potential for paralytic ileus, hyperthermia and heat stroke). Products include:

- Ditropan 1516

Perphenazine (Potential for paralytic ileus, hyperthermia and heat stroke). Products include:

- Etrafon 2355
- Triavil Tablets 1757
- Trilafon 2389

Pimozide (Potential for paralytic ileus, hyperthermia and heat stroke). Products include:

- Orap Tablets 1050

Prochlorperazine (Potential for paralytic ileus, hyperthermia and heat stroke). Products include:

- Compazine 2470

Procyclidine Hydrochloride (Potential for paralytic ileus, hyperthermia and heat stroke). Products include:

- Kemadrin Tablets 1112

Promethazine Hydrochloride (Potential for paralytic ileus, hyperthermia and heat stroke). Products include:

- Mepergan Injection 2753
- Phenergan with Codeine 2777
- Phenergan with Dextromethorphan 2778
- Phenergan Injection 2773
- Phenergan Suppositories 2775
- Phenergan Syrup 2774
- Phenergan Tablets 2775
- Phenergan VC 2779
- Phenergan VC with Codeine 2781

Propantheline Bromide (Potential for paralytic ileus, hyperthermia and heat stroke). Products include:

- Pro-Banthīne Tablets 2052

Protriptyline Hydrochloride (Potential for paralytic ileus, hyperthermia and heat stroke). Products include:

- Vivactil Tablets 1774

Scopolamine (Potential for paralytic ileus, hyperthermia and heat stroke). Products include:

- Transderm Scōp Transdermal Therapeutic System 869

Scopolamine Hydrobromide (Potential for paralytic ileus, hyperthermia and heat stroke). Products include:

- Atrohist Plus Tablets 454
- Donnatal 2060
- Donnatal Extentabs 2061
- Donnatal Tablets 2060

Thioridazine Hydrochloride (Potential for paralytic ileus, hyperthermia and heat stroke). Products include:

- Mellaril 2269

Tridihexethyl Chloride (Potential for paralytic ileus, hyperthermia and heat stroke).

No products indexed under this heading.

Trifluoperazine Hydrochloride (Potential for paralytic ileus, hyperthermia and heat stroke). Products include:

- Stelazine 2514

Trihexyphenidyl Hydrochloride (Potential for paralytic ileus, hyperthermia and heat stroke). Products include:

- Artane 1368

Trimipramine Maleate (Potential for paralytic ileus, hyperthermia and heat stroke). Products include:

- Surmontil Capsules 2811

COGENTIN TABLETS

(Benztropine Mesylate) 1621

See **Cogentin Injection**

COGNEX CAPSULES

(Tacrine Hydrochloride) 1901

May interact with xanthine bronchodilators, non-steroidal anti-inflammatory agents, cholinergic agents, anticholinergics, and certain other agents. Compounds in these categories include:

Aminophylline (Co-administration increases theophylline elimination half-life and average plasma theophylline concentrations by approximately 2-fold).

No products indexed under this heading.

Atropine Sulfate (Tacrine has potential to interfere with the activity of anticholinergic drugs). Products include:

- Arco-Lase Plus Tablets 512
- Atrohist Plus Tablets 454
- Atropine Sulfate Sterile Ophthalmic Solution .... ◎ 233
- Donnatal 2060
- Donnatal Extentabs 2061
- Donnatal Tablets 2060
- Lomotil 2439
- Motofen Tablets 784
- Urised Tablets 1964

Belladonna Alkaloids (Tacrine has potential to interfere with the activity of anticholinergic drugs). Products include:

- Bellergal-S Tablets 2250
- Hyland's Bed Wetting Tablets .... ▣ 828
- Hyland's EnurAid Tablets .... ▣ 829
- Hyland's Teething Tablets .... ▣ 830

Benztropine Mesylate (Tacrine has potential to interfere with the activity of anticholinergic drugs). Products include:

- Cogentin 1621

Bethanechol Chloride (Concurrent administration with cholinergic agonist may result in synergistic effect). Products include:

- Duvoid 2044
- Urecholine 1761

Biperiden Hydrochloride (Tacrine has potential to interfere with the activity of anticholinergic drugs). Products include:

- Akineton 1333

Cimetidine (Increases C_{max} and AUC of tacrine by approximately 54% and 64% respectively). Products include:

- Tagamet Tablets 2516

Cimetidine Hydrochloride (Increases C_{max} and AUC of tacrine by approximately 54% and 64% respectively). Products include:

- Tagamet 2516

Clidinium Bromide (Tacrine has potential to interfere with the activity of anticholinergic drugs). Products include:

- Librax Capsules 2176
- Quarzan Capsules 2181

Diclofenac Potassium (Patients receiving concurrent nonsteroidal anti-inflammatory agents are at increased risk for developing ulcers since tacrine may be expected to increase gastric acid secretion due to increased cholinergic activity). Products include:

- Cataflam 816

Diclofenac Sodium (Patients receiving concurrent nonsteroidal anti-inflammatory agents are at increased risk for developing ulcers since tacrine may be expected to increase gastric acid secretion due to increased cholinergic activity). Products include:

- Voltaren Ophthalmic Sterile Ophthalmic Solution .... ◎ 272
- Voltaren Tablets 861

Dicyclomine Hydrochloride (Tacrine has potential to interfere with the activity of anticholinergic drugs). Products include:

- Bentyl 1501

Dyphylline (Co-administration increases theophylline elimination half-life and average plasma theophylline concentrations by approximately 2-fold). Products include:

- Lufyllin & Lufyllin-400 Tablets 2670
- Lufyllin-GG Elixir & Tablets 2671

Edrophonium Chloride (Concurrent administration may result in synergistic effect). Products include:

- Tensilon Injectable 1261

Etodolac (Patients receiving concurrent nonsteroidal anti-inflammatory agents are at increased risk for developing ulcers since tacrine may be expected to increase gastric acid secretion due to increased cholinergic activity). Products include:

- Lodine Capsules and Tablets 2743

Fenoprofen Calcium (Patients receiving concurrent nonsteroidal anti-inflammatory agents are at increased risk for developing ulcers since tacrine may be expected to increase gastric acid secretion due to increased cholinergic activity). Products include:

- Nalfon 200 Pulvules & Nalfon Tablets 917

Flurbiprofen (Patients receiving concurrent nonsteroidal anti-inflammatory agents are at increased risk for developing ulcers since tacrine may be expected to increase gastric acid secretion due to increased cholinergic activity). Products include:

- Ansaid Tablets 2579

Glycopyrrolate (Tacrine has potential to interfere with the activity of anticholinergic drugs). Products include:

- Robinul Forte Tablets 2072
- Robinul Injectable 2072
- Robinul Tablets 2072

Hyoscyamine (Tacrine has potential to interfere with the activity of anticholinergic drugs). Products include:

- Cystospaz Tablets 1963
- Urised Tablets 1964

Hyoscyamine Sulfate (Tacrine has potential to interfere with the activity of anticholinergic drugs). Products include:

- Arco-Lase Plus Tablets 512
- Atrohist Plus Tablets 454
- Cystospaz-M Capsules 1963
- Donnatal 2060
- Donnatal Extentabs 2061
- Donnatal Tablets 2060
- Kutrase Capsules 2402
- Levsin/Levsinex/Levbid 2405

Ibuprofen (Patients receiving concurrent nonsteroidal anti-inflammatory agents are at increased risk for developing ulcers since tacrine may be expected to increase gastric acid secretion due to increased cholinergic activity). Products include:

- Advil Cold and Sinus Caplets and Tablets (formerly CoAdvil) .... ▣ 870
- Advil Ibuprofen Tablets and Caplets .... ▣ 870
- Children's Advil Suspension 2692
- Arthritis Foundation Ibuprofen Tablets .... ▣ 674
- Bayer Select Ibuprofen Pain Relief Formula .... ▣ 715
- Cramp End Tablets .... ▣ 735
- Dimetapp Sinus Caplets .... ▣ 775
- Haltran Tablets .... ▣ 771
- IBU Tablets 1342
- Ibuprohm .... ▣ 735
- Children's Motrin Ibuprofen Oral Suspension 1546
- Motrin Tablets 2625
- Motrin IB Caplets, Tablets, and Geltabs .... ▣ 838
- Motrin IB Sinus .... ▣ 838
- Motrin Ibuprofen Suspension, Oral Drops, Chewable Tablets, Caplets 1546
- Nuprin Ibuprofen/Analgesic Tablets & Caplets .... ▣ 622
- Sine-Aid IB Caplets 1554
- Vicks DayQuil SINUS Pressure & PAIN Relief with IBUPROFEN .... ▣ 762

Indomethacin (Patients receiving concurrent nonsteroidal anti-inflammatory agents are at increased risk for developing ulcers since tacrine may be expected to increase gastric acid secretion due to increased cholinergic activity). Products include:

- Indocin 1680

Indomethacin Sodium Trihydrate (Patients receiving concurrent nonsteroidal anti-inflammatory agents are at increased risk for developing ulcers since tacrine may be expected to increase gastric acid secretion due to increased cholinergic activity). Products include:

- Indocin I.V. 1684

Ipratropium Bromide (Tacrine has potential to interfere with the activity of anticholinergic drugs). Products include:

- Atrovent Inhalation Aerosol 671
- Atrovent Inhalation Solution 673

Ketoprofen (Patients receiving concurrent nonsteroidal anti-inflammatory agents are at increased risk for developing ulcers since tacrine may be expected to increase gastric acid secretion due to increased cholinergic activity). Products include:

- Orudis Capsules 2766
- Oruvail Capsules 2766

Ketorolac Tromethamine (Patients receiving concurrent nonsteroidal anti-inflammatory agents are at increased risk for developing ulcers since tacrine may be expected to increase gastric acid secretion due to increased cholinergic activity). Products include:

- Acular 474
- Acular .... ◎ 277
- Toradol 2159

Meclofenamate Sodium (Patients receiving concurrent nonsteroidal anti-inflammatory agents are at increased risk for developing ulcers since tacrine may be expected to increase gastric acid secretion due to increased cholinergic activity).

No products indexed under this heading.

IMPORTANT NOTE: Always consult each drug listing in the patient's regimen for possible interactions.

Cognex **Interactions Index** **188**

Mefenamic Acid (Patients receiving concurrent nonsteroidal anti-inflammatory agents are at increased risk for developing ulcers since tacrine may be expected to increase gastric acid secretion due to increased cholinergic activity). Products include:
Ponstel ... 1925

Mepenzolate Bromide (Tacrine has potential to interfere with the activity of anticholinergic drugs).
No products indexed under this heading.

Nabumetone (Patients receiving concurrent nonsteroidal anti-inflammatory agents are at increased risk for developing ulcers since tacrine may be expected to increase gastric acid secretion due to increased cholinergic activity). Products include:
Relafen Tablets ... 2510

Naproxen (Patients receiving concurrent nonsteroidal anti-inflammatory agents are at increased risk for developing ulcers since tacrine may be expected to increase gastric acid secretion due to increased cholinergic activity). Products include:
Anaprox/Naprosyn ... 2117

Naproxen Sodium (Patients receiving concurrent nonsteroidal anti-inflammatory agents are at increased risk for developing ulcers since tacrine may be expected to increase gastric acid secretion due to increased cholinergic activity). Products include:
Aleve ... 1975
Anaprox/Naprosyn ... 2117

Neostigmine Bromide (Concurrent administration may result in synergistic effect). Products include:
Prostigmin Tablets ... 1261

Neostigmine Methylsulfate (Concurrent administration may result in synergistic effect). Products include:
Prostigmin Injectable ... 1260

Oxaprozin (Patients receiving concurrent nonsteroidal anti-inflammatory agents are at increased risk for developing ulcers since tacrine may be expected to increase gastric acid secretion due to increased cholinergic activity). Products include:
Daypro Caplets ... 2426

Oxybutynin Chloride (Tacrine has potential to interfere with the activity of anticholinergic drugs). Products include:
Ditropan ... 1516

Phenylbutazone (Patients receiving concurrent nonsteroidal anti-inflammatory agents are at increased risk for developing ulcers since tacrine may be expected to increase gastric acid secretion due to increased cholinergic activity).
No products indexed under this heading.

Piroxicam (Patients receiving concurrent nonsteroidal anti-inflammatory agents are at increased risk for developing ulcers since tacrine may be expected to increase gastric acid secretion due to increased cholinergic activity). Products include:
Feldene Capsules ... 1965

Procyclidine Hydrochloride (Tacrine has potential to interfere with the activity of anticholinergic drugs). Products include:
Kemadrin Tablets ... 1112

Propantheline Bromide (Tacrine has potential to interfere with the activity of anticholinergic drugs). Products include:
Pro-Banthīne Tablets ... 2052

Pyridostigmine Bromide (Concurrent administration may result in synergistic effect). Products include:
Mestinon Injectable ... 1253
Mestinon ... 1254

Scopolamine (Tacrine has potential to interfere with the activity of anticholinergic drugs). Products include:
Transderm Scōp Transdermal Therapeutic System ... 869

Scopolamine Hydrobromide (Tacrine has potential to interfere with the activity of anticholinergic drugs). Products include:
Atrohist Plus Tablets ... 454
Donnatal ... 2060
Donnatal Extentabs ... 2061
Donnatal Tablets ... 2060

Succinylcholine Chloride (Tacrine, as a cholinesterase inhibitor, may exaggerate succinylcholine-type muscle relaxation during anesthesia). Products include:
Anectine ... 1073

Sulindac (Patients receiving concurrent nonsteroidal anti-inflammatory agents are at increased risk for developing ulcers since tacrine may be expected to increase gastric acid secretion due to increased cholinergic activity). Products include:
Clinoril Tablets ... 1618

Theophylline (Co-administration increases theophylline elimination half-life and average plasma theophylline concentrations by approximately 2-fold). Products include:
Marax Tablets & DF Syrup ... 2200
Quibron ... 2053

Theophylline Anhydrous (Co-administration increases theophylline elimination half-life and average plasma theophylline concentrations by approximately 2-fold). Products include:
Aerolate ... 1004
Primatene Dual Action Formula ... ▣ 872
Primatene Tablets ... ▣ 873
Respbid Tablets ... 682
Slo-bid Gyrocaps ... 2033
Theo-24 Extended Release Capsules ... 2568
Theo-Dur Extended-Release Tablets ... 1327
Theo-X Extended-Release Tablets ... 788
Uni-Dur Extended-Release Tablets ... 1331
Uniphyl 400 mg Tablets ... 2001

Theophylline Calcium Salicylate (Co-administration increases theophylline elimination half-life and average plasma theophylline concentrations by approximately 2-fold). Products include:
Quadrinal Tablets ... 1350

Theophylline Sodium Glycinate (Co-administration increases theophylline elimination half-life and average plasma theophylline concentrations by approximately 2-fold).
No products indexed under this heading.

Tolmetin Sodium (Patients receiving concurrent nonsteroidal anti-inflammatory agents are at increased risk for developing ulcers since tacrine may be expected to increase gastric acid secretion due to increase cholinergic activity). Products include:
Tolectin (200, 400 and 600 mg) ... 1581

Tridihexethyl Chloride (Tacrine has potential to interfere with the activity of anticholinergic drugs).
No products indexed under this heading.

Trihexyphenidyl Hydrochloride (Tacrine has potential to interfere with the activity of anticholinergic drugs). Products include:
Artane ... 1368

Food Interactions

Food, unspecified (Food reduces tacrine bioavailability by approximately 30% to 40%; no effect if tacrine is administered at least one hour before meals).

COLACE
(Docusate Sodium) ... 2044
None cited in PDR database.

COLBENEMID TABLETS
(Probenecid, Colchicine) ... 1622
May interact with penicillins, salicylates, sulfonamides, sulfonylureas, and certain other agents. Compounds in these categories include:

Acetaminophen (Increased plasma concentrations of acetaminophen). Products include:
Actifed Plus Caplets ... ▣ 845
Actifed Plus Tablets ... ▣ 845
Actifed Sinus Daytime/Nighttime Tablets and Caplets ... ▣ 846
Alka-Seltzer Plus Cold Medicine Liqui-Gels ... ▣ 706
Alka-Seltzer Plus Cold & Cough Medicine Liqui-Gels ... ▣ 705
Alka-Seltzer Plus Night-Time Cold Medicine Liqui-Gels ... ▣ 706
Allerest Headache Strength Tablets ... ▣ 627
Allerest No Drowsiness Tablets ... ▣ 627
Allerest Sinus Pain Formula ... ▣ 627
Anexsia 5/500 Elixir ... 1781
Anexia Tablets ... 1782
Arthritis Foundation Aspirin Free Caplets ... ▣ 673
Arthritis Foundation NightTime Caplets ... ▣ 674
Bayer Select Headache Pain Relief Formula ... ▣ 716
Bayer Select Menstrual Multi-Symptom Formula ... ▣ 716
Bayer Select Night Time Pain Relief Formula ... ▣ 716
Bayer Select Sinus Pain Relief Formula ... ▣ 717
Benadryl Allergy Sinus Headache Formula Caplets ... ▣ 849
Comtrex Multi-Symptom Cold Reliever Tablets/Caplets/Liqui-Gels/Liquid ... ▣ 615
Allergy-Sinus Comtrex Multi-Symptom Allergy-Sinus Formula Tablets ... ▣ 617
Comtrex Non-Drowsy ... ▣ 618
Contac Day Allergy/Sinus Caplets ... ▣ 812
Contac Day & Night ... ▣ 812
Contac Night Allergy/Sinus Caplets ... ▣ 812
Contac Severe Cold and Flu Formula Caplets ... ▣ 814
Contac Severe Cold & Flu Non-Drowsy ... ▣ 815
Coricidin 'D' Decongestant Tablets ... ▣ 800
Coricidin Tablets ... ▣ 800
DHCplus Capsules ... 1993
Darvon-N/Darvocet-N ... 1433
Drixoral Cold and Flu Extended-Release Tablets ... ▣ 803
Drixoral Cough + Sore Throat Liquid Caps ... ▣ 802
Drixoral Allergy/Sinus Extended Release Tablets ... ▣ 804
Esgic-plus Tablets ... 1013
Aspirin Free Excedrin Analgesic Caplets and Geltabs ... 732
Excedrin Extra-Strength Analgesic Tablets & Caplets ... 732
Excedrin P.M. Analgesic/Sleeping Aid Tablets, Caplets, Liquigels ... 733
Fioricet Tablets ... 2258
Fioricet with Codeine Capsules ... 2260
Hycomine Compound Tablets ... 932
Hydrocet Capsules ... 782
Legatrin PM ... ▣ 651
Lorcet 10/650 ... 1018
Lortab ... 2566
Lurline PMS Tablets ... 982
Maximum Strength Multi-Symptom Formula Midol ... ▣ 722
PMS Multi-Symptom Formula Midol ... ▣ 723
Teen Multi-Symptom Formula Midol ... ▣ 722
Midrin Capsules ... 783
Migralam Capsules ... 2038
Panodol Tablets and Caplets ... ▣ 824
Children's Panadol Chewable Tablets, Liquid, Infant's Drops ... ▣ 824
Percocet Tablets ... 938
Percogesic Analgesic Tablets ... ▣ 754
Phrenilin ... 785
Pyrroxate Caplets ... ▣ 772
Sedapap Tablets 50 mg/650 mg ... 1543
Sinarest Tablets ... ▣ 648
Sinarest Extra Strength Tablets ... ▣ 648
Sinarest No Drowsiness Tablets ... ▣ 648
Sine-Aid Maximum Strength Sinus Medication Gelcaps, Caplets and Tablets ... 1554
Sine-Off No Drowsiness Formula Caplets ... ▣ 824
Sine-Off Sinus Medicine ... ▣ 825
Singlet Tablets ... ▣ 825
Sinulin Tablets ... 787
Sinutab Sinus Allergy Medication, Maximum Strength Tablets and Caplets ... ▣ 860
Sinutab Sinus Medication, Maximum Strength Without Drowsiness Formula, Tablets & Caplets ... ▣ 860
Sinutab Sinus Medication, Regular Strength Without Drowsiness Formula ... ▣ 859
Sudafed Cold and Cough Liquidcaps ... ▣ 862
Sudafed Severe Cold Formula Caplets ... ▣ 863
Sudafed Severe Cold Formula Tablets ... ▣ 864
Sudafed Sinus Caplets ... ▣ 864
Sudafed Sinus Tablets ... ▣ 864
Talacen ... 2333
TheraFlu ... ▣ 787
TheraFlu Maximum Strength Nighttime Flu, Cold & Cough Medicine ... ▣ 788
TheraFlu Maximum Strength Non-Drowsy Formula Flu, Cold & Cough Medicine ... ▣ 788
Thera Flu Maximum Strength, Non-Drowsy Formula Flu, Cold and Cough Caplets ... ▣ 789
Triaminic Sore Throat Formula ... ▣ 791
Triaminicin Tablets ... ▣ 793
Children's TYLENOL acetaminophen Chewable Tablets, Elixir, Suspension Liquid ... 1555
Children's TYLENOL Cold Multi-Symptom Liquid Formula and Chewable Tablets ... 1561
Children's TYLENOL Cold Plus Cough Multi Symptom Tablets and Liquid ... ▣ 681
Infants' TYLENOL acetaminophen Drops and Suspension Drops ... 1555
Infants' TYLENOL Cold Decongestant & Fever-Reducer Drops ... 1556
TYLENOL Extended Relief Caplets ... 1558
TYLENOL, Extra Strength, Acetaminophen Adult Liquid Pain Reliever ... 1560
TYLENOL, Extra Strength, acetaminophen Gelcaps, Geltabs, Caplets, Tablets ... 1559
TYLENOL, Extra Strength, Headache Plus Pain Reliever with Antacid Caplets ... 1559
TYLENOL, Junior Strength, acetaminophen Coated Caplets, Grape and Fruit Chewable Tablets ... 1557
TYLENOL Maximum Strength Allergy Sinus Medication Gelcaps and Caplets ... 1563
TYLENOL Maximum Strength Allergy Sinus NightTime Medication Caplets ... 1555
TYLENOL Flu Maximum Strength Gelcaps ... 1565
TYLENOL Flu NightTime, Maximum Strength, Gelcaps ... 1566

(▣ Described in PDR For Nonprescription Drugs) (◉ Described in PDR For Ophthalmology)

Interactions Index

Colestid Tablets

TYLENOL Maximum Strength Flu NightTime Hot Medication Packets 1562

TYLENOL, Maximum Strength, Sinus Medication Geltabs, Gelcaps, Caplets and Tablets 1566

TYLENOL Cold Multi-Symptom Formula Medication Tablets and Caplets 1561

TYLENOL Cold Medication No Drowsiness Formula Gelcaps and Caplets 1562

TYLENOL Cold Multi-Symptom Hot Medication Liquid Packets.............. 1557

TYLENOL Cough Multi-Symptom Medication 1564

TYLENOL Cough Multi-Symptom Medication with Decongestant 1565

TYLENOL, Regular Strength, acetaminophen Caplets and Tablets .. 1558

TYLENOL PM, Extra Strength Pain Reliever/Sleep Aid Caplets, Geltabs, Gelcaps... 1560

TYLENOL Severe Allergy Medication Caplets 1564

Tylenol with Codeine 1583

Tylox Capsules 1584

Unisom With Pain Relief-Nighttime Sleep Aid and Pain Reliever............ 1934

Vanquish Analgesic Caplets .... ⊞ 731

Vicks 44 LiquiCaps Cough, Cold & Flu Relief... ⊞ 755

Vicks 44M Cough, Cold & Flu Relief... ⊞ 756

Vicks DayQuil .... ⊞ 761

Vicks Nyquil Hot Therapy.................. ⊞ 762

Vicks NyQuil LiquiCaps Multi-Symptom Cold/Flu Relief .... ⊞ 763

Vicks NyQuil Multi-Symptom Cold/Flu Relief - (Original & Cherry Flavor) .... ⊞ 763

Vicodin Tablets... 1356

Vicodin ES Tablets 1357

Wygesic Tablets 2827

Zydone Capsules 949

Amoxicillin Trihydrate (Elevated plasma concentration of amoxicillin). Products include:

Amoxil... 2464

Augmentin 2468

Ampicillin Sodium (Elevated plasma concentration of ampicillin). Products include:

Unasyn 2212

Aspirin (Uricosuric action of probenecid antagonized). Products include:

Alka-Seltzer Effervescent Antacid and Pain Reliever .... ⊞ 701

Alka-Seltzer Extra Strength Effervescent Antacid and Pain Reliever .... ⊞ 703

Alka-Seltzer Lemon Lime Effervescent Antacid and Pain Reliever .... ⊞ 703

Alka-Seltzer Plus Cold Medicine .... ⊞ 705

Alka-Seltzer Plus Cold & Cough Medicine .... ⊞ 708

Alka-Seltzer Plus Night-Time Cold Medicine .... ⊞ 707

Alka Seltzer Plus Sinus Medicine .. ⊞ 707

Arthritis Foundation Safety Coated Aspirin Tablets .... ⊞ 675

Arthritis Pain Ascriptin .... ⊞ 631

Maximum Strength Ascriptin .... ⊞ 630

Regular Strength Ascriptin Tablets .... ⊞ 629

Arthritis Strength BC Powder.......... ⊞ 609

BC Cold Powder Multi-Symptom Formula (Cold-Sinus-Allergy) ...... ⊞ 609

BC Cold Powder Non-Drowsy Formula (Cold-Sinus) .... ⊞ 609

BC Powder .... ⊞ 609

Bayer Children's Chewable Aspirin... ⊞ 711

Genuine Bayer Aspirin Tablets & Caplets .... ⊞ 713

Extra Strength Bayer Arthritis Pain Regimen Formula .... ⊞ 711

Extra Strength Bayer Aspirin Caplets & Tablets .... ⊞ 712

Extended-Release Bayer 8-Hour Aspirin .... ⊞ 712

Extra Strength Bayer Plus Aspirin Caplets .... ⊞ 713

Extra Strength Bayer PM Aspirin .. ⊞ 713

Bayer Enteric Aspirin .... ⊞ 709

Bufferin Analgesic Tablets and Caplets .... ⊞ 613

Arthritis Strength Bufferin Analgesic Caplets .... ⊞ 614

Extra Strength Bufferin Analgesic Tablets .... ⊞ 615

Cama Arthritis Pain Reliever............ ⊞ 785

Darvon Compound-65 Pulvules 1435

Easprin... 1914

Ecotrin 2455

Ecotrin Enteric Coated Aspirin Maximum Strength Tablets and Caplets .... ⊞ 816

Ecotrin Enteric Coated Aspirin Regular Strength Tablets 2455

Empirin Aspirin Tablets .... ⊞ 854

Empirin with Codeine Tablets............ 1093

Excedrin Extra-Strength Analgesic Tablets & Caplets 732

Fiorinal Capsules 2261

Fiorinal with Codeine Capsules 2262

Fiorinal Tablets... 2261

Halfprin 1362

Healthprin Aspirin 2455

Norgesic... 1496

Percodan Tablets... 939

Percodan-Demi Tablets........................ 940

Robaxisal Tablets... 2071

Soma Compound w/Codeine Tablets 2676

Soma Compound Tablets 2675

St. Joseph Adult Chewable Aspirin (81 mg.) .... ⊞ 808

Talwin Compound 2335

Ursinus Inlay-Tabs................................ ⊞ 794

Vanquish Analgesic Caplets .... ⊞ 731

Azlocillin Sodium (Elevated plasma concentration of azlocillin).

No products indexed under this heading.

Bacampicillin Hydrochloride (Elevated plasma concentration of bacampicillin). Products include:

Spectrobid Tablets 2206

Carbenicillin Disodium (Elevated plasma concentration of carbenicillin).

No products indexed under this heading.

Carbenicillin Indanyl Sodium (Elevated plasma concentration of carbenicillin). Products include:

Geocillin Tablets... 2199

Chlorpropamide (Prolonged or enhanced action of oral sulfonylureas). Products include:

Diabinese Tablets 1935

Choline Magnesium Trisalicylate (Uricosuric action of probenecid antagonized). Products include:

Trilisate 2000

Dicloxacillin Sodium (Elevated plasma concentration of amoxicillin).

No products indexed under this heading.

Diflunisal (Uricosuric action of probenecid antagonized). Products include:

Dolobid Tablets... 1654

Glipizide (Prolonged or enhanced action of oral sulfonylureas). Products include:

Glucotrol Tablets 1967

Glucotrol XL Extended Release Tablets 1968

Glyburide (Prolonged or enhanced action of oral sulfonylureas). Products include:

DiaBeta Tablets 1239

Glynase PresTab Tablets 2609

Micronase Tablets 2623

Indomethacin (Increased plasma levels of indomethacin). Products include:

Indocin 1680

Indomethacin Sodium Trihydrate (Increased plasma levels of indomethacin). Products include:

Indocin I.V. 1684

Ketamine Hydrochloride (Anesthesia prolonged).

No products indexed under this heading.

Ketoprofen (Increased plasma concentrations of ketoprofen). Products include:

Orudis Capsules 2766

Oruvail Capsules 2766

Lorazepam (Increased plasma concentrations of lorazepam). Products include:

Ativan Injection... 2698

Ativan Tablets 2700

Magnesium Salicylate (Uricosuric action of probenecid antagonized). Products include:

Backache Caplets .... ⊞ 613

Bayer Select Backache Pain Relief Formula .... ⊞ 715

Doan's Extra-Strength Analgesic.... ⊞ 633

Extra Strength Doan's P.M................ ⊞ 633

Doan's Regular Strength Analgesic... ⊞ 634

Mobigesic Tablets .... ⊞ 602

Meclofenamate Sodium (Increased plasma concentrations of meclofenamate).

No products indexed under this heading.

Methotrexate Sodium (In concurrent administration methotrexate dosage should be reduced). Products include:

Methotrexate Sodium Tablets, Injection, for Injection and LPF Injection 1275

Mezlocillin Sodium (Elevated plasma concentration of mezlocillin). Products include:

Mezlin... 601

Mezlin Pharmacy Bulk Package........ 604

Nafcillin Sodium (Elevated plasma concentration of nafcillin).

No products indexed under this heading.

Naproxen (Increased plasma concentrations of naproxen). Products include:

Anaprox/Naprosyn 2117

Naproxen Sodium (Increased plasma concentrations of naproxen). Products include:

Aleve 1975

Anaprox/Naprosyn 2117

Penicillin G Benzathine (Elevated plasma concentration of penicillin). Products include:

Bicillin C-R Injection 2704

Bicillin C-R 900/300 Injection 2706

Bicillin L-A Injection 2707

Penicillin G Potassium (Elevated plasma concentration of penicillin). Products include:

Pfizerpen for Injection 2203

Penicillin G Procaine (Elevated plasma concentration of penicillin). Products include:

Bicillin C-R Injection 2704

Bicillin C-R 900/300 Injection 2706

Penicillin G Sodium (Elevated plasma concentration of penicillin).

No products indexed under this heading.

Penicillin V Potassium (Elevated plasma concentration of penicillin). Products include:

Pen•Vee K... 2772

Pyrazinamide (Uricosuric action of probenecid antagonized). Products include:

Pyrazinamide Tablets 1398

Rifater... 1532

Rifampin (Increased plasma concentrations of rifampin). Products include:

Rifadin 1528

Rifamate Capsules 1530

Rifater... 1532

Rimactane Capsules 847

Salsalate (Uricosuric action of probenecid antagonized). Products include:

Mono-Gesic Tablets 792

Salflex Tablets... 786

Sulfamethizole (Significant increase in total sulfonamide plasma levels). Products include:

Urobiotic-250 Capsules 2214

Sulfamethoxazole (Significant increase in total sulfonamide plasma levels). Products include:

Azo Gantanol Tablets............................ 2080

Bactrim DS Tablets................................ 2084

Bactrim I.V. Infusion 2082

Bactrim 2084

Gantanol Tablets 2119

Septra... 1174

Septra I.V. Infusion 1169

Septra I.V. Infusion ADD-Vantage Vials... 1171

Septra 1174

Sulfasalazine (Significant increase in total sulfonamide plasma levels). Products include:

Azulfidine 1949

Sulfinpyrazone (Significant increase in total sulfonamide plasma levels). Products include:

Anturane 807

Sulfisoxazole (Significant increase in total sulfonamide plasma levels). Products include:

Azo Gantrisin Tablets............................ 2081

Gantrisin Tablets 2120

Sulfisoxazole Diolamine (Significant increase in total sulfonamide plasma levels).

No products indexed under this heading.

Sulindac (Increased plasma levels of sulindac; modest reduction in uricosuric action of probenecid). Products include:

Clinoril Tablets 1618

Ticarcillin Disodium (Elevated plasma concentration of ticarcillin). Products include:

Ticar for Injection 2526

Timentin for Injection............................ 2528

Tolazamide (Prolonged or enhanced action of oral sulfonylureas).

No products indexed under this heading.

Tolbutamide (Prolonged or enhanced action of oral sulfonylureas).

No products indexed under this heading.

COLESTID TABLETS

(Colestipol Hydrochloride) 2591

May interact with cardiac glycosides and certain other agents. Compounds in these categories include:

Chlorothiazide (Absorption of chlorothiazide is markedly decreased). Products include:

Aldoclor Tablets 1598

Diupres Tablets 1650

Diuril Oral 1653

Deslanoside (Potential for binding of digitalis glycosides).

No products indexed under this heading.

Digitoxin (Potential for binding of digitalis glycosides). Products include:

Crystodigin Tablets................................ 1433

Digoxin (Potential for binding of digitalis glycosides). Products include:

Lanoxicaps 1117

Lanoxin Elixir Pediatric 1120

Lanoxin Injection 1123

Lanoxin Injection Pediatric.................. 1126

Lanoxin Tablets 1128

IMPORTANT NOTE: Always consult each drug listing in the patient's regimen for possible interactions.

Folic Acid (Colestipol may reduce absorption of folic acid). Products include:

- Cefol Filmtab 412
- Fero-Folic-500 Filmtab 429
- Iberet-Folic-500 Filmtab 429
- Materna Tablets 1379
- Mega-B 512
- Megadose 512
- Nephro-Fer Rx Tablets 2005
- Nephro-Vite + Fe Tablets 2006
- Nephro-Vite Rx Tablets 2006
- Niferex-150 Forte Capsules 794
- Niferex Forte Elixir 794
- Sigtab Tablets .... ▣ 772
- Slow Fe with Folic Acid 869
- Stuart Prenatal Tablets .... ▣ 881
- The Stuart Formula Tablets .... ▣ 663
- Trinsicon Capsules 2570
- Zymacap Capsules .... ▣ 772

Furosemide (Absorption of furosemide is significantly decreased). Products include:

- Lasix Injection, Oral Solution and Tablets 1240

Gemfibrozil (Absorption of gemfibrizil is significantly decreased). Products include:

- Lopid Tablets 1917

Hydrochlorothiazide (Absorption of hydrochlorothiazide is significantly decreased). Products include:

- Aldactazide 2413
- Aldoril Tablets 1604
- Apresazide Capsules 808
- Capozide 742
- Dyazide 2479
- Esidrix Tablets 821
- Esimil Tablets 822
- HydroDIURIL Tablets 1674
- Hydropres Tablets 1675
- Hyzaar Tablets 1677
- Inderide Tablets 2732
- Inderide LA Long Acting Capsules 2734
- Lopressor HCT Tablets 832
- Lotensin HCT 837
- Maxzide 1380
- Moduretic Tablets 1705
- Oretic Tablets 443
- Prinzide Tablets 1737
- Ser-Ap-Es Tablets 849
- Timolide Tablets 1748
- Vaseretic Tablets 1765
- Zestoretic 2850
- Ziac 1415

Penicillin V Potassium (Absorption of penicillin G is significantly decreased). Products include:

- Pen•Vee K 2772

Phytonadione (Colestipol may reduce absorption of vitamin K). Products include:

- AquaMEPHYTON Injection 1608
- Konakion Injection 2127
- Mephyton Tablets 1696

Propranolol Hydrochloride (Potential for decreased propranolol absorption). Products include:

- Inderal 2728
- Inderal LA Long Acting Capsules 2730
- Inderide Tablets 2732
- Inderide LA Long Acting Capsules 2734

Vitamin A (Colestipol may reduce absorption of vitamin A). Products include:

- Aquasol A Vitamin A Capsules, USP 534
- Aquasol A Parenteral 534
- Materna Tablets 1379
- Megadose 512
- Nature Made Antioxidant Formula .... ▣ 748
- One-A-Day Extras Antioxidant .... ▣ 728
- Theragran Antioxidant .... ▣ 623
- Zymacap Capsules .... ▣ 772

Vitamin D (Colestipol may reduce absorption of vitamin D). Products include:

- Caltrate PLUS .... ▣ 665
- Caltrate 600 + D .... ▣ 665
- Citracal Caplets + D 1780
- Dical-D Tablets & Wafers 420
- Drisdol .... ▣ 794
- Materna Tablets 1379
- Megadose 512
- Zymacap Capsules .... ▣ 772

Vitamin K (Colestipol may reduce absorption of vitamin K).

No products indexed under this heading.

COLLAGEN PLUGS (INTRACANALICULAR)

(Collagen, bovine) .... ⊙ 284
None cited in PDR database.

COLLAGENASE SANTYL OINTMENT

(Collagenase) 1334
May interact with:

Cortisone Acetate (Chronic concurrent use may result in systemic manifestations of hypersensitivity to collagenase). Products include:

- Cortone Acetate Sterile Suspension 1623
- Cortone Acetate Tablets 1624

COLLYRIUM FOR FRESH EYES

(Boric Acid, Sodium Borate) .... ▣ 878
May interact with:

Polyvinyl Alcohol (Avoid concurrent use). Products include:

- Hypotears .... ⊙ 265
- Liquifilm Wetting Solution .... ⊙ 337
- Murine Lubricant Eye Drops .... ▣ 781
- Murine Plus Lubricant Redness Reliever Eye Drops .... ▣ 781
- Murine Tears Lubricant Eye Drops ⊙ 316
- Murine Tears Plus Lubricant Redness Reliever Eye Drops .... ⊙ 316
- Total All-In-One Hard Contact Lens Solution .... ⊙ 342
- Wet-N-Soak Plus Wetting and Soaking Solution .... ⊙ 345

COLLYRIUM FRESH

(Tetrahydrozoline Hydrochloride, Glycerin) .... ▣ 879
None cited in PDR database.

COLY-MYCIN M PARENTERAL

(Colistimethate Sodium) 1905
May interact with:

Decamethonium (Potentiation of neuromuscular blocking effect of Coly-Mycin M).

Dihydrostreptomycin (Interference with nerve transmission at the neuromuscular junction).

Ether (Potentiation of neuromuscular blocking effect of Coly-Mycin M).

Gallamine (Potentiation of neuromuscular blocking effect of Coly-Mycin M).

Kanamycin Sulfate (Interference with nerve transmission at the neuromuscular junction).

No products indexed under this heading.

Neomycin, oral (Interference with nerve transmission at the neuromuscular junction).

Polymyxin Preparations (Interference with nerve transmission at the neuromuscular junction).

Sodium Citrate (Potentiation of neuromuscular blocking effect of Coly-Mycin M). Products include:

- Bicitra 578
- Citrocarbonate Antacid .... ▣ 770
- Polycitra 578
- Salix SST Lozenges Saliva Stimulant .... ▣ 797

Streptomycin Sulfate (Interference with nerve transmission at the neuromuscular junction). Products include:

- Streptomycin Sulfate Injection 2208

Succinylcholine Chloride (Potentiation of neuromuscular blocking effect of Coly-Mycin M). Products include:

- Anectine 1073

Tubocurarine Chloride (Potentiation of neuromuscular blocking effect of Coly-Mycin M).

No products indexed under this heading.

COLY-MYCIN S OTIC W/NEOMYCIN & HYDROCORTISONE

(Colistin Sulfate, Neomycin Sulfate, Hydrocortisone Acetate) 1906
None cited in PDR database.

COLYTE AND COLYTE-FLAVORED

(Polyethylene Glycol) 2396
May interact with:

Oral Medications, unspecified (Those administered within one hour of Colyte usage may be flushed from the gastrointestinal tract and not absorbed).

COMBIPRES TABLETS

(Clonidine Hydrochloride, Chlorthalidone) 677
May interact with tricyclic antidepressants, barbiturates, hypnotics and sedatives, cardiac glycosides, antihypertensives, insulin, oral hypoglycemic agents, lithium preparations, narcotic analgesics, and certain other agents. Compounds in these categories include:

Acarbose (Higher dosage of oral hypoglycemic agents may be required).

No products indexed under this heading.

Acebutolol Hydrochloride (Chlorthalidone may add to or potentiate the action of other antihypertensive drugs). Products include:

- Sectral Capsules 2807

Alfentanil Hydrochloride (Orthostatic hypotension). Products include:

- Alfenta Injection 1286

Amitriptyline Hydrochloride (Enhanced manifestation of corneal lesions (in rats); reduced effect of clonidine). Products include:

- Elavil 2838
- Endep Tablets 2174
- Etrafon 2355
- Limbitrol 2180
- Triavil Tablets 1757

Amlodipine Besylate (Chlorthalidone may add to or potentiate the action of other antihypertensive drugs). Products include:

- Lotrel Capsules 840
- Norvasc Tablets 1940

Amoxapine (Reduced effect of clonidine). Products include:

- Asendin Tablets 1369

Aprobarbital (Orthostatic hypotension; enhanced CNS-depressive effects).

No products indexed under this heading.

Atenolol (Chlorthalidone may add to or potentiate the action of other antihypertensive drugs). Products include:

- Tenoretic Tablets 2845
- Tenormin Tablets and I.V. Injection 2847

Benazepril Hydrochloride (Chlorthalidone may add to or potentiate the action of other antihypertensive drugs). Products include:

- Lotensin Tablets 834
- Lotensin HCT 837
- Lotrel Capsules 840

Bendroflumethiazide (Chlorthalidone may add to or potentiate the action of other antihypertensive drugs).

No products indexed under this heading.

Betaxolol Hydrochloride (Chlorthalidone may add to or potentiate the action of other antihypertensive drugs). Products include:

- Betoptic Ophthalmic Solution 469
- Betoptic S Ophthalmic Suspension 471
- Kerlone Tablets 2436

Bisoprolol Fumarate (Chlorthalidone may add to or potentiate the action of other antihypertensive drugs). Products include:

- Zebeta Tablets 1413
- Ziac 1415

Buprenorphine (Orthostatic hypotension). Products include:

- Buprenex Injectable 2006

Butabarbital (Orthostatic hypotension; enhanced CNS-depressive effects).

No products indexed under this heading.

Butalbital (Orthostatic hypotension; enhanced CNS-depressive effects). Products include:

- Esgic-plus Tablets 1013
- Fioricet Tablets 2258
- Fioricet with Codeine Capsules 2260
- Fiorinal Capsules 2261
- Fiorinal with Codeine Capsules 2262
- Fiorinal Tablets 2261
- Phrenilin 785
- Sedapap Tablets 50 mg/650 mg 1543

Captopril (Chlorthalidone may add to or potentiate the action of other antihypertensive drugs). Products include:

- Capoten 739
- Capozide 742

Carteolol Hydrochloride (Chlorthalidone may add to or potentiate the action of other antihypertensive drugs). Products include:

- Cartrol Tablets 410
- Ocupress Ophthalmic Solution, 1% Sterile .... ⊙ 309

Chlorothiazide (Chlorthalidone may add to or potentiate the action of other antihypertensive drugs). Products include:

- Aldoclor Tablets 1598
- Diupres Tablets 1650
- Diuril Oral 1653

Chlorothiazide Sodium (Chlorthalidone may add to or potentiate the action of other antihypertensive drugs). Products include:

- Diuril Sodium Intravenous 1652

Chlorpropamide (Higher dosage of oral hypoglycemic agents may be required). Products include:

- Diabinese Tablets 1935

Clomipramine Hydrochloride (Enhanced manifestation of corneal lesions (in rats); reduced effect of clonidine). Products include:

- Anafranil Capsules 803

Clonidine (Chlorthalidone may add to or potentiate the action of other antihypertensive drugs). Products include:

- Catapres-TTS 675

Codeine Phosphate (Orthostatic hypotension). Products include:

- Actifed with Codeine Cough Syrup 1067
- Brontex 1981
- Deconsal C Expectorant Syrup 456
- Deconsal Pediatric Syrup 457
- Dimetane-DC Cough Syrup 2059
- Empirin with Codeine Tablets 1093
- Fioricet with Codeine Capsules 2260
- Fiorinal with Codeine Capsules 2262
- Isoclor Expectorant 990
- Novahistine DH 2462
- Novahistine Expectorant 2463
- Nucofed 2051

(▣ Described in PDR For Nonprescription Drugs) (⊙ Described in PDR For Ophthalmology)

191 **Interactions Index** **Combipres**

Phenergan with Codeine 2777
Phenergan VC with Codeine 2781
Robitussin A-C Syrup 2073
Robitussin-DAC Syrup 2074
Ryna 841
Soma Compound w/Codeine Tablets 2676
Tussi-Organidin NR Liquid and S NR Liquid 2677
Tylenol with Codeine 1583

Deserpidine (Chlorthalidone may add to or potentiate the action of other antihypertensive drugs).
No products indexed under this heading.

Desipramine Hydrochloride (Reduced effect of clonidine). Products include:
Norpramin Tablets 1526

Deslanoside (Sinus bradycardia and atrioventricular block (rare)).
No products indexed under this heading.

Dezocine (Orthostatic hypotension). Products include:
Dalgan Injection 538

Diazoxide (Chlorthalidone may add to or potentiate the action of other antihypertensive drugs). Products include:
Hyperstat I.V. Injection 2363
Proglycem 580

Digitoxin (Sinus bradycardia and atrioventricular block (rare)). Products include:
Crystodigin Tablets 1433

Digoxin (Sinus bradycardia and atrioventricular block (rare)). Products include:
Lanoxicaps 1117
Lanoxin Elixir Pediatric 1120
Lanoxin Injection 1123
Lanoxin Injection Pediatric 1126
Lanoxin Tablets 1128

Diltiazem Hydrochloride (Chlorthalidone may add to or potentiate the action of other antihypertensive drugs). Products include:
Cardizem CD Capsules 1506
Cardizem SR Capsules 1510
Cardizem Injectable 1508
Cardizem Tablets 1512
Dilacor XR Extended-release Capsules 2018

Doxazosin Mesylate (Chlorthalidone may add to or potentiate the action of other antihypertensive drugs). Products include:
Cardura Tablets 2186

Doxepin Hydrochloride (Reduced effect of clonidine). Products include:
Sinequan 2205
Zonalon Cream 1055

Enalapril Maleate (Chlorthalidone may add to or potentiate the action of other antihypertensive drugs). Products include:
Vaseretic Tablets 1765
Vasotec Tablets 1771

Enalaprilat (Chlorthalidone may add to or potentiate the action of other antihypertensive drugs). Products include:
Vasotec I.V. 1768

Esmolol Hydrochloride (Chlorthalidone may add to or potentiate the action of other antihypertensive drugs). Products include:
Brevibloc Injection 1808

Estazolam (Enhanced CNS-depressive effects). Products include:
ProSom Tablets 449

Ethchlorvynol (Enhanced CNS-depressive effects). Products include:
Placidyl Capsules 448

Ethinamate (Enhanced CNS-depressive effects).
No products indexed under this heading.

Felodipine (Chlorthalidone may add to or potentiate the action of other antihypertensive drugs). Products include:
Plendil Extended-Release Tablets 527

Fentanyl (Orthostatic hypotension). Products include:
Duragesic Transdermal System 1288

Fentanyl Citrate (Orthostatic hypotension). Products include:
Sublimaze Injection 1307

Flurazepam Hydrochloride (Enhanced CNS-depressive effects). Products include:
Dalmane Capsules 2173

Fosinopril Sodium (Chlorthalidone may add to or potentiate the action of other antihypertensive drugs). Products include:
Monopril Tablets 757

Furosemide (Chlorthalidone may add to or potentiate the action of other antihypertensive drugs). Products include:
Lasix Injection, Oral Solution and Tablets 1240

Glipizide (Higher dosage of oral hypoglycemic agents may be required). Products include:
Glucotrol Tablets 1967
Glucotrol XL Extended Release Tablets 1968

Glutethimide (Enhanced CNS-depressive effects).
No products indexed under this heading.

Glyburide (Higher dosage of oral hypoglycemic agents may be required). Products include:
DiaBeta Tablets 1239
Glynase PresTab Tablets 2609
Micronase Tablets 2623

Guanabenz Acetate (Chlorthalidone may add to or potentiate the action of other antihypertensive drugs).
No products indexed under this heading.

Guanethidine Monosulfate (Chlorthalidone may add to or potentiate the action of other antihypertensive drugs). Products include:
Esimil Tablets 822
Ismelin Tablets 827

Hydralazine Hydrochloride (Chlorthalidone may add to or potentiate the action of other antihypertensive drugs). Products include:
Apresazide Capsules 808
Apresoline Hydrochloride Tablets 809
Ser-Ap-Es Tablets 849

Hydrochlorothiazide (Chlorthalidone may add to or potentiate the action of other antihypertensive drugs). Products include:
Aldactazide 2413
Aldoril Tablets 1604
Apresazide Capsules 808
Capozide 742
Dyazide 2479
Esidrix Tablets 821
Esimil Tablets 822
HydroDIURIL Tablets 1674
Hydropres Tablets 1675
Hyzaar Tablets 1677
Inderide Tablets 2732
Inderide LA Long Acting Capsules 2734
Lopressor HCT Tablets 832
Lotensin HCT 837
Maxzide 1380
Moduretic Tablets 1705
Oretic Tablets 443
Prinzide Tablets 1737
Ser-Ap-Es Tablets 849
Timolide Tablets 1748
Vaseretic Tablets 1765
Zestoretic 2850
Ziac 1415

Hydrocodone Bitartrate (Orthostatic hypotension). Products include:
Anexsia 5/500 Elixir 1781
Anexia Tablets 1782
Codiclear DH Syrup 791
Deconamine CX Cough and Cold Liquid and Tablets 1319
Duratuss HD Elixir 2565
Hycodan Tablets and Syrup 930
Hycomine Compound Tablets 932
Hycomine 931
Hycotuss Expectorant Syrup 933
Hydrocet Capsules 782
Lorcet 10/650 1018
Lortab 2566
Tussend 1783
Tussend Expectorant 1785
Vicodin Tablets 1356
Vicodin ES Tablets 1357
Vicodin Tuss Expectorant 1358
Zydone Capsules 949

Hydrocodone Polistirex (Orthostatic hypotension). Products include:
Tussionex Pennkinetic Extended-Release Suspension 998

Hydroflumethiazide (Chlorthalidone may add to or potentiate the action of other antihypertensive drugs). Products include:
Diucardin Tablets 2718

Imipramine Hydrochloride (Reduced effect of clonidine). Products include:
Tofranil Ampuls 854
Tofranil Tablets 856

Imipramine Pamoate (Reduced effect of clonidine). Products include:
Tofranil-PM Capsules 857

Indapamide (Chlorthalidone may add to or potentiate the action of other antihypertensive drugs). Products include:
Lozol Tablets 2022

Insulin, Human (Insulin requirements in diabetic patients may be increased, decreased or unchanged).
No products indexed under this heading.

Insulin, Human Isophane Suspension (Insulin requirements in diabetic patients may be increased, decreased or unchanged). Products include:
Novolin N Human Insulin 10 ml Vials 1795

Insulin, Human NPH (Insulin requirements in diabetic patients may be increased, decreased or unchanged). Products include:
Humulin N, 100 Units 1448
Novolin N PenFill Cartridges Durable Insulin Delivery System 1798
Novolin N Prefilled Syringe Disposable Insulin Delivery System 1798

Insulin, Human Regular (Insulin requirements in diabetic patients may be increased, decreased or unchanged). Products include:
Humulin R, 100 Units 1449
Novolin R Human Insulin 10 ml Vials 1795
Novolin R PenFill Cartridges Durable Insulin Delivery System 1798
Novolin R Prefilled Syringe Disposable Insulin Delivery System 1798
Velosulin BR Human Insulin 10 ml Vials 1795

Insulin, Human, Zinc Suspension (Insulin requirements in diabetic patients may be increased, decreased or unchanged). Products include:
Humulin L, 100 Units 1446
Humulin U, 100 Units 1450
Novolin L Human Insulin 10 ml Vials 1795

Insulin, NPH (Insulin requirements in diabetic patients may be increased, decreased or unchanged). Products include:
NPH, 100 Units 1450
Pork NPH, 100 Units 1452
Purified Pork NPH Isophane Insulin 1801

Insulin, Regular (Insulin requirements in diabetic patients may be increased, decreased or unchanged). Products include:
Regular, 100 Units 1450
Pork Regular, 100 Units 1452
Pork Regular (Concentrated), 500 Units 1453
Purified Pork Regular Insulin 1801

Insulin, Zinc Crystals (Insulin requirements in diabetic patients may be increased, decreased or unchanged). Products include:
NPH, 100 Units 1450

Insulin, Zinc Suspension (Insulin requirements in diabetic patients may be increased, decreased or unchanged). Products include:
Iletin I 1450
Lente, 100 Units 1450
Iletin II 1452
Pork Lente, 100 Units 1452
Purified Pork Lente Insulin 1801

Isradipine (Chlorthalidone may add to or potentiate the action of other antihypertensive drugs). Products include:
DynaCirc Capsules 2256

Labetalol Hydrochloride (Chlorthalidone may add to or potentiate the action of other antihypertensive drugs). Products include:
Normodyne Injection 2377
Normodyne Tablets 2379
Trandate 1185

Levorphanol Tartrate (Orthostatic hypotension). Products include:
Levo-Dromoran 2129

Lisinopril (Chlorthalidone may add to or potentiate the action of other antihypertensive drugs). Products include:
Prinivil Tablets 1733
Prinzide Tablets 1737
Zestoretic 2850
Zestril Tablets 2854

Lithium Carbonate (Reduced renal lithium clearance and increased risk of lithium toxicity). Products include:
Eskalith 2485
Lithium Carbonate Capsules & Tablets 2230
Lithonate/Lithotabs/Lithobid 2543

Lithium Citrate (Reduced renal lithium clearance and increased risk of lithium toxicity).
No products indexed under this heading.

Lorazepam (Enhanced CNS-depressive effects). Products include:
Ativan Injection 2698
Ativan Tablets 2700

Losartan Potassium (Chlorthalidone may add to or potentiate the action of other antihypertensive drugs). Products include:
Cozaar Tablets 1628
Hyzaar Tablets 1677

Maprotiline Hydrochloride (Reduced effect of clonidine). Products include:
Ludiomil Tablets 843

Mecamylamine Hydrochloride (Chlorthalidone may add to or potentiate the action of other antihypertensive drugs). Products include:
Inversine Tablets 1686

IMPORTANT NOTE: Always consult each drug listing in the patient's regimen for possible interactions.

Combipres Interactions Index 192

Meperidine Hydrochloride (Orthostatic hypotension). Products include:
- Demerol ... 2308
- Mepergan Injection ... 2753

Mephobarbital (Orthostatic hypotension; enhanced CNS-depressive effects). Products include:
- Mebaral Tablets ... 2322

Metformin Hydrochloride (Higher dosage of oral hypoglycemic agents may be required). Products include:
- Glucophage ... 752

Methadone Hydrochloride (Orthostatic hypotension). Products include:
- Methadone Hydrochloride Oral Concentrate ... 2233
- Methadone Hydrochloride Oral Solution & Tablets ... 2235

Methyclothiazide (Chlorthalidone may add to or potentiate the action of other antihypertensive drugs). Products include:
- Enduron Tablets ... 420

Methyldopa (Chlorthalidone may add to or potentiate the action of other antihypertensive drugs). Products include:
- Aldoclor Tablets ... 1598
- Aldomet Oral ... 1600
- Aldoril Tablets ... 1604

Methyldopate Hydrochloride (Chlorthalidone may add to or potentiate the action of other antihypertensive drugs). Products include:
- Aldomet Ester HCl Injection ... 1602

Metolazone (Chlorthalidone may add to or potentiate the action of other antihypertensive drugs). Products include:
- Mykrox Tablets ... 993
- Zaroxolyn Tablets ... 1000

Metoprolol Succinate (Chlorthalidone may add to or potentiate the action of other antihypertensive drugs). Products include:
- Toprol-XL Tablets ... 565

Metoprolol Tartrate (Chlorthalidone may add to or potentiate the action of other antihypertensive drugs). Products include:
- Lopressor Ampuls ... 830
- Lopressor HCT Tablets ... 832
- Lopressor Tablets ... 830

Metyrosine (Chlorthalidone may add to or potentiate the action of other antihypertensive drugs). Products include:
- Demser Capsules ... 1649

Midazolam Hydrochloride (Enhanced CNS-depressive effects). Products include:
- Versed Injection ... 2170

Minoxidil (Chlorthalidone may add to or potentiate the action of other antihypertensive drugs). Products include:
- Loniten Tablets ... 2618
- Rogaine Topical Solution ... 2637

Moexipril Hydrochloride (Chlorthalidone may add to or potentiate the action of other antihypertensive drugs). Products include:
- Univasc Tablets ... 2410

Morphine Sulfate (Orthostatic hypotension). Products include:
- Astramorph/PF Injection, USP (Preservative-Free) ... 535
- Duramorph ... 962
- Infumorph 200 and Infumorph 500 Sterile Solutions ... 965
- MS Contin Tablets ... 1994
- MSIR ... 1997
- Oramorph SR (Morphine Sulfate Sustained Release Tablets) ... 2236
- RMS Suppositories ... 2657
- Roxanol ... 2243

Nadolol (Chlorthalidone may add to or potentiate the action of other antihypertensive drugs).
- No products indexed under this heading.

Nicardipine Hydrochloride (Chlorthalidone may add to or potentiate the action of other antihypertensive drugs). Products include:
- Cardene Capsules ... 2095
- Cardene I.V. ... 2709
- Cardene SR Capsules ... 2097

Nifedipine (Chlorthalidone may add to or potentiate the action of other antihypertensive drugs). Products include:
- Adalat Capsules (10 mg and 20 mg) ... 587
- Adalat CC ... 589
- Procardia Capsules ... 1971
- Procardia XL Extended Release Tablets ... 1972

Nisoldipine (Chlorthalidone may add to or potentiate the action of other antihypertensive drugs).
- No products indexed under this heading.

Nitroglycerin (Chlorthalidone may add to or potentiate the action of other antihypertensive drugs). Products include:
- Deponit NTG Transdermal Delivery System ... 2397
- Nitro-Bid IV ... 1523
- Nitro-Bid Ointment ... 1524
- Nitrodisc ... 2047
- Nitro-Dur (nitroglycerin) Transdermal Infusion System ... 1326
- Nitrolingual Spray ... 2027
- Nitrostat Tablets ... 1925
- Transderm-Nitro Transdermal Therapeutic System ... 859

Norepinephrine Bitartrate (Decreased arterial responsiveness to norepinephrine). Products include:
- Levophed Bitartrate Injection ... 2315

Nortriptyline Hydrochloride (Reduced effect of clonidine). Products include:
- Pamelor ... 2280

Opium Alkaloids (Orthostatic hypotension).
- No products indexed under this heading.

Oxycodone Hydrochloride (Orthostatic hypotension). Products include:
- Percocet Tablets ... 938
- Percodan Tablets ... 939
- Percodan-Demi Tablets ... 940
- Roxicodone Tablets, Oral Solution & Intensol (Oxycodone) ... 2244
- Tylox Capsules ... 1584

Papaverine (Drug-induced hepatitis (one case)).

Penbutolol Sulfate (Chlorthalidone may add to or potentiate the action of other antihypertensive drugs). Products include:
- Levatol ... 2403

Pentobarbital Sodium (Orthostatic hypotension; enhanced CNS-depressive effects). Products include:
- Nembutal Sodium Capsules ... 436
- Nembutal Sodium Solution ... 438
- Nembutal Sodium Suppositories ... 440

Phenobarbital (Orthostatic hypotension; enhanced CNS-depressive effects). Products include:
- Arco-Lase Plus Tablets ... 512
- Bellergal-S Tablets ... 2250
- Donnatal ... 2060
- Donnatal Extentabs ... 2061
- Donnatal Tablets ... 2060
- Phenobarbital Elixir and Tablets ... 1469
- Quadrinal Tablets ... 1350

Phenoxybenzamine Hydrochloride (Chlorthalidone may add to or potentiate the action of other antihypertensive drugs). Products include:
- Dibenzyline Capsules ... 2476

Phentolamine Mesylate (Chlorthalidone may add to or potentiate the action of other antihypertensive drugs). Products include:
- Regitine ... 846

Pindolol (Chlorthalidone may add to or potentiate the action of other antihypertensive drugs). Products include:
- Visken Tablets ... 2299

Polythiazide (Chlorthalidone may add to or potentiate the action of other antihypertensive drugs). Products include:
- Minizide Capsules ... 1938

Prazosin Hydrochloride (Chlorthalidone may add to or potentiate the action of other antihypertensive drugs). Products include:
- Minipress Capsules ... 1937
- Minizide Capsules ... 1938

Propofol (Enhanced CNS-depressive effects). Products include:
- Diprivan Injection ... 2833

Propoxyphene Hydrochloride (Orthostatic hypotension). Products include:
- Darvon ... 1435
- Wygesic Tablets ... 2827

Propoxyphene Napsylate (Orthostatic hypotension). Products include:
- Darvon-N/Darvocet-N ... 1433

Propranolol Hydrochloride (Chlorthalidone may add to or potentiate the action of other antihypertensive drugs). Products include:
- Inderal ... 2728
- Inderal LA Long Acting Capsules ... 2730
- Inderide Tablets ... 2732
- Inderide LA Long Acting Capsules ... 2734

Protriptyline Hydrochloride (Reduced effect of clonidine). Products include:
- Vivactil Tablets ... 1774

Quazepam (Enhanced CNS-depressive effects). Products include:
- Doral Tablets ... 2664

Quinapril Hydrochloride (Chlorthalidone may add to or potentiate the action of other antihypertensive drugs). Products include:
- Accupril Tablets ... 1893

Ramipril (Chlorthalidone may add to or potentiate the action of other antihypertensive drugs). Products include:
- Altace Capsules ... 1232

Rauwolfia Serpentina (Chlorthalidone may add to or potentiate the action of other antihypertensive drugs).
- No products indexed under this heading.

Rescinnamine (Chlorthalidone may add to or potentiate the action of other antihypertensive drugs).
- No products indexed under this heading.

Reserpine (Chlorthalidone may add to or potentiate the action of other antihypertensive drugs). Products include:
- Diupres Tablets ... 1650
- Hydropres Tablets ... 1675
- Ser-Ap-Es Tablets ... 849

Secobarbital Sodium (Orthostatic hypotension; enhanced CNS-depressive effects). Products include:
- Seconal Sodium Pulvules ... 1474

Sodium Nitroprusside (Chlorthalidone may add to or potentiate the action of other antihypertensive drugs).
- No products indexed under this heading.

Sotalol Hydrochloride (Chlorthalidone may add to or potentiate the action of other antihypertensive drugs). Products include:
- Betapace Tablets ... 641

Spirapril Hydrochloride (Chlorthalidone may add to or potentiate the action of other antihypertensive drugs).
- No products indexed under this heading.

Sufentanil Citrate (Orthostatic hypotension). Products include:
- Sufenta Injection ... 1309

Temazepam (Enhanced CNS-depressive effects). Products include:
- Restoril Capsules ... 2284

Terazosin Hydrochloride (Chlorthalidone may add to or potentiate the action of other antihypertensive drugs). Products include:
- Hytrin Capsules ... 430

Thiamylal Sodium (Orthostatic hypotension; enhanced CNS-depressive effects).
- No products indexed under this heading.

Timolol Maleate (Chlorthalidone may add to or potentiate the action of other antihypertensive drugs). Products include:
- Blocadren Tablets ... 1614
- Timolide Tablets ... 1748
- Timoptic in Ocudose ... 1753
- Timoptic Sterile Ophthalmic Solution ... 1751
- Timoptic-XE ... 1755

Tolazamide (Higher dosage of oral hypoglycemic agents may be required).
- No products indexed under this heading.

Tolbutamide (Higher dosage of oral hypoglycemic agents may be required).
- No products indexed under this heading.

Torsemide (Chlorthalidone may add to or potentiate the action of other antihypertensive drugs). Products include:
- Demadex Tablets and Injection ... 686

Triazolam (Enhanced CNS-depressive effects). Products include:
- Halcion Tablets ... 2611

Trimethaphan Camsylate (Chlorthalidone may add to or potentiate the action of other antihypertensive drugs). Products include:
- Arfonad Ampuls ... 2080

Trimipramine Maleate (Reduced effect of clonidine). Products include:
- Surmontil Capsules ... 2811

Tubocurarine Chloride (Increased responsiveness to tubocurarine).
- No products indexed under this heading.

Verapamil Hydrochloride (Chlorthalidone may add to or potentiate the action of other antihypertensive drugs). Products include:
- Calan SR Caplets ... 2422
- Calan Tablets ... 2419
- Isoptin Injectable ... 1344
- Isoptin Oral Tablets ... 1346
- Isoptin SR Tablets ... 1348
- Verelan Capsules ... 1410
- Verelan Capsules ... 2824

(Described in PDR For Nonprescription Drugs) (⊙ Described in PDR For Ophthalmology)

193 **Interactions Index** **Compazine**

Zolpidem Tartrate (Enhanced CNS-depressive effects). Products include:
Ambien Tablets 2416

Food Interactions

Alcohol (Orthostatic hypotension; enhanced CNS-depressive effects).

COMHIST LA CAPSULES

(Chlorpheniramine Maleate, Phenyltoloxamine Citrate, Phenylephrine Hydrochloride) 2038
May interact with hypnotics and sedatives, tranquilizers, monoamine oxidase inhibitors, and certain other agents. Compounds in these categories include:

Alprazolam (Sedative effects additive to CNS depressant effects). Products include:
Xanax Tablets 2649

Buspirone Hydrochloride (Sedative effects additive to CNS depressant effects). Products include:
BuSpar 737

Chlordiazepoxide (Sedative effects additive to CNS depressant effects). Products include:
Libritabs Tablets 2177
Limbitrol 2180

Chlordiazepoxide Hydrochloride (Sedative effects additive to CNS depressant effects). Products include:
Librax Capsules 2176
Librium Capsules 2178
Librium Injectable 2179

Chlorpromazine (Sedative effects additive to CNS depressant effects). Products include:
Thorazine Suppositories 2523

Clorazepate Dipotassium (Sedative effects additive to CNS depressant effects). Products include:
Tranxene 451

Diazepam (Sedative effects additive to CNS depressant effects). Products include:
Dizac 1809
Valium Injectable 2182
Valium Tablets 2183
Valrelease Capsules 2169

Droperidol (Sedative effects additive to CNS depressant effects). Products include:
Inapsine Injection 1296

Estazolam (Sedative effects additive to CNS depressant effects). Products include:
ProSom Tablets 449

Ethchlorvynol (Sedative effects additive to CNS depressant effects). Products include:
Placidyl Capsules 448

Ethinamate (Sedative effects additive to CNS depressant effects).
No products indexed under this heading.

Fluphenazine Decanoate (Sedative effects additive to CNS depressant effects). Products include:
Prolixin Decanoate 509

Fluphenazine Enanthate (Sedative effects additive to CNS depressant effects). Products include:
Prolixin Enanthate 509

Fluphenazine Hydrochloride (Sedative effects additive to CNS depressant effects). Products include:
Prolixin 509

Flurazepam Hydrochloride (Sedative effects additive to CNS depressant effects). Products include:
Dalmane Capsules 2173

Furazolidone (Concurrent use is not recommended). Products include:
Furoxone 2046

Glutethimide (Sedative effects additive to CNS depressant effects).
No products indexed under this heading.

Haloperidol (Sedative effects additive to CNS depressant effects). Products include:
Haldol Injection, Tablets and Concentrate 1575

Haloperidol Decanoate (Sedative effects additive to CNS depressant effects). Products include:
Haldol Decanoate 1577

Hydroxyzine Hydrochloride (Sedative effects additive to CNS depressant effects). Products include:
Atarax Tablets & Syrup 2185
Marax Tablets & DF Syrup 2200
Vistaril Intramuscular Solution 2216

Isocarboxazid (Concurrent use is not recommended).
No products indexed under this heading.

Lorazepam (Sedative effects additive to CNS depressant effects). Products include:
Ativan Injection 2698
Ativan Tablets 2700

Loxapine Hydrochloride (Sedative effects additive to CNS depressant effects). Products include:
Loxitane 1378

Loxapine Succinate (Sedative effects additive to CNS depressant effects). Products include:
Loxitane Capsules 1378

Meprobamate (Sedative effects additive to CNS depressant effects). Products include:
Miltown Tablets 2672
PMB 200 and PMB 400 2783

Mesoridazine Besylate (Sedative effects additive to CNS depressant effects). Products include:
Serentil 684

Midazolam Hydrochloride (Sedative effects additive to CNS depressant effects). Products include:
Versed Injection 2170

Molindone Hydrochloride (Sedative effects additive to CNS depressant effects). Products include:
Moban Tablets and Concentrate 1048

Oxazepam (Sedative effects additive to CNS depressant effects). Products include:
Serax Capsules 2810
Serax Tablets 2810

Perphenazine (Sedative effects additive to CNS depressant effects). Products include:
Etrafon 2355
Triavil Tablets 1757
Trilafon 2389

Phenelzine Sulfate (Concurrent use is not recommended). Products include:
Nardil 1920

Prazepam (Sedative effects additive to CNS depressant effects).
No products indexed under this heading.

Prochlorperazine (Sedative effects additive to CNS depressant effects). Products include:
Compazine 2470

Promethazine Hydrochloride (Sedative effects additive to CNS depressant effects). Products include:
Mepergan Injection 2753
Phenergan with Codeine 2777
Phenergan with Dextromethorphan 2778
Phenergan Injection 2773
Phenergan Suppositories 2775
Phenergan Syrup 2774
Phenergan Tablets 2775
Phenergan VC 2779
Phenergan VC with Codeine 2781

Propofol (Sedative effects additive to CNS depressant effects). Products include:
Diprivan Injection 2833

Quazepam (Sedative effects additive to CNS depressant effects). Products include:
Doral Tablets 2664

Secobarbital Sodium (Sedative effects additive to CNS depressant effects). Products include:
Seconal Sodium Pulvules 1474

Selegiline Hydrochloride (Concurrent use is not recommended). Products include:
Eldepryl Tablets 2550

Temazepam (Sedative effects additive to CNS depressant effects). Products include:
Restoril Capsules 2284

Thioridazine Hydrochloride (Sedative effects additive to CNS depressant effects). Products include:
Mellaril 2269

Tranylcypromine Sulfate (Concurrent use is not recommended). Products include:
Parnate Tablets 2503

Triazolam (Sedative effects additive to CNS depressant effects). Products include:
Halcion Tablets 2611

Trifluoperazine Hydrochloride (Sedative effects additive to CNS depressant effects). Products include:
Stelazine 2514

Zolpidem Tartrate (Sedative effects additive to CNS depressant effects). Products include:
Ambien Tablets 2416

Food Interactions

Alcohol (Sedative effects additive to CNS depressant effects).

COMHIST TABLETS

(Chlorpheniramine Maleate, Phenylephrine Hydrochloride, Phenyltoloxamine Citrate) 2038
See **Comhist LA Capsules**

COMPAZINE INJECTION

(Prochlorperazine) 2470
See **Compazine Tablets**

COMPAZINE MULTI-DOSE VIALS

(Prochlorperazine) 2470
See **Compazine Tablets**

COMPAZINE PREFILLED DISPOSABLE SYRINGES

(Prochlorperazine) 2470
See **Compazine Tablets**

COMPAZINE SPANSULE CAPSULES

(Prochlorperazine) 2470
See **Compazine Tablets**

COMPAZINE SUPPOSITORIES

(Prochlorperazine) 2470
See **Compazine Tablets**

COMPAZINE SYRUP

(Prochlorperazine) 2470
See **Compazine Tablets**

COMPAZINE TABLETS

(Prochlorperazine) 2470
May interact with central nervous system depressants, narcotic analgesics, general anesthetics, antihistamines, barbiturates, oral anticoagulants, thiazides, anticonvulsants, antineoplastics, and certain other agents. Compounds in these categories include:

Acrivastine (Phenothiazines may intensify or prolong the action of other central nervous system depressants). Products include:
Semprex-D Capsules 463
Semprex-D Capsules 1167

Alfentanil Hydrochloride (Phenothiazines may intensify or prolong the action of other central nervous system depressants). Products include:
Alfenta Injection 1286

Alprazolam (Phenothiazines may intensify or prolong the action of other central nervous system depressants). Products include:
Xanax Tablets 2649

Altretamine (Vomiting as a sign of toxicity of antineoplastic agents may be obscured by the antiemetic effect of Compazine). Products include:
Hexalen Capsules 2571

Aprobarbital (Phenothiazines may intensify or prolong the action of other central nervous system depressants).
No products indexed under this heading.

Asparaginase (Vomiting as a sign of toxicity of antineoplastic agents may be obscured by the antiemetic effect of Compazine). Products include:
Elspar 1659

Astemizole (Phenothiazines may intensify or prolong the action of other central nervous system depressants). Products include:
Hismanal Tablets 1293

Atropine Sulfate (Phenothiazines may intensify or prolong the action of atropine). Products include:
Arco-Lase Plus Tablets 512
Atrohist Plus Tablets 454
Atropine Sulfate Sterile Ophthalmic Solution ◉ 233
Donnatal 2060
Donnatal Extentabs 2061
Donnatal Tablets 2060
Lomotil 2439
Motofen Tablets 784
Urised Tablets 1964

Azatadine Maleate (Phenothiazines may intensify or prolong the action of other central nervous system depressants). Products include:
Trinalin Repetabs Tablets 1330

Bendroflumethiazide (Accentuates the orthostatic hypotension that may occur with phenothiazines).
No products indexed under this heading.

Bleomycin Sulfate (Vomiting as a sign of toxicity of antineoplastic agents may be obscured by the antiemetic effect of Compazine). Products include:
Blenoxane 692

Bromodiphenhydramine Hydrochloride (Phenothiazines may intensify or prolong the action of other central nervous system depressants).
No products indexed under this heading.

IMPORTANT NOTE: Always consult each drug listing in the patient's regimen for possible interactions.

Compazine **Interactions Index** **194**

Brompheniramine Maleate (Phenothiazines may intensify or prolong the action of other central nervous system depressants). Products include:
Alka Seltzer Plus Sinus Medicine ▣ 707
Bromfed Capsules (Extended-Release) 1785
Bromfed Syrup ▣ 733
Bromfed Tablets 1785
Bromfed-DM Cough Syrup 1786
Bromfed-PD Capsules (Extended-Release) 1785
Dimetane-DC Cough Syrup 2059
Dimetane-DX Cough Syrup 2059
Dimetapp Elixir ▣ 773
Dimetapp Extentabs ▣ 774
Dimetapp Tablets/Liqui-Gels ▣ 775
Dimetapp Cold & Allergy Chewable Tablets ▣ 773
Dimetapp DM Elixir ▣ 774
Vicks DayQuil Allergy Relief 12-Hour Extended Release Tablets ▣ 760
Vicks DayQuil Allergy Relief 4-Hour Tablets ▣ 760

Buprenorphine (Phenothiazines may intensify or prolong the action of other central nervous system depressants). Products include:
Buprenex Injectable 2006

Buspirone Hydrochloride (Phenothiazines may intensify or prolong the action of other central nervous system depressants). Products include:
BuSpar 737

Busulfan (Vomiting as a sign of toxicity of antineoplastic agents may be obscured by the antiemetic effect of Compazine). Products include:
Myleran Tablets 1143

Butabarbital (Phenothiazines may intensify or prolong the action of other central nervous system depressants).
No products indexed under this heading.

Butalbital (Phenothiazines may intensify or prolong the action of other central nervous system depressants). Products include:
Esgic-plus Tablets 1013
Fioricet Tablets 2258
Fioricet with Codeine Capsules 2260
Fiorinal Capsules 2261
Fiorinal with Codeine Capsules 2262
Fiorinal Tablets 2261
Phrenilin 785
Sedapap Tablets 50 mg/650 mg 1543

Carbamazepine (Phenothiazines may lower convulsive threshold; dosage adjustments of anticonvulsant may be necessary). Products include:
Atretol Tablets 573
Tegretol Chewable Tablets 852
Tegretol Suspension 852
Tegretol Tablets 852

Carboplatin (Vomiting as a sign of toxicity of antineoplastic agents may be obscured by the antiemetic effect of Compazine). Products include:
Paraplatin for Injection 705

Carmustine (BCNU) (Vomiting as a sign of toxicity of antineoplastic agents may be obscured by the antiemetic effect of Compazine). Products include:
BiCNU 691

Chlorambucil (Vomiting as a sign of toxicity of antineoplastic agents may be obscured by the antiemetic effect of Compazine). Products include:
Leukeran Tablets 1133

Chlordiazepoxide (Phenothiazines may intensify or prolong the action of other central nervous system depressants). Products include:
Libritabs Tablets 2177
Limbitrol 2180

Chlordiazepoxide Hydrochloride (Phenothiazines may intensify or prolong the action of other central nervous system depressants). Products include:
Librax Capsules 2176
Librium Capsules 2178
Librium Injectable 2179

Chlorothiazide (Accentuates the orthostatic hypotension that may occur with phenothiazines). Products include:
Aldoclor Tablets 1598
Diupres Tablets 1650
Diuril Oral 1653

Chlorothiazide Sodium (Accentuates the orthostatic hypotension that may occur with phenothiazines). Products include:
Diuril Sodium Intravenous 1652

Chlorpheniramine Maleate (Phenothiazines may intensify or prolong the action of other central nervous system depressants). Products include:
Alka-Seltzer Plus Cold Medicine ▣ 705
Alka-Seltzer Plus Cold Medicine Liqui-Gels ▣ 706
Alka-Seltzer Plus Cold & Cough Medicine ▣ 708
Alka-Seltzer Plus Cold & Cough Medicine Liqui-Gels ▣ 705
Allerest Children's Chewable Tablets ▣ 627
Allerest Headache Strength Tablets ▣ 627
Allerest Maximum Strength Tablets ▣ 627
Allerest Sinus Pain Formula ▣ 627
Allerest 12 Hour Caplets ▣ 627
Ana-Kit Anaphylaxis Emergency Treatment Kit 617
Atrohist Pediatric Capsules 453
Atrohist Plus Tablets 454
BC Cold Powder Multi-Symptom Formula (Cold-Sinus-Allergy) ▣ 609
Cerose DM ▣ 878
Cheracol Plus Head Cold/Cough Formula ▣ 769
Children's Vicks DayQuil Allergy Relief ▣ 757
Children's Vicks NyQuil Cold/Cough Relief ▣ 758
Chlor-Trimeton Allergy Decongestant Tablets ▣ 799
Chlor-Trimeton Allergy Tablets ▣ 798
Comhist 2038
Comtrex Multi-Symptom Cold Reliever Tablets/Caplets/Liqui-Gels/Liquid ▣ 615
Allergy-Sinus Comtrex Multi-Symptom Allergy-Sinus Formula Tablets ▣ 617
Contac Continuous Action Nasal Decongestant/Antihistamine 12 Hour Capsules ▣ 813
Contac Maximum Strength Continuous Action Decongestant/Antihistamine 12 Hour Caplets ▣ 813
Contac Severe Cold and Flu Formula Caplets ▣ 814
Coricidin 'D' Decongestant Tablets ▣ 800
Coricidin Tablets ▣ 800
D.A. Chewable Tablets 951
Deconamine 1320
Dura-Tap/PD Capsules 2867
Dura-Vent/DA Tablets 953
Extendryl 1005
Fedahist Gyrocaps 2401
Fedahist Timecaps 2401
Hycomine Compound Tablets 932
Isoclor Timesule Capsules ▣ 637
Kronofed-A 977
Nolamine Timed-Release Tablets 785
Novahistine DH 2462
Novahistine Elixir ▣ 823
Ornade Spansule Capsules 2502
PediaCare Cold Allergy Chewable Tablets ▣ 677
PediaCare Cough-Cold Chewable Tablets 1553
PediaCare Cough-Cold Liquid 1553
PediaCare NightRest Cough-Cold Liquid 1553
Pediatric Vicks 44m Cough & Cold Relief ▣ 764
Pyrroxate Caplets ▣ 772
Ryna ▣ 841
Sinarest Tablets ▣ 648
Sinarest Extra Strength Tablets ▣ 648
Sine-Off Sinus Medicine ▣ 825
Singlet Tablets ▣ 825
Sinulin Tablets 787
Sinutab Sinus Allergy Medication, Maximum Strength Tablets and Caplets ▣ 860
Sudafed Plus Liquid ▣ 862
Sudafed Plus Tablets ▣ 863
Teldrin 12 Hour Antihistamine/Nasal Decongestant Allergy Relief Capsules ▣ 826
TheraFlu ▣ 787
TheraFlu Maximum Strength Nighttime Flu, Cold & Cough Medicine ▣ 788
Triaminic Allergy Tablets ▣ 789
Triaminic Cold Tablets ▣ 790
Triaminic Nite Light ▣ 791
Triaminic Syrup ▣ 792
Triaminic-12 Tablets ▣ 792
Triaminicin Tablets ▣ 793
Triaminicol Multi-Symptom Cold Tablets ▣ 793
Triaminicol Multi-Symptom Relief ▣ 794
Tussend 1783
Children's TYLENOL Cold Multi-Symptom Liquid Formula and Chewable Tablets 1561
Children's TYLENOL Cold Plus Cough Multi Symptom Tablets and Liquid ▣ 681
TYLENOL Maximum Strength Allergy Sinus Medication Gelcaps and Caplets 1563
TYLENOL Cold Multi-Symptom Formula Medication Tablets and Caplets 1561
TYLENOL Cold Multi-Symptom Hot Medication Liquid Packets 1557
Vicks 44 LiquiCaps Cough, Cold & Flu Relief ▣ 755
Vicks 44M Cough, Cold & Flu Relief ▣ 756

Chlorpheniramine Polistirex (Phenothiazines may intensify or prolong the action of other central nervous system depressants). Products include:
Tussionex Pennkinetic Extended-Release Suspension 998

Chlorpheniramine Tannate (Phenothiazines may intensify or prolong the action of other central nervous system depressants). Products include:
Atrohist Pediatric Suspension 454
Ricobid Tablets and Pediatric Suspension 2038
Rynatan 2673
Rynatuss 2673

Chlorpromazine (Phenothiazines may intensify or prolong the action of other central nervous system depressants). Products include:
Thorazine Suppositories 2523

Chlorpromazine Hydrochloride (Phenothiazines may intensify or prolong the action of other central nervous system depressants). Products include:
Thorazine 2523

Chlorprothixene (Phenothiazines may intensify or prolong the action of other central nervous system depressants).
No products indexed under this heading.

Chlorprothixene Hydrochloride (Phenothiazines may intensify or prolong the action of other central nervous system depressants).
No products indexed under this heading.

Cisplatin (Vomiting as a sign of toxicity of antineoplastic agents may be obscured by the antiemetic effect of Compazine). Products include:
Platinol 708
Platinol-AQ Injection 710

Clemastine Fumarate (Phenothiazines may intensify or prolong the action of other central nervous system depressants). Products include:
Tavist Syrup 2297
Tavist Tablets 2298
Tavist-1 12 Hour Relief Tablets ▣ 787
Tavist-D 12 Hour Relief Tablets ▣ 787

Clorazepate Dipotassium (Phenothiazines may intensify or prolong the action of other central nervous system depressants). Products include:
Tranxene 451

Clozapine (Phenothiazines may intensify or prolong the action of other central nervous system depressants). Products include:
Clozaril Tablets 2252

Codeine Phosphate (Phenothiazines may intensify or prolong the action of other central nervous system depressants). Products include:
Actifed with Codeine Cough Syrup 1067
Brontex 1981
Deconsal C Expectorant Syrup 456
Deconsal Pediatric Syrup 457
Dimetane-DC Cough Syrup 2059
Empirin with Codeine Tablets 1093
Fioricet with Codeine Capsules 2260
Fiorinal with Codeine Capsules 2262
Isoclor Expectorant 990
Novahistine DH 2462
Novahistine Expectorant 2463
Nucofed 2051
Phenergan with Codeine 2777
Phenergan VC with Codeine 2781
Robitussin A-C Syrup 2073
Robitussin-DAC Syrup 2074
Ryna ▣ 841
Soma Compound w/Codeine Tablets 2676
Tussi-Organidin NR Liquid and S NR Liquid 2677
Tylenol with Codeine 1583

Cyclophosphamide (Vomiting as a sign of toxicity of antineoplastic agents may be obscured by the antiemetic effect of Compazine). Products include:
Cytoxan 694
NEOSAR Lyophilized/Neosar 1959

Cyproheptadine Hydrochloride (Phenothiazines may intensify or prolong the action of other central nervous system depressants). Products include:
Periactin 1724

Dacarbazine (Vomiting as a sign of toxicity of antineoplastic agents may be obscured by the antiemetic effect of Compazine). Products include:
DTIC-Dome 600

Daunorubicin Hydrochloride (Vomiting as a sign of toxicity of antineoplastic agents may be obscured by the antiemetic effect of Compazine). Products include:
Cerubidine 795

Desflurane (Phenothiazines may intensify or prolong the action of other central nervous system depressants). Products include:
Suprane 1813

Dexchlorpheniramine Maleate (Phenothiazines may intensify or prolong the action of other central nervous system depressants).
No products indexed under this heading.

Dezocine (Phenothiazines may intensify or prolong the action of other central nervous system depressants). Products include:
Dalgan Injection 538

Diazepam (Phenothiazines may intensify or prolong the action of other central nervous system depressants). Products include:
Dizac 1809

(▣ Described in PDR For Nonprescription Drugs) (◉ Described in PDR For Ophthalmology)

Valium Injectable 2182
Valium Tablets 2183
Valrelease Capsules 2169

Dicumarol (Diminished effect of oral anticoagulants).

No products indexed under this heading.

Diphenhydramine Citrate (Phenothiazines may intensify or prolong the action of other central nervous system depressants). Products include:

Excedrin P.M. Analgesic/Sleeping Aid Tablets, Caplets, Liquigels...... 733

Diphenhydramine Hydrochloride (Phenothiazines may intensify or prolong the action of other central nervous system depressants). Products include:

Actifed Allergy Daytime/Nighttime Caplets.. ◻ 844
Actifed Sinus Daytime/Nighttime Tablets and Caplets .... ◻ 846
Arthritis Foundation NightTime Caplets.. ◻ 674
Extra Strength Bayer PM Aspirin .. ◻ 713
Bayer Select Night Time Pain Relief Formula................................... ◻ 716
Benadryl Allergy Decongestant Liquid Medication .... ◻ 848
Benadryl Allergy Decongestant Tablets .... ◻ 848
Benadryl Allergy Liquid Medication.. ◻ 849
Benadryl Allergy .... ◻ 848
Benadryl Allergy Sinus Headache Formula Caplets .... ◻ 849
Benadryl Capsules............................ 1898
Benadryl Dye-Free Allergy Liquigel Softgels.. ◻ 850
Benadryl Dye-Free Allergy Liquid Medication .... ◻ 850
Benadryl Itch Relief Cream, Children's Formula and Maximum Strength 2% .... ◻ 851
Benadryl Itch Relief Spray, Children's Formula and Maximum Strength 2% .... ◻ 851
Benadryl Itch Relief Stick Maximum Strength 2% .... ◻ 850
Benadryl Itch Stopping Gel, Children's Formula and Maximum Strength 2% .... ◻ 851
Benadryl Kapseals............................ 1898
Benadryl Injection 1898
Contac Day & Night Cold/Flu Night Caplets.................................... ◻ 812
Contac Night Allergy/Sinus Caplets .... ◻ 812
Extra Strength Doan's P.M. .... ◻ 633
Legatrin PM .... ◻ 651
Miles Nervine Nighttime Sleep-Aid ◻ 723
Nytol QuickCaps Caplets .... ◻ 610
Sleepinal Night-time Sleep Aid Capsules and Softgels .... ◻ 834
TYLENOL Maximum Strength Allergy Sinus NightTime Medication Caplets 1555
TYLENOL Flu NightTime, Maximum Strength, Gelcaps 1566
TYLENOL Maximum Strength Flu NightTime Hot Medication Packets 1562
TYLENOL PM, Extra Strength Pain Reliever/Sleep Aid Caplets, Geltabs, Gelcaps................................... 1560
TYLENOL Severe Allergy Medication Caplets 1564
Maximum Strength Unisom Sleepgels 1934
Unisom With Pain Relief-Nighttime Sleep Aid and Pain Reliever............ 1934

Divalproex Sodium (Phenothiazines may lower convulsive threshold; dosage adjustments of anticonvulsant may be necessary). Products include:

Depakote Tablets............................... 415

Doxorubicin Hydrochloride (Vomiting as a sign of toxicity of antineoplastic agents may be obscured by the antiemetic effect of Compazine). Products include:

Adriamycin PFS 1947
Adriamycin RDF 1947
Doxorubicin Astra 540
Rubex 712

Droperidol (Phenothiazines may intensify or prolong the action of other central nervous system depressants). Products include:

Inapsine Injection.............................. 1296

Enflurane (Phenothiazines may intensify or prolong the action of other central nervous system depressants).

No products indexed under this heading.

Epinephrine (Potential for paradoxical lowering of blood pressure). Products include:

Bronkaid Mist .... ◻ 717
EPIFRIN .... ◻ 239
EpiPen 790
Marcaine Hydrochloride with Epinephrine 1:200,000 2316
Primatene Mist .... ◻ 873
Sensorcaine with Epinephrine Injection... 559
Sus-Phrine Injection 1019
Xylocaine with Epinephrine Injections... 567

Epinephrine Hydrochloride (Potential for paradoxical lowering of blood pressure). Products include:

Ana-Kit Anaphylaxis Emergency Treatment Kit 617

Estazolam (Phenothiazines may intensify or prolong the action of other central nervous system depressants). Products include:

ProSom Tablets 449

Estramustine Phosphate Sodium (Vomiting as a sign of toxicity of antineoplastic agents may be obscured by the antiemetic effect of Compazine). Products include:

Emcyt Capsules 1953

Ethchlorvynol (Phenothiazines may intensify or prolong the action of other central nervous system depressants). Products include:

Placidyl Capsules............................... 448

Ethinamate (Phenothiazines may intensify or prolong the action of other central nervous system depressants).

No products indexed under this heading.

Ethosuximide (Phenothiazines may lower convulsive threshold; dosage adjustments of anticonvulsant may be necessary). Products include:

Zarontin Capsules 1928
Zarontin Syrup 1929

Ethotoin (Phenothiazines may lower convulsive threshold; dosage adjustments of anticonvulsant may be necessary). Products include:

Peganone Tablets 446

Etoposide (Vomiting as a sign of toxicity of antineoplastic agents may be obscured by the antiemetic effect of Compazine). Products include:

VePesid Capsules and Injection........ 718

Felbamate (Phenothiazines may lower convulsive threshold; dosage adjustments of anticonvulsant may be necessary). Products include:

Felbatol 2666

Fentanyl (Phenothiazines may intensify or prolong the action of other central nervous system depressants). Products include:

Duragesic Transdermal System........ 1288

Fentanyl Citrate (Phenothiazines may intensify or prolong the action of other central nervous system depressants). Products include:

Sublimaze Injection........................... 1307

Floxuridine (Vomiting as a sign of toxicity of antineoplastic agents may be obscured by the antiemetic effect of Compazine). Products include:

Sterile FUDR 2118

Fluorouracil (Vomiting as a sign of toxicity of antineoplastic agents may be obscured by the antiemetic effect of Compazine). Products include:

Efudex 2113
Fluoroplex Topical Solution & Cream 1% 479
Fluorouracil Injection 2116

Fluphenazine Decanoate (Phenothiazines may intensify or prolong the action of other central nervous system depressants). Products include:

Prolixin Decanoate 509

Fluphenazine Enanthate (Phenothiazines may intensify or prolong the action of other central nervous system depressants). Products include:

Prolixin Enanthate 509

Fluphenazine Hydrochloride (Phenothiazines may intensify or prolong the action of other central nervous system depressants). Products include:

Prolixin... 509

Flurazepam Hydrochloride (Phenothiazines may intensify or prolong the action of other central nervous system depressants). Products include:

Dalmane Capsules.............................. 2173

Flutamide (Vomiting as a sign of toxicity of antineoplastic agents may be obscured by the antiemetic effect of Compazine). Products include:

Eulexin Capsules 2358

Glutethimide (Phenothiazines may intensify or prolong the action of other central nervous system depressants).

No products indexed under this heading.

Guanadrel Sulfate (Co-administration may counteract antihypertensive effects of guanadrel). Products include:

Hylorel Tablets 985

Guanethidine Monosulfate (Co-administration may counteract antihypertensive effects of guanethidine). Products include:

Esimil Tablets 822
Ismelin Tablets 827

Haloperidol (Phenothiazines may intensify or prolong the action of other central nervous system depressants). Products include:

Haldol Injection, Tablets and Concentrate 1575

Haloperidol Decanoate (Phenothiazines may intensify or prolong the action of other central nervous system depressants). Products include:

Haldol Decanoate............................... 1577

Hydrochlorothiazide (Accentuates the orthostatic hypotension that may occur with phenothiazines). Products include:

Aldactazide... 2413
Aldoril Tablets.................................... 1604
Apresazide Capsules 808
Capozide 742
Dyazide 2479
Esidrix Tablets 821
Esimil Tablets 822
HydroDIURIL Tablets 1674
Hydropres Tablets.............................. 1675
Hyzaar Tablets 1677
Inderide Tablets 2732
Inderide LA Long Acting Capsules .. 2734
Lopressor HCT Tablets 832
Lotensin HCT..................................... 837
Maxzide 1380
Moduretic Tablets 1705
Oretic Tablets 443
Prinzide Tablets 1737
Ser-Ap-Es Tablets 849

Timolide Tablets................................. 1748
Vaseretic Tablets 1765
Zestoretic 2850
Ziac 1415

Hydrocodone Bitartrate (Phenothiazines may intensify or prolong the action of other central nervous system depressants). Products include:

Anexsia 5/500 Elixir 1781
Anexia Tablets................................... 1782
Codiclear DH Syrup 791
Deconamine CX Cough and Cold Liquid and Tablets.............................. 1319
Duratuss HD Elixir............................. 2565
Hycodan Tablets and Syrup 930
Hycomine Compound Tablets 932
Hycomine 931
Hycotuss Expectorant Syrup 933
Hydrocet Capsules 782
Lorcet 10/650.................................... 1018
Lortab... 2566
Tussend 1783
Tussend Expectorant 1785
Vicodin Tablets.................................. 1356
Vicodin ES Tablets 1357
Vicodin Tuss Expectorant 1358
Zydone Capsules 949

Hydrocodone Polistirex (Phenothiazines may intensify or prolong the action of other central nervous system depressants). Products include:

Tussionex Pennkinetic Extended-Release Suspension 998

Hydroflumethiazide (Accentuates the orthostatic hypotension that may occur with phenothiazines). Products include:

Diucardin Tablets............................... 2718

Hydroxyurea (Vomiting as a sign of toxicity of antineoplastic agents may be obscured by the antiemetic effect of Compazine). Products include:

Hydrea Capsules 696

Hydroxyzine Hydrochloride (Phenothiazines may intensify or prolong the action of other central nervous system depressants). Products include:

Atarax Tablets & Syrup...................... 2185
Marax Tablets & DF Syrup................. 2200
Vistaril Intramuscular Solution.......... 2216

Idarubicin Hydrochloride (Vomiting as a sign of toxicity of antineoplastic agents may be obscured by the antiemetic effect of Compazine). Products include:

Idamycin 1955

Ifosfamide (Vomiting as a sign of toxicity of antineoplastic agents may be obscured by the antiemetic effect of Compazine). Products include:

IFEX 697

Interferon alfa-2A, Recombinant (Vomiting as a sign of toxicity of antineoplastic agents may be obscured by the antiemetic effect of Compazine). Products include:

Roferon-A Injection 2145

Interferon alfa-2B, Recombinant (Vomiting as a sign of toxicity of antineoplastic agents may be obscured by the antiemetic effect of Compazine). Products include:

Intron A 2364

Isoflurane (Phenothiazines may intensify or prolong the action of other central nervous system depressants).

No products indexed under this heading.

Ketamine Hydrochloride (Phenothiazines may intensify or prolong the action of other central nervous system depressants).

No products indexed under this heading.

IMPORTANT NOTE: Always consult each drug listing in the patient's regimen for possible interactions.

Compazine Interactions Index 196

Lamotrigine (Phenothiazines may lower convulsive threshold; dosage adjustments of anticonvulsant may be necessary). Products include:
Lamictal Tablets ... 1112
Levamisole Hydrochloride (Vomiting as a sign of toxicity of antineoplastic agents may be obscured by the antiemetic effect of Compazine). Products include:
Ergamisol Tablets ... 1292
Levomethadyl Acetate Hydrochloride (Phenothiazines may intensify or prolong the action of other central nervous system depressants). Products include:
Orlamm ... 2239
Levorphanol Tartrate (Phenothiazines may intensify or prolong the action of other central nervous system depressants). Products include:
Levo-Dromoran ... 2129
Lomustine (CCNU) (Vomiting as a sign of toxicity of antineoplastic agents may be obscured by the antiemetic effect of Compazine). Products include:
CeeNU ... 693
Loratadine (Phenothiazines may intensify or prolong the action of other central nervous system depressants). Products include:
Claritin ... 2349
Claritin-D ... 2350
Lorazepam (Phenothiazines may intensify or prolong the action of other central nervous system depressants). Products include:
Ativan Injection ... 2698
Ativan Tablets ... 2700
Loxapine Hydrochloride (Phenothiazines may intensify or prolong the action of other central nervous system depressants). Products include:
Loxitane ... 1378
Loxapine Succinate (Phenothiazines may intensify or prolong the action of other central nervous system depressants). Products include:
Loxitane Capsules ... 1378
Mechlorethamine Hydrochloride (Vomiting as a sign of toxicity of antineoplastic agents may be obscured by the antiemetic effect of Compazine). Products include:
Mustargen ... 1709
Megestrol Acetate (Vomiting as a sign of toxicity of antineoplastic agents may be obscured by the antiemetic effect of Compazine). Products include:
Megace Oral Suspension ... 699
Megace Tablets ... 701
Melphalan (Vomiting as a sign of toxicity of antineoplastic agents may be obscured by the antiemetic effect of Compazine). Products include:
Alkeran Tablets ... 1071
Meperidine Hydrochloride (Phenothiazines may intensify or prolong the action of other central nervous system depressants). Products include:
Demerol ... 2308
Mepergan Injection ... 2753
Mephenytoin (Phenothiazines may lower convulsive threshold; dosage adjustments of anticonvulsant may be necessary). Products include:
Mesantoin Tablets ... 2272
Mephobarbital (Phenothiazines may intensify or prolong the action of other central nervous system depressants). Products include:
Mebaral Tablets ... 2322
Meprobamate (Phenothiazines may intensify or prolong the action of other central nervous system depressants). Products include:
Miltown Tablets ... 2672
PMB 200 and PMB 400 ... 2783
Mercaptopurine (Vomiting as a sign of toxicity of antineoplastic agents may be obscured by the antiemetic effect of Compazine). Products include:
Purinethol Tablets ... 1156
Mesoridazine (Phenothiazines may intensify or prolong the action of other central nervous system depressants).
Methadone Hydrochloride (Phenothiazines may intensify or prolong the action of other central nervous system depressants). Products include:
Methadone Hydrochloride Oral Concentrate ... 2233
Methadone Hydrochloride Oral Solution & Tablets ... 2235
Methdilazine Hydrochloride (Phenothiazines may intensify or prolong the action of other central nervous system depressants).
No products indexed under this heading.
Methohexital Sodium (Phenothiazines may intensify or prolong the action of other central nervous system depressants). Products include:
Brevital Sodium Vials ... 1429
Methotrexate Sodium (Vomiting as a sign of toxicity of antineoplastic agents may be obscured by the antiemetic effect of Compazine). Products include:
Methotrexate Sodium Tablets, Injection, for Injection and LPF Injection ... 1275
Methotrimeprazine (Phenothiazines may intensify or prolong the action of other central nervous system depressants). Products include:
Levoprome ... 1274
Methoxyflurane (Phenothiazines may intensify or prolong the action of other central nervous system depressants).
No products indexed under this heading.
Methsuximide (Phenothiazines may lower convulsive threshold; dosage adjustments of anticonvulsant may be necessary). Products include:
Celontin Kapseals ... 1899
Methyclothiazide (Accentuates the orthostatic hypotension that may occur with phenothiazines). Products include:
Enduron Tablets ... 420
Metrizamide (Concurrent use is not recommended; Compazine should be discontinued at least 48 hours before myelography and should not be resumed for at least 24 hours).
Midazolam Hydrochloride (Phenothiazines may intensify or prolong the action of other central nervous system depressants). Products include:
Versed Injection ... 2170
Mitomycin (Mitomycin-C) (Vomiting as a sign of toxicity of antineoplastic agents may be obscured by the antiemetic effect of Compazine). Products include:
Mutamycin ... 703
Mitotane (Vomiting as a sign of toxicity of antineoplastic agents may be obscured by the antiemetic effect of Compazine). Products include:
Lysodren ... 698
Mitoxantrone Hydrochloride (Vomiting as a sign of toxicity of antineoplastic agents may be obscured by the antiemetic effect of Compazine). Products include:
Novantrone ... 1279
Molindone Hydrochloride (Phenothiazines may intensify or prolong the action of other central nervous system depressants). Products include:
Moban Tablets and Concentrate ... 1048
Morphine Sulfate (Phenothiazines may intensify or prolong the action of other central nervous system depressants). Products include:
Astramorph/PF Injection, USP (Preservative-Free) ... 535
Duramorph ... 962
Infumorph 200 and Infumorph 500 Sterile Solutions ... 965
MS Contin Tablets ... 1994
MSIR ... 1997
Oramorph SR (Morphine Sulfate Sustained Release Tablets) ... 2236
RMS Suppositories ... 2657
Roxanol ... 2243
Oxazepam (Phenothiazines may intensify or prolong the action of other central nervous system depressants). Products include:
Serax Capsules ... 2810
Serax Tablets ... 2810
Oxycodone Hydrochloride (Phenothiazines may intensify or prolong the action of other central nervous system depressants). Products include:
Percocet Tablets ... 938
Percodan Tablets ... 939
Percodan-Demi Tablets ... 940
Roxicodone Tablets, Oral Solution & Intensol (Oxycodone) ... 2244
Tylox Capsules ... 1584
Paclitaxel (Vomiting as a sign of toxicity of antineoplastic agents may be obscured by the antiemetic effect of Compazine). Products include:
Taxol ... 714
Paramethadione (Phenothiazines may lower convulsive threshold; dosage adjustments of anticonvulsant may be necessary).
No products indexed under this heading.
Pentobarbital Sodium (Phenothiazines may intensify or prolong the action of other central nervous system depressants). Products include:
Nembutal Sodium Capsules ... 436
Nembutal Sodium Solution ... 438
Nembutal Sodium Suppositories ... 440
Perphenazine (Phenothiazines may intensify or prolong the action of other central nervous system depressants). Products include:
Etrafon ... 2355
Triavil Tablets ... 1757
Trilafon ... 2389
Phenacemide (Phenothiazines may lower convulsive threshold; dosage adjustments of anticonvulsant may be necessary). Products include:
Phenurone Tablets ... 447
Phenobarbital (Phenothiazines may lower convulsive threshold; dosage adjustments of anticonvulsant may be necessary; phenothiazines may intensify or prolong the action of other central nervous system depressants). Products include:
Arco-Lase Plus Tablets ... 512
Bellergal-S Tablets ... 2250
Donnatal ... 2060
Donnatal Extentabs ... 2061
Donnatal Tablets ... 2060
Phenobarbital Elixir and Tablets ... 1469
Quadrinal Tablets ... 1350
Phensuximide (Phenothiazines may lower convulsive threshold; dosage adjustments of anticonvulsant may be necessary). Products include:
Milontin Kapseals ... 1920
Phenytoin (Phenothiazines may lower convulsive threshold; dosage adjustments of anticonvulsant may be necessary; interference with the metabolism of phenytoin precipitating in the phenytoin toxicity). Products include:
Dilantin Infatabs ... 1908
Dilantin-125 Suspension ... 1911
Phenytoin Sodium (Phenothiazines may lower convulsive threshold; dosage adjustments of anticonvulsant may be necessary; interference with the metabolism of phenytoin precipitating in the phenytoin toxicity). Products include:
Dilantin Kapseals ... 1906
Dilantin Parenteral ... 1910
Polythiazide (Accentuates the orthostatic hypotension that may occur with phenothiazines). Products include:
Minizide Capsules ... 1938
Prazepam (Phenothiazines may intensify or prolong the action of other central nervous system depressants).
No products indexed under this heading.
Primidone (Phenothiazines may lower convulsive threshold; dosage adjustments of anticonvulsant may be necessary). Products include:
Mysoline ... 2754
Procarbazine Hydrochloride (Vomiting as a sign of toxicity of antineoplastic agents may be obscured by the antiemetic effect of Compazine). Products include:
Matulane Capsules ... 2131
Promethazine Hydrochloride (Phenothiazines may intensify or prolong the action of other central nervous system depressants). Products include:
Mepergan Injection ... 2753
Phenergan with Codeine ... 2777
Phenergan with Dextromethorphan 2778
Phenergan Injection ... 2773
Phenergan Suppositories ... 2775
Phenergan Syrup ... 2774
Phenergan Tablets ... 2775
Phenergan VC ... 2779
Phenergan VC with Codeine ... 2781
Propofol (Phenothiazines may intensify or prolong the action of other central nervous system depressants). Products include:
Diprivan Injection ... 2833
Propoxyphene Hydrochloride (Phenothiazines may intensify or prolong the action of other central nervous system depressants). Products include:
Darvon ... 1435
Wygesic Tablets ... 2827
Propoxyphene Napsylate (Phenothiazines may intensify or prolong the action of other central nervous system depressants). Products include:
Darvon-N/Darvocet-N ... 1433
Propranolol Hydrochloride (Co-administration results in increased plasma levels of both drugs). Products include:
Inderal ... 2728
Inderal LA Long Acting Capsules ... 2730
Inderide Tablets ... 2732
Inderide LA Long Acting Capsules .. 2734

(▣ Described in PDR For Nonprescription Drugs) (◉ Described in PDR For Ophthalmology)

Pyrilamine Maleate (Phenothiazines may intensify or prolong the action of other central nervous system depressants). Products include:

4-Way Fast Acting Nasal Spray (regular & mentholated) .... ◼️ 621
Maximum Strength Multi-Symptom Formula Midol .... ◼️ 722
PMS Multi-Symptom Formula Midol .... ◼️ 723

Pyrilamine Tannate (Phenothiazines may intensify or prolong the action of other central nervous system depressants). Products include:

Atrohist Pediatric Suspension 454
Rynatan 2673

Quazepam (Phenothiazines may intensify or prolong the action of other central nervous system depressants). Products include:

Doral Tablets 2664

Risperidone (Phenothiazines may intensify or prolong the action of other central nervous system depressants). Products include:

Risperdal 1301

Secobarbital Sodium (Phenothiazines may intensify or prolong the action of other central nervous system depressants). Products include:

Seconal Sodium Pulvules 1474

Streptozocin (Vomiting as a sign of toxicity of antineoplastic agents may be obscured by the antiemetic effect of Compazine). Products include:

Zanosar Sterile Powder 2653

Sufentanil Citrate (Phenothiazines may intensify or prolong the action of other central nervous system depressants). Products include:

Sufenta Injection 1309

Tamoxifen Citrate (Vomiting as a sign of toxicity of antineoplastic agents may be obscured by the antiemetic effect of Compazine). Products include:

Nolvadex Tablets 2841

Temazepam (Phenothiazines may intensify or prolong the action of other central nervous system depressants). Products include:

Restoril Capsules 2284

Teniposide (Vomiting as a sign of toxicity of antineoplastic agents may be obscured by the antiemetic effect of Compazine). Products include:

Vumon 727

Terfenadine (Phenothiazines may intensify or prolong the action of other central nervous system depressants). Products include:

Seldane Tablets 1536
Seldane-D Extended-Release Tablets 1538

Thiamylal Sodium (Phenothiazines may intensify or prolong the action of other central nervous system depressants).

No products indexed under this heading.

Thioguanine (Vomiting as a sign of toxicity of antineoplastic agents may be obscured by the antiemetic effect of Compazine). Products include:

Thioguanine Tablets, Tabloid Brand 1181

Thioridazine Hydrochloride (Phenothiazines may intensify or prolong the action of other central nervous system depressants). Products include:

Mellaril 2269

Thiotepa (Vomiting as a sign of toxicity of antineoplastic agents may be obscured by the antiemetic effect of Compazine). Products include:

Thioplex (Thiotepa For Injection) 1281

Thiothixene (Phenothiazines may intensify or prolong the action of other central nervous system depressants). Products include:

Navane Capsules and Concentrate 2201
Navane Intramuscular 2202

Triazolam (Phenothiazines may intensify or prolong the action of other central nervous system depressants). Products include:

Halcion Tablets 2611

Trifluoperazine Hydrochloride (Phenothiazines may intensify or prolong the action of other central nervous system depressants). Products include:

Stelazine 2514

Trimeprazine Tartrate (Phenothiazines may intensify or prolong the action of other central nervous system depressants). Products include:

Temaril Tablets, Syrup and Spansule Extended-Release Capsules.. 483

Trimethadione (Phenothiazines may lower convulsive threshold; dosage adjustments of anticonvulsant may be necessary).

No products indexed under this heading.

Tripelennamine Hydrochloride (Phenothiazines may intensify or prolong the action of other central nervous system depressants). Products include:

PBZ Tablets 845
PBZ-SR Tablets 844

Triprolidine Hydrochloride (Phenothiazines may intensify or prolong the action of other central nervous system depressants). Products include:

Actifed Plus Caplets .... ◼️ 845
Actifed Plus Tablets .... ◼️ 845
Actifed with Codeine Cough Syrup.. 1067
Actifed Syrup .... ◼️ 846
Actifed Tablets .... ◼️ 844

Valproic Acid (Phenothiazines may lower convulsive threshold; dosage adjustments of anticonvulsant may be necessary). Products include:

Depakene 413

Vincristine Sulfate (Vomiting as a sign of toxicity of antineoplastic agents may be obscured by the antiemetic effect of Compazine). Products include:

Oncovin Solution Vials & Hyporets 1466

Vinorelbine Tartrate (Vomiting as a sign of toxicity of antineoplastic agents may be obscured by the antiemetic effect of Compazine). Products include:

Navelbine Injection 1145

Warfarin Sodium (Diminished effect of oral anticoagulants). Products include:

Coumadin 926

Zolpidem Tartrate (Phenothiazines may intensify or prolong the action of other central nervous system depressants). Products include:

Ambien Tablets 2416

Food Interactions

Alcohol (Phenothiazines may intensify or prolong the action of other central nervous system depressants).

COMPLEX 15 THERAPEUTIC MOISTURIZING FACE CREAM

(Dimethicone, Lecithin) .... ◼️ 800
None cited in PDR database.

COMPLEX 15 THERAPEUTIC MOISTURIZING LOTION

(Dimethicone, Lecithin) .... ◼️ 799
None cited in PDR database.

COMTREX MULTI-SYMPTOM COLD RELIEVER TABLETS/CAPLETS/ LIQUI-GELS/LIQUID

(Acetaminophen, Chlorpheniramine Maleate, Dextromethorphan Hydrobromide, Pseudoephedrine Hydrochloride) .... ◼️ 615

May interact with monoamine oxidase inhibitors, hypnotics and sedatives, tranquilizers, and certain other agents. Compounds in these categories include:

Alprazolam (May increase drowsiness effect). Products include:

Xanax Tablets 2649

Buspirone Hydrochloride (May increase drowsiness effect). Products include:

BuSpar 737

Chlordiazepoxide (May increase drowsiness effect). Products include:

Libritabs Tablets 2177
Limbitrol 2180

Chlordiazepoxide Hydrochloride (May increase drowsiness effect). Products include:

Librax Capsules 2176
Librium Capsules 2178
Librium Injectable 2179

Chlorpromazine (May increase drowsiness effect). Products include:

Thorazine Suppositories 2523

Chlorpromazine Hydrochloride (May increase drowsiness effect). Products include:

Thorazine 2523

Chlorprothixene (May increase drowsiness effect).

No products indexed under this heading.

Chlorprothixene Hydrochloride (May increase drowsiness effect).

No products indexed under this heading.

Clorazepate Dipotassium (May increase drowsiness effect). Products include:

Tranxene 451

Diazepam (May increase drowsiness effect). Products include:

Dizac 1809
Valium Injectable 2182
Valium Tablets 2183
Valrelease Capsules 2169

Droperidol (May increase drowsiness effect). Products include:

Inapsine Injection 1296

Estazolam (May increase drowsiness effect). Products include:

ProSom Tablets 449

Ethchlorvynol (May increase drowsiness effect). Products include:

Placidyl Capsules 448

Ethinamate (May increase drowsiness effect).

No products indexed under this heading.

Fluphenazine Decanoate (May increase drowsiness effect). Products include:

Prolixin Decanoate 509

Fluphenazine Enanthate (May increase drowsiness effect). Products include:

Prolixin Enanthate 509

Fluphenazine Hydrochloride (May increase drowsiness effect). Products include:

Prolixin 509

Flurazepam Hydrochloride (May increase drowsiness effect). Products include:

Dalmane Capsules 2173

Furazolidone (Concurrent and/or sequential use is not recommended). Products include:

Furoxone 2046

Glutethimide (May increase drowsiness effect).

No products indexed under this heading.

Haloperidol (May increase drowsiness effect). Products include:

Haldol Injection, Tablets and Concentrate 1575

Haloperidol Decanoate (May increase drowsiness effect). Products include:

Haldol Decanoate 1577

Hydroxyzine Hydrochloride (May increase drowsiness effect). Products include:

Atarax Tablets & Syrup 2185
Marax Tablets & DF Syrup 2200
Vistaril Intramuscular Solution 2216

Isocarboxazid (Concurrent and/or sequential use is not recommended).

No products indexed under this heading.

Lorazepam (May increase drowsiness effect). Products include:

Ativan Injection 2698
Ativan Tablets 2700

Loxapine Hydrochloride (May increase drowsiness effect). Products include:

Loxitane 1378

Loxapine Succinate (May increase drowsiness effect). Products include:

Loxitane Capsules 1378

Meprobamate (May increase drowsiness effect). Products include:

Miltown Tablets 2672
PMB 200 and PMB 400 2783

Mesoridazine Besylate (May increase drowsiness effect). Products include:

Serentil 684

Midazolam Hydrochloride (May increase drowsiness effect). Products include:

Versed Injection 2170

Molindone Hydrochloride (May increase drowsiness effect). Products include:

Moban Tablets and Concentrate 1048

Oxazepam (May increase drowsiness effect). Products include:

Serax Capsules 2810
Serax Tablets 2810

Perphenazine (May increase drowsiness effect). Products include:

Etrafon 2355
Triavil Tablets 1757
Trilafon 2389

Phenelzine Sulfate (Concurrent and/or sequential use is not recommended). Products include:

Nardil 1920

Prazepam (May increase drowsiness effect).

No products indexed under this heading.

Prochlorperazine (May increase drowsiness effect). Products include:

Compazine 2470

Promethazine Hydrochloride (May increase drowsiness effect). Products include:

Mepergan Injection 2753
Phenergan with Codeine 2777
Phenergan with Dextromethorphan 2778
Phenergan Injection 2773
Phenergan Suppositories 2775
Phenergan Syrup 2774
Phenergan Tablets 2775
Phenergan VC 2779

IMPORTANT NOTE: Always consult each drug listing in the patient's regimen for possible interactions.

Phenergan VC with Codeine 2781

Propofol (May increase drowsiness effect). Products include:

Diprivan Injection 2833

Quazepam (May increase drowsiness effect). Products include:

Doral Tablets 2664

Secobarbital Sodium (May increase drowsiness effect). Products include:

Seconal Sodium Pulvules 1474

Selegiline Hydrochloride (Concurrent and/or sequential use is not recommended). Products include:

Eldepryl Tablets 2550

Temazepam (May increase drowsiness effect). Products include:

Restoril Capsules 2284

Thioridazine Hydrochloride (May increase drowsiness effect). Products include:

Mellaril 2269

Thiothixene (May increase drowsiness effect). Products include:

Navane Capsules and Concentrate 2201
Navane Intramuscular 2202

Tranylcypromine Sulfate (Concurrent and/or sequential use is not recommended). Products include:

Parnate Tablets 2503

Triazolam (May increase drowsiness effect). Products include:

Halcion Tablets 2611

Trifluoperazine Hydrochloride (May increase drowsiness effect). Products include:

Stelazine 2514

Zolpidem Tartrate (May increase drowsiness effect). Products include:

Ambien Tablets 2416

Food Interactions

Alcohol (May increase drowsiness effect).

ALLERGY-SINUS COMTREX MULTI-SYMPTOM ALLERGY-SINUS FORMULA TABLETS

(Acetaminophen, Chlorpheniramine Maleate, Pseudoephedrine Hydrochloride) .... ▣ 617

May interact with:

Alprazolam (Increases drowsiness effect). Products include:

Xanax Tablets 2649

Antidepressant Medications, unspecified (Effect not specified).

Blood Pressure Medications, unspecified (Effect not specified).

No products indexed under this heading.

Buspirone Hydrochloride (Increases drowsiness effect). Products include:

BuSpar 737

Chlordiazepoxide (Increases drowsiness effect). Products include:

Libritabs Tablets 2177
Limbitrol 2180

Chlordiazepoxide Hydrochloride (Increases drowsiness effect). Products include:

Librax Capsules 2176
Librium Capsules 2178
Librium Injectable 2179

Chlorpromazine (Increases drowsiness effect). Products include:

Thorazine Suppositories 2523

Chlorprothixene (Increases drowsiness effect).

No products indexed under this heading.

Chlorprothixene Hydrochloride (Increases drowsiness effect).

No products indexed under this heading.

Clorazepate Dipotassium (Increases drowsiness effect). Products include:

Tranxene 451

Diazepam (Increases drowsiness effect). Products include:

Dizac 1809
Valium Injectable 2182
Valium Tablets 2183
Valrelease Capsules 2169

Droperidol (Increases drowsiness effect). Products include:

Inapsine Injection 1296

Estazolam (Increases drowsiness effect). Products include:

ProSom Tablets 449

Ethchlorvynol (Increases drowsiness effect). Products include:

Placidyl Capsules 448

Ethinamate (Increases drowsiness effect).

No products indexed under this heading.

Fluphenazine Decanoate (Increases drowsiness effect). Products include:

Prolixin Decanoate 509

Fluphenazine Enanthate (Increases drowsiness effect). Products include:

Prolixin Enanthate 509

Fluphenazine Hydrochloride (Increases drowsiness effect). Products include:

Prolixin 509

Flurazepam Hydrochloride (Increases drowsiness effect). Products include:

Dalmane Capsules 2173

Glutethimide (Increases drowsiness effect).

No products indexed under this heading.

Haloperidol (Increases drowsiness effect). Products include:

Haldol Injection, Tablets and Concentrate 1575

Haloperidol Decanoate (Increases drowsiness effect). Products include:

Haldol Decanoate 1577

Hydroxyzine Hydrochloride (Increases drowsiness effect). Products include:

Atarax Tablets & Syrup 2185
Marax Tablets & DF Syrup 2200
Vistaril Intramuscular Solution 2216

Lorazepam (Increases drowsiness effect). Products include:

Ativan Injection 2698
Ativan Tablets 2700

Loxapine Hydrochloride (Increases drowsiness effect). Products include:

Loxitane 1378

Loxapine Succinate (Increases drowsiness effect). Products include:

Loxitane Capsules 1378

Meprobamate (Increases drowsiness effect). Products include:

Miltown Tablets 2672
PMB 200 and PMB 400 2783

Mesoridazine Besylate (Increases drowsiness effect). Products include:

Serentil 684

Midazolam Hydrochloride (Increases drowsiness effect). Products include:

Versed Injection 2170

Molindone Hydrochloride (Increases drowsiness effect). Products include:

Moban Tablets and Concentrate 1048

Oxazepam (Increases drowsiness effect). Products include:

Serax Capsules 2810
Serax Tablets 2810

Perphenazine (Increases drowsiness effect). Products include:

Etrafon 2355
Triavil Tablets 1757
Trilafon 2389

Prazepam (Increases drowsiness effect).

No products indexed under this heading.

Prochlorperazine (Increases drowsiness effect). Products include:

Compazine 2470

Promethazine Hydrochloride (Increases drowsiness effect). Products include:

Mepergan Injection 2753
Phenergan with Codeine 2777
Phenergan with Dextromethorphan 2778
Phenergan Injection 2773
Phenergan Suppositories 2775
Phenergan Syrup 2774
Phenergan Tablets 2775
Phenergan VC 2779
Phenergan VC with Codeine 2781

Propofol (Increases drowsiness effect). Products include:

Diprivan Injection 2833

Quazepam (Increases drowsiness effect). Products include:

Doral Tablets 2664

Secobarbital Sodium (Increases drowsiness effect). Products include:

Seconal Sodium Pulvules 1474

Temazepam (Increases drowsiness effect). Products include:

Restoril Capsules 2284

Thioridazine Hydrochloride (Increases drowsiness effect). Products include:

Mellaril 2269

Thiothixene (Increases drowsiness effect). Products include:

Navane Capsules and Concentrate 2201
Navane Intramuscular 2202

Triazolam (Increases drowsiness effect). Products include:

Halcion Tablets 2611

Trifluoperazine Hydrochloride (Increases drowsiness effect). Products include:

Stelazine 2514

Zolpidem Tartrate (Increases drowsiness effect). Products include:

Ambien Tablets 2416

Food Interactions

Alcohol (Increases drowsiness effect).

COMTREX MULTI-SYMPTOM NON-DROWSY CAPLETS

(Acetaminophen, Dextromethorphan Hydrobromide, Pseudoephedrine Hydrochloride) .... ▣ 618

May interact with monoamine oxidase inhibitors. Compounds in this category include:

Furazolidone (Concurrent and/or sequential use is not recommended). Products include:

Furoxone 2046

Isocarboxazid (Concurrent and/or sequential use is not recommended).

No products indexed under this heading.

Phenelzine Sulfate (Concurrent and/or sequential use is not recommended). Products include:

Nardil 1920

Selegiline Hydrochloride (Concurrent and/or sequential use is not recommended). Products include:

Eldepryl Tablets 2550

Tranylcypromine Sulfate (Concurrent and/or sequential use is not recommended). Products include:

Parnate Tablets 2503

COMTREX MULTI-SYMPTOM NON-DROWSY LIQUI-GELS

(Acetaminophen, Dextromethorphan Hydrobromide, Phenylpropanolamine Hydrochloride) .... ▣ 618

See **Comtrex Multi-Symptom Non-Drowsy Caplets**

CONCEPT ANTIMICROBIAL SKIN CLEANSER

(Chloroxylenol) .... ▣ 625

None cited in PDR database.

CONCEPTROL CONTRACEPTIVE GEL SINGLE USE APPLICATORS

(Nonoxynol-9) .... ▣ 736

None cited in PDR database.

CONCEPTROL CONTRACEPTIVE INSERTS

(Nonoxynol-9) .... ▣ 737

None cited in PDR database.

CONDYLOX

(Podofilox) 1802

None cited in PDR database.

CONGESS JR. T.D. CAPSULES

(Guaifenesin, Pseudoephedrine Hydrochloride) 1004

May interact with monoamine oxidase inhibitors. Compounds in this category include:

Furazolidone (Concurrent administration is contraindicated). Products include:

Furoxone 2046

Isocarboxazid (Concurrent administration is contraindicated).

No products indexed under this heading.

Phenelzine Sulfate (Concurrent administration is contraindicated). Products include:

Nardil 1920

Selegiline Hydrochloride (Concurrent administration is contraindicated). Products include:

Eldepryl Tablets 2550

Tranylcypromine Sulfate (Concurrent administration is contraindicated). Products include:

Parnate Tablets 2503

CONGESS SR. T.D. CAPSULES

(Guaifenesin, Pseudoephedrine Hydrochloride) 1004

May interact with monoamine oxidase inhibitors. Compounds in this category include:

Furazolidone (Concurrent administration is contraindicated). Products include:

Furoxone 2046

Isocarboxazid (Concurrent administration is contraindicated).

No products indexed under this heading.

Phenelzine Sulfate (Concurrent administration is contraindicated). Products include:

Nardil 1920

Selegiline Hydrochloride (Concurrent administration is contraindicated). Products include:

Eldepryl Tablets 2550

199 **Interactions Index** **Contac Day & Night**

Tranylcypromine Sulfate (Concurrent administration is contraindicated). Products include:
Parnate Tablets 2503

CONTAC CONTINUOUS ACTION NASAL DECONGESTANT/ANTIHISTAMINE 12 HOUR CAPSULES
(Chlorpheniramine Maleate, Phenylpropanolamine Hydrochloride)........ 813
May interact with monoamine oxidase inhibitors, tranquilizers, hypnotics and sedatives, and certain other agents. Compounds in these categories include:

Alprazolam (May increase drowsiness effect; concurrent use should be avoided). Products include:
Xanax Tablets 2649

Buspirone Hydrochloride (May increase drowsiness effect; concurrent use should be avoided). Products include:
BuSpar 737

Chlordiazepoxide (May increase drowsiness effect; concurrent use should be avoided). Products include:
Libritabs Tablets 2177
Limbitrol 2180

Chlordiazepoxide Hydrochloride (May increase drowsiness effect; concurrent use should be avoided). Products include:
Librax Capsules 2176
Librium Capsules 2178
Librium Injectable 2179

Chlorpromazine (May increase drowsiness effect; concurrent use should be avoided). Products include:
Thorazine Suppositories 2523

Chlorpromazine Hydrochloride (May increase drowsiness effect; concurrent use should be avoided). Products include:
Thorazine 2523

Chlorprothixene (May increase drowsiness effect; concurrent use should be avoided).
No products indexed under this heading.

Chlorprothixene Hydrochloride (May increase drowsiness effect; concurrent use should be avoided).
No products indexed under this heading.

Clorazepate Dipotassium (May increase drowsiness effect; concurrent use should be avoided). Products include:
Tranxene 451

Diazepam (May increase drowsiness effect; concurrent use should be avoided). Products include:
Dizac 1809
Valium Injectable 2182
Valium Tablets 2183
Valrelease Capsules 2169

Droperidol (May increase drowsiness effect; concurrent use should be avoided). Products include:
Inapsine Injection 1296

Estazolam (May increase drowsiness effect; concurrent use should be avoided). Products include:
ProSom Tablets 449

Ethchlorvynol (May increase drowsiness effect; concurrent use should be avoided). Products include:
Placidyl Capsules 448

Ethinamate (May increase drowsiness effect; concurrent use should be avoided).
No products indexed under this heading.

Fluphenazine Decanoate (May increase drowsiness effect; concurrent use should be avoided). Products include:
Prolixin Decanoate 509

Fluphenazine Enanthate (May increase drowsiness effect; concurrent use should be avoided). Products include:
Prolixin Enanthate 509

Fluphenazine Hydrochloride (May increase drowsiness effect; concurrent use should be avoided). Products include:
Prolixin 509

Flurazepam Hydrochloride (May increase drowsiness effect; concurrent use should be avoided). Products include:
Dalmane Capsules 2173

Furazolidone (Concurrent and/or sequential use is not recommended unless directed by a doctor). Products include:
Furoxone 2046

Glutethimide (May increase drowsiness effect; concurrent use should be avoided).
No products indexed under this heading.

Haloperidol (May increase drowsiness effect; concurrent use should be avoided). Products include:
Haldol Injection, Tablets and Concentrate 1575

Haloperidol Decanoate (May increase drowsiness effect; concurrent use should be avoided). Products include:
Haldol Decanoate 1577

Hydroxyzine Hydrochloride (May increase drowsiness effect; concurrent use should be avoided). Products include:
Atarax Tablets & Syrup 2185
Marax Tablets & DF Syrup 2200
Vistaril Intramuscular Solution 2216

Isocarboxazid (Concurrent and/or sequential use is not recommended unless directed by a doctor).
No products indexed under this heading.

Lorazepam (May increase drowsiness effect; concurrent use should be avoided). Products include:
Ativan Injection 2698
Ativan Tablets 2700

Loxapine Hydrochloride (May increase drowsiness effect; concurrent use should be avoided). Products include:
Loxitane 1378

Loxapine Succinate (May increase drowsiness effect; concurrent use should be avoided). Products include:
Loxitane Capsules 1378

Meprobamate (May increase drowsiness effect; concurrent use should be avoided). Products include:
Miltown Tablets 2672
PMB 200 and PMB 400 2783

Mesoridazine Besylate (May increase drowsiness effect; concurrent use should be avoided). Products include:
Serentil 684

Midazolam Hydrochloride (May increase drowsiness effect; concurrent use should be avoided). Products include:
Versed Injection 2170

Molindone Hydrochloride (May increase drowsiness effect; concurrent use should be avoided). Products include:
Moban Tablets and Concentrate 1048

Oxazepam (May increase drowsiness effect; concurrent use should be avoided). Products include:
Serax Capsules 2810
Serax Tablets 2810

Perphenazine (May increase drowsiness effect; concurrent use should be avoided). Products include:
Etrafon 2355
Triavil Tablets 1757
Trilafon 2389

Phenelzine Sulfate (Concurrent and/or sequential use is not recommended unless directed by a doctor). Products include:
Nardil 1920

Prazepam (May increase drowsiness effect; concurrent use should be avoided).
No products indexed under this heading.

Prochlorperazine (May increase drowsiness effect; concurrent use should be avoided). Products include:
Compazine 2470

Promethazine Hydrochloride (May increase drowsiness effect; concurrent use should be avoided). Products include:
Mepergan Injection 2753
Phenergan with Codeine 2777
Phenergan with Dextromethorphan 2778
Phenergan Injection 2773
Phenergan Suppositories 2775
Phenergan Syrup 2774
Phenergan Tablets 2775
Phenergan VC 2779
Phenergan VC with Codeine 2781

Propofol (May increase drowsiness effect; concurrent use should be avoided). Products include:
Diprivan Injection 2833

Quazepam (May increase drowsiness effect; concurrent use should be avoided). Products include:
Doral Tablets 2664

Secobarbital Sodium (May increase drowsiness effect; concurrent use should be avoided). Products include:
Seconal Sodium Pulvules 1474

Selegiline Hydrochloride (Concurrent and/or sequential use is not recommended unless directed by a doctor). Products include:
Eldepryl Tablets 2550

Temazepam (May increase drowsiness effect; concurrent use should be avoided). Products include:
Restoril Capsules 2284

Thioridazine Hydrochloride (May increase drowsiness effect; concurrent use should be avoided). Products include:
Mellaril 2269

Thiothixene (May increase drowsiness effect; concurrent use should be avoided). Products include:
Navane Capsules and Concentrate 2201
Navane Intramuscular 2202

Tranylcypromine Sulfate (Concurrent and/or sequential use is not recommended unless directed by a doctor). Products include:
Parnate Tablets 2503

Triazolam (May increase drowsiness effect; concurrent use should be avoided). Products include:
Halcion Tablets 2611

Trifluoperazine Hydrochloride (May increase drowsiness effect; concurrent use should be avoided). Products include:
Stelazine 2514

Zolpidem Tartrate (May increase drowsiness effect; concurrent use should be avoided). Products include:
Ambien Tablets 2416

Food Interactions

Alcohol (May increase drowsiness effect; concurrent use should be avoided).

CONTAC DAY ALLERGY/SINUS CAPLETS
(Acetaminophen)........ 812
See **Contac Night Allergy/Sinus Caplets**

CONTAC DAY & NIGHT COLD/FLU CAPLETS
(Acetaminophen, Pseudoephedrine Hydrochloride, Dextromethorphan Hydrobromide) 812
See **Contac Day & Night Cold/Flu Night Caplets**

CONTAC DAY & NIGHT COLD/FLU NIGHT CAPLETS
(Acetaminophen, Pseudoephedrine Hydrochloride, Diphenhydramine Hydrochloride)........ 812
May interact with monoamine oxidase inhibitors, tranquilizers, hypnotics and sedatives, and certain other agents. Compounds in these categories include:

Alprazolam (May increase the drowsiness effect). Products include:
Xanax Tablets 2649

Buspirone Hydrochloride (May increase the drowsiness effect). Products include:
BuSpar 737

Chlordiazepoxide (May increase the drowsiness effect). Products include:
Libritabs Tablets 2177
Limbitrol 2180

Chlordiazepoxide Hydrochloride (May increase the drowsiness effect). Products include:
Librax Capsules 2176
Librium Capsules 2178
Librium Injectable 2179

Chlorpromazine (May increase the drowsiness effect). Products include:
Thorazine Suppositories 2523

Chlorpromazine Hydrochloride (May increase the drowsiness effect). Products include:
Thorazine 2523

Chlorprothixene (May increase the drowsiness effect).
No products indexed under this heading.

Chlorprothixene Hydrochloride (May increase the drowsiness effect).
No products indexed under this heading.

Clorazepate Dipotassium (May increase the drowsiness effect). Products include:
Tranxene 451

Diazepam (May increase the drowsiness effect). Products include:
Dizac 1809
Valium Injectable 2182
Valium Tablets 2183
Valrelease Capsules 2169

Droperidol (May increase the drowsiness effect). Products include:
Inapsine Injection 1296

IMPORTANT NOTE: Always consult each drug listing in the patient's regimen for possible interactions.

Estazolam (May increase the drowsiness effect). Products include:
ProSom Tablets ... 449
Ethchlorvynol (May increase the drowsiness effect). Products include:
Placidyl Capsules ... 448
Ethinamate (May increase the drowsiness effect).
No products indexed under this heading.
Fluphenazine Decanoate (May increase the drowsiness effect). Products include:
Prolixin Decanoate ... 509
Fluphenazine Enanthate (May increase the drowsiness effect). Products include:
Prolixin Enanthate ... 509
Fluphenazine Hydrochloride (May increase the drowsiness effect). Products include:
Prolixin ... 509
Flurazepam Hydrochloride (May increase the drowsiness effect). Products include:
Dalmane Capsules ... 2173
Furazolidone (Concurrent and/or sequential use is not recommended). Products include:
Furoxone ... 2046
Glutethimide (May increase the drowsiness effect).
No products indexed under this heading.
Haloperidol (May increase the drowsiness effect). Products include:
Haldol Injection, Tablets and Concentrate ... 1575
Haloperidol Decanoate (May increase the drowsiness effect). Products include:
Haldol Decanoate ... 1577
Hydroxyzine Hydrochloride (May increase the drowsiness effect). Products include:
Atarax Tablets & Syrup ... 2185
Marax Tablets & DF Syrup ... 2200
Vistaril Intramuscular Solution ... 2216
Isocarboxazid (Concurrent and/or sequential use is not recommended).
No products indexed under this heading.
Lorazepam (May increase the drowsiness effect). Products include:
Ativan Injection ... 2698
Ativan Tablets ... 2700
Loxapine Hydrochloride (May increase the drowsiness effect). Products include:
Loxitane ... 1378
Loxapine Succinate (May increase the drowsiness effect). Products include:
Loxitane Capsules ... 1378
Meprobamate (May increase the drowsiness effect). Products include:
Miltown Tablets ... 2672
PMB 200 and PMB 400 ... 2783
Mesoridazine Besylate (May increase the drowsiness effect). Products include:
Serentil ... 684
Midazolam Hydrochloride (May increase the drowsiness effect). Products include:
Versed Injection ... 2170
Molindone Hydrochloride (May increase the drowsiness effect). Products include:
Moban Tablets and Concentrate ... 1048
Oxazepam (May increase the drowsiness effect). Products include:
Serax Capsules ... 2810
Serax Tablets ... 2810
Perphenazine (May increase the drowsiness effect). Products include:
Etrafon ... 2355
Triavil Tablets ... 1757
Trilafon ... 2389
Phenelzine Sulfate (Concurrent and/or sequential use is not recommended). Products include:
Nardil ... 1920
Prazepam (May increase the drowsiness effect).
No products indexed under this heading.
Prochlorperazine (May increase the drowsiness effect). Products include:
Compazine ... 2470
Promethazine Hydrochloride (May increase the drowsiness effect). Products include:
Mepergan Injection ... 2753
Phenergan with Codeine ... 2777
Phenergan with Dextromethorphan 2778
Phenergan Injection ... 2773
Phenergan Suppositories ... 2775
Phenergan Syrup ... 2774
Phenergan Tablets ... 2775
Phenergan VC ... 2779
Phenergan VC with Codeine ... 2781
Propofol (May increase the drowsiness effect). Products include:
Diprivan Injection ... 2833
Quazepam (May increase the drowsiness effect). Products include:
Doral Tablets ... 2664
Secobarbital Sodium (May increase the drowsiness effect). Products include:
Seconal Sodium Pulvules ... 1474
Selegiline Hydrochloride (Concurrent and/or sequential use is not recommended). Products include:
Eldepryl Tablets ... 2550
Temazepam (May increase the drowsiness effect). Products include:
Restoril Capsules ... 2284
Thioridazine Hydrochloride (May increase the drowsiness effect). Products include:
Mellaril ... 2269
Thiothixene (May increase the drowsiness effect). Products include:
Navane Capsules and Concentrate 2201
Navane Intramuscular ... 2202
Tranylcypromine Sulfate (Concurrent and/or sequential use is not recommended). Products include:
Parnate Tablets ... 2503
Triazolam (May increase the drowsiness effect). Products include:
Halcion Tablets ... 2611
Trifluoperazine Hydrochloride (May increase the drowsiness effect). Products include:
Stelazine ... 2514
Zolpidem Tartrate (May increase the drowsiness effect). Products include:
Ambien Tablets ... 2416

Food Interactions

Alcohol (Increases drowsiness effect).

CONTAC MAXIMUM STRENGTH CONTINUOUS ACTION DECONGESTANT/ ANTIHISTAMINE 12 HOUR CAPLETS

(Chlorpheniramine Maleate, Phenylpropanolamine Hydrochloride) ... ▣ 813
May interact with monoamine oxidase inhibitors, tranquilizers, hypnotics and sedatives, and certain other agents. Compounds in these categories include:
Alprazolam (May increase drowsiness effect; concurrent use should be avoided). Products include:
Xanax Tablets ... 2649
Buspirone Hydrochloride (May increase drowsiness effect; concurrent use should be avoided). Products include:
BuSpar ... 737
Chlordiazepoxide (May increase drowsiness effect; concurrent use should be avoided). Products include:
Libritabs Tablets ... 2177
Limbitrol ... 2180
Chlordiazepoxide Hydrochloride (May increase drowsiness effect; concurrent use should be avoided). Products include:
Librax Capsules ... 2176
Librium Capsules ... 2178
Librium Injectable ... 2179
Chlorpromazine (May increase drowsiness effect; concurrent use should be avoided). Products include:
Thorazine Suppositories ... 2523
Chlorpromazine Hydrochloride (May increase drowsiness effect; concurrent use should be avoided). Products include:
Thorazine ... 2523
Chlorprothixene (May increase drowsiness effect; concurrent use should be avoided).
No products indexed under this heading.
Chlorprothixene Hydrochloride (May increase drowsiness effect; concurrent use should be avoided).
No products indexed under this heading.
Clorazepate Dipotassium (May increase drowsiness effect; concurrent use should be avoided). Products include:
Tranxene ... 451
Diazepam (May increase drowsiness effect; concurrent use should be avoided). Products include:
Dizac ... 1809
Valium Injectable ... 2182
Valium Tablets ... 2183
Valrelease Capsules ... 2169
Droperidol (May increase drowsiness effect; concurrent use should be avoided). Products include:
Inapsine Injection ... 1296
Estazolam (May increase drowsiness effect; concurrent use should be avoided). Products include:
ProSom Tablets ... 449
Ethchlorvynol (May increase drowsiness effect; concurrent use should be avoided). Products include:
Placidyl Capsules ... 448
Ethinamate (May increase drowsiness effect; concurrent use should be avoided).
No products indexed under this heading.
Fluphenazine Decanoate (May increase drowsiness effect; concurrent use should be avoided). Products include:
Prolixin Decanoate ... 509
Fluphenazine Enanthate (May increase drowsiness effect; concurrent use should be avoided). Products include:
Prolixin Enanthate ... 509
Fluphenazine Hydrochloride (May increase drowsiness effect; concurrent use should be avoided). Products include:
Prolixin ... 509
Flurazepam Hydrochloride (May increase drowsiness effect; concurrent use should be avoided). Products include:
Dalmane Capsules ... 2173
Furazolidone (Concurrent and/or sequential use is not recommended unless directed by a doctor). Products include:
Furoxone ... 2046
Glutethimide (May increase drowsiness effect; concurrent use should be avoided).
No products indexed under this heading.
Haloperidol (May increase drowsiness effect; concurrent use should be avoided). Products include:
Haldol Injection, Tablets and Concentrate ... 1575
Haloperidol Decanoate (May increase drowsiness effect; concurrent use should be avoided). Products include:
Haldol Decanoate ... 1577
Hydroxyzine Hydrochloride (May increase drowsiness effect; concurrent use should be avoided). Products include:
Atarax Tablets & Syrup ... 2185
Marax Tablets & DF Syrup ... 2200
Vistaril Intramuscular Solution ... 2216
Isocarboxazid (Concurrent and/or sequential use is not recommended unless directed by a doctor).
No products indexed under this heading.
Lorazepam (May increase drowsiness effect; concurrent use should be avoided). Products include:
Ativan Injection ... 2698
Ativan Tablets ... 2700
Loxapine Hydrochloride (May increase drowsiness effect; concurrent use should be avoided). Products include:
Loxitane ... 1378
Loxapine Succinate (May increase drowsiness effect; concurrent use should be avoided). Products include:
Loxitane Capsules ... 1378
Meprobamate (May increase drowsiness effect; concurrent use should be avoided). Products include:
Miltown Tablets ... 2672
PMB 200 and PMB 400 ... 2783
Mesoridazine Besylate (May increase drowsiness effect; concurrent use should be avoided). Products include:
Serentil ... 684
Midazolam Hydrochloride (May increase drowsiness effect; concurrent use should be avoided). Products include:
Versed Injection ... 2170
Molindone Hydrochloride (May increase drowsiness effect; concurrent use should be avoided). Products include:
Moban Tablets and Concentrate ... 1048
Oxazepam (May increase drowsiness effect; concurrent use should be avoided). Products include:
Serax Capsules ... 2810
Serax Tablets ... 2810
Perphenazine (May increase drowsiness effect; concurrent use should be avoided). Products include:
Etrafon ... 2355
Triavil Tablets ... 1757
Trilafon ... 2389
Phenelzine Sulfate (Concurrent and/or sequential use is not recommended unless directed by a doctor). Products include:
Nardil ... 1920

(▣ Described in PDR For Nonprescription Drugs) (◉ Described in PDR For Ophthalmology)

201 Interactions Index Contact Severe Cold Formula

Prazepam (May increase drowsiness effect; concurrent use should be avoided).
No products indexed under this heading.

Prochlorperazine (May increase drowsiness effect; concurrent use should be avoided). Products include:
Compazine 2470

Promethazine Hydrochloride (May increase drowsiness effect; concurrent use should be avoided). Products include:
Mepergan Injection 2753
Phenergan with Codeine 2777
Phenergan with Dextromethorphan 2778
Phenergan Injection 2773
Phenergan Suppositories 2775
Phenergan Syrup 2774
Phenergan Tablets 2775
Phenergan VC 2779
Phenergan VC with Codeine 2781

Propofol (May increase drowsiness effect; concurrent use should be avoided). Products include:
Diprivan Injection 2833

Quazepam (May increase drowsiness effect; concurrent use should be avoided). Products include:
Doral Tablets 2664

Secobarbital Sodium (May increase drowsiness effect; concurrent use should be avoided). Products include:
Seconal Sodium Pulvules 1474

Selegiline Hydrochloride (Concurrent and/or sequential use is not recommended unless directed by a doctor). Products include:
Eldepryl Tablets 2550

Temazepam (May increase drowsiness effect; concurrent use should be avoided). Products include:
Restoril Capsules 2284

Thioridazine Hydrochloride (May increase drowsiness effect; concurrent use should be avoided). Products include:
Mellaril 2269

Thiothixene (May increase drowsiness effect; concurrent use should be avoided). Products include:
Navane Capsules and Concentrate 2201
Navane Intramuscular 2202

Tranylcypromine Sulfate (Concurrent and/or sequential use is not recommended unless directed by a doctor). Products include:
Parnate Tablets 2503

Triazolam (May increase drowsiness effect; concurrent use should be avoided). Products include:
Halcion Tablets 2611

Trifluoperazine Hydrochloride (May increase drowsiness effect; concurrent use should be avoided). Products include:
Stelazine 2514

Zolpidem Tartrate (May increase drowsiness effect; concurrent use should be avoided). Products include:
Ambien Tablets 2416

Food Interactions

Alcohol (May increase drowsiness effect; concurrent use should be avoided).

CONTAC NIGHT ALLERGY/SINUS CAPLETS

(Acetaminophen, Pseudoephedrine Hydrochloride, Diphenhydramine Hydrochloride) 812
May interact with monoamine oxidase inhibitors, hypnotics and sedatives, tranquilizers, and certain other agents. Compounds in these categories include:

Alprazolam (May increase the drowsiness effect; avoid concurrent use). Products include:
Xanax Tablets 2649

Buspirone Hydrochloride (May increase the drowsiness effect; avoid concurrent use). Products include:
BuSpar 737

Chlordiazepoxide (May increase the drowsiness effect; avoid concurrent use). Products include:
Libritabs Tablets 2177
Limbitrol 2180

Chlordiazepoxide Hydrochloride (May increase the drowsiness effect; avoid concurrent use). Products include:
Librax Capsules 2176
Librium Capsules 2178
Librium Injectable 2179

Chlorpromazine (May increase the drowsiness effect; avoid concurrent use). Products include:
Thorazine Suppositories 2523

Chlorpromazine Hydrochloride (May increase the drowsiness effect; avoid concurrent use). Products include:
Thorazine 2523

Chlorprothixene (May increase the drowsiness effect; avoid concurrent use).
No products indexed under this heading.

Chlorprothixene Hydrochloride (May increase the drowsiness effect; avoid concurrent use).
No products indexed under this heading.

Clorazepate Dipotassium (May increase the drowsiness effect; avoid concurrent use). Products include:
Tranxene 451

Diazepam (May increase the drowsiness effect; avoid concurrent use). Products include:
Dizac 1809
Valium Injectable 2182
Valium Tablets 2183
Valrelease Capsules 2169

Droperidol (May increase the drowsiness effect; avoid concurrent use). Products include:
Inapsine Injection 1296

Estazolam (May increase the drowsiness effect; avoid concurrent use). Products include:
ProSom Tablets 449

Ethchlorvynol (May increase the drowsiness effect; avoid concurrent use). Products include:
Placidyl Capsules 448

Ethinamate (May increase the drowsiness effect; avoid concurrent use).
No products indexed under this heading.

Fluphenazine Decanoate (May increase the drowsiness effect; avoid concurrent use). Products include:
Prolixin Decanoate 509

Fluphenazine Enanthate (May increase the drowsiness effect; avoid concurrent use). Products include:
Prolixin Enanthate 509

Fluphenazine Hydrochloride (May increase the drowsiness effect; avoid concurrent use). Products include:
Prolixin 509

Flurazepam Hydrochloride (May increase the drowsiness effect; avoid concurrent use). Products include:
Dalmane Capsules 2173

Furazolidone (Concurrent and/or sequential use is not recommended). Products include:
Furoxone 2046

Glutethimide (May increase the drowsiness effect; avoid concurrent use).
No products indexed under this heading.

Haloperidol (May increase the drowsiness effect; avoid concurrent use). Products include:
Haldol Injection, Tablets and Concentrate 1575

Haloperidol Decanoate (May increase the drowsiness effect; avoid concurrent use). Products include:
Haldol Decanoate 1577

Hydroxyzine Hydrochloride (May increase the drowsiness effect; avoid concurrent use). Products include:
Atarax Tablets & Syrup 2185
Marax Tablets & DF Syrup 2200
Vistaril Intramuscular Solution 2216

Isocarboxazid (Concurrent and/or sequential use is not recommended).
No products indexed under this heading.

Lorazepam (May increase the drowsiness effect; avoid concurrent use). Products include:
Ativan Injection 2698
Ativan Tablets 2700

Loxapine Hydrochloride (May increase the drowsiness effect; avoid concurrent use). Products include:
Loxitane 1378

Loxapine Succinate (May increase the drowsiness effect; avoid concurrent use). Products include:
Loxitane Capsules 1378

Meprobamate (May increase the drowsiness effect; avoid concurrent use). Products include:
Miltown Tablets 2672
PMB 200 and PMB 400 2783

Mesoridazine Besylate (May increase the drowsiness effect; avoid concurrent use). Products include:
Serentil 684

Midazolam Hydrochloride (May increase the drowsiness effect; avoid concurrent use). Products include:
Versed Injection 2170

Molindone Hydrochloride (May increase the drowsiness effect; avoid concurrent use). Products include:
Moban Tablets and Concentrate 1048

Oxazepam (May increase the drowsiness effect; avoid concurrent use). Products include:
Serax Capsules 2810
Serax Tablets 2810

Perphenazine (May increase the drowsiness effect; avoid concurrent use). Products include:
Etrafon 2355
Triavil Tablets 1757
Trilafon 2389

Phenelzine Sulfate (Concurrent and/or sequential use is not recommended). Products include:
Nardil 1920

Prazepam (May increase the drowsiness effect; avoid concurrent use).
No products indexed under this heading.

Prochlorperazine (May increase the drowsiness effect; avoid concurrent use). Products include:
Compazine 2470

Promethazine Hydrochloride (May increase the drowsiness effect; avoid concurrent use). Products include:
Mepergan Injection 2753
Phenergan with Codeine 2777
Phenergan with Dextromethorphan 2778
Phenergan Injection 2773
Phenergan Suppositories 2775
Phenergan Syrup 2774
Phenergan Tablets 2775
Phenergan VC 2779
Phenergan VC with Codeine 2781

Propofol (May increase the drowsiness effect; avoid concurrent use). Products include:
Diprivan Injection 2833

Quazepam (May increase the drowsiness effect; avoid concurrent use). Products include:
Doral Tablets 2664

Secobarbital Sodium (May increase the drowsiness effect; avoid concurrent use). Products include:
Seconal Sodium Pulvules 1474

Selegiline Hydrochloride (Concurrent and/or sequential use is not recommended). Products include:
Eldepryl Tablets 2550

Temazepam (May increase the drowsiness effect; avoid concurrent use). Products include:
Restoril Capsules 2284

Thioridazine Hydrochloride (May increase the drowsiness effect; avoid concurrent use). Products include:
Mellaril 2269

Thiothixene (May increase the drowsiness effect; avoid concurrent use). Products include:
Navane Capsules and Concentrate 2201
Navane Intramuscular 2202

Tranylcypromine Sulfate (Concurrent and/or sequential use is not recommended). Products include:
Parnate Tablets 2503

Triazolam (May increase the drowsiness effect; avoid concurrent use). Products include:
Halcion Tablets 2611

Trifluoperazine Hydrochloride (May increase the drowsiness effect; avoid concurrent use). Products include:
Stelazine 2514

Zolpidem Tartrate (May increase the drowsiness effect; avoid concurrent use). Products include:
Ambien Tablets 2416

Food Interactions

Alcohol (May increase the drowsiness effect; avoid concurrent use).

CONTAC SEVERE COLD AND FLU FORMULA CAPLETS

(Acetaminophen, Chlorpheniramine Maleate, Dextromethorphan Hydrobromide, Phenylpropanolamine Hydrochloride) 814
May interact with monoamine oxidase inhibitors, tranquilizers, hypnotics and sedatives, and certain other agents. Compounds in these categories include:

Alprazolam (May increase drowsiness effect; concurrent use should be avoided). Products include:
Xanax Tablets 2649

Buspirone Hydrochloride (May increase drowsiness effect; concurrent use should be avoided). Products include:
BuSpar 737

Chlordiazepoxide (May increase drowsiness effect; concurrent use should be avoided). Products include:
Libritabs Tablets 2177
Limbitrol 2180

Chlordiazepoxide Hydrochloride (May increase drowsiness effect; concurrent use should be avoided). Products include:

- Librax Capsules ... 2176
- Librium Capsules ... 2178
- Librium Injectable ... 2179

Chlorpromazine (May increase drowsiness effect; concurrent use should be avoided). Products include:

- Thorazine Suppositories ... 2523

Chlorpromazine Hydrochloride (May increase drowsiness effect; concurrent use should be avoided). Products include:

- Thorazine ... 2523

Chlorprothixene (May increase drowsiness effect; concurrent use should be avoided).

- No products indexed under this heading.

Chlorprothixene Hydrochloride (May increase drowsiness effect; concurrent use should be avoided).

- No products indexed under this heading.

Clorazepate Dipotassium (May increase drowsiness effect; concurrent use should be avoided). Products include:

- Tranxene ... 451

Diazepam (May increase drowsiness effect; concurrent use should be avoided). Products include:

- Dizac ... 1809
- Valium Injectable ... 2182
- Valium Tablets ... 2183
- Valrelease Capsules ... 2169

Droperidol (May increase drowsiness effect; concurrent use should be avoided). Products include:

- Inapsine Injection ... 1296

Estazolam (May increase drowsiness effect; concurrent use should be avoided). Products include:

- ProSom Tablets ... 449

Ethchlorvynol (May increase drowsiness effect; concurrent use should be avoided). Products include:

- Placidyl Capsules ... 448

Ethinamate (May increase drowsiness effect; concurrent use should be avoided).

- No products indexed under this heading.

Fluphenazine Decanoate (May increase drowsiness effect; concurrent use should be avoided). Products include:

- Prolixin Decanoate ... 509

Fluphenazine Enanthate (May increase drowsiness effect; concurrent use should be avoided). Products include:

- Prolixin Enanthate ... 509

Fluphenazine Hydrochloride (May increase drowsiness effect; concurrent use should be avoided). Products include:

- Prolixin ... 509

Flurazepam Hydrochloride (May increase drowsiness effect; concurrent use should be avoided). Products include:

- Dalmane Capsules ... 2173

Furazolidone (Concurrent and/or sequential use is not recommended unless directed by a doctor). Products include:

- Furoxone ... 2046

Glutethimide (May increase drowsiness effect; concurrent use should be avoided).

- No products indexed under this heading.

Haloperidol (May increase drowsiness effect; concurrent use should be avoided). Products include:

- Haldol Injection, Tablets and Concentrate ... 1575

Haloperidol Decanoate (May increase drowsiness effect; concurrent use should be avoided). Products include:

- Haldol Decanoate ... 1577

Hydroxyzine Hydrochloride (May increase drowsiness effect; concurrent use should be avoided). Products include:

- Atarax Tablets & Syrup ... 2185
- Marax Tablets & DF Syrup ... 2200
- Vistaril Intramuscular Solution ... 2216

Isocarboxazid (Concurrent and/or sequential use is not recommended unless directed by a doctor).

- No products indexed under this heading.

Lorazepam (May increase drowsiness effect; concurrent use should be avoided). Products include:

- Ativan Injection ... 2698
- Ativan Tablets ... 2700

Loxapine Hydrochloride (May increase drowsiness effect; concurrent use should be avoided). Products include:

- Loxitane ... 1378

Loxapine Succinate (May increase drowsiness effect; concurrent use should be avoided). Products include:

- Loxitane Capsules ... 1378

Meprobamate (May increase drowsiness effect; concurrent use should be avoided). Products include:

- Miltown Tablets ... 2672
- PMB 200 and PMB 400 ... 2783

Mesoridazine Besylate (May increase drowsiness effect; concurrent use should be avoided). Products include:

- Serentil ... 684

Midazolam Hydrochloride (May increase drowsiness effect; concurrent use should be avoided). Products include:

- Versed Injection ... 2170

Molindone Hydrochloride (May increase drowsiness effect; concurrent use should be avoided). Products include:

- Moban Tablets and Concentrate ... 1048

Oxazepam (May increase drowsiness effect; concurrent use should be avoided). Products include:

- Serax Capsules ... 2810
- Serax Tablets ... 2810

Perphenazine (May increase drowsiness effect; concurrent use should be avoided). Products include:

- Etrafon ... 2355
- Triavil Tablets ... 1757
- Trilafon ... 2389

Phenelzine Sulfate (Concurrent and/or sequential use is not recommended unless directed by a doctor). Products include:

- Nardil ... 1920

Prazepam (May increase drowsiness effect; concurrent use should be avoided).

- No products indexed under this heading.

Prochlorperazine (May increase drowsiness effect; concurrent use should be avoided). Products include:

- Compazine ... 2470

Promethazine Hydrochloride (May increase drowsiness effect; concurrent use should be avoided). Products include:

- Mepergan Injection ... 2753
- Phenergan with Codeine ... 2777
- Phenergan with Dextromethorphan 2778
- Phenergan Injection ... 2773
- Phenergan Suppositories ... 2775
- Phenergan Syrup ... 2774
- Phenergan Tablets ... 2775
- Phenergan VC ... 2779
- Phenergan VC with Codeine ... 2781

Propofol (May increase drowsiness effect; concurrent use should be avoided). Products include:

- Diprivan Injection ... 2833

Quazepam (May increase drowsiness effect; concurrent use should be avoided). Products include:

- Doral Tablets ... 2664

Secobarbital Sodium (May increase drowsiness effect; concurrent use should be avoided). Products include:

- Seconal Sodium Pulvules ... 1474

Selegiline Hydrochloride (Concurrent and/or sequential use is not recommended unless directed by a doctor). Products include:

- Eldepryl Tablets ... 2550

Temazepam (May increase drowsiness effect; concurrent use should be avoided). Products include:

- Restoril Capsules ... 2284

Thioridazine Hydrochloride (May increase drowsiness effect; concurrent use should be avoided). Products include:

- Mellaril ... 2269

Thiothixene (May increase drowsiness effect; concurrent use should be avoided). Products include:

- Navane Capsules and Concentrate 2201
- Navane Intramuscular ... 2202

Tranylcypromine Sulfate (Concurrent and/or sequential use is not recommended unless directed by a doctor). Products include:

- Parnate Tablets ... 2503

Triazolam (May increase drowsiness effect; concurrent use should be avoided). Products include:

- Halcion Tablets ... 2611

Trifluoperazine Hydrochloride (May increase drowsiness effect; concurrent use should be avoided). Products include:

- Stelazine ... 2514

Zolpidem Tartrate (May increase drowsiness effect; concurrent use should be avoided). Products include:

- Ambien Tablets ... 2416

Food Interactions

Alcohol (May increase drowsiness effect; concurrent use should be avoided).

CONTAC SEVERE COLD & FLU NON-DROWSY

(Acetaminophen, Dextromethorphan Hydrobromide, Pseudoephedrine Hydrochloride) ... ▣ 815

May interact with monoamine oxidase inhibitors. Compounds in this category include:

Furazolidone (Concurrent and/or sequential use is not recommended). Products include:

- Furoxone ... 2046

Isocarboxazid (Concurrent and/or sequential use is not recommended).

- No products indexed under this heading.

Phenelzine Sulfate (Concurrent and/or sequential use is not recommended). Products include:

- Nardil ... 1920

Selegiline Hydrochloride (Concurrent and/or sequential use is not recommended). Products include:

- Eldepryl Tablets ... 2550

Tranylcypromine Sulfate (Concurrent and/or sequential use is not recommended). Products include:

- Parnate Tablets ... 2503

CORDARONE INTRAVENOUS

(Amiodarone Hydrochloride) ... 2715

May interact with beta blockers, calcium channel blockers, and certain other agents. Compounds in these categories include:

Acebutolol Hydrochloride (Increased risk of hypotension and bradycardia). Products include:

- Sectral Capsules ... 2807

Amlodipine Besylate (Increased risk of AV block and hypotension). Products include:

- Lotrel Capsules ... 840
- Norvasc Tablets ... 1940

Atenolol (Increased risk of hypotension and bradycardia). Products include:

- Tenoretic Tablets ... 2845
- Tenormin Tablets and I.V. Injection 2847

Bepridil Hydrochloride (Increased risk of AV block and hypotension). Products include:

- Vascor (200, 300 and 400 mg) Tablets ... 1587

Betaxolol Hydrochloride (Increased risk of hypotension and bradycardia). Products include:

- Betoptic Ophthalmic Solution ... 469
- Betoptic S Ophthalmic Suspension 471
- Kerlone Tablets ... 2436

Bisoprolol Fumarate (Increased risk of hypotension and bradycardia). Products include:

- Zebeta Tablets ... 1413
- Ziac ... 1415

Carteolol Hydrochloride (Increased risk of hypotension and bradycardia). Products include:

- Cartrol Tablets ... 410
- Ocupress Ophthalmic Solution, 1% Sterile ... ⊙ 309

Cholestyramine (Increases enterohepatic elimination of amiodarone and may reduce serum levels and t½). Products include:

- Questran Light ... 769
- Questran Powder ... 770

Cimetidine (Increases serum amiodarone levels). Products include:

- Tagamet Tablets ... 2516

Cimetidine Hydrochloride (Increases serum amiodarone levels). Products include:

- Tagamet ... 2516

Cyclosporine (Elevated plasma concentrations of cyclosporine resulting in elevated creatinine, despite reduction in dose of cyclosporine). Products include:

- Neoral ... 2276
- Sandimmune ... 2286

Dextromethorphan Hydrobromide (Chronic oral amiodarone administration impairs metabolism of dextromethorphan). Products include:

- Alka-Seltzer Plus Cold & Cough Medicine ... ▣ 708
- Alka-Seltzer Plus Cold & Cough Medicine Liqui-Gels ... ▣ 705
- Alka-Seltzer Plus Night-Time Cold Medicine ... ▣ 707
- Alka-Seltzer Plus Night-Time Cold Medicine Liqui-Gels ... ▣ 706

Interactions Index

Cordarone Tablets

Benylin Adult Formula Cough Suppressant....................................... ℞ 852
Benylin Expectorant .... ℞ 852
Benylin Multisymptom........................... ℞ 852
Benylin Pediatric Cough Suppressant .... ℞ 853
Bromfed-DM Cough Syrup.................. 1786
Buckley's Mixture .... ℞ 624
Cerose DM .... ℞ 878
Cheracol-D Cough Formula .... ℞ 769
Cheracol Plus Head Cold/Cough Formula .... ℞ 769
Children's Vicks NyQuil Cold/ Cough Relief.. ℞ 758
Comtrex Multi-Symptom Cold Reliever Tablets/Caplets/Liqui-Gels/Liquid... ℞ 615
Comtrex Non-Drowsy............................. ℞ 618
Contac Day & Night Cold/Flu Caplets .... ℞ 812
Contac Severe Cold and Flu Formula Caplets .... ℞ 814
Contac Severe Cold & Flu Non-Drowsy .... ℞ 815
Cough-X Lozenges.................................. ℞ 602
Diabe-Tuss DM Syrup 1891
Dimetane-DX Cough Syrup 2059
Dimetapp DM Elixir............................... ℞ 774
Dorcol Children's Cough Syrup ...... ℞ 785
Drixoral Cough Liquid Caps................ ℞ 801
Drixoral Cough + Congestion Liquid Caps .... ℞ 802
Drixoral Cough + Sore Throat Liquid Caps .... ℞ 802
Humibid 462
Novahistine DMX .... ℞ 822
PediaCare Cough-Cold Chewable Tablets 1553
PediaCare Cough-Cold Liquid............ 1553
PediCare Infant's Drops Decongestant Plus Cough 1553
PediaCare NightRest Cough-Cold Liquid 1553
Pediatric Vicks 44d Dry Hacking Cough & Head Congestion............ ℞ 763
Pediatric Vicks 44e Chest Cough & Chest Congestion .... ℞ 764
Pediatric Vicks 44m Cough & Cold Relief .... ℞ 764
Phenergan with Dextromethorphan 2778
Robitussin Cold & Cough Liqui-Gels .... ℞ 776
Robitussin Maximum Strength Cough Suppressant .... ℞ 778
Robitussin Maximum Strength Cough & Cold .... ℞ 778
Robitussin Pediatric Cough & Cold Formula... ℞ 779
Robitussin Pediatric Cough Suppressant.. ℞ 779
Robitussin-CF .... ℞ 777
Robitussin-DM.. ℞ 777
Rondec-DM Oral Drops 954
Rondec-DM Syrup 954
Safe Tussin 30 1363
Sucrets 4-Hour Cough Suppressant .... ℞ 826
Sudafed Cold and Cough Liquidcaps... ℞ 862
Sudafed Cough Syrup .... ℞ 862
Sudafed Severe Cold Formula Caplets .... ℞ 863
Sudafed Severe Cold Formula Tablets .... ℞ 864
Syn-Rx DM Tablets 466
TheraFlu Flu, Cold and Cough Medicine .... ℞ 787
TheraFlu Maximum Strength Nighttime Flu, Cold & Cough Medicine .... ℞ 788
TheraFlu Maximum Strength Non-Drowsy Formula Flu, Cold & Cough Medicine .... ℞ 788
Thera Flu Maximum Strength, Non-Drowsy Formula Flu, Cold and Cough Caplets .... ℞ 789
Triaminic AM Cough and Decongestant Formula................................. ℞ 789
Triaminic Nite Light............................... ℞ 791
Triaminic Sore Throat Formula ...... ℞ 791
Triaminic-DM Syrup .... ℞ 792
Triaminicol Multi-Symptom Cold Tablets .... ℞ 793
Triaminicol Multi-Symptom Relief ℞ 794
Tussi-Organidin DM NR Liquid and DM-S NR Liquid 2677
Children's TYLENOL Cold Plus Cough Multi Symptom Tablets and Liquid... ℞ 681
TYLENOL Flu Maximum Strength Gelcaps 1565

TYLENOL Cold Multi-Symptom Formula Medication Tablets and Caplets 1561
TYLENOL Cold Medication No Drowsiness Formula Gelcaps and Caplets 1562
TYLENOL Cold Multi-Symptom Hot Medication Liquid Packets.............. 1557
TYLENOL Cough Multi-Symptom Medication 1564
TYLENOL Cough Multi-Symptom Medication with Decongestant...... 1565
Vicks 44 Dry Hacking Cough .... ℞ 755
Vicks 44 LiquiCaps Cough, Cold & Flu Relief.. ℞ 755
Vicks 44 LiquiCaps Non-Drowsy Cough & Cold Relief .... ℞ 756
Vicks 44D Dry Hacking Cough & Head Congestion .... ℞ 755
Vicks 44E Chest Cough & Chest Congestion .... ℞ 756
Vicks 44M Cough, Cold & Flu Relief... ℞ 756
Vicks DayQuil .... ℞ 761
Vicks Nyquil Hot Therapy................... ℞ 762
Vicks NyQuil LiquiCaps Multi-Symptom Cold/Flu Relief............... ℞ 763
Vicks NyQuil Multi-Symptom Cold/Flu Relief - (Original & Cherry Flavor) .... ℞ 763

Digoxin (Amiodarone increases serum concentration and effects of digoxin). Products include:

Lanoxicaps 1117
Lanoxin Elixir Pediatric 1120
Lanoxin Injection 1123
Lanoxin Injection Pediatric.................. 1126
Lanoxin Tablets 1128

Diltiazem Hydrochloride (Increased risk of AV block and hypotension). Products include:

Cardizem CD Capsules 1506
Cardizem SR Capsules 1510
Cardizem Injectable 1508
Cardizem Tablets.................................... 1512
Dilacor XR Extended-release Capsules 2018

Disopyramide Phosphate (Increased QT prolongation which would cause arrhythmia). Products include:

Norpace 2444

Esmolol Hydrochloride (Increased risk of hypotension and bradycardia). Products include:

Brevibloc Injection.................................. 1808

Felodipine (Increased risk of AV block and hypotension). Products include:

Plendil Extended-Release Tablets.... 527

Fentanyl (Potential for hypotension, bradycardia, decreased cardiac output). Products include:

Duragesic Transdermal System........ 1288

Fentanyl Citrate (Potential for hypotension, bradycardia, decreased cardiac output). Products include:

Sublimaze Injection................................ 1307

Flecainide Acetate (Increased effects of flecainide; reduces the dose of flecainide needed to maintain therapeutic plasma concentrations). Products include:

Tambocor Tablets 1497

Isradipine (Increased risk of AV block and hypotension). Products include:

DynaCirc Capsules 2256

Labetalol Hydrochloride (Increased risk of hypotension and bradycardia). Products include:

Normodyne Injection 2377
Normodyne Tablets 2379
Trandate 1185

Levobunolol Hydrochloride (Increased risk of hypotension and bradycardia). Products include:

Betagan .... © 233

Lidocaine Hydrochloride (Potential for seizure associated with increased lidocaine concentrations; sinus bradycardia has been observed with oral amiodarone and lidocaine for anesthesia). Products include:

Bactine Antiseptic/Anesthetic First Aid Liquid .... ℞ 708
Campho-Phenique Maximum Strength First Aid Antibiotic Plus Pain Reliever Ointment .... ℞ 719
Decadron Phosphate with Xylocaine Injection, Sterile 1639
Xylocaine Injections 567

Methotrexate Sodium (Chronic oral amiodarone administration impairs metabolism of methotrexate). Products include:

Methotrexate Sodium Tablets, Injection, for Injection and LPF Injection 1275

Metipranolol Hydrochloride (Increased risk of hypotension and bradycardia). Products include:

OptiPranolol (Metipranolol 0.3%) Sterile Ophthalmic Solution.......... © 258

Metoprolol Succinate (Increased risk of hypotension and bradycardia). Products include:

Toprol-XL Tablets 565

Metoprolol Tartrate (Increased risk of hypotension and bradycardia). Products include:

Lopressor Ampuls................................... 830
Lopressor HCT Tablets 832
Lopressor Tablets 830

Nadolol (Increased risk of hypotension and bradycardia).
No products indexed under this heading.

Nicardipine Hydrochloride (Increased risk of AV block and hypotension). Products include:

Cardene Capsules 2095
Cardene I.V. 2709
Cardene SR Capsules............................. 2097

Nifedipine (Increased risk of AV block and hypotension). Products include:

Adalat Capsules (10 mg and 20 mg) 587
Adalat CC 589
Procardia Capsules................................. 1971
Procardia XL Extended Release Tablets 1972

Nimodipine (Increased risk of AV block and hypotension). Products include:

Nimotop Capsules................................... 610

Nisoldipine (Increased risk of AV block and hypotension).
No products indexed under this heading.

Penbutolol Sulfate (Increased risk of hypotension and bradycardia). Products include:

Levatol 2403

Phenytoin (Decreases serum amiodarone levels; chronic oral amiodarone administration impairs metabolism of phenytoin). Products include:

Dilantin Infatabs 1908
Dilantin-125 Suspension 1911

Phenytoin Sodium (Decreases serum amiodarone levels; chronic oral amiodarone administration impairs metabolism of phenytoin). Products include:

Dilantin Kapseals 1906
Dilantin Parenteral 1910

Pindolol (Increased risk of hypotension and bradycardia). Products include:

Visken Tablets.. 2299

Procainamide Hydrochloride (Amiodarone increases serum concentration of procainamide and N-acetylprocainamide; increased effects of procainamide). Products include:

Procan SR Tablets................................... 1926

Propranolol Hydrochloride (Increased risk of hypotension and bradycardia). Products include:

Inderal 2728
Inderal LA Long Acting Capsules 2730
Inderide Tablets 2732
Inderide LA Long Acting Capsules .. 2734

Quinidine Gluconate (Amiodarone increases serum concentration and effects of quinidine). Products include:

Quinaglute Dura-Tabs Tablets 649

Quinidine Polygalacturonate (Amiodarone increases serum concentration and effects of quinidine).
No products indexed under this heading.

Quinidine Sulfate (Amiodarone increases serum concentration and effects of quinidine). Products include:

Quinidex Extentabs 2067

Sotalol Hydrochloride (Increased risk of hypotension and bradycardia). Products include:

Betapace Tablets 641

Timolol Hemihydrate (Increased risk of hypotension and bradycardia). Products include:

Betimol 0.25%, 0.5% .... © 261

Timolol Maleate (Increased risk of hypotension and bradycardia). Products include:

Blocadren Tablets 1614
Timolide Tablets...................................... 1748
Timoptic in Ocudose 1753
Timoptic Sterile Ophthalmic Solution... 1751
Timoptic-XE 1755

Verapamil Hydrochloride (Increased risk of AV block and hypotension). Products include:

Calan SR Caplets 2422
Calan Tablets.. 2419
Isoptin Injectable 1344
Isoptin Oral Tablets 1346
Isoptin SR Tablets................................... 1348
Verelan Capsules..................................... 1410
Verelan Capsules..................................... 2824

Warfarin Sodium (Increased prothrombin time; amiodarone increases effects of warfarin). Products include:

Coumadin 926

CORDARONE TABLETS

(Amiodarone Hydrochloride) 2712
May interact with antiarrhythmics, oral anticoagulants, beta blockers, calcium channel blockers, cardiac glycosides, and certain other agents. Compounds in these categories include:

Acebutolol Hydrochloride (Bradycardia, sinus arrest, and AV block potentiated; potentially serious toxicity). Products include:

Sectral Capsules 2807

Adenosine (Bradycardia, sinus arrest, and AV block potentiated; potentially serious toxicity). Products include:

Adenocard Injection 1021
Adenoscan 1024

Amlodipine Besylate (Bradycardia, sinus arrest, and AV block potentiated). Products include:

Lotrel Capsules.. 840
Norvasc Tablets 1940

Atenolol (Bradycardia, sinus arrest, and AV block potentiated). Products include:

Tenoretic Tablets..................................... 2845

IMPORTANT NOTE: Always consult each drug listing in the patient's regimen for possible interactions.

Cordarone Tablets | **Interactions Index** | **204**

Tenormin Tablets and I.V. Injection 2847

Bepridil Hydrochloride (Bradycardia, sinus arrest, and AV block potentiated). Products include:

- Vascor (200, 300 and 400 mg) Tablets 1587

Betaxolol Hydrochloride (Bradycardia, sinus arrest, and AV block potentiated; potentially serious toxicity). Products include:

- Betoptic Ophthalmic Solution 469
- Betoptic S Ophthalmic Suspension 471
- Kerlone Tablets 2436

Bisoprolol Fumarate (Bradycardia, sinus arrest, and AV block potentiated; potentially serious toxicity). Products include:

- Zebeta Tablets 1413
- Ziac 1415

Bretylium Tosylate (Potentially serious toxicity).

- No products indexed under this heading.

Carteolol Hydrochloride (Bradycardia, sinus arrest, and AV block potentiated; potentially serious toxicity). Products include:

- Cartrol Tablets 410
- Ocupress Ophthalmic Solution, 1% Sterile .... ◉ 309

Cyclosporine (Concomitant use has reported to produce persistently elevated plasma concentrations of cyclosporine resulting in elevated creatinine, despite reduction in dose of cyclosporine). Products include:

- Neoral 2276
- Sandimmune 2286

Deslanoside (Increased in serum digitalis glycoside levels resulting in clinical toxicity; discontinue or reduce digitalis dosage by 50%).

- No products indexed under this heading.

Dicumarol (Potentiated; serious or fatal bleeding).

- No products indexed under this heading.

Digitoxin (Increased in serum digitalis glycoside levels resulting in clinical toxicity; discontinue or reduce digitalis dosage by 50%). Products include:

- Crystodigin Tablets 1433

Digoxin (Increased in serum digitalis glycoside levels resulting in clinical toxicity; discontinue or reduce digitalis dosage by 50%). Products include:

- Lanoxicaps 1117
- Lanoxin Elixir Pediatric 1120
- Lanoxin Injection 1123
- Lanoxin Injection Pediatric 1126
- Lanoxin Tablets 1128

Diltiazem Hydrochloride (Bradycardia, sinus arrest, and AV block potentiated). Products include:

- Cardizem CD Capsules 1506
- Cardizem SR Capsules 1510
- Cardizem Injectable 1508
- Cardizem Tablets 1512
- Dilacor XR Extended-release Capsules 2018

Disopyramide Phosphate (Potentially serious toxicity). Products include:

- Norpace 2444

Esmolol Hydrochloride (Bradycardia, sinus arrest, and AV block potentiated). Products include:

- Brevibloc Injection 1808

Felodipine (Bradycardia, sinus arrest, and AV block potentiated). Products include:

- Plendil Extended-Release Tablets 527

Isradipine (Bradycardia, sinus arrest, and AV block potentiated). Products include:

- DynaCirc Capsules 2256

Labetalol Hydrochloride (Bradycardia, sinus arrest, and AV block potentiated). Products include:

- Normodyne Injection 2377
- Normodyne Tablets 2379
- Trandate 1185

Levobunolol Hydrochloride (Bradycardia, sinus arrest, and AV block potentiated; potentially serious toxicity). Products include:

- Betagan .... ◉ 233

Lidocaine Hydrochloride (Potentially serious toxicity). Products include:

- Bactine Antiseptic/Anesthetic First Aid Liquid .... ◙ 708
- Campho-Phenique Maximum Strength First Aid Antibiotic Plus Pain Reliever Ointment .... ◙ 719
- Decadron Phosphate with Xylocaine Injection, Sterile 1639
- Xylocaine Injections 567

Metipranolol Hydrochloride (Bradycardia, sinus arrest, and AV block potentiated; potentially serious toxicity). Products include:

- OptiPranolol (Metipranolol 0.3%) Sterile Ophthalmic Solution .... ◉ 258

Metoprolol Succinate (Bradycardia, sinus arrest, and AV block potentiated; potentially serious toxicity). Products include:

- Toprol-XL Tablets 565

Metoprolol Tartrate (Bradycardia, sinus arrest, and AV block potentiated). Products include:

- Lopressor Ampuls 830
- Lopressor HCT Tablets 832
- Lopressor Tablets 830

Mexiletine Hydrochloride (Potentially serious toxicity). Products include:

- Mexitil Capsules 678

Moricizine Hydrochloride (Bradycardia, sinus arrest, and AV block potentiated; potentially serious toxicity). Products include:

- Ethmozine Tablets 2041

Nadolol (Bradycardia, sinus arrest, and AV block potentiated).

- No products indexed under this heading.

Nicardipine Hydrochloride (Bradycardia, sinus arrest, and AV block potentiated). Products include:

- Cardene Capsules 2095
- Cardene I.V. 2709
- Cardene SR Capsules 2097

Nifedipine (Bradycardia, sinus arrest, and AV block potentiated). Products include:

- Adalat Capsules (10 mg and 20 mg) 587
- Adalat CC 589
- Procardia Capsules 1971
- Procardia XL Extended Release Tablets 1972

Nimodipine (Bradycardia, sinus arrest, and AV block potentiated). Products include:

- Nimotop Capsules 610

Nisoldipine (Bradycardia, sinus arrest, and AV block potentiated).

- No products indexed under this heading.

Penbutolol Sulfate (Bradycardia, sinus arrest, and AV block potentiated; potentially serious toxicity). Products include:

- Levatol 2403

Phenytoin (Increased steady state levels). Products include:

- Dilantin Infatabs 1908
- Dilantin-125 Suspension 1911

Phenytoin Sodium (Increased steady state levels). Products include:

- Dilantin Kapseals 1906
- Dilantin Parenteral 1910

Pindolol (Bradycardia, sinus arrest, and AV block potentiated). Products include:

- Visken Tablets 2299

Procainamide Hydrochloride (Increased steady state levels; bradycardia, sinus arrest, and AV block potentiated; potentially serious toxicity). Products include:

- Procan SR Tablets 1926

Propafenone Hydrochloride (Bradycardia, sinus arrest, and AV block potentiated; potentially serious toxicity). Products include:

- Rythmol Tablets–150mg, 225mg, 300mg 1352

Propranolol Hydrochloride (Bradycardia, sinus arrest, and AV block potentiated; potentially serious toxicity). Products include:

- Inderal 2728
- Inderal LA Long Acting Capsules 2730
- Inderide Tablets 2732
- Inderide LA Long Acting Capsules .. 2734

Quinidine Gluconate (Potentially serious toxicity; increases serum concentration by 33%). Products include:

- Quinaglute Dura-Tabs Tablets 649

Quinidine Polygalacturonate (Potentially serious toxicity; increases serum concentration by 33%).

- No products indexed under this heading.

Quinidine Sulfate (Potentially serious toxicity; increases serum concentration by 33%). Products include:

- Quinidex Extentabs 2067

Sotalol Hydrochloride (Bradycardia, sinus arrest, and AV block potentiated; potentially serious toxicity). Products include:

- Betapace Tablets 641

Timolol Hemihydrate (Bradycardia, sinus arrest, and AV block potentiated; potentially serious toxicity). Products include:

- Betimol 0.25%, 0.5% .... ◉ 261

Timolol Maleate (Bradycardia, sinus arrest, and AV block potentiated). Products include:

- Blocadren Tablets 1614
- Timolide Tablets 1748
- Timoptic in Ocudose 1753
- Timoptic Sterile Ophthalmic Solution 1751
- Timoptic-XE 1755

Tocainide Hydrochloride (Potentially serious toxicity). Products include:

- Tonocard Tablets 531

Verapamil Hydrochloride (Bradycardia, sinus arrest, and AV block potentiated; potentially serious toxicity). Products include:

- Calan SR Caplets 2422
- Calan Tablets 2419
- Isoptin Injectable 1344
- Isoptin Oral Tablets 1346
- Isoptin SR Tablets 1348
- Verelan Capsules 1410
- Verelan Capsules 2824

Warfarin Sodium (Potentiated; serious or fatal bleeding; increased prothrombin time by 100%). Products include:

- Coumadin 926

CORDRAN LOTION

(Flurandrenolide) 1803

None cited in PDR database.

CORDRAN TAPE

(Flurandrenolide) 1804

None cited in PDR database.

CORICIDIN 'D' DECONGESTANT TABLETS

(Acetaminophen, Chlorpheniramine Maleate, Phenylpropanolamine Hydrochloride) .... ◙ 800

May interact with phenylpropanolamine containing anorectics, hypnotics and sedatives, tranquilizers, monoamine oxidase inhibitors, and certain other agents. Compounds in these categories include:

Alprazolam (May increase drowsiness effect). Products include:

- Xanax Tablets 2649

Buspirone Hydrochloride (May increase drowsiness effect). Products include:

- BuSpar 737

Chlordiazepoxide (May increase drowsiness effect). Products include:

- Libritabs Tablets 2177
- Limbitrol 2180

Chlordiazepoxide Hydrochloride (May increase drowsiness effect). Products include:

- Librax Capsules 2176
- Librium Capsules 2178
- Librium Injectable 2179

Chlorpromazine (May increase drowsiness effect). Products include:

- Thorazine Suppositories 2523

Chlorpromazine Hydrochloride (May increase drowsiness effect). Products include:

- Thorazine 2523

Chlorprothixene (May increase drowsiness effect).

- No products indexed under this heading.

Chlorprothixene Hydrochloride (May increase drowsiness effect).

- No products indexed under this heading.

Clorazepate Dipotassium (May increase drowsiness effect). Products include:

- Tranxene 451

Diazepam (May increase drowsiness effect). Products include:

- Dizac 1809
- Valium Injectable 2182
- Valium Tablets 2183
- Valrelease Capsules 2169

Droperidol (May increase drowsiness effect). Products include:

- Inapsine Injection 1296

Estazolam (May increase drowsiness effect). Products include:

- ProSom Tablets 449

Ethchlorvynol (May increase drowsiness effect). Products include:

- Placidyl Capsules 448

Ethinamate (May increase drowsiness effect).

- No products indexed under this heading.

Fluphenazine Decanoate (May increase drowsiness effect). Products include:

- Prolixin Decanoate 509

Fluphenazine Enanthate (May increase drowsiness effect). Products include:

- Prolixin Enanthate 509

Fluphenazine Hydrochloride (May increase drowsiness effect). Products include:

- Prolixin 509

Flurazepam Hydrochloride (May increase drowsiness effect). Products include:

- Dalmane Capsules 2173

Furazolidone (Concurrent use is not recommended). Products include:

- Furoxone 2046

Glutethimide (May increase drowsiness effect).

No products indexed under this heading.

Haloperidol (May increase drowsiness effect). Products include:

Haldol Injection, Tablets and Concentrate 1575

Haloperidol Decanoate (May increase drowsiness effect). Products include:

Haldol Decanoate..................................... 1577

Hydroxyzine Hydrochloride (May increase drowsiness effect). Products include:

Atarax Tablets & Syrup......................... 2185
Marax Tablets & DF Syrup.................. 2200
Vistaril Intramuscular Solution.......... 2216

Isocarboxazid (Concurrent use is not recommended).

No products indexed under this heading.

Lorazepam (May increase drowsiness effect). Products include:

Ativan Injection.. 2698
Ativan Tablets... 2700

Loxapine Hydrochloride (May increase drowsiness effect). Products include:

Loxitane 1378

Loxapine Succinate (May increase drowsiness effect). Products include:

Loxitane Capsules 1378

Meprobamate (May increase drowsiness effect). Products include:

Miltown Tablets 2672
PMB 200 and PMB 400 2783

Mesoridazine Besylate (May increase drowsiness effect). Products include:

Serentil.. 684

Midazolam Hydrochloride (May increase drowsiness effect). Products include:

Versed Injection 2170

Molindone Hydrochloride (May increase drowsiness effect). Products include:

Moban Tablets and Concentrate...... 1048

Oxazepam (May increase drowsiness effect). Products include:

Serax Capsules 2810
Serax Tablets... 2810

Perphenazine (May increase drowsiness effect). Products include:

Etrafon 2355
Triavil Tablets 1757
Trilafon... 2389

Phenelzine Sulfate (Concurrent use is not recommended). Products include:

Nardil 1920

Phenylpropanolamine Containing Anorectics (Product labeling recommends physician's supervision for concurrent administration of these drugs).

Prazepam (May increase drowsiness effect).

No products indexed under this heading.

Prochlorperazine (May increase drowsiness effect). Products include:

Compazine 2470

Promethazine Hydrochloride (May increase drowsiness effect). Products include:

Mepergan Injection 2753
Phenergan with Codeine....................... 2777
Phenergan with Dextromethorphan 2778
Phenergan Injection 2773
Phenergan Suppositories 2775
Phenergan Syrup..................................... 2774
Phenergan Tablets................................... 2775
Phenergan VC... 2779
Phenergan VC with Codeine............... 2781

Propofol (May increase drowsiness effect). Products include:

Diprivan Injection.................................... 2833

Quazepam (May increase drowsiness effect). Products include:

Doral Tablets 2664

Secobarbital Sodium (May increase drowsiness effect). Products include:

Seconal Sodium Pulvules 1474

Selegiline Hydrochloride (Concurrent use is not recommended). Products include:

Eldepryl Tablets 2550

Temazepam (May increase drowsiness effect). Products include:

Restoril Capsules 2284

Thioridazine Hydrochloride (May increase drowsiness effect). Products include:

Mellaril 2269

Thiothixene (May increase drowsiness effect). Products include:

Navane Capsules and Concentrate 2201
Navane Intramuscular 2202

Tranylcypromine Sulfate (Concurrent use is not recommended). Products include:

Parnate Tablets 2503

Triazolam (May increase drowsiness effect). Products include:

Halcion Tablets... 2611

Trifluoperazine Hydrochloride (May increase drowsiness effect). Products include:

Stelazine 2514

Zolpidem Tartrate (May increase drowsiness effect). Products include:

Ambien Tablets... 2416

Food Interactions

Alcohol (May increase drowsiness effect).

CORICIDIN TABLETS

(Acetaminophen, Chlorpheniramine Maleate) .... ⊞ 800

See Coricidin 'D' Decongestant Tablets

CORRECTOL EXTRA GENTLE STOOL SOFTENER

(Docusate Sodium) .... ⊞ 801
None cited in PDR database.

CORRECTOL LAXATIVE TABLETS & CAPLETS

(Docusate Sodium, Phenolphthalein) .... ⊞ 801
None cited in PDR database.

CORTAID CREAM WITH ALOE

(Hydrocortisone Acetate).................... ⊞ 836
None cited in PDR database.

CORTAID LOTION

(Hydrocortisone Acetate).................... ⊞ 836
None cited in PDR database.

CORTAID OINTMENT WITH ALOE

(Hydrocortisone Acetate).................... ⊞ 836
None cited in PDR database.

CORTAID SPRAY

(Hydrocortisone) .... ⊞ 836
None cited in PDR database.

MAXIMUM STRENGTH CORTAID CREAM

(Hydrocortisone Acetate).................... ⊞ 836
None cited in PDR database.

MAXIMUM STRENGTH CORTAID OINTMENT

(Hydrocortisone Acetate).................... ⊞ 836
None cited in PDR database.

MAXIMUM STRENGTH CORTAID SPRAY

(Hydrocortisone) .... ⊞ 836
None cited in PDR database.

CORTENEMA

(Hydrocortisone) 2535
May interact with:

Aspirin (Concurrent use requires caution in hypoprothrombinemia). Products include:

Alka-Seltzer Effervescent Antacid and Pain Reliever............................... ⊞ 701
Alka-Seltzer Extra Strength Effervescent Antacid and Pain Reliever .... ⊞ 703
Alka-Seltzer Lemon Lime Effervescent Antacid and Pain Reliever .... ⊞ 703
Alka-Seltzer Plus Cold Medicine .... ⊞ 705
Alka-Seltzer Plus Cold & Cough Medicine .... ⊞ 708
Alka-Seltzer Plus Night-Time Cold Medicine .... ⊞ 707
Alka Seltzer Plus Sinus Medicine .. ⊞ 707
Arthritis Foundation Safety Coated Aspirin Tablets .... ⊞ 675
Arthritis Pain Ascriptin .... ⊞ 631
Maximum Strength Ascriptin .... ⊞ 630
Regular Strength Ascriptin Tablets .... ⊞ 629
Arthritis Strength BC Powder.......... ⊞ 609
BC Cold Powder Multi-Symptom Formula (Cold-Sinus-Allergy) ...... ⊞ 609
BC Cold Powder Non-Drowsy Formula (Cold-Sinus) .... ⊞ 609
BC Powder .... ⊞ 609
Bayer Children's Chewable Aspirin .... ⊞ 711
Genuine Bayer Aspirin Tablets & Caplets .... ⊞ 713
Extra Strength Bayer Arthritis Pain Regimen Formula .... ⊞ 711
Extra Strength Bayer Aspirin Caplets & Tablets .... ⊞ 712
Extended-Release Bayer 8-Hour Aspirin .... ⊞ 712
Extra Strength Bayer Plus Aspirin Caplets .... ⊞ 713
Extra Strength Bayer PM Aspirin .. ⊞ 713
Bayer Enteric Aspirin .... ⊞ 709
Bufferin Analgesic Tablets and Caplets .... ⊞ 613
Arthritis Strength Bufferin Analgesic Caplets .... ⊞ 614
Extra Strength Bufferin Analgesic Tablets .... ⊞ 615
Cama Arthritis Pain Reliever........... ⊞ 785
Darvon Compound-65 Pulvules 1435
Easprin.. 1914
Ecotrin 2455
Ecotrin Enteric Coated Aspirin Maximum Strength Tablets and Caplets .... ⊞ 816
Ecotrin Enteric Coated Aspirin Regular Strength Tablets 2455
Empirin Aspirin Tablets .... ⊞ 854
Empirin with Codeine Tablets........... 1093
Excedrin Extra-Strength Analgesic Tablets & Caplets 732
Fiorinal Capsules 2261
Fiorinal with Codeine Capsules 2262
Fiorinal Tablets.. 2261
Halfprin 1362
Healthprin Aspirin 2455
Norgesic.. 1496
Percodan Tablets..................................... 939
Percodan-Demi Tablets......................... 940
Robaxisal Tablets.................................... 2071
Soma Compound w/Codeine Tablets 2676
Soma Compound Tablets...................... 2675
St. Joseph Adult Chewable Aspirin (81 mg.) .... ⊞ 808
Talwin Compound 2335
Ursinus Inlay-Tabs................................. ⊞ 794
Vanquish Analgesic Caplets .... ⊞ 731

Immunization (Possible hazards of neurological complications and a lack of antibody response, especially in patients on high dose of corticosteroid).

Smallpox Vaccine (Possible hazards of neurological complications and a lack of antibody response, especially in patients on high dose of corticosteroid).

CORTIFOAM

(Hydrocortisone Acetate) 2396
None cited in PDR database.

CORTISPORIN CREAM

(Polymyxin B Sulfate, Neomycin Sulfate, Hydrocortisone Acetate)........1084
None cited in PDR database.

CORTISPORIN OINTMENT

(Polymyxin B Sulfate, Bacitracin Zinc, Neomycin Sulfate, Hydrocortisone) 1085
None cited in PDR database.

CORTISPORIN OPHTHALMIC OINTMENT STERILE

(Polymyxin B Sulfate, Bacitracin Zinc, Neomycin Sulfate, Hydrocortisone) 1085
None cited in PDR database.

CORTISPORIN OPHTHALMIC SUSPENSION STERILE

(Hydrocortisone, Polymyxin B Sulfate, Neomycin Sulfate) 1086
None cited in PDR database.

CORTISPORIN OTIC SOLUTION STERILE

(Polymyxin B Sulfate, Neomycin Sulfate, Hydrocortisone)....................1087
None cited in PDR database.

CORTISPORIN OTIC SUSPENSION STERILE

(Polymyxin B Sulfate, Neomycin Sulfate, Hydrocortisone)....................1088
None cited in PDR database.

CORTIZONE FOR KIDS

(Hydrocortisone) .... ⊞ 831
None cited in PDR database.

CORTIZONE-5 CREME AND OINTMENT

(Hydrocortisone) .... ⊞ 831
None cited in PDR database.

CORTIZONE-10 CREME AND OINTMENT

(Hydrocortisone) .... ⊞ 831
None cited in PDR database.

CORTIZONE-10 EXTERNAL ANAL ITCH RELIEF

(Hydrocortisone) .... ⊞ 831
None cited in PDR database.

CORTIZONE-10 SCALP ITCH FORMULA

(Hydrocortisone) .... ⊞ 831
None cited in PDR database.

CORTONE ACETATE STERILE SUSPENSION

(Cortisone Acetate) 1623

May interact with oral anticoagulants, potassium sparing diuretics, and certain other agents. Compounds in these categories include:

Amiloride Hydrochloride (Hypokalemia). Products include:

Midamor Tablets 1703
Moduretic Tablets 1705

Aspirin (Aspirin should be used cautiously in conjunction with corticosteroids in hypoprothrombinemia). Products include:

Alka-Seltzer Effervescent Antacid and Pain Reliever............................... ⊞ 701
Alka-Seltzer Extra Strength Effervescent Antacid and Pain Reliever .... ⊞ 703

IMPORTANT NOTE: Always consult each drug listing in the patient's regimen for possible interactions.

Cortone Acetate Injection

Alka-Seltzer Lemon Lime Effervescent Antacid and Pain Reliever .... ✦D 703
Alka-Seltzer Plus Cold Medicine .... ✦D 705
Alka-Seltzer Plus Cold & Cough Medicine .... ✦D 708
Alka-Seltzer Plus Night-Time Cold Medicine .... ✦D 707
Alka Seltzer Plus Sinus Medicine .. ✦D 707
Arthritis Foundation Safety Coated Aspirin Tablets .... ✦D 675
Arthritis Pain Ascriptin .... ✦D 631
Maximum Strength Ascriptin .... ✦D 630
Regular Strength Ascriptin Tablets .... ✦D 629
Arthritis Strength BC Powder......... ✦D 609
BC Cold Powder Multi-Symptom Formula (Cold-Sinus-Allergy) ...... ✦D 609
BC Cold Powder Non-Drowsy Formula (Cold-Sinus) .... ✦D 609
BC Powder .... ✦D 609
Bayer Children's Chewable Aspirin .... ✦D 711
Genuine Bayer Aspirin Tablets & Caplets .... ✦D 713
Extra Strength Bayer Arthritis Pain Regimen Formula .... ✦D 711
Extra Strength Bayer Aspirin Caplets & Tablets .... ✦D 712
Extended-Release Bayer 8-Hour Aspirin .... ✦D 712
Extra Strength Bayer Plus Aspirin Caplets .... ✦D 713
Extra Strength Bayer PM Aspirin .. ✦D 713
Bayer Enteric Aspirin .... ✦D 709
Bufferin Analgesic Tablets and Caplets .... ✦D 613
Arthritis Strength Bufferin Analgesic Caplets .... ✦D 614
Extra Strength Bufferin Analgesic Tablets .... ✦D 615
Cama Arthritis Pain Reliever........... ✦D 785
Darvon Compound-65 Pulvules 1435
Easprin 1914
Ecotrin 2455
Ecotrin Enteric Coated Aspirin Maximum Strength Tablets and Caplets .... ✦D 816
Ecotrin Enteric Coated Aspirin Regular Strength Tablets 2455
Empirin Aspirin Tablets .... ✦D 854
Empirin with Codeine Tablets.......... 1093
Excedrin Extra-Strength Analgesic Tablets & Caplets 732
Fiorinal Capsules 2261
Fiorinal with Codeine Capsules 2262
Fiorinal Tablets 2261
Halfprin 1362
Healthprin Aspirin 2455
Norgesic... 1496
Percodan Tablets................................ 939
Percodan-Demi Tablets..................... 940
Robaxisal Tablets............................... 2071
Soma Compound w/Codeine Tablets 2676
Soma Compound Tablets................... 2675
St. Joseph Adult Chewable Aspirin (81 mg.) .... ✦D 808
Talwin Compound 2335
Ursinus Inlay-Tabs............................. ✦D 794
Vanquish Analgesic Caplets .... ✦D 731

Dicumarol (Response to dicumarol inhibited).

No products indexed under this heading.

Ephedrine Hydrochloride (Enhanced metabolic clearance of corticosteroids). Products include:

Primatene Dual Action Formula...... ✦D 872
Primatene Tablets .... ✦D 873
Quadrinal Tablets 1350

Ephedrine Sulfate (Enhanced metabolic clearance of corticosteroids). Products include:

Bronkaid Caplets .... ✦D 717
Marax Tablets & DF Syrup................ 2200

Ephedrine Tannate (Enhanced metabolic clearance of corticosteroids). Products include:

Rynatuss 2673

Phenobarbital (Enhanced metabolic clearance of corticosteroids). Products include:

Arco-Lase Plus Tablets 512
Bellergal-S Tablets 2250
Donnatal 2060
Donnatal Extentabs.............................. 2061
Donnatal Tablets 2060

Phenobarbital Elixir and Tablets 1469
Quadrinal Tablets 1350

Phenytoin (Enhanced metabolic clearance of corticosteroids). Products include:

Dilantin Infatabs 1908
Dilantin-125 Suspension 1911

Phenytoin Sodium (Enhanced metabolic clearance of corticosteroids). Products include:

Dilantin Kapseals 1906
Dilantin Parenteral 1910

Rifampin (Enhanced metabolic clearance of corticosteroids). Products include:

Rifadin 1528
Rifamate Capsules 1530
Rifater.. 1532
Rimactane Capsules 847

Spironolactone (Hypokalemia). Products include:

Aldactazide... 2413
Aldactone 2414

Triamterene (Hypokalemia). Products include:

Dyazide 2479
Dyrenium Capsules.............................. 2481
Maxzide 1380

Warfarin Sodium (Response to warfarin inhibited). Products include:

Coumadin 926

CORTONE ACETATE TABLETS

(Cortisone Acetate) 1624

May interact with oral anticoagulants, potassium sparing diuretics, and certain other agents. Compounds in these categories include:

Amiloride Hydrochloride (Hypokalemia). Products include:

Midamor Tablets 1703
Moduretic Tablets 1705

Aspirin (Aspirin should be used cautiously in conjunction with corticosteroids in hypoprothrombinemia). Products include:

Alka-Seltzer Effervescent Antacid and Pain Reliever................................ ✦D 701
Alka-Seltzer Extra Strength Effervescent Antacid and Pain Reliever .... ✦D 703
Alka-Seltzer Lemon Lime Effervescent Antacid and Pain Reliever .... ✦D 703
Alka-Seltzer Plus Cold Medicine .... ✦D 705
Alka-Seltzer Plus Cold & Cough Medicine .... ✦D 708
Alka-Seltzer Plus Night-Time Cold Medicine .... ✦D 707
Alka Seltzer Plus Sinus Medicine .. ✦D 707
Arthritis Foundation Safety Coated Aspirin Tablets .... ✦D 675
Arthritis Pain Ascriptin .... ✦D 631
Maximum Strength Ascriptin .... ✦D 630
Regular Strength Ascriptin Tablets .... ✦D 629
Arthritis Strength BC Powder......... ✦D 609
BC Cold Powder Multi-Symptom Formula (Cold-Sinus-Allergy) ...... ✦D 609
BC Cold Powder Non-Drowsy Formula (Cold-Sinus) .... ✦D 609
BC Powder .... ✦D 609
Bayer Children's Chewable Aspirin .... ✦D 711
Genuine Bayer Aspirin Tablets & Caplets .... ✦D 713
Extra Strength Bayer Arthritis Pain Regimen Formula .... ✦D 711
Extra Strength Bayer Aspirin Caplets & Tablets .... ✦D 712
Extended-Release Bayer 8-Hour Aspirin .... ✦D 712
Extra Strength Bayer Plus Aspirin Caplets .... ✦D 713
Extra Strength Bayer PM Aspirin .. ✦D 713
Bayer Enteric Aspirin .... ✦D 709
Bufferin Analgesic Tablets and Caplets .... ✦D 613
Arthritis Strength Bufferin Analgesic Caplets .... ✦D 614
Extra Strength Bufferin Analgesic Tablets .... ✦D 615
Cama Arthritis Pain Reliever........... ✦D 785
Darvon Compound-65 Pulvules 1435

Easprin 1914
Ecotrin 2455
Ecotrin Enteric Coated Aspirin Maximum Strength Tablets and Caplets .... ✦D 816
Ecotrin Enteric Coated Aspirin Regular Strength Tablets 2455
Empirin Aspirin Tablets .... ✦D 854
Empirin with Codeine Tablets........... 1093
Excedrin Extra-Strength Analgesic Tablets & Caplets 732
Fiorinal Capsules 2261
Fiorinal with Codeine Capsules 2262
Fiorinal Tablets 2261
Halfprin 1362
Healthprin Aspirin 2455
Norgesic... 1496
Percodan Tablets.................................. 939
Percodan-Demi Tablets....................... 940
Robaxisal Tablets................................. 2071
Soma Compound w/Codeine Tablets 2676
Soma Compound Tablets.................... 2675
St. Joseph Adult Chewable Aspirin (81 mg.) .... ✦D 808
Talwin Compound 2335
Ursinus Inlay-Tabs.............................. ✦D 794
Vanquish Analgesic Caplets .... ✦D 731

Dicumarol (Response to dicumarol inhibited).

No products indexed under this heading.

Ephedrine Hydrochloride (Enhanced metabolic clearance of corticosteroids). Products include:

Primatene Dual Action Formula...... ✦D 872
Primatene Tablets .... ✦D 873
Quadrinal Tablets 1350

Ephedrine Sulfate (Enhanced metabolic clearance of corticosteroids). Products include:

Bronkaid Caplets .... ✦D 717
Marax Tablets & DF Syrup................. 2200

Ephedrine Tannate (Enhanced metabolic clearance of corticosteroids). Products include:

Rynatuss 2673

Phenobarbital (Enhanced metabolic clearance of corticosteroids). Products include:

Arco-Lase Plus Tablets 512
Bellergal-S Tablets 2250
Donnatal 2060
Donnatal Extentabs.............................. 2061
Donnatal Tablets 2060
Phenobarbital Elixir and Tablets 1469
Quadrinal Tablets 1350

Phenytoin (Enhanced metabolic clearance of corticosteroids). Products include:

Dilantin Infatabs 1908
Dilantin-125 Suspension 1911

Phenytoin Sodium (Enhanced metabolic clearance of corticosteroids). Products include:

Dilantin Kapseals 1906
Dilantin Parenteral 1910

Rifampin (Enhanced metabolic clearance of corticosteroids). Products include:

Rifadin 1528
Rifamate Capsules 1530
Rifater.. 1532
Rimactane Capsules 847

Spironolactone (Hypokalemia). Products include:

Aldactazide... 2413
Aldactone 2414

Triamterene (Hypokalemia). Products include:

Dyazide 2479
Dyrenium Capsules.............................. 2481
Maxzide 1380

Warfarin Sodium (Response to warfarin inhibited). Products include:

Coumadin 926

COSMEGEN INJECTION

(Dactinomycin) 1626

None cited in PDR database.

COTAZYM

(Pancrelipase) 1817

None cited in PDR database.

COUGH-X LOZENGES

(Dextromethorphan Hydrobromide, Benzocaine) .... ✦D 602

May interact with monoamine oxidase inhibitors. Compounds in this category include:

Furazolidone (Concurrent use is not recommended). Products include:

Furoxone 2046

Isocarboxazid (Concurrent use is not recommended).

No products indexed under this heading.

Phenelzine Sulfate (Concurrent use is not recommended). Products include:

Nardil 1920

Selegiline Hydrochloride (Concurrent use is not recommended). Products include:

Eldepryl Tablets 2550

Tranylcypromine Sulfate (Concurrent use is not recommended). Products include:

Parnate Tablets 2503

COUMADIN FOR INJECTION

(Warfarin Sodium) 926

See Coumadin Tablets

COUMADIN TABLETS

(Warfarin Sodium) 926

May interact with antihistamines, diuretics, androgens, monoamine oxidase inhibitors, salicylates, sulfonamides, thyroid preparations, barbiturates, non-steroidal anti-inflammatory agents, oral contraceptives, inhalant anesthetics, corticosteroids, narcotic analgesics, antacids, fluoroquinolone antibiotics, pyrazolon derivatives, and certain other agents. Compounds in these categories include:

Acetaminophen (May be responsible for increased prothrombin time response). Products include:

Actifed Plus Caplets .... ✦D 845
Actifed Plus Tablets .... ✦D 845
Actifed Sinus Daytime/Nighttime Tablets and Caplets .... ✦D 846
Alka-Seltzer Plus Cold Medicine Liqui-Gels .... ✦D 706
Alka-Seltzer Plus Cold & Cough Medicine Liqui-Gels.......................... ✦D 705
Alka-Seltzer Plus Night-Time Cold Medicine Liqui-Gels.......................... ✦D 706
Allerest Headache Strength Tablets .... ✦D 627
Allerest No Drowsiness Tablets ...... ✦D 627
Allerest Sinus Pain Formula .... ✦D 627
Anexsia 5/500 Elixir 1781
Anexia Tablets...................................... 1782
Arthritis Foundation Aspirin Free Caplets .... ✦D 673
Arthritis Foundation NightTime Caplets .... ✦D 674
Bayer Select Headache Pain Relief Formula .... ✦D 716
Bayer Select Menstrual Multi-Symptom Formula............................. ✦D 716
Bayer Select Night Time Pain Relief Formula..................................... ✦D 716
Bayer Select Sinus Pain Relief Formula .... ✦D 717
Benadryl Allergy Sinus Headache Formula Caplets................................ ✦D 849
Comtrex Multi-Symptom Cold Reliever Tablets/Caplets/Liqui-Gels/Liquid.. ✦D 615
Allergy-Sinus Comtrex Multi-Symptom Allergy-Sinus Formula Tablets .... ✦D 617
Comtrex Non-Drowsy .... ✦D 618
Contac Day Allergy/Sinus Caplets ✦D 812
Contac Day & Night .... ✦D 812
Contac Night Allergy/Sinus Caplets .... ✦D 812
Contac Severe Cold and Flu Formula Caplets .... ✦D 814

(✦D Described in PDR For Nonprescription Drugs)

(◎ Described in PDR For Ophthalmology)

Interactions Index — Coumadin

Contac Severe Cold & Flu Non-Drowsy .... ✦D 815
Coricidin 'D' Decongestant Tablets .... ✦D 800
Coricidin Tablets .... ✦D 800
DHCplus Capsules............................... 1993
Darvon-N/Darvocet-N 1433
Drixoral Cold and Flu Extended-Release Tablets.............................. ✦D 803
Drixoral Cough + Sore Throat Liquid Caps .... ✦D 802
Drixoral Allergy/Sinus Extended Release Tablets................................ ✦D 804
Esgic-plus Tablets 1013
Aspirin Free Excedrin Analgesic Caplets and Geltabs 732
Excedrin Extra-Strength Analgesic Tablets & Caplets 732
Excedrin P.M. Analgesic/Sleeping Aid Tablets, Caplets, Liquigels 733
Fioricet Tablets.................................... 2258
Fioricet with Codeine Capsules 2260
Hycomine Compound Tablets 932
Hydrocet Capsules 782
Legatrin PM .... ✦D 651
Lorcet 10/650...................................... 1018
Lortab 2566
Lurline PMS Tablets 982
Maximum Strength Multi-Symptom Formula Midol .... ✦D 722
PMS Multi-Symptom Formula Midol .... ✦D 723
Teen Multi-Symptom Formula Midol .... ✦D 722
Midrin Capsules 783
Migralam Capsules 2038
Panodol Tablets and Caplets .... ✦D 824
Children's Panadol Chewable Tablets, Liquid, Infant's Drops .... ✦D 824
Percocet Tablets 938
Percogesic Analgesic Tablets .... ✦D 754
Phrenilin 785
Pyrroxate Caplets .... ✦D 772
Sedapap Tablets 50 mg/650 mg .. 1543
Sinarest Tablets .... ✦D 648
Sinarest Extra Strength Tablets...... ✦D 648
Sinarest No Drowsiness Tablets .... ✦D 648
Sine-Aid Maximum Strength Sinus Medication Gelcaps, Caplets and Tablets 1554
Sine-Off No Drowsiness Formula Caplets .... ✦D 824
Sine-Off Sinus Medicine .... ✦D 825
Singlet Tablets .... ✦D 825
Sinulin Tablets 787
Sinutab Sinus Allergy Medication, Maximum Strength Tablets and Caplets .... ✦D 860
Sinutab Sinus Medication, Maximum Strength Without Drowsiness Formula, Tablets & Caplets .... ✦D 860
Sinutab Sinus Medication, Regular Strength Without Drowsiness Formula .... ✦D 859
Sudafed Cold and Cough Liquidcaps .... ✦D 862
Sudafed Severe Cold Formula Caplets .... ✦D 863
Sudafed Severe Cold Formula Tablets .... ✦D 864
Sudafed Sinus Caplets......................... ✦D 864
Sudafed Sinus Tablets.......................... ✦D 864
Talacen... 2333
TheraFlu... ✦D 787
TheraFlu Maximum Strength Nighttime Flu, Cold & Cough Medicine .... ✦D 788
TheraFlu Maximum Strength Non-Drowsy Formula Flu, Cold & Cough Medicine .... ✦D 788
Thera Flu Maximum Strength, Non-Drowsy Formula Flu, Cold and Cough Caplets .... ✦D 789
Triaminic Sore Throat Formula ...... ✦D 791
Triaminicin Tablets .... ✦D 793
Children's TYLENOL acetaminophen Chewable Tablets, Elixir, Suspension Liquid 1555
Children's TYLENOL Cold Multi Symptom Liquid Formula and Chewable Tablets............................... 1561
Children's TYLENOL Cold Plus Cough Multi Symptom Tablets and Liquid... ✦D 681
Infants' TYLENOL acetaminophen Drops and Suspension Drops 1555
Infants' TYLENOL Cold Decongestant & Fever-Reducer Drops 1556
TYLENOL Extended Relief Caplets.. 1558

TYLENOL, Extra Strength, Acetaminophen Adult Liquid Pain Reliever 1560
TYLENOL, Extra Strength, acetaminophen Gelcaps, Geltabs, Caplets, Tablets 1559
TYLENOL, Extra Strength, Headache Plus Pain Reliever with Antacid Caplets 1559
TYLENOL, Junior Strength, acetaminophen Coated Caplets, Grape and Fruit Chewable Tablets 1557
TYLENOL Maximum Strength Allergy Sinus Medication Gelcaps and Caplets 1563
TYLENOL Maximum Strength Allergy Sinus NightTime Medication Caplets 1555
TYLENOL Flu Maximum Strength Gelcaps 1565
TYLENOL Flu NightTime, Maximum Strength, Gelcaps 1566
TYLENOL Maximum Strength Flu NightTime Hot Medication Packets 1562
TYLENOL, Maximum Strength, Sinus Medication Geltabs, Gelcaps, Caplets and Tablets 1566
TYLENOL Cold Multi-Symptom Formula Medication Tablets and Caplets 1561
TYLENOL Cold Medication No Drowsiness Formula Gelcaps and Caplets 1562
TYLENOL Cold Multi-Symptom Hot Medication Liquid Packets.............. 1557
TYLENOL Cough Multi-Symptom Medication 1564
TYLENOL Cough Multi-Symptom Medication with Decongestant...... 1565
TYLENOL, Regular Strength, acetaminophen Caplets and Tablets .. 1558
TYLENOL PM, Extra Strength Pain Reliever/Sleep Aid Caplets, Geltabs, Gelcaps 1560
TYLENOL Severe Allergy Medication Caplets 1564
Tylenol with Codeine 1583
Tylox Capsules 1584
Unisom With Pain Relief-Nighttime Sleep Aid and Pain Reliever............ 1934
Vanquish Analgesic Caplets .... ✦D 731
Vicks 44 LiquiCaps Cough, Cold & Flu Relief.. ✦D 755
Vicks 44M Cough, Cold & Flu Relief .... ✦D 756
Vicks DayQuil .... ✦D 761
Vicks Nyquil Hot Therapy................... ✦D 762
Vicks NyQuil LiquiCaps Multi-Symptom Cold/Flu Relief .... ✦D 763
Vicks NyQuil Multi-Symptom Cold/Flu Relief - (Original & Cherry Flavor) .... ✦D 763
Vicodin Tablets.................................... 1356
Vicodin ES Tablets 1357
Wygesic Tablets 2827
Zydone Capsules 949

Acrivastine (Decreased prothrombin time response). Products include:

Semprex-D Capsules 463
Semprex-D Capsules 1167

Alfentanil Hydrochloride (Increased prothrombin time response with prolonged use). Products include:

Alfenta Injection 1286

Allopurinol (Increased prothrombin time response). Products include:

Zyloprim Tablets 1226

Aluminum Carbonate Gel (Decreased prothrombin time response). Products include:

Basaljel... 2703

Aluminum Hydroxide (Decreased prothrombin response). Products include:

ALternaGEL Liquid 1316
Maximum Strength Ascriptin .... ✦D 630
Cama Arthritis Pain Reliever.............. ✦D 785
Gaviscon Extra Strength Relief Formula Antacid Tablets.................. ✦D 819
Gaviscon Extra Strength Relief Formula Liquid Antacid.................... ✦D 819
Gaviscon Liquid Antacid .... ✦D 820

Gelusil Liquid & Tablets .... ✦D 855
Maalox Heartburn Relief Suspension .... ✦D 642
Maalox Heartburn Relief Tablets.... ✦D 641
Maalox Magnesia and Alumina Oral Suspension .... ✦D 642
Maalox Plus Tablets .... ✦D 643
Extra Strength Maalox Antacid Plus Antigas Liquid and Tablets ✦D 638
Tempo Soft Antacid .... ✦D 835

Aluminum Hydroxide Gel (Decreased prothrombin time response). Products include:

ALternaGEL Liquid .... ✦D 659
Aludrox Oral Suspension 2695
Amphojel Suspension 2695
Amphojel Suspension without Flavor 2695
Amphojel Tablets................................. 2695
Arthritis Pain Ascriptin .... ✦D 631
Regular Strength Ascriptin Tablets .... ✦D 629
Gaviscon Antacid Tablets................... ✦D 819
Gaviscon-2 Antacid Tablets .... ✦D 820
Mylanta Liquid 1317
Mylanta Tablets .... ✦D 660
Mylanta Double Strength Liquid 1317
Mylanta Double Strength Tablets .. ✦D 660
Nephrox Suspension .... ✦D 655

Amiloride Hydrochloride (Decreased or increased prothrombin time response). Products include:

Midamor Tablets 1703
Moduretic Tablets 1705

Aminoglutethimide (Decreased prothrombin time response). Products include:

Cytadren Tablets 819

p-Aminosalicylic Acid (Increased prothrombin time response).

No products indexed under this heading.

Amiodarone Hydrochloride (Increased prothrombin time response). Products include:

Cordarone Intravenous 2715
Cordarone Tablets............................... 2712

Antibiotics, unspecified (Increased prothrombin time response).

Antipyrine (Increased prothrombin time response). Products include:

Auralgan Otic Solution........................ 2703
Tympagesic Ear Drops 2342

Aprobarbital (Decreased prothrombin time response).

No products indexed under this heading.

Aspirin (Increased prothrombin time response). Products include:

Alka-Seltzer Effervescent Antacid and Pain Reliever .... ✦D 701
Alka-Seltzer Extra Strength Effervescent Antacid and Pain Reliever .... ✦D 703
Alka-Seltzer Lemon Lime Effervescent Antacid and Pain Reliever .... ✦D 703
Alka-Seltzer Plus Cold Medicine .... ✦D 705
Alka-Seltzer Plus Cold & Cough Medicine .... ✦D 708
Alka-Seltzer Plus Night-Time Cold Medicine .... ✦D 707
Alka Seltzer Plus Sinus Medicine .. ✦D 707
Arthritis Foundation Safety Coated Aspirin Tablets .... ✦D 675
Arthritis Pain Ascriptin .... ✦D 631
Maximum Strength Ascriptin .... ✦D 630
Regular Strength Ascriptin Tablets .... ✦D 629
Arthritis Strength BC Powder........... ✦D 609
BC Cold Powder Multi-Symptom Formula (Cold-Sinus-Allergy) ...... ✦D 609
BC Cold Powder Non-Drowsy Formula (Cold-Sinus) .... ✦D 609
BC Powder .... ✦D 609
Bayer Children's Chewable Aspirin .... ✦D 711
Genuine Bayer Aspirin Tablets & Caplets .... ✦D 713
Extra Strength Bayer Arthritis Pain Regimen Formula .... ✦D 711
Extra Strength Bayer Aspirin Caplets & Tablets .... ✦D 712

Extended-Release Bayer 8-Hour Aspirin .... ✦D 712
Extra Strength Bayer Plus Aspirin Caplets .... ✦D 713
Extra Strength Bayer PM Aspirin .. ✦D 713
Bayer Enteric Aspirin.......................... ✦D 709
Bufferin Analgesic Tablets and Caplets .... ✦D 613
Arthritis Strength Bufferin Analgesic Caplets .... ✦D 614
Extra Strength Bufferin Analgesic Tablets .... ✦D 615
Cama Arthritis Pain Reliever............ ✦D 785
Darvon Compound-65 Pulvules 1435
Easprin.. 1914
Ecotrin 2455
Ecotrin Enteric Coated Aspirin Maximum Strength Tablets and Caplets .... ✦D 816
Ecotrin Enteric Coated Aspirin Regular Strength Tablets 2455
Empirin Aspirin Tablets .... ✦D 854
Empirin with Codeine Tablets........... 1093
Excedrin Extra-Strength Analgesic Tablets & Caplets 732
Fiorinal Capsules 2261
Fiorinal with Codeine Capsules 2262
Fiorinal Tablets 2261
Halfprin 1362
Healthprin Aspirin............................... 2455
Norgesic.. 1496
Percodan Tablets................................. 939
Percodan-Demi Tablets....................... 940
Robaxisal Tablets................................. 2071
Soma Compound w/Codeine Tablets 2676
Soma Compound Tablets................... 2675
St. Joseph Adult Chewable Aspirin (81 mg.) .... ✦D 808
Talwin Compound 2335
Ursinus Inlay-Tabs.............................. ✦D 794
Vanquish Analgesic Caplets .... ✦D 731

Astemizole (Decreased prothrombin time response). Products include:

Hismanal Tablets 1293

Azatadine Maleate (Decreased prothrombin time response). Products include:

Trinalin Repetabs Tablets 1330

Bendroflumethiazide (Decreased or increased prothrombin time response).

No products indexed under this heading.

Betamethasone Acetate (Decreased prothrombin time response). Products include:

Celestone Soluspan Suspension 2347

Betamethasone Sodium Phosphate (Decreased prothrombin time response). Products include:

Celestone Soluspan Suspension 2347

Bromelains (Increased prothrombin time response). Products include:

Wobenzym N .... ✦D 673

Bromodiphenhydramine Hydrochloride (Decreased prothrombin time response).

No products indexed under this heading.

Brompheniramine Maleate (Decreased prothrombin time response). Products include:

Alka Seltzer Plus Sinus Medicine .. ✦D 707
Bromfed Capsules (Extended-Release) 1785
Bromfed Syrup .... ✦D 733
Bromfed Tablets 1785
Bromfed-DM Cough Syrup................. 1786
Bromfed-PD Capsules (Extended-Release).. 1785
Dimetane-DC Cough Syrup 2059
Dimetane-DX Cough Syrup 2059
Dimetapp Elixir.................................... ✦D 773
Dimetapp Extentabs .... ✦D 774
Dimetapp Tablets/Liqui-Gels .... ✦D 775
Dimetapp Cold & Allergy Chewable Tablets .... ✦D 773
Dimetapp DM Elixir............................. ✦D 774
Vicks DayQuil Allergy Relief 12-Hour Extended Release Tablets.. ✦D 760
Vicks DayQuil Allergy Relief 4-Hour Tablets .... ✦D 760

IMPORTANT NOTE: Always consult each drug listing in the patient's regimen for possible interactions.

Coumadin **Interactions Index** **208**

Bumetanide (Decreased or increased prothrombin time response). Products include:
Bumex ... 2093

Buprenorphine (Increased prothrombin time response with prolonged use). Products include:
Buprenex Injectable ... 2006

Butabarbital (Decreased prothrombin time response).
No products indexed under this heading.

Butalbital (Decreased prothrombin time response). Products include:
Esgic-plus Tablets ... 1013
Fioricet Tablets ... 2258
Fioricet with Codeine Capsules ... 2260
Fiorinal Capsules ... 2261
Fiorinal with Codeine Capsules ... 2262
Fiorinal Tablets ... 2261
Phrenilin ... 785
Sedapap Tablets 50 mg/650 mg ... 1543

Carbamazepine (Decreased prothrombin time response). Products include:
Atretol Tablets ... 573
Tegretol Chewable Tablets ... 852
Tegretol Suspension ... 852
Tegretol Tablets ... 852

Chenodiol (Increased prothrombin time response).
No products indexed under this heading.

Chloral Hydrate (Decreased or increased prothrombin time response).
No products indexed under this heading.

Chlordiazepoxide (Decreased prothrombin time response). Products include:
Libritabs Tablets ... 2177
Limbitrol ... 2180

Chlordiazepoxide Hydrochloride (Decreased prothrombin time response). Products include:
Librax Capsules ... 2176
Librium Capsules ... 2178
Librium Injectable ... 2179

Chlorothiazide (Decreased or increased prothrombin time response). Products include:
Aldoclor Tablets ... 1598
Diupres Tablets ... 1650
Diuril Oral ... 1653

Chlorothiazide Sodium (Decreased or increased prothrombin time response). Products include:
Diuril Sodium Intravenous ... 1652

Chlorpheniramine Maleate (Decreased prothrombin time response). Products include:
Alka-Seltzer Plus Cold Medicine ... ▣ 705
Alka-Seltzer Plus Cold Medicine Liqui-Gels ... ▣ 706
Alka-Seltzer Plus Cold & Cough Medicine ... ▣ 708
Alka-Seltzer Plus Cold & Cough Medicine Liqui-Gels ... ▣ 705
Allerest Children's Chewable Tablets ... ▣ 627
Allerest Headache Strength Tablets ... ▣ 627
Allerest Maximum Strength Tablets ... ▣ 627
Allerest Sinus Pain Formula ... ▣ 627
Allerest 12 Hour Caplets ... ▣ 627
Ana-Kit Anaphylaxis Emergency Treatment Kit ... 617
Atrohist Pediatric Capsules ... 453
Atrohist Plus Tablets ... 454
BC Cold Powder Multi-Symptom Formula (Cold-Sinus-Allergy) ... ▣ 609
Cerose DM ... ▣ 878
Cheracol Plus Head Cold/Cough Formula ... ▣ 769
Children's Vicks DayQuil Allergy Relief ... ▣ 757
Children's Vicks NyQuil Cold/Cough Relief ... ▣ 758
Chlor-Trimeton Allergy Decongestant Tablets ... ▣ 799
Chlor-Trimeton Allergy Tablets ... ▣ 798
Comhist ... 2038
Comtrex Multi-Symptom Cold Reliever Tablets/Caplets/Liqui-Gels/Liquid ... ▣ 615
Allergy-Sinus Comtrex Multi-Symptom Allergy-Sinus Formula Tablets ... ▣ 617
Contac Continuous Action Nasal Decongestant/Antihistamine 12 Hour Capsules ... ▣ 813
Contac Maximum Strength Continuous Action Decongestant/Antihistamine 12 Hour Caplets ... ▣ 813
Contac Severe Cold and Flu Formula Caplets ... ▣ 814
Coricidin 'D' Decongestant Tablets ... ▣ 800
Coricidin Tablets ... ▣ 800
D.A. Chewable Tablets ... 951
Deconamine ... 1320
Dura-Tap/PD Capsules ... 2867
Dura-Vent/DA Tablets ... 953
Extendryl ... 1005
Fedahist Gyrocaps ... 2401
Fedahist Timecaps ... 2401
Hycomine Compound Tablets ... 932
Isoclor Timesule Capsules ... ▣ 637
Kronofed-A ... 977
Nolamine Timed-Release Tablets ... 785
Novahistine DH ... 2462
Novahistine Elixir ... ▣ 823
Ornade Spansule Capsules ... 2502
PediaCare Cold Allergy Chewable Tablets ... ▣ 677
PediaCare Cough-Cold Chewable Tablets ... 1553
PediaCare Cough-Cold Liquid ... 1553
PediaCare NightRest Cough-Cold Liquid ... 1553
Pediatric Vicks 44m Cough & Cold Relief ... ▣ 764
Pyrroxate Caplets ... ▣ 772
Ryna ... ▣ 841
Sinarest Tablets ... ▣ 648
Sinarest Extra Strength Tablets ... ▣ 648
Sine-Off Sinus Medicine ... ▣ 825
Singlet Tablets ... ▣ 825
Sinulin Tablets ... 787
Sinutab Sinus Allergy Medication, Maximum Strength Tablets and Caplets ... ▣ 860
Sudafed Plus Liquid ... ▣ 862
Sudafed Plus Tablets ... ▣ 863
Teldrin 12 Hour Antihistamine/Nasal Decongestant Allergy Relief Capsules ... ▣ 826
TheraFlu ... ▣ 787
TheraFlu Maximum Strength Nighttime Flu, Cold & Cough Medicine ... ▣ 788
Triaminic Allergy Tablets ... ▣ 789
Triaminic Cold Tablets ... ▣ 790
Triaminic Nite Light ... ▣ 791
Triaminic Syrup ... ▣ 792
Triaminic-12 Tablets ... ▣ 792
Triaminicin Tablets ... ▣ 793
Triaminicol Multi-Symptom Cold Tablets ... ▣ 793
Triaminicol Multi-Symptom Relief ... ▣ 794
Tussend ... 1783
Children's TYLENOL Cold Multi-Symptom Liquid Formula and Chewable Tablets ... 1561
Children's TYLENOL Cold Plus Cough Multi Symptom Tablets and Liquid ... ▣ 681
TYLENOL Maximum Strength Allergy Sinus Medication Gelcaps and Caplets ... 1563
TYLENOL Cold Multi-Symptom Formula Medication Tablets and Caplets ... 1561
TYLENOL Cold Multi-Symptom Hot Medication Liquid Packets ... 1557
Vicks 44 LiquiCaps Cough, Cold & Flu Relief ... ▣ 755
Vicks 44M Cough, Cold & Flu Relief ... ▣ 756

Chlorpheniramine Polistirex (Decreased prothrombin time response). Products include:
Tussionex Pennkinetic Extended-Release Suspension ... 998

Chlorpheniramine Tannate (Decreased prothrombin time response). Products include:
Atrohist Pediatric Suspension ... 454
Ricobid Tablets and Pediatric Suspension ... 2038
Rynatan ... 2673
Rynatuss ... 2673

Chlorpropamide (Increased prothrombin time response; accumulation of chlorpropamide). Products include:
Diabinese Tablets ... 1935

Chlorthalidone (Decreased or increased prothrombin time response). Products include:
Combipres Tablets ... 677
Tenoretic Tablets ... 2845
Thalitone ... 1245

Cholestyramine (Decreased prothrombin time response). Products include:
Questran Light ... 769
Questran Powder ... 770

Choline Magnesium Trisalicylate (Increased prothrombin time response). Products include:
Trilisate ... 2000

Chymotrypsin (Increased prothrombin time response). Products include:
Wobenzym N ... ▣ 673

Cimetidine (Increased prothrombin time response). Products include:
Tagamet Tablets ... 2516

Cimetidine Hydrochloride (Increased prothrombin time response). Products include:
Tagamet ... 2516

Ciprofloxacin (Increased prothrombin time response). Products include:
Cipro I.V. ... 595
Cipro I.V. Pharmacy Bulk Package ... 597

Ciprofloxacin Hydrochloride (Increased prothrombin time response). Products include:
Ciloxan Ophthalmic Solution ... 472
Cipro Tablets ... 592

Clemastine Fumarate (Decreased prothrombin time response). Products include:
Tavist Syrup ... 2297
Tavist Tablets ... 2298
Tavist-1 12 Hour Relief Tablets ... ▣ 787
Tavist-D 12 Hour Relief Tablets ... ▣ 787

Clofibrate (Increased prothrombin time response). Products include:
Atromid-S Capsules ... 2701

Codeine Phosphate (Increased prothrombin time response with prolonged use). Products include:
Actifed with Codeine Cough Syrup ... 1067
Brontex ... 1981
Deconsal C Expectorant Syrup ... 456
Deconsal Pediatric Syrup ... 457
Dimetane-DC Cough Syrup ... 2059
Empirin with Codeine Tablets ... 1093
Fioricet with Codeine Capsules ... 2260
Fiorinal with Codeine Capsules ... 2262
Isoclor Expectorant ... 990
Novahistine DH ... 2462
Novahistine Expectorant ... 2463
Nucofed ... 2051
Phenergan with Codeine ... 2777
Phenergan VC with Codeine ... 2781
Robitussin A-C Syrup ... 2073
Robitussin-DAC Syrup ... 2074
Ryna ... ▣ 841
Soma Compound w/Codeine Tablets ... 2676
Tussi-Organidin NR Liquid and S NR Liquid ... 2677
Tylenol with Codeine ... 1583

Cortisone Acetate (Decreased prothrombin time response). Products include:
Cortone Acetate Sterile Suspension ... 1623
Cortone Acetate Tablets ... 1624

Cyproheptadine Hydrochloride (Decreased prothrombin time response). Products include:
Periactin ... 1724

Desflurane (Increased prothrombin time response). Products include:
Suprane ... 1813

Desogestrel (Decreased prothrombin time response). Products include:
Desogen Tablets ... 1817
Ortho-Cept ... 1851

Dexamethasone (Decreased prothrombin time response). Products include:
AK-Trol Ointment & Suspension ... ⊙ 205
Decadron Elixir ... 1633
Decadron Tablets ... 1635
Decaspray Topical Aerosol ... 1648
Dexacidin Ointment ... ⊙ 263
Maxitrol Ophthalmic Ointment and Suspension ... ⊙ 224
TobraDex Ophthalmic Suspension and Ointment ... 473

Dexamethasone Acetate (Decreased prothrombin time response). Products include:
Dalalone D.P. Injectable ... 1011
Decadron-LA Sterile Suspension ... 1646

Dexamethasone Sodium Phosphate (Decreased prothrombin time response). Products include:
Decadron Phosphate Injection ... 1637
Decadron Phosphate Respihaler ... 1642
Decadron Phosphate Sterile Ophthalmic Ointment ... 1641
Decadron Phosphate Sterile Ophthalmic Solution ... 1642
Decadron Phosphate Topical Cream ... 1644
Decadron Phosphate Turbinaire ... 1645
Decadron Phosphate with Xylocaine Injection, Sterile ... 1639
Dexacort Phosphate in Respihaler ... 458
Dexacort Phosphate in Turbinaire ... 459
NeoDecadron Sterile Ophthalmic Ointment ... 1712
NeoDecadron Sterile Ophthalmic Solution ... 1713
NeoDecadron Topical Cream ... 1714

Dexchlorpheniramine Maleate (Decreased prothrombin time response).
No products indexed under this heading.

Dextrans (Low Molecular Weight) (Increased prothrombin time response).
No products indexed under this heading.

Dextrothyroxine Sodium (Increased prothrombin time response).
No products indexed under this heading.

Dezocine (Increased prothrombin time response with prolonged use). Products include:
Dalgan Injection ... 538

Diazoxide (Increased prothrombin time response). Products include:
Hyperstat I.V. Injection ... 2363
Proglycem ... 580

Diclofenac Potassium (Increased prothrombin time response; caution should be observed when used concurrently). Products include:
Cataflam ... 816

Diclofenac Sodium (Increased prothrombin time response; caution should be observed when used concurrently). Products include:
Voltaren Ophthalmic Sterile Ophthalmic Solution ... ⊙ 272
Voltaren Tablets ... 861

Diflunisal (Increased prothrombin time response). Products include:
Dolobid Tablets ... 1654

Dihydroxyaluminum Sodium Carbonate (Decreased prothrombin time response).
No products indexed under this heading.

(▣ Described in PDR For Nonprescription Drugs) (⊙ Described in PDR For Ophthalmology)

Interactions Index — Coumadin

Diphenhydramine Citrate (Decreased prothrombin time response). Products include:

Excedrin P.M. Analgesic/Sleeping Aid Tablets, Caplets, Liquigels...... 733

Diphenhydramine Hydrochloride (Decreased prothrombin time response). Products include:

Actifed Allergy Daytime/Nighttime Caplets....................................... ᴮᴰ 844
Actifed Sinus Daytime/Nighttime Tablets and Caplets........................ ᴮᴰ 846
Arthritis Foundation NightTime Caplets... ᴮᴰ 674
Extra Strength Bayer PM Aspirin.. ᴮᴰ 713
Bayer Select Night Time Pain Relief Formula.................................... ᴮᴰ 716
Benadryl Allergy Decongestant Liquid Medication.............................. ᴮᴰ 848
Benadryl Allergy Decongestant Tablets.. ᴮᴰ 848
Benadryl Allergy Liquid Medication.. ᴮᴰ 848
Benadryl Allergy.. ᴮᴰ 848
Benadryl Allergy Sinus Headache Formula Caplets............................ ᴮᴰ 849
Benadryl Capsules................................... 1898
Benadryl Dye-Free Allergy Liquigel Softgels...................................... ᴮᴰ 850
Benadryl Dye-Free Allergy Liquid Medication..................................... ᴮᴰ 850
Benadryl Itch Relief Cream, Children's Formula and Maximum Strength 2%....................................... ᴮᴰ 851
Benadryl Itch Relief Spray, Children's Formula and Maximum Strength 2%...................................... ᴮᴰ 851
Benadryl Itch Relief Stick Maximum Strength 2%.............................. ᴮᴰ 850
Benadryl Itch Stopping Gel, Children's Formula and Maximum Strength 2%...................................... ᴮᴰ 851
Benadryl Kapseals.................................. 1898
Benadryl Injection................................... 1898
Contac Day & Night Cold/Flu Night Caplets....................................... ᴮᴰ 812
Contac Night Allergy/Sinus Caplets.. ᴮᴰ 812
Extra Strength Doan's P.M............... ᴮᴰ 633
Legatrin PM... ᴮᴰ 651
Miles Nervine Nighttime Sleep-Aid ᴮᴰ 723
Nytol QuickCaps Caplets.................... ᴮᴰ 610
Sleepinal Night-time Sleep Aid Capsules and Softgels........................ ᴮᴰ 834
TYLENOL Maximum Strength Allergy Sinus NightTime Medication Caplets... 1555
TYLENOL Flu NightTime, Maximum Strength, Gelcaps..................... 1566
TYLENOL Maximum Strength Flu NightTime Hot Medication Packets.. 1562
TYLENOL PM, Extra Strength Pain Reliever/Sleep Aid Caplets, Geltabs, Gelcaps...................................... 1560
TYLENOL Severe Allergy Medication Caplets...................................... 1564
Maximum Strength Unisom Sleepgels.. 1934
Unisom With Pain Relief-Nighttime Sleep Aid and Pain Reliever............. 1934

Diphenylpyraline Hydrochloride (Decreased prothrombin time response).

No products indexed under this heading.

Disulfiram (Increased prothrombin time response). Products include:

Antabuse Tablets..................................... 2695

Enflurane (Increased prothrombin time response).

No products indexed under this heading.

Enoxacin (Increased prothrombin time response). Products include:

Penetrex Tablets...................................... 2031

Ethacrynic Acid (Increased prothrombin time response). Products include:

Edecrin Tablets... 1657

Ethchlorvynol (Decreased prothrombin time response). Products include:

Placidyl Capsules..................................... 448

Ethinyl Estradiol (Decreased prothrombin time response). Products include:

Brevicon.. 2088
Demulen.. 2428
Desogen Tablets....................................... 1817
Levlen/Tri-Levlen.................................... 651
Lo/Ovral Tablets...................................... 2746
Lo/Ovral-28 Tablets................................. 2751
Modicon... 1872
Nordette-21 Tablets.................................. 2755
Nordette-28 Tablets.................................. 2758
Norinyl... 2088
Ortho-Cept... 1851
Ortho-Cyclen/Ortho-Tri-Cyclen........ 1858
Ortho-Novum... 1872
Ortho-Cyclen/Ortho Tri-Cyclen........ 1858
Ovcon... 760
Ovral Tablets.. 2770
Ovral-28 Tablets...................................... 2770
Levlen/Tri-Levlen.................................... 651
Tri-Norinyl... 2164
Triphasil-21 Tablets................................. 2814
Triphasil-28 Tablets................................. 2819

Ethynodiol Diacetate (Decreased prothrombin time response). Products include:

Demulen... 2428

Etodolac (Increased prothrombin time response; caution should be observed when used concurrently). Products include:

Lodine Capsules and Tablets............. 2743

Fenoprofen Calcium (Increased prothrombin time response; caution should be observed when used concurrently). Products include:

Nalfon 200 Pulvules & Nalfon Tablets.. 917

Fentanyl (Increased prothrombin time response with prolonged use). Products include:

Duragesic Transdermal System........ 1288

Fentanyl Citrate (Increased prothrombin time response with prolonged use). Products include:

Sublimaze Injection................................. 1307

Fludrocortisone Acetate (Decreased prothrombin time response). Products include:

Florinef Acetate Tablets.......................... 505

Fluoxymesterone (Increased prothrombin time response). Products include:

Halotestin Tablets.................................... 2614

Flurbiprofen (Increased prothrombin time response; caution should be observed when used concurrently). Products include:

Ansaid Tablets.. 2579

Furazolidone (Increased prothrombin time response). Products include:

Furoxone.. 2046

Furosemide (Decreased or increased prothrombin time response). Products include:

Lasix Injection, Oral Solution and Tablets.. 1240

Glipizide (Increased prothrombin time response). Products include:

Glucotrol Tablets...................................... 1967
Glucotrol XL Extended Release Tablets.. 1968

Glucagon (Increased prothrombin time response). Products include:

Glucagon for Injection Vials and Emergency Kit.. 1440

Glutethimide (Decreased prothrombin time response).

No products indexed under this heading.

Glyburide (Increased prothrombin time response). Products include:

DiaBeta Tablets.. 1239
Glynase PresTab Tablets.......................... 2609
Micronase Tablets.................................... 2623

Griseofulvin (Decreased prothrombin time response). Products include:

Fulvicin P/G Tablets................................ 2359
Fulvicin P/G 165 & 330 Tablets.... 2359
Grifulvin V (griseofulvin tablets) Microsize (griseofulvin oral suspension) Microsize............................. 1888
Gris-PEG Tablets, 125 mg & 250 mg... 479

Haloperidol (Decreased prothrombin time response). Products include:

Haldol Injection, Tablets and Concentrate... 1575

Haloperidol Decanoate (Decreased prothrombin time response). Products include:

Haldol Decanoate..................................... 1577

Halothane (Increased prothrombin time response). Products include:

Fluothane... 2724

Heparin Calcium (Concomitant administration prolongs one-stage prothrombin time response).

No products indexed under this heading.

Heparin Sodium (Concomitant administration prolongs one-stage prothrombin time response). Products include:

Heparin Lock Flush Solution.............. 2725
Heparin Sodium Injection...................... 2726
Heparin Sodium Injection, USP, Sterile Solution...................................... 2615
Heparin Sodium Vials............................. 1441

Hepatotoxic Drugs, unspecified (Increased prothrombin time response).

Hydrochlorothiazide (Decreased or increased prothrombin time response). Products include:

Aldactazide... 2413
Aldoril Tablets.. 1604
Apresazide Capsules................................ 808
Capozide... 742
Dyazide... 2479
Esidrix Tablets.. 821
Esimil Tablets... 822
HydroDIURIL Tablets.............................. 1674
Hydropres Tablets.................................... 1675
Hyzaar Tablets... 1677
Inderide Tablets....................................... 2732
Inderide LA Long Acting Capsules.. 2734
Lopressor HCT Tablets........................... 832
Lotensin HCT... 837
Maxzide.. 1380
Moduretic Tablets.................................... 1705
Oretic Tablets... 443
Prinzide Tablets....................................... 1737
Ser-Ap-Es Tablets.................................... 849
Timolide Tablets....................................... 1748
Vaseretic Tablets...................................... 1765
Zestoretic.. 2850
Ziac... 1415

Hydrocodone Bitartrate (Increased prothrombin time response with prolonged use). Products include:

Anexsia 5/500 Elixir............................... 1781
Anexia Tablets.. 1782
Codiclear DH Syrup................................ 791
Deconamine CX Cough and Cold Liquid and Tablets................................... 1319
Duratuss HD Elixir.................................. 2565
Hycodan Tablets and Syrup................... 930
Hycomine Compound Tablets........... 932
Hycomine.. 931
Hycotuss Expectorant Syrup.............. 933
Hydrocet Capsules.................................. 782
Lorcet 10/650.. 1018
Lortab... 2566
Tussend... 1783
Tussend Expectorant............................... 1785
Vicodin Tablets... 1356
Vicodin ES Tablets................................... 1357
Vicodin Tuss Expectorant...................... 1358
Zydone Capsules...................................... 949

Hydrocodone Polistirex (Increased prothrombin time response with prolonged use). Products include:

Tussionex Pennkinetic Extended-Release Suspension.............................. 998

Hydrocortisone (Decreased prothrombin time response). Products include:

Anusol-HC Cream 2.5%........................ 1896
Aquanil HC Lotion.................................. 1931
Bactine Hydrocortisone Anti-Itch Cream... ᴮᴰ 709
Caldecort Anti-Itch Hydrocortisone Spray... ᴮᴰ 631
Cortaid.. ᴮᴰ 836
CORTENEMA... 2535
Cortisporin Ointment.............................. 1085
Cortisporin Ophthalmic Ointment Sterile... 1085
Cortisporin Ophthalmic Suspension Sterile... 1086
Cortisporin Otic Solution Sterile...... 1087
Cortisporin Otic Suspension Sterile 1088
Cortizone-5.. ᴮᴰ 831
Cortizone-10.. ᴮᴰ 831
Hydrocortone Tablets............................. 1672
Hytone.. 907
Massengill Medicated Soft Cloth Towelettes... 2458
PediOtic Suspension Sterile............... 1153
Preparation H Hydrocortisone 1% Cream.. ᴮᴰ 872
ProctoCream-HC 2.5%........................... 2408
VōSoL HC Otic Solution......................... 2678

Hydrocortisone Acetate (Decreased prothrombin time response). Products include:

Analpram-HC Rectal Cream 1% and 2.5%.. 977
Anusol HC-1 Anti-Itch Hydrocortisone Ointment...................................... ᴮᴰ 847
Anusol-HC Suppositories...................... 1897
Caldecort... ᴮᴰ 631
Carmol HC.. 924
Coly-Mycin S Otic w/Neomycin & Hydrocortisone...................................... 1906
Cortaid.. ᴮᴰ 836
Cortifoam.. 2396
Cortisporin Cream................................... 1084
Epifoam.. 2399
Hydrocortone Acetate Sterile Suspension... 1669
Mantadil Cream....................................... 1135
Nupercainal Hydrocortisone 1% Cream... ᴮᴰ 645
Ophthocort... ⊙ 311
Pramosone Cream, Lotion & Ointment.. 978
ProctoCream-HC..................................... 2408
ProctoFoam-HC...................................... 2409
Terra-Cortril Ophthalmic Suspension... 2210

Hydrocortisone Sodium Phosphate (Decreased prothrombin time response). Products include:

Hydrocortone Phosphate Injection, Sterile... 1670

Hydrocortisone Sodium Succinate (Decreased prothrombin time response). Products include:

Solu-Cortef Sterile Powder.................... 2641

Hydroflumethiazide (Decreased or increased prothrombin time response). Products include:

Diucardin Tablets..................................... 2718

Ibuprofen (Increased prothrombin time response; caution should be observed when used concurrently). Products include:

Advil Cold and Sinus Caplets and Tablets (formerly CoAdvil).......... ᴮᴰ 870
Advil Ibuprofen Tablets and Caplets.. ᴮᴰ 870
Children's Advil Suspension.............. 2692
Arthritis Foundation Ibuprofen Tablets.. ᴮᴰ 674
Bayer Select Ibuprofen Pain Relief Formula.. ᴮᴰ 715
Cramp End Tablets.................................. ᴮᴰ 735
Dimetapp Sinus Caplets......................... ᴮᴰ 775
Haltran Tablets.. ᴮᴰ 771
IBU Tablets... 1342
Ibuprohm.. ᴮᴰ 735
Children's Motrin Ibuprofen Oral Suspension.. 1546
Motrin Tablets.. 2625
Motrin IB Caplets, Tablets, and Geltabs... ᴮᴰ 838
Motrin IB Sinus.. ᴮᴰ 838
Motrin Ibuprofen Suspension, Oral Drops, Chewable Tablets, Caplets.. 1546

IMPORTANT NOTE: Always consult each drug listing in the patient's regimen for possible interactions.

Coumadin Interactions Index 210

Nuprin Ibuprofen/Analgesic Tablets & Caplets ■ 622
Sine-Aid IB Caplets 1554
Vicks DayQuil SINUS Pressure & PAIN Relief with IBUPROFEN ■ 762

Indapamide (Decreased or increased prothrombin time response). Products include:
Lozol Tablets 2022

Indomethacin (Increased prothrombin time response; caution should be observed when used concurrently). Products include:
Indocin 1680

Indomethacin Sodium Trihydrate (Increased prothrombin time response; caution should be observed when used concurrently). Products include:
Indocin I.V. 1684

Influenza Virus Vaccine (Increased prothrombin time response). Products include:
Fluvirin 460
Influenza Virus Vaccine, Trivalent, Types A and B (chromatograph- and filter-purified subviron antigen) FluShield, 1995-1996 Formula 2736

Isocarboxazid (Increased prothrombin time response).
No products indexed under this heading.

Isoflurane (Increased prothrombin time response).
No products indexed under this heading.

Ketoprofen (Increased prothrombin time response; caution should be observed when used concurrently). Products include:
Orudis Capsules 2766
Oruvail Capsules 2766

Ketorolac Tromethamine (Increased prothrombin time response; caution should be observed when used concurrently). Products include:
Acular 474
Acular ⊙ 277
Toradol 2159

Levonorgestrel (Decreased prothrombin time response). Products include:
Levlen/Tri-Levlen 651
Nordette-21 Tablets 2755
Nordette-28 Tablets 2758
Norplant System 2759
Levlen/Tri-Levlen 651
Triphasil-21 Tablets 2814
Triphasil-28 Tablets 2819

Levorphanol Tartrate (Increased prothrombin response with prolonged use). Products include:
Levo-Dromoran 2129

Levothyroxine Sodium (Increased prothrombin time response). Products include:
Levothroid Tablets 1016
Levoxyl Tablets 903
Synthroid 1359

Liothyronine Sodium (Increased prothrombin time response). Products include:
Cytomel Tablets 2473
Triostat Injection 2530

Liotrix (Increased prothrombin time response).
No products indexed under this heading.

Lomefloxacin Hydrochloride (Increased prothrombin time response). Products include:
Maxaquin Tablets 2440

Loratadine (Decreased prothrombin time response). Products include:
Claritin 2349
Claritin-D 2350

Lovastatin (Increased prothrombin time response). Products include:
Mevacor Tablets 1699

Magaldrate (Decreased prothrombin time response).
No products indexed under this heading.

Magnesium Hydroxide (Decreased prothrombin time response). Products include:
Aludrox Oral Suspension 2695
Arthritis Pain Ascriptin ■ 631
Maximum Strength Ascriptin ■ 630
Regular Strength Ascriptin Tablets ■ 629
Di-Gel Antacid/Anti-Gas ■ 801
Gelusil Liquid & Tablets ■ 855
Maalox Magnesia and Alumina Oral Suspension ■ 642
Maalox Plus Tablets ■ 643
Extra Strength Maalox Antacid Plus Antigas Liquid and Tablets ■ 638
Mylanta Calcium Carbonate and Magnesium Hydroxide Tablets 1318
Mylanta Liquid 1317
Mylanta Tablets ■ 660
Mylanta Double Strength Liquid 1317
Mylanta Double Strength Tablets ■ 660
Phillips' Milk of Magnesia Liquid ■ 729
Rolaids Tablets ■ 843
Tempo Soft Antacid ■ 835

Magnesium Oxide (Decreased prothrombin time response). Products include:
Beelith Tablets 639
Bufferin Analgesic Tablets and Caplets ■ 613
Caltrate PLUS ■ 665
Cama Arthritis Pain Reliever ■ 785
Mag-Ox 400 668
Uro-Mag 668

Magnesium Salicylate (Increased prothrombin time response). Products include:
Backache Caplets ■ 613
Bayer Select Backache Pain Relief Formula ■ 715
Doan's Extra-Strength Analgesic ■ 633
Extra Strength Doan's P.M. ■ 633
Doan's Regular Strength Analgesic ■ 634
Mobigesic Tablets ■ 602

Meclofenamate Sodium (Increased prothrombin time response; caution should be observed when used concurrently).
No products indexed under this heading.

Mefenamic Acid (Increased prothrombin time response; caution should be observed when used concurrently). Products include:
Ponstel 1925

Meperidine Hydrochloride (Increased prothrombin time response with prolonged use). Products include:
Demerol 2308
Mepergan Injection 2753

Mephobarbital (Decreased prothrombin time response). Products include:
Mebaral Tablets 2322

Meprobamate (Decreased prothrombin time response). Products include:
Miltown Tablets 2672
PMB 200 and PMB 400 2783

Mestranol (Decreased prothrombin time response). Products include:
Norinyl 2088
Ortho-Novum 1872

Methadone Hydrochloride (Increased prothrombin time response with prolonged use). Products include:
Methadone Hydrochloride Oral Concentrate 2233
Methadone Hydrochloride Oral Solution & Tablets 2235

Methdilazine Hydrochloride (Decreased prothrombin time response).
No products indexed under this heading.

Methoxyflurane (Increased prothrombin time response).
No products indexed under this heading.

Methyclothiazide (Decreased or increased prothrombin time response). Products include:
Enduron Tablets 420

Methyldopa (Increased prothrombin time response). Products include:
Aldoclor Tablets 1598
Aldomet Oral 1600
Aldoril Tablets 1604

Methyldopate Hydrochloride (Increased prothrombin time response). Products include:
Aldomet Ester HCl Injection 1602

Methylphenidate Hydrochloride (Increased prothrombin time response). Products include:
Ritalin 848

Methylprednisolone Acetate (Decreased prothrombin time response). Products include:
Depo-Medrol Single-Dose Vial 2600
Depo-Medrol Sterile Aqueous Suspension 2597

Methylprednisolone Sodium Succinate (Decreased prothrombin time response). Products include:
Solu-Medrol Sterile Powder 2643

Methyltestosterone (Increased prothrombin time response). Products include:
Android Capsules, 10 mg 1250
Android 1251
Estratest 2539
Oreton Methyl 1255
Premarin with Methyltestosterone 2794
Testred Capsules 1262

Metolazone (Decreased or increased prothrombin time response). Products include:
Mykrox Tablets 993
Zaroxolyn Tablets 1000

Metronidazole (Increased prothrombin time response). Products include:
Flagyl 375 Capsules 2434
Flagyl I.V. RTU 2247
MetroGel 1047
MetroGel-Vaginal 902
Protostat Tablets 1883

Metronidazole Hydrochloride (Increased prothrombin time response). Products include:
Flagyl I.V. 2247

Miconazole (Increased prothrombin time response).
No products indexed under this heading.

Moricizine Hydrochloride (Decreased or increased prothrombin time response). Products include:
Ethmozine Tablets 2041

Morphine Sulfate (Increased prothrombin time response with prolonged use). Products include:
Astramorph/PF Injection, USP (Preservative-Free) 535
Duramorph 962
Infumorph 200 and Infumorph 500 Sterile Solutions 965
MS Contin Tablets 1994
MSIR 1997
Oramorph SR (Morphine Sulfate Sustained Release Tablets) 2236
RMS Suppositories 2657
Roxanol 2243

Nabumetone (Increased prothrombin time response; caution should be observed when used concurrently). Products include:
Relafen Tablets 2510

Nafcillin Sodium (Decreased prothrombin time response).
No products indexed under this heading.

Nalidixic Acid (Increased prothrombin time response). Products include:
NegGram 2323

Naproxen (Increased prothrombin time response; caution should be observed when used concurrently). Products include:
Anaprox/Naprosyn 2117

Naproxen Sodium (Increased prothrombin time response; caution should be observed when used concurrently). Products include:
Aleve 1975
Anaprox/Naprosyn 2117

Norethindrone (Decreased prothrombin time response). Products include:
Brevicon 2088
Micronor Tablets 1872
Modicon 1872
Norinyl 2088
Nor-Q D Tablets 2135
Ortho-Novum 1872
Ovcon 760
Tri-Norinyl 2164

Norethynodrel (Decreased prothrombin time response).
No products indexed under this heading.

Norfloxacin (Increased prothrombin time response). Products include:
Chibroxin Sterile Ophthalmic Solution 1617
Noroxin Tablets 1715
Noroxin Tablets 2048

Norgestimate (Decreased prothrombin time response). Products include:
Ortho-Cyclen/Ortho-Tri-Cyclen 1858
Ortho-Cyclen/Ortho Tri-Cyclen 1858

Norgestrel (Decreased prothrombin time response). Products include:
Lo/Ovral Tablets 2746
Lo/Ovral-28 Tablets 2751
Ovral Tablets 2770
Ovral-28 Tablets 2770
Ovrette Tablets 2771

Ofloxacin (Increased prothrombin time response). Products include:
Floxin I.V. 1571
Floxin Tablets (200 mg, 300 mg, 400 mg) 1567
Ocuflox 481
Ocuflox ⊙ 246

Opium Alkaloids (Increased prothrombin time response with prolonged use).
No products indexed under this heading.

Oxandrolone (Increased prothrombin time response). Products include:
Oxandrin 2862

Oxaprozin (Increased prothrombin time response; caution should be observed when used concurrently). Products include:
Daypro Caplets 2426

Oxycodone Hydrochloride (Increased prothrombin time response with prolonged use). Products include:
Percocet Tablets 938
Percodan Tablets 939
Percodan-Demi Tablets 940
Roxicodone Tablets, Oral Solution & Intensol (Oxycodone) 2244
Tylox Capsules 1584

Oxymetholone (Increased prothrombin time response).
No products indexed under this heading.

(■ Described in PDR For Nonprescription Drugs) (⊙ Described in PDR For Ophthalmology)

Interactions Index — Coumadin

Oxyphenbutazone (Increased prothrombin time response).

Paraldehyde (Decreased prothrombin time response).

Pentobarbital Sodium (Decreased prothrombin time response). Products include:

Nembutal Sodium Capsules 436
Nembutal Sodium Solution 438
Nembutal Sodium Suppositories...... 440

Pentoxifylline (Increased prothrombin time response). Products include:

Trental Tablets 1244

Phenelzine Sulfate (Increased prothrombin time response). Products include:

Nardil 1920

Phenobarbital (Decreased prothrombin time response; accumulation of phenobarbital). Products include:

Arco-Lase Plus Tablets 512
Bellergal-S Tablets 2250
Donnatal 2060
Donnatal Extentabs............................... 2061
Donnatal Tablets 2060
Phenobarbital Elixir and Tablets 1469
Quadrinal Tablets 1350

Phenylbutazone (Increased prothrombin time response; caution should be observed when used concurrently).

No products indexed under this heading.

Phenytoin (Accumulation of phenytoin; increased prothrombin time response). Products include:

Dilantin Infatabs 1908
Dilantin-125 Suspension 1911

Phenytoin Sodium (Accumulation of phenytoin; increased prothrombin time response). Products include:

Dilantin Kapseals 1906
Dilantin Parenteral 1910

Piroxicam (Increased prothrombin time response; caution should be observed when used concurrently). Products include:

Feldene Capsules................................... 1965

Polythiazide (Decreased or increased prothrombin time response). Products include:

Minizide Capsules 1938

Prednisolone Acetate (Decreased prothrombin time response). Products include:

AK-CIDE.. ⊘ 202
AK-CIDE Ointment................................. ⊘ 202
Blephamide Liquifilm Sterile Ophthalmic Suspension.............................. 476
Blephamide Ointment .... ⊘ 237
Econopred & Econopred Plus Ophthalmic Suspensions .... ⊘ 217
Poly-Pred Liquifilm .... ⊘ 248
Pred Forte... ⊘ 250
Pred Mild... ⊘ 253
Pred-G Liquifilm Sterile Ophthalmic Suspension .... ⊘ 251
Pred-G S.O.P. Sterile Ophthalmic Ointment .... ⊘ 252
Vasocidin Ointment .... ⊘ 268

Prednisolone Sodium Phosphate (Decreased prothrombin time response). Products include:

AK-Pred .... ⊘ 204
Hydeltrasol Injection, Sterile.............. 1665
Inflamase... ⊘ 265
Pediapred Oral Liquid 995
Vasocidin Ophthalmic Solution ...... ⊘ 270

Prednisolone Tebutate (Decreased prothrombin time response). Products include:

Hydeltra-T.B.A. Sterile Suspension 1667

Prednisone (Decreased prothrombin time response). Products include:

Deltasone Tablets 2595

Primidone (Decreased prothrombin time response). Products include:

Mysoline... 2754

Promethazine Hydrochloride (Decreased prothrombin time response). Products include:

Mepergan Injection 2753
Phenergan with Codeine...................... 2777
Phenergan with Dextromethorphan 2778
Phenergan Injection 2773
Phenergan Suppositories 2775
Phenergan Syrup 2774
Phenergan Tablets 2775
Phenergan VC 2779
Phenergan VC with Codeine 2781

Propafenone Hydrochloride (Increased prothrombin time response). Products include:

Rythmol Tablets–150mg, 225mg, 300mg.. 1352

Propoxyphene Hydrochloride (Increased prothrombin time response with prolonged use). Products include:

Darvon 1435
Wygesic Tablets 2827

Propoxyphene Napsylate (Increased prothrombin time response with prolonged use). Products include:

Darvon-N/Darvocet-N 1433

Pyrazolones (Increased prothrombin time response).

Pyrilamine Maleate (Decreased prothrombin time response). Products include:

4-Way Fast Acting Nasal Spray (regular & mentholated) .... ⊕ 621
Maximum Strength Multi-Symptom Formula Midol .... ⊕ 722
PMS Multi-Symptom Formula Midol .... ⊕ 723

Pyrilamine Tannate (Decreased prothrombin time response). Products include:

Atrohist Pediatric Suspension 454
Rynatan 2673

Quinidine Gluconate (Increased prothrombin time response). Products include:

Quinaglute Dura-Tabs Tablets 649

Quinidine Polygalacturonate (Increased prothrombin time response).

No products indexed under this heading.

Quinidine Sulfate (Increased prothrombin time response). Products include:

Quinidex Extentabs 2067

Quinine Sulfate (Increased prothrombin time response).

No products indexed under this heading.

Ranitidine Hydrochloride (Decreased or increased prothrombin time response). Products include:

Zantac.. 1209
Zantac Injection 1207
Zantac Syrup 1209

Rifampin (Decreased prothrombin time response). Products include:

Rifadin 1528
Rifamate Capsules 1530
Rifater.. 1532
Rimactane Capsules............................... 847

Salsalate (Increased prothrombin time response). Products include:

Mono-Gesic Tablets 792
Salflex Tablets.. 786

Secobarbital Sodium (Decreased prothrombin time response). Products include:

Seconal Sodium Pulvules 1474

Selegiline Hydrochloride (Increased prothrombin time response). Products include:

Eldepryl Tablets 2550

Sodium Bicarbonate (Decreased prothrombin time response). Products include:

Alka-Seltzer Effervescent Antacid and Pain Reliever .... ⊕ 701
Alka-Seltzer Extra Strength Effervescent Antacid and Pain Reliever .... ⊕ 703
Alka-Seltzer Gold Effervescent Antacid .... ⊕ 703
Alka-Seltzer Lemon Lime Effervescent Antacid and Pain Reliever .... ⊕ 703
Arm & Hammer Pure Baking Soda .... ⊕ 627
Ceo-Two Rectal Suppositories 666
Citrocarbonate Antacid .... ⊕ 770
Massengill Disposable Douches....... ⊕ 820
Massengill Liquid Concentrate......... ⊕ 820
NuLYTELY... 689
Cherry Flavor NuLYTELY 689

Spironolactone (Decreased or increased prothrombin time response). Products include:

Aldactazide.. 2413
Aldactone 2414

Stanozolol (Increased prothrombin time response). Products include:

Winstrol Tablets 2337

Streptokinase (Concurrent use is not recommended and may be hazardous). Products include:

Streptase for Infusion 562

Sucralfate (Decreased prothrombin time response). Products include:

Carafate Suspension 1505
Carafate Tablets...................................... 1504

Sufentanil Citrate (Increased prothrombin time response with prolonged use). Products include:

Sufenta Injection 1309

Sulfacytine (Increased prothrombin time response).

Sulfamethizole (Increased prothrombin time response). Products include:

Urobiotic-250 Capsules 2214

Sulfamethoxazole (Increased prothrombin time response). Products include:

Azo Gantanol Tablets............................ 2080
Bactrim DS Tablets................................. 2084
Bactrim I.V. Infusion............................. 2082
Bactrim 2084
Gantanol Tablets 2119
Septra... 1174
Septra I.V. Infusion 1169
Septra I.V. Infusion ADD-Vantage Vials.. 1171
Septra... 1174

Sulfasalazine (Increased prothrombin time response). Products include:

Azulfidine 1949

Sulfinpyrazone (Increased prothrombin time response). Products include:

Anturane 807

Sulfisoxazole (Increased prothrombin time response). Products include:

Azo Gantrisin Tablets............................ 2081
Gantrisin Tablets 2120

Sulfisoxazole Diolamine (Increased prothrombin time response).

No products indexed under this heading.

Sulindac (Increased prothrombin time response; caution should be observed when used concurrently). Products include:

Clinoril Tablets 1618

Tamoxifen Citrate (Increased prothrombin time response). Products include:

Nolvadex Tablets 2841

Temafloxacin Hydrochloride (Increased prothrombin time response).

No products indexed under this heading.

Terfenadine (Decreased prothrombin time response). Products include:

Seldane Tablets 1536
Seldane-D Extended-Release Tablets... 1538

Thiamylal Sodium (Decreased prothrombin time response).

No products indexed under this heading.

Thyroglobulin (Increased prothrombin time response).

No products indexed under this heading.

Thyroid (Increased prothrombin time response).

No products indexed under this heading.

Thyroxine (Increased prothrombin time response).

No products indexed under this heading.

Thyroxine Sodium (Increased prothrombin time response).

No products indexed under this heading.

Ticlopidine Hydrochloride (Concomitant administration may be associated with cholestatic hepatitis). Products include:

Ticlid Tablets 2156

Tolazamide (Increased prothrombin time response).

No products indexed under this heading.

Tolbutamide (Increased prothrombin time response; accumulation of tolbutamide).

No products indexed under this heading.

Tolmetin Sodium (Increased prothrombin time response; caution should be observed when used concurrently). Products include:

Tolectin (200, 400 and 600 mg) .. 1581

Torsemide (Decreased or increased prothrombin time response). Products include:

Demadex Tablets and Injection 686

Tranylcypromine Sulfate (Increased prothrombin time response). Products include:

Parnate Tablets 2503

Trazodone Hydrochloride (Decreased prothrombin time response). Products include:

Desyrel and Desyrel Dividose 503

Triamcinolone (Decreased prothrombin time response). Products include:

Aristocort Tablets 1022

Triamcinolone Acetonide (Decreased prothrombin time response). Products include:

Aristocort A 0.025% Cream 1027
Aristocort A 0.5% Cream 1031
Aristocort A 0.1% Cream 1029
Aristocort A 0.1% Ointment 1030
Azmacort Oral Inhaler 2011
Nasacort Nasal Inhaler 2024

Triamcinolone Diacetate (Decreased prothrombin time response). Products include:

Aristocort Suspension (Forte Parenteral).. 1027
Aristocort Suspension (Intralesional) 1025

Triamcinolone Hexacetonide (Decreased prothrombin time response). Products include:

Aristospan Suspension (Intra-articular) 1033
Aristospan Suspension (Intralesional) 1032

IMPORTANT NOTE: Always consult each drug listing in the patient's regimen for possible interactions.

Triamterene (Decreased or increased prothrombin time response). Products include:

Dyazide ... 2479
Dyrenium Capsules ... 2481
Maxzide ... 1380

Trimeprazine Tartrate (Decreased prothrombin time response). Products include:

Temaril Tablets, Syrup and Spansule Extended-Release Capsules.. 483

Trimethoprim (Increased prothrombin time response). Products include:

Bactrim DS Tablets ... 2084
Bactrim I.V. Infusion ... 2082
Bactrim ... 2084
Proloprim Tablets ... 1155
Septra ... 1174
Septra I.V. Infusion ... 1169
Septra I.V. Infusion ADD-Vantage Vials ... 1171
Septra ... 1174
Trimpex Tablets ... 2163

Tripelennamine Hydrochloride (Decreased prothrombin time response). Products include:

PBZ Tablets ... 845
PBZ-SR Tablets ... 844

Triprolidine Hydrochloride (Decreased prothrombin time response). Products include:

Actifed Plus Caplets ... ▣ 845
Actifed Plus Tablets ... ▣ 845
Actifed with Codeine Cough Syrup.. 1067
Actifed Syrup ... ▣ 846
Actifed Tablets ... ▣ 844

Urokinase (Concurrent use is not recommended and may be hazardous). Products include:

Abbokinase ... 403
Abbokinase Open-Cath ... 405

Vitamin C (Decreased prothrombin time response). Products include:

ANTIOX Capsules ... 1543
C-Buff ... 667
Centrum Singles Vitamin C ... ▣ 669
Chromagen Capsules ... 2339
Dexatrim Maximum Strength Plus Vitamin C/Caffeine-free Caplets ▣ 832
Ester-C Mineral Ascorbates Powder ... ▣ 658
Fero-Folic-500 Filmtab ... 429
Fero-Grad-500 Filmtab ... 429
Halls Vitamin C Drops ... ▣ 843
Hyland's Vitamin C for Children ... ▣ 830
Irospan ... 982
Materna Tablets ... 1379
Nature Made Antioxidant Formula ▣ 748
Niferex w/Vitamin C Tablets ... 793
One-A-Day Extras Antioxidant ... ▣ 728
One-A-Day Extras Vitamin C ... ▣ 728
Protegra Antioxidant Vitamin & Mineral Supplement ... ▣ 670
Stuart Prenatal Tablets ... ▣ 881
The Stuart Formula Tablets ... ▣ 663
Sunkist Children's Chewable Multivitamins - Plus Extra C ... ▣ 649
Sunkist Vitamin C ... ▣ 649
Theragran Antioxidant ... ▣ 623
Trinsicon Capsules ... 2570
Vitron-C Tablets ... ▣ 650

Food Interactions

Alcohol (Decreased or increased prothrombin time response).

Diet high in vitamin K (Decreased prothrombin time).

Vegetables, green leafy (Large amounts of green leafy vegetables may affect Coumadin therapy).

COZAAR TABLETS

(Losartan Potassium) ... 1628
May interact with:

Cimetidine (Co-administration leads to an increase of about 18% in AUC of losartan with no effect on pharmacokinetics of its active metabolites). Products include:

Tagamet Tablets ... 2516

Cimetidine Hydrochloride (Co-administration leads to an increase of about 18% in AUC of losartan with no effect on pharmacokinetics of its active metabolites). Products include:

Tagamet ... 2516

Gestodene (*In Vitro* studies show significant inhibition of the formation of the active metabolite by inhibitors of P450 3A4 such as gestodene; pharmacodynamic consequences of concomitant use is undefined).

No products indexed under this heading.

Ketoconazole (*In Vitro* studies show significant inhibition of the formation of the active metabolite by inhibitors of P450 3A4 such as ketoconazole or complete inhibition by the combination of ketoconazole and sulfaphenazole; pharmacodynamic consequences of concomitant use is undefined). Products include:

Nizoral 2% Cream ... 1297
Nizoral 2% Shampoo ... 1298
Nizoral Tablets ... 1298

Phenobarbital (Co-administration leads to a reduction of about 20% in AUC of losartan and that of its active metabolites). Products include:

Arco-Lase Plus Tablets ... 512
Bellergal-S Tablets ... 2250
Donnatal ... 2060
Donnatal Extentabs ... 2061
Donnatal Tablets ... 2060
Phenobarbital Elixir and Tablets ... 1469
Quadrinal Tablets ... 1350

Sulfaphenazole (*In Vitro* studies show significant inhibition of the formation of the active metabolite by inhibitors of P450 3A4 such as sulfaphenazole; pharmacodynamic consequences of concomitant use is undefined).

No products indexed under this heading.

Troleandomycin (*In Vitro* studies show significant inhibition of the formation of the active metabolite by inhibitors of P450 3A4 such as troleandomycin; pharmacodynamic consequences of concomitant use is undefined). Products include:

Tao Capsules ... 2209

Food Interactions

Meal, unspecified (Meal slows absorption and decreases C_{max} but has minor effects on losartan AUC or on the AUC of the metabolite).

CRAMP END TABLETS

(Ibuprofen) ... ▣ 735
None cited in PDR database.

CREON 5 CAPSULES

(Pancrelipase) ... 2536

Food Interactions

Food having a pH greater than 5.5 (Can dissolve the protective coating resulting in early release of enzymes, irritation of oral mucosa, and/or loss of enzyme activity).

CREON 10 CAPSULES

(Pancrelipase) ... 2536
See **CREON 5 Capsules**

CREON 20 CAPSULES

(Pancrelipase) ... 2536
See **CREON 5 Capsules**

CREST SENSITIVITY PROTECTION TOOTHPASTE

(Potassium Nitrate, Sodium Fluoride) ... ▣ 750
None cited in PDR database.

CRITIC-AID, ANTIMICROBIAL SKIN PASTE

(Zinc Oxide, Benzethonium Chloride) 2554
None cited in PDR database.

CROLOM

(Cromolyn Sodium) ... ⊙ 257
None cited in PDR database.

CRUEX ANTIFUNGAL CREAM

(Undecylenic Acid, Zinc Undecylenate) ... ▣ 632
None cited in PDR database.

CRUEX ANTIFUNGAL POWDER

(Calcium Undecylenate) ... ▣ 632
None cited in PDR database.

CRUEX ANTIFUNGAL SPRAY POWDER

(Undecylenic Acid, Zinc Undecylenate) ... ▣ 632
None cited in PDR database.

CRYSTODIGIN TABLETS

(Digitoxin) ... 1433
May interact with antihistamines, anticonvulsants, barbiturates, oral hypoglycemic agents, diuretics, and certain other agents. Compounds in these categories include:

Acarbose (Digitoxin metabolism stimulated).

No products indexed under this heading.

Acrivastine (Digitoxin metabolism stimulated). Products include:

Semprex-D Capsules ... 463
Semprex-D Capsules ... 1167

Amphotericin B (Increased potassium excretion). Products include:

Fungizone Intravenous ... 506

Aprobarbital (Digitoxin metabolism stimulated).

No products indexed under this heading.

Astemizole (Digitoxin metabolism stimulated). Products include:

Hismanal Tablets ... 1293

Azatadine Maleate (Digitoxin metabolism stimulated). Products include:

Trinalin Repetabs Tablets ... 1330

Bendroflumethiazide (Hypokalemia).

No products indexed under this heading.

Bromodiphenhydramine Hydrochloride (Digitoxin metabolism stimulated).

No products indexed under this heading.

Brompheniramine Maleate (Digitoxin metabolism stimulated). Products include:

Alka Seltzer Plus Sinus Medicine .. ▣ 707
Bromfed Capsules (Extended-Release) ... 1785
Bromfed Syrup ... ▣ 733
Bromfed Tablets ... 1785
Bromfed-DM Cough Syrup ... 1786
Bromfed-PD Capsules (Extended-Release) ... 1785
Dimetane-DC Cough Syrup ... 2059
Dimetane-DX Cough Syrup ... 2059
Dimetapp Elixir ... ▣ 773
Dimetapp Extentabs ... ▣ 774
Dimetapp Tablets/Liqui-Gels ... ▣ 775
Dimetapp Cold & Allergy Chewable Tablets ... ▣ 773
Dimetapp DM Elixir ... ▣ 774
Vicks DayQuil Allergy Relief 12-Hour Extended Release Tablets.. ▣ 760
Vicks DayQuil Allergy Relief 4-Hour Tablets ... ▣ 760

Bumetanide (Hypokalemia). Products include:

Bumex ... 2093

Butabarbital (Digitoxin metabolism stimulated).

No products indexed under this heading.

Butalbital (Digitoxin metabolism stimulated). Products include:

Esgic-plus Tablets ... 1013
Fioricet Tablets ... 2258
Fioricet with Codeine Capsules ... 2260
Fiorinal Capsules ... 2261
Fiorinal with Codeine Capsules ... 2262
Fiorinal Tablets ... 2261
Phrenilin ... 785
Sedapap Tablets 50 mg/650 mg .. 1543

Calcium, intravenous (Concurrent use is contraindicated).

No products indexed under this heading.

Carbamazepine (Digitoxin metabolism stimulated). Products include:

Atretol Tablets ... 573
Tegretol Chewable Tablets ... 852
Tegretol Suspension ... 852
Tegretol Tablets ... 852

Chlorothiazide (Hypokalemia). Products include:

Aldoclor Tablets ... 1598
Diupres Tablets ... 1650
Diuril Oral ... 1653

Chlorothiazide Sodium (Hypokalemia). Products include:

Diuril Sodium Intravenous ... 1652

Chlorpheniramine Maleate (Digitoxin metabolism stimulated). Products include:

Alka-Seltzer Plus Cold Medicine ... ▣ 705
Alka-Seltzer Plus Cold Medicine Liqui-Gels ... ▣ 706
Alka-Seltzer Plus Cold & Cough Medicine ... ▣ 708
Alka-Seltzer Plus Cold & Cough Medicine Liqui-Gels ... ▣ 705
Allerest Children's Chewable Tablets ... ▣ 627
Allerest Headache Strength Tablets ... ▣ 627
Allerest Maximum Strength Tablets ... ▣ 627
Allerest Sinus Pain Formula ... ▣ 627
Allerest 12 Hour Caplets ... ▣ 627
Ana-Kit Anaphylaxis Emergency Treatment Kit ... 617
Atrohist Pediatric Capsules ... 453
Atrohist Plus Tablets ... 454
BC Cold Powder Multi-Symptom Formula (Cold-Sinus-Allergy) ... ▣ 609
Cerose DM ... ▣ 878
Cheracol Plus Head Cold/Cough Formula ... ▣ 769
Children's Vicks DayQuil Allergy Relief ... ▣ 757
Children's Vicks NyQuil Cold/Cough Relief ... ▣ 758
Chlor-Trimeton Allergy Decongestant Tablets ... ▣ 799
Chlor-Trimeton Allergy Tablets ... ▣ 798
Comhist ... 2038
Comtrex Multi-Symptom Cold Reliever Tablets/Caplets/Liqui-Gels/Liquid ... ▣ 615
Allergy-Sinus Comtrex Multi-Symptom Allergy-Sinus Formula Tablets ... ▣ 617
Contac Continuous Action Nasal Decongestant/Antihistamine 12 Hour Capsules ... ▣ 813
Contac Maximum Strength Continuous Action Decongestant/Antihistamine 12 Hour Caplets.. ▣ 813
Contac Severe Cold and Flu Formula Caplets ... ▣ 814
Coricidin 'D' Decongestant Tablets ... ▣ 800
Coricidin Tablets ... ▣ 800
D.A. Chewable Tablets ... 951
Deconamine ... 1320
Dura-Tap/PD Capsules ... 2867
Dura-Vent/DA Tablets ... 953
Extendryl ... 1005
Fedahist Gyrocaps ... 2401
Fedahist Timecaps ... 2401
Hycomine Compound Tablets ... 932
Isoclor Timesule Capsules ... ▣ 637
Kronofed-A ... 977

(▣ Described in PDR For Nonprescription Drugs) (⊙ Described in PDR For Ophthalmology)

Interactions Index — Cuprimine

Nolamine Timed-Release Tablets 785
Novahistine DH....................................... 2462
Novahistine Elixir .... ⊞ 823
Ornade Spansule Capsules 2502
PediaCare Cold Allergy Chewable Tablets .... ⊞ 677
PediaCare Cough-Cold Chewable Tablets 1553
PediaCare Cough-Cold Liquid............ 1553
PediaCare NightRest Cough-Cold Liquid 1553
Pediatric Vicks 44m Cough & Cold Relief .... ⊞ 764
Pyrroxate Caplets .... ⊞ 772
Ryna .... ⊞ 841
Sinarest Tablets .... ⊞ 648
Sinarest Extra Strength Tablets...... ⊞ 648
Sine-Off Sinus Medicine .... ⊞ 825
Singlet Tablets .... ⊞ 825
Sinulin Tablets 787
Sinutab Sinus Allergy Medication, Maximum Strength Tablets and Caplets .... ⊞ 860
Sudafed Plus Liquid .... ⊞ 862
Sudafed Plus Tablets............................. ⊞ 863
Teldrin 12 Hour Antihistamine/ Nasal Decongestant Allergy Relief Capsules .... ⊞ 826
TheraFlu.. ⊞ 787
TheraFlu Maximum Strength Nighttime Flu, Cold & Cough Medicine .... ⊞ 788
Triaminic Allergy Tablets .... ⊞ 789
Triaminic Cold Tablets .... ⊞ 790
Triaminic Nite Light .... ⊞ 791
Triaminic Syrup .... ⊞ 792
Triaminic-12 Tablets .... ⊞ 792
Triaminicin Tablets................................. ⊞ 793
Triaminicol Multi-Symptom Cold Tablets .... ⊞ 793
Triaminicol Multi-Symptom Relief ⊞ 794
Tussend 1783
Children's TYLENOL Cold Multi-Symptom Liquid Formula and Chewable Tablets................................ 1561
Children's TYLENOL Cold Plus Cough Multi Symptom Tablets and Liquid .... ⊞ 681
TYLENOL Maximum Strength Allergy Sinus Medication Gelcaps and Caplets 1563
TYLENOL Cold Multi-Symptom Formula Medication Tablets and Caplets 1561
TYLENOL Cold Multi-Symptom Hot Medication Liquid Packets.............. 1557
Vicks 44 LiquiCaps Cough, Cold & Flu Relief... ⊞ 755
Vicks 44M Cough, Cold & Flu Relief... ⊞ 756

Chlorpheniramine Polistirex (Digitoxin metabolism stimulated). Products include:

Tussionex Pennkinetic Extended-Release Suspension 998

Chlorpheniramine Tannate (Digitoxin metabolism stimulated). Products include:

Atrohist Pediatric Suspension 454
Ricobid Tablets and Pediatric Suspension.. 2038
Rynatan 2673
Rynatuss 2673

Chlorpropamide (Digitoxin metabolism stimulated). Products include:

Diabinese Tablets 1935

Chlorthalidone (Hypokalemia). Products include:

Combipres Tablets 677
Tenoretic Tablets.................................... 2845
Thalitone 1245

Clemastine Fumarate (Digitoxin metabolism stimulated). Products include:

Tavist Syrup... 2297
Tavist Tablets 2298
Tavist-1 12 Hour Relief Tablets .... ⊞ 787
Tavist-D 12 Hour Relief Tablets .... ⊞ 787

Cyproheptadine Hydrochloride (Digitoxin metabolism stimulated). Products include:

Periactin 1724

Dexchlorpheniramine Maleate (Digitoxin metabolism stimulated).

No products indexed under this heading.

Diphenhydramine Citrate (Digitoxin metabolism stimulated). Products include:

Excedrin P.M. Analgesic/Sleeping Aid Tablets, Caplets, Liquigels...... 733

Diphenylpyraline Hydrochloride (Digitoxin metabolism stimulated).

No products indexed under this heading.

Divalproex Sodium (Digitoxin metabolism stimulated). Products include:

Depakote Tablets..................................... 415

Ethacrynic Acid (Hypokalemia). Products include:

Edecrin Tablets.. 1657

Ethosuximide (Digitoxin metabolism stimulated). Products include:

Zarontin Capsules 1928
Zarontin Syrup 1929

Ethotoin (Digitoxin metabolism stimulated). Products include:

Peganone Tablets 446

Felbamate (Digitoxin metabolism stimulated). Products include:

Felbatol 2666

Furosemide (Hypokalemia). Products include:

Lasix Injection, Oral Solution and Tablets 1240

Glipizide (Digitoxin metabolism stimulated). Products include:

Glucotrol Tablets 1967
Glucotrol XL Extended Release Tablets 1968

Glyburide (Digitoxin metabolism stimulated). Products include:

DiaBeta Tablets 1239
Glynase PresTab Tablets 2609
Micronase Tablets 2623

Hydrochlorothiazide (Hypokalemia). Products include:

Aldactazide... 2413
Aldoril Tablets... 1604
Apresazide Capsules 808
Capozide 742
Dyazide 2479
Esidrix Tablets 821
Esimil Tablets 822
HydroDIURIL Tablets 1674
Hydropres Tablets................................... 1675
Hyzaar Tablets 1677
Inderide Tablets 2732
Inderide LA Long Acting Capsules .. 2734
Lopressor HCT Tablets 832
Lotensin HCT... 837
Maxzide 1380
Moduretic Tablets 1705
Oretic Tablets 443
Prinzide Tablets 1737
Ser-Ap-Es Tablets 849
Timolide Tablets...................................... 1748
Vaseretic Tablets 1765
Zestoretic 2850
Ziac 1415

Hydroflumethiazide (Hypokalemia). Products include:

Diucardin Tablets.................................... 2718

Indapamide (Hypokalemia). Products include:

Lozol Tablets 2022

Lamotrigine (Digitoxin metabolism stimulated). Products include:

Lamictal Tablets...................................... 1112

Loratadine (Digitoxin metabolism stimulated). Products include:

Claritin 2349
Claritin-D 2350

Mephenytoin (Digitoxin metabolism stimulated). Products include:

Mesantoin Tablets................................... 2272

Mephobarbital (Digitoxin metabolism stimulated). Products include:

Mebaral Tablets 2322

Metformin Hydrochloride (Digitoxin metabolism stimulated). Products include:

Glucophage 752

Methdilazine Hydrochloride (Digitoxin metabolism stimulated).

No products indexed under this heading.

Methsuximide (Digitoxin metabolism stimulated). Products include:

Celontin Kapseals 1899

Methyclothiazide (Hypokalemia). Products include:

Enduron Tablets....................................... 420

Metolazone (Hypokalemia). Products include:

Mykrox Tablets.. 993
Zaroxolyn Tablets 1000

Paramethadione (Digitoxin metabolism stimulated).

No products indexed under this heading.

Pentobarbital Sodium (Digitoxin metabolism stimulated). Products include:

Nembutal Sodium Capsules 436
Nembutal Sodium Solution 438
Nembutal Sodium Suppositories...... 440

Phenacemide (Digitoxin metabolism stimulated). Products include:

Phenurone Tablets 447

Phenobarbital (Increases rate of metabolism of digitoxin). Products include:

Arco-Lase Plus Tablets 512
Bellergal-S Tablets 2250
Donnatal 2060
Donnatal Extentabs................................ 2061
Donnatal Tablets 2060
Phenobarbital Elixir and Tablets 1469
Quadrinal Tablets 1350

Phensuximide (Digitoxin metabolism stimulated). Products include:

Milontin Kapseals................................... 1920

Phenylbutazone (Increased rate of digitoxin metabolism).

No products indexed under this heading.

Phenytoin (Increased rate of digitoxin metabolism). Products include:

Dilantin Infatabs..................................... 1908
Dilantin-125 Suspension 1911

Phenytoin Sodium (Increased rate of digitoxin metabolism). Products include:

Dilantin Kapseals 1906
Dilantin Parenteral 1910

Polythiazide (Hypokalemia). Products include:

Minizide Capsules 1938

Prednisone (Increased potassium excretion). Products include:

Deltasone Tablets 2595

Primidone (Digitoxin metabolism stimulated). Products include:

Mysoline... 2754

Promethazine Hydrochloride (Digitoxin metabolism stimulated). Products include:

Mepergan Injection 2753
Phenergan with Codeine...................... 2777
Phenergan with Dextromethorphan 2778
Phenergan Injection 2773
Phenergan Suppositories 2775
Phenergan Syrup.................................... 2774
Phenergan Tablets 2775
Phenergan VC 2779
Phenergan VC with Codeine 2781

Pyrilamine Maleate (Digitoxin metabolism stimulated). Products include:

4-Way Fast Acting Nasal Spray (regular & mentholated) .... ⊞ 621
Maximum Strength Multi-Symptom Formula Midol .... ⊞ 722
PMS Multi-Symptom Formula Midol .... ⊞ 723

Pyrilamine Tannate (Digitoxin metabolism stimulated). Products include:

Atrohist Pediatric Suspension 454
Rynatan 2673

Secobarbital Sodium (Digitoxin metabolism stimulated). Products include:

Seconal Sodium Pulvules 1474

Terfenadine (Digitoxin metabolism stimulated). Products include:

Seldane Tablets 1536
Seldane-D Extended-Release Tablets 1538

Thiamylal Sodium (Digitoxin metabolism stimulated).

No products indexed under this heading.

Tolazamide (Digitoxin metabolism stimulated).

No products indexed under this heading.

Tolbutamide (Digitoxin metabolism stimulated).

No products indexed under this heading.

Torsemide (Hypokalemia). Products include:

Demadex Tablets and Injection 686

Trimeprazine Tartrate (Digitoxin metabolism stimulated). Products include:

Temaril Tablets, Syrup and Spansule Extended-Release Capsules.. 483

Trimethadione (Digitoxin metabolism stimulated).

No products indexed under this heading.

Tripelennamine Hydrochloride (Digitoxin metabolism stimulated). Products include:

PBZ Tablets 845
PBZ-SR Tablets.. 844

Triprolidine Hydrochloride (Digitoxin metabolism stimulated). Products include:

Actifed Plus Caplets .... ⊞ 845
Actifed Plus Tablets .... ⊞ 845
Actifed with Codeine Cough Syrup.. 1067
Actifed Syrup... ⊞ 846
Actifed Tablets .... ⊞ 844

Valproic Acid (Digitoxin metabolism stimulated). Products include:

Depakene 413

CUPRIMINE CAPSULES

(Penicillamine) 1630

May interact with cytotoxic drugs, antimalarials, and certain other agents. Compounds in these categories include:

Auranofin (Concurrent use not recommended). Products include:

Ridaura Capsules.................................... 2513

Aurothioglucose (Concurrent use not recommended). Products include:

Solganal Suspension............................... 2388

Bleomycin Sulfate (Concurrent use not recommended). Products include:

Blenoxane 692

Chloroquine Hydrochloride (Concurrent use not recommended). Products include:

Aralen Hydrochloride Injection 2301

Chloroquine Phosphate (Concurrent use not recommended). Products include:

Aralen Phosphate Tablets 2301

Daunorubicin Hydrochloride (Concurrent use not recommended). Products include:

Cerubidine 795

Doxorubicin Hydrochloride (Concurrent use not recommended). Products include:

Adriamycin PFS 1947
Adriamycin RDF 1947
Doxorubicin Astra 540
Rubex 712

IMPORTANT NOTE: Always consult each drug listing in the patient's regimen for possible interactions.

Cuprimine | Interactions Index | 214

Fluorouracil (Concurrent use not recommended). Products include:
- Efudex 2113
- Fluoroplex Topical Solution & Cream 1% 479
- Fluorouracil Injection 2116

Hydroxychloroquine Sulfate (Concurrent use not recommended). Products include:
- Plaquenil Sulfate Tablets 2328

Hydroxyurea (Concurrent use not recommended). Products include:
- Hydrea Capsules 696

Mefloquine Hydrochloride (Concurrent use not recommended). Products include:
- Lariam Tablets 2128

Methotrexate Sodium (Concurrent use not recommended). Products include:
- Methotrexate Sodium Tablets, Injection, for Injection and LPF Injection 1275

Mineral Supplements (Block response).

Mitotane (Concurrent use not recommended). Products include:
- Lysodren 698

Mitoxantrone Hydrochloride (Concurrent use not recommended). Products include:
- Novantrone 1279

Oxyphenbutazone (Concurrent use not recommended).

Phenylbutazone (Concurrent use not recommended).
- No products indexed under this heading.

Procarbazine Hydrochloride (Concurrent use not recommended). Products include:
- Matulane Capsules 2131

Pyridoxine (Penicillamine increases pyridoxine requirement).

Pyrimethamine (Concurrent use not recommended). Products include:
- Daraprim Tablets 1090
- Fansidar Tablets 2114

Tamoxifen Citrate (Concurrent use not recommended). Products include:
- Nolvadex Tablets 2841

Vincristine Sulfate (Concurrent use not recommended). Products include:
- Oncovin Solution Vials & Hyporets 1466

CUREL LOTION AND CREAM
(Moisturizing formula) .... ▣ 606
None cited in PDR database.

CUTIVATE CREAM
(Fluticasone Propionate) 1088
None cited in PDR database.

CUTIVATE OINTMENT
(Fluticasone Propionate) 1089
None cited in PDR database.

CYCLOCORT TOPICAL CREAM 0.1%
(Amcinonide) 1037
None cited in PDR database.

CYCLOCORT TOPICAL LOTION 0.1%
(Amcinonide) 1037
None cited in PDR database.

CYCLOCORT TOPICAL OINTMENT 0.1%
(Amcinonide) 1037
None cited in PDR database.

CYCRIN TABLETS
(Medroxyprogesterone Acetate) 975
May interact with estrogens and certain other agents. Compounds in these categories include:

Aminoglutethimide (Concomitant administration may depress the bioavailability of Amen). Products include:
- Cytadren Tablets 819

Chlorotrianisene (Potential for adverse effects on carbohydrate and lipid metabolism).
- No products indexed under this heading.

Dienestrol (Potential for adverse effects on carbohydrate and lipid metabolism). Products include:
- Ortho Dienestrol Cream 1866

Diethylstilbestrol (Potential for adverse effects on carbohydrate and lipid metabolism). Products include:
- Diethylstilbestrol Tablets 1437

Estradiol (Potential for adverse effects on carbohydrate and lipid metabolism). Products include:
- Climara Transdermal System 645
- Estrace Cream and Tablets 749
- Estraderm Transdermal System 824

Estrogens, Conjugated (Potential for adverse effects on carbohydrate and lipid metabolism). Products include:
- PMB 200 and PMB 400 2783
- Premarin Intravenous 2787
- Premarin with Methyltestosterone .. 2794
- Premarin Tablets 2789
- Premarin Vaginal Cream 2791
- Premphase 2797
- Prempro 2801

Estrogens, Esterified (Potential for adverse effects on carbohydrate and lipid metabolism). Products include:
- ESTRATAB Tablets (0.3, 0.625, 1.25, 2.5 mg) 2536
- Estratest 2539
- Menest Tablets 2494

Estropipate (Potential for adverse effects on carbohydrate and lipid metabolism). Products include:
- Ogen Tablets 2627
- Ogen Vaginal Cream 2630
- Ortho-Est 1869

Ethinyl Estradiol (Potential for adverse effects on carbohydrate and lipid metabolism). Products include:
- Brevicon 2088
- Demulen 2428
- Desogen Tablets 1817
- Levlen/Tri-Levlen 651
- Lo/Ovral Tablets 2746
- Lo/Ovral-28 Tablets 2751
- Modicon 1872
- Nordette-21 Tablets 2755
- Nordette-28 Tablets 2758
- Norinyl 2088
- Ortho-Cept 1851
- Ortho-Cyclen/Ortho-Tri-Cyclen 1858
- Ortho-Novum 1872
- Ortho-Cyclen/Ortho Tri-Cyclen 1858
- Ovcon 760
- Ovral Tablets 2770
- Ovral-28 Tablets 2770
- Levlen/Tri-Levlen 651
- Tri-Norinyl 2164
- Triphasil-21 Tablets 2814
- Triphasil-28 Tablets 2819

Polyestradiol Phosphate (Potential for adverse effects on carbohydrate and lipid metabolism).
- No products indexed under this heading.

Quinestrol (Potential for adverse effects on carbohydrate and lipid metabolism).
- No products indexed under this heading.

CYKLOKAPRON TABLETS AND INJECTION
(Tranexamic Acid) 1950
None cited in PDR database.

CYLERT CHEWABLE TABLETS
(Pemoline) 412
See **Cylert Tablets**

CYLERT TABLETS
(Pemoline) 412
May interact with anticonvulsants and central nervous system stimulants. Compounds in these categories include:

Amphetamine Resins (Effects not specified). Products include:
- Biphetamine Capsules 983

Carbamazepine (Decreased seizure threshold). Products include:
- Atretol Tablets 573
- Tegretol Chewable Tablets 852
- Tegretol Suspension 852
- Tegretol Tablets 852

Dextroamphetamine Sulfate (Effects not specified). Products include:
- Dexedrine 2474
- DextroStat Dextroamphetamine Tablets 2036

Divalproex Sodium (Decreased seizure threshold). Products include:
- Depakote Tablets 415

Ethosuximide (Decreased seizure threshold). Products include:
- Zarontin Capsules 1928
- Zarontin Syrup 1929

Ethotoin (Decreased seizure threshold). Products include:
- Peganone Tablets 446

Felbamate (Decreased seizure threshold). Products include:
- Felbatol 2666

Lamotrigine (Decreased seizure threshold). Products include:
- Lamictal Tablets 1112

Mephenytoin (Decreased seizure threshold). Products include:
- Mesantoin Tablets 2272

Methamphetamine Hydrochloride (Effects not specified). Products include:
- Desoxyn Gradumet Tablets 419

Methsuximide (Decreased seizure threshold). Products include:
- Celontin Kapseals 1899

Methylphenidate Hydrochloride (Effects not specified). Products include:
- Ritalin 848

Paramethadione (Decreased seizure threshold).
- No products indexed under this heading.

Phenacemide (Decreased seizure threshold). Products include:
- Phenurone Tablets 447

Phenobarbital (Decreased seizure threshold). Products include:
- Arco-Lase Plus Tablets 512
- Bellergal-S Tablets 2250
- Donnatal 2060
- Donnatal Extentabs 2061
- Donnatal Tablets 2060
- Phenobarbital Elixir and Tablets 1469
- Quadrinal Tablets 1350

Phensuximide (Decreased seizure threshold). Products include:
- Milontin Kapseals 1920

Phenytoin (Decreased seizure threshold). Products include:
- Dilantin Infatabs 1908
- Dilantin-125 Suspension 1911

Phenytoin Sodium (Decreased seizure threshold). Products include:
- Dilantin Kapseals 1906
- Dilantin Parenteral 1910

Primidone (Decreased seizure threshold). Products include:
- Mysoline 2754

Trimethadione (Decreased seizure threshold).
- No products indexed under this heading.

Valproic Acid (Decreased seizure threshold). Products include:
- Depakene 413

CYSTOSPAZ TABLETS
(Hyoscyamine) 1963
May interact with phenothiazines, monoamine oxidase inhibitors, tricyclic antidepressants, antihistamines, antimuscarinic drugs, antacids, and certain other agents. Compounds in these categories include:

Acrivastine (Additive adverse effects resulting from cholinergic blockade). Products include:
- Semprex-D Capsules 463
- Semprex-D Capsules 1167

Aluminum Carbonate Gel (Interferes with absorption). Products include:
- Basaljel 2703

Aluminum Hydroxide (Interferes with absorption). Products include:
- ALternaGEL Liquid 1316
- Maximum Strength Ascriptin .... ▣ 630
- Cama Arthritis Pain Reliever .... ▣ 785
- Gaviscon Extra Strength Relief Formula Antacid Tablets .... ▣ 819
- Gaviscon Extra Strength Relief Formula Liquid Antacid .... ▣ 819
- Gaviscon Liquid Antacid .... ▣ 820
- Gelusil Liquid & Tablets .... ▣ 855
- Maalox Heartburn Relief Suspension .... ▣ 642
- Maalox Heartburn Relief Tablets .... ▣ 641
- Maalox Magnesia and Alumina Oral Suspension .... ▣ 642
- Maalox Plus Tablets .... ▣ 643
- Extra Strength Maalox Antacid Plus Antigas Liquid and Tablets ▣ 638
- Tempo Soft Antacid .... ▣ 835

Aluminum Hydroxide Gel (Interferes with absorption). Products include:
- ALternaGEL Liquid .... ▣ 659
- Aludrox Oral Suspension 2695
- Amphojel Suspension 2695
- Amphojel Suspension without Flavor 2695
- Amphojel Tablets 2695
- Arthritis Pain Ascriptin .... ▣ 631
- Regular Strength Ascriptin Tablets .... ▣ 629
- Gaviscon Antacid Tablets .... ▣ 819
- Gaviscon-2 Antacid Tablets .... ▣ 820
- Mylanta Liquid 1317
- Mylanta Tablets .... ▣ 660
- Mylanta Double Strength Liquid 1317
- Mylanta Double Strength Tablets .. ▣ 660
- Nephrox Suspension .... ▣ 655

Aluminum Hydroxide Gel, Dried (Interferes with absorption).

Amantadine Hydrochloride (Additive adverse effects resulting from cholinergic blockade). Products include:
- Symmetrel Capsules and Syrup 946

Amitriptyline Hydrochloride (Additive adverse effects resulting from cholinergic blockade). Products include:
- Elavil 2838
- Endep Tablets 2174
- Etrafon 2355
- Limbitrol 2180
- Triavil Tablets 1757

Amoxapine (Additive adverse effects resulting from cholinergic blockade). Products include:
- Asendin Tablets 1369

Astemizole (Additive adverse effects resulting from cholinergic blockade). Products include:
- Hismanal Tablets 1293

(▣ Described in PDR For Nonprescription Drugs) (◉ Described in PDR For Ophthalmology)

Interactions Index

Atropine Sulfate (Additive adverse effects resulting from cholinergic blockade). Products include:

Arco-Lase Plus Tablets 512
Atrohist Plus Tablets 454
Atropine Sulfate Sterile Ophthalmic Solution .... ◉ 233
Donnatal 2060
Donnatal Extentabs................................ 2061
Donnatal Tablets 2060
Lomotil 2439
Motofen Tablets 784
Urised Tablets.. 1964

Azatadine Maleate (Additive adverse effects resulting from cholinergic blockade). Products include:

Trinalin Repetabs Tablets 1330

Belladonna Alkaloids (Additive adverse effects resulting from cholinergic blockade). Products include:

Bellergal-S Tablets 2250
Hyland's Bed Wetting Tablets .... 🔲 828
Hyland's EnurAid Tablets................... 🔲 829
Hyland's Teething Tablets .... 🔲 830

Bromodiphenhydramine Hydrochloride (Additive adverse effects resulting from cholinergic blockade).

No products indexed under this heading.

Brompheniramine Maleate (Additive adverse effects resulting from cholinergic blockade). Products include:

Alka Seltzer Plus Sinus Medicine .. 🔲 707
Bromfed Capsules (Extended-Release) 1785
Bromfed Syrup .... 🔲 733
Bromfed Tablets 1785
Bromfed-DM Cough Syrup................. 1786
Bromfed-PD Capsules (Extended-Release) 1785
Dimetane-DC Cough Syrup 2059
Dimetane-DX Cough Syrup 2059
Dimetapp Elixir .... 🔲 773
Dimetapp Extentabs .... 🔲 774
Dimetapp Tablets/Liqui-Gels .... 🔲 775
Dimetapp Cold & Allergy Chewable Tablets .... 🔲 773
Dimetapp DM Elixir................................ 🔲 774
Vicks DayQuil Allergy Relief 12-Hour Extended Release Tablets.. 🔲 760
Vicks DayQuil Allergy Relief 4-Hour Tablets .... 🔲 760

Chlorpheniramine Maleate (Additive adverse effects resulting from cholinergic blockade). Products include:

Alka-Seltzer Plus Cold Medicine .... 🔲 705
Alka-Seltzer Plus Cold Medicine Liqui-Gels .... 🔲 706
Alka-Seltzer Plus Cold & Cough Medicine .... 🔲 708
Alka-Seltzer Plus Cold & Cough Medicine Liqui-Gels........................... 🔲 705
Allerest Children's Chewable Tablets .... 🔲 627
Allerest Headache Strength Tablets .... 🔲 627
Allerest Maximum Strength Tablets .... 🔲 627
Allerest Sinus Pain Formula .... 🔲 627
Allerest 12 Hour Caplets .... 🔲 627
Ana-Kit Anaphylaxis Emergency Treatment Kit 617
Atrohist Pediatric Capsules............... 453
Atrohist Plus Tablets 454
BC Cold Powder Multi-Symptom Formula (Cold-Sinus-Allergy) ...... 🔲 609
Cerose DM .... 🔲 878
Cheracol Plus Head Cold/Cough Formula .... 🔲 769
Children's Vicks DayQuil Allergy Relief .... 🔲 757
Children's Vicks NyQuil Cold/Cough Relief... 🔲 758
Chlor-Trimeton Allergy Decongestant Tablets .... 🔲 799
Chlor-Trimeton Allergy Tablets ...... 🔲 798
Comhist 2038
Comtrex Multi-Symptom Cold Reliever Tablets/Caplets/Liqui-Gels/Liquid... 🔲 615
Allergy-Sinus Comtrex Multi-Symptom Allergy-Sinus Formula Tablets .... 🔲 617

Contac Continuous Action Nasal Decongestant/Antihistamine 12 Hour Capsules...................................... 🔲 813
Contac Maximum Strength Continuous Action Decongestant/Antihistamine 12 Hour Caplets.. 🔲 813
Contac Severe Cold and Flu Formula Caplets .... 🔲 814
Coricidin 'D' Decongestant Tablets .... 🔲 800
Coricidin Tablets .... 🔲 800
D.A. Chewable Tablets.......................... 951
Deconamine 1320
Dura-Tap/PD Capsules 2867
Dura-Vent/DA Tablets 953
Extendryl 1005
Fedahist Gyrocaps.................................. 2401
Fedahist Timecaps 2401
Hycomine Compound Tablets 932
Isoclor Timesule Capsules .... 🔲 637
Kronofed-A 977
Nolamine Timed-Release Tablets 785
Novahistine DH.. 2462
Novahistine Elixir .... 🔲 823
Ornade Spansule Capsules 2502
PediaCare Cold Allergy Chewable Tablets .... 🔲 677
PediaCare Cough-Cold Chewable Tablets 1553
PediaCare Cough-Cold Liquid........... 1553
PediaCare NightRest Cough-Cold Liquid 1553
Pediatric Vicks 44m Cough & Cold Relief .... 🔲 764
Pyroxate Caplets .... 🔲 772
Ryna .... 🔲 841
Sinarest Tablets .... 🔲 648
Sinarest Extra Strength Tablets...... 🔲 648
Sine-Off Sinus Medicine .... 🔲 825
Singlet Tablets .... 🔲 825
Sinutin Tablets 787
Sinutab Sinus Allergy Medication, Maximum Strength Tablets and Caplets .... 🔲 860
Sudafed Plus Liquid .... 🔲 862
Sudafed Plus Tablets .... 🔲 863
Teldrin 12 Hour Antihistamine/Nasal Decongestant Allergy Relief Capsules .... 🔲 826
TheraFlu.. 🔲 787
TheraFlu Maximum Strength Nighttime Flu, Cold & Cough Medicine .... 🔲 788
Triaminic Allergy Tablets .... 🔲 789
Triaminic Cold Tablets .... 🔲 790
Triaminic Nite Light .... 🔲 791
Triaminic Syrup .... 🔲 792
Triaminic-12 Tablets .... 🔲 792
Triaminicin Tablets .... 🔲 793
Triaminicol Multi-Symptom Cold Tablets .... 🔲 793
Triaminicol Multi-Symptom Relief 🔲 794
Tussend 1783
Children's TYLENOL Cold Multi-Symptom Liquid Formula and Chewable Tablets.................................. 1561
Children's TYLENOL Cold Plus Cough Multi Symptom Tablets and Liquid .... 🔲 681
TYLENOL Maximum Strength Allergy Sinus Medication Gelcaps and Caplets 1563
TYLENOL Cold Multi-Symptom Formula Medication Tablets and Caplets 1561
TYLENOL Cold Multi-Symptom Hot Medication Liquid Packets.............. 1557
Vicks 44 LiquiCaps Cough, Cold & Flu Relief... 🔲 755
Vicks 44M Cough, Cold & Flu Relief .... 🔲 756

Chlorpheniramine Polistirex (Additive adverse effects resulting from cholinergic blockade). Products include:

Tussionex Pennkinetic Extended-Release Suspension 998

Chlorpheniramine Tannate (Additive adverse effects resulting from cholinergic blockade). Products include:

Atrohist Pediatric Suspension .... ' 454
Ricobid Tablets and Pediatric Suspension... 2038
Rynatan 2673
Rynatuss 2673

Chlorpromazine (Additive adverse effects resulting from cholinergic blockade). Products include:

Thorazine Suppositories 2523

Chlorpromazine Hydrochloride (Additive adverse effects resulting from cholinergic blockade). Products include:

Thorazine 2523

Clemastine Fumarate (Additive adverse effects resulting from cholinergic blockade). Products include:

Tavist Syrup 2297
Tavist Tablets 2298
Tavist-1 12 Hour Relief Tablets .... 🔲 787
Tavist-D 12 Hour Relief Tablets .... 🔲 787

Clidinium Bromide (Additive adverse effects resulting from cholinergic blockade). Products include:

Librax Capsules 2176
Quarzan Capsules 2181

Clomipramine Hydrochloride (Additive adverse effects resulting from cholinergic blockade). Products include:

Anafranil Capsules 803

Cyproheptadine Hydrochloride (Additive adverse effects resulting from cholinergic blockade). Products include:

Periactin 1724

Desipramine Hydrochloride (Additive adverse effects resulting from cholinergic blockade). Products include:

Norpramin Tablets 1526

Dexchlorpheniramine Maleate (Additive adverse effects resulting from cholinergic blockade).

No products indexed under this heading.

Dicyclomine Hydrochloride (Additive adverse effects resulting from cholinergic blockade). Products include:

Bentyl 1501

Dihydroxyaluminum Sodium Carbonate (Interferes with absorption).

No products indexed under this heading.

Diphenhydramine Citrate (Additive adverse effects resulting from cholinergic blockade). Products include:

Excedrin P.M. Analgesic/Sleeping Aid Tablets, Caplets, Liquigels...... 733

Diphenhydramine Hydrochloride (Additive adverse effects resulting from cholinergic blockade). Products include:

Actifed Allergy Daytime/Nighttime Caplets.. 🔲 844
Actifed Sinus Daytime/Nighttime Tablets and Caplets .... 🔲 846
Arthritis Foundation NightTime Caplets .... 🔲 674
Extra Strength Bayer PM Aspirin .. 🔲 713
Bayer Select Night Time Pain Relief Formula... 🔲 716
Benadryl Allergy Decongestant Liquid Medication .... 🔲 848
Benadryl Allergy Decongestant Tablets .... 🔲 848
Benadryl Allergy Liquid Medication.. 🔲 849
Benadryl Allergy .... 🔲 848
Benadryl Allergy Sinus Headache Formula Caplets .... 🔲 849
Benadryl Capsules.................................. 1898
Benadryl Dye-Free Allergy Liquigel Softgels.. 🔲 850
Benadryl Dye-Free Allergy Liquid Medication .... 🔲 850
Benadryl Itch Relief Cream, Children's Formula and Maximum Strength 2% .... 🔲 851
Benadryl Itch Relief Spray, Children's Formula and Maximum Strength 2% .... 🔲 851
Benadryl Itch Relief Stick Maximum Strength 2% .... 🔲 850

Benadryl Itch Stopping Gel, Children's Formula and Maximum Strength 2% .... 🔲 851
Benadryl Kapseals.................................. 1898
Benadryl Injection 1898
Contac Day & Night Cold/Flu Night Caplets.. 🔲 812
Contac Night Allergy/Sinus Caplets .... 🔲 812
Extra Strength Doan's P.M. .... 🔲 633
Legatrin PM .... 🔲 651
Miles Nervine Nighttime Sleep-Aid 🔲 723
Nytol QuickCaps Caplets .... 🔲 610
Sleepinal Night-time Sleep Aid Capsules and Softgels .... 🔲 834
TYLENOL Maximum Strength Allergy Sinus NightTime Medication Caplets 1555
TYLENOL Flu NightTime, Maximum Strength, Gelcaps 1566
TYLENOL Maximum Strength Flu NightTime Hot Medication Packets 1562
TYLENOL PM, Extra Strength Pain Reliever/Sleep Aid Caplets, Geltabs, Gelcaps.. 1560
TYLENOL Severe Allergy Medication Caplets 1564
Maximum Strength Unisom Sleepgels 1934
Unisom With Pain Relief-Nighttime Sleep Aid and Pain Reliever............. 1934

Diphenylpyraline Hydrochloride (Additive adverse effects resulting from cholinergic blockade).

No products indexed under this heading.

Doxepin Hydrochloride (Additive adverse effects resulting from cholinergic blockade). Products include:

Sinequan 2205
Zonalon Cream 1055

Fluphenazine Decanoate (Additive adverse effects resulting from cholinergic blockade). Products include:

Prolixin Decanoate 509

Fluphenazine Enanthate (Additive adverse effects resulting from cholinergic blockade). Products include:

Prolixin Enanthate 509

Fluphenazine Hydrochloride (Additive adverse effects resulting from cholinergic blockade). Products include:

Prolixin 509

Furazolidone (Additive adverse effects resulting from cholinergic blockade). Products include:

Furoxone 2046

Glycopyrrolate (Additive adverse effects resulting from cholinergic blockade). Products include:

Robinul Forte Tablets............................. 2072
Robinul Injectable 2072
Robinul Tablets.. 2072

Haloperidol (Additive adverse effects resulting from cholinergic blockade). Products include:

Haldol Injection, Tablets and Concentrate 1575

Haloperidol Decanoate (Additive adverse effects resulting from cholinergic blockade). Products include:

Haldol Decanoate..................................... 1577

Hyoscyamine Sulfate (Additive adverse effects resulting from cholinergic blockade). Products include:

Arco-Lase Plus Tablets 512
Atrohist Plus Tablets 454
Cystospaz-M Capsules 1963
Donnatal 2060
Donnatal Extentabs................................ 2061
Donnatal Tablets 2060
Kutrase Capsules..................................... 2402
Levsin/Levsinex/Levbid 2405

Imipramine Hydrochloride (Additive adverse effects resulting from cholinergic blockade). Products include:

Tofranil Ampuls 854
Tofranil Tablets 856

IMPORTANT NOTE: Always consult each drug listing in the patient's regimen for possible interactions.

Cystospaz | Interactions Index | 216

Imipramine Pamoate (Additive adverse effects resulting from cholinergic blockade). Products include:
- Tofranil-PM Capsules 857

Ipratropium Bromide (Additive adverse effects resulting from cholinergic blockade). Products include:
- Atrovent Inhalation Aerosol 671
- Atrovent Inhalation Solution 673

Isocarboxazid (Additive adverse effects resulting from cholinergic blockade).
- No products indexed under this heading.

Loratadine (Additive adverse effects resulting from cholinergic blockade). Products include:
- Claritin 2349
- Claritin-D 2350

Magaldrate (Interferes with absorption).
- No products indexed under this heading.

Magnesium Hydroxide (Interferes with absorption). Products include:
- Aludrox Oral Suspension 2695
- Arthritis Pain Ascriptin .... ■ 631
- Maximum Strength Ascriptin .... ■ 630
- Regular Strength Ascriptin Tablets .... ■ 629
- Di-Gel Antacid/Anti-Gas .... ■ 801
- Gelusil Liquid & Tablets .... ■ 855
- Maalox Magnesia and Alumina Oral Suspension .... ■ 642
- Maalox Plus Tablets .... ■ 643
- Extra Strength Maalox Antacid Plus Antigas Liquid and Tablets ■ 638
- Mylanta Calcium Carbonate and Magnesium Hydroxide Tablets 1318
- Mylanta Liquid 1317
- Mylanta Tablets .... ■ 660
- Mylanta Double Strength Liquid 1317
- Mylanta Double Strength Tablets .... ■ 660
- Phillips' Milk of Magnesia Liquid .... ■ 729
- Rolaids Tablets .... ■ 843
- Tempo Soft Antacid .... ■ 835

Magnesium Oxide (Interferes with absorption). Products include:
- Beelith Tablets 639
- Bufferin Analgesic Tablets and Caplets .... ■ 613
- Caltrate PLUS .... ■ 665
- Cama Arthritis Pain Reliever .... ■ 785
- Mag-Ox 400 668
- Uro-Mag 668

Maprotiline Hydrochloride (Additive adverse effects resulting from cholinergic blockade). Products include:
- Ludiomil Tablets 843

Mepenzolate Bromide (Additive adverse effects resulting from cholinergic blockade).
- No products indexed under this heading.

Mesoridazine Besylate (Additive adverse effects resulting from cholinergic blockade). Products include:
- Serentil 684

Methdilazine Hydrochloride (Additive adverse effects resulting from cholinergic blockade).
- No products indexed under this heading.

Methotrimeprazine (Additive adverse effects resulting from cholinergic blockade). Products include:
- Levoprome 1274

Nortriptyline Hydrochloride (Additive adverse effects resulting from cholinergic blockade). Products include:
- Pamelor 2280

Oxyphenonium Bromide (Additive adverse effects resulting from cholinergic blockade).

Perphenazine (Additive adverse effects resulting from cholinergic blockade). Products include:
- Etrafon 2355
- Triavil Tablets 1757
- Trilafon 2389

Phenelzine Sulfate (Additive adverse effects resulting from cholinergic blockade). Products include:
- Nardil 1920

Prochlorperazine (Additive adverse effects resulting from cholinergic blockade). Products include:
- Compazine 2470

Promethazine Hydrochloride (Additive adverse effects resulting from cholinergic blockade). Products include:
- Mepergan Injection 2753
- Phenergan with Codeine 2777
- Phenergan with Dextromethorphan 2778
- Phenergan Injection 2773
- Phenergan Suppositories 2775
- Phenergan Syrup 2774
- Phenergan Tablets 2775
- Phenergan VC 2779
- Phenergan VC with Codeine 2781

Propantheline Bromide (Additive adverse effects resulting from cholinergic blockade). Products include:
- Pro-Banthīne Tablets 2052

Protriptyline Hydrochloride (Additive adverse effects resulting from cholinergic blockade). Products include:
- Vivactil Tablets 1774

Pyrilamine Maleate (Additive adverse effects resulting from cholinergic blockade). Products include:
- 4-Way Fast Acting Nasal Spray (regular & mentholated) .... ■ 621
- Maximum Strength Multi-Symptom Formula Midol .... ■ 722
- PMS Multi-Symptom Formula Midol .... ■ 723

Pyrilamine Tannate (Additive adverse effects resulting from cholinergic blockade). Products include:
- Atrohist Pediatric Suspension 454
- Rynatan 2673

Scopolamine (Additive adverse effects resulting from cholinergic blockade). Products include:
- Transderm Scōp Transdermal Therapeutic System 869

Scopolamine Hydrobromide (Additive adverse effects resulting from cholinergic blockade). Products include:
- Atrohist Plus Tablets 454
- Donnatal 2060
- Donnatal Extentabs 2061
- Donnatal Tablets 2060

Selegiline Hydrochloride (Additive adverse effects resulting from cholinergic blockade). Products include:
- Eldepryl Tablets 2550

Sodium Bicarbonate (Interferes with absorption). Products include:
- Alka-Seltzer Effervescent Antacid and Pain Reliever .... ■ 701
- Alka-Seltzer Extra Strength Effervescent Antacid and Pain Reliever .... ■ 703
- Alka-Seltzer Gold Effervescent Antacid .... ■ 703
- Alka-Seltzer Lemon Lime Effervescent Antacid and Pain Reliever .... ■ 703
- Arm & Hammer Pure Baking Soda .... ■ 627
- Ceo-Two Rectal Suppositories 666
- Citrocarbonate Antacid .... ■ 770
- Massengill Disposable Douches .... ■ 820
- Massengill Liquid Concentrate .... ■ 820
- NuLYTELY 689
- Cherry Flavor NuLYTELY 689

Terfenadine (Additive adverse effects resulting from cholinergic blockade). Products include:
- Seldane Tablets 1536
- Seldane-D Extended-Release Tablets 1538

Thioridazine Hydrochloride (Additive adverse effects resulting from cholinergic blockade). Products include:
- Mellaril 2269

Tranylcypromine Sulfate (Additive adverse effects resulting from cholinergic blockade). Products include:
- Parnate Tablets 2503

Tridihexethyl Chloride (Additive adverse effects resulting from cholinergic blockade).
- No products indexed under this heading.

Trifluoperazine Hydrochloride (Additive adverse effects resulting from cholinergic blockade). Products include:
- Stelazine 2514

Trimeprazine Tartrate (Additive adverse effects resulting from cholinergic blockade). Products include:
- Temaril Tablets, Syrup and Spansule Extended-Release Capsules 483

Trimipramine Maleate (Additive adverse effects resulting from cholinergic blockade). Products include:
- Surmontil Capsules 2811

Tripelennamine Hydrochloride (Additive adverse effects resulting from cholinergic blockade). Products include:
- PBZ Tablets 845
- PBZ-SR Tablets 844

Triprolidine Hydrochloride (Additive adverse effects resulting from cholinergic blockade). Products include:
- Actifed Plus Caplets .... ■ 845
- Actifed Plus Tablets .... ■ 845
- Actifed with Codeine Cough Syrup 1067
- Actifed Syrup .... ■ 846
- Actifed Tablets .... ■ 844

CYSTOSPAZ-M CAPSULES
(Hyoscyamine Sulfate) 1963

See **Cystospaz Tablets**

CYTADREN TABLETS
(Aminoglutethimide) 819

May interact with oral anticoagulants and certain other agents. Compounds in these categories include:

Dexamethasone (Accelerates metabolism of dexamethasone). Products include:
- AK-Trol Ointment & Suspension .... ◉ 205
- Decadron Elixir 1633
- Decadron Tablets 1635
- Decaspray Topical Aerosol 1648
- Dexacidin Ointment .... ◉ 263
- Maxitrol Ophthalmic Ointment and Suspension .... ◉ 224
- TobraDex Ophthalmic Suspension and Ointment 473

Dexamethasone Acetate (Accelerates metabolism of dexamethasone). Products include:
- Dalalone D.P. Injectable 1011
- Decadron-LA Sterile Suspension 1646

Dexamethasone Phosphate (Accelerates metabolism of dexamethasone).
- No products indexed under this heading.

Dexamethasone Sodium Phosphate (Accelerates metabolism of dexamethasone). Products include:
- Decadron Phosphate Injection 1637
- Decadron Phosphate Respihaler 1642
- Decadron Phosphate Sterile Ophthalmic Ointment 1641
- Decadron Phosphate Sterile Ophthalmic Solution 1642
- Decadron Phosphate Topical Cream 1644
- Decadron Phosphate Turbinaire 1645
- Decadron Phosphate with Xylocaine Injection, Sterile 1639
- Dexacort Phosphate in Respihaler 458
- Dexacort Phosphate in Turbinaire 459
- NeoDecadron Sterile Ophthalmic Ointment 1712
- NeoDecadron Sterile Ophthalmic Solution 1713
- NeoDecadron Topical Cream 1714

Dicumarol (Diminishes anticoagulant effect).
- No products indexed under this heading.

Warfarin Sodium (Diminishes anticoagulant effect). Products include:
- Coumadin 926

Food Interactions

Alcohol (Effects of alcohol potentiated).

CYTOGAM
(Cytomegalovirus Immune Globulin) 1593

May interact with:

Measles, Mumps & Rubella Virus Vaccine Live (May interfere with the immune response to live virus vaccine). Products include:
- M-M-R II 1687

CYTOMEL TABLETS
(Liothyronine Sodium) 2473

May interact with oral anticoagulants, insulin, oral hypoglycemic agents, estrogens, oral contraceptives, tricyclic antidepressants, cardiac glycosides, and certain other agents. Compounds in these categories include:

Acarbose (Possible increase in oral hypoglycemic requirements).
- No products indexed under this heading.

Amitriptyline Hydrochloride (Enhanced antidepressant and thyroid activities). Products include:
- Elavil 2838
- Endep Tablets 2174
- Etrafon 2355
- Limbitrol 2180
- Triavil Tablets 1757

Amoxapine (Enhanced antidepressant and thyroid activities). Products include:
- Asendin Tablets 1369

Chlorpropamide (Possible increase in oral hypoglycemic requirements). Products include:
- Diabinese Tablets 1935

Cholestyramine (Impaired absorption of T4 and T3). Products include:
- Questran Light 769
- Questran Powder 770

Clomipramine Hydrochloride (Enhanced antidepressant and thyroid activities). Products include:
- Anafranil Capsules 803

Desipramine Hydrochloride (Enhanced antidepressant and thyroid activities). Products include:
- Norpramin Tablets 1526

Deslanoside (Toxic effects of digitalis glycosides potentiated).
- No products indexed under this heading.

Desogestrel (Increases thyroid requirements). Products include:
- Desogen Tablets 1817
- Ortho-Cept 1851

Dicumarol (Reduction of anticoagulant dosage may be necessary).
- No products indexed under this heading.

Dienestrol (Increases thyroid requirements). Products include:
- Ortho Dienestrol Cream 1866

Diethylstilbestrol (Increases thyroid requirements). Products include:
- Diethylstilbestrol Tablets 1437

(■ Described in PDR For Nonprescription Drugs) (◉ Described in PDR For Ophthalmology)

Digitoxin (Toxic effects of digitalis glycosides potentiated). Products include:

Crystodigin Tablets 1433

Digoxin (Toxic effects of digitalis glycosides potentiated). Products include:

Lanoxicaps 1117
Lanoxin Elixir Pediatric 1120
Lanoxin Injection 1123
Lanoxin Injection Pediatric 1126
Lanoxin Tablets 1128

Doxepin Hydrochloride (Enhanced antidepressant and thyroid activities). Products include:

Sinequan 2205
Zonalon Cream 1055

Epinephrine (Increased adrenergic effect; increased risk of precipitating coronary insufficiency). Products include:

Bronkaid Mist .... ▣ 717
EPIFRIN .... ⊙ 239
EpiPen 790
Marcaine Hydrochloride with Epinephrine 1:200,000 2316
Primatene Mist .... ▣ 873
Sensorcaine with Epinephrine Injection 559
Sus-Phrine Injection 1019
Xylocaine with Epinephrine Injections 567

Epinephrine Bitartrate (Increased adrenergic effect; increased risk of precipitating coronary insufficiency). Products include:

Bronkaid Mist Suspension .... ▣ 718
Sensorcaine-MPF with Epinephrine Injection 559

Estradiol (Increases thyroid requirements). Products include:

Climara Transdermal System 645
Estrace Cream and Tablets 749
Estraderm Transdermal System 824

Estrogens, Conjugated (Increases thyroid requirements). Products include:

PMB 200 and PMB 400 2783
Premarin Intravenous 2787
Premarin with Methyltestosterone 2794
Premarin Tablets 2789
Premarin Vaginal Cream 2791
Premphase 2797
Prempro 2801

Estrogens, Esterified (Increases thyroid requirements). Products include:

ESTRATAB Tablets (0.3, 0.625, 1.25, 2.5 mg) 2536
Estratest 2539
Menest Tablets 2494

Estropipate (Increases thyroid requirements). Products include:

Ogen Tablets 2627
Ogen Vaginal Cream 2630
Ortho-Est 1869

Ethinyl Estradiol (Increases thyroid requirements). Products include:

Brevicon 2088
Demulen 2428
Desogen Tablets 1817
Levlen/Tri-Levlen 651
Lo/Ovral Tablets 2746
Lo/Ovral-28 Tablets 2751
Modicon 1872
Nordette-21 Tablets 2755
Nordette-28 Tablets 2758
Norinyl 2088
Ortho-Cept 1851
Ortho-Cyclen/Ortho-Tri-Cyclen 1858
Ortho-Novum 1872
Ortho-Cyclen/Ortho Tri-Cyclen 1858
Ovcon 760
Ovral Tablets 2770
Ovral-28 Tablets 2770
Levlen/Tri-Levlen 651
Tri-Norinyl 2164
Triphasil-21 Tablets 2814
Triphasil-28 Tablets 2819

Ethynodiol Diacetate (Increases thyroid requirements). Products include:

Demulen 2428

Glipizide (Possible increase in oral hypoglycemic requirements). Products include:

Glucotrol Tablets 1967
Glucotrol XL Extended Release Tablets 1968

Glyburide (Possible increase in oral hypoglycemic requirements). Products include:

DiaBeta Tablets 1239
Glynase PresTab Tablets 2609
Micronase Tablets 2623

Imipramine Hydrochloride (Enhanced antidepressant and thyroid activities). Products include:

Tofranil Ampuls 854
Tofranil Tablets 856

Imipramine Pamoate (Enhanced antidepressant and thyroid activities). Products include:

Tofranil-PM Capsules 857

Insulin, Human (Possible increase in insulin requirements).

No products indexed under this heading.

Insulin, Human Isophane Suspension (Possible increase in insulin requirements). Products include:

Novolin N Human Insulin 10 ml Vials 1795

Insulin, Human NPH (Possible increase in insulin requirements). Products include:

Humulin N, 100 Units 1448
Novolin N PenFill Cartridges Durable Insulin Delivery System 1798
Novolin N Prefilled Syringe Disposable Insulin Delivery System 1798

Insulin, Human Regular (Possible increase in insulin requirements). Products include:

Humulin R, 100 Units 1449
Novolin R Human Insulin 10 ml Vials 1795
Novolin R PenFill Cartridges Durable Insulin Delivery System 1798
Novolin R Prefilled Syringe Disposable Insulin Delivery System 1798
Velosulin BR Human Insulin 10 ml Vials 1795

Insulin, Human, Zinc Suspension (Possible increase in insulin requirements). Products include:

Humulin L, 100 Units 1446
Humulin U, 100 Units 1450
Novolin L Human Insulin 10 ml Vials 1795

Insulin, NPH (Possible increase in insulin requirements). Products include:

NPH, 100 Units 1450
Pork NPH, 100 Units 1452
Purified Pork NPH Isophane Insulin 1801

Insulin, Regular (Possible increase in insulin requirements). Products include:

Regular, 100 Units 1450
Pork Regular, 100 Units 1452
Pork Regular (Concentrated), 500 Units 1453
Purified Pork Regular Insulin 1801

Insulin, Zinc Crystals (Possible increase in insulin requirements). Products include:

NPH, 100 Units 1450

Insulin, Zinc Suspension (Possible increase in insulin requirements). Products include:

Iletin I 1450
Lente, 100 Units 1450
Iletin II 1452
Pork Lente, 100 Units 1452
Purified Pork Lente Insulin 1801

Ketamine Hydrochloride (May cause hypertension, and tachycardia).

No products indexed under this heading.

Levonorgestrel (Increases thyroid requirements). Products include:

Levlen/Tri-Levlen 651
Nordette-21 Tablets 2755
Nordette-28 Tablets 2758
Norplant System 2759
Levlen/Tri-Levlen 651
Triphasil-21 Tablets 2814
Triphasil-28 Tablets 2819

Maprotiline Hydrochloride (Enhanced antidepressant and thyroid activities). Products include:

Ludiomil Tablets 843

Mestranol (Increases thyroid requirements). Products include:

Norinyl 2088
Ortho-Novum 1872

Metformin Hydrochloride (Possible increase in oral hypoglycemic requirements). Products include:

Glucophage 752

Norepinephrine Bitartrate (Increased adrenergic effect; increased risk of precipitating coronary insufficiency). Products include:

Levophed Bitartrate Injection 2315

Norethindrone (Increases thyroid requirements). Products include:

Brevicon 2088
Micronor Tablets 1872
Modicon 1872
Norinyl 2088
Nor-Q D Tablets 2135
Ortho-Novum 1872
Ovcon 760
Tri-Norinyl 2164

Norethynodrel (Increases thyroid requirements).

No products indexed under this heading.

Norgestimate (Increases thyroid requirements). Products include:

Ortho-Cyclen/Ortho-Tri-Cyclen 1858
Ortho-Cyclen/Ortho Tri-Cyclen 1858

Norgestrel (Increases thyroid requirements). Products include:

Lo/Ovral Tablets 2746
Lo/Ovral-28 Tablets 2751
Ovral Tablets 2770
Ovral-28 Tablets 2770
Ovrette Tablets 2771

Nortriptyline Hydrochloride (Enhanced antidepressant and thyroid activities). Products include:

Pamelor 2280

Polyestradiol Phosphate (Increases thyroid requirements).

No products indexed under this heading.

Protriptyline Hydrochloride (Enhanced antidepressant and thyroid activities). Products include:

Vivactil Tablets 1774

Quinestrol (Increases thyroid requirements).

No products indexed under this heading.

Tolazamide (Possible increase in oral hypoglycemic requirements).

No products indexed under this heading.

Tolbutamide (Possible increase in oral hypoglycemic requirements).

No products indexed under this heading.

Trimipramine Maleate (Enhanced antidepressant and thyroid activities). Products include:

Surmontil Capsules 2811

Warfarin Sodium (Reduction of anticoagulant dosage may be necessary). Products include:

Coumadin 926

CYTOSAR-U STERILE POWDER

(Cytarabine) 2592

May interact with:

Asparaginase (May result in acute pancreatitis). Products include:

Elspar 1659

Cyclophosphamide (Increased cardiomyopathy). Products include:

Cytoxan 694
NEOSAR Lyophilized/Neosar 1959

Digoxin (A reversible decrease in steady-state plasma digoxin concentrations and renal glycoside excretion in patients receiving beta-acetyldigoxin and combination chemotherapy regimens). Products include:

Lanoxicaps 1117
Lanoxin Elixir Pediatric 1120
Lanoxin Injection 1123
Lanoxin Injection Pediatric 1126
Lanoxin Tablets 1128

Flucytosine (Possible inhibition of flucytosine efficacy). Products include:

Ancobon Capsules 2079

Gentamicin Sulfate (Possible lack of antibacterial therapeutic response). Products include:

Garamycin Injectable 2360
Genoptic Sterile Ophthalmic Solution .... ⊙ 243
Genoptic Sterile Ophthalmic Ointment .... ⊙ 243
Gentacidin Ointment .... ⊙ 264
Gentacidin Solution .... ⊙ 264
Gentak .... ⊙ 208
Pred-G Liquifilm Sterile Ophthalmic Suspension .... ⊙ 251
Pred-G S.O.P. Sterile Ophthalmic Ointment .... ⊙ 252

CYTOTEC

(Misoprostol) 2424

May interact with antacids containing aluminium, calcium and magnesium. Compounds in this category include:

Aluminum Carbonate Gel (Total availability of misoprostol is reduced by use of concomitant antacid). Products include:

Basaljel 2703

Aluminum Hydroxide (Total availability of misoprostol is reduced by use of concomitant antacid). Products include:

ALternaGEL Liquid 1316
Maximum Strength Ascriptin .... ▣ 630
Cama Arthritis Pain Reliever .... ▣ 785
Gaviscon Extra Strength Relief Formula Antacid Tablets .... ▣ 819
Gaviscon Extra Strength Relief Formula Liquid Antacid .... ▣ 819
Gaviscon Liquid Antacid .... ▣ 820
Gelusil Liquid & Tablets .... ▣ 855
Maalox Heartburn Relief Suspension .... ▣ 642
Maalox Heartburn Relief Tablets .... ▣ 641
Maalox Magnesia and Alumina Oral Suspension .... ▣ 642
Maalox Plus Tablets .... ▣ 643
Extra Strength Maalox Antacid Plus Antigas Liquid and Tablets ▣ 638
Tempo Soft Antacid .... ▣ 835

Aluminum Hydroxide Gel (Total availability of misoprostol is reduced by use of concomitant antacid). Products include:

ALternaGEL Liquid .... ▣ 659
Aludrox Oral Suspension 2695
Amphojel Suspension 2695
Amphojel Suspension without Flavor 2695
Amphojel Tablets 2695
Arthritis Pain Ascriptin .... ▣ 631
Regular Strength Ascriptin Tablets .... ▣ 629
Gaviscon Antacid Tablets .... ▣ 819
Gaviscon-2 Antacid Tablets .... ▣ 820
Mylanta Liquid 1317

IMPORTANT NOTE: Always consult each drug listing in the patient's regimen for possible interactions.

Mylanta Tablets ▣ 660
Mylanta Double Strength Liquid 1317
Mylanta Double Strength Tablets ▣ 660
Nephrox Suspension ▣ 655

Aluminum Hydroxide Gel, Dried (Total availability of misoprostol is reduced by use of concomitant antacid).

Dihydroxyaluminum Sodium Carbonate (Total availability of misoprostol is reduced by use of concomitant antacid).
No products indexed under this heading.

Magaldrate (Avoid coadministration with magnesium containing antacids; total availability of misoprostol is reduced by use of concomitant antacid).
No products indexed under this heading.

Magnesium Carbonate (Avoid coadministration with magnesium containing antacids). Products include:
Gaviscon Extra Strength Relief Formula Antacid Tablets ▣ 819
Gaviscon Extra Strength Relief Formula Liquid Antacid ▣ 819
Gaviscon Liquid Antacid ▣ 820
Maalox Heartburn Relief Suspension ▣ 642
Maalox Heartburn Relief Tablets ▣ 641
Marblen ▣ 655
Mylanta Gelcaps Antacid ▣ 662

Magnesium Hydroxide (Avoid coadministration with magnesium containing antacids; total availability of misoprostol is reduced by use of concomitant antacid). Products include:
Aludrox Oral Suspension 2695
Arthritis Pain Ascriptin ▣ 631
Maximum Strength Ascriptin ▣ 630
Regular Strength Ascriptin Tablets ▣ 629
Di-Gel Antacid/Anti-Gas ▣ 801
Gelusil Liquid & Tablets ▣ 855
Maalox Magnesia and Alumina Oral Suspension ▣ 642
Maalox Plus Tablets ▣ 643
Extra Strength Maalox Antacid Plus Antigas Liquid and Tablets ▣ 638
Mylanta Calcium Carbonate and Magnesium Hydroxide Tablets 1318
Mylanta Liquid 1317
Mylanta Tablets ▣ 660
Mylanta Double Strength Liquid 1317
Mylanta Double Strength Tablets ▣ 660
Phillips' Milk of Magnesia Liquid ▣ 729
Rolaids Tablets ▣ 843
Tempo Soft Antacid ▣ 835

Magnesium Oxide (Total availability of misoprostol is reduced by use of concomitant antacid). Products include:
Beelith Tablets 639
Bufferin Analgesic Tablets and Caplets ▣ 613
Caltrate PLUS ▣ 665
Cama Arthritis Pain Reliever ▣ 785
Mag-Ox 400 668
Uro-Mag 668

Food Interactions

Food, unspecified (Diminishes maximum plasma concentrations).

CYTOVENE CAPSULES

(Ganciclovir Sodium) 2103
May interact with drugs inhibiting replication of cell populations of bone marrow, spermatogonia, and germinal layers of skin and gi mucosa, nucleoside analogues, and certain other agents. Compounds in these categories include:

Acyclovir (Potential for additive toxicity). Products include:
Zovirax Capsules 1219
Zovirax Ointment 5% 1223
Zovirax 1219

Acyclovir Sodium (Potential for additive toxicity). Products include:
Zovirax Sterile Powder 1223

Amphotericin B (Potential for additive toxicity; increases in serum creatinine and may result in increased nephrotoxicity). Products include:
Fungizone Intravenous 506

Cyclosporine (Increases in serum creatinine and may result in increased nephrotoxicity). Products include:
Neoral 2276
Sandimmune 2286

Dapsone (Potential for additive toxicity). Products include:
Dapsone Tablets USP 1284

Didanosine (When administered concurrently or 2 hours prior to oral Cytovene, the steady-state didanosine AUC_{0-12} increased 111 +/− 114%; a decrease in ganciclovir steady-state AUC of 21 +/− 17%). Products include:
Videx Tablets, Powder for Oral Solution, & Pediatric Powder for Oral Solution 720

Doxorubicin Hydrochloride (Potential for additive toxicity). Products include:
Adriamycin PFS 1947
Adriamycin RDF 1947
Doxorubicin Astra 540
Rubex 712

Flucytosine (Potential for additive toxicity). Products include:
Ancobon Capsules 2079

Imipenem-Cilastatin Sodium (Co-administration results in generalized seizures). Products include:
Primaxin I.M. 1727
Primaxin I.V. 1729

Pentamidine Isethionate (Potential for additive toxicity). Products include:
NebuPent for Inhalation Solution 1040
Pentam 300 Injection 1041

Probenecid (Increases AUC_{0-8} 53 +/− 91%, decreases renal clearance 22 +/− 20%). Products include:
Benemid Tablets 1611
ColBENEMID Tablets 1622

Sulfamethoxazole (Potential for additive toxicity). Products include:
Azo Gantanol Tablets 2080
Bactrim DS Tablets 2084
Bactrim I.V. Infusion 2082
Bactrim 2084
Gantanol Tablets 2119
Septra 1174
Septra I.V. Infusion 1169
Septra I.V. Infusion ADD-Vantage Vials 1171
Septra 1174

Trimethoprim (Potential for additive toxicity). Products include:
Bactrim DS Tablets 2084
Bactrim I.V. Infusion 2082
Bactrim 2084
Proloprim Tablets 1155
Septra 1174
Septra I.V. Infusion 1169
Septra I.V. Infusion ADD-Vantage Vials 1171
Septra 1174
Trimpex Tablets 2163

Vinblastine Sulfate (Potential for additive toxicity). Products include:
Velban Vials 1484

Vincristine Sulfate (Potential for additive toxicity). Products include:
Oncovin Solution Vials & Hyporets 1466

Zidovudine (Man steady-state ganciclovir AUC_{0-8} decreases 17 +/− 25% in presence of zidovudine; steady-state zidovudine AUC_{0-4} increases 19 +/− 27%; both have potential to cause anemia and neutropenia). Products include:
Retrovir Capsules 1158
Retrovir I.V. Infusion 1163
Retrovir Syrup 1158

Food Interactions

Meal, unspecified (Meal containing 46.5% fat increases the steady-state AUC of oral Cytovene by 22% +/− 22% and significant prolongation of time T_{max} and a higher C_{max}).

CYTOVENE-IV

(Ganciclovir Sodium) 2103
See **Cytovene Capsules**

CYTOXAN FOR INJECTION

(Cyclophosphamide) 694
May interact with cytotoxic drugs, general anesthetics, and certain other agents. Compounds in these categories include:

Bleomycin Sulfate (Concurrent use may require reduction in dose of Cytoxan as well as that of other cytotoxic drugs). Products include:
Blenoxane 692

Daunorubicin Hydrochloride (Concurrent use may require reduction in dose of Cytoxan as well as that of other cytotoxic drugs). Products include:
Cerubidine 795

Doxorubicin Hydrochloride (Potentiation of doxorubicin-induced cardiotoxicity; concurrent use may require reduction in dose of Cytoxan as well as that of other cytotoxic drugs). Products include:
Adriamycin PFS 1947
Adriamycin RDF 1947
Doxorubicin Astra 540
Rubex 712

Enflurane (Anesthesiologist should be alerted if patient has been treated with cyclophosphamide within 10 days).
No products indexed under this heading.

Fluorouracil (Concurrent use may require reduction in dose of Cytoxan as well as that of other cytotoxic drugs). Products include:
Efudex 2113
Fluoroplex Topical Solution & Cream 1% 479
Fluorouracil Injection 2116

Hydroxyurea (Concurrent use may require reduction in dose of Cytoxan as well as that of other cytotoxic drugs). Products include:
Hydrea Capsules 696

Isoflurane (Anesthesiologist should be alerted if patient has been treated with cyclophosphamide within 10 days).
No products indexed under this heading.

Ketamine Hydrochloride (Anesthesiologist should be alerted if patient has been treated with cyclophosphamide within 10 days).
No products indexed under this heading.

Methohexital Sodium (Anesthesiologist should be alerted if patient has been treated with cyclophosphamide within 10 days). Products include:
Brevital Sodium Vials 1429

Methotrexate Sodium (Concurrent use may require reduction in dose of Cytoxan as well as that of other cytotoxic drugs). Products include:
Methotrexate Sodium Tablets, Injection, for Injection and LPF Injection 1275

Methoxyflurane (Anesthesiologist should be alerted if patient has been treated with cyclophosphamide within 10 days).
No products indexed under this heading.

Mitotane (Concurrent use may require reduction in dose of Cytoxan as well as that of other cytotoxic drugs). Products include:
Lysodren 698

Mitoxantrone Hydrochloride (Concurrent use may require reduction in dose of Cytoxan as well as that of other cytotoxic drugs). Products include:
Novantrone 1279

Phenobarbital (Increased rate of metabolism and leukopenic activity of cyclophosphamide). Products include:
Arco-Lase Plus Tablets 512
Bellergal-S Tablets 2250
Donnatal 2060
Donnatal Extentabs 2061
Donnatal Tablets 2060
Phenobarbital Elixir and Tablets 1469
Quadrinal Tablets 1350

Procarbazine Hydrochloride (Concurrent use may require reduction in dose of Cytoxan as well as that of other cytotoxic drugs). Products include:
Matulane Capsules 2131

Propofol (Anesthesiologist should be alerted if patient has been treated with cyclophosphamide within 10 days). Products include:
Diprivan Injection 2833

Succinylcholine Chloride (Inhibition of cholinesterase activity and potentiation of succinylcholine chloride's effect). Products include:
Anectine 1073

Tamoxifen Citrate (Concurrent use may require reduction in dose of Cytoxan as well as that of other cytotoxic drugs). Products include:
Nolvadex Tablets 2841

Vincristine Sulfate (Concurrent use may require reduction in dose of Cytoxan as well as that of other cytotoxic drugs). Products include:
Oncovin Solution Vials & Hyporets 1466

CYTOXAN TABLETS

(Cyclophosphamide) 694
See **Cytoxan for Injection**

D.A. CHEWABLE TABLETS

(Chlorpheniramine Maleate, Phenylephrine Hydrochloride, Methscopolamine Nitrate) 951
May interact with monoamine oxidase inhibitors, beta blockers, hypnotics and sedatives, tricyclic antidepressants, barbiturates, central nervous system depressants, tranquilizers, and certain other agents. Compounds in these categories include:

Acebutolol Hydrochloride (Increases the effects of sympathomimetics). Products include:
Sectral Capsules 2807

Alfentanil Hydrochloride (Potential for additive effects). Products include:
Alfenta Injection 1286

219 Interactions Index D.A. Chewable

Alprazolam (Potential for additive effects). Products include:
Xanax Tablets 2649

Amitriptyline Hydrochloride (Potential for additive effects). Products include:
Elavil 2838
Endep Tablets 2174
Etrafon 2355
Limbitrol 2180
Triavil Tablets 1757

Amoxapine (Potential for additive effects). Products include:
Asendin Tablets 1369

Aprobarbital (Potential for additive effects).
No products indexed under this heading.

Atenolol (Increases the effects of sympathomimetics). Products include:
Tenoretic Tablets 2845
Tenormin Tablets and I.V. Injection 2847

Betaxolol Hydrochloride (Increases the effects of sympathomimetics). Products include:
Betoptic Ophthalmic Solution 469
Betoptic S Ophthalmic Suspension 471
Kerlone Tablets 2436

Bisoprolol Fumarate (Increases the effects of sympathomimetics). Products include:
Zebeta Tablets 1413
Ziac 1415

Buprenorphine (Potential for additive effects). Products include:
Buprenex Injectable 2006

Buspirone Hydrochloride (Potential for additive effects). Products include:
BuSpar 737

Butabarbital (Potential for additive effects).
No products indexed under this heading.

Butalbital (Potential for additive effects). Products include:
Esgic-plus Tablets 1013
Fioricet Tablets 2258
Fioricet with Codeine Capsules 2260
Fiorinal Capsules 2261
Fiorinal with Codeine Capsules 2262
Fiorinal Tablets 2261
Phrenilin 785
Sedapap Tablets 50 mg/650 mg 1543

Carteolol Hydrochloride (Increases the effects of sympathomimetics). Products include:
Cartrol Tablets 410
Ocupress Ophthalmic Solution, 1% Sterile ⊙ 309

Chlordiazepoxide (Potential for additive effects). Products include:
Libritabs Tablets 2177
Limbitrol 2180

Chlordiazepoxide Hydrochloride (Potential for additive effects). Products include:
Librax Capsules 2176
Librium Capsules 2178
Librium Injectable 2179

Chlorpromazine (Potential for additive effects). Products include:
Thorazine Suppositories 2523

Chlorpromazine Hydrochloride (Potential for additive effects). Products include:
Thorazine 2523

Chlorprothixene (Potential for additive effects).
No products indexed under this heading.

Chlorprothixene Hydrochloride (Potential for additive effects).
No products indexed under this heading.

Clomipramine Hydrochloride (Potential for additive effects). Products include:
Anafranil Capsules 803

Clorazepate Dipotassium (Potential for additive effects). Products include:
Tranxene 451

Clozapine (Potential for additive effects). Products include:
Clozaril Tablets 2252

Codeine Phosphate (Potential for additive effects). Products include:
Actifed with Codeine Cough Syrup 1067
Brontex 1981
Deconsal C Expectorant Syrup 456
Deconsal Pediatric Syrup 457
Dimetane-DC Cough Syrup 2059
Empirin with Codeine Tablets 1093
Fioricet with Codeine Capsules 2260
Fiorinal with Codeine Capsules 2262
Isoclor Expectorant 990
Novahistine DH 2462
Novahistine Expectorant 2463
Nucofed 2051
Phenergan with Codeine 2777
Phenergan VC with Codeine 2781
Robitussin A-C Syrup 2073
Robitussin-DAC Syrup 2074
Ryna ▣ 841
Soma Compound w/Codeine Tablets 2676
Tussi-Organidin NR Liquid and S NR Liquid 2677
Tylenol with Codeine 1583

Desflurane (Potential for additive effects). Products include:
Suprane 1813

Desipramine Hydrochloride (Potential for additive effects). Products include:
Norpramin Tablets 1526

Dezocine (Potential for additive effects). Products include:
Dalgan Injection 538

Diazepam (Potential for additive effects). Products include:
Dizac 1809
Valium Injectable 2182
Valium Tablets 2183
Valrelease Capsules 2169

Doxepin Hydrochloride (Potential for additive effects). Products include:
Sinequan 2205
Zonalon Cream 1055

Droperidol (Potential for additive effects). Products include:
Inapsine Injection 1296

Enflurane (Potential for additive effects).
No products indexed under this heading.

Esmolol Hydrochloride (Increases the effects of sympathomimetics). Products include:
Brevibloc Injection 1808

Estazolam (Potential for additive effects). Products include:
ProSom Tablets 449

Ethchlorvynol (Potential for additive effects). Products include:
Placidyl Capsules 448

Ethinamate (Potential for additive effects).
No products indexed under this heading.

Fentanyl (Potential for additive effects). Products include:
Duragesic Transdermal System 1288

Fentanyl Citrate (Potential for additive effects). Products include:
Sublimaze Injection 1307

Fluphenazine Decanoate (Potential for additive effects). Products include:
Prolixin Decanoate 509

Fluphenazine Enanthate (Potential for additive effects). Products include:
Prolixin Enanthate 509

Fluphenazine Hydrochloride (Potential for additive effects). Products include:
Prolixin 509

Flurazepam Hydrochloride (Potential for additive effects). Products include:
Dalmane Capsules 2173

Furazolidone (Increases the effects of sympathomimetics; concurrent and/or sequential use is contraindicated). Products include:
Furoxone 2046

Glutethimide (Potential for additive effects).
No products indexed under this heading.

Haloperidol (Potential for additive effects). Products include:
Haldol Injection, Tablets and Concentrate 1575

Haloperidol Decanoate (Potential for additive effects). Products include:
Haldol Decanoate 1577

Hydrocodone Bitartrate (Potential for additive effects). Products include:
Anexsia 5/500 Elixir 1781
Anexia Tablets 1782
Codiclear DH Syrup 791
Deconamine CX Cough and Cold Liquid and Tablets 1319
Duratuss HD Elixir 2565
Hycodan Tablets and Syrup 930
Hycomine Compound Tablets 932
Hycomine 931
Hycotuss Expectorant Syrup 933
Hydrocet Capsules 782
Lorcet 10/650 1018
Lortab 2566
Tussend 1783
Tussend Expectorant 1785
Vicodin Tablets 1356
Vicodin ES Tablets 1357
Vicodin Tuss Expectorant 1358
Zydone Capsules 949

Hydrocodone Polistirex (Potential for additive effects). Products include:
Tussionex Pennkinetic Extended-Release Suspension 998

Hydroxyzine Hydrochloride (Potential for additive effects). Products include:
Atarax Tablets & Syrup 2185
Marax Tablets & DF Syrup 2200
Vistaril Intramuscular Solution 2216

Imipramine Hydrochloride (Potential for additive effects). Products include:
Tofranil Ampuls 854
Tofranil Tablets 856

Imipramine Pamoate (Potential for additive effects). Products include:
Tofranil-PM Capsules 857

Isocarboxazid (Increases the effects of sympathomimetics; concurrent and/or sequential use is contraindicated).
No products indexed under this heading.

Isoflurane (Potential for additive effects).
No products indexed under this heading.

Ketamine Hydrochloride (Potential for additive effects).
No products indexed under this heading.

Labetalol Hydrochloride (Increases the effects of sympathomimetics). Products include:
Normodyne Injection 2377
Normodyne Tablets 2379
Trandate 1185

Levobunolol Hydrochloride (Increases the effects of sympathomimetics). Products include:
Betagan ⊙ 233

Levorphanol Tartrate (Potential for additive effects). Products include:
Levo-Dromoran 2129

Lorazepam (Potential for additive effects). Products include:
Ativan Injection 2698
Ativan Tablets 2700

Loxapine Hydrochloride (Potential for additive effects). Products include:
Loxitane 1378

Loxapine Succinate (Potential for additive effects). Products include:
Loxitane Capsules 1378

Maprotiline Hydrochloride (Potential for additive effects). Products include:
Ludiomil Tablets 843

Mecamylamine Hydrochloride (Sympathomimetic may reduce the antihypertensive effects). Products include:
Inversine Tablets 1686

Meperidine Hydrochloride (Potential for additive effects). Products include:
Demerol 2308
Mepergan Injection 2753

Mephobarbital (Potential for additive effects). Products include:
Mebaral Tablets 2322

Meprobamate (Potential for additive effects). Products include:
Miltown Tablets 2672
PMB 200 and PMB 400 2783

Mesoridazine Besylate (Potential for additive effects). Products include:
Serentil 684

Methadone Hydrochloride (Potential for additive effects). Products include:
Methadone Hydrochloride Oral Concentrate 2233
Methadone Hydrochloride Oral Solution & Tablets 2235

Methohexital Sodium (Potential for additive effects). Products include:
Brevital Sodium Vials 1429

Methotrimeprazine (Potential for additive effects). Products include:
Levoprome 1274

Methoxyflurane (Potential for additive effects).
No products indexed under this heading.

Methyldopa (Sympathomimetic may reduce the antihypertensive effects). Products include:
Aldoclor Tablets 1598
Aldomet Oral 1600
Aldoril Tablets 1604

Methyldopate Hydrochloride (Sympathomimetic may reduce the antihypertensive effects). Products include:
Aldomet Ester HCl Injection 1602

Metipranolol Hydrochloride (Increases the effects of sympathomimetics). Products include:
OptiPranolol (Metipranolol 0.3%) Sterile Ophthalmic Solution ⊙ 258

Metoprolol Succinate (Increases the effects of sympathomimetics). Products include:
Toprol-XL Tablets 565

Metoprolol Tartrate (Increases the effects of sympathomimetics). Products include:
Lopressor Ampuls 830
Lopressor HCT Tablets 832
Lopressor Tablets 830

Midazolam Hydrochloride (Potential for additive effects). Products include:
Versed Injection 2170

IMPORTANT NOTE: Always consult each drug listing in the patient's regimen for possible interactions.

D.A. Chewable Interactions Index 220

Molindone Hydrochloride (Potential for additive effects). Products include:
Moban Tablets and Concentrate...... 1048

Morphine Sulfate (Potential for additive effects). Products include:
Astramorph/PF Injection, USP (Preservative-Free)........ 535
Duramorph........ 962
Infumorph 200 and Infumorph 500 Sterile Solutions........ 965
MS Contin Tablets........ 1994
MSIR........ 1997
Oramorph SR (Morphine Sulfate Sustained Release Tablets)........ 2236
RMS Suppositories........ 2657
Roxanol........ 2243

Nadolol (Increases the effects of sympathomimetics).
No products indexed under this heading.

Nortriptyline Hydrochloride (Potential for additive effects). Products include:
Pamelor........ 2280

Opium Alkaloids (Potential for additive effects).
No products indexed under this heading.

Oxazepam (Potential for additive effects). Products include:
Serax Capsules........ 2810
Serax Tablets........ 2810

Oxycodone Hydrochloride (Potential for additive effects). Products include:
Percocet Tablets........ 938
Percodan Tablets........ 939
Percodan-Demi Tablets........ 940
Roxicodone Tablets, Oral Solution & Intensol (Oxycodone)........ 2244
Tylox Capsules........ 1584

Penbutolol Sulfate (Increases the effects of sympathomimetics). Products include:
Levatol........ 2403

Pentobarbital Sodium (Potential for additive effects). Products include:
Nembutal Sodium Capsules........ 436
Nembutal Sodium Solution........ 438
Nembutal Sodium Suppositories...... 440

Perphenazine (Potential for additive effects). Products include:
Etrafon........ 2355
Triavil Tablets........ 1757
Trilafon........ 2389

Phenelzine Sulfate (Increases the effects of sympathomimetics; concurrent and/or sequential use is contraindicated). Products include:
Nardil........ 1920

Phenobarbital (Potential for additive effects). Products include:
Arco-Lase Plus Tablets........ 512
Bellergal-S Tablets........ 2250
Donnatal........ 2060
Donnatal Extentabs........ 2061
Donnatal Tablets........ 2060
Phenobarbital Elixir and Tablets...... 1469
Quadrinal Tablets........ 1350

Pindolol (Increases the effects of sympathomimetics). Products include:
Visken Tablets........ 2299

Prazepam (Potential for additive effects).
No products indexed under this heading.

Prochlorperazine (Potential for additive effects). Products include:
Compazine........ 2470

Promethazine Hydrochloride (Potential for additive effects). Products include:
Mepergan Injection........ 2753
Phenergan with Codeine........ 2777
Phenergan with Dextromethorphan 2778
Phenergan Injection........ 2773
Phenergan Suppositories........ 2775
Phenergan Syrup........ 2774
Phenergan Tablets........ 2775
Phenergan VC........ 2779
Phenergan VC with Codeine........ 2781

Propofol (Potential for additive effects). Products include:
Diprivan Injection........ 2833

Propoxyphene Hydrochloride (Potential for additive effects). Products include:
Darvon........ 1435
Wygesic Tablets........ 2827

Propoxyphene Napsylate (Potential for additive effects). Products include:
Darvon-N/Darvocet-N........ 1433

Propranolol Hydrochloride (Increases the effects of sympathomimetics). Products include:
Inderal........ 2728
Inderal LA Long Acting Capsules 2730
Inderide Tablets........ 2732
Inderide LA Long Acting Capsules .. 2734

Protriptyline Hydrochloride (Potential for additive effects). Products include:
Vivactil Tablets........ 1774

Quazepam (Potential for additive effects). Products include:
Doral Tablets........ 2664

Reserpine (Sympathomimetic may reduce the antihypertensive effects). Products include:
Diupres Tablets........ 1650
Hydropres Tablets........ 1675
Ser-Ap-Es Tablets........ 849

Risperidone (Potential for additive effects). Products include:
Risperdal........ 1301

Secobarbital Sodium (Potential for additive effects). Products include:
Seconal Sodium Pulvules........ 1474

Selegiline Hydrochloride (Increases the effects of sympathomimetics; concurrent and/or sequential use is contraindicated). Products include:
Eldepryl Tablets........ 2550

Sotalol Hydrochloride (Increases the effects of sympathomimetics). Products include:
Betapace Tablets........ 641

Sufentanil Citrate (Potential for additive effects). Products include:
Sufenta Injection........ 1309

Temazepam (Potential for additive effects). Products include:
Restoril Capsules........ 2284

Thiamylal Sodium (Potential for additive effects).
No products indexed under this heading.

Thioridazine Hydrochloride (Potential for additive effects). Products include:
Mellaril........ 2269

Thiothixene (Potential for additive effects). Products include:
Navane Capsules and Concentrate 2201
Navane Intramuscular........ 2202

Timolol Maleate (Increases the effects of sympathomimetics). Products include:
Blocadren Tablets........ 1614
Timolide Tablets........ 1748
Timoptic in Ocudose........ 1753
Timoptic Sterile Ophthalmic Solution........ 1751
Timoptic-XE........ 1755

Tranylcypromine Sulfate (Increases the effects of sympathomimetics; concurrent and/or sequential use is contraindicated). Products include:
Parnate Tablets........ 2503

Triazolam (Potential for additive effects). Products include:
Halcion Tablets........ 2611

Trifluoperazine Hydrochloride (Potential for additive effects). Products include:
Stelazine........ 2514

Trimipramine Maleate (Potential for additive effects). Products include:
Surmontil Capsules........ 2811

Zolpidem Tartrate (Potential for additive effects). Products include:
Ambien Tablets........ 2416

Food Interactions

Alcohol (Potential for additive effects).

DDAVP INJECTION
(Desmopressin Acetate)........2014
May interact with vasopressors. Compounds in this category include:

Dopamine Hydrochloride (Possible additive effects; use only with careful monitoring).
No products indexed under this heading.

Epinephrine Hydrochloride (Possible additive effects; use only with careful monitoring). Products include:
Ana-Kit Anaphylaxis Emergency Treatment Kit........ 617

Metaraminol Bitartrate (Possible additive effects; use only with careful monitoring). Products include:
Aramine Injection........ 1609

Methoxamine Hydrochloride (Possible additive effects; use only with careful monitoring). Products include:
Vasoxyl Injection........ 1196

Norepinephrine Bitartrate (Possible additive effects; use only with careful monitoring). Products include:
Levophed Bitartrate Injection........ 2315

Phenylephrine Hydrochloride (Possible additive effects; use only with careful monitoring). Products include:
Atrohist Plus Tablets........ 454
Cerose DM........ ▣ 878
Comhist........ 2038
D.A. Chewable Tablets........ 951
Deconsal Pediatric Capsules........ 454
Dura-Vent/DA Tablets........ 953
Entex Capsules........ 1986
Entex Liquid........ 1986
Extendryl........ 1005
4-Way Fast Acting Nasal Spray (regular & mentholated)........ ▣ 621
Hemorid For Women........ ▣ 834
Hycomine Compound Tablets........ 932
Neo-Synephrine Hydrochloride 1% Carpuject........ 2324
Neo-Synephrine Hydrochloride 1% Injection........ 2324
Neo-Synephrine Hydrochloride (Ophthalmic)........ 2325
Neo-Synephrine........ ▣ 726
Nōstril........ ▣ 644
Novahistine Elixir........ ▣ 823
Phenergan VC........ 2779
Phenergan VC with Codeine........ 2781
Preparation H........ ▣ 871
Tympagesic Ear Drops........ 2342
Vasosulf........ ⊙ 271
Vicks Sinex Nasal Spray and Ultra Fine Mist........ ▣ 765

DDAVP INJECTION 15 MCG/ML
(Desmopressin Acetate)........2015
May interact with vasopressors. Compounds in this category include:

Dopamine Hydrochloride (Use of doses as large as 0.3ug/kg of DDAVP with other vasopressor agents should be done only with careful patient monitoring).
No products indexed under this heading.

Epinephrine Bitartrate (Use of doses as large as 0.3ug/kg of DDAVP with other vasopressor agents should be done only with careful patient monitoring). Products include:
Bronkaid Mist Suspension........ ▣ 718
Sensorcaine-MPF with Epinephrine Injection........ 559

Epinephrine Hydrochloride (Use of doses as large as 0.3ug/kg of DDAVP with other vasopressor agents should be done only with careful patient monitoring). Products include:
Ana-Kit Anaphylaxis Emergency Treatment Kit........ 617

Metaraminol Bitartrate (Use of doses as large as 0.3ug/kg of DDAVP with other vasopressor agents should be done only with careful patient monitoring). Products include:
Aramine Injection........ 1609

Methoxamine Hydrochloride (Use of doses as large as 0.3ug/kg of DDAVP with other vasopressor agents should be done only with careful patient monitoring). Products include:
Vasoxyl Injection........ 1196

Norepinephrine Bitartrate (Use of doses as large as 0.3ug/kg of DDAVP with other vasopressor agents should be done only with careful patient monitoring). Products include:
Levophed Bitartrate Injection........ 2315

Phenylephrine Hydrochloride (Use of doses as large as 0.3ug/kg of DDAVP with other vasopressor agents should be done only with careful patient monitoring). Products include:
Atrohist Plus Tablets........ 454
Cerose DM........ ▣ 878
Comhist........ 2038
D.A. Chewable Tablets........ 951
Deconsal Pediatric Capsules........ 454
Dura-Vent/DA Tablets........ 953
Entex Capsules........ 1986
Entex Liquid........ 1986
Extendryl........ 1005
4-Way Fast Acting Nasal Spray (regular & mentholated)........ ▣ 621
Hemorid For Women........ ▣ 834
Hycomine Compound Tablets........ 932
Neo-Synephrine Hydrochloride 1% Carpuject........ 2324
Neo-Synephrine Hydrochloride 1% Injection........ 2324
Neo-Synephrine Hydrochloride (Ophthalmic)........ 2325
Neo-Synephrine........ ▣ 726
Nōstril........ ▣ 644
Novahistine Elixir........ ▣ 823
Phenergan VC........ 2779
Phenergan VC with Codeine........ 2781
Preparation H........ ▣ 871
Tympagesic Ear Drops........ 2342
Vasosulf........ ⊙ 271
Vicks Sinex Nasal Spray and Ultra Fine Mist........ ▣ 765

DDAVP NASAL SPRAY
(Desmopressin Acetate)........2017
See **DDAVP Rhinal Tube**

DDAVP RHINAL TUBE
(Desmopressin Acetate)........2017
May interact with vasopressors. Compounds in this category include:

Dopamine Hydrochloride (Possible additive effects; use only with careful monitoring).
No products indexed under this heading.

(▣ Described in PDR For Nonprescription Drugs) (⊙ Described in PDR For Ophthalmology)

Epinephrine Hydrochloride (Possible additive effects; use only with careful monitoring). Products include:
- Ana-Kit Anaphylaxis Emergency Treatment Kit 617

Metaraminol Bitartrate (Possible additive effects; use only with careful monitoring). Products include:
- Aramine Injection 1609

Methoxamine Hydrochloride (Possible additive effects; use only with careful monitoring). Products include:
- Vasoxyl Injection 1196

Norepinephrine Bitartrate (Possible additive effects; use only with careful monitoring). Products include:
- Levophed Bitartrate Injection 2315

Phenylephrine Hydrochloride (Possible additive effects; use only with careful monitoring). Products include:
- Atrohist Plus Tablets 454
- Cerose DM .... ▣ 878
- Comhist 2038
- D.A. Chewable Tablets 951
- Deconsal Pediatric Capsules 454
- Dura-Vent/DA Tablets 953
- Entex Capsules 1986
- Entex Liquid 1986
- Extendryl 1005
- 4-Way Fast Acting Nasal Spray (regular & mentholated) .... ▣ 621
- Hemorid For Women .... ▣ 834
- Hycomine Compound Tablets 932
- Neo-Synephrine Hydrochloride 1% Carpuject 2324
- Neo-Synephrine Hydrochloride 1% Injection 2324
- Neo-Synephrine Hydrochloride (Ophthalmic) 2325
- Neo-Synephrine .... ▣ 726
- Nōstril .... ▣ 644
- Novahistine Elixir .... ▣ 823
- Phenergan VC 2779
- Phenergan VC with Codeine 2781
- Preparation H .... ▣ 871
- Tympagesic Ear Drops 2342
- Vasosulf .... ⊙ 271
- Vicks Sinex Nasal Spray and Ultra Fine Mist .... ▣ 765

DDS-ACIDOPHILUS

(Lactobacillus Acidophilus) .... ▣ 835

None cited in PDR database.

DHCPLUS CAPSULES

(Dihydrocodeine Bitartrate, Acetaminophen, Caffeine) 1993

May interact with central nervous system depressants, beta-adrenergic stimulating agents, fluoroquinolone antibiotics, and certain other agents. Compounds in these categories include:

Albuterol (Caffeine may enhance the cardiac inotropic effects of beta-adrenergic stimulating agents). Products include:
- Proventil Inhalation Aerosol 2382
- Ventolin Inhalation Aerosol and Refill 1197

Albuterol Sulfate (Caffeine may enhance the cardiac inotropic effects of beta-adrenergic stimulating agents). Products include:
- Airet Solution for Inhalation 452
- Proventil Inhalation Solution 0.083% 2384
- Proventil Repetabs Tablets 2386
- Proventil Solution for Inhalation 0.5% 2383
- Proventil Syrup 2385
- Proventil Tablets 2386
- Ventolin Inhalation Solution 1198
- Ventolin Nebules Inhalation Solution 1199
- Ventolin Rotacaps for Inhalation 1200
- Ventolin Syrup 1202
- Ventolin Tablets 1203
- Volmax Extended-Release Tablets 1788

Alfentanil Hydrochloride (Potential for additive CNS depression). Products include:
- Alfenta Injection 1286

Alprazolam (Potential for additive CNS depression). Products include:
- Xanax Tablets 2649

Aprobarbital (Potential for additive CNS depression).
- No products indexed under this heading.

Aspirin (Caffeine may increase the metabolism of aspirin). Products include:
- Alka-Seltzer Effervescent Antacid and Pain Reliever .... ▣ 701
- Alka-Seltzer Extra Strength Effervescent Antacid and Pain Reliever .... ▣ 703
- Alka-Seltzer Lemon Lime Effervescent Antacid and Pain Reliever .... ▣ 703
- Alka-Seltzer Plus Cold Medicine .... ▣ 705
- Alka-Seltzer Plus Cold & Cough Medicine .... ▣ 708
- Alka-Seltzer Plus Night-Time Cold Medicine .... ▣ 707
- Alka Seltzer Plus Sinus Medicine .... ▣ 707
- Arthritis Foundation Safety Coated Aspirin Tablets .... ▣ 675
- Arthritis Pain Ascriptin .... ▣ 631
- Maximum Strength Ascriptin .... ▣ 630
- Regular Strength Ascriptin Tablets .... ▣ 629
- Arthritis Strength BC Powder .... ▣ 609
- BC Cold Powder Multi-Symptom Formula (Cold-Sinus-Allergy) .... ▣ 609
- BC Cold Powder Non-Drowsy Formula (Cold-Sinus) .... ▣ 609
- BC Powder .... ▣ 609
- Bayer Children's Chewable Aspirin .... ▣ 711
- Genuine Bayer Aspirin Tablets & Caplets .... ▣ 713
- Extra Strength Bayer Arthritis Pain Regimen Formula .... ▣ 711
- Extra Strength Bayer Aspirin Caplets & Tablets .... ▣ 712
- Extended-Release Bayer 8-Hour Aspirin .... ▣ 712
- Extra Strength Bayer Plus Aspirin Caplets .... ▣ 713
- Extra Strength Bayer PM Aspirin .... ▣ 713
- Bayer Enteric Aspirin .... ▣ 709
- Bufferin Analgesic Tablets and Caplets .... ▣ 613
- Arthritis Strength Bufferin Analgesic Caplets .... ▣ 614
- Extra Strength Bufferin Analgesic Tablets .... ▣ 615
- Cama Arthritis Pain Reliever .... ▣ 785
- Darvon Compound-65 Pulvules 1435
- Easprin 1914
- Ecotrin 2455
- Ecotrin Enteric Coated Aspirin Maximum Strength Tablets and Caplets .... ▣ 816
- Ecotrin Enteric Coated Aspirin Regular Strength Tablets 2455
- Empirin Aspirin Tablets .... ▣ 854
- Empirin with Codeine Tablets 1093
- Excedrin Extra-Strength Analgesic Tablets & Caplets 732
- Fiorinal Capsules 2261
- Fiorinal with Codeine Capsules 2262
- Fiorinal Tablets 2261
- Halfprin 1362
- Healthprin Aspirin 2455
- Norgesic 1496
- Percodan Tablets 939
- Percodan-Demi Tablets 940
- Robaxisal Tablets 2071
- Soma Compound w/Codeine Tablets 2676
- Soma Compound Tablets 2675
- St. Joseph Adult Chewable Aspirin (81 mg.) .... ▣ 808
- Talwin Compound 2335
- Ursinus Inlay-Tabs .... ▣ 794
- Vanquish Analgesic Caplets .... ▣ 731

Bitolterol Mesylate (Caffeine may enhance the cardiac inotropic effects of beta-adrenergic stimulating agents). Products include:
- Tornalate Solution for Inhalation, 0.2% 956
- Tornalate Metered Dose Inhaler 957

Buprenorphine (Potential for additive CNS depression). Products include:
- Buprenex Injectable 2006

Buspirone Hydrochloride (Potential for additive CNS depression). Products include:
- BuSpar 737

Butabarbital (Potential for additive CNS depression).
- No products indexed under this heading.

Butalbital (Potential for additive CNS depression). Products include:
- Esgic-plus Tablets 1013
- Fioricet Tablets 2258
- Fioricet with Codeine Capsules 2260
- Fiorinal Capsules 2261
- Fiorinal with Codeine Capsules 2262
- Fiorinal Tablets 2261
- Phrenilin 785
- Sedapap Tablets 50 mg/650 mg 1543

Chlordiazepoxide (Potential for additive CNS depression). Products include:
- Libritabs Tablets 2177
- Limbitrol 2180

Chlordiazepoxide Hydrochloride (Potential for additive CNS depression). Products include:
- Librax Capsules 2176
- Librium Capsules 2178
- Librium Injectable 2179

Chlorpromazine (Potential for additive CNS depression). Products include:
- Thorazine Suppositories 2523

Chlorpromazine Hydrochloride (Potential for additive CNS depression). Products include:
- Thorazine 2523

Chlorprothixene (Potential for additive CNS depression).
- No products indexed under this heading.

Chlorprothixene Hydrochloride (Potential for additive CNS depression).
- No products indexed under this heading.

Ciprofloxacin (Concomitant use may result in caffeine accumulation when DHC Plus is consumed with quinolones). Products include:
- Cipro I.V. 595
- Cipro I.V. Pharmacy Bulk Package 597

Ciprofloxacin Hydrochloride (Concomitant use may result in caffeine accumulation when DHC Plus is consumed with quinolones). Products include:
- Ciloxan Ophthalmic Solution 472
- Cipro Tablets 592

Clorazepate Dipotassium (Potential for additive CNS depression). Products include:
- Tranxene 451

Clozapine (Potential for additive CNS depression). Products include:
- Clozaril Tablets 2252

Codeine Phosphate (Potential for additive CNS depression). Products include:
- Actifed with Codeine Cough Syrup 1067
- Brontex 1981
- Deconsal C Expectorant Syrup 456
- Deconsal Pediatric Syrup 457
- Dimetane-DC Cough Syrup 2059
- Empirin with Codeine Tablets 1093
- Fioricet with Codeine Capsules 2260
- Fiorinal with Codeine Capsules 2262
- Isoclor Expectorant 990
- Novahistine DH 2462
- Novahistine Expectorant 2463
- Nucofed 2051
- Phenergan with Codeine 2777
- Phenergan VC with Codeine 2781
- Robitussin A-C Syrup 2073
- Robitussin-DAC Syrup 2074
- Ryna .... ▣ 841
- Soma Compound w/Codeine Tablets 2676
- Tussi-Organidin NR Liquid and S NR Liquid 2677
- Tylenol with Codeine 1583

Desflurane (Potential for additive CNS depression). Products include:
- Suprane 1813

Dezocine (Potential for additive CNS depression). Products include:
- Dalgan Injection 538

Diazepam (Potential for additive CNS depression). Products include:
- Dizac 1809
- Valium Injectable 2182
- Valium Tablets 2183
- Valrelease Capsules 2169

Disulfiram (Co-administration may lead to a substantial decrease in caffeine clearance). Products include:
- Antabuse Tablets 2695

Droperidol (Potential for additive CNS depression). Products include:
- Inapsine Injection 1296

Enflurane (Potential for additive CNS depression).
- No products indexed under this heading.

Enoxacin (Concomitant use may result in caffeine accumulation when DHC Plus is consumed with quinolones). Products include:
- Penetrex Tablets 2031

Ephedrine Hydrochloride (Caffeine may enhance the cardiac inotropic effects of beta-adrenergic stimulating agents). Products include:
- Primatene Dual Action Formula .... ▣ 872
- Primatene Tablets .... ▣ 873
- Quadrinal Tablets 1350

Ephedrine Sulfate (Caffeine may enhance the cardiac inotropic effects of beta-adrenergic stimulating agents). Products include:
- Bronkaid Caplets .... ▣ 717
- Marax Tablets & DF Syrup 2200

Ephedrine Tannate (Caffeine may enhance the cardiac inotropic effects of beta-adrenergic stimulating agents). Products include:
- Rynatuss 2673

Epinephrine (Caffeine may enhance the cardiac inotropic effects of beta-adrenergic stimulating agents). Products include:
- Bronkaid Mist .... ▣ 717
- EPIFRIN .... ⊙ 239
- EpiPen 790
- Marcaine Hydrochloride with Epinephrine 1:200,000 2316
- Primatene Mist .... ▣ 873
- Sensorcaine with Epinephrine Injection 559
- Sus-Phrine Injection 1019
- Xylocaine with Epinephrine Injections 567

Epinephrine Hydrochloride (Caffeine may enhance the cardiac inotropic effects of beta-adrenergic stimulating agents). Products include:
- Ana-Kit Anaphylaxis Emergency Treatment Kit 617

Estazolam (Potential for additive CNS depression). Products include:
- ProSom Tablets 449

Ethchlorvynol (Potential for additive CNS depression). Products include:
- Placidyl Capsules 448

Ethinamate (Potential for additive CNS depression).
- No products indexed under this heading.

IMPORTANT NOTE: Always consult each drug listing in the patient's regimen for possible interactions.

DHC Plus Interactions Index 222

Ethylnorepinephrine Hydrochloride (Caffeine may enhance the cardiac inotropic effects of beta-adrenergic stimulating agents).
No products indexed under this heading.

Fentanyl (Potential for additive CNS depression). Products include:
Duragesic Transdermal System........ 1288

Fentanyl Citrate (Potential for additive CNS depression). Products include:
Sublimaze Injection........ 1307

Fluphenazine Decanoate (Potential for additive CNS depression). Products include:
Prolixin Decanoate........ 509

Fluphenazine Enanthate (Potential for additive CNS depression). Products include:
Prolixin Enanthate........ 509

Fluphenazine Hydrochloride (Potential for additive CNS depression). Products include:
Prolixin........ 509

Flurazepam Hydrochloride (Potential for additive CNS depression). Products include:
Dalmane Capsules........ 2173

Glutethimide (Potential for additive CNS depression).
No products indexed under this heading.

Haloperidol (Potential for additive CNS depression). Products include:
Haldol Injection, Tablets and Concentrate........ 1575

Haloperidol Decanoate (Potential for additive CNS depression). Products include:
Haldol Decanoate........ 1577

Hydrocodone Bitartrate (Potential for additive CNS depression). Products include:
Anexsia 5/500 Elixir........ 1781
Anexia Tablets........ 1782
Codiclear DH Syrup........ 791
Deconamine CX Cough and Cold Liquid and Tablets........ 1319
Duratuss HD Elixir........ 2565
Hycodan Tablets and Syrup........ 930
Hycomine Compound Tablets........ 932
Hycomine........ 931
Hycotuss Expectorant Syrup........ 933
Hydrocet Capsules........ 782
Lorcet 10/650........ 1018
Lortab........ 2566
Tussend........ 1783
Tussend Expectorant........ 1785
Vicodin Tablets........ 1356
Vicodin ES Tablets........ 1357
Vicodin Tuss Expectorant........ 1358
Zydone Capsules........ 949

Hydrocodone Polistirex (Potential for additive CNS depression). Products include:
Tussionex Pennkinetic Extended-Release Suspension........ 998

Hydroxyzine Hydrochloride (Potential for additive CNS depression). Products include:
Atarax Tablets & Syrup........ 2185
Marax Tablets & DF Syrup........ 2200
Vistaril Intramuscular Solution........ 2216

Isoetharine (Caffeine may enhance the cardiac inotropic effects of beta-adrenergic stimulating agents). Products include:
Bronkometer Aerosol........ 2302
Bronkosol Solution........ 2302
Isoetharine Inhalation Solution, USP, Arm-a-Med........ 551

Isoflurane (Potential for additive CNS depression).
No products indexed under this heading.

Isoproterenol Hydrochloride (Caffeine may enhance the cardiac inotropic effects of beta-adrenergic stimulating agents). Products include:
Isuprel Hydrochloride Injection 1:5000........ 2311
Isuprel Hydrochloride Solution 1:200 & 1:100........ 2313
Isuprel Mistometer........ 2312

Isoproterenol Sulfate (Caffeine may enhance the cardiac inotropic effects of beta-adrenergic stimulating agents). Products include:
Norisodrine with Calcium Iodide Syrup........ 442

Ketamine Hydrochloride (Potential for additive CNS depression).
No products indexed under this heading.

Levomethadyl Acetate Hydrochloride (Potential for additive CNS depression). Products include:
Orlamm........ 2239

Levorphanol Tartrate (Potential for additive CNS depression). Products include:
Levo-Dromoran........ 2129

Lomefloxacin Hydrochloride (Concomitant use may result in caffeine accumulation when DHC Plus is consumed with quinolones). Products include:
Maxaquin Tablets........ 2440

Lorazepam (Potential for additive CNS depression). Products include:
Ativan Injection........ 2698
Ativan Tablets........ 2700

Loxapine Hydrochloride (Potential for additive CNS depression). Products include:
Loxitane........ 1378

Loxapine Succinate (Potential for additive CNS depression). Products include:
Loxitane Capsules........ 1378

Meperidine Hydrochloride (Potential for additive CNS depression). Products include:
Demerol........ 2308
Mepergan Injection........ 2753

Mephobarbital (Potential for additive CNS depression). Products include:
Mebaral Tablets........ 2322

Meprobamate (Potential for additive CNS depression). Products include:
Miltown Tablets........ 2672
PMB 200 and PMB 400........ 2783

Mesoridazine (Potential for additive CNS depression).

Metaproterenol Sulfate (Caffeine may enhance the cardiac inotropic effects of beta-adrenergic stimulating agents). Products include:
Alupent........ 669
Metaproterenol Sulfate Inhalation Solution, USP, Arm-a-Med........ 552

Methadone Hydrochloride (Potential for additive CNS depression). Products include:
Methadone Hydrochloride Oral Concentrate........ 2233
Methadone Hydrochloride Oral Solution & Tablets........ 2235

Methohexital Sodium (Potential for additive CNS depression). Products include:
Brevital Sodium Vials........ 1429

Methotrimeprazine (Potential for additive CNS depression). Products include:
Levoprome........ 1274

Methoxyflurane (Potential for additive CNS depression).
No products indexed under this heading.

Midazolam Hydrochloride (Potential for additive CNS depression). Products include:
Versed Injection........ 2170

Molindone Hydrochloride (Potential for additive CNS depression). Products include:
Moban Tablets and Concentrate........ 1048

Morphine Sulfate (Potential for additive CNS depression). Products include:
Astramorph/PF Injection, USP (Preservative-Free)........ 535
Duramorph........ 962
Infumorph 200 and Infumorph 500 Sterile Solutions........ 965
MS Contin Tablets........ 1994
MSIR........ 1997
Oramorph SR (Morphine Sulfate Sustained Release Tablets)........ 2236
RMS Suppositories........ 2657
Roxanol........ 2243

Norfloxacin (Concomitant use may result in caffeine accumulation when DHC Plus is consumed with quinolones). Products include:
Chibroxin Sterile Ophthalmic Solution........ 1617
Noroxin Tablets........ 1715
Noroxin Tablets........ 2048

Ofloxacin (Concomitant use may result in caffeine accumulation when DHC Plus is consumed with quinolones). Products include:
Floxin I.V........ 1571
Floxin Tablets (200 mg, 300 mg, 400 mg)........ 1567
Ocuflox........ 481
Ocuflox........ ⊙ 246

Opium Alkaloids (Potential for additive CNS depression).
No products indexed under this heading.

Oxazepam (Potential for additive CNS depression). Products include:
Serax Capsules........ 2810
Serax Tablets........ 2810

Oxycodone Hydrochloride (Potential for additive CNS depression). Products include:
Percocet Tablets........ 938
Percodan Tablets........ 939
Percodan-Demi Tablets........ 940
Roxicodone Tablets, Oral Solution & Intensol (Oxycodone)........ 2244
Tylox Capsules........ 1584

Pentobarbital Sodium (Potential for additive CNS depression). Products include:
Nembutal Sodium Capsules........ 436
Nembutal Sodium Solution........ 438
Nembutal Sodium Suppositories........ 440

Perphenazine (Potential for additive CNS depression). Products include:
Etrafon........ 2355
Triavil Tablets........ 1757
Trilafon........ 2389

Phenobarbital (Potential for additive CNS depression; caffeine may increase the metabolism of phenobarbital). Products include:
Arco-Lase Plus Tablets........ 512
Bellergal-S Tablets........ 2250
Donnatal........ 2060
Donnatal Extentabs........ 2061
Donnatal Tablets........ 2060
Phenobarbital Elixir and Tablets........ 1469
Quadrinal Tablets........ 1350

Pirbuterol Acetate (Caffeine may enhance the cardiac inotropic effects of beta-adrenergic stimulating agents). Products include:
Maxair Autohaler........ 1492
Maxair Inhaler........ 1494

Prazepam (Potential for additive CNS depression).
No products indexed under this heading.

Prochlorperazine (Potential for additive CNS depression). Products include:
Compazine........ 2470

Promethazine Hydrochloride (Potential for additive CNS depression). Products include:
Mepergan Injection........ 2753
Phenergan with Codeine........ 2777
Phenergan with Dextromethorphan 2778
Phenergan Injection........ 2773
Phenergan Suppositories........ 2775
Phenergan Syrup........ 2774
Phenergan Tablets........ 2775
Phenergan VC........ 2779
Phenergan VC with Codeine........ 2781

Propofol (Potential for additive CNS depression). Products include:
Diprivan Injection........ 2833

Propoxyphene Hydrochloride (Potential for additive CNS depression). Products include:
Darvon........ 1435
Wygesic Tablets........ 2827

Propoxyphene Napsylate (Potential for additive CNS depression). Products include:
Darvon-N/Darvocet-N........ 1433

Quazepam (Potential for additive CNS depression). Products include:
Doral Tablets........ 2664

Risperidone (Potential for additive CNS depression). Products include:
Risperdal........ 1301

Salmeterol Xinafoate (Caffeine may enhance the cardiac inotropic effects of beta-adrenergic stimulating agents). Products include:
Serevent Inhalation Aerosol........ 1176

Secobarbital Sodium (Potential for additive CNS depression). Products include:
Seconal Sodium Pulvules........ 1474

Sufentanil Citrate (Potential for additive CNS depression). Products include:
Sufenta Injection........ 1309

Temafloxacin Hydrochloride (Concomitant use may result in caffeine accumulation when DHC Plus is consumed with quinolones).
No products indexed under this heading.

Temazepam (Potential for additive CNS depression). Products include:
Restoril Capsules........ 2284

Terbutaline Sulfate (Caffeine may enhance the cardiac inotropic effects of beta-adrenergic stimulating agents). Products include:
Brethaire Inhaler........ 813
Brethine Ampuls........ 815
Brethine Tablets........ 814
Bricanyl Subcutaneous Injection........ 1502
Bricanyl Tablets........ 1503

Thiamylal Sodium (Potential for additive CNS depression).
No products indexed under this heading.

Thioridazine Hydrochloride (Potential for additive CNS depression). Products include:
Mellaril........ 2269

Thiothixene (Potential for additive CNS depression). Products include:
Navane Capsules and Concentrate 2201
Navane Intramuscular........ 2202

Triazolam (Potential for additive CNS depression). Products include:
Halcion Tablets........ 2611

Trifluoperazine Hydrochloride (Potential for additive CNS depression). Products include:
Stelazine........ 2514

Zolpidem Tartrate (Potential for additive CNS depression). Products include:

Ambien Tablets....................................... 2416

Food Interactions

Alcohol (Potential for additive CNS depression).

Food, caffeine containing (Concomitant use may result in caffeine accumulation when DHC Plus is consumed with caffeine-containing foods).

D.H.E. 45 INJECTION

(Dihydroergotamine Mesylate)............2255 May interact with vasopressors, macrolide antibiotics, and certain other agents. Compounds in these categories include:

Azithromycin (Potential for increased plasma levels of unchanged alkaloids and peripheral vasoconstriction; vasospastic reactions may result from concurrent use). Products include:

Zithromax 1944

Clarithromycin (Potential for increased plasma levels of unchanged alkaloids and peripheral vasoconstriction; vasospastic reactions may result from concurrent use). Products include:

Biaxin 405

Dopamine Hydrochloride (Concurrent administration may cause extreme elevation of blood pressure).

No products indexed under this heading.

Epinephrine Bitartrate (Concurrent administration may cause extreme elevation of blood pressure). Products include:

Bronkaid Mist Suspension .... ⊕ 718

Sensorcaine-MPF with Epinephrine Injection 559

Epinephrine Hydrochloride (Concurrent administration may cause extreme elevation of blood pressure). Products include:

Ana-Kit Anaphylaxis Emergency Treatment Kit 617

Erythromycin (Potential for increased plasma levels of unchanged alkaloids and peripheral vasoconstriction; vasospastic reactions may result from concurrent use). Products include:

A/T/S 2% Acne Topical Gel and Solution .... 1234 Benzamycin Topical Gel .... 905 E-Mycin Tablets .... 1341 Emgel 2% Topical Gel.......................... 1093 ERYC .... 1915 Erycette (erythromycin 2%) Topical Solution... 1888 Ery-Tab Tablets .... 422 Erythromycin Base Filmtab .... 426 Erythromycin Delayed-Release Capsules, USP.................................... 427 Ilotycin Ophthalmic Ointment........... 912 PCE Dispertab Tablets .... 444 T-Stat 2.0% Topical Solution and Pads .... 2688 Theramycin Z Topical Solution 2% 1592

Erythromycin Estolate (Potential for increased plasma levels of unchanged alkaloids and peripheral vasoconstriction; vasospastic reactions may result from concurrent use). Products include:

Ilosone 911

Erythromycin Ethylsuccinate (Potential for increased plasma levels of unchanged alkaloids and peripheral vasoconstriction; vasospastic reactions may result from concurrent use). Products include:

E.E.S.. 424 EryPed 421

Erythromycin Gluceptate (Potential for increased plasma levels of unchanged alkaloids and peripheral vasoconstriction; vasospastic reactions may result from concurrent use). Products include:

Ilotycin Gluceptate, IV, Vials 913

Erythromycin Stearate (Potential for increased plasma levels of unchanged alkaloids and peripheral vasoconstriction; vasospastic reactions may result from concurrent use). Products include:

Erythrocin Stearate Filmtab 425

Metaraminol Bitartrate (Concurrent administration may cause extreme elevation of blood pressure). Products include:

Aramine Injection................................... 1609

Methoxamine Hydrochloride (Concurrent administration may cause extreme elevation of blood pressure). Products include:

Vasoxyl Injection 1196

Nicotine (Nicotine may provoke vasoconstriction in some patients, predisposing to a greater ischemic response to ergot therapy). Products include:

Habitrol Nicotine Transdermal System .... 865 Nicoderm (nicotine transdermal system) .... 1518 Nicotrol Nicotine Transdermal System .... 1550 Prostep (nicotine transdermal system) 1394

Nicotine Polacrilex (Nicotine may provoke vasoconstriction in some patients, predisposing to a greater ischemic response to ergot therapy). Products include:

Nicorette 2458

Norepinephrine Bitartrate (Concurrent administration may cause extreme elevation of blood pressure). Products include:

Levophed Bitartrate Injection 2315

Phenylephrine Hydrochloride (Concurrent administration may cause extreme elevation of blood pressure). Products include:

Atrohist Plus Tablets .... 454 Cerose DM .... ⊕ 878 Comhist .... 2038 D.A. Chewable Tablets.......................... 951 Deconsal Pediatric Capsules............... 454 Dura-Vent/DA Tablets .... 953 Entex Capsules .... 1986 Entex Liquid .... 1986 Extendryl .... 1005 4-Way Fast Acting Nasal Spray (regular & mentholated) .... ⊕ 621 Hemorid For Women .... ⊕ 834 Hycomine Compound Tablets .... 932 Neo-Synephrine Hydrochloride 1% Carpuject... 2324 Neo-Synephrine Hydrochloride 1% Injection.. 2324 Neo-Synephrine Hydrochloride (Ophthalmic) .... 2325 Neo-Synephrine .... ⊕ 726 Nōstril .... ⊕ 644 Novahistine Elixir .... ⊕ 823 Phenergan VC .... 2779 Phenergan VC with Codeine .... 2781 Preparation H .... ⊕ 871 Tympagesic Ear Drops .... 2342 Vasosulf .... © 271 Vicks Sinex Nasal Spray and Ultra Fine Mist .... ⊕ 765

Propranolol Hydrochloride (Potentiates the vasoconstrictive action of ergotamine). Products include:

Inderal .... 2728 Inderal LA Long Acting Capsules .... 2730 Inderide Tablets .... 2732 Inderide LA Long Acting Capsules .. 2734

Troleandomycin (Potential for increased plasma levels of unchanged alkaloids and peripheral vasoconstriction; vasospastic reactions may result from concurrent use). Products include:

Tao Capsules 2209

DHS TAR GEL SHAMPOO

(Coal Tar) ....1932 None cited in PDR database.

DHS TAR SHAMPOO

(Coal Tar) ....1932 None cited in PDR database.

DHS ZINC DANDRUFF SHAMPOO

(Pyrithione Zinc) ....1932 None cited in PDR database.

DHT (DIHYDROTACHYSTEROL) TABLETS & INTENSOL

(Dihydrotachysterol) ....2229 May interact with thiazides. Compounds in this category include:

Bendroflumethiazide (May cause hypercalcemia in hypoparathyroid patients).

No products indexed under this heading.

Chlorothiazide (May cause hypercalcemia in hypoparathyroid patients). Products include:

Aldoclor Tablets .... 1598 Diupres Tablets .... 1650 Diuril Oral 1653

Chlorothiazide Sodium (May cause hypercalcemia in hypoparathyroid patients). Products include:

Diuril Sodium Intravenous 1652

Hydrochlorothiazide (May cause hypercalcemia in hypoparathyroid patients). Products include:

Aldactazide.. 2413 Aldoril Tablets .... 1604 Apresazide Capsules .... 808 Capozide .... 742 Dyazide .... 2479 Esidrix Tablets .... 821 Esimil Tablets .... 822 HydroDIURIL Tablets .... 1674 Hydropres Tablets.................................. 1675 Hyzaar Tablets .... 1677 Inderide Tablets .... 2732 Inderide LA Long Acting Capsules .. 2734 Lopressor HCT Tablets........................ 832 Lotensin HCT... 837 Maxzide .... 1380 Moduretic Tablets .... 1705 Oretic Tablets .... 443 Prinzide Tablets .... 1737 Ser-Ap-Es Tablets .... 849 Timolide Tablets..................................... 1748 Vaseretic Tablets .... 1765 Zestoretic .... 2850 Ziac 1415

Hydroflumethiazide (May cause hypercalcemia in hypoparathyroid patients). Products include:

Diucardin Tablets................................... 2718

Methyclothiazide (May cause hypercalcemia in hypoparathyroid patients). Products include:

Enduron Tablets...................................... 420

Polythiazide (May cause hypercalcemia in hypoparathyroid patients). Products include:

Minizide Capsules 1938

DML FACIAL MOISTURIZER WITH SUNSCREEN

(Glycerin, Hyaluronic Acid, Octyl Methoxycinnamate, Oxybenzone) .....1932 None cited in PDR database.

DML FORTE CREAM

(Petrolatum) 1932

None cited in PDR database.

DTIC-DOME

(Dacarbazine) .... 600 May interact with antineoplastics. Compounds in this category include:

Altretamine (Hepatic toxicity). Products include:

Hexalen Capsules 2571

Asparaginase (Hepatic toxicity). Products include:

Elspar 1659

Bleomycin Sulfate (Hepatic toxicity). Products include:

Blenoxane 692

Busulfan (Hepatic toxicity). Products include:

Myleran Tablets 1143

Carboplatin (Hepatic toxicity). Products include:

Paraplatin for Injection 705

Carmustine (BCNU) (Hepatic toxicity). Products include:

BiCNU... 691

Chlorambucil (Hepatic toxicity). Products include:

Leukeran Tablets 1133

Cisplatin (Hepatic toxicity). Products include:

Platinol .... 708 Platinol-AQ Injection 710

Cyclophosphamide (Hepatic toxicity). Products include:

Cytoxan .... 694 NEOSAR Lyophilized/Neosar 1959

Daunorubicin Hydrochloride (Hepatic toxicity). Products include:

Cerubidine 795

Doxorubicin Hydrochloride (Hepatic toxicity). Products include:

Adriamycin PFS .... 1947 Adriamycin RDF .... 1947 Doxorubicin Astra .... 540 Rubex 712

Estramustine Phosphate Sodium (Hepatic toxicity). Products include:

Emcyt Capsules 1953

Etoposide (Hepatic toxicity). Products include:

VePesid Capsules and Injection........ 718

Floxuridine (Hepatic toxicity). Products include:

Sterile FUDR 2118

Fluorouracil (Hepatic toxicity). Products include:

Efudex .... 2113 Fluoroplex Topical Solution & Cream 1% .... 479 Fluorouracil Injection 2116

Flutamide (Hepatic toxicity). Products include:

Eulexin Capsules 2358

Hydroxyurea (Hepatic toxicity). Products include:

Hydrea Capsules 696

Idarubicin Hydrochloride (Hepatic toxicity). Products include:

Idamycin 1955

Ifosfamide (Hepatic toxicity). Products include:

IFEX 697

Interferon alfa-2A, Recombinant (Hepatic toxicity). Products include:

Roferon-A Injection 2145

Interferon alfa-2B, Recombinant (Hepatic toxicity). Products include:

Intron A 2364

Levamisole Hydrochloride (Hepatic toxicity). Products include:

Ergamisol Tablets 1292

Lomustine (CCNU) (Hepatic toxicity). Products include:

CeeNU 693

IMPORTANT NOTE: Always consult each drug listing in the patient's regimen for possible interactions.

Mechlorethamine Hydrochloride (Hepatic toxicity). Products include:
- Mustargen 1709

Megestrol Acetate (Hepatic toxicity). Products include:
- Megace Oral Suspension 699
- Megace Tablets 701

Melphalan (Hepatic toxicity). Products include:
- Alkeran Tablets 1071

Mercaptopurine (Hepatic toxicity). Products include:
- Purinethol Tablets 1156

Methotrexate Sodium (Hepatic toxicity). Products include:
- Methotrexate Sodium Tablets, Injection, for Injection and LPF Injection 1275

Mitomycin (Mitomycin-C) (Hepatic toxicity). Products include:
- Mutamycin 703

Mitotane (Hepatic toxicity). Products include:
- Lysodren 698

Mitoxantrone Hydrochloride (Hepatic Toxicity). Products include:
- Novantrone 1279

Paclitaxel (Hepatic toxicity). Products include:
- Taxol 714

Procarbazine Hydrochloride (Hepatic toxicity). Products include:
- Matulane Capsules 2131

Streptozocin (Hepatic toxicity). Products include:
- Zanosar Sterile Powder 2653

Tamoxifen Citrate (Hepatic toxicity). Products include:
- Nolvadex Tablets 2841

Teniposide (Hepatic toxicity). Products include:
- Vumon 727

Thioguanine (Hepatic toxicity). Products include:
- Thioguanine Tablets, Tabloid Brand 1181

Thiotepa (Hepatic toxicity). Products include:
- Thioplex (Thiotepa For Injection) 1281

Vincristine Sulfate (Hepatic toxicity). Products include:
- Oncovin Solution Vials & Hyporets 1466

Vinorelbine Tartrate (Hepatic toxicity). Products include:
- Navelbine Injection 1145

DAILY CARE FROM DESITIN

(Zinc Oxide) .... ▣ 742

None cited in PDR database.

DAIRY EASE CAPLETS AND TABLETS

(Lactase (beta-d-Galactosidase)) .... ▣ 720

None cited in PDR database.

DAIRY EASE DROPS

(Lactase (beta-d-Galactosidase)) .... ▣ 720

None cited in PDR database.

DALALONE D.P. INJECTABLE

(Dexamethasone Acetate) 1011

May interact with oral anticoagulants, potassium-depleting diuretics, and certain other agents. Compounds in these categories include:

Bendroflumethiazide (Potential for hypokalemia).
- No products indexed under this heading.

Chlorothiazide (Potential for hypokalemia). Products include:
- Aldoclor Tablets 1598
- Diupres Tablets 1650
- Diuril Oral 1653

Chlorothiazide Sodium (Potential for hypokalemia). Products include:
- Diuril Sodium Intravenous 1652

Dicumarol (Corticosteroids may alter the response to this anticoagulant).
- No products indexed under this heading.

Ephedrine (May alter cortisol metabolism).

Ephedrine Hydrochloride (May alter cortisol metabolism). Products include:
- Primatene Dual Action Formula .... ▣ 872
- Primatene Tablets .... ▣ 873
- Quadrinal Tablets 1350

Ephedrine Sulfate (May alter cortisol metabolism). Products include:
- Bronkaid Caplets .... ▣ 717
- Marax Tablets & DF Syrup 2200

Ephedrine Tannate (May alter cortisol metabolism). Products include:
- Rynatuss 2673

Flucytosine (Neurological complications and lack of antibody response). Products include:
- Ancobon Capsules 2079

Hydrochlorothiazide (Potential for hypokalemia). Products include:
- Aldactazide 2413
- Aldoril Tablets 1604
- Apresazide Capsules 808
- Capozide 742
- Dyazide 2479
- Esidrix Tablets 821
- Esimil Tablets 822
- HydroDIURIL Tablets 1674
- Hydropres Tablets 1675
- Hyzaar Tablets 1677
- Inderide Tablets 2732
- Inderide LA Long Acting Capsules 2734
- Lopressor HCT Tablets 832
- Lotensin HCT 837
- Maxzide 1380
- Moduretic Tablets 1705
- Oretic Tablets 443
- Prinzide Tablets 1737
- Ser-Ap-Es Tablets 849
- Timolide Tablets 1748
- Vaseretic Tablets 1765
- Zestoretic 2850
- Ziac 1415

Hydroflumethiazide (Potential for hypokalemia). Products include:
- Diucardin Tablets 2718

Live Virus Vaccines (Potential for neurological complications and loss of antibody response).

Methyclothiazide (Potential for hypokalemia). Products include:
- Enduron Tablets 420

Phenobarbital (May enhance the metabolic clearance of corticosteroids resulting in decreased blood levels and lessened physiologic activity). Products include:
- Arco-Lase Plus Tablets 512
- Bellergal-S Tablets 2250
- Donnatal 2060
- Donnatal Extentabs 2061
- Donnatal Tablets 2060
- Phenobarbital Elixir and Tablets 1469
- Quadrinal Tablets 1350

Phenytoin (May enhance the metabolic clearance of corticosteroids resulting in decreased blood levels and lessened physiologic activity). Products include:
- Dilantin Infatabs 1908
- Dilantin-125 Suspension 1911

Phenytoin Sodium (May enhance the metabolic clearance of corticosteroids resulting in decreased blood levels and lessened physiologic activity). Products include:
- Dilantin Kapseals 1906
- Dilantin Parenteral 1910

Polythiazide (Potential for hypokalemia). Products include:
- Minizide Capsules 1938

Rifampin (May enhance the metabolic cleearance of corticosteroids resulting in decreased blood levels and lessened physiologic activity). Products include:
- Rifadin 1528
- Rifamate Capsules 1530
- Rifater 1532
- Rimactane Capsules 847

Smallpox Vaccine (Neurological complications and lack of antibody response).

Warfarin Sodium (Corticosteroids may alter the response to this anticoagulant). Products include:
- Coumadin 926

DALGAN INJECTION

(Dezocine) 538

May interact with central nervous system depressants, general anesthetics, hypnotics and sedatives, tranquilizers, narcotic analgesics, and certain other agents. Compounds in these categories include:

Alfentanil Hydrochloride (Concomitant administration may have an additive effect). Products include:
- Alfenta Injection 1286

Alprazolam (Concomitant administration may have an additive effect). Products include:
- Xanax Tablets 2649

Aprobarbital (Concomitant administration may have an additive effect).
- No products indexed under this heading.

Buprenorphine (Concomitant administration may have an additive effect). Products include:
- Buprenex Injectable 2006

Buspirone Hydrochloride (Concomitant administration may have an additive effect). Products include:
- BuSpar 737

Butabarbital (Concomitant administration may have an additive effect).
- No products indexed under this heading.

Butalbital (Concomitant administration may have an additive effect). Products include:
- Esgic-plus Tablets 1013
- Fioricet Tablets 2258
- Fioricet with Codeine Capsules 2260
- Fiorinal Capsules 2261
- Fiorinal with Codeine Capsules 2262
- Fiorinal Tablets 2261
- Phrenilin 785
- Sedapap Tablets 50 mg/650 mg 1543

Chlordiazepoxide (Concomitant administration may have an additive effect). Products include:
- Libritabs Tablets 2177
- Limbitrol 2180

Chlordiazepoxide Hydrochloride (Concomitant administration may have an additive effect). Products include:
- Librax Capsules 2176
- Librium Capsules 2178
- Librium Injectable 2179

Chlorpromazine (Concomitant administration may have an additive effect). Products include:
- Thorazine Suppositories 2523

Chlorprothixene (Concomitant administration may have an additive effect).
- No products indexed under this heading.

Chlorprothixene Hydrochloride (Concomitant administration may have an additive effect).
- No products indexed under this heading.

Clorazepate Dipotassium (Concomitant administration may have an additive effect). Products include:
- Tranxene 451

Clozapine (Concomitant administration may have an additive effect). Products include:
- Clozaril Tablets 2252

Codeine Phosphate (Concomitant administration may have an additive effect). Products include:
- Actifed with Codeine Cough Syrup 1067
- Brontex 1981
- Deconsal C Expectorant Syrup 456
- Deconsal Pediatric Syrup 457
- Dimetane-DC Cough Syrup 2059
- Empirin with Codeine Tablets 1093
- Fioricet with Codeine Capsules 2260
- Fiorinal with Codeine Capsules 2262
- Isoclor Expectorant 990
- Novahistine DH 2462
- Novahistine Expectorant 2463
- Nucofed 2051
- Phenergan with Codeine 2777
- Phenergan VC with Codeine 2781
- Robitussin A-C Syrup 2073
- Robitussin-DAC Syrup 2074
- Ryna .... ▣ 841
- Soma Compound w/Codeine Tablets 2676
- Tussi-Organidin NR Liquid and S NR Liquid 2677
- Tylenol with Codeine 1583

Desflurane (Concomitant administration may have an additive effect). Products include:
- Suprane 1813

Diazepam (Concomitant administration may have an additive effect). Products include:
- Dizac 1809
- Valium Injectable 2182
- Valium Tablets 2183
- Valrelease Capsules 2169

Droperidol (Concomitant administration may have an additive effect). Products include:
- Inapsine Injection 1296

Enflurane (Concomitant administration may have an additive effect).
- No products indexed under this heading.

Estazolam (Concomitant administration may have an additive effect). Products include:
- ProSom Tablets 449

Ethchlorvynol (Concomitant administration may have an additive effect). Products include:
- Placidyl Capsules 448

Ethinamate (Concomitant administration may have an additive effect).
- No products indexed under this heading.

Fentanyl (Concomitant administration may have an additive effect). Products include:
- Duragesic Transdermal System 1288

Fentanyl Citrate (Concomitant administration may have an additive effect). Products include:
- Sublimaze Injection 1307

Fluphenazine Decanoate (Concomitant administration may have an additive effect). Products include:
- Prolixin Decanoate 509

Fluphenazine Enanthate (Concomitant administration may have an additive effect). Products include:
- Prolixin Enanthate 509

Fluphenazine Hydrochloride (Concomitant administration may have an additive effect). Products include:
- Prolixin 509

(▣ Described in PDR For Nonprescription Drugs) (◉ Described in PDR For Ophthalmology)

Flurazepam Hydrochloride (Concomitant administration may have an additive effect). Products include:
- Dalmane Capsules ... 2173

Glutethimide (Concomitant administration may have an additive effect).
- No products indexed under this heading.

Haloperidol (Concomitant administration may have an additive effect). Products include:
- Haldol Injection, Tablets and Concentrate ... 1575

Haloperidol Decanoate (Concomitant administration may have an additive effect). Products include:
- Haldol Decanoate ... 1577

Hydrocodone Bitartrate (Concomitant administration may have an additive effect). Products include:
- Anexsia 5/500 Elixir ... 1781
- Anexia Tablets ... 1782
- Codiclear DH Syrup ... 791
- Deconamine CX Cough and Cold Liquid and Tablets ... 1319
- Duratuss HD Elixir ... 2565
- Hycodan Tablets and Syrup ... 930
- Hycomine Compound Tablets ... 932
- Hycomine ... 931
- Hycotuss Expectorant Syrup ... 933
- Hydrocet Capsules ... 782
- Lorcet 10/650 ... 1018
- Lortab ... 2566
- Tussend ... 1783
- Tussend Expectorant ... 1785
- Vicodin Tablets ... 1356
- Vicodin ES Tablets ... 1357
- Vicodin Tuss Expectorant ... 1358
- Zydone Capsules ... 949

Hydrocodone Polistirex (Concomitant administration may have an additive effect). Products include:
- Tussionex Pennkinetic Extended-Release Suspension ... 998

Hydroxyzine Hydrochloride (Concomitant administration may have an additive effect). Products include:
- Atarax Tablets & Syrup ... 2185
- Marax Tablets & DF Syrup ... 2200
- Vistaril Intramuscular Solution ... 2216

Isoflurane (Concomitant administration may have an additive effect).
- No products indexed under this heading.

Ketamine Hydrochloride (Concomitant administration may have an additive effect).
- No products indexed under this heading.

Levomethadyl Acetate Hydrochloride (Concomitant administration may have an additive effect). Products include:
- Orlamm ... 2239

Levorphanol Tartrate (Concomitant administration may have an additive effect). Products include:
- Levo-Dromoran ... 2129

Lorazepam (Concomitant administration may have an additive effect). Products include:
- Ativan Injection ... 2698
- Ativan Tablets ... 2700

Loxapine Hydrochloride (Concomitant administration may have an additive effect). Products include:
- Loxitane ... 1378

Loxapine Succinate (Concomitant administration may have an additive effect). Products include:
- Loxitane Capsules ... 1378

Meperidine Hydrochloride (Concomitant administration may have an additive effect). Products include:
- Demerol ... 2308
- Mepergan Injection ... 2753

Mephobarbital (Concomitant administration may have an additive effect). Products include:
- Mebaral Tablets ... 2322

Meprobamate (Concomitant administration may have an additive effect). Products include:
- Miltown Tablets ... 2672
- PMB 200 and PMB 400 ... 2783

Mesoridazine Besylate (Concomitant administration may have an additive effect). Products include:
- Serentil ... 684

Methadone Hydrochloride (Concomitant administration may have an additive effect). Products include:
- Methadone Hydrochloride Oral Concentrate ... 2233
- Methadone Hydrochloride Oral Solution & Tablets ... 2235

Methohexital Sodium (Concomitant administration may have an additive effect). Products include:
- Brevital Sodium Vials ... 1429

Methotrimeprazine (Concomitant administration may have an additive effect). Products include:
- Levoprome ... 1274

Methoxyflurane (Concomitant administration may have an additive effect).
- No products indexed under this heading.

Midazolam Hydrochloride (Concomitant administration may have an additive effect). Products include:
- Versed Injection ... 2170

Molindone Hydrochloride (Concomitant administration may have an additive effect). Products include:
- Moban Tablets and Concentrate ... 1048

Morphine Sulfate (Concomitant administration may have an additive effect). Products include:
- Astramorph/PF Injection, USP (Preservative-Free) ... 535
- Duramorph ... 962
- Infumorph 200 and Infumorph 500 Sterile Solutions ... 965
- MS Contin Tablets ... 1994
- MSIR ... 1997
- Oramorph SR (Morphine Sulfate Sustained Release Tablets) ... 2236
- RMS Suppositories ... 2657
- Roxanol ... 2243

Opium Alkaloids (Concomitant administration may have an additive effect).
- No products indexed under this heading.

Oxazepam (Concomitant administration may have an additive effect). Products include:
- Serax Capsules ... 2810
- Serax Tablets ... 2810

Oxycodone Hydrochloride (Concomitant administration may have an additive effect). Products include:
- Percocet Tablets ... 938
- Percodan Tablets ... 939
- Percodan-Demi Tablets ... 940
- Roxicodone Tablets, Oral Solution & Intensol (Oxycodone) ... 2244
- Tylox Capsules ... 1584

Pentobarbital Sodium (Concomitant administration may have an additive effect). Products include:
- Nembutal Sodium Capsules ... 436
- Nembutal Sodium Solution ... 438
- Nembutal Sodium Suppositories ... 440

Perphenazine (Concomitant administration may have an additive effect). Products include:
- Etrafon ... 2355
- Triavil Tablets ... 1757
- Trilafon ... 2389

Phenobarbital (Concomitant administration may have an additive effect). Products include:
- Arco-Lase Plus Tablets ... 512
- Bellergal-S Tablets ... 2250
- Donnatal ... 2060
- Donnatal Extentabs ... 2061
- Donnatal Tablets ... 2060
- Phenobarbital Elixir and Tablets ... 1469
- Quadrinal Tablets ... 1350

Prazepam (Concomitant administration may have an additive effect).
- No products indexed under this heading.

Prochlorperazine (Concomitant administration may have an additive effect). Products include:
- Compazine ... 2470

Promethazine Hydrochloride (Concomitant administration may have an additive effect). Products include:
- Mepergan Injection ... 2753
- Phenergan with Codeine ... 2777
- Phenergan with Dextromethorphan 2778
- Phenergan Injection ... 2773
- Phenergan Suppositories ... 2775
- Phenergan Syrup ... 2774
- Phenergan Tablets ... 2775
- Phenergan VC ... 2779
- Phenergan VC with Codeine ... 2781

Propofol (Concomitant administration may have an additive effect). Products include:
- Diprivan Injection ... 2833

Propoxyphene Hydrochloride (Concomitant administration may have an additive effect). Products include:
- Darvon ... 1435
- Wygesic Tablets ... 2827

Propoxyphene Napsylate (Concomitant administration may have an additive effect). Products include:
- Darvon-N/Darvocet-N ... 1433

Quazepam (Concomitant administration may have an additive effect). Products include:
- Doral Tablets ... 2664

Risperidone (Concomitant administration may have an additive effect). Products include:
- Risperdal ... 1301

Secobarbital Sodium (Concomitant administration may have an additive effect). Products include:
- Seconal Sodium Pulvules ... 1474

Sufentanil Citrate (Concomitant administration may have an additive effect). Products include:
- Sufenta Injection ... 1309

Temazepam (Concomitant administration may have an additive effect). Products include:
- Restoril Capsules ... 2284

Thiamylal Sodium (Concomitant administration may have an additive effect).
- No products indexed under this heading.

Thioridazine Hydrochloride (Concomitant administration may have an additive effect). Products include:
- Mellaril ... 2269

Thiothixene (Concomitant administration may have an additive effect). Products include:
- Navane Capsules and Concentrate 2201
- Navane Intramuscular ... 2202

Triazolam (Concomitant administration may have an additive effect). Products include:
- Halcion Tablets ... 2611

Trifluoperazine Hydrochloride (Concomitant administration may have an additive effect). Products include:
- Stelazine ... 2514

Zolpidem Tartrate (Concomitant administration may have an additive effect). Products include:
- Ambien Tablets ... 2416

Food Interactions

Alcohol (Concomitant administration may have an additive effect).

DALMANE CAPSULES

(Flurazepam Hydrochloride) ... 2173

May interact with central nervous system depressants and certain other agents. Compounds in these categories include:

Alfentanil Hydrochloride (Additive effects). Products include:
- Alfenta Injection ... 1286

Alprazolam (Additive effects). Products include:
- Xanax Tablets ... 2649

Aprobarbital (Additive effects).
- No products indexed under this heading.

Buprenorphine (Additive effects). Products include:
- Buprenex Injectable ... 2006

Buspirone Hydrochloride (Additive effects). Products include:
- BuSpar ... 737

Butabarbital (Additive effects).
- No products indexed under this heading.

Butalbital (Additive effects). Products include:
- Esgic-plus Tablets ... 1013
- Fioricet Tablets ... 2258
- Fioricet with Codeine Capsules ... 2260
- Fiorinal Capsules ... 2261
- Fiorinal with Codeine Capsules ... 2262
- Fiorinal Tablets ... 2261
- Phrenilin ... 785
- Sedapap Tablets 50 mg/650 mg .. 1543

Chlordiazepoxide (Additive effects). Products include:
- Libritabs Tablets ... 2177
- Limbitrol ... 2180

Chlordiazepoxide Hydrochloride (Additive effects). Products include:
- Librax Capsules ... 2176
- Librium Capsules ... 2178
- Librium Injectable ... 2179

Chlorpromazine (Additive effects). Products include:
- Thorazine Suppositories ... 2523

Chlorprothixene (Additive effects).
- No products indexed under this heading.

Chlorprothixene Hydrochloride (Additive effects).
- No products indexed under this heading.

Clorazepate Dipotassium (Additive effects). Products include:
- Tranxene ... 451

Clozapine (Additive effects). Products include:
- Clozaril Tablets ... 2252

Codeine Phosphate (Additive effects). Products include:
- Actifed with Codeine Cough Syrup.. 1067
- Brontex ... 1981
- Deconsal C Expectorant Syrup ... 456
- Deconsal Pediatric Syrup ... 457
- Dimetane-DC Cough Syrup ... 2059
- Empirin with Codeine Tablets ... 1093
- Fioricet with Codeine Capsules ... 2260
- Fiorinal with Codeine Capsules ... 2262
- Isoclor Expectorant ... 990
- Novahistine DH ... 2462
- Novahistine Expectorant ... 2463
- Nucofed ... 2051
- Phenergan with Codeine ... 2777
- Phenergan VC with Codeine ... 2781
- Robitussin A-C Syrup ... 2073
- Robitussin-DAC Syrup ... 2074
- Ryna ... 841
- Soma Compound w/Codeine Tablets ... 2676

IMPORTANT NOTE: Always consult each drug listing in the patient's regimen for possible interactions.

Dalmane Interactions Index 226

Tussi-Organidin NR Liquid and S NR Liquid 2677
Tylenol with Codeine 1583

Desflurane (Additive effects). Products include:
Suprane 1813

Dezocine (Additive effects). Products include:
Dalgan Injection 538

Diazepam (Additive effects). Products include:
Dizac 1809
Valium Injectable 2182
Valium Tablets 2183
Valrelease Capsules 2169

Droperidol (Additive effects). Products include:
Inapsine Injection 1296

Enflurane (Additive effects).
No products indexed under this heading.

Estazolam (Additive effects). Products include:
ProSom Tablets 449

Ethchlorvynol (Additive effects). Products include:
Placidyl Capsules 448

Ethinamate (Additive effects).
No products indexed under this heading.

Fentanyl (Additive effects). Products include:
Duragesic Transdermal System 1288

Fentanyl Citrate (Additive effects). Products include:
Sublimaze Injection 1307

Fluphenazine Decanoate (Additive effects). Products include:
Prolixin Decanoate 509

Fluphenazine Enanthate (Additive effects). Products include:
Prolixin Enanthate 509

Fluphenazine Hydrochloride (Additive effects). Products include:
Prolixin 509

Glutethimide (Additive effects).
No products indexed under this heading.

Haloperidol (Additive effects). Products include:
Haldol Injection, Tablets and Concentrate 1575

Haloperidol Decanoate (Additive effects). Products include:
Haldol Decanoate 1577

Hydrocodone Bitartrate (Additive effects). Products include:
Anexsia 5/500 Elixir 1781
Anexia Tablets 1782
Codiclear DH Syrup 791
Deconamine CX Cough and Cold Liquid and Tablets 1319
Duratuss HD Elixir 2565
Hycodan Tablets and Syrup 930
Hycomine Compound Tablets 932
Hycomine 931
Hycotuss Expectorant Syrup 933
Hydrocet Capsules 782
Lorcet 10/650 1018
Lortab 2566
Tussend 1783
Tussend Expectorant 1785
Vicodin Tablets 1356
Vicodin ES Tablets 1357
Vicodin Tuss Expectorant 1358
Zydone Capsules 949

Hydrocodone Polistirex (Additive effects). Products include:
Tussionex Pennkinetic Extended-Release Suspension 998

Hydroxyzine Hydrochloride (Additive effects). Products include:
Atarax Tablets & Syrup 2185
Marax Tablets & DF Syrup 2200
Vistaril Intramuscular Solution 2216

Isoflurane (Additive effects).
No products indexed under this heading.

Ketamine Hydrochloride (Additive effects).
No products indexed under this heading.

Levomethadyl Acetate Hydrochloride (Additive effects). Products include:
Orlamm 2239

Levorphanol Tartrate (Additive effects). Products include:
Levo-Dromoran 2129

Lorazepam (Additive effects). Products include:
Ativan Injection 2698
Ativan Tablets 2700

Loxapine Hydrochloride (Additive effects). Products include:
Loxitane 1378

Loxapine Succinate (Additive effects). Products include:
Loxitane Capsules 1378

Meperidine Hydrochloride (Additive effects). Products include:
Demerol 2308
Mepergan Injection 2753

Mephobarbital (Additive effects). Products include:
Mebaral Tablets 2322

Meprobamate (Additive effects). Products include:
Miltown Tablets 2672
PMB 200 and PMB 400 2783

Mesoridazine Besylate (Additive effects). Products include:
Serentil 684

Methadone Hydrochloride (Additive effects). Products include:
Methadone Hydrochloride Oral Concentrate 2233
Methadone Hydrochloride Oral Solution & Tablets 2235

Methohexital Sodium (Additive effects). Products include:
Brevital Sodium Vials 1429

Methotrimeprazine (Additive effects). Products include:
Levoprome 1274

Methoxyflurane (Additive effects).
No products indexed under this heading.

Midazolam Hydrochloride (Additive effects). Products include:
Versed Injection 2170

Molindone Hydrochloride (Additive effects). Products include:
Moban Tablets and Concentrate 1048

Morphine Sulfate (Additive effects). Products include:
Astramorph/PF Injection, USP (Preservative-Free) 535
Duramorph 962
Infumorph 200 and Infumorph 500 Sterile Solutions 965
MS Contin Tablets 1994
MSIR 1997
Oramorph SR (Morphine Sulfate Sustained Release Tablets) 2236
RMS Suppositories 2657
Roxanol 2243

Opium Alkaloids (Additive effects).
No products indexed under this heading.

Oxazepam (Additive effects). Products include:
Serax Capsules 2810
Serax Tablets 2810

Oxycodone Hydrochloride (Additive effects). Products include:
Percocet Tablets 938
Percodan Tablets 939
Percodan-Demi Tablets 940
Roxicodone Tablets, Oral Solution & Intensol (Oxycodone) 2244
Tylox Capsules 1584

Pentobarbital Sodium (Additive effects). Products include:
Nembutal Sodium Capsules 436
Nembutal Sodium Solution 438
Nembutal Sodium Suppositories 440

Perphenazine (Additive effects). Products include:
Etrafon 2355
Triavil Tablets 1757
Trilafon 2389

Phenobarbital (Additive effects). Products include:
Arco-Lase Plus Tablets 512
Bellergal-S Tablets 2250
Donnatal 2060
Donnatal Extentabs 2061
Donnatal Tablets 2060
Phenobarbital Elixir and Tablets 1469
Quadrinal Tablets 1350

Prazepam (Additive effects).
No products indexed under this heading.

Prochlorperazine (Additive effects). Products include:
Compazine 2470

Promethazine Hydrochloride (Additive effects). Products include:
Mepergan Injection 2753
Phenergan with Codeine 2777
Phenergan with Dextromethorphan 2778
Phenergan Injection 2773
Phenergan Suppositories 2775
Phenergan Syrup 2774
Phenergan Tablets 2775
Phenergan VC 2779
Phenergan VC with Codeine 2781

Propofol (Additive effects). Products include:
Diprivan Injection 2833

Propoxyphene Hydrochloride (Additive effects). Products include:
Darvon 1435
Wygesic Tablets 2827

Propoxyphene Napsylate (Additive effects). Products include:
Darvon-N/Darvocet-N 1433

Quazepam (Additive effects). Products include:
Doral Tablets 2664

Risperidone (Additive effects). Products include:
Risperdal 1301

Secobarbital Sodium (Additive effects). Products include:
Seconal Sodium Pulvules 1474

Sufentanil Citrate (Additive effects). Products include:
Sufenta Injection 1309

Temazepam (Additive effects). Products include:
Restoril Capsules 2284

Thiamylal Sodium (Additive effects).
No products indexed under this heading.

Thioridazine Hydrochloride (Additive effects). Products include:
Mellaril 2269

Thiothixene (Additive effects). Products include:
Navane Capsules and Concentrate 2201
Navane Intramuscular 2202

Triazolam (Additive effects). Products include:
Halcion Tablets 2611

Trifluoperazine Hydrochloride (Additive effects). Products include:
Stelazine 2514

Zolpidem Tartrate (Additive effects). Products include:
Ambien Tablets 2416

Food Interactions

Alcohol (Additive effects; potential for continuation of interaction after discontinuance of flurazepam).

DANOCRINE CAPSULES
(Danazol) 2307
May interact with insulin and certain other agents. Compounds in these categories include:

Carbamazepine (May result in increased carbamazepine levels). Products include:
Atretol Tablets 573
Tegretol Chewable Tablets 852
Tegretol Suspension 852
Tegretol Tablets 852

Insulin, Human (Insulin requirement may be increased in diabetic patients).
No products indexed under this heading.

Insulin, Human Isophane Suspension (Insulin requirement may be increased in diabetic patients). Products include:
Novolin N Human Insulin 10 ml Vials 1795

Insulin, Human NPH (Insulin requirement may be increased in diabetic patients). Products include:
Humulin N, 100 Units 1448
Novolin N PenFill Cartridges Durable Insulin Delivery System 1798
Novolin N Prefilled Syringe Disposable Insulin Delivery System 1798

Insulin, Human Regular (Insulin requirement may be increased in diabetic patients). Products include:
Humulin R, 100 Units 1449
Novolin R Human Insulin 10 ml Vials 1795
Novolin R PenFill Cartridges Durable Insulin Delivery System 1798
Novolin R Prefilled Syringe Disposable Insulin Delivery System 1798
Velosulin BR Human Insulin 10 ml Vials 1795

Insulin, Human, Zinc Suspension (Insulin requirement may be increased in diabetic patients). Products include:
Humulin L, 100 Units 1446
Humulin U, 100 Units 1450
Novolin L Human Insulin 10 ml Vials 1795

Insulin, NPH (Insulin requirement may be increased in diabetic patients). Products include:
NPH, 100 Units 1450
Pork NPH, 100 Units 1452
Purified Pork NPH Isophane Insulin 1801

Insulin, Regular (Insulin requirement may be increased in diabetic patients). Products include:
Regular, 100 Units 1450
Pork Regular, 100 Units 1452
Pork Regular (Concentrated), 500 Units 1453
Purified Pork Regular Insulin 1801

Insulin, Zinc Crystals (Insulin requirement may be increased in diabetic patients). Products include:
NPH, 100 Units 1450

Insulin, Zinc Suspension (Insulin requirement may be increased in diabetic patients). Products include:
Iletin I 1450
Lente, 100 Units 1450
Iletin II 1452
Pork Lente, 100 Units 1452
Purified Pork Lente Insulin 1801

Warfarin Sodium (Prolongation of prothrombin time in patients stabilized on warfarin). Products include:
Coumadin 926

DANTRIUM CAPSULES
(Dantrolene Sodium) 1982
May interact with estrogens and certain other agents. Compounds in these categories include:

Chlorotrianisene (Potential for hepatotoxicity).
No products indexed under this heading.

Dienestrol (Potential for hepatotoxicity). Products include:

Ortho Dienestrol Cream 1866

Diethylstilbestrol (Potential for hepatotoxicity). Products include:

Diethylstilbestrol Tablets 1437

Estradiol (Potential for hepatotoxicity). Products include:

Climara Transdermal System............. 645
Estrace Cream and Tablets................. 749
Estraderm Transdermal System 824

Estrogens, Conjugated (Potential for hepatotoxicity). Products include:

PMB 200 and PMB 400 2783
Premarin Intravenous 2787
Premarin with Methyltestosterone.. 2794
Premarin Tablets 2789
Premarin Vaginal Cream.................... 2791
Premphase 2797
Prempro.. 2801

Estrogens, Esterified (Potential for hepatotoxicity). Products include:

ESTRATAB Tablets (0.3, 0.625, 1.25, 2.5 mg) 2536
Estratest 2539
Menest Tablets 2494

Estropipate (Potential for hepatotoxicity). Products include:

Ogen Tablets 2627
Ogen Vaginal Cream............................. 2630
Ortho-Est.. 1869

Ethinyl Estradiol (Potential for hepatotoxicity). Products include:

Brevicon... 2088
Demulen 2428
Desogen Tablets..................................... 1817
Levlen/Tri-Levlen 651
Lo/Ovral Tablets 2746
Lo/Ovral-28 Tablets.............................. 2751
Modicon 1872
Nordette-21 Tablets............................... 2755
Nordette-28 Tablets............................... 2758
Norinyl 2088
Ortho-Cept 1851
Ortho-Cyclen/Ortho-Tri-Cyclen 1858
Ortho-Novum... 1872
Ortho-Cyclen/Ortho Tri-Cyclen 1858
Ovcon 760
Ovral Tablets 2770
Ovral-28 Tablets 2770
Levlen/Tri-Levlen 651
Tri-Norinyl.. 2164
Triphasil-21 Tablets 2814
Triphasil-28 Tablets 2819

Polyestradiol Phosphate (Potential for hepatotoxicity).

No products indexed under this heading.

Quinestrol (Potential for hepatotoxicity).

No products indexed under this heading.

Verapamil Hydrochloride (The combination of therapeutic doses of intravenous dantrolene sodium and verapamil in halothane anesthetized subjects has resulted in ventricular fibrillation and cardiovascular collapse; this combination is not recommended during the management of malignant hyperthermia). Products include:

Calan SR Caplets 2422
Calan Tablets... 2419
Isoptin Injectable 1344
Isoptin Oral Tablets 1346
Isoptin SR Tablets 1348
Verelan Capsules 1410
Verelan Capsules 2824

DANTRIUM INTRAVENOUS

(Dantrolene Sodium) 1983

May interact with hepatic microsomal enzyme inducers and certain other agents. Compounds in these categories include:

Carbamazepine (Theoretical possibility that the metabolism of dantrolene may be enhanced by drugs known to induce hepatic microsomal enzymes). Products include:

Atretol Tablets 573
Tegretol Chewable Tablets 852
Tegretol Suspension.............................. 852
Tegretol Tablets 852

Chlorpropamide (Theoretical possibility that the metabolism of dantrolene may be enhanced by drugs known to induce hepatic microsomal enzymes). Products include:

Diabinese Tablets 1935

Clofibrate (Reduces binding of dantrolene to plasma proteins). Products include:

Atromid-S Capsules 2701

Glipizide (Theoretical possibility that the metabolism of dantrolene may be enhanced by drugs known to induce hepatic microsomal enzymes). Products include:

Glucotrol Tablets.................................... 1967
Glucotrol XL Extended Release Tablets 1968

Glyburide (Theoretical possibility that the metabolism of dantrolene may be enhanced by drugs known to induce hepatic microsomal enzymes). Products include:

DiaBeta Tablets 1239
Glynase PresTab Tablets 2609
Micronase Tablets 2623

Phenobarbital (Theoretical possibility that the metabolism of dantrolene may be enhanced by drugs known to induce hepatic microsomal enzymes; phenobarbital does not appear to affect Dantrium metabolism). Products include:

Arco-Lase Plus Tablets 512
Bellergal-S Tablets 2250
Donnatal 2060
Donnatal Extentabs............................... 2061
Donnatal Tablets 2060
Phenobarbital Elixir and Tablets 1469
Quadrinal Tablets 1350

Phenylbutazone (Theoretical possibility that the metabolism of dantrolene may be enhanced by drugs known to induce hepatic microsomal enzymes).

No products indexed under this heading.

Phenytoin (Theoretical possibility that the metabolism of dantrolene may be enhanced by drugs known to induce hepatic microsomal enzymes). Products include:

Dilantin Infatabs 1908
Dilantin-125 Suspension 1911

Phenytoin Sodium (Theoretical possibility that the metabolism of dantrolene may be enhanced by drugs known to induce hepatic microsomal enzymes). Products include:

Dilantin Kapseals 1906
Dilantin Parenteral 1910

Rifampin (Theoretical possibility that the metabolism of dantrolene may be enhanced by drugs known to induce hepatic microsomal enzymes). Products include:

Rifadin 1528
Rifamate Capsules 1530
Rifater... 1532
Rimactane Capsules 847

Tolazamide (Theoretical possibility that the metabolism of dantrolene may be enhanced by drugs known to induce hepatic microsomal enzymes).

No products indexed under this heading.

Tolbutamide (Increases binding of dantrolene to plasma proteins).

No products indexed under this heading.

Verapamil Hydrochloride (The combination of therapeutic doses of intravenous dantrolene sodium and verapamil in halothane/alpha-chloralose anesthetized swine has resulted in ventricular collapse in association with marked hyperkalemia; this combination should not be used during the management of malignant hyperthermia crisis). Products include:

Calan SR Caplets 2422
Calan Tablets... 2419
Isoptin Injectable 1344
Isoptin Oral Tablets 1346
Isoptin SR Tablets 1348
Verelan Capsules 1410
Verelan Capsules 2824

Warfarin Sodium (Reduces binding of dantrolene to plasma proteins). Products include:

Coumadin 926

DAPSONE TABLETS USP

(Dapsone) 1284

May interact with:

Pyrimethamine (Agranulocytosis; increased likelihood of hematological reactions). Products include:

Daraprim Tablets 1090
Fansidar Tablets..................................... 2114

Rifampin (Lowered Dapsone levels). Products include:

Rifadin 1528
Rifamate Capsules 1530
Rifater... 1532
Rimactane Capsules 847

Trimethoprim (Mutual interaction between Dapsone and trimethoprim in which each raises the level of the other about 1.5 times). Products include:

Bactrim DS Tablets................................ 2084
Bactrim I.V. Infusion............................. 2082
Bactrim 2084
Proloprim Tablets 1155
Septra.. 1174
Septra I.V. Infusion 1169
Septra I.V. Infusion ADD-Vantage Vials.. 1171
Septra.. 1174
Trimpex Tablets 2163

DARANIDE TABLETS

(Dichlorphenamide) 1633

May interact with corticosteroids and certain other agents. Compounds in these categories include:

ACTH (Hypokalemia may develop).

No products indexed under this heading.

Aspirin (Concomitant high-dose aspirin may produce anorexia, tachypnea, lethargy and coma). Products include:

Alka-Seltzer Effervescent Antacid and Pain Reliever.................................... ⊞ 701
Alka-Seltzer Extra Strength Effervescent Antacid and Pain Reliever .... ⊞ 703
Alka-Seltzer Lemon Lime Effervescent Antacid and Pain Reliever .... ⊞ 703
Alka-Seltzer Plus Cold Medicine .... ⊞ 705
Alka-Seltzer Plus Cold & Cough Medicine .... ⊞ 708
Alka-Seltzer Plus Night-Time Cold Medicine .... ⊞ 707
Alka Seltzer Plus Sinus Medicine .. ⊞ 707
Arthritis Foundation Safety Coated Aspirin Tablets .... ⊞ 675
Arthritis Pain Ascriptin .... ⊞ 631
Maximum Strength Ascriptin .... ⊞ 630
Regular Strength Ascriptin Tablets .... ⊞ 629
Arthritis Strength BC Powder........... ⊞ 609
BC Cold Powder Multi-Symptom Formula (Cold-Sinus-Allergy) ...... ⊞ 609
BC Cold Powder Non-Drowsy Formula (Cold-Sinus) .... ⊞ 609
BC Powder .... ⊞ 609
Bayer Children's Chewable Aspirin... ⊞ 711
Genuine Bayer Aspirin Tablets & Caplets .... ⊞ 713
Extra Strength Bayer Arthritis Pain Regimen Formula .... ⊞ 711
Extra Strength Bayer Aspirin Caplets & Tablets .... ⊞ 712
Extended-Release Bayer 8-Hour Aspirin .... ⊞ 712
Extra Strength Bayer Plus Aspirin Caplets .... ⊞ 713
Extra Strength Bayer PM Aspirin .. ⊞ 713
Bayer Enteric Aspirin .... ⊞ 709
Bufferin Analgesic Tablets and Caplets .... ⊞ 613
Arthritis Strength Bufferin Analgesic Caplets .... ⊞ 614
Extra Strength Bufferin Analgesic Tablets .... ⊞ 615
Cama Arthritis Pain Reliever............ ⊞ 785
Darvon Compound-65 Pulvules 1435
Easprin 1914
Ecotrin 2455
Ecotrin Enteric Coated Aspirin Maximum Strength Tablets and Caplets .... ⊞ 816
Ecotrin Enteric Coated Aspirin Regular Strength Tablets 2455
Empirin Aspirin Tablets .... ⊞ 854
Empirin with Codeine Tablets.......... 1093
Excedrin Extra-Strength Analgesic Tablets & Caplets 732
Fiorinal Capsules 2261
Fiorinal with Codeine Capsules 2262
Fiorinal Tablets 2261
Halfprin 1362
Healthprin Aspirin 2455
Norgesic.. 1496
Percodan Tablets.................................... 939
Percodan-Demi Tablets........................ 940
Robaxisal Tablets................................... 2071
Soma Compound w/Codeine Tablets 2676
Soma Compound Tablets..................... 2675
St. Joseph Adult Chewable Aspirin (81 mg.) .... ⊞ 808
Talwin Compound 2335
Ursinus Inlay-Tabs................................. ⊞ 794
Vanquish Analgesic Caplets .... ⊞ 731

Aspirin, Enteric Coated (Concomitant high-dose aspirin may produce anorexia, tachypnea, lethargy and coma). Products include:

Bayer Enteric Aspirin .... ⊞ 709
Ecotrin 2455

Betamethasone Acetate (Hypokalemia may develop). Products include:

Celestone Soluspan Suspension 2347

Betamethasone Sodium Phosphate (Hypokalemia may develop). Products include:

Celestone Soluspan Suspension 2347

Cortisone Acetate (Hypokalemia may develop). Products include:

Cortone Acetate Sterile Suspension 1623
Cortone Acetate Tablets 1624

Dexamethasone (Hypokalemia may develop). Products include:

AK-Trol Ointment & Suspension .... ◎ 205
Decadron Elixir 1633
Decadron Tablets.................................... 1635
Decaspray Topical Aerosol 1648
Dexacidin Ointment .... ◎ 263
Maxitrol Ophthalmic Ointment and Suspension .... ◎ 224
TobraDex Ophthalmic Suspension and Ointment.. 473

Dexamethasone Acetate (Hypokalemia may develop). Products include:

Dalalone D.P. Injectable 1011
Decadron-LA Sterile Suspension...... 1646

IMPORTANT NOTE: Always consult each drug listing in the patient's regimen for possible interactions.

Dexamethasone Sodium Phosphate (Hypokalemia may develop). Products include:
- Decadron Phosphate Injection ... 1637
- Decadron Phosphate Respihaler ... 1642
- Decadron Phosphate Sterile Ophthalmic Ointment ... 1641
- Decadron Phosphate Sterile Ophthalmic Solution ... 1642
- Decadron Phosphate Topical Cream ... 1644
- Decadron Phosphate Turbinaire ... 1645
- Decadron Phosphate with Xylocaine Injection, Sterile ... 1639
- Dexacort Phosphate in Respihaler ... 458
- Dexacort Phosphate in Turbinaire ... 459
- NeoDecadron Sterile Ophthalmic Ointment ... 1712
- NeoDecadron Sterile Ophthalmic Solution ... 1713
- NeoDecadron Topical Cream ... 1714

Fludrocortisone Acetate (Hypokalemia may develop). Products include:
- Florinef Acetate Tablets ... 505

Hydrocortisone (Hypokalemia may develop). Products include:
- Anusol-HC Cream 2.5% ... 1896
- Aquanil HC Lotion ... 1931
- Bactine Hydrocortisone Anti-Itch Cream ... ▣ 709
- Caldecort Anti-Itch Hydrocortisone Spray ... ▣ 631
- Cortaid ... ▣ 836
- CORTENEMA ... 2535
- Cortisporin Ointment ... 1085
- Cortisporin Ophthalmic Ointment Sterile ... 1085
- Cortisporin Ophthalmic Suspension Sterile ... 1086
- Cortisporin Otic Solution Sterile ... 1087
- Cortisporin Otic Suspension Sterile ... 1088
- Cortizone-5 ... ▣ 831
- Cortizone-10 ... ▣ 831
- Hydrocortone Tablets ... 1672
- Hytone ... 907
- Massengill Medicated Soft Cloth Towelettes ... 2458
- PediOtic Suspension Sterile ... 1153
- Preparation H Hydrocortisone 1% Cream ... ▣ 872
- ProctoCream-HC 2.5% ... 2408
- VōSoL HC Otic Solution ... 2678

Hydrocortisone Acetate (Hypokalemia may develop). Products include:
- Analpram-HC Rectal Cream 1% and 2.5% ... 977
- Anusol HC-1 Anti-Itch Hydrocortisone Ointment ... ▣ 847
- Anusol-HC Suppositories ... 1897
- Caldecort ... ▣ 631
- Carmol HC ... 924
- Coly-Mycin S Otic w/Neomycin & Hydrocortisone ... 1906
- Cortaid ... ▣ 836
- Cortifoam ... 2396
- Cortisporin Cream ... 1084
- Epifoam ... 2399
- Hydrocortone Acetate Sterile Suspension ... 1669
- Mantadil Cream ... 1135
- Nupercainal Hydrocortisone 1% Cream ... ▣ 645
- Ophthocort ... ⊙ 311
- Pramosone Cream, Lotion & Ointment ... 978
- ProctoCream-HC ... 2408
- ProctoFoam-HC ... 2409
- Terra-Cortril Ophthalmic Suspension ... 2210

Hydrocortisone Sodium Phosphate (Hypokalemia may develop). Products include:
- Hydrocortone Phosphate Injection, Sterile ... 1670

Hydrocortisone Sodium Succinate (Hypokalemia may develop). Products include:
- Solu-Cortef Sterile Powder ... 2641

Methylprednisolone Acetate (Hypokalemia may develop). Products include:
- Depo-Medrol Single-Dose Vial ... 2600
- Depo-Medrol Sterile Aqueous Suspension ... 2597

Methylprednisolone Sodium Succinate (Hypokalemia may develop). Products include:
- Solu-Medrol Sterile Powder ... 2643

Prednisolone Acetate (Hypokalemia may develop). Products include:
- AK-CIDE ... ⊙ 202
- AK-CIDE Ointment ... ⊙ 202
- Blephamide Liquifilm Sterile Ophthalmic Suspension ... 476
- Blephamide Ointment ... ⊙ 237
- Econopred & Econopred Plus Ophthalmic Suspensions ... ⊙ 217
- Poly-Pred Liquifilm ... ⊙ 248
- Pred Forte ... ⊙ 250
- Pred Mild ... ⊙ 253
- Pred-G Liquifilm Sterile Ophthalmic Suspension ... ⊙ 251
- Pred-G S.O.P. Sterile Ophthalmic Ointment ... ⊙ 252
- Vasocidin Ointment ... ⊙ 268

Prednisolone Sodium Phosphate (Hypokalemia may develop). Products include:
- AK-Pred ... ⊙ 204
- Hydeltrasol Injection, Sterile ... 1665
- Inflamase ... ⊙ 265
- Pediapred Oral Liquid ... 995
- Vasocidin Ophthalmic Solution ... ⊙ 270

Prednisolone Tebutate (Hypokalemia may develop). Products include:
- Hydeltra-T.B.A. Sterile Suspension ... 1667

Prednisone (Hypokalemia may develop). Products include:
- Deltasone Tablets ... 2595

Triamcinolone (Hypokalemia may develop). Products include:
- Aristocort Tablets ... 1022

Triamcinolone Acetonide (Hypokalemia may develop). Products include:
- Aristocort A 0.025% Cream ... 1027
- Aristocort A 0.5% Cream ... 1031
- Aristocort A 0.1% Cream ... 1029
- Aristocort A 0.1% Ointment ... 1030
- Azmacort Oral Inhaler ... 2011
- Nasacort Nasal Inhaler ... 2024

Triamcinolone Diacetate (Hypokalemia may develop). Products include:
- Aristocort Suspension (Forte Parenteral) ... 1027
- Aristocort Suspension (Intralesional) ... 1025

Triamcinolone Hexacetonide (Hypokalemia may develop). Products include:
- Aristospan Suspension (Intra-articular) ... 1033
- Aristospan Suspension (Intralesional) ... 1032

DARAPRIM TABLETS

(Pyrimethamine) ... 1090

May interact with sulfonamides and certain other agents. Compounds in these categories include:

Lorazepam (Concomitant therapy may result in mild hepatotoxicity). Products include:
- Ativan Injection ... 2698
- Ativan Tablets ... 2700

Phenytoin (Daraprim should be used with caution). Products include:
- Dilantin Infatabs ... 1908
- Dilantin-125 Suspension ... 1911

Phenytoin Sodium (Daraprim should be used with caution). Products include:
- Dilantin Kapseals ... 1906
- Dilantin Parenteral ... 1910

Sulfamethizole (Increased risk of bone marrow suppression and hypersensitivity reactions). Products include:
- Urobiotic-250 Capsules ... 2214

Sulfamethoxazole (Increased risk of bone marrow suppression and hypersensitivity reactions). Products include:
- Azo Gantanol Tablets ... 2080
- Bactrim DS Tablets ... 2084
- Bactrim I.V. Infusion ... 2082
- Bactrim ... 2084
- Gantanol Tablets ... 2119
- Septra ... 1174
- Septra I.V. Infusion ... 1169
- Septra I.V. Infusion ADD-Vantage Vials ... 1171
- Septra ... 1174

Sulfasalazine (Increased risk of bone marrow suppression and hypersensitivity reactions). Products include:
- Azulfidine ... 1949

Sulfinpyrazone (Increased risk of bone marrow suppression and hypersensitivity reactions). Products include:
- Anturane ... 807

Sulfisoxazole (Increased risk of bone marrow suppression and hypersensitivity reactions). Products include:
- Azo Gantrisin Tablets ... 2081
- Gantrisin Tablets ... 2120

Sulfisoxazole Diolamine (Increased risk of bone marrow suppression and hypersensitivity reactions).
- No products indexed under this heading.

Trimethoprim (Increased risk of bone marrow suppression and hypersensitivity reactions). Products include:
- Bactrim DS Tablets ... 2084
- Bactrim I.V. Infusion ... 2082
- Bactrim ... 2084
- Proloprim Tablets ... 1155
- Septra ... 1174
- Septra I.V. Infusion ... 1169
- Septra I.V. Infusion ADD-Vantage Vials ... 1171
- Septra ... 1174
- Trimpex Tablets ... 2163

DARVOCET-N 50 TABLETS

(Propoxyphene Napsylate, Acetaminophen) ... 1433

May interact with central nervous system depressants, tricyclic antidepressants, anticonvulsants, oral anticoagulants, and certain other agents. Compounds in these categories include:

Alfentanil Hydrochloride (Additive CNS depression). Products include:
- Alfenta Injection ... 1286

Alprazolam (Additive CNS depression). Products include:
- Xanax Tablets ... 2649

Amitriptyline Hydrochloride (Propoxyphene may slow metabolism). Products include:
- Elavil ... 2838
- Endep Tablets ... 2174
- Etrafon ... 2355
- Limbitrol ... 2180
- Triavil Tablets ... 1757

Amoxapine (Propoxyphene may slow metabolism). Products include:
- Asendin Tablets ... 1369

Aprobarbital (Additive CNS depression).
- No products indexed under this heading.

Buprenorphine (Additive CNS depression). Products include:
- Buprenex Injectable ... 2006

Buspirone Hydrochloride (Additive CNS depression). Products include:
- BuSpar ... 737

Butabarbital (Additive CNS depression).
- No products indexed under this heading.

Butalbital (Additive CNS depression). Products include:
- Esgic-plus Tablets ... 1013
- Fioricet Tablets ... 2258
- Fioricet with Codeine Capsules ... 2260
- Fiorinal Capsules ... 2261
- Fiorinal with Codeine Capsules ... 2262
- Fiorinal Tablets ... 2261
- Phrenilin ... 785
- Sedapap Tablets 50 mg/650 mg ... 1543

Carbamazepine (Concurrent use may result in severe neurological signs, including coma). Products include:
- Atretol Tablets ... 573
- Tegretol Chewable Tablets ... 852
- Tegretol Suspension ... 852
- Tegretol Tablets ... 852

Chlordiazepoxide (Additive CNS depression). Products include:
- Libritabs Tablets ... 2177
- Limbitrol ... 2180

Chlordiazepoxide Hydrochloride (Additive CNS depression). Products include:
- Librax Capsules ... 2176
- Librium Capsules ... 2178
- Librium Injectable ... 2179

Chlorpromazine (Additive CNS depression). Products include:
- Thorazine Suppositories ... 2523

Chlorprothixene (Additive CNS depression).
- No products indexed under this heading.

Chlorprothixene Hydrochloride (Additive CNS depression).
- No products indexed under this heading.

Clomipramine Hydrochloride (Propoxyphene may slow metabolism). Products include:
- Anafranil Capsules ... 803

Clorazepate Dipotassium (Additive CNS depression). Products include:
- Tranxene ... 451

Clozapine (Additive CNS depression). Products include:
- Clozaril Tablets ... 2252

Codeine Phosphate (Additive CNS depression). Products include:
- Actifed with Codeine Cough Syrup ... 1067
- Brontex ... 1981
- Deconsal C Expectorant Syrup ... 456
- Deconsal Pediatric Syrup ... 457
- Dimetane-DC Cough Syrup ... 2059
- Empirin with Codeine Tablets ... 1093
- Fioricet with Codeine Capsules ... 2260
- Fiorinal with Codeine Capsules ... 2262
- Isoclor Expectorant ... 990
- Novahistine DH ... 2462
- Novahistine Expectorant ... 2463
- Nucofed ... 2051
- Phenergan with Codeine ... 2777
- Phenergan VC with Codeine ... 2781
- Robitussin A-C Syrup ... 2073
- Robitussin-DAC Syrup ... 2074
- Ryna ... ▣ 841
- Soma Compound w/Codeine Tablets ... 2676
- Tussi-Organidin NR Liquid and S NR Liquid ... 2677
- Tylenol with Codeine ... 1583

Desflurane (Additive CNS depression). Products include:
- Suprane ... 1813

Desipramine Hydrochloride (Propoxyphene may slow metabolism). Products include:
- Norpramin Tablets ... 1526

Dezocine (Additive CNS depression). Products include:
- Dalgan Injection ... 538

Diazepam (Additive CNS depression). Products include:
- Dizac ... 1809
- Valium Injectable ... 2182

(▣ Described in PDR For Nonprescription Drugs) (⊙ Described in PDR For Ophthalmology)

Valium Tablets 2183
Valrelease Capsules 2169

Dicumarol (Propoxyphene may slow metabolism).

No products indexed under this heading.

Divalproex Sodium (Propoxyphene may slow metabolism). Products include:

Depakote Tablets 415

Doxepin Hydrochloride (Propoxyphene may slow metabolism). Products include:

Sinequan 2205
Zonalon Cream 1055

Droperidol (Additive CNS depression). Products include:

Inapsine Injection 1296

Enflurane (Additive CNS depression).

No products indexed under this heading.

Estazolam (Additive CNS depression). Products include:

ProSom Tablets 449

Ethchlorvynol (Additive CNS depression). Products include:

Placidyl Capsules 448

Ethinamate (Additive CNS depression).

No products indexed under this heading.

Ethosuximide (Propoxyphene may slow metabolism). Products include:

Zarontin Capsules 1928
Zarontin Syrup 1929

Ethotoin (Propoxyphene may slow metabolism). Products include:

Peganone Tablets 446

Felbamate (Concurrent use may result in severe neurological signs, including coma). Products include:

Felbatol 2666

Fentanyl (Additive CNS depression). Products include:

Duragesic Transdermal System 1288

Fentanyl Citrate (Additive CNS depression). Products include:

Sublimaze Injection 1307

Fluphenazine Decanoate (Additive CNS depression). Products include:

Prolixin Decanoate 509

Fluphenazine Enanthate (Additive CNS depression). Products include:

Prolixin Enanthate 509

Fluphenazine Hydrochloride (Additive CNS depression). Products include:

Prolixin 509

Flurazepam Hydrochloride (Additive CNS depression). Products include:

Dalmane Capsules 2173

Glutethimide (Additive CNS depression).

No products indexed under this heading.

Haloperidol (Additive CNS depression). Products include:

Haldol Injection, Tablets and Concentrate 1575

Haloperidol Decanoate (Additive CNS depression). Products include:

Haldol Decanoate 1577

Hydrocodone Bitartrate (Additive CNS depression). Products include:

Anexsia 5/500 Elixir 1781
Anexia Tablets 1782
Codiclear DH Syrup 791
Deconamine CX Cough and Cold Liquid and Tablets 1319
Duratuss HD Elixir 2565
Hycodan Tablets and Syrup 930
Hycomine Compound Tablets 932

Hycomine 931
Hycotuss Expectorant Syrup 933
Hydrocet Capsules 782
Lorcet 10/650 1018
Lortab 2566
Tussend 1783
Tussend Expectorant 1785
Vicodin Tablets 1356
Vicodin ES Tablets 1357
Vicodin Tuss Expectorant 1358
Zydone Capsules 949

Hydrocodone Polistirex (Additive CNS depression). Products include:

Tussionex Pennkinetic Extended-Release Suspension 998

Hydroxyzine Hydrochloride (Additive CNS depression). Products include:

Atarax Tablets & Syrup 2185
Marax Tablets & DF Syrup 2200
Vistaril Intramuscular Solution 2216

Imipramine Hydrochloride (Propoxyphene may slow metabolism). Products include:

Tofranil Ampuls 854
Tofranil Tablets 856

Imipramine Pamoate (Propoxyphene may slow metabolism). Products include:

Tofranil-PM Capsules 857

Isoflurane (Additive CNS depression).

No products indexed under this heading.

Ketamine Hydrochloride (Additive CNS depression).

No products indexed under this heading.

Lamotrigine (Propoxyphene may slow the metabolism of anticonvulsants). Products include:

Lamictal Tablets 1112

Levomethadyl Acetate Hydrochloride (Additive CNS depression). Products include:

Orlaam 2239

Levorphanol Tartrate (Additive CNS depression). Products include:

Levo-Dromoran 2129

Lorazepam (Additive CNS depression). Products include:

Ativan Injection 2698
Ativan Tablets 2700

Loxapine Hydrochloride (Additive CNS depression). Products include:

Loxitane 1378

Loxapine Succinate (Additive CNS depression). Products include:

Loxitane Capsules 1378

Maprotiline Hydrochloride (Propoxyphene may slow metabolism). Products include:

Ludiomil Tablets 843

Meperidine Hydrochloride (Additive CNS depression). Products include:

Demerol 2308
Mepergan Injection 2753

Mephenytoin (Propoxyphene may slow metabolism). Products include:

Mesantoin Tablets 2272

Mephobarbital (Additive CNS depression). Products include:

Mebaral Tablets 2322

Meprobamate (Additive CNS depression). Products include:

Miltown Tablets 2672
PMB 200 and PMB 400 2783

Mesoridazine Besylate (Additive CNS depression). Products include:

Serentil 684

Methadone Hydrochloride (Additive CNS depression). Products include:

Methadone Hydrochloride Oral Concentrate 2233

Methadone Hydrochloride Oral Solution & Tablets 2235

Methohexital Sodium (Additive CNS depression). Products include:

Brevital Sodium Vials 1429

Methotrimeprazine (Additive CNS depression). Products include:

Levoprome 1274

Methoxyflurane (Additive CNS depression).

No products indexed under this heading.

Methsuximide (Propoxyphene may slow metabolism). Products include:

Celontin Kapseals 1899

Midazolam Hydrochloride (Additive CNS depression). Products include:

Versed Injection 2170

Molindone Hydrochloride (Additive CNS depression). Products include:

Moban Tablets and Concentrate 1048

Morphine Sulfate (Additive CNS depression). Products include:

Astramorph/PF Injection, USP (Preservative-Free) 535
Duramorph 962
Infumorph 200 and Infumorph 500 Sterile Solutions 965
MS Contin Tablets 1994
MSIR 1997
Oramorph SR (Morphine Sulfate Sustained Release Tablets) 2236
RMS Suppositories 2657
Roxanol 2243

Nortriptyline Hydrochloride (Propoxyphene may slow metabolism). Products include:

Pamelor 2280

Opium Alkaloids (Additive CNS depression).

No products indexed under this heading.

Oxazepam (Additive CNS depression). Products include:

Serax Capsules 2810
Serax Tablets 2810

Oxycodone Hydrochloride (Additive CNS depression). Products include:

Percocet Tablets 938
Percodan Tablets 939
Percodan-Demi Tablets 940
Roxicodone Tablets, Oral Solution & Intensol (Oxycodone) 2244
Tylox Capsules 1584

Paramethadione (Propoxyphene may slow metabolism).

No products indexed under this heading.

Pentobarbital Sodium (Additive CNS depression). Products include:

Nembutal Sodium Capsules 436
Nembutal Sodium Solution 438
Nembutal Sodium Suppositories 440

Perphenazine (Additive CNS depression). Products include:

Etrafon 2355
Triavil Tablets 1757
Trilafon 2389

Phenacemide (Propoxyphene may slow metabolism). Products include:

Phenurone Tablets 447

Phenobarbital (Additive CNS depression; propoxyphene may slow metabolism). Products include:

Arco-Lase Plus Tablets 512
Bellergal-S Tablets 2250
Donnatal 2060
Donnatal Extentabs 2061
Donnatal Tablets 2060
Phenobarbital Elixir and Tablets 1469
Quadrinal Tablets 1350

Phensuximide (Propoxyphene may slow metabolism). Products include:

Milontin Kapseals 1920

Phenytoin (Propoxyphene may slow metabolism). Products include:

Dilantin Infatabs 1908
Dilantin-125 Suspension 1911

Phenytoin Sodium (Propoxyphene may slow metabolism). Products include:

Dilantin Kapseals 1906
Dilantin Parenteral 1910

Prazepam (Additive CNS depression).

No products indexed under this heading.

Primidone (Propoxyphene may slow metabolism). Products include:

Mysoline 2754

Prochlorperazine (Additive CNS depression). Products include:

Compazine 2470

Promethazine Hydrochloride (Additive CNS depression). Products include:

Mepergan Injection 2753
Phenergan with Codeine 2777
Phenergan with Dextromethorphan 2778
Phenergan Injection 2773
Phenergan Suppositories 2775
Phenergan Syrup 2774
Phenergan Tablets 2775
Phenergan VC 2779
Phenergan VC with Codeine 2781

Propofol (Additive CNS depression). Products include:

Diprivan Injection 2833

Propoxyphene Hydrochloride (Additive CNS depression). Products include:

Darvon 1435
Wygesic Tablets 2827

Protriptyline Hydrochloride (Propoxyphene may slow metabolism). Products include:

Vivactil Tablets 1774

Quazepam (Additive CNS depression). Products include:

Doral Tablets 2664

Risperidone (Additive CNS depression). Products include:

Risperdal 1301

Secobarbital Sodium (Additive CNS depression). Products include:

Seconal Sodium Pulvules 1474

Sufentanil Citrate (Additive CNS depression). Products include:

Sufenta Injection 1309

Temazepam (Additive CNS depression). Products include:

Restoril Capsules 2284

Thiamylal Sodium (Additive CNS depression).

No products indexed under this heading.

Thioridazine Hydrochloride (Additive CNS depression). Products include:

Mellaril 2269

Thiothixene (Additive CNS depression). Products include:

Navane Capsules and Concentrate 2201
Navane Intramuscular 2202

Triazolam (Additive CNS depression). Products include:

Halcion Tablets 2611

Trifluoperazine Hydrochloride (Additive CNS depression). Products include:

Stelazine 2514

Trimethadione (Propoxyphene may slow metabolism).

No products indexed under this heading.

Trimipramine Maleate (Propoxyphene may slow metabolism). Products include:

Surmontil Capsules 2811

Valproic Acid (Propoxyphene may slow metabolism). Products include:

Depakene 413

IMPORTANT NOTE: Always consult each drug listing in the patient's regimen for possible interactions.

Darvon-N/Darvocet-N

Warfarin Sodium (Propoxyphene may slow metabolism). Products include:

Coumadin 926

Zolpidem Tartrate (Additive CNS depression). Products include:

Ambien Tablets... 2416

Food Interactions

Alcohol (Additive CNS depression).

DARVOCET-N 100 TABLETS

(Propoxyphene Napsylate, Acetaminophen) 1433

See Darvocet-N 50 Tablets

DARVON COMPOUND-65 PULVULES

(Propoxyphene Hydrochloride, Aspirin, Caffeine) 1435

May interact with central nervous system depressants, oral anticoagulants, antigout agents, antidepressant drugs, anticonvulsants, and certain other agents. Compounds in these categories include:

Alfentanil Hydrochloride (Additive CNS-depressant effect). Products include:

Alfenta Injection 1286

Allopurinol (Uricosuric effect inhibited). Products include:

Zyloprim Tablets 1226

Alprazolam (Additive CNS-depressant effect). Products include:

Xanax Tablets 2649

Amitriptyline Hydrochloride (Propoxyphene slows the metabolism). Products include:

Elavil	2838
Endep Tablets	2174
Etrafon	2355
Limbitrol	2180
Triavil Tablets	1757

Amoxapine (Propoxyphene slows the metabolism). Products include:

Asendin Tablets 1369

Aprobarbital (Additive CNS-depressant effect).

No products indexed under this heading.

Buprenorphine (Additive CNS-depressant effect). Products include:

Buprenex Injectable 2006

Bupropion Hydrochloride (Propoxyphene slows the metabolism). Products include:

Wellbutrin Tablets 1204

Buspirone Hydrochloride (Additive CNS-depressant effect). Products include:

BuSpar 737

Butabarbital (Additive CNS-depressant effect).

No products indexed under this heading.

Butalbital (Additive CNS-depressant effect). Products include:

Esgic-plus Tablets	1013
Fioricet Tablets	2258
Fioricet with Codeine Capsules	2260
Fiorinal Capsules	2261
Fiorinal with Codeine Capsules	2262
Fiorinal Tablets	2261
Phrenilin	785
Sedapap Tablets 50 mg/650 mg	1543

Carbamazepine (Concurrent use may result in severe neurological signs, including coma). Products include:

Atretol Tablets	573
Tegretol Chewable Tablets	852
Tegretol Suspension	852
Tegretol Tablets	852

Chlordiazepoxide (Additive CNS-depressant effect). Products include:

Libritabs Tablets 2177

Limbitrol 2180

Chlordiazepoxide Hydrochloride (Additive CNS-depressant effect). Products include:

Librax Capsules	2176
Librium Capsules	2178
Librium Injectable	2179

Chlorpromazine (Additive CNS-depressant effect). Products include:

Thorazine Suppositories 2523

Chlorprothixene (Additive CNS-depressant effect).

No products indexed under this heading.

Chlorprothixene Hydrochloride (Additive CNS-depressant effect).

No products indexed under this heading.

Clorazepate Dipotassium (Additive CNS-depressant effect). Products include:

Tranxene 451

Clozapine (Additive CNS-depressant effect). Products include:

Clozaril Tablets.. 2252

Codeine Phosphate (Additive CNS-depressant effect). Products include:

Actifed with Codeine Cough Syrup..	1067
Brontex	1981
Deconsal C Expectorant Syrup	456
Deconsal Pediatric Syrup	457
Dimetane-DC Cough Syrup	2059
Empirin with Codeine Tablets	1093
Fioricet with Codeine Capsules	2260
Fiorinal with Codeine Capsules	2262
Isoclor Expectorant	990
Novahistine DH	2462
Novahistine Expectorant	2463
Nucofed	2051
Phenergan with Codeine	2777
Phenergan VC with Codeine	2781
Robitussin A-C Syrup	2073
Robitussin-DAC Syrup	2074
Ryna	ᴮᴰ 841
Soma Compound w/Codeine Tablets	2676
Tussi-Organidin NR Liquid and S NR Liquid	2677
Tylenol with Codeine	1583

Desflurane (Additive CNS-depressant effect). Products include:

Suprane 1813

Desipramine Hydrochloride (Propoxyphene slows the metabolism). Products include:

Norpramin Tablets 1526

Dezocine (Additive CNS-depressant effect). Products include:

Dalgan Injection 538

Diazepam (Additive CNS-depressant effect). Products include:

Dizac	1809
Valium Injectable	2182
Valium Tablets	2183
Valrelease Capsules	2169

Dicumarol (Enhanced anticoagulant effect).

No products indexed under this heading.

Divalproex Sodium (Propoxyphene slows the metabolism). Products include:

Depakote Tablets...................................... 415

Doxepin Hydrochloride (Propoxyphene slows the metabolism). Products include:

Sinequan	2205
Zonalon Cream	1055

Droperidol (Additive CNS-depressant effect). Products include:

Inapsine Injection..................................... 1296

Enflurane (Additive CNS-depressant effect).

No products indexed under this heading.

Estazolam (Additive CNS-depressant effect). Products include:

ProSom Tablets 449

Ethchlorvynol (Additive CNS-depressant effect). Products include:

Placidyl Capsules 448

Ethinamate (Additive CNS-depressant effect).

No products indexed under this heading.

Ethosuximide (Propoxyphene slows the metabolism). Products include:

Zarontin Capsules	1928
Zarontin Syrup	1929

Ethotoin (Propoxyphene slows the metabolism). Products include:

Peganone Tablets 446

Felbamate (Concurrent use may result in severe neurological signs, including coma). Products include:

Felbatol 2666

Fentanyl (Additive CNS-depressant effect). Products include:

Duragesic Transdermal System........ 1288

Fentanyl Citrate (Additive CNS-depressant effect). Products include:

Sublimaze Injection.................................. 1307

Fluoxetine Hydrochloride (Propoxyphene slows the metabolism). Products include:

Prozac Pulvules & Liquid, Oral Solution 919

Fluphenazine Decanoate (Additive CNS-depressant effect). Products include:

Prolixin Decanoate 509

Fluphenazine Enanthate (Additive CNS-depressant effect). Products include:

Prolixin Enanthate 509

Fluphenazine Hydrochloride (Additive CNS-depressant effect). Products include:

Prolixin 509

Flurazepam Hydrochloride (Additive CNS-depressant effect). Products include:

Dalmane Capsules 2173

Glutethimide (Additive CNS-depressant effect).

No products indexed under this heading.

Haloperidol (Additive CNS-depressant effect). Products include:

Haldol Injection, Tablets and Concentrate 1575

Haloperidol Decanoate (Additive CNS-depressant effect). Products include:

Haldol Decanoate..................................... 1577

Hydrocodone Bitartrate (Additive CNS-depressant effect). Products include:

Anexsia 5/500 Elixir	1781
Anexia Tablets	1782
Codiclear DH Syrup	791
Deconamine CX Cough and Cold Liquid and Tablets	1319
Duratuss HD Elixir	2565
Hycodan Tablets and Syrup	930
Hycomine Compound Tablets	932
Hycomine	931
Hycotuss Expectorant Syrup	933
Hydrocet Capsules	782
Lorcet 10/650	1018
Lortab	2566
Tussend	1783
Tussend Expectorant	1785
Vicodin Tablets	1356
Vicodin ES Tablets	1357
Vicodin Tuss Expectorant	1358
Zydone Capsules	949

Hydrocodone Polistirex (Additive CNS-depressant effect). Products include:

Tussionex Pennkinetic Extended-Release Suspension 998

Hydroxyzine Hydrochloride (Additive CNS-depressant effect). Products include:

Atarax Tablets & Syrup............................ 2185

Marax Tablets & DF Syrup.................... 2200

Vistaril Intramuscular Solution.......... 2216

Imipramine Hydrochloride (Propoxyphene slows the metabolism). Products include:

Tofranil Ampuls	854
Tofranil Tablets	856

Imipramine Pamoate (Propoxyphene slows the metabolism). Products include:

Tofranil-PM Capsules.............................. 857

Isocarboxazid (Propoxyphene slows the metabolism).

No products indexed under this heading.

Isoflurane (Additive CNS-depressant effect).

No products indexed under this heading.

Ketamine Hydrochloride (Additive CNS-depressant effect).

No products indexed under this heading.

Lamotrigine (Propoxyphene may slow the metabolism of anticonvulsants). Products include:

Lamictal Tablets....................................... 1112

Levomethadyl Acetate Hydrochloride (Additive CNS-depressant effect). Products include:

Orlamm 2239

Levorphanol Tartrate (Additive CNS-depressant effect). Products include:

Levo-Dromoran 2129

Lorazepam (Additive CNS-depressant effect). Products include:

Ativan Injection	2698
Ativan Tablets	2700

Loxapine Hydrochloride (Additive CNS-depressant effect). Products include:

Loxitane 1378

Loxapine Succinate (Additive CNS-depressant effect). Products include:

Loxitane Capsules 1378

Maprotiline Hydrochloride (Propoxyphene slows the metabolism). Products include:

Ludiomil Tablets....................................... 843

Meperidine Hydrochloride (Additive CNS-depressant effect). Products include:

Demerol	2308
Mepergan Injection	2753

Mephenytoin (Propoxyphene slows the metabolism). Products include:

Mesantoin Tablets 2272

Mephobarbital (Additive CNS-depressant effect). Products include:

Mebaral Tablets 2322

Meprobamate (Additive CNS-depressant effect). Products include:

Miltown Tablets	2672
PMB 200 and PMB 400	2783

Mesoridazine Besylate (Additive CNS-depressant effect). Products include:

Serentil... 684

Methadone Hydrochloride (Additive CNS-depressant effect). Products include:

Methadone Hydrochloride Oral Concentrate	2233
Methadone Hydrochloride Oral Solution & Tablets	2235

Methohexital Sodium (Additive CNS-depressant effect). Products include:

Brevital Sodium Vials 1429

Methotrimeprazine (Additive CNS-depressant effect). Products include:

Levoprome 1274

(ᴮᴰ Described in PDR For Nonprescription Drugs) (◎ Described in PDR For Ophthalmology)

Methoxyflurane (Additive CNS-depressant effect).
- No products indexed under this heading.

Methsuximide (Propoxyphene slows the metabolism). Products include:
- Celontin Kapseals 1899

Midazolam Hydrochloride (Additive CNS-depressant effect). Products include:
- Versed Injection 2170

Molindone Hydrochloride (Additive CNS-depressant effect). Products include:
- Moban Tablets and Concentrate 1048

Morphine Sulfate (Additive CNS-depressant effect). Products include:
- Astramorph/PF Injection, USP (Preservative-Free) 535
- Duramorph 962
- Infumorph 200 and Infumorph 500 Sterile Solutions 965
- MS Contin Tablets 1994
- MSIR 1997
- Oramorph SR (Morphine Sulfate Sustained Release Tablets) 2236
- RMS Suppositories 2657
- Roxanol 2243

Nefazodone Hydrochloride (Propoxyphene slows the metabolism). Products include:
- Serzone Tablets 771

Nortriptyline Hydrochloride (Propoxyphene slows the metabolism). Products include:
- Pamelor 2280

Opium Alkaloids (Additive CNS-depressant effect).
- No products indexed under this heading.

Oxazepam (Additive CNS-depressant effect). Products include:
- Serax Capsules 2810
- Serax Tablets 2810

Oxycodone Hydrochloride (Additive CNS-depressant effect). Products include:
- Percocet Tablets 938
- Percodan Tablets 939
- Percodan-Demi Tablets 940
- Roxicodone Tablets, Oral Solution & Intensol (Oxycodone) 2244
- Tylox Capsules 1584

Paramethadione (Propoxyphene slows the metabolism).
- No products indexed under this heading.

Paroxetine Hydrochloride (Propoxyphene slows the metabolism). Products include:
- Paxil Tablets 2505

Pentobarbital Sodium (Additive CNS-depressant effect). Products include:
- Nembutal Sodium Capsules 436
- Nembutal Sodium Solution 438
- Nembutal Sodium Suppositories 440

Perphenazine (Additive CNS-depressant effect). Products include:
- Etrafon 2355
- Triavil Tablets 1757
- Trilafon 2389

Phenacemide (Propoxyphene slows the metabolism). Products include:
- Phenurone Tablets 447

Phenelzine Sulfate (Propoxyphene slows the metabolism). Products include:
- Nardil 1920

Phenobarbital (Propoxyphene slows the metabolism; additive CNS-depressant effect). Products include:
- Arco-Lase Plus Tablets 512
- Bellergal-S Tablets 2250
- Donnatal 2060
- Donnatal Extentabs 2061
- Donnatal Tablets 2060
- Phenobarbital Elixir and Tablets 1469
- Quadrinal Tablets 1350

Phensuximide (Propoxyphene slows the metabolism). Products include:
- Milontin Kapseals 1920

Phenytoin (Propoxyphene slows the metabolism). Products include:
- Dilantin Infatabs 1908
- Dilantin-125 Suspension 1911

Phenytoin Sodium (Propoxyphene slows the metabolism). Products include:
- Dilantin Kapseals 1906
- Dilantin Parenteral 1910

Prazepam (Additive CNS-depressant effect).
- No products indexed under this heading.

Primidone (Propoxyphene slows the metabolism). Products include:
- Mysoline 2754

Probenecid (Uricosuric effect inhibited). Products include:
- Benemid Tablets 1611
- ColBENEMID Tablets 1622

Prochlorperazine (Additive CNS-depressant effect). Products include:
- Compazine 2470

Promethazine Hydrochloride (Additive CNS-depressant effect). Products include:
- Mepergan Injection 2753
- Phenergan with Codeine 2777
- Phenergan with Dextromethorphan 2778
- Phenergan Injection 2773
- Phenergan Suppositories 2775
- Phenergan Syrup 2774
- Phenergan Tablets 2775
- Phenergan VC 2779
- Phenergan VC with Codeine 2781

Propofol (Additive CNS-depressant effect). Products include:
- Diprivan Injection 2833

Propoxyphene Napsylate (Additive CNS-depressant effect). Products include:
- Darvon-N/Darvocet-N 1433

Protriptyline Hydrochloride (Propoxyphene slows the metabolism). Products include:
- Vivactil Tablets 1774

Quazepam (Additive CNS-depressant effect). Products include:
- Doral Tablets 2664

Risperidone (Additive CNS-depressant effect). Products include:
- Risperdal 1301

Secobarbital Sodium (Additive CNS-depressant effect). Products include:
- Seconal Sodium Pulvules 1474

Sertraline Hydrochloride (Propoxyphene slows the metabolism). Products include:
- Zoloft Tablets 2217

Sufentanil Citrate (Additive CNS-depressant effect). Products include:
- Sufenta Injection 1309

Sulfinpyrazone (Uricosuric effect inhibited). Products include:
- Anturane 807

Temazepam (Additive CNS-depressant effect). Products include:
- Restoril Capsules 2284

Thiamylal Sodium (Additive CNS-depressant effect).
- No products indexed under this heading.

Thioridazine Hydrochloride (Additive CNS-depressant effect). Products include:
- Mellaril 2269

Thiothixene (Additive CNS-depressant effect). Products include:
- Navane Capsules and Concentrate 2201
- Navane Intramuscular 2202

Tranylcypromine Sulfate (Propoxyphene slows the metabolism). Products include:
- Parnate Tablets 2503

Trazodone Hydrochloride (Propoxyphene slows the metabolism). Products include:
- Desyrel and Desyrel Dividose 503

Triazolam (Additive CNS-depressant effect). Products include:
- Halcion Tablets 2611

Trifluoperazine Hydrochloride (Additive CNS-depressant effect). Products include:
- Stelazine 2514

Trimethadione (Propoxyphene slows the metabolism).
- No products indexed under this heading.

Trimipramine Maleate (Propoxyphene slows the metabolism). Products include:
- Surmontil Capsules 2811

Valproic Acid (Propoxyphene slows the metabolism). Products include:
- Depakene 413

Venlafaxine Hydrochloride (Propoxyphene slows the metabolism). Products include:
- Effexor 2719

Warfarin Sodium (Enhanced anticoagulant effect). Products include:
- Coumadin 926

Zolpidem Tartrate (Additive CNS-depressant effect). Products include:
- Ambien Tablets 2416

Food Interactions

Alcohol (Additive CNS-depressant effect).

DARVON PULVULES

(Propoxyphene Hydrochloride) 1435

See **Darvocet-N 50 Tablets**

DARVON-N SUSPENSION & TABLETS

(Propoxyphene Napsylate) 1433

See **Darvocet-N 50 Tablets**

DAYPRO CAPLETS

(Oxaprozin) 2426

May interact with salicylates, oral anticoagulants, beta blockers, and certain other agents. Compounds in these categories include:

Acebutolol Hydrochloride (Potential for statistically significant but transient increase in blood pressure). Products include:
- Sectral Capsules 2807

Aspirin (Oxaprozin displaces salicylates from plasma protein binding sites; coadministration would be expected to increase the risk of salicylate toxicity). Products include:
- Alka-Seltzer Effervescent Antacid and Pain Reliever 701
- Alka-Seltzer Extra Strength Effervescent Antacid and Pain Reliever 703
- Alka-Seltzer Lemon Lime Effervescent Antacid and Pain Reliever 703
- Alka-Seltzer Plus Cold Medicine 705
- Alka-Seltzer Plus Cold & Cough Medicine 708
- Alka-Seltzer Plus Night-Time Cold Medicine 707
- Alka Seltzer Plus Sinus Medicine 707
- Arthritis Foundation Safety Coated Aspirin Tablets 675
- Arthritis Pain Ascriptin 631
- Maximum Strength Ascriptin 630
- Regular Strength Ascriptin Tablets 629
- Arthritis Strength BC Powder 609
- BC Cold Powder Multi-Symptom Formula (Cold-Sinus-Allergy) 609
- BC Cold Powder Non-Drowsy Formula (Cold-Sinus) 609
- BC Powder 609
- Bayer Children's Chewable Aspirin 711
- Genuine Bayer Aspirin Tablets & Caplets 713
- Extra Strength Bayer Arthritis Pain Regimen Formula 711
- Extra Strength Bayer Aspirin Caplets & Tablets 712
- Extended-Release Bayer 8-Hour Aspirin 712
- Extra Strength Bayer Plus Aspirin Caplets 713
- Extra Strength Bayer PM Aspirin 713
- Bayer Enteric Aspirin 709
- Bufferin Analgesic Tablets and Caplets 613
- Arthritis Strength Bufferin Analgesic Caplets 614
- Extra Strength Bufferin Analgesic Tablets 615
- Cama Arthritis Pain Reliever 785
- Darvon Compound-65 Pulvules 1435
- Easprin 1914
- Ecotrin 2455
- Ecotrin Enteric Coated Aspirin Maximum Strength Tablets and Caplets 816
- Ecotrin Enteric Coated Aspirin Regular Strength Tablets 2455
- Empirin Aspirin Tablets 854
- Empirin with Codeine Tablets 1093
- Excedrin Extra-Strength Analgesic Tablets & Caplets 732
- Fiorinal Capsules 2261
- Fiorinal with Codeine Capsules 2262
- Fiorinal Tablets 2261
- Halfprin 1362
- Healthprin Aspirin 2455
- Norgesic 1496
- Percodan Tablets 939
- Percodan-Demi Tablets 940
- Robaxisal Tablets 2071
- Soma Compound w/Codeine Tablets 2676
- Soma Compound Tablets 2675
- St. Joseph Adult Chewable Aspirin (81 mg.) 808
- Talwin Compound 2335
- Ursinus Inlay-Tabs 794
- Vanquish Analgesic Caplets 731

Atenolol (Potential for statistically significant but transient increase in blood pressure). Products include:
- Tenoretic Tablets 2845
- Tenormin Tablets and I.V. Injection 2847

Betaxolol Hydrochloride (Potential for statistically significant but transient increase in blood pressure). Products include:
- Betoptic Ophthalmic Solution 469
- Betoptic S Ophthalmic Suspension 471
- Kerlone Tablets 2436

Bisoprolol Fumarate (Potential for statistically significant but transient increase in blood pressure). Products include:
- Zebeta Tablets 1413
- Ziac 1415

Carteolol Hydrochloride (Potential for statistically significant but transient increase in blood pressure). Products include:
- Cartrol Tablets 410
- Ocupress Ophthalmic Solution, 1% Sterile ⊙ 309

Choline Magnesium Trisalicylate (Oxaprozin displaces salicylates from plasma protein binding sites; coadministration would be expected to increase the risk of salicylate toxicity). Products include:
- Trilisate 2000

Cimetidine (Concurrent use may reduce the total body clearance of oxaprozin). Products include:
- Tagamet Tablets 2516

Cimetidine Hydrochloride (Concurrent use may reduce the total body clearance of oxaprozin). Products include:
- Tagamet 2516

IMPORTANT NOTE: Always consult each drug listing in the patient's regimen for possible interactions.

Daypro

Dicumarol (Caution should be exercised if used concurrently).

No products indexed under this heading.

Diflunisal (Oxaprozin displaces salicylates from plasma protein binding sites; coadministration would be expected to increase the risk of salicylate toxicity). Products include:

Dolobid Tablets....................................... 1654

Esmolol Hydrochloride (Potential for statistically significant but transient increase in blood pressure). Products include:

Brevibloc Injection................................. 1808

Labetalol Hydrochloride (Potential for statistically significant but transient increase in blood pressure). Products include:

Normodyne Injection 2377
Normodyne Tablets 2379
Trandate 1185

Levobunolol Hydrochloride (Potential for statistically significant but transient increase in blood pressure). Products include:

Betagan .... ◉ 233

Magnesium Salicylate (Oxaprozin displaces salicylates from plasma protein binding sites; coadministration would be expected to increase the risk of salicylate toxicity). Products include:

Backache Caplets .... ®D 613
Bayer Select Backache Pain Relief Formula .... ®D 715
Doan's Extra-Strength Analgesic.... ®D 633
Extra Strength Doan's P.M. .... ®D 633
Doan's Regular Strength Analgesic .... ®D 634
Mobigesic Tablets .... ®D 602

Metipranolol Hydrochloride (Potential for statistically significant but transient increase in blood pressure). Products include:

OptiPranolol (Metipranolol 0.3%) Sterile Ophthalmic Solution........... ◉ 258

Metoprolol Succinate (Potential for statistically significant but transient increase in blood pressure). Products include:

Toprol-XL Tablets 565

Metoprolol Tartrate (Potential for statistically significant but transient increase in blood pressure). Products include:

Lopressor Ampuls 830
Lopressor HCT Tablets 832
Lopressor Tablets 830

Nadolol (Potential for statistically significant but transient increase in blood pressure).

No products indexed under this heading.

Penbutolol Sulfate (Potential for statistically but transient increase in blood pressure). Products include:

Levatol 2403

Pindolol (Potential for statistically significant but transient increase in blood pressure). Products include:

Visken Tablets... 2299

Propranolol Hydrochloride (Potential for statistically significant but transient increase in blood pressure). Products include:

Inderal 2728
Inderal LA Long Acting Capsules 2730
Inderide Tablets 2732
Inderide LA Long Acting Capsules .. 2734

Ranitidine Hydrochloride (Concurrent use may reduce the total body clearance of oxaprozin). Products include:

Zantac.. 1209
Zantac Injection 1207
Zantac Syrup 1209

Salsalate (Oxaprozin displaces salicylates from plasma protein binding sites; coadministration would be expected to increase the risk of salicylate toxicity). Products include:

Mono-Gesic Tablets 792
Salflex Tablets... 786

Sotalol Hydrochloride (Potential for statistically significant but transient increase in blood pressure). Products include:

Betapace Tablets 641

Timolol Hemihydrate (Potential for statistically significant but transient increase in blood pressure). Products include:

Betimol 0.25%, 0.5% .... ◉ 261

Timolol Maleate (Potential for statistically significant but transient increase in blood pressure). Products include:

Blocadren Tablets 1614
Timolide Tablets..................................... 1748
Timoptic in Ocudose 1753
Timoptic Sterile Ophthalmic Solution.. 1751
Timoptic-XE 1755

Warfarin Sodium (Caution should be exercised if used concurrently). Products include:

Coumadin 926

Food Interactions

Food, unspecified (Reduces the rate of absorption of oxaprozin, but the extent of absorption is unchanged).

DEBROX DROPS

(Carbamide Peroxide) .... ®D 815
None cited in PDR database.

DECADRON ELIXIR

(Dexamethasone)...................................1633
May interact with oral anticoagulants, potassium sparing diuretics, and certain other agents. Compounds in these categories include:

Amiloride Hydrochloride (Hypokalemia). Products include:

Midamor Tablets 1703
Moduretic Tablets 1705

Aspirin (Aspirin should be used cautiously in conjunction with corticosteroids in hypoprothrombinemia). Products include:

Alka-Seltzer Effervescent Antacid and Pain Reliever.................................. ®D 701
Alka-Seltzer Extra Strength Effervescent Antacid and Pain Reliever .... ®D 703
Alka-Seltzer Lemon Lime Effervescent Antacid and Pain Reliever .... ®D 703
Alka-Seltzer Plus Cold Medicine .... ®D 705
Alka-Seltzer Plus Cold & Cough Medicine .... ®D 708
Alka-Seltzer Plus Night-Time Cold Medicine .... ®D 707
Alka Seltzer Plus Sinus Medicine .. ®D 707
Arthritis Foundation Safety Coated Aspirin Tablets .... ®D 675
Arthritis Pain Ascriptin .... ®D 631
Maximum Strength Ascriptin .... ®D 630
Regular Strength Ascriptin Tablets .... ®D 629
Arthritis Strength BC Powder........... ®D 609
BC Cold Powder Multi-Symptom Formula (Cold-Sinus-Allergy) ...... ®D 609
BC Cold Powder Non-Drowsy Formula (Cold-Sinus) .... ®D 609
BC Powder .... ®D 609
Bayer Children's Chewable Aspirin.. ®D 711
Genuine Bayer Aspirin Tablets & Caplets .... ®D 713
Extra Strength Bayer Arthritis Pain Regimen Formula .... ®D 711
Extra Strength Bayer Aspirin Caplets & Tablets .... ®D 712
Extended-Release Bayer 8-Hour Aspirin .... ®D 712
Extra Strength Bayer Plus Aspirin Caplets .... ®D 713
Extra Strength Bayer PM Aspirin .. ®D 713
Bayer Enteric Aspirin .... ®D 709
Bufferin Analgesic Tablets and Caplets .... ®D 613
Arthritis Strength Bufferin Analgesic Caplets .... ®D 614
Extra Strength Bufferin Analgesic Tablets .... ®D 615
Cama Arthritis Pain Reliever............ ®D 785
Darvon Compound-65 Pulvules 1435
Easprin 1914
Ecotrin 2455
Ecotrin Enteric Coated Aspirin Maximum Strength Tablets and Caplets .... ®D 816
Ecotrin Enteric Coated Aspirin Regular Strength Tablets 2455
Empirin Aspirin Tablets .... ®D 854
Empirin with Codeine Tablets........... 1093
Excedrin Extra-Strength Analgesic Tablets & Caplets 732
Fiorinal Capsules 2261
Fiorinal with Codeine Capsules 2262
Fiorinal Tablets 2261
Halfprin 1362
Healthprin Aspirin 2455
Norgesic... 1496
Percodan Tablets.................................... 939
Percodan-Demi Tablets........................ 940
Robaxisal Tablets................................... 2071
Soma Compound w/Codeine Tablets 2676
Soma Compound Tablets..................... 2675
St. Joseph Adult Chewable Aspirin (81 mg.) .... ®D 808
Talwin Compound 2335
Ursinus Inlay-Tabs................................ ®D 794
Vanquish Analgesic Caplets .... ®D 731

Dicumarol (Response to dicumarol inhibited).

No products indexed under this heading.

Ephedrine (Enhanced metabolic clearance of corticosteroids).

Ephedrine Hydrochloride (Enhanced metabolic clearance of corticosteroids). Products include:

Primatene Dual Action Formula...... ®D 872
Primatene Tablets .... ®D 873
Quadrinal Tablets 1350

Ephedrine Sulfate (Enhanced metabolic clearance of corticosteroids). Products include:

Bronkaid Caplets .... ®D 717
Marax Tablets & DF Syrup.................. 2200

Ephedrine Tannate (Enhanced metabolic clearance of corticosteroids). Products include:

Rynatuss 2673

Live Virus Vaccines (Contraindicated).

Phenobarbital (Enhanced metabolic clearance of corticosteroids). Products include:

Arco-Lase Plus Tablets 512
Bellergal-S Tablets 2250
Donnatal 2060
Donnatal Extentabs............................... 2061
Donnatal Tablets 2060
Phenobarbital Elixir and Tablets 1469
Quadrinal Tablets 1350

Phenytoin (Enhanced metabolic clearance of corticosteroids). Products include:

Dilantin Infatabs.................................... 1908
Dilantin-125 Suspension 1911

Phenytoin Sodium (Enhanced metabolic clearance of corticosteroids). Products include:

Dilantin Kapseals................................... 1906
Dilantin Parenteral 1910

Rifampin (Enhanced metabolic clearance of corticosteroids). Products include:

Rifadin 1528
Rifamate Capsules 1530
Rifater... 1532
Rimactane Capsules 847

Spironolactone (Hypokalemia). Products include:

Aldactazide... 2413
Aldactone 2414

Triamterene (Hypokalemia). Products include:

Dyazide 2479
Dyrenium Capsules 2481
Maxzide 1380

Warfarin Sodium (Response to warfarin inhibited). Products include:

Coumadin 926

DECADRON PHOSPHATE INJECTION

(Dexamethasone Sodium Phosphate) **1637**
May interact with potassium sparing diuretics, oral anticoagulants, and certain other agents. Compounds in these categories include:

Amiloride Hydrochloride (Hypokalemia). Products include:

Midamor Tablets 1703
Moduretic Tablets 1705

Aspirin (Aspirin should be used cautiously in conjunction with corticosteroids in hypoprothrombinemia). Products include:

Alka-Seltzer Effervescent Antacid and Pain Reliever.................................. ®D 701
Alka-Seltzer Extra Strength Effervescent Antacid and Pain Reliever .... ®D 703
Alka-Seltzer Lemon Lime Effervescent Antacid and Pain Reliever .... ®D 703
Alka-Seltzer Plus Cold Medicine .... ®D 705
Alka-Seltzer Plus Cold & Cough Medicine .... ®D 708
Alka-Seltzer Plus Night-Time Cold Medicine .... ®D 707
Alka Seltzer Plus Sinus Medicine .. ®D 707
Arthritis Foundation Safety Coated Aspirin Tablets .... ®D 675
Arthritis Pain Ascriptin .... ®D 631
Maximum Strength Ascriptin .... ®D 630
Regular Strength Ascriptin Tablets .... ®D 629
Arthritis Strength BC Powder........... ®D 609
BC Cold Powder Multi-Symptom Formula (Cold-Sinus-Allergy) ...... ®D 609
BC Cold Powder Non-Drowsy Formula (Cold-Sinus) .... ®D 609
BC Powder .... ®D 609
Bayer Children's Chewable Aspirin.. ®D 711
Genuine Bayer Aspirin Tablets & Caplets .... ®D 713
Extra Strength Bayer Arthritis Pain Regimen Formula .... ®D 711
Extra Strength Bayer Aspirin Caplets & Tablets .... ®D 712
Extended-Release Bayer 8-Hour Aspirin .... ®D 712
Extra Strength Bayer Plus Aspirin Caplets .... ®D 713
Extra Strength Bayer PM Aspirin .. ®D 713
Bayer Enteric Aspirin .... ®D 709
Bufferin Analgesic Tablets and Caplets .... ®D 613
Arthritis Strength Bufferin Analgesic Caplets .... ®D 614
Extra Strength Bufferin Analgesic Tablets .... ®D 615
Cama Arthritis Pain Reliever............ ®D 785
Darvon Compound-65 Pulvules 1435
Easprin 1914
Ecotrin 2455
Ecotrin Enteric Coated Aspirin Maximum Strength Tablets and Caplets .... ®D 816
Ecotrin Enteric Coated Aspirin Regular Strength Tablets 2455
Empirin Aspirin Tablets .... ®D 854
Empirin with Codeine Tablets........... 1093
Excedrin Extra-Strength Analgesic Tablets & Caplets 732
Fiorinal Capsules 2261
Fiorinal with Codeine Capsules 2262
Fiorinal Tablets 2261
Halfprin 1362
Healthprin Aspirin 2455
Norgesic... 1496
Percodan Tablets.................................... 939
Percodan-Demi Tablets........................ 940
Robaxisal Tablets................................... 2071
Soma Compound w/Codeine Tablets 2676
Soma Compound Tablets..................... 2675
St. Joseph Adult Chewable Aspirin (81 mg.) .... ®D 808

(®D Described in PDR For Nonprescription Drugs) (◉ Described in PDR For Ophthalmology)

Interactions Index — Decadron Turbinaire

Talwin Compound 2335
Ursinus Inlay-Tabs................................. ⊕ 794
Vanquish Analgesic Caplets .... ⊕ 731

Dicumarol (Response to dicumarol inhibited).

No products indexed under this heading.

Ephedrine (Enhanced metabolic clearance of corticosteroids).

Ephedrine Hydrochloride (Enhanced metabolic clearance of corticosteroids). Products include:

Primatene Dual Action Formula...... ⊕ 872
Primatene Tablets .... ⊕ 873
Quadrinal Tablets 1350

Ephedrine Sulfate (Enhanced metabolic clearance of corticosteroids). Products include:

Bronkaid Caplets .... ⊕ 717
Marax Tablets & DF Syrup.................. 2200

Ephedrine Tannate (Enhanced metabolic clearance of corticosteroids). Products include:

Rynatuss 2673

Live Virus Vaccines (Contraindicated).

Phenobarbital (Enhanced metabolic clearance of corticosteroids). Products include:

Arco-Lase Plus Tablets 512
Bellergal-S Tablets 2250
Donnatal 2060
Donnatal Extentabs............................... 2061
Donnatal Tablets 2060
Phenobarbital Elixir and Tablets 1469
Quadrinal Tablets 1350

Phenytoin (Enhanced metabolic clearance of corticosteroids). Products include:

Dilantin Infatabs.................................... 1908
Dilantin-125 Suspension 1911

Phenytoin Sodium (Enhanced metabolic clearance of corticosteroids). Products include:

Dilantin Kapseals 1906
Dilantin Parenteral 1910

Rifampin (Enhanced metabolic clearance of corticosteroids). Products include:

Rifadin 1528
Rifamate Capsules 1530
Rifater.. 1532
Rimactane Capsules 847

Spironolactone (Hypokalemia). Products include:

Aldactazide... 2413
Aldactone 2414

Triamterene (Hypokalemia). Products include:

Dyazide 2479
Dyrenium Capsules................................ 2481
Maxzide 1380

Warfarin Sodium (Response to warfarin inhibited). Products include:

Coumadin 926

DECADRON PHOSPHATE RESPIHALER

(Dexamethasone Sodium Phosphate) 1642
May interact with oral anticoagulants, potassium sparing diuretics, and certain other agents. Compounds in these categories include:

Amiloride Hydrochloride (Hypokalemia). Products include:

Midamor Tablets 1703
Moduretic Tablets 1705

Aspirin (Concomitant administration requires caution). Products include:

Alka-Seltzer Effervescent Antacid and Pain Reliever .... ⊕ 701
Alka-Seltzer Extra Strength Effervescent Antacid and Pain Reliever .... ⊕ 703
Alka-Seltzer Lemon Lime Effervescent Antacid and Pain Reliever .... ⊕ 703
Alka-Seltzer Plus Cold Medicine .... ⊕ 705
Alka-Seltzer Plus Cold & Cough Medicine .... ⊕ 708
Alka-Seltzer Plus Night-Time Cold Medicine .... ⊕ 707
Alka Seltzer Plus Sinus Medicine .. ⊕ 707
Arthritis Foundation Safety Coated Aspirin Tablets .... ⊕ 675
Arthritis Pain Ascriptin .... ⊕ 631
Maximum Strength Ascriptin .... ⊕ 630
Regular Strength Ascriptin Tablets .... ⊕ 629
Arthritis Strength BC Powder.......... ⊕ 609
BC Cold Powder Multi-Symptom Formula (Cold-Sinus-Allergy) ...... ⊕ 609
BC Cold Powder Non-Drowsy Formula (Cold-Sinus) .... ⊕ 609
BC Powder .... ⊕ 609
Bayer Children's Chewable Aspirin .... ⊕ 711
Genuine Bayer Aspirin Tablets & Caplets .... ⊕ 713
Extra Strength Bayer Arthritis Pain Regimen Formula .... ⊕ 711
Extra Strength Bayer Aspirin Caplets & Tablets .... ⊕ 712
Extended-Release Bayer 8-Hour Aspirin .... ⊕ 712
Extra Strength Bayer Plus Aspirin Caplets .... ⊕ 713
Extra Strength Bayer PM Aspirin .. ⊕ 713
Bayer Enteric Aspirin.......................... ⊕ 709
Bufferin Analgesic Tablets and Caplets .... ⊕ 613
Arthritis Strength Bufferin Analgesic Caplets .... ⊕ 614
Extra Strength Bufferin Analgesic Tablets .... ⊕ 615
Cama Arthritis Pain Reliever............ ⊕ 785
Darvon Compound-65 Pulvules 1435
Easprin... 1914
Ecotrin 2455
Ecotrin Enteric Coated Aspirin Maximum Strength Tablets and Caplets .... ⊕ 816
Ecotrin Enteric Coated Aspirin Regular Strength Tablets 2455
Empirin Aspirin Tablets .... ⊕ 854
Empirin with Codeine Tablets........... 1093
Excedrin Extra-Strength Analgesic Tablets & Caplets 732
Fiorinal Capsules 2261
Fiorinal with Codeine Capsules 2262
Fiorinal Tablets 2261
Halfprin 1362
Healthprin Aspirin 2455
Norgesic... 1496
Percodan Tablets................................... 939
Percodan-Demi Tablets........................ 940
Robaxisal Tablets................................... 2071
Soma Compound w/Codeine Tablets 2676
Soma Compound Tablets..................... 2675
St. Joseph Adult Chewable Aspirin (81 mg.) .... ⊕ 808
Talwin Compound 2335
Ursinus Inlay-Tabs................................ ⊕ 794
Vanquish Analgesic Caplets .... ⊕ 731

Dicumarol (Response to dicumarol inhibited).

No products indexed under this heading.

Ephedrine (Enhanced metabolic clearance of corticosteroids).

Ephedrine Hydrochloride (Enhanced metabolic clearance of corticosteroids). Products include:

Primatene Dual Action Formula...... ⊕ 872
Primatene Tablets .... ⊕ 873
Quadrinal Tablets 1350

Ephedrine Sulfate (Enhanced metabolic clearance of corticosteroids). Products include:

Bronkaid Caplets .... ⊕ 717
Marax Tablets & DF Syrup.................. 2200

Ephedrine Tannate (Enhanced metabolic clearance of corticosteroids). Products include:

Rynatuss 2673

Live Virus Vaccines (Contraindicated).

Phenobarbital (Enhanced metabolic clearance of corticosteroids). Products include:

Arco-Lase Plus Tablets 512
Bellergal-S Tablets 2250
Donnatal 2060
Donnatal Extentabs............................... 2061

Donnatal Tablets 2060
Phenobarbital Elixir and Tablets 1469
Quadrinal Tablets 1350

Phenytoin (Enhanced metabolic clearance of corticosteroids). Products include:

Dilantin Infatabs.................................... 1908
Dilantin-125 Suspension 1911

Phenytoin Sodium (Enhanced metabolic clearance of corticosteroids). Products include:

Dilantin Kapseals 1906
Dilantin Parenteral 1910

Rifampin (Enhanced metabolic clearance of corticosteroids). Products include:

Rifadin 1528
Rifamate Capsules 1530
Rifater.. 1532
Rimactane Capsules 847

Spironolactone (Hypokalemia). Products include:

Aldactazide... 2413
Aldactone 2414

Triamterene (Hypokalemia). Products include:

Dyazide 2479
Dyrenium Capsules................................ 2481
Maxzide 1380

Warfarin Sodium (Response to warfarin inhibited). Products include:

Coumadin 926

DECADRON PHOSPHATE STERILE OPHTHALMIC OINTMENT

(Dexamethasone Sodium Phosphate) 1641
None cited in PDR database.

DECADRON PHOSPHATE STERILE OPHTHALMIC SOLUTION

(Dexamethasone Sodium Phosphate) 1642
None cited in PDR database.

DECADRON PHOSPHATE TOPICAL CREAM

(Dexamethasone Sodium Phosphate) 1644
None cited in PDR database.

DECADRON PHOSPHATE TURBINAIRE

(Dexamethasone Sodium Phosphate) 1645
May interact with potassium sparing diuretics, oral anticoagulants, and certain other agents. Compounds in these categories include:

Amiloride Hydrochloride (Hypokalemia). Products include:

Midamor Tablets 1703
Moduretic Tablets 1705

Aspirin (Concomitant administration requires caution). Products include:

Alka-Seltzer Effervescent Antacid and Pain Reliever .... ⊕ 701
Alka-Seltzer Extra Strength Effervescent Antacid and Pain Reliever .... ⊕ 703
Alka-Seltzer Lemon Lime Effervescent Antacid and Pain Reliever .... ⊕ 703
Alka-Seltzer Plus Cold Medicine .... ⊕ 705
Alka-Seltzer Plus Cold & Cough Medicine .... ⊕ 708
Alka-Seltzer Plus Night-Time Cold Medicine .... ⊕ 707
Alka Seltzer Plus Sinus Medicine .. ⊕ 707
Arthritis Foundation Safety Coated Aspirin Tablets .... ⊕ 675
Arthritis Pain Ascriptin .... ⊕ 631
Maximum Strength Ascriptin .... ⊕ 630
Regular Strength Ascriptin Tablets .... ⊕ 629
Arthritis Strength BC Powder.......... ⊕ 609
BC Cold Powder Multi-Symptom Formula (Cold-Sinus-Allergy) ...... ⊕ 609
BC Cold Powder Non-Drowsy Formula (Cold-Sinus) .... ⊕ 609
BC Powder .... ⊕ 609
Bayer Children's Chewable Aspirin .... ⊕ 711
Genuine Bayer Aspirin Tablets & Caplets .... ⊕ 713
Extra Strength Bayer Arthritis Pain Regimen Formula .... ⊕ 711
Extra Strength Bayer Aspirin Caplets & Tablets .... ⊕ 712
Extended-Release Bayer 8-Hour Aspirin .... ⊕ 712
Extra Strength Bayer Plus Aspirin Caplets .... ⊕ 713
Extra Strength Bayer PM Aspirin .. ⊕ 713
Bayer Enteric Aspirin.......................... ⊕ 709
Bufferin Analgesic Tablets and Caplets .... ⊕ 613
Arthritis Strength Bufferin Analgesic Caplets .... ⊕ 614
Extra Strength Bufferin Analgesic Tablets .... ⊕ 615
Cama Arthritis Pain Reliever............ ⊕ 785
Darvon Compound-65 Pulvules 1435
Easprin... 1914
Ecotrin 2455
Ecotrin Enteric Coated Aspirin Maximum Strength Tablets and Caplets .... ⊕ 816
Ecotrin Enteric Coated Aspirin Regular Strength Tablets 2455
Empirin Aspirin Tablets .... ⊕ 854
Empirin with Codeine Tablets........... 1093
Excedrin Extra-Strength Analgesic Tablets & Caplets 732
Fiorinal Capsules 2261
Fiorinal with Codeine Capsules 2262
Fiorinal Tablets 2261
Halfprin 1362
Healthprin Aspirin 2455
Norgesic... 1496
Percodan Tablets................................... 939
Percodan-Demi Tablets........................ 940
Robaxisal Tablets................................... 2071
Soma Compound w/Codeine Tablets 2676
Soma Compound Tablets..................... 2675
St. Joseph Adult Chewable Aspirin (81 mg.) .... ⊕ 808
Talwin Compound 2335
Ursinus Inlay-Tabs................................ ⊕ 794
Vanquish Analgesic Caplets .... ⊕ 731

Dicumarol (Response to dicumarol inhibited).

No products indexed under this heading.

Ephedrine (Enhanced metabolic clearance of corticosteroids).

Ephedrine Hydrochloride (Enhanced metabolic clearance of corticosteroids). Products include:

Primatene Dual Action Formula...... ⊕ 872
Primatene Tablets .... ⊕ 873
Quadrinal Tablets 1350

Ephedrine Sulfate (Enhanced metabolic clearance of corticosteroids). Products include:

Bronkaid Caplets .... ⊕ 717
Marax Tablets & DF Syrup.................. 2200

Ephedrine Tannate (Enhanced metabolic clearance of corticosteroids). Products include:

Rynatuss 2673

Live Virus Vaccines (Contraindicated).

Phenobarbital (Enhanced metabolic clearance of corticosteroids). Products include:

Arco-Lase Plus Tablets 512
Bellergal-S Tablets 2250
Donnatal 2060
Donnatal Extentabs............................... 2061
Donnatal Tablets 2060
Phenobarbital Elixir and Tablets 1469
Quadrinal Tablets 1350

Phenytoin (Enhanced metabolic clearance of corticosteroids). Products include:

Dilantin Infatabs.................................... 1908
Dilantin-125 Suspension 1911

Phenytoin Sodium (Enhanced metabolic clearance of corticosteroids). Products include:

Dilantin Kapseals 1906
Dilantin Parenteral 1910

Rifampin (Enhanced metabolic clearance of corticosteroids). Products include:

Rifadin 1528

IMPORTANT NOTE: Always consult each drug listing in the patient's regimen for possible interactions.

Decadron Turbinaire

Rifamate Capsules 1530
Rifater.. 1532
Rimactane Capsules................................... 847

Spironolactone (Hypokalemia). Products include:

Aldactazide.. 2413
Aldactone 2414

Triamterene (Hypokalemia). Products include:

Dyazide 2479
Dyrenium Capsules.................................... 2481
Maxzide 1380

Warfarin Sodium (Response to warfarin inhibited). Products include:

Coumadin 926

DECADRON PHOSPHATE WITH XYLOCAINE INJECTION, STERILE

(Dexamethasone Sodium Phosphate, Lidocaine Hydrochloride) 1639

May interact with potassium sparing diuretics, oral anticoagulants, and certain other agents. Compounds in these categories include:

Amiloride Hydrochloride (Hypokalemia). Products include:

Midamor Tablets 1703
Moduretic Tablets 1705

Aspirin (Aspirin should be used cautiously in conjunction with corticosteroids in hypoprothrombinemia). Products include:

Alka-Seltzer Effervescent Antacid and Pain Reliever .... ⊕D 701
Alka-Seltzer Extra Strength Effervescent Antacid and Pain Reliever .... ⊕D 703
Alka-Seltzer Lemon Lime Effervescent Antacid and Pain Reliever .... ⊕D 703
Alka-Seltzer Plus Cold Medicine .... ⊕D 705
Alka-Seltzer Plus Cold & Cough Medicine .... ⊕D 708
Alka-Seltzer Plus Night-Time Cold Medicine .... ⊕D 707
Alka Seltzer Plus Sinus Medicine .. ⊕D 707
Arthritis Foundation Safety Coated Aspirin Tablets .... ⊕D 675
Arthritis Pain Ascriptin .... ⊕D 631
Maximum Strength Ascriptin .... ⊕D 630
Regular Strength Ascriptin Tablets .... ⊕D 629
Arthritis Strength BC Powder.......... ⊕D 609
BC Cold Powder Multi-Symptom Formula (Cold-Sinus-Allergy) ...... ⊕D 609
BC Cold Powder Non-Drowsy Formula (Cold-Sinus) .... ⊕D 609
BC Powder .... ⊕D 609
Bayer Children's Chewable Aspirin... ⊕D 711
Genuine Bayer Aspirin Tablets & Caplets.. ⊕D 713
Extra Strength Bayer Arthritis Pain Regimen Formula .... ⊕D 711
Extra Strength Bayer Aspirin Caplets & Tablets .... ⊕D 712
Extended-Release Bayer 8-Hour Aspirin .... ⊕D 712
Extra Strength Bayer Plus Aspirin Caplets.. ⊕D 713
Extra Strength Bayer PM Aspirin .. ⊕D 713
Bayer Enteric Aspirin .... ⊕D 709
Bufferin Analgesic Tablets and Caplets.. ⊕D 613
Arthritis Strength Bufferin Analgesic Caplets .... ⊕D 614
Extra Strength Bufferin Analgesic Tablets .... ⊕D 615
Cama Arthritis Pain Reliever............ ⊕D 785
Darvon Compound-65 Pulvules 1435
Easprin.. 1914
Ecotrin 2455
Ecotrin Enteric Coated Aspirin Maximum Strength Tablets and Caplets.. ⊕D 816
Ecotrin Enteric Coated Aspirin Regular Strength Tablets 2455
Empirin Aspirin Tablets .... ⊕D 854
Empirin with Codeine Tablets........... 1093
Excedrin Extra-Strength Analgesic Tablets & Caplets 732
Fiorinal Capsules 2261
Fiorinal with Codeine Capsules 2262
Fiorinal Tablets...................................... 2261
Halfprin 1362

Healthprin Aspirin 2455
Norgesic.. 1496
Percodan Tablets.................................... 939
Percodan-Demi Tablets......................... 940
Robaxisal Tablets................................... 2071
Soma Compound w/Codeine Tablets 2676
Soma Compound Tablets..................... 2675
St. Joseph Adult Chewable Aspirin (81 mg.) .... ⊕D 808
Talwin Compound 2335
Ursinus Inlay-Tabs................................. ⊕D 794
Vanquish Analgesic Caplets .... ⊕D 731

Dicumarol (Response to dicumarol inhibited).

No products indexed under this heading.

Ephedrine Hydrochloride (Enhanced metabolic clearance of corticosteroids). Products include:

Primatene Dual Action Formula...... ⊕D 872
Primatene Tablets .... ⊕D 873
Quadrinal Tablets 1350

Ephedrine Sulfate (Enhanced metabolic clearance of corticosteroids). Products include:

Bronkaid Caplets .... ⊕D 717
Marax Tablets & DF Syrup................... 2200

Ephedrine Tannate (Enhanced metabolic clearance of corticosteroids). Products include:

Rynatuss 2673

Live Virus Vaccines (Contraindicated).

Phenobarbital (Enhanced metabolic clearance of corticosteroids). Products include:

Arco-Lase Plus Tablets 512
Bellergal-S Tablets 2250
Donnatal 2060
Donnatal Extentabs............................... 2061
Donnatal Tablets 2060
Phenobarbital Elixir and Tablets 1469
Quadrinal Tablets 1350

Phenytoin (Enhanced metabolic clearance of corticosteroids). Products include:

Dilantin Infatabs..................................... 1908
Dilantin-125 Suspension 1911

Phenytoin Sodium (Enhanced metabolic clearance of corticosteroids). Products include:

Dilantin Kapseals 1906
Dilantin Parenteral 1910

Rifampin (Enhanced metabolic clearance of corticosteroids). Products include:

Rifadin 1528
Rifamate Capsules 1530
Rifater.. 1532
Rimactane Capsules.............................. 847

Spironolactone (Hypokalemia). Products include:

Aldactazide... 2413
Aldactone 2414

Triamterene (Hypokalemia). Products include:

Dyazide 2479
Dyrenium Capsules................................ 2481
Maxzide 1380

Warfarin Sodium (Response to warfarin inhibited). Products include:

Coumadin 926

DECADRON TABLETS

(Dexamethasone)..................................1635

May interact with oral anticoagulants, potassium sparing diuretics, and certain other agents. Compounds in these categories include:

Amiloride Hydrochloride (Possible hypokalemia). Products include:

Midamor Tablets 1703
Moduretic Tablets 1705

Aspirin (Use cautiously with dexamethasone in hypoprothrombinemia). Products include:

Alka-Seltzer Effervescent Antacid and Pain Reliever .... ⊕D 701

Alka-Seltzer Extra Strength Effervescent Antacid and Pain Reliever .... ⊕D 703
Alka-Seltzer Lemon Lime Effervescent Antacid and Pain Reliever .... ⊕D 703
Alka-Seltzer Plus Cold Medicine .... ⊕D 705
Alka-Seltzer Plus Cold & Cough Medicine .... ⊕D 708
Alka-Seltzer Plus Night-Time Cold Medicine .... ⊕D 707
Alka Seltzer Plus Sinus Medicine .. ⊕D 707
Arthritis Foundation Safety Coated Aspirin Tablets .... ⊕D 675
Arthritis Pain Ascriptin .... ⊕D 631
Maximum Strength Ascriptin .... ⊕D 630
Regular Strength Ascriptin Tablets .... ⊕D 629
Arthritis Strength BC Powder.......... ⊕D 609
BC Cold Powder Multi-Symptom Formula (Cold-Sinus-Allergy) ...... ⊕D 609
BC Cold Powder Non-Drowsy Formula (Cold-Sinus) .... ⊕D 609
BC Powder .... ⊕D 609
Bayer Children's Chewable Aspirin... ⊕D 711
Genuine Bayer Aspirin Tablets & Caplets.. ⊕D 713
Extra Strength Bayer Arthritis Pain Regimen Formula .... ⊕D 711
Extra Strength Bayer Aspirin Caplets & Tablets .... ⊕D 712
Extended-Release Bayer 8-Hour Aspirin .... ⊕D 712
Extra Strength Bayer Plus Aspirin Caplets.. ⊕D 713
Extra Strength Bayer PM Aspirin .. ⊕D 713
Bayer Enteric Aspirin .... ⊕D 709
Bufferin Analgesic Tablets and Caplets.. ⊕D 613
Arthritis Strength Bufferin Analgesic Caplets .... ⊕D 614
Extra Strength Bufferin Analgesic Tablets .... ⊕D 615
Cama Arthritis Pain Reliever............ ⊕D 785
Darvon Compound-65 Pulvules 1435
Easprin.. 1914
Ecotrin 2455
Ecotrin Enteric Coated Aspirin Maximum Strength Tablets and Caplets.. ⊕D 816
Ecotrin Enteric Coated Aspirin Regular Strength Tablets 2455
Empirin Aspirin Tablets .... ⊕D 854
Empirin with Codeine Tablets........... 1093
Excedrin Extra-Strength Analgesic Tablets & Caplets 732
Fiorinal Capsules 2261
Fiorinal with Codeine Capsules 2262
Fiorinal Tablets...................................... 2261
Halfprin 1362
Healthprin Aspirin 2455
Norgesic.. 1496
Percodan Tablets.................................... 939
Percodan-Demi Tablets......................... 940
Robaxisal Tablets................................... 2071
Soma Compound w/Codeine Tablets 2676
Soma Compound Tablets..................... 2675
St. Joseph Adult Chewable Aspirin (81 mg.) .... ⊕D 808
Talwin Compound 2335
Ursinus Inlay-Tabs................................. ⊕D 794
Vanquish Analgesic Caplets .... ⊕D 731

Dicumarol (Altered response to dicumarol).

No products indexed under this heading.

Ephedrine Hydrochloride (Decreases blood levels of dexamethasone). Products include:

Primatene Dual Action Formula...... ⊕D 872
Primatene Tablets .... ⊕D 873
Quadrinal Tablets 1350

Ephedrine Sulfate (Decreases blood levels of dexamethasone). Products include:

Bronkaid Caplets .... ⊕D 717
Marax Tablets & DF Syrup................... 2200

Ephedrine Tannate (Decreases blood levels of dexamethasone). Products include:

Rynatuss 2673

Live virus vaccines; smallpox (Contraindicated).

Phenobarbital (Decreases blood levels of dexamethasone). Products include:

Arco-Lase Plus Tablets 512
Bellergal-S Tablets 2250
Donnatal 2060
Donnatal Extentabs............................... 2061
Donnatal Tablets 2060
Phenobarbital Elixir and Tablets 1469
Quadrinal Tablets 1350

Phenytoin (Decreases blood levels of dexamethasone). Products include:

Dilantin Infatabs..................................... 1908
Dilantin-125 Suspension 1911

Phenytoin Sodium (Decreases blood levels of dexamethasone). Products include:

Dilantin Kapseals 1906
Dilantin Parenteral 1910

Rifampin (Decreases blood levels of dexamethasone). Products include:

Rifadin 1528
Rifamate Capsules 1530
Rifater.. 1532
Rimactane Capsules.............................. 847

Spironolactone (Possible hypokalemia). Products include:

Aldactazide... 2413
Aldactone 2414

Triamterene (Possible hypokalemia). Products include:

Dyazide 2479
Dyrenium Capsules................................ 2481
Maxzide 1380

Warfarin Sodium (Altered response to warfarin). Products include:

Coumadin 926

DECADRON-LA STERILE SUSPENSION

(Dexamethasone Acetate)....................1646

May interact with oral anticoagulants, potassium sparing diuretics, and certain other agents. Compounds in these categories include:

Amiloride Hydrochloride (Possible hypokalemia). Products include:

Midamor Tablets 1703
Moduretic Tablets 1705

Aspirin (Use cautiously with dexamethasone in hypoprothrombinemia). Products include:

Alka-Seltzer Effervescent Antacid and Pain Reliever .... ⊕D 701
Alka-Seltzer Extra Strength Effervescent Antacid and Pain Reliever .... ⊕D 703
Alka-Seltzer Lemon Lime Effervescent Antacid and Pain Reliever .... ⊕D 703
Alka-Seltzer Plus Cold Medicine .... ⊕D 705
Alka-Seltzer Plus Cold & Cough Medicine .... ⊕D 708
Alka-Seltzer Plus Night-Time Cold Medicine .... ⊕D 707
Alka Seltzer Plus Sinus Medicine .. ⊕D 707
Arthritis Foundation Safety Coated Aspirin Tablets .... ⊕D 675
Arthritis Pain Ascriptin .... ⊕D 631
Maximum Strength Ascriptin .... ⊕D 630
Regular Strength Ascriptin Tablets .... ⊕D 629
Arthritis Strength BC Powder.......... ⊕D 609
BC Cold Powder Multi-Symptom Formula (Cold-Sinus-Allergy) ...... ⊕D 609
BC Cold Powder Non-Drowsy Formula (Cold-Sinus) .... ⊕D 609
BC Powder .... ⊕D 609
Bayer Children's Chewable Aspirin... ⊕D 711
Genuine Bayer Aspirin Tablets & Caplets.. ⊕D 713
Extra Strength Bayer Arthritis Pain Regimen Formula .... ⊕D 711
Extra Strength Bayer Aspirin Caplets & Tablets .... ⊕D 712
Extended-Release Bayer 8-Hour Aspirin .... ⊕D 712
Extra Strength Bayer Plus Aspirin Caplets.. ⊕D 713
Extra Strength Bayer PM Aspirin .. ⊕D 713

Bayer Enteric Aspirin .... ᴾᴰ 709
Bufferin Analgesic Tablets and Caplets .... ᴾᴰ 613
Arthritis Strength Bufferin Analgesic Caplets .... ᴾᴰ 614
Extra Strength Bufferin Analgesic Tablets .... ᴾᴰ 615
Cama Arthritis Pain Reliever .... ᴾᴰ 785
Darvon Compound-65 Pulvules 1435
Easprin 1914
Ecotrin 2455
Ecotrin Enteric Coated Aspirin Maximum Strength Tablets and Caplets .... ᴾᴰ 816
Ecotrin Enteric Coated Aspirin Regular Strength Tablets 2455
Empirin Aspirin Tablets .... ᴾᴰ 854
Empirin with Codeine Tablets........... 1093
Excedrin Extra-Strength Analgesic Tablets & Caplets 732
Fiorinal Capsules 2261
Fiorinal with Codeine Capsules 2262
Fiorinal Tablets 2261
Halfprin 1362
Healthprin Aspirin 2455
Norgesic.. 1496
Percodan Tablets................................. 939
Percodan-Demi Tablets...................... 940
Robaxisal Tablets................................ 2071
Soma Compound w/Codeine Tablets 2676
Soma Compound Tablets 2675
St. Joseph Adult Chewable Aspirin (81 mg.) .... ᴾᴰ 808
Talwin Compound 2335
Ursinus Inlay-Tabs.............................. ᴾᴰ 794
Vanquish Analgesic Caplets .... ᴾᴰ 731

Dicumarol (Altered response to dicumarol).

No products indexed under this heading.

Ephedrine Hydrochloride (Decreases blood levels of dexamethasone). Products include:

Primatene Dual Action Formula...... ᴾᴰ 872
Primatene Tablets .... ᴾᴰ 873
Quadrinal Tablets 1350

Ephedrine Sulfate (Decreases blood levels of dexamethasone). Products include:

Bronkaid Caplets .... ᴾᴰ 717
Marax Tablets & DF Syrup................ 2200

Ephedrine Tannate (Decreases blood levels of dexamethasone). Products include:

Rynatuss 2673

Live virus vaccines; smallpox (Contraindicated).

Phenobarbital (Decreases blood levels of dexamethasone). Products include:

Arco-Lase Plus Tablets 512
Bellergal-S Tablets 2250
Donnatal 2060
Donnatal Extentabs............................. 2061
Donnatal Tablets 2060
Phenobarbital Elixir and Tablets 1469
Quadrinal Tablets 1350

Phenytoin (Decreases blood levels of dexamethasone). Products include:

Dilantin Infatabs 1908
Dilantin-125 Suspension 1911

Phenytoin Sodium (Decreases blood levels of dexamethasone). Products include:

Dilantin Kapseals 1906
Dilantin Parenteral 1910

Rifampin (Decreases blood levels of dexamethasone). Products include:

Rifadin 1528
Rifamate Capsules 1530
Rifater.. 1532
Rimactane Capsules 847

Spironolactone (Possible hypokalemia). Products include:

Aldactazide... 2413
Aldactone 2414

Triamterene (Possible hypokalemia). Products include:

Dyazide 2479
Dyrenium Capsules............................. 2481

Maxzide 1380

Warfarin Sodium (Altered response to warfarin). Products include:

Coumadin 926

DECASPRAY TOPICAL AEROSOL

(Dexamethasone) 1648

None cited in PDR database.

DECLOMYCIN TABLETS

(Demeclocycline Hydrochloride) 1371

May interact with anticoagulants, penicillins, antacids, oral contraceptives, and certain other agents. Compounds in these categories include:

Aluminum Carbonate Gel (Tetracycline absorption impaired). Products include:

Basaljel.. 2703

Aluminum Hydroxide (Tetracycline absorption impaired). Products include:

ALternaGEL Liquid 1316
Maximum Strength Ascriptin .... ᴾᴰ 630
Cama Arthritis Pain Reliever............ ᴾᴰ 785
Gaviscon Extra Strength Relief Formula Antacid Tablets.................. ᴾᴰ 819
Gaviscon Extra Strength Relief Formula Liquid Antacid .... ᴾᴰ 819
Gaviscon Liquid Antacid .... ᴾᴰ 820
Gelusil Liquid & Tablets .... ᴾᴰ 855
Maalox Heartburn Relief Suspension .... ᴾᴰ 642
Maalox Heartburn Relief Tablets.... ᴾᴰ 641
Maalox Magnesia and Alumina Oral Suspension .... ᴾᴰ 642
Maalox Plus Tablets .... ᴾᴰ 643
Extra Strength Maalox Antacid Plus Antigas Liquid and Tablets ᴾᴰ 638
Tempo Soft Antacid .... ᴾᴰ 835

Aluminum Hydroxide Gel (Tetracycline absorption impaired). Products include:

ALternaGEL Liquid .... ᴾᴰ 659
Aludrox Oral Suspension 2695
Amphojel Suspension 2695
Amphojel Suspension without Flavor 2695
Amphojel Tablets................................. 2695
Arthritis Pain Ascriptin .... ᴾᴰ 631
Regular Strength Ascriptin Tablets .... ᴾᴰ 629
Gaviscon Antacid Tablets................... ᴾᴰ 819
Gaviscon-2 Antacid Tablets .... ᴾᴰ 820
Mylanta Liquid 1317
Mylanta Tablets .... ᴾᴰ 660
Mylanta Double Strength Liquid 1317
Mylanta Double Strength Tablets .. ᴾᴰ 660
Nephrox Suspension .... ᴾᴰ 655

Aluminum Hydroxide Gel, Dried (Tetracycline absorption impaired).

Amoxicillin Trihydrate (Interference with bactericidal action of penicillin). Products include:

Amoxil.. 2464
Augmentin 2468

Ampicillin Sodium (Interference with bactericidal action of penicillin). Products include:

Unasyn 2212

Azlocillin Sodium (Interference with bactericidal action of penicillin).

No products indexed under this heading.

Bacampicillin Hydrochloride (Interference with bactericidal action of penicillin). Products include:

Spectrobid Tablets 2206

Carbenicillin Disodium (Interference with bactericidal action of penicillin).

No products indexed under this heading.

Carbenicillin Indanyl Sodium (Interference with bactericidal action of penicillin). Products include:

Geocillin Tablets.................................. 2199

Dalteparin Sodium (Plasma prothrombin activity depressed; downward adjustment of anticoagulant dosage may be necessary). Products include:

Fragmin 1954

Desogestrel (Reduced efficacy and increased breakthrough bleeding). Products include:

Desogen Tablets................................... 1817
Ortho-Cept 1851

Dicloxacillin Sodium (Interference with bactericidal action of penicillin).

No products indexed under this heading.

Dicumarol (Plasma prothrombin activity depressed; downward adjustment of anticoagulant dosage may be necessary).

No products indexed under this heading.

Dihydroxyaluminum Sodium Carbonate (Tetracycline absorption impaired).

No products indexed under this heading.

Enoxaparin (Plasma prothrombin activity depressed; downward adjustment of anticoagulant dosage may be necessary). Products include:

Lovenox Injection................................ 2020

Ethinyl Estradiol (Reduced efficacy and increased breakthrough bleeding). Products include:

Brevicon... 2088
Demulen 2428
Desogen Tablets................................... 1817
Levlen/Tri-Levlen................................ 651
Lo/Ovral Tablets 2746
Lo/Ovral-28 Tablets............................ 2751
Modicon.. 1872
Nordette-21 Tablets............................. 2755
Nordette-28 Tablets............................. 2758
Norinyl.. 2088
Ortho-Cept.. 1851
Ortho-Cyclen/Ortho-Tri-Cyclen 1858
Ortho-Novum.. 1872
Ortho-Cyclen/Ortho Tri-Cyclen 1858
Ovcon 760
Ovral Tablets 2770
Ovral-28 Tablets 2770
Levlen/Tri-Levlen................................ 651
Tri-Norinyl.. 2164
Triphasil-21 Tablets............................ 2814
Triphasil-28 Tablets............................ 2819

Ethynodiol Diacetate (Reduced efficacy and increased breakthrough bleeding). Products include:

Demulen 2428

Heparin Calcium (Plasma prothrombin activity depressed; downward adjustment of anticoagulant dosage may be necessary).

No products indexed under this heading.

Heparin Sodium (Plasma prothrombin activity depressed; downward adjustment of anticoagulant dosage may be necessary). Products include:

Heparin Lock Flush Solution 2725
Heparin Sodium Injection.................. 2726
Heparin Sodium Injection, USP, Sterile Solution 2615
Heparin Sodium Vials......................... 1441

Levonorgestrel (Reduced efficacy and increased breakthrough bleeding). Products include:

Levlen/Tri-Levlen................................ 651
Nordette-21 Tablets............................. 2755
Nordette-28 Tablets............................. 2758
Norplant System 2759
Levlen/Tri-Levlen................................ 651
Triphasil-21 Tablets............................ 2814
Triphasil-28 Tablets............................ 2819

Magaldrate (Tetracycline absorption impaired).

No products indexed under this heading.

Magnesium Hydroxide (Tetracycline absorption impaired). Products include:

Aludrox Oral Suspension 2695
Arthritis Pain Ascriptin .... ᴾᴰ 631
Maximum Strength Ascriptin .... ᴾᴰ 630
Regular Strength Ascriptin Tablets .... ᴾᴰ 629
Di-Gel Antacid/Anti-Gas .... ᴾᴰ 801
Gelusil Liquid & Tablets .... ᴾᴰ 855
Maalox Magnesia and Alumina Oral Suspension .... ᴾᴰ 642
Maalox Plus Tablets .... ᴾᴰ 643
Extra Strength Maalox Antacid Plus Antigas Liquid and Tablets ᴾᴰ 638
Mylanta Calcium Carbonate and Magnesium Hydroxide Tablets...... 1318
Mylanta Liquid 1317
Mylanta Tablets .... ᴾᴰ 660
Mylanta Double Strength Liquid 1317
Mylanta Double Strength Tablets .. ᴾᴰ 660
Phillips' Milk of Magnesia Liquid.... ᴾᴰ 729
Rolaids Tablets .... ᴾᴰ 843
Tempo Soft Antacid .... ᴾᴰ 835

Magnesium Oxide (Tetracycline absorption impaired). Products include:

Beelith Tablets 639
Bufferin Analgesic Tablets and Caplets .... ᴾᴰ 613
Caltrate PLUS .... ᴾᴰ 665
Cama Arthritis Pain Reliever............ ᴾᴰ 785
Mag-Ox 400 668
Uro-Mag.. 668

Mestranol (Reduced efficacy and increased breakthrough bleeding). Products include:

Norinyl.. 2088
Ortho-Novum.. 1872

Mezlocillin Sodium (Interference with bactericidal action of penicillin). Products include:

Mezlin 601
Mezlin Pharmacy Bulk Package........ 604

Nafcillin Sodium (Interference with bactericidal action of penicillin).

No products indexed under this heading.

Norethindrone (Reduced efficacy and increased breakthrough bleeding). Products include:

Brevicon... 2088
Micronor Tablets 1872
Modicon.. 1872
Norinyl 2088
Nor-Q D Tablets 2135
Ortho-Novum.. 1872
Ovcon 760
Tri-Norinyl.. 2164

Norethynodrel (Reduced efficacy and increased breakthrough bleeding).

No products indexed under this heading.

Norgestimate (Reduced efficacy and increased breakthrough bleeding). Products include:

Ortho-Cyclen/Ortho-Tri-Cyclen 1858
Ortho-Cyclen/Ortho Tri-Cyclen 1858

Norgestrel (Reduced efficacy and increased breakthrough bleeding). Products include:

Lo/Ovral Tablets 2746
Lo/Ovral-28 Tablets............................ 2751
Ovral Tablets 2770
Ovral-28 Tablets 2770
Ovrette Tablets..................................... 2771

Penicillin G Benzathine (Interference with bactericidal action of penicillin). Products include:

Bicillin C-R Injection 2704
Bicillin C-R 900/300 Injection 2706
Bicillin L-A Injection 2707

Penicillin G Potassium (Interference with bactericidal action of penicillin). Products include:

Pfizerpen for Injection 2203

Penicillin G Procaine (Interference with bactericidal action of penicillin). Products include:

Bicillin C-R Injection 2704
Bicillin C-R 900/300 Injection 2706

IMPORTANT NOTE: Always consult each drug listing in the patient's regimen for possible interactions.

Declomycin

Penicillin V Potassium (Interference with bactericidal action of penicillin). Products include:

Pen•Vee K 2772

Ticarcillin Disodium (Interference with bactericidal action of penicillin). Products include:

Ticar for Injection 2526
Timentin for Injection................................. 2528

Warfarin Sodium (Plasma prothrombin activity depressed; downward adjustment of anticoagulant dosage may be necessary). Products include:

Coumadin 926

Food Interactions

Dairy products (Interferes with absorption).

Food, unspecified (Interferes with absorption).

DECONAMINE CHEWABLE TABLETS

(Chlorpheniramine Maleate, Pseudoephedrine Hydrochloride) 1320

See Deconamine SR Capsules

DECONAMINE CX COUGH AND COLD LIQUID AND TABLETS

(Hydrocodone Bitartrate, Pseudoephedrine Hydrochloride, Guaifenesin) 1319

May interact with narcotic analgesics, general anesthetics, tranquilizers, hypnotics and sedatives, tricyclic antidepressants, central nervous system depressants, monoamine oxidase inhibitors, beta blockers, veratrum alkaloids, and certain other agents. Compounds in these categories include:

Acebutolol Hydrochloride (Potentiates the sympathomimetic effects of pseudoephedrine). Products include:

Sectral Capsules 2807

Alfentanil Hydrochloride (Hydrocodone may potentiate CNS depressant effects). Products include:

Alfenta Injection 1286

Alprazolam (Hydrocodone may potentiate CNS depressant effects). Products include:

Xanax Tablets 2649

Amitriptyline Hydrochloride (Hydrocodone may potentiate CNS depressant effects). Products include:

Elavil 2838
Endep Tablets 2174
Etrafon 2355
Limbitrol 2180
Triavil Tablets 1757

Amoxapine (Hydrocodone may potentiate CNS depressant effects). Products include:

Asendin Tablets 1369

Aprobarbital (Hydrocodone may potentiate CNS depressant effects).

No products indexed under this heading.

Atenolol (Potentiates the sympathomimetic effects of pseudoephedrine). Products include:

Tenoretic Tablets 2845
Tenormin Tablets and I.V. Injection 2847

Betaxolol Hydrochloride (Potentiates the sympathomimetic effects of pseudoephedrine). Products include:

Betoptic Ophthalmic Solution........... 469
Betoptic S Ophthalmic Suspension 471
Kerlone Tablets... 2436

Bisoprolol Fumarate (Potentiates the sympathomimetic effects of pseudoephedrine). Products include:

Zebeta Tablets 1413

Ziac 1415

Buprenorphine (Hydrocodone may potentiate CNS depressant effects). Products include:

Buprenex Injectable 2006

Buspirone Hydrochloride (Hydrocodone may potentiate CNS depressant effects). Products include:

BuSpar 737

Butabarbital (Hydrocodone may potentiate CNS depressant effects).

No products indexed under this heading.

Butalbital (Hydrocodone may potentiate CNS depressant effects). Products include:

Esgic-plus Tablets 1013
Fioricet Tablets 2258
Fioricet with Codeine Capsules 2260
Fiorinal Capsules 2261
Fiorinal with Codeine Capsules 2262
Fiorinal Tablets 2261
Phrenilin 785
Sedapap Tablets 50 mg/650 mg.. 1543

Carteolol Hydrochloride (Potentiates the sympathomimetic effects of pseudoephedrine). Products include:

Cartrol Tablets 410
Ocupress Ophthalmic Solution, 1% Sterile... ◉ 309

Chlordiazepoxide (Hydrocodone may potentiate CNS depressant effects). Products include:

Libritabs Tablets 2177
Limbitrol 2180

Chlordiazepoxide Hydrochloride (Hydrocodone may potentiate CNS depressant effects). Products include:

Librax Capsules 2176
Librium Capsules.. 2178
Librium Injectable 2179

Chlorpromazine (Hydrocodone may potentiate CNS depressant effects). Products include:

Thorazine Suppositories............................ 2523

Chlorpromazine Hydrochloride (Hydrocodone may potentiate CNS depressant effects). Products include:

Thorazine 2523

Chlorprothixene (Hydrocodone may potentiate CNS depressant effects).

No products indexed under this heading.

Chlorprothixene Hydrochloride (Hydrocodone may potentiate CNS depressant effects).

No products indexed under this heading.

Clomipramine Hydrochloride (Hydrocodone may potentiate CNS depressant effects). Products include:

Anafranil Capsules 803

Clorazepate Dipotassium (Hydrocodone may potentiate CNS depressant effects). Products include:

Tranxene 451

Clozapine (Hydrocodone may potentiate CNS depressant effects). Products include:

Clozaril Tablets... 2252

Codeine Phosphate (Hydrocodone may potentiate CNS depressant effects). Products include:

Actifed with Codeine Cough Syrup.. 1067
Brontex 1981
Deconsal C Expectorant Syrup 456
Deconsal Pediatric Syrup 457
Dimetane-DC Cough Syrup 2059
Empirin with Codeine Tablets............ 1093
Fioricet with Codeine Capsules 2260
Fiorinal with Codeine Capsules 2262
Isoclor Expectorant.................................... 990
Novahistine DH.. 2462
Novahistine Expectorant........................... 2463
Nucofed 2051

Phenergan with Codeine........................... 2777
Phenergan VC with Codeine 2781
Robitussin A-C Syrup................................. 2073
Robitussin-DAC Syrup................................ 2074
Ryna .... ◙ 841
Soma Compound w/Codeine Tablets 2676
Tussi-Organidin NR Liquid and S NR Liquid 2677
Tylenol with Codeine 1583

Cryptenamine Preparations (Sympathomimetic may reduce the antihypertensive effects of veratrum alkaloids).

Desflurane (Hydrocodone may potentiate CNS depressant effects). Products include:

Suprane 1813

Desipramine Hydrochloride (Hydrocodone may potentiate CNS depressant effects). Products include:

Norpramin Tablets 1526

Dezocine (Hydrocodone may potentiate CNS depressant effects). Products include:

Dalgan Injection 538

Diazepam (Hydrocodone may potentiate CNS depressant effects). Products include:

Dizac 1809
Valium Injectable 2182
Valium Tablets 2183
Valrelease Capsules 2169

Doxepin Hydrochloride (Hydrocodone may potentiate CNS depressant effects). Products include:

Sinequan 2205
Zonalon Cream 1055

Droperidol (Hydrocodone may potentiate CNS depressant effects). Products include:

Inapsine Injection....................................... 1296

Enflurane (Hydrocodone may potentiate CNS depressant effects).

No products indexed under this heading.

Esmolol Hydrochloride (Potentiates the sympathomimetic effects of pseudoephedrine). Products include:

Brevibloc Injection...................................... 1808

Estazolam (Hydrocodone may potentiate CNS depressant effects). Products include:

ProSom Tablets 449

Ethchlorvynol (Hydrocodone may potentiate CNS depressant effects). Products include:

Placidyl Capsules.. 448

Ethinamate (Hydrocodone may potentiate CNS depressant effects).

No products indexed under this heading.

Fentanyl (Hydrocodone may potentiate CNS depressant effects). Products include:

Duragesic Transdermal System........ 1288

Fentanyl Citrate (Hydrocodone may potentiate CNS depressant effects). Products include:

Sublimaze Injection.................................... 1307

Fluphenazine Decanoate (Hydrocodone may potentiate CNS depressant effects). Products include:

Prolixin Decanoate 509

Fluphenazine Enanthate (Hydrocodone may potentiate CNS depressant effects). Products include:

Prolixin Enanthate 509

Fluphenazine Hydrochloride (Hydrocodone may potentiate CNS depressant effects). Products include:

Prolixin 509

Flurazepam Hydrochloride (Hydrocodone may potentiate CNS depressant effects). Products include:

Dalmane Capsules...................................... 2173

Furazolidone (Potentiates the sympathomimetic effects of pseudoephedrine). Products include:

Furoxone 2046

Glutethimide (Hydrocodone may potentiate CNS depressant effects).

No products indexed under this heading.

Haloperidol (Hydrocodone may potentiate CNS depressant effects). Products include:

Haldol Injection, Tablets and Concentrate 1575

Haloperidol Decanoate (Hydrocodone may potentiate CNS depressant effects). Products include:

Haldol Decanoate.. 1577

Hydrocodone Polistirex (Hydrocodone may potentiate CNS depressant effects). Products include:

Tussionex Pennkinetic Extended-Release Suspension 998

Hydroxyzine Hydrochloride (Hydrocodone may potentiate CNS depressant effects). Products include:

Atarax Tablets & Syrup.............................. 2185
Marax Tablets & DF Syrup.................. 2200
Vistaril Intramuscular Solution......... 2216

Imipramine Hydrochloride (Hydrocodone may potentiate CNS depressant effects). Products include:

Tofranil Ampuls 854
Tofranil Tablets 856

Imipramine Pamoate (Hydrocodone may potentiate CNS depressant effects). Products include:

Tofranil-PM Capsules................................. 857

Isocarboxazid (Potentiates the sympathomimetic effects of pseudoephedrine).

No products indexed under this heading.

Isoflurane (Hydrocodone may potentiate CNS depressant effects).

No products indexed under this heading.

Ketamine Hydrochloride (Hydrocodone may potentiate CNS depressant effects).

No products indexed under this heading.

Labetalol Hydrochloride (Potentiates the sympathomimetic effects of pseudoephedrine). Products include:

Normodyne Injection 2377
Normodyne Tablets 2379
Trandate 1185

Levobunolol Hydrochloride (Potentiates the sympathomimetic effects of pseudoephedrine). Products include:

Betagan .... ◉ 233

Levomethadyl Acetate Hydrochloride (Hydrocodone may potentiate CNS depressant effects). Products include:

Orlaam 2239

Levorphanol Tartrate (Hydrocodone may potentiate CNS depressant effects). Products include:

Levo-Dromoran.. 2129

Lorazepam (Hydrocodone may potentiate CNS depressant effects). Products include:

Ativan Injection... 2698
Ativan Tablets.. 2700

Loxapine Hydrochloride (Hydrocodone may potentiate CNS depressant effects). Products include:

Loxitane 1378

Loxapine Succinate (Hydrocodone may potentiate CNS depressant effects). Products include:

Loxitane Capsules 1378

(◙ Described in PDR For Nonprescription Drugs) (◉ Described in PDR For Ophthalmology)

Maprotiline Hydrochloride (Hydrocodone may potentiate CNS depressant effects). Products include:
Ludiomil Tablets 843
Mecamylamine Hydrochloride (Sympathomimetic may reduce the antihypertensive effects). Products include:
Inversine Tablets 1686
Meperidine Hydrochloride (Hydrocodone may potentiate CNS depressant effects). Products include:
Demerol 2308
Mepergan Injection 2753
Mephobarbital (Hydrocodone may potentiate CNS depressant effects). Products include:
Mebaral Tablets 2322
Meprobamate (Hydrocodone may potentiate CNS depressant effects). Products include:
Miltown Tablets 2672
PMB 200 and PMB 400 2783
Mesoridazine Besylate (Hydrocodone may potentiate CNS depressant effects). Products include:
Serentil 684
Methadone Hydrochloride (Hydrocodone may potentiate CNS depressant effects). Products include:
Methadone Hydrochloride Oral Concentrate 2233
Methadone Hydrochloride Oral Solution & Tablets 2235
Methohexital Sodium (Hydrocodone may potentiate CNS depressant effects). Products include:
Brevital Sodium Vials 1429
Methotrimeprazine (Hydrocodone may potentiate CNS depressant effects). Products include:
Levoprome 1274
Methoxyflurane (Hydrocodone may potentiate CNS depressant effects).
No products indexed under this heading.
Methyldopa (Sympathomimetic may reduce the antihypertensive effects). Products include:
Aldoclor Tablets 1598
Aldomet Oral 1600
Aldoril Tablets 1604
Methyldopate Hydrochloride (Sympathomimetic may reduce the antihypertensive effects). Products include:
Aldomet Ester HCl Injection 1602
Metipranolol Hydrochloride (Potentiates the sympathomimetic effects of pseudoephedrine). Products include:
OptiPranolol (Metipranolol 0.3%) Sterile Ophthalmic Solution .... ◉ 258
Metoprolol Succinate (Potentiates the sympathomimetic effects of pseudoephedrine). Products include:
Toprol-XL Tablets 565
Metoprolol Tartrate (Potentiates the sympathomimetic effects of pseudoephedrine). Products include:
Lopressor Ampuls 830
Lopressor HCT Tablets 832
Lopressor Tablets 830
Midazolam Hydrochloride (Hydrocodone may potentiate CNS depressant effects). Products include:
Versed Injection 2170
Molindone Hydrochloride (Hydrocodone may potentiate CNS depressant effects). Products include:
Moban Tablets and Concentrate 1048
Morphine Sulfate (Hydrocodone may potentiate CNS depressant effects). Products include:
Astramorph/PF Injection, USP (Preservative-Free) 535
Duramorph 962
Infumorph 200 and Infumorph 500 Sterile Solutions 965
MS Contin Tablets 1994
MSIR 1997
Oramorph SR (Morphine Sulfate Sustained Release Tablets) 2236
RMS Suppositories 2657
Roxanol 2243
Nadolol (Potentiates the sympathomimetic effects of pseudoephedrine).
No products indexed under this heading.
Nortriptyline Hydrochloride (Hydrocodone may potentiate CNS depressant effects). Products include:
Pamelor 2280
Opium Alkaloids (Hydrocodone may potentiate CNS depressant effects).
No products indexed under this heading.
Oxazepam (Hydrocodone may potentiate CNS depressant effects). Products include:
Serax Capsules 2810
Serax Tablets 2810
Oxycodone Hydrochloride (Hydrocodone may potentiate CNS depressant effects). Products include:
Percocet Tablets 938
Percodan Tablets 939
Percodan-Demi Tablets 940
Roxicodone Tablets, Oral Solution & Intensol (Oxycodone) 2244
Tylox Capsules 1584
Penbutolol Sulfate (Potentiates the sympathomimetic effects of pseudoephedrine). Products include:
Levatol 2403
Pentobarbital Sodium (Hydrocodone may potentiate CNS depressant effects). Products include:
Nembutal Sodium Capsules 436
Nembutal Sodium Solution 438
Nembutal Sodium Suppositories 440
Perphenazine (Hydrocodone may potentiate CNS depressant effects). Products include:
Etrafon 2355
Triavil Tablets 1757
Trilafon 2389
Phenelzine Sulfate (Potentiates the sympathomimetic effects of pseudoephedrine). Products include:
Nardil 1920
Phenobarbital (Hydrocodone may potentiate CNS depressant effects). Products include:
Arco-Lase Plus Tablets 512
Bellergal-S Tablets 2250
Donnatal 2060
Donnatal Extentabs 2061
Donnatal Tablets 2060
Phenobarbital Elixir and Tablets 1469
Quadrinal Tablets 1350
Pindolol (Potentiates the sympathomimetic effects of pseudoephedrine). Products include:
Visken Tablets 2299
Prazepam (Hydrocodone may potentiate CNS depressant effects).
No products indexed under this heading.
Prochlorperazine (Hydrocodone may potentiate CNS depressant effects). Products include:
Compazine 2470
Promethazine Hydrochloride (Hydrocodone may potentiate CNS depressant effects). Products include:
Mepergan Injection 2753
Phenergan with Codeine 2777
Phenergan with Dextromethorphan 2778
Phenergan Injection 2773
Phenergan Suppositories 2775
Phenergan Syrup 2774
Phenergan Tablets 2775
Phenergan VC 2779
Phenergan VC with Codeine 2781
Propofol (Hydrocodone may potentiate CNS depressant effects). Products include:
Diprivan Injection 2833
Propoxyphene Hydrochloride (Hydrocodone may potentiate CNS depressant effects). Products include:
Darvon 1435
Wygesic Tablets 2827
Propoxyphene Napsylate (Hydrocodone may potentiate CNS depressant effects). Products include:
Darvon-N/Darvocet-N 1433
Propranolol Hydrochloride (Potentiates the sympathomimetic effects of pseudoephedrine). Products include:
Inderal 2728
Inderal LA Long Acting Capsules 2730
Inderide Tablets 2732
Inderide LA Long Acting Capsules 2734
Protriptyline Hydrochloride (Hydrocodone may potentiate CNS depressant effects). Products include:
Vivactil Tablets 1774
Quazepam (Hydrocodone may potentiate CNS depressant effects). Products include:
Doral Tablets 2664
Reserpine (Sympathomimetic may reduce the antihypertensive effects). Products include:
Diupres Tablets 1650
Hydropres Tablets 1675
Ser-Ap-Es Tablets 849
Risperidone (Hydrocodone may potentiate CNS depressant effects). Products include:
Risperdal 1301
Secobarbital Sodium (Hydrocodone may potentiate CNS depressant effects). Products include:
Seconal Sodium Pulvules 1474
Selegiline Hydrochloride (Potentiates the sympathomimetic effects of pseudoephedrine). Products include:
Eldepryl Tablets 2550
Sotalol Hydrochloride (Potentiates the sympathomimetic effects of pseudoephedrine). Products include:
Betapace Tablets 641
Sufentanil Citrate (Hydrocodone may potentiate CNS depressant effects). Products include:
Sufenta Injection 1309
Temazepam (Hydrocodone may potentiate CNS depressant effects). Products include:
Restoril Capsules 2284
Thiamylal Sodium (Hydrocodone may potentiate CNS depressant effects).
No products indexed under this heading.
Thioridazine Hydrochloride (Hydrocodone may potentiate CNS depressant effects). Products include:
Mellaril 2269
Thiothixene (Hydrocodone may potentiate CNS depressant effects). Products include:
Navane Capsules and Concentrate 2201
Navane Intramuscular 2202
Timolol Hemihydrate (Potentiates the sympathomimetic effects of pseudoephedrine). Products include:
Betimol 0.25%, 0.5% .... ◉ 261
Timolol Maleate (Potentiates the sympathomimetic effects of pseudoephedrine). Products include:
Blocadren Tablets 1614
Timolide Tablets 1748
Timoptic in Ocudose 1753
Timoptic Sterile Ophthalmic Solution 1751
Timoptic-XE 1755
Tranylcypromine Sulfate (Potentiates the sympathomimetic effects of pseudoephedrine). Products include:
Parnate Tablets 2503
Triazolam (Hydrocodone may potentiate CNS depressant effects). Products include:
Halcion Tablets 2611
Trifluoperazine Hydrochloride (Hydrocodone may potentiate CNS depressant effects). Products include:
Stelazine 2514
Trimipramine Maleate (Hydrocodone may potentiate CNS depressant effects). Products include:
Surmontil Capsules 2811
Zolpidem Tartrate (Hydrocodone may potentiate CNS depressant effects). Products include:
Ambien Tablets 2416

Food Interactions

Alcohol (Hydrocodone may potentiate CNS depressant effects).

DECONAMINE SR CAPSULES

(Chlorpheniramine Maleate, Pseudoephedrine Hydrochloride) 1320

May interact with hypnotics and sedatives, tranquilizers, monoamine oxidase inhibitors, veratrum alkaloids, sympathomimetics, and certain other agents. Compounds in these categories include:

Albuterol (Potentially harmful combined effect on cardiovascular system). Products include:
Proventil Inhalation Aerosol 2382
Ventolin Inhalation Aerosol and Refill 1197
Albuterol Sulfate (Potentially harmful combined effect on cardiovascular system). Products include:
Airet Solution for Inhalation 452
Proventil Inhalation Solution 0.083% 2384
Proventil Repetabs Tablets 2386
Proventil Solution for Inhalation 0.5% 2383
Proventil Syrup 2385
Proventil Tablets 2386
Ventolin Inhalation Solution 1198
Ventolin Nebules Inhalation Solution 1199
Ventolin Rotacaps for Inhalation 1200
Ventolin Syrup 1202
Ventolin Tablets 1203
Volmax Extended-Release Tablets 1788
Alprazolam (Additive effects). Products include:
Xanax Tablets 2649
Buspirone Hydrochloride (Additive effects). Products include:
BuSpar 737
Chlordiazepoxide (Additive effects). Products include:
Libritabs Tablets 2177
Limbitrol 2180
Chlordiazepoxide Hydrochloride (Additive effects). Products include:
Librax Capsules 2176
Librium Capsules 2178
Librium Injectable 2179
Chlorpromazine (Additive effects). Products include:
Thorazine Suppositories 2523
Chlorpromazine Hydrochloride (Additive effects). Products include:
Thorazine 2523
Chlorprothixene (Additive effects).
No products indexed under this heading.

IMPORTANT NOTE: Always consult each drug listing in the patient's regimen for possible interactions.

Deconamine **Interactions Index** **238**

Chlorprothixene Hydrochloride (Additive effects).
No products indexed under this heading.

Clorazepate Dipotassium (Additive effects). Products include:
Tranxene ... 451

Cryptenamine Preparations (Reduced antihypertensive effect of cryptenamine).

Diazepam (Additive effects). Products include:
Dizac ... 1809
Valium Injectable ... 2182
Valium Tablets ... 2183
Valrelease Capsules ... 2169

Dobutamine Hydrochloride (Potentially harmful combined effect on cardiovascular system). Products include:
Dobutrex Solution Vials ... 1439

Dopamine Hydrochloride (Potentially harmful combined effect on cardiovascular system).
No products indexed under this heading.

Droperidol (Additive effects). Products include:
Inapsine Injection ... 1296

Ephedrine Hydrochloride (Potentially harmful combined effect on cardiovascular system). Products include:
Primatene Dual Action Formula ... ◘ 872
Primatene Tablets ... ◘ 873
Quadrinal Tablets ... 1350

Ephedrine Sulfate (Potentially harmful combined effect on cardiovascular system). Products include:
Bronkaid Caplets ... ◘ 717
Marax Tablets & DF Syrup ... 2200

Ephedrine Tannate (Potentially harmful combined effect on cardiovascular system). Products include:
Rynatuss ... 2673

Epinephrine (Potentially harmful combined effect on cardiovascular system). Products include:
Bronkaid Mist ... ◘ 717
EPIFRIN ... ⊙ 239
EpiPen ... 790
Marcaine Hydrochloride with Epinephrine 1:200,000 ... 2316
Primatene Mist ... ◘ 873
Sensorcaine with Epinephrine Injection ... 559
Sus-Phrine Injection ... 1019
Xylocaine with Epinephrine Injections ... 567

Epinephrine Bitartrate (Potentially harmful combined effect on cardiovascular system). Products include:
Bronkaid Mist Suspension ... ◘ 718
Sensorcaine-MPF with Epinephrine Injection ... 559

Epinephrine Hydrochloride (Potentially harmful combined effect on cardiovascular system). Products include:
Ana-Kit Anaphylaxis Emergency Treatment Kit ... 617

Estazolam (Additive effects). Products include:
ProSom Tablets ... 449

Ethchlorvynol (Additive effects). Products include:
Placidyl Capsules ... 448

Ethinamate (Additive effects).
No products indexed under this heading.

Fluphenazine Decanoate (Additive effects). Products include:
Prolixin Decanoate ... 509

Fluphenazine Enanthate (Additive effects). Products include:
Prolixin Enanthate ... 509

Fluphenazine Hydrochloride (Additive effects). Products include:
Prolixin ... 509

Flurazepam Hydrochloride (Additive effects). Products include:
Dalmane Capsules ... 2173

Furazolidone (May precipitate hypertensive crisis; prolong and intensify anticholinergic effects of antihistamines; contraindication). Products include:
Furoxone ... 2046

Glutethimide (Additive effects).
No products indexed under this heading.

Haloperidol (Additive effects). Products include:
Haldol Injection, Tablets and Concentrate ... 1575

Haloperidol Decanoate (Additive effects). Products include:
Haldol Decanoate ... 1577

Hydroxyzine Hydrochloride (Additive effects). Products include:
Atarax Tablets & Syrup ... 2185
Marax Tablets & DF Syrup ... 2200
Vistaril Intramuscular Solution ... 2216

Isocarboxazid (May precipitate hypertensive crisis; prolong and intensify anticholinergic effects of antihistamines; contraindication).
No products indexed under this heading.

Isoproterenol Hydrochloride (Potentially harmful combined effect on cardiovascular system). Products include:
Isuprel Hydrochloride Injection 1:5000 ... 2311
Isuprel Hydrochloride Solution 1:200 & 1:100 ... 2313
Isuprel Mistometer ... 2312

Isoproterenol Sulfate (Potentially harmful combined effect on cardiovascular system). Products include:
Norisodrine with Calcium Iodide Syrup ... 442

Lorazepam (Additive effects). Products include:
Ativan Injection ... 2698
Ativan Tablets ... 2700

Loxapine Hydrochloride (Additive effects). Products include:
Loxitane ... 1378

Loxapine Succinate (Additive effects). Products include:
Loxitane Capsules ... 1378

Mecamylamine Hydrochloride (Reduced antihypertensive effect of mecamylamine). Products include:
Inversine Tablets ... 1686

Meprobamate (Additive effects). Products include:
Miltown Tablets ... 2672
PMB 200 and PMB 400 ... 2783

Mesoridazine Besylate (Additive effects). Products include:
Serentil ... 684

Metaproterenol Sulfate (Potentially harmful combined effect on cardiovascular system). Products include:
Alupent ... 669
Metaproterenol Sulfate Inhalation Solution, USP, Arm-a-Med ... 552

Metaraminol Bitartrate (Potentially harmful combined effect on cardiovascular system). Products include:
Aramine Injection ... 1609

Methoxamine Hydrochloride (Potentially harmful combined effect on cardiovascular system). Products include:
Vasoxyl Injection ... 1196

Methyldopa (Reduced antihypertensive effect of methyldopa). Products include:
Aldoclor Tablets ... 1598
Aldomet Oral ... 1600
Aldoril Tablets ... 1604

Methyldopate Hydrochloride (Reduced antihypertensive effect of methyldopate hydrochloride). Products include:
Aldomet Ester HCl Injection ... 1602

Midazolam Hydrochloride (Additive effects). Products include:
Versed Injection ... 2170

Molindone Hydrochloride (Additive effects). Products include:
Moban Tablets and Concentrate ... 1048

Norepinephrine Bitartrate (Potentially harmful combined effect on cardiovascular system). Products include:
Levophed Bitartrate Injection ... 2315

Oxazepam (Additive effects). Products include:
Serax Capsules ... 2810
Serax Tablets ... 2810

Perphenazine (Additive effects). Products include:
Etrafon ... 2355
Triavil Tablets ... 1757
Trilafon ... 2389

Phenelzine Sulfate (May precipitate hypertensive crisis; prolong and intensify anticholinergic effects of antihistamines; contraindication). Products include:
Nardil ... 1920

Phenylephrine Bitartrate (Potentially harmful combined effect on cardiovascular system).
No products indexed under this heading.

Phenylephrine Hydrochloride (Potentially harmful combined effect on cardiovascular system). Products include:
Atrohist Plus Tablets ... 454
Cerose DM ... ◘ 878
Comhist ... 2038
D.A. Chewable Tablets ... 951
Deconsal Pediatric Capsules ... 454
Dura-Vent/DA Tablets ... 953
Entex Capsules ... 1986
Entex Liquid ... 1986
Extendryl ... 1005
4-Way Fast Acting Nasal Spray (regular & mentholated) ... ◘ 621
Hemorid For Women ... ◘ 834
Hycomine Compound Tablets ... 932
Neo-Synephrine Hydrochloride 1% Carpuject ... 2324
Neo-Synephrine Hydrochloride 1% Injection ... 2324
Neo-Synephrine Hydrochloride (Ophthalmic) ... 2325
Neo-Synephrine ... ◘ 726
Nōstril ... ◘ 644
Novahistine Elixir ... ◘ 823
Phenergan VC ... 2779
Phenergan VC with Codeine ... 2781
Preparation H ... ◘ 871
Tympagesic Ear Drops ... 2342
Vasosulf ... ⊙ 271
Vicks Sinex Nasal Spray and Ultra Fine Mist ... ◘ 765

Phenylephrine Tannate (Potentially harmful combined effect on cardiovascular system). Products include:
Atrohist Pediatric Suspension ... 454
Ricobid-D Pediatric Suspension ... 2038
Ricobid Tablets and Pediatric Suspension ... 2038
Rynatan ... 2673
Rynatuss ... 2673

Phenylpropanolamine Hydrochloride (Potentially harmful combined effect on cardiovascular system). Products include:
Acutrim ... ◘ 628
Allerest Children's Chewable Tablets ... ◘ 627
Allerest 12 Hour Caplets ... ◘ 627
Atrohist Plus Tablets ... 454
BC Cold Powder Multi-Symptom Formula (Cold-Sinus-Allergy) ... ◘ 609
BC Cold Powder Non-Drowsy Formula (Cold-Sinus) ... ◘ 609
Cheracol Plus Head Cold/Cough Formula ... ◘ 769
Comtrex Multi-Symptom Non-Drowsy Liqui-gels ... ◘ 618
Contac Continuous Action Nasal Decongestant/Antihistamine 12 Hour Capsules ... ◘ 813
Contac Maximum Strength Continuous Action Decongestant/Antihistamine 12 Hour Caplets ... ◘ 813
Contac Severe Cold and Flu Formula Caplets ... ◘ 814
Coricidin 'D' Decongestant Tablets ... ◘ 800
Dexatrim ... ◘ 832
Dexatrim Plus Vitamins Caplets ... ◘ 832
Dimetane-DC Cough Syrup ... 2059
Dimetapp Elixir ... ◘ 773
Dimetapp Extentabs ... ◘ 774
Dimetapp Tablets/Liqui-Gels ... ◘ 775
Dimetapp Cold & Allergy Chewable Tablets ... ◘ 773
Dimetapp DM Elixir ... ◘ 774
Dura-Vent Tablets ... 952
Entex Capsules ... 1986
Entex LA Tablets ... 1987
Entex Liquid ... 1986
Exgest LA Tablets ... 782
Hycomine ... 931
Isoclor Timesule Capsules ... ◘ 637
Nolamine Timed-Release Tablets ... 785
Ornade Spansule Capsules ... 2502
Propagest Tablets ... 786
Pyrroxate Caplets ... ◘ 772
Robitussin-CF ... ◘ 777
Sinulin Tablets ... 787
Tavist-D 12 Hour Relief Tablets ... ◘ 787
Teldrin 12 Hour Antihistamine/Nasal Decongestant Allergy Relief Capsules ... ◘ 826
Triaminic Allergy Tablets ... ◘ 789
Triaminic Cold Tablets ... ◘ 790
Triaminic Expectorant ... ◘ 790
Triaminic Syrup ... ◘ 792
Triaminic-12 Tablets ... ◘ 792
Triaminic-DM Syrup ... ◘ 792
Triaminicin Tablets ... ◘ 793
Triaminicol Multi-Symptom Cold Tablets ... ◘ 793
Triaminicol Multi-Symptom Relief ... ◘ 794
Vicks DayQuil Allergy Relief 12-Hour Extended Release Tablets ... ◘ 760
Vicks DayQuil Allergy Relief 4-Hour Tablets ... ◘ 760
Vicks DayQuil SINUS Pressure & CONGESTION Relief ... ◘ 761

Pirbuterol Acetate (Potentially harmful combined effect on cardiovascular system). Products include:
Maxair Autohaler ... 1492
Maxair Inhaler ... 1494

Prazepam (Additive effects).
No products indexed under this heading.

Prochlorperazine (Additive effects). Products include:
Compazine ... 2470

Promethazine Hydrochloride (Additive effects). Products include:
Mepergan Injection ... 2753
Phenergan with Codeine ... 2777
Phenergan with Dextromethorphan ... 2778
Phenergan Injection ... 2773
Phenergan Suppositories ... 2775
Phenergan Syrup ... 2774
Phenergan Tablets ... 2775
Phenergan VC ... 2779
Phenergan VC with Codeine ... 2781

Propofol (Additive effects). Products include:
Diprivan Injection ... 2833

Pseudoephedrine Sulfate (Potentially harmful combined effect on cardiovascular system). Products include:
Cheracol Sinus ... ◘ 768
Chlor-Trimeton Allergy Decongestant Tablets ... ◘ 799
Claritin-D ... 2350
Drixoral Cold and Allergy Sustained-Action Tablets ... ◘ 802
Drixoral Cold and Flu Extended-Release Tablets ... ◘ 803
Drixoral Non-Drowsy Formula Extended-Release Tablets ... ◘ 803
Drixoral Allergy/Sinus Extended Release Tablets ... ◘ 804
Trinalin Repetabs Tablets ... 1330

(◘ Described in PDR For Nonprescription Drugs) (⊙ Described in PDR For Ophthalmology)

Quazepam (Additive effects). Products include:

Doral Tablets 2664

Reserpine (Reduced antihypertensive effect of reserpine). Products include:

Diupres Tablets 1650
Hydropres Tablets 1675
Ser-Ap-Es Tablets 849

Salmeterol Xinafoate (Potentially harmful combined effect on cardiovascular system). Products include:

Serevent Inhalation Aerosol 1176

Secobarbital Sodium (Additive effects). Products include:

Seconal Sodium Pulvules 1474

Selegiline Hydrochloride (May precipitate hypertensive crisis; prolong and intensify anticholinergic effects of antihistamines; contraindication). Products include:

Eldepryl Tablets 2550

Temazepam (Additive effects). Products include:

Restoril Capsules 2284

Terbutaline Sulfate (Potentially harmful combined effect on cardiovascular system). Products include:

Brethaire Inhaler 813
Brethine Ampuls 815
Brethine Tablets 814
Bricanyl Subcutaneous Injection 1502
Bricanyl Tablets 1503

Thioridazine Hydrochloride (Additive effects). Products include:

Mellaril 2269

Thiothixene (Additive effects). Products include:

Navane Capsules and Concentrate 2201
Navane Intramuscular 2202

Tranylcypromine Sulfate (May precipitate hypertensive crisis; prolong and intensify anticholinergic effects of antihistamines; contraindication). Products include:

Parnate Tablets 2503

Triazolam (Additive effects). Products include:

Halcion Tablets 2611

Trifluoperazine Hydrochloride (Additive effects). Products include:

Stelazine 2514

Zolpidem Tartrate (Additive effects). Products include:

Ambien Tablets 2416

Food Interactions

Alcohol (Additive effects; potentiates the sedative effects of chlorpheniramine).

DECONAMINE SYRUP

(Chlorpheniramine Maleate, Pseudoephedrine Hydrochloride) 1320

See **Deconamine SR Capsules**

DECONAMINE TABLETS

(Chlorpheniramine Maleate, Pseudoephedrine Hydrochloride) 1320

See **Deconamine SR Capsules**

DECONSAL C EXPECTORANT SYRUP

(Codeine Phosphate, Pseudoephedrine Hydrochloride, Guaifenesin) 456

May interact with beta blockers, cardiac glycosides, monoamine oxidase inhibitors, sympathomimetics, tricyclic antidepressants, anticholinergics, central nervous system depressants, general anesthetics, and certain other agents. Compounds in these categories include:

Acebutolol Hydrochloride (Concurrent use may increase the pressor effect of pseudoephedrine). Products include:

Sectral Capsules 2807

Albuterol (Concurrent use may increase the effects of either of these agents thereby increasing the potential for side effects). Products include:

Proventil Inhalation Aerosol 2382
Ventolin Inhalation Aerosol and Refill 1197

Albuterol Sulfate (Concurrent use may increase the effects of either of these agents thereby increasing the potential for side effects). Products include:

Airet Solution for Inhalation 452
Proventil Inhalation Solution 0.083% 2384
Proventil Repetabs Tablets 2386
Proventil Solution for Inhalation 0.5% 2383
Proventil Syrup 2385
Proventil Tablets 2386
Ventolin Inhalation Solution 1198
Ventolin Nebules Inhalation Solution 1199
Ventolin Rotacaps for Inhalation 1200
Ventolin Syrup 1202
Ventolin Tablets 1203
Volmax Extended-Release Tablets 1788

Alfentanil Hydrochloride (Effects of concurrent use not specified). Products include:

Alfenta Injection 1286

Alprazolam (Effects of concurrent use not specified). Products include:

Xanax Tablets 2649

Amitriptyline Hydrochloride (May antagonize the effects of pseudoephedrine and may increase the effects either of the antidepressants themselves or of the codeine). Products include:

Elavil 2838
Endep Tablets 2174
Etrafon 2355
Limbitrol 2180
Triavil Tablets 1757

Amoxapine (May antagonize the effects of pseudoephedrine and may increase the effects either of the antidepressants themselves or of the codeine). Products include:

Asendin Tablets 1369

Aprobarbital (Effects of concurrent use not specified).

No products indexed under this heading.

Atenolol (Concurrent use may increase the pressor effect of pseudoephedrine). Products include:

Tenoretic Tablets 2845
Tenormin Tablets and I.V. Injection 2847

Atropine Sulfate (Concurrent use may result in paralytic ileus). Products include:

Arco-Lase Plus Tablets 512
Atrohist Plus Tablets 454
Atropine Sulfate Sterile Ophthalmic Solution ◉ 233
Donnatal 2060
Donnatal Extentabs 2061
Donnatal Tablets 2060
Lomotil 2439
Motofen Tablets 784
Urised Tablets 1964

Belladonna Alkaloids (Concurrent use may result in paralytic ileus). Products include:

Bellergal-S Tablets 2250
Hyland's Bed Wetting Tablets ▣ 828
Hyland's EnurAid Tablets ▣ 829
Hyland's Teething Tablets ▣ 830

Benztropine Mesylate (Concurrent use may result in paralytic ileus). Products include:

Cogentin 1621

Betaxolol Hydrochloride (Concurrent use may increase the pressor effect of pseudoephedrine). Products include:

Betoptic Ophthalmic Solution 469
Betoptic S Ophthalmic Suspension 471
Kerlone Tablets 2436

Biperiden Hydrochloride (Concurrent use may result in paralytic ileus). Products include:

Akineton 1333

Bisoprolol Fumarate (Concurrent use may increase the pressor effect of pseudoephedrine). Products include:

Zebeta Tablets 1413
Ziac 1415

Buprenorphine (Effects of concurrent use not specified). Products include:

Buprenex Injectable 2006

Buspirone Hydrochloride (Effects of concurrent use not specified). Products include:

BuSpar 737

Butabarbital (Effects of concurrent use not specified).

No products indexed under this heading.

Butalbital (Effects of concurrent use not specified). Products include:

Esgic-plus Tablets 1013
Fioricet Tablets 2258
Fioricet with Codeine Capsules 2260
Fiorinal Capsules 2261
Fiorinal with Codeine Capsules 2262
Fiorinal Tablets 2261
Phrenilin 785
Sedapap Tablets 50 mg/650 mg 1543

Carteolol Hydrochloride (Concurrent use may increase the pressor effect of pseudoephedrine). Products include:

Cartrol Tablets 410
Ocupress Ophthalmic Solution, 1% Sterile ◉ 309

Chlordiazepoxide (Effects of concurrent use not specified). Products include:

Libritabs Tablets 2177
Limbitrol 2180

Chlordiazepoxide Hydrochloride (Effects of concurrent use not specified). Products include:

Librax Capsules 2176
Librium Capsules 2178
Librium Injectable 2179

Chlorpromazine (Effects of concurrent use not specified). Products include:

Thorazine Suppositories 2523

Chlorpromazine Hydrochloride (Effects of concurrent use not specified). Products include:

Thorazine 2523

Chlorprothixene (Effects of concurrent use not specified).

No products indexed under this heading.

Chlorprothixene Hydrochloride (Effects of concurrent use not specified).

No products indexed under this heading.

Clidinium Bromide (Concurrent use may result in paralytic ileus). Products include:

Librax Capsules 2176
Quarzan Capsules 2181

Clomipramine Hydrochloride (May antagonize the effects of pseudoephedrine and may increase the effects either of the antidepressants themselves or of the codeine). Products include:

Anafranil Capsules 803

Clorazepate Dipotassium (Effects of concurrent use not specified). Products include:

Tranxene 451

Clozapine (Effects of concurrent use not specified). Products include:

Clozaril Tablets 2252

Desflurane (Effects of concurrent use not specified). Products include:

Suprane 1813

Desipramine Hydrochloride (May antagonize the effects of pseudoephedrine and may increase the effects either of the antidepressants themselves or of the codeine). Products include:

Norpramin Tablets 1526

Deslanoside (Concurrent use with pseudoephedrine may increase the possibility of cardiac arrhythmias).

No products indexed under this heading.

Dezocine (Effects of concurrent use not specified). Products include:

Dalgan Injection 538

Diazepam (Effects of concurrent use not specified). Products include:

Dizac 1809
Valium Injectable 2182
Valium Tablets 2183
Valrelease Capsules 2169

Dicyclomine Hydrochloride (Concurrent use may result in paralytic ileus). Products include:

Bentyl 1501

Digitoxin (Concurrent use with pseudoephedrine may increase the possibility of cardiac arrhythmias). Products include:

Crystodigin Tablets 1433

Digoxin (Concurrent use with pseudoephedrine may increase the possibility of cardiac arrhythmias). Products include:

Lanoxicaps 1117
Lanoxin Elixir Pediatric 1120
Lanoxin Injection 1123
Lanoxin Injection Pediatric 1126
Lanoxin Tablets 1128

Dobutamine Hydrochloride (Concurrent use may increase the effects of either of these agents thereby increasing the potential for side effects). Products include:

Dobutrex Solution Vials 1439

Dopamine Hydrochloride (Concurrent use may increase the effects of either of these agents thereby increasing the potential for side effects).

No products indexed under this heading.

Doxepin Hydrochloride (May antagonize the effects of pseudoephedrine and may increase the effects either of the antidepressants themselves or of the codeine). Products include:

Sinequan 2205
Zonalon Cream 1055

Droperidol (Effects of concurrent use not specified). Products include:

Inapsine Injection 1296

Enflurane (Effects of concurrent use not specified).

No products indexed under this heading.

Ephedrine Hydrochloride (Concurrent use may increase the effects of either of these agents thereby increasing the potential for side effects). Products include:

Primatene Dual Action Formula ▣ 872
Primatene Tablets ▣ 873
Quadrinal Tablets 1350

Ephedrine Sulfate (Concurrent use may increase the effects of either of these agents thereby increasing the potential for side effects). Products include:

Bronkaid Caplets ▣ 717
Marax Tablets & DF Syrup 2200

Ephedrine Tannate (Concurrent use may increase the effects of either of these agents thereby increasing the potential for side effects). Products include:

Rynatuss 2673

IMPORTANT NOTE: Always consult each drug listing in the patient's regimen for possible interactions.

Deconsal C Interactions Index 240

Epinephrine (Concurrent use may increase the effects of either of these agents thereby increasing the potential for side effects). Products include:
Bronkaid Mist ▣ 717
EPIFRIN ⊙ 239
EpiPen 790
Marcaine Hydrochloride with Epinephrine 1:200,000 2316
Primatene Mist ▣ 873
Sensorcaine with Epinephrine Injection 559
Sus-Phrine Injection 1019
Xylocaine with Epinephrine Injections 567

Epinephrine Bitartrate (Concurrent use may increase the effects of either of these agents thereby increasing the potential for side effects). Products include:
Bronkaid Mist Suspension ▣ 718
Sensorcaine-MPF with Epinephrine Injection 559

Epinephrine Hydrochloride (Concurrent use may increase the effects of either of these agents thereby increasing the potential for side effects). Products include:
Ana-Kit Anaphylaxis Emergency Treatment Kit 617

Esmolol Hydrochloride (Concurrent use may increase the pressor effect of pseudoephedrine). Products include:
Brevibloc Injection 1808

Estazolam (Effects of concurrent use not specified). Products include:
ProSom Tablets 449

Ethchlorvynol (Effects of concurrent use not specified). Products include:
Placidyl Capsules 448

Ethinamate (Effects of concurrent use not specified).
No products indexed under this heading.

Fentanyl (Effects of concurrent use not specified). Products include:
Duragesic Transdermal System 1288

Fentanyl Citrate (Effects of concurrent use not specified). Products include:
Sublimaze Injection 1307

Fluphenazine Decanoate (Effects of concurrent use not specified). Products include:
Prolixin Decanoate 509

Fluphenazine Enanthate (Effects of concurrent use not specified). Products include:
Prolixin Enanthate 509

Fluphenazine Hydrochloride (Effects of concurrent use not specified). Products include:
Prolixin 509

Flurazepam Hydrochloride (Effects of concurrent use not specified). Products include:
Dalmane Capsules 2173

Furazolidone (Potentiates the pressor effect of pseudoephedrine resulting in hypertensive crisis; concurrent and/or sequential use is not recommended). Products include:
Furoxone 2046

Glutethimide (Effects of concurrent use not specified).
No products indexed under this heading.

Glycopyrrolate (Concurrent use may result in paralytic ileus). Products include:
Robinul Forte Tablets 2072
Robinul Injectable 2072
Robinul Tablets 2072

Haloperidol (Effects of concurrent use not specified). Products include:
Haldol Injection, Tablets and Concentrate 1575

Haloperidol Decanoate (Effects of concurrent use not specified). Products include:
Haldol Decanoate 1577

Hydrocodone Bitartrate (Effects of concurrent use not specified). Products include:
Anexsia 5/500 Elixir 1781
Anexia Tablets 1782
Codiclear DH Syrup 791
Deconamine CX Cough and Cold Liquid and Tablets 1319
Duratuss HD Elixir 2565
Hycodan Tablets and Syrup 930
Hycomine Compound Tablets 932
Hycomine 931
Hycotuss Expectorant Syrup 933
Hydrocet Capsules 782
Lorcet 10/650 1018
Lortab 2566
Tussend 1783
Tussend Expectorant 1785
Vicodin Tablets 1356
Vicodin ES Tablets 1357
Vicodin Tuss Expectorant 1358
Zydone Capsules 949

Hydrocodone Polistirex (Effects of concurrent use not specified). Products include:
Tussionex Pennkinetic Extended-Release Suspension 998

Hydroxyzine Hydrochloride (Effects of concurrent use not specified). Products include:
Atarax Tablets & Syrup 2185
Marax Tablets & DF Syrup 2200
Vistaril Intramuscular Solution 2216

Hyoscyamine (Concurrent use may result in paralytic ileus). Products include:
Cystospaz Tablets 1963
Urised Tablets 1964

Hyoscyamine Sulfate (Concurrent use may result in paralytic ileus). Products include:
Arco-Lase Plus Tablets 512
Atrohist Plus Tablets 454
Cystospaz-M Capsules 1963
Donnatal 2060
Donnatal Extentabs 2061
Donnatal Tablets 2060
Kutrase Capsules 2402
Levsin/Levsinex/Levbid 2405

Imipramine Hydrochloride (May antagonize the effects of pseudoephedrine and may increase the effects either of the antidepressants themselves or of the codeine). Products include:
Tofranil Ampuls 854
Tofranil Tablets 856

Imipramine Pamoate (May antagonize the effects of pseudoephedrine and may increase the effects either of the antidepressants themselves or of the codeine). Products include:
Tofranil-PM Capsules 857

Ipratropium Bromide (Concurrent use may result in paralytic ileus). Products include:
Atrovent Inhalation Aerosol 671
Atrovent Inhalation Solution 673

Isocarboxazid (Potentiates the pressor effect of pseudoephedrine resulting in hypertensive crisis; concurrent and/or sequential use is not recommended).
No products indexed under this heading.

Isoflurane (Effects of concurrent use not specified).
No products indexed under this heading.

Isoproterenol Hydrochloride (Concurrent use may increase the effects of either of these agents thereby increasing the potential for side effects). Products include:
Isuprel Hydrochloride Injection 1:5000 2311
Isuprel Hydrochloride Solution 1:200 & 1:100 2313
Isuprel Mistometer 2312

Isoproterenol Sulfate (Concurrent use may increase the effects of either of these agents thereby increasing the potential for side effects). Products include:
Norisodrine with Calcium Iodide Syrup 442

Ketamine Hydrochloride (Effects of concurrent use not specified).
No products indexed under this heading.

Labetalol Hydrochloride (Concurrent use may increase the pressor effect of pseudoephedrine). Products include:
Normodyne Injection 2377
Normodyne Tablets 2379
Trandate 1185

Levobunolol Hydrochloride (Concurrent use may increase the pressor effect of pseudoephedrine). Products include:
Betagan ⊙ 233

Levomethadyl Acetate Hydrochloride (Effects of concurrent use not specified). Products include:
Orlamm 2239

Levorphanol Tartrate (Effects of concurrent use not specified). Products include:
Levo-Dromoran 2129

Lorazepam (Effects of concurrent use not specified). Products include:
Ativan Injection 2698
Ativan Tablets 2700

Loxapine Hydrochloride (Effects of concurrent use not specified). Products include:
Loxitane 1378

Loxapine Succinate (Effects of concurrent use not specified). Products include:
Loxitane Capsules 1378

Maprotiline Hydrochloride (May antagonize the effects of pseudoephedrine and may increase the effects either of the antidepressants themselves or of the codeine). Products include:
Ludiomil Tablets 843

Mepenzolate Bromide (Concurrent use may result in paralytic ileus).
No products indexed under this heading.

Meperidine Hydrochloride (Effects of concurrent use not specified). Products include:
Demerol 2308
Mepergan Injection 2753

Mephobarbital (Effects of concurrent use not specified). Products include:
Mebaral Tablets 2322

Meprobamate (Effects of concurrent use not specified). Products include:
Miltown Tablets 2672
PMB 200 and PMB 400 2783

Mesoridazine (Effects of concurrent use not specified).

Metaproterenol Sulfate (Concurrent use may increase the effects of either of these agents thereby increasing the potential for side effects). Products include:
Alupent 669
Metaproterenol Sulfate Inhalation Solution, USP, Arm-a-Med 552

Metaraminol Bitartrate (Concurrent use may increase the effects of either of these agents thereby increasing the potential for side effects). Products include:
Aramine Injection 1609

Methadone Hydrochloride (Effects of concurrent use not specified). Products include:
Methadone Hydrochloride Oral Concentrate 2233
Methadone Hydrochloride Oral Solution & Tablets 2235

Methohexital Sodium (Effects of concurrent use not specified). Products include:
Brevital Sodium Vials 1429

Methotrimeprazine (Effects of concurrent use not specified). Products include:
Levoprome 1274

Methoxamine Hydrochloride (Concurrent use may increase the effects of either of these agents thereby increasing the potential for side effects). Products include:
Vasoxyl Injection 1196

Methoxyflurane (Effects of concurrent use not specified).
No products indexed under this heading.

Metipranolol Hydrochloride (Concurrent use may increase the pressor effect of pseudoephedrine). Products include:
OptiPranolol (Metipranolol 0.3%) Sterile Ophthalmic Solution ⊙ 258

Metoprolol Succinate (Concurrent use may increase the pressor effect of pseudoephedrine). Products include:
Toprol-XL Tablets 565

Metoprolol Tartrate (Concurrent use may increase the pressor effect of pseudoephedrine). Products include:
Lopressor Ampuls 830
Lopressor HCT Tablets 832
Lopressor Tablets 830

Midazolam Hydrochloride (Effects of concurrent use not specified). Products include:
Versed Injection 2170

Molindone Hydrochloride (Effects of concurrent use not specified). Products include:
Moban Tablets and Concentrate 1048

Morphine Sulfate (Effects of concurrent use not specified). Products include:
Astramorph/PF Injection, USP (Preservative-Free) 535
Duramorph 962
Infumorph 200 and Infumorph 500 Sterile Solutions 965
MS Contin Tablets 1994
MSIR 1997
Oramorph SR (Morphine Sulfate Sustained Release Tablets) 2236
RMS Suppositories 2657
Roxanol 2243

Nadolol (Concurrent use may increase the pressor effect of pseudoephedrine).
No products indexed under this heading.

Norepinephrine Bitartrate (Concurrent use may increase the effects of either of these agents thereby increasing the potential for side effects). Products include:
Levophed Bitartrate Injection 2315

(▣ Described in PDR For Nonprescription Drugs) (⊙ Described in PDR For Ophthalmology)

Interactions Index — Deconsal C

Nortriptyline Hydrochloride (May antagonize the effects of pseudoephedrine and may increase the effects either of the antidepressants themselves or of the codeine). Products include:

Pamelor 2280

Opium Alkaloids (Effects of concurrent use not specified).

No products indexed under this heading.

Oxazepam (Effects of concurrent use not specified). Products include:

Serax Capsules 2810
Serax Tablets.. 2810

Oxybutynin Chloride (Concurrent use may result in paralytic ileus). Products include:

Ditropan.. 1516

Oxycodone Hydrochloride (Effects of concurrent use not specified). Products include:

Percocet Tablets 938
Percodan Tablets...................................... 939
Percodan-Demi Tablets............................ 940
Roxicodone Tablets, Oral Solution & Intensol (Oxycodone) 2244
Tylox Capsules 1584

Penbutolol Sulfate (Concurrent use may increase the pressor effect of pseudoephedrine). Products include:

Levatol 2403

Pentobarbital Sodium (Effects of concurrent use not specified). Products include:

Nembutal Sodium Capsules 436
Nembutal Sodium Solution 438
Nembutal Sodium Suppositories...... 440

Perphenazine (Effects of concurrent use not specified). Products include:

Etrafon 2355
Triavil Tablets 1757
Trilafon.. 2389

Phenelzine Sulfate (Potentiates the pressor effect of pseudoephedrine resulting in hypertensive crisis; concurrent and/or sequential use is not recommended). Products include:

Nardil 1920

Phenobarbital (Effects of concurrent use not specified). Products include:

Arco-Lase Plus Tablets 512
Bellergal-S Tablets 2250
Donnatal 2060
Donnatal Extentabs................................ 2061
Donnatal Tablets 2060
Phenobarbital Elixir and Tablets 1469
Quadrinal Tablets 1350

Phenylephrine Bitartrate (Concurrent use may increase the effects of either of these agents thereby increasing the potential for side effects).

No products indexed under this heading.

Phenylephrine Hydrochloride (Concurrent use may increase the effects of either of these agents thereby increasing the potential for side effects). Products include:

Atrohist Plus Tablets 454
Cerose DM .... ⊕ 878
Comhist 2038
D.A. Chewable Tablets........................... 951
Deconsal Pediatric Capsules.............. 454
Dura-Vent/DA Tablets 953
Entex Capsules 1986
Entex Liquid 1986
Extendryl 1005
4-Way Fast Acting Nasal Spray (regular & mentholated) .... ⊕ 621
Hemorid For Women .... ⊕ 834
Hycomine Compound Tablets 932
Neo-Synephrine Hydrochloride 1% Carpuject... 2324
Neo-Synephrine Hydrochloride 1% Injection 2324

Neo-Synephrine Hydrochloride (Ophthalmic) 2325
Neo-Synephrine .... ⊕ 726
Nōstril.. ⊕ 644
Novahistine Elixir .... ⊕ 823
Phenergan VC 2779
Phenergan VC with Codeine 2781
Preparation H .... ⊕ 871
Tympagesic Ear Drops 2342
Vasosulf .... © 271
Vicks Sinex Nasal Spray and Ultra Fine Mist .... ⊕ 765

Phenylephrine Tannate (Concurrent use may increase the effects of either of these agents thereby increasing the potential for side effects). Products include:

Atrohist Pediatric Suspension 454
Ricobid-D Pediatric Suspension........ 2038
Ricobid Tablets and Pediatric Suspension.. 2038
Rynatan 2673
Rynatuss 2673

Phenylpropanolamine Hydrochloride (Concurrent use may increase the effects of either of these agents thereby increasing the potential for side effects). Products include:

Acutrim .... ⊕ 628
Allerest Children's Chewable Tablets .... ⊕ 627
Allerest 12 Hour Caplets .... ⊕ 627
Atrohist Plus Tablets 454
BC Cold Powder Multi-Symptom Formula (Cold-Sinus-Allergy) ...... ⊕ 609
BC Cold Powder Non-Drowsy Formula (Cold-Sinus) .... ⊕ 609
Cheracol Plus Head Cold/Cough Formula .... ⊕ 769
Comtrex Multi-Symptom Non-Drowsy Liqui-gels................................ ⊕ 618
Contac Continuous Action Nasal Decongestant/Antihistamine 12 Hour Capsules..................................... ⊕ 813
Contac Maximum Strength Continuous Action Decongestant/Antihistamine 12 Hour Caplets.. ⊕ 813
Contac Severe Cold and Flu Formula Caplets .... ⊕ 814
Coricidin 'D' Decongestant Tablets .... ⊕ 800
Dexatrim .... ⊕ 832
Dexatrim Plus Vitamins Caplets .... ⊕ 832
Dimetane-DC Cough Syrup 2059
Dimetapp Elixir..................................... ⊕ 773
Dimetapp Extentabs .... ⊕ 774
Dimetapp Tablets/Liqui-Gels .... ⊕ 775
Dimetapp Cold & Allergy Chewable Tablets .... ⊕ 773
Dimetapp DM Elixir .... ⊕ 774
Dura-Vent Tablets 952
Entex Capsules 1986
Entex LA Tablets 1987
Entex Liquid 1986
Exgest LA Tablets 782
Hycomine 931
Isoclor Timesule Capsules .... ⊕ 637
Nolamine Timed-Release Tablets 785
Ornade Spansule Capsules 2502
Propagest Tablets 786
Pyrroxate Caplets .... ⊕ 772
Robitussin-CF .... ⊕ 777
Sinulin Tablets 787
Tavist-D 12 Hour Relief Tablets .... ⊕ 787
Teldrin 12 Hour Antihistamine/Nasal Decongestant Allergy Relief Capsules .... ⊕ 826
Triaminic Allergy Tablets .... ⊕ 789
Triaminic Cold Tablets .... ⊕ 790
Triaminic Expectorant .... ⊕ 790
Triaminic Syrup .... ⊕ 792
Triaminic-12 Tablets .... ⊕ 792
Triaminic-DM Syrup .... ⊕ 792
Triaminicin Tablets .... ⊕ 793
Triaminicol Multi-Symptom Cold Tablets .... ⊕ 793
Triaminicol Multi-Symptom Relief ⊕ 794
Vicks DayQuil Allergy Relief 12-Hour Extended Release Tablets.. ⊕ 760
Vicks DayQuil Allergy Relief 4-Hour Tablets .... ⊕ 760
Vicks DayQuil SINUS Pressure & CONGESTION Relief........................ ⊕ 761

Pindolol (Concurrent use may increase the pressor effect of pseudoephedrine). Products include:

Visken Tablets... 2299

Pirbuterol Acetate (Concurrent use may increase the effects of either of these agents thereby increasing the potential for side effects). Products include:

Maxair Autohaler 1492
Maxair Inhaler 1494

Prazepam (Effects of concurrent use not specified).

No products indexed under this heading.

Prochlorperazine (Effects of concurrent use not specified). Products include:

Compazine 2470

Procyclidine Hydrochloride (Concurrent use may result in paralytic ileus). Products include:

Kemadrin Tablets 1112

Promethazine Hydrochloride (Effects of concurrent use not specified). Products include:

Mepergan Injection 2753
Phenergan with Codeine 2777
Phenergan with Dextromethorphan 2778
Phenergan Injection 2773
Phenergan Suppositories 2775
Phenergan Syrup 2774
Phenergan Tablets 2775
Phenergan VC 2779
Phenergan VC with Codeine 2781

Propantheline Bromide (Concurrent use may result in paralytic ileus). Products include:

Pro-Banthine Tablets............................. 2052

Propofol (Effects of concurrent use not specified). Products include:

Diprivan Injection................................... 2833

Propoxyphene Hydrochloride (Effects of concurrent use not specified). Products include:

Darvon 1435
Wygesic Tablets 2827

Propoxyphene Napsylate (Effects of concurrent use not specified). Products include:

Darvon-N/Darvocet-N 1433

Propranolol Hydrochloride (Concurrent use may increase the pressor effect of pseudoephedrine). Products include:

Inderal 2728
Inderal LA Long Acting Capsules 2730
Inderide Tablets 2732
Inderide LA Long Acting Capsules .. 2734

Protriptyline Hydrochloride (May antagonize the effects of pseudoephedrine and may increase the effects either of the antidepressants themselves or of the codeine). Products include:

Vivactil Tablets 1774

Pseudoephedrine Sulfate (Concurrent use may increase the effects of either of these agents thereby increasing the potential for side effects). Products include:

Cheracol Sinus .... ⊕ 768
Chlor-Trimeton Allergy Decongestant Tablets .... ⊕ 799
Claritin-D 2350
Drixoral Cold and Allergy Sustained-Action Tablets .... ⊕ 802
Drixoral Cold and Flu Extended-Release Tablets................................... ⊕ 803
Drixoral Non-Drowsy Formula Extended-Release Tablets .... ⊕ 803
Drixoral Allergy/Sinus Extended Release Tablets................................... ⊕ 804
Trinalin Repetabs Tablets 1330

Quazepam (Effects of concurrent use not specified). Products include:

Doral Tablets 2664

Risperidone (Effects of concurrent use not specified). Products include:

Risperdal 1301

Salmeterol Xinafoate (Concurrent use may increase the effects of either of these agents thereby increasing the potential for side effects). Products include:

Serevent Inhalation Aerosol................ 1176

Scopolamine (Concurrent use may result in paralytic ileus). Products include:

Transderm Scōp Transdermal Therapeutic System 869

Scopolamine Hydrobromide (Concurrent use may result in paralytic ileus). Products include:

Atrohist Plus Tablets 454
Donnatal 2060
Donnatal Extentabs................................ 2061
Donnatal Tablets 2060

Secobarbital Sodium (Effects of concurrent use not specified). Products include:

Seconal Sodium Pulvules 1474

Selegiline Hydrochloride (Potentiates the pressor effect of pseudoephedrine resulting in hypertensive crisis; concurrent and/or sequential use is not recommended). Products include:

Eldepryl Tablets 2550

Sotalol Hydrochloride (Concurrent use may increase the pressor effect of pseudoephedrine). Products include:

Betapace Tablets 641

Sufentanil Citrate (Effects of concurrent use not specified). Products include:

Sufenta Injection 1309

Temazepam (Effects of concurrent use not specified). Products include:

Restoril Capsules.................................... 2284

Terbutaline Sulfate (Concurrent use may increase the effects of either of these agents thereby increasing the potential for side effects). Products include:

Brethaire Inhaler 813
Brethine Ampuls 815
Brethine Tablets...................................... 814
Bricanyl Subcutaneous Injection 1502
Bricanyl Tablets 1503

Thiamylal Sodium (Effects of concurrent use not specified).

No products indexed under this heading.

Thioridazine Hydrochloride (Effects of concurrent use not specified). Products include:

Mellaril 2269

Thiothixene (Effects of concurrent use not specified). Products include:

Navane Capsules and Concentrate 2201
Navane Intramuscular........................... 2202

Timolol Hemihydrate (Concurrent use may increase the pressor effect of pseudoephedrine). Products include:

Betimol 0.25%, 0.5% .... © 261

Timolol Maleate (Concurrent use may increase the pressor effect of pseudoephedrine). Products include:

Blocadren Tablets 1614
Timolide Tablets...................................... 1748
Timoptic in Ocudose 1753
Timoptic Sterile Ophthalmic Solution.. 1751
Timoptic-XE 1755

Tranylcypromine Sulfate (Potentiates the pressor effect of pseudoephedrine resulting in hypertensive crisis; concurrent and/or sequential use is not recommended). Products include:

Parnate Tablets 2503

Triazolam (Effects of concurrent use not specified). Products include:

Halcion Tablets.. 2611

IMPORTANT NOTE: Always consult each drug listing in the patient's regimen for possible interactions.

Tridihexethyl Chloride (Concurrent use may result in paralytic ileus).
No products indexed under this heading.

Trifluoperazine Hydrochloride (Effects of concurrent use not specified). Products include:
Stelazine ... 2514

Trihexyphenidyl Hydrochloride (Concurrent use may result in paralytic ileus). Products include:
Artane ... 1368

Trimipramine Maleate (May antagonize the effects of pseudoephedrine and may increase the effects either of the antidepressants themselves or of the codeine). Products include:
Surmontil Capsules ... 2811

Zolpidem Tartrate (Effects of concurrent use not specified). Products include:
Ambien Tablets ... 2416

Food Interactions

Alcohol (Effects of concurrent use not specified).

DECONSAL PEDIATRIC CAPSULES

(Guaifenesin, Phenylephrine Hydrochloride) ... **454**
See **Deconsal II Tablets**

DECONSAL PEDIATRIC SYRUP

(Codeine Phosphate, Pseudoephedrine Hydrochloride, Guaifenesin) ... **457**

May interact with beta blockers, cardiac glycosides, antihypertensives, veratrum alkaloids, monoamine oxidase inhibitors, sympathomimetics, tricyclic antidepressants, central nervous system depressants, general anesthetics, anticholinergics, and certain other agents. Compounds in these categories include:

Acebutolol Hydrochloride (Decreased hypotensive effect; beta blockers increase the pressor effect of pseudoephedrine). Products include:
Sectral Capsules ... 2807

Albuterol (May increase the effects of either of these agents thereby increasing the potential of side effects). Products include:
Proventil Inhalation Aerosol ... 2382
Ventolin Inhalation Aerosol and Refill ... 1197

Albuterol Sulfate (May increase the effects of either of these agents thereby increasing the potential of side effects). Products include:
Airet Solution for Inhalation ... 452
Proventil Inhalation Solution 0.083% ... 2384
Proventil Repetabs Tablets ... 2386
Proventil Solution for Inhalation 0.5% ... 2383
Proventil Syrup ... 2385
Proventil Tablets ... 2386
Ventolin Inhalation Solution ... 1198
Ventolin Nebules Inhalation Solution ... 1199
Ventolin Rotacaps for Inhalation ... 1200
Ventolin Syrup ... 1202
Ventolin Tablets ... 1203
Volmax Extended-Release Tablets .. 1788

Alfentanil Hydrochloride (Potential for unspecified CNS effect). Products include:
Alfenta Injection ... 1286

Alprazolam (Potential for unspecified CNS effect). Products include:
Xanax Tablets ... 2649

Amitriptyline Hydrochloride (May antagonize the effect of pseudoephedrine and may increase the effects of either antidepressant or codeine component). Products include:
Elavil ... 2838
Endep Tablets ... 2174
Etrafon ... 2355
Limbitrol ... 2180
Triavil Tablets ... 1757

Amlodipine Besylate (Decreased hypotensive effect). Products include:
Lotrel Capsules ... 840
Norvasc Tablets ... 1940

Amoxapine (May antagonize the effect of pseudoephedrine and may increase the effects of either antidepressant or codeine component). Products include:
Asendin Tablets ... 1369

Aprobarbital (Potential for unspecified CNS effect).
No products indexed under this heading.

Atenolol (Decreased hypotensive effect; beta blockers increase the pressor effect of pseudoephedrine). Products include:
Tenoretic Tablets ... 2845
Tenormin Tablets and I.V. Injection 2847

Atropine Sulfate (Concurrent use may result in paralytic ileus). Products include:
Arco-Lase Plus Tablets ... 512
Atrohist Plus Tablets ... 454
Atropine Sulfate Sterile Ophthalmic Solution ... ⊙ 233
Donnatal ... 2060
Donnatal Extentabs ... 2061
Donnatal Tablets ... 2060
Lomotil ... 2439
Motofen Tablets ... 784
Urised Tablets ... 1964

Belladonna Alkaloids (Concurrent use may result in paralytic ileus). Products include:
Bellergal-S Tablets ... 2250
Hyland's Bed Wetting Tablets ... ▣ 828
Hyland's EnurAid Tablets ... ▣ 829
Hyland's Teething Tablets ... ▣ 830

Benazepril Hydrochloride (Decreased hypotensive effect). Products include:
Lotensin Tablets ... 834
Lotensin HCT ... 837
Lotrel Capsules ... 840

Bendroflumethiazide (Decreased hypotensive effect).
No products indexed under this heading.

Benztropine Mesylate (Concurrent use may result in paralytic ileus). Products include:
Cogentin ... 1621

Betaxolol Hydrochloride (Decreased hypotensive effect; beta blockers increase the pressor effect of pseudoephedrine). Products include:
Betoptic Ophthalmic Solution ... 469
Betoptic S Ophthalmic Suspension 471
Kerlone Tablets ... 2436

Biperiden Hydrochloride (Concurrent use may result in paralytic ileus). Products include:
Akineton ... 1333

Bisoprolol Fumarate (Decreased hypotensive effect; beta blockers increase the pressor effect of pseudoephedrine). Products include:
Zebeta Tablets ... 1413
Ziac ... 1415

Buprenorphine (Potential for unspecified CNS effect). Products include:
Buprenex Injectable ... 2006

Buspirone Hydrochloride (Potential for unspecified CNS effect). Products include:
BuSpar ... 737

Butabarbital (Potential for unspecified CNS effect).
No products indexed under this heading.

Butalbital (Potential for unspecified CNS effect). Products include:
Esgic-plus Tablets ... 1013
Fioricet Tablets ... 2258
Fioricet with Codeine Capsules ... 2260
Fiorinal Capsules ... 2261
Fiorinal with Codeine Capsules ... 2262
Fiorinal Tablets ... 2261
Phrenilin ... 785
Sedapap Tablets 50 mg/650 mg .. 1543

Captopril (Decreased hypotensive effect). Products include:
Capoten ... 739
Capozide ... 742

Carteolol Hydrochloride (Decreased hypotensive effect; beta blockers increase the pressor effect of pseudoephedrine). Products include:
Cartrol Tablets ... 410
Ocupress Ophthalmic Solution, 1% Sterile ... ⊙ 309

Chlordiazepoxide (Potential for unspecified CNS effect). Products include:
Libritabs Tablets ... 2177
Limbitrol ... 2180

Chlordiazepoxide Hydrochloride (Potential for unspecified CNS effect). Products include:
Librax Capsules ... 2176
Librium Capsules ... 2178
Librium Injectable ... 2179

Chlorothiazide (Decreased hypotensive effect). Products include:
Aldoclor Tablets ... 1598
Diupres Tablets ... 1650
Diuril Oral ... 1653

Chlorothiazide Sodium (Decreased hypotensive effect). Products include:
Diuril Sodium Intravenous ... 1652

Chlorpromazine (Potential for unspecified CNS effect). Products include:
Thorazine Suppositories ... 2523

Chlorpromazine Hydrochloride (Potential for unspecified CNS effect). Products include:
Thorazine ... 2523

Chlorprothixene (Potential for unspecified CNS effect).
No products indexed under this heading.

Chlorprothixene Hydrochloride (Potential for unspecified CNS effect).
No products indexed under this heading.

Chlorthalidone (Decreased hypotensive effect). Products include:
Combipres Tablets ... 677
Tenoretic Tablets ... 2845
Thalitone ... 1245

Clidinium Bromide (Concurrent use may result in paralytic ileus). Products include:
Librax Capsules ... 2176
Quarzan Capsules ... 2181

Clomipramine Hydrochloride (May antagonize the effect of pseudoephedrine and may increase the effects of either antidepressant or codeine component). Products include:
Anafranil Capsules ... 803

Clonidine (Decreased hypotensive effect). Products include:
Catapres-TTS ... 675

Clonidine Hydrochloride (Decreased hypotensive effect). Products include:
Catapres Tablets ... 674
Combipres Tablets ... 677

Clorazepate Dipotassium (Potential for unspecified CNS effect). Products include:
Tranxene ... 451

Clozapine (Potential for unspecified CNS effect). Products include:
Clozaril Tablets ... 2252

Cryptenamine Preparations (Decreased hypotensive effect).

Deserpidine (Decreased hypotensive effect).
No products indexed under this heading.

Desflurane (Potential for unspecified CNS effect). Products include:
Suprane ... 1813

Desipramine Hydrochloride (May antagonize the effect of pseudoephedrine and may increase the effects of either antidepressant or codeine component). Products include:
Norpramin Tablets ... 1526

Deslanoside (Concurrent use may increase the possibility of cardiac arrhythmias).
No products indexed under this heading.

Dezocine (Potential for unspecified CNS effect). Products include:
Dalgan Injection ... 538

Diazepam (Potential for unspecified CNS effect). Products include:
Dizac ... 1809
Valium Injectable ... 2182
Valium Tablets ... 2183
Valrelease Capsules ... 2169

Diazoxide (Decreased hypotensive effect). Products include:
Hyperstat I.V. Injection ... 2363
Proglycem ... 580

Dicyclomine Hydrochloride (Concurrent use may result in paralytic ileus). Products include:
Bentyl ... 1501

Digitoxin (Concurrent use may increase the possibility of cardiac arrhythmias). Products include:
Crystodigin Tablets ... 1433

Digoxin (Concurrent use may increase the possibility of cardiac arrhythmias). Products include:
Lanoxicaps ... 1117
Lanoxin Elixir Pediatric ... 1120
Lanoxin Injection ... 1123
Lanoxin Injection Pediatric ... 1126
Lanoxin Tablets ... 1128

Diltiazem Hydrochloride (Decreased hypotensive effect). Products include:
Cardizem CD Capsules ... 1506
Cardizem SR Capsules ... 1510
Cardizem Injectable ... 1508
Cardizem Tablets ... 1512
Dilacor XR Extended-release Capsules ... 2018

Dobutamine Hydrochloride (May increase the effects of either of these agents thereby increasing the potential of side effects). Products include:
Dobutrex Solution Vials ... 1439

Dopamine Hydrochloride (May increase the effects of either of these agents thereby increasing the potential of side effects).
No products indexed under this heading.

Doxazosin Mesylate (Decreased hypotensive effect). Products include:
Cardura Tablets ... 2186

(▣ Described in PDR For Nonprescription Drugs) (⊙ Described in PDR For Ophthalmology)

243 Interactions Index Deconsal Pediatric Syrup

Doxepin Hydrochloride (May antagonize the effect of pseudoephedrine and may increase the effects of either antidepressant or codeine component). Products include:
Sinequan ... 2205
Zonalon Cream ... 1055

Droperidol (Potential for unspecified CNS effect). Products include:
Inapsine Injection ... 1296

Enalapril Maleate (Decreased hypotensive effect). Products include:
Vaseretic Tablets ... 1765
Vasotec Tablets ... 1771

Enalaprilat (Decreased hypotensive effect). Products include:
Vasotec I.V. ... 1768

Enflurane (Potential for unspecified CNS effect).
No products indexed under this heading.

Ephedrine Hydrochloride (May increase the effects of either of these agents thereby increasing the potential of side effects). Products include:
Primatene Dual Action Formula ... ▣ 872
Primatene Tablets ... ▣ 873
Quadrinal Tablets ... 1350

Ephedrine Sulfate (May increase the effects of either of these agents thereby increasing the potential of side effects). Products include:
Bronkaid Caplets ... ▣ 717
Marax Tablets & DF Syrup ... 2200

Ephedrine Tannate (May increase the effects of either of these agents thereby increasing the potential of side effects). Products include:
Rynatuss ... 2673

Epinephrine (May increase the effects of either of these agents thereby increasing the potential of side effects). Products include:
Bronkaid Mist ... ▣ 717
EPIFRIN ... ◉ 239
EpiPen ... 790
Marcaine Hydrochloride with Epinephrine 1:200,000 ... 2316
Primatene Mist ... ▣ 873
Sensorcaine with Epinephrine Injection ... 559
Sus-Phrine Injection ... 1019
Xylocaine with Epinephrine Injections ... 567

Epinephrine Bitartrate (May increase the effects of either of these agents thereby increasing the potential of side effects). Products include:
Bronkaid Mist Suspension ... ▣ 718
Sensorcaine-MPF with Epinephrine Injection ... 559

Epinephrine Hydrochloride (May increase the effects of either of these agents thereby increasing the potential of side effects). Products include:
Ana-Kit Anaphylaxis Emergency Treatment Kit ... 617

Esmolol Hydrochloride (Decreased hypotensive effect; beta blockers increase the pressor effect of pseudoephedrine). Products include:
Brevibloc Injection ... 1808

Estazolam (Potential for unspecified CNS effect). Products include:
ProSom Tablets ... 449

Ethchlorvynol (Potential for unspecified CNS effect). Products include:
Placidyl Capsules ... 448

Ethinamate (Potential for unspecified CNS effect).
No products indexed under this heading.

Felodipine (Decreased hypotensive effect). Products include:
Plendil Extended-Release Tablets ... 527

Fentanyl (Potential for unspecified CNS effect). Products include:
Duragesic Transdermal System ... 1288

Fentanyl Citrate (Potential for unspecified CNS effect). Products include:
Sublimaze Injection ... 1307

Fluphenazine Decanoate (Potential for unspecified CNS effect). Products include:
Prolixin Decanoate ... 509

Fluphenazine Enanthate (Potential for unspecified CNS effect). Products include:
Prolixin Enanthate ... 509

Fluphenazine Hydrochloride (Potential for unspecified CNS effect). Products include:
Prolixin ... 509

Flurazepam Hydrochloride (Potential for unspecified CNS effect). Products include:
Dalmane Capsules ... 2173

Fosinopril Sodium (Decreased hypotensive effect). Products include:
Monopril Tablets ... 757

Furazolidone (Potentiates the pressor effect; concurrent and/or sequential use is not recommended). Products include:
Furoxone ... 2046

Furosemide (Decreased hypotensive effect). Products include:
Lasix Injection, Oral Solution and Tablets ... 1240

Glutethimide (Potential for unspecified CNS effect).
No products indexed under this heading.

Glycopyrrolate (Concurrent use may result in paralytic ileus). Products include:
Robinul Forte Tablets ... 2072
Robinul Injectable ... 2072
Robinul Tablets ... 2072

Guanabenz Acetate (Decreased hypotensive effect).
No products indexed under this heading.

Guanethidine Monosulfate (Decreased hypotensive effect). Products include:
Esimil Tablets ... 822
Ismelin Tablets ... 827

Haloperidol (Potential for unspecified CNS effect). Products include:
Haldol Injection, Tablets and Concentrate ... 1575

Haloperidol Decanoate (Potential for unspecified CNS effect). Products include:
Haldol Decanoate ... 1577

Hydralazine Hydrochloride (Decreased hypotensive effect). Products include:
Apresazide Capsules ... 808
Apresoline Hydrochloride Tablets ... 809
Ser-Ap-Es Tablets ... 849

Hydrochlorothiazide (Decreased hypotensive effect). Products include:
Aldactazide ... 2413
Aldoril Tablets ... 1604
Apresazide Capsules ... 808
Capozide ... 742
Dyazide ... 2479
Esidrix Tablets ... 821
Esimil Tablets ... 822
HydroDIURIL Tablets ... 1674
Hydropres Tablets ... 1675
Hyzaar Tablets ... 1677
Inderide Tablets ... 2732
Inderide LA Long Acting Capsules ... 2734
Lopressor HCT Tablets ... 832
Lotensin HCT ... 837
Maxzide ... 1380
Moduretic Tablets ... 1705
Oretic Tablets ... 443
Prinzide Tablets ... 1737
Ser-Ap-Es Tablets ... 849
Timolide Tablets ... 1748
Vaseretic Tablets ... 1765
Zestoretic ... 2850
Ziac ... 1415

Hydrocodone Bitartrate (Potential for unspecified CNS effect). Products include:
Anexsia 5/500 Elixir ... 1781
Anexia Tablets ... 1782
Codiclear DH Syrup ... 791
Deconamine CX Cough and Cold Liquid and Tablets ... 1319
Duratuss HD Elixir ... 2565
Hycodan Tablets and Syrup ... 930
Hycomine Compound Tablets ... 932
Hycomine ... 931
Hycotuss Expectorant Syrup ... 933
Hydrocet Capsules ... 782
Lorcet 10/650 ... 1018
Lortab ... 2566
Tussend ... 1783
Tussend Expectorant ... 1785
Vicodin Tablets ... 1356
Vicodin ES Tablets ... 1357
Vicodin Tuss Expectorant ... 1358
Zydone Capsules ... 949

Hydrocodone Polistirex (Potential for unspecified CNS effect). Products include:
Tussionex Pennkinetic Extended-Release Suspension ... 998

Hydroflumethiazide (Decreased hypotensive effect). Products include:
Diucardin Tablets ... 2718

Hydroxyzine Hydrochloride (Potential for unspecified CNS effect). Products include:
Atarax Tablets & Syrup ... 2185
Marax Tablets & DF Syrup ... 2200
Vistaril Intramuscular Solution ... 2216

Hyoscyamine (Concurrent use may result in paralytic ileus). Products include:
Cystospaz Tablets ... 1963
Urised Tablets ... 1964

Hyoscyamine Sulfate (Concurrent use may result in paralytic ileus). Products include:
Arco-Lase Plus Tablets ... 512
Atrohist Plus Tablets ... 454
Cystospaz-M Capsules ... 1963
Donnatal ... 2060
Donnatal Extentabs ... 2061
Donnatal Tablets ... 2060
Kutrase Capsules ... 2402
Levsin/Levsinex/Levbid ... 2405

Imipramine Hydrochloride (May antagonize the effect of pseudoephedrine and may increase the effects of either antidepressant or codeine component). Products include:
Tofranil Ampuls ... 854
Tofranil Tablets ... 856

Imipramine Pamoate (May antagonize the effect of pseudoephedrine and may increase the effects of either antidepressant or codeine component). Products include:
Tofranil-PM Capsules ... 857

Indapamide (Decreased hypotensive effect). Products include:
Lozol Tablets ... 2022

Ipratropium Bromide (Concurrent use may result in paralytic ileus). Products include:
Atrovent Inhalation Aerosol ... 671
Atrovent Inhalation Solution ... 673

Isocarboxazid (Potentiates the pressor effect; concurrent and/or sequential use is not recommended).
No products indexed under this heading.

Isoflurane (Potential for unspecified CNS effect).
No products indexed under this heading.

Isoproterenol Hydrochloride (May increase the effects of either of these agents thereby increasing the potential of side effects). Products include:
Isuprel Hydrochloride Injection 1:5000 ... 2311
Isuprel Hydrochloride Solution 1:200 & 1:100 ... 2313
Isuprel Mistometer ... 2312

Isradipine (Decreased hypotensive effect). Products include:
DynaCirc Capsules ... 2256

Ketamine Hydrochloride (Potential for unspecified CNS effect).
No products indexed under this heading.

Labetalol Hydrochloride (Decreased hypotensive effect; beta blockers increase the pressor effect of pseudoephedrine). Products include:
Normodyne Injection ... 2377
Normodyne Tablets ... 2379
Trandate ... 1185

Levobunolol Hydrochloride (Decreased hypotensive effect; beta blockers increase the pressor effect of pseudoephedrine). Products include:
Betagan ... ◉ 233

Levomethadyl Acetate Hydrochloride (Potential for unspecified CNS effect). Products include:
Orlamm ... 2239

Levorphanol Tartrate (Potential for unspecified CNS effect). Products include:
Levo-Dromoran ... 2129

Lisinopril (Decreased hypotensive effect). Products include:
Prinivil Tablets ... 1733
Prinzide Tablets ... 1737
Zestoretic ... 2850
Zestril Tablets ... 2854

Lorazepam (Potential for unspecified CNS effect). Products include:
Ativan Injection ... 2698
Ativan Tablets ... 2700

Losartan Potassium (Decreased hypotensive effect). Products include:
Cozaar Tablets ... 1628
Hyzaar Tablets ... 1677

Loxapine Hydrochloride (Potential for unspecified CNS effect). Products include:
Loxitane ... 1378

Loxapine Succinate (Potential for unspecified CNS effect). Products include:
Loxitane Capsules ... 1378

Maprotiline Hydrochloride (May antagonize the effect of pseudoephedrine and may increase the effects of either antidepressant or codeine component). Products include:
Ludiomil Tablets ... 843

Mecamylamine Hydrochloride (Decreased hypotensive effect). Products include:
Inversine Tablets ... 1686

Mepenzolate Bromide (Concurrent use may result in paralytic ileus).
No products indexed under this heading.

Meperidine Hydrochloride (Potential for unspecified CNS effect). Products include:
Demerol ... 2308
Mepergan Injection ... 2753

IMPORTANT NOTE: Always consult each drug listing in the patient's regimen for possible interactions.

Deconsal Pediatric Syrup **Interactions Index** **244**

Mephobarbital (Potential for unspecified CNS effect). Products include:
- Mebaral Tablets ... 2322

Meprobamate (Potential for unspecified CNS effect). Products include:
- Miltown Tablets ... 2672
- PMB 200 and PMB 400 ... 2783

Mesoridazine (Potential for unspecified CNS effect).

Metaproterenol Sulfate (May increase the effects of either of these agents thereby increasing the potential of side effects). Products include:
- Alupent ... 669
- Metaproterenol Sulfate Inhalation Solution, USP, Arm-a-Med ... 552

Metaraminol Bitartrate (May increase the effects of either of these agents thereby increasing the potential of side effects). Products include:
- Aramine Injection ... 1609

Methadone Hydrochloride (Potential for unspecified CNS effect). Products include:
- Methadone Hydrochloride Oral Concentrate ... 2233
- Methadone Hydrochloride Oral Solution & Tablets ... 2235

Methohexital Sodium (Potential for unspecified CNS effect). Products include:
- Brevital Sodium Vials ... 1429

Methotrimeprazine (Potential for unspecified CNS effect). Products include:
- Levoprome ... 1274

Methoxamine Hydrochloride (May increase the effects of either of these agents thereby increasing the potential of side effects). Products include:
- Vasoxyl Injection ... 1196

Methoxyflurane (Potential for unspecified CNS effect).
- No products indexed under this heading.

Methyclothiazide (Decreased hypotensive effect). Products include:
- Enduron Tablets ... 420

Methyldopa (Decreased hypotensive effect). Products include:
- Aldoclor Tablets ... 1598
- Aldomet Oral ... 1600
- Aldoril Tablets ... 1604

Methyldopate Hydrochloride (Decreased hypotensive effect). Products include:
- Aldomet Ester HCl Injection ... 1602

Metipranolol Hydrochloride (Decreased hypotensive effect; beta blockers increase the pressor effect of pseudoephedrine). Products include:
- OptiPranolol (Metipranolol 0.3%) Sterile Ophthalmic Solution ... ◉ 258

Metolazone (Decreased hypotensive effect). Products include:
- Mykrox Tablets ... 993
- Zaroxolyn Tablets ... 1000

Metoprolol Succinate (Decreased hypotensive effect; beta blockers increase the pressor effect of pseudoephedrine). Products include:
- Toprol-XL Tablets ... 565

Metoprolol Tartrate (Decreased hypotensive effect; beta blockers increase the pressor effect of pseudoephedrine). Products include:
- Lopressor Ampuls ... 830
- Lopressor HCT Tablets ... 832
- Lopressor Tablets ... 830

Metyrosine (Decreased hypotensive effect). Products include:
- Demser Capsules ... 1649

Midazolam Hydrochloride (Potential for unspecified CNS effect). Products include:
- Versed Injection ... 2170

Minoxidil (Decreased hypotensive effect). Products include:
- Loniten Tablets ... 2618
- Rogaine Topical Solution ... 2637

Moexipril Hydrochloride (Decreased hypotensive effect). Products include:
- Univasc Tablets ... 2410

Molindone Hydrochloride (Potential for unspecified CNS effect). Products include:
- Moban Tablets and Concentrate ... 1048

Morphine Sulfate (Potential for unspecified CNS effect). Products include:
- Astramorph/PF Injection, USP (Preservative-Free) ... 535
- Duramorph ... 962
- Infumorph 200 and Infumorph 500 Sterile Solutions ... 965
- MS Contin Tablets ... 1994
- MSIR ... 1997
- Oramorph SR (Morphine Sulfate Sustained Release Tablets) ... 2236
- RMS Suppositories ... 2657
- Roxanol ... 2243

Nadolol (Decreased hypotensive effect; beta blockers increase the pressor effect of pseudoephedrine).
- No products indexed under this heading.

Nicardipine Hydrochloride (Decreased hypotensive effect). Products include:
- Cardene Capsules ... 2095
- Cardene I.V. ... 2709
- Cardene SR Capsules ... 2097

Nifedipine (Decreased hypotensive effect). Products include:
- Adalat Capsules (10 mg and 20 mg) ... 587
- Adalat CC ... 589
- Procardia Capsules ... 1971
- Procardia XL Extended Release Tablets ... 1972

Nisoldipine (Decreased hypotensive effect).
- No products indexed under this heading.

Nitroglycerin (Decreased hypotensive effect). Products include:
- Deponit NTG Transdermal Delivery System ... 2397
- Nitro-Bid IV ... 1523
- Nitro-Bid Ointment ... 1524
- Nitrodisc ... 2047
- Nitro-Dur (nitroglycerin) Transdermal Infusion System ... 1326
- Nitrolingual Spray ... 2027
- Nitrostat Tablets ... 1925
- Transderm-Nitro Transdermal Therapeutic System ... 859

Norepinephrine Bitartrate (May increase the effects of either of these agents thereby increasing the potential of side effects). Products include:
- Levophed Bitartrate Injection ... 2315

Nortriptyline Hydrochloride (May antagonize the effect of pseudoephedrine and may increase the effects of either antidepressant or codeine component). Products include:
- Pamelor ... 2280

Opium Alkaloids (Potential for unspecified CNS effect).
- No products indexed under this heading.

Oxazepam (Potential for unspecified CNS effect). Products include:
- Serax Capsules ... 2810
- Serax Tablets ... 2810

Oxybutynin Chloride (Concurrent use may result in paralytic ileus). Products include:
- Ditropan ... 1516

Oxycodone Hydrochloride (Potential for unspecified CNS effect). Products include:
- Percocet Tablets ... 938
- Percodan Tablets ... 939
- Percodan-Demi Tablets ... 940
- Roxicodone Tablets, Oral Solution & Intensol (Oxycodone) ... 2244
- Tylox Capsules ... 1584

Penbutolol Sulfate (Decreased hypotensive effect; beta blockers increase the pressor effect of pseudoephedrine). Products include:
- Levatol ... 2403

Pentobarbital Sodium (Potential for unspecified CNS effect). Products include:
- Nembutal Sodium Capsules ... 436
- Nembutal Sodium Solution ... 438
- Nembutal Sodium Suppositories ... 440

Perphenazine (Potential for unspecified CNS effect). Products include:
- Etrafon ... 2355
- Triavil Tablets ... 1757
- Trilafon ... 2389

Phenelzine Sulfate (Potentiates the pressor effect; concurrent and/or sequential use is not recommended). Products include:
- Nardil ... 1920

Phenobarbital (Potential for unspecified CNS effect). Products include:
- Arco-Lase Plus Tablets ... 512
- Bellergal-S Tablets ... 2250
- Donnatal ... 2060
- Donnatal Extentabs ... 2061
- Donnatal Tablets ... 2060
- Phenobarbital Elixir and Tablets ... 1469
- Quadrinal Tablets ... 1350

Phenoxybenzamine Hydrochloride (Decreased hypotensive effect). Products include:
- Dibenzyline Capsules ... 2476

Phentolamine Mesylate (Decreased hypotensive effect). Products include:
- Regitine ... 846

Phenylephrine Bitartrate (May increase the effects of either of these agents thereby increasing the potential of side effects).
- No products indexed under this heading.

Phenylephrine Hydrochloride (May increase the effects of either of these agents thereby increasing the potential of side effects). Products include:
- Atrohist Plus Tablets ... 454
- Cerose DM ... ▣ 878
- Comhist ... 2038
- D.A. Chewable Tablets ... 951
- Deconsal Pediatric Capsules ... 454
- Dura-Vent/DA Tablets ... 953
- Entex Capsules ... 1986
- Entex Liquid ... 1986
- Extendryl ... 1005
- 4-Way Fast Acting Nasal Spray (regular & mentholated) ... ▣ 621
- Hemorid For Women ... ▣ 834
- Hycomine Compound Tablets ... 932
- Neo-Synephrine Hydrochloride 1% Carpuject ... 2324
- Neo-Synephrine Hydrochloride 1% Injection ... 2324
- Neo-Synephrine Hydrochloride (Ophthalmic) ... 2325
- Neo-Synephrine ... ▣ 726
- Nōstril ... ▣ 644
- Novahistine Elixir ... ▣ 823
- Phenergan VC ... 2779
- Phenergan VC with Codeine ... 2781
- Preparation H ... ▣ 871
- Tympagesic Ear Drops ... 2342
- Vasosulf ... ◉ 271
- Vicks Sinex Nasal Spray and Ultra Fine Mist ... ▣ 765

Phenylephrine Tannate (May increase the effects of either of these agents thereby increasing the potential of side effects). Products include:
- Atrohist Pediatric Suspension ... 454
- Ricobid-D Pediatric Suspension ... 2038
- Ricobid Tablets and Pediatric Suspension ... 2038
- Rynatan ... 2673
- Rynatuss ... 2673

Phenylpropanolamine Hydrochloride (May increase the effects of either of these agents thereby increasing the potential of side effects). Products include:
- Acutrim ... ▣ 628
- Allerest Children's Chewable Tablets ... ▣ 627
- Allerest 12 Hour Caplets ... ▣ 627
- Atrohist Plus Tablets ... 454
- BC Cold Powder Multi-Symptom Formula (Cold-Sinus-Allergy) ... ▣ 609
- BC Cold Powder Non-Drowsy Formula (Cold-Sinus) ... ▣ 609
- Cheracol Plus Head Cold/Cough Formula ... ▣ 769
- Comtrex Multi-Symptom Non-Drowsy Liqui-gels ... ▣ 618
- Contac Continuous Action Nasal Decongestant/Antihistamine 12 Hour Capsules ... ▣ 813
- Contac Maximum Strength Continuous Action Decongestant/Antihistamine 12 Hour Caplets ... ▣ 813
- Contac Severe Cold and Flu Formula Caplets ... ▣ 814
- Coricidin 'D' Decongestant Tablets ... ▣ 800
- Dexatrim ... ▣ 832
- Dexatrim Plus Vitamins Caplets ... ▣ 832
- Dimetane-DC Cough Syrup ... 2059
- Dimetapp Elixir ... ▣ 773
- Dimetapp Extentabs ... ▣ 774
- Dimetapp Tablets/Liqui-Gels ... ▣ 775
- Dimetapp Cold & Allergy Chewable Tablets ... ▣ 773
- Dimetapp DM Elixir ... ▣ 774
- Dura-Vent Tablets ... 952
- Entex Capsules ... 1986
- Entex LA Tablets ... 1987
- Entex Liquid ... 1986
- Exgest LA Tablets ... 782
- Hycomine ... 931
- Isoclor Timesule Capsules ... ▣ 637
- Nolamine Timed-Release Tablets ... 785
- Ornade Spansule Capsules ... 2502
- Propagest Tablets ... 786
- Pyrroxate Caplets ... ▣ 772
- Robitussin-CF ... ▣ 777
- Sinulin Tablets ... 787
- Tavist-D 12 Hour Relief Tablets ... ▣ 787
- Teldrin 12 Hour Antihistamine/Nasal Decongestant Allergy Relief Capsules ... ▣ 826
- Triaminic Allergy Tablets ... ▣ 789
- Triaminic Cold Tablets ... ▣ 790
- Triaminic Expectorant ... ▣ 790
- Triaminic Syrup ... ▣ 792
- Triaminic-12 Tablets ... ▣ 792
- Triaminic-DM Syrup ... ▣ 792
- Triaminicin Tablets ... ▣ 793
- Triaminicol Multi-Symptom Cold Tablets ... ▣ 793
- Triaminicol Multi-Symptom Relief ... ▣ 794
- Vicks DayQuil Allergy Relief 12-Hour Extended Release Tablets ... ▣ 760
- Vicks DayQuil Allergy Relief 4-Hour Tablets ... ▣ 760
- Vicks DayQuil SINUS Pressure & CONGESTION Relief ... ▣ 761

Pindolol (Decreased hypotensive effect; beta blockers increase the pressor effect of pseudoephedrine). Products include:
- Visken Tablets ... 2299

Pirbuterol Acetate (May increase the effects of either of these agents thereby increasing the potential of side effects). Products include:
- Maxair Autohaler ... 1492
- Maxair Inhaler ... 1494

Polythiazide (Decreased hypotensive effect). Products include:
- Minizide Capsules ... 1938

(▣ Described in PDR For Nonprescription Drugs) (◉ Described in PDR For Ophthalmology)

245 **Interactions Index** **Deconsal**

Prazepam (Potential for unspecified CNS effect).
No products indexed under this heading.

Prazosin Hydrochloride (Decreased hypotensive effect). Products include:
Minipress Capsules 1937
Minizide Capsules 1938

Prochlorperazine (Potential for unspecified CNS effect). Products include:
Compazine 2470

Procyclidine Hydrochloride (Concurrent use may result in paralytic ileus). Products include:
Kemadrin Tablets 1112

Promethazine Hydrochloride (Potential for unspecified CNS effect). Products include:
Mepergan Injection 2753
Phenergan with Codeine 2777
Phenergan with Dextromethorphan 2778
Phenergan Injection 2773
Phenergan Suppositories 2775
Phenergan Syrup 2774
Phenergan Tablets 2775
Phenergan VC 2779
Phenergan VC with Codeine 2781

Propantheline Bromide (Concurrent use may result in paralytic ileus). Products include:
Pro-Banthīne Tablets 2052

Propofol (Potential for unspecified CNS effect). Products include:
Diprivan Injection 2833

Propoxyphene Hydrochloride (Potential for unspecified CNS effect). Products include:
Darvon 1435
Wygesic Tablets 2827

Propoxyphene Napsylate (Potential for unspecified CNS effect). Products include:
Darvon-N/Darvocet-N 1433

Propranolol Hydrochloride (Decreased hypotensive effect; beta blockers increase the pressor effect of pseudoephedrine). Products include:
Inderal 2728
Inderal LA Long Acting Capsules 2730
Inderide Tablets 2732
Inderide LA Long Acting Capsules .. 2734

Protriptyline Hydrochloride (May antagonize the effect of pseudoephedrine and may increase the effects of either antidepressant or codeine component). Products include:
Vivactil Tablets 1774

Pseudoephedrine Sulfate (May increase the effects of either of these agents thereby increasing the potential of side effects). Products include:
Cheracol Sinus .... ▣ 768
Chlor-Trimeton Allergy Decongestant Tablets .... ▣ 799
Claritin-D 2350
Drixoral Cold and Allergy Sustained-Action Tablets .... ▣ 802
Drixoral Cold and Flu Extended-Release Tablets .... ▣ 803
Drixoral Non-Drowsy Formula Extended-Release Tablets .... ▣ 803
Drixoral Allergy/Sinus Extended Release Tablets .... ▣ 804
Trinalin Repetabs Tablets 1330

Quazepam (Potential for unspecified CNS effect). Products include:
Doral Tablets 2664

Quinapril Hydrochloride (Decreased hypotensive effect). Products include:
Accupril Tablets 1893

Ramipril (Decreased hypotensive effect). Products include:
Altace Capsules 1232

Rauwolfia Serpentina (Decreased hypotensive effect).
No products indexed under this heading.

Rescinnamine (Decreased hypotensive effect).
No products indexed under this heading.

Reserpine (Decreased hypotensive effect). Products include:
Diupres Tablets 1650
Hydropres Tablets 1675
Ser-Ap-Es Tablets 849

Risperidone (Potential for unspecified CNS effect). Products include:
Risperdal 1301

Salmeterol Xinafoate (May increase the effects of either of these agents thereby increasing the potential of side effects). Products include:
Serevent Inhalation Aerosol 1176

Scopolamine (Concurrent use may result in paralytic ileus). Products include:
Transderm Scōp Transdermal Therapeutic System 869

Scopolamine Hydrobromide (Concurrent use may result in paralytic ileus). Products include:
Atrohist Plus Tablets 454
Donnatal 2060
Donnatal Extentabs 2061
Donnatal Tablets 2060

Secobarbital Sodium (Potential for unspecified CNS effect). Products include:
Seconal Sodium Pulvules 1474

Selegiline Hydrochloride (Potentiates the pressor effect; concurrent and/or sequential use is not recommended). Products include:
Eldepryl Tablets 2550

Sodium Nitroprusside (Decreased hypotensive effect).
No products indexed under this heading.

Sotalol Hydrochloride (Decreased hypotensive effect; beta blockers increase the pressor effect of pseudoephedrine). Products include:
Betapace Tablets 641

Spirapril Hydrochloride (Decreased hypotensive effect).
No products indexed under this heading.

Sufentanil Citrate (Potential for unspecified CNS effect). Products include:
Sufenta Injection 1309

Temazepam (Potential for unspecified CNS effect). Products include:
Restoril Capsules 2284

Terazosin Hydrochloride (Decreased hypotensive effect). Products include:
Hytrin Capsules 430

Terbutaline Sulfate (May increase the effects of either of these agents thereby increasing the potential of side effects). Products include:
Brethaire Inhaler 813
Brethine Ampuls 815
Brethine Tablets 814
Bricanyl Subcutaneous Injection 1502
Bricanyl Tablets 1503

Thiamylal Sodium (Potential for unspecified CNS effect).
No products indexed under this heading.

Thioridazine Hydrochloride (Potential for unspecified CNS effect). Products include:
Mellaril 2269

Thiothixene (Potential for unspecified CNS effect). Products include:
Navane Capsules and Concentrate 2201
Navane Intramuscular 2202

Timolol Hemihydrate (Decreased hypotensive effect; beta blockers increase the pressor effect of pseudoephedrine). Products include:
Betimol 0.25%, 0.5% .... ⊙ 261

Timolol Maleate (Decreased hypotensive effect; beta blockers increase the pressor effect of pseudoephedrine). Products include:
Blocadren Tablets 1614
Timolide Tablets 1748
Timoptic in Ocudose 1753
Timoptic Sterile Ophthalmic Solution 1751
Timoptic-XE 1755

Torsemide (Decreased hypotensive effect). Products include:
Demadex Tablets and Injection 686

Tranylcypromine Sulfate (Potentiates the pressor effect; concurrent and/or sequential use is not recommended). Products include:
Parnate Tablets 2503

Triazolam (Potential for unspecified CNS effect). Products include:
Halcion Tablets 2611

Tridihexethyl Chloride (Concurrent use may result in paralytic ileus).
No products indexed under this heading.

Trifluoperazine Hydrochloride (Potential for unspecified CNS effect). Products include:
Stelazine 2514

Trihexyphenidyl Hydrochloride (Concurrent use may result in paralytic ileus rwn). Products include:
Artane 1368

Trimethaphan Camsylate (Decreased hypotensive effect). Products include:
Arfonad Ampuls 2080

Trimipramine Maleate (May antagonize the effect of pseudoephedrine and may increase the effects of either antidepressant or codeine component). Products include:
Surmontil Capsules 2811

Verapamil Hydrochloride (Decreased hypotensive effect). Products include:
Calan SR Caplets 2422
Calan Tablets 2419
Isoptin Injectable 1344
Isoptin Oral Tablets 1346
Isoptin SR Tablets 1348
Verelan Capsules 1410
Verelan Capsules 2824

Zolpidem Tartrate (Potential for unspecified CNS effect). Products include:
Ambien Tablets 2416

Food Interactions

Alcohol (Potential for unspecified CNS effect).

DECONSAL II TABLETS

(Pseudoephedrine Hydrochloride, Guaifenesin) 454

May interact with monoamine oxidase inhibitors, beta blockers, cardiac glycosides, veratrum alkaloids, tricyclic antidepressants, and certain other agents. Compounds in these categories include:

Acebutolol Hydrochloride (Potentiates the pressor effect of sympathomimetic amines). Products include:
Sectral Capsules 2807

Amitriptyline Hydrochloride (Antagonizes the effects of sympathomimetic amines). Products include:
Elavil 2838
Endep Tablets 2174
Etrafon 2355
Limbitrol 2180
Triavil Tablets 1757

Amoxapine (Antagonizes the effects of sympathomimetic amines). Products include:
Asendin Tablets 1369

Atenolol (Potentiates the pressor effect of sympathomimetic amines). Products include:
Tenoretic Tablets 2845
Tenormin Tablets and I.V. Injection 2847

Betaxolol Hydrochloride (Potentiates the pressor effect of sympathomimetic amines). Products include:
Betoptic Ophthalmic Solution 469
Betoptic S Ophthalmic Suspension 471
Kerlone Tablets 2436

Bisoprolol Fumarate (Potentiates the pressor effect of sympathomimetic amines). Products include:
Zebeta Tablets 1413
Ziac 1415

Carteolol Hydrochloride (Potentiates the pressor effect of sympathomimetic amines). Products include:
Cartrol Tablets 410
Ocupress Ophthalmic Solution, 1% Sterile .... ⊙ 309

Clomipramine Hydrochloride (Antagonizes the effects of sympathomimetic amines). Products include:
Anafranil Capsules 803

Cryptenamine Preparations (Reduced hypotensive effect).

Deserpidine (Reduced hypotensive effect).
No products indexed under this heading.

Desipramine Hydrochloride (Antagonizes the effects of sympathomimetic amines). Products include:
Norpramin Tablets 1526

Deslanoside (Increased possibility of cardiac arrhythmias).
No products indexed under this heading.

Digitoxin (Increased possibility of cardiac arrhythmias). Products include:
Crystodigin Tablets 1433

Digoxin (Increased possibility of cardiac arrhythmias). Products include:
Lanoxicaps 1117
Lanoxin Elixir Pediatric 1120
Lanoxin Injection 1123
Lanoxin Injection Pediatric 1126
Lanoxin Tablets 1128

Doxepin Hydrochloride (Antagonizes the effects of sympathomimetic amines). Products include:
Sinequan 2205
Zonalon Cream 1055

Esmolol Hydrochloride (Potentiates the pressor effect of sympathomimetic amines). Products include:
Brevibloc Injection 1808

Furazolidone (Potentiates the pressor effect of sympathomimetic amines; concurrent use is contraindicated). Products include:
Furoxone 2046

Guanethidine Monosulfate (Reduced hypotensive effect). Products include:
Esimil Tablets 822
Ismelin Tablets 827

IMPORTANT NOTE: Always consult each drug listing in the patient's regimen for possible interactions.

Deconsal **Interactions Index** **246**

Imipramine Hydrochloride (Antagonizes the effects of sympathomimetic amines). Products include:
Tofranil Ampuls 854
Tofranil Tablets 856

Imipramine Pamoate (Antagonizes the effects of sympathomimetic amines). Products include:
Tofranil-PM Capsules 857

Isocarboxazid (Potentiates the pressor effect of sympathomimetic amines; concurrent use is contraindicated).
No products indexed under this heading.

Labetalol Hydrochloride (Potentiates the pressor effect of sympathomimetic amines). Products include:
Normodyne Injection 2377
Normodyne Tablets 2379
Trandate 1185

Levobunolol Hydrochloride (Potentiates the pressor effect of sympathomimetic amines). Products include:
Betagan ◉ 233

Maprotiline Hydrochloride (Antagonizes the effects of sympathomimetic amines). Products include:
Ludiomil Tablets 843

Mecamylamine Hydrochloride (Reduced hypotensive effect). Products include:
Inversine Tablets 1686

Methyldopa (Reduced hypotensive effect). Products include:
Aldoclor Tablets 1598
Aldomet Oral 1600
Aldoril Tablets 1604

Methyldopate Hydrochloride (Reduced hypotensive effect). Products include:
Aldomet Ester HCl Injection 1602

Metipranolol Hydrochloride (Potentiates the pressor effect of sympathomimetic amines). Products include:
OptiPranolol (Metipranolol 0.3%) Sterile Ophthalmic Solution ◉ 258

Metoprolol Succinate (Potentiates the pressor effect of sympathomimetic amines). Products include:
Toprol-XL Tablets 565

Metoprolol Tartrate (Potentiates the pressor effect of sympathomimetic amines). Products include:
Lopressor Ampuls 830
Lopressor HCT Tablets 832
Lopressor Tablets 830

Nadolol (Potentiates the pressor effect of sympathomimetic amines).
No products indexed under this heading.

Nortriptyline Hydrochloride (Antagonizes the effects of sympathomimetic amines). Products include:
Pamelor 2280

Penbutolol Sulfate (Potentiates the pressor effect of sympathomimetic amines). Products include:
Levatol 2403

Phenelzine Sulfate (Potentiates the pressor effect of sympathomimetic amines; concurrent use is contraindicated). Products include:
Nardil 1920

Pindolol (Potentiates the pressor effect of sympathomimetic amines). Products include:
Visken Tablets 2299

Propranolol Hydrochloride (Potentiates the pressor effect of sympathomimetic amines). Products include:
Inderal 2728
Inderal LA Long Acting Capsules 2730
Inderide Tablets 2732
Inderide LA Long Acting Capsules 2734

Protriptyline Hydrochloride (Antagonizes the effects of sympathomimetic amines). Products include:
Vivactil Tablets 1774

Rauwolfia Serpentina (Reduced hypotensive effect).
No products indexed under this heading.

Rescinnamine (Reduced hypotensive effect).
No products indexed under this heading.

Reserpine (Reduced hypotensive effect). Products include:
Diupres Tablets 1650
Hydropres Tablets 1675
Ser-Ap-Es Tablets 849

Selegiline Hydrochloride (Potentiates the pressor effect of sympathomimetic amines; concurrent use is contraindicated). Products include:
Eldepryl Tablets 2550

Sotalol Hydrochloride (Potentiates the pressor effect of sympathomimetic amines). Products include:
Betapace Tablets 641

Timolol Hemihydrate (Potentiates the pressor effect of sympathomimetic amines). Products include:
Betimol 0.25%, 0.5% ◉ 261

Timolol Maleate (Potentiates the pressor effect of sympathomimetic amines). Products include:
Blocadren Tablets 1614
Timolide Tablets 1748
Timoptic in Ocudose 1753
Timoptic Sterile Ophthalmic Solution 1751
Timoptic-XE 1755

Tranylcypromine Sulfate (Potentiates the pressor effect of sympathomimetic amines; concurrent use is contraindicated). Products include:
Parnate Tablets 2503

Trimipramine Maleate (Antagonizes the effects of sympathomimetic amines). Products include:
Surmontil Capsules 2811

DELATESTRYL INJECTION

(Testosterone Enanthate) 2860
May interact with oral anticoagulants, oral hypoglycemic agents, insulin, corticosteroids, and certain other agents. Compounds in these categories include:

Acarbose (In diabetic patients the metabolic effects of androgens may decrease blood glucose).
No products indexed under this heading.

ACTH (Enhanced tendency toward edema).
No products indexed under this heading.

Betamethasone Acetate (Enhanced tendency toward edema). Products include:
Celestone Soluspan Suspension 2347

Betamethasone Sodium Phosphate (Enhanced tendency toward edema). Products include:
Celestone Soluspan Suspension 2347

Chlorpropamide (In diabetic patients the metabolic effects of androgens may decrease blood glucose). Products include:
Diabinese Tablets 1935

Cortisone Acetate (Enhanced tendency toward edema). Products include:
Cortone Acetate Sterile Suspension 1623
Cortone Acetate Tablets 1624

Dexamethasone (Enhanced tendency toward edema). Products include:
AK-Trol Ointment & Suspension ◉ 205
Decadron Elixir 1633
Decadron Tablets 1635
Decaspray Topical Aerosol 1648
Dexacidin Ointment ◉ 263
Maxitrol Ophthalmic Ointment and Suspension ◉ 224
TobraDex Ophthalmic Suspension and Ointment 473

Dexamethasone Acetate (Enhanced tendency toward edema). Products include:
Dalalone D.P. Injectable 1011
Decadron-LA Sterile Suspension 1646

Dexamethasone Sodium Phosphate (Enhanced tendency toward edema). Products include:
Decadron Phosphate Injection 1637
Decadron Phosphate Respihaler 1642
Decadron Phosphate Sterile Ophthalmic Ointment 1641
Decadron Phosphate Sterile Ophthalmic Solution 1642
Decadron Phosphate Topical Cream 1644
Decadron Phosphate Turbinaire 1645
Decadron Phosphate with Xylocaine Injection, Sterile 1639
Dexacort Phosphate in Respihaler 458
Dexacort Phosphate in Turbinaire 459
NeoDecadron Sterile Ophthalmic Ointment 1712
NeoDecadron Sterile Ophthalmic Solution 1713
NeoDecadron Topical Cream 1714

Dicumarol (C-17 substituted derivatives of testosterone may decrease the oral anticoagulant requirements).
No products indexed under this heading.

Fludrocortisone Acetate (Enhanced tendency toward edema). Products include:
Florinef Acetate Tablets 505

Glipizide (In diabetic patients the metabolic effects of androgens may decrease blood glucose). Products include:
Glucotrol Tablets 1967
Glucotrol XL Extended Release Tablets 1968

Glyburide (In diabetic patients the metabolic effects of androgens may decrease blood glucose). Products include:
DiaBeta Tablets 1239
Glynase PresTab Tablets 2609
Micronase Tablets 2623

Hydrocortisone (Enhanced tendency toward edema). Products include:
Anusol-HC Cream 2.5% 1896
Aquanil HC Lotion 1931
Bactine Hydrocortisone Anti-Itch Cream ■ 709
Caldecort Anti-Itch Hydrocortisone Spray ■ 631
Cortaid ■ 836
CORTENEMA 2535
Cortisporin Ointment 1085
Cortisporin Ophthalmic Ointment Sterile 1085
Cortisporin Ophthalmic Suspension Sterile 1086
Cortisporin Otic Solution Sterile 1087
Cortisporin Otic Suspension Sterile 1088
Cortizone-5 ■ 831
Cortizone-10 ■ 831
Hydrocortone Tablets 1672
Hytone 907
Massengill Medicated Soft Cloth Towelettes 2458
PediOtic Suspension Sterile 1153
Preparation H Hydrocortisone 1% Cream ■ 872
ProctoCream-HC 2.5% 2408
VōSoL HC Otic Solution 2678

Hydrocortisone Acetate (Enhanced tendency toward edema). Products include:
Analpram-HC Rectal Cream 1% and 2.5% 977
Anusol HC-1 Anti-Itch Hydrocortisone Ointment ■ 847
Anusol-HC Suppositories 1897
Caldecort ■ 631
Carmol HC 924
Coly-Mycin S Otic w/Neomycin & Hydrocortisone 1906
Cortaid ■ 836
Cortifoam 2396
Cortisporin Cream 1084
Epifoam 2399
Hydrocortone Acetate Sterile Suspension 1669
Mantadil Cream 1135
Nupercainal Hydrocortisone 1% Cream ■ 645
Ophthocort ◉ 311
Pramosone Cream, Lotion & Ointment 978
ProctoCream-HC 2408
ProctoFoam-HC 2409
Terra-Cortril Ophthalmic Suspension 2210

Hydrocortisone Sodium Phosphate (Enhanced tendency toward edema). Products include:
Hydrocortone Phosphate Injection, Sterile 1670

Hydrocortisone Sodium Succinate (Enhanced tendency toward edema). Products include:
Solu-Cortef Sterile Powder 2641

Insulin, Human (In diabetic patients the metabolic effects of androgens may decrease blood glucose and insulin requirements).
No products indexed under this heading.

Insulin, Human Isophane Suspension (In diabetic patients the metabolic effects of androgens may decrease blood glucose and insulin requirements). Products include:
Novolin N Human Insulin 10 ml Vials 1795

Insulin, Human NPH (In diabetic patients the metabolic effects of androgens may decrease blood glucose and insulin requirements). Products include:
Humulin N, 100 Units 1448
Novolin N PenFill Cartridges Durable Insulin Delivery System 1798
Novolin N Prefilled Syringe Disposable Insulin Delivery System 1798

Insulin, Human Regular (In diabetic patients the metabolic effects of androgens may decrease blood glucose and insulin requirements). Products include:
Humulin R, 100 Units 1449
Novolin R Human Insulin 10 ml Vials 1795
Novolin R PenFill Cartridges Durable Insulin Delivery System 1798
Novolin R Prefilled Syringe Disposable Insulin Delivery System 1798
Velosulin BR Human Insulin 10 ml Vials 1795

Insulin, Human, Zinc Suspension (In diabetic patients the metabolic effects of androgens may decrease blood glucose and insulin requirements). Products include:
Humulin L, 100 Units 1446
Humulin U, 100 Units 1450
Novolin L Human Insulin 10 ml Vials 1795

Insulin, NPH (In diabetic patients the metabolic effects of androgens may decrease blood glucose and insulin requirements). Products include:
NPH, 100 Units 1450
Pork NPH, 100 Units 1452
Purified Pork NPH Isophane Insulin 1801

Insulin, Regular (In diabetic patients the metabolic effects of androgens may decrease blood glucose and insulin requirements). Products include:
Regular, 100 Units 1450

247 **Interactions Index** **Deltasone**

Pork Regular, 100 Units 1452
Pork Regular (Concentrated), 500 Units 1453
Purified Pork Regular Insulin 1801

Insulin, Zinc Crystals (In diabetic patients the metabolic effects of androgens may decrease blood glucose and insulin requirements). Products include:
NPH, 100 Units 1450

Insulin, Zinc Suspension (In diabetic patients the metabolic effects of androgens may decrease blood glucose and insulin requirements). Products include:
Iletin I 1450
Lente, 100 Units 1450
Iletin II 1452
Pork Lente, 100 Units 1452
Purified Pork Lente Insulin 1801

Metformin Hydrochloride (In diabetic patients the metabolic effects of androgens may decrease blood glucose). Products include:
Glucophage 752

Methylprednisolone Acetate (Enhanced tendency toward edema). Products include:
Depo-Medrol Single-Dose Vial 2600
Depo-Medrol Sterile Aqueous Suspension 2597

Methylprednisolone Sodium Succinate (Enhanced tendency toward edema). Products include:
Solu-Medrol Sterile Powder 2643

Oxyphenbutazone (Elevated serum levels of oxyphenbutazone).

Prednisolone Acetate (Enhanced tendency toward edema). Products include:
AK-CIDE .... ⊙ 202
AK-CIDE Ointment .... ⊙ 202
Blephamide Liquifilm Sterile Ophthalmic Suspension 476
Blephamide Ointment .... ⊙ 237
Econopred & Econopred Plus Ophthalmic Suspensions .... ⊙ 217
Poly-Pred Liquifilm .... ⊙ 248
Pred Forte .... ⊙ 250
Pred Mild .... ⊙ 253
Pred-G Liquifilm Sterile Ophthalmic Suspension .... ⊙ 251
Pred-G S.O.P. Sterile Ophthalmic Ointment .... ⊙ 252
Vasocidin Ointment .... ⊙ 268

Prednisolone Sodium Phosphate (Enhanced tendency toward edema). Products include:
AK-Pred .... ⊙ 204
Hydeltrasol Injection, Sterile 1665
Inflamase .... ⊙ 265
Pediapred Oral Liquid 995
Vasocidin Ophthalmic Solution .... ⊙ 270

Prednisolone Tebutate (Enhanced tendency toward edema). Products include:
Hydeltra-T.B.A. Sterile Suspension 1667

Prednisone (Enhanced tendency toward edema). Products include:
Deltasone Tablets 2595

Tolazamide (In diabetic patients the metabolic effects of androgens may decrease blood glucose).
No products indexed under this heading.

Tolbutamide (In diabetic patients the metabolic effects of androgens may decrease blood glucose).
No products indexed under this heading.

Triamcinolone (Enhanced tendency toward edema). Products include:
Aristocort Tablets 1022

Triamcinolone Acetonide (Enhanced tendency toward edema). Products include:
Aristocort A 0.025% Cream 1027
Aristocort A 0.5% Cream 1031
Aristocort A 0.1% Cream 1029
Aristocort A 0.1% Ointment 1030
Azmacort Oral Inhaler 2011
Nasacort Nasal Inhaler 2024

Triamcinolone Diacetate (Enhanced tendency toward edema). Products include:
Aristocort Suspension (Forte Parenteral) 1027
Aristocort Suspension (Intralesional) 1025

Triamcinolone Hexacetonide (Enhanced tendency toward edema). Products include:
Aristospan Suspension (Intra-articular) 1033
Aristospan Suspension (Intralesional) 1032

Warfarin Sodium (C-17 substituted derivatives of testosterone may decrease the oral anticoagulant requirements). Products include:
Coumadin 926

DELFEN CONTRACEPTIVE FOAM
(Nonoxynol-9) .... ▣ 737
None cited in PDR database.

DELSYM EXTENDED-RELEASE SUSPENSION
(Dextromethorphan Polistirex) .... ▣ 654
May interact with monoamine oxidase inhibitors. Compounds in this category include:

Furazolidone (Concurrent and/or sequential use is not recommended). Products include:
Furoxone 2046

Isocarboxazid (Concurrent and/or sequential use is not recommended).
No products indexed under this heading.

Phenelzine Sulfate (Concurrent and/or sequential use is not recommended). Products include:
Nardil 1920

Selegiline Hydrochloride (Concurrent and/or sequential use is not recommended). Products include:
Eldepryl Tablets 2550

Tranylcypromine Sulfate (Concurrent and/or sequential use is not recommended). Products include:
Parnate Tablets 2503

DELTASONE TABLETS
(Prednisone) 2595
May interact with oral anticoagulants, oral hypoglycemic agents, insulin, and certain other agents. Compounds in these categories include:

Acarbose (Increased requirements for oral hypoglycemic agents in diabetes).
No products indexed under this heading.

Aspirin (Increased clearance of chronic high dose aspirin leading to decreased salicylate serum levels or increased risk of salicylate toxicity when corticosteroid is withdrawn). Products include:
Alka-Seltzer Effervescent Antacid and Pain Reliever .... ▣ 701
Alka-Seltzer Extra Strength Effervescent Antacid and Pain Reliever .... ▣ 703
Alka-Seltzer Lemon Lime Effervescent Antacid and Pain Reliever .... ▣ 703
Alka-Seltzer Plus Cold Medicine .... ▣ 705
Alka-Seltzer Plus Cold & Cough Medicine .... ▣ 708
Alka-Seltzer Plus Night-Time Cold Medicine .... ▣ 707
Alka Seltzer Plus Sinus Medicine .... ▣ 707
Arthritis Foundation Safety Coated Aspirin Tablets .... ▣ 675
Arthritis Pain Ascriptin .... ▣ 631
Maximum Strength Ascriptin .... ▣ 630
Regular Strength Ascriptin Tablets .... ▣ 629
Arthritis Strength BC Powder .... ▣ 609
BC Cold Powder Multi-Symptom Formula (Cold-Sinus-Allergy) .... ▣ 609
BC Cold Powder Non-Drowsy Formula (Cold-Sinus) .... ▣ 609
BC Powder .... ▣ 609
Bayer Children's Chewable Aspirin .... ▣ 711
Genuine Bayer Aspirin Tablets & Caplets .... ▣ 713
Extra Strength Bayer Arthritis Pain Regimen Formula .... ▣ 711
Extra Strength Bayer Aspirin Caplets & Tablets .... ▣ 712
Extended-Release Bayer 8-Hour Aspirin .... ▣ 712
Extra Strength Bayer Plus Aspirin Caplets .... ▣ 713
Extra Strength Bayer PM Aspirin .. ▣ 713
Bayer Enteric Aspirin .... ▣ 709
Bufferin Analgesic Tablets and Caplets .... ▣ 613
Arthritis Strength Bufferin Analgesic Caplets .... ▣ 614
Extra Strength Bufferin Analgesic Tablets .... ▣ 615
Cama Arthritis Pain Reliever .... ▣ 785
Darvon Compound-65 Pulvules 1435
Easprin 1914
Ecotrin 2455
Ecotrin Enteric Coated Aspirin Maximum Strength Tablets and Caplets .... ▣ 816
Ecotrin Enteric Coated Aspirin Regular Strength Tablets 2455
Empirin Aspirin Tablets .... ▣ 854
Empirin with Codeine Tablets 1093
Excedrin Extra-Strength Analgesic Tablets & Caplets 732
Fiorinal Capsules 2261
Fiorinal with Codeine Capsules 2262
Fiorinal Tablets 2261
Halfprin 1362
Healthprin Aspirin 2455
Norgesic 1496
Percodan Tablets 939
Percodan-Demi Tablets 940
Robaxisal Tablets 2071
Soma Compound w/Codeine Tablets 2676
Soma Compound Tablets 2675
St. Joseph Adult Chewable Aspirin (81 mg.) .... ▣ 808
Talwin Compound 2335
Ursinus Inlay-Tabs .... ▣ 794
Vanquish Analgesic Caplets .... ▣ 731

Chlorpropamide (Increased requirements for oral hypoglycemic agents in diabetes). Products include:
Diabinese Tablets 1935

Cyclosporine (Potential for convulsions). Products include:
Neoral 2276
Sandimmune 2286

Dicumarol (Potential for variable effect; concurrent use may result in enhanced as well as diminished effects of anticoagulant).
No products indexed under this heading.

Glipizide (Increased requirements for oral hypoglycemic agents in diabetes). Products include:
Glucotrol Tablets 1967
Glucotrol XL Extended Release Tablets 1968

Glyburide (Increased requirements for oral hypoglycemic agents in diabetes). Products include:
DiaBeta Tablets 1239
Glynase PresTab Tablets 2609
Micronase Tablets 2623

Insulin, Human (Increased requirements for insulin in diabetes).
No products indexed under this heading.

Insulin, Human Isophane Suspension (Increased requirements for insulin in diabetes). Products include:
Novolin N Human Insulin 10 ml Vials 1795

Insulin, Human NPH (Increased requirements for insulin in diabetes). Products include:
Humulin N, 100 Units 1448
Novolin N PenFill Cartridges Durable Insulin Delivery System 1798
Novolin N Prefilled Syringe Disposable Insulin Delivery System 1798

Insulin, Human Regular (Increased requirements for insulin in diabetes). Products include:
Humulin R, 100 Units 1449
Novolin R Human Insulin 10 ml Vials 1795
Novolin R PenFill Cartridges Durable Insulin Delivery System 1798
Novolin R Prefilled Syringe Disposable Insulin Delivery System 1798
Velosulin BR Human Insulin 10 ml Vials 1795

Insulin, Human, Zinc Suspension (Increased requirements for insulin in diabetes). Products include:
Humulin L, 100 Units 1446
Humulin U, 100 Units 1450
Novolin L Human Insulin 10 ml Vials 1795

Insulin, NPH (Increased requirements for insulin in diabetes). Products include:
NPH, 100 Units 1450
Pork NPH, 100 Units 1452
Purified Pork NPH Isophane Insulin 1801

Insulin, Regular (Increased requirements for insulin in diabetes). Products include:
Regular, 100 Units 1450
Pork Regular, 100 Units 1452
Pork Regular (Concentrated), 500 Units 1453
Purified Pork Regular Insulin 1801

Insulin, Zinc Crystals (Increased requirements for insulin in diabetes). Products include:
NPH, 100 Units 1450

Insulin, Zinc Suspension (Increased requirements for insulin in diabetes). Products include:
Iletin I 1450
Lente, 100 Units 1450
Iletin II 1452
Pork Lente, 100 Units 1452
Purified Pork Lente Insulin 1801

Ketoconazole (May inhibit the metabolism of corticosteroid and thus decrease its clearance; the dose of corticosteroid should be titrated to avoid toxicity). Products include:
Nizoral 2% Cream 1297
Nizoral 2% Shampoo 1298
Nizoral Tablets 1298

Metformin Hydrochloride (Increased requirements for oral hypoglycemic agents in diabetes). Products include:
Glucophage 752

Phenobarbital (Increases clearance of corticosteroid and may require increase in dose of corticosteroid to achieve the desired response). Products include:
Arco-Lase Plus Tablets 512
Bellergal-S Tablets 2250
Donnatal 2060
Donnatal Extentabs 2061
Donnatal Tablets 2060
Phenobarbital Elixir and Tablets 1469
Quadrinal Tablets 1350

Phenytoin (Increases clearance of corticosteroid and may require increase in dose of corticosteroid to achieve the desired response). Products include:
Dilantin Infatabs 1908
Dilantin-125 Suspension 1911

IMPORTANT NOTE: Always consult each drug listing in the patient's regimen for possible interactions.

Deltasone Interactions Index 248

Phenytoin Sodium (Increases clearance of corticosteroid and may require increase in dose of corticosteroid to achieve the desired response). Products include:

Dilantin Kapseals 1906
Dilantin Parenteral 1910

Rifampin (Increases clearance of corticosteroid and may require increase in dose of corticosteroid to achieve the desired response). Products include:

Rifadin 1528
Rifamate Capsules 1530
Rifater 1532
Rimactane Capsules 847

Tolazamide (Increased requirements for oral hypoglycemic agents in diabetes).

No products indexed under this heading.

Tolbutamide (Increased requirements for oral hypoglycemic agents in diabetes).

No products indexed under this heading.

Troleandomycin (May inhibit the metabolism of corticosteroid and thus decrease its clearance; the dose of corticosteroid should be titrated to avoid toxicity). Products include:

Tao Capsules 2209

Vaccines (Live) (Administration of live or live attenuated vaccines is contraindicated).

Warfarin Sodium (Potential for variable effect; concurrent use may result in enhanced as well as diminished effects of anticoagulant). Products include:

Coumadin 926

DEMADEX TABLETS AND INJECTION
(Torsemide) 686

May interact with salicylates, nonsteroidal anti-inflammatory agents, and certain other agents. Compounds in these categories include:

Aspirin (Coadministration in patients receiving high dose of salicylates may be associated with salicylate toxicity due to competition for secretion by renal tubule). Products include:

Alka-Seltzer Effervescent Antacid and Pain Reliever ▣ 701
Alka-Seltzer Extra Strength Effervescent Antacid and Pain Reliever ▣ 703
Alka-Seltzer Lemon Lime Effervescent Antacid and Pain Reliever ▣ 703
Alka-Seltzer Plus Cold Medicine ▣ 705
Alka-Seltzer Plus Cold & Cough Medicine ▣ 708
Alka-Seltzer Plus Night-Time Cold Medicine ▣ 707
Alka Seltzer Plus Sinus Medicine ▣ 707
Arthritis Foundation Safety Coated Aspirin Tablets ▣ 675
Arthritis Pain Ascriptin ▣ 631
Maximum Strength Ascriptin ▣ 630
Regular Strength Ascriptin Tablets ▣ 629
Arthritis Strength BC Powder ▣ 609
BC Cold Powder Multi-Symptom Formula (Cold-Sinus-Allergy) ▣ 609
BC Cold Powder Non-Drowsy Formula (Cold-Sinus) ▣ 609
BC Powder ▣ 609
Bayer Children's Chewable Aspirin ▣ 711
Genuine Bayer Aspirin Tablets & Caplets ▣ 713
Extra Strength Bayer Arthritis Pain Regimen Formula ▣ 711
Extra Strength Bayer Aspirin Caplets & Tablets ▣ 712
Extended-Release Bayer 8-Hour Aspirin ▣ 712
Extra Strength Bayer Plus Aspirin Caplets ▣ 713
Extra Strength Bayer PM Aspirin ▣ 713
Bayer Enteric Aspirin ▣ 709
Bufferin Analgesic Tablets and Caplets ▣ 613
Arthritis Strength Bufferin Analgesic Caplets ▣ 614
Extra Strength Bufferin Analgesic Tablets ▣ 615
Cama Arthritis Pain Reliever ▣ 785
Darvon Compound-65 Pulvules 1435
Easprin 1914
Ecotrin 2455
Ecotrin Enteric Coated Aspirin Maximum Strength Tablets and Caplets ▣ 816
Ecotrin Enteric Coated Aspirin Regular Strength Tablets 2455
Empirin Aspirin Tablets ▣ 854
Empirin with Codeine Tablets 1093
Excedrin Extra-Strength Analgesic Tablets & Caplets 732
Fiorinal Capsules 2261
Fiorinal with Codeine Capsules 2262
Fiorinal Tablets 2261
Halfprin 1362
Healthprin Aspirin 2455
Norgesic 1496
Percodan Tablets 939
Percodan-Demi Tablets 940
Robaxisal Tablets 2071
Soma Compound w/Codeine Tablets 2676
Soma Compound Tablets 2675
St. Joseph Adult Chewable Aspirin (81 mg.) ▣ 808
Talwin Compound 2335
Ursinus Inlay-Tabs ▣ 794
Vanquish Analgesic Caplets ▣ 731

Cholestyramine (Possibility of decreased oral absorption of torsemide; simultaneous administration is not recommended). Products include:

Questran Light 769
Questran Powder 770

Choline Magnesium Trisalicylate (Coadministration in patients receiving high dose of salicylates may be associated with salicylate toxicity due to competition for secretion by renal tubule). Products include:

Trilisate 2000

Diclofenac Potassium (Possible inhibition of natriuretic effect; potential for renal dysfunction). Products include:

Cataflam 816

Diclofenac Sodium (Possible inhibition of natriuretic effect; potential for renal dysfunction). Products include:

Voltaren Ophthalmic Sterile Ophthalmic Solution ◉ 272
Voltaren Tablets 861

Diflunisal (Coadministration in patients receiving high dose of salicylates may be associated with salicylate toxicity due to competition for secretion by renal tubule). Products include:

Dolobid Tablets 1654

Digoxin (Coadministration of digoxin is reported to increase the AUC for torsemide by 50%). Products include:

Lanoxicaps 1117
Lanoxin Elixir Pediatric 1120
Lanoxin Injection 1123
Lanoxin Injection Pediatric 1126
Lanoxin Tablets 1128

Etodolac (Possible inhibition of natriuretic effect; potential for renal dysfunction). Products include:

Lodine Capsules and Tablets 2743

Fenoprofen Calcium (Possible inhibition of natriuretic effect; potential for renal dysfunction). Products include:

Nalfon 200 Pulvules & Nalfon Tablets 917

Flurbiprofen (Possible inhibition of natriuretic effect; potential for renal dysfunction). Products include:

Ansaid Tablets 2579

Ibuprofen (Possible inhibition of natriuretic effect; potential for renal dysfunction). Products include:

Advil Cold and Sinus Caplets and Tablets (formerly CoAdvil) ▣ 870
Advil Ibuprofen Tablets and Caplets ▣ 870
Children's Advil Suspension 2692
Arthritis Foundation Ibuprofen Tablets ▣ 674
Bayer Select Ibuprofen Pain Relief Formula ▣ 715
Cramp End Tablets ▣ 735
Dimetapp Sinus Caplets ▣ 775
Haltran Tablets ▣ 771
IBU Tablets 1342
Ibuprohm ▣ 735
Children's Motrin Ibuprofen Oral Suspension 1546
Motrin Tablets 2625
Motrin IB Caplets, Tablets, and Geltabs ▣ 838
Motrin IB Sinus ▣ 838
Motrin Ibuprofen Suspension, Oral Drops, Chewable Tablets, Caplets 1546
Nuprin Ibuprofen/Analgesic Tablets & Caplets ▣ 622
Sine-Aid IB Caplets 1554
Vicks DayQuil SINUS Pressure & PAIN Relief with IBUPROFEN ▣ 762

Indomethacin (Possible inhibition of natriuretic effect; potential for renal dysfunction). Products include:

Indocin 1680

Indomethacin Sodium Trihydrate (Possible inhibition of natriuretic effect; potential for renal dysfunction). Products include:

Indocin I.V. 1684

Ketoprofen (Possible inhibition of natriuretic effect; potential for renal dysfunction). Products include:

Orudis Capsules 2766
Oruvail Capsules 2766

Ketorolac Tromethamine (Possible inhibition of natriuretic effect; potential for renal dysfunction). Products include:

Acular 474
Acular ◉ 277
Toradol 2159

Magnesium Salicylate (Coadministration in patients receiving high dose of salicylates may be associated with salicylate toxicity due to competition for secretion by renal tubule). Products include:

Backache Caplets ▣ 613
Bayer Select Backache Pain Relief Formula ▣ 715
Doan's Extra-Strength Analgesic ▣ 633
Extra Strength Doan's P.M. ▣ 633
Doan's Regular Strength Analgesic ▣ 634
Mobigesic Tablets ▣ 602

Meclofenamate Sodium (Possible inhibition of natriuretic effect; potential for renal dysfunction).

No products indexed under this heading.

Mefenamic Acid (Possible inhibition of natriuretic effect; potential for renal dysfunction). Products include:

Ponstel 1925

Nabumetone (Possible inhibition of natriuretic effect; potential for renal dysfunction). Products include:

Relafen Tablets 2510

Naproxen (Possible inhibition of natriuretic effect; potential for renal dysfunction). Products include:

Anaprox/Naprosyn 2117

Naproxen Sodium (Possible inhibition of natriuretic effect; potential for renal dysfunction). Products include:

Aleve 1975
Anaprox/Naprosyn 2117

Oxaprozin (Possible inhibition of natriuretic effect; potential for renal dysfunction). Products include:

Daypro Caplets 2426

Phenylbutazone (Possible inhibition of natriuretic effect; potential for renal dysfunction).

No products indexed under this heading.

Piroxicam (Possible inhibition of natriuretic effect; potential for renal dysfunction). Products include:

Feldene Capsules 1965

Probenecid (Reduces secretion of torsemide into the proximal tubule and thereby decreases diuretic effect). Products include:

Benemid Tablets 1611
ColBENEMID Tablets 1622

Salsalate (Coadministration in patients receiving high dose of salicylates may be associated with salicylate toxicity due to competition for secretion by renal tubule). Products include:

Mono-Gesic Tablets 792
Salflex Tablets 786

Spironolactone (Coadministration may be associated with significant reduction in the renal clearance of spironolactone, with corresponding increase in the AUC). Products include:

Aldactazide 2413
Aldactone 2414

Sulindac (Possible inhibition of natriuretic effect; potential for renal dysfunction). Products include:

Clinoril Tablets 1618

Tolmetin Sodium (Possible inhibition of natriuretic effect; potential for renal dysfunction). Products include:

Tolectin (200, 400 and 600 mg) 1581

DEMEROL HYDROCHLORIDE CARPUJECT
(Meperidine Hydrochloride) 2308

May interact with narcotic analgesics, general anesthetics, phenothiazines, tranquilizers, hypnotics and sedatives, tricyclic antidepressants, central nervous system depressants, monoamine oxidase inhibitors, and certain other agents. Compounds in these categories include:

Alfentanil Hydrochloride (Respiratory depression, hypotension, profound sedation or coma). Products include:

Alfenta Injection 1286

Alprazolam (Respiratory depression, hypotension, profound sedation or coma). Products include:

Xanax Tablets 2649

Amitriptyline Hydrochloride (Respiratory depression, hypotension, profound sedation or coma). Products include:

Elavil 2838
Endep Tablets 2174
Etrafon 2355
Limbitrol 2180
Triavil Tablets 1757

Amoxapine (Respiratory depression, hypotension, profound sedation or coma). Products include:

Asendin Tablets 1369

(▣ Described in PDR For Nonprescription Drugs) (◉ Described in PDR For Ophthalmology)

249 **Interactions Index** **Demerol**

Aprobarbital (Respiratory depression, hypotension, profound sedation or coma).
No products indexed under this heading.

Buprenorphine (Respiratory depression, hypotension, profound sedation or coma). Products include:
Buprenex Injectable ... 2006

Buspirone Hydrochloride (Respiratory depression, hypotension, profound sedation or coma). Products include:
BuSpar ... 737

Butabarbital (Respiratory depression, hypotension, profound sedation or coma).
No products indexed under this heading.

Butalbital (Respiratory depression, hypotension, profound sedation or coma). Products include:
Esgic-plus Tablets ... 1013
Fioricet Tablets ... 2258
Fioricet with Codeine Capsules ... 2260
Fiorinal Capsules ... 2261
Fiorinal with Codeine Capsules ... 2262
Fiorinal Tablets ... 2261
Phrenilin ... 785
Sedapap Tablets 50 mg/650 mg ... 1543

Chlordiazepoxide (Respiratory depression, hypotension, profound sedation or coma). Products include:
Libritabs Tablets ... 2177
Limbitrol ... 2180

Chlordiazepoxide Hydrochloride (Respiratory depression, hypotension, profound sedation or coma). Products include:
Librax Capsules ... 2176
Librium Capsules ... 2178
Librium Injectable ... 2179

Chlorpromazine (Respiratory depression, hypotension, profound sedation or coma). Products include:
Thorazine Suppositories ... 2523

Chlorprothixene (Respiratory depression, hypotension, profound sedation or coma).
No products indexed under this heading.

Chlorprothixene Hydrochloride (Respiratory depression, hypotension, profound sedation or coma).
No products indexed under this heading.

Clomipramine Hydrochloride (Respiratory depression, hypotension, profound sedation or coma). Products include:
Anafranil Capsules ... 803

Clorazepate Dipotassium (Respiratory depression, hypotension, profound sedation or coma). Products include:
Tranxene ... 451

Clozapine (Respiratory depression, hypotension, profound sedation or coma). Products include:
Clozaril Tablets ... 2252

Codeine Phosphate (Respiratory depression, hypotension, profound sedation or coma). Products include:
Actifed with Codeine Cough Syrup ... 1067
Brontex ... 1981
Deconsal C Expectorant Syrup ... 456
Deconsal Pediatric Syrup ... 457
Dimetane-DC Cough Syrup ... 2059
Empirin with Codeine Tablets ... 1093
Fioricet with Codeine Capsules ... 2260
Fiorinal with Codeine Capsules ... 2262
Isoclor Expectorant ... 990
Novahistine DH ... 2462
Novahistine Expectorant ... 2463
Nucofed ... 2051
Phenergan with Codeine ... 2777
Phenergan VC with Codeine ... 2781
Robitussin A-C Syrup ... 2073
Robitussin-DAC Syrup ... 2074
Ryna ... 841
Soma Compound w/Codeine Tablets ... 2676
Tussi-Organidin NR Liquid and S NR Liquid ... 2677
Tylenol with Codeine ... 1583

Desflurane (Respiratory depression, hypotension, profound sedation or coma). Products include:
Suprane ... 1813

Desipramine Hydrochloride (Respiratory depression, hypotension, profound sedation or coma). Products include:
Norpramin Tablets ... 1526

Dezocine (Respiratory depression, hypotension, profound sedation or coma). Products include:
Dalgan Injection ... 538

Diazepam (Respiratory depression, hypotension, profound sedation or coma). Products include:
Dizac ... 1809
Valium Injectable ... 2182
Valium Tablets ... 2183
Valrelease Capsules ... 2169

Doxepin Hydrochloride (Respiratory depression, hypotension, profound sedation or coma). Products include:
Sinequan ... 2205
Zonalon Cream ... 1055

Droperidol (Respiratory depression, hypotension, profound sedation or coma). Products include:
Inapsine Injection ... 1296

Enflurane (Respiratory depression, hypotension, profound sedation or coma).
No products indexed under this heading.

Estazolam (Respiratory depression, hypotension, profound sedation or coma). Products include:
ProSom Tablets ... 449

Ethchlorvynol (Respiratory depression, hypotension, profound sedation or coma). Products include:
Placidyl Capsules ... 448

Ethinamate (Respiratory depression, hypotension, profound sedation or coma).
No products indexed under this heading.

Fentanyl (Respiratory depression, hypotension, profound sedation or coma). Products include:
Duragesic Transdermal System ... 1288

Fentanyl Citrate (Respiratory depression, hypotension, profound sedation or coma). Products include:
Sublimaze Injection ... 1307

Fluphenazine Decanoate (Respiratory depression, hypotension, profound sedation or coma). Products include:
Prolixin Decanoate ... 509

Fluphenazine Enanthate (Respiratory depression, hypotension, profound sedation or coma). Products include:
Prolixin Enanthate ... 509

Fluphenazine Hydrochloride (Respiratory depression, hypotension, profound sedation or coma). Products include:
Prolixin ... 509

Flurazepam Hydrochloride (Respiratory depression, hypotension, profound sedation or coma). Products include:
Dalmane Capsules ... 2173

Furazolidone (Contraindicated: unpredictable, severe, and occasionally fatal reactions when given within 14 days). Products include:
Furoxone ... 2046

Glutethimide (Respiratory depression, hypotension, profound sedation or coma).
No products indexed under this heading.

Haloperidol (Respiratory depression, hypotension, profound sedation or coma). Products include:
Haldol Injection, Tablets and Concentrate ... 1575

Haloperidol Decanoate (Respiratory depression, hypotension, profound sedation or coma). Products include:
Haldol Decanoate ... 1577

Hydrocodone Bitartrate (Respiratory depression, hypotension, profound sedation or coma). Products include:
Anexsia 5/500 Elixir ... 1781
Anexia Tablets ... 1782
Codiclear DH Syrup ... 791
Deconamine CX Cough and Cold Liquid and Tablets ... 1319
Duratuss HD Elixir ... 2565
Hycodan Tablets and Syrup ... 930
Hycomine Compound Tablets ... 932
Hycomine ... 931
Hycotuss Expectorant Syrup ... 933
Hydrocet Capsules ... 782
Lorcet 10/650 ... 1018
Lortab ... 2566
Tussend ... 1783
Tussend Expectorant ... 1785
Vicodin Tablets ... 1356
Vicodin ES Tablets ... 1357
Vicodin Tuss Expectorant ... 1358
Zydone Capsules ... 949

Hydrocodone Polistirex (Respiratory depression, hypotension, profound sedation or coma). Products include:
Tussionex Pennkinetic Extended-Release Suspension ... 998

Hydroxyzine Hydrochloride (Respiratory depression, hypotension, profound sedation or coma). Products include:
Atarax Tablets & Syrup ... 2185
Marax Tablets & DF Syrup ... 2200
Vistaril Intramuscular Solution ... 2216

Imipramine Hydrochloride (Respiratory depression, hypotension, profound sedation or coma). Products include:
Tofranil Ampuls ... 854
Tofranil Tablets ... 856

Imipramine Pamoate (Respiratory depression, hypotension, profound sedation or coma). Products include:
Tofranil-PM Capsules ... 857

Isocarboxazid (Contraindicated: unpredictable, severe, and occasionally fatal reactions when given within 14 days).
No products indexed under this heading.

Isoflurane (Respiratory depression, hypotension, profound sedation or coma).
No products indexed under this heading.

Ketamine Hydrochloride (Respiratory depression, hypotension, profound sedation or coma).
No products indexed under this heading.

Levomethadyl Acetate Hydrochloride (Respiratory depression, hypotension, profound sedation or coma). Products include:
Orlamm ... 2239

Levorphanol Tartrate (Respiratory depression, hypotension, profound sedation or coma). Products include:
Levo-Dromoran ... 2129

Lorazepam (Respiratory depression, hypotension, profound sedation or coma). Products include:
Ativan Injection ... 2698
Ativan Tablets ... 2700

Loxapine Hydrochloride (Respiratory depression, hypotension, profound sedation or coma). Products include:
Loxitane ... 1378

Loxapine Succinate (Respiratory depression, hypotension, profound sedation or coma). Products include:
Loxitane Capsules ... 1378

Maprotiline Hydrochloride (Respiratory depression, hypotension, profound sedation or coma). Products include:
Ludiomil Tablets ... 843

Mephobarbital (Respiratory depression, hypotension, profound sedation or coma). Products include:
Mebaral Tablets ... 2322

Meprobamate (Respiratory depression, hypotension, profound sedation or coma). Products include:
Miltown Tablets ... 2672
PMB 200 and PMB 400 ... 2783

Mesoridazine Besylate (Respiratory depression, hypotension, profound sedation or coma). Products include:
Serentil ... 684

Methadone Hydrochloride (Respiratory depression, hypotension, profound sedation or coma). Products include:
Methadone Hydrochloride Oral Concentrate ... 2233
Methadone Hydrochloride Oral Solution & Tablets ... 2235

Methohexital Sodium (Respiratory depression, hypotension, profound sedation or coma). Products include:
Brevital Sodium Vials ... 1429

Methotrimeprazine (Respiratory depression, hypotension, profound sedation or coma). Products include:
Levoprome ... 1274

Methoxyflurane (Respiratory depression, hypotension, profound sedation or coma).
No products indexed under this heading.

Midazolam Hydrochloride (Respiratory depression, hypotension, profound sedation or coma). Products include:
Versed Injection ... 2170

Molindone Hydrochloride (Respiratory depression, hypotension, profound sedation or coma). Products include:
Moban Tablets and Concentrate ... 1048

Morphine Sulfate (Respiratory depression, hypotension, profound sedation or coma). Products include:
Astramorph/PF Injection, USP (Preservative-Free) ... 535
Duramorph ... 962
Infumorph 200 and Infumorph 500 Sterile Solutions ... 965
MS Contin Tablets ... 1994
MSIR ... 1997
Oramorph SR (Morphine Sulfate Sustained Release Tablets) ... 2236
RMS Suppositories ... 2657
Roxanol ... 2243

Nortriptyline Hydrochloride (Respiratory depression, hypotension, profound sedation or coma). Products include:
Pamelor ... 2280

Opium Alkaloids (Respiratory depression, hypotension, profound sedation or coma).
No products indexed under this heading.

IMPORTANT NOTE: Always consult each drug listing in the patient's regimen for possible interactions.

Oxazepam (Respiratory depression, hypotension, profound sedation or coma). Products include:
- Serax Capsules ... 2810
- Serax Tablets ... 2810

Oxycodone Hydrochloride (Respiratory depression, hypotension, profound sedation or coma). Products include:
- Percocet Tablets ... 938
- Percodan Tablets ... 939
- Percodan-Demi Tablets ... 940
- Roxicodone Tablets, Oral Solution & Intensol (Oxycodone) ... 2244
- Tylox Capsules ... 1584

Pentobarbital Sodium (Respiratory depression, hypotension, profound sedation or coma). Products include:
- Nembutal Sodium Capsules ... 436
- Nembutal Sodium Solution ... 438
- Nembutal Sodium Suppositories ... 440

Perphenazine (Respiratory depression, hypotension, profound sedation or coma). Products include:
- Etrafon ... 2355
- Triavil Tablets ... 1757
- Trilafon ... 2389

Phenelzine Sulfate (Contraindicated: unpredictable, severe, and occasionally fatal reactions when given within 14 days). Products include:
- Nardil ... 1920

Phenobarbital (Respiratory depression, hypotension, profound sedation or coma). Products include:
- Arco-Lase Plus Tablets ... 512
- Bellergal-S Tablets ... 2250
- Donnatal ... 2060
- Donnatal Extentabs ... 2061
- Donnatal Tablets ... 2060
- Phenobarbital Elixir and Tablets ... 1469
- Quadrinal Tablets ... 1350

Prazepam (Respiratory depression, hypotension, profound sedation or coma).
- No products indexed under this heading.

Prochlorperazine (Respiratory depression, hypotension, profound sedation or coma). Products include:
- Compazine ... 2470

Promethazine Hydrochloride (Respiratory depression, hypotension, profound sedation or coma). Products include:
- Mepergan Injection ... 2753
- Phenergan with Codeine ... 2777
- Phenergan with Dextromethorphan 2778
- Phenergan Injection ... 2773
- Phenergan Suppositories ... 2775
- Phenergan Syrup ... 2774
- Phenergan Tablets ... 2775
- Phenergan VC ... 2779
- Phenergan VC with Codeine ... 2781

Propofol (Respiratory depression, hypotension, profound sedation or coma). Products include:
- Diprivan Injection ... 2833

Propoxyphene Hydrochloride (Respiratory depression, hypotension, profound sedation or coma). Products include:
- Darvon ... 1435
- Wygesic Tablets ... 2827

Propoxyphene Napsylate (Respiratory depression, hypotension, profound sedation or coma). Products include:
- Darvon-N/Darvocet-N ... 1433

Protriptyline Hydrochloride (Respiratory depression, hypotension, profound sedation or coma). Products include:
- Vivactil Tablets ... 1774

Quazepam (Respiratory depression, hypotension, profound sedation or coma). Products include:
- Doral Tablets ... 2664

Risperidone (Respiratory depression, hypotension, profound sedation or coma). Products include:
- Risperdal ... 1301

Secobarbital Sodium (Respiratory depression, hypotension, profound sedation or coma). Products include:
- Seconal Sodium Pulvules ... 1474

Selegiline Hydrochloride (Contraindicated: unpredictable, severe, and occasionally fatal reactions when given within 14 days). Products include:
- Eldepryl Tablets ... 2550

Sufentanil Citrate (Respiratory depression, hypotension, profound sedation or coma). Products include:
- Sufenta Injection ... 1309

Temazepam (Respiratory depression, hypotension, profound sedation or coma). Products include:
- Restoril Capsules ... 2284

Thiamylal Sodium (Respiratory depression, hypotension, profound sedation or coma).
- No products indexed under this heading.

Thioridazine Hydrochloride (Respiratory depression, hypotension, profound sedation or coma). Products include:
- Mellaril ... 2269

Thiothixene (Respiratory depression, hypotension, profound sedation or coma). Products include:
- Navane Capsules and Concentrate 2201
- Navane Intramuscular ... 2202

Tranylcypromine Sulfate (Contraindicated: unpredictable, severe, and occasionally fatal reactions when given within 14 days). Products include:
- Parnate Tablets ... 2503

Triazolam (Respiratory depression, hypotension, profound sedation or coma). Products include:
- Halcion Tablets ... 2611

Trifluoperazine Hydrochloride (Respiratory depression, hypotension, profound sedation or coma). Products include:
- Stelazine ... 2514

Trimipramine Maleate (Respiratory depression, hypotension, profound sedation or coma). Products include:
- Surmontil Capsules ... 2811

Zolpidem Tartrate (Respiratory depression, hypotension, profound sedation or coma). Products include:
- Ambien Tablets ... 2416

Food Interactions

Alcohol (Respiratory depression, hypotension, profound sedation or coma).

DEMEROL HYDROCHLORIDE INJECTION

(Meperidine Hydrochloride) ... 2308

See **Demerol Hydrochloride Carpuject**

DEMEROL HYDROCHLORIDE SYRUP

(Meperidine Hydrochloride) ... 2308

See **Demerol Hydrochloride Carpuject**

DEMEROL HYDROCHLORIDE TABLETS

(Meperidine Hydrochloride) ... 2308

See **Demerol Hydrochloride Carpuject**

DEMEROL HYDROCHLORIDE UNI-AMP

(Meperidine Hydrochloride) ... 2308

See **Demerol Hydrochloride Carpuject**

DEMSER CAPSULES

(Metyrosine) ... 1649

May interact with central nervous system depressants, phenothiazines, butyrophenones, and certain other agents. Compounds in these categories include:

Alfentanil Hydrochloride (Additive sedative effects). Products include:
- Alfenta Injection ... 1286

Alprazolam (Additive sedative effects). Products include:
- Xanax Tablets ... 2649

Aprobarbital (Additive sedative effects).
- No products indexed under this heading.

Buprenorphine (Additive sedative effects). Products include:
- Buprenex Injectable ... 2006

Buspirone Hydrochloride (Additive sedative effects). Products include:
- BuSpar ... 737

Butabarbital (Additive sedative effects).
- No products indexed under this heading.

Butalbital (Additive sedative effects). Products include:
- Esgic-plus Tablets ... 1013
- Fioricet Tablets ... 2258
- Fioricet with Codeine Capsules ... 2260
- Fiorinal Capsules ... 2261
- Fiorinal with Codeine Capsules ... 2262
- Fiorinal Tablets ... 2261
- Phrenilin ... 785
- Sedapap Tablets 50 mg/650 mg .. 1543

Chlordiazepoxide (Additive sedative effects). Products include:
- Libritabs Tablets ... 2177
- Limbitrol ... 2180

Chlordiazepoxide Hydrochloride (Additive sedative effects). Products include:
- Librax Capsules ... 2176
- Librium Capsules ... 2178
- Librium Injectable ... 2179

Chlorpromazine (Potentiation of extrapyramidal effects of chlorpromazine). Products include:
- Thorazine Suppositories ... 2523

Chlorprothixene (Additive sedative effects).
- No products indexed under this heading.

Chlorprothixene Hydrochloride (Additive sedative effects).
- No products indexed under this heading.

Chlorprothixene Lactate (Additive sedative effects).
- No products indexed under this heading.

Clorazepate Dipotassium (Additive sedative effects). Products include:
- Tranxene ... 451

Clozapine (Additive sedative effects). Products include:
- Clozaril Tablets ... 2252

Codeine Phosphate (Additive sedative effects). Products include:
- Actifed with Codeine Cough Syrup.. 1067
- Brontex ... 1981
- Deconsal C Expectorant Syrup ... 456
- Deconsal Pediatric Syrup ... 457
- Dimetane-DC Cough Syrup ... 2059
- Empirin with Codeine Tablets ... 1093
- Fioricet with Codeine Capsules ... 2260
- Fiorinal with Codeine Capsules ... 2262
- Isoclor Expectorant ... 990
- Novahistine DH ... 2462
- Novahistine Expectorant ... 2463
- Nucofed ... 2051
- Phenergan with Codeine ... 2777
- Phenergan VC with Codeine ... 2781
- Robitussin A-C Syrup ... 2073
- Robitussin-DAC Syrup ... 2074
- Ryna ... ▣ 841
- Soma Compound w/Codeine Tablets ... 2676
- Tussi-Organidin NR Liquid and S NR Liquid ... 2677
- Tylenol with Codeine ... 1583

Desflurane (Additive sedative effects). Products include:
- Suprane ... 1813

Dezocine (Additive sedative effects). Products include:
- Dalgan Injection ... 538

Diazepam (Additive sedative effects). Products include:
- Dizac ... 1809
- Valium Injectable ... 2182
- Valium Tablets ... 2183
- Valrelease Capsules ... 2169

Droperidol (Additive sedative effects). Products include:
- Inapsine Injection ... 1296

Enflurane (Additive sedative effects).
- No products indexed under this heading.

Estazolam (Additive sedative effects). Products include:
- ProSom Tablets ... 449

Ethchlorvynol (Additive sedative effects). Products include:
- Placidyl Capsules ... 448

Ethinamate (Additive sedative effects).
- No products indexed under this heading.

Fentanyl (Additive sedative effects). Products include:
- Duragesic Transdermal System ... 1288

Fentanyl Citrate (Additive sedative effects). Products include:
- Sublimaze Injection ... 1307

Fluphenazine Decanoate (Potentiation of extrapyramidal effects of fluphenazine). Products include:
- Prolixin Decanoate ... 509

Fluphenazine Enanthate (Potentiation of extrapyramidal effects of fluphenazine). Products include:
- Prolixin Enanthate ... 509

Fluphenazine Hydrochloride (Potentiation of extrapyramidal effects of fluphenazine). Products include:
- Prolixin ... 509

Flurazepam Hydrochloride (Additive sedative effects). Products include:
- Dalmane Capsules ... 2173

Glutethimide (Additive sedative effects).
- No products indexed under this heading.

Haloperidol (Potentiation of extrapyramidal effects of haloperidol; additive sedative effects). Products include:
- Haldol Injection, Tablets and Concentrate ... 1575

Haloperidol Decanoate (Potentiation of extrapyramidal effects of haloperidol; additive sedative effects). Products include:
- Haldol Decanoate ... 1577

Hydrocodone Bitartrate (Additive sedative effects). Products include:
- Anexsia 5/500 Elixir ... 1781
- Anexia Tablets ... 1782
- Codiclear DH Syrup ... 791
- Deconamine CX Cough and Cold Liquid and Tablets ... 1319
- Duratuss HD Elixir ... 2565
- Hycodan Tablets and Syrup ... 930

(▣ Described in PDR For Nonprescription Drugs) (⊙ Described in PDR For Ophthalmology)

Hycomine Compound Tablets ... 932
Hycomine ... 931
Hycotuss Expectorant Syrup ... 933
Hydrocet Capsules ... 782
Lorcet 10/650 ... 1018
Lortab ... 2566
Tussend ... 1783
Tussend Expectorant ... 1785
Vicodin Tablets ... 1356
Vicodin ES Tablets ... 1357
Vicodin Tuss Expectorant ... 1358
Zydone Capsules ... 949

Hydrocodone Polistirex (Additive sedative effects). Products include:
Tussionex Pennkinetic Extended-Release Suspension ... 998

Hydroxyzine Hydrochloride (Additive sedative effects). Products include:
Atarax Tablets & Syrup ... 2185
Marax Tablets & DF Syrup ... 2200
Vistaril Intramuscular Solution ... 2216

Isoflurane (Additive sedative effects).
No products indexed under this heading.

Ketamine Hydrochloride (Additive sedative effects).
No products indexed under this heading.

Levomethadyl Acetate Hydrochloride (Additive sedative effects). Products include:
Orlamm ... 2239

Levorphanol Tartrate (Additive sedative effects). Products include:
Levo-Dromoran ... 2129

Lorazepam (Additive sedative effects). Products include:
Ativan Injection ... 2698
Ativan Tablets ... 2700

Loxapine Hydrochloride (Additive sedative effects). Products include:
Loxitane ... 1378

Loxapine Succinate (Additive sedative effects). Products include:
Loxitane Capsules ... 1378

Meperidine Hydrochloride (Additive sedative effects). Products include:
Demerol ... 2308
Mepergan Injection ... 2753

Mephobarbital (Additive sedative effects). Products include:
Mebaral Tablets ... 2322

Meprobamate (Additive sedative effects). Products include:
Miltown Tablets ... 2672
PMB 200 and PMB 400 ... 2783

Mesoridazine Besylate (Potentiation of extrapyramidal effects of mesoridazine). Products include:
Serentil ... 684

Methadone Hydrochloride (Additive sedative effects). Products include:
Methadone Hydrochloride Oral Concentrate ... 2233
Methadone Hydrochloride Oral Solution & Tablets ... 2235

Methohexital Sodium (Additive sedative effects). Products include:
Brevital Sodium Vials ... 1429

Methotrimeprazine (Additive sedative effects). Products include:
Levoprome ... 1274

Methoxyflurane (Additive sedative effects).
No products indexed under this heading.

Midazolam Hydrochloride (Additive sedative effects). Products include:
Versed Injection ... 2170

Molindone Hydrochloride (Additive sedative effects). Products include:
Moban Tablets and Concentrate ... 1048

Morphine Sulfate (Additive sedative effects). Products include:
Astramorph/PF Injection, USP (Preservative-Free) ... 535
Duramorph ... 962
Infumorph 200 and Infumorph 500 Sterile Solutions ... 965
MS Contin Tablets ... 1994
MSIR ... 1997
Oramorph SR (Morphine Sulfate Sustained Release Tablets) ... 2236
RMS Suppositories ... 2657
Roxanol ... 2243

Opium Alkaloids (Additive sedative effects).
No products indexed under this heading.

Oxazepam (Additive sedative effects). Products include:
Serax Capsules ... 2810
Serax Tablets ... 2810

Oxycodone Hydrochloride (Additive sedative effects). Products include:
Percocet Tablets ... 938
Percodan Tablets ... 939
Percodan-Demi Tablets ... 940
Roxicodone Tablets, Oral Solution & Intensol (Oxycodone) ... 2244
Tylox Capsules ... 1584

Pentobarbital Sodium (Additive sedative effects). Products include:
Nembutal Sodium Capsules ... 436
Nembutal Sodium Solution ... 438
Nembutal Sodium Suppositories ... 440

Perphenazine (Potentiation of extrapyramidal effects of perphenazine). Products include:
Etrafon ... 2355
Triavil Tablets ... 1757
Trilafon ... 2389

Phenobarbital (Additive sedative effects). Products include:
Arco-Lase Plus Tablets ... 512
Bellergal-S Tablets ... 2250
Donnatal ... 2060
Donnatal Extentabs ... 2061
Donnatal Tablets ... 2060
Phenobarbital Elixir and Tablets ... 1469
Quadrinal Tablets ... 1350

Prazepam (Additive sedative effects).
No products indexed under this heading.

Prochlorperazine (Potentiation of extrapyramidal effects of chlorpromazine). Products include:
Compazine ... 2470

Promethazine Hydrochloride (Potentiation of extrapyramidal effects of promethazine). Products include:
Mepergan Injection ... 2753
Phenergan with Codeine ... 2777
Phenergan with Dextromethorphan ... 2778
Phenergan Injection ... 2773
Phenergan Suppositories ... 2775
Phenergan Syrup ... 2774
Phenergan Tablets ... 2775
Phenergan VC ... 2779
Phenergan VC with Codeine ... 2781

Propofol (Additive sedative effects). Products include:
Diprivan Injection ... 2833

Propoxyphene Hydrochloride (Additive sedative effects). Products include:
Darvon ... 1435
Wygesic Tablets ... 2827

Propoxyphene Napsylate (Additive sedative effects). Products include:
Darvon-N/Darvocet-N ... 1433

Quazepam (Additive sedative effects). Products include:
Doral Tablets ... 2664

Risperidone (Additive sedative effects). Products include:
Risperdal ... 1301

Secobarbital Sodium (Additive sedative effects). Products include:
Seconal Sodium Pulvules ... 1474

Sufentanil Citrate (Additive sedative effects). Products include:
Sufenta Injection ... 1309

Temazepam (Additive sedative effects). Products include:
Restoril Capsules ... 2284

Thiamylal Sodium (Additive sedative effects).
No products indexed under this heading.

Thioridazine Hydrochloride (Potentiation of extrapyramidal effects of thioridazine). Products include:
Mellaril ... 2269

Thiothixene (Additive sedative effects). Products include:
Navane Capsules and Concentrate ... 2201
Navane Intramuscular ... 2202

Triazolam (Additive sedative effects). Products include:
Halcion Tablets ... 2611

Trifluoperazine Hydrochloride (Potentiation of extrapyramidal effects of trifluoperazine). Products include:
Stelazine ... 2514

Zolpidem Tartrate (Additive sedative effects). Products include:
Ambien Tablets ... 2416

Food Interactions

Alcohol (Additive sedative effects).

DEMULEN 1/35-21

(Ethynodiol Diacetate, Ethinyl Estradiol) ... 2428
May interact with barbiturates, tetracyclines, and certain other agents. Compounds in these categories include:

Ampicillin Sodium (Reduces efficacy and increased incidence of breakthrough bleeding and menstrual irregularities). Products include:
Unasyn ... 2212

Aprobarbital (Reduces efficacy and increased incidence of breakthrough bleeding and menstrual irregularities).
No products indexed under this heading.

Butabarbital (Reduces efficacy and increased incidence of breakthrough bleeding and menstrual irregularities).
No products indexed under this heading.

Butalbital (Reduces efficacy and increased incidence of breakthrough bleeding and menstrual irregularities). Products include:
Esgic-plus Tablets ... 1013
Fioricet Tablets ... 2258
Fioricet with Codeine Capsules ... 2260
Fiorinal Capsules ... 2261
Fiorinal with Codeine Capsules ... 2262
Fiorinal Tablets ... 2261
Phrenilin ... 785
Sedapap Tablets 50 mg/650 mg ... 1543

Demeclocycline Hydrochloride (Reduces efficacy and increased incidence of breakthrough bleeding and menstrual irregularities). Products include:
Declomycin Tablets ... 1371

Doxycycline Calcium (Reduces efficacy and increased incidence of breakthrough bleeding and menstrual irregularities). Products include:
Vibramycin Calcium Oral Suspension Syrup ... 1941

Doxycycline Hyclate (Reduces efficacy and increased incidence of breakthrough bleeding and menstrual irregularities). Products include:
Doryx Capsules ... 1913
Vibramycin Hyclate Capsules ... 1941
Vibramycin Hyclate Intravenous ... 2215
Vibra-Tabs Film Coated Tablets ... 1941

Doxycycline Monohydrate (Reduces efficacy and increased incidence of breakthrough bleeding and menstrual irregularities). Products include:
Monodox Capsules ... 1805
Vibramycin Monohydrate for Oral Suspension ... 1941

Griseofulvin (Reduces efficacy and increased incidence of breakthrough bleeding and menstrual irregularities). Products include:
Fulvicin P/G Tablets ... 2359
Fulvicin P/G 165 & 330 Tablets ... 2359
Grifulvin V (griseofulvin tablets) Microsize (griseofulvin oral suspension) Microsize ... 1888
Gris-PEG Tablets, 125 mg & 250 mg ... 479

Mephobarbital (Reduces efficacy and increased incidence of breakthrough bleeding and menstrual irregularities). Products include:
Mebaral Tablets ... 2322

Methacycline Hydrochloride (Reduces efficacy and increased incidence of breakthrough bleeding and menstrual irregularities).
No products indexed under this heading.

Minocycline Hydrochloride (Reduces efficacy and increased incidence of breakthrough bleeding and menstrual irregularities). Products include:
Dynacin Capsules ... 1590
Minocin Intravenous ... 1382
Minocin Oral Suspension ... 1385
Minocin Pellet-Filled Capsules ... 1383

Oxytetracycline Hydrochloride (Reduces efficacy and increased incidence of breakthrough bleeding and menstrual irregularities). Products include:
TERAK Ointment ... ◉ 209
Terra-Cortril Ophthalmic Suspension ... 2210
Terramycin with Polymyxin B Sulfate Ophthalmic Ointment ... 2211
Urobiotic-250 Capsules ... 2214

Pentobarbital Sodium (Reduces efficacy and increased incidence of breakthrough bleeding and menstrual irregularities). Products include:
Nembutal Sodium Capsules ... 436
Nembutal Sodium Solution ... 438
Nembutal Sodium Suppositories ... 440

Phenobarbital (Reduces efficacy and increased incidence of breakthrough bleeding and menstrual irregularities). Products include:
Arco-Lase Plus Tablets ... 512
Bellergal-S Tablets ... 2250
Donnatal ... 2060
Donnatal Extentabs ... 2061
Donnatal Tablets ... 2060
Phenobarbital Elixir and Tablets ... 1469
Quadrinal Tablets ... 1350

Phenylbutazone (Reduces efficacy and increased incidence of breakthrough bleeding and menstrual irregularities).
No products indexed under this heading.

IMPORTANT NOTE: Always consult each drug listing in the patient's regimen for possible interactions.

Phenytoin (Reduces efficacy and increased incidence of breakthrough bleeding and menstrual irregularities). Products include:
- Dilantin Infatabs ... 1908
- Dilantin-125 Suspension ... 1911

Phenytoin Sodium (Reduces efficacy and increased incidence of breakthrough bleeding and menstrual irregularities). Products include:
- Dilantin Kapseals ... 1906
- Dilantin Parenteral ... 1910

Rifampin (Reduces efficacy and increased incidence of breakthrough bleeding and menstrual irregularities). Products include:
- Rifadin ... 1528
- Rifamate Capsules ... 1530
- Rifater ... 1532
- Rimactane Capsules ... 847

Secobarbital Sodium (Reduces efficacy and increased incidence of breakthrough bleeding and menstrual irregularities). Products include:
- Seconal Sodium Pulvules ... 1474

Tetracycline Hydrochloride (Reduces efficacy and increased incidence of breakthrough bleeding and menstrual irregularities). Products include:
- Achromycin V Capsules ... 1367

Thiamylal Sodium (Reduces efficacy and increased incidence of breakthrough bleeding and menstrual irregularities).
- No products indexed under this heading.

DEMULEN 1/35-28
(Ethynodiol Diacetate, Ethinyl Estradiol) ... 2428
See **Demulen 1/35-21**

DEMULEN 1/50-21
(Ethynodiol Diacetate, Ethinyl Estradiol) ... 2428
See **Demulen 1/35-21**

DEMULEN 1/50-28
(Ethynodiol Diacetate, Ethinyl Estradiol) ... 2428
See **Demulen 1/35-21**

DEPAKENE CAPSULES
(Valproic Acid) ... 413
May interact with oral anticoagulants, central nervous system depressants, benzodiazepines, oral contraceptives, and certain other agents. Compounds in these categories include:

Alfentanil Hydrochloride (Valproate may potentiate the action of CNS depressants). Products include:
- Alfenta Injection ... 1286

Alprazolam (Valproate may potentiate the action of CNS depressants). Products include:
- Xanax Tablets ... 2649

Aprobarbital (Valproate may potentiate the action of CNS depressants).
- No products indexed under this heading.

Aspirin (Altered serum drug levels). Products include:
- Alka-Seltzer Effervescent Antacid and Pain Reliever ... ▣ 701
- Alka-Seltzer Extra Strength Effervescent Antacid and Pain Reliever ... ▣ 703
- Alka-Seltzer Lemon Lime Effervescent Antacid and Pain Reliever ... ▣ 703
- Alka-Seltzer Plus Cold Medicine ... ▣ 705
- Alka-Seltzer Plus Cold & Cough Medicine ... ▣ 708
- Alka-Seltzer Plus Night-Time Cold Medicine ... ▣ 707
- Alka Seltzer Plus Sinus Medicine ... ▣ 707
- Arthritis Foundation Safety Coated Aspirin Tablets ... ▣ 675
- Arthritis Pain Ascriptin ... ▣ 631
- Maximum Strength Ascriptin ... ▣ 630
- Regular Strength Ascriptin Tablets ... ▣ 629
- Arthritis Strength BC Powder ... ▣ 609
- BC Cold Powder Multi-Symptom Formula (Cold-Sinus-Allergy) ... ▣ 609
- BC Cold Powder Non-Drowsy Formula (Cold-Sinus) ... ▣ 609
- BC Powder ... ▣ 609
- Bayer Children's Chewable Aspirin ... ▣ 711
- Genuine Bayer Aspirin Tablets & Caplets ... ▣ 713
- Extra Strength Bayer Arthritis Pain Regimen Formula ... ▣ 711
- Extra Strength Bayer Aspirin Caplets & Tablets ... ▣ 712
- Extended-Release Bayer 8-Hour Aspirin ... ▣ 712
- Extra Strength Bayer Plus Aspirin Caplets ... ▣ 713
- Extra Strength Bayer PM Aspirin ... ▣ 713
- Bayer Enteric Aspirin ... ▣ 709
- Bufferin Analgesic Tablets and Caplets ... ▣ 613
- Arthritis Strength Bufferin Analgesic Caplets ... ▣ 614
- Extra Strength Bufferin Analgesic Tablets ... ▣ 615
- Cama Arthritis Pain Reliever ... ▣ 785
- Darvon Compound-65 Pulvules ... 1435
- Easprin ... 1914
- Ecotrin ... 2455
- Ecotrin Enteric Coated Aspirin Maximum Strength Tablets and Caplets ... ▣ 816
- Ecotrin Enteric Coated Aspirin Regular Strength Tablets ... 2455
- Empirin Aspirin Tablets ... ▣ 854
- Empirin with Codeine Tablets ... 1093
- Excedrin Extra-Strength Analgesic Tablets & Caplets ... 732
- Fiorinal Capsules ... 2261
- Fiorinal with Codeine Capsules ... 2262
- Fiorinal Tablets ... 2261
- Halfprin ... 1362
- Healthprin Aspirin ... 2455
- Norgesic ... 1496
- Percodan Tablets ... 939
- Percodan-Demi Tablets ... 940
- Robaxisal Tablets ... 2071
- Soma Compound w/Codeine Tablets ... 2676
- Soma Compound Tablets ... 2675
- St. Joseph Adult Chewable Aspirin (81 mg.) ... ▣ 808
- Talwin Compound ... 2335
- Ursinus Inlay-Tabs ... ▣ 794
- Vanquish Analgesic Caplets ... ▣ 731

Buprenorphine (Valproate may potentiate the action of CNS depressants). Products include:
- Buprenex Injectable ... 2006

Buspirone Hydrochloride (Valproate may potentiate the action of CNS depressants). Products include:
- BuSpar ... 737

Butabarbital (Valproate may potentiate the action of CNS depressants).
- No products indexed under this heading.

Butalbital (Valproate may potentiate the action of CNS depressants). Products include:
- Esgic-plus Tablets ... 1013
- Fioricet Tablets ... 2258
- Fioricet with Codeine Capsules ... 2260
- Fiorinal Capsules ... 2261
- Fiorinal with Codeine Capsules ... 2262
- Fiorinal Tablets ... 2261
- Phrenilin ... 785
- Sedapap Tablets 50 mg/650 mg ... 1543

Carbamazepine (Altered serum drug levels). Products include:
- Atretol Tablets ... 573
- Tegretol Chewable Tablets ... 852
- Tegretol Suspension ... 852
- Tegretol Tablets ... 852

Chlordiazepoxide (Valproate may potentiate the action of CNS depressants). Products include:
- Libritabs Tablets ... 2177
- Limbitrol ... 2180

Chlordiazepoxide Hydrochloride (Valproate may potentiate the action of CNS depressants). Products include:
- Librax Capsules ... 2176
- Librium Capsules ... 2178
- Librium Injectable ... 2179

Chlorpromazine (Valproate may potentiate the action of CNS depressants). Products include:
- Thorazine Suppositories ... 2523

Chlorprothixene (Valproate may potentiate the action of CNS depressants).
- No products indexed under this heading.

Chlorprothixene Hydrochloride (Valproate may potentiate the action of CNS depressants).
- No products indexed under this heading.

Clonazepam (Concomitant use may produce absence status in patients with a history of absence type seizures). Products include:
- Klonopin Tablets ... 2126

Clorazepate Dipotassium (Valproate may potentiate the action of CNS depressants). Products include:
- Tranxene ... 451

Clozapine (Valproate may potentiate the action of CNS depressants). Products include:
- Clozaril Tablets ... 2252

Codeine Phosphate (Valproate may potentiate the action of CNS depressants). Products include:
- Actifed with Codeine Cough Syrup ... 1067
- Brontex ... 1981
- Deconsal C Expectorant Syrup ... 456
- Deconsal Pediatric Syrup ... 457
- Dimetane-DC Cough Syrup ... 2059
- Empirin with Codeine Tablets ... 1093
- Fioricet with Codeine Capsules ... 2260
- Fiorinal with Codeine Capsules ... 2262
- Isoclor Expectorant ... 990
- Novahistine DH ... 2462
- Novahistine Expectorant ... 2463
- Nucofed ... 2051
- Phenergan with Codeine ... 2777
- Phenergan VC with Codeine ... 2781
- Robitussin A-C Syrup ... 2073
- Robitussin-DAC Syrup ... 2074
- Ryna ... ▣ 841
- Soma Compound w/Codeine Tablets ... 2676
- Tussi-Organidin NR Liquid and S NR Liquid ... 2677
- Tylenol with Codeine ... 1583

Desflurane (Valproate may potentiate the action of CNS depressants). Products include:
- Suprane ... 1813

Desogestrel (Possible oral contraceptive failure). Products include:
- Desogen Tablets ... 1817
- Ortho-Cept ... 1851

Dezocine (Valproate may potentiate the action of CNS depressants). Products include:
- Dalgan Injection ... 538

Diazepam (Valproate may potentiate the action of CNS depressants). Products include:
- Dizac ... 1809
- Valium Injectable ... 2182
- Valium Tablets ... 2183
- Valrelease Capsules ... 2169

Dicumarol (Altered serum drug levels).
- No products indexed under this heading.

Droperidol (Valproate may potentiate the action of CNS depressants). Products include:
- Inapsine Injection ... 1296

Enflurane (Valproate may potentiate the action of CNS depressants).
- No products indexed under this heading.

Estazolam (Valproate may potentiate the action of CNS depressants). Products include:
- ProSom Tablets ... 449

Ethchlorvynol (Valproate may potentiate the action of CNS depressants). Products include:
- Placidyl Capsules ... 448

Ethinamate (Valproate may potentiate the action of CNS depressants).
- No products indexed under this heading.

Ethinyl Estradiol (Possible oral contraceptive failure). Products include:
- Brevicon ... 2088
- Demulen ... 2428
- Desogen Tablets ... 1817
- Levlen/Tri-Levlen ... 651
- Lo/Ovral Tablets ... 2746
- Lo/Ovral-28 Tablets ... 2751
- Modicon ... 1872
- Nordette-21 Tablets ... 2755
- Nordette-28 Tablets ... 2758
- Norinyl ... 2088
- Ortho-Cept ... 1851
- Ortho-Cyclen/Ortho-Tri-Cyclen ... 1858
- Ortho-Novum ... 1872
- Ortho-Cyclen/Ortho Tri-Cyclen ... 1858
- Ovcon ... 760
- Ovral Tablets ... 2770
- Ovral-28 Tablets ... 2770
- Levlen/Tri-Levlen ... 651
- Tri-Norinyl ... 2164
- Triphasil-21 Tablets ... 2814
- Triphasil-28 Tablets ... 2819

Ethosuximide (Altered serum concentrations of both drugs). Products include:
- Zarontin Capsules ... 1928
- Zarontin Syrup ... 1929

Ethynodiol Diacetate (Possible oral contraceptive failure). Products include:
- Demulen ... 2428

Fentanyl (Valproate may potentiate the action of CNS depressants). Products include:
- Duragesic Transdermal System ... 1288

Fentanyl Citrate (Valproate may potentiate the action of CNS depressants). Products include:
- Sublimaze Injection ... 1307

Fluphenazine Decanoate (Valproate may potentiate the action of CNS depressants). Products include:
- Prolixin Decanoate ... 509

Fluphenazine Enanthate (Valproate may potentiate the action of CNS depressants). Products include:
- Prolixin Enanthate ... 509

Fluphenazine Hydrochloride (Valproate may potentiate the action of CNS depressants). Products include:
- Prolixin ... 509

Flurazepam Hydrochloride (Valproate may potentiate the action of CNS depressants). Products include:
- Dalmane Capsules ... 2173

Glutethimide (Valproate may potentiate the action of CNS depressants).
- No products indexed under this heading.

Halazepam (Valproate may potentiate the action of CNS depressants).
- No products indexed under this heading.

Haloperidol (Valproate may potentiate the action of CNS depressants). Products include:
- Haldol Injection, Tablets and Concentrate ... 1575

Haloperidol Decanoate (Valproate may potentiate the action of CNS depressants). Products include:
- Haldol Decanoate ... 1577

Hydrocodone Bitartrate (Valproate may potentiate the action of CNS depressants). Products include:

Anexsia 5/500 Elixir 1781
Anexia Tablets....................................... 1782
Codiclear DH Syrup 791
Deconamine CX Cough and Cold Liquid and Tablets.............................. 1319
Duratuss HD Elixir................................. 2565
Hycodan Tablets and Syrup 930
Hycomine Compound Tablets 932
Hycomine 931
Hycotuss Expectorant Syrup 933
Hydrocet Capsules 782
Lorcet 10/650.. 1018
Lortab 2566
Tussend 1783
Tussend Expectorant 1785
Vicodin Tablets...................................... 1356
Vicodin ES Tablets 1357
Vicodin Tuss Expectorant 1358
Zydone Capsules 949

Hydrocodone Polistirex (Valproate may potentiate the action of CNS depressants). Products include:

Tussionex Pennkinetic Extended-Release Suspension 998

Hydroxyzine Hydrochloride (Valproate may potentiate the action of CNS depressants). Products include:

Atarax Tablets & Syrup......................... 2185
Marax Tablets & DF Syrup.................... 2200
Vistaril Intramuscular Solution.......... 2216

Isoflurane (Valproate may potentiate the action of CNS depressants).

No products indexed under this heading.

Ketamine Hydrochloride (Valproate may potentiate the action of CNS depressants).

No products indexed under this heading.

Levomethadyl Acetate Hydrochloride (Valproate may potentiate the action of CNS depressants). Products include:

Orlaam 2239

Levonorgestrel (Possible oral contraceptive failure). Products include:

Levlen/Tri-Levlen.................................. 651
Nordette-21 Tablets............................... 2755
Nordette-28 Tablets............................... 2758
Norplant System 2759
Levlen/Tri-Levlen.................................. 651
Triphasil-21 Tablets............................... 2814
Triphasil-28 Tablets............................... 2819

Levorphanol Tartrate (Valproate may potentiate the action of CNS depressants). Products include:

Levo-Dromoran...................................... 2129

Lorazepam (Valproate may potentiate the action of CNS depressants). Products include:

Ativan Injection..................................... 2698
Ativan Tablets.. 2700

Loxapine Hydrochloride (Valproate may potentiate the action of CNS depressants). Products include:

Loxitane 1378

Loxapine Succinate (Valproate may potentiate the action of CNS depressants). Products include:

Loxitane Capsules 1378

Meperidine Hydrochloride (Valproate may potentiate the action of CNS depressants). Products include:

Demerol 2308
Mepergan Injection 2753

Mephobarbital (Valproate may potentiate the action of CNS depressants). Products include:

Mebaral Tablets 2322

Meprobamate (Valproate may potentiate the action of CNS depressants). Products include:

Miltown Tablets 2672
PMB 200 and PMB 400 2783

Mesoridazine Besylate (Valproate may potentiate the action of CNS depressants). Products include:

Serentil... 684

Mestranol (Possible oral contraceptive failure). Products include:

Norinyl 2088
Ortho-Novum... 1872

Methadone Hydrochloride (Valproate may potentiate the action of CNS depressants). Products include:

Methadone Hydrochloride Oral Concentrate 2233
Methadone Hydrochloride Oral Solution & Tablets................................. 2235

Methohexital Sodium (Valproate may potentiate the action of CNS depressants). Products include:

Brevital Sodium Vials............................ 1429

Methotrimeprazine (Valproate may potentiate the action of CNS depressants). Products include:

Levoprome 1274

Methoxyflurane (Valproate may potentiate the action of CNS depressants).

No products indexed under this heading.

Midazolam Hydrochloride (Valproate may potentiate the action of CNS depressants). Products include:

Versed Injection 2170

Molindone Hydrochloride (Valproate may potentiate the action of CNS depressants). Products include:

Moban Tablets and Concentrate...... 1048

Morphine Sulfate (Valproate may potentiate the action of CNS depressants). Products include:

Astramorph/PF Injection, USP (Preservative-Free) 535
Duramorph... 962
Infumorph 200 and Infumorph 500 Sterile Solutions........................... 965
MS Contin Tablets.................................. 1994
MSIR 1997
Oramorph SR (Morphine Sulfate Sustained Release Tablets) 2236
RMS Suppositories 2657
Roxanol 2243

Norethindrone (Possible oral contraceptive failure). Products include:

Brevicon.. 2088
Micronor Tablets 1872
Modicon 1872
Norinyl 2088
Nor-Q D Tablets 2135
Ortho-Novum... 1872
Ovcon 760
Tri-Norinyl... 2164

Norethynodrel (Possible oral contraceptive failure).

No products indexed under this heading.

Norgestimate (Possible oral contraceptive failure). Products include:

Ortho-Cyclen/Ortho-Tri-Cyclen 1858
Ortho-Cyclen/Ortho Tri-Cyclen 1858

Norgestrel (Possible oral contraceptive failure). Products include:

Lo/Ovral Tablets 2746
Lo/Ovral-28 Tablets............................... 2751
Ovral Tablets 2770
Ovral-28 Tablets 2770
Ovrette Tablets...................................... 2771

Opium Alkaloids (Valproate may potentiate the action of CNS depressants).

No products indexed under this heading.

Oxazepam (Valproate may potentiate the action of CNS depressants). Products include:

Serax Capsules 2810
Serax Tablets.. 2810

Oxycodone Hydrochloride (Valproate may potentiate the action of CNS depressants). Products include:

Percocet Tablets 938
Percodan Tablets................................... 939
Percodan-Demi Tablets......................... 940
Roxicodone Tablets, Oral Solution & Intensol (Oxycodone) 2244
Tylox Capsules 1584

Pentobarbital Sodium (Valproate may potentiate the action of CNS depressants). Products include:

Nembutal Sodium Capsules 436
Nembutal Sodium Solution 438
Nembutal Sodium Suppositories...... 440

Perphenazine (Valproate may potentiate the action of CNS depressants). Products include:

Etrafon 2355
Triavil Tablets 1757
Trilafon... 2389

Phenobarbital (Increased serum phenobarbital levels; potential for increased CNS depression; monitor for neurological toxicity). Products include:

Arco-Lase Plus Tablets 512
Bellergal-S Tablets 2250
Donnatal 2060
Donnatal Extentabs............................... 2061
Donnatal Tablets 2060
Phenobarbital Elixir and Tablets...... 1469
Quadrinal Tablets 1350

Phenytoin (Potential for breakthrough seizures; potential for alteration in serum drug concentrations; dosage of phenytoin should be adjusted). Products include:

Dilantin Infatabs 1908
Dilantin-125 Suspension 1911

Phenytoin Sodium (Potential for breakthrough seizures; potential for alteration in serum drug concentrations; dosage of phenytoin should be adjusted). Products include:

Dilantin Kapseals 1906
Dilantin Parenteral 1910

Prazepam (Valproate may potentiate the action of CNS depressants).

No products indexed under this heading.

Primidone (Potential for neurological toxicity). Products include:

Mysoline... 2754

Prochlorperazine (Valproate may potentiate the action of CNS depressants). Products include:

Compazine 2470

Promethazine Hydrochloride (Valproate may potentiate the action of CNS depressants). Products include:

Mepergan Injection 2753
Phenergan with Codeine....................... 2777
Phenergan with Dextromethorphan 2778
Phenergan Injection 2773
Phenergan Suppositories 2775
Phenergan Syrup 2774
Phenergan Tablets 2775
Phenergan VC.. 2779
Phenergan VC with Codeine 2781

Propofol (Valproate may potentiate the action of CNS depressants). Products include:

Diprivan Injection.................................. 2833

Propoxyphene Hydrochloride (Valproate may potentiate the action of CNS depressants). Products include:

Darvon 1435
Wygesic Tablets 2827

Propoxyphene Napsylate (Valproate may potentiate the action of CNS depressants). Products include:

Darvon-N/Darvocet-N 1433

Quazepam (Valproate may potentiate the action of CNS depressants). Products include:

Doral Tablets 2664

Risperidone (Valproate may potentiate the action of CNS depressants). Products include:

Risperdal 1301

Secobarbital Sodium (Valproate may potentiate the action of CNS depressants). Products include:

Seconal Sodium Pulvules 1474

Sufentanil Citrate (Valproate may potentiate the action of CNS depressants). Products include:

Sufenta Injection 1309

Temazepam (Valproate may potentiate the action of CNS depressants). Products include:

Restoril Capsules 2284

Thiamylal Sodium (Valproate may potentiate the action of CNS depressants).

No products indexed under this heading.

Thioridazine Hydrochloride (Valproate may potentiate the action of CNS depressants). Products include:

Mellaril 2269

Thiothixene (Valproate may potentiate the action of CNS depressants). Products include:

Navane Capsules and Concentrate 2201
Navane Intramuscular 2202

Triazolam (Valproate may potentiate the action of CNS depressants). Products include:

Halcion Tablets...................................... 2611

Trifluoperazine Hydrochloride (Valproate may potentiate the action of CNS depressants). Products include:

Stelazine 2514

Warfarin Sodium (Altered bleeding time). Products include:

Coumadin 926

Zolpidem Tartrate (Valproate may potentiate the action of CNS depressants). Products include:

Ambien Tablets...................................... 2416

Food Interactions

Alcohol (Depakene may potentiate CNS depressant activity).

DEPAKENE SYRUP

(Valproic Acid) 413

See **Depakene Capsules**

DEPAKOTE TABLETS

(Divalproex Sodium) 415

May interact with central nervous system depressants, drugs that elevate levels of glucuronosyl transferase, and certain other agents. Compounds in these categories include:

Alfentanil Hydrochloride (May result in additive CNS depression). Products include:

Alfenta Injection 1286

Alprazolam (May result in additive CNS depression). Products include:

Xanax Tablets 2649

Amitriptyline Hydrochloride (Decreased plasma clearance of amitriptyline). Products include:

Elavil 2838
Endep Tablets 2174
Etrafon 2355
Limbitrol 2180
Triavil Tablets 1757

Aprobarbital (May result in additive CNS depression).

No products indexed under this heading.

Aspirin (Decrease in protein binding and an inhibition of metabolism of valproate thereby increasing free fraction of free valproate). Products include:

Alka-Seltzer Effervescent Antacid and Pain Reliever .... ⊕ 701
Alka-Seltzer Extra Strength Effervescent Antacid and Pain Reliever .... ⊕ 703

IMPORTANT NOTE: Always consult each drug listing in the patient's regimen for possible interactions.

Depakote **Interactions Index** **254**

Alka-Seltzer Lemon Lime Effervescent Antacid and Pain Reliever ▣ 703
Alka-Seltzer Plus Cold Medicine ▣ 705
Alka-Seltzer Plus Cold & Cough Medicine ▣ 708
Alka-Seltzer Plus Night-Time Cold Medicine ▣ 707
Alka Seltzer Plus Sinus Medicine ▣ 707
Arthritis Foundation Safety Coated Aspirin Tablets ▣ 675
Arthritis Pain Ascriptin ▣ 631
Maximum Strength Ascriptin ▣ 630
Regular Strength Ascriptin Tablets ▣ 629
Arthritis Strength BC Powder ▣ 609
BC Cold Powder Multi-Symptom Formula (Cold-Sinus-Allergy) ▣ 609
BC Cold Powder Non-Drowsy Formula (Cold-Sinus) ▣ 609
BC Powder ▣ 609
Bayer Children's Chewable Aspirin ▣ 711
Genuine Bayer Aspirin Tablets & Caplets ▣ 713
Extra Strength Bayer Arthritis Pain Regimen Formula ▣ 711
Extra Strength Bayer Aspirin Caplets & Tablets ▣ 712
Extended-Release Bayer 8-Hour Aspirin ▣ 712
Extra Strength Bayer Plus Aspirin Caplets ▣ 713
Extra Strength Bayer PM Aspirin ▣ 713
Bayer Enteric Aspirin ▣ 709
Bufferin Analgesic Tablets and Caplets ▣ 613
Arthritis Strength Bufferin Analgesic Caplets ▣ 614
Extra Strength Bufferin Analgesic Tablets ▣ 615
Cama Arthritis Pain Reliever ▣ 785
Darvon Compound-65 Pulvules 1435
Easprin 1914
Ecotrin 2455
Ecotrin Enteric Coated Aspirin Maximum Strength Tablets and Caplets ▣ 816
Ecotrin Enteric Coated Aspirin Regular Strength Tablets 2455
Empirin Aspirin Tablets ▣ 854
Empirin with Codeine Tablets 1093
Excedrin Extra-Strength Analgesic Tablets & Caplets ▣ 732
Fiorinal Capsules 2261
Fiorinal with Codeine Capsules 2262
Fiorinal Tablets 2261
Halfprin 1362
Healthprin Aspirin 2455
Norgesic 1496
Percodan Tablets 939
Percodan-Demi Tablets 940
Robaxisal Tablets 2071
Soma Compound w/Codeine Tablets 2676
Soma Compound Tablets 2675
St. Joseph Adult Chewable Aspirin (81 mg.) ▣ 808
Talwin Compound 2335
Ursinus Inlay-Tabs ▣ 794
Vanquish Analgesic Caplets ▣ 731

Buprenorphine (May result in additive CNS depression). Products include:
Buprenex Injectable 2006

Buspirone Hydrochloride (May result in additive CNS depression). Products include:
BuSpar 737

Butabarbital (May result in additive CNS depression).
No products indexed under this heading.

Butalbital (May result in additive CNS depression). Products include:
Esgic-plus Tablets 1013
Fioricet Tablets 2258
Fioricet with Codeine Capsules 2260
Fiorinal Capsules 2261
Fiorinal with Codeine Capsules 2262
Fiorinal Tablets 2261
Phrenilin 785
Sedapap Tablets 50 mg/650 mg 1543

Carbamazepine (Drugs that affect the level of expression of hepatic enzymes, particularly those that elevate glucuronosyl transferases, may increase the clearance of valproate; decreased serum levels of carbamazepine and carbamazepine epoxide). Products include:
Atretol Tablets 573
Tegretol Chewable Tablets 852
Tegretol Suspension 852
Tegretol Tablets 852

Chlordiazepoxide (May result in additive CNS depression). Products include:
Libritabs Tablets 2177
Limbitrol 2180

Chlordiazepoxide Hydrochloride (May result in additive CNS depression). Products include:
Librax Capsules 2176
Librium Capsules 2178
Librium Injectable 2179

Chlorpromazine (Concurrent use in schizophrenic patients already receiving valproate results in 15% increase in trough plasma levels of valproate). Products include:
Thorazine Suppositories 2523

Chlorpromazine Hydrochloride (Concurrent use in schizophrenic patients already receiving valproate results in 15% increase in trough plasma levels of valproate). Products include:
Thorazine 2523

Chlorprothixene (May result in additive CNS depression).
No products indexed under this heading.

Chlorprothixene Hydrochloride (May result in additive CNS depression).
No products indexed under this heading.

Clonazepam (Concomitant use may induce absence status in patients with a history of absence type seizures). Products include:
Klonopin Tablets 2126

Clorazepate Dipotassium (May result in additive CNS depression). Products include:
Tranxene 451

Clozapine (May result in additive CNS depression). Products include:
Clozaril Tablets 2252

Codeine Phosphate (May result in additive CNS depression). Products include:
Actifed with Codeine Cough Syrup 1067
Brontex 1981
Deconsal C Expectorant Syrup 456
Deconsal Pediatric Syrup 457
Dimetane-DC Cough Syrup 2059
Empirin with Codeine Tablets 1093
Fioricet with Codeine Capsules 2260
Fiorinal with Codeine Capsules 2262
Isoclor Expectorant 990
Novahistine DH 2462
Novahistine Expectorant 2463
Nucofed 2051
Phenergan with Codeine 2777
Phenergan VC with Codeine 2781
Robitussin A-C Syrup 2073
Robitussin-DAC Syrup 2074
Ryna ▣ 841
Soma Compound w/Codeine Tablets 2676
Tussi-Organidin NR Liquid and S NR Liquid 2677
Tylenol with Codeine 1583

Desflurane (May result in additive CNS depression). Products include:
Suprane 1813

Dezocine (May result in additive CNS depression). Products include:
Dalgan Injection 538

Diazepam (Valproate displaces diazepam from its plasma albumin sites and inhibits its metabolism). Products include:
Dizac 1809
Valium Injectable 2182
Valium Tablets 2183
Valrelease Capsules 2169

Droperidol (May result in additive CNS depression). Products include:
Inapsine Injection 1296

Enflurane (May result in additive CNS depression).
No products indexed under this heading.

Estazolam (May result in additive CNS depression). Products include:
ProSom Tablets 449

Ethchlorvynol (May result in additive CNS depression). Products include:
Placidyl Capsules 448

Ethinamate (May result in additive CNS depression).
No products indexed under this heading.

Ethosuximide (Valproate inhibits the metabolism of ethosuximide). Products include:
Zarontin Capsules 1928
Zarontin Syrup 1929

Felbamate (Increase in mean valproate concentration; a decrease in valproate dose may be necessary when felbamate therapy is initiated). Products include:
Felbatol 2666

Fentanyl (May result in additive CNS depression). Products include:
Duragesic Transdermal System 1288

Fentanyl Citrate (May result in additive CNS depression). Products include:
Sublimaze Injection 1307

Fluphenazine Decanoate (May result in additive CNS depression). Products include:
Prolixin Decanoate 509

Fluphenazine Enanthate (May result in additive CNS depression). Products include:
Prolixin Enanthate 509

Fluphenazine Hydrochloride (May result in additive CNS depression). Products include:
Prolixin 509

Flurazepam Hydrochloride (May result in additive CNS depression). Products include:
Dalmane Capsules 2173

Glutethimide (May result in additive CNS depression).
No products indexed under this heading.

Haloperidol (May result in additive CNS depression). Products include:
Haldol Injection, Tablets and Concentrate 1575

Haloperidol Decanoate (May result in additive CNS depression). Products include:
Haldol Decanoate 1577

Hydrocodone Bitartrate (May result in additive CNS depression). Products include:
Anexsia 5/500 Elixir 1781
Anexia Tablets 1782
Codiclear DH Syrup 791
Deconamine CX Cough and Cold Liquid and Tablets 1319
Duratuss HD Elixir 2565
Hycodan Tablets and Syrup 930
Hycomine Compound Tablets 932
Hycomine 931
Hycotuss Expectorant Syrup 933
Hydrocet Capsules 782
Lorcet 10/650 1018
Lortab 2566
Tussend 1783
Tussend Expectorant 1785
Vicodin Tablets 1356
Vicodin ES Tablets 1357
Vicodin Tuss Expectorant 1358
Zydone Capsules 949

Hydrocodone Polistirex (May result in additive CNS depression). Products include:
Tussionex Pennkinetic Extended-Release Suspension 998

Hydroxyzine Hydrochloride (May result in additive CNS depression). Products include:
Atarax Tablets & Syrup 2185
Marax Tablets & DF Syrup 2200
Vistaril Intramuscular Solution 2216

Isoflurane (May result in additive CNS depression).
No products indexed under this heading.

Ketamine Hydrochloride (May result in additive CNS depression).
No products indexed under this heading.

Lamotrigine (Increased elimination half-life of lamotrigine; dosage of lamotrigine should be reduced when co-administered). Products include:
Lamictal Tablets 1112

Levorphanol Tartrate (May result in additive CNS depression). Products include:
Levo-Dromoran 2129

Lorazepam (Potential for decreased lorazepam clearance). Products include:
Ativan Injection 2698
Ativan Tablets 2700

Loxapine Hydrochloride (May result in additive CNS depression). Products include:
Loxitane 1378

Loxapine Succinate (May result in additive CNS depression). Products include:
Loxitane Capsules 1378

Meperidine Hydrochloride (May result in additive CNS depression). Products include:
Demerol 2308
Mepergan Injection 2753

Mephobarbital (May result in additive CNS depression). Products include:
Mebaral Tablets 2322

Meprobamate (May result in additive CNS depression). Products include:
Miltown Tablets 2672
PMB 200 and PMB 400 2783

Mesoridazine Besylate (May result in additive CNS depression). Products include:
Serentil 684

Methadone Hydrochloride (May result in additive CNS depression). Products include:
Methadone Hydrochloride Oral Concentrate 2233
Methadone Hydrochloride Oral Solution & Tablets 2235

Methohexital Sodium (May result in additive CNS depression). Products include:
Brevital Sodium Vials 1429

Methotrimeprazine (May result in additive CNS depression). Products include:
Levoprome 1274

Methoxyflurane (May result in additive CNS depression).
No products indexed under this heading.

Midazolam Hydrochloride (May result in additive CNS depression). Products include:
Versed Injection 2170

(▣ Described in PDR For Nonprescription Drugs) (◉ Described in PDR For Ophthalmology)

Molindone Hydrochloride (May result in additive CNS depression). Products include:

Moban Tablets and Concentrate 1048

Morphine Sulfate (May result in additive CNS depression). Products include:

Astramorph/PF Injection, USP (Preservative-Free) 535
Duramorph 962
Infumorph 200 and Infumorph 500 Sterile Solutions 965
MS Contin Tablets 1994
MSIR 1997
Oramorph SR (Morphine Sulfate Sustained Release Tablets) 2236
RMS Suppositories 2657
Roxanol 2243

Nortriptyline Hydrochloride (Decreased plasma clearance of nortriptyline). Products include:

Pamelor 2280

Opium Alkaloids (May result in additive CNS depression).

No products indexed under this heading.

Oxazepam (May result in additive CNS depression). Products include:

Serax Capsules 2810
Serax Tablets 2810

Oxycodone Hydrochloride (May result in additive CNS depression). Products include:

Percocet Tablets 938
Percodan Tablets 939
Percodan-Demi Tablets 940
Roxicodone Tablets, Oral Solution & Intensol (Oxycodone) 2244
Tylox Capsules 1584

Pentobarbital Sodium (May result in additive CNS depression). Products include:

Nembutal Sodium Capsules 436
Nembutal Sodium Solution 438
Nembutal Sodium Suppositories 440

Perphenazine (May result in additive CNS depression). Products include:

Etrafon 2355
Triavil Tablets 1757
Trilafon 2389

Phenobarbital (Drugs that affect the level of expression of hepatic enzymes, particularly those that elevate glucuronosyl transferases, may increase the clearance of valproate; valproate may inhibit the metabolism of phenobarbital; may result in additive CNS depression). Products include:

Arco-Lase Plus Tablets 512
Bellergal-S Tablets 2250
Donnatal 2060
Donnatal Extentabs 2061
Donnatal Tablets 2060
Phenobarbital Elixir and Tablets 1469
Quadrinal Tablets 1350

Phenytoin (Drugs that affect the level of expression of hepatic enzymes, particularly those that elevate glucuronosyl transferases, may increase the clearance of valproate; valproate displaces phenytoin from its plasma albumin binding sites and inhibits its hepatic metabolism; potential for breakthrough seizures). Products include:

Dilantin Infatabs 1908
Dilantin-125 Suspension 1911

Phenytoin Sodium (Drugs that affect the level of expression of hepatic enzymes, particularly those that elevate glucuronosyl transferases, may increase the clearance of valproate; valproate displaces phenytoin from its plasma albumin binding sites and inhibits its hepatic metabolism; potential for breakthrough seizures). Products include:

Dilantin Kapseals 1906
Dilantin Parenteral 1910

Prazepam (May result in additive CNS depression).

No products indexed under this heading.

Primidone (Drugs that affect the level of expression of hepatic enzymes, particularly those that elevate glucuronosyl transferases, may increase the clearance of valproate; metabolism of primidone may be inhibited). Products include:

Mysoline 2754

Prochlorperazine (May result in additive CNS depression). Products include:

Compazine 2470

Promethazine Hydrochloride (May result in additive CNS depression). Products include:

Mepergan Injection 2753
Phenergan with Codeine 2777
Phenergan with Dextromethorphan 2778
Phenergan Injection 2773
Phenergan Suppositories 2775
Phenergan Syrup 2774
Phenergan Tablets 2775
Phenergan VC 2779
Phenergan VC with Codeine 2781

Propofol (May result in additive CNS depression). Products include:

Diprivan Injection 2833

Propoxyphene Hydrochloride (May result in additive CNS depression). Products include:

Darvon 1435
Wygesic Tablets 2827

Propoxyphene Napsylate (May result in additive CNS depression). Products include:

Darvon-N/Darvocet-N 1433

Quazepam (May result in additive CNS depression). Products include:

Doral Tablets 2664

Rifampin (Increases oral clearance of valproate). Products include:

Rifadin 1528
Rifamate Capsules 1530
Rifater 1532
Rimactane Capsules 847

Risperidone (May result in additive CNS depression). Products include:

Risperdal 1301

Secobarbital Sodium (May result in additive CNS depression). Products include:

Seconal Sodium Pulvules 1474

Sufentanil Citrate (May result in additive CNS depression). Products include:

Sufenta Injection 1309

Temazepam (May result in additive CNS depression). Products include:

Restoril Capsules 2284

Thiamylal Sodium (May result in additive CNS depression).

No products indexed under this heading.

Thioridazine Hydrochloride (May result in additive CNS depression). Products include:

Mellaril 2269

Thiothixene (May result in additive CNS depression). Products include:

Navane Capsules and Concentrate 2201
Navane Intramuscular 2202

Tolbutamide (Potential for increased unbound fraction of tolbutamide based on *in vitro* studies).

No products indexed under this heading.

Triazolam (May result in additive CNS depression). Products include:

Halcion Tablets 2611

Trifluoperazine Hydrochloride (May result in additive CNS depression). Products include:

Stelazine 2514

Warfarin Sodium (Potential exits for valproate to displace warfarin from its binding site on plasma albumin). Products include:

Coumadin 926

Zidovudine (Potential for decreased zidovudine clearance). Products include:

Retrovir Capsules 1158
Retrovir I.V. Infusion 1163
Retrovir Syrup 1158

Zolpidem Tartrate (May result in additive CNS depression). Products include:

Ambien Tablets 2416

Food Interactions

Alcohol (May result in additive CNS depression).

DEPEN TITRATABLE TABLETS

(Penicillamine) 2662

May interact with cytotoxic drugs, antimalarials, and certain other agents. Compounds in these categories include:

Auranofin (Serious hematologic and/or renal adverse reactions). Products include:

Ridaura Capsules 2513

Aurothioglucose (Serious hematologic and/or renal adverse reactions). Products include:

Solganal Suspension 2388

Bleomycin Sulfate (Hematologic and renal reactions). Products include:

Blenoxane 692

Chloroquine Hydrochloride (Serious hematologic and/or renal adverse reactions). Products include:

Aralen Hydrochloride Injection 2301

Chloroquine Phosphate (Serious hematologic and/or renal adverse reactions). Products include:

Aralen Phosphate Tablets 2301

Daunorubicin Hydrochloride (Hematologic and renal reactions). Products include:

Cerubidine 795

Doxorubicin Hydrochloride (Hematologic and renal reactions). Products include:

Adriamycin PFS 1947
Adriamycin RDF 1947
Doxorubicin Astra 540
Rubex 712

Fluorouracil (Hematologic and renal reactions). Products include:

Efudex 2113
Fluoroplex Topical Solution & Cream 1 % 479
Fluorouracil Injection 2116

Gold Sodium Thiomalate (Serious hematologic and/or renal adverse reactions). Products include:

Myochrysine Injection 1711

Hydroxyurea (Hematologic and renal reactions). Products include:

Hydrea Capsules 696

Iron Supplements (Reduced effects of penicillamine with orally administered iron).

Mefloquine Hydrochloride (Serious hematologic and/or renal adverse reactions). Products include:

Lariam Tablets 2128

Methotrexate Sodium (Hematologic and renal reactions). Products include:

Methotrexate Sodium Tablets, Injection, for Injection and LPF Injection 1275

Mineral Supplements (Blocked response to penicillamine).

Mitotane (Hematologic and renal reactions). Products include:

Lysodren 698

Mitoxantrone Hydrochloride (Hematologic and renal reactions). Products include:

Novantrone 1279

Oxyphenbutazone (Hematologic and renal reactions).

Phenylbutazone (Hematologic and renal reactions).

No products indexed under this heading.

Primaquine Phosphate (Serious hematologic and/or renal adverse reactions).

No products indexed under this heading.

Procarbazine Hydrochloride (Hematologic and renal reactions). Products include:

Matulane Capsules 2131

Pyrimethamine (Serious hematologic and/or renal adverse reactions). Products include:

Daraprim Tablets 1090
Fansidar Tablets 2114

Tamoxifen Citrate (Hematologic and renal reactions). Products include:

Nolvadex Tablets 2841

Vincristine Sulfate (Hematologic and renal reactions). Products include:

Oncovin Solution Vials & Hyporets 1466

Food Interactions

Meal, unspecified (Potential for reduced absorption and the likelihood of inactivation by metal binding in the GI tract; Depen should be given on an empty stomach).

DEPO-MEDROL SINGLE-DOSE VIAL

(Methylprednisolone Acetate) 2600

May interact with oral anticoagulants, oral hypoglycemic agents, insulin, and certain other agents. Compounds in these categories include:

Acarbose (Increased requirements for oral hypoglycemic agents in diabetes).

No products indexed under this heading.

Aspirin (Increased clearance of chronic high dose aspirin leading to decreased salicylate serum levels or increase the risk of salicylate toxicity when methylprednisolone is withdrawn). Products include:

Alka-Seltzer Effervescent Antacid and Pain Reliever .... ◾◻ 701
Alka-Seltzer Extra Strength Effervescent Antacid and Pain Reliever .... ◾◻ 703
Alka-Seltzer Lemon Lime Effervescent Antacid and Pain Reliever .... ◾◻ 703
Alka-Seltzer Plus Cold Medicine .... ◾◻ 705
Alka-Seltzer Plus Cold & Cough Medicine .... ◾◻ 708
Alka-Seltzer Plus Night-Time Cold Medicine .... ◾◻ 707
Alka Seltzer Plus Sinus Medicine .. ◾◻ 707
Arthritis Foundation Safety Coated Aspirin Tablets .... ◾◻ 675
Arthritis Pain Ascriptin .... ◾◻ 631
Maximum Strength Ascriptin .... ◾◻ 630
Regular Strength Ascriptin Tablets .... ◾◻ 629
Arthritis Strength BC Powder .... ◾◻ 609
BC Cold Powder Multi-Symptom Formula (Cold-Sinus-Allergy) ...... ◾◻ 609
BC Cold Powder Non-Drowsy Formula (Cold-Sinus) .... ◾◻ 609
BC Powder .... ◾◻ 609
Bayer Children's Chewable Aspirin .... ◾◻ 711

IMPORTANT NOTE: Always consult each drug listing in the patient's regimen for possible interactions.

Depo-Medrol Single-Dose

Interactions Index

Genuine Bayer Aspirin Tablets & Caplets .... ᴹᴰ 713
Extra Strength Bayer Arthritis Pain Regimen Formula .... ᴹᴰ 711
Extra Strength Bayer Aspirin Caplets & Tablets .... ᴹᴰ 712
Extended-Release Bayer 8-Hour Aspirin .... ᴹᴰ 712
Extra Strength Bayer Plus Aspirin Caplets .... ᴹᴰ 713
Extra Strength Bayer PM Aspirin .. ᴹᴰ 713
Bayer Enteric Aspirin .... ᴹᴰ 709
Bufferin Analgesic Tablets and Caplets .... ᴹᴰ 613
Arthritis Strength Bufferin Analgesic Caplets .... ᴹᴰ 614
Extra Strength Bufferin Analgesic Tablets .... ᴹᴰ 615
Cama Arthritis Pain Reliever .... ᴹᴰ 785
Darvon Compound-65 Pulvules 1435
Easprin 1914
Ecotrin 2455
Ecotrin Enteric Coated Aspirin Maximum Strength Tablets and Caplets .... ᴹᴰ 816
Ecotrin Enteric Coated Aspirin Regular Strength Tablets 2455
Empirin Aspirin Tablets .... ᴹᴰ 854
Empirin with Codeine Tablets........... 1093
Excedrin Extra-Strength Analgesic Tablets & Caplets 732
Fiorinal Capsules 2261
Fiorinal with Codeine Capsules 2262
Fiorinal Tablets 2261
Halfprin 1362
Healthprin Aspirin 2455
Norgesic... 1496
Percodan Tablets.................................. 939
Percodan-Demi Tablets 940
Robaxisal Tablets.................................. 2071
Soma Compound w/Codeine Tablets 2676
Soma Compound Tablets 2675
St. Joseph Adult Chewable Aspirin (81 mg.) .... ᴹᴰ 808
Talwin Compound 2335
Ursinus Inlay-Tabs................................ ᴹᴰ 794
Vanquish Analgesic Caplets .... ᴹᴰ 731

Chlorpropamide (Increased requirements for oral hypoglycemic agents in diabetes). Products include:

Diabinese Tablets 1935

Cyclosporine (Potential for convulsions; concurrent use results in mutual inhibition of metabolism). Products include:

Neoral 2276
Sandimmune 2286

Dicumarol (Potential for variable effect; concurrent use may result in enhanced as well as diminished effects of anticoagulant).

No products indexed under this heading.

Glipizide (Increased requirements for oral hypoglycemic agents in diabetes). Products include:

Glucotrol Tablets 1967
Glucotrol XL Extended Release Tablets 1968

Glyburide (Increased requirements for oral hypoglycemic agents in diabetes). Products include:

DiaBeta Tablets 1239
Glynase PresTab Tablets 2609
Micronase Tablets 2623

Insulin, Human (Increased requirements for insulin in diabetes).

No products indexed under this heading.

Insulin, Human Isophane Suspension (Increased requirements for insulin in diabetes). Products include:

Novolin N Human Insulin 10 ml Vials.. 1795

Insulin, Human NPH (Increased requirements for insulin in diabetes). Products include:

Humulin N, 100 Units 1448
Novolin N PenFill Cartridges Durable Insulin Delivery System 1798
Novolin N Prefilled Syringe Disposable Insulin Delivery System 1798

Insulin, Human Regular (Increased requirements for insulin in diabetes). Products include:

Humulin R, 100 Units 1449
Novolin R Human Insulin 10 ml Vials.. 1795
Novolin R PenFill Cartridges Durable Insulin Delivery System 1798
Novolin R Prefilled Syringe Disposable Insulin Delivery System 1798
Velosulin BR Human Insulin 10 ml Vials.. 1795

Insulin, Human, Zinc Suspension (Increased requirements for insulin in diabetes). Products include:

Humulin L, 100 Units 1446
Humulin U, 100 Units 1450
Novolin L Human Insulin 10 ml Vials.. 1795

Insulin, NPH (Increased requirements for insulin in diabetes). Products include:

NPH, 100 Units 1450
Pork NPH, 100 Units............................. 1452
Purified Pork NPH Isophane Insulin 1801

Insulin, Regular (Increased requirements for insulin in diabetes). Products include:

Regular, 100 Units 1450
Pork Regular, 100 Units 1452
Pork Regular (Concentrated), 500 Units 1453
Purified Pork Regular Insulin 1801

Insulin, Zinc Crystals (Increased requirements for insulin in diabetes). Products include:

NPH, 100 Units 1450

Insulin, Zinc Suspension (Increased requirements for insulin in diabetes). Products include:

Iletin I 1450
Lente, 100 Units 1450
Iletin II.. 1452
Pork Lente, 100 Units........................... 1452
Purified Pork Lente Insulin 1801

Ketoconazole (May inhibit the metabolism of methylprednisolone and thus decrease its clearance; the dose of methylprednisolone should be titrated to avoid toxicity). Products include:

Nizoral 2% Cream 1297
Nizoral 2% Shampoo............................. 1298
Nizoral Tablets 1298

Metformin Hydrochloride (Increased requirements for oral hypoglycemic agents in diabetes). Products include:

Glucophage 752

Phenobarbital (Increases clearance of methylprednisolone and may require increase in dose of methylprednisolone to achieve the desired response). Products include:

Arco-Lase Plus Tablets 512
Bellergal-S Tablets 2250
Donnatal 2060
Donnatal Extentabs................................ 2061
Donnatal Tablets 2060
Phenobarbital Elixir and Tablets 1469
Quadrinal Tablets 1350

Phenytoin (Increases clearance of methylprednisolone and may require increase in dose of methylprednisolone to achieve the desired response). Products include:

Dilantin Infatabs...................................... 1908
Dilantin-125 Suspension 1911

Phenytoin Sodium (Increases clearance of methylprednisolone and may require increase in dose of methylprednisolone to achieve the desired response). Products include:

Dilantin Kapseals 1906
Dilantin Parenteral 1910

Rifampin (Increases clearance of methylprednisolone and may require increase in dose of methylprednisolone to achieve the desired response). Products include:

Rifadin 1528
Rifamate Capsules 1530
Rifater.. 1532
Rimactane Capsules 847

Smallpox Vaccine (Possible hazards of neurological complications; patients on corticosteroid therapy should not be vaccinated against smallpox).

Tolazamide (Increased requirements for oral hypoglycemic agents in diabetes).

No products indexed under this heading.

Tolbutamide (Increased requirements for oral hypoglycemic agents in diabetes).

No products indexed under this heading.

Troleandomycin (May inhibit the metabolism of methylprednisolone and thus decrease its clearance; the dose of methylprednisolone should be titrated to avoid toxicity). Products include:

Tao Capsules 2209

Vaccines (Live) (Administration of live or live attenuated vaccines is contraindicated).

Warfarin Sodium (Potential for variable effect; concurrent use may result in enhanced as well as diminished effects of anticoagulant). Products include:

Coumadin 926

DEPO-MEDROL STERILE AQUEOUS SUSPENSION

(Methylprednisolone Acetate) 2597

May interact with oral hypoglycemic agents, insulin, and certain other agents. Compounds in these categories include:

Acarbose (Increased requirements for oral hypoglycemic agents in diabetes).

No products indexed under this heading.

Aspirin (Increased clearance of chronic high dose aspirin leading to decreased salicylate serum levels or increased risk of salicylate toxicity when methylprednisolone is withdrawn). Products include:

Alka-Seltzer Effervescent Antacid and Pain Reliever .... ᴹᴰ 701
Alka-Seltzer Extra Strength Effervescent Antacid and Pain Reliever .... ᴹᴰ 703
Alka-Seltzer Lemon Lime Effervescent Antacid and Pain Reliever .... ᴹᴰ 703
Alka-Seltzer Plus Cold Medicine .... ᴹᴰ 705
Alka-Seltzer Plus Cold & Cough Medicine .... ᴹᴰ 708
Alka-Seltzer Plus Night-Time Cold Medicine .... ᴹᴰ 707
Alka Seltzer Plus Sinus Medicine .. ᴹᴰ 707
Arthritis Foundation Safety Coated Aspirin Tablets .... ᴹᴰ 675
Arthritis Pain Ascriptin .... ᴹᴰ 631
Maximum Strength Ascriptin .... ᴹᴰ 630
Regular Strength Ascriptin Tablets .... ᴹᴰ 629
Arthritis Strength BC Powder.......... ᴹᴰ 609
BC Cold Powder Multi-Symptom Formula (Cold-Sinus-Allergy) ...... ᴹᴰ 609
BC Cold Powder Non-Drowsy Formula (Cold-Sinus) .... ᴹᴰ 609
BC Powder .... ᴹᴰ 609
Bayer Children's Chewable Aspirin.. ᴹᴰ 711
Genuine Bayer Aspirin Tablets & Caplets .... ᴹᴰ 713
Extra Strength Bayer Arthritis Pain Regimen Formula .... ᴹᴰ 711

Extra Strength Bayer Aspirin Caplets & Tablets .... ᴹᴰ 712
Extended-Release Bayer 8-Hour Aspirin .... ᴹᴰ 712
Extra Strength Bayer Plus Aspirin Caplets .... ᴹᴰ 713
Extra Strength Bayer PM Aspirin .. ᴹᴰ 713
Bayer Enteric Aspirin .... ᴹᴰ 709
Bufferin Analgesic Tablets and Caplets .... ᴹᴰ 613
Arthritis Strength Bufferin Analgesic Caplets .... ᴹᴰ 614
Extra Strength Bufferin Analgesic Tablets .... ᴹᴰ 615
Cama Arthritis Pain Reliever .... ᴹᴰ 785
Darvon Compound-65 Pulvules 1435
Easprin 1914
Ecotrin 2455
Ecotrin Enteric Coated Aspirin Maximum Strength Tablets and Caplets .... ᴹᴰ 816
Ecotrin Enteric Coated Aspirin Regular Strength Tablets 2455
Empirin Aspirin Tablets .... ᴹᴰ 854
Empirin with Codeine Tablets........... 1093
Excedrin Extra-Strength Analgesic Tablets & Caplets 732
Fiorinal Capsules 2261
Fiorinal with Codeine Capsules 2262
Fiorinal Tablets 2261
Halfprin 1362
Healthprin Aspirin 2455
Norgesic... 1496
Percodan Tablets.................................. 939
Percodan-Demi Tablets 940
Robaxisal Tablets.................................. 2071
Soma Compound w/Codeine Tablets 2676
Soma Compound Tablets 2675
St. Joseph Adult Chewable Aspirin (81 mg.) .... ᴹᴰ 808
Talwin Compound 2335
Ursinus Inlay-Tabs................................ ᴹᴰ 794
Vanquish Analgesic Caplets .... ᴹᴰ 731

Chlorpropamide (Increased requirements for oral hypoglycemic agents in diabetes). Products include:

Diabinese Tablets 1935

Cyclosporine (Potential for convulsions; concurrent use results in mutual inhibition of metabolism). Products include:

Neoral 2276
Sandimmune 2286

Dicumarol (Potential for variable effect; concurrent use may result in enhanced as well as diminished effects of anticoagulant).

No products indexed under this heading.

Glipizide (Increased requirements for oral hypoglycemic agents in diabetes). Products include:

Glucotrol Tablets 1967
Glucotrol XL Extended Release Tablets 1968

Glyburide (Increased requirements for oral hypoglycemic agents in diabetes). Products include:

DiaBeta Tablets 1239
Glynase PresTab Tablets 2609
Micronase Tablets 2623

Insulin, Human (Increased requirements for insulin in diabetes).

No products indexed under this heading.

Insulin, Human Isophane Suspension (Increased requirements for insulin in diabetes). Products include:

Novolin N Human Insulin 10 ml Vials.. 1795

Insulin, Human NPH (Increased requirements for insulin in diabetes). Products include:

Humulin N, 100 Units 1448
Novolin N PenFill Cartridges Durable Insulin Delivery System 1798
Novolin N Prefilled Syringe Disposable Insulin Delivery System 1798

Insulin, Human Regular (Increased requirements for insulin in diabetes). Products include:

Humulin R, 100 Units 1449

(ᴹᴰ Described in PDR For Nonprescription Drugs)   (◉ Described in PDR For Ophthalmology)

Novolin R Human Insulin 10 ml Vials 1795
Novolin R PenFill Cartridges Durable Insulin Delivery System 1798
Novolin R Prefilled Syringe Disposable Insulin Delivery System 1798
Velosulin BR Human Insulin 10 ml Vials 1795

Insulin, Human, Zinc Suspension (Increased requirements for insulin in diabetes). Products include:
Humulin L, 100 Units 1446
Humulin U, 100 Units 1450
Novolin L Human Insulin 10 ml Vials 1795

Insulin, NPH (Increased requirements for insulin in diabetes). Products include:
NPH, 100 Units 1450
Pork NPH, 100 Units 1452
Purified Pork NPH Isophane Insulin 1801

Insulin, Regular (Increased requirements for insulin in diabetes). Products include:
Regular, 100 Units 1450
Pork Regular, 100 Units 1452
Pork Regular (Concentrated), 500 Units 1453
Purified Pork Regular Insulin 1801

Insulin, Zinc Crystals (Increased requirements for insulin in diabetes). Products include:
NPH, 100 Units 1450

Insulin, Zinc Suspension (Increased requirements for insulin in diabetes). Products include:
Iletin I 1450
Lente, 100 Units 1450
Iletin II 1452
Pork Lente, 100 Units 1452
Purified Pork Lente Insulin 1801

Ketoconazole (May inhibit the metabolism of methylprednisolone and thus decrease its clearance; the dose of methylprednisolone should be titrated to avoid toxicity). Products include:
Nizoral 2% Cream 1297
Nizoral 2% Shampoo 1298
Nizoral Tablets 1298

Metformin Hydrochloride (Increased requirements for oral hypoglycemic agents in diabetes). Products include:
Glucophage 752

Phenobarbital (Increases clearance of methylprednisolone and may require increase in dose of methylprednisolone to achieve the desired response). Products include:
Arco-Lase Plus Tablets 512
Bellergal-S Tablets 2250
Donnatal 2060
Donnatal Extentabs 2061
Donnatal Tablets 2060
Phenobarbital Elixir and Tablets 1469
Quadrinal Tablets 1350

Phenytoin (Increases clearance of methylprednisolone and may require increase in dose of methylprednisolone to achieve the desired response). Products include:
Dilantin Infatabs 1908
Dilantin-125 Suspension 1911

Phenytoin Sodium (Increases clearance of methylprednisolone and may require increase in dose of methylprednisolone to achieve the desired response). Products include:
Dilantin Kapseals 1906
Dilantin Parenteral 1910

Rifampin (Increases clearance of methylprednisolone and may require increase in dose of methylprednisolone to achieve the desired response). Products include:
Rifadin 1528
Rifamate Capsules 1530
Rifater 1532
Rimactane Capsules 847

Smallpox Vaccine (Possible neurological complications).

Tolazamide (Increased requirements for oral hypoglycemic agents in diabetes).
No products indexed under this heading.

Tolbutamide (Increased requirements for oral hypoglycemic agents in diabetes).
No products indexed under this heading.

Troleandomycin (May inhibit the metabolism of methylprednisolone and thus decrease its clearance; the dose of methylprednisolone should be titrated to avoid toxicity). Products include:
Tao Capsules 2209

Vaccines (Live) (Administration of live or live attenuated vaccines is contraindicated).

Warfarin Sodium (Potential for variable effect; concurrent use may result in enhanced as well as diminished effects of anticoagulant). Products include:
Coumadin 926

DEPO-PROVERA CONTRACEPTIVE INJECTION

(Medroxyprogesterone Acetate) 2602
May interact with:

Aminoglutethimide (Significantly depresses the serum concentrations of medroxyprogesterone acetate). Products include:
Cytadren Tablets 819

DEPO-PROVERA STERILE AQUEOUS SUSPENSION

(Medroxyprogesterone Acetate) 2606
May interact with estrogens and certain other agents. Compounds in these categories include:

Aminoglutethimide (Significantly depresses the bioavailability of Depo-Provera). Products include:
Cytadren Tablets 819

Chlorotrianisene (Potential adverse effects on carbohydrate and lipid metabolism).
No products indexed under this heading.

Dienestrol (Potential adverse effects on carbohydrate and lipid metabolism). Products include:
Ortho Dienestrol Cream 1866

Diethylstilbestrol (Potential adverse effects on carbohydrate and lipid metabolism). Products include:
Diethylstilbestrol Tablets 1437

Estradiol (Potential adverse effects on carbohydrate and lipid metabolism). Products include:
Climara Transdermal System 645
Estrace Cream and Tablets 749
Estraderm Transdermal System 824

Estrogens, Conjugated (Potential adverse effects on carbohydrate and lipid metabolism). Products include:
PMB 200 and PMB 400 2783
Premarin Intravenous 2787
Premarin with Methyltestosterone 2794
Premarin Tablets 2789
Premarin Vaginal Cream 2791
Premphase 2797
Prempro 2801

Estrogens, Esterified (Potential adverse effects on carbohydrate and lipid metabolism). Products include:
ESTRATAB Tablets (0.3, 0.625, 1.25, 2.5 mg) 2536
Estratest 2539
Menest Tablets 2494

Estropipate (Potential adverse effects on carbohydrate and lipid metabolism). Products include:
Ogen Tablets 2627
Ogen Vaginal Cream 2630
Ortho-Est 1869

Ethinyl Estradiol (Potential adverse effects on carbohydrate and lipid metabolism). Products include:
Brevicon 2088
Demulen 2428
Desogen Tablets 1817
Levlen/Tri-Levlen 651
Lo/Ovral Tablets 2746
Lo/Ovral-28 Tablets 2751
Modicon 1872
Nordette-21 Tablets 2755
Nordette-28 Tablets 2758
Norinyl 2088
Ortho-Cept 1851
Ortho-Cyclen/Ortho-Tri-Cyclen 1858
Ortho-Novum 1872
Ortho-Cyclen/Ortho Tri-Cyclen 1858
Ovcon 760
Ovral Tablets 2770
Ovral-28 Tablets 2770
Levlen/Tri-Levlen 651
Tri-Norinyl 2164
Triphasil-21 Tablets 2814
Triphasil-28 Tablets 2819

Polyestradiol Phosphate (Potential adverse effects on carbohydrate and lipid metabolism).
No products indexed under this heading.

Quinestrol (Potential adverse effects on carbohydrate and lipid metabolism).
No products indexed under this heading.

DEPONIT NTG TRANSDERMAL DELIVERY SYSTEM

(Nitroglycerin) 2397
May interact with vasodilators and certain other agents. Compounds in these categories include:

Diazoxide (Additive vasodilating effects). Products include:
Hyperstat I.V. Injection 2363
Proglycem 580

Hydralazine Hydrochloride (Additive vasodilating effects). Products include:
Apresazide Capsules 808
Apresoline Hydrochloride Tablets 809
Ser-Ap-Es Tablets 849

Minoxidil (Additive vasodilating effects). Products include:
Loniten Tablets 2618
Rogaine Topical Solution 2637

Food Interactions

Alcohol (Additive vasodilating effects).

DERIFIL TABLETS

(Chlorophyllin Copper Complex) 2246
None cited in PDR database.

DERMAFLEX TOPICAL ANESTHETIC GEL

(Lidocaine) 882
None cited in PDR database.

DERMASIL DRY SKIN CONCENTRATED TREATMENT

(Glycerin, Dimethicone) 627
None cited in PDR database.

DERMASIL DRY SKIN TREATMENT CREAM

(Dimethicone) 626
None cited in PDR database.

DERMASIL DRY SKIN TREATMENT LOTION

(Dimethicone) 626
None cited in PDR database.

DERMASORB SPIRAL WOUND DRESSING

(Hydrocolloids) 2863
None cited in PDR database.

DERMATOP EMOLLIENT CREAM 0.1%

(Prednicarbate) 1238
None cited in PDR database.

DESENEX ANTIFUNGAL CREAM

(Undecylenic Acid, Zinc Undecylenate) 632
None cited in PDR database.

DESENEX ANTIFUNGAL OINTMENT

(Undecylenic Acid, Zinc Undecylenate) 632
None cited in PDR database.

DESENEX ANTIFUNGAL POWDER

(Undecylenic Acid, Zinc Undecylenate) 632
None cited in PDR database.

DESENEX ANTIFUNGAL SPRAY LIQUID

(Tolnaftate) 632
None cited in PDR database.

DESENEX ANTIFUNGAL SPRAY POWDER

(Undecylenic Acid, Zinc Undecylenate) 632
None cited in PDR database.

DESENEX FOOT & SNEAKER DEODORANT SPRAY

(Aluminum Chlorohydrate) 633
None cited in PDR database.

PRESCRIPTION STRENGTH DESENEX CREAM

(Clotrimazole) 633
None cited in PDR database.

PRESCRIPTION STRENGTH DESENEX SPRAY POWDER AND SPRAY LIQUID

(Mineral Supplements) 633
None cited in PDR database.

DESFERAL VIALS

(Deferoxamine Mesylate) 820
None cited in PDR database.

DESITIN CORNSTARCH BABY POWDER

(Zinc Oxide, Corn Starch) 742
None cited in PDR database.

DESITIN OINTMENT

(Cod Liver Oil, Zinc Oxide) 742
None cited in PDR database.

DESMOPRESSIN ACETATE RHINAL TUBE

(Desmopressin Acetate) 979
May interact with vasopressors and certain other agents. Compounds in these categories include:

Dopamine Hydrochloride (The pressor activity of desmopressin is very low, use of large doses of desmopressin with pressor agents should only be done with careful monitoring).
No products indexed under this heading.

IMPORTANT NOTE: Always consult each drug listing in the patient's regimen for possible interactions.

Epinephrine Bitartrate (The pressor activity of desmopressin is very low, use of large doses of desmopressin with pressor agents should only be done with careful monitoring). Products include:

- Bronkaid Mist Suspension ▣ 718
- Sensorcaine-MPF with Epinephrine Injection 559

Epinephrine Hydrochloride (The pressor activity of desmopressin is very low, use of large doses of desmopressin with pressor agents should only be done with careful monitoring). Products include:

- Ana-Kit Anaphylaxis Emergency Treatment Kit 617

Metaraminol Bitartrate (The pressor activity of desmopressin is very low, use of large doses of desmopressin with pressor agents should only be done with careful monitoring). Products include:

- Aramine Injection 1609

Methoxamine Hydrochloride (The pressor activity of desmopressin is very low, use of large doses of desmopressin with pressor agents should only be done with careful monitoring). Products include:

- Vasoxyl Injection 1196

Norepinephrine Bitartrate (The pressor activity of desmopressin is very low, use of large doses of desmopressin with pressor agents should only be done with careful monitoring). Products include:

- Levophed Bitartrate Injection 2315

Phenylephrine Hydrochloride (The pressor activity of desmopressin is very low, use of large doses of desmopressin with pressor agents should only be done with careful monitoring). Products include:

- Atrohist Plus Tablets 454
- Cerose DM ▣ 878
- Comhist 2038
- D.A. Chewable Tablets 951
- Deconsal Pediatric Capsules 454
- Dura-Vent/DA Tablets 953
- Entex Capsules 1986
- Entex Liquid 1986
- Extendryl 1005
- 4-Way Fast Acting Nasal Spray (regular & mentholated) ▣ 621
- Hemorid For Women ▣ 834
- Hycomine Compound Tablets 932
- Neo-Synephrine Hydrochloride 1% Carpuject 2324
- Neo-Synephrine Hydrochloride 1% Injection 2324
- Neo-Synephrine Hydrochloride (Ophthalmic) 2325
- Neo-Synephrine ▣ 726
- Nōstril ▣ 644
- Novahistine Elixir ▣ 823
- Phenergan VC 2779
- Phenergan VC with Codeine 2781
- Preparation H ▣ 871
- Tympagesic Ear Drops 2342
- Vasosulf ◎ 271
- Vicks Sinex Nasal Spray and Ultra Fine Mist ▣ 765

DESOGEN TABLETS

(Desogestrel, Ethinyl Estradiol) 1817
May interact with barbiturates and tetracyclines. Compounds in these categories include:

Ampicillin (Potential for reduced efficacy and increased incidence of breakthrough bleeding and menstrual irregularities). Products include:

- Omnipen Capsules 2764
- Omnipen for Oral Suspension 2765

Ampicillin Sodium (Potential for reduced efficacy and increased incidence of breakthrough bleeding and menstrual irregularities). Products include:

- Unasyn 2212

Aprobarbital (Potential for reduced efficacy and increased incidence of breakthrough bleeding and menstrual irregularities).

No products indexed under this heading.

Butabarbital (Potential for reduced efficacy and increased incidence of breakthrough bleeding and menstrual irregularities).

No products indexed under this heading.

Butalbital (Potential for reduced efficacy and increased incidence of breakthrough bleeding and menstrual irregularities). Products include:

- Esgic-plus Tablets 1013
- Fioricet Tablets 2258
- Fioricet with Codeine Capsules 2260
- Fiorinal Capsules 2261
- Fiorinal with Codeine Capsules 2262
- Fiorinal Tablets 2261
- Phrenilin 785
- Sedapap Tablets 50 mg/650 mg 1543

Demeclocycline Hydrochloride (Potential for reduced efficacy and increased incidence of breakthrough bleeding and menstrual irregularities). Products include:

- Declomycin Tablets 1371

Doxycycline Calcium (Potential for reduced efficacy and increased incidence of breakthrough bleeding and menstrual irregularities). Products include:

- Vibramycin Calcium Oral Suspension Syrup 1941

Doxycycline Hyclate (Potential for reduced efficacy and increased incidence of breakthrough bleeding and menstrual irregularities). Products include:

- Doryx Capsules 1913
- Vibramycin Hyclate Capsules 1941
- Vibramycin Hyclate Intravenous 2215
- Vibra-Tabs Film Coated Tablets 1941

Doxycycline Monohydrate (Potential for reduced efficacy and increased incidence of breakthrough bleeding and menstrual irregularities). Products include:

- Monodox Capsules 1805
- Vibramycin Monohydrate for Oral Suspension 1941

Griseofulvin (Potential for reduced efficacy and increased incidence of breakthrough bleeding and menstrual irregularities). Products include:

- Fulvicin P/G Tablets 2359
- Fulvicin P/G 165 & 330 Tablets 2359
- Grifulvin V (griseofulvin tablets) Microsize (griseofulvin oral suspension) Microsize 1888
- Gris-PEG Tablets, 125 mg & 250 mg 479

Mephobarbital (Potential for reduced efficacy and increased incidence of breakthrough bleeding and menstrual irregularities). Products include:

- Mebaral Tablets 2322

Methacycline Hydrochloride (Potential for reduced efficacy and increased incidence of breakthrough bleeding and menstrual irregularities).

No products indexed under this heading.

Minocycline Hydrochloride (Potential for reduced efficacy and increased incidence of breakthrough bleeding and menstrual irregularities). Products include:

- Dynacin Capsules 1590
- Minocin Intravenous 1382
- Minocin Oral Suspension 1385
- Minocin Pellet-Filled Capsules 1383

Oxytetracycline Hydrochloride (Potential for reduced efficacy and increased incidence of breakthrough bleeding and menstrual irregularities). Products include:

- TERAK Ointment ◎ 209
- Terra-Cortril Ophthalmic Suspension 2210
- Terramycin with Polymyxin B Sulfate Ophthalmic Ointment 2211
- Urobiotic-250 Capsules 2214

Pentobarbital Sodium (Potential for reduced efficacy and increased incidence of breakthrough bleeding and menstrual irregularities). Products include:

- Nembutal Sodium Capsules 436
- Nembutal Sodium Solution 438
- Nembutal Sodium Suppositories 440

Phenobarbital (Potential for reduced efficacy and increased incidence of breakthrough bleeding and menstrual irregularities). Products include:

- Arco-Lase Plus Tablets 512
- Bellergal-S Tablets 2250
- Donnatal 2060
- Donnatal Extentabs 2061
- Donnatal Tablets 2060
- Phenobarbital Elixir and Tablets 1469
- Quadrinal Tablets 1350

Phenylbutazone (Potential for reduced efficacy and increased incidence of breakthrough bleeding and menstrual irregularities).

No products indexed under this heading.

Phenytoin Sodium (Potential for reduced efficacy and increased incidence of breakthrough bleeding and menstrual irregularities). Products include:

- Dilantin Kapseals 1906
- Dilantin Parenteral 1910

Rifampin (Potential for reduced efficacy and increased incidence of breakthrough bleeding and menstrual irregularities). Products include:

- Rifadin 1528
- Rifamate Capsules 1530
- Rifater 1532
- Rimactane Capsules 847

Secobarbital Sodium (Potential for reduced efficacy and increased incidence of breakthrough bleeding and menstrual irregularities). Products include:

- Seconal Sodium Pulvules 1474

Tetracycline Hydrochloride (Potential for reduced efficacy and increased incidence of breakthrough bleeding and menstrual irregularities). Products include:

- Achromycin V Capsules 1367

Thiamylal Sodium (Potential for reduced efficacy and increased incidence of breakthrough bleeding and menstrual irregularities).

No products indexed under this heading.

DESOWEN CREAM, OINTMENT AND LOTION

(Desonide) 1046
None cited in PDR database.

DESOXYN GRADUMET TABLETS

(Methamphetamine Hydrochloride) 419
May interact with insulin, monoamine oxidase inhibitors, phenothiazines, tricyclic antidepressants, and certain other agents. Compounds in these categories include:

Amitriptyline Hydrochloride (Concurrent administration should be closely supervised and dosage carefully adjusted). Products include:

- Elavil 2838
- Endep Tablets 2174
- Etrafon 2355
- Limbitrol 2180
- Triavil Tablets 1757

Amoxapine (Concurrent administration should be closely supervised and dosage carefully adjusted). Products include:

- Asendin Tablets 1369

Chlorpromazine (May antagonize the CNS stimulant action of the amphetamine). Products include:

- Thorazine Suppositories 2523

Clomipramine Hydrochloride (Concurrent administration should be closely supervised and dosage carefully adjusted). Products include:

- Anafranil Capsules 803

Desipramine Hydrochloride (Concurrent administration should be closely supervised and dosage carefully adjusted). Products include:

- Norpramin Tablets 1526

Doxepin Hydrochloride (Concurrent administration should be closely supervised and dosage carefully adjusted). Products include:

- Sinequan 2205
- Zonalon Cream 1055

Fluphenazine Decanoate (May antagonize the CNS stimulant action of the amphetamine). Products include:

- Prolixin Decanoate 509

Fluphenazine Enanthate (May antagonize the CNS stimulant action of the amphetamine). Products include:

- Prolixin Enanthate 509

Fluphenazine Hydrochloride (May antagonize the CNS stimulant action of the amphetamine). Products include:

- Prolixin 509

Furazolidone (Concurrent or sequential administration is contraindicated). Products include:

- Furoxone 2046

Guanethidine Monosulfate (Decreased hypotensive effect). Products include:

- Esimil Tablets 822
- Ismelin Tablets 827

Imipramine Hydrochloride (Concurrent administration should be closely supervised and dosage carefully adjusted). Products include:

- Tofranil Ampuls 854
- Tofranil Tablets 856

Imipramine Pamoate (Concurrent administration should be closely supervised and dosage carefully adjusted). Products include:

- Tofranil-PM Capsules 857

Insulin, Human (Insulin requirement in diabetics may be altered).

No products indexed under this heading.

Insulin, Human Isophane Suspension (Insulin requirement in diabetics may be altered). Products include:

- Novolin N Human Insulin 10 ml Vials 1795

Insulin, Human NPH (Insulin requirement in diabetics may be altered). Products include:

- Humulin N, 100 Units 1448
- Novolin N PenFill Cartridges Durable Insulin Delivery System 1798
- Novolin N Prefilled Syringe Disposable Insulin Delivery System 1798

259 Interactions Index Desyrel

Insulin, Human Regular (Insulin requirement in diabetics may be altered). Products include:
- Humulin R, 100 Units ... 1449
- Novolin R Human Insulin 10 ml Vials ... 1795
- Novolin R PenFill Cartridges Durable Insulin Delivery System ... 1798
- Novolin R Prefilled Syringe Disposable Insulin Delivery System ... 1798
- Velosulin BR Human Insulin 10 ml Vials ... 1795

Insulin, Human, Zinc Suspension (Insulin requirement in diabetics may be altered). Products include:
- Humulin L, 100 Units ... 1446
- Humulin U, 100 Units ... 1450
- Novolin L Human Insulin 10 ml Vials ... 1795

Insulin, NPH (Insulin requirement in diabetics may be altered). Products include:
- NPH, 100 Units ... 1450
- Pork NPH, 100 Units ... 1452
- Purified Pork NPH Isophane Insulin ... 1801

Insulin, Regular (Insulin requirement in diabetics may be altered). Products include:
- Regular, 100 Units ... 1450
- Pork Regular, 100 Units ... 1452
- Pork Regular (Concentrated), 500 Units ... 1453
- Purified Pork Regular Insulin ... 1801

Insulin, Zinc Crystals (Insulin requirement in diabetics may be altered). Products include:
- NPH, 100 Units ... 1450

Insulin, Zinc Suspension (Insulin requirement in diabetics may be altered). Products include:
- Iletin I ... 1450
- Lente, 100 Units ... 1450
- Iletin II ... 1452
- Pork Lente, 100 Units ... 1452
- Purified Pork Lente Insulin ... 1801

Isocarboxazid (Concurrent or sequential administration is contraindicated).
- No products indexed under this heading.

Maprotiline Hydrochloride (Concurrent administration should be closely supervised and dosage carefully adjusted). Products include:
- Ludiomil Tablets ... 843

Mesoridazine Besylate (May antagonize the CNS stimulant action of the amphetamine). Products include:
- Serentil ... 684

Methotrimeprazine (May antagonize the CNS stimulant action of the amphetamine). Products include:
- Levoprome ... 1274

Nortriptyline Hydrochloride (Concurrent administration should be closely supervised and dosage carefully adjusted). Products include:
- Pamelor ... 2280

Perphenazine (May antagonize the CNS stimulant action of the amphetamine). Products include:
- Etrafon ... 2355
- Triavil Tablets ... 1757
- Trilafon ... 2389

Phenelzine Sulfate (Concurrent or sequential administration is contraindicated). Products include:
- Nardil ... 1920

Prochlorperazine (May antagonize the CNS stimulant action of the amphetamine). Products include:
- Compazine ... 2470

Promethazine Hydrochloride (May antagonize the CNS stimulant action of the amphetamine). Products include:
- Mepergan Injection ... 2753
- Phenergan with Codeine ... 2777
- Phenergan with Dextromethorphan ... 2778
- Phenergan Injection ... 2773
- Phenergan Suppositories ... 2775
- Phenergan Syrup ... 2774
- Phenergan Tablets ... 2775
- Phenergan VC ... 2779
- Phenergan VC with Codeine ... 2781

Protriptyline Hydrochloride (Concurrent administration should be closely supervised and dosage carefully adjusted). Products include:
- Vivactil Tablets ... 1774

Selegiline Hydrochloride (Concurrent or sequential administration is contraindicated). Products include:
- Eldepryl Tablets ... 2550

Thioridazine Hydrochloride (May antagonize the CNS stimulant action of the amphetamine). Products include:
- Mellaril ... 2269

Tranylcypromine Sulfate (Concurrent or sequential administration is contraindicated). Products include:
- Parnate Tablets ... 2503

Trifluoperazine Hydrochloride (May antagonize the CNS stimulant action of the amphetamine). Products include:
- Stelazine ... 2514

Trimipramine Maleate (Concurrent administration should be closely supervised and dosage carefully adjusted). Products include:
- Surmontil Capsules ... 2811

DESQUAM-E 2.5 EMOLLIENT GEL
(Benzoyl Peroxide) ... 2684
May interact with:

Octyl Dimethyl PABA (Concurrent use with PABA-containing sunscreens may result in transient discoloration of the skin).
- No products indexed under this heading.

DESQUAM-E 5 EMOLLIENT GEL
(Benzoyl Peroxide) ... 2684
See **Desquam-E 2.5 Emollient Gel**

DESQUAM-E 10 EMOLLIENT GEL
(Benzoyl Peroxide) ... 2684
See **Desquam-E 2.5 Emollient Gel**

DESQUAM-X 5 GEL
(Benzoyl Peroxide) ... 2684
See **Desquam-E 2.5 Emollient Gel**

DESQUAM-X 10 GEL
(Benzoyl Peroxide) ... 2684
See **Desquam-E 2.5 Emollient Gel**

DESQUAM-X 10 BAR
(Benzoyl Peroxide) ... 2684
See **Desquam-E 2.5 Emollient Gel**

DESQUAM-X 5 WASH
(Benzoyl Peroxide) ... 2684
See **Desquam-E 2.5 Emollient Gel**

DESQUAM-X 10 WASH
(Benzoyl Peroxide) ... 2684
See **Desquam-E 2.5 Emollient Gel**

DESYREL AND DESYREL DIVIDOSE
(Trazodone Hydrochloride) ... 503
May interact with monoamine oxidase inhibitors, central nervous system depressants, antihypertensives, oral anticoagulants, and certain other agents. Compounds in these categories include:

Acebutolol Hydrochloride (Concomitant administration may require a reduction in the dose of the antihypertensive). Products include:
- Sectral Capsules ... 2807

Alfentanil Hydrochloride (Enhanced response to CNS depressants). Products include:
- Alfenta Injection ... 1286

Alprazolam (Enhanced response to CNS depressants). Products include:
- Xanax Tablets ... 2649

Amlodipine Besylate (Concomitant administration may require a reduction in the dose of the antihypertensive). Products include:
- Lotrel Capsules ... 840
- Norvasc Tablets ... 1940

Aprobarbital (Enhanced response to CNS depressants).
- No products indexed under this heading.

Atenolol (Concomitant administration may require a reduction in the dose of the antihypertensive). Products include:
- Tenoretic Tablets ... 2845
- Tenormin Tablets and I.V. Injection ... 2847

Benazepril Hydrochloride (Concomitant administration may require a reduction in the dose of the antihypertensive). Products include:
- Lotensin Tablets ... 834
- Lotensin HCT ... 837
- Lotrel Capsules ... 840

Bendroflumethiazide (Concomitant administration may require a reduction in the dose of the antihypertensive).
- No products indexed under this heading.

Betaxolol Hydrochloride (Concomitant administration may require a reduction in the dose of the antihypertensive). Products include:
- Betoptic Ophthalmic Solution ... 469
- Betoptic S Ophthalmic Suspension ... 471
- Kerlone Tablets ... 2436

Bisoprolol Fumarate (Concomitant administration may require a reduction in the dose of the antihypertensive). Products include:
- Zebeta Tablets ... 1413
- Ziac ... 1415

Buprenorphine (Enhanced response to CNS depressants). Products include:
- Buprenex Injectable ... 2006

Buspirone Hydrochloride (Enhanced response to CNS depressants). Products include:
- BuSpar ... 737

Butabarbital (Enhanced response to CNS depressants).
- No products indexed under this heading.

Butalbital (Enhanced response to CNS depressants). Products include:
- Esgic-plus Tablets ... 1013
- Fioricet Tablets ... 2258
- Fioricet with Codeine Capsules ... 2260
- Fiorinal Capsules ... 2261
- Fiorinal with Codeine Capsules ... 2262
- Fiorinal Tablets ... 2261
- Phrenilin ... 785
- Sedapap Tablets 50 mg/650 mg ... 1543

Captopril (Concomitant administration may require a reduction in the dose of the antihypertensive). Products include:
- Capoten ... 739
- Capozide ... 742

Carteolol Hydrochloride (Concomitant administration may require a reduction in the dose of the antihypertensive). Products include:
- Cartrol Tablets ... 410
- Ocupress Ophthalmic Solution, 1% Sterile ... ⊙ 309

Chlordiazepoxide (Enhanced response to CNS depressants). Products include:
- Libritabs Tablets ... 2177
- Limbitrol ... 2180

Chlordiazepoxide Hydrochloride (Enhanced response to CNS depressants). Products include:
- Librax Capsules ... 2176
- Librium Capsules ... 2178
- Librium Injectable ... 2179

Chlorothiazide (Concomitant administration may require a reduction in the dose of the antihypertensive). Products include:
- Aldoclor Tablets ... 1598
- Diupres Tablets ... 1650
- Diuril Oral ... 1653

Chlorothiazide Sodium (Concomitant administration may require a reduction in the dose of the antihypertensive). Products include:
- Diuril Sodium Intravenous ... 1652

Chlorpromazine (Enhanced response to CNS depressants). Products include:
- Thorazine Suppositories ... 2523

Chlorpromazine Hydrochloride (Enhanced response to CNS depressants). Products include:
- Thorazine ... 2523

Chlorprothixene (Enhanced response to CNS depressants).
- No products indexed under this heading.

Chlorprothixene Hydrochloride (Enhanced response to CNS depressants).
- No products indexed under this heading.

Chlorthalidone (Concomitant administration may require a reduction in the dose of the antihypertensive). Products include:
- Combipres Tablets ... 677
- Tenoretic Tablets ... 2845
- Thalitone ... 1245

Clonidine (Concomitant administration may require a reduction in the dose of the antihypertensive). Products include:
- Catapres-TTS ... 675

Clonidine Hydrochloride (Concomitant administration may require a reduction in the dose of the antihypertensive). Products include:
- Catapres Tablets ... 674
- Combipres Tablets ... 677

Clorazepate Dipotassium (Enhanced response to CNS depressants). Products include:
- Tranxene ... 451

Clozapine (Enhanced response to CNS depressants). Products include:
- Clozaril Tablets ... 2252

Codeine Phosphate (Enhanced response to CNS depressants). Products include:
- Actifed with Codeine Cough Syrup ... 1067
- Brontex ... 1981
- Deconsal C Expectorant Syrup ... 456
- Deconsal Pediatric Syrup ... 457
- Dimetane-DC Cough Syrup ... 2059
- Empirin with Codeine Tablets ... 1093
- Fioricet with Codeine Capsules ... 2260
- Fiorinal with Codeine Capsules ... 2262
- Isoclor Expectorant ... 990

IMPORTANT NOTE: Always consult each drug listing in the patient's regimen for possible interactions.

Desyrel **Interactions Index** 260

Novahistine DH ... 2462
Novahistine Expectorant ... 2463
Nucofed ... 2051
Phenergan with Codeine ... 2777
Phenergan VC with Codeine ... 2781
Robitussin A-C Syrup ... 2073
Robitussin-DAC Syrup ... 2074
Ryna ... ▣ 841
Soma Compound w/Codeine Tablets ... 2676
Tussi-Organidin NR Liquid and S NR Liquid ... 2677
Tylenol with Codeine ... 1583

Deserpidine (Concomitant administration may require a reduction in the dose of the antihypertensive).
No products indexed under this heading.

Desflurane (Enhanced response to CNS depressants). Products include:
Suprane ... 1813

Dezocine (Enhanced response to CNS depressants). Products include:
Dalgan Injection ... 538

Diazepam (Enhanced response to CNS depressants). Products include:
Dizac ... 1809
Valium Injectable ... 2182
Valium Tablets ... 2183
Valrelease Capsules ... 2169

Diazoxide (Concomitant administration may require a reduction in the dose of the antihypertensive). Products include:
Hyperstat I.V. Injection ... 2363
Proglycem ... 580

Dicumarol (Increased or decreased prothrombin time).
No products indexed under this heading.

Digoxin (Increased serum levels of digoxin). Products include:
Lanoxicaps ... 1117
Lanoxin Elixir Pediatric ... 1120
Lanoxin Injection ... 1123
Lanoxin Injection Pediatric ... 1126
Lanoxin Tablets ... 1128

Diltiazem Hydrochloride (Concomitant administration may require a reduction in the dose of the antihypertensive). Products include:
Cardizem CD Capsules ... 1506
Cardizem SR Capsules ... 1510
Cardizem Injectable ... 1508
Cardizem Tablets ... 1512
Dilacor XR Extended-release Capsules ... 2018

Doxazosin Mesylate (Concomitant administration may require a reduction in the dose of the antihypertensive). Products include:
Cardura Tablets ... 2186

Droperidol (Enhanced response to CNS depressants). Products include:
Inapsine Injection ... 1296

Enalapril Maleate (Concomitant administration may require a reduction in the dose of the antihypertensive). Products include:
Vaseretic Tablets ... 1765
Vasotec Tablets ... 1771

Enalaprilat (Concomitant administration may require a reduction in the dose of the antihypertensive). Products include:
Vasotec I.V. ... 1768

Enflurane (Enhanced response to CNS depressants).
No products indexed under this heading.

Esmolol Hydrochloride (Concomitant administration may require a reduction in the dose of the antihypertensive). Products include:
Brevibloc Injection ... 1808

Estazolam (Enhanced response to CNS depressants). Products include:
ProSom Tablets ... 449

Ethchlorvynol (Enhanced response to CNS depressants). Products include:
Placidyl Capsules ... 448

Ethinamate (Enhanced response to CNS depressants).
No products indexed under this heading.

Felodipine (Concomitant administration may require a reduction in the dose of the antihypertensive). Products include:
Plendil Extended-Release Tablets ... 527

Fentanyl (Enhanced response to CNS depressants). Products include:
Duragesic Transdermal System ... 1288

Fentanyl Citrate (Enhanced response to CNS depressants). Products include:
Sublimaze Injection ... 1307

Fluphenazine Decanoate (Enhanced response to CNS depressants). Products include:
Prolixin Decanoate ... 509

Fluphenazine Enanthate (Enhanced response to CNS depressants). Products include:
Prolixin Enanthate ... 509

Fluphenazine Hydrochloride (Enhanced response to CNS depressants). Products include:
Prolixin ... 509

Flurazepam Hydrochloride (Enhanced response to CNS depressants). Products include:
Dalmane Capsules ... 2173

Fosinopril Sodium (Concomitant administration may require a reduction in the dose of the antihypertensive). Products include:
Monopril Tablets ... 757

Furazolidone (Initiate Desyrel cautiously). Products include:
Furoxone ... 2046

Furosemide (Concomitant administration may require a reduction in the dose of the antihypertensive). Products include:
Lasix Injection, Oral Solution and Tablets ... 1240

Glutethimide (Enhanced response to CNS depressants).
No products indexed under this heading.

Guanabenz Acetate (Concomitant administration may require a reduction in the dose of the antihypertensive).
No products indexed under this heading.

Guanethidine Monosulfate (Concomitant administration may require a reduction in the dose of the antihypertensive). Products include:
Esimil Tablets ... 822
Ismelin Tablets ... 827

Haloperidol (Enhanced response to CNS depressants). Products include:
Haldol Injection, Tablets and Concentrate ... 1575

Haloperidol Decanoate (Enhanced response to CNS depressants). Products include:
Haldol Decanoate ... 1577

Hydralazine Hydrochloride (Concomitant administration may require a reduction in the dose of the antihypertensive). Products include:
Apresazide Capsules ... 808
Apresoline Hydrochloride Tablets ... 809
Ser-Ap-Es Tablets ... 849

Hydrochlorothiazide (Concomitant administration may require a reduction in the dose of the antihypertensive). Products include:
Aldactazide ... 2413
Aldoril Tablets ... 1604
Apresazide Capsules ... 808
Capozide ... 742
Dyazide ... 2479
Esidrix Tablets ... 821
Esimil Tablets ... 822
HydroDIURIL Tablets ... 1674
Hydropres Tablets ... 1675
Hyzaar Tablets ... 1677
Inderide Tablets ... 2732
Inderide LA Long Acting Capsules ... 2734
Lopressor HCT Tablets ... 832
Lotensin HCT ... 837
Maxzide ... 1380
Moduretic Tablets ... 1705
Oretic Tablets ... 443
Prinzide Tablets ... 1737
Ser-Ap-Es Tablets ... 849
Timolide Tablets ... 1748
Vaseretic Tablets ... 1765
Zestoretic ... 2850
Ziac ... 1415

Hydrocodone Bitartrate (Enhanced response to CNS depressants). Products include:
Anexsia 5/500 Elixir ... 1781
Anexia Tablets ... 1782
Codiclear DH Syrup ... 791
Deconamine CX Cough and Cold Liquid and Tablets ... 1319
Duratuss HD Elixir ... 2565
Hycodan Tablets and Syrup ... 930
Hycomine Compound Tablets ... 932
Hycomine ... 931
Hycotuss Expectorant Syrup ... 933
Hydrocet Capsules ... 782
Lorcet 10/650 ... 1018
Lortab ... 2566
Tussend ... 1783
Tussend Expectorant ... 1785
Vicodin Tablets ... 1356
Vicodin ES Tablets ... 1357
Vicodin Tuss Expectorant ... 1358
Zydone Capsules ... 949

Hydrocodone Polistirex (Enhanced response to CNS depressants). Products include:
Tussionex Pennkinetic Extended-Release Suspension ... 998

Hydroflumethiazide (Concomitant administration may require a reduction in the dose of the antihypertensive). Products include:
Diucardin Tablets ... 2718

Hydroxyzine Hydrochloride (Enhanced response to CNS depressants). Products include:
Atarax Tablets & Syrup ... 2185
Marax Tablets & DF Syrup ... 2200
Vistaril Intramuscular Solution ... 2216

Indapamide (Concomitant administration may require a reduction in the dose of the antihypertensive). Products include:
Lozol Tablets ... 2022

Isocarboxazid (Initiate Desyrel cautiously).
No products indexed under this heading.

Isoflurane (Enhanced response to CNS depressants).
No products indexed under this heading.

Isradipine (Concomitant administration may require a reduction in the dose of the antihypertensive). Products include:
DynaCirc Capsules ... 2256

Ketamine Hydrochloride (Enhanced response to CNS depressants).
No products indexed under this heading.

Labetalol Hydrochloride (Concomitant administration may require a reduction in the dose of the antihypertensive). Products include:
Normodyne Injection ... 2377
Normodyne Tablets ... 2379
Trandate ... 1185

Levobunolol Hydrochloride (Concomitant administration may require a reduction in the dose of the antihypertensive). Products include:
Betagan ... ◉ 233

Levomethadyl Acetate Hydrochloride (Enhanced response to CNS depressants). Products include:
Orlamm ... 2239

Levorphanol Tartrate (Enhanced response to CNS depressants). Products include:
Levo-Dromoran ... 2129

Lisinopril (Concomitant administration may require a reduction in the dose of the antihypertensive). Products include:
Prinivil Tablets ... 1733
Prinzide Tablets ... 1737
Zestoretic ... 2850
Zestril Tablets ... 2854

Lorazepam (Enhanced response to CNS depressants). Products include:
Ativan Injection ... 2698
Ativan Tablets ... 2700

Losartan Potassium (Concomitant administration may require a reduction in the dose of the antihypertensive). Products include:
Cozaar Tablets ... 1628
Hyzaar Tablets ... 1677

Loxapine Hydrochloride (Enhanced response to CNS depressants). Products include:
Loxitane ... 1378

Loxapine Succinate (Enhanced response to CNS depressants). Products include:
Loxitane Capsules ... 1378

Mecamylamine Hydrochloride (Concomitant administration may require a reduction in the dose of the antihypertensive). Products include:
Inversine Tablets ... 1686

Meperidine Hydrochloride (Enhanced response to CNS depressants). Products include:
Demerol ... 2308
Mepergan Injection ... 2753

Mephobarbital (Enhanced response to CNS depressants). Products include:
Mebaral Tablets ... 2322

Meprobamate (Enhanced response to CNS depressants). Products include:
Miltown Tablets ... 2672
PMB 200 and PMB 400 ... 2783

Mesoridazine Besylate (Enhanced response to CNS depressants). Products include:
Serentil ... 684

Methadone Hydrochloride (Enhanced response to CNS depressants). Products include:
Methadone Hydrochloride Oral Concentrate ... 2233
Methadone Hydrochloride Oral Solution & Tablets ... 2235

Methohexital Sodium (Enhanced response to CNS depressants). Products include:
Brevital Sodium Vials ... 1429

Methotrimeprazine (Enhanced response to CNS depressants). Products include:
Levoprome ... 1274

Methoxyflurane (Enhanced response to CNS depressants).
No products indexed under this heading.

Methyclothiazide (Concomitant administration may require a reduction in the dose of the antihypertensive). Products include:
Enduron Tablets ... 420

(▣ Described in PDR For Nonprescription Drugs) (◉ Described in PDR For Ophthalmology)

261 **Interactions Index** **Desyrel**

Methyldopa (Concomitant administration may require a reduction in the dose of the antihypertensive). Products include:

- Aldoclor Tablets ... 1598
- Aldomet Oral ... 1600
- Aldoril Tablets ... 1604

Methyldopate Hydrochloride (Concomitant administration may require a reduction in the dose of the antihypertensive). Products include:

- Aldomet Ester HCl Injection ... 1602

Metipranolol Hydrochloride (Concomitant administration may require a reduction in the dose of the antihypertensive). Products include:

- OptiPranolol (Metipranolol 0.3%) Sterile Ophthalmic Solution ... ⊕ 258

Metolazone (Concomitant administration may require a reduction in the dose of the antihypertensive). Products include:

- Mykrox Tablets ... 993
- Zaroxolyn Tablets ... 1000

Metoprolol Succinate (Concomitant administration may require a reduction in the dose of the antihypertensive). Products include:

- Toprol-XL Tablets ... 565

Metoprolol Tartrate (Concomitant administration may require a reduction in the dose of the antihypertensive). Products include:

- Lopressor Ampuls ... 830
- Lopressor HCT Tablets ... 832
- Lopressor Tablets ... 830

Metyrosine (Concomitant administration may require a reduction in the dose of the antihypertensive). Products include:

- Demser Capsules ... 1649

Midazolam Hydrochloride (Enhanced response to CNS depressants). Products include:

- Versed Injection ... 2170

Minoxidil (Concomitant administration may require a reduction in the dose of the antihypertensive). Products include:

- Loniten Tablets ... 2618
- Rogaine Topical Solution ... 2637

Moexipril Hydrochloride (Concomitant administration may require a reduction in the dose of the antihypertensive). Products include:

- Univasc Tablets ... 2410

Molindone Hydrochloride (Enhanced response to CNS depressants). Products include:

- Moban Tablets and Concentrate ... 1048

Morphine Sulfate (Enhanced response to CNS depressants). Products include:

- Astramorph/PF Injection, USP (Preservative-Free) ... 535
- Duramorph ... 962
- Infumorph 200 and Infumorph 500 Sterile Solutions ... 965
- MS Contin Tablets ... 1994
- MSIR ... 1997
- Oramorph SR (Morphine Sulfate Sustained Release Tablets) ... 2236
- RMS Suppositories ... 2657
- Roxanol ... 2243

Nadolol (Concomitant administration may require a reduction in the dose of the antihypertensive).

- No products indexed under this heading.

Nicardipine Hydrochloride (Concomitant administration may require a reduction in the dose of the antihypertensive). Products include:

- Cardene Capsules ... 2095
- Cardene I.V. ... 2709
- Cardene SR Capsules ... 2097

Nifedipine (Concomitant administration may require a reduction in the dose of the antihypertensive). Products include:

- Adalat Capsules (10 mg and 20 mg) ... 587
- Adalat CC ... 589
- Procardia Capsules ... 1971
- Procardia XL Extended Release Tablets ... 1972

Nisoldipine (Concomitant administration may require a reduction in the dose of the antihypertensive).

- No products indexed under this heading.

Nitroglycerin (Concomitant administration may require a reduction in the dose of the antihypertensive). Products include:

- Deponit NTG Transdermal Delivery System ... 2397
- Nitro-Bid IV ... 1523
- Nitro-Bid Ointment ... 1524
- Nitrodisc ... 2047
- Nitro-Dur (nitroglycerin) Transdermal Infusion System ... 1326
- Nitrolingual Spray ... 2027
- Nitrostat Tablets ... 1925
- Transderm-Nitro Transdermal Therapeutic System ... 859

Opium Alkaloids (Enhanced response to CNS depressants).

- No products indexed under this heading.

Oxazepam (Enhanced response to CNS depressants). Products include:

- Serax Capsules ... 2810
- Serax Tablets ... 2810

Oxycodone Hydrochloride (Enhanced response to CNS depressants). Products include:

- Percocet Tablets ... 938
- Percodan Tablets ... 939
- Percodan-Demi Tablets ... 940
- Roxicodone Tablets, Oral Solution & Intensol (Oxycodone) ... 2244
- Tylox Capsules ... 1584

Penbutolol Sulfate (Concomitant administration may require a reduction in the dose of the antihypertensive). Products include:

- Levatol ... 2403

Pentobarbital Sodium (Enhanced response to CNS depressants). Products include:

- Nembutal Sodium Capsules ... 436
- Nembutal Sodium Solution ... 438
- Nembutal Sodium Suppositories ... 440

Perphenazine (Enhanced response to CNS depressants). Products include:

- Etrafon ... 2355
- Triavil Tablets ... 1757
- Trilafon ... 2389

Phenelzine Sulfate (Initiate Desyrel cautiously). Products include:

- Nardil ... 1920

Phenobarbital (Enhanced response to CNS depressants). Products include:

- Arco-Lase Plus Tablets ... 512
- Bellergal-S Tablets ... 2250
- Donnatal ... 2060
- Donnatal Extentabs ... 2061
- Donnatal Tablets ... 2060
- Phenobarbital Elixir and Tablets ... 1469
- Quadrinal Tablets ... 1350

Phenoxybenzamine Hydrochloride (Concomitant administration may require a reduction in the dose of the antihypertensive). Products include:

- Dibenzyline Capsules ... 2476

Phentolamine Mesylate (Concomitant administration may require a reduction in the dose of the antihypertensive). Products include:

- Regitine ... 846

Phenytoin (Increased serum levels of phenytoin). Products include:

- Dilantin Infatabs ... 1908
- Dilantin-125 Suspension ... 1911

Phenytoin Sodium (Increased serum levels of phenytoin). Products include:

- Dilantin Kapseals ... 1906
- Dilantin Parenteral ... 1910

Pindolol (Concomitant administration may require a reduction in the dose of the antihypertensive). Products include:

- Visken Tablets ... 2299

Polythiazide (Concomitant administration may require a reduction in the dose of the antihypertensive). Products include:

- Minizide Capsules ... 1938

Prazepam (Enhanced response to CNS depressants).

- No products indexed under this heading.

Prazosin Hydrochloride (Concomitant administration may require a reduction in the dose of the antihypertensive). Products include:

- Minipress Capsules ... 1937
- Minizide Capsules ... 1938

Prochlorperazine (Enhanced response to CNS depressants). Products include:

- Compazine ... 2470

Promethazine Hydrochloride (Enhanced response to CNS depressants). Products include:

- Mepergan Injection ... 2753
- Phenergan with Codeine ... 2777
- Phenergan with Dextromethorphan 2778
- Phenergan Injection ... 2773
- Phenergan Suppositories ... 2775
- Phenergan Syrup ... 2774
- Phenergan Tablets ... 2775
- Phenergan VC ... 2779
- Phenergan VC with Codeine ... 2781

Propofol (Enhanced response to CNS depressants). Products include:

- Diprivan Injection ... 2833

Propoxyphene Hydrochloride (Enhanced response to CNS depressants). Products include:

- Darvon ... 1435
- Wygesic Tablets ... 2827

Propoxyphene Napsylate (Enhanced response to CNS depressants). Products include:

- Darvon-N/Darvocet-N ... 1433

Propranolol Hydrochloride (Concomitant administration may require a reduction in the dose of the antihypertensive). Products include:

- Inderal ... 2728
- Inderal LA Long Acting Capsules ... 2730
- Inderide Tablets ... 2732
- Inderide LA Long Acting Capsules .. 2734

Quazepam (Enhanced response to CNS depressants). Products include:

- Doral Tablets ... 2664

Quinapril Hydrochloride (Concomitant administration may require a reduction in the dose of the antihypertensive). Products include:

- Accupril Tablets ... 1893

Ramipril (Concomitant administration may require a reduction in the dose of the antihypertensive). Products include:

- Altace Capsules ... 1232

Rauwolfia Serpentina (Concomitant administration may require a reduction in the dose of the antihypertensive).

- No products indexed under this heading.

Rescinnamine (Concomitant administration may require a reduction in the dose of the antihypertensive).

- No products indexed under this heading.

Reserpine (Concomitant administration may require a reduction in the dose of the antihypertensive). Products include:

- Diupres Tablets ... 1650
- Hydropres Tablets ... 1675
- Ser-Ap-Es Tablets ... 849

Risperidone (Enhanced response to CNS depressants). Products include:

- Risperdal ... 1301

Secobarbital Sodium (Enhanced response to CNS depressants). Products include:

- Seconal Sodium Pulvules ... 1474

Selegiline Hydrochloride (Initiate Desyrel cautiously). Products include:

- Eldepryl Tablets ... 2550

Sodium Nitroprusside (Concomitant administration may require a reduction in the dose of the antihypertensive).

- No products indexed under this heading.

Sotalol Hydrochloride (Concomitant administration may require a reduction in the dose of the antihypertensive). Products include:

- Betapace Tablets ... 641

Spirapril Hydrochloride (Concomitant administration may require a reduction in the dose of the antihypertensive).

- No products indexed under this heading.

Sufentanil Citrate (Enhanced response to CNS depressants). Products include:

- Sufenta Injection ... 1309

Temazepam (Enhanced response to CNS depressants). Products include:

- Restoril Capsules ... 2284

Terazosin Hydrochloride (Concomitant administration may require a reduction in the dose of the antihypertensive). Products include:

- Hytrin Capsules ... 430

Thiamylal Sodium (Enhanced response to CNS depressants).

- No products indexed under this heading.

Thioridazine Hydrochloride (Enhanced response to CNS depressants). Products include:

- Mellaril ... 2269

Thiothixene (Enhanced response to CNS depressants). Products include:

- Navane Capsules and Concentrate 2201
- Navane Intramuscular ... 2202

Timolol Maleate (Concomitant administration may require a reduction in the dose of the antihypertensive). Products include:

- Blocadren Tablets ... 1614
- Timolide Tablets ... 1748
- Timoptic in Ocudose ... 1753
- Timoptic Sterile Ophthalmic Solution ... 1751
- Timoptic-XE ... 1755

Torsemide (Concomitant administration may require a reduction in the dose of the antihypertensive). Products include:

- Demadex Tablets and Injection ... 686

Tranylcypromine Sulfate (Initiate Desyrel cautiously). Products include:

- Parnate Tablets ... 2503

Triazolam (Enhanced response to CNS depressants). Products include:

- Halcion Tablets ... 2611

Trifluoperazine Hydrochloride (Enhanced response to CNS depressants). Products include:

- Stelazine ... 2514

IMPORTANT NOTE: Always consult each drug listing in the patient's regimen for possible interactions.

Desyrel

Trimethaphan Camsylate (Concomitant administration may require a reduction in the dose of the antihypertensive). Products include:

Arfonad Ampuls 2080

Verapamil Hydrochloride (Concomitant administration may require a reduction in the dose of the antihypertensive). Products include:

Calan SR Caplets 2422
Calan Tablets... 2419
Isoptin Injectable 1344
Isoptin Oral Tablets 1346
Isoptin SR Tablets 1348
Verelan Capsules 1410
Verelan Capsules 2824

Warfarin Sodium (Increased or decreased prothrombin time). Products include:

Coumadin 926

Zolpidem Tartrate (Enhanced response to CNS depressants). Products include:

Ambien Tablets.. 2416

Food Interactions

Alcohol (Enhanced response to alcohol).

Food, unspecified (Total drug absorption may be up to 20% higher when the drug is taken with food rather than on an empty stomach; the risk of dizziness, lightheadedness may increase under fasting conditions).

DEVROM CHEWABLE TABLETS

(Bismuth Subgallate) .... ⊕D 741
None cited in PDR database.

DEXACIDIN OINTMENT

(Dexamethasone, Neomycin Sulfate, Polymyxin B Sulfate) .... ◎ 263
None cited in PDR database.

DEXACORT PHOSPHATE IN RESPIHALER

(Dexamethasone Sodium Phosphate) 458
May interact with oral anticoagulants, potassium sparing diuretics, and certain other agents. Compounds in these categories include:

Amiloride Hydrochloride (Potential for hypokalemia). Products include:

Midamor Tablets 1703
Moduretic Tablets 1705

Aspirin (Aspirin should be used cautiously in conjunction with Dexacort in hypoprothrombinemia). Products include:

Alka-Seltzer Effervescent Antacid and Pain Reliever............................... ⊕D 701
Alka-Seltzer Extra Strength Effervescent Antacid and Pain Reliever .... ⊕D 703
Alka-Seltzer Lemon Lime Effervescent Antacid and Pain Reliever .... ⊕D 703
Alka-Seltzer Plus Cold Medicine .... ⊕D 705
Alka-Seltzer Plus Cold & Cough Medicine .... ⊕D 708
Alka-Seltzer Plus Night-Time Cold Medicine .... ⊕D 707
Alka Seltzer Plus Sinus Medicine .. ⊕D 707
Arthritis Foundation Safety Coated Aspirin Tablets .... ⊕D 675
Arthritis Pain Ascriptin .... ⊕D 631
Maximum Strength Ascriptin .... ⊕D 630
Regular Strength Ascriptin Tablets .... ⊕D 629
Arthritis Strength BC Powder .... ⊕D 609
BC Cold Powder Multi-Symptom Formula (Cold-Sinus-Allergy) ...... ⊕D 609
BC Cold Powder Non-Drowsy Formula (Cold-Sinus) .... ⊕D 609
BC Powder .... ⊕D 609
Bayer Children's Chewable Aspirin .... ⊕D 711
Genuine Bayer Aspirin Tablets & Caplets .... ⊕D 713
Extra Strength Bayer Arthritis Pain Regimen Formula .... ⊕D 711
Extra Strength Bayer Aspirin Caplets & Tablets .... ⊕D 712
Extended-Release Bayer 8-Hour Aspirin .... ⊕D 712
Extra Strength Bayer Plus Aspirin Caplets .... ⊕D 713
Extra Strength Bayer PM Aspirin .. ⊕D 713
Bayer Enteric Aspirin .... ⊕D 709
Bufferin Analgesic Tablets and Caplets .... ⊕D 613
Arthritis Strength Bufferin Analgesic Caplets .... ⊕D 614
Extra Strength Bufferin Analgesic Tablets .... ⊕D 615
Cama Arthritis Pain Reliever............ ⊕D 785
Darvon Compound-65 Pulvules 1435
Easprin 1914
Ecotrin 2455
Ecotrin Enteric Coated Aspirin Maximum Strength Tablets and Caplets .... ⊕D 816
Ecotrin Enteric Coated Aspirin Regular Strength Tablets 2455
Empirin Aspirin Tablets .... ⊕D 854
Empirin with Codeine Tablets........... 1093
Excedrin Extra-Strength Analgesic Tablets & Caplets 732
Fiorinal Capsules 2261
Fiorinal with Codeine Capsules 2262
Fiorinal Tablets 2261
Halfprin 1362
Healthprin Aspirin 2455
Norgesic.. 1496
Percodan Tablets...................................... 939
Percodan-Demi Tablets.......................... 940
Robaxisal Tablets..................................... 2071
Soma Compound w/Codeine Tablets 2676
Soma Compound Tablets....................... 2675
St. Joseph Adult Chewable Aspirin (81 mg.) .... ⊕D 808
Talwin Compound 2335
Ursinus Inlay-Tabs.................................. ⊕D 794
Vanquish Analgesic Caplets .... ⊕D 731

Dicumarol (Corticosteroid may alter the response to coumarin anticoagulant).

No products indexed under this heading.

Ephedrine (May enhance the metabolic clearance of dexamethasone, resulting in decreased blood levels and lessened physiologic activity).

Ephedrine Hydrochloride (May enhance the metabolic clearance of dexamethasone, resulting in decreased blood levels and lessened physiologic activity). Products include:

Primatene Dual Action Formula...... ⊕D 872
Primatene Tablets .... ⊕D 873
Quadrinal Tablets 1350

Ephedrine Sulfate (May enhance the metabolic clearance of dexamethasone, resulting in decreased blood levels and lessened physiologic activity). Products include:

Bronkaid Caplets .... ⊕D 717
Marax Tablets & DF Syrup................... 2200

Phenobarbital (May enhance the metabolic clearance of dexamethasone, resulting in decreased blood levels and lessened physiologic activity). Products include:

Arco-Lase Plus Tablets 512
Bellergal-S Tablets 2250
Donnatal 2060
Donnatal Extentabs................................ 2061
Donnatal Tablets 2060
Phenobarbital Elixir and Tablets 1469
Quadrinal Tablets 1350

Phenytoin (May enhance the metabolic clearance of dexamethasone, resulting in decreased blood levels and lessened physiologic activity). Products include:

Dilantin Infatabs...................................... 1908
Dilantin-125 Suspension 1911

Phenytoin Sodium (May enhance the metabolic clearance of dexamethasone, resulting in decreased blood levels and lessened physiologic activity). Products include:

Dilantin Kapseals 1906
Dilantin Parenteral 1910

Rifampin (May enhance the metabolic clearance of dexamethasone, resulting in decreased blood levels and lessened physiologic activity). Products include:

Rifadin 1528
Rifamate Capsules 1530
Rifater.. 1532
Rimactane Capsules................................ 847

Smallpox Vaccine (The expected serum antibody response may not be obtained in individuals receiving immunosuppressive doses of corticosteroid).

Spironolactone (Potential for hypokalemia). Products include:

Aldactazide... 2413
Aldactone 2414

Triamterene (Potential for hypokalemia). Products include:

Dyazide 2479
Dyrenium Capsules.................................. 2481
Maxzide 1380

Warfarin Sodium (Corticosteroid may alter the response to coumarin anticoagulant). Products include:

Coumadin 926

DEXACORT PHOSPHATE IN TURBINAIRE

(Dexamethasone Sodium Phosphate) 459
May interact with oral anticoagulants, potassium sparing diuretics, and certain other agents. Compounds in these categories include:

Amiloride Hydrochloride (Potential for hypokalemia). Products include:

Midamor Tablets 1703
Moduretic Tablets 1705

Aspirin (Aspirin should be used cautiously in conjunction with Dexacort in hypoprothrombinemia). Products include:

Alka-Seltzer Effervescent Antacid and Pain Reliever............................... ⊕D 701
Alka-Seltzer Extra Strength Effervescent Antacid and Pain Reliever .... ⊕D 703
Alka-Seltzer Lemon Lime Effervescent Antacid and Pain Reliever .... ⊕D 703
Alka-Seltzer Plus Cold Medicine .... ⊕D 705
Alka-Seltzer Plus Cold & Cough Medicine .... ⊕D 708
Alka-Seltzer Plus Night-Time Cold Medicine .... ⊕D 707
Alka Seltzer Plus Sinus Medicine .. ⊕D 707
Arthritis Foundation Safety Coated Aspirin Tablets .... ⊕D 675
Arthritis Pain Ascriptin .... ⊕D 631
Maximum Strength Ascriptin .... ⊕D 630
Regular Strength Ascriptin Tablets .... ⊕D 629
Arthritis Strength BC Powder.......... ⊕D 609
BC Cold Powder Multi-Symptom Formula (Cold-Sinus-Allergy) ...... ⊕D 609
BC Cold Powder Non-Drowsy Formula (Cold-Sinus) .... ⊕D 609
BC Powder .... ⊕D 609
Bayer Children's Chewable Aspirin .... ⊕D 711
Genuine Bayer Aspirin Tablets & Caplets .... ⊕D 713
Extra Strength Bayer Arthritis Pain Regimen Formula .... ⊕D 711
Extra Strength Bayer Aspirin Caplets & Tablets .... ⊕D 712
Extended-Release Bayer 8-Hour Aspirin .... ⊕D 712
Extra Strength Bayer Plus Aspirin Caplets .... ⊕D 713
Extra Strength Bayer PM Aspirin .. ⊕D 713
Bayer Enteric Aspirin .... ⊕D 709
Bufferin Analgesic Tablets and Caplets .... ⊕D 613
Arthritis Strength Bufferin Analgesic Caplets .... ⊕D 614
Extra Strength Bufferin Analgesic Tablets .... ⊕D 615
Cama Arthritis Pain Reliever............ ⊕D 785
Darvon Compound-65 Pulvules 1435
Easprin 1914
Ecotrin 2455
Ecotrin Enteric Coated Aspirin Maximum Strength Tablets and Caplets .... ⊕D 816
Ecotrin Enteric Coated Aspirin Regular Strength Tablets 2455
Empirin Aspirin Tablets .... ⊕D 854
Empirin with Codeine Tablets........... 1093
Excedrin Extra-Strength Analgesic Tablets & Caplets 732
Fiorinal Capsules 2261
Fiorinal with Codeine Capsules 2262
Fiorinal Tablets 2261
Halfprin 1362
Healthprin Aspirin 2455
Norgesic.. 1496
Percodan Tablets...................................... 939
Percodan-Demi Tablets.......................... 940
Robaxisal Tablets..................................... 2071
Soma Compound w/Codeine Tablets 2676
Soma Compound Tablets....................... 2675
St. Joseph Adult Chewable Aspirin (81 mg.) .... ⊕D 808
Talwin Compound 2335
Ursinus Inlay-Tabs.................................. ⊕D 794
Vanquish Analgesic Caplets .... ⊕D 731

Dicumarol (Corticosteroid may alter the response to coumarin anticoagulant).

No products indexed under this heading.

Ephedrine (May enhance the metabolic clearance of dexamethasone, resulting in decreased blood levels and lessened physiologic activity).

Ephedrine Hydrochloride (May enhance the metabolic clearance of dexamethasone, resulting in decreased blood levels and lessened physiologic activity). Products include:

Primatene Dual Action Formula...... ⊕D 872
Primatene Tablets .... ⊕D 873
Quadrinal Tablets 1350

Ephedrine Sulfate (May enhance the metabolic clearance of dexamethasone, resulting in decreased blood levels and lessened physiologic activity). Products include:

Bronkaid Caplets .... ⊕D 717
Marax Tablets & DF Syrup................... 2200

Phenobarbital (May enhance the metabolic clearance of dexamethasone, resulting in decreased blood levels and lessened physiologic activity). Products include:

Arco-Lase Plus Tablets 512
Bellergal-S Tablets 2250
Donnatal 2060
Donnatal Extentabs................................ 2061
Donnatal Tablets 2060
Phenobarbital Elixir and Tablets 1469
Quadrinal Tablets 1350

Phenytoin (May enhance the metabolic clearance of dexamethasone, resulting in decreased blood levels and lessened physiologic activity). Products include:

Dilantin Infatabs...................................... 1908
Dilantin-125 Suspension 1911

Phenytoin Sodium (May enhance the metabolic clearance of dexamethasone, resulting in decreased blood levels and lessened physiologic activity). Products include:

Dilantin Kapseals 1906
Dilantin Parenteral 1910

Rifampin (May enhance the metabolic clearance of dexamethasone, resulting in decreased blood levels and lessened physiologic activity). Products include:

Rifadin 1528
Rifamate Capsules 1530
Rifater.. 1532
Rimactane Capsules................................ 847

Smallpox Vaccine (The expected serum antibody response may not be obtained in individuals receiving immunosuppressive doses of corticosteroid).

(⊕D Described in PDR For Nonprescription Drugs) (◎ Described in PDR For Ophthalmology)

Spironolactone (Potential for hypokalemia). Products include:

Aldactazide 2413
Aldactone 2414

Triamterene (Potential for hypokalemia). Products include:

Dyazide 2479
Dyrenium Capsules 2481
Maxzide 1380

Warfarin Sodium (Corticosteroid may alter the response to coumarin anticoagulant). Products include:

Coumadin 926

DEXATRIM MAXIMUM STRENGTH CAFFEINE-FREE CAPLETS

(Phenylpropanolamine Hydrochloride) .... ⓢⓓ 832

May interact with monoamine oxidase inhibitors. Compounds in this category include:

Furazolidone (Concurrent and/or sequential use is not recommended). Products include:

Furoxone 2046

Isocarboxazid (Concurrent and/or sequential use is not recommended).

No products indexed under this heading.

Phenelzine Sulfate (Concurrent and/or sequential use is not recommended). Products include:

Nardil 1920

Phenylpropanolamine Containing Anorectics (Concurrent use with phenylpropanolamine-containing products should be avoided).

Selegiline Hydrochloride (Concurrent and/or sequential use is not recommended). Products include:

Eldepryl Tablets 2550

Tranylcypromine Sulfate (Concurrent and/or sequential use is not recommended). Products include:

Parnate Tablets 2503

DEXATRIM MAXIMUM STRENGTH EXTENDED DURATION TIME TABLETS

(Phenylpropanolamine Hydrochloride) .... ⓢⓓ 832

See Dexatrim Maximum Strength Caffeine-Free Caplets

DEXATRIM MAXIMUM STRENGTH PLUS VITAMIN C/CAFFEINE-FREE CAPLETS

(Phenylpropanolamine Hydrochloride, Vitamin C) .... ⓢⓓ 832

See Dexatrim Maximum Strength Caffeine-Free Caplets

DEXATRIM PLUS VITAMINS CAPLETS

(Phenylpropanolamine Hydrochloride, Vitamins with Minerals) .... ⓢⓓ 832

May interact with monoamine oxidase inhibitors and certain other agents. Compounds in these categories include:

Furazolidone (Concurrent and/or sequential use is not recommended). Products include:

Furoxone 2046

Isocarboxazid (Concurrent and/or sequential use is not recommended).

No products indexed under this heading.

Phenelzine Sulfate (Concurrent and/or sequential use is not recommended). Products include:

Nardil 1920

Phenylpropanolamine (Concurrent use with any form of phenylpropanolamine is not recommended).

Selegiline Hydrochloride (Concurrent and/or sequential use is not recommended). Products include:

Eldepryl Tablets 2550

Tranylcypromine Sulfate (Concurrent and/or sequential use is not recommended). Products include:

Parnate Tablets 2503

DEXEDRINE SPANSULE CAPSULES

(Dextroamphetamine Sulfate) 2474

May interact with monoamine oxidase inhibitors, tricyclic antidepressants, antihistamines, antihypertensives, beta blockers, veratrum alkaloids, thiazides, urinary alkalizing agents, and certain other agents. Compounds in these categories include:

Acebutolol Hydrochloride (Amphetamine may antagonize the hypotensive effects of antihypertensives; adrenergic blockers are inhibited by amphetamines). Products include:

Sectral Capsules 2807

Acetazolamide (Increases the concentration of the non-ionized species of the amphetamine molecule, thereby decreasing urinary excretion; increases amphetamines blood levels and thereby potentiates the actions of amphetamines). Products include:

Diamox Sequels (Sustained Release) 1373
Diamox Sequels (Sustained Release) .... ⓒ 319
Diamox Tablets 1372
Diamox Tablets .... ⓒ 317

Acetazolamide Sodium (Increases the concentration of the non-ionized species of the amphetamine molecule, thereby decreasing urinary excretion; increases amphetamines blood levels and thereby potentiates the actions of amphetamines). Products include:

Diamox Intravenous 1372
Diamox Intravenous .... ⓒ 317

Acrivastine (Amphetamines may counteract the sedative effect of antihistamine). Products include:

Semprex-D Capsules 463
Semprex-D Capsules 1167

Amitriptyline Hydrochloride (Enhanced activity of tricyclic or sympathomimetics; possible increases in the brain concentration of d-amphetamine in the brain; cardiovascular effect may be potentiated). Products include:

Elavil 2838
Endep Tablets 2174
Etrafon 2355
Limbitrol 2180
Triavil Tablets 1757

Amlodipine Besylate (Amphetamine may antagonize the hypotensive effects of antihypertensives). Products include:

Lotrel Capsules 840
Norvasc Tablets 1940

Ammonium Chloride (Increases the concentration of the ionized species of the amphetamine molecule, thereby increasing urinary excretion; lowers amphetamines blood levels and efficacy).

No products indexed under this heading.

Amoxapine (Enhanced activity of tricyclic or sympathomimetics; possible increases in the brain concentration of d-amphetamine in the brain; cardiovascular effect may be potentiated). Products include:

Asendin Tablets 1369

Astemizole (Amphetamines may counteract the sedative effect of antihistamine). Products include:

Hismanal Tablets 1293

Atenolol (Amphetamine may antagonize the hypotensive effects of antihypertensives; adrenergic blockers are inhibited by amphetamines). Products include:

Tenoretic Tablets 2845
Tenormin Tablets and I.V. Injection 2847

Azatadine Maleate (Amphetamines may counteract the sedative effect of antihistamine). Products include:

Trinalin Repetabs Tablets 1330

Benazepril Hydrochloride (Amphetamine may antagonize the hypotensive effects of antihypertensives). Products include:

Lotensin Tablets 834
Lotensin HCT 837
Lotrel Capsules 840

Bendroflumethiazide (Increases the concentration of the non-ionized species of the amphetamine molecule, thereby decreasing urinary excretion; increases amphetamines blood levels and thereby potentiates the actions of amphetamines).

No products indexed under this heading.

Betaxolol Hydrochloride (Amphetamine may antagonize the hypotensive effects of antihypertensives; adrenergic blockers are inhibited by amphetamines). Products include:

Betoptic Ophthalmic Solution............ 469
Betoptic S Ophthalmic Suspension 471
Kerlone Tablets 2436

Bisoprolol Fumarate (Amphetamine may antagonize the hypotensive effects of antihypertensives; adrenergic blockers are inhibited by amphetamines). Products include:

Zebeta Tablets 1413
Ziac 1415

Bromodiphenhydramine Hydrochloride (Amphetamines may counteract the sedative effect of antihistamine).

No products indexed under this heading.

Brompheniramine Maleate (Amphetamines may counteract the sedative effect of antihistamine). Products include:

Alka Seltzer Plus Sinus Medicine .. ⓢⓓ 707
Bromfed Capsules (Extended-Release) 1785
Bromfed Syrup .... ⓢⓓ 733
Bromfed Tablets 1785
Bromfed-DM Cough Syrup 1786
Bromfed-PD Capsules (Extended-Release) 1785
Dimetane-DC Cough Syrup 2059
Dimetane-DX Cough Syrup 2059
Dimetapp Elixir .... ⓢⓓ 773
Dimetapp Extentabs .... ⓢⓓ 774
Dimetapp Tablets/Liqui-Gels .... ⓢⓓ 775
Dimetapp Cold & Allergy Chewable Tablets .... ⓢⓓ 773
Dimetapp DM Elixir .... ⓢⓓ 774
Vicks DayQuil Allergy Relief 12-Hour Extended Release Tablets.. ⓢⓓ 760
Vicks DayQuil Allergy Relief 4-Hour Tablets .... ⓢⓓ 760

Captopril (Amphetamine may antagonize the hypotensive effects of antihypertensives). Products include:

Capoten 739
Capozide 742

Carteolol Hydrochloride (Amphetamine may antagonize the hypotensive effects of antihypertensives; adrenergic blockers are inhibited by amphetamines). Products include:

Cartrol Tablets 410
Ocupress Ophthalmic Solution, 1% Sterile .... ⓒ 309

Chlorothiazide (Increases the concentration of the non-ionized species of the amphetamine molecule, thereby decreasing urinary excretion; increases amphetamines blood levels and thereby potentiates the actions of amphetamines). Products include:

Aldoclor Tablets 1598
Diupres Tablets 1650
Diuril Oral 1653

Chlorothiazide Sodium (Increases the concentration of the non-ionized species of the amphetamine molecule, thereby decreasing urinary excretion; increases amphetamines blood levels and thereby potentiates the actions of amphetamines). Products include:

Diuril Sodium Intravenous 1652

Chlorpheniramine Maleate (Amphetamines may counteract the sedative effect of antihistamine). Products include:

Alka-Seltzer Plus Cold Medicine .... ⓢⓓ 705
Alka-Seltzer Plus Cold Medicine Liqui-Gels .... ⓢⓓ 706
Alka-Seltzer Plus Cold & Cough Medicine .... ⓢⓓ 708
Alka-Seltzer Plus Cold & Cough Medicine Liqui-Gels .... ⓢⓓ 705
Allerest Children's Chewable Tablets .... ⓢⓓ 627
Allerest Headache Strength Tablets .... ⓢⓓ 627
Allerest Maximum Strength Tablets .... ⓢⓓ 627
Allerest Sinus Pain Formula .... ⓢⓓ 627
Allerest 12 Hour Caplets .... ⓢⓓ 627
Ana-Kit Anaphylaxis Emergency Treatment Kit 617
Atrohist Pediatric Capsules 453
Atrohist Plus Tablets 454
BC Cold Powder Multi-Symptom Formula (Cold-Sinus-Allergy) ...... ⓢⓓ 609
Cerose DM .... ⓢⓓ 878
Cheracol Plus Head Cold/Cough Formula .... ⓢⓓ 769
Children's Vicks DayQuil Allergy Relief .... ⓢⓓ 757
Children's Vicks NyQuil Cold/Cough Relief .... ⓢⓓ 758
Chlor-Trimeton Allergy Decongestant Tablets .... ⓢⓓ 799
Chlor-Trimeton Allergy Tablets ...... ⓢⓓ 798
Comhist 2038
Comtrex Multi-Symptom Cold Reliever Tablets/Caplets/Liqui-Gels/Liquid .... ⓢⓓ 615
Allergy-Sinus Comtrex Multi-Symptom Allergy-Sinus Formula Tablets .... ⓢⓓ 617
Contac Continuous Action Nasal Decongestant/Antihistamine 12 Hour Capsules .... ⓢⓓ 813
Contac Maximum Strength Continuous Action Decongestant/Antihistamine 12 Hour Caplets.. ⓢⓓ 813
Contac Severe Cold and Flu Formula Caplets .... ⓢⓓ 814
Coricidin 'D' Decongestant Tablets .... ⓢⓓ 800
Coricidin Tablets .... ⓢⓓ 800
D.A. Chewable Tablets 951
Deconamine 1320
Dura-Tap/PD Capsules 2867
Dura-Vent/DA Tablets 953
Extendryl 1005
Fedahist Gyrocaps 2401
Fedahist Timecaps 2401
Hycomine Compound Tablets 932
Isoclor Timesule Capsules .... ⓢⓓ 637
Kronofed-A 977
Nolamine Timed-Release Tablets 785
Novahistine DH 2462
Novahistine Elixir .... ⓢⓓ 823
Ornade Spansule Capsules 2502
PediaCare Cold Allergy Chewable Tablets .... ⓢⓓ 677

IMPORTANT NOTE: Always consult each drug listing in the patient's regimen for possible interactions.

PediaCare Cough-Cold Chewable Tablets 1553
PediaCare Cough-Cold Liquid 1553
PediaCare NightRest Cough-Cold Liquid 1553
Pediatric Vicks 44m Cough & Cold Relief .... ◘ 764
Pyrroxate Caplets .... ◘ 772
Ryna .... ◘ 841
Sinarest Tablets .... ◘ 648
Sinarest Extra Strength Tablets .... ◘ 648
Sine-Off Sinus Medicine .... ◘ 825
Singlet Tablets .... ◘ 825
Sinulin Tablets 787
Sinutab Sinus Allergy Medication, Maximum Strength Tablets and Caplets .... ◘ 860
Sudafed Plus Liquid .... ◘ 862
Sudafed Plus Tablets .... ◘ 863
Teldrin 12 Hour Antihistamine/Nasal Decongestant Allergy Relief Capsules .... ◘ 826
TheraFlu .... ◘ 787
TheraFlu Maximum Strength Nighttime Flu, Cold & Cough Medicine .... ◘ 788
Triaminic Allergy Tablets .... ◘ 789
Triaminic Cold Tablets .... ◘ 790
Triaminic Nite Light .... ◘ 791
Triaminic Syrup .... ◘ 792
Triaminic-12 Tablets .... ◘ 792
Triaminicin Tablets .... ◘ 793
Triaminicol Multi-Symptom Cold Tablets .... ◘ 793
Triaminicol Multi-Symptom Relief ◘ 794
Tussend 1783
Children's TYLENOL Cold Multi-Symptom Liquid Formula and Chewable Tablets 1561
Children's TYLENOL Cold Plus Cough Multi Symptom Tablets and Liquid .... ◘ 681
TYLENOL Maximum Strength Allergy Sinus Medication Gelcaps and Caplets 1563
TYLENOL Cold Multi-Symptom Formula Medication Tablets and Caplets 1561
TYLENOL Cold Multi-Symptom Hot Medication Liquid Packets 1557
Vicks 44 LiquiCaps Cough, Cold & Flu Relief .... ◘ 755
Vicks 44M Cough, Cold & Flu Relief .... ◘ 756

Chlorpheniramine Polistirex (Amphetamines may counteract the sedative effect of antihistamine). Products include:
Tussionex Pennkinetic Extended-Release Suspension 998

Chlorpheniramine Tannate (Amphetamines may counteract the sedative effect of antihistamine). Products include:
Atrohist Pediatric Suspension 454
Ricobid Tablets and Pediatric Suspension 2038
Rynatan 2673
Rynatuss 2673

Chlorpromazine (Blocks dopamine and norepinephrine reuptake resulting in inhibition of central stimulating effects). Products include:
Thorazine Suppositories 2523

Chlorpromazine Hydrochloride (Blocks dopamine and norepinephrine reuptake resulting in inhibition of central stimulating effects). Products include:
Thorazine 2523

Chlorthalidone (Amphetamine may antagonize the hypotensive effects of antihypertensives). Products include:
Combipres Tablets 677
Tenoretic Tablets 2845
Thalitone 1245

Clemastine Fumarate (Amphetamines may counteract the sedative effect of antihistamine). Products include:
Tavist Syrup 2297
Tavist Tablets 2298
Tavist-1 12 Hour Relief Tablets .... ◘ 787
Tavist-D 12 Hour Relief Tablets .... ◘ 787

Clomipramine Hydrochloride (Enhanced activity of tricyclic or sympathomimetics; possible increases in the brain concentration of d-amphetamine in the brain; cardiovascular effect may be potentiated). Products include:
Anafranil Capsules 803

Clonidine (Amphetamine may antagonize the hypotensive effects of antihypertensives). Products include:
Catapres-TTS 675

Clonidine Hydrochloride (Amphetamine may antagonize the hypotensive effects of antihypertensives). Products include:
Catapres Tablets 674
Combipres Tablets 677

Cryptenamine Preparations (Amphetamines inhibit the hypotensive effect of veratrum alkaloids).

Cyproheptadine Hydrochloride (Amphetamines may counteract the sedative effect of antihistamine). Products include:
Periactin 1724

Deserpidine (Amphetamine may antagonize the hypotensive effects of antihypertensives).
No products indexed under this heading.

Desipramine Hydrochloride (Enhanced activity of tricyclic or sympathomimetics; possible increases in the brain concentration of d-amphetamine in the brain; cardiovascular effect may be potentiated). Products include:
Norpramin Tablets 1526

Dexchlorpheniramine Maleate (Amphetamines may counteract the sedative effect of antihistamine).
No products indexed under this heading.

Diazoxide (Amphetamine may antagonize the hypotensive effects of antihypertensives). Products include:
Hyperstat I.V. Injection 2363
Proglycem 580

Diltiazem Hydrochloride (Amphetamine may antagonize the hypotensive effects of antihypertensives). Products include:
Cardizem CD Capsules 1506
Cardizem SR Capsules 1510
Cardizem Injectable 1508
Cardizem Tablets 1512
Dilacor XR Extended-release Capsules 2018

Diphenhydramine Citrate (Amphetamines may counteract the sedative effect of antihistamine). Products include:
Excedrin P.M. Analgesic/Sleeping Aid Tablets, Caplets, Liquigels 733

Diphenhydramine Hydrochloride (Amphetamines may counteract the sedative effect of antihistamine). Products include:
Actifed Allergy Daytime/Nighttime Caplets .... ◘ 844
Actifed Sinus Daytime/Nighttime Tablets and Caplets .... ◘ 846
Arthritis Foundation NightTime Caplets .... ◘ 674
Extra Strength Bayer PM Aspirin .. ◘ 713
Bayer Select Night Time Pain Relief Formula .... ◘ 716
Benadryl Allergy Decongestant Liquid Medication .... ◘ 848
Benadryl Allergy Decongestant Tablets .... ◘ 848
Benadryl Allergy Liquid Medication .... ◘ 849
Benadryl Allergy .... ◘ 848
Benadryl Allergy Sinus Headache Formula Caplets .... ◘ 849
Benadryl Capsules 1898
Benadryl Dye-Free Allergy Liquigel Softgels .... ◘ 850
Benadryl Dye-Free Allergy Liquid Medication .... ◘ 850
Benadryl Itch Relief Cream, Children's Formula and Maximum Strength 2% .... ◘ 851
Benadryl Itch Relief Spray, Children's Formula and Maximum Strength 2% .... ◘ 851
Benadryl Itch Relief Stick Maximum Strength 2% .... ◘ 850
Benadryl Itch Stopping Gel, Children's Formula and Maximum Strength 2% .... ◘ 851
Benadryl Kapseals 1898
Benadryl Injection 1898
Contac Day & Night Cold/Flu Night Caplets .... ◘ 812
Contac Night Allergy/Sinus Caplets .... ◘ 812
Extra Strength Doan's P.M. .... ◘ 633
Legatrin PM .... ◘ 651
Miles Nervine Nighttime Sleep-Aid ◘ 723
Nytol QuickCaps Caplets .... ◘ 610
Sleepinal Night-time Sleep Aid Capsules and Softgels .... ◘ 834
TYLENOL Maximum Strength Allergy Sinus NightTime Medication Caplets 1555
TYLENOL Flu NightTime, Maximum Strength, Gelcaps 1566
TYLENOL Maximum Strength Flu NightTime Hot Medication Packets 1562
TYLENOL PM, Extra Strength Pain Reliever/Sleep Aid Caplets, Geltabs, Gelcaps 1560
TYLENOL Severe Allergy Medication Caplets 1564
Maximum Strength Unisom Sleepgels 1934
Unisom With Pain Relief-Nighttime Sleep Aid and Pain Reliever 1934

Diphenylpyraline Hydrochloride (Amphetamines may counteract the sedative effect of antihistamine).
No products indexed under this heading.

Doxazosin Mesylate (Amphetamine may antagonize the hypotensive effects of antihypertensives). Products include:
Cardura Tablets 2186

Doxepin Hydrochloride (Enhanced activity of tricyclic or sympathomimetics; possible increases in the brain concentration of d-amphetamine in the brain; cardiovascular effect may be potentiated). Products include:
Sinequan 2205
Zonalon Cream 1055

Enalapril Maleate (Amphetamine may antagonize the hypotensive effects of antihypertensives). Products include:
Vaseretic Tablets 1765
Vasotec Tablets 1771

Enalaprilat (Amphetamine may antagonize the hypotensive effects of antihypertensives). Products include:
Vasotec I.V. 1768

Esmolol Hydrochloride (Amphetamine may antagonize the hypotensive effects of antihypertensives; adrenergic blockers are inhibited by amphetamines). Products include:
Brevibloc Injection 1808

Ethosuximide (Amphetamine may delay intestinal absorption of ethosuximide). Products include:
Zarontin Capsules 1928
Zarontin Syrup 1929

Felodipine (Amphetamine may antagonize the hypotensive effects of antihypertensives). Products include:
Plendil Extended-Release Tablets 527

Fosinopril Sodium (Amphetamine may antagonize the hypotensive effects of antihypertensives). Products include:
Monopril Tablets 757

Furazolidone (Concurrent and/or sequential use is contraindicated; hypertensive crisis may result). Products include:
Furoxone 2046

Furosemide (Amphetamine may antagonize the hypotensive effects of antihypertensives). Products include:
Lasix Injection, Oral Solution and Tablets 1240

Glutamic Acid Hydrochloride (Lowers absorption of amphetamines).
No products indexed under this heading.

Guanabenz Acetate (Amphetamine may antagonize the hypotensive effects of antihypertensives).
No products indexed under this heading.

Guanethidine Monosulfate (Lowers absorption of amphetamines). Products include:
Esimil Tablets 822
Ismelin Tablets 827

Haloperidol (Blocks dopamine and norepinephrine reuptake resulting in inhibition of central stimulating effects). Products include:
Haldol Injection, Tablets and Concentrate 1575

Haloperidol Decanoate (Blocks dopamine and norepinephrine reuptake resulting in inhibition of central stimulating effects). Products include:
Haldol Decanoate 1577

Hydralazine Hydrochloride (Amphetamine may antagonize the hypotensive effects of antihypertensives). Products include:
Apresazide Capsules 808
Apresoline Hydrochloride Tablets .. 809
Ser-Ap-Es Tablets 849

Hydrochlorothiazide (Increases the concentration of the non-ionized species of the amphetamine molecule, thereby decreasing urinary excretion; increases amphetamines blood levels and thereby potentiates the actions of amphetamines). Products include:
Aldactazide 2413
Aldoril Tablets 1604
Apresazide Capsules 808
Capozide 742
Dyazide 2479
Esidrix Tablets 821
Esimil Tablets 822
HydroDIURIL Tablets 1674
Hydropres Tablets 1675
Hyzaar Tablets 1677
Inderide Tablets 2732
Inderide LA Long Acting Capsules .. 2734
Lopressor HCT Tablets 832
Lotensin HCT 837
Maxzide 1380
Moduretic Tablets 1705
Oretic Tablets 443
Prinzide Tablets 1737
Ser-Ap-Es Tablets 849
Timolide Tablets 1748
Vaseretic Tablets 1765
Zestoretic 2850
Ziac 1415

Hydroflumethiazide (Increases the concentration of the non-ionized species of the amphetamine molecule, thereby decreasing urinary excretion; increases amphetamines blood levels and thereby potentiates the actions of amphetamines). Products include:
Diucardin Tablets 2718

(◘ Described in PDR For Nonprescription Drugs) (⊙ Described in PDR For Ophthalmology)

265 Interactions Index Dexedrine

Imipramine Hydrochloride (Enhanced activity of tricyclic or sympathomimetics; possible increases in the brain concentration of d-amphetamine in the brain; cardiovascular effect may be potentiated). Products include:

Tofranil Ampuls ... 854
Tofranil Tablets ... 856

Imipramine Pamoate (Enhanced activity of tricyclic or sympathomimetics; possible increases in the brain concentration of d-amphetamine in the brain; cardiovascular effect may be potentiated). Products include:

Tofranil-PM Capsules ... 857

Indapamide (Amphetamine may antagonize the hypotensive effects of antihypertensives). Products include:

Lozol Tablets ... 2022

Isocarboxazid (Concurrent and/or sequential use is contraindicated; hypertensive crisis may result).

No products indexed under this heading.

Isradipine (Amphetamine may antagonize the hypotensive effects of antihypertensives). Products include:

DynaCirc Capsules ... 2256

Labetalol Hydrochloride (Amphetamine may antagonize the hypotensive effects of antihypertensives; adrenergic blockers are inhibited by amphetamines). Products include:

Normodyne Injection ... 2377
Normodyne Tablets ... 2379
Trandate ... 1185

Levobunolol Hydrochloride (Amphetamine may antagonize the hypotensive effects of antihypertensives; adrenergic blockers are inhibited by amphetamines). Products include:

Betagan ... ◉ 233

Lisinopril (Amphetamine may antagonize the hypotensive effects of antihypertensives). Products include:

Prinivil Tablets ... 1733
Prinzide Tablets ... 1737
Zestoretic ... 2850
Zestril Tablets ... 2854

Lithium Carbonate (Inhibits anti-obesity and stimulatory effects of amphetamines). Products include:

Eskalith ... 2485
Lithium Carbonate Capsules & Tablets ... 2230
Lithonate/Lithotabs/Lithobid ... 2543

Loratadine (Amphetamines may counteract the sedative effect of antihistamine). Products include:

Claritin ... 2349
Claritin-D ... 2350

Losartan Potassium (Amphetamine may antagonize the hypotensive effects of antihypertensives). Products include:

Cozaar Tablets ... 1628
Hyzaar Tablets ... 1677

Maprotiline Hydrochloride (Enhanced activity of tricyclic or sympathomimetics; possible increases in the brain concentration of d-amphetamine in the brain; cardiovascular effect may be potentiated). Products include:

Ludiomil Tablets ... 843

Mecamylamine Hydrochloride (Amphetamine may antagonize the hypotensive effects of antihypertensives). Products include:

Inversine Tablets ... 1686

Meperidine Hydrochloride (Amphetamine potentiates the analgesic effect of meperidine). Products include:

Demerol ... 2308
Mepergan Injection ... 2753

Methdilazine Hydrochloride (Amphetamines may counteract the sedative effect of antihistamine).

No products indexed under this heading.

Methenamine (Acidifying agents used in methenamine therapy increases the urinary excretion and reduces the efficacy of amphetamine). Products include:

Urised Tablets ... 1964

Methenamine Hippurate (Acidifying agents used in methenamine therapy increases the urinary excretion and reduces the efficacy of amphetamine).

No products indexed under this heading.

Methenamine Mandelate (Acidifying agents used in methenamine therapy increases the urinary excretion and reduces the efficacy of amphetamine). Products include:

Uroqid-Acid No. 2 Tablets ... 640

Methyclothiazide (Increases the concentration of the non-ionized species of the amphetamine molecule, thereby decreasing urinary excretion; increases amphetamines blood levels and thereby potentiates the actions of amphetamines). Products include:

Enduron Tablets ... 420

Methyldopa (Amphetamine may antagonize the hypotensive effects of antihypertensives). Products include:

Aldoclor Tablets ... 1598
Aldomet Oral ... 1600
Aldoril Tablets ... 1604

Methyldopate Hydrochloride (Amphetamine may antagonize the hypotensive effects of antihypertensives). Products include:

Aldomet Ester HCl Injection ... 1602

Metipranolol Hydrochloride (Amphetamine may antagonize the hypotensive effects of antihypertensives; adrenergic blockers are inhibited by amphetamines). Products include:

OptiPranolol (Metipranolol 0.3%) Sterile Ophthalmic Solution ... ◉ 258

Metolazone (Amphetamine may antagonize the hypotensive effects of antihypertensives). Products include:

Mykrox Tablets ... 993
Zaroxolyn Tablets ... 1000

Metoprolol Succinate (Amphetamine may antagonize the hypotensive effects of antihypertensives; adrenergic blockers are inhibited by amphetamines). Products include:

Toprol-XL Tablets ... 565

Metoprolol Tartrate (Amphetamine may antagonize the hypotensive effects of antihypertensives; adrenergic blockers are inhibited by amphetamines). Products include:

Lopressor Ampuls ... 830
Lopressor HCT Tablets ... 832
Lopressor Tablets ... 830

Metyrosine (Amphetamine may antagonize the hypotensive effects of antihypertensives). Products include:

Demser Capsules ... 1649

Minoxidil (Amphetamine may antagonize the hypotensive effects of antihypertensives). Products include:

Loniten Tablets ... 2618
Rogaine Topical Solution ... 2637

Moexipril Hydrochloride (Amphetamine may antagonize the hypotensive effects of antihypertensives). Products include:

Univasc Tablets ... 2410

Nadolol (Amphetamine may antagonize the hypotensive effects of antihypertensives; adrenergic blockers are inhibited by amphetamines).

No products indexed under this heading.

Nicardipine Hydrochloride (Amphetamine may antagonize the hypotensive effects of antihypertensives). Products include:

Cardene Capsules ... 2095
Cardene I.V. ... 2709
Cardene SR Capsules ... 2097

Nifedipine (Amphetamine may antagonize the hypotensive effects of antihypertensives). Products include:

Adalat Capsules (10 mg and 20 mg) ... 587
Adalat CC ... 589
Procardia Capsules ... 1971
Procardia XL Extended Release Tablets ... 1972

Nisoldipine (Amphetamine may antagonize the hypotensive effects of antihypertensives).

No products indexed under this heading.

Nitroglycerin (Amphetamine may antagonize the hypotensive effects of antihypertensives). Products include:

Deponit NTG Transdermal Delivery System ... 2397
Nitro-Bid IV ... 1523
Nitro-Bid Ointment ... 1524
Nitrodisc ... 2047
Nitro-Dur (nitroglycerin) Transdermal Infusion System ... 1326
Nitrolingual Spray ... 2027
Nitrostat Tablets ... 1925
Transderm-Nitro Transdermal Therapeutic System ... 859

Norepinephrine Hydrochloride (Enhances adenergic effect of norepinephrine).

Nortriptyline Hydrochloride (Enhanced activity of tricyclic or sympathomimetics; possible increases in the brain concentration of d-amphetamine in the brain; cardiovascular effect may be potentiated). Products include:

Pamelor ... 2280

Penbutolol Sulfate (Amphetamine may antagonize the hypotensive effects of antihypertensives; adrenergic blockers are inhibited by amphetamines). Products include:

Levatol ... 2403

Phenelzine Sulfate (Concurrent and/or sequential use is contraindicated; hypertensive crisis may result). Products include:

Nardil ... 1920

Phenobarbital (Amphetamine delays intestinal absorption of phenobarbital; co-administration may produce synergistic anticonvulsant action). Products include:

Arco-Lase Plus Tablets ... 512
Bellergal-S Tablets ... 2250
Donnatal ... 2060
Donnatal Extentabs ... 2061
Donnatal Tablets ... 2060
Phenobarbital Elixir and Tablets ... 1469
Quadrinal Tablets ... 1350

Phenoxybenzamine Hydrochloride (Amphetamine may antagonize the hypotensive effects of antihypertensives). Products include:

Dibenzyline Capsules ... 2476

Phentolamine Mesylate (Amphetamine may antagonize the hypotensive effects of antihypertensives). Products include:

Regitine ... 846

Phenytoin (Amphetamine delays intestinal absorption of phenytoin; co-administration may produce synergistic anticonvulsant action). Products include:

Dilantin Infatabs ... 1908
Dilantin-125 Suspension ... 1911

Phenytoin Sodium (Amphetamine delays intestinal absorption of phenytoin; co-administration may produce synergistic anticonvulsant action). Products include:

Dilantin Kapseals ... 1906
Dilantin Parenteral ... 1910

Pindolol (Amphetamine may antagonize the hypotensive effects of antihypertensives; adrenergic blockers are inhibited by amphetamines). Products include:

Visken Tablets ... 2299

Polythiazide (Increases the concentration of the non-ionized species of the amphetamine molecule, thereby decreasing urinary excretion; increases amphetamines blood levels and thereby potentiates the actions of amphetamines). Products include:

Minizide Capsules ... 1938

Potassium Citrate (Increases the concentration of the non-ionized species of the amphetamine molecule, thereby decreasing urinary excretion; increases amphetamines blood levels and thereby potentiates the actions of amphetamines). Products include:

Polycitra Syrup ... 578
Polycitra-K Crystals ... 579
Polycitra-K Oral Solution ... 579
Polycitra-LC ... 578

Prazosin Hydrochloride (Amphetamine may antagonize the hypotensive effects of antihypertensives). Products include:

Minipress Capsules ... 1937
Minizide Capsules ... 1938

Promethazine Hydrochloride (Amphetamines may counteract the sedative effect of antihistamine). Products include:

Mepergan Injection ... 2753
Phenergan with Codeine ... 2777
Phenergan with Dextromethorphan ... 2778
Phenergan Injection ... 2773
Phenergan Suppositories ... 2775
Phenergan Syrup ... 2774
Phenergan Tablets ... 2775
Phenergan VC ... 2779
Phenergan VC with Codeine ... 2781

Propoxyphene Hydrochloride (In cases of propoxyphene overdosage, amphetamine CNS stimulation is potentiated and fatal convulsions can occur). Products include:

Darvon ... 1435
Wygesic Tablets ... 2827

Propoxyphene Napsylate (In cases of propoxyphene overdosage, amphetamine CNS stimulation is potentiated and fatal convulsions can occur). Products include:

Darvon-N/Darvocet-N ... 1433

Propranolol Hydrochloride (Amphetamine may antagonize the hypotensive effects of antihypertensives; adrenergic blockers are inhibited by amphetamines). Products include:

Inderal ... 2728
Inderal LA Long Acting Capsules ... 2730
Inderide Tablets ... 2732
Inderide LA Long Acting Capsules .. 2734

IMPORTANT NOTE: Always consult each drug listing in the patient's regimen for possible interactions.

Protriptyline Hydrochloride (Enhanced activity of tricyclic or sympathomimetics; possible increases in the brain concentration of d-amphetamine in the brain; cardiovascular effect may be potentiated). Products include:
- Vivactil Tablets 1774

Pyrilamine Maleate (Amphetamines may counteract the sedative effect of antihistamine). Products include:
- 4-Way Fast Acting Nasal Spray (regular & mentholated) ▣ 621
- Maximum Strength Multi-Symptom Formula Midol ▣ 722
- PMS Multi-Symptom Formula Midol ▣ 723

Pyrilamine Tannate (Amphetamines may counteract the sedative effect of antihistamine). Products include:
- Atrohist Pediatric Suspension 454
- Rynatan 2673

Quinapril Hydrochloride (Amphetamine may antagonize the hypotensive effects of antihypertensives). Products include:
- Accupril Tablets 1893

Ramipril (Amphetamine may antagonize the hypotensive effects of antihypertensives). Products include:
- Altace Capsules 1232

Rauwolfia Serpentina (Amphetamine may antagonize the hypotensive effects of antihypertensives).
- No products indexed under this heading.

Rescinnamine (Amphetamine may antagonize the hypotensive effects of antihypertensives).
- No products indexed under this heading.

Reserpine (Lowers absorption of amphetamines). Products include:
- Diupres Tablets 1650
- Hydropres Tablets 1675
- Ser-Ap-Es Tablets 849

Selegiline Hydrochloride (Concurrent and/or sequential use is contraindicated; hypertensive crisis may result). Products include:
- Eldepryl Tablets 2550

Sodium Acid Phosphate (Increases the concentration of the ionized species of the amphetamine molecule, thereby increasing urinary excretion; lowers amphetamines blood levels and efficacy). Products include:
- Uroqid-Acid No. 2 Tablets 640

Sodium Bicarbonate (Increases absorption of amphetamines). Products include:
- Alka-Seltzer Effervescent Antacid and Pain Reliever ▣ 701
- Alka-Seltzer Extra Strength Effervescent Antacid and Pain Reliever ▣ 703
- Alka-Seltzer Gold Effervescent Antacid ▣ 703
- Alka-Seltzer Lemon Lime Effervescent Antacid and Pain Reliever ▣ 703
- Arm & Hammer Pure Baking Soda ▣ 627
- Ceo-Two Rectal Suppositories 666
- Citrocarbonate Antacid ▣ 770
- Massengill Disposable Douches ▣ 820
- Massengill Liquid Concentrate ▣ 820
- NuLYTELY 689
- Cherry Flavor NuLYTELY 689

Sodium Citrate (Increases the concentration of the non-ionized species of the amphetamine molecule, thereby decreasing urinary excretion; increases amphetamines blood levels and thereby potentiates the actions of amphetamines). Products include:
- Bicitra 578
- Citrocarbonate Antacid ▣ 770
- Polycitra 578
- Salix SST Lozenges Saliva Stimulant ▣ 797

Sodium Nitroprusside (Amphetamine may antagonize the hypotensive effects of antihypertensives).
- No products indexed under this heading.

Sotalol Hydrochloride (Amphetamine may antagonize the hypotensive effects of antihypertensives; adrenergic blockers are inhibited by amphetamines). Products include:
- Betapace Tablets 641

Spirapril Hydrochloride (Amphetamine may antagonize the hypotensive effects of antihypertensives).
- No products indexed under this heading.

Terazosin Hydrochloride (Amphetamine may antagonize the hypotensive effects of antihypertensives). Products include:
- Hytrin Capsules 430

Terfenadine (Amphetamines may counteract the sedative effect of antihistamine). Products include:
- Seldane Tablets 1536
- Seldane-D Extended-Release Tablets 1538

Timolol Hemihydrate (Amphetamine may antagonize the hypotensive effects of antihypertensives; adrenergic blockers are inhibited by amphetamines). Products include:
- Betimol 0.25%, 0.5% ◉ 261

Timolol Maleate (Amphetamine may antagonize the hypotensive effects of antihypertensives; adrenergic blockers are inhibited by amphetamines). Products include:
- Blocadren Tablets 1614
- Timolide Tablets 1748
- Timoptic in Ocudose 1753
- Timoptic Sterile Ophthalmic Solution 1751
- Timoptic-XE 1755

Torsemide (Amphetamine may antagonize the hypotensive effects of antihypertensives). Products include:
- Demadex Tablets and Injection 686

Tranylcypromine Sulfate (Concurrent and/or sequential use is contraindicated; hypertensive crisis may result). Products include:
- Parnate Tablets 2503

Trimeprazine Tartrate (Amphetamines may counteract the sedative effect of antihistamine). Products include:
- Temaril Tablets, Syrup and Spansule Extended-Release Capsules 483

Trimethaphan Camsylate (Amphetamine may antagonize the hypotensive effects of antihypertensives). Products include:
- Arfonad Ampuls 2080

Trimipramine Maleate (Enhanced activity of tricyclic or sympathomimetics; possible increases in the brain concentration of d-amphetamine in the brain; cardiovascular effect may be potentiated). Products include:
- Surmontil Capsules 2811

Tripelennamine Hydrochloride (Amphetamines may counteract the sedative effect of antihistamine). Products include:
- PBZ Tablets 845
- PBZ-SR Tablets 844

Triprolidine Hydrochloride (Amphetamines may counteract the sedative effect of antihistamine). Products include:
- Actifed Plus Caplets ▣ 845
- Actifed Plus Tablets ▣ 845
- Actifed with Codeine Cough Syrup 1067
- Actifed Syrup ▣ 846
- Actifed Tablets ▣ 844

Verapamil Hydrochloride (Amphetamine may antagonize the hypotensive effects of antihypertensives). Products include:
- Calan SR Caplets 2422
- Calan Tablets 2419
- Isoptin Injectable 1344
- Isoptin Oral Tablets 1346
- Isoptin SR Tablets 1348
- Verelan Capsules 1410
- Verelan Capsules 2824

Vitamin C (Lowers absorption of amphetamines). Products include:
- ANTIOX Capsules 1543
- C-Buff 667
- Centrum Singles Vitamin C ▣ 669
- Chromagen Capsules 2339
- Dexatrim Maximum Strength Plus Vitamin C/Caffeine-free Caplets ▣ 832
- Ester-C Mineral Ascorbates Powder ▣ 658
- Fero-Folic-500 Filmtab 429
- Fero-Grad-500 Filmtab 429
- Halls Vitamin C Drops ▣ 843
- Hyland's Vitamin C for Children ▣ 830
- Irospan 982
- Materna Tablets 1379
- Nature Made Antioxidant Formula ▣ 748
- Niferex w/Vitamin C Tablets 793
- One-A-Day Extras Antioxidant ▣ 728
- One-A-Day Extras Vitamin C ▣ 728
- Protegra Antioxidant Vitamin & Mineral Supplement ▣ 670
- Stuart Prenatal Tablets ▣ 881
- The Stuart Formula Tablets ▣ 663
- Sunkist Children's Chewable Multivitamins - Plus Extra C ▣ 649
- Sunkist Vitamin C ▣ 649
- Theragran Antioxidant ▣ 623
- Trinsicon Capsules 2570
- Vitron-C Tablets ▣ 650

Food Interactions

Fruit juices, unspecified (Lowers absorption of amphetamines).

DEXEDRINE TABLETS

(Dextroamphetamine Sulfate) 2474

See **Dexedrine Spansule Capsules**

DEXTROSTAT DEXTROAMPHETAMINE TABLETS

(Dextroamphetamine Sulfate) 2036

May interact with monoamine oxidase inhibitors, antihypertensives, beta blockers, alpha adrenergic blockers, urinary alkalizing agents, thiazides, tricyclic antidepressants, sympathomimetics, antihistamines, veratrum alkaloids, and certain other agents. Compounds in these categories include:

Acebutolol Hydrochloride (Adrenergic blockers are inhibited by amphetamines; amphetamines may antagonize the hypotensive effects of antihypertensives). Products include:
- Sectral Capsules 2807

Acetazolamide (Increases the concentration of the non-ionized species of the amphetamine molecule thereby decreasing urinary excretion; increases blood levels and potentiates the action of amphetamines). Products include:
- Diamox Sequels (Sustained Release) 1373
- Diamox Sequels (Sustained Release) ◉ 319
- Diamox Tablets 1372
- Diamox Tablets ◉ 317

Acetazolamide Sodium (Increases the concentration of the non-ionized species of the amphetamine molecule thereby decreasing urinary excretion; increases blood levels and potentiates the action of amphetamines). Products include:
- Diamox Intravenous 1372
- Diamox Intravenous ◉ 317

Acrivastine (Amphetamines may counteract the sedative effect of antihistamines). Products include:
- Semprex-D Capsules 463
- Semprex-D Capsules 1167

Albuterol (Enhanced activity of sympathomimetics). Products include:
- Proventil Inhalation Aerosol 2382
- Ventolin Inhalation Aerosol and Refill 1197

Albuterol Sulfate (Enhanced activity of sympathomimetics). Products include:
- Airet Solution for Inhalation 452
- Proventil Inhalation Solution 0.083% 2384
- Proventil Repetabs Tablets 2386
- Proventil Solution for Inhalation 0.5% 2383
- Proventil Syrup 2385
- Proventil Tablets 2386
- Ventolin Inhalation Solution 1198
- Ventolin Nebules Inhalation Solution 1199
- Ventolin Rotacaps for Inhalation 1200
- Ventolin Syrup 1202
- Ventolin Tablets 1203
- Volmax Extended-Release Tablets 1788

Amitriptyline Hydrochloride (Enhanced activity of tricyclic antidepressants; cardiovascular effects can be potentiated). Products include:
- Elavil 2838
- Endep Tablets 2174
- Etrafon 2355
- Limbitrol 2180
- Triavil Tablets 1757

Amlodipine Besylate (Amphetamines may antagonize the hypotensive effects of antihypertensives). Products include:
- Lotrel Capsules 840
- Norvasc Tablets 1940

Ammonium Chloride (Increases the concentration of ionized species of the amphetamine molecule thereby increasing urinary excretion; lowers blood levels and efficacy of amphetamines).
- No products indexed under this heading.

Amoxapine (Enhanced activity of tricyclic antidepressants; cardiovascular effects can be potentiated). Products include:
- Asendin Tablets 1369

Astemizole (Amphetamines may counteract the sedative effect of antihistamines). Products include:
- Hismanal Tablets 1293

Atenolol (Adrenergic blockers are inhibited by amphetamines; amphetamines may antagonize the hypotensive effects of antihypertensives). Products include:
- Tenoretic Tablets 2845
- Tenormin Tablets and I.V. Injection 2847

Azatadine Maleate (Amphetamines may counteract the sedative effect of antihistamines). Products include:
- Trinalin Repetabs Tablets 1330

Benazepril Hydrochloride (Amphetamines may antagonize the hypotensive effects of antihypertensives). Products include:
- Lotensin Tablets 834
- Lotensin HCT 837
- Lotrel Capsules 840

(▣ Described in PDR For Nonprescription Drugs) (◉ Described in PDR For Ophthalmology)

Interactions Index

Bendroflumethiazide (Some thiazide diuretics increase concentration of the non-ionized species of the amphetamine molecule thereby decreasing urinary excretion; increases blood levels and potentiates the action of amphetamines; amphetamines may antagonize the hypotensive effects of antihypertensives).

No products indexed under this heading.

Betaxolol Hydrochloride (Adrenergic blockers are inhibited by amphetamines; amphetamines may antagonize the hypotensive effects of antihypertensives). Products include:

Betoptic Ophthalmic Solution.......... 469
Betoptic S Ophthalmic Suspension 471
Kerlone Tablets.................................... 2436

Bisoprolol Fumarate (Adrenergic blockers are inhibited by amphetamines; amphetamines may antagonize the hypotensive effects of antihypertensives). Products include:

Zebeta Tablets 1413
Ziac 1415

Bromodiphenhydramine Hydrochloride (Amphetamines may counteract the sedative effect of antihistamines).

No products indexed under this heading.

Brompheniramine Maleate (Amphetamines may counteract the sedative effect of antihistamines). Products include:

Alka Seltzer Plus Sinus Medicine .. ⊞ 707
Bromfed Capsules (Extended-Release) 1785
Bromfed Syrup .... ⊞ 733
Bromfed Tablets 1785
Bromfed-DM Cough Syrup................ 1786
Bromfed-PD Capsules (Extended-Release).. 1785
Dimetane-DC Cough Syrup 2059
Dimetane-DX Cough Syrup 2059
Dimetapp Elixir .... ⊞ 773
Dimetapp Extentabs .... ⊞ 774
Dimetapp Tablets/Liqui-Gels .... ⊞ 775
Dimetapp Cold & Allergy Chewable Tablets .... ⊞ 773
Dimetapp DM Elixir .... ⊞ 774
Vicks DayQuil Allergy Relief 12-Hour Extended Release Tablets.. ⊞ 760
Vicks DayQuil Allergy Relief 4-Hour Tablets .... ⊞ 760

Captopril (Amphetamines may antagonize the hypotensive effects of antihypertensives). Products include:

Capoten 739
Capozide 742

Carteolol Hydrochloride (Adrenergic blockers are inhibited by amphetamines; amphetamines may antagonize the hypotensive effects of antihypertensives). Products include:

Cartrol Tablets 410
Ocupress Ophthalmic Solution, 1% Sterile.. ⊞ 309

Chlorothiazide (Some thiazide diuretics increase concentration of the non-ionized species of the amphetamine molecule thereby decreasing urinary excretion; increases blood levels and potentiates the action of amphetamines; amphetamines may antagonize the hypotensive effects of antihypertensives). Products include:

Aldoclor Tablets 1598
Diupres Tablets 1650
Diuril Oral 1653

Chlorothiazide Sodium (Some thiazide diuretics increase concentration of the non-ionized species of the amphetamine molecule thereby decreasing urinary excretion; increases blood levels and potentiates the action of amphetamines; amphetamines may antagonize the hypotensive effects of antihypertensives). Products include:

Diuril Sodium Intravenous 1652

Chlorpheniramine Maleate (Amphetamines may counteract the sedative effect of antihistamines). Products include:

Alka-Seltzer Plus Cold Medicine .... ⊞ 705
Alka-Seltzer Plus Cold Medicine Liqui-Gels .... ⊞ 706
Alka-Seltzer Plus Cold & Cough Medicine .... ⊞ 708
Alka-Seltzer Plus Cold & Cough Medicine Liqui-Gels........................ ⊞ 705
Allerest Children's Chewable Tablets .... ⊞ 627
Allerest Headache Strength Tablets .... ⊞ 627
Allerest Maximum Strength Tablets .... ⊞ 627
Allerest Sinus Pain Formula .... ⊞ 627
Allerest 12 Hour Caplets .... ⊞ 627
Ana-Kit Anaphylaxis Emergency Treatment Kit 617
Atrorhist Pediatric Capsules 453
Atrorhist Plus Tablets 454
BC Cold Powder Multi-Symptom Formula (Cold-Sinus-Allergy) ...... ⊞ 609
Cerose DM .... ⊞ 878
Cheracol Plus Head Cold/Cough Formula .... ⊞ 769
Children's Vicks DayQuil Allergy Relief.. ⊞ 757
Children's Vicks NyQuil Cold/Cough Relief...................................... ⊞ 758
Chlor-Trimeton Allergy Decongestant Tablets .... ⊞ 799
Chlor-Trimeton Allergy Tablets ...... ⊞ 798
Comhist 2038
Comtrex Multi-Symptom Cold Reliever Tablets/Caplets/Liqui-Gels/Liquid.. ⊞ 615
Allergy-Sinus Comtrex Multi-Symptom Allergy-Sinus Formula Tablets .... ⊞ 617
Contac Continuous Action Nasal Decongestant/Antihistamine 12 Hour Capsules.................................. ⊞ 813
Contac Maximum Strength Continuous Action Decongestant/Antihistamine 12 Hour Caplets.. ⊞ 813
Contac Severe Cold and Flu Formula Caplets .... ⊞ 814
Coricidin 'D' Decongestant Tablets .... ⊞ 800
Coricidin Tablets .... ⊞ 800
D.A. Chewable Tablets........................ 951
Deconamine 1320
Dura-Tap/PD Capsules 2867
Dura-Vent/DA Tablets 953
Extendryl 1005
Fedahist Gyrocaps................................ 2401
Fedahist Timecaps 2401
Hycomine Compound Tablets 932
Isoclor Timesule Capsules .... ⊞ 637
Kronofed-A 977
Nolamine Timed-Release Tablets 785
Novahistine DH.................................... 2462
Novahistine Elixir .... ⊞ 823
Ornade Spansule Capsules 2502
PediaCare Cold Allergy Chewable Tablets .... ⊞ 677
PediaCare Cough-Cold Chewable Tablets 1553
PediaCare Cough-Cold Liquid............ 1553
PediaCare NightRest Cough-Cold Liquid 1553
Pediatric Vicks 44m Cough & Cold Relief .... ⊞ 764
Pyrroxate Caplets .... ⊞ 772
Ryna .... ⊞ 841
Sinarest Tablets .... ⊞ 648
Sinarest Extra Strength Tablets........ ⊞ 648
Sine-Off Sinus Medicine .... ⊞ 825
Singlet Tablets .... ⊞ 825
Sinulin Tablets 787
Sinutab Sinus Allergy Medication, Maximum Strength Tablets and Caplets .... ⊞ 860
Sudafed Plus Liquid .... ⊞ 862
Sudafed Plus Tablets .... ⊞ 863

Teldrin 12 Hour Antihistamine/Nasal Decongestant Allergy Relief Capsules .... ⊞ 826
TheraFlu.. ⊞ 787
TheraFlu Maximum Strength Nighttime Flu, Cold & Cough Medicine .... ⊞ 788
Triaminic Allergy Tablets .... ⊞ 789
Triaminic Cold Tablets .... ⊞ 790
Triaminic Nite Light .... ⊞ 791
Triaminic Syrup .... ⊞ 792
Triaminic-12 Tablets .... ⊞ 792
Triaminicin Tablets .... ⊞ 793
Triaminicol Multi-Symptom Cold Tablets .... ⊞ 793
Triaminicol Multi-Symptom Relief ⊞ 794
Tussend 1783
Children's TYLENOL Cold Multi-Symptom Liquid Formula and Chewable Tablets................................ 1561
Children's TYLENOL Cold Plus Cough Multi Symptom Tablets and Liquid .... ⊞ 681
TYLENOL Maximum Strength Allergy Sinus Medication Gelcaps and Caplets 1563
TYLENOL Cold Multi-Symptom Formula Medication Tablets and Caplets 1561
TYLENOL Cold Multi-Symptom Hot Medication Liquid Packets.............. 1557
Vicks 44 LiquiCaps Cough, Cold & Flu Relief .... ⊞ 755
Vicks 44M Cough, Cold & Flu Relief.. ⊞ 756

Chlorpheniramine Polistirex (Amphetamines may counteract the sedative effect of antihistamines). Products include:

Tussionex Pennkinetic Extended-Release Suspension 998

Chlorpheniramine Tannate (Amphetamines may counteract the sedative effect of antihistamines). Products include:

Atrorhist Pediatric Suspension 454
Ricobid Tablets and Pediatric Suspension.. 2038
Rynatan 2673
Rynatuss 2673

Chlorpromazine (Inhibits central stimulant effects of amphetamines). Products include:

Thorazine Suppositories 2523

Chlorpromazine Hydrochloride (Inhibits central stimulant effects of amphetamines). Products include:

Thorazine 2523

Chlorthalidone (Amphetamines may antagonize the hypotensive effects of antihypertensives). Products include:

Combipres Tablets 677
Tenoretic Tablets.................................. 2845
Thalitone 1245

Clemastine Fumarate (Amphetamines may counteract the sedative effect of antihistamines). Products include:

Tavist Syrup.. 2297
Tavist Tablets 2298
Tavist-1 12 Hour Relief Tablets .... ⊞ 787
Tavist-D 12 Hour Relief Tablets .... ⊞ 787

Clomipramine Hydrochloride (Enhanced activity of tricyclic antidepressants; cardiovascular effects can be potentiated). Products include:

Anafranil Capsules 803

Clonidine (Amphetamines may antagonize the hypotensive effects of antihypertensives). Products include:

Catapres-TTS.. 675

Clonidine Hydrochloride (Amphetamines may antagonize the hypotensive effects of antihypertensives). Products include:

Catapres Tablets 674
Combipres Tablets 677

Cryptenamine Preparations (Amphetamines may inhibit the hypotensive effects of veratrum alkaloids).

Cyproheptadine Hydrochloride (Amphetamines may counteract the sedative effect of antihistamines). Products include:

Periactin 1724

Deserpidine (Amphetamines may antagonize the hypotensive effects of antihypertensives).

No products indexed under this heading.

Desipramine Hydrochloride (Enhanced activity of tricyclic antidepressants; cardiovascular effects can be potentiated). Products include:

Norpramin Tablets 1526

Dexchlorpheniramine Maleate (Amphetamines may counteract the sedative effect of antihistamines).

No products indexed under this heading.

Diazoxide (Amphetamines may antagonize the hypotensive effects of antihypertensives). Products include:

Hyperstat I.V. Injection 2363
Proglycem.. 580

Diltiazem Hydrochloride (Amphetamines may antagonize the hypotensive effects of antihypertensives). Products include:

Cardizem CD Capsules 1506
Cardizem SR Capsules 1510
Cardizem Injectable 1508
Cardizem Tablets.................................. 1512
Dilacor XR Extended-release Capsules 2018

Diphenhydramine Citrate (Amphetamines may counteract the sedative effect of antihistamines). Products include:

Excedrin P.M. Analgesic/Sleeping Aid Tablets, Caplets, Liquigels...... 733

Diphenhydramine Hydrochloride (Amphetamines may counteract the sedative effect of antihistamines). Products include:

Actifed Allergy Daytime/Nighttime Caplets.. ⊞ 844
Actifed Sinus Daytime/Nighttime Tablets and Caplets .... ⊞ 846
Arthritis Foundation NightTime Caplets .... ⊞ 674
Extra Strength Bayer PM Aspirin .. ⊞ 713
Bayer Select Night Time Pain Relief Formula...................................... ⊞ 716
Benadryl Allergy Decongestant Liquid Medication .... ⊞ 848
Benadryl Allergy Decongestant Tablets .... ⊞ 848
Benadryl Allergy Liquid Medication.. ⊞ 849
Benadryl Allergy .... ⊞ 848
Benadryl Allergy Sinus Headache Formula Caplets .... ⊞ 849
Benadryl Capsules................................ 1898
Benadryl Dye-Free Allergy Liquigel Softgels.. ⊞ 850
Benadryl Dye-Free Allergy Liquid Medication .... ⊞ 850
Benadryl Itch Relief Cream, Children's Formula and Maximum Strength 2% .... ⊞ 851
Benadryl Itch Relief Spray, Children's Formula and Maximum Strength 2% .... ⊞ 851
Benadryl Itch Relief Stick Maximum Strength 2% .... ⊞ 850
Benadryl Itch Stopping Gel, Children's Formula and Maximum Strength 2% .... ⊞ 851
Benadryl Kapseals................................ 1898
Benadryl Injection 1898
Contac Day & Night Cold/Flu Night Caplets...................................... ⊞ 812
Contac Night Allergy/Sinus Caplets .... ⊞ 812
Extra Strength Doan's P.M................ ⊞ 633
Legatrin PM .... ⊞ 651
Miles Nervine Nighttime Sleep-Aid ⊞ 723
Nytol QuickCaps Caplets .... ⊞ 610
Sleepinal Night-time Sleep Aid Capsules and Softgels .... ⊞ 834
TYLENOL Maximum Strength Allergy Sinus NightTime Medication Caplets 1555

IMPORTANT NOTE: Always consult each drug listing in the patient's regimen for possible interactions.

DextroStat Interactions Index 268

TYLENOL Flu NightTime, Maximum Strength, Gelcaps ... 1566
TYLENOL Maximum Strength Flu NightTime Hot Medication Packets ... 1562
TYLENOL PM, Extra Strength Pain Reliever/Sleep Aid Caplets, Geltabs, Gelcaps ... 1560
TYLENOL Severe Allergy Medication Caplets ... 1564
Maximum Strength Unisom Sleepgels ... 1934
Unisom With Pain Relief-Nighttime Sleep Aid and Pain Reliever ... 1934

Diphenylpyraline Hydrochloride (Amphetamines may counteract the sedative effect of antihistamines).
No products indexed under this heading.

Dobutamine Hydrochloride (Enhanced activity of sympathomimetics). Products include:
Dobutrex Solution Vials ... 1439

Dopamine Hydrochloride (Enhanced activity of sympathomimetics).
No products indexed under this heading.

Doxazosin Mesylate (Adrenergic blockers are inhibited by amphetamines; amphetamines may antagonize the hypotensive effects of antihypertensives). Products include:
Cardura Tablets ... 2186

Doxepin Hydrochloride (Enhanced activity of tricyclic antidepressants; cardiovascular effects can be potentiated). Products include:
Sinequan ... 2205
Zonalon Cream ... 1055

Enalapril Maleate (Amphetamines may antagonize the hypotensive effects of antihypertensives). Products include:
Vaseretic Tablets ... 1765
Vasotec Tablets ... 1771

Enalaprilat (Amphetamines may antagonize the hypotensive effects of antihypertensives). Products include:
Vasotec I.V. ... 1768

Ephedrine Hydrochloride (Enhanced activity of sympathomimetics). Products include:
Primatene Dual Action Formula ... ▣ 872
Primatene Tablets ... ▣ 873
Quadrinal Tablets ... 1350

Ephedrine Sulfate (Enhanced activity of sympathomimetics). Products include:
Bronkaid Caplets ... ▣ 717
Marax Tablets & DF Syrup ... 2200

Ephedrine Tannate (Enhanced activity of sympathomimetics). Products include:
Rynatuss ... 2673

Epinephrine (Enhanced activity of sympathomimetics). Products include:
Bronkaid Mist ... ▣ 717
EPIFRIN ... ◉ 239
EpiPen ... 790
Marcaine Hydrochloride with Epinephrine 1:200,000 ... 2316
Primatene Mist ... ▣ 873
Sensorcaine with Epinephrine Injection ... 559
Sus-Phrine Injection ... 1019
Xylocaine with Epinephrine Injections ... 567

Epinephrine Bitartrate (Enhanced activity of sympathomimetics). Products include:
Bronkaid Mist Suspension ... ▣ 718
Sensorcaine-MPF with Epinephrine Injection ... 559

Epinephrine Hydrochloride (Enhanced activity of sympathomimetics). Products include:
Ana-Kit Anaphylaxis Emergency Treatment Kit ... 617

Esmolol Hydrochloride (Adrenergic blockers are inhibited by amphetamines; amphetamines may antagonize the hypotensive effects of antihypertensives). Products include:
Brevibloc Injection ... 1808

Ethosuximide (Delayed intestinal absorption of ethosuximide). Products include:
Zarontin Capsules ... 1928
Zarontin Syrup ... 1929

Felodipine (Amphetamines may antagonize the hypotensive effects of antihypertensives). Products include:
Plendil Extended-Release Tablets ... 527

Fosinopril Sodium (Amphetamines may antagonize the hypotensive effects of antihypertensives). Products include:
Monopril Tablets ... 757

Furazolidone (Potential for hypertensive crisis; slows amphetamine metabolism; concurrent and/or sequential use is contraindicated). Products include:
Furoxone ... 2046

Furosemide (Amphetamines may antagonize the hypotensive effects of antihypertensives). Products include:
Lasix Injection, Oral Solution and Tablets ... 1240

Glutamic Acid Hydrochloride (Lowers absorption of amphetamines by acting as gastrointestinal acidifying agent).
No products indexed under this heading.

Guanabenz Acetate (Amphetamines may antagonize the hypotensive effects of antihypertensives).
No products indexed under this heading.

Guanethidine Monosulfate (Lowers absorption of amphetamines by acting as gastrointestinal acidifying agent; amphetamines may antagonize the hypotensive effects of antihypertensives). Products include:
Esimil Tablets ... 822
Ismelin Tablets ... 827

Haloperidol (Inhibits central stimulant effects of amphetamines). Products include:
Haldol Injection, Tablets and Concentrate ... 1575

Haloperidol Decanoate (Inhibits central stimulant effects of amphetamines). Products include:
Haldol Decanoate ... 1577

Hydralazine Hydrochloride (Amphetamines may antagonize the hypotensive effects of antihypertensives). Products include:
Apresazide Capsules ... 808
Apresoline Hydrochloride Tablets ... 809
Ser-Ap-Es Tablets ... 849

Hydrochlorothiazide (Some thiazide diuretics increase concentration of the non-ionized species of the amphetamine molecule thereby decreasing urinary excretion; increases blood levels and potentiates the action of amphetamines; amphetamines may antagonize the hypotensive effects of antihypertensives). Products include:
Aldactazide ... 2413
Aldoril Tablets ... 1604
Apresazide Capsules ... 808
Capozide ... 742
Dyazide ... 2479
Esidrix Tablets ... 821
Esimil Tablets ... 822
HydroDIURIL Tablets ... 1674
Hydropres Tablets ... 1675
Hyzaar Tablets ... 1677
Inderide Tablets ... 2732
Inderide LA Long Acting Capsules ... 2734
Lopressor HCT Tablets ... 832
Lotensin HCT ... 837
Maxzide ... 1380
Moduretic Tablets ... 1705
Oretic Tablets ... 443
Prinzide Tablets ... 1737
Ser-Ap-Es Tablets ... 849
Timolide Tablets ... 1748
Vaseretic Tablets ... 1765
Zestoretic ... 2850
Ziac ... 1415

Hydroflumethiazide (Some thiazide diuretics increase concentration of the non-ionized species of the amphetamine molecule thereby decreasing urinary excretion; increases blood levels and potentiates the action of amphetamines; amphetamines may antagonize the hypotensive effects of antihypertensives). Products include:
Diucardin Tablets ... 2718

Imipramine Hydrochloride (Enhanced activity of tricyclic antidepressants; cardiovascular effects can be potentiated). Products include:
Tofranil Ampuls ... 854
Tofranil Tablets ... 856

Imipramine Pamoate (Enhanced activity of tricyclic antidepressants; cardiovascular effects can be potentiated). Products include:
Tofranil-PM Capsules ... 857

Indapamide (Amphetamines may antagonize the hypotensive effects of antihypertensives). Products include:
Lozol Tablets ... 2022

Isocarboxazid (Potential for hypertensive crisis; slows amphetamine metabolism; concurrent and/or sequential use is contraindicated).
No products indexed under this heading.

Isoproterenol Hydrochloride (Enhanced activity of sympathomimetics). Products include:
Isuprel Hydrochloride Injection 1:5000 ... 2311
Isuprel Hydrochloride Solution 1:200 & 1:100 ... 2313
Isuprel Mistometer ... 2312

Isoproterenol Sulfate (Enhanced activity of sympathomimetics). Products include:
Norisodrine with Calcium Iodide Syrup ... 442

Isradipine (Amphetamines may antagonize the hypotensive effects of antihypertensives). Products include:
DynaCirc Capsules ... 2256

Labetalol Hydrochloride (Adrenergic blockers are inhibited by amphetamines; amphetamines may antagonize the hypotensive effects of antihypertensives). Products include:
Normodyne Injection ... 2377
Normodyne Tablets ... 2379
Trandate ... 1185

Levobunolol Hydrochloride (Adrenergic blockers are inhibited by amphetamines; amphetamines may antagonize the hypotensive effects of antihypertensives). Products include:
Betagan ... ◉ 233

Lisinopril (Amphetamines may antagonize the hypotensive effects of antihypertensives). Products include:
Prinivil Tablets ... 1733
Prinzide Tablets ... 1737
Zestoretic ... 2850
Zestril Tablets ... 2854

Lithium Carbonate (Inhibits anti-obesity and stimulatory effects). Products include:
Eskalith ... 2485
Lithium Carbonate Capsules & Tablets ... 2230
Lithonate/Lithotabs/Lithobid ... 2543

Loratadine (Amphetamines may counteract the sedative effect of antihistamines). Products include:
Claritin ... 2349
Claritin-D ... 2350

Losartan Potassium (Amphetamines may antagonize the hypotensive effects of antihypertensives). Products include:
Cozaar Tablets ... 1628
Hyzaar Tablets ... 1677

Maprotiline Hydrochloride (Enhanced activity of tricyclic antidepressants; cardiovascular effects can be potentiated). Products include:
Ludiomil Tablets ... 843

Mecamylamine Hydrochloride (Amphetamines may antagonize the hypotensive effects of antihypertensives). Products include:
Inversine Tablets ... 1686

Meperidine Hydrochloride (Analgesic effect of meperidine potentiated). Products include:
Demerol ... 2308
Mepergan Injection ... 2753

Metaproterenol Sulfate (Enhanced activity of sympathomimetics). Products include:
Alupent ... 669
Metaproterenol Sulfate Inhalation Solution, USP, Arm-a-Med ... 552

Metaraminol Bitartrate (Enhanced activity of sympathomimetics). Products include:
Aramine Injection ... 1609

Methdilazine Hydrochloride (Amphetamines may counteract the sedative effect of antihistamines).
No products indexed under this heading.

Methenamine (Increases urinary excretion and efficacy is reduced by acidifying agents used in methenamine therapy). Products include:
Urised Tablets ... 1964

Methenamine Hippurate (Increases urinary excretion and efficacy is reduced by acidifying agents used in methenamine therapy).
No products indexed under this heading.

Methenamine Mandelate (Increases urinary excretion and efficacy is reduced by acidifying agents used in methenamine therapy). Products include:
Uroqid-Acid No. 2 Tablets ... 640

Methoxamine Hydrochloride (Enhanced activity of sympathomimetics). Products include:
Vasoxyl Injection ... 1196

Methyclothiazide (Some thiazide diuretics increase concentration of the non-ionized species of the amphetamine molecule thereby decreasing urinary excretion; increases blood levels and potentiates the action of amphetamines; amphetamines may antagonize the hypotensive effects of antihypertensives). Products include:
Enduron Tablets ... 420

Methyldopa (Amphetamines may antagonize the hypotensive effects of antihypertensives). Products include:
Aldoclor Tablets ... 1598
Aldomet Oral ... 1600
Aldoril Tablets ... 1604

(▣ Described in PDR For Nonprescription Drugs) (◉ Described in PDR For Ophthalmology)

Methyldopate Hydrochloride (Amphetamines may antagonize the hypotensive effects of antihypertensives). Products include:

Aldomet Ester HCl Injection 1602

Metipranolol Hydrochloride (Adrenergic blockers are inhibited by amphetamines; amphetamines may antagonize the hypotensive effects of antihypertensives). Products include:

OptiPranolol (Metipranolol 0.3%) Sterile Ophthalmic Solution.......... ◉ 258

Metolazone (Amphetamines may antagonize the hypotensive effects of antihypertensives). Products include:

Mykrox Tablets 993
Zaroxolyn Tablets 1000

Metoprolol Succinate (Adrenergic blockers are inhibited by amphetamines; amphetamines may antagonize the hypotensive effects of antihypertensives). Products include:

Toprol-XL Tablets 565

Metoprolol Tartrate (Adrenergic blockers are inhibited by amphetamines; amphetamines may antagonize the hypotensive effects of antihypertensives). Products include:

Lopressor Ampuls 830
Lopressor HCT Tablets 832
Lopressor Tablets 830

Metyrosine (Amphetamines may antagonize the hypotensive effects of antihypertensives). Products include:

Demser Capsules 1649

Minoxidil (Amphetamines may antagonize the hypotensive effects of antihypertensives). Products include:

Loniten Tablets 2618
Rogaine Topical Solution 2637

Moexipril Hydrochloride (Amphetamines may antagonize the hypotensive effects of antihypertensives). Products include:

Univasc Tablets 2410

Nadolol (Adrenergic blockers are inhibited by amphetamines; amphetamines may antagonize the hypotensive effects of antihypertensives).

No products indexed under this heading.

Nicardipine Hydrochloride (Amphetamines may antagonize the hypotensive effects of antihypertensives). Products include:

Cardene Capsules 2095
Cardene I.V. 2709
Cardene SR Capsules............................... 2097

Nifedipine (Amphetamines may antagonize the hypotensive effects of antihypertensives). Products include:

Adalat Capsules (10 mg and 20 mg) 587
Adalat CC 589
Procardia Capsules................................... 1971
Procardia XL Extended Release Tablets 1972

Nisoldipine (Amphetamines may antagonize the hypotensive effects of antihypertensives).

No products indexed under this heading.

Nitroglycerin (Amphetamines may antagonize the hypotensive effects of antihypertensives). Products include:

Deponit NTG Transdermal Delivery System 2397
Nitro-Bid IV... 1523
Nitro-Bid Ointment 1524
Nitrodisc 2047
Nitro-Dur (nitroglycerin) Transdermal Infusion System 1326
Nitrolingual Spray 2027
Nitrostat Tablets 1925
Transderm-Nitro Transdermal Therapeutic System 859

Norepinephrine Bitartrate (Enhanced activity of sympathomimetics). Products include:

Levophed Bitartrate Injection 2315

Norepinephrine Hydrochloride (Enhanced adrenergic effect of norepinephrine).

Nortriptyline Hydrochloride (Enhanced activity of tricyclic antidepressants; cardiovascular effects can be potentiated). Products include:

Pamelor 2280

Penbutolol Sulfate (Adrenergic blockers are inhibited by amphetamines; amphetamines may antagonize the hypotensive effects of antihypertensives). Products include:

Levatol 2403

Phenelzine Sulfate (Potential for hypertensive crisis; slows amphetamine metabolism; concurrent and/or sequential use is contraindicated). Products include:

Nardil 1920

Phenobarbital (Delayed intestinal absorption of phenobarbital; synergistic anticonvulsant action may be produced). Products include:

Arco-Lase Plus Tablets 512
Bellergal-S Tablets 2250
Donnatal 2060
Donnatal Extentabs.................................. 2061
Donnatal Tablets 2060
Phenobarbital Elixir and Tablets 1469
Quadrinal Tablets 1350

Phenoxybenzamine Hydrochloride (Amphetamines may antagonize the hypotensive effects of antihypertensives). Products include:

Dibenzyline Capsules 2476

Phentolamine Mesylate (Amphetamines may antagonize the hypotensive effects of antihypertensives). Products include:

Regitine 846

Phenylephrine Bitartrate (Enhanced activity of sympathomimetics).

No products indexed under this heading.

Phenylephrine Hydrochloride (Enhanced activity of sympathomimetics). Products include:

Atrohist Plus Tablets 454
Cerose DM .... ◙ 878
Comhist 2038
D.A. Chewable Tablets............................. 951
Deconsal Pediatric Capsules.................. 454
Dura-Vent/DA Tablets 953
Entex Capsules 1986
Entex Liquid 1986
Extendryl 1005
4-Way Fast Acting Nasal Spray (regular & mentholated).................. ◙ 621
Hemorid For Women .... ◙ 834
Hycomine Compound Tablets 932
Neo-Synephrine Hydrochloride 1% Carpuject.. 2324
Neo-Synephrine Hydrochloride 1% Injection 2324
Neo-Synephrine Hydrochloride (Ophthalmic) 2325
Neo-Synephrine .... ◙ 726
Nōstril.. ◙ 644
Novahistine Elixir .... ◙ 823
Phenergan VC 2779
Phenergan VC with Codeine 2781
Preparation H .... ◙ 871
Tympagesic Ear Drops 2342
Vasosulf .... ◉ 271
Vicks Sinex Nasal Spray and Ultra Fine Mist .... ◙ 765

Phenylephrine Tannate (Enhanced activity of sympathomimetics). Products include:

Atrohist Pediatric Suspension 454
Ricobid-D Pediatric Suspension........ 2038

Ricobid Tablets and Pediatric Suspension... 2038
Rynatan 2673
Rynatuss 2673

Phenylpropanolamine Hydrochloride (Enhanced activity of sympathomimetics). Products include:

Acutrim .... ◙ 628
Allerest Children's Chewable Tablets .... ◙ 627
Allerest 12 Hour Caplets .... ◙ 627
Atrohist Plus Tablets 454
BC Cold Powder Multi-Symptom Formula (Cold-Sinus-Allergy) ...... ◙ 609
BC Cold Powder Non-Drowsy Formula (Cold-Sinus) .... ◙ 609
Cheracol Plus Head Cold/Cough Formula .... ◙ 769
Comtrex Multi-Symptom Non-Drowsy Liqui-gels.................................. ◙ 618
Contac Continuous Action Nasal Decongestant/Antihistamine 12 Hour Capsules..................................... ◙ 813
Contac Maximum Strength Continuous Action Decongestant/ Antihistamine 12 Hour Caplets.. ◙ 813
Contac Severe Cold and Flu Formula Caplets .... ◙ 814
Coricidin 'D' Decongestant Tablets .... ◙ 800
Dexatrim .... ◙ 832
Dexatrim Plus Vitamins Caplets .... ◙ 832
Dimetane-DC Cough Syrup 2059
Dimetapp Elixir .... ◙ 773
Dimetapp Extentabs .... ◙ 774
Dimetapp Tablets/Liqui-Gels .... ◙ 775
Dimetapp Cold & Allergy Chewable Tablets .... ◙ 773
Dimetapp DM Elixir .... ◙ 774
Dura-Vent Tablets 952
Entex Capsules 1986
Entex LA Tablets 1987
Entex Liquid 1986
Exgest LA Tablets 782
Hycomine 931
Isoclor Timesule Capsules .... ◙ 637
Nolamine Timed-Release Tablets 785
Ornade Spansule Capsules 2502
Propagest Tablets 786
Pyrroxate Caplets .... ◙ 772
Robitussin-CF .... ◙ 777
Sinulin Tablets 787
Tavist-D 12 Hour Relief Tablets .... ◙ 787
Teldrin 12 Hour Antihistamine/ Nasal Decongestant Allergy Relief Capsules..................................... ◙ 826
Triaminic Allergy Tablets .... ◙ 789
Triaminic Cold Tablets .... ◙ 790
Triaminic Expectorant .... ◙ 790
Triaminic Syrup .... ◙ 792
Triaminic-12 Tablets .... ◙ 792
Triaminic-DM Syrup .... ◙ 792
Triaminicin Tablets .... ◙ 793
Triaminicol Multi-Symptom Cold Tablets .... ◙ 793
Triaminicol Multi-Symptom Relief ◙ 794
Vicks DayQuil Allergy Relief 12-Hour Extended Release Tablets.. ◙ 760
Vicks DayQuil Allergy Relief 4-Hour Tablets .... ◙ 760
Vicks DayQuil SINUS Pressure & CONGESTION Relief.......................... ◙ 761

Phenytoin (Delayed intestinal absorption of phenobarbital; synergistic anticonvulsant action may be produced). Products include:

Dilantin Infatabs.. 1908
Dilantin-125 Suspension 1911

Phenytoin Sodium (Delayed intestinal absorption of phenobarbital; synergistic anticonvulsant action may be produced). Products include:

Dilantin Kapseals 1906
Dilantin Parenteral 1910

Pindolol (Adrenergic blockers are inhibited by amphetamines; amphetamines may antagonize the hypotensive effects of antihypertensives). Products include:

Visken Tablets.. 2299

Pirbuterol Acetate (Enhanced activity of sympathomimetics). Products include:

Maxair Autohaler 1492
Maxair Inhaler 1494

Polythiazide (Some thiazide diuretics increase concentration of the non-ionized species of the amphetamine molecule thereby decreasing urinary excretion; increases blood levels and potentiates the action of amphetamines; amphetamines may antagonize the hypotensive effects of antihypertensives). Products include:

Minizide Capsules 1938

Potassium Citrate (Increases the concentration of the non-ionized species of the amphetamine molecule thereby decreasing urinary excretion; increases blood levels and potentiates the action of amphetamines). Products include:

Polycitra Syrup 578
Polycitra-K Crystals 579
Polycitra-K Oral Solution 579
Polycitra-LC 578

Prazosin Hydrochloride (Adrenergic blockers are inhibited by amphetamines; amphetamines may antagonize the hypotensive effects of antihypertensives). Products include:

Minipress Capsules................................... 1937
Minizide Capsules 1938

Promethazine Hydrochloride (Amphetamines may counteract the sedative effect of antihistamines). Products include:

Mepergan Injection 2753
Phenergan with Codeine 2777
Phenergan with Dextromethorphan 2778
Phenergan Injection 2773
Phenergan Suppositories 2775
Phenergan Syrup 2774
Phenergan Tablets 2775
Phenergan VC 2779
Phenergan VC with Codeine 2781

Propoxyphene Hydrochloride (In cases of propoxyphene overdosage, amphetamine CNS stimulation is potentiated and fatal convulsions can occur). Products include:

Darvon 1435
Wygesic Tablets 2827

Propoxyphene Napsylate (In cases of propoxyphene overdosage, amphetamine CNS stimulation is potentiated and fatal convulsions can occur). Products include:

Darvon-N/Darvocet-N 1433

Propranolol Hydrochloride (Adrenergic blockers are inhibited by amphetamines; amphetamines may antagonize the hypotensive effects of antihypertensives). Products include:

Inderal 2728
Inderal LA Long Acting Capsules 2730
Inderide Tablets 2732
Inderide LA Long Acting Capsules .. 2734

Protriptyline Hydrochloride (Enhanced activity of tricyclic antidepressants; cardiovascular effects can be potentiated). Products include:

Vivactil Tablets 1774

Pseudoephedrine Hydrochloride (Enhanced activity of sympathomimetics). Products include:

Actifed Allergy Daytime/Nighttime Caplets .... ◙ 844
Actifed Plus Caplets .... ◙ 845
Actifed Plus Tablets .... ◙ 845
Actifed with Codeine Cough Syrup.. 1067
Actifed Sinus Daytime/Nighttime Tablets and Caplets .... ◙ 846
Actifed Syrup.. ◙ 846
Actifed Tablets .... ◙ 844
Advil Cold and Sinus Caplets and Tablets (formerly CoAdvil) .... ◙ 870
Alka-Seltzer Plus Cold Medicine Liqui-Gels .... ◙ 706
Alka-Seltzer Plus Cold & Cough Medicine Liqui-Gels............................ ◙ 705
Alka-Seltzer Plus Night-Time Cold Medicine Liqui-Gels............................ ◙ 706

IMPORTANT NOTE: Always consult each drug listing in the patient's regimen for possible interactions.

DextroStat **Interactions Index** 270

Allerest Headache Strength Tablets ■ 627
Allerest Maximum Strength Tablets ■ 627
Allerest No Drowsiness Tablets ■ 627
Allerest Sinus Pain Formula ■ 627
Anatuss LA Tablets 1542
Atrohist Pediatric Capsules 453
Bayer Select Sinus Pain Relief Formula ■ 717
Benadryl Allergy Decongestant Liquid Medication ■ 848
Benadryl Allergy Decongestant Tablets ■ 848
Benadryl Allergy Sinus Headache Formula Caplets ■ 849
Benylin Multisymptom ■ 852
Bromfed Capsules (Extended-Release) 1785
Bromfed Syrup ■ 733
Bromfed Tablets 1785
Bromfed-DM Cough Syrup 1786
Bromfed-PD Capsules (Extended-Release) 1785
Children's Vicks DayQuil Allergy Relief ■ 757
Children's Vicks NyQuil Cold/Cough Relief ■ 758
Comtrex Multi-Symptom Cold Reliever Tablets/Caplets/Liqui-Gels/Liquid ■ 615
Allergy-Sinus Comtrex Multi-Symptom Allergy-Sinus Formula Tablets ■ 617
Comtrex Multi-Symptom Non-Drowsy Caplets ■ 618
Congess 1004
Contac Day Allergy/Sinus Caplets ■ 812
Contac Day & Night ■ 812
Contac Night Allergy/Sinus Caplets ■ 812
Contac Severe Cold & Flu Non-Drowsy ■ 815
Deconamine Chewable Tablets 1320
Deconamine CX Cough and Cold Liquid and Tablets 1319
Deconamine 1320
Deconsal C Expectorant Syrup 456
Deconsal Pediatric Syrup 457
Deconsal II Tablets 454
Dimetane-DX Cough Syrup 2059
Dimetapp Sinus Caplets ■ 775
Dorcol Children's Cough Syrup ■ 785
Drixoral Cough + Congestion Liquid Caps ■ 802
Dura-Tap/PD Capsules 2867
Duratuss Tablets 2565
Duratuss HD Elixir 2565
Efidac/24 ■ 635
Entex PSE Tablets 1987
Fedahist Gyrocaps 2401
Fedahist Timecaps 2401
Guaifed 1787
Guaifed Syrup ■ 734
Guaimax-D Tablets 792
Guaitab Tablets ■ 734
Isoclor Expectorant 990
Kronofed-A 977
Motrin IB Sinus ■ 838
Novahistine DH 2462
Novahistine DMX ■ 822
Novahistine Expectorant 2463
Nucofed 2051
PediaCare Cold Allergy Chewable Tablets ■ 677
PediaCare Cough-Cold Chewable Tablets 1553
PediaCare 1553
PediaCare Infants' Decongestant Drops ■ 677
PediCare Infant's Drops Decongestant Plus Cough 1553
PediaCare NightRest Cough-Cold Liquid 1553
Pediatric Vicks 44d Dry Hacking Cough & Head Congestion ■ 763
Pediatric Vicks 44m Cough & Cold Relief ■ 764
Robitussin Cold & Cough Liqui-Gels ■ 776
Robitussin Maximum Strength Cough & Cold ■ 778
Robitussin Pediatric Cough & Cold Formula ■ 779
Robitussin Severe Congestion Liqui-Gels ■ 776
Robitussin-DAC Syrup 2074
Robitussin-PE ■ 778
Rondec Oral Drops 953
Rondec Syrup 953
Rondec Tablet 953
Rondec-DM Oral Drops 954
Rondec-DM Syrup 954
Rondec-TR Tablet 953
Ryna ■ 841
Seldane-D Extended-Release Tablets 1538
Semprex-D Capsules 463
Semprex-D Capsules 1167
Sinarest Tablets ■ 648
Sinarest Extra Strength Tablets ■ 648
Sinarest No Drowsiness Tablets ■ 648
Sine-Aid IB Caplets 1554
Sine-Aid Maximum Strength Sinus Medication Gelcaps, Caplets and Tablets 1554
Sine-Off No Drowsiness Formula Caplets ■ 824
Sine-Off Sinus Medicine ■ 825
Singlet Tablets ■ 825
Sinutab Non-Drying Liquid Caps ■ 859
Sinutab Sinus Allergy Medication, Maximum Strength Tablets and Caplets ■ 860
Sinutab Sinus Medication, Maximum Strength Without Drowsiness Formula, Tablets & Caplets ■ 860
Sinutab Sinus Medication, Regular Strength Without Drowsiness Formula ■ 859
Sudafed Children's Liquid ■ 861
Sudafed Cold and Cough Liquidcaps ■ 862
Sudafed Cough Syrup ■ 862
Sudafed Plus Liquid ■ 862
Sudafed Plus Tablets ■ 863
Sudafed Severe Cold Formula Caplets ■ 863
Sudafed Severe Cold Formula Tablets ■ 864
Sudafed Sinus Caplets ■ 864
Sudafed Sinus Tablets ■ 864
Sudafed Tablets, 30 mg ■ 861
Sudafed Tablets, 60 mg ■ 861
Sudafed 12 Hour Caplets ■ 861
Syn-Rx Tablets 465
Syn-Rx DM Tablets 466
TheraFlu ■ 787
TheraFlu Maximum Strength Nighttime Flu, Cold & Cough Medicine ■ 788
TheraFlu Maximum Strength Non-Drowsy Formula Flu, Cold & Cough Medicine ■ 788
Thera Flu Maximum Strength, Non-Drowsy Formula Flu, Cold and Cough Caplets ■ 789
Triaminic AM Cough and Decongestant Formula ■ 789
Triaminic AM Decongestant Formula ■ 790
Triaminic Nite Light ■ 791
Triaminic Sore Throat Formula ■ 791
Tussend 1783
Tussend Expectorant 1785
Children's TYLENOL Cold Multi-Symptom Liquid Formula and Chewable Tablets 1561
Children's TYLENOL Cold Plus Cough Multi Symptom Tablets and Liquid ■ 681
Infants' TYLENOL Cold Decongestant & Fever-Reducer Drops 1556
TYLENOL Maximum Strength Allergy Sinus Medication Gelcaps and Caplets 1563
TYLENOL Maximum Strength Allergy Sinus NightTime Medication Caplets 1555
TYLENOL Flu Maximum Strength Gelcaps 1565
TYLENOL Flu NightTime, Maximum Strength, Gelcaps 1566
TYLENOL Maximum Strength Flu NightTime Hot Medication Packets 1562
TYLENOL, Maximum Strength, Sinus Medication Geltabs, Gelcaps, Caplets and Tablets 1566
TYLENOL Cold Multi-Symptom Formula Medication Tablets and Caplets 1561
TYLENOL Cold Medication No Drowsiness Formula Gelcaps and Caplets 1562
TYLENOL Cold Multi-Symptom Hot Medication Liquid Packets 1557
TYLENOL Cough Multi-Symptom Medication with Decongestant 1565
Ursinus Inlay-Tabs ■ 794
Vicks 44 LiquiCaps Cough, Cold & Flu Relief ■ 755
Vicks 44 LiquiCaps Non-Drowsy Cough & Cold Relief ■ 756
Vicks 44D Dry Hacking Cough & Head Congestion ■ 755
Vicks 44M Cough, Cold & Flu Relief ■ 756
Vicks DayQuil ■ 761
Vicks DayQuil SINUS Pressure & PAIN Relief with IBUPROFEN ■ 762
Vicks Nyquil Hot Therapy ■ 762
Vicks NyQuil LiquiCaps Multi-Symptom Cold/Flu Relief ■ 763
Vicks NyQuil Multi-Symptom Cold/Flu Relief - (Original & Cherry Flavor) ■ 763

Pseudoephedrine Sulfate (Enhanced activity of sympathomimetics). Products include:
Cheracol Sinus ■ 768
Chlor-Trimeton Allergy Decongestant Tablets ■ 799
Claritin-D 2350
Drixoral Cold and Allergy Sustained-Action Tablets ■ 802
Drixoral Cold and Flu Extended-Release Tablets ■ 803
Drixoral Non-Drowsy Formula Extended-Release Tablets ■ 803
Drixoral Allergy/Sinus Extended Release Tablets ■ 804
Trinalin Repetabs Tablets 1330

Pyrilamine Maleate (Amphetamines may counteract the sedative effect of antihistamines). Products include:
4-Way Fast Acting Nasal Spray (regular & mentholated) ■ 621
Maximum Strength Multi-Symptom Formula Midol ■ 722
PMS Multi-Symptom Formula Midol ■ 723

Pyrilamine Tannate (Amphetamines may counteract the sedative effect of antihistamines). Products include:
Atrohist Pediatric Suspension 454
Rynatan 2673

Quinapril Hydrochloride (Amphetamines may antagonize the hypotensive effects of antihypertensives). Products include:
Accupril Tablets 1893

Ramipril (Amphetamines may antagonize the hypotensive effects of antihypertensives). Products include:
Altace Capsules 1232

Rauwolfia Serpentina (Amphetamines may antagonize the hypotensive effects of antihypertensives).
No products indexed under this heading.

Rescinnamine (Amphetamines may antagonize the hypotensive effects of antihypertensives).
No products indexed under this heading.

Reserpine (Lowers absorption of amphetamines by acting as gastrointestinal acidifying agent; amphetamines may antagonize the hypotensive effects of antihypertensives). Products include:
Diupres Tablets 1650
Hydropres Tablets 1675
Ser-Ap-Es Tablets 849

Salmeterol Xinafoate (Enhanced activity of sympathomimetics). Products include:
Serevent Inhalation Aerosol 1176

Selegiline Hydrochloride (Potential for hypertensive crisis; slows amphetamine metabolism; concurrent and/or sequential use is contraindicated). Products include:
Eldepryl Tablets 2550

Sodium Acid Phosphate (Increases the concentration of ionized species of the amphetamine molecule thereby increasing urinary excretion; lowers blood levels and efficacy of amphetamines). Products include:
Uroqid-Acid No. 2 Tablets 640

Sodium Bicarbonate (Increases absorption of amphetamines; increases blood levels and potentiates the action of amphetamines). Products include:
Alka-Seltzer Effervescent Antacid and Pain Reliever ■ 701
Alka-Seltzer Extra Strength Effervescent Antacid and Pain Reliever ■ 703
Alka-Seltzer Gold Effervescent Antacid ■ 703
Alka-Seltzer Lemon Lime Effervescent Antacid and Pain Reliever ■ 703
Arm & Hammer Pure Baking Soda ■ 627
Ceo-Two Rectal Suppositories 666
Citrocarbonate Antacid ■ 770
Massengill Disposable Douches ■ 820
Massengill Liquid Concentrate ■ 820
NuLYTELY 689
Cherry Flavor NuLYTELY 689

Sodium Citrate (Increases the concentration of the non-ionized species of the amphetamine molecule thereby decreasing urinary excretion; increases blood levels and potentiates the action of amphetamines). Products include:
Bicitra 578
Citrocarbonate Antacid ■ 770
Polycitra 578
Salix SST Lozenges Saliva Stimulant ■ 797

Sodium Nitroprusside (Amphetamines may antagonize the hypotensive effects of antihypertensives).
No products indexed under this heading.

Sotalol Hydrochloride (Adrenergic blockers are inhibited by amphetamines; amphetamines may antagonize the hypotensive effects of antihypertensives). Products include:
Betapace Tablets 641

Spirapril Hydrochloride (Amphetamines may antagonize the hypotensive effects of antihypertensives).
No products indexed under this heading.

Terazosin Hydrochloride (Adrenergic blockers are inhibited by amphetamines; amphetamines may antagonize the hypotensive effects of antihypertensives). Products include:
Hytrin Capsules 430

Terbutaline Sulfate (Enhanced activity of sympathomimetics). Products include:
Brethaire Inhaler 813
Brethine Ampuls 815
Brethine Tablets 814
Bricanyl Subcutaneous Injection 1502
Bricanyl Tablets 1503

Terfenadine (Amphetamines may counteract the sedative effect of antihistamines). Products include:
Seldane Tablets 1536
Seldane-D Extended-Release Tablets 1538

Timolol Hemihydrate (Adrenergic blockers are inhibited by amphetamines; amphetamines may antagonize the hypotensive effects of antihypertensives). Products include:
Betimol 0.25%, 0.5% ⊙ 261

(■ Described in PDR For Nonprescription Drugs) (⊙ Described in PDR For Ophthalmology)

Timolol Maleate (Adrenergic blockers are inhibited by amphetamines; amphetamines may antagonize the hypotensive effects of antihypertensives). Products include:

Blocadren Tablets 1614
Timolide Tablets...................................... 1748
Timoptic in Ocudose 1753
Timoptic Sterile Ophthalmic Solution... 1751
Timoptic-XE 1755

Torsemide (Amphetamines may antagonize the hypotensive effects of antihypertensives). Products include:

Demadex Tablets and Injection 686

Tranylcypromine Sulfate (Potential for hypertensive crisis; slows amphetamine metabolism; concurrent and/or sequential use is contraindicated). Products include:

Parnate Tablets 2503

Trimeprazine Tartrate (Amphetamines may counteract the sedative effect of antihistamines). Products include:

Temaril Tablets, Syrup and Spansule Extended-Release Capsules.. 483

Trimethaphan Camsylate (Amphetamines may antagonize the hypotensive effects of antihypertensives). Products include:

Arfonad Ampuls 2080

Trimipramine Maleate (Enhanced activity of tricyclic antidepressants; cardiovascular effects can be potentiated). Products include:

Surmontil Capsules................................ 2811

Tripelennamine Hydrochloride (Amphetamines may counteract the sedative effect of antihistamines). Products include:

PBZ Tablets 845
PBZ-SR Tablets... 844

Triprolidine Hydrochloride (Amphetamines may counteract the sedative effect of antihistamines). Products include:

Actifed Plus Caplets .... ◾ 845
Actifed Plus Tablets .... ◾ 845
Actifed with Codeine Cough Syrup.. 1067
Actifed Syrup.. ◾ 846
Actifed Tablets .... ◾ 844

Verapamil Hydrochloride (Amphetamines may antagonize the hypotensive effects of antihypertensives). Products include:

Calan SR Caplets 2422
Calan Tablets... 2419
Isoptin Injectable 1344
Isoptin Oral Tablets 1346
Isoptin SR Tablets 1348
Verelan Capsules 1410
Verelan Capsules 2824

Vitamin C (Lowers absorption of amphetamines by acting as gastrointestinal acidifying agent). Products include:

ANTIOX Capsules 1543
C-Buff 667
Centrum Singles Vitamin C .... ◾ 669
Chromagen Capsules.............................. 2339
Dexatrim Maximum Strength Plus Vitamin C/Caffeine-free Caplets ◾ 832
Ester-C Mineral Ascorbates Powder .... ◾ 658
Fero-Folic-500 Filmtab 429
Fero-Grad-500 Filmtab......................... 429
Halls Vitamin C Drops .... ◾ 843
Hyland's Vitamin C for Children .... ◾ 830
Irospan 982
Materna Tablets 1379
Nature Made Antioxidant Formula ◾ 748
Niferex w/Vitamin C Tablets.............. 793
One-A-Day Extras Antioxidant .... ◾ 728
One-A-Day Extras Vitamin C .... ◾ 728
Protegra Antioxidant Vitamin & Mineral Supplement .... ◾ 670
Stuart Prenatal Tablets .... ◾ 881
The Stuart Formula Tablets................ ◾ 663
Sunkist Children's Chewable Multivitamins - Plus Extra C .... ◾ 649
Sunkist Vitamin C .... ◾ 649
Theragran Antioxidant........................... ◾ 623
Trinsicon Capsules 2570
Vitron-C Tablets .... ◾ 650

Food Interactions

Fruit juices, unspecified (Lowers absorption of amphetamines by acting as gastrointestinal acidifying agent).

DIABETA TABLETS

(Glyburide) 1239

May interact with salicylates, sulfonamides, oral anticoagulants, monoamine oxidase inhibitors, beta blockers, thiazides, diuretics, corticosteroids, phenothiazines, thyroid preparations, estrogens, oral contraceptives, sympathomimetics, calcium channel blockers, non-steroidal anti-inflammatory agents, highly protein bound drugs (selected), fluoroquinolone antibiotics, and certain other agents. Compounds in these categories include:

Acebutolol Hydrochloride (Potentiates the hypoglycemic action; patients should be observed for hypoglycemia or loss of control). Products include:

Sectral Capsules 2807

Albuterol (Potential for hyperglycemia leading to loss of control). Products include:

Proventil Inhalation Aerosol 2382
Ventolin Inhalation Aerosol and Refill 1197

Albuterol Sulfate (Potential for hyperglycemia leading to loss of control). Products include:

Airet Solution for Inhalation 452
Proventil Inhalation Solution 0.083% 2384
Proventil Repetabs Tablets 2386
Proventil Solution for Inhalation 0.5% 2383
Proventil Syrup 2385
Proventil Tablets 2386
Ventolin Inhalation Solution................ 1198
Ventolin Nebules Inhalation Solution 1199
Ventolin Rotacaps for Inhalation 1200
Ventolin Syrup... 1202
Ventolin Tablets 1203
Volmax Extended-Release Tablets .. 1788

Amiloride Hydrochloride (Potential for hyperglycemia leading to loss of control). Products include:

Midamor Tablets 1703
Moduretic Tablets 1705

Amiodarone Hydrochloride (Potentiates the hypoglycemic action; patients should be observed for hypoglycemia or loss of control). Products include:

Cordarone Intravenous 2715
Cordarone Tablets.................................... 2712

Amitriptyline Hydrochloride (Potentiates the hypoglycemic action; patients should be observed for hypoglycemia or loss of control). Products include:

Elavil 2838
Endep Tablets 2174
Etrafon 2355
Limbitrol 2180
Triavil Tablets 1757

Amlodipine Besylate (Potential for hyperglycemia leading to loss of control). Products include:

Lotrel Capsules.. 840
Norvasc Tablets 1940

Aspirin (Potentiates the hypoglycemic action; patients should be observed for hypoglycemia or loss of control). Products include:

Alka-Seltzer Effervescent Antacid and Pain Reliever .... ◾ 701
Alka-Seltzer Extra Strength Effervescent Antacid and Pain Reliever .... ◾ 703
Alka-Seltzer Lemon Lime Effervescent Antacid and Pain Reliever .... ◾ 703
Alka-Seltzer Plus Cold Medicine .... ◾ 705
Alka-Seltzer Plus Cold & Cough Medicine .... ◾ 708
Alka-Seltzer Plus Night-Time Cold Medicine .... ◾ 707
Alka Seltzer Plus Sinus Medicine .. ◾ 707
Arthritis Foundation Safety Coated Aspirin Tablets .... ◾ 675
Arthritis Pain Ascriptin .... ◾ 631
Maximum Strength Ascriptin .... ◾ 630
Regular Strength Ascriptin Tablets .... ◾ 629
Arthritis Strength BC Powder.......... ◾ 609
BC Cold Powder Multi-Symptom Formula (Cold-Sinus-Allergy) ...... ◾ 609
BC Cold Powder Non-Drowsy Formula (Cold-Sinus) .... ◾ 609
BC Powder .... ◾ 609
Bayer Children's Chewable Aspirin .... ◾ 711
Genuine Bayer Aspirin Tablets & Caplets .... ◾ 713
Extra Strength Bayer Arthritis Pain Regimen Formula .... ◾ 711
Extra Strength Bayer Aspirin Caplets & Tablets .... ◾ 712
Extended-Release Bayer 8-Hour Aspirin .... ◾ 712
Extra Strength Bayer Plus Aspirin Caplets .... ◾ 713
Extra Strength Bayer PM Aspirin .. ◾ 713
Bayer Enteric Aspirin .... ◾ 709
Bufferin Analgesic Tablets and Caplets .... ◾ 613
Arthritis Strength Bufferin Analgesic Caplets .... ◾ 614
Extra Strength Bufferin Analgesic Tablets .... ◾ 615
Cama Arthritis Pain Reliever............ ◾ 785
Darvon Compound-65 Pulvules 1435
Easprin 1914
Ecotrin 2455
Ecotrin Enteric Coated Aspirin Maximum Strength Tablets and Caplets .... ◾ 816
Ecotrin Enteric Coated Aspirin Regular Strength Tablets 2455
Empirin Aspirin Tablets .... ◾ 854
Empirin with Codeine Tablets........... 1093
Excedrin Extra-Strength Analgesic Tablets & Caplets 732
Fiorinal Capsules 2261
Fiorinal with Codeine Capsules 2262
Fiorinal Tablets 2261
Halfprin 1362
Healthprin Aspirin 2455
Norgesic.. 1496
Percodan Tablets...................................... 939
Percodan-Demi Tablets......................... 940
Robaxisal Tablets..................................... 2071
Soma Compound w/Codeine Tablets 2676
Soma Compound Tablets...................... 2675
St. Joseph Adult Chewable Aspirin (81 mg.) .... ◾ 808
Talwin Compound 2335
Ursinus Inlay-Tabs.................................. ◾ 794
Vanquish Analgesic Caplets .... ◾ 731

Atenolol (Potentiates the hypoglycemic action; patients should be observed for hypoglycemia or loss of control). Products include:

Tenoretic Tablets...................................... 2845
Tenormin Tablets and I.V. Injection 2847

Atovaquone (Potentiates the hypoglycemic action; patients should be observed for hypoglycemia or loss of control). Products include:

Mepron Suspension 1135

Bendroflumethiazide (Potentiates the hypoglycemic action; patients should be observed for hypoglycemia or loss of control; potential for hyperglycemia leading to loss of control).

No products indexed under this heading.

Bepridil Hydrochloride (Potential for hyperglycemia leading to loss of control). Products include:

Vascor (200, 300 and 400 mg) Tablets 1587

Betamethasone Acetate (Potential for hyperglycemia leading to loss of control). Products include:

Celestone Soluspan Suspension 2347

Betamethasone Sodium Phosphate (Potential for hyperglycemia leading to loss of control). Products include:

Celestone Soluspan Suspension 2347

Betaxolol Hydrochloride (Potentiates the hypoglycemic action; patients should be observed for hypoglycemia or loss of control). Products include:

Betoptic Ophthalmic Solution............ 469
Betoptic S Ophthalmic Suspension 471
Kerlone Tablets.. 2436

Bisoprolol Fumarate (Potentiates the hypoglycemic action; patients should be observed for hypoglycemia or loss of control). Products include:

Zebeta Tablets 1413
Ziac 1415

Bumetanide (Potential for hyperglycemia leading to loss of control). Products include:

Bumex 2093

Carteolol Hydrochloride (Potentiates the hypoglycemic action; patients should be observed for hypoglycemia or loss of control). Products include:

Cartrol Tablets 410
Ocupress Ophthalmic Solution, 1% Sterile.. ◎ 309

Cefonicid Sodium (Potentiates the hypoglycemic action; patients should be observed for hypoglycemia or loss of control). Products include:

Monocid Injection 2497

Chloramphenicol (Potentiates the hypoglycemic action; patients should be observed for hypoglycemia or loss of control). Products include:

Chloromycetin Ophthalmic Ointment, 1% .... ◎ 310
Chloromycetin Ophthalmic Solution .... ◎ 310
Chloroptic S.O.P. .... ◎ 239
Chloroptic Sterile Ophthalmic Solution .... ◎ 239
Elase-Chloromycetin Ointment 1040
Ophthocort .... ◎ 311

Chloramphenicol Palmitate (Potentiates the hypoglycemic action; patients should be observed for hypoglycemia or loss of control).

No products indexed under this heading.

Chloramphenicol Sodium Succinate (Potentiates the hypoglycemic action; patients should be observed for hypoglycemia or loss of control). Products include:

Chloromycetin Sodium Succinate.... 1900

Chlordiazepoxide (Potentiates the hypoglycemic action; patients should be observed for hypoglycemia or loss of control). Products include:

Libritabs Tablets 2177
Limbitrol 2180

Chlordiazepoxide Hydrochloride (Potentiates the hypoglycemic action; patients should be observed for hypoglycemia or loss of control). Products include:

Librax Capsules 2176
Librium Capsules 2178
Librium Injectable 2179

Chlorothiazide (Potentiates the hypoglycemic action; patients should be observed for hypoglycemia or loss of control; potential for hyperglycemia leading to loss of control). Products include:

Aldoclor Tablets 1598
Diupres Tablets 1650
Diuril Oral 1653

IMPORTANT NOTE: Always consult each drug listing in the patient's regimen for possible interactions.

DiaBeta **Interactions Index** 272

Chlorothiazide Sodium (Potentiates the hypoglycemic action; patients should be observed for hypoglycemia or loss of control; potential for hyperglycemia leading to loss of control). Products include:
Diuril Sodium Intravenous 1652
Chlorotrianisene (Potential for hyperglycemia leading to loss of control).
No products indexed under this heading.
Chlorpromazine (Potentiates the hypoglycemic action; patients should be observed for hypoglycemia or loss of control; potential for hyperglycemia leading to loss of control). Products include:
Thorazine Suppositories 2523
Chlorpromazine Hydrochloride (Potentiates the hypoglycemic action; patients should be observed for hypoglycemia or loss of control; potential for hyperglycemia leading to loss of control). Products include:
Thorazine 2523
Chlorpropamide (Potentiates the hypoglycemic action; patients should be observed for hypoglycemia or loss of control). Products include:
Diabinese Tablets 1935
Chlorthalidone (Potential for hyperglycemia leading to loss of control). Products include:
Combipres Tablets 677
Tenoretic Tablets 2845
Thalitone 1245
Choline Magnesium Trisalicylate (Potentiates the hypoglycemic action; patients should be observed for hypoglycemia or loss of control). Products include:
Trilisate 2000
Ciprofloxacin (Potentiates the hypoglycemic action). Products include:
Cipro I.V. 595
Cipro I.V. Pharmacy Bulk Package.. 597
Ciprofloxacin Hydrochloride (Potentiates the hypoglycemic action). Products include:
Ciloxan Ophthalmic Solution........ 472
Cipro Tablets 592
Clomipramine Hydrochloride (Potentiates the hypoglycemic action; patients should be observed for hypoglycemia or loss of control). Products include:
Anafranil Capsules 803
Clozapine (Potentiates the hypoglycemic action; patients should be observed for hypoglycemia or loss of control). Products include:
Clozaril Tablets 2252
Cortisone Acetate (Potential for hyperglycemia leading to loss of control). Products include:
Cortone Acetate Sterile Suspension 1623
Cortone Acetate Tablets 1624
Cyclosporine (Potentiates the hypoglycemic action; patients should be observed for hypoglycemia or loss of control). Products include:
Neoral 2276
Sandimmune 2286
Desogestrel (Potential for hyperglycemia leading to loss of control). Products include:
Desogen Tablets 1817
Ortho-Cept 1851
Dexamethasone (Potential for hyperglycemia leading to loss of control). Products include:
AK-Trol Ointment & Suspension .... ◉ 205
Decadron Elixir 1633
Decadron Tablets 1635
Decaspray Topical Aerosol 1648
Dexacidin Ointment .... ◉ 263
Maxitrol Ophthalmic Ointment and Suspension .... ◉ 224
TobraDex Ophthalmic Suspension and Ointment 473
Dexamethasone Acetate (Potential for hyperglycemia leading to loss of control). Products include:
Dalalone D.P. Injectable 1011
Decadron-LA Sterile Suspension...... 1646
Dexamethasone Sodium Phosphate (Potential for hyperglycemia leading to loss of control). Products include:
Decadron Phosphate Injection 1637
Decadron Phosphate Respihaler 1642
Decadron Phosphate Sterile Ophthalmic Ointment 1641
Decadron Phosphate Sterile Ophthalmic Solution 1642
Decadron Phosphate Topical Cream 1644
Decadron Phosphate Turbinaire 1645
Decadron Phosphate with Xylocaine Injection, Sterile 1639
Dexacort Phosphate in Respihaler .. 458
Dexacort Phosphate in Turbinaire .. 459
NeoDecadron Sterile Ophthalmic Ointment 1712
NeoDecadron Sterile Ophthalmic Solution 1713
NeoDecadron Topical Cream 1714
Diazepam (Potentiates the hypoglycemic action; patients should be observed for hypoglycemia or loss of control). Products include:
Dizac 1809
Valium Injectable 2182
Valium Tablets 2183
Valrelease Capsules 2169
Diclofenac Potassium (Potentiates the hypoglycemic action; patients should be observed for hypoglycemia or loss of control). Products include:
Cataflam 816
Diclofenac Sodium (Potentiates the hypoglycemic action; patients should be observed for hypoglycemia or loss of control). Products include:
Voltaren Ophthalmic Sterile Ophthalmic Solution .... ◉ 272
Voltaren Tablets 861
Dicumarol (Potentiates the hypoglycemic action; patients should be observed for hypoglycemia or loss of control).
No products indexed under this heading.
Dienestrol (Potential for hyperglycemia leading to loss of control). Products include:
Ortho Dienestrol Cream 1866
Diethylstilbestrol (Potential for hyperglycemia leading to loss of control). Products include:
Diethylstilbestrol Tablets 1437
Diflunisal (Potentiates the hypoglycemic action; patients should be observed for hypoglycemia or loss of control). Products include:
Dolobid Tablets 1654
Diltiazem Hydrochloride (Potential for hyperglycemia leading to loss of control). Products include:
Cardizem CD Capsules 1506
Cardizem SR Capsules 1510
Cardizem Injectable 1508
Cardizem Tablets 1512
Dilacor XR Extended-release Capsules 2018
Dipyridamole (Potentiates the hypoglycemic action; patients should be observed for hypoglycemia or loss of control). Products include:
Persantine Tablets 681
Dobutamine Hydrochloride (Potential for hyperglycemia leading to loss of control). Products include:
Dobutrex Solution Vials 1439
Dopamine Hydrochloride (Potential for hyperglycemia leading to loss of control).
No products indexed under this heading.
Enoxacin (Potentiates the hypoglycemic action). Products include:
Penetrex Tablets 2031
Ephedrine Hydrochloride (Potential for hyperglycemia leading to loss of control). Products include:
Primatene Dual Action Formula...... ▣ 872
Primatene Tablets .... ▣ 873
Quadrinal Tablets 1350
Ephedrine Sulfate (Potential for hyperglycemia leading to loss of control). Products include:
Bronkaid Caplets .... ▣ 717
Marax Tablets & DF Syrup........ 2200
Ephedrine Tannate (Potential for hyperglycemia leading to loss of control). Products include:
Rynatuss 2673
Epinephrine (Potential for hyperglycemia leading to loss of control). Products include:
Bronkaid Mist .... ▣ 717
EPIFRIN .... ◉ 239
EpiPen 790
Marcaine Hydrochloride with Epinephrine 1:200,000 2316
Primatene Mist .... ▣ 873
Sensorcaine with Epinephrine Injection 559
Sus-Phrine Injection 1019
Xylocaine with Epinephrine Injections 567
Epinephrine Bitartrate (Potential for hyperglycemia leading to loss of control). Products include:
Bronkaid Mist Suspension .... ▣ 718
Sensorcaine-MPF with Epinephrine Injection 559
Epinephrine Hydrochloride (Potential for hyperglycemia leading to loss of control). Products include:
Ana-Kit Anaphylaxis Emergency Treatment Kit 617
Esmolol Hydrochloride (Potentiates the hypoglycemic action; patients should be observed for hypoglycemia or loss of control). Products include:
Brevibloc Injection 1808
Estradiol (Potential for hyperglycemia leading to loss of control). Products include:
Climara Transdermal System 645
Estrace Cream and Tablets 749
Estraderm Transdermal System 824
Estrogens, Conjugated (Potential for hyperglycemia leading to loss of control). Products include:
PMB 200 and PMB 400 2783
Premarin Intravenous 2787
Premarin with Methyltestosterone .. 2794
Premarin Tablets 2789
Premarin Vaginal Cream........ 2791
Premphase 2797
Prempro 2801
Estrogens, Esterified (Potential for hyperglycemia leading to loss of control). Products include:
ESTRATAB Tablets (0.3, 0.625, 1.25, 2.5 mg) 2536
Estratest 2539
Menest Tablets 2494
Estropipate (Potential for hyperglycemia leading to loss of control). Products include:
Ogen Tablets 2627
Ogen Vaginal Cream........ 2630
Ortho-Est 1869
Ethacrynic Acid (Potential for hyperglycemia leading to loss of control). Products include:
Edecrin Tablets 1657
Ethinyl Estradiol (Potential for hyperglycemia leading to loss of control). Products include:
Brevicon 2088
Demulen 2428
Desogen Tablets 1817
Levlen/Tri-Levlen 651
Lo/Ovral Tablets 2746
Lo/Ovral-28 Tablets 2751
Modicon 1872
Nordette-21 Tablets 2755
Nordette-28 Tablets 2758
Norinyl 2088
Ortho-Cept 1851
Ortho-Cyclen/Ortho-Tri-Cyclen 1858
Ortho-Novum 1872
Ortho-Cyclen/Ortho Tri-Cyclen 1858
Ovcon 760
Ovral Tablets 2770
Ovral-28 Tablets 2770
Levlen/Tri-Levlen 651
Tri-Norinyl 2164
Triphasil-21 Tablets 2814
Triphasil-28 Tablets 2819
Ethynodiol Diacetate (Potential for hyperglycemia leading to loss of control). Products include:
Demulen 2428
Etodolac (Potentiates the hypoglycemic action; patients should be observed for hypoglycemia or loss of control). Products include:
Lodine Capsules and Tablets 2743
Felodipine (Potential for hyperglycemia leading to loss of control). Products include:
Plendil Extended-Release Tablets.... 527
Fenoprofen Calcium (Potentiates the hypoglycemic action; patients should be observed for hypoglycemia or loss of control). Products include:
Nalfon 200 Pulvules & Nalfon Tablets 917
Fludrocortisone Acetate (Potential for hyperglycemia leading to loss of control). Products include:
Florinef Acetate Tablets 505
Fluphenazine Decanoate (Potential for hyperglycemia leading to loss of control). Products include:
Prolixin Decanoate 509
Fluphenazine Enanthate (Potential for hyperglycemia leading to loss of control). Products include:
Prolixin Enanthate 509
Fluphenazine Hydrochloride (Potential for hyperglycemia leading to loss of control). Products include:
Prolixin 509
Flurazepam Hydrochloride (Potentiates the hypoglycemic action; patients should be observed for hypoglycemia or loss of control). Products include:
Dalmane Capsules 2173
Flurbiprofen (Potentiates the hypoglycemic action; patients should be observed for hypoglycemia or loss of control). Products include:
Ansaid Tablets 2579
Furazolidone (Potentiates the hypoglycemic action; patients should be observed for hypoglycemia or loss of control). Products include:
Furoxone 2046
Furosemide (Potential for hyperglycemia leading to loss of control). Products include:
Lasix Injection, Oral Solution and Tablets 1240
Glipizide (Potentiates the hypoglycemic action; patients should be observed for hypoglycemia or loss of control). Products include:
Glucotrol Tablets 1967
Glucotrol XL Extended Release Tablets 1968

(▣ Described in PDR For Nonprescription Drugs) (◉ Described in PDR For Ophthalmology)

273 **Interactions Index** **DiaBeta**

Hydrochlorothiazide (Potentiates the hypoglycemic action; patients should be observed for hypoglycemia or loss of control; potential for hyperglycemia leading to loss of control). Products include:

- Aldactazide 2413
- Aldoril Tablets 1604
- Apresazide Capsules 808
- Capozide 742
- Dyazide 2479
- Esidrix Tablets 821
- Esimil Tablets 822
- HydroDIURIL Tablets 1674
- Hydropres Tablets 1675
- Hyzaar Tablets 1677
- Inderide Tablets 2732
- Inderide LA Long Acting Capsules .. 2734
- Lopressor HCT Tablets 832
- Lotensin HCT 837
- Maxzide 1380
- Moduretic Tablets 1705
- Oretic Tablets 443
- Prinzide Tablets 1737
- Ser-Ap-Es Tablets 849
- Timolide Tablets 1748
- Vaseretic Tablets 1765
- Zestoretic 2850
- Ziac 1415

Hydrocortisone (Potential for hyperglycemia leading to loss of control). Products include:

- Anusol-HC Cream 2.5% 1896
- Aquanil HC Lotion 1931
- Bactine Hydrocortisone Anti-Itch Cream .... ▣ 709
- Caldecort Anti-Itch Hydrocortisone Spray .... ▣ 631
- Cortaid .... ▣ 836
- CORTENEMA 2535
- Cortisporin Ointment 1085
- Cortisporin Ophthalmic Ointment Sterile 1085
- Cortisporin Ophthalmic Suspension Sterile 1086
- Cortisporin Otic Solution Sterile 1087
- Cortisporin Otic Suspension Sterile 1088
- Cortizone-5 .... ▣ 831
- Cortizone-10 .... ▣ 831
- Hydrocortone Tablets 1672
- Hytone 907
- Massengill Medicated Soft Cloth Towelettes 2458
- PediOtic Suspension Sterile 1153
- Preparation H Hydrocortisone 1% Cream .... ▣ 872
- ProctoCream-HC 2.5% 2408
- VōSoL HC Otic Solution 2678

Hydrocortisone Acetate (Potential for hyperglycemia leading to loss of control). Products include:

- Analpram-HC Rectal Cream 1% and 2.5% 977
- Anusol HC-1 Anti-Itch Hydrocortisone Ointment .... ▣ 847
- Anusol-HC Suppositories 1897
- Caldecort .... ▣ 631
- Carmol HC 924
- Coly-Mycin S Otic w/Neomycin & Hydrocortisone 1906
- Cortaid .... ▣ 836
- Cortifoam 2396
- Cortisporin Cream 1084
- Epifoam 2399
- Hydrocortone Acetate Sterile Suspension 1669
- Mantadil Cream 1135
- Nupercainal Hydrocortisone 1% Cream .... ▣ 645
- Ophthocort .... ◉ 311
- Pramosone Cream, Lotion & Ointment 978
- ProctoCream-HC 2408
- ProctoFoam-HC 2409
- Terra-Cortril Ophthalmic Suspension 2210

Hydrocortisone Sodium Phosphate (Potential for hyperglycemia leading to loss of control). Products include:

- Hydrocortone Phosphate Injection, Sterile 1670

Hydrocortisone Sodium Succinate (Potential for hyperglycemia leading to loss of control). Products include:

- Solu-Cortef Sterile Powder 2641

Hydroflumethiazide (Potentiates the hypoglycemic action; patients should be observed for hypoglycemia or loss of control; potential for hyperglycemia leading to loss of control). Products include:

- Diucardin Tablets 2718

Ibuprofen (Potentiates the hypoglycemic action; patients should be observed for hypoglycemia or loss of control). Products include:

- Advil Cold and Sinus Caplets and Tablets (formerly CoAdvil) .... ▣ 870
- Advil Ibuprofen Tablets and Caplets .... ▣ 870
- Children's Advil Suspension 2692
- Arthritis Foundation Ibuprofen Tablets .... ▣ 674
- Bayer Select Ibuprofen Pain Relief Formula .... ▣ 715
- Cramp End Tablets .... ▣ 735
- Dimetapp Sinus Caplets .... ▣ 775
- Haltran Tablets .... ▣ 771
- IBU Tablets 1342
- Ibuprohm .... ▣ 735
- Children's Motrin Ibuprofen Oral Suspension 1546
- Motrin Tablets 2625
- Motrin IB Caplets, Tablets, and Geltabs .... ▣ 838
- Motrin IB Sinus .... ▣ 838
- Motrin Ibuprofen Suspension, Oral Drops, Chewable Tablets, Caplets 1546
- Nuprin Ibuprofen/Analgesic Tablets & Caplets .... ▣ 622
- Sine-Aid IB Caplets 1554
- Vicks DayQuil SINUS Pressure & PAIN Relief with IBUPROFEN .... ▣ 762

Imipramine Hydrochloride (Potentiates the hypoglycemic action; patients should be observed for hypoglycemia or loss of control). Products include:

- Tofranil Ampuls 854
- Tofranil Tablets 856

Imipramine Pamoate (Potentiates the hypoglycemic action; patients should be observed for hypoglycemia or loss of control). Products include:

- Tofranil-PM Capsules 857

Indapamide (Potential for hyperglycemia leading to loss of control). Products include:

- Lozol Tablets 2022

Indomethacin (Potentiates the hypoglycemic action; patients should be observed for hypoglycemia or loss of control). Products include:

- Indocin 1680

Indomethacin Sodium Trihydrate (Potentiates the hypoglycemic action; patients should be observed for hypoglycemia or loss of control). Products include:

- Indocin I.V. 1684

Isocarboxazid (Potentiates the hypoglycemic action; patients should be observed for hypoglycemia or loss of control).

No products indexed under this heading.

Isoniazid (Potential for hyperglycemia leading to loss of control). Products include:

- Nydrazid Injection 508
- Rifamate Capsules 1530
- Rifater 1532

Isoproterenol Hydrochloride (Potential for hyperglycemia leading to loss of control). Products include:

- Isuprel Hydrochloride Injection 1:5000 2311
- Isuprel Hydrochloride Solution 1:200 & 1:100 2313
- Isuprel Mistometer 2312

Isoproterenol Sulfate (Potential for hyperglycemia leading to loss of control). Products include:

- Norisodrine with Calcium Iodide Syrup 442

Isradipine (Potential for hyperglycemia leading to loss of control). Products include:

- DynaCirc Capsules 2256

Ketoprofen (Potentiates the hypoglycemic action; patients should be observed for hypoglycemia or loss of control). Products include:

- Orudis Capsules 2766
- Oruvail Capsules 2766

Ketorolac Tromethamine (Potentiates the hypoglycemic action; patients should be observed for hypoglycemia or loss of control). Products include:

- Acular 474
- Acular .... ◉ 277
- Toradol 2159

Labetalol Hydrochloride (Potentiates the hypoglycemic action; patients should be observed for hypoglycemia or loss of control). Products include:

- Normodyne Injection 2377
- Normodyne Tablets 2379
- Trandate 1185

Levobunolol Hydrochloride (Potentiates the hypoglycemic action; patients should be observed for hypoglycemia or loss of control). Products include:

- Betagan .... ◉ 233

Levonorgestrel (Potential for hyperglycemia leading to loss of control). Products include:

- Levlen/Tri-Levlen 651
- Nordette-21 Tablets 2755
- Nordette-28 Tablets 2758
- Norplant System 2759
- Levlen/Tri-Levlen 651
- Triphasil-21 Tablets 2814
- Triphasil-28 Tablets 2819

Levothyroxine Sodium (Potential for hyperglycemia leading to loss of control). Products include:

- Levothroid Tablets 1016
- Levoxyl Tablets 903
- Synthroid 1359

Liothyronine Sodium (Potential for hyperglycemia leading to loss of control). Products include:

- Cytomel Tablets 2473
- Triostat Injection 2530

Liotrix (Potential for hyperglycemia leading to loss of control).

No products indexed under this heading.

Lomefloxacin Hydrochloride (Potentiates the hypoglycemic action). Products include:

- Maxaquin Tablets 2440

Magnesium Salicylate (Potentiates the hypoglycemic action; patients should be observed for hypoglycemia or loss of control). Products include:

- Backache Caplets .... ▣ 613
- Bayer Select Backache Pain Relief Formula .... ▣ 715
- Doan's Extra-Strength Analgesic.... ▣ 633
- Extra Strength Doan's P.M. .... ▣ 633
- Doan's Regular Strength Analgesic .... ▣ 634
- Mobigesic Tablets .... ▣ 602

Meclofenamate Sodium (Potentiates the hypoglycemic action; patients should be observed for hypoglycemia or loss of control).

No products indexed under this heading.

Mefenamic Acid (Potentiates the hypoglycemic action; patients should be observed for hypoglycemia or loss of control). Products include:

- Ponstel 1925

Mesoridazine Besylate (Potential for hyperglycemia leading to loss of control). Products include:

- Serentil 684

Mestranol (Potential for hyperglycemia leading to loss of control). Products include:

- Norinyl 2088
- Ortho-Novum 1872

Metaproterenol Sulfate (Potential for hyperglycemia leading to loss of control). Products include:

- Alupent 669
- Metaproterenol Sulfate Inhalation Solution, USP, Arm-a-Med 552

Metaraminol Bitartrate (Potential for hyperglycemia leading to loss of control). Products include:

- Aramine Injection 1609

Methotrimeprazine (Potential for hyperglycemia leading to loss of control). Products include:

- Levoprome 1274

Methoxamine Hydrochloride (Potential for hyperglycemia leading to loss of control). Products include:

- Vasoxyl Injection 1196

Methyclothiazide (Potentiates the hypoglycemic action; patients should be observed for hypoglycemia or loss of control; potential for hyperglycemia leading to loss of control). Products include:

- Enduron Tablets 420

Methylprednisolone Acetate (Potential for hyperglycemia leading to loss of control). Products include:

- Depo-Medrol Single-Dose Vial 2600
- Depo-Medrol Sterile Aqueous Suspension 2597

Methylprednisolone Sodium Succinate (Potential for hyperglycemia leading to loss of control). Products include:

- Solu-Medrol Sterile Powder 2643

Metipranolol Hydrochloride (Potentiates the hypoglycemic action; patients should be observed for hypoglycemia or loss of control). Products include:

- OptiPranolol (Metipranolol 0.3%) Sterile Ophthalmic Solution .... ◉ 258

Metolazone (Potential for hyperglycemia leading to loss of control). Products include:

- Mykrox Tablets 993
- Zaroxolyn Tablets 1000

Metoprolol Succinate (Potentiates the hypoglycemic action; patients should be observed for hypoglycemia or loss of control). Products include:

- Toprol-XL Tablets 565

Metoprolol Tartrate (Potentiates the hypoglycemic action; patients should be observed for hypoglycemia or loss of control). Products include:

- Lopressor Ampuls 830
- Lopressor HCT Tablets 832
- Lopressor Tablets 830

Miconazole (Potential for severe hypoglycemia when co-administered with oral miconazole).

No products indexed under this heading.

Midazolam Hydrochloride (Potentiates the hypoglycemic action; patients should be observed for hypoglycemia or loss of control). Products include:

- Versed Injection 2170

Nabumetone (Potentiates the hypoglycemic action; patients should be observed for hypoglycemia or loss of control). Products include:

- Relafen Tablets 2510

IMPORTANT NOTE: Always consult each drug listing in the patient's regimen for possible interactions.

Nadolol (Potentiates the hypoglycemic action; patients should be observed for hypoglycemia or loss of control).

No products indexed under this heading.

Naproxen (Potentiates the hypoglycemic action; patients should be observed for hypoglycemia or loss of control). Products include:

Anaprox/Naprosyn 2117

Naproxen Sodium (Potentiates the hypoglycemic action; patients should be observed for hypoglycemia or loss of control). Products include:

Aleve 1975
Anaprox/Naprosyn 2117

Niacin (Potential for hyperglycemia leading to loss of control). Products include:

Nicobid 2026
Nicolar Tablets 2026
Nicotinex Elixir .... ■ 655
Sigtab Tablets .... ■ 772
Slo-Niacin Tablets 2659
Stuart Prenatal Tablets .... ■ 881
The Stuart Formula Tablets .... ■ 663
Zymacap Capsules .... ■ 772

Nicardipine Hydrochloride (Potential for hyperglycemia leading to loss of control). Products include:

Cardene Capsules 2095
Cardene I.V. 2709
Cardene SR Capsules 2097

Nicotinic Acid (Potential for hyperglycemia leading to loss of control).

No products indexed under this heading.

Nifedipine (Potential for hyperglycemia leading to loss of control). Products include:

Adalat Capsules (10 mg and 20 mg) 587
Adalat CC 589
Procardia Capsules 1971
Procardia XL Extended Release Tablets 1972

Nimodipine (Potential for hyperglycemia leading to loss of control). Products include:

Nimotop Capsules 610

Nisoldipine (Potential for hyperglycemia leading to loss of control).

No products indexed under this heading.

Norepinephrine Bitartrate (Potential for hyperglycemia leading to loss of control). Products include:

Levophed Bitartrate Injection 2315

Norethindrone (Potential for hyperglycemia leading to loss of control). Products include:

Brevicon 2088
Micronor Tablets 1872
Modicon 1872
Norinyl 2088
Nor-Q D Tablets 2135
Ortho-Novum 1872
Ovcon 760
Tri-Norinyl 2164

Norethynodrel (Potential for hyperglycemia leading to loss of control).

No products indexed under this heading.

Norfloxacin (Potentiates the hypoglycemic action). Products include:

Chibroxin Sterile Ophthalmic Solution 1617
Noroxin Tablets 1715
Noroxin Tablets 2048

Norgestimate (Potential for hyperglycemia leading to loss of control). Products include:

Ortho-Cyclen/Ortho-Tri-Cyclen 1858
Ortho-Cyclen/Ortho Tri-Cyclen 1858

Norgestrel (Potential for hyperglycemia leading to loss of control). Products include:

Lo/Ovral Tablets 2746
Lo/Ovral-28 Tablets 2751
Ovral Tablets 2770
Ovral-28 Tablets 2770
Ovrette Tablets 2771

Nortriptyline Hydrochloride (Potentiates the hypoglycemic action; patients should be observed for hypoglycemia or loss of control). Products include:

Pamelor 2280

Ofloxacin (Potentiates the hypoglycemic action). Products include:

Floxin I.V. 1571
Floxin Tablets (200 mg, 300 mg, 400 mg) 1567
Ocuflox 481
Ocuflox .... ⊙ 246

Oxaprozin (Potentiates the hypoglycemic action; patients should be observed for hypoglycemia or loss of control). Products include:

Daypro Caplets 2426

Oxazepam (Potentiates the hypoglycemic action; patients should be observed for hypoglycemia or loss of control). Products include:

Serax Capsules 2810
Serax Tablets 2810

Penbutolol Sulfate (Potentiates the hypoglycemic action; patients should be observed for hypoglycemia or loss of control). Products include:

Levatol 2403

Perphenazine (Potential for hyperglycemia leading to loss of control). Products include:

Etrafon 2355
Triavil Tablets 1757
Trilafon 2389

Phenelzine Sulfate (Potentiates the hypoglycemic action; patients should be observed for hypoglycemia or loss of control). Products include:

Nardil 1920

Phenylbutazone (Potentiates the hypoglycemic action; patients should be observed for hypoglycemia or loss of control).

No products indexed under this heading.

Phenylephrine Bitartrate (Potential for hyperglycemia leading to loss of control).

No products indexed under this heading.

Phenylephrine Hydrochloride (Potential for hyperglycemia leading to loss of control). Products include:

Atrohist Plus Tablets 454
Cerose DM .... ■ 878
Comhist 2038
D.A. Chewable Tablets 951
Deconsal Pediatric Capsules 454
Dura-Vent/DA Tablets 953
Entex Capsules 1986
Entex Liquid 1986
Extendryl 1005
4-Way Fast Acting Nasal Spray (regular & mentholated) .... ■ 621
Hemorid For Women .... ■ 834
Hycomine Compound Tablets 932
Neo-Synephrine Hydrochloride 1% Carpuject 2324
Neo-Synephrine Hydrochloride 1% Injection 2324
Neo-Synephrine Hydrochloride (Ophthalmic) 2325
Neo-Synephrine .... ■ 726
Nōstril .... ■ 644
Novahistine Elixir .... ■ 823
Phenergan VC 2779
Phenergan VC with Codeine 2781
Preparation H .... ■ 871
Tympagesic Ear Drops 2342
Vasosulf .... ⊙ 271
Vicks Sinex Nasal Spray and Ultra Fine Mist .... ■ 765

Phenylephrine Tannate (Potential for hyperglycemia leading to loss of control). Products include:

Atrohist Pediatric Suspension 454
Ricobid-D Pediatric Suspension 2038
Ricobid Tablets and Pediatric Suspension 2038
Rynatan 2673
Rynatuss 2673

Phenylpropanolamine Hydrochloride (Potential for hyperglycemia leading to loss of control). Products include:

Acutrim .... ■ 628
Allerest Children's Chewable Tablets .... ■ 627
Allerest 12 Hour Caplets .... ■ 627
Atrohist Plus Tablets 454
BC Cold Powder Multi-Symptom Formula (Cold-Sinus-Allergy) .... ■ 609
BC Cold Powder Non-Drowsy Formula (Cold-Sinus) .... ■ 609
Cheracol Plus Head Cold/Cough Formula .... ■ 769
Comtrex Multi-Symptom Non-Drowsy Liqui-gels .... ■ 618
Contac Continuous Action Nasal Decongestant/Antihistamine 12 Hour Capsules .... ■ 813
Contac Maximum Strength Continuous Action Decongestant/Antihistamine 12 Hour Caplets .... ■ 813
Contac Severe Cold and Flu Formula Caplets .... ■ 814
Coricidin 'D' Decongestant Tablets .... ■ 800
Dexatrim .... ■ 832
Dexatrim Plus Vitamins Caplets .... ■ 832
Dimetane-DC Cough Syrup 2059
Dimetapp Elixir .... ■ 773
Dimetapp Extentabs .... ■ 774
Dimetapp Tablets/Liqui-Gels .... ■ 775
Dimetapp Cold & Allergy Chewable Tablets .... ■ 773
Dimetapp DM Elixir .... ■ 774
Dura-Vent Tablets 952
Entex Capsules 1986
Entex LA Tablets 1987
Entex Liquid 1986
Exgest LA Tablets 782
Hycomine 931
Isoclor Timesule Capsules .... ■ 637
Nolamine Timed-Release Tablets 785
Ornade Spansule Capsules 2502
Propagest Tablets 786
Pyrroxate Caplets .... ■ 772
Robitussin-CF .... ■ 777
Sinulin Tablets 787
Tavist-D 12 Hour Relief Tablets .... ■ 787
Teldrin 12 Hour Antihistamine/Nasal Decongestant Allergy Relief Capsules .... ■ 826
Triaminic Allergy Tablets .... ■ 789
Triaminic Cold Tablets .... ■ 790
Triaminic Expectorant .... ■ 790
Triaminic Syrup .... ■ 792
Triaminic-12 Tablets .... ■ 792
Triaminic-DM Syrup .... ■ 792
Triaminicin Tablets .... ■ 793
Triaminicol Multi-Symptom Cold Tablets .... ■ 793
Triaminicol Multi-Symptom Relief .... ■ 794
Vicks DayQuil Allergy Relief 12-Hour Extended Release Tablets .... ■ 760
Vicks DayQuil Allergy Relief 4-Hour Tablets .... ■ 760
Vicks DayQuil SINUS Pressure & CONGESTION Relief .... ■ 761

Phenytoin (Potential for hyperglycemia leading to loss of control). Products include:

Dilantin Infatabs 1908
Dilantin-125 Suspension 1911

Phenytoin Sodium (Potential for hyperglycemia leading to loss of control). Products include:

Dilantin Kapseals 1906
Dilantin Parenteral 1910

Pindolol (Potentiates the hypoglycemic action; patients should be observed for hypoglycemia or loss of control). Products include:

Visken Tablets 2299

Pirbuterol Acetate (Potential for hyperglycemia leading to loss of control). Products include:

Maxair Autohaler 1492
Maxair Inhaler 1494

Piroxicam (Potentiates the hypoglycemic action; patients should be observed for hypoglycemia or loss of control). Products include:

Feldene Capsules 1965

Polyestradiol Phosphate (Potential for hyperglycemia leading to loss of control).

No products indexed under this heading.

Polythiazide (Potentiates the hypoglycemic action; patients should be observed for hypoglycemia or loss of control; potential for hyperglycemia leading to loss of control). Products include:

Minizide Capsules 1938

Prednisolone Acetate (Potential for hyperglycemia leading to loss of control). Products include:

AK-CIDE .... ⊙ 202
AK-CIDE Ointment .... ⊙ 202
Blephamide Liquifilm Sterile Ophthalmic Suspension 476
Blephamide Ointment .... ⊙ 237
Econopred & Econopred Plus Ophthalmic Suspensions .... ⊙ 217
Poly-Pred Liquifilm .... ⊙ 248
Pred Forte .... ⊙ 250
Pred Mild .... ⊙ 253
Pred-G Liquifilm Sterile Ophthalmic Suspension .... ⊙ 251
Pred-G S.O.P. Sterile Ophthalmic Ointment .... ⊙ 252
Vasocidin Ointment .... ⊙ 268

Prednisolone Sodium Phosphate (Potential for hyperglycemia leading to loss of control). Products include:

AK-Pred .... ⊙ 204
Hydeltrasol Injection, Sterile 1665
Inflamase .... ⊙ 265
Pediapred Oral Liquid 995
Vasocidin Ophthalmic Solution .... ⊙ 270

Prednisolone Tebutate (Potential for hyperglycemia leading to loss of control). Products include:

Hydeltra-T.B.A. Sterile Suspension 1667

Prednisone (Potential for hyperglycemia leading to loss of control). Products include:

Deltasone Tablets 2595

Probenecid (Potentiates the hypoglycemic action; patients should be observed for hypoglycemia or loss of control; potential for hyperglycemia leading to loss of control). Products include:

Benemid Tablets 1611
ColBENEMID Tablets 1622

Prochlorperazine (Potential for hyperglycemia leading to loss of control). Products include:

Compazine 2470

Promethazine Hydrochloride (Potential for hyperglycemia leading to loss of control). Products include:

Mepergan Injection 2753
Phenergan with Codeine 2777
Phenergan with Dextromethorphan 2778
Phenergan Injection 2773
Phenergan Suppositories 2775
Phenergan Syrup 2774
Phenergan Tablets 2775
Phenergan VC 2779
Phenergan VC with Codeine 2781

Propranolol Hydrochloride (Potentiates the hypoglycemic action; patients should be observed for hypoglycemia or loss of control). Products include:

Inderal 2728
Inderal LA Long Acting Capsules 2730
Inderide Tablets 2732
Inderide LA Long Acting Capsules .. 2734

Pseudoephedrine Hydrochloride (Potential for hyperglycemia leading to loss of control). Products include:

Actifed Allergy Daytime/Nighttime Caplets .... ■ 844

Interactions Index — DiaBeta

Actifed Plus Caplets .... ✦D 845
Actifed Plus Tablets .... ✦D 845
Actifed with Codeine Cough Syrup.. 1067
Actifed Sinus Daytime/Nighttime Tablets and Caplets .... ✦D 846
Actifed Syrup.. ✦D 846
Actifed Tablets .... ✦D 844
Advil Cold and Sinus Caplets and Tablets (formerly CoAdvil) .... ✦D 870
Alka-Seltzer Plus Cold Medicine Liqui-Gels .... ✦D 706
Alka-Seltzer Plus Cold & Cough Medicine Liqui-Gels........................... ✦D 705
Alka-Seltzer Plus Night-Time Cold Medicine Liqui-Gels........................... ✦D 706
Allerest Headache Strength Tablets .... ✦D 627
Allerest Maximum Strength Tablets .... ✦D 627
Allerest No Drowsiness Tablets...... ✦D 627
Allerest Sinus Pain Formula .... ✦D 627
Anatuss LA Tablets................................ 1542
Atrohist Pediatric Capsules................ 453
Bayer Select Sinus Pain Relief Formula .... ✦D 717
Benadryl Allergy Decongestant Liquid Medication .... ✦D 848
Benadryl Allergy Decongestant Tablets .... ✦D 848
Benadryl Allergy Sinus Headache Formula Caplets .... ✦D 849
Benylin Multisymptom .... ✦D 852
Bromfed Capsules (Extended-Release) 1785
Bromfed Syrup .... ✦D 733
Bromfed Tablets 1785
Bromfed-DM Cough Syrup.................. 1786
Bromfed-PD Capsules (Extended-Release) 1785
Children's Vicks DayQuil Allergy Relief... ✦D 757
Children's Vicks NyQuil Cold/Cough Relief.. ✦D 758
Comtrex Multi-Symptom Cold Reliever Tablets/Caplets/Liqui-Gels/Liquid... ✦D 615
Allergy-Sinus Comtrex Multi-Symptom Allergy-Sinus Formula Tablets .... ✦D 617
Comtrex Multi-Symptom Non-Drowsy Caplets................................... ✦D 618
Congess 1004
Contac Day Allergy/Sinus Caplets ✦D 812
Contac Day & Night .... ✦D 812
Contac Night Allergy/Sinus Caplets .... ✦D 812
Contac Severe Cold & Flu Non-Drowsy .... ✦D 815
Deconamine Chewable Tablets 1320
Deconamine CX Cough and Cold Liquid and Tablets............................... 1319
Deconamine 1320
Deconsal C Expectorant Syrup 456
Deconsal Pediatric Syrup.................... 457
Deconsal II Tablets 454
Dimetane-DX Cough Syrup 2059
Dimetapp Sinus Caplets .... ✦D 775
Dorcol Children's Cough Syrup ...... ✦D 785
Drixoral Cough + Congestion Liquid Caps .... ✦D 802
Dura-Tap/PD Capsules 2867
Duratuss Tablets 2565
Duratuss HD Elixir.................................. 2565
Efidac/24 .... ✦D 635
Entex PSE Tablets................................... 1987
Fedahist Gyrocaps.................................. 2401
Fedahist Timecaps 2401
Guaifed.. 1787
Guaifed Syrup .... ✦D 734
Guaimax-D Tablets 792
Guaitab Tablets .... ✦D 734
Isoclor Expectorant................................ 990
Kronofed-A 977
Motrin IB Sinus.. ✦D 838
Novahistine DH.. 2462
Novahistine DMX .... ✦D 822
Novahistine Expectorant...................... 2463
Nucofed 2051
PediaCare Cold Allergy Chewable Tablets .... ✦D 677
PediaCare Cough-Cold Chewable Tablets 1553
PediaCare 1553
PediaCare Infants' Decongestant Drops .... ✦D 677
PediCare Infant's Drops Decongestant Plus Cough 1553
PediaCare NightRest Cough-Cold Liquid 1553
Pediatric Vicks 44d Dry Hacking Cough & Head Congestion............. ✦D 763
Pediatric Vicks 44m Cough & Cold Relief .... ✦D 764
Robitussin Cold & Cough Liqui-Gels .... ✦D 776
Robitussin Maximum Strength Cough & Cold .... ✦D 778
Robitussin Pediatric Cough & Cold Formula .... ✦D 779
Robitussin Severe Congestion Liqui-Gels .... ✦D 776
Robitussin-DAC Syrup 2074
Robitussin-PE .... ✦D 778
Rondec Oral Drops 953
Rondec Syrup 953
Rondec Tablet... 953
Rondec-DM Oral Drops 954
Rondec-DM Syrup 954
Rondec-TR Tablet 953
Ryna .... ✦D 841
Seldane-D Extended-Release Tablets 1538
Semprex-D Capsules 463
Semprex-D Capsules 1167
Sinarest Tablets....................................... ✦D 648
Sinarest Extra Strength Tablets...... ✦D 648
Sinarest No Drowsiness Tablets .... ✦D 648
Sine-Aid IB Caplets 1554
Sine-Aid Maximum Strength Sinus Medication Gelcaps, Caplets and Tablets 1554
Sine-Off No Drowsiness Formula Caplets .... ✦D 824
Sine-Off Sinus Medicine .... ✦D 825
Singlet Tablets .... ✦D 825
Sinutab Non-Drying Liquid Caps .... ✦D 859
Sinutab Sinus Allergy Medication, Maximum Strength Tablets and Caplets .... ✦D 860
Sinutab Sinus Medication, Maximum Strength Without Drowsiness Formula, Tablets & Caplets .... ✦D 860
Sinutab Sinus Medication, Regular Strength Without Drowsiness Formula .... ✦D 859
Sudafed Children's Liquid .... ✦D 861
Sudafed Cold and Cough Liquidcaps... ✦D 862
Sudafed Cough Syrup .... ✦D 862
Sudafed Plus Liquid .... ✦D 862
Sudafed Plus Tablets .... ✦D 863
Sudafed Severe Cold Formula Caplets .... ✦D 863
Sudafed Severe Cold Formula Tablets .... ✦D 864
Sudafed Sinus Caplets.......................... ✦D 864
Sudafed Sinus Tablets........................... ✦D 864
Sudafed Tablets, 30 mg........................ ✦D 861
Sudafed Tablets, 60 mg........................ ✦D 861
Sudafed 12 Hour Caplets .... ✦D 861
Syn-Rx Tablets 465
Syn-Rx DM Tablets 466
TheraFlu... ✦D 787
TheraFlu Maximum Strength Nighttime Flu, Cold & Cough Medicine .... ✦D 788
TheraFlu Maximum Strength Non-Drowsy Formula Flu, Cold & Cough Medicine .... ✦D 788
Thera Flu Maximum Strength, Non-Drowsy Formula Flu, Cold and Cough Caplets .... ✦D 789
Triaminic AM Cough and Decongestant Formula .... ✦D 789
Triaminic AM Decongestant Formula .... ✦D 790
Triaminic Nite Light .... ✦D 791
Triaminic Sore Throat Formula ...... ✦D 791
Tussend 1783
Tussend Expectorant............................. 1785
Children's TYLENOL Cold Multi-Symptom Liquid Formula and Chewable Tablets................................. 1561
Children's TYLENOL Cold Plus Cough Multi Symptom Tablets and Liquid .... ✦D 681
Infants' TYLENOL Cold Decongestant & Fever-Reducer Drops 1556
TYLENOL Maximum Strength Allergy Sinus Medication Gelcaps and Caplets 1563
TYLENOL Maximum Strength Allergy Sinus NightTime Medication Caplets 1555
TYLENOL Flu Maximum Strength Gelcaps 1565
TYLENOL Flu NightTime, Maximum Strength, Gelcaps 1566
TYLENOL Maximum Strength Flu NightTime Hot Medication Packets 1562
TYLENOL, Maximum Strength, Sinus Medication Geltabs, Gelcaps, Caplets and Tablets 1566
TYLENOL Cold Multi-Symptom Formula Medication Tablets and Caplets 1561
TYLENOL Cold Medication No Drowsiness Formula Gelcaps and Caplets 1562
TYLENOL Cold Multi-Symptom Hot Medication Liquid Packets.............. 1557
TYLENOL Cough Multi-Symptom Medication with Decongestant...... 1565
Ursinus Inlay-Tabs.................................. ✦D 794
Vicks 44 LiquiCaps Cough, Cold & Flu Relief... ✦D 755
Vicks 44 LiquiCaps Non-Drowsy Cough & Cold Relief .... ✦D 756
Vicks 44D Dry Hacking Cough & Head Congestion .... ✦D 755
Vicks 44M Cough, Cold & Flu Relief... ✦D 756
Vicks DayQuil .... ✦D 761
Vicks DayQuil SINUS Pressure & PAIN Relief with IBUPROFEN ...... ✦D 762
Vicks Nyquil Hot Therapy.................... ✦D 762
Vicks NyQuil LiquiCaps Multi-Symptom Cold/Flu Relief .... ✦D 763
Vicks NyQuil Multi-Symptom Cold/Flu Relief - (Original & Cherry Flavor) .... ✦D 763

Pseudoephedrine Sulfate (Potential for hyperglycemia leading to loss of control). Products include:

Cheracol Sinus .... ✦D 768
Chlor-Trimeton Allergy Decongestant Tablets .... ✦D 799
Claritin-D 2350
Drixoral Cold and Allergy Sustained-Action Tablets .... ✦D 802
Drixoral Cold and Flu Extended-Release Tablets................................... ✦D 803
Drixoral Non-Drowsy Formula Extended-Release Tablets .... ✦D 803
Drixoral Allergy/Sinus Extended Release Tablets................................... ✦D 804
Trinalin Repetabs Tablets 1330

Quinestrol (Potential for hyperglycemia leading to loss of control).

No products indexed under this heading.

Salmeterol Xinafoate (Potential for hyperglycemia leading to loss of control). Products include:

Serevent Inhalation Aerosol............... 1176

Salsalate (Potentiates the hypoglycemic action; patients should be observed for hypoglycemia or loss of control). Products include:

Mono-Gesic Tablets 792
Salflex Tablets.. 786

Selegiline Hydrochloride (Potentiates the hypoglycemic action; patients should be observed for hypoglycemia or loss of control). Products include:

Eldepryl Tablets 2550

Sotalol Hydrochloride (Potentiates the hypoglycemic action; patients should be observed for hypoglycemia or loss of control). Products include:

Betapace Tablets 641

Spironolactone (Potential for hyperglycemia leading to loss of control). Products include:

Aldactazide... 2413
Aldactone 2414

Sulfacytine (Potentiates the hypoglycemic action; patients should be observed for hypoglycemia or loss of control).

Sulfamethizole (Potentiates the hypoglycemic action; patients should be observed for hypoglycemia or loss of control). Products include:

Urobiotic-250 Capsules 2214

Sulfamethoxazole (Potentiates the hypoglycemic action; patients should be observed for hypoglycemia or loss of control). Products include:

Azo Gantanol Tablets............................. 2080
Bactrim DS Tablets.................................. 2084
Bactrim I.V. Infusion.............................. 2082
Bactrim 2084
Gantanol Tablets 2119
Septra 1174
Septra I.V. Infusion 1169
Septra I.V. Infusion ADD-Vantage Vials.. 1171
Septra 1174

Sulfasalazine (Potentiates the hypoglycemic action; patients should be observed for hypoglycemia or loss of control). Products include:

Azulfidine 1949

Sulfinpyrazone (Potentiates the hypoglycemic action; patients should be observed for hypoglycemia or loss of control). Products include:

Anturane 807

Sulfisoxazole (Potentiates the hypoglycemic action; patients should be observed for hypoglycemia or loss of control). Products include:

Azo Gantrisin Tablets.............................. 2081
Gantrisin Tablets 2120

Sulfisoxazole Diolamine (Potentiates the hypoglycemic action; patients should be observed for hypoglycemia or loss of control).

No products indexed under this heading.

Sulindac (Potentiates the hypoglycemic action; patients should be observed for hypoglycemia or loss of control). Products include:

Clinoril Tablets 1618

Temafloxacin Hydrochloride (Potentiates the hypoglycemic action).

No products indexed under this heading.

Temazepam (Potentiates the hypoglycemic action; patients should be observed for hypoglycemia or loss of control). Products include:

Restoril Capsules...................................... 2284

Terbutaline Sulfate (Potential for hyperglycemia leading to loss of control). Products include:

Brethaire Inhaler 813
Brethine Ampuls 815
Brethine Tablets.. 814
Bricanyl Subcutaneous Injection...... 1502
Bricanyl Tablets 1503

Thioridazine Hydrochloride (Potential for hyperglycemia leading to loss of control). Products include:

Mellaril 2269

Thyroglobulin (Potential for hyperglycemia leading to loss of control).

No products indexed under this heading.

Thyroid (Potential for hyperglycemia leading to loss of control).

No products indexed under this heading.

Thyroxine (Potential for hyperglycemia leading to loss of control).

No products indexed under this heading.

Thyroxine Sodium (Potential for hyperglycemia leading to loss of control).

No products indexed under this heading.

Timolol Hemihydrate (Potentiates the hypoglycemic action; patients should be observed for hypoglycemia or loss of control). Products include:

Betimol 0.25%, 0.5% .... ◉ 261

Timolol Maleate (Potentiates the hypoglycemic action; patients should be observed for hypoglycemia or loss of control). Products include:

Blocadren Tablets 1614
Timolide Tablets.. 1748
Timoptic in Ocudose 1753

IMPORTANT NOTE: Always consult each drug listing in the patient's regimen for possible interactions.

DiaBeta **Interactions Index** **276**

Timoptic Sterile Ophthalmic Solution 1751
Timoptic-XE 1755

Tolazamide (Potentiates the hypoglycemic action; patients should be observed for hypoglycemia or loss of control).
No products indexed under this heading.

Tolbutamide (Potentiates the hypoglycemic action; patients should be observed for hypoglycemia or loss of control).
No products indexed under this heading.

Tolmetin Sodium (Potentiates the hypoglycemic action; patients should be observed for hypoglycemia or loss of control). Products include:
Tolectin (200, 400 and 600 mg) .. 1581

Torsemide (Potential for hyperglycemia leading to loss of control). Products include:
Demadex Tablets and Injection 686

Tranylcypromine Sulfate (Potentiates the hypoglycemic action; patients should be observed for hypoglycemia or loss of control). Products include:
Parnate Tablets 2503

Triamcinolone (Potential for hyperglycemia leading to loss of control). Products include:
Aristocort Tablets 1022

Triamcinolone Acetonide (Potential for hyperglycemia leading to loss of control). Products include:
Aristocort A 0.025% Cream 1027
Aristocort A 0.5% Cream 1031
Aristocort A 0.1% Cream 1029
Aristocort A 0.1% Ointment 1030
Azmacort Oral Inhaler 2011
Nasacort Nasal Inhaler 2024

Triamcinolone Diacetate (Potential for hyperglycemia leading to loss of control). Products include:
Aristocort Suspension (Forte Parenteral) 1027
Aristocort Suspension (Intralesional) 1025

Triamcinolone Hexacetonide (Potential for hyperglycemia leading to loss of control). Products include:
Aristospan Suspension (Intra-articular) 1033
Aristospan Suspension (Intralesional) 1032

Triamterene (Potential for hyperglycemia leading to loss of control). Products include:
Dyazide 2479
Dyrenium Capsules 2481
Maxzide 1380

Trifluoperazine Hydrochloride (Potential for hyperglycemia leading to loss of control). Products include:
Stelazine 2514

Trimipramine Maleate (Potentiates the hypoglycemic action; patients should be observed for hypoglycemia or loss of control). Products include:
Surmontil Capsules 2811

Verapamil Hydrochloride (Potential for hyperglycemia leading to loss of control). Products include:
Calan SR Caplets 2422
Calan Tablets 2419
Isoptin Injectable 1344
Isoptin Oral Tablets 1346
Isoptin SR Tablets 1348
Verelan Capsules 1410
Verelan Capsules 2824

Warfarin Sodium (Potentiates the hypoglycemic action; patients should be observed for hypoglycemia or loss of control). Products include:
Coumadin 926

Food Interactions

Alcohol (Potential for hypoglycemia).

DIABE-TUSS DM SYRUP

(Dextromethorphan Hydrobromide) .. 1891
None cited in PDR database.

DIABINESE TABLETS

(Chlorpropamide) 1935
May interact with sympathomimetics, calcium channel blockers, barbiturates, non-steroidal anti-inflammatory agents, salicylates, sulfonamides, oral anticoagulants, monoamine oxidase inhibitors, beta blockers, thiazides, diuretics, corticosteroids, phenothiazines, oral contraceptives, thyroid preparations, estrogens, and certain other agents. Compounds in these categories include:

Acebutolol Hydrochloride (Potentiation of hypoglycemic action). Products include:
Sectral Capsules 2807

Albuterol (Co-administration may result in hyperglycemia leading to loss of control). Products include:
Proventil Inhalation Aerosol 2382
Ventolin Inhalation Aerosol and Refill 1197

Albuterol Sulfate (Co-administration may result in hyperglycemia leading to loss of control). Products include:
Airet Solution for Inhalation 452
Proventil Inhalation Solution 0.083% 2384
Proventil Repetabs Tablets 2386
Proventil Solution for Inhalation 0.5% 2383
Proventil Syrup 2385
Proventil Tablets 2386
Ventolin Inhalation Solution 1198
Ventolin Nebules Inhalation Solution 1199
Ventolin Rotacaps for Inhalation 1200
Ventolin Syrup 1202
Ventolin Tablets 1203
Volmax Extended-Release Tablets .. 1788

Amiloride Hydrochloride (Co-administration may result in hyperglycemia leading to loss of control). Products include:
Midamor Tablets 1703
Moduretic Tablets 1705

Amlodipine Besylate (Co-administration may result in hyperglycemia leading to loss of control). Products include:
Lotrel Capsules 840
Norvasc Tablets 1940

Aprobarbital (Prolonged barbiturate action).
No products indexed under this heading.

Aspirin (Potentiation of hypoglycemic action). Products include:
Alka-Seltzer Effervescent Antacid and Pain Reliever .... ▣ 701
Alka-Seltzer Extra Strength Effervescent Antacid and Pain Reliever .... ▣ 703
Alka-Seltzer Lemon Lime Effervescent Antacid and Pain Reliever .... ▣ 703
Alka-Seltzer Plus Cold Medicine .... ▣ 705
Alka-Seltzer Plus Cold & Cough Medicine .... ▣ 708
Alka-Seltzer Plus Night-Time Cold Medicine .... ▣ 707
Alka Seltzer Plus Sinus Medicine .. ▣ 707
Arthritis Foundation Safety Coated Aspirin Tablets .... ▣ 675
Arthritis Pain Ascriptin .... ▣ 631
Maximum Strength Ascriptin .... ▣ 630
Regular Strength Ascriptin Tablets .... ▣ 629
Arthritis Strength BC Powder .... ▣ 609
BC Cold Powder Multi-Symptom Formula (Cold-Sinus-Allergy) .... ▣ 609
BC Cold Powder Non-Drowsy Formula (Cold-Sinus) .... ▣ 609
BC Powder .... ▣ 609
Bayer Children's Chewable Aspirin .... ▣ 711
Genuine Bayer Aspirin Tablets & Caplets .... ▣ 713
Extra Strength Bayer Arthritis Pain Regimen Formula .... ▣ 711
Extra Strength Bayer Aspirin Caplets & Tablets .... ▣ 712
Extended-Release Bayer 8-Hour Aspirin .... ▣ 712
Extra Strength Bayer Plus Aspirin Caplets .... ▣ 713
Extra Strength Bayer PM Aspirin .. ▣ 713
Bayer Enteric Aspirin .... ▣ 709
Bufferin Analgesic Tablets and Caplets .... ▣ 613
Arthritis Strength Bufferin Analgesic Caplets .... ▣ 614
Extra Strength Bufferin Analgesic Tablets .... ▣ 615
Cama Arthritis Pain Reliever .... ▣ 785
Darvon Compound-65 Pulvules 1435
Easprin 1914
Ecotrin 2455
Ecotrin Enteric Coated Aspirin Maximum Strength Tablets and Caplets .... ▣ 816
Ecotrin Enteric Coated Aspirin Regular Strength Tablets 2455
Empirin Aspirin Tablets .... ▣ 854
Empirin with Codeine Tablets 1093
Excedrin Extra-Strength Analgesic Tablets & Caplets 732
Fiorinal Capsules 2261
Fiorinal with Codeine Capsules 2262
Fiorinal Tablets 2261
Halfprin 1362
Healthprin Aspirin 2455
Norgesic 1496
Percodan Tablets 939
Percodan-Demi Tablets 940
Robaxisal Tablets 2071
Soma Compound w/Codeine Tablets 2676
Soma Compound Tablets 2675
St. Joseph Adult Chewable Aspirin (81 mg.) .... ▣ 808
Talwin Compound 2335
Ursinus Inlay-Tabs .... ▣ 794
Vanquish Analgesic Caplets .... ▣ 731

Atenolol (Potentiation of hypoglycemic action). Products include:
Tenoretic Tablets 2845
Tenormin Tablets and I.V. Injection 2847

Bendroflumethiazide (Co-administration may result in hyperglycemia leading to loss of control).
No products indexed under this heading.

Bepridil Hydrochloride (Co-administration may result in hyperglycemia leading to loss of control). Products include:
Vascor (200, 300 and 400 mg) Tablets 1587

Betamethasone Acetate (Co-administration may result in hyperglycemia leading to loss of control). Products include:
Celestone Soluspan Suspension 2347

Betamethasone Sodium Phosphate (Co-administration may result in hyperglycemia leading to loss of control). Products include:
Celestone Soluspan Suspension 2347

Betaxolol Hydrochloride (Potentiation of hypoglycemic action). Products include:
Betoptic Ophthalmic Solution 469
Betoptic S Ophthalmic Suspension 471
Kerlone Tablets 2436

Bisoprolol Fumarate (Potentiation of hypoglycemic action). Products include:
Zebeta Tablets 1413
Ziac 1415

Bumetanide (Co-administration may result in hyperglycemia leading to loss of control). Products include:
Bumex 2093

Butabarbital (Prolonged barbiturate action).
No products indexed under this heading.

Butalbital (Prolonged barbiturate action). Products include:
Esgic-plus Tablets 1013
Fioricet Tablets 2258
Fioricet with Codeine Capsules 2260
Fiorinal Capsules 2261
Fiorinal with Codeine Capsules 2262
Fiorinal Tablets 2261
Phrenilin 785
Sedapap Tablets 50 mg/650 mg .. 1543

Carteolol Hydrochloride (Potentiation of hypoglycemic action). Products include:
Cartrol Tablets 410
Ocupress Ophthalmic Solution, 1% Sterile .... ⊙ 309

Chloramphenicol (Potentiation of hypoglycemic action). Products include:
Chloromycetin Ophthalmic Ointment, 1% .... ⊙ 310
Chloromycetin Ophthalmic Solution .... ⊙ 310
Chloroptic S.O.P. .... ⊙ 239
Chloroptic Sterile Ophthalmic Solution .... ⊙ 239
Elase-Chloromycetin Ointment 1040
Ophthocort .... ⊙ 311

Chloramphenicol Palmitate (Potentiation of hypoglycemic action).
No products indexed under this heading.

Chloramphenicol Sodium Succinate (Potentiation of hypoglycemic action). Products include:
Chloromycetin Sodium Succinate 1900

Chlorothiazide (Co-administration may result in hyperglycemia leading to loss of control). Products include:
Aldoclor Tablets 1598
Diupres Tablets 1650
Diuril Oral 1653

Chlorothiazide Sodium (Co-administration may result in hyperglycemia leading to loss of control). Products include:
Diuril Sodium Intravenous 1652

Chlorotrianisene (Co-administration may result in hyperglycemia leading to loss of control).
No products indexed under this heading.

Chlorpromazine (Co-administration may result in hyperglycemia leading to loss of control). Products include:
Thorazine Suppositories 2523

Chlorpromazine Hydrochloride (Co-administration may result in hyperglycemia leading to loss of control). Products include:
Thorazine 2523

Chlorthalidone (Co-administration may result in hyperglycemia leading to loss of control). Products include:
Combipres Tablets 677
Tenoretic Tablets 2845
Thalitone 1245

Choline Magnesium Trisalicylate (Potentiation of hypoglycemic action). Products include:
Trilisate 2000

Cortisone Acetate (Co-administration may result in hyperglycemia leading to loss of control). Products include:
Cortone Acetate Sterile Suspension 1623
Cortone Acetate Tablets 1624

Desogestrel (Co-administration may result in hyperglycemia leading to loss of control). Products include:
Desogen Tablets 1817
Ortho-Cept 1851

Dexamethasone (Co-administration may result in hyperglycemia leading to loss of control). Products include:
AK-Trol Ointment & Suspension .... ⊙ 205

(▣ Described in PDR For Nonprescription Drugs) (⊙ Described in PDR For Ophthalmology)

277 **Interactions Index** **Diabinese**

Decadron Elixir ... 1633
Decadron Tablets ... 1635
Decaspray Topical Aerosol ... 1648
Dexacidin Ointment ... ⊙ 263
Maxitrol Ophthalmic Ointment and Suspension ... ⊙ 224
TobraDex Ophthalmic Suspension and Ointment ... 473

Dexamethasone Acetate (Co-administration may result in hyperglycemia leading to loss of control). Products include:
Dalalone D.P. Injectable ... 1011
Decadron-LA Sterile Suspension ... 1646

Dexamethasone Sodium Phosphate (Co-administration may result in hyperglycemia leading to loss of control). Products include:
Decadron Phosphate Injection ... 1637
Decadron Phosphate Respihaler ... 1642
Decadron Phosphate Sterile Ophthalmic Ointment ... 1641
Decadron Phosphate Sterile Ophthalmic Solution ... 1642
Decadron Phosphate Topical Cream ... 1644
Decadron Phosphate Turbinaire ... 1645
Decadron Phosphate with Xylocaine Injection, Sterile ... 1639
Dexacort Phosphate in Respihaler .. 458
Dexacort Phosphate in Turbinaire .. 459
NeoDecadron Sterile Ophthalmic Ointment ... 1712
NeoDecadron Sterile Ophthalmic Solution ... 1713
NeoDecadron Topical Cream ... 1714

Diclofenac Potassium (Potentiation of hypoglycemic action). Products include:
Cataflam ... 816

Diclofenac Sodium (Potentiation of hypoglycemic action). Products include:
Voltaren Ophthalmic Sterile Ophthalmic Solution ... ⊙ 272
Voltaren Tablets ... 861

Dicumarol (Potentiation of hypoglycemic action).
No products indexed under this heading.

Dienestrol (Co-administration may result in hyperglycemia leading to loss of control). Products include:
Ortho Dienestrol Cream ... 1866

Diethylstilbestrol (Co-administration may result in hyperglycemia leading to loss of control). Products include:
Diethylstilbestrol Tablets ... 1437

Diflunisal (Potentiation of hypoglycemic action). Products include:
Dolobid Tablets ... 1654

Diltiazem Hydrochloride (Co-administration may result in hyperglycemia leading to loss of control). Products include:
Cardizem CD Capsules ... 1506
Cardizem SR Capsules ... 1510
Cardizem Injectable ... 1508
Cardizem Tablets ... 1512
Dilacor XR Extended-release Capsules ... 2018

Dobutamine Hydrochloride (Co-administration may result in hyperglycemia leading to loss of control). Products include:
Dobutrex Solution Vials ... 1439

Dopamine Hydrochloride (Co-administration may result in hyperglycemia leading to loss of control).
No products indexed under this heading.

Ephedrine Hydrochloride (Co-administration may result in hyperglycemia leading to loss of control). Products include:
Primatene Dual Action Formula ... ▣ 872
Primatene Tablets ... ▣ 873
Quadrinal Tablets ... 1350

Ephedrine Sulfate (Co-administration may result in hyperglycemia leading to loss of control). Products include:
Bronkaid Caplets ... ▣ 717
Marax Tablets & DF Syrup ... 2200

Ephedrine Tannate (Co-administration may result in hyperglycemia leading to loss of control). Products include:
Rynatuss ... 2673

Epinephrine (Co-administration may result in hyperglycemia leading to loss of control). Products include:
Bronkaid Mist ... ▣ 717
EPIFRIN ... ⊙ 239
EpiPen ... 790
Marcaine Hydrochloride with Epinephrine 1:200,000 ... 2316
Primatene Mist ... ▣ 873
Sensorcaine with Epinephrine Injection ... 559
Sus-Phrine Injection ... 1019
Xylocaine with Epinephrine Injections ... 567

Epinephrine Bitartrate (Co-administration may result in hyperglycemia leading to loss of control). Products include:
Bronkaid Mist Suspension ... ▣ 718
Sensorcaine-MPF with Epinephrine Injection ... 559

Epinephrine Hydrochloride (Co-administration may result in hyperglycemia leading to loss of control). Products include:
Ana-Kit Anaphylaxis Emergency Treatment Kit ... 617

Esmolol Hydrochloride (Potentiation of hypoglycemic action). Products include:
Brevibloc Injection ... 1808

Estradiol (Co-administration may result in hyperglycemia leading to loss of control). Products include:
Climara Transdermal System ... 645
Estrace Cream and Tablets ... 749
Estraderm Transdermal System ... 824

Estrogens, Conjugated (Co-administration may result in hyperglycemia leading to loss of control). Products include:
PMB 200 and PMB 400 ... 2783
Premarin Intravenous ... 2787
Premarin with Methyltestosterone .. 2794
Premarin Tablets ... 2789
Premarin Vaginal Cream ... 2791
Premphase ... 2797
Prempro ... 2801

Estrogens, Esterified (Co-administration may result in hyperglycemia leading to loss of control). Products include:
ESTRATAB Tablets (0.3, 0.625, 1.25, 2.5 mg) ... 2536
Estratest ... 2539
Menest Tablets ... 2494

Estropipate (Co-administration may result in hyperglycemia leading to loss of control). Products include:
Ogen Tablets ... 2627
Ogen Vaginal Cream ... 2630
Ortho-Est ... 1869

Ethacrynic Acid (Co-administration may result in hyperglycemia leading to loss of control). Products include:
Edecrin Tablets ... 1657

Ethinyl Estradiol (Co-administration may result in hyperglycemia leading to loss of control). Products include:
Brevicon ... 2088
Demulen ... 2428
Desogen Tablets ... 1817
Levlen/Tri-Levlen ... 651
Lo/Ovral Tablets ... 2746
Lo/Ovral-28 Tablets ... 2751
Modicon ... 1872
Nordette-21 Tablets ... 2755
Nordette-28 Tablets ... 2758
Norinyl ... 2088
Ortho-Cept ... 1851
Ortho-Cyclen/Ortho-Tri-Cyclen ... 1858
Ortho-Novum ... 1872
Ortho-Cyclen/Ortho Tri-Cyclen ... 1858
Ovcon ... 760
Ovral Tablets ... 2770
Ovral-28 Tablets ... 2770
Levlen/Tri-Levlen ... 651
Tri-Norinyl ... 2164
Triphasil-21 Tablets ... 2814
Triphasil-28 Tablets ... 2819

Ethynodiol Diacetate (Co-administration may result in hyperglycemia leading to loss of control). Products include:
Demulen ... 2428

Etodolac (Potentiation of hypoglycemic action). Products include:
Lodine Capsules and Tablets ... 2743

Felodipine (Co-administration may result in hyperglycemia leading to loss of control). Products include:
Plendil Extended-Release Tablets ... 527

Fenoprofen Calcium (Potentiation of hypoglycemic action). Products include:
Nalfon 200 Pulvules & Nalfon Tablets ... 917

Fludrocortisone Acetate (Co-administration may result in hyperglycemia leading to loss of control). Products include:
Florinef Acetate Tablets ... 505

Fluphenazine Decanoate (Co-administration may result in hyperglycemia leading to loss of control). Products include:
Prolixin Decanoate ... 509

Fluphenazine Enanthate (Co-administration may result in hyperglycemia leading to loss of control). Products include:
Prolixin Enanthate ... 509

Fluphenazine Hydrochloride (Co-administration may result in hyperglycemia leading to loss of control). Products include:
Prolixin ... 509

Flurbiprofen (Potentiation of hypoglycemic action). Products include:
Ansaid Tablets ... 2579

Furazolidone (Potentiation of hypoglycemic action). Products include:
Furoxone ... 2046

Furosemide (Co-administration may result in hyperglycemia leading to loss of control). Products include:
Lasix Injection, Oral Solution and Tablets ... 1240

Glipizide (Potentiation of hypoglycemic action). Products include:
Glucotrol Tablets ... 1967
Glucotrol XL Extended Release Tablets ... 1968

Glyburide (Potentiation of hypoglycemic action). Products include:
DiaBeta Tablets ... 1239
Glynase PresTab Tablets ... 2609
Micronase Tablets ... 2623

Hydrochlorothiazide (Co-administration may result in hyperglycemia leading to loss of control). Products include:
Aldactazide ... 2413
Aldoril Tablets ... 1604
Apresazide Capsules ... 808
Capozide ... 742
Dyazide ... 2479
Esidrix Tablets ... 821
Esimil Tablets ... 822
HydroDIURIL Tablets ... 1674
Hydropres Tablets ... 1675
Hyzaar Tablets ... 1677
Inderide Tablets ... 2732
Inderide LA Long Acting Capsules .. 2734
Lopressor HCT Tablets ... 832
Lotensin HCT ... 837
Maxzide ... 1380
Moduretic Tablets ... 1705
Oretic Tablets ... 443
Prinzide Tablets ... 1737
Ser-Ap-Es Tablets ... 849
Timolide Tablets ... 1748
Vaseretic Tablets ... 1765
Zestoretic ... 2850
Ziac ... 1415

Hydrocortisone (Co-administration may result in hyperglycemia leading to loss of control). Products include:
Anusol-HC Cream 2.5% ... 1896
Aquanil HC Lotion ... 1931
Bactine Hydrocortisone Anti-Itch Cream ... ▣ 709
Caldecort Anti-Itch Hydrocortisone Spray ... ▣ 631
Cortaid ... ▣ 836
CORTENEMA ... 2535
Cortisporin Ointment ... 1085
Cortisporin Ophthalmic Ointment Sterile ... 1085
Cortisporin Ophthalmic Suspension Sterile ... 1086
Cortisporin Otic Solution Sterile ... 1087
Cortisporin Otic Suspension Sterile 1088
Cortizone-5 ... ▣ 831
Cortizone-10 ... ▣ 831
Hydrocortone Tablets ... 1672
Hytone ... 907
Massengill Medicated Soft Cloth Towelettes ... 2458
PediOtic Suspension Sterile ... 1153
Preparation H Hydrocortisone 1% Cream ... ▣ 872
ProctoCream-HC 2.5% ... 2408
VōSoL HC Otic Solution ... 2678

Hydrocortisone Acetate (Co-administration may result in hyperglycemia leading to loss of control). Products include:
Analpram-HC Rectal Cream 1% and 2.5% ... 977
Anusol HC-1 Anti-Itch Hydrocortisone Ointment ... ▣ 847
Anusol-HC Suppositories ... 1897
Caldecort ... ▣ 631
Carmol HC ... 924
Coly-Mycin S Otic w/Neomycin & Hydrocortisone ... 1906
Cortaid ... ▣ 836
Cortifoam ... 2396
Cortisporin Cream ... 1084
Epifoam ... 2399
Hydrocortone Acetate Sterile Suspension ... 1669
Mantadil Cream ... 1135
Nupercainal Hydrocortisone 1% Cream ... ▣ 645
Ophthocort ... ⊙ 311
Pramosone Cream, Lotion & Ointment ... 978
ProctoCream-HC ... 2408
ProctoFoam-HC ... 2409
Terra-Cortril Ophthalmic Suspension ... 2210

Hydrocortisone Sodium Phosphate (Co-administration may result in hyperglycemia leading to loss of control). Products include:
Hydrocortone Phosphate Injection, Sterile ... 1670

Hydrocortisone Sodium Succinate (Co-administration may result in hyperglycemia leading to loss of control). Products include:
Solu-Cortef Sterile Powder ... 2641

Hydroflumethiazide (Co-administration may result in hyperglycemia leading to loss of control). Products include:
Diucardin Tablets ... 2718

Ibuprofen (Potentiation of hypoglycemic action). Products include:
Advil Cold and Sinus Caplets and Tablets (formerly CoAdvil) ... ▣ 870
Advil Ibuprofen Tablets and Caplets ... ▣ 870
Children's Advil Suspension ... 2692
Arthritis Foundation Ibuprofen Tablets ... ▣ 674
Bayer Select Ibuprofen Pain Relief Formula ... ▣ 715
Cramp End Tablets ... ▣ 735
Dimetapp Sinus Caplets ... ▣ 775
Haltran Tablets ... ▣ 771
IBU Tablets ... 1342
Ibuprohm ... ▣ 735

IMPORTANT NOTE: Always consult each drug listing in the patient's regimen for possible interactions.

Diabinese **Interactions Index** **278**

Children's Motrin Ibuprofen Oral Suspension 1546
Motrin Tablets 2625
Motrin IB Caplets, Tablets, and Geltabs .... ◙ 838
Motrin IB Sinus .... ◙ 838
Motrin Ibuprofen Suspension, Oral Drops, Chewable Tablets, Caplets 1546
Nuprin Ibuprofen/Analgesic Tablets & Caplets .... ◙ 622
Sine-Aid IB Caplets 1554
Vicks DayQuil SINUS Pressure & PAIN Relief with IBUPROFEN .... ◙ 762

Indapamide (Co-administration may result in hyperglycemia leading to loss of control). Products include:
Lozol Tablets 2022

Indomethacin (Potentiation of hypoglycemic action). Products include:
Indocin 1680

Indomethacin Sodium Trihydrate (Potentiation of hypoglycemic action). Products include:
Indocin I.V. 1684

Isocarboxazid (Potentiation of hypoglycemic action).
No products indexed under this heading.

Isoniazid (Co-administration may result in hyperglycemia leading to loss of control). Products include:
Nydrazid Injection 508
Rifamate Capsules 1530
Rifater 1532

Isoproterenol Hydrochloride (Co-administration may result in hyperglycemia leading to loss of control). Products include:
Isuprel Hydrochloride Injection 1:5000 2311
Isuprel Hydrochloride Solution 1:200 & 1:100 2313
Isuprel Mistometer 2312

Isoproterenol Sulfate (Co-administration may result in hyperglycemia leading to loss of control). Products include:
Norisodrine with Calcium Iodide Syrup 442

Isradipine (Co-administration may result in hyperglycemia leading to loss of control). Products include:
DynaCirc Capsules 2256

Ketoprofen (Potentiation of hypoglycemic action). Products include:
Orudis Capsules 2766
Oruvail Capsules 2766

Ketorolac Tromethamine (Potentiation of hypoglycemic action). Products include:
Acular 474
Acular .... ⊙ 277
Toradol 2159

Labetalol Hydrochloride (Potentiation of hypoglycemic action). Products include:
Normodyne Injection 2377
Normodyne Tablets 2379
Trandate 1185

Levobunolol Hydrochloride (Potentiation of hypoglycemic action). Products include:
Betagan .... ⊙ 233

Levonorgestrel (Co-administration may result in hyperglycemia leading to loss of control). Products include:
Levlen/Tri-Levlen 651
Nordette-21 Tablets 2755
Nordette-28 Tablets 2758
Norplant System 2759
Levlen/Tri-Levlen 651
Triphasil-21 Tablets 2814
Triphasil-28 Tablets 2819

Levothyroxine Sodium (Co-administration may result in hyperglycemia leading to loss of control). Products include:
Levothroid Tablets 1016
Levoxyl Tablets 903
Synthroid 1359

Liothyronine Sodium (Co-administration may result in hyperglycemia leading to loss of control). Products include:
Cytomel Tablets 2473
Triostat Injection 2530

Liotrix (Co-administration may result in hyperglycemia leading to loss of control).
No products indexed under this heading.

Magnesium Salicylate (Potentiation of hypoglycemic action). Products include:
Backache Caplets .... ◙ 613
Bayer Select Backache Pain Relief Formula .... ◙ 715
Doan's Extra-Strength Analgesic .... ◙ 633
Extra Strength Doan's P.M. .... ◙ 633
Doan's Regular Strength Analgesic .... ◙ 634
Mobigesic Tablets .... ◙ 602

Meclofenamate Sodium (Potentiation of hypoglycemic action).
No products indexed under this heading.

Mefenamic Acid (Potentiation of hypoglycemic action). Products include:
Ponstel 1925

Mephobarbital (Prolonged barbiturate action). Products include:
Mebaral Tablets 2322

Mesoridazine Besylate (Co-administration may result in hyperglycemia leading to loss of control). Products include:
Serentil 684

Mestranol (Co-administration may result in hyperglycemia leading to loss of control). Products include:
Norinyl 2088
Ortho-Novum 1872

Metaproterenol Sulfate (Co-administration may result in hyperglycemia leading to loss of control). Products include:
Alupent 669
Metaproterenol Sulfate Inhalation Solution, USP, Arm-a-Med 552

Metaraminol Bitartrate (Co-administration may result in hyperglycemia leading to loss of control). Products include:
Aramine Injection 1609

Methotrimeprazine (Co-administration may result in hyperglycemia leading to loss of control). Products include:
Levoprome 1274

Methoxamine Hydrochloride (Co-administration may result in hyperglycemia leading to loss of control). Products include:
Vasoxyl Injection 1196

Methyclothiazide (Co-administration may result in hyperglycemia leading to loss of control). Products include:
Enduron Tablets 420

Methylprednisolone (Co-administration may result in hyperglycemia leading to loss of control). Products include:
Medrol 2621

Methylprednisolone Acetate (Co-administration may result in hyperglycemia leading to loss of control). Products include:
Depo-Medrol Single-Dose Vial 2600
Depo-Medrol Sterile Aqueous Suspension 2597

Methylprednisolone Sodium Succinate (Co-administration may result in hyperglycemia leading to loss of control). Products include:
Solu-Medrol Sterile Powder 2643

Metipranolol Hydrochloride (Potentiation of hypoglycemic action). Products include:
OptiPranolol (Metipranolol 0.3%) Sterile Ophthalmic Solution .... ⊙ 258

Metolazone (Co-administration may result in hyperglycemia leading to loss of control). Products include:
Mykrox Tablets 993
Zaroxolyn Tablets 1000

Metoprolol Succinate (Potentiation of hypoglycemic action). Products include:
Toprol-XL Tablets 565

Metoprolol Tartrate (Potentiation of hypoglycemic action). Products include:
Lopressor Ampuls 830
Lopressor HCT Tablets 832
Lopressor Tablets 830

Miconazole (Potential for severe hypoglycemia when co-administered with oral miconazole).
No products indexed under this heading.

Nabumetone (Potentiation of hypoglycemic action). Products include:
Relafen Tablets 2510

Nadolol (Potentiation of hypoglycemic action).
No products indexed under this heading.

Naproxen (Potentiation of hypoglycemic action). Products include:
Anaprox/Naprosyn 2117

Naproxen Sodium (Potentiation of hypoglycemic action). Products include:
Aleve 1975
Anaprox/Naprosyn 2117

Niacin (Co-administration may result in hyperglycemia leading to loss of control). Products include:
Nicobid 2026
Nicolar Tablets 2026
Nicotinex Elixir .... ◙ 655
Sigtab Tablets .... ◙ 772
Slo-Niacin Tablets 2659
Stuart Prenatal Tablets .... ◙ 881
The Stuart Formula Tablets .... ◙ 663
Zymacap Capsules .... ◙ 772

Nicardipine Hydrochloride (Co-administration may result in hyperglycemia leading to loss of control). Products include:
Cardene Capsules 2095
Cardene I.V. 2709
Cardene SR Capsules 2097

Nifedipine (Co-administration may result in hyperglycemia leading to loss of control). Products include:
Adalat Capsules (10 mg and 20 mg) 587
Adalat CC 589
Procardia Capsules 1971
Procardia XL Extended Release Tablets 1972

Nimodipine (Co-administration may result in hyperglycemia leading to loss of control). Products include:
Nimotop Capsules 610

Nisoldipine (Co-administration may result in hyperglycemia leading to loss of control).
No products indexed under this heading.

Norepinephrine Bitartrate (Co-administration may result in hyperglycemia leading to loss of control). Products include:
Levophed Bitartrate Injection 2315

Norethindrone (Co-administration may result in hyperglycemia leading to loss of control). Products include:
Brevicon 2088
Micronor Tablets 1872
Modicon 1872
Norinyl 2088
Nor-Q D Tablets 2135
Ortho-Novum 1872
Ovcon 760
Tri-Norinyl 2164

Norethynodrel (Co-administration may result in hyperglycemia leading to loss of control).
No products indexed under this heading.

Norgestimate (Co-administration may result in hyperglycemia leading to loss of control). Products include:
Ortho-Cyclen/Ortho-Tri-Cyclen 1858
Ortho-Cyclen/Ortho Tri-Cyclen 1858

Norgestrel (Co-administration may result in hyperglycemia leading to loss of control). Products include:
Lo/Ovral Tablets 2746
Lo/Ovral-28 Tablets 2751
Ovral Tablets 2770
Ovral-28 Tablets 2770
Ovrette Tablets 2771

Oxaprozin (Potentiation of hypoglycemic action). Products include:
Daypro Caplets 2426

Penbutolol Sulfate (Potentiation of hypoglycemic action). Products include:
Levatol 2403

Pentobarbital Sodium (Prolonged barbiturate action). Products include:
Nembutal Sodium Capsules 436
Nembutal Sodium Solution 438
Nembutal Sodium Suppositories 440

Perphenazine (Co-administration may result in hyperglycemia leading to loss of control). Products include:
Etrafon 2355
Triavil Tablets 1757
Trilafon 2389

Phenelzine Sulfate (Potentiation of hypoglycemic action). Products include:
Nardil 1920

Phenobarbital (Prolonged barbiturate action). Products include:
Arco-Lase Plus Tablets 512
Bellergal-S Tablets 2250
Donnatal 2060
Donnatal Extentabs 2061
Donnatal Tablets 2060
Phenobarbital Elixir and Tablets 1469
Quadrinal Tablets 1350

Phenylbutazone (Potentiation of hypoglycemic action).
No products indexed under this heading.

Phenylephrine Bitartrate (Co-administration may result in hyperglycemia leading to loss of control).
No products indexed under this heading.

Phenylephrine Hydrochloride (Co-administration may result in hyperglycemia leading to loss of control). Products include:
Atrohist Plus Tablets 454
Cerose DM .... ◙ 878
Comhist 2038
D.A. Chewable Tablets 951
Deconsal Pediatric Capsules 454
Dura-Vent/DA Tablets 953
Entex Capsules 1986
Entex Liquid 1986
Extendryl 1005
4-Way Fast Acting Nasal Spray (regular & mentholated) .... ◙ 621
Hemorid For Women .... ◙ 834
Hycomine Compound Tablets 932
Neo-Synephrine Hydrochloride 1% Carpuject 2324
Neo-Synephrine Hydrochloride 1% Injection 2324
Neo-Synephrine Hydrochloride (Ophthalmic) 2325
Neo-Synephrine .... ◙ 726
Nōstril .... ◙ 644
Novahistine Elixir .... ◙ 823
Phenergan VC 2779
Phenergan VC with Codeine 2781
Preparation H .... ◙ 871
Tympagesic Ear Drops 2342
Vasosulf .... ⊙ 271

(◙ Described in PDR For Nonprescription Drugs) (⊙ Described in PDR For Ophthalmology)

279 **Interactions Index** **Diabinese**

Vicks Sinex Nasal Spray and Ultra Fine Mist ... 765

Phenylephrine Tannate (Co-administration may result in hyperglycemia leading to loss of control). Products include:

Atrohist Pediatric Suspension ... 454
Ricobid-D Pediatric Suspension ... 2038
Ricobid Tablets and Pediatric Suspension ... 2038
Rynatan ... 2673
Rynatuss ... 2673

Phenylpropanolamine Hydrochloride (Co-administration may result in hyperglycemia leading to loss of control). Products include:

Acutrim ... 628
Allerest Children's Chewable Tablets ... 627
Allerest 12 Hour Caplets ... 627
Atrohist Plus Tablets ... 454
BC Cold Powder Multi-Symptom Formula (Cold-Sinus-Allergy) ... 609
BC Cold Powder Non-Drowsy Formula (Cold-Sinus) ... 609
Cheracol Plus Head Cold/Cough Formula ... 769
Comtrex Multi-Symptom Non-Drowsy Liqui-gels ... 618
Contac Continuous Action Nasal Decongestant/Antihistamine 12 Hour Capsules ... 813
Contac Maximum Strength Continuous Action Decongestant/Antihistamine 12 Hour Caplets ... 813
Contac Severe Cold and Flu Formula Caplets ... 814
Coricidin 'D' Decongestant Tablets ... 800
Dexatrim ... 832
Dexatrim Plus Vitamins Caplets ... 832
Dimetane-DC Cough Syrup ... 2059
Dimetapp Elixir ... 773
Dimetapp Extentabs ... 774
Dimetapp Tablets/Liqui-Gels ... 775
Dimetapp Cold & Allergy Chewable Tablets ... 773
Dimetapp DM Elixir ... 774
Dura-Vent Tablets ... 952
Entex Capsules ... 1986
Entex LA Tablets ... 1987
Entex Liquid ... 1986
Exgest LA Tablets ... 782
Hycomine ... 931
Isoclor Timesule Capsules ... 637
Nolamine Timed-Release Tablets ... 785
Ornade Spansule Capsules ... 2502
Propagest Tablets ... 786
Pyrroxate Caplets ... 772
Robitussin-CF ... 777
Sinulin Tablets ... 787
Tavist-D 12 Hour Relief Tablets ... 787
Teldrin 12 Hour Antihistamine/Nasal Decongestant Allergy Relief Capsules ... 826
Triaminic Allergy Tablets ... 789
Triaminic Cold Tablets ... 790
Triaminic Expectorant ... 790
Triaminic Syrup ... 792
Triaminic-12 Tablets ... 792
Triaminic-DM Syrup ... 792
Triaminicin Tablets ... 793
Triaminicol Multi-Symptom Cold Tablets ... 793
Triaminicol Multi-Symptom Relief ... 794
Vicks DayQuil Allergy Relief 12-Hour Extended Release Tablets ... 760
Vicks DayQuil Allergy Relief 4-Hour Tablets ... 760
Vicks DayQuil SINUS Pressure & CONGESTION Relief ... 761

Phenytoin (Co-administration may result in hyperglycemia leading to loss of control). Products include:

Dilantin Infatabs ... 1908
Dilantin-125 Suspension ... 1911

Phenytoin Sodium (Co-administration may result in hyperglycemia leading to loss of control). Products include:

Dilantin Kapseals ... 1906
Dilantin Parenteral ... 1910

Pindolol (Potentiation of hypoglycemic action). Products include:

Visken Tablets ... 2299

Pirbuterol Acetate (Co-administration may result in hyperglycemia leading to loss of control). Products include:

Maxair Autohaler ... 1492
Maxair Inhaler ... 1494

Piroxicam (Potentiation of hypoglycemic action). Products include:

Feldene Capsules ... 1965

Polyestradiol Phosphate (Co-administration may result in hyperglycemia leading to loss of control).

No products indexed under this heading.

Polythiazide (Co-administration may result in hyperglycemia leading to loss of control). Products include:

Minizide Capsules ... 1938

Prednisolone Acetate (Co-administration may result in hyperglycemia leading to loss of control). Products include:

AK-CIDE ... 202
AK-CIDE Ointment ... 202
Blephamide Liquifilm Sterile Ophthalmic Suspension ... 476
Blephamide Ointment ... 237
Econopred & Econopred Plus Ophthalmic Suspensions ... 217
Poly-Pred Liquifilm ... 248
Pred Forte ... 250
Pred Mild ... 253
Pred-G Liquifilm Sterile Ophthalmic Suspension ... 251
Pred-G S.O.P. Sterile Ophthalmic Ointment ... 252
Vasocidin Ointment ... 268

Prednisolone Sodium Phosphate (Co-administration may result in hyperglycemia leading to loss of control). Products include:

AK-Pred ... 204
Hydeltrasol Injection, Sterile ... 1665
Inflamase ... 265
Pediapred Oral Liquid ... 995
Vasocidin Ophthalmic Solution ... 270

Prednisolone Tebutate (Co-administration may result in hyperglycemia leading to loss of control). Products include:

Hydeltra-T.B.A. Sterile Suspension 1667

Prednisone (Co-administration may result in hyperglycemia leading to loss of control). Products include:

Deltasone Tablets ... 2595

Probenecid (Potentiation of hypoglycemic action). Products include:

Benemid Tablets ... 1611
ColBENEMID Tablets ... 1622

Prochlorperazine (Co-administration may result in hyperglycemia leading to loss of control). Products include:

Compazine ... 2470

Promethazine Hydrochloride (Co-administration may result in hyperglycemia leading to loss of control). Products include:

Mepergan Injection ... 2753
Phenergan with Codeine ... 2777
Phenergan with Dextromethorphan 2778
Phenergan Injection ... 2773
Phenergan Suppositories ... 2775
Phenergan Syrup ... 2774
Phenergan Tablets ... 2775
Phenergan VC ... 2779
Phenergan VC with Codeine ... 2781

Propranolol Hydrochloride (Potentiation of hypoglycemic action). Products include:

Inderal ... 2728
Inderal LA Long Acting Capsules ... 2730
Inderide Tablets ... 2732
Inderide LA Long Acting Capsules .. 2734

Pseudoephedrine Hydrochloride (Co-administration may result in hyperglycemia leading to loss of control). Products include:

Actifed Allergy Daytime/Nighttime Caplets ... 844
Actifed Plus Caplets ... 845
Actifed Plus Tablets ... 845
Actifed with Codeine Cough Syrup .. 1067
Actifed Sinus Daytime/Nighttime Tablets and Caplets ... 846
Actifed Syrup ... 846
Actifed Tablets ... 844
Advil Cold and Sinus Caplets and Tablets (formerly CoAdvil) ... 870
Alka-Seltzer Plus Cold Medicine Liqui-Gels ... 706
Alka-Seltzer Plus Cold & Cough Medicine Liqui-Gels ... 705
Alka-Seltzer Plus Night-Time Cold Medicine Liqui-Gels ... 706
Allerest Headache Strength Tablets ... 627
Allerest Maximum Strength Tablets ... 627
Allerest No Drowsiness Tablets ... 627
Allerest Sinus Pain Formula ... 627
Anatuss LA Tablets ... 1542
Atrohist Pediatric Capsules ... 453
Bayer Select Sinus Pain Relief Formula ... 717
Benadryl Allergy Decongestant Liquid Medication ... 848
Benadryl Allergy Decongestant Tablets ... 848
Benadryl Allergy Sinus Headache Formula Caplets ... 849
Benylin Multisymptom ... 852
Bromfed Capsules (Extended-Release) ... 1785
Bromfed Syrup ... 733
Bromfed Tablets ... 1785
Bromfed-DM Cough Syrup ... 1786
Bromfed-PD Capsules (Extended-Release) ... 1785
Children's Vicks DayQuil Allergy Relief ... 757
Children's Vicks NyQuil Cold/Cough Relief ... 758
Comtrex Multi-Symptom Cold Reliever Tablets/Caplets/Liqui-Gels/Liquid ... 615
Allergy-Sinus Comtrex Multi-Symptom Allergy-Sinus Formula Tablets ... 617
Comtrex Multi-Symptom Non-Drowsy Caplets ... 618
Congess ... 1004
Contac Day Allergy/Sinus Caplets ... 812
Contac Day & Night ... 812
Contac Night Allergy/Sinus Caplets ... 812
Contac Severe Cold & Flu Non-Drowsy ... 815
Deconamine Chewable Tablets ... 1320
Deconamine CX Cough and Cold Liquid and Tablets ... 1319
Deconamine ... 1320
Deconsal C Expectorant Syrup ... 456
Deconsal Pediatric Syrup ... 457
Deconsal II Tablets ... 454
Dimetane-DX Cough Syrup ... 2059
Dimetapp Sinus Caplets ... 775
Dorcol Children's Cough Syrup ... 785
Drixoral Cough + Congestion Liquid Caps ... 802
Dura-Tap/PD Capsules ... 2867
Duratuss Tablets ... 2565
Duratuss HD Elixir ... 2565
Efidac/24 ... 635
Entex PSE Tablets ... 1987
Fedahist Gyrocaps ... 2401
Fedahist Timecaps ... 2401
Guaifed ... 1787
Guaifed Syrup ... 734
Guaimax-D Tablets ... 792
Guaitab Tablets ... 734
Isoclor Expectorant ... 990
Kronofed-A ... 977
Motrin IB Sinus ... 838
Novahistine DH ... 2462
Novahistine DMX ... 822
Novahistine Expectorant ... 2463
Nucofed ... 2051
PediaCare Cold Allergy Chewable Tablets ... 677
PediaCare Cough-Cold Chewable Tablets ... 1553
PediaCare ... 1553
PediaCare Infants' Decongestant Drops ... 677
PediCare Infant's Drops Decongestant Plus Cough ... 1553
PediaCare NightRest Cough-Cold Liquid ... 1553
Pediatric Vicks 44d Dry Hacking Cough & Head Congestion ... 763
Pediatric Vicks 44m Cough & Cold Relief ... 764
Robitussin Cold & Cough Liqui-Gels ... 776
Robitussin Maximum Strength Cough & Cold ... 778
Robitussin Pediatric Cough & Cold Formula ... 779
Robitussin Severe Congestion Liqui-Gels ... 776
Robitussin-DAC Syrup ... 2074
Robitussin-PE ... 778
Rondec Oral Drops ... 953
Rondec Syrup ... 953
Rondec Tablet ... 953
Rondec-DM Oral Drops ... 954
Rondec-DM Syrup ... 954
Rondec-TR Tablet ... 953
Ryna ... 841
Seldane-D Extended-Release Tablets ... 1538
Semprex-D Capsules ... 463
Semprex-D Capsules ... 1167
Sinarest Tablets ... 648
Sinarest Extra Strength Tablets ... 648
Sinarest No Drowsiness Tablets ... 648
Sine-Aid IB Caplets ... 1554
Sine-Aid Maximum Strength Sinus Medication Gelcaps, Caplets and Tablets ... 1554
Sine-Off No Drowsiness Formula Caplets ... 824
Sine-Off Sinus Medicine ... 825
Singlet Tablets ... 825
Sinutab Non-Drying Liquid Caps ... 859
Sinutab Sinus Allergy Medication, Maximum Strength Tablets and Caplets ... 860
Sinutab Sinus Medication, Maximum Strength Without Drowsiness Formula, Tablets & Caplets ... 860
Sinutab Sinus Medication, Regular Strength Without Drowsiness Formula ... 859
Sudafed Children's Liquid ... 861
Sudafed Cold and Cough Liquidcaps ... 862
Sudafed Cough Syrup ... 862
Sudafed Plus Liquid ... 862
Sudafed Plus Tablets ... 863
Sudafed Severe Cold Formula Caplets ... 863
Sudafed Severe Cold Formula Tablets ... 864
Sudafed Sinus Caplets ... 864
Sudafed Sinus Tablets ... 864
Sudafed Tablets, 30 mg ... 861
Sudafed Tablets, 60 mg ... 861
Sudafed 12 Hour Caplets ... 861
Syn-Rx Tablets ... 465
Syn-Rx DM Tablets ... 466
TheraFlu ... 787
TheraFlu Maximum Strength Nighttime Flu, Cold & Cough Medicine ... 788
TheraFlu Maximum Strength Non-Drowsy Formula Flu, Cold & Cough Medicine ... 788
Thera Flu Maximum Strength, Non-Drowsy Formula Flu, Cold and Cough Caplets ... 789
Triaminic AM Cough and Decongestant Formula ... 789
Triaminic AM Decongestant Formula ... 790
Triaminic Nite Light ... 791
Triaminic Sore Throat Formula ... 791
Tussend ... 1783
Tussend Expectorant ... 1785
Children's TYLENOL Cold Multi-Symptom Liquid Formula and Chewable Tablets ... 1561
Children's TYLENOL Cold Plus Cough Multi Symptom Tablets and Liquid ... 681
Infants' TYLENOL Cold Decongestant & Fever-Reducer Drops ... 1556
TYLENOL Maximum Strength Allergy Sinus Medication Gelcaps and Caplets ... 1563
TYLENOL Maximum Strength Allergy Sinus NightTime Medication Caplets ... 1555
TYLENOL Flu Maximum Strength Gelcaps ... 1565
TYLENOL Flu NightTime, Maximum Strength, Gelcaps ... 1566
TYLENOL Maximum Strength Flu NightTime Hot Medication Packets ... 1562

IMPORTANT NOTE: Always consult each drug listing in the patient's regimen for possible interactions.

Diabinese **Interactions Index** **280**

TYLENOL, Maximum Strength, Sinus Medication Geltabs, Gelcaps, Caplets and Tablets 1566
TYLENOL Cold Multi-Symptom Formula Medication Tablets and Caplets 1561
TYLENOL Cold Medication No Drowsiness Formula Gelcaps and Caplets 1562
TYLENOL Cold Multi-Symptom Hot Medication Liquid Packets 1557
TYLENOL Cough Multi-Symptom Medication with Decongestant 1565
Ursinus Inlay-Tabs .... ▣ 794
Vicks 44 LiquiCaps Cough, Cold & Flu Relief .... ▣ 755
Vicks 44 LiquiCaps Non-Drowsy Cough & Cold Relief .... ▣ 756
Vicks 44D Dry Hacking Cough & Head Congestion .... ▣ 755
Vicks 44M Cough, Cold & Flu Relief .... ▣ 756
Vicks DayQuil .... ▣ 761
Vicks DayQuil SINUS Pressure & PAIN Relief with IBUPROFEN .... ▣ 762
Vicks Nyquil Hot Therapy .... ▣ 762
Vicks NyQuil LiquiCaps Multi-Symptom Cold/Flu Relief .... ▣ 763
Vicks NyQuil Multi-Symptom Cold/Flu Relief - (Original & Cherry Flavor) .... ▣ 763

Pseudoephedrine Sulfate (Co-administration may result in hyperglycemia leading to loss of control). Products include:
Cheracol Sinus .... ▣ 768
Chlor-Trimeton Allergy Decongestant Tablets .... ▣ 799
Claritin-D 2350
Drixoral Cold and Allergy Sustained-Action Tablets .... ▣ 802
Drixoral Cold and Flu Extended-Release Tablets .... ▣ 803
Drixoral Non-Drowsy Formula Extended-Release Tablets .... ▣ 803
Drixoral Allergy/Sinus Extended Release Tablets .... ▣ 804
Trinalin Repetabs Tablets 1330

Quinestrol (Co-administration may result in hyperglycemia leading to loss of control).
No products indexed under this heading.

Salmeterol Xinafoate (Co-administration may result in hyperglycemia leading to loss of control). Products include:
Serevent Inhalation Aerosol 1176

Salsalate (Potentiation of hypoglycemic action). Products include:
Mono-Gesic Tablets 792
Salflex Tablets 786

Secobarbital Sodium (Prolonged barbiturate action). Products include:
Seconal Sodium Pulvules 1474

Selegiline Hydrochloride (Potentiation of hypoglycemic action). Products include:
Eldepryl Tablets 2550

Sotalol Hydrochloride (Potentiation of hypoglycemic action). Products include:
Betapace Tablets 641

Spironolactone (Co-administration may result in hyperglycemia leading to loss of control). Products include:
Aldactazide 2413
Aldactone 2414

Sulfamethizole (Potentiation of hypoglycemic action). Products include:
Urobiotic-250 Capsules 2214

Sulfamethoxazole (Potentiation of hypoglycemic action). Products include:
Azo Gantanol Tablets 2080
Bactrim DS Tablets 2084
Bactrim I.V. Infusion 2082
Bactrim 2084
Gantanol Tablets 2119
Septra 1174
Septra I.V. Infusion 1169
Septra I.V. Infusion ADD-Vantage Vials 1171
Septra 1174

Sulfasalazine (Potentiation of hypoglycemic action). Products include:
Azulfidine 1949

Sulfinpyrazone (Potentiation of hypoglycemic action). Products include:
Anturane 807

Sulfisoxazole (Potentiation of hypoglycemic action). Products include:
Azo Gantrisin Tablets 2081
Gantrisin Tablets 2120

Sulfisoxazole Diolamine (Potentiation of hypoglycemic action).
No products indexed under this heading.

Sulindac (Potentiation of hypoglycemic action). Products include:
Clinoril Tablets 1618

Terbutaline Sulfate (Co-administration may result in hyperglycemia leading to loss of control). Products include:
Brethaire Inhaler 813
Brethine Ampuls 815
Brethine Tablets 814
Bricanyl Subcutaneous Injection 1502
Bricanyl Tablets 1503

Thiamylal Sodium (Prolonged barbiturate action).
No products indexed under this heading.

Thioridazine Hydrochloride (Co-administration may result in hyperglycemia leading to loss of control). Products include:
Mellaril 2269

Thyroglobulin (Co-administration may result in hyperglycemia leading to loss of control).
No products indexed under this heading.

Thyroid (Co-administration may result in hyperglycemia leading to loss of control).
No products indexed under this heading.

Thyroxine (Co-administration may result in hyperglycemia leading to loss of control).
No products indexed under this heading.

Thyroxine Sodium (Co-administration may result in hyperglycemia leading to loss of control).
No products indexed under this heading.

Timolol Hemihydrate (Potentiation of hypoglycemic action). Products include:
Betimol 0.25%, 0.5% .... ⊙ 261

Timolol Maleate (Potentiation of hypoglycemic action). Products include:
Blocadren Tablets 1614
Timolide Tablets 1748
Timoptic in Ocudose 1753
Timoptic Sterile Ophthalmic Solution 1751
Timoptic-XE 1755

Tolazamide (Potentiation of hypoglycemic action).
No products indexed under this heading.

Tolbutamide (Potentiation of hypoglycemic action).
No products indexed under this heading.

Tolmetin Sodium (Potentiation of hypoglycemic action). Products include:
Tolectin (200, 400 and 600 mg) .. 1581

Torsemide (Co-administration may result in hyperglycemia leading to loss of control). Products include:
Demadex Tablets and Injection 686

Tranylcypromine Sulfate (Potentiation of hypoglycemic action). Products include:
Parnate Tablets 2503

Triamcinolone (Co-administration may result in hyperglycemia leading to loss of control). Products include:
Aristocort Tablets 1022

Triamcinolone Acetonide (Co-administration may result in hyperglycemia leading to loss of control). Products include:
Aristocort A 0.025% Cream 1027
Aristocort A 0.5% Cream 1031
Aristocort A 0.1% Cream 1029
Aristocort A 0.1% Ointment 1030
Azmacort Oral Inhaler 2011
Nasacort Nasal Inhaler 2024

Triamcinolone Diacetate (Co-administration may result in hyperglycemia leading to loss of control). Products include:
Aristocort Suspension (Forte Parenteral) 1027
Aristocort Suspension (Intralesional) 1025

Triamcinolone Hexacetonide (Co-administration may result in hyperglycemia leading to loss of control). Products include:
Aristospan Suspension (Intra-articular) 1033
Aristospan Suspension (Intralesional) 1032

Triamterene (Co-administration may result in hyperglycemia leading to loss of control). Products include:
Dyazide 2479
Dyrenium Capsules 2481
Maxzide 1380

Trifluoperazine Hydrochloride (Co-administration may result in hyperglycemia leading to loss of control). Products include:
Stelazine 2514

Verapamil Hydrochloride (Co-administration may result in hyperglycemia leading to loss of control). Products include:
Calan SR Caplets 2422
Calan Tablets 2419
Isoptin Injectable 1344
Isoptin Oral Tablets 1346
Isoptin SR Tablets 1348
Verelan Capsules 1410
Verelan Capsules 2824

Warfarin Sodium (Potentiation of hypoglycemic action). Products include:
Coumadin 926

Food Interactions

Alcohol (Potential for disulfiram-like reaction).

DIALOSE TABLETS
(Docusate Sodium) 1317
May interact with:

Mineral Oil (Effect not specified). Products include:
Anusol Ointment .... ▣ 847
Aquaphor Healing Ointment 640
Aquaphor Healing Ointment, Original Formula 640
Eucerin Original Moisturizing Creme (Unscented) 641
Eucerin Original Moisturizing Lotion 641
Eucerin Plus Dry Skin Care Moisturizing Lotion 641
Eucerin Plus Moisturizing Creme 641
Fleet Mineral Oil Enema 1002
Hemorid For Women Creme .... ▣ 834
Keri Lotion - Original Formula .... ▣ 622
Kondremul .... ▣ 637
Lubriderm Bath and Shower Oil .... ▣ 856
Nephrox Suspension .... ▣ 655
Preparation H Hemorrhoidal Ointment .... ▣ 871
Refresh PM Lubricant Eye Ointment .... ⊙ 254
Replens Vaginal Moisturizer .... ▣ 859
Tears Renewed Ointment .... ⊙ 209

Prescription Drugs, unspecified (Effect not specified).

DIALOSE PLUS TABLETS
(Docusate Sodium, Phenolphthalein) 1317
May interact with:

Mineral Oil (Effect not specified). Products include:
Anusol Ointment .... ▣ 847
Aquaphor Healing Ointment 640
Aquaphor Healing Ointment, Original Formula 640
Eucerin Original Moisturizing Creme (Unscented) 641
Eucerin Original Moisturizing Lotion 641
Eucerin Plus Dry Skin Care Moisturizing Lotion 641
Eucerin Plus Moisturizing Creme 641
Fleet Mineral Oil Enema 1002
Hemorid For Women Creme .... ▣ 834
Keri Lotion - Original Formula .... ▣ 622
Kondremul .... ▣ 637
Lubriderm Bath and Shower Oil .... ▣ 856
Nephrox Suspension .... ▣ 655
Preparation H Hemorrhoidal Ointment .... ▣ 871
Refresh PM Lubricant Eye Ointment .... ⊙ 254
Replens Vaginal Moisturizer .... ▣ 859
Tears Renewed Ointment .... ⊙ 209

Prescription Drugs, unspecified (Effect not specified).

DIAMOX INTRAVENOUS
(Acetazolamide) 1372
See **Diamox Tablets**

DIAMOX SEQUELS (SUSTAINED RELEASE)
(Acetazolamide) 1373
May interact with:

Aspirin (Concomitant administration with high-dose aspirin may result in anorexia, tachypnea, lethargy, coma and death). Products include:
Alka-Seltzer Effervescent Antacid and Pain Reliever .... ▣ 701
Alka-Seltzer Extra Strength Effervescent Antacid and Pain Reliever .... ▣ 703
Alka-Seltzer Lemon Lime Effervescent Antacid and Pain Reliever .... ▣ 703
Alka-Seltzer Plus Cold Medicine .... ▣ 705
Alka-Seltzer Plus Cold & Cough Medicine .... ▣ 708
Alka-Seltzer Plus Night-Time Cold Medicine .... ▣ 707
Alka Seltzer Plus Sinus Medicine .... ▣ 707
Arthritis Foundation Safety Coated Aspirin Tablets .... ▣ 675
Arthritis Pain Ascriptin .... ▣ 631
Maximum Strength Ascriptin .... ▣ 630
Regular Strength Ascriptin Tablets .... ▣ 629
Arthritis Strength BC Powder .... ▣ 609
BC Cold Powder Multi-Symptom Formula (Cold-Sinus-Allergy) .... ▣ 609
BC Cold Powder Non-Drowsy Formula (Cold-Sinus) .... ▣ 609
BC Powder .... ▣ 609
Bayer Children's Chewable Aspirin .... ▣ 711
Genuine Bayer Aspirin Tablets & Caplets .... ▣ 713
Extra Strength Bayer Arthritis Pain Regimen Formula .... ▣ 711
Extra Strength Bayer Aspirin Caplets & Tablets .... ▣ 712
Extended-Release Bayer 8-Hour Aspirin .... ▣ 712
Extra Strength Bayer Plus Aspirin Caplets .... ▣ 713
Extra Strength Bayer PM Aspirin .. ▣ 713
Bayer Enteric Aspirin .... ▣ 709
Bufferin Analgesic Tablets and Caplets .... ▣ 613
Arthritis Strength Bufferin Analgesic Caplets .... ▣ 614

(▣ Described in PDR For Nonprescription Drugs) (⊙ Described in PDR For Ophthalmology)

281 Interactions Index Didrex

Extra Strength Bufferin Analgesic Tablets ... 615
Cama Arthritis Pain Reliever ... 785
Darvon Compound-65 Pulvules ... 1435
Easprin ... 1914
Ecotrin ... 2455
Ecotrin Enteric Coated Aspirin Maximum Strength Tablets and Caplets ... 816
Ecotrin Enteric Coated Aspirin Regular Strength Tablets ... 2455
Empirin Aspirin Tablets ... 854
Empirin with Codeine Tablets ... 1093
Excedrin Extra-Strength Analgesic Tablets & Caplets ... 732
Fiorinal Capsules ... 2261
Fiorinal with Codeine Capsules ... 2262
Fiorinal Tablets ... 2261
Halfprin ... 1362
Healthprin Aspirin ... 2455
Norgesic ... 1496
Percodan Tablets ... 939
Percodan-Demi Tablets ... 940
Robaxisal Tablets ... 2071
Soma Compound w/Codeine Tablets ... 2676
Soma Compound Tablets ... 2675
St. Joseph Adult Chewable Aspirin (81 mg.) ... 808
Talwin Compound ... 2335
Ursinus Inlay-Tabs ... 794
Vanquish Analgesic Caplets ... 731

DIAMOX TABLETS

(Acetazolamide) ... 1372
May interact with:

Aspirin (Concomitant administration with high-dose aspirin may result in anorexia, tachypnea, lethargy, coma and death). Products include:

Alka-Seltzer Effervescent Antacid and Pain Reliever ... 701
Alka-Seltzer Extra Strength Effervescent Antacid and Pain Reliever ... 703
Alka-Seltzer Lemon Lime Effervescent Antacid and Pain Reliever ... 703
Alka-Seltzer Plus Cold Medicine ... 705
Alka-Seltzer Plus Cold & Cough Medicine ... 708
Alka-Seltzer Plus Night-Time Cold Medicine ... 707
Alka Seltzer Plus Sinus Medicine ... 707
Arthritis Foundation Safety Coated Aspirin Tablets ... 675
Arthritis Pain Ascriptin ... 631
Maximum Strength Ascriptin ... 630
Regular Strength Ascriptin Tablets ... 629
Arthritis Strength BC Powder ... 609
BC Cold Powder Multi-Symptom Formula (Cold-Sinus-Allergy) ... 609
BC Cold Powder Non-Drowsy Formula (Cold-Sinus) ... 609
BC Powder ... 609
Bayer Children's Chewable Aspirin ... 711
Genuine Bayer Aspirin Tablets & Caplets ... 713
Extra Strength Bayer Arthritis Pain Regimen Formula ... 711
Extra Strength Bayer Aspirin Caplets & Tablets ... 712
Extended-Release Bayer 8-Hour Aspirin ... 712
Extra Strength Bayer Plus Aspirin Caplets ... 713
Extra Strength Bayer PM Aspirin ... 713
Bayer Enteric Aspirin ... 709
Bufferin Analgesic Tablets and Caplets ... 613
Arthritis Strength Bufferin Analgesic Caplets ... 614
Extra Strength Bufferin Analgesic Tablets ... 615
Cama Arthritis Pain Reliever ... 785
Darvon Compound-65 Pulvules ... 1435
Easprin ... 1914
Ecotrin ... 2455
Ecotrin Enteric Coated Aspirin Maximum Strength Tablets and Caplets ... 816
Ecotrin Enteric Coated Aspirin Regular Strength Tablets ... 2455
Empirin Aspirin Tablets ... 854
Empirin with Codeine Tablets ... 1093
Excedrin Extra-Strength Analgesic Tablets & Caplets ... 732
Fiorinal Capsules ... 2261
Fiorinal with Codeine Capsules ... 2262
Fiorinal Tablets ... 2261
Halfprin ... 1362
Healthprin Aspirin ... 2455
Norgesic ... 1496
Percodan Tablets ... 939
Percodan-Demi Tablets ... 940
Robaxisal Tablets ... 2071
Soma Compound w/Codeine Tablets ... 2676
Soma Compound Tablets ... 2675
St. Joseph Adult Chewable Aspirin (81 mg.) ... 808
Talwin Compound ... 2335
Ursinus Inlay-Tabs ... 794
Vanquish Analgesic Caplets ... 731

DIASORB LIQUID

(Attapulgite, Nonfibrous Activated) 650
None cited in PDR database.

DIASORB TABLETS

(Attapulgite, Nonfibrous Activated) 650
None cited in PDR database.

DIBENZYLINE CAPSULES

(Phenoxybenzamine Hydrochloride) .. 2476
May interact with:

Alpha and Beta Adrenergic Stimulators (Exaggerated hypotensive response; tachycardia).

Epinephrine (Exaggerated hypotensive response; tachycardia). Products include:

Bronkaid Mist ... 717
EPIFRIN ... ◉ 239
EpiPen ... 790
Marcaine Hydrochloride with Epinephrine 1:200,000 ... 2316
Primatene Mist ... 873
Sensorcaine with Epinephrine Injection ... 559
Sus-Phrine Injection ... 1019
Xylocaine with Epinephrine Injections ... 567

Epinephrine Bitartrate (Exaggerated hypotensive response; tachycardia). Products include:

Bronkaid Mist Suspension ... 718
Sensorcaine-MPF with Epinephrine Injection ... 559

Norepinephrine Bitartrate (Hyperthermia production of levarterenol blocked by dibenzyline). Products include:

Levophed Bitartrate Injection ... 2315

Reserpine (Hypothermia production of reserpine blocked by dibenzyline). Products include:

Diupres Tablets ... 1650
Hydropres Tablets ... 1675
Ser-Ap-Es Tablets ... 849

DICAL-D TABLETS & WAFERS

(Calcium Phosphate, Dibasic, Vitamin D) ... 420
None cited in PDR database.

DIDREX TABLETS

(Benzphetamine Hydrochloride) ... 2607
May interact with monoamine oxidase inhibitors, central nervous system stimulants, tricyclic antidepressants, urinary alkalizing agents, antihypertensives, insulin, and certain other agents. Compounds in these categories include:

Acebutolol Hydrochloride (Amphetamine-type drugs may decrease the hypotensive effect of antihypertensives). Products include:

Sectral Capsules ... 2807

Amitriptyline Hydrochloride (Amphetamine-type drugs may enhance the effects of tricyclic antidepressants). Products include:

Elavil ... 2838
Endep Tablets ... 2174
Etrafon ... 2355
Limbitrol ... 2180
Triavil Tablets ... 1757

Amlodipine Besylate (Amphetamine-type drugs may decrease the hypotensive effect of antihypertensives). Products include:

Lotrel Capsules ... 840
Norvasc Tablets ... 1940

Ammonium Chloride (Urinary acidifying agents decrease blood levels and increase excretion of amphetamine-type drugs).

No products indexed under this heading.

Amoxapine (Amphetamine-type drugs may enhance the effects of tricyclic antidepressants). Products include:

Asendin Tablets ... 1369

Amphetamine Resins (Concurrent use with other central nervous system stimulants is not recommended). Products include:

Biphetamine Capsules ... 983

Atenolol (Amphetamine-type drugs may decrease the hypotensive effect of antihypertensives). Products include:

Tenoretic Tablets ... 2845
Tenormin Tablets and I.V. Injection ... 2847

Benazepril Hydrochloride (Amphetamine-type drugs may decrease the hypotensive effect of antihypertensives). Products include:

Lotensin Tablets ... 834
Lotensin HCT ... 837
Lotrel Capsules ... 840

Bendroflumethiazide (Amphetamine-type drugs may decrease the hypotensive effect of antihypertensives).

No products indexed under this heading.

Betaxolol Hydrochloride (Amphetamine-type drugs may decrease the hypotensive effect of antihypertensives). Products include:

Betoptic Ophthalmic Solution ... 469
Betoptic S Ophthalmic Suspension ... 471
Kerlone Tablets ... 2436

Bisoprolol Fumarate (Amphetamine-type drugs may decrease the hypotensive effect of antihypertensives). Products include:

Zebeta Tablets ... 1413
Ziac ... 1415

Captopril (Amphetamine-type drugs may decrease the hypotensive effect of antihypertensives). Products include:

Capoten ... 739
Capozide ... 742

Carteolol Hydrochloride (Amphetamine-type drugs may decrease the hypotensive effect of antihypertensives). Products include:

Cartrol Tablets ... 410
Ocupress Ophthalmic Solution, 1% Sterile ... ◉ 309

Chlorothiazide (Amphetamine-type drugs may decrease the hypotensive effect of antihypertensives). Products include:

Aldoclor Tablets ... 1598
Diupres Tablets ... 1650
Diuril Oral ... 1653

Chlorothiazide Sodium (Amphetamine-type drugs may decrease the hypotensive effect of antihypertensives). Products include:

Diuril Sodium Intravenous ... 1652

Chlorthalidone (Amphetamine-type drugs may decrease the hypotensive effect of antihypertensives). Products include:

Combipres Tablets ... 677
Tenoretic Tablets ... 2845
Thalitone ... 1245

Clomipramine Hydrochloride (Amphetamine-type drugs may enhance the effects of tricyclic antidepressants). Products include:

Anafranil Capsules ... 803

Clonidine (Amphetamine-type drugs may decrease the hypotensive effect of antihypertensives). Products include:

Catapres-TTS ... 675

Clonidine Hydrochloride (Amphetamine-type drugs may decrease the hypotensive effect of antihypertensives). Products include:

Catapres Tablets ... 674
Combipres Tablets ... 677

Deserpidine (Amphetamine-type drugs may decrease the hypotensive effect of antihypertensives).

No products indexed under this heading.

Desipramine Hydrochloride (Amphetamine-type drugs may enhance the effects of tricyclic antidepressants). Products include:

Norpramin Tablets ... 1526

Dextroamphetamine Sulfate (Concurrent use with other central nervous system stimulants is not recommended). Products include:

Dexedrine ... 2474
DextroStat Dextroamphetamine Tablets ... 2036

Diazoxide (Amphetamine-type drugs may decrease the hypotensive effect of antihypertensives). Products include:

Hyperstat I.V. Injection ... 2363
Proglycem ... 580

Diltiazem Hydrochloride (Amphetamine-type drugs may decrease the hypotensive effect of antihypertensives). Products include:

Cardizem CD Capsules ... 1506
Cardizem SR Capsules ... 1510
Cardizem Injectable ... 1508
Cardizem Tablets ... 1512
Dilacor XR Extended-release Capsules ... 2018

Doxazosin Mesylate (Amphetamine-type drugs may decrease the hypotensive effect of antihypertensives). Products include:

Cardura Tablets ... 2186

Doxepin Hydrochloride (Amphetamine-type drugs may enhance the effects of tricyclic antidepressants). Products include:

Sinequan ... 2205
Zonalon Cream ... 1055

Enalapril Maleate (Amphetamine-type drugs may decrease the hypotensive effect of antihypertensives). Products include:

Vaseretic Tablets ... 1765
Vasotec Tablets ... 1771

Enalaprilat (Amphetamine-type drugs may decrease the hypotensive effect of antihypertensives). Products include:

Vasotec I.V. ... 1768

Esmolol Hydrochloride (Amphetamine-type drugs may decrease the hypotensive effect of antihypertensives). Products include:

Brevibloc Injection ... 1808

Felodipine (Amphetamine-type drugs may decrease the hypotensive effect of antihypertensives). Products include:

Plendil Extended-Release Tablets ... 527

Fosinopril Sodium (Amphetamine-type drugs may decrease the hypotensive effect of antihypertensives). Products include:

Monopril Tablets ... 757

IMPORTANT NOTE: Always consult each drug listing in the patient's regimen for possible interactions.

Didrex **Interactions Index** 282

Furazolidone (Potential for hypertensive crises; concomitant use is contraindicated). Products include:
Furoxone 2046

Furosemide (Amphetamine-type drugs may decrease the hypotensive effect of antihypertensives). Products include:
Lasix Injection, Oral Solution and Tablets 1240

Guanabenz Acetate (Amphetamine-type drugs may decrease the hypotensive effect of antihypertensives).
No products indexed under this heading.

Guanethidine Monosulfate (Amphetamine-type drugs may decrease the hypotensive effect of antihypertensives). Products include:
Esimil Tablets 822
Ismelin Tablets 827

Hydralazine Hydrochloride (Amphetamine-type drugs may decrease the hypotensive effect of antihypertensives). Products include:
Apresazide Capsules 808
Apresoline Hydrochloride Tablets .. 809
Ser-Ap-Es Tablets 849

Hydrochlorothiazide (Amphetamine-type drugs may decrease the hypotensive effect of antihypertensives). Products include:
Aldactazide 2413
Aldoril Tablets 1604
Apresazide Capsules 808
Capozide 742
Dyazide 2479
Esidrix Tablets 821
Esimil Tablets 822
HydroDIURIL Tablets 1674
Hydropres Tablets 1675
Hyzaar Tablets 1677
Inderide Tablets 2732
Inderide LA Long Acting Capsules .. 2734
Lopressor HCT Tablets 832
Lotensin HCT 837
Maxzide 1380
Moduretic Tablets 1705
Oretic Tablets 443
Prinzide Tablets 1737
Ser-Ap-Es Tablets 849
Timolide Tablets 1748
Vaseretic Tablets 1765
Zestoretic 2850
Ziac 1415

Hydroflumethiazide (Amphetamine-type drugs may decrease the hypotensive effect of antihypertensives). Products include:
Diucardin Tablets 2718

Imipramine Hydrochloride (Amphetamine-type drugs may enhance the effects of tricyclic antidepressants). Products include:
Tofranil Ampuls 854
Tofranil Tablets 856

Imipramine Pamoate (Amphetamine-type drugs may enhance the effects of tricyclic antidepressants). Products include:
Tofranil-PM Capsules 857

Indapamide (Amphetamine-type drugs may decrease the hypotensive effect of antihypertensives). Products include:
Lozol Tablets 2022

Insulin, Human (Insulin requirements in diabetes mellitus may be altered in association with use of anorexigenic drugs and concomitant dietary restrictions).
No products indexed under this heading.

Insulin, Human Isophane Suspension (Insulin requirements in diabetes mellitus may be altered in association with use of anorexigenic drugs and concomitant dietary restrictions). Products include:
Novolin N Human Insulin 10 ml Vials 1795

Insulin, Human NPH (Insulin requirements in diabetes mellitus may be altered in association with use of anorexigenic drugs and concomitant dietary restrictions). Products include:
Humulin N, 100 Units 1448
Novolin N PenFill Cartridges Durable Insulin Delivery System 1798
Novolin N Prefilled Syringe Disposable Insulin Delivery System 1798

Insulin, Human Regular (Insulin requirements in diabetes mellitus may be altered in association with use of anorexigenic drugs and concomitant dietary restrictions). Products include:
Humulin R, 100 Units 1449
Novolin R Human Insulin 10 ml Vials 1795
Novolin R PenFill Cartridges Durable Insulin Delivery System 1798
Novolin R Prefilled Syringe Disposable Insulin Delivery System 1798
Velosulin BR Human Insulin 10 ml Vials 1795

Insulin, Human, Zinc Suspension (Insulin requirements in diabetes mellitus may be altered in association with use of anorexigenic drugs and concomitant dietary restrictions). Products include:
Humulin L, 100 Units 1446
Humulin U, 100 Units 1450
Novolin L Human Insulin 10 ml Vials 1795

Insulin, NPH (Insulin requirements in diabetes mellitus may be altered in association with use of anorexigenic drugs and concomitant dietary restrictions). Products include:
NPH, 100 Units 1450
Pork NPH, 100 Units 1452
Purified Pork NPH Isophane Insulin 1801

Insulin, Regular (Insulin requirements in diabetes mellitus may be altered in association with use of anorexigenic drugs and concomitant dietary restrictions). Products include:
Regular, 100 Units 1450
Pork Regular, 100 Units 1452
Pork Regular (Concentrated), 500 Units 1453
Purified Pork Regular Insulin 1801

Insulin, Zinc Crystals (Insulin requirements in diabetes mellitus may be altered in association with use of anorexigenic drugs and concomitant dietary restrictions). Products include:
NPH, 100 Units 1450

Insulin, Zinc Suspension (Insulin requirements in diabetes mellitus may be altered in association with use of anorexigenic drugs and concomitant dietary restrictions). Products include:
Iletin I 1450
Lente, 100 Units 1450
Iletin II 1452
Pork Lente, 100 Units 1452
Purified Pork Lente Insulin 1801

Isocarboxazid (Potential for hypertensive crises; concomitant use is contraindicated).
No products indexed under this heading.

Isradipine (Amphetamine-type drugs may decrease the hypotensive effect of antihypertensives). Products include:
DynaCirc Capsules 2256

Labetalol Hydrochloride (Amphetamine-type drugs may decrease the hypotensive effect of antihypertensives). Products include:
Normodyne Injection 2377
Normodyne Tablets 2379
Trandate 1185

Levobunolol Hydrochloride (Amphetamine-type drugs may decrease the hypotensive effect of antihypertensives). Products include:
Betagan .... ◉ 233

Lisinopril (Amphetamine-type drugs may decrease the hypotensive effect of antihypertensives). Products include:
Prinivil Tablets 1733
Prinzide Tablets 1737
Zestoretic 2850
Zestril Tablets 2854

Losartan Potassium (Amphetamine-type drugs may decrease the hypotensive effect of antihypertensives). Products include:
Cozaar Tablets 1628
Hyzaar Tablets 1677

Maprotiline Hydrochloride (Amphetamine-type drugs may enhance the effects of tricyclic antidepressants). Products include:
Ludiomil Tablets 843

Mecamylamine Hydrochloride (Amphetamine-type drugs may decrease the hypotensive effect of antihypertensives). Products include:
Inversine Tablets 1686

Methamphetamine Hydrochloride (Concurrent use with other central nervous system stimulants is not recommended). Products include:
Desoxyn Gradumet Tablets 419

Methyclothiazide (Amphetamine-type drugs may decrease the hypotensive effect of antihypertensives). Products include:
Enduron Tablets 420

Methyldopa (Amphetamine-type drugs may decrease the hypotensive effect of antihypertensives). Products include:
Aldoclor Tablets 1598
Aldomet Oral 1600
Aldoril Tablets 1604

Methyldopate Hydrochloride (Amphetamine-type drugs may decrease the hypotensive effect of antihypertensives). Products include:
Aldomet Ester HCl Injection 1602

Methylphenidate Hydrochloride (Concurrent use with other central nervous system stimulants is not recommended). Products include:
Ritalin 848

Metipranolol Hydrochloride (Amphetamine-type drugs may decrease the hypotensive effect of antihypertensives). Products include:
OptiPranolol (Metipranolol 0.3%) Sterile Ophthalmic Solution .... ◉ 258

Metolazone (Amphetamine-type drugs may decrease the hypotensive effect of antihypertensives). Products include:
Mykrox Tablets 993
Zaroxolyn Tablets 1000

Metoprolol Succinate (Amphetamine-type drugs may decrease the hypotensive effect of antihypertensives). Products include:
Toprol-XL Tablets 565

Metoprolol Tartrate (Amphetamine-type drugs may decrease the hypotensive effect of antihypertensives). Products include:
Lopressor Ampuls 830
Lopressor HCT Tablets 832
Lopressor Tablets 830

Metyrosine (Amphetamine-type drugs may decrease the hypotensive effect of antihypertensives). Products include:
Demser Capsules 1649

Minoxidil (Amphetamine-type drugs may decrease the hypotensive effect of antihypertensives). Products include:
Loniten Tablets 2618
Rogaine Topical Solution 2637

Moexipril Hydrochloride (Amphetamine-type drugs may decrease the hypotensive effect of antihypertensives). Products include:
Univasc Tablets 2410

Nadolol (Amphetamine-type drugs may decrease the hypotensive effect of antihypertensives).
No products indexed under this heading.

Nicardipine Hydrochloride (Amphetamine-type drugs may decrease the hypotensive effect of antihypertensives). Products include:
Cardene Capsules 2095
Cardene I.V. 2709
Cardene SR Capsules 2097

Nifedipine (Amphetamine-type drugs may decrease the hypotensive effect of antihypertensives). Products include:
Adalat Capsules (10 mg and 20 mg) 587
Adalat CC 589
Procardia Capsules 1971
Procardia XL Extended Release Tablets 1972

Nisoldipine (Amphetamine-type drugs may decrease the hypotensive effect of antihypertensives).
No products indexed under this heading.

Nitroglycerin (Amphetamine-type drugs may decrease the hypotensive effect of antihypertensives). Products include:
Deponit NTG Transdermal Delivery System 2397
Nitro-Bid IV 1523
Nitro-Bid Ointment 1524
Nitrodisc 2047
Nitro-Dur (nitroglycerin) Transdermal Infusion System 1326
Nitrolingual Spray 2027
Nitrostat Tablets 1925
Transderm-Nitro Transdermal Therapeutic System 859

Nortriptyline Hydrochloride (Amphetamine-type drugs may enhance the effects of tricyclic antidepressants). Products include:
Pamelor 2280

Pemoline (Concurrent use with other central nervous system stimulants is not recommended). Products include:
Cylert Tablets 412

Penbutolol Sulfate (Amphetamine-type drugs may decrease the hypotensive effect of antihypertensives). Products include:
Levatol 2403

Phenelzine Sulfate (Potential for hypertensive crises; concomitant use is contraindicated). Products include:
Nardil 1920

Phenoxybenzamine Hydrochloride (Amphetamine-type drugs may decrease the hypotensive effect of antihypertensives). Products include:
Dibenzyline Capsules 2476

(▣ Described in PDR For Nonprescription Drugs) (◉ Described in PDR For Ophthalmology)

Interactions Index — Diflucan

Phentolamine Mesylate (Amphetamine-type drugs may decrease the hypotensive effect of antihypertensives). Products include:

Regitine 846

Pindolol (Amphetamine-type drugs may decrease the hypotensive effect of antihypertensives). Products include:

Visken Tablets... 2299

Polythiazide (Amphetamine-type drugs may decrease the hypotensive effect of antihypertensives). Products include:

Minizide Capsules 1938

Potassium Citrate (Urinary alkalinizing agents increase the blood levels and decrease excretion of amphetamine-type drugs). Products include:

Polycitra Syrup 578
Polycitra-K Crystals 579
Polycitra-K Oral Solution 579
Polycitra-LC 578

Prazosin Hydrochloride (Amphetamine-type drugs may decrease the hypotensive effect of antihypertensives). Products include:

Minipress Capsules................................... 1937
Minizide Capsules 1938

Propranolol Hydrochloride (Amphetamine-type drugs may decrease the hypotensive effect of antihypertensives). Products include:

Inderal 2728
Inderal LA Long Acting Capsules 2730
Inderide Tablets 2732
Inderide LA Long Acting Capsules .. 2734

Protriptyline Hydrochloride (Amphetamine-type drugs may enhance the effects of tricyclic antidepressants). Products include:

Vivactil Tablets 1774

Quinapril Hydrochloride (Amphetamine-type drugs may decrease the hypotensive effect of antihypertensives). Products include:.

Accupril Tablets 1893

Ramipril (Amphetamine-type drugs may decrease the hypotensive effect of antihypertensives). Products include:

Altace Capsules 1232

Rauwolfia Serpentina (Amphetamine-type drugs may decrease the hypotensive effect of antihypertensives).

No products indexed under this heading.

Rescinnamine (Amphetamine-type drugs may decrease the hypotensive effect of antihypertensives).

No products indexed under this heading.

Reserpine (Amphetamine-type drugs may decrease the hypotensive effect of antihypertensives). Products include:

Diupres Tablets 1650
Hydropres Tablets..................................... 1675
Ser-Ap-Es Tablets 849

Selegiline Hydrochloride (Potential for hypertensive crises; concomitant use is contraindicated). Products include:

Eldepryl Tablets 2550

Sodium Acid Phosphate (Urinary acidifying agents decrease blood levels and increase excretion of amphetamine-type drugs). Products include:

Uroqid-Acid No. 2 Tablets 640

Sodium Citrate (Urinary alkalinizing agents increase the blood levels and decrease excretion of amphetamine-type drugs). Products include:

Bicitra 578

Citrocarbonate Antacid .... ✦D 770
Polycitra... 578
Salix SST Lozenges Saliva Stimulant... ✦D 797

Sodium Nitroprusside (Amphetamine-type drugs may decrease the hypotensive effect of antihypertensives).

No products indexed under this heading.

Sotalol Hydrochloride (Amphetamine-type drugs may decrease the hypotensive effect of antihypertensives). Products include:

Betapace Tablets 641

Spirapril Hydrochloride (Amphetamine-type drugs may decrease the hypotensive effect of antihypertensives).

No products indexed under this heading.

Terazosin Hydrochloride (Amphetamine-type drugs may decrease the hypotensive effect of antihypertensives). Products include:

Hytrin Capsules 430

Timolol Maleate (Amphetamine-type drugs may decrease the hypotensive effect of antihypertensives). Products include:

Blocadren Tablets 1614
Timolide Tablets.. 1748
Timoptic in Ocudose 1753
Timoptic Sterile Ophthalmic Solution.. 1751
Timoptic-XE 1755

Torsemide (Amphetamine-type drugs may decrease the hypotensive effect of antihypertensives). Products include:

Demadex Tablets and Injection 686

Tranylcypromine Sulfate (Potential for hypertensive crises; concomitant use is contraindicated). Products include:

Parnate Tablets 2503

Trimethaphan Camsylate (Amphetamine-type drugs may decrease the hypotensive effect of antihypertensives). Products include:

Arfonad Ampuls 2080

Trimipramine Maleate (Amphetamine-type drugs may enhance the effects of tricyclic antidepressants). Products include:

Surmontil Capsules................................... 2811

Verapamil Hydrochloride (Amphetamine-type drugs may decrease the hypotensive effect of antihypertensives). Products include:

Calan SR Caplets 2422
Calan Tablets... 2419
Isoptin Injectable 1344
Isoptin Oral Tablets 1346
Isoptin SR Tablets 1348
Verelan Capsules 1410
Verelan Capsules 2824

DIDRONEL I.V. INFUSION

(Etidronate Disodium (Biphosphonate)) 1488

May interact with:

Nephrotoxic Drugs (Potential for excessive depression of renal function).

DIDRONEL TABLETS

(Etidronate Disodium (Diphosphonate)) 1984

None cited in PDR database.

DIETHYLSTILBESTROL TABLETS

(Diethylstilbestrol) 1437

None cited in PDR database.

DIFLUCAN INJECTION, TABLETS, AND ORAL SUSPENSION

(Fluconazole) 2194

May interact with oral contraceptives, oral hypoglycemic agents, oral anticoagulants, xanthine bronchodilators, and certain other agents. Compounds in these categories include:

Acarbose (Co-administration may precipitate clinically significant hypoglycemia; potential for reduced metabolism of sulfonylurea).

No products indexed under this heading.

Aminophylline (Increased serum concentrations of theophylline).

No products indexed under this heading.

Chlorpropamide (Co-administration may precipitate clinically significant hypoglycemia; potential for reduced metabolism of sulfonylurea). Products include:

Diabinese Tablets 1935

Cimetidine (Potential for a significant decrease in fluconazole AUC (13% +/- 11%) and C_{max} (19% +/- 14%) after oral dose). Products include:

Tagamet Tablets 2516

Cimetidine Hydrochloride (Potential for a significant decrease in fluconazole AUC (13% +/- 11%) and C_{max} (19% +/- 14%) after oral dose). Products include:

Tagamet... 2516

Cyclosporine (Fluconazole may significantly increase cyclosporine levels in renal transplant patients with or without renal impairment). Products include:

Neoral 2276
Sandimmune 2286

Dicumarol (Increased prothrombin time; monitoring of prothrombin time is recommended).

No products indexed under this heading.

Dyphylline (Increased serum concentrations of theophylline). Products include:

Lufyllin & Lufyllin-400 Tablets 2670
Lufyllin-GG Elixir & Tablets 2671

Ethinyl Estradiol (Co-administration with ethinyl estradiol and levonorgestrel-containing oral contraceptive produces an overall mean increase in ethinyl estradiol and levonorgestrel levels; however, in some patients there may be a decrease in these levels; clinical significance unknown). Products include:

Brevicon... 2088
Demulen 2428
Desogen Tablets.. 1817
Levlen/Tri-Levlen...................................... 651
Lo/Ovral Tablets 2746
Lo/Ovral-28 Tablets.................................. 2751
Modicon 1872
Nordette-21 Tablets.................................. 2755
Nordette-28 Tablets.................................. 2758
Norinyl 2088
Ortho-Cept 1851
Ortho-Cyclen/Ortho-Tri-Cyclen 1858
Ortho-Novum... 1872
Ortho-Cyclen/Ortho Tri-Cyclen 1858
Ovcon 760
Ovral Tablets 2770
Ovral-28 Tablets 2770
Levlen/Tri-Levlen...................................... 651
Tri-Norinyl.. 2164
Triphasil-21 Tablets.................................. 2814
Triphasil-28 Tablets.................................. 2819

Glipizide (Co-administration may precipitate clinically significant hypoglycemia; potential for reduced metabolism of sulfonylurea). Products include:

Glucotrol Tablets 1967

Glucotrol XL Extended Release Tablets 1968

Glyburide (Co-administration may precipitate clinically significant hypoglycemia; potential for reduced metabolism of sulfonylurea). Products include:

DiaBeta Tablets 1239
Glynase PresTab Tablets 2609
Micronase Tablets 2623

Hydrochlorothiazide (Potential for a significant increase in fluconazole AUC (45% +/- 31%) and C_{max} (43% +/- 31%) attributable to reduction in renal clearance of 30% +/- 12%). Products include:

Aldactazide... 2413
Aldoril Tablets.. 1604
Apresazide Capsules 808
Capozide 742
Dyazide 2479
Esidrix Tablets 821
Esimil Tablets 822
HydroDIURIL Tablets 1674
Hydropres Tablets...................................... 1675
Hyzaar Tablets 1677
Inderide Tablets 2732
Inderide LA Long Acting Capsules .. 2734
Lopressor HCT Tablets 832
Lotensin HCT... 837
Maxzide 1380
Moduretic Tablets 1705
Oretic Tablets 443
Prinzide Tablets 1737
Ser-Ap-Es Tablets 849
Timolide Tablets... 1748
Vaseretic Tablets 1765
Zestoretic 2850
Ziac 1415

Isoniazid (The incidence of abnormally elevated serum transaminase was greater in patients taking Diflucan concomitantly with isoniazid). Products include:

Nydrazid Injection 508
Rifamate Capsules 1530
Rifater.. 1532

Levonorgestrel (Co-administration with ethinyl estradiol and levonorgestrel-containing oral contraceptive produces an overall mean increase in ethinyl estradiol and levonorgestrel levels; however, in some patients there may be a decrease in these levels; clinical significance unknown). Products include:

Levlen/Tri-Levlen...................................... 651
Nordette-21 Tablets.................................. 2755
Nordette-28 Tablets.................................. 2758
Norplant System 2759
Levlen/Tri-Levlen...................................... 651
Triphasil-21 Tablets.................................. 2814
Triphasil-28 Tablets.................................. 2819

Metformin Hydrochloride (Co-administration may precipitate clinically significant hypoglycemia; potential for reduced metabolism of sulfonylurea). Products include:

Glucophage 752

Phenytoin (Increased plasma concentrations of phenytoin; monitor phenytoin concentration). Products include:

Dilantin Infatabs.. 1908
Dilantin-125 Suspension 1911

Phenytoin Sodium (Increased plasma concentrations of phenytoin; monitor phenytoin concentration). Products include:

Dilantin Kapseals 1906
Dilantin Parenteral 1910

Rifampin (Enhances the metabolism of concurrently administered fluconazole and significantly decreases in fluconazole AUC). Products include:

Rifadin 1528
Rifamate Capsules 1530
Rifater.. 1532
Rimactane Capsules 847

IMPORTANT NOTE: Always consult each drug listing in the patient's regimen for possible interactions.

Terfenadine (Potential for increase in terfenadine acid metabolite AUC (36%) from day 8 to day 15 with concomitant fluconazole administration; no change in cardiac repolization as measured by Holter QTc interval). Products include:

Seldane Tablets 1536
Seldane-D Extended-Release Tablets 1538

Theophylline (Increased serum concentrations of theophylline). Products include:

Marax Tablets & DF Syrup 2200
Quibron 2053

Theophylline Anhydrous (Increased serum concentrations of theophylline). Products include:

Aerolate 1004
Primatene Dual Action Formula ..... ▣ 872
Primatene Tablets ..... ▣ 873
Respbid Tablets 682
Slo-bid Gyrocaps 2033
Theo-24 Extended Release Capsules 2568
Theo-Dur Extended-Release Tablets 1327
Theo-X Extended-Release Tablets .. 788
Uni-Dur Extended-Release Tablets .. 1331
Uniphyl 400 mg Tablets 2001

Theophylline Calcium Salicylate (Increased serum concentrations of theophylline). Products include:

Quadrinal Tablets 1350

Theophylline Sodium Glycinate (Increased serum concentrations of theophylline).

No products indexed under this heading.

Tolazamide (Co-administration may precipitate clinically significant hypoglycemia; potential for reduced metabolism of sulfonylurea).

No products indexed under this heading.

Tolbutamide (Co-administration may precipitate clinically significant hypoglycemia; potential for reduced metabolism of sulfonylurea).

No products indexed under this heading.

Valproic Acid (The incidence of abnormally elevated serum transaminase was greater in patients taking Diflucan concomitantly with isoniazid). Products include:

Depakene 413

Warfarin Sodium (Increased prothrombin time; monitoring of prothrombin time is recommended). Products include:

Coumadin 926

Zidovudine (Potential for a significant increase in zidovudine AUC (20% +/- 32%) following the administration of fluconazole). Products include:

Retrovir Capsules 1158
Retrovir I.V. Infusion 1163
Retrovir Syrup 1158

DI-GEL ANTACID/ANTI-GAS

(Calcium Carbonate, Magnesium Hydroxide, Simethicone) ..... ▣ 801
May interact with tetracyclines. Compounds in this category include:

Demeclocycline Hydrochloride (Concurrent use with Di-Gel Liquid is not recommended). Products include:

Declomycin Tablets 1371

Doxycycline Calcium (Concurrent use with Di-Gel Liquid is not recommended). Products include:

Vibramycin Calcium Oral Suspension Syrup 1941

Doxycycline Hyclate (Concurrent use with Di-Gel Liquid is not recommended). Products include:

Doryx Capsules 1913
Vibramycin Hyclate Capsules 1941
Vibramycin Hyclate Intravenous 2215
Vibra-Tabs Film Coated Tablets 1941

Doxycycline Monohydrate (Concurrent use with Di-Gel Liquid is not recommended). Products include:

Monodox Capsules 1805
Vibramycin Monohydrate for Oral Suspension 1941

Methacycline Hydrochloride (Concurrent use with Di-Gel Liquid is not recommended).

No products indexed under this heading.

Minocycline Hydrochloride (Concurrent use with Di-Gel Liquid is not recommended). Products include:

Dynacin Capsules 1590
Minocin Intravenous 1382
Minocin Oral Suspension 1385
Minocin Pellet-Filled Capsules 1383

Oxytetracycline Hydrochloride (Concurrent use with Di-Gel Liquid is not recommended). Products include:

TERAK Ointment ..... ◉ 209
Terra-Cortril Ophthalmic Suspension 2210
Terramycin with Polymyxin B Sulfate Ophthalmic Ointment 2211
Urobiotic-250 Capsules 2214

Tetracycline Hydrochloride (Concurrent use with Di-Gel Liquid is not recommended). Products include:

Achromycin V Capsules 1367

DIGIBIND

(Digoxin Immune Fab (Ovine)) 1091
None cited in PDR database.

DILACOR XR EXTENDED-RELEASE CAPSULES

(Diltiazem Hydrochloride) 2018
May interact with beta blockers, cardiac glycosides, anesthetics, and certain other agents. Compounds in these categories include:

Acebutolol Hydrochloride (Possible additive effects in prolonging AV conduction). Products include:

Sectral Capsules 2807

Alfentanil Hydrochloride (Depression of cardiac contractility, conductivity, automaticity, and vasodilation associated with anesthetic may be potentiated). Products include:

Alfenta Injection 1286

Atenolol (Possible additive effects in prolonging AV conduction). Products include:

Tenoretic Tablets 2845
Tenormin Tablets and I.V. Injection 2847

Betaxolol Hydrochloride (Possible additive effects in prolonging AV conduction). Products include:

Betoptic Ophthalmic Solution 469
Betoptic S Ophthalmic Suspension 471
Kerlone Tablets 2436

Bisoprolol Fumarate (Possible additive effects in prolonging AV conduction). Products include:

Zebeta Tablets 1413
Ziac 1415

Carteolol Hydrochloride (Possible additive effects in prolonging AV conduction). Products include:

Cartrol Tablets 410
Ocupress Ophthalmic Solution, 1% Sterile ..... ◉ 309

Cimetidine (Significant increase in peak diltiazem plasma levels and area under the curve). Products include:

Tagamet Tablets 2516

Cimetidine Hydrochloride (Significant increase in peak diltiazem plasma levels and area under the curve). Products include:

Tagamet 2516

Cyclosporine (May result in competitive inhibition of metabolism; dosage of cyclosporin may need to be adjusted). Products include:

Neoral 2276
Sandimmune 2286

Deslanoside (Possible additive effects in prolonging AV conduction; potential for increased digoxin serum levels).

No products indexed under this heading.

Digitoxin (Possible additive effects in prolonging AV conduction; potential for increased digoxin serum levels). Products include:

Crystodigin Tablets 1433

Digoxin (Possible additive effects in prolonging AV conduction; potential for increased digoxin serum levels). Products include:

Lanoxicaps 1117
Lanoxin Elixir Pediatric 1120
Lanoxin Injection 1123
Lanoxin Injection Pediatric 1126
Lanoxin Tablets 1128

Drugs which undergo biotransformation by cytochrome P-450 mixed function oxidase (Coadministration may result in the competitive inhibition of metabolism).

Enflurane (Depression of cardiac contractility, conductivity, automaticity, and vasodilation associated with anesthetic may be potentiated).

No products indexed under this heading.

Esmolol Hydrochloride (Possible additive effects in prolonging AV conduction). Products include:

Brevibloc Injection 1808

Fentanyl Citrate (Depression of cardiac contractility, conductivity, automaticity, and vasodilation associated with anesthetic may be potentiated). Products include:

Sublimaze Injection 1307

Halothane (Depression of cardiac contractility, conductivity, automaticity, and vasodilation associated with anesthetic may be potentiated). Products include:

Fluothane 2724

Isoflurane (Depression of cardiac contractility, conductivity, automaticity, and vasodilation associated with anesthetic may be potentiated).

No products indexed under this heading.

Ketamine Hydrochloride (Depression of cardiac contractility, conductivity, automaticity, and vasodilation associated with anesthetic may be potentiated).

No products indexed under this heading.

Labetalol Hydrochloride (Possible additive effects in prolonging AV conduction). Products include:

Normodyne Injection 2377
Normodyne Tablets 2379
Trandate 1185

Levobunolol Hydrochloride (Possible additive effects in prolonging AV conduction). Products include:

Betagan ..... ◉ 233

Methohexital Sodium (Depression of cardiac contractility, conductivity, automaticity, and vasodilation associated with anesthetic may be potentiated). Products include:

Brevital Sodium Vials 1429

Metipranolol Hydrochloride (Possible additive effects in prolonging AV conduction). Products include:

OptiPranolol (Metipranolol 0.3%) Sterile Ophthalmic Solution ..... ◉ 258

Metoprolol Succinate (Possible additive effects in prolonging AV conduction). Products include:

Toprol-XL Tablets 565

Metoprolol Tartrate (Possible additive effects in prolonging AV conduction). Products include:

Lopressor Ampuls 830
Lopressor HCT Tablets 832
Lopressor Tablets 830

Midazolam Hydrochloride (Depression of cardiac contractility, conductivity, automaticity, and vasodilation associated with anesthetic may be potentiated). Products include:

Versed Injection 2170

Nadolol (Possible additive effects in prolonging AV conduction).

No products indexed under this heading.

Penbutolol Sulfate (Possible additive effects in prolonging AV conduction). Products include:

Levatol 2403

Pindolol (Possible additive effects in prolonging AV conduction). Products include:

Visken Tablets 2299

Propofol (Depression of cardiac contractility, conductivity, automaticity, and vasodilation associated with anesthetic may be potentiated). Products include:

Diprivan Injection 2833

Propranolol Hydrochloride (Possible additive effects in prolonging AV conduction). Products include:

Inderal 2728
Inderal LA Long Acting Capsules 2730
Inderide Tablets 2732
Inderide LA Long Acting Capsules .. 2734

Ranitidine Hydrochloride (Produces smaller, nonsignificant increase in diltiazem plasma levels). Products include:

Zantac 1209
Zantac Injection 1207
Zantac Syrup 1209

Sotalol Hydrochloride (Possible additive effects in prolonging AV conduction). Products include:

Betapace Tablets 641

Sufentanil Citrate (Depression of cardiac contractility, conductivity, automaticity, and vasodilation associated with anesthetic may be potentiated). Products include:

Sufenta Injection 1309

Thiamylal Sodium (Depression of cardiac contractility, conductivity, automaticity, and vasodilation associated with anesthetic may be potentiated).

No products indexed under this heading.

Timolol Hemihydrate (Possible additive effects in prolonging AV conduction). Products include:

Betimol 0.25%, 0.5% ..... ◉ 261

Timolol Maleate (Possible additive effects in prolonging AV conduction). Products include:

Blocadren Tablets 1614
Timolide Tablets 1748

(▣ Described in PDR For Nonprescription Drugs) (◉ Described in PDR For Ophthalmology)

285 **Interactions Index** **Dilantin Infatabs**

Timoptic in Ocudose 1753
Timoptic Sterile Ophthalmic Solution 1751
Timoptic-XE 1755

Food Interactions

Diet, high-lipid (Simultaneous administration of Dilacor XR with a high-fat breakfast has a modest effect on diltiazem bioavailability).

DILANTIN INFATABS

(Phenytoin) 1908

May interact with oral anticoagulants, corticosteroids, tricyclic antidepressants, oral contraceptives, salicylates, phenothiazines, estrogens, sulfonamides, histamine h2-receptor antagonists, succinimides, xanthine bronchodilators, and certain other agents. Compounds in these categories include:

Aminophylline (Efficacy impaired by phenytoin).
No products indexed under this heading.

Amiodarone Hydrochloride (Increases phenytoin serum levels). Products include:
Cordarone Intravenous 2715
Cordarone Tablets 2712

Amitriptyline Hydrochloride (Tricyclic antidepressants may precipitate seizures in some patients; phenytoin dosage may need to be adjusted). Products include:
Elavil 2838
Endep Tablets 2174
Etrafon 2355
Limbitrol 2180
Triavil Tablets 1757

Amoxapine (Tricyclic antidepressants may precipitate seizures in some patients; phenytoin dosage may need to be adjusted). Products include:
Asendin Tablets 1369

Aspirin (Increased phenytoin levels). Products include:
Alka-Seltzer Effervescent Antacid and Pain Reliever ..... ▣ 701
Alka-Seltzer Extra Strength Effervescent Antacid and Pain Reliever ..... ▣ 703
Alka-Seltzer Lemon Lime Effervescent Antacid and Pain Reliever ..... ▣ 703
Alka-Seltzer Plus Cold Medicine ..... ▣ 705
Alka-Seltzer Plus Cold & Cough Medicine ..... ▣ 708
Alka-Seltzer Plus Night-Time Cold Medicine ..... ▣ 707
Alka Seltzer Plus Sinus Medicine ..... ▣ 707
Arthritis Foundation Safety Coated Aspirin Tablets ..... ▣ 675
Arthritis Pain Ascriptin ..... ▣ 631
Maximum Strength Ascriptin ..... ▣ 630
Regular Strength Ascriptin Tablets ..... ▣ 629
Arthritis Strength BC Powder ..... ▣ 609
BC Cold Powder Multi-Symptom Formula (Cold-Sinus-Allergy) ..... ▣ 609
BC Cold Powder Non-Drowsy Formula (Cold-Sinus) ..... ▣ 609
BC Powder ..... ▣ 609
Bayer Children's Chewable Aspirin ..... ▣ 711
Genuine Bayer Aspirin Tablets & Caplets ..... ▣ 713
Extra Strength Bayer Arthritis Pain Regimen Formula ..... ▣ 711
Extra Strength Bayer Aspirin Caplets & Tablets ..... ▣ 712
Extended-Release Bayer 8-Hour Aspirin ..... ▣ 712
Extra Strength Bayer Plus Aspirin Caplets ..... ▣ 713
Extra Strength Bayer PM Aspirin ..... ▣ 713
Bayer Enteric Aspirin ..... ▣ 709
Bufferin Analgesic Tablets and Caplets ..... ▣ 613
Arthritis Strength Bufferin Analgesic Caplets ..... ▣ 614
Extra Strength Bufferin Analgesic Tablets ..... ▣ 615
Cama Arthritis Pain Reliever ..... ▣ 785
Darvon Compound-65 Pulvules 1435
Easprin 1914
Ecotrin 2455
Ecotrin Enteric Coated Aspirin Maximum Strength Tablets and Caplets ..... ▣ 816
Ecotrin Enteric Coated Aspirin Regular Strength Tablets 2455
Empirin Aspirin Tablets ..... ▣ 854
Empirin with Codeine Tablets 1093
Excedrin Extra-Strength Analgesic Tablets & Caplets 732
Fiorinal Capsules 2261
Fiorinal with Codeine Capsules 2262
Fiorinal Tablets 2261
Halfprin 1362
Healthprin Aspirin 2455
Norgesic 1496
Percodan Tablets 939
Percodan-Demi Tablets 940
Robaxisal Tablets 2071
Soma Compound w/Codeine Tablets 2676
Soma Compound Tablets 2675
St. Joseph Adult Chewable Aspirin (81 mg.) ..... ▣ 808
Talwin Compound 2335
Ursinus Inlay-Tabs ..... ▣ 794
Vanquish Analgesic Caplets ..... ▣ 731

Bendroflumethiazide (Increased phenytoin levels).
No products indexed under this heading.

Betamethasone Acetate (Efficacy impaired by phenytoin). Products include:
Celestone Soluspan Suspension 2347

Betamethasone Sodium Phosphate (Efficacy impaired by phenytoin). Products include:
Celestone Soluspan Suspension 2347

Calcium Carbonate (Ingestion times of phenytoin and antacids containing calcium should be staggered to prevent absorption problems). Products include:
Alka-Mints Chewable Antacid ..... ▣ 701
Arthritis Pain Ascriptin ..... ▣ 631
Maximum Strength Ascriptin ..... ▣ 630
Regular Strength Ascriptin Tablets ..... ▣ 629
Extra Strength Bayer Plus Aspirin Caplets ..... ▣ 713
Bufferin Analgesic Tablets and Caplets ..... ▣ 613
Calci-Chew Tablets 2004
Calci-Mix Capsules 2004
Caltrate 600 ..... ▣ 665
Caltrate PLUS ..... ▣ 665
Caltrate 600 + D ..... ▣ 665
Centrum Singles Calcium ..... ▣ 669
Chooz Antacid Gum ..... ▣ 799
Di-Gel Antacid/Anti-Gas ..... ▣ 801
Gerimed Tablets 982
Maalox Antacid Caplets ..... ▣ 638
Marblen ..... ▣ 655
Materna Tablets 1379
Mylanta Calcium Carbonate and Magnesium Hydroxide Tablets 1318
Mylanta Gelcaps Antacid ..... ▣ 662
Mylanta Soothing Lozenges 1319
Nephro-Calci Tablets 2004
Rolaids Tablets ..... ▣ 843
Rolaids (Calcium Rich/Sodium Free) Tablets ..... ▣ 843
Tempo Soft Antacid ..... ▣ 835
Titralac ..... ▣ 672
Titralac Plus ..... ▣ 672
Tums Antacid Tablets ..... ▣ 827
Tums Anti-gas/Antacid Formula Tablets, Assorted Fruit ..... ▣ 827
Tums E-X Antacid Tablets ..... ▣ 827
Tums 500 Calcium Supplement ..... ▣ 828
Tums ULTRA Antacid Tablets ..... ▣ 827
TYLENOL, Extra Strength, Headache Plus Pain Reliever with Antacid Caplets 1559

Calcium Carbonate, Precipitated (Ingestion times of phenytoin and antacids containing calcium should be staggered to prevent absorption problems).

Carbamazepine (Decreased phenytoin levels). Products include:
Atretol Tablets 573
Tegretol Chewable Tablets 852
Tegretol Suspension 852
Tegretol Tablets 852

Chloramphenicol (Increased phenytoin levels). Products include:
Chloromycetin Ophthalmic Ointment, 1% ..... ◉ 310
Chloromycetin Ophthalmic Solution ..... ◉ 310
Chloroptic S.O.P. ..... ◉ 239
Chloroptic Sterile Ophthalmic Solution ..... ◉ 239
Elase-Chloromycetin Ointment 1040
Ophthocort ..... ◉ 311

Chloramphenicol Palmitate (Increased phenytoin levels).
No products indexed under this heading.

Chloramphenicol Sodium Succinate (Increased phenytoin levels). Products include:
Chloromycetin Sodium Succinate 1900

Chlordiazepoxide (Increased phenytoin levels). Products include:
Libritabs Tablets 2177
Limbitrol 2180

Chlordiazepoxide Hydrochloride (Increased phenytoin levels). Products include:
Librax Capsules 2176
Librium Capsules 2178
Librium Injectable 2179

Chlorothiazide (Increased phenytoin levels). Products include:
Aldoclor Tablets 1598
Diupres Tablets 1650
Diuril Oral 1653

Chlorothiazide Sodium (Increased phenytoin levels). Products include:
Diuril Sodium Intravenous 1652

Chlorotrianisene (Increased phenytoin levels; efficacy impaired by phenytoin).
No products indexed under this heading.

Chlorpromazine (Increased phenytoin levels). Products include:
Thorazine Suppositories 2523

Chlorpropamide (Increased phenytoin levels). Products include:
Diabinese Tablets 1935

Choline Magnesium Trisalicylate (Increased phenytoin levels). Products include:
Trilisate 2000

Cimetidine (Increases phenytoin levels). Products include:
Tagamet Tablets 2516

Cimetidine Hydrochloride (Increases phenytoin serum levels). Products include:
Tagamet 2516

Clomipramine Hydrochloride (Tricyclic antidepressants may precipitate seizures in some patients; phenytoin dosage may need to be adjusted). Products include:
Anafranil Capsules 803

Cortisone Acetate (Efficacy impaired by phenytoin). Products include:
Cortone Acetate Sterile Suspension 1623
Cortone Acetate Tablets 1624

Desipramine Hydrochloride (Tricyclic antidepressants may precipitate seizures in some patients; phenytoin dosage may need to be adjusted). Products include:
Norpramin Tablets 1526

Desogestrel (Increased phenytoin levels; efficacy impaired by phenytoin). Products include:
Desogen Tablets 1817
Ortho-Cept 1851

Dexamethasone (Efficacy impaired by phenytoin). Products include:
AK-Trol Ointment & Suspension ..... ◉ 205
Decadron Elixir 1633
Decadron Tablets 1635
Decaspray Topical Aerosol 1648
Dexacidin Ointment ..... ◉ 263
Maxitrol Ophthalmic Ointment and Suspension ..... ◉ 224
TobraDex Ophthalmic Suspension and Ointment 473

Dexamethasone Acetate (Efficacy impaired by phenytoin). Products include:
Dalalone D.P. Injectable 1011
Decadron-LA Sterile Suspension 1646

Dexamethasone Phosphate (Efficacy impaired by phenytoin).
No products indexed under this heading.

Dexamethasone Sodium Phosphate (Efficacy impaired by phenytoin). Products include:
Decadron Phosphate Injection 1637
Decadron Phosphate Respihaler 1642
Decadron Phosphate Sterile Ophthalmic Ointment 1641
Decadron Phosphate Sterile Ophthalmic Solution 1642
Decadron Phosphate Topical Cream 1644
Decadron Phosphate Turbinaire 1645
Decadron Phosphate with Xylocaine Injection, Sterile 1639
Dexacort Phosphate in Respihaler 458
Dexacort Phosphate in Turbinaire 459
NeoDecadron Sterile Ophthalmic Ointment 1712
NeoDecadron Sterile Ophthalmic Solution 1713
NeoDecadron Topical Cream 1714

Diazepam (Increased phenytoin levels). Products include:
Dizac 1809
Valium Injectable 2182
Valium Tablets 2183
Valrelease Capsules 2169

Dicumarol (Efficacy impaired by phenytoin; increases phenytoin serum levels).
No products indexed under this heading.

Dienestrol (Increased phenytoin levels; efficacy impaired by phenytoin). Products include:
Ortho Dienestrol Cream 1866

Diethylstilbestrol (Increased phenytoin levels; efficacy impaired by phenytoin). Products include:
Diethylstilbestrol Tablets 1437

Diflunisal (Increased phenytoin levels). Products include:
Dolobid Tablets 1654

Digitoxin (Efficacy impaired by phenytoin). Products include:
Crystodigin Tablets 1433

Dihydroxyaluminum Sodium Carbonate (Interferes with absorption of phenytoin).
No products indexed under this heading.

Disulfiram (Increased phenytoin levels). Products include:
Antabuse Tablets 2695

Divalproex Sodium (Increased or decreased phenytoin levels). Products include:
Depakote Tablets 415

Doxepin Hydrochloride (Tricyclic antidepressants may precipitate seizures in some patients; phenytoin dosage may need to be adjusted). Products include:
Sinequan 2205
Zonalon Cream 1055

Doxycycline Calcium (Efficacy impaired by phenytoin). Products include:
Vibramycin Calcium Oral Suspension Syrup 1941

Doxycycline Hyclate (Efficacy impaired by phenytoin). Products include:
Doryx Capsules 1913
Vibramycin Hyclate Capsules 1941

IMPORTANT NOTE: Always consult each drug listing in the patient's regimen for possible interactions.

Dilantin Infatabs

Vibramycin Hyclate Intravenous 2215
Vibra-Tabs Film Coated Tablets 1941

Doxycycline Monohydrate (Efficacy impaired by phenytoin). Products include:

Monodox Capsules 1805
Vibramycin Monohydrate for Oral Suspension 1941

Dyphylline (Efficacy impaired by phenytoin). Products include:

Lufyllin & Lufyllin-400 Tablets 2670
Lufyllin-GG Elixir & Tablets 2671

Estradiol (Increased phenytoin levels; efficacy impaired by phenytoin). Products include:

Climara Transdermal System............ 645
Estrace Cream and Tablets.................. 749
Estraderm Transdermal System 824

Estrogens, Conjugated (Increased phenytoin levels; efficacy impaired by phenytoin). Products include:

PMB 200 and PMB 400 2783
Premarin Intravenous 2787
Premarin with Methyltestosterone.. 2794
Premarin Tablets 2789
Premarin Vaginal Cream........................ 2791
Premphase 2797
Prempro.. 2801

Estrogens, Esterified (Increased phenytoin levels; efficacy impaired by phenytoin). Products include:

ESTRATAB Tablets (0.3, 0.625, 1.25, 2.5 mg).. 2536
Estratest 2539
Menest Tablets 2494

Estropipate (Increased phenytoin levels; efficacy impaired by phenytoin). Products include:

Ogen Tablets 2627
Ogen Vaginal Cream................................ 2630
Ortho-Est.. 1869

Ethinyl Estradiol (Increased phenytoin levels; efficacy impaired by phenytoin). Products include:

Brevicon.. 2088
Demulen 2428
Desogen Tablets.. 1817
Levlen/Tri-Levlen 651
Lo/Ovral Tablets 2746
Lo/Ovral-28 Tablets.................................. 2751
Modicon 1872
Nordette-21 Tablets.................................. 2755
Nordette-28 Tablets.................................. 2758
Norinyl 2088
Ortho-Cept 1851
Ortho-Cyclen/Ortho-Tri-Cyclen 1858
Ortho-Novum.. 1872
Ortho-Cyclen/Ortho Tri-Cyclen 1858
Ovcon 760
Ovral Tablets.. 2770
Ovral-28 Tablets 2770
Levlen/Tri-Levlen 651
Tri-Norinyl.. 2164
Triphasil-21 Tablets.................................. 2814
Triphasil-28 Tablets.................................. 2819

Ethosuximide (Increases phenytoin levels). Products include:

Zarontin Capsules 1928
Zarontin Syrup 1929

Ethynodiol Diacetate (Efficacy impaired by phenytoin). Products include:

Demulen 2428

Famotidine (Increases phenytoin serum levels). Products include:

Pepcid AC 1319
Pepcid Injection 1722
Pepcid.. 1720

Fludrocortisone Acetate (Efficacy impaired by phenytoin). Products include:

Florinef Acetate Tablets 505

Fluphenazine Enanthate (Increased phenytoin levels). Products include:

Prolixin Enanthate 509

Fluphenazine Hydrochloride (Increased phenytoin levels). Products include:

Prolixin 509

Interactions Index

Furosemide (Efficacy impaired by phenytoin). Products include:

Lasix Injection, Oral Solution and Tablets 1240

Glipizide (Increased phenytoin levels). Products include:

Glucotrol Tablets 1967
Glucotrol XL Extended Release Tablets 1968

Glyburide (Increased phenytoin levels). Products include:

DiaBeta Tablets 1239
Glynase PresTab Tablets 2609
Micronase Tablets...................................... 2623

Halothane (Increased phenytoin levels). Products include:

Fluothane 2724

Hydrochlorothiazide (Increased phenytoin levels). Products include:

Aldactazide.. 2413
Aldoril Tablets.. 1604
Apresazide Capsules 808
Capozide 742
Dyazide 2479
Esidrix Tablets 821
Esimil Tablets 822
HydroDIURIL Tablets 1674
Hydropres Tablets...................................... 1675
Hyzaar Tablets.. 1677
Inderide Tablets.. 2732
Inderide LA Long Acting Capsules.. 2734
Lopressor HCT Tablets 832
Lotensin HCT.. 837
Maxzide 1380
Moduretic Tablets 1705
Oretic Tablets 443
Prinzide Tablets 1737
Ser-Ap-Es Tablets 849
Timolide Tablets.. 1748
Vaseretic Tablets 1765
Zestoretic 2850
Ziac 1415

Hydrocortisone (Efficacy impaired by phenytoin). Products include:

Anusol-HC Cream 2.5% 1896
Aquanil HC Lotion 1931
Bactine Hydrocortisone Anti-Itch Cream.. ᴹᴰ 709
Caldecort Anti-Itch Hydrocortisone Spray .... ᴹᴰ 631
Cortaid .... ᴹᴰ 836
CORTENEMA.. 2535
Cortisporin Ointment................................ 1085
Cortisporin Ophthalmic Ointment Sterile 1085
Cortisporin Ophthalmic Suspension Sterile 1086
Cortisporin Otic Solution Sterile 1087
Cortisporin Otic Suspension Sterile 1088
Cortizone-5 .... ᴹᴰ 831
Cortizone-10 .... ᴹᴰ 831
Hydrocortone Tablets 1672
Hytone 907
Massengill Medicated Soft Cloth Towelettes.. 2458
PediOtic Suspension Sterile 1153
Preparation H Hydrocortisone 1% Cream .... ᴹᴰ 872
ProctoCream-HC 2.5% 2408
VōSoL HC Otic Solution.......................... 2678

Hydrocortisone Acetate (Efficacy impaired by phenytoin). Products include:

Analpram-HC Rectal Cream 1% and 2.5% 977
Anusol HC-1 Anti-Itch Hydrocortisone Ointment.. ᴹᴰ 847
Anusol-HC Suppositories 1897
Caldecort.. ᴹᴰ 631
Carmol HC 924
Coly-Mycin S Otic w/Neomycin & Hydrocortisone 1906
Cortaid .... ᴹᴰ 836
Cortifoam 2396
Cortisporin Cream...................................... 1084
Epifoam 2399
Hydrocortone Acetate Sterile Suspension.. 1669
Mantadil Cream 1135
Nupercainal Hydrocortisone 1% Cream.. ᴹᴰ 645
Ophthocort.. ◉ 311
Pramosone Cream, Lotion & Ointment 978
ProctoCream-HC 2408

ProctoFoam-HC 2409
Terra-Cortril Ophthalmic Suspension 2210

Hydrocortisone Sodium Phosphate (Efficacy impaired by phenytoin). Products include:

Hydrocortone Phosphate Injection, Sterile 1670

Hydrocortisone Sodium Succinate (Efficacy impaired by phenytoin). Products include:

Solu-Cortef Sterile Powder.................... 2641

Hydroflumethiazide (Increased phenytoin levels). Products include:

Diucardin Tablets.. 2718

Imipramine Hydrochloride (Tricyclic antidepressants may precipitate seizures in some patients; phenytoin dosage may need to be adjusted). Products include:

Tofranil Ampuls 854
Tofranil Tablets 856

Imipramine Pamoate (Tricyclic antidepressants may precipitate seizures in some patients; phenytoin dosage may need to be adjusted). Products include:

Tofranil-PM Capsules................................ 857

Isoniazid (Increased phenytoin levels). Products include:

Nydrazid Injection 508
Rifamate Capsules 1530
Rifater.. 1532

Levonorgestrel (Efficacy impaired by phenytoin). Products include:

Levlen/Tri-Levlen.. 651
Nordette-21 Tablets.................................. 2755
Nordette-28 Tablets.................................. 2758
Norplant System 2759
Levlen/Tri-Levlen.. 651
Triphasil-21 Tablets.................................. 2814
Triphasil-28 Tablets.................................. 2819

Magnesium Salicylate (Increased phenytoin levels). Products include:

Backache Caplets .... ᴹᴰ 613
Bayer Select Backache Pain Relief Formula .... ᴹᴰ 715
Doan's Extra-Strength Analgesic.... ᴹᴰ 633
Extra Strength Doan's P.M. .... ᴹᴰ 633
Doan's Regular Strength Analgesic.. ᴹᴰ 634
Mobigesic Tablets .... ᴹᴰ 602

Maprotiline Hydrochloride (Tricyclic antidepressants may precipitate seizures in some patients; phenytoin dosage may need to be adjusted). Products include:

Ludiomil Tablets.. 843

Mesoridazine Besylate (Increased phenytoin levels). Products include:

Serentil.. 684

Mestranol (Efficacy impaired by phenytoin). Products include:

Norinyl 2088
Ortho-Novum.. 1872

Methotrimeprazine (Increased phenytoin levels). Products include:

Levoprome 1274

Methsuximide (Increases phenytoin serum levels). Products include:

Celontin Kapseals 1899

Methyclothiazide (Increased phenytoin levels). Products include:

Enduron Tablets.. 420

Methylphenidate Hydrochloride (Increased phenytoin levels). Products include:

Ritalin 848

Methylprednisolone Acetate (Efficacy impaired by phenytoin). Products include:

Depo-Medrol Single-Dose Vial 2600
Depo-Medrol Sterile Aqueous Suspension.. 2597

Methylprednisolone Sodium Succinate (Efficacy impaired by phenytoin). Products include:

Solu-Medrol Sterile Powder 2643

Molindone Hydrochloride (Interferes with absorption of phenytoin). Products include:

Moban Tablets and Concentrate...... 1048

Nizatidine (Increases phenytoin serum levels). Products include:

Axid Pulvules 1427

Norethindrone (Efficacy impaired by phenytoin). Products include:

Brevicon.. 2088
Micronor Tablets 1872
Modicon 1872
Norinyl 2088
Nor-Q D Tablets 2135
Ortho-Novum.. 1872
Ovcon 760
Tri-Norinyl.. 2164

Norethynodrel (Efficacy impaired by phenytoin).

No products indexed under this heading.

Norgestimate (Increased phenytoin levels; efficacy impaired by phenytoin). Products include:

Ortho-Cyclen/Ortho-Tri-Cyclen 1858
Ortho-Cyclen/Ortho Tri-Cyclen 1858

Norgestrel (Efficacy impaired by phenytoin). Products include:

Lo/Ovral Tablets 2746
Lo/Ovral-28 Tablets.................................. 2751
Ovral Tablets 2770
Ovral-28 Tablets 2770
Ovrette Tablets.. 2771

Nortriptyline Hydrochloride (Tricyclic antidepressants may precipitate seizures in some patients; phenytoin dosage may need to be adjusted). Products include:

Pamelor 2280

Perphenazine (Increased phenytoin levels). Products include:

Etrafon 2355
Triavil Tablets 1757
Trilafon.. 2389

Phenobarbital (Increased or decreased phenytoin levels). Products include:

Arco-Lase Plus Tablets 512
Bellergal-S Tablets 2250
Donnatal 2060
Donnatal Extentabs.................................. 2061
Donnatal Tablets 2060
Phenobarbital Elixir and Tablets 1469
Quadrinal Tablets 1350

Phensuximide (Increases phenytoin serum levels). Products include:

Milontin Kapseals.. 1920

Phenylbutazone (Increased phenytoin levels).

No products indexed under this heading.

Polyestradiol Phosphate (Increased phenytoin levels; efficacy impaired by phenytoin).

No products indexed under this heading.

Polythiazide (Increased phenytoin levels). Products include:

Minizide Capsules 1938

Prednisolone (Efficacy impaired by phenytoin). Products include:

Prelone Syrup 1787

Prednisolone Acetate (Efficacy impaired by phenytoin). Products include:

AK-CIDE .... ◉ 202
AK-CIDE Ointment...................................... ◉ 202
Blephamide Liquifilm Sterile Ophthalmic Suspension.................................. 476
Blephamide Ointment .... ◉ 237
Econopred & Econopred Plus Ophthalmic Suspensions .... ◉ 217
Poly-Pred Liquifilm .... ◉ 248
Pred Forte.. ◉ 250
Pred Mild.. ◉ 253
Pred-G Liquifilm Sterile Ophthalmic Suspension .... ◉ 251
Pred-G S.O.P. Sterile Ophthalmic Ointment .... ◉ 252
Vasocidin Ointment .... ◉ 268

(ᴹᴰ Described in PDR For Nonprescription Drugs) (◉ Described in PDR For Ophthalmology)

287 Interactions Index Dilantin Kapseals

Prednisolone Sodium Phosphate (Efficacy impaired by phenytoin). Products include:
- AK-Pred ◎ 204
- Hydeltrasol Injection, Sterile 1665
- Inflamase ◎ 265
- Pediapred Oral Liquid 995
- Vasocidin Ophthalmic Solution ◎ 270

Prednisolone Tebutate (Efficacy impaired by phenytoin). Products include:
- Hydeltra-T.B.A. Sterile Suspension 1667

Prednisone (Efficacy impaired by phenytoin). Products include:
- Deltasone Tablets 2595

Prochlorperazine (Increased phenytoin levels). Products include:
- Compazine 2470

Promethazine Hydrochloride (Increased phenytoin levels). Products include:
- Mepergan Injection 2753
- Phenergan with Codeine 2777
- Phenergan with Dextromethorphan 2778
- Phenergan Injection 2773
- Phenergan Suppositories 2775
- Phenergan Syrup 2774
- Phenergan Tablets 2775
- Phenergan VC 2779
- Phenergan VC with Codeine 2781

Protriptyline Hydrochloride (Tricyclic antidepressants may precipitate seizures in some patients; phenytoin dosage may need to be adjusted). Products include:
- Vivactil Tablets 1774

Quinestrol (Increased phenytoin levels; efficacy impaired by phenytoin).
- No products indexed under this heading.

Quinidine Gluconate (Efficacy impaired by phenytoin). Products include:
- Quinaglute Dura-Tabs Tablets 649

Quinidine Polygalacturonate (Efficacy impaired by phenytoin).
- No products indexed under this heading.

Quinidine Sulfate (Efficacy impaired by phenytoin). Products include:
- Quinidex Extentabs 2067

Ranitidine Hydrochloride (Increases phenytoin serum levels). Products include:
- Zantac 1209
- Zantac Injection 1207
- Zantac Syrup 1209

Reserpine (Decreased phenytoin levels). Products include:
- Diupres Tablets 1650
- Hydropres Tablets 1675
- Ser-Ap-Es Tablets 849

Rifampin (Efficacy impaired by phenytoin). Products include:
- Rifadin 1528
- Rifamate Capsules 1530
- Rifater 1532
- Rimactane Capsules 847

Salsalate (Increased phenytoin levels). Products include:
- Mono-Gesic Tablets 792
- Salflex Tablets 786

Sodium Valproate (Increased or decreased phenytoin levels).

Sucralfate (Decreases phenytoin serum levels). Products include:
- Carafate Suspension 1505
- Carafate Tablets 1504

Sulfamethizole (Increased phenytoin levels). Products include:
- Urobiotic-250 Capsules 2214

Sulfamethoxazole (Increased phenytoin levels). Products include:
- Azo Gantanol Tablets 2080
- Bactrim DS Tablets 2084
- Bactrim I.V. Infusion 2082
- Bactrim 2084
- Gantanol Tablets 2119
- Septra 1174
- Septra I.V. Infusion 1169
- Septra I.V. Infusion ADD-Vantage Vials 1171
- Septra 1174

Sulfasalazine (Increased phenytoin levels). Products include:
- Azulfidine 1949

Sulfinpyrazone (Increased phenytoin levels). Products include:
- Anturane 807

Sulfisoxazole (Increased phenytoin levels). Products include:
- Azo Gantrisin Tablets 2081
- Gantrisin Tablets 2120

Sulfisoxazole Diolamine (Increased phenytoin levels).
- No products indexed under this heading.

Theophylline (Efficacy impaired by phenytoin). Products include:
- Marax Tablets & DF Syrup 2200
- Quibron 2053

Theophylline Anhydrous (Efficacy impaired by phenytoin). Products include:
- Aerolate 1004
- Primatene Dual Action Formula ◙ 872
- Primatene Tablets ◙ 873
- Respbid Tablets 682
- Slo-bid Gyrocaps 2033
- Theo-24 Extended Release Capsules 2568
- Theo-Dur Extended-Release Tablets 1327
- Theo-X Extended-Release Tablets 788
- Uni-Dur Extended-Release Tablets 1331
- Uniphyl 400 mg Tablets 2001

Theophylline Calcium Salicylate (Efficacy impaired by phenytoin). Products include:
- Quadrinal Tablets 1350

Theophylline Sodium Glycinate (Efficacy impaired by phenytoin).
- No products indexed under this heading.

Thioridazine Hydrochloride (Increased phenytoin levels). Products include:
- Mellaril 2269

Tolazamide (Increased phenytoin levels).
- No products indexed under this heading.

Tolbutamide (Increased phenytoin levels).
- No products indexed under this heading.

Trazodone Hydrochloride (Increased phenytoin levels). Products include:
- Desyrel and Desyrel Dividose 503

Triamcinolone (Efficacy impaired by phenytoin). Products include:
- Aristocort Tablets 1022

Triamcinolone Acetonide (Efficacy impaired by phenytoin). Products include:
- Aristocort A 0.025% Cream 1027
- Aristocort A 0.5% Cream 1031
- Aristocort A 0.1% Cream 1029
- Aristocort A 0.1% Ointment 1030
- Azmacort Oral Inhaler 2011
- Nasacort Nasal Inhaler 2024

Triamcinolone Diacetate (Efficacy impaired by phenytoin). Products include:
- Aristocort Suspension (Forte Parenteral) 1027
- Aristocort Suspension (Intralesional) 1025

Triamcinolone Hexacetonide (Efficacy impaired by phenytoin). Products include:
- Aristospan Suspension (Intra-articular) 1033
- Aristospan Suspension (Intralesional) 1032

Trifluoperazine Hydrochloride (Increased phenytoin levels). Products include:
- Stelazine 2514

Trimipramine Maleate (Tricyclic antidepressants may precipitate seizures in some patients; phenytoin dosage may need to be adjusted). Products include:
- Surmontil Capsules 2811

Valproic Acid (Increased or decreased phenytoin levels). Products include:
- Depakene 413

Vitamin D (Efficacy impaired by phenytoin). Products include:
- Caltrate PLUS ◙ 665
- Caltrate 600 + D ◙ 665
- Citracal Caplets + D 1780
- Dical-D Tablets & Wafers 420
- Drisdol ◙ 794
- Materna Tablets 1379
- Megadose 512
- Zymacap Capsules ◙ 772

Warfarin Sodium (Efficacy impaired by phenytoin). Products include:
- Coumadin 926

Food Interactions

Alcohol (Increased phenytoin serum levels with acute alcohol intake; decreased levels with chronic alcohol intake).

DILANTIN KAPSEALS

(Phenytoin Sodium) 1906

May interact with oral anticoagulants, corticosteroids, oral contraceptives, salicylates, phenothiazines, estrogens, sulfonamides, tricyclic antidepressants, histamine h2-receptor antagonists, succinimides, xanthine bronchodilators, and certain other agents. Compounds in these categories include:

Aminophylline (Efficacy impaired by phenytoin).
- No products indexed under this heading.

Amiodarone Hydrochloride (Increases phenytoin serum levels). Products include:
- Cordarone Intravenous 2715
- Cordarone Tablets 2712

Amitriptyline Hydrochloride (Tricyclic antidepressants may precipitate seizures in some patients; phenytoin dosage may need to be adjusted). Products include:
- Elavil 2838
- Endep Tablets 2174
- Etrafon 2355
- Limbitrol 2180
- Triavil Tablets 1757

Amoxapine (Tricyclic antidepressants may precipitate seizures in some patients; phenytoin dosage may need to be adjusted). Products include:
- Asendin Tablets 1369

Aspirin (Increased phenytoin serum levels). Products include:
- Alka-Seltzer Effervescent Antacid and Pain Reliever ◙ 701
- Alka-Seltzer Extra Strength Effervescent Antacid and Pain Reliever ◙ 703
- Alka-Seltzer Lemon Lime Effervescent Antacid and Pain Reliever ◙ 703
- Alka-Seltzer Plus Cold Medicine ◙ 705
- Alka-Seltzer Plus Cold & Cough Medicine ◙ 708
- Alka-Seltzer Plus Night-Time Cold Medicine ◙ 707
- Alka Seltzer Plus Sinus Medicine ◙ 707
- Arthritis Foundation Safety Coated Aspirin Tablets ◙ 675
- Arthritis Pain Ascriptin ◙ 631
- Maximum Strength Ascriptin ◙ 630
- Regular Strength Ascriptin Tablets ◙ 629
- Arthritis Strength BC Powder ◙ 609
- BC Cold Powder Multi-Symptom Formula (Cold-Sinus-Allergy) ◙ 609
- BC Cold Powder Non-Drowsy Formula (Cold-Sinus) ◙ 609
- BC Powder ◙ 609
- Bayer Children's Chewable Aspirin ◙ 711
- Genuine Bayer Aspirin Tablets & Caplets ◙ 713
- Extra Strength Bayer Arthritis Pain Regimen Formula ◙ 711
- Extra Strength Bayer Aspirin Caplets & Tablets ◙ 712
- Extended-Release Bayer 8-Hour Aspirin ◙ 712
- Extra Strength Bayer Plus Aspirin Caplets ◙ 713
- Extra Strength Bayer PM Aspirin ◙ 713
- Bayer Enteric Aspirin ◙ 709
- Bufferin Analgesic Tablets and Caplets ◙ 613
- Arthritis Strength Bufferin Analgesic Caplets ◙ 614
- Extra Strength Bufferin Analgesic Tablets ◙ 615
- Cama Arthritis Pain Reliever ◙ 785
- Darvon Compound-65 Pulvules 1435
- Easprin 1914
- Ecotrin 2455
- Ecotrin Enteric Coated Aspirin Maximum Strength Tablets and Caplets ◙ 816
- Ecotrin Enteric Coated Aspirin Regular Strength Tablets 2455
- Empirin Aspirin Tablets ◙ 854
- Empirin with Codeine Tablets 1093
- Excedrin Extra-Strength Analgesic Tablets & Caplets 732
- Fiorinal Capsules 2261
- Fiorinal with Codeine Capsules 2262
- Fiorinal Tablets 2261
- Halfprin 1362
- Healthprin Aspirin 2455
- Norgesic 1496
- Percodan Tablets 939
- Percodan-Demi Tablets 940
- Robaxisal Tablets 2071
- Soma Compound w/Codeine Tablets 2676
- Soma Compound Tablets 2675
- St. Joseph Adult Chewable Aspirin (81 mg.) ◙ 808
- Talwin Compound 2335
- Ursinus Inlay-Tabs ◙ 794
- Vanquish Analgesic Caplets ◙ 731

Bendroflumethiazide (Increased phenytoin serum levels).
- No products indexed under this heading.

Betamethasone Acetate (Efficacy impaired by phenytoin). Products include:
- Celestone Soluspan Suspension 2347

Betamethasone Sodium Phosphate (Efficacy impaired by phenytoin). Products include:
- Celestone Soluspan Suspension 2347

Calcium Carbonate (Ingestion times of phenytoin and antacids containing calcium should be staggered to prevent absorption problems). Products include:
- Alka-Mints Chewable Antacid ◙ 701
- Arthritis Pain Ascriptin ◙ 631
- Maximum Strength Ascriptin ◙ 630
- Regular Strength Ascriptin Tablets ◙ 629
- Extra Strength Bayer Plus Aspirin Caplets ◙ 713
- Bufferin Analgesic Tablets and Caplets ◙ 613
- Calci-Chew Tablets 2004
- Calci-Mix Capsules 2004
- Caltrate 600 ◙ 665
- Caltrate PLUS ◙ 665
- Caltrate 600 + D ◙ 665
- Centrum Singles Calcium ◙ 669
- Chooz Antacid Gum ◙ 799
- Di-Gel Antacid/Anti-Gas ◙ 801
- Gerimed Tablets 982
- Maalox Antacid Caplets ◙ 638
- Marblen ◙ 655
- Materna Tablets 1379
- Mylanta Calcium Carbonate and Magnesium Hydroxide Tablets 1318
- Mylanta Gelcaps Antacid ◙ 662
- Mylanta Soothing Lozenges 1319

IMPORTANT NOTE: Always consult each drug listing in the patient's regimen for possible interactions.

Dilantin Kapseals

Nephro-Calci Tablets 2004
Rolaids Tablets .... ᴹᴰ 843
Rolaids (Calcium Rich/Sodium Free) Tablets .... ᴹᴰ 843
Tempo Soft Antacid .... ᴹᴰ 835
Titralac .... ᴹᴰ 672
Titralac Plus .... ᴹᴰ 672
Tums Antacid Tablets .... ᴹᴰ 827
Tums Anti-gas/Antacid Formula Tablets, Assorted Fruit .... ᴹᴰ 827
Tums E-X Antacid Tablets .... ᴹᴰ 827
Tums 500 Calcium Supplement .... ᴹᴰ 828
Tums ULTRA Antacid Tablets .... ᴹᴰ 827
TYLENOL, Extra Strength, Headache Plus Pain Reliever with Antacid Caplets 1559

Calcium Carbonate, Precipitated (Ingestion times of phenytoin and antacids containing calcium should be staggered to prevent absorption problems).

Carbamazepine (Decreased phenytoin levels). Products include:

Atretol Tablets 573
Tegretol Chewable Tablets 852
Tegretol Suspension 852
Tegretol Tablets 852

Chloramphenicol (Increased phenytoin serum levels). Products include:

Chloromycetin Ophthalmic Ointment, 1% .... ⊙ 310
Chloromycetin Ophthalmic Solution .... ⊙ 310
Chloroptic S.O.P. .... ⊙ 239
Chloroptic Sterile Ophthalmic Solution .... ⊙ 239
Elase-Chloromycetin Ointment 1040
Ophthocort .... ⊙ 311

Chloramphenicol Palmitate (Increased phenytoin serum levels).

No products indexed under this heading.

Chloramphenicol Sodium Succinate (Increased phenytoin serum levels). Products include:

Chloromycetin Sodium Succinate 1900

Chlordiazepoxide (Increased phenytoin serum levels). Products include:

Libritabs Tablets 2177
Limbitrol 2180

Chlordiazepoxide Hydrochloride (Increased phenytoin serum levels). Products include:

Librax Capsules 2176
Librium Capsules 2178
Librium Injectable 2179

Chlorothiazide (Increased phenytoin serum levels). Products include:

Aldoclor Tablets 1598
Diupres Tablets 1650
Diuril Oral 1653

Chlorothiazide Sodium (Increased phenytoin serum levels). Products include:

Diuril Sodium Intravenous 1652

Chlorotrianisene (Increased phenytoin serum levels; efficacy impaired by phenytoin).

No products indexed under this heading.

Chlorpromazine (Increased phenytoin serum levels). Products include:

Thorazine Suppositories 2523

Chlorpromazine Hydrochloride (Increased phenytoin serum levels). Products include:

Thorazine 2523

Chlorpropamide (Increased phenytoin serum levels). Products include:

Diabinese Tablets 1935

Choline Magnesium Trisalicylate (Increased phenytoin serum levels). Products include:

Trilisate 2000

Cimetidine (Increased phenytoin serum levels). Products include:

Tagamet Tablets 2516

Cimetidine Hydrochloride (Increased phenytoin serum levels). Products include:

Tagamet 2516

Clomipramine Hydrochloride (Tricyclic antidepressants may precipitate seizures in some patients; phenytoin dosage may need to be adjusted). Products include:

Anafranil Capsules 803

Cortisone Acetate (Efficacy impaired by phenytoin). Products include:

Cortone Acetate Sterile Suspension 1623
Cortone Acetate Tablets 1624

Desipramine Hydrochloride (Tricyclic antidepressants may precipitate seizures in some patients; phenytoin dosage may need to be adjusted). Products include:

Norpramin Tablets 1526

Desogestrel (Increased phenytoin serum levels; efficacy impaired by phenytoin). Products include:

Desogen Tablets 1817
Ortho-Cept 1851

Dexamethasone (Efficacy impaired by phenytoin). Products include:

AK-Trol Ointment & Suspension .... ⊙ 205
Decadron Elixir 1633
Decadron Tablets 1635
Decaspray Topical Aerosol 1648
Dexacidin Ointment .... ⊙ 263
Maxitrol Ophthalmic Ointment and Suspension .... ⊙ 224
TobraDex Ophthalmic Suspension and Ointment 473

Dexamethasone Acetate (Efficacy impaired by phenytoin). Products include:

Dalalone D.P. Injectable 1011
Decadron-LA Sterile Suspension 1646

Dexamethasone Sodium Phosphate (Efficacy impaired by phenytoin). Products include:

Decadron Phosphate Injection 1637
Decadron Phosphate Respihaler 1642
Decadron Phosphate Sterile Ophthalmic Ointment 1641
Decadron Phosphate Sterile Ophthalmic Solution 1642
Decadron Phosphate Topical Cream 1644
Decadron Phosphate Turbinaire 1645
Decadron Phosphate with Xylocaine Injection, Sterile 1639
Dexacort Phosphate in Respihaler .. 458
Dexacort Phosphate in Turbinaire .. 459
NeoDecadron Sterile Ophthalmic Ointment 1712
NeoDecadron Sterile Ophthalmic Solution 1713
NeoDecadron Topical Cream 1714

Diazepam (Increased phenytoin serum levels). Products include:

Dizac 1809
Valium Injectable 2182
Valium Tablets 2183
Valrelease Capsules 2169

Dicumarol (Efficacy impaired by phenytoin; increased phenytoin serum levels).

No products indexed under this heading.

Dienestrol (Increased phenytoin serum levels; efficacy impaired by phenytoin). Products include:

Ortho Dienestrol Cream 1866

Diethylstilbestrol (Increased phenytoin serum levels; efficacy impaired by phenytoin). Products include:

Diethylstilbestrol Tablets 1437

Diflunisal (Increased phenytoin serum levels). Products include:

Dolobid Tablets 1654

Digitoxin (Efficacy impaired by phenytoin). Products include:

Crystodigin Tablets 1433

Disulfiram (Increased phenytoin serum levels). Products include:

Antabuse Tablets 2695

Divalproex Sodium (Increased or decreased phenytoin serum levels). Products include:

Depakote Tablets 415

Doxepin Hydrochloride (Tricyclic antidepressants may precipitate seizures in some patients; phenytoin dosage may need to be adjusted). Products include:

Sinequan 2205
Zonalon Cream 1055

Doxycycline Calcium (Efficacy impaired by phenytoin). Products include:

Vibramycin Calcium Oral Suspension Syrup 1941

Doxycycline Hyclate (Efficacy impaired by phenytoin). Products include:

Doryx Capsules 1913
Vibramycin Hyclate Capsules 1941
Vibramycin Hyclate Intravenous 2215
Vibra-Tabs Film Coated Tablets 1941

Doxycycline Monohydrate (Efficacy impaired by phenytoin). Products include:

Monodox Capsules 1805
Vibramycin Monohydrate for Oral Suspension 1941

Dyphylline (Efficacy impaired by phenytoin). Products include:

Lufyllin & Lufyllin-400 Tablets 2670
Lufyllin-GG Elixir & Tablets 2671

Estradiol (Increased phenytoin serum levels; efficacy impaired by phenytoin). Products include:

Climara Transdermal System 645
Estrace Cream and Tablets 749
Estraderm Transdermal System 824

Estrogens, Conjugated (Increased phenytoin serum levels; efficacy impaired by phenytoin). Products include:

PMB 200 and PMB 400 2783
Premarin Intravenous 2787
Premarin with Methyltestosterone .. 2794
Premarin Tablets 2789
Premarin Vaginal Cream 2791
Premphase 2797
Prempro 2801

Estrogens, Esterified (Increased phenytoin serum levels; efficacy impaired by phenytoin). Products include:

ESTRATAB Tablets (0.3, 0.625, 1.25, 2.5 mg) 2536
Estratest 2539
Menest Tablets 2494

Estropipate (Increased phenytoin serum levels; efficacy impaired by phenytoin). Products include:

Ogen Tablets 2627
Ogen Vaginal Cream 2630
Ortho-Est 1869

Ethinyl Estradiol (Increased phenytoin serum levels; efficacy impaired by phenytoin). Products include:

Brevicon 2088
Demulen 2428
Desogen Tablets 1817
Levlen/Tri-Levlen 651
Lo/Ovral Tablets 2746
Lo/Ovral-28 Tablets 2751
Modicon 1872
Nordette-21 Tablets 2755
Nordette-28 Tablets 2758
Norinyl 2088
Ortho-Cept 1851
Ortho-Cyclen/Ortho-Tri-Cyclen 1858
Ortho-Novum 1872
Ortho-Cyclen/Ortho Tri-Cyclen 1858
Ovcon 760
Ovral Tablets 2770
Ovral-28 Tablets 2770
Levlen/Tri-Levlen 651
Tri-Norinyl 2164
Triphasil-21 Tablets 2814
Triphasil-28 Tablets 2819

Ethosuximide (Increased phenytoin serum levels). Products include:

Zarontin Capsules 1928
Zarontin Syrup 1929

Ethynodiol Diacetate (Efficacy impaired by phenytoin). Products include:

Demulen 2428

Famotidine (Increased phenytoin serum levels). Products include:

Pepcid AC 1319
Pepcid Injection 1722
Pepcid 1720

Fludrocortisone Acetate (Efficacy impaired by phenytoin). Products include:

Florinef Acetate Tablets 505

Fluphenazine Decanoate (Increased phenytoin serum levels). Products include:

Prolixin Decanoate 509

Fluphenazine Enanthate (Increased phenytoin serum levels). Products include:

Prolixin Enanthate 509

Fluphenazine Hydrochloride (Increased phenytoin serum levels). Products include:

Prolixin 509

Furosemide (Efficacy impaired by phenytoin). Products include:

Lasix Injection, Oral Solution and Tablets 1240

Glipizide (Increased phenytoin serum levels). Products include:

Glucotrol Tablets 1967
Glucotrol XL Extended Release Tablets 1968

Glyburide (Increased phenytoin serum levels). Products include:

DiaBeta Tablets 1239
Glynase PresTab Tablets 2609
Micronase Tablets 2623

Halothane (Increased phenytoin serum levels). Products include:

Fluothane 2724

Hydrochlorothiazide (Increased phenytoin serum levels). Products include:

Aldactazide 2413
Aldoril Tablets 1604
Apresazide Capsules 808
Capozide 742
Dyazide 2479
Esidrix Tablets 821
Esimil Tablets 822
HydroDIURIL Tablets 1674
Hydropres Tablets 1675
Hyzaar Tablets 1677
Inderide Tablets 2732
Inderide LA Long Acting Capsules .. 2734
Lopressor HCT Tablets 832
Lotensin HCT 837
Maxzide 1380
Moduretic Tablets 1705
Oretic Tablets 443
Prinzide Tablets 1737
Ser-Ap-Es Tablets 849
Timolide Tablets 1748
Vaseretic Tablets 1765
Zestoretic 2850
Ziac 1415

Hydrocortisone (Efficacy impaired by phenytoin). Products include:

Anusol-HC Cream 2.5% 1896
Aquanil HC Lotion 1931
Bactine Hydrocortisone Anti-Itch Cream .... ᴹᴰ 709
Caldecort Anti-Itch Hydrocortisone Spray .... ᴹᴰ 631
Cortaid .... ᴹᴰ 836
CORTENEMA 2535
Cortisporin Ointment 1085
Cortisporin Ophthalmic Ointment Sterile 1085
Cortisporin Ophthalmic Suspension Sterile 1086
Cortisporin Otic Solution Sterile 1087
Cortisporin Otic Suspension Sterile 1088
Cortizone-5 .... ᴹᴰ 831
Cortizone-10 .... ᴹᴰ 831
Hydrocortone Tablets 1672

(ᴹᴰ Described in PDR For Nonprescription Drugs)

(⊙ Described in PDR For Ophthalmology)

Hytone 907
Massengill Medicated Soft Cloth Towelettes... 2458
PediOtic Suspension Sterile 1153
Preparation H Hydrocortisone 1% Cream .... ⊕ 872
ProctoCream-HC 2.5% 2408
VōSoL HC Otic Solution........................ 2678

Hydrocortisone Acetate (Efficacy impaired by phenytoin). Products include:

Analpram-HC Rectal Cream 1% and 2.5% 977
Anusol HC-1 Anti-Itch Hydrocortisone Ointment...................................... ⊕ 847
Anusol-HC Suppositories 1897
Caldecort... ⊕ 631
Carmol HC 924
Coly-Mycin S Otic w/Neomycin & Hydrocortisone 1906
Cortaid .... ⊕ 836
Cortifoam 2396
Cortisporin Cream............................... 1084
Epifoam 2399
Hydrocortone Acetate Sterile Suspension... 1669
Mantadil Cream 1135
Nupercainal Hydrocortisone 1% Cream... ⊕ 645
Ophthocort .... © 311
Pramosone Cream, Lotion & Ointment 978
ProctoCream-HC 2408
ProctoFoam-HC 2409
Terra-Cortril Ophthalmic Suspension 2210

Hydrocortisone Sodium Phosphate (Efficacy impaired by phenytoin). Products include:

Hydrocortone Phosphate Injection, Sterile 1670

Hydrocortisone Sodium Succinate (Efficacy impaired by phenytoin). Products include:

Solu-Cortef Sterile Powder.................. 2641

Hydroflumethiazide (Increased phenytoin serum levels). Products include:

Diucardin Tablets.................................. 2718

Imipramine Hydrochloride (Tricyclic antidepressants may precipitate seizures in some patients; phenytoin dosage may need to be adjusted). Products include:

Tofranil Ampuls 854
Tofranil Tablets 856

Imipramine Pamoate (Tricyclic antidepressants may precipitate seizures in some patients; phenytoin dosage may need to be adjusted). Products include:

Tofranil-PM Capsules........................... 857

Isoniazid (Increased phenytoin serum levels). Products include:

Nydrazid Injection 508
Rifamate Capsules 1530
Rifater.. 1532

Levonorgestrel (Efficacy impaired by phenytoin). Products include:

Levlen/Tri-Levlen 651
Nordette-21 Tablets.............................. 2755
Nordette-28 Tablets.............................. 2758
Norplant System 2759
Levlen/Tri-Levlen.................................. 651
Triphasil-21 Tablets.............................. 2814
Triphasil-28 Tablets.............................. 2819

Magnesium Salicylate (Increased phenytoin serum levels). Products include:

Backache Caplets .... ⊕ 613
Bayer Select Backache Pain Relief Formula .... ⊕ 715
Doan's Extra-Strength Analgesic.... ⊕ 633
Extra Strength Doan's P.M. .... ⊕ 633
Doan's Regular Strength Analgesic.. ⊕ 634
Mobigesic Tablets .... ⊕ 602

Maprotiline Hydrochloride (Tricyclic antidepressants may precipitate seizures in some patients; phenytoin dosage may need to be adjusted). Products include:

Ludiomil Tablets................................... 843

Mesoridazine Besylate (Increased phenytoin serum levels). Products include:

Serentil 684

Mestranol (Efficacy impaired by phenytoin). Products include:

Norinyl 2088
Ortho-Novum....................................... 1872

Methotrimeprazine (Increased phenytoin serum levels). Products include:

Levoprome 1274

Methsuximide (Increased phenytoin serum levels). Products include:

Celontin Kapseals 1899

Methyclothiazide (Increased phenytoin serum levels). Products include:

Enduron Tablets.................................... 420

Methylphenidate Hydrochloride (Increased phenytoin serum levels). Products include:

Ritalin 848

Methylprednisolone Acetate (Efficacy impaired by phenytoin). Products include:

Depo-Medrol Single-Dose Vial 2600
Depo-Medrol Sterile Aqueous Suspension... 2597

Methylprednisolone Sodium Succinate (Efficacy impaired by phenytoin). Products include:

Solu-Medrol Sterile Powder 2643

Molindone Hydrochloride (Interferes with absorption of phenytoin). Products include:

Moban Tablets and Concentrate...... 1048

Nizatidine (Increased phenytoin serum levels). Products include:

Axid Pulvules....................................... 1427

Norethindrone (Efficacy impaired by phenytoin). Products include:

Brevicon.. 2088
Micronor Tablets 1872
Modicon 1872
Norinyl 2088
Nor-Q D Tablets 2135
Ortho-Novum....................................... 1872
Ovcon 760
Tri-Norinyl.. 2164

Norethynodrel (Efficacy impaired by phenytoin).

No products indexed under this heading.

Norgestimate (Efficacy impaired by phenytoin). Products include:

Ortho-Cyclen/Ortho-Tri-Cyclen 1858
Ortho-Cyclen/Ortho Tri-Cyclen 1858

Norgestrel (Efficacy impaired by phenytoin). Products include:

Lo/Ovral Tablets 2746
Lo/Ovral-28 Tablets............................. 2751
Ovral Tablets 2770
Ovral-28 Tablets 2770
Ovrette Tablets..................................... 2771

Nortriptyline Hydrochloride (Tricyclic antidepressants may precipitate seizures in some patients; phenytoin dosage may need to be adjusted). Products include:

Pamelor 2280

Perphenazine (Increased phenytoin serum levels). Products include:

Etrafon 2355
Triavil Tablets 1757
Trilafon.. 2389

Phenobarbital (Increased or decreased phenytoin serum levels). Products include:

Arco-Lase Plus Tablets 512
Bellergal-S Tablets 2250
Donnatal 2060
Donnatal Extentabs.............................. 2061
Donnatal Tablets 2060
Phenobarbital Elixir and Tablets 1469
Quadrinal Tablets 1350

Phensuximide (Increased phenytoin serum levels). Products include:

Milontin Kapseals................................. 1920

Phenylbutazone (Increased phenytoin serum levels).

No products indexed under this heading.

Polyestradiol Phosphate (Increased phenytoin serum levels; efficacy impaired by phenytoin).

No products indexed under this heading.

Polythiazide (Increased phenytoin serum levels). Products include:

Minizide Capsules 1938

Prednisolone Acetate (Efficacy impaired by phenytoin). Products include:

AK-CIDE... © 202
AK-CIDE Ointment............................... © 202
Blephamide Liquifilm Sterile Ophthalmic Suspension.............................. 476
Blephamide Ointment .... © 237
Econopred & Econopred Plus Ophthalmic Suspensions .... © 217
Poly-Pred Liquifilm .... © 248
Pred Forte... © 250
Pred Mild... © 253
Pred-G Liquifilm Sterile Ophthalmic Suspension .... © 251
Pred-G S.O.P. Sterile Ophthalmic Ointment .... © 252
Vasocidin Ointment .... © 268

Prednisolone Sodium Phosphate (Efficacy impaired by phenytoin). Products include:

AK-Pred .... © 204
Hydeltrasol Injection, Sterile.............. 1665
Inflamase.. © 265
Pediapred Oral Liquid 995
Vasocidin Ophthalmic Solution ...... © 270

Prednisolone Tebutate (Efficacy impaired by phenytoin). Products include:

Hydeltra-T.B.A. Sterile Suspension 1667

Prednisone (Efficacy impaired by phenytoin). Products include:

Deltasone Tablets 2595

Prochlorperazine (Increased phenytoin serum levels). Products include:

Compazine 2470

Promethazine Hydrochloride (Increased phenytoin serum levels). Products include:

Mepergan Injection 2753
Phenergan with Codeine...................... 2777
Phenergan with Dextromethorphan 2778
Phenergan Injection 2773
Phenergan Suppositories 2775
Phenergan Syrup 2774
Phenergan Tablets 2775
Phenergan VC 2779
Phenergan VC with Codeine 2781

Protriptyline Hydrochloride (Tricyclic antidepressants may precipitate seizures in some patients; phenytoin dosage may need to be adjusted). Products include:

Vivactil Tablets 1774

Quinestrol (Increased phenytoin serum levels; efficacy impaired by phenytoin).

No products indexed under this heading.

Quinidine Gluconate (Efficacy impaired by phenytoin). Products include:

Quinaglute Dura-Tabs Tablets 649

Quinidine Polygalacturonate (Efficacy impaired by phenytoin).

No products indexed under this heading.

Quinidine Sulfate (Efficacy impaired by phenytoin). Products include:

Quinidex Extentabs.............................. 2067

Ranitidine Hydrochloride (Increased phenytoin serum levels). Products include:

Zantac.. 1209
Zantac Injection 1207

Zantac Syrup 1209

Reserpine (Decreased phenytoin levels). Products include:

Diupres Tablets 1650
Hydropres Tablets................................. 1675
Ser-Ap-Es Tablets 849

Rifampin (Efficacy impaired by phenytoin). Products include:

Rifadin 1528
Rifamate Capsules 1530
Rifater.. 1532
Rimactane Capsules............................. 847

Salsalate (Increased phenytoin serum levels). Products include:

Mono-Gesic Tablets 792
Salflex Tablets...................................... 786

Sodium Valproate (Increased or decreased phenytoin levels).

Sucralfate (Decreased phenytoin serum levels). Products include:

Carafate Suspension 1505
Carafate Tablets................................... 1504

Sulfacytine (Increased phenytoin serum levels).

Sulfamethizole (Increased phenytoin serum levels). Products include:

Urobiotic-250 Capsules 2214

Sulfamethoxazole (Increased phenytoin serum levels). Products include:

Azo Gantanol Tablets........................... 2080
Bactrim DS Tablets............................... 2084
Bactrim I.V. Infusion............................ 2082
Bactrim 2084
Gantanol Tablets 2119
Septra.. 1174
Septra I.V. Infusion 1169
Septra I.V. Infusion ADD-Vantage Vials... 1171
Septra.. 1174

Sulfasalazine (Increased phenytoin serum levels). Products include:

Azulfidine 1949

Sulfinpyrazone (Increased phenytoin serum levels). Products include:

Anturane 807

Sulfisoxazole (Increased phenytoin serum levels). Products include:

Azo Gantrisin Tablets........................... 2081
Gantrisin Tablets 2120

Sulfisoxazole Diolamine (Increased phenytoin serum levels).

No products indexed under this heading.

Theophylline (Efficacy impaired by phenytoin). Products include:

Marax Tablets & DF Syrup................... 2200
Quibron 2053

Theophylline Anhydrous (Efficacy impaired by phenytoin). Products include:

Aerolate 1004
Primatene Dual Action Formula...... ⊕ 872
Primatene Tablets .... ⊕ 873
Respbid Tablets 682
Slo-bid Gyrocaps 2033
Theo-24 Extended Release Capsules 2568
Theo-Dur Extended-Release Tablets 1327
Theo-X Extended-Release Tablets .. 788
Uni-Dur Extended-Release Tablets.. 1331
Uniphyl 400 mg Tablets....................... 2001

Theophylline Calcium Salicylate (Efficacy impaired by phenytoin). Products include:

Quadrinal Tablets 1350

Theophylline Sodium Glycinate (Efficacy impaired by phenytoin).

No products indexed under this heading.

Thioridazine Hydrochloride (Increased phenytoin serum levels). Products include:

Mellaril 2269

Tolazamide (Increased phenytoin serum levels).

No products indexed under this heading.

IMPORTANT NOTE: Always consult each drug listing in the patient's regimen for possible interactions.

Dilantin Kapseals

Interactions Index

Tolbutamide (Increased phenytoin serum levels).

No products indexed under this heading.

Trazodone Hydrochloride (Increased phenytoin serum levels). Products include:

Desyrel and Desyrel Dividose 503

Triamcinolone (Efficacy impaired by phenytoin). Products include:

Aristocort Tablets 1022

Triamcinolone Acetonide (Efficacy impaired by phenytoin). Products include:

Aristocort A 0.025% Cream 1027
Aristocort A 0.5% Cream 1031
Aristocort A 0.1% Cream 1029
Aristocort A 0.1% Ointment 1030
Azmacort Oral Inhaler 2011
Nasacort Nasal Inhaler 2024

Triamcinolone Diacetate (Efficacy impaired by phenytoin). Products include:

Aristocort Suspension (Forte Parenteral).. 1027
Aristocort Suspension (Intralesional) 1025

Triamcinolone Hexacetonide (Efficacy impaired by phenytoin). Products include:

Aristospan Suspension (Intra-articular) 1033
Aristospan Suspension (Intralesional) 1032

Trifluoperazine Hydrochloride (Increased phenytoin serum levels). Products include:

Stelazine 2514

Trimipramine Maleate (Tricyclic antidepressants may precipitate seizures in some patients; phenytoin dosage may need to be adjusted). Products include:

Surmontil Capsules................................ 2811

Valproic Acid (Increased or decreased phenytoin serum levels). Products include:

Depakene 413

Vitamin D (Efficacy impaired by phenytoin). Products include:

Caltrate PLUS .... ᴾᴰ 665
Caltrate 600 + D .... ᴾᴰ 665
Citracal Caplets + D 1780
Dical-D Tablets & Wafers 420
Drisdol .... ᴾᴰ 794
Materna Tablets 1379
Megadose 512
Zymacap Capsules .... ᴾᴰ 772

Warfarin Sodium (Efficacy impaired by phenytoin). Products include:

Coumadin 926

Food Interactions

Alcohol (Increased phenytoin serum levels with acute alcohol intake; decreased levels with chronic alcohol intake).

DILANTIN PARENTERAL

(Phenytoin Sodium) 1910

May interact with antacids containing aluminium, calcium and magnesium, oral anticoagulants, corticosteroids, oral contraceptives, salicylates, phenothiazines, estrogens, sulfonamides, tricyclic antidepressants, and certain other agents. Compounds in these categories include:

Aluminum Carbonate Gel (Interferes with absorption of phenytoin). Products include:

Basaljel 2703

Aluminum Hydroxide (Interferes with absorption of phenytoin). Products include:

ALternaGEL Liquid 1316
Maximum Strength Ascriptin .... ᴾᴰ 630
Cama Arthritis Pain Reliever .... ᴾᴰ 785

Gaviscon Extra Strength Relief Formula Antacid Tablets.................. ᴾᴰ 819
Gaviscon Extra Strength Relief Formula Liquid Antacid .... ᴾᴰ 819
Gaviscon Liquid Antacid .... ᴾᴰ 820
Gelusil Liquid & Tablets .... ᴾᴰ 855
Maalox Heartburn Relief Suspension .... ᴾᴰ 642
Maalox Heartburn Relief Tablets.... ᴾᴰ 641
Maalox Magnesia and Alumina Oral Suspension .... ᴾᴰ 642
Maalox Plus Tablets .... ᴾᴰ 643
Extra Strength Maalox Antacid Plus Antigas Liquid and Tablets ᴾᴰ 638
Tempo Soft Antacid .... ᴾᴰ 835

Aluminum Hydroxide Gel (Interferes with absorption of phenytoin). Products include:

ALternaGEL Liquid .... ᴾᴰ 659
Aludrox Oral Suspension 2695
Amphojel Suspension 2695
Amphojel Suspension without Flavor 2695
Amphojel Tablets 2695
Arthritis Pain Ascriptin .... ᴾᴰ 631
Regular Strength Ascriptin Tablets .... ᴾᴰ 629
Gaviscon Antacid Tablets.................... ᴾᴰ 819
Gaviscon-2 Antacid Tablets .... ᴾᴰ 820
Mylanta Liquid 1317
Mylanta Tablets .... ᴾᴰ 660
Mylanta Double Strength Liquid 1317
Mylanta Double Strength Tablets .. ᴾᴰ 660
Nephrox Suspension .... ᴾᴰ 655

Amitriptyline Hydrochloride (Tricyclic antidepressants may precipitate seizures in some patients; phenytoin dosage may need to be adjusted). Products include:

Elavil 2838
Endep Tablets 2174
Etrafon 2355
Limbitrol 2180
Triavil Tablets 1757

Amoxapine (Tricyclic antidepressants may precipitate seizures in some patients; phenytoin dosage may need to be adjusted). Products include:

Asendin Tablets 1369

Aspirin (Increased phenytoin levels). Products include:

Alka-Seltzer Effervescent Antacid and Pain Reliever .... ᴾᴰ 701
Alka-Seltzer Extra Strength Effervescent Antacid and Pain Reliever .... ᴾᴰ 703
Alka-Seltzer Lemon Lime Effervescent Antacid and Pain Reliever .... ᴾᴰ 703
Alka-Seltzer Plus Cold Medicine .... ᴾᴰ 705
Alka-Seltzer Plus Cold & Cough Medicine .... ᴾᴰ 708
Alka-Seltzer Plus Night-Time Cold Medicine .... ᴾᴰ 707
Alka Seltzer Plus Sinus Medicine .. ᴾᴰ 707
Arthritis Foundation Safety Coated Aspirin Tablets .... ᴾᴰ 675
Arthritis Pain Ascriptin .... ᴾᴰ 631
Maximum Strength Ascriptin .... ᴾᴰ 630
Regular Strength Ascriptin Tablets .... ᴾᴰ 629
Arthritis Strength BC Powder.......... ᴾᴰ 609
BC Cold Powder Multi-Symptom Formula (Cold-Sinus-Allergy) ...... ᴾᴰ 609
BC Cold Powder Non-Drowsy Formula (Cold-Sinus) .... ᴾᴰ 609
BC Powder .... ᴾᴰ 609
Bayer Children's Chewable Aspirin .... ᴾᴰ 711
Genuine Bayer Aspirin Tablets & Caplets .... ᴾᴰ 713
Extra Strength Bayer Arthritis Pain Regimen Formula .... ᴾᴰ 711
Extra Strength Bayer Aspirin Caplets & Tablets .... ᴾᴰ 712
Extended-Release Bayer 8-Hour Aspirin .... ᴾᴰ 712
Extra Strength Bayer Plus Aspirin Caplets .... ᴾᴰ 713
Extra Strength Bayer PM Aspirin .. ᴾᴰ 713
Bayer Enteric Aspirin .... ᴾᴰ 709
Bufferin Analgesic Tablets and Caplets .... ᴾᴰ 613
Arthritis Strength Bufferin Analgesic Caplets .... ᴾᴰ 614
Extra Strength Bufferin Analgesic Tablets .... ᴾᴰ 615

Cama Arthritis Pain Reliever .... ᴾᴰ 785
Darvon Compound-65 Pulvules 1435
Easprin 1914
Ecotrin 2455
Ecotrin Enteric Coated Aspirin Maximum Strength Tablets and Caplets .... ᴾᴰ 816
Ecotrin Enteric Coated Aspirin Regular Strength Tablets 2455
Empirin Aspirin Tablets .... ᴾᴰ 854
Empirin with Codeine Tablets........... 1093
Excedrin Extra-Strength Analgesic Tablets & Caplets 732
Fiorinal Capsules 2261
Fiorinal with Codeine Capsules 2262
Fiorinal Tablets 2261
Halfprin 1362
Healthprin Aspirin 2455
Norgesic.. 1496
Percodan Tablets 939
Percodan-Demi Tablets......................... 940
Robaxisal Tablets.................................... 2071
Soma Compound w/Codeine Tablets 2676
Soma Compound Tablets..................... 2675
St. Joseph Adult Chewable Aspirin (81 mg.) .... ᴾᴰ 808
Talwin Compound 2335
Ursinus Inlay-Tabs................................. ᴾᴰ 794
Vanquish Analgesic Caplets .... ᴾᴰ 731

Bendroflumethiazide (Increased phenytoin levels).

No products indexed under this heading.

Betamethasone Acetate (Efficacy impaired by phenytoin). Products include:

Celestone Soluspan Suspension 2347

Betamethasone Sodium Phosphate (Efficacy impaired by phenytoin). Products include:

Celestone Soluspan Suspension 2347

Carbamazepine (Decreased phenytoin levels). Products include:

Atretol Tablets 573
Tegretol Chewable Tablets 852
Tegretol Suspension.............................. 852
Tegretol Tablets 852

Chloramphenicol (Increased phenytoin levels). Products include:

Chloromycetin Ophthalmic Ointment, 1% .... ⊙ 310
Chloromycetin Ophthalmic Solution.. ⊙ 310
Chloroptic S.O.P. .... ⊙ 239
Chloroptic Sterile Ophthalmic Solution .... ⊙ 239
Elase-Chloromycetin Ointment 1040
Ophthocort .... ⊙ 311

Chloramphenicol Palmitate (Increased phenytoin levels).

No products indexed under this heading.

Chloramphenicol Sodium Succinate (Increased phenytoin levels). Products include:

Chloromycetin Sodium Succinate.... 1900

Chlordiazepoxide (Increased phenytoin levels). Products include:

Libritabs Tablets 2177
Limbitrol 2180

Chlordiazepoxide Hydrochloride (Increased phenytoin levels). Products include:

Librax Capsules 2176
Librium Capsules 2178
Librium Injectable 2179

Chlorothiazide (Increased phenytoin levels). Products include:

Aldoclor Tablets 1598
Diupres Tablets 1650
Diuril Oral 1653

Chlorothiazide Sodium (Increased phenytoin levels). Products include:

Diuril Sodium Intravenous 1652

Chlorotrianisene (Increased phenytoin levels).

No products indexed under this heading.

Chlorpromazine (Increased phenytoin levels). Products include:

Thorazine Suppositories 2523

Chlorpromazine Hydrochloride (Increased phenytoin levels). Products include:

Thorazine 2523

Chlorpropamide (Increased phenytoin levels). Products include:

Diabinese Tablets 1935

Choline Magnesium Trisalicylate (Increased phenytoin levels). Products include:

Trilisate 2000

Cimetidine (Increased phenytoin levels). Products include:

Tagamet Tablets 2516

Cimetidine Hydrochloride (Increased phenytoin levels). Products include:

Tagamet.. 2516

Clomipramine Hydrochloride (Tricyclic antidepressants may precipitate seizures in some patients; phenytoin dosage may need to be adjusted). Products include:

Anafranil Capsules 803

Cortisone Acetate (Efficacy impaired by phenytoin). Products include:

Cortone Acetate Sterile Suspension 1623
Cortone Acetate Tablets....................... 1624

Desipramine Hydrochloride (Tricyclic antidepressants may precipitate seizures in some patients; phenytoin dosage may need to be adjusted). Products include:

Norpramin Tablets 1526

Desogestrel (Increased phenytoin levels; efficacy impaired by phenytoin). Products include:

Desogen Tablets....................................... 1817
Ortho-Cept 1851

Dexamethasone (Efficacy impaired by phenytoin). Products include:

AK-Trol Ointment & Suspension .... ⊙ 205
Decadron Elixir 1633
Decadron Tablets..................................... 1635
Decaspray Topical Aerosol 1648
Dexacidin Ointment .... ⊙ 263
Maxitrol Ophthalmic Ointment and Suspension .... ⊙ 224
TobraDex Ophthalmic Suspension and Ointment.. 473

Dexamethasone Acetate (Efficacy impaired by phenytoin). Products include:

Dalalone D.P. Injectable 1011
Decadron-LA Sterile Suspension...... 1646

Dexamethasone Sodium Phosphate (Efficacy impaired by phenytoin). Products include:

Decadron Phosphate Injection 1637
Decadron Phosphate Respihaler 1642
Decadron Phosphate Sterile Ophthalmic Ointment.................................. 1641
Decadron Phosphate Sterile Ophthalmic Solution 1642
Decadron Phosphate Topical Cream.. 1644
Decadron Phosphate Turbinaire 1645
Decadron Phosphate with Xylocaine Injection, Sterile 1639
Dexacort Phosphate in Respihaler .. 458
Dexacort Phosphate in Turbinaire .. 459
NeoDecadron Sterile Ophthalmic Ointment 1712
NeoDecadron Sterile Ophthalmic Solution 1713
NeoDecadron Topical Cream 1714

Diazepam (Increased phenytoin levels). Products include:

Dizac 1809
Valium Injectable 2182
Valium Tablets 2183
Valrelease Capsules 2169

Dicumarol (Increased phenytoin levels; efficacy impaired by phenytoin).

No products indexed under this heading.

(ᴾᴰ Described in PDR For Nonprescription Drugs) (⊙ Described in PDR For Ophthalmology)

Interactions Index

Dilantin Parenteral

Dienestrol (Increased phenytoin levels; efficacy impaired by phenytoin). Products include:

Ortho Dienestrol Cream 1866

Diethylstilbestrol (Increased phenytoin levels; efficacy impaired by phenytoin). Products include:

Diethylstilbestrol Tablets 1437

Diflunisal (Increased phenytoin levels). Products include:

Dolobid Tablets....................................... 1654

Digitoxin (Efficacy impaired by phenytoin). Products include:

Crystodigin Tablets................................ 1433

Dihydroxyaluminum Sodium Carbonate (Interferes with absorption of phenytoin).

No products indexed under this heading.

Disulfiram (Increased phenytoin levels). Products include:

Antabuse Tablets.................................... 2695

Divalproex Sodium (Increased or decreased phenytoin serum levels). Products include:

Depakote Tablets.................................... 415

Doxepin Hydrochloride (Tricyclic antidepressants may precipitate seizures in some patients; phenytoin dosage may need to be adjusted). Products include:

Sinequan	2205
Zonalon Cream	1055

Doxycycline Calcium (Efficacy impaired by phenytoin). Products include:

Vibramycin Calcium Oral Suspension Syrup... 1941

Doxycycline Hyclate (Efficacy impaired by phenytoin). Products include:

Doryx Capsules	1913
Vibramycin Hyclate Capsules	1941
Vibramycin Hyclate Intravenous	2215
Vibra-Tabs Film Coated Tablets	1941

Doxycycline Monohydrate (Efficacy impaired by phenytoin). Products include:

Monodox Capsules	1805
Vibramycin Monohydrate for Oral Suspension	1941

Estradiol (Increased phenytoin levels; efficacy impaired by phenytoin). Products include:

Climara Transdermal System	645
Estrace Cream and Tablets	749
Estraderm Transdermal System	824

Estrogens, Conjugated (Increased phenytoin levels; efficacy impaired by phenytoin). Products include:

PMB 200 and PMB 400	2783
Premarin Intravenous	2787
Premarin with Methyltestosterone	2794
Premarin Tablets	2789
Premarin Vaginal Cream	2791
Premphase	2797
Prempro	2801

Estrogens, Esterified (Increased phenytoin levels; efficacy impaired by phenytoin). Products include:

ESTRATAB Tablets (0.3, 0.625, 1.25, 2.5 mg)	2536
Estratest	2539
Menest Tablets	2494

Estropipate (Increased phenytoin levels; efficacy impaired by phenytoin). Products include:

Ogen Tablets	2627
Ogen Vaginal Cream	2630
Ortho-Est	1869

Ethinyl Estradiol (Increased phenytoin levels; efficacy impaired by phenytoin). Products include:

Brevicon	2088
Demulen	2428
Desogen Tablets	1817
Levlen/Tri-Levlen	651
Lo/Ovral Tablets	2746
Lo/Ovral-28 Tablets	2751
Modicon	1872
Nordette-21 Tablets	2755
Nordette-28 Tablets	2758
Norinyl	2088
Ortho-Cept	1851
Ortho-Cyclen/Ortho-Tri-Cyclen	1858
Ortho-Novum	1872
Ortho-Cyclen/Ortho Tri-Cyclen	1858
Ovcon	760
Ovral Tablets	2770
Ovral-28 Tablets	2770
Levlen/Tri-Levlen	651
Tri-Norinyl	2164
Triphasil-21 Tablets	2814
Triphasil-28 Tablets	2819

Ethosuximide (Increased phenytoin levels). Products include:

Zarontin Capsules	1928
Zarontin Syrup	1929

Ethynodiol Diacetate (Efficacy impaired by phenytoin). Products include:

Demulen 2428

Fludrocortisone Acetate (Efficacy impaired by phenytoin). Products include:

Florinef Acetate Tablets 505

Fluoxetine Hydrochloride (Increased phenytoin levels). Products include:

Prozac Pulvules & Liquid, Oral Solution 919

Fluphenazine Decanoate (Increased phenytoin levels). Products include:

Prolixin Decanoate 509

Fluphenazine Enanthate (Increased phenytoin levels). Products include:

Prolixin Enanthate 509

Fluphenazine Hydrochloride (Increased phenytoin levels). Products include:

Prolixin 509

Furosemide (Efficacy impaired by phenytoin). Products include:

Lasix Injection, Oral Solution and Tablets 1240

Glipizide (Increased phenytoin levels). Products include:

Glucotrol Tablets	1967
Glucotrol XL Extended Release Tablets	1968

Glyburide (Increased phenytoin levels). Products include:

DiaBeta Tablets	1239
Glynase PresTab Tablets	2609
Micronase Tablets	2623

Halothane (Increased phenytoin levels). Products include:

Fluothane 2724

Hydrochlorothiazide (Increased phenytoin levels). Products include:

Aldactazide	2413
Aldoril Tablets	1604
Apresazide Capsules	808
Capozide	742
Dyazide	2479
Esidrix Tablets	821
Esmil Tablets	822
HydroDIURIL Tablets	1674
Hydropres Tablets	1675
Hyzaar Tablets	1677
Inderide Tablets	2732
Inderide LA Long Acting Capsules	2734
Lopressor HCT Tablets	832
Lotensin HCT	837
Maxzide	1380
Moduretic Tablets	1705
Oretic Tablets	443
Prinzide Tablets	1737
Ser-Ap-Es Tablets	849
Timolide Tablets	1748
Vaseretic Tablets	1765
Zestoretic	2850
Ziac	1415

Hydrocortisone (Efficacy impaired by phenytoin). Products include:

Anusol-HC Cream 2.5%	1896
Aquanil HC Lotion	1931
Bactine Hydrocortisone Anti-Itch Cream	ᴴᴰ 709

Caldecort Anti-Itch Hydrocortisone Spray .... ᴴᴰ 631

Cortaid	ᴴᴰ 836
CORTENEMA	2535
Cortisporin Ointment	1085
Cortisporin Ophthalmic Ointment Sterile	1085
Cortisporin Ophthalmic Suspension Sterile	1086
Cortisporin Otic Solution Sterile	1087
Cortisporin Otic Suspension Sterile	1088
Cortizone-5	ᴴᴰ 831
Cortizone-10	ᴴᴰ 831
Hydrocortone Tablets	1672
Hytone	907
Massengill Medicated Soft Cloth Towelettes	2458
PediOtic Suspension Sterile	1153
Preparation H Hydrocortisone 1% Cream	ᴴᴰ 872
ProctoCream-HC 2.5%	2408
VōSoL HC Otic Solution	2678

Hydrocortisone Acetate (Efficacy impaired by phenytoin). Products include:

Analpram-HC Rectal Cream 1% and 2.5%	977
Anusol HC-1 Anti-Itch Hydrocortisone Ointment	ᴴᴰ 847
Anusol-HC Suppositories	1897
Caldecort	ᴴᴰ 631
Carmol HC	924
Coly-Mycin S Otic w/Neomycin & Hydrocortisone	1906
Cortaid	ᴴᴰ 836
Cortifoam	2396
Cortisporin Cream	1084
Epifoam	2399
Hydrocortone Acetate Sterile Suspension	1669
Mantadil Cream	1135
Nupercainal Hydrocortisone 1% Cream	ᴴᴰ 645
Ophthocort	© 311
Pramosone Cream, Lotion & Ointment	978
ProctoCream-HC	2408
ProctoFoam-HC	2409
Terra-Cortril Ophthalmic Suspension	2210

Hydrocortisone Sodium Phosphate (Efficacy impaired by phenytoin). Products include:

Hydrocortone Phosphate Injection, Sterile 1670

Hydrocortisone Sodium Succinate (Efficacy impaired by phenytoin). Products include:

Solu-Cortef Sterile Powder................. 2641

Hydroflumethiazide (Increased phenytoin levels). Products include:

Diucardin Tablets................................... 2718

Imipramine Hydrochloride (Tricyclic antidepressants may precipitate seizures in some patients; phenytoin dosage may need to be adjusted). Products include:

Tofranil Ampuls	854
Tofranil Tablets	856

Imipramine Pamoate (Tricyclic antidepressants may precipitate seizures in some patients; phenytoin dosage may need to be adjusted). Products include:

Tofranil-PM Capsules........................... 857

Isoniazid (Increased phenytoin levels). Products include:

Nydrazid Injection	508
Rifamate Capsules	1530
Rifater	1532

Levonorgestrel (Efficacy impaired by phenytoin). Products include:

Levlen/Tri-Levlen	651
Nordette-21 Tablets	2755
Nordette-28 Tablets	2758
Norplant System	2759
Levlen/Tri-Levlen	651
Triphasil-21 Tablets	2814
Triphasil-28 Tablets	2819

Magaldrate (Interferes with absorption of phenytoin).

No products indexed under this heading.

Magnesium Hydroxide (Interferes with absorption of phenytoin). Products include:

Aludrox Oral Suspension	2695
Arthritis Pain Ascriptin	ᴴᴰ 631
Maximum Strength Ascriptin	ᴴᴰ 630
Regular Strength Ascriptin Tablets	ᴴᴰ 629
Di-Gel Antacid/Anti-Gas	ᴴᴰ 801
Gelusil Liquid & Tablets	ᴴᴰ 855
Maalox Magnesia and Alumina Oral Suspension	ᴴᴰ 642
Maalox Plus Tablets	ᴴᴰ 643
Extra Strength Maalox Antacid Plus Antigas Liquid and Tablets	ᴴᴰ 638
Mylanta Calcium Carbonate and Magnesium Hydroxide Tablets	1318
Mylanta Liquid	1317
Mylanta Tablets	ᴴᴰ 660
Mylanta Double Strength Liquid	1317
Mylanta Double Strength Tablets	ᴴᴰ 660
Phillips' Milk of Magnesia Liquid	ᴴᴰ 729
Rolaids Tablets	ᴴᴰ 843
Tempo Soft Antacid	ᴴᴰ 835

Magnesium Oxide (Interferes with absorption of phenytoin). Products include:

Beelith Tablets	639
Bufferin Analgesic Tablets and Caplets	ᴴᴰ 613
Caltrate PLUS	ᴴᴰ 665
Cama Arthritis Pain Reliever	ᴴᴰ 785
Mag-Ox 400	668
Uro-Mag	668

Magnesium Salicylate (Increased phenytoin levels). Products include:

Backache Caplets	ᴴᴰ 613
Bayer Select Backache Pain Relief Formula	ᴴᴰ 715
Doan's Extra-Strength Analgesic	ᴴᴰ 633
Extra Strength Doan's P.M.	ᴴᴰ 633
Doan's Regular Strength Analgesic	ᴴᴰ 634
Mobigesic Tablets	ᴴᴰ 602

Maprotiline Hydrochloride (Tricyclic antidepressants may precipitate seizures in some patients; phenytoin dosage may need to be adjusted). Products include:

Ludiomil Tablets.................................... 843

Mesoridazine Besylate (Increased phenytoin levels). Products include:

Serentil 684

Mestranol (Efficacy impaired by phenytoin). Products include:

Norinyl	2088
Ortho-Novum	1872

Methotrimeprazine (Increased phenytoin levels). Products include:

Levoprome 1274

Methyclothiazide (Increased phenytoin levels). Products include:

Enduron Tablets...................................... 420

Methylphenidate Hydrochloride (Increased phenytoin levels). Products include:

Ritalin 848

Methylprednisolone Acetate (Efficacy impaired by phenytoin). Products include:

Depo-Medrol Single-Dose Vial	2600
Depo-Medrol Sterile Aqueous Suspension	2597

Methylprednisolone Sodium Succinate (Efficacy impaired by phenytoin). Products include:

Solu-Medrol Sterile Powder 2643

Molindone Hydrochloride (Moban brand interferes with absorption of phenytoin). Products include:

Moban Tablets and Concentrate 1048

Norethindrone (Efficacy impaired by phenytoin). Products include:

Brevicon	2088
Micronor Tablets	1872
Modicon	1872
Norinyl	2088
Nor-Q D Tablets	2135
Ortho-Novum	1872
Ovcon	760
Tri-Norinyl	2164

IMPORTANT NOTE: Always consult each drug listing in the patient's regimen for possible interactions.

Norethynodrel (Efficacy impaired by phenytoin).
No products indexed under this heading.

Norgestimate (Increased phenytoin levels; efficacy impaired by phenytoin). Products include:
Ortho-Cyclen/Ortho-Tri-Cyclen 1858
Ortho-Cyclen/Ortho Tri-Cyclen 1858

Norgestrel (Efficacy impaired by phenytoin). Products include:
Lo/Ovral Tablets 2746
Lo/Ovral-28 Tablets 2751
Ovral Tablets 2770
Ovral-28 Tablets 2770
Ovrette Tablets 2771

Nortriptyline Hydrochloride (Tricyclic antidepressants may precipitate seizures in some patients; phenytoin dosage may need to be adjusted). Products include:
Pamelor 2280

Perphenazine (Increased phenytoin levels). Products include:
Etrafon 2355
Triavil Tablets 1757
Trilafon 2389

Phenobarbital (Increased or decreased phenytoin serum levels). Products include:
Arco-Lase Plus Tablets 512
Bellergal-S Tablets 2250
Donnatal 2060
Donnatal Extentabs 2061
Donnatal Tablets 2060
Phenobarbital Elixir and Tablets 1469
Quadrinal Tablets 1350

Phenylbutazone (Increased phenytoin levels).
No products indexed under this heading.

Polyestradiol Phosphate (Increased phenytoin levels; efficacy impaired by phenytoin).
No products indexed under this heading.

Polythiazide (Increased phenytoin levels). Products include:
Minizide Capsules 1938

Prednisolone Acetate (Efficacy impaired by phenytoin). Products include:
AK-CIDE .... ⊙ 202
AK-CIDE Ointment .... ⊙ 202
Blephamide Liquifilm Sterile Ophthalmic Suspension 476
Blephamide Ointment .... ⊙ 237
Econopred & Econopred Plus Ophthalmic Suspensions .... ⊙ 217
Poly-Pred Liquifilm .... ⊙ 248
Pred Forte .... ⊙ 250
Pred Mild .... ⊙ 253
Pred-G Liquifilm Sterile Ophthalmic Suspension .... ⊙ 251
Pred-G S.O.P. Sterile Ophthalmic Ointment .... ⊙ 252
Vasocidin Ointment .... ⊙ 268

Prednisolone Sodium Phosphate (Efficacy impaired by phenytoin). Products include:
AK-Pred .... ⊙ 204
Hydeltrasol Injection, Sterile 1665
Inflamase .... ⊙ 265
Pediapred Oral Liquid 995
Vasocidin Ophthalmic Solution .... ⊙ 270

Prednisolone Tebutate (Efficacy impaired by phenytoin). Products include:
Hydeltra-T.B.A. Sterile Suspension 1667

Prednisone (Efficacy impaired by phenytoin). Products include:
Deltasone Tablets 2595

Prochlorperazine (Increased phenytoin levels). Products include:
Compazine 2470

Promethazine Hydrochloride (Increased phenytoin levels). Products include:
Mepergan Injection 2753
Phenergan with Codeine 2777
Phenergan with Dextromethorphan 2778
Phenergan Injection 2773
Phenergan Suppositories 2775
Phenergan Syrup 2774
Phenergan Tablets 2775
Phenergan VC 2779
Phenergan VC with Codeine 2781

Protriptyline Hydrochloride (Tricyclic antidepressants may precipitate seizures in some patients; phenytoin dosage may need to be adjusted). Products include:
Vivactil Tablets 1774

Quinestrol (Increased phenytoin levels).
No products indexed under this heading.

Quinidine Gluconate (Efficacy impaired by phenytoin). Products include:
Quinaglute Dura-Tabs Tablets 649

Quinidine Polygalacturonate (Efficacy impaired by phenytoin).
No products indexed under this heading.

Quinidine Sulfate (Efficacy impaired by phenytoin). Products include:
Quinidex Extentabs 2067

Reserpine (Decreased phenytoin levels). Products include:
Diupres Tablets 1650
Hydropres Tablets 1675
Ser-Ap-Es Tablets 849

Rifampin (Efficacy impaired by phenytoin). Products include:
Rifadin 1528
Rifamate Capsules 1530
Rifater 1532
Rimactane Capsules 847

Salsalate (Increased phenytoin levels). Products include:
Mono-Gesic Tablets 792
Salflex Tablets 786

Sodium Valproate (Increased or decreased phenytoin levels).

Sulfacytine (Increased phenytoin levels).

Sulfamethizole (Increased phenytoin levels). Products include:
Urobiotic-250 Capsules 2214

Sulfamethoxazole (Increased phenytoin levels). Products include:
Azo Gantanol Tablets 2080
Bactrim DS Tablets 2084
Bactrim I.V. Infusion 2082
Bactrim 2084
Gantanol Tablets 2119
Septra 1174
Septra I.V. Infusion 1169
Septra I.V. Infusion ADD-Vantage Vials 1171
Septra 1174

Sulfasalazine (Increased phenytoin levels). Products include:
Azulfidine 1949

Sulfinpyrazone (Increased phenytoin levels). Products include:
Anturane 807

Sulfisoxazole (Increased phenytoin levels). Products include:
Azo Gantrisin Tablets 2081
Gantrisin Tablets 2120

Sulfisoxazole Diolamine (Increased phenytoin levels).
No products indexed under this heading.

Thioridazine Hydrochloride (Increased phenytoin levels). Products include:
Mellaril 2269

Tolazamide (Increased phenytoin levels).
No products indexed under this heading.

Tolbutamide (Increased phenytoin levels).
No products indexed under this heading.

Trazodone Hydrochloride (Increased phenytoin levels). Products include:
Desyrel and Desyrel Dividose 503

Triamcinolone (Efficacy impaired by phenytoin). Products include:
Aristocort Tablets 1022

Triamcinolone Acetonide (Efficacy impaired by phenytoin). Products include:
Aristocort A 0.025% Cream 1027
Aristocort A 0.5% Cream 1031
Aristocort A 0.1% Cream 1029
Aristocort A 0.1% Ointment 1030
Azmacort Oral Inhaler 2011
Nasacort Nasal Inhaler 2024

Triamcinolone Diacetate (Efficacy impaired by phenytoin). Products include:
Aristocort Suspension (Forte Parenteral) 1027
Aristocort Suspension (Intralesional) 1025

Triamcinolone Hexacetonide (Efficacy impaired by phenytoin). Products include:
Aristospan Suspension (Intra-articular) 1033
Aristospan Suspension (Intralesional) 1032

Trifluoperazine Hydrochloride (Increased phenytoin levels). Products include:
Stelazine 2514

Trimipramine Maleate (Tricyclic antidepressants may precipitate seizures in some patients; phenytoin dosage may need to be adjusted). Products include:
Surmontil Capsules 2811

Valproic Acid (Increased or decreased phenytoin serum levels). Products include:
Depakene 413

Vitamin D (Efficacy impaired by phenytoin). Products include:
Caltrate PLUS .... ▣ 665
Caltrate 600 + D .... ▣ 665
Citracal Caplets + D 1780
Dical-D Tablets & Wafers 420
Drisdol .... ▣ 794
Materna Tablets 1379
Megadose 512
Zymacap Capsules .... ▣ 772

Warfarin Sodium (Efficacy impaired by phenytoin). Products include:
Coumadin 926

Food Interactions

Alcohol (Increased phenytoin levels with acute alcohol intake; decreased levels with chronic alcohol intake).

DILANTIN-125 SUSPENSION

(Phenytoin) 1911
May interact with salicylates, phenothiazines, estrogens, sulfonamides, corticosteroids, oral anticoagulants, histamine h2-receptor antagonists, succinimides, tricyclic antidepressants, xanthine bronchodilators, oral contraceptives, and certain other agents. Compounds in these categories include:

Aminophylline (Efficacy impaired by phenytoin).
No products indexed under this heading.

Amiodarone Hydrochloride (Increased phenytoin serum levels). Products include:
Cordarone Intravenous 2715
Cordarone Tablets 2712

Amitriptyline Hydrochloride (Tricyclic antidepressants may precipitate seizures in some patients; phenytoin dosage may need to be adjusted). Products include:
Elavil 2838
Endep Tablets 2174
Etrafon 2355
Limbitrol 2180
Triavil Tablets 1757

Amoxapine (Tricyclic antidepressants may precipitate seizures in some patients; phenytoin dosage may need to be adjusted). Products include:
Asendin Tablets 1369

Aspirin (Increased phenytoin serum levels). Products include:
Alka-Seltzer Effervescent Antacid and Pain Reliever .... ▣ 701
Alka-Seltzer Extra Strength Effervescent Antacid and Pain Reliever .... ▣ 703
Alka-Seltzer Lemon Lime Effervescent Antacid and Pain Reliever .... ▣ 703
Alka-Seltzer Plus Cold Medicine .... ▣ 705
Alka-Seltzer Plus Cold & Cough Medicine .... ▣ 708
Alka-Seltzer Plus Night-Time Cold Medicine .... ▣ 707
Alka Seltzer Plus Sinus Medicine .... ▣ 707
Arthritis Foundation Safety Coated Aspirin Tablets .... ▣ 675
Arthritis Pain Ascriptin .... ▣ 631
Maximum Strength Ascriptin .... ▣ 630
Regular Strength Ascriptin Tablets .... ▣ 629
Arthritis Strength BC Powder .... ▣ 609
BC Cold Powder Multi-Symptom Formula (Cold-Sinus-Allergy) .... ▣ 609
BC Cold Powder Non-Drowsy Formula (Cold-Sinus) .... ▣ 609
BC Powder .... ▣ 609
Bayer Children's Chewable Aspirin .... ▣ 711
Genuine Bayer Aspirin Tablets & Caplets .... ▣ 713
Extra Strength Bayer Arthritis Pain Regimen Formula .... ▣ 711
Extra Strength Bayer Aspirin Caplets & Tablets .... ▣ 712
Extended-Release Bayer 8-Hour Aspirin .... ▣ 712
Extra Strength Bayer Plus Aspirin Caplets .... ▣ 713
Extra Strength Bayer PM Aspirin .... ▣ 713
Bayer Enteric Aspirin .... ▣ 709
Bufferin Analgesic Tablets and Caplets .... ▣ 613
Arthritis Strength Bufferin Analgesic Caplets .... ▣ 614
Extra Strength Bufferin Analgesic Tablets .... ▣ 615
Cama Arthritis Pain Reliever .... ▣ 785
Darvon Compound-65 Pulvules 1435
Easprin 1914
Ecotrin 2455
Ecotrin Enteric Coated Aspirin Maximum Strength Tablets and Caplets .... ▣ 816
Ecotrin Enteric Coated Aspirin Regular Strength Tablets 2455
Empirin Aspirin Tablets .... ▣ 854
Empirin with Codeine Tablets 1093
Excedrin Extra-Strength Analgesic Tablets & Caplets 732
Fiorinal Capsules 2261
Fiorinal with Codeine Capsules 2262
Fiorinal Tablets 2261
Halfprin 1362
Healthprin Aspirin 2455
Norgesic 1496
Percodan Tablets 939
Percodan-Demi Tablets 940
Robaxisal Tablets 2071
Soma Compound w/Codeine Tablets 2676
Soma Compound Tablets 2675
St. Joseph Adult Chewable Aspirin (81 mg.) .... ▣ 808
Talwin Compound 2335
Ursinus Inlay-Tabs .... ▣ 794
Vanquish Analgesic Caplets .... ▣ 731

Bendroflumethiazide (Increased phenytoin serum levels).
No products indexed under this heading.

(▣ Described in PDR For Nonprescription Drugs) (⊙ Described in PDR For Ophthalmology)

Betamethasone Acetate (Efficacy impaired by phenytoin). Products include:
- Celestone Soluspan Suspension 2347

Betamethasone Sodium Phosphate (Efficacy impaired by phenytoin). Products include:
- Celestone Soluspan Suspension 2347

Calcium Carbonate (Ingestion times of phenytoin and antacids containing calcium should be staggered to prevent absorption problems). Products include:
- Alka-Mints Chewable Antacid ...... ▣ 701
- Arthritis Pain Ascriptin ...... ▣ 631
- Maximum Strength Ascriptin ...... ▣ 630
- Regular Strength Ascriptin Tablets ...... ▣ 629
- Extra Strength Bayer Plus Aspirin Caplets ...... ▣ 713
- Bufferin Analgesic Tablets and Caplets ...... ▣ 613
- Calci-Chew Tablets 2004
- Calci-Mix Capsules 2004
- Caltrate 600 ...... ▣ 665
- Caltrate PLUS ...... ▣ 665
- Caltrate 600 + D ...... ▣ 665
- Centrum Singles Calcium ...... ▣ 669
- Chooz Antacid Gum ...... ▣ 799
- Di-Gel Antacid/Anti-Gas ...... ▣ 801
- Gerimed Tablets 982
- Maalox Antacid Caplets ...... ▣ 638
- Marblen ...... ▣ 655
- Materna Tablets 1379
- Mylanta Calcium Carbonate and Magnesium Hydroxide Tablets 1318
- Mylanta Gelcaps Antacid ...... ▣ 662
- Mylanta Soothing Lozenges 1319
- Nephro-Calci Tablets 2004
- Rolaids Tablets ...... ▣ 843
- Rolaids (Calcium Rich/Sodium Free) Tablets ...... ▣ 843
- Tempo Soft Antacid ...... ▣ 835
- Titralac ...... ▣ 672
- Titralac Plus ...... ▣ 672
- Tums Antacid Tablets ...... ▣ 827
- Tums Anti-gas/Antacid Formula Tablets, Assorted Fruit ...... ▣ 827
- Tums E-X Antacid Tablets ...... ▣ 827
- Tums 500 Calcium Supplement ...... ▣ 828
- Tums ULTRA Antacid Tablets ...... ▣ 827
- TYLENOL, Extra Strength, Headache Plus Pain Reliever with Antacid Caplets 1559

Calcium Carbonate, Precipitated (Ingestion times of phenytoin and antacids containing calcium should be staggered to prevent absorption problems).

Carbamazepine (Decreased phenytoin serum levels). Products include:
- Atretol Tablets 573
- Tegretol Chewable Tablets 852
- Tegretol Suspension 852
- Tegretol Tablets 852

Chloramphenicol (Increased phenytoin serum levels). Products include:
- Chloromycetin Ophthalmic Ointment, 1% ...... ⊙ 310
- Chloromycetin Ophthalmic Solution ...... ⊙ 310
- Chloroptic S.O.P. ...... ⊙ 239
- Chloroptic Sterile Ophthalmic Solution ...... ⊙ 239
- Elase-Chloromycetin Ointment 1040
- Ophthocort ...... ⊙ 311

Chloramphenicol Palmitate (Increased phenytoin serum levels).
- No products indexed under this heading.

Chloramphenicol Sodium Succinate (Increased phenytoin serum levels). Products include:
- Chloromycetin Sodium Succinate 1900

Chlordiazepoxide (Increased phenytoin serum levels). Products include:
- Libritabs Tablets 2177
- Limbitrol 2180

Chlordiazepoxide Hydrochloride (Increased phenytoin serum levels). Products include:
- Librax Capsules 2176
- Librium Capsules 2178
- Librium Injectable 2179

Chlorothiazide (Increased phenytoin serum levels). Products include:
- Aldoclor Tablets 1598
- Diupres Tablets 1650
- Diuril Oral 1653

Chlorothiazide Sodium (Increased phenytoin serum levels). Products include:
- Diuril Sodium Intravenous 1652

Chlorotrianisene (Increased phenytoin serum levels; efficacy impaired by phenytoin).
- No products indexed under this heading.

Chlorpromazine (Increased phenytoin serum levels). Products include:
- Thorazine Suppositories 2523

Chlorpromazine Hydrochloride (Increased phenytoin serum levels). Products include:
- Thorazine 2523

Chlorpropamide (Increased phenytoin serum levels). Products include:
- Diabinese Tablets 1935

Choline Magnesium Trisalicylate (Increased phenytoin serum levels). Products include:
- Trilisate 2000

Cimetidine (Increased phenytoin serum levels). Products include:
- Tagamet Tablets 2516

Cimetidine Hydrochloride (Increased phenytoin serum levels). Products include:
- Tagamet 2516

Clomipramine Hydrochloride (Tricyclic antidepressants may precipitate seizures in some patients; phenytoin dosage may need to be adjusted). Products include:
- Anafranil Capsules 803

Cortisone Acetate (Efficacy impaired by phenytoin). Products include:
- Cortone Acetate Sterile Suspension 1623
- Cortone Acetate Tablets 1624

Desipramine Hydrochloride (Tricyclic antidepressants may precipitate seizures in some patients; phenytoin dosage may need to be adjusted). Products include:
- Norpramin Tablets 1526

Desogestrel (Increased phenytoin serum levels; efficacy impaired by phenytoin). Products include:
- Desogen Tablets 1817
- Ortho-Cept 1851

Dexamethasone (Efficacy impaired by phenytoin). Products include:
- AK-Trol Ointment & Suspension ...... ⊙ 205
- Decadron Elixir 1633
- Decadron Tablets 1635
- Decaspray Topical Aerosol 1648
- Dexacidin Ointment ...... ⊙ 263
- Maxitrol Ophthalmic Ointment and Suspension ...... ⊙ 224
- TobraDex Ophthalmic Suspension and Ointment 473

Dexamethasone Acetate (Efficacy impaired by phenytoin). Products include:
- Dalalone D.P. Injectable 1011
- Decadron-LA Sterile Suspension 1646

Dexamethasone Sodium Phosphate (Efficacy impaired by phenytoin). Products include:
- Decadron Phosphate Injection 1637
- Decadron Phosphate Respihaler 1642
- Decadron Phosphate Sterile Ophthalmic Ointment 1641
- Decadron Phosphate Sterile Ophthalmic Solution 1642
- Decadron Phosphate Topical Cream 1644
- Decadron Phosphate Turbinaire 1645
- Decadron Phosphate with Xylocaine Injection, Sterile 1639
- Dexacort Phosphate in Respihaler .. 458
- Dexacort Phosphate in Turbinaire .. 459
- NeoDecadron Sterile Ophthalmic Ointment 1712
- NeoDecadron Sterile Ophthalmic Solution 1713
- NeoDecadron Topical Cream 1714

Diazepam (Increased phenytoin serum levels). Products include:
- Dizac 1809
- Valium Injectable 2182
- Valium Tablets 2183
- Valrelease Capsules 2169

Dicumarol (Efficacy impaired by phenytoin; increases phenytoin serum levels).
- No products indexed under this heading.

Dienestrol (Increased phenytoin serum levels; efficacy impaired by phenytoin). Products include:
- Ortho Dienestrol Cream 1866

Diethylstilbestrol (Increased phenytoin serum levels; efficacy impaired by phenytoin). Products include:
- Diethylstilbestrol Tablets 1437

Diflunisal (Increased phenytoin serum levels). Products include:
- Dolobid Tablets 1654

Digitoxin (Efficacy impaired by phenytoin). Products include:
- Crystodigin Tablets 1433

Disulfiram (Increased phenytoin serum levels). Products include:
- Antabuse Tablets 2695

Divalproex Sodium (Increased or decreased phenytoin levels). Products include:
- Depakote Tablets 415

Doxepin Hydrochloride (Tricyclic antidepressants may precipitate seizures in some patients; phenytoin dosage may need to be adjusted). Products include:
- Sinequan 2205
- Zonalon Cream 1055

Doxycycline Calcium (Efficacy impaired by phenytoin). Products include:
- Vibramycin Calcium Oral Suspension Syrup 1941

Doxycycline Hyclate (Efficacy impaired by phenytoin). Products include:
- Doryx Capsules 1913
- Vibramycin Hyclate Capsules 1941
- Vibramycin Hyclate Intravenous 2215
- Vibra-Tabs Film Coated Tablets 1941

Doxycycline Monohydrate (Efficacy impaired by phenytoin). Products include:
- Monodox Capsules 1805
- Vibramycin Monohydrate for Oral Suspension 1941

Dyphylline (Efficacy impaired by phenytoin). Products include:
- Lufyllin & Lufyllin-400 Tablets 2670
- Lufyllin-GG Elixir & Tablets 2671

Estradiol (Increased phenytoin serum levels; efficacy impaired by phenytoin). Products include:
- Climara Transdermal System 645
- Estrace Cream and Tablets 749
- Estraderm Transdermal System 824

Estrogens, Conjugated (Increased phenytoin serum levels; efficacy impaired by phenytoin). Products include:
- PMB 200 and PMB 400 2783
- Premarin Intravenous 2787
- Premarin with Methyltestosterone .. 2794
- Premarin Tablets 2789
- Premarin Vaginal Cream 2791
- Premphase 2797
- Prempro 2801

Estrogens, Esterified (Increased phenytoin serum levels; efficacy impaired by phenytoin). Products include:
- ESTRATAB Tablets (0.3, 0.625, 1.25, 2.5 mg) 2536
- Estratest 2539
- Menest Tablets 2494

Estropipate (Increased phenytoin serum levels; efficacy impaired by phenytoin). Products include:
- Ogen Tablets 2627
- Ogen Vaginal Cream 2630
- Ortho-Est 1869

Ethinyl Estradiol (Increased phenytoin serum levels; efficacy impaired by phenytoin). Products include:
- Brevicon 2088
- Demulen 2428
- Desogen Tablets 1817
- Levlen/Tri-Levlen 651
- Lo/Ovral Tablets 2746
- Lo/Ovral-28 Tablets 2751
- Modicon 1872
- Nordette-21 Tablets 2755
- Nordette-28 Tablets 2758
- Norinyl 2088
- Ortho-Cept 1851
- Ortho-Cyclen/Ortho-Tri-Cyclen 1858
- Ortho-Novum 1872
- Ortho-Cyclen/Ortho Tri-Cyclen 1858
- Ovcon 760
- Ovral Tablets 2770
- Ovral-28 Tablets 2770
- Levlen/Tri-Levlen 651
- Tri-Norinyl 2164
- Triphasil-21 Tablets 2814
- Triphasil-28 Tablets 2819

Ethosuximide (Increased phenytoin serum levels). Products include:
- Zarontin Capsules 1928
- Zarontin Syrup 1929

Ethynodiol Diacetate (Efficacy impaired by phenytoin). Products include:
- Demulen 2428

Famotidine (Increased phenytoin serum levels). Products include:
- Pepcid AC 1319
- Pepcid Injection 1722
- Pepcid 1720

Fludrocortisone Acetate (Efficacy impaired by phenytoin). Products include:
- Florinef Acetate Tablets 505

Fluoxetine Hydrochloride (Increased phenytoin serum levels). Products include:
- Prozac Pulvules & Liquid, Oral Solution 919

Fluphenazine Decanoate (Increased phenytoin serum levels). Products include:
- Prolixin Decanoate 509

Fluphenazine Enanthate (Increased phenytoin serum levels). Products include:
- Prolixin Enanthate 509

Fluphenazine Hydrochloride (Increased phenytoin serum levels). Products include:
- Prolixin 509

Furosemide (Efficacy impaired by phenytoin). Products include:
- Lasix Injection, Oral Solution and Tablets 1240

Glipizide (Increased phenytoin serum levels). Products include:
- Glucotrol Tablets 1967
- Glucotrol XL Extended Release Tablets 1968

Glyburide (Increased phenytoin serum levels). Products include:
- DiaBeta Tablets 1239
- Glynase PresTab Tablets 2609
- Micronase Tablets 2623

IMPORTANT NOTE: Always consult each drug listing in the patient's regimen for possible interactions.

Dilantin Suspension

Interactions Index

Halothane (Increased phenytoin serum levels). Products include:

Fluothane 2724

Hydrochlorothiazide (Increased phenytoin serum levels). Products include:

Aldactazide... 2413
Aldoril Tablets... 1604
Apresazide Capsules 808
Capozide 742
Dyazide 2479
Esidrix Tablets 821
Esimil Tablets 822
HydroDIURIL Tablets.................................. 1674
Hydropres Tablets...................................... 1675
Hyzaar Tablets.. 1677
Inderide Tablets 2732
Inderide LA Long Acting Capsules .. 2734
Lopressor HCT Tablets 832
Lotensin HCT.. 837
Maxzide 1380
Moduretic Tablets 1705
Oretic Tablets 443
Prinzide Tablets 1737
Ser-Ap-Es Tablets 849
Timolide Tablets.. 1748
Vaseretic Tablets 1765
Zestoretic 2850
Ziac 1415

Hydrocortisone (Efficacy impaired by phenytoin). Products include:

Anusol-HC Cream 2.5% 1896
Aquanil HC Lotion 1931
Bactine Hydrocortisone Anti-Itch Cream.. ᴹᴰ 709
Caldecort Anti-Itch Hydrocortisone Spray .... ᴹᴰ 631
Cortaid .... ᴹᴰ 836
CORTENEMA... 2535
Cortisporin Ointment 1085
Cortisporin Ophthalmic Ointment Sterile 1085
Cortisporin Ophthalmic Suspension Sterile 1086
Cortisporin Otic Solution Sterile 1087
Cortisporin Otic Suspension Sterile 1088
Cortizone-5 .... ᴹᴰ 831
Cortizone-10 .... ᴹᴰ 831
Hydrocortone Tablets 1672
Hytone 907
Massengill Medicated Soft Cloth Towelettes... 2458
PediOtic Suspension Sterile 1153
Preparation H Hydrocortisone 1% Cream .... ᴹᴰ 872
ProctoCream-HC 2.5% 2408
VōSoL HC Otic Solution............................ 2678

Hydrocortisone Acetate (Efficacy impaired by phenytoin). Products include:

Analpram-HC Rectal Cream 1% and 2.5% 977
Anusol HC-1 Anti-Itch Hydrocortisone Ointment..................................... ᴹᴰ 847
Anusol-HC Suppositories 1897
Caldecort.. ᴹᴰ 631
Carmol HC 924
Coly-Mycin S Otic w/Neomycin & Hydrocortisone 1906
Cortaid .... ᴹᴰ 836
Cortifoam 2396
Cortisporin Cream..................................... 1084
Epifoam 2399
Hydrocortone Acetate Sterile Suspension... 1669
Mantadil Cream 1135
Nupercainal Hydrocortisone 1% Cream.. ᴹᴰ 645
Ophthocort .... ◎ 311
Pramosone Cream, Lotion & Ointment 978
ProctoCream-HC 2408
ProctoFoam-HC 2409
Terra-Cortril Ophthalmic Suspension 2210

Hydrocortisone Sodium Phosphate (Efficacy impaired by phenytoin). Products include:

Hydrocortone Phosphate Injection, Sterile 1670

Hydrocortisone Sodium Succinate (Efficacy impaired by phenytoin). Products include:

Solu-Cortef Sterile Powder.................. 2641

Hydroflumethiazide (Increased phenytoin serum levels). Products include:

Diucardin Tablets...................................... 2718

Imipramine Hydrochloride (Tricyclic antidepressants may precipitate seizures in some patients; phenytoin dosage may need to be adjusted). Products include:

Tofranil Ampuls 854
Tofranil Tablets 856

Imipramine Pamoate (Tricyclic antidepressants may precipitate seizures in some patients; phenytoin dosage may need to be adjusted). Products include:

Tofranil-PM Capsules................................ 857

Isoniazid (Increased phenytoin serum levels). Products include:

Nydrazid Injection 508
Rifamate Capsules 1530
Rifater.. 1532

Levonorgestrel (Efficacy impaired by phenytoin). Products include:

Levlen/Tri-Levlen...................................... 651
Nordette-21 Tablets................................... 2755
Nordette-28 Tablets................................... 2758
Norplant System 2759
Levlen/Tri-Levlen...................................... 651
Triphasil-21 Tablets................................... 2814
Triphasil-28 Tablets................................... 2819

Magnesium Salicylate (Increased phenytoin serum levels). Products include:

Backache Caplets .... ᴹᴰ 613
Bayer Select Backache Pain Relief Formula .... ᴹᴰ 715
Doan's Extra-Strength Analgesic.... ᴹᴰ 633
Extra Strength Doan's P.M. .... ᴹᴰ 633
Doan's Regular Strength Analgesic.. ᴹᴰ 634
Mobigesic Tablets .... ᴹᴰ 602

Maprotiline Hydrochloride (Tricyclic antidepressants may precipitate seizures in some patients; phenytoin dosage may need to be adjusted). Products include:

Ludiomil Tablets....................................... 843

Mesoridazine Besylate (Increased phenytoin serum levels). Products include:

Serentil.. 684

Mestranol (Efficacy impaired by phenytoin). Products include:

Norinyl 2088
Ortho-Novum.. 1872

Methotrimeprazine (Increased phenytoin serum levels). Products include:

Levoprome 1274

Methsuximide (Increased phenytoin serum levels). Products include:

Celontin Kapseals 1899

Methylclothiazide (Increased phenytoin serum levels). Products include:

Enduron Tablets.. 420

Methylphenidate Hydrochloride (Increased phenytoin serum levels). Products include:

Ritalin 848

Methylprednisolone Acetate (Efficacy impaired by phenytoin). Products include:

Depo-Medrol Single-Dose Vial 2600
Depo-Medrol Sterile Aqueous Suspension.. 2597

Methylprednisolone Sodium Succinate (Efficacy impaired by phenytoin). Products include:

Solu-Medrol Sterile Powder 2643

Molindone Hydrochloride (Interferes with absorption of phenytoin). Products include:

Moban Tablets and Concentrate...... 1048

Nizatidine (Increased phenytoin serum levels). Products include:

Axid Pulvules 1427

Norethindrone (Efficacy impaired by phenytoin). Products include:

Brevicon... 2088
Micronor Tablets 1872
Modicon 1872
Norinyl 2088
Nor-Q D Tablets 2135
Ortho-Novum.. 1872
Ovcon 760
Tri-Norinyl.. 2164

Norethynodrel (Efficacy impaired by phenytoin).

No products indexed under this heading.

Norgestimate (Increased phenytoin serum levels; efficacy impaired by phenytoin). Products include:

Ortho-Cyclen/Ortho-Tri-Cyclen 1858
Ortho-Cyclen/Ortho Tri-Cyclen 1858

Norgestrel (Efficacy impaired by phenytoin). Products include:

Lo/Ovral Tablets 2746
Lo/Ovral-28 Tablets................................... 2751
Ovral Tablets... 2770
Ovral-28 Tablets 2770
Ovrette Tablets... 2771

Nortriptyline Hydrochloride (Tricyclic antidepressants may precipitate seizures in some patients; phenytoin dosage may need to be adjusted). Products include:

Pamelor 2280

Perphenazine (Increased phenytoin serum levels). Products include:

Etrafon 2355
Triavil Tablets 1757
Trilafon... 2389

Phenobarbital (Increased or decreased phenytoin levels). Products include:

Arco-Lase Plus Tablets 512
Bellergal-S Tablets 2250
Donnatal 2060
Donnatal Extentabs................................... 2061
Donnatal Tablets 2060
Phenobarbital Elixir and Tablets 1469
Quadrinal Tablets 1350

Phensuximide (Increased phenytoin serum levels). Products include:

Milontin Kapseals...................................... 1920

Phenylbutazone (Increased phenytoin serum levels).

No products indexed under this heading.

Polyestradiol Phosphate (Increased phenytoin serum levels; efficacy impaired by phenytoin).

No products indexed under this heading.

Polythiazide (Increased phenytoin serum levels). Products include:

Minizide Capsules 1938

Prednisolone Acetate (Efficacy impaired by phenytoin). Products include:

AK-CIDE .... ◎ 202
AK-CIDE Ointment.................................... ◎ 202
Blephamide Liquifilm Sterile Ophthalmic Suspension.............................. 476
Blephamide Ointment .... ◎ 237
Econopred & Econopred Plus Ophthalmic Suspensions .... ◎ 217
Poly-Pred Liquifilm .... ◎ 248
Pred Forte.. ◎ 250
Pred Mild.. ◎ 253
Pred-G Liquifilm Sterile Ophthalmic Suspension .... ◎ 251
Pred-G S.O.P. Sterile Ophthalmic Ointment .... ◎ 252
Vasocidin Ointment .... ◎ 268

Prednisolone Sodium Phosphate (Efficacy impaired by phenytoin). Products include:

AK-Pred .... ◎ 204
Hydeltrasol Injection, Sterile.............. 1665
Inflamase.. ◎ 265
Pediapred Oral Liquid 995
Vasocidin Ophthalmic Solution ...... ◎ 270

Prednisolone Tebutate (Efficacy impaired by phenytoin). Products include:

Hydeltra-T.B.A. Sterile Suspension 1667

Prednisone (Efficacy impaired by phenytoin). Products include:

Deltasone Tablets 2595

Prochlorperazine (Increased phenytoin levels). Products include:

Compazine 2470

Promethazine Hydrochloride (Increased phenytoin serum levels). Products include:

Mepergan Injection 2753
Phenergan with Codeine............................ 2777
Phenergan with Dextromethorphan 2778
Phenergan Injection 2773
Phenergan Suppositories 2775
Phenergan Syrup 2774
Phenergan Tablets 2775
Phenergan VC 2779
Phenergan VC with Codeine 2781

Protriptyline Hydrochloride (Tricyclic antidepressants may precipitate seizures in some patients; phenytoin dosage may need to be adjusted). Products include:

Vivactil Tablets 1774

Quinestrol (Increased phenytoin serum levels; efficacy impaired by phenytoin).

No products indexed under this heading.

Quinidine Gluconate (Efficacy impaired by phenytoin). Products include:

Quinaglute Dura-Tabs Tablets 649

Quinidine Polygalacturonate (Efficacy impaired by phenytoin).

No products indexed under this heading.

Quinidine Sulfate (Efficacy impaired by phenytoin). Products include:

Quinidex Extentabs................................... 2067

Ranitidine Hydrochloride (Increased phenytoin serum levels). Products include:

Zantac.. 1209
Zantac Injection 1207
Zantac Syrup 1209

Reserpine (Decreased phenytoin serum levels). Products include:

Diupres Tablets 1650
Hydropres Tablets...................................... 1675
Ser-Ap-Es Tablets 849

Rifampin (Efficacy impaired by phenytoin). Products include:

Rifadin 1528
Rifamate Capsules 1530
Rifater.. 1532
Rimactane Capsules 847

Salsalate (Increased phenytoin serum levels). Products include:

Mono-Gesic Tablets 792
Salflex Tablets... 786

Sodium Valproate (Increased or decreased phenytoin levels).

Sucralfate (Decreased phenytoin serum levels). Products include:

Carafate Suspension 1505
Carafate Tablets.. 1504

Sulfacytine (Increased phenytoin serum levels).

Sulfamethizole (Increased phenytoin serum levels). Products include:

Urobiotic-250 Capsules 2214

Sulfamethoxazole (Increased phenytoin serum levels). Products include:

Azo Gantanol Tablets................................. 2080
Bactrim DS Tablets.................................... 2084
Bactrim I.V. Infusion.................................. 2082
Bactrim 2084
Gantanol Tablets 2119
Septra 1174
Septra I.V. Infusion 1169
Septra I.V. Infusion ADD-Vantage Vials.. 1171
Septra 1174

Sulfasalazine (Increased phenytoin serum levels). Products include:

Azulfidine 1949

(ᴹᴰ Described in PDR For Nonprescription Drugs) (◎ Described in PDR For Ophthalmology)

Sulfinpyrazone (Increased phenytoin serum levels). Products include:

Anturane 807

Sulfisoxazole (Increased phenytoin serum levels). Products include:

Azo Gantrisin Tablets............................ 2081
Gantrisin Tablets 2120

Sulfisoxazole Diolamine (Increased phenytoin serum levels).

No products indexed under this heading.

Theophylline (Efficacy impaired by phenytoin). Products include:

Marax Tablets & DF Syrup.................. 2200
Quibron 2053

Theophylline Anhydrous (Efficacy impaired by phenytoin). Products include:

Aerolate 1004
Primatene Dual Action Formula...... ◙ 872
Primatene Tablets .... ◙ 873
Respbid Tablets 682
Slo-bid Gyrocaps 2033
Theo-24 Extended Release Capsules 2568
Theo-Dur Extended-Release Tablets 1327
Theo-X Extended-Release Tablets .. 788
Uni-Dur Extended-Release Tablets.. 1331
Uniphyl 400 mg Tablets...................... 2001

Theophylline Calcium Salicylate (Efficacy impaired by phenytoin). Products include:

Quadrinal Tablets 1350

Theophylline Sodium Glycinate (Efficacy impaired by phenytoin).

No products indexed under this heading.

Thioridazine Hydrochloride (Increased phenytoin serum levels). Products include:

Mellaril 2269

Tolazamide (Increased phenytoin serum levels).

No products indexed under this heading.

Tolbutamide (Increased phenytoin serum levels).

No products indexed under this heading.

Trazodone Hydrochloride (Increased phenytoin serum levels). Products include:

Desyrel and Desyrel Dividose 503

Triamcinolone (Efficacy impaired by phenytoin). Products include:

Aristocort Tablets 1022

Triamcinolone Acetonide (Efficacy impaired by phenytoin). Products include:

Aristocort A 0.025% Cream 1027
Aristocort A 0.5% Cream 1031
Aristocort A 0.1% Cream 1029
Aristocort A 0.1% Ointment 1030
Azmacort Oral Inhaler 2011
Nasacort Nasal Inhaler 2024

Triamcinolone Diacetate (Efficacy impaired by phenytoin). Products include:

Aristocort Suspension (Forte Parenteral).. 1027
Aristocort Suspension (Intralesional).. 1025

Triamcinolone Hexacetonide (Efficacy impaired by phenytoin). Products include:

Aristospan Suspension (Intra-articular).. 1033
Aristospan Suspension (Intralesional).. 1032

Trifluoperazine Hydrochloride (Increased phenytoin serum levels). Products include:

Stelazine 2514

Trimipramine Maleate (Tricyclic antidepressants may precipitate seizures in some patients; phenytoin dosage may need to be adjusted). Products include:

Surmontil Capsules............................... 2811

Valproic Acid (Increased or decreased phenytoin levels). Products include:

Depakene 413

Vitamin D (Efficacy impaired by phenytoin). Products include:

Caltrate PLUS .... ◙ 665
Caltrate 600 + D .... ◙ 665
Citracal Caplets + D 1780
Dical-D Tablets & Wafers 420
Drisdol .... ◙ 794
Materna Tablets 1379
Megadose 512
Zymacap Capsules .... ◙ 772

Warfarin Sodium (Efficacy impaired by phenytoin). Products include:

Coumadin 926

Food Interactions

Alcohol (Increased phenytoin serum levels with acute alcohol intake; decreased levels with chronic alcohol intake).

DILATRATE-SR

(Isosorbide Dinitrate) 2398

May interact with calcium channel blockers and certain other agents. Compounds in these categories include:

Amlodipine Besylate (Marked orthostatic hypotension). Products include:

Lotrel Capsules....................................... 840
Norvasc Tablets 1940

Bepridil Hydrochloride (Marked orthostatic hypotension). Products include:

Vascor (200, 300 and 400 mg) Tablets 1587

Diltiazem Hydrochloride (Marked orthostatic hypotension). Products include:

Cardizem CD Capsules 1506
Cardizem SR Capsules 1510
Cardizem Injectable 1508
Cardizem Tablets................................... 1512
Dilacor XR Extended-release Capsules 2018

Felodipine (Marked orthostatic hypotension). Products include:

Plendil Extended-Release Tablets.... 527

Isradipine (Marked orthostatic hypotension). Products include:

DynaCirc Capsules 2256

Nicardipine Hydrochloride (Marked orthostatic hypotension). Products include:

Cardene Capsules 2095
Cardene I.V. 2709
Cardene SR Capsules............................ 2097

Nifedipine (Marked orthostatic hypotension). Products include:

Adalat Capsules (10 mg and 20 mg) 587
Adalat CC 589
Procardia Capsules................................ 1971
Procardia XL Extended Release Tablets 1972

Nimodipine (Marked orthostatic hypotension). Products include:

Nimotop Capsules.................................. 610

Nisoldipine (Marked orthostatic hypotension).

No products indexed under this heading.

Verapamil Hydrochloride (Marked orthostatic hypotension). Products include:

Calan SR Caplets 2422
Calan Tablets.. 2419
Isoptin Injectable 1344
Isoptin Oral Tablets 1346
Isoptin SR Tablets 1348
Verelan Capsules 1410
Verelan Capsules 2824

Food Interactions

Alcohol (Enhanced hypotensive effects).

DILAUDID AMPULES

(Hydromorphone Hydrochloride) 1335

May interact with central nervous system depressants, tricyclic antidepressants, and certain other agents. Compounds in these categories include:

Alfentanil Hydrochloride (Additive CNS depression). Products include:

Alfenta Injection 1286

Alprazolam (Additive CNS depression). Products include:

Xanax Tablets 2649

Amitriptyline Hydrochloride (Additive CNS depression). Products include:

Elavil 2838
Endep Tablets 2174
Etrafon 2355
Limbitrol 2180
Triavil Tablets 1757

Amoxapine (Additive CNS depression). Products include:

Asendin Tablets 1369

Aprobarbital (Additive CNS depression).

No products indexed under this heading.

Buprenorphine (Additive CNS depression). Products include:

Buprenex Injectable 2006

Buspirone Hydrochloride (Additive CNS depression). Products include:

BuSpar 737

Butabarbital (Additive CNS depression).

No products indexed under this heading.

Butalbital (Additive CNS depression). Products include:

Esgic-plus Tablets 1013
Fioricet Tablets....................................... 2258
Fioricet with Codeine Capsules 2260
Fiorinal Capsules 2261
Fiorinal with Codeine Capsules 2262
Fiorinal Tablets 2261
Phrenilin 785
Sedapap Tablets 50 mg/650 mg .. 1543

Chlordiazepoxide (Additive CNS depression). Products include:

Libritabs Tablets 2177
Limbitrol 2180

Chlordiazepoxide Hydrochloride (Additive CNS depression). Products include:

Librax Capsules 2176
Librium Capsules................................... 2178
Librium Injectable 2179

Chlorpromazine (Additive CNS depression). Products include:

Thorazine Suppositories...................... 2523

Chlorprothixene (Additive CNS depression).

No products indexed under this heading.

Chlorprothixene Hydrochloride (Additive CNS depression).

No products indexed under this heading.

Chlorprothixene Lactate (Additive CNS depression).

No products indexed under this heading.

Clomipramine Hydrochloride (Additive CNS depression). Products include:

Anafranil Capsules 803

Clorazepate Dipotassium (Additive CNS depression). Products include:

Tranxene 451

Clozapine (Additive CNS depression). Products include:

Clozaril Tablets....................................... 2252

Codeine Phosphate (Additive CNS depression). Products include:

Actifed with Codeine Cough Syrup.. 1067

Brontex 1981
Deconsal C Expectorant Syrup 456
Deconsal Pediatric Syrup 457
Dimetane-DC Cough Syrup 2059
Empirin with Codeine Tablets............ 1093
Fioricet with Codeine Capsules 2260
Fiorinal with Codeine Capsules 2262
Isoclor Expectorant............................... 990
Novahistine DH...................................... 2462
Novahistine Expectorant...................... 2463
Nucofed 2051
Phenergan with Codeine...................... 2777
Phenergan VC with Codeine 2781
Robitussin A-C Syrup 2073
Robitussin-DAC Syrup 2074
Ryna .... ◙ 841
Soma Compound w/Codeine Tablets 2676
Tussi-Organidin NR Liquid and S NR Liquid 2677
Tylenol with Codeine 1583

Desflurane (Additive CNS depression). Products include:

Suprane 1813

Desipramine Hydrochloride (Additive CNS depression). Products include:

Norpramin Tablets 1526

Dezocine (Additive CNS depression). Products include:

Dalgan Injection 538

Diazepam (Additive CNS depression). Products include:

Dizac 1809
Valium Injectable 2182
Valium Tablets 2183
Valrelease Capsules 2169

Doxepin Hydrochloride (Additive CNS depression). Products include:

Sinequan 2205
Zonalon Cream 1055

Droperidol (Additive CNS depression). Products include:

Inapsine Injection.................................. 1296

Enflurane (Additive CNS depression).

No products indexed under this heading.

Estazolam (Additive CNS depression). Products include:

ProSom Tablets 449

Ethchlorvynol (Additive CNS depression). Products include:

Placidyl Capsules................................... 448

Ethinamate (Additive CNS depression).

No products indexed under this heading.

Fentanyl (Additive CNS depression). Products include:

Duragesic Transdermal System........ 1288

Fentanyl Citrate (Additive CNS depression). Products include:

Sublimaze Injection............................... 1307

Fluphenazine Decanoate (Additive CNS depression). Products include:

Prolixin Decanoate 509

Fluphenazine Enanthate (Additive CNS depression). Products include:

Prolixin Enanthate 509

Fluphenazine Hydrochloride (Additive CNS depression). Products include:

Prolixin 509

Flurazepam Hydrochloride (Additive CNS depression). Products include:

Dalmane Capsules.................................. 2173

Glutethimide (Additive CNS depression).

No products indexed under this heading.

Haloperidol (Additive CNS depression). Products include:

Haldol Injection, Tablets and Concentrate 1575

IMPORTANT NOTE: Always consult each drug listing in the patient's regimen for possible interactions.

Dilaudid Interactions Index 296

Haloperidol Decanoate (Additive CNS depression). Products include:
Haldol Decanoate ... 1577
Hydrocodone Bitartrate (Additive CNS depression). Products include:
Anexsia 5/500 Elixir ... 1781
Anexia Tablets ... 1782
Codiclear DH Syrup ... 791
Deconamine CX Cough and Cold Liquid and Tablets ... 1319
Duratuss HD Elixir ... 2565
Hycodan Tablets and Syrup ... 930
Hycomine Compound Tablets ... 932
Hycomine ... 931
Hycotuss Expectorant Syrup ... 933
Hydrocet Capsules ... 782
Lorcet 10/650 ... 1018
Lortab ... 2566
Tussend ... 1783
Tussend Expectorant ... 1785
Vicodin Tablets ... 1356
Vicodin ES Tablets ... 1357
Vicodin Tuss Expectorant ... 1358
Zydone Capsules ... 949
Hydrocodone Polistirex (Additive CNS depression). Products include:
Tussionex Pennkinetic Extended-Release Suspension ... 998
Hydroxyzine Hydrochloride (Additive CNS depression). Products include:
Atarax Tablets & Syrup ... 2185
Marax Tablets & DF Syrup ... 2200
Vistaril Intramuscular Solution ... 2216
Imipramine Hydrochloride (Additive CNS depression). Products include:
Tofranil Ampuls ... 854
Tofranil Tablets ... 856
Imipramine Pamoate (Additive CNS depression). Products include:
Tofranil-PM Capsules ... 857
Isoflurane (Additive CNS depression).
No products indexed under this heading.
Ketamine Hydrochloride (Additive CNS depression).
No products indexed under this heading.
Levomethadyl Acetate Hydrochloride (Additive CNS depression). Products include:
Orlamm ... 2239
Levorphanol Tartrate (Additive CNS depression). Products include:
Levo-Dromoran ... 2129
Lorazepam (Additive CNS depression). Products include:
Ativan Injection ... 2698
Ativan Tablets ... 2700
Loxapine Hydrochloride (Additive CNS depression). Products include:
Loxitane ... 1378
Loxapine Succinate (Additive CNS depression). Products include:
Loxitane Capsules ... 1378
Maprotiline Hydrochloride (Additive CNS depression). Products include:
Ludiomil Tablets ... 843
Meperidine Hydrochloride (Additive CNS depression). Products include:
Demerol ... 2308
Mepergan Injection ... 2753
Mephobarbital (Additive CNS depression). Products include:
Mebaral Tablets ... 2322
Meprobamate (Additive CNS depression). Products include:
Miltown Tablets ... 2672
PMB 200 and PMB 400 ... 2783
Mesoridazine Besylate (Additive CNS depression). Products include:
Serentil ... 684
Methadone Hydrochloride (Additive CNS depression). Products include:
Methadone Hydrochloride Oral Concentrate ... 2233
Methadone Hydrochloride Oral Solution & Tablets ... 2235
Methohexital Sodium (Additive CNS depression). Products include:
Brevital Sodium Vials ... 1429
Methotrimeprazine (Additive CNS depression). Products include:
Levoprome ... 1274
Methoxyflurane (Additive CNS depression).
No products indexed under this heading.
Midazolam Hydrochloride (Additive CNS depression). Products include:
Versed Injection ... 2170
Molindone Hydrochloride (Additive CNS depression). Products include:
Moban Tablets and Concentrate ... 1048
Morphine Sulfate (Additive CNS depression). Products include:
Astramorph/PF Injection, USP (Preservative-Free) ... 535
Duramorph ... 962
Infumorph 200 and Infumorph 500 Sterile Solutions ... 965
MS Contin Tablets ... 1994
MSIR ... 1997
Oramorph SR (Morphine Sulfate Sustained Release Tablets) ... 2236
RMS Suppositories ... 2657
Roxanol ... 2243
Nortriptyline Hydrochloride (Additive CNS depression). Products include:
Pamelor ... 2280
Opium Alkaloids (Additive CNS depression).
No products indexed under this heading.
Oxazepam (Additive CNS depression). Products include:
Serax Capsules ... 2810
Serax Tablets ... 2810
Oxycodone Hydrochloride (Additive CNS depression). Products include:
Percocet Tablets ... 938
Percodan Tablets ... 939
Percodan-Demi Tablets ... 940
Roxicodone Tablets, Oral Solution & Intensol (Oxycodone) ... 2244
Tylox Capsules ... 1584
Pentobarbital Sodium (Additive CNS depression). Products include:
Nembutal Sodium Capsules ... 436
Nembutal Sodium Solution ... 438
Nembutal Sodium Suppositories ... 440
Perphenazine (Additive CNS depression). Products include:
Etrafon ... 2355
Triavil Tablets ... 1757
Trilafon ... 2389
Phenobarbital (Additive CNS depression). Products include:
Arco-Lase Plus Tablets ... 512
Bellergal-S Tablets ... 2250
Donnatal ... 2060
Donnatal Extentabs ... 2061
Donnatal Tablets ... 2060
Phenobarbital Elixir and Tablets ... 1469
Quadrinal Tablets ... 1350
Prazepam (Additive CNS depression).
No products indexed under this heading.
Prochlorperazine (Additive CNS depression). Products include:
Compazine ... 2470
Promethazine Hydrochloride (Additive CNS depression). Products include:
Mepergan Injection ... 2753
Phenergan with Codeine ... 2777
Phenergan with Dextromethorphan ... 2778
Phenergan Injection ... 2773
Phenergan Suppositories ... 2775
Phenergan Syrup ... 2774
Phenergan Tablets ... 2775
Phenergan VC ... 2779
Phenergan VC with Codeine ... 2781
Propofol (Additive CNS depression). Products include:
Diprivan Injection ... 2833
Propoxyphene Hydrochloride (Additive CNS depression). Products include:
Darvon ... 1435
Wygesic Tablets ... 2827
Propoxyphene Napsylate (Additive CNS depression). Products include:
Darvon-N/Darvocet-N ... 1433
Protriptyline Hydrochloride (Additive CNS depression). Products include:
Vivactil Tablets ... 1774
Quazepam (Additive CNS depression). Products include:
Doral Tablets ... 2664
Risperidone (Additive CNS depression). Products include:
Risperdal ... 1301
Secobarbital Sodium (Additive CNS depression). Products include:
Seconal Sodium Pulvules ... 1474
Sufentanil Citrate (Additive CNS depression). Products include:
Sufenta Injection ... 1309
Temazepam (Additive CNS depression). Products include:
Restoril Capsules ... 2284
Thiamylal Sodium (Additive CNS depression).
No products indexed under this heading.
Thioridazine Hydrochloride (Additive CNS depression). Products include:
Mellaril ... 2269
Thiothixene (Additive CNS depression). Products include:
Navane Capsules and Concentrate ... 2201
Navane Intramuscular ... 2202
Triazolam (Additive CNS depression). Products include:
Halcion Tablets ... 2611
Trifluoperazine Hydrochloride (Additive CNS depression). Products include:
Stelazine ... 2514
Trimipramine Maleate (Additive CNS depression). Products include:
Surmontil Capsules ... 2811
Zolpidem Tartrate (Additive CNS depression). Products include:
Ambien Tablets ... 2416

Food Interactions

Alcohol (Additive CNS depression).

DILAUDID COUGH SYRUP
(Hydromorphone Hydrochloride) ... 1336
May interact with central nervous system depressants, tricyclic antidepressants, and certain other agents. Compounds in these categories include:

Alfentanil Hydrochloride (Additive CNS depression). Products include:
Alfenta Injection ... 1286
Alprazolam (Additive CNS depression). Products include:
Xanax Tablets ... 2649
Amitriptyline Hydrochloride (Additive CNS depression). Products include:
Elavil ... 2838
Endep Tablets ... 2174
Etrafon ... 2355
Limbitrol ... 2180
Triavil Tablets ... 1757
Amoxapine (Additive CNS depression). Products include:
Asendin Tablets ... 1369
Aprobarbital (Additive CNS depression).
No products indexed under this heading.
Buprenorphine (Additive CNS depression). Products include:
Buprenex Injectable ... 2006
Buspirone Hydrochloride (Additive CNS depression). Products include:
BuSpar ... 737
Butabarbital (Additive CNS depression).
No products indexed under this heading.
Butalbital (Additive CNS depression). Products include:
Esgic-plus Tablets ... 1013
Fioricet Tablets ... 2258
Fioricet with Codeine Capsules ... 2260
Fiorinal Capsules ... 2261
Fiorinal with Codeine Capsules ... 2262
Fiorinal Tablets ... 2261
Phrenilin ... 785
Sedapap Tablets 50 mg/650 mg ... 1543
Chlordiazepoxide (Additive CNS depression). Products include:
Libritabs Tablets ... 2177
Limbitrol ... 2180
Chlordiazepoxide Hydrochloride (Additive CNS depression). Products include:
Librax Capsules ... 2176
Librium Capsules ... 2178
Librium Injectable ... 2179
Chlorpromazine (Additive CNS depression). Products include:
Thorazine Suppositories ... 2523
Chlorprothixene (Additive CNS depression).
No products indexed under this heading.
Chlorprothixene Hydrochloride (Additive CNS depression).
No products indexed under this heading.
Chlorprothixene Lactate (Additive CNS depression).
No products indexed under this heading.
Clomipramine Hydrochloride (Additive CNS depression). Products include:
Anafranil Capsules ... 803
Clorazepate Dipotassium (Additive CNS depression). Products include:
Tranxene ... 451
Clozapine (Additive CNS depression). Products include:
Clozaril Tablets ... 2252
Codeine Phosphate (Additive CNS depression). Products include:
Actifed with Codeine Cough Syrup ... 1067
Brontex ... 1981
Deconsal C Expectorant Syrup ... 456
Deconsal Pediatric Syrup ... 457
Dimetane-DC Cough Syrup ... 2059
Empirin with Codeine Tablets ... 1093
Fioricet with Codeine Capsules ... 2260
Fiorinal with Codeine Capsules ... 2262
Isoclor Expectorant ... 990
Novahistine DH ... 2462
Novahistine Expectorant ... 2463
Nucofed ... 2051
Phenergan with Codeine ... 2777
Phenergan VC with Codeine ... 2781
Robitussin A-C Syrup ... 2073
Robitussin-DAC Syrup ... 2074
Ryna ... ▣ 841
Soma Compound w/Codeine Tablets ... 2676
Tussi-Organidin NR Liquid and S NR Liquid ... 2677
Tylenol with Codeine ... 1583
Desflurane (Additive CNS depression). Products include:
Suprane ... 1813

(▣ Described in PDR For Nonprescription Drugs) (◉ Described in PDR For Ophthalmology)

Desipramine Hydrochloride (Additive CNS depression). Products include:
Norpramin Tablets ... 1526

Dezocine (Additive CNS depression). Products include:
Dalgan Injection ... 538

Diazepam (Additive CNS depression). Products include:
Dizac ... 1809
Valium Injectable ... 2182
Valium Tablets ... 2183
Valrelease Capsules ... 2169

Doxepin Hydrochloride (Additive CNS depression). Products include:
Sinequan ... 2205
Zonalon Cream ... 1055

Droperidol (Additive CNS depression). Products include:
Inapsine Injection ... 1296

Enflurane (Additive CNS depression).
No products indexed under this heading.

Estazolam (Additive CNS depression). Products include:
ProSom Tablets ... 449

Ethchlorvynol (Additive CNS depression). Products include:
Placidyl Capsules ... 448

Ethinamate (Additive CNS depression).
No products indexed under this heading.

Fentanyl (Additive CNS depression). Products include:
Duragesic Transdermal System ... 1288

Fentanyl Citrate (Additive CNS depression). Products include:
Sublimaze Injection ... 1307

Fluphenazine Decanoate (Additive CNS depression). Products include:
Prolixin Decanoate ... 509

Fluphenazine Enanthate (Additive CNS depression). Products include:
Prolixin Enanthate ... 509

Fluphenazine Hydrochloride (Additive CNS depression). Products include:
Prolixin ... 509

Flurazepam Hydrochloride (Additive CNS depression). Products include:
Dalmane Capsules ... 2173

Glutethimide (Additive CNS depression).
No products indexed under this heading.

Haloperidol (Additive CNS depression). Products include:
Haldol Injection, Tablets and Concentrate ... 1575

Haloperidol Decanoate (Additive CNS depression). Products include:
Haldol Decanoate ... 1577

Hydrocodone Bitartrate (Additive CNS depression). Products include:
Anexsia 5/500 Elixir ... 1781
Anexia Tablets ... 1782
Codiclear DH Syrup ... 791
Deconamine CX Cough and Cold Liquid and Tablets ... 1319
Duratuss HD Elixir ... 2565
Hycodan Tablets and Syrup ... 930
Hycomine Compound Tablets ... 932
Hycomine ... 931
Hycotuss Expectorant Syrup ... 933
Hydrocet Capsules ... 782
Lorcet 10/650 ... 1018
Lortab ... 2566
Tussend ... 1783
Tussend Expectorant ... 1785
Vicodin Tablets ... 1356
Vicodin ES Tablets ... 1357
Vicodin Tuss Expectorant ... 1358
Zydone Capsules ... 949

Hydrocodone Polistirex (Additive CNS depression). Products include:
Tussionex Pennkinetic Extended-Release Suspension ... 998

Hydroxyzine Hydrochloride (Additive CNS depression). Products include:
Atarax Tablets & Syrup ... 2185
Marax Tablets & DF Syrup ... 2200
Vistaril Intramuscular Solution ... 2216

Imipramine Hydrochloride (Additive CNS depression). Products include:
Tofranil Ampuls ... 854
Tofranil Tablets ... 856

Imipramine Pamoate (Additive CNS depression). Products include:
Tofranil-PM Capsules ... 857

Isoflurane (Additive CNS depression).
No products indexed under this heading.

Ketamine Hydrochloride (Additive CNS depression).
No products indexed under this heading.

Levomethadyl Acetate Hydrochloride (Additive CNS depression). Products include:
Orlamm ... 2239

Levorphanol Tartrate (Additive CNS depression). Products include:
Levo-Dromoran ... 2129

Lorazepam (Additive CNS depression). Products include:
Ativan Injection ... 2698
Ativan Tablets ... 2700

Loxapine Hydrochloride (Additive CNS depression). Products include:
Loxitane ... 1378

Loxapine Succinate (Additive CNS depression). Products include:
Loxitane Capsules ... 1378

Maprotiline Hydrochloride (Additive CNS depression). Products include:
Ludiomil Tablets ... 843

Meperidine Hydrochloride (Additive CNS depression). Products include:
Demerol ... 2308
Mepergan Injection ... 2753

Mephobarbital (Additive CNS depression). Products include:
Mebaral Tablets ... 2322

Meprobamate (Additive CNS depression). Products include:
Miltown Tablets ... 2672
PMB 200 and PMB 400 ... 2783

Mesoridazine Besylate (Additive CNS depression). Products include:
Serentil ... 684

Methadone Hydrochloride (Additive CNS depression). Products include:
Methadone Hydrochloride Oral Concentrate ... 2233
Methadone Hydrochloride Oral Solution & Tablets ... 2235

Methohexital Sodium (Additive CNS depression). Products include:
Brevital Sodium Vials ... 1429

Methotrimeprazine (Additive CNS depression). Products include:
Levoprome ... 1274

Methoxyflurane (Additive CNS depression).
No products indexed under this heading.

Midazolam Hydrochloride (Additive CNS depression). Products include:
Versed Injection ... 2170

Molindone Hydrochloride (Additive CNS depression). Products include:
Moban Tablets and Concentrate ... 1048

Morphine Sulfate (Additive CNS depression). Products include:
Astramorph/PF Injection, USP (Preservative-Free) ... 535
Duramorph ... 962
Infumorph 200 and Infumorph 500 Sterile Solutions ... 965
MS Contin Tablets ... 1994
MSIR ... 1997
Oramorph SR (Morphine Sulfate Sustained Release Tablets) ... 2236
RMS Suppositories ... 2657
Roxanol ... 2243

Nortriptyline Hydrochloride (Additive CNS depression). Products include:
Pamelor ... 2280

Opium Alkaloids (Additive CNS depression).
No products indexed under this heading.

Oxazepam (Additive CNS depression). Products include:
Serax Capsules ... 2810
Serax Tablets ... 2810

Oxycodone Hydrochloride (Additive CNS depression). Products include:
Percocet Tablets ... 938
Percodan Tablets ... 939
Percodan-Demi Tablets ... 940
Roxicodone Tablets, Oral Solution & Intensol (Oxycodone) ... 2244
Tylox Capsules ... 1584

Pentobarbital Sodium (Additive CNS depression). Products include:
Nembutal Sodium Capsules ... 436
Nembutal Sodium Solution ... 438
Nembutal Sodium Suppositories ... 440

Perphenazine (Additive CNS depression). Products include:
Etrafon ... 2355
Triavil Tablets ... 1757
Trilafon ... 2389

Phenobarbital (Additive CNS depression). Products include:
Arco-Lase Plus Tablets ... 512
Bellergal-S Tablets ... 2250
Donnatal ... 2060
Donnatal Extentabs ... 2061
Donnatal Tablets ... 2060
Phenobarbital Elixir and Tablets ... 1469
Quadrinal Tablets ... 1350

Prazepam (Additive CNS depression).
No products indexed under this heading.

Prochlorperazine (Additive CNS depression). Products include:
Compazine ... 2470

Promethazine Hydrochloride (Additive CNS depression). Products include:
Mepergan Injection ... 2753
Phenergan with Codeine ... 2777
Phenergan with Dextromethorphan ... 2778
Phenergan Injection ... 2773
Phenergan Suppositories ... 2775
Phenergan Syrup ... 2774
Phenergan Tablets ... 2775
Phenergan VC ... 2779
Phenergan VC with Codeine ... 2781

Propofol (Additive CNS depression). Products include:
Diprivan Injection ... 2833

Propoxyphene Hydrochloride (Additive CNS depression). Products include:
Darvon ... 1435
Wygesic Tablets ... 2827

Propoxyphene Napsylate (Additive CNS depression). Products include:
Darvon-N/Darvocet-N ... 1433

Protriptyline Hydrochloride (Additive CNS depression). Products include:
Vivactil Tablets ... 1774

Quazepam (Additive CNS depression). Products include:
Doral Tablets ... 2664

Risperidone (Additive CNS depression). Products include:
Risperdal ... 1301

Secobarbital Sodium (Additive CNS depression). Products include:
Seconal Sodium Pulvules ... 1474

Sufentanil Citrate (Additive CNS depression). Products include:
Sufenta Injection ... 1309

Temazepam (Additive CNS depression). Products include:
Restoril Capsules ... 2284

Thiamylal Sodium (Additive CNS depression).
No products indexed under this heading.

Thioridazine Hydrochloride (Additive CNS depression). Products include:
Mellaril ... 2269

Thiothixene (Additive CNS depression). Products include:
Navane Capsules and Concentrate ... 2201
Navane Intramuscular ... 2202

Triazolam (Additive CNS depression). Products include:
Halcion Tablets ... 2611

Trifluoperazine Hydrochloride (Additive CNS depression). Products include:
Stelazine ... 2514

Trimipramine Maleate (Additive CNS depression). Products include:
Surmontil Capsules ... 2811

Zolpidem Tartrate (Additive CNS depression). Products include:
Ambien Tablets ... 2416

Food Interactions

Alcohol (Additive CNS depression).

DILAUDID-HP INJECTION

(Hydromorphone Hydrochloride) ... 1337

May interact with central nervous system depressants, nondepolarizing neuromuscular blocking agents, general anesthetics, tranquilizers, phenothiazines, hypnotics and sedatives, and certain other agents. Compounds in these categories include:

Alfentanil Hydrochloride (Additive depressant effects). Products include:
Alfenta Injection ... 1286

Alprazolam (Additive depressant effects). Products include:
Xanax Tablets ... 2649

Aprobarbital (Additive depressant effects).
No products indexed under this heading.

Atracurium Besylate (Increased respiratory depression; enhanced action of neuromuscular blocking agents). Products include:
Tracrium Injection ... 1183

Buprenorphine (Additive depressant effects). Products include:
Buprenex Injectable ... 2006

Buspirone Hydrochloride (Additive depressant effects). Products include:
BuSpar ... 737

Butabarbital (Additive depressant effects).
No products indexed under this heading.

Butalbital (Additive depressant effects). Products include:
Esgic-plus Tablets ... 1013
Fioricet Tablets ... 2258
Fioricet with Codeine Capsules ... 2260
Fiorinal Capsules ... 2261
Fiorinal with Codeine Capsules ... 2262
Fiorinal Tablets ... 2261

IMPORTANT NOTE: Always consult each drug listing in the patient's regimen for possible interactions.

Dilaudid-HP Injection

Phrenilin 785
Sedapap Tablets 50 mg/650 mg .. 1543

Chlordiazepoxide (Additive depressant effects). Products include:

Libritabs Tablets 2177
Limbitrol 2180

Chlordiazepoxide Hydrochloride (Additive depressant effects). Products include:

Librax Capsules 2176
Librium Capsules 2178
Librium Injectable 2179

Chlorpromazine (Additive depressant effects). Products include:

Thorazine Suppositories 2523

Chlorpromazine Hydrochloride (Additive depressant effects). Products include:

Thorazine 2523

Chlorprothixene (Additive depressant effects).

No products indexed under this heading.

Chlorprothixene Hydrochloride (Additive depressant effects).

No products indexed under this heading.

Chlorprothixene Lactate (Additive depressant effects).

No products indexed under this heading.

Clorazepate Dipotassium (Additive depressant effects). Products include:

Tranxene 451

Clozapine (Additive depressant effects). Products include:

Clozaril Tablets 2252

Codeine Phosphate (Additive depressant effects). Products include:

Actifed with Codeine Cough Syrup.. 1067
Brontex 1981
Deconsal C Expectorant Syrup 456
Deconsal Pediatric Syrup 457
Dimetane-DC Cough Syrup 2059
Empirin with Codeine Tablets............ 1093
Fioricet with Codeine Capsules 2260
Fiorinal with Codeine Capsules 2262
Isoclor Expectorant 990
Novahistine DH 2462
Novahistine Expectorant 2463
Nucofed 2051
Phenergan with Codeine 2777
Phenergan VC with Codeine 2781
Robitussin A-C Syrup 2073
Robitussin-DAC Syrup 2074
Ryna .... ⊕ 841
Soma Compound w/Codeine Tablets 2676
Tussi-Organidin NR Liquid and S NR Liquid 2677
Tylenol with Codeine 1583

Desflurane (Additive depressant effects). Products include:

Suprane 1813

Dezocine (Additive depressant effects). Products include:

Dalgan Injection 538

Diazepam (Additive depressant effects). Products include:

Dizac 1809
Valium Injectable 2182
Valium Tablets 2183
Valrelease Capsules 2169

Droperidol (Additive depressant effects). Products include:

Inapsine Injection 1296

Enflurane (Additive depressant effects).

No products indexed under this heading.

Estazolam (Additive depressant effects). Products include:

ProSom Tablets 449

Ethchlorvynol (Additive depressant effects). Products include:

Placidyl Capsules 448

Ethinamate (Additive depressant effects).

No products indexed under this heading.

Fentanyl (Additive depressant effects). Products include:

Duragesic Transdermal System........ 1288

Fentanyl Citrate (Additive depressant effects). Products include:

Sublimaze Injection 1307

Fluphenazine Decanoate (Additive depressant effects). Products include:

Prolixin Decanoate 509

Fluphenazine Enanthate (Additive depressant effects). Products include:

Prolixin Enanthate 509

Fluphenazine Hydrochloride (Additive depressant effects). Products include:

Prolixin 509

Flurazepam Hydrochloride (Additive depressant effects). Products include:

Dalmane Capsules 2173

Glutethimide (Additive depressant effects).

No products indexed under this heading.

Haloperidol (Additive depressant effects). Products include:

Haldol Injection, Tablets and Concentrate 1575

Haloperidol Decanoate (Additive depressant effects). Products include:

Haldol Decanoate 1577

Hydrocodone Bitartrate (Additive depressant effects). Products include:

Anexsia 5/500 Elixir 1781
Anexia Tablets 1782
Codiclear DH Syrup 791
Deconamine CX Cough and Cold Liquid and Tablets 1319
Duratuss HD Elixir 2565
Hycodan Tablets and Syrup 930
Hycomine Compound Tablets 932
Hycomine 931
Hycotuss Expectorant Syrup 933
Hydrocet Capsules 782
Lorcet 10/650 1018
Lortab 2566
Tussend 1783
Tussend Expectorant 1785
Vicodin Tablets 1356
Vicodin ES Tablets 1357
Vicodin Tuss Expectorant 1358
Zydone Capsules 949

Hydrocodone Polistirex (Additive depressant effects). Products include:

Tussionex Pennkinetic Extended-Release Suspension 998

Hydroxyzine Hydrochloride (Additive depressant effects). Products include:

Atarax Tablets & Syrup 2185
Marax Tablets & DF Syrup 2200
Vistaril Intramuscular Solution 2216

Isoflurane (Additive depressant effects).

No products indexed under this heading.

Ketamine Hydrochloride (Additive depressant effects).

No products indexed under this heading.

Levomethadyl Acetate Hydrochloride (Additive depressant effects). Products include:

Orlaam 2239

Levorphanol Tartrate (Additive depressant effects). Products include:

Levo-Dromoran 2129

Lorazepam (Additive depressant effects). Products include:

Ativan Injection 2698

Ativan Tablets 2700

Loxapine Hydrochloride (Additive depressant effects). Products include:

Loxitane 1378

Loxapine Succinate (Additive depressant effects). Products include:

Loxitane Capsules 1378

Meperidine Hydrochloride (Additive depressant effects). Products include:

Demerol 2308
Mepergan Injection 2753

Mephobarbital (Additive depressant effects). Products include:

Mebaral Tablets 2322

Meprobamate (Additive depressant effects). Products include:

Miltown Tablets 2672
PMB 200 and PMB 400 2783

Mesoridazine Besylate (Additive depressant effects). Products include:

Serentil 684

Methadone Hydrochloride (Additive depressant effects). Products include:

Methadone Hydrochloride Oral Concentrate 2233
Methadone Hydrochloride Oral Solution & Tablets 2235

Methohexital Sodium (Additive depressant effects). Products include:

Brevital Sodium Vials 1429

Methotrimeprazine (Additive depressant effects). Products include:

Levoprome 1274

Methoxyflurane (Additive depressant effects).

No products indexed under this heading.

Metocurine Iodide (Increased respiratory depression; enhanced action of neuromuscular blocking agents). Products include:

Metubine Iodide Vials 916

Midazolam Hydrochloride (Additive depressant effects). Products include:

Versed Injection 2170

Mivacurium Chloride (Increased respiratory depression; enhanced action of neuromuscular blocking agents). Products include:

Mivacron 1138

Molindone Hydrochloride (Additive depressant effects). Products include:

Moban Tablets and Concentrate 1048

Morphine Sulfate (Additive depressant effects). Products include:

Astramorph/PF Injection, USP (Preservative-Free) 535
Duramorph 962
Infumorph 200 and Infumorph 500 Sterile Solutions 965
MS Contin Tablets 1994
MSIR 1997
Oramorph SR (Morphine Sulfate Sustained Release Tablets) 2236
RMS Suppositories 2657
Roxanol 2243

Opium Alkaloids (Additive depressant effects).

No products indexed under this heading.

Oxazepam (Additive depressant effects). Products include:

Serax Capsules 2810
Serax Tablets 2810

Oxycodone Hydrochloride (Additive depressant effects). Products include:

Percocet Tablets 938
Percodan Tablets 939
Percodan-Demi Tablets 940

Roxicodone Tablets, Oral Solution & Intensol (Oxycodone) 2244
Tylox Capsules 1584

Pancuronium Bromide Injection (Increased respiratory depression; enhanced action of neuromuscular blocking agents).

No products indexed under this heading.

Pentobarbital Sodium (Additive depressant effects). Products include:

Nembutal Sodium Capsules 436
Nembutal Sodium Solution 438
Nembutal Sodium Suppositories 440

Perphenazine (Additive depressant effects). Products include:

Etrafon 2355
Triavil Tablets 1757
Trilafon 2389

Phenobarbital (Additive depressant effects). Products include:

Arco-Lase Plus Tablets 512
Bellergal-S Tablets 2250
Donnatal 2060
Donnatal Extentabs 2061
Donnatal Tablets 2060
Phenobarbital Elixir and Tablets 1469
Quadrinal Tablets 1350

Prazepam (Additive depressant effects).

No products indexed under this heading.

Prochlorperazine (Additive depressant effects). Products include:

Compazine 2470

Promethazine Hydrochloride (Additive depressant effects). Products include:

Mepergan Injection 2753
Phenergan with Codeine 2777
Phenergan with Dextromethorphan 2778
Phenergan Injection 2773
Phenergan Suppositories 2775
Phenergan Syrup 2774
Phenergan Tablets 2775
Phenergan VC 2779
Phenergan VC with Codeine 2781

Propofol (Additive depressant effects). Products include:

Diprivan Injection 2833

Propoxyphene Hydrochloride (Additive depressant effects). Products include:

Darvon 1435
Wygesic Tablets 2827

Propoxyphene Napsylate (Additive depressant effects). Products include:

Darvon-N/Darvocet-N 1433

Quazepam (Additive depressant effects). Products include:

Doral Tablets 2664

Risperidone (Additive depressant effects). Products include:

Risperdal 1301

Rocuronium Bromide (Increased respiratory depression; enhanced action of neuromuscular blocking agents). Products include:

Zemuron 1830

Secobarbital Sodium (Additive depressant effects). Products include:

Seconal Sodium Pulvules 1474

Sufentanil Citrate (Additive depressant effects). Products include:

Sufenta Injection 1309

Temazepam (Additive depressant effects). Products include:

Restoril Capsules 2284

Thiamylal Sodium (Additive depressant effects).

No products indexed under this heading.

Thioridazine Hydrochloride (Additive depressant effects). Products include:

Mellaril 2269

(⊕ Described in PDR For Nonprescription Drugs) (◉ Described in PDR For Ophthalmology)

Thiothixene (Additive depressant effects). Products include:

Navane Capsules and Concentrate ... 2201
Navane Intramuscular ... 2202

Triazolam (Additive depressant effects). Products include:

Halcion Tablets ... 2611

Trifluoperazine Hydrochloride (Additive depressant effects). Products include:

Stelazine ... 2514

Vecuronium Bromide (Increased respiratory depression; enhanced action of neuromuscular blocking agents). Products include:

Norcuron ... 1826

Zolpidem Tartrate (Additive depressant effects). Products include:

Ambien Tablets ... 2416

Food Interactions

Alcohol (Additive depressant effects).

DILAUDID-HP LYOPHILIZED POWDER 250 MG

(Hydromorphone Hydrochloride) ...1337
See **Dilaudid-HP Injection**

DILAUDID INJECTION

(Hydromorphone Hydrochloride) ...1335
See **Dilaudid Ampules**

DILAUDID MULTIPLE DOSE VIALS (STERILE SOLUTION)

(Hydromorphone Hydrochloride) ...1335
See **Dilaudid Ampules**

DILAUDID ORAL LIQUID

(Hydromorphone Hydrochloride) ...1339

May interact with central nervous system depressants, hypnotics and sedatives, general anesthetics, phenothiazines, tranquilizers, neuromuscular blocking agents, and certain other agents. Compounds in these categories include:

Alfentanil Hydrochloride (May produce additive depressant effects; respiratory depression, hypotension and profound sedation or coma may occur; the dose of one or both agents should be reduced). Products include:

Alfenta Injection ... 1286

Alprazolam (May produce additive depressant effects; respiratory depression, hypotension and profound sedation or coma may occur; the dose of one or both agents should be reduced). Products include:

Xanax Tablets ... 2649

Aprobarbital (May produce additive depressant effects; respiratory depression, hypotension and profound sedation or coma may occur; the dose of one or both agents should be reduced).

No products indexed under this heading.

Atracurium Besylate (Enhanced action of neuromuscular blocking agents and produce an excessive degree of respiratory depression). Products include:

Tracrium Injection ... 1183

Buprenorphine (May produce additive depressant effects; respiratory depression, hypotension and profound sedation or coma may occur; the dose of one or both agents should be reduced). Products include:

Buprenex Injectable ... 2006

Buspirone Hydrochloride (May produce additive depressant effects; respiratory depression, hypotension and profound sedation or coma may occur; the dose of one or both agents should be reduced). Products include:

BuSpar ... 737

Butabarbital (May produce additive depressant effects; respiratory depression, hypotension and profound sedation or coma may occur; the dose of one or both agents should be reduced).

No products indexed under this heading.

Butalbital (May produce additive depressant effects; respiratory depression, hypotension and profound sedation or coma may occur; the dose of one or both agents should be reduced). Products include:

Esgic-plus Tablets ... 1013
Fioricet Tablets ... 2258
Fioricet with Codeine Capsules ... 2260
Fiorinal Capsules ... 2261
Fiorinal with Codeine Capsules ... 2262
Fiorinal Tablets ... 2261
Phrenilin ... 785
Sedapap Tablets 50 mg/650 mg .. 1543

Chlordiazepoxide (May produce additive depressant effects; respiratory depression, hypotension and profound sedation or coma may occur; the dose of one or both agents should be reduced). Products include:

Libritabs Tablets ... 2177
Limbitrol ... 2180

Chlordiazepoxide Hydrochloride (May produce additive depressant effects; respiratory depression, hypotension and profound sedation or coma may occur; the dose of one or both agents should be reduced). Products include:

Librax Capsules ... 2176
Librium Capsules ... 2178
Librium Injectable ... 2179

Chlorpromazine (May produce additive depressant effects; respiratory depression, hypotension and profound sedation or coma may occur; the dose of one or both agents should be reduced). Products include:

Thorazine Suppositories ... 2523

Chlorpromazine Hydrochloride (May produce additive depressant effects; respiratory depression, hypotension and profound sedation or coma may occur; the dose of one or both agents should be reduced). Products include:

Thorazine ... 2523

Chlorprothixene (May produce additive depressant effects; respiratory depression, hypotension and profound sedation or coma may occur; the dose of one or both agents should be reduced).

No products indexed under this heading.

Chlorprothixene Hydrochloride (May produce additive depressant effects; respiratory depression, hypotension and profound sedation or coma may occur; the dose of one or both agents should be reduced).

No products indexed under this heading.

Clorazepate Dipotassium (May produce additive depressant effects; respiratory depression, hypotension and profound sedation or coma may occur; the dose of one or both agents should be reduced). Products include:

Tranxene ... 451

Clozapine (May produce additive depressant effects; respiratory depression, hypotension and profound sedation or coma may occur; the dose of one or both agents should be reduced). Products include:

Clozaril Tablets ... 2252

Codeine Phosphate (May produce additive depressant effects; respiratory depression, hypotension and profound sedation or coma may occur; the dose of one or both agents should be reduced). Products include:

Actifed with Codeine Cough Syrup.. 1067
Brontex ... 1981
Deconsal C Expectorant Syrup ... 456
Deconsal Pediatric Syrup ... 457
Dimetane-DC Cough Syrup ... 2059
Empirin with Codeine Tablets ... 1093
Fioricet with Codeine Capsules ... 2260
Fiorinal with Codeine Capsules ... 2262
Isoclor Expectorant ... 990
Novahistine DH ... 2462
Novahistine Expectorant ... 2463
Nucofed ... 2051
Phenergan with Codeine ... 2777
Phenergan VC with Codeine ... 2781
Robitussin A-C Syrup ... 2073
Robitussin-DAC Syrup ... 2074
Ryna ... 841
Soma Compound w/Codeine Tablets ... 2676
Tussi-Organidin NR Liquid and S NR Liquid ... 2677
Tylenol with Codeine ... 1583

Desflurane (May produce additive depressant effects; respiratory depression, hypotension and profound sedation or coma may occur; the dose of one or both agents should be reduced). Products include:

Suprane ... 1813

Dezocine (May produce additive depressant effects; respiratory depression, hypotension and profound sedation or coma may occur; the dose of one or both agents should be reduced). Products include:

Dalgan Injection ... 538

Diazepam (May produce additive depressant effects; respiratory depression, hypotension and profound sedation or coma may occur; the dose of one or both agents should be reduced). Products include:

Dizac ... 1809
Valium Injectable ... 2182
Valium Tablets ... 2183
Valrelease Capsules ... 2169

Doxacurium Chloride (Enhanced action of neuromuscular blocking agents and produce an excessive degree of respiratory depression). Products include:

Nuromax Injection ... 1149

Droperidol (May produce additive depressant effects; respiratory depression, hypotension and profound sedation or coma may occur; the dose of one or both agents should be reduced). Products include:

Inapsine Injection ... 1296

Enflurane (May produce additive depressant effects; respiratory depression, hypotension and profound sedation or coma may occur; the dose of one or both agents should be reduced).

No products indexed under this heading.

Estazolam (May produce additive depressant effects; respiratory depression, hypotension and profound sedation or coma may occur; the dose of one or both agents should be reduced). Products include:

ProSom Tablets ... 449

Ethchlorvynol (May produce additive depressant effects; respiratory depression, hypotension and profound sedation or coma may occur; the dose of one or both agents should be reduced). Products include:

Placidyl Capsules ... 448

Ethinamate (May produce additive depressant effects; respiratory depression, hypotension and profound sedation or coma may occur; the dose of one or both agents should be reduced).

No products indexed under this heading.

Fentanyl (May produce additive depressant effects; respiratory depression, hypotension and profound sedation or coma may occur; the dose of one or both agents should be reduced). Products include:

Duragesic Transdermal System ... 1288

Fentanyl Citrate (May produce additive depressant effects; respiratory depression, hypotension and profound sedation or coma may occur; the dose of one or both agents should be reduced). Products include:

Sublimaze Injection ... 1307

Fluphenazine Decanoate (May produce additive depressant effects; respiratory depression, hypotension and profound sedation or coma may occur; the dose of one or both agents should be reduced). Products include:

Prolixin Decanoate ... 509

Fluphenazine Enanthate (May produce additive depressant effects; respiratory depression, hypotension and profound sedation or coma may occur; the dose of one or both agents should be reduced). Products include:

Prolixin Enanthate ... 509

Fluphenazine Hydrochloride (May produce additive depressant effects; respiratory depression, hypotension and profound sedation or coma may occur; the dose of one or both agents should be reduced). Products include:

Prolixin ... 509

Flurazepam Hydrochloride (May produce additive depressant effects; respiratory depression, hypotension and profound sedation or coma may occur; the dose of one or both agents should be reduced). Products include:

Dalmane Capsules ... 2173

Glutethimide (May produce additive depressant effects; respiratory depression, hypotension and profound sedation or coma may occur; the dose of one or both agents should be reduced).

No products indexed under this heading.

Haloperidol (May produce additive depressant effects; respiratory depression, hypotension and profound sedation or coma may occur; the dose of one or both agents should be reduced). Products include:

Haldol Injection, Tablets and Concentrate ... 1575

Haloperidol Decanoate (May produce additive depressant effects; respiratory depression, hypotension and profound sedation or coma may occur; the dose of one or both agents should be reduced). Products include:

Haldol Decanoate ... 1577

IMPORTANT NOTE: Always consult each drug listing in the patient's regimen for possible interactions.

Dilaudid Tablets and Liquid Interactions Index 300

Hydrocodone Bitartrate (May produce additive depressant effects; respiratory depression, hypotension and profound sedation or coma may occur; the dose of one or both agents should be reduced). Products include:

Anexsia 5/500 Elixir ... 1781
Anexia Tablets ... 1782
Codiclear DH Syrup ... 791
Deconamine CX Cough and Cold Liquid and Tablets ... 1319
Duratuss HD Elixir ... 2565
Hycodan Tablets and Syrup ... 930
Hycomine Compound Tablets ... 932
Hycomine ... 931
Hycotuss Expectorant Syrup ... 933
Hydrocet Capsules ... 782
Lorcet 10/650 ... 1018
Lortab ... 2566
Tussend ... 1783
Tussend Expectorant ... 1785
Vicodin Tablets ... 1356
Vicodin ES Tablets ... 1357
Vicodin Tuss Expectorant ... 1358
Zydone Capsules ... 949

Hydrocodone Polistirex (May produce additive depressant effects; respiratory depression, hypotension and profound sedation or coma may occur; the dose of one or both agents should be reduced). Products include:

Tussionex Pennkinetic Extended-Release Suspension ... 998

Hydroxyzine Hydrochloride (May produce additive depressant effects; respiratory depression, hypotension and profound sedation or coma may occur; the dose of one or both agents should be reduced). Products include:

Atarax Tablets & Syrup ... 2185
Marax Tablets & DF Syrup ... 2200
Vistaril Intramuscular Solution ... 2216

Isoflurane (May produce additive depressant effects; respiratory depression, hypotension and profound sedation or coma may occur; the dose of one or both agents should be reduced).

No products indexed under this heading.

Ketamine Hydrochloride (May produce additive depressant effects; respiratory depression, hypotension and profound sedation or coma may occur; the dose of one or both agents should be reduced).

No products indexed under this heading.

Levomethadyl Acetate Hydrochloride (May produce additive depressant effects; respiratory depression, hypotension and profound sedation or coma may occur; the dose of one or both agents should be reduced). Products include:

Orlamm ... 2239

Levorphanol Tartrate (May produce additive depressant effects; respiratory depression, hypotension and profound sedation or coma may occur; the dose of one or both agents should be reduced). Products include:

Levo-Dromoran ... 2129

Lorazepam (May produce additive depressant effects; respiratory depression, hypotension and profound sedation or coma may occur; the dose of one or both agents should be reduced). Products include:

Ativan Injection ... 2698
Ativan Tablets ... 2700

Loxapine Hydrochloride (May produce additive depressant effects; respiratory depression, hypotension and profound sedation or coma may occur; the dose of one or both agents should be reduced). Products include:

Loxitane ... 1378

Loxapine Succinate (May produce additive depressant effects; respiratory depression, hypotension and profound sedation or coma may occur; the dose of one or both agents should be reduced). Products include:

Loxitane Capsules ... 1378

Meperidine Hydrochloride (May produce additive depressant effects; respiratory depression, hypotension and profound sedation or coma may occur; the dose of one or both agents should be reduced). Products include:

Demerol ... 2308
Mepergan Injection ... 2753

Mephobarbital (May produce additive depressant effects; respiratory depression, hypotension and profound sedation or coma may occur; the dose of one or both agents should be reduced). Products include:

Mebaral Tablets ... 2322

Meprobamate (May produce additive depressant effects; respiratory depression, hypotension and profound sedation or coma may occur; the dose of one or both agents should be reduced). Products include:

Miltown Tablets ... 2672
PMB 200 and PMB 400 ... 2783

Mesoridazine (May produce additive depressant effects; respiratory depression, hypotension and profound sedation or coma may occur; the dose of one or both agents should be reduced).

Mesoridazine Besylate (May produce additive depressant effects; respiratory depression, hypotension and profound sedation or coma may occur; the dose of one or both agents should be reduced). Products include:

Serentil ... 684

Methadone Hydrochloride (May produce additive depressant effects; respiratory depression, hypotension and profound sedation or coma may occur; the dose of one or both agents should be reduced). Products include:

Methadone Hydrochloride Oral Concentrate ... 2233
Methadone Hydrochloride Oral Solution & Tablets ... 2235

Methohexital Sodium (May produce additive depressant effects; respiratory depression, hypotension and profound sedation or coma may occur; the dose of one or both agents should be reduced). Products include:

Brevital Sodium Vials ... 1429

Methotrimeprazine (May produce additive depressant effects; respiratory depression, hypotension and profound sedation or coma may occur; the dose of one or both agents should be reduced). Products include:

Levoprome ... 1274

Methoxyflurane (May produce additive depressant effects; respiratory depression, hypotension and profound sedation or coma may occur; the dose of one or both agents should be reduced).

No products indexed under this heading.

Metocurine Iodide (Enhanced action of neuromuscular blocking agents and produce an excessive degree of respiratory depression). Products include:

Metubine Iodide Vials ... 916

Midazolam Hydrochloride (May produce additive depressant effects; respiratory depression, hypotension and profound sedation or coma may occur; the dose of one or both agents should be reduced). Products include:

Versed Injection ... 2170

Mivacurium Chloride (Enhanced action of neuromuscular blocking agents and produce an excessive degree of respiratory depression). Products include:

Mivacron ... 1138

Molindone Hydrochloride (May produce additive depressant effects; respiratory depression, hypotension and profound sedation or coma may occur; the dose of one or both agents should be reduced). Products include:

Moban Tablets and Concentrate ... 1048

Morphine Sulfate (May produce additive depressant effects; respiratory depression, hypotension and profound sedation or coma may occur; the dose of one or both agents should be reduced). Products include:

Astramorph/PF Injection, USP (Preservative-Free) ... 535
Duramorph ... 962
Infumorph 200 and Infumorph 500 Sterile Solutions ... 965
MS Contin Tablets ... 1994
MSIR ... 1997
Oramorph SR (Morphine Sulfate Sustained Release Tablets) ... 2236
RMS Suppositories ... 2657
Roxanol ... 2243

Opium Alkaloids (May produce additive depressant effects; respiratory depression, hypotension and profound sedation or coma may occur; the dose of one or both agents should be reduced).

No products indexed under this heading.

Oxazepam (May produce additive depressant effects; respiratory depression, hypotension and profound sedation or coma may occur; the dose of one or both agents should be reduced). Products include:

Serax Capsules ... 2810
Serax Tablets ... 2810

Oxycodone Hydrochloride (May produce additive depressant effects; respiratory depression, hypotension and profound sedation or coma may occur; the dose of one or both agents should be reduced). Products include:

Percocet Tablets ... 938
Percodan Tablets ... 939
Percodan-Demi Tablets ... 940
Roxicodone Tablets, Oral Solution & Intensol (Oxycodone) ... 2244
Tylox Capsules ... 1584

Pancuronium Bromide Injection (Enhanced action of neuromuscular blocking agents and produce an excessive degree of respiratory depression).

No products indexed under this heading.

Pentobarbital Sodium (May produce additive depressant effects; respiratory depression, hypotension and profound sedation or coma may occur; the dose of one or both agents should be reduced). Products include:

Nembutal Sodium Capsules ... 436
Nembutal Sodium Solution ... 438
Nembutal Sodium Suppositories ... 440

Perphenazine (May produce additive depressant effects; respiratory depression, hypotension and profound sedation or coma may occur; the dose of one or both agents should be reduced). Products include:

Etrafon ... 2355
Triavil Tablets ... 1757
Trilafon ... 2389

Phenobarbital (May produce additive depressant effects; respiratory depression, hypotension and profound sedation or coma may occur; the dose of one or both agents should be reduced). Products include:

Arco-Lase Plus Tablets ... 512
Bellergal-S Tablets ... 2250
Donnatal ... 2060
Donnatal Extentabs ... 2061
Donnatal Tablets ... 2060
Phenobarbital Elixir and Tablets ... 1469
Quadrinal Tablets ... 1350

Prazepam (May produce additive depressant effects; respiratory depression, hypotension and profound sedation or coma may occur; the dose of one or both agents should be reduced).

No products indexed under this heading.

Prochlorperazine (May produce additive depressant effects; respiratory depression, hypotension and profound sedation or coma may occur; the dose of one or both agents should be reduced). Products include:

Compazine ... 2470

Promethazine Hydrochloride (May produce additive depressant effects; respiratory depression, hypotension and profound sedation or coma may occur; the dose of one or both agents should be reduced). Products include:

Mepergan Injection ... 2753
Phenergan with Codeine ... 2777
Phenergan with Dextromethorphan 2778
Phenergan Injection ... 2773
Phenergan Suppositories ... 2775
Phenergan Syrup ... 2774
Phenergan Tablets ... 2775
Phenergan VC ... 2779
Phenergan VC with Codeine ... 2781

Propofol (May produce additive depressant effects; respiratory depression, hypotension and profound sedation or coma may occur; the dose of one or both agents should be reduced). Products include:

Diprivan Injection ... 2833

Propoxyphene Hydrochloride (May produce additive depressant effects; respiratory depression, hypotension and profound sedation or coma may occur; the dose of one or both agents should be reduced). Products include:

Darvon ... 1435
Wygesic Tablets ... 2827

Propoxyphene Napsylate (May produce additive depressant effects; respiratory depression, hypotension and profound sedation or coma may occur; the dose of one or both agents should be reduced). Products include:

Darvon-N/Darvocet-N ... 1433

(Described in PDR For Nonprescription Drugs) (◉ Described in PDR For Ophthalmology)

301 Interactions Index Dimetane-DC

Quazepam (May produce additive depressant effects; respiratory depression, hypotension and profound sedation or coma may occur; the dose of one or both agents should be reduced). Products include:
Doral Tablets 2664
Risperidone (May produce additive depressant effects; respiratory depression, hypotension and profound sedation or coma may occur; the dose of one or both agents should be reduced). Products include:
Risperdal 1301
Rocuronium Bromide (Enhanced action of neuromuscular blocking agents and produce an excessive degree of respiratory depression). Products include:
Zemuron 1830
Secobarbital Sodium (May produce additive depressant effects; respiratory depression, hypotension and profound sedation or coma may occur; the dose of one or both agents should be reduced). Products include:
Seconal Sodium Pulvules 1474
Succinylcholine Chloride (Enhanced action of neuromuscular blocking agents and produce an excessive degree of respiratory depression). Products include:
Anectine 1073
Sufentanil Citrate (May produce additive depressant effects; respiratory depression, hypotension and profound sedation or coma may occur; the dose of one or both agents should be reduced). Products include:
Sufenta Injection 1309
Temazepam (May produce additive depressant effects; respiratory depression, hypotension and profound sedation or coma may occur; the dose of one or both agents should be reduced). Products include:
Restoril Capsules 2284
Thiamylal Sodium (May produce additive depressant effects; respiratory depression, hypotension and profound sedation or coma may occur; the dose of one or both agents should be reduced).
No products indexed under this heading.
Thioridazine Hydrochloride (May produce additive depressant effects; respiratory depression, hypotension and profound sedation or coma may occur; the dose of one or both agents should be reduced). Products include:
Mellaril 2269
Thiothixene (May produce additive depressant effects; respiratory depression, hypotension and profound sedation or coma may occur; the dose of one or both agents should be reduced). Products include:
Navane Capsules and Concentrate 2201
Navane Intramuscular 2202
Triazolam (May produce additive depressant effects; respiratory depression, hypotension and profound sedation or coma may occur; the dose of one or both agents should be reduced). Products include:
Halcion Tablets 2611
Trifluoperazine Hydrochloride (May produce additive depressant effects; respiratory depression, hypotension and profound sedation or coma may occur; the dose of one or both agents should be reduced). Products include:
Stelazine 2514
Vecuronium Bromide (Enhanced action of neuromuscular blocking agents and produce an excessive degree of respiratory depression). Products include:
Norcuron 1826
Zolpidem Tartrate (May produce additive depressant effects; respiratory depression, hypotension and profound sedation or coma may occur; the dose of one or both agents should be reduced). Products include:
Ambien Tablets 2416

Food Interactions
Alcohol (May exhibit an additive CNS depression).

DILAUDID POWDER
(Hydromorphone Hydrochloride) 1335
See **Dilaudid Ampules**

DILAUDID RECTAL SUPPOSITORIES
(Hydromorphone Hydrochloride) 1335
See **Dilaudid Ampules**

DILAUDID TABLETS 2MG AND 4MG
(Hydromorphone Hydrochloride) 1335
See **Dilaudid Ampules**

DILAUDID TABLETS - 8 MG
(Hydromorphone Hydrochloride) 1339
See **Dilaudid Oral Liquid**

DIMETANE-DC COUGH SYRUP
(Brompheniramine Maleate, Phenylpropanolamine Hydrochloride, Codeine Phosphate) 2059
May interact with hypnotics and sedatives, tranquilizers, benzodiazepines, monoamine oxidase inhibitors, antihypertensives, central nervous system depressants, and certain other agents. Compounds in these categories include:
Acebutolol Hydrochloride (Reduced antihypertensive effects). Products include:
Sectral Capsules 2807
Alfentanil Hydrochloride (Additive effects). Products include:
Alfenta Injection 1286
Alprazolam (Additive effects). Products include:
Xanax Tablets 2649
Amlodipine Besylate (Reduced antihypertensive effects). Products include:
Lotrel Capsules 840
Norvasc Tablets 1940
Aprobarbital (Additive effects).
No products indexed under this heading.
Atenolol (Reduced antihypertensive effects). Products include:
Tenoretic Tablets 2845
Tenormin Tablets and I.V. Injection 2847
Benazepril Hydrochloride (Reduced antihypertensive effects). Products include:
Lotensin Tablets 834
Lotensin HCT 837
Lotrel Capsules 840
Bendroflumethiazide (Reduced antihypertensive effects).
No products indexed under this heading.
Betaxolol Hydrochloride (Reduced antihypertensive effects). Products include:
Betoptic Ophthalmic Solution 469
Betoptic S Ophthalmic Suspension 471
Kerlone Tablets 2436
Bisoprolol Fumarate (Reduced antihypertensive effects). Products include:
Zebeta Tablets 1413
Ziac 1415
Buprenorphine (Additive effects). Products include:
Buprenex Injectable 2006
Buspirone Hydrochloride (Additive effects). Products include:
BuSpar 737
Butabarbital (Additive effects).
No products indexed under this heading.
Butalbital (Additive effects). Products include:
Esgic-plus Tablets 1013
Fioricet Tablets 2258
Fioricet with Codeine Capsules 2260
Fiorinal Capsules 2261
Fiorinal with Codeine Capsules 2262
Fiorinal Tablets 2261
Phrenilin 785
Sedapap Tablets 50 mg/650 mg .. 1543
Captopril (Reduced antihypertensive effects). Products include:
Capoten 739
Capozide 742
Carteolol Hydrochloride (Reduced antihypertensive effects). Products include:
Cartrol Tablets 410
Ocupress Ophthalmic Solution, 1% Sterile .... ⊙ 309
Chlordiazepoxide (Additive effects). Products include:
Libritabs Tablets 2177
Limbitrol 2180
Chlordiazepoxide Hydrochloride (Additive effects). Products include:
Librax Capsules 2176
Librium Capsules 2178
Librium Injectable 2179
Chlorothiazide (Reduced antihypertensive effects). Products include:
Aldoclor Tablets 1598
Diupres Tablets 1650
Diuril Oral 1653
Chlorothiazide Sodium (Reduced antihypertensive effects). Products include:
Diuril Sodium Intravenous 1652
Chlorpromazine (Additive effects). Products include:
Thorazine Suppositories 2523
Chlorprothixene (Additive effects).
No products indexed under this heading.
Chlorprothixene Hydrochloride (Additive effects).
No products indexed under this heading.
Chlorthalidone (Reduced antihypertensive effects). Products include:
Combipres Tablets 677
Tenoretic Tablets 2845
Thalitone 1245
Clonidine (Reduced antihypertensive effects). Products include:
Catapres-TTS 675
Clonidine Hydrochloride (Additive effects; reduced antihypertensive effects). Products include:
Catapres Tablets 674
Combipres Tablets 677
Clorazepate Dipotassium (Additive effects). Products include:
Tranxene 451
Clozapine (Additive effects). Products include:
Clozaril Tablets 2252
Deserpidine (Reduced antihypertensive effects).
No products indexed under this heading.
Desflurane (Additive effects). Products include:
Suprane 1813
Dezocine (Additive effects). Products include:
Dalgan Injection 538
Diazepam (Additive effects). Products include:
Dizac 1809
Valium Injectable 2182
Valium Tablets 2183
Valrelease Capsules 2169
Diazoxide (Reduced antihypertensive effects). Products include:
Hyperstat I.V. Injection 2363
Proglycem 580
Diltiazem Hydrochloride (Reduced antihypertensive effects). Products include:
Cardizem CD Capsules 1506
Cardizem SR Capsules 1510
Cardizem Injectable 1508
Cardizem Tablets 1512
Dilacor XR Extended-release Capsules 2018
Doxazosin Mesylate (Reduced antihypertensive effects). Products include:
Cardura Tablets 2186
Droperidol (Additive effects). Products include:
Inapsine Injection 1296
Enalapril Maleate (Reduced antihypertensive effects). Products include:
Vaseretic Tablets 1765
Vasotec Tablets 1771
Enalaprilat (Reduced antihypertensive effects). Products include:
Vasotec I.V. 1768
Enflurane (Additive effects).
No products indexed under this heading.
Esmolol Hydrochloride (Reduced antihypertensive effects). Products include:
Brevibloc Injection 1808
Estazolam (Additive effects). Products include:
ProSom Tablets 449
Ethchlorvynol (Additive effects). Products include:
Placidyl Capsules 448
Ethinamate (Additive effects).
No products indexed under this heading.
Felodipine (Reduced antihypertensive effects). Products include:
Plendil Extended-Release Tablets 527
Fentanyl (Additive effects). Products include:
Duragesic Transdermal System 1288
Fentanyl Citrate (Additive effects). Products include:
Sublimaze Injection 1307
Fluphenazine Decanoate (Additive effects). Products include:
Prolixin Decanoate 509
Fluphenazine Enanthate (Additive effects). Products include:
Prolixin Enanthate 509
Fluphenazine Hydrochloride (Additive effects). Products include:
Prolixin 509
Flurazepam Hydrochloride (Additive effects). Products include:
Dalmane Capsules 2173

IMPORTANT NOTE: Always consult each drug listing in the patient's regimen for possible interactions.

Dimetane-DC Interactions Index 302

Fosinopril Sodium (Reduced antihypertensive effects). Products include:
Monopril Tablets ... 757

Furazolidone (Enhances phenylpropanolamine's effect and anticholinergic effects of antihistamines). Products include:
Furoxone ... 2046

Furosemide (Reduced antihypertensive effects). Products include:
Lasix Injection, Oral Solution and Tablets ... 1240

Glutethimide (Additive effects).
No products indexed under this heading.

Guanabenz Acetate (Reduced antihypertensive effects).
No products indexed under this heading.

Guanethidine Monosulfate (Reduced antihypertensive effects). Products include:
Esimil Tablets ... 822
Ismelin Tablets ... 827

Halazepam (Additive effects).
No products indexed under this heading.

Haloperidol (Additive effects). Products include:
Haldol Injection, Tablets and Concentrate ... 1575

Haloperidol Decanoate (Additive effects). Products include:
Haldol Decanoate ... 1577

Hydralazine Hydrochloride (Reduced antihypertensive effects). Products include:
Apresazide Capsules ... 808
Apresoline Hydrochloride Tablets ... 809
Ser-Ap-Es Tablets ... 849

Hydrochlorothiazide (Reduced antihypertensive effects). Products include:
Aldactazide ... 2413
Aldoril Tablets ... 1604
Apresazide Capsules ... 808
Capozide ... 742
Dyazide ... 2479
Esidrix Tablets ... 821
Esimil Tablets ... 822
HydroDIURIL Tablets ... 1674
Hydropres Tablets ... 1675
Hyzaar Tablets ... 1677
Inderide Tablets ... 2732
Inderide LA Long Acting Capsules ... 2734
Lopressor HCT Tablets ... 832
Lotensin HCT ... 837
Maxzide ... 1380
Moduretic Tablets ... 1705
Oretic Tablets ... 443
Prinzide Tablets ... 1737
Ser-Ap-Es Tablets ... 849
Timolide Tablets ... 1748
Vaseretic Tablets ... 1765
Zestoretic ... 2850
Ziac ... 1415

Hydrocodone Bitartrate (Additive effects). Products include:
Anexsia 5/500 Elixir ... 1781
Anexia Tablets ... 1782
Codiclear DH Syrup ... 791
Deconamine CX Cough and Cold Liquid and Tablets ... 1319
Duratuss HD Elixir ... 2565
Hycodan Tablets and Syrup ... 930
Hycomine Compound Tablets ... 932
Hycomine ... 931
Hycotuss Expectorant Syrup ... 933
Hydrocet Capsules ... 782
Lorcet 10/650 ... 1018
Lortab ... 2566
Tussend ... 1783
Tussend Expectorant ... 1785
Vicodin Tablets ... 1356
Vicodin ES Tablets ... 1357
Vicodin Tuss Expectorant ... 1358
Zydone Capsules ... 949

Hydrocodone Polistirex (Additive effects). Products include:
Tussionex Pennkinetic Extended-Release Suspension ... 998

Hydroflumethiazide (Reduced antihypertensive effects). Products include:
Diucardin Tablets ... 2718

Hydroxyzine Hydrochloride (Additive effects). Products include:
Atarax Tablets & Syrup ... 2185
Marax Tablets & DF Syrup ... 2200
Vistaril Intramuscular Solution ... 2216

Indapamide (Reduced antihypertensive effects). Products include:
Lozol Tablets ... 2022

Isocarboxazid (Enhances phenylpropanolamine's effect and anticholinergic effects of antihistamines).
No products indexed under this heading.

Isoflurane (Additive effects).
No products indexed under this heading.

Isoproterenol Hydrochloride (Reduced effects of antihypertensive drugs). Products include:
Isuprel Hydrochloride Injection 1:5000 ... 2311
Isuprel Hydrochloride Solution 1:200 & 1:100 ... 2313
Isuprel Mistometer ... 2312

Isoproterenol Sulfate (Reduced effects of antihypeertensive drugs). Products include:
Norisodrine with Calcium Iodide Syrup ... 442

Isradipine (Reduced antihypertensive effects). Products include:
DynaCirc Capsules ... 2256

Ketamine Hydrochloride (Additive effects).
No products indexed under this heading.

Labetalol Hydrochloride (Reduced antihypertensive effects). Products include:
Normodyne Injection ... 2377
Normodyne Tablets ... 2379
Trandate ... 1185

Levomethadyl Acetate Hydrochloride (Additive effects). Products include:
Orlamm ... 2239

Levorphanol Tartrate (Additive effects). Products include:
Levo-Dromoran ... 2129

Lisinopril (Reduced antihypertensive effects). Products include:
Prinivil Tablets ... 1733
Prinzide Tablets ... 1737
Zestoretic ... 2850
Zestril Tablets ... 2854

Lorazepam (Additive effects). Products include:
Ativan Injection ... 2698
Ativan Tablets ... 2700

Losartan Potassium (Reduced antihypertensive effects). Products include:
Cozaar Tablets ... 1628
Hyzaar Tablets ... 1677

Loxapine Hydrochloride (Additive effects). Products include:
Loxitane ... 1378

Loxapine Succinate (Additive effects). Products include:
Loxitane Capsules ... 1378

Mecamylamine Hydrochloride (Reduced antihypertensive effects). Products include:
Inversine Tablets ... 1686

Meperidine Hydrochloride (Additive effects). Products include:
Demerol ... 2308
Mepergan Injection ... 2753

Mephobarbital (Additive effects). Products include:
Mebaral Tablets ... 2322

Meprobamate (Additive effects). Products include:
Miltown Tablets ... 2672
PMB 200 and PMB 400 ... 2783

Mesoridazine Besylate (Additive effects). Products include:
Serentil ... 684

Methadone Hydrochloride (Additive effects). Products include:
Methadone Hydrochloride Oral Concentrate ... 2233
Methadone Hydrochloride Oral Solution & Tablets ... 2235

Methohexital Sodium (Additive effects). Products include:
Brevital Sodium Vials ... 1429

Methotrimeprazine (Additive effects). Products include:
Levoprome ... 1274

Methoxyflurane (Additive effects).
No products indexed under this heading.

Methyclothiazide (Reduced antihypertensive effects). Products include:
Enduron Tablets ... 420

Methyldopa (Reduced antihypertensive effects). Products include:
Aldoclor Tablets ... 1598
Aldomet Oral ... 1600
Aldoril Tablets ... 1604

Methyldopate Hydrochloride (Reduced antihypertensive effects). Products include:
Aldomet Ester HCl Injection ... 1602

Metolazone (Reduced antihypertensive effects). Products include:
Mykrox Tablets ... 993
Zaroxolyn Tablets ... 1000

Metoprolol Succinate (Reduced antihypertensive effects). Products include:
Toprol-XL Tablets ... 565

Metoprolol Tartrate (Reduced antihypertensive effects). Products include:
Lopressor Ampuls ... 830
Lopressor HCT Tablets ... 832
Lopressor Tablets ... 830

Midazolam Hydrochloride (Additive effects). Products include:
Versed Injection ... 2170

Minoxidil (Reduced antihypertensive effects). Products include:
Loniten Tablets ... 2618
Rogaine Topical Solution ... 2637

Moexipril Hydrochloride (Reduced antihypertensive effects). Products include:
Univasc Tablets ... 2410

Molindone Hydrochloride (Additive effects). Products include:
Moban Tablets and Concentrate ... 1048

Morphine Sulfate (Additive effects). Products include:
Astramorph/PF Injection, USP (Preservative-Free) ... 535
Duramorph ... 962
Infumorph 200 and Infumorph 500 Sterile Solutions ... 965
MS Contin Tablets ... 1994
MSIR ... 1997
Oramorph SR (Morphine Sulfate Sustained Release Tablets) ... 2236
RMS Suppositories ... 2657
Roxanol ... 2243

Nadolol (Reduced antihypertensive effects).
No products indexed under this heading.

Nicardipine Hydrochloride (Reduced antihypertensive effects). Products include:
Cardene Capsules ... 2095
Cardene I.V. ... 2709
Cardene SR Capsules ... 2097

Nifedipine (Reduced antihypertensive effects). Products include:
Adalat Capsules (10 mg and 20 mg) ... 587
Adalat CC ... 589
Procardia Capsules ... 1971
Procardia XL Extended Release Tablets ... 1972

Nisoldipine (Reduced antihypertensive effects).
No products indexed under this heading.

Nitroglycerin (Reduced antihypertensive effects). Products include:
Deponit NTG Transdermal Delivery System ... 2397
Nitro-Bid IV ... 1523
Nitro-Bid Ointment ... 1524
Nitrodisc ... 2047
Nitro-Dur (nitroglycerin) Transdermal Infusion System ... 1326
Nitrolingual Spray ... 2027
Nitrostat Tablets ... 1925
Transderm-Nitro Transdermal Therapeutic System ... 859

Opium Alkaloids (Additive effects).
No products indexed under this heading.

Oxazepam (Additive effects). Products include:
Serax Capsules ... 2810
Serax Tablets ... 2810

Oxycodone Hydrochloride (Additive effects). Products include:
Percocet Tablets ... 938
Percodan Tablets ... 939
Percodan-Demi Tablets ... 940
Roxicodone Tablets, Oral Solution & Intensol (Oxycodone) ... 2244
Tylox Capsules ... 1584

Penbutolol Sulfate (Reduced antihypertensive effects). Products include:
Levatol ... 2403

Pentobarbital Sodium (Additive effects). Products include:
Nembutal Sodium Capsules ... 436
Nembutal Sodium Solution ... 438
Nembutal Sodium Suppositories ... 440

Perphenazine (Additive effects). Products include:
Etrafon ... 2355
Triavil Tablets ... 1757
Trilafon ... 2389

Phenelzine Sulfate (Enhances phenylpropanolamine's effect and anticholinergic effects of antihistamines). Products include:
Nardil ... 1920

Phenobarbital (Additive effects). Products include:
Arco-Lase Plus Tablets ... 512
Bellergal-S Tablets ... 2250
Donnatal ... 2060
Donnatal Extentabs ... 2061
Donnatal Tablets ... 2060
Phenobarbital Elixir and Tablets ... 1469
Quadrinal Tablets ... 1350

Phenoxybenzamine Hydrochloride (Reduced antihypertensive effects). Products include:
Dibenzyline Capsules ... 2476

Phentolamine Mesylate (Reduced antihypertensive effects). Products include:
Regitine ... 846

Pindolol (Reduced antihypertensive effects). Products include:
Visken Tablets ... 2299

Polythiazide (Reduced antihypertensive effects). Products include:
Minizide Capsules ... 1938

Prazepam (Additive effects).
No products indexed under this heading.

Prazosin Hydrochloride (Reduced antihypertensive effects). Products include:
Minipress Capsules ... 1937
Minizide Capsules ... 1938

Prochlorperazine (Additive effects). Products include:
Compazine ... 2470

Promethazine Hydrochloride (Additive effects). Products include:
Mepergan Injection ... 2753
Phenergan with Codeine ... 2777
Phenergan with Dextromethorphan 2778

303 **Interactions Index** **Dimetane-DX**

Phenergan Injection 2773
Phenergan Suppositories 2775
Phenergan Syrup 2774
Phenergan Tablets 2775
Phenergan VC 2779
Phenergan VC with Codeine 2781

Propofol (Additive effects). Products include:
Diprivan Injection 2833

Propoxyphene Hydrochloride (Additive effects). Products include:
Darvon 1435
Wygesic Tablets 2827

Propoxyphene Napsylate (Additive effects). Products include:
Darvon-N/Darvocet-N 1433

Propranolol Hydrochloride (Reduced antihypertensive effects). Products include:
Inderal 2728
Inderal LA Long Acting Capsules 2730
Inderide Tablets 2732
Inderide LA Long Acting Capsules 2734

Quazepam (Additive effects). Products include:
Doral Tablets 2664

Quinapril Hydrochloride (Reduced antihypertensive effects). Products include:
Accupril Tablets 1893

Ramipril (Reduced antihypertensive effects). Products include:
Altace Capsules 1232

Rauwolfia Serpentina (Reduced antihypertensive effects).
No products indexed under this heading.

Rescinnamine (Reduced antihypertensive effects).
No products indexed under this heading.

Reserpine (Reduced antihypertensive effects). Products include:
Diupres Tablets 1650
Hydropres Tablets 1675
Ser-Ap-Es Tablets 849

Risperidone (Additive effects). Products include:
Risperdal 1301

Secobarbital Sodium (Additive effects). Products include:
Seconal Sodium Pulvules 1474

Selegiline Hydrochloride (Enhances phenylpropanolamine's effect and anticholinergic effects of antihistamines). Products include:
Eldepryl Tablets 2550

Sodium Nitroprusside (Reduced antihypertensive effects).
No products indexed under this heading.

Sotalol Hydrochloride (Reduced antihypertensive effects). Products include:
Betapace Tablets 641

Spirapril Hydrochloride (Reduced antihypertensive effects).
No products indexed under this heading.

Sufentanil Citrate (Additive effects). Products include:
Sufenta Injection 1309

Temazepam (Additive effects). Products include:
Restoril Capsules 2284

Terazosin Hydrochloride (Reduced antihypertensive effects). Products include:
Hytrin Capsules 430

Thiamylal Sodium (Additive effects).
No products indexed under this heading.

Thioridazine Hydrochloride (Additive effects). Products include:
Mellaril 2269

Thiothixene (Additive effects). Products include:
Navane Capsules and Concentrate 2201
Navane Intramuscular 2202

Timolol Maleate (Reduced antihypertensive effects). Products include:
Blocadren Tablets 1614
Timolide Tablets 1748
Timoptic in Ocudose 1753
Timoptic Sterile Ophthalmic Solution 1751
Timoptic-XE 1755

Torsemide (Reduced antihypertensive effects). Products include:
Demadex Tablets and Injection 686

Tranylcypromine Sulfate (Enhances phenylpropanolamine's effect and anticholinergic effects of antihistamines). Products include:
Parnate Tablets 2503

Triazolam (Additive effects). Products include:
Halcion Tablets 2611

Trifluoperazine Hydrochloride (Additive effects). Products include:
Stelazine 2514

Trimethaphan Camsylate (Reduced antihypertensive effects). Products include:
Arfonad Ampuls 2080

Verapamil Hydrochloride (Reduced antihypertensive effects). Products include:
Calan SR Caplets 2422
Calan Tablets 2419
Isoptin Injectable 1344
Isoptin Oral Tablets 1346
Isoptin SR Tablets 1348
Verelan Capsules 1410
Verelan Capsules 2824

Zolpidem Tartrate (Additive effects). Products include:
Ambien Tablets 2416

Food Interactions

Alcohol (Additive effects).

DIMETANE-DX COUGH SYRUP

(Brompheniramine Maleate, Pseudoephedrine Hydrochloride, Dextromethorphan Hydrobromide)....2059
May interact with monoamine oxidase inhibitors, central nervous system depressants, and antihypertensives. Compounds in these categories include:

Acebutolol Hydrochloride (Decreased antihypertensive effect). Products include:
Sectral Capsules 2807

Alfentanil Hydrochloride (Additive effect). Products include:
Alfenta Injection 1286

Alprazolam (Additive effect). Products include:
Xanax Tablets 2649

Amlodipine Besylate (Decreased antihypertensive effect). Products include:
Lotrel Capsules 840
Norvasc Tablets 1940

Aprobarbital (Additive effect).
No products indexed under this heading.

Atenolol (Decreased antihypertensive effect). Products include:
Tenoretic Tablets 2845
Tenormin Tablets and I.V. Injection 2847

Benazepril Hydrochloride (Decreased antihypertensive effect). Products include:
Lotensin Tablets 834
Lotensin HCT 837
Lotrel Capsules 840

Bendroflumethiazide (Decreased antihypertensive effect).
No products indexed under this heading.

Betaxolol Hydrochloride (Decreased antihypertensive effect). Products include:
Betoptic Ophthalmic Solution 469
Betoptic S Ophthalmic Suspension 471
Kerlone Tablets 2436

Bisoprolol Fumarate (Decreased antihypertensive effect). Products include:
Zebeta Tablets 1413
Ziac 1415

Buprenorphine (Additive effect). Products include:
Buprenex Injectable 2006

Buspirone Hydrochloride (Additive effect). Products include:
BuSpar 737

Butabarbital (Additive effect).
No products indexed under this heading.

Butalbital (Additive effect). Products include:
Esgic-plus Tablets 1013
Fioricet Tablets 2258
Fioricet with Codeine Capsules 2260
Fiorinal Capsules 2261
Fiorinal with Codeine Capsules 2262
Fiorinal Tablets 2261
Phrenilin 785
Sedapap Tablets 50 mg/650 mg 1543

Captopril (Decreased antihypertensive effect). Products include:
Capoten 739
Capozide 742

Carteolol Hydrochloride (Decreased antihypertensive effect). Products include:
Cartrol Tablets 410
Ocupress Ophthalmic Solution, 1% Sterile .... ◉ 309

Chlordiazepoxide (Additive effect). Products include:
Libritabs Tablets 2177
Limbitrol 2180

Chlordiazepoxide Hydrochloride (Additive effect). Products include:
Librax Capsules 2176
Librium Capsules 2178
Librium Injectable 2179

Chlorothiazide (Decreased antihypertensive effect). Products include:
Aldoclor Tablets 1598
Diupres Tablets 1650
Diuril Oral 1653

Chlorothiazide Sodium (Decreased antihypertensive effect). Products include:
Diuril Sodium Intravenous 1652

Chlorpromazine (Additive effect). Products include:
Thorazine Suppositories 2523

Chlorprothixene (Additive effect).
No products indexed under this heading.

Chlorprothixene Hydrochloride (Additive effect).
No products indexed under this heading.

Chlorthalidone (Decreased antihypertensive effect). Products include:
Combipres Tablets 677
Tenoretic Tablets 2845
Thalitone 1245

Clonidine (Decreased antihypertensive effect). Products include:
Catapres-TTS 675

Clonidine Hydrochloride (Decreased antihypertensive effect). Products include:
Catapres Tablets 674
Combipres Tablets 677

Clorazepate Dipotassium (Additive effect). Products include:
Tranxene 451

Clozapine (Additive effect). Products include:
Clozaril Tablets 2252

Codeine Phosphate (Additive effect). Products include:
Actifed with Codeine Cough Syrup 1067
Brontex 1981
Deconsal C Expectorant Syrup 456
Deconsal Pediatric Syrup 457
Dimetane-DC Cough Syrup 2059
Empirin with Codeine Tablets 1093
Fioricet with Codeine Capsules 2260
Fiorinal with Codeine Capsules 2262
Isoclor Expectorant 990
Novahistine DH 2462
Novahistine Expectorant 2463
Nucofed 2051
Phenergan with Codeine 2777
Phenergan VC with Codeine 2781
Robitussin A-C Syrup 2073
Robitussin-DAC Syrup 2074
Ryna .... ▣ 841
Soma Compound w/Codeine Tablets 2676
Tussi-Organidin NR Liquid and S NR Liquid 2677
Tylenol with Codeine 1583

Deserpidine (Decreased antihypertensive effect).
No products indexed under this heading.

Desflurane (Additive effect). Products include:
Suprane 1813

Dezocine (Additive effect). Products include:
Dalgan Injection 538

Diazepam (Additive effect). Products include:
Dizac 1809
Valium Injectable 2182
Valium Tablets 2183
Valrelease Capsules 2169

Diazoxide (Decreased antihypertensive effect). Products include:
Hyperstat I.V. Injection 2363
Proglycem 580

Diltiazem Hydrochloride (Decreased antihypertensive effect). Products include:
Cardizem CD Capsules 1506
Cardizem SR Capsules 1510
Cardizem Injectable 1508
Cardizem Tablets 1512
Dilacor XR Extended-release Capsules 2018

Doxazosin Mesylate (Decreased antihypertensive effect). Products include:
Cardura Tablets 2186

Droperidol (Additive effect). Products include:
Inapsine Injection 1296

Enalapril Maleate (Decreased antihypertensive effect). Products include:
Vaseretic Tablets 1765
Vasotec Tablets 1771

Enalaprilat (Decreased antihypertensive effect). Products include:
Vasotec I.V. 1768

Enflurane (Additive effect).
No products indexed under this heading.

Esmolol Hydrochloride (Decreased antihypertensive effect). Products include:
Brevibloc Injection 1808

Estazolam (Additive effect). Products include:
ProSom Tablets 449

Ethchlorvynol (Additive effect). Products include:
Placidyl Capsules 448

Ethinamate (Additive effect).
No products indexed under this heading.

Felodipine (Decreased antihypertensive effect). Products include:
Plendil Extended-Release Tablets 527

IMPORTANT NOTE: Always consult each drug listing in the patient's regimen for possible interactions.

Dimetane-DX **Interactions Index** **304**

Fentanyl (Additive effect). Products include:
Duragesic Transdermal System 1288

Fentanyl Citrate (Additive effect). Products include:
Sublimaze Injection 1307

Fluphenazine Decanoate (Additive effect). Products include:
Prolixin Decanoate 509

Fluphenazine Enanthate (Additive effect). Products include:
Prolixin Enanthate 509

Fluphenazine Hydrochloride (Additive effect). Products include:
Prolixin 509

Flurazepam Hydrochloride (Additive effect). Products include:
Dalmane Capsules 2173

Fosinopril Sodium (Decreased antihypertensive effect). Products include:
Monopril Tablets 757

Furazolidone (Prolonged anticholinergic effect). Products include:
Furoxone 2046

Furosemide (Decreased antihypertensive effect). Products include:
Lasix Injection, Oral Solution and Tablets 1240

Glutethimide (Additive effect).
No products indexed under this heading.

Guanabenz Acetate (Decreased antihypertensive effect).
No products indexed under this heading.

Guanethidine Monosulfate (Decreased antihypertensive effect). Products include:
Esimil Tablets 822
Ismelin Tablets 827

Haloperidol (Additive effect). Products include:
Haldol Injection, Tablets and Concentrate 1575

Haloperidol Decanoate (Additive effect). Products include:
Haldol Decanoate 1577

Hydralazine Hydrochloride (Decreased antihypertensive effect). Products include:
Apresazide Capsules 808
Apresoline Hydrochloride Tablets .. 809
Ser-Ap-Es Tablets 849

Hydrochlorothiazide (Decreased antihypertensive effect). Products include:
Aldactazide 2413
Aldoril Tablets 1604
Apresazide Capsules 808
Capozide 742
Dyazide 2479
Esidrix Tablets 821
Esimil Tablets 822
HydroDIURIL Tablets 1674
Hydropres Tablets 1675
Hyzaar Tablets 1677
Inderide Tablets 2732
Inderide LA Long Acting Capsules .. 2734
Lopressor HCT Tablets 832
Lotensin HCT 837
Maxzide 1380
Moduretic Tablets 1705
Oretic Tablets 443
Prinzide Tablets 1737
Ser-Ap-Es Tablets 849
Timolide Tablets 1748
Vaseretic Tablets 1765
Zestoretic 2850
Ziac 1415

Hydrocodone Bitartrate (Additive effect). Products include:
Anexsia 5/500 Elixir 1781
Anexia Tablets 1782
Codiclear DH Syrup 791
Deconamine CX Cough and Cold Liquid and Tablets 1319
Duratuss HD Elixir 2565
Hycodan Tablets and Syrup 930
Hycomine Compound Tablets 932
Hycomine 931
Hycotuss Expectorant Syrup 933
Hydrocet Capsules 782
Lorcet 10/650 1018
Lortab 2566
Tussend 1783
Tussend Expectorant 1785
Vicodin Tablets 1356
Vicodin ES Tablets 1357
Vicodin Tuss Expectorant 1358
Zydone Capsules 949

Hydrocodone Polistirex (Additive effect). Products include:
Tussionex Pennkinetic Extended-Release Suspension 998

Hydroflumethiazide (Decreased antihypertensive effect). Products include:
Diucardin Tablets 2718

Hydroxyzine Hydrochloride (Additive effect). Products include:
Atarax Tablets & Syrup 2185
Marax Tablets & DF Syrup 2200
Vistaril Intramuscular Solution 2216

Indapamide (Decreased antihypertensive effect). Products include:
Lozol Tablets 2022

Isocarboxazid (Prolonged anticholinergic effect).
No products indexed under this heading.

Isoflurane (Additive effect).
No products indexed under this heading.

Isradipine (Decreased antihypertensive effect). Products include:
DynaCirc Capsules 2256

Ketamine Hydrochloride (Additive effect).
No products indexed under this heading.

Labetalol Hydrochloride (Decreased antihypertensive effect). Products include:
Normodyne Injection 2377
Normodyne Tablets 2379
Trandate 1185

Levomethadyl Acetate Hydrochloride (Additive effect). Products include:
Orlamm 2239

Levorphanol Tartrate (Additive effect). Products include:
Levo-Dromoran 2129

Lisinopril (Decreased antihypertensive effect). Products include:
Prinivil Tablets 1733
Prinzide Tablets 1737
Zestoretic 2850
Zestril Tablets 2854

Lorazepam (Additive effect). Products include:
Ativan Injection 2698
Ativan Tablets 2700

Losartan Potassium (Decreased antihypertensive effect). Products include:
Cozaar Tablets 1628
Hyzaar Tablets 1677

Loxapine Hydrochloride (Additive effect). Products include:
Loxitane 1378

Loxapine Succinate (Additive effect). Products include:
Loxitane Capsules 1378

Mecamylamine Hydrochloride (Decreased antihypertensive effect). Products include:
Inversine Tablets 1686

Meperidine Hydrochloride (Additive effect). Products include:
Demerol 2308
Mepergan Injection 2753

Mephobarbital (Additive effect). Products include:
Mebaral Tablets 2322

Meprobamate (Additive effect). Products include:
Miltown Tablets 2672
PMB 200 and PMB 400 2783

Mesoridazine Besylate (Additive effect). Products include:
Serentil 684

Methadone Hydrochloride (Additive effect). Products include:
Methadone Hydrochloride Oral Concentrate 2233
Methadone Hydrochloride Oral Solution & Tablets 2235

Methohexital Sodium (Additive effect). Products include:
Brevital Sodium Vials 1429

Methotrimeprazine (Additive effect). Products include:
Levoprome 1274

Methoxyflurane (Additive effect).
No products indexed under this heading.

Methyclothiazide (Decreased antihypertensive effect). Products include:
Enduron Tablets 420

Methyldopa (Decreased antihypertensive effect). Products include:
Aldoclor Tablets 1598
Aldomet Oral 1600
Aldoril Tablets 1604

Methyldopate Hydrochloride (Decreased antihypertensive effect). Products include:
Aldomet Ester HCl Injection 1602

Metolazone (Decreased antihypertensive effect). Products include:
Mykrox Tablets 993
Zaroxolyn Tablets 1000

Metoprolol Succinate (Decreased antihypertensive effect). Products include:
Toprol-XL Tablets 565

Metoprolol Tartrate (Decreased antihypertensive effect). Products include:
Lopressor Ampuls 830
Lopressor HCT Tablets 832
Lopressor Tablets 830

Metyrosine (Decreased antihypertensive effect). Products include:
Demser Capsules 1649

Midazolam Hydrochloride (Additive effect). Products include:
Versed Injection 2170

Minoxidil (Decreased antihypertensive effect). Products include:
Loniten Tablets 2618
Rogaine Topical Solution 2637

Moexipril Hydrochloride (Decreased antihypertensive effect). Products include:
Univasc Tablets 2410

Molindone Hydrochloride (Additive effect). Products include:
Moban Tablets and Concentrate 1048

Morphine Sulfate (Additive effect). Products include:
Astramorph/PF Injection, USP (Preservative-Free) 535
Duramorph 962
Infumorph 200 and Infumorph 500 Sterile Solutions 965
MS Contin Tablets 1994
MSIR 1997
Oramorph SR (Morphine Sulfate Sustained Release Tablets) 2236
RMS Suppositories 2657
Roxanol 2243

Nadolol (Decreased antihypertensive effect).
No products indexed under this heading.

Nicardipine Hydrochloride (Decreased antihypertensive effect). Products include:
Cardene Capsules 2095
Cardene I.V. 2709
Cardene SR Capsules 2097

Nifedipine (Decreased antihypertensive effect). Products include:
Adalat Capsules (10 mg and 20 mg) 587
Adalat CC 589
Procardia Capsules 1971
Procardia XL Extended Release Tablets 1972

Nisoldipine (Decreased antihypertensive effect).
No products indexed under this heading.

Nitroglycerin (Decreased antihypertensive effect). Products include:
Deponit NTG Transdermal Delivery System 2397
Nitro-Bid IV 1523
Nitro-Bid Ointment 1524
Nitrodisc 2047
Nitro-Dur (nitroglycerin) Transdermal Infusion System 1326
Nitrolingual Spray 2027
Nitrostat Tablets 1925
Transderm-Nitro Transdermal Therapeutic System 859

Opium Alkaloids (Additive effect).
No products indexed under this heading.

Oxazepam (Additive effect). Products include:
Serax Capsules 2810
Serax Tablets 2810

Oxycodone Hydrochloride (Additive effect). Products include:
Percocet Tablets 938
Percodan Tablets 939
Percodan-Demi Tablets 940
Roxicodone Tablets, Oral Solution & Intensol (Oxycodone) 2244
Tylox Capsules 1584

Penbutolol Sulfate (Decreased antihypertensive effect). Products include:
Levatol 2403

Pentobarbital Sodium (Additive effect). Products include:
Nembutal Sodium Capsules 436
Nembutal Sodium Solution 438
Nembutal Sodium Suppositories 440

Perphenazine (Additive effect). Products include:
Etrafon 2355
Triavil Tablets 1757
Trilafon 2389

Phenelzine Sulfate (Prolonged anticholinergic effect). Products include:
Nardil 1920

Phenobarbital (Additive effect). Products include:
Arco-Lase Plus Tablets 512
Bellergal-S Tablets 2250
Donnatal 2060
Donnatal Extentabs 2061
Donnatal Tablets 2060
Phenobarbital Elixir and Tablets 1469
Quadrinal Tablets 1350

Phenoxybenzamine Hydrochloride (Decreased antihypertensive effect). Products include:
Dibenzyline Capsules 2476

Phentolamine Mesylate (Decreased antihypertensive effect). Products include:
Regitine 846

Pindolol (Decreased antihypertensive effect). Products include:
Visken Tablets 2299

Polythiazide (Decreased antihypertensive effect). Products include:
Minizide Capsules 1938

Prazepam (Additive effect).
No products indexed under this heading.

Prazosin Hydrochloride (Decreased antihypertensive effect). Products include:
Minipress Capsules 1937
Minizide Capsules 1938

Prochlorperazine (Additive effect). Products include:
Compazine 2470

Promethazine Hydrochloride (Additive effect). Products include:
Mepergan Injection 2753

(▣ Described in PDR For Nonprescription Drugs) (◉ Described in PDR For Ophthalmology)

Phenergan with Codeine 2777
Phenergan with Dextromethorphan 2778
Phenergan Injection 2773
Phenergan Suppositories 2775
Phenergan Syrup 2774
Phenergan Tablets 2775
Phenergan VC 2779
Phenergan VC with Codeine 2781

Propofol (Additive effect). Products include:
Diprivan Injection 2833

Propoxyphene Hydrochloride (Additive effect). Products include:
Darvon 1435
Wygesic Tablets 2827

Propoxyphene Napsylate (Additive effect). Products include:
Darvon-N/Darvocet-N 1433

Propranolol Hydrochloride (Decreased antihypertensive effect). Products include:
Inderal 2728
Inderal LA Long Acting Capsules 2730
Inderide Tablets 2732
Inderide LA Long Acting Capsules .. 2734

Quazepam (Additive effect). Products include:
Doral Tablets 2664

Quinapril Hydrochloride (Decreased antihypertensive effect). Products include:
Accupril Tablets 1893

Ramipril (Decreased antihypertensive effect). Products include:
Altace Capsules 1232

Rauwolfia Serpentina (Decreased antihypertensive effect).
No products indexed under this heading.

Rescinnamine (Decreased antihypertensive effect).
No products indexed under this heading.

Reserpine (Decreased antihypertensive effect). Products include:
Diupres Tablets 1650
Hydropres Tablets 1675
Ser-Ap-Es Tablets 849

Risperidone (Additive effect). Products include:
Risperdal 1301

Secobarbital Sodium (Additive effect). Products include:
Seconal Sodium Pulvules 1474

Selegiline Hydrochloride (Prolonged anticholinergic effect). Products include:
Eldepryl Tablets 2550

Sodium Nitroprusside (Decreased antihypertensive effect).
No products indexed under this heading.

Sotalol Hydrochloride (Decreased antihypertensive effect). Products include:
Betapace Tablets 641

Spirapril Hydrochloride (Decreased antihypertensive effect).
No products indexed under this heading.

Sufentanil Citrate (Additive effect). Products include:
Sufenta Injection 1309

Temazepam (Additive effect). Products include:
Restoril Capsules 2284

Terazosin Hydrochloride (Decreased antihypertensive effect). Products include:
Hytrin Capsules 430

Thiamylal Sodium (Additive effect).
No products indexed under this heading.

Thioridazine Hydrochloride (Additive effect). Products include:
Mellaril 2269

Thiothixene (Additive effect). Products include:
Navane Capsules and Concentrate 2201
Navane Intramuscular 2202

Timolol Maleate (Decreased antihypertensive effect). Products include:
Blocadren Tablets 1614
Timolide Tablets 1748
Timoptic in Ocudose 1753
Timoptic Sterile Ophthalmic Solution 1751
Timoptic-XE 1755

Torsemide (Decreased antihypertensive effect). Products include:
Demadex Tablets and Injection 686

Tranylcypromine Sulfate (Prolonged anticholinergic effect). Products include:
Parnate Tablets 2503

Triazolam (Additive effect). Products include:
Halcion Tablets 2611

Trifluoperazine Hydrochloride (Additive effect). Products include:
Stelazine 2514

Trimethaphan Camsylate (Decreased antihypertensive effect). Products include:
Arfonad Ampuls 2080

Verapamil Hydrochloride (Decreased antihypertensive effect). Products include:
Calan SR Caplets 2422
Calan Tablets 2419
Isoptin Injectable 1344
Isoptin Oral Tablets 1346
Isoptin SR Tablets 1348
Verelan Capsules 1410
Verelan Capsules 2824

Zolpidem Tartrate (Additive effect). Products include:
Ambien Tablets 2416

Food Interactions

Alcohol (Additive effect).

DIMETAPP ELIXIR

(Brompheniramine Maleate, Phenylpropanolamine Hydrochloride) .... ☞ 773

May interact with monoamine oxidase inhibitors, hypnotics and sedatives, tranquilizers, and certain other agents. Compounds in these categories include:

Alprazolam (May increase drowsiness effect). Products include:
Xanax Tablets 2649

Buspirone Hydrochloride (May increase drowsiness effect). Products include:
BuSpar 737

Chlordiazepoxide (May increase drowsiness effect). Products include:
Libritabs Tablets 2177
Limbitrol 2180

Chlordiazepoxide Hydrochloride (May increase drowsiness effect). Products include:
Librax Capsules 2176
Librium Capsules 2178
Librium Injectable 2179

Chlorpromazine (May increase drowsiness effect). Products include:
Thorazine Suppositories 2523

Chlorpromazine Hydrochloride (May increase drowsiness effect). Products include:
Thorazine 2523

Chlorprothixene (May increase drowsiness effect).
No products indexed under this heading.

Chlorprothixene Hydrochloride (May increase drowsiness effect).
No products indexed under this heading.

Clorazepate Dipotassium (May increase drowsiness effect). Products include:
Tranxene 451

Diazepam (May increase drowsiness effect). Products include:
Dizac 1809
Valium Injectable 2182
Valium Tablets 2183
Valrelease Capsules 2169

Droperidol (May increase drowsiness effect). Products include:
Inapsine Injection 1296

Estazolam (May increase drowsiness effect). Products include:
ProSom Tablets 449

Ethchlorvynol (May increase drowsiness effect). Products include:
Placidyl Capsules 448

Ethinamate (May increase drowsiness effect).
No products indexed under this heading.

Fluphenazine Decanoate (May increase drowsiness effect). Products include:
Prolixin Decanoate 509

Fluphenazine Enanthate (May increase drowsiness effect). Products include:
Prolixin Enanthate 509

Fluphenazine Hydrochloride (May increase drowsiness effect). Products include:
Prolixin 509

Flurazepam Hydrochloride (May increase drowsiness effect). Products include:
Dalmane Capsules 2173

Furazolidone (Concurrent and/or sequential use is not recommended). Products include:
Furoxone 2046

Glutethimide (May increase drowsiness effect).
No products indexed under this heading.

Haloperidol (May increase drowsiness effect). Products include:
Haldol Injection, Tablets and Concentrate 1575

Haloperidol Decanoate (May increase drowsiness effect). Products include:
Haldol Decanoate 1577

Hydroxyzine Hydrochloride (May increase drowsiness effect). Products include:
Atarax Tablets & Syrup 2185
Marax Tablets & DF Syrup 2200
Vistaril Intramuscular Solution 2216

Isocarboxazid (Concurrent and/or sequential use is not recommended).
No products indexed under this heading.

Lorazepam (May increase drowsiness effect). Products include:
Ativan Injection 2698
Ativan Tablets 2700

Loxapine Hydrochloride (May increase drowsiness effect). Products include:
Loxitane 1378

Loxapine Succinate (May increase drowsiness effect). Products include:
Loxitane Capsules 1378

Meprobamate (May increase drowsiness effect). Products include:
Miltown Tablets 2672
PMB 200 and PMB 400 2783

Mesoridazine Besylate (May increase drowsiness effect). Products include:
Serentil 684

Midazolam Hydrochloride (May increase drowsiness effect). Products include:
Versed Injection 2170

Molindone Hydrochloride (May increase drowsiness effect). Products include:
Moban Tablets and Concentrate 1048

Oxazepam (May increase drowsiness effect). Products include:
Serax Capsules 2810
Serax Tablets 2810

Perphenazine (May increase drowsiness effect). Products include:
Etrafon 2355
Triavil Tablets 1757
Trilafon 2389

Phenelzine Sulfate (Concurrent and/or sequential use is not recommended). Products include:
Nardil 1920

Prazepam (May increase drowsiness effect).
No products indexed under this heading.

Prochlorperazine (May increase drowsiness effect). Products include:
Compazine 2470

Promethazine Hydrochloride (May increase drowsiness effect). Products include:
Mepergan Injection 2753
Phenergan with Codeine 2777
Phenergan with Dextromethorphan 2778
Phenergan Injection 2773
Phenergan Suppositories 2775
Phenergan Syrup 2774
Phenergan Tablets 2775
Phenergan VC 2779
Phenergan VC with Codeine 2781

Propofol (May increase drowsiness effect). Products include:
Diprivan Injection 2833

Quazepam (May increase drowsiness effect). Products include:
Doral Tablets 2664

Secobarbital Sodium (May increase drowsiness effect). Products include:
Seconal Sodium Pulvules 1474

Selegiline Hydrochloride (Concurrent and/or sequential use is not recommended). Products include:
Eldepryl Tablets 2550

Temazepam (May increase drowsiness effect). Products include:
Restoril Capsules 2284

Thioridazine Hydrochloride (May increase drowsiness effect). Products include:
Mellaril 2269

Thiothixene (May increase drowsiness effect). Products include:
Navane Capsules and Concentrate 2201
Navane Intramuscular 2202

Tranylcypromine Sulfate (Concurrent and/or sequential use is not recommended). Products include:
Parnate Tablets 2503

Triazolam (May increase drowsiness effect). Products include:
Halcion Tablets 2611

Trifluoperazine Hydrochloride (May increase drowsiness effect). Products include:
Stelazine 2514

Zolpidem Tartrate (May increase drowsiness effect). Products include:
Ambien Tablets 2416

Food Interactions

Alcohol (May increase drowsiness effect).

DIMETAPP EXTENTABS

(Brompheniramine Maleate, Phenylpropanolamine Hydrochloride) .... ☞ 774

May interact with sympathomimet-

IMPORTANT NOTE: Always consult each drug listing in the patient's regimen for possible interactions.

Dimetapp Extentabs

ics, monoamine oxidase inhibitors, and certain other agents. Compounds in these categories include:

Albuterol (May produce additive effects). Products include:

Proventil Inhalation Aerosol 2382
Ventolin Inhalation Aerosol and Refill 1197

Albuterol Sulfate (May produce additive effects). Products include:

Airet Solution for Inhalation 452
Proventil Inhalation Solution 0.083% 2384
Proventil Repetabs Tablets 2386
Proventil Solution for Inhalation 0.5% 2383
Proventil Syrup 2385
Proventil Tablets 2386
Ventolin Inhalation Solution................ 1198
Ventolin Nebules Inhalation Solution 1199
Ventolin Rotacaps for Inhalation 1200
Ventolin Syrup.. 1202
Ventolin Tablets 1203
Volmax Extended-Release Tablets .. 1788

Antihypertensive agents, unspecified (Diminished antihypertensive effect).

Dobutamine Hydrochloride (May produce additive effects). Products include:

Dobutrex Solution Vials......................... 1439

Dopamine Hydrochloride (May produce additive effects).

No products indexed under this heading.

Ephedrine Hydrochloride (May produce additive effects). Products include:

Primatene Dual Action Formula...... ᴮᴰ 872
Primatene Tablets .... ᴮᴰ 873
Quadrinal Tablets 1350

Ephedrine Sulfate (May produce additive effects). Products include:

Bronkaid Caplets .... ᴮᴰ 717
Marax Tablets & DF Syrup.................. 2200

Ephedrine Tannate (May produce additive effects). Products include:

Rynatuss 2673

Epinephrine (May produce additive effects). Products include:

Bronkaid Mist .... ᴮᴰ 717
EPIFRIN .... ⊚ 239
EpiPen 790
Marcaine Hydrochloride with Epinephrine 1:200,000 2316
Primatene Mist .... ᴮᴰ 873
Sensorcaine with Epinephrine Injection... 559
Sus-Phrine Injection 1019
Xylocaine with Epinephrine Injections... 567

Epinephrine Bitartrate (May produce additive effects). Products include:

Bronkaid Mist Suspension .... ᴮᴰ 718
Sensorcaine-MPF with Epinephrine Injection 559

Epinephrine Hydrochloride (May produce additive effects). Products include:

Ana-Kit Anaphylaxis Emergency Treatment Kit 617

Furazolidone (May produce hypertensive crisis). Products include:

Furoxone 2046

Isocarboxazid (May produce hypertensive crisis).

No products indexed under this heading.

Isoproterenol Hydrochloride (May produce additive effects). Products include:

Isuprel Hydrochloride Injection 1:5000 2311
Isuprel Hydrochloride Solution 1:200 & 1:100 2313
Isuprel Mistometer 2312

Isoproterenol Sulfate (May produce additive effects). Products include:

Norisodrine with Calcium Iodide Syrup... 442

Metaproterenol Sulfate (May produce additive effects). Products include:

Alupent... 669
Metaproterenol Sulfate Inhalation Solution, USP, Arm-a-Med 552

Metaraminol Bitartrate (May produce additive effects). Products include:

Aramine Injection.................................... 1609

Methoxamine Hydrochloride (May produce additive effects). Products include:

Vasoxyl Injection 1196

Norepinephrine Bitartrate (May produce additive effects). Products include:

Levophed Bitartrate Injection 2315

Phenelzine Sulfate (May produce hypertensive crisis). Products include:

Nardil 1920

Phenylephrine Bitartrate (May produce additive effects).

No products indexed under this heading.

Phenylephrine Hydrochloride (May produce additive effects). Products include:

Atrohist Plus Tablets 454
Cerose DM .... ᴮᴰ 878
Comhist 2038
D.A. Chewable Tablets.......................... 951
Deconsal Pediatric Capsules.............. 454
Dura-Vent/DA Tablets 953
Entex Capsules.. 1986
Entex Liquid 1986
Extendryl 1005
4-Way Fast Acting Nasal Spray (regular & mentholated) .... ᴮᴰ 621
Hemorrhoid For Women .... ᴮᴰ 834
Hycomine Compound Tablets 932
Neo-Synephrine Hydrochloride 1% Carpuject.. 2324
Neo-Synephrine Hydrochloride 1% Injection 2324
Neo-Synephrine Hydrochloride (Ophthalmic) 2325
Neo-Synephrine .... ᴮᴰ 726
Nöstril... ᴮᴰ 644
Novahistine Elixir .... ᴮᴰ 823
Phenergan VC 2779
Phenergan VC with Codeine 2781
Preparation H .... ᴮᴰ 871
Tympagesic Ear Drops 2342
Vasosulf .... ⊚ 271
Vicks Sinex Nasal Spray and Ultra Fine Mist .... ᴮᴰ 765

Phenylephrine Tannate (May produce additive effects). Products include:

Atrohist Pediatric Suspension 454
Ricobid-D Pediatric Suspension........ 2038
Ricobid Tablets and Pediatric Suspension.. 2038
Rynatan 2673
Rynatuss 2673

Pirbuterol Acetate (May produce additive effects). Products include:

Maxair Autohaler 1492
Maxair Inhaler 1494

Pseudoephedrine Hydrochloride (May produce additive effects). Products include:

Actifed Allergy Daytime/Nighttime Caplets .... ᴮᴰ 844
Actifed Plus Caplets .... ᴮᴰ 845
Actifed Plus Tablets .... ᴮᴰ 845
Actifed with Codeine Cough Syrup.. 1067
Actifed Sinus Daytime/Nighttime Tablets and Caplets .... ᴮᴰ 846
Actifed Syrup.. ᴮᴰ 846
Actifed Tablets .... ᴮᴰ 844
Advil Cold and Sinus Caplets and Tablets (formerly CoAdvil) .... ᴮᴰ 870
Alka-Seltzer Plus Cold Medicine Liqui-Gels .... ᴮᴰ 706
Alka-Seltzer Plus Cold & Cough Medicine Liqui-Gels............................ ᴮᴰ 705

Alka-Seltzer Plus Night-Time Cold Medicine Liqui-Gels............................ ᴮᴰ 706
Allerest Headache Strength Tablets .... ᴮᴰ 627
Allerest Maximum Strength Tablets .... ᴮᴰ 627
Allerest No Drowsiness Tablets .... ᴮᴰ 627
Allerest Sinus Pain Formula .... ᴮᴰ 627
Anatuss LA Tablets.................................. 1542
Atrohist Pediatric Capsules................ 453
Bayer Select Sinus Pain Relief Formula .... ᴮᴰ 717
Benadryl Allergy Decongestant Liquid Medication .... ᴮᴰ 848
Benadryl Allergy Decongestant Tablets .... ᴮᴰ 848
Benadryl Allergy Sinus Headache Formula Caplets .... ᴮᴰ 849
Benylin Multisymptom .... ᴮᴰ 852
Bromfed Capsules (Extended-Release) 1785
Bromfed Syrup .... ᴮᴰ 733
Bromfed Tablets 1785
Bromfed-DM Cough Syrup.................. 1786
Bromfed-PD Capsules (Extended-Release).. 1785
Children's Vicks DayQuil Allergy Relief .... ᴮᴰ 757
Children's Vicks NyQuil Cold/ Cough Relief.. ᴮᴰ 758
Comtrex Multi-Symptom Cold Reliever Tablets/Caplets/Liqui-Gels/Liquid.. ᴮᴰ 615
Allergy-Sinus Comtrex Multi-Symptom Allergy-Sinus Formula Tablets .... ᴮᴰ 617
Comtrex Multi-Symptom Non-Drowsy Caplets...................................... ᴮᴰ 618
Congess 1004
Contac Day Allergy/Sinus Caplets ᴮᴰ 812
Contac Day & Night .... ᴮᴰ 812
Contac Night Allergy/Sinus Caplets .... ᴮᴰ 812
Contac Severe Cold & Flu Non-Drowsy .... ᴮᴰ 815
Deconamine Chewable Tablets 1320
Deconamine CX Cough and Cold Liquid and Tablets.................................. 1319
Deconamine 1320
Deconsal C Expectorant Syrup 456
Deconsal Pediatric Syrup 457
Deconsal II Tablets 454
Dimetane-DX Cough Syrup 2059
Dimetapp Sinus Caplets .... ᴮᴰ 775
Dorcol Children's Cough Syrup ...... ᴮᴰ 785
Drixoral Cough + Congestion Liquid Caps .... ᴮᴰ 802
Dura-Tap/PD Capsules 2867
Duratuss Tablets 2565
Duratuss HD Elixir.................................... 2565
Efidac/24 .... ᴮᴰ 635
Entex PSE Tablets 1987
Fedahist Gyrocaps................................... 2401
Fedahist Timecaps 2401
Guaifed... 1787
Guaifed Syrup .... ᴮᴰ 734
Guaimax-D Tablets 792
Guaitab Tablets .... ᴮᴰ 734
Isoclor Expectorant.................................. 990
Kronofed-A 977
Motrin IB Sinus.. ᴮᴰ 838
Novahistine DH.. 2462
Novahistine DMX .... ᴮᴰ 822
Novahistine Expectorant...................... 2463
Nucofed 2051
PediaCare Cold Allergy Chewable Tablets .... ᴮᴰ 677
PediaCare Cough-Cold Chewable Tablets 1553
PediaCare 1553
PediaCare Infants' Decongestant Drops .... ᴮᴰ 677
PediCare Infant's Drops Decongestant Plus Cough 1553
PediaCare NightRest Cough-Cold Liquid 1553
Pediatric Vicks 44d Dry Hacking Cough & Head Congestion................ ᴮᴰ 763
Pediatric Vicks 44m Cough & Cold Relief .... ᴮᴰ 764
Robitussin Cold & Cough Liqui-Gels .... ᴮᴰ 776
Robitussin Maximum Strength Cough & Cold .... ᴮᴰ 778
Robitussin Pediatric Cough & Cold Formula .... ᴮᴰ 779
Robitussin Severe Congestion Liqui-Gels .... ᴮᴰ 776
Robitussin-DAC Syrup 2074
Robitussin-PE .... ᴮᴰ 778
Rondec Oral Drops 953

Rondec Syrup 953
Rondec Tablet.. 953
Rondec-DM Oral Drops.......................... 954
Rondec-DM Syrup 954
Rondec-TR Tablet 953
Ryna .... ᴮᴰ 841
Seldane-D Extended-Release Tablets 1538
Semprex-D Capsules 463
Semprex-D Capsules 1167
Sinarest Tablets .... ᴮᴰ 648
Sinarest Extra Strength Tablets...... ᴮᴰ 648
Sinarest No Drowsiness Tablets .... ᴮᴰ 648
Sine-Aid IB Caplets 1554
Sine-Aid Maximum Strength Sinus Medication Gelcaps, Caplets and Tablets 1554
Sine-Off No Drowsiness Formula Caplets .... ᴮᴰ 824
Sine-Off Sinus Medicine .... ᴮᴰ 825
Singlet Tablets .... ᴮᴰ 825
Sinutab Non-Drying Liquid Caps.... ᴮᴰ 859
Sinutab Sinus Allergy Medication, Maximum Strength Tablets and Caplets .... ᴮᴰ 860
Sinutab Sinus Medication, Maximum Strength Without Drowsiness Formula, Tablets & Caplets .... ᴮᴰ 860
Sinutab Sinus Medication, Regular Strength Without Drowsiness Formula .... ᴮᴰ 859
Sudafed Children's Liquid .... ᴮᴰ 861
Sudafed Cold and Cough Liquidcaps .... ᴮᴰ 862
Sudafed Cough Syrup .... ᴮᴰ 862
Sudafed Plus Liquid .... ᴮᴰ 862
Sudafed Plus Tablets .... ᴮᴰ 863
Sudafed Severe Cold Formula Caplets .... ᴮᴰ 863
Sudafed Severe Cold Formula Tablets .... ᴮᴰ 864
Sudafed Sinus Caplets............................ ᴮᴰ 864
Sudafed Sinus Tablets............................ ᴮᴰ 864
Sudafed Tablets, 30 mg.......................... ᴮᴰ 861
Sudafed Tablets, 60 mg.......................... ᴮᴰ 861
Sudafed 12 Hour Caplets .... ᴮᴰ 861
Syn-Rx Tablets 465
Syn-Rx DM Tablets 466
TheraFlu.. ᴮᴰ 787
TheraFlu Maximum Strength Nighttime Flu, Cold & Cough Medicine .... ᴮᴰ 788
TheraFlu Maximum Strength Non-Drowsy Formula Flu, Cold & Cough Medicine .... ᴮᴰ 788
Thera Flu Maximum Strength, Non-Drowsy Formula Flu, Cold and Cough Caplets .... ᴮᴰ 789
Triaminic AM Cough and Decongestant Formula .... ᴮᴰ 789
Triaminic AM Decongestant Formula .... ᴮᴰ 790
Triaminic Nite Light .... ᴮᴰ 791
Triaminic Sore Throat Formula ...... ᴮᴰ 791
Tussend 1783
Tussend Expectorant 1785
Children's TYLENOL Cold Multi-Symptom Liquid Formula and Chewable Tablets.................................... 1561
Children's TYLENOL Cold Plus Cough Multi Symptom Tablets and Liquid .... ᴮᴰ 681
Infants' TYLENOL Cold Decongestant & Fever-Reducer Drops 1556
TYLENOL Maximum Strength Allergy Sinus Medication Gelcaps and Caplets 1563
TYLENOL Maximum Strength Allergy Sinus NightTime Medication Caplets 1555
TYLENOL Flu Maximum Strength Gelcaps 1565
TYLENOL Flu NightTime, Maximum Strength, Gelcaps 1566
TYLENOL Maximum Strength Flu NightTime Hot Medication Packets 1562
TYLENOL, Maximum Strength, Sinus Medication Geltabs, Gelcaps, Caplets and Tablets 1566
TYLENOL Cold Multi-Symptom Formula Medication Tablets and Caplets 1561
TYLENOL Cold Medication No Drowsiness Formula Gelcaps and Caplets 1562
TYLENOL Cold Multi-Symptom Hot Medication Liquid Packets.............. 1557
TYLENOL Cough Multi-Symptom Medication with Decongestant...... 1565

(ᴮᴰ Described in PDR For Nonprescription Drugs) (⊚ Described in PDR For Ophthalmology)

Ursinus Inlay-Tabs .... ⊕ 794
Vicks 44 LiquiCaps Cough, Cold & Flu Relief .... ⊕ 755
Vicks 44 LiquiCaps Non-Drowsy Cough & Cold Relief .... ⊕ 756
Vicks 44D Dry Hacking Cough & Head Congestion .... ⊕ 755
Vicks 44M Cough, Cold & Flu Relief .... ⊕ 756
Vicks DayQuil .... ⊕ 761
Vicks DayQuil SINUS Pressure & PAIN Relief with IBUPROFEN ..... ⊕ 762
Vicks Nyquil Hot Therapy .... ⊕ 762
Vicks NyQuil LiquiCaps Multi-Symptom Cold/Flu Relief .... ⊕ 763
Vicks NyQuil Multi-Symptom Cold/Flu Relief - (Original & Cherry Flavor) .... ⊕ 763

Pseudoephedrine Sulfate (May produce additive effects). Products include:

Cheracol Sinus .... ⊕ 768
Chlor-Trimeton Allergy Decongestant Tablets .... ⊕ 799
Claritin-D 2350
Drixoral Cold and Allergy Sustained-Action Tablets .... ⊕ 802
Drixoral Cold and Flu Extended-Release Tablets .... ⊕ 803
Drixoral Non-Drowsy Formula Extended-Release Tablets .... ⊕ 803
Drixoral Allergy/Sinus Extended Release Tablets .... ⊕ 804
Trinalin Repetabs Tablets 1330

Salmeterol Xinafoate (May produce additive effects). Products include:

Serevent Inhalation Aerosol 1176

Selegiline Hydrochloride (May produce hypertensive crisis). Products include:

Eldepryl Tablets 2550

Terbutaline Sulfate (May produce additive effects). Products include:

Brethaire Inhaler 813
Brethine Ampuls 815
Brethine Tablets 814
Bricanyl Subcutaneous Injection 1502
Bricanyl Tablets 1503

Tranylcypromine Sulfate (May produce hypertensive crisis). Products include:

Parnate Tablets 2503

Food Interactions

Alcohol (Do not use concomitantly).

DIMETAPP LIQUI-GELS

(Brompheniramine Maleate, Phenylpropanolamine Hydrochloride) .... ⊕ 775

May interact with hypnotics and sedatives, tranquilizers, monoamine oxidase inhibitors, and certain other agents. Compounds in these categories include:

Alprazolam (Increases drowsiness effect). Products include:

Xanax Tablets 2649

Buspirone Hydrochloride (Increases drowsiness effect). Products include:

BuSpar 737

Chlordiazepoxide (Increases drowsiness effect). Products include:

Libritabs Tablets 2177
Limbitrol 2180

Chlordiazepoxide Hydrochloride (Increases drowsiness effect). Products include:

Librax Capsules 2176
Librium Capsules 2178
Librium Injectable 2179

Chlorpromazine (Increases drowsiness effect). Products include:

Thorazine Suppositories 2523

Chlorpromazine Hydrochloride (Increases drowsiness effect). Products include:

Thorazine 2523

Chlorprothixene (Increases drowsiness effect).

No products indexed under this heading.

Chlorprothixene Hydrochloride (Increases drowsiness effect).

No products indexed under this heading.

Clorazepate Dipotassium (Increases drowsiness effect). Products include:

Tranxene 451

Diazepam (Increases drowsiness effect). Products include:

Dizac 1809
Valium Injectable 2182
Valium Tablets 2183
Valrelease Capsules 2169

Droperidol (Increases drowsiness effect). Products include:

Inapsine Injection 1296

Estazolam (Increases drowsiness effect). Products include:

ProSom Tablets 449

Ethchlorvynol (Increases drowsiness effect). Products include:

Placidyl Capsules 448

Ethinamate (Increases drowsiness effect).

No products indexed under this heading.

Fluphenazine Decanoate (Increases drowsiness effect). Products include:

Prolixin Decanoate 509

Fluphenazine Enanthate (Increases drowsiness effect). Products include:

Prolixin Enanthate 509

Fluphenazine Hydrochloride (Increases drowsiness effect). Products include:

Prolixin 509

Flurazepam Hydrochloride (Increases drowsiness effect). Products include:

Dalmane Capsules 2173

Furazolidone (Concurrent and/or sequential use is contraindicated). Products include:

Furoxone 2046

Glutethimide (Increases drowsiness effect).

No products indexed under this heading.

Haloperidol (Increases drowsiness effect). Products include:

Haldol Injection, Tablets and Concentrate 1575

Haloperidol Decanoate (Increases drowsiness effect). Products include:

Haldol Decanoate 1577

Hydroxyzine Hydrochloride (Increases drowsiness effect). Products include:

Atarax Tablets & Syrup 2185
Marax Tablets & DF Syrup 2200
Vistaril Intramuscular Solution 2216

Isocarboxazid (Concurrent and/or sequential use is contraindicated).

No products indexed under this heading.

Lorazepam (Increases drowsiness effect). Products include:

Ativan Injection 2698
Ativan Tablets 2700

Loxapine Hydrochloride (Increases drowsiness effect). Products include:

Loxitane 1378

Loxapine Succinate (Increases drowsiness effect). Products include:

Loxitane Capsules 1378

Meprobamate (Increases drowsiness effect). Products include:

Miltown Tablets 2672

PMB 200 and PMB 400 2783

Mesoridazine Besylate (Increases drowsiness effect). Products include:

Serentil 684

Midazolam Hydrochloride (Increases drowsiness effect). Products include:

Versed Injection 2170

Molindone Hydrochloride (Increases drowsiness effect). Products include:

Moban Tablets and Concentrate 1048

Oxazepam (Increases drowsiness effect). Products include:

Serax Capsules 2810
Serax Tablets 2810

Perphenazine (Increases drowsiness effect). Products include:

Etrafon 2355
Triavil Tablets 1757
Trilafon 2389

Phenelzine Sulfate (Concurrent and/or sequential use is contraindicated). Products include:

Nardil 1920

Prazepam (Increases drowsiness effect).

No products indexed under this heading.

Prochlorperazine (Increases drowsiness effect). Products include:

Compazine 2470

Promethazine Hydrochloride (Increases drowsiness effect). Products include:

Mepergan Injection 2753
Phenergan with Codeine 2777
Phenergan with Dextromethorphan 2778
Phenergan Injection 2773
Phenergan Suppositories 2775
Phenergan Syrup 2774
Phenergan Tablets 2775
Phenergan VC 2779
Phenergan VC with Codeine 2781

Propofol (Increases drowsiness effect). Products include:

Diprivan Injection 2833

Quazepam (Increases drowsiness effect). Products include:

Doral Tablets 2664

Secobarbital Sodium (Increases drowsiness effect). Products include:

Seconal Sodium Pulvules 1474

Selegiline Hydrochloride (Concurrent and/or sequential use is contraindicated). Products include:

Eldepryl Tablets 2550

Temazepam (Increases drowsiness effect). Products include:

Restoril Capsules 2284

Thioridazine Hydrochloride (Increases drowsiness effect). Products include:

Mellaril 2269

Thiothixene (Increases drowsiness effect). Products include:

Navane Capsules and Concentrate 2201
Navane Intramuscular 2202

Tranylcypromine Sulfate (Concurrent and/or sequential use is contraindicated). Products include:

Parnate Tablets 2503

Triazolam (Increases drowsiness effect). Products include:

Halcion Tablets 2611

Trifluoperazine Hydrochloride (Increases drowsiness effect). Products include:

Stelazine 2514

Zolpidem Tartrate (Increases drowsiness effect). Products include:

Ambien Tablets 2416

Food Interactions

Alcohol (Increases drowsiness effect; avoid concurrent use).

DIMETAPP TABLETS

(Brompheniramine Maleate, Phenylpropanolamine Hydrochloride) .... ⊕ 775

See Dimetapp Liqui-Gels

DIMETAPP COLD & ALLERGY CHEWABLE TABLETS

(Brompheniramine Maleate, Phenylpropanolamine Hydrochloride) .... ⊕ 773

May interact with hypnotics and sedatives, monoamine oxidase inhibitors, and tranquilizers. Compounds in these categories include:

Alprazolam (May increase drowsiness effect). Products include:

Xanax Tablets 2649

Buspirone Hydrochloride (May increase drowsiness effect). Products include:

BuSpar 737

Chlordiazepoxide (May increase drowsiness effect). Products include:

Libritabs Tablets 2177
Limbitrol 2180

Chlordiazepoxide Hydrochloride (May increase drowsiness effect). Products include:

Librax Capsules 2176
Librium Capsules 2178
Librium Injectable 2179

Chlorpromazine (May increase drowsiness effect). Products include:

Thorazine Suppositories 2523

Chlorpromazine Hydrochloride (May increase drowsiness effect). Products include:

Thorazine 2523

Chlorprothixene (May increase drowsiness effect).

No products indexed under this heading.

Chlorprothixene Hydrochloride (May increase drowsiness effect).

No products indexed under this heading.

Clorazepate Dipotassium (May increase drowsiness effect). Products include:

Tranxene 451

Diazepam (May increase drowsiness effect). Products include:

Dizac 1809
Valium Injectable 2182
Valium Tablets 2183
Valrelease Capsules 2169

Droperidol (May increase drowsiness effect). Products include:

Inapsine Injection 1296

Estazolam (May increase drowsiness effect). Products include:

ProSom Tablets 449

Ethchlorvynol (May increase drowsiness effect). Products include:

Placidyl Capsules 448

Ethinamate (May increase drowsiness effect).

No products indexed under this heading.

Fluphenazine Decanoate (May increase drowsiness effect). Products include:

Prolixin Decanoate 509

Fluphenazine Enanthate (May increase drowsiness effect). Products include:

Prolixin Enanthate 509

Fluphenazine Hydrochloride (May increase drowsiness effect). Products include:

Prolixin 509

Flurazepam Hydrochloride (May increase drowsiness effect). Products include:

Dalmane Capsules 2173

IMPORTANT NOTE: Always consult each drug listing in the patient's regimen for possible interactions.

Furazolidone (Concurrent and/or sequential use is not recommended). Products include:

Furoxone 2046

Glutethimide (May increase drowsiness effect).

No products indexed under this heading.

Haloperidol (May increase drowsiness effect). Products include:

Haldol Injection, Tablets and Concentrate 1575

Haloperidol Decanoate (May increase drowsiness effect). Products include:

Haldol Decanoate 1577

Hydroxyzine Hydrochloride (May increase drowsiness effect). Products include:

Atarax Tablets & Syrup 2185
Marax Tablets & DF Syrup 2200
Vistaril Intramuscular Solution 2216

Isocarboxazid (Concurrent and/or sequential use is not recommended).

No products indexed under this heading.

Lorazepam (May increase drowsiness effect). Products include:

Ativan Injection 2698
Ativan Tablets 2700

Loxapine Hydrochloride (May increase drowsiness effect). Products include:

Loxitane 1378

Loxapine Succinate (May increase drowsiness effect). Products include:

Loxitane Capsules 1378

Meprobamate (May increase drowsiness effect). Products include:

Miltown Tablets 2672
PMB 200 and PMB 400 2783

Mesoridazine Besylate (May increase drowsiness effect). Products include:

Serentil 684

Midazolam Hydrochloride (May increase drowsiness effect). Products include:

Versed Injection 2170

Molindone Hydrochloride (May increase drowsiness effect). Products include:

Moban Tablets and Concentrate 1048

Oxazepam (May increase drowsiness effect). Products include:

Serax Capsules 2810
Serax Tablets 2810

Perphenazine (May increase drowsiness effect). Products include:

Etrafon 2355
Triavil Tablets 1757
Trilafon 2389

Phenelzine Sulfate (Concurrent and/or sequential use is not recommended). Products include:

Nardil 1920

Prazepam (May increase drowsiness effect).

No products indexed under this heading.

Prochlorperazine (May increase drowsiness effect). Products include:

Compazine 2470

Promethazine Hydrochloride (May increase drowsiness effect). Products include:

Mepergan Injection 2753
Phenergan with Codeine 2777
Phenergan with Dextromethorphan 2778
Phenergan Injection 2773
Phenergan Suppositories 2775
Phenergan Syrup 2774
Phenergan Tablets 2775
Phenergan VC 2779
Phenergan VC with Codeine 2781

Propofol (May increase drowsiness effect). Products include:

Diprivan Injection 2833

Quazepam (May increase drowsiness effect). Products include:

Doral Tablets 2664

Secobarbital Sodium (May increase drowsiness effect). Products include:

Seconal Sodium Pulvules 1474

Selegiline Hydrochloride (Concurrent and/or sequential use is not recommended). Products include:

Eldepryl Tablets 2550

Temazepam (May increase drowsiness effect). Products include:

Restoril Capsules 2284

Thioridazine Hydrochloride (May increase drowsiness effect). Products include:

Mellaril 2269

Thiothixene (May increase drowsiness effect). Products include:

Navane Capsules and Concentrate 2201
Navane Intramuscular 2202

Tranylcypromine Sulfate (Concurrent and/or sequential use is not recommended). Products include:

Parnate Tablets 2503

Triazolam (May increase drowsiness effect). Products include:

Halcion Tablets 2611

Trifluoperazine Hydrochloride (May increase drowsiness effect). Products include:

Stelazine 2514

Zolpidem Tartrate (May increase drowsiness effect). Products include:

Ambien Tablets 2416

DIMETAPP DM ELIXIR

(Brompheniramine Maleate, Dextromethorphan Hydrobromide) ◙ 774

May interact with monoamine oxidase inhibitors, tranquilizers, hypnotics and sedatives, and certain other agents. Compounds in these categories include:

Alprazolam (Increases drowsiness effect). Products include:

Xanax Tablets 2649

Buspirone Hydrochloride (Increases drowsiness effect). Products include:

BuSpar 737

Chlordiazepoxide (Increases drowsiness effect). Products include:

Libritabs Tablets 2177
Limbitrol 2180

Chlordiazepoxide Hydrochloride (Increases drowsiness effect). Products include:

Librax Capsules 2176
Librium Capsules 2178
Librium Injectable 2179

Chlorpromazine (Increases drowsiness effect). Products include:

Thorazine Suppositories 2523

Chlorpromazine Hydrochloride (Increases drowsiness effect). Products include:

Thorazine 2523

Chlorprothixene (Increases drowsiness effect).

No products indexed under this heading.

Chlorprothixene Hydrochloride (Increases drowsiness effect).

No products indexed under this heading.

Clorazepate Dipotassium (Increases drowsiness effect). Products include:

Tranxene 451

Diazepam (Increases drowsiness effect). Products include:

Dizac 1809
Valium Injectable 2182
Valium Tablets 2183
Valrelease Capsules 2169

Droperidol (Increases drowsiness effect). Products include:

Inapsine Injection 1296

Estazolam (Increases drowsiness effect). Products include:

ProSom Tablets 449

Ethchlorvynol (Increases drowsiness effect). Products include:

Placidyl Capsules 448

Ethinamate (Increases drowsiness effect).

No products indexed under this heading.

Fluphenazine Decanoate (Increases drowsiness effect). Products include:

Prolixin Decanoate 509

Fluphenazine Enanthate (Increases drowsiness effect). Products include:

Prolixin Enanthate 509

Fluphenazine Hydrochloride (Increases drowsiness effect). Products include:

Prolixin 509

Flurazepam Hydrochloride (Increases drowsiness effect). Products include:

Dalmane Capsules 2173

Furazolidone (Concurrent and/or sequential use is contraindicated). Products include:

Furoxone 2046

Glutethimide (Increases drowsiness effect).

No products indexed under this heading.

Haloperidol (Increases drowsiness effect). Products include:

Haldol Injection, Tablets and Concentrate 1575

Haloperidol Decanoate (Increases drowsiness effect). Products include:

Haldol Decanoate 1577

Hydroxyzine Hydrochloride (Increases drowsiness effect). Products include:

Atarax Tablets & Syrup 2185
Marax Tablets & DF Syrup 2200
Vistaril Intramuscular Solution 2216

Isocarboxazid (Concurrent and/or sequential use is contraindicated).

No products indexed under this heading.

Lorazepam (Increases drowsiness effect). Products include:

Ativan Injection 2698
Ativan Tablets 2700

Loxapine Hydrochloride (Increases drowsiness effect). Products include:

Loxitane 1378

Loxapine Succinate (Increases drowsiness effect). Products include:

Loxitane Capsules 1378

Meprobamate (Increases drowsiness effect). Products include:

Miltown Tablets 2672
PMB 200 and PMB 400 2783

Mesoridazine Besylate (Increases drowsiness effect). Products include:

Serentil 684

Midazolam Hydrochloride (Increases drowsiness effect). Products include:

Versed Injection 2170

Molindone Hydrochloride (Increases drowsiness effect). Products include:

Moban Tablets and Concentrate 1048

Oxazepam (Increases drowsiness effect). Products include:

Serax Capsules 2810
Serax Tablets 2810

Perphenazine (Increases drowsiness effect). Products include:

Etrafon 2355
Triavil Tablets 1757
Trilafon 2389

Phenelzine Sulfate (Concurrent and/or sequential use is contraindicated). Products include:

Nardil 1920

Prazepam (Increases drowsiness effect).

No products indexed under this heading.

Prochlorperazine (Increases drowsiness effect). Products include:

Compazine 2470

Promethazine Hydrochloride (Increases drowsiness effect). Products include:

Mepergan Injection 2753
Phenergan with Codeine 2777
Phenergan with Dextromethorphan 2778
Phenergan Injection 2773
Phenergan Suppositories 2775
Phenergan Syrup 2774
Phenergan Tablets 2775
Phenergan VC 2779
Phenergan VC with Codeine 2781

Propofol (Increases drowsiness effect). Products include:

Diprivan Injection 2833

Quazepam (Increases drowsiness effect). Products include:

Doral Tablets 2664

Secobarbital Sodium (Increases drowsiness effect). Products include:

Seconal Sodium Pulvules 1474

Selegiline Hydrochloride (Concurrent and/or sequential use is contraindicated). Products include:

Eldepryl Tablets 2550

Temazepam (Increases drowsiness effect). Products include:

Restoril Capsules 2284

Thioridazine Hydrochloride (Increases drowsiness effect). Products include:

Mellaril 2269

Thiothixene (Increases drowsiness effect). Products include:

Navane Capsules and Concentrate 2201
Navane Intramuscular 2202

Tranylcypromine Sulfate (Concurrent and/or sequential use is contraindicated). Products include:

Parnate Tablets 2503

Triazolam (Increases drowsiness effect). Products include:

Halcion Tablets 2611

Trifluoperazine Hydrochloride (Increases drowsiness effect). Products include:

Stelazine 2514

Zolpidem Tartrate (Increases drowsiness effect). Products include:

Ambien Tablets 2416

Food Interactions

Alcohol (Increases drowsiness effect; avoid concurrent use).

DIMETAPP SINUS CAPLETS

(Ibuprofen, Pseudoephedrine Hydrochloride) .... ◙ 775

May interact with antidepressant drugs and sympathomimetics. Compounds in these categories include:

Albuterol (Concurrent use is not recommended unless directed by a doctor). Products include:

Proventil Inhalation Aerosol 2382
Ventolin Inhalation Aerosol and Refill 1197

Albuterol Sulfate (Concurrent use is not recommended unless directed by a doctor). Products include:

Airet Solution for Inhalation 452

(◙ Described in PDR For Nonprescription Drugs) (◉ Described in PDR For Ophthalmology)

309 Interactions Index Dimetapp Sinus

Proventil Inhalation Solution 0.083% 2384
Proventil Repetabs Tablets 2386
Proventil Solution for Inhalation 0.5% 2383
Proventil Syrup 2385
Proventil Tablets 2386
Ventolin Inhalation Solution 1198
Ventolin Nebules Inhalation Solution 1199
Ventolin Rotacaps for Inhalation 1200
Ventolin Syrup 1202
Ventolin Tablets 1203
Volmax Extended-Release Tablets 1788

Amitriptyline Hydrochloride (Concurrent use is not recommended unless directed by a doctor). Products include:
Elavil 2838
Endep Tablets 2174
Etrafon 2355
Limbitrol 2180
Triavil Tablets 1757

Amoxapine (Concurrent use is not recommended unless directed by a doctor). Products include:
Asendin Tablets 1369

Bupropion Hydrochloride (Concurrent use is not recommended unless directed by a doctor). Products include:
Wellbutrin Tablets 1204

Desipramine Hydrochloride (Concurrent use is not recommended unless directed by a doctor). Products include:
Norpramin Tablets 1526

Dobutamine Hydrochloride (Concurrent use is not recommended unless directed by a doctor). Products include:
Dobutrex Solution Vials 1439

Dopamine Hydrochloride (Concurrent use is not recommended unless directed by a doctor).
No products indexed under this heading.

Doxepin Hydrochloride (Concurrent use is not recommended unless directed by a doctor). Products include:
Sinequan 2205
Zonalon Cream 1055

Ephedrine Hydrochloride (Concurrent use is not recommended unless directed by a doctor). Products include:
Primatene Dual Action Formula ▣ 872
Primatene Tablets ▣ 873
Quadrinal Tablets 1350

Ephedrine Sulfate (Concurrent use is not recommended unless directed by a doctor). Products include:
Bronkaid Caplets ▣ 717
Marax Tablets & DF Syrup 2200

Ephedrine Tannate (Concurrent use is not recommended unless directed by a doctor). Products include:
Rynatuss 2673

Epinephrine (Concurrent use is not recommended unless directed by a doctor). Products include:
Bronkaid Mist ▣ 717
EPIFRIN ◎ 239
EpiPen 790
Marcaine Hydrochloride with Epinephrine 1:200,000 2316
Primatene Mist ▣ 873
Sensorcaine with Epinephrine Injection 559
Sus-Phrine Injection 1019
Xylocaine with Epinephrine Injections 567

Epinephrine Bitartrate (Concurrent use is not recommended unless directed by a doctor). Products include:
Bronkaid Mist Suspension ▣ 718
Sensorcaine-MPF with Epinephrine Injection 559

Epinephrine Hydrochloride (Concurrent use is not recommended unless directed by a doctor). Products include:
Ana-Kit Anaphylaxis Emergency Treatment Kit 617

Fluoxetine Hydrochloride (Concurrent use is not recommended unless directed by a doctor). Products include:
Prozac Pulvules & Liquid, Oral Solution 919

Imipramine Hydrochloride (Concurrent use is not recommended unless directed by a doctor). Products include:
Tofranil Ampuls 854
Tofranil Tablets 856

Imipramine Pamoate (Concurrent use is not recommended unless directed by a doctor). Products include:
Tofranil-PM Capsules 857

Isocarboxazid (Concurrent use is not recommended unless directed by a doctor).
No products indexed under this heading.

Isoproterenol Hydrochloride (Concurrent use is not recommended unless directed by a doctor). Products include:
Isuprel Hydrochloride Injection 1:5000 2311
Isuprel Hydrochloride Solution 1:200 & 1:100 2313
Isuprel Mistometer 2312

Isoproterenol Sulfate (Concurrent use is not recommended unless directed by a doctor). Products include:
Norisodrine with Calcium Iodide Syrup 442

Maprotiline Hydrochloride (Concurrent use is not recommended unless directed by a doctor). Products include:
Ludiomil Tablets 843

Metaproterenol Sulfate (Concurrent use is not recommended unless directed by a doctor). Products include:
Alupent 669
Metaproterenol Sulfate Inhalation Solution, USP, Arm-a-Med 552

Metaraminol Bitartrate (Concurrent use is not recommended unless directed by a doctor). Products include:
Aramine Injection 1609

Methoxamine Hydrochloride (Concurrent use is not recommended unless directed by a doctor). Products include:
Vasoxyl Injection 1196

Nefazodone Hydrochloride (Concurrent use is not recommended unless directed by a doctor). Products include:
Serzone Tablets 771

Norepinephrine Bitartrate (Concurrent use is not recommended unless directed by a doctor). Products include:
Levophed Bitartrate Injection 2315

Nortriptyline Hydrochloride (Concurrent use is not recommended unless directed by a doctor). Products include:
Pamelor 2280

Paroxetine Hydrochloride (Concurrent use is not recommended unless directed by a doctor). Products include:
Paxil Tablets 2505

Phenelzine Sulfate (Concurrent use is not recommended unless directed by a doctor). Products include:
Nardil 1920

Phenylephrine Bitartrate (Concurrent use is not recommended unless directed by a doctor).
No products indexed under this heading.

Phenylephrine Hydrochloride (Concurrent use is not recommended unless directed by a doctor). Products include:
Atrohist Plus Tablets 454
Cerose DM ▣ 878
Comhist 2038
D.A. Chewable Tablets 951
Deconsal Pediatric Capsules 454
Dura-Vent/DA Tablets 953
Entex Capsules 1986
Entex Liquid 1986
Extendryl 1005
4-Way Fast Acting Nasal Spray (regular & mentholated) ▣ 621
Hemorid For Women ▣ 834
Hycomine Compound Tablets 932
Neo-Synephrine Hydrochloride 1% Carpuject 2324
Neo-Synephrine Hydrochloride 1% Injection 2324
Neo-Synephrine Hydrochloride (Ophthalmic) 2325
Neo-Synephrine ▣ 726
Nōstril ▣ 644
Novahistine Elixir ▣ 823
Phenergan VC 2779
Phenergan VC with Codeine 2781
Preparation H ▣ 871
Tympagesic Ear Drops 2342
Vasosulf ◎ 271
Vicks Sinex Nasal Spray and Ultra Fine Mist ▣ 765

Phenylephrine Tannate (Concurrent use is not recommended unless directed by a doctor). Products include:
Atrohist Pediatric Suspension 454
Ricobid-D Pediatric Suspension 2038
Ricobid Tablets and Pediatric Suspension 2038
Rynatan 2673
Rynatuss 2673

Phenylpropanolamine Hydrochloride (Concurrent use is not recommended unless directed by a doctor). Products include:
Acutrim ▣ 628
Allerest Children's Chewable Tablets ▣ 627
Allerest 12 Hour Caplets ▣ 627
Atrohist Plus Tablets 454
BC Cold Powder Multi-Symptom Formula (Cold-Sinus-Allergy) ▣ 609
BC Cold Powder Non-Drowsy Formula (Cold-Sinus) ▣ 609
Cheracol Plus Head Cold/Cough Formula ▣ 769
Comtrex Multi-Symptom Non-Drowsy Liqui-gels ▣ 618
Contac Continuous Action Nasal Decongestant/Antihistamine 12 Hour Capsules ▣ 813
Contac Maximum Strength Continuous Action Decongestant/Antihistamine 12 Hour Caplets ▣ 813
Contac Severe Cold and Flu Formula Caplets ▣ 814
Coricidin 'D' Decongestant Tablets ▣ 800
Dexatrim ▣ 832
Dexatrim Plus Vitamins Caplets ▣ 832
Dimetane-DC Cough Syrup 2059
Dimetapp Elixir ▣ 773
Dimetapp Extentabs ▣ 774
Dimetapp Tablets/Liqui-Gels ▣ 775
Dimetapp Cold & Allergy Chewable Tablets ▣ 773
Dimetapp DM Elixir ▣ 774
Dura-Vent Tablets 952
Entex Capsules 1986
Entex LA Tablets 1987
Entex Liquid 1986
Exgest LA Tablets 782
Hycomine 931
Isoclor Timesule Capsules ▣ 637
Nolamine Timed-Release Tablets 785
Ornade Spansule Capsules 2502
Propagest Tablets 786
Pyrroxate Caplets ▣ 772
Robitussin-CF ▣ 777
Sinulin Tablets 787
Tavist-D 12 Hour Relief Tablets ▣ 787
Teldrin 12 Hour Antihistamine/Nasal Decongestant Allergy Relief Capsules ▣ 826
Triaminic Allergy Tablets ▣ 789
Triaminic Cold Tablets ▣ 790
Triaminic Expectorant ▣ 790
Triaminic Syrup ▣ 792
Triaminic-12 Tablets ▣ 792
Triaminic-DM Syrup ▣ 792
Triaminicin Tablets ▣ 793
Triaminicol Multi-Symptom Cold Tablets ▣ 793
Triaminicol Multi-Symptom Relief ▣ 794
Vicks DayQuil Allergy Relief 12-Hour Extended Release Tablets ▣ 760
Vicks DayQuil Allergy Relief 4-Hour Tablets ▣ 760
Vicks DayQuil SINUS Pressure & CONGESTION Relief ▣ 761

Pirbuterol Acetate (Concurrent use is not recommended unless directed by a doctor). Products include:
Maxair Autohaler 1492
Maxair Inhaler 1494

Protriptyline Hydrochloride (Concurrent use is not recommended unless directed by a doctor). Products include:
Vivactil Tablets 1774

Pseudoephedrine Sulfate (Concurrent use is not recommended unless directed by a doctor). Products include:
Cheracol Sinus ▣ 768
Chlor-Trimeton Allergy Decongestant Tablets ▣ 799
Claritin-D 2350
Drixoral Cold and Allergy Sustained-Action Tablets ▣ 802
Drixoral Cold and Flu Extended-Release Tablets ▣ 803
Drixoral Non-Drowsy Formula Extended-Release Tablets ▣ 803
Drixoral Allergy/Sinus Extended Release Tablets ▣ 804
Trinalin Repetabs Tablets 1330

Salmeterol Xinafoate (Concurrent use is not recommended unless directed by a doctor). Products include:
Serevent Inhalation Aerosol 1176

Sertraline Hydrochloride (Concurrent use is not recommended unless directed by a doctor). Products include:
Zoloft Tablets 2217

Terbutaline Sulfate (Concurrent use is not recommended unless directed by a doctor). Products include:
Brethaire Inhaler 813
Brethine Ampuls 815
Brethine Tablets 814
Bricanyl Subcutaneous Injection 1502
Bricanyl Tablets 1503

Tranylcypromine Sulfate (Concurrent use is not recommended unless directed by a doctor). Products include:
Parnate Tablets 2503

Trazodone Hydrochloride (Concurrent use is not recommended unless directed by a doctor). Products include:
Desyrel and Desyrel Dividose 503

Trimipramine Maleate (Concurrent use is not recommended unless directed by a doctor). Products include:
Surmontil Capsules 2811

Venlafaxine Hydrochloride (Concurrent use is not recommended unless directed by a doctor). Products include:
Effexor 2719

IMPORTANT NOTE: Always consult each drug listing in the patient's regimen for possible interactions.

Dipentum | Interactions Index | 310

DIPENTUM CAPSULES
(Olsalazine Sodium)............................1951
May interact with oral anticoagulants. Compounds in this category include:

Dicumarol (Potential for increased prothrombin time).
No products indexed under this heading.

Warfarin Sodium (Potential for increased prothrombin time). Products include:
Coumadin 926

DIPHTHERIA & TETANUS TOXOIDS ADSORBED PUROGENATED
(Diphtheria & Tetanus Toxoids Adsorbed, (For Pediatric Use)) 1374
None cited in PDR database.

DIPHTHERIA AND TETANUS TOXOIDS AND PERTUSSIS VACCINE ADSORBED
(Diphtheria & Tetanus Toxoids w/Pertussis Vaccine Combined, Aluminum Phosphate Adsorbed)........2477
May interact with immunosuppressive agents, corticosteroids, cytotoxic drugs, alkylating agents, anticoagulants, and certain other agents. Compounds in these categories include:

Azathioprine (Reduces response to active immunization procedure). Products include:
Imuran 1110

Betamethasone Acetate (Reduces response to active immunization procedure). Products include:
Celestone Soluspan Suspension 2347

Betamethasone Sodium Phosphate (Reduces response to active immunization procedure). Products include:
Celestone Soluspan Suspension 2347

Bleomycin Sulfate (Reduces response to active immunization procedure). Products include:
Blenoxane 692

Busulfan (Reduces response to active immunization procedure). Products include:
Myleran Tablets 1143

Carmustine (BCNU) (Reduces response to active immunization procedure). Products include:
BiCNU 691

Chlorambucil (Reduces response to active immunization procedure). Products include:
Leukeran Tablets 1133

Cortisone Acetate (Reduces response to active immunization procedure). Products include:
Cortone Acetate Sterile Suspension 1623
Cortone Acetate Tablets 1624

Cyclophosphamide (Reduces response to active immunization procedure). Products include:
Cytoxan 694
NEOSAR Lyophilized/Neosar 1959

Cyclosporine (Reduces response to active immunization procedure). Products include:
Neoral 2276
Sandimmune 2286

Dacarbazine (Reduces response to active immunization procedure). Products include:
DTIC-Dome 600

Dalteparin Sodium (Caution should be exercised). Products include:
Fragmin 1954

Daunorubicin Hydrochloride (Reduces response to active immunization procedure). Products include:
Cerubidine 795

Dexamethasone (Reduces response to active immunization procedure). Products include:
AK-Trol Ointment & Suspension .... ◉ 205
Decadron Elixir 1633
Decadron Tablets 1635
Decaspray Topical Aerosol 1648
Dexacidin Ointment .... ◉ 263
Maxitrol Ophthalmic Ointment and Suspension .... ◉ 224
TobraDex Ophthalmic Suspension and Ointment 473

Dexamethasone Acetate (Reduces response to active immunization procedure). Products include:
Dalalone D.P. Injectable 1011
Decadron-LA Sterile Suspension 1646

Dexamethasone Sodium Phosphate (Reduces response to active immunization procedure). Products include:
Decadron Phosphate Injection 1637
Decadron Phosphate Respihaler 1642
Decadron Phosphate Sterile Ophthalmic Ointment 1641
Decadron Phosphate Sterile Ophthalmic Solution 1642
Decadron Phosphate Topical Cream 1644
Decadron Phosphate Turbinaire 1645
Decadron Phosphate with Xylocaine Injection, Sterile 1639
Dexacort Phosphate in Respihaler .. 458
Dexacort Phosphate in Turbinaire .. 459
NeoDecadron Sterile Ophthalmic Ointment 1712
NeoDecadron Sterile Ophthalmic Solution 1713
NeoDecadron Topical Cream 1714

Dicumarol (Caution should be exercised).
No products indexed under this heading.

Doxorubicin Hydrochloride (Reduces response to active immunization procedure). Products include:
Adriamycin PFS 1947
Adriamycin RDF 1947
Doxorubicin Astra 540
Rubex 712

Enoxaparin (Caution should be exercised). Products include:
Lovenox Injection 2020

Fludrocortisone Acetate (Reduces response to active immunization procedure). Products include:
Florinef Acetate Tablets 505

Fluorouracil (Reduces response to active immunization procedure). Products include:
Efudex 2113
Fluoroplex Topical Solution & Cream 1% 479
Fluorouracil Injection 2116

Heparin Calcium (Caution should be exercised).
No products indexed under this heading.

Heparin Sodium (Caution should be exercised). Products include:
Heparin Lock Flush Solution 2725
Heparin Sodium Injection 2726
Heparin Sodium Injection, USP, Sterile Solution 2615
Heparin Sodium Vials 1441

Hydrocortisone (Reduces response to active immunization procedure). Products include:
Anusol-HC Cream 2.5% 1896
Aquanil HC Lotion 1931
Bactine Hydrocortisone Anti-Itch Cream .... ▣ 709
Caldecort Anti-Itch Hydrocortisone Spray .... ▣ 631
Cortaid .... ▣ 836
CORTENEMA 2535
Cortisporin Ointment 1085
Cortisporin Ophthalmic Ointment Sterile 1085
Cortisporin Ophthalmic Suspension Sterile 1086
Cortisporin Otic Solution Sterile 1087
Cortisporin Otic Suspension Sterile 1088
Cortizone-5 .... ▣ 831
Cortizone-10 .... ▣ 831
Hydrocortone Tablets 1672
Hytone 907
Massengill Medicated Soft Cloth Towelettes 2458
PediOtic Suspension Sterile 1153
Preparation H Hydrocortisone 1% Cream .... ▣ 872
ProctoCream-HC 2.5% 2408
VōSoL HC Otic Solution 2678

Hydrocortisone Acetate (Reduces response to active immunization procedure). Products include:
Analpram-HC Rectal Cream 1% and 2.5% 977
Anusol HC-1 Anti-Itch Hydrocortisone Ointment .... ▣ 847
Anusol-HC Suppositories 1897
Caldecort .... ▣ 631
Carmol HC 924
Coly-Mycin S Otic w/Neomycin & Hydrocortisone 1906
Cortaid .... ▣ 836
Cortifoam 2396
Cortisporin Cream 1084
Epifoam 2399
Hydrocortone Acetate Sterile Suspension 1669
Mantadil Cream 1135
Nupercainal Hydrocortisone 1% Cream .... ▣ 645
Ophthocort .... ◉ 311
Pramosone Cream, Lotion & Ointment 978
ProctoCream-HC 2408
ProctoFoam-HC 2409
Terra-Cortril Ophthalmic Suspension 2210

Hydrocortisone Sodium Phosphate (Reduces response to active immunization procedure). Products include:
Hydrocortone Phosphate Injection, Sterile 1670

Hydrocortisone Sodium Succinate (Reduces response to active immunization procedure). Products include:
Solu-Cortef Sterile Powder 2641

Hydroxyurea (Reduces response to active immunization procedure). Products include:
Hydrea Capsules 696

Immune Globulin (Human) (Reduces response to active immunization procedure).
No products indexed under this heading.

Influenza Virus Vaccine (Influenza Virus Vaccine should not be given within 3 days of immunization). Products include:
Fluvirin 460
Influenza Virus Vaccine, Trivalent, Types A and B (chromatograph- and filter-purified subviron antigen) FluShield, 1995-1996 Formula 2736

Lomustine (CCNU) (Reduces response to active immunization procedure). Products include:
CeeNU 693

Mechlorethamine Hydrochloride (Reduces response to active immunization procedure). Products include:
Mustargen 1709

Melphalan (Reduces response to active immunization procedure). Products include:
Alkeran Tablets 1071

Methotrexate Sodium (Reduces response to active immunization procedure). Products include:
Methotrexate Sodium Tablets, Injection, for Injection and LPF Injection 1275

Methylprednisolone Acetate (Reduces response to active immunization procedure). Products include:
Depo-Medrol Single-Dose Vial 2600
Depo-Medrol Sterile Aqueous Suspension 2597

Methylprednisolone Sodium Succinate (Reduces response to active immunization procedure). Products include:
Solu-Medrol Sterile Powder 2643

Mitotane (Reduces response to active immunization procedure). Products include:
Lysodren 698

Mitoxantrone Hydrochloride (Reduces response to active immunization procedure). Products include:
Novantrone 1279

Muromonab-CD3 (Reduces response to active immunization procedure). Products include:
Orthoclone OKT3 Sterile Solution .. 1837

Mycophenolate Mofetil (Reduces response to active immunization procedure). Products include:
CellCept Capsules 2099

Prednisolone Acetate (Reduces response to active immunization procedure). Products include:
AK-CIDE .... ◉ 202
AK-CIDE Ointment .... ◉ 202
Blephamide Liquifilm Sterile Ophthalmic Suspension 476
Blephamide Ointment .... ◉ 237
Econopred & Econopred Plus Ophthalmic Suspensions .... ◉ 217
Poly-Pred Liquifilm .... ◉ 248
Pred Forte .... ◉ 250
Pred Mild .... ◉ 253
Pred-G Liquifilm Sterile Ophthalmic Suspension .... ◉ 251
Pred-G S.O.P. Sterile Ophthalmic Ointment .... ◉ 252
Vasocidin Ointment .... ◉ 268

Prednisolone Sodium Phosphate (Reduces response to active immunization procedure). Products include:
AK-Pred .... ◉ 204
Hydeltrasol Injection, Sterile 1665
Inflamase .... ◉ 265
Pediapred Oral Liquid 995
Vasocidin Ophthalmic Solution ...... ◉ 270

Prednisolone Tebutate (Reduces response to active immunization procedure). Products include:
Hydeltra-T.B.A. Sterile Suspension 1667

Prednisone (Reduces response to active immunization procedure). Products include:
Deltasone Tablets 2595

Procarbazine Hydrochloride (Reduces response to active immunization procedure). Products include:
Matulane Capsules 2131

Tacrolimus (Reduces response to active immunization procedure). Products include:
Prograf 1042

Tamoxifen Citrate (Reduces response to active immunization procedure). Products include:
Nolvadex Tablets 2841

Thiotepa (Reduces response to active immunization procedure). Products include:
Thioplex (Thiotepa For Injection) 1281

Triamcinolone (Reduces response to active immunization procedure). Products include:
Aristocort Tablets 1022

Triamcinolone Acetonide (Reduces response to active immunization procedure). Products include:
Aristocort A 0.025% Cream 1027
Aristocort A 0.5% Cream 1031
Aristocort A 0.1% Cream 1029
Aristocort A 0.1% Ointment 1030
Azmacort Oral Inhaler 2011

(▣ Described in PDR For Nonprescription Drugs) (◉ Described in PDR For Ophthalmology)

Nasacort Nasal Inhaler 2024

Triamcinolone Diacetate (Reduces response to active immunization procedure). Products include:

Aristocort Suspension (Forte Parenteral) 1027
Aristocort Suspension (Intralesional) 1025

Triamcinolone Hexacetonide (Reduces response to active immunization procedure). Products include:

Aristospan Suspension (Intra-articular) 1033
Aristospan Suspension (Intralesional) 1032

Vincristine Sulfate (Reduces response to active immunization procedure). Products include:

Oncovin Solution Vials & Hyporets 1466

Warfarin Sodium (Caution should be exercised). Products include:

Coumadin 926

DIPHTHERIA AND TETANUS TOXOIDS AND PERTUSSIS VACCINE ADSORBED USP (FOR PEDIATRIC USE)

(Diphtheria & Tetanus Toxoids w/Pertussis Vaccine Combined, Aluminum Potassium Sulfate Adsorbed) 875

May interact with immunosuppressive agents, corticosteroids, antineoplastics, cytotoxic drugs, alkylating agents, and anticoagulants. Compounds in these categories include:

Altretamine (May reduce immune response to vaccines). Products include:

Hexalen Capsules 2571

Asparaginase (May reduce immune response to vaccines). Products include:

Elspar 1659

Azathioprine (May reduce immune response to vaccines). Products include:

Imuran 1110

Betamethasone Acetate (May reduce immune response to vaccines). Products include:

Celestone Soluspan Suspension 2347

Betamethasone Sodium Phosphate (May reduce immune response to vaccines). Products include:

Celestone Soluspan Suspension 2347

Bleomycin Sulfate (May reduce immune response to vaccines). Products include:

Blenoxane 692

Busulfan (May reduce immune response to vaccines). Products include:

Myleran Tablets 1143

Carboplatin (May reduce immune response to vaccines). Products include:

Paraplatin for Injection 705

Carmustine (BCNU) (May reduce immune response to vaccines). Products include:

BiCNU 691

Chlorambucil (May reduce immune response to vaccines). Products include:

Leukeran Tablets 1133

Cisplatin (May reduce immune response to vaccines). Products include:

Platinol 708
Platinol-AQ Injection 710

Cortisone Acetate (May reduce immune response to vaccines). Products include:

Cortone Acetate Sterile Suspension 1623

Cortone Acetate Tablets 1624

Cyclophosphamide (May reduce immune response to vaccines). Products include:

Cytoxan 694
NEOSAR Lyophilized/Neosar 1959

Cyclosporine (May reduce immune response to vaccines). Products include:

Neoral 2276
Sandimmune 2286

Dacarbazine (May reduce immune response to vaccines). Products include:

DTIC-Dome 600

Dalteparin Sodium (Use DTP with caution in patients on anticoagulant therapy). Products include:

Fragmin 1954

Daunorubicin Hydrochloride (May reduce immune response to vaccines). Products include:

Cerubidine 795

Dexamethasone (May reduce immune response to vaccines). Products include:

AK-Trol Ointment & Suspension .... ⊙ 205
Decadron Elixir 1633
Decadron Tablets................................... 1635
Decaspray Topical Aerosol 1648
Dexacidin Ointment .... ⊙ 263
Maxitrol Ophthalmic Ointment and Suspension .... ⊙ 224
TobraDex Ophthalmic Suspension and Ointment.. 473

Dexamethasone Acetate (May reduce immune response to vaccines). Products include:

Dalalone D.P. Injectable 1011
Decadron-LA Sterile Suspension 1646

Dexamethasone Sodium Phosphate (May reduce immune response to vaccines). Products include:

Decadron Phosphate Injection 1637
Decadron Phosphate Respihaler 1642
Decadron Phosphate Sterile Ophthalmic Ointment 1641
Decadron Phosphate Sterile Ophthalmic Solution 1642
Decadron Phosphate Topical Cream 1644
Decadron Phosphate Turbinaire 1645
Decadron Phosphate with Xylocaine Injection, Sterile 1639
Dexacort Phosphate in Respihaler .. 458
Dexacort Phosphate in Turbinaire .. 459
NeoDecadron Sterile Ophthalmic Ointment 1712
NeoDecadron Sterile Ophthalmic Solution 1713
NeoDecadron Topical Cream 1714

Dicumarol (Use DTP with caution in patients on anticoagulant therapy).

No products indexed under this heading.

Doxorubicin Hydrochloride (May reduce immune response to vaccines). Products include:

Adriamycin PFS 1947
Adriamycin RDF 1947
Doxorubicin Astra 540
Rubex 712

Enoxaparin (Use DTP with caution in patients on anticoagulant therapy). Products include:

Lovenox Injection 2020

Estramustine Phosphate Sodium (May reduce immune response to vaccines). Products include:

Emcyt Capsules 1953

Etoposide (May reduce immune response to vaccines). Products include:

VePesid Capsules and Injection 718

Floxuridine (May reduce immune response to vaccines). Products include:

Sterile FUDR 2118

Fludrocortisone Acetate (May reduce immune response to vaccines). Products include:

Florinef Acetate Tablets 505

Fluorouracil (May reduce immune response to vaccines). Products include:

Efudex 2113
Fluoroplex Topical Solution & Cream 1% 479
Fluorouracil Injection 2116

Flutamide (May reduce immune response to vaccines). Products include:

Eulexin Capsules 2358

Heparin Calcium (Use DTP with caution in patients on anticoagulant therapy).

No products indexed under this heading.

Heparin Sodium (Use DTP with caution in patients on anticoagulant therapy). Products include:

Heparin Lock Flush Solution 2725
Heparin Sodium Injection.................... 2726
Heparin Sodium Injection, USP, Sterile Solution 2615
Heparin Sodium Vials........................... 1441

Hydrocortisone (May reduce immune response to vaccines). Products include:

Anusol-HC Cream 2.5% 1896
Aquanil HC Lotion 1931
Bactine Hydrocortisone Anti-Itch Cream .... ⊞ 709
Caldecort Anti-Itch Hydrocortisone Spray .... ⊞ 631
Cortaid .... ⊞ 836
CORTENEMA 2535
Cortisporin Ointment 1085
Cortisporin Ophthalmic Ointment Sterile 1085
Cortisporin Ophthalmic Suspension Sterile 1086
Cortisporin Otic Solution Sterile 1087
Cortisporin Otic Suspension Sterile 1088
Cortizone-5 .... ⊞ 831
Cortizone-10 .... ⊞ 831
Hydrocortone Tablets 1672
Hytone 907
Massengill Medicated Soft Cloth Towelettes... 2458
PediOtic Suspension Sterile 1153
Preparation H Hydrocortisone 1% Cream .... ⊞ 872
ProctoCream-HC 2.5% 2408
VōSoL HC Otic Solution....................... 2678

Hydrocortisone Acetate (May reduce immune response to vaccines). Products include:

Analpram-HC Rectal Cream 1% and 2.5% 977
Anusol HC-1 Anti-Itch Hydrocortisone Ointment.. ⊞ 847
Anusol-HC Suppositories 1897
Caldecort .... ⊞ 631
Carmol HC 924
Coly-Mycin S Otic w/Neomycin & Hydrocortisone 1906
Cortaid .... ⊞ 836
Cortifoam 2396
Cortisporin Cream................................. 1084
Epifoam 2399
Hydrocortone Acetate Sterile Suspension... 1669
Mantadil Cream 1135
Nupercainal Hydrocortisone 1% Cream .... ⊞ 645
Ophthocort .... ⊙ 311
Pramosone Cream, Lotion & Ointment 978
ProctoCream-HC 2408
ProctoFoam-HC 2409
Terra-Cortril Ophthalmic Suspension 2210

Hydrocortisone Sodium Phosphate (May reduce immune response to vaccines). Products include:

Hydrocortone Phosphate Injection, Sterile 1670

Hydrocortisone Sodium Succinate (May reduce immune response to vaccines). Products include:

Solu-Cortef Sterile Powder................. 2641

Hydroxyurea (May reduce immune response to vaccines). Products include:

Hydrea Capsules 696

Idarubicin Hydrochloride (May reduce immune response to vaccines). Products include:

Idamycin 1955

Ifosfamide (May reduce immune response to vaccines). Products include:

IFEX 697

Immune Globulin (Human) (May reduce immune response to vaccines).

No products indexed under this heading.

Interferon alfa-2A, Recombinant (May reduce immune response to vaccines). Products include:

Roferon-A Injection 2145

Interferon alfa-2B, Recombinant (May reduce immune response to vaccines). Products include:

Intron A 2364

Levamisole Hydrochloride (May reduce immune response to vaccines). Products include:

Ergamisol Tablets 1292

Lomustine (CCNU) (May reduce immune response to vaccines). Products include:

CeeNU 693

Mechlorethamine Hydrochloride (May reduce immune response to vaccines). Products include:

Mustargen... 1709

Megestrol Acetate (May reduce immune response to vaccines). Products include:

Megace Oral Suspension 699
Megace Tablets 701

Melphalan (May reduce immune response to vaccines). Products include:

Alkeran Tablets...................................... 1071

Mercaptopurine (May reduce immune response to vaccines). Products include:

Purinethol Tablets 1156

Methotrexate Sodium (May reduce immune response to vaccines). Products include:

Methotrexate Sodium Tablets, Injection, for Injection and LPF Injection 1275

Methylprednisolone Acetate (May reduce immune response to vaccines). Products include:

Depo-Medrol Single-Dose Vial 2600
Depo-Medrol Sterile Aqueous Suspension... 2597

Methylprednisolone Sodium Succinate (May reduce immune response to vaccines). Products include:

Solu-Medrol Sterile Powder 2643

Mitomycin (Mitomycin-C) (May reduce immune response to vaccines). Products include:

Mutamycin 703

Mitotane (May reduce immune response to vaccines). Products include:

Lysodren 698

Mitoxantrone Hydrochloride (May reduce immune response to vaccines). Products include:

Novantrone... 1279

Muromonab-CD3 (May reduce immune response to vaccines). Products include:

Orthoclone OKT3 Sterile Solution .. 1837

Mycophenolate Mofetil (May reduce immune response to vaccines). Products include:

CellCept Capsules 2099

IMPORTANT NOTE: Always consult each drug listing in the patient's regimen for possible interactions.

Paclitaxel (May reduce immune response to vaccines). Products include:
- Taxol ... 714

Prednisolone Acetate (May reduce immune response to vaccines). Products include:
- AK-CIDE ... ⊙ 202
- AK-CIDE Ointment ... ⊙ 202
- Blephamide Liquifilm Sterile Ophthalmic Suspension ... 476
- Blephamide Ointment ... ⊙ 237
- Econopred & Econopred Plus Ophthalmic Suspensions ... ⊙ 217
- Poly-Pred Liquifilm ... ⊙ 248
- Pred Forte ... ⊙ 250
- Pred Mild ... ⊙ 253
- Pred-G Liquifilm Sterile Ophthalmic Suspension ... ⊙ 251
- Pred-G S.O.P. Sterile Ophthalmic Ointment ... ⊙ 252
- Vasocidin Ointment ... ⊙ 268

Prednisolone Sodium Phosphate (May reduce immune response to vaccines). Products include:
- AK-Pred ... ⊙ 204
- Hydeltrasol Injection, Sterile ... 1665
- Inflamase ... ⊙ 265
- Pediapred Oral Liquid ... 995
- Vasocidin Ophthalmic Solution ... ⊙ 270

Prednisolone Tebutate (May reduce immune response to vaccines). Products include:
- Hydeltra-T.B.A. Sterile Suspension 1667

Prednisone (May reduce immune response to vaccines). Products include:
- Deltasone Tablets ... 2595

Procarbazine Hydrochloride (May reduce immune response to vaccines). Products include:
- Matulane Capsules ... 2131

Streptozocin (May reduce immune response to vaccines). Products include:
- Zanosar Sterile Powder ... 2653

Tacrolimus (May reduce immune response to vaccines). Products include:
- Prograf ... 1042

Tamoxifen Citrate (May reduce immune response to vaccines). Products include:
- Nolvadex Tablets ... 2841

Teniposide (May reduce immune response to vaccines). Products include:
- Vumon ... 727

Thioguanine (May reduce immune response to vaccines). Products include:
- Thioguanine Tablets, Tabloid Brand ... 1181

Thiotepa (May reduce immune response to vaccines). Products include:
- Thioplex (Thiotepa For Injection) ... 1281

Triamcinolone (May reduce immune response to vaccines). Products include:
- Aristocort Tablets ... 1022

Triamcinolone Acetonide (May reduce immune response to vaccines). Products include:
- Aristocort A 0.025% Cream ... 1027
- Aristocort A 0.5% Cream ... 1031
- Aristocort A 0.1% Cream ... 1029
- Aristocort A 0.1% Ointment ... 1030
- Azmacort Oral Inhaler ... 2011
- Nasacort Nasal Inhaler ... 2024

Triamcinolone Diacetate (May reduce immune response to vaccines). Products include:
- Aristocort Suspension (Forte Parenteral) ... 1027
- Aristocort Suspension (Intralesional) ... 1025

Triamcinolone Hexacetonide (May reduce immune response to vaccines). Products include:
- Aristospan Suspension (Intra-articular) ... 1033
- Aristospan Suspension (Intralesional) ... 1032

Vincristine Sulfate (May reduce immune response to vaccines). Products include:
- Oncovin Solution Vials & Hyporets 1466

Vinorelbine Tartrate (May reduce immune response to vaccines). Products include:
- Navelbine Injection ... 1145

Warfarin Sodium (Use DTP with caution in patients on anticoagulant therapy). Products include:
- Coumadin ... 926

DIPRIVAN INJECTION
(Propofol) ... 2833

May interact with narcotic analgesics, hypnotics and sedatives, benzodiazepines, barbiturates, inhalant anesthetics, and certain other agents. Compounds in these categories include:

Alfentanil Hydrochloride (Increases anesthetic or sedative effects; may also result in pronounced decreases in systolic, diastolic, and mean arterial pressure and cardiac output). Products include:
- Alfenta Injection ... 1286

Alprazolam (Increases anesthetic or sedative effects; may also result in pronounced decreases in systolic, diastolic, and mean arterial pressure and cardiac output). Products include:
- Xanax Tablets ... 2649

Aprobarbital (Increases anesthetic or sedative effects; may also result in pronounced decreases in systolic, diastolic, and mean arterial pressure and cardiac output).
- No products indexed under this heading.

Buprenorphine (Increases anesthetic or sedative effects; may also result in pronounced decreases in systolic, diastolic, and mean arterial pressure and cardiac output). Products include:
- Buprenex Injectable ... 2006

Butabarbital (Increases anesthetic or sedative effects; may also result in pronounced decreases in systolic, diastolic, and mean arterial pressure and cardiac output).
- No products indexed under this heading.

Butalbital (Increases anesthetic or sedative effects; may also result in pronounced decreases in systolic, diastolic, and mean arterial pressure and cardiac output). Products include:
- Esgic-plus Tablets ... 1013
- Fioricet Tablets ... 2258
- Fioricet with Codeine Capsules ... 2260
- Fiorinal Capsules ... 2261
- Fiorinal with Codeine Capsules ... 2262
- Fiorinal Tablets ... 2261
- Phrenilin ... 785
- Sedapap Tablets 50 mg/650 mg .. 1543

Chloral Hydrate (Increases anesthetic or sedative effects; may also result in pronounced decreases in systolic, diastolic, and mean arterial pressure and cardiac output).
- No products indexed under this heading.

Chlordiazepoxide (Increases anesthetic or sedative effects; may also result in pronounced decreases in systolic, diastolic, and mean arterial pressure and cardiac output). Products include:
- Libritabs Tablets ... 2177
- Limbitrol ... 2180

Chlordiazepoxide Hydrochloride (Increases anesthetic or sedative effects; may also result in pronounced decreases in systolic, diastolic, and mean arterial pressure and cardiac output). Products include:
- Librax Capsules ... 2176
- Librium Capsules ... 2178
- Librium Injectable ... 2179

Clorazepate Dipotassium (Increases anesthetic or sedative effects; may also result in pronounced decreases in systolic, diastolic, and mean arterial pressure and cardiac output). Products include:
- Tranxene ... 451

Codeine Phosphate (Increases anesthetic or sedative effects; may also result in pronounced decreases in systolic, diastolic, and mean arterial pressure and cardiac output). Products include:
- Actifed with Codeine Cough Syrup.. 1067
- Brontex ... 1981
- Deconsal C Expectorant Syrup ... 456
- Deconsal Pediatric Syrup ... 457
- Dimetane-DC Cough Syrup ... 2059
- Empirin with Codeine Tablets ... 1093
- Fioricet with Codeine Capsules ... 2260
- Fiorinal with Codeine Capsules ... 2262
- Isoclor Expectorant ... 990
- Novahistine DH ... 2462
- Novahistine Expectorant ... 2463
- Nucofed ... 2051
- Phenergan with Codeine ... 2777
- Phenergan VC with Codeine ... 2781
- Robitussin A-C Syrup ... 2073
- Robitussin-DAC Syrup ... 2074
- Ryna ... ▣ 841
- Soma Compound w/Codeine Tablets ... 2676
- Tussi-Organidin NR Liquid and S NR Liquid ... 2677
- Tylenol with Codeine ... 1583

Desflurane (Increases anesthetic or sedative and cardiorespiratory effects). Products include:
- Suprane ... 1813

Dezocine (Increases anesthetic or sedative effects; may also result in pronounced decreases in systolic, diastolic, and mean arterial pressure and cardiac output). Products include:
- Dalgan Injection ... 538

Diazepam (Increases anesthetic or sedative effects; may also result in pronounced decreases in systolic, diastolic, and mean arterial pressure and cardiac output). Products include:
- Dizac ... 1809
- Valium Injectable ... 2182
- Valium Tablets ... 2183
- Valrelease Capsules ... 2169

Droperidol (Increases anesthetic or sedative effects; may also result in pronounced decreases in systolic, diastolic, and mean arterial pressure and cardiac output). Products include:
- Inapsine Injection ... 1296

Enflurane (Increases anesthetic or sedative and cardiorespiratory effects).
- No products indexed under this heading.

Estazolam (Increases anesthetic or sedative effects; may also result in pronounced decreases in systolic, diastolic, and mean arterial pressure and cardiac output). Products include:
- ProSom Tablets ... 449

Ethchlorvynol (Increases anesthetic or sedative effects; may also result in pronounced decreases in systolic, diastolic, and mean arterial pressure and cardiac output). Products include:
- Placidyl Capsules ... 448

Ethinamate (Increases anesthetic or sedative effects; may also result in pronounced decreases in systolic, diastolic, and mean arterial pressure and cardiac output).
- No products indexed under this heading.

Fentanyl (Increases anesthetic or sedative effects; may also result in pronounced decreases in systolic, diastolic, and mean arterial pressure and cardiac output). Products include:
- Duragesic Transdermal System ... 1288

Fentanyl Citrate (Increases anesethetic or sedative effects; may also result in pronounced decreases in systolic, diastolic, and mean arterial pressure and cardiac output). Products include:
- Sublimaze Injection ... 1307

Flurazepam Hydrochloride (Increases anesthetic or sedative effects; may also result in pronounced decreases in systolic, diastolic, and mean arterial pressure and cardiac output). Products include:
- Dalmane Capsules ... 2173

Glutethimide (Increases anesthetic or sedative effects; may also result in pronounced decreases in systolic, diastolic, and mean arterial pressure and cardiac output).
- No products indexed under this heading.

Halazepam (Increases anesthetic or sedative effects; may also result in pronounced decreases in systolic, diastolic, and mean arterial pressure and cardiac output).
- No products indexed under this heading.

Halothane (Increases anesthetic or sedative and cardiorespiratory effects). Products include:
- Fluothane ... 2724

Hydrocodone Bitartrate (Increases anesthetic or sedative effects; may also result in pronounced decreases in systolic, diastolic, and mean arterial pressure and cardiac output). Products include:
- Anexsia 5/500 Elixir ... 1781
- Anexia Tablets ... 1782
- Codiclear DH Syrup ... 791
- Deconamine CX Cough and Cold Liquid and Tablets ... 1319
- Duratuss HD Elixir ... 2565
- Hycodan Tablets and Syrup ... 930
- Hycomine Compound Tablets ... 932
- Hycomine ... 931
- Hycotuss Expectorant Syrup ... 933
- Hydrocet Capsules ... 782
- Lorcet 10/650 ... 1018
- Lortab ... 2566
- Tussend ... 1783
- Tussend Expectorant ... 1785
- Vicodin Tablets ... 1356
- Vicodin ES Tablets ... 1357
- Vicodin Tuss Expectorant ... 1358
- Zydone Capsules ... 949

(▣ Described in PDR For Nonprescription Drugs) (⊙ Described in PDR For Ophthalmology)

Hydrocodone Polistirex (Increases anesthetic or sedative effects; may also result in pronounced decreases in systolic, diastolic, and mean arterial pressure and cardiac output). Products include:

Tussionex Pennkinetic Extended-Release Suspension 998

Isoflurane (Increases anesthetic or sedative and cardiorespiratory effects).

No products indexed under this heading.

Levorphanol Tartrate (Increases anesthetic or sedative effects; may also result in pronounced decreases in systolic, diastolic, and mean arterial pressure and cardiac output). Products include:

Levo-Dromoran 2129

Lorazepam (Increases anesthetic or sedative effects; may also result in pronounced decreases in systolic, diastolic, and mean arterial pressure and cardiac output). Products include:

Ativan Injection 2698
Ativan Tablets 2700

Meperidine Hydrochloride (Increases anesthetic or sedative effects; may also result in pronounced decreases in systolic, diastolic, and mean arterial pressure and cardiac output). Products include:

Demerol 2308
Mepergan Injection 2753

Mephobarbital (Increases anesthetic or sedative effects; may also result in pronounced decreases in systolic, diastolic, and mean arterial pressure and cardiac output). Products include:

Mebaral Tablets 2322

Methadone Hydrochloride (Increases anesthetic or sedative effects; may also result in pronounced decreases in systolic, diastolic, and mean arterial pressure and cardiac output). Products include:

Methadone Hydrochloride Oral Concentrate 2233
Methadone Hydrochloride Oral Solution & Tablets 2235

Methoxyflurane (Increases anesthetic or sedative and cardiorespiratory effects).

No products indexed under this heading.

Midazolam Hydrochloride (Increases anesthetic or sedative effects; may also result in pronounced decreases in systolic, diastolic, and mean arterial pressure and cardiac output). Products include:

Versed Injection 2170

Morphine Sulfate (Increases anesthetic or sedative effects; may also result in pronounced decreases in systolic, diastolic, and mean arterial pressure and cardiac output). Products include:

Astramorph/PF Injection, USP (Preservative-Free) 535
Duramorph 962
Infumorph 200 and Infumorph 500 Sterile Solutions 965
MS Contin Tablets 1994
MSIR 1997
Oramorph SR (Morphine Sulfate Sustained Release Tablets) 2236
RMS Suppositories 2657
Roxanol 2243

Nitrous Oxide (Rate of administration requires adjustment).

Opium Alkaloids (Increases anesthetic or sedative effects; may also result in pronounced decreases in systolic, diastolic, and mean arterial pressure and cardiac output).

No products indexed under this heading.

Oxazepam (Increases anesthetic or sedative effects; may also result in pronounced decreases in systolic, diastolic, and mean arterial pressure and cardiac output). Products include:

Serax Capsules 2810
Serax Tablets 2810

Oxycodone Hydrochloride (Increases anesthetic or sedative effects; may also result in pronounced decreases in systolic, diastolic, and mean arterial pressure and cardiac output). Products include:

Percocet Tablets 938
Percodan Tablets 939
Percodan-Demi Tablets 940
Roxicodone Tablets, Oral Solution & Intensol (Oxycodone) 2244
Tylox Capsules 1584

Pentobarbital Sodium (Increases anesthetic or sedative effects; may also result in pronounced decreases in systolic, diastolic, and mean arterial pressure and cardiac output). Products include:

Nembutal Sodium Capsules 436
Nembutal Sodium Solution 438
Nembutal Sodium Suppositories 440

Phenobarbital (Increases anesthetic or sedative effects; may also result in pronounced decreases in systolic, diastolic, and mean arterial pressure and cardiac output). Products include:

Arco-Lase Plus Tablets 512
Bellergal-S Tablets 2250
Donnatal 2060
Donnatal Extentabs 2061
Donnatal Tablets 2060
Phenobarbital Elixir and Tablets 1469
Quadrinal Tablets 1350

Prazepam (Increases anesthetic or sedative effects; may also result in pronounced decreases in systolic, diastolic, and mean arterial pressure and cardiac output).

No products indexed under this heading.

Propoxyphene Hydrochloride (Increases anesthetic or sedative effects; may also result in pronounced decreases in systolic, diastolic, and mean arterial pressure and cardiac output). Products include:

Darvon 1435
Wygesic Tablets 2827

Propoxyphene Napsylate (Increases anesthetic or sedative effects; may also result in pronounced decreases in systolic, diastolic, and mean arterial pressure and cardiac output). Products include:

Darvon-N/Darvocet-N 1433

Quazepam (Increases anesthetic or sedative effects; may also result in pronounced decreases in systolic, diastolic, and mean arterial pressure and cardiac output). Products include:

Doral Tablets 2664

Secobarbital Sodium (Increases anesthetic or sedative effects; may also result in pronounced decreases in systolic, diastolic, and mean arterial pressure and cardiac output). Products include:

Seconal Sodium Pulvules 1474

Sufentanil Citrate (Increases anesthetic or sedative effects; may also result in pronounced decreases in systolic, diastolic, and mean arterial pressure and cardiac output). Products include:

Sufenta Injection 1309

Temazepam (Increases anesthetic or sedative effects; may also result in pronounced decreases in systolic, diastolic, and mean arterial pressure and cardiac output). Products include:

Restoril Capsules 2284

Thiamylal Sodium (Increases anesthetic or sedative effects; may also result in pronounced decreases in systolic, diastolic, and mean arterial pressure and cardiac output).

No products indexed under this heading.

Triazolam (Increases anesthetic or sedative effects; may also result in pronounced decreases in systolic, diastolic, and mean arterial pressure and cardiac output). Products include:

Halcion Tablets 2611

Zolpidem Tartrate (Increases anesthetic or sedative effects; may also result in pronounced decreases in systolic, diastolic, and mean arterial pressure and cardiac output). Products include:

Ambien Tablets 2416

DIPROLENE AF CREAM

(Betamethasone Dipropionate) 2352
None cited in PDR database.

DIPROLENE GEL 0.05%

(Betamethasone Dipropionate) 2353
None cited in PDR database.

DIPROLENE LOTION 0.05%

(Betamethasone Dipropionate) 2352
None cited in PDR database.

DIPROLENE OINTMENT 0.05%

(Betamethasone Dipropionate) 2352
None cited in PDR database.

DITROPAN SYRUP

(Oxybutynin Chloride) 1516
See **Ditropan Tablets**

DITROPAN TABLETS

(Oxybutynin Chloride) 1516
May interact with hypnotics and sedatives and certain other agents. Compounds in these categories include:

Estazolam (Enhances the drowsiness effect). Products include:

ProSom Tablets 449

Ethchlorvynol (Enhances the drowsiness effect). Products include:

Placidyl Capsules 448

Ethinamate (Enhances the drowsiness effect).

No products indexed under this heading.

Flurazepam Hydrochloride (Enhances the drowsiness effect). Products include:

Dalmane Capsules 2173

Glutethimide (Enhances the drowsiness effect).

No products indexed under this heading.

Lorazepam (Enhances the drowsiness effect). Products include:

Ativan Injection 2698
Ativan Tablets 2700

Midazolam Hydrochloride (Enhances the drowsiness effect). Products include:

Versed Injection 2170

Propofol (Enhances the drowsiness effect). Products include:

Diprivan Injection 2833

Quazepam (Enhances the drowsiness effect). Products include:

Doral Tablets 2664

Secobarbital Sodium (Enhances the drowsiness effect). Products include:

Seconal Sodium Pulvules 1474

Temazepam (Enhances the drowsiness effect). Products include:

Restoril Capsules 2284

Triazolam (Enhances the drowsiness effect). Products include:

Halcion Tablets 2611

Zolpidem Tartrate (Enhances the drowsiness effect). Products include:

Ambien Tablets 2416

Food Interactions

Alcohol (Enhances the drowsiness effect).

DIUCARDIN TABLETS

(Hydroflumethiazide) 2718
May interact with antihypertensives, corticosteroids, insulin, lithium preparations, general anesthetics, preanesthetic medications, nondepolarizing neuromuscular blocking agents, cardiac glycosides, oral hypoglycemic agents, oral anticoagulants, barbiturates, narcotic analgesics, non-steroidal anti-inflammatory agents, and certain other agents. Compounds in these categories include:

Acarbose (Thiazides may raise blood glucose levels).

No products indexed under this heading.

Acebutolol Hydrochloride (Effects may be potentiated when used concurrently with thiazide diuretics). Products include:

Sectral Capsules 2807

ACTH (Concurrent use with thiazide diuretics may intensify electrolyte imbalance, particularly hypokalemia).

No products indexed under this heading.

Alfentanil Hydrochloride (Orthostatic hypotension may be aggravated). Products include:

Alfenta Injection 1286

Allopurinol (Thiazide diuretics may raise the level of blood uric acid). Products include:

Zyloprim Tablets 1226

Amlodipine Besylate (Effects may be potentiated when used concurrently with thiazide diuretics). Products include:

Lotrel Capsules 840
Norvasc Tablets 1940

Amphotericin B (Concurrent use with thiazide diuretics may intensify electrolyte imbalance, particularly hypokalemia). Products include:

Fungizone Intravenous 506

Aprobarbital (Orthostatic hypotension may be aggravated).

No products indexed under this heading.

Atenolol (Effects may be potentiated when used concurrently with thiazide diuretics). Products include:

Tenoretic Tablets 2845
Tenormin Tablets and I.V. Injection 2847

IMPORTANT NOTE: Always consult each drug listing in the patient's regimen for possible interactions.

Diucardin Interactions Index 314

Atracurium Besylate (Effects may be potentiated when used concurrently with thiazide diuretics). Products include:
- Tracrium Injection 1183

Benazepril Hydrochloride (Effects may be potentiated when used concurrently with thiazide diuretics). Products include:
- Lotensin Tablets 834
- Lotensin HCT 837
- Lotrel Capsules 840

Bendroflumethiazide (Effects may be potentiated when used concurrently with thiazide diuretics).
- No products indexed under this heading.

Betamethasone Acetate (Concurrent use with thiazide diuretics may intensify electrolyte imbalance, particularly hypokalemia). Products include:
- Celestone Soluspan Suspension 2347

Betamethasone Sodium Phosphate (Concurrent use with thiazide diuretics may intensify electrolyte imbalance, particularly hypokalemia). Products include:
- Celestone Soluspan Suspension 2347

Betaxolol Hydrochloride (Effects may be potentiated when used concurrently with thiazide diuretics). Products include:
- Betoptic Ophthalmic Solution 469
- Betoptic S Ophthalmic Suspension 471
- Kerlone Tablets 2436

Bisoprolol Fumarate (Effects may be potentiated when used concurrently with thiazide diuretics). Products include:
- Zebeta Tablets 1413
- Ziac 1415

Buprenorphine (Orthostatic hypotension may be aggravated). Products include:
- Buprenex Injectable 2006

Butabarbital (Orthostatic hypotension may be aggravated).
- No products indexed under this heading.

Butalbital (Orthostatic hypotension may be aggravated). Products include:
- Esgic-plus Tablets 1013
- Fioricet Tablets 2258
- Fioricet with Codeine Capsules 2260
- Fiorinal Capsules 2261
- Fiorinal with Codeine Capsules 2262
- Fiorinal Tablets 2261
- Phrenilin 785
- Sedapap Tablets 50 mg/650 mg .. 1543

Captopril (Effects may be potentiated when used concurrently with thiazide diuretics). Products include:
- Capoten 739
- Capozide 742

Carteolol Hydrochloride (Effects may be potentiated when used concurrently with thiazide diuretics). Products include:
- Cartrol Tablets 410
- Ocupress Ophthalmic Solution, 1% Sterile .... ◉ 309

Chlorothiazide (Effects may be potentiated when used concurrently with thiazide diuretics). Products include:
- Aldoclor Tablets 1598
- Diupres Tablets 1650
- Diuril Oral 1653

Chlorothiazide Sodium (Effects may be potentiated when used concurrently with thiazide diuretics). Products include:
- Diuril Sodium Intravenous 1652

Chlorpropamide (Thiazides may raise blood glucose levels). Products include:
- Diabinese Tablets 1935

Chlorthalidone (Effects may be potentiated when used concurrently with thiazide diuretics). Products include:
- Combipres Tablets 677
- Tenoretic Tablets 2845
- Thalitone 1245

Clonidine (Effects may be potentiated when used concurrently with thiazide diuretics). Products include:
- Catapres-TTS 675

Clonidine Hydrochloride (Effects may be potentiated when used concurrently with thiazide diuretics). Products include:
- Catapres Tablets 674
- Combipres Tablets 677

Codeine Phosphate (Orthostatic hypotension may be aggravated). Products include:
- Actifed with Codeine Cough Syrup.. 1067
- Brontex 1981
- Deconsal C Expectorant Syrup 456
- Deconsal Pediatric Syrup 457
- Dimetane-DC Cough Syrup 2059
- Empirin with Codeine Tablets 1093
- Fioricet with Codeine Capsules 2260
- Fiorinal with Codeine Capsules 2262
- Isoclor Expectorant 990
- Novahistine DH 2462
- Novahistine Expectorant 2463
- Nucofed 2051
- Phenergan with Codeine 2777
- Phenergan VC with Codeine 2781
- Robitussin A-C Syrup 2073
- Robitussin-DAC Syrup 2074
- Ryna .... ▣ 841
- Soma Compound w/Codeine Tablets 2676
- Tussi-Organidin NR Liquid and S NR Liquid 2677
- Tylenol with Codeine 1583

Colestipol Hydrochloride (May inhibit gastrointestinal absorption of the thiazide diuretics). Products include:
- Colestid Tablets 2591

Cortisone Acetate (Concurrent use with thiazide diuretics may intensify electrolyte imbalance, particularly hypokalemia). Products include:
- Cortone Acetate Sterile Suspension 1623
- Cortone Acetate Tablets 1624

Deserpidine (Effects may be potentiated when used concurrently with thiazide diuretics).
- No products indexed under this heading.

Deslanoside (Enhanced possibility of digitalis toxicity associated with hypokalemia).
- No products indexed under this heading.

Dexamethasone (Concurrent use with thiazide diuretics may intensify electrolyte imbalance, particularly hypokalemia). Products include:
- AK-Trol Ointment & Suspension .... ◉ 205
- Decadron Elixir 1633
- Decadron Tablets 1635
- Decaspray Topical Aerosol 1648
- Dexacidin Ointment .... ◉ 263
- Maxitrol Ophthalmic Ointment and Suspension .... ◉ 224
- TobraDex Ophthalmic Suspension and Ointment 473

Dexamethasone Acetate (Concurrent use with thiazide diuretics may intensify electrolyte imbalance, particularly hypokalemia). Products include:
- Dalalone D.P. Injectable 1011
- Decadron-LA Sterile Suspension 1646

Dexamethasone Sodium Phosphate (Concurrent use with thiazide diuretics may intensify electrolyte imbalance, particularly hypokalemia). Products include:
- Decadron Phosphate Injection 1637
- Decadron Phosphate Respihaler 1642
- Decadron Phosphate Sterile Ophthalmic Ointment 1641
- Decadron Phosphate Sterile Ophthalmic Solution 1642
- Decadron Phosphate Topical Cream 1644
- Decadron Phosphate Turbinaire 1645
- Decadron Phosphate with Xylocaine Injection, Sterile 1639
- Dexacort Phosphate in Respihaler .. 458
- Dexacort Phosphate in Turbinaire .. 459
- NeoDecadron Sterile Ophthalmic Ointment 1712
- NeoDecadron Sterile Ophthalmic Solution 1713
- NeoDecadron Topical Cream 1714

Dezocine (Orthostatic hypotension may be aggravated). Products include:
- Dalgan Injection 538

Diazepam (Effects may be potentiated when used concurrently with thiazide diuretics). Products include:
- Dizac 1809
- Valium Injectable 2182
- Valium Tablets 2183
- Valrelease Capsules 2169

Diazoxide (Effects may be potentiated when used concurrently with thiazide diuretics). Products include:
- Hyperstat I.V. Injection 2363
- Proglycem 580

Diclofenac Potassium (Reduces the diuretic, natriuretic, and antihypertensive effects). Products include:
- Cataflam 816

Diclofenac Sodium (Reduces the diuretic, natriuretic, and antihypertensive effects). Products include:
- Voltaren Ophthalmic Sterile Ophthalmic Solution .... ◉ 272
- Voltaren Tablets 861

Dicumarol (Effects may be decreased when used concurrently with thiazide diuretics; dosage adjustment may be necessary).
- No products indexed under this heading.

Digitoxin (Enhanced possibility of digitalis toxicity associated with hypokalemia). Products include:
- Crystodigin Tablets 1433

Digoxin (Enhanced possibility of digitalis toxicity associated with hypokalemia). Products include:
- Lanoxicaps 1117
- Lanoxin Elixir Pediatric 1120
- Lanoxin Injection 1123
- Lanoxin Injection Pediatric 1126
- Lanoxin Tablets 1128

Diltiazem Hydrochloride (Effects may be potentiated when used concurrently with thiazide diuretics). Products include:
- Cardizem CD Capsules 1506
- Cardizem SR Capsules 1510
- Cardizem Injectable 1508
- Cardizem Tablets 1512
- Dilacor XR Extended-release Capsules 2018

Doxazosin Mesylate (Effects may be potentiated when used concurrently with thiazide diuretics). Products include:
- Cardura Tablets 2186

Droperidol (Effects may be potentiated when used concurrently with thiazide diuretics). Products include:
- Inapsine Injection 1296

Enalapril Maleate (Effects may be potentiated when used concurrently with thiazide diuretics). Products include:
- Vaseretic Tablets 1765
- Vasotec Tablets 1771

Enalaprilat (Effects may be potentiated when used concurrently with thiazide diuretics). Products include:
- Vasotec I.V. 1768

Enflurane (Effects may be potentiated when used concurrently with thiazide diuretics).
- No products indexed under this heading.

Esmolol Hydrochloride (Effects may be potentiated when used concurrently with thiazide diuretics). Products include:
- Brevibloc Injection 1808

Etodolac (Reduces the diuretic, natriuretic, and antihypertensive effects). Products include:
- Lodine Capsules and Tablets 2743

Felodipine (Effects may be potentiated when used concurrently with thiazide diuretics). Products include:
- Plendil Extended-Release Tablets 527

Fenoprofen Calcium (Reduces the diuretic, natriuretic, and antihypertensive effects). Products include:
- Nalfon 200 Pulvules & Nalfon Tablets 917

Fentanyl (Orthostatic hypotension may be aggravated). Products include:
- Duragesic Transdermal System 1288

Fentanyl Citrate (Effects may be potentiated when used concurrently with thiazide diuretics; orthostatic hypotension may be aggravated). Products include:
- Sublimaze Injection 1307

Fludrocortisone Acetate (Concurrent use with thiazide diuretics may intensify electrolyte imbalance, particularly hypokalemia). Products include:
- Florinef Acetate Tablets 505

Flurbiprofen (Reduces the diuretic, natriuretic, and antihypertensive effects). Products include:
- Ansaid Tablets 2579

Fosinopril Sodium (Effects may be potentiated when used concurrently with thiazide diuretics). Products include:
- Monopril Tablets 757

Furosemide (Effects may be potentiated when used concurrently with thiazide diuretics). Products include:
- Lasix Injection, Oral Solution and Tablets 1240

Glipizide (Thiazides may raise blood glucose levels). Products include:
- Glucotrol Tablets 1967
- Glucotrol XL Extended Release Tablets 1968

Glyburide (Thiazides may raise blood glucose levels). Products include:
- DiaBeta Tablets 1239
- Glynase PresTab Tablets 2609
- Micronase Tablets 2623

Guanabenz Acetate (Effects may be potentiated when used concurrently with thiazide diuretics).
- No products indexed under this heading.

Guanethidine Monosulfate (Effects may be potentiated when used concurrently with thiazide diuretics). Products include:
- Esimil Tablets 822
- Ismelin Tablets 827

Hydralazine Hydrochloride (Effects may be potentiated when used concurrently with thiazide diuretics). Products include:
- Apresazide Capsules 808
- Apresoline Hydrochloride Tablets .. 809
- Ser-Ap-Es Tablets 849

(▣ Described in PDR For Nonprescription Drugs) (◉ Described in PDR For Ophthalmology)

Interactions Index

Hydrochlorothiazide (Effects may be potentiated when used concurrently with thiazide diuretics). Products include:

Aldactazide 2413
Aldoril Tablets 1604
Apresazide Capsules 808
Capozide 742
Dyazide 2479
Esidrix Tablets 821
Esimil Tablets 822
HydroDIURIL Tablets 1674
Hydropres Tablets...................................... 1675
Hyzaar Tablets 1677
Inderide Tablets 2732
Inderide LA Long Acting Capsules .. 2734
Lopressor HCT Tablets 832
Lotensin HCT... 837
Maxzide 1380
Moduretic Tablets 1705
Oretic Tablets 443
Prinzide Tablets 1737
Ser-Ap-Es Tablets 849
Timolide Tablets... 1748
Vaseretic Tablets 1765
Zestoretic 2850
Ziac 1415

Hydrocodone Bitartrate (Orthostatic hypotension may be aggravated). Products include:

Anexsia 5/500 Elixir 1781
Anexia Tablets.. 1782
Codiclear DH Syrup 791
Deconamine CX Cough and Cold Liquid and Tablets................................... 1319
Duratuss HD Elixir..................................... 2565
Hycodan Tablets and Syrup 930
Hycomine Compound Tablets 932
Hycomine 931
Hycotuss Expectorant Syrup 933
Hydrocet Capsules 782
Lorcet 10/650.. 1018
Lortab 2566
Tussend 1783
Tussend Expectorant 1785
Vicodin Tablets 1356
Vicodin ES Tablets 1357
Vicodin Tuss Expectorant 1358
Zydone Capsules 949

Hydrocodone Polistirex (Orthostatic hypotension may be aggravated). Products include:

Tussionex Pennkinetic Extended-Release Suspension 998

Hydrocortisone (Concurrent use with thiazide diuretics may intensify electrolyte imbalance, particularly hypokalemia). Products include:

Anusol-HC Cream 2.5% 1896
Aquanil HC Lotion 1931
Bactine Hydrocortisone Anti-Itch Cream.. ᴴᴰ 709
Caldecort Anti-Itch Hydrocortisone Spray .... ᴴᴰ 631
Cortaid .... ᴴᴰ 836
CORTENEMA.. 2535
Cortisporin Ointment................................. 1085
Cortisporin Ophthalmic Ointment Sterile 1085
Cortisporin Ophthalmic Suspension Sterile 1086
Cortisporin Otic Solution Sterile 1087
Cortisporin Otic Suspension Sterile 1088
Cortizone-5 .... ᴴᴰ 831
Cortizone-10 .... ᴴᴰ 831
Hydrocortone Tablets 1672
Hytone 907
Massengill Medicated Soft Cloth Towelettes... 2458
PediOtic Suspension Sterile 1153
Preparation H Hydrocortisone 1% Cream .... ᴴᴰ 872
ProctoCream-HC 2.5% 2408
VōSoL HC Otic Solution............................ 2678

Hydrocortisone Acetate (Concurrent use with thiazide diuretics may intensify electrolyte imbalance, particularly hypokalemia). Products include:

Analpram-HC Rectal Cream 1% and 2.5% 977
Anusol HC-1 Anti-Itch Hydrocortisone Ointment..................................... ᴴᴰ 847
Anusol-HC Suppositories 1897
Caldecort.. ᴴᴰ 631
Carmol HC 924

Coly-Mycin S Otic w/Neomycin & Hydrocortisone 1906
Cortaid .... ᴴᴰ 836
Cortifoam 2396
Cortisporin Cream..................................... 1084
Epifoam 2399
Hydrocortone Acetate Sterile Suspension.. 1669
Mantadil Cream 1135
Nupercainal Hydrocortisone 1% Cream.. ᴴᴰ 645
Ophthocort .... © 311
Pramosone Cream, Lotion & Ointment 978
ProctoCream-HC 2408
ProctoFoam-HC 2409
Terra-Cortril Ophthalmic Suspension 2210

Hydrocortisone Sodium Phosphate (Concurrent use with thiazide diuretics may intensify electrolyte imbalance, particularly hypokalemia). Products include:

Hydrocortone Phosphate Injection, Sterile 1670

Hydrocortisone Sodium Succinate (Concurrent use with thiazide diuretics may intensify electrolyte imbalance, particularly hypokalemia). Products include:

Solu-Cortef Sterile Powder................. 2641

Hydroxyzine Hydrochloride (Effects may be potentiated when used concurrently with thiazide diuretics). Products include:

Atarax Tablets & Syrup.............................. 2185
Marax Tablets & DF Syrup......................... 2200
Vistaril Intramuscular Solution.......... 2216

Ibuprofen (Reduces the diuretic, natriuretic, and antihypertensive effects). Products include:

Advil Cold and Sinus Caplets and Tablets (formerly CoAdvil) .... ᴴᴰ 870
Advil Ibuprofen Tablets and Caplets .... ᴴᴰ 870
Children's Advil Suspension 2692
Arthritis Foundation Ibuprofen Tablets .... ᴴᴰ 674
Bayer Select Ibuprofen Pain Relief Formula .... ᴴᴰ 715
Cramp End Tablets .... ᴴᴰ 735
Dimetapp Sinus Caplets .... ᴴᴰ 775
Haltran Tablets.. ᴴᴰ 771
IBU Tablets... 1342
Ibuprohm... ᴴᴰ 735
Children's Motrin Ibuprofen Oral Suspension 1546
Motrin Tablets.. 2625
Motrin IB Caplets, Tablets, and Geltabs .... ᴴᴰ 838
Motrin IB Sinus .... ᴴᴰ 838
Motrin Ibuprofen Suspension, Oral Drops, Chewable Tablets, Caplets 1546
Nuprin Ibuprofen/Analgesic Tablets & Caplets .... ᴴᴰ 622
Sine-Aid IB Caplets 1554
Vicks DayQuil SINUS Pressure & PAIN Relief with IBUPROFEN ...... ᴴᴰ 762

Indapamide (Effects may be potentiated when used concurrently with thiazide diuretics). Products include:

Lozol Tablets 2022

Indomethacin (Reduces the diuretic, natriuretic, and antihypertensive effects). Products include:

Indocin 1680

Indomethacin Sodium Trihydrate (Reduces the diuretic, natriuretic, and antihypertensive effects). Products include:

Indocin I.V. 1684

Insulin, Human (Insulin requirements may be increased, decreased, or unchanged).

No products indexed under this heading.

Insulin, Human Isophane Suspension (Insulin requirements may be increased, decreased, or unchanged). Products include:

Novolin N Human Insulin 10 ml Vials.. 1795

Insulin, Human NPH (Insulin requirements may be increased, decreased, or unchanged). Products include:

Humulin N, 100 Units 1448
Novolin N PenFill Cartridges Durable Insulin Delivery System 1798
Novolin N Prefilled Syringe Disposable Insulin Delivery System 1798

Insulin, Human Regular (Insulin requirements may be increased, decreased, or unchanged). Products include:

Humulin R, 100 Units 1449
Novolin R Human Insulin 10 ml Vials.. 1795
Novolin R PenFill Cartridges Durable Insulin Delivery System 1798
Novolin R Prefilled Syringe Disposable Insulin Delivery System 1798
Velosulin BR Human Insulin 10 ml Vials.. 1795

Insulin, Human, Zinc Suspension (Insulin requirements may be increased, decreased, or unchanged). Products include:

Humulin L, 100 Units 1446
Humulin U, 100 Units 1450
Novolin L Human Insulin 10 ml Vials.. 1795

Insulin, NPH (Insulin requirements may be increased, decreased, or unchanged). Products include:

NPH, 100 Units 1450
Pork NPH, 100 Units................................. 1452
Purified Pork NPH Isophane Insulin 1801

Insulin, Regular (Insulin requirements may be increased, decreased, or unchanged). Products include:

Regular, 100 Units 1450
Pork Regular, 100 Units 1452
Pork Regular (Concentrated), 500 Units 1453
Purified Pork Regular Insulin 1801

Insulin, Zinc Crystals (Insulin requirements may be increased, decreased, or unchanged). Products include:

NPH, 100 Units 1450

Insulin, Zinc Suspension (Insulin requirements may be increased, decreased, or unchanged). Products include:

Iletin I 1450
Lente, 100 Units 1450
Iletin II 1452
Pork Lente, 100 Units................................ 1452
Purified Pork Lente Insulin 1801

Isoflurane (Effects may be potentiated when used concurrently with thiazide diuretics).

No products indexed under this heading.

Isradipine (Effects may be potentiated when used concurrently with thiazide diuretics). Products include:

DynaCirc Capsules 2256

Ketamine Hydrochloride (Effects may be potentiated when used concurrently with thiazide diuretics).

No products indexed under this heading.

Ketoprofen (Reduces the diuretic, natriuretic, and antihypertensive effects). Products include:

Orudis Capsules... 2766
Oruvail Capsules 2766

Ketorolac Tromethamine (Reduces the diuretic, natriuretic, and antihypertensive effects). Products include:

Acular 474
Acular .... © 277
Toradol... 2159

Labetalol Hydrochloride (Effects may be potentiated when used concurrently with thiazide diuretics). Products include:

Normodyne Injection 2377
Normodyne Tablets 2379
Trandate 1185

Levorphanol Tartrate (Orthostatic hypotension may be aggravated). Products include:

Levo-Dromoran 2129

Lisinopril (Effects may be potentiated when used concurrently with thiazide diuretics). Products include:

Prinivil Tablets 1733
Prinzide Tablets 1737
Zestoretic 2850
Zestril Tablets 2854

Lithium Carbonate (Potential for lithium toxicity because of reduced renal clearance). Products include:

Eskalith 2485
Lithium Carbonate Capsules & Tablets 2230
Lithonate/Lithotabs/Lithobid 2543

Lithium Citrate (Potential for lithium toxicity because of reduced renal clearance).

No products indexed under this heading.

Lorazepam (Effects may be potentiated when used concurrently with thiazide diuretics). Products include:

Ativan Injection.. 2698
Ativan Tablets 2700

Losartan Potassium (Effects may be potentiated when used concurrently with thiazide diuretics). Products include:

Cozaar Tablets 1628
Hyzaar Tablets 1677

Mecamylamine Hydrochloride (Effects may be potentiated when used concurrently with thiazide diuretics). Products include:

Inversine Tablets 1686

Meclofenamate Sodium (Reduces the diuretic, natriuretic, and antihypertensive effects).

No products indexed under this heading.

Mefenamic Acid (Reduces the diuretic, natriuretic, and antihypertensive effects). Products include:

Ponstel 1925

Meperidine Hydrochloride (Effects may be potentiated when used concurrently with thiazide diuretics; orthostatic hypotension may be aggravated). Products include:

Demerol 2308
Mepergan Injection 2753

Mephobarbital (Orthostatic hypotension may be aggravated). Products include:

Mebaral Tablets 2322

Metformin Hydrochloride (Thiazides may raise blood glucose levels). Products include:

Glucophage 752

Methadone Hydrochloride (Orthostatic hypotension may be aggravated). Products include:

Methadone Hydrochloride Oral Concentrate 2233
Methadone Hydrochloride Oral Solution & Tablets................................. 2235

Methenamine (Reduced effectiveness because of alkalinization of urine). Products include:

Urised Tablets.. 1964

Methenamine Hippurate (Reduced effectiveness because of alkalinization of urine).

No products indexed under this heading.

Methenamine Mandelate (Reduced effectiveness because of alkalinization of urine). Products include:

Uroqid-Acid No. 2 Tablets 640

Methohexital Sodium (Effects may be potentiated when used concurrently with thiazide diuretics). Products include:

Brevital Sodium Vials................................ 1429

IMPORTANT NOTE: Always consult each drug listing in the patient's regimen for possible interactions.

Diucardin | Interactions Index | 316

Methoxyflurane (Effects may be potentiated when used concurrently with thiazide diuretics).
No products indexed under this heading.

Methyclothiazide (Effects may be potentiated when used concurrently with thiazide diuretics). Products include:
Enduron Tablets ... 420

Methyldopa (Effects may be potentiated when used concurrently with thiazide diuretics). Products include:
Aldoclor Tablets ... 1598
Aldomet Oral ... 1600
Aldoril Tablets ... 1604

Methyldopate Hydrochloride (Effects may be potentiated when used concurrently with thiazide diuretics). Products include:
Aldomet Ester HCl Injection ... 1602

Methylprednisolone Acetate (Concurrent use with thiazide diuretics may intensify electrolyte imbalance, particularly hypokalemia). Products include:
Depo-Medrol Single-Dose Vial ... 2600
Depo-Medrol Sterile Aqueous Suspension ... 2597

Methylprednisolone Sodium Succinate (Concurrent use with thiazide diuretics may intensify electrolyte imbalance, particularly hypokalemia). Products include:
Solu-Medrol Sterile Powder ... 2643

Metocurine Iodide (Effects may be potentiated when used concurrently with thiazide diuretics). Products include:
Metubine Iodide Vials ... 916

Metolazone (Effects may be potentiated when used concurrently with thiazide diuretics). Products include:
Mykrox Tablets ... 993
Zaroxolyn Tablets ... 1000

Metoprolol Succinate (Effects may be potentiated when used concurrently with thiazide diuretics). Products include:
Toprol-XL Tablets ... 565

Metoprolol Tartrate (Effects may be potentiated when used concurrently with thiazide diuretics). Products include:
Lopressor Ampuls ... 830
Lopressor HCT Tablets ... 832
Lopressor Tablets ... 830

Metyrosine (Effects may be potentiated when used concurrently with thiazide diuretics). Products include:
Demser Capsules ... 1649

Minoxidil (Effects may be potentiated when used concurrently with thiazide diuretics). Products include:
Loniten Tablets ... 2618
Rogaine Topical Solution ... 2637

Mivacurium Chloride (Effects may be potentiated when used concurrently with thiazide diuretics). Products include:
Mivacron ... 1138

Moexipril Hydrochloride (Effects may be potentiated when used concurrently with thiazide diuretics). Products include:
Univasc Tablets ... 2410

Morphine Sulfate (Effects may be potentiated when used concurrently with thiazide diuretics; orthostatic hypotension may be aggravated). Products include:
Astramorph/PF Injection, USP (Preservative-Free) ... 535
Duramorph ... 962
Infumorph 200 and Infumorph 500 Sterile Solutions ... 965
MS Contin Tablets ... 1994
MSIR ... 1997
Oramorph SR (Morphine Sulfate Sustained Release Tablets) ... 2236
RMS Suppositories ... 2657
Roxanol ... 2243

Nabumetone (Reduces the diuretic, natriuretic, and antihypertensive effects). Products include:
Relafen Tablets ... 2510

Nadolol (Effects may be potentiated when used concurrently with thiazide diuretics).
No products indexed under this heading.

Naproxen (Reduces the diuretic, natriuretic, and antihypertensive effects). Products include:
Anaprox/Naprosyn ... 2117

Naproxen Sodium (Reduces the diuretic, natriuretic, and antihypertensive effects). Products include:
Aleve ... 1975
Anaprox/Naprosyn ... 2117

Nicardipine Hydrochloride (Effects may be potentiated when used concurrently with thiazide diuretics). Products include:
Cardene Capsules ... 2095
Cardene I.V. ... 2709
Cardene SR Capsules ... 2097

Nifedipine (Effects may be potentiated when used concurrently with thiazide diuretics). Products include:
Adalat Capsules (10 mg and 20 mg) ... 587
Adalat CC ... 589
Procardia Capsules ... 1971
Procardia XL Extended Release Tablets ... 1972

Nisoldipine (Effects may be potentiated when used concurrently with thiazide diuretics).
No products indexed under this heading.

Nitroglycerin (Effects may be potentiated when used concurrently with thiazide diuretics). Products include:
Deponit NTG Transdermal Delivery System ... 2397
Nitro-Bid IV ... 1523
Nitro-Bid Ointment ... 1524
Nitrodisc ... 2047
Nitro-Dur (nitroglycerin) Transdermal Infusion System ... 1326
Nitrolingual Spray ... 2027
Nitrostat Tablets ... 1925
Transderm-Nitro Transdermal Therapeutic System ... 859

Norepinephrine Bitartrate (Decreased arterial responsiveness to norepinephrine). Products include:
Levophed Bitartrate Injection ... 2315

Opium Alkaloids (Orthostatic hypotension may be aggravated).
No products indexed under this heading.

Oxaprozin (Reduces the diuretic, natriuretic, and antihypertensive effects). Products include:
Daypro Caplets ... 2426

Oxycodone Hydrochloride (Orthostatic hypotension may be aggravated). Products include:
Percocet Tablets ... 938
Percodan Tablets ... 939
Percodan-Demi Tablets ... 940
Roxicodone Tablets, Oral Solution & Intensol (Oxycodone) ... 2244
Tylox Capsules ... 1584

Pancuronium Bromide Injection (Effects may be potentiated when used concurrently with thiazide diuretics).
No products indexed under this heading.

Penbutolol Sulfate (Effects may be potentiated when used concurrently with thiazide diuretics). Products include:
Levatol ... 2403

Pentobarbital Sodium (Effects may be potentiated when used concurrently with thiazide diuretics; orthostatic hypotension may be aggravated). Products include:
Nembutal Sodium Capsules ... 436
Nembutal Sodium Solution ... 438
Nembutal Sodium Suppositories ... 440

Phenobarbital (Orthostatic hypotension may be aggravated). Products include:
Arco-Lase Plus Tablets ... 512
Bellergal-S Tablets ... 2250
Donnatal ... 2060
Donnatal Extentabs ... 2061
Donnatal Tablets ... 2060
Phenobarbital Elixir and Tablets ... 1469
Quadrinal Tablets ... 1350

Phenoxybenzamine Hydrochloride (Effects may be potentiated when used concurrently with thiazide diuretics). Products include:
Dibenzyline Capsules ... 2476

Phentolamine Mesylate (Effects may be potentiated when used concurrently with thiazide diuretics). Products include:
Regitine ... 846

Phenylbutazone (Reduces the diuretic, natriuretic, and antihypertensive effects).
No products indexed under this heading.

Pindolol (Effects may be potentiated when used concurrently with thiazide diuretics). Products include:
Visken Tablets ... 2299

Piroxicam (Reduces the diuretic, natriuretic, and antihypertensive effects). Products include:
Feldene Capsules ... 1965

Polythiazide (Effects may be potentiated when used concurrently with thiazide diuretics). Products include:
Minizide Capsules ... 1938

Prazosin Hydrochloride (Effects may be potentiated when used concurrently with thiazide diuretics). Products include:
Minipress Capsules ... 1937
Minizide Capsules ... 1938

Prednisolone Acetate (Concurrent use with thiazide diuretics may intensify electrolyte imbalance, particularly hypokalemia). Products include:
AK-CIDE ... ⊙ 202
AK-CIDE Ointment ... ⊙ 202
Blephamide Liquifilm Sterile Ophthalmic Suspension ... 476
Blephamide Ointment ... ⊙ 237
Econopred & Econopred Plus Ophthalmic Suspensions ... ⊙ 217
Poly-Pred Liquifilm ... ⊙ 248
Pred Forte ... ⊙ 250
Pred Mild ... ⊙ 253
Pred-G Liquifilm Sterile Ophthalmic Suspension ... ⊙ 251
Pred-G S.O.P. Sterile Ophthalmic Ointment ... ⊙ 252
Vasocidin Ointment ... ⊙ 268

Prednisolone Sodium Phosphate (Concurrent use with thiazide diuretics may intensify electrolyte imbalance, particularly hypokalemia). Products include:
AK-Pred ... ⊙ 204
Hydeltrasol Injection, Sterile ... 1665
Inflamase ... ⊙ 265
Pediapred Oral Liquid ... 995
Vasocidin Ophthalmic Solution ... ⊙ 270

Prednisolone Tebutate (Concurrent use with thiazide diuretics may intensify electrolyte imbalance, particularly hypokalemia). Products include:
Hydeltra-T.B.A. Sterile Suspension 1667

Prednisone (Concurrent use with thiazide diuretics may intensify electrolyte imbalance, particularly hypokalemia). Products include:
Deltasone Tablets ... 2595

Probenecid (Thiazide diuretics may raise the level of blood uric acid). Products include:
Benemid Tablets ... 1611
ColBENEMID Tablets ... 1622

Promethazine Hydrochloride (Effects may be potentiated when used concurrently with thiazide diuretics). Products include:
Mepergan Injection ... 2753
Phenergan with Codeine ... 2777
Phenergan with Dextromethorphan 2778
Phenergan Injection ... 2773
Phenergan Suppositories ... 2775
Phenergan Syrup ... 2774
Phenergan Tablets ... 2775
Phenergan VC ... 2779
Phenergan VC with Codeine ... 2781

Propofol (Effects may be potentiated when used concurrently with thiazide diuretics). Products include:
Diprivan Injection ... 2833

Propoxyphene Hydrochloride (Orthostatic hypotension may be aggravated). Products include:
Darvon ... 1435
Wygesic Tablets ... 2827

Propoxyphene Napsylate (Orthostatic hypotension may be aggravated). Products include:
Darvon-N/Darvocet-N ... 1433

Propranolol Hydrochloride (Effects may be potentiated when used concurrently with thiazide diuretics). Products include:
Inderal ... 2728
Inderal LA Long Acting Capsules ... 2730
Inderide Tablets ... 2732
Inderide LA Long Acting Capsules .. 2734

Quinapril Hydrochloride (Effects may be potentiated when used concurrently with thiazide diuretics). Products include:
Accupril Tablets ... 1893

Ramipril (Effects may be potentiated when used concurrently with thiazide diuretics). Products include:
Altace Capsules ... 1232

Rauwolfia Serpentina (Effects may be potentiated when used concurrently with thiazide diuretics).
No products indexed under this heading.

Rescinnamine (Effects may be potentiated when used concurrently with thiazide diuretics).
No products indexed under this heading.

Reserpine (Effects may be potentiated when used concurrently with thiazide diuretics). Products include:
Diupres Tablets ... 1650
Hydropres Tablets ... 1675
Ser-Ap-Es Tablets ... 849

Rocuronium Bromide (Effects may be potentiated when used concurrently with thiazide diuretics). Products include:
Zemuron ... 1830

Secobarbital Sodium (Orthostatic hypotension may be aggravated). Products include:
Seconal Sodium Pulvules ... 1474

Sodium Nitroprusside (Effects may be potentiated when used concurrently with thiazide diuretics).
No products indexed under this heading.

Sotalol Hydrochloride (Effects may be potentiated when used concurrently with thiazide diuretics). Products include:
Betapace Tablets ... 641

(▣ Described in PDR For Nonprescription Drugs) (⊙ Described in PDR For Ophthalmology)

317 Interactions Index Diupres

Spirapril Hydrochloride (Effects may be potentiated when used concurrently with thiazide diuretics).
No products indexed under this heading.

Sufentanil Citrate (Orthostatic hypotension may be aggravated). Products include:
Sufenta Injection ... 1309

Sulfinpyrazone (Thiazide diuretics may raise the level of blood uric acid). Products include:
Anturane ... 807

Sulindac (Reduces the diuretic, natriuretic, and antihypertensive effects). Products include:
Clinoril Tablets ... 1618

Terazosin Hydrochloride (Effects may be potentiated when used concurrently with thiazide diuretics). Products include:
Hytrin Capsules ... 430

Thiamylal Sodium (Orthostatic hypotension may be aggravated).
No products indexed under this heading.

Timolol Maleate (Effects may be potentiated when used concurrently with thiazide diuretics). Products include:
Blocadren Tablets ... 1614
Timolide Tablets ... 1748
Timoptic in Ocudose ... 1753
Timoptic Sterile Ophthalmic Solution ... 1751
Timoptic-XE ... 1755

Tolazamide (Thiazides may raise blood glucose levels).
No products indexed under this heading.

Tolbutamide (Thiazides may raise blood glucose levels).
No products indexed under this heading.

Tolmetin Sodium (Reduces the diuretic, natriuretic, and antihypertensive effects). Products include:
Tolectin (200, 400 and 600 mg) .. 1581

Torsemide (Effects may be potentiated when used concurrently with thiazide diuretics). Products include:
Demadex Tablets and Injection ... 686

Triamcinolone (Concurrent use with thiazide diuretics may intensify electrolyte imbalance, particularly hypokalemia). Products include:
Aristocort Tablets ... 1022

Triamcinolone Acetonide (Concurrent use with thiazide diuretics may intensify electrolyte imbalance, particularly hypokalemia). Products include:
Aristocort A 0.025% Cream ... 1027
Aristocort A 0.5% Cream ... 1031
Aristocort A 0.1% Cream ... 1029
Aristocort A 0.1% Ointment ... 1030
Azmacort Oral Inhaler ... 2011
Nasacort Nasal Inhaler ... 2024

Triamcinolone Diacetate (Concurrent use with thiazide diuretics may intensify electrolyte imbalance, particularly hypokalemia). Products include:
Aristocort Suspension (Forte Parenteral) ... 1027
Aristocort Suspension (Intralesional) ... 1025

Triamcinolone Hexacetonide (Concurrent use with thiazide diuretics may intensify electrolyte imbalance, particularly hypokalemia). Products include:
Aristospan Suspension (Intra-articular) ... 1033
Aristospan Suspension (Intralesional) ... 1032

Trimethaphan Camsylate (Effects may be potentiated when used concurrently with thiazide diuretics). Products include:
Arfonad Ampuls ... 2080

Tubocurarine Chloride (Increased responsiveness to tubocurarine).
No products indexed under this heading.

Vecuronium Bromide (Effects may be potentiated when used concurrently with thiazide diuretics). Products include:
Norcuron ... 1826

Verapamil Hydrochloride (Effects may be potentiated when used concurrently with thiazide diuretics). Products include:
Calan SR Caplets ... 2422
Calan Tablets ... 2419
Isoptin Injectable ... 1344
Isoptin Oral Tablets ... 1346
Isoptin SR Tablets ... 1348
Verelan Capsules ... 1410
Verelan Capsules ... 2824

Warfarin Sodium (Effects may be decreased when used concurrently with thiazide diuretics; dosage adjustment may be necessary). Products include:
Coumadin ... 926

DIUPRES TABLETS
(Reserpine, Chlorothiazide) ... 1650
May interact with antihypertensives, lithium preparations, cardiac glycosides, corticosteroids, insulin, nonsteroidal anti-inflammatory agents, barbiturates, monoamine oxidase inhibitors, narcotic analgesics, oral hypoglycemic agents, general anesthetics, bile acid sequestering agents, and certain other agents. Compounds in these categories include:

Acarbose (Dosage adjustment of the antidiabetic drug may be required).
No products indexed under this heading.

Acebutolol Hydrochloride (Potentiated; additive effects). Products include:
Sectral Capsules ... 2807

ACTH (Hypokalemia).
No products indexed under this heading.

Alfentanil Hydrochloride (Orthostatic hypotension may be aggravated). Products include:
Alfenta Injection ... 1286

Amlodipine Besylate (Potentiated; additive effects). Products include:
Lotrel Capsules ... 840
Norvasc Tablets ... 1940

Aprobarbital (Orthostatic hypotension may be aggravated).
No products indexed under this heading.

Atenolol (Potentiated; additive effects). Products include:
Tenoretic Tablets ... 2845
Tenormin Tablets and I.V. Injection 2847

Benazepril Hydrochloride (Potentiated; additive effects). Products include:
Lotensin Tablets ... 834
Lotensin HCT ... 837
Lotrel Capsules ... 840

Bendroflumethiazide (Potentiated; additive effects).
No products indexed under this heading.

Betamethasone Acetate (Hypokalemia). Products include:
Celestone Soluspan Suspension ... 2347

Betamethasone Sodium Phosphate (Hypokalemia). Products include:
Celestone Soluspan Suspension ... 2347

Betaxolol Hydrochloride (Potentiated; additive effects). Products include:
Betoptic Ophthalmic Solution ... 469
Betoptic S Ophthalmic Suspension ... 471
Kerlone Tablets ... 2436

Bisoprolol Fumarate (Potentiated; additive effects). Products include:
Zebeta Tablets ... 1413
Ziac ... 1415

Buprenorphine (Orthostatic hypotension may be aggravated). Products include:
Buprenex Injectable ... 2006

Butabarbital (Orthostatic hypotension may be aggravated).
No products indexed under this heading.

Butalbital (Orthostatic hypotension may be aggravated). Products include:
Esgic-plus Tablets ... 1013
Fioricet Tablets ... 2258
Fioricet with Codeine Capsules ... 2260
Fiorinal Capsules ... 2261
Fiorinal with Codeine Capsules ... 2262
Fiorinal Tablets ... 2261
Phrenilin ... 785
Sedapap Tablets 50 mg/650 mg .. 1543

Captopril (Potentiated; additive effects). Products include:
Capoten ... 739
Capozide ... 742

Carteolol Hydrochloride (Potentiated; additive effects). Products include:
Cartrol Tablets ... 410
Ocupress Ophthalmic Solution, 1% Sterile ... ⊙ 309

Chlorothiazide Sodium (Potentiated; additive effects). Products include:
Diuril Sodium Intravenous ... 1652

Chlorpropamide (Dosage adjustment of the antidiabetic drug may be required). Products include:
Diabinese Tablets ... 1935

Chlorthalidone (Potentiated; additive effects). Products include:
Combipres Tablets ... 677
Tenoretic Tablets ... 2845
Thalitone ... 1245

Cholestyramine (Cholestyramine resin has potential of binding thiazide diuretics and reducing diuretic absorption from the GI tract). Products include:
Questran Light ... 769
Questran Powder ... 770

Clonidine (Potentiated; additive effects). Products include:
Catapres-TTS ... 675

Clonidine Hydrochloride (Potentiated; additive effects). Products include:
Catapres Tablets ... 674
Combipres Tablets ... 677

Codeine Phosphate (Orthostatic hypotension may be aggravated). Products include:
Actifed with Codeine Cough Syrup.. 1067
Brontex ... 1981
Deconsal C Expectorant Syrup ... 456
Deconsal Pediatric Syrup ... 457
Dimetane-DC Cough Syrup ... 2059
Empirin with Codeine Tablets ... 1093
Fioricet with Codeine Capsules ... 2260
Fiorinal with Codeine Capsules ... 2262
Isoclor Expectorant ... 990
Novahistine DH ... 2462
Novahistine Expectorant ... 2463
Nucofed ... 2051
Phenergan with Codeine ... 2777
Phenergan VC with Codeine ... 2781
Robitussin A-C Syrup ... 2073
Robitussin-DAC Syrup ... 2074
Ryna ... 841
Soma Compound w/Codeine Tablets ... 2676
Tussi-Organidin NR Liquid and S NR Liquid ... 2677
Tylenol with Codeine ... 1583

Colestipol Hydrochloride (Colestipol resin has potential of binding thiazide diuretics and reducing diuretic absorption from the GI tract). Products include:
Colestid Tablets ... 2591

Cortisone Acetate (Hypokalemia). Products include:
Cortone Acetate Sterile Suspension ... 1623
Cortone Acetate Tablets ... 1624

Deserpidine (Potentiated; additive effects).
No products indexed under this heading.

Deslanoside (Cardiac arrhythmias; increased ventricular irritability).
No products indexed under this heading.

Dexamethasone (Hypokalemia). Products include:
AK-Trol Ointment & Suspension ... ⊙ 205
Decadron Elixir ... 1633
Decadron Tablets ... 1635
Decaspray Topical Aerosol ... 1648
Dexacidin Ointment ... ⊙ 263
Maxitrol Ophthalmic Ointment and Suspension ... ⊙ 224
TobraDex Ophthalmic Suspension and Ointment ... 473

Dexamethasone Acetate (Hypokalemia). Products include:
Dalalone D.P. Injectable ... 1011
Decadron-LA Sterile Suspension ... 1646

Dexamethasone Sodium Phosphate (Hypokalemia). Products include:
Decadron Phosphate Injection ... 1637
Decadron Phosphate Respihaler ... 1642
Decadron Phosphate Sterile Ophthalmic Ointment ... 1641
Decadron Phosphate Sterile Ophthalmic Solution ... 1642
Decadron Phosphate Topical Cream ... 1644
Decadron Phosphate Turbinaire ... 1645
Decadron Phosphate with Xylocaine Injection, Sterile ... 1639
Dexacort Phosphate in Respihaler .. 458
Dexacort Phosphate in Turbinaire .. 459
NeoDecadron Sterile Ophthalmic Ointment ... 1712
NeoDecadron Sterile Ophthalmic Solution ... 1713
NeoDecadron Topical Cream ... 1714

Dezocine (Orthostatic hypotension may be aggravated). Products include:
Dalgan Injection ... 538

Diazoxide (Potentiated; additive effects). Products include:
Hyperstat I.V. Injection ... 2363
Proglycem ... 580

Diclofenac Potassium (Reduced diuretic, natriuretic, and antihypertensive effects of chlorothiazide). Products include:
Cataflam ... 816

Diclofenac Sodium (Reduced diuretic, natriuretic, and antihypertensive effects of chlorothiazide). Products include:
Voltaren Ophthalmic Sterile Ophthalmic Solution ... ⊙ 272
Voltaren Tablets ... 861

Digitoxin (Cardiac arrhythmias; increased ventricular irritability). Products include:
Crystodigin Tablets ... 1433

Digoxin (Cardiac arrhythmias; increased ventricular irritability). Products include:
Lanoxicaps ... 1117
Lanoxin Elixir Pediatric ... 1120
Lanoxin Injection ... 1123
Lanoxin Injection Pediatric ... 1126
Lanoxin Tablets ... 1128

IMPORTANT NOTE: Always consult each drug listing in the patient's regimen for possible interactions.

Diupres Interactions Index 318

Diltiazem Hydrochloride (Potentiated; additive effects). Products include:
- Cardizem CD Capsules ... 1506
- Cardizem SR Capsules ... 1510
- Cardizem Injectable ... 1508
- Cardizem Tablets ... 1512
- Dilacor XR Extended-release Capsules ... 2018

Doxazosin Mesylate (Potentiated; additive effects). Products include:
- Cardura Tablets ... 2186

Enalapril Maleate (Potentiated; additive effects). Products include:
- Vaseretic Tablets ... 1765
- Vasotec Tablets ... 1771

Enalaprilat (Potentiation of antihypertensive effect). Products include:
- Vasotec I.V. ... 1768

Enflurane (Significant hypotension; bradycardia).
- No products indexed under this heading.

Esmolol Hydrochloride (Potentiated; additive effects). Products include:
- Brevibloc Injection ... 1808

Etodolac (Reduced diuretic, natriuretic, and antihypertensive effects of chlorothiazide). Products include:
- Lodine Capsules and Tablets ... 2743

Felodipine (Potentiated; additive effects). Products include:
- Plendil Extended-Release Tablets ... 527

Fenoprofen Calcium (Reduced diuretic, natriuretic, and antihypertensive effects of chlorothiazide). Products include:
- Nalfon 200 Pulvules & Nalfon Tablets ... 917

Fentanyl (Orthostatic hypotension may be aggravated). Products include:
- Duragesic Transdermal System ... 1288

Fentanyl Citrate (Orthostatic hypotension may be aggravated). Products include:
- Sublimaze Injection ... 1307

Fludrocortisone Acetate (Hypokalemia). Products include:
- Florinef Acetate Tablets ... 505

Flurbiprofen (Reduced diuretic, natriuretic, and antihypertensive effects of chlorothiazide). Products include:
- Ansaid Tablets ... 2579

Fosinopril Sodium (Potentiated; additive effects). Products include:
- Monopril Tablets ... 757

Furazolidone (Concurrent use is contraindicated). Products include:
- Furoxone ... 2046

Furosemide (Potentiated; additive effects). Products include:
- Lasix Injection, Oral Solution and Tablets ... 1240

Glipizide (Dosage adjustment of the antidiabetic drug may be required). Products include:
- Glucotrol Tablets ... 1967
- Glucotrol XL Extended Release Tablets ... 1968

Glyburide (Dosage adjustment of the antidiabetic drug may be required). Products include:
- DiaBeta Tablets ... 1239
- Glynase PresTab Tablets ... 2609
- Micronase Tablets ... 2623

Guanabenz Acetate (Potentiated; additive effects).
- No products indexed under this heading.

Guanethidine Monosulfate (Potentiated; additive effects). Products include:
- Esimil Tablets ... 822
- Ismelin Tablets ... 827

Hydralazine Hydrochloride (Potentiated; additive effects). Products include:
- Apresazide Capsules ... 808
- Apresoline Hydrochloride Tablets ... 809
- Ser-Ap-Es Tablets ... 849

Hydrochlorothiazide (Potentiated; additive effects). Products include:
- Aldactazide ... 2413
- Aldoril Tablets ... 1604
- Apresazide Capsules ... 808
- Capozide ... 742
- Dyazide ... 2479
- Esidrix Tablets ... 821
- Esimil Tablets ... 822
- HydroDIURIL Tablets ... 1674
- Hydropres Tablets ... 1675
- Hyzaar Tablets ... 1677
- Inderide Tablets ... 2732
- Inderide LA Long Acting Capsules ... 2734
- Lopressor HCT Tablets ... 832
- Lotensin HCT ... 837
- Maxzide ... 1380
- Moduretic Tablets ... 1705
- Oretic Tablets ... 443
- Prinzide Tablets ... 1737
- Ser-Ap-Es Tablets ... 849
- Timolide Tablets ... 1748
- Vaseretic Tablets ... 1765
- Zestoretic ... 2850
- Ziac ... 1415

Hydrocodone Bitartrate (Orthostatic hypotension may be aggravated). Products include:
- Anexsia 5/500 Elixir ... 1781
- Anexia Tablets ... 1782
- Codiclear DH Syrup ... 791
- Deconamine CX Cough and Cold Liquid and Tablets ... 1319
- Duratuss HD Elixir ... 2565
- Hycodan Tablets and Syrup ... 930
- Hycomine Compound Tablets ... 932
- Hycomine ... 931
- Hycotuss Expectorant Syrup ... 933
- Hydrocet Capsules ... 782
- Lorcet 10/650 ... 1018
- Lortab ... 2566
- Tussend ... 1783
- Tussend Expectorant ... 1785
- Vicodin Tablets ... 1356
- Vicodin ES Tablets ... 1357
- Vicodin Tuss Expectorant ... 1358
- Zydone Capsules ... 949

Hydrocodone Polistirex (Orthostatic hypotension may be aggravated). Products include:
- Tussionex Pennkinetic Extended-Release Suspension ... 998

Hydrocortisone (Hypokalemia). Products include:
- Anusol-HC Cream 2.5% ... 1896
- Aquanil HC Lotion ... 1931
- Bactine Hydrocortisone Anti-Itch Cream ... ▣ 709
- Caldecort Anti-Itch Hydrocortisone Spray ... ▣ 631
- Cortaid ... ▣ 836
- CORTENEMA ... 2535
- Cortisporin Ointment ... 1085
- Cortisporin Ophthalmic Ointment Sterile ... 1085
- Cortisporin Ophthalmic Suspension Sterile ... 1086
- Cortisporin Otic Solution Sterile ... 1087
- Cortisporin Otic Suspension Sterile ... 1088
- Cortizone-5 ... ▣ 831
- Cortizone-10 ... ▣ 831
- Hydrocortone Tablets ... 1672
- Hytone ... 907
- Massengill Medicated Soft Cloth Towelettes ... 2458
- PediOtic Suspension Sterile ... 1153
- Preparation H Hydrocortisone 1% Cream ... ▣ 872
- ProctoCream-HC 2.5% ... 2408
- VōSoL HC Otic Solution ... 2678

Hydrocortisone Acetate (Hypokalemia). Products include:
- Analpram-HC Rectal Cream 1% and 2.5% ... 977
- Anusol HC-1 Anti-Itch Hydrocortisone Ointment ... ▣ 847
- Anusol-HC Suppositories ... 1897
- Caldecort ... ▣ 631
- Carmol HC ... 924
- Coly-Mycin S Otic w/Neomycin & Hydrocortisone ... 1906
- Cortaid ... ▣ 836
- Cortifoam ... 2396
- Cortisporin Cream ... 1084
- Epifoam ... 2399
- Hydrocortone Acetate Sterile Suspension ... 1669
- Mantadil Cream ... 1135
- Nupercainal Hydrocortisone 1% Cream ... ▣ 645
- Ophthocort ... ⊙ 311
- Pramosone Cream, Lotion & Ointment ... 978
- ProctoCream-HC ... 2408
- ProctoFoam-HC ... 2409
- Terra-Cortril Ophthalmic Suspension ... 2210

Hydrocortisone Sodium Phosphate (Hypokalemia). Products include:
- Hydrocortone Phosphate Injection, Sterile ... 1670

Hydrocortisone Sodium Succinate (Hypokalemia). Products include:
- Solu-Cortef Sterile Powder ... 2641

Hydroflumethiazide (Potentiated; additive effects). Products include:
- Diucardin Tablets ... 2718

Ibuprofen (Reduced diuretic, natriuretic, and antihypertensive effects of chlorothiazide). Products include:
- Advil Cold and Sinus Caplets and Tablets (formerly CoAdvil) ... ▣ 870
- Advil Ibuprofen Tablets and Caplets ... ▣ 870
- Children's Advil Suspension ... 2692
- Arthritis Foundation Ibuprofen Tablets ... ▣ 674
- Bayer Select Ibuprofen Pain Relief Formula ... ▣ 715
- Cramp End Tablets ... ▣ 735
- Dimetapp Sinus Caplets ... ▣ 775
- Haltran Tablets ... ▣ 771
- IBU Tablets ... 1342
- Ibuprohm ... ▣ 735
- Children's Motrin Ibuprofen Oral Suspension ... 1546
- Motrin Tablets ... 2625
- Motrin IB Caplets, Tablets, and Geltabs ... ▣ 838
- Motrin IB Sinus ... ▣ 838
- Motrin Ibuprofen Suspension, Oral Drops, Chewable Tablets, Caplets ... 1546
- Nuprin Ibuprofen/Analgesic Tablets & Caplets ... ▣ 622
- Sine-Aid IB Caplets ... 1554
- Vicks DayQuil SINUS Pressure & PAIN Relief with IBUPROFEN ... ▣ 762

Indapamide (Potentiated; additive effects). Products include:
- Lozol Tablets ... 2022

Indomethacin (Reduced diuretic, natriuretic, and antihypertensive effects of chlorothiazide). Products include:
- Indocin ... 1680

Indomethacin Sodium Trihydrate (Reduced diuretic, natriuretic, and antihypertensive effects of chlorothiazide). Products include:
- Indocin I.V. ... 1684

Insulin, Human (Insulin requirements may be altered).
- No products indexed under this heading.

Insulin, Human Isophane Suspension (Insulin requirements may be altered). Products include:
- Novolin N Human Insulin 10 ml Vials ... 1795

Insulin, Human NPH (Insulin requirements may be altered). Products include:
- Humulin N, 100 Units ... 1448
- Novolin N PenFill Cartridges Durable Insulin Delivery System ... 1798
- Novolin N Prefilled Syringe Disposable Insulin Delivery System ... 1798

Insulin, Human Regular (Insulin requirements may be altered). Products include:
- Humulin R, 100 Units ... 1449
- Novolin R Human Insulin 10 ml Vials ... 1795
- Novolin R PenFill Cartridges Durable Insulin Delivery System ... 1798
- Novolin R Prefilled Syringe Disposable Insulin Delivery System ... 1798
- Velosulin BR Human Insulin 10 ml Vials ... 1795

Insulin, Human, Zinc Suspension (Insulin requirements may be altered). Products include:
- Humulin L, 100 Units ... 1446
- Humulin U, 100 Units ... 1450
- Novolin L Human Insulin 10 ml Vials ... 1795

Insulin, NPH (Insulin requirements may be altered). Products include:
- NPH, 100 Units ... 1450
- Pork NPH, 100 Units ... 1452
- Purified Pork NPH Isophane Insulin ... 1801

Insulin, Regular (Insulin requirements may be altered). Products include:
- Regular, 100 Units ... 1450
- Pork Regular, 100 Units ... 1452
- Pork Regular (Concentrated), 500 Units ... 1453
- Purified Pork Regular Insulin ... 1801

Insulin, Zinc Crystals (Insulin requirements may be altered). Products include:
- NPH, 100 Units ... 1450

Insulin, Zinc Suspension (Insulin requirements may be altered). Products include:
- Iletin I ... 1450
- Lente, 100 Units ... 1450
- Iletin II ... 1452
- Pork Lente, 100 Units ... 1452
- Purified Pork Lente Insulin ... 1801

Isocarboxazid (Concurrent use is contraindicated).
- No products indexed under this heading.

Isoflurane (Significant hypotension; bradycardia).
- No products indexed under this heading.

Isradipine (Potentiated; additive effects). Products include:
- DynaCirc Capsules ... 2256

Ketamine Hydrochloride (May require reduced dose of anesthetics).
- No products indexed under this heading.

Ketoprofen (Reduced diuretic, natriuretic, and antihypertensive effects of chlorothiazide). Products include:
- Orudis Capsules ... 2766
- Oruvail Capsules ... 2766

Ketorolac Tromethamine (Reduced diuretic, natriuretic, and antihypertensive effects of chlorothiazide). Products include:
- Acular ... 474
- Acular ... ⊙ 277
- Toradol ... 2159

Labetalol Hydrochloride (Potentiated; additive effects). Products include:
- Normodyne Injection ... 2377
- Normodyne Tablets ... 2379
- Trandate ... 1185

Levorphanol Tartrate (Orthostatic hypotension may be aggravated). Products include:
- Levo-Dromoran ... 2129

Lisinopril (Potentiation of antihypertensive effect). Products include:
- Prinivil Tablets ... 1733
- Prinzide Tablets ... 1737
- Zestoretic ... 2850
- Zestril Tablets ... 2854

Lithium Carbonate (High risk of lithium toxicity). Products include:
- Eskalith ... 2485
- Lithium Carbonate Capsules & Tablets ... 2230

(▣ Described in PDR For Nonprescription Drugs) (⊙ Described in PDR For Ophthalmology)

319 **Interactions Index** **Diupres**

Lithonate/Lithotabs/Lithobid 2543

Lithium Citrate (High risk of lithium toxicity).
No products indexed under this heading.

Losartan Potassium (Potentiated; additive effects). Products include:
Cozaar Tablets 1628
Hyzaar Tablets 1677

Mecamylamine Hydrochloride (Potentiated; additive effects). Products include:
Inversine Tablets 1686

Meclofenamate Sodium (Reduced diuretic, natriuretic, and antihypertensive effects of chlorothiazide).
No products indexed under this heading.

Mefenamic Acid (Reduced diuretic, natriuretic, and antihypertensive effects of chlorothiazide). Products include:
Ponstel 1925

Meperidine Hydrochloride (Orthostatic hypotension may be aggravated). Products include:
Demerol 2308
Mepergan Injection 2753

Mephobarbital (Orthostatic hypotension may be aggravated). Products include:
Mebaral Tablets 2322

Metformin Hydrochloride (Dosage adjustment of the antidiabetic drug may be required). Products include:
Glucophage 752

Methadone Hydrochloride (Orthostatic hypotension may be aggravated). Products include:
Methadone Hydrochloride Oral Concentrate 2233
Methadone Hydrochloride Oral Solution & Tablets 2235

Methohexital Sodium (Significant hypotension; bradycardia). Products include:
Brevital Sodium Vials 1429

Methoxyflurane (Significant hypotension; bradycardia).
No products indexed under this heading.

Methyclothiazide (Potentiated; additive effects). Products include:
Enduron Tablets 420

Methyldopa (Potentiated; additive effects). Products include:
Aldoclor Tablets 1598
Aldomet Oral 1600
Aldoril Tablets 1604

Methyldopate Hydrochloride (Potentiated; additive effects). Products include:
Aldomet Ester HCl Injection 1602

Methylprednisolone Acetate (Hypokalemia). Products include:
Depo-Medrol Single-Dose Vial 2600
Depo-Medrol Sterile Aqueous Suspension 2597

Methylprednisolone Sodium Succinate (Hypokalemia). Products include:
Solu-Medrol Sterile Powder 2643

Metolazone (Potentiated; additive effects). Products include:
Mykrox Tablets 993
Zaroxolyn Tablets 1000

Metoprolol Succinate (Potentiated; additive effects). Products include:
Toprol-XL Tablets 565

Metoprolol Tartrate (Potentiated; additive effects). Products include:
Lopressor Ampuls 830
Lopressor HCT Tablets 832
Lopressor Tablets 830

Metyrosine (Potentiated; additive effects). Products include:
Demser Capsules 1649

Minoxidil (Potentiated; additive effects). Products include:
Loniten Tablets 2618
Rogaine Topical Solution 2637

Moexipril Hydrochloride (Potentiated; additive effects). Products include:
Univasc Tablets 2410

Morphine Sulfate (Orthostatic hypotension may be aggravated). Products include:
Astramorph/PF Injection, USP (Preservative-Free) 535
Duramorph 962
Infumorph 200 and Infumorph 500 Sterile Solutions 965
MS Contin Tablets 1994
MSIR 1997
Oramorph SR (Morphine Sulfate Sustained Release Tablets) 2236
RMS Suppositories 2657
Roxanol 2243

Nabumetone (Reduced diuretic, natriuretic, and antihypertensive effects of chlorothiazide). Products include:
Relafen Tablets 2510

Nadolol (Potentiated; additive effects).
No products indexed under this heading.

Naproxen (Reduced diuretic natriuretic, and antihypertensive effects of chlorothiazide). Products include:
Anaprox/Naprosyn 2117

Naproxen Sodium (Reduced diuretic, natriuretic, and antihypertensive effects of chlorothiazide). Products include:
Aleve 1975
Anaprox/Naprosyn 2117

Nicardipine Hydrochloride (Potentiated; additive effects). Products include:
Cardene Capsules 2095
Cardene I.V. 2709
Cardene SR Capsules 2097

Nifedipine (Potentiated; additive effects). Products include:
Adalat Capsules (10 mg and 20 mg) 587
Adalat CC 589
Procardia Capsules 1971
Procardia XL Extended Release Tablets 1972

Nisoldipine (Potentiated; additive effects).
No products indexed under this heading.

Nitroglycerin (Potentiated; additive effects). Products include:
Deponit NTG Transdermal Delivery System 2397
Nitro-Bid IV 1523
Nitro-Bid Ointment 1524
Nitrodisc 2047
Nitro-Dur (nitroglycerin) Transdermal Infusion System 1326
Nitrolingual Spray 2027
Nitrostat Tablets 1925
Transderm-Nitro Transdermal Therapeutic System 859

Norepinephrine Bitartrate (Decreased arterial responsiveness to norepinephrine). Products include:
Levophed Bitartrate Injection 2315

Opium Alkaloids (Orthostatic hypotension may be aggravated).
No products indexed under this heading.

Oxaprozin (Reduced diuretic, natriuretic, and antihypertensive effects of chlorothiazide). Products include:
Daypro Caplets 2426

Oxycodone Hydrochloride (Orthostatic hypotension may be aggravated). Products include:
Percocet Tablets 938
Percodan Tablets 939
Percodan-Demi Tablets 940
Roxicodone Tablets, Oral Solution & Intensol (Oxycodone) 2244
Tylox Capsules 1584

Penbutolol Sulfate (Potentiated; additive effects). Products include:
Levatol 2403

Pentobarbital Sodium (Orthostatic hypotension may be aggrevated). Products include:
Nembutal Sodium Capsules 436
Nembutal Sodium Solution 438
Nembutal Sodium Suppositories 440

Phenelzine Sulfate (Concurrent use is contraindicated). Products include:
Nardil 1920

Phenobarbital (Orthostatic hypotension may be aggravated). Products include:
Arco-Lase Plus Tablets 512
Bellergal-S Tablets 2250
Donnatal 2060
Donnatal Extentabs 2061
Donnatal Tablets 2060
Phenobarbital Elixir and Tablets 1469
Quadrinal Tablets 1350

Phenoxybenzamine Hydrochloride (Potentiated; additive effects). Products include:
Dibenzyline Capsules 2476

Phentolamine Mesylate (Potentiated; additive effects). Products include:
Regitine 846

Phenylbutazone (Reduced diuretic, natriuretic, and antihypertensive effects of chlorothiazide).
No products indexed under this heading.

Pindolol (Potentiated; additive effects). Products include:
Visken Tablets 2299

Piroxicam (Reduced diuretic, natriuretic, and antihypertensive effects of chlorothiazide). Products include:
Feldene Capsules 1965

Polythiazide (Potentiated; additive effects). Products include:
Minizide Capsules 1938

Prazosin Hydrochloride (Potentiated; additive effects). Products include:
Minipress Capsules 1937
Minizide Capsules 1938

Prednisolone Acetate (Hypokalemia). Products include:
AK-CIDE .... ◉ 202
AK-CIDE Ointment .... ◉ 202
Blephamide Liquifilm Sterile Ophthalmic Suspension 476
Blephamide Ointment .... ◉ 237
Econopred & Econopred Plus Ophthalmic Suspensions .... ◉ 217
Poly-Pred Liquifilm .... ◉ 248
Pred Forte .... ◉ 250
Pred Mild .... ◉ 253
Pred-G Liquifilm Sterile Ophthalmic Suspension .... ◉ 251
Pred-G S.O.P. Sterile Ophthalmic Ointment .... ◉ 252
Vasocidin Ointment .... ◉ 268

Prednisolone Sodium Phosphate (Hypokalemia). Products include:
AK-Pred .... ◉ 204
Hydeltrasol Injection, Sterile 1665
Inflamase .... ◉ 265
Pediapred Oral Liquid 995
Vasocidin Ophthalmic Solution .... ◉ 270

Prednisolone Tebutate (Hypokalemia). Products include:
Hydeltra-T.B.A. Sterile Suspension 1667

Prednisone (Hypokalemia). Products include:
Deltasone Tablets 2595

Propofol (Significant hypotension; bradycardia). Products include:
Diprivan Injection 2833

Propoxyphene Hydrochloride (Orthostatic hypotension may be aggravated). Products include:
Darvon 1435
Wygesic Tablets 2827

Propoxyphene Napsylate (Orthostatic hypotension may be aggravated). Products include:
Darvon-N/Darvocet-N 1433

Propranolol Hydrochloride (Potentiated; additive effects). Products include:
Inderal 2728
Inderal LA Long Acting Capsules 2730
Inderide Tablets 2732
Inderide LA Long Acting Capsules 2734

Quinapril Hydrochloride (Potentiated; additive effects). Products include:
Accupril Tablets 1893

Quinidine Gluconate (Cardiac arrhythmias). Products include:
Quinaglute Dura-Tabs Tablets 649

Quinidine Polygalacturonate (Cardiac arrhythmias).
No products indexed under this heading.

Quinidine Sulfate (Cardiac arrhythmias). Products include:
Quinidex Extentabs 2067

Ramipril (Potentiated; additive effects). Products include:
Altace Capsules 1232

Rauwolfia Serpentina (Potentiated; additive effects).
No products indexed under this heading.

Rescinnamine (Potentiated; additive effects).
No products indexed under this heading.

Secobarbital Sodium (Orthostatic hypotension may be aggravated). Products include:
Seconal Sodium Pulvules 1474

Selegiline Hydrochloride (Concurrent use is contraindicated). Products include:
Eldepryl Tablets 2550

Sodium Nitroprusside (Potentiated; additive effects).
No products indexed under this heading.

Sotalol Hydrochloride (Potentiated; additive effects). Products include:
Betapace Tablets 641

Spirapril Hydrochloride (Potentiated; additive effects).
No products indexed under this heading.

Sufentanil Citrate (Orthostatic hypotension may be aggravated). Products include:
Sufenta Injection 1309

Sulindac (Reduced diuretic, natriuretic, and antihypertensive effects of chlorothiazide). Products include:
Clinoril Tablets 1618

Terazosin Hydrochloride (Potentiated; additive effects). Products include:
Hytrin Capsules 430

Thiamylal Sodium (Orthostatic hypotension may be aggravated).
No products indexed under this heading.

Timolol Maleate (Potentiated; additive effects). Products include:
Blocadren Tablets 1614
Timolide Tablets 1748
Timoptic in Ocudose 1753
Timoptic Sterile Ophthalmic Solution 1751
Timoptic-XE 1755

IMPORTANT NOTE: Always consult each drug listing in the patient's regimen for possible interactions.

Diupres **Interactions Index** **320**

Tolazamide (Dosage adjustment of the antidiabetic drug may be required).
No products indexed under this heading.

Tolbutamide (Dosage adjustment of the antidiabetic drug may be required).
No products indexed under this heading.

Tolmetin Sodium (Reduced diuretic, natriuretic, and antihypertensive effects of chlorothiazide). Products include:
Tolectin (200, 400 and 600 mg) .. 1581

Torsemide (Potentiated; additive effects). Products include:
Demadex Tablets and Injection 686

Tranylcypromine Sulfate (Concurrent use is contraindicated). Products include:
Parnate Tablets 2503

Triamcinolone (Hypokalemia). Products include:
Aristocort Tablets 1022

Triamcinolone Acetonide (Hypokalemia). Products include:
Aristocort A 0.025% Cream 1027
Aristocort A 0.5% Cream 1031
Aristocort A 0.1% Cream 1029
Aristocort A 0.1% Ointment 1030
Azmacort Oral Inhaler 2011
Nasacort Nasal Inhaler 2024

Triamcinolone Diacetate (Hypokalemia). Products include:
Aristocort Suspension (Forte Parenteral) 1027
Aristocort Suspension (Intralesional) 1025

Triamcinolone Hexacetonide (Hypokalemia). Products include:
Aristospan Suspension (Intra-articular) 1033
Aristospan Suspension (Intralesional) 1032

Trimethaphan Camsylate (Potentiated; additive effects). Products include:
Arfonad Ampuls 2080

Tubocurarine Chloride (Increased responsiveness to tubocurarine).
No products indexed under this heading.

Verapamil Hydrochloride (Potentiated; additive effects). Products include:
Calan SR Caplets 2422
Calan Tablets 2419
Isoptin Injectable 1344
Isoptin Oral Tablets 1346
Isoptin SR Tablets 1348
Verelan Capsules 1410
Verelan Capsules 2824

Food Interactions

Alcohol (Orthostatic hypotension may be aggravated).

DIURIL ORAL SUSPENSION

(Chlorothiazide) 1653
May interact with lithium preparations, corticosteroids, insulin, nonsteroidal anti-inflammatory agents, barbiturates, narcotic analgesics, cardiac glycosides, antihypertensives, oral hypoglycemic agents, bile acid sequestering agents, and certain other agents. Compounds in these categories include:

Acarbose (Dosage adjustment of the antidiabetic drug may be required).
No products indexed under this heading.

Acebutolol Hydrochloride (Potentiated or additive effects). Products include:
Sectral Capsules 2807

ACTH (Hypokalemia).
No products indexed under this heading.

Alfentanil Hydrochloride (Orthostatic hypotension may be aggravated). Products include:
Alfenta Injection 1286

Amlodipine Besylate (Potentiated or additive effects). Products include:
Lotrel Capsules 840
Norvasc Tablets 1940

Aprobarbital (Orthostatic hypotension may be aggravated).
No products indexed under this heading.

Atenolol (Potentiated or additive effects). Products include:
Tenoretic Tablets 2845
Tenormin Tablets and I.V. Injection 2847

Benazepril Hydrochloride (Potentiated or additive effects). Products include:
Lotensin Tablets 834
Lotensin HCT 837
Lotrel Capsules 840

Bendroflumethiazide (Potentiated or additive effects).
No products indexed under this heading.

Betamethasone Acetate (Hypokalemia). Products include:
Celestone Soluspan Suspension 2347

Betamethasone Sodium Phosphate (Hypokalemia). Products include:
Celestone Soluspan Suspension 2347

Betaxolol Hydrochloride (Potentiated or additive effects). Products include:
Betoptic Ophthalmic Solution 469
Betoptic S Ophthalmic Suspension 471
Kerlone Tablets 2436

Bisoprolol Fumarate (Potentiated or additive effects). Products include:
Zebeta Tablets 1413
Ziac 1415

Buprenorphine (Orthostatic hypotension may be aggravated). Products include:
Buprenex Injectable 2006

Butabarbital (Orthostatic hypotension may be aggravated).
No products indexed under this heading.

Butalbital (Orthostatic hypotension may be aggravated). Products include:
Esgic-plus Tablets 1013
Fioricet Tablets 2258
Fioricet with Codeine Capsules 2260
Fiorinal Capsules 2261
Fiorinal with Codeine Capsules 2262
Fiorinal Tablets 2261
Phrenilin 785
Sedapap Tablets 50 mg/650 mg .. 1543

Captopril (Potentiated or additive effects). Products include:
Capoten 739
Capozide 742

Carteolol Hydrochloride (Potentiated or additive effects). Products include:
Cartrol Tablets 410
Ocupress Ophthalmic Solution, 1% Sterile .... ⊙ 309

Chlorothiazide Sodium (Potentiated or additive effects). Products include:
Diuril Sodium Intravenous 1652

Chlorpropamide (Dosage adjustment of the antidiabetic drug may be required). Products include:
Diabinese Tablets 1935

Chlorthalidone (Potentiated or additive effects). Products include:
Combipres Tablets 677
Tenoretic Tablets 2845
Thalitone 1245

Cholestyramine (Cholestyramine resin has the potential of binding thiazide diuretics and reducing diuretic absorption from the GI tract). Products include:
Questran Light 769
Questran Powder 770

Clonidine (Potentiated or additive effects). Products include:
Catapres-TTS 675

Clonidine Hydrochloride (Potentiated or additive effects). Products include:
Catapres Tablets 674
Combipres Tablets 677

Codeine Phosphate (Orthostatic hypotension may be aggravated). Products include:
Actifed with Codeine Cough Syrup.. 1067
Brontex 1981
Deconsal C Expectorant Syrup 456
Deconsal Pediatric Syrup 457
Dimetane-DC Cough Syrup 2059
Empirin with Codeine Tablets 1093
Fioricet with Codeine Capsules 2260
Fiorinal with Codeine Capsules 2262
Isoclor Expectorant 990
Novahistine DH 2462
Novahistine Expectorant 2463
Nucofed 2051
Phenergan with Codeine 2777
Phenergan VC with Codeine 2781
Robitussin A-C Syrup 2073
Robitussin-DAC Syrup 2074
Ryna .... ▣ 841
Soma Compound w/Codeine Tablets 2676
Tussi-Organidin NR Liquid and S NR Liquid 2677
Tylenol with Codeine 1583

Colestipol Hydrochloride (Colestipol resin has the potential of binding thiazide diuretics and reducing diuretic absorption from the GI tract). Products include:
Colestid Tablets 2591

Cortisone Acetate (Hypokalemia). Products include:
Cortone Acetate Sterile Suspension 1623
Cortone Acetate Tablets 1624

Deserpidine (Potentiated or additive effects).
No products indexed under this heading.

Deslanoside (Increased ventricular irritability).
No products indexed under this heading.

Dexamethasone (Hypokalemia). Products include:
AK-Trol Ointment & Suspension .... ⊙ 205
Decadron Elixir 1633
Decadron Tablets 1635
Decaspray Topical Aerosol 1648
Dexacidin Ointment .... ⊙ 263
Maxitrol Ophthalmic Ointment and Suspension .... ⊙ 224
TobraDex Ophthalmic Suspension and Ointment 473

Dexamethasone Acetate (Hypokalemia). Products include:
Dalalone D.P. Injectable 1011
Decadron-LA Sterile Suspension 1646

Dexamethasone Sodium Phosphate (Hypokalemia). Products include:
Decadron Phosphate Injection 1637
Decadron Phosphate Respihaler 1642
Decadron Phosphate Sterile Ophthalmic Ointment 1641
Decadron Phosphate Sterile Ophthalmic Solution 1642
Decadron Phosphate Topical Cream 1644
Decadron Phosphate Turbinaire 1645
Decadron Phosphate with Xylocaine Injection, Sterile 1639
Dexacort Phosphate in Respihaler .. 458
Dexacort Phosphate in Turbinaire .. 459
NeoDecadron Sterile Ophthalmic Ointment 1712
NeoDecadron Sterile Ophthalmic Solution 1713
NeoDecadron Topical Cream 1714

Dezocine (Orthostatic hypotension may be aggravated). Products include:
Dalgan Injection 538

Diazoxide (Potentiated or additive effects). Products include:
Hyperstat I.V. Injection 2363
Proglycem 580

Diclofenac Potassium (Reduces diuretic, natriuretic, and antihypertensive effects). Products include:
Cataflam 816

Diclofenac Sodium (Reduces diuretic, natriuretic, and antihypertensive effects). Products include:
Voltaren Ophthalmic Sterile Ophthalmic Solution .... ⊙ 272
Voltaren Tablets 861

Digitoxin (Increased ventricular irritability). Products include:
Crystodigin Tablets 1433

Digoxin (Increased ventricular irritability). Products include:
Lanoxicaps 1117
Lanoxin Elixir Pediatric 1120
Lanoxin Injection 1123
Lanoxin Injection Pediatric 1126
Lanoxin Tablets 1128

Diltiazem Hydrochloride (Potentiated or additive effects). Products include:
Cardizem CD Capsules 1506
Cardizem SR Capsules 1510
Cardizem Injectable 1508
Cardizem Tablets 1512
Dilacor XR Extended-release Capsules 2018

Doxazosin Mesylate (Potentiated or additive effects). Products include:
Cardura Tablets 2186

Enalapril Maleate (Potentiated or additive effects). Products include:
Vaseretic Tablets 1765
Vasotec Tablets 1771

Enalaprilat (Potentiation of antihypertensive effect). Products include:
Vasotec I.V. 1768

Esmolol Hydrochloride (Potentiated or additive effects). Products include:
Brevibloc Injection 1808

Etodolac (Reduces diuretic, natriuretic, and antihypertensive effects). Products include:
Lodine Capsules and Tablets 2743

Felodipine (Potentiated or additive effects). Products include:
Plendil Extended-Release Tablets 527

Fenoprofen Calcium (Reduces diuretic, natriuretic, and antihypertensive effects). Products include:
Nalfon 200 Pulvules & Nalfon Tablets 917

Fentanyl (Orthostatic hypotension may be aggravated). Products include:
Duragesic Transdermal System 1288

Fentanyl Citrate (Orthostatic hypotension may be aggravated). Products include:
Sublimaze Injection 1307

Fludrocortisone Acetate (Hypokalemia). Products include:
Florinef Acetate Tablets 505

Flurbiprofen (Reduces diuretic, natriuretic, and antihypertensive effects). Products include:
Ansaid Tablets 2579

Fosinopril Sodium (Potentiated or additive effects). Products include:
Monopril Tablets 757

Furosemide (Potentiated or additive effects). Products include:

Lasix Injection, Oral Solution and Tablets 1240

Glipizide (Dosage adjustment of the antidiabetic drug may be required). Products include:

Glucotrol Tablets 1967
Glucotrol XL Extended Release Tablets 1968

Glyburide (Dosage adjustment of the antidiabetic drug may be required). Products include:

DiaBeta Tablets 1239
Glynase PresTab Tablets 2609
Micronase Tablets 2623

Guanabenz Acetate (Potentiated or additive effects).

No products indexed under this heading.

Guanethidine Monosulfate (Potentiated or additive effects). Products include:

Esimil Tablets 822
Ismelin Tablets 827

Hydralazine Hydrochloride (Potentiated or additive effects). Products include:

Apresazide Capsules 808
Apresoline Hydrochloride Tablets .. 809
Ser-Ap-Es Tablets 849

Hydrochlorothiazide (Potentiated or additive effects). Products include:

Aldactazide 2413
Aldoril Tablets 1604
Apresazide Capsules 808
Capozide 742
Dyazide 2479
Esidrix Tablets 821
Esimil Tablets 822
HydroDIURIL Tablets 1674
Hydropres Tablets 1675
Hyzaar Tablets 1677
Inderide Tablets 2732
Inderide LA Long Acting Capsules .. 2734
Lopressor HCT Tablets 832
Lotensin HCT 837
Maxzide 1380
Moduretic Tablets 1705
Oretic Tablets 443
Prinzide Tablets 1737
Ser-Ap-Es Tablets 849
Timolide Tablets 1748
Vaseretic Tablets 1765
Zestoretic 2850
Ziac 1415

Hydrocodone Bitartrate (Orthostatic hypotension may be aggravated). Products include:

Anexsia 5/500 Elixir 1781
Anexia Tablets 1782
Codiclear DH Syrup 791
Deconamine CX Cough and Cold Liquid and Tablets 1319
Duratuss HD Elixir 2565
Hycodan Tablets and Syrup 930
Hycomine Compound Tablets 932
Hycomine 931
Hycotuss Expectorant Syrup 933
Hydrocet Capsules 782
Lorcet 10/650 1018
Lortab 2566
Tussend 1783
Tussend Expectorant 1785
Vicodin Tablets 1356
Vicodin ES Tablets 1357
Vicodin Tuss Expectorant 1358
Zydone Capsules 949

Hydrocodone Polistirex (Orthostatic hypotension may be aggravated). Products include:

Tussionex Pennkinetic Extended-Release Suspension 998

Hydrocortisone (Hypokalemia). Products include:

Anusol-HC Cream 2.5% 1896
Aquanil HC Lotion 1931
Bactine Hydrocortisone Anti-Itch Cream .... ®D 709
Caldecort Anti-Itch Hydrocortisone Spray .... ®D 631
Cortaid .... ®D 836
CORTENEMA 2535
Cortisporin Ointment 1085
Cortisporin Ophthalmic Ointment Sterile 1085
Cortisporin Ophthalmic Suspension Sterile 1086
Cortisporin Otic Solution Sterile 1087
Cortisporin Otic Suspension Sterile 1088
Cortizone-5 .... ®D 831
Cortizone-10 .... ®D 831
Hydrocortone Tablets 1672
Hytone 907
Massengill Medicated Soft Cloth Towelettes 2458
PediOtic Suspension Sterile 1153
Preparation H Hydrocortisone 1% Cream .... ®D 872
ProctoCream-HC 2.5% 2408
VöSoL HC Otic Solution 2678

Hydrocortisone Acetate (Hypokalemia). Products include:

Analpram-HC Rectal Cream 1% and 2.5% 977
Anusol HC-1 Anti-Itch Hydrocortisone Ointment .... ®D 847
Anusol-HC Suppositories 1897
Caldecort .... ®D 631
Carmol HC 924
Coly-Mycin S Otic w/Neomycin & Hydrocortisone 1906
Cortaid .... ®D 836
Cortifoam 2396
Cortisporin Cream 1084
Epifoam 2399
Hydrocortone Acetate Sterile Suspension 1669
Mantadil Cream 1135
Nupercainal Hydrocortisone 1% Cream .... ®D 645
Ophthocort .... © 311
Pramosone Cream, Lotion & Ointment 978
ProctoCream-HC 2408
ProctoFoam-HC 2409
Terra-Cortril Ophthalmic Suspension 2210

Hydrocortisone Sodium Phosphate (Hypokalemia). Products include:

Hydrocortone Phosphate Injection, Sterile 1670

Hydrocortisone Sodium Succinate (Hypokalemia). Products include:

Solu-Cortef Sterile Powder 2641

Hydroflumethiazide (Potentiated or additive effects). Products include:

Diucardin Tablets 2718

Ibuprofen (Reduces diuretic, natriuretic, and antihypertensive effects). Products include:

Advil Cold and Sinus Caplets and Tablets (formerly CoAdvil) .... ®D 870
Advil Ibuprofen Tablets and Caplets .... ®D 870
Children's Advil Suspension 2692
Arthritis Foundation Ibuprofen Tablets .... ®D 674
Bayer Select Ibuprofen Pain Relief Formula .... ®D 715
Cramp End Tablets .... ®D 735
Dimetapp Sinus Caplets .... ®D 775
Haltran Tablets .... ®D 771
IBU Tablets 1342
Ibuprohm .... ®D 735
Children's Motrin Ibuprofen Oral Suspension 1546
Motrin Tablets 2625
Motrin IB Caplets, Tablets, and Geltabs .... ®D 838
Motrin IB Sinus .... ®D 838
Motrin Ibuprofen Suspension, Oral Drops, Chewable Tablets, Caplets 1546
Nuprin Ibuprofen/Analgesic Tablets & Caplets .... ®D 622
Sine-Aid IB Caplets 1554
Vicks DayQuil SINUS Pressure & PAIN Relief with IBUPROFEN ...... ®D 762

Indapamide (Potentiated or additive effects). Products include:

Lozol Tablets 2022

Indomethacin (Reduces diuretic, natriuretic, and antihypertensive effects). Products include:

Indocin 1680

Indomethacin Sodium Trihydrate (Reduces diuretic, natriuretic, and antihypertensive effects). Products include:

Indocin I.V. 1684

Insulin, Human (Altered insulin requirements).

No products indexed under this heading.

Insulin, Human Isophane Suspension (Altered insulin requirements). Products include:

Novolin N Human Insulin 10 ml Vials 1795

Insulin, Human NPH (Altered insulin requirements). Products include:

Humulin N, 100 Units 1448
Novolin N PenFill Cartridges Durable Insulin Delivery System 1798
Novolin N Prefilled Syringe Disposable Insulin Delivery System 1798

Insulin, Human Regular (Altered insulin requirements). Products include:

Humulin R, 100 Units 1449
Novolin R Human Insulin 10 ml Vials 1795
Novolin R PenFill Cartridges Durable Insulin Delivery System 1798
Novolin R Prefilled Syringe Disposable Insulin Delivery System 1798
Velosulin BR Human Insulin 10 ml Vials 1795

Insulin, Human, Zinc Suspension (Altered insulin requirements). Products include:

Humulin L, 100 Units 1446
Humulin U, 100 Units 1450
Novolin L Human Insulin 10 ml Vials 1795

Insulin, NPH (Altered insulin requirements). Products include:

NPH, 100 Units 1450
Pork NPH, 100 Units 1452
Purified Pork NPH Isophane Insulin 1801

Insulin, Regular (Altered insulin requirements). Products include:

Regular, 100 Units 1450
Pork Regular, 100 Units 1452
Pork Regular (Concentrated), 500 Units 1453
Purified Pork Regular Insulin 1801

Insulin, Zinc Crystals (Altered insulin requirements). Products include:

NPH, 100 Units 1450

Insulin, Zinc Suspension (Altered insulin requirements). Products include:

Iletin I 1450
Lente, 100 Units 1450
Iletin II 1452
Pork Lente, 100 Units 1452
Purified Pork Lente Insulin 1801

Isradipine (Potentiated or additive effects). Products include:

DynaCirc Capsules 2256

Ketoprofen (Reduces diuretic, natriuretic, and antihypertensive effects). Products include:

Orudis Capsules 2766
Oruvail Capsules 2766

Ketorolac Tromethamine (Reduces diuretic, natriuretic, and antihypertensive effects). Products include:

Acular 474
Acular .... © 277
Toradol 2159

Labetalol Hydrochloride (Potentiated or additive effects). Products include:

Normodyne Injection 2377
Normodyne Tablets 2379
Trandate 1185

Levorphanol Tartrate (Orthostatic hypotension may be aggravated). Products include:

Levo-Dromoran 2129

Lisinopril (Potentiation of antihypertensive effect). Products include:

Prinivil Tablets 1733
Prinzide Tablets 1737
Zestoretic 2850
Zestril Tablets 2854

Lithium Carbonate (High risk of lithium toxicity). Products include:

Eskalith 2485
Lithium Carbonate Capsules & Tablets 2230
Lithonate/Lithotabs/Lithobid 2543

Lithium Citrate (High risk of lithium toxicity).

No products indexed under this heading.

Losartan Potassium (Potentiated or additive effects). Products include:

Cozaar Tablets 1628
Hyzaar Tablets 1677

Mecamylamine Hydrochloride (Potentiated or additive effects). Products include:

Inversine Tablets 1686

Meclofenamate Sodium (Reduced diuretic, natriuretic, and antihypertensive effects of chlorothiazide).

No products indexed under this heading.

Mefenamic Acid (Reduced diuretic, natriuretic, and antihypertensive effects of chlorothiazide). Products include:

Ponstel 1925

Meperidine Hydrochloride (Orthostatic hypotension may be aggravated). Products include:

Demerol 2308
Mepergan Injection 2753

Mephobarbital (Orthostatic hypotension may be aggravated). Products include:

Mebaral Tablets 2322

Metformin Hydrochloride (Dosage adjustment of the antidiabetic drug may be required). Products include:

Glucophage 752

Methadone Hydrochloride (Orthostatic hypotension may be aggravated). Products include:

Methadone Hydrochloride Oral Concentrate 2233
Methadone Hydrochloride Oral Solution & Tablets 2235

Methyclothiazide (Potentiated or additive effects). Products include:

Enduron Tablets 420

Methyldopa (Potentiated or additive effects). Products include:

Aldoclor Tablets 1598
Aldomet Oral 1600
Aldoril Tablets 1604

Methyldopate Hydrochloride (Potentiated or additive effects). Products include:

Aldomet Ester HCl Injection 1602

Methylprednisolone (Hypokalemia). Products include:

Medrol 2621

Methylprednisolone Acetate (Hypokalemia). Products include:

Depo-Medrol Single-Dose Vial 2600
Depo-Medrol Sterile Aqueous Suspension 2597

Methylprednisolone Sodium Succinate (Hypokalemia). Products include:

Solu-Medrol Sterile Powder 2643

Metolazone (Potentiated or additive effects). Products include:

Mykrox Tablets 993
Zaroxolyn Tablets 1000

Metoprolol Succinate (Potentiated or additive effects). Products include:

Toprol-XL Tablets 565

IMPORTANT NOTE: Always consult each drug listing in the patient's regimen for possible interactions.

Metoprolol Tartrate (Potentiated or additive effects). Products include:
- Lopressor Ampuls 830
- Lopressor HCT Tablets 832
- Lopressor Tablets 830

Metyrosine (Potentiated or additive effects). Products include:
- Demser Capsules 1649

Minoxidil (Potentiated or additive effects). Products include:
- Loniten Tablets 2618
- Rogaine Topical Solution 2637

Moexipril Hydrochloride (Potentiated or additive effects). Products include:
- Univasc Tablets 2410

Morphine Sulfate (Orthostatic hypotension may be aggravated). Products include:
- Astramorph/PF Injection, USP (Preservative-Free) 535
- Duramorph 962
- Infumorph 200 and Infumorph 500 Sterile Solutions 965
- MS Contin Tablets 1994
- MSIR 1997
- Oramorph SR (Morphine Sulfate Sustained Release Tablets) 2236
- RMS Suppositories 2657
- Roxanol 2243

Nabumetone (Reduces diuretic, natriuretic, and antihypertensive effects). Products include:
- Relafen Tablets 2510

Nadolol (Potentiated or additive effects).
- No products indexed under this heading.

Naproxen (Reduces diuretic, natriuretic, and antihypertensive effects). Products include:
- Anaprox/Naprosyn 2117

Naproxen Sodium (Reduces diuretic, natriuretic, and antihypertensive effects). Products include:
- Aleve 1975
- Anaprox/Naprosyn 2117

Nicardipine Hydrochloride (Potentiated or additive effects). Products include:
- Cardene Capsules 2095
- Cardene I.V. 2709
- Cardene SR Capsules 2097

Nifedipine (Potentiated or additive effects). Products include:
- Adalat Capsules (10 mg and 20 mg) 587
- Adalat CC 589
- Procardia Capsules 1971
- Procardia XL Extended Release Tablets 1972

Nisoldipine (Potentiated or additive effects).
- No products indexed under this heading.

Nitroglycerin (Potentiated or additive effects). Products include:
- Deponit NTG Transdermal Delivery System 2397
- Nitro-Bid IV 1523
- Nitro-Bid Ointment 1524
- Nitrodisc 2047
- Nitro-Dur (nitroglycerin) Transdermal Infusion System 1326
- Nitrolingual Spray 2027
- Nitrostat Tablets 1925
- Transderm-Nitro Transdermal Therapeutic System 859

Norepinephrine Bitartrate (Decreased arterial responsiveness to norepinephrine). Products include:
- Levophed Bitartrate Injection 2315

Opium Alkaloids (Orthostatic hypotension may be aggravated).
- No products indexed under this heading.

Oxaprozin (Reduces diuretic, natriuretic, and antihypertensive effects). Products include:
- Daypro Caplets 2426

Oxycodone Hydrochloride (Orthostatic hypotension may be aggravated). Products include:
- Percocet Tablets 938
- Percodan Tablets 939
- Percodan-Demi Tablets 940
- Roxicodone Tablets, Oral Solution & Intensol (Oxycodone) 2244
- Tylox Capsules 1584

Penbutolol Sulfate (Potentiated or additive effects). Products include:
- Levatol 2403

Pentobarbital Sodium (Orthostatic hypotension may be aggravated). Products include:
- Nembutal Sodium Capsules 436
- Nembutal Sodium Solution 438
- Nembutal Sodium Suppositories 440

Phenobarbital (Orthostatic hypotension may be aggravated). Products include:
- Arco-Lase Plus Tablets 512
- Bellergal-S Tablets 2250
- Donnatal 2060
- Donnatal Extentabs 2061
- Donnatal Tablets 2060
- Phenobarbital Elixir and Tablets 1469
- Quadrinal Tablets 1350

Phenoxybenzamine Hydrochloride (Potentiated or additive effects). Products include:
- Dibenzyline Capsules 2476

Phentolamine Mesylate (Potentiated or additive effects). Products include:
- Regitine 846

Phenylbutazone (Reduces diuretic, natriuretic, and antihypertensive effects).
- No products indexed under this heading.

Pindolol (Potentiated or additive effects). Products include:
- Visken Tablets 2299

Piroxicam (Reduces diuretic, natriuretic, and antihypertensive effects). Products include:
- Feldene Capsules 1965

Polythiazide (Potentiated or additive effects). Products include:
- Minizide Capsules 1938

Prazosin Hydrochloride (Potentiated or additive effects). Products include:
- Minipress Capsules 1937
- Minizide Capsules 1938

Prednisolone Acetate (Hypokalemia). Products include:
- AK-CIDE .... ◉ 202
- AK-CIDE Ointment .... ◉ 202
- Blephamide Liquifilm Sterile Ophthalmic Suspension 476
- Blephamide Ointment .... ◉ 237
- Econopred & Econopred Plus Ophthalmic Suspensions .... ◉ 217
- Poly-Pred Liquifilm .... ◉ 248
- Pred Forte .... ◉ 250
- Pred Mild .... ◉ 253
- Pred-G Liquifilm Sterile Ophthalmic Suspension .... ◉ 251
- Pred-G S.O.P. Sterile Ophthalmic Ointment .... ◉ 252
- Vasocidin Ointment .... ◉ 268

Prednisolone Sodium Phosphate (Hypokalemia). Products include:
- AK-Pred .... ◉ 204
- Hydeltrasol Injection, Sterile 1665
- Inflamase .... ◉ 265
- Pediapred Oral Liquid 995
- Vasocidin Ophthalmic Solution .... ◉ 270

Prednisolone Tebutate (Hypokalemia). Products include:
- Hydeltra-T.B.A. Sterile Suspension 1667

Prednisone (Hypokalemia). Products include:
- Deltasone Tablets 2595

Propoxyphene Hydrochloride (Orthostatic hypotension may be aggravated). Products include:
- Darvon 1435
- Wygesic Tablets 2827

Propoxyphene Napsylate (Orthostatic hypotension may be aggravated). Products include:
- Darvon-N/Darvocet-N 1433

Propranolol Hydrochloride (Potentiated or additive effects). Products include:
- Inderal 2728
- Inderal LA Long Acting Capsules 2730
- Inderide Tablets 2732
- Inderide LA Long Acting Capsules 2734

Quinapril Hydrochloride (Potentiated or additive effects). Products include:
- Accupril Tablets 1893

Ramipril (Potentiated or additive effects). Products include:
- Altace Capsules 1232

Rauwolfia Serpentina (Potentiated or additive effects).
- No products indexed under this heading.

Rescinnamine (Potentiated or additive effects).
- No products indexed under this heading.

Reserpine (Potentiated or additive effects). Products include:
- Diupres Tablets 1650
- Hydropres Tablets 1675
- Ser-Ap-Es Tablets 849

Secobarbital Sodium (Orthostatic hypotension may be aggravated). Products include:
- Seconal Sodium Pulvules 1474

Sodium Nitroprusside (Potentiated or additive effects).
- No products indexed under this heading.

Sotalol Hydrochloride (Potentiated or additive effects). Products include:
- Betapace Tablets 641

Spirapril Hydrochloride (Potentiated or additive effects).
- No products indexed under this heading.

Sufentanil Citrate (Orthostatic hypotension may be aggravated). Products include:
- Sufenta Injection 1309

Sulindac (Reduces diuretic, natriuretic, and antihypertensive effects). Products include:
- Clinoril Tablets 1618

Terazosin Hydrochloride (Potentiated or additive effects). Products include:
- Hytrin Capsules 430

Thiamylal Sodium (Orthostatic hypotension may be aggravated).
- No products indexed under this heading.

Timolol Maleate (Potentiated or additive effects). Products include:
- Blocadren Tablets 1614
- Timolide Tablets 1748
- Timoptic in Ocudose 1753
- Timoptic Sterile Ophthalmic Solution 1751
- Timoptic-XE 1755

Tolazamide (Dosage adjustment of the antidiabetic drug may be required).
- No products indexed under this heading.

Tolbutamide (Dosage adjustment of the antidiabetic drug may be required).
- No products indexed under this heading.

Tolmetin Sodium (Reduces diuretic, natriuretic, and antihypertensive effects). Products include:
- Tolectin (200, 400 and 600 mg) .. 1581

Torsemide (Potentiated or additive effects). Products include:
- Demadex Tablets and Injection 686

Triamcinolone (Hypokalemia). Products include:
- Aristocort Tablets 1022

Triamcinolone Acetonide (Hypokalemia). Products include:
- Aristocort A 0.025% Cream 1027
- Aristocort A 0.5% Cream 1031
- Aristocort A 0.1% Cream 1029
- Aristocort A 0.1% Ointment 1030
- Azmacort Oral Inhaler 2011
- Nasacort Nasal Inhaler 2024

Triamcinolone Diacetate (Hypokalemia). Products include:
- Aristocort Suspension (Forte Parenteral) 1027
- Aristocort Suspension (Intralesional) 1025

Triamcinolone Hexacetonide (Hypokalemia). Products include:
- Aristospan Suspension (Intra-articular) 1033
- Aristospan Suspension (Intralesional) 1032

Trimethaphan Camsylate (Potentiated or additive effects). Products include:
- Arfonad Ampuls 2080

Tubocurarine Chloride (Increased responsiveness to tubocurarine).
- No products indexed under this heading.

Verapamil Hydrochloride (Potentiated or additive effects). Products include:
- Calan SR Caplets 2422
- Calan Tablets 2419
- Isoptin Injectable 1344
- Isoptin Oral Tablets 1346
- Isoptin SR Tablets 1348
- Verelan Capsules 1410
- Verelan Capsules 2824

Food Interactions

Alcohol (Orthostatic hypotension may be aggravated).

DIURIL SODIUM INTRAVENOUS

(Chlorothiazide Sodium) 1652

May interact with lithium preparations, corticosteroids, insulin, nonsteroidal anti-inflammatory agents, barbiturates, narcotic analgesics, cardiac glycosides, antihypertensives, oral hypoglycemic agents, and certain other agents. Compounds in these categories include:

Acarbose (Dosage adjustment of oral hypoglycemic agent may be necessary).
- No products indexed under this heading.

Acebutolol Hydrochloride (Potentiated or additive effects). Products include:
- Sectral Capsules 2807

ACTH (Hypokalemia).
- No products indexed under this heading.

Alfentanil Hydrochloride (Potentiation of orthostatic hypotension). Products include:
- Alfenta Injection 1286

Amlodipine Besylate (Potentiated or additive effects). Products include:
- Lotrel Capsules 840
- Norvasc Tablets 1940

Aprobarbital (Potentiation of orthostatic hypotension).
- No products indexed under this heading.

(▭ Described in PDR For Nonprescription Drugs) (◉ Described in PDR For Ophthalmology)

Atenolol (Potentiated or additive effects). Products include:
Tenoretic Tablets ... 2845
Tenormin Tablets and I.V. Injection 2847

Benazepril Hydrochloride (Potentiated or additive effects). Products include:
Lotensin Tablets ... 834
Lotensin HCT ... 837
Lotrel Capsules ... 840

Bendroflumethiazide (Potentiated or additive effects).
No products indexed under this heading.

Betamethasone Acetate (Hypokalemia). Products include:
Celestone Soluspan Suspension ... 2347

Betamethasone Sodium Phosphate (Hypokalemia). Products include:
Celestone Soluspan Suspension ... 2347

Betaxolol Hydrochloride (Potentiated or additive effects). Products include:
Betoptic Ophthalmic Solution ... 469
Betoptic S Ophthalmic Suspension ... 471
Kerlone Tablets ... 2436

Bisoprolol Fumarate (Potentiated or additive effects). Products include:
Zebeta Tablets ... 1413
Ziac ... 1415

Buprenorphine (Potentiation of orthostatic hypotension). Products include:
Buprenex Injectable ... 2006

Butabarbital (Potentiation of orthostatic hypotension).
No products indexed under this heading.

Butalbital (Potentiation of orthostatic hypotension aggravated). Products include:
Esgic-plus Tablets ... 1013
Fioricet Tablets ... 2258
Fioricet with Codeine Capsules ... 2260
Fiorinal Capsules ... 2261
Fiorinal with Codeine Capsules ... 2262
Fiorinal Tablets ... 2261
Phrenilin ... 785
Sedapap Tablets 50 mg/650 mg ... 1543

Captopril (Potentiated or additive effects). Products include:
Capoten ... 739
Capozide ... 742

Carteolol Hydrochloride (Potentiated or additive effects). Products include:
Cartrol Tablets ... 410
Ocupress Ophthalmic Solution, 1% Sterile ... ◉ 309

Chlorpropamide (Dosage adjustment of oral hypoglycemic agent may be necessary). Products include:
Diabinese Tablets ... 1935

Chlorthalidone (Potentiated or additive effects). Products include:
Combipres Tablets ... 677
Tenoretic Tablets ... 2845
Thalitone ... 1245

Clonidine (Potentiated or additive effects). Products include:
Catapres-TTS ... 675

Clonidine Hydrochloride (Potentiated or additive effects). Products include:
Catapres Tablets ... 674
Combipres Tablets ... 677

Codeine Phosphate (Potentiation of orthostatic hypotension). Products include:
Actifed with Codeine Cough Syrup ... 1067
Brontex ... 1981
Deconsal C Expectorant Syrup ... 456
Deconsal Pediatric Syrup ... 457
Dimetane-DC Cough Syrup ... 2059
Empirin with Codeine Tablets ... 1093
Fioricet with Codeine Capsules ... 2260
Fiorinal with Codeine Capsules ... 2262
Isoclor Expectorant ... 990
Novahistine DH ... 2462
Novahistine Expectorant ... 2463
Nucofed ... 2051
Phenergan with Codeine ... 2777
Phenergan VC with Codeine ... 2781
Robitussin A-C Syrup ... 2073
Robitussin-DAC Syrup ... 2074
Ryna ... ▣ 841
Soma Compound w/Codeine Tablets ... 2676
Tussi-Organidin NR Liquid and S NR Liquid ... 2677
Tylenol with Codeine ... 1583

Cortisone Acetate (Hypokalemia). Products include:
Cortone Acetate Sterile Suspension ... 1623
Cortone Acetate Tablets ... 1624

Deserpidine (Potentiated or additive effects).
No products indexed under this heading.

Deslanoside (Increased ventricular irritability).
No products indexed under this heading.

Dexamethasone (Hypokalemia). Products include:
AK-Trol Ointment & Suspension ... ◉ 205
Decadron Elixir ... 1633
Decadron Tablets ... 1635
Decaspray Topical Aerosol ... 1648
Dexacidin Ointment ... ◉ 263
Maxitrol Ophthalmic Ointment and Suspension ... ◉ 224
TobraDex Ophthalmic Suspension and Ointment ... 473

Dexamethasone Acetate (Hypokalemia). Products include:
Dalalone D.P. Injectable ... 1011
Decadron-LA Sterile Suspension ... 1646

Dexamethasone Sodium Phosphate (Hypokalemia). Products include:
Decadron Phosphate Injection ... 1637
Decadron Phosphate Respihaler ... 1642
Decadron Phosphate Sterile Ophthalmic Ointment ... 1641
Decadron Phosphate Sterile Ophthalmic Solution ... 1642
Decadron Phosphate Topical Cream ... 1644
Decadron Phosphate Turbinaire ... 1645
Decadron Phosphate with Xylocaine Injection, Sterile ... 1639
Dexacort Phosphate in Respihaler ... 458
Dexacort Phosphate in Turbinaire ... 459
NeoDecadron Sterile Ophthalmic Ointment ... 1712
NeoDecadron Sterile Ophthalmic Solution ... 1713
NeoDecadron Topical Cream ... 1714

Dezocine (Potentiation of orthostatic hypotension). Products include:
Dalgan Injection ... 538

Diazoxide (Potentiated or additive effects). Products include:
Hyperstat I.V. Injection ... 2363
Proglycem ... 580

Diclofenac Potassium (Reduces diuretic, natriuretic, and antihypertensive effects). Products include:
Cataflam ... 816

Diclofenac Sodium (Reduces diuretic, natriuretic, and antihypertensive effects). Products include:
Voltaren Ophthalmic Sterile Ophthalmic Solution ... ◉ 272
Voltaren Tablets ... 861

Digitoxin (Increased ventricular irritability). Products include:
Crystodigin Tablets ... 1433

Digoxin (Increased ventricular irritability). Products include:
Lanoxicaps ... 1117
Lanoxin Elixir Pediatric ... 1120
Lanoxin Injection ... 1123
Lanoxin Injection Pediatric ... 1126
Lanoxin Tablets ... 1128

Diltiazem Hydrochloride (Potentiated or additive effects). Products include:
Cardizem CD Capsules ... 1506
Cardizem SR Capsules ... 1510
Cardizem Injectable ... 1508
Cardizem Tablets ... 1512
Dilacor XR Extended-release Capsules ... 2018

Doxazosin Mesylate (Potentiated or additive effects). Products include:
Cardura Tablets ... 2186

Enalapril Maleate (Potentiated or additive effects). Products include:
Vaseretic Tablets ... 1765
Vasotec Tablets ... 1771

Enalaprilat (Potentiated or additive effects). Products include:
Vasotec I.V. ... 1768

Esmolol Hydrochloride (Potentiated or additive effects). Products include:
Brevibloc Injection ... 1808

Etodolac (Reduces diuretic, natriuretic, and antihypertensive effects). Products include:
Lodine Capsules and Tablets ... 2743

Felodipine (Potentiated or additive effects). Products include:
Plendil Extended-Release Tablets ... 527

Fenoprofen Calcium (Reduces diuretic, natriuretic, and antihypertensive effects). Products include:
Nalfon 200 Pulvules & Nalfon Tablets ... 917

Fentanyl (Potentiation of orthostatic hypotension). Products include:
Duragesic Transdermal System ... 1288

Fentanyl Citrate (Potentiation of orthostatic hypotension). Products include:
Sublimaze Injection ... 1307

Fludrocortisone Acetate (Hypokalemia). Products include:
Florinef Acetate Tablets ... 505

Flurbiprofen (Reduces diuretic, natriuretic, and antihypertensive effects). Products include:
Ansaid Tablets ... 2579

Fosinopril Sodium (Potentiated or additive effects). Products include:
Monopril Tablets ... 757

Furosemide (Potentiated or additive effects). Products include:
Lasix Injection, Oral Solution and Tablets ... 1240

Glipizide (Dosage adjustment of oral hypoglycemic agent may be necessary). Products include:
Glucotrol Tablets ... 1967
Glucotrol XL Extended Release Tablets ... 1968

Glyburide (Dosage adjustment of oral hypoglycemic agent may be necessary). Products include:
DiaBeta Tablets ... 1239
Glynase PresTab Tablets ... 2609
Micronase Tablets ... 2623

Guanabenz Acetate (Potentiated or additive effects).
No products indexed under this heading.

Guanethidine Monosulfate (Potentiated or additive effects). Products include:
Esimil Tablets ... 822
Ismelin Tablets ... 827

Hydralazine Hydrochloride (Potentiated or additive effects). Products include:
Apresazide Capsules ... 808
Apresoline Hydrochloride Tablets ... 809
Ser-Ap-Es Tablets ... 849

Hydrochlorothiazide (Potentiated or additive effects). Products include:
Aldactazide ... 2413
Aldoril Tablets ... 1604
Apresazide Capsules ... 808
Capozide ... 742
Dyazide ... 2479
Esidrix Tablets ... 821
Esimil Tablets ... 822
HydroDIURIL Tablets ... 1674
Hydropres Tablets ... 1675
Hyzaar Tablets ... 1677
Inderide Tablets ... 2732
Inderide LA Long Acting Capsules ... 2734
Lopressor HCT Tablets ... 832
Lotensin HCT ... 837
Maxzide ... 1380
Moduretic Tablets ... 1705
Oretic Tablets ... 443
Prinzide Tablets ... 1737
Ser-Ap-Es Tablets ... 849
Timolide Tablets ... 1748
Vaseretic Tablets ... 1765
Zestoretic ... 2850
Ziac ... 1415

Hydrocodone Bitartrate (Potentiation of orthostatic hypotension). Products include:
Anexsia 5/500 Elixir ... 1781
Anexia Tablets ... 1782
Codiclear DH Syrup ... 791
Deconamine CX Cough and Cold Liquid and Tablets ... 1319
Duratuss HD Elixir ... 2565
Hycodan Tablets and Syrup ... 930
Hycomine Compound Tablets ... 932
Hycomine ... 931
Hycotuss Expectorant Syrup ... 933
Hydrocet Capsules ... 782
Lorcet 10/650 ... 1018
Lortab ... 2566
Tussend ... 1783
Tussend Expectorant ... 1785
Vicodin Tablets ... 1356
Vicodin ES Tablets ... 1357
Vicodin Tuss Expectorant ... 1358
Zydone Capsules ... 949

Hydrocodone Polistirex (Potentiation of orthostatic hypotension). Products include:
Tussionex Pennkinetic Extended-Release Suspension ... 998

Hydrocortisone (Hypokalemia). Products include:
Anusol-HC Cream 2.5% ... 1896
Aquanil HC Lotion ... 1931
Bactine Hydrocortisone Anti-Itch Cream ... ▣ 709
Caldecort Anti-Itch Hydrocortisone Spray ... ▣ 631
Cortaid ... ▣ 836
CORTENEMA ... 2535
Cortisporin Ointment ... 1085
Cortisporin Ophthalmic Ointment Sterile ... 1085
Cortisporin Ophthalmic Suspension Sterile ... 1086
Cortisporin Otic Solution Sterile ... 1087
Cortisporin Otic Suspension Sterile 1088
Cortizone-5 ... ▣ 831
Cortizone-10 ... ▣ 831
Hydrocortone Tablets ... 1672
Hytone ... 907
Massengill Medicated Soft Cloth Towelettes ... 2458
PediOtic Suspension Sterile ... 1153
Preparation H Hydrocortisone 1% Cream ... ▣ 872
ProctoCream-HC 2.5% ... 2408
VōSoL HC Otic Solution ... 2678

Hydrocortisone Acetate (Hypokalemia). Products include:
Analpram-HC Rectal Cream 1% and 2.5% ... 977
Anusol HC-1 Anti-Itch Hydrocortisone Ointment ... ▣ 847
Anusol-HC Suppositories ... 1897
Caldecort ... ▣ 631
Carmol HC ... 924
Coly-Mycin S Otic w/Neomycin & Hydrocortisone ... 1906
Cortaid ... ▣ 836
Cortifoam ... 2396
Cortisporin Cream ... 1084
Epifoam ... 2399
Hydrocortone Acetate Sterile Suspension ... 1669

IMPORTANT NOTE: Always consult each drug listing in the patient's regimen for possible interactions.

Diuril Intravenous **Interactions Index** **324**

- Mantadil Cream 1135
- Nupercainal Hydrocortisone 1% Cream .... ■ 645
- Ophthocort .... ◉ 311
- Pramosone Cream, Lotion & Ointment 978
- ProctoCream-HC 2408
- ProctoFoam-HC 2409
- Terra-Cortril Ophthalmic Suspension 2210

Hydrocortisone Sodium Phosphate (Hypokalemia). Products include:
- Hydrocortone Phosphate Injection, Sterile 1670

Hydrocortisone Sodium Succinate (Hypokalemia). Products include:
- Solu-Cortef Sterile Powder 2641

Hydroflumethiazide (Potentiated or additive effects). Products include:
- Diucardin Tablets 2718

Ibuprofen (Reduces diuretic, natriuretic, and antihypertensive effects). Products include:
- Advil Cold and Sinus Caplets and Tablets (formerly CoAdvil) .... ■ 870
- Advil Ibuprofen Tablets and Caplets .... ■ 870
- Children's Advil Suspension 2692
- Arthritis Foundation Ibuprofen Tablets .... ■ 674
- Bayer Select Ibuprofen Pain Relief Formula .... ■ 715
- Cramp End Tablets .... ■ 735
- Dimetapp Sinus Caplets .... ■ 775
- Haltran Tablets .... ■ 771
- IBU Tablets 1342
- Ibuprohm .... ■ 735
- Children's Motrin Ibuprofen Oral Suspension 1546
- Motrin Tablets 2625
- Motrin IB Caplets, Tablets, and Geltabs .... ■ 838
- Motrin IB Sinus .... ■ 838
- Motrin Ibuprofen Suspension, Oral Drops, Chewable Tablets, Caplets 1546
- Nuprin Ibuprofen/Analgesic Tablets & Caplets .... ■ 622
- Sine-Aid IB Caplets 1554
- Vicks DayQuil SINUS Pressure & PAIN Relief with IBUPROFEN .... ■ 762

Indapamide (Potentiated or additive effects). Products include:
- Lozol Tablets 2022

Indomethacin (Reduces diuretic, natriuretic, and antihypertensive effects). Products include:
- Indocin 1680

Indomethacin Sodium Trihydrate (Reduces diuretic, natriuretic, and antihypertensive effects). Products include:
- Indocin I.V. 1684

Insulin, Human (Altered insulin requirements).
- No products indexed under this heading.

Insulin, Human Isophane Suspension (Altered insulin requirements). Products include:
- Novolin N Human Insulin 10 ml Vials 1795

Insulin, Human NPH (Altered insulin requirements). Products include:
- Humulin N, 100 Units 1448
- Novolin N PenFill Cartridges Durable Insulin Delivery System 1798
- Novolin N Prefilled Syringe Disposable Insulin Delivery System 1798

Insulin, Human Regular (Altered insulin requirements). Products include:
- Humulin R, 100 Units 1449
- Novolin R Human Insulin 10 ml Vials 1795
- Novolin R PenFill Cartridges Durable Insulin Delivery System 1798
- Novolin R Prefilled Syringe Disposable Insulin Delivery System 1798
- Velosulin BR Human Insulin 10 ml Vials 1795

Insulin, Human, Zinc Suspension (Altered insulin requirements). Products include:
- Humulin L, 100 Units 1446
- Humulin U, 100 Units 1450
- Novolin L Human Insulin 10 ml Vials 1795

Insulin, NPH (Altered insulin requirements). Products include:
- NPH, 100 Units 1450
- Pork NPH, 100 Units 1452
- Purified Pork NPH Isophane Insulin 1801

Insulin, Regular (Altered insulin requirements). Products include:
- Regular, 100 Units 1450
- Pork Regular, 100 Units 1452
- Pork Regular (Concentrated), 500 Units 1453
- Purified Pork Regular Insulin 1801

Insulin, Zinc Crystals (Altered insulin requirements). Products include:
- NPH, 100 Units 1450

Insulin, Zinc Suspension (Altered insulin requirements). Products include:
- Iletin I 1450
- Lente, 100 Units 1450
- Iletin II 1452
- Pork Lente, 100 Units 1452
- Purified Pork Lente Insulin 1801

Isradipine (Potentiated or additive effects). Products include:
- DynaCirc Capsules 2256

Ketoprofen (Reduces diuretic, natriuretic, and antihypertensive effects). Products include:
- Orudis Capsules 2766
- Oruvail Capsules 2766

Ketorolac Tromethamine (Reduces diuretic, natriuretic, and antihypertensive effects). Products include:
- Acular 474
- Acular .... ◉ 277
- Toradol 2159

Labetalol Hydrochloride (Potentiated or additive effects). Products include:
- Normodyne Injection 2377
- Normodyne Tablets 2379
- Trandate 1185

Levorphanol Tartrate (Potentiation of orthostatic hypotension). Products include:
- Levo-Dromoran 2129

Lisinopril (Potentiated or additive effects). Products include:
- Prinivil Tablets 1733
- Prinzide Tablets 1737
- Zestoretic 2850
- Zestril Tablets 2854

Lithium Carbonate (High risk of lithium toxicity). Products include:
- Eskalith 2485
- Lithium Carbonate Capsules & Tablets 2230
- Lithonate/Lithotabs/Lithobid 2543

Lithium Citrate (High risk of lithium toxicity).
- No products indexed under this heading.

Losartan Potassium (Potentiated or additive effects). Products include:
- Cozaar Tablets 1628
- Hyzaar Tablets 1677

Mecamylamine Hydrochloride (Potentiated or additive effects). Products include:
- Inversine Tablets 1686

Meclofenamate Sodium (Reduces diuretic, natriuretic, and antihypertensive effects).
- No products indexed under this heading.

Mefenamic Acid (Reduces diuretic, natriuretic, and antihypertensive effects). Products include:
- Ponstel 1925

Meperidine Hydrochloride (Potentiation of orthostatic hypotension). Products include:
- Demerol 2308
- Mepergan Injection 2753

Mephobarbital (Potentiation of orthostatic hypotension). Products include:
- Mebaral Tablets 2322

Metformin Hydrochloride (Dosage adjustment of oral hypoglycemic agent may be necessary). Products include:
- Glucophage 752

Methadone Hydrochloride (Potentiation of orthostatic hypotension). Products include:
- Methadone Hydrochloride Oral Concentrate 2233
- Methadone Hydrochloride Oral Solution & Tablets 2235

Methyclothiazide (Potentiated or additive effects). Products include:
- Enduron Tablets 420

Methyldopa (Potentiated or additive effects). Products include:
- Aldoclor Tablets 1598
- Aldomet Oral 1600
- Aldoril Tablets 1604

Methyldopate Hydrochloride (Potentiated or additive effects). Products include:
- Aldomet Ester HCl Injection 1602

Methylprednisolone Acetate (Hypokalemia). Products include:
- Depo-Medrol Single-Dose Vial 2600
- Depo-Medrol Sterile Aqueous Suspension 2597

Methylprednisolone Sodium Succinate (Hypokalemia). Products include:
- Solu-Medrol Sterile Powder 2643

Metolazone (Potentiated or additive effects). Products include:
- Mykrox Tablets 993
- Zaroxolyn Tablets 1000

Metoprolol Succinate (Potentiated or additive effects). Products include:
- Toprol-XL Tablets 565

Metoprolol Tartrate (Potentiated or additive effects). Products include:
- Lopressor Ampuls 830
- Lopressor HCT Tablets 832
- Lopressor Tablets 830

Metyrosine (Potentiated or additive effects). Products include:
- Demser Capsules 1649

Minoxidil (Potentiated or additive effects). Products include:
- Loniten Tablets 2618
- Rogaine Topical Solution 2637

Moexipril Hydrochloride (Potentiated or additive effects). Products include:
- Univasc Tablets 2410

Morphine Sulfate (Potentiation of orthostatic hypotension). Products include:
- Astramorph/PF Injection, USP (Preservative-Free) 535
- Duramorph 962
- Infumorph 200 and Infumorph 500 Sterile Solutions 965
- MS Contin Tablets 1994
- MSIR 1997
- Oramorph SR (Morphine Sulfate Sustained Release Tablets) 2236
- RMS Suppositories 2657
- Roxanol 2243

Nabumetone (Reduces diuretic, natriuretic, and antihypertensive effects). Products include:
- Relafen Tablets 2510

Nadolol (Potentiated or additive effects).
- No products indexed under this heading.

Naproxen (Reduces diuretic, natriuretic, and antihypertensive effects). Products include:
- Anaprox/Naprosyn 2117

Naproxen Sodium (Reduces diuretic, natriuretic, and antihypertensive effects). Products include:
- Aleve 1975
- Anaprox/Naprosyn 2117

Nicardipine Hydrochloride (Potentiated or additive effects). Products include:
- Cardene Capsules 2095
- Cardene I.V. 2709
- Cardene SR Capsules 2097

Nifedipine (Potentiated or additive effects). Products include:
- Adalat Capsules (10 mg and 20 mg) 587
- Adalat CC 589
- Procardia Capsules 1971
- Procardia XL Extended Release Tablets 1972

Nisoldipine (Potentiated or additive effects).
- No products indexed under this heading.

Nitroglycerin (Potentiated or additive effects). Products include:
- Deponit NTG Transdermal Delivery System 2397
- Nitro-Bid IV 1523
- Nitro-Bid Ointment 1524
- Nitrodisc 2047
- Nitro-Dur (nitroglycerin) Transdermal Infusion System 1326
- Nitrolingual Spray 2027
- Nitrostat Tablets 1925
- Transderm-Nitro Transdermal Therapeutic System 859

Norepinephrine Bitartrate (Decreased arterial responsiveness to norepinephrine). Products include:
- Levophed Bitartrate Injection 2315

Opium Alkaloids (Potentiation of orthostatic hypotension).
- No products indexed under this heading.

Oxaprozin (Reduces diuretic, natriuretic, and antihypertensive effects). Products include:
- Daypro Caplets 2426

Oxycodone Hydrochloride (Potentiation of orthostatic hypotension). Products include:
- Percocet Tablets 938
- Percodan Tablets 939
- Percodan-Demi Tablets 940
- Roxicodone Tablets, Oral Solution & Intensol (Oxycodone) 2244
- Tylox Capsules 1584

Penbutolol Sulfate (Potentiated or additive effects). Products include:
- Levatol 2403

Pentobarbital Sodium (Potentiation of orthostatic hypotension). Products include:
- Nembutal Sodium Capsules 436
- Nembutal Sodium Solution 438
- Nembutal Sodium Suppositories 440

Phenobarbital (Potentiation of orthostatic hypotension). Products include:
- Arco-Lase Plus Tablets 512
- Bellergal-S Tablets 2250
- Donnatal 2060
- Donnatal Extentabs 2061
- Donnatal Tablets 2060
- Phenobarbital Elixir and Tablets 1469
- Quadrinal Tablets 1350

Phenoxybenzamine Hydrochloride (Potentiated or additive effects). Products include:
- Dibenzyline Capsules 2476

(■ Described in PDR For Nonprescription Drugs) (◉ Described in PDR For Ophthalmology)

Phentolamine Mesylate (Potentiated or additive effects). Products include:
- Regitine ... 846

Phenylbutazone (Reduces diuretic, natriuretic, and antihypertensive effects).
- No products indexed under this heading.

Pindolol (Potentiated or additive effects). Products include:
- Visken Tablets ... 2299

Piroxicam (Reduces diuretic, natriuretic, and antihypertensive effects). Products include:
- Feldene Capsules ... 1965

Polythiazide (Potentiated or additive effects). Products include:
- Minizide Capsules ... 1938

Prazosin Hydrochloride (Potentiated or additive effects). Products include:
- Minipress Capsules ... 1937
- Minizide Capsules ... 1938

Prednisolone Acetate (Hypokalemia). Products include:
- AK-CIDE ... ◉ 202
- AK-CIDE Ointment ... ◉ 202
- Blephamide Liquifilm Sterile Ophthalmic Suspension ... 476
- Blephamide Ointment ... ◉ 237
- Econopred & Econopred Plus Ophthalmic Suspensions ... ◉ 217
- Poly-Pred Liquifilm ... ◉ 248
- Pred Forte ... ◉ 250
- Pred Mild ... ◉ 253
- Pred-G Liquifilm Sterile Ophthalmic Suspension ... ◉ 251
- Pred-G S.O.P. Sterile Ophthalmic Ointment ... ◉ 252
- Vasocidin Ointment ... ◉ 268

Prednisolone Sodium Phosphate (Hypokalemia). Products include:
- AK-Pred ... ◉ 204
- Hydeltrasol Injection, Sterile ... 1665
- Inflamase ... ◉ 265
- Pediapred Oral Liquid ... 995
- Vasocidin Ophthalmic Solution ... ◉ 270

Prednisolone Tebutate (Hypokalemia). Products include:
- Hydeltra-T.B.A. Sterile Suspension 1667

Prednisone (Hypokalemia). Products include:
- Deltasone Tablets ... 2595

Propoxyphene Hydrochloride (Potentiation of orthostatic hypotension). Products include:
- Darvon ... 1435
- Wygesic Tablets ... 2827

Propoxyphene Napsylate (Potentiation of orthostatic hypotension). Products include:
- Darvon-N/Darvocet-N ... 1433

Propranolol Hydrochloride (Potentiated or additive effects). Products include:
- Inderal ... 2728
- Inderal LA Long Acting Capsules ... 2730
- Inderide Tablets ... 2732
- Inderide LA Long Acting Capsules .. 2734

Quinapril Hydrochloride (Potentiated or additive effects). Products include:
- Accupril Tablets ... 1893

Ramipril (Potentiated or additive effects). Products include:
- Altace Capsules ... 1232

Rauwolfia Serpentina (Potentiated or additive effects).
- No products indexed under this heading.

Rescinnamine (Potentiated or additive effects).
- No products indexed under this heading.

Reserpine (Potentiated or additive effects). Products include:
- Diupres Tablets ... 1650
- Hydropres Tablets ... 1675
- Ser-Ap-Es Tablets ... 849

Secobarbital Sodium (Potentiation of orthostatic hypotension). Products include:
- Seconal Sodium Pulvules ... 1474

Sodium Nitroprusside (Potentiated or additive effects).
- No products indexed under this heading.

Sotalol Hydrochloride (Potentiated or additive effects). Products include:
- Betapace Tablets ... 641

Spirapril Hydrochloride (Potentiated or additive effects).
- No products indexed under this heading.

Sufentanil Citrate (Potentiation of orthostatic hypotension). Products include:
- Sufenta Injection ... 1309

Sulindac (Reduces diuretic, natriuretic, and antihypertensive effects). Products include:
- Clinoril Tablets ... 1618

Terazosin Hydrochloride (Potentiated or additive effects). Products include:
- Hytrin Capsules ... 430

Thiamylal Sodium (Potentiation of orthostatic hypotension).
- No products indexed under this heading.

Timolol Maleate (Potentiated or additive effects). Products include:
- Blocadren Tablets ... 1614
- Timolide Tablets ... 1748
- Timoptic in Ocudose ... 1753
- Timoptic Sterile Ophthalmic Solution ... 1751
- Timoptic-XE ... 1755

Tolazamide (Dosage adjustment of oral hypoglycemic agent may be necessary).
- No products indexed under this heading.

Tolbutamide (Dosage adjustment of oral hypoglycemic agent may be necessary).
- No products indexed under this heading.

Tolmetin Sodium (Reduces diuretic, natriuretic, and antihypertensive effects). Products include:
- Tolectin (200, 400 and 600 mg) .. 1581

Torsemide (Potentiated or additive effects). Products include:
- Demadex Tablets and Injection ... 686

Triamcinolone (Hypokalemia). Products include:
- Aristocort Tablets ... 1022

Triamcinolone Acetonide (Hypokalemia). Products include:
- Aristocort A 0.025% Cream ... 1027
- Aristocort A 0.5% Cream ... 1031
- Aristocort A 0.1% Cream ... 1029
- Aristocort A 0.1% Ointment ... 1030
- Azmacort Oral Inhaler ... 2011
- Nasacort Nasal Inhaler ... 2024

Triamcinolone Diacetate (Hypokalemia). Products include:
- Aristocort Suspension (Forte Parenteral) ... 1027
- Aristocort Suspension (Intralesional) ... 1025

Triamcinolone Hexacetonide (Hypokalemia). Products include:
- Aristospan Suspension (Intra-articular) ... 1033
- Aristospan Suspension (Intralesional) ... 1032

Trimethaphan Camsylate (Potentiated or additive effects). Products include:
- Arfonad Ampuls ... 2080

Tubocurarine Chloride (Increased responsiveness to tubocurarine).
- No products indexed under this heading.

Verapamil Hydrochloride (Potentiated or additive effects). Products include:
- Calan SR Caplets ... 2422
- Calan Tablets ... 2419
- Isoptin Injectable ... 1344
- Isoptin Oral Tablets ... 1346
- Isoptin SR Tablets ... 1348
- Verelan Capsules ... 1410
- Verelan Capsules ... 2824

Food Interactions

Alcohol (Potentiation of orthostatic hypotension).

DIURIL TABLETS

(Chlorothiazide) ... 1653

See **Diuril Oral Suspension**

DIZAC

(Diazepam) ... 1809

May interact with central nervous system depressants, barbiturates, narcotic analgesics, phenothiazines, monoamine oxidase inhibitors, antidepressant drugs, and certain other agents. Compounds in these categories include:

Alfentanil Hydrochloride (Concomitant use increases depression with increased risk of apnea; dosage of narcotic analgesic should be reduced by at least one-third and administered in small increments; potentiates the action of diazepam). Products include:
- Alfenta Injection ... 1286

Alprazolam (Concomitant use increases depression with increased risk of apnea). Products include:
- Xanax Tablets ... 2649

Amitriptyline Hydrochloride (Potentiates the action of diazepam). Products include:
- Elavil ... 2838
- Endep Tablets ... 2174
- Etrafon ... 2355
- Limbitrol ... 2180
- Triavil Tablets ... 1757

Amoxapine (Potentiates the action of diazepam). Products include:
- Asendin Tablets ... 1369

Aprobarbital (Concomitant use increases depression with increased risk of apnea; potentiates the action of diazepam).
- No products indexed under this heading.

Buprenorphine (Concomitant use increases depression with increased risk of apnea; dosage of narcotic analgesic should be reduced by at least one-third and administered in small increments; potentiates the action of diazepam). Products include:
- Buprenex Injectable ... 2006

Bupropion Hydrochloride (Potentiates the action of diazepam). Products include:
- Wellbutrin Tablets ... 1204

Buspirone Hydrochloride (Concomitant use increases depression with increased risk of apnea). Products include:
- BuSpar ... 737

Butabarbital (Concomitant use increases depression with increased risk of apnea; potentiates the action of diazepam).
- No products indexed under this heading.

Butalbital (Concomitant use increases depression with increased risk of apnea; potentiates the action of diazepam). Products include:
- Esgic-plus Tablets ... 1013
- Fioricet Tablets ... 2258
- Fioricet with Codeine Capsules ... 2260
- Fiorinal Capsules ... 2261
- Fiorinal with Codeine Capsules ... 2262
- Fiorinal Tablets ... 2261
- Phrenilin ... 785
- Sedapap Tablets 50 mg/650 mg .. 1543

Chlordiazepoxide (Concomitant use increases depression with increased risk of apnea). Products include:
- Libritabs Tablets ... 2177
- Limbitrol ... 2180

Chlordiazepoxide Hydrochloride (Concomitant use increases depression with increased risk of apnea). Products include:
- Librax Capsules ... 2176
- Librium Capsules ... 2178
- Librium Injectable ... 2179

Chlorpromazine (Potentiates the action of diazepam). Products include:
- Thorazine Suppositories ... 2523

Chlorpromazine Hydrochloride (Potentiates the action of diazepam). Products include:
- Thorazine ... 2523

Chlorprothixene (Concomitant use increases depression with increased risk of apnea).
- No products indexed under this heading.

Chlorprothixene Hydrochloride (Concomitant use increases depression with increased risk of apnea).
- No products indexed under this heading.

Cimetidine (The clearance of diazepam is delayed by concurrent use of cimetidine; clinical significance is unknown). Products include:
- Tagamet Tablets ... 2516

Cimetidine Hydrochloride (The clearance of diazepam is delayed by concurrent use of cimetidine; clinical significance is unknown). Products include:
- Tagamet ... 2516

Clorazepate Dipotassium (Concomitant use increases depression with increased risk of apnea). Products include:
- Tranxene ... 451

Clozapine (Concomitant use increases depression with increased risk of apnea). Products include:
- Clozaril Tablets ... 2252

Codeine Phosphate (Concomitant use increases depression with increased risk of apnea; dosage of narcotic analgesic should be reduced by at least one-third and administered in small increments; potentiates the action of diazepam). Products include:
- Actifed with Codeine Cough Syrup .. 1067
- Brontex ... 1981
- Deconsal C Expectorant Syrup ... 456
- Deconsal Pediatric Syrup ... 457
- Dimetane-DC Cough Syrup ... 2059
- Empirin with Codeine Tablets ... 1093
- Fioricet with Codeine Capsules ... 2260
- Fiorinal with Codeine Capsules ... 2262
- Isoclor Expectorant ... 990
- Novahistine DH ... 2462
- Novahistine Expectorant ... 2463
- Nucofed ... 2051
- Phenergan with Codeine ... 2777
- Phenergan VC with Codeine ... 2781
- Robitussin A-C Syrup ... 2073
- Robitussin-DAC Syrup ... 2074
- Ryna ... ▣ 841
- Soma Compound w/Codeine Tablets ... 2676

IMPORTANT NOTE: Always consult each drug listing in the patient's regimen for possible interactions.

Tussi-Organidin NR Liquid and S NR Liquid 2677
Tylenol with Codeine 1583

Desflurane (Concomitant use increases depression with increased risk of apnea). Products include:
Suprane 1813

Desipramine Hydrochloride (Potentiates the action of diazepam). Products include:
Norpramin Tablets 1526

Dezocine (Concomitant use increases depression with increased risk of apnea; dosage of narcotic analgesic should be reduced by at least one-third and administered in small increments; potentiates the action of diazepam). Products include:
Dalgan Injection 538

Doxepin Hydrochloride (Potentiates the action of diazepam). Products include:
Sinequan 2205
Zonalon Cream 1055

Droperidol (Concomitant use increases depression with increased risk of apnea). Products include:
Inapsine Injection 1296

Enflurane (Concomitant use increases depression with increased risk of apnea).
No products indexed under this heading.

Estazolam (Concomitant use increases depression with increased risk of apnea). Products include:
ProSom Tablets 449

Ethchlorvynol (Concomitant use increases depression with increased risk of apnea). Products include:
Placidyl Capsules 448

Ethinamate (Concomitant use increases depression with increased risk of apnea).
No products indexed under this heading.

Fentanyl (Concomitant use increases depression with increased risk of apnea; dosage of narcotic analgesic should be reduced by at least one-third and administered in small increments; potentiates the action of diazepam). Products include:
Duragesic Transdermal System 1288

Fentanyl Citrate (Concomitant use increases depression with increased risk of apnea; dosage of narcotic analgesic should be reduced by at least one-third and administered in small increments; potentiates the action of diazepam). Products include:
Sublimaze Injection 1307

Fluoxetine Hydrochloride (Potentiates the action of diazepam). Products include:
Prozac Pulvules & Liquid, Oral Solution 919

Fluphenazine Decanoate (Potentiates the action of diazepam). Products include:
Prolixin Decanoate 509

Fluphenazine Enanthate (Potentiates the action of diazepam). Products include:
Prolixin Enanthate 509

Fluphenazine Hydrochloride (Potentiates the action of diazepam). Products include:
Prolixin 509

Flurazepam Hydrochloride (Concomitant use increases depression with increased risk of apnea). Products include:
Dalmane Capsules 2173

Furazolidone (Potentiates the action of diazepam). Products include:
Furoxone 2046

Glutethimide (Concomitant use increases depression with increased risk of apnea).
No products indexed under this heading.

Haloperidol (Concomitant use increases depression with increased risk of apnea). Products include:
Haldol Injection, Tablets and Concentrate 1575

Haloperidol Decanoate (Concomitant use increases depression with increased risk of apnea). Products include:
Haldol Decanoate 1577

Hydrocodone Bitartrate (Concomitant use increases depression with increased risk of apnea; dosage of narcotic analgesic should be reduced by at least one-third and administered in small increments; potentiates the action of diazepam). Products include:
Anexsia 5/500 Elixir 1781
Anexia Tablets 1782
Codiclear DH Syrup 791
Deconamine CX Cough and Cold Liquid and Tablets 1319
Duratuss HD Elixir 2565
Hycodan Tablets and Syrup 930
Hycomine Compound Tablets 932
Hycomine 931
Hycotuss Expectorant Syrup 933
Hydrocet Capsules 782
Lorcet 10/650 1018
Lortab 2566
Tussend 1783
Tussend Expectorant 1785
Vicodin Tablets 1356
Vicodin ES Tablets 1357
Vicodin Tuss Expectorant 1358
Zydone Capsules 949

Hydrocodone Polistirex (Concomitant use increases depression with increased risk of apnea; dosage of narcotic analgesic should be reduced by at least one-third and administered in small increments; potentiates the action of diazepam). Products include:
Tussionex Pennkinetic Extended-Release Suspension 998

Hydroxyzine Hydrochloride (Concomitant use increases depression with increased risk of apnea). Products include:
Atarax Tablets & Syrup 2185
Marax Tablets & DF Syrup 2200
Vistaril Intramuscular Solution 2216

Imipramine Hydrochloride (Potentiates the action of diazepam). Products include:
Tofranil Ampuls 854
Tofranil Tablets 856

Imipramine Pamoate (Potentiates the action of diazepam). Products include:
Tofranil-PM Capsules 857

Isocarboxazid (Potentiates the action of diazepam).
No products indexed under this heading.

Isoflurane (Concomitant use increases depression with increased risk of apnea).
No products indexed under this heading.

Ketamine Hydrochloride (Concomitant use increases depression with increased risk of apnea).
No products indexed under this heading.

Levomethadyl Acetate Hydrochloride (Concomitant use increases depression with increased risk of apnea). Products include:
Orlamm 2239

Levorphanol Tartrate (Concomitant use increases depression with increased risk of apnea; dosage of narcotic analgesic should be reduced by at least one-third and administered in small increments; potentiates the action of diazepam). Products include:
Levo-Dromoran 2129

Lorazepam (Concomitant use increases depression with increased risk of apnea). Products include:
Ativan Injection 2698
Ativan Tablets 2700

Loxapine Hydrochloride (Concomitant use increases depression with increased risk of apnea). Products include:
Loxitane 1378

Loxapine Succinate (Concomitant use increases depression with increased risk of apnea). Products include:
Loxitane Capsules 1378

Maprotiline Hydrochloride (Potentiates the action of diazepam). Products include:
Ludiomil Tablets 843

Meperidine Hydrochloride (Concomitant use increases depression with increased risk of apnea; dosage of narcotic analgesic should be reduced by at least one-third and administered in small increments; potentiates the action of diazepam). Products include:
Demerol 2308
Mepergan Injection 2753

Mephobarbital (Concomitant use increases depression with increased risk of apnea; potentiates the action of diazepam). Products include:
Mebaral Tablets 2322

Meprobamate (Concomitant use increases depression with increased risk of apnea). Products include:
Miltown Tablets 2672
PMB 200 and PMB 400 2783

Mesoridazine Besylate (Potentiates the action of diazepam). Products include:
Serentil 684

Methadone Hydrochloride (Concomitant use increases depression with increased risk of apnea; dosage of narcotic analgesic should be reduced by at least one-third and administered in small increments; potentiates the action of diazepam). Products include:
Methadone Hydrochloride Oral Concentrate 2233
Methadone Hydrochloride Oral Solution & Tablets 2235

Methohexital Sodium (Concomitant use increases depression with increased risk of apnea). Products include:
Brevital Sodium Vials 1429

Methotrimeprazine (Potentiates the action of diazepam). Products include:
Levoprome 1274

Methoxyflurane (Concomitant use increases depression with increased risk of apnea).
No products indexed under this heading.

Midazolam Hydrochloride (Concomitant use increases depression with increased risk of apnea). Products include:
Versed Injection 2170

Molindone Hydrochloride (Concomitant use increases depression with increased risk of apnea). Products include:
Moban Tablets and Concentrate 1048

Morphine Sulfate (Concomitant use increases depression with increased risk of apnea; dosage of narcotic analgesic should be reduced by at least one-third and administered in small increments; potentiates the action of diazepam). Products include:
Astramorph/PF Injection, USP (Preservative-Free) 535
Duramorph 962
Infumorph 200 and Infumorph 500 Sterile Solutions 965
MS Contin Tablets 1994
MSIR 1997
Oramorph SR (Morphine Sulfate Sustained Release Tablets) 2236
RMS Suppositories 2657
Roxanol 2243

Nefazodone Hydrochloride (Potentiates the action of diazepam). Products include:
Serzone Tablets 771

Nortriptyline Hydrochloride (Potentiates the action of diazepam). Products include:
Pamelor 2280

Opium Alkaloids (Concomitant use increases depression with increased risk of apnea; dosage of narcotic analgesic should be reduced by at least one-third and administered in small increments; potentiates the action of diazepam).
No products indexed under this heading.

Oxazepam (Concomitant use increases depression with increased risk of apnea). Products include:
Serax Capsules 2810
Serax Tablets 2810

Oxycodone Hydrochloride (Concomitant use increases depression with increased risk of apnea; dosage of narcotic analgesic should be reduced by at least one-third and administered in small increments; potentiates the action of diazepam). Products include:
Percocet Tablets 938
Percodan Tablets 939
Percodan-Demi Tablets 940
Roxicodone Tablets, Oral Solution & Intensol (Oxycodone) 2244
Tylox Capsules 1584

Paroxetine Hydrochloride (Potentiates the action of diazepam). Products include:
Paxil Tablets 2505

Pentobarbital Sodium (Concomitant use increases depression with increased risk of apnea; potentiates the action of diazepam). Products include:
Nembutal Sodium Capsules 436
Nembutal Sodium Solution 438
Nembutal Sodium Suppositories 440

Perphenazine (Potentiates the action of diazepam). Products include:
Etrafon 2355
Triavil Tablets 1757
Trilafon 2389

Phenelzine Sulfate (Potentiates the action of diazepam). Products include:
Nardil 1920

Phenobarbital (Concomitant use increases depression with increased risk of apnea; potentiates the action of diazepam). Products include:
Arco-Lase Plus Tablets 512
Bellergal-S Tablets 2250
Donnatal 2060
Donnatal Extentabs 2061
Donnatal Tablets 2060
Phenobarbital Elixir and Tablets 1469
Quadrinal Tablets 1350

Interactions Index — Doan's Original

Prazepam (Concomitant use increases depression with increased risk of apnea).

No products indexed under this heading.

Prochlorperazine (Potentiates the action of diazepam). Products include:

Compazine 2470

Promethazine Hydrochloride (Potentiates the action of diazepam). Products include:

Mepergan Injection 2753
Phenergan with Codeine 2777
Phenergan with Dextromethorphan 2778
Phenergan Injection 2773
Phenergan Suppositories 2775
Phenergan Syrup 2774
Phenergan Tablets 2775
Phenergan VC 2779
Phenergan VC with Codeine 2781

Propofol (Concomitant use increases depression with increased risk of apnea). Products include:

Diprivan Injection............................... 2833

Propoxyphene Hydrochloride (Concomitant use increases depression with increased risk of apnea; dosage of narcotic analgesic should be reduced by at least one-third and administered in small increments; potentiates the action of diazepam). Products include:

Darvon 1435
Wygesic Tablets 2827

Propoxyphene Napsylate (Concomitant use increases depression with increased risk of apnea; dosage of narcotic analgesic should be reduced by at least one-third and administered in small increments; potentiates the action of diazepam). Products include:

Darvon-N/Darvocet-N 1433

Protriptyline Hydrochloride (Potentiates the action of diazepam). Products include:

Vivactil Tablets 1774

Quazepam (Concomitant use increases depression with increased risk of apnea). Products include:

Doral Tablets 2664

Risperidone (Concomitant use increases depression with increased risk of apnea). Products include:

Risperdal 1301

Secobarbital Sodium (Concomitant use increases depression with increased risk of apnea; potentiates the action of diazepam). Products include:

Seconal Sodium Pulvules 1474

Selegiline Hydrochloride (Potentiates the action of diazepam). Products include:

Eldepryl Tablets 2550

Sertraline Hydrochloride (Potentiates the action of diazepam). Products include:

Zoloft Tablets 2217

Sufentanil Citrate (Concomitant use increases depression with increased risk of apnea; dosage of narcotic analgesic should be reduced by at least one-third and administered in small increments; potentiates the action of diazepam). Products include:

Sufenta Injection 1309

Temazepam (Concomitant use increases depression with increased risk of apnea). Products include:

Restoril Capsules 2284

Thiamylal Sodium (Concomitant use increases depression with increased risk of apnea; potentiates the action of diazepam).

No products indexed under this heading.

Thioridazine Hydrochloride (Potentiates the action of diazepam). Products include:

Mellaril 2269

Thiothixene (Concomitant use increases depression with increased risk of apnea). Products include:

Navane Capsules and Concentrate 2201
Navane Intramuscular 2202

Tranylcypromine Sulfate (Potentiates the action of diazepam). Products include:

Parnate Tablets 2503

Trazodone Hydrochloride (Potentiates the action of diazepam). Products include:

Desyrel and Desyrel Dividose 503

Triazolam (Concomitant use increases depression with increased risk of apnea). Products include:

Halcion Tablets.................................. 2611

Trifluoperazine Hydrochloride (Potentiates the action of diazepam). Products include:

Stelazine 2514

Trimipramine Maleate (Potentiates the action of diazepam). Products include:

Surmontil Capsules............................ 2811

Venlafaxine Hydrochloride (Potentiates the action of diazepam). Products include:

Effexor 2719

Zolpidem Tartrate (Concomitant use increases depression with increased risk of apnea). Products include:

Ambien Tablets.................................. 2416

Food Interactions

Alcohol (Potentiates the action of diazepam; concomitant use increases depression with increased risk of apnea).

DOAN'S EXTRA-STRENGTH ANALGESIC

(Magnesium Salicylate) ....✪ 633

May interact with oral anticoagulants and certain other agents. Compounds in these categories include:

Antiarthritic Drugs, unspecified (Concurrent use is not recommended).

Antidiabetic Drugs, unspecified (Concurrent use is not recommended).

Antigout Drugs, unspecified (Concurrent use is not recommended).

Dicumarol (Concurrent use is not recommended).

No products indexed under this heading.

Warfarin Sodium (Concurrent use is not recommended). Products include:

Coumadin 926

EXTRA STRENGTH DOAN'S P.M.

(Magnesium Salicylate, Diphenhydramine Hydrochloride)....✪ 633

May interact with hypnotics and sedatives, tranquilizers, and certain other agents. Compounds in these categories include:

Alprazolam (Effect not specified). Products include:

Xanax Tablets 2649

Antiarthritic Drugs, unspecified (Concurrent use is not recommended).

Antidiabetic Drugs, unspecified (Concurrent use is not recommended).

Antigout Drugs, unspecified (Concurrent use is not recommended).

Buspirone Hydrochloride (Effect not specified). Products include:

BuSpar 737

Chlordiazepoxide (Effect not specified). Products include:

Libritabs Tablets 2177
Limbitrol 2180

Chlordiazepoxide Hydrochloride (Effect not specified). Products include:

Librax Capsules 2176
Librium Capsules 2178
Librium Injectable 2179

Chlorpromazine (Effect not specified). Products include:

Thorazine Suppositories..................... 2523

Chlorprothixene (Effect not specified).

No products indexed under this heading.

Chlorprothixene Hydrochloride (Effect not specified).

No products indexed under this heading.

Clorazepate Dipotassium (Effect not specified). Products include:

Tranxene 451

Diazepam (Effect not specified). Products include:

Dizac 1809
Valium Injectable 2182
Valium Tablets 2183
Valrelease Capsules 2169

Dicumarol (Concurrent use is not recommended).

No products indexed under this heading.

Droperidol (Effect not specified). Products include:

Inapsine Injection............................... 1296

Estazolam (Effect not specified). Products include:

ProSom Tablets 449

Ethchlorvynol (Effect not specified). Products include:

Placidyl Capsules 448

Ethinamate (Effect not specified).

No products indexed under this heading.

Fluphenazine Decanoate (Effect not specified). Products include:

Prolixin Decanoate 509

Fluphenazine Enanthate (Effect not specified). Products include:

Prolixin Enanthate 509

Fluphenazine Hydrochloride (Effect not specified). Products include:

Prolixin 509

Flurazepam Hydrochloride (Effect not specified). Products include:

Dalmane Capsules.............................. 2173

Glutethimide (Effect not specified).

No products indexed under this heading.

Haloperidol (Effect not specified). Products include:

Haldol Injection, Tablets and Concentrate 1575

Haloperidol Decanoate (Effect not specified). Products include:

Haldol Decanoate............................... 1577

Hydroxyzine Hydrochloride (Effect not specified). Products include:

Atarax Tablets & Syrup....................... 2185
Marax Tablets & DF Syrup.................. 2200
Vistaril Intramuscular Solution........... 2216

Lorazepam (Effect not specified). Products include:

Ativan Injection 2698
Ativan Tablets 2700

Loxapine Hydrochloride (Effect not specified). Products include:

Loxitane 1378

Loxapine Succinate (Effect not specified). Products include:

Loxitane Capsules 1378

Meprobamate (Effect not specified). Products include:

Miltown Tablets 2672
PMB 200 and PMB 400 2783

Mesoridazine Besylate (Effect not specified). Products include:

Serentil 684

Midazolam Hydrochloride (Effect not specified). Products include:

Versed Injection 2170

Molindone Hydrochloride (Effect not specified). Products include:

Moban Tablets and Concentrate...... 1048

Oxazepam (Effect not specified). Products include:

Serax Capsules 2810
Serax Tablets..................................... 2810

Perphenazine (Effect not specified). Products include:

Etrafon 2355
Triavil Tablets 1757
Trilafon.. 2389

Prazepam (Effect not specified).

No products indexed under this heading.

Prochlorperazine (Effect not specified). Products include:

Compazine 2470

Promethazine Hydrochloride (Effect not specified). Products include:

Mepergan Injection 2753
Phenergan with Codeine 2777
Phenergan with Dextromethorphan 2778
Phenergan Injection 2773
Phenergan Suppositories 2775
Phenergan Syrup 2774
Phenergan Tablets 2775
Phenergan VC 2779
Phenergan VC with Codeine 2781

Propofol (Effect not specified). Products include:

Diprivan Injection............................... 2833

Quazepam (Effect not specified). Products include:

Doral Tablets 2664

Secobarbital Sodium (Effect not specified). Products include:

Seconal Sodium Pulvules 1474

Temazepam (Effect not specified). Products include:

Restoril Capsules 2284

Thioridazine Hydrochloride (Effect not specified). Products include:

Mellaril 2269

Thiothixene (Effect not specified). Products include:

Navane Capsules and Concentrate 2201
Navane Intramuscular 2202

Triazolam (Effect not specified). Products include:

Halcion Tablets.................................. 2611

Trifluoperazine Hydrochloride (Effect not specified). Products include:

Stelazine 2514

Warfarin Sodium (Concurrent use is not recommended). Products include:

Coumadin 926

Zolpidem Tartrate (Effect not specified). Products include:

Ambien Tablets.................................. 2416

Food Interactions

Alcohol (Avoid concomitant use).

DOAN'S REGULAR STRENGTH ANALGESIC

(Magnesium Salicylate) ....✪ 634

May interact with oral anticoagulants

IMPORTANT NOTE: Always consult each drug listing in the patient's regimen for possible interactions.

Doan's Original | **Interactions Index** | **328**

and certain other agents. Compounds in these categories include:

Antiarthritic Drugs, unspecified (Concurrent use is not recommended unless directed by a doctor).

Antidiabetic Drugs, unspecified (Concurrent use is not recommended unless directed by a doctor).

Antigout Drugs, unspecified (Concurrent use is not recommended unless directed by a doctor).

Dicumarol (Concurrent use is not recommended unless directed by a doctor).

No products indexed under this heading.

Warfarin Sodium (Concurrent use is not recommended unless directed by a doctor). Products include:

Coumadin 926

DOBUTREX SOLUTION VIALS

(Dobutamine Hydrochloride) 1439

May interact with beta blockers and certain other agents. Compounds in these categories include:

Acebutolol Hydrochloride (Based on animal studies, dobutamine may be ineffective in patients recently on beta blocker; potential for increased peripheral vascular resistance). Products include:

Sectral Capsules 2807

Atenolol (Based on animal studies, dobutamine may be ineffective in patients recently on beta blocker; potential for increased peripheral vascular resistance). Products include:

Tenoretic Tablets 2845
Tenormin Tablets and I.V. Injection 2847

Betaxolol Hydrochloride (Based on animal studies, dobutamine may be ineffective in patients recently on beta blocker; potential for increased peripheral vascular resistance). Products include:

Betoptic Ophthalmic Solution 469
Betoptic S Ophthalmic Suspension 471
Kerlone Tablets 2436

Bisoprolol Fumarate (Based on animal studies, dobutamine may be ineffective in patients recently on beta blocker; potential for increased peripheral vascular resistance). Products include:

Zebeta Tablets 1413
Ziac 1415

Carteolol Hydrochloride (Based on animal studies, dobutamine may be ineffective in patients recently on beta blocker; potential for increased peripheral vascular resistance). Products include:

Cartrol Tablets 410
Ocupress Ophthalmic Solution, 1% Sterile .... ⊙ 309

Esmolol Hydrochloride (Based on animal studies, dobutamine may be ineffective in patients recently on beta blocker; potential for increased peripheral vascular resistance). Products include:

Brevibloc Injection 1808

Labetalol Hydrochloride (Based on animal studies, dobutamine may be ineffective in patients recently on beta blocker; potential for increased peripheral vascular resistance). Products include:

Normodyne Injection 2377
Normodyne Tablets 2379
Trandate 1185

Levobunolol Hydrochloride (Based on animal studies, dobutamine may be ineffective in patients recently on beta blocker; potential for increased peripheral vascular resistance). Products include:

Betagan .... ⊙ 233

Metipranolol Hydrochloride (Based on animal studies, dobutamine may be ineffective in patients recently on beta blocker; potential for increased peripheral vascular resistance). Products include:

OptiPranolol (Metipranolol 0.3%) Sterile Ophthalmic Solution .... ⊙ 258

Metoprolol Succinate (Based on animal studies, dobutamine may be ineffective in patients recently on beta blocker; potential for increased peripheral vascular resistance). Products include:

Toprol-XL Tablets 565

Metoprolol Tartrate (Based on animal studies, dobutamine may be ineffective in patients recently on beta blocker; potential for increased peripheral vascular resistance). Products include:

Lopressor Ampuls 830
Lopressor HCT Tablets 832
Lopressor Tablets 830

Nadolol (Based on animal studies, dobutamine may be ineffective in patients recently on beta blocker; potential for increased peripheral vascular resistance).

No products indexed under this heading.

Penbutolol Sulfate (Based on animal studies, dobutamine may be ineffective in patients recently on beta blocker; potential for increased peripheral vascular resistance). Products include:

Levatol 2403

Pindolol (Based on animal studies, dobutamine may be ineffective in patients recently on beta blocker; potential for increased peripheral vascular resistance). Products include:

Visken Tablets 2299

Propranolol Hydrochloride (Based on animal studies, dobutamine may be ineffective in patients recently on beta blocker; potential for increased peripheral vascular resistance). Products include:

Inderal 2728
Inderal LA Long Acting Capsules 2730
Inderide Tablets 2732
Inderide LA Long Acting Capsules .. 2734

Sodium Nitroprusside (Concomitant use results in a higher cardiac output and, usually, a lower pulmonary wedge pressure).

No products indexed under this heading.

Sotalol Hydrochloride (Based on animal studies, dobutamine may be ineffective in patients recently on beta blocker; potential for increased peripheral vascular resistance). Products include:

Betapace Tablets 641

Timolol Hemihydrate (Based on animal studies, dobutamine may be ineffective in patients recently on beta blocker; potential for increased peripheral vascular resistance). Products include:

Betimol 0.25%, 0.5% .... ⊙ 261

Timolol Maleate (Based on animal studies, dobutamine may be ineffective in patients recently on beta blocker; potential for increased peripheral vascular resistance). Products include:

Blocadren Tablets 1614
Timolide Tablets 1748
Timoptic in Ocudose 1753
Timoptic Sterile Ophthalmic Solution 1751
Timoptic-XE 1755

DOLOBID TABLETS

(Diflunisal) 1654

May interact with oral anticoagulants, antacids, and certain other agents. Compounds in these categories include:

Acetaminophen (Increased plasma levels of acetaminophen). Products include:

Actifed Plus Caplets .... ◘ 845
Actifed Plus Tablets .... ◘ 845
Actifed Sinus Daytime/Nighttime Tablets and Caplets .... ◘ 846
Alka-Seltzer Plus Cold Medicine Liqui-Gels .... ◘ 706
Alka-Seltzer Plus Cold & Cough Medicine Liqui-Gels .... ◘ 705
Alka-Seltzer Plus Night-Time Cold Medicine Liqui-Gels .... ◘ 706
Allerest Headache Strength Tablets .... ◘ 627
Allerest No Drowsiness Tablets .... ◘ 627
Allerest Sinus Pain Formula .... ◘ 627
Anexsia 5/500 Elixir 1781
Anexia Tablets 1782
Arthritis Foundation Aspirin Free Caplets .... ◘ 673
Arthritis Foundation NightTime Caplets .... ◘ 674
Bayer Select Headache Pain Relief Formula .... ◘ 716
Bayer Select Menstrual Multi-Symptom Formula .... ◘ 716
Bayer Select Night Time Pain Relief Formula .... ◘ 716
Bayer Select Sinus Pain Relief Formula .... ◘ 717
Benadryl Allergy Sinus Headache Formula Caplets .... ◘ 849
Comtrex Multi-Symptom Cold Reliever Tablets/Caplets/Liqui-Gels/Liquid .... ◘ 615
Allergy-Sinus Comtrex Multi-Symptom Allergy-Sinus Formula Tablets .... ◘ 617
Comtrex Non-Drowsy .... ◘ 618
Contac Day Allergy/Sinus Caplets ◘ 812
Contac Day & Night .... ◘ 812
Contac Night Allergy/Sinus Caplets .... ◘ 812
Contac Severe Cold and Flu Formula Caplets .... ◘ 814
Contac Severe Cold & Flu Non-Drowsy .... ◘ 815
Coricidin 'D' Decongestant Tablets .... ◘ 800
Coricidin Tablets .... ◘ 800
DHCplus Capsules 1993
Darvon-N/Darvocet-N 1433
Drixoral Cold and Flu Extended-Release Tablets .... ◘ 803
Drixoral Cough + Sore Throat Liquid Caps .... ◘ 802
Drixoral Allergy/Sinus Extended Release Tablets .... ◘ 804
Esgic-plus Tablets 1013
Aspirin Free Excedrin Analgesic Caplets and Geltabs 732
Excedrin Extra-Strength Analgesic Tablets & Caplets 732
Excedrin P.M. Analgesic/Sleeping Aid Tablets, Caplets, Liquigels 733
Fioricet Tablets 2258
Fioricet with Codeine Capsules 2260
Hycomine Compound Tablets 932
Hydrocet Capsules 782
Legatrin PM .... ◘ 651
Lorcet 10/650 1018
Lortab 2566
Lurline PMS Tablets 982
Maximum Strength Multi-Symptom Formula Midol .... ◘ 722
PMS Multi-Symptom Formula Midol .... ◘ 723
Teen Multi-Symptom Formula Midol .... ◘ 722
Midrin Capsules 783
Migralam Capsules 2038
Panodol Tablets and Caplets .... ◘ 824
Children's Panadol Chewable Tablets, Liquid, Infant's Drops .... ◘ 824
Percocet Tablets 938
Percogesic Analgesic Tablets .... ◘ 754
Phrenilin 785
Pyrroxate Caplets .... ◘ 772
Sedapap Tablets 50 mg/650 mg .. 1543
Sinarest Tablets .... ◘ 648
Sinarest Extra Strength Tablets .... ◘ 648
Sinarest No Drowsiness Tablets .... ◘ 648
Sine-Aid Maximum Strength Sinus Medication Gelcaps, Caplets and Tablets 1554
Sine-Off No Drowsiness Formula Caplets .... ◘ 824
Sine-Off Sinus Medicine .... ◘ 825
Singlet Tablets .... ◘ 825
Sinulin Tablets 787
Sinutab Sinus Allergy Medication, Maximum Strength Tablets and Caplets .... ◘ 860
Sinutab Sinus Medication, Maximum Strength Without Drowsiness Formula, Tablets & Caplets .... ◘ 860
Sinutab Sinus Medication, Regular Strength Without Drowsiness Formula .... ◘ 859
Sudafed Cold and Cough Liquidcaps .... ◘ 862
Sudafed Severe Cold Formula Caplets .... ◘ 863
Sudafed Severe Cold Formula Tablets .... ◘ 864
Sudafed Sinus Caplets .... ◘ 864
Sudafed Sinus Tablets .... ◘ 864
Talacen 2333
TheraFlu .... ◘ 787
TheraFlu Maximum Strength Nighttime Flu, Cold & Cough Medicine .... ◘ 788
TheraFlu Maximum Strength Non-Drowsy Formula Flu, Cold & Cough Medicine .... ◘ 788
Thera Flu Maximum Strength, Non-Drowsy Formula Flu, Cold and Cough Caplets .... ◘ 789
Triaminic Sore Throat Formula .... ◘ 791
Triaminicin Tablets .... ◘ 793
Children's TYLENOL acetaminophen Chewable Tablets, Elixir, Suspension Liquid 1555
Children's TYLENOL Cold Multi-Symptom Liquid Formula and Chewable Tablets 1561
Children's TYLENOL Cold Plus Cough Multi Symptom Tablets and Liquid .... ◘ 681
Infants' TYLENOL acetaminophen Drops and Suspension Drops 1555
Infants' TYLENOL Cold Decongestant & Fever-Reducer Drops 1556
TYLENOL Extended Relief Caplets .. 1558
TYLENOL, Extra Strength, Acetaminophen Adult Liquid Pain Reliever 1560
TYLENOL, Extra Strength, acetaminophen Gelcaps, Geltabs, Caplets, Tablets 1559
TYLENOL, Extra Strength, Headache Plus Pain Reliever with Antacid Caplets 1559
TYLENOL, Junior Strength, acetaminophen Coated Caplets, Grape and Fruit Chewable Tablets 1557
TYLENOL Maximum Strength Allergy Sinus Medication Gelcaps and Caplets 1563
TYLENOL Maximum Strength Allergy Sinus NightTime Medication Caplets 1555
TYLENOL Flu Maximum Strength Gelcaps 1565
TYLENOL Flu NightTime, Maximum Strength, Gelcaps 1566
TYLENOL Maximum Strength Flu NightTime Hot Medication Packets 1562
TYLENOL, Maximum Strength, Sinus Medication Geltabs, Gelcaps, Caplets and Tablets 1566
TYLENOL Cold Multi-Symptom Formula Medication Tablets and Caplets 1561
TYLENOL Cold Medication No Drowsiness Formula Gelcaps and Caplets 1562
TYLENOL Cold Multi-Symptom Hot Medication Liquid Packets 1557
TYLENOL Cough Multi-Symptom Medication 1564
TYLENOL Cough Multi-Symptom Medication with Decongestant 1565

(◘ Described in PDR For Nonprescription Drugs) (⊙ Described in PDR For Ophthalmology)

TYLENOL, Regular Strength, acetaminophen Caplets and Tablets .. 1558
TYLENOL PM, Extra Strength Pain Reliever/Sleep Aid Caplets, Geltabs, Gelcaps 1560
TYLENOL Severe Allergy Medication Caplets 1564
Tylenol with Codeine 1583
Tylox Capsules 1584
Unisom With Pain Relief-Nighttime Sleep Aid and Pain Reliever........... 1934
Vanquish Analgesic Caplets .... ⊞ 731
Vicks 44 LiquiCaps Cough, Cold & Flu Relief.. ⊞ 755
Vicks 44M Cough, Cold & Flu Relief... ⊞ 756
Vicks DayQuil .... ⊞ 761
Vicks Nyquil Hot Therapy................... ⊞ 762
Vicks NyQuil LiquiCaps Multi-Symptom Cold/Flu Relief............... ⊞ 763
Vicks NyQuil Multi-Symptom Cold/Flu Relief - (Original & Cherry Flavor).. ⊞ 763
Vicodin Tablets.. 1356
Vicodin ES Tablets 1357
Wygesic Tablets 2827
Zydone Capsules 949

Aluminum Carbonate Gel (Reduced plasma levels of Dolobid). Products include:

Basaljel... 2703

Aluminum Hydroxide (Reduced plasma levels of Dolobid). Products include:

ALternaGEL Liquid 1316
Maximum Strength Ascriptin .... ⊞ 630
Cama Arthritis Pain Reliever............ ⊞ 785
Gaviscon Extra Strength Relief Formula Antacid Tablets................. ⊞ 819
Gaviscon Extra Strength Relief Formula Liquid Antacid................... ⊞ 819
Gaviscon Liquid Antacid .... ⊞ 820
Gelusil Liquid & Tablets .... ⊞ 855
Maalox Heartburn Relief Suspension .... ⊞ 642
Maalox Heartburn Relief Tablets.... ⊞ 641
Maalox Magnesia and Alumina Oral Suspension .... ⊞ 642
Maalox Plus Tablets .... ⊞ 643
Extra Strength Maalox Antacid Plus Antigas Liquid and Tablets ⊞ 638
Tempo Soft Antacid .... ⊞ 835

Aluminum Hydroxide Gel (Reduced plasma levels of Dolobid). Products include:

ALternaGEL Liquid .... ⊞ 659
Aludrox Oral Suspension 2695
Amphojel Suspension 2695
Amphojel Suspension without Flavor 2695
Amphojel Tablets.. 2695
Arthritis Pain Ascriptin .... ⊞ 631
Regular Strength Ascriptin Tablets .... ⊞ 629
Gaviscon Antacid Tablets.................... ⊞ 819
Gaviscon-2 Antacid Tablets .... ⊞ 820
Mylanta Liquid 1317
Mylanta Tablets .... ⊞ 660
Mylanta Double Strength Liquid 1317
Mylanta Double Strength Tablets .. ⊞ 660
Nephrox Suspension .... ⊞ 655

Aluminum Hydroxide Gel, Dried (Reduced plasma levels of Dolobid).

Aspirin (Small decrease in diflunisal levels). Products include:

Alka-Seltzer Effervescent Antacid and Pain Reliever................................ ⊞ 701
Alka-Seltzer Extra Strength Effervescent Antacid and Pain Reliever .... ⊞ 703
Alka-Seltzer Lemon Lime Effervescent Antacid and Pain Reliever .... ⊞ 703
Alka-Seltzer Plus Cold Medicine .... ⊞ 705
Alka-Seltzer Plus Cold & Cough Medicine .... ⊞ 708
Alka-Seltzer Plus Night-Time Cold Medicine .... ⊞ 707
Alka Seltzer Plus Sinus Medicine .. ⊞ 707
Arthritis Foundation Safety Coated Aspirin Tablets .... ⊞ 675
Arthritis Pain Ascriptin .... ⊞ 631
Maximum Strength Ascriptin .... ⊞ 630
Regular Strength Ascriptin Tablets .... ⊞ 629
Arthritis Strength BC Powder.......... ⊞ 609

BC Cold Powder Multi-Symptom Formula (Cold-Sinus-Allergy) ...... ⊞ 609
BC Cold Powder Non-Drowsy Formula (Cold-Sinus) .... ⊞ 609
BC Powder .... ⊞ 609
Bayer Children's Chewable Aspirin.. ⊞ 711
Genuine Bayer Aspirin Tablets & Caplets .... ⊞ 713
Extra Strength Bayer Arthritis Pain Regimen Formula .... ⊞ 711
Extra Strength Bayer Aspirin Caplets & Tablets .... ⊞ 712
Extended-Release Bayer 8-Hour Aspirin .... ⊞ 712
Extra Strength Bayer Plus Aspirin Caplets .... ⊞ 713
Extra Strength Bayer PM Aspirin .. ⊞ 713
Bayer Enteric Aspirin........................... ⊞ 709
Bufferin Analgesic Tablets and Caplets .... ⊞ 613
Arthritis Strength Bufferin Analgesic Caplets .... ⊞ 614
Extra Strength Bufferin Analgesic Tablets .... ⊞ 615
Cama Arthritis Pain Reliever............ ⊞ 785
Darvon Compound-65 Pulvules 1435
Easprin... 1914
Ecotrin 2455
Ecotrin Enteric Coated Aspirin Maximum Strength Tablets and Caplets .... ⊞ 816
Ecotrin Enteric Coated Aspirin Regular Strength Tablets 2455
Empirin Aspirin Tablets .... ⊞ 854
Empirin with Codeine Tablets........... 1093
Excedrin Extra-Strength Analgesic Tablets & Caplets 732
Fiorinal Capsules 2261
Fiorinal with Codeine Capsules 2262
Fiorinal Tablets.. 2261
Halfprin 1362
Healthprin Aspirin.................................. 2455
Norgesic... 1496
Percodan Tablets.. 939
Percodan-Demi Tablets.......................... 940
Robaxisal Tablets.................................... 2071
Soma Compound w/Codeine Tablets 2676
Soma Compound Tablets 2675
St. Joseph Adult Chewable Aspirin (81 mg.) .... ⊞ 808
Talwin Compound 2335
Ursinus Inlay-Tabs................................. ⊞ 794
Vanquish Analgesic Caplets .... ⊞ 731

Cyclosporine (Increased cyclosporine-induced toxicity). Products include:

Neoral 2276
Sandimmune 2286

Dicumarol (Prolonged prothrombin time; adjustment of dosage of oral anticoagulants may be required).

No products indexed under this heading.

Dihydroxyaluminum Sodium Carbonate (Reduced plasma levels of Dolobid).

No products indexed under this heading.

Furosemide (Decreased hyperuricemic effect). Products include:

Lasix Injection, Oral Solution and Tablets 1240

Hydrochlorothiazide (Decreased hyperuricemic effect; increased plasma levels). Products include:

Aldactazide.. 2413
Aldoril Tablets.. 1604
Apresazide Capsules 808
Capozide 742
Dyazide 2479
Esidrix Tablets 821
Esimil Tablets 822
HydroDIURIL Tablets 1674
Hydropres Tablets................................... 1675
Hyzaar Tablets 1677
Inderide Tablets 2732
Inderide LA Long Acting Capsules .. 2734
Lopressor HCT Tablets 832
Lotensin HCT.. 837
Maxzide 1380
Moduretic Tablets 1705
Oretic Tablets 443
Prinzide Tablets.. 1737
Ser-Ap-Es Tablets 849
Timolide Tablets....................................... 1748
Vaseretic Tablets 1765

Zestoretic 2850
Ziac 1415

Indomethacin (Fatal gastrointestinal hemorrhage; concomitant use is not recommended). Products include:

Indocin 1680

Indomethacin Sodium Trihydrate (Fatal gastrointestinal hemorrhage; concomitant use is not recommended). Products include:

Indocin I.V. 1684

Magaldrate (Reduced plasma levels of Dolobid).

No products indexed under this heading.

Magnesium Hydroxide (Reduced plasma levels of Dolobid). Products include:

Aludrox Oral Suspension 2695
Arthritis Pain Ascriptin .... ⊞ 631
Maximum Strength Ascriptin .... ⊞ 630
Regular Strength Ascriptin Tablets .... ⊞ 629
Di-Gel Antacid/Anti-Gas .... ⊞ 801
Gelusil Liquid & Tablets .... ⊞ 855
Maalox Magnesia and Alumina Oral Suspension .... ⊞ 642
Maalox Plus Tablets .... ⊞ 643
Extra Strength Maalox Antacid Plus Antigas Liquid and Tablets ⊞ 638
Mylanta Calcium Carbonate and Magnesium Hydroxide Tablets...... 1318
Mylanta Liquid 1317
Mylanta Tablets .... ⊞ 660
Mylanta Double Strength Liquid 1317
Mylanta Double Strength Tablets .. ⊞ 660
Phillips' Milk of Magnesia Liquid.... ⊞ 729
Rolaids Tablets .... ⊞ 843
Tempo Soft Antacid .... ⊞ 835

Magnesium Oxide (Reduced plasma levels of Dolobid). Products include:

Beelith Tablets 639
Bufferin Analgesic Tablets and Caplets .... ⊞ 613
Caltrate PLUS .... ⊞ 665
Cama Arthritis Pain Reliever............ ⊞ 785
Mag-Ox 400 668
Uro-Mag... 668

Methotrexate Sodium (Decreased tubular secretion of methotrexate and potentiation of its toxicity). Products include:

Methotrexate Sodium Tablets, Injection, for Injection and LPF Injection 1275

Naproxen (Decreased urinary excretion of naproxen and its glucuronide metabolite). Products include:

Anaprox/Naprosyn 2117

Naproxen Sodium (Decreased urinary excretion of naproxen and its glucoronide metabolite). Products include:

Aleve 1975
Anaprox/Naprosyn 2117

Nephrotoxic Drugs (Overt renal decompensation).

Phenprocoumon (Prolonged prothrombin time).

Sulindac (Decreased plasma levels of active sulindac sulfide metabolite). Products include:

Clinoril Tablets 1618

Warfarin Sodium (Prolonged prothrombin time; adjustment of dosage of oral anticoagulants may be required). Products include:

Coumadin 926

DOLORAC

(Capsaicin) 1054
None cited in PDR database.

DOMEBORO ASTRINGENT SOLUTION EFFERVESCENT TABLETS

(Aluminum Acetate, Calcium Acetate) .... ⊞ 721
None cited in PDR database.

DOMEBORO ASTRINGENT SOLUTION POWDER PACKETS

(Aluminum Acetate, Calcium Acetate) .... ⊞ 720
None cited in PDR database.

DONNAGEL LIQUID AND DONNAGEL CHEWABLE TABLETS

(Attapulgite).. ⊞ 879
None cited in PDR database.

DONNATAL CAPSULES

(Phenobarbital, Belladonna Alkaloids) 2060
May interact with oral anticoagulants. Compounds in this category include:

Dicumarol (Decreased phenobarbital effect).

No products indexed under this heading.

Warfarin Sodium (Decreased phenobarbital effect). Products include:

Coumadin 926

DONNATAL ELIXIR

(Phenobarbital, Belladonna Alkaloids) 2060
See Donnatal Capsules

DONNATAL EXTENTABS

(Phenobarbital, Belladonna Alkaloids) 2061
May interact with oral anticoagulants. Compounds in this category include:

Dicumarol (Decreased phenobarbital effect).

No products indexed under this heading.

Warfarin Sodium (Decreased phenobarbital effect). Products include:

Coumadin 926

DONNATAL TABLETS

(Phenobarbital, Belladonna Alkaloids) 2060
See Donnatal Capsules

DONNAZYME TABLETS

(Pancreatin) 2061
None cited in PDR database.

DOPRAM INJECTABLE

(Doxapram Hydrochloride)..................2061
May interact with sympathomimetics, monoamine oxidase inhibitors, muscle relaxants, inhalant anesthetics, and certain other agents. Compounds in these categories include:

Albuterol (Additive pressor effect). Products include:

Proventil Inhalation Aerosol 2382
Ventolin Inhalation Aerosol and Refill 1197

Albuterol Sulfate (Additive pressor effect). Products include:

Airet Solution for Inhalation 452
Proventil Inhalation Solution 0.083% 2384
Proventil Repetabs Tablets 2386
Proventil Solution for Inhalation 0.5% 2383
Proventil Syrup.. 2385
Proventil Tablets 2386
Ventolin Inhalation Solution................ 1198
Ventolin Nebules Inhalation Solution... 1199
Ventolin Rotacaps for Inhalation 1200
Ventolin Syrup.. 1202
Ventolin Tablets 1203
Volmax Extended-Release Tablets .. 1788

Atracurium Besylate (Residual effects masked by Dopram). Products include:

Tracrium Injection 1183

IMPORTANT NOTE: Always consult each drug listing in the patient's regimen for possible interactions.

Dopram **Interactions Index** 330

Baclofen (Residual effects masked by Dopram). Products include:
- Lioresal Intrathecal ... 1596
- Lioresal Tablets ... 829

Carisoprodol (Residual effects masked by Dopram). Products include:
- Soma Compound w/Codeine Tablets ... 2676
- Soma Compound Tablets ... 2675
- Soma Tablets ... 2674

Chlorzoxazone (Residual effects masked by Dopram). Products include:
- Paraflex Caplets ... 1580
- Parafon Forte DSC Caplets ... 1581

Cyclobenzaprine Hydrochloride (Residual effects masked by Dopram). Products include:
- Flexeril Tablets ... 1661

Dantrolene Sodium (Residual effects masked by Dopram). Products include:
- Dantrium Capsules ... 1982
- Dantrium Intravenous ... 1983

Desflurane (Increased epinephrine release). Products include:
- Suprane ... 1813

Dobutamine Hydrochloride (Additive pressor effect). Products include:
- Dobutrex Solution Vials ... 1439

Dopamine Hydrochloride (Additive pressor effect).
- No products indexed under this heading.

Doxacurium Chloride (Residual effects masked by Dopram). Products include:
- Nuromax Injection ... 1149

Enflurane (Increased epinephrine release).
- No products indexed under this heading.

Ephedrine Hydrochloride (Additive pressor effect). Products include:
- Primatene Dual Action Formula ... ▣ 872
- Primatene Tablets ... ▣ 873
- Quadrinal Tablets ... 1350

Ephedrine Sulfate (Additive pressor effect). Products include:
- Bronkaid Caplets ... ▣ 717
- Marax Tablets & DF Syrup ... 2200

Ephedrine Tannate (Additive pressor effect). Products include:
- Rynatuss ... 2673

Epinephrine (Additive pressor effect). Products include:
- Bronkaid Mist ... ▣ 717
- EPIFRIN ... ⊙ 239
- EpiPen ... 790
- Marcaine Hydrochloride with Epinephrine 1:200,000 ... 2316
- Primatene Mist ... ▣ 873
- Sensorcaine with Epinephrine Injection ... 559
- Sus-Phrine Injection ... 1019
- Xylocaine with Epinephrine Injections ... 567

Epinephrine Bitartrate (Additive pressor effect). Products include:
- Bronkaid Mist Suspension ... ▣ 718
- Sensorcaine-MPF with Epinephrine Injection ... 559

Epinephrine Hydrochloride (Additive pressor effect). Products include:
- Ana-Kit Anaphylaxis Emergency Treatment Kit ... 617

Furazolidone (Additive pressor effect). Products include:
- Furoxone ... 2046

Halothane (Increased epinephrine release). Products include:
- Fluothane ... 2724

Isocarboxazid (Additive pressor effect).
- No products indexed under this heading.

Isoflurane (Increased epinephrine release).
- No products indexed under this heading.

Isoproterenol Hydrochloride (Additive pressor effect). Products include:
- Isuprel Hydrochloride Injection 1:5000 ... 2311
- Isuprel Hydrochloride Solution 1:200 & 1:100 ... 2313
- Isuprel Mistometer ... 2312

Isoproterenol Sulfate (Additive pressor effect). Products include:
- Norisodrine with Calcium Iodide Syrup ... 442

Metaproterenol Sulfate (Additive pressor effect). Products include:
- Alupent ... 669
- Metaproterenol Sulfate Inhalation Solution, USP, Arm-a-Med ... 552

Metaraminol Bitartrate (Additive pressor effect). Products include:
- Aramine Injection ... 1609

Metaxalone (Residual effects masked by Dopram). Products include:
- Skelaxin Tablets ... 788

Methocarbamol (Residual effects masked by Dopram). Products include:
- Robaxin Injectable ... 2070
- Robaxin Tablets ... 2071
- Robaxisal Tablets ... 2071

Methoxamine Hydrochloride (Additive pressor effect). Products include:
- Vasoxyl Injection ... 1196

Methoxyflurane (Increased epinephrine release).
- No products indexed under this heading.

Metocurine Iodide (Residual effects masked by Dopram). Products include:
- Metubine Iodide Vials ... 916

Norepinephrine Bitartrate (Additive pressor effect). Products include:
- Levophed Bitartrate Injection ... 2315

Orphenadrine Citrate (Residual effects masked by Dopram). Products include:
- Norflex ... 1496
- Norgesic ... 1496

Pancuronium Bromide Injection (Residual effects masked by Dopram).
- No products indexed under this heading.

Phenelzine Sulfate (Additive pressor effect). Products include:
- Nardil ... 1920

Phenylephrine Bitartrate (Additive pressor effect).
- No products indexed under this heading.

Phenylephrine Hydrochloride (Additive pressor effect). Products include:
- Atrohist Plus Tablets ... 454
- Cerose DM ... ▣ 878
- Comhist ... 2038
- D.A. Chewable Tablets ... 951
- Deconsal Pediatric Capsules ... 454
- Dura-Vent/DA Tablets ... 953
- Entex Capsules ... 1986
- Entex Liquid ... 1986
- Extendryl ... 1005
- 4-Way Fast Acting Nasal Spray (regular & mentholated) ... ▣ 621
- Hemorid For Women ... ▣ 834
- Hycomine Compound Tablets ... 932
- Neo-Synephrine Hydrochloride 1% Carpuject ... 2324
- Neo-Synephrine Hydrochloride 1% Injection ... 2324
- Neo-Synephrine Hydrochloride (Ophthalmic) ... 2325
- Neo-Synephrine ... ▣ 726
- Nōstril ... ▣ 644
- Novahistine Elixir ... ▣ 823
- Phenergan VC ... 2779
- Phenergan VC with Codeine ... 2781
- Preparation H ... ▣ 871
- Tympagesic Ear Drops ... 2342
- Vasosulf ... ⊙ 271
- Vicks Sinex Nasal Spray and Ultra Fine Mist ... ▣ 765

Phenylephrine Tannate (Additive pressor effect). Products include:
- Atrohist Pediatric Suspension ... 454
- Ricobid-D Pediatric Suspension ... 2038
- Ricobid Tablets and Pediatric Suspension ... 2038
- Rynatan ... 2673
- Rynatuss ... 2673

Phenylpropanolamine Hydrochloride (Additive pressor effect). Products include:
- Acutrim ... ▣ 628
- Allerest Children's Chewable Tablets ... ▣ 627
- Allerest 12 Hour Caplets ... ▣ 627
- Atrohist Plus Tablets ... 454
- BC Cold Powder Multi-Symptom Formula (Cold-Sinus-Allergy) ... ▣ 609
- BC Cold Powder Non-Drowsy Formula (Cold-Sinus) ... ▣ 609
- Cheracol Plus Head Cold/Cough Formula ... ▣ 769
- Comtrex Multi-Symptom Non-Drowsy Liqui-gels ... ▣ 618
- Contac Continuous Action Nasal Decongestant/Antihistamine 12 Hour Capsules ... ▣ 813
- Contac Maximum Strength Continuous Action Decongestant/Antihistamine 12 Hour Caplets ... ▣ 813
- Contac Severe Cold and Flu Formula Caplets ... ▣ 814
- Coricidin 'D' Decongestant Tablets ... ▣ 800
- Dexatrim ... ▣ 832
- Dexatrim Plus Vitamins Caplets ... ▣ 832
- Dimetane-DC Cough Syrup ... 2059
- Dimetapp Elixir ... ▣ 773
- Dimetapp Extentabs ... ▣ 774
- Dimetapp Tablets/Liqui-Gels ... ▣ 775
- Dimetapp Cold & Allergy Chewable Tablets ... ▣ 773
- Dimetapp DM Elixir ... ▣ 774
- Dura-Vent Tablets ... 952
- Entex Capsules ... 1986
- Entex LA Tablets ... 1987
- Entex Liquid ... 1986
- Exgest LA Tablets ... 782
- Hycomine ... 931
- Isoclor Timesule Capsules ... ▣ 637
- Nolamine Timed-Release Tablets ... 785
- Ornade Spansule Capsules ... 2502
- Propagest Tablets ... 786
- Pyrroxate Caplets ... ▣ 772
- Robitussin-CF ... ▣ 777
- Sinulin Tablets ... 787
- Tavist-D 12 Hour Relief Tablets ... ▣ 787
- Teldrin 12 Hour Antihistamine/Nasal Decongestant Allergy Relief Capsules ... ▣ 826
- Triaminic Allergy Tablets ... ▣ 789
- Triaminic Cold Tablets ... ▣ 790
- Triaminic Expectorant ... ▣ 790
- Triaminic Syrup ... ▣ 792
- Triaminic-12 Tablets ... ▣ 792
- Triaminic-DM Syrup ... ▣ 792
- Triaminicin Tablets ... ▣ 793
- Triaminicol Multi-Symptom Cold Tablets ... ▣ 793
- Triaminicol Multi-Symptom Relief ... ▣ 794
- Vicks DayQuil Allergy Relief 12-Hour Extended Release Tablets ... ▣ 760
- Vicks DayQuil Allergy Relief 4-Hour Tablets ... ▣ 760
- Vicks DayQuil SINUS Pressure & CONGESTION Relief ... ▣ 761

Pirbuterol Acetate (Additive pressor effect). Products include:
- Maxair Autohaler ... 1492
- Maxair Inhaler ... 1494

Pseudoephedrine Hydrochloride (Additive pressor effect). Products include:
- Actifed Allergy Daytime/Nighttime Caplets ... ▣ 844
- Actifed Plus Caplets ... ▣ 845
- Actifed Plus Tablets ... ▣ 845
- Actifed with Codeine Cough Syrup ... 1067
- Actifed Sinus Daytime/Nighttime Tablets and Caplets ... ▣ 846
- Actifed Syrup ... ▣ 846
- Actifed Tablets ... ▣ 844
- Advil Cold and Sinus Caplets and Tablets (formerly CoAdvil) ... ▣ 870
- Alka-Seltzer Plus Cold Medicine Liqui-Gels ... ▣ 706
- Alka-Seltzer Plus Cold & Cough Medicine Liqui-Gels ... ▣ 705
- Alka-Seltzer Plus Night-Time Cold Medicine Liqui-Gels ... ▣ 706
- Allerest Headache Strength Tablets ... ▣ 627
- Allerest Maximum Strength Tablets ... ▣ 627
- Allerest No Drowsiness Tablets ... ▣ 627
- Allerest Sinus Pain Formula ... ▣ 627
- Anatuss LA Tablets ... 1542
- Atrohist Pediatric Capsules ... 453
- Bayer Select Sinus Pain Relief Formula ... ▣ 717
- Benadryl Allergy Decongestant Liquid Medication ... ▣ 848
- Benadryl Allergy Decongestant Tablets ... ▣ 848
- Benadryl Allergy Sinus Headache Formula Caplets ... ▣ 849
- Benylin Multisymptom ... ▣ 852
- Bromfed Capsules (Extended-Release) ... 1785
- Bromfed Syrup ... ▣ 733
- Bromfed Tablets ... 1785
- Bromfed-DM Cough Syrup ... 1786
- Bromfed-PD Capsules (Extended-Release) ... 1785
- Children's Vicks DayQuil Allergy Relief ... ▣ 757
- Children's Vicks NyQuil Cold/Cough Relief ... ▣ 758
- Comtrex Multi-Symptom Cold Reliever Tablets/Caplets/Liqui-Gels/Liquid ... ▣ 615
- Allergy-Sinus Comtrex Multi-Symptom Allergy-Sinus Formula Tablets ... ▣ 617
- Comtrex Multi-Symptom Non-Drowsy Caplets ... ▣ 618
- Congess ... 1004
- Contac Day Allergy/Sinus Caplets ▣ 812
- Contac Day & Night ... ▣ 812
- Contac Night Allergy/Sinus Caplets ... ▣ 812
- Contac Severe Cold & Flu Non-Drowsy ... ▣ 815
- Deconamine Chewable Tablets ... 1320
- Deconamine CX Cough and Cold Liquid and Tablets ... 1319
- Deconamine ... 1320
- Deconsal C Expectorant Syrup ... 456
- Deconsal Pediatric Syrup ... 457
- Deconsal II Tablets ... 454
- Dimetane-DX Cough Syrup ... 2059
- Dimetapp Sinus Caplets ... ▣ 775
- Dorcol Children's Cough Syrup ... ▣ 785
- Drixoral Cough + Congestion Liquid Caps ... ▣ 802
- Dura-Tap/PD Capsules ... 2867
- Duratuss Tablets ... 2565
- Duratuss HD Elixir ... 2565
- Efidac/24 ... ▣ 635
- Entex PSE Tablets ... 1987
- Fedahist Gyrocaps ... 2401
- Fedahist Timecaps ... 2401
- Guaifed ... 1787
- Guaifed Syrup ... ▣ 734
- Guaimax-D Tablets ... 792
- Guaitab Tablets ... ▣ 734
- Isoclor Expectorant ... 990
- Kronofed-A ... 977
- Motrin IB Sinus ... ▣ 838
- Novahistine DH ... 2462
- Novahistine DMX ... ▣ 822
- Novahistine Expectorant ... 2463
- Nucofed ... 2051
- PediaCare Cold Allergy Chewable Tablets ... ▣ 677
- PediaCare Cough-Cold Chewable Tablets ... 1553
- PediaCare ... 1553
- PediaCare Infants' Decongestant Drops ... ▣ 677
- PediCare Infant's Drops Decongestant Plus Cough ... 1553
- PediaCare NightRest Cough-Cold Liquid ... 1553
- Pediatric Vicks 44d Dry Hacking Cough & Head Congestion ... ▣ 763
- Pediatric Vicks 44m Cough & Cold Relief ... ▣ 764
- Robitussin Cold & Cough Liqui-Gels ... ▣ 776

(▣ Described in PDR For Nonprescription Drugs) (⊙ Described in PDR For Ophthalmology)

Interactions Index

Robitussin Maximum Strength Cough & Cold .... ◻ 778
Robitussin Pediatric Cough & Cold Formula .... ◻ 779
Robitussin Severe Congestion Liqui-Gels .... ◻ 776
Robitussin-DAC Syrup 2074
Robitussin-PE .... ◻ 778
Rondec Oral Drops 953
Rondec Syrup 953
Rondec Tablet 953
Rondec-DM Oral Drops 954
Rondec-DM Syrup 954
Rondec-TR Tablet 953
Ryna .... ◻ 841
Seldane-D Extended-Release Tablets 1538
Semprex-D Capsules 463
Semprex-D Capsules 1167
Sinarest Tablets .... ◻ 648
Sinarest Extra Strength Tablets...... ◻ 648
Sinarest No Drowsiness Tablets .... ◻ 648
Sine-Aid IB Caplets 1554
Sine-Aid Maximum Strength Sinus Medication Gelcaps, Caplets and Tablets 1554
Sine-Off No Drowsiness Formula Caplets .... ◻ 824
Sine-Off Sinus Medicine .... ◻ 825
Singlet Tablets .... ◻ 825
Sinutab Non-Drying Liquid Caps .... ◻ 859
Sinutab Sinus Allergy Medication, Maximum Strength Tablets and Caplets .... ◻ 860
Sinutab Sinus Medication, Maximum Strength Without Drowsiness Formula, Tablets & Caplets .... ◻ 860
Sinutab Sinus Medication, Regular Strength Without Drowsiness Formula .... ◻ 859
Sudafed Children's Liquid .... ◻ 861
Sudafed Cold and Cough Liquidcaps .... ◻ 862
Sudafed Cough Syrup .... ◻ 862
Sudafed Plus Liquid .... ◻ 862
Sudafed Plus Tablets .... ◻ 863
Sudafed Severe Cold Formula Caplets .... ◻ 863
Sudafed Severe Cold Formula Tablets .... ◻ 864
Sudafed Sinus Caplets.......................... ◻ 864
Sudafed Sinus Tablets........................... ◻ 864
Sudafed Tablets, 30 mg........................ ◻ 861
Sudafed Tablets, 60 mg........................ ◻ 861
Sudafed 12 Hour Caplets .... ◻ 861
Syn-Rx Tablets 465
Syn-Rx DM Tablets 466
TheraFlu... ◻ 787
TheraFlu Maximum Strength Nighttime Flu, Cold & Cough Medicine .... ◻ 788
TheraFlu Maximum Strength Non-Drowsy Formula Flu, Cold & Cough Medicine .... ◻ 788
Thera Flu Maximum Strength, Non-Drowsy Formula Flu, Cold and Cough Caplets .... ◻ 789
Triaminic AM Cough and Decongestant Formula .... ◻ 789
Triaminic AM Decongestant Formula .... ◻ 790
Triaminic Nite Light .... ◻ 791
Triaminic Sore Throat Formula ...... ◻ 791
Tussend 1783
Tussend Expectorant 1785
Children's TYLENOL Cold Multi-Symptom Liquid Formula and Chewable Tablets................................. 1561
Children's TYLENOL Cold Plus Cough Multi Symptom Tablets and Liquid .... ◻ 681
Infants' TYLENOL Cold Decongestant & Fever-Reducer Drops 1556
TYLENOL Maximum Strength Allergy Sinus Medication Gelcaps and Caplets 1563
TYLENOL Maximum Strength Allergy Sinus NightTime Medication Caplets 1555
TYLENOL Flu Maximum Strength Gelcaps 1565
TYLENOL Flu NightTime, Maximum Strength, Gelcaps 1566
TYLENOL Maximum Strength Flu NightTime Hot Medication Packets 1562
TYLENOL, Maximum Strength, Sinus Medication Geltabs, Gelcaps, Caplets and Tablets 1566

TYLENOL Cold Multi-Symptom Formula Medication Tablets and Caplets 1561
TYLENOL Cold Medication No Drowsiness Formula Gelcaps and Caplets 1562
TYLENOL Cold Multi-Symptom Hot Medication Liquid Packets.............. 1557
TYLENOL Cough Multi-Symptom Medication with Decongestant 1565
Ursinus Inlay-Tabs................................ ◻ 794
Vicks 44 LiquiCaps Cough, Cold & Flu Relief .... ◻ 755
Vicks 44 LiquiCaps Non-Drowsy Cough & Cold Relief .... ◻ 756
Vicks 44D Dry Hacking Cough & Head Congestion .... ◻ 755
Vicks 44M Cough, Cold & Flu Relief .... ◻ 756
Vicks DayQuil .... ◻ 761
Vicks DayQuil SINUS Pressure & PAIN Relief with IBUPROFEN ...... ◻ 762
Vicks Nyquil Hot Therapy.................... ◻ 762
Vicks NyQuil LiquiCaps Multi-Symptom Cold/Flu Relief .... ◻ 763
Vicks NyQuil Multi-Symptom Cold/Flu Relief - (Original & Cherry Flavor) .... ◻ 763

Pseudoephedrine Sulfate (Additive pressor effect). Products include:

Cheracol Sinus .... ◻ 768
Chlor-Trimeton Allergy Decongestant Tablets .... ◻ 799
Claritin-D 2350
Drixoral Cold and Allergy Sustained-Action Tablets........................ ◻ 802
Drixoral Cold and Flu Extended-Release Tablets................................... ◻ 803
Drixoral Non-Drowsy Formula Extended-Release Tablets .... ◻ 803
Drixoral Allergy/Sinus Extended Release Tablets................................... ◻ 804
Trinalin Repetabs Tablets 1330

Rocuronium Bromide (Residual effects masked by Dopram). Products include:

Zemuron 1830

Salmeterol Xinafoate (Additive pressor effect). Products include:

Serevent Inhalation Aerosol............... 1176

Selegiline Hydrochloride (Additive pressor effect). Products include:

Eldepryl Tablets 2550

Succinylcholine Chloride (Residual effects masked by Dopram). Products include:

Anectine... 1073

Terbutaline Sulfate (Additive pressor effect). Products include:

Brethaire Inhaler 813
Brethine Ampuls 815
Brethine Tablets.................................... 814
Bricanyl Subcutaneous Injection 1502
Bricanyl Tablets 1503

Tranylcypromine Sulfate (Additive pressor effect). Products include:

Parnate Tablets 2503

Vecuronium Bromide (Residual effects masked by Dopram). Products include:

Norcuron 1826

DORAL TABLETS

(Quazepam) 2664
May interact with central nervous system depressants, anticonvulsants, psychotropics, and certain other agents. Compounds in these categories include:

Alfentanil Hydrochloride (Additive CNS depressant effects). Products include:

Alfenta Injection 1286

Alprazolam (Additive CNS depressant effects). Products include:

Xanax Tablets 2649

Amitriptyline Hydrochloride (Additive CNS depressant effects). Products include:

Elavil 2838

Endep Tablets 2174
Etrafon 2355
Limbitrol 2180
Triavil Tablets 1757

Amoxapine (Additive CNS depressant effects). Products include:

Asendin Tablets 1369

Aprobarbital (Additive CNS depressant effects).

No products indexed under this heading.

Buprenorphine (Additive CNS depressant effects). Products include:

Buprenex Injectable 2006

Buspirone Hydrochloride (Additive CNS depressant effects). Products include:

BuSpar 737

Butabarbital (Additive CNS depressant effects).

No products indexed under this heading.

Butalbital (Additive CNS depressant effects). Products include:

Esgic-plus Tablets 1013
Fioricet Tablets 2258
Fioricet with Codeine Capsules 2260
Fiorinal Capsules 2261
Fiorinal with Codeine Capsules 2262
Fiorinal Tablets 2261
Phrenilin 785
Sedapap Tablets 50 mg/650 mg .. 1543

Carbamazepine (Additive CNS depressant effects). Products include:

Atretol Tablets 573
Tegretol Chewable Tablets 852
Tegretol Suspension.............................. 852
Tegretol Tablets 852

Chlordiazepoxide (Additive CNS depressant effects). Products include:

Libritabs Tablets 2177
Limbitrol 2180

Chlordiazepoxide Hydrochloride (Additive CNS depressant effects). Products include:

Librax Capsules 2176
Librium Capsules................................... 2178
Librium Injectable 2179

Chlorpromazine (Additive CNS depressant effects). Products include:

Thorazine Suppositories 2523

Chlorprothixene (Additive CNS depressant effects).

No products indexed under this heading.

Chlorprothixene Hydrochloride (Additive CNS depressant effects).

No products indexed under this heading.

Clorazepate Dipotassium (Additive CNS depressant effects). Products include:

Tranxene 451

Clozapine (Additive CNS depressant effects). Products include:

Clozaril Tablets 2252

Codeine Phosphate (Additive CNS depressant effects). Products include:

Actifed with Codeine Cough Syrup.. 1067
Brontex 1981
Deconsal C Expectorant Syrup 456
Deconsal Pediatric Syrup.................... 457
Dimetane-DC Cough Syrup 2059
Empirin with Codeine Tablets............ 1093
Fioricet with Codeine Capsules 2260
Fiorinal with Codeine Capsules 2262
Isoclor Expectorant 990
Novahistine DH...................................... 2462
Novahistine Expectorant...................... 2463
Nucofed 2051
Phenergan with Codeine 2777
Phenergan VC with Codeine 2781
Robitussin A-C Syrup 2073
Robitussin-DAC Syrup 2074
Ryna .... ◻ 841

Soma Compound w/Codeine Tablets 2676
Tussi-Organidin NR Liquid and S NR Liquid 2677
Tylenol with Codeine 1583

Desflurane (Additive CNS depressant effects). Products include:

Suprane 1813

Desipramine Hydrochloride (Additive CNS depressant effects). Products include:

Norpramin Tablets 1526

Dezocine (Additive CNS depressant effects). Products include:

Dalgan Injection 538

Diazepam (Additive CNS depressant effects). Products include:

Dizac 1809
Valium Injectable 2182
Valium Tablets 2183
Valrelease Capsules 2169

Divalproex Sodium (Additive CNS depressant effects). Products include:

Depakote Tablets................................... 415

Doxepin Hydrochloride (Additive CNS depressant effects). Products include:

Sinequan 2205
Zonalon Cream 1055

Droperidol (Additive CNS depressant effects). Products include:

Inapsine Injection................................. 1296

Enflurane (Additive CNS depressant effects).

No products indexed under this heading.

Estazolam (Additive CNS depressant effects). Products include:

ProSom Tablets 449

Ethchlorvynol (Additive CNS depressant effects). Products include:

Placidyl Capsules.................................. 448

Ethinamate (Additive CNS depressant effects).

No products indexed under this heading.

Ethosuximide (Additive CNS depressant effects). Products include:

Zarontin Capsules 1928
Zarontin Syrup 1929

Ethotoin (Additive CNS depressant effects). Products include:

Peganone Tablets 446

Felbamate (Additive CNS depressant effects). Products include:

Felbatol 2666

Fentanyl (Additive CNS depressant effects). Products include:

Duragesic Transdermal System........ 1288

Fentanyl Citrate (Additive CNS depressant effects). Products include:

Sublimaze Injection............................... 1307

Fluphenazine Decanoate (Additive CNS depressant effects). Products include:

Prolixin Decanoate 509

Fluphenazine Enanthate (Additive CNS depressant effects). Products include:

Prolixin Enanthate 509

Fluphenazine Hydrochloride (Additive CNS depressant effects). Products include:

Prolixin 509

Flurazepam Hydrochloride (Additive CNS depressant effects). Products include:

Dalmane Capsules................................. 2173

Glutethimide (Additive CNS depressant effects).

No products indexed under this heading.

Haloperidol (Additive CNS depressant effects). Products include:

Haldol Injection, Tablets and Concentrate 1575

IMPORTANT NOTE: Always consult each drug listing in the patient's regimen for possible interactions.

Haloperidol Decanoate (Additive CNS depressant effects). Products include:
- Haldol Decanoate ... 1577

Hydrocodone Bitartrate (Additive CNS depressant effects). Products include:
- Anexsia 5/500 Elixir ... 1781
- Anexia Tablets ... 1782
- Codiclear DH Syrup ... 791
- Deconamine CX Cough and Cold Liquid and Tablets ... 1319
- Duratuss HD Elixir ... 2565
- Hycodan Tablets and Syrup ... 930
- Hycomine Compound Tablets ... 932
- Hycomine ... 931
- Hycotuss Expectorant Syrup ... 933
- Hydrocet Capsules ... 782
- Lorcet 10/650 ... 1018
- Lortab ... 2566
- Tussend ... 1783
- Tussend Expectorant ... 1785
- Vicodin Tablets ... 1356
- Vicodin ES Tablets ... 1357
- Vicodin Tuss Expectorant ... 1358
- Zydone Capsules ... 949

Hydrocodone Polistirex (Additive CNS depressant effects). Products include:
- Tussionex Pennkinetic Extended-Release Suspension ... 998

Hydroxyzine Hydrochloride (Additive CNS depressant effects). Products include:
- Atarax Tablets & Syrup ... 2185
- Marax Tablets & DF Syrup ... 2200
- Vistaril Intramuscular Solution ... 2216

Imipramine Hydrochloride (Additive CNS depressant effects). Products include:
- Tofranil Ampuls ... 854
- Tofranil Tablets ... 856

Imipramine Pamoate (Additive CNS depressant effects). Products include:
- Tofranil-PM Capsules ... 857

Isocarboxazid (Additive CNS depressant effects).
- No products indexed under this heading.

Isoflurane (Additive CNS depressant effects).
- No products indexed under this heading.

Ketamine Hydrochloride (Additive CNS depressant effects).
- No products indexed under this heading.

Lamotrigine (Additive CNS depressant effects). Products include:
- Lamictal Tablets ... 1112

Levomethadyl Acetate Hydrochloride (Additive CNS depressant effects). Products include:
- Orlamm ... 2239

Levorphanol Tartrate (Additive CNS depressant effects). Products include:
- Levo-Dromoran ... 2129

Lithium Carbonate (Additive CNS depressant effects). Products include:
- Eskalith ... 2485
- Lithium Carbonate Capsules & Tablets ... 2230
- Lithonate/Lithotabs/Lithobid ... 2543

Lithium Citrate (Additive CNS depressant effects).
- No products indexed under this heading.

Lorazepam (Additive CNS depressant effects). Products include:
- Ativan Injection ... 2698
- Ativan Tablets ... 2700

Loxapine Hydrochloride (Additive CNS depressant effects). Products include:
- Loxitane ... 1378

Loxapine Succinate (Additive CNS depressant effects). Products include:
- Loxitane Capsules ... 1378

Maprotiline Hydrochloride (Additive CNS depressant effects). Products include:
- Ludiomil Tablets ... 843

Meperidine Hydrochloride (Additive CNS depressant effects). Products include:
- Demerol ... 2308
- Mepergan Injection ... 2753

Mephenytoin (Additive CNS depressant effects). Products include:
- Mesantoin Tablets ... 2272

Mephobarbital (Additive CNS depressant effects). Products include:
- Mebaral Tablets ... 2322

Meprobamate (Additive CNS depressant effects). Products include:
- Miltown Tablets ... 2672
- PMB 200 and PMB 400 ... 2783

Mesoridazine Besylate (Additive CNS depressant effects). Products include:
- Serentil ... 684

Methadone Hydrochloride (Additive CNS depressant effects). Products include:
- Methadone Hydrochloride Oral Concentrate ... 2233
- Methadone Hydrochloride Oral Solution & Tablets ... 2235

Methohexital Sodium (Additive CNS depressant effects). Products include:
- Brevital Sodium Vials ... 1429

Methotrimeprazine (Additive CNS depressant effects). Products include:
- Levoprome ... 1274

Methoxyflurane (Additive CNS depressant effects).
- No products indexed under this heading.

Methsuximide (Additive CNS depressant effects). Products include:
- Celontin Kapseals ... 1899

Midazolam Hydrochloride (Additive CNS depressant effects). Products include:
- Versed Injection ... 2170

Molindone Hydrochloride (Additive CNS depressant effects). Products include:
- Moban Tablets and Concentrate ... 1048

Morphine Sulfate (Additive CNS depressant effects). Products include:
- Astramorph/PF Injection, USP (Preservative-Free) ... 535
- Duramorph ... 962
- Infumorph 200 and Infumorph 500 Sterile Solutions ... 965
- MS Contin Tablets ... 1994
- MSIR ... 1997
- Oramorph SR (Morphine Sulfate Sustained Release Tablets) ... 2236
- RMS Suppositories ... 2657
- Roxanol ... 2243

Nortriptyline Hydrochloride (Additive CNS depressant effects). Products include:
- Pamelor ... 2280

Opium Alkaloids (Additive CNS depressant effects).
- No products indexed under this heading.

Oxazepam (Additive CNS depressant effects). Products include:
- Serax Capsules ... 2810
- Serax Tablets ... 2810

Oxycodone Hydrochloride (Additive CNS depressant effects). Products include:
- Percocet Tablets ... 938
- Percodan Tablets ... 939
- Percodan-Demi Tablets ... 940
- Roxicodone Tablets, Oral Solution & Intensol (Oxycodone) ... 2244
- Tylox Capsules ... 1584

Paramethadione (Additive CNS depressant effects).
- No products indexed under this heading.

Pentobarbital Sodium (Additive CNS depressant effects). Products include:
- Nembutal Sodium Capsules ... 436
- Nembutal Sodium Solution ... 438
- Nembutal Sodium Suppositories ... 440

Perphenazine (Additive CNS depressant effects). Products include:
- Etrafon ... 2355
- Triavil Tablets ... 1757
- Trilafon ... 2389

Phenacemide (Additive CNS depressant effects). Products include:
- Phenurone Tablets ... 447

Phenelzine Sulfate (Additive CNS depressant effects). Products include:
- Nardil ... 1920

Phenobarbital (Additive CNS depressant effects). Products include:
- Arco-Lase Plus Tablets ... 512
- Bellergal-S Tablets ... 2250
- Donnatal ... 2060
- Donnatal Extentabs ... 2061
- Donnatal Tablets ... 2060
- Phenobarbital Elixir and Tablets ... 1469
- Quadrinal Tablets ... 1350

Phensuximide (Additive CNS depressant effects). Products include:
- Milontin Kapseals ... 1920

Phenytoin (Additive CNS depressant effects). Products include:
- Dilantin Infatabs ... 1908
- Dilantin-125 Suspension ... 1911

Phenytoin Sodium (Additive CNS depressant effects). Products include:
- Dilantin Kapseals ... 1906
- Dilantin Parenteral ... 1910

Prazepam (Additive CNS depressant effects).
- No products indexed under this heading.

Primidone (Additive CNS depressant effects). Products include:
- Mysoline ... 2754

Prochlorperazine (Additive CNS depressant effects). Products include:
- Compazine ... 2470

Promethazine Hydrochloride (Additive CNS depressant effects). Products include:
- Mepergan Injection ... 2753
- Phenergan with Codeine ... 2777
- Phenergan with Dextromethorphan ... 2778
- Phenergan Injection ... 2773
- Phenergan Suppositories ... 2775
- Phenergan Syrup ... 2774
- Phenergan Tablets ... 2775
- Phenergan VC ... 2779
- Phenergan VC with Codeine ... 2781

Propofol (Additive CNS depressant effects). Products include:
- Diprivan Injection ... 2833

Propoxyphene Hydrochloride (Additive CNS depressant effects). Products include:
- Darvon ... 1435
- Wygesic Tablets ... 2827

Propoxyphene Napsylate (Additive CNS depressant effects). Products include:
- Darvon-N/Darvocet-N ... 1433

Protriptyline Hydrochloride (Additive CNS depressant effects). Products include:
- Vivactil Tablets ... 1774

Risperidone (Additive CNS depressant effects). Products include:
- Risperdal ... 1301

Secobarbital Sodium (Additive CNS depressant effects). Products include:
- Seconal Sodium Pulvules ... 1474

Sufentanil Citrate (Additive CNS depressant effects). Products include:
- Sufenta Injection ... 1309

Temazepam (Additive CNS depressant effects). Products include:
- Restoril Capsules ... 2284

Thiamylal Sodium (Additive CNS depressant effects).
- No products indexed under this heading.

Thioridazine Hydrochloride (Additive CNS depressant effects). Products include:
- Mellaril ... 2269

Thiothixene (Additive CNS depressant effects). Products include:
- Navane Capsules and Concentrate 2201
- Navane Intramuscular ... 2202

Tranylcypromine Sulfate (Additive CNS depressant effects). Products include:
- Parnate Tablets ... 2503

Triazolam (Additive CNS depressant effects). Products include:
- Halcion Tablets ... 2611

Trifluoperazine Hydrochloride (Additive CNS depressant effects). Products include:
- Stelazine ... 2514

Trimethadione (Additive CNS depressant effects).
- No products indexed under this heading.

Trimipramine Maleate (Additive CNS depressant effects). Products include:
- Surmontil Capsules ... 2811

Valproic Acid (Additive CNS depressant effects). Products include:
- Depakene ... 413

Zolpidem Tartrate (Additive CNS depressant effects). Products include:
- Ambien Tablets ... 2416

Food Interactions

Alcohol (Additive CNS depressant effects).

DORCOL CHILDREN'S COUGH SYRUP

(Pseudoephedrine Hydrochloride, Guaifenesin, Dextromethorphan Hydrobromide) ... (▣) 785

May interact with monoamine oxidase inhibitors. Compounds in this category include:

Furazolidone (Concurrent and/or sequential use is not recommended). Products include:
- Furoxone ... 2046

Isocarboxazid (Concurrent and/or sequential use is not recommended).
- No products indexed under this heading.

Phenelzine Sulfate (Concurrent and/or sequential use is not recommended). Products include:
- Nardil ... 1920

Selegiline Hydrochloride (Concurrent and/or sequential use is not recommended). Products include:
- Eldepryl Tablets ... 2550

Tranylcypromine Sulfate (Concurrent and/or sequential use is not recommended). Products include:
- Parnate Tablets ... 2503

DORYX CAPSULES

(Doxycycline Hyclate) ... 1913

May interact with penicillins, antacids, anticoagulants, iron containing oral preparations, and certain other agents. Compounds in these categories include:

Aluminum Carbonate Gel (Should not be given concurrently). Products include:

Basaljel 2703

Aluminum Hydroxide (Should not be given concurrently). Products include:

ALternaGEL Liquid 1316
Maximum Strength Ascriptin .... ✪ 630
Cama Arthritis Pain Reliever........... ✪ 785
Gaviscon Extra Strength Relief Formula Antacid Tablets................ ✪ 819
Gaviscon Extra Strength Relief Formula Liquid Antacid .... ✪ 819
Gaviscon Liquid Antacid .... ✪ 820
Gelusil Liquid & Tablets .... ✪ 855
Maalox Heartburn Relief Suspension .... ✪ 642
Maalox Heartburn Relief Tablets.... ✪ 641
Maalox Magnesia and Alumina Oral Suspension .... ✪ 642
Maalox Plus Tablets .... ✪ 643
Extra Strength Maalox Antacid Plus Antigas Liquid and Tablets ✪ 638
Tempo Soft Antacid .... ✪ 835

Aluminum Hydroxide Gel (Should not be given concurrently). Products include:

ALternaGEL Liquid .... ✪ 659
Aludrox Oral Suspension 2695
Amphojel Suspension 2695
Amphojel Suspension without Flavor 2695
Amphojel Tablets.................................. 2695
Arthritis Pain Ascriptin .... ✪ 631
Regular Strength Ascriptin Tablets .... ✪ 629
Gaviscon Antacid Tablets................... ✪ 819
Gaviscon-2 Antacid Tablets .... ✪ 820
Mylanta Liquid 1317
Mylanta Tablets .... ✪ 660
Mylanta Double Strength Liquid 1317
Mylanta Double Strength Tablets .. ✪ 660
Nephrox Suspension .... ✪ 655

Amoxicillin Trihydrate (Interference with bactericidal action of penicillins). Products include:

Amoxil.. 2464
Augmentin 2468

Ampicillin (Interference with bactericidal action of penicillins). Products include:

Omnipen Capsules 2764
Omnipen for Oral Suspension 2765

Ampicillin Sodium (Interference with bactericidal action of penicillins). Products include:

Unasyn 2212

Azlocillin Sodium (Interference with bactericidal action of penicillins).

No products indexed under this heading.

Bacampicillin Hydrochloride (Interference with bactericidal action of penicillins). Products include:

Spectrobid Tablets 2206

Carbenicillin Disodium (Interference with bactericidal action of penicillins).

No products indexed under this heading.

Carbenicillin Indanyl Sodium (Interference with bactericidal action of penicillins). Products include:

Geocillin Tablets.................................... 2199

Dalteparin Sodium (Downward adjustment of anticoagulant dosage may be necessary). Products include:

Fragmin 1954

Dicloxacillin Sodium (Interference with bactericidal action of penicillins).

No products indexed under this heading.

Dicumarol (Downward adjustment of anticoagulant dosage may be necessary).

No products indexed under this heading.

Dihydroxyaluminum Sodium Carbonate (Should not be given concurrently).

No products indexed under this heading.

Enoxaparin (Downward adjustment of anticoagulant dosage may be necessary). Products include:

Lovenox Injection.................................. 2020

Ferrous Fumarate (Should not be given concurrently). Products include:

Chromagen Capsules............................ 2339
Ferro-Sequels .... ✪ 669
Nephro-Fer Tablets............................... 2004
Nephro-Fer Rx Tablets......................... 2005
Nephro-Vite + Fe Tablets 2006
Sigtab-M Tablets .... ✪ 772
Stresstabs + Iron .... ✪ 671
The Stuart Formula Tablets............... ✪ 663
Theragran-M Tablets with Beta Carotene .... ✪ 623
Trinsicon Capsules 2570
Vitron-C Tablets .... ✪ 650

Ferrous Gluconate (Should not be given concurrently). Products include:

Fergon Iron Supplement Tablets.... ✪ 721
Megadose 512

Ferrous Sulfate (Should not be given concurrently). Products include:

Feosol Capsules 2456
Feosol Elixir 2456
Feosol Tablets 2457
Fero-Folic-500 Filmtab 429
Fero-Grad-500 Filmtab 429
Fero-Gradumet Filmtab....................... 429
Iberet Tablets 433
Iberet-500 Liquid 433
Iberet-Folic-500 Filmtab..................... 429
Iberet-Liquid... 433
Irospan 982
Slow Fe Tablets...................................... 869
Slow Fe with Folic Acid 869

Heparin Calcium (Downward adjustment of anticoagulant dosage may be necessary).

No products indexed under this heading.

Heparin Sodium (Downward adjustment of anticoagulant dosage may be necessary). Products include:

Heparin Lock Flush Solution 2725
Heparin Sodium Injection.................... 2726
Heparin Sodium Injection, USP, Sterile Solution 2615
Heparin Sodium Vials........................... 1441

Magaldrate (Should not be given concurrently).

No products indexed under this heading.

Magnesium Hydroxide (Should not be given concurrently). Products include:

Aludrox Oral Suspension 2695
Arthritis Pain Ascriptin .... ✪ 631
Maximum Strength Ascriptin .... ✪ 630
Regular Strength Ascriptin Tablets .... ✪ 629
Di-Gel Antacid/Anti-Gas .... ✪ 801
Gelusil Liquid & Tablets .... ✪ 855
Maalox Magnesia and Alumina Oral Suspension .... ✪ 642
Maalox Plus Tablets .... ✪ 643
Extra Strength Maalox Antacid Plus Antigas Liquid and Tablets ✪ 638
Mylanta Calcium Carbonate and Magnesium Hydroxide Tablets...... 1318
Mylanta Liquid 1317
Mylanta Tablets .... ✪ 660
Mylanta Double Strength Liquid 1317
Mylanta Double Strength Tablets.. ✪ 660
Phillips' Milk of Magnesia Liquid.... ✪ 729
Rolaids Tablets....................................... ✪ 843
Tempo Soft Antacid .... ✪ 835

Magnesium Oxide (Should not be given concurrently). Products include:

Beelith Tablets 639
Bufferin Analgesic Tablets and Caplets .... ✪ 613
Caltrate PLUS .... ✪ 665
Cama Arthritis Pain Reliever............ ✪ 785
Mag-Ox 400 668
Uro-Mag.. 668

Mezlocillin Sodium (Interference with bactericidal action of penicillins). Products include:

Mezlin 601
Mezlin Pharmacy Bulk Package....... 604

Nafcillin Sodium (Interference with bactericidal action of penicillins).

No products indexed under this heading.

Penicillin G Benzathine (Interference with bactericidal action of penicillin). Products include:

Bicillin C-R Injection 2704
Bicillin C-R 900/300 Injection 2706
Bicillin L-A Injection 2707

Penicillin G Potassium (Interference with bactericidal action of penicillin). Products include:

Pfizerpen for Injection 2203

Penicillin G Procaine (Interference with bactericidal action of penicillin). Products include:

Bicillin C-R Injection 2704
Bicillin C-R 900/300 Injection 2706

Penicillin G Sodium (Interference with bactericidal action of penicillin).

No products indexed under this heading.

Penicillin V Potassium (Interference with bactericidal action of penicillin). Products include:

Pen•Vee K... 2772

Polysaccharide-Iron Complex (Should not be given concurrently). Products include:

Niferex-150 Capsules 793
Niferex Elixir 793
Niferex-150 Forte Capsules 794
Niferex Forte Elixir 794
Niferex 793
Niferex-PN Tablets 794
Nu-Iron 150 Capsules.......................... 1543
Nu-Iron Elixir 1543
Sunkist Children's Chewable Multivitamins - Plus Iron......................... ✪ 649

Ticarcillin Disodium (Interference with bactericidal action of penicillins). Products include:

Ticar for Injection 2526
Timentin for Injection........................... 2528

Warfarin Sodium (Downward adjustment of anticoagulant dosage may be necessary). Products include:

Coumadin 926

DOVE BAR

(Sodium Tallowate).............................. ✪ 672
None cited in PDR database.

LIQUID DOVE BEAUTY WASH

(Sodium Tallowate).............................. ✪ 672
None cited in PDR database.

DOVONEX OINTMENT 0.005%

(Calcipotriene) 2684
None cited in PDR database.

DOXIDAN LIQUI-GELS

(Docusate Calcium, Phenolphthalein)................................... ✪ 836
None cited in PDR database.

DOXORUBICIN HYDROCHLORIDE INJECTION

(Doxorubicin Hydrochloride) 540

See Doxorubicin Hydrochloride for Injection, USP.

DOXORUBICIN HYDROCHLORIDE FOR INJECTION, USP

(Doxorubicin Hydrochloride) 540
May interact with antineoplastics and certain other agents. Compounds in these categories include:

Altretamine (Toxicity of other anticancer therapies potentiated). Products include:

Hexalen Capsules 2571

Asparaginase (Toxicity of other anticancer therapies potentiated). Products include:

Elspar 1659

Bleomycin Sulfate (Toxicity of other anticancer therapies potentiated). Products include:

Blenoxane 692

Busulfan (Toxicity of other anticancer therapies potentiated). Products include:

Myleran Tablets 1143

Carboplatin (Toxicity of other anticancer therapies potentiated). Products include:

Paraplatin for Injection 705

Carmustine (BCNU) (Toxicity of other anticancer therapies potentiated). Products include:

BiCNU... 691

Chlorambucil (Toxicity of other anticancer therapies potentiated). Products include:

Leukeran Tablets 1133

Cisplatin (Toxicity of other anticancer therapies potentiated). Products include:

Platinol 708
Platinol-AQ Injection............................ 710

Cyclophosphamide (Toxicity of other anticancer therapies potentiated; exacerbation of cyclophosphamide-induced hemorrhagic cystitis). Products include:

Cytoxan 694
NEOSAR Lyophilized/Neosar 1959

Dacarbazine (Toxicity of other anticancer therapies potentiated). Products include:

DTIC-Dome 600

Daunorubicin Hydrochloride (Toxicity of other anticancer therapies potentiated). Products include:

Cerubidine 795

Estramustine Phosphate Sodium (Toxicity of other anticancer therapies potentiated). Products include:

Emcyt Capsules 1953

Etoposide (Toxicity of other anticancer therapies potentiated). Products include:

VePesid Capsules and Injection........ 718

Floxuridine (Toxicity of other anticancer therapies potentiated). Products include:

Sterile FUDR 2118

Fluorouracil (Toxicity of other anticancer therapies potentiated). Products include:

Efudex 2113
Fluoroplex Topical Solution & Cream 1% 479
Fluorouracil Injection 2116

Flutamide (Toxicity of other anticancer therapies potentiated). Products include:

Eulexin Capsules 2358

Hydroxyurea (Toxicity of other anticancer therapies potentiated). Products include:

Hydrea Capsules 696

IMPORTANT NOTE: Always consult each drug listing in the patient's regimen for possible interactions.

Idarubicin Hydrochloride (Toxicity of other anticancer therapies potentiated). Products include:
- Idamycin 1955

Ifosfamide (Toxicity of other anticancer therapies potentiated). Products include:
- IFEX 697

Interferon alfa-2A, Recombinant (Toxicity of other anticancer therapies potentiated). Products include:
- Roferon-A Injection 2145

Interferon alfa-2B, Recombinant (Toxicity of other anticancer therapies potentiated). Products include:
- Intron A 2364

Levamisole Hydrochloride (Toxicity of other anticancer therapies potentiated). Products include:
- Ergamisol Tablets 1292

Lomustine (CCNU) (Toxicity of other anticancer therapies potentiated). Products include:
- CeeNU 693

Mechlorethamine Hydrochloride (Toxicity of other anticancer therapies potentiated). Products include:
- Mustargen 1709

Megestrol Acetate (Toxicity of other anticancer therapies potentiated). Products include:
- Megace Oral Suspension 699
- Megace Tablets 701

Melphalan (Toxicity of other anticancer therapies potentiated). Products include:
- Alkeran Tablets 1071

Mercaptopurine (Toxicity of other anticancer therapies potentiated; enhancement of the hepatotoxicity of 6-mercaptopurine). Products include:
- Purinethol Tablets 1156

Methotrexate Sodium (Toxicity of other anticancer therapies potentiated). Products include:
- Methotrexate Sodium Tablets, Injection, for Injection and LPF Injection 1275

Mitomycin (Mitomycin-C) (Toxicity of other anticancer therapies potentiated). Products include:
- Mutamycin 703

Mitotane (Toxicity of other anticancer therapies potentiated). Products include:
- Lysodren 698

Mitoxantrone Hydrochloride (Toxicity of other anticancer therapies potentiated). Products include:
- Novantrone 1279

Paclitaxel (Toxicity of other anticancer therapies potentiated). Products include:
- Taxol 714

Procarbazine Hydrochloride (Toxicity of other anticancer therapies potentiated). Products include:
- Matulane Capsules 2131

Streptozocin (Toxicity of other anticancer therapies potentiated). Products include:
- Zanosar Sterile Powder 2653

Tamoxifen Citrate (Toxicity of other anticancer therapies potentiated). Products include:
- Nolvadex Tablets 2841

Teniposide (Toxicity of other anticancer therapies potentiated). Products include:
- Vumon 727

Thioguanine (Toxicity of other anticancer therapies potentiated). Products include:
- Thioguanine Tablets, Tabloid Brand 1181

Thiotepa (Toxicity of other anticancer therapies potentiated). Products include:
- Thioplex (Thiotepa For Injection) 1281

Vincristine Sulfate (Toxicity of other anticancer therapies potentiated). Products include:
- Oncovin Solution Vials & Hyporets 1466

Vinorelbine Tartrate (Toxicity of other anticancer therapies potentiated). Products include:
- Navelbine Injection 1145

DRAMAMINE CHEWABLE TABLETS
(Dimenhydrinate) .... ◙ 836

See **Dramamine Tablets**

CHILDREN'S DRAMAMINE LIQUID
(Dimenhydrinate) .... ◙ 836

See **Dramamine Tablets**

DRAMAMINE TABLETS
(Dimenhydrinate) .... ◙ 836

May interact with hypnotics and sedatives, tranquilizers, and certain other agents. Compounds in these categories include:

Alprazolam (May increase drowsiness effect). Products include:
- Xanax Tablets 2649

Buspirone Hydrochloride (May increase drowsiness effect). Products include:
- BuSpar 737

Chlordiazepoxide (May increase drowsiness effect). Products include:
- Libritabs Tablets 2177
- Limbitrol 2180

Chlordiazepoxide Hydrochloride (May increase drowsiness effect). Products include:
- Librax Capsules 2176
- Librium Capsules 2178
- Librium Injectable 2179

Chlorpromazine (May increase drowsiness effect). Products include:
- Thorazine Suppositories 2523

Chlorpromazine Hydrochloride (May increase drowsiness effect). Products include:
- Thorazine 2523

Chlorprothixene (May increase drowsiness effect).
- No products indexed under this heading.

Chlorprothixene Hydrochloride (May increase drowsiness effect).
- No products indexed under this heading.

Clorazepate Dipotassium (May increase drowsiness effect). Products include:
- Tranxene 451

Diazepam (May increase drowsiness effect). Products include:
- Dizac 1809
- Valium Injectable 2182
- Valium Tablets 2183
- Valrelease Capsules 2169

Droperidol (May increase drowsiness effect). Products include:
- Inapsine Injection 1296

Estazolam (May increase drowsiness effect). Products include:
- ProSom Tablets 449

Ethchlorvynol (May increase drowsiness effect). Products include:
- Placidyl Capsules 448

Ethinamate (May increase drowsiness effect).
- No products indexed under this heading.

Fluphenazine Decanoate (May increase drowsiness effect). Products include:
- Prolixin Decanoate 509

Fluphenazine Enanthate (May increase drowsiness effect). Products include:
- Prolixin Enanthate 509

Fluphenazine Hydrochloride (May increase drowsiness effect). Products include:
- Prolixin 509

Flurazepam Hydrochloride (May increase drowsiness effect). Products include:
- Dalmane Capsules 2173

Glutethimide (May increase drowsiness effect).
- No products indexed under this heading.

Haloperidol (May increase drowsiness effect). Products include:
- Haldol Injection, Tablets and Concentrate 1575

Haloperidol Decanoate (May increase drowsiness effect). Products include:
- Haldol Decanoate 1577

Hydroxyzine Hydrochloride (May increase drowsiness effect). Products include:
- Atarax Tablets & Syrup 2185
- Marax Tablets & DF Syrup 2200
- Vistaril Intramuscular Solution 2216

Lorazepam (May increase drowsiness effect). Products include:
- Ativan Injection 2698
- Ativan Tablets 2700

Loxapine Hydrochloride (May increase drowsiness effect). Products include:
- Loxitane 1378

Loxapine Succinate (May increase drowsiness effect). Products include:
- Loxitane Capsules 1378

Meprobamate (May increase drowsiness effect). Products include:
- Miltown Tablets 2672
- PMB 200 and PMB 400 2783

Mesoridazine Besylate (May increase drowsiness effect). Products include:
- Serentil 684

Midazolam Hydrochloride (May increase drowsiness effect). Products include:
- Versed Injection 2170

Molindone Hydrochloride (May increase drowsiness effect). Products include:
- Moban Tablets and Concentrate 1048

Oxazepam (May increase drowsiness effect). Products include:
- Serax Capsules 2810
- Serax Tablets 2810

Perphenazine (May increase drowsiness effect). Products include:
- Etrafon 2355
- Triavil Tablets 1757
- Trilafon 2389

Prazepam (May increase drowsiness effect).
- No products indexed under this heading.

Prochlorperazine (May increase drowsiness effect). Products include:
- Compazine 2470

Promethazine Hydrochloride (May increase drowsiness effect). Products include:
- Mepergan Injection 2753
- Phenergan with Codeine 2777
- Phenergan with Dextromethorphan 2778
- Phenergan Injection 2773
- Phenergan Suppositories 2775
- Phenergan Syrup 2774
- Phenergan Tablets 2775
- Phenergan VC 2779
- Phenergan VC with Codeine 2781

Propofol (May increase drowsiness effect). Products include:
- Diprivan Injection 2833

Quazepam (May increase drowsiness effect). Products include:
- Doral Tablets 2664

Secobarbital Sodium (May increase drowsiness effect). Products include:
- Seconal Sodium Pulvules 1474

Temazepam (May increase drowsiness effect). Products include:
- Restoril Capsules 2284

Thioridazine Hydrochloride (May increase drowsiness effect). Products include:
- Mellaril 2269

Thiothixene (May increase drowsiness effect). Products include:
- Navane Capsules and Concentrate 2201
- Navane Intramuscular 2202

Triazolam (May increase drowsiness effect). Products include:
- Halcion Tablets 2611

Trifluoperazine Hydrochloride (May increase drowsiness effect). Products include:
- Stelazine 2514

Zolpidem Tartrate (May increase drowsiness effect). Products include:
- Ambien Tablets 2416

Food Interactions

Alcohol (May increase drowsiness effect).

DRAMAMINE II TABLETS
(Meclizine Hydrochloride) .... ◙ 837

May interact with hypnotics and sedatives, tranquilizers, and certain other agents. Compounds in these categories include:

Alprazolam (May increase drowsiness effect). Products include:
- Xanax Tablets 2649

Buspirone Hydrochloride (May increase drowsiness effect). Products include:
- BuSpar 737

Chlordiazepoxide (May increase drowsiness effect). Products include:
- Libritabs Tablets 2177
- Limbitrol 2180

Chlordiazepoxide Hydrochloride (May increase drowsiness effect). Products include:
- Librax Capsules 2176
- Librium Capsules 2178
- Librium Injectable 2179

Chlorpromazine (May increase drowsiness effect). Products include:
- Thorazine Suppositories 2523

Chlorpromazine Hydrochloride (May increase drowsiness effect). Products include:
- Thorazine 2523

Chlorprothixene (May increase drowsiness effect).
- No products indexed under this heading.

Chlorprothixene Hydrochloride (May increase drowsiness effect).
- No products indexed under this heading.

Clorazepate Dipotassium (May increase drowsiness effect). Products include:
- Tranxene 451

Diazepam (May increase drowsiness effect). Products include:
- Dizac 1809
- Valium Injectable 2182

(◙ Described in PDR For Nonprescription Drugs) (◎ Described in PDR For Ophthalmology)

Valium Tablets 2183
Valrelease Capsules 2169

Droperidol (May increase drowsiness effect). Products include:
Inapsine Injection 1296

Estazolam (May increase drowsiness effect). Products include:
ProSom Tablets 449

Ethchlorvynol (May increase drowsiness effect). Products include:
Placidyl Capsules 448

Ethinamate (May increase drowsiness effect).
No products indexed under this heading.

Fluphenazine Decanoate (May increase drowsiness effect). Products include:
Prolixin Decanoate 509

Fluphenazine Enanthate (May increase drowsiness effect). Products include:
Prolixin Enanthate 509

Fluphenazine Hydrochloride (May increase drowsiness effect). Products include:
Prolixin 509

Flurazepam Hydrochloride (May increase drowsiness effect). Products include:
Dalmane Capsules 2173

Glutethimide (May increase drowsiness effect).
No products indexed under this heading.

Haloperidol (May increase drowsiness effect). Products include:
Haldol Injection, Tablets and Concentrate 1575

Haloperidol Decanoate (May increase drowsiness effect). Products include:
Haldol Decanoate 1577

Hydroxyzine Hydrochloride (May increase drowsiness effect). Products include:
Atarax Tablets & Syrup 2185
Marax Tablets & DF Syrup 2200
Vistaril Intramuscular Solution 2216

Lorazepam (May increase drowsiness effect). Products include:
Ativan Injection 2698
Ativan Tablets 2700

Loxapine Hydrochloride (May increase drowsiness effect). Products include:
Loxitane 1378

Loxapine Succinate (May increase drowsiness effect). Products include:
Loxitane Capsules 1378

Meprobamate (May increase drowsiness effect). Products include:
Miltown Tablets 2672
PMB 200 and PMB 400 2783

Mesoridazine Besylate (May increase drowsiness effect). Products include:
Serentil 684

Midazolam Hydrochloride (May increase drowsiness effect). Products include:
Versed Injection 2170

Molindone Hydrochloride (May increase drowsiness effect). Products include:
Moban Tablets and Concentrate 1048

Oxazepam (May increase drowsiness effect). Products include:
Serax Capsules 2810
Serax Tablets 2810

Perphenazine (May increase drowsiness effect). Products include:
Etrafon 2355
Triavil Tablets 1757
Trilafon 2389

Prazepam (May increase drowsiness effect).
No products indexed under this heading.

Prochlorperazine (May increase drowsiness effect). Products include:
Compazine 2470

Promethazine Hydrochloride (May increase drowsiness effect). Products include:
Mepergan Injection 2753
Phenergan with Codeine 2777
Phenergan with Dextromethorphan 2778
Phenergan Injection 2773
Phenergan Suppositories 2775
Phenergan Syrup 2774
Phenergan Tablets 2775
Phenergan VC 2779
Phenergan VC with Codeine 2781

Propofol (May increase drowsiness effect). Products include:
Diprivan Injection 2833

Quazepam (May increase drowsiness effect). Products include:
Doral Tablets 2664

Secobarbital Sodium (May increase drowsiness effect). Products include:
Seconal Sodium Pulvules 1474

Temazepam (May increase drowsiness effect). Products include:
Restoril Capsules 2284

Thioridazine Hydrochloride (May increase drowsiness effect). Products include:
Mellaril 2269

Thiothixene (May increase drowsiness effect). Products include:
Navane Capsules and Concentrate 2201
Navane Intramuscular 2202

Triazolam (May increase drowsiness effect). Products include:
Halcion Tablets 2611

Trifluoperazine Hydrochloride (May increase drowsiness effect). Products include:
Stelazine 2514

Zolpidem Tartrate (May increase drowsiness effect). Products include:
Ambien Tablets 2416

Food Interactions

Alcohol (May increase drowsiness effect).

DRISDOL

(Vitamin D) .... ᴴᴰ 794
None cited in PDR database.

DRITHOCREME 0.1%, 0.25%, 0.5%, 1.0% (HP)

(Anthralin) 905
May interact with:

Corticosteroids, Topical, Unspecified (Withdrawal of topical corticosteroids may give rise to a "rebound" phenomenon, an interval of at least one week should be allowed between the discontinuance of such steroids and the commencement of Drithocreme).

DRITHO-SCALP 0.25%, 0.5%

(Anthralin) 906
May interact with:

Corticosteroids, Topical, Unspecified (Withdrawal of topical corticosteroids may give rise to a "rebound" phenomenon, an interval of at least one week should be allowed between the discontinuance of such steroids and the commencement of Drithocreme).
No products indexed under this heading.

DRIXORAL COLD AND ALLERGY SUSTAINED-ACTION TABLETS

(Dexbrompheniramine Maleate, Pseudoephedrine Sulfate) .... ᴴᴰ 802
May interact with monoamine oxidase inhibitors and certain other agents. Compounds in these categories include:

Furazolidone (Concurrent and/or sequential use is not recommended). Products include:
Furoxone 2046

Isocarboxazid (Concurrent and/or sequential use is not recommended).
No products indexed under this heading.

Phenelzine Sulfate (Concurrent and/or sequential use is not recommended). Products include:
Nardil 1920

Selegiline Hydrochloride (Concurrent and/or sequential use is not recommended). Products include:
Eldepryl Tablets 2550

Tranylcypromine Sulfate (Concurrent and/or sequential use is not recommended). Products include:
Parnate Tablets 2503

Food Interactions

Alcohol (Increases drowsiness effect).

DRIXORAL COLD AND FLU EXTENDED-RELEASE TABLETS

(Acetaminophen, Dexbrompheniramine Maleate, Pseudoephedrine Sulfate) .... ᴴᴰ 803
May interact with antihypertensives, antidepressant drugs, hypnotics and sedatives, tranquilizers, and certain other agents. Compounds in these categories include:

Acebutolol Hydrochloride (Concurrent use is not recommended). Products include:
Sectral Capsules 2807

Alprazolam (Concurrent use is not recommended). Products include:
Xanax Tablets 2649

Amitriptyline Hydrochloride (Concurrent use is not recommended). Products include:
Elavil 2838
Endep Tablets 2174
Etrafon 2355
Limbitrol 2180
Triavil Tablets 1757

Amlodipine Besylate (Concurrent use is not recommended). Products include:
Lotrel Capsules 840
Norvasc Tablets 1940

Amoxapine (Concurrent use is not recommended). Products include:
Asendin Tablets 1369

Atenolol (Concurrent use is not recommended). Products include:
Tenoretic Tablets 2845

Tenormin Tablets and I.V. Injection 2847

Benazepril Hydrochloride (Concurrent use is not recommended). Products include:
Lotensin Tablets 834
Lotensin HCT 837
Lotrel Capsules 840

Bendroflumethiazide (Concurrent use is not recommended).
No products indexed under this heading.

Betaxolol Hydrochloride (Concurrent use is not recommended). Products include:
Betoptic Ophthalmic Solution 469
Betoptic S Ophthalmic Suspension 471
Kerlone Tablets 2436

Bisoprolol Fumarate (Concurrent use is not recommended). Products include:
Zebeta Tablets 1413
Ziac 1415

Bupropion Hydrochloride (Concurrent use is not recommended). Products include:
Wellbutrin Tablets 1204

Buspirone Hydrochloride (Concurrent use is not recommended). Products include:
BuSpar 737

Captopril (Concurrent use is not recommended). Products include:
Capoten 739
Capozide 742

Carteolol Hydrochloride (Concurrent use is not recommended). Products include:
Cartrol Tablets 410
Ocupress Ophthalmic Solution, 1% Sterile .... ⊙ 309

Chlordiazepoxide (Concurrent use is not recommended). Products include:
Libritabs Tablets 2177
Limbitrol 2180

Chlordiazepoxide Hydrochloride (Concurrent use is not recommended). Products include:
Librax Capsules 2176
Librium Capsules 2178
Librium Injectable 2179

Chlorothiazide (Concurrent use is not recommended). Products include:
Aldoclor Tablets 1598
Diupres Tablets 1650
Diuril Oral 1653

Chlorothiazide Sodium (Concurrent use is not recommended). Products include:
Diuril Sodium Intravenous 1652

Chlorpromazine (Concurrent use is not recommended). Products include:
Thorazine Suppositories 2523

Chlorprothixene (Concurrent use is not recommended).
No products indexed under this heading.

Chlorprothixene Hydrochloride (Concurrent use is not recommended).
No products indexed under this heading.

Chlorthalidone (Concurrent use is not recommended). Products include:
Combipres Tablets 677
Tenoretic Tablets 2845
Thalitone 1245

Clonidine (Concurrent use is not recommended). Products include:
Catapres-TTS 675

Clonidine Hydrochloride (Concurrent use is not recommended). Products include:
Catapres Tablets 674
Combipres Tablets 677

IMPORTANT NOTE: Always consult each drug listing in the patient's regimen for possible interactions.

Drixoral Cold and Flu Interactions Index 336

Clorazepate Dipotassium (Concurrent use is not recommended). Products include:
Tranxene ... 451
Deserpidine (Concurrent use is not recommended).
No products indexed under this heading.
Desipramine Hydrochloride (Concurrent use is not recommended). Products include:
Norpramin Tablets ... 1526
Diazepam (Concurrent use is not recommended). Products include:
Dizac ... 1809
Valium Injectable ... 2182
Valium Tablets ... 2183
Valrelease Capsules ... 2169
Diazoxide (Concurrent use is not recommended). Products include:
Hyperstat I.V. Injection ... 2363
Proglycem ... 580
Diltiazem Hydrochloride (Concurrent use is not recommended). Products include:
Cardizem CD Capsules ... 1506
Cardizem SR Capsules ... 1510
Cardizem Injectable ... 1508
Cardizem Tablets ... 1512
Dilacor XR Extended-release Capsules ... 2018
Doxazosin Mesylate (Concurrent use is not recommended). Products include:
Cardura Tablets ... 2186
Doxepin Hydrochloride (Concurrent use is not recommended). Products include:
Sinequan ... 2205
Zonalon Cream ... 1055
Droperidol (Concurrent use is not recommended). Products include:
Inapsine Injection ... 1296
Enalapril Maleate (Concurrent use is not recommended). Products include:
Vaseretic Tablets ... 1765
Vasotec Tablets ... 1771
Enalaprilat (Concurrent use is not recommended). Products include:
Vasotec I.V. ... 1768
Esmolol Hydrochloride (Concurrent use is not recommended). Products include:
Brevibloc Injection ... 1808
Estazolam (Concurrent use is not recommended). Products include:
ProSom Tablets ... 449
Ethchlorvynol (Concurrent use is not recommended). Products include:
Placidyl Capsules ... 448
Ethinamate (Concurrent use is not recommended).
No products indexed under this heading.
Felodipine (Concurrent use is not recommended). Products include:
Plendil Extended-Release Tablets ... 527
Fluoxetine Hydrochloride (Concurrent use is not recommended). Products include:
Prozac Pulvules & Liquid, Oral Solution ... 919
Fluphenazine Decanoate (Concurrent use is not recommended). Products include:
Prolixin Decanoate ... 509
Fluphenazine Enanthate (Concurrent use is not recommended). Products include:
Prolixin Enanthate ... 509
Fluphenazine Hydrochloride (Concurrent use is not recommended). Products include:
Prolixin ... 509
Flurazepam Hydrochloride (Concurrent use is not recommended). Products include:
Dalmane Capsules ... 2173
Fosinopril Sodium (Concurrent use is not recommended). Products include:
Monopril Tablets ... 757
Furosemide (Concurrent use is not recommended). Products include:
Lasix Injection, Oral Solution and Tablets ... 1240
Glutethimide (Concurrent use is not recommended).
No products indexed under this heading.
Guanabenz Acetate (Concurrent use is not recommended).
No products indexed under this heading.
Guanethidine Monosulfate (Concurrent use is not recommended). Products include:
Esimil Tablets ... 822
Ismelin Tablets ... 827
Haloperidol (Concurrent use is not recommended). Products include:
Haldol Injection, Tablets and Concentrate ... 1575
Haloperidol Decanoate (Concurrent use is not recommended). Products include:
Haldol Decanoate ... 1577
Hydralazine Hydrochloride (Concurrent use is not recommended). Products include:
Apresazide Capsules ... 808
Apresoline Hydrochloride Tablets ... 809
Ser-Ap-Es Tablets ... 849
Hydrochlorothiazide (Concurrent use is not recommended). Products include:
Aldactazide ... 2413
Aldoril Tablets ... 1604
Apresazide Capsules ... 808
Capozide ... 742
Dyazide ... 2479
Esidrix Tablets ... 821
Esimil Tablets ... 822
HydroDIURIL Tablets ... 1674
Hydropres Tablets ... 1675
Hyzaar Tablets ... 1677
Inderide Tablets ... 2732
Inderide LA Long Acting Capsules ... 2734
Lopressor HCT Tablets ... 832
Lotensin HCT ... 837
Maxzide ... 1380
Moduretic Tablets ... 1705
Oretic Tablets ... 443
Prinzide Tablets ... 1737
Ser-Ap-Es Tablets ... 849
Timolide Tablets ... 1748
Vaseretic Tablets ... 1765
Zestoretic ... 2850
Ziac ... 1415
Hydroflumethiazide (Concurrent use is not recommended). Products include:
Diucardin Tablets ... 2718
Hydroxyzine Hydrochloride (Concurrent use is not recommended). Products include:
Atarax Tablets & Syrup ... 2185
Marax Tablets & DF Syrup ... 2200
Vistaril Intramuscular Solution ... 2216
Imipramine Hydrochloride (Concurrent use is not recommended). Products include:
Tofranil Ampuls ... 854
Tofranil Tablets ... 856
Imipramine Pamoate (Concurrent use is not recommended). Products include:
Tofranil-PM Capsules ... 857
Indapamide (Concurrent use is not recommended). Products include:
Lozol Tablets ... 2022
Isocarboxazid (Concurrent use is not recommended).
No products indexed under this heading.
Isradipine (Concurrent use is not recommended). Products include:
DynaCirc Capsules ... 2256
Labetalol Hydrochloride (Concurrent use is not recommended). Products include:
Normodyne Injection ... 2377
Normodyne Tablets ... 2379
Trandate ... 1185
Lisinopril (Concurrent use is not recommended). Products include:
Prinivil Tablets ... 1733
Prinzide Tablets ... 1737
Zestoretic ... 2850
Zestril Tablets ... 2854
Lorazepam (Concurrent use is not recommended). Products include:
Ativan Injection ... 2698
Ativan Tablets ... 2700
Losartan Potassium (Concurrent use is not recommended). Products include:
Cozaar Tablets ... 1628
Hyzaar Tablets ... 1677
Loxapine Hydrochloride (Concurrent use is not recommended). Products include:
Loxitane ... 1378
Loxapine Succinate (Concurrent use is not recommended). Products include:
Loxitane Capsules ... 1378
Maprotiline Hydrochloride (Concurrent use is not recommended). Products include:
Ludiomil Tablets ... 843
Mecamylamine Hydrochloride (Concurrent use is not recommended). Products include:
Inversine Tablets ... 1686
Meprobamate (Concurrent use is not recommended). Products include:
Miltown Tablets ... 2672
PMB 200 and PMB 400 ... 2783
Mesoridazine Besylate (Concurrent use is not recommended). Products include:
Serentil ... 684
Methyclothiazide (Concurrent use is not recommended). Products include:
Enduron Tablets ... 420
Methyldopa (Concurrent use is not recommended). Products include:
Aldoclor Tablets ... 1598
Aldomet Oral ... 1600
Aldoril Tablets ... 1604
Methyldopate Hydrochloride (Concurrent use is not recommended). Products include:
Aldomet Ester HCl Injection ... 1602
Metolazone (Concurrent use is not recommended). Products include:
Mykrox Tablets ... 993
Zaroxolyn Tablets ... 1000
Metoprolol Succinate (Concurrent use is not recommended). Products include:
Toprol-XL Tablets ... 565
Metoprolol Tartrate (Concurrent use is not recommended). Products include:
Lopressor Ampuls ... 830
Lopressor HCT Tablets ... 832
Lopressor Tablets ... 830
Metyrosine (Concurrent use is not recommended). Products include:
Demser Capsules ... 1649
Midazolam Hydrochloride (Concurrent use is not recommended). Products include:
Versed Injection ... 2170
Minoxidil (Concurrent use is not recommended). Products include:
Loniten Tablets ... 2618
Rogaine Topical Solution ... 2637
Moexipril Hydrochloride (Concurrent use is not recommended). Products include:
Univasc Tablets ... 2410
Molindone Hydrochloride (Concurrent use is not recommended). Products include:
Moban Tablets and Concentrate ... 1048
Nadolol (Concurrent use is not recommended).
No products indexed under this heading.
Nefazodone Hydrochloride (Concurrent use is not recommended). Products include:
Serzone Tablets ... 771
Nicardipine Hydrochloride (Concurrent use is not recommended). Products include:
Cardene Capsules ... 2095
Cardene I.V. ... 2709
Cardene SR Capsules ... 2097
Nifedipine (Concurrent use is not recommended). Products include:
Adalat Capsules (10 mg and 20 mg) ... 587
Adalat CC ... 589
Procardia Capsules ... 1971
Procardia XL Extended Release Tablets ... 1972
Nisoldipine (Concurrent use is not recommended).
No products indexed under this heading.
Nitroglycerin (Concurrent use is not recommended). Products include:
Deponit NTG Transdermal Delivery System ... 2397
Nitro-Bid IV ... 1523
Nitro-Bid Ointment ... 1524
Nitrodisc ... 2047
Nitro-Dur (nitroglycerin) Transdermal Infusion System ... 1326
Nitrolingual Spray ... 2027
Nitrostat Tablets ... 1925
Transderm-Nitro Transdermal Therapeutic System ... 859
Nortriptyline Hydrochloride (Concurrent use is not recommended). Products include:
Pamelor ... 2280
Oxazepam (Concurrent use is not recommended). Products include:
Serax Capsules ... 2810
Serax Tablets ... 2810
Paroxetine Hydrochloride (Concurrent use is not recommended). Products include:
Paxil Tablets ... 2505
Penbutolol Sulfate (Concurrent use is not recommended). Products include:
Levatol ... 2403
Perphenazine (Concurrent use is not recommended). Products include:
Etrafon ... 2355
Triavil Tablets ... 1757
Trilafon ... 2389
Phenelzine Sulfate (Concurrent use is not recommended). Products include:
Nardil ... 1920
Phenoxybenzamine Hydrochloride (Concurrent use is not recommended). Products include:
Dibenzyline Capsules ... 2476
Phentolamine Mesylate (Concurrent use is not recommended). Products include:
Regitine ... 846
Pindolol (Concurrent use is not recommended). Products include:
Visken Tablets ... 2299
Polythiazide (Concurrent use is not recommended). Products include:
Minizide Capsules ... 1938

Prazepam (Concurrent use is not recommended).

No products indexed under this heading.

Prazosin Hydrochloride (Concurrent use is not recommended). Products include:

Minipress Capsules................................. 1937
Minizide Capsules................................... 1938

Prochlorperazine (Concurrent use is not recommended). Products include:

Compazine... 2470

Promethazine Hydrochloride (Concurrent use is not recommended). Products include:

Mepergan Injection................................. 2753
Phenergan with Codeine....................... 2777
Phenergan with Dextromethorphan 2778
Phenergan Injection............................... 2773
Phenergan Suppositories...................... 2775
Phenergan Syrup.................................... 2774
Phenergan Tablets.................................. 2775
Phenergan VC... 2779
Phenergan VC with Codeine................ 2781

Propofol (Concurrent use is not recommended). Products include:

Diprivan Injection.................................... 2833

Propranolol Hydrochloride (Concurrent use is not recommended). Products include:

Inderal... 2728
Inderal LA Long Acting Capsules..... 2730
Inderide Tablets...................................... 2732
Inderide LA Long Acting Capsules.. 2734

Protriptyline Hydrochloride (Concurrent use is not recommended). Products include:

Vivactil Tablets.. 1774

Quazepam (Concurrent use is not recommended). Products include:

Doral Tablets.. 2664

Quinapril Hydrochloride (Concurrent use is not recommended). Products include:

Accupril Tablets...................................... 1893

Ramipril (Concurrent use is not recommended). Products include:

Altace Capsules...................................... 1232

Rauwolfia Serpentina (Concurrent use is not recommended).

No products indexed under this heading.

Rescinnamine (Concurrent use is not recommended).

No products indexed under this heading.

Reserpine (Concurrent use is not recommended). Products include:

Diupres Tablets....................................... 1650
Hydropres Tablets................................... 1675
Ser-Ap-Es Tablets................................... 849

Secobarbital Sodium (Concurrent use is not recommended). Products include:

Seconal Sodium Pulvules..................... 1474

Sertraline Hydrochloride (Concurrent use is not recommended). Products include:

Zoloft Tablets... 2217

Sodium Nitroprusside (Concurrent use is not recommended).

No products indexed under this heading.

Sotalol Hydrochloride (Concurrent use is not recommended). Products include:

Betapace Tablets..................................... 641

Spirapril Hydrochloride (Concurrent use is not recommended).

No products indexed under this heading.

Temazepam (Concurrent use is not recommended). Products include:

Restoril Capsules.................................... 2284

Terazosin Hydrochloride (Concurrent use is not recommended). Products include:

Hytrin Capsules....................................... 430

Thioridazine Hydrochloride (Concurrent use is not recommended). Products include:

Mellaril... 2269

Thiothixene (Concurrent use is not recommended). Products include:

Navane Capsules and Concentrate 2201
Navane Intramuscular........................... 2202

Timolol Maleate (Concurrent use is not recommended). Products include:

Blocadren Tablets................................... 1614
Timolide Tablets...................................... 1748
Timoptic in Ocudose............................. 1753
Timoptic Sterile Ophthalmic Solution.. 1751
Timoptic-XE... 1755

Torsemide (Concurrent use is not recommended). Products include:

Demadex Tablets and Injection......... 686

Tranylcypromine Sulfate (Concurrent use is not recommended). Products include:

Parnate Tablets....................................... 2503

Trazodone Hydrochloride (Concurrent use is not recommended). Products include:

Desyrel and Desyrel Dividose............ 503

Triazolam (Concurrent use is not recommended). Products include:

Halcion Tablets.. 2611

Trifluoperazine Hydrochloride (Concurrent use is not recommended). Products include:

Stelazine.. 2514

Trimethaphan Camsylate (Concurrent use is not recommended). Products include:

Arfonad Ampuls...................................... 2080

Trimipramine Maleate (Concurrent use is not recommended). Products include:

Surmontil Capsules................................ 2811

Venlafaxine Hydrochloride (Concurrent use is not recommended). Products include:

Effexor... 2719

Verapamil Hydrochloride (Concurrent use is not recommended). Products include:

Calan SR Caplets.................................... 2422
Calan Tablets... 2419
Isoptin Injectable.................................... 1344
Isoptin Oral Tablets................................ 1346
Isoptin SR Tablets................................... 1348
Verelan Capsules.................................... 1410
Verelan Capsules.................................... 2824

Zolpidem Tartrate (Concurrent use is not recommended). Products include:

Ambien Tablets.. 2416

Food Interactions

Alcohol (Increases drowsiness effect).

DRIXORAL COUGH LIQUID CAPS

(Dextromethorphan Hydrobromide).................................... ✦ 801

May interact with monoamine oxidase inhibitors. Compounds in this category include:

Furazolidone (Concurrent use not recommended; consult your doctor). Products include:

Furoxone.. 2046

Isocarboxazid (Concurrent use not recommended; consult your doctor).

No products indexed under this heading.

Phenelzine Sulfate (Concurrent use not recommended; consult your doctor). Products include:

Nardil.. 1920

Selegiline Hydrochloride (Concurrent use not recommended; consult your doctor). Products include:

Eldepryl Tablets....................................... 2550

Tranylcypromine Sulfate (Concurrent use not recommended; consult your doctor). Products include:

Parnate Tablets....................................... 2503

DRIXORAL COUGH + CONGESTION LIQUID CAPS

(Dextromethorphan Hydrobromide, Pseudoephedrine Hydrochloride).... ✦ 802

May interact with monoamine oxidase inhibitors. Compounds in this category include:

Furazolidone (Concurrent use not recommended; consult your doctor). Products include:

Furoxone.. 2046

Isocarboxazid (Concurrent use not recommended; consult your doctor).

No products indexed under this heading.

Phenelzine Sulfate (Concurrent use not recommended; consult your doctor). Products include:

Nardil.. 1920

Selegiline Hydrochloride (Concurrent use not recommended; consult your doctor). Products include:

Eldepryl Tablets....................................... 2550

Tranylcypromine Sulfate (Concurrent use not recommended; consult your doctor). Products include:

Parnate Tablets....................................... 2503

DRIXORAL COUGH + SORE THROAT LIQUID CAPS

(Dextromethorphan Hydrobromide, Acetaminophen).................................... ✦ 802

May interact with monoamine oxidase inhibitors. Compounds in this category include:

Furazolidone (Concurrent use not recommended; consult your doctor). Products include:

Furoxone.. 2046

Isocarboxazid (Concurrent use not recommended; consult your doctor).

No products indexed under this heading.

Phenelzine Sulfate (Concurrent use not recommended; consult your doctor). Products include:

Nardil.. 1920

Selegiline Hydrochloride (Concurrent use not recommended; consult your doctor). Products include:

Eldepryl Tablets....................................... 2550

Tranylcypromine Sulfate (Concurrent use not recommended; consult your doctor). Products include:

Parnate Tablets....................................... 2503

DRIXORAL NON-DROWSY FORMULA EXTENDED-RELEASE TABLETS

(Pseudoephedrine Sulfate)................ ✦ 803

May interact with:

Antidepressant Medications, unspecified (Effects not specified).

Blood Pressure Medications, unspecified (Effects not specified).

No products indexed under this heading.

DRIXORAL ALLERGY/SINUS EXTENDED RELEASE TABLETS

(Acetaminophen, Pseudoephedrine Sulfate, Dexbrompheniramine Maleate).. ✦ 804

May interact with hypnotics and sedatives, tranquilizers, monoamine oxidase inhibitors, and certain other agents. Compounds in these categories include:

Alprazolam (May increase the drowsiness effect). Products include:

Xanax Tablets.. 2649

Buspirone Hydrochloride (May increase the drowsiness effect). Products include:

BuSpar... 737

Chlordiazepoxide (May increase the drowsiness effect). Products include:

Libritabs Tablets...................................... 2177
Limbitrol... 2180

Chlordiazepoxide Hydrochloride (May increase the drowsiness effect). Products include:

Librax Capsules....................................... 2176
Librium Capsules.................................... 2178
Librium Injectable................................... 2179

Chlorpromazine (May increase the drowsiness effect). Products include:

Thorazine Suppositories....................... 2523

Chlorpromazine Hydrochloride (May increase the drowsiness effect). Products include:

Thorazine... 2523

Chlorprothixene (May increase the drowsiness effect).

No products indexed under this heading.

Chlorprothixene Hydrochloride (May increase the drowsiness effect).

No products indexed under this heading.

Clorazepate Dipotassium (May increase the drowsiness effect). Products include:

Tranxene.. 451

Diazepam (May increase the drowsiness effect). Products include:

Dizac... 1809
Valium Injectable.................................... 2182
Valium Tablets... 2183
Valrelease Capsules............................... 2169

Droperidol (May increase the drowsiness effect). Products include:

Inapsine Injection................................... 1296

Estazolam (May increase the drowsiness effect). Products include:

ProSom Tablets....................................... 449

Ethchlorvynol (May increase the drowsiness effect). Products include:

Placidyl Capsules.................................... 448

Ethinamate (May increase the drowsiness effect).

No products indexed under this heading.

Fluphenazine Decanoate (May increase the drowsiness effect). Products include:

Prolixin Decanoate.................................. 509

Fluphenazine Enanthate (May increase the drowsiness effect). Products include:

Prolixin Enanthate.................................. 509

Fluphenazine Hydrochloride (May increase the drowsiness effect). Products include:

Prolixin... 509

Flurazepam Hydrochloride (May increase the drowsiness effect). Products include:

Dalmane Capsules.................................. 2173

IMPORTANT NOTE: Always consult each drug listing in the patient's regimen for possible interactions.

Furazolidone (Concurrent and/or sequential use is not recommended). Products include:
- Furoxone ... 2046

Glutethimide (May increase the drowsiness effect).
- No products indexed under this heading.

Haloperidol (May increase the drowsiness effect). Products include:
- Haldol Injection, Tablets and Concentrate ... 1575

Haloperidol Decanoate (May increase the drowsiness effect). Products include:
- Haldol Decanoate ... 1577

Hydroxyzine Hydrochloride (May increase the drowsiness effect). Products include:
- Atarax Tablets & Syrup ... 2185
- Marax Tablets & DF Syrup ... 2200
- Vistaril Intramuscular Solution ... 2216

Isocarboxazid (Concurrent and/or sequential use is not recommended).
- No products indexed under this heading.

Lorazepam (May increase the drowsiness effect). Products include:
- Ativan Injection ... 2698
- Ativan Tablets ... 2700

Loxapine Hydrochloride (May increase the drowsiness effect). Products include:
- Loxitane ... 1378

Loxapine Succinate (May increase the drowsiness effect). Products include:
- Loxitane Capsules ... 1378

Meprobamate (May increase the drowsiness effect). Products include:
- Miltown Tablets ... 2672
- PMB 200 and PMB 400 ... 2783

Mesoridazine Besylate (May increase the drowsiness effect). Products include:
- Serentil ... 684

Midazolam Hydrochloride (May increase the drowsiness effect). Products include:
- Versed Injection ... 2170

Molindone Hydrochloride (May increase the drowsiness effect). Products include:
- Moban Tablets and Concentrate ... 1048

Oxazepam (May increase the drowsiness effect). Products include:
- Serax Capsules ... 2810
- Serax Tablets ... 2810

Perphenazine (May increase the drowsiness effect). Products include:
- Etrafon ... 2355
- Triavil Tablets ... 1757
- Trilafon ... 2389

Phenelzine Sulfate (Concurrent and/or sequential use is not recommended). Products include:
- Nardil ... 1920

Prazepam (May increase the drowsiness effect).
- No products indexed under this heading.

Prochlorperazine (May increase the drowsiness effect). Products include:
- Compazine ... 2470

Promethazine Hydrochloride (May increase the drowsiness effect). Products include:
- Mepergan Injection ... 2753
- Phenergan with Codeine ... 2777
- Phenergan with Dextromethorphan 2778
- Phenergan Injection ... 2773
- Phenergan Suppositories ... 2775
- Phenergan Syrup ... 2774
- Phenergan Tablets ... 2775
- Phenergan VC ... 2779
- Phenergan VC with Codeine ... 2781

Propofol (May increase the drowsiness effect). Products include:
- Diprivan Injection ... 2833

Quazepam (May increase the drowsiness effect). Products include:
- Doral Tablets ... 2664

Secobarbital Sodium (May increase the drowsiness effect). Products include:
- Seconal Sodium Pulvules ... 1474

Selegiline Hydrochloride (Concurrent and/or sequential use is not recommended). Products include:
- Eldepryl Tablets ... 2550

Temazepam (May increase the drowsiness effect). Products include:
- Restoril Capsules ... 2284

Thioridazine Hydrochloride (May increase the drowsiness effect). Products include:
- Mellaril ... 2269

Thiothixene (May increase the drowsiness effect). Products include:
- Navane Capsules and Concentrate 2201
- Navane Intramuscular ... 2202

Tranylcypromine Sulfate (Concurrent and/or sequential use is not recommended). Products include:
- Parnate Tablets ... 2503

Triazolam (May increase the drowsiness effect). Products include:
- Halcion Tablets ... 2611

Trifluoperazine Hydrochloride (May increase the drowsiness effect). Products include:
- Stelazine ... 2514

Zolpidem Tartrate (May increase the drowsiness effect). Products include:
- Ambien Tablets ... 2416

Food Interactions

Alcohol (May increase the drowsiness effect).

DRYSOL
(Aluminum Chloride) ... 1932
None cited in PDR database.

DULCOLAX SUPPOSITORIES
(Bisacodyl) ... 864
None cited in PDR database.

DULCOLAX TABLETS
(Bisacodyl) ... 864
None cited in PDR database.

DUODERM CGF CONTROL GEL FORMULA DRESSING
(Hydrocolloids) ... 2864
None cited in PDR database.

DUODERM CGF CONTROL GEL FORMULA BORDER DRESSING
(Hydrocolloids) ... 2864
None cited in PDR database.

DUODERM EXTRA THIN CGF DRESSING
(Hydrocolloids) ... 2863
None cited in PDR database.

DUODERM GEL
(Dressings, sterile) ... 2863
None cited in PDR database.

DUODERM HYDROACTIVE DRESSING
(Hydrocolloids) ... 2865
None cited in PDR database.

DUODERM SCB SUSTAINED COMPRESSION BANDAGE
(Hydrocolloids) ... 2865
None cited in PDR database.

DUOFILM LIQUID WART REMOVER
(Salicylic Acid) ... ◘ 804
None cited in PDR database.

DUOFILM PATCH WART REMOVER
(Salicylic Acid) ... ◘ 804
None cited in PDR database.

DUOPLANT GEL PLANTAR WART REMOVER
(Salicylic Acid) ... ◘ 804
None cited in PDR database.

DURAGESIC TRANSDERMAL SYSTEM
(Fentanyl) ... 1288
May interact with central nervous system depressants, narcotic analgesics, hypnotics and sedatives, tranquilizers, phenothiazines, antihistamines, and certain other agents. Compounds in these categories include:

Acrivastine (May produce additive depressant effects, hypoventilation, hypotension and profound sedation or coma may occur). Products include:
- Semprex-D Capsules ... 463
- Semprex-D Capsules ... 1167

Alfentanil Hydrochloride (May produce additive depressant effects, hypoventilation, hypotension and profound sedation or coma may occur). Products include:
- Alfenta Injection ... 1286

Alprazolam (May produce additive depressant effects, hypoventilation, hypotension and profound sedation or coma may occur). Products include:
- Xanax Tablets ... 2649

Aprobarbital (May produce additive depressant effects, hypoventilation, hypotension and profound sedation or coma may occur).
- No products indexed under this heading.

Astemizole (May produce additive depressant effects, hypoventilation, hypotension and profound sedation or coma may occur). Products include:
- Hismanal Tablets ... 1293

Azatadine Maleate (May produce additive depressant effects, hypoventilation, hypotension and profound sedation or coma may occur). Products include:
- Trinalin Repetabs Tablets ... 1330

Bromodiphenhydramine Hydrochloride (May produce additive depressant effects, hypoventilation, hypotension and profound sedation or coma may occur).
- No products indexed under this heading.

Brompheniramine Maleate (May produce additive depressant effects, hypoventilation, hypotension and profound sedation or coma may occur). Products include:
- Alka Seltzer Plus Sinus Medicine .. ◘ 707
- Bromfed Capsules (Extended-Release) ... 1785
- Bromfed Syrup ... ◘ 733
- Bromfed Tablets ... 1785
- Bromfed-DM Cough Syrup ... 1786
- Bromfed-PD Capsules (Extended-Release) ... 1785
- Dimetane-DC Cough Syrup ... 2059
- Dimetane-DX Cough Syrup ... 2059
- Dimetapp Elixir ... ◘ 773
- Dimetapp Extentabs ... ◘ 774
- Dimetapp Tablets/Liqui-Gels ... ◘ 775
- Dimetapp Cold & Allergy Chewable Tablets ... ◘ 773
- Dimetapp DM Elixir ... ◘ 774
- Vicks DayQuil Allergy Relief 12-Hour Extended Release Tablets.. ◘ 760
- Vicks DayQuil Allergy Relief 4-Hour Tablets ... ◘ 760

Buprenorphine (May produce additive depressant effects, hypoventilation, hypotension and profound sedation or coma may occur). Products include:
- Buprenex Injectable ... 2006

Buspirone Hydrochloride (May produce additive depressant effects, hypoventilation, hypotension and profound sedation or coma may occur). Products include:
- BuSpar ... 737

Butabarbital (May produce additive depressant effects, hypoventilation, hypotension and profound sedation or coma may occur).
- No products indexed under this heading.

Butalbital (May produce additive depressant effects, hypoventilation, hypotension and profound sedation or coma may occur). Products include:
- Esgic-plus Tablets ... 1013
- Fioricet Tablets ... 2258
- Fioricet with Codeine Capsules ... 2260
- Fiorinal Capsules ... 2261
- Fiorinal with Codeine Capsules ... 2262
- Fiorinal Tablets ... 2261
- Phrenilin ... 785
- Sedapap Tablets 50 mg/650 mg .. 1543

Chlordiazepoxide (May produce additive depressant effects, hypoventilation, hypotension and profound sedation or coma may occur). Products include:
- Libritabs Tablets ... 2177
- Limbitrol ... 2180

Chlordiazepoxide Hydrochloride (May produce additive depressant effects, hypoventilation, hypotension and profound sedation or coma may occur). Products include:
- Librax Capsules ... 2176
- Librium Capsules ... 2178
- Librium Injectable ... 2179

Chlorpheniramine Maleate (May produce additive depressant effects, hypoventilation, hypotension and profound sedation or coma may occur). Products include:
- Alka-Seltzer Plus Cold Medicine ... ◘ 705
- Alka-Seltzer Plus Cold Medicine Liqui-Gels ... ◘ 706
- Alka-Seltzer Plus Cold & Cough Medicine ... ◘ 708
- Alka-Seltzer Plus Cold & Cough Medicine Liqui-Gels ... ◘ 705
- Allerest Children's Chewable Tablets ... ◘ 627
- Allerest Headache Strength Tablets ... ◘ 627
- Allerest Maximum Strength Tablets ... ◘ 627
- Allerest Sinus Pain Formula ... ◘ 627
- Allerest 12 Hour Caplets ... ◘ 627
- Ana-Kit Anaphylaxis Emergency Treatment Kit ... 617
- Atrohist Pediatric Capsules ... 453
- Atrohist Plus Tablets ... 454
- BC Cold Powder Multi-Symptom Formula (Cold-Sinus-Allergy) ... ◘ 609
- Cerose DM ... ◘ 878
- Cheracol Plus Head Cold/Cough Formula ... ◘ 769
- Children's Vicks DayQuil Allergy Relief ... ◘ 757
- Children's Vicks NyQuil Cold/Cough Relief ... ◘ 758
- Chlor-Trimeton Allergy Decongestant Tablets ... ◘ 799
- Chlor-Trimeton Allergy Tablets ... ◘ 798
- Comhist ... 2038
- Comtrex Multi-Symptom Cold Reliever Tablets/Caplets/Liqui-Gels/Liquid ... ◘ 615

(◘ Described in PDR For Nonprescription Drugs) (◉ Described in PDR For Ophthalmology)

Interactions Index

Duragesic

Allergy-Sinus Comtrex Multi-Symptom Allergy-Sinus Formula Tablets .... ◾ 617

Contac Continuous Action Nasal Decongestant/Antihistamine 12 Hour Capsules .... ◾ 813

Contac Maximum Strength Continuous Action Decongestant/Antihistamine 12 Hour Caplets.. ◾ 813

Contac Severe Cold and Flu Formula Caplets .... ◾ 814

Coricidin 'D' Decongestant Tablets .... ◾ 800

Coricidin Tablets .... ◾ 800

D.A. Chewable Tablets 951

Deconamine 1320

Dura-Tap/PD Capsules 2867

Dura-Vent/DA Tablets 953

Extendryl 1005

Fedahist Gyrocaps 2401

Fedahist Timecaps 2401

Hycomine Compound Tablets 932

Isoclor Timesule Capsules .... ◾ 637

Kronofed-A 977

Nolamine Timed-Release Tablets 785

Novahistine DH 2462

Novahistine Elixir .... ◾ 823

Ornade Spansule Capsules 2502

PediaCare Cold Allergy Chewable Tablets .... ◾ 677

PediaCare Cough-Cold Chewable Tablets 1553

PediaCare Cough-Cold Liquid 1553

PediaCare NightRest Cough-Cold Liquid 1553

Pediatric Vicks 44m Cough & Cold Relief .... ◾ 764

Pyrroxate Caplets .... ◾ 772

Ryna .... ◾ 841

Sinarest Tablets .... ◾ 648

Sinarest Extra Strength Tablets ...... ◾ 648

Sine-Off Sinus Medicine .... ◾ 825

Singlet Tablets .... ◾ 825

Sinulin Tablets 787

Sinutab Sinus Allergy Medication, Maximum Strength Tablets and Caplets .... ◾ 860

Sudafed Plus Liquid .... ◾ 862

Sudafed Plus Tablets .... ◾ 863

Teldrin 12 Hour Antihistamine/Nasal Decongestant Allergy Relief Capsules .... ◾ 826

TheraFlu .... ◾ 787

TheraFlu Maximum Strength Nighttime Flu, Cold & Cough Medicine .... ◾ 788

Triaminic Allergy Tablets .... ◾ 789

Triaminic Cold Tablets .... ◾ 790

Triaminic Nite Light .... ◾ 791

Triaminic Syrup .... ◾ 792

Triaminic-12 Tablets .... ◾ 792

Triaminicin Tablets .... ◾ 793

Triaminicol Multi-Symptom Cold Tablets .... ◾ 793

Triaminicol Multi-Symptom Relief ◾ 794

Tussend 1783

Children's TYLENOL Cold Multi-Symptom Liquid Formula and Chewable Tablets 1561

Children's TYLENOL Cold Plus Cough Multi Symptom Tablets and Liquid .... ◾ 681

TYLENOL Maximum Strength Allergy Sinus Medication Gelcaps and Caplets 1563

TYLENOL Cold Multi-Symptom Formula Medication Tablets and Caplets 1561

TYLENOL Cold Multi-Symptom Hot Medication Liquid Packets 1557

Vicks 44 LiquiCaps Cough, Cold & Flu Relief .... ◾ 755

Vicks 44M Cough, Cold & Flu Relief .... ◾ 756

Chlorpheniramine Polistirex (May produce additive depressant effects, hypoventilation, hypotension and profound sedation or coma may occur). Products include:

Tussionex Pennkinetic Extended-Release Suspension 998

Chlorpheniramine Tannate (May produce additive depressant effects, hypoventilation, hypotension and profound sedation or coma may occur). Products include:

Atrohist Pediatric Suspension 454

Ricobid Tablets and Pediatric Suspension 2038

Rynatan 2673

Rynatuss 2673

Chlorpromazine (May produce additive depressant effects, hypoventilation, hypotension and profound sedation or coma may occur). Products include:

Thorazine Suppositories 2523

Chlorprothixene (May produce additive depressant effects, hypoventilation, hypotension and profound sedation or coma may occur).

No products indexed under this heading.

Chlorprothixene Hydrochloride (May produce additive depressant effects, hypoventilation, hypotension and profound sedation or coma may occur).

No products indexed under this heading.

Clemastine Fumarate (May produce additive depressant effects, hypoventilation, hypotension and profound sedation or coma may occur). Products include:

Tavist Syrup 2297

Tavist Tablets 2298

Tavist-1 12 Hour Relief Tablets .... ◾ 787

Tavist-D 12 Hour Relief Tablets .... ◾ 787

Clorazepate Dipotassium (May produce additive depressant effects, hypoventilation, hypotension and profound sedation or coma may occur). Products include:

Tranxene 451

Clozapine (May produce additive depressant effects, hypoventilation, hypotension and profound sedation or coma may occur). Products include:

Clozaril Tablets 2252

Codeine Phosphate (May produce additive depressant effects, hypoventilation, hypotension and profound sedation or coma may occur). Products include:

Actifed with Codeine Cough Syrup.. 1067

Brontex 1981

Deconsal C Expectorant Syrup 456

Deconsal Pediatric Syrup 457

Dimetane-DC Cough Syrup 2059

Empirin with Codeine Tablets 1093

Fioricet with Codeine Capsules 2260

Fiorinal with Codeine Capsules 2262

Isoclor Expectorant 990

Novahistine DH 2462

Novahistine Expectorant 2463

Nucofed 2051

Phenergan with Codeine 2777

Phenergan VC with Codeine 2781

Robitussin A-C Syrup 2073

Robitussin-DAC Syrup 2074

Ryna .... ◾ 841

Soma Compound w/Codeine Tablets 2676

Tussi-Organidin NR Liquid and S NR Liquid 2677

Tylenol with Codeine 1583

Cyproheptadine Hydrochloride (May produce additive depressant effects, hypoventilation, hypotension and profound sedation or coma may occur). Products include:

Periactin 1724

Desflurane (May produce additive depressant effects, hypoventilation, hypotension and profound sedation or coma may occur). Products include:

Suprane 1813

Dexchlorpheniramine Maleate (May produce additive depressant effects, hypoventilation, hypotension and profound sedation or coma may occur).

No products indexed under this heading.

Dezocine (May produce additive depressant effects, hypoventilation, hypotension and profound sedation or coma may occur). Products include:

Dalgan Injection 538

Diazepam (May produce additive depressant effects, hypoventilation, hypotension and profound sedation or coma may occur). Products include:

Dizac 1809

Valium Injectable 2182

Valium Tablets 2183

Valrelease Capsules 2169

Diphenhydramine Citrate (May produce additive depressant effects, hypoventilation, hypotension and profound sedation or coma may occur). Products include:

Excedrin P.M. Analgesic/Sleeping Aid Tablets, Caplets, Liquigels 733

Diphenhydramine Hydrochloride (May produce additive depressant effects, hypoventilation, hypotension and profound sedation or coma may occur). Products include:

Actifed Allergy Daytime/Nighttime Caplets .... ◾ 844

Actifed Sinus Daytime/Nighttime Tablets and Caplets .... ◾ 846

Arthritis Foundation NightTime Caplets .... ◾ 674

Extra Strength Bayer PM Aspirin .. ◾ 713

Bayer Select Night Time Pain Relief Formula .... ◾ 716

Benadryl Allergy Decongestant Liquid Medication .... ◾ 848

Benadryl Allergy Decongestant Tablets .... ◾ 848

Benadryl Allergy Liquid Medication .... ◾ 849

Benadryl Allergy .... ◾ 848

Benadryl Allergy Sinus Headache Formula Caplets .... ◾ 849

Benadryl Capsules 1898

Benadryl Dye-Free Allergy Liquigel Softgels .... ◾ 850

Benadryl Dye-Free Allergy Liquid Medication .... ◾ 850

Benadryl Itch Relief Cream, Children's Formula and Maximum Strength 2% .... ◾ 851

Benadryl Itch Relief Spray, Children's Formula and Maximum Strength 2% .... ◾ 851

Benadryl Itch Relief Stick Maximum Strength 2% .... ◾ 850

Benadryl Itch Stopping Gel, Children's Formula and Maximum Strength 2% .... ◾ 851

Benadryl Kapseals 1898

Benadryl Injection 1898

Contac Day & Night Cold/Flu Night Caplets .... ◾ 812

Contac Night Allergy/Sinus Caplets .... ◾ 812

Extra Strength Doan's P.M. .... ◾ 633

Legatrin PM .... ◾ 651

Miles Nervine Nighttime Sleep-Aid ◾ 723

Nytol QuickCaps Caplets .... ◾ 610

Sleepinal Night-time Sleep Aid Capsules and Softgels .... ◾ 834

TYLENOL Maximum Strength Allergy Sinus NightTime Medication Caplets 1555

TYLENOL Flu NightTime, Maximum Strength, Gelcaps 1566

TYLENOL Maximum Strength Flu NightTime Hot Medication Packets 1562

TYLENOL PM, Extra Strength Pain Reliever/Sleep Aid Caplets, Geltabs, Gelcaps 1560

TYLENOL Severe Allergy Medication Caplets 1564

Maximum Strength Unisom Sleepgels 1934

Unisom With Pain Relief-Nighttime Sleep Aid and Pain Reliever 1934

Droperidol (May produce additive depressant effects, hypoventilation, hypotension and profound sedation or coma may occur). Products include:

Inapsine Injection 1296

Enflurane (May produce additive depressant effects, hypoventilation, hypotension and profound sedation or coma may occur).

No products indexed under this heading.

Estazolam (May produce additive depressant effects, hypoventilation, hypotension and profound sedation or coma may occur). Products include:

ProSom Tablets 449

Ethchlorvynol (May produce additive depressant effects, hypoventilation, hypotension and profound sedation or coma may occur). Products include:

Placidyl Capsules 448

Ethinamate (May produce additive depressant effects, hypoventilation, hypotension and profound sedation or coma may occur).

No products indexed under this heading.

Fentanyl Citrate (May produce additive depressant effects, hypoventilation, hypotension and profound sedation or coma may occur). Products include:

Sublimaze Injection 1307

Fluphenazine Decanoate (May produce additive depressant effects, hypoventilation, hypotension and profound sedation or coma may occur). Products include:

Prolixin Decanoate 509

Fluphenazine Enanthate (May produce additive depressant effects, hypoventilation, hypotension and profound sedation or coma may occur). Products include:

Prolixin Enanthate 509

Fluphenazine Hydrochloride (May produce additive depressant effects, hypoventilation, hypotension and profound sedation or coma may occur). Products include:

Prolixin 509

Flurazepam Hydrochloride (May produce additive depressant effects, hypoventilation, hypotension and profound sedation or coma may occur). Products include:

Dalmane Capsules 2173

Glutethimide (May produce additive depressant effects, hypoventilation, hypotension and profound sedation or coma may occur).

No products indexed under this heading.

Haloperidol (May produce additive depressant effects, hypoventilation, hypotension and profound sedation or coma may occur). Products include:

Haldol Injection, Tablets and Concentrate 1575

Haloperidol Decanoate (May produce additive depressant effects, hypoventilation, hypotension and profound sedation or coma may occur). Products include:

Haldol Decanoate 1577

Hydrocodone Bitartrate (May produce additive depressant effects, hypoventilation, hypotension and profound sedation or coma may occur). Products include:

Anexsia 5/500 Elixir 1781

Anexia Tablets 1782

Codiclear DH Syrup 791

Deconamine CX Cough and Cold Liquid and Tablets 1319

Duratuss HD Elixir 2565

Hycodan Tablets and Syrup 930

Hycomine Compound Tablets 932

Hycomine 931

Hycotuss Expectorant Syrup 933

Hydrocet Capsules 782

IMPORTANT NOTE: Always consult each drug listing in the patient's regimen for possible interactions.

Duragesic

Lorcet 10/650 1018
Lortab 2566
Tussend 1783
Tussend Expectorant 1785
Vicodin Tablets 1356
Vicodin ES Tablets 1357
Vicodin Tuss Expectorant 1358
Zydone Capsules 949

Hydrocodone Polistirex (May produce additive depressant effects, hypoventilation, hypotension and profound sedation or coma may occur). Products include:

Tussionex Pennkinetic Extended-Release Suspension 998

Hydroxyzine Hydrochloride (May produce additive depressant effects, hypoventilation, hypotension and profound sedation or coma may occur). Products include:

Atarax Tablets & Syrup......................... 2185
Marax Tablets & DF Syrup................... 2200
Vistaril Intramuscular Solution.......... 2216

Isoflurane (May produce additive depressant effects, hypoventilation, hypotension and profound sedation or coma may occur).

No products indexed under this heading.

Ketamine Hydrochloride (May produce additive depressant effects, hypoventilation, hypotension and profound sedation or coma may occur).

No products indexed under this heading.

Levomethadyl Acetate Hydrochloride (May produce additive depressant effects, hypoventilation, hypotension and profound sedation or coma may occur). Products include:

Orlamm 2239

Levorphanol Tartrate (May produce additive depressant effects, hypoventilation, hypotension and profound sedation or coma may occur). Products include:

Levo-Dromoran 2129

Loratadine (May produce additive depressant effects, hypoventilation, hypotension and profound sedation or coma may occur). Products include:

Claritin 2349
Claritin-D 2350

Lorazepam (May produce additive depressant effects, hypoventilation, hypotension and profound sedation or coma may occur). Products include:

Ativan Injection....................................... 2698
Ativan Tablets 2700

Loxapine Hydrochloride (May produce additive depressant effects, hypoventilation, hypotension and profound sedation or coma may occur). Products include:

Loxitane 1378

Loxapine Succinate (May produce additive depressant effects, hypoventilation, hypotension and profound sedation or coma may occur). Products include:

Loxitane Capsules 1378

Meperidine Hydrochloride (May produce additive depressant effects, hypoventilation, hypotension and profound sedation or coma may occur). Products include:

Demerol 2308
Mepergan Injection 2753

Mephobarbital (May produce additive depressant effects, hypoventilation, hypotension and profound sedation or coma may occur). Products include:

Mebaral Tablets 2322

Meprobamate (May produce additive depressant effects, hypoventilation, hypotension and profound sedation or coma may occur). Products include:

Miltown Tablets 2672
PMB 200 and PMB 400 2783

Mesoridazine Besylate (May produce additive depressant effects, hypoventilation, hypotension and profound sedation or coma may occur). Products include:

Serentil 684

Methadone Hydrochloride (May produce additive depressant effects, hypoventilation, hypotension and profound sedation or coma may occur). Products include:

Methadone Hydrochloride Oral Concentrate 2233
Methadone Hydrochloride Oral Solution & Tablets................................ 2235

Methdilazine Hydrochloride (May produce additive depressant effects, hypoventilation, hypotension and profound sedation or coma may occur).

No products indexed under this heading.

Methohexital Sodium (May produce additive depressant effects, hypoventilation, hypotension and profound sedation or coma may occur). Products include:

Brevital Sodium Vials............................ 1429

Methotrimeprazine (May produce additive depressant effects, hypoventilation, hypotension and profound sedation or coma may occur). Products include:

Levoprome 1274

Methoxyflurane (May produce additive depressant effects, hypoventilation, hypotension and profound sedation or coma may occur).

No products indexed under this heading.

Midazolam Hydrochloride (May produce additive depressant effects, hypoventilation, hypotension and profound sedation or coma may occur). Products include:

Versed Injection 2170

Molindone Hydrochloride (May produce additive depressant effects, hypoventilation, hypotension and profound sedation or coma may occur). Products include:

Moban Tablets and Concentrate 1048

Morphine Sulfate (May produce additive depressant effects, hypoventilation, hypotension and profound sedation or coma may occur). Products include:

Astramorph/PF Injection, USP (Preservative-Free) 535
Duramorph 962
Infumorph 200 and Infumorph 500 Sterile Solutions............................ 965
MS Contin Tablets.................................. 1994
MSIR 1997
Oramorph SR (Morphine Sulfate Sustained Release Tablets) 2236
RMS Suppositories 2657
Roxanol 2243

Opium Alkaloids (May produce additive depressant effects, hypoventilation, hypotension and profound sedation or coma may occur).

No products indexed under this heading.

Oxazepam (May produce additive depressant effects, hypoventilation, hypotension and profound sedation or coma may occur). Products include:

Serax Capsules 2810
Serax Tablets.. 2810

Oxycodone Hydrochloride (May produce additive depressant effects, hypoventilation, hypotension and profound sedation or coma may occur). Products include:

Percocet Tablets 938
Percodan Tablets..................................... 939
Percodan-Demi Tablets......................... 940
Roxicodone Tablets, Oral Solution & Intensol (Oxycodone) 2244
Tylox Capsules 1584

Pentobarbital Sodium (May produce additive depressant effects, hypoventilation, hypotension and profound sedation or coma may occur). Products include:

Nembutal Sodium Capsules 436
Nembutal Sodium Solution 438
Nembutal Sodium Suppositories...... 440

Perphenazine (May produce additive depressant effects, hypoventilation, hypotension and profound sedation or coma may occur). Products include:

Etrafon 2355
Triavil Tablets 1757
Trilafon... 2389

Phenobarbital (May produce additive depressant effects, hypoventilation, hypotension and profound sedation or coma may occur). Products include:

Arco-Lase Plus Tablets 512
Bellergal-S Tablets 2250
Donnatal 2060
Donnatal Extentabs................................ 2061
Donnatal Tablets 2060
Phenobarbital Elixir and Tablets 1469
Quadrinal Tablets 1350

Prazepam (May produce additive depressant effects, hypoventilation, hypotension and profound sedation or coma may occur).

No products indexed under this heading.

Prochlorperazine (May produce additive depressant effects, hypoventilation, hypotension and profound sedation or coma may occur). Products include:

Compazine 2470

Promethazine Hydrochloride (May produce additive depressant effects, hypoventilation, hypotension and profound sedation or coma may occur). Products include:

Mepergan Injection 2753
Phenergan with Codeine 2777
Phenergan with Dextromethorphan 2778
Phenergan Injection 2773
Phenergan Suppositories 2775
Phenergan Syrup 2774
Phenergan Tablets 2775
Phenergan VC 2779
Phenergan VC with Codeine 2781

Propofol (May produce additive depressant effects, hypoventilation, hypotension and profound sedation or coma may occur). Products include:

Diprivan Injection................................... 2833

Propoxyphene Hydrochloride (May produce additive depressant effects, hypoventilation, hypotension and profound sedation or coma may occur). Products include:

Darvon 1435
Wygesic Tablets 2827

Propoxyphene Napsylate (May produce additive depressant effects, hypoventilation, hypotension and profound sedation or coma may occur). Products include:

Darvon-N/Darvocet-N 1433

Pyrilamine Maleate (May produce additive depressant effects, hypoventilation, hypotension and profound sedation or coma may occur). Products include:

4-Way Fast Acting Nasal Spray (regular & mentholated) ....ⓑⓓ 621

Maximum Strength Multi-Symptom Formula Midol ....ⓑⓓ 722
PMS Multi-Symptom Formula Midol ....ⓑⓓ 723

Pyrilamine Tannate (May produce additive depressant effects, hypoventilation, hypotension and profound sedation or coma may occur). Products include:

Atrohist Pediatric Suspension 454
Rynatan 2673

Quazepam (May produce additive depressant effects, hypoventilation, hypotension and profound sedation or coma may occur). Products include:

Doral Tablets 2664

Risperidone (May produce additive depressant effects, hypoventilation, hypotension and profound sedation or coma may occur). Products include:

Risperdal 1301

Secobarbital Sodium (May produce additive depressant effects, hypoventilation, hypotension and profound sedation or coma may occur). Products include:

Seconal Sodium Pulvules 1474

Sufentanil Citrate (May produce additive depressant effects, hypoventilation, hypotension and profound sedation or coma may occur). Products include:

Sufenta Injection 1309

Temazepam (May produce additive depressant effects, hypoventilation, hypotension and profound sedation or coma may occur). Products include:

Restoril Capsules 2284

Terfenadine (May produce additive depressant effects, hypoventilation, hypotension and profound sedation or coma may occur). Products include:

Seldane Tablets 1536
Seldane-D Extended-Release Tablets 1538

Thiamylal Sodium (May produce additive depressant effects, hypoventilation, hypotension and profound sedation or coma may occur).

No products indexed under this heading.

Thioridazine Hydrochloride (May produce additive depressant effects, hypoventilation, hypotension and profound sedation or coma may occur). Products include:

Mellaril 2269

Thiothixene (May produce additive depressant effects, hypoventilation, hypotension and profound sedation or coma may occur). Products include:

Navane Capsules and Concentrate 2201
Navane Intramuscular 2202

Triazolam (May produce additive depressant effects, hypoventilation, hypotension and profound sedation or coma may occur). Products include:

Halcion Tablets.. 2611

Trifluoperazine Hydrochloride (May produce additive depressant effects, hypoventilation, hypotension and profound sedation or coma may occur). Products include:

Stelazine 2514

Trimeprazine Tartrate (May produce additive depressant effects, hypoventilation, hypotension and profound sedation or coma may occur). Products include:

Temaril Tablets, Syrup and Spansule Extended-Release Capsules.. 483

(ⓑⓓ Described in PDR For Nonprescription Drugs) (◉ Described in PDR For Ophthalmology)

Interactions Index — Duramorph

Tripelennamine Hydrochloride (May produce additive depressant effects, hypoventilation, hypotension and profound sedation or coma may occur). Products include:

PBZ Tablets 845
PBZ-SR Tablets 844

Triprolidine Hydrochloride (May produce additive depressant effects, hypoventilation, hypotension and profound sedation or coma may occur). Products include:

Actifed Plus Caplets .... ⊞ 845
Actifed Plus Tablets .... ⊞ 845
Actifed with Codeine Cough Syrup.. 1067
Actifed Syrup .... ⊞ 846
Actifed Tablets .... ⊞ 844

Zolpidem Tartrate (May produce additive depressant effects, hypoventilation, hypotension and profound sedation or coma may occur). Products include:

Ambien Tablets 2416

Food Interactions

Alcohol (May produce additive depressant effects).

DURAMORPH

(Morphine Sulfate) 962

May interact with hypnotics and sedatives, monoamine oxidase inhibitors, tricyclic antidepressants, butyrophenones, anticoagulants, antihistamines, psychotropics, phenothiazines, antipsychotic agents, and certain other agents. Compounds in these categories include:

Acrivastine (Potentiation of depressant effect). Products include:

Semprex-D Capsules 463
Semprex-D Capsules 1167

Alfentanil Hydrochloride (Potentiation of depressant effect). Products include:

Alfenta Injection 1286

Alprazolam (Potentiation of depressant effect). Products include:

Xanax Tablets 2649

Amitriptyline Hydrochloride (Potentiation of depressant effect). Products include:

Elavil 2838
Endep Tablets 2174
Etrafon 2355
Limbitrol 2180
Triavil Tablets 1757

Amoxapine (Potentiation of depressant effect). Products include:

Asendin Tablets 1369

Aprobarbital (Potentiation of depressant effect).

No products indexed under this heading.

Astemizole (Potentiation of depressant effect). Products include:

Hismanal Tablets 1293

Azatadine Maleate (Potentiation of depressant effect). Products include:

Trinalin Repetabs Tablets 1330

Bromodiphenhydramine Hydrochloride (Potentiation of depressant effect).

No products indexed under this heading.

Brompheniramine Maleate (Potentiation of depressant effect). Products include:

Alka Seltzer Plus Sinus Medicine .. ⊞ 707
Bromfed Capsules (Extended-Release) 1785
Bromfed Syrup .... ⊞ 733
Bromfed Tablets 1785
Bromfed-DM Cough Syrup 1786
Bromfed-PD Capsules (Extended-Release) 1785
Dimetane-DC Cough Syrup 2059
Dimetane-DX Cough Syrup 2059

Dimetapp Elixir .... ⊞ 773
Dimetapp Extentabs .... ⊞ 774
Dimetapp Tablets/Liqui-Gels .... ⊞ 775
Dimetapp Cold & Allergy Chewable Tablets .... ⊞ 773
Dimetapp DM Elixir .... ⊞ 774
Vicks DayQuil Allergy Relief 12-Hour Extended Release Tablets.. ⊞ 760
Vicks DayQuil Allergy Relief 4-Hour Tablets .... ⊞ 760

Buprenorphine (Potentiation of depressant effect). Products include:

Buprenex Injectable 2006

Buspirone Hydrochloride (Potentiation of depressant effect). Products include:

BuSpar 737

Butabarbital (Potentiation of depressant effect).

No products indexed under this heading.

Butalbital (Potentiation of depressant effect). Products include:

Esgic-plus Tablets 1013
Fioricet Tablets 2258
Fioricet with Codeine Capsules 2260
Fiorinal Capsules 2261
Fiorinal with Codeine Capsules 2262
Fiorinal Tablets 2261
Phrenilin 785
Sedapap Tablets 50 mg/650 mg .. 1543

Chlordiazepoxide (Potentiation of depressant effect). Products include:

Libritabs Tablets 2177
Limbitrol 2180

Chlordiazepoxide Hydrochloride (Potentiation of depressant effect). Products include:

Librax Capsules 2176
Librium Capsules 2178
Librium Injectable 2179

Chlorpheniramine Maleate (Potentiation of depressant effect). Products include:

Alka-Seltzer Plus Cold Medicine .... ⊞ 705
Alka-Seltzer Plus Cold Medicine Liqui-Gels .... ⊞ 706
Alka-Seltzer Plus Cold & Cough Medicine .... ⊞ 708
Alka-Seltzer Plus Cold & Cough Medicine Liqui-Gels .... ⊞ 705
Allerest Children's Chewable Tablets .... ⊞ 627
Allerest Headache Strength Tablets .... ⊞ 627
Allerest Maximum Strength Tablets .... ⊞ 627
Allerest Sinus Pain Formula .... ⊞ 627
Allerest 12 Hour Caplets .... ⊞ 627
Ana-Kit Anaphylaxis Emergency Treatment Kit 617
Atrohist Pediatric Capsules 453
Atrohist Plus Tablets 454
BC Cold Powder Multi-Symptom Formula (Cold-Sinus-Allergy) ...... ⊞ 609
Cerose DM .... ⊞ 878
Cheracol Plus Head Cold/Cough Formula .... ⊞ 769
Children's Vicks DayQuil Allergy Relief .... ⊞ 757
Children's Vicks NyQuil Cold/Cough Relief .... ⊞ 758
Chlor-Trimeton Allergy Decongestant Tablets .... ⊞ 799
Chlor-Trimeton Allergy Tablets ...... ⊞ 798
Comhist 2038
Comtrex Multi-Symptom Cold Reliever Tablets/Caplets/Liqui-Gels/Liquid .... ⊞ 615
Allergy-Sinus Comtrex Multi-Symptom Allergy-Sinus Formula Tablets .... ⊞ 617
Contac Continuous Action Nasal Decongestant/Antihistamine 12 Hour Capsules .... ⊞ 813
Contac Maximum Strength Continuous Action Decongestant/Antihistamine 12 Hour Caplets.. ⊞ 813
Contac Severe Cold and Flu Formula Caplets .... ⊞ 814
Coricidin 'D' Decongestant Tablets .... ⊞ 800
Coricidin Tablets .... ⊞ 800
D.A. Chewable Tablets 951
Deconamine 1320
Dura-Tap/PD Capsules 2867

Dura-Vent/DA Tablets 953
Extendryl 1005
Fedahist Gyrocaps 2401
Fedahist Timecaps 2401
Hycomine Compound Tablets 932
Isoclor Timesule Capsules .... ⊞ 637
Kronofed-A 977
Nolamine Timed-Release Tablets 785
Novahistine DH 2462
Novahistine Elixir .... ⊞ 823
Ornade Spansule Capsules 2502
PediaCare Cold Allergy Chewable Tablets .... ⊞ 677
PediaCare Cough-Cold Chewable Tablets 1553
PediaCare Cough-Cold Liquid 1553
PediaCare NightRest Cough-Cold Liquid 1553
Pediatric Vicks 44m Cough & Cold Relief .... ⊞ 764
Pyrroxate Caplets .... ⊞ 772
Ryna .... ⊞ 841
Sinarest Tablets .... ⊞ 648
Sinarest Extra Strength Tablets ...... ⊞ 648
Sine-Off Sinus Medicine .... ⊞ 825
Singlet Tablets .... ⊞ 825
Sinulin Tablets 787
Sinutab Sinus Allergy Medication, Maximum Strength Tablets and Caplets .... ⊞ 860
Sudafed Plus Liquid .... ⊞ 862
Sudafed Plus Tablets .... ⊞ 863
Teldrin 12 Hour Antihistamine/Nasal Decongestant Allergy Relief Capsules .... ⊞ 826
TheraFlu .... ⊞ 787
TheraFlu Maximum Strength Nighttime Flu, Cold & Cough Medicine .... ⊞ 788
Triaminic Allergy Tablets .... ⊞ 789
Triaminic Cold Tablets .... ⊞ 790
Triaminic Nite Light .... ⊞ 791
Triaminic Syrup .... ⊞ 792
Triaminic-12 Tablets .... ⊞ 792
Triaminicin Tablets .... ⊞ 793
Triaminicol Multi-Symptom Cold Tablets .... ⊞ 793
Triaminicol Multi-Symptom Relief ⊞ 794
Tussend 1783
Children's TYLENOL Cold Multi-Symptom Liquid Formula and Chewable Tablets 1561
Children's TYLENOL Cold Plus Cough Multi Symptom Tablets and Liquid .... ⊞ 681
TYLENOL Maximum Strength Allergy Sinus Medication Gelcaps and Caplets 1563
TYLENOL Cold Multi-Symptom Formula Medication Tablets and Caplets 1561
TYLENOL Cold Multi-Symptom Hot Medication Liquid Packets 1557
Vicks 44 LiquiCaps Cough, Cold & Flu Relief .... ⊞ 755
Vicks 44M Cough, Cold & Flu Relief .... ⊞ 756

Chlorpheniramine Polistirex (Potentiation of depressant effect). Products include:

Tussionex Pennkinetic Extended-Release Suspension 998

Chlorpheniramine Tannate (Potentiation of depressant effect). Products include:

Atrohist Pediatric Suspension 454
Ricobid Tablets and Pediatric Suspension 2038
Rynatan 2673
Rynatuss 2673

Chlorpromazine (Potentiation of depressant effect; increased risk of respiratory depression). Products include:

Thorazine Suppositories 2523

Chlorpromazine Hydrochloride (Potentiation of depressant effect; increased risk of respiratory depression). Products include:

Thorazine 2523

Chlorprothixene (Potentiation of depressant effect; increased risk of respiratory depression).

No products indexed under this heading.

Chlorprothixene Hydrochloride (Potentiation of depressant effect; increased risk of respiratory depression).

No products indexed under this heading.

Clemastine Fumarate (Potentiation of depressant effect). Products include:

Tavist Syrup 2297
Tavist Tablets 2298
Tavist-1 12 Hour Relief Tablets .... ⊞ 787
Tavist-D 12 Hour Relief Tablets .... ⊞ 787

Clomipramine Hydrochloride (Potentiation of depressant effect). Products include:

Anafranil Capsules 803

Clorazepate Dipotassium (Potentiation of depressant effect). Products include:

Tranxene 451

Clozapine (Potentiation of depressant effect; increased risk of respiratory depression). Products include:

Clozaril Tablets 2252

Codeine Phosphate (Potentiation of depressant effect). Products include:

Actifed with Codeine Cough Syrup.. 1067
Brontex 1981
Deconsal C Expectorant Syrup 456
Deconsal Pediatric Syrup 457
Dimetane-DC Cough Syrup 2059
Empirin with Codeine Tablets 1093
Fioricet with Codeine Capsules 2260
Fiorinal with Codeine Capsules 2262
Isoclor Expectorant 990
Novahistine DH 2462
Novahistine Expectorant 2463
Nucofed 2051
Phenergan with Codeine 2777
Phenergan VC with Codeine 2781
Robitussin A-C Syrup 2073
Robitussin-DAC Syrup 2074
Ryna .... ⊞ 841
Soma Compound w/Codeine Tablets 2676
Tussi-Organidin NR Liquid and S NR Liquid 2677
Tylenol with Codeine 1583

Cyproheptadine Hydrochloride (Potentiation of depressant effect). Products include:

Periactin 1724

Dalteparin Sodium (Concurrent use by epidural or intrathecal route is contraindicated with anticoagulant therapy). Products include:

Fragmin 1954

Desipramine Hydrochloride (Potentiation of depressant effect). Products include:

Norpramin Tablets 1526

Dexchlorpheniramine Maleate (Potentiation of depressant effect).

No products indexed under this heading.

Diazepam (Potentiation of depressant effect). Products include:

Dizac 1809
Valium Injectable 2182
Valium Tablets 2183
Valrelease Capsules 2169

Dicumarol (Concurrent use by epidural or intrathecal route is contraindicated with anticoagulant therapy).

No products indexed under this heading.

Diphenhydramine Citrate (Potentiation of depressant effect). Products include:

Excedrin P.M. Analgesic/Sleeping Aid Tablets, Caplets, Liquigels 733

Diphenhydramine Hydrochloride (Potentiation of depressant effect). Products include:

Actifed Allergy Daytime/Nighttime Caplets .... ⊞ 844
Actifed Sinus Daytime/Nighttime Tablets and Caplets .... ⊞ 846

IMPORTANT NOTE: Always consult each drug listing in the patient's regimen for possible interactions.

Duramorph | Interactions Index | 342

Arthritis Foundation NightTime Caplets ▣ 674
Extra Strength Bayer PM Aspirin ▣ 713
Bayer Select Night Time Pain Relief Formula ▣ 716
Benadryl Allergy Decongestant Liquid Medication ▣ 848
Benadryl Allergy Decongestant Tablets ▣ 848
Benadryl Allergy Liquid Medication ▣ 849
Benadryl Allergy ▣ 848
Benadryl Allergy Sinus Headache Formula Caplets ▣ 849
Benadryl Capsules 1898
Benadryl Dye-Free Allergy Liqui-gel Softgels ▣ 850
Benadryl Dye-Free Allergy Liquid Medication ▣ 850
Benadryl Itch Relief Cream, Children's Formula and Maximum Strength 2% ▣ 851
Benadryl Itch Relief Spray, Children's Formula and Maximum Strength 2% ▣ 851
Benadryl Itch Relief Stick Maximum Strength 2% ▣ 850
Benadryl Itch Stopping Gel, Children's Formula and Maximum Strength 2% ▣ 851
Benadryl Kapseals 1898
Benadryl Injection 1898
Contac Day & Night Cold/Flu Night Caplets ▣ 812
Contac Night Allergy/Sinus Caplets ▣ 812
Extra Strength Doan's P.M. ▣ 633
Legatrin PM ▣ 651
Miles Nervine Nighttime Sleep-Aid ▣ 723
Nytol QuickCaps Caplets ▣ 610
Sleepinal Night-time Sleep Aid Capsules and Softgels ▣ 834
TYLENOL Maximum Strength Allergy Sinus NightTime Medication Caplets 1555
TYLENOL Flu NightTime, Maximum Strength, Gelcaps 1566
TYLENOL Maximum Strength Flu NightTime Hot Medication Packets 1562
TYLENOL PM, Extra Strength Pain Reliever/Sleep Aid Caplets, Geltabs, Gelcaps 1560
TYLENOL Severe Allergy Medication Caplets 1564
Maximum Strength Unisom Sleepgels 1934
Unisom With Pain Relief-Nighttime Sleep Aid and Pain Reliever 1934

Diphenylpyraline Hydrochloride (Potentiation of depressant effect).
No products indexed under this heading.

Doxepin Hydrochloride (Potentiation of depressant effect). Products include:
Sinequan 2205
Zonalon Cream 1055

Droperidol (Potentiation of depressant effect). Products include:
Inapsine Injection 1296

Enflurane (Potentiation of depressant effect).
No products indexed under this heading.

Enoxaparin (Concurrent use by epidural or intrathecal route is contraindicated with anticoagulant therapy). Products include:
Lovenox Injection 2020

Estazolam (Potentiation of depressant effect). Products include:
ProSom Tablets 449

Ethchlorvynol (Potentiation of depressant effect). Products include:
Placidyl Capsules 448

Ethinamate (Potentiation of depressant effect).
No products indexed under this heading.

Fentanyl Citrate (Potentiation of depressant effect). Products include:
Sublimaze Injection 1307

Fluphenazine Decanoate (Potentiation of depressant effect; increased risk of respiratory depression). Products include:
Prolixin Decanoate 509

Fluphenazine Enanthate (Potentiation of depressant effect; increased risk of respiratory depression). Products include:
Prolixin Enanthate 509

Fluphenazine Hydrochloride (Potentiation of depressant effect; increased risk of respiratory depression). Products include:
Prolixin 509

Flurazepam Hydrochloride (Potentiation of depressant effect). Products include:
Dalmane Capsules 2173

Furazolidone (Potentiation of depressant effect). Products include:
Furoxone 2046

Glutethimide (Potentiation of depressant effect).
No products indexed under this heading.

Haloperidol (Potentiation of depressant effect; increased risk of respiratory depression). Products include:
Haldol Injection, Tablets and Concentrate 1575

Haloperidol Decanoate (Potentiation of depressant effect; increased risk of respiratory depression). Products include:
Haldol Decanoate 1577

Heparin Calcium (Concurrent use by epidural or intrathecal route is contraindicated with anticoagulant therapy).
No products indexed under this heading.

Heparin Sodium (Concurrent use by epidural or intrathecal route is contraindicated with anticoagulant therapy). Products include:
Heparin Lock Flush Solution 2725
Heparin Sodium Injection 2726
Heparin Sodium Injection, USP, Sterile Solution 2615
Heparin Sodium Vials 1441

Hydrocodone Bitartrate (Potentiation of depressant effect). Products include:
Anexsia 5/500 Elixir 1781
Anexia Tablets 1782
Codiclear DH Syrup 791
Deconamine CX Cough and Cold Liquid and Tablets 1319
Duratuss HD Elixir 2565
Hycodan Tablets and Syrup 930
Hycomine Compound Tablets 932
Hycomine 931
Hycotuss Expectorant Syrup 933
Hydrocet Capsules 782
Lorcet 10/650 1018
Lortab 2566
Tussend 1783
Tussend Expectorant 1785
Vicodin Tablets 1356
Vicodin ES Tablets 1357
Vicodin Tuss Expectorant 1358
Zydone Capsules 949

Hydrocodone Polistirex (Potentiation of depressant effect). Products include:
Tussionex Pennkinetic Extended-Release Suspension 998

Hydroxyzine Hydrochloride (Potentiation of depressant effect). Products include:
Atarax Tablets & Syrup 2185
Marax Tablets & DF Syrup 2200
Vistaril Intramuscular Solution 2216

Imipramine Hydrochloride (Potentiation of depressant effect). Products include:
Tofranil Ampuls 854
Tofranil Tablets 856

Imipramine Pamoate (Potentiation of depressant effect). Products include:
Tofranil-PM Capsules 857

Isocarboxazid (Potentiation of depressant effect).
No products indexed under this heading.

Isoflurane (Potentiation of depressant effect).
No products indexed under this heading.

Ketamine Hydrochloride (Potentiation of depressant effect).
No products indexed under this heading.

Levorphanol Tartrate (Potentiation of depressant effect). Products include:
Levo-Dromoran 2129

Lithium Carbonate (Potentiation of depressant effect; increased risk of respiratory depression). Products include:
Eskalith 2485
Lithium Carbonate Capsules & Tablets 2230
Lithonate/Lithotabs/Lithobid 2543

Lithium Citrate (Potentiation of depressant effect; increased risk of respiratory depression).
No products indexed under this heading.

Loratadine (Potentiation of depressant effect). Products include:
Claritin 2349
Claritin-D 2350

Lorazepam (Potentiation of depressant effect). Products include:
Ativan Injection 2698
Ativan Tablets 2700

Loxapine Hydrochloride (Potentiation of depressant effect; increased risk of respiratory depression). Products include:
Loxitane 1378

Loxapine Succinate (Potentiation of depressant effect; increased risk of respiratory depression). Products include:
Loxitane Capsules 1378

Maprotiline Hydrochloride (Potentiation of depressant effect). Products include:
Ludiomil Tablets 843

Meperidine Hydrochloride (Potentiation of depressant effect). Products include:
Demerol 2308
Mepergan Injection 2753

Mephobarbital (Potentiation of depressant effect). Products include:
Mebaral Tablets 2322

Meprobamate (Potentiation of depressant effect). Products include:
Miltown Tablets 2672
PMB 200 and PMB 400 2783

Mesoridazine Besylate (Potentiation of depressant effect; increased risk of respiratory depression). Products include:
Serentil 684

Methadone Hydrochloride (Potentiation of depressant effect). Products include:
Methadone Hydrochloride Oral Concentrate 2233
Methadone Hydrochloride Oral Solution & Tablets 2235

Methdilazine Hydrochloride (Potentiation of depressant effect).
No products indexed under this heading.

Methohexital Sodium (Potentiation of depressant effect). Products include:
Brevital Sodium Vials 1429

Methotrimeprazine (Potentiation of depressant effect; increased risk of respiratory depression). Products include:
Levoprome 1274

Methoxyflurane (Potentiation of depressant effect).
No products indexed under this heading.

Midazolam Hydrochloride (Potentiation of depressant effect). Products include:
Versed Injection 2170

Molindone Hydrochloride (Potentiation of depressant effect; increased risk of respiratory depression). Products include:
Moban Tablets and Concentrate 1048

Nortriptyline Hydrochloride (Potentiation of depressant effect). Products include:
Pamelor 2280

Opium Alkaloids (Potentiation of depressant effect).
No products indexed under this heading.

Oxazepam (Potentiation of depressant effect). Products include:
Serax Capsules 2810
Serax Tablets 2810

Oxycodone Hydrochloride (Potentiation of depressant effect). Products include:
Percocet Tablets 938
Percodan Tablets 939
Percodan-Demi Tablets 940
Roxicodone Tablets, Oral Solution & Intensol (Oxycodone) 2244
Tylox Capsules 1584

Pentobarbital Sodium (Potentiation of depressant effect). Products include:
Nembutal Sodium Capsules 436
Nembutal Sodium Solution 438
Nembutal Sodium Suppositories 440

Perphenazine (Potentiation of depressant effect; increased risk of respiratory depression). Products include:
Etrafon 2355
Triavil Tablets 1757
Trilafon 2389

Phenelzine Sulfate (Potentiation of depressant effect). Products include:
Nardil 1920

Phenobarbital (Potentiation of depressant effect). Products include:
Arco-Lase Plus Tablets 512
Bellergal-S Tablets 2250
Donnatal 2060
Donnatal Extentabs 2061
Donnatal Tablets 2060
Phenobarbital Elixir and Tablets 1469
Quadrinal Tablets 1350

Pimozide (Potentiation of depressant effect; increased risk of respiratory depression). Products include:
Orap Tablets 1050

Prazepam (Potentiation of depressant effect).
No products indexed under this heading.

Prochlorperazine (Potentiation of depressant effect; increased risk of respiratory depression). Products include:
Compazine 2470

Promethazine Hydrochloride (Potentiation of depressant effect; increased risk of respiratory depression). Products include:
Mepergan Injection 2753
Phenergan with Codeine 2777
Phenergan with Dextromethorphan 2778
Phenergan Injection 2773
Phenergan Suppositories 2775
Phenergan Syrup 2774
Phenergan Tablets 2775
Phenergan VC 2779

(▣ Described in PDR For Nonprescription Drugs) (◉ Described in PDR For Ophthalmology)

Phenergan VC with Codeine 2781

Propofol (Potentiation of depressant effect). Products include:

Diprivan Injection.................................... 2833

Propoxyphene Hydrochloride (Potentiation of depressant effect). Products include:

Darvon 1435
Wygesic Tablets 2827

Propoxyphene Napsylate (Potentiation of depressant effect). Products include:

Darvon-N/Darvocet-N 1433

Protriptyline Hydrochloride (Potentiation of depressant effect). Products include:

Vivactil Tablets 1774

Pyrilamine Maleate (Potentiation of depressant effect). Products include:

4-Way Fast Acting Nasal Spray (regular & mentholated) ....◆⊡ 621
Maximum Strength Multi-Symptom Formula Midol ....◆⊡ 722
PMS Multi-Symptom Formula Midol ....◆⊡ 723

Pyrilamine Tannate (Potentiation of depressant effect). Products include:

Atrohist Pediatric Suspension 454
Rynatan 2673

Quazepam (Potentiation of depressant effect). Products include:

Doral Tablets 2664

Risperidone (Potentiation of depressant effect; increased risk of respiratory depression). Products include:

Risperdal 1301

Secobarbital Sodium (Potentiation of depressant effect). Products include:

Seconal Sodium Pulvules 1474

Selegiline Hydrochloride (Potentiation of depressant effect). Products include:

Eldepryl Tablets 2550

Sufentanil Citrate (Potentiation of depressant effect). Products include:

Sufenta Injection 1309

Temazepam (Potentiation of depressant effect). Products include:

Restoril Capsules 2284

Terfenadine (Potentiation of depressant effect). Products include:

Seldane Tablets 1536
Seldane-D Extended-Release Tablets 1538

Thiamylal Sodium (Potentiation of depressant effect).

No products indexed under this heading.

Thioridazine Hydrochloride (Potentiation of depressant effect; increased risk of respiratory depression). Products include:

Mellaril 2269

Thiothixene (Potentiation of depressant effect; increased risk of respiratory depression). Products include:

Navane Capsules and Concentrate 2201
Navane Intramuscular 2202

Tranylcypromine Sulfate (Potentiation of depressant effect). Products include:

Parnate Tablets 2503

Triazolam (Potentiation of depressant effect). Products include:

Halcion Tablets....................................... 2611

Trifluoperazine Hydrochloride (Potentiation of depressant effect; increased risk of respiratory depression). Products include:

Stelazine 2514

Trimeprazine Tartrate (Potentiation of depressant effect). Products include:

Temaril Tablets, Syrup and Spansule Extended-Release Capsules.. 483

Trimipramine Maleate (Potentiation of depressant effect). Products include:

Surmontil Capsules................................ 2811

Tripelennamine Hydrochloride (Potentiation of depressant effect). Products include:

PBZ Tablets 845
PBZ-SR Tablets....................................... 844

Triprolidine Hydrochloride (Potentiation of depressant effect). Products include:

Actifed Plus Caplets ....◆⊡ 845
Actifed Plus Tablets ....◆⊡ 845
Actifed with Codeine Cough Syrup.. 1067
Actifed Syrup...◆⊡ 846
Actifed Tablets ....◆⊡ 844

Warfarin Sodium (Concurrent use by epidural or intrathecal route is contraindicated with anticoagulant therapy). Products include:

Coumadin 926

Zolpidem Tartrate (Potentiation of depressant effect). Products include:

Ambien Tablets.. 2416

Food Interactions

Alcohol (Potentiation of depressant effect).

DURANEST INJECTIONS

(Etidocaine Hydrochloride).................... 542

May interact with monoamine oxidase inhibitors, tricyclic antidepressants, phenothiazines, and ergot-type oxytocic drugs. Compounds in these categories include:

Amitriptyline Hydrochloride (Concurrent use of Duranest Injection containing epinephrine with tricyclic antidepressant may produce severe, prolonged hypotension or hypertension; concurrent use should be avoided). Products include:

Elavil 2838
Endep Tablets 2174
Etrafon 2355
Limbitrol 2180
Triavil Tablets 1757

Amoxapine (Concurrent use of Duranest Injection containing epinephrine with tricyclic antidepressant may produce severe, prolonged hypotension or hypertension; concurrent use should be avoided). Products include:

Asendin Tablets 1369

Chlorpromazine (Concurrent use of Duranest Injection containing epinephrine with phenothiazine may produce severe, prolonged hypotension or hypertension; concurrent use should be avoided). Products include:

Thorazine Suppositories 2523

Chlorpromazine Hydrochloride (Concurrent use of Duranest Injection containing epinephrine with phenothiazine may produce severe, prolonged hypotension or hypertension; concurrent use should be avoided). Products include:

Thorazine 2523

Clomipramine Hydrochloride (Concurrent use of Duranest Injection containing epinephrine with tricyclic antidepressant may produce severe, prolonged hypotension or hypertension; concurrent use should be avoided). Products include:

Anafranil Capsules 803

Desipramine Hydrochloride (Concurrent use of Duranest Injection containing epinephrine with tricyclic antidepressant may produce severe, prolonged hypotension or hypertension; concurrent use should be avoided). Products include:

Norpramin Tablets 1526

Doxepin Hydrochloride (Concurrent use of Duranest Injection containing epinephrine with tricyclic antidepressant may produce severe, prolonged hypotension or hypertension; concurrent use should be avoided). Products include:

Sinequan 2205
Zonalon Cream 1055

Fluphenazine Decanoate (Concurrent use of Duranest Injection containing epinephrine with phenothiazine may produce severe, prolonged hypotension or hypertension; concurrent use should be avoided). Products include:

Prolixin Decanoate 509

Fluphenazine Enanthate (Concurrent use of Duranest Injection containing epinephrine with phenothiazine may produce severe, prolonged hypotension or hypertension; concurrent use should be avoided). Products include:

Prolixin Enanthate.................................. 509

Fluphenazine Hydrochloride (Concurrent use of Duranest Injection containing epinephrine with phenothiazine may produce severe, prolonged hypotension or hypertension; concurrent use should be avoided). Products include:

Prolixin 509

Furazolidone (Concurrent use of Duranest Injection containing epinephrine with MAOI may produce severe, prolonged hypotension or hypertension; concurrent use should be avoided). Products include:

Furoxone 2046

Imipramine Hydrochloride (Concurrent use of Duranest Injection containing epinephrine with tricyclic antidepressant may produce severe, prolonged hypotension or hypertension; concurrent use should be avoided). Products include:

Tofranil Ampuls 854
Tofranil Tablets 856

Imipramine Pamoate (Concurrent use of Duranest Injection containing epinephrine with tricyclic antidepressant may produce severe, prolonged hypotension or hypertension; concurrent use should be avoided). Products include:

Tofranil-PM Capsules............................. 857

Isocarboxazid (Concurrent use of Duranest Injection containing epinephrine with MAOI may produce severe, prolonged hypotension or hypertension; concurrent use should be avoided).

No products indexed under this heading.

Maprotiline Hydrochloride (Concurrent use of Duranest Injection containing epinephrine with tricyclic antidepressant may produce severe, prolonged hypotension or hypertension; concurrent use should be avoided). Products include:

Ludiomil Tablets...................................... 843

Mesoridazine Besylate (Concurrent use of Duranest Injection containing epinephrine with phenothiazine may produce severe, prolonged hypotension or hypertension; concurrent use should be avoided). Products include:

Serentil... 684

Methotrimeprazine (Concurrent use of Duranest Injection containing epinephrine with phenothiazine may produce severe, prolonged hypotension or hypertension; concurrent use should be avoided). Products include:

Levoprome 1274

Methylergonovine Maleate (Concurrent use of vasopressor drugs, for the treatment of hypotension related to epidural blocks, and ergot-type oxytocic drugs may cause severe, persistent hypertension or cerebrovascular accidents). Products include:

Methergine 2272

Nortriptyline Hydrochloride (Concurrent use of Duranest Injection containing epinephrine with tricyclic antidepressant may produce severe, prolonged hypotension or hypertension; concurrent use should be avoided). Products include:

Pamelor 2280

Perphenazine (Concurrent use of Duranest Injection containing epinephrine with phenothiazine may produce severe, prolonged hypotension or hypertension; concurrent use should be avoided). Products include:

Etrafon 2355
Triavil Tablets 1757
Trilafon... 2389

Phenelzine Sulfate (Concurrent use of Duranest Injection containing epinephrine with MAOI may produce severe, prolonged hypotension or hypertension; concurrent use should be avoided). Products include:

Nardil 1920

Prochlorperazine (Concurrent use of Duranest Injection containing epinephrine with phenothiazine may produce severe, prolonged hypotension or hypertension; concurrent use should be avoided). Products include:

Compazine 2470

Promethazine Hydrochloride (Concurrent use of Duranest Injection containing epinephrine with phenothiazine may produce severe, prolonged hypotension or hypertension; concurrent use should be avoided). Products include:

Mepergan Injection 2753
Phenergan with Codeine......................... 2777
Phenergan with Dextromethorphan 2778
Phenergan Injection 2773
Phenergan Suppositories 2775
Phenergan Syrup 2774
Phenergan Tablets 2775
Phenergan VC 2779
Phenergan VC with Codeine 2781

Protriptyline Hydrochloride (Concurrent use of Duranest Injection containing epinephrine with tricyclic antidepressant may produce severe, prolonged hypotension or hypertension; concurrent use should be avoided). Products include:

Vivactil Tablets 1774

IMPORTANT NOTE: Always consult each drug listing in the patient's regimen for possible interactions.

Duranest | **Interactions Index** | **344**

Selegiline Hydrochloride (Concurrent use of Duranest Injection containing epinephrine with MAOI may produce severe, prolonged hypotension or hypertension; concurrent use should be avoided). Products include:
Eldepryl Tablets 2550

Thioridazine Hydrochloride (Concurrent use of Duranest Injection containing epinephrine with phenothiazine may produce severe, prolonged hypotension or hypertension; concurrent use should be avoided). Products include:
Mellaril 2269

Tranylcypromine Sulfate (Concurrent use of Duranest Injection containing epinephrine with MAOI may produce severe, prolonged hypotension or hypertension; concurrent use should be avoided). Products include:
Parnate Tablets 2503

Trifluoperazine Hydrochloride (Concurrent use of Duranest Injection containing epinephrine with phenothiazine may produce severe, prolonged hypotension or hypertension; concurrent use should be avoided). Products include:
Stelazine 2514

Trimipramine Maleate (Concurrent use of Duranest Injection containing epinephrine with tricyclic antidepressant may produce severe, prolonged hypotension or hypertension; concurrent use should be avoided). Products include:
Surmontil Capsules 2811

DURA-TAP/PD CAPSULES
(Chlorpheniramine Maleate, Pseudoephedrine Hydrochloride) 2867
May interact with monoamine oxidase inhibitors, beta blockers, hypnotics and sedatives, tricyclic antidepressants, barbiturates, central nervous system depressants, tranquilizers, and certain other agents. Compounds in these categories include:

Acebutolol Hydrochloride (Increases the effects of sympathomimetics). Products include:
Sectral Capsules 2807

Alfentanil Hydrochloride (Potential for additive effects). Products include:
Alfenta Injection 1286

Alprazolam (Potential for additive effects). Products include:
Xanax Tablets 2649

Amitriptyline Hydrochloride (Potential for additive effects). Products include:
Elavil 2838
Endep Tablets 2174
Etrafon 2355
Limbitrol 2180
Triavil Tablets 1757

Amoxapine (Potential for additive effects). Products include:
Asendin Tablets 1369

Aprobarbital (Potential for additive effects).
No products indexed under this heading.

Atenolol (Increases the effects of sympathomimetics). Products include:
Tenoretic Tablets 2845
Tenormin Tablets and I.V. Injection 2847

Betaxolol Hydrochloride (Increases the effects of sympathomimetics). Products include:
Betoptic Ophthalmic Solution 469
Betoptic S Ophthalmic Suspension 471
Kerlone Tablets 2436

Bisoprolol Fumarate (Increases the effects of sympathomimetics). Products include:
Zebeta Tablets 1413
Ziac 1415

Buprenorphine (Potential for additive effects). Products include:
Buprenex Injectable 2006

Buspirone Hydrochloride (Potential for additive effects). Products include:
BuSpar 737

Butabarbital (Potential for additive effects).
No products indexed under this heading.

Butalbital (Potential for additive effects). Products include:
Esgic-plus Tablets 1013
Fioricet Tablets 2258
Fioricet with Codeine Capsules 2260
Fiorinal Capsules 2261
Fiorinal with Codeine Capsules 2262
Fiorinal Tablets 2261
Phrenilin 785
Sedapap Tablets 50 mg/650 mg .. 1543

Carteolol Hydrochloride (Increases the effects of sympathomimetics). Products include:
Cartrol Tablets 410
Ocupress Ophthalmic Solution, 1% Sterile .... ◉ 309

Chlordiazepoxide (Potential for additive effects). Products include:
Libritabs Tablets 2177
Limbitrol 2180

Chlordiazepoxide Hydrochloride (Potential for additive effects). Products include:
Librax Capsules 2176
Librium Capsules 2178
Librium Injectable 2179

Chlorpromazine (Potential for additive effects). Products include:
Thorazine Suppositories 2523

Chlorpromazine Hydrochloride (Potential for additive effects). Products include:
Thorazine 2523

Chlorprothixene (Potential for additive effects).
No products indexed under this heading.

Chlorprothixene Hydrochloride (Potential for additive effects).
No products indexed under this heading.

Clomipramine Hydrochloride (Potential for additive effects). Products include:
Anafranil Capsules 803

Clorazepate Dipotassium (Potential for additive effects). Products include:
Tranxene 451

Clozapine (Potential for additive effects). Products include:
Clozaril Tablets 2252

Codeine Phosphate (Potential for additive effects). Products include:
Actifed with Codeine Cough Syrup.. 1067
Brontex 1981
Deconsal C Expectorant Syrup 456
Deconsal Pediatric Syrup 457
Dimetane-DC Cough Syrup 2059
Empirin with Codeine Tablets 1093
Fioricet with Codeine Capsules 2260
Fiorinal with Codeine Capsules 2262
Isoclor Expectorant 990
Novahistine DH 2462
Novahistine Expectorant 2463
Nucofed 2051
Phenergan with Codeine 2777
Phenergan VC with Codeine 2781
Robitussin A-C Syrup 2073
Robitussin-DAC Syrup 2074
Ryna .... ■ 841
Soma Compound w/Codeine Tablets 2676
Tussi-Organidin NR Liquid and S NR Liquid 2677
Tylenol with Codeine 1583

Desflurane (Potential for additive effects). Products include:
Suprane 1813

Desipramine Hydrochloride (Potential for additive effects). Products include:
Norpramin Tablets 1526

Dezocine (Potential for additive effects). Products include:
Dalgan Injection 538

Diazepam (Potential for additive effects). Products include:
Dizac 1809
Valium Injectable 2182
Valium Tablets 2183
Valrelease Capsules 2169

Doxepin Hydrochloride (Potential for additive effects). Products include:
Sinequan 2205
Zonalon Cream 1055

Droperidol (Potential for additive effects). Products include:
Inapsine Injection 1296

Enflurane (Potential for additive effects).
No products indexed under this heading.

Esmolol Hydrochloride (Increases the effects of sympathomimetics). Products include:
Brevibloc Injection 1808

Estazolam (Potential for additive effects). Products include:
ProSom Tablets 449

Ethchlorvynol (Potential for additive effects). Products include:
Placidyl Capsules 448

Ethinamate (Potential for additive effects).
No products indexed under this heading.

Fentanyl (Potential for additive effects). Products include:
Duragesic Transdermal System 1288

Fentanyl Citrate (Potential for additive effects). Products include:
Sublimaze Injection 1307

Fluphenazine Decanoate (Potential for additive effects). Products include:
Prolixin Decanoate 509

Fluphenazine Enanthate (Potential for additive effects). Products include:
Prolixin Enanthate 509

Fluphenazine Hydrochloride (Potential for additive effects). Products include:
Prolixin 509

Flurazepam Hydrochloride (Potential for additive effects). Products include:
Dalmane Capsules 2173

Furazolidone (Increases the effects of sympathomimetics; concurrent and/or sequential use is contraindicated). Products include:
Furoxone 2046

Glutethimide (Potential for additive effects).
No products indexed under this heading.

Haloperidol (Potential for additive effects). Products include:
Haldol Injection, Tablets and Concentrate 1575

Haloperidol Decanoate (Potential for additive effects). Products include:
Haldol Decanoate 1577

Hydrocodone Bitartrate (Potential for additive effects). Products include:
Anexsia 5/500 Elixir 1781
Anexia Tablets 1782
Codiclear DH Syrup 791
Deconamine CX Cough and Cold Liquid and Tablets 1319
Duratuss HD Elixir 2565
Hycodan Tablets and Syrup 930
Hycomine Compound Tablets 932
Hycomine 931
Hycotuss Expectorant Syrup 933
Hydrocet Capsules 782
Lorcet 10/650 1018
Lortab 2566
Tussend 1783
Tussend Expectorant 1785
Vicodin Tablets 1356
Vicodin ES Tablets 1357
Vicodin Tuss Expectorant 1358
Zydone Capsules 949

Hydrocodone Polistirex (Potential for additive effects). Products include:
Tussionex Pennkinetic Extended-Release Suspension 998

Hydroxyzine Hydrochloride (Potential for additive effects). Products include:
Atarax Tablets & Syrup 2185
Marax Tablets & DF Syrup 2200
Vistaril Intramuscular Solution 2216

Imipramine Hydrochloride (Potential for additive effects). Products include:
Tofranil Ampuls 854
Tofranil Tablets 856

Imipramine Pamoate (Potential for additive effects). Products include:
Tofranil-PM Capsules 857

Isocarboxazid (Increases the effects of sympathomimetics; concurrent and/or sequential use is contraindicated).
No products indexed under this heading.

Isoflurane (Potential for additive effects).
No products indexed under this heading.

Ketamine Hydrochloride (Potential for additive effects).
No products indexed under this heading.

Labetalol Hydrochloride (Increases the effects of sympathomimetics). Products include:
Normodyne Injection 2377
Normodyne Tablets 2379
Trandate 1185

Levobunolol Hydrochloride (Increases the effects of sympathomimetics). Products include:
Betagan .... ◉ 233

Levomethadyl Acetate Hydrochloride (Potential for additive effects). Products include:
Orlamm 2239

Levorphanol Tartrate (Potential for additive effects). Products include:
Levo-Dromoran 2129

Lorazepam (Potential for additive effects). Products include:
Ativan Injection 2698
Ativan Tablets 2700

Loxapine Hydrochloride (Potential for additive effects). Products include:
Loxitane 1378

Loxapine Succinate (Potential for additive effects). Products include:
Loxitane Capsules 1378

Maprotiline Hydrochloride (Potential for additive effects). Products include:
Ludiomil Tablets 843

Mecamylamine Hydrochloride (Sympathomimetic may reduce the antihypertensive effects). Products include:
Inversine Tablets 1686

(■ Described in PDR For Nonprescription Drugs) (◉ Described in PDR For Ophthalmology)

345 **Interactions Index** **Dura-Vent/DA**

Meperidine Hydrochloride (Potential for additive effects). Products include:
- Demerol 2308
- Mepergan Injection 2753

Mephobarbital (Potential for additive effects). Products include:
- Mebaral Tablets 2322

Meprobamate (Potential for additive effects). Products include:
- Miltown Tablets 2672
- PMB 200 and PMB 400 2783

Mesoridazine Besylate (Potential for additive effects). Products include:
- Serentil 684

Methadone Hydrochloride (Potential for additive effects). Products include:
- Methadone Hydrochloride Oral Concentrate 2233
- Methadone Hydrochloride Oral Solution & Tablets 2235

Methohexital Sodium (Potential for additive effects). Products include:
- Brevital Sodium Vials 1429

Methotrimeprazine (Potential for additive effects). Products include:
- Levoprome 1274

Methoxyflurane (Potential for additive effects).
- No products indexed under this heading.

Methyldopa (Sympathomimetic may reduce the antihypertensive effects). Products include:
- Aldoclor Tablets 1598
- Aldomet Oral 1600
- Aldoril Tablets 1604

Methyldopate Hydrochloride (Sympathomimetic may reduce the antihypertensive effects). Products include:
- Aldomet Ester HCl Injection 1602

Metipranolol Hydrochloride (Increases the effects of sympathomimetics). Products include:
- OptiPranolol (Metipranolol 0.3%) Sterile Ophthalmic Solution .... ◉ 258

Metoprolol Succinate (Increases the effects of sympathomimetics). Products include:
- Toprol-XL Tablets 565

Metoprolol Tartrate (Increases the effects of sympathomimetics). Products include:
- Lopressor Ampuls 830
- Lopressor HCT Tablets 832
- Lopressor Tablets 830

Midazolam Hydrochloride (Potential for additive effects). Products include:
- Versed Injection 2170

Molindone Hydrochloride (Potential for additive effects). Products include:
- Moban Tablets and Concentrate 1048

Morphine Sulfate (Potential for additive effects). Products include:
- Astramorph/PF Injection, USP (Preservative-Free) 535
- Duramorph 962
- Infumorph 200 and Infumorph 500 Sterile Solutions 965
- MS Contin Tablets 1994
- MSIR 1997
- Oramorph SR (Morphine Sulfate Sustained Release Tablets) 2236
- RMS Suppositories 2657
- Roxanol 2243

Nadolol (Increases the effects of sympathomimetics).
- No products indexed under this heading.

Nortriptyline Hydrochloride (Potential for additive effects). Products include:
- Pamelor 2280

Opium Alkaloids (Potential for additive effects).
- No products indexed under this heading.

Oxazepam (Potential for additive effects). Products include:
- Serax Capsules 2810
- Serax Tablets 2810

Oxycodone Hydrochloride (Potential for additive effects). Products include:
- Percocet Tablets 938
- Percodan Tablets 939
- Percodan-Demi Tablets 940
- Roxicodone Tablets, Oral Solution & Intensol (Oxycodone) 2244
- Tylox Capsules 1584

Penbutolol Sulfate (Increases the effects of sympathomimetics). Products include:
- Levatol 2403

Pentobarbital Sodium (Potential for additive effects). Products include:
- Nembutal Sodium Capsules 436
- Nembutal Sodium Solution 438
- Nembutal Sodium Suppositories 440

Perphenazine (Potential for additive effects). Products include:
- Etrafon 2355
- Triavil Tablets 1757
- Trilafon 2389

Phenelzine Sulfate (Increases the effects of sympathomimetics; concurrent and/or sequential use is contraindicated). Products include:
- Nardil 1920

Phenobarbital (Potential for additive effects). Products include:
- Arco-Lase Plus Tablets 512
- Bellergal-S Tablets 2250
- Donnatal 2060
- Donnatal Extentabs 2061
- Donnatal Tablets 2060
- Phenobarbital Elixir and Tablets 1469
- Quadrinal Tablets 1350

Pindolol (Increases the effects of sympathomimetics). Products include:
- Visken Tablets 2299

Prazepam (Potential for additive effects).
- No products indexed under this heading.

Prochlorperazine (Potential for additive effects). Products include:
- Compazine 2470

Promethazine Hydrochloride (Potential for additive effects). Products include:
- Mepergan Injection 2753
- Phenergan with Codeine 2777
- Phenergan with Dextromethorphan 2778
- Phenergan Injection 2773
- Phenergan Suppositories 2775
- Phenergan Syrup 2774
- Phenergan Tablets 2775
- Phenergan VC 2779
- Phenergan VC with Codeine 2781

Propofol (Potential for additive effects). Products include:
- Diprivan Injection 2833

Propoxyphene Hydrochloride (Potential for additive effects). Products include:
- Darvon 1435
- Wygesic Tablets 2827

Propoxyphene Napsylate (Potential for additive effects). Products include:
- Darvon-N/Darvocet-N 1433

Propranolol Hydrochloride (Increases the effects of sympathomimetics). Products include:
- Inderal 2728
- Inderal LA Long Acting Capsules 2730
- Inderide Tablets 2732
- Inderide LA Long Acting Capsules 2734

Protriptyline Hydrochloride (Potential for additive effects). Products include:
- Vivactil Tablets 1774

Quazepam (Potential for additive effects). Products include:
- Doral Tablets 2664

Reserpine (Sympathomimetic may reduce the antihypertensive effects). Products include:
- Diupres Tablets 1650
- Hydropres Tablets 1675
- Ser-Ap-Es Tablets 849

Risperidone (Potential for additive effects). Products include:
- Risperdal 1301

Secobarbital Sodium (Potential for additive effects). Products include:
- Seconal Sodium Pulvules 1474

Selegiline Hydrochloride (Increases the effects of sympathomimetics; concurrent and/or sequential use is contraindicated). Products include:
- Eldepryl Tablets 2550

Sotalol Hydrochloride (Increases the effects of sympathomimetics). Products include:
- Betapace Tablets 641

Sufentanil Citrate (Potential for additive effects). Products include:
- Sufenta Injection 1309

Temazepam (Potential for additive effects). Products include:
- Restoril Capsules 2284

Thiamylal Sodium (Potential for additive effects).
- No products indexed under this heading.

Thioridazine Hydrochloride (Potential for additive effects). Products include:
- Mellaril 2269

Thiothixene (Potential for additive effects). Products include:
- Navane Capsules and Concentrate 2201
- Navane Intramuscular 2202

Timolol Hemihydrate (Increases the effects of sympathomimetics). Products include:
- Betimol 0.25%, 0.5% .... ◉ 261

Timolol Maleate (Increases the effects of sympathomimetics). Products include:
- Blocadren Tablets 1614
- Timolide Tablets 1748
- Timoptic in Ocudose 1753
- Timoptic Sterile Ophthalmic Solution 1751
- Timoptic-XE 1755

Tranylcypromine Sulfate (Increases the effects of sympathomimetics; concurrent and/or sequential use is contraindicated). Products include:
- Parnate Tablets 2503

Triazolam (Potential for additive effects). Products include:
- Halcion Tablets 2611

Trifluoperazine Hydrochloride (Potential for additive effects). Products include:
- Stelazine 2514

Trimipramine Maleate (Potential for additive effects). Products include:
- Surmontil Capsules 2811

Zolpidem Tartrate (Potential for additive effects). Products include:
- Ambien Tablets 2416

Food Interactions

Alcohol (Potential for additive effects).

DURATION 12 HOUR NASAL SPRAY
(Oxymetazoline Hydrochloride) .... ▣ 805
None cited in PDR database.

DURATUSS TABLETS
(Pseudoephedrine Hydrochloride, Guaifenesin) 2565
May interact with monoamine oxidase inhibitors. Compounds in this category include:

Furazolidone (Concurrent use is contraindicated). Products include:
- Furoxone 2046

Isocarboxazid (Concurrent use is contraindicated).
- No products indexed under this heading.

Phenelzine Sulfate (Concurrent use is contraindicated). Products include:
- Nardil 1920

Selegiline Hydrochloride (Concurrent use is contraindicated). Products include:
- Eldepryl Tablets 2550

Tranylcypromine Sulfate (Concurrent use is contraindicated). Products include:
- Parnate Tablets 2503

DURA-VENT/DA TABLETS
(Chlorpheniramine Maleate, Phenylephrine Hydrochloride, Methscopolamine Nitrate) 953
May interact with monoamine oxidase inhibitors, beta blockers, hypnotics and sedatives, tricyclic antidepressants, barbiturates, central nervous system depressants, tranquilizers, and certain other agents. Compounds in these categories include:

Acebutolol Hydrochloride (Increases the effects of sympathomimetics). Products include:
- Sectral Capsules 2807

Alfentanil Hydrochloride (Potential for additive effects). Products include:
- Alfenta Injection 1286

Alprazolam (Potential for additive effects). Products include:
- Xanax Tablets 2649

Amitriptyline Hydrochloride (Potential for additive effects). Products include:
- Elavil 2838
- Endep Tablets 2174
- Etrafon 2355
- Limbitrol 2180
- Triavil Tablets 1757

Amoxapine (Potential for additive effects). Products include:
- Asendin Tablets 1369

Aprobarbital (Potential for additive effects).
- No products indexed under this heading.

Atenolol (Increases the effects of sympathomimetics). Products include:
- Tenoretic Tablets 2845
- Tenormin Tablets and I.V. Injection 2847

Betaxolol Hydrochloride (Increases the effects of sympathomimetics). Products include:
- Betoptic Ophthalmic Solution 469
- Betoptic S Ophthalmic Suspension 471
- Kerlone Tablets 2436

Bisoprolol Fumarate (Increases the effects of sympathomimetics). Products include:
- Zebeta Tablets 1413
- Ziac 1415

Buprenorphine (Potential for additive effects). Products include:
- Buprenex Injectable 2006

IMPORTANT NOTE: Always consult each drug listing in the patient's regimen for possible interactions.

Dura-Vent/DA **Interactions Index** 346

Buspirone Hydrochloride (Potential for additive effects). Products include:
- BuSpar ... 737

Butabarbital (Potential for additive effects).
- No products indexed under this heading.

Butalbital (Potential for additive effects). Products include:
- Esgic-plus Tablets ... 1013
- Fioricet Tablets ... 2258
- Fioricet with Codeine Capsules ... 2260
- Fiorinal Capsules ... 2261
- Fiorinal with Codeine Capsules ... 2262
- Fiorinal Tablets ... 2261
- Phrenilin ... 785
- Sedapap Tablets 50 mg/650 mg .. 1543

Carteolol Hydrochloride (Increases the effects of sympathomimetics). Products include:
- Cartrol Tablets ... 410
- Ocupress Ophthalmic Solution, 1% Sterile ... ⊙ 309

Chlordiazepoxide (Potential for additive effects). Products include:
- Libritabs Tablets ... 2177
- Limbitrol ... 2180

Chlordiazepoxide Hydrochloride (Potential for additive effects). Products include:
- Librax Capsules ... 2176
- Librium Capsules ... 2178
- Librium Injectable ... 2179

Chlorpromazine (Potential for additive effects). Products include:
- Thorazine Suppositories ... 2523

Chlorpromazine Hydrochloride (Potential for additive effects). Products include:
- Thorazine ... 2523

Chlorprothixene (Potential for additive effects).
- No products indexed under this heading.

Chlorprothixene Hydrochloride (Potential for additive effects).
- No products indexed under this heading.

Clomipramine Hydrochloride (Potential for additive effects). Products include:
- Anafranil Capsules ... 803

Clorazepate Dipotassium (Potential for additive effects). Products include:
- Tranxene ... 451

Clozapine (Potential for additive effects). Products include:
- Clozaril Tablets ... 2252

Codeine Phosphate (Potential for additive effects). Products include:
- Actifed with Codeine Cough Syrup.. 1067
- Brontex ... 1981
- Deconsal C Expectorant Syrup ... 456
- Deconsal Pediatric Syrup ... 457
- Dimetane-DC Cough Syrup ... 2059
- Empirin with Codeine Tablets ... 1093
- Fioricet with Codeine Capsules ... 2260
- Fiorinal with Codeine Capsules ... 2262
- Isoclor Expectorant ... 990
- Novahistine DH ... 2462
- Novahistine Expectorant ... 2463
- Nucofed ... 2051
- Phenergan with Codeine ... 2777
- Phenergan VC with Codeine ... 2781
- Robitussin A-C Syrup ... 2073
- Robitussin-DAC Syrup ... 2074
- Ryna ... ▣ 841
- Soma Compound w/Codeine Tablets ... 2676
- Tussi-Organidin NR Liquid and S NR Liquid ... 2677
- Tylenol with Codeine ... 1583

Desflurane (Potential for additive effects). Products include:
- Suprane ... 1813

Desipramine Hydrochloride (Potential for additive effects). Products include:
- Norpramin Tablets ... 1526

Dezocine (Potential for additive effects). Products include:
- Dalgan Injection ... 538

Diazepam (Potential for additive effects). Products include:
- Dizac ... 1809
- Valium Injectable ... 2182
- Valium Tablets ... 2183
- Valrelease Capsules ... 2169

Doxepin Hydrochloride (Potential for additive effects). Products include:
- Sinequan ... 2205
- Zonalon Cream ... 1055

Droperidol (Potential for additive effects). Products include:
- Inapsine Injection ... 1296

Enflurane (Potential for additive effects).
- No products indexed under this heading.

Esmolol Hydrochloride (Increases the effects of sympathomimetics). Products include:
- Brevibloc Injection ... 1808

Estazolam (Potential for additive effects). Products include:
- ProSom Tablets ... 449

Ethchlorvynol (Potential for additive effects). Products include:
- Placidyl Capsules ... 448

Ethinamate (Potential for additive effects).
- No products indexed under this heading.

Fentanyl (Potential for additive effects). Products include:
- Duragesic Transdermal System ... 1288

Fentanyl Citrate (Potential for additive effects). Products include:
- Sublimaze Injection ... 1307

Fluphenazine Decanoate (Potential for additive effects). Products include:
- Prolixin Decanoate ... 509

Fluphenazine Enanthate (Potential for additive effects). Products include:
- Prolixin Enanthate ... 509

Fluphenazine Hydrochloride (Potential for additive effects). Products include:
- Prolixin ... 509

Flurazepam Hydrochloride (Potential for additive effects). Products include:
- Dalmane Capsules ... 2173

Furazolidone (Increases the effects of sympathomimetics; concurrent and/or sequential use is contraindicated). Products include:
- Furoxone ... 2046

Glutethimide (Potential for additive effects).
- No products indexed under this heading.

Haloperidol (Potential for additive effects). Products include:
- Haldol Injection, Tablets and Concentrate ... 1575

Haloperidol Decanoate (Potential for additive effects). Products include:
- Haldol Decanoate ... 1577

Hydrocodone Bitartrate (Potential for additive effects). Products include:
- Anexsia 5/500 Elixir ... 1781
- Anexia Tablets ... 1782
- Codiclear DH Syrup ... 791
- Deconamine CX Cough and Cold Liquid and Tablets ... 1319
- Duratuss HD Elixir ... 2565
- Hycodan Tablets and Syrup ... 930
- Hycomine Compound Tablets ... 932
- Hycomine ... 931
- Hycotuss Expectorant Syrup ... 933
- Hydrocet Capsules ... 782
- Lorcet 10/650 ... 1018
- Lortab ... 2566
- Tussend ... 1783
- Tussend Expectorant ... 1785
- Vicodin Tablets ... 1356
- Vicodin ES Tablets ... 1357
- Vicodin Tuss Expectorant ... 1358
- Zydone Capsules ... 949

Hydrocodone Polistirex (Potential for additive effects). Products include:
- Tussionex Pennkinetic Extended-Release Suspension ... 998

Hydroxyzine Hydrochloride (Potential for additive effects). Products include:
- Atarax Tablets & Syrup ... 2185
- Marax Tablets & DF Syrup ... 2200
- Vistaril Intramuscular Solution ... 2216

Imipramine Hydrochloride (Potential for additive effects). Products include:
- Tofranil Ampuls ... 854
- Tofranil Tablets ... 856

Imipramine Pamoate (Potential for additive effects). Products include:
- Tofranil-PM Capsules ... 857

Isocarboxazid (Increases the effects of sympathomimetics; concurrent and/or sequential use is contraindicated).
- No products indexed under this heading.

Isoflurane (Potential for additive effects).
- No products indexed under this heading.

Ketamine Hydrochloride (Potential for additive effects).
- No products indexed under this heading.

Labetalol Hydrochloride (Increases the effects of sympathomimetics). Products include:
- Normodyne Injection ... 2377
- Normodyne Tablets ... 2379
- Trandate ... 1185

Levobunolol Hydrochloride (Increases the effects of sympathomimetics). Products include:
- Betagan ... ⊙ 233

Levomethadyl Acetate Hydrochloride (Potential for additive effects). Products include:
- Orlamm ... 2239

Levorphanol Tartrate (Potential for additive effects). Products include:
- Levo-Dromoran ... 2129

Lorazepam (Potential for additive effects). Products include:
- Ativan Injection ... 2698
- Ativan Tablets ... 2700

Loxapine Hydrochloride (Potential for additive effects). Products include:
- Loxitane ... 1378

Loxapine Succinate (Potential for additive effects). Products include:
- Loxitane Capsules ... 1378

Maprotiline Hydrochloride (Potential for additive effects). Products include:
- Ludiomil Tablets ... 843

Mecamylamine Hydrochloride (Sympathomimetic may reduce the antihypertensive effects). Products include:
- Inversine Tablets ... 1686

Meperidine Hydrochloride (Potential for additive effects). Products include:
- Demerol ... 2308
- Mepergan Injection ... 2753

Mephobarbital (Potential for additive effects). Products include:
- Mebaral Tablets ... 2322

Meprobamate (Potential for additive effects). Products include:
- Miltown Tablets ... 2672
- PMB 200 and PMB 400 ... 2783

Mesoridazine Besylate (Potential for additive effects). Products include:
- Serentil ... 684

Methadone Hydrochloride (Potential for additive effects). Products include:
- Methadone Hydrochloride Oral Concentrate ... 2233
- Methadone Hydrochloride Oral Solution & Tablets ... 2235

Methohexital Sodium (Potential for additive effects). Products include:
- Brevital Sodium Vials ... 1429

Methotrimeprazine (Potential for additive effects). Products include:
- Levoprome ... 1274

Methoxyflurane (Potential for additive effects).
- No products indexed under this heading.

Methyldopa (Sympathomimetic may reduce the antihypertensive effects). Products include:
- Aldoclor Tablets ... 1598
- Aldomet Oral ... 1600
- Aldoril Tablets ... 1604

Methyldopate Hydrochloride (Sympathomimetic may reduce the antihypertensive effects). Products include:
- Aldomet Ester HCl Injection ... 1602

Metipranolol Hydrochloride (Increases the effects of sympathomimetics). Products include:
- OptiPranolol (Metipranolol 0.3%) Sterile Ophthalmic Solution ... ⊙ 258

Metoprolol Succinate (Increases the effects of sympathomimetics). Products include:
- Toprol-XL Tablets ... 565

Metoprolol Tartrate (Increases the effects of sympathomimetics). Products include:
- Lopressor Ampuls ... 830
- Lopressor HCT Tablets ... 832
- Lopressor Tablets ... 830

Midazolam Hydrochloride (Potential for additive effects). Products include:
- Versed Injection ... 2170

Molindone Hydrochloride (Potential for additive effects). Products include:
- Moban Tablets and Concentrate ... 1048

Morphine Sulfate (Potential for additive effects). Products include:
- Astramorph/PF Injection, USP (Preservative-Free) ... 535
- Duramorph ... 962
- Infumorph 200 and Infumorph 500 Sterile Solutions ... 965
- MS Contin Tablets ... 1994
- MSIR ... 1997
- Oramorph SR (Morphine Sulfate Sustained Release Tablets) ... 2236
- RMS Suppositories ... 2657
- Roxanol ... 2243

Nadolol (Increases the effects of sympathomimetics).
- No products indexed under this heading.

Nortriptyline Hydrochloride (Potential for additive effects). Products include:
- Pamelor ... 2280

Opium Alkaloids (Potential for additive effects).
- No products indexed under this heading.

Oxazepam (Potential for additive effects). Products include:
- Serax Capsules ... 2810
- Serax Tablets ... 2810

(▣ Described in PDR For Nonprescription Drugs) (⊙ Described in PDR For Ophthalmology)

Oxycodone Hydrochloride (Potential for additive effects). Products include:

Percocet Tablets 938
Percodan Tablets.. 939
Percodan-Demi Tablets.............................. 940
Roxicodone Tablets, Oral Solution & Intensol (Oxycodone) 2244
Tylox Capsules 1584

Penbutolol Sulfate (Increases the effects of sympathomimetics). Products include:

Levatol 2403

Pentobarbital Sodium (Potential for additive effects). Products include:

Nembutal Sodium Capsules 436
Nembutal Sodium Solution 438
Nembutal Sodium Suppositories...... 440

Perphenazine (Potential for additive effects). Products include:

Etrafon 2355
Triavil Tablets 1757
Trilafon... 2389

Phenelzine Sulfate (Increases the effects of sympathomimetics; concurrent and/or sequential use is contraindicated). Products include:

Nardil 1920

Phenobarbital (Potential for additive effects). Products include:

Arco-Lase Plus Tablets 512
Bellergal-S Tablets 2250
Donnatal 2060
Donnatal Extentabs................................ 2061
Donnatal Tablets 2060
Phenobarbital Elixir and Tablets 1469
Quadrinal Tablets 1350

Pindolol (Increases the effects of sympathomimetics). Products include:

Visken Tablets.. 2299

Prazepam (Potential for additive effects).

No products indexed under this heading.

Prochlorperazine (Potential for additive effects). Products include:

Compazine 2470

Promethazine Hydrochloride (Potential for additive effects). Products include:

Mepergan Injection 2753
Phenergan with Codeine 2777
Phenergan with Dextromethorphan 2778
Phenergan Injection 2773
Phenergan Suppositories 2775
Phenergan Syrup 2774
Phenergan Tablets 2775
Phenergan VC 2779
Phenergan VC with Codeine 2781

Propofol (Potential for additive effects). Products include:

Diprivan Injection.................................... 2833

Propoxyphene Hydrochloride (Potential for additive effects). Products include:

Darvon 1435
Wygesic Tablets 2827

Propoxyphene Napsylate (Potential for additive effects). Products include:

Darvon-N/Darvocet-N 1433

Propranolol Hydrochloride (Increases the effects of sympathomimetics). Products include:

Inderal 2728
Inderal LA Long Acting Capsules 2730
Inderide Tablets 2732
Inderide LA Long Acting Capsules .. 2734

Protriptyline Hydrochloride (Potential for additive effects). Products include:

Vivactil Tablets 1774

Quazepam (Potential for additive effects). Products include:

Doral Tablets 2664

Reserpine (Sympathomimetic may reduce the antihypertensive effects). Products include:

Diupres Tablets 1650
Hydropres Tablets................................... 1675
Ser-Ap-Es Tablets 849

Risperidone (Potential for additive effects). Products include:

Risperdal 1301

Secobarbital Sodium (Potential for additive effects). Products include:

Seconal Sodium Pulvules 1474

Selegiline Hydrochloride (Increases the effects of sympathomimetics; concurrent and/or sequential use is contraindicated). Products include:

Eldepryl Tablets 2550

Sotalol Hydrochloride (Increases the effects of sympathomimetics). Products include:

Betapace Tablets 641

Sufentanil Citrate (Potential for additive effects). Products include:

Sufenta Injection 1309

Temazepam (Potential for additive effects). Products include:

Restoril Capsules..................................... 2284

Thiamylal Sodium (Potential for additive effects).

No products indexed under this heading.

Thioridazine Hydrochloride (Potential for additive effects). Products include:

Mellaril 2269

Thiothixene (Potential for additive effects). Products include:

Navane Capsules and Concentrate 2201
Navane Intramuscular 2202

Timolol Hemihydrate (Increases the effects of sympathomimetics). Products include:

Betimol 0.25%, 0.5% .... ⊙ 261

Timolol Maleate (Increases the effects of sympathomimetics). Products include:

Blocadren Tablets 1614
Timolide Tablets....................................... 1748
Timoptic in Ocudose 1753
Timoptic Sterile Ophthalmic Solution... 1751
Timoptic-XE 1755

Tranylcypromine Sulfate (Increases the effects of sympathomimetics; concurrent and/or sequential use is contraindicated). Products include:

Parnate Tablets 2503

Triazolam (Potential for additive effects). Products include:

Halcion Tablets 2611

Trifluoperazine Hydrochloride (Potential for additive effects). Products include:

Stelazine 2514

Trimipramine Maleate (Potential for additive effects). Products include:

Surmontil Capsules................................. 2811

Zolpidem Tartrate (Potential for additive effects). Products include:

Ambien Tablets... 2416

Food Interactions

Alcohol (Potential for additive effects).

DURATUSS HD ELIXIR

(Hydrocodone Bitartrate, Pseudoephedrine Hydrochloride, Guaifenesin) 2565

May interact with central nervous system depressants, narcotic analgesics, general anesthetics, hypnotics and sedatives, tranquilizers, tricyclic antidepressants, monoamine oxidase inhibitors, beta blockers, veratrum alkaloids, and certain other agents. Compounds in these categories include:

Acebutolol Hydrochloride (Potentiation of sympathomimetic effects of pseudoephedrine). Products include:

Sectral Capsules 2807

Alfentanil Hydrochloride (Potentiation of central nervous system effects). Products include:

Alfenta Injection 1286

Alprazolam (Potentiation of central nervous system effects). Products include:

Xanax Tablets 2649

Amitriptyline Hydrochloride (Potentiation of central nervous system effects). Products include:

Elavil 2838
Endep Tablets 2174
Etrafon 2355
Limbitrol 2180
Triavil Tablets.. 1757

Amoxapine (Potentiation of central nervous system effects). Products include:

Asendin Tablets 1369

Aprobarbital (Potentiation of central nervous system effects).

No products indexed under this heading.

Atenolol (Potentiation of sympathomimetic effects of pseudoephedrine). Products include:

Tenoretic Tablets...................................... 2845
Tenormin Tablets and I.V. Injection 2847

Betaxolol Hydrochloride (Potentiation of sympathomimetic effects of pseudoephedrine). Products include:

Betoptic Ophthalmic Solution............ 469
Betoptic S Ophthalmic Suspension 471
Kerlone Tablets... 2436

Bisoprolol Fumarate (Potentiation of sympathomimetic effects of pseudoephedrine). Products include:

Zebeta Tablets 1413
Ziac 1415

Buprenorphine (Potentiation of central nervous system effects). Products include:

Buprenex Injectable 2006

Buspirone Hydrochloride (Potentiation of central nervous system effects). Products include:

BuSpar 737

Butabarbital (Potentiation of central nervous system effects).

No products indexed under this heading.

Butalbital (Potentiation of central nervous system effects). Products include:

Esgic-plus Tablets 1013
Fioricet Tablets... 2258
Fioricet with Codeine Capsules 2260
Fiorinal Capsules 2261
Fiorinal with Codeine Capsules 2262
Fiorinal Tablets... 2261
Phrenilin 785
Sedapap Tablets 50 mg/650 mg .. 1543

Carteolol Hydrochloride (Potentiation of sympathomimetic effects of pseudoephedrine). Products include:

Cartrol Tablets 410
Ocupress Ophthalmic Solution, 1% Sterile... ⊙ 309

Chlordiazepoxide (Potentiation of central nervous system effects). Products include:

Libritabs Tablets 2177
Limbitrol 2180

Chlordiazepoxide Hydrochloride (Potentiation of central nervous system effects). Products include:

Librax Capsules 2176

Librium Capsules..................................... 2178
Librium Injectable 2179

Chlorpromazine (Potentiation of central nervous system effects). Products include:

Thorazine Suppositories 2523

Chlorpromazine Hydrochloride (Potentiation of central nervous system effects). Products include:

Thorazine 2523

Chlorprothixene (Potentiation of central nervous system effects).

No products indexed under this heading.

Chlorprothixene Hydrochloride (Potentiation of central nervous system effects).

No products indexed under this heading.

Clomipramine Hydrochloride (Potentiation of central nervous system effects). Products include:

Anafranil Capsules 803

Clorazepate Dipotassium (Potentiation of central nervous system effects). Products include:

Tranxene 451

Clozapine (Potentiation of central nervous system effects). Products include:

Clozaril Tablets... 2252

Codeine Phosphate (Potentiation of central nervous system effects). Products include:

Actifed with Codeine Cough Syrup.. 1067
Brontex 1981
Deconsal C Expectorant Syrup 456
Deconsal Pediatric Syrup 457
Dimetane-DC Cough Syrup 2059
Empirin with Codeine Tablets............ 1093
Fioricet with Codeine Capsules 2260
Fiorinal with Codeine Capsules 2262
Isoclor Expectorant................................. 990
Novahistine DH.. 2462
Novahistine Expectorant....................... 2463
Nucofed 2051
Phenergan with Codeine 2777
Phenergan VC with Codeine 2781
Robitussin A-C Syrup 2073
Robitussin-DAC Syrup 2074
Ryna .... ⊞ 841
Soma Compound w/Codeine Tablets 2676
Tussi-Organidin NR Liquid and S NR Liquid 2677
Tylenol with Codeine 1583

Cryptenamine Preparations (Reduced antihypertensive effects).

Desflurane (Potentiation of central nervous system effects). Products include:

Suprane 1813

Desipramine Hydrochloride (Potentiation of central nervous system effects). Products include:

Norpramin Tablets 1526

Dezocine (Potentiation of central nervous system effects). Products include:

Dalgan Injection 538

Diazepam (Potentiation of central nervous system effects). Products include:

Dizac 1809
Valium Injectable 2182
Valium Tablets 2183
Valrelease Capsules 2169

Doxepin Hydrochloride (Potentiation of central nervous system effects). Products include:

Sinequan 2205
Zonalon Cream 1055

Droperidol (Potentiation of central nervous system effects). Products include:

Inapsine Injection.................................... 1296

Enflurane (Potentiation of central nervous system effects).

No products indexed under this heading.

IMPORTANT NOTE: Always consult each drug listing in the patient's regimen for possible interactions.

Duratuss HD Interactions Index 348

Esmolol Hydrochloride (Potentiation of sympathomimetic effects of pseudoephedrine). Products include:
Brevibloc Injection ... 1808
Estazolam (Potentiation of central nervous system effects). Products include:
ProSom Tablets ... 449
Ethchlorvynol (Potentiation of central nervous system effects). Products include:
Placidyl Capsules ... 448
Ethinamate (Potentiation of central nervous system effects).
No products indexed under this heading.
Fentanyl (Potentiation of central nervous system effects). Products include:
Duragesic Transdermal System ... 1288
Fentanyl Citrate (Potentiation of central nervous system effects). Products include:
Sublimaze Injection ... 1307
Fluphenazine Decanoate (Potentiation of central nervous system effects). Products include:
Prolixin Decanoate ... 509
Fluphenazine Enanthate (Potentiation of central nervous system effects). Products include:
Prolixin Enanthate ... 509
Fluphenazine Hydrochloride (Potentiation of central nervous system effects). Products include:
Prolixin ... 509
Flurazepam Hydrochloride (Potentiation of central nervous system effects). Products include:
Dalmane Capsules ... 2173
Furazolidone (Concurrent use is contraindicated; potentiation of central nervous system effects of hydrocodone and potentiation of sympathomimetic effects of pseudoephedrine). Products include:
Furoxone ... 2046
Glutethimide (Potentiation of central nervous system effects).
No products indexed under this heading.
Haloperidol (Potentiation of central nervous system effects). Products include:
Haldol Injection, Tablets and Concentrate ... 1575
Haloperidol Decanoate (Potentiation of central nervous system effects). Products include:
Haldol Decanoate ... 1577
Hydrocodone Polistirex (Potentiation of central nervous system effects). Products include:
Tussionex Pennkinetic Extended-Release Suspension ... 998
Hydroxyzine Hydrochloride (Potentiation of central nervous system effects). Products include:
Atarax Tablets & Syrup ... 2185
Marax Tablets & DF Syrup ... 2200
Vistaril Intramuscular Solution ... 2216
Imipramine Hydrochloride (Potentiation of central nervous system effects). Products include:
Tofranil Ampuls ... 854
Tofranil Tablets ... 856
Imipramine Pamoate (Potentiation of central nervous system effects). Products include:
Tofranil-PM Capsules ... 857
Isocarboxazid (Concurrent use is contraindicated; potentiation of central nervous system effects of hydrocodone and potentiation of sympathomimetic effects of pseudoephedrine).
No products indexed under this heading.
Isoflurane (Potentiation of central nervous system effects).
No products indexed under this heading.
Ketamine Hydrochloride (Potentiation of central nervous system effects).
No products indexed under this heading.
Labetalol Hydrochloride (Potentiation of sympathomimetic effects of pseudoephedrine). Products include:
Normodyne Injection ... 2377
Normodyne Tablets ... 2379
Trandate ... 1185
Levobunolol Hydrochloride (Potentiation of sympathomimetic effects of pseudoephedrine). Products include:
Betagan ... ◉ 233
Levomethadyl Acetate Hydrochloride (Potentiation of central nervous system effects). Products include:
Orlamm ... 2239
Levorphanol Tartrate (Potentiation of central nervous system effects). Products include:
Levo-Dromoran ... 2129
Lorazepam (Potentiation of central nervous system effects). Products include:
Ativan Injection ... 2698
Ativan Tablets ... 2700
Loxapine Hydrochloride (Potentiation of central nervous system effects). Products include:
Loxitane ... 1378
Loxapine Succinate (Potentiation of central nervous system effects). Products include:
Loxitane Capsules ... 1378
Maprotiline Hydrochloride (Potentiation of central nervous system effects). Products include:
Ludiomil Tablets ... 843
Mecamylamine Hydrochloride (Reduced antihypertensive effects). Products include:
Inversine Tablets ... 1686
Meperidine Hydrochloride (Potentiation of central nervous system effects). Products include:
Demerol ... 2308
Mepergan Injection ... 2753
Mephobarbital (Potentiation of central nervous system effects). Products include:
Mebaral Tablets ... 2322
Meprobamate (Potentiation of central nervous system effects). Products include:
Miltown Tablets ... 2672
PMB 200 and PMB 400 ... 2783
Mesoridazine (Potentiation of central nervous system effects).
Methadone Hydrochloride (Potentiation of central nervous system effects). Products include:
Methadone Hydrochloride Oral Concentrate ... 2233
Methadone Hydrochloride Oral Solution & Tablets ... 2235
Methohexital Sodium (Potentiation of central nervous system effects). Products include:
Brevital Sodium Vials ... 1429
Methotrimeprazine (Potentiation of central nervous system effects). Products include:
Levoprome ... 1274
Methoxyflurane (Potentiation of central nervous system effects).
No products indexed under this heading.
Methyldopa (Reduced antihypertensive effects). Products include:
Aldoclor Tablets ... 1598
Aldomet Oral ... 1600
Aldoril Tablets ... 1604
Methyldopate Hydrochloride (Reduced antihypertensive effects). Products include:
Aldomet Ester HCl Injection ... 1602
Metipranolol Hydrochloride (Potentiation of sympathomimetic effects of pseudoephedrine). Products include:
OptiPranolol (Metipranolol 0.3%) Sterile Ophthalmic Solution ... ◉ 258
Metoprolol Succinate (Potentiation of sympathomimetic effects of pseudoephedrine). Products include:
Toprol-XL Tablets ... 565
Metoprolol Tartrate (Potentiation of sympathomimetic effects of pseudoephedrine). Products include:
Lopressor Ampuls ... 830
Lopressor HCT Tablets ... 832
Lopressor Tablets ... 830
Midazolam Hydrochloride (Potentiation of central nervous system effects). Products include:
Versed Injection ... 2170
Molindone Hydrochloride (Potentiation of central nervous system effects). Products include:
Moban Tablets and Concentrate ... 1048
Morphine Sulfate (Potentiation of central nervous system effects). Products include:
Astramorph/PF Injection, USP (Preservative-Free) ... 535
Duramorph ... 962
Infumorph 200 and Infumorph 500 Sterile Solutions ... 965
MS Contin Tablets ... 1994
MSIR ... 1997
Oramorph SR (Morphine Sulfate Sustained Release Tablets) ... 2236
RMS Suppositories ... 2657
Roxanol ... 2243
Nadolol (Potentiation of sympathomimetic effects of pseudoephedrine).
No products indexed under this heading.
Nortriptyline Hydrochloride (Potentiation of central nervous system effects). Products include:
Pamelor ... 2280
Opium Alkaloids (Potentiation of central nervous system effects).
No products indexed under this heading.
Oxazepam (Potentiation of central nervous system effects). Products include:
Serax Capsules ... 2810
Serax Tablets ... 2810
Oxycodone Hydrochloride (Potentiation of central nervous system effects). Products include:
Percocet Tablets ... 938
Percodan Tablets ... 939
Percodan-Demi Tablets ... 940
Roxicodone Tablets, Oral Solution & Intensol (Oxycodone) ... 2244
Tylox Capsules ... 1584
Penbutolol Sulfate (Potentiation of sympathomimetic effects of pseudoephedrine). Products include:
Levatol ... 2403
Pentobarbital Sodium (Potentiation of central nervous system effects). Products include:
Nembutal Sodium Capsules ... 436
Nembutal Sodium Solution ... 438
Nembutal Sodium Suppositories ... 440
Perphenazine (Potentiation of central nervous system effects). Products include:
Etrafon ... 2355
Triavil Tablets ... 1757
Trilafon ... 2389
Phenelzine Sulfate (Concurrent use is contraindicated; potentiation of central nervous system effects of hydrocodone and potentiation of sympathomimetic effects of pseudoephedrine). Products include:
Nardil ... 1920
Phenobarbital (Potentiation of central nervous system effects). Products include:
Arco-Lase Plus Tablets ... 512
Bellergal-S Tablets ... 2250
Donnatal ... 2060
Donnatal Extentabs ... 2061
Donnatal Tablets ... 2060
Phenobarbital Elixir and Tablets ... 1469
Quadrinal Tablets ... 1350
Pindolol (Potentiation of sympathomimetic effects of pseudoephedrine). Products include:
Visken Tablets ... 2299
Prazepam (Potentiation of central nervous system effects).
No products indexed under this heading.
Prochlorperazine (Potentiation of central nervous system effects). Products include:
Compazine ... 2470
Promethazine Hydrochloride (Potentiation of central nervous system effects). Products include:
Mepergan Injection ... 2753
Phenergan with Codeine ... 2777
Phenergan with Dextromethorphan ... 2778
Phenergan Injection ... 2773
Phenergan Suppositories ... 2775
Phenergan Syrup ... 2774
Phenergan Tablets ... 2775
Phenergan VC ... 2779
Phenergan VC with Codeine ... 2781
Propofol (Potentiation of central nervous system effects). Products include:
Diprivan Injection ... 2833
Propoxyphene Hydrochloride (Potentiation of central nervous system effects). Products include:
Darvon ... 1435
Wygesic Tablets ... 2827
Propoxyphene Napsylate (Potentiation of central nervous system effects). Products include:
Darvon-N/Darvocet-N ... 1433
Propranolol Hydrochloride (Potentiation of sympathomimetic effects of pseudoephedrine). Products include:
Inderal ... 2728
Inderal LA Long Acting Capsules ... 2730
Inderide Tablets ... 2732
Inderide LA Long Acting Capsules ... 2734
Protriptyline Hydrochloride (Potentiation of central nervous system effects). Products include:
Vivactil Tablets ... 1774
Quazepam (Potentiation of central nervous system effects). Products include:
Doral Tablets ... 2664
Reserpine (Reduced antihypertensive effects). Products include:
Diupres Tablets ... 1650
Hydropres Tablets ... 1675
Ser-Ap-Es Tablets ... 849
Risperidone (Potentiation of central nervous system effects). Products include:
Risperdal ... 1301
Secobarbital Sodium (Potentiation of central nervous system effects). Products include:
Seconal Sodium Pulvules ... 1474
Selegiline Hydrochloride (Concurrent use is contraindicated; potentiation of central nervous system effects of hydrocodone and potentiation of sympathomimetic effects of pseudoephedrine). Products include:
Eldepryl Tablets ... 2550

349 **Interactions Index** **Dyazide**

Sotalol Hydrochloride (Potentiation of sympathomimetic effects of pseudoephedrine). Products include:
Betapace Tablets ... 641
Sufentanil Citrate (Potentiation of central nervous system effects). Products include:
Sufenta Injection ... 1309
Temazepam (Potentiation of central nervous system effects). Products include:
Restoril Capsules ... 2284
Thiamylal Sodium (Potentiation of central nervous system effects).
No products indexed under this heading.
Thioridazine Hydrochloride (Potentiation of central nervous system effects). Products include:
Mellaril ... 2269
Thiothixene (Potentiation of central nervous system effects). Products include:
Navane Capsules and Concentrate 2201
Navane Intramuscular ... 2202
Timolol Hemihydrate (Potentiation of sympathomimetic effects of pseudoephedrine). Products include:
Betimol 0.25%, 0.5% ... ◉ 261
Timolol Maleate (Potentiation of sympathomimetic effects of pseudoephedrine). Products include:
Blocadren Tablets ... 1614
Timolide Tablets ... 1748
Timoptic in Ocudose ... 1753
Timoptic Sterile Ophthalmic Solution ... 1751
Timoptic-XE ... 1755
Tranylcypromine Sulfate (Concurrent use is contraindicated; potentiation of central nervous system effects of hydrocodone and potentiation of sympathomimetic effects of pseudoephedrine). Products include:
Parnate Tablets ... 2503
Triazolam (Potentiation of central nervous system effects). Products include:
Halcion Tablets ... 2611
Trifluoperazine Hydrochloride (Potentiation of central nervous system effects). Products include:
Stelazine ... 2514
Trimipramine Maleate (Potentiation of central nervous system effects). Products include:
Surmontil Capsules ... 2811
Zolpidem Tartrate (Potentiation of central nervous system effects). Products include:
Ambien Tablets ... 2416

Food Interactions

Alcohol (Potentiation of central nervous system effects).

DURA-VENT TABLETS

(Phenylpropanolamine Hydrochloride, Guaifenesin) ... 952
May interact with monoamine oxidase inhibitors, beta blockers, and certain other agents. Compounds in these categories include:

Acebutolol Hydrochloride (Increases the effects of sympathomimetics). Products include:
Sectral Capsules ... 2807
Atenolol (Increases the effects of sympathomimetics). Products include:
Tenoretic Tablets ... 2845
Tenormin Tablets and I.V. Injection 2847
Betaxolol Hydrochloride (Increases the effects of sympathomimetics). Products include:
Betoptic Ophthalmic Solution ... 469
Betoptic S Ophthalmic Suspension 471
Kerlone Tablets ... 2436
Bisoprolol Fumarate (Increases the effects of sympathomimetics). Products include:
Zebeta Tablets ... 1413
Ziac ... 1415
Carteolol Hydrochloride (Increases the effects of sympathomimetics). Products include:
Cartrol Tablets ... 410
Ocupress Ophthalmic Solution, 1% Sterile ... ◉ 309
Esmolol Hydrochloride (Increases the effects of sympathomimetics). Products include:
Brevibloc Injection ... 1808
Furazolidone (Increases the effects of sympathomimetics; concurrent and/or sequential use is contraindicated). Products include:
Furoxone ... 2046
Isocarboxazid (Increases the effects of sympathomimetics; concurrent and/or sequential use is contraindicated).
No products indexed under this heading.
Labetalol Hydrochloride (Increases the effects of sympathomimetics). Products include:
Normodyne Injection ... 2377
Normodyne Tablets ... 2379
Trandate ... 1185
Levobunolol Hydrochloride (Increases the effects of sympathomimetics). Products include:
Betagan ... ◉ 233
Mecamylamine Hydrochloride (Sympathomimetic may reduce the antihypertensive effects). Products include:
Inversine Tablets ... 1686
Methyldopa (Sympathomimetic may reduce the antihypertensive effects). Products include:
Aldoclor Tablets ... 1598
Aldomet Oral ... 1600
Aldoril Tablets ... 1604
Methyldopate Hydrochloride (Sympathomimetic may reduce the antihypertensive effects). Products include:
Aldomet Ester HCl Injection ... 1602
Metipranolol Hydrochloride (Increases the effects of sympathomimetics). Products include:
OptiPranolol (Metipranolol 0.3%) Sterile Ophthalmic Solution ... ◉ 258
Metoprolol Succinate (Increases the effects of sympathomimetics). Products include:
Toprol-XL Tablets ... 565
Metoprolol Tartrate (Increases the effects of sympathomimetics). Products include:
Lopressor Ampuls ... 830
Lopressor HCT Tablets ... 832
Lopressor Tablets ... 830
Nadolol (Increases the effects of sympathomimetics).
No products indexed under this heading.
Penbutolol Sulfate (Increases the effects of sympathomimetics). Products include:
Levatol ... 2403
Phenelzine Sulfate (Increases the effects of sympathomimetics; concurrent and/or sequential use is contraindicated). Products include:
Nardil ... 1920
Pindolol (Increases the effects of sympathomimetics). Products include:
Visken Tablets ... 2299
Propranolol Hydrochloride (Increases the effects of sympathomimetics). Products include:
Inderal ... 2728
Inderal LA Long Acting Capsules ... 2730
Inderide Tablets ... 2732
Inderide LA Long Acting Capsules .. 2734
Reserpine (Sympathomimetic may reduce the antihypertensive effects). Products include:
Diupres Tablets ... 1650
Hydropres Tablets ... 1675
Ser-Ap-Es Tablets ... 849
Selegiline Hydrochloride (Increases the effects of sympathomimetics; concurrent and/or sequential use is contraindicated). Products include:
Eldepryl Tablets ... 2550
Sotalol Hydrochloride (Increases the effects of sympathomimetics). Products include:
Betapace Tablets ... 641
Timolol Hemihydrate (Increases the effects of sympathomimetics). Products include:
Betimol 0.25%, 0.5% ... ◉ 261
Timolol Maleate (Increases the effects of sympathomimetics). Products include:
Blocadren Tablets ... 1614
Timolide Tablets ... 1748
Timoptic in Ocudose ... 1753
Timoptic Sterile Ophthalmic Solution ... 1751
Timoptic-XE ... 1755
Tranylcypromine Sulfate (Increases the effects of sympathomimetics; concurrent and/or sequential use is contraindicated). Products include:
Parnate Tablets ... 2503

DURICEF

(Cefadroxil Monohydrate) ... 748
None cited in PDR database.

DUVOID

(Bethanechol Chloride) ... 2044
May interact with ganglionic blocking agents. Compounds in this category include:

Mecamylamine Hydrochloride (Potential for critical fall in blood pressure may occur; exercise caution). Products include:
Inversine Tablets ... 1686
Trimethaphan Camsylate (Potential for critical fall in blood pressure may occur; exercise caution). Products include:
Arfonad Ampuls ... 2080

DYAZIDE

(Triamterene, Hydrochlorothiazide) .. 2479
May interact with potassium sparing diuretics, potassium preparations, ACE inhibitors, non-steroidal anti-inflammatory agents, lithium preparations, corticosteroids, antihypertensives, oral anticoagulants, antigout agents, nondepolarizing neuromuscular blocking agents, and certain other agents. Compounds in these categories include:

Acarbose (Increased risk of severe hyponatremia).
No products indexed under this heading.
Acebutolol Hydrochloride (May add to potentiate the action of other hypertensives). Products include:
Sectral Capsules ... 2807
ACTH (May intensify electrolyte imbalance, particularly hypokalemia).
No products indexed under this heading.
Allopurinol (Dyazide may raise the level of blood uric acid; may require dosage adjustment of antigout agent). Products include:
Zyloprim Tablets ... 1226
Amiloride Hydrochloride (Concurrent use is contraindicated). Products include:
Midamor Tablets ... 1703
Moduretic Tablets ... 1705
Amlodipine Besylate (May add to potentiate the action of other hypertensives). Products include:
Lotrel Capsules ... 840
Norvasc Tablets ... 1940
Amphotericin B (May intensify electrolyte imbalance, particularly hypokalemia). Products include:
Fungizone Intravenous ... 506
Atenolol (May add to potentiate the action of other hypertensives). Products include:
Tenoretic Tablets ... 2845
Tenormin Tablets and I.V. Injection 2847
Atracurium Besylate (Increased paralyzing effect). Products include:
Tracrium Injection ... 1183
Benazepril Hydrochloride (May add to potentiate the action of other hypertensives; increased risk of hyperkalemia). Products include:
Lotensin Tablets ... 834
Lotensin HCT ... 837
Lotrel Capsules ... 840
Bendroflumethiazide (May add to potentiate the action of other hypertensives).
No products indexed under this heading.
Betamethasone Acetate (May intensify electrolyte imbalance, particularly hypokalemia). Products include:
Celestone Soluspan Suspension ... 2347
Betamethasone Sodium Phosphate (May intensify electrolyte imbalance, particularly hypokalemia). Products include:
Celestone Soluspan Suspension ... 2347
Betaxolol Hydrochloride (May add to potentiate the action of other hypertensives). Products include:
Betoptic Ophthalmic Solution ... 469
Betoptic S Ophthalmic Suspension 471
Kerlone Tablets ... 2436
Bisoprolol Fumarate (May add to potentiate the action of other hypertensives). Products include:
Zebeta Tablets ... 1413
Ziac ... 1415
Blood, whole (Concurrent use of whole blood from blood bank with triamterene may result in hyperkalemia, especially in patients with renal insufficiency).
No products indexed under this heading.
Captopril (May add to potentiate the action of other hypertensives; increased risk of hyperkalemia). Products include:
Capoten ... 739
Capozide ... 742
Carteolol Hydrochloride (May add to potentiate the action of other hypertensives). Products include:
Cartrol Tablets ... 410
Ocupress Ophthalmic Solution, 1% Sterile ... ◉ 309
Chlorothiazide (May add to potentiate the action of other hypertensives). Products include:
Aldoclor Tablets ... 1598
Diupres Tablets ... 1650
Diuril Oral ... 1653
Chlorothiazide Sodium (May add to potentiate the action of other hypertensives). Products include:
Diuril Sodium Intravenous ... 1652
Chlorpropamide (Increased risk of severe hyponatremia). Products include:
Diabinese Tablets ... 1935

IMPORTANT NOTE: Always consult each drug listing in the patient's regimen for possible interactions.

Dyazide **Interactions Index** 350

Chlorthalidone (May add to potentiate the action of other hypertensives). Products include:
- Combipres Tablets ... 677
- Tenoretic Tablets ... 2845
- Thalitone ... 1245

Clonidine (May add to potentiate the action of other hypertensives). Products include:
- Catapres-TTS ... 675

Clonidine Hydrochloride (May add to potentiate the action of other hypertensives). Products include:
- Catapres Tablets ... 674
- Combipres Tablets ... 677

Cortisone Acetate (May intensify electrolyte imbalance, particularly hypokalemia). Products include:
- Cortone Acetate Sterile Suspension ... 1623
- Cortone Acetate Tablets ... 1624

Deserpidine (May add to potentiate the action of other hypertensives).
- No products indexed under this heading.

Dexamethasone (May intensify electrolyte imbalance, particularly hypokalemia). Products include:
- AK-Trol Ointment & Suspension ... ⊙ 205
- Decadron Elixir ... 1633
- Decadron Tablets ... 1635
- Decaspray Topical Aerosol ... 1648
- Dexacidin Ointment ... ⊙ 263
- Maxitrol Ophthalmic Ointment and Suspension ... ⊙ 224
- TobraDex Ophthalmic Suspension and Ointment ... 473

Dexamethasone Acetate (May intensify electrolyte imbalance, particularly hypokalemia). Products include:
- Dalalone D.P. Injectable ... 1011
- Decadron-LA Sterile Suspension ... 1646

Dexamethasone Sodium Phosphate (May intensify electrolyte imbalance, particularly hypokalemia). Products include:
- Decadron Phosphate Injection ... 1637
- Decadron Phosphate Respihaler ... 1642
- Decadron Phosphate Sterile Ophthalmic Ointment ... 1641
- Decadron Phosphate Sterile Ophthalmic Solution ... 1642
- Decadron Phosphate Topical Cream ... 1644
- Decadron Phosphate Turbinaire ... 1645
- Decadron Phosphate with Xylocaine Injection, Sterile ... 1639
- Dexacort Phosphate in Respihaler ... 458
- Dexacort Phosphate in Turbinaire ... 459
- NeoDecadron Sterile Ophthalmic Ointment ... 1712
- NeoDecadron Sterile Ophthalmic Solution ... 1713
- NeoDecadron Topical Cream ... 1714

Diazoxide (May add to potentiate the action of other hypertensives). Products include:
- Hyperstat I.V. Injection ... 2363
- Proglycem ... 580

Diclofenac Potassium (Potential for acute renal failure). Products include:
- Cataflam ... 816

Diclofenac Sodium (Potential for acute renal failure). Products include:
- Voltaren Ophthalmic Sterile Ophthalmic Solution ... ⊙ 272
- Voltaren Tablets ... 861

Dicumarol (Effects of oral anticoagulants may be decreased).
- No products indexed under this heading.

Diltiazem Hydrochloride (May add to potentiate the action of other hypertensives). Products include:
- Cardizem CD Capsules ... 1506
- Cardizem SR Capsules ... 1510
- Cardizem Injectable ... 1508
- Cardizem Tablets ... 1512
- Dilacor XR Extended-release Capsules ... 2018

Doxazosin Mesylate (May add to potentiate the action of other hypertensives). Products include:
- Cardura Tablets ... 2186

Enalapril Maleate (May add to potentiate the action of other hypertensives; increased risk of hyperkalemia). Products include:
- Vaseretic Tablets ... 1765
- Vasotec Tablets ... 1771

Enalaprilat (May add to potentiate the action of other hypertensives; increased risk of hyperkalemia). Products include:
- Vasotec I.V. ... 1768

Esmolol Hydrochloride (May add to potentiate the action of other hypertensives). Products include:
- Brevibloc Injection ... 1808

Etodolac (Potential for acute renal failure). Products include:
- Lodine Capsules and Tablets ... 2743

Felodipine (May add to potentiate the action of other hypertensives). Products include:
- Plendil Extended-Release Tablets ... 527

Fenoprofen Calcium (Potential for acute renal failure). Products include:
- Nalfon 200 Pulvules & Nalfon Tablets ... 917

Fludrocortisone Acetate (May intensify electrolyte imbalance, particularly hypokalemia). Products include:
- Florinef Acetate Tablets ... 505

Flurbiprofen (Potential for acute renal failure). Products include:
- Ansaid Tablets ... 2579

Fosinopril Sodium (May add to potentiate the action of other hypertensives; increased risk of hyperkalemia). Products include:
- Monopril Tablets ... 757

Furosemide (May add to potentiate the action of other hypertensives). Products include:
- Lasix Injection, Oral Solution and Tablets ... 1240

Guanabenz Acetate (May add to potentiate the action of other hypertensives).
- No products indexed under this heading.

Guanethidine Monosulfate (May add to potentiate the action of other hypertensives). Products include:
- Esimil Tablets ... 822
- Ismelin Tablets ... 827

Hydralazine Hydrochloride (May add to potentiate the action of other hypertensives). Products include:
- Apresazide Capsules ... 808
- Apresoline Hydrochloride Tablets ... 809
- Ser-Ap-Es Tablets ... 849

Hydrocortisone (May intensify electrolyte imbalance, particularly hypokalemia). Products include:
- Anusol-HC Cream 2.5% ... 1896
- Aquanil HC Lotion ... 1931
- Bactine Hydrocortisone Anti-Itch Cream ... ▣ 709
- Caldecort Anti-Itch Hydrocortisone Spray ... ▣ 631
- Cortaid ... ▣ 836
- CORTENEMA ... 2535
- Cortisporin Ointment ... 1085
- Cortisporin Ophthalmic Ointment Sterile ... 1085
- Cortisporin Ophthalmic Suspension Sterile ... 1086
- Cortisporin Otic Solution Sterile ... 1087
- Cortisporin Otic Suspension Sterile ... 1088
- Cortizone-5 ... ▣ 831
- Cortizone-10 ... ▣ 831
- Hydrocortone Tablets ... 1672
- Hytone ... 907
- Massengill Medicated Soft Cloth Towelettes ... 2458
- PediOtic Suspension Sterile ... 1153
- Preparation H Hydrocortisone 1% Cream ... ▣ 872
- ProctoCream-HC 2.5% ... 2408
- VōSoL HC Otic Solution ... 2678

Hydrocortisone Acetate (May intensify electrolyte imbalance, particularly hypokalemia). Products include:
- Analpram-HC Rectal Cream 1% and 2.5% ... 977
- Anusol HC-1 Anti-Itch Hydrocortisone Ointment ... ▣ 847
- Anusol-HC Suppositories ... 1897
- Caldecort ... ▣ 631
- Carmol HC ... 924
- Coly-Mycin S Otic w/Neomycin & Hydrocortisone ... 1906
- Cortaid ... ▣ 836
- Cortifoam ... 2396
- Cortisporin Cream ... 1084
- Epifoam ... 2399
- Hydrocortone Acetate Sterile Suspension ... 1669
- Mantadil Cream ... 1135
- Nupercainal Hydrocortisone 1% Cream ... ▣ 645
- Ophthocort ... ⊙ 311
- Pramosone Cream, Lotion & Ointment ... 978
- ProctoCream-HC ... 2408
- ProctoFoam-HC ... 2409
- Terra-Cortril Ophthalmic Suspension ... 2210

Hydrocortisone Sodium Phosphate (May intensify electrolyte imbalance, particularly hypokalemia). Products include:
- Hydrocortone Phosphate Injection, Sterile ... 1670

Hydrocortisone Sodium Succinate (May intensify electrolyte imbalance, particularly hypokalemia). Products include:
- Solu-Cortef Sterile Powder ... 2641

Hydroflumethiazide (May add to potentiate the action of other hypertensives). Products include:
- Diucardin Tablets ... 2718

Ibuprofen (Potential for acute renal failure). Products include:
- Advil Cold and Sinus Caplets and Tablets (formerly CoAdvil) ... ▣ 870
- Advil Ibuprofen Tablets and Caplets ... ▣ 870
- Children's Advil Suspension ... 2692
- Arthritis Foundation Ibuprofen Tablets ... ▣ 674
- Bayer Select Ibuprofen Pain Relief Formula ... ▣ 715
- Cramp End Tablets ... ▣ 735
- Dimetapp Sinus Caplets ... ▣ 775
- Haltran Tablets ... ▣ 771
- IBU Tablets ... 1342
- Ibuprohm ... ▣ 735
- Children's Motrin Ibuprofen Oral Suspension ... 1546
- Motrin Tablets ... 2625
- Motrin IB Caplets, Tablets, and Geltabs ... ▣ 838
- Motrin IB Sinus ... ▣ 838
- Motrin Ibuprofen Suspension, Oral Drops, Chewable Tablets, Caplets ... 1546
- Nuprin Ibuprofen/Analgesic Tablets & Caplets ... ▣ 622
- Sine-Aid IB Caplets ... 1554
- Vicks DayQuil SINUS Pressure & PAIN Relief with IBUPROFEN ... ▣ 762

Indapamide (May add to potentiate the action of other hypertensives). Products include:
- Lozol Tablets ... 2022

Indomethacin (Potential for acute renal failure). Products include:
- Indocin ... 1680

Indomethacin Sodium Trihydrate (Potential for acute renal failure). Products include:
- Indocin I.V. ... 1684

Isradipine (May add to potentiate the action of other hypertensives). Products include:
- DynaCirc Capsules ... 2256

Ketoprofen (Potential for acute renal failure). Products include:
- Orudis Capsules ... 2766
- Oruvail Capsules ... 2766

Ketorolac Tromethamine (Potential for acute renal failure). Products include:
- Acular ... 474
- Acular ... ⊙ 277
- Toradol ... 2159

Labetalol Hydrochloride (May add to potentiate the action of other hypertensives). Products include:
- Normodyne Injection ... 2377
- Normodyne Tablets ... 2379
- Trandate ... 1185

Laxatives, unspecified (Interferes with the potassium-retaining effects of triamterene; chronic or overuse of laxatives may reduce serum potassium).
- No products indexed under this heading.

Levobunolol Hydrochloride (May add to potentiate the action of other hypertensives). Products include:
- Betagan ... ⊙ 233

Lisinopril (May add to potentiate the action of other hypertensives; increased risk of hyperkalemia). Products include:
- Prinivil Tablets ... 1733
- Prinzide Tablets ... 1737
- Zestoretic ... 2850
- Zestril Tablets ... 2854

Lithium Carbonate (Reduced renal clearance and increased risk of lithium toxicity). Products include:
- Eskalith ... 2485
- Lithium Carbonate Capsules & Tablets ... 2230
- Lithonate/Lithotabs/Lithobid ... 2543

Lithium Citrate (Reduced renal clearance and increased risk of lithium toxicity).
- No products indexed under this heading.

Losartan Potassium (May add to potentiate the action of other hypertensives). Products include:
- Cozaar Tablets ... 1628
- Hyzaar Tablets ... 1677

Mecamylamine Hydrochloride (May add to potentiate the action of other hypertensives). Products include:
- Inversine Tablets ... 1686

Meclofenamate Sodium (Potential for acute renal failure).
- No products indexed under this heading.

Mefenamic Acid (Potential for acute renal failure). Products include:
- Ponstel ... 1925

Metformin Hydrochloride (Increased risk of severe hyponatremia). Products include:
- Glucophage ... 752

Methenamine (Decreased effectiveness of methenamine due to alkalinization of urine). Products include:
- Urised Tablets ... 1964

Methenamine Hippurate (Decreased effectiveness of methenamine due to alkalinization of urine).
- No products indexed under this heading.

Methenamine Mandelate (Decreased effectiveness of methenamine due to alkalinization of urine). Products include:
- Uroqid-Acid No. 2 Tablets ... 640

(▣ Described in PDR For Nonprescription Drugs) (⊙ Described in PDR For Ophthalmology)

Interactions Index — Dyazide

Methyclothiazide (May add to potentiate the action of other hypertensives). Products include:

Enduron Tablets 420

Methyldopa (May add to potentiate the action of other hypertensives). Products include:

Aldoclor Tablets 1598
Aldomet Oral 1600
Aldoril Tablets 1604

Methyldopate Hydrochloride (May add to potentiate the action of other hypertensives). Products include:

Aldomet Ester HCl Injection 1602

Methylprednisolone Acetate (May intensify electrolyte imbalance, particularly hypokalemia). Products include:

Depo-Medrol Single-Dose Vial 2600
Depo-Medrol Sterile Aqueous Suspension 2597

Methylprednisolone Sodium Succinate (May intensify electrolyte imbalance, particularly hypokalemia). Products include:

Solu-Medrol Sterile Powder 2643

Metipranolol Hydrochloride (May add to potentiate the action of other hypertensives). Products include:

OptiPranolol (Metipranolol 0.3%) Sterile Ophthalmic Solution .... ◉ 258

Metocurine Iodide (Increased paralyzing effect). Products include:

Metubine Iodide Vials 916

Metolazone (May add to potentiate the action of other hypertensives). Products include:

Mykrox Tablets 993
Zaroxolyn Tablets 1000

Metoprolol Succinate (May add to potentiate the action of other hypertensives). Products include:

Toprol-XL Tablets 565

Metoprolol Tartrate (May add to potentiate the action of other hypertensives). Products include:

Lopressor Ampuls 830
Lopressor HCT Tablets 832
Lopressor Tablets 830

Metyrosine (May add to potentiate the action of other hypertensives). Products include:

Demser Capsules 1649

Minoxidil (May add to potentiate the action of other hypertensives). Products include:

Loniten Tablets 2618
Rogaine Topical Solution 2637

Mivacurium Chloride (Increased paralyzing effect). Products include:

Mivacron 1138

Moexipril Hydrochloride (May add to potentiate the action of other hypertensives; increased risk of hyperkalemia). Products include:

Univasc Tablets 2410

Nabumetone (Potential for acute renal failure). Products include:

Relafen Tablets 2510

Nadolol (May add to potentiate the action of other hypertensives).

No products indexed under this heading.

Naproxen (Potential for acute renal failure). Products include:

Anaprox/Naprosyn 2117

Naproxen Sodium (Potential for acute renal failure). Products include:

Aleve 1975
Anaprox/Naprosyn 2117

Nicardipine Hydrochloride (May add to potentiate the action of other hypertensives). Products include:

Cardene Capsules 2095
Cardene I.V. 2709
Cardene SR Capsules 2097

Nifedipine (May add to potentiate the action of other hypertensives). Products include:

Adalat Capsules (10 mg and 20 mg) 587
Adalat CC 589
Procardia Capsules 1971
Procardia XL Extended Release Tablets 1972

Nisoldipine (May add to potentiate the action of other hypertensives).

No products indexed under this heading.

Nitroglycerin (May add to potentiate the action of other hypertensives). Products include:

Deponit NTG Transdermal Delivery System 2397
Nitro-Bid IV 1523
Nitro-Bid Ointment 1524
Nitrodisc 2047
Nitro-Dur (nitroglycerin) Transdermal Infusion System 1326
Nitrolingual Spray 2027
Nitrostat Tablets 1925
Transderm-Nitro Transdermal Therapeutic System 859

Norepinephrine Bitartrate (Decreased arterial responsiveness to norepinephrine). Products include:

Levophed Bitartrate Injection 2315

Oxaprozin (Potential for acute renal failure). Products include:

Daypro Caplets 2426

Pancuronium Bromide Injection (Increased paralyzing effect).

No products indexed under this heading.

Penbutolol Sulfate (May add to potentiate the action of other hypertensives). Products include:

Levatol 2403

Penicillin G Potassium (Concurrent use of parenteral penicillin G potassium with triamterene may result in hyperkalemia, especially in patients with renal insufficiency). Products include:

Pfizerpen for Injection 2203

Phenoxybenzamine Hydrochloride (May add to potentiate the action of other hypertensives). Products include:

Dibenzyline Capsules 2476

Phentolamine Mesylate (May add to potentiate the action of other hypertensives). Products include:

Regitine 846

Phenylbutazone (Potential for acute renal failure).

No products indexed under this heading.

Pindolol (May add to potentiate the action of other hypertensives). Products include:

Visken Tablets 2299

Piroxicam (Potential for acute renal failure). Products include:

Feldene Capsules 1965

Polythiazide (May add to potentiate the action of other hypertensives). Products include:

Minizide Capsules 1938

Potassium Acid Phosphate (Potential for hyperkalemia; concomitant use should be avoided). Products include:

K-Phos Original Formula 'Sodium Free' Tablets 639

Potassium Bicarbonate (Potential for hyperkalemia; concomitant use should be avoided). Products include:

Alka-Seltzer Gold Effervescent Antacid ....ⓐⓓ 703

Potassium Chloride (Potential for hyperkalemia; concomitant use should be avoided). Products include:

Chlor-3 Condiment 1004
K-Dur Microburst Release System (potassium chloride, USP) E.R. Tablets 1325
K-Lor Powder Packets 434
K-Norm Extended-Release Capsules 991
K-Tab Filmtab 434
Kolyum Liquid 992
Micro-K 2063
Micro-K LS Packets 2064
NuLYTELY 689
Cherry Flavor NuLYTELY 689
Rum-K Syrup 1005
Slow-K Extended-Release Tablets 851

Potassium Citrate (Potential for hyperkalemia; concomitant use should be avoided). Products include:

Polycitra Syrup 578
Polycitra-K Crystals 579
Polycitra-K Oral Solution 579
Polycitra-LC 578

Potassium Gluconate (Potential for hyperkalemia; concomitant use should be avoided). Products include:

Kolyum Liquid 992

Potassium Phosphate, Dibasic (Potential for hyperkalemia; concomitant use should be avoided).

No products indexed under this heading.

Potassium Phosphate, Monobasic (Potential for hyperkalemia; concomitant use should be avoided). Products include:

K-Phos Neutral Tablets 639
K-Phos Original Formula 'Sodium Free' Tablets 639

Prazosin Hydrochloride (May add to potentiate the action of other hypertensives). Products include:

Minipress Capsules 1937
Minizide Capsules 1938

Prednisolone Acetate (May intensify electrolyte imbalance, particularly hypokalemia). Products include:

AK-CIDE .... ◉ 202
AK-CIDE Ointment .... ◉ 202
Blephamide Liquifilm Sterile Ophthalmic Suspension 476
Blephamide Ointment .... ◉ 237
Econopred & Econopred Plus Ophthalmic Suspensions .... ◉ 217
Poly-Pred Liquifilm .... ◉ 248
Pred Forte .... ◉ 250
Pred Mild .... ◉ 253
Pred-G Liquifilm Sterile Ophthalmic Suspension .... ◉ 251
Pred-G S.O.P. Sterile Ophthalmic Ointment .... ◉ 252
Vasocidin Ointment .... ◉ 268

Prednisolone Sodium Phosphate (May intensify electrolyte imbalance, particularly hypokalemia). Products include:

AK-Pred .... ◉ 204
Hydeltrasol Injection, Sterile 1665
Inflamase .... ◉ 265
Pediapred Oral Liquid 995
Vasocidin Ophthalmic Solution .... ◉ 270

Prednisolone Tebutate (May intensify electrolyte imbalance, particularly hypokalemia). Products include:

Hydeltra-T.B.A. Sterile Suspension 1667

Prednisone (May intensify electrolyte imbalance, particularly hypokalemia). Products include:

Deltasone Tablets 2595

Probenecid (Dyazide may raise the level of blood uric acid; may require dosage adjustment of antigout agent). Products include:

Benemid Tablets 1611
ColBENEMID Tablets 1622

Propranolol Hydrochloride (May add to potentiate the action of other hypertensives). Products include:

Inderal 2728
Inderal LA Long Acting Capsules 2730
Inderide Tablets 2732
Inderide LA Long Acting Capsules .. 2734

Quinapril Hydrochloride (May add to potentiate the action of other hypertensives; increased risk of hyperkalemia). Products include:

Accupril Tablets 1893

Ramipril (May add to potentiate the action of other hypertensives; increased risk of hyperkalemia). Products include:

Altace Capsules 1232

Rauwolfia Serpentina (May add to potentiate the action of other hypertensives).

No products indexed under this heading.

Rescinnamine (May add to potentiate the action of other hypertensives).

No products indexed under this heading.

Reserpine (May add to potentiate the action of other hypertensives). Products include:

Diupres Tablets 1650
Hydropres Tablets 1675
Ser-Ap-Es Tablets 849

Rocuronium Bromide (Increased paralyzing effect). Products include:

Zemuron 1830

Salt Substitutes (Concurrent use of salt substitues with triamterene may result in hyperkalemia, especially in patients with renal insufficiency).

No products indexed under this heading.

Sodium Nitroprusside (May add to potentiate the action of other hypertensives).

No products indexed under this heading.

Sodium Polystyrene Sulfonate (May result in fluid retention). Products include:

Kayexalate 2314
Sodium Polystyrene Sulfonate Suspension 2244

Sotalol Hydrochloride (May add to potentiate the action of other hypertensives). Products include:

Betapace Tablets 641

Spirapril Hydrochloride (May add to potentiate the action of other hypertensives; increased risk of hyperkalemia).

No products indexed under this heading.

Spironolactone (Concurrent use is contraindicated). Products include:

Aldactazide 2413
Aldactone 2414

Sulfinpyrazone (Dyazide may raise the level of blood uric acid; may require dosage adjustment of antigout agent). Products include:

Anturane 807

Sulindac (Potential for acute renal failure). Products include:

Clinoril Tablets 1618

Terazosin Hydrochloride (May add to potentiate the action of other hypertensives). Products include:

Hytrin Capsules 430

Timolol Maleate (May add to potentiate the action of other hypertensives). Products include:

Blocadren Tablets 1614
Timolide Tablets 1748
Timoptic in Ocudose 1753

IMPORTANT NOTE: Always consult each drug listing in the patient's regimen for possible interactions.

Timoptic Sterile Ophthalmic Solution ... 1751
Timoptic-XE ... 1755

Tolmetin Sodium (Potential for acute renal failure). Products include:
Tolectin (200, 400 and 600 mg) .. 1581

Torsemide (May add to potentiate the action of other hypertensives). Products include:
Demadex Tablets and Injection ... 686

Triamcinolone (May intensify electrolyte imbalance, particularly hypokalemia). Products include:
Aristocort Tablets ... 1022

Triamcinolone Acetonide (May intensify electrolyte imbalance, particularly hypokalemia). Products include:
Aristocort A 0.025% Cream ... 1027
Aristocort A 0.5% Cream ... 1031
Aristocort A 0.1% Cream ... 1029
Aristocort A 0.1% Ointment ... 1030
Azmacort Oral Inhaler ... 2011
Nasacort Nasal Inhaler ... 2024

Triamcinolone Diacetate (May intensify electrolyte imbalance, particularly hypokalemia). Products include:
Aristocort Suspension (Forte Parenteral) ... 1027
Aristocort Suspension (Intralesional) ... 1025

Triamcinolone Hexacetonide (May intensify electrolyte imbalance, particularly hypokalemia). Products include:
Aristospan Suspension (Intra-articular) ... 1033
Aristospan Suspension (Intralesional) ... 1032

Trimethaphan Camsylate (May add to potentiate the action of other hypertensives). Products include:
Arfonad Ampuls ... 2080

Tubocurarine Chloride (Increased paralyzing effect).
No products indexed under this heading.

Vecuronium Bromide (Increased paralyzing effect). Products include:
Norcuron ... 1826

Verapamil Hydrochloride (May add to potentiate the action of other hypertensives). Products include:
Calan SR Caplets ... 2422
Calan Tablets ... 2419
Isoptin Injectable ... 1344
Isoptin Oral Tablets ... 1346
Isoptin SR Tablets ... 1348
Verelan Capsules ... 1410
Verelan Capsules ... 2824

Warfarin Sodium (Effects of oral anticoagulants may be decreased). Products include:
Coumadin ... 926

Food Interactions

Milk, low fat (Concurrent use of low-salt milk with triamterene may result in hyperkalemia, especially in patients with renal insufficiency).

DYCLONE 0.5% AND 1% TOPICAL SOLUTIONS, USP
(Dyclonine Hydrochloride) ... 544

Food Interactions

Food, unspecified (Topical anesthesia may impair swallowing and thus enhance the danger of aspiration; food should not be ingested for 60 minutes).

DYNACIN CAPSULES
(Minocycline Hydrochloride) ... 1590
May interact with oral anticoagulants, penicillins, antacids containing aluminium, calcium and magnesium, iron containing oral preparations, oral contraceptives, and certain other agents. Compounds in these categories include:

Aluminum Carbonate Gel (Absorption of tetracyclines is impaired by antacids). Products include:
Basaljel ... 2703

Aluminum Hydroxide (Absorption of tetracyclines is impaired by antacids). Products include:
ALternaGEL Liquid ... 1316
Maximum Strength Ascriptin ... ▣ 630
Cama Arthritis Pain Reliever ... ▣ 785
Gaviscon Extra Strength Relief Formula Antacid Tablets ... ▣ 819
Gaviscon Extra Strength Relief Formula Liquid Antacid ... ▣ 819
Gaviscon Liquid Antacid ... ▣ 820
Gelusil Liquid & Tablets ... ▣ 855
Maalox Heartburn Relief Suspension ... ▣ 642
Maalox Heartburn Relief Tablets ... ▣ 641
Maalox Magnesia and Alumina Oral Suspension ... ▣ 642
Maalox Plus Tablets ... ▣ 643
Extra Strength Maalox Antacid Plus Antigas Liquid and Tablets ▣ 638
Tempo Soft Antacid ... ▣ 835

Aluminum Hydroxide Gel (Absorption of tetracyclines is impaired by antacids). Products include:
ALternaGEL Liquid ... ▣ 659
Aludrox Oral Suspension ... 2695
Amphojel Suspension ... 2695
Amphojel Suspension without Flavor ... 2695
Amphojel Tablets ... 2695
Arthritis Pain Ascriptin ... ▣ 631
Regular Strength Ascriptin Tablets ... ▣ 629
Gaviscon Antacid Tablets ... ▣ 819
Gaviscon-2 Antacid Tablets ... ▣ 820
Mylanta Liquid ... 1317
Mylanta Tablets ... ▣ 660
Mylanta Double Strength Liquid ... 1317
Mylanta Double Strength Tablets .. ▣ 660
Nephrox Suspension ... ▣ 655

Aluminum Hydroxide Gel, Dried (Absorption of tetracyclines is impaired by antacids).

Amoxicillin Trihydrate (Interference with bactericidal action of penicillin; avoid giving tetracycline-class drugs in conjunction with penicillin). Products include:
Amoxil ... 2464
Augmentin ... 2468

Ampicillin (Interference with bactericidal action of penicillin; avoid giving tetracycline-class drugs in conjunction with penicillin). Products include:
Omnipen Capsules ... 2764
Omnipen for Oral Suspension ... 2765

Ampicillin Sodium (Interference with bactericidal action of penicillin; avoid giving tetracycline-class drugs in conjunction with penicillin). Products include:
Unasyn ... 2212

Ampicillin Trihydrate (Interference with bactericidal action of penicillin; avoid giving tetracycline-class drugs in conjunction with penicillin).
No products indexed under this heading.

Azlocillin Sodium (Interference with bactericidal action of penicillin; avoid giving tetracycline-class drugs in conjunction with penicillin).
No products indexed under this heading.

Bacampicillin Hydrochloride (Interference with bactericidal action of penicillin; avoid giving tetracycline-class drugs in conjunction with penicillin). Products include:
Spectrobid Tablets ... 2206

Carbenicillin Disodium (Interference with bactericidal action of penicillin; avoid giving tetracycline-class drugs in conjunction with penicillin).
No products indexed under this heading.

Carbenicillin Indanyl Sodium (Interference with bactericidal action of penicillin; avoid giving tetracycline-class drugs in conjunction with penicillin). Products include:
Geocillin Tablets ... 2199

Desogestrel (Concurrent use may render oral contraceptives less effective and breakthrough bleeding may occur). Products include:
Desogen Tablets ... 1817
Ortho-Cept ... 1851

Dicloxacillin Sodium (Interference with bactericidal action of penicillin; avoid giving tetracycline-class drugs in conjunction with penicillin).
No products indexed under this heading.

Dicumarol (Tetracyclines have shown to depress plasma prothrombin activity; patients on anticoagulant may require downward adjustments of their anticoagulant dosage).
No products indexed under this heading.

Dihydroxyaluminum Sodium Carbonate (Absorption of tetracyclines is impaired by antacids).
No products indexed under this heading.

Ethinyl Estradiol (Concurrent use may render oral contraceptives less effective and breakthrough bleeding may occur). Products include:
Brevicon ... 2088
Demulen ... 2428
Desogen Tablets ... 1817
Levlen/Tri-Levlen ... 651
Lo/Ovral Tablets ... 2746
Lo/Ovral-28 Tablets ... 2751
Modicon ... 1872
Nordette-21 Tablets ... 2755
Nordette-28 Tablets ... 2758
Norinyl ... 2088
Ortho-Cept ... 1851
Ortho-Cyclen/Ortho-Tri-Cyclen ... 1858
Ortho-Novum ... 1872
Ortho-Cyclen/Ortho Tri-Cyclen ... 1858
Ovcon ... 760
Ovral Tablets ... 2770
Ovral-28 Tablets ... 2770
Levlen/Tri-Levlen ... 651
Tri-Norinyl ... 2164
Triphasil-21 Tablets ... 2814
Triphasil-28 Tablets ... 2819

Ethynodiol Diacetate (Concurrent use may render oral contraceptives less effective and breakthrough bleeding may occur). Products include:
Demulen ... 2428

Ferrous Fumarate (Absorption of tetracyclines is impaired by iron-containing preparations). Products include:
Chromagen Capsules ... 2339
Ferro-Sequels ... ▣ 669
Nephro-Fer Tablets ... 2004
Nephro-Fer Rx Tablets ... 2005
Nephro-Vite + Fe Tablets ... 2006
Sigtab-M Tablets ... ▣ 772
Stresstabs + Iron ... ▣ 671
The Stuart Formula Tablets ... ▣ 663
Theragran-M Tablets with Beta Carotene ... ▣ 623
Trinsicon Capsules ... 2570
Vitron-C Tablets ... ▣ 650

Ferrous Gluconate (Absorption of tetracyclines is impaired by iron-containing preparations). Products include:
Fergon Iron Supplement Tablets ... ▣ 721
Megadose ... 512

Ferrous Sulfate (Absorption of tetracyclines is impaired by iron-containing preparations). Products include:
Feosol Capsules ... 2456
Feosol Elixir ... 2456
Feosol Tablets ... 2457
Fero-Folic-500 Filmtab ... 429
Fero-Grad-500 Filmtab ... 429
Fero-Gradumet Filmtab ... 429
Iberet Tablets ... 433
Iberet-500 Liquid ... 433
Iberet-Folic-500 Filmtab ... 429
Iberet-Liquid ... 433
Irospan ... 982
Slow Fe Tablets ... 869
Slow Fe with Folic Acid ... 869

Levonorgestrel (Concurrent use may render oral contraceptives less effective and breakthrough bleeding may occur). Products include:
Levlen/Tri-Levlen ... 651
Nordette-21 Tablets ... 2755
Nordette-28 Tablets ... 2758
Norplant System ... 2759
Levlen/Tri-Levlen ... 651
Triphasil-21 Tablets ... 2814
Triphasil-28 Tablets ... 2819

Magaldrate (Absorption of tetracyclines is impaired by antacids).
No products indexed under this heading.

Magnesium Hydroxide (Absorption of tetracyclines is impaired by antacids). Products include:
Aludrox Oral Suspension ... 2695
Arthritis Pain Ascriptin ... ▣ 631
Maximum Strength Ascriptin ... ▣ 630
Regular Strength Ascriptin Tablets ... ▣ 629
Di-Gel Antacid/Anti-Gas ... ▣ 801
Gelusil Liquid & Tablets ... ▣ 855
Maalox Magnesia and Alumina Oral Suspension ... ▣ 642
Maalox Plus Tablets ... ▣ 643
Extra Strength Maalox Antacid Plus Antigas Liquid and Tablets ▣ 638
Mylanta Calcium Carbonate and Magnesium Hydroxide Tablets ... 1318
Mylanta Liquid ... 1317
Mylanta Tablets ... ▣ 660
Mylanta Double Strength Liquid ... 1317
Mylanta Double Strength Tablets .. ▣ 660
Phillips' Milk of Magnesia Liquid ... ▣ 729
Rolaids Tablets ... ▣ 843
Tempo Soft Antacid ... ▣ 835

Magnesium Oxide (Absorption of tetracyclines is impaired by antacids). Products include:
Beelith Tablets ... 639
Bufferin Analgesic Tablets and Caplets ... ▣ 613
Caltrate PLUS ... ▣ 665
Cama Arthritis Pain Reliever ... ▣ 785
Mag-Ox 400 ... 668
Uro-Mag ... 668

Mestranol (Concurrent use may render oral contraceptives less effective and breakthrough bleeding may occur). Products include:
Norinyl ... 2088
Ortho-Novum ... 1872

Methoxyflurane (Potential for fatal renal toxicity).
No products indexed under this heading.

Mezlocillin Sodium (Interference with bactericidal action of penicillin; avoid giving tetracycline-class drugs in conjunction with penicillin). Products include:
Mezlin ... 601
Mezlin Pharmacy Bulk Package ... 604

Nafcillin Sodium (Interference with bactericidal action of penicillin; avoid giving tetracycline-class drugs in conjunction with penicillin).
No products indexed under this heading.

Norethindrone (Concurrent use may render oral contraceptives less effective and breakthrough bleeding may occur). Products include:
Brevicon ... 2088

353 **Interactions Index** **Dyrenium**

Micronor Tablets ... 1872
Modicon ... 1872
Norinyl ... 2088
Nor-Q D Tablets ... 2135
Ortho-Novum ... 1872
Ovcon ... 760
Tri-Norinyl ... 2164

Norethynodrel (Concurrent use may render oral contraceptives less effective and breakthrough bleeding may occur).
No products indexed under this heading.

Norgestimate (Concurrent use may render oral contraceptives less effective and breakthrough bleeding may occur). Products include:
Ortho-Cyclen/Ortho-Tri-Cyclen ... 1858
Ortho-Cyclen/Ortho Tri-Cyclen ... 1858

Norgestrel (Concurrent use may render oral contraceptives less effective and breakthrough bleeding may occur). Products include:
Lo/Ovral Tablets ... 2746
Lo/Ovral-28 Tablets ... 2751
Ovral Tablets ... 2770
Ovral-28 Tablets ... 2770
Ovrette Tablets ... 2771

Penicillin G Benzathine (Interference with bactericidal action of penicillin; avoid giving tetracycline-class drugs in conjunction with penicillin). Products include:
Bicillin C-R Injection ... 2704
Bicillin C-R 900/300 Injection ... 2706
Bicillin L-A Injection ... 2707

Penicillin G Potassium (Interference with bactericidal action of penicillin; avoid giving tetracycline-class drugs in conjunction with penicillin). Products include:
Pfizerpen for Injection ... 2203

Penicillin G Procaine (Interference with bactericidal action of penicillin; avoid giving tetracycline-class drugs in conjunction with penicillin). Products include:
Bicillin C-R Injection ... 2704
Bicillin C-R 900/300 Injection ... 2706

Penicillin G Sodium (Interference with bactericidal action of penicillin; avoid giving tetracycline-class drugs in conjunction with penicillin).
No products indexed under this heading.

Penicillin V Potassium (Interference with bactericidal action of penicillin; avoid giving tetracycline-class drugs in conjunction with penicillin). Products include:
Pen•Vee K ... 2772

Polysaccharide-Iron Complex (Absorption of tetracyclines is impaired by iron-containing preparations). Products include:
Niferex-150 Capsules ... 793
Niferex Elixir ... 793
Niferex-150 Forte Capsules ... 794
Niferex Forte Elixir ... 794
Niferex ... 793
Niferex-PN Tablets ... 794
Nu-Iron 150 Capsules ... 1543
Nu-Iron Elixir ... 1543
Sunkist Children's Chewable Multivitamins - Plus Iron ... 649

Ticarcillin Disodium (Interference with bactericidal action of penicillin; avoid giving tetracycline-class drugs in conjunction with penicillin). Products include:
Ticar for Injection ... 2526
Timentin for Injection ... 2528

Warfarin Sodium (Tetracyclines have shown to depress plasma prothrombin activity; patients on anticoagulant may require downward adjustments of their anticoagulant dosage). Products include:
Coumadin ... 926

DYNACIRC CAPSULES

(Isradipine) ... 2256
May interact with:

Cimetidine (Potential for increase in isradipine mean peak plasma concentration and significant increase in the AUC). Products include:
Tagamet Tablets ... 2516

Cimetidine Hydrochloride (Potential for increase in isradipine mean peak plasma concentration and significant increase in the AUC). Products include:
Tagamet ... 2516

Fentanyl (Severe hypotension has been reported during fentanyl anesthesia with concomitant use of beta blocker and calcium channel blocker). Products include:
Duragesic Transdermal System ... 1288

Fentanyl Citrate (Severe hypotension has been reported during fentanyl anesthesia with concomitant use of beta blocker and calcium channel blocker). Products include:
Sublimaze Injection ... 1307

Hydrochlorothiazide (Potential for additive antihypertensive effect). Products include:
Aldactazide ... 2413
Aldoril Tablets ... 1604
Apresazide Capsules ... 808
Capozide ... 742
Dyazide ... 2479
Esidrix Tablets ... 821
Esimil Tablets ... 822
HydroDIURIL Tablets ... 1674
Hydropres Tablets ... 1675
Hyzaar Tablets ... 1677
Inderide Tablets ... 2732
Inderide LA Long Acting Capsules ... 2734
Lopressor HCT Tablets ... 832
Lotensin HCT ... 837
Maxzide ... 1380
Moduretic Tablets ... 1705
Oretic Tablets ... 443
Prinzide Tablets ... 1737
Ser-Ap-Es Tablets ... 849
Timolide Tablets ... 1748
Vaseretic Tablets ... 1765
Zestoretic ... 2850
Ziac ... 1415

Propranolol Hydrochloride (Coadministration of DynaCirc resulted in significant increases in AUC and C_{max} and decreases in t_{max} of propranolol). Products include:
Inderal ... 2728
Inderal LA Long Acting Capsules ... 2730
Inderide Tablets ... 2732
Inderide LA Long Acting Capsules ... 2734

Rifampin (Potential for reduction in isradipine levels to below detectable limits). Products include:
Rifadin ... 1528
Rifamate Capsules ... 1530
Rifater ... 1532
Rimactane Capsules ... 847

Food Interactions

Food, unspecified (Coadministration significantly increases the time to peak by about an hour with no effect on AUC).

DYRENIUM CAPSULES

(Triamterene) ... 2481
May interact with potassium preparations, lithium preparations, nonsteroidal anti-inflammatory agents, antihypertensives, diuretics, preanesthetic medications, general anesthetics, nondepolarizing neuromuscular blocking agents, ACE inhibitors, oral hypoglycemic agents, potassium sparing diuretics, and certain other agents. Compounds in these categories include:

Acarbose (Concurrent use may increase the risk of severe hyponatremia; triamterene may raise blood glucose levels; for adult-onset diabetes, dosage adjustments of hypoglycemic agents may be necessary).
No products indexed under this heading.

Acebutolol Hydrochloride (Potentiation of antihypertensive effect). Products include:
Sectral Capsules ... 2807

Amiloride Hydrochloride (Potentiation of diuretic effect; concomitant administration is contraindicated). Products include:
Midamor Tablets ... 1703
Moduretic Tablets ... 1705

Amlodipine Besylate (Potentiation of antihypertensive effect). Products include:
Lotrel Capsules ... 840
Norvasc Tablets ... 1940

Atenolol (Potentiation of antihypertensive effect). Products include:
Tenoretic Tablets ... 2845
Tenormin Tablets and I.V. Injection ... 2847

Atracurium Besylate (The effects of nondepolarizing skeletal muscle relaxants may be potentiated). Products include:
Tracrium Injection ... 1183

Benazepril Hydrochloride (Potential for antihypertensive effect and increased risk of hyperkalemia). Products include:
Lotensin Tablets ... 834
Lotensin HCT ... 837
Lotrel Capsules ... 840

Bendroflumethiazide (Potentiation of diuretic effect).
No products indexed under this heading.

Betaxolol Hydrochloride (Potentiation of antihypertensive effect). Products include:
Betoptic Ophthalmic Solution ... 469
Betoptic S Ophthalmic Suspension ... 471
Kerlone Tablets ... 2436

Bisoprolol Fumarate (Potentiation of antihypertensive effect). Products include:
Zebeta Tablets ... 1413
Ziac ... 1415

Blood, whole (Co-administration with blood from blood bank may promote serum potassium accumulation and possibly resulting in hyperkalemia).
No products indexed under this heading.

Bumetanide (Potentiation of diuretic effect). Products include:
Bumex ... 2093

Captopril (Potential for antihypertensive effect and increased risk of hyperkalemia). Products include:
Capoten ... 739
Capozide ... 742

Carteolol Hydrochloride (Potentiation of antihypertensive effect). Products include:
Cartrol Tablets ... 410
Ocupress Ophthalmic Solution, 1% Sterile ... ◉ 309

Chlorothiazide (Potentiation of diuretic effect). Products include:
Aldoclor Tablets ... 1598
Diupres Tablets ... 1650
Diuril Oral ... 1653

Chlorothiazide Sodium (Potentiation of antihypertensive and/or diuretic effect). Products include:
Diuril Sodium Intravenous ... 1652

Chlorpropamide (Concurrent use may increase the risk of severe hyponatremia; triamterene may raise blood glucose levels; for adult-onset diabetes, dosage adjustments of hypoglycemic agents may be necessary). Products include:
Diabinese Tablets ... 1935

Chlorthalidone (Potentiation of antihypertensive and/or diuretic effect). Products include:
Combipres Tablets ... 677
Tenoretic Tablets ... 2845
Thalitone ... 1245

Clonidine (Potentiation of antihypertensive effect). Products include:
Catapres-TTS ... 675

Clonidine Hydrochloride (Potentiation of antihypertensive effect). Products include:
Catapres Tablets ... 674
Combipres Tablets ... 677

Deserpidine (Potentiation of antihypertensive effect).
No products indexed under this heading.

Diazepam (The effects of preanesthetic agents may be potentiated). Products include:
Dizac ... 1809
Valium Injectable ... 2182
Valium Tablets ... 2183
Valrelease Capsules ... 2169

Diazoxide (Potentiation of antihypertensive effect). Products include:
Hyperstat I.V. Injection ... 2363
Proglycem ... 580

Diclofenac Potassium (Possibility for acute renal failure). Products include:
Cataflam ... 816

Diclofenac Sodium (Possibility for acute renal failure). Products include:
Voltaren Ophthalmic Sterile Ophthalmic Solution ... ◉ 272
Voltaren Tablets ... 861

Diltiazem Hydrochloride (Potentiation of antihypertensive effect). Products include:
Cardizem CD Capsules ... 1506
Cardizem SR Capsules ... 1510
Cardizem Injectable ... 1508
Cardizem Tablets ... 1512
Dilacor XR Extended-release Capsules ... 2018

Doxazosin Mesylate (Potentiation of antihypertensive effect). Products include:
Cardura Tablets ... 2186

Droperidol (The effects of preanesthetic agents may be potentiated). Products include:
Inapsine Injection ... 1296

Enalapril Maleate (Potential for increased antihypertensive effect and risk of hyperkalemia). Products include:
Vaseretic Tablets ... 1765
Vasotec Tablets ... 1771

Enalaprilat (Potential for increased antihypertensive effect and risk of hyperkalemia). Products include:
Vasotec I.V. ... 1768

Enflurane (The effects of anesthetic agents may be potentiated).
No products indexed under this heading.

Esmolol Hydrochloride (Potentiation of antihypertensive effect). Products include:
Brevibloc Injection ... 1808

Ethacrynic Acid (Potentiation of diuretic effect). Products include:
Edecrin Tablets ... 1657

Etodolac (Possibility for acute renal failure). Products include:
Lodine Capsules and Tablets ... 2743

IMPORTANT NOTE: Always consult each drug listing in the patient's regimen for possible interactions.

Dyrenium Interactions Index 354

Felodipine (Potentiation of antihypertensive effect). Products include:
Plendil Extended-Release Tablets 527

Fenoprofen Calcium (Possibility for acute renal failure). Products include:
Nalfon 200 Pulvules & Nalfon Tablets 917

Fentanyl Citrate (The effects of preanesthetic agents may be potentiated). Products include:
Sublimaze Injection 1307

Flurbiprofen (Possibility for acute renal failure). Products include:
Ansaid Tablets 2579

Fosinopril Sodium (Potential for antihypertensive effect and increased risk of hyperkalemia). Products include:
Monopril Tablets 757

Furosemide (Potentiation of antihypertensive and/or diuretic effect). Products include:
Lasix Injection, Oral Solution and Tablets 1240

Glipizide (Triamterene may raise blood glucose levels; for adult-onset diabetes, dosage adjustments of hypoglycemic agents may be necessary). Products include:
Glucotrol Tablets 1967
Glucotrol XL Extended Release Tablets 1968

Glyburide (Triamterene may raise blood glucose levels; for adult-onset diabetes, dosage adjustments of hypoglycemic agents may be necessary). Products include:
DiaBeta Tablets 1239
Glynase PresTab Tablets 2609
Micronase Tablets 2623

Guanabenz Acetate (Potentiation of antihypertensive effect).
No products indexed under this heading.

Guanethidine Monosulfate (Potentiation of antihypertensive effect). Products include:
Esimil Tablets 822
Ismelin Tablets 827

Hydralazine Hydrochloride (Potentiation of antihypertensive effect). Products include:
Apresazide Capsules 808
Apresoline Hydrochloride Tablets .. 809
Ser-Ap-Es Tablets 849

Hydrochlorothiazide (Potentiation of antihypertensive and/or diuretic effect). Products include:
Aldactazide 2413
Aldoril Tablets 1604
Apresazide Capsules 808
Capozide 742
Dyazide 2479
Esidrix Tablets 821
Esimil Tablets 822
HydroDIURIL Tablets 1674
Hydropres Tablets 1675
Hyzaar Tablets 1677
Inderide Tablets 2732
Inderide LA Long Acting Capsules .. 2734
Lopressor HCT Tablets 832
Lotensin HCT 837
Maxzide 1380
Moduretic Tablets 1705
Oretic Tablets 443
Prinzide Tablets 1737
Ser-Ap-Es Tablets 849
Timolide Tablets 1748
Vaseretic Tablets 1765
Zestoretic 2850
Ziac 1415

Hydroflumethiazide (Potentiation of antihypertensive and/or diuretic effect). Products include:
Diucardin Tablets 2718

Hydroxyzine Hydrochloride (The effects of preanesthetic agents may be potentiated). Products include:
Atarax Tablets & Syrup 2185
Marax Tablets & DF Syrup 2200
Vistaril Intramuscular Solution 2216

Ibuprofen (Possibility for acute renal failure). Products include:
Advil Cold and Sinus Caplets and Tablets (formerly CoAdvil) .... ◘ 870
Advil Ibuprofen Tablets and Caplets .... ◘ 870
Children's Advil Suspension 2692
Arthritis Foundation Ibuprofen Tablets .... ◘ 674
Bayer Select Ibuprofen Pain Relief Formula .... ◘ 715
Cramp End Tablets .... ◘ 735
Dimetapp Sinus Caplets .... ◘ 775
Haltran Tablets .... ◘ 771
IBU Tablets 1342
Ibuprohm .... ◘ 735
Children's Motrin Ibuprofen Oral Suspension 1546
Motrin Tablets 2625
Motrin IB Caplets, Tablets, and Geltabs .... ◘ 838
Motrin IB Sinus .... ◘ 838
Motrin Ibuprofen Suspension, Oral Drops, Chewable Tablets, Caplets 1546
Nuprin Ibuprofen/Analgesic Tablets & Caplets .... ◘ 622
Sine-Aid IB Caplets 1554
Vicks DayQuil SINUS Pressure & PAIN Relief with IBUPROFEN .... ◘ 762

Indapamide (Potentiation of antihypertensive and/or diuretic effect). Products include:
Lozol Tablets 2022

Indomethacin (Possibility for acute renal failure). Products include:
Indocin 1680

Indomethacin Sodium Trihydrate (Possibility for acute renal failure). Products include:
Indocin I.V. 1684

Isoflurane (The effects of anesthetic agents may be potentiated).
No products indexed under this heading.

Isradipine (Potentiation of antihypertensive effect). Products include:
DynaCirc Capsules 2256

Ketamine Hydrochloride (The effects of anesthetic agents may be potentiated).
No products indexed under this heading.

Ketoprofen (Possibility for acute renal failure). Products include:
Orudis Capsules 2766
Oruvail Capsules 2766

Ketorolac Tromethamine (Possibility for acute renal failure). Products include:
Acular 474
Acular .... ⊙ 277
Toradol 2159

Labetalol Hydrochloride (Potentiation of antihypertensive effect). Products include:
Normodyne Injection 2377
Normodyne Tablets 2379
Trandate 1185

Levobunolol Hydrochloride (Potentiation of antihypertensive effect). Products include:
Betagan .... ⊙ 233

Lisinopril (Potential for antihypertensive effect and increased risk of hyperkalemia). Products include:
Prinivil Tablets 1733
Prinzide Tablets 1737
Zestoretic 2850
Zestril Tablets 2854

Lithium Carbonate (Diuretic-induced sodium loss may reduce the renal clearance of lithium and increase serum lithium levels with the risk of lithium toxicity). Products include:
Eskalith 2485
Lithium Carbonate Capsules & Tablets 2230
Lithonate/Lithotabs/Lithobid 2543

Lithium Citrate (Diuretic-induced sodium loss may reduce the renal clearance of lithium and increase serum lithium levels with the risk of lithium toxicity).
No products indexed under this heading.

Lorazepam (The effects of preanesthetic agents may be potentiated). Products include:
Ativan Injection 2698
Ativan Tablets 2700

Losartan Potassium (Potentiation of antihypertensive effect). Products include:
Cozaar Tablets 1628
Hyzaar Tablets 1677

Mecamylamine Hydrochloride (Potentiation of antihypertensive effect). Products include:
Inversine Tablets 1686

Meclofenamate Sodium (Possibility for acute renal failure).
No products indexed under this heading.

Mefenamic Acid (Possibility for acute renal failure). Products include:
Ponstel 1925

Meperidine Hydrochloride (The effects of preanesthetic agents may be potentiated). Products include:
Demerol 2308
Mepergan Injection 2753

Metformin Hydrochloride (Concurrent use may increase the risk of severe hyponatremia; triamterene may raise blood glucose levels; for adult-onset diabetes, dosage adjustments of hypoglycemic agents may be necessary). Products include:
Glucophage 752

Methohexital Sodium (The effects of anesthetic agents may be potentiated). Products include:
Brevital Sodium Vials 1429

Methoxyflurane (The effects of anesthetic agents may be potentiated).
No products indexed under this heading.

Methyclothiazide (Potentiation of antihypertensive and/or diuretic effect). Products include:
Enduron Tablets 420

Methyldopa (Potentiation of antihypertensive effect). Products include:
Aldoclor Tablets 1598
Aldomet Oral 1600
Aldoril Tablets 1604

Methyldopate Hydrochloride (Potentiation of antihypertensive effect). Products include:
Aldomet Ester HCl Injection 1602

Metipranolol Hydrochloride (Potentiation of antihypertensive effect). Products include:
OptiPranolol (Metipranolol 0.3%) Sterile Ophthalmic Solution .... ⊙ 258

Metocurine Iodide (The effects of nondepolarizing skeletal muscle relaxants may be potentiated). Products include:
Metubine Iodide Vials 916

Metolazone (Potentiation of antihypertensive and/or diuretic effect). Products include:
Mykrox Tablets 993
Zaroxolyn Tablets 1000

Metoprolol Succinate (Potentiation of antihypertensive effect). Products include:
Toprol-XL Tablets 565

Metoprolol Tartrate (Potentiation of antihypertensive effect). Products include:
Lopressor Ampuls 830
Lopressor HCT Tablets 832
Lopressor Tablets 830

Metyrosine (Potentiation of antihypertensive effect). Products include:
Demser Capsules 1649

Minoxidil (Potentiation of antihypertensive effect). Products include:
Loniten Tablets 2618
Rogaine Topical Solution 2637

Mivacurium Chloride (The effects of nondepolarizing skeletal muscle relaxants may be potentiated). Products include:
Mivacron 1138

Moexipril Hydrochloride (Potential for antihypertensive effect and increased risk of hyperkalemia). Products include:
Univasc Tablets 2410

Morphine Sulfate (The effects of preanesthetic agents may be potentiated). Products include:
Astramorph/PF Injection, USP (Preservative-Free) 535
Duramorph 962
Infumorph 200 and Infumorph 500 Sterile Solutions 965
MS Contin Tablets 1994
MSIR 1997
Oramorph SR (Morphine Sulfate Sustained Release Tablets) 2236
RMS Suppositories 2657
Roxanol 2243

Nabumetone (Possibility for acute renal failure). Products include:
Relafen Tablets 2510

Nadolol (Potentiation of antihypertensive effect).
No products indexed under this heading.

Naproxen (Possibility for acute renal failure). Products include:
Anaprox/Naprosyn 2117

Naproxen Sodium (Possibility for acute renal failure). Products include:
Aleve 1975
Anaprox/Naprosyn 2117

Nicardipine Hydrochloride (Potentiation of antihypertensive effect). Products include:
Cardene Capsules 2095
Cardene I.V. 2709
Cardene SR Capsules 2097

Nifedipine (Potentiation of antihypertensive effect). Products include:
Adalat Capsules (10 mg and 20 mg) 587
Adalat CC 589
Procardia Capsules 1971
Procardia XL Extended Release Tablets 1972

Nisoldipine (Potentiation of antihypertensive effect).
No products indexed under this heading.

Nitroglycerin (Potentiation of antihypertensive effect). Products include:
Deponit NTG Transdermal Delivery System 2397
Nitro-Bid IV 1523
Nitro-Bid Ointment 1524
Nitrodisc 2047
Nitro-Dur (nitroglycerin) Transdermal Infusion System 1326
Nitrolingual Spray 2027
Nitrostat Tablets 1925
Transderm-Nitro Transdermal Therapeutic System 859

Oxaprozin (Possibility for acute renal failure). Products include:
Daypro Caplets 2426

(◘ Described in PDR For Nonprescription Drugs) (⊙ Described in PDR For Ophthalmology)

Interactions Index

Pancuronium Bromide Injection
(The effects of nondepolarizing skeletal muscle relaxants may be potentiated).

No products indexed under this heading.

Penbutolol Sulfate (Potentiation of antihypertensive effect). Products include:

Levatol 2403

Penicillin G Potassium (Co-administration may promote serum potassium accumulation and possibly resulting in hyperkalemia). Products include:

Pfizerpen for Injection 2203

Pentobarbital Sodium (The effects of preanesthetic agents may be potentiated). Products include:

Nembutal Sodium Capsules 436
Nembutal Sodium Solution 438
Nembutal Sodium Suppositories........ 440

Phenoxybenzamine Hydrochloride (Potentiation of antihypertensive effect). Products include:

Dibenzyline Capsules 2476

Phentolamine Mesylate (Potentiation of antihypertensive effect). Products include:

Regitine 846

Phenylbutazone (Possibility for acute renal failure).

No products indexed under this heading.

Pindolol (Potentiation of antihypertensive effect). Products include:

Visken Tablets................................... 2299

Piroxicam (Possibility for acute renal failure). Products include:

Feldene Capsules 1965

Polythiazide (Potentiation of antihypertensive and/or diuretic effect). Products include:

Minizide Capsules 1938

Potassium Acid Phosphate (Concomitant administration is contraindicated). Products include:

K-Phos Original Formula 'Sodium Free' Tablets 639

Potassium Bicarbonate (Concomitant administration is contraindicated). Products include:

Alka-Seltzer Gold Effervescent Antacid .... ◻ 703

Potassium Chloride (Concomitant administration is contraindicated). Products include:

Chlor-3 Condiment 1004
K-Dur Microburst Release System (potassium chloride, USP) E.R. Tablets 1325
K-Lor Powder Packets 434
K-Norm Extended-Release Capsules 991
K-Tab Filmtab 434
Kolyum Liquid 992
Micro-K... 2063
Micro-K LS Packets........................... 2064
NuLYTELY... 689
Cherry Flavor NuLYTELY 689
Rum-K Syrup 1005
Slow-K Extended-Release Tablets...... 851

Potassium Citrate (Concomitant administration is contraindicated). Products include:

Polycitra Syrup 578
Polycitra-K Crystals 579
Polycitra-K Oral Solution 579
Polycitra-LC 578

Potassium Gluconate (Concomitant administration is contraindicated). Products include:

Kolyum Liquid 992

Potassium Phosphate, Dibasic (Concomitant administration is contraindicated).

No products indexed under this heading.

Potassium Phosphate, Monobasic (Concomitant administration is contraindicated). Products include:

K-Phos Neutral Tablets 639
K-Phos Original Formula 'Sodium Free' Tablets 639

Prazosin Hydrochloride (Potentiation of antihypertensive effect). Products include:

Minipress Capsules............................ 1937
Minizide Capsules 1938

Promethazine Hydrochloride (The effects of preanesthetic agents may be potentiated). Products include:

Mepergan Injection 2753
Phenergan with Codeine 2777
Phenergan with Dextromethorphan 2778
Phenergan Injection 2773
Phenergan Suppositories 2775
Phenergan Syrup 2774
Phenergan Tablets 2775
Phenergan VC 2779
Phenergan VC with Codeine 2781

Propofol (The effects of anesthetic agents may be potentiated). Products include:

Diprivan Injection............................... 2833

Propranolol Hydrochloride (Potentiation of antihypertensive effect). Products include:

Inderal 2728
Inderal LA Long Acting Capsules 2730
Inderide Tablets 2732
Inderide LA Long Acting Capsules .. 2734

Quinapril Hydrochloride (Potential for antihypertensive effect and increased risk of hyperkalemia). Products include:

Accupril Tablets 1893

Ramipril (Potential for increased risk of hyperkalemia). Products include:

Altace Capsules 1232

Rauwolfia Serpentina (Potentiation of antihypertensive effect).

No products indexed under this heading.

Rescinnamine (Potentiation of antihypertensive effect).

No products indexed under this heading.

Reserpine (Potentiation of antihypertensive effect). Products include:

Diupres Tablets 1650
Hydropres Tablets.............................. 1675
Ser-Ap-Es Tablets 849

Rocuronium Bromide (The effects of nondepolarizing skeletal muscle relaxants may be potentiated). Products include:

Zemuron 1830

Secobarbital Sodium (The effects of preanesthetic agents may be potentiated). Products include:

Seconal Sodium Pulvules 1474

Sodium Nitroprusside (Potentiation of antihypertensive effect).

No products indexed under this heading.

Sotalol Hydrochloride (Potentiation of antihypertensive effect). Products include:

Betapace Tablets 641

Spirapril Hydrochloride (Potential for antihypertensive effect and increased risk of hyperkalemia).

No products indexed under this heading.

Spironolactone (Concomitant use has resulted in fatalities; co-administration is contraindicated). Products include:

Aldactazide 2413
Aldactone 2414

Sulindac (Possibility for acute renal failure). Products include:

Clinoril Tablets 1618

Terazosin Hydrochloride (Potentiation of antihypertensive effect). Products include:

Hytrin Capsules 430

Timolol Maleate (Potentiation of antihypertensive effect). Products include:

Blocadren Tablets 1614
Timolide Tablets................................. 1748
Timoptic in Ocudose 1753
Timoptic Sterile Ophthalmic Solution.. 1751
Timoptic-XE 1755

Tolazamide (Triamterene may raise blood glucose levels; for adult-onset diabetes, dosage adjustments of hypoglycemic agents may be necessary).

No products indexed under this heading.

Tolbutamide (Triamterene may raise blood glucose levels; for adult-onset diabetes, dosage adjustments of hypoglycemic agents may be necessary).

No products indexed under this heading.

Tolmetin Sodium (Possibility for acute renal failure). Products include:

Tolectin (200, 400 and 600 mg) .. 1581

Torsemide (Potentiation of diuretic effect). Products include:

Demadex Tablets and Injection 686

Trimethaphan Camsylate (Potentiation of antihypertensive effect). Products include:

Arfonad Ampuls 2080

Vecuronium Bromide (The effects of nondepolarizing skeletal muscle relaxants may be potentiated). Products include:

Norcuron 1826

Verapamil Hydrochloride (Potentiation of antihypertensive effect). Products include:

Calan SR Caplets 2422
Calan Tablets..................................... 2419
Isoptin Injectable 1344
Isoptin Oral Tablets 1346
Isoptin SR Tablets 1348
Verelan Capsules 1410
Verelan Capsules 2824

Food Interactions

Milk, low salt (Co-administration may promote serum potassium accumulation and possibly resulting in hyperkalemia).

E.E.S. 400 FILMTAB

(Erythromycin Ethylsuccinate)............ 424

May interact with xanthine bronchodilators, oral anticoagulants, and certain other agents. Compounds in these categories include:

Aminophylline (Concomitant administration with high doses of theophylline may be associated with increased theophylline levels and potential toxicity).

No products indexed under this heading.

Carbamazepine (Elevations in serum erythromycin and carbamazepine concentration). Products include:

Atretol Tablets 573
Tegretol Chewable Tablets 852
Tegretol Suspension........................... 852
Tegretol Tablets 852

Cyclosporine (Elevations in serum erythromycin and cyclosporine concentration). Products include:

Neoral 2276
Sandimmune 2286

Dicumarol (Increased anticoagulant effects).

No products indexed under this heading.

Digoxin (Elevated digoxin serum levels). Products include:

Lanoxicaps 1117
Lanoxin Elixir Pediatric 1120
Lanoxin Injection 1123
Lanoxin Injection Pediatric................. 1126
Lanoxin Tablets 1128

Dihydroergotamine Mesylate (Potential for acute ergot toxicity characterized by severe peripheral vasospasm and dysesthesia). Products include:

D.H.E. 45 Injection 2255

Dyphylline (Concomitant administration with high doses of theophylline may be associated with increased theophylline levels and potential toxicity). Products include:

Lufyllin & Lufyllin-400 Tablets 2670
Lufyllin-GG Elixir & Tablets 2671

Ergotamine Tartrate (Potential for acute ergot toxicity characterized by severe peripheral vasospasm and dysesthesia). Products include:

Bellergal-S Tablets 2250
Cafergot... 2251
Ergomar.. 1486
Wigraine Tablets & Suppositories .. 1829

Hexobarbital (Elevations in serum erythromycin and hexobarbital concentration).

Lovastatin (Potential for rhabdomyolysis in seriously ill patients). Products include:

Mevacor Tablets................................. 1699

Phenytoin (Elevations in serum erythromycin and phenytoin concentration). Products include:

Dilantin Infatabs................................. 1908
Dilantin-125 Suspension 1911

Phenytoin Sodium (Elevations in serum erythromycin and phenytoin concentration). Products include:

Dilantin Kapseals 1906
Dilantin Parenteral 1910

Terfenadine (Potential for altered terfenadine metabolism). Products include:

Seldane Tablets 1536
Seldane-D Extended-Release Tablets 1538

Theophylline (Concomitant administration with high doses of theophylline may be associated with increased theophylline levels and potential toxicity). Products include:

Marax Tablets & DF Syrup.................. 2200
Quibron 2053

Theophylline Anhydrous (Concomitant administration with high doses of theophylline may be associated with increased theophylline levels and potential toxicity). Products include:

Aerolate 1004
Primatene Dual Action Formula...... ◻ 872
Primatene Tablets .... ◻ 873
Respbid Tablets 682
Slo-bid Gyrocaps 2033
Theo-24 Extended Release Capsules 2568
Theo-Dur Extended-Release Tablets 1327
Theo-X Extended-Release Tablets .. 788
Uni-Dur Extended-Release Tablets.. 1331
Uniphyl 400 mg Tablets..................... 2001

Theophylline Calcium Salicylate (Concomitant administration with high doses of theophylline may be associated with increased theophylline levels and potential toxicity). Products include:

Quadrinal Tablets 1350

Theophylline Sodium Glycinate (Concomitant administration with high doses of theophylline may be associated with increased theophylline levels and potential toxicity).

No products indexed under this heading.

IMPORTANT NOTE: Always consult each drug listing in the patient's regimen for possible interactions.

E.E.S. **Interactions Index** 356

Triazolam (Decreased clearance of triazolam and increased the pharmacologic effect of triazolam). Products include:
Halcion Tablets ... 2611

Warfarin Sodium (Increased anticoagulant effects). Products include:
Coumadin ... 926

E.E.S. GRANULES
(Erythromycin Ethylsuccinate) ... 424
See **E.E.S. 400 Filmtab**

E.E.S. 200 LIQUID
(Erythromycin Ethylsuccinate) ... 424
See **E.E.S. 400 Filmtab**

E.E.S. 400 LIQUID
(Erythromycin Ethylsuccinate) ... 424
See **E.E.S. 400 Filmtab**

E-MYCIN TABLETS
(Erythromycin) ... 1341
May interact with xanthine bronchodilators, oral anticoagulants, drugs which undergo biotransformation by cytochrome p-450 mixed function oxidase, and certain other agents. Compounds in these categories include:

Alfentanil Hydrochloride (Concurrent use may be associated with elevation in serum level of alfentanil; monitor serum levels closely). Products include:
Alfenta Injection ... 1286

Aminophylline (Co-administration with high doses of theophylline may be associated with increased serum theophylline levels and potential theophylline toxicity).
No products indexed under this heading.

Bromocriptine Mesylate (Concurrent use may be associated with elevation in serum level of bromcriptine; monitor serum levels closely). Products include:
Parlodel ... 2281

Carbamazepine (Concurrent use may be associated with elevation in serum level of carbamazepine; monitor serum levels closely). Products include:
Atretol Tablets ... 573
Tegretol Chewable Tablets ... 852
Tegretol Suspension ... 852
Tegretol Tablets ... 852

Cyclosporine (Concurrent use may be associated with elevation in serum level of cyclosporine; monitor serum levels closely). Products include:
Neoral ... 2276
Sandimmune ... 2286

Dicumarol (Concomitant therapy may result in increased anticoagulant effects).
No products indexed under this heading.

Digoxin (Co-administration may result in elevated digoxin serum levels). Products include:
Lanoxicaps ... 1117
Lanoxin Elixir Pediatric ... 1120
Lanoxin Injection ... 1123
Lanoxin Injection Pediatric ... 1126
Lanoxin Tablets ... 1128

Dihydroergotamine Mesylate (Concurrent use has been associated with acute ergot toxicity characterized by severe peripheral vasospasm and dysesthesia). Products include:
D.H.E. 45 Injection ... 2255

Disopyramide Phosphate (Concurrent use may be associated with elevation in serum level of disopyramide; monitor serum levels closely). Products include:
Norpace ... 2444

Drugs which undergo biotransformation by cytochrome P-450 mixed function oxidase (Concurrent use may be associated with elevation in serum level of drugs metabolized by the cytochrome P450 system).

Dyphylline (Co-administration with high doses of theophylline may be associated with increased serum theophylline levels and potential theophylline toxicity). Products include:
Lufyllin & Lufyllin-400 Tablets ... 2670
Lufyllin-GG Elixir & Tablets ... 2671

Ergotamine Tartrate (Concurrent use has been associated with acute ergot toxicity characterized by severe peripheral vasospasm and dysesthesia). Products include:
Bellergal-S Tablets ... 2250
Cafergot ... 2251
Ergomar ... 1486
Wigraine Tablets & Suppositories ... 1829

Hexobarbital (Concurrent use may be associated with elevation in serum level of hexobarbital; monitor serum levels closely).

Lovastatin (Potential for rhabdomyolysis with or without renal impairment in seriously ill patients; concurrent use may be associated with elevation in serum level of lovastatin; monitor serum levels closely). Products include:
Mevacor Tablets ... 1699

Midazolam Hydrochloride (Decrease clearance of midazolam; potential for increased pharmacologic effect of midazolam). Products include:
Versed Injection ... 2170

Phenytoin (Concurrent use may be associated with elevation in serum level of phenytoin; monitor serum levels closely). Products include:
Dilantin Infatabs ... 1908
Dilantin-125 Suspension ... 1911

Phenytoin Sodium (Concurrent use may be associated with elevation in serum level of phenytoin; monitor serum levels closely). Products include:
Dilantin Kapseals ... 1906
Dilantin Parenteral ... 1910

Terfenadine (Concomitant use may significantly alter the metabolism of terfenadine; rare cases of serious cardiovascular adverse events, including death, cardiac arrest, torsades de pointes and other ventricular arrhythmias have been reported; concurrent use is contraindicated). Products include:
Seldane Tablets ... 1536
Seldane-D Extended-Release Tablets ... 1538

Theophylline (Co-administration with high doses of theophylline may be associated with increased serum theophylline levels and potential theophylline toxicity). Products include:
Marax Tablets & DF Syrup ... 2200
Quibron ... 2053

Theophylline Anhydrous (Co-administration with high doses of theophylline may be associated with increased serum theophylline levels and potential theophylline toxicity). Products include:
Aerolate ... 1004
Primatene Dual Action Formula ... ■ 872
Primatene Tablets ... ■ 873
Respbid Tablets ... 682
Slo-bid Gyrocaps ... 2033
Theo-24 Extended Release Capsules ... 2568
Theo-Dur Extended-Release Tablets ... 1327
Theo-X Extended-Release Tablets ... 788
Uni-Dur Extended-Release Tablets ... 1331
Uniphyl 400 mg Tablets ... 2001

Theophylline Calcium Salicylate (Co-administration with high doses of theophylline may be associated with increased serum theophylline levels and potential theophylline toxicity). Products include:
Quadrinal Tablets ... 1350

Theophylline Sodium Glycinate (Co-administration with high doses of theophylline may be associated with increased serum theophylline levels and potential theophylline toxicity).
No products indexed under this heading.

Triazolam (Decrease clearance of triazolam; potential for increased pharmacologic effect of triazolam). Products include:
Halcion Tablets ... 2611

Warfarin Sodium (Concomitant therapy may result in increased anticoagulant effects). Products include:
Coumadin ... 926

E.P.T. EARLY PREGNANCY TEST
(HCG Monoclonal Antibody) ... ■ 854
None cited in PDR database.

EASPRIN
(Aspirin) ... 1914
May interact with anticoagulants, oral hypoglycemic agents, antigout agents, corticosteroids, insulin, urinary alkalizing agents, antacids, pyrazolon derivatives, and certain other agents. Compounds in these categories include:

Acarbose (Enhanced effect of hypoglycemics).
No products indexed under this heading.

Aluminum Carbonate Gel (Increases stomach pH; affects enteric coating of tablets). Products include:
Basaljel ... 2703

Aluminum Hydroxide (Increases stomach pH; affects enteric coating of tablets). Products include:
ALternaGEL Liquid ... 1316
Maximum Strength Ascriptin ... ■ 630
Cama Arthritis Pain Reliever ... ■ 785
Gaviscon Extra Strength Relief Formula Antacid Tablets ... ■ 819
Gaviscon Extra Strength Relief Formula Liquid Antacid ... ■ 819
Gaviscon Liquid Antacid ... ■ 820
Gelusil Liquid & Tablets ... ■ 855
Maalox Heartburn Relief Suspension ... ■ 642
Maalox Heartburn Relief Tablets ... ■ 641
Maalox Magnesia and Alumina Oral Suspension ... ■ 642
Maalox Plus Tablets ... ■ 643
Extra Strength Maalox Antacid Plus Antigas Liquid and Tablets ■ 638
Tempo Soft Antacid ... ■ 835

Aluminum Hydroxide Gel (Increases stomach pH; affects enteric coating of tablets). Products include:
ALternaGEL Liquid ... ■ 659
Aludrox Oral Suspension ... 2695
Amphojel Suspension ... 2695
Amphojel Suspension without Flavor ... 2695
Amphojel Tablets ... 2695
Arthritis Pain Ascriptin ... ■ 631
Regular Strength Ascriptin Tablets ... ■ 629
Gaviscon Antacid Tablets ... ■ 819
Gaviscon-2 Antacid Tablets ... ■ 820
Mylanta Liquid ... 1317
Mylanta Tablets ... ■ 660
Mylanta Double Strength Liquid ... 1317
Mylanta Double Strength Tablets ... ■ 660
Nephrox Suspension ... ■ 655

Antipyrine (Increased risk of gastrointestinal ulceration). Products include:
Auralgan Otic Solution ... 2703
Tympagesic Ear Drops ... 2342

Betamethasone Acetate (Increased risk of gastrointestinal ulceration; may reduce serum salicylate levels). Products include:
Celestone Soluspan Suspension ... 2347

Betamethasone Sodium Phosphate (Increased risk of gastrointestinal ulceration; may reduce serum salicylate levels). Products include:
Celestone Soluspan Suspension ... 2347

Chlorpropamide (Enhanced effect of hypoglycemics). Products include:
Diabinese Tablets ... 1935

Cortisone Acetate (Increased risk of gastrointestinal ulceration; may reduce serum salicylate levels). Products include:
Cortone Acetate Sterile Suspension ... 1623
Cortone Acetate Tablets ... 1624

Dalteparin Sodium (Increased bleeding time). Products include:
Fragmin ... 1954

Dexamethasone (Increased risk of gastrointestinal ulceration; may reduce serum salicylate levels). Products include:
AK-Trol Ointment & Suspension ... ⊙ 205
Decadron Elixir ... 1633
Decadron Tablets ... 1635
Decaspray Topical Aerosol ... 1648
Dexacidin Ointment ... ⊙ 263
Maxitrol Ophthalmic Ointment and Suspension ... ⊙ 224
TobraDex Ophthalmic Suspension and Ointment ... 473

Dexamethasone Acetate (Increased risk of gastrointestinal ulceration; may reduce serum salicylate levels). Products include:
Dalalone D.P. Injectable ... 1011
Decadron-LA Sterile Suspension ... 1646

Dexamethasone Sodium Phosphate (Increased risk of gastrointestinal ulceration; may reduce serum salicylate levels). Products include:
Decadron Phosphate Injection ... 1637
Decadron Phosphate Respihaler ... 1642
Decadron Phosphate Sterile Ophthalmic Ointment ... 1641
Decadron Phosphate Sterile Ophthalmic Solution ... 1642
Decadron Phosphate Topical Cream ... 1644
Decadron Phosphate Turbinaire ... 1645
Decadron Phosphate with Xylocaine Injection, Sterile ... 1639
Dexacort Phosphate in Respihaler ... 458
Dexacort Phosphate in Turbinaire ... 459
NeoDecadron Sterile Ophthalmic Ointment ... 1712
NeoDecadron Sterile Ophthalmic Solution ... 1713
NeoDecadron Topical Cream ... 1714

Dicumarol (Increased bleeding time).
No products indexed under this heading.

Dihydroxyaluminum Sodium Carbonate (Increases stomach pH; affects enteric coating of tablets).
No products indexed under this heading.

Dipyrone (Possible increase in gastrointestinal ulceration).

Enoxaparin (Increased bleeding time). Products include:
Lovenox Injection ... 2020

(■ Described in PDR For Nonprescription Drugs) (⊙ Described in PDR For Ophthalmology)

357 **Interactions Index** **Easprin**

Fludrocortisone Acetate (Increased risk of gastrointestinal ulceration; may reduce serum salicylate levels). Products include:
- Florinef Acetate Tablets ... 505

Glipizide (Enhanced effect of hypoglycemics). Products include:
- Glucotrol Tablets ... 1967
- Glucotrol XL Extended Release Tablets ... 1968

Glyburide (Enhanced effect of hypoglycemics). Products include:
- DiaBeta Tablets ... 1239
- Glynase PresTab Tablets ... 2609
- Micronase Tablets ... 2623

Heparin Calcium (Increased bleeding time).
- No products indexed under this heading.

Heparin Sodium (Increased bleeding time). Products include:
- Heparin Lock Flush Solution ... 2725
- Heparin Sodium Injection ... 2726
- Heparin Sodium Injection, USP, Sterile Solution ... 2615
- Heparin Sodium Vials ... 1441

Hydrocortisone (Increased risk of gastrointestinal ulceration; may reduce serum salicylate levels). Products include:
- Anusol-HC Cream 2.5% ... 1896
- Aquanil HC Lotion ... 1931
- Bactine Hydrocortisone Anti-Itch Cream ... ▣ 709
- Caldecort Anti-Itch Hydrocortisone Spray ... ▣ 631
- Cortaid ... ▣ 836
- CORTENEMA ... 2535
- Cortisporin Ointment ... 1085
- Cortisporin Ophthalmic Ointment Sterile ... 1085
- Cortisporin Ophthalmic Suspension Sterile ... 1086
- Cortisporin Otic Solution Sterile ... 1087
- Cortisporin Otic Suspension Sterile ... 1088
- Cortizone-5 ... ▣ 831
- Cortizone-10 ... ▣ 831
- Hydrocortone Tablets ... 1672
- Hytone ... 907
- Massengill Medicated Soft Cloth Towelettes ... 2458
- PediOtic Suspension Sterile ... 1153
- Preparation H Hydrocortisone 1% Cream ... ▣ 872
- ProctoCream-HC 2.5% ... 2408
- VōSoL HC Otic Solution ... 2678

Hydrocortisone Acetate (Increased risk of gastrointestinal ulceration; may reduce serum salicylate levels). Products include:
- Analpram-HC Rectal Cream 1% and 2.5% ... 977
- Anusol HC-1 Anti-Itch Hydrocortisone Ointment ... ▣ 847
- Anusol-HC Suppositories ... 1897
- Caldecort ... ▣ 631
- Carmol HC ... 924
- Coly-Mycin S Otic w/Neomycin & Hydrocortisone ... 1906
- Cortaid ... ▣ 836
- Cortifoam ... 2396
- Cortisporin Cream ... 1084
- Epifoam ... 2399
- Hydrocortone Acetate Sterile Suspension ... 1669
- Mantadil Cream ... 1135
- Nupercainal Hydrocortisone 1% Cream ... ▣ 645
- Ophthocort ... ◉ 311
- Pramosone Cream, Lotion & Ointment ... 978
- ProctoCream-HC ... 2408
- ProctoFoam-HC ... 2409
- Terra-Cortril Ophthalmic Suspension ... 2210

Hydrocortisone Sodium Phosphate (Increased risk of gastrointestinal ulceration; may reduce serum salicylate levels). Products include:
- Hydrocortone Phosphate Injection, Sterile ... 1670

Hydrocortisone Sodium Succinate (Increased risk of gastrointestinal ulceration; may reduce serum salicylate levels). Products include:
- Solu-Cortef Sterile Powder ... 2641

Insulin, Human (Altered insulin requirements).
- No products indexed under this heading.

Insulin, Human Isophane Suspension (Altered insulin requirements). Products include:
- Novolin N Human Insulin 10 ml Vials ... 1795

Insulin, Human NPH (Altered insulin requirements). Products include:
- Humulin N, 100 Units ... 1448
- Novolin N PenFill Cartridges Durable Insulin Delivery System ... 1798
- Novolin N Prefilled Syringe Disposable Insulin Delivery System ... 1798

Insulin, Human Regular (Altered insulin requirements). Products include:
- Humulin R, 100 Units ... 1449
- Novolin R Human Insulin 10 ml Vials ... 1795
- Novolin R PenFill Cartridges Durable Insulin Delivery System ... 1798
- Novolin R Prefilled Syringe Disposable Insulin Delivery System ... 1798
- Velosulin BR Human Insulin 10 ml Vials ... 1795

Insulin, Human, Zinc Suspension (Altered insulin requirements). Products include:
- Humulin L, 100 Units ... 1446
- Humulin U, 100 Units ... 1450
- Novolin L Human Insulin 10 ml Vials ... 1795

Insulin, NPH (Altered insulin requirements). Products include:
- NPH, 100 Units ... 1450
- Pork NPH, 100 Units ... 1452
- Purified Pork NPH Isophane Insulin ... 1801

Insulin, Regular (Altered insulin requirements). Products include:
- Regular, 100 Units ... 1450
- Pork Regular, 100 Units ... 1452
- Pork Regular (Concentrated), 500 Units ... 1453
- Purified Pork Regular Insulin ... 1801

Insulin, Zinc Crystals (Altered insulin requirements). Products include:
- NPH, 100 Units ... 1450

Insulin, Zinc Suspension (Altered insulin requirements). Products include:
- Iletin I ... 1450
- Lente, 100 Units ... 1450
- Iletin II ... 1452
- Pork Lente, 100 Units ... 1452
- Purified Pork Lente Insulin ... 1801

Magaldrate (Increases stomach pH; affects enteric coating of tablets).
- No products indexed under this heading.

Magnesium Hydroxide (Increases stomach pH; affects enteric coating of tablets). Products include:
- Aludrox Oral Suspension ... 2695
- Arthritis Pain Ascriptin ... ▣ 631
- Maximum Strength Ascriptin ... ▣ 630
- Regular Strength Ascriptin Tablets ... ▣ 629
- Di-Gel Antacid/Anti-Gas ... ▣ 801
- Gelusil Liquid & Tablets ... ▣ 855
- Maalox Magnesia and Alumina Oral Suspension ... ▣ 642
- Maalox Plus Tablets ... ▣ 643
- Extra Strength Maalox Antacid Plus Antigas Liquid and Tablets ▣ 638
- Mylanta Calcium Carbonate and Magnesium Hydroxide Tablets ... 1318
- Mylanta Liquid ... 1317
- Mylanta Tablets ... ▣ 660
- Mylanta Double Strength Liquid ... 1317
- Mylanta Double Strength Tablets .. ▣ 660
- Phillips' Milk of Magnesia Liquid ... ▣ 729
- Rolaids Tablets ... ▣ 843
- Tempo Soft Antacid ... ▣ 835

Magnesium Oxide (Increases stomach pH; affects enteric coating of tablets). Products include:
- Beelith Tablets ... 639
- Bufferin Analgesic Tablets and Caplets ... ▣ 613
- Caltrate PLUS ... ▣ 665
- Cama Arthritis Pain Reliever ... ▣ 785
- Mag-Ox 400 ... 668
- Uro-Mag ... 668

Metformin Hydrochloride (Enhanced effect of hypoglycemics). Products include:
- Glucophage ... 752

Methylprednisolone Acetate (Increased risk of gastrointestinal ulceration; may reduce serum salicylate levels). Products include:
- Depo-Medrol Single-Dose Vial ... 2600
- Depo-Medrol Sterile Aqueous Suspension ... 2597

Methylprednisolone Sodium Succinate (Increased risk of gastrointestinal ulceration; may reduce serum salicylate levels). Products include:
- Solu-Medrol Sterile Powder ... 2643

Oxyphenbutazone (Increased risk of gastrointestinal ulceration).

Phenobarbital (Decreases aspirin effectiveness). Products include:
- Arco-Lase Plus Tablets ... 512
- Bellergal-S Tablets ... 2250
- Donnatal ... 2060
- Donnatal Extentabs ... 2061
- Donnatal Tablets ... 2060
- Phenobarbital Elixir and Tablets ... 1469
- Quadrinal Tablets ... 1350

Phenylbutazone (Decreased effects of phenylbutazone; increased risk of gastrointestinal ulceration).
- No products indexed under this heading.

Phenytoin (Increased serum phenytoin levels). Products include:
- Dilantin Infatabs ... 1908
- Dilantin-125 Suspension ... 1911

Phenytoin Sodium (Increased phenytoin levels). Products include:
- Dilantin Kapseals ... 1906
- Dilantin Parenteral ... 1910

Potassium Citrate (Decreased aspirin effectiveness). Products include:
- Polycitra Syrup ... 578
- Polycitra-K Crystals ... 579
- Polycitra-K Oral Solution ... 579
- Polycitra-LC ... 578

Prednisolone Acetate (Increased risk of gastrointestinal ulceration; may reduce serum salicylate levels). Products include:
- AK-CIDE ... ◉ 202
- AK-CIDE Ointment ... ◉ 202
- Blephamide Liquifilm Sterile Ophthalmic Suspension ... 476
- Blephamide Ointment ... ◉ 237
- Econopred & Econopred Plus Ophthalmic Suspensions ... ◉ 217
- Poly-Pred Liquifilm ... ◉ 248
- Pred Forte ... ◉ 250
- Pred Mild ... ◉ 253
- Pred-G Liquifilm Sterile Ophthalmic Suspension ... ◉ 251
- Pred-G S.O.P. Sterile Ophthalmic Ointment ... ◉ 252
- Vasocidin Ointment ... ◉ 268

Prednisolone Sodium Phosphate (Increased risk of gastrointestinal ulceration; may reduce serum salicylate levels). Products include:
- AK-Pred ... ◉ 204
- Hydeltrasol Injection, Sterile ... 1665
- Inflamase ... ◉ 265
- Pediapred Oral Liquid ... 995
- Vasocidin Ophthalmic Solution ... ◉ 270

Prednisolone Tebutate (Increased risk of gastrointestinal ulceration; may reduce serum salicylate levels). Products include:
- Hydeltra-T.B.A. Sterile Suspension 1667

Prednisone (Increased risk of gastrointestinal ulceration; may reduce serum salicylate levels). Products include:
- Deltasone Tablets ... 2595

Probenecid (Decreased effects of probenecid). Products include:
- Benemid Tablets ... 1611
- ColBENEMID Tablets ... 1622

Propranolol Hydrochloride (Decreases anti-inflammatory action of aspirin). Products include:
- Inderal ... 2728
- Inderal LA Long Acting Capsules ... 2730
- Inderide Tablets ... 2732
- Inderide LA Long Acting Capsules .. 2734

Sodium Bicarbonate (Increases stomach pH affects enteric coating of tablets). Products include:
- Alka-Seltzer Effervescent Antacid and Pain Reliever ... ▣ 701
- Alka-Seltzer Extra Strength Effervescent Antacid and Pain Reliever ... ▣ 703
- Alka-Seltzer Gold Effervescent Antacid ... ▣ 703
- Alka-Seltzer Lemon Lime Effervescent Antacid and Pain Reliever ... ▣ 703
- Arm & Hammer Pure Baking Soda ... ▣ 627
- Ceo-Two Rectal Suppositories ... 666
- Citrocarbonate Antacid ... ▣ 770
- Massengill Disposable Douches ... ▣ 820
- Massengill Liquid Concentrate ... ▣ 820
- NuLYTELY ... 689
- Cherry Flavor NuLYTELY ... 689

Sodium Citrate (Decreased aspirin effectiveness). Products include:
- Bicitra ... 578
- Citrocarbonate Antacid ... ▣ 770
- Polycitra ... 578
- Salix SST Lozenges Saliva Stimulant ... ▣ 797

Spironolactone (Decreased sodium excretion). Products include:
- Aldactazide ... 2413
- Aldactone ... 2414

Sulfinpyrazone (Decreased effects of sulfinpyrazone). Products include:
- Anturane ... 807

Tolazamide (Enhanced effect of hypoglycemics).
- No products indexed under this heading.

Tolbutamide (Enhanced effect of hypoglycemics).
- No products indexed under this heading.

Triamcinolone (Increased risk of gastrointestinal ulceration; may reduce serum salicylate levels). Products include:
- Aristocort Tablets ... 1022

Triamcinolone Acetonide (Increased risk of gastrointestinal ulceration; may reduce serum salicylate levels). Products include:
- Aristocort A 0.025% Cream ... 1027
- Aristocort A 0.5% Cream ... 1031
- Aristocort A 0.1% Cream ... 1029
- Aristocort A 0.1% Ointment ... 1030
- Azmacort Oral Inhaler ... 2011
- Nasacort Nasal Inhaler ... 2024

Triamcinolone Diacetate (Increased risk of gastrointestinal ulceration; may reduce serum salicylate levels). Products include:
- Aristocort Suspension (Forte Parenteral) ... 1027
- Aristocort Suspension (Intralesional) ... 1025

IMPORTANT NOTE: Always consult each drug listing in the patient's regimen for possible interactions.

Easprin
Interactions Index
358

Triamcinolone Hexacetonide (Increased risk of gastrointestinal ulceration; may reduce serum salicylate levels). Products include:
Aristospan Suspension (Intra-articular) ... 1033
Aristospan Suspension (Intralesional) ... 1032

Warfarin Sodium (Increased bleeding time). Products include:
Coumadin ... 926

Food Interactions

Alcohol (Synergism; gastrointestinal bleeding).

EC-NAPROSYN DELAYED-RELEASE TABLETS

(Naproxen) ... 2117

May interact with oral anticoagulants, sulfonamides, oral hypoglycemic agents, hydantoin anticonvulsants, lithium preparations, beta blockers, histamine h2-receptor antagonists, antacids, and certain other agents. Compounds in these categories include:

Acarbose (Potential for sulfonylurea toxicity).
No products indexed under this heading.

Acebutolol Hydrochloride (Reduced antihypertensive effect of beta blockers). Products include:
Sectral Capsules ... 2807

Aluminum Carbonate Gel (Due to the gastric pH elevating effects of H_2-blockers concomitant administration of EC-Naprosyn is not recommended). Products include:
Basaljel ... 2703

Aluminum Hydroxide (Due to the gastric pH elevating effects of H_2-blockers concomitant administration of EC-Naprosyn is not recommended). Products include:
ALternaGEL Liquid ... 1316
Maximum Strength Ascriptin ... ▣ 630
Cama Arthritis Pain Reliever ... ▣ 785
Gaviscon Extra Strength Relief Formula Antacid Tablets ... ▣ 819
Gaviscon Extra Strength Relief Formula Liquid Antacid ... ▣ 819
Gaviscon Liquid Antacid ... ▣ 820
Gelusil Liquid & Tablets ... ▣ 855
Maalox Heartburn Relief Suspension ... ▣ 642
Maalox Heartburn Relief Tablets ... ▣ 641
Maalox Magnesia and Alumina Oral Suspension ... ▣ 642
Maalox Plus Tablets ... ▣ 643
Extra Strength Maalox Antacid Plus Antigas Liquid and Tablets ▣ 638
Tempo Soft Antacid ... ▣ 835

Aluminum Hydroxide Gel (Due to the gastric pH elevating effects of H_2-blockers concomitant administration of EC-Naprosyn is not recommended). Products include:
ALternaGEL Liquid ... ▣ 659
Aludrox Oral Suspension ... 2695
Amphojel Suspension ... 2695
Amphojel Suspension without Flavor ... 2695
Amphojel Tablets ... 2695
Arthritis Pain Ascriptin ... ▣ 631
Regular Strength Ascriptin Tablets ... ▣ 629
Gaviscon Antacid Tablets ... ▣ 819
Gaviscon-2 Antacid Tablets ... ▣ 820
Mylanta Liquid ... 1317
Mylanta Tablets ... ▣ 660
Mylanta Double Strength Liquid ... 1317
Mylanta Double Strength Tablets .. ▣ 660
Nephrox Suspension ... ▣ 655

Aspirin (Naproxen is displaced from its binding sites during the concomitant administration of aspirin resulting in lower plasma concentrations and peak plasma levels; concurrent use is not recommended). Products include:
Alka-Seltzer Effervescent Antacid and Pain Reliever ... ▣ 701
Alka-Seltzer Extra Strength Effervescent Antacid and Pain Reliever ... ▣ 703
Alka-Seltzer Lemon Lime Effervescent Antacid and Pain Reliever ... ▣ 703
Alka-Seltzer Plus Cold Medicine ... ▣ 705
Alka-Seltzer Plus Cold & Cough Medicine ... ▣ 708
Alka-Seltzer Plus Night-Time Cold Medicine ... ▣ 707
Alka Seltzer Plus Sinus Medicine .. ▣ 707
Arthritis Foundation Safety Coated Aspirin Tablets ... ▣ 675
Arthritis Pain Ascriptin ... ▣ 631
Maximum Strength Ascriptin ... ▣ 630
Regular Strength Ascriptin Tablets ... ▣ 629
Arthritis Strength BC Powder ... ▣ 609
BC Cold Powder Multi-Symptom Formula (Cold-Sinus-Allergy) ... ▣ 609
BC Cold Powder Non-Drowsy Formula (Cold-Sinus) ... ▣ 609
BC Powder ... ▣ 609
Bayer Children's Chewable Aspirin ... ▣ 711
Genuine Bayer Aspirin Tablets & Caplets ... ▣ 713
Extra Strength Bayer Arthritis Pain Regimen Formula ... ▣ 711
Extra Strength Bayer Aspirin Caplets & Tablets ... ▣ 712
Extended-Release Bayer 8-Hour Aspirin ... ▣ 712
Extra Strength Bayer Plus Aspirin Caplets ... ▣ 713
Extra Strength Bayer PM Aspirin .. ▣ 713
Bayer Enteric Aspirin ... ▣ 709
Bufferin Analgesic Tablets and Caplets ... ▣ 613
Arthritis Strength Bufferin Analgesic Caplets ... ▣ 614
Extra Strength Bufferin Analgesic Tablets ... ▣ 615
Cama Arthritis Pain Reliever ... ▣ 785
Darvon Compound-65 Pulvules ... 1435
Easprin ... 1914
Ecotrin ... 2455
Ecotrin Enteric Coated Aspirin Maximum Strength Tablets and Caplets ... ▣ 816
Ecotrin Enteric Coated Aspirin Regular Strength Tablets ... 2455
Empirin Aspirin Tablets ... ▣ 854
Empirin with Codeine Tablets ... 1093
Excedrin Extra-Strength Analgesic Tablets & Caplets ... 732
Fiorinal Capsules ... 2261
Fiorinal with Codeine Capsules ... 2262
Fiorinal Tablets ... 2261
Halfprin ... 1362
Healthprin Aspirin ... 2455
Norgesic ... 1496
Percodan Tablets ... 939
Percodan-Demi Tablets ... 940
Robaxisal Tablets ... 2071
Soma Compound w/Codeine Tablets ... 2676
Soma Compound Tablets ... 2675
St. Joseph Adult Chewable Aspirin (81 mg.) ... ▣ 808
Talwin Compound ... 2335
Ursinus Inlay-Tabs ... ▣ 794
Vanquish Analgesic Caplets ... ▣ 731

Atenolol (Reduced antihypertensive effect of beta blockers). Products include:
Tenoretic Tablets ... 2845
Tenormin Tablets and I.V. Injection 2847

Bendroflumethiazide (Potential for sulfonamide toxicity).
No products indexed under this heading.

Betaxolol Hydrochloride (Reduced antihypertensive effect of beta blockers). Products include:
Betoptic Ophthalmic Solution ... 469
Betoptic S Ophthalmic Suspension 471
Kerlone Tablets ... 2436

Bisoprolol Fumarate (Reduced antihypertensive effect of beta blockers). Products include:
Zebeta Tablets ... 1413
Ziac ... 1415

Carteolol Hydrochloride (Reduced antihypertensive effect of beta blockers). Products include:
Cartrol Tablets ... 410
Ocupress Ophthalmic Solution, 1% Sterile ... ◉ 309

Chlorothiazide (Potential for sulfonamide toxicity). Products include:
Aldoclor Tablets ... 1598
Diupres Tablets ... 1650
Diuril Oral ... 1653

Chlorothiazide Sodium (Potential for sulfonamide toxicity). Products include:
Diuril Sodium Intravenous ... 1652

Chlorpropamide (Potential for sulfonylurea toxicity). Products include:
Diabinese Tablets ... 1935

Cimetidine (Due to the gastric pH elevating effects of H_2-blockers concomitant administration of EC-Naprosyn is not recommended). Products include:
Tagamet Tablets ... 2516

Cimetidine Hydrochloride (Due to the gastric pH elevating effects of H_2-blockers concomitant administration of EC-Naprosyn is not recommended). Products include:
Tagamet ... 2516

Dicumarol (Short-term studies have failed to show any significant effect of concurrent use on prothrombin time; caution is advised since interactions have been seen with other NSAIDs).
No products indexed under this heading.

Dihydroxyaluminum Sodium Carbonate (Due to the gastric pH elevating effects of H_2-blockers concomitant administration of EC-Naprosyn is not recommended).
No products indexed under this heading.

Esmolol Hydrochloride (Reduced antihypertensive effect of beta blockers). Products include:
Brevibloc Injection ... 1808

Ethotoin (Potential for hydantoin toxicity). Products include:
Peganone Tablets ... 446

Famotidine (Due to the gastric pH elevating effects of H_2-blockers concomitant administration of EC-Naprosyn is not recommended). Products include:
Pepcid AC ... 1319
Pepcid Injection ... 1722
Pepcid ... 1720

Furosemide (Inhibition of natriuretic effect of furosemide). Products include:
Lasix Injection, Oral Solution and Tablets ... 1240

Glipizide (Potential for sulfonylurea toxicity). Products include:
Glucotrol Tablets ... 1967
Glucotrol XL Extended Release Tablets ... 1968

Glyburide (Potential for sulfonylurea toxicity). Products include:
DiaBeta Tablets ... 1239
Glynase PresTab Tablets ... 2609
Micronase Tablets ... 2623

Hydrochlorothiazide (Potential for sulfonamide toxicity). Products include:
Aldactazide ... 2413
Aldoril Tablets ... 1604
Apresazide Capsules ... 808
Capozide ... 742
Dyazide ... 2479
Esidrix Tablets ... 821
Esimil Tablets ... 822
HydroDIURIL Tablets ... 1674
Hydropres Tablets ... 1675
Hyzaar Tablets ... 1677
Inderide Tablets ... 2732
Inderide LA Long Acting Capsules .. 2734
Lopressor HCT Tablets ... 832
Lotensin HCT ... 837
Maxzide ... 1380
Moduretic Tablets ... 1705
Oretic Tablets ... 443
Prinzide Tablets ... 1737
Ser-Ap-Es Tablets ... 849
Timolide Tablets ... 1748
Vaseretic Tablets ... 1765
Zestoretic ... 2850
Ziac ... 1415

Hydroflumethiazide (Potential for sulfonamide toxicity). Products include:
Diucardin Tablets ... 2718

Labetalol Hydrochloride (Reduced antihypertensive effect of beta blockers). Products include:
Normodyne Injection ... 2377
Normodyne Tablets ... 2379
Trandate ... 1185

Levobunolol Hydrochloride (Reduced antihypertensive effect of beta blockers). Products include:
Betagan ... ◉ 233

Lithium Carbonate (Inhibition of lithium renal clearance leading to increase in plasma lithium concentrations). Products include:
Eskalith ... 2485
Lithium Carbonate Capsules & Tablets ... 2230
Lithonate/Lithotabs/Lithobid ... 2543

Lithium Citrate (Inhibition of lithium renal clearance leading to increase in plasma lithium concentrations).
No products indexed under this heading.

Magaldrate (Due to the gastric pH elevating effects of H_2-blockers concomitant administration of EC-Naprosyn is not recommended).
No products indexed under this heading.

Magnesium Hydroxide (Due to the gastric pH elevating effects of H_2-blockers concomitant administration of EC-Naprosyn is not recommended). Products include:
Aludrox Oral Suspension ... 2695
Arthritis Pain Ascriptin ... ▣ 631
Maximum Strength Ascriptin ... ▣ 630
Regular Strength Ascriptin Tablets ... ▣ 629
Di-Gel Antacid/Anti-Gas ... ▣ 801
Gelusil Liquid & Tablets ... ▣ 855
Maalox Magnesia and Alumina Oral Suspension ... ▣ 642
Maalox Plus Tablets ... ▣ 643
Extra Strength Maalox Antacid Plus Antigas Liquid and Tablets ▣ 638
Mylanta Calcium Carbonate and Magnesium Hydroxide Tablets ... 1318
Mylanta Liquid ... 1317
Mylanta Tablets ... ▣ 660
Mylanta Double Strength Liquid ... 1317
Mylanta Double Strength Tablets .. ▣ 660
Phillips' Milk of Magnesia Liquid ... ▣ 729
Rolaids Tablets ... ▣ 843
Tempo Soft Antacid ... ▣ 835

Magnesium Oxide (Due to the gastric pH elevating effects of H_2-blockers concomitant administration of EC-Naprosyn is not recommended). Products include:
Beelith Tablets ... 639
Bufferin Analgesic Tablets and Caplets ... ▣ 613
Caltrate PLUS ... ▣ 665
Cama Arthritis Pain Reliever ... ▣ 785
Mag-Ox 400 ... 668
Uro-Mag ... 668

Mephenytoin (Potential for hydantoin toxicity). Products include:
Mesantoin Tablets ... 2272

(▣ Described in PDR For Nonprescription Drugs)
(◉ Described in PDR For Ophthalmology)

Metformin Hydrochloride (Potential for sulfonylurea toxicity). Products include:

Glucophage 752

Methotrexate Sodium (Potential for reduced tubular secretion of methotrexate and possible increased methotrexate toxicity as shown in animal model; caution is recommended). Products include:

Methotrexate Sodium Tablets, Injection, for Injection and LPF Injection 1275

Methyclothiazide (Potential for sulfonamide toxicity). Products include:

Enduron Tablets.................................... 420

Metipranolol Hydrochloride (Reduced antihypertensive effect of beta blockers). Products include:

OptiPranolol (Metipranolol 0.3%) Sterile Ophthalmic Solution.......... ◆ 258

Metoprolol Succinate (Reduced antihypertensive effect of beta blockers). Products include:

Toprol-XL Tablets 565

Metoprolol Tartrate (Reduced antihypertensive effect of beta blockers). Products include:

Lopressor Ampuls.................................. 830
Lopressor HCT Tablets 832
Lopressor Tablets 830

Nadolol (Reduced antihypertensive effect of beta blockers).

No products indexed under this heading.

Naproxen Sodium (Concurrent use of naproxen or naproxen sodium in any dosage form is not recommended since they all circulate in the plasma as the naproxen anion). Products include:

Aleve 1975
Anaprox/Naprosyn 2117

Nizatidine (Due to the gastric pH elevating effects of H_2-blockers concomitant administration of EC-Naprosyn is not recommended). Products include:

Axid Pulvules 1427

Penbutolol Sulfate (Reduced antihypertensive effect of beta blockers). Products include:

Levatol 2403

Phenytoin (Potential for hydantoin toxicity). Products include:

Dilantin Infatabs 1908
Dilantin-125 Suspension 1911

Phenytoin Sodium (Potential for hydantoin toxicity). Products include:

Dilantin Kapseals 1906
Dilantin Parenteral 1910

Pindolol (Reduced antihypertensive effect of beta blockers). Products include:

Visken Tablets....................................... 2299

Polythiazide (Potential for sulfonamide toxicity). Products include:

Minizide Capsules 1938

Probenecid (Probenecid given concurrently increases naproxen anion plasma levels and extends its plasma half-life significantly). Products include:

Benemid Tablets 1611
ColBENEMID Tablets 1622

Propranolol Hydrochloride (Reduced antihypertensive effect of beta blockers). Products include:

Inderal 2728
Inderal LA Long Acting Capsules 2730
Inderide Tablets 2732
Inderide LA Long Acting Capsules .. 2734

Ranitidine Hydrochloride (Due to the gastric pH elevating effects of H_2-blockers concomitant administration of EC-Naprosyn is not recommended). Products include:

Zantac.. 1209
Zantac Injection 1207
Zantac Syrup 1209

Sodium Bicarbonate (Due to the gastric pH elevating effects of H_2-blockers concomitant administration of EC-Naprosyn is not recommended). Products include:

Alka-Seltzer Effervescent Antacid and Pain Reliever................................ ⊞ 701
Alka-Seltzer Extra Strength Effervescent Antacid and Pain Reliever .... ⊞ 703
Alka-Seltzer Gold Effervescent Antacid.. ⊞ 703
Alka-Seltzer Lemon Lime Effervescent Antacid and Pain Reliever .... ⊞ 703
Arm & Hammer Pure Baking Soda .... ⊞ 627
Ceo-Two Rectal Suppositories 666
Citrocarbonate Antacid .... ⊞ 770
Massengill Disposable Douches...... ⊞ 820
Massengill Liquid Concentrate .... ⊞ 820
NuLYTELY.. 689
Cherry Flavor NuLYTELY 689

Sotalol Hydrochloride (Reduced antihypertensive effect of beta blockers). Products include:

Betapace Tablets 641

Sucralfate (Due to the gastric pH elevating effects of H_2-blockers concomitant administration of EC-Naprosyn is not recommended). Products include:

Carafate Suspension 1505
Carafate Tablets.................................... 1504

Sulfacytine (Potential for sulfonamide toxicity).

Sulfamethizole (Potential for sulfonamide toxicity). Products include:

Urobiotic-250 Capsules 2214

Sulfamethoxazole (Potential for sulfonamide toxicity). Products include:

Azo Gantanol Tablets............................ 2080
Bactrim DS Tablets................................ 2084
Bactrim I.V. Infusion 2082
Bactrim 2084
Gantanol Tablets 2119
Septra... 1174
Septra I.V. Infusion 1169
Septra I.V. Infusion ADD-Vantage Vials.. 1171
Septra... 1174

Sulfasalazine (Potential for sulfonamide toxicity). Products include:

Azulfidine 1949

Sulfinpyrazone (Potential for sulfonamide toxicity). Products include:

Anturane 807

Sulfisoxazole (Potential for sulfonamide toxicity). Products include:

Azo Gantrisin Tablets............................ 2081
Gantrisin Tablets 2120

Sulfisoxazole Diolamine (Potential for sulfonamide toxicity).

No products indexed under this heading.

Timolol Hemihydrate (Reduced antihypertensive effect of beta blockers). Products include:

Betimol 0.25%, 0.5% .... ◆ 261

Timolol Maleate (Reduced antihypertensive effect of beta blockers). Products include:

Blocadren Tablets 1614
Timolide Tablets.................................... 1748
Timoptic in Ocudose 1753
Timoptic Sterile Ophthalmic Solution... 1751
Timoptic-XE 1755

Tolazamide (Potential for sulfonylurea toxicity).

No products indexed under this heading.

Tolbutamide (Potential for sulfonylurea toxicity).

No products indexed under this heading.

Warfarin Sodium (Short-term studies have failed to show any significant effect of concurrent use on prothrombin time; caution is advised since interactions have been seen with other NSAIDs). Products include:

Coumadin 926

Food Interactions

Food, unspecified (The presence of food prolonged the time the EC-Naprosyn remained in the stomach, time to first detectable serum naproxen levels, and time to maximal naproxen levels (T_{max}), but did not affect peak naproxen levels (C_{max})).

ECONOPRED & ECONOPRED PLUS OPHTHALMIC SUSPENSIONS

(Prednisolone Acetate)........................ ◆ 217

None cited in PDR database.

ECOTRIN ENTERIC COATED ASPIRIN LOW STRENGTH TABLETS

(Aspirin, Enteric Coated) 2455

See Ecotrin Enteric Coated Aspirin Maximum Strength Tablets and Caplets

ECOTRIN ENTERIC COATED ASPIRIN MAXIMUM STRENGTH TABLETS AND CAPLETS

(Aspirin, Enteric Coated) 2455

May interact with antacids containing aluminium, calcium and magnesium and certain other agents. Compounds in these categories include:

Aluminum Carbonate Gel (Concurrent administration of nonabsorbable antacids may alter the rate of absorption of aspirin). Products include:

Basaljel.. 2703

Aluminum Hydroxide (Concurrent administration of nonabsorbable antacids may alter the rate of absorption of aspirin). Products include:

ALternaGEL Liquid 1316
Maximum Strength Ascriptin .... ⊞ 630
Cama Arthritis Pain Reliever........... ⊞ 785
Gaviscon Extra Strength Relief Formula Antacid Tablets................ ⊞ 819
Gaviscon Extra Strength Relief Formula Liquid Antacid.................. ⊞ 819
Gaviscon Liquid Antacid.................... ⊞ 820
Gelusil Liquid & Tablets .... ⊞ 855
Maalox Heartburn Relief Suspension .... ⊞ 642
Maalox Heartburn Relief Tablets.... ⊞ 641
Maalox Magnesia and Alumina Oral Suspension .... ⊞ 642
Maalox Plus Tablets .... ⊞ 643
Extra Strength Maalox Antacid Plus Antigas Liquid and Tablets ⊞ 638
Tempo Soft Antacid .... ⊞ 835

Aluminum Hydroxide Gel (Concurrent administration of nonabsorbable antacids may alter the rate of absorption of aspirin). Products include:

ALternaGEL Liquid .... ⊞ 659
Aludrox Oral Suspension 2695
Amphojel Suspension 2695
Amphojel Suspension without Flavor 2695
Amphojel Tablets.................................. 2695
Arthritis Pain Ascriptin .... ⊞ 631
Regular Strength Ascriptin Tablets .... ⊞ 629

Gaviscon Antacid Tablets.................. ⊞ 819
Gaviscon-2 Antacid Tablets .... ⊞ 820
Mylanta Liquid 1317
Mylanta Tablets .... ⊞ 660
Mylanta Double Strength Liquid 1317
Mylanta Double Strength Tablets.. ⊞ 660
Nephrox Suspension .... ⊞ 655

Aluminum Hydroxide Gel, Dried (Concurrent administration of nonabsorbable antacids may alter the rate of absorption of aspirin).

Antiarthritic Drugs, unspecified (Effect not specified).

Anticoagulant Drugs, unspecified (Effect not specified).

Antidiabetic Drugs, unspecified (Effect not specified).

Antigout Drugs, unspecified (Effect not specified).

Dihydroxyaluminum Sodium Carbonate (Concurrent administration of nonabsorbable antacids may alter the rate of absorption of aspirin).

No products indexed under this heading.

Magaldrate (Concurrent administration of nonabsorbable antacids may alter the rate of absorption of aspirin).

No products indexed under this heading.

Magnesium Hydroxide (Concurrent administration of nonabsorbable antacids may alter the rate of absorption of aspirin). Products include:

Aludrox Oral Suspension 2695
Arthritis Pain Ascriptin .... ⊞ 631
Maximum Strength Ascriptin .... ⊞ 630
Regular Strength Ascriptin Tablets .... ⊞ 629
Di-Gel Antacid/Anti-Gas .... ⊞ 801
Gelusil Liquid & Tablets .... ⊞ 855
Maalox Magnesia and Alumina Oral Suspension .... ⊞ 642
Maalox Plus Tablets .... ⊞ 643
Extra Strength Maalox Antacid Plus Antigas Liquid and Tablets ⊞ 638
Mylanta Calcium Carbonate and Magnesium Hydroxide Tablets...... 1318
Mylanta Liquid 1317
Mylanta Tablets .... ⊞ 660
Mylanta Double Strength Liquid 1317
Mylanta Double Strength Tablets.. ⊞ 660
Phillips' Milk of Magnesia Liquid.... ⊞ 729
Rolaids Tablets .... ⊞ 843
Tempo Soft Antacid .... ⊞ 835

Magnesium Oxide (Concurrent administration of nonabsorbable antacids may alter the rate of absorption of aspirin). Products include:

Beelith Tablets 639
Bufferin Analgesic Tablets and Caplets.. ⊞ 613
Caltrate PLUS .... ⊞ 665
Cama Arthritis Pain Reliever........... ⊞ 785
Mag-Ox 400 668
Uro-Mag.. 668

Sodium Bicarbonate (Concurrent administration with absorbable antacids may increase the clearance of salicylates). Products include:

Alka-Seltzer Effervescent Antacid and Pain Reliever................................ ⊞ 701
Alka-Seltzer Extra Strength Effervescent Antacid and Pain Reliever .... ⊞ 703
Alka-Seltzer Gold Effervescent Antacid.. ⊞ 703
Alka-Seltzer Lemon Lime Effervescent Antacid and Pain Reliever .... ⊞ 703
Arm & Hammer Pure Baking Soda .... ⊞ 627
Ceo-Two Rectal Suppositories 666
Citrocarbonate Antacid .... ⊞ 770
Massengill Disposable Douches...... ⊞ 820
Massengill Liquid Concentrate .... ⊞ 820
NuLYTELY.. 689
Cherry Flavor NuLYTELY 689

IMPORTANT NOTE: Always consult each drug listing in the patient's regimen for possible interactions.

Ecotrin | Interactions Index | 360

ECOTRIN ENTERIC COATED ASPIRIN REGULAR STRENGTH TABLETS
(Aspirin, Enteric Coated) 2455
See **Ecotrin Enteric Coated Aspirin Maximum Strength Tablets and Caplets**

EDECRIN SODIUM INTRAVENOUS
(Ethacrynate Sodium) 1657
May interact with aminoglycosides, cephalosporins, non-steroidal anti-inflammatory agents, cardiac glycosides, and certain other agents. Compounds in these categories include:

Amikacin Sulfate (Increased ototoxic potential of aminoglycosides). Products include:
- Amikacin Sulfate Injection, USP 960
- Amikin Injectable 501

Cefaclor (Increased ototoxic potential of cephalosporins). Products include:
- Ceclor Pulvules & Suspension 1431

Cefadroxil Monohydrate (Increased ototoxic potential of cephalosporins). Products include:
- Duricef 748

Cefamandole Nafate (Increased ototoxic potential of cephalosporins). Products include:
- Mandol Vials, Faspak & ADD-Vantage 1461

Cefazolin Sodium (Increased ototoxic potential of cephalosporins). Products include:
- Ancef Injection 2465
- Kefzol Vials, Faspak & ADD-Vantage 1456

Cefixime (Increased ototoxic potential of cephalosporins). Products include:
- Suprax 1399

Cefmetazole Sodium (Increased ototoxic potential of cephalosporins). Products include:
- Zefazone 2654

Cefonicid Sodium (Increased ototoxic potential of cephalosporins). Products include:
- Monocid Injection 2497

Cefoperazone Sodium (Increased ototoxic potential of cephalosporins). Products include:
- Cefobid Intravenous/Intramuscular 2189
- Cefobid Pharmacy Bulk Package - Not for Direct Infusion 2192

Ceforanide (Increased ototoxic potential of cephalosporins).
- No products indexed under this heading.

Cefotaxime Sodium (Increased ototoxic potential of cephalosporins). Products include:
- Claforan Sterile and Injection 1235

Cefotetan (Increased ototoxic potential of cephalosporins). Products include:
- Cefotan 2829

Cefoxitin Sodium (Increased ototoxic potential of cephalosporins). Products include:
- Mefoxin 1691
- Mefoxin Premixed Intravenous Solution 1694

Cefpodoxime Proxetil (Increased ototoxic potential of cephalosporins). Products include:
- Vantin for Oral Suspension and Vantin Tablets 2646

Cefprozil (Increased ototoxic potential of cephalosporins). Products include:
- Cefzil Tablets and Oral Suspension 746

Ceftazidime (Increased ototoxic potential of cephalosporins). Products include:
- Ceptaz 1081
- Fortaz 1100
- Tazicef for Injection 2519
- Tazidime Vials, Faspak & ADD-Vantage 1478

Ceftizoxime Sodium (Increased ototoxic potential of cephalosporins). Products include:
- Cefizox for Intramuscular or Intravenous Use 1034

Ceftriaxone Sodium (Increased ototoxic potential of cephalosporins). Products include:
- Rocephin Injectable Vials, ADD-Vantage, Galaxy Container 2142

Cefuroxime Axetil (Increased ototoxic potential of cephalosporins). Products include:
- Ceftin 1078

Cefuroxime Sodium (Increased ototoxic potential of cephalosporins). Products include:
- Kefurox Vials, Faspak & ADD-Vantage 1454
- Zinacef 1211

Cephalexin (Increased ototoxic potential of cephalosporins). Products include:
- Keflex Pulvules & Oral Suspension 914

Cephalothin Sodium (Increased ototoxic potential of cephalosporins).

Cephapirin Sodium (Increased ototoxic potential of cephalosporins).
- No products indexed under this heading.

Cephradine (Increased ototoxic potential of cephalosporins).
- No products indexed under this heading.

Deslanoside (Excessive potassium loss may precipitate digitalis toxicity).
- No products indexed under this heading.

Diclofenac Potassium (Reduces diuretic, natriuretic, and antihypertensive effects). Products include:
- Cataflam 816

Diclofenac Sodium (Reduces diuretic, natriuretic, and antihypertensive effects). Products include:
- Voltaren Ophthalmic Sterile Ophthalmic Solution ...... ⊙ 272
- Voltaren Tablets 861

Digitoxin (Excessive potassium loss may precipitate digitalis toxicity). Products include:
- Crystodigin Tablets 1433

Digoxin (Excessive potassium loss may precipitate digitalis toxicity). Products include:
- Lanoxicaps 1117
- Lanoxin Elixir Pediatric 1120
- Lanoxin Injection 1123
- Lanoxin Injection Pediatric 1126
- Lanoxin Tablets 1128

Etodolac (Reduces diuretic, natriuretic, and antihypertensive effects). Products include:
- Lodine Capsules and Tablets 2743

Fenoprofen Calcium (Reduces diuretic, natriuretic, and antihypertensive effects). Products include:
- Nalfon 200 Pulvules & Nalfon Tablets 917

Flurbiprofen (Reduces diuretic, natriuretic, and antihypertensive effects). Products include:
- Ansaid Tablets 2579

Gentamicin Sulfate (Increased ototoxic potential of aminoglycosides). Products include:
- Garamycin Injectable 2360
- Genoptic Sterile Ophthalmic Solution ...... ⊙ 243
- Genoptic Sterile Ophthalmic Ointment ...... ⊙ 243
- Gentacidin Ointment ...... ⊙ 264
- Gentacidin Solution ...... ⊙ 264
- Gentak ...... ⊙ 208
- Pred-G Liquifilm Sterile Ophthalmic Suspension ...... ⊙ 251
- Pred-G S.O.P. Sterile Ophthalmic Ointment ...... ⊙ 252

Ibuprofen (Reduces diuretic, natriuretic, and antihypertensive effects). Products include:
- Advil Cold and Sinus Caplets and Tablets (formerly CoAdvil) ...... ▣ 870
- Advil Ibuprofen Tablets and Caplets ...... ▣ 870
- Children's Advil Suspension 2692
- Arthritis Foundation Ibuprofen Tablets ...... ▣ 674
- Bayer Select Ibuprofen Pain Relief Formula ...... ▣ 715
- Cramp End Tablets ...... ▣ 735
- Dimetapp Sinus Caplets ...... ▣ 775
- Haltran Tablets ...... ▣ 771
- IBU Tablets 1342
- Ibuprohm ...... ▣ 735
- Children's Motrin Ibuprofen Oral Suspension 1546
- Motrin Tablets 2625
- Motrin IB Caplets, Tablets, and Geltabs ...... ▣ 838
- Motrin IB Sinus ...... ▣ 838
- Motrin Ibuprofen Suspension, Oral Drops, Chewable Tablets, Caplets 1546
- Nuprin Ibuprofen/Analgesic Tablets & Caplets ...... ▣ 622
- Sine-Aid IB Caplets 1554
- Vicks DayQuil SINUS Pressure & PAIN Relief with IBUPROFEN ...... ▣ 762

Indomethacin (Reduces diuretic, natriuretic, and antihypertensive effects). Products include:
- Indocin 1680

Indomethacin Sodium Trihydrate (Reduces diuretic, natriuretic, and antihypertensive effects). Products include:
- Indocin I.V. 1684

Isoproterenol Hydrochloride (Careful adjustment of dosages required). Products include:
- Isuprel Hydrochloride Injection 1:5000 2311
- Isuprel Hydrochloride Solution 1:200 & 1:100 2313
- Isuprel Mistometer 2312

Kanamycin Sulfate (Increased ototoxic potential of aminoglycosides).
- No products indexed under this heading.

Ketoprofen (Reduces diuretic, natriuretic, and antihypertensive effects). Products include:
- Orudis Capsules 2766
- Oruvail Capsules 2766

Ketorolac Tromethamine (Reduces diuretic, natriuretic, and antihypertensive effects). Products include:
- Acular 474
- Acular ...... ⊙ 277
- Toradol 2159

Lithium Carbonate (High risk of lithium toxicity). Products include:
- Eskalith 2485
- Lithium Carbonate Capsules & Tablets 2230
- Lithonate/Lithotabs/Lithobid 2543

Lithium Citrate (High risk of lithium toxicity).
- No products indexed under this heading.

Loracarbef (Increased ototoxic potential of cephalosporins). Products include:
- Lorabid Suspension and Pulvules 1459

Meclofenamate Sodium (Reduces diuretic, natriuretic, and antihypertensive effects).
- No products indexed under this heading.

Mefenamic Acid (Reduces diuretic, natriuretic, and antihypertensive effects). Products include:
- Ponstel 1925

Nabumetone (Reduces diuretic, natriuretic, and antihypertensive effects). Products include:
- Relafen Tablets 2510

Naproxen (Reduces diuretic, natriuretic, and antihypertensive effects). Products include:
- Anaprox/Naprosyn 2117

Naproxen Sodium (Reduces diuretic, natriuretic, and antihypertensive effects). Products include:
- Aleve 1975
- Anaprox/Naprosyn 2117

Oxaprozin (Reduces diuretic, natriuretic, and antihypertensive effects). Products include:
- Daypro Caplets 2426

Phenylbutazone (Reduces diuretic, natriuretic, and antihypertensive effects).
- No products indexed under this heading.

Piroxicam (Reduces diuretic, natriuretic, and antihypertensive effects). Products include:
- Feldene Capsules 1965

Streptomycin Sulfate (Increased ototoxic potential of aminoglycosides). Products include:
- Streptomycin Sulfate Injection 2208

Sulindac (Reduces diuretic, natriuretic, and antihypertensive effects). Products include:
- Clinoril Tablets 1618

Tobramycin Sulfate (Increased ototoxic potential of aminoglycosides). Products include:
- Nebcin Vials, Hyporets & ADD-Vantage 1464
- Tobramycin Sulfate Injection 968

Tolmetin Sodium (Reduces diuretic, natriuretic, and antihypertensive effects). Products include:
- Tolectin (200, 400 and 600 mg) 1581

Warfarin Sodium (Warfarin displaced from plasma protein; reduction in warfarin dosage may be required). Products include:
- Coumadin 926

EDECRIN TABLETS
(Ethacrynic Acid) 1657
See **Edecrin Sodium Intravenous**

EFFEXOR
(Venlafaxine Hydrochloride) 2719
May interact with monoamine oxidase inhibitors and certain other agents. Compounds in these categories include:

Cimetidine (Inhibition of first-pass metabolism of venlafaxine; reduces the oral clearance by 43% and the AUC and C_{max} of venlafaxine were increased by about 60%). Products include:
- Tagamet Tablets 2516

Cimetidine Hydrochloride (Inhibition of first-pass metabolism of venlafaxine; reduces the oral clearance by 43% and the AUC and C_{max} of venlafaxine were increased by about 60%). Products include:
- Tagamet 2516

Furazolidone (Potential for serious, sometimes fatal reactions including hyperthermia, rigidity, myoclonus, autonomic instability; concurrent and or sequential use within 14 days is contraindicated). Products include:
- Furoxone 2046

(▣ Described in PDR For Nonprescription Drugs) (⊙ Described in PDR For Ophthalmology)

Isocarboxazid (Potential for serious, sometimes fatal reactions including hyperthermia, rigidity, myoclonus, autonomic instability; concurrent and or sequential use within 14 days is contraindicated).
No products indexed under this heading.

Phenelzine Sulfate (Potential for serious, sometimes fatal reactions including hyperthermia, rigidity, myoclonus, autonomic instability; concurrent and or sequential use within 14 days is contraindicated). Products include:
Nardil 1920

Selegiline Hydrochloride (Potential for serious, sometimes fatal reactions including hyperthermia, rigidity, myoclonus, autonomic instability; concurrent and or sequential use within 14 days is contraindicated). Products include:
Eldepryl Tablets 2550

Tranylcypromine Sulfate (Potential for serious, sometimes fatal reactions including hyperthermia, rigidity, myoclonus, autonomic instability; concurrent and or sequential use within 14 days is contraindicated). Products include:
Parnate Tablets 2503

Food Interactions

Alcohol (Concurrent use should be avoided).

EFIDAC/24

(Pseudoephedrine Hydrochloride) .. ▭ 635
May interact with antihypertensives, antidepressant drugs, and certain other agents. Compounds in these categories include:

Acebutolol Hydrochloride (Concurrent use is not recommended; consult your doctor). Products include:
Sectral Capsules 2807

Amitriptyline Hydrochloride (Concurrent use is not recommended; consult your doctor). Products include:
Elavil 2838
Endep Tablets 2174
Etrafon 2355
Limbitrol 2180
Triavil Tablets 1757

Amlodipine Besylate (Concurrent use is not recommended; consult your doctor). Products include:
Lotrel Capsules 840
Norvasc Tablets 1940

Amoxapine (Concurrent use is not recommended; consult your doctor). Products include:
Asendin Tablets 1369

Atenolol (Concurrent use is not recommended; consult your doctor). Products include:
Tenoretic Tablets 2845
Tenormin Tablets and I.V. Injection 2847

Benazepril Hydrochloride (Concurrent use is not recommended; consult your doctor). Products include:
Lotensin Tablets 834
Lotensin HCT 837
Lotrel Capsules 840

Bendroflumethiazide (Concurrent use is not recommended; consult your doctor).
No products indexed under this heading.

Betaxolol Hydrochloride (Concurrent use is not recommended; consult your doctor). Products include:
Betoptic Ophthalmic Solution 469
Betoptic S Ophthalmic Suspension 471
Kerlone Tablets 2436

Bisoprolol Fumarate (Concurrent use is not recommended; consult your doctor). Products include:
Zebeta Tablets 1413
Ziac 1415

Bupropion Hydrochloride (Concurrent use is not recommended; consult your doctor). Products include:
Wellbutrin Tablets 1204

Captopril (Concurrent use is not recommended; consult your doctor). Products include:
Capoten 739
Capozide 742

Carteolol Hydrochloride (Concurrent use is not recommended; consult your doctor). Products include:
Cartrol Tablets 410
Ocupress Ophthalmic Solution, 1% Sterile .... ⊙ 309

Chlorothiazide (Concurrent use is not recommended; consult your doctor). Products include:
Aldoclor Tablets 1598
Diupres Tablets 1650
Diuril Oral 1653

Chlorothiazide Sodium (Concurrent use is not recommended; consult your doctor). Products include:
Diuril Sodium Intravenous 1652

Chlorthalidone (Concurrent use is not recommended; consult your doctor). Products include:
Combipres Tablets 677
Tenoretic Tablets 2845
Thalitone 1245

Clonidine (Concurrent use is not recommended; consult your doctor). Products include:
Catapres-TTS 675

Clonidine Hydrochloride (Concurrent use is not recommended; consult your doctor). Products include:
Catapres Tablets 674
Combipres Tablets 677

Deserpidine (Concurrent use is not recommended; consult your doctor).
No products indexed under this heading.

Desipramine Hydrochloride (Concurrent use is not recommended; consult your doctor). Products include:
Norpramin Tablets 1526

Diazoxide (Concurrent use is not recommended; consult your doctor). Products include:
Hyperstat I.V. Injection 2363
Proglycem 580

Diltiazem Hydrochloride (Concurrent use is not recommended; consult your doctor). Products include:
Cardizem CD Capsules 1506
Cardizem SR Capsules 1510
Cardizem Injectable 1508
Cardizem Tablets 1512
Dilacor XR Extended-release Capsules 2018

Doxazosin Mesylate (Concurrent use is not recommended; consult your doctor). Products include:
Cardura Tablets 2186

Doxepin Hydrochloride (Concurrent use is not recommended; consult your doctor). Products include:
Sinequan 2205
Zonalon Cream 1055

Enalapril Maleate (Concurrent use is not recommended; consult your doctor). Products include:
Vaseretic Tablets 1765
Vasotec Tablets 1771

Enalaprilat (Concurrent use is not recommended; consult your doctor). Products include:
Vasotec I.V. 1768

Esmolol Hydrochloride (Concurrent use is not recommended; consult your doctor). Products include:
Brevibloc Injection 1808

Felodipine (Concurrent use is not recommended; consult your doctor). Products include:
Plendil Extended-Release Tablets.... 527

Fluoxetine Hydrochloride (Concurrent use is not recommended; consult your doctor). Products include:
Prozac Pulvules & Liquid, Oral Solution 919

Fosinopril Sodium (Concurrent use is not recommended; consult your doctor). Products include:
Monopril Tablets 757

Furosemide (Concurrent use is not recommended; consult your doctor). Products include:
Lasix Injection, Oral Solution and Tablets 1240

Guanabenz Acetate (Concurrent use is not recommended; consult your doctor).
No products indexed under this heading.

Guanethidine Monosulfate (Concurrent use is not recommended; consult your doctor). Products include:
Esimil Tablets 822
Ismelin Tablets 827

Hydralazine Hydrochloride (Concurrent use is not recommended; consult your doctor). Products include:
Apresazide Capsules 808
Apresoline Hydrochloride Tablets .. 809
Ser-Ap-Es Tablets 849

Hydrochlorothiazide (Concurrent use is not recommended; consult your doctor). Products include:
Aldactazide 2413
Aldoril Tablets 1604
Apresazide Capsules 808
Capozide 742
Dyazide 2479
Esidrix Tablets 821
Esimil Tablets 822
HydroDIURIL Tablets 1674
Hydropres Tablets 1675
Hyzaar Tablets 1677
Inderide Tablets 2732
Inderide LA Long Acting Capsules .. 2734
Lopressor HCT Tablets 832
Lotensin HCT 837
Maxzide 1380
Moduretic Tablets 1705
Oretic Tablets 443
Prinzide Tablets 1737
Ser-Ap-Es Tablets 849
Timolide Tablets 1748
Vaseretic Tablets 1765
Zestoretic 2850
Ziac 1415

Hydroflumethiazide (Concurrent use is not recommended; consult your doctor). Products include:
Diucardin Tablets 2718

Imipramine Hydrochloride (Concurrent use is not recommended; consult your doctor). Products include:
Tofranil Ampuls 854
Tofranil Tablets 856

Imipramine Pamoate (Concurrent use is not recommended; consult your doctor). Products include:
Tofranil-PM Capsules 857

Indapamide (Concurrent use is not recommended; consult your doctor). Products include:
Lozol Tablets 2022

Isocarboxazid (Concurrent use is not recommended; consult your doctor).
No products indexed under this heading.

Isradipine (Concurrent use is not recommended; consult your doctor). Products include:
DynaCirc Capsules 2256

Labetalol Hydrochloride (Concurrent use is not recommended; consult your doctor). Products include:
Normodyne Injection 2377
Normodyne Tablets 2379
Trandate 1185

Lisinopril (Concurrent use is not recommended; consult your doctor). Products include:
Prinivil Tablets 1733
Prinzide Tablets 1737
Zestoretic 2850
Zestril Tablets 2854

Losartan Potassium (Concurrent use is not recommended; consult your doctor). Products include:
Cozaar Tablets 1628
Hyzaar Tablets 1677

Maprotiline Hydrochloride (Concurrent use is not recommended; consult your doctor). Products include:
Ludiomil Tablets 843

Mecamylamine Hydrochloride (Concurrent use is not recommended; consult your doctor). Products include:
Inversine Tablets 1686

Methyclothiazide (Concurrent use is not recommended; consult your doctor). Products include:
Enduron Tablets 420

Methyldopa (Concurrent use is not recommended; consult your doctor). Products include:
Aldoclor Tablets 1598
Aldomet Oral 1600
Aldoril Tablets 1604

Methyldopate Hydrochloride (Concurrent use is not recommended; consult your doctor). Products include:
Aldomet Ester HCl Injection 1602

Metolazone (Concurrent use is not recommended; consult your doctor). Products include:
Mykrox Tablets 993
Zaroxolyn Tablets 1000

Metoprolol Succinate (Concurrent use is not recommended; consult your doctor). Products include:
Toprol-XL Tablets 565

Metoprolol Tartrate (Concurrent use is not recommended; consult your doctor). Products include:
Lopressor Ampuls 830
Lopressor HCT Tablets 832
Lopressor Tablets 830

Metyrosine (Concurrent use is not recommended; consult your doctor). Products include:
Demser Capsules 1649

Minoxidil (Concurrent use is not recommended; consult your doctor). Products include:
Loniten Tablets 2618
Rogaine Topical Solution 2637

Moexipril Hydrochloride (Concurrent use is not recommended; consult your doctor). Products include:
Univasc Tablets 2410

Nadolol (Concurrent use is not recommended; consult your doctor).
No products indexed under this heading.

IMPORTANT NOTE: Always consult each drug listing in the patient's regimen for possible interactions.

Nefazodone Hydrochloride (Concurrent use is not recommended; consult your doctor). Products include:
Serzone Tablets 771

Nicardipine Hydrochloride (Concurrent use is not recommended; consult your doctor). Products include:
Cardene Capsules 2095
Cardene I.V. 2709
Cardene SR Capsules 2097

Nifedipine (Concurrent use is not recommended; consult your doctor). Products include:
Adalat Capsules (10 mg and 20 mg) 587
Adalat CC 589
Procardia Capsules 1971
Procardia XL Extended Release Tablets 1972

Nisoldipine (Concurrent use is not recommended; consult your doctor).
No products indexed under this heading.

Nitroglycerin (Concurrent use is not recommended; consult your doctor). Products include:
Deponit NTG Transdermal Delivery System 2397
Nitro-Bid IV 1523
Nitro-Bid Ointment 1524
Nitrodisc 2047
Nitro-Dur (nitroglycerin) Transdermal Infusion System 1326
Nitrolingual Spray 2027
Nitrostat Tablets 1925
Transderm-Nitro Transdermal Therapeutic System 859

Nortriptyline Hydrochloride (Concurrent use is not recommended; consult your doctor). Products include:
Pamelor 2280

Paroxetine Hydrochloride (Concurrent use is not recommended; consult your doctor). Products include:
Paxil Tablets 2505

Penbutolol Sulfate (Concurrent use is not recommended; consult your doctor). Products include:
Levatol 2403

Phenelzine Sulfate (Concurrent use is not recommended; consult your doctor). Products include:
Nardil 1920

Phenoxybenzamine Hydrochloride (Concurrent use is not recommended; consult your doctor). Products include:
Dibenzyline Capsules 2476

Phentolamine Mesylate (Concurrent use is not recommended; consult your doctor). Products include:
Regitine 846

Pindolol (Concurrent use is not recommended; consult your doctor). Products include:
Visken Tablets 2299

Polythiazide (Concurrent use is not recommended; consult your doctor). Products include:
Minizide Capsules 1938

Prazosin Hydrochloride (Concurrent use is not recommended; consult your doctor). Products include:
Minipress Capsules 1937
Minizide Capsules 1938

Propranolol Hydrochloride (Concurrent use is not recommended; consult your doctor). Products include:
Inderal 2728
Inderal LA Long Acting Capsules 2730
Inderide Tablets 2732
Inderide LA Long Acting Capsules 2734

Protriptyline Hydrochloride (Concurrent use is not recommended; consult your doctor). Products include:
Vivactil Tablets 1774

Quinapril Hydrochloride (Concurrent use is not recommended; consult your doctor). Products include:
Accupril Tablets 1893

Ramipril (Concurrent use is not recommended; consult your doctor). Products include:
Altace Capsules 1232

Rauwolfia Serpentina (Concurrent use is not recommended; consult your doctor).
No products indexed under this heading.

Rescinnamine (Concurrent use is not recommended; consult your doctor).
No products indexed under this heading.

Reserpine (Concurrent use is not recommended; consult your doctor). Products include:
Diupres Tablets 1650
Hydropres Tablets 1675
Ser-Ap-Es Tablets 849

Sertraline Hydrochloride (Concurrent use is not recommended; consult your doctor). Products include:
Zoloft Tablets 2217

Sodium Nitroprusside (Concurrent use is not recommended; consult your doctor).
No products indexed under this heading.

Sotalol Hydrochloride (Concurrent use is not recommended; consult your doctor). Products include:
Betapace Tablets 641

Spirapril Hydrochloride (Concurrent use is not recommended; consult your doctor).
No products indexed under this heading.

Terazosin Hydrochloride (Concurrent use is not recommended; consult your doctor). Products include:
Hytrin Capsules 430

Timolol Maleate (Concurrent use is not recommended; consult your doctor). Products include:
Blocadren Tablets 1614
Timolide Tablets 1748
Timoptic in Ocudose 1753
Timoptic Sterile Ophthalmic Solution 1751
Timoptic-XE 1755

Torsemide (Concurrent use is not recommended; consult your doctor). Products include:
Demadex Tablets and Injection 686

Tranylcypromine Sulfate (Concurrent use is not recommended; consult your doctor). Products include:
Parnate Tablets 2503

Trazodone Hydrochloride (Concurrent use is not recommended; consult your doctor). Products include:
Desyrel and Desyrel Dividose 503

Trimethaphan Camsylate (Concurrent use is not recommended; consult your doctor). Products include:
Arfonad Ampuls 2080

Trimipramine Maleate (Concurrent use is not recommended; consult your doctor). Products include:
Surmontil Capsules 2811

Venlafaxine Hydrochloride (Concurrent use is not recommended; consult your doctor). Products include:
Effexor 2719

Verapamil Hydrochloride (Concurrent use is not recommended; consult your doctor). Products include:
Calan SR Caplets 2422
Calan Tablets 2419
Isoptin Injectable 1344
Isoptin Oral Tablets 1346
Isoptin SR Tablets 1348
Verelan Capsules 1410
Verelan Capsules 2824

EFUDEX CREAM
(Fluorouracil) 2113
None cited in PDR database.

EFUDEX SOLUTIONS
(Fluorouracil) 2113
None cited in PDR database.

ELASE OINTMENT
(Desoxyribonuclease, Fibrinolysin) 1039
None cited in PDR database.

ELASE VIALS
(Fibrinolysin, Desoxyribonuclease) 1038
None cited in PDR database.

ELASE-CHLOROMYCETIN OINTMENT
(Fibrinolysin, Desoxyribonuclease, Chloramphenicol) 1040
None cited in PDR database.

ELAVIL INJECTION
(Amitriptyline Hydrochloride) 2838
May interact with barbiturates, central nervous system depressants, anticholinergics, antipsychotic agents, sympathomimetics, monoamine oxidase inhibitors, thyroid preparations, drugs that inhibit cytochrome p450iid6, antidepressant drugs, phenothiazines, selective serotonin reuptake inhibitors, and certain other agents. Compounds in these categories include:

Albuterol (Effects of concurrent use not specified; careful adjustment of dosage and close supervision are required). Products include:
Proventil Inhalation Aerosol 2382
Ventolin Inhalation Aerosol and Refill 1197

Albuterol Sulfate (Effects of concurrent use not specified; careful adjustment of dosage and close supervision are required). Products include:
Airet Solution for Inhalation 452
Proventil Inhalation Solution 0.083% 2384
Proventil Repetabs Tablets 2386
Proventil Solution for Inhalation 0.5% 2383
Proventil Syrup 2385
Proventil Tablets 2386
Ventolin Inhalation Solution 1198
Ventolin Nebules Inhalation Solution 1199
Ventolin Rotacaps for Inhalation 1200
Ventolin Syrup 1202
Ventolin Tablets 1203
Volmax Extended-Release Tablets .. 1788

Alfentanil Hydrochloride (Amitriptyline may enhance the response to CNS depressants). Products include:
Alfenta Injection 1286

Alprazolam (Amitriptyline may enhance the response to CNS depressants). Products include:
Xanax Tablets 2649

Amoxapine (Concurrent use with drugs that are substrate for cytochrome $P_{450}IID_6$ may make normal metabolizer resemble poor metabolizer leading to higher than expected plasma concentrations of TCA with resultant toxicity). Products include:
Asendin Tablets 1369

Aprobarbital (Amitriptyline may enhance the response to barbiturates).
No products indexed under this heading.

Atropine Sulfate (Concurrent use may result in hyperpyrexia, particularly in hot weather; potential for paralytic ileus). Products include:
Arco-Lase Plus Tablets 512
Atrohist Plus Tablets 454
Atropine Sulfate Sterile Ophthalmic Solution .... ◉ 233
Donnatal 2060
Donnatal Extentabs 2061
Donnatal Tablets 2060
Lomotil 2439
Motofen Tablets 784
Urised Tablets 1964

Belladonna Alkaloids (Concurrent use may result in hyperpyrexia, particularly in hot weather; potential for paralytic ileus). Products include:
Bellergal-S Tablets 2250
Hyland's Bed Wetting Tablets .... ▣ 828
Hyland's EnurAid Tablets .... ▣ 829
Hyland's Teething Tablets .... ▣ 830

Benztropine Mesylate (Concurrent use may result in hyperpyrexia, particularly in hot weather; potential for paralytic ileus). Products include:
Cogentin 1621

Biperiden Hydrochloride (Concurrent use may result in hyperpyrexia, particularly in hot weather; potential for paralytic ileus). Products include:
Akineton 1333

Buprenorphine (Amitriptyline may enhance the response to CNS depressants). Products include:
Buprenex Injectable 2006

Bupropion Hydrochloride (Concurrent use with drugs that are substrate for cytochrome $P_{450}IID_6$ may make normal metabolizer resemble poor metabolizer leading to higher than expected plasma concentrations of TCA with resultant toxicity). Products include:
Wellbutrin Tablets 1204

Buspirone Hydrochloride (Amitriptyline may enhance the response to CNS depressants). Products include:
BuSpar 737

Butabarbital (Amitriptyline may enhance the response to barbiturates).
No products indexed under this heading.

Butalbital (Amitriptyline may enhance the response to barbiturates). Products include:
Esgic-plus Tablets 1013
Fioricet Tablets 2258
Fioricet with Codeine Capsules 2260
Fiorinal Capsules 2261
Fiorinal with Codeine Capsules 2262
Fiorinal Tablets 2261
Phrenilin 785
Sedapap Tablets 50 mg/650 mg .. 1543

Chlordiazepoxide (Amitriptyline may enhance the response to CNS depressants). Products include:
Libritabs Tablets 2177
Limbitrol 2180

Chlordiazepoxide Hydrochloride (Amitriptyline may enhance the response to CNS depressants). Products include:
Librax Capsules 2176

(▣ Described in PDR For Nonprescription Drugs) (◉ Described in PDR For Ophthalmology)

Librium Capsules 2178
Librium Injectable 2179

Chlorpromazine (Concurrent use with drugs that are substrate for cytochrome $P_{450}IID_6$ may make normal metabolizer resemble poor metabolizer leading to higher than expected plasma concentrations of TCA with resultant toxicity; concurrent use with neuroleptics may result in hyperpyrexia, particularly in hot weather). Products include:

Thorazine Suppositories 2523

Chlorpromazine Hydrochloride (Concurrent use with drugs that are substrate for cytochrome $P_{450}IID_6$ may make normal metabolizer resemble poor metabolizer leading to higher than expected plasma concentrations of TCA with resultant toxicity; concurrent use with neuroleptics may result in hyperpyrexia, particularly in hot weather). Products include:

Thorazine 2523

Chlorprothixene (Concurrent use with neuroleptics may result in hyperpyrexia, particularly in hot weather).

No products indexed under this heading.

Chlorprothixene Hydrochloride (Concurrent use with neuroleptics may result in hyperpyrexia, particularly in hot weather).

No products indexed under this heading.

Cimetidine (Reduces the hepatic metabolism of certain tricylic antidepressants, thereby delaying elimination and increasing steady-state concentrations resulting in frequency and severity of side effects, particularly anticholinergic). Products include:

Tagamet Tablets 2516

Cimetidine Hydrochloride (Reduces the hepatic metabolism of certain tricylic antidepressants, thereby delaying elimination and increasing steady-state concentrations resulting in frequency and severity of side effects, particularly anticholinergic). Products include:

Tagamet 2516

Clidinium Bromide (Concurrent use may result in hyperpyrexia, particularly in hot weather; potential for paralytic ileus). Products include:

Librax Capsules 2176
Quarzan Capsules 2181

Clonidine (Amitriptyline may block the antihypertensive effect). Products include:

Catapres-TTS 675

Clonidine Hydrochloride (Amitriptyline may block the antihypertensive effect). Products include:

Catapres Tablets 674
Combipres Tablets 677

Clorazepate Dipotassium (Amitriptyline may enhance the response to CNS depressants). Products include:

Tranxene 451

Clozapine (Concurrent use with neuroleptics may result in hyperpyrexia, particularly in hot weather). Products include:

Clozaril Tablets 2252

Codeine Phosphate (Amitriptyline may enhance the response to CNS depressants). Products include:

Actifed with Codeine Cough Syrup.. 1067
Brontex 1981
Deconsal C Expectorant Syrup 456
Deconsal Pediatric Syrup 457
Dimetane-DC Cough Syrup 2059

Empirin with Codeine Tablets........... 1093
Fioricet with Codeine Capsules 2260
Fiorinal with Codeine Capsules 2262
Isoclor Expectorant 990
Novahistine DH 2462
Novahistine Expectorant...................... 2463
Nucofed 2051
Phenergan with Codeine 2777
Phenergan VC with Codeine 2781
Robitussin A-C Syrup 2073
Robitussin-DAC Syrup 2074
Ryna .... ◙ 841
Soma Compound w/Codeine Tablets 2676
Tussi-Organidin NR Liquid and S NR Liquid 2677
Tylenol with Codeine 1583

Desflurane (Amitriptyline may enhance the response to CNS depressants). Products include:

Suprane 1813

Desipramine Hydrochloride (Concurrent use with drugs that are substrate for cytochrome $P_{450}IID_6$ may make normal metabolizer resemble poor metabolizer leading to higher than expected plasma concentrations of TCA with resultant toxicity). Products include:

Norpramin Tablets 1526

Dezocine (Amitriptyline may enhance the response to CNS depressants). Products include:

Dalgan Injection 538

Diazepam (Amitriptyline may enhance the response to CNS depressants). Products include:

Dizac 1809
Valium Injectable 2182
Valium Tablets 2183
Valrelease Capsules 2169

Dicyclomine Hydrochloride (Concurrent use may result in hyperpyrexia, particularly in hot weather; potential for paralytic ileus). Products include:

Bentyl 1501

Disulfiram (Concurrent administration may produce delirium). Products include:

Antabuse Tablets 2695

Dobutamine Hydrochloride (Effects of concurrent use not specified; careful adjustment of dosage and close supervision are required). Products include:

Dobutrex Solution Vials 1439

Dopamine Hydrochloride (Effects of concurrent use not specified; careful adjustment of dosage and close supervision are required).

No products indexed under this heading.

Doxepin Hydrochloride (Concurrent use with drugs that are substrate for cytochrome $P_{450}IID_6$ may make normal metabolizer resemble poor metabolizer leading to higher than expected plasma concentrations of TCA with resultant toxicity). Products include:

Sinequan 2205
Zonalon Cream 1055

Droperidol (Amitriptyline may enhance the response to CNS depressants). Products include:

Inapsine Injection 1296

Enflurane (Amitriptyline may enhance the response to CNS depressants).

No products indexed under this heading.

Ephedrine Hydrochloride (Effects of concurrent use not specified; careful adjustment of dosage and close supervision are required). Products include:

Primatene Dual Action Formula ...... ◙ 872
Primatene Tablets .... ◙ 873
Quadrinal Tablets 1350

Ephedrine Sulfate (Effects of concurrent use not specified; careful adjustment of dosage and close supervision are required). Products include:

Bronkaid Caplets .... ◙ 717
Marax Tablets & DF Syrup................... 2200

Ephedrine Tannate (Effects of concurrent use not specified; careful adjustment of dosage and close supervision are required). Products include:

Rynatuss 2673

Epinephrine (Effects of concurrent use of epinephrine (combined with local anesthetics) not specified; careful adjustment of dosage and close supervision are required). Products include:

Bronkaid Mist .... ◙ 717
EPIFRIN .... © 239
EpiPen 790
Marcaine Hydrochloride with Epinephrine 1:200,000 2316
Primatene Mist .... ◙ 873
Sensorcaine with Epinephrine Injection 559
Sus-Phrine Injection 1019
Xylocaine with Epinephrine Injections 567

Epinephrine Bitartrate (Effects of concurrent use of epinephrine (combined with local anesthetics) not specified; careful adjustment of dosage and close supervision are required). Products include:

Bronkaid Mist Suspension .... ◙ 718
Sensorcaine-MPF with Epinephrine Injection 559

Epinephrine Hydrochloride (Effects of concurrent use of epinephrine (combined with local anesthetics) not specified; careful adjustment of dosage and close supervision are required). Products include:

Ana-Kit Anaphylaxis Emergency Treatment Kit 617

Estazolam (Amitriptyline may enhance the response to CNS depressants). Products include:

ProSom Tablets 449

Ethchlorvynol (Concurrent use of high dose of ethchlorvynol may produce transient delirium). Products include:

Placidyl Capsules 448

Ethinamate (Amitriptyline may enhance the response to CNS depressants).

No products indexed under this heading.

Fentanyl (Amitriptyline may enhance the response to CNS depressants). Products include:

Duragesic Transdermal System....... 1288

Fentanyl Citrate (Amitriptyline may enhance the response to CNS depressants). Products include:

Sublimaze Injection 1307

Flecainide Acetate (Concurrent use with drugs that are substrate for cytochrome $P_{450}IID_6$ may make normal metabolizer resemble poor metabolizer leading to higher than expected plasma concentrations of TCA with resultant toxicity). Products include:

Tambocor Tablets 1497

Fluoxetine Hydrochloride (Concurrent use with drugs that are substrate for cytochrome $P_{450}IID_6$ may make normal metabolizer resemble poor metabolizer leading to higher than expected plasma concentrations of TCA with resultant toxicity; due to variation in the extent of inhibition of $P_{450}IID_6$ and long half-life of the parent (fluoxetine) and active metabolite sufficient time should/must elapse, at least 5 weeks before switching to TCA). Products include:

Prozac Pulvules & Liquid, Oral Solution 919

Fluphenazine Decanoate (Concurrent use with drugs that are substrate for cytochrome $P_{450}IID_6$ may make normal metabolizer resemble poor metabolizer leading to higher than expected plasma concentrations of TCA with resultant toxicity; concurrent use with neuroleptics may result in hyperpyrexia, particularly in hot weather). Products include:

Prolixin Decanoate 509

Fluphenazine Enanthate (Concurrent use with drugs that are substrate for cytochrome $P_{450}IID_6$ may make normal metabolizer resemble poor metabolizer leading to higher than expected plasma concentrations of TCA with resultant toxicity; concurrent use with neuroleptics may result in hyperpyrexia, particularly in hot weather). Products include:

Prolixin Enanthate 509

Fluphenazine Hydrochloride (Concurrent use with drugs that are substrate for cytochrome $P_{450}IID_6$ may make normal metabolizer resemble poor metabolizer leading to higher than expected plasma concentrations of TCA with resultant toxicity; concurrent use with neuroleptics may result in hyperpyrexia, particularly in hot weather). Products include:

Prolixin 509

Flurazepam Hydrochloride (Amitriptyline may enhance the response to CNS depressants). Products include:

Dalmane Capsules 2173

Fluvoxamine Maleate (Concurrent use with drugs that are substrate for cytochrome $P_{450}IID_6$ may make normal metabolizer resemble poor metabolizer leading to higher than expected plasma concentrations of TCA with resultant toxicity; due to variation in the extent of inhibition of $P_{450}IID_6$ and long half-life of the parent (fluoxetine) and active metabolite sufficient time must elapse, at least 5 weeks before switching to TCA). Products include:

Luvox Tablets 2544

Furazolidone (Potential for hyperpyretic crises, severe convulsions, and deaths; concurrent and/or sequential use is contraindicated). Products include:

Furoxone 2046

Glutethimide (Amitriptyline may enhance the response to CNS depressants).

No products indexed under this heading.

Glycopyrrolate (Concurrent use may result in hyperpyrexia, particularly in hot weather; potential for paralytic ileus). Products include:

Robinul Forte Tablets 2072
Robinul Injectable 2072
Robinul Tablets 2072

IMPORTANT NOTE: Always consult each drug listing in the patient's regimen for possible interactions.

Guanadrel Sulfate (Amitriptyline may block the antihypertensive effect). Products include:

- Hylorel Tablets ... 985

Guanethidine Monosulfate (Amitriptyline may block the antihypertensive effect of guanethidine or similarly acting compounds). Products include:

- Esimil Tablets ... 822
- Ismelin Tablets ... 827

Haloperidol (Concurrent use with neuroleptics may result in hyperpyrexia, particularly in hot weather). Products include:

- Haldol Injection, Tablets and Concentrate ... 1575

Haloperidol Decanoate (Concurrent use with neuroleptics may result in hyperpyrexia, particularly in hot weather). Products include:

- Haldol Decanoate ... 1577

Hydrocodone Bitartrate (Amitriptyline may enhance the response to CNS depressants). Products include:

- Anexsia 5/500 Elixir ... 1781
- Anexia Tablets ... 1782
- Codiclear DH Syrup ... 791
- Deconamine CX Cough and Cold Liquid and Tablets ... 1319
- Duratuss HD Elixir ... 2565
- Hycodan Tablets and Syrup ... 930
- Hycomine Compound Tablets ... 932
- Hycomine ... 931
- Hycotuss Expectorant Syrup ... 933
- Hydrocet Capsules ... 782
- Lorcet 10/650 ... 1018
- Lortab ... 2566
- Tussend ... 1783
- Tussend Expectorant ... 1785
- Vicodin Tablets ... 1356
- Vicodin ES Tablets ... 1357
- Vicodin Tuss Expectorant ... 1358
- Zydone Capsules ... 949

Hydrocodone Polistirex (Amitriptyline may enhance the response to CNS depressants). Products include:

- Tussionex Pennkinetic Extended-Release Suspension ... 998

Hydroxyzine Hydrochloride (Amitriptyline may enhance the response to CNS depressants). Products include:

- Atarax Tablets & Syrup ... 2185
- Marax Tablets & DF Syrup ... 2200
- Vistaril Intramuscular Solution ... 2216

Hyoscyamine (Concurrent use may result in hyperpyrexia, particularly in hot weather; potential for paralytic ileus). Products include:

- Cystospaz Tablets ... 1963
- Urised Tablets ... 1964

Hyoscyamine Sulfate (Concurrent use may result in hyperpyrexia, particularly in hot weather; potential for paralytic ileus). Products include:

- Arco-Lase Plus Tablets ... 512
- Atrohist Plus Tablets ... 454
- Cystospaz-M Capsules ... 1963
- Donnatal ... 2060
- Donnatal Extentabs ... 2061
- Donnatal Tablets ... 2060
- Kutrase Capsules ... 2402
- Levsin/Levsinex/Levbid ... 2405

Imipramine Hydrochloride (Concurrent use with drugs that are substrate for cytochrome $P_{450}IID_6$ may make normal metabolizer resemble poor metabolizer leading to higher than expected plasma concentrations of TCA with resultant toxicity). Products include:

- Tofranil Ampuls ... 854
- Tofranil Tablets ... 856

Imipramine Pamoate (Concurrent use with drugs that are substrate for cytochrome $P_{450}IID_6$ may make normal metabolizer resemble poor metabolizer leading to higher than expected plasma concentrations of TCA with resultant toxicity). Products include:

- Tofranil-PM Capsules ... 857

Ipratropium Bromide (Concurrent use may result in hyperpyrexia, particularly in hot weather; potential for paralytic ileus). Products include:

- Atrovent Inhalation Aerosol ... 671
- Atrovent Inhalation Solution ... 673

Isocarboxazid (Potential for hyperpyretic crises, severe convulsions, and deaths; concurrent and/or sequential use is contraindicated).

- No products indexed under this heading.

Isoflurane (Amitriptyline may enhance the response to CNS depressants).

- No products indexed under this heading.

Isoproterenol Hydrochloride (Effects of concurrent use not specified; careful adjustment of dosage and close supervision are required). Products include:

- Isuprel Hydrochloride Injection 1:5000 ... 2311
- Isuprel Hydrochloride Solution 1:200 & 1:100 ... 2313
- Isuprel Mistometer ... 2312

Isoproterenol Sulfate (Effects of concurrent use not specified; careful adjustment of dosage and close supervision are required). Products include:

- Norisodrine with Calcium Iodide Syrup ... 442

Ketamine Hydrochloride (Amitriptyline may enhance the response to CNS depressants).

- No products indexed under this heading.

Levomethadyl Acetate Hydrochloride (Amitriptyline may enhance the response to CNS depressants). Products include:

- Orlamm ... 2239

Levorphanol Tartrate (Amitriptyline may enhance the response to CNS depressants). Products include:

- Levo-Dromoran ... 2129

Levothyroxine Sodium (On rare occasions, co-administration may produce arrhythmias). Products include:

- Levothroid Tablets ... 1016
- Levoxyl Tablets ... 903
- Synthroid ... 1359

Liothyronine Sodium (On rare occasions, co-administration may produce arrhythmias). Products include:

- Cytomel Tablets ... 2473
- Triostat Injection ... 2530

Liotrix (On rare occasions, co-administration may produce arrhythmias).

- No products indexed under this heading.

Lorazepam (Amitriptyline may enhance the response to CNS depressants). Products include:

- Ativan Injection ... 2698
- Ativan Tablets ... 2700

Loxapine Hydrochloride (Concurrent use with neuroleptics may result in hyperpyrexia, particularly in hot weather). Products include:

- Loxitane ... 1378

Loxapine Succinate (Concurrent use with neuroleptics may result in hyperpyrexia, particularly in hot weather). Products include:

- Loxitane Capsules ... 1378

Maprotiline Hydrochloride (Concurrent use with drugs that are substrate for cytochrome $P_{450}IID_6$ may make normal metabolizer resemble poor metabolizer leading to higher than expected plasma concentrations of TCA with resultant toxicity). Products include:

- Ludiomil Tablets ... 843

Mepenzolate Bromide (Concurrent use may result in hyperpyrexia, particularly in hot weather; potential for paralytic ileus).

- No products indexed under this heading.

Meperidine Hydrochloride (Amitriptyline may enhance the response to CNS depressants). Products include:

- Demerol ... 2308
- Mepergan Injection ... 2753

Mephobarbital (Amitriptyline may enhance the response to barbiturates). Products include:

- Mebaral Tablets ... 2322

Meprobamate (Amitriptyline may enhance the response to CNS depressants). Products include:

- Miltown Tablets ... 2672
- PMB 200 and PMB 400 ... 2783

Mesoridazine (Amitriptyline may enhance the response to CNS depressants).

Mesoridazine Besylate (Concurrent use with drugs that are substrate for cytochrome $P_{450}IID_6$ may make normal metabolizer resemble poor metabolizer leading to higher than expected plasma concentrations of TCA with resultant toxicity; concurrent use with neuroleptics may result in hyperpyrexia, particularly in hot weather). Products include:

- Serentil ... 684

Metaproterenol Sulfate (Effects of concurrent use not specified; careful adjustment of dosage and close supervision are required). Products include:

- Alupent ... 669
- Metaproterenol Sulfate Inhalation Solution, USP, Arm-a-Med ... 552

Metaraminol Bitartrate (Effects of concurrent use not specified; careful adjustment of dosage and close supervision are required). Products include:

- Aramine Injection ... 1609

Methadone Hydrochloride (Amitriptyline may enhance the response to CNS depressants). Products include:

- Methadone Hydrochloride Oral Concentrate ... 2233
- Methadone Hydrochloride Oral Solution & Tablets ... 2235

Methohexital Sodium (Amitriptyline may enhance the response to CNS depressants). Products include:

- Brevital Sodium Vials ... 1429

Methotrimeprazine (Concurrent use with drugs that are substrate for cytochrome $P_{450}IID_6$ may make normal metabolizer resemble poor metabolizer leading to higher than expected plasma concentrations of TCA with resultant toxicity; concurrent use with neuroleptics may result in hyperpyrexia, particularly in hot weather). Products include:

- Levoprome ... 1274

Methoxamine Hydrochloride (Effects of concurrent use not specified; careful adjustment of dosage and close supervision are required). Products include:

- Vasoxyl Injection ... 1196

Methoxyflurane (Amitriptyline may enhance the response to CNS depressants).

- No products indexed under this heading.

Midazolam Hydrochloride (Amitriptyline may enhance the response to CNS depressants). Products include:

- Versed Injection ... 2170

Molindone Hydrochloride (Concurrent use with neuroleptics may result in hyperpyrexia, particularly in hot weather). Products include:

- Moban Tablets and Concentrate ... 1048

Morphine Sulfate (Amitriptyline may enhance the response to CNS depressants). Products include:

- Astramorph/PF Injection, USP (Preservative-Free) ... 535
- Duramorph ... 962
- Infumorph 200 and Infumorph 500 Sterile Solutions ... 965
- MS Contin Tablets ... 1994
- MSIR ... 1997
- Oramorph SR (Morphine Sulfate Sustained Release Tablets) ... 2236
- RMS Suppositories ... 2657
- Roxanol ... 2243

Nefazodone Hydrochloride (Concurrent use with drugs that are substrate for cytochrome $P_{450}IID_6$ may make normal metabolizer resemble poor metabolizer leading to higher than expected plasma concentrations of TCA with resultant toxicity). Products include:

- Serzone Tablets ... 771

Norepinephrine Bitartrate (Effects of concurrent use not specified; careful adjustment of dosage and close supervision are required). Products include:

- Levophed Bitartrate Injection ... 2315

Nortriptyline Hydrochloride (Concurrent use with drugs that are substrate for cytochrome $P_{450}IID_6$ may make normal metabolizer resemble poor metabolizer leading to higher than expected plasma concentrations of TCA with resultant toxicity). Products include:

- Pamelor ... 2280

Opium Alkaloids (Amitriptyline may enhance the response to CNS depressants).

- No products indexed under this heading.

Oxazepam (Amitriptyline may enhance the response to CNS depressants). Products include:

- Serax Capsules ... 2810
- Serax Tablets ... 2810

Oxybutynin Chloride (Concurrent use may result in hyperpyrexia, particularly in hot weather; potential for paralytic ileus). Products include:

- Ditropan ... 1516

Oxycodone Hydrochloride (Amitriptyline may enhance the response to CNS depressants). Products include:

- Percocet Tablets ... 938
- Percodan Tablets ... 939
- Percodan-Demi Tablets ... 940
- Roxicodone Tablets, Oral Solution & Intensol (Oxycodone) ... 2244
- Tylox Capsules ... 1584

Paroxetine Hydrochloride (Concurrent use with drugs that are substrate for cytochrome $P_{450}IID_6$ may make normal metabolizer resemble poor metabolizer leading to higher than expected plasma concentrations of TCA with resultant toxicity; due to variation in the extent of inhibition of $P_{450}IID_6$ caution is indicated, if coadministered sufficient time should/must elapse). Products include:

Paxil Tablets 2505

Pentobarbital Sodium (Amitriptyline may enhance the response to barbiturates). Products include:

Nembutal Sodium Capsules 436
Nembutal Sodium Solution 438
Nembutal Sodium Suppositories....... 440

Perphenazine (Concurrent use with drugs that are substrate for cytochrome $P_{450}IID_6$ may make normal metabolizer resemble poor metabolizer leading to higher than expected plasma concentrations of TCA with resultant toxicity; concurrent use with neuroleptics may result in hyperpyrexia, particularly in hot weather). Products include:

Etrafon 2355
Triavil Tablets 1757
Trilafon 2389

Phenelzine Sulfate (Potential for hyperpyretic crises, severe convulsions, and deaths; concurrent and/or sequential use is contraindicated). Products include:

Nardil 1920

Phenobarbital (Amitriptyline may enhance the response to barbiturates). Products include:

Arco-Lase Plus Tablets 512
Bellergal-S Tablets 2250
Donnatal 2060
Donnatal Extentabs............................. 2061
Donnatal Tablets 2060
Phenobarbital Elixir and Tablets....... 1469
Quadrinal Tablets 1350

Phenylephrine Bitartrate (Effects of concurrent use not specified; careful adjustment of dosage and close supervision are required).

No products indexed under this heading.

Phenylephrine Hydrochloride (Effects of concurrent use not specified; careful adjustment of dosage and close supervision are required). Products include:

Atrohist Plus Tablets 454
Cerose DM .... ⊞ 878
Comhist 2038
D.A. Chewable Tablets........................ 951
Deconsal Pediatric Capsules............... 454
Dura-Vent/DA Tablets 953
Entex Capsules 1986
Entex Liquid 1986
Extendryl 1005
4-Way Fast Acting Nasal Spray (regular & mentholated) .... ⊞ 621
Hemorid For Women .... ⊞ 834
Hycomine Compound Tablets 932
Neo-Synephrine Hydrochloride 1% Carpuject... 2324
Neo-Synephrine Hydrochloride 1% Injection 2324
Neo-Synephrine Hydrochloride (Ophthalmic) 2325
Neo-Synephrine .... ⊞ 726
Nōstril .... ⊞ 644
Novahistine Elixir .... ⊞ 823
Phenergan VC 2779
Phenergan VC with Codeine 2781
Preparation H .... ⊞ 871
Tympagesic Ear Drops 2342
Vasosulf .... ⓒ 271
Vicks Sinex Nasal Spray and Ultra Fine Mist .... ⊞ 765

Phenylephrine Tannate (Effects of concurrent use not specified; careful adjustment of dosage and close supervision are required). Products include:

Atrohist Pediatric Suspension 454
Ricobid-D Pediatric Suspension........ 2038
Ricobid Tablets and Pediatric Suspension... 2038
Rynatan 2673
Rynatuss 2673

Phenylpropanolamine Hydrochloride (Effects of concurrent use not specified; careful adjustment of dosage and close supervision are required). Products include:

Acutrim .... ⊞ 628
Allerest Children's Chewable Tablets .... ⊞ 627
Allerest 12 Hour Caplets .... ⊞ 627
Atrohist Plus Tablets 454
BC Cold Powder Multi-Symptom Formula (Cold-Sinus-Allergy) ...... ⊞ 609
BC Cold Powder Non-Drowsy Formula (Cold-Sinus) .... ⊞ 609
Cheracol Plus Head Cold/Cough Formula .... ⊞ 769
Comtrex Multi-Symptom Non-Drowsy Liqui-gels............................... ⊞ 618
Contac Continuous Action Nasal Decongestant/Antihistamine 12 Hour Capsules...................................... ⊞ 813
Contac Maximum Strength Continuous Action Decongestant/Antihistamine 12 Hour Caplets.. ⊞ 813
Contac Severe Cold and Flu Formula Caplets .... ⊞ 814
Coricidin 'D' Decongestant Tablets .... ⊞ 800
Dexatrim .... ⊞ 832
Dexatrim Plus Vitamins Caplets .... ⊞ 832
Dimetane-DC Cough Syrup 2059
Dimetapp Elixir .... ⊞ 773
Dimetapp Extentabs........................... ⊞ 774
Dimetapp Tablets/Liqui-Gels .... ⊞ 775
Dimetapp Cold & Allergy Chewable Tablets .... ⊞ 773
Dimetapp DM Elixir........................... ⊞ 774
Dura-Vent Tablets 952
Entex Capsules 1986
Entex LA Tablets 1987
Entex Liquid 1986
Exgest LA Tablets................................ 782
Hycomine 931
Isoclor Timesule Capsules .... ⊞ 637
Nolamine Timed-Release Tablets 785
Ornade Spansule Capsules 2502
Propagest Tablets 786
Pyrroxate Caplets .... ⊞ 772
Robitussin-CF .... ⊞ 777
Sinulin Tablets..................................... 787
Tavist-D 12 Hour Relief Tablets .... ⊞ 787
Teldrin 12 Hour Antihistamine/Nasal Decongestant Allergy Relief Capsules .... ⊞ 826
Triaminic Allergy Tablets .... ⊞ 789
Triaminic Cold Tablets .... ⊞ 790
Triaminic Expectorant .... ⊞ 790
Triaminic Syrup .... ⊞ 792
Triaminic-12 Tablets........................... ⊞ 792
Triaminic-DM Syrup .... ⊞ 792
Triaminicin Tablets............................. ⊞ 793
Triaminicol Multi-Symptom Cold Tablets .... ⊞ 793
Triaminicol Multi-Symptom Relief ⊞ 794
Vicks DayQuil Allergy Relief 12-Hour Extended Release Tablets.. ⊞ 760
Vicks DayQuil Allergy Relief 4-Hour Tablets .... ⊞ 760
Vicks DayQuil SINUS Pressure & CONGESTION Relief.......................... ⊞ 761

Pimozide (Concurrent use with neuroleptics may result in hyperpyrexia, particularly in hot weather). Products include:

Orap Tablets 1050

Pirbuterol Acetate (Effects of concurrent use not specified; careful adjustment of dosage and close supervision are required). Products include:

Maxair Autohaler 1492
Maxair Inhaler 1494

Prazepam (Amitriptyline may enhance the response to CNS depressants).

No products indexed under this heading.

Prochlorperazine (Concurrent use with drugs that are substrate for cytochrome $P_{450}IID_6$ may make normal metabolizer resemble poor metabolizer leading to higher than expected plasma concentrations of TCA with resultant toxicity; concurrent use with neuroleptics may result in hyperpyrexia, particularly in hot weather). Products include:

Compazine 2470

Procyclidine Hydrochloride (Concurrent use may result in hyperpyrexia, particularly in hot weather; potential for paralytic ileus). Products include:

Kemadrin Tablets 1112

Promethazine Hydrochloride (Concurrent use with drugs that are substrate for cytochrome $P_{450}IID_6$ may make normal metabolizer resemble poor metabolizer leading to higher than expected plasma concentrations of TCA with resultant toxicity; concurrent use with neuroleptics may result in hyperpyrexia, particularly in hot weather). Products include:

Mepergan Injection 2753
Phenergan with Codeine..................... 2777
Phenergan with Dextromethorphan 2778
Phenergan Injection 2773
Phenergan Suppositories 2775
Phenergan Syrup 2774
Phenergan Tablets 2775
Phenergan VC 2779
Phenergan VC with Codeine 2781

Propafenone Hydrochloride (Concurrent use with drugs that are substrate for cytochrome $P_{450}IID_6$ may make normal metabolizer resemble poor metabolizer leading to higher than expected plasma concentrations of TCA with resultant toxicity). Products include:

Rythmol Tablets–150mg, 225mg, 300mg... 1352

Propantheline Bromide (Concurrent use may result in hyperpyrexia, particularly in hot weather; potential for paralytic ileus). Products include:

Pro-Banthine Tablets........................... 2052

Propofol (Amitriptyline may enhance the response to CNS depressants). Products include:

Diprivan Injection............................... 2833

Propoxyphene Hydrochloride (Amitriptyline may enhance the response to CNS depressants). Products include:

Darvon 1435
Wygesic Tablets 2827

Propoxyphene Napsylate (Amitriptyline may enhance the response to CNS depressants). Products include:

Darvon-N/Darvocet-N 1433

Protriptyline Hydrochloride (Concurrent use with drugs that are substrate for cytochrome $P_{450}IID_6$ may make normal metabolizer resemble poor metabolizer leading to higher than expected plasma concentrations of TCA with resultant toxicity). Products include:

Vivactil Tablets 1774

Pseudoephedrine Hydrochloride (Effects of concurrent use not specified; careful adjustment of dosage and close supervision are required). Products include:

Actifed Allergy Daytime/Nighttime Caplets... ⊞ 844
Actifed Plus Caplets .... ⊞ 845
Actifed Plus Tablets .... ⊞ 845
Actifed with Codeine Cough Syrup.. 1067
Actifed Sinus Daytime/Nighttime Tablets and Caplets .... ⊞ 846
Actifed Syrup...................................... ⊞ 846
Actifed Tablets .... ⊞ 844
Advil Cold and Sinus Caplets and Tablets (formerly CoAdvil) .... ⊞ 870
Alka-Seltzer Plus Cold Medicine Liqui-Gels .... ⊞ 706
Alka-Seltzer Plus Cold & Cough Medicine Liqui-Gels.......................... ⊞ 705
Alka-Seltzer Plus Night-Time Cold Medicine Liqui-Gels.......................... ⊞ 706
Allerest Headache Strength Tablets .... ⊞ 627
Allerest Maximum Strength Tablets .... ⊞ 627
Allerest No Drowsiness Tablets...... ⊞ 627
Allerest Sinus Pain Formula .... ⊞ 627
Anatuss LA Tablets.............................. 1542
Atrohist Pediatric Capsules................ 453
Bayer Select Sinus Pain Relief Formula .... ⊞ 717
Benadryl Allergy Decongestant Liquid Medication .... ⊞ 848
Benadryl Allergy Decongestant Tablets .... ⊞ 848
Benadryl Allergy Sinus Headache Formula Caplets................................ ⊞ 849
Benylin Multisymptom...................... ⊞ 852
Bromfed Capsules (Extended-Release) 1785
Bromfed Syrup................................... ⊞ 733
Bromfed Tablets 1785
Bromfed-DM Cough Syrup................. 1786
Bromfed-PD Capsules (Extended-Release) 1785
Children's Vicks DayQuil Allergy Relief .... ⊞ 757
Children's Vicks NyQuil Cold/Cough Relief... ⊞ 758
Comtrex Multi-Symptom Cold Reliever Tablets/Caplets/Liqui-Gels/Liquid... ⊞ 615
Allergy-Sinus Comtrex Multi-Symptom Allergy-Sinus Formula Tablets .... ⊞ 617
Comtrex Multi-Symptom Non-Drowsy Caplets................................... ⊞ 618
Congess 1004
Contac Day Allergy/Sinus Caplets ⊞ 812
Contac Day & Night .... ⊞ 812
Contac Night Allergy/Sinus Caplets .... ⊞ 812
Contac Severe Cold & Flu Non-Drowsy .... ⊞ 815
Deconamine Chewable Tablets 1320
Deconamine CX Cough and Cold Liquid and Tablets............................... 1319
Deconamine 1320
Deconsal C Expectorant Syrup 456
Deconsal Pediatric Syrup 457
Deconsal II Tablets 454
Dimetane-DX Cough Syrup 2059
Dimetapp Sinus Caplets .... ⊞ 775
Dorcol Children's Cough Syrup ...... ⊞ 785
Drixoral Cough + Congestion Liquid Caps .... ⊞ 802
Dura-Tap/PD Capsules 2867
Duratuss Tablets 2565
Duratuss HD Elixir.............................. 2565
Efidac/24 .... ⊞ 635
Entex PSE Tablets 1987
Fedahist Gyrocaps............................... 2401
Fedahist Timecaps 2401
Guaifed... 1787
Guaifed Syrup .... ⊞ 734
Guaimax-D Tablets 792
Guaitab Tablets .... ⊞ 734
Isoclor Expectorant............................. 990
Kronofed-A 977
Motrin IB Sinus.................................. ⊞ 838
Novahistine DH................................... 2462
Novahistine DMX .... ⊞ 822
Novahistine Expectorant..................... 2463
Nucofed 2051
PediaCare Cold Allergy Chewable Tablets .... ⊞ 677
PediaCare Cough-Cold Chewable Tablets 1553
PediaCare 1553
PediaCare Infants' Decongestant Drops .... ⊞ 677
PediCare Infant's Drops Decongestant Plus Cough 1553
PediaCare NightRest Cough-Cold Liquid 1553
Pediatric Vicks 44d Dry Hacking Cough & Head Congestion............. ⊞ 763
Pediatric Vicks 44m Cough & Cold Relief .... ⊞ 764

IMPORTANT NOTE: Always consult each drug listing in the patient's regimen for possible interactions.

Elavil — Interactions Index — 366

Robitussin Cold & Cough Liqui-Gels ◼ 776
Robitussin Maximum Strength Cough & Cold ◼ 778
Robitussin Pediatric Cough & Cold Formula ◼ 779
Robitussin Severe Congestion Liqui-Gels ◼ 776
Robitussin-DAC Syrup 2074
Robitussin-PE ◼ 778
Rondec Oral Drops 953
Rondec Syrup 953
Rondec Tablet 953
Rondec-DM Oral Drops 954
Rondec-DM Syrup 954
Rondec-TR Tablet 953
Ryna ◼ 841
Seldane-D Extended-Release Tablets 1538
Semprex-D Capsules 463
Semprex-D Capsules 1167
Sinarest Tablets ◼ 648
Sinarest Extra Strength Tablets ◼ 648
Sinarest No Drowsiness Tablets ◼ 648
Sine-Aid IB Caplets 1554
Sine-Aid Maximum Strength Sinus Medication Gelcaps, Caplets and Tablets 1554
Sine-Off No Drowsiness Formula Caplets ◼ 824
Sine-Off Sinus Medicine ◼ 825
Singlet Tablets ◼ 825
Sinutab Non-Drying Liquid Caps ◼ 859
Sinutab Sinus Allergy Medication, Maximum Strength Tablets and Caplets ◼ 860
Sinutab Sinus Medication, Maximum Strength Without Drowsiness Formula, Tablets & Caplets ◼ 860
Sinutab Sinus Medication, Regular Strength Without Drowsiness Formula ◼ 859
Sudafed Children's Liquid ◼ 861
Sudafed Cold and Cough Liquidcaps ◼ 862
Sudafed Cough Syrup ◼ 862
Sudafed Plus Liquid ◼ 862
Sudafed Plus Tablets ◼ 863
Sudafed Severe Cold Formula Caplets ◼ 863
Sudafed Severe Cold Formula Tablets ◼ 864
Sudafed Sinus Caplets ◼ 864
Sudafed Sinus Tablets ◼ 864
Sudafed Tablets, 30 mg ◼ 861
Sudafed Tablets, 60 mg ◼ 861
Sudafed 12 Hour Caplets ◼ 861
Syn-Rx Tablets 465
Syn-Rx DM Tablets 466
TheraFlu ◼ 787
TheraFlu Maximum Strength Nighttime Flu, Cold & Cough Medicine ◼ 788
TheraFlu Maximum Strength Non-Drowsy Formula Flu, Cold & Cough Medicine ◼ 788
Thera Flu Maximum Strength, Non-Drowsy Formula Flu, Cold and Cough Caplets ◼ 789
Triaminic AM Cough and Decongestant Formula ◼ 789
Triaminic AM Decongestant Formula ◼ 790
Triaminic Nite Light ◼ 791
Triaminic Sore Throat Formula ◼ 791
Tussend 1783
Tussend Expectorant 1785
Children's TYLENOL Cold Multi-Symptom Liquid Formula and Chewable Tablets 1561
Children's TYLENOL Cold Plus Cough Multi Symptom Tablets and Liquid ◼ 681
Infants' TYLENOL Cold Decongestant & Fever-Reducer Drops 1556
TYLENOL Maximum Strength Allergy Sinus Medication Gelcaps and Caplets 1563
TYLENOL Maximum Strength Allergy Sinus NightTime Medication Caplets 1555
TYLENOL Flu Maximum Strength Gelcaps 1565
TYLENOL Flu NightTime, Maximum Strength, Gelcaps 1566
TYLENOL Maximum Strength Flu NightTime Hot Medication Packets 1562
TYLENOL, Maximum Strength, Sinus Medication Geltabs, Gelcaps, Caplets and Tablets 1566
TYLENOL Cold Multi-Symptom Formula Medication Tablets and Caplets 1561
TYLENOL Cold Medication No Drowsiness Formula Gelcaps and Caplets 1562
TYLENOL Cold Multi-Symptom Hot Medication Liquid Packets 1557
TYLENOL Cough Multi-Symptom Medication with Decongestant 1565
Ursinus Inlay-Tabs ◼ 794
Vicks 44 LiquiCaps Cough, Cold & Flu Relief ◼ 755
Vicks 44 LiquiCaps Non-Drowsy Cough & Cold Relief ◼ 756
Vicks 44D Dry Hacking Cough & Head Congestion ◼ 755
Vicks 44M Cough, Cold & Flu Relief ◼ 756
Vicks DayQuil ◼ 761
Vicks DayQuil SINUS Pressure & PAIN Relief with IBUPROFEN ◼ 762
Vicks Nyquil Hot Therapy ◼ 762
Vicks NyQuil LiquiCaps Multi-Symptom Cold/Flu Relief ◼ 763
Vicks NyQuil Multi-Symptom Cold/Flu Relief - (Original & Cherry Flavor) ◼ 763

Pseudoephedrine Sulfate (Effects of concurrent use not specified; careful adjustment of dosage and close supervision are required). Products include:
Cheracol Sinus ◼ 768
Chlor-Trimeton Allergy Decongestant Tablets ◼ 799
Claritin-D 2350
Drixoral Cold and Allergy Sustained-Action Tablets ◼ 802
Drixoral Cold and Flu Extended-Release Tablets ◼ 803
Drixoral Non-Drowsy Formula Extended-Release Tablets ◼ 803
Drixoral Allergy/Sinus Extended Release Tablets ◼ 804
Trinalin Repetabs Tablets 1330

Quazepam (Amitriptyline may enhance the response to CNS depressants). Products include:
Doral Tablets 2664

Quinidine Gluconate (Concurrent use with drugs that inhibit cytochrome $P_{450}IID_6$ may make normal metabolizer resemble poor metabolizer leading to higher than expected plasma concentrations of TCA with resultant toxicity). Products include:
Quinaglute Dura-Tabs Tablets 649

Quinidine Polygalacturonate (Concurrent use with drugs that inhibit cytochrome $P_{450}IID_6$ may make normal metabolizer resemble poor metabolizer leading to higher than expected plasma concentrations of TCA with resultant toxicity).
No products indexed under this heading.

Quinidine Sulfate (Concurrent use with drugs that inhibit cytochrome $P_{450}IID_6$ may make normal metabolizer resemble poor metabolizer leading to higher than expected plasma concentrations of TCA with resultant toxicity). Products include:
Quinidex Extentabs 2067

Risperidone (Concurrent use with neuroleptics may result in hyperpyrexia, particularly in hot weather). Products include:
Risperdal 1301

Salmeterol Xinafoate (Effects of concurrent use not specified; careful adjustment of dosage and close supervision are required). Products include:
Serevent Inhalation Aerosol 1176

Scopolamine (Concurrent use may result in hyperpyrexia, particularly in hot weather; potential for paralytic ileus). Products include:
Transderm Scōp Transdermal Therapeutic System 869

Scopolamine Hydrobromide (Concurrent use may result in hyperpyrexia, particularly in hot weather; potential for paralytic ileus). Products include:
Atrohist Plus Tablets 454
Donnatal 2060
Donnatal Extentabs 2061
Donnatal Tablets 2060

Secobarbital Sodium (Amitriptyline may enhance the response to barbiturates). Products include:
Seconal Sodium Pulvules 1474

Selegiline Hydrochloride (Potential for hyperpyretic crises, severe convulsions, and deaths; concurrent and/or sequential use is contraindicated). Products include:
Eldepryl Tablets 2550

Sertraline Hydrochloride (Concurrent use with drugs that are substrate for cytochrome $P_{450}IID_6$ may make normal metabolizer resemble poor metabolizer leading to higher than expected plasma concentrations of TCA with resultant toxicity; due to variation in the extent of inhibition of $P_{450}IID_6$ caution is indicated, if co-administered sufficient time should/must elapse). Products include:
Zoloft Tablets 2217

Sufentanil Citrate (Amitriptyline may enhance the response to CNS depressants). Products include:
Sufenta Injection 1309

Temazepam (Amitriptyline may enhance the response to CNS depressants). Products include:
Restoril Capsules 2284

Terbutaline Sulfate (Effects of concurrent use not specified; careful adjustment of dosage and close supervision are required). Products include:
Brethaire Inhaler 813
Brethine Ampuls 815
Brethine Tablets 814
Bricanyl Subcutaneous Injection 1502
Bricanyl Tablets 1503

Thiamylal Sodium (Amitriptyline may enhance the response to barbiturates).
No products indexed under this heading.

Thioridazine Hydrochloride (Concurrent use with drugs that are substrate for cytochrome $P_{450}IID_6$ may make normal metabolizer resemble poor metabolizer leading to higher than expected plasma concentrations of TCA with resultant toxicity; concurrent use with neuroleptics may result in hyperpyrexia, particularly in hot weather). Products include:
Mellaril 2269

Thiothixene (Concurrent use with neuroleptics may result in hyperpyrexia, particularly in hot weather). Products include:
Navane Capsules and Concentrate 2201
Navane Intramuscular 2202

Thyroglobulin (On rare occasions, co-administration may produce arrhythmias).
No products indexed under this heading.

Thyroid (On rare occasions, co-administration may produce arrhythmias).
No products indexed under this heading.

Thyroxine (On rare occasions, co-administration may produce arrhythmias).
No products indexed under this heading.

Thyroxine Sodium (On rare occasions, co-administration may produce arrhythmias).
No products indexed under this heading.

Tranylcypromine Sulfate (Potential for hyperpyretic crises, severe convulsions, and deaths; concurrent and/or sequential use is contraindicated). Products include:
Parnate Tablets 2503

Trazodone Hydrochloride (Concurrent use with drugs that are substrate for cytochrome $P_{450}IID_6$ may make normal metabolizer resemble poor metabolizer leading to higher than expected plasma concentrations of TCA with resultant toxicity). Products include:
Desyrel and Desyrel Dividose 503

Triazolam (Amitriptyline may enhance the response to CNS depressants). Products include:
Halcion Tablets 2611

Tridihexethyl Chloride (Concurrent use may result in hyperpyrexia, particularly in hot weather; potential for paralytic ileus).
No products indexed under this heading.

Trifluoperazine Hydrochloride (Concurrent use with drugs that are substrate for cytochrome $P_{450}IID_6$ may make normal metabolizer resemble poor metabolizer leading to higher than expected plasma concentrations of TCA with resultant toxicity; concurrent use with neuroleptics may result in hyperpyrexia, particularly in hot weather). Products include:
Stelazine 2514

Trihexyphenidyl Hydrochloride (Concurrent use may result in hyperpyrexia, particularly in hot weather; potential for paralytic ileus). Products include:
Artane 1368

Trimipramine Maleate (Concurrent use with drugs that are substrate for cytochrome $P_{450}IID_6$ may make normal metabolizer resemble poor metabolizer leading to higher than expected plasma concentrations of TCA with resultant toxicity). Products include:
Surmontil Capsules 2811

Venlafaxine Hydrochloride (Concurrent use with drugs that are substrate for cytochrome $P_{450}IID_6$ may make normal metabolizer resemble poor metabolizer leading to higher than expected plasma concentrations of TCA with resultant toxicity; due to variation in the extent of inhibition of $P_{450}IID_6$ caution is indicated, if co-administered sufficient time should/must elapse). Products include:
Effexor 2719

Zolpidem Tartrate (Amitriptyline may enhance the response to CNS depressants). Products include:
Ambien Tablets 2416

Food Interactions

Alcohol (Amitriptyline may enhance the response to alcohol).

ELAVIL TABLETS
(Amitriptyline Hydrochloride) 2838
See **Elavil Injection**

367 Interactions Index Elspar

ELDEPRYL TABLETS
(Selegiline Hydrochloride) 2550
May interact with narcotic analgesics, tricyclic antidepressants, selective serotonin reuptake inhibitors, and certain other agents. Compounds in these categories include:

Alfentanil Hydrochloride (Contraindication warning for meperidine is extended to other opioids). Products include:
Alfenta Injection 1286

Amitriptyline Hydrochloride (Potential for hypertension, syncope, asystole, diaphoresis, seizures, changes in behavior and mental status, and muscular rigidity; concurrent and/or sequential use should be avoided; severe CNS toxicity associated with hyperpyrexia and fatality has been reported with concurrent use in a single case). Products include:
Elavil 2838
Endep Tablets 2174
Etrafon 2355
Limbitrol 2180
Triavil Tablets 1757

Amoxapine (Potential for hypertension, syncope, asystole, diaphoresis, seizures, changes in behavior and mental status, and muscular rigidity; concurrent and/or sequential use should be avoided). Products include:
Asendin Tablets 1369

Buprenorphine (Contraindication warning for meperidine is extended to other opioids). Products include:
Buprenex Injectable 2006

Clomipramine Hydrochloride (Potential for hypertension, syncope, asystole, diaphoresis, seizures, changes in behavior and mental status, and muscular rigidity; concurrent and/or sequential use should be avoided). Products include:
Anafranil Capsules 803

Codeine Phosphate (Contraindication warning for meperidine is extended to other opioids). Products include:
Actifed with Codeine Cough Syrup.. 1067
Brontex 1981
Deconsal C Expectorant Syrup 456
Deconsal Pediatric Syrup 457
Dimetane-DC Cough Syrup 2059
Empirin with Codeine Tablets.... 1093
Fioricet with Codeine Capsules 2260
Fiorinal with Codeine Capsules 2262
Isoclor Expectorant 990
Novahistine DH 2462
Novahistine Expectorant 2463
Nucofed 2051
Phenergan with Codeine 2777
Phenergan VC with Codeine 2781
Robitussin A-C Syrup 2073
Robitussin-DAC Syrup 2074
Ryna 841
Soma Compound w/Codeine Tablets 2676
Tussi-Organidin NR Liquid and S NR Liquid 2677
Tylenol with Codeine 1583

Desipramine Hydrochloride (Potential for hypertension, syncope, asystole, diaphoresis, seizures, changes in behavior and mental status, and muscular rigidity; concurrent and/or sequential use should be avoided). Products include:
Norpramin Tablets 1526

Dezocine (Contraindication warning for meperidine is extended to other opioids). Products include:
Dalgan Injection 538

Doxepin Hydrochloride (Potential for hypertension, syncope, asystole, diaphoresis, seizures, changes in behavior and mental status, and muscular rigidity; concurrent and/or sequential use should be avoided). Products include:
Sinequan 2205
Zonalon Cream 1055

Fentanyl (Contraindication warning for meperidine is extended to other opioids). Products include:
Duragesic Transdermal System.... 1288

Fentanyl Citrate (Contraindication warning for meperidine is extended to other opioids). Products include:
Sublimaze Injection 1307

Fluoxetine Hydrochloride (Potential for serious, sometimes fatal, reactions including hyperthermia, rigidity, myoclonus, autonomic instability, extreme agitation progressing to delirium and coma; concurrent and/or sequential use should be avoided). Products include:
Prozac Pulvules & Liquid, Oral Solution 919

Fluvoxamine Maleate (Potential for serious, sometimes fatal, reactions including hyperthermia, rigidity, myoclonus, autonomic instability, extreme agitation progressing to delirium and coma; concurrent and/or sequential use should be avoided). Products include:
Luvox Tablets 2544

Hydrocodone Bitartrate (Contraindication warning for meperidine is extended to other opioids). Products include:
Anexsia 5/500 Elixir 1781
Anexia Tablets 1782
Codiclear DH Syrup 791
Deconamine CX Cough and Cold Liquid and Tablets 1319
Duratuss HD Elixir 2565
Hycodan Tablets and Syrup 930
Hycomine Compound Tablets 932
Hycomine 931
Hycotuss Expectorant Syrup 933
Hydrocet Capsules 782
Lorcet 10/650 1018
Lortab 2566
Tussend 1783
Tussend Expectorant 1785
Vicodin Tablets 1356
Vicodin ES Tablets 1357
Vicodin Tuss Expectorant 1358
Zydone Capsules 949

Hydrocodone Polistirex (Contraindication warning for meperidine is extended to other opioids). Products include:
Tussionex Pennkinetic Extended-Release Suspension 998

Imipramine Hydrochloride (Potential for hypertension, syncope, asystole, diaphoresis, seizures, changes in behavior and mental status, and muscular rigidity; concurrent and/or sequential use should be avoided). Products include:
Tofranil Ampuls 854
Tofranil Tablets 856

Imipramine Pamoate (Potential for hypertension, syncope, asystole, diaphoresis, seizures, changes in behavior and mental status, and muscular rigidity; concurrent and/or sequential use should be avoided). Products include:
Tofranil-PM Capsules 857

Levodopa (Potential exacerbation of levodopa associated side effects). Products include:
Atamet 572
Larodopa Tablets 2129
Sinemet Tablets 943
Sinemet CR Tablets 944

Levorphanol Tartrate (Contraindication warning for meperidine is extended to other opioids). Products include:
Levo-Dromoran 2129

Maprotiline Hydrochloride (Potential for hypertension, syncope, asystole, diaphoresis, seizures, changes in behavior and mental status, and muscular rigidity; concurrent and/or sequential use should be avoided). Products include:
Ludiomil Tablets 843

Meperidine Hydrochloride (Concurrent use is contraindicated; potential for muscular rigidity, stupor, severe agitation, and elevated temperature). Products include:
Demerol 2308
Mepergan Injection 2753

Methadone Hydrochloride (Contraindication warning for meperidine is extended to other opioids). Products include:
Methadone Hydrochloride Oral Concentrate 2233
Methadone Hydrochloride Oral Solution & Tablets 2235

Morphine Sulfate (Contraindication warning for meperidine is extended to other opioids). Products include:
Astramorph/PF Injection, USP (Preservative-Free) 535
Duramorph 962
Infumorph 200 and Infumorph 500 Sterile Solutions 965
MS Contin Tablets 1994
MSIR 1997
Oramorph SR (Morphine Sulfate Sustained Release Tablets) 2236
RMS Suppositories 2657
Roxanol 2243

Nortriptyline Hydrochloride (Potential for hypertension, syncope, asystole, diaphoresis, seizures, changes in behavior and mental status, and muscular rigidity; concurrent and/or sequential use should be avoided). Products include:
Pamelor 2280

Opium Alkaloids (Contraindication warning for meperidine is extended to other opioids).
No products indexed under this heading.

Oxycodone Hydrochloride (Contraindication warning for meperidine is extended to other opioids). Products include:
Percocet Tablets 938
Percodan Tablets 939
Percodan-Demi Tablets 940
Roxicodone Tablets, Oral Solution & Intensol (Oxycodone) 2244
Tylox Capsules 1584

Paroxetine Hydrochloride (Potential for serious, sometimes fatal, reactions including hyperthermia, rigidity, myoclonus, autonomic instability, extreme agitation progressing to delirium and coma; concurrent and/or sequential use should be avoided). Products include:
Paxil Tablets 2505

Propoxyphene Hydrochloride (Contraindication warning for meperidine is extended to other opioids). Products include:
Darvon 1435
Wygesic Tablets 2827

Propoxyphene Napsylate (Contraindication warning for meperidine is extended to other opioids). Products include:
Darvon-N/Darvocet-N 1433

Protriptyline Hydrochloride (Potential for hypertension, syncope, asystole, diaphoresis, seizures, changes in behavior and mental status, and muscular rigidity; concurrent and/or sequential use should be avoided; tremors, agitation, and restlessness followed by unresponsiveness and fatality has been reported with concurrent use in a single case). Products include:
Vivactil Tablets 1774

Sertraline Hydrochloride (Potential for serious, sometimes fatal, reactions including hyperthermia, rigidity, myoclonus, autonomic instability, extreme agitation progressing to delirium and coma; concurrent and/or sequential use should be avoided). Products include:
Zoloft Tablets 2217

Sufentanil Citrate (Contraindication warning for meperidine is extended to other opioids). Products include:
Sufenta Injection 1309

Trimipramine Maleate (Potential for hypertension, syncope, asystole, diaphoresis, seizures, changes in behavior and mental status, and muscular rigidity; concurrent and/or sequential use should be avoided). Products include:
Surmontil Capsules 2811

Venlafaxine Hydrochloride (Potential for serious, sometimes fatal, reactions including hyperthermia, rigidity, myoclonus, autonomic instability, extreme agitation progressing to delirium and coma; concurrent and/or sequential use should be avoided). Products include:
Effexor 2719

Food Interactions

Food with high concentration of tyramine (Potential for "cheese reaction" if attention is not paid to the dose dependent nature of selegine's selectivity).

ELDERTONIC
(Vitamins with Minerals) 1543
None cited in PDR database.

ELDOPAQUE FORTE 4% CREAM
(Hydroquinone) 1252
None cited in PDR database.

ELDOQUIN FORTE 4% CREAM
(Hydroquinone) 1252
None cited in PDR database.

ELIMITE (PERMETHRIN) 5% CREAM
(Permethrin) 478
None cited in PDR database.

ELOCON CREAM 0.1%
(Mometasone Furoate) 2354
None cited in PDR database.

ELOCON LOTION 0.1%
(Mometasone Furoate) 2354
None cited in PDR database.

ELOCON OINTMENT 0.1%
(Mometasone Furoate) 2354
None cited in PDR database.

IMPORTANT NOTE: Always consult each drug listing in the patient's regimen for possible interactions.

ELSPAR
(Asparaginase) 1659
May interact with:

Methotrexate Sodium (Diminished or abolished effect of methotrexate on malignant cells). Products include:
- Methotrexate Sodium Tablets, Injection, for Injection and LPF Injection 1275

Prednisone (Increased toxicity). Products include:
- Deltasone Tablets 2595

Vincristine Sulfate (Increased toxicity). Products include:
- Oncovin Solution Vials & Hyporets 1466

EMCYT CAPSULES
(Estramustine Phosphate Sodium) 1953
May interact with calcium preparations. Compounds in this category include:

Calcium Carbonate (Impaired absorption of Emcyt). Products include:
- Alka-Mints Chewable Antacid .... ■ 701
- Arthritis Pain Ascriptin .... ■ 631
- Maximum Strength Ascriptin .... ■ 630
- Regular Strength Ascriptin Tablets .... ■ 629
- Extra Strength Bayer Plus Aspirin Caplets .... ■ 713
- Bufferin Analgesic Tablets and Caplets .... ■ 613
- Calci-Chew Tablets 2004
- Calci-Mix Capsules 2004
- Caltrate 600 .... ■ 665
- Caltrate PLUS .... ■ 665
- Caltrate 600 + D .... ■ 665
- Centrum Singles Calcium .... ■ 669
- Chooz Antacid Gum .... ■ 799
- Di-Gel Antacid/Anti-Gas .... ■ 801
- Gerimed Tablets 982
- Maalox Antacid Caplets .... ■ 638
- Marblen .... ■ 655
- Materna Tablets 1379
- Mylanta Calcium Carbonate and Magnesium Hydroxide Tablets 1318
- Mylanta Gelcaps Antacid .... ■ 662
- Mylanta Soothing Lozenges 1319
- Nephro-Calci Tablets 2004
- Rolaids Tablets .... ■ 843
- Rolaids (Calcium Rich/Sodium Free) Tablets .... ■ 843
- Tempo Soft Antacid .... ■ 835
- Titralac .... ■ 672
- Titralac Plus .... ■ 672
- Tums Antacid Tablets .... ■ 827
- Tums Anti-gas/Antacid Formula Tablets, Assorted Fruit .... ■ 827
- Tums E-X Antacid Tablets .... ■ 827
- Tums 500 Calcium Supplement .... ■ 828
- Tums ULTRA Antacid Tablets .... ■ 827
- TYLENOL, Extra Strength, Headache Plus Pain Reliever with Antacid Caplets 1559

Calcium Chloride (Impaired absorption of Emcyt).
- No products indexed under this heading.

Calcium Citrate (Impaired absorption of Emcyt). Products include:
- Citracal 1779
- Citracal Caplets + D 1780
- Citracal Liquitab 1780

Calcium Glubionate (Impaired absorption of Emcyt).
- No products indexed under this heading.

Food Interactions

Dairy products (Impairs the absorption of Emcyt).

Food, calcium-rich (Impairs the absorption of Emcyt).

EMETE-CON INTRAMUSCULAR/ INTRAVENOUS
(Benzquinamide Hydrochloride) 2198
May interact with preanesthetic medications, vasopressors, and sympathomimetics. Compounds in these categories include:

Albuterol (In simultaneous use, benzquinamide should be decreased). Products include:
- Proventil Inhalation Aerosol 2382
- Ventolin Inhalation Aerosol and Refill 1197

Albuterol Sulfate (In simultaneous use, benzquinamide should be decreased). Products include:
- Airet Solution for Inhalation 452
- Proventil Inhalation Solution 0.083% 2384
- Proventil Repetabs Tablets 2386
- Proventil Solution for Inhalation 0.5% 2383
- Proventil Syrup 2385
- Proventil Tablets 2386
- Ventolin Inhalation Solution 1198
- Ventolin Nebules Inhalation Solution 1199
- Ventolin Rotacaps for Inhalation 1200
- Ventolin Syrup 1202
- Ventolin Tablets 1203
- Volmax Extended-Release Tablets .. 1788

Diazepam (Do not administer benzquinamide by IV route). Products include:
- Dizac 1809
- Valium Injectable 2182
- Valium Tablets 2183
- Valrelease Capsules 2169

Dobutamine Hydrochloride (In simultaneous use, benzquinamide should be decreased). Products include:
- Dobutrex Solution Vials 1439

Dopamine Hydrochloride (In simultaneous use, benzquinamide should be decreased).
- No products indexed under this heading.

Droperidol (Do not administer benzquinamide by IV route). Products include:
- Inapsine Injection 1296

Ephedrine Hydrochloride (In simultaneous use, benzquinamide should be decreased). Products include:
- Primatene Dual Action Formula .... ■ 872
- Primatene Tablets .... ■ 873
- Quadrinal Tablets 1350

Ephedrine Sulfate (In simultaneous use, benzquinamide should be decreased). Products include:
- Bronkaid Caplets .... ■ 717
- Marax Tablets & DF Syrup 2200

Ephedrine Tannate (In simultaneous use, benzquinamide should be decreased). Products include:
- Rynatuss 2673

Epinephrine Bitartrate (In simultaneous use, benzquinamide should be decreased). Products include:
- Bronkaid Mist Suspension .... ■ 718
- Sensorcaine-MPF with Epinephrine Injection 559

Epinephrine Hydrochloride (In simultaneous use, benzquinamide should be decreased). Products include:
- Ana-Kit Anaphylaxis Emergency Treatment Kit 617

Fentanyl Citrate (Do not administer benzquinamide by IV route). Products include:
- Sublimaze Injection 1307

Hydroxyzine Hydrochloride (Do not administer benzquinamide by IV route). Products include:
- Atarax Tablets & Syrup 2185
- Marax Tablets & DF Syrup 2200
- Vistaril Intramuscular Solution 2216

Isoproterenol Hydrochloride (In simultaneous use, benzquinamide should be decreased; careful dosage adjustment required). Products include:
- Isuprel Hydrochloride Injection 1:5000 2311
- Isuprel Hydrochloride Solution 1:200 & 1:100 2313
- Isuprel Mistometer 2312

Isoproterenol Sulfate (In simultaneous use, benzquinamide should be decreased; careful dosage adjustment required). Products include:
- Norisodrine with Calcium Iodide Syrup 442

Lorazepam (Do not administer benzquinamide by IV route). Products include:
- Ativan Injection 2698
- Ativan Tablets 2700

Meperidine Hydrochloride (Do not administer benzquinamide by IV route). Products include:
- Demerol 2308
- Mepergan Injection 2753

Metaproterenol Sulfate (In simultaneous use, benzquinamide should be decreased). Products include:
- Alupent 669
- Metaproterenol Sulfate Inhalation Solution, USP, Arm-a-Med 552

Metaraminol Bitartrate (In simultaneous use, benzquinamide should be decreased). Products include:
- Aramine Injection 1609

Methoxamine Hydrochloride (In simultaneous use, benzquinamide should be decreased). Products include:
- Vasoxyl Injection 1196

Morphine Sulfate (Do not administer benzquinamide by IV route). Products include:
- Astramorph/PF Injection, USP (Preservative-Free) 535
- Duramorph 962
- Infumorph 200 and Infumorph 500 Sterile Solutions 965
- MS Contin Tablets 1994
- MSIR 1997
- Oramorph SR (Morphine Sulfate Sustained Release Tablets) 2236
- RMS Suppositories 2657
- Roxanol 2243

Norepinephrine Bitartrate (I.V. use not with cardiovascular drugs; in simultaneous use, benzquinamide should be decreased). Products include:
- Levophed Bitartrate Injection 2315

Pentobarbital Sodium (Do not administer benzquinamide by IV route). Products include:
- Nembutal Sodium Capsules 436
- Nembutal Sodium Solution 438
- Nembutal Sodium Suppositories 440

Phenylephrine Bitartrate (In simultaneous use, benzquinamide should be decreased).
- No products indexed under this heading.

Phenylephrine Hydrochloride (In simultaneous use, benzquinamide should be decreased). Products include:
- Atrohist Plus Tablets 454
- Cerose DM .... ■ 878
- Comhist 2038
- D.A. Chewable Tablets 951
- Deconsal Pediatric Capsules 454
- Dura-Vent/DA Tablets 953
- Entex Capsules 1986
- Entex Liquid 1986
- Extendryl 1005
- 4-Way Fast Acting Nasal Spray (regular & mentholated) .... ■ 621
- Hemorid For Women .... ■ 834
- Hycomine Compound Tablets 932
- Neo-Synephrine Hydrochloride 1% Carpuject 2324
- Neo-Synephrine Hydrochloride 1% Injection 2324
- Neo-Synephrine Hydrochloride (Ophthalmic) 2325
- Neo-Synephrine .... ■ 726
- Nōstril .... ■ 644
- Novahistine Elixir .... ■ 823
- Phenergan VC 2779
- Phenergan VC with Codeine 2781
- Preparation H .... ■ 871
- Tympagesic Ear Drops 2342
- Vasosulf .... ⊙ 271
- Vicks Sinex Nasal Spray and Ultra Fine Mist .... ■ 765

Phenylephrine Tannate (In simultaneous use, benzquinamide should be decreased). Products include:
- Atrohist Pediatric Suspension 454
- Ricobid-D Pediatric Suspension 2038
- Ricobid Tablets and Pediatric Suspension 2038
- Rynatan 2673
- Rynatuss 2673

Phenylpropanolamine Hydrochloride (In simultaneous use, benzquinamide should be decreased). Products include:
- Acutrim .... ■ 628
- Allerest Children's Chewable Tablets .... ■ 627
- Allerest 12 Hour Caplets .... ■ 627
- Atrohist Plus Tablets 454
- BC Cold Powder Multi-Symptom Formula (Cold-Sinus-Allergy) .... ■ 609
- BC Cold Powder Non-Drowsy Formula (Cold-Sinus) .... ■ 609
- Cheracol Plus Head Cold/Cough Formula .... ■ 769
- Comtrex Multi-Symptom Non-Drowsy Liqui-gels .... ■ 618
- Contac Continuous Action Nasal Decongestant/Antihistamine 12 Hour Capsules .... ■ 813
- Contac Maximum Strength Continuous Action Decongestant/ Antihistamine 12 Hour Caplets .. ■ 813
- Contac Severe Cold and Flu Formula Caplets .... ■ 814
- Coricidin 'D' Decongestant Tablets .... ■ 800
- Dexatrim .... ■ 832
- Dexatrim Plus Vitamins Caplets .... ■ 832
- Dimetane-DC Cough Syrup 2059
- Dimetapp Elixir .... ■ 773
- Dimetapp Extentabs .... ■ 774
- Dimetapp Tablets/Liqui-Gels .... ■ 775
- Dimetapp Cold & Allergy Chewable Tablets .... ■ 773
- Dimetapp DM Elixir .... ■ 774
- Dura-Vent Tablets 952
- Entex Capsules 1986
- Entex LA Tablets 1987
- Entex Liquid 1986
- Exgest LA Tablets 782
- Hycomine 931
- Isoclor Timesule Capsules .... ■ 637
- Nolamine Timed-Release Tablets 785
- Ornade Spansule Capsules 2502
- Propagest Tablets 786
- Pyrroxate Caplets .... ■ 772
- Robitussin-CF .... ■ 777
- Sinulin Tablets 787
- Tavist-D 12 Hour Relief Tablets .... ■ 787
- Teldrin 12 Hour Antihistamine/ Nasal Decongestant Allergy Relief Capsules .... ■ 826
- Triaminic Allergy Tablets .... ■ 789
- Triaminic Cold Tablets .... ■ 790
- Triaminic Expectorant .... ■ 790
- Triaminic Syrup .... ■ 792
- Triaminic-12 Tablets .... ■ 792
- Triaminic-DM Syrup .... ■ 792
- Triaminicin Tablets .... ■ 793
- Triaminicol Multi-Symptom Cold Tablets .... ■ 793
- Triaminicol Multi-Symptom Relief .... ■ 794
- Vicks DayQuil Allergy Relief 12-Hour Extended Release Tablets .... ■ 760
- Vicks DayQuil Allergy Relief 4-Hour Tablets .... ■ 760
- Vicks DayQuil SINUS Pressure & CONGESTION Relief .... ■ 761

Pirbuterol Acetate (In simultaneous use, benzquinamide should be decreased). Products include:
- Maxair Autohaler 1492

(■ Described in PDR For Nonprescription Drugs) (⊙ Described in PDR For Ophthalmology)

Maxair Inhaler 1494

Promethazine (Do not administer benzquinamide by IV route).

No products indexed under this heading.

Promethazine Hydrochloride (Do not administer benzquinamide by IV route). Products include:

Mepergan Injection 2753
Phenergan with Codeine 2777
Phenergan with Dextromethorphan 2778
Phenergan Injection 2773
Phenergan Suppositories 2775
Phenergan Syrup 2774
Phenergan Tablets 2775
Phenergan VC 2779
Phenergan VC with Codeine 2781

Pseudoephedrine Hydrochloride (In simultaneous use, benzquinamide should be decreased). Products include:

Actifed Allergy Daytime/Nighttime Caplets .... ⊕ 844
Actifed Plus Caplets .... ⊕ 845
Actifed Plus Tablets .... ⊕ 845
Actifed with Codeine Cough Syrup.. 1067
Actifed Sinus Daytime/Nighttime Tablets and Caplets .... ⊕ 846
Actifed Syrup... ⊕ 846
Actifed Tablets .... ⊕ 844
Advil Cold and Sinus Caplets and Tablets (formerly CoAdvil) .... ⊕ 870
Alka-Seltzer Plus Cold Medicine Liqui-Gels .... ⊕ 706
Alka-Seltzer Plus Cold & Cough Medicine Liqui-Gels.......................... ⊕ 705
Alka-Seltzer Plus Night-Time Cold Medicine Liqui-Gels.......................... ⊕ 706
Allerest Headache Strength Tablets .... ⊕ 627
Allerest Maximum Strength Tablets .... ⊕ 627
Allerest No Drowsiness Tablets...... ⊕ 627
Allerest Sinus Pain Formula .... ⊕ 627
Anatuss LA Tablets................................. 1542
Atrohist Pediatric Capsules.................. 453
Bayer Select Sinus Pain Relief Formula .... ⊕ 717
Benadryl Allergy Decongestant Liquid Medication .... ⊕ 848
Benadryl Allergy Decongestant Tablets .... ⊕ 848
Benadryl Allergy Sinus Headache Formula Caplets................................. ⊕ 849
Benylin Multisymptom......................... ⊕ 852
Bromfed Capsules (Extended-Release) 1785
Bromfed Syrup .... ⊕ 733
Bromfed Tablets 1785
Bromfed-DM Cough Syrup.................. 1786
Bromfed-PD Capsules (Extended-Release) 1785
Children's Vicks DayQuil Allergy Relief... ⊕ 757
Children's Vicks NyQuil Cold/ Cough Relief.. ⊕ 758
Comtrex Multi-Symptom Cold Reliever Tablets/Caplets/Liqui-Gels/Liquid.. ⊕ 615
Allergy-Sinus Comtrex Multi-Symptom Allergy-Sinus Formula Tablets .... ⊕ 617
Comtrex Multi-Symptom Non-Drowsy Caplets................................... ⊕ 618
Congess 1004
Contac Day Allergy/Sinus Caplets ⊕ 812
Contac Day & Night .... ⊕ 812
Contac Night Allergy/Sinus Caplets .... ⊕ 812
Contac Severe Cold & Flu Non-Drowsy .... ⊕ 815
Deconamine Chewable Tablets 1320
Deconamine CX Cough and Cold Liquid and Tablets............................... 1319
Deconamine 1320
Deconsal C Expectorant Syrup 456
Deconsal Pediatric Syrup..................... 457
Deconsal II Tablets 454
Dimetane-DX Cough Syrup 2059
Dimetapp Sinus Caplets .... ⊕ 775
Dorcol Children's Cough Syrup ...... ⊕ 785
Drixoral Cough + Congestion Liquid Caps .... ⊕ 802
Dura-Tap/PD Capsules 2867
Duratuss Tablets 2565
Duratuss HD Elixir................................. 2565
Efidac/24 .... ⊕ 635
Entex PSE Tablets.................................. 1987

Fedahist Gyrocaps.................................. 2401
Fedahist Timecaps 2401
Guaifed.. 1787
Guaifed Syrup .... ⊕ 734
Guaimax-D Tablets 792
Guaitab Tablets .... ⊕ 734
Isoclor Expectorant............................... 990
Kronofed-A 977
Motrin IB Sinus .... ⊕ 838
Novahistine DH....................................... 2462
Novahistine DMX .... ⊕ 822
Novahistine Expectorant...................... 2463
Nucofed 2051
PediaCare Cold Allergy Chewable Tablets .... ⊕ 677
PediaCare Cough-Cold Chewable Tablets 1553
PediaCare 1553
PediaCare Infants' Decongestant Drops .... ⊕ 677
PediCare Infant's Drops Decongestant Plus Cough 1553
PediaCare NightRest Cough-Cold Liquid 1553
Pediatric Vicks 44d Dry Hacking Cough & Head Congestion............. ⊕ 763
Pediatric Vicks 44m Cough & Cold Relief .... ⊕ 764
Robitussin Cold & Cough Liqui-Gels .... ⊕ 776
Robitussin Maximum Strength Cough & Cold .... ⊕ 778
Robitussin Pediatric Cough & Cold Formula .... ⊕ 779
Robitussin Severe Congestion Liqui-Gels .... ⊕ 776
Robitussin-DAC Syrup 2074
Robitussin-PE .... ⊕ 778
Rondec Oral Drops 953
Rondec Syrup 953
Rondec Tablet 953
Rondec-DM Oral Drops 954
Rondec-DM Syrup 954
Rondec-TR Tablet 953
Ryna .... ⊕ 841
Seldane-D Extended-Release Tablets 1538
Semprex-D Capsules 463
Semprex-D Capsules 1167
Sinarest Tablets .... ⊕ 648
Sinarest Extra Strength Tablets....... ⊕ 648
Sinarest No Drowsiness Tablets .... ⊕ 648
Sine-Aid IB Caplets 1554
Sine-Aid Maximum Strength Sinus Medication Gelcaps, Caplets and Tablets.. 1554
Sine-Off No Drowsiness Formula Caplets .... ⊕ 824
Sine-Off Sinus Medicine .... ⊕ 825
Singlet Tablets .... ⊕ 825
Sinutab Non-Drying Liquid Caps.... ⊕ 859
Sinutab Sinus Allergy Medication, Maximum Strength Tablets and Caplets .... ⊕ 860
Sinutab Sinus Medication, Maximum Strength Without Drowsiness Formula, Tablets & Caplets.. ⊕ 860
Sinutab Sinus Medication, Regular Strength Without Drowsiness Formula .... ⊕ 859
Sudafed Children's Liquid .... ⊕ 861
Sudafed Cold and Cough Liquidcaps .... ⊕ 862
Sudafed Cough Syrup .... ⊕ 862
Sudafed Plus Liquid .... ⊕ 862
Sudafed Plus Tablets .... ⊕ 863
Sudafed Severe Cold Formula Caplets .... ⊕ 863
Sudafed Severe Cold Formula Tablets .... ⊕ 864
Sudafed Sinus Caplets......................... ⊕ 864
Sudafed Sinus Tablets.......................... ⊕ 864
Sudafed Tablets, 30 mg....................... ⊕ 861
Sudafed Tablets, 60 mg....................... ⊕ 861
Sudafed 12 Hour Caplets .... ⊕ 861
Syn-Rx Tablets 465
Syn-Rx DM Tablets 466
TheraFlu... ⊕ 787
TheraFlu Maximum Strength Nighttime Flu, Cold & Cough Medicine .... ⊕ 788
TheraFlu Maximum Strength Non-Drowsy Formula Flu, Cold & Cough Medicine .... ⊕ 788
Thera Flu Maximum Strength, Non-Drowsy Formula Flu, Cold and Cough Caplets .... ⊕ 789
Triaminic AM Cough and Decongestant Formula .... ⊕ 789

Triaminic AM Decongestant Formula .... ⊕ 790
Triaminic Nite Light .... ⊕ 791
Triaminic Sore Throat Formula ...... ⊕ 791
Tussend 1783
Tussend Expectorant 1785
Children's TYLENOL Cold Multi-Symptom Liquid Formula and Chewable Tablets................................. 1561
Children's TYLENOL Cold Plus Cough Multi Symptom Tablets and Liquid .... ⊕ 681
Infants' TYLENOL Cold Decongestant & Fever-Reducer Drops 1556
TYLENOL Maximum Strength Allergy Sinus Medication Gelcaps and Caplets 1563
TYLENOL Maximum Strength Allergy Sinus NightTime Medication Caplets 1555
TYLENOL Flu Maximum Strength Gelcaps 1565
TYLENOL Flu NightTime, Maximum Strength, Gelcaps 1566
TYLENOL Maximum Strength Flu NightTime Hot Medication Packets 1562
TYLENOL, Maximum Strength, Sinus Medication Geltabs, Gelcaps, Caplets and Tablets 1566
TYLENOL Cold Multi-Symptom Formula Medication Tablets and Caplets 1561
TYLENOL Cold Medication No Drowsiness Formula Gelcaps and Caplets 1562
TYLENOL Cold Multi-Symptom Hot Medication Liquid Packets........... 1557
TYLENOL Cough Multi-Symptom Medication with Decongestant...... 1565
Ursinus Inlay-Tabs................................. ⊕ 794
Vicks 44 LiquiCaps Cough, Cold & Flu Relief.. ⊕ 755
Vicks 44 LiquiCaps Non-Drowsy Cough & Cold Relief .... ⊕ 756
Vicks 44D Dry Hacking Cough & Head Congestion .... ⊕ 755
Vicks 44M Cough, Cold & Flu Relief... ⊕ 756
Vicks DayQuil .... ⊕ 761
Vicks DayQuil SINUS Pressure & PAIN Relief with IBUPROFEN .... ⊕ 762
Vicks Nyquil Hot Therapy.................... ⊕ 762
Vicks NyQuil LiquiCaps Multi-Symptom Cold/Flu Relief .... ⊕ 763
Vicks NyQuil Multi-Symptom Cold/Flu Relief - (Original & Cherry Flavor) .... ⊕ 763

Pseudoephedrine Sulfate (In simultaneous use, benzquinamide should be decreased). Products include:

Cheracol Sinus .... ⊕ 768
Chlor-Trimeton Allergy Decongestant Tablets .... ⊕ 799
Claritin-D 2350
Drixoral Cold and Allergy Sustained-Action Tablets .... ⊕ 802
Drixoral Cold and Flu Extended-Release Tablets.................................... ⊕ 803
Drixoral Non-Drowsy Formula Extended-Release Tablets .... ⊕ 803
Drixoral Allergy/Sinus Extended Release Tablets.................................... ⊕ 804
Trinalin Repetabs Tablets 1330

Salmeterol Xinafoate (In simultaneous use, benzquinamide should be decreased). Products include:

Serevent Inhalation Aerosol............... 1176

Secobarbital Sodium (Do not administer benzquinamide by IV route). Products include:

Seconal Sodium Pulvules 1474

Terbutaline Sulfate (In simultaneous use, benzquinamide should be decreased). Products include:

Brethaire Inhaler 813
Brethine Ampuls 815
Brethine Tablets 814
Bricanyl Subcutaneous Injection 1502
Bricanyl Tablets 1503

EMETROL

(Dextrose, Phosphoric Acid, Levulose) .... ⊕ 612

None cited in PDR database.

EMGEL 2% TOPICAL GEL

(Erythromycin) 1093

May interact with:

Concomitant Topical Acne Therapy (Possible cumulative irritancy effect).

EMINASE

(Anistreplase) 2039

May interact with anticoagulants, platelet inhibitors, and certain other agents. Compounds in these categories include:

Aspirin (Increases risk of bleeding and bleeding events). Products include:

Alka-Seltzer Effervescent Antacid and Pain Reliever .... ⊕ 701
Alka-Seltzer Extra Strength Effervescent Antacid and Pain Reliever .... ⊕ 703
Alka-Seltzer Lemon Lime Effervescent Antacid and Pain Reliever .... ⊕ 703
Alka-Seltzer Plus Cold Medicine .... ⊕ 705
Alka-Seltzer Plus Cold & Cough Medicine .... ⊕ 708
Alka-Seltzer Plus Night-Time Cold Medicine .... ⊕ 707
Alka Seltzer Plus Sinus Medicine .. ⊕ 707
Arthritis Foundation Safety Coated Aspirin Tablets .... ⊕ 675
Arthritis Pain Ascriptin .... ⊕ 631
Maximum Strength Ascriptin .... ⊕ 630
Regular Strength Ascriptin Tablets .... ⊕ 629
Arthritis Strength BC Powder........... ⊕ 609
BC Cold Powder Multi-Symptom Formula (Cold-Sinus-Allergy) ...... ⊕ 609
BC Cold Powder Non-Drowsy Formula (Cold-Sinus) .... ⊕ 609
BC Powder .... ⊕ 609
Bayer Children's Chewable Aspirin... ⊕ 711
Genuine Bayer Aspirin Tablets & Caplets .... ⊕ 713
Extra Strength Bayer Arthritis Pain Regimen Formula .... ⊕ 711
Extra Strength Bayer Aspirin Caplets & Tablets .... ⊕ 712
Extended-Release Bayer 8-Hour Aspirin .... ⊕ 712
Extra Strength Bayer Plus Aspirin Caplets .... ⊕ 713
Extra Strength Bayer PM Aspirin .. ⊕ 713
Bayer Enteric Aspirin .... ⊕ 709
Bufferin Analgesic Tablets and Caplets .... ⊕ 613
Arthritis Strength Bufferin Analgesic Caplets .... ⊕ 614
Extra Strength Bufferin Analgesic Tablets .... ⊕ 615
Cama Arthritis Pain Reliever............ ⊕ 785
Darvon Compound-65 Pulvules 1435
Easprin.. 1914
Ecotrin 2455
Ecotrin Enteric Coated Aspirin Maximum Strength Tablets and Caplets .... ⊕ 816
Ecotrin Enteric Coated Aspirin Regular Strength Tablets 2455
Empirin Aspirin Tablets .... ⊕ 854
Empirin with Codeine Tablets........... 1093
Excedrin Extra-Strength Analgesic Tablets & Caplets 732
Fiorinal Capsules 2261
Fiorinal with Codeine Capsules 2262
Fiorinal Tablets 2261
Halfprin 1362
Healthprin Aspirin 2455
Norgesic.. 1496
Percodan Tablets.................................... 939
Percodan-Demi Tablets........................ 940
Robaxisal Tablets.................................... 2071
Soma Compound w/Codeine Tablets 2676
Soma Compound Tablets..................... 2675
St. Joseph Adult Chewable Aspirin (81 mg.) .... ⊕ 808
Talwin Compound 2335
Ursinus Inlay-Tabs................................. ⊕ 794
Vanquish Analgesic Caplets .... ⊕ 731

Azlocillin Sodium (Increases risk of bleeding and bleeding events).

No products indexed under this heading.

IMPORTANT NOTE: Always consult each drug listing in the patient's regimen for possible interactions.

Carbenicillin Indanyl Sodium (Increases risk of bleeding and bleeding events). Products include:

- Geocillin Tablets ... 2199

Choline Magnesium Trisalicylate (Increases risk of bleeding and bleeding events). Products include:

- Trilisate ... 2000

Dalteparin Sodium (Potential for bleeding and bleeding complications). Products include:

- Fragmin ... 1954

Diclofenac Potassium (Increases risk of bleeding and bleeding events). Products include:

- Cataflam ... 816

Diclofenac Sodium (Increases risk of bleeding and bleeding events). Products include:

- Voltaren Ophthalmic Sterile Ophthalmic Solution ... ◉ 272
- Voltaren Tablets ... 861

Dicumarol (Potential for bleeding and bleeding complications).

- No products indexed under this heading.

Diflunisal (Increases risk of bleeding and bleeding events). Products include:

- Dolobid Tablets ... 1654

Dipyridamole (Increases risk of bleeding and bleeding events). Products include:

- Persantine Tablets ... 681

Enoxaparin (Potential for bleeding and bleeding complications). Products include:

- Lovenox Injection ... 2020

Fenoprofen Calcium (Increases risk of bleeding and bleeding events). Products include:

- Nalfon 200 Pulvules & Nalfon Tablets ... 917

Flurbiprofen (Increases risk of bleeding and bleeding events). Products include:

- Ansaid Tablets ... 2579

Heparin Calcium (Potential for bleeding and bleeding complications).

- No products indexed under this heading.

Heparin Sodium (Potential for bleeding and bleeding complications). Products include:

- Heparin Lock Flush Solution ... 2725
- Heparin Sodium Injection ... 2726
- Heparin Sodium Injection, USP, Sterile Solution ... 2615
- Heparin Sodium Vials ... 1441

Ibuprofen (Increases risk of bleeding and bleeding events). Products include:

- Advil Cold and Sinus Caplets and Tablets (formerly CoAdvil) ... ▣ 870
- Advil Ibuprofen Tablets and Caplets ... ▣ 870
- Children's Advil Suspension ... 2692
- Arthritis Foundation Ibuprofen Tablets ... ▣ 674
- Bayer Select Ibuprofen Pain Relief Formula ... ▣ 715
- Cramp End Tablets ... ▣ 735
- Dimetapp Sinus Caplets ... ▣ 775
- Haltran Tablets ... ▣ 771
- IBU Tablets ... 1342
- Ibuprohm ... ▣ 735
- Children's Motrin Ibuprofen Oral Suspension ... 1546
- Motrin Tablets ... 2625
- Motrin IB Caplets, Tablets, and Geltabs ... ▣ 838
- Motrin IB Sinus ... ▣ 838
- Motrin Ibuprofen Suspension, Oral Drops, Chewable Tablets, Caplets ... 1546
- Nuprin Ibuprofen/Analgesic Tablets & Caplets ... ▣ 622
- Sine-Aid IB Caplets ... 1554
- Vicks DayQuil SINUS Pressure & PAIN Relief with IBUPROFEN ... ▣ 762

Indomethacin (Increases risk of bleeding and bleeding events). Products include:

- Indocin ... 1680

Indomethacin Sodium Trihydrate (Increases risk of bleeding and bleeding events). Products include:

- Indocin I.V. ... 1684

Ketoprofen (Increases risk of bleeding and bleeding events). Products include:

- Orudis Capsules ... 2766
- Oruvail Capsules ... 2766

Magnesium Salicylate (Increases risk of bleeding and bleeding events). Products include:

- Backache Caplets ... ▣ 613
- Bayer Select Backache Pain Relief Formula ... ▣ 715
- Doan's Extra-Strength Analgesic ... ▣ 633
- Extra Strength Doan's P.M. ... ▣ 633
- Doan's Regular Strength Analgesic ... ▣ 634
- Mobigesic Tablets ... ▣ 602

Meclofenamate Sodium (Increases risk of bleeding and bleeding events).

- No products indexed under this heading.

Mefenamic Acid (Increases risk of bleeding and bleeding events). Products include:

- Ponstel ... 1925

Mezlocillin Sodium (Increases risk of bleeding and bleeding events). Products include:

- Mezlin ... 601
- Mezlin Pharmacy Bulk Package ... 604

Nafcillin Sodium (Increases risk of bleeding and bleeding events).

- No products indexed under this heading.

Naproxen (Increases risk of bleeding and bleeding events). Products include:

- Anaprox/Naprosyn ... 2117

Naproxen Sodium (Increases risk of bleeding and bleeding events). Products include:

- Aleve ... 1975
- Anaprox/Naprosyn ... 2117

Penicillin G Benzathine (Increases risk of bleeding and bleeding events). Products include:

- Bicillin C-R Injection ... 2704
- Bicillin C-R 900/300 Injection ... 2706
- Bicillin L-A Injection ... 2707

Penicillin G Procaine (Increases risk of bleeding and bleeding events). Products include:

- Bicillin C-R Injection ... 2704
- Bicillin C-R 900/300 Injection ... 2706

Phenylbutazone (Increases risk of bleeding and bleeding events).

- No products indexed under this heading.

Piroxicam (Increases risk of bleeding and bleeding events). Products include:

- Feldene Capsules ... 1965

Salsalate (Increases risk of bleeding and bleeding events). Products include:

- Mono-Gesic Tablets ... 792
- Salflex Tablets ... 786

Sulindac (Increases risk of bleeding and bleeding events). Products include:

- Clinoril Tablets ... 1618

Ticarcillin Disodium (Increases risk of bleeding and bleeding events). Products include:

- Ticar for Injection ... 2526
- Timentin for Injection ... 2528

Ticlopidine Hydrochloride (Increases risk of bleeding and bleeding events). Products include:

- Ticlid Tablets ... 2156

Tolmetin Sodium (Increases risk of bleeding and bleeding events). Products include:

- Tolectin (200, 400 and 600 mg) ... 1581

Warfarin Sodium (Potential for bleeding and bleeding complications). Products include:

- Coumadin ... 926

EMLA CREAM

(Prilocaine, Lidocaine) ... 545

May interact with methemoglobinemia-inducing drugs and certain other agents. Compounds in these categories include:

Acetaminophen (Potential for greater risk of developing methemoglobinemia). Products include:

- Actifed Plus Caplets ... ▣ 845
- Actifed Plus Tablets ... ▣ 845
- Actifed Sinus Daytime/Nighttime Tablets and Caplets ... ▣ 846
- Alka-Seltzer Plus Cold Medicine Liqui-Gels ... ▣ 706
- Alka-Seltzer Plus Cold & Cough Medicine Liqui-Gels ... ▣ 705
- Alka-Seltzer Plus Night-Time Cold Medicine Liqui-Gels ... ▣ 706
- Allerest Headache Strength Tablets ... ▣ 627
- Allerest No Drowsiness Tablets ... ▣ 627
- Allerest Sinus Pain Formula ... ▣ 627
- Anexsia 5/500 Elixir ... 1781
- Anexia Tablets ... 1782
- Arthritis Foundation Aspirin Free Caplets ... ▣ 673
- Arthritis Foundation NightTime Caplets ... ▣ 674
- Bayer Select Headache Pain Relief Formula ... ▣ 716
- Bayer Select Menstrual Multi-Symptom Formula ... ▣ 716
- Bayer Select Night Time Pain Relief Formula ... ▣ 716
- Bayer Select Sinus Pain Relief Formula ... ▣ 717
- Benadryl Allergy Sinus Headache Formula Caplets ... ▣ 849
- Comtrex Multi-Symptom Cold Reliever Tablets/Caplets/Liqui-Gels/Liquid ... ▣ 615
- Allergy-Sinus Comtrex Multi-Symptom Allergy-Sinus Formula Tablets ... ▣ 617
- Comtrex Non-Drowsy ... ▣ 618
- Contac Day Allergy/Sinus Caplets ▣ 812
- Contac Day & Night ... ▣ 812
- Contac Night Allergy/Sinus Caplets ... ▣ 812
- Contac Severe Cold and Flu Formula Caplets ... ▣ 814
- Contac Severe Cold & Flu Non-Drowsy ... ▣ 815
- Coricidin 'D' Decongestant Tablets ... ▣ 800
- Coricidin Tablets ... ▣ 800
- DHCplus Capsules ... 1993
- Darvon-N/Darvocet-N ... 1433
- Drixoral Cold and Flu Extended-Release Tablets ... ▣ 803
- Drixoral Cough + Sore Throat Liquid Caps ... ▣ 802
- Drixoral Allergy/Sinus Extended Release Tablets ... ▣ 804
- Esgic-plus Tablets ... 1013
- Aspirin Free Excedrin Analgesic Caplets and Geltabs ... 732
- Excedrin Extra-Strength Analgesic Tablets & Caplets ... 732
- Excedrin P.M. Analgesic/Sleeping Aid Tablets, Caplets, Liquigels ... 733
- Fioricet Tablets ... 2258
- Fioricet with Codeine Capsules ... 2260
- Hycomine Compound Tablets ... 932
- Hydrocet Capsules ... 782
- Legatrin PM ... ▣ 651
- Lorcet 10/650 ... 1018
- Lortab ... 2566
- Lurline PMS Tablets ... 982
- Maximum Strength Multi-Symptom Formula Midol ... ▣ 722
- PMS Multi-Symptom Formula Midol ... ▣ 723
- Teen Multi-Symptom Formula Midol ... ▣ 722
- Midrin Capsules ... 783
- Migralam Capsules ... 2038
- Panodol Tablets and Caplets ... ▣ 824
- Children's Panadol Chewable Tablets, Liquid, Infant's Drops ... ▣ 824
- Percocet Tablets ... 938
- Percogesic Analgesic Tablets ... ▣ 754
- Phrenilin ... 785
- Pyrroxate Caplets ... ▣ 772
- Sedapap Tablets 50 mg/650 mg .. 1543
- Sinarest Tablets ... ▣ 648
- Sinarest Extra Strength Tablets ... ▣ 648
- Sinarest No Drowsiness Tablets ... ▣ 648
- Sine-Aid Maximum Strength Sinus Medication Gelcaps, Caplets and Tablets ... 1554
- Sine-Off No Drowsiness Formula Caplets ... ▣ 824
- Sine-Off Sinus Medicine ... ▣ 825
- Singlet Tablets ... ▣ 825
- Sinulin Tablets ... 787
- Sinutab Sinus Allergy Medication, Maximum Strength Tablets and Caplets ... ▣ 860
- Sinutab Sinus Medication, Maximum Strength Without Drowsiness Formula, Tablets & Caplets ... ▣ 860
- Sinutab Sinus Medication, Regular Strength Without Drowsiness Formula ... ▣ 859
- Sudafed Cold and Cough Liquidcaps ... ▣ 862
- Sudafed Severe Cold Formula Caplets ... ▣ 863
- Sudafed Severe Cold Formula Tablets ... ▣ 864
- Sudafed Sinus Caplets ... ▣ 864
- Sudafed Sinus Tablets ... ▣ 864
- Talacen ... 2333
- TheraFlu ... ▣ 787
- TheraFlu Maximum Strength Nighttime Flu, Cold & Cough Medicine ... ▣ 788
- TheraFlu Maximum Strength Non-Drowsy Formula Flu, Cold & Cough Medicine ... ▣ 788
- Thera Flu Maximum Strength, Non-Drowsy Formula Flu, Cold and Cough Caplets ... ▣ 789
- Triaminic Sore Throat Formula ... ▣ 791
- Triaminicin Tablets ... ▣ 793
- Children's TYLENOL acetaminophen Chewable Tablets, Elixir, Suspension Liquid ... 1555
- Children's TYLENOL Cold Multi-Symptom Liquid Formula and Chewable Tablets ... 1561
- Children's TYLENOL Cold Plus Cough Multi Symptom Tablets and Liquid ... ▣ 681
- Infants' TYLENOL acetaminophen Drops and Suspension Drops ... 1555
- Infants' TYLENOL Cold Decongestant & Fever-Reducer Drops ... 1556
- TYLENOL Extended Relief Caplets .. 1558
- TYLENOL, Extra Strength, Acetaminophen Adult Liquid Pain Reliever ... 1560
- TYLENOL, Extra Strength, acetaminophen Gelcaps, Geltabs, Caplets, Tablets ... 1559
- TYLENOL, Extra Strength, Headache Plus Pain Reliever with Antacid Caplets ... 1559
- TYLENOL, Junior Strength, acetaminophen Coated Caplets, Grape and Fruit Chewable Tablets ... 1557
- TYLENOL Maximum Strength Allergy Sinus Medication Gelcaps and Caplets ... 1563
- TYLENOL Maximum Strength Allergy Sinus NightTime Medication Caplets ... 1555
- TYLENOL Flu Maximum Strength Gelcaps ... 1565
- TYLENOL Flu NightTime, Maximum Strength, Gelcaps ... 1566
- TYLENOL Maximum Strength Flu NightTime Hot Medication Packets ... 1562
- TYLENOL, Maximum Strength, Sinus Medication Geltabs, Gelcaps, Caplets and Tablets ... 1566
- TYLENOL Cold Multi-Symptom Formula Medication Tablets and Caplets ... 1561
- TYLENOL Cold Medication No Drowsiness Formula Gelcaps and Caplets ... 1562
- TYLENOL Cold Multi-Symptom Hot Medication Liquid Packets ... 1557

(▣ Described in PDR For Nonprescription Drugs) (◉ Described in PDR For Ophthalmology)

Interactions Index — Empirin with Codeine

TYLENOL Cough Multi-Symptom Medication 1564
TYLENOL Cough Multi-Symptom Medication with Decongestant 1565
TYLENOL, Regular Strength, acetaminophen Caplets and Tablets .. 1558
TYLENOL PM, Extra Strength Pain Reliever/Sleep Aid Caplets, Geltabs, Gelcaps 1560
TYLENOL Severe Allergy Medication Caplets 1564
Tylenol with Codeine 1583
Tylox Capsules 1584
Unisom With Pain Relief-Nighttime Sleep Aid and Pain Reliever............ 1934
Vanquish Analgesic Caplets .... ⊕ 731
Vicks 44 LiquiCaps Cough, Cold & Flu Relief .... ⊕ 755
Vicks 44M Cough, Cold & Flu Relief .... ⊕ 756
Vicks DayQuil .... ⊕ 761
Vicks Nyquil Hot Therapy................... ⊕ 762
Vicks NyQuil LiquiCaps Multi-Symptom Cold/Flu Relief .... ⊕ 763
Vicks NyQuil Multi-Symptom Cold/Flu Relief - (Original & Cherry Flavor) .... ⊕ 763
Vicodin Tablets 1356
Vicodin ES Tablets 1357
Wygesic Tablets 2827
Zydone Capsules 949

Amyl Nitrite (Potential for greater risk of developing methemoglobinemia).

No products indexed under this heading.

Bendroflumethiazide (Potential for greater risk of developing methemoglobinemia).

No products indexed under this heading.

Benzocaine (Potential for greater risk of developing methemoglobinemia). Products include:

Americaine Anesthetic Lubricant 983
Americaine Hemorrhoidal Ointment .... ⊕ 629
Americaine Otic Topical Anesthetic Ear Drops 983
Americaine .... ⊕ 629
Auralgan Otic Solution........................ 2703
BiCozene Creme................................... ⊕ 785
Cēpacol Anesthetic Lozenges .... ⊕ 875
Cetacaine Topical Anesthetic 794
Children's Vicks Chloraseptic Sore Throat Lozenges .... ⊕ 757
Cough-X Lozenges................................ ⊕ 602
Hurricaine 666
Hurricaine Topical 666
Baby Orajel Teething Pain Medicine .... ⊕ 652
Orajel Maximum Strength Toothache Medication .... ⊕ 652
Orajel Mouth-Aid for Canker and Cold Sores .... ⊕ 652
Tanac No Sting Liquid .... ⊕ 653
Tympagesic Ear Drops 2342
Vicks Chloraseptic Sore Throat Lozenges .... ⊕ 759
Zilactin-B Medicated Gel with Benzocaine .... ⊕ 882

Chloroquine (Potential for greater risk of developing methemoglobinemia).

Chloroquine Hydrochloride (Potential for greater risk of developing methemoglobinemia). Products include:

Aralen Hydrochloride Injection 2301

Chloroquine Phosphate (Potential for greater risk of developing methemoglobinemia). Products include:

Aralen Phosphate Tablets 2301

Chlorothiazide (Potential for greater risk of developing methemoglobinemia). Products include:

Aldoclor Tablets 1598
Diupres Tablets 1650
Diuril Oral 1653

Chlorothiazide Sodium (Potential for greater risk of developing methemoglobinemia). Products include:

Diuril Sodium Intravenous 1652

Chlorpropamide (Potential for greater risk of developing methemoglobinemia). Products include:

Diabinese Tablets 1935

Dapsone (Potential for greater risk of developing methemoglobinemia). Products include:

Dapsone Tablets USP 1284

Erythrityl Tetranitrate (Potential for greater risk of developing methemoglobinemia).

No products indexed under this heading.

Glipizide (Potential for greater risk of developing methemoglobinemia). Products include:

Glucotrol Tablets 1967
Glucotrol XL Extended Release Tablets 1968

Glyburide (Potential for greater risk of developing methemoglobinemia). Products include:

DiaBeta Tablets.................................... 1239
Glynase PresTab Tablets 2609
Micronase Tablets 2623

Hydrochlorothiazide (Potential for greater risk of developing methemoglobinemia). Products include:

Aldactazide... 2413
Aldoril Tablets...................................... 1604
Apresazide Capsules 808
Capozide 742
Dyazide 2479
Esidrix Tablets 821
Esimil Tablets 822
HydroDIURIL Tablets 1674
Hydropres Tablets................................ 1675
Hyzaar Tablets 1677
Inderide Tablets 2732
Inderide LA Long Acting Capsules .. 2734
Lopressor HCT Tablets 832
Lotensin HCT.. 837
Maxzide 1380
Moduretic Tablets 1705
Oretic Tablets 443
Prinzide Tablets 1737
Ser-Ap-Es Tablets 849
Timolide Tablets................................... 1748
Vaseretic Tablets 1765
Zestoretic 2850
Ziac 1415

Hydroflumethiazide (Potential for greater risk of developing methemoglobinemia). Products include:

Diucardin Tablets................................. 2718

Isosorbide Dinitrate (Potential for greater risk of developing methemoglobinemia). Products include:

Dilatrate-SR 2398
Isordil Sublingual Tablets................... 2739
Isordil Tembids..................................... 2741
Isordil Titradose Tablets..................... 2742
Sorbitrate 2843

Isosorbide Mononitrate (Potential for greater risk of developing methemoglobinemia). Products include:

Imdur 1323
Ismo Tablets 2738
Monoket... 2406

Methyclothiazide (Potential for greater risk of developing methemoglobinemia). Products include:

Enduron Tablets................................... 420

Mexiletine Hydrochloride (Potential for additive or synergistic toxic effects). Products include:

Mexitil Capsules 678

Nitrofurantoin (Potential for greater risk of developing methemoglobinemia). Products include:

Macrodantin Capsules 1989

Nitrofurantoin Monohydrate (Potential for greater risk of developing methemoglobinemia). Products include:

Macrobid Capsules 1988

Nitroglycerin (Potential for greater risk of developing methemoglobinemia). Products include:

Deponit NTG Transdermal Delivery System 2397
Nitro-Bid IV... 1523
Nitro-Bid Ointment 1524
Nitrodisc 2047
Nitro-Dur (nitroglycerin) Transdermal Infusion System 1326
Nitrolingual Spray 2027
Nitrostat Tablets 1925
Transderm-Nitro Transdermal Therapeutic System 859

Para-Aminosalicylic Acid (Potential for greater risk of developing methemoglobinemia).

Pentaerythritol Tetranitrate (Potential for greater risk of developing methemoglobinemia).

No products indexed under this heading.

Phenacetin (Potential for greater risk of developing methemoglobinemia).

Phenobarbital (Potential for greater risk of developing methemoglobinemia). Products include:

Arco-Lase Plus Tablets 512
Bellergal-S Tablets 2250
Donnatal 2060
Donnatal Extentabs............................. 2061
Donnatal Tablets 2060
Phenobarbital Elixir and Tablets 1469
Quadrinal Tablets 1350

Phenytoin (Potential for greater risk of developing methemoglobinemia). Products include:

Dilantin Infatabs 1908
Dilantin-125 Suspension 1911

Phenytoin Sodium (Potential for greater risk of developing methemoglobinemia). Products include:

Dilantin Kapseals 1906
Dilantin Parenteral 1910

Polythiazide (Potential for greater risk of developing methemoglobinemia). Products include:

Minizide Capsules 1938

Primaquine Phosphate (Potential for greater risk of developing methemoglobinemia).

No products indexed under this heading.

Quinine Sulfate (Potential for greater risk of developing methemoglobinemia).

No products indexed under this heading.

Sodium Nitroprusside (Potential for greater risk of developing methemoglobinemia).

No products indexed under this heading.

Sulfacytine (Potential for greater risk of developing methemoglobinemia).

Sulfamethizole (Potential for greater risk of developing methemoglobinemia). Products include:

Urobiotic-250 Capsules 2214

Sulfamethoxazole (Potential for greater risk of developing methemoglobinemia). Products include:

Azo Gantanol Tablets.......................... 2080
Bactrim DS Tablets.............................. 2084
Bactrim I.V. Infusion........................... 2082
Bactrim 2084
Gantanol Tablets 2119
Septra 1174
Septra I.V. Infusion 1169
Septra I.V. Infusion ADD-Vantage Vials... 1171
Septra 1174

Sulfasalazine (Potential for greater risk of developing methemoglobinemia). Products include:

Azulfidine 1949

Sulfinpyrazone (Potential for greater risk of developing methemoglobinemia). Products include:

Anturane 807

Sulfisoxazole (Potential for greater risk of developing methemoglobinemia). Products include:

Azo Gantrisin Tablets.......................... 2081
Gantrisin Tablets 2120

Sulfisoxazole Diolamine (Potential for greater risk of developing methemoglobinemia).

No products indexed under this heading.

Tocainide Hydrochloride (Potential for additive or synergistic toxic effects). Products include:

Tonocard Tablets.................................. 531

Tolazamide (Potential for greater risk of developing methemoglobinemia).

No products indexed under this heading.

Tolbutamide (Potential for greater risk of developing methemoglobinemia).

No products indexed under this heading.

EMPIRIN ASPIRIN TABLETS

(Aspirin) .... ⊕ 854

May interact with oral anticoagulants. Compounds in this category include:

Dicumarol (Concurrent administration is not recommended).

No products indexed under this heading.

Warfarin Sodium (Concurrent administration is not recommended). Products include:

Coumadin 926

EMPIRIN WITH CODEINE TABLETS

(Aspirin, Codeine Phosphate) 1093

May interact with central nervous system depressants, monoamine oxidase inhibitors, oral anticoagulants, oral hypoglycemic agents, penicillins, sulfonamides, non-steroidal anti-inflammatory agents, narcotic analgesics, general anesthetics, tranquilizers, corticosteroids, hypnotics and sedatives, and certain other agents. Compounds in these categories include:

Acarbose (May result in hypoglycemia).

No products indexed under this heading.

Alfentanil Hydrochloride (Increased CNS depression). Products include:

Alfenta Injection 1286

Alprazolam (Increased CNS depression). Products include:

Xanax Tablets 2649

Amoxicillin Trihydrate (Enhanced effect). Products include:

Amoxil.. 2464
Augmentin 2468

Ampicillin Sodium (Enhanced effect). Products include:

Unasyn 2212

Aprobarbital (Increased CNS depression).

No products indexed under this heading.

Azlocillin Sodium (Enhanced effect).

No products indexed under this heading.

Bacampicillin Hydrochloride (Enhanced effect). Products include:

Spectrobid Tablets 2206

IMPORTANT NOTE: Always consult each drug listing in the patient's regimen for possible interactions.

Empirin with Codeine — Interactions Index — 372

Betamethasone Acetate (Steroid effects potentiated). Products include:
Celestone Soluspan Suspension 2347

Betamethasone Sodium Phosphate (Steroid effects potentiated). Products include:
Celestone Soluspan Suspension 2347

Buprenorphine (Increased CNS depression). Products include:
Buprenex Injectable 2006

Buspirone Hydrochloride (Increased CNS depression). Products include:
BuSpar 737

Butabarbital (Increased CNS depression).
No products indexed under this heading.

Butalbital (Increased CNS depression). Products include:
Esgic-plus Tablets 1013
Fioricet Tablets 2258
Fioricet with Codeine Capsules 2260
Fiorinal Capsules 2261
Fiorinal with Codeine Capsules 2262
Fiorinal Tablets 2261
Phrenilin 785
Sedapap Tablets 50 mg/650 mg .. 1543

Carbenicillin Disodium (Enhanced effect).
No products indexed under this heading.

Carbenicillin Indanyl Sodium (Enhanced effect). Products include:
Geocillin Tablets 2199

Chlordiazepoxide (Increased CNS depression). Products include:
Libritabs Tablets 2177
Limbitrol 2180

Chlordiazepoxide Hydrochloride (Increased CNS depression). Products include:
Librax Capsules 2176
Librium Capsules 2178
Librium Injectable 2179

Chlorpromazine (Increased CNS depression). Products include:
Thorazine Suppositories 2523

Chlorpropamide (May result in hypoglycemia). Products include:
Diabinese Tablets 1935

Chlorprothixene (Increased CNS depression).
No products indexed under this heading.

Chlorprothixene Hydrochloride (Increased CNS depression).
No products indexed under this heading.

Chlorprothixene Lactate (Increased CNS depression).
No products indexed under this heading.

Clorazepate Dipotassium (Increased CNS depression). Products include:
Tranxene 451

Clozapine (Increased CNS depression). Products include:
Clozaril Tablets 2252

Colchicine (Diminished uricosoric effect). Products include:
ColBENEMID Tablets 1622

Cortisone Acetate (Steroid effects potentiated). Products include:
Cortone Acetate Sterile Suspension 1623
Cortone Acetate Tablets 1624

Desflurane (Increased CNS depression). Products include:
Suprane 1813

Dexamethasone (Steroid effects potentiated). Products include:
AK-Trol Ointment & Suspension .... ⊙ 205
Decadron Elixir 1633
Decadron Tablets 1635
Decaspray Topical Aerosol 1648
Dexacidin Ointment ...... ⊙ 263
Maxitrol Ophthalmic Ointment and Suspension ...... ⊙ 224
TobraDex Ophthalmic Suspension and Ointment 473

Dexamethasone Acetate (Steroid effects potentiated). Products include:
Dalalone D.P. Injectable 1011
Decadron-LA Sterile Suspension 1646

Dexamethasone Sodium Phosphate (Steroid effects potentiated). Products include:
Decadron Phosphate Injection 1637
Decadron Phosphate Respihaler 1642
Decadron Phosphate Sterile Ophthalmic Ointment 1641
Decadron Phosphate Sterile Ophthalmic Solution 1642
Decadron Phosphate Topical Cream 1644
Decadron Phosphate Turbinaire 1645
Decadron Phosphate with Xylocaine Injection, Sterile 1639
Dexacort Phosphate in Respihaler .. 458
Dexacort Phosphate in Turbinaire .. 459
NeoDecadron Sterile Ophthalmic Ointment 1712
NeoDecadron Sterile Ophthalmic Solution 1713
NeoDecadron Topical Cream 1714

Dezocine (Increased CNS depression). Products include:
Dalgan Injection 538

Diazepam (Increased CNS depression). Products include:
Dizac 1809
Valium Injectable 2182
Valium Tablets 2183
Valrelease Capsules 2169

Diclofenac Potassium (Enhanced effect of NSAID). Products include:
Cataflam 816

Diclofenac Sodium (Enhanced effect of NSAID). Products include:
Voltaren Ophthalmic Sterile Ophthalmic Solution ...... ⊙ 272
Voltaren Tablets 861

Dicloxacillin Sodium (Enhanced effect).
No products indexed under this heading.

Dicumarol (Enhanced effect, bleeding).
No products indexed under this heading.

Droperidol (Increased CNS depression). Products include:
Inapsine Injection 1296

Enflurane (Increased CNS depression).
No products indexed under this heading.

Estazolam (Increased CNS depression). Products include:
ProSom Tablets 449

Ethchlorvynol (Increased CNS depression). Products include:
Placidyl Capsules 448

Ethinamate (Increased CNS depression).
No products indexed under this heading.

Etodolac (Enhanced effect of NSAID). Products include:
Lodine Capsules and Tablets 2743

Fenoprofen Calcium (Enhanced effect of NSAID). Products include:
Nalfon 200 Pulvules & Nalfon Tablets 917

Fentanyl (Increased CNS depression). Products include:
Duragesic Transdermal System 1288

Fentanyl Citrate (Increased CNS depression). Products include:
Sublimaze Injection 1307

Fludrocortisone Acetate (Steroid effects potentiated). Products include:
Florinef Acetate Tablets 505

Fluphenazine Decanoate (Increased CNS depression). Products include:
Prolixin Decanoate 509

Fluphenazine Enanthate (Increased CNS depression). Products include:
Prolixin Enanthate 509

Fluphenazine Hydrochloride (Increased CNS depression). Products include:
Prolixin 509

Flurazepam Hydrochloride (Increased CNS depression). Products include:
Dalmane Capsules 2173

Flurbiprofen (Enhanced effect of NSAID). Products include:
Ansaid Tablets 2579

Furazolidone (Enhanced effect). Products include:
Furoxone 2046

Furosemide (Causes aspirin accumulation). Products include:
Lasix Injection, Oral Solution and Tablets 1240

Glipizide (May result in hypoglycemia). Products include:
Glucotrol Tablets 1967
Glucotrol XL Extended Release Tablets 1968

Glutethimide (Increased CNS depression).
No products indexed under this heading.

Glyburide (May result in hypoglycemia). Products include:
DiaBeta Tablets 1239
Glynase PresTab Tablets 2609
Micronase Tablets 2623

Haloperidol (Increased CNS depression). Products include:
Haldol Injection, Tablets and Concentrate 1575

Haloperidol Decanoate (Increased CNS depression). Products include:
Haldol Decanoate 1577

Hydrocodone Bitartrate (Increased CNS depression). Products include:
Anexsia 5/500 Elixir 1781
Anexia Tablets 1782
Codiclear DH Syrup 791
Deconamine CX Cough and Cold Liquid and Tablets 1319
Duratuss HD Elixir 2565
Hycodan Tablets and Syrup 930
Hycomine Compound Tablets 932
Hycomine 931
Hycotuss Expectorant Syrup 933
Hydrocet Capsules 782
Lorcet 10/650 1018
Lortab 2566
Tussend 1783
Tussend Expectorant 1785
Vicodin Tablets 1356
Vicodin ES Tablets 1357
Vicodin Tuss Expectorant 1358
Zydone Capsules 949

Hydrocodone Polistirex (Increased CNS depression). Products include:
Tussionex Pennkinetic Extended-Release Suspension 998

Hydrocortisone Acetate (Steroid effects potentiated). Products include:
Analpram-HC Rectal Cream 1% and 2.5% 977
Anusol HC-1 Anti-Itch Hydrocortisone Ointment ...... ▣ 847
Anusol-HC Suppositories 1897
Caldecort ...... ▣ 631
Carmol HC 924
Coly-Mycin S Otic w/Neomycin & Hydrocortisone 1906
Cortaid ...... ▣ 836
Cortifoam 2396
Cortisporin Cream 1084
Epifoam 2399
Hydrocortone Acetate Sterile Suspension 1669
Mantadil Cream 1135
Nupercainal Hydrocortisone 1% Cream ...... ▣ 645
Ophthocort ...... ⊙ 311
Pramosone Cream, Lotion & Ointment 978
ProctoCream-HC 2408
ProctoFoam-HC 2409
Terra-Cortril Ophthalmic Suspension 2210

Hydrocortisone Sodium Phosphate (Steroid effects potentiated). Products include:
Hydrocortone Phosphate Injection, Sterile 1670

Hydrocortisone Sodium Succinate (Steroid effects potentiated). Products include:
Solu-Cortef Sterile Powder 2641

Hydroxyzine Hydrochloride (Increased CNS depression). Products include:
Atarax Tablets & Syrup 2185
Marax Tablets & DF Syrup 2200
Vistaril Intramuscular Solution 2216

Ibuprofen (Enhanced effect of NSAID). Products include:
Advil Cold and Sinus Caplets and Tablets (formerly CoAdvil) ...... ▣ 870
Advil Ibuprofen Tablets and Caplets ...... ▣ 870
Children's Advil Suspension 2692
Arthritis Foundation Ibuprofen Tablets ...... ▣ 674
Bayer Select Ibuprofen Pain Relief Formula ...... ▣ 715
Cramp End Tablets ...... ▣ 735
Dimetapp Sinus Caplets ...... ▣ 775
Haltran Tablets ...... ▣ 771
IBU Tablets 1342
Ibuprohm ...... ▣ 735
Children's Motrin Ibuprofen Oral Suspension 1546
Motrin Tablets 2625
Motrin IB Caplets, Tablets, and Geltabs ...... ▣ 838
Motrin IB Sinus ...... ▣ 838
Motrin Ibuprofen Suspension, Oral Drops, Chewable Tablets, Caplets 1546
Nuprin Ibuprofen/Analgesic Tablets & Caplets ...... ▣ 622
Sine-Aid IB Caplets 1554
Vicks DayQuil SINUS Pressure & PAIN Relief with IBUPROFEN ...... ▣ 762

Indomethacin (Enhanced effect of NSAID). Products include:
Indocin 1680

Indomethacin Sodium Trihydrate (Enhanced effect of NSAID). Products include:
Indocin I.V. 1684

Isocarboxazid (Enhanced effect).
No products indexed under this heading.

Isoflurane (Increased CNS depression).
No products indexed under this heading.

Ketamine Hydrochloride (Increased CNS depression).
No products indexed under this heading.

Ketoprofen (Enhanced effect of NSAID). Products include:
Orudis Capsules 2766
Oruvail Capsules 2766

Ketorolac Tromethamine (Enhanced effect of NSAID). Products include:
Acular 474
Acular ...... ⊙ 277
Toradol 2159

Levomethadyl Acetate Hydrochloride (Increased CNS depression). Products include:
Orlamm 2239

Levorphanol Tartrate (Increased CNS depression). Products include:
Levo-Dromoran 2129

(▣ Described in PDR For Nonprescription Drugs) (⊙ Described in PDR For Ophthalmology)

373 Interactions Index Empirin with Codeine

Lorazepam (Increased CNS depression). Products include:
- Ativan Injection ... 2698
- Ativan Tablets ... 2700

Loxapine Hydrochloride (Increased CNS depression). Products include:
- Loxitane ... 1378

Loxapine Succinate (Increased CNS depression). Products include:
- Loxitane Capsules ... 1378

Meclofenamate Sodium (Enhanced effect of NSAID).
- No products indexed under this heading.

Mefenamic Acid (Enhanced effect of NSAIDS). Products include:
- Ponstel ... 1925

Meperidine Hydrochloride (Increased CNS depression). Products include:
- Demerol ... 2308
- Mepergan Injection ... 2753

Mephobarbital (Increased CNS depression). Products include:
- Mebaral Tablets ... 2322

Meprobamate (Increased CNS depression). Products include:
- Miltown Tablets ... 2672
- PMB 200 and PMB 400 ... 2783

Mercaptopurine (Enhanced bone marrow toxicity and blood dyscrasias). Products include:
- Purinethol Tablets ... 1156

Mesoridazine Besylate (Increased CNS depression). Products include:
- Serentil ... 684

Metformin Hydrochloride (May result in hypoglycemia). Products include:
- Glucophage ... 752

Methadone Hydrochloride (Increased CNS depression). Products include:
- Methadone Hydrochloride Oral Concentrate ... 2233
- Methadone Hydrochloride Oral Solution & Tablets ... 2235

Methohexital Sodium (Increased CNS depression). Products include:
- Brevital Sodium Vials ... 1429

Methotrimeprazine (Increased CNS depression). Products include:
- Levoprome ... 1274

Methoxyflurane (Increased CNS depression).
- No products indexed under this heading.

Methylprednisolone (Steroid effects potentiated). Products include:
- Medrol ... 2621

Methylprednisolone Acetate (Steroid effects potentiated). Products include:
- Depo-Medrol Single-Dose Vial ... 2600
- Depo-Medrol Sterile Aqueous Suspension ... 2597

Methylprednisolone Sodium Succinate (Steroid effects potentiated). Products include:
- Solu-Medrol Sterile Powder ... 2643

Mezlocillin Sodium (Enhanced effect). Products include:
- Mezlin ... 601
- Mezlin Pharmacy Bulk Package ... 604

Midazolam Hydrochloride (Increased CNS depression). Products include:
- Versed Injection ... 2170

Molindone Hydrochloride (Increased CNS depression). Products include:
- Moban Tablets and Concentrate ... 1048

Morphine Sulfate (Increased CNS depression). Products include:
- Astramorph/PF Injection, USP (Preservative-Free) ... 535
- Duramorph ... 962
- Infumorph 200 and Infumorph 500 Sterile Solutions ... 965
- MS Contin Tablets ... 1994
- MSIR ... 1997
- Oramorph SR (Morphine Sulfate Sustained Release Tablets) ... 2236
- RMS Suppositories ... 2657
- Roxanol ... 2243

Nabumetone (Enhanced effect of NSAID). Products include:
- Relafen Tablets ... 2510

Nafcillin Sodium (Enhanced effect).
- No products indexed under this heading.

Naproxen (Enhanced effect of NSAID). Products include:
- Anaprox/Naprosyn ... 2117

Naproxen Sodium (Enhanced effect of NSAID). Products include:
- Aleve ... 1975
- Anaprox/Naprosyn ... 2117

Opium Alkaloids (Increased CNS depression).
- No products indexed under this heading.

Oxaprozin (Enhanced effect of NSAID). Products include:
- Daypro Caplets ... 2426

Oxazepam (Increased CNS depression). Products include:
- Serax Capsules ... 2810
- Serax Tablets ... 2810

Oxycodone Hydrochloride (Increased CNS depression). Products include:
- Percocet Tablets ... 938
- Percodan Tablets ... 939
- Percodan-Demi Tablets ... 940
- Roxicodone Tablets, Oral Solution & Intensol (Oxycodone) ... 2244
- Tylox Capsules ... 1584

Penicillin G Benzathine (Enhanced effect). Products include:
- Bicillin C-R Injection ... 2704
- Bicillin C-R 900/300 Injection ... 2706
- Bicillin L-A Injection ... 2707

Penicillin G Potassium (Enhanced effect). Products include:
- Pfizerpen for Injection ... 2203

Penicillin G Procaine (Enhanced effect). Products include:
- Bicillin C-R Injection ... 2704
- Bicillin C-R 900/300 Injection ... 2706

Penicillin G Sodium (Enhanced effect).
- No products indexed under this heading.

Penicillin V Potassium (Enhanced effect). Products include:
- Pen•Vee K ... 2772

Pentobarbital Sodium (Increased CNS depression). Products include:
- Nembutal Sodium Capsules ... 436
- Nembutal Sodium Solution ... 438
- Nembutal Sodium Suppositories ... 440

Perphenazine (Increased CNS depression). Products include:
- Etrafon ... 2355
- Triavil Tablets ... 1757
- Trilafon ... 2389

Phenelzine Sulfate (Enhanced effect). Products include:
- Nardil ... 1920

Phenobarbital (Increased CNS depression). Products include:
- Arco-Lase Plus Tablets ... 512
- Bellergal-S Tablets ... 2250
- Donnatal ... 2060
- Donnatal Extentabs ... 2061
- Donnatal Tablets ... 2060
- Phenobarbital Elixir and Tablets ... 1469
- Quadrinal Tablets ... 1350

Phenylbutazone (Enhanced effect of NSAID).
- No products indexed under this heading.

Piroxicam (Enhanced effect of NSAID). Products include:
- Feldene Capsules ... 1965

Prazepam (Increased CNS depression).
- No products indexed under this heading.

Prednisolone Acetate (Steroid effects potentiated). Products include:
- AK-CIDE ... ◉ 202
- AK-CIDE Ointment ... ◉ 202
- Blephamide Liquifilm Sterile Ophthalmic Suspension ... 476
- Blephamide Ointment ... ◉ 237
- Econopred & Econopred Plus Ophthalmic Suspensions ... ◉ 217
- Poly-Pred Liquifilm ... ◉ 248
- Pred Forte ... ◉ 250
- Pred Mild ... ◉ 253
- Pred-G Liquifilm Sterile Ophthalmic Suspension ... ◉ 251
- Pred-G S.O.P. Sterile Ophthalmic Ointment ... ◉ 252
- Vasocidin Ointment ... ◉ 268

Prednisolone Sodium Phosphate (Steroid effects potentiated). Products include:
- AK-Pred ... ◉ 204
- Hydeltrasol Injection, Sterile ... 1665
- Inflamase ... ◉ 265
- Pediapred Oral Liquid ... 995
- Vasocidin Ophthalmic Solution ... ◉ 270

Prednisolone Tebutate (Steroid effects potentiated). Products include:
- Hydeltra-T.B.A. Sterile Suspension 1667

Prednisone (Steroid effects potentiated). Products include:
- Deltasone Tablets ... 2595

Probenecid (Diminished uricosuric effect). Products include:
- Benemid Tablets ... 1611
- ColBENEMID Tablets ... 1622

Prochlorperazine (Increased CNS depression). Products include:
- Compazine ... 2470

Promethazine Hydrochloride (Increased CNS depression). Products include:
- Mepergan Injection ... 2753
- Phenergan with Codeine ... 2777
- Phenergan with Dextromethorphan 2778
- Phenergan Injection ... 2773
- Phenergan Suppositories ... 2775
- Phenergan Syrup ... 2774
- Phenergan Tablets ... 2775
- Phenergan VC ... 2779
- Phenergan VC with Codeine ... 2781

Propofol (Increased CNS depression). Products include:
- Diprivan Injection ... 2833

Propoxyphene Hydrochloride (Increased CNS depression). Products include:
- Darvon ... 1435
- Wygesic Tablets ... 2827

Propoxyphene Napsylate (Increased CNS depression). Products include:
- Darvon-N/Darvocet-N ... 1433

Quazepam (Increased CNS depression). Products include:
- Doral Tablets ... 2664

Risperidone (Increased CNS depression). Products include:
- Risperdal ... 1301

Secobarbital Sodium (Increased CNS depression). Products include:
- Seconal Sodium Pulvules ... 1474

Selegiline Hydrochloride (Enhanced effect). Products include:
- Eldepryl Tablets ... 2550

Sufentanil Citrate (Increased CNS depression). Products include:
- Sufenta Injection ... 1309

Sulfamethizole (Enhanced effect of sulfonamides). Products include:
- Urobiotic-250 Capsules ... 2214

Sulfamethoxazole (Enhanced effect of sulfonamides). Products include:
- Azo Gantanol Tablets ... 2080
- Bactrim DS Tablets ... 2084
- Bactrim I.V. Infusion ... 2082
- Bactrim ... 2084
- Gantanol Tablets ... 2119
- Septra ... 1174
- Septra I.V. Infusion ... 1169
- Septra I.V. Infusion ADD-Vantage Vials ... 1171
- Septra ... 1174

Sulfasalazine (Enhanced effect of sulfonamides). Products include:
- Azulfidine ... 1949

Sulfinpyrazone (Diminished uricosuric effect). Products include:
- Anturane ... 807

Sulfisoxazole (Enhanced effect of sulfonamides). Products include:
- Azo Gantrisin Tablets ... 2081
- Gantrisin Tablets ... 2120

Sulfisoxazole Diolamine (Enhanced effect of sulfonamides).
- No products indexed under this heading.

Sulindac (Enhanced effect of NSAID). Products include:
- Clinoril Tablets ... 1618

Temazepam (Increased CNS depression). Products include:
- Restoril Capsules ... 2284

Thiamylal Sodium (Increased CNS depression).
- No products indexed under this heading.

Thioridazine Hydrochloride (Increased CNS depression). Products include:
- Mellaril ... 2269

Thiothixene (Increased CNS depression). Products include:
- Navane Capsules and Concentrate 2201
- Navane Intramuscular ... 2202

Ticarcillin Disodium (Enhanced effect). Products include:
- Ticar for Injection ... 2526
- Timentin for Injection ... 2528

Tolazamide (May result in hypoglycemia).
- No products indexed under this heading.

Tolbutamide (May result in hypoglycemia).
- No products indexed under this heading.

Tolmetin Sodium (Enhanced effect of NSAID). Products include:
- Tolectin (200, 400 and 600 mg) .. 1581

Tranylcypromine Sulfate (Enhanced effect). Products include:
- Parnate Tablets ... 2503

Triamcinolone (Steroid effects potentiated). Products include:
- Aristocort Tablets ... 1022

Triamcinolone Acetonide (Steroid effects potentiated). Products include:
- Aristocort A 0.025% Cream ... 1027
- Aristocort A 0.5% Cream ... 1031
- Aristocort A 0.1% Cream ... 1029
- Aristocort A 0.1% Ointment ... 1030
- Azmacort Oral Inhaler ... 2011
- Nasacort Nasal Inhaler ... 2024

Triamcinolone Diacetate (Steroid effects potentiated). Products include:
- Aristocort Suspension (Forte Parenteral) ... 1027
- Aristocort Suspension (Intralesional) ... 1025

Triamcinolone Hexacetonide (Steroid effects potentiated). Products include:
- Aristospan Suspension (Intra-articular) ... 1033

IMPORTANT NOTE: Always consult each drug listing in the patient's regimen for possible interactions.

Aristospan Suspension (Intralesional) ... 1032

Triazolam (Increased CNS depression). Products include:

Halcion Tablets ... 2611

Trifluoperazine Hydrochloride (Increased CNS depression). Products include:

Stelazine ... 2514

Vitamin C (Causes aspirin accumulation). Products include:

ANTIOX Capsules ... 1543
C-Buff ... 667
Centrum Singles Vitamin C ... ▣ 669
Chromagen Capsules ... 2339
Dexatrim Maximum Strength Plus Vitamin C/Caffeine-free Caplets ▣ 832
Ester-C Mineral Ascorbates Powder ... ▣ 658
Fero-Folic-500 Filmtab ... 429
Fero-Grad-500 Filmtab ... 429
Halls Vitamin C Drops ... ▣ 843
Hyland's Vitamin C for Children ... ▣ 830
Irospan ... 982
Materna Tablets ... 1379
Nature Made Antioxidant Formula ▣ 748
Niferex w/Vitamin C Tablets ... 793
One-A-Day Extras Antioxidant ... ▣ 728
One-A-Day Extras Vitamin C ... ▣ 728
Protegra Antioxidant Vitamin & Mineral Supplement ... ▣ 670
Stuart Prenatal Tablets ... ▣ 881
The Stuart Formula Tablets ... ▣ 663
Sunkist Children's Chewable Multivitamins - Plus Extra C ... ▣ 649
Sunkist Vitamin C ... ▣ 649
Theragran Antioxidant ... ▣ 623
Trinsicon Capsules ... 2570
Vitron-C Tablets ... ▣ 650

Warfarin Sodium (Enhanced effect, bleeding). Products include:

Coumadin ... 926

Zolpidem Tartrate (Increased CNS depression). Products include:

Ambien Tablets ... 2416

Food Interactions

Alcohol (Increased CNS depressant).

Food, unspecified (The presence of food slightly delays absorption).

ENCARE VAGINAL CONTRACEPTIVE SUPPOSITORIES

(Nonoxynol-9) ... ▣ 833
None cited in PDR database.

ENDEP TABLETS

(Amitriptyline Hydrochloride) ... 2174
May interact with monoamine oxidase inhibitors, central nervous system depressants, anticholinergics, sympathomimetics, thyroid preparations, drugs that inhibit cytochrome p450iid6, selective serotonin reuptake inhibitors, antidepressant drugs, phenothiazines, and certain other agents. Compounds in these categories include:

Albuterol (Careful dosage adjustments required). Products include:

Proventil Inhalation Aerosol ... 2382
Ventolin Inhalation Aerosol and Refill ... 1197

Albuterol Sulfate (Careful dosage adjustments required). Products include:

Airet Solution for Inhalation ... 452
Proventil Inhalation Solution 0.083% ... 2384
Proventil Repetabs Tablets ... 2386
Proventil Solution for Inhalation 0.5% ... 2383
Proventil Syrup ... 2385
Proventil Tablets ... 2386
Ventolin Inhalation Solution ... 1198
Ventolin Nebules Inhalation Solution ... 1199
Ventolin Rotacaps for Inhalation ... 1200
Ventolin Syrup ... 1202
Ventolin Tablets ... 1203
Volmax Extended-Release Tablets .. 1788

Alfentanil Hydrochloride (Increased response to the effects of CNS depressants). Products include:

Alfenta Injection ... 1286

Alprazolam (Increased response to the effects of CNS depressants). Products include:

Xanax Tablets ... 2649

Amoxapine (Concomitant use of amitryptyline with drugs that can inhibit cytochrome P_{450}IID6 may require lower than usually prescribed for either the tricyclic antidepressant or the other drug). Products include:

Asendin Tablets ... 1369

Aprobarbital (Increased response to the effects of CNS depressants).

No products indexed under this heading.

Atropine Sulfate (Paralytic ileus). Products include:

Arco-Lase Plus Tablets ... 512
Atrohist Plus Tablets ... 454
Atropine Sulfate Sterile Ophthalmic Solution ... ◉ 233
Donnatal ... 2060
Donnatal Extentabs ... 2061
Donnatal Tablets ... 2060
Lomotil ... 2439
Motofen Tablets ... 784
Urised Tablets ... 1964

Belladonna Alkaloids (Paralytic ileus). Products include:

Bellergal-S Tablets ... 2250
Hyland's Bed Wetting Tablets ... ▣ 828
Hyland's EnurAid Tablets ... ▣ 829
Hyland's Teething Tablets ... ▣ 830

Benztropine Mesylate (Paralytic ileus). Products include:

Cogentin ... 1621

Biperiden Hydrochloride (Paralytic ileus). Products include:

Akineton ... 1333

Buprenorphine (Increased response to the effects of CNS depressants). Products include:

Buprenex Injectable ... 2006

Bupropion Hydrochloride (Concomitant use of amitryptyline with drugs that can inhibit cytochrome P_{450}IID6 may require lower than usually prescribed for either the tricyclic antidepressant or the other drug). Products include:

Wellbutrin Tablets ... 1204

Buspirone Hydrochloride (Increased response to the effects of CNS depressants). Products include:

BuSpar ... 737

Butabarbital (Increased response to the effects of CNS depressants).

No products indexed under this heading.

Butalbital (Increased response to the effects of CNS depressants). Products include:

Esgic-plus Tablets ... 1013
Fioricet Tablets ... 2258
Fioricet with Codeine Capsules ... 2260
Fiorinal Capsules ... 2261
Fiorinal with Codeine Capsules ... 2262
Fiorinal Tablets ... 2261
Phrenilin ... 785
Sedapap Tablets 50 mg/650 mg .. 1543

Chlordiazepoxide (Increased response to the effects of CNS depressants). Products include:

Libritabs Tablets ... 2177
Limbitrol ... 2180

Chlordiazepoxide Hydrochloride (Increased response to the effects of CNS depressants). Products include:

Librax Capsules ... 2176
Librium Capsules ... 2178
Librium Injectable ... 2179

Chlorpromazine (Increased response to the effects of CNS depressants). Products include:

Thorazine Suppositories ... 2523

Chlorpromazine Hydrochloride (Increased response to the effects of CNS depressants). Products include:

Thorazine ... 2523

Chlorprothixene (Increased response to the effects of CNS depressants).

No products indexed under this heading.

Chlorprothixene Hydrochloride (Increased response to the effects of CNS depressants).

No products indexed under this heading.

Cimetidine (Concomitant use of amitryptyline with drugs that can inhibit cytochrome P_{450}IID6 may require lower than usually prescribed for either the tricyclic antidepressant or the other drug; increased plasma levels of tricyclic antidepressants; increased frequency of anticholinergic side effects). Products include:

Tagamet Tablets ... 2516

Cimetidine Hydrochloride (Concomitant use of amitryptyline with drugs that can inhibit cytochrome P450 IID6 may require lower than usually prescribed for either the tricyclic antidepressant or the other drug; increased plasma levels of tricyclic antidepressants; increased frequency of anitcholinergic side effects). Products include:

Tagamet ... 2516

Clidinium Bromide (Paralytic ileus). Products include:

Librax Capsules ... 2176
Quarzan Capsules ... 2181

Clorazepate Dipotassium (Increased response to the effects of CNS depressants). Products include:

Tranxene ... 451

Clozapine (Increased response to the effects of CNS depressants). Products include:

Clozaril Tablets ... 2252

Codeine Phosphate (Increased response to the effects of CNS depressants). Products include:

Actifed with Codeine Cough Syrup.. 1067
Brontex ... 1981
Deconsal C Expectorant Syrup ... 456
Deconsal Pediatric Syrup ... 457
Dimetane-DC Cough Syrup ... 2059
Empirin with Codeine Tablets ... 1093
Fioricet with Codeine Capsules ... 2260
Fiorinal with Codeine Capsules ... 2262
Isoclor Expectorant ... 990
Novahistine DH ... 2462
Novahistine Expectorant ... 2463
Nucofed ... 2051
Phenergan with Codeine ... 2777
Phenergan VC with Codeine ... 2781
Robitussin A-C Syrup ... 2073
Robitussin-DAC Syrup ... 2074
Ryna ... ▣ 841
Soma Compound w/Codeine Tablets ... 2676
Tussi-Organidin NR Liquid and S NR Liquid ... 2677
Tylenol with Codeine ... 1583

Desflurane (Increased response to the effects of CNS depressants). Products include:

Suprane ... 1813

Desipramine Hydrochloride (Concomitant use of amitryptyline with drugs that can inhibit cytochrome P_{450}IID6 may require lower than usually prescribed for either the tricyclic antidepressant or the other drug). Products include:

Norpramin Tablets ... 1526

Dezocine (Increased response to the effects of CNS depressants). Products include:

Dalgan Injection ... 538

Diazepam (Increased response to the effects of CNS depressants). Products include:

Dizac ... 1809
Valium Injectable ... 2182
Valium Tablets ... 2183
Valrelease Capsules ... 2169

Dicyclomine Hydrochloride (Paralytic ileus). Products include:

Bentyl ... 1501

Disulfiram (Delirium may result). Products include:

Antabuse Tablets ... 2695

Dobutamine Hydrochloride (Careful dosage adjustments required). Products include:

Dobutrex Solution Vials ... 1439

Dopamine Hydrochloride (Careful dosage adjustments required).

No products indexed under this heading.

Doxepin Hydrochloride (Concomitant use of amitryptyline with drugs that can inhibit cytochrome P_{450}IID6 may require lower than usually prescribed for either the tricyclic antidepressant or the other drug). Products include:

Sinequan ... 2205
Zonalon Cream ... 1055

Droperidol (Increased response to the effects of CNS depressants). Products include:

Inapsine Injection ... 1296

Enflurane (Increased response to the effects of CNS depressants).

No products indexed under this heading.

Ephedrine Hydrochloride (Careful dosage adjustments required). Products include:

Primatene Dual Action Formula ... ▣ 872
Primatene Tablets ... ▣ 873
Quadrinal Tablets ... 1350

Ephedrine Sulfate (Careful dosage adjustments required). Products include:

Bronkaid Caplets ... ▣ 717
Marax Tablets & DF Syrup ... 2200

Ephedrine Tannate (Careful dosage adjustments required). Products include:

Rynatuss ... 2673

Epinephrine (Careful dosage adjustments required). Products include:

Bronkaid Mist ... ▣ 717
EPIFRIN ... ◉ 239
EpiPen ... 790
Marcaine Hydrochloride with Epinephrine 1:200,000 ... 2316
Primatene Mist ... ▣ 873
Sensorcaine with Epinephrine Injection ... 559
Sus-Phrine Injection ... 1019
Xylocaine with Epinephrine Injections ... 567

Epinephrine Bitartrate (Careful dosage adjustments required). Products include:

Bronkaid Mist Suspension ... ▣ 718
Sensorcaine-MPF with Epinephrine Injection ... 559

Epinephrine Hydrochloride (Careful dosage adjustments required). Products include:

Ana-Kit Anaphylaxis Emergency Treatment Kit ... 617

Estazolam (Increased response to the effects of CNS depressants). Products include:

ProSom Tablets ... 449

Ethchlorvynol (Transient delirium; increased response to the effects of CNS depressants). Products include:

Placidyl Capsules ... 448

Ethinamate (Increased response to the effects of CNS depressants).

No products indexed under this heading.

(▣ Described in PDR For Nonprescription Drugs) (◉ Described in PDR For Ophthalmology)

375 Interactions Index Endep

Fentanyl (Increased response to the effects of CNS depressants). Products include:
Duragesic Transdermal System........ 1288

Fentanyl Citrate (Increased response to the effects of CNS depressants). Products include:
Sublimaze Injection.............................. 1307

Flecainide Acetate (Concomitant use of amitryptyline with drugs that can inhibit cytochrome P_{450}IID6 may require lower than usually prescribed for either the tricyclic antidepressant or the other drug). Products include:
Tambocor Tablets 1497

Fluoxetine Hydrochloride (Concomitant use of amitryptyline with drugs that can inhibit cytochrome P_{450}IID6 may require lower than usually prescribed for either the tricyclic antidepressant or the other drug; sufficient time must elapse before initiating amitriptyline therapy in a patient being withdrawn from fluoxetine due to its long half-life). Products include:
Prozac Pulvules & Liquid, Oral Solution 919

Fluphenazine Decanoate (Increased response to the effects of CNS depressants). Products include:
Prolixin Decanoate 509

Fluphenazine Enanthate (Increased response to the effects of CNS depressants). Products include:
Prolixin Enanthate 509

Fluphenazine Hydrochloride (Increased response to the effects of CNS depressants). Products include:
Prolixin 509

Flurazepam Hydrochloride (Increased response to the effects of CNS depressants). Products include:
Dalmane Capsules 2173

Fluvoxamine Maleate (Concomitant use of amitryptyline with drugs that can inhibit cytochrome P_{450}IID6 may require lower than usually prescribed for either the tricyclic antidepressant or the other drug; sufficient time must elapse before initiating amitriptyline therapy in a patient being withdrawn from fluoxetine due to its long half-life). Products include:
Luvox Tablets 2544

Furazolidone (Hyperpyretic crisis; concurrent or sequential use within 14 days is contraindicated). Products include:
Furoxone 2046

Glutethimide (Increased response to the effects of CNS depressants).
No products indexed under this heading.

Glycopyrrolate (Paralytic ileus). Products include:
Robinul Forte Tablets 2072
Robinul Injectable 2072
Robinul Tablets 2072

Guanethidine Sulfate (Decreased antihypertensive action of guanethidine).

Haloperidol (Increased response to the effects of CNS depressants). Products include:
Haldol Injection, Tablets and Concentrate 1575

Haloperidol Decanoate (Increased response to the effects of CNS depressants). Products include:
Haldol Decanoate 1577

Hydrocodone Bitartrate (Increased response to the effects of CNS depressants). Products include:
Anexsia 5/500 Elixir 1781
Anexia Tablets 1782
Codiclear DH Syrup 791
Deconamine CX Cough and Cold Liquid and Tablets 1319
Duratuss HD Elixir 2565
Hycodan Tablets and Syrup 930
Hycomine Compound Tablets 932
Hycomine 931
Hycotuss Expectorant Syrup 933
Hydrocet Capsules 782
Lorcet 10/650 1018
Lortab 2566
Tussend 1783
Tussend Expectorant 1785
Vicodin Tablets 1356
Vicodin ES Tablets 1357
Vicodin Tuss Expectorant 1358
Zydone Capsules 949

Hydrocodone Polistirex (Increased response to the effects of CNS depressants). Products include:
Tussionex Pennkinetic Extended-Release Suspension 998

Hydroxyzine Hydrochloride (Increased response to the effects of CNS depressants). Products include:
Atarax Tablets & Syrup 2185
Marax Tablets & DF Syrup 2200
Vistaril Intramuscular Solution 2216

Hyoscyamine (Paralytic ileus). Products include:
Cystospaz Tablets 1963
Urised Tablets 1964

Hyoscyamine Sulfate (Paralytic ileus). Products include:
Arco-Lase Plus Tablets 512
Atrohist Plus Tablets 454
Cystospaz-M Capsules 1963
Donnatal 2060
Donnatal Extentabs 2061
Donnatal Tablets 2060
Kutrase Capsules 2402
Levsin/Levsinex/Levbid 2405

Imipramine Hydrochloride (Concomitant use of amitryptyline with drugs that can inhibit cytochrome P_{450}IID6 may require lower than usually prescribed for either the tricyclic antidepressant or the other drug). Products include:
Tofranil Ampuls 854
Tofranil Tablets 856

Imipramine Pamoate (Concomitant use of amitryptyline with drugs that can inhibit cytochrome P_{450}IID6 may require lower than usually prescribed for either the tricyclic antidepressant or the other drug). Products include:
Tofranil-PM Capsules 857

Ipratropium Bromide (Paralytic ileus). Products include:
Atrovent Inhalation Aerosol 671
Atrovent Inhalation Solution 673

Isocarboxazid (Hyperpyretic crisis; concurrent or sequential use within 14 days is contraindicated).
No products indexed under this heading.

Isoflurane (Increased response to the effects of CNS depressants).
No products indexed under this heading.

Isoproterenol Hydrochloride (Careful dosage adjustments required). Products include:
Isuprel Hydrochloride Injection 1:5000 2311
Isuprel Hydrochloride Solution 1:200 & 1:100 2313
Isuprel Mistometer 2312

Isoproterenol Sulfate (Careful dosage adjustments required). Products include:
Norisodrine with Calcium Iodide Syrup 442

Ketamine Hydrochloride (Increased response to the effects of CNS depressants).
No products indexed under this heading.

Levomethadyl Acetate Hydrochloride (Increased response to the effects of CNS depressants). Products include:
Orlamm 2239

Levorphanol Tartrate (Increased response to the effects of CNS depressants). Products include:
Levo-Dromoran 2129

Levothyroxine Sodium (Careful dosage adjustments required). Products include:
Levothroid Tablets 1016
Levoxyl Tablets 903
Synthroid 1359

Liothyronine Sodium (Careful dosage adjustments required). Products include:
Cytomel Tablets 2473
Triostat Injection 2530

Liotrix (Careful dosage adjustments required).
No products indexed under this heading.

Lorazepam (Increased response to the effects of CNS depressants). Products include:
Ativan Injection 2698
Ativan Tablets 2700

Loxapine Hydrochloride (Increased response to the effects of CNS depressants). Products include:
Loxitane 1378

Loxapine Succinate (Increased response to the effects of CNS depressants). Products include:
Loxitane Capsules 1378

Maprotiline Hydrochloride (Concomitant use of amitryptyline with drugs that can inhibit cytochrome P_{450}IID6 may require lower than usually prescribed for either the tricyclic antidepressant or the other drug). Products include:
Ludiomil Tablets 843

Mepenzolate Bromide (Paralytic ileus).
No products indexed under this heading.

Meperidine Hydrochloride (Increased response to the effects of CNS depressants). Products include:
Demerol 2308
Mepergan Injection 2753

Mephobarbital (Increased response to the effects of CNS depressants). Products include:
Mebaral Tablets 2322

Meprobamate (Increased response to the effects of CNS depressants). Products include:
Miltown Tablets 2672
PMB 200 and PMB 400 2783

Mesoridazine Besylate (Increased response to the effects of CNS depressants). Products include:
Serentil 684

Metaproterenol Sulfate (Careful dosage adjustments required). Products include:
Alupent 669
Metaproterenol Sulfate Inhalation Solution, USP, Arm-a-Med 552

Metaraminol Bitartrate (Careful dosage adjustments required). Products include:
Aramine Injection 1609

Methadone Hydrochloride (Increased response to the effects of CNS depressants). Products include:
Methadone Hydrochloride Oral Concentrate 2233
Methadone Hydrochloride Oral Solution & Tablets 2235

Methohexital Sodium (Increased response to the effects of CNS depressants). Products include:
Brevital Sodium Vials 1429

Methotrimeprazine (Increased response to the effects of CNS depressants). Products include:
Levoprome 1274

Methoxamine Hydrochloride (Careful dosage adjustments required). Products include:
Vasoxyl Injection 1196

Methoxyflurane (Increased response to the effects of CNS depressants).
No products indexed under this heading.

Midazolam Hydrochloride (Increased response to the effects of CNS depressants). Products include:
Versed Injection 2170

Molindone Hydrochloride (Increased response to the effects of CNS depressants). Products include:
Moban Tablets and Concentrate 1048

Morphine Sulfate (Increased response to the effects of CNS depressants). Products include:
Astramorph/PF Injection, USP (Preservative-Free) 535
Duramorph 962
Infumorph 200 and Infumorph 500 Sterile Solutions 965
MS Contin Tablets 1994
MSIR 1997
Oramorph SR (Morphine Sulfate Sustained Release Tablets) 2236
RMS Suppositories 2657
Roxanol 2243

Nefazodone Hydrochloride (Concomitant use of amitryptyline with drugs that can inhibit cytochrome P_{450}IID6 may require lower than usually prescribed for either the tricyclic antidepressant or the other drug). Products include:
Serzone Tablets 771

Norepinephrine Bitartrate (Careful dosage adjustments required). Products include:
Levophed Bitartrate Injection 2315

Nortriptyline Hydrochloride (Concomitant use of amitryptyline with drugs that can inhibit cytochrome P_{450}IID6 may require lower than usually prescribed for either the tricyclic antidepressant or the other drug). Products include:
Pamelor 2280

Opium Alkaloids (Increased response to the effects of CNS depressants).
No products indexed under this heading.

Oxazepam (Increased response to the effects of CNS depressants). Products include:
Serax Capsules 2810
Serax Tablets 2810

Oxycodone Hydrochloride (Increased response to the effects of CNS depressants). Products include:
Percocet Tablets 938
Percodan Tablets 939
Percodan-Demi Tablets 940
Roxicodone Tablets, Oral Solution & Intensol (Oxycodone) 2244
Tylox Capsules 1584

Oxyphenonium Bromide (Paralytic ileus).

Paroxetine Hydrochloride (Concomitant use of amitryptyline with drugs that can inhibit cytochrome P_{450}IID6 may require lower than usually prescribed for either the tricyclic antidepressant or the other drug). Products include:
Paxil Tablets 2505

Pentobarbital Sodium (Increased response to the effects of CNS depressants). Products include:
Nembutal Sodium Capsules 436
Nembutal Sodium Solution 438
Nembutal Sodium Suppositories 440

IMPORTANT NOTE: Always consult each drug listing in the patient's regimen for possible interactions.

Endep | Interactions Index | 376

Perphenazine (Increased response to the effects of CNS depressants). Products include:

Etrafon 2355
Triavil Tablets 1757
Trilafon 2389

Phenelzine Sulfate (Hyperpyretic crisis; concurrent or sequential use within 14 days is contraindicated). Products include:

Nardil 1920

Phenobarbital (Increased response to the effects of CNS depressants). Products include:

Arco-Lase Plus Tablets 512
Bellergal-S Tablets 2250
Donnatal 2060
Donnatal Extentabs 2061
Donnatal Tablets 2060
Phenobarbital Elixir and Tablets 1469
Quadrinal Tablets 1350

Phenylephrine Bitartrate (Careful dosage adjustments required).

No products indexed under this heading.

Phenylephrine Hydrochloride (Careful dosage adjustments required). Products include:

Atrohist Plus Tablets 454
Cerose DM ▣ 878
Comhist 2038
D.A. Chewable Tablets 951
Deconsal Pediatric Capsules 454
Dura-Vent/DA Tablets 953
Entex Capsules 1986
Entex Liquid 1986
Extendryl 1005
4-Way Fast Acting Nasal Spray (regular & mentholated) ▣ 621
Hemorid For Women ▣ 834
Hycomine Compound Tablets 932
Neo-Synephrine Hydrochloride 1% Carpuject 2324
Neo-Synephrine Hydrochloride 1% Injection 2324
Neo-Synephrine Hydrochloride (Ophthalmic) 2325
Neo-Synephrine ▣ 726
Nōstril ▣ 644
Novahistine Elixir ▣ 823
Phenergan VC 2779
Phenergan VC with Codeine 2781
Preparation H ▣ 871
Tympagesic Ear Drops 2342
Vasosulf ◉ 271
Vicks Sinex Nasal Spray and Ultra Fine Mist ▣ 765

Phenylephrine Tannate (Careful dosage adjustments required). Products include:

Atrohist Pediatric Suspension 454
Ricobid-D Pediatric Suspension 2038
Ricobid Tablets and Pediatric Suspension 2038
Rynatan 2673
Rynatuss 2673

Phenylpropanolamine Hydrochloride (Careful dosage adjustments required). Products include:

Acutrim ▣ 628
Allerest Children's Chewable Tablets ▣ 627
Allerest 12 Hour Caplets ▣ 627
Atrohist Plus Tablets 454
BC Cold Powder Multi-Symptom Formula (Cold-Sinus-Allergy) ▣ 609
BC Cold Powder Non-Drowsy Formula (Cold-Sinus) ▣ 609
Cheracol Plus Head Cold/Cough Formula ▣ 769
Comtrex Multi-Symptom Non-Drowsy Liqui-gels ▣ 618
Contac Continuous Action Nasal Decongestant/Antihistamine 12 Hour Capsules ▣ 813
Contac Maximum Strength Continuous Action Decongestant/Antihistamine 12 Hour Caplets ▣ 813
Contac Severe Cold and Flu Formula Caplets ▣ 814
Coricidin 'D' Decongestant Tablets ▣ 800
Dexatrim ▣ 832
Dexatrim Plus Vitamins Caplets ▣ 832
Dimetane-DC Cough Syrup 2059
Dimetapp Elixir ▣ 773
Dimetapp Extentabs ▣ 774
Dimetapp Tablets/Liqui-Gels ▣ 775
Dimetapp Cold & Allergy Chewable Tablets ▣ 773
Dimetapp DM Elixir ▣ 774
Dura-Vent Tablets 952
Entex Capsules 1986
Entex LA Tablets 1987
Entex Liquid 1986
Exgest LA Tablets 782
Hycomine 931
Isoclor Timesule Capsules ▣ 637
Nolamine Timed-Release Tablets 785
Ornade Spansule Capsules 2502
Propagest Tablets 786
Pyrroxate Caplets ▣ 772
Robitussin-CF ▣ 777
Sinulin Tablets 787
Tavist-D 12 Hour Relief Tablets ▣ 787
Teldrin 12 Hour Antihistamine/Nasal Decongestant Allergy Relief Capsules ▣ 826
Triaminic Allergy Tablets ▣ 789
Triaminic Cold Tablets ▣ 790
Triaminic Expectorant ▣ 790
Triaminic Syrup ▣ 792
Triaminic-12 Tablets ▣ 792
Triaminic-DM Syrup ▣ 792
Triaminicin Tablets ▣ 793
Triaminicol Multi-Symptom Cold Tablets ▣ 793
Triaminicol Multi-Symptom Relief ▣ 794
Vicks DayQuil Allergy Relief 12-Hour Extended Release Tablets ▣ 760
Vicks DayQuil Allergy Relief 4-Hour Tablets ▣ 760
Vicks DayQuil SINUS Pressure & CONGESTION Relief ▣ 761

Pirbuterol Acetate (Careful dosage adjustments required). Products include:

Maxair Autohaler 1492
Maxair Inhaler 1494

Prazepam (Increased response to the effects of CNS depressants).

No products indexed under this heading.

Prochlorperazine (Increased response to the effects of CNS depressants). Products include:

Compazine 2470

Procyclidine Hydrochloride (Paralytic ileus). Products include:

Kemadrin Tablets 1112

Promethazine Hydrochloride (Increased response to the effects of CNS depressants). Products include:

Mepergan Injection 2753
Phenergan with Codeine 2777
Phenergan with Dextromethorphan 2778
Phenergan Injection 2773
Phenergan Suppositories 2775
Phenergan Syrup 2774
Phenergan Tablets 2775
Phenergan VC 2779
Phenergan VC with Codeine 2781

Propafenone Hydrochloride (Concomitant use of amitryptyline with drugs that can inhibit cytochrome P_{450}IID6 may require lower than usually prescribed for either the tricyclic antidepressant or the other drug; potential for increased CNS depression). Products include:

Rythmol Tablets–150mg, 225mg, 300mg 1352

Propantheline Bromide (Paralytic ileus). Products include:

Pro-Banthīne Tablets 2052

Propofol (Increased response to the effects of CNS depressants). Products include:

Diprivan Injection 2833

Propoxyphene Hydrochloride (Increased response to the effects of CNS depressants). Products include:

Darvon 1435
Wygesic Tablets 2827

Propoxyphene Napsylate (Increased response to the effects of CNS depressants). Products include:

Darvon-N/Darvocet-N 1433

Protriptyline Hydrochloride (Concomitant use of amitryptyline with drugs that can inhibit cytochrome P_{450}IID6 may require lower than usually prescribed for either the tricyclic antidepressant or the other drug). Products include:

Vivactil Tablets 1774

Pseudoephedrine Hydrochloride (Careful dosage adjustments required). Products include:

Actifed Allergy Daytime/Nighttime Caplets ▣ 844
Actifed Plus Caplets ▣ 845
Actifed Plus Tablets ▣ 845
Actifed with Codeine Cough Syrup 1067
Actifed Sinus Daytime/Nighttime Tablets and Caplets ▣ 846
Actifed Syrup ▣ 846
Actifed Tablets ▣ 844
Advil Cold and Sinus Caplets and Tablets (formerly CoAdvil) ▣ 870
Alka-Seltzer Plus Cold Medicine Liqui-Gels ▣ 706
Alka-Seltzer Plus Cold & Cough Medicine Liqui-Gels ▣ 705
Alka-Seltzer Plus Night-Time Cold Medicine Liqui-Gels ▣ 706
Allerest Headache Strength Tablets ▣ 627
Allerest Maximum Strength Tablets ▣ 627
Allerest No Drowsiness Tablets ▣ 627
Allerest Sinus Pain Formula ▣ 627
Anatuss LA Tablets 1542
Atrohist Pediatric Capsules 453
Bayer Select Sinus Pain Relief Formula ▣ 717
Benadryl Allergy Decongestant Liquid Medication ▣ 848
Benadryl Allergy Decongestant Tablets ▣ 848
Benadryl Allergy Sinus Headache Formula Caplets ▣ 849
Benylin Multisymptom ▣ 852
Bromfed Capsules (Extended-Release) 1785
Bromfed Syrup ▣ 733
Bromfed Tablets 1785
Bromfed-DM Cough Syrup 1786
Bromfed-PD Capsules (Extended-Release) 1785
Children's Vicks DayQuil Allergy Relief ▣ 757
Children's Vicks NyQuil Cold/Cough Relief ▣ 758
Comtrex Multi-Symptom Cold Reliever Tablets/Caplets/Liqui-Gels/Liquid ▣ 615
Allergy-Sinus Comtrex Multi-Symptom Allergy-Sinus Formula Tablets ▣ 617
Comtrex Multi-Symptom Non-Drowsy Caplets ▣ 618
Congess 1004
Contac Day Allergy/Sinus Caplets ▣ 812
Contac Day & Night ▣ 812
Contac Night Allergy/Sinus Caplets ▣ 812
Contac Severe Cold & Flu Non-Drowsy ▣ 815
Deconamine Chewable Tablets 1320
Deconamine CX Cough and Cold Liquid and Tablets 1319
Deconamine 1320
Deconsal C Expectorant Syrup 456
Deconsal Pediatric Syrup 457
Deconsal II Tablets 454
Dimetane-DX Cough Syrup 2059
Dimetapp Sinus Caplets ▣ 775
Dorcol Children's Cough Syrup ▣ 785
Drixoral Cough + Congestion Liquid Caps ▣ 802
Dura-Tap/PD Capsules 2867
Duratuss Tablets 2565
Duratuss HD Elixir 2565
Efidac/24 ▣ 635
Entex PSE Tablets 1987
Fedahist Gyrocaps 2401
Fedahist Timecaps 2401
Guaifed 1787
Guaifed Syrup ▣ 734
Guaimax-D Tablets 792
Guaitab Tablets ▣ 734
Isoclor Expectorant 990
Kronofed-A 977
Motrin IB Sinus ▣ 838
Novahistine DH 2462
Novahistine DMX ▣ 822
Novahistine Expectorant 2463
Nucofed 2051
PediaCare Cold Allergy Chewable Tablets ▣ 677
PediaCare Cough-Cold Chewable Tablets 1553
PediaCare 1553
PediaCare Infants' Decongestant Drops ▣ 677
PediCare Infant's Drops Decongestant Plus Cough 1553
PediaCare NightRest Cough-Cold Liquid 1553
Pediatric Vicks 44d Dry Hacking Cough & Head Congestion ▣ 763
Pediatric Vicks 44m Cough & Cold Relief ▣ 764
Robitussin Cold & Cough Liqui-Gels ▣ 776
Robitussin Maximum Strength Cough & Cold ▣ 778
Robitussin Pediatric Cough & Cold Formula ▣ 779
Robitussin Severe Congestion Liqui-Gels ▣ 776
Robitussin-DAC Syrup 2074
Robitussin-PE ▣ 778
Rondec Oral Drops 953
Rondec Syrup 953
Rondec Tablet 953
Rondec-DM Oral Drops 954
Rondec-DM Syrup 954
Rondec-TR Tablet 953
Ryna ▣ 841
Seldane-D Extended-Release Tablets 1538
Semprex-D Capsules 463
Semprex-D Capsules 1167
Sinarest Tablets ▣ 648
Sinarest Extra Strength Tablets ▣ 648
Sinarest No Drowsiness Tablets ▣ 648
Sine-Aid IB Caplets 1554
Sine-Aid Maximum Strength Sinus Medication Gelcaps, Caplets and Tablets 1554
Sine-Off No Drowsiness Formula Caplets ▣ 824
Sine-Off Sinus Medicine ▣ 825
Singlet Tablets ▣ 825
Sinutab Non-Drying Liquid Caps ▣ 859
Sinutab Sinus Allergy Medication, Maximum Strength Tablets and Caplets ▣ 860
Sinutab Sinus Medication, Maximum Strength Without Drowsiness Formula, Tablets & Caplets ▣ 860
Sinutab Sinus Medication, Regular Strength Without Drowsiness Formula ▣ 859
Sudafed Children's Liquid ▣ 861
Sudafed Cold and Cough Liquidcaps ▣ 862
Sudafed Cough Syrup ▣ 862
Sudafed Plus Liquid ▣ 862
Sudafed Plus Tablets ▣ 863
Sudafed Severe Cold Formula Caplets ▣ 863
Sudafed Severe Cold Formula Tablets ▣ 864
Sudafed Sinus Caplets ▣ 864
Sudafed Sinus Tablets ▣ 864
Sudafed Tablets, 30 mg ▣ 861
Sudafed Tablets, 60 mg ▣ 861
Sudafed 12 Hour Caplets ▣ 861
Syn-Rx Tablets 465
Syn-Rx DM Tablets 466
TheraFlu ▣ 787
TheraFlu Maximum Strength Nighttime Flu, Cold & Cough Medicine ▣ 788
TheraFlu Maximum Strength Non-Drowsy Formula Flu, Cold & Cough Medicine ▣ 788
Thera Flu Maximum Strength, Non-Drowsy Formula Flu, Cold and Cough Caplets ▣ 789
Triaminic AM Cough and Decongestant Formula ▣ 789
Triaminic AM Decongestant Formula ▣ 790
Triaminic Nite Light ▣ 791
Triaminic Sore Throat Formula ▣ 791
Tussend 1783
Tussend Expectorant 1785
Children's TYLENOL Cold Multi-Symptom Liquid Formula and Chewable Tablets 1561
Children's TYLENOL Cold Plus Cough Multi Symptom Tablets and Liquid ▣ 681

(▣ Described in PDR For Nonprescription Drugs) (◉ Described in PDR For Ophthalmology)

Infants' TYLENOL Cold Decongestant & Fever-Reducer Drops.......... 1556
TYLENOL Maximum Strength Allergy Sinus Medication Gelcaps and Caplets 1563
TYLENOL Maximum Strength Allergy Sinus NightTime Medication Caplets 1555
TYLENOL Flu Maximum Strength Gelcaps 1565
TYLENOL Flu NightTime, Maximum Strength, Gelcaps 1566
TYLENOL Maximum Strength Flu NightTime Hot Medication Packets 1562
TYLENOL, Maximum Strength, Sinus Medication Geltabs, Gelcaps, Caplets and Tablets 1566
TYLENOL Cold Multi-Symptom Formula Medication Tablets and Caplets 1561
TYLENOL Cold Medication No Drowsiness Formula Gelcaps and Caplets 1562
TYLENOL Cold Multi-Symptom Hot Medication Liquid Packets.............. 1557
TYLENOL Cough Multi-Symptom Medication with Decongestant 1565
Ursinus Inlay-Tabs................................ ⊕ 794
Vicks 44 LiquiCaps Cough, Cold & Flu Relief.. ⊕ 755
Vicks 44 LiquiCaps Non-Drowsy Cough & Cold Relief .... ⊕ 756
Vicks 44D Dry Hacking Cough & Head Congestion .... ⊕ 755
Vicks 44M Cough, Cold & Flu Relief.. ⊕ 756
Vicks DayQuil .... ⊕ 761
Vicks DayQuil SINUS Pressure & PAIN Relief with IBUPROFEN ..... ⊕ 762
Vicks Nyquil Hot Therapy.................. ⊕ 762
Vicks NyQuil LiquiCaps Multi-Symptom Cold/Flu Relief .... ⊕ 763
Vicks NyQuil Multi-Symptom Cold/Flu Relief - (Original & Cherry Flavor) .... ⊕ 763

Pseudoephedrine Sulfate (Careful dosage adjustments required). Products include:

Cheracol Sinus .... ⊕ 768
Chlor-Trimeton Allergy Decongestant Tablets .... ⊕ 799
Claritin-D 2350
Drixoral Cold and Allergy Sustained-Action Tablets .... ⊕ 802
Drixoral Cold and Flu Extended-Release Tablets................................... ⊕ 803
Drixoral Non-Drowsy Formula Extended-Release Tablets .... ⊕ 803
Drixoral Allergy/Sinus Extended Release Tablets................................... ⊕ 804
Trinalin Repetabs Tablets 1330

Quazepam (Increased response to the effects of CNS depressants). Products include:

Doral Tablets 2664

Quinidine Gluconate (Concomitant use of amitryptyline with drugs that can inhibit cytochrome P_{450}IID6 may require lower than usually prescribed for either the tricyclic antidepressant or the other drug). Products include:

Quinaglute Dura-Tabs Tablets 649

Quinidine Polygalacturonate (Concomitant use of amitryptyline with drugs that can inhibit cytochrome P_{450}IID6 may require lower than usually prescribed for either the tricyclic antidepressant or the other drug).

No products indexed under this heading.

Quinidine Sulfate (Concomitant use of amitryptyline with drugs that can inhibit cytochrome P_{450}IID6 may require lower than usually prescribed for either the tricyclic antidepressant or the other drug). Products include:

Quinidex Extentabs................................ 2067

Risperidone (Increased response to the effects of CNS depressants). Products include:

Risperdal 1301

Salmeterol Xinafoate (Careful dosage adjustments required). Products include:

Serevent Inhalation Aerosol................. 1176

Scopolamine (Paralytic ileus). Products include:

Transderm Scōp Transdermal Therapeutic System 869

Scopolamine Hydrobromide (Paralytic ileus). Products include:

Atrohist Plus Tablets 454
Donnatal 2060
Donnatal Extentabs................................ 2061
Donnatal Tablets 2060

Secobarbital Sodium (Increased response to the effects of CNS depressants). Products include:

Seconal Sodium Pulvules 1474

Selegiline Hydrochloride (Hyperpyretic crisis; concurrent or sequential use within 14 days is contraindicated). Products include:

Eldepryl Tablets 2550

Sertraline Hydrochloride (Concomitant use of amitryptyline with drugs that can inhibit cytochrome P_{450}IID6 may require lower than usually prescribed for either the tricyclic antidepressant or the other drug). Products include:

Zoloft Tablets 2217

Sufentanil Citrate (Increased response to the effects of CNS depressants). Products include:

Sufenta Injection 1309

Temazepam (Increased response to the effects of CNS depressants). Products include:

Restoril Capsules 2284

Terbutaline Sulfate (Careful dosage adjustments required). Products include:

Brethaire Inhaler 813
Brethine Ampuls 815
Brethine Tablets...................................... 814
Bricanyl Subcutaneous Injection...... 1502
Bricanyl Tablets 1503

Thiamylal Sodium (Increased response to the effects of CNS depressants).

No products indexed under this heading.

Thioridazine Hydrochloride (Increased response to the effects of CNS depressants). Products include:

Mellaril 2269

Thiothixene (Increased response to the effects of CNS depressants). Products include:

Navane Capsules and Concentrate 2201
Navane Intramuscular 2202

Thyroglobulin (Careful dosage adjustments required).

No products indexed under this heading.

Thyroid (Careful dosage adjustments required).

No products indexed under this heading.

Thyroxine (Careful dosage adjustments required).

No products indexed under this heading.

Thyroxine Sodium (Careful dosage adjustments required).

No products indexed under this heading.

Tranylcypromine Sulfate (Hyperpyretic crisis; concurrent or sequential use within 14 days is contraindicated). Products include:

Parnate Tablets 2503

Trazodone Hydrochloride (Concomitant use of amitryptyline with drugs that can inhibit cytochrome P_{450}IID6 may require lower than usually prescribed for either the tricyclic antidepressant or the other drug). Products include:

Desyrel and Desyrel Dividose 503

Triazolam (Increased response to the effects of CNS depressants). Products include:

Halcion Tablets... 2611

Tridihexethyl Chloride (Paralytic ileus).

No products indexed under this heading.

Trifluoperazine Hydrochloride (Increased response to the effects of CNS depressants). Products include:

Stelazine 2514

Trihexyphenidyl Hydrochloride (Paralytic ileus). Products include:

Artane... 1368

Trimipramine Maleate (Concomitant use of amitryptyline with drugs that can inhibit cytochrome P_{450}IID6 may require lower than usually prescribed for either the tricyclic antidepressant or the other drug). Products include:

Surmontil Capsules................................. 2811

Venlafaxine Hydrochloride (Concomitant use of amitryptyline with drugs that can inhibit cytochrome P_{450}IID6 may require lower than usually prescribed for either the tricyclic antidepressant or the other drug). Products include:

Effexor 2719

Zolpidem Tartrate (Increased response to the effects of CNS depressants). Products include:

Ambien Tablets... 2416

Food Interactions

Alcohol (Increased response).

ENDURON TABLETS

(Methyclothiazide) 420

May interact with antihypertensives, beta blockers, corticosteroids, insulin, barbiturates, narcotic analgesics, cardiac glycosides, lithium preparations, and certain other agents. Compounds in these categories include:

Acebutolol Hydrochloride (Additive action). Products include:

Sectral Capsules 2807

ACTH (Hypokalemia).

No products indexed under this heading.

Alfentanil Hydrochloride (Potentiates orthostatic hypotension). Products include:

Alfenta Injection 1286

Amlodipine Besylate (Additive action). Products include:

Lotrel Capsules... 840
Norvasc Tablets 1940

Aprobarbital (Potentiates orthostatic hypotension).

No products indexed under this heading.

Atenolol (Additive action). Products include:

Tenoretic Tablets...................................... 2845
Tenormin Tablets and I.V. Injection 2847

Benazepril Hydrochloride (Additive action). Products include:

Lotensin Tablets.. 834
Lotensin HCT.. 837
Lotrel Capsules... 840

Bendroflumethiazide (Additive action).

No products indexed under this heading.

Betamethasone Acetate (Hypokalemia). Products include:

Celestone Soluspan Suspension 2347

Betamethasone Sodium Phosphate (Hypokalemia). Products include:

Celestone Soluspan Suspension 2347

Betaxolol Hydrochloride (Additive action). Products include:

Betoptic Ophthalmic Solution............. 469
Betoptic S Ophthalmic Suspension 471
Kerlone Tablets... 2436

Bisoprolol Fumarate (Additive action). Products include:

Zebeta Tablets 1413
Ziac 1415

Buprenorphine (Potentiates orthostatic hypotension). Products include:

Buprenex Injectable 2006

Butabarbital (Potentiates orthostatic hypotension).

No products indexed under this heading.

Butalbital (Potentiates orthostatic hypotension). Products include:

Esgic-plus Tablets 1013
Fioricet Tablets... 2258
Fioricet with Codeine Capsules 2260
Fiorinal Capsules 2261
Fiorinal with Codeine Capsules 2262
Fiorinal Tablets... 2261
Phrenilin 785
Sedapap Tablets 50 mg/650 mg .. 1543

Captopril (Additive action). Products include:

Capoten 739
Capozide 742

Carteolol Hydrochloride (Additive action). Products include:

Cartrol Tablets 410
Ocupress Ophthalmic Solution, 1 % Sterile... ⊚ 309

Chlorothiazide (Additive action). Products include:

Aldoclor Tablets.. 1598
Diupres Tablets 1650
Diuril Oral 1653

Chlorothiazide Sodium (Additive action). Products include:

Diuril Sodium Intravenous 1652

Chlorthalidone (Additive action). Products include:

Combipres Tablets 677
Tenoretic Tablets...................................... 2845
Thalitone 1245

Clonidine (Additive action). Products include:

Catapres-TTS.. 675

Clonidine Hydrochloride (Additive action). Products include:

Catapres Tablets 674
Combipres Tablets 677

Codeine Phosphate (Potentiates orthostatic hypotension). Products include:

Actifed with Codeine Cough Syrup.. 1067
Brontex 1981
Deconsal C Expectorant Syrup 456
Deconsal Pediatric Syrup 457
Dimetane-DC Cough Syrup 2059
Empirin with Codeine Tablets............ 1093
Fioricet with Codeine Capsules 2260
Fiorinal with Codeine Capsules 2262
Isoclor Expectorant................................. 990
Novahistine DH.. 2462
Novahistine Expectorant....................... 2463
Nucofed 2051
Phenergan with Codeine 2777
Phenergan VC with Codeine 2781
Robitussin A-C Syrup............................. 2073
Robitussin-DAC Syrup 2074
Ryna .... ⊕ 841
Soma Compound w/Codeine Tablets 2676
Tussi-Organidin NR Liquid and S NR Liquid 2677
Tylenol with Codeine 1583

Cortisone Acetate (Hypokalemia). Products include:

Cortone Acetate Sterile Suspension 1623

IMPORTANT NOTE: Always consult each drug listing in the patient's regimen for possible interactions.

Enduron Interactions Index 378

Cortone Acetate Tablets 1624

Deserpidine (Additive or potentiative action).
No products indexed under this heading.

Deslanoside (Thiazide-induced hypokalemia may exaggerate the response of the heart to the toxic effects of digitalis).
No products indexed under this heading.

Dexamethasone (Hypokalemia). Products include:
AK-Trol Ointment & Suspension ..... ◉ 205
Decadron Elixir 1633
Decadron Tablets 1635
Decaspray Topical Aerosol 1648
Dexacidin Ointment ..... ◉ 263
Maxitrol Ophthalmic Ointment and Suspension ..... ◉ 224
TobraDex Ophthalmic Suspension and Ointment 473

Dexamethasone Acetate (Hypokalemia). Products include:
Dalalone D.P. Injectable 1011
Decadron-LA Sterile Suspension 1646

Dexamethasone Sodium Phosphate (Hypokalemia). Products include:
Decadron Phosphate Injection 1637
Decadron Phosphate Respihaler 1642
Decadron Phosphate Sterile Ophthalmic Ointment 1641
Decadron Phosphate Sterile Ophthalmic Solution 1642
Decadron Phosphate Topical Cream 1644
Decadron Phosphate Turbinaire 1645
Decadron Phosphate with Xylocaine Injection, Sterile 1639
Dexacort Phosphate in Respihaler .. 458
Dexacort Phosphate in Turbinaire .. 459
NeoDecadron Sterile Ophthalmic Ointment 1712
NeoDecadron Sterile Ophthalmic Solution 1713
NeoDecadron Topical Cream 1714

Dezocine (Potentiates orthostatic hypotension). Products include:
Dalgan Injection 538

Diazoxide (Additive action). Products include:
Hyperstat I.V. Injection 2363
Proglycem 580

Digitoxin (Thiazide-induced hypokalemia may exaggerate the response of the heart to the toxic effects of digitalis). Products include:
Crystodigin Tablets 1433

Digoxin (Thiazide-induced hypokalemia may exaggerate the response of the heart to the toxic effects of digitalis). Products include:
Lanoxicaps 1117
Lanoxin Elixir Pediatric 1120
Lanoxin Injection 1123
Lanoxin Injection Pediatric 1126
Lanoxin Tablets 1128

Diltiazem Hydrochloride (Additive action). Products include:
Cardizem CD Capsules 1506
Cardizem SR Capsules 1510
Cardizem Injectable 1508
Cardizem Tablets 1512
Dilacor XR Extended-release Capsules 2018

Doxazosin Mesylate (Additive action). Products include:
Cardura Tablets 2186

Enalapril Maleate (Additive action). Products include:
Vaseretic Tablets 1765
Vasotec Tablets 1771

Enalaprilat (Additive action). Products include:
Vasotec I.V. 1768

Esmolol Hydrochloride (Additive action). Products include:
Brevibloc Injection 1808

Felodipine (Additive action). Products include:
Plendil Extended-Release Tablets 527

Fentanyl (Potentiates orthostatic hypotension). Products include:
Duragesic Transdermal System 1288

Fentanyl Citrate (Potentiates orthostatic hypotension). Products include:
Sublimaze Injection 1307

Fludrocortisone Acetate (Hypokalemia). Products include:
Florinef Acetate Tablets 505

Fosinopril Sodium (Additive action). Products include:
Monopril Tablets 757

Furosemide (Additive action). Products include:
Lasix Injection, Oral Solution and Tablets 1240

Guanabenz Acetate (Additive action).
No products indexed under this heading.

Guanethidine Monosulfate (Additive or potentiative action). Products include:
Esimil Tablets 822
Ismelin Tablets 827

Hydralazine Hydrochloride (Additive action). Products include:
Apresazide Capsules 808
Apresoline Hydrochloride Tablets .. 809
Ser-Ap-Es Tablets 849

Hydrochlorothiazide (Additive action). Products include:
Aldactazide 2413
Aldoril Tablets 1604
Apresazide Capsules 808
Capozide 742
Dyazide 2479
Esidrix Tablets 821
Esimil Tablets 822
HydroDIURIL Tablets 1674
Hydropres Tablets 1675
Hyzaar Tablets 1677
Inderide Tablets 2732
Inderide LA Long Acting Capsules .. 2734
Lopressor HCT Tablets 832
Lotensin HCT 837
Maxzide 1380
Moduretic Tablets 1705
Oretic Tablets 443
Prinzide Tablets 1737
Ser-Ap-Es Tablets 849
Timolide Tablets 1748
Vaseretic Tablets 1765
Zestoretic 2850
Ziac 1415

Hydrocodone Bitartrate (Potentiates orthostatic hypotension). Products include:
Anexsia 5/500 Elixir 1781
Anexia Tablets 1782
Codiclear DH Syrup 791
Deconamine CX Cough and Cold Liquid and Tablets 1319
Duratuss HD Elixir 2565
Hycodan Tablets and Syrup 930
Hycomine Compound Tablets 932
Hycomine 931
Hycotuss Expectorant Syrup 933
Hydrocet Capsules 782
Lorcet 10/650 1018
Lortab 2566
Tussend 1783
Tussend Expectorant 1785
Vicodin Tablets 1356
Vicodin ES Tablets 1357
Vicodin Tuss Expectorant 1358
Zydone Capsules 949

Hydrocodone Polistirex (Potentiates orthostatic hypotension). Products include:
Tussionex Pennkinetic Extended-Release Suspension 998

Hydrocortisone (Hypokalemia). Products include:
Anusol-HC Cream 2.5% 1896
Aquanil HC Lotion 1931
Bactine Hydrocortisone Anti-Itch Cream ..... ▣ 709
Caldecort Anti-Itch Hydrocortisone Spray ..... ▣ 631
Cortaid ..... ▣ 836
CORTENEMA 2535
Cortisporin Ointment 1085
Cortisporin Ophthalmic Ointment Sterile 1085
Cortisporin Ophthalmic Suspension Sterile 1086
Cortisporin Otic Solution Sterile 1087
Cortisporin Otic Suspension Sterile 1088
Cortizone-5 ..... ▣ 831
Cortizone-10 ..... ▣ 831
Hydrocortone Tablets 1672
Hytone 907
Massengill Medicated Soft Cloth Towelettes 2458
PediOtic Suspension Sterile 1153
Preparation H Hydrocortisone 1% Cream ..... ▣ 872
ProctoCream-HC 2.5% 2408
VōSoL HC Otic Solution 2678

Hydrocortisone Acetate (Hypokalemia). Products include:
Analpram-HC Rectal Cream 1% and 2.5% 977
Anusol HC-1 Anti-Itch Hydrocortisone Ointment ..... ▣ 847
Anusol-HC Suppositories 1897
Caldecort ..... ▣ 631
Carmol HC 924
Coly-Mycin S Otic w/Neomycin & Hydrocortisone 1906
Cortaid ..... ▣ 836
Cortifoam 2396
Cortisporin Cream 1084
Epifoam 2399
Hydrocortone Acetate Sterile Suspension 1669
Mantadil Cream 1135
Nupercainal Hydrocortisone 1% Cream ..... ▣ 645
Ophthocort ..... ◉ 311
Pramosone Cream, Lotion & Ointment 978
ProctoCream-HC 2408
ProctoFoam-HC 2409
Terra-Cortril Ophthalmic Suspension 2210

Hydrocortisone Sodium Phosphate (Hypokalemia). Products include:
Hydrocortone Phosphate Injection, Sterile 1670

Hydrocortisone Sodium Succinate (Hypokalemia). Products include:
Solu-Cortef Sterile Powder 2641

Hydroflumethiazide (Additive action). Products include:
Diucardin Tablets 2718

Indapamide (Additive action). Products include:
Lozol Tablets 2022

Insulin, Human (Changes in insulin requirements).
No products indexed under this heading.

Insulin, Human Isophane Suspension (Changes in insulin requirements). Products include:
Novolin N Human Insulin 10 ml Vials 1795

Insulin, Human NPH (Changes in insulin requirements). Products include:
Humulin N, 100 Units 1448
Novolin N PenFill Cartridges Durable Insulin Delivery System 1798
Novolin N Prefilled Syringe Disposable Insulin Delivery System 1798

Insulin, Human Regular (Changes in insulin requirements). Products include:
Humulin R, 100 Units 1449
Novolin R Human Insulin 10 ml Vials 1795
Novolin R PenFill Cartridges Durable Insulin Delivery System 1798
Novolin R Prefilled Syringe Disposable Insulin Delivery System 1798
Velosulin BR Human Insulin 10 ml Vials 1795

Insulin, Human, Zinc Suspension (Changes in insulin requirements). Products include:
Humulin L, 100 Units 1446
Humulin U, 100 Units 1450
Novolin L Human Insulin 10 ml Vials 1795

Insulin, NPH (Changes in insulin requirements). Products include:
NPH, 100 Units 1450
Pork NPH, 100 Units 1452
Purified Pork NPH Isophane Insulin 1801

Insulin, Regular (Changes in insulin requirements). Products include:
Regular, 100 Units 1450
Pork Regular, 100 Units 1452
Pork Regular (Concentrated), 500 Units 1453
Purified Pork Regular Insulin 1801

Insulin, Zinc Crystals (Changes in insulin requirements). Products include:
NPH, 100 Units 1450

Insulin, Zinc Suspension (Changes in insulin requirements). Products include:
Iletin I 1450
Lente, 100 Units 1450
Iletin II 1452
Pork Lente, 100 Units 1452
Purified Pork Lente Insulin 1801

Isradipine (Additive action). Products include:
DynaCirc Capsules 2256

Labetalol Hydrochloride (Additive action). Products include:
Normodyne Injection 2377
Normodyne Tablets 2379
Trandate 1185

Levobunolol Hydrochloride (Additive action). Products include:
Betagan ..... ◉ 233

Levorphanol Tartrate (Potentiates orthostatic hypotension). Products include:
Levo-Dromoran 2129

Lisinopril (Additive action). Products include:
Prinivil Tablets 1733
Prinzide Tablets 1737
Zestoretic 2850
Zestril Tablets 2854

Lithium Carbonate (Increased risk of lithium toxicity). Products include:
Eskalith 2485
Lithium Carbonate Capsules & Tablets 2230
Lithonate/Lithotabs/Lithobid 2543

Lithium Citrate (Increased risk of lithium toxicity).
No products indexed under this heading.

Losartan Potassium (Additive action). Products include:
Cozaar Tablets 1628
Hyzaar Tablets 1677

Mecamylamine Hydrochloride (Additive or potentiative action). Products include:
Inversine Tablets 1686

Meperidine Hydrochloride (Potentiates orthostatic hypotension). Products include:
Demerol 2308
Mepergan Injection 2753

Mephobarbital (Potentiates orthostatic hypotension). Products include:
Mebaral Tablets 2322

Methadone Hydrochloride (Potentiates orthostatic hypotension). Products include:
Methadone Hydrochloride Oral Concentrate 2233
Methadone Hydrochloride Oral Solution & Tablets 2235

Methyldopa (Additive action). Products include:
Aldoclor Tablets 1598
Aldomet Oral 1600
Aldoril Tablets 1604

Methyldopate Hydrochloride (Additive action). Products include:
Aldomet Ester HCl Injection 1602

(▣ Described in PDR For Nonprescription Drugs) (◉ Described in PDR For Ophthalmology)

379 Interactions Index Entex

Methylprednisolone (Hypokalemia). Products include:
Medrol ... 2621
Methylprednisolone Acetate (Hypokalemia). Products include:
Depo-Medrol Single-Dose Vial ... 2600
Depo-Medrol Sterile Aqueous Suspension ... 2597
Methylprednisolone Sodium Succinate (Hypokalemia). Products include:
Solu-Medrol Sterile Powder ... 2643
Metipranolol Hydrochloride (Additive action). Products include:
OptiPranolol (Metipranolol 0.3%) Sterile Ophthalmic Solution ... ◉ 258
Metolazone (Additive action). Products include:
Mykrox Tablets ... 993
Zaroxolyn Tablets ... 1000
Metoprolol Succinate (Additive action). Products include:
Toprol-XL Tablets ... 565
Metoprolol Tartrate (Additive action). Products include:
Lopressor Ampuls ... 830
Lopressor HCT Tablets ... 832
Lopressor Tablets ... 830
Metyrosine (Additive action). Products include:
Demser Capsules ... 1649
Minoxidil (Additive action). Products include:
Loniten Tablets ... 2618
Rogaine Topical Solution ... 2637
Moexipril Hydrochloride (Additive action). Products include:
Univasc Tablets ... 2410
Morphine Sulfate (Potentiates orthostatic hypotension). Products include:
Astramorph/PF Injection, USP (Preservative-Free) ... 535
Duramorph ... 962
Infumorph 200 and Infumorph 500 Sterile Solutions ... 965
MS Contin Tablets ... 1994
MSIR ... 1997
Oramorph SR (Morphine Sulfate Sustained Release Tablets) ... 2236
RMS Suppositories ... 2657
Roxanol ... 2243
Nadolol (Additive action).
No products indexed under this heading.
Nicardipine Hydrochloride (Additive action). Products include:
Cardene Capsules ... 2095
Cardene I.V. ... 2709
Cardene SR Capsules ... 2097
Nifedipine (Additive action). Products include:
Adalat Capsules (10 mg and 20 mg) ... 587
Adalat CC ... 589
Procardia Capsules ... 1971
Procardia XL Extended Release Tablets ... 1972
Nisoldipine (Additive action).
No products indexed under this heading.
Nitroglycerin (Additive action). Products include:
Deponit NTG Transdermal Delivery System ... 2397
Nitro-Bid IV ... 1523
Nitro-Bid Ointment ... 1524
Nitrodisc ... 2047
Nitro-Dur (nitroglycerin) Transdermal Infusion System ... 1326
Nitrolingual Spray ... 2027
Nitrostat Tablets ... 1925
Transderm-Nitro Transdermal Therapeutic System ... 859
Norepinephrine Bitartrate (Decreased arterial responsiveness). Products include:
Levophed Bitartrate Injection ... 2315
Opium Alkaloids (Potentiates orthostatic hypotension).
No products indexed under this heading.
Oxycodone Hydrochloride (Potentiates orthostatic hypotension). Products include:
Percocet Tablets ... 938
Percodan Tablets ... 939
Percodan-Demi Tablets ... 940
Roxicodone Tablets, Oral Solution & Intensol (Oxycodone) ... 2244
Tylox Capsules ... 1584
Pancuronium Bromide Injection (Decreased serum levels).
No products indexed under this heading.
Penbutolol Sulfate (Additive action). Products include:
Levatol ... 2403
Pentobarbital Sodium (Potentiates orthostatic hypotension). Products include:
Nembutal Sodium Capsules ... 436
Nembutal Sodium Solution ... 438
Nembutal Sodium Suppositories ... 440
Phenobarbital (Potentiates orthostatic hypotension). Products include:
Arco-Lase Plus Tablets ... 512
Bellergal-S Tablets ... 2250
Donnatal ... 2060
Donnatal Extentabs ... 2061
Donnatal Tablets ... 2060
Phenobarbital Elixir and Tablets ... 1469
Quadrinal Tablets ... 1350
Phenoxybenzamine Hydrochloride (Additive action). Products include:
Dibenzyline Capsules ... 2476
Phentolamine Mesylate (Additive action). Products include:
Regitine ... 846
Pindolol (Additive action). Products include:
Visken Tablets ... 2299
Polythiazide (Additive action). Products include:
Minizide Capsules ... 1938
Prazosin Hydrochloride (Additive or potentiative action). Products include:
Minipress Capsules ... 1937
Minizide Capsules ... 1938
Prednisolone Acetate (Hypokalemia). Products include:
AK-CIDE ... ◉ 202
AK-CIDE Ointment ... ◉ 202
Blephamide Liquifilm Sterile Ophthalmic Suspension ... 476
Blephamide Ointment ... ◉ 237
Econopred & Econopred Plus Ophthalmic Suspensions ... ◉ 217
Poly-Pred Liquifilm ... ◉ 248
Pred Forte ... ◉ 250
Pred Mild ... ◉ 253
Pred-G Liquifilm Sterile Ophthalmic Suspension ... ◉ 251
Pred-G S.O.P. Sterile Ophthalmic Ointment ... ◉ 252
Vasocidin Ointment ... ◉ 268
Prednisolone Sodium Phosphate (Hypokalemia). Products include:
AK-Pred ... ◉ 204
Hydeltrasol Injection, Sterile ... 1665
Inflamase ... ◉ 265
Pediapred Oral Liquid ... 995
Vasocidin Ophthalmic Solution ... ◉ 270
Prednisolone Tebutate (Hypokalemia). Products include:
Hydeltra-T.B.A. Sterile Suspension 1667
Prednisone (Hypokalemia). Products include:
Deltasone Tablets ... 2595
Propoxyphene Hydrochloride (Potentiates orthostatic hypotension). Products include:
Darvon ... 1435
Wygesic Tablets ... 2827
Propoxyphene Napsylate (Potentiates orthostatic hypotension). Products include:
Darvon-N/Darvocet-N ... 1433
Propranolol Hydrochloride (Additive action). Products include:
Inderal ... 2728
Inderal LA Long Acting Capsules ... 2730
Inderide Tablets ... 2732
Inderide LA Long Acting Capsules .. 2734
Quinapril Hydrochloride (Additive action). Products include:
Accupril Tablets ... 1893
Ramipril (Additive action). Products include:
Altace Capsules ... 1232
Rauwolfia Serpentina (Additive or potentiative action).
No products indexed under this heading.
Rescinnamine (Additive or potentiative action).
No products indexed under this heading.
Reserpine (Additive or potentiative action). Products include:
Diupres Tablets ... 1650
Hydropres Tablets ... 1675
Ser-Ap-Es Tablets ... 849
Secobarbital Sodium (Potentiates orthostatic hypotension). Products include:
Seconal Sodium Pulvules ... 1474
Sodium Nitroprusside (Additive action).
No products indexed under this heading.
Sotalol Hydrochloride (Additive action). Products include:
Betapace Tablets ... 641
Spirapril Hydrochloride (Additive action).
No products indexed under this heading.
Sufentanil Citrate (Potentiates orthostatic hypotension). Products include:
Sufenta Injection ... 1309
Terazosin Hydrochloride (Additive or potentiative action). Products include:
Hytrin Capsules ... 430
Thiamylal Sodium (Potentiates orthostatic hypotension).
No products indexed under this heading.
Timolol Hemihydrate (Additive action). Products include:
Betimol 0.25%, 0.5% ... ◉ 261
Timolol Maleate (Additive action). Products include:
Blocadren Tablets ... 1614
Timolide Tablets ... 1748
Timoptic in Ocudose ... 1753
Timoptic Sterile Ophthalmic Solution ... 1751
Timoptic-XE ... 1755
Torsemide (Additive action). Products include:
Demadex Tablets and Injection ... 686
Triamcinolone Acetonide (Hypokalemia). Products include:
Aristocort A 0.025% Cream ... 1027
Aristocort A 0.5% Cream ... 1031
Aristocort A 0.1% Cream ... 1029
Aristocort A 0.1% Ointment ... 1030
Azmacort Oral Inhaler ... 2011
Nasacort Nasal Inhaler ... 2024
Triamcinolone Diacetate (Hypokalemia). Products include:
Aristocort Suspension (Forte Parenteral) ... 1027
Aristocort Suspension (Intralesional) ... 1025
Triamcinolone Hexacetonide (Hypokalemia). Products include:
Aristospan Suspension (Intra-articular) ... 1033
Aristospan Suspension (Intralesional) ... 1032
Trimethaphan Camsylate (Additive or potentiative action). Products include:
Arfonad Ampuls ... 2080
Tubocurarine Chloride (Increase responsiveness).
No products indexed under this heading.
Verapamil Hydrochloride (Additive action). Products include:
Calan SR Caplets ... 2422
Calan Tablets ... 2419
Isoptin Injectable ... 1344
Isoptin Oral Tablets ... 1346
Isoptin SR Tablets ... 1348
Verelan Capsules ... 1410
Verelan Capsules ... 2824

Food Interactions
Alcohol (Potentiates orthostatic hypotension).

ENER-B VITAMIN B_{12} NASAL GEL DIETARY SUPPLEMENT
(Vitamin B_{12}) ... 1792
None cited in PDR database.

ENGERIX-B UNIT-DOSE VIALS
(Hepatitis B Vaccine) ... 2482
None cited in PDR database.

ENSURE COMPLETE BALANCED NUTRITION
(Nutritional Supplement) ... 2221
None cited in PDR database.

ENSURE HIGH PROTEIN COMPLETE BALANCED NUTRITION
(Nutritional Beverage) ... 2220
None cited in PDR database.

ENSURE PLUS HIGH CALORIE COMPLETE NUTRITION
(Nutritional Supplement) ... 2221
None cited in PDR database.

ENSURE WITH FIBER COMPLETE, BALANCED NUTRITION
(Nutritional Supplement) ... 2221
None cited in PDR database.

ENTEX CAPSULES
(Phenylephrine Hydrochloride, Phenylpropanolamine Hydrochloride, Guaifenesin) ... 1986
May interact with monoamine oxidase inhibitors and sympathomimetics. Compounds in these categories include:

Albuterol (Concurrent usage not recommended). Products include:
Proventil Inhalation Aerosol ... 2382
Ventolin Inhalation Aerosol and Refill ... 1197
Albuterol Sulfate (Concurrent usage not recommended). Products include:
Airet Solution for Inhalation ... 452
Proventil Inhalation Solution 0.083% ... 2384
Proventil Repetabs Tablets ... 2386
Proventil Solution for Inhalation 0.5% ... 2383
Proventil Syrup ... 2385
Proventil Tablets ... 2386
Ventolin Inhalation Solution ... 1198
Ventolin Nebules Inhalation Solution ... 1199
Ventolin Rotacaps for Inhalation ... 1200
Ventolin Syrup ... 1202
Ventolin Tablets ... 1203
Volmax Extended-Release Tablets .. 1788

IMPORTANT NOTE: Always consult each drug listing in the patient's regimen for possible interactions.

Entex

Dobutamine Hydrochloride (Concurrent usage not recommended). Products include:

Dobutrex Solution Vials 1439

Dopamine Hydrochloride (Concurrent usage not recommended).

No products indexed under this heading.

Ephedrine Hydrochloride (Concurrent usage not recommended). Products include:

Primatene Dual Action Formula ...... ᴾᴰ 872
Primatene Tablets .... ᴾᴰ 873
Quadrinal Tablets 1350

Ephedrine Sulfate (Concurrent usage not recommended). Products include:

Bronkaid Caplets .... ᴾᴰ 717
Marax Tablets & DF Syrup.................. 2200

Ephedrine Tannate (Concurrent usage not recommended). Products include:

Rynatuss 2673

Epinephrine (Concurrent usage not recommended). Products include:

Bronkaid Mist .... ᴾᴰ 717
EPIFRIN .... ⊙ 239
EpiPen 790
Marcaine Hydrochloride with Epinephrine 1:200,000 2316
Primatene Mist .... ᴾᴰ 873
Sensorcaine with Epinephrine Injection 559
Sus-Phrine Injection 1019
Xylocaine with Epinephrine Injections 567

Epinephrine Bitartrate (Concurrent usage not recommended). Products include:

Bronkaid Mist Suspension .... ᴾᴰ 718
Sensorcaine-MPF with Epinephrine Injection 559

Epinephrine Hydrochloride (Concurrent usage not recommended). Products include:

Ana-Kit Anaphylaxis Emergency Treatment Kit 617

Furazolidone (Concurrent usage not recommended). Products include:

Furoxone 2046

Isocarboxazid (Concurrent usage not recommended).

No products indexed under this heading.

Isoproterenol Hydrochloride (Concurrent usage not recommended). Products include:

Isuprel Hydrochloride Injection 1:5000 2311
Isuprel Hydrochloride Solution 1:200 & 1:100 2313
Isuprel Mistometer 2312

Isoproterenol Sulfate (Concurrent usage not recommended). Products include:

Norisodrine with Calcium Iodide Syrup... 442

Metaproterenol Sulfate (Concurrent usage not recommended). Products include:

Alupent 669
Metaproterenol Sulfate Inhalation Solution, USP, Arm-a-Med 552

Metaraminol Bitartrate (Concurrent usage not recommended). Products include:

Aramine Injection 1609

Methoxamine Hydrochloride (Concurrent usage not recommended). Products include:

Vasoxyl Injection 1196

Norepinephrine Bitartrate (Concurrent usage not recommended). Products include:

Levophed Bitartrate Injection 2315

Phenelzine Sulfate (Concurrent usage not recommended). Products include:

Nardil 1920

Phenylephrine Bitartrate (Concurrent usage not recommended).

No products indexed under this heading.

Phenylephrine Tannate (Concurrent usage not recommended). Products include:

Atrohist Pediatric Suspension 454
Ricobid-D Pediatric Suspension 2038
Ricobid Tablets and Pediatric Suspension 2038
Rynatan 2673
Rynatuss 2673

Pirbuterol Acetate (Concurrent usage not recommended). Products include:

Maxair Autohaler 1492
Maxair Inhaler 1494

Pseudoephedrine Hydrochloride (Concurrent usage not recommended). Products include:

Actifed Allergy Daytime/Nighttime Caplets... ᴾᴰ 844
Actifed Plus Caplets .... ᴾᴰ 845
Actifed Plus Tablets .... ᴾᴰ 845
Actifed with Codeine Cough Syrup.. 1067
Actifed Sinus Daytime/Nighttime Tablets and Caplets .... ᴾᴰ 846
Actifed Syrup.. ᴾᴰ 846
Actifed Tablets .... ᴾᴰ 844
Advil Cold and Sinus Caplets and Tablets (formerly CoAdvil) .... ᴾᴰ 870
Alka-Seltzer Plus Cold Medicine Liqui-Gels .... ᴾᴰ 706
Alka-Seltzer Plus Cold & Cough Medicine Liqui-Gels........................ ᴾᴰ 705
Alka-Seltzer Plus Night-Time Cold Medicine Liqui-Gels........................ ᴾᴰ 706
Allerest Headache Strength Tablets .... ᴾᴰ 627
Allerest Maximum Strength Tablets .... ᴾᴰ 627
Allerest No Drowsiness Tablets ...... ᴾᴰ 627
Allerest Sinus Pain Formula .... ᴾᴰ 627
Anatuss LA Tablets.............................. 1542
Atrohist Pediatric Capsules................ 453
Bayer Select Sinus Pain Relief Formula .... ᴾᴰ 717
Benadryl Allergy Decongestant Liquid Medication .... ᴾᴰ 848
Benadryl Allergy Decongestant Tablets .... ᴾᴰ 848
Benadryl Allergy Sinus Headache Formula Caplets.............................. ᴾᴰ 849
Benylin Multisymptom...................... ᴾᴰ 852
Bromfed Capsules (Extended-Release) 1785
Bromfed Syrup .... ᴾᴰ 733
Bromfed Tablets 1785
Bromfed-DM Cough Syrup................ 1786
Bromfed-PD Capsules (Extended-Release) 1785
Children's Vicks DayQuil Allergy Relief .... ᴾᴰ 757
Children's Vicks NyQuil Cold/ Cough Relief..................................... ᴾᴰ 758
Comtrex Multi-Symptom Cold Reliever Tablets/Caplets/Liqui-Gels/Liquid..................................... ᴾᴰ 615
Allergy-Sinus Comtrex Multi-Symptom Allergy-Sinus Formula Tablets .... ᴾᴰ 617
Comtrex Multi-Symptom Non-Drowsy Caplets................................ ᴾᴰ 618
Congess 1004
Contac Day Allergy/Sinus Caplets ᴾᴰ 812
Contac Day & Night .... ᴾᴰ 812
Contac Night Allergy/Sinus Caplets .... ᴾᴰ 812
Contac Severe Cold & Flu Non-Drowsy .... ᴾᴰ 815
Deconamine Chewable Tablets 1320
Deconamine CX Cough and Cold Liquid and Tablets.............................. 1319
Deconamine 1320
Deconsal C Expectorant Syrup 456
Deconsal Pediatric Syrup 457
Deconsal II Tablets 454
Dimetane-DX Cough Syrup 2059
Dimetapp Sinus Caplets .... ᴾᴰ 775
Dorcol Children's Cough Syrup ...... ᴾᴰ 785
Drixoral Cough + Congestion Liquid Caps .... ᴾᴰ 802

Dura-Tap/PD Capsules 2867
Duratuss Tablets 2565
Duratuss HD Elixir................................ 2565
Efidac/24 .... ᴾᴰ 635
Entex PSE Tablets 1987
Fedahist Gyrocaps................................ 2401
Fedahist Timecaps 2401
Guaifed... 1787
Guaifed Syrup .... ᴾᴰ 734
Guaimax-D Tablets 792
Guaitab Tablets .... ᴾᴰ 734
Isoclor Expectorant.............................. 990
Kronofed-A 977
Motrin IB Sinus .... ᴾᴰ 838
Novahistine DH.................................... 2462
Novahistine DMX .... ᴾᴰ 822
Novahistine Expectorant...................... 2463
Nucofed 2051
PediaCare Cold Allergy Chewable Tablets .... ᴾᴰ 677
PediaCare Cough-Cold Chewable Tablets 1553
PediaCare 1553
PediaCare Infants' Decongestant Drops .... ᴾᴰ 677
PediCare Infant's Drops Decongestant Plus Cough 1553
PediaCare NightRest Cough-Cold Liquid 1553
Pediatric Vicks 44d Dry Hacking Cough & Head Congestion.............. ᴾᴰ 763
Pediatric Vicks 44m Cough & Cold Relief .... ᴾᴰ 764
Robitussin Cold & Cough Liqui-Gels .... ᴾᴰ 776
Robitussin Maximum Strength Cough & Cold .... ᴾᴰ 778
Robitussin Pediatric Cough & Cold Formula...................................... ᴾᴰ 779
Robitussin Severe Congestion Liqui-Gels .... ᴾᴰ 776
Robitussin-DAC Syrup 2074
Robitussin-PE .... ᴾᴰ 778
Rondec Oral Drops 953
Rondec Syrup 953
Rondec Tablet.. 953
Rondec-DM Oral Drops 954
Rondec-DM Syrup 954
Rondec-TR Tablet 953
Ryna .... ᴾᴰ 841
Seldane-D Extended-Release Tablets 1538
Semprex-D Capsules 463
Semprex-D Capsules 1167
Sinarest Tablets .... ᴾᴰ 648
Sinarest Extra Strength Tablets...... ᴾᴰ 648
Sinarest No Drowsiness Tablets .... ᴾᴰ 648
Sine-Aid IB Caplets 1554
Sine-Aid Maximum Strength Sinus Medication Gelcaps, Caplets and Tablets 1554
Sine-Off No Drowsiness Formula Caplets .... ᴾᴰ 824
Sine-Off Sinus Medicine .... ᴾᴰ 825
Singlet Tablets .... ᴾᴰ 825
Sinutab Non-Drying Liquid Caps .. ᴾᴰ 859
Sinutab Sinus Allergy Medication, Maximum Strength Tablets and Caplets .... ᴾᴰ 860
Sinutab Sinus Medication, Maximum Strength Without Drowsiness Formula, Tablets & Caplets .... ᴾᴰ 860
Sinutab Sinus Medication, Regular Strength Without Drowsiness Formula .... ᴾᴰ 859
Sudafed Children's Liquid .... ᴾᴰ 861
Sudafed Cold and Cough Liquidcaps .... ᴾᴰ 862
Sudafed Cough Syrup .... ᴾᴰ 862
Sudafed Plus Liquid .... ᴾᴰ 862
Sudafed Plus Tablets .... ᴾᴰ 863
Sudafed Severe Cold Formula Caplets .... ᴾᴰ 863
Sudafed Severe Cold Formula Tablets .... ᴾᴰ 864
Sudafed Sinus Caplets...................... ᴾᴰ 864
Sudafed Sinus Tablets...................... ᴾᴰ 864
Sudafed Tablets, 30 mg .... ᴾᴰ 861
Sudafed Tablets, 60 mg.................... ᴾᴰ 861
Sudafed 12 Hour Caplets .... ᴾᴰ 861
Syn-Rx Tablets 465
Syn-Rx DM Tablets 466
TheraFlu.. ᴾᴰ 787
TheraFlu Maximum Strength Nighttime Flu, Cold & Cough Medicine .... ᴾᴰ 788
TheraFlu Maximum Strength Non-Drowsy Formula Flu, Cold & Cough Medicine.............................. ᴾᴰ 788

Thera Flu Maximum Strength, Non-Drowsy Formula Flu, Cold and Cough Caplets .... ᴾᴰ 789
Triaminic AM Cough and Decongestant Formula .... ᴾᴰ 789
Triaminic AM Decongestant Formula .... ᴾᴰ 790
Triaminic Nite Light .... ᴾᴰ 791
Triaminic Sore Throat Formula .... ᴾᴰ 791
Tussend 1783
Tussend Expectorant 1785
Children's TYLENOL Cold Multi-Symptom Liquid Formula and Chewable Tablets................................ 1561
Children's TYLENOL Cold Plus Cough Multi Symptom Tablets and Liquid.. ᴾᴰ 681
Infants' TYLENOL Cold Decongestant & Fever-Reducer Drops 1556
TYLENOL Maximum Strength Allergy Sinus Medication Gelcaps and Caplets 1563
TYLENOL Maximum Strength Allergy Sinus NightTime Medication Caplets 1555
TYLENOL Flu Maximum Strength Gelcaps 1565
TYLENOL Flu NightTime, Maximum Strength, Gelcaps 1566
TYLENOL Maximum Strength Flu NightTime Hot Medication Packets 1562
TYLENOL, Maximum Strength, Sinus Medication Geltabs, Gelcaps, Caplets and Tablets 1566
TYLENOL Cold Multi-Symptom Formula Medication Tablets and Caplets 1561
TYLENOL Cold Medication No Drowsiness Formula Gelcaps and Caplets 1562
TYLENOL Cold Multi-Symptom Hot Medication Liquid Packets.............. 1557
TYLENOL Cough Multi-Symptom Medication with Decongestant 1565
Ursinus Inlay-Tabs.............................. ᴾᴰ 794
Vicks 44 LiquiCaps Cough, Cold & Flu Relief.. ᴾᴰ 755
Vicks 44 LiquiCaps Non-Drowsy Cough & Cold Relief .... ᴾᴰ 756
Vicks 44D Dry Hacking Cough & Head Congestion .... ᴾᴰ 755
Vicks 44M Cough, Cold & Flu Relief.. ᴾᴰ 756
Vicks DayQuil .... ᴾᴰ 761
Vicks DayQuil SINUS Pressure & PAIN Relief with IBUPROFEN ...... ᴾᴰ 762
Vicks Nyquil Hot Therapy.................. ᴾᴰ 762
Vicks NyQuil LiquiCaps Multi-Symptom Cold/Flu Relief.............. ᴾᴰ 763
Vicks NyQuil Multi-Symptom Cold/Flu Relief - (Original & Cherry Flavor).................................... ᴾᴰ 763

Pseudoephedrine Sulfate (Concurrent usage not recommended). Products include:

Chlorcol Sinus .... ᴾᴰ 768
Chlor-Trimeton Allergy Decongestant Tablets .... ᴾᴰ 799
Claritin-D.. 2350
Drixoral Cold and Allergy Sustained-Action Tablets .... ᴾᴰ 802
Drixoral Cold and Flu Extended-Release Tablets.................................. ᴾᴰ 803
Drixoral Non-Drowsy Formula Extended-Release Tablets .... ᴾᴰ 803
Drixoral Allergy/Sinus Extended Release Tablets................................ ᴾᴰ 804
Trinalin Repetabs Tablets 1330

Salmeterol Xinafoate (Concurrent usage not recommended). Products include:

Serevent Inhalation Aerosol................ 1176

Selegiline Hydrochloride (Concurrent usage not recommended). Products include:

Eldepryl Tablets 2550

Terbutaline Sulfate (Concurrent usage not recommended). Products include:

Brethaire Inhaler 813
Brethine Ampuls 815
Brethine Tablets.................................... 814
Bricanyl Subcutaneous Injection 1502
Bricanyl Tablets 1503

(ᴾᴰ Described in PDR For Nonprescription Drugs) (⊙ Described in PDR For Ophthalmology)

381 **Interactions Index** **Entex LA**

Tranylcypromine Sulfate (Concurrent usage not recommended). Products include:
Parnate Tablets 2503

ENTEX LA TABLETS
(Phenylpropanolamine Hydrochloride, Guaifenesin) 1987
May interact with monoamine oxidase inhibitors and sympathomimetics. Compounds in these categories include:

Albuterol (Concurrent usage not recommended). Products include:
Proventil Inhalation Aerosol 2382
Ventolin Inhalation Aerosol and Refill 1197

Albuterol Sulfate (Concurrent usage not recommended). Products include:
Airet Solution for Inhalation 452
Proventil Inhalation Solution 0.083% 2384
Proventil Repetabs Tablets 2386
Proventil Solution for Inhalation 0.5% 2383
Proventil Syrup 2385
Proventil Tablets 2386
Ventolin Inhalation Solution 1198
Ventolin Nebules Inhalation Solution 1199
Ventolin Rotacaps for Inhalation 1200
Ventolin Syrup 1202
Ventolin Tablets 1203
Volmax Extended-Release Tablets 1788

Dobutamine Hydrochloride (Concurrent usage not recommended). Products include:
Dobutrex Solution Vials 1439

Dopamine Hydrochloride (Concurrent usage not recommended).
No products indexed under this heading.

Ephedrine Hydrochloride (Concurrent usage not recommended). Products include:
Primatene Dual Action Formula 872
Primatene Tablets 873
Quadrinal Tablets 1350

Ephedrine Sulfate (Concurrent usage not recommended). Products include:
Bronkaid Caplets 717
Marax Tablets & DF Syrup 2200

Ephedrine Tannate (Concurrent usage not recommended). Products include:
Rynatuss 2673

Epinephrine (Concurrent usage not recommended). Products include:
Bronkaid Mist 717
EPIFRIN ⊙ 239
EpiPen 790
Marcaine Hydrochloride with Epinephrine 1:200,000 2316
Primatene Mist 873
Sensorcaine with Epinephrine Injection 559
Sus-Phrine Injection 1019
Xylocaine with Epinephrine Injections 567

Epinephrine Bitartrate (Concurrent usage not recommended). Products include:
Bronkaid Mist Suspension 718
Sensorcaine-MPF with Epinephrine Injection 559

Epinephrine Hydrochloride (Concurrent usage not recommended). Products include:
Ana-Kit Anaphylaxis Emergency Treatment Kit 617

Furazolidone (Concurrent usage not recommended). Products include:
Furoxone 2046

Isocarboxazid (Concurrent usage not recommended).
No products indexed under this heading.

Isoproterenol Hydrochloride (Concurrent usage not recommended). Products include:
Isuprel Hydrochloride Injection 1:5000 2311
Isuprel Hydrochloride Solution 1:200 & 1:100 2313
Isuprel Mistometer 2312

Isoproterenol Sulfate (Concurrent usage not recommended). Products include:
Norisodrine with Calcium Iodide Syrup 442

Metaproterenol Sulfate (Concurrent usage not recommended). Products include:
Alupent 669
Metaproterenol Sulfate Inhalation Solution, USP, Arm-a-Med 552

Metaraminol Bitartrate (Concurrent usage not recommended). Products include:
Aramine Injection 1609

Methoxamine Hydrochloride (Concurrent usage not recommended). Products include:
Vasoxyl Injection 1196

Norepinephrine Bitartrate (Concurrent usage not recommended). Products include:
Levophed Bitartrate Injection 2315

Phenelzine Sulfate (Concurrent usage not recommended). Products include:
Nardil 1920

Phenylephrine Bitartrate (Concurrent usage not recommended).
No products indexed under this heading.

Phenylephrine Hydrochloride (Concurrent usage not recommended). Products include:
Atrohist Plus Tablets 454
Cerose DM 878
Comhist 2038
D.A. Chewable Tablets 951
Deconsal Pediatric Capsules 454
Dura-Vent/DA Tablets 953
Entex Capsules 1986
Entex Liquid 1986
Extendryl 1005
4-Way Fast Acting Nasal Spray (regular & mentholated) 621
Hemorid For Women 834
Hycomine Compound Tablets 932
Neo-Synephrine Hydrochloride 1% Carpuject 2324
Neo-Synephrine Hydrochloride 1% Injection 2324
Neo-Synephrine Hydrochloride (Ophthalmic) 2325
Neo-Synephrine 726
Nōstril 644
Novahistine Elixir 823
Phenergan VC 2779
Phenergan VC with Codeine 2781
Preparation H 871
Tympagesic Ear Drops 2342
Vasosulf ⊙ 271
Vicks Sinex Nasal Spray and Ultra Fine Mist 765

Phenylephrine Tannate (Concurrent usage not recommended). Products include:
Atrohist Pediatric Suspension 454
Ricobid-D Pediatric Suspension 2038
Ricobid Tablets and Pediatric Suspension 2038
Rynatan 2673
Rynatuss 2673

Pirbuterol Acetate (Concurrent usage not recommended). Products include:
Maxair Autohaler 1492
Maxair Inhaler 1494

Pseudoephedrine Hydrochloride (Concurrent usage not recommended). Products include:
Actifed Allergy Daytime/Nighttime Caplets 844
Actifed Plus Caplets 845
Actifed Plus Tablets 845
Actifed with Codeine Cough Syrup 1067
Actifed Sinus Daytime/Nighttime Tablets and Caplets 846
Actifed Syrup 846
Actifed Tablets 844
Advil Cold and Sinus Caplets and Tablets (formerly CoAdvil) 870
Alka-Seltzer Plus Cold Medicine Liqui-Gels 706
Alka-Seltzer Plus Cold & Cough Medicine Liqui-Gels 705
Alka-Seltzer Plus Night-Time Cold Medicine Liqui-Gels 706
Allerest Headache Strength Tablets 627
Allerest Maximum Strength Tablets 627
Allerest No Drowsiness Tablets 627
Allerest Sinus Pain Formula 627
Anatuss LA Tablets 1542
Atrohist Pediatric Capsules 453
Bayer Select Sinus Pain Relief Formula 717
Benadryl Allergy Decongestant Liquid Medication 848
Benadryl Allergy Decongestant Tablets 848
Benadryl Allergy Sinus Headache Formula Caplets 849
Benylin Multisymptom 852
Bromfed Capsules (Extended-Release) 1785
Bromfed Syrup 733
Bromfed Tablets 1785
Bromfed-DM Cough Syrup 1786
Bromfed-PD Capsules (Extended-Release) 1785
Children's Vicks DayQuil Allergy Relief 757
Children's Vicks NyQuil Cold/Cough Relief 758
Comtrex Multi-Symptom Cold Reliever Tablets/Caplets/Liqui-Gels/Liquid 615
Allergy-Sinus Comtrex Multi-Symptom Allergy-Sinus Formula Tablets 617
Comtrex Multi-Symptom Non-Drowsy Caplets 618
Congess 1004
Contac Day Allergy/Sinus Caplets 812
Contac Day & Night 812
Contac Night Allergy/Sinus Caplets 812
Contac Severe Cold & Flu Non-Drowsy 815
Deconamine Chewable Tablets 1320
Deconamine CX Cough and Cold Liquid and Tablets 1319
Deconamine 1320
Deconsal C Expectorant Syrup 456
Deconsal Pediatric Syrup 457
Deconsal II Tablets 454
Dimetane-DX Cough Syrup 2059
Dimetapp Sinus Caplets 775
Dorcol Children's Cough Syrup 785
Drixoral Cough + Congestion Liquid Caps 802
Dura-Tap/PD Capsules 2867
Duratuss Tablets 2565
Duratuss HD Elixir 2565
Efidac/24 635
Entex PSE Tablets 1987
Fedahist Gyrocaps 2401
Fedahist Timecaps 2401
Guaifed 1787
Guaifed Syrup 734
Guaimax-D Tablets 792
Guaitab Tablets 734
Isoclor Expectorant 990
Kronofed-A 977
Motrin IB Sinus 838
Novahistine DH 2462
Novahistine DMX 822
Novahistine Expectorant 2463
Nucofed 2051
PediaCare Cold Allergy Chewable Tablets 677
PediaCare Cough-Cold Chewable Tablets 1553
PediaCare 1553
PediaCare Infants' Decongestant Drops 677
PediCare Infant's Drops Decongestant Plus Cough 1553
PediaCare NightRest Cough-Cold Liquid 1553
Pediatric Vicks 44d Dry Hacking Cough & Head Congestion 763
Pediatric Vicks 44m Cough & Cold Relief 764
Robitussin Cold & Cough Liqui-Gels 776
Robitussin Maximum Strength Cough & Cold 778
Robitussin Pediatric Cough & Cold Formula 779
Robitussin Severe Congestion Liqui-Gels 776
Robitussin-DAC Syrup 2074
Robitussin-PE 778
Rondec Oral Drops 953
Rondec Syrup 953
Rondec Tablet 953
Rondec-DM Oral Drops 954
Rondec-DM Syrup 954
Rondec-TR Tablet 953
Ryna 841
Seldane-D Extended-Release Tablets 1538
Semprex-D Capsules 463
Semprex-D Capsules 1167
Sinarest Tablets 648
Sinarest Extra Strength Tablets 648
Sinarest No Drowsiness Tablets 648
Sine-Aid IB Caplets 1554
Sine-Aid Maximum Strength Sinus Medication Gelcaps, Caplets and Tablets 1554
Sine-Off No Drowsiness Formula Caplets 824
Sine-Off Sinus Medicine 825
Singlet Tablets 825
Sinutab Non-Drying Liquid Caps 859
Sinutab Sinus Allergy Medication, Maximum Strength Tablets and Caplets 860
Sinutab Sinus Medication, Maximum Strength Without Drowsiness Formula, Tablets & Caplets 860
Sinutab Sinus Medication, Regular Strength Without Drowsiness Formula 859
Sudafed Children's Liquid 861
Sudafed Cold and Cough Liquidcaps 862
Sudafed Cough Syrup 862
Sudafed Plus Liquid 862
Sudafed Plus Tablets 863
Sudafed Severe Cold Formula Caplets 863
Sudafed Severe Cold Formula Tablets 864
Sudafed Sinus Caplets 864
Sudafed Sinus Tablets 864
Sudafed Tablets, 30 mg 861
Sudafed Tablets, 60 mg 861
Sudafed 12 Hour Caplets 861
Syn-Rx Tablets 465
Syn-Rx DM Tablets 466
TheraFlu 787
TheraFlu Maximum Strength Nighttime Flu, Cold & Cough Medicine 788
TheraFlu Maximum Strength Non-Drowsy Formula Flu, Cold & Cough Medicine 788
Thera Flu Maximum Strength, Non-Drowsy Formula Flu, Cold and Cough Caplets 789
Triaminic AM Cough and Decongestant Formula 789
Triaminic AM Decongestant Formula 790
Triaminic Nite Light 791
Triaminic Sore Throat Formula 791
Tussend 1783
Tussend Expectorant 1785
Children's TYLENOL Cold Multi-Symptom Liquid Formula and Chewable Tablets 1561
Children's TYLENOL Cold Plus Cough Multi Symptom Tablets and Liquid 681
Infants' TYLENOL Cold Decongestant & Fever-Reducer Drops 1556
TYLENOL Maximum Strength Allergy Sinus Medication Gelcaps and Caplets 1563
TYLENOL Maximum Strength Allergy Sinus NightTime Medication Caplets 1555
TYLENOL Flu Maximum Strength Gelcaps 1565
TYLENOL Flu NightTime, Maximum Strength, Gelcaps 1566
TYLENOL Maximum Strength Flu NightTime Hot Medication Packets 1562

IMPORTANT NOTE: Always consult each drug listing in the patient's regimen for possible interactions.

- TYLENOL, Maximum Strength, Sinus Medication Geltabs, Gelcaps, Caplets and Tablets 1566
- TYLENOL Cold Multi-Symptom Formula Medication Tablets and Caplets 1561
- TYLENOL Cold Medication No Drowsiness Formula Gelcaps and Caplets 1562
- TYLENOL Cold Multi-Symptom Hot Medication Liquid Packets 1557
- TYLENOL Cough Multi-Symptom Medication with Decongestant 1565
- Ursinus Inlay-Tabs ▣ 794
- Vicks 44 LiquiCaps Cough, Cold & Flu Relief ▣ 755
- Vicks 44 LiquiCaps Non-Drowsy Cough & Cold Relief ▣ 756
- Vicks 44D Dry Hacking Cough & Head Congestion ▣ 755
- Vicks 44M Cough, Cold & Flu Relief ▣ 756
- Vicks DayQuil ▣ 761
- Vicks DayQuil SINUS Pressure & PAIN Relief with IBUPROFEN ▣ 762
- Vicks Nyquil Hot Therapy ▣ 762
- Vicks NyQuil LiquiCaps Multi-Symptom Cold/Flu Relief ▣ 763
- Vicks NyQuil Multi-Symptom Cold/Flu Relief - (Original & Cherry Flavor) ▣ 763

Pseudoephedrine Sulfate (Concurrent usage not recommended). Products include:

- Cheracol Sinus ▣ 768
- Chlor-Trimeton Allergy Decongestant Tablets ▣ 799
- Claritin-D 2350
- Drixoral Cold and Allergy Sustained-Action Tablets ▣ 802
- Drixoral Cold and Flu Extended-Release Tablets ▣ 803
- Drixoral Non-Drowsy Formula Extended-Release Tablets ▣ 803
- Drixoral Allergy/Sinus Extended Release Tablets ▣ 804
- Trinalin Repetabs Tablets 1330

Salmeterol Xinafoate (Concurrent usage not recommended). Products include:

- Serevent Inhalation Aerosol 1176

Selegiline Hydrochloride (Concurrent usage not recommended). Products include:

- Eldepryl Tablets 2550

Terbutaline Sulfate (Concurrent usage not recommended). Products include:

- Brethaire Inhaler 813
- Brethine Ampuls 815
- Brethine Tablets 814
- Bricanyl Subcutaneous Injection 1502
- Bricanyl Tablets 1503

Tranylcypromine Sulfate (Concurrent usage not recommended). Products include:

- Parnate Tablets 2503

ENTEX LIQUID

(Phenylephrine Hydrochloride, Phenylpropanolamine Hydrochloride, Guaifenesin) 1986

May interact with monoamine oxidase inhibitors and sympathomimetics. Compounds in these categories include:

Albuterol (Concurrent usage not recommended). Products include:

- Proventil Inhalation Aerosol 2382
- Ventolin Inhalation Aerosol and Refill 1197

Albuterol Sulfate (Concurrent usage not recommended). Products include:

- Airet Solution for Inhalation 452
- Proventil Inhalation Solution 0.083% 2384
- Proventil Repetabs Tablets 2386
- Proventil Solution for Inhalation 0.5% 2383
- Proventil Syrup 2385
- Proventil Tablets 2386
- Ventolin Inhalation Solution 1198
- Ventolin Nebules Inhalation Solution 1199
- Ventolin Rotacaps for Inhalation 1200
- Ventolin Syrup 1202
- Ventolin Tablets 1203
- Volmax Extended-Release Tablets 1788

Dobutamine Hydrochloride (Concurrent usage not recommended). Products include:

- Dobutrex Solution Vials 1439

Dopamine Hydrochloride (Concurrent usage not recommended).

- No products indexed under this heading.

Ephedrine Hydrochloride (Concurrent usage not recommended). Products include:

- Primatene Dual Action Formula ▣ 872
- Primatene Tablets ▣ 873
- Quadrinal Tablets 1350

Ephedrine Sulfate (Concurrent usage not recommended). Products include:

- Bronkaid Caplets ▣ 717
- Marax Tablets & DF Syrup 2200

Ephedrine Tannate (Concurrent usage not recommended). Products include:

- Rynatuss 2673

Epinephrine (Concurrent usage not recommended). Products include:

- Bronkaid Mist ▣ 717
- EPIFRIN ⊙ 239
- EpiPen 790
- Marcaine Hydrochloride with Epinephrine 1:200,000 2316
- Primatene Mist ▣ 873
- Sensorcaine with Epinephrine Injection 559
- Sus-Phrine Injection 1019
- Xylocaine with Epinephrine Injections 567

Epinephrine Bitartrate (Concurrent usage not recommended). Products include:

- Bronkaid Mist Suspension ▣ 718
- Sensorcaine-MPF with Epinephrine Injection 559

Epinephrine Hydrochloride (Concurrent usage not recommended). Products include:

- Ana-Kit Anaphylaxis Emergency Treatment Kit 617

Furazolidone (Concurrent usage not recommended). Products include:

- Furoxone 2046

Isocarboxazid (Concurrent usage not recommended).

- No products indexed under this heading.

Isoproterenol Hydrochloride (Concurrent usage not recommended). Products include:

- Isuprel Hydrochloride Injection 1:5000 2311
- Isuprel Hydrochloride Solution 1:200 & 1:100 2313
- Isuprel Mistometer 2312

Isoproterenol Sulfate (Concurrent usage not recommended). Products include:

- Norisodrine with Calcium Iodide Syrup 442

Metaproterenol Sulfate (Concurrent usage not recommended). Products include:

- Alupent 669
- Metaproterenol Sulfate Inhalation Solution, USP, Arm-a-Med 552

Metaraminol Bitartrate (Concurrent usage not recommended). Products include:

- Aramine Injection 1609

Methoxamine Hydrochloride (Concurrent usage not recommended). Products include:

- Vasoxyl Injection 1196

Norepinephrine Bitartrate (Concurrent usage not recommended). Products include:

- Levophed Bitartrate Injection 2315

Phenelzine Sulfate (Concurrent usage not recommended). Products include:

- Nardil 1920

Phenylephrine Bitartrate (Concurrent usage not recommended).

- No products indexed under this heading.

Phenylephrine Tannate (Concurrent usage not recommended). Products include:

- Atrohist Pediatric Suspension 454
- Ricobid-D Pediatric Suspension 2038
- Ricobid Tablets and Pediatric Suspension 2038
- Rynatan 2673
- Rynatuss 2673

Pirbuterol Acetate (Concurrent usage not recommended). Products include:

- Maxair Autohaler 1492
- Maxair Inhaler 1494

Pseudoephedrine Hydrochloride (Concurrent usage not recommended). Products include:

- Actifed Allergy Daytime/Nighttime Caplets ▣ 844
- Actifed Plus Caplets ▣ 845
- Actifed Plus Tablets ▣ 845
- Actifed with Codeine Cough Syrup 1067
- Actifed Sinus Daytime/Nighttime Tablets and Caplets ▣ 846
- Actifed Syrup ▣ 846
- Actifed Tablets ▣ 844
- Advil Cold and Sinus Caplets and Tablets (formerly CoAdvil) ▣ 870
- Alka-Seltzer Plus Cold Medicine Liqui-Gels ▣ 706
- Alka-Seltzer Plus Cold & Cough Medicine Liqui-Gels ▣ 705
- Alka-Seltzer Plus Night-Time Cold Medicine Liqui-Gels ▣ 706
- Allerest Headache Strength Tablets ▣ 627
- Allerest Maximum Strength Tablets ▣ 627
- Allerest No Drowsiness Tablets ▣ 627
- Allerest Sinus Pain Formula ▣ 627
- Anatuss LA Tablets 1542
- Atrohist Pediatric Capsules 453
- Bayer Select Sinus Pain Relief Formula ▣ 717
- Benadryl Allergy Decongestant Liquid Medication ▣ 848
- Benadryl Allergy Decongestant Tablets ▣ 848
- Benadryl Allergy Sinus Headache Formula Caplets ▣ 849
- Benylin Multisymptom ▣ 852
- Bromfed Capsules (Extended-Release) 1785
- Bromfed Syrup ▣ 733
- Bromfed Tablets 1785
- Bromfed-DM Cough Syrup 1786
- Bromfed-PD Capsules (Extended-Release) 1785
- Children's Vicks DayQuil Allergy Relief ▣ 757
- Children's Vicks NyQuil Cold/Cough Relief ▣ 758
- Comtrex Multi-Symptom Cold Reliever Tablets/Caplets/Liqui-Gels/Liquid ▣ 615
- Allergy-Sinus Comtrex Multi-Symptom Allergy-Sinus Formula Tablets ▣ 617
- Comtrex Multi-Symptom Non-Drowsy Caplets ▣ 618
- Congess 1004
- Contac Day Allergy/Sinus Caplets ▣ 812
- Contac Day & Night ▣ 812
- Contac Night Allergy/Sinus Caplets ▣ 812
- Contac Severe Cold & Flu Non-Drowsy ▣ 815
- Deconamine Chewable Tablets 1320
- Deconamine CX Cough and Cold Liquid and Tablets 1319
- Deconamine 1320
- Deconsal C Expectorant Syrup 456
- Deconsal Pediatric Syrup 457
- Deconsal II Tablets 454
- Dimetane-DX Cough Syrup 2059
- Dimetapp Sinus Caplets ▣ 775
- Dorcol Children's Cough Syrup ▣ 785
- Drixoral Cough + Congestion Liquid Caps ▣ 802
- Dura-Tap/PD Capsules 2867
- Duratuss Tablets 2565
- Duratuss HD Elixir 2565
- Efidac/24 ▣ 635
- Entex PSE Tablets 1987
- Fedahist Gyrocaps 2401
- Fedahist Timecaps 2401
- Guaifed 1787
- Guaifed Syrup ▣ 734
- Guaimax-D Tablets 792
- Guaitab Tablets ▣ 734
- Isoclor Expectorant 990
- Kronofed-A 977
- Motrin IB Sinus ▣ 838
- Novahistine DH 2462
- Novahistine DMX ▣ 822
- Novahistine Expectorant 2463
- Nucofed 2051
- PediaCare Cold Allergy Chewable Tablets ▣ 677
- PediaCare Cough-Cold Chewable Tablets 1553
- PediaCare 1553
- PediaCare Infants' Decongestant Drops ▣ 677
- PediCare Infant's Drops Decongestant Plus Cough 1553
- PediaCare NightRest Cough-Cold Liquid 1553
- Pediatric Vicks 44d Dry Hacking Cough & Head Congestion ▣ 763
- Pediatric Vicks 44m Cough & Cold Relief ▣ 764
- Robitussin Cold & Cough Liqui-Gels ▣ 776
- Robitussin Maximum Strength Cough & Cold ▣ 778
- Robitussin Pediatric Cough & Cold Formula ▣ 779
- Robitussin Severe Congestion Liqui-Gels ▣ 776
- Robitussin-DAC Syrup 2074
- Robitussin-PE ▣ 778
- Rondec Oral Drops 953
- Rondec Syrup 953
- Rondec Tablet 953
- Rondec-DM Oral Drops 954
- Rondec-DM Syrup 954
- Rondec-TR Tablet 953
- Ryna ▣ 841
- Seldane-D Extended-Release Tablets 1538
- Semprex-D Capsules 463
- Semprex-D Capsules 1167
- Sinarest Tablets ▣ 648
- Sinarest Extra Strength Tablets ▣ 648
- Sinarest No Drowsiness Tablets ▣ 648
- Sine-Aid IB Caplets 1554
- Sine-Aid Maximum Strength Sinus Medication Gelcaps, Caplets and Tablets 1554
- Sine-Off No Drowsiness Formula Caplets ▣ 824
- Sine-Off Sinus Medicine ▣ 825
- Singlet Tablets ▣ 825
- Sinutab Non-Drying Liquid Caps ▣ 859
- Sinutab Sinus Allergy Medication, Maximum Strength Tablets and Caplets ▣ 860
- Sinutab Sinus Medication, Maximum Strength Without Drowsiness Formula, Tablets & Caplets ▣ 860
- Sinutab Sinus Medication, Regular Strength Without Drowsiness Formula ▣ 859
- Sudafed Children's Liquid ▣ 861
- Sudafed Cold and Cough Liquidcaps ▣ 862
- Sudafed Cough Syrup ▣ 862
- Sudafed Plus Liquid ▣ 862
- Sudafed Plus Tablets ▣ 863
- Sudafed Severe Cold Formula Caplets ▣ 863
- Sudafed Severe Cold Formula Tablets ▣ 864
- Sudafed Sinus Caplets ▣ 864
- Sudafed Sinus Tablets ▣ 864
- Sudafed Tablets, 30 mg ▣ 861
- Sudafed Tablets, 60 mg ▣ 861
- Sudafed 12 Hour Caplets ▣ 861
- Syn-Rx Tablets 465
- Syn-Rx DM Tablets 466
- TheraFlu ▣ 787
- TheraFlu Maximum Strength Nighttime Flu, Cold & Cough Medicine ▣ 788
- TheraFlu Maximum Strength Non-Drowsy Formula Flu, Cold & Cough Medicine ▣ 788

(▣ Described in PDR For Nonprescription Drugs) (⊙ Described in PDR For Ophthalmology)

Thera Flu Maximum Strength, Non-Drowsy Formula Flu, Cold and Cough Caplets ◙ 789
Triaminic AM Cough and Decongestant Formula ◙ 789
Triaminic AM Decongestant Formula ◙ 790
Triaminic Nite Light ◙ 791
Triaminic Sore Throat Formula ◙ 791
Tussend 1783
Tussend Expectorant 1785
Children's TYLENOL Cold Multi-Symptom Liquid Formula and Chewable Tablets 1561
Children's TYLENOL Cold Plus Cough Multi Symptom Tablets and Liquid ◙ 681
Infants' TYLENOL Cold Decongestant & Fever-Reducer Drops 1556
TYLENOL Maximum Strength Allergy Sinus Medication Gelcaps and Caplets 1563
TYLENOL Maximum Strength Allergy Sinus NightTime Medication Caplets 1555
TYLENOL Flu Maximum Strength Gelcaps 1565
TYLENOL Flu NightTime, Maximum Strength, Gelcaps 1566
TYLENOL Maximum Strength Flu NightTime Hot Medication Packets 1562
TYLENOL, Maximum Strength, Sinus Medication Geltabs, Gelcaps, Caplets and Tablets 1566
TYLENOL Cold Multi-Symptom Formula Medication Tablets and Caplets 1561
TYLENOL Cold Medication No Drowsiness Formula Gelcaps and Caplets 1562
TYLENOL Cold Multi-Symptom Hot Medication Liquid Packets 1557
TYLENOL Cough Multi-Symptom Medication with Decongestant 1565
Ursinus Inlay-Tabs ◙ 794
Vicks 44 LiquiCaps Cough, Cold & Flu Relief ◙ 755
Vicks 44 LiquiCaps Non-Drowsy Cough & Cold Relief ◙ 756
Vicks 44D Dry Hacking Cough & Head Congestion ◙ 755
Vicks 44M Cough, Cold & Flu Relief ◙ 756
Vicks DayQuil ◙ 761
Vicks DayQuil SINUS Pressure & PAIN Relief with IBUPROFEN ◙ 762
Vicks Nyquil Hot Therapy ◙ 762
Vicks NyQuil LiquiCaps Multi-Symptom Cold/Flu Relief ◙ 763
Vicks NyQuil Multi-Symptom Cold/Flu Relief - (Original & Cherry Flavor) ◙ 763

Pseudoephedrine Sulfate (Concurrent usage not recommended). Products include:
Cheracol Sinus ◙ 768
Chlor-Trimeton Allergy Decongestant Tablets ◙ 799
Claritin-D 2350
Drixoral Cold and Allergy Sustained-Action Tablets ◙ 802
Drixoral Cold and Flu Extended-Release Tablets ◙ 803
Drixoral Non-Drowsy Formula Extended-Release Tablets ◙ 803
Drixoral Allergy/Sinus Extended Release Tablets ◙ 804
Trinalin Repetabs Tablets 1330

Salmeterol Xinafoate (Concurrent usage not recommended). Products include:
Serevent Inhalation Aerosol 1176

Selegiline Hydrochloride (Concurrent usage not recommended). Products include:
Eldepryl Tablets 2550

Terbutaline Sulfate (Concurrent usage not recommended). Products include:
Brethaire Inhaler 813
Brethine Ampuls 815
Brethine Tablets 814
Bricanyl Subcutaneous Injection 1502
Bricanyl Tablets 1503

Tranylcypromine Sulfate (Concurrent usage not recommended). Products include:
Parnate Tablets 2503

ENTEX PSE TABLETS
(Pseudoephedrine Hydrochloride, Guaifenesin) 1987
May interact with monoamine oxidase inhibitors, beta blockers, veratrum alkaloids, catecholamine depleting drugs, and certain other agents. Compounds in these categories include:

Acebutolol Hydrochloride (Increases effects of sympathomimetics). Products include:
Sectral Capsules 2807

Atenolol (Increases effects of sympathomimetics). Products include:
Tenoretic Tablets 2845
Tenormin Tablets and I.V. Injection 2847

Betaxolol Hydrochloride (Increases effects of sympathomimetics). Products include:
Betoptic Ophthalmic Solution 469
Betoptic S Ophthalmic Suspension 471
Kerlone Tablets 2436

Bisoprolol Fumarate (Increases effects of sympathomimetics). Products include:
Zebeta Tablets 1413
Ziac 1415

Carteolol Hydrochloride (Increases effects of sympathomimetics). Products include:
Cartrol Tablets 410
Ocupress Ophthalmic Solution, 1% Sterile ⊙ 309

Cryptenamine Preparations (Reduced antihypertensive effects).

Deserpidine (Reduced antihypertensive effects).
No products indexed under this heading.

Esmolol Hydrochloride (Increases effects of sympathomimetics). Products include:
Brevibloc Injection 1808

Furazolidone (Increases effects of sympathomimetics; concurrent administration is contraindicated). Products include:
Furoxone 2046

Guanethidine Monosulfate (Reduced antihypertensive effects). Products include:
Esimil Tablets 822
Ismelin Tablets 827

Isocarboxazid (Increases effects of sympathomimetics; concurrent administration is contraindicated).
No products indexed under this heading.

Labetalol Hydrochloride (Increases effects of sympathomimetics). Products include:
Normodyne Injection 2377
Normodyne Tablets 2379
Trandate 1185

Levobunolol Hydrochloride (Increases effects of sympathomimetics). Products include:
Betagan ⊙ 233

Mecamylamine Hydrochloride (Reduced antihypertensive effects). Products include:
Inversine Tablets 1686

Methyldopa (Reduced antihypertensive effects). Products include:
Aldoclor Tablets 1598
Aldomet Oral 1600
Aldoril Tablets 1604

Metipranolol Hydrochloride (Increases effects of sympathomimetics). Products include:
OptiPranolol (Metipranolol 0.3%) Sterile Ophthalmic Solution ⊙ 258

Metoprolol Succinate (Increases effects of sympathomimetics). Products include:
Toprol-XL Tablets 565

Metoprolol Tartrate (Increases effects of sympathomimetics). Products include:
Lopressor Ampuls 830
Lopressor HCT Tablets 832
Lopressor Tablets 830

Nadolol (Increases effects of sympathomimetics).
No products indexed under this heading.

Penbutolol Sulfate (Increases effects of sympathomimetics). Products include:
Levatol 2403

Phenelzine Sulfate (Increases effects of sympathomimetics; concurrent administration is contraindicated). Products include:
Nardil 1920

Pindolol (Increases effects of sympathomimetics). Products include:
Visken Tablets 2299

Propranolol Hydrochloride (Increases effects of sympathomimetics). Products include:
Inderal 2728
Inderal LA Long Acting Capsules 2730
Inderide Tablets 2732
Inderide LA Long Acting Capsules 2734

Rauwolfia Serpentina (Reduced antihypertensive effects).
No products indexed under this heading.

Rescinnamine (Reduced antihypertensive effects).
No products indexed under this heading.

Reserpine (Reduced antihypertensive effects). Products include:
Diupres Tablets 1650
Hydropres Tablets 1675
Ser-Ap-Es Tablets 849

Selegiline Hydrochloride (Increases effects of sympathomimetics; concurrent administration is contraindicated). Products include:
Eldepryl Tablets 2550

Sotalol Hydrochloride (Increases effects of sympathomimetics). Products include:
Betapace Tablets 641

Timolol Hemihydrate (Increases effects of sympathomimetics). Products include:
Betimol 0.25%, 0.5% ⊙ 261

Timolol Maleate (Increases effects of sympathomimetics). Products include:
Blocadren Tablets 1614
Timolide Tablets 1748
Timoptic in Ocudose 1753
Timoptic Sterile Ophthalmic Solution 1751
Timoptic-XE 1755

Tranylcypromine Sulfate (Increases effects of sympathomimetics; concurrent administration is contraindicated). Products include:
Parnate Tablets 2503

ENUCLENE CLEANING, LUBRICATING SOLUTION FOR ARTIFICIAL EYES
(Benzalkonium Chloride, Tyloxapol) ⊙ 218
None cited in PDR database.

EPIFOAM
(Hydrocortisone Acetate, Pramoxine Hydrochloride) 2399
None cited in PDR database.

EPIFRIN
(Epinephrine) ⊙ 239
None cited in PDR database.

EPIPEN JR.
(Epinephrine) 790
See **EpiPen—Epinephrine Auto-Injector**

EPIPEN—EPINEPHRINE AUTO-INJECTOR
(Epinephrine) 790
May interact with tricyclic antidepressants, monoamine oxidase inhibitors, cardiac glycosides, and certain other agents. Compounds in these categories include:

Amitriptyline Hydrochloride (Potentiation of epinephrine). Products include:
Elavil 2838
Endep Tablets 2174
Etrafon 2355
Limbitrol 2180
Triavil Tablets 1757

Amoxapine (Potentiation of epinephrine). Products include:
Asendin Tablets 1369

Clomipramine Hydrochloride (Potentiation of epinephrine). Products include:
Anafranil Capsules 803

Desipramine Hydrochloride (Potentiation of epinephrine). Products include:
Norpramin Tablets 1526

Deslanoside (Concurrent use is not recommended).
No products indexed under this heading.

Digitoxin (Concurrent use is not recommended). Products include:
Crystodigin Tablets 1433

Digoxin (Concurrent use is not recommended). Products include:
Lanoxicaps 1117
Lanoxin Elixir Pediatric 1120
Lanoxin Injection 1123
Lanoxin Injection Pediatric 1126
Lanoxin Tablets 1128

Doxepin Hydrochloride (Potentiation of epinephrine). Products include:
Sinequan 2205
Zonalon Cream 1055

Furazolidone (Potentiation of epinephrine). Products include:
Furoxone 2046

Imipramine Hydrochloride (Potentiation of epinephrine). Products include:
Tofranil Ampuls 854
Tofranil Tablets 856

Imipramine Pamoate (Potentiation of epinephrine). Products include:
Tofranil-PM Capsules 857

Isocarboxazid (Potentiation of epinephrine).
No products indexed under this heading.

Maprotiline Hydrochloride (Potentiation of epinephrine). Products include:
Ludiomil Tablets 843

Nortriptyline Hydrochloride (Potentiation of epinephrine). Products include:
Pamelor 2280

Phenelzine Sulfate (Potentiation of epinephrine). Products include:
Nardil 1920

Protriptyline Hydrochloride (Potentiation of epinephrine). Products include:
Vivactil Tablets 1774

Quinidine Gluconate (Concurrent use is not recommended). Products include:
Quinaglute Dura-Tabs Tablets 649

IMPORTANT NOTE: Always consult each drug listing in the patient's regimen for possible interactions.

Quinidine Polygalacturonate (Concurrent use is not recommended).
No products indexed under this heading.

Quinidine Sulfate (Concurrent use is not recommended). Products include:
Quinidex Extentabs 2067

Selegiline Hydrochloride (Potentiation of epinephrine). Products include:
Eldepryl Tablets 2550

Tranylcypromine Sulfate (Potentiation of epinephrine). Products include:
Parnate Tablets 2503

Trimipramine Maleate (Potentiation of epinephrine). Products include:
Surmontil Capsules 2811

EPOGEN FOR INJECTION
(Epoetin Alfa) 489
None cited in PDR database.

ERGAMISOL TABLETS
(Levamisole Hydrochloride) 1292
May interact with oral anticoagulants and certain other agents. Compounds in these categories include:

Dicumarol (Prolongation of the prothrombin time beyond the therapeutic range when co-administered; monitor PT and the dose of warfarin or other coumarin-like drugs should be adjusted accordingly).
No products indexed under this heading.

Fluorouracil (Combination therapy may result in marked elevation in triglyceride levels). Products include:
Efudex 2113
Fluoroplex Topical Solution & Cream 1% 479
Fluorouracil Injection 2116

Phenytoin (Concomitant administration of phenytoin and Ergamisol plus fluorouracil has led to increased plasma levels of phenytoin). Products include:
Dilantin Infatabs 1908
Dilantin-125 Suspension 1911

Phenytoin Sodium (Concomitant administration of phenytoin and Ergamisol plus fluorouracil has led to increased plasma levels of phenytoin). Products include:
Dilantin Kapseals 1906
Dilantin Parenteral 1910

Warfarin Sodium (Prolongation of the prothrombin time beyond the therapeutic range when co-administered; monitor PT and the dose of warfarin or other coumarin-like drugs should be adjusted accordingly). Products include:
Coumadin 926

Food Interactions

Alcohol (May result in ANTABUSE-like side effects).

ERGOMAR
(Ergotamine Tartrate) 1486
May interact with vasopressors and certain other agents. Compounds in these categories include:

Dopamine Hydrochloride (The pressor effects of Ergomar and other vasoconstrictor drugs can combine to cause dangerous hypertension).
No products indexed under this heading.

Epinephrine Bitartrate (The pressor effects of Ergomar and other vasoconstrictor drugs can combine to cause dangerous hypertension). Products include:
Bronkaid Mist Suspension .... ▣ 718
Sensorcaine-MPF with Epinephrine Injection 559

Epinephrine Hydrochloride (The pressor effects of Ergomar and other vasoconstrictor drugs can combine to cause dangerous hypertension). Products include:
Ana-Kit Anaphylaxis Emergency Treatment Kit 617

Metaraminol Bitartrate (The pressor effects of Ergomar and other vasoconstrictor drugs can combine to cause dangerous hypertension). Products include:
Aramine Injection 1609

Methoxamine Hydrochloride (The pressor effects of Ergomar and other vasoconstrictor drugs can combine to cause dangerous hypertension). Products include:
Vasoxyl Injection 1196

Norepinephrine Bitartrate (The pressor effects of Ergomar and other vasoconstrictor drugs can combine to cause dangerous hypertension). Products include:
Levophed Bitartrate Injection 2315

Phenylephrine Hydrochloride (The pressor effects of Ergomar and other vasoconstrictor drugs can combine to cause dangerous hypertension). Products include:
Atrohist Plus Tablets 454
Cerose DM .... ▣ 878
Comhist 2038
D.A. Chewable Tablets 951
Deconsal Pediatric Capsules 454
Dura-Vent/DA Tablets 953
Entex Capsules 1986
Entex Liquid 1986
Extendryl 1005
4-Way Fast Acting Nasal Spray (regular & mentholated) .... ▣ 621
Hemorid For Women .... ▣ 834
Hycomine Compound Tablets 932
Neo-Synephrine Hydrochloride 1% Carpuject 2324
Neo-Synephrine Hydrochloride 1% Injection 2324
Neo-Synephrine Hydrochloride (Ophthalmic) 2325
Neo-Synephrine .... ▣ 726
Nōstril .... ▣ 644
Novahistine Elixir .... ▣ 823
Phenergan VC 2779
Phenergan VC with Codeine 2781
Preparation H .... ▣ 871
Tympagesic Ear Drops 2342
Vasosulf .... ◉ 271
Vicks Sinex Nasal Spray and Ultra Fine Mist .... ▣ 765

Troleandomycin (Triacetyloleandomycin inhibits the metabolism of ergotamine; potentiates the effects of Ergomar). Products include:
Tao Capsules 2209

ERYC
(Erythromycin) 1915
May interact with xanthine bronchodilators, oral anticoagulants, drugs which undergo biotransformation by cytochrome p-450 mixed function oxidase, and certain other agents. Compounds in these categories include:

Aminophylline (Co-administration with high doses of theophylline may be associated with increased serum theophylline levels and potential theophylline toxicity).
No products indexed under this heading.

Carbamazepine (Concurrent use may be associated with elevation in serum level of carbamazepine; monitor serum levels closely). Products include:
Atretol Tablets 573
Tegretol Chewable Tablets 852
Tegretol Suspension 852
Tegretol Tablets 852

Cyclosporine (Concurrent use may be associated with elevation in serum level of cyclosporine; monitor serum levels closely). Products include:
Neoral 2276
Sandimmune 2286

Dicumarol (Concomitant therapy may result in increased anticoagulant effects).
No products indexed under this heading.

Digoxin (Co-administration may result in elevated digoxin serum levels). Products include:
Lanoxicaps 1117
Lanoxin Elixir Pediatric 1120
Lanoxin Injection 1123
Lanoxin Injection Pediatric 1126
Lanoxin Tablets 1128

Dihydroergotamine Mesylate (Concurrent use has been associated with acute ergot toxicity characterized by severe peripheral vasospasm and dysesthesia). Products include:
D.H.E. 45 Injection 2255

Drugs which undergo biotransformation by cytochrome P-450 mixed function oxidase (Concurrent use may be associated with elevation in serum level of drugs metabolized by the cytochrome P450 system).

Dyphylline (Co-administration with high doses of theophylline may be associated with increased serum theophylline levels and potential theophylline toxicity). Products include:
Lufyllin & Lufyllin-400 Tablets 2670
Lufyllin-GG Elixir & Tablets 2671

Ergotamine Tartrate (Concurrent use has been associated with acute ergot toxicity characterized by severe peripheral vasospasm and dysesthesia). Products include:
Bellergal-S Tablets 2250
Cafergot 2251
Ergomar 1486
Wigraine Tablets & Suppositories 1829

Hexobarbital (Concurrent use may be associated with elevation in serum level of hexobarbital; monitor serum levels closely).

Phenytoin (Concurrent use may be associated with elevation in serum level of phenytoin; monitor serum levels closely). Products include:
Dilantin Infatabs 1908
Dilantin-125 Suspension 1911

Phenytoin Sodium (Concurrent use may be associated with elevation in serum level of phenytoin; monitor serum levels closely). Products include:
Dilantin Kapseals 1906
Dilantin Parenteral 1910

Terfenadine (Erythromycin significantly alters the metabolism of terfenadine when used concomitantly; potential for rare cases of serious cardiovascular adverse events, including death, cardiac arrest, torsade de pointes and other ventricular arrhythmias; concurrent use is contraindicated). Products include:
Seldane Tablets 1536
Seldane-D Extended-Release Tablets 1538

Theophylline (Co-administration with high doses of theophylline may be associated with increased serum theophylline levels and potential theophylline toxicity). Products include:
Marax Tablets & DF Syrup 2200
Quibron 2053

Theophylline Anhydrous (Co-administration with high doses of theophylline may be associated with increased serum theophylline levels and potential theophylline toxicity). Products include:
Aerolate 1004
Primatene Dual Action Formula .... ▣ 872
Primatene Tablets .... ▣ 873
Respbid Tablets 682
Slo-bid Gyrocaps 2033
Theo-24 Extended Release Capsules 2568
Theo-Dur Extended-Release Tablets 1327
Theo-X Extended-Release Tablets 788
Uni-Dur Extended-Release Tablets 1331
Uniphyl 400 mg Tablets 2001

Theophylline Calcium Salicylate (Co-administration with high doses of theophylline may be associated with increased serum theophylline levels and potential theophylline toxicity). Products include:
Quadrinal Tablets 1350

Theophylline Sodium Glycinate (Co-administration with high doses of theophylline may be associated with increased serum theophylline levels and potential theophylline toxicity).
No products indexed under this heading.

Triazolam (Decrease clearance of triazolam; potential for increased pharmacologic effect of triazolam). Products include:
Halcion Tablets 2611

Warfarin Sodium (Concomitant therapy may result in increased anticoagulant effects). Products include:
Coumadin 926

Food Interactions

Meal, unspecified (Optimum blood levels are obtained on a fasting stomach; administration is preferable one-half hour pre- or two hours post-meal).

ERYCETTE (ERYTHROMYCIN 2%) TOPICAL SOLUTION
(Erythromycin) 1888
None cited in PDR database.

ERYPED DROPS AND CHEWABLE TABLETS
(Erythromycin Ethylsuccinate) 421
May interact with xanthine bronchodilators, oral anticoagulants, and certain other agents. Compounds in these categories include:

Aminophylline (Concomitant administration with high doses of theophylline may be associated with increased theophylline levels and potential toxicity).
No products indexed under this heading.

Carbamazepine (Elevations in serum erythromycin and carbamazepine concentration). Products include:
Atretol Tablets 573
Tegretol Chewable Tablets 852
Tegretol Suspension 852
Tegretol Tablets 852

Cyclosporine (Elevations in serum erythromycin and cyclosporine concentration). Products include:
Neoral 2276

Sandimmune 2286

Dicumarol (Increased anticoagulant effects).

No products indexed under this heading.

Digoxin (Elevated digoxin serum levels). Products include:

Lanoxicaps 1117
Lanoxin Elixir Pediatric 1120
Lanoxin Injection 1123
Lanoxin Injection Pediatric.................... 1126
Lanoxin Tablets 1128

Dihydroergotamine Mesylate (Potential for acute ergot toxicity characterized by severe peripheral vasospasm and dysesthesia). Products include:

D.H.E. 45 Injection 2255

Dyphylline (Concomitant administration with high doses of theophylline may be associated with increased theophylline levels and potential toxicity). Products include:

Lufyllin & Lufyllin-400 Tablets 2670
Lufyllin-GG Elixir & Tablets 2671

Ergotamine Tartrate (Potential for acute ergot toxicity characterized by severe peripheral vasospasm and dysesthesia). Products include:

Bellergal-S Tablets 2250
Cafergot 2251
Ergomar 1486
Wigraine Tablets & Suppositories .. 1829

Hexobarbital (Elevations in serum erythromycin and hexobarbital concentration).

Lovastatin (Potential for rhabdomyolysis in seriously ill patients). Products include:

Mevacor Tablets.................................... 1699

Phenytoin (Elevations in serum erythromycin and phenytoin concentration). Products include:

Dilantin Infatabs 1908
Dilantin-125 Suspension 1911

Phenytoin Sodium (Elevations in serum erythromycin and phenytoin concentration). Products include:

Dilantin Kapseals 1906
Dilantin Parenteral 1910

Terfenadine (Potential for altered terfenadine metabolism). Products include:

Seldane Tablets 1536
Seldane-D Extended-Release Tablets 1538

Theophylline (Concomitant administration with high doses of theophylline may be associated with increased theophylline levels and potential toxicity). Products include:

Marax Tablets & DF Syrup.................... 2200
Quibron 2053

Theophylline Anhydrous (Concomitant administration with high doses of theophylline may be associated with increased theophylline levels and potential toxicity). Products include:

Aerolate 1004
Primatene Dual Action Formula...... ◉ 872
Primatene Tablets .... ◉ 873
Respbid Tablets 682
Slo-bid Gyrocaps 2033
Theo-24 Extended Release Capsules 2568
Theo-Dur Extended-Release Tablets 1327
Theo-X Extended-Release Tablets .. 788
Uni-Dur Extended-Release Tablets.. 1331
Uniphyl 400 mg Tablets........................ 2001

Theophylline Calcium Salicylate (Concomitant administration with high doses of theophylline may be associated with increased theophylline levels and potential toxicity). Products include:

Quadrinal Tablets 1350

Theophylline Sodium Glycinate (Concomitant administration with high doses of theophylline may be associated with increased theophylline levels and potential toxicity).

No products indexed under this heading.

Triazolam (Decreased clearance of triazolam and increased the pharmacologic effect of triazolam). Products include:

Halcion Tablets...................................... 2611

Warfarin Sodium (Increased anticoagulant effects). Products include:

Coumadin 926

ERYPED 200 & ERYPED 400 GRANULES

(Erythromycin Ethylsuccinate)............. 421

See **EryPed Drops and Chewable Tablets**

ERY-TAB TABLETS

(Erythromycin) 422

May interact with xanthine bronchodilators, oral anticoagulants, and certain other agents. Compounds in these categories include:

Aminophylline (Concomitant administration with high doses of theophylline may be associated with increased theophylline levels and potential toxicity).

No products indexed under this heading.

Carbamazepine (Elevations in serum erythromycin and carbamazepine concentration). Products include:

Atretol Tablets 573
Tegretol Chewable Tablets 852
Tegretol Suspension 852
Tegretol Tablets 852

Cyclosporine (Elevations in serum erythromycin and cyclosporine concentration). Products include:

Neoral 2276
Sandimmune 2286

Dicumarol (Increased anticoagulant effects).

No products indexed under this heading.

Digoxin (Elevated digoxin serum levels). Products include:

Lanoxicaps 1117
Lanoxin Elixir Pediatric 1120
Lanoxin Injection 1123
Lanoxin Injection Pediatric.................... 1126
Lanoxin Tablets 1128

Dihydroergotamine Mesylate (Potential for acute ergot toxicity characterized by severe peripheral vasospasm and dysesthesia). Products include:

D.H.E. 45 Injection 2255

Dyphylline (Concomitant administration with high doses of theophylline may be associated with increased theophylline levels and potential toxicity). Products include:

Lufyllin & Lufyllin-400 Tablets 2670
Lufyllin-GG Elixir & Tablets 2671

Ergotamine Tartrate (Potential for acute ergot toxicity characterized by severe peripheral vasospasm and dysesthesia). Products include:

Bellergal-S Tablets 2250
Cafergot 2251
Ergomar 1486
Wigraine Tablets & Suppositories .. 1829

Hexobarbital (Elevations in serum erythromycin and hexobarbital concentration).

Lovastatin (Potential for rhabdomyolysis in seriously ill patients). Products include:

Mevacor Tablets..................................... 1699

Phenytoin (Elevations in serum erythromycin and phenytoin concentration). Products include:

Dilantin Infatabs 1908
Dilantin-125 Suspension 1911

Phenytoin Sodium (Elevations in serum erythromycin and phenytoin concentration). Products include:

Dilantin Kapseals 1906
Dilantin Parenteral 1910

Terfenadine (Potential for altered terfenadine metabolism). Products include:

Seldane Tablets 1536
Seldane-D Extended-Release Tablets 1538

Theophylline (Concomitant administration with high doses of theophylline may be associated with increased theophylline levels and potential toxicity). Products include:

Marax Tablets & DF Syrup.................... 2200
Quibron 2053

Theophylline Anhydrous (Concomitant administration with high doses of theophylline may be associated with increased theophylline levels and potential toxicity). Products include:

Aerolate 1004
Primatene Dual Action Formula...... ◉ 872
Primatene Tablets .... ◉ 873
Respbid Tablets 682
Slo-bid Gyrocaps 2033
Theo-24 Extended Release Capsules 2568
Theo-Dur Extended-Release Tablets 1327
Theo-X Extended-Release Tablets .. 788
Uni-Dur Extended-Release Tablets.. 1331
Uniphyl 400 mg Tablets......................... 2001

Theophylline Calcium Salicylate (Concomitant administration with high doses of theophylline may be associated with increased theophylline levels and potential toxicity). Products include:

Quadrinal Tablets 1350

Theophylline Sodium Glycinate (Concomitant administration with high doses of theophylline may be associated with increased theophylline levels and potential toxicity).

No products indexed under this heading.

Triazolam (Decreased clearance of triazolam and increased the pharmacologic effect of triazolam). Products include:

Halcion Tablets....................................... 2611

Warfarin Sodium (Increased anticoagulant effects). Products include:

Coumadin 926

ERYTHROCIN STEARATE FILMTAB

(Erythromycin Stearate) 425

May interact with xanthine bronchodilators, oral anticoagulants, and certain other agents. Compounds in these categories include:

Aminophylline (Concomitant administration with high doses of theophylline may be associated with increased theophylline levels and potential toxicity).

No products indexed under this heading.

Carbamazepine (Elevations in serum erythromycin and carbamazepine concentration). Products include:

Atretol Tablets 573
Tegretol Chewable Tablets 852
Tegretol Suspension 852
Tegretol Tablets 852

Cyclosporine (Elevations in serum erythromycin and cyclosporine concentration). Products include:

Neoral 2276

Sandimmune 2286

Dicumarol (Increased anticoagulant effects).

No products indexed under this heading.

Digoxin (Elevated digoxin serum levels). Products include:

Lanoxicaps 1117
Lanoxin Elixir Pediatric 1120
Lanoxin Injection 1123
Lanoxin Injection Pediatric.................... 1126
Lanoxin Tablets 1128

Dihydroergotamine Mesylate (Potential for acute ergot toxicity characterized by severe peripheral vasospasm and dysesthesia). Products include:

D.H.E. 45 Injection 2255

Dyphylline (Concomitant administration with high doses of theophylline may be associated with increased theophylline levels and potential toxicity). Products include:

Lufyllin & Lufyllin-400 Tablets 2670
Lufyllin-GG Elixir & Tablets 2671

Ergotamine Tartrate (Potential for acute ergot toxicity characterized by severe peripheral vasospasm and dysesthesia). Products include:

Bellergal-S Tablets 2250
Cafergot 2251
Ergomar 1486
Wigraine Tablets & Suppositories .. 1829

Hexobarbital (Elevations in serum erythromycin and hexobarbital concentration).

Lovastatin (Potential for rhabdomyolysis in seriously ill patients). Products include:

Mevacor Tablets..................................... 1699

Phenytoin (Elevations in serum erythromycin and phenytoin concentration). Products include:

Dilantin Infatabs 1908
Dilantin-125 Suspension 1911

Phenytoin Sodium (Elevations in serum erythromycin and phenytoin concentration). Products include:

Dilantin Kapseals 1906
Dilantin Parenteral 1910

Terfenadine (Potential for altered terfenadine metabolism). Products include:

Seldane Tablets 1536
Seldane-D Extended-Release Tablets 1538

Theophylline (Concomitant administration with high doses of theophylline may be associated with increased theophylline levels and potential toxicity). Products include:

Marax Tablets & DF Syrup.................... 2200
Quibron 2053

Theophylline Anhydrous (Concomitant administration with high doses of theophylline may be associated with increased theophylline levels and potential toxicity). Products include:

Aerolate 1004
Primatene Dual Action Formula...... ◉ 872
Primatene Tablets .... ◉ 873
Respbid Tablets 682
Slo-bid Gyrocaps 2033
Theo-24 Extended Release Capsules 2568
Theo-Dur Extended-Release Tablets 1327
Theo-X Extended-Release Tablets .. 788
Uni-Dur Extended-Release Tablets.. 1331
Uniphyl 400 mg Tablets......................... 2001

Theophylline Calcium Salicylate (Concomitant administration with high doses of theophylline may be associated with increased theophylline levels and potential toxicity). Products include:

Quadrinal Tablets 1350

IMPORTANT NOTE: Always consult each drug listing in the patient's regimen for possible interactions.

Theophylline Sodium Glycinate (Concomitant administration with high doses of theophylline may be associated with increased theophylline levels and potential toxicity).
No products indexed under this heading.

Triazolam (Decreased clearance of triazolam and increased the pharmacologic effect of triazolam). Products include:
Halcion Tablets ... 2611

Warfarin Sodium (Increased anticoagulant effects). Products include:
Coumadin ... 926

ERYTHROMYCIN BASE FILMTAB

(Erythromycin) ... 426
May interact with xanthine bronchodilators, oral anticoagulants, and certain other agents. Compounds in these categories include:

Aminophylline (Concomitant administration with high doses of theophylline may be associated with increased theophylline levels and potential toxicity).
No products indexed under this heading.

Carbamazepine (Elevations in serum erythromycin and carbamazepine concentration). Products include:
Atretol Tablets ... 573
Tegretol Chewable Tablets ... 852
Tegretol Suspension ... 852
Tegretol Tablets ... 852

Cyclosporine (Elevations in serum erythromycin and cyclosporine concentration). Products include:
Neoral ... 2276
Sandimmune ... 2286

Dicumarol (Increased anticoagulant effects).
No products indexed under this heading.

Digoxin (Elevated digoxin serum levels). Products include:
Lanoxicaps ... 1117
Lanoxin Elixir Pediatric ... 1120
Lanoxin Injection ... 1123
Lanoxin Injection Pediatric ... 1126
Lanoxin Tablets ... 1128

Dihydroergotamine Mesylate (Potential for acute ergot toxicity characterized by severe peripheral vasospasm and dysesthesia). Products include:
D.H.E. 45 Injection ... 2255

Dyphylline (Concomitant administration with high doses of theophylline may be associated with increased theophylline levels and potential toxicity). Products include:
Lufyllin & Lufyllin-400 Tablets ... 2670
Lufyllin-GG Elixir & Tablets ... 2671

Ergotamine Tartrate (Potential for acute ergot toxicity characterized by severe peripheral vasospasm and dysesthesia). Products include:
Bellergal-S Tablets ... 2250
Cafergot ... 2251
Ergomar ... 1486
Wigraine Tablets & Suppositories ... 1829

Hexobarbital (Elevations in serum erythromycin and hexobarbital concentration).

Lovastatin (Potential for rhabdomyolysis in seriously ill patients). Products include:
Mevacor Tablets ... 1699

Phenytoin (Elevations in serum erythromycin and phenytoin concentration). Products include:
Dilantin Infatabs ... 1908
Dilantin-125 Suspension ... 1911

Phenytoin Sodium (Elevations in serum erythromycin and phenytoin concentration). Products include:
Dilantin Kapseals ... 1906
Dilantin Parenteral ... 1910

Terfenadine (Potential for altered terfenadine metabolism). Products include:
Seldane Tablets ... 1536
Seldane-D Extended-Release Tablets ... 1538

Theophylline (Concomitant administration with high doses of theophylline may be associated with increased theophylline levels and potential toxicity). Products include:
Marax Tablets & DF Syrup ... 2200
Quibron ... 2053

Theophylline Anhydrous (Concomitant administration with high doses of theophylline may be associated with increased theophylline levels and potential toxicity). Products include:
Aerolate ... 1004
Primatene Dual Action Formula ... ▣ 872
Primatene Tablets ... ▣ 873
Respbid Tablets ... 682
Slo-bid Gyrocaps ... 2033
Theo-24 Extended Release Capsules ... 2568
Theo-Dur Extended-Release Tablets ... 1327
Theo-X Extended-Release Tablets ... 788
Uni-Dur Extended-Release Tablets ... 1331
Uniphyl 400 mg Tablets ... 2001

Theophylline Calcium Salicylate (Concomitant administration with high doses of theophylline may be associated with increased theophylline levels and potential toxicity). Products include:
Quadrinal Tablets ... 1350

Theophylline Sodium Glycinate (Concomitant administration with high doses of theophylline may be associated with increased theophylline levels and potential toxicity).
No products indexed under this heading.

Triazolam (Decreased clearance of triazolam and increased the pharmacologic effect of triazolam). Products include:
Halcion Tablets ... 2611

Warfarin Sodium (Increased anticoagulant effects). Products include:
Coumadin ... 926

ERYTHROMYCIN DELAYED-RELEASE CAPSULES, USP

(Erythromycin) ... 427
May interact with xanthine bronchodilators, oral anticoagulants, and certain other agents. Compounds in these categories include:

Aminophylline (Concomitant administration with high doses of theophylline may be associated with increased theophylline levels and potential toxicity).
No products indexed under this heading.

Carbamazepine (Elevations in serum erythromycin and carbamazepine concentration). Products include:
Atretol Tablets ... 573
Tegretol Chewable Tablets ... 852
Tegretol Suspension ... 852
Tegretol Tablets ... 852

Cyclosporine (Elevations in serum erythromycin and cyclosporine concentration). Products include:
Neoral ... 2276
Sandimmune ... 2286

Dicumarol (Increased anticoagulant effects).
No products indexed under this heading.

Digoxin (Elevated digoxin serum levels). Products include:
Lanoxicaps ... 1117
Lanoxin Elixir Pediatric ... 1120
Lanoxin Injection ... 1123
Lanoxin Injection Pediatric ... 1126
Lanoxin Tablets ... 1128

Dihydroergotamine Mesylate (Potential for acute ergot toxicity characterized by severe peripheral vasospasm and dysesthesia). Products include:
D.H.E. 45 Injection ... 2255

Drugs which undergo biotransformation by cytochrome P-450 mixed function oxidase (Potential for elevation in serum levels).

Dyphylline (Concomitant administration with high doses of theophylline may be associated with increased theophylline levels and potential toxicity). Products include:
Lufyllin & Lufyllin-400 Tablets ... 2670
Lufyllin-GG Elixir & Tablets ... 2671

Ergotamine Tartrate (Potential for acute ergot toxicity characterized by severe peripheral vasospasm and dysesthesia). Products include:
Bellergal-S Tablets ... 2250
Cafergot ... 2251
Ergomar ... 1486
Wigraine Tablets & Suppositories ... 1829

Hexobarbital (Elevations in serum erythromycin and hexobarbital concentration).

Lovastatin (Potential for rhabdomyolysis in seriously ill patients). Products include:
Mevacor Tablets ... 1699

Phenytoin (Elevations in serum erythromycin and phenytoin concentration). Products include:
Dilantin Infatabs ... 1908
Dilantin-125 Suspension ... 1911

Phenytoin Sodium (Elevations in serum erythromycin and phenytoin concentration). Products include:
Dilantin Kapseals ... 1906
Dilantin Parenteral ... 1910

Terfenadine (Potential for altered terfenadine metabolism). Products include:
Seldane Tablets ... 1536
Seldane-D Extended-Release Tablets ... 1538

Theophylline (Concomitant administration with high doses of theophylline may be associated with increased theophylline levels and potential toxicity). Products include:
Marax Tablets & DF Syrup ... 2200
Quibron ... 2053

Theophylline Anhydrous (Concomitant administration with high doses of theophylline may be associated with increased theophylline levels and potential toxicity). Products include:
Aerolate ... 1004
Primatene Dual Action Formula ... ▣ 872
Primatene Tablets ... ▣ 873
Respbid Tablets ... 682
Slo-bid Gyrocaps ... 2033
Theo-24 Extended Release Capsules ... 2568
Theo-Dur Extended-Release Tablets ... 1327
Theo-X Extended-Release Tablets ... 788
Uni-Dur Extended-Release Tablets ... 1331
Uniphyl 400 mg Tablets ... 2001

Theophylline Calcium Salicylate (Concomitant administration with high doses of theophylline may be associated with increased theophylline levels and potential toxicity). Products include:
Quadrinal Tablets ... 1350

Theophylline Sodium Glycinate (Concomitant administration with high doses of theophylline may be associated with increased theophylline levels and potential toxicity).
No products indexed under this heading.

Triazolam (Decreased clearance of triazolam and increased the pharmacologic effect of triazolam). Products include:
Halcion Tablets ... 2611

Warfarin Sodium (Increased anticoagulant effects). Products include:
Coumadin ... 926

Food Interactions

Food, unspecified (Lowers the blood levels of systemically available erythromycin).

ESGIC-PLUS TABLETS

(Butalbital, Acetaminophen, Caffeine) ... 1013
May interact with monoamine oxidase inhibitors, general anesthetics, barbiturates, benzodiazepines, hypnotics and sedatives, central nervous system depressants, narcotic analgesics, tricyclic antidepressants, antihistamines, tranquilizers, and certain other agents. Compounds in these categories include:

Acrivastine (May exhibit additive CNS depressant effects). Products include:
Semprex-D Capsules ... 463
Semprex-D Capsules ... 1167

Alfentanil Hydrochloride (May exhibit additive CNS depressant effects). Products include:
Alfenta Injection ... 1286

Alprazolam (May exhibit additive CNS depressant effects). Products include:
Xanax Tablets ... 2649

Amitriptyline Hydrochloride (May exhibit additive CNS depressant effects). Products include:
Elavil ... 2838
Endep Tablets ... 2174
Etrafon ... 2355
Limbitrol ... 2180
Triavil Tablets ... 1757

Amoxapine (May exhibit additive CNS depressant effects). Products include:
Asendin Tablets ... 1369

Aprobarbital (May exhibit additive CNS depressant effects).
No products indexed under this heading.

Astemizole (May exhibit additive CNS depressant effects). Products include:
Hismanal Tablets ... 1293

Azatadine Maleate (May exhibit additive CNS depressant effects). Products include:
Trinalin Repetabs Tablets ... 1330

Bromodiphenhydramine Hydrochloride (May exhibit additive CNS depressant effects).
No products indexed under this heading.

Brompheniramine Maleate (May exhibit additive CNS depressant effects). Products include:
Alka Seltzer Plus Sinus Medicine ... ▣ 707
Bromfed Capsules (Extended-Release) ... 1785
Bromfed Syrup ... ▣ 733

(▣ Described in PDR For Nonprescription Drugs) (⊙ Described in PDR For Ophthalmology)

Interactions Index

Esgic-Plus Tablets

Bromfed Tablets 1785
Bromfed-DM Cough Syrup................. 1786
Bromfed-PD Capsules (Extended-Release) 1785
Dimetane-DC Cough Syrup 2059
Dimetane-DX Cough Syrup 2059
Dimetapp Elixir .... ⊕D 773
Dimetapp Extentabs .... ⊕D 774
Dimetapp Tablets/Liqui-Gels .... ⊕D 775
Dimetapp Cold & Allergy Chewable Tablets .... ⊕D 773
Dimetapp DM Elixir .... ⊕D 774
Vicks DayQuil Allergy Relief 12-Hour Extended Release Tablets.. ⊕D 760
Vicks DayQuil Allergy Relief 4-Hour Tablets .... ⊕D 760

Buprenorphine (May exhibit additive CNS depressant effects). Products include:

Buprenex Injectable 2006

Buspirone Hydrochloride (May exhibit additive CNS depressant effects). Products include:

BuSpar 737

Butabarbital (May exhibit additive CNS depressant effects).

No products indexed under this heading.

Chlordiazepoxide (May exhibit additive CNS depressant effects). Products include:

Libritabs Tablets 2177
Limbitrol 2180

Chlordiazepoxide Hydrochloride (May exhibit additive CNS depressant effects). Products include:

Librax Capsules 2176
Librium Capsules 2178
Librium Injectable 2179

Chlorpheniramine Maleate (May exhibit additive CNS depressant effects). Products include:

Alka-Seltzer Plus Cold Medicine .... ⊕D 705
Alka-Seltzer Plus Cold Medicine Liqui-Gels .... ⊕D 706
Alka-Seltzer Plus Cold & Cough Medicine .... ⊕D 708
Alka-Seltzer Plus Cold & Cough Medicine Liqui-Gels.......................... ⊕D 705
Allerest Children's Chewable Tablets .... ⊕D 627
Allerest Headache Strength Tablets .... ⊕D 627
Allerest Maximum Strength Tablets .... ⊕D 627
Allerest Sinus Pain Formula .... ⊕D 627
Allerest 12 Hour Caplets .... ⊕D 627
Ana-Kit Anaphylaxis Emergency Treatment Kit 617
Atrohist Pediatric Capsules.................. 453
Atrohist Plus Tablets 454
BC Cold Powder Multi-Symptom Formula (Cold-Sinus-Allergy) ...... ⊕D 609
Cerose DM .... ⊕D 878
Cheracol Plus Head Cold/Cough Formula .... ⊕D 769
Children's Vicks DayQuil Allergy Relief .... ⊕D 757
Children's Vicks NyQuil Cold/Cough Relief.. ⊕D 758
Chlor-Trimeton Allergy Decongestant Tablets .... ⊕D 799
Chlor-Trimeton Allergy Tablets ...... ⊕D 798
Comhist 2038
Comtrex Multi-Symptom Cold Reliever Tablets/Caplets/Liqui-Gels/Liquid.. ⊕D 615
Allergy-Sinus Comtrex Multi-Symptom Allergy-Sinus Formula Tablets .... ⊕D 617
Contac Continuous Action Nasal Decongestant/Antihistamine 12 Hour Capsules..................................... ⊕D 813
Contac Maximum Strength Continuous Action Decongestant/Antihistamine 12 Hour Caplets.. ⊕D 813
Contac Severe Cold and Flu Formula Caplets .... ⊕D 814
Coricidin 'D' Decongestant Tablets .... ⊕D 800
Coricidin Tablets .... ⊕D 800
D.A. Chewable Tablets.......................... 951
Deconamine 1320
Dura-Tap/PD Capsules 2867
Dura-Vent/DA Tablets.......................... 953
Extendryl 1005
Fedahist Gyrocaps.................................. 2401
Fedahist Timecaps 2401
Hycomine Compound Tablets 932
Isoclor Timesule Capsules .... ⊕D 637
Kronofed-A 977
Nalamine Timed-Release Tablets 785
Novahistine DH...................................... 2462
Novahistine Elixir .... ⊕D 823
Ornade Spansule Capsules 2502
PediaCare Cold Allergy Chewable Tablets .... ⊕D 677
PediaCare Cough-Cold Chewable Tablets 1553
PediaCare Cough-Cold Liquid............ 1553
PediaCare NightRest Cough-Cold Liquid 1553
Pediatric Vicks 44m Cough & Cold Relief .... ⊕D 764
Pyrroxate Caplets .... ⊕D 772
Ryna .... ⊕D 841
Sinarest Tablets .... ⊕D 648
Sinarest Extra Strength Tablets...... ⊕D 648
Sine-Off Sinus Medicine .... ⊕D 825
Singlet Tablets .... ⊕D 825
Sinulin Tablets 787
Sinutab Sinus Allergy Medication, Maximum Strength Tablets and Caplets .... ⊕D 860
Sudafed Plus Liquid .... ⊕D 862
Sudafed Plus Tablets .... ⊕D 863
Teldrin 12 Hour Antihistamine/Nasal Decongestant Allergy Relief Capsules .... ⊕D 826
TheraFlu.. ⊕D 787
TheraFlu Maximum Strength Nighttime Flu, Cold & Cough Medicine .... ⊕D 788
Triaminic Allergy Tablets .... ⊕D 789
Triaminic Cold Tablets .... ⊕D 790
Triaminic Nite Light .... ⊕D 791
Triaminic Syrup .... ⊕D 792
Triaminic-12 Tablets .... ⊕D 792
Triaminicin Tablets .... ⊕D 793
Triaminicol Multi-Symptom Cold Tablets .... ⊕D 793
Triaminicol Multi-Symptom Relief ⊕D 794
Tussend 1783
Children's TYLENOL Cold Multi-Symptom Liquid Formula and Chewable Tablets............................... 1561
Children's TYLENOL Cold Plus Cough Multi Symptom Tablets and Liquid .... ⊕D 681
TYLENOL Maximum Strength Allergy Sinus Medication Gelcaps and Caplets 1563
TYLENOL Cold Multi-Symptom Formula Medication Tablets and Caplets 1561
TYLENOL Cold Multi-Symptom Hot Medication Liquid Packets.............. 1557
Vicks 44 LiquiCaps Cough, Cold & Flu Relief.. ⊕D 755
Vicks 44M Cough, Cold & Flu Relief .... ⊕D 756

Chlorpheniramine Polistirex (May exhibit additive CNS depressant effects). Products include:

Tussionex Pennkinetic Extended-Release Suspension 998

Chlorpheniramine Tannate (May exhibit additive CNS depressant effects). Products include:

Atrohist Pediatric Suspension 454
Ricobid Tablets and Pediatric Suspension.. 2038
Rynatan 2673
Rynatuss 2673

Chlorpromazine (May exhibit additive CNS depressant effects). Products include:

Thorazine Suppositories 2523

Chlorpromazine Hydrochloride (May exhibit additive CNS depressant effects). Products include:

Thorazine 2523

Chlorprothixene (May exhibit additive CNS depressant effects).

No products indexed under this heading.

Chlorprothixene Hydrochloride (May exhibit additive CNS depressant effects).

No products indexed under this heading.

Chlorprothixene Lactate (May exhibit additive CNS depressant effects).

No products indexed under this heading.

Clemastine Fumarate (May exhibit additive CNS depressant effects). Products include:

Tavist Syrup.. 2297
Tavist Tablets 2298
Tavist-1 12 Hour Relief Tablets .... ⊕D 787
Tavist-D 12 Hour Relief Tablets .... ⊕D 787

Clomipramine Hydrochloride (May exhibit additive CNS depressant effects). Products include:

Anafranil Capsules 803

Clorazepate Dipotassium (May exhibit additive CNS depressant effects). Products include:

Tranxene 451

Clozapine (May exhibit additive CNS depressant effects). Products include:

Clozaril Tablets....................................... 2252

Codeine Phosphate (May exhibit additive CNS depressant effects). Products include:

Actifed with Codeine Cough Syrup.. 1067
Brontex 1981
Deconsal C Expectorant Syrup 456
Deconsal Pediatric Syrup 457
Dimetane-DC Cough Syrup 2059
Empirin with Codeine Tablets........... 1093
Fioricet with Codeine Capsules 2260
Fiorinal with Codeine Capsules 2262
Isoclor Expectorant............................... 990
Novahistine DH....................................... 2462
Novahistine Expectorant..................... 2463
Nucofed 2051
Phenergan with Codeine..................... 2777
Phenergan VC with Codeine 2781
Robitussin A-C Syrup 2073
Robitussin-DAC Syrup 2074
Ryna .... ⊕D 841
Soma Compound w/Codeine Tablets 2676
Tussi-Organidin NR Liquid and S NR Liquid 2677
Tylenol with Codeine 1583

Cyproheptadine Hydrochloride (May exhibit additive CNS depressant effects). Products include:

Periactin 1724

Desflurane (May exhibit additive CNS depressant effects). Products include:

Suprane 1813

Desipramine Hydrochloride (May exhibit additive CNS depressant effects). Products include:

Norpramin Tablets 1526

Dexchlorpheniramine Maleate (May exhibit additive CNS depressant effects).

No products indexed under this heading.

Dezocine (May exhibit additive CNS depressant effects). Products include:

Dalgan Injection 538

Diazepam (May exhibit additive CNS depressant effects). Products include:

Dizac 1809
Valium Injectable 2182
Valium Tablets 2183
Valrelease Capsules 2169

Diphenhydramine Citrate (May exhibit additive CNS depressant effects). Products include:

Excedrin P.M. Analgesic/Sleeping Aid Tablets, Caplets, Liquigels...... 733

Diphenhydramine Hydrochloride (May exhibit additive CNS depressant effects). Products include:

Actifed Allergy Daytime/Nighttime Caplets .... ⊕D 844
Actifed Sinus Daytime/Nighttime Tablets and Caplets .... ⊕D 846
Arthritis Foundation NightTime Caplets .... ⊕D 674
Extra Strength Bayer PM Aspirin .. ⊕D 713
Bayer Select Night Time Pain Relief Formula...................................... ⊕D 716
Benadryl Allergy Decongestant Liquid Medication .... ⊕D 848
Benadryl Allergy Decongestant Tablets .... ⊕D 848
Benadryl Allergy Liquid Medication.. ⊕D 849
Benadryl Allergy .... ⊕D 848
Benadryl Allergy Sinus Headache Formula Caplets .... ⊕D 849
Benadryl Capsules.................................. 1898
Benadryl Dye-Free Allergy Liquigel Softgels.. ⊕D 850
Benadryl Dye-Free Allergy Liquid Medication .... ⊕D 850
Benadryl Itch Relief Cream, Children's Formula and Maximum Strength 2% .... ⊕D 851
Benadryl Itch Relief Spray, Children's Formula and Maximum Strength 2% .... ⊕D 851
Benadryl Itch Relief Stick Maximum Strength 2% .... ⊕D 850
Benadryl Itch Stopping Gel, Children's Formula and Maximum Strength 2% .... ⊕D 851
Benadryl Kapseals.................................. 1898
Benadryl Injection 1898
Contac Day & Night Cold/Flu Night Caplets .... ⊕D 812
Contac Night Allergy/Sinus Caplets .... ⊕D 812
Extra Strength Doan's P.M. .... ⊕D 633
Legatrin PM .... ⊕D 651
Miles Nervine Nighttime Sleep-Aid ⊕D 723
Nytol QuickCaps Caplets .... ⊕D 610
Sleepinal Night-time Sleep Aid Capsules and Softgels .... ⊕D 834
TYLENOL Maximum Strength Allergy Sinus NightTime Medication Caplets 1555
TYLENOL Flu NightTime, Maximum Strength, Gelcaps 1566
TYLENOL Maximum Strength Flu NightTime Hot Medication Packets 1562
TYLENOL PM, Extra Strength Pain Reliever/Sleep Aid Caplets, Geltabs, Gelcaps 1560
TYLENOL Severe Allergy Medication Caplets 1564
Maximum Strength Unisom Sleepgels 1934
Unisom With Pain Relief-Nighttime Sleep Aid and Pain Reliever........... 1934

Diphenylpyraline Hydrochloride (May exhibit additive CNS depressant effects).

No products indexed under this heading.

Doxepin Hydrochloride (May exhibit additive CNS depressant effects). Products include:

Sinequan 2205
Zonalon Cream 1055

Droperidol (May exhibit additive CNS depressant effects). Products include:

Inapsine Injection................................... 1296

Enflurane (May exhibit additive CNS depressant effects).

No products indexed under this heading.

Estazolam (May exhibit additive CNS depressant effects). Products include:

ProSom Tablets 449

Ethchlorvynol (May exhibit additive CNS depressant effects). Products include:

Placidyl Capsules.................................... 448

Ethinamate (May exhibit additive CNS depressant effects).

No products indexed under this heading.

Fentanyl (May exhibit additive CNS depressant effects). Products include:

Duragesic Transdermal System........ 1288

Fentanyl Citrate (May exhibit additive CNS depressant effects). Products include:

Sublimaze Injection................................ 1307

IMPORTANT NOTE: Always consult each drug listing in the patient's regimen for possible interactions.

Esgic-Plus Tablets | Interactions Index | 388

Fluphenazine Decanoate (May exhibit additive CNS depressant effects). Products include:
- Prolixin Decanoate 509

Fluphenazine Enanthate (May exhibit additive CNS depressant effects). Products include:
- Prolixin Enanthate 509

Fluphenazine Hydrochloride (May exhibit additive CNS depressant effects). Products include:
- Prolixin 509

Flurazepam Hydrochloride (May exhibit additive CNS depressant effects). Products include:
- Dalmane Capsules 2173

Furazolidone (CNS effects of butalbital may be enhanced). Products include:
- Furoxone 2046

Glutethimide (May exhibit additive CNS depressant effects).
- No products indexed under this heading.

Halazepam (May exhibit additive CNS depressant effects).
- No products indexed under this heading.

Haloperidol (May exhibit additive CNS depressant effects). Products include:
- Haldol Injection, Tablets and Concentrate 1575

Haloperidol Decanoate (May exhibit additive CNS depressant effects). Products include:
- Haldol Decanoate 1577

Hydrocodone Bitartrate (May exhibit additive CNS depressant effects). Products include:
- Anexsia 5/500 Elixir 1781
- Anexia Tablets 1782
- Codiclear DH Syrup 791
- Deconamine CX Cough and Cold Liquid and Tablets 1319
- Duratuss HD Elixir 2565
- Hycodan Tablets and Syrup 930
- Hycomine Compound Tablets 932
- Hycomine 931
- Hycotuss Expectorant Syrup 933
- Hydrocet Capsules 782
- Lorcet 10/650 1018
- Lortab 2566
- Tussend 1783
- Tussend Expectorant 1785
- Vicodin Tablets 1356
- Vicodin ES Tablets 1357
- Vicodin Tuss Expectorant 1358
- Zydone Capsules 949

Hydrocodone Polistirex (May exhibit additive CNS depressant effects). Products include:
- Tussionex Pennkinetic Extended-Release Suspension 998

Hydroxyzine Hydrochloride (May exhibit additive CNS depressant effects). Products include:
- Atarax Tablets & Syrup 2185
- Marax Tablets & DF Syrup 2200
- Vistaril Intramuscular Solution 2216

Imipramine Hydrochloride (May exhibit additive CNS depressant effects). Products include:
- Tofranil Ampuls 854
- Tofranil Tablets 856

Imipramine Pamoate (May exhibit additive CNS depressant effects). Products include:
- Tofranil-PM Capsules 857

Isocarboxazid (CNS effects of butalbital may be enhanced).
- No products indexed under this heading.

Isoflurane (May exhibit additive CNS depressant effects).
- No products indexed under this heading.

Ketamine Hydrochloride (May exhibit additive CNS depressant effects).
- No products indexed under this heading.

Levomethadyl Acetate Hydrochloride (May exhibit additive CNS depressant effects). Products include:
- Orlamm 2239

Levorphanol Tartrate (May exhibit additive CNS depressant effects). Products include:
- Levo-Dromoran 2129

Loratadine (May exhibit additive CNS depressant effects). Products include:
- Claritin 2349
- Claritin-D 2350

Lorazepam (May exhibit additive CNS depressant effects). Products include:
- Ativan Injection 2698
- Ativan Tablets 2700

Loxapine Hydrochloride (May exhibit additive CNS depressant effects). Products include:
- Loxitane 1378

Loxapine Succinate (May exhibit additive CNS depressant effects). Products include:
- Loxitane Capsules 1378

Maprotiline Hydrochloride (May exhibit additive CNS depressant effects). Products include:
- Ludiomil Tablets 843

Meperidine Hydrochloride (May exhibit additive CNS depressant effects). Products include:
- Demerol 2308
- Mepergan Injection 2753

Mephobarbital (May exhibit additive CNS depressant effects). Products include:
- Mebaral Tablets 2322

Meprobamate (May exhibit additive CNS depressant effects). Products include:
- Miltown Tablets 2672
- PMB 200 and PMB 400 2783

Mesoridazine Besylate (May exhibit additive CNS depressant effects). Products include:
- Serentil 684

Methadone Hydrochloride (May exhibit additive CNS depressant effects). Products include:
- Methadone Hydrochloride Oral Concentrate 2233
- Methadone Hydrochloride Oral Solution & Tablets 2235

Methdilazine Hydrochloride (May exhibit additive CNS depressant effects).
- No products indexed under this heading.

Methohexital Sodium (May exhibit additive CNS depressant effects). Products include:
- Brevital Sodium Vials 1429

Methotrimeprazine (May exhibit additive CNS depressant effects). Products include:
- Levoprome 1274

Methoxyflurane (May exhibit additive CNS depressant effects).
- No products indexed under this heading.

Midazolam Hydrochloride (May exhibit additive CNS depressant effects). Products include:
- Versed Injection 2170

Molindone Hydrochloride (May exhibit additive CNS depressant effects). Products include:
- Moban Tablets and Concentrate 1048

Morphine Sulfate (May exhibit additive CNS depressant effects). Products include:
- Astramorph/PF Injection, USP (Preservative-Free) 535
- Duramorph 962
- Infumorph 200 and Infumorph 500 Sterile Solutions 965
- MS Contin Tablets 1994
- MSIR 1997
- Oramorph SR (Morphine Sulfate Sustained Release Tablets) 2236
- RMS Suppositories 2657
- Roxanol 2243

Nortriptyline Hydrochloride (May exhibit additive CNS depressant effects). Products include:
- Pamelor 2280

Opium Alkaloids (May exhibit additive CNS depressant effects).
- No products indexed under this heading.

Oxazepam (May exhibit additive CNS depressant effects). Products include:
- Serax Capsules 2810
- Serax Tablets 2810

Oxycodone Hydrochloride (May exhibit additive CNS depressant effects). Products include:
- Percocet Tablets 938
- Percodan Tablets 939
- Percodan-Demi Tablets 940
- Roxicodone Tablets, Oral Solution & Intensol (Oxycodone) 2244
- Tylox Capsules 1584

Pentobarbital Sodium (May exhibit additive CNS depressant effects). Products include:
- Nembutal Sodium Capsules 436
- Nembutal Sodium Solution 438
- Nembutal Sodium Suppositories 440

Perphenazine (May exhibit additive CNS depressant effects). Products include:
- Etrafon 2355
- Triavil Tablets 1757
- Trilafon 2389

Phenelzine Sulfate (CNS effects of butalbital may be enhanced). Products include:
- Nardil 1920

Phenobarbital (May exhibit additive CNS depressant effects). Products include:
- Arco-Lase Plus Tablets 512
- Bellergal-S Tablets 2250
- Donnatal 2060
- Donnatal Extentabs 2061
- Donnatal Tablets 2060
- Phenobarbital Elixir and Tablets 1469
- Quadrinal Tablets 1350

Prazepam (May exhibit additive CNS depressant effects).
- No products indexed under this heading.

Prochlorperazine (May exhibit additive CNS depressant effects). Products include:
- Compazine 2470

Promethazine Hydrochloride (May exhibit additive CNS depressant effects). Products include:
- Mepergan Injection 2753
- Phenergan with Codeine 2777
- Phenergan with Dextromethorphan 2778
- Phenergan Injection 2773
- Phenergan Suppositories 2775
- Phenergan Syrup 2774
- Phenergan Tablets 2775
- Phenergan VC 2779
- Phenergan VC with Codeine 2781

Propofol (May exhibit additive CNS depressant effects). Products include:
- Diprivan Injection 2833

Propoxyphene Hydrochloride (May exhibit additive CNS depressant effects). Products include:
- Darvon 1435
- Wygesic Tablets 2827

Propoxyphene Napsylate (May exhibit additive CNS depressant effects). Products include:
- Darvon-N/Darvocet-N 1433

Protriptyline Hydrochloride (May exhibit additive CNS depressant effects). Products include:
- Vivactil Tablets 1774

Pyrilamine Maleate (May exhibit additive CNS depressant effects). Products include:
- 4-Way Fast Acting Nasal Spray (regular & mentholated) .... ▣ 621
- Maximum Strength Multi-Symptom Formula Midol .... ▣ 722
- PMS Multi-Symptom Formula Midol .... ▣ 723

Pyrilamine Tannate (May exhibit additive CNS depressant effects). Products include:
- Atrohist Pediatric Suspension 454
- Rynatan 2673

Quazepam (May exhibit additive CNS depressant effects). Products include:
- Doral Tablets 2664

Risperidone (May exhibit additive CNS depressant effects). Products include:
- Risperdal 1301

Secobarbital Sodium (May exhibit additive CNS depressant effects). Products include:
- Seconal Sodium Pulvules 1474

Selegiline Hydrochloride (CNS effects of butalbital may be enhanced). Products include:
- Eldepryl Tablets 2550

Sufentanil Citrate (May exhibit additive CNS depressant effects). Products include:
- Sufenta Injection 1309

Temazepam (May exhibit additive CNS depressant effects). Products include:
- Restoril Capsules 2284

Terfenadine (May exhibit additive CNS depressant effects). Products include:
- Seldane Tablets 1536
- Seldane-D Extended-Release Tablets 1538

Thiamylal Sodium (May exhibit additive CNS depressant effects).
- No products indexed under this heading.

Thioridazine Hydrochloride (May exhibit additive CNS depressant effects). Products include:
- Mellaril 2269

Thiothixene (May exhibit additive CNS depressant effects). Products include:
- Navane Capsules and Concentrate 2201
- Navane Intramuscular 2202

Tranylcypromine Sulfate (CNS effects of butalbital may be enhanced). Products include:
- Parnate Tablets 2503

Triazolam (May exhibit additive CNS depressant effects). Products include:
- Halcion Tablets 2611

Trifluoperazine Hydrochloride (May exhibit additive CNS depressant effects). Products include:
- Stelazine 2514

Trimeprazine Tartrate (May exhibit additive CNS depressant effects). Products include:
- Temaril Tablets, Syrup and Spansule Extended-Release Capsules 483

Trimipramine Maleate (May exhibit additive CNS depressant effects). Products include:
- Surmontil Capsules 2811

389 **Interactions Index** **Esidrix**

Tripelennamine Hydrochloride (May exhibit additive CNS depressant effects). Products include:

- PBZ Tablets ... 845
- PBZ-SR Tablets ... 844

Triprolidine Hydrochloride (May exhibit additive CNS depressant effects). Products include:

- Actifed Plus Caplets ... ▣ 845
- Actifed Plus Tablets ... ▣ 845
- Actifed with Codeine Cough Syrup.. 1067
- Actifed Syrup ... ▣ 846
- Actifed Tablets ... ▣ 844

Zolpidem Tartrate (May exhibit additive CNS depressant effects). Products include:

- Ambien Tablets ... 2416

Food Interactions

Alcohol (May exhibit additive CNS depressant effects).

ESIDRIX TABLETS

(Hydrochlorothiazide) ... 821

May interact with corticosteroids, insulin, antihypertensives, barbiturates, cardiac glycosides, lithium preparations, narcotic analgesics, non-steroidal anti-inflammatory agents, and certain other agents. Compounds in these categories include:

Acebutolol Hydrochloride (Additive or potentiated action). Products include:

- Sectral Capsules ... 2807

ACTH (Hypokalemia may develop during concomitant use of ACTH).

- No products indexed under this heading.

Alfentanil Hydrochloride (May potentiate orthostatic hypotension). Products include:

- Alfenta Injection ... 1286

Amlodipine Besylate (Additive or potentiated action). Products include:

- Lotrel Capsules ... 840
- Norvasc Tablets ... 1940

Aprobarbital (May potentiate orthostatic hypotension).

- No products indexed under this heading.

Atenolol (Additive or potentiated action). Products include:

- Tenoretic Tablets ... 2845
- Tenormin Tablets and I.V. Injection 2847

Benazepril Hydrochloride (Additive or potentiated action). Products include:

- Lotensin Tablets ... 834
- Lotensin HCT ... 837
- Lotrel Capsules ... 840

Bendroflumethiazide (Additive or potentiated action).

- No products indexed under this heading.

Betamethasone Acetate (Hypokalemia may develop during concomitant use of steroid). Products include:

- Celestone Soluspan Suspension ... 2347

Betamethasone Sodium Phosphate (Hypokalemia may develop during concomitant use of steroid). Products include:

- Celestone Soluspan Suspension ... 2347

Betaxolol Hydrochloride (Additive or potentiated action). Products include:

- Betoptic Ophthalmic Solution ... 469
- Betoptic S Ophthalmic Suspension ... 471
- Kerlone Tablets ... 2436

Bisoprolol Fumarate (Additive or potentiated action). Products include:

- Zebeta Tablets ... 1413
- Ziac ... 1415

Buprenorphine (May potentiate orthostatic hypotension). Products include:

- Buprenex Injectable ... 2006

Butabarbital (May potentiate orthostatic hypotension).

- No products indexed under this heading.

Butalbital (May potentiate orthostatic hypotension). Products include:

- Esgic-plus Tablets ... 1013
- Fioricet Tablets ... 2258
- Fioricet with Codeine Capsules ... 2260
- Fiorinal Capsules ... 2261
- Fiorinal with Codeine Capsules ... 2262
- Fiorinal Tablets ... 2261
- Phrenilin ... 785
- Sedapap Tablets 50 mg/650 mg .. 1543

Captopril (Additive or potentiated action). Products include:

- Capoten ... 739
- Capozide ... 742

Carteolol Hydrochloride (Additive or potentiated action). Products include:

- Cartrol Tablets ... 410
- Ocupress Ophthalmic Solution, 1% Sterile ... ◉ 309

Chlorothiazide (Additive or potentiated action). Products include:

- Aldoclor Tablets ... 1598
- Diupres Tablets ... 1650
- Diuril Oral ... 1653

Chlorothiazide Sodium (Additive or potentiated action). Products include:

- Diuril Sodium Intravenous ... 1652

Chlorthalidone (Additive or potentiated action). Products include:

- Combipres Tablets ... 677
- Tenoretic Tablets ... 2845
- Thalitone ... 1245

Cholestyramine (Impairs the oral absorption of hydrochlorothiazide from gastrointestinal tract by up to 85%). Products include:

- Questran Light ... 769
- Questran Powder ... 770

Clonidine (Additive or potentiated action). Products include:

- Catapres-TTS ... 675

Clonidine Hydrochloride (Additive or potentiated action). Products include:

- Catapres Tablets ... 674
- Combipres Tablets ... 677

Codeine Phosphate (May potentiate orthostatic hypotension). Products include:

- Actifed with Codeine Cough Syrup.. 1067
- Brontex ... 1981
- Deconsal C Expectorant Syrup ... 456
- Deconsal Pediatric Syrup ... 457
- Dimetane-DC Cough Syrup ... 2059
- Empirin with Codeine Tablets ... 1093
- Fioricet with Codeine Capsules ... 2260
- Fiorinal with Codeine Capsules ... 2262
- Isoclor Expectorant ... 990
- Novahistine DH ... 2462
- Novahistine Expectorant ... 2463
- Nucofed ... 2051
- Phenergan with Codeine ... 2777
- Phenergan VC with Codeine ... 2781
- Robitussin A-C Syrup ... 2073
- Robitussin-DAC Syrup ... 2074
- Ryna ... ▣ 841
- Soma Compound w/Codeine Tablets ... 2676
- Tussi-Organidin NR Liquid and S NR Liquid ... 2677
- Tylenol with Codeine ... 1583

Colestipol Hydrochloride (Impairs the oral absorption of hydrochlorothiazide from gastrointestinal tract by up to 43%). Products include:

- Colestid Tablets ... 2591

Cortisone Acetate (Hypokalemia may develop during concomitant use of steroid). Products include:

- Cortone Acetate Sterile Suspension ... 1623
- Cortone Acetate Tablets ... 1624

Deserpidine (Additive or potentiated action).

- No products indexed under this heading.

Deslanoside (Thiazide-induced hypokalemia can sensitize or exaggerate the response of the heart to the toxic effects of digitalis, e.g., increased ventricular irritability).

- No products indexed under this heading.

Dexamethasone (Hypokalemia may develop during concomitant use of steroid). Products include:

- AK-Trol Ointment & Suspension ... ◉ 205
- Decadron Elixir ... 1633
- Decadron Tablets ... 1635
- Decaspray Topical Aerosol ... 1648
- Dexacidin Ointment ... ◉ 263
- Maxitrol Ophthalmic Ointment and Suspension ... ◉ 224
- TobraDex Ophthalmic Suspension and Ointment ... 473

Dexamethasone Acetate (Hypokalemia may develop during concomitant use of steroid). Products include:

- Dalalone D.P. Injectable ... 1011
- Decadron-LA Sterile Suspension ... 1646

Dexamethasone Sodium Phosphate (Hypokalemia may develop during concomitant use of steroid). Products include:

- Decadron Phosphate Injection ... 1637
- Decadron Phosphate Respihaler ... 1642
- Decadron Phosphate Sterile Ophthalmic Ointment ... 1641
- Decadron Phosphate Sterile Ophthalmic Solution ... 1642
- Decadron Phosphate Topical Cream ... 1644
- Decadron Phosphate Turbinaire ... 1645
- Decadron Phosphate with Xylocaine Injection, Sterile ... 1639
- Dexacort Phosphate in Respihaler .. 458
- Dexacort Phosphate in Turbinaire .. 459
- NeoDecadron Sterile Ophthalmic Ointment ... 1712
- NeoDecadron Sterile Ophthalmic Solution ... 1713
- NeoDecadron Topical Cream ... 1714

Dezocine (May potentiate orthostatic hypotension). Products include:

- Dalgan Injection ... 538

Diazoxide (Additive or potentiated action). Products include:

- Hyperstat I.V. Injection ... 2363
- Proglycem ... 580

Diclofenac Potassium (May reduce diuretic, natriuretic, and antihypertensive effects of thiazide diuretics). Products include:

- Cataflam ... 816

Diclofenac Sodium (May reduce diuretic, natriuretic, and antihypertensive effects of thiazide diuretics). Products include:

- Voltaren Ophthalmic Sterile Ophthalmic Solution ... ◉ 272
- Voltaren Tablets ... 861

Digitoxin (Thiazide-induced hypokalemia can sensitize or exaggerate the response of the heart to the toxic effects of digitalis, e.g., increased ventricular irritability). Products include:

- Crystodigin Tablets ... 1433

Digoxin (Thiazide-induced hypokalemia can sensitize or exaggerate the response of the heart to the toxic effects of digitalis, e.g., increased ventricular irritability). Products include:

- Lanoxicaps ... 1117
- Lanoxin Elixir Pediatric ... 1120
- Lanoxin Injection ... 1123
- Lanoxin Injection Pediatric ... 1126
- Lanoxin Tablets ... 1128

Diltiazem Hydrochloride (Additive or potentiated action). Products include:

- Cardizem CD Capsules ... 1506
- Cardizem SR Capsules ... 1510
- Cardizem Injectable ... 1508
- Cardizem Tablets ... 1512
- Dilacor XR Extended-release Capsules ... 2018

Doxazosin Mesylate (Additive or potentiated action). Products include:

- Cardura Tablets ... 2186

Enalapril Maleate (Additive or potentiated action). Products include:

- Vaseretic Tablets ... 1765
- Vasotec Tablets ... 1771

Enalaprilat (Additive or potentiated action). Products include:

- Vasotec I.V. ... 1768

Esmolol Hydrochloride (Additive or potentiated action). Products include:

- Brevibloc Injection ... 1808

Etodolac (May reduce diuretic, natriuretic, and antihypertensive effects of thiazide diuretics). Products include:

- Lodine Capsules and Tablets ... 2743

Felodipine (Additive or potentiated action). Products include:

- Plendil Extended-Release Tablets ... 527

Fenoprofen Calcium (May reduce diuretic, natriuretic, and antihypertensive effects of thiazide diuretics). Products include:

- Nalfon 200 Pulvules & Nalfon Tablets ... 917

Fentanyl (May potentiate orthostatic hypotension). Products include:

- Duragesic Transdermal System ... 1288

Fentanyl Citrate (May potentiate orthostatic hypotension). Products include:

- Sublimaze Injection ... 1307

Fludrocortisone Acetate (Hypokalemia may develop during concomitant use of steroid). Products include:

- Florinef Acetate Tablets ... 505

Flurbiprofen (May reduce diuretic, natriuretic, and antihypertensive effects of thiazide diuretics). Products include:

- Ansaid Tablets ... 2579

Fosinopril Sodium (Additive or potentiated action). Products include:

- Monopril Tablets ... 757

Furosemide (Additive or potentiated action). Products include:

- Lasix Injection, Oral Solution and Tablets ... 1240

Guanabenz Acetate (Additive or potentiated action).

- No products indexed under this heading.

Guanethidine Monosulfate (Additive or potentiated action). Products include:

- Esimil Tablets ... 822
- Ismelin Tablets ... 827

Hydralazine Hydrochloride (Additive or potentiated action). Products include:

- Apresazide Capsules ... 808
- Apresoline Hydrochloride Tablets .. 809
- Ser-Ap-Es Tablets ... 849

Hydrocodone Bitartrate (May potentiate orthostatic hypotension). Products include:

- Anexsia 5/500 Elixir ... 1781
- Anexia Tablets ... 1782

IMPORTANT NOTE: Always consult each drug listing in the patient's regimen for possible interactions.

Esidrix

Codiclear DH Syrup 791
Deconamine CX Cough and Cold Liquid and Tablets.............................. 1319
Duratuss HD Elixir.................................. 2565
Hycodan Tablets and Syrup 930
Hycomine Compound Tablets 932
Hycomine 931
Hycotuss Expectorant Syrup 933
Hydrocet Capsules 782
Lorcet 10/650.. 1018
Lortab 2566
Tussend 1783
Tussend Expectorant 1785
Vicodin Tablets 1356
Vicodin ES Tablets 1357
Vicodin Tuss Expectorant 1358
Zydone Capsules 949

Hydrocodone Polistirex (May potentiate orthostatic hypotension). Products include:

Tussionex Pennkinetic Extended-Release Suspension 998

Hydrocortisone (Hypokalemia may develop during concomitant use of steroid). Products include:

Anusol-HC Cream 2.5% 1896
Aquanil HC Lotion 1931
Bactine Hydrocortisone Anti-Itch Cream... ᴹᴰ 709
Caldecort Anti-Itch Hydrocortisone Spray .... ᴹᴰ 631
Cortaid .... ᴹᴰ 836
CORTENEMA... 2535
Cortisporin Ointment 1085
Cortisporin Ophthalmic Ointment Sterile 1085
Cortisporin Ophthalmic Suspension Sterile 1086
Cortisporin Otic Solution Sterile 1087
Cortisporin Otic Suspension Sterile 1088
Cortizone-5 .... ᴹᴰ 831
Cortizone-10 .... ᴹᴰ 831
Hydrocortone Tablets 1672
Hytone 907
Massengill Medicated Soft Cloth Towelettes.. 2458
PediOtic Suspension Sterile 1153
Preparation H Hydrocortisone 1% Cream .... ᴹᴰ 872
ProctoCream-HC 2.5% 2408
VōSoL HC Otic Solution 2678

Hydrocortisone Acetate (Hypokalemia may develop during concomitant use of steroid). Products include:

Analpram-HC Rectal Cream 1% and 2.5% 977
Anusol HC-1 Anti-Itch Hydrocortisone Ointment...................................... ᴹᴰ 847
Anusol-HC Suppositories 1897
Caldecort... ᴹᴰ 631
Carmol HC 924
Coly-Mycin S Otic w/Neomycin & Hydrocortisone 1906
Cortaid .... ᴹᴰ 836
Cortifoam 2396
Cortisporin Cream.................................. 1084
Epifoam 2399
Hydrocortone Acetate Sterile Suspension... 1669
Mantadil Cream 1135
Nupercainal Hydrocortisone 1% Cream... ᴹᴰ 645
Ophthocort .... ◉ 311
Pramosone Cream, Lotion & Ointment 978
ProctoCream-HC 2408
ProctoFoam-HC 2409
Terra-Cortril Ophthalmic Suspension 2210

Hydrocortisone Sodium Phosphate (Hypokalemia may develop during concomitant use of steroid). Products include:

Hydrocortone Phosphate Injection, Sterile 1670

Hydrocortisone Sodium Succinate (Hypokalemia may develop during concomitant use of steroid). Products include:

Solu-Cortef Sterile Powder.................. 2641

Hydroflumethiazide (Additive or potentiated action). Products include:

Diucardin Tablets..................................... 2718

Ibuprofen (May reduce diuretic, natriuretic, and antihypertensive effects of thiazide diuretics). Products include:

Advil Cold and Sinus Caplets and Tablets (formerly CoAdvil) .... ᴹᴰ 870
Advil Ibuprofen Tablets and Caplets .... ᴹᴰ 870
Children's Advil Suspension 2692
Arthritis Foundation Ibuprofen Tablets .... ᴹᴰ 674
Bayer Select Ibuprofen Pain Relief Formula .... ᴹᴰ 715
Cramp End Tablets................................. ᴹᴰ 735
Dimetapp Sinus Caplets .... ᴹᴰ 775
Haltran Tablets... ᴹᴰ 771
IBU Tablets... 1342
Ibuprohm.. ᴹᴰ 735
Children's Motrin Ibuprofen Oral Suspension 1546
Motrin Tablets... 2625
Motrin IB Caplets, Tablets, and Geltabs .... ᴹᴰ 838
Motrin IB Sinus .... ᴹᴰ 838
Motrin Ibuprofen Suspension, Oral Drops, Chewable Tablets, Caplets 1546
Nuprin Ibuprofen/Analgesic Tablets & Caplets .... ᴹᴰ 622
Sine-Aid IB Caplets 1554
Vicks DayQuil SINUS Pressure & PAIN Relief with IBUPROFEN ...... ᴹᴰ 762

Indapamide (Additive or potentiated action). Products include:

Lozol Tablets 2022

Indomethacin (May reduce diuretic, natriuretic, and antihypertensive effects of thiazide diuretics). Products include:

Indocin 1680

Indomethacin Sodium Trihydrate (May reduce diuretic, natriuretic, and antihypertensive effects of thiazide diuretics). Products include:

Indocin I.V. 1684

Insulin, Human (Insulin requirements may be altered).

No products indexed under this heading.

Insulin, Human Isophane Suspension (Insulin requirements may be altered). Products include:

Novolin N Human Insulin 10 ml Vials... 1795

Insulin, Human NPH (Insulin requirements may be altered). Products include:

Humulin N, 100 Units 1448
Novolin N PenFill Cartridges Durable Insulin Delivery System 1798
Novolin N Prefilled Syringe Disposable Insulin Delivery System 1798

Insulin, Human Regular (Insulin requirements may be altered). Products include:

Humulin R, 100 Units 1449
Novolin R Human Insulin 10 ml Vials... 1795
Novolin R PenFill Cartridges Durable Insulin Delivery System 1798
Novolin R Prefilled Syringe Disposable Insulin Delivery System 1798
Velosulin BR Human Insulin 10 ml Vials... 1795

Insulin, Human, Zinc Suspension (Insulin requirements may be altered). Products include:

Humulin L, 100 Units 1446
Humulin U, 100 Units 1450
Novolin L Human Insulin 10 ml Vials... 1795

Insulin, NPH (Insulin requirements may be altered). Products include:

NPH, 100 Units 1450
Pork NPH, 100 Units............................ 1452
Purified Pork NPH Isophane Insulin 1801

Insulin, Regular (Insulin requirements may be altered). Products include:

Regular, 100 Units 1450
Pork Regular, 100 Units 1452
Pork Regular (Concentrated), 500 Units 1453
Purified Pork Regular Insulin 1801

Insulin, Zinc Crystals (Insulin requirements may be altered). Products include:

NPH, 100 Units 1450

Insulin, Zinc Suspension (Insulin requirements may be altered). Products include:

Iletin I 1450
Lente, 100 Units 1450
Iletin II... 1452
Pork Lente, 100 Units........................... 1452
Purified Pork Lente Insulin 1801

Isradipine (Additive or potentiated action). Products include:

DynaCirc Capsules 2256

Ketoprofen (May reduce diuretic, natriuretic, and antihypertensive effects of thiazide diuretics). Products include:

Orudis Capsules 2766
Oruvail Capsules 2766

Ketorolac Tromethamine (May reduce diuretic, natriuretic, and antihypertensive effects of thiazide diuretics). Products include:

Acular 474
Acular .... ◉ 277
Toradol... 2159

Labetalol Hydrochloride (Additive or potentiated action). Products include:

Normodyne Injection 2377
Normodyne Tablets 2379
Trandate 1185

Levorphanol Tartrate (May potentiate orthostatic hypotension). Products include:

Levo-Dromoran 2129

Lisinopril (Additive or potentiated action). Products include:

Prinivil Tablets 1733
Prinzide Tablets 1737
Zestoretic 2850
Zestril Tablets 2854

Lithium Carbonate (Increased risk of lithium toxicity). Products include:

Eskalith 2485
Lithium Carbonate Capsules & Tablets 2230
Lithonate/Lithotabs/Lithobid 2543

Lithium Citrate (Increased risk of lithium toxicity).

No products indexed under this heading.

Losartan Potassium (Additive or potentiated action). Products include:

Cozaar Tablets 1628
Hyzaar Tablets 1677

Mecamylamine Hydrochloride (Additive or potentiated action). Products include:

Inversine Tablets 1686

Meclofenamate Sodium (May reduce diuretic, natriuretic, and antihypertensive effects of thiazide diuretics).

No products indexed under this heading.

Mefenamic Acid (May reduce diuretic, natriuretic, and antihypertensive effects of thiazide diuretics). Products include:

Ponstel 1925

Meperidine Hydrochloride (May potentiate orthostatic hypotension). Products include:

Demerol 2308
Mepergan Injection 2753

Mephobarbital (May potentiate orthostatic hypotension). Products include:

Mebaral Tablets 2322

Methadone Hydrochloride (May potentiate orthostatic hypotension). Products include:

Methadone Hydrochloride Oral Concentrate 2233
Methadone Hydrochloride Oral Solution & Tablets................................ 2235

Methyclothiazide (Additive or potentiated action). Products include:

Enduron Tablets.. 420

Methyldopa (Additive or potentiated action; potential for hemolytic anemia). Products include:

Aldoclor Tablets 1598
Aldomet Oral 1600
Aldoril Tablets... 1604

Methyldopate Hydrochloride (Additive or potentiated action). Products include:

Aldomet Ester HCl Injection 1602

Methylprednisolone Acetate (Hypokalemia may develop during concomitant use of steroid). Products include:

Depo-Medrol Single-Dose Vial 2600
Depo-Medrol Sterile Aqueous Suspension... 2597

Methylprednisolone Sodium Succinate (Hypokalemia may develop during concomitant use of steroid). Products include:

Solu-Medrol Sterile Powder 2643

Metolazone (Additive or potentiated action). Products include:

Mykrox Tablets 993
Zaroxolyn Tablets 1000

Metoprolol Succinate (Additive or potentiated action). Products include:

Toprol-XL Tablets 565

Metoprolol Tartrate (Additive or potentiated action). Products include:

Lopressor Ampuls 830
Lopressor HCT Tablets 832
Lopressor Tablets 830

Metyrosine (Additive or potentiated action). Products include:

Demser Capsules...................................... 1649

Minoxidil (Additive or potentiated action). Products include:

Loniten Tablets.. 2618
Rogaine Topical Solution 2637

Moexipril Hydrochloride (Additive or potentiated action). Products include:

Univasc Tablets 2410

Morphine Sulfate (May potentiate orthostatic hypotension). Products include:

Astramorph/PF Injection, USP (Preservative-Free) 535
Duramorph 962
Infumorph 200 and Infumorph 500 Sterile Solutions.......................... 965
MS Contin Tablets................................... 1994
MSIR 1997
Oramorph SR (Morphine Sulfate Sustained Release Tablets) 2236
RMS Suppositories 2657
Roxanol 2243

Nabumetone (May reduce diuretic, natriuretic, and antihypertensive effects of thiazide diuretics). Products include:

Relafen Tablets.. 2510

Nadolol (Additive or potentiated action).

No products indexed under this heading.

Naproxen (May reduce diuretic, natriuretic, and antihypertensive effects of thiazide diuretics). Products include:

Anaprox/Naprosyn 2117

(ᴹᴰ Described in PDR For Nonprescription Drugs) (◉ Described in PDR For Ophthalmology)

Naproxen Sodium (May reduce diuretic, natriuretic, and antihypertensive effects of thiazide diuretics). Products include:

Aleve 1975
Anaprox/Naprosyn 2117

Nicardipine Hydrochloride (Additive or potentiated action). Products include:

Cardene Capsules 2095
Cardene I.V. 2709
Cardene SR Capsules 2097

Nifedipine (Additive or potentiated action). Products include:

Adalat Capsules (10 mg and 20 mg) 587
Adalat CC 589
Procardia Capsules 1971
Procardia XL Extended Release Tablets 1972

Nisoldipine (Additive or potentiated action).

No products indexed under this heading.

Nitroglycerin (Additive or potentiated action). Products include:

Deponit NTG Transdermal Delivery System 2397
Nitro-Bid IV 1523
Nitro-Bid Ointment 1524
Nitrodisc 2047
Nitro-Dur (nitroglycerin) Transdermal Infusion System 1326
Nitrolingual Spray 2027
Nitrostat Tablets 1925
Transderm-Nitro Transdermal Therapeutic System 859

Norepinephrine Bitartrate (Decreased arterial response to norepinephrine). Products include:

Levophed Bitartrate Injection 2315

Opium Alkaloids (May potentiate orthostatic hypotension).

No products indexed under this heading.

Oxaprozin (May reduce diuretic, natriuretic, and antihypertensive effects of thiazide diuretics). Products include:

Daypro Caplets 2426

Oxycodone Hydrochloride (May potentiate orthostatic hypotension). Products include:

Percocet Tablets 938
Percodan Tablets 939
Percodan-Demi Tablets 940
Roxicodone Tablets, Oral Solution & Intensol (Oxycodone) 2244
Tylox Capsules 1584

Penbutolol Sulfate (Additive or potentiated action). Products include:

Levatol 2403

Pentobarbital Sodium (May potentiate orthostatic hypotension). Products include:

Nembutal Sodium Capsules 436
Nembutal Sodium Solution 438
Nembutal Sodium Suppositories 440

Phenobarbital (May potentiate orthostatic hypotension). Products include:

Arco-Lase Plus Tablets 512
Bellergal-S Tablets 2250
Donnatal 2060
Donnatal Extentabs 2061
Donnatal Tablets 2060
Phenobarbital Elixir and Tablets 1469
Quadrinal Tablets 1350

Phenoxybenzamine Hydrochloride (Additive or potentiated action). Products include:

Dibenzyline Capsules 2476

Phentolamine Mesylate (Additive or potentiated action). Products include:

Regitine 846

Phenylbutazone (May reduce diuretic, natriuretic, and antihypertensive effects of thiazide diuretics).

No products indexed under this heading.

Pindolol (Additive or potentiated action). Products include:

Visken Tablets 2299

Piroxicam (May reduce diuretic, natriuretic, and antihypertensive effects of thiazide diuretics). Products include:

Feldene Capsules 1965

Polythiazide (Additive or potentiated action). Products include:

Minizide Capsules 1938

Prazosin Hydrochloride (Additive or potentiated action). Products include:

Minipress Capsules 1937
Minizide Capsules 1938

Prednisolone Acetate (Hypokalemia may develop during concomitant use of steroid). Products include:

AK-CIDE .... ◉ 202
AK-CIDE Ointment .... ◉ 202
Blephamide Liquifilm Sterile Ophthalmic Suspension 476
Blephamide Ointment .... ◉ 237
Econopred & Econopred Plus Ophthalmic Suspensions .... ◉ 217
Poly-Pred Liquifilm .... ◉ 248
Pred Forte .... ◉ 250
Pred Mild .... ◉ 253
Pred-G Liquifilm Sterile Ophthalmic Suspension .... ◉ 251
Pred-G S.O.P. Sterile Ophthalmic Ointment .... ◉ 252
Vasocidin Ointment .... ◉ 268

Prednisolone Sodium Phosphate (Hypokalemia may develop during concomitant use of steroid). Products include:

AK-Pred .... ◉ 204
Hydeltrasol Injection, Sterile 1665
Inflamase .... ◉ 265
Pediapred Oral Liquid 995
Vasocidin Ophthalmic Solution .... ◉ 270

Prednisolone Tebutate (Hypokalemia may develop during concomitant use of steroid). Products include:

Hydeltra-T.B.A. Sterile Suspension 1667

Prednisone (Hypokalemia may develop during concomitant use of steroid). Products include:

Deltasone Tablets 2595

Propoxyphene Hydrochloride (May potentiate orthostatic hypotension). Products include:

Darvon 1435
Wygesic Tablets 2827

Propoxyphene Napsylate (May potentiate orthostatic hypotension). Products include:

Darvon-N/Darvocet-N 1433

Propranolol Hydrochloride (Additive or potentiated action). Products include:

Inderal 2728
Inderal LA Long Acting Capsules 2730
Inderide Tablets 2732
Inderide LA Long Acting Capsules .. 2734

Quinapril Hydrochloride (Additive or potentiated action). Products include:

Accupril Tablets 1893

Ramipril (Additive or potentiated action). Products include:

Altace Capsules 1232

Rauwolfia Serpentina (Additive or potentiated action).

No products indexed under this heading.

Rescinnamine (Additive or potentiated action).

No products indexed under this heading.

Reserpine (Additive or potentiated action). Products include:

Diupres Tablets 1650
Hydropres Tablets 1675
Ser-Ap-Es Tablets 849

Secobarbital Sodium (May potentiate orthostatic hypotension). Products include:

Seconal Sodium Pulvules 1474

Sodium Nitroprusside (Additive or potentiated action).

No products indexed under this heading.

Sotalol Hydrochloride (Additive or potentiated action). Products include:

Betapace Tablets 641

Spirapril Hydrochloride (Additive or potentiated action).

No products indexed under this heading.

Sufentanil Citrate (May potentiate orthostatic hypotension). Products include:

Sufenta Injection 1309

Sulindac (May reduce diuretic, natriuretic, and antihypertensive effects of thiazide diuretics). Products include:

Clinoril Tablets 1618

Terazosin Hydrochloride (Additive or potentiated action). Products include:

Hytrin Capsules 430

Thiamylal Sodium (May potentiate orthostatic hypotension).

No products indexed under this heading.

Timolol Maleate (Additive or potentiated action). Products include:

Blocadren Tablets 1614
Timolide Tablets 1748
Timoptic in Ocudose 1753
Timoptic Sterile Ophthalmic Solution 1751
Timoptic-XE 1755

Tolmetin Sodium (May reduce diuretic, natriuretic, and antihypertensive effects of thiazide diuretics). Products include:

Tolectin (200, 400 and 600 mg) .. 1581

Torsemide (Additive or potentiated action). Products include:

Demadex Tablets and Injection 686

Triamcinolone (Hypokalemia may develop during concomitant use of steroid). Products include:

Aristocort Tablets 1022

Triamcinolone Acetonide (Hypokalemia may develop during concomitant use of steroid). Products include:

Aristocort A 0.025% Cream 1027
Aristocort A 0.5% Cream 1031
Aristocort A 0.1% Cream 1029
Aristocort A 0.1% Ointment 1030
Azmacort Oral Inhaler 2011
Nasacort Nasal Inhaler 2024

Triamcinolone Diacetate (Hypokalemia may develop during concomitant use of steroid). Products include:

Aristocort Suspension (Forte Parenteral) 1027
Aristocort Suspension (Intralesional) 1025

Triamcinolone Hexacetonide (Hypokalemia may develop during concomitant use of steroid). Products include:

Aristospan Suspension (Intra-articular) 1033
Aristospan Suspension (Intralesional) 1032

Trimethaphan Camsylate (Additive or potentiated action). Products include:

Arfonad Ampuls 2080

Tubocurarine Chloride (Increased responsiveness to tubocurarine).

No products indexed under this heading.

Verapamil Hydrochloride (Additive or potentiated action). Products include:

Calan SR Caplets 2422
Calan Tablets 2419
Isoptin Injectable 1344
Isoptin Oral Tablets 1346
Isoptin SR Tablets 1348
Verelan Capsules 1410
Verelan Capsules 2824

Food Interactions

Alcohol (May potentiate orthostatic hypotension).

ESIMIL TABLETS

(Guanethidine Monosulfate, Hydrochlorothiazide) 822

May interact with monoamine oxidase inhibitors, tricyclic antidepressants, phenothiazines, estrogens, corticosteroids, lithium preparations, insulin, non-steroidal anti-inflammatory agents, antihypertensives, oral contraceptives, cardiac glycosides, barbiturates, narcotic analgesics, and certain other agents. Compounds in these categories include:

Acebutolol Hydrochloride (Additive or potentiated action). Products include:

Sectral Capsules 2807

ACTH (Hypokalemia).

No products indexed under this heading.

Alfentanil Hydrochloride (May potentiate orthostatic hypotension). Products include:

Alfenta Injection 1286

Amitriptyline Hydrochloride (Reduces hypotensive effect). Products include:

Elavil 2838
Endep Tablets 2174
Etrafon 2355
Limbitrol 2180
Triavil Tablets 1757

Amlodipine Besylate (Additive or potentiated action). Products include:

Lotrel Capsules 840
Norvasc Tablets 1940

Amoxapine (Reduces hypotensive effect). Products include:

Asendin Tablets 1369

Aprobarbital (May potentiate orthostatic hypotension).

No products indexed under this heading.

Atenolol (Additive or potentiated action). Products include:

Tenoretic Tablets 2845
Tenormin Tablets and I.V. Injection 2847

Benazepril Hydrochloride (Additive or potentiated action). Products include:

Lotensin Tablets 834
Lotensin HCT 837
Lotrel Capsules 840

Bendroflumethiazide (Additive or potentiated action).

No products indexed under this heading.

Betamethasone Acetate (Hypokalemia). Products include:

Celestone Soluspan Suspension 2347

Betamethasone Dipropionate (Hypokalemia). Products include:

Diprolene AF Cream 2352
Diprolene Gel 0.05% 2353
Diprolene 2352
Lotrisone Cream 2372

IMPORTANT NOTE: Always consult each drug listing in the patient's regimen for possible interactions.

Esimil Interactions Index 392

Betamethasone Sodium Phosphate (Hypokalemia). Products include:
- Celestone Soluspan Suspension 2347

Betaxolol Hydrochloride (Additive or potentiated action). Products include:
- Betoptic Ophthalmic Solution 469
- Betoptic S Ophthalmic Suspension 471
- Kerlone Tablets 2436

Bisoprolol Fumarate (Additive or potentiated action). Products include:
- Zebeta Tablets 1413
- Ziac 1415

Buprenorphine (May potentiate orthostatic hypotension). Products include:
- Buprenex Injectable 2006

Butabarbital (May potentiate orthostatic hypotension).
- No products indexed under this heading.

Butalbital (May potentiate orthostatic hypotension). Products include:
- Esgic-plus Tablets 1013
- Fioricet Tablets 2258
- Fioricet with Codeine Capsules 2260
- Fiorinal Capsules 2261
- Fiorinal with Codeine Capsules 2262
- Fiorinal Tablets 2261
- Phrenilin 785
- Sedapap Tablets 50 mg/650 mg .. 1543

Captopril (Additive or potentiated action). Products include:
- Capoten 739
- Capozide 742

Carteolol Hydrochloride (Additive or potentiated action). Products include:
- Cartrol Tablets 410
- Ocupress Ophthalmic Solution, 1% Sterile .... ◉ 309

Chlorothiazide (Additive or potentiated action). Products include:
- Aldoclor Tablets 1598
- Diupres Tablets 1650
- Diuril Oral 1653

Chlorothiazide Sodium (Additive or potentiated action). Products include:
- Diuril Sodium Intravenous 1652

Chlorotrianisene (Reduces hypotensive effect).
- No products indexed under this heading.

Chlorpromazine (Reduces hypotensive effect). Products include:
- Thorazine Suppositories 2523

Chlorthalidone (Additive or potentiated action). Products include:
- Combipres Tablets 677
- Tenoretic Tablets 2845
- Thalitone 1245

Cholestyramine (Impairs the oral absorption of hydrochlorothiazide from gastrointestinal tract by up to 85%). Products include:
- Questran Light 769
- Questran Powder 770

Clomipramine Hydrochloride (Reduces hypotensive effect). Products include:
- Anafranil Capsules 803

Clonidine (Additive or potentiated action). Products include:
- Catapres-TTS 675

Clonidine Hydrochloride (Additive or potentiated action). Products include:
- Catapres Tablets 674
- Combipres Tablets 677

Codeine Phosphate (May potentiate orthostatic hypotension). Products include:
- Actifed with Codeine Cough Syrup .. 1067
- Brontex 1981
- Deconsal C Expectorant Syrup 456
- Deconsal Pediatric Syrup 457
- Dimetane-DC Cough Syrup 2059
- Empirin with Codeine Tablets 1093
- Fioricet with Codeine Capsules 2260
- Fiorinal with Codeine Capsules 2262
- Isoclor Expectorant 990
- Novahistine DH 2462
- Novahistine Expectorant 2463
- Nucofed 2051
- Phenergan with Codeine 2777
- Phenergan VC with Codeine 2781
- Robitussin A-C Syrup 2073
- Robitussin-DAC Syrup 2074
- Ryna .... ■□ 841
- Soma Compound w/Codeine Tablets 2676
- Tussi-Organidin NR Liquid and S NR Liquid 2677
- Tylenol with Codeine 1583

Colestipol Hydrochloride (Impairs the oral absorption of hydrochlorothiazide from gastrointestinal tract by up to 43%). Products include:
- Colestid Tablets 2591

Cortisone Acetate (Hypokalemia). Products include:
- Cortone Acetate Sterile Suspension 1623
- Cortone Acetate Tablets 1624

Deserpidine (May result in excessive postural hypotension, bradycardia and mental depression).
- No products indexed under this heading.

Desipramine Hydrochloride (Reduces hypotensive effect). Products include:
- Norpramin Tablets 1526

Deslanoside (Increased ventricular irritability; slow heart).
- No products indexed under this heading.

Desogestrel (Reduces hypotensive effect). Products include:
- Desogen Tablets 1817
- Ortho-Cept 1851

Dexamethasone Acetate (Hypokalemia). Products include:
- Dalalone D.P. Injectable 1011
- Decadron-LA Sterile Suspension 1646

Dexamethasone Sodium Phosphate (Hypokalemia). Products include:
- Decadron Phosphate Injection 1637
- Decadron Phosphate Respihaler 1642
- Decadron Phosphate Sterile Ophthalmic Ointment 1641
- Decadron Phosphate Sterile Ophthalmic Solution 1642
- Decadron Phosphate Topical Cream 1644
- Decadron Phosphate Turbinaire 1645
- Decadron Phosphate with Xylocaine Injection, Sterile 1639
- Dexacort Phosphate in Respihaler .. 458
- Dexacort Phosphate in Turbinaire .. 459
- NeoDecadron Sterile Ophthalmic Ointment 1712
- NeoDecadron Sterile Ophthalmic Solution 1713
- NeoDecadron Topical Cream 1714

Dezocine (May potentiate orthostatic hypotension). Products include:
- Dalgan Injection 538

Diazoxide (Additive or potentiated action). Products include:
- Hyperstat I.V. Injection 2363
- Proglycem 580

Diclofenac Potassium (May reduce diuretic, natriuretic, and antihypertensive effects of thiazide diuretics). Products include:
- Cataflam 816

Diclofenac Sodium (May reduce diuretic, natriuretic, and antihypertensive effects of thiazide diuretics). Products include:
- Voltaren Ophthalmic Sterile Ophthalmic Solution .... ◉ 272
- Voltaren Tablets 861

Dienestrol (Reduces hypotensive effect). Products include:
- Ortho Dienestrol Cream 1866

Diethylstilbestrol (Reduces hypotensive effect). Products include:
- Diethylstilbestrol Tablets 1437

Digitoxin (Increased ventricular irritability; slow heart). Products include:
- Crystodigin Tablets 1433

Digoxin (Increased ventricular irritability; slow heart). Products include:
- Lanoxicaps 1117
- Lanoxin Elixir Pediatric 1120
- Lanoxin Injection 1123
- Lanoxin Injection Pediatric 1126
- Lanoxin Tablets 1128

Diltiazem Hydrochloride (Additive or potentiated action). Products include:
- Cardizem CD Capsules 1506
- Cardizem SR Capsules 1510
- Cardizem Injectable 1508
- Cardizem Tablets 1512
- Dilacor XR Extended-release Capsules 2018

Doxazosin Mesylate (Additive or potentiated action). Products include:
- Cardura Tablets 2186

Doxepin Hydrochloride (Reduces hypotensive effect). Products include:
- Sinequan 2205
- Zonalon Cream 1055

Enalapril Maleate (Additive or potentiated action). Products include:
- Vaseretic Tablets 1765
- Vasotec Tablets 1771

Enalaprilat (Additive or potentiated action). Products include:
- Vasotec I.V. 1768

Ephedrine Hydrochloride (Reduces hypotensive effect). Products include:
- Primatene Dual Action Formula ...... ■□ 872
- Primatene Tablets .... ■□ 873
- Quadrinal Tablets 1350

Ephedrine Sulfate (Reduces hypotensive effect). Products include:
- Bronkaid Caplets .... ■□ 717
- Marax Tablets & DF Syrup 2200

Ephedrine Tannate (Reduces hypotensive effect). Products include:
- Rynatuss 2673

Esmolol Hydrochloride (Additive or potentiated action). Products include:
- Brevibloc Injection 1808

Estradiol (Reduces hypotensive effect). Products include:
- Climara Transdermal System 645
- Estrace Cream and Tablets 749
- Estraderm Transdermal System 824

Estrogens, Conjugated (Reduces hypotensive effect). Products include:
- PMB 200 and PMB 400 2783
- Premarin Intravenous 2787
- Premarin with Methyltestosterone .. 2794
- Premarin Tablets 2789
- Premarin Vaginal Cream 2791
- Premphase 2797
- Prempro 2801

Estrogens, Esterified (Reduces hypotensive effect). Products include:
- ESTRATAB Tablets (0.3, 0.625, 1.25, 2.5 mg) 2536
- Estratest 2539
- Menest Tablets 2494

Estropipate (Reduces hypotensive effect). Products include:
- Ogen Tablets 2627
- Ogen Vaginal Cream 2630
- Ortho-Est 1869

Ethinyl Estradiol (Reduces hypotensive effect). Products include:
- Brevicon 2088
- Demulen 2428
- Desogen Tablets 1817
- Levlen/Tri-Levlen 651
- Lo/Ovral Tablets 2746
- Lo/Ovral-28 Tablets 2751
- Modicon 1872
- Nordette-21 Tablets 2755
- Nordette-28 Tablets 2758
- Norinyl 2088
- Ortho-Cept 1851
- Ortho-Cyclen/Ortho-Tri-Cyclen 1858
- Ortho-Novum 1872
- Ortho-Cyclen/Ortho Tri-Cyclen 1858
- Ovcon 760
- Ovral Tablets 2770
- Ovral-28 Tablets 2770
- Levlen/Tri-Levlen 651
- Tri-Norinyl 2164
- Triphasil-21 Tablets 2814
- Triphasil-28 Tablets 2819

Ethynodiol Diacetate (Reduces hypotensive effect). Products include:
- Demulen 2428

Etodolac (May reduce diuretic, natriuretic, and antihypertensive effects of thiazide diuretics). Products include:
- Lodine Capsules and Tablets 2743

Felodipine (Additive or potentiated action). Products include:
- Plendil Extended-Release Tablets 527

Fenoprofen Calcium (May reduce the diuretic, natriuretic, and antihypertensive effects of thiazide diuretics). Products include:
- Nalfon 200 Pulvules & Nalfon Tablets 917

Fentanyl (May potentiate orthostatic hypotension). Products include:
- Duragesic Transdermal System 1288

Fentanyl Citrate (May potentiate orthostatic hypotension). Products include:
- Sublimaze Injection 1307

Fludrocortisone Acetate (Hypokalemia). Products include:
- Florinef Acetate Tablets 505

Fluphenazine Decanoate (Reduces hypotensive effect). Products include:
- Prolixin Decanoate 509

Fluphenazine Enanthate (Reduces hypotensive effect). Products include:
- Prolixin Enanthate 509

Fluphenazine Hydrochloride (Reduces hypotensive effect). Products include:
- Prolixin 509

Flurbiprofen (May reduce diuretic, natriuretic, and antihypertensive effects of thiazide diuretics). Products include:
- Ansaid Tablets 2579

Fosinopril Sodium (Additive or potentiated action). Products include:
- Monopril Tablets 757

Furazolidone (Concurrent use contraindicated). Products include:
- Furoxone 2046

Furosemide (Additive or potentiated action). Products include:
- Lasix Injection, Oral Solution and Tablets 1240

Guanabenz Acetate (Additive or potentiated action).
- No products indexed under this heading.

Hydralazine Hydrochloride (Additive or potentiated action). Products include:
- Apresazide Capsules 808
- Apresoline Hydrochloride Tablets .. 809
- Ser-Ap-Es Tablets 849

(■□ Described in PDR For Nonprescription Drugs) (◉ Described in PDR For Ophthalmology)

Interactions Index

Hydrocodone Bitartrate (May potentiate orthostatic hypotension). Products include:

Anexsia 5/500 Elixir 1781
Anexia Tablets 1782
Codiclear DH Syrup 791
Deconamine CX Cough and Cold Liquid and Tablets 1319
Duratuss HD Elixir 2565
Hycodan Tablets and Syrup 930
Hycomine Compound Tablets 932
Hycomine 931
Hycotuss Expectorant Syrup 933
Hydrocet Capsules 782
Lorcet 10/650 1018
Lortab 2566
Tussend 1783
Tussend Expectorant 1785
Vicodin Tablets 1356
Vicodin ES Tablets 1357
Vicodin Tuss Expectorant 1358
Zydone Capsules 949

Hydrocodone Polistirex (May potentiate orthostatic hypotension). Products include:

Tussionex Pennkinetic Extended-Release Suspension 998

Hydrocortisone (Hypokalemia). Products include:

Anusol-HC Cream 2.5% 1896
Aquanil HC Lotion 1931
Bactine Hydrocortisone Anti-Itch Cream .... ✦⊘ 709
Caldecort Anti-Itch Hydrocortisone Spray .... ✦⊘ 631
Cortaid .... ✦⊘ 836
CORTENEMA 2535
Cortisporin Ointment 1085
Cortisporin Ophthalmic Ointment Sterile 1085
Cortisporin Ophthalmic Suspension Sterile 1086
Cortisporin Otic Solution Sterile 1087
Cortisporin Otic Suspension Sterile 1088
Cortizone-5 .... ✦⊘ 831
Cortizone-10 .... ✦⊘ 831
Hydrocortone Tablets 1672
Hytone 907
Massengill Medicated Soft Cloth Towelettes 2458
PediOtic Suspension Sterile 1153
Preparation H Hydrocortisone 1% Cream .... ✦⊘ 872
ProctoCream-HC 2.5% 2408
VōSoL HC Otic Solution 2678

Hydrocortisone Acetate (Hypokalemia). Products include:

Analpram-HC Rectal Cream 1% and 2.5% 977
Anusol HC-1 Anti-Itch Hydrocortisone Ointment .... ✦⊘ 847
Anusol-HC Suppositories 1897
Caldecort .... ✦⊘ 631
Carmol HC 924
Coly-Mycin S Otic w/Neomycin & Hydrocortisone 1906
Cortaid .... ✦⊘ 836
Cortifoam 2396
Cortisporin Cream 1084
Epifoam 2399
Hydrocortone Acetate Sterile Suspension 1669
Mantadil Cream 1135
Nupercainal Hydrocortisone 1% Cream .... ✦⊘ 645
Ophthocort .... ◎ 311
Pramosone Cream, Lotion & Ointment 978
ProctoCream-HC 2408
ProctoFoam-HC 2409
Terra-Cortril Ophthalmic Suspension 2210

Hydrocortisone Sodium Phosphate (Hypokalemia). Products include:

Hydrocortone Phosphate Injection, Sterile 1670

Hydrocortisone Sodium Succinate (Hypokalemia). Products include:

Solu-Cortef Sterile Powder 2641

Hydroflumethiazide (Additive or potentiated action). Products include:

Diucardin Tablets 2718

Ibuprofen (May reduce the diuretic, natriuretic, and antihypertensive effects of thiazide diuretics). Products include:

Advil Cold and Sinus Caplets and Tablets (formerly CoAdvil) .... ✦⊘ 870
Advil Ibuprofen Tablets and Caplets .... ✦⊘ 870
Children's Advil Suspension 2692
Arthritis Foundation Ibuprofen Tablets .... ✦⊘ 674
Bayer Select Ibuprofen Pain Relief Formula .... ✦⊘ 715
Cramp End Tablets .... ✦⊘ 735
Dimetapp Sinus Caplets .... ✦⊘ 775
Haltran Tablets .... ✦⊘ 771
IBU Tablets 1342
Ibuprohm .... ✦⊘ 735
Children's Motrin Ibuprofen Oral Suspension 1546
Motrin Tablets 2625
Motrin IB Caplets, Tablets, and Geltabs .... ✦⊘ 838
Motrin IB Sinus .... ✦⊘ 838
Motrin Ibuprofen Suspension, Oral Drops, Chewable Tablets, Caplets 1546
Nuprin Ibuprofen/Analgesic Tablets & Caplets .... ✦⊘ 622
Sine-Aid IB Caplets 1554
Vicks DayQuil SINUS Pressure & PAIN Relief with IBUPROFEN ...... ✦⊘ 762

Imipramine Hydrochloride (Reduces hypotensive effect). Products include:

Tofranil Ampuls 854
Tofranil Tablets 856

Imipramine Pamoate (Reduces hypotensive effect). Products include:

Tofranil-PM Capsules 857

Indapamide (Additive or potentiated action). Products include:

Lozol Tablets 2022

Indomethacin (May reduce the diuretic, natriuretic, and antihypertensive effects of thiazide diuretics). Products include:

Indocin 1680

Indomethacin Sodium Trihydrate (May reduce the diuretic, natriuretic, and antihypertensive effects of thiazide diuretics). Products include:

Indocin I.V. 1684

Insulin, Human (Insulin requirements may be altered).

No products indexed under this heading.

Insulin, Human Isophane Suspension (Insulin requirements may be altered). Products include:

Novolin N Human Insulin 10 ml Vials 1795

Insulin, Human NPH (Insulin requirements may be altered). Products include:

Humulin N, 100 Units 1448
Novolin N PenFill Cartridges Durable Insulin Delivery System 1798
Novolin N Prefilled Syringe Disposable Insulin Delivery System 1798

Insulin, Human Regular (Insulin requirements may be altered). Products include:

Humulin R, 100 Units 1449
Novolin R Human Insulin 10 ml Vials 1795
Novolin R PenFill Cartridges Durable Insulin Delivery System 1798
Novolin R Prefilled Syringe Disposable Insulin Delivery System 1798
Velosulin BR Human Insulin 10 ml Vials 1795

Insulin, Human, Zinc Suspension (Insulin requirements may be altered). Products include:

Humulin L, 100 Units 1446
Humulin U, 100 Units 1450
Novolin L Human Insulin 10 ml Vials 1795

Insulin, NPH (Insulin requirements may be altered). Products include:

NPH, 100 Units 1450
Pork NPH, 100 Units 1452
Purified Pork NPH Isophane Insulin 1801

Insulin, Regular (Insulin requirements may be altered). Products include:

Regular, 100 Units 1450
Pork Regular, 100 Units 1452
Pork Regular (Concentrated), 500 Units 1453
Purified Pork Regular Insulin 1801

Insulin, Zinc Crystals (Insulin requirements may be altered). Products include:

NPH, 100 Units 1450

Insulin, Zinc Suspension (Insulin requirements may be altered). Products include:

Iletin I 1450
Lente, 100 Units 1450
Iletin II 1452
Pork Lente, 100 Units 1452
Purified Pork Lente Insulin 1801

Isocarboxazid (Concurrent use contraindicated).

No products indexed under this heading.

Isradipine (Additive or potentiated action). Products include:

DynaCirc Capsules 2256

Ketoprofen (May reduce the diuretic, natriuretic, and antihypertensive effects of thiazide diuretics). Products include:

Orudis Capsules 2766
Oruvail Capsules 2766

Ketorolac Tromethamine (May reduce diuretic, natriuretic, and antihypertensive effects of thiazide diuretics). Products include:

Acular 474
Acular .... ◎ 277
Toradol 2159

Labetalol Hydrochloride (Additive or potentiated action). Products include:

Normodyne Injection 2377
Normodyne Tablets 2379
Trandate 1185

Levonorgestrel (Reduces hypotensive effect). Products include:

Levlen/Tri-Levlen 651
Nordette-21 Tablets 2755
Nordette-28 Tablets 2758
Norplant System 2759
Levlen/Tri-Levlen 651
Triphasil-21 Tablets 2814
Triphasil-28 Tablets 2819

Levorphanol Tartrate (May potentiate orthostatic hypotension). Products include:

Levo-Dromoran 2129

Lisinopril (Additive or potentiated action). Products include:

Prinivil Tablets 1733
Prinzide Tablets 1737
Zestoretic 2850
Zestril Tablets 2854

Lithium Carbonate (Increased risk of lithium toxicity). Products include:

Eskalith 2485
Lithium Carbonate Capsules & Tablets 2230
Lithonate/Lithotabs/Lithobid 2543

Lithium Citrate (Increases risk of lithium toxicity).

No products indexed under this heading.

Losartan Potassium (Additive or potentiated action). Products include:

Cozaar Tablets 1628
Hyzaar Tablets 1677

Maprotiline Hydrochloride (Reduces hypotensive effect). Products include:

Ludiomil Tablets 843

Mecamylamine Hydrochloride (Additive or potentiated action). Products include:

Inversine Tablets 1686

Meclofenamate Sodium (May reduce the diuretic, natriuretic, and antihypertensive effects of thiazide diuretics).

No products indexed under this heading.

Mefenamic Acid (May reduce the diuretic, natriuretic, and antihypertensive effects of thiazide diuretics). Products include:

Ponstel 1925

Meperidine Hydrochloride (May potentiate orthostatic hypotension). Products include:

Demerol 2308
Mepergan Injection 2753

Mephobarbital (May potentiate orthostatic hypotension). Products include:

Mebaral Tablets 2322

Mesoridazine Besylate (Reduces hypotensive effect). Products include:

Serentil 684

Mestranol (Reduces hypotensive effect). Products include:

Norinyl 2088
Ortho-Novum 1872

Methadone Hydrochloride (May potentiate orthostatic hypotension). Products include:

Methadone Hydrochloride Oral Concentrate 2233
Methadone Hydrochloride Oral Solution & Tablets 2235

Methotrimeprazine (Reduces hypotensive effect). Products include:

Levoprome 1274

Methyclothiazide (Additive or potentiated action). Products include:

Enduron Tablets 420

Methyldopa (Additive or potentiated action; hemolytic anemia). Products include:

Aldoclor Tablets 1598
Aldomet Oral 1600
Aldoril Tablets 1604

Methyldopate Hydrochloride (Additive or potentiated action; hemolytic anemia). Products include:

Aldomet Ester HCl Injection 1602

Methylphenidate Hydrochloride (Reduces hypotensive effect). Products include:

Ritalin 848

Methylprednisolone (Hypokalemia). Products include:

Medrol 2621

Methylprednisolone Acetate (Hypokalemia). Products include:

Depo-Medrol Single-Dose Vial 2600
Depo-Medrol Sterile Aqueous Suspension 2597

Methylprednisolone Sodium Succinate (Hypokalemia). Products include:

Solu-Medrol Sterile Powder 2643

Metolazone (Additive or potentiated action). Products include:

Mykrox Tablets 993
Zaroxolyn Tablets 1000

Metoprolol Succinate (Additive or potentiated action). Products include:

Toprol-XL Tablets 565

Metoprolol Tartrate (Additive or potentiated action). Products include:

Lopressor Ampuls 830
Lopressor HCT Tablets 832
Lopressor Tablets 830

IMPORTANT NOTE: Always consult each drug listing in the patient's regimen for possible interactions.

Esimil **Interactions Index** 394

Metyrosine (Additive or potentiated action). Products include:
- Demser Capsules ... 1649

Minoxidil (Additive or potentiated action). Products include:
- Loniten Tablets ... 2618
- Rogaine Topical Solution ... 2637

Moexipril Hydrochloride (Additive or potentiated action). Products include:
- Univasc Tablets ... 2410

Morphine Sulfate (May potentiate orthostatic hypotension). Products include:
- Astramorph/PF Injection, USP (Preservative-Free) ... 535
- Duramorph ... 962
- Infumorph 200 and Infumorph 500 Sterile Solutions ... 965
- MS Contin Tablets ... 1994
- MSIR ... 1997
- Oramorph SR (Morphine Sulfate Sustained Release Tablets) ... 2236
- RMS Suppositories ... 2657
- Roxanol ... 2243

Nabumetone (May reduce diuretic, natriuretic, and antihypertensive effects of thiazide diuretics). Products include:
- Relafen Tablets ... 2510

Nadolol (Additive or potentiated action).
- No products indexed under this heading.

Naproxen (May reduce the diuretic, natriuretic, and antihypertensive effects of thiazide diuretics). Products include:
- Anaprox/Naprosyn ... 2117

Naproxen Sodium (May reduce the diuretic, natriuretic, and antihypertensive effects of thiazide diuretics). Products include:
- Aleve ... 1975
- Anaprox/Naprosyn ... 2117

Nicardipine Hydrochloride (Additive or potentiated action). Products include:
- Cardene Capsules ... 2095
- Cardene I.V. ... 2709
- Cardene SR Capsules ... 2097

Nifedipine (Additive or potentiated action). Products include:
- Adalat Capsules (10 mg and 20 mg) ... 587
- Adalat CC ... 589
- Procardia Capsules ... 1971
- Procardia XL Extended Release Tablets ... 1972

Nisoldipine (Additive or potentiated action).
- No products indexed under this heading.

Nitroglycerin (Additive or potentiated action). Products include:
- Deponit NTG Transdermal Delivery System ... 2397
- Nitro-Bid IV ... 1523
- Nitro-Bid Ointment ... 1524
- Nitrodisc ... 2047
- Nitro-Dur (nitroglycerin) Transdermal Infusion System ... 1326
- Nitrolingual Spray ... 2027
- Nitrostat Tablets ... 1925
- Transderm-Nitro Transdermal Therapeutic System ... 859

Norepinephrine Bitartrate (Decreased arterial response to norepinephrine). Products include:
- Levophed Bitartrate Injection ... 2315

Norethindrone (Reduces hypotensive effect). Products include:
- Brevicon ... 2088
- Micronor Tablets ... 1872
- Modicon ... 1872
- Norinyl ... 2088
- Nor-Q D Tablets ... 2135
- Ortho-Novum ... 1872
- Ovcon ... 760
- Tri-Norinyl ... 2164

Norethynodrel (Reduces hypotensive effect).
- No products indexed under this heading.

Norgestimate (Reduces hypotensive effect). Products include:
- Ortho-Cyclen/Ortho-Tri-Cyclen ... 1858
- Ortho-Cyclen/Ortho Tri-Cyclen ... 1858

Norgestrel (Reduces hypotensive effect). Products include:
- Lo/Ovral Tablets ... 2746
- Lo/Ovral-28 Tablets ... 2751
- Ovral Tablets ... 2770
- Ovral-28 Tablets ... 2770
- Ovrette Tablets ... 2771

Nortriptyline Hydrochloride (Reduces hypotensive effect). Products include:
- Pamelor ... 2280

Opium Alkaloids (May potentiate orthostatic hypotension).
- No products indexed under this heading.

Oxaprozin (May reduce diuretic, natriuretic, and antihypertensive effects of thiazide diuretics). Products include:
- Daypro Caplets ... 2426

Oxycodone Hydrochloride (May potentiate orthostatic hypotension). Products include:
- Percocet Tablets ... 938
- Percodan Tablets ... 939
- Percodan-Demi Tablets ... 940
- Roxicodone Tablets, Oral Solution & Intensol (Oxycodone) ... 2244
- Tylox Capsules ... 1584

Penbutolol Sulfate (Additive or potentiated action). Products include:
- Levatol ... 2403

Pentobarbital Sodium (May potentiate orthostatic hypotension). Products include:
- Nembutal Sodium Capsules ... 436
- Nembutal Sodium Solution ... 438
- Nembutal Sodium Suppositories ... 440

Perphenazine (Reduces hypotensive effect). Products include:
- Etrafon ... 2355
- Triavil Tablets ... 1757
- Trilafon ... 2389

Phenelzine Sulfate (Concurrent use contraindicated). Products include:
- Nardil ... 1920

Phenobarbital (May potentiate orthostatic hypotension). Products include:
- Arco-Lase Plus Tablets ... 512
- Bellergal-S Tablets ... 2250
- Donnatal ... 2060
- Donnatal Extentabs ... 2061
- Donnatal Tablets ... 2060
- Phenobarbital Elixir and Tablets ... 1469
- Quadrinal Tablets ... 1350

Phenoxybenzamine Hydrochloride (Additive or potentiated action). Products include:
- Dibenzyline Capsules ... 2476

Phentolamine Mesylate (Additive or potentiated action). Products include:
- Regitine ... 846

Phenylbutazone (May reduce the diuretic, natriuretic, and antihypertensive effects of thiazide diuretics).
- No products indexed under this heading.

Pindolol (Additive or potentiated action). Products include:
- Visken Tablets ... 2299

Piroxicam (May reduce the diuretic, natriuretic, and antihypertensive effects of thiazide diuretics). Products include:
- Feldene Capsules ... 1965

Polythiazide (Additive or potentiated action). Products include:
- Minizide Capsules ... 1938

Prazosin Hydrochloride (Additive or potentiated action). Products include:
- Minipress Capsules ... 1937
- Minizide Capsules ... 1938

Prednisolone Acetate (Hypokalemia). Products include:
- AK-CIDE ... ◉ 202
- AK-CIDE Ointment ... ◉ 202
- Blephamide Liquifilm Sterile Ophthalmic Suspension ... 476
- Blephamide Ointment ... ◉ 237
- Econopred & Econopred Plus Ophthalmic Suspensions ... ◉ 217
- Poly-Pred Liquifilm ... ◉ 248
- Pred Forte ... ◉ 250
- Pred Mild ... ◉ 253
- Pred-G Liquifilm Sterile Ophthalmic Suspension ... ◉ 251
- Pred-G S.O.P. Sterile Ophthalmic Ointment ... ◉ 252
- Vasocidin Ointment ... ◉ 268

Prednisolone Sodium Phosphate (Hypokalemia). Products include:
- AK-Pred ... ◉ 204
- Hydeltrasol Injection, Sterile ... 1665
- Inflamase ... ◉ 265
- Pediapred Oral Liquid ... 995
- Vasocidin Ophthalmic Solution ... ◉ 270

Prednisolone Tebutate (Hypokalemia). Products include:
- Hydeltra-T.B.A. Sterile Suspension 1667

Prednisone (Hypokalemia). Products include:
- Deltasone Tablets ... 2595

Prochlorperazine (Reduced hypotensive effect). Products include:
- Compazine ... 2470

Promethazine Hydrochloride (Reduces hypotensive effect). Products include:
- Mepergan Injection ... 2753
- Phenergan with Codeine ... 2777
- Phenergan with Dextromethorphan 2778
- Phenergan Injection ... 2773
- Phenergan Suppositories ... 2775
- Phenergan Syrup ... 2774
- Phenergan Tablets ... 2775
- Phenergan VC ... 2779
- Phenergan VC with Codeine ... 2781

Propoxyphene Hydrochloride (May potentiate orthostatic hypotension). Products include:
- Darvon ... 1435
- Wygesic Tablets ... 2827

Propoxyphene Napsylate (May potentiate orthostatic hypotension). Products include:
- Darvon-N/Darvocet-N ... 1433

Propranolol Hydrochloride (Additive or potentiated action). Products include:
- Inderal ... 2728
- Inderal LA Long Acting Capsules ... 2730
- Inderide Tablets ... 2732
- Inderide LA Long Acting Capsules .. 2734

Protriptyline Hydrochloride (Reduces hypotensive effect). Products include:
- Vivactil Tablets ... 1774

Quinapril Hydrochloride (Additive or potentiated action). Products include:
- Accupril Tablets ... 1893

Quinestrol (Reduces hypotensive effect).
- No products indexed under this heading.

Ramipril (Additive or potentiated action). Products include:
- Altace Capsules ... 1232

Rauwolfia Serpentina (May result in excessive postural hypotension, bradycardia and mental depression).
- No products indexed under this heading.

Rescinnamine (May result in excessive postural hypotension, bradycardia and mental depression).
- No products indexed under this heading.

Reserpine (May result in excessive postural hypotension, bradycardia and mental depression). Products include:
- Diupres Tablets ... 1650
- Hydropres Tablets ... 1675
- Ser-Ap-Es Tablets ... 849

Secobarbital Sodium (May potentiate orthostatic hypotension). Products include:
- Seconal Sodium Pulvules ... 1474

Selegiline Hydrochloride (Concurrent use contraindicated). Products include:
- Eldepryl Tablets ... 2550

Sodium Nitroprusside (Additive or potentiated action).
- No products indexed under this heading.

Sotalol Hydrochloride (Additive or potentiated action). Products include:
- Betapace Tablets ... 641

Spirapril Hydrochloride (Additive or potentiated action).
- No products indexed under this heading.

Sufentanil Citrate (May potentiate orthostatic hypotension). Products include:
- Sufenta Injection ... 1309

Sulindac (May reduce the diuretic, natriuretic, and antihypertensive effects of thiazide diuretics). Products include:
- Clinoril Tablets ... 1618

Terazosin Hydrochloride (Additive or potentiated action). Products include:
- Hytrin Capsules ... 430

Thiamylal Sodium (May potentiate orthostatic hypotension).
- No products indexed under this heading.

Thioridazine Hydrochloride (Reduces hypotensive effect). Products include:
- Mellaril ... 2269

Timolol Maleate (Additive or potentiated action). Products include:
- Blocadren Tablets ... 1614
- Timolide Tablets ... 1748
- Timoptic in Ocudose ... 1753
- Timoptic Sterile Ophthalmic Solution ... 1751
- Timoptic-XE ... 1755

Tolmetin Sodium (May reduce the diuretic, natriuretic, and antihypertensive effects of thiazide diuretics). Products include:
- Tolectin (200, 400 and 600 mg) .. 1581

Torsemide (Additive or potentiated action). Products include:
- Demadex Tablets and Injection ... 686

Tranylcypromine Sulfate (Concurrent use contraindicated). Products include:
- Parnate Tablets ... 2503

Triamcinolone (Hypokalemia). Products include:
- Aristocort Tablets ... 1022

Triamcinolone Acetonide (Hypokalemia). Products include:
- Aristocort A 0.025% Cream ... 1027
- Aristocort A 0.5% Cream ... 1031
- Aristocort A 0.1% Cream ... 1029
- Aristocort A 0.1% Ointment ... 1030
- Azmacort Oral Inhaler ... 2011
- Nasacort Nasal Inhaler ... 2024

Triamcinolone Diacetate (Hypokalemia). Products include:
- Aristocort Suspension (Forte Parenteral) ... 1027

(▣ Described in PDR For Nonprescription Drugs) (◉ Described in PDR For Ophthalmology)

395 **Interactions Index** **Eskalith**

Aristocort Suspension (Intralesional) 1025

Triamcinolone Hexacetonide (Hypokalemia). Products include:

Aristospan Suspension (Intra-articular) 1033
Aristospan Suspension (Intralesional) 1032

Trifluoperazine Hydrochloride (Reduces hypotensive effect). Products include:

Stelazine 2514

Trimethaphan Camsylate (Additive or potentiated action). Products include:

Arfonad Ampuls 2080

Trimipramine Maleate (Reduces hypotensive effect). Products include:

Surmontil Capsules 2811

Tubocurarine Chloride (Increased response to tubocurarine).

No products indexed under this heading.

Verapamil Hydrochloride (Additive or potentiated action). Products include:

Calan SR Caplets 2422
Calan Tablets 2419
Isoptin Injectable 1344
Isoptin Oral Tablets 1346
Isoptin SR Tablets 1348
Verelan Capsules 1410
Verelan Capsules 2824

Food Interactions

Alcohol (Orthostatic hypotension aggravated).

Food, unspecified (Enhances gastrointestinal absorption of hydrochlorothiazide).

ESKALITH CAPSULES

(Lithium Carbonate) 2485

May interact with nondepolarizing neuromuscular blocking agents, diuretics, urinary alkalizing agents, xanthine bronchodilators, antipsychotic agents, non-steroidal anti-inflammatory agents, calcium channel blockers, ACE inhibitors, and certain other agents. Compounds in these categories include:

Acetazolamide (Increases urinary lithium excretion). Products include:

Diamox Sequels (Sustained Release) 1373
Diamox Sequels (Sustained Release) .... ⊙ 319
Diamox Tablets 1372
Diamox Tablets .... ⊙ 317

Amiloride Hydrochloride (Increased risk of lithium toxicity). Products include:

Midamor Tablets 1703
Moduretic Tablets 1705

Aminophylline (Lowers serum lithium concentrations).

No products indexed under this heading.

Amlodipine Besylate (Increases the risk of neurotoxicity). Products include:

Lotrel Capsules 840
Norvasc Tablets 1940

Atracurium Besylate (Effects may be prolonged). Products include:

Tracrium Injection 1183

Benazepril Hydrochloride (May substantially increase steady-state plasma lithium levels resulting in lithium toxicity). Products include:

Lotensin Tablets 834
Lotensin HCT 837
Lotrel Capsules 840

Bendroflumethiazide (Increased risk of lithium toxicity).

No products indexed under this heading.

Bepridil Hydrochloride (Increases the risk of neurotoxicity). Products include:

Vascor (200, 300 and 400 mg) Tablets 1587

Bumetanide (Increases risk of lithium toxicity). Products include:

Bumex 2093

Captopril (May substantially increase steady-state plasma lithium levels resulting in lithium toxicity). Products include:

Capoten 739
Capozide 742

Chlorothiazide (Increases risk of lithium toxicity). Products include:

Aldoclor Tablets 1598
Diupres Tablets 1650
Diuril Oral 1653

Chlorothiazide Sodium (Increases risk of lithium toxicity). Products include:

Diuril Sodium Intravenous 1652

Chlorpromazine (Neurologic toxicity). Products include:

Thorazine Suppositories 2523

Chlorprothixene (Neurologic toxicity).

No products indexed under this heading.

Chlorprothixene Hydrochloride (Neurological toxicity).

No products indexed under this heading.

Chlorthalidone (Increased risk of lithium toxicity). Products include:

Combipres Tablets 677
Tenoretic Tablets 2845
Thalitone 1245

Clozapine (Neurologic toxicity). Products include:

Clozaril Tablets 2252

Diclofenac Potassium (Increases lithium toxicity). Products include:

Cataflam 816

Diclofenac Sodium (Increases lithium toxicity). Products include:

Voltaren Ophthalmic Sterile Ophthalmic Solution .... ⊙ 272
Voltaren Tablets 861

Diltiazem Hydrochloride (Increases the risk of neurotoxicity). Products include:

Cardizem CD Capsules 1506
Cardizem SR Capsules 1510
Cardizem Injectable 1508
Cardizem Tablets 1512
Dilacor XR Extended-release Capsules 2018

Dyphylline (Lowers serum lithium concentrations). Products include:

Lufyllin & Lufyllin-400 Tablets 2670
Lufyllin-GG Elixir & Tablets 2671

Enalapril Maleate (May substantially increase steady-state plasma lithium levels resulting in lithium toxicity). Products include:

Vaseretic Tablets 1765
Vasotec Tablets 1771

Enalaprilat (May substantially increase steady-state plasma lithium levels resulting in lithium toxicity). Products include:

Vasotec I.V. 1768

Ethacrynic Acid (Increases risk of lithium toxicity). Products include:

Edecrin Tablets 1657

Etodolac (Increases lithium toxicity). Products include:

Lodine Capsules and Tablets 2743

Felodipine (Increases the risk of neurotoxicity). Products include:

Plendil Extended-Release Tablets 527

Fenoprofen Calcium (Increases lithium toxicity). Products include:

Nalfon 200 Pulvules & Nalfon Tablets 917

Fluphenazine Decanoate (Neurologic toxicity). Products include:

Prolixin Decanoate 509

Fluphenazine Enanthate (Neurologic toxicity). Products include:

Prolixin Enanthate 509

Fluphenazine Hydrochloride (Neurologic toxicity). Products include:

Prolixin 509

Flurbiprofen (Increases lithium toxicity). Products include:

Ansaid Tablets 2579

Fosinopril Sodium (May substantially increase steady-state plasma lithium levels resulting in lithium toxicity). Products include:

Monopril Tablets 757

Furosemide (Increases risk of lithium toxicity). Products include:

Lasix Injection, Oral Solution and Tablets 1240

Haloperidol (Neurologic toxicity). Products include:

Haldol Injection, Tablets and Concentrate 1575

Haloperidol Decanoate (Neurologic toxicity). Products include:

Haldol Decanoate 1577

Hydrochlorothiazide (Increases risk of lithium toxicity). Products include:

Aldactazide 2413
Aldoril Tablets 1604
Apresazide Capsules 808
Capozide 742
Dyazide 2479
Esidrix Tablets 821
Esimil Tablets 822
HydroDIURIL Tablets 1674
Hydropres Tablets 1675
Hyzaar Tablets 1677
Inderide Tablets 2732
Inderide LA Long Acting Capsules 2734
Lopressor HCT Tablets 832
Lotensin HCT 837
Maxzide 1380
Moduretic Tablets 1705
Oretic Tablets 443
Prinzide Tablets 1737
Ser-Ap-Es Tablets 849
Timolide Tablets 1748
Vaseretic Tablets 1765
Zestoretic 2850
Ziac 1415

Hydroflumethiazide (Increases risk of lithium toxicity). Products include:

Diucardin Tablets 2718

Ibuprofen (Increases lithium toxicity). Products include:

Advil Cold and Sinus Caplets and Tablets (formerly CoAdvil) .... ▣ 870
Advil Ibuprofen Tablets and Caplets .... ▣ 870
Children's Advil Suspension 2692
Arthritis Foundation Ibuprofen Tablets .... ▣ 674
Bayer Select Ibuprofen Pain Relief Formula .... ▣ 715
Cramp End Tablets .... ▣ 735
Dimetapp Sinus Caplets .... ▣ 775
Haltran Tablets .... ▣ 771
IBU Tablets 1342
Ibuprohm .... ▣ 735
Children's Motrin Ibuprofen Oral Suspension 1546
Motrin Tablets 2625
Motrin IB Caplets, Tablets, and Geltabs .... ▣ 838
Motrin IB Sinus .... ▣ 838
Motrin Ibuprofen Suspension, Oral Drops, Chewable Tablets, Caplets 1546
Nuprin Ibuprofen/Analgesic Tablets & Caplets .... ▣ 622
Sine-Aid IB Caplets 1554
Vicks DayQuil SINUS Pressure & PAIN Relief with IBUPROFEN .... ▣ 762

Indapamide (Increases risk of lithium toxicity). Products include:

Lozol Tablets 2022

Indomethacin (Increases lithium toxicity). Products include:

Indocin 1680

Indomethacin Sodium Trihydrate (Increases lithium toxicity). Products include:

Indocin I.V. 1684

Isradipine (Increases the risk of neurotoxicity). Products include:

DynaCirc Capsules 2256

Ketoprofen (Increases lithium toxicity). Products include:

Orudis Capsules 2766
Oruvail Capsules 2766

Ketorolac Tromethamine (Increases lithium toxicity). Products include:

Acular 474
Acular .... ⊙ 277
Toradol 2159

Lisinopril (May substantially increase steady-state plasma lithium levels resulting in lithium toxicity). Products include:

Prinivil Tablets 1733
Prinzide Tablets 1737
Zestoretic 2850
Zestril Tablets 2854

Loxapine Hydrochloride (Neurologic toxicity). Products include:

Loxitane 1378

Loxapine Succinate (Neurologic toxicity). Products include:

Loxitane Capsules 1378

Meclofenamate Sodium (Increases lithium toxicity).

No products indexed under this heading.

Mefenamic Acid (Increases lithium toxicity). Products include:

Ponstel 1925

Mesoridazine Besylate (Neurologic toxicity). Products include:

Serentil 684

Methyclothiazide (Increases risk of lithium toxicity). Products include:

Enduron Tablets 420

Metocurine Iodide (Effects of neuromuscular blockers may be prolonged). Products include:

Metubine Iodide Vials 916

Metolazone (Increases risk of lithium toxicity). Products include:

Mykrox Tablets 993
Zaroxolyn Tablets 1000

Metronidazole (May provoke lithium toxicity due to reduced renal clearance). Products include:

Flagyl 375 Capsules 2434
Flagyl I.V. RTU 2247
MetroGel 1047
MetroGel-Vaginal 902
Protostat Tablets 1883

Metronidazole Hydrochloride (May provoke lithium toxicity due to reduced renal clearance). Products include:

Flagyl I.V. 2247

Mivacurium Chloride (Effects may be prolonged). Products include:

Mivacron 1138

Moexipril Hydrochloride (May substantially increase steady-state plasma lithium levels resulting in lithium toxicity). Products include:

Univasc Tablets 2410

Molindone Hydrochloride (Neurologic toxicity). Products include:

Moban Tablets and Concentrate 1048

Nabumetone (Increases lithium toxicity). Products include:

Relafen Tablets 2510

Naproxen (Increases lithium toxicity). Products include:

Anaprox/Naprosyn 2117

IMPORTANT NOTE: Always consult each drug listing in the patient's regimen for possible interactions.

Eskalith — Interactions Index — 396

Naproxen Sodium (Increases lithium toxicity). Products include:
- Aleve 1975
- Anaprox/Naprosyn 2117

Nicardipine Hydrochloride (Increases the risk of neurotoxicity). Products include:
- Cardene Capsules 2095
- Cardene I.V. 2709
- Cardene SR Capsules 2097

Nifedipine (Increases the risk of neurotoxicity). Products include:
- Adalat Capsules (10 mg and 20 mg) 587
- Adalat CC 589
- Procardia Capsules 1971
- Procardia XL Extended Release Tablets 1972

Nimodipine (Increases the risk of neurotoxicity). Products include:
- Nimotop Capsules 610

Nisoldipine (Increases the risk of neurotoxicity).
- No products indexed under this heading.

Oxaprozin (Increases lithium toxicity). Products include:
- Daypro Caplets 2426

Pancuronium Bromide Injection (Effects of neuromuscular blockers may be prolonged).
- No products indexed under this heading.

Perphenazine (Neurologic toxicity). Products include:
- Etrafon 2355
- Triavil Tablets 1757
- Trilafon 2389

Phenylbutazone (Increases lithium toxicity).
- No products indexed under this heading.

Pimozide (Neurologic toxicity). Products include:
- Orap Tablets 1050

Piroxicam (Increases lithium toxicity). Products include:
- Feldene Capsules 1965

Polythiazide (Increases risk of lithium toxicity). Products include:
- Minizide Capsules 1938

Potassium Citrate (Increases urinary lithium excretion). Products include:
- Polycitra Syrup 578
- Polycitra-K Crystals 579
- Polycitra-K Oral Solution 579
- Polycitra-LC 578

Prochlorperazine (Neurologic toxicity). Products include:
- Compazine 2470

Promethazine Hydrochloride (Neurologic toxicity). Products include:
- Mepergan Injection 2753
- Phenergan with Codeine 2777
- Phenergan with Dextromethorphan 2778
- Phenergan Injection 2773
- Phenergan Suppositories 2775
- Phenergan Syrup 2774
- Phenergan Tablets 2775
- Phenergan VC 2779
- Phenergan VC with Codeine 2781

Quinapril Hydrochloride (May substantially increase steady-state plasma lithium levels resulting in lithium toxicity). Products include:
- Accupril Tablets 1893

Ramipril (May substantially increase steady-state plasma lithium levels resulting in lithium toxicity). Products include:
- Altace Capsules 1232

Risperidone (Neurologic toxicity). Products include:
- Risperdal 1301

Rocuronium Bromide (Effects may be prolonged). Products include:
- Zemuron 1830

Sodium Bicarbonate (Increases urinary lithium excretion). Products include:
- Alka-Seltzer Effervescent Antacid and Pain Reliever ▣ 701
- Alka-Seltzer Extra Strength Effervescent Antacid and Pain Reliever ▣ 703
- Alka-Seltzer Gold Effervescent Antacid ▣ 703
- Alka-Seltzer Lemon Lime Effervescent Antacid and Pain Reliever ▣ 703
- Arm & Hammer Pure Baking Soda ▣ 627
- Ceo-Two Rectal Suppositories 666
- Citrocarbonate Antacid ▣ 770
- Massengill Disposable Douches ▣ 820
- Massengill Liquid Concentrate ▣ 820
- NuLYTELY 689
- Cherry Flavor NuLYTELY 689

Sodium Citrate (Increases urinary lithium excretion). Products include:
- Bicitra 578
- Citrocarbonate Antacid ▣ 770
- Polycitra 578
- Salix SST Lozenges Saliva Stimulant ▣ 797

Spirapril Hydrochloride (May substantially increase steady-state plasma lithium levels resulting in lithium toxicity).
- No products indexed under this heading.

Spironolactone (Increases risk of lithium toxicity). Products include:
- Aldactazide 2413
- Aldactone 2414

Sulindac (Increases lithium toxicity). Products include:
- Clinoril Tablets 1618

Theophylline (Lowers serum lithium concentrations). Products include:
- Marax Tablets & DF Syrup 2200
- Quibron 2053

Theophylline Anhydrous (Lowers serum lithium concentrations). Products include:
- Aerolate 1004
- Primatene Dual Action Formula ▣ 872
- Primatene Tablets ▣ 873
- Respbid Tablets 682
- Slo-bid Gyrocaps 2033
- Theo-24 Extended Release Capsules 2568
- Theo-Dur Extended-Release Tablets 1327
- Theo-X Extended-Release Tablets 788
- Uni-Dur Extended-Release Tablets 1331
- Uniphyl 400 mg Tablets 2001

Theophylline Calcium Salicylate (Lowers serum lithium concentrations). Products include:
- Quadrinal Tablets 1350

Theophylline Sodium Glycinate (Lowers serum lithium concentrations).
- No products indexed under this heading.

Thioridazine Hydrochloride (Neurologic toxicity). Products include:
- Mellaril 2269

Thiothixene (Neurologic toxicity). Products include:
- Navane Capsules and Concentrate 2201
- Navane Intramuscular 2202

Tolmetin Sodium (Increases lithium toxicity). Products include:
- Tolectin (200, 400 and 600 mg) 1581

Torsemide (Increases risk of lithium toxicity). Products include:
- Demadex Tablets and Injection 686

Triamterene (Increases risk of lithium toxicity). Products include:
- Dyazide 2479
- Dyrenium Capsules 2481
- Maxzide 1380

Trifluoperazine Hydrochloride (Neurologic toxicity). Products include:
- Stelazine 2514

Urea (Lowers serum lithium concentrations). Products include:
- Amino-Cerv 1779
- Atrac-Tain, Moisturizing Cream 2554
- Eucerin Plus Dry Skin Care Moisturizing Lotion 641
- Eucerin Plus Moisturizing Creme 641
- Panafil Ointment 2246
- Panafil-White Ointment 2247
- Pen•Kera Creme ▣ 603
- Ultra Mide 25 Lotion ▣ 605

Vecuronium Bromide (Effects of neuromuscular blockers may be prolonged). Products include:
- Norcuron 1826

Verapamil Hydrochloride (Increases the risk of neurotoxicity). Products include:
- Calan SR Caplets 2422
- Calan Tablets 2419
- Isoptin Injectable 1344
- Isoptin Oral Tablets 1346
- Isoptin SR Tablets 1348
- Verelan Capsules 1410
- Verelan Capsules 2824

ESKALITH CR CONTROLLED RELEASE TABLETS
(Lithium Carbonate) 2485
See **Eskalith Capsules**

ESTER-C MINERAL ASCORBATES POWDER
(Calcium Ascorbate) ▣ 658
None cited in PDR database.

ESTRACE CREAM AND TABLETS
(Estradiol) 749
None cited in PDR database.

ESTRADERM TRANSDERMAL SYSTEM
(Estradiol) 824
May interact with progestins. Compounds in this category include:

Desogestrel (Potential for adverse effects on carbohydrate and lipid metabolism). Products include:
- Desogen Tablets 1817
- Ortho-Cept 1851

Medroxyprogesterone Acetate (Potential for adverse effects on carbohydrate and lipid metabolism). Products include:
- Amen Tablets 780
- Cycrin Tablets 975
- Depo-Provera Contraceptive Injection 2602
- Depo-Provera Sterile Aqueous Suspension 2606
- Premphase 2797
- Prempro 2801
- Provera Tablets 2636

Megestrol Acetate (Potential for adverse effects on carbohydrate and lipid metabolism). Products include:
- Megace Oral Suspension 699
- Megace Tablets 701

Norgestimate (Potential for adverse effects on carbohydrate and lipid metabolism). Products include:
- Ortho-Cyclen/Ortho-Tri-Cyclen 1858
- Ortho-Cyclen/Ortho Tri-Cyclen 1858

ESTRATAB TABLETS (0.3, 0.625, 1.25, 2.5 MG)
(Estrogens, Esterified) 2536
May interact with progestins. Compounds in this category include:

Desogestrel (Potential adverse effects on carbohydrate and lipid metabolism). Products include:
- Desogen Tablets 1817
- Ortho-Cept 1851

Medroxyprogesterone Acetate (Potential adverse effects on carbohydrate and lipid metabolism). Products include:
- Amen Tablets 780
- Cycrin Tablets 975
- Depo-Provera Contraceptive Injection 2602
- Depo-Provera Sterile Aqueous Suspension 2606
- Premphase 2797
- Prempro 2801
- Provera Tablets 2636

Megestrol Acetate (Potential adverse effects on carbohydrate and lipid metabolism). Products include:
- Megace Oral Suspension 699
- Megace Tablets 701

Norgestimate (Potential adverse effects on carbohydrate and lipid metabolism). Products include:
- Ortho-Cyclen/Ortho-Tri-Cyclen 1858
- Ortho-Cyclen/Ortho Tri-Cyclen 1858

ESTRATEST TABLETS
(Estrogens, Esterified, Methyltestosterone) 2539
See **ESTRATEST H.S. Tablets**

ESTRATEST H.S. TABLETS
(Estrogens, Esterified, Methyltestosterone) 2539
May interact with oral anticoagulants, insulin, and certain other agents. Compounds in these categories include:

Dicumarol (Decreased anticoagulant requirements).
- No products indexed under this heading.

Insulin, Human (Decreased blood glucose and insulin requirements).
- No products indexed under this heading.

Insulin, Human Isophane Suspension (Decreased blood glucose and insulin requirements). Products include:
- Novolin N Human Insulin 10 ml Vials 1795

Insulin, Human NPH (Decreased blood glucose and insulin requirements). Products include:
- Humulin N, 100 Units 1448
- Novolin N PenFill Cartridges Durable Insulin Delivery System 1798
- Novolin N Prefilled Syringe Disposable Insulin Delivery System 1798

Insulin, Human Regular (Decreased blood glucose and insulin requirements). Products include:
- Humulin R, 100 Units 1449
- Novolin R Human Insulin 10 ml Vials 1795
- Novolin R PenFill Cartridges Durable Insulin Delivery System 1798
- Novolin R Prefilled Syringe Disposable Insulin Delivery System 1798
- Velosulin BR Human Insulin 10 ml Vials 1795

Insulin, Human, Zinc Suspension (Decreased blood glucose and insulin requirements). Products include:
- Humulin L, 100 Units 1446
- Humulin U, 100 Units 1450
- Novolin L Human Insulin 10 ml Vials 1795

(▣ Described in PDR For Nonprescription Drugs) (◉ Described in PDR For Ophthalmology)

Insulin, NPH (Decreased blood glucose and insulin requirements). Products include:

NPH, 100 Units 1450
Pork NPH, 100 Units.............................. 1452
Purified Pork NPH Isophane Insulin 1801

Insulin, Regular (Decreased blood glucose and insulin requirements). Products include:

Regular, 100 Units 1450
Pork Regular, 100 Units 1452
Pork Regular (Concentrated), 500 Units 1453
Purified Pork Regular Insulin 1801

Insulin, Zinc Crystals (Decreased blood glucose and insulin requirements). Products include:

NPH, 100 Units 1450

Insulin, Zinc Suspension (Decreased blood glucose and insulin requirements). Products include:

Iletin I 1450
Lente, 100 Units 1450
Iletin II... 1452
Pork Lente, 100 Units............................ 1452
Purified Pork Lente Insulin 1801

Oxyphenbutazone (Concurrent use may result in elevated serum levels of oxyphenbutazone).

Warfarin Sodium (Decreased anticoagulant requirements). Products include:

Coumadin 926

ETHAMOLIN

(Ethanolamine Oleate)...........................2400
None cited in PDR database.

ETHIODOL

(Ethiodized Oil) 2340
None cited in PDR database.

ETHMOZINE TABLETS

(Moricizine Hydrochloride)..................2041
May interact with xanthine bronchodilators and certain other agents. Compounds in these categories include:

Aminophylline (Theophylline clearance and plasma half-life significantly affected).

No products indexed under this heading.

Cimetidine (Concomitant use results in a decrease in Ethmozine clearance of 49% and a 1.4 fold increase in plasma levels). Products include:

Tagamet Tablets 2516

Cimetidine Hydrochloride (Concomitant use results in a decrease in Ethmozine clearance of 49% and a 1.4 fold increase in plasma levels). Products include:

Tagamet... 2516

Digoxin (Potential for additive prolongation of the PR interval). Products include:

Lanoxicaps 1117
Lanoxin Elixir Pediatric 1120
Lanoxin Injection 1123
Lanoxin Injection Pediatric.................. 1126
Lanoxin Tablets 1128

Dyphylline (Theophylline clearance and plasma half-life significantly affected). Products include:

Lufyllin & Lufyllin-400 Tablets 2670
Lufyllin-GG Elixir & Tablets 2671

Propranolol Hydrochloride (Small additive increase in the PR interval). Products include:

Inderal 2728
Inderal LA Long Acting Capsules 2730
Inderide Tablets 2732
Inderide LA Long Acting Capsules .. 2734

Theophylline (Theophylline clearance and plasma half-life significantly affected). Products include:

Marax Tablets & DF Syrup................... 2200
Quibron 2053

Theophylline Anhydrous (Theophylline clearance and plasma half-life significantly affected). Products include:

Aerolate 1004
Primatene Dual Action Formula...... ᴿᴰ 872
Primatene Tablets .... ᴿᴰ 873
Respbid Tablets 682
Slo-bid Gyrocaps 2033
Theo-24 Extended Release Capsules 2568
Theo-Dur Extended-Release Tablets 1327
Theo-X Extended-Release Tablets .. 788
Uni-Dur Extended-Release Tablets.. 1331
Uniphyl 400 mg Tablets........................ 2001

Theophylline Calcium Salicylate (Theophylline clearance and plasma half-life significantly affected). Products include:

Quadrinal Tablets 1350

Theophylline Sodium Glycinate (Theophylline clearance and plasma half-life significantly affected).

No products indexed under this heading.

Warfarin Sodium (Isolated reports of the need to either increase or decrease warfarin doses after initiation of Ethmozine; potential for excessive prolongation of prothrombin time following initiation of Ethmozine in patients with stable prothrombin time). Products include:

Coumadin 926

Food Interactions

Meal, unspecified (Administration 30 minutes after a meal delays the rate of absorption but the extent of absorption is not altered).

ETHYL CHLORIDE, U.S.P.

(Chloroethane, Ethyl Chloride)...........1052
None cited in PDR database.

ETRAFON FORTE TABLETS (4-25)

(Perphenazine, Amitriptyline Hydrochloride) 2355
See Etrafon Tablets (2-25)

ETRAFON 2-10 TABLETS (2-10)

(Perphenazine, Amitriptyline Hydrochloride) 2355
See Etrafon Tablets (2-25)

ETRAFON TABLETS (2-25)

(Perphenazine, Amitriptyline Hydrochloride) 2355
May interact with barbiturates, central nervous system depressants, narcotic analgesics, anticholinergics, antihistamines, sympathomimetics, monoamine oxidase inhibitors, thyroid preparations, drugs that inhibit cytochrome p450iid6, antidepressant drugs, phenothiazines, selective serotonin reuptake inhibitors, and certain other agents. Compounds in these categories include:

Acrivastine (Since phenothiazines and antihistamines are CNS depressants, each can potentiate each other). Products include:

Semprex-D Capsules 463
Semprex-D Capsules 1167

Albuterol (Effects of concurrent use not specified; close supervision and careful adjustment of dosages are required). Products include:

Proventil Inhalation Aerosol 2382
Ventolin Inhalation Aerosol and Refill 1197

Albuterol Sulfate (Effects of concurrent use not specified; close supervision and careful adjustment of dosages are required). Products include:

Airet Solution for Inhalation 452
Proventil Inhalation Solution 0.083% 2384
Proventil Repetabs Tablets 2386
Proventil Solution for Inhalation 0.5% 2383
Proventil Syrup... 2385
Proventil Tablets 2386
Ventolin Inhalation Solution................ 1198
Ventolin Nebules Inhalation Solution... 1199
Ventolin Rotacaps for Inhalation 1200
Ventolin Syrup... 1202
Ventolin Tablets 1203
Volmax Extended-Release Tablets .. 1788

Alfentanil Hydrochloride (Enhanced response to the effects of central nervous system depressants). Products include:

Alfenta Injection 1286

Alprazolam (Enhanced response to the effects of central nervous system depressants). Products include:

Xanax Tablets 2649

Amoxapine (Concurrent use with drugs that are substrate for cytochrome $P_{450}IID_6$ may make normal metabolizer resemble poor metabolizer leading to higher than expected plasma concentrations of TCA with resultant toxicity). Products include:

Asendin Tablets 1369

Aprobarbital (Enhanced response to barbiturates).

No products indexed under this heading.

Astemizole (Since phenothiazines and antihistamines are CNS depressants, each can potentiate each other). Products include:

Hismanal Tablets 1293

Atropine Sulfate (Concurrent use may result in additive anticholinergic effects including paralytic ileus). Products include:

Arco-Lase Plus Tablets 512
Atrohist Plus Tablets 454
Atropine Sulfate Sterile Ophthalmic Solution .... © 233
Donnatal 2060
Donnatal Extentabs................................. 2061
Donnatal Tablets 2060
Lomotil 2439
Motofen Tablets 784
Urised Tablets.. 1964

Azatadine Maleate (Since phenothiazines and antihistamines are CNS depressants, each can potentiate each other). Products include:

Trinalin Repetabs Tablets 1330

Belladonna Alkaloids (Concurrent use may result in additive anticholinergic effects including paralytic ileus). Products include:

Bellergal-S Tablets 2250
Hyland's Bed Wetting Tablets .... ᴿᴰ 828
Hyland's EnurAid Tablets.................. ᴿᴰ 829
Hyland's Teething Tablets .... ᴿᴰ 830

Benztropine Mesylate (Concurrent use may result in additive anticholinergic effects including paralytic ileus). Products include:

Cogentin 1621

Biperiden Hydrochloride (Concurrent use may result in additive anticholinergic effects including paralytic ileus). Products include:

Akineton 1333

Bromodiphenhydramine Hydrochloride (Since phenothiazines and antihistamines are CNS depressants, each can potentiate each other).

No products indexed under this heading.

Brompheniramine Maleate (Since phenothiazines and antihistamines are CNS depressants, each can potentiate each other). Products include:

Alka Seltzer Plus Sinus Medicine .. ᴿᴰ 707
Bromfed Capsules (Extended-Release) 1785
Bromfed Syrup .... ᴿᴰ 733
Bromfed Tablets 1785
Bromfed-DM Cough Syrup.................. 1786
Bromfed-PD Capsules (Extended-Release) 1785
Dimetane-DC Cough Syrup 2059
Dimetane-DX Cough Syrup 2059
Dimetapp Elixir .... ᴿᴰ 773
Dimetapp Extentabs .... ᴿᴰ 774
Dimetapp Tablets/Liqui-Gels .... ᴿᴰ 775
Dimetapp Cold & Allergy Chewable Tablets .... ᴿᴰ 773
Dimetapp DM Elixir................................ ᴿᴰ 774
Vicks DayQuil Allergy Relief 12-Hour Extended Release Tablets.. ᴿᴰ 760
Vicks DayQuil Allergy Relief 4-Hour Tablets .... ᴿᴰ 760

Buprenorphine (Enhanced response to the effects of central nervous system depressants). Products include:

Buprenex Injectable 2006

Bupropion Hydrochloride (Concurrent use with drugs that are substrate for cytochrome $P_{450}IID_6$ may make normal metabolizer resemble poor metabolizer leading to higher than expected plasma concentrations of TCA with resultant toxicity). Products include:

Wellbutrin Tablets 1204

Buspirone Hydrochloride (Enhanced response to the effects of central nervous system depressants). Products include:

BuSpar 737

Butabarbital (Enhanced response to barbiturates).

No products indexed under this heading.

Butalbital (Enhanced response to barbiturates). Products include:

Esgic-plus Tablets 1013
Fioricet Tablets.. 2258
Fioricet with Codeine Capsules 2260
Fiorinal Capsules 2261
Fiorinal with Codeine Capsules 2262
Fiorinal Tablets 2261
Phrenilin 785
Sedapap Tablets 50 mg/650 mg .. 1543

Chlordiazepoxide (Enhanced response to the effects of central nervous system depressants). Products include:

Libritabs Tablets 2177
Limbitrol 2180

Chlordiazepoxide Hydrochloride (Enhanced response to the effects of central nervous system depressants). Products include:

Librax Capsules 2176
Librium Capsules...................................... 2178
Librium Injectable 2179

Chlorpheniramine Maleate (Since phenothiazines and antihistamines are CNS depressants, each can potentiate each other). Products include:

Alka-Seltzer Plus Cold Medicine .... ᴿᴰ 705
Alka-Seltzer Plus Cold Medicine Liqui-Gels .... ᴿᴰ 706
Alka-Seltzer Plus Cold & Cough Medicine .... ᴿᴰ 708
Alka-Seltzer Plus Cold & Cough Medicine Liqui-Gels........................... ᴿᴰ 705
Allerest Children's Chewable Tablets .... ᴿᴰ 627
Allerest Headache Strength Tablets .... ᴿᴰ 627
Allerest Maximum Strength Tablets .... ᴿᴰ 627
Allerest Sinus Pain Formula .... ᴿᴰ 627
Allerest 12 Hour Caplets .... ᴿᴰ 627
Ana-Kit Anaphylaxis Emergency Treatment Kit 617
Atrohist Pediatric Capsules 453

IMPORTANT NOTE: Always consult each drug listing in the patient's regimen for possible interactions.

Etrafon
Interactions Index
398

Atrohist Plus Tablets 454
BC Cold Powder Multi-Symptom Formula (Cold-Sinus-Allergy) .... ▣ 609
Cerose DM .... ▣ 878
Cheracol Plus Head Cold/Cough Formula .... ▣ 769
Children's Vicks DayQuil Allergy Relief .... ▣ 757
Children's Vicks NyQuil Cold/Cough Relief .... ▣ 758
Chlor-Trimeton Allergy Decongestant Tablets .... ▣ 799
Chlor-Trimeton Allergy Tablets .... ▣ 798
Comhist 2038
Comtrex Multi-Symptom Cold Reliever Tablets/Caplets/Liqui-Gels/Liquid .... ▣ 615
Allergy-Sinus Comtrex Multi-Symptom Allergy-Sinus Formula Tablets .... ▣ 617
Contac Continuous Action Nasal Decongestant/Antihistamine 12 Hour Capsules .... ▣ 813
Contac Maximum Strength Continuous Action Decongestant/Antihistamine 12 Hour Caplets .... ▣ 813
Contac Severe Cold and Flu Formula Caplets .... ▣ 814
Coricidin 'D' Decongestant Tablets .... ▣ 800
Coricidin Tablets .... ▣ 800
D.A. Chewable Tablets 951
Deconamine 1320
Dura-Tap/PD Capsules 2867
Dura-Vent/DA Tablets 953
Extendryl 1005
Fedahist Gyrocaps 2401
Fedahist Timecaps 2401
Hycomine Compound Tablets 932
Isoclor Timesule Capsules .... ▣ 637
Kronofed-A 977
Nolamine Timed-Release Tablets 785
Novahistine DH 2462
Novahistine Elixir .... ▣ 823
Ornade Spansule Capsules 2502
PediaCare Cold Allergy Chewable Tablets .... ▣ 677
PediaCare Cough-Cold Chewable Tablets 1553
PediaCare Cough-Cold Liquid 1553
PediaCare NightRest Cough-Cold Liquid 1553
Pediatric Vicks 44m Cough & Cold Relief .... ▣ 764
Pyrroxate Caplets .... ▣ 772
Ryna .... ▣ 841
Sinarest Tablets .... ▣ 648
Sinarest Extra Strength Tablets .... ▣ 648
Sine-Off Sinus Medicine .... ▣ 825
Singlet Tablets .... ▣ 825
Sinulin Tablets 787
Sinutab Sinus Allergy Medication, Maximum Strength Tablets and Caplets .... ▣ 860
Sudafed Plus Liquid .... ▣ 862
Sudafed Plus Tablets .... ▣ 863
Teldrin 12 Hour Antihistamine/Nasal Decongestant Allergy Relief Capsules .... ▣ 826
TheraFlu .... ▣ 787
TheraFlu Maximum Strength Nighttime Flu, Cold & Cough Medicine .... ▣ 788
Triaminic Allergy Tablets .... ▣ 789
Triaminic Cold Tablets .... ▣ 790
Triaminic Nite Light .... ▣ 791
Triaminic Syrup .... ▣ 792
Triaminic-12 Tablets .... ▣ 792
Triaminicin Tablets .... ▣ 793
Triaminicol Multi-Symptom Cold Tablets .... ▣ 793
Triaminicol Multi-Symptom Relief ▣ 794
Tussend 1783
Children's TYLENOL Cold Multi-Symptom Liquid Formula and Chewable Tablets 1561
Children's TYLENOL Cold Plus Cough Multi Symptom Tablets and Liquid .... ▣ 681
TYLENOL Maximum Strength Allergy Sinus Medication Gelcaps and Caplets 1563
TYLENOL Cold Multi-Symptom Formula Medication Tablets and Caplets 1561
TYLENOL Cold Multi-Symptom Hot Medication Liquid Packets 1557
Vicks 44 LiquiCaps Cough, Cold & Flu Relief .... ▣ 755
Vicks 44M Cough, Cold & Flu Relief .... ▣ 756

Chlorpheniramine Polistirex (Since phenothiazines and antihistamines are CNS depressants, each can potentiate each other). Products include:
Tussionex Pennkinetic Extended-Release Suspension 998

Chlorpheniramine Tannate (Since phenothiazines and antihistamines are CNS depressants, each can potentiate each other). Products include:
Atrohist Pediatric Suspension 454
Ricobid Tablets and Pediatric Suspension 2038
Rynatan 2673
Rynatuss 2673

Chlorpromazine (Enhanced response to the effects of central nervous system depressants; concurrent use with drugs that are substrate for cytochrome $P_{450}IID_6$ may make normal metabolizer resemble poor metabolizer leading to higher than expected plasma concentrations of TCA with resultant toxicity). Products include:
Thorazine Suppositories 2523

Chlorpromazine Hydrochloride (Enhanced response to the effects of central nervous system depressants; concurrent use with drugs that are substrate for cytochrome $P_{450}IID_6$ may make normal metabolizer resemble poor metabolizer leading to higher than expected plasma concentrations of TCA with resultant toxicity). Products include:
Thorazine 2523

Chlorprothixene (Enhanced response to the effects of central nervous system depressants).
No products indexed under this heading.

Chlorprothixene Hydrochloride (Enhanced response to the effects of central nervous system depressants).
No products indexed under this heading.

Cimetidine (Co-administration can produce clinically significant increases in plasma concentrations of tricyclic antidepressants resulting in severe anticholinergic symptoms including dry mouth, urinary retention and blurred vision). Products include:
Tagamet Tablets 2516

Cimetidine Hydrochloride (Co-administration can produce clinically significant increases in plasma concentrations of tricyclic antidepressants resulting in severe anticholinergic symptoms including dry mouth, urinary retention and blurred vision). Products include:
Tagamet 2516

Clidinium Bromide (Concurrent use may result in additive anticholinergic effects including paralytic ileus). Products include:
Librax Capsules 2176
Quarzan Capsules 2181

Clonidine (Amitriptyline may block the antihypertensive effect). Products include:
Catapres-TTS 675

Clonidine Hydrochloride (Amitriptyline may block the antihypertensive effect). Products include:
Catapres Tablets 674
Combipres Tablets 677

Clorazepate Dipotassium (Enhanced response to the effects of central nervous system depressants). Products include:
Tranxene 451

Clozapine (Enhanced response to the effects of central nervous system depressants). Products include:
Clozaril Tablets 2252

Codeine Phosphate (Enhanced response to the effects of central nervous system depressants; enhanced response to central nervous system depressants). Products include:
Actifed with Codeine Cough Syrup 1067
Brontex 1981
Deconsal C Expectorant Syrup 456
Deconsal Pediatric Syrup 457
Dimetane-DC Cough Syrup 2059
Empirin with Codeine Tablets 1093
Fioricet with Codeine Capsules 2260
Fiorinal with Codeine Capsules 2262
Isoclor Expectorant 990
Novahistine DH 2462
Novahistine Expectorant 2463
Nucofed 2051
Phenergan with Codeine 2777
Phenergan VC with Codeine 2781
Robitussin A-C Syrup 2073
Robitussin-DAC Syrup 2074
Ryna .... ▣ 841
Soma Compound w/Codeine Tablets 2676
Tussi-Organidin NR Liquid and S NR Liquid 2677
Tylenol with Codeine 1583

Cyproheptadine Hydrochloride (Since phenothiazines and antihistamines are CNS depressants, each can potentiate each other). Products include:
Periactin 1724

Desflurane (Enhanced response to the effects of central nervous system depressants). Products include:
Suprane 1813

Desipramine Hydrochloride (Concurrent use with drugs that are substrate for cytochrome $P_{450}IID_6$ may make normal metabolizer resemble poor metabolizer leading to higher than expected plasma concentrations of TCA with resultant toxicity). Products include:
Norpramin Tablets 1526

Dexchlorpheniramine Maleate (Since phenothiazines and antihistamines are CNS depressants, each can potentiate each other).
No products indexed under this heading.

Dezocine (Enhanced response to the effects of central nervous system depressants). Products include:
Dalgan Injection 538

Diazepam (Enhanced response to the effects of central nervous system depressants). Products include:
Dizac 1809
Valium Injectable 2182
Valium Tablets 2183
Valrelease Capsules 2169

Dicyclomine Hydrochloride (Concurrent use may result in additive anticholinergic effects including paralytic ileus). Products include:
Bentyl 1501

Diphenhydramine Citrate (Since phenothiazines and antihistamines are CNS depressants, each can potentiate each other). Products include:
Excedrin P.M. Analgesic/Sleeping Aid Tablets, Caplets, Liquigels 733

Diphenhydramine Hydrochloride (Since phenothiazines and antihistamines are CNS depressants, each can potentiate each other). Products include:
Actifed Allergy Daytime/Nighttime Caplets .... ▣ 844
Actifed Sinus Daytime/Nighttime Tablets and Caplets .... ▣ 846
Arthritis Foundation NightTime Caplets .... ▣ 674
Extra Strength Bayer PM Aspirin .... ▣ 713
Bayer Select Night Time Pain Relief Formula .... ▣ 716
Benadryl Allergy Decongestant Liquid Medication .... ▣ 848
Benadryl Allergy Decongestant Tablets .... ▣ 848
Benadryl Allergy Liquid Medication .... ▣ 849
Benadryl Allergy .... ▣ 848
Benadryl Allergy Sinus Headache Formula Caplets .... ▣ 849
Benadryl Capsules 1898
Benadryl Dye-Free Allergy Liqui-gel Softgels .... ▣ 850
Benadryl Dye-Free Allergy Liquid Medication .... ▣ 850
Benadryl Itch Relief Cream, Children's Formula and Maximum Strength 2% .... ▣ 851
Benadryl Itch Relief Spray, Children's Formula and Maximum Strength 2% .... ▣ 851
Benadryl Itch Relief Stick Maximum Strength 2% .... ▣ 850
Benadryl Itch Stopping Gel, Children's Formula and Maximum Strength 2% .... ▣ 851
Benadryl Kapseals 1898
Benadryl Injection 1898
Contac Day & Night Cold/Flu Night Caplets .... ▣ 812
Contac Night Allergy/Sinus Caplets .... ▣ 812
Extra Strength Doan's P.M. .... ▣ 633
Legatrin PM .... ▣ 651
Miles Nervine Nighttime Sleep-Aid ▣ 723
Nytol QuickCaps Caplets .... ▣ 610
Sleepinal Night-time Sleep Aid Capsules and Softgels .... ▣ 834
TYLENOL Maximum Strength Allergy Sinus NightTime Medication Caplets 1555
TYLENOL Flu NightTime, Maximum Strength, Gelcaps 1566
TYLENOL Maximum Strength Flu NightTime Hot Medication Packets 1562
TYLENOL PM, Extra Strength Pain Reliever/Sleep Aid Caplets, Geltabs, Gelcaps 1560
TYLENOL Severe Allergy Medication Caplets 1564
Maximum Strength Unisom Sleepgels 1934
Unisom With Pain Relief-Nighttime Sleep Aid and Pain Reliever 1934

Diphenylpyraline Hydrochloride (Since phenothiazines and antihistamines are CNS depressants, each can potentiate each other).
No products indexed under this heading.

Dobutamine Hydrochloride (Effects of concurrent use not specified; close supervision and careful adjustment of dosages are required). Products include:
Dobutrex Solution Vials 1439

Dopamine Hydrochloride (Effects of concurrent use not specified; close supervision and careful adjustment of dosages are required).
No products indexed under this heading.

Doxepin Hydrochloride (Concurrent use with drugs that are substrate for cytochrome $P_{450}IID_6$ may make normal metabolizer resemble poor metabolizer leading to higher than expected plasma concentrations of TCA with resultant toxicity). Products include:
Sinequan 2205
Zonalon Cream 1055

Droperidol (Enhanced response to the effects of central nervous system depressants). Products include:
Inapsine Injection 1296

Enflurane (Enhanced response to the effects of central nervous system depressants).
No products indexed under this heading.

(▣ Described in PDR For Nonprescription Drugs) (⊙ Described in PDR For Ophthalmology)

Interactions Index

Ephedrine Hydrochloride (Effects of concurrent use not specified; close supervision and careful adjustment of dosages are required). Products include:

Primatene Dual Action Formula...... ⊞ 872
Primatene Tablets................................. ⊞ 873
Quadrinal Tablets.................................. 1350

Ephedrine Sulfate (Effects of concurrent use not specified; close supervision and careful adjustment of dosages are required). Products include:

Bronkaid Caplets................................... ⊞ 717
Marax Tablets & DF Syrup.................. 2200

Ephedrine Tannate (Effects of concurrent use not specified; close supervision and careful adjustment of dosages are required). Products include:

Rynatuss.. 2673

Epinephrine (Effects of concurrent use of epinephrine (combined with local anesthetics) not specified; close supervision and careful adjustment of dosages are required). Products include:

Bronkaid Mist.. ⊞ 717
EPIFRIN.. ⊙ 239
EpiPen... 790
Marcaine Hydrochloride with Epinephrine 1:200,000.......................... 2316
Primatene Mist...................................... ⊞ 873
Sensorcaine with Epinephrine Injection.. 559
Sus-Phrine Injection.............................. 1019
Xylocaine with Epinephrine Injections.. 567

Epinephrine Bitartrate (Effects of concurrent use not specified; close supervision and careful adjustment of dosages are required). Products include:

Bronkaid Mist Suspension................... ⊞ 718
Sensorcaine-MPF with Epinephrine Injection.. 559

Epinephrine Hydrochloride (Effects of concurrent use of epinephrine (combined with local anesthetics) not specified). Products include:

Ana-Kit Anaphylaxis Emergency Treatment Kit.. 617

Estazolam (Enhanced response to the effects of central nervous system depressants). Products include:

ProSom Tablets...................................... 449

Ethchlorvynol (Concurrent use of high dose of ethchlorvynol may produce transient delirium; enhanced response to central nervous system depressants). Products include:

Placidyl Capsules................................... 448

Ethinamate (Enhanced response to the effects of central nervous system depressants).

No products indexed under this heading.

Fentanyl (Enhanced response to the effects of central nervous system depressants). Products include:

Duragesic Transdermal System...... 1288

Fentanyl Citrate (Enhanced response to the effects of central nervous system depressants). Products include:

Sublimaze Injection............................... 1307

Flecainide Acetate (Concurrent use with drugs that are substrate for cytochrome $P_{450}IID_6$ may make normal metabolizer resemble poor metabolizer leading to higher than expected plasma concentrations of TCA with resultant toxicity). Products include:

Tambocor Tablets.................................. 1497

Fluoxetine Hydrochloride (Concurrent use with drugs that are substrate for cytochrome $P_{450}IID_6$ may make normal metabolizer resemble poor metabolizer leading to higher than expected plasma concentrations of TCA with resultant toxicity; due to variation in the extent of inhibition of $P_{450}IID_6$ and long half-life of the parent (fluoxetine) and active metabolite sufficient time must elapse at least 5 weeks before switching to TCA). Products include:

Prozac Pulvules & Liquid, Oral Solution.. 919

Fluphenazine Decanoate (Enhanced response to the effects of central nervous system depressants; concurrent use with drugs that are substrate for cytochrome $P_{450}IID_6$ may make normal metabolizer resemble poor metabolizer leading to higher than expected plasma concentrations of TCA with resultant toxicity). Products include:

Prolixin Decanoate................................. 509

Fluphenazine Enanthate (Enhanced response to the effects of central nervous system depressants; concurrent use with drugs that are substrate for cytochrome $P_{450}IID_6$ may make normal metabolizer resemble poor metabolizer leading to higher than expected plasma concentrations of TCA with resultant toxicity). Products include:

Prolixin Enanthate................................. 509

Fluphenazine Hydrochloride (Enhanced response to the effects of central nervous system depressants; concurrent use with drugs that are substrate for cytochrome $P_{450}IID_6$ may make normal metabolizer resemble poor metabolizer leading to higher than expected plasma concentrations of TCA with resultant toxicity). Products include:

Prolixin.. 509

Flurazepam Hydrochloride (Enhanced response to the effects of central nervous system depressants). Products include:

Dalmane Capsules................................. 2173

Fluvoxamine Maleate (Concurrent use with drugs that are substrate for cytochrome $P_{450}IID_6$ may make normal metabolizer resemble poor metabolizer leading to higher than expected plasma concentrations of TCA with resultant toxicity; due to variation in the extent of inhibition of $P_{450}IID_6$ caution is indicated if co-administered sufficient time must elapse). Products include:

Luvox Tablets... 2544

Furazolidone (Potential for hyperpyretic crises, severe convulsions and death; concurrent and/or sequential use is contraindicated). Products include:

Furoxone... 2046

Glutethimide (Enhanced response to the effects of central nervous system depressants).

No products indexed under this heading.

Glycopyrrolate (Concurrent use may result in additive anticholinergic effects including paralytic ileus). Products include:

Robinul Forte Tablets............................ 2072
Robinul Injectable.................................. 2072
Robinul Tablets...................................... 2072

Guanadrel Sulfate (Amitriptyline may block the antihypertensive effect). Products include:

Hylorel Tablets....................................... 985

Guanethidine Monosulfate (Amitriptyline may block the antihypertensive effect of guanethidine or similarly acting compounds). Products include:

Esimil Tablets... 822
Ismelin Tablets....................................... 827

Haloperidol (Enhanced response to the effects of central nervous system depressants). Products include:

Haldol Injection, Tablets and Concentrate.. 1575

Haloperidol Decanoate (Enhanced response to the effects of central nervous system depressants). Products include:

Haldol Decanoate................................... 1577

Hydrocodone Bitartrate (Enhanced response to the effects of central nervous system depressants). Products include:

Anexsia 5/500 Elixir............................. 1781
Anexia Tablets.. 1782
Codiclear DH Syrup.............................. 791
Deconamine CX Cough and Cold Liquid and Tablets............................... 1319
Duratuss HD Elixir................................ 2565
Hycodan Tablets and Syrup................ 930
Hycomine Compound Tablets............ 932
Hycomine.. 931
Hycotuss Expectorant Syrup.............. 933
Hydrocet Capsules................................ 782
Lorcet 10/650.. 1018
Lortab.. 2566
Tussend... 1783
Tussend Expectorant............................ 1785
Vicodin Tablets....................................... 1356
Vicodin ES Tablets................................. 1357
Vicodin Tuss Expectorant.................... 1358
Zydone Capsules................................... 949

Hydrocodone Polistirex (Enhanced response to the effects of central nervous system depressants). Products include:

Tussionex Pennkinetic Extended-Release Suspension.............................. 998

Hydroxyzine Hydrochloride (Enhanced response to the effects of central nervous system depressants). Products include:

Atarax Tablets & Syrup........................ 2185
Marax Tablets & DF Syrup.................. 2200
Vistaril Intramuscular Solution.......... 2216

Hyoscyamine (Concurrent use may result in additive anticholinergic effects including paralytic ileus). Products include:

Cystospaz Tablets.................................. 1963
Urised Tablets.. 1964

Hyoscyamine Sulfate (Concurrent use may result in additive anticholinergic effects including paralytic ileus). Products include:

Arco-Lase Plus Tablets......................... 512
Atrohist Plus Tablets............................ 454
Cystospaz-M Capsules......................... 1963
Donnatal.. 2060
Donnatal Extentabs............................... 2061
Donnatal Tablets.................................... 2060
Kutrase Capsules................................... 2402
Levsin/Levsinex/Levbid....................... 2405

Imipramine Hydrochloride (Concurrent use with drugs that are substrate for cytochrome $P_{450}IID_6$ may make normal metabolizer resemble poor metabolizer leading to higher than expected plasma concentrations of TCA with resultant toxicity). Products include:

Tofranil Ampuls..................................... 854
Tofranil Tablets...................................... 856

Imipramine Pamoate (Concurrent use with drugs that are substrate for cytochrome $P_{450}IID_6$ may make normal metabolizer resemble poor metabolizer leading to higher than expected plasma concentrations of TCA with resultant toxicity). Products include:

Tofranil-PM Capsules........................... 857

Ipratropium Bromide (Concurrent use may result in additive anticholinergic effects including paralytic ileus). Products include:

Atrovent Inhalation Aerosol................ 671
Atrovent Inhalation Solution.............. 673

Isocarboxazid (Potential for hyperpyretic crises, severe convulsions and death; concurrent and/or sequential use is contraindicated).

No products indexed under this heading.

Isoflurane (Enhanced response to the effects of central nervous system depressants).

No products indexed under this heading.

Isoproterenol Hydrochloride (Effects of concurrent use not specified; close supervision and careful adjustment of dosages are required). Products include:

Isuprel Hydrochloride Injection 1:5000.. 2311
Isuprel Hydrochloride Solution 1:200 & 1:100...................................... 2313
Isuprel Mistometer................................ 2312

Isoproterenol Sulfate (Effects of concurrent use not specified; close supervision and careful adjustment of dosages are required). Products include:

Norisodrine with Calcium Iodide Syrup.. 442

Ketamine Hydrochloride (Enhanced response to the effects of central nervous system depressants).

No products indexed under this heading.

Levomethadyl Acetate Hydrochloride (Enhanced response to the effects of central nervous system depressants). Products include:

Orlaam... 2239

Levorphanol Tartrate (cnsd; Enhanced response to central nervous system depressants). Products include:

Levo-Dromoran...................................... 2129

Levothyroxine Sodium (On rare occasions, co-administration may produce arrhythmias). Products include:

Levothroid Tablets................................. 1016
Levoxyl Tablets...................................... 903
Synthroid... 1359

Liothyronine Sodium (On rare occasions, co-administration may produce arrhythmias). Products include:

Cytomel Tablets..................................... 2473
Triostat Injection................................... 2530

Liotrix (On rare occasions, co-administration may produce arrhythmias).

No products indexed under this heading.

Loratadine (Since phenothiazines and antihistamines are CNS depressants, each can potentiate each other). Products include:

Claritin... 2349
Claritin-D... 2350

Lorazepam (Enhanced response to the effects of central nervous system depressants). Products include:

Ativan Injection...................................... 2698
Ativan Tablets... 2700

Loxapine Hydrochloride (Enhanced response to the effects of central nervous system depressants). Products include:

Loxitane... 1378

Loxapine Succinate (Enhanced response to the effects of central nervous system depressants). Products include:

Loxitane Capsules.................................. 1378

IMPORTANT NOTE: Always consult each drug listing in the patient's regimen for possible interactions.

Etrafon
Interactions Index
400

Maprotiline Hydrochloride (Concurrent use with drugs that are substrate for cytochrome $P_{450}IID_6$ may make normal metabolizer resemble poor metabolizer leading to higher than expected plasma concentrations of TCA with resultant toxicity). Products include:
- Ludiomil Tablets 843

Mepenzolate Bromide (Concurrent use may result in additive anticholinergic effects including paralytic ileus).
- No products indexed under this heading.

Meperidine Hydrochloride (Enhanced response to central nervous system depressants). Products include:
- Demerol 2308
- Mepergan Injection 2753

Mephobarbital (Enhanced response to barbiturates). Products include:
- Mebaral Tablets 2322

Meprobamate (Enhanced response to the effects of central nervous system depressants). Products include:
- Miltown Tablets 2672
- PMB 200 and PMB 400 2783

Mesoridazine (Enhanced response to the effects of central nervous system depressants).

Mesoridazine Besylate (Concurrent use with drugs that are substrate for cytochrome $P_{450}IID_6$ may make normal metabolizer resemble poor metabolizer leading to higher than expected plasma concentrations of TCA with resultant toxicity). Products include:
- Serentil 684

Metaproterenol Sulfate (Effects of concurrent use not specified; close supervision and careful adjustment of dosages are required). Products include:
- Alupent 669
- Metaproterenol Sulfate Inhalation Solution, USP, Arm-a-Med 552

Metaraminol Bitartrate (Effects of concurrent use not specified; close supervision and careful adjustment of dosages are required). Products include:
- Aramine Injection 1609

Methadone Hydrochloride (Enhanced response to central nervous system depressants). Products include:
- Methadone Hydrochloride Oral Concentrate 2233
- Methadone Hydrochloride Oral Solution & Tablets 2235

Methdilazine Hydrochloride (Since phenothiazines and antihistamines are CNS depressants, each can potentiate each other).
- No products indexed under this heading.

Methohexital Sodium (Enhanced response to the effects of central nervous system depressants). Products include:
- Brevital Sodium Vials 1429

Methotrimeprazine (Enhanced response to the effects of central nervous system depressants; concurrent use with drugs that are substrate for cytochrome $P_{450}IID_6$ may make normal metabolizer resemble poor metabolizer leading to higher than expected plasma concentrations of TCA with resultant toxicity). Products include:
- Levoprome 1274

Methoxamine Hydrochloride (Effects of concurrent use not specified; close supervision and careful adjustment of dosages are required). Products include:
- Vasoxyl Injection 1196

Methoxyflurane (Enhanced response to the effects of central nervous system depressants).
- No products indexed under this heading.

Midazolam Hydrochloride (Enhanced response to the effects of central nervous system depressants). Products include:
- Versed Injection 2170

Molindone Hydrochloride (Enhanced response to the effects of central nervous system depressants). Products include:
- Moban Tablets and Concentrate 1048

Morphine Sulfate (Enhanced response to central nervous system depressants). Products include:
- Astramorph/PF Injection, USP (Preservative-Free) 535
- Duramorph 962
- Infumorph 200 and Infumorph 500 Sterile Solutions 965
- MS Contin Tablets 1994
- MSIR 1997
- Oramorph SR (Morphine Sulfate Sustained Release Tablets) 2236
- RMS Suppositories 2657
- Roxanol 2243

Nefazodone Hydrochloride (Concurrent use with drugs that are substrate for cytochrome $P_{450}IID_6$ may make normal metabolizer resemble poor metabolizer leading to higher than expected plasma concentrations of TCA with resultant toxicity). Products include:
- Serzone Tablets 771

Norepinephrine Bitartrate (Effects of concurrent use not specified; close supervision and careful adjustment of dosages are required). Products include:
- Levophed Bitartrate Injection 2315

Nortriptyline Hydrochloride (Concurrent use with drugs that are substrate for cytochrome $P_{450}IID_6$ may make normal metabolizer resemble poor metabolizer leading to higher than expected plasma concentrations of TCA with resultant toxicity). Products include:
- Pamelor 2280

Opium Alkaloids (Enhanced response to central nervous system depressants).
- No products indexed under this heading.

Oxazepam (Enhanced response to the effects of central nervous system depressants). Products include:
- Serax Capsules 2810
- Serax Tablets 2810

Oxybutynin Chloride (Concurrent use may result in additive anticholinergic effects including paralytic ileus). Products include:
- Ditropan 1516

Oxycodone Hydrochloride (Enhanced response to central nervous system depressants). Products include:
- Percocet Tablets 938
- Percodan Tablets 939
- Percodan-Demi Tablets 940
- Roxicodone Tablets, Oral Solution & Intensol (Oxycodone) 2244
- Tylox Capsules 1584

Paroxetine Hydrochloride (Concurrent use with drugs that are substrate for cytochrome $P_{450}IID_6$ may make normal metabolizer resemble poor metabolizer leading to higher than expected plasma concentrations of TCA with resultant toxicity; due to variation in the extent of inhibition of $P_{450}IID_6$ caution is indicated if co-administered sufficient time must elapse). Products include:
- Paxil Tablets 2505

Pentobarbital Sodium (Enhanced response to barbiturates). Products include:
- Nembutal Sodium Capsules 436
- Nembutal Sodium Solution 438
- Nembutal Sodium Suppositories 440

Phenelzine Sulfate (Potential for hyperpyretic crises, severe convulsions and death; concurrent and/or sequential use is contraindicated). Products include:
- Nardil 1920

Phenobarbital (Enhanced response to barbiturates). Products include:
- Arco-Lase Plus Tablets 512
- Bellergal-S Tablets 2250
- Donnatal 2060
- Donnatal Extentabs 2061
- Donnatal Tablets 2060
- Phenobarbital Elixir and Tablets 1469
- Quadrinal Tablets 1350

Phenylephrine Bitartrate (Effects of concurrent use not specified; close supervision and careful adjustment of dosages are required).
- No products indexed under this heading.

Phenylephrine Hydrochloride (Effects of concurrent use not specified; close supervision and careful adjustment of dosages are required). Products include:
- Atrohist Plus Tablets 454
- Cerose DM ..... ◘ 878
- Comhist 2038
- D.A. Chewable Tablets 951
- Deconsal Pediatric Capsules 454
- Dura-Vent/DA Tablets 953
- Entex Capsules 1986
- Entex Liquid 1986
- Extendryl 1005
- 4-Way Fast Acting Nasal Spray (regular & mentholated) ..... ◘ 621
- Hemorid For Women ..... ◘ 834
- Hycomine Compound Tablets 932
- Neo-Synephrine Hydrochloride 1% Carpuject 2324
- Neo-Synephrine Hydrochloride 1% Injection 2324
- Neo-Synephrine Hydrochloride (Ophthalmic) 2325
- Neo-Synephrine ..... ◘ 726
- Nōstril ..... ◘ 644
- Novahistine Elixir ..... ◘ 823
- Phenergan VC 2779
- Phenergan VC with Codeine 2781
- Preparation H ..... ◘ 871
- Tympagesic Ear Drops 2342
- Vasosulf ..... ⊙ 271
- Vicks Sinex Nasal Spray and Ultra Fine Mist ..... ◘ 765

Phenylephrine Tannate (Effects of concurrent use not specified; close supervision and careful adjustment of dosages are required). Products include:
- Atrohist Pediatric Suspension 454
- Ricobid-D Pediatric Suspension 2038
- Ricobid Tablets and Pediatric Suspension 2038
- Rynatan 2673
- Rynatuss 2673

Phenylpropanolamine Hydrochloride (Effects of concurrent use not specified; close supervision and careful adjustment of dosages are required). Products include:
- Acutrim ..... ◘ 628
- Allerest Children's Chewable Tablets ..... ◘ 627
- Allerest 12 Hour Caplets ..... ◘ 627
- Atrohist Plus Tablets 454
- BC Cold Powder Multi-Symptom Formula (Cold-Sinus-Allergy) ..... ◘ 609
- BC Cold Powder Non-Drowsy Formula (Cold-Sinus) ..... ◘ 609
- Cheracol Plus Head Cold/Cough Formula ..... ◘ 769
- Comtrex Multi-Symptom Non-Drowsy Liqui-gels ..... ◘ 618
- Contac Continuous Action Nasal Decongestant/Antihistamine 12 Hour Capsules ..... ◘ 813
- Contac Maximum Strength Continuous Action Decongestant/Antihistamine 12 Hour Caplets ..... ◘ 813
- Contac Severe Cold and Flu Formula Caplets ..... ◘ 814
- Coricidin 'D' Decongestant Tablets ..... ◘ 800
- Dexatrim ..... ◘ 832
- Dexatrim Plus Vitamins Caplets ..... ◘ 832
- Dimetane-DC Cough Syrup 2059
- Dimetapp Elixir ..... ◘ 773
- Dimetapp Extentabs ..... ◘ 774
- Dimetapp Tablets/Liqui-Gels ..... ◘ 775
- Dimetapp Cold & Allergy Chewable Tablets ..... ◘ 773
- Dimetapp DM Elixir ..... ◘ 774
- Dura-Vent Tablets 952
- Entex Capsules 1986
- Entex LA Tablets 1987
- Entex Liquid 1986
- Exgest LA Tablets 782
- Hycomine 931
- Isoclor Timesule Capsules ..... ◘ 637
- Nolamine Timed-Release Tablets 785
- Ornade Spansule Capsules 2502
- Propagest Tablets 786
- Pyrroxate Caplets ..... ◘ 772
- Robitussin-CF ..... ◘ 777
- Sinulin Tablets 787
- Tavist-D 12 Hour Relief Tablets ..... ◘ 787
- Teldrin 12 Hour Antihistamine/Nasal Decongestant Allergy Relief Capsules ..... ◘ 826
- Triaminic Allergy Tablets ..... ◘ 789
- Triaminic Cold Tablets ..... ◘ 790
- Triaminic Expectorant ..... ◘ 790
- Triaminic Syrup ..... ◘ 792
- Triaminic-12 Tablets ..... ◘ 792
- Triaminic-DM Syrup ..... ◘ 792
- Triaminicin Tablets ..... ◘ 793
- Triaminicol Multi-Symptom Cold Tablets ..... ◘ 793
- Triaminicol Multi-Symptom Relief ..... ◘ 794
- Vicks DayQuil Allergy Relief 12-Hour Extended Release Tablets ..... ◘ 760
- Vicks DayQuil Allergy Relief 4-Hour Tablets ..... ◘ 760
- Vicks DayQuil SINUS Pressure & CONGESTION Relief ..... ◘ 761

Pirbuterol Acetate (Effects of concurrent use not specified; close supervision and careful adjustment of dosages are required). Products include:
- Maxair Autohaler 1492
- Maxair Inhaler 1494

Prazepam (Enhanced response to the effects of central nervous system depressants).
- No products indexed under this heading.

Prochlorperazine (Enhanced response to the effects of central nervous system depressants; concurrent use with drugs that are substrate for cytochrome $P_{450}IID_6$ may make normal metabolizer resemble poor metabolizer leading to higher than expected plasma concentrations of TCA with resultant toxicity). Products include:
- Compazine 2470

Procyclidine Hydrochloride (Concurrent use may result in additive anticholinergic effects including paralytic ileus). Products include:
- Kemadrin Tablets 1112

(◘ Described in PDR For Nonprescription Drugs)
(⊙ Described in PDR For Ophthalmology)

Interactions Index

Promethazine Hydrochloride (Enhanced response to the effects of central nervous system depressants; concurrent use with drugs that are substrate for cytochrome $P_{450}IID_6$ may make normal metabolizer resemble poor metabolizer leading to higher than expected plasma concentrations of TCA with resultant toxicity). Products include:

Mepergan Injection 2753
Phenergan with Codeine 2777
Phenergan with Dextromethorphan 2778
Phenergan Injection 2773
Phenergan Suppositories 2775
Phenergan Syrup 2774
Phenergan Tablets 2775
Phenergan VC 2779
Phenergan VC with Codeine 2781

Propafenone Hydrochloride (Concurrent use with drugs that are substrate for cytochrome $P_{450}IID_6$ may make normal metabolizer resemble poor metabolizer leading to higher than expected plasma concentrations of TCA with resultant toxicity). Products include:

Rythmol Tablets–150mg, 225mg, 300mg 1352

Propantheline Bromide (Concurrent use may result in additive anticholinergic effects including paralytic ileus). Products include:

Pro-Banthine Tablets 2052

Propofol (Enhanced response to the effects of central nervous system depressants). Products include:

Diprivan Injection 2833

Propoxyphene Hydrochloride (Enhanced response to central nervous system depressants). Products include:

Darvon 1435
Wygesic Tablets 2827

Propoxyphene Napsylate (Enhanced response to central nervous system depressants). Products include:

Darvon-N/Darvocet-N 1433

Protriptyline Hydrochloride (Concurrent use with drugs that are substrate for cytochrome $P_{450}IID_6$ may make normal metabolizer resemble poor metabolizer leading to higher than expected plasma concentrations of TCA with resultant toxicity). Products include:

Vivactil Tablets 1774

Pseudoephedrine Hydrochloride (Effects of concurrent use not specified; close supervision and careful adjustment of dosages are required). Products include:

Actifed Allergy Daytime/Nighttime Caplets .... ⊞ 844
Actifed Plus Caplets .... ⊞ 845
Actifed Plus Tablets .... ⊞ 845
Actifed with Codeine Cough Syrup.. 1067
Actifed Sinus Daytime/Nighttime Tablets and Caplets .... ⊞ 846
Actifed Syrup .... ⊞ 846
Actifed Tablets .... ⊞ 844
Advil Cold and Sinus Caplets and Tablets (formerly CoAdvil) .... ⊞ 870
Alka-Seltzer Plus Cold Medicine Liqui-Gels .... ⊞ 706
Alka-Seltzer Plus Cold & Cough Medicine Liqui-Gels .... ⊞ 705
Alka-Seltzer Plus Night-Time Cold Medicine Liqui-Gels .... ⊞ 706
Allerest Headache Strength Tablets .... ⊞ 627
Allerest Maximum Strength Tablets .... ⊞ 627
Allerest No Drowsiness Tablets ...... ⊞ 627
Allerest Sinus Pain Formula .... ⊞ 627
Anatuss LA Tablets 1542
Atrohist Pediatric Capsules 453
Bayer Select Sinus Pain Relief Formula .... ⊞ 717
Benadryl Allergy Decongestant Liquid Medication .... ⊞ 848
Benadryl Allergy Decongestant Tablets .... ⊞ 848
Benadryl Allergy Sinus Headache Formula Caplets .... ⊞ 849
Benylin Multisymptom .... ⊞ 852
Bromfed Capsules (Extended-Release) 1785
Bromfed Syrup .... ⊞ 733
Bromfed Tablets 1785
Bromfed-DM Cough Syrup 1786
Bromfed-PD Capsules (Extended-Release) 1785
Children's Vicks DayQuil Allergy Relief .... ⊞ 757
Children's Vicks NyQuil Cold/Cough Relief .... ⊞ 758
Comtrex Multi-Symptom Cold Reliever Tablets/Caplets/Liqui-Gels/Liquid .... ⊞ 615
Allergy-Sinus Comtrex Multi-Symptom Allergy-Sinus Formula Tablets .... ⊞ 617
Comtrex Multi-Symptom Non-Drowsy Caplets .... ⊞ 618
Congess 1004
Contac Day Allergy/Sinus Caplets ⊞ 812
Contac Day & Night .... ⊞ 812
Contac Night Allergy/Sinus Caplets .... ⊞ 812
Contac Severe Cold & Flu Non-Drowsy .... ⊞ 815
Deconamine Chewable Tablets 1320
Deconamine CX Cough and Cold Liquid and Tablets 1319
Deconamine 1320
Deconsal C Expectorant Syrup 456
Deconsal Pediatric Syrup 457
Deconsal II Tablets 454
Dimetane-DX Cough Syrup 2059
Dimetapp Sinus Caplets .... ⊞ 775
Dorcol Children's Cough Syrup ...... ⊞ 785
Drixoral Cough + Congestion Liquid Caps .... ⊞ 802
Dura-Tap/PD Capsules 2867
Duratuss Tablets 2565
Duratuss HD Elixir 2565
Efidac/24 .... ⊞ 635
Entex PSE Tablets 1987
Fedahist Gyrocaps 2401
Fedahist Timecaps 2401
Guaifed 1787
Guaifed Syrup .... ⊞ 734
Guaimax-D Tablets 792
Guaitab Tablets .... ⊞ 734
Isoclor Expectorant 990
Kronofed-A 977
Motrin IB Sinus .... ⊞ 838
Novahistine DH 2462
Novahistine DMX .... ⊞ 822
Novahistine Expectorant 2463
Nucofed 2051
PediaCare Cold Allergy Chewable Tablets .... ⊞ 677
PediaCare Cough-Cold Chewable Tablets 1553
PediaCare 1553
PediaCare Infants' Decongestant Drops .... ⊞ 677
PediaCare Infant's Drops Decongestant Plus Cough 1553
PediaCare NightRest Cough-Cold Liquid 1553
Pediatric Vicks 44d Dry Hacking Cough & Head Congestion .... ⊞ 763
Pediatric Vicks 44m Cough & Cold Relief .... ⊞ 764
Robitussin Cold & Cough Liqui-Gels .... ⊞ 776
Robitussin Maximum Strength Cough & Cold .... ⊞ 778
Robitussin Pediatric Cough & Cold Formula .... ⊞ 779
Robitussin Severe Congestion Liqui-Gels .... ⊞ 776
Robitussin-DAC Syrup 2074
Robitussin-PE .... ⊞ 778
Rondec Oral Drops 953
Rondec Syrup 953
Rondec Tablet 953
Rondec-DM Oral Drops 954
Rondec-DM Syrup 954
Rondec-TR Tablet 953
Ryna .... ⊞ 841
Seldane-D Extended-Release Tablets 1538
Semprex-D Capsules 463
Semprex-D Capsules 1167
Sinarest Tablets .... ⊞ 648
Sinarest Extra Strength Tablets ...... ⊞ 648
Sinarest No Drowsiness Tablets .... ⊞ 648
Sine-Aid IB Caplets 1554
Sine-Aid Maximum Strength Sinus Medication Gelcaps, Caplets and Tablets 1554
Sine-Off No Drowsiness Formula Caplets .... ⊞ 824
Sine-Off Sinus Medicine .... ⊞ 825
Singlet Tablets .... ⊞ 825
Sinutab Non-Drying Liquid Caps .... ⊞ 859
Sinutab Sinus Allergy Medication, Maximum Strength Tablets and Caplets .... ⊞ 860
Sinutab Sinus Medication, Maximum Strength Without Drowsiness Formula, Tablets & Caplets .... ⊞ 860
Sinutab Sinus Medication, Regular Strength Without Drowsiness Formula .... ⊞ 859
Sudafed Children's Liquid .... ⊞ 861
Sudafed Cold and Cough Liquidcaps .... ⊞ 862
Sudafed Cough Syrup .... ⊞ 862
Sudafed Plus Liquid .... ⊞ 862
Sudafed Plus Tablets .... ⊞ 863
Sudafed Severe Cold Formula Caplets .... ⊞ 863
Sudafed Severe Cold Formula Tablets .... ⊞ 864
Sudafed Sinus Caplets .... ⊞ 864
Sudafed Sinus Tablets .... ⊞ 864
Sudafed Tablets, 30 mg .... ⊞ 861
Sudafed Tablets, 60 mg .... ⊞ 861
Sudafed 12 Hour Caplets .... ⊞ 861
Syn-Rx Tablets 465
Syn-Rx DM Tablets 466
TheraFlu .... ⊞ 787
TheraFlu Maximum Strength Nighttime Flu, Cold & Cough Medicine .... ⊞ 788
TheraFlu Maximum Strength Non-Drowsy Formula Flu, Cold & Cough Medicine .... ⊞ 788
Thera Flu Maximum Strength, Non-Drowsy Formula Flu, Cold and Cough Caplets .... ⊞ 789
Triaminic AM Cough and Decongestant Formula .... ⊞ 789
Triaminic AM Decongestant Formula .... ⊞ 790
Triaminic Nite Light .... ⊞ 791
Triaminic Sore Throat Formula ...... ⊞ 791
Tussend 1783
Tussend Expectorant 1785
Children's TYLENOL Cold Multi-Symptom Liquid Formula and Chewable Tablets 1561
Children's TYLENOL Cold Plus Cough Multi Symptom Tablets and Liquid .... ⊞ 681
Infants' TYLENOL Cold Decongestant & Fever-Reducer Drops 1556
TYLENOL Maximum Strength Allergy Sinus Medication Gelcaps and Caplets 1563
TYLENOL Maximum Strength Allergy Sinus NightTime Medication Caplets 1555
TYLENOL Flu Maximum Strength Gelcaps 1565
TYLENOL Flu NightTime, Maximum Strength, Gelcaps 1566
TYLENOL Maximum Strength Flu NightTime Hot Medication Packets 1562
TYLENOL, Maximum Strength, Sinus Medication Geltabs, Gelcaps, Caplets and Tablets 1566
TYLENOL Cold Multi-Symptom Formula Medication Tablets and Caplets 1561
TYLENOL Cold Medication No Drowsiness Formula Gelcaps and Caplets 1562
TYLENOL Cold Multi-Symptom Hot Medication Liquid Packets 1557
TYLENOL Cough Multi-Symptom Medication with Decongestant 1565
Ursinus Inlay-Tabs .... ⊞ 794
Vicks 44 LiquiCaps Cough, Cold & Flu Relief .... ⊞ 755
Vicks 44 LiquiCaps Non-Drowsy Cough & Cold Relief .... ⊞ 756
Vicks 44D Dry Hacking Cough & Head Congestion .... ⊞ 755
Vicks 44M Cough, Cold & Flu Relief .... ⊞ 756
Vicks DayQuil .... ⊞ 761
Vicks DayQuil SINUS Pressure & PAIN Relief with IBUPROFEN .... ⊞ 762
Vicks Nyquil Hot Therapy .... ⊞ 762
Vicks NyQuil LiquiCaps Multi-Symptom Cold/Flu Relief .... ⊞ 763
Vicks NyQuil Multi-Symptom Cold/Flu Relief - (Original & Cherry Flavor) .... ⊞ 763

Pseudoephedrine Sulfate (Effects of concurrent use not specified; close supervision and careful adjustment of dosages are required). Products include:

Cheracol Sinus .... ⊞ 768
Chlor-Trimeton Allergy Decongestant Tablets .... ⊞ 799
Claritin-D 2350
Drixoral Cold and Allergy Sustained-Action Tablets .... ⊞ 802
Drixoral Cold and Flu Extended-Release Tablets .... ⊞ 803
Drixoral Non-Drowsy Formula Extended-Release Tablets .... ⊞ 803
Drixoral Allergy/Sinus Extended Release Tablets .... ⊞ 804
Trinalin Repetabs Tablets 1330

Pyrilamine Maleate (Since phenothiazines and antihistamines are CNS depressants, each can potentiate each other). Products include:

4-Way Fast Acting Nasal Spray (regular & mentholated) .... ⊞ 621
Maximum Strength Multi-Symptom Formula Midol .... ⊞ 722
PMS Multi-Symptom Formula Midol .... ⊞ 723

Pyrilamine Tannate (Since phenothiazines and antihistamines are CNS depressants, each can potentiate each other). Products include:

Atrohist Pediatric Suspension 454
Rynatan 2673

Quazepam (Enhanced response to the effects of central nervous system depressants). Products include:

Doral Tablets 2664

Quinidine Gluconate (Concurrent use with drugs that inhibit cytochrome $P_{450}IID_6$ may make normal metabolizer resemble poor metabolizer leading to higher than expected plasma concentrations of TCA with resultant toxicity). Products include:

Quinaglute Dura-Tabs Tablets 649

Quinidine Polygalacturonate (Concurrent use with drugs that inhibit cytochrome $P_{450}IID_6$ may make normal metabolizer resemble poor metabolizer leading to higher than expected plasma concentrations of TCA with resultant toxicity).

No products indexed under this heading.

Quinidine Sulfate (Concurrent use with drugs that inhibit cytochrome $P_{450}IID_6$ may make normal metabolizer resemble poor metabolizer leading to higher than expected plasma concentrations of TCA with resultant toxicity). Products include:

Quinidex Extentabs 2067

Risperidone (Enhanced response to the effects of central nervous system depressants). Products include:

Risperdal 1301

Salmeterol Xinafoate (Effects of concurrent use not specified; close supervision and careful adjustment of dosages are required). Products include:

Serevent Inhalation Aerosol 1176

Scopolamine (Concurrent use may result in additive anticholinergic effects including paralytic ileus). Products include:

Transderm Scōp Transdermal Therapeutic System 869

Scopolamine Hydrobromide (Concurrent use may result in additive anticholinergic effects including paralytic ileus). Products include:

Atrohist Plus Tablets 454
Donnatal 2060

IMPORTANT NOTE: Always consult each drug listing in the patient's regimen for possible interactions.

Etrafon

Donnatal Extentabs................................. 2061
Donnatal Tablets 2060

Secobarbital Sodium (Enhanced response to barbiturates). Products include:

Seconal Sodium Pulvules 1474

Selegiline Hydrochloride (Potential for hyperpyretic crises, severe convulsions and death; concurrent and/or sequential use is contraindicated). Products include:

Eldepryl Tablets 2550

Sertraline Hydrochloride (Concurrent use with drugs that are substrate for cytochrome $P_{450}IID_6$ may make normal metabolizer resemble poor metabolizer leading to higher than expected plasma concentrations of TCA with resultant toxicity; due to variation in the extent of inhibition of $P_{450}IID_6$ caution is indicated if co-administered sufficient time must elapse). Products include:

Zoloft Tablets 2217

Sufentanil Citrate (Enhanced response to central nervous system depressants). Products include:

Sufenta Injection 1309

Temazepam (Enhanced response to the effects of central nervous system depressants). Products include:

Restoril Capsules 2284

Terbutaline Sulfate (Effects of concurrent use not specified; close supervision and careful adjustment of dosages are required). Products include:

Brethaire Inhaler 813
Brethine Ampuls 815
Brethine Tablets...................................... 814
Bricanyl Subcutaneous Injection 1502
Bricanyl Tablets 1503

Terfenadine (Since phenothiazines and antihistamines are CNS depressants, each can potentiate each other). Products include:

Seldane Tablets 1536
Seldane-D Extended-Release Tablets 1538

Thiamylal Sodium (Enhanced response to barbiturates).

No products indexed under this heading.

Thioridazine Hydrochloride (Enhanced response to the effects of central nervous system depressants; concurrent use with drugs that are substrate for cytochrome $P_{450}IID_6$ may make normal metabolizer resemble poor metabolizer leading to higher than expected plasma concentrations of TCA with resultant toxicity). Products include:

Mellaril 2269

Thiothixene (Enhanced response to the effects of central nervous system depressants). Products include:

Navane Capsules and Concentrate 2201
Navane Intramuscular 2202

Thyroglobulin (On rare occasions, co-administration may produce arrhythmias).

No products indexed under this heading.

Thyroid (On rare occasions, co-administration may produce arrhythmias).

No products indexed under this heading.

Thyroxine (On rare occasions, co-administration may produce arrhythmias).

No products indexed under this heading.

Thyroxine Sodium (On rare occasions, co-administration may produce arrhythmias).

No products indexed under this heading.

Tranylcypromine Sulfate (Potential for hyperpyretic crises, severe convulsions and death; concurrent and/or sequential use is contraindicated). Products include:

Parnate Tablets 2503

Trazodone Hydrochloride (Concurrent use with drugs that are substrate for cytochrome $P_{450}IID_6$ may make normal metabolizer resemble poor metabolizer leading to higher than expected plasma concentrations of TCA with resultant toxicity). Products include:

Desyrel and Desyrel Dividose 503

Triazolam (Enhanced response to the effects of central nervous system depressants). Products include:

Halcion Tablets.. 2611

Tridihexethyl Chloride (Concurrent use may result in additive anticholinergic effects including paralytic ileus).

No products indexed under this heading.

Trifluoperazine Hydrochloride (Enhanced response to the effects of central nervous system depressants; concurrent use with drugs that are substrate for cytochrome $P_{450}IID_6$ may make normal metabolizer resemble poor metabolizer leading to higher than expected plasma concentrations of TCA with resultant toxicity). Products include:

Stelazine 2514

Trihexyphenidyl Hydrochloride (Concurrent use may result in additive anticholinergic effects including paralytic ileus). Products include:

Artane 1368

Trimeprazine Tartrate (Since phenothiazines and antihistamines are CNS depressants, each can potentiate each other). Products include:

Temaril Tablets, Syrup and Spansule Extended-Release Capsules.. 483

Trimipramine Maleate (Concurrent use with drugs that are substrate for cytochrome $P_{450}IID_6$ may make normal metabolizer resemble poor metabolizer leading to higher than expected plasma concentrations of TCA with resultant toxicity). Products include:

Surmontil Capsules 2811

Tripelennamine Hydrochloride (Since phenothiazines and antihistamines are CNS depressants, each can potentiate each other). Products include:

PBZ Tablets 845
PBZ-SR Tablets.. 844

Triprolidine Hydrochloride (Since phenothiazines and antihistamines are CNS depressants, each can potentiate each other). Products include:

Actifed Plus Caplets .... ⊕ 845
Actifed Plus Tablets .... ⊕ 845
Actifed with Codeine Cough Syrup.. 1067
Actifed Syrup... ⊕ 846
Actifed Tablets .... ⊕ 844

Venlafaxine Hydrochloride (Concurrent use with drugs that are substrate for cytochrome $P_{450}IID_6$ may make normal metabolizer resemble poor metabolizer leading to higher than expected plasma concentrations of TCA with resultant toxicity; due to variation in the extent of inhibition of $P_{450}IID_6$ caution is indicated if co-administered sufficient time must elapse). Products include:

Effexor 2719

Zolpidem Tartrate (Enhanced response to the effects of central nervous system depressants). Products include:

Ambien Tablets.. 2416

Food Interactions

Alcohol (Amitriptyline may enhance the response to alcohol; potential for additive effects and hypotension; concurrent use should be avoided).

EUCALYPTAMINT ARTHRITIS PAIN RELIEVER (EXTERNAL ANALGESIC)

(Menthol) .... ⊕ 635
None cited in PDR database.

EUCALYPTAMINT MUSCLE PAIN RELIEF FORMULA

(Menthol) .... ⊕ 636
None cited in PDR database.

EUCERIN DRY SKIN THERAPY CLEANSING BAR

(Eucerite) 641
None cited in PDR database.

EUCERIN ORIGINAL MOISTURIZING CREME (UNSCENTED)

(Mineral Oil, Petrolatum) 641
None cited in PDR database.

EUCERIN FACIAL MOISTURIZING LOTION SPF 25

(Phenylbenzimidazole-5-Sulfonic Acid, Titanium Dioxide, 2-Ethylhexyl-p-Methoxycinnamate, 2-Ethylhexyl Salicylate) 641
None cited in PDR database.

EUCERIN ORIGINAL MOISTURIZING LOTION

(Isopropyl Myristate, Mineral Oil) 641
None cited in PDR database.

EUCERIN PLUS DRY SKIN CARE MOISTURIZING LOTION

(Mineral Oil, Urea) 641
None cited in PDR database.

EUCERIN PLUS MOISTURIZING CREME

(Urea, Mineral Oil) 641
None cited in PDR database.

EULEXIN CAPSULES

(Flutamide) 2358
May interact with:

Warfarin Sodium (Increases in prothrombin time have been noted in patients receiving long-term warfarin therapy after flutamide was initiated). Products include:

Coumadin 926

EURAX CREAM & LOTION

(Crotamiton) 2685
None cited in PDR database.

EXACT VANISHING AND TINTED CREAMS

(Benzoyl Peroxide) .... ⊕ 749
None cited in PDR database.

ASPIRIN FREE EXCEDRIN ANALGESIC CAPLETS AND GELTABS

(Acetaminophen, Caffeine) 732
None cited in PDR database.

EXCEDRIN EXTRA-STRENGTH ANALGESIC TABLETS & CAPLETS

(Acetaminophen, Aspirin, Caffeine) .. 732
May interact with:

Antiarthritic Drugs, unspecified (Effect not specified).

Anticoagulant Drugs, unspecified (Effect not specified).

Antidiabetic Drugs, unspecified (Effect not specified).

Antigout Drugs, unspecified (Effect not specified).

EXCEDRIN P.M. ANALGESIC/SLEEPING AID TABLETS, CAPLETS, LIQUIGELS

(Acetaminophen, Diphenhydramine Citrate) 733
May interact with hypnotics and sedatives, tranquilizers, and certain other agents. Compounds in these categories include:

Alprazolam (Effect not specified). Products include:

Xanax Tablets 2649

Buspirone Hydrochloride (Effect not specified). Products include:

BuSpar 737

Chlordiazepoxide (Effect not specified). Products include:

Libritabs Tablets 2177
Limbitrol 2180

Chlordiazepoxide Hydrochloride (Effect not specified). Products include:

Librax Capsules 2176
Librium Capsules.................................... 2178
Librium Injectable 2179

Chlorpromazine (Effect not specified). Products include:

Thorazine Suppositories 2523

Chlorprothixene (Effect not specified).

No products indexed under this heading.

Chlorprothixene Hydrochloride (Effect not specified).

No products indexed under this heading.

Clorazepate Dipotassium (Effect not specified). Products include:

Tranxene 451

Diazepam (Effect not specified). Products include:

Dizac 1809
Valium Injectable 2182
Valium Tablets 2183
Valrelease Capsules 2169

Droperidol (Effect not specified). Products include:

Inapsine Injection 1296

Estazolam (Effect not specified). Products include:

ProSom Tablets 449

Ethchlorvynol (Effect not specified). Products include:

Placidyl Capsules 448

Ethinamate (Effect not specified).

No products indexed under this heading.

(⊕ Described in PDR For Nonprescription Drugs) (◎ Described in PDR For Ophthalmology)

Fluphenazine Decanoate (Effect not specified). Products include:

Prolixin Decanoate 509

Fluphenazine Enanthate (Effect not specified). Products include:

Prolixin Enanthate 509

Fluphenazine Hydrochloride (Effect not specified). Products include:

Prolixin 509

Flurazepam Hydrochloride (Effect not specified). Products include:

Dalmane Capsules 2173

Glutethimide (Effect not specified).

No products indexed under this heading.

Haloperidol (Effect not specified). Products include:

Haldol Injection, Tablets and Concentrate 1575

Haloperidol Decanoate (Effect not specified). Products include:

Haldol Decanoate..................................... 1577

Hydroxyzine Hydrochloride (Effect not specified). Products include:

Atarax Tablets & Syrup......................... 2185
Marax Tablets & DF Syrup................... 2200
Vistaril Intramuscular Solution.......... 2216

Lorazepam (Effect not specified). Products include:

Ativan Injection....................................... 2698
Ativan Tablets 2700

Loxapine Hydrochloride (Effect not specified). Products include:

Loxitane 1378

Loxapine Succinate (Effect not specified). Products include:

Loxitane Capsules 1378

Meprobamate (Effect not specified). Products include:

Miltown Tablets 2672
PMB 200 and PMB 400 2783

Mesoridazine Besylate (Effect not specified). Products include:

Serentil 684

Midazolam Hydrochloride (Effect not specified). Products include:

Versed Injection 2170

Molindone Hydrochloride (Effect not specified). Products include:

Moban Tablets and Concentrate 1048

Oxazepam (Effect not specified). Products include:

Serax Capsules 2810
Serax Tablets... 2810

Perphenazine (Effect not specified). Products include:

Etrafon 2355
Triavil Tablets 1757
Trilafon... 2389

Prazepam (Effect not specified).

No products indexed under this heading.

Prochlorperazine (Effect not specified). Products include:

Compazine 2470

Promethazine Hydrochloride (Effect not specified). Products include:

Mepergan Injection 2753
Phenergan with Codeine 2777
Phenergan with Dextromethorphan 2778
Phenergan Injection 2773
Phenergan Suppositories 2775
Phenergan Syrup 2774
Phenergan Tablets 2775
Phenergan VC 2779
Phenergan VC with Codeine 2781

Propofol (Effect not specified). Products include:

Diprivan Injection.................................... 2833

Quazepam (Effect not specified). Products include:

Doral Tablets 2664

Secobarbital Sodium (Effect not specified). Products include:

Seconal Sodium Pulvules 1474

Temazepam (Effect not specified). Products include:

Restoril Capsules 2284

Thioridazine Hydrochloride (Effect not specified). Products include:

Mellaril 2269

Thiothixene (Effect not specified). Products include:

Navane Capsules and Concentrate 2201
Navane Intramuscular 2202

Triazolam (Effect not specified). Products include:

Halcion Tablets 2611

Trifluoperazine Hydrochloride (Effect not specified). Products include:

Stelazine 2514

Zolpidem Tartrate (Effect not specified). Products include:

Ambien Tablets... 2416

Food Interactions

Alcohol (Effect not specified).

EXELDERM CREAM 1.0%

(Sulconazole Nitrate)..............................2685

None cited in PDR database.

EXELDERM SOLUTION 1.0%

(Sulconazole Nitrate)..............................2686

None cited in PDR database.

EXGEST LA TABLETS

(Phenylpropanolamine Hydrochloride, Guaifenesin)................. 782

May interact with monoamine oxidase inhibitors and sympathomimetics. Compounds in these categories include:

Albuterol (Concurrent use is not recommended). Products include:

Proventil Inhalation Aerosol 2382
Ventolin Inhalation Aerosol and Refill 1197

Albuterol Sulfate (Concurrent use is not recommended). Products include:

Airet Solution for Inhalation 452
Proventil Inhalation Solution 0.083% 2384
Proventil Repetabs Tablets 2386
Proventil Solution for Inhalation 0.5% 2383
Proventil Syrup.. 2385
Proventil Tablets 2386
Ventolin Inhalation Solution................ 1198
Ventolin Nebules Inhalation Solution.. 1199
Ventolin Rotacaps for Inhalation 1200
Ventolin Syrup.. 1202
Ventolin Tablets 1203
Volmax Extended-Release Tablets .. 1788

Dobutamine Hydrochloride (Concurrent use is not recommended). Products include:

Dobutrex Solution Vials........................ 1439

Dopamine Hydrochloride (Concurrent use is not recommended).

No products indexed under this heading.

Ephedrine Hydrochloride (Concurrent use is not recommended). Products include:

Primatene Dual Action Formula...... ⊞ 872
Primatene Tablets .... ⊞ 873
Quadrinal Tablets 1350

Ephedrine Sulfate (Concurrent use is not recommended). Products include:

Bronkaid Caplets .... ⊞ 717
Marax Tablets & DF Syrup................... 2200

Ephedrine Tannate (Concurrent use is not recommended). Products include:

Rynatuss 2673

Epinephrine (Concurrent use is not recommended). Products include:

Bronkaid Mist .... ⊞ 717
EPIFRIN .... ◉ 239
EpiPen 790
Marcaine Hydrochloride with Epinephrine 1:200,000 2316
Primatene Mist .... ⊞ 873
Sensorcaine with Epinephrine Injection... 559
Sus-Phrine Injection 1019
Xylocaine with Epinephrine Injections.. 567

Epinephrine Bitartrate (Concurrent use is not recommended). Products include:

Bronkaid Mist Suspension .... ⊞ 718
Sensorcaine-MPF with Epinephrine Injection... 559

Epinephrine Hydrochloride (Concurrent use is not recommended). Products include:

Ana-Kit Anaphylaxis Emergency Treatment Kit 617

Furazolidone (Concurrent use is contraindicated). Products include:

Furoxone 2046

Isocarboxazid (Concurrent use is contraindicated).

No products indexed under this heading.

Isoproterenol Hydrochloride (Concurrent use is not recommended). Products include:

Isuprel Hydrochloride Injection 1:5000 2311
Isuprel Hydrochloride Solution 1:200 & 1:100 2313
Isuprel Mistometer 2312

Isoproterenol Sulfate (Concurrent use is not recommended). Products include:

Norisodrine with Calcium Iodide Syrup.. 442

Metaproterenol Sulfate (Concurrent use is not recommended). Products include:

Alupent.. 669
Metaproterenol Sulfate Inhalation Solution, USP, Arm-a-Med 552

Metaraminol Bitartrate (Concurrent use is not recommended). Products include:

Aramine Injection.................................... 1609

Methoxamine Hydrochloride (Concurrent use is not recommended). Products include:

Vasoxyl Injection 1196

Norepinephrine Bitartrate (Concurrent use is not recommended). Products include:

Levophed Bitartrate Injection 2315

Phenelzine Sulfate (Concurrent use is contraindicated). Products include:

Nardil 1920

Phenylephrine Bitartrate (Concurrent use is not recommended).

No products indexed under this heading.

Phenylephrine Hydrochloride (Concurrent use is not recommended). Products include:

Atrohist Plus Tablets 454
Cerose DM .... ⊞ 878
Comhist 2038
D.A. Chewable Tablets........................... 951
Deconsal Pediatric Capsules................ 454
Dura-Vent/DA Tablets 953
Entex Capsules 1986
Entex Liquid 1986
Extendryl 1005
4-Way Fast Acting Nasal Spray (regular & mentholated) .... ⊞ 621
Hemorid For Women .... ⊞ 834
Hycomine Compound Tablets 932
Neo-Synephrine Hydrochloride 1% Carpuject... 2324
Neo-Synephrine Hydrochloride 1% Injection 2324

Neo-Synephrine Hydrochloride (Ophthalmic) 2325
Neo-Synephrine .... ⊞ 726
Nōstril .... ⊞ 644
Novahistine Elixir .... ⊞ 823
Phenergan VC 2779
Phenergan VC with Codeine 2781
Preparation H .... ⊞ 871
Tympagesic Ear Drops 2342
Vasosulf .... ◉ 271
Vicks Sinex Nasal Spray and Ultra Fine Mist .... ⊞ 765

Phenylephrine Tannate (Concurrent use is not recommended). Products include:

Atrohist Pediatric Suspension 454
Ricobid-D Pediatric Suspension........ 2038
Ricobid Tablets and Pediatric Suspension... 2038
Rynatan 2673
Rynatuss 2673

Pirbuterol Acetate (Concurrent use is not recommended). Products include:

Maxair Autohaler 1492
Maxair Inhaler 1494

Pseudoephedrine Hydrochloride (Concurrent use is not recommended). Products include:

Actifed Allergy Daytime/Nighttime Caplets .... ⊞ 844
Actifed Plus Caplets .... ⊞ 845
Actifed Plus Tablets .... ⊞ 845
Actifed with Codeine Cough Syrup.. 1067
Actifed Sinus Daytime/Nighttime Tablets and Caplets .... ⊞ 846
Actifed Syrup.. ⊞ 846
Actifed Tablets .... ⊞ 844
Advil Cold and Sinus Caplets and Tablets (formerly CoAdvil) .... ⊞ 870
Alka-Seltzer Plus Cold Medicine Liqui-Gels .... ⊞ 706
Alka-Seltzer Plus Cold & Cough Medicine Liqui-Gels........................... ⊞ 705
Alka-Seltzer Plus Night-Time Cold Medicine Liqui-Gels........................... ⊞ 706
Allerest Headache Strength Tablets .... ⊞ 627
Allerest Maximum Strength Tablets .... ⊞ 627
Allerest No Drowsiness Tablets .... ⊞ 627
Allerest Sinus Pain Formula .... ⊞ 627
Anatuss LA Tablets.................................. 1542
Atrohist Pediatric Capsules.................. 453
Bayer Select Sinus Pain Relief Formula .... ⊞ 717
Benadryl Allergy Decongestant Liquid Medication .... ⊞ 848
Benadryl Allergy Decongestant Tablets .... ⊞ 848
Benadryl Allergy Sinus Headache Formula Caplets .... ⊞ 849
Benylin Multisymptom .... ⊞ 852
Bromfed Capsules (Extended-Release) 1785
Bromfed Syrup .... ⊞ 733
Bromfed Tablets 1785
Bromfed-DM Cough Syrup................... 1786
Bromfed-PD Capsules (Extended-Release) 1785
Children's Vicks DayQuil Allergy Relief .... ⊞ 757
Children's Vicks NyQuil Cold/ Cough Relief... ⊞ 758
Comtrex Multi-Symptom Cold Reliever Tablets/Caplets/Liqui-Gels/Liquid... ⊞ 615
Allergy-Sinus Comtrex Multi-Symptom Allergy-Sinus Formula Tablets .... ⊞ 617
Comtrex Multi-Symptom Non-Drowsy Caplets.................................... ⊞ 618
Congess 1004
Contac Day Allergy/Sinus Caplets ⊞ 812
Contac Day & Night .... ⊞ 812
Contac Night Allergy/Sinus Caplets .... ⊞ 812
Contac Severe Cold & Flu Non-Drowsy .... ⊞ 815
Deconamine Chewable Tablets 1320
Deconamine CX Cough and Cold Liquid and Tablets............................... 1319
Deconamine 1320
Deconsal C Expectorant Syrup 456
Deconsal Pediatric Syrup...................... 457
Deconsal II Tablets 454
Dimetane-DX Cough Syrup 2059
Dimetapp Sinus Caplets .... ⊞ 775
Dorcol Children's Cough Syrup ...... ⊞ 785

IMPORTANT NOTE: Always consult each drug listing in the patient's regimen for possible interactions.

Exgest LA — Interactions Index — 404

Drixoral Cough + Congestion Liquid Caps ▣ 802
Dura-Tap/PD Capsules 2867
Duratuss Tablets 2565
Duratuss HD Elixir 2565
Efidac/24 ▣ 635
Entex PSE Tablets 1987
Fedahist Gyrocaps 2401
Fedahist Timecaps 2401
Guaifed 1787
Guaifed Syrup ▣ 734
Guaimax-D Tablets 792
Guaitab Tablets ▣ 734
Isoclor Expectorant 990
Kronofed-A 977
Motrin IB Sinus ▣ 838
Novahistine DH 2462
Novahistine DMX ▣ 822
Novahistine Expectorant 2463
Nucofed 2051
PediaCare Cold Allergy Chewable Tablets ▣ 677
PediaCare Cough-Cold Chewable Tablets 1553
PediaCare 1553
PediaCare Infants' Decongestant Drops ▣ 677
PediCare Infant's Drops Decongestant Plus Cough 1553
PediaCare NightRest Cough-Cold Liquid 1553
Pediatric Vicks 44d Dry Hacking Cough & Head Congestion ▣ 763
Pediatric Vicks 44m Cough & Cold Relief ▣ 764
Robitussin Cold & Cough Liqui-Gels ▣ 776
Robitussin Maximum Strength Cough & Cold ▣ 778
Robitussin Pediatric Cough & Cold Formula ▣ 779
Robitussin Severe Congestion Liqui-Gels ▣ 776
Robitussin-DAC Syrup 2074
Robitussin-PE ▣ 778
Rondec Oral Drops 953
Rondec Syrup 953
Rondec Tablet 953
Rondec-DM Oral Drops 954
Rondec-DM Syrup 954
Rondec-TR Tablet 953
Ryna ▣ 841
Seldane-D Extended-Release Tablets 1538
Semprex-D Capsules 463
Semprex-D Capsules 1167
Sinarest Tablets ▣ 648
Sinarest Extra Strength Tablets ▣ 648
Sinarest No Drowsiness Tablets ▣ 648
Sine-Aid IB Caplets 1554
Sine-Aid Maximum Strength Sinus Medication Gelcaps, Caplets and Tablets 1554
Sine-Off No Drowsiness Formula Caplets ▣ 824
Sine-Off Sinus Medicine ▣ 825
Singlet Tablets ▣ 825
Sinutab Non-Drying Liquid Caps ▣ 859
Sinutab Sinus Allergy Medication, Maximum Strength Tablets and Caplets ▣ 860
Sinutab Sinus Medication, Maximum Strength Without Drowsiness Formula, Tablets & Caplets ▣ 860
Sinutab Sinus Medication, Regular Strength Without Drowsiness Formula ▣ 859
Sudafed Children's Liquid ▣ 861
Sudafed Cold and Cough Liquidcaps ▣ 862
Sudafed Cough Syrup ▣ 862
Sudafed Plus Liquid ▣ 862
Sudafed Plus Tablets ▣ 863
Sudafed Severe Cold Formula Caplets ▣ 863
Sudafed Severe Cold Formula Tablets ▣ 864
Sudafed Sinus Caplets ▣ 864
Sudafed Sinus Tablets ▣ 864
Sudafed Tablets, 30 mg ▣ 861
Sudafed Tablets, 60 mg ▣ 861
Sudafed 12 Hour Caplets ▣ 861
Syn-Rx Tablets 465
Syn-Rx DM Tablets 466
TheraFlu ▣ 787
TheraFlu Maximum Strength Nighttime Flu, Cold & Cough Medicine ▣ 788
TheraFlu Maximum Strength Non-Drowsy Formula Flu, Cold & Cough Medicine ▣ 788
Thera Flu Maximum Strength, Non-Drowsy Formula Flu, Cold and Cough Caplets ▣ 789
Triaminic AM Cough and Decongestant Formula ▣ 789
Triaminic AM Decongestant Formula ▣ 790
Triaminic Nite Light ▣ 791
Triaminic Sore Throat Formula ▣ 791
Tussend 1783
Tussend Expectorant 1785
Children's TYLENOL Cold Multi-Symptom Liquid Formula and Chewable Tablets 1561
Children's TYLENOL Cold Plus Cough Multi Symptom Tablets and Liquid ▣ 681
Infants' TYLENOL Cold Decongestant & Fever-Reducer Drops 1556
TYLENOL Maximum Strength Allergy Sinus Medication Gelcaps and Caplets 1563
TYLENOL Maximum Strength Allergy Sinus NightTime Medication Caplets 1555
TYLENOL Flu Maximum Strength Gelcaps 1565
TYLENOL Flu NightTime, Maximum Strength, Gelcaps 1566
TYLENOL Maximum Strength Flu NightTime Hot Medication Packets 1562
TYLENOL, Maximum Strength, Sinus Medication Geltabs, Gelcaps, Caplets and Tablets 1566
TYLENOL Cold Multi-Symptom Formula Medication Tablets and Caplets 1561
TYLENOL Cold Medication No Drowsiness Formula Gelcaps and Caplets 1562
TYLENOL Cold Multi-Symptom Hot Medication Liquid Packets 1557
TYLENOL Cough Multi-Symptom Medication with Decongestant 1565
Ursinus Inlay-Tabs ▣ 794
Vicks 44 LiquiCaps Cough, Cold & Flu Relief ▣ 755
Vicks 44 LiquiCaps Non-Drowsy Cough & Cold Relief ▣ 756
Vicks 44D Dry Hacking Cough & Head Congestion ▣ 755
Vicks 44M Cough, Cold & Flu Relief ▣ 756
Vicks DayQuil ▣ 761
Vicks DayQuil SINUS Pressure & PAIN Relief with IBUPROFEN ▣ 762
Vicks Nyquil Hot Therapy ▣ 762
Vicks NyQuil LiquiCaps Multi-Symptom Cold/Flu Relief ▣ 763
Vicks NyQuil Multi-Symptom Cold/Flu Relief (Original & Cherry Flavor) ▣ 763

Pseudoephedrine Sulfate (Concurrent use is not recommended). Products include:
Cheracol Sinus ▣ 768
Chlor-Trimeton Allergy Decongestant Tablets ▣ 799
Claritin-D 2350
Drixoral Cold and Allergy Sustained-Action Tablets ▣ 802
Drixoral Cold and Flu Extended-Release Tablets ▣ 803
Drixoral Non-Drowsy Formula Extended-Release Tablets ▣ 803
Drixoral Allergy/Sinus Extended Release Tablets ▣ 804
Trinalin Repetabs Tablets 1330

Salmeterol Xinafoate (Concurrent use is not recommended). Products include:
Serevent Inhalation Aerosol 1176

Selegiline Hydrochloride (Concurrent use is contraindicated). Products include:
Eldepryl Tablets 2550

Terbutaline Sulfate (Concurrent use is not recommended). Products include:
Brethaire Inhaler 813
Brethine Ampuls 815
Brethine Tablets 814
Bricanyl Subcutaneous Injection 1502
Bricanyl Tablets 1503

Tranylcypromine Sulfate (Concurrent use is contraindicated). Products include:
Parnate Tablets 2503

EX-LAX CHOCOLATED LAXATIVE TABLETS
(Phenolphthalein) ▣ 786
None cited in PDR database.

EXTRA GENTLE EX-LAX LAXATIVE PILLS
(Docusate Sodium, Phenolphthalein) ▣ 786
None cited in PDR database.

MAXIMUM RELIEF FORMULA EX-LAX LAXATIVE PILLS
(Phenolphthalein) ▣ 786
None cited in PDR database.

REGULAR STRENGTH EX-LAX LAXATIVE PILLS
(Phenolphthalein) ▣ 786
None cited in PDR database.

EX-LAX GENTLE NATURE LAXATIVE PILLS
(Senna Concentrates) ▣ 786
None cited in PDR database.

EXOSURF NEONATAL FOR INTRATRACHEAL SUSPENSION
(Colfosceril Palmitate) 1095
None cited in PDR database.

EXTENDRYL CHEWABLE TABLETS
(Chlorpheniramine Maleate, Methscopolamine Nitrate, Phenylephrine Hydrochloride) 1005
None cited in PDR database.

EXTENDRYL SR. & JR. T.D. CAPSULES
(Chlorpheniramine Maleate, Methscopolamine Nitrate, Phenylephrine Hydrochloride) 1005
None cited in PDR database.

EXTENDRYL SYRUP
(Chlorpheniramine Maleate, Methscopolamine Nitrate, Phenylephrine Hydrochloride) 1005
None cited in PDR database.

EXTRA STRENGTH VICKS COUGH DROPS
(Menthol) ▣ 760
None cited in PDR database.

EYE-SCRUB
(Cleanser) ⊙ 263
None cited in PDR database.

EYE-STREAM EYE IRRIGATING SOLUTION
(Balanced Salt Solution) 473
None cited in PDR database.

4-WAY FAST ACTING NASAL SPRAY (REGULAR & MENTHOLATED)
(Naphazoline Hydrochloride, Phenylephrine Hydrochloride, Pyrilamine Maleate) ▣ 621
None cited in PDR database.

4-WAY LONG LASTING NASAL SPRAY
(Oxymetazoline Hydrochloride) ▣ 621
None cited in PDR database.

FML FORTE LIQUIFILM
(Fluorometholone) ⊙ 240
None cited in PDR database.

FML LIQUIFILM
(Fluorometholone) ⊙ 241
None cited in PDR database.

FML S.O.P.
(Fluorometholone) ⊙ 241
None cited in PDR database.

FML-S LIQUIFILM
(Sulfacetamide Sodium, Fluorometholone) ⊙ 242
May interact with silver preparations. Compounds in this category include:

Silver Nitrate (Physical incompatibility).
No products indexed under this heading.

FACTREL
(Gonadorelin Hydrochloride) 2877
May interact with androgens, estrogens, progestins, corticosteroids, oral contraceptives, phenothiazines, dopamine antagonists, and certain other agents. Compounds in these categories include:

Betamethasone Acetate (Pituitary secretion of gonadotropins affected). Products include:
Celestone Soluspan Suspension 2347

Betamethasone Sodium Phosphate (Pituitary secretion of gonadotropins affected). Products include:
Celestone Soluspan Suspension 2347

Chlorotrianisene (Pituitary secretion of gonadotropins affected).
No products indexed under this heading.

Chlorpromazine (Rise in prolactin; response to Factrel may be blunted). Products include:
Thorazine Suppositories 2523

Chlorpromazine Hydrochloride (Rise in prolactin; response to Factrel may be blunted). Products include:
Thorazine 2523

Clozapine (Rise in prolactin; response to Factrel may be blunted). Products include:
Clozaril Tablets 2252

Cortisone Acetate (Pituitary secretion of gonadotropins affected). Products include:
Cortone Acetate Sterile Suspension 1623
Cortone Acetate Tablets 1624

Desogestrel (Pituitary secretion of gonadotropins affected; gonadotropin levels suppressed). Products include:
Desogen Tablets 1817
Ortho-Cept 1851

Dexamethasone (Pituitary secretion of gonadotropins affected). Products include:
AK-Trol Ointment & Suspension ⊙ 205
Decadron Elixir 1633
Decadron Tablets 1635
Decaspray Topical Aerosol 1648
Dexacidin Ointment ⊙ 263
Maxitrol Ophthalmic Ointment and Suspension ⊙ 224
TobraDex Ophthalmic Suspension and Ointment 473

Dexamethasone Acetate (Pituitary secretion of gonadotropins affected). Products include:
Dalalone D.P. Injectable 1011
Decadron-LA Sterile Suspension 1646

Dexamethasone Sodium Phosphate (Pituitary secretion of gonadotropins affected). Products include:
Decadron Phosphate Injection 1637
Decadron Phosphate Respihaler 1642
Decadron Phosphate Sterile Ophthalmic Ointment 1641

(▣ Described in PDR For Nonprescription Drugs) (⊙ Described in PDR For Ophthalmology)

405 **Interactions Index** **Factrel**

Decadron Phosphate Sterile Ophthalmic Solution 1642
Decadron Phosphate Topical Cream 1644
Decadron Phosphate Turbinaire 1645
Decadron Phosphate with Xylocaine Injection, Sterile 1639
Dexacort Phosphate in Respihaler .. 458
Dexacort Phosphate in Turbinaire .. 459
NeoDecadron Sterile Ophthalmic Ointment 1712
NeoDecadron Sterile Ophthalmic Solution 1713
NeoDecadron Topical Cream 1714

Dienestrol (Pituitary secretion of gonadotropins affected). Products include:
Ortho Dienestrol Cream 1866

Diethylstilbestrol (Pituitary secretion of gonadotropins affected). Products include:
Diethylstilbestrol Tablets 1437

Digitoxin (Gonadotropin levels suppressed). Products include:
Crystodigin Tablets 1433

Digoxin (Gonadotropin levels suppressed). Products include:
Lanoxicaps 1117
Lanoxin Elixir Pediatric 1120
Lanoxin Injection 1123
Lanoxin Injection Pediatric 1126
Lanoxin Tablets 1128

Estradiol (Pituitary secretion of gonadotropins affected). Products include:
Climara Transdermal System 645
Estrace Cream and Tablets 749
Estraderm Transdermal System 824

Estrogens, Conjugated (Pituitary secretion of gonadotropins affected). Products include:
PMB 200 and PMB 400 2783
Premarin Intravenous 2787
Premarin with Methyltestosterone .. 2794
Premarin Tablets 2789
Premarin Vaginal Cream 2791
Premphase 2797
Prempro 2801

Estrogens, Esterified (Pituitary secretion of gonadotropins affected). Products include:
ESTRATAB Tablets (0.3, 0.625, 1.25, 2.5 mg) 2536
Estratest 2539
Menest Tablets 2494

Estropipate (Pituitary secretion of gonadotropins affected). Products include:
Ogen Tablets 2627
Ogen Vaginal Cream 2630
Ortho-Est 1869

Ethinyl Estradiol (Pituitary secretion of gonadotropins affected; gonadotropin levels suppressed). Products include:
Brevicon 2088
Demulen 2428
Desogen Tablets 1817
Levlen/Tri-Levlen 651
Lo/Ovral Tablets 2746
Lo/Ovral-28 Tablets 2751
Modicon 1872
Nordette-21 Tablets 2755
Nordette-28 Tablets 2758
Norinyl 2088
Ortho-Cept 1851
Ortho-Cyclen/Ortho-Tri-Cyclen 1858
Ortho-Novum 1872
Ortho-Cyclen/Ortho Tri-Cyclen 1858
Ovcon 760
Ovral Tablets 2770
Ovral-28 Tablets 2770
Levlen/Tri-Levlen 651
Tri-Norinyl 2164
Triphasil-21 Tablets 2814
Triphasil-28 Tablets 2819

Ethynodiol Diacetate (Gonadotropin levels suppressed). Products include:
Demulen 2428

Fludrocortisone Acetate (Pituitary secretion of gonadotropins affected). Products include:
Florinef Acetate Tablets 505

Fluoxymesterone (Pituitary secretion of gonadotropins affected). Products include:
Halotestin Tablets 2614

Fluphenazine Decanoate (Rise in prolactin; response to Factrel may be blunted). Products include:
Prolixin Decanoate 509

Fluphenazine Enanthate (Rise in prolactin; response to Factrel may be blunted). Products include:
Prolixin Enanthate 509

Fluphenazine Hydrochloride (Rise in prolactin; response to Factrel may be blunted). Products include:
Prolixin 509

Haloperidol (Rise in prolactin; response to Factrel may be blunted). Products include:
Haldol Injection, Tablets and Concentrate 1575

Haloperidol Decanoate (Rise in prolactin; response to Factrel may be blunted). Products include:
Haldol Decanoate 1577

Hydrocortisone (Pituitary secretion of gonadotropins affected). Products include:
Anusol-HC Cream 2.5% 1896
Aquanil HC Lotion 1931
Bactine Hydrocortisone Anti-Itch Cream .... ▣ 709
Caldecort Anti-Itch Hydrocortisone Spray .... ▣ 631
Cortaid .... ▣ 836
CORTENEMA 2535
Cortisporin Ointment 1085
Cortisporin Ophthalmic Ointment Sterile 1085
Cortisporin Ophthalmic Suspension Sterile 1086
Cortisporin Otic Solution Sterile 1087
Cortisporin Otic Suspension Sterile 1088
Cortizone-5 .... ▣ 831
Cortizone-10 .... ▣ 831
Hydrocortone Tablets 1672
Hytone 907
Massengill Medicated Soft Cloth Towelettes 2458
PediOtic Suspension Sterile 1153
Preparation H Hydrocortisone 1% Cream .... ▣ 872
ProctoCream-HC 2.5% 2408
VōSoL HC Otic Solution 2678

Hydrocortisone Acetate (Pituitary secretion of gonadotropins affected). Products include:
Analpram-HC Rectal Cream 1% and 2.5% 977
Anusol HC-1 Anti-Itch Hydrocortisone Ointment .... ▣ 847
Anusol-HC Suppositories 1897
Caldecort .... ▣ 631
Carmol HC 924
Coly-Mycin S Otic w/Neomycin & Hydrocortisone 1906
Cortaid .... ▣ 836
Cortifoam 2396
Cortisporin Cream 1084
Epifoam 2399
Hydrocortone Acetate Sterile Suspension 1669
Mantadil Cream 1135
Nupercainal Hydrocortisone 1% Cream .... ▣ 645
Ophthocort .... ⊙ 311
Pramosone Cream, Lotion & Ointment 978
ProctoCream-HC 2408
ProctoFoam-HC 2409
Terra-Cortril Ophthalmic Suspension 2210

Hydrocortisone Sodium Phosphate (Pituitary secretion of gonadotropins affected). Products include:
Hydrocortone Phosphate Injection, Sterile 1670

Hydrocortisone Sodium Succinate (Pituitary secretion of gonadotropins affected). Products include:
Solu-Cortef Sterile Powder 2641

Levodopa (Minimal elevation of gonadotropin levels). Products include:
Atamet 572
Larodopa Tablets 2129
Sinemet Tablets 943
Sinemet CR Tablets 944

Levonorgestrel (Gonadotropin levels suppressed). Products include:
Levlen/Tri-Levlen 651
Nordette-21 Tablets 2755
Nordette-28 Tablets 2758
Norplant System 2759
Levlen/Tri-Levlen 651
Triphasil-21 Tablets 2814
Triphasil-28 Tablets 2819

Medroxyprogesterone Acetate (Pituitary secretion of gonadotropins affected). Products include:
Amen Tablets 780
Cycrin Tablets 975
Depo-Provera Contraceptive Injection 2602
Depo-Provera Sterile Aqueous Suspension 2606
Premphase 2797
Prempro 2801
Provera Tablets 2636

Megestrol Acetate (Pituitary secretion of gonadotropins affected). Products include:
Megace Oral Suspension 699
Megace Tablets 701

Mesoridazine Besylate (Rise in prolactin; response to Factrel may be blunted). Products include:
Serentil 684

Mestranol (Gonadotropin levels suppressed). Products include:
Norinyl 2088
Ortho-Novum 1872

Methotrimeprazine (Rise in prolactin; response to Factrel may be blunted). Products include:
Levoprome 1274

Methylprednisolone Acetate (Pituitary secretion of gonadotropins affected). Products include:
Depo-Medrol Single-Dose Vial 2600
Depo-Medrol Sterile Aqueous Suspension 2597

Methylprednisolone Sodium Succinate (Pituitary secretion of gonadotropins affected). Products include:
Solu-Medrol Sterile Powder 2643

Methyltestosterone (Pituitary secretion of gonadotropins affected). Products include:
Android Capsules, 10 mg 1250
Android 1251
Estratest 2539
Oreton Methyl 1255
Premarin with Methyltestosterone .. 2794
Testred Capsules 1262

Metoclopramide Hydrochloride (Rise in prolactin; response to Factrel may be blunted). Products include:
Reglan 2068

Norethindrone (Gonadotropin levels suppressed). Products include:
Brevicon 2088
Micronor Tablets 1872
Modicon 1872
Norinyl 2088
Nor-Q D Tablets 2135
Ortho-Novum 1872
Ovcon 760
Tri-Norinyl 2164

Norethynodrel (Gonadotropin levels suppressed).
No products indexed under this heading.

Norgestimate (Pituitary secretion of gonadotropins affected; gonadotropin levels suppressed). Products include:
Ortho-Cyclen/Ortho-Tri-Cyclen 1858
Ortho-Cyclen/Ortho Tri-Cyclen 1858

Norgestrel (Gonadotropin levels suppressed). Products include:
Lo/Ovral Tablets 2746
Lo/Ovral-28 Tablets 2751
Ovral Tablets 2770
Ovral-28 Tablets 2770
Ovrette Tablets 2771

Oxandrolone (Pituitary secretion of gonadotropins affected). Products include:
Oxandrin 2862

Oxymetholone (Pituitary secretion of gonadotropins affected).
No products indexed under this heading.

Perphenazine (Rise in prolactin; response to Factrel may be blunted). Products include:
Etrafon 2355
Triavil Tablets 1757
Trilafon 2389

Pimozide (Rise in prolactin; response to Factrel may be blunted). Products include:
Orap Tablets 1050

Polyestradiol Phosphate (Pituitary secretion of gonadotropins affected).
No products indexed under this heading.

Prednisolone Acetate (Pituitary secretion of gonadotropins affected). Products include:
AK-CIDE .... ⊙ 202
AK-CIDE Ointment .... ⊙ 202
Blephamide Liquifilm Sterile Ophthalmic Suspension 476
Blephamide Ointment .... ⊙ 237
Econopred & Econopred Plus Ophthalmic Suspensions .... ⊙ 217
Poly-Pred Liquifilm .... ⊙ 248
Pred Forte .... ⊙ 250
Pred Mild .... ⊙ 253
Pred-G Liquifilm Sterile Ophthalmic Suspension .... ⊙ 251
Pred-G S.O.P. Sterile Ophthalmic Ointment .... ⊙ 252
Vasocidin Ointment .... ⊙ 268

Prednisolone Sodium Phosphate (Pituitary secretion of gonadotropins affected). Products include:
AK-Pred .... ⊙ 204
Hydeltrasol Injection, Sterile 1665
Inflamase .... ⊙ 265
Pediapred Oral Liquid 995
Vasocidin Ophthalmic Solution .... ⊙ 270

Prednisolone Tebutate (Pituitary secretion of gonadotropins affected). Products include:
Hydeltra-T.B.A. Sterile Suspension 1667

Prednisone (Pituitary secretion of gonadotropins affected). Products include:
Deltasone Tablets 2595

Prochlorperazine (Rise in prolactin; response to Factrel may be blunted). Products include:
Compazine 2470

Promethazine Hydrochloride (Rise in prolactin; response to Factrel may be blunted). Products include:
Mepergan Injection 2753
Phenergan with Codeine 2777
Phenergan with Dextromethorphan 2778
Phenergan Injection 2773
Phenergan Suppositories 2775
Phenergan Syrup 2774
Phenergan Tablets 2775
Phenergan VC 2779
Phenergan VC with Codeine 2781

Quinestrol (Pituitary secretion of gonadotropins affected).
No products indexed under this heading.

Spironolactone (Gonadotropin levels transiently elevated). Products include:
Aldactazide 2413
Aldactone 2414

IMPORTANT NOTE: Always consult each drug listing in the patient's regimen for possible interactions.

Factrel Interactions Index 406

Stanozolol (Pituitary secretion of gonadotropins affected). Products include:
Winstrol Tablets 2337
Thioridazine Hydrochloride (Rise in prolactin; response to Factrel may be blunted). Products include:
Mellaril 2269
Triamcinolone (Pituitary secretion of gonadotropins affected). Products include:
Aristocort Tablets 1022
Triamcinolone Acetonide (Pituitary secretion of gonadotropins affected). Products include:
Aristocort A 0.025% Cream 1027
Aristocort A 0.5% Cream 1031
Aristocort A 0.1% Cream 1029
Aristocort A 0.1% Ointment 1030
Azmacort Oral Inhaler 2011
Nasacort Nasal Inhaler 2024
Triamcinolone Diacetate (Pituitary secretion of gonadotropins affected). Products include:
Aristocort Suspension (Forte Parenteral) 1027
Aristocort Suspension (Intralesional) 1025
Triamcinolone Hexacetonide (Pituitary secretion of gonadotropins affected). Products include:
Aristospan Suspension (Intra-articular) 1033
Aristospan Suspension (Intralesional) 1032
Trifluoperazine Hydrochloride (Rise in prolactin; response to Factrel may be blunted). Products include:
Stelazine 2514

FAMVIR
(Famciclovir) 2486
May interact with xanthine bronchodilators and certain other agents. Compounds in these categories include:

Aminophylline (Potential for increase in penciclovir AUC and C_{max} and decrease in renal clearance; the magnitude of this effect is considered to be of no clinical importance).
No products indexed under this heading.
Cimetidine (Increase in penciclovir AUC and urinary recovery; the magnitude of this effect is considered to be of no clinical importance). Products include:
Tagamet Tablets 2516
Cimetidine Hydrochloride (Increase in penciclovir AUC and urinary recovery; the magnitude of this effect is considered to be of no clinical importance). Products include:
Tagamet 2516
Digoxin (Potential for increase in C_{max} of digoxin). Products include:
Lanoxicaps 1117
Lanoxin Elixir Pediatric 1120
Lanoxin Injection 1123
Lanoxin Injection Pediatric 1126
Lanoxin Tablets 1128
Dyphylline (Potential for increase in penciclovir AUC and C_{max} and decrease in renal clearance; the magnitude of this effect is considered to be of no clinical importance). Products include:
Lufyllin & Lufyllin-400 Tablets 2670
Lufyllin-GG Elixir & Tablets 2671
Probenecid (Concurrent use may result in increased plasma concentration of penciclovir). Products include:
Benemid Tablets 1611
ColBENEMID Tablets 1622
Theophylline (Potential for increase in penciclovir AUC and C_{max} and decrease in renal clearance; the magnitude of this effect is considered to be of no clinical importance). Products include:
Marax Tablets & DF Syrup 2200
Quibron 2053
Theophylline Anhydrous (Potential for increase in penciclovir AUC and C_{max} and decrease in renal clearance; the magnitude of this effect is considered to be of no clinical importance). Products include:
Aerolate 1004
Primatene Dual Action Formula ..... ▣ 872
Primatene Tablets ..... ▣ 873
Respbid Tablets 682
Slo-bid Gyrocaps 2033
Theo-24 Extended Release Capsules 2568
Theo-Dur Extended-Release Tablets 1327
Theo-X Extended-Release Tablets .. 788
Uni-Dur Extended-Release Tablets .. 1331
Uniphyl 400 mg Tablets 2001
Theophylline Calcium Salicylate (Potential for increase in penciclovir AUC and C_{max} and decrease in renal clearance; the magnitude of this effect is considered to be of no clinical importance). Products include:
Quadrinal Tablets 1350
Theophylline Sodium Glycinate (Potential for increase in penciclovir AUC and C_{max} and decrease in renal clearance; the magnitude of this effect is considered to be of no clinical importance).
No products indexed under this heading.

Food Interactions
Meal, unspecified (Penciclovir C_{max} decreased approximately 50% and T_{max} was delayed by 1.5 hours when a capsule formulation of famciclovir was administered with food; there is no effect on the extent of availability (AUC) of penciclovir).

FANSIDAR TABLETS
(Sulfadoxine, Pyrimethamine) 2114
May interact with sulfonamides and certain other agents. Compounds in these categories include:

Chloroquine (Increased incidence and severity of adverse reactions).
Sulfamethizole (Interferes with antimalarial prophylaxis). Products include:
Urobiotic-250 Capsules 2214
Sulfamethoxazole (Interferes with antimalarial prophylaxis). Products include:
Azo Gantanol Tablets 2080
Bactrim DS Tablets 2084
Bactrim I.V. Infusion 2082
Bactrim 2084
Gantanol Tablets 2119
Septra 1174
Septra I.V. Infusion 1169
Septra I.V. Infusion ADD-Vantage Vials 1171
Septra 1174
Sulfasalazine (Interferes with antimalarial prophylaxis). Products include:
Azulfidine 1949
Sulfinpyrazone (Interferes with antimalarial prophylaxis). Products include:
Anturane 807
Sulfisoxazole (Interferes with antimalarial prophylaxis). Products include:
Azo Gantrisin Tablets 2081
Gantrisin Tablets 2120
Sulfisoxazole Diolamine (Interferes with antimalarial prophylaxis).
No products indexed under this heading.

FASTIN CAPSULES
(Phentermine Hydrochloride) 2488
May interact with monoamine oxidase inhibitors, insulin, and certain other agents. Compounds in these categories include:

Furazolidone (Hypertensive crises may result). Products include:
Furoxone 2046
Guanethidine Monosulfate (May decrease hypotensive effect of guanethidine). Products include:
Esimil Tablets 822
Ismelin Tablets 827
Insulin, Human (Insulin requirements may be altered).
No products indexed under this heading.
Insulin, Human Isophane Suspension (Insulin requirements may be altered). Products include:
Novolin N Human Insulin 10 ml Vials 1795
Insulin, Human NPH (Insulin requirements may be altered). Products include:
Humulin N, 100 Units 1448
Novolin N PenFill Cartridges Durable Insulin Delivery System 1798
Novolin N Prefilled Syringe Disposable Insulin Delivery System 1798
Insulin, Human Regular (Insulin requirements may be altered). Products include:
Humulin R, 100 Units 1449
Novolin R Human Insulin 10 ml Vials 1795
Novolin R PenFill Cartridges Durable Insulin Delivery System 1798
Novolin R Prefilled Syringe Disposable Insulin Delivery System 1798
Velosulin BR Human Insulin 10 ml Vials 1795
Insulin, Human, Zinc Suspension (Insulin requirements may be altered). Products include:
Humulin L, 100 Units 1446
Humulin U, 100 Units 1450
Novolin L Human Insulin 10 ml Vials 1795
Insulin, NPH (Insulin requirements may be altered). Products include:
NPH, 100 Units 1450
Pork NPH, 100 Units 1452
Purified Pork NPH Isophane Insulin 1801
Insulin, Regular (Insulin requirements may be altered). Products include:
Regular, 100 Units 1450
Pork Regular, 100 Units 1452
Pork Regular (Concentrated), 500 Units 1453
Purified Pork Regular Insulin 1801
Insulin, Zinc Crystals (Insulin requirements may be altered). Products include:
NPH, 100 Units 1450
Insulin, Zinc Suspension (Insulin requirements may be altered). Products include:
Iletin I 1450
Lente, 100 Units 1450
Iletin II 1452
Pork Lente, 100 Units 1452
Purified Pork Lente Insulin 1801
Isocarboxazid (Hypertensive crises may result).
No products indexed under this heading.
Phenelzine Sulfate (Hypertensive crises may result). Products include:
Nardil 1920
Selegiline Hydrochloride (Hypertensive crises may result). Products include:
Eldepryl Tablets 2550
Tranylcypromine Sulfate (Hypertensive crises may result). Products include:
Parnate Tablets 2503

Food Interactions
Alcohol (Concomitant use may result in adverse drug interaction).

FEDAHIST GYROCAPS
(Pseudoephedrine Hydrochloride, Chlorpheniramine Maleate) 2401
May interact with monoamine oxidase inhibitors, beta blockers, veratrum alkaloids, tricyclic antidepressants, barbiturates, central nervous system depressants, and certain other agents. Compounds in these categories include:

Acebutolol Hydrochloride (Increases the effect of sympathomimetics). Products include:
Sectral Capsules 2807
Alfentanil Hydrochloride (May have an additive CNS depressant effect). Products include:
Alfenta Injection 1286
Alprazolam (May have an additive CNS depressant effect). Products include:
Xanax Tablets 2649
Amitriptyline Hydrochloride (May have an additive CNS depressant effect). Products include:
Elavil 2838
Endep Tablets 2174
Etrafon 2355
Limbitrol 2180
Triavil Tablets 1757
Amoxapine (May have an additive CNS depressant effect). Products include:
Asendin Tablets 1369
Aprobarbital (May have an additive CNS depressant effect).
No products indexed under this heading.
Atenolol (Increases the effect of sympathomimetics). Products include:
Tenoretic Tablets 2845
Tenormin Tablets and I.V. Injection 2847
Betaxolol Hydrochloride (Increases the effect of sympathomimetics). Products include:
Betoptic Ophthalmic Solution 469
Betoptic S Ophthalmic Suspension 471
Kerlone Tablets 2436
Bisoprolol Fumarate (Increases the effect of sympathomimetics). Products include:
Zebeta Tablets 1413
Ziac 1415
Buprenorphine (May have an additive CNS depressant effect). Products include:
Buprenex Injectable 2006
Buspirone Hydrochloride (May have an additive CNS depressant effect). Products include:
BuSpar 737
Butabarbital (May have an additive CNS depressant effect).
No products indexed under this heading.
Butalbital (May have an additive CNS depressant effect). Products include:
Esgic-plus Tablets 1013
Fioricet Tablets 2258
Fioricet with Codeine Capsules 2260
Fiorinal Capsules 2261
Fiorinal with Codeine Capsules 2262
Fiorinal Tablets 2261
Phrenilin 785

(▣ Described in PDR For Nonprescription Drugs) (◉ Described in PDR For Ophthalmology)

407 **Interactions Index** **Fedahist GyroCaps/Timecaps**

Sedapap Tablets 50 mg/650 mg .. 1543

Carteolol Hydrochloride (Increases the effect of sympathomimetics). Products include:
- Cartrol Tablets 410
- Ocupress Ophthalmic Solution, 1% Sterile .... ◉ 309

Chlordiazepoxide (May have an additive CNS depressant effect). Products include:
- Libritabs Tablets 2177
- Limbitrol 2180

Chlordiazepoxide Hydrochloride (May have an additive CNS depressant effect). Products include:
- Librax Capsules 2176
- Librium Capsules 2178
- Librium Injectable 2179

Chlorpromazine (May have an additive CNS depressant effect). Products include:
- Thorazine Suppositories 2523

Chlorprothixene (May have an additive CNS depressant effect).
- No products indexed under this heading.

Chlorprothixene Hydrochloride (May have an additive CNS depressant effect).
- No products indexed under this heading.

Clomipramine Hydrochloride (May have an additive CNS depressant effect). Products include:
- Anafranil Capsules 803

Clorazepate Dipotassium (May have an additive CNS depressant effect). Products include:
- Tranxene 451

Clozapine (May have an additive CNS depressant effect). Products include:
- Clozaril Tablets 2252

Codeine Phosphate (May have an additive CNS depressant effect). Products include:
- Actifed with Codeine Cough Syrup.. 1067
- Brontex 1981
- Deconsal C Expectorant Syrup 456
- Deconsal Pediatric Syrup 457
- Dimetane-DC Cough Syrup 2059
- Empirin with Codeine Tablets 1093
- Fioricet with Codeine Capsules 2260
- Fiorinal with Codeine Capsules 2262
- Isoclor Expectorant 990
- Novahistine DH 2462
- Novahistine Expectorant 2463
- Nucofed 2051
- Phenergan with Codeine 2777
- Phenergan VC with Codeine 2781
- Robitussin A-C Syrup 2073
- Robitussin-DAC Syrup 2074
- Ryna .... ▣ 841
- Soma Compound w/Codeine Tablets 2676
- Tussi-Organidin NR Liquid and S NR Liquid 2677
- Tylenol with Codeine 1583

Cryptenamine Preparations (Reduced antihypertensive effect).

Desflurane (May have an additive CNS depressant effect). Products include:
- Suprane 1813

Desipramine Hydrochloride (May have an additive CNS depressant effect). Products include:
- Norpramin Tablets 1526

Dezocine (May have an additive CNS depressant effect). Products include:
- Dalgan Injection 538

Diazepam (May have an additive CNS depressant effect). Products include:
- Dizac 1809
- Valium Injectable 2182
- Valium Tablets 2183
- Valrelease Capsules 2169

Doxepin Hydrochloride (May have an additive CNS depressant effect). Products include:
- Sinequan 2205
- Zonalon Cream 1055

Droperidol (May have an additive CNS depressant effect). Products include:
- Inapsine Injection 1296

Enflurane (May have an additive CNS depressant effect).
- No products indexed under this heading.

Esmolol Hydrochloride (Increases the effect of sympathomimetics). Products include:
- Brevibloc Injection 1808

Estazolam (May have an additive CNS depressant effect). Products include:
- ProSom Tablets 449

Ethchlorvynol (May have an additive CNS depressant effect). Products include:
- Placidyl Capsules 448

Ethinamate (May have an additive CNS depressant effect).
- No products indexed under this heading.

Fentanyl (May have an additive CNS depressant effect). Products include:
- Duragesic Transdermal System 1288

Fentanyl Citrate (May have an additive CNS depressant effect). Products include:
- Sublimaze Injection 1307

Fluphenazine Decanoate (May have an additive CNS depressant effect). Products include:
- Prolixin Decanoate 509

Fluphenazine Enanthate (May have an additive CNS depressant effect). Products include:
- Prolixin Enanthate 509

Fluphenazine Hydrochloride (May have an additive CNS depressant effect). Products include:
- Prolixin 509

Flurazepam Hydrochloride (May have an additive CNS depressant effect). Products include:
- Dalmane Capsules 2173

Furazolidone (Increases the effect of sympathomimetics; concurrent use is contraindicated). Products include:
- Furoxone 2046

Glutethimide (May have an additive CNS depressant effect).
- No products indexed under this heading.

Haloperidol (May have an additive CNS depressant effect). Products include:
- Haldol Injection, Tablets and Concentrate 1575

Haloperidol Decanoate (May have an additive CNS depressant effect). Products include:
- Haldol Decanoate 1577

Hydrocodone Bitartrate (May have an additive CNS depressant effect). Products include:
- Anexsia 5/500 Elixir 1781
- Anexia Tablets 1782
- Codiclear DH Syrup 791
- Deconamine CX Cough and Cold Liquid and Tablets 1319
- Duratuss HD Elixir 2565
- Hycodan Tablets and Syrup 930
- Hycomine Compound Tablets 932
- Hycomine 931
- Hycotuss Expectorant Syrup 933
- Hydrocet Capsules 782
- Lorcet 10/650 1018
- Lortab 2566
- Tussend 1783
- Tussend Expectorant 1785
- Vicodin Tablets 1356
- Vicodin ES Tablets 1357
- Vicodin Tuss Expectorant 1358
- Zydone Capsules 949

Hydrocodone Polistirex (May have an additive CNS depressant effect). Products include:
- Tussionex Pennkinetic Extended-Release Suspension 998

Hydroxyzine Hydrochloride (May have an additive CNS depressant effect). Products include:
- Atarax Tablets & Syrup 2185
- Marax Tablets & DF Syrup 2200
- Vistaril Intramuscular Solution 2216

Imipramine Hydrochloride (May have an additive CNS depressant effect). Products include:
- Tofranil Ampuls 854
- Tofranil Tablets 856

Imipramine Pamoate (May have an additive CNS depressant effect). Products include:
- Tofranil-PM Capsules 857

Isocarboxazid (Increases the effect of sympathomimetics; concurrent use is contraindicated).
- No products indexed under this heading.

Isoflurane (May have an additive CNS depressant effect).
- No products indexed under this heading.

Ketamine Hydrochloride (May have an additive CNS depressant effect).
- No products indexed under this heading.

Labetalol Hydrochloride (Increases the effect of sympathomimetics). Products include:
- Normodyne Injection 2377
- Normodyne Tablets 2379
- Trandate 1185

Levobunolol Hydrochloride (Increases the effect of sympathomimetics). Products include:
- Betagan .... ◉ 233

Levomethadyl Acetate Hydrochloride (May have an additive CNS depressant effect). Products include:
- Orlamm 2239

Levorphanol Tartrate (May have an additive CNS depressant effect). Products include:
- Levo-Dromoran 2129

Lorazepam (May have an additive CNS depressant effect). Products include:
- Ativan Injection 2698
- Ativan Tablets 2700

Loxapine Hydrochloride (May have an additive CNS depressant effect). Products include:
- Loxitane 1378

Loxapine Succinate (May have an additive CNS depressant effect). Products include:
- Loxitane Capsules 1378

Maprotiline Hydrochloride (May have an additive CNS depressant effect). Products include:
- Ludiomil Tablets 843

Mecamylamine Hydrochloride (Reduced antihypertensive effect). Products include:
- Inversine Tablets 1686

Meperidine Hydrochloride (May have an additive CNS depressant effect). Products include:
- Demerol 2308
- Mepergan Injection 2753

Mephobarbital (May have an additive CNS depressant effect). Products include:
- Mebaral Tablets 2322

Meprobamate (May have an additive CNS depressant effect). Products include:
- Miltown Tablets 2672
- PMB 200 and PMB 400 2783

Mesoridazine Besylate (May have an additive CNS depressant effect). Products include:
- Serentil 684

Methadone Hydrochloride (May have an additive CNS depressant effect). Products include:
- Methadone Hydrochloride Oral Concentrate 2233
- Methadone Hydrochloride Oral Solution & Tablets 2235

Methohexital Sodium (May have an additive CNS depressant effect). Products include:
- Brevital Sodium Vials 1429

Methotrimeprazine (May have an additive CNS depressant effect). Products include:
- Levoprome 1274

Methoxyflurane (May have an additive CNS depressant effect).
- No products indexed under this heading.

Methyldopa (Reduced antihypertensive effect). Products include:
- Aldoclor Tablets 1598
- Aldomet Oral 1600
- Aldoril Tablets 1604

Methyldopate Hydrochloride (Reduced antihypertensive effect). Products include:
- Aldomet Ester HCl Injection 1602

Metipranolol Hydrochloride (Increases the effect of sympathomimetics). Products include:
- OptiPranolol (Metipranolol 0.3%) Sterile Ophthalmic Solution .... ◉ 258

Metoprolol Succinate (Increases the effect of sympathomimetics). Products include:
- Toprol-XL Tablets 565

Metoprolol Tartrate (Increases the effect of sympathomimetics). Products include:
- Lopressor Ampuls 830
- Lopressor HCT Tablets 832
- Lopressor Tablets 830

Midazolam Hydrochloride (May have an additive CNS depressant effect). Products include:
- Versed Injection 2170

Molindone Hydrochloride (May have an additive CNS depressant effect). Products include:
- Moban Tablets and Concentrate 1048

Morphine Sulfate (May have an additive CNS depressant effect). Products include:
- Astramorph/PF Injection, USP (Preservative-Free) 535
- Duramorph 962
- Infumorph 200 and Infumorph 500 Sterile Solutions 965
- MS Contin Tablets 1994
- MSIR 1997
- Oramorph SR (Morphine Sulfate Sustained Release Tablets) 2236
- RMS Suppositories 2657
- Roxanol 2243

Nadolol (Increases the effect of sympathomimetics).
- No products indexed under this heading.

Nortriptyline Hydrochloride (May have an additive CNS depressant effect). Products include:
- Pamelor 2280

Opium Alkaloids (May have an additive CNS depressant effect).
- No products indexed under this heading.

Oxazepam (May have an additive CNS depressant effect). Products include:
- Serax Capsules 2810

IMPORTANT NOTE: Always consult each drug listing in the patient's regimen for possible interactions.

Serax Tablets 2810

Oxycodone Hydrochloride (May have an additive CNS depressant effect). Products include:

Percocet Tablets 938
Percodan Tablets 939
Percodan-Demi Tablets 940
Roxicodone Tablets, Oral Solution & Intensol (Oxycodone) 2244
Tylox Capsules 1584

Penbutolol Sulfate (Increases the effect of sympathomimetics). Products include:

Levatol 2403

Pentobarbital Sodium (May have an additive CNS depressant effect). Products include:

Nembutal Sodium Capsules 436
Nembutal Sodium Solution 438
Nembutal Sodium Suppositories 440

Perphenazine (May have an additive CNS depressant effect). Products include:

Etrafon 2355
Triavil Tablets 1757
Trilafon 2389

Phenelzine Sulfate (Increases the effect of sympathomimetics; concurrent use is contraindicated). Products include:

Nardil 1920

Phenobarbital (May have an additive CNS depressant effect). Products include:

Arco-Lase Plus Tablets 512
Bellergal-S Tablets 2250
Donnatal 2060
Donnatal Extentabs 2061
Donnatal Tablets 2060
Phenobarbital Elixir and Tablets 1469
Quadrinal Tablets 1350

Pindolol (Increases the effect of sympathomimetics). Products include:

Visken Tablets 2299

Prazepam (May have an additive CNS depressant effect).

No products indexed under this heading.

Prochlorperazine (May have an additive CNS depressant effect). Products include:

Compazine 2470

Promethazine Hydrochloride (May have an additive CNS depressant effect). Products include:

Mepergan Injection 2753
Phenergan with Codeine 2777
Phenergan with Dextromethorphan 2778
Phenergan Injection 2773
Phenergan Suppositories 2775
Phenergan Syrup 2774
Phenergan Tablets 2775
Phenergan VC 2779
Phenergan VC with Codeine 2781

Propofol (May have an additive CNS depressant effect). Products include:

Diprivan Injection 2833

Propoxyphene Hydrochloride (May have an additive CNS depressant effect). Products include:

Darvon 1435
Wygesic Tablets 2827

Propoxyphene Napsylate (May have an additive CNS depressant effect). Products include:

Darvon-N/Darvocet-N 1433

Propranolol Hydrochloride (Increases the effect of sympathomimetics). Products include:

Inderal 2728
Inderal LA Long Acting Capsules 2730
Inderide Tablets 2732
Inderide LA Long Acting Capsules 2734

Protriptyline Hydrochloride (May have an additive CNS depressant effect). Products include:

Vivactil Tablets 1774

Quazepam (May have an additive CNS depressant effect). Products include:

Doral Tablets 2664

Rauwolfia Serpentina (Reduced antihypertensive effect).

No products indexed under this heading.

Reserpine (Reduced antihypertensive effect). Products include:

Diupres Tablets 1650
Hydropres Tablets 1675
Ser-Ap-Es Tablets 849

Risperidone (May have an additive CNS depressant effect). Products include:

Risperdal 1301

Secobarbital Sodium (May have an additive CNS depressant effect). Products include:

Seconal Sodium Pulvules 1474

Selegiline Hydrochloride (Increases the effect of sympathomimetics; concurrent use is contraindicated). Products include:

Eldepryl Tablets 2550

Sotalol Hydrochloride (Increases the effect of sympathomimetics). Products include:

Betapace Tablets 641

Sufentanil Citrate (May have an additive CNS depressant effect). Products include:

Sufenta Injection 1309

Temazepam (May have an additive CNS depressant effect). Products include:

Restoril Capsules 2284

Thiamylal Sodium (May have an additive CNS depressant effect).

No products indexed under this heading.

Thioridazine Hydrochloride (May have an additive CNS depressant effect). Products include:

Mellaril 2269

Thiothixene (May have an additive CNS depressant effect). Products include:

Navane Capsules and Concentrate 2201
Navane Intramuscular 2202

Timolol Hemihydrate (Increases the effect of sympathomimetics). Products include:

Betimol 0.25%, 0.5% .... ⊙ 261

Timolol Maleate (Increases the effect of sympathomimetics). Products include:

Blocadren Tablets 1614
Timolide Tablets 1748
Timoptic in Ocudose 1753
Timoptic Sterile Ophthalmic Solution 1751
Timoptic-XE 1755

Tranylcypromine Sulfate (Increases the effect of sympathomimetics; concurrent use is contraindicated). Products include:

Parnate Tablets 2503

Triazolam (May have an additive CNS depressant effect). Products include:

Halcion Tablets 2611

Trifluoperazine Hydrochloride (May have an additive CNS depressant effect). Products include:

Stelazine 2514

Trimipramine Maleate (May have an additive CNS depressant effect). Products include:

Surmontil Capsules 2811

Zolpidem Tartrate (May have an additive CNS depressant effect). Products include:

Ambien Tablets 2416

Food Interactions

Alcohol (May have an additive CNS depressant effect).

FEDAHIST TIMECAPS

(Pseudoephedrine Hydrochloride, Chlorpheniramine Maleate) 2401

See **Fedahist Gyrocaps**

FEEN-A-MINT GUM

(Phenolphthalein) .... ▣ 805

None cited in PDR database.

FEEN-A-MINT LAXATIVE PILLS

(Phenolphthalein, Docusate Sodium) .... ▣ 805

None cited in PDR database.

FELBATOL

(Felbamate) 2666

May interact with:

Carbamazepine (Causes an approximate 50% increase in the clearance of felbamate; decrease in steady-state carbamazepine plasma concentration and an increase in the steady-state carbamazepine epoxide plasma concentration caused by felbamate). Products include:

Atretol Tablets 573
Tegretol Chewable Tablets 852
Tegretol Suspension 852
Tegretol Tablets 852

Divalproex Sodium (Felbamate causes an increase in steady-state valproate concentrations). Products include:

Depakote Tablets 415

Phenytoin (Causes an approximate doubling of the clearance of felbamate; increase in steady-state phenytoin plasma concentration caused by felbamate). Products include:

Dilantin Infatabs 1908
Dilantin-125 Suspension 1911

Phenytoin Sodium (Causes an approximate doubling of the clearance of felbamate; increase in steady-state phenytoin plasma concentration caused by felbamate). Products include:

Dilantin Kapseals 1906
Dilantin Parenteral 1910

Valproic Acid (Felbamate causes an increase in steady-state valproate concentrations). Products include:

Depakene 413

FELDENE CAPSULES

(Piroxicam) 1965

May interact with oral anticoagulants, lithium preparations, highly protein bound drugs (selected), and certain other agents. Compounds in these categories include:

Amiodarone Hydrochloride (Feldene might displace other highly protein bound drugs). Products include:

Cordarone Intravenous 2715
Cordarone Tablets 2712

Amitriptyline Hydrochloride (Feldene might displace other highly protein bound drugs). Products include:

Elavil 2838
Endep Tablets 2174
Etrafon 2355
Limbitrol 2180
Triavil Tablets 1757

Aspirin (Aspirin (3900 mg/day) depresses plasma levels of piroxicam). Products include:

Alka-Seltzer Effervescent Antacid and Pain Reliever .... ▣ 701
Alka-Seltzer Extra Strength Effervescent Antacid and Pain Reliever .... ▣ 703
Alka-Seltzer Lemon Lime Effervescent Antacid and Pain Reliever .... ▣ 703
Alka-Seltzer Plus Cold Medicine .... ▣ 705
Alka-Seltzer Plus Cold & Cough Medicine .... ▣ 708
Alka-Seltzer Plus Night-Time Cold Medicine .... ▣ 707
Alka Seltzer Plus Sinus Medicine .... ▣ 707
Arthritis Foundation Safety Coated Aspirin Tablets .... ▣ 675
Arthritis Pain Ascriptin .... ▣ 631
Maximum Strength Ascriptin .... ▣ 630
Regular Strength Ascriptin Tablets .... ▣ 629
Arthritis Strength BC Powder .... ▣ 609
BC Cold Powder Multi-Symptom Formula (Cold-Sinus-Allergy) .... ▣ 609
BC Cold Powder Non-Drowsy Formula (Cold-Sinus) .... ▣ 609
BC Powder .... ▣ 609
Bayer Children's Chewable Aspirin .... ▣ 711
Genuine Bayer Aspirin Tablets & Caplets .... ▣ 713
Extra Strength Bayer Arthritis Pain Regimen Formula .... ▣ 711
Extra Strength Bayer Aspirin Caplets & Tablets .... ▣ 712
Extended-Release Bayer 8-Hour Aspirin .... ▣ 712
Extra Strength Bayer Plus Aspirin Caplets .... ▣ 713
Extra Strength Bayer PM Aspirin .... ▣ 713
Bayer Enteric Aspirin .... ▣ 709
Bufferin Analgesic Tablets and Caplets .... ▣ 613
Arthritis Strength Bufferin Analgesic Caplets .... ▣ 614
Extra Strength Bufferin Analgesic Tablets .... ▣ 615
Cama Arthritis Pain Reliever .... ▣ 785
Darvon Compound-65 Pulvules 1435
Easprin 1914
Ecotrin 2455
Ecotrin Enteric Coated Aspirin Maximum Strength Tablets and Caplets .... ▣ 816
Ecotrin Enteric Coated Aspirin Regular Strength Tablets 2455
Empirin Aspirin Tablets .... ▣ 854
Empirin with Codeine Tablets 1093
Excedrin Extra-Strength Analgesic Tablets & Caplets 732
Fiorinal Capsules 2261
Fiorinal with Codeine Capsules 2262
Fiorinal Tablets 2261
Halfprin 1362
Healthprin Aspirin 2455
Norgesic 1496
Percodan Tablets 939
Percodan-Demi Tablets 940
Robaxisal Tablets 2071
Soma Compound w/Codeine Tablets 2676
Soma Compound Tablets 2675
St. Joseph Adult Chewable Aspirin (81 mg.) .... ▣ 808
Talwin Compound 2335
Ursinus Inlay-Tabs .... ▣ 794
Vanquish Analgesic Caplets .... ▣ 731

Aspirin, Enteric Coated (Aspirin (3900 mg/day) depresses plasma levels of piroxicam). Products include:

Bayer Enteric Aspirin .... ▣ 709
Ecotrin 2455

Atovaquone (Feldene might displace other highly protein bound drugs). Products include:

Mepron Suspension 1135

Cefonicid Sodium (Feldene might displace other highly protein bound drugs). Products include:

Monocid Injection 2497

Chlordiazepoxide (Feldene might displace other highly protein bound drugs). Products include:

Libritabs Tablets 2177
Limbitrol 2180

Chlordiazepoxide Hydrochloride (Feldene might displace other highly protein bound drugs). Products include:

Librax Capsules 2176
Librium Capsules 2178
Librium Injectable 2179

(▣ Described in PDR For Nonprescription Drugs) (⊙ Described in PDR For Ophthalmology)

Interactions Index

Chlorpromazine (Feldene might displace other highly protein bound drugs). Products include:

Thorazine Suppositories 2523

Chlorpromazine Hydrochloride (Feldene might displace other highly protein bound drugs). Products include:

Thorazine 2523

Clomipramine Hydrochloride (Feldene might displace other highly protein bound drugs). Products include:

Anafranil Capsules 803

Clozapine (Feldene might displace other highly protein bound drugs). Products include:

Clozaril Tablets..................................... 2252

Cyclosporine (Feldene might displace other highly protein bound drugs). Products include:

Neoral 2276
Sandimmune 2286

Diazepam (Feldene might displace other highly protein bound drugs). Products include:

Dizac 1809
Valium Injectable 2182
Valium Tablets 2183
Valrelease Capsules 2169

Diclofenac Potassium (Feldene might displace other highly protein bound drugs). Products include:

Cataflam 816

Diclofenac Sodium (Feldene might displace other highly protein bound drugs). Products include:

Voltaren Ophthalmic Sterile Ophthalmic Solution .... ◉ 272
Voltaren Tablets 861

Dicumarol (Altered dosage requirements).

No products indexed under this heading.

Dipyridamole (Feldene might displace other highly protein bound drugs). Products include:

Persantine Tablets 681

Fenoprofen Calcium (Feldene might displace other highly protein bound drugs). Products include:

Nalfon 200 Pulvules & Nalfon Tablets 917

Flurazepam Hydrochloride (Feldene might displace other highly protein bound drugs). Products include:

Dalmane Capsules.................................. 2173

Flurbiprofen (Feldene might displace other highly protein bound drugs). Products include:

Ansaid Tablets 2579

Glipizide (Feldene might displace other highly protein bound drugs). Products include:

Glucotrol Tablets 1967
Glucotrol XL Extended Release Tablets 1968

Ibuprofen (Feldene might displace other highly protein bound drugs). Products include:

Advil Cold and Sinus Caplets and Tablets (formerly CoAdvil) .... ⊞ 870
Advil Ibuprofen Tablets and Caplets .... ⊞ 870
Children's Advil Suspension 2692
Arthritis Foundation Ibuprofen Tablets .... ⊞ 674
Bayer Select Ibuprofen Pain Relief Formula .... ⊞ 715
Cramp End Tablets .... ⊞ 735
Dimetapp Sinus Caplets .... ⊞ 775
Haltran Tablets...................................... ⊞ 771
IBU Tablets.. 1342
Ibuprohm... ⊞ 735
Children's Motrin Ibuprofen Oral Suspension 1546
Motrin Tablets.. 2625
Motrin IB Caplets, Tablets, and Geltabs .... ⊞ 838

Motrin IB Sinus..................................... ⊞ 838
Motrin Ibuprofen Suspension, Oral Drops, Chewable Tablets, Caplets 1546
Nuprin Ibuprofen/Analgesic Tablets & Caplets .... ⊞ 622
Sine-Aid IB Caplets 1554
Vicks DayQuil SINUS Pressure & PAIN Relief with IBUPROFEN ...... ⊞ 762

Imipramine Hydrochloride (Feldene might displace other highly protein bound drugs). Products include:

Tofranil Ampuls 854
Tofranil Tablets 856

Imipramine Pamoate (Feldene might displace other highly protein bound drugs). Products include:

Tofranil-PM Capsules............................ 857

Indomethacin (Feldene might displace other highly protein bound drugs). Products include:

Indocin 1680

Indomethacin Sodium Trihydrate (Feldene might displace other highly protein bound drugs). Products include:

Indocin I.V. 1684

Ketoprofen (Feldene might displace other highly protein bound drugs). Products include:

Orudis Capsules 2766
Oruvail Capsules 2766

Ketorolac Tromethamine (Feldene might displace other highly protein bound drugs). Products include:

Acular 474
Acular .... ◉ 277
Toradol... 2159

Lithium Carbonate (Increased plasma lithium levels). Products include:

Eskalith 2485
Lithium Carbonate Capsules & Tablets 2230
Lithonate/Lithotabs/Lithobid 2543

Lithium Citrate (Increased plasma lithium levels).

No products indexed under this heading.

Meclofenamate Sodium (Feldene might displace other highly protein bound drugs).

No products indexed under this heading.

Mefenamic Acid (Feldene might displace other highly protein bound drugs). Products include:

Ponstel 1925

Midazolam Hydrochloride (Feldene might displace other highly protein bound drugs). Products include:

Versed Injection 2170

Naproxen (Feldene might displace other highly protein bound drugs). Products include:

Anaprox/Naprosyn 2117

Naproxen Sodium (Feldene might displace other highly protein bound drugs). Products include:

Aleve 1975
Anaprox/Naprosyn 2117

Nortriptyline Hydrochloride (Feldene might displace other highly protein bound drugs). Products include:

Pamelor 2280

Oxaprozin (Feldene might displace other highly protein bound drugs). Products include:

Daypro Caplets 2426

Oxazepam (Feldene might displace other highly protein bound drugs). Products include:

Serax Capsules 2810

Serax Tablets... 2810

Phenylbutazone (Feldene might displace other highly protein bound drugs).

No products indexed under this heading.

Propranolol Hydrochloride (Feldene might displace other highly protein bound drugs). Products include:

Inderal 2728
Inderal LA Long Acting Capsules 2730
Inderide Tablets 2732
Inderide LA Long Acting Capsules .. 2734

Sulindac (Feldene might displace other highly protein bound drugs). Products include:

Clinoril Tablets 1618

Temazepam (Feldene might displace other highly protein bound drugs). Products include:

Restoril Capsules 2284

Tolbutamide (Feldene might displace other highly protein bound drugs).

No products indexed under this heading.

Tolmetin Sodium (Feldene might displace other highly protein bound drugs). Products include:

Tolectin (200, 400 and 600 mg) .. 1581

Trimipramine Maleate (Feldene might displace other highly protein bound drugs). Products include:

Surmontil Capsules................................ 2811

Warfarin Sodium (Altered dosage requirements; Feldene might displace other highly protein bound drugs). Products include:

Coumadin 926

FEMSTAT PREFILL VAGINAL CREAM 2%

(Butoconazole Nitrate) 2116

None cited in PDR database.

FEMSTAT VAGINAL CREAM 2%

(Butoconazole Nitrate) 2115

None cited in PDR database.

FEOSOL CAPSULES

(Ferrous Sulfate) 2456

May interact with tetracyclines. Compounds in this category include:

Demeclocycline Hydrochloride (Interference with absorption of oral tetracycline products). Products include:

Declomycin Tablets................................ 1371

Doxycycline Calcium (Interference with absorption of oral tetracycline products). Products include:

Vibramycin Calcium Oral Suspension Syrup.. 1941

Doxycycline Hyclate (Interference with absorption of oral tetracycline products). Products include:

Doryx Capsules...................................... 1913
Vibramycin Hyclate Capsules 1941
Vibramycin Hyclate Intravenous 2215
Vibra-Tabs Film Coated Tablets 1941

Doxycycline Monohydrate (Interference with absorption of oral tetracycline products). Products include:

Monodox Capsules 1805
Vibramycin Monohydrate for Oral Suspension 1941

Methacycline Hydrochloride (Interference with absorption of oral tetracycline products).

No products indexed under this heading.

Minocycline Hydrochloride (Interference with absorption of oral tetracycline products). Products include:

Dynacin Capsules 1590
Minocin Intravenous.............................. 1382
Minocin Oral Suspension 1385
Minocin Pellet-Filled Capsules 1383

Oxytetracycline (Interference with absorption of oral tetracycline products). Products include:

Terramycin Intramuscular Solution 2210

Oxytetracycline Hydrochloride (Interference with absorption of oral tetracycline products). Products include:

TERAK Ointment .... ◉ 209
Terra-Cortril Ophthalmic Suspension 2210
Terramycin with Polymyxin B Sulfate Ophthalmic Ointment 2211
Urobiotic-250 Capsules 2214

Tetracycline Hydrochloride (Interference with absorption of oral tetracycline products). Products include:

Achromycin V Capsules 1367

FEOSOL ELIXIR

(Ferrous Sulfate) 2456

May interact with tetracyclines. Compounds in this category include:

Demeclocycline Hydrochloride (Interference with absorption of oral tetracycline products). Products include:

Declomycin Tablets................................ 1371

Doxycycline Calcium (Interference with absorption of oral tetracycline products). Products include:

Vibramycin Calcium Oral Suspension Syrup.. 1941

Doxycycline Hyclate (Interference with absorption of oral tetracycline products). Products include:

Doryx Capsules...................................... 1913
Vibramycin Hyclate Capsules 1941
Vibramycin Hyclate Intravenous 2215
Vibra-Tabs Film Coated Tablets 1941

Doxycycline Monohydrate (Interference with absorption of oral tetracycline products). Products include:

Monodox Capsules 1805
Vibramycin Monohydrate for Oral Suspension 1941

Methacycline Hydrochloride (Interference with absorption of oral tetracycline products).

No products indexed under this heading.

Minocycline Hydrochloride (Interference with absorption of oral tetracycline products). Products include:

Dynacin Capsules 1590
Minocin Intravenous.............................. 1382
Minocin Oral Suspension 1385
Minocin Pellet-Filled Capsules 1383

Oxytetracycline (Interference with absorption of oral tetracycline products). Products include:

Terramycin Intramuscular Solution 2210

Oxytetracycline Hydrochloride (Interference with absorption of oral tetracycline products). Products include:

TERAK Ointment .... ◉ 209
Terra-Cortril Ophthalmic Suspension 2210
Terramycin with Polymyxin B Sulfate Ophthalmic Ointment 2211
Urobiotic-250 Capsules 2214

Tetracycline Hydrochloride (Interference with absorption of oral tetracycline products). Products include:

Achromycin V Capsules 1367

IMPORTANT NOTE: Always consult each drug listing in the patient's regimen for possible interactions.

FEOSOL TABLETS
(Ferrous Sulfate) ... 2457
May interact with tetracyclines. Compounds in this category include:

Demeclocycline Hydrochloride (Interference with absorption of oral tetracycline products; should not be taken within two hours of each other). Products include:
- Declomycin Tablets ... 1371

Doxycycline Calcium (Interference with absorption of oral tetracycline products; should not be taken within two hours of each other). Products include:
- Vibramycin Calcium Oral Suspension Syrup ... 1941

Doxycycline Hyclate (Interference with absorption of oral tetracycline products; should not be taken within two hours of each other). Products include:
- Doryx Capsules ... 1913
- Vibramycin Hyclate Capsules ... 1941
- Vibramycin Hyclate Intravenous ... 2215
- Vibra-Tabs Film Coated Tablets ... 1941

Doxycycline Monohydrate (Interference with absorption of oral tetracycline products; should not be taken within two hours of each other). Products include:
- Monodox Capsules ... 1805
- Vibramycin Monohydrate for Oral Suspension ... 1941

Methacycline Hydrochloride (Interference with absorption of oral tetracycline products; should not be taken within two hours of each other).
- No products indexed under this heading.

Minocycline Hydrochloride (Interference with absorption of oral tetracycline products; should not be taken within two hours of each other). Products include:
- Dynacin Capsules ... 1590
- Minocin Intravenous ... 1382
- Minocin Oral Suspension ... 1385
- Minocin Pellet-Filled Capsules ... 1383

Oxytetracycline (Interference with absorption of oral tetracycline products; should not be taken within two hours of each other). Products include:
- Terramycin Intramuscular Solution 2210

Oxytetracycline Hydrochloride (Interference with absorption of oral tetracycline products; should not be taken within two hours of each other). Products include:
- TERAK Ointment ... ⊙ 209
- Terra-Cortril Ophthalmic Suspension ... 2210
- Terramycin with Polymyxin B Sulfate Ophthalmic Ointment ... 2211
- Urobiotic-250 Capsules ... 2214

Tetracycline Hydrochloride (Interference with absorption of oral tetracycline products; should not be taken within two hours of each other). Products include:
- Achromycin V Capsules ... 1367

FERGON IRON SUPPLEMENT TABLETS
(Ferrous Gluconate) ... ▣ 721
None cited in PDR database.

FERO-FOLIC-500 FILMTAB
(Ferrous Sulfate, Folic Acid, Vitamin C) ... 429
May interact with tetracyclines and certain other agents. Compounds in these categories include:

Calcium Carbonate (Inhibits iron absorption). Products include:
- Alka-Mints Chewable Antacid ... ▣ 701
- Arthritis Pain Ascriptin ... ▣ 631
- Maximum Strength Ascriptin ... ▣ 630
- Regular Strength Ascriptin Tablets ... ▣ 629
- Extra Strength Bayer Plus Aspirin Caplets ... ▣ 713
- Bufferin Analgesic Tablets and Caplets ... ▣ 613
- Calci-Chew Tablets ... 2004
- Calci-Mix Capsules ... 2004
- Caltrate 600 ... ▣ 665
- Caltrate PLUS ... ▣ 665
- Caltrate 600 + D ... ▣ 665
- Centrum Singles Calcium ... ▣ 669
- Chooz Antacid Gum ... ▣ 799
- Di-Gel Antacid/Anti-Gas ... ▣ 801
- Gerimed Tablets ... 982
- Maalox Antacid Caplets ... ▣ 638
- Marblen ... ▣ 655
- Materna Tablets ... 1379
- Mylanta Calcium Carbonate and Magnesium Hydroxide Tablets ... 1318
- Mylanta Gelcaps Antacid ... ▣ 662
- Mylanta Soothing Lozenges ... 1319
- Nephro-Calci Tablets ... 2004
- Rolaids Tablets ... ▣ 843
- Rolaids (Calcium Rich/Sodium Free) Tablets ... ▣ 843
- Tempo Soft Antacid ... ▣ 835
- Titralac ... ▣ 672
- Titralac Plus ... ▣ 672
- Tums Antacid Tablets ... ▣ 827
- Tums Anti-gas/Antacid Formula Tablets, Assorted Fruit ... ▣ 827
- Tums E-X Antacid Tablets ... ▣ 827
- Tums 500 Calcium Supplement ... ▣ 828
- Tums ULTRA Antacid Tablets ... ▣ 827
- TYLENOL, Extra Strength, Headache Plus Pain Reliever with Antacid Caplets ... 1559

Demeclocycline Hydrochloride (Ferrous sulfate may interfere with absorption of tetracycline). Products include:
- Declomycin Tablets ... 1371

Doxycycline Calcium (Ferrous sulfate may interfere with absorption of tetracycline). Products include:
- Vibramycin Calcium Oral Suspension Syrup ... 1941

Doxycycline Hyclate (Ferrous sulfate may interfere with absorption of tetracycline). Products include:
- Doryx Capsules ... 1913
- Vibramycin Hyclate Capsules ... 1941
- Vibramycin Hyclate Intravenous ... 2215
- Vibra-Tabs Film Coated Tablets ... 1941

Doxycycline Monohydrate (Ferrous sulfate may interfere with absorption of tetracycline). Products include:
- Monodox Capsules ... 1805
- Vibramycin Monohydrate for Oral Suspension ... 1941

Levodopa (Antiparkinsonism effects of levodopa may be reversed by pyridoxine). Products include:
- Atamet ... 572
- Larodopa Tablets ... 2129
- Sinemet Tablets ... 943
- Sinemet CR Tablets ... 944

Magnesium Trisilicate (Inhibits absorption of iron). Products include:
- Gaviscon Antacid Tablets ... ▣ 819
- Gaviscon-2 Antacid Tablets ... ▣ 820

Methacycline Hydrochloride (Ferrous sulfate may interfere with absorption of tetracycline).
- No products indexed under this heading.

Minocycline Hydrochloride (Ferrous sulfate may interfere with absorption of tetracycline). Products include:
- Dynacin Capsules ... 1590
- Minocin Intravenous ... 1382
- Minocin Oral Suspension ... 1385
- Minocin Pellet-Filled Capsules ... 1383

Oxytetracycline (Ferrous sulfate may interfere with absorption of tetracycline). Products include:
- Terramycin Intramuscular Solution 2210

Oxytetracycline Hydrochloride (Ferrous sulfate may interfere with absorption of tetracycline). Products include:
- TERAK Ointment ... ⊙ 209
- Terra-Cortril Ophthalmic Suspension ... 2210
- Terramycin with Polymyxin B Sulfate Ophthalmic Ointment ... 2211
- Urobiotic-250 Capsules ... 2214

Sodium Bicarbonate (Inhibits iron absorption). Products include:
- Alka-Seltzer Effervescent Antacid and Pain Reliever ... ▣ 701
- Alka-Seltzer Extra Strength Effervescent Antacid and Pain Reliever ... ▣ 703
- Alka-Seltzer Gold Effervescent Antacid ... ▣ 703
- Alka-Seltzer Lemon Lime Effervescent Antacid and Pain Reliever ... ▣ 703
- Arm & Hammer Pure Baking Soda ... ▣ 627
- Ceo-Two Rectal Suppositories ... 666
- Citrocarbonate Antacid ... ▣ 770
- Massengill Disposable Douches ... ▣ 820
- Massengill Liquid Concentrate ... ▣ 820
- NuLYTELY ... 689
- Cherry Flavor NuLYTELY ... 689

Tetracycline Hydrochloride (Ferrous sulfate may interfere with absorption of tetracycline). Products include:
- Achromycin V Capsules ... 1367

Food Interactions

Dairy products (Ingestion of milk inhibits iron absorption).

Eggs (Ingestion of eggs inhibits iron absorption).

FERO-GRAD-500 FILMTAB
(Ferrous Sulfate, Vitamin C) ... 429
None cited in PDR database.

FERO-GRADUMET FILMTAB
(Ferrous Sulfate) ... 429
None cited in PDR database.

FERRO-SEQUELS
(Ferrous Fumarate, Docusate Sodium) ... ▣ 669
None cited in PDR database.

FIBERALL CHEWABLE TABLETS, LEMON CREME FLAVOR
(Calcium Polycarbophil) ... ▣ 636
May interact with:

Oxytetracycline (Give 1 hour before or 2 to 3 hours after Fiberall). Products include:
- Terramycin Intramuscular Solution 2210

Oxytetracycline Hydrochloride (Give 1 hour before or 2 to 3 hours after Fiberall). Products include:
- TERAK Ointment ... ⊙ 209
- Terra-Cortril Ophthalmic Suspension ... 2210
- Terramycin with Polymyxin B Sulfate Ophthalmic Ointment ... 2211
- Urobiotic-250 Capsules ... 2214

Tetracycline Hydrochloride (Give 1 hour before or 2 to 3 hours after Fiberall). Products include:
- Achromycin V Capsules ... 1367

FIBERALL FIBER WAFERS - FRUIT & NUT
(Psyllium Preparations) ... ▣ 636
None cited in PDR database.

FIBERALL FIBER WAFERS - OATMEAL RAISIN
(Psyllium Preparations) ... ▣ 636
None cited in PDR database.

FIBERALL POWDER, NATURAL FLAVOR
(Psyllium Preparations) ... ▣ 637
None cited in PDR database.

FIBERALL POWDER, ORANGE FLAVOR
(Psyllium Preparations) ... ▣ 637
None cited in PDR database.

FIBERCON CAPLETS
(Calcium Polycarbophil) ... ▣ 670
May interact with tetracyclines. Compounds in this category include:

Demeclocycline Hydrochloride (Fibercon should be taken at least one hour before or two hours after you have taken any form of tetracycline). Products include:
- Declomycin Tablets ... 1371

Doxycycline Calcium (Fibercon should be taken at least one hour before or two hours after you have taken any form of tetracycline). Products include:
- Vibramycin Calcium Oral Suspension Syrup ... 1941

Doxycycline Hyclate (Fibercon should be taken at least one hour before or two hours after you have taken any form of tetracycline). Products include:
- Doryx Capsules ... 1913
- Vibramycin Hyclate Capsules ... 1941
- Vibramycin Hyclate Intravenous ... 2215
- Vibra-Tabs Film Coated Tablets ... 1941

Doxycycline Monohydrate (Fibercon should be taken at least one hour before or two hours after you have taken any form of tetracycline). Products include:
- Monodox Capsules ... 1805
- Vibramycin Monohydrate for Oral Suspension ... 1941

Methacycline Hydrochloride (Fibercon should be taken at least one hour before or two hours after you have taken any form of tetracycline).
- No products indexed under this heading.

Minocycline Hydrochloride (Fibercon should be taken at least one hour before or two hours after you have taken any form of tetracycline). Products include:
- Dynacin Capsules ... 1590
- Minocin Intravenous ... 1382
- Minocin Oral Suspension ... 1385
- Minocin Pellet-Filled Capsules ... 1383

Oxytetracycline Hydrochloride (Fibercon should be taken at least one hour before or two hours after you have taken any form of tetracycline). Products include:
- TERAK Ointment ... ⊙ 209
- Terra-Cortril Ophthalmic Suspension ... 2210
- Terramycin with Polymyxin B Sulfate Ophthalmic Ointment ... 2211
- Urobiotic-250 Capsules ... 2214

Tetracycline Hydrochloride (Fibercon should be taken at least one hour before or two hours after you have taken any form of tetracycline). Products include:
- Achromycin V Capsules ... 1367

FIORICET TABLETS
(Butalbital, Acetaminophen, Caffeine) ... 2258
May interact with narcotic analgesics, tranquilizers, central nervous system depressants, monoamine oxidase inhibitors, general anesthetics, hypnotics and sedatives, and certain other agents. Compounds in these categories include:

Acrivastine (Additive CNS depressant effects). Products include:
- Semprex-D Capsules ... 463

Interactions Index — Fioricet

Semprex-D Capsules 1167

Alfentanil Hydrochloride (Additive CNS depressant effects). Products include:

Alfenta Injection 1286

Alprazolam (Additive CNS depressant effects). Products include:

Xanax Tablets 2649

Aprobarbital (Additive CNS depressant effects).

No products indexed under this heading.

Buprenorphine (Additive CNS depressant effects). Products include:

Buprenex Injectable 2006

Buspirone Hydrochloride (Additive CNS depressant effects). Products include:

BuSpar 737

Butabarbital (Additive CNS depressant effects).

No products indexed under this heading.

Chlordiazepoxide (Additive CNS depressant effects). Products include:

Libritabs Tablets 2177
Limbitrol 2180

Chlordiazepoxide Hydrochloride (Additive CNS depressant effects). Products include:

Librax Capsules 2176
Librium Capsules 2178
Librium Injectable 2179

Chlorpromazine (Additive CNS depressant effects). Products include:

Thorazine Suppositories 2523

Chlorpromazine Hydrochloride (Additive CNS depressant). Products include:

Thorazine 2523

Chlorprothixene (Additive CNS depressant effects).

No products indexed under this heading.

Chlorprothixene Hydrochloride (Additive CNS depressant effects).

No products indexed under this heading.

Clomipramine Hydrochloride (Decreased blood levels of the antidepressant). Products include:

Anafranil Capsules 803

Clorazepate Dipotassium (Additive CNS depressant effects). Products include:

Tranxene 451

Clozapine (Additive CNS depressant effects). Products include:

Clozaril Tablets 2252

Codeine Phosphate (Additive CNS depressant effects). Products include:

Actifed with Codeine Cough Syrup.. 1067
Brontex 1981
Deconsal C Expectorant Syrup 456
Deconsal Pediatric Syrup 457
Dimetane-DC Cough Syrup 2059
Empirin with Codeine Tablets............ 1093
Fioricet with Codeine Capsules 2260
Fiorinal with Codeine Capsules 2262
Isoclor Expectorant 990
Novahistine DH 2462
Novahistine Expectorant 2463
Nucofed 2051
Phenergan with Codeine 2777
Phenergan VC with Codeine 2781
Robitussin A-C Syrup 2073
Robitussin-DAC Syrup 2074
Ryna .... ⊕ 841
Soma Compound w/Codeine Tablets 2676
Tussi-Organidin NR Liquid and S NR Liquid 2677
Tylenol with Codeine 1583

Desflurane (Additive CNS depressant effects). Products include:

Suprane 1813

Dezocine (Additive CNS depressant effects). Products include:

Dalgan Injection 538

Diazepam (Additive CNS depressant effects). Products include:

Dizac 1809
Valium Injectable 2182
Valium Tablets 2183
Valrelease Capsules 2169

Doxepin Hydrochloride (Decreased blood levels of the antidepressant). Products include:

Sinequan 2205
Zonalon Cream 1055

Droperidol (Additive CNS depressant effects). Products include:

Inapsine Injection 1296

Enflurane (Additive CNS depressant effects).

No products indexed under this heading.

Estazolam (Additive CNS depressant effects). Products include:

ProSom Tablets 449

Ethchlorvynol (Additive CNS depressant effects). Products include:

Placidyl Capsules 448

Ethinamate (Additive CNS depressant effects).

No products indexed under this heading.

Fentanyl (Additive CNS depressant effects). Products include:

Duragesic Transdermal System........ 1288

Fentanyl Citrate (Additive CNS depressant effects). Products include:

Sublimaze Injection 1307

Fluphenazine Decanoate (Additive CNS depressant effects). Products include:

Prolixin Decanoate 509

Fluphenazine Enanthate (Additive CNS depressant effects). Products include:

Prolixin Enanthate 509

Fluphenazine Hydrochloride (Additive CNS depressant effects). Products include:

Prolixin 509

Flurazepam Hydrochloride (Additive CNS depressant effects). Products include:

Dalmane Capsules 2173

Furazolidone (Enhances the CNS effects of butalbital). Products include:

Furoxone 2046

Glutethimide (Additive CNS depressant effects).

No products indexed under this heading.

Haloperidol (Additive CNS depressant effects). Products include:

Haldol Injection, Tablets and Concentrate 1575

Haloperidol Decanoate (Additive CNS depressant effects). Products include:

Haldol Decanoate 1577

Hydrocodone Bitartrate (Additive CNS depressant effects). Products include:

Anexsia 5/500 Elixir 1781
Anexia Tablets 1782
Codiclear DH Syrup 791
Deconamine CX Cough and Cold Liquid and Tablets 1319
Duratuss HD Elixir 2565
Hycodan Tablets and Syrup 930
Hycomine Compound Tablets 932
Hycomine 931
Hycotuss Expectorant Syrup 933
Hydrocet Capsules 782
Lorcet 10/650 1018
Lortab 2566
Tussend 1783
Tussend Expectorant 1785

Vicodin Tablets 1356
Vicodin ES Tablets 1357
Vicodin Tuss Expectorant 1358
Zydone Capsules 949

Hydrocodone Polistirex (Additive CNS depressant effects). Products include:

Tussionex Pennkinetic Extended-Release Suspension 998

Hydroxyzine Hydrochloride (Additive CNS depressant effects). Products include:

Atarax Tablets & Syrup 2185
Marax Tablets & DF Syrup 2200
Vistaril Intramuscular Solution......... 2216

Isocarboxazid (Enhances the CNS effects of butalbital).

No products indexed under this heading.

Isoflurane (Additive CNS depressant effects).

No products indexed under this heading.

Ketamine Hydrochloride (Additive CNS depressant effects).

No products indexed under this heading.

Levomethadyl Acetate Hydrochloride (Additive CNS depressant effects). Products include:

Orlamm 2239

Levorphanol Tartrate (Additive CNS depressant effects). Products include:

Levo-Dromoran 2129

Lorazepam (Additive CNS depressant effects). Products include:

Ativan Injection 2698
Ativan Tablets 2700

Loxapine Hydrochloride (Additive CNS depressant effects). Products include:

Loxitane 1378

Loxapine Succinate (Additive CNS depressant effects). Products include:

Loxitane Capsules 1378

Meperidine Hydrochloride (Additive CNS depressant effects). Products include:

Demerol 2308
Mepergan Injection 2753

Mephobarbital (Additive CNS depressant effects). Products include:

Mebaral Tablets 2322

Meprobamate (Additive CNS depressant effects). Products include:

Miltown Tablets 2672
PMB 200 and PMB 400 2783

Mesoridazine Besylate (Additive CNS depressant effects). Products include:

Serentil 684

Methadone Hydrochloride (Additive CNS depressant effects). Products include:

Methadone Hydrochloride Oral Concentrate 2233
Methadone Hydrochloride Oral Solution & Tablets 2235

Methohexital Sodium (Additive CNS depressant effects). Products include:

Brevital Sodium Vials 1429

Methotrimeprazine (Additive CNS depressant effects). Products include:

Levoprome 1274

Methoxyflurane (Additive CNS depressant effects).

No products indexed under this heading.

Midazolam Hydrochloride (Additive CNS depressant effects). Products include:

Versed Injection 2170

Molindone Hydrochloride (Additive CNS depressant effects). Products include:

Moban Tablets and Concentrate 1048

Morphine Sulfate (Additive CNS depressant effects). Products include:

Astramorph/PF Injection, USP (Preservative-Free) 535
Duramorph 962
Infumorph 200 and Infumorph 500 Sterile Solutions 965
MS Contin Tablets 1994
MSIR 1997
Oramorph SR (Morphine Sulfate Sustained Release Tablets) 2236
RMS Suppositories 2657
Roxanol 2243

Opium Alkaloids (Additive CNS depressant effects).

No products indexed under this heading.

Oxazepam (Additive CNS depressant effects). Products include:

Serax Capsules 2810
Serax Tablets 2810

Oxycodone Hydrochloride (Additive CNS depressant effects). Products include:

Percocet Tablets 938
Percodan Tablets 939
Percodan-Demi Tablets 940
Roxicodone Tablets, Oral Solution & Intensol (Oxycodone) 2244
Tylox Capsules 1584

Pentobarbital Sodium (Additive CNS depressant effects). Products include:

Nembutal Sodium Capsules 436
Nembutal Sodium Solution 438
Nembutal Sodium Suppositories 440

Perphenazine (Additive CNS depressant effects). Products include:

Etrafon 2355
Triavil Tablets 1757
Trilafon 2389

Phenelzine Sulfate (Enhances the CNS effects of butalbital). Products include:

Nardil 1920

Phenobarbital (Additive CNS depressant effects). Products include:

Arco-Lase Plus Tablets 512
Bellergal-S Tablets 2250
Donnatal 2060
Donnatal Extentabs 2061
Donnatal Tablets 2060
Phenobarbital Elixir and Tablets 1469
Quadrinal Tablets 1350

Prazepam (Additive CNS depressant effects).

No products indexed under this heading.

Propofol (Additive CNS depressant effects). Products include:

Diprivan Injection 2833

Propoxyphene Hydrochloride (Additive CNS depressant effects). Products include:

Darvon 1435
Wygesic Tablets 2827

Propoxyphene Napsylate (Additive CNS depressant effects). Products include:

Darvon-N/Darvocet-N 1433

Quazepam (Additive CNS depressant effects). Products include:

Doral Tablets 2664

Risperidone (Additive CNS depressant effects). Products include:

Risperdal 1301

Secobarbital Sodium (Additive CNS depressant effects). Products include:

Seconal Sodium Pulvules 1474

Selegiline Hydrochloride (Enhances the CNS effects of butalbital). Products include:

Eldepryl Tablets 2550

IMPORTANT NOTE: Always consult each drug listing in the patient's regimen for possible interactions.

Sufentanil Citrate (Additive CNS depressant effects). Products include:
Sufenta Injection ... 1309
Temazepam (Additive CNS depressant effects). Products include:
Restoril Capsules ... 2284
Thiamylal Sodium (Additive CNS depressant effects).
No products indexed under this heading.
Tranylcypromine Sulfate (Enhances the CNS effects of butalbital). Products include:
Parnate Tablets ... 2503
Triazolam (Additive CNS depressant effects). Products include:
Halcion Tablets ... 2611
Trifluoperazine Hydrochloride (Additive CNS depressant effects). Products include:
Stelazine ... 2514
Zolpidem Tartrate (Additive CNS depressant effects). Products include:
Ambien Tablets ... 2416

Food Interactions

Alcohol (Additive CNS depressant effects).

FIORICET WITH CODEINE CAPSULES

(Butalbital, Acetaminophen, Caffeine, Codeine Phosphate) ... 2260
May interact with monoamine oxidase inhibitors, narcotic analgesics, tranquilizers, general anesthetics, hypnotics and sedatives, central nervous system depressants, and certain other agents. Compounds in these categories include:

Alfentanil Hydrochloride (Enhanced effect of central nervous system depressant and narcotic analgesic). Products include:
Alfenta Injection ... 1286
Alprazolam (Enhanced effect of central nervous system depressant and tranquilizer). Products include:
Xanax Tablets ... 2649
Aprobarbital (Enhanced effect of central nervous system depressant).
No products indexed under this heading.
Buprenorphine (Enhanced effect of central nervous system depressant and narcotic analgesic). Products include:
Buprenex Injectable ... 2006
Buspirone Hydrochloride (Enhanced effect of central nervous system depressant and tranquilizer). Products include:
BuSpar ... 737
Butabarbital (Enhanced effect of central nervous system depressant).
No products indexed under this heading.
Chlordiazepoxide (Enhanced effect of central nervous system depressant and tranquilizer). Products include:
Libritabs Tablets ... 2177
Limbitrol ... 2180
Chlordiazepoxide Hydrochloride (Enhanced effect of central nervous system depressant and tranquilizer). Products include:
Librax Capsules ... 2176
Librium Capsules ... 2178
Librium Injectable ... 2179
Chlorpromazine (Enhanced effect of central nervous system depressant and tranquilizer). Products include:
Thorazine Suppositories ... 2523
Chlorprothixene (Enhanced effect of central nervous system depressant and tranquilizer).
No products indexed under this heading.
Chlorprothixene Hydrochloride (Enhanced effect of central nervous system depressant and tranquilizer).
No products indexed under this heading.
Clorazepate Dipotassium (Enhanced effect of central nervous system depressant and tranquilizer). Products include:
Tranxene ... 451
Clozapine (Enhanced effect of central nervous system depressant and narcotic analgesic). Products include:
Clozaril Tablets ... 2252
Desflurane (Enhanced effect of central nervous system depressant and narcotic analgesic). Products include:
Suprane ... 1813
Dezocine (Enhanced effect of central nervous system depressant and narcotic analgesic). Products include:
Dalgan Injection ... 538
Diazepam (Enhanced effect of central nervous system depressant and tranquilizer). Products include:
Dizac ... 1809
Valium Injectable ... 2182
Valium Tablets ... 2183
Valrelease Capsules ... 2169
Droperidol (Enhanced effect of central nervous system depressant and tranquilizer). Products include:
Inapsine Injection ... 1296
Enflurane (Enhanced effect of central nervous system depressant and anesthetic).
No products indexed under this heading.
Estazolam (Enhanced effect of central nervous system depressant and sedative-hypnotic). Products include:
ProSom Tablets ... 449
Ethchlorvynol (Enhanced effect of central nervous system depressant and sedative-hypnotic). Products include:
Placidyl Capsules ... 448
Ethinamate (Enhanced effect of central nervous system depressant and sedative-hypnotic).
No products indexed under this heading.
Fentanyl (Enhanced effect of central nervous system depressant and narcotic analgesic). Products include:
Duragesic Transdermal System ... 1288
Fentanyl Citrate (Enhanced effect of central nervous system depressant and narcotic analgesic). Products include:
Sublimaze Injection ... 1307
Fluphenazine Decanoate (Enhanced effect of central nervous system depressant and tranquilizer). Products include:
Prolixin Decanoate ... 509
Fluphenazine Enanthate (Enhanced effect of central nervous system depressant and tranquilizer). Products include:
Prolixin Enanthate ... 509
Fluphenazine Hydrochloride (Enhanced effect of central nervous system depressant and tranquilizer). Products include:
Prolixin ... 509
Flurazepam Hydrochloride (Enhanced effect of central nervous system depressant and sedative-hypnotic). Products include:
Dalmane Capsules ... 2173
Furazolidone (Enhanced CNS effects of butalbital). Products include:
Furoxone ... 2046
Glutethimide (Enhanced effect of central nervous system depressant and sedative-hypnotic).
No products indexed under this heading.
Haloperidol (Enhanced effect of central nervous system depressant and tranquilizer). Products include:
Haldol Injection, Tablets and Concentrate ... 1575
Haloperidol Decanoate (Enhanced effect of central nervous system depressant and tranquilizer). Products include:
Haldol Decanoate ... 1577
Hydrocodone Bitartrate (Enhanced effect of central nervous system depressant and narcotic analgesic). Products include:
Anexsia 5/500 Elixir ... 1781
Anexia Tablets ... 1782
Codiclear DH Syrup ... 791
Deconamine CX Cough and Cold Liquid and Tablets ... 1319
Duratuss HD Elixir ... 2565
Hycodan Tablets and Syrup ... 930
Hycomine Compound Tablets ... 932
Hycomine ... 931
Hycotuss Expectorant Syrup ... 933
Hydrocet Capsules ... 782
Lorcet 10/650 ... 1018
Lortab ... 2566
Tussend ... 1783
Tussend Expectorant ... 1785
Vicodin Tablets ... 1356
Vicodin ES Tablets ... 1357
Vicodin Tuss Expectorant ... 1358
Zydone Capsules ... 949
Hydrocodone Polistirex (Enhanced effect of central nervous system depressant and narcotic analgesic). Products include:
Tussionex Pennkinetic Extended-Release Suspension ... 998
Hydroxyzine Hydrochloride (Enhanced effect of central nervous system depressant and tranquilizer). Products include:
Atarax Tablets & Syrup ... 2185
Marax Tablets & DF Syrup ... 2200
Vistaril Intramuscular Solution ... 2216
Isocarboxazid (Enhanced CNS effects of butalbital).
No products indexed under this heading.
Isoflurane (Enhanced effect of central nervous system depressant and anesthetic).
No products indexed under this heading.
Ketamine Hydrochloride (Enhanced effect of central nervous system depressant and anesthetic).
No products indexed under this heading.
Levomethadyl Acetate Hydrochloride (Enhanced effect of central nervous system depressant and narcotic analgesic). Products include:
Orlamm ... 2239
Levorphanol Tartrate (Enhanced effect of central nervous system depressant and narcotic analgesic). Products include:
Levo-Dromoran ... 2129
Lorazepam (Enhanced effect of central nervous system depressant, sedative-hypnotic and tranquilizer). Products include:
Ativan Injection ... 2698
Ativan Tablets ... 2700
Loxapine Hydrochloride (Enhanced effect of central nervous system depressant and tranquilizer). Products include:
Loxitane ... 1378
Loxapine Succinate (Enhanced effect of central nervous system depressant and tranquilizer). Products include:
Loxitane Capsules ... 1378
Meperidine Hydrochloride (Enhanced effect of central nervous system depressant and narcotic analgesic). Products include:
Demerol ... 2308
Mepergan Injection ... 2753
Mephobarbital (Enhanced effect of central nervous system depressant). Products include:
Mebaral Tablets ... 2322
Meprobamate (Enhanced effect of central nervous system depressant and tranquilizer). Products include:
Miltown Tablets ... 2672
PMB 200 and PMB 400 ... 2783
Mesoridazine Besylate (Enhanced effect of tranquilizer). Products include:
Serentil ... 684
Methadone Hydrochloride (Enhanced effect of central nervous system depressant and narcotic analgesic). Products include:
Methadone Hydrochloride Oral Concentrate ... 2233
Methadone Hydrochloride Oral Solution & Tablets ... 2235
Methohexital Sodium (Enhanced effect of central nervous system depressant and anesthetic). Products include:
Brevital Sodium Vials ... 1429
Methotrimeprazine (Enhanced effect of central nervous system depressant and narcotic analgesic). Products include:
Levoprome ... 1274
Methoxyflurane (Enhanced effect of central nervous system depressant and anesthetic).
No products indexed under this heading.
Midazolam Hydrochloride (Enhanced effect of central nervous system depressant and sedative-hypnotic). Products include:
Versed Injection ... 2170
Molindone Hydrochloride (Enhanced effect of central nervous system depressant and tranquilizer). Products include:
Moban Tablets and Concentrate ... 1048
Morphine Sulfate (Enhanced effect of central nervous system depressant and narcotic analgesic). Products include:
Astramorph/PF Injection, USP (Preservative-Free) ... 535
Duramorph ... 962
Infumorph 200 and Infumorph 500 Sterile Solutions ... 965
MS Contin Tablets ... 1994
MSIR ... 1997
Oramorph SR (Morphine Sulfate Sustained Release Tablets) ... 2236
RMS Suppositories ... 2657
Roxanol ... 2243
Opium Alkaloids (Enhanced effect of central nervous system depressant and narcotic analgesic).
No products indexed under this heading.
Oxazepam (Enhanced effect of central nervous system depressant and tranquilizer). Products include:
Serax Capsules ... 2810
Serax Tablets ... 2810

Oxycodone Hydrochloride (Enhanced effect of central nervous system depressant and narcotic analgesic). Products include:

- Percocet Tablets ... 938
- Percodan Tablets ... 939
- Percodan-Demi Tablets ... 940
- Roxicodone Tablets, Oral Solution & Intensol (Oxycodone) ... 2244
- Tylox Capsules ... 1584

Pentobarbital Sodium (Enhanced effect of central nervous system depressant). Products include:

- Nembutal Sodium Capsules ... 436
- Nembutal Sodium Solution ... 438
- Nembutal Sodium Suppositories ... 440

Perphenazine (Enhanced effect of central nervous system depressant and tranquilizer). Products include:

- Etrafon ... 2355
- Triavil Tablets ... 1757
- Trilafon ... 2389

Phenelzine Sulfate (Enhanced CNS effects of butalbital). Products include:

- Nardil ... 1920

Phenobarbital (Enhanced effect of central nervous system depressant). Products include:

- Arco-Lase Plus Tablets ... 512
- Bellergal-S Tablets ... 2250
- Donnatal ... 2060
- Donnatal Extentabs ... 2061
- Donnatal Tablets ... 2060
- Phenobarbital Elixir and Tablets ... 1469
- Quadrinal Tablets ... 1350

Prazepam (Enhanced effect of central nervous system depressant and tranquilizer).

No products indexed under this heading.

Prochlorperazine (Enhanced effect of central nervous system depressant and tranquilizer). Products include:

- Compazine ... 2470

Promethazine Hydrochloride (Enhanced effect of central nervous system depressant and tranquilizer). Products include:

- Mepergan Injection ... 2753
- Phenergan with Codeine ... 2777
- Phenergan with Dextromethorphan 2778
- Phenergan Injection ... 2773
- Phenergan Suppositories ... 2775
- Phenergan Syrup ... 2774
- Phenergan Tablets ... 2775
- Phenergan VC ... 2779
- Phenergan VC with Codeine ... 2781

Propofol (Enhanced effect of central nervous system depressant, sedative-hypnotic and anesthetic). Products include:

- Diprivan Injection ... 2833

Propoxyphene Hydrochloride (Enhanced effect of central nervous system depressant and narcotic analgesic). Products include:

- Darvon ... 1435
- Wygesic Tablets ... 2827

Propoxyphene Napsylate (Enhanced effect of central nervous system depressant and narcotic analgesic). Products include:

- Darvon-N/Darvocet-N ... 1433

Quazepam (Enhanced effect of central nervous system depressant and sedative-hypnotic). Products include:

- Doral Tablets ... 2664

Risperidone (Enhanced effect of central nervous system depressant and narcotic analgesic). Products include:

- Risperdal ... 1301

Secobarbital Sodium (Enhanced effect of central nervous system depressant and sedative-hypnotic). Products include:

- Seconal Sodium Pulvules ... 1474

Selegiline Hydrochloride (Enhanced CNS effects of butalbital). Products include:

- Eldepryl Tablets ... 2550

Sufentanil Citrate (Enhanced effect of central nervous system depressant and narcotic analgesic). Products include:

- Sufenta Injection ... 1309

Temazepam (Enhanced effect of central nervous system depressant and sedative-hypnotic). Products include:

- Restoril Capsules ... 2284

Thiamylal Sodium (Enhanced effect of central nervous system depressant).

No products indexed under this heading.

Thioridazine Hydrochloride (Enhanced effect of central nervous system depressant and tranquilizer). Products include:

- Mellaril ... 2269

Thiothixene (Enhanced effect of central nervous system depressant and tranquilizer). Products include:

- Navane Capsules and Concentrate 2201
- Navane Intramuscular ... 2202

Tranylcypromine Sulfate (Enhanced CNS effects of butalbital). Products include:

- Parnate Tablets ... 2503

Triazolam (Enhanced effect of central nervous system depressant and sedative-hypnotic). Products include:

- Halcion Tablets ... 2611

Trifluoperazine Hydrochloride (Enhanced effect of central nervous system depressant and tranquilizer). Products include:

- Stelazine ... 2514

Zolpidem Tartrate (Enhanced effect of central nervous system depressant and narcotic analgesic). Products include:

- Ambien Tablets ... 2416

Food Interactions

Alcohol (Enhanced effect of central nervous system depressant).

FIORINAL CAPSULES

(Butalbital, Aspirin) ... 2261

May interact with monoamine oxidase inhibitors, corticosteroids, oral anticoagulants, oral hypoglycemic agents, insulin, non-steroidal anti-inflammatory agents, narcotic analgesics, general anesthetics, hypnotics and sedatives, tranquilizers, central nervous system depressants, and certain other agents. Compounds in these categories include:

Acarbose (Potential for enhanced effects of oral antidiabetic agents causing hypoglycemia).

No products indexed under this heading.

Alfentanil Hydrochloride (Increased CNS depression). Products include:

- Alfenta Injection ... 1286

Alprazolam (Increased CNS depression). Products include:

- Xanax Tablets ... 2649

Aprobarbital (Increased CNS depression).

No products indexed under this heading.

Betamethasone Acetate (Concomitant corticosteroids and chronic use of aspirin may result in salicylism upon withdrawal of corticosteroid because corticosteroids enhance renal clearance of salicylates). Products include:

- Celestone Soluspan Suspension ... 2347

Betamethasone Sodium Phosphate (Concomitant corticosteroids and chronic use of aspirin may result in salicylism upon withdrawal of corticosteroid because corticosteroids enhance renal clearance of salicylates). Products include:

- Celestone Soluspan Suspension ... 2347

Buprenorphine (Increased CNS depression). Products include:

- Buprenex Injectable ... 2006

Buspirone Hydrochloride (Increased CNS depression). Products include:

- BuSpar ... 737

Butabarbital (Increased CNS depression).

No products indexed under this heading.

Chlordiazepoxide (Increased CNS depression). Products include:

- Libritabs Tablets ... 2177
- Limbitrol ... 2180

Chlordiazepoxide Hydrochloride (Increased CNS depression). Products include:

- Librax Capsules ... 2176
- Librium Capsules ... 2178
- Librium Injectable ... 2179

Chlorpromazine (Increased CNS depression). Products include:

- Thorazine Suppositories ... 2523

Chlorpromazine Hydrochloride (Increased CNS depression). Products include:

- Thorazine ... 2523

Chlorpropamide (Potential for enhanced effects of oral antidiabetic agents causing hypoglycemia). Products include:

- Diabinese Tablets ... 1935

Chlorprothixene (Increased CNS depression).

No products indexed under this heading.

Chlorprothixene Hydrochloride (Increased CNS depression).

No products indexed under this heading.

Clorazepate Dipotassium (Increased CNS depression). Products include:

- Tranxene ... 451

Clozapine (Increased CNS depression). Products include:

- Clozaril Tablets ... 2252

Codeine Phosphate (Increased CNS depression). Products include:

- Actifed with Codeine Cough Syrup.. 1067
- Brontex ... 1981
- Deconsal C Expectorant Syrup ... 456
- Deconsal Pediatric Syrup ... 457
- Dimetane-DC Cough Syrup ... 2059
- Empirin with Codeine Tablets ... 1093
- Fioricet with Codeine Capsules ... 2260
- Fiorinal with Codeine Capsules ... 2262
- Isoclor Expectorant ... 990
- Novahistine DH ... 2462
- Novahistine Expectorant ... 2463
- Nucofed ... 2051
- Phenergan with Codeine ... 2777
- Phenergan VC with Codeine ... 2781
- Robitussin A-C Syrup ... 2073
- Robitussin-DAC Syrup ... 2074
- Ryna ... ⊡ 841
- Soma Compound w/Codeine Tablets ... 2676
- Tussi-Organidin NR Liquid and S NR Liquid ... 2677
- Tylenol with Codeine ... 1583

Cortisone Acetate (Concomitant corticosteroids and chronic use of aspirin may result in salicylism upon withdrawal of corticosteroid because corticosteroids enhance renal clearance of salicylates). Products include:

- Cortone Acetate Sterile Suspension ... 1623
- Cortone Acetate Tablets ... 1624

Desflurane (Increased CNS depression). Products include:

- Suprane ... 1813

Dexamethasone (Concomitant corticosteroids and chronic use of aspirin may result in salicylism upon withdrawal of corticosteroid because corticosteroids enhance renal clearance of salicylates). Products include:

- AK-Trol Ointment & Suspension ... ◉ 205
- Decadron Elixir ... 1633
- Decadron Tablets ... 1635
- Decaspray Topical Aerosol ... 1648
- Dexacidin Ointment ... ◉ 263
- Maxitrol Ophthalmic Ointment and Suspension ... ◉ 224
- TobraDex Ophthalmic Suspension and Ointment ... 473

Dexamethasone Acetate (Concomitant corticosteroids and chronic use of aspirin may result in salicylism upon withdrawal of corticosteroid because corticosteroids enhance renal clearance of salicylates). Products include:

- Dalalone D.P. Injectable ... 1011
- Decadron-LA Sterile Suspension ... 1646

Dexamethasone Sodium Phosphate (Concomitant corticosteroids and chronic use of aspirin may result in salicylism upon withdrawal of corticosteroid because corticosteroids enhance renal clearance of salicylates). Products include:

- Decadron Phosphate Injection ... 1637
- Decadron Phosphate Respihaler ... 1642
- Decadron Phosphate Sterile Ophthalmic Ointment ... 1641
- Decadron Phosphate Sterile Ophthalmic Solution ... 1642
- Decadron Phosphate Topical Cream ... 1644
- Decadron Phosphate Turbinaire ... 1645
- Decadron Phosphate with Xylocaine Injection, Sterile ... 1639
- Dexacort Phosphate in Respihaler .. 458
- Dexacort Phosphate in Turbinaire .. 459
- NeoDecadron Sterile Ophthalmic Ointment ... 1712
- NeoDecadron Sterile Ophthalmic Solution ... 1713
- NeoDecadron Topical Cream ... 1714

Dezocine (Increased CNS depression). Products include:

- Dalgan Injection ... 538

Diazepam (Increased CNS depression). Products include:

- Dizac ... 1809
- Valium Injectable ... 2182
- Valium Tablets ... 2183
- Valrelease Capsules ... 2169

Diclofenac Potassium (Enhanced effects of non-steroidal anti-inflammatory agents thereby increasing the risk of peptic ulceration and bleeding). Products include:

- Cataflam ... 816

Diclofenac Sodium (Enhanced effects of non-steroidal anti-inflammatory agents thereby increasing the risk of peptic ulceration and bleeding). Products include:

- Voltaren Ophthalmic Sterile Ophthalmic Solution ... ◉ 272
- Voltaren Tablets ... 861

IMPORTANT NOTE: Always consult each drug listing in the patient's regimen for possible interactions.

Fiorinal | Interactions Index | 414

Dicumarol (Enhanced effects of oral coagulants causing bleeding by prothrombin formation in the liver and displacing anticoagulants from plasma protein binding sites).
No products indexed under this heading.

Droperidol (Increased CNS depression). Products include:
Inapsine Injection ... 1296

Enflurane (Increased CNS depression).
No products indexed under this heading.

Estazolam (Increased CNS depression). Products include:
ProSom Tablets ... 449

Ethchlorvynol (Increased CNS depression). Products include:
Placidyl Capsules ... 448

Ethinamate (Increased CNS depression).
No products indexed under this heading.

Etodolac (Enhanced effects of non-steroidal anti-inflammatory agents thereby increasing the risk of peptic ulceration and bleeding). Products include:
Lodine Capsules and Tablets ... 2743

Fenoprofen Calcium (Enhanced effects of non-steroidal anti-inflammatory agents thereby increasing the risk of peptic ulceration and bleeding). Products include:
Nalfon 200 Pulvules & Nalfon Tablets ... 917

Fentanyl (Increased CNS depression). Products include:
Duragesic Transdermal System ... 1288

Fentanyl Citrate (Increased CNS depression). Products include:
Sublimaze Injection ... 1307

Fludrocortisone Acetate (Concomitant corticosteroids and chronic use of aspirin may result in salicylism upon withdrawal of corticosteroid because corticosteroids enhance renal clearance of salicylates). Products include:
Florinef Acetate Tablets ... 505

Fluphenazine Decanoate (Increased CNS depression). Products include:
Prolixin Decanoate ... 509

Fluphenazine Enanthate (Increased CNS depression). Products include:
Prolixin Enanthate ... 509

Fluphenazine Hydrochloride (Increased CNS depression). Products include:
Prolixin ... 509

Flurazepam Hydrochloride (Increased CNS depression). Products include:
Dalmane Capsules ... 2173

Flurbiprofen (Enhanced effects of non-steroidal anti-inflammatory agents thereby increasing the risk of peptic ulceration and bleeding). Products include:
Ansaid Tablets ... 2579

Furazolidone (The CNS effects of butalbital may be enhanced by monoamine oxidase inhibitors). Products include:
Furoxone ... 2046

Glipizide (Potential for enhanced effects of oral antidiabetic agents causing hypoglycemia). Products include:
Glucotrol Tablets ... 1967
Glucotrol XL Extended Release Tablets ... 1968

Glutethimide (Increased CNS depression).
No products indexed under this heading.

Glyburide (Potential for enhanced effects of oral antidiabetic agents causing hypoglycemia). Products include:
DiaBeta Tablets ... 1239
Glynase PresTab Tablets ... 2609
Micronase Tablets ... 2623

Haloperidol (Increased CNS depression). Products include:
Haldol Injection, Tablets and Concentrate ... 1575

Haloperidol Decanoate (Increased CNS depression). Products include:
Haldol Decanoate ... 1577

Hydrocodone Bitartrate (Increased CNS depression). Products include:
Anexsia 5/500 Elixir ... 1781
Anexia Tablets ... 1782
Codiclear DH Syrup ... 791
Deconamine CX Cough and Cold Liquid and Tablets ... 1319
Duratuss HD Elixir ... 2565
Hycodan Tablets and Syrup ... 930
Hycomine Compound Tablets ... 932
Hycomine ... 931
Hycotuss Expectorant Syrup ... 933
Hydrocet Capsules ... 782
Lorcet 10/650 ... 1018
Lortab ... 2566
Tussend ... 1783
Tussend Expectorant ... 1785
Vicodin Tablets ... 1356
Vicodin ES Tablets ... 1357
Vicodin Tuss Expectorant ... 1358
Zydone Capsules ... 949

Hydrocodone Polistirex (Increased CNS depression). Products include:
Tussionex Pennkinetic Extended-Release Suspension ... 998

Hydrocortisone (Concomitant corticosteroids and chronic use of aspirin may result in salicylism upon withdrawal of corticosteroid because corticosteroids enhance renal clearance of salicylates). Products include:
Anusol-HC Cream 2.5% ... 1896
Aquanil HC Lotion ... 1931
Bactine Hydrocortisone Anti-Itch Cream ... ■ 709
Caldecort Anti-Itch Hydrocortisone Spray ... ■ 631
Cortaid ... ■ 836
CORTENEMA ... 2535
Cortisporin Ointment ... 1085
Cortisporin Ophthalmic Ointment Sterile ... 1085
Cortisporin Ophthalmic Suspension Sterile ... 1086
Cortisporin Otic Solution Sterile ... 1087
Cortisporin Otic Suspension Sterile 1088
Cortizone-5 ... ■ 831
Cortizone-10 ... ■ 831
Hydrocortone Tablets ... 1672
Hytone ... 907
Massengill Medicated Soft Cloth Towelettes ... 2458
PediOtic Suspension Sterile ... 1153
Preparation H Hydrocortisone 1% Cream ... ■ 872
ProctoCream-HC 2.5% ... 2408
VōSoL HC Otic Solution ... 2678

Hydrocortisone Acetate (Concomitant corticosteroids and chronic use of aspirin may result in salicylism upon withdrawal of corticosteroid because corticosteroids enhance renal clearance of salicylates). Products include:
Analpram-HC Rectal Cream 1% and 2.5% ... 977
Anusol HC-1 Anti-Itch Hydrocortisone Ointment ... ■ 847
Anusol-HC Suppositories ... 1897
Caldecort ... ■ 631
Carmol HC ... 924
Coly-Mycin S Otic w/Neomycin & Hydrocortisone ... 1906
Cortaid ... ■ 836
Cortifoam ... 2396
Cortisporin Cream ... 1084
Epifoam ... 2399
Hydrocortone Acetate Sterile Suspension ... 1669
Mantadil Cream ... 1135
Nupercainal Hydrocortisone 1% Cream ... ■ 645
Ophthocort ... ⊙ 311
Pramosone Cream, Lotion & Ointment ... 978
ProctoCream-HC ... 2408
ProctoFoam-HC ... 2409
Terra-Cortril Ophthalmic Suspension ... 2210

Hydrocortisone Sodium Phosphate (Concomitant corticosteroids and chronic use of aspirin may result in salicylism upon withdrawal of corticosteroid because corticosteroids enhance renal clearance of salicylates). Products include:
Hydrocortone Phosphate Injection, Sterile ... 1670

Hydrocortisone Sodium Succinate (Concomitant corticosteroids and chronic use of aspirin may result in salicylism upon withdrawal of corticosteroid because corticosteroids enhance renal clearance of salicylates). Products include:
Solu-Cortef Sterile Powder ... 2641

Hydroxyzine Hydrochloride (Increased CNS depression). Products include:
Atarax Tablets & Syrup ... 2185
Marax Tablets & DF Syrup ... 2200
Vistaril Intramuscular Solution ... 2216

Ibuprofen (Enhanced effects of non-steroidal anti-inflammatory agents thereby increasing the risk of peptic ulceration and bleeding). Products include:
Advil Cold and Sinus Caplets and Tablets (formerly CoAdvil) ... ■ 870
Advil Ibuprofen Tablets and Caplets ... ■ 870
Children's Advil Suspension ... 2692
Arthritis Foundation Ibuprofen Tablets ... ■ 674
Bayer Select Ibuprofen Pain Relief Formula ... ■ 715
Cramp End Tablets ... ■ 735
Dimetapp Sinus Caplets ... ■ 775
Haltran Tablets ... ■ 771
IBU Tablets ... 1342
Ibuprohm ... ■ 735
Children's Motrin Ibuprofen Oral Suspension ... 1546
Motrin Tablets ... 2625
Motrin IB Caplets, Tablets, and Geltabs ... ■ 838
Motrin IB Sinus ... ■ 838
Motrin Ibuprofen Suspension, Oral Drops, Chewable Tablets, Caplets ... 1546
Nuprin Ibuprofen/Analgesic Tablets & Caplets ... ■ 622
Sine-Aid IB Caplets ... 1554
Vicks DayQuil SINUS Pressure & PAIN Relief with IBUPROFEN ... ■ 762

Indomethacin (Enhanced effects of non-steroidal anti-inflammatory agents thereby increasing the risk of peptic ulceration and bleeding). Products include:
Indocin ... 1680

Indomethacin Sodium Trihydrate (Enhanced effects of non-steroidal anti-inflammatory agents thereby increasing the risk of peptic ulceration and bleeding). Products include:
Indocin I.V. ... 1684

Insulin, Human (Potential for enhanced effects of insulin causing hypoglycemia).
No products indexed under this heading.

Insulin, Human Isophane Suspension (Potential for enhanced effects of insulin causing hypoglycemia). Products include:
Novolin N Human Insulin 10 ml Vials ... 1795

Insulin, Human NPH (Potential for enhanced effects of insulin causing hypoglycemia). Products include:
Humulin N, 100 Units ... 1448
Novolin N PenFill Cartridges Durable Insulin Delivery System ... 1798
Novolin N Prefilled Syringe Disposable Insulin Delivery System ... 1798

Insulin, Human Regular (Potential for enhanced effects of insulin causing hypoglycemia). Products include:
Humulin R, 100 Units ... 1449
Novolin R Human Insulin 10 ml Vials ... 1795
Novolin R PenFill Cartridges Durable Insulin Delivery System ... 1798
Novolin R Prefilled Syringe Disposable Insulin Delivery System ... 1798
Velosulin BR Human Insulin 10 ml Vials ... 1795

Insulin, Human, Zinc Suspension (Potential for enhanced effects of insulin causing hypoglycemia). Products include:
Humulin L, 100 Units ... 1446
Humulin U, 100 Units ... 1450
Novolin L Human Insulin 10 ml Vials ... 1795

Insulin, NPH (Potential for enhanced effects of insulin causing hypoglycemia). Products include:
NPH, 100 Units ... 1450
Pork NPH, 100 Units ... 1452
Purified Pork NPH Isophane Insulin ... 1801

Insulin, Regular (Potential for enhanced effects of insulin causing hypoglycemia). Products include:
Regular, 100 Units ... 1450
Pork Regular, 100 Units ... 1452
Pork Regular (Concentrated), 500 Units ... 1453
Purified Pork Regular Insulin ... 1801

Insulin, Zinc Crystals (Potential for enhanced effects of insulin causing hypoglycemia). Products include:
NPH, 100 Units ... 1450

Insulin, Zinc Suspension (Potential for enhanced effects of insulin causing hypoglycemia). Products include:
Iletin I ... 1450
Lente, 100 Units ... 1450
Iletin II ... 1452
Pork Lente, 100 Units ... 1452
Purified Pork Lente Insulin ... 1801

Isocarboxazid (The CNS effects of butalbital may be enhanced by monoamine oxidase inhibitors).
No products indexed under this heading.

Isoflurane (Increased CNS depression).
No products indexed under this heading.

Ketamine Hydrochloride (Increased CNS depression).
No products indexed under this heading.

Ketoprofen (Enhanced effects of non-steroidal anti-inflammatory agents thereby increasing the risk of peptic ulceration and bleeding). Products include:
Orudis Capsules ... 2766
Oruvail Capsules ... 2766

Ketorolac Tromethamine (Enhanced effects of non-steroidal anti-inflammatory agents thereby increasing the risk of peptic ulceration and bleeding). Products include:
Acular ... 474
Acular ... ⊙ 277
Toradol ... 2159

Levomethadyl Acetate Hydrochloride (Increased CNS depression). Products include:
- Orlamm ... 2239

Levorphanol Tartrate (Increased CNS depression). Products include:
- Levo-Dromoran ... 2129

Lorazepam (Increased CNS depression). Products include:
- Ativan Injection ... 2698
- Ativan Tablets ... 2700

Loxapine Hydrochloride (Increased CNS depression). Products include:
- Loxitane ... 1378

Loxapine Succinate (Increased CNS depression). Products include:
- Loxitane Capsules ... 1378

Meclofenamate Sodium (Enhanced effects of non-steroidal anti-inflammatory agents thereby increasing the risk of peptic ulceration and bleeding).
- No products indexed under this heading.

Mefenamic Acid (Enhanced effects of non-steroidal anti-inflammatory agents thereby increasing the risk of peptic ulceration and bleeding). Products include:
- Ponstel ... 1925

Meperidine Hydrochloride (Increased CNS depression). Products include:
- Demerol ... 2308
- Mepergan Injection ... 2753

Mephobarbital (Increased CNS depression). Products include:
- Mebaral Tablets ... 2322

Meprobamate (Increased CNS depression). Products include:
- Miltown Tablets ... 2672
- PMB 200 and PMB 400 ... 2783

Mercaptopurine (Enhanced effects of 6-mercaptopurine causing bone marrow toxicity and blood dyscrasias by displacing it from secondary binding sites). Products include:
- Purinethol Tablets ... 1156

Mesoridazine (Increased CNS depression).

Mesoridazine Besylate (Increased CNS depression). Products include:
- Serentil ... 684

Metformin Hydrochloride (Potential for enhanced effects of oral antidiabetic agents causing hypoglycemia). Products include:
- Glucophage ... 752

Methadone Hydrochloride (Increased CNS depression). Products include:
- Methadone Hydrochloride Oral Concentrate ... 2233
- Methadone Hydrochloride Oral Solution & Tablets ... 2235

Methohexital Sodium (Increased CNS depression). Products include:
- Brevital Sodium Vials ... 1429

Methotrexate Sodium (Enhanced effects of 6-mercaptopurine causing bone marrow toxicity and blood dyscrasias by displacing it from secondary binding sites and reducing its excretion). Products include:
- Methotrexate Sodium Tablets, Injection, for Injection and LPF Injection ... 1275

Methotrimeprazine (Increased CNS depression). Products include:
- Levoprome ... 1274

Methoxyflurane (Increased CNS depression).
- No products indexed under this heading.

Methylprednisolone Acetate (Concomitant corticosteroids and chronic use of aspirin may result in salicylism upon withdrawal of corticosteroid because corticosteroids enhance renal clearance of salicylates). Products include:
- Depo-Medrol Single-Dose Vial ... 2600
- Depo-Medrol Sterile Aqueous Suspension ... 2597

Methylprednisolone Sodium Succinate (Concomitant corticosteroids and chronic use of aspirin may result in salicylism upon withdrawal of corticosteroid because corticosteroids enhance renal clearance of salicylates). Products include:
- Solu-Medrol Sterile Powder ... 2643

Midazolam Hydrochloride (Increased CNS depression). Products include:
- Versed Injection ... 2170

Molindone Hydrochloride (Increased CNS depression). Products include:
- Moban Tablets and Concentrate ... 1048

Morphine Sulfate (Increased CNS depression). Products include:
- Astramorph/PF Injection, USP (Preservative-Free) ... 535
- Duramorph ... 962
- Infumorph 200 and Infumorph 500 Sterile Solutions ... 965
- MS Contin Tablets ... 1994
- MSIR ... 1997
- Oramorph SR (Morphine Sulfate Sustained Release Tablets) ... 2236
- RMS Suppositories ... 2657
- Roxanol ... 2243

Nabumetone (Enhanced effects of non-steroidal anti-inflammatory agents thereby increasing the risk of peptic ulceration and bleeding). Products include:
- Relafen Tablets ... 2510

Naproxen (Enhanced effects of non-steroidal anti-inflammatory agents thereby increasing the risk of peptic ulceration and bleeding). Products include:
- Anaprox/Naprosyn ... 2117

Naproxen Sodium (Enhanced effects of non-steroidal anti-inflammatory agents thereby increasing the risk of peptic ulceration and bleeding). Products include:
- Aleve ... 1975
- Anaprox/Naprosyn ... 2117

Opium Alkaloids (Increased CNS depression).
- No products indexed under this heading.

Oxaprozin (Enhanced effects of non-steroidal anti-inflammatory agents thereby increasing the risk of peptic ulceration and bleeding). Products include:
- Daypro Caplets ... 2426

Oxazepam (Increased CNS depression). Products include:
- Serax Capsules ... 2810
- Serax Tablets ... 2810

Oxycodone Hydrochloride (Increased CNS depression). Products include:
- Percocet Tablets ... 938
- Percodan Tablets ... 939
- Percodan-Demi Tablets ... 940
- Roxicodone Tablets, Oral Solution & Intensol (Oxycodone) ... 2244
- Tylox Capsules ... 1584

Pentobarbital Sodium (Increased CNS depression). Products include:
- Nembutal Sodium Capsules ... 436
- Nembutal Sodium Solution ... 438
- Nembutal Sodium Suppositories ... 440

Perphenazine (Increased CNS depression). Products include:
- Etrafon ... 2355
- Triavil Tablets ... 1757
- Trilafon ... 2389

Phenelzine Sulfate (The CNS effects of butalbital may be enhanced by monoamine oxidase inhibitors). Products include:
- Nardil ... 1920

Phenobarbital (Increased CNS depression). Products include:
- Arco-Lase Plus Tablets ... 512
- Bellergal-S Tablets ... 2250
- Donnatal ... 2060
- Donnatal Extentabs ... 2061
- Donnatal Tablets ... 2060
- Phenobarbital Elixir and Tablets ... 1469
- Quadrinal Tablets ... 1350

Phenylbutazone (Enhanced effects of non-steroidal anti-inflammatory agents thereby increasing the risk of peptic ulceration and bleeding).
- No products indexed under this heading.

Piroxicam (Enhanced effects of non-steroidal anti-inflammatory agents thereby increasing the risk of peptic ulceration and bleeding). Products include:
- Feldene Capsules ... 1965

Prazepam (Increased CNS depression).
- No products indexed under this heading.

Prednisolone Acetate (Concomitant corticosteroids and chronic use of aspirin may result in salicylism upon withdrawal of corticosteroid because corticosteroids enhance renal clearance of salicylates). Products include:
- AK-CIDE ... ◉ 202
- AK-CIDE Ointment ... ◉ 202
- Blephamide Liquifilm Sterile Ophthalmic Suspension ... 476
- Blephamide Ointment ... ◉ 237
- Econopred & Econopred Plus Ophthalmic Suspensions ... ◉ 217
- Poly-Pred Liquifilm ... ◉ 248
- Pred Forte ... ◉ 250
- Pred Mild ... ◉ 253
- Pred-G Liquifilm Sterile Ophthalmic Suspension ... ◉ 251
- Pred-G S.O.P. Sterile Ophthalmic Ointment ... ◉ 252
- Vasocidin Ointment ... ◉ 268

Prednisolone Sodium Phosphate (Concomitant corticosteroids and chronic use of aspirin may result in salicylism upon withdrawal of corticosteroid because corticosteroids enhance renal clearance of salicylates). Products include:
- AK-Pred ... ◉ 204
- Hydeltrasol Injection, Sterile ... 1665
- Inflamase ... ◉ 265
- Pediapred Oral Liquid ... 995
- Vasocidin Ophthalmic Solution ... ◉ 270

Prednisolone Tebutate (Concomitant corticosteroids and chronic use of aspirin may result in salicylism upon withdrawal of corticosteroid because corticosteroids enhance renal clearance of salicylates). Products include:
- Hydeltra-T.B.A. Sterile Suspension 1667

Prednisone (Concomitant corticosteroids and chronic use of aspirin may result in salicylism upon withdrawal of corticosteroid because corticosteroids enhance renal clearance of salicylates). Products include:
- Deltasone Tablets ... 2595

Probenecid (Diminished effects of uricosuric agent, probenecid, thereby reducing its effectiveness in the treatment of gout). Products include:
- Benemid Tablets ... 1611
- ColBENEMID Tablets ... 1622

Prochlorperazine (Increased CNS depression). Products include:
- Compazine ... 2470

Promethazine Hydrochloride (Increased CNS depression). Products include:
- Mepergan Injection ... 2753
- Phenergan with Codeine ... 2777
- Phenergan with Dextromethorphan 2778
- Phenergan Injection ... 2773
- Phenergan Suppositories ... 2775
- Phenergan Syrup ... 2774
- Phenergan Tablets ... 2775
- Phenergan VC ... 2779
- Phenergan VC with Codeine ... 2781

Propofol (Increased CNS depression). Products include:
- Diprivan Injection ... 2833

Propoxyphene Hydrochloride (Increased CNS depression). Products include:
- Darvon ... 1435
- Wygesic Tablets ... 2827

Propoxyphene Napsylate (Increased CNS depression). Products include:
- Darvon-N/Darvocet-N ... 1433

Quazepam (Increased CNS depression). Products include:
- Doral Tablets ... 2664

Risperidone (Increased CNS depression). Products include:
- Risperdal ... 1301

Secobarbital Sodium (Increased CNS depression). Products include:
- Seconal Sodium Pulvules ... 1474

Selegiline Hydrochloride (The CNS effects of butalbital may be enhanced by monoamine oxidase inhibitors). Products include:
- Eldepryl Tablets ... 2550

Sufentanil Citrate (Increased CNS depression). Products include:
- Sufenta Injection ... 1309

Sulfinpyrazone (Diminished effects of uricosuric agent, sulfinpyrazone, thereby reducing its effectiveness in the treatment of gout). Products include:
- Anturane ... 807

Sulindac (Enhanced effects of non-steroidal anti-inflammatory agents thereby increasing the risk of peptic ulceration and bleeding). Products include:
- Clinoril Tablets ... 1618

Temazepam (Increased CNS depression). Products include:
- Restoril Capsules ... 2284

Thiamylal Sodium (Increased CNS depression).
- No products indexed under this heading.

Thioridazine Hydrochloride (Increased CNS depression). Products include:
- Mellaril ... 2269

Thiothixene (Increased CNS depression). Products include:
- Navane Capsules and Concentrate 2201
- Navane Intramuscular ... 2202

Tolazamide (Potential for enhanced effects of oral antidiabetic agents causing hypoglycemia).
- No products indexed under this heading.

Tolbutamide (Potential for enhanced effects of oral antidiabetic agents causing hypoglycemia).
- No products indexed under this heading.

Tolmetin Sodium (Enhanced effects of non-steroidal anti-inflammatory agents thereby increasing the risk of peptic ulceration and bleeding). Products include:
- Tolectin (200, 400 and 600 mg) .. 1581

IMPORTANT NOTE: Always consult each drug listing in the patient's regimen for possible interactions.

Tranylcypromine Sulfate (The CNS effects of butalbital may be enhanced by monoamine oxidase inhibitors). Products include:

Parnate Tablets ... 2503

Triamcinolone (Concomitant corticosteroids and chronic use of aspirin may result in salicylism upon withdrawal of corticosteroid because corticosteroids enhance renal clearance of salicylates). Products include:

Aristocort Tablets ... 1022

Triamcinolone Acetonide (Concomitant corticosteroids and chronic use of aspirin may result in salicylism upon withdrawal of corticosteroid because corticosteroids enhance renal clearance of salicylates). Products include:

Aristocort A 0.025% Cream ... 1027
Aristocort A 0.5% Cream ... 1031
Aristocort A 0.1% Cream ... 1029
Aristocort A 0.1% Ointment ... 1030
Azmacort Oral Inhaler ... 2011
Nasacort Nasal Inhaler ... 2024

Triamcinolone Diacetate (Concomitant corticosteroids and chronic use of aspirin may result in salicylism upon withdrawal of corticosteroid because corticosteroids enhance renal clearance of salicylates). Products include:

Aristocort Suspension (Forte Parenteral) ... 1027
Aristocort Suspension (Intralesional) ... 1025

Triamcinolone Hexacetonide (Concomitant corticosteroids and chronic use of aspirin may result in salicylism upon withdrawal of corticosteroid because corticosteroids enhance renal clearance of salicylates). Products include:

Aristospan Suspension (Intra-articular) ... 1033
Aristospan Suspension (Intralesional) ... 1032

Triazolam (Increased CNS depression). Products include:

Halcion Tablets ... 2611

Trifluoperazine Hydrochloride (Increased CNS depression). Products include:

Stelazine ... 2514

Warfarin Sodium (Enhanced effects of oral coagulants causing bleeding by prothrombin formation in the liver and displacing anticoagulants from plasma protein binding sites). Products include:

Coumadin ... 926

Zolpidem Tartrate (Increased CNS depression). Products include:

Ambien Tablets ... 2416

Food Interactions

Alcohol (Increased CNS depression).

FIORINAL WITH CODEINE CAPSULES

(Codeine Phosphate, Butalbital, Caffeine, Aspirin) ... 2262

May interact with central nervous system depressants, hypnotics and sedatives, monoamine oxidase inhibitors, corticosteroids, oral anticoagulants, oral hypoglycemic agents, insulin, tranquilizers, narcotic analgesics, non-steroidal anti-inflammatory agents, general anesthetics, and certain other agents. Compounds in these categories include:

Acarbose (Potential for hypoglycemia).

No products indexed under this heading.

Alfentanil Hydrochloride (Increased CNS depression). Products include:

Alfenta Injection ... 1286

Alprazolam (Increased CNS depression). Products include:

Xanax Tablets ... 2649

Aprobarbital (Increased CNS depression).

No products indexed under this heading.

Betamethasone Acetate (Potential for salicylism when corticosteroids therapy is stopped). Products include:

Celestone Soluspan Suspension ... 2347

Betamethasone Sodium Phosphate (Potential for salicylism when corticosteroids therapy is stopped). Products include:

Celestone Soluspan Suspension ... 2347

Buprenorphine (Increased CNS depression). Products include:

Buprenex Injectable ... 2006

Buspirone Hydrochloride (Increased CNS depression). Products include:

BuSpar ... 737

Butabarbital (Increased CNS depression).

No products indexed under this heading.

Chlordiazepoxide (Increased CNS depression). Products include:

Libritabs Tablets ... 2177
Limbitrol ... 2180

Chlordiazepoxide Hydrochloride (Increased CNS depression). Products include:

Librax Capsules ... 2176
Librium Capsules ... 2178
Librium Injectable ... 2179

Chlorpromazine (Increased CNS depression). Products include:

Thorazine Suppositories ... 2523

Chlorpromazine Hydrochloride (Increased CNS depression). Products include:

Thorazine ... 2523

Chlorpropamide (Potential for hypoglycemia). Products include:

Diabinese Tablets ... 1935

Chlorprothixene (Increased CNS depression).

No products indexed under this heading.

Chlorprothixene Hydrochloride (Increased CNS depression).

No products indexed under this heading.

Clorazepate Dipotassium (Increased CNS depression). Products include:

Tranxene ... 451

Clozapine (Increased CNS depression). Products include:

Clozaril Tablets ... 2252

Cortisone Acetate (Potential for salicylism when corticosteroids therapy is stopped). Products include:

Cortone Acetate Sterile Suspension ... 1623
Cortone Acetate Tablets ... 1624

Desflurane (Increased CNS depression). Products include:

Suprane ... 1813

Dexamethasone (Potential for salicylism when corticosteroids therapy is stopped). Products include:

AK-Trol Ointment & Suspension ... ◉ 205
Decadron Elixir ... 1633
Decadron Tablets ... 1635
Decaspray Topical Aerosol ... 1648
Dexacidin Ointment ... ◉ 263
Maxitrol Ophthalmic Ointment and Suspension ... ◉ 224
TobraDex Ophthalmic Suspension and Ointment ... 473

Dexamethasone Acetate (Potential for salicylism when corticosteroids therapy is stopped). Products include:

Dalalone D.P. Injectable ... 1011
Decadron-LA Sterile Suspension ... 1646

Dexamethasone Sodium Phosphate (Potential for salicylism when corticosteroids therapy is stopped). Products include:

Decadron Phosphate Injection ... 1637
Decadron Phosphate Respihaler ... 1642
Decadron Phosphate Sterile Ophthalmic Ointment ... 1641
Decadron Phosphate Sterile Ophthalmic Solution ... 1642
Decadron Phosphate Topical Cream ... 1644
Decadron Phosphate Turbinaire ... 1645
Decadron Phosphate with Xylocaine Injection, Sterile ... 1639
Dexacort Phosphate in Respihaler ... 458
Dexacort Phosphate in Turbinaire ... 459
NeoDecadron Sterile Ophthalmic Ointment ... 1712
NeoDecadron Sterile Ophthalmic Solution ... 1713
NeoDecadron Topical Cream ... 1714

Dezocine (Increased CNS depression). Products include:

Dalgan Injection ... 538

Diazepam (Increased CNS depression). Products include:

Dizac ... 1809
Valium Injectable ... 2182
Valium Tablets ... 2183
Valrelease Capsules ... 2169

Diclofenac Potassium (Increased risk of peptic ulceration and bleeding). Products include:

Cataflam ... 816

Diclofenac Sodium (Increased risk of peptic ulceration and bleeding). Products include:

Voltaren Ophthalmic Sterile Ophthalmic Solution ... ◉ 272
Voltaren Tablets ... 861

Dicumarol (Enhanced effects of anticoagulants).

No products indexed under this heading.

Droperidol (Increased CNS depression). Products include:

Inapsine Injection ... 1296

Enflurane (Increased CNS depression).

No products indexed under this heading.

Estazolam (Increased CNS depression). Products include:

ProSom Tablets ... 449

Ethchlorvynol (Increased CNS depression). Products include:

Placidyl Capsules ... 448

Ethinamate (Increased CNS depression).

No products indexed under this heading.

Etodolac (Increased risk of peptic ulceration and bleeding). Products include:

Lodine Capsules and Tablets ... 2743

Fenoprofen Calcium (Increased risk of peptic ulceration and bleeding). Products include:

Nalfon 200 Pulvules & Nalfon Tablets ... 917

Fentanyl (Increased CNS depression). Products include:

Duragesic Transdermal System ... 1288

Fentanyl Citrate (Increased CNS depression). Products include:

Sublimaze Injection ... 1307

Fludrocortisone Acetate (Potential for salicylism when corticosteroids therapy is stopped). Products include:

Florinef Acetate Tablets ... 505

Fluphenazine Decanoate (Increased CNS depression). Products include:

Prolixin Decanoate ... 509

Fluphenazine Enanthate (Increased CNS depression). Products include:

Prolixin Enanthate ... 509

Fluphenazine Hydrochloride (Increased CNS depression). Products include:

Prolixin ... 509

Flurazepam Hydrochloride (Increased CNS depression). Products include:

Dalmane Capsules ... 2173

Flurbiprofen (Increased risk of peptic ulceration and bleeding). Products include:

Ansaid Tablets ... 2579

Furazolidone (Enhances CNS effects of butalbital). Products include:

Furoxone ... 2046

Glipizide (Potential for hypoglycemia). Products include:

Glucotrol Tablets ... 1967
Glucotrol XL Extended Release Tablets ... 1968

Glutethimide (Increased CNS depression).

No products indexed under this heading.

Glyburide (Potential for hypoglycemia). Products include:

DiaBeta Tablets ... 1239
Glynase PresTab Tablets ... 2609
Micronase Tablets ... 2623

Haloperidol (Increased CNS depression). Products include:

Haldol Injection, Tablets and Concentrate ... 1575

Haloperidol Decanoate (Increased CNS depression). Products include:

Haldol Decanoate ... 1577

Hydrocodone Bitartrate (Increased CNS depression). Products include:

Anexsia 5/500 Elixir ... 1781
Anexia Tablets ... 1782
Codiclear DH Syrup ... 791
Deconamine CX Cough and Cold Liquid and Tablets ... 1319
Duratuss HD Elixir ... 2565
Hycodan Tablets and Syrup ... 930
Hycomine Compound Tablets ... 932
Hycomine ... 931
Hycotuss Expectorant Syrup ... 933
Hydrocet Capsules ... 782
Lorcet 10/650 ... 1018
Lortab ... 2566
Tussend ... 1783
Tussend Expectorant ... 1785
Vicodin Tablets ... 1356
Vicodin ES Tablets ... 1357
Vicodin Tuss Expectorant ... 1358
Zydone Capsules ... 949

Hydrocodone Polistirex (Increased CNS depression). Products include:

Tussionex Pennkinetic Extended-Release Suspension ... 998

Hydrocortisone (Potential for salicylism when corticosteroids therapy is stopped). Products include:

Anusol-HC Cream 2.5% ... 1896
Aquanil HC Lotion ... 1931
Bactine Hydrocortisone Anti-Itch Cream ... ▣ 709
Caldecort Anti-Itch Hydrocortisone Spray ... ▣ 631
Cortaid ... ▣ 836
CORTENEMA ... 2535
Cortisporin Ointment ... 1085
Cortisporin Ophthalmic Ointment Sterile ... 1085
Cortisporin Ophthalmic Suspension Sterile ... 1086
Cortisporin Otic Solution Sterile ... 1087
Cortisporin Otic Suspension Sterile ... 1088
Cortizone-5 ... ▣ 831
Cortizone-10 ... ▣ 831

(▣ Described in PDR For Nonprescription Drugs) (◉ Described in PDR For Ophthalmology)

417 **Interactions Index** **Fiorinal with Codeine**

Hydrocortone Tablets 1672
Hytone 907
Massengill Medicated Soft Cloth Towelettes 2458
PediOtic Suspension Sterile 1153
Preparation H Hydrocortisone 1% Cream .... ▣ 872
ProctoCream-HC 2.5% 2408
VōSoL HC Otic Solution 2678

Hydrocortisone Acetate (Potential for salicylism when corticosteroids therapy is stopped). Products include:
Analpram-HC Rectal Cream 1% and 2.5% 977
Anusol HC-1 Anti-Itch Hydrocortisone Ointment .... ▣ 847
Anusol-HC Suppositories 1897
Caldecort .... ▣ 631
Carmol HC 924
Coly-Mycin S Otic w/Neomycin & Hydrocortisone 1906
Cortaid .... ▣ 836
Cortifoam 2396
Cortisporin Cream 1084
Epifoam 2399
Hydrocortone Acetate Sterile Suspension 1669
Mantadil Cream 1135
Nupercainal Hydrocortisone 1% Cream .... ▣ 645
Ophthocort .... ⊙ 311
Pramosone Cream, Lotion & Ointment 978
ProctoCream-HC 2408
ProctoFoam-HC 2409
Terra-Cortril Ophthalmic Suspension 2210

Hydrocortisone Sodium Phosphate (Potential for salicylism when corticosteroids therapy is stopped). Products include:
Hydrocortone Phosphate Injection, Sterile 1670

Hydrocortisone Sodium Succinate (Potential for salicylism when corticosteroids therapy is stopped). Products include:
Solu-Cortef Sterile Powder 2641

Hydroxyzine Hydrochloride (Increased CNS depression). Products include:
Atarax Tablets & Syrup 2185
Marax Tablets & DF Syrup 2200
Vistaril Intramuscular Solution 2216

Ibuprofen (Increased risk of peptic ulceration and bleeding). Products include:
Advil Cold and Sinus Caplets and Tablets (formerly CoAdvil) .... ▣ 870
Advil Ibuprofen Tablets and Caplets .... ▣ 870
Children's Advil Suspension 2692
Arthritis Foundation Ibuprofen Tablets .... ▣ 674
Bayer Select Ibuprofen Pain Relief Formula .... ▣ 715
Cramp End Tablets .... ▣ 735
Dimetapp Sinus Caplets .... ▣ 775
Haltran Tablets .... ▣ 771
IBU Tablets 1342
Ibuprohm .... ▣ 735
Children's Motrin Ibuprofen Oral Suspension 1546
Motrin Tablets 2625
Motrin IB Caplets, Tablets, and Geltabs .... ▣ 838
Motrin IB Sinus .... ▣ 838
Motrin Ibuprofen Suspension, Oral Drops, Chewable Tablets, Caplets 1546
Nuprin Ibuprofen/Analgesic Tablets & Caplets .... ▣ 622
Sine-Aid IB Caplets 1554
Vicks DayQuil SINUS Pressure & PAIN Relief with IBUPROFEN .... ▣ 762

Indomethacin (Increased risk of peptic ulceration and bleeding). Products include:
Indocin 1680

Indomethacin Sodium Trihydrate (Increased risk of peptic ulceration and bleeding). Products include:
Indocin I.V. 1684

Insulin, Human (Potential for hypoglycemia).
No products indexed under this heading.

Insulin, Human Isophane Suspension (Potential for hypoglycemia). Products include:
Novolin N Human Insulin 10 ml Vials 1795

Insulin, Human NPH (Potential for hypoglycemia). Products include:
Humulin N, 100 Units 1448
Novolin N PenFill Cartridges Durable Insulin Delivery System 1798
Novolin N Prefilled Syringe Disposable Insulin Delivery System 1798

Insulin, Human Regular (Potential for hypoglycemia). Products include:
Humulin R, 100 Units 1449
Novolin R Human Insulin 10 ml Vials 1795
Novolin R PenFill Cartridges Durable Insulin Delivery System 1798
Novolin R Prefilled Syringe Disposable Insulin Delivery System 1798
Velosulin BR Human Insulin 10 ml Vials 1795

Insulin, Human, Zinc Suspension (Potential for hypoglycemia). Products include:
Humulin L, 100 Units 1446
Humulin U, 100 Units 1450
Novolin L Human Insulin 10 ml Vials 1795

Insulin, NPH (Potential for hypoglycemia). Products include:
NPH, 100 Units 1450
Pork NPH, 100 Units 1452
Purified Pork NPH Isophane Insulin 1801

Insulin, Regular (Potential for hypoglycemia). Products include:
Regular, 100 Units 1450
Pork Regular, 100 Units 1452
Pork Regular (Concentrated), 500 Units 1453
Purified Pork Regular Insulin 1801

Insulin, Zinc Crystals (Potential for hypoglycemia). Products include:
NPH, 100 Units 1450

Insulin, Zinc Suspension (Potential for hypoglycemia). Products include:
Iletin I 1450
Lente, 100 Units 1450
Iletin II 1452
Pork Lente, 100 Units 1452
Purified Pork Lente Insulin 1801

Isocarboxazid (Enhances CNS effects of butalbital).
No products indexed under this heading.

Isoflurane (Increased CNS depression).
No products indexed under this heading.

Ketamine Hydrochloride (Increased CNS depression).
No products indexed under this heading.

Ketoprofen (Increased risk of peptic ulceration and bleeding). Products include:
Orudis Capsules 2766
Oruvail Capsules 2766

Ketorolac Tromethamine (Increased risk of peptic ulceration and bleeding). Products include:
Acular 474
Acular .... ⊙ 277
Toradol 2159

Levomethadyl Acetate Hydrochloride (Increased CNS depression). Products include:
Orlamm 2239

Levorphanol Tartrate (Increased CNS depression). Products include:
Levo-Dromoran 2129

Lorazepam (Increased CNS depression). Products include:
Ativan Injection 2698
Ativan Tablets 2700

Loxapine Hydrochloride (Increased CNS depression). Products include:
Loxitane 1378

Loxapine Succinate (Increased CNS depression). Products include:
Loxitane Capsules 1378

Meclofenamate Sodium (Increased risk of peptic ulceration and bleeding).
No products indexed under this heading.

Mefenamic Acid (Increased risk of peptic ulceration and bleeding). Products include:
Ponstel 1925

Meperidine Hydrochloride (Increased CNS depression). Products include:
Demerol 2308
Mepergan Injection 2753

Mephobarbital (Increased CNS depression). Products include:
Mebaral Tablets 2322

Meprobamate (Increased CNS depression). Products include:
Miltown Tablets 2672
PMB 200 and PMB 400 2783

Mercaptopurine (Enhanced effects of 6-mercaptopurine and potential for bone marrow toxicity and blood dyscrasias). Products include:
Purinethol Tablets 1156

Mesoridazine Besylate (Increased CNS depression). Products include:
Serentil 684

Metformin Hydrochloride (Potential for hypoglycemia). Products include:
Glucophage 752

Methadone Hydrochloride (Increased CNS depression). Products include:
Methadone Hydrochloride Oral Concentrate 2233
Methadone Hydrochloride Oral Solution & Tablets 2235

Methohexital Sodium (Increased CNS depression). Products include:
Brevital Sodium Vials 1429

Methotrexate Sodium (Enhanced effects of methotrexate and potential for bone marrow toxicity and blood dyscrasias). Products include:
Methotrexate Sodium Tablets, Injection, for Injection and LPF Injection 1275

Methotrimeprazine (Increased CNS depression). Products include:
Levoprome 1274

Methoxyflurane (Increased CNS depression).
No products indexed under this heading.

Methylprednisolone Acetate (Potential for salicylism when corticosteroids therapy is stopped). Products include:
Depo-Medrol Single-Dose Vial 2600
Depo-Medrol Sterile Aqueous Suspension 2597

Methylprednisolone Sodium Succinate (Potential for salicylism when corticosteroids therapy is stopped). Products include:
Solu-Medrol Sterile Powder 2643

Midazolam Hydrochloride (Increased CNS depression). Products include:
Versed Injection 2170

Molindone Hydrochloride (Increased CNS depression). Products include:
Moban Tablets and Concentrate 1048

Morphine Sulfate (Increased CNS depression). Products include:
Astramorph/PF Injection, USP (Preservative-Free) 535
Duramorph 962
Infumorph 200 and Infumorph 500 Sterile Solutions 965
MS Contin Tablets 1994
MSIR 1997
Oramorph SR (Morphine Sulfate Sustained Release Tablets) 2236
RMS Suppositories 2657
Roxanol 2243

Nabumetone (Increased risk of peptic ulceration and bleeding). Products include:
Relafen Tablets 2510

Naproxen (Increased risk of peptic ulceration and bleeding). Products include:
Anaprox/Naprosyn 2117

Naproxen Sodium (Increased risk of peptic ulceration and bleeding). Products include:
Aleve 1975
Anaprox/Naprosyn 2117

Opium Alkaloids (Increased CNS depression).
No products indexed under this heading.

Oxaprozin (Increased risk of peptic ulceration and bleeding). Products include:
Daypro Caplets 2426

Oxazepam (Increased CNS depression). Products include:
Serax Capsules 2810
Serax Tablets 2810

Oxycodone Hydrochloride (Increased CNS depression). Products include:
Percocet Tablets 938
Percodan Tablets 939
Percodan-Demi Tablets 940
Roxicodone Tablets, Oral Solution & Intensol (Oxycodone) 2244
Tylox Capsules 1584

Pentobarbital Sodium (Increased CNS depression). Products include:
Nembutal Sodium Capsules 436
Nembutal Sodium Solution 438
Nembutal Sodium Suppositories 440

Perphenazine (Increased CNS depression). Products include:
Etrafon 2355
Triavil Tablets 1757
Trilafon 2389

Phenelzine Sulfate (Enhances CNS effects of butalbital). Products include:
Nardil 1920

Phenobarbital (Increased CNS depression). Products include:
Arco-Lase Plus Tablets 512
Bellergal-S Tablets 2250
Donnatal 2060
Donnatal Extentabs 2061
Donnatal Tablets 2060
Phenobarbital Elixir and Tablets 1469
Quadrinal Tablets 1350

Phenylbutazone (Increased risk of peptic ulceration and bleeding).
No products indexed under this heading.

Piroxicam (Increased risk of peptic ulceration and bleeding). Products include:
Feldene Capsules 1965

Prazepam (Increased CNS depression).
No products indexed under this heading.

IMPORTANT NOTE: Always consult each drug listing in the patient's regimen for possible interactions.

Prednisolone Acetate (Potential for salicylism when corticosteroids therapy is stopped). Products include:
- AK-CIDE ⊙ 202
- AK-CIDE Ointment ⊙ 202
- Blephamide Liquifilm Sterile Ophthalmic Suspension 476
- Blephamide Ointment ⊙ 237
- Econopred & Econopred Plus Ophthalmic Suspensions ⊙ 217
- Poly-Pred Liquifilm ⊙ 248
- Pred Forte ⊙ 250
- Pred Mild ⊙ 253
- Pred-G Liquifilm Sterile Ophthalmic Suspension ⊙ 251
- Pred-G S.O.P. Sterile Ophthalmic Ointment ⊙ 252
- Vasocidin Ointment ⊙ 268

Prednisolone Sodium Phosphate (Potential for salicylism when corticosteroids therapy is stopped). Products include:
- AK-Pred ⊙ 204
- Hydeltrasol Injection, Sterile 1665
- Inflamase ⊙ 265
- Pediapred Oral Liquid 995
- Vasocidin Ophthalmic Solution ⊙ 270

Prednisolone Tebutate (Potential for salicylism when corticosteroids therapy is stopped). Products include:
- Hydeltra-T.B.A. Sterile Suspension 1667

Prednisone (Potential for salicylism when corticosteroids therapy is stopped). Products include:
- Deltasone Tablets 2595

Probenecid (Reduced uricosuric effects). Products include:
- Benemid Tablets 1611
- ColBENEMID Tablets 1622

Prochlorperazine (Increased CNS depression). Products include:
- Compazine 2470

Promethazine Hydrochloride (Increased CNS depression). Products include:
- Mepergan Injection 2753
- Phenergan with Codeine 2777
- Phenergan with Dextromethorphan 2778
- Phenergan Injection 2773
- Phenergan Suppositories 2775
- Phenergan Syrup 2774
- Phenergan Tablets 2775
- Phenergan VC 2779
- Phenergan VC with Codeine 2781

Propofol (Increased CNS depression). Products include:
- Diprivan Injection 2833

Propoxyphene Hydrochloride (Increased CNS depression). Products include:
- Darvon 1435
- Wygesic Tablets 2827

Propoxyphene Napsylate (Increased CNS depression). Products include:
- Darvon-N/Darvocet-N 1433

Quazepam (Increased CNS depression). Products include:
- Doral Tablets 2664

Risperidone (Increased CNS depression). Products include:
- Risperdal 1301

Secobarbital Sodium (Increased CNS depression). Products include:
- Seconal Sodium Pulvules 1474

Selegiline Hydrochloride (Enhances CNS effects of butalbital). Products include:
- Eldepryl Tablets 2550

Sufentanil Citrate (Increased CNS depression). Products include:
- Sufenta Injection 1309

Sulfinpyrazone (Reduced uricosuric effects). Products include:
- Anturane 807

Sulindac (Increased risk of peptic ulceration and bleeding). Products include:
- Clinoril Tablets 1618

Temazepam (Increased CNS depression). Products include:
- Restoril Capsules 2284

Thiamylal Sodium (Increased CNS depression).
- No products indexed under this heading.

Thioridazine Hydrochloride (Increased CNS depression). Products include:
- Mellaril 2269

Thiothixene (Increased CNS depression). Products include:
- Navane Capsules and Concentrate 2201
- Navane Intramuscular 2202

Tolazamide (Potential for hypoglycemia).
- No products indexed under this heading.

Tolbutamide (Potential for hypoglycemia).
- No products indexed under this heading.

Tolmetin Sodium (Increased risk of peptic ulceration and bleeding). Products include:
- Tolectin (200, 400 and 600 mg) 1581

Tranylcypromine Sulfate (Enhances CNS effects of butalbital). Products include:
- Parnate Tablets 2503

Triamcinolone (Potential for salicylism when corticosteroids therapy is stopped). Products include:
- Aristocort Tablets 1022

Triamcinolone Acetonide (Potential for salicylism when corticosteroids therapy is stopped). Products include:
- Aristocort A 0.025% Cream 1027
- Aristocort A 0.5% Cream 1031
- Aristocort A 0.1% Cream 1029
- Aristocort A 0.1% Ointment 1030
- Azmacort Oral Inhaler 2011
- Nasacort Nasal Inhaler 2024

Triamcinolone Diacetate (Potential for salicylism when corticosteroids therapy is stopped). Products include:
- Aristocort Suspension (Forte Parenteral) 1027
- Aristocort Suspension (Intralesional) 1025

Triamcinolone Hexacetonide (Potential for salicylism when corticosteroids therapy is stopped). Products include:
- Aristospan Suspension (Intra-articular) 1033
- Aristospan Suspension (Intralesional) 1032

Triazolam (Increased CNS depression). Products include:
- Halcion Tablets 2611

Trifluoperazine Hydrochloride (Increased CNS depression). Products include:
- Stelazine 2514

Warfarin Sodium (Enhanced effects of anticoagulants). Products include:
- Coumadin 926

Zolpidem Tartrate (Increased CNS depression). Products include:
- Ambien Tablets 2416

Food Interactions

Alcohol (Increased CNS depression).

FIORINAL TABLETS
(Butalbital, Aspirin) 2261
See **Fiorinal Capsules**

FLAGYL 375 CAPSULES
(Metronidazole) 2434

May interact with oral anticoagulants, lithium preparations, and certain other agents. Compounds in these categories include:

Cimetidine (May prolong the half-life and decrease plasma clearance of metronidazole). Products include:
- Tagamet Tablets 2516

Dicumarol (Metronidazole may potentiate the anticoagulant effect resulting in prolongation of prothrombin time).
- No products indexed under this heading.

Disulfiram (Psychotic reactions have been reported in alcoholic patients who are using metronidazole and disulfiram concurrently, do not give metronidazole to patients who have taken disulfiram within the last 2 weeks). Products include:
- Antabuse Tablets 2695

Lithium Carbonate (In patients stabilized on relatively high-dose of lithium, short-term metronidazole therapy has been associated with elevation of serum lithium resulting in lithium toxicity). Products include:
- Eskalith 2485
- Lithium Carbonate Capsules & Tablets 2230
- Lithonate/Lithotabs/Lithobid 2543

Lithium Citrate (In patients stabilized on relatively high-dose of lithium, short-term metronidazole therapy has been associated with elevation of serum lithium resulting in lithium toxicity).
- No products indexed under this heading.

Phenobarbital (May accelerate the elimination of metronidazole, resulting in reduced plasma levels). Products include:
- Arco-Lase Plus Tablets 512
- Bellergal-S Tablets 2250
- Donnatal 2060
- Donnatal Extentabs 2061
- Donnatal Tablets 2060
- Phenobarbital Elixir and Tablets 1469
- Quadrinal Tablets 1350

Phenytoin (May accelerate the elimination of metronidazole, resulting in reduced plasma levels; impaired phenytoin clearance has been reported). Products include:
- Dilantin Infatabs 1908
- Dilantin-125 Suspension 1911

Phenytoin Sodium (May accelerate the elimination of metronidazole, resulting in reduced plasma levels; impaired phenytoin clearance has been reported). Products include:
- Dilantin Kapseals 1906
- Dilantin Parenteral 1910

Warfarin Sodium (Metronidazole may potentiate the anticoagulant effect resulting in prolongation of prothrombin time). Products include:
- Coumadin 926

Food Interactions

Alcohol (Alcohol should not be consumed during metronidazole therapy and for at least three days afterward because abdominal cramps, nausea, vomiting, headaches, and flushing may occur).

FLAGYL I.V.
(Metronidazole Hydrochloride) 2247

May interact with oral anticoagulants and certain other agents. Compounds in these categories include:

Cimetidine (Decreases plasma clearance of metronidazole). Products include:
- Tagamet Tablets 2516

Cimetidine Hydrochloride (Decreases plasma clearance of metronidazole). Products include:
- Tagamet 2516

Dicumarol (Potentiation of anticoagulant effect).
- No products indexed under this heading.

Disulfiram (Psychotic reactions have been reported in alcoholic patients who are using metronidazole and disulfiram concurrently). Products include:
- Antabuse Tablets 2695

Phenobarbital (Reduces metronidazole plasma levels). Products include:
- Arco-Lase Plus Tablets 512
- Bellergal-S Tablets 2250
- Donnatal 2060
- Donnatal Extentabs 2061
- Donnatal Tablets 2060
- Phenobarbital Elixir and Tablets 1469
- Quadrinal Tablets 1350

Phenytoin (Reduces metronidazole plasma levels; impaired clearance of phenytoin). Products include:
- Dilantin Infatabs 1908
- Dilantin-125 Suspension 1911

Phenytoin Sodium (Reduces metronidazole plasma levels; impaired clearance of phenytoin). Products include:
- Dilantin Kapseals 1906
- Dilantin Parenteral 1910

Warfarin Sodium (Potentiation of anticoagulant effect). Products include:
- Coumadin 926

Food Interactions

Alcohol (Potential for abdominal cramps, nausea, vomiting, and headaches, and flushing).

FLAGYL I.V. RTU
(Metronidazole) 2247
See **Flagyl I.V.**

FLAREX OPHTHALMIC SUSPENSION
(Fluorometholone Acetate) ⊙ 218
None cited in PDR database.

FLEET BABYLAX
(Glycerin) 1001
None cited in PDR database.

FLEET BISACODYL ENEMA
(Bisacodyl) 1002
None cited in PDR database.

FLEET CHILDREN'S ENEMA
(Sodium Phosphate, Dibasic, Sodium Phosphate, Monobasic) 1002
See **Fleet Enema**

FLEET ENEMA
(Sodium Phosphate, Dibasic, Sodium Phosphate, Monobasic) 1002
May interact with:

Calcium Channel Blockers, Unspecified (Effect not specified).

Diuretics, Unspecified (Effect not specified).

FLEET GLYCERIN LAXATIVE RECTAL APPLICATORS
(Glycerin) 1001
None cited in PDR database.

FLEET MINERAL OIL ENEMA
(Mineral Oil) 1002
None cited in PDR database.

(▭ Described in PDR For Nonprescription Drugs) (⊙ Described in PDR For Ophthalmology)

FLEET PAIN RELIEF PADS
(Pramoxine Hydrochloride) 1003
None cited in PDR database.

FLEET PHOSPHO-SODA
(Sodium Phosphate, Dibasic, Sodium Phosphate, Monobasic)........................1003
None cited in PDR database.

FLEET PREP KITS
(Sodium Phosphate, Dibasic, Sodium Phosphate, Monobasic)........................1003
May interact with antacids and certain other agents. Compounds in these categories include:

Aluminum Carbonate Gel (Concurrent use within one-hour should be avoided). Products include:
- Basaljel................................... 2703

Aluminum Hydroxide (Concurrent use within one-hour should be avoided). Products include:
- ALternaGEL Liquid 1316
- Maximum Strength Ascriptin .... ▣ 630
- Cama Arthritis Pain Reliever.......... ▣ 785
- Gaviscon Extra Strength Relief Formula Antacid Tablets.............. ▣ 819
- Gaviscon Extra Strength Relief Formula Liquid Antacid .... ▣ 819
- Gaviscon Liquid Antacid .... ▣ 820
- Gelusil Liquid & Tablets .... ▣ 855
- Maalox Heartburn Relief Suspension .... ▣ 642
- Maalox Heartburn Relief Tablets.... ▣ 641
- Maalox Magnesia and Alumina Oral Suspension .... ▣ 642
- Maalox Plus Tablets .... ▣ 643
- Extra Strength Maalox Antacid Plus Antigas Liquid and Tablets ▣ 638
- Tempo Soft Antacid .... ▣ 835

Aluminum Hydroxide Gel (Concurrent use within one-hour should be avoided). Products include:
- ALternaGEL Liquid .... ▣ 659
- Aludrox Oral Suspension 2695
- Amphojel Suspension 2695
- Amphojel Suspension without Flavor 2695
- Amphojel Tablets.............................. 2695
- Arthritis Pain Ascriptin .... ▣ 631
- Regular Strength Ascriptin Tablets .... ▣ 629
- Gaviscon Antacid Tablets................ ▣ 819
- Gaviscon-2 Antacid Tablets .... ▣ 820
- Mylanta Liquid 1317
- Mylanta Tablets .... ▣ 660
- Mylanta Double Strength Liquid 1317
- Mylanta Double Strength Tablets .. ▣ 660
- Nephrox Suspension .... ▣ 655

Dihydroxyaluminum Sodium Carbonate (Concurrent use within one-hour should be avoided).
- No products indexed under this heading.

Magaldrate (Concurrent use within one-hour should be avoided).
- No products indexed under this heading.

Magnesium Hydroxide (Concurrent use within one-hour should be avoided). Products include:
- Aludrox Oral Suspension 2695
- Arthritis Pain Ascriptin .... ▣ 631
- Maximum Strength Ascriptin .... ▣ 630
- Regular Strength Ascriptin Tablets .... ▣ 629
- Di-Gel Antacid/Anti-Gas .... ▣ 801
- Gelusil Liquid & Tablets .... ▣ 855
- Maalox Magnesia and Alumina Oral Suspension .... ▣ 642
- Maalox Plus Tablets .... ▣ 643
- Extra Strength Maalox Antacid Plus Antigas Liquid and Tablets ▣ 638
- Mylanta Calcium Carbonate and Magnesium Hydroxide Tablets...... 1318
- Mylanta Liquid 1317
- Mylanta Tablets .... ▣ 660
- Mylanta Double Strength Liquid 1317
- Mylanta Double Strength Tablets .. ▣ 660
- Phillips' Milk of Magnesia Liquid.... ▣ 729
- Rolaids Tablets .... ▣ 843
- Tempo Soft Antacid .... ▣ 835

Magnesium Oxide (Concurrent use within one-hour should be avoided). Products include:
- Beelith Tablets 639
- Bufferin Analgesic Tablets and Caplets .... ▣ 613
- Caltrate PLUS .... ▣ 665
- Cama Arthritis Pain Reliever........... ▣ 785
- Mag-Ox 400 668
- Uro-Mag... 668

Sodium Bicarbonate (Concurrent use within one-hour should be avoided). Products include:
- Alka-Seltzer Effervescent Antacid and Pain Reliever .... ▣ 701
- Alka-Seltzer Extra Strength Effervescent Antacid and Pain Reliever .... ▣ 703
- Alka-Seltzer Gold Effervescent Antacid .... ▣ 703
- Alka-Seltzer Lemon Lime Effervescent Antacid and Pain Reliever .... ▣ 703
- Arm & Hammer Pure Baking Soda .... ▣ 627
- Ceo-Two Rectal Suppositories 666
- Citrocarbonate Antacid .... ▣ 770
- Massengill Disposable Douches....... ▣ 820
- Massengill Liquid Concentrate........ ▣ 820
- NuLYTELY... 689
- Cherry Flavor NuLYTELY 689

Food Interactions

Dairy products (Concurrent use within one-hour should be avoided).

FLEET SOF-LAX
(Docusate Sodium) 1004
None cited in PDR database.

FLEET SOF-LAX OVERNIGHT
(Docusate Sodium, Casanthranol)......1004
None cited in PDR database.

FLEXERIL TABLETS
(Cyclobenzaprine Hydrochloride) 1661
May interact with central nervous system depressants, anticholinergics, monoamine oxidase inhibitors, barbiturates, and certain other agents. Compounds in these categories include:

Alfentanil Hydrochloride (Enhanced effect of CNS depressants). Products include:
- Alfenta Injection 1286

Alprazolam (Enhanced effect of CNS depressants). Products include:
- Xanax Tablets 2649

Aprobarbital (Enhanced effect of barbiturates).
- No products indexed under this heading.

Atropine Sulfate (Use cyclobenzaprine with caution). Products include:
- Arco-Lase Plus Tablets 512
- Atrohist Plus Tablets 454
- Atropine Sulfate Sterile Ophthalmic Solution .... ⊙ 233
- Donnatal 2060
- Donnatal Extentabs.......................... 2061
- Donnatal Tablets 2060
- Lomotil 2439
- Motofen Tablets 784
- Urised Tablets................................... 1964

Belladonna Alkaloids (Use cyclobenzaprine with caution). Products include:
- Bellergal-S Tablets 2250
- Hyland's Bed Wetting Tablets .... ▣ 828
- Hyland's EnurAid Tablets................ ▣ 829
- Hyland's Teething Tablets .... ▣ 830

Benztropine Mesylate (Use cyclobenzaprine with caution). Products include:
- Cogentin 1621

Biperiden Hydrochloride (Use cyclobenzaprine with caution). Products include:
- Akineton 1333

Buprenorphine (Enhanced effect of CNS depressants). Products include:
- Buprenex Injectable 2006

Buspirone Hydrochloride (Enhanced effect of CNS depressants). Products include:
- BuSpar 737

Butabarbital (Enhanced effect of barbiturates).
- No products indexed under this heading.

Butalbital (Enhanced effect of barbiturates). Products include:
- Esgic-plus Tablets 1013
- Fioricet Tablets................................. 2258
- Fioricet with Codeine Capsules 2260
- Fiorinal Capsules 2261
- Fiorinal with Codeine Capsules 2262
- Fiorinal Tablets................................. 2261
- Phrenilin 785
- Sedapap Tablets 50 mg/650 mg .. 1543

Chlordiazepoxide (Enhanced effect of CNS depressants). Products include:
- Libritabs Tablets 2177
- Limbitrol 2180

Chlordiazepoxide Hydrochloride (Enhanced effect of CNS depressants). Products include:
- Librax Capsules 2176
- Librium Capsules 2178
- Librium Injectable 2179

Chlorpromazine (Enhanced effect of CNS depressants). Products include:
- Thorazine Suppositories.................... 2523

Chlorprothixene (Enhanced effect of CNS depressants).
- No products indexed under this heading.

Chlorprothixene Hydrochloride (Enhanced effect of CNS depressants).
- No products indexed under this heading.

Clidinium Bromide (Use cyclobenzaprine with caution). Products include:
- Librax Capsules 2176
- Quarzan Capsules 2181

Clorazepate Dipotassium (Enhanced effect of CNS depressants). Products include:
- Tranxene 451

Clozapine (Enhanced effect of CNS depressants). Products include:
- Clozaril Tablets................................. 2252

Codeine Phosphate (Enhanced effect of CNS depressants). Products include:
- Actifed with Codeine Cough Syrup.. 1067
- Brontex 1981
- Deconsal C Expectorant Syrup 456
- Deconsal Pediatric Syrup 457
- Dimetane-DC Cough Syrup 2059
- Empirin with Codeine Tablets........... 1093
- Fioricet with Codeine Capsules 2260
- Fiorinal with Codeine Capsules 2262
- Isoclor Expectorant............................ 990
- Novahistine DH................................. 2462
- Novahistine Expectorant.................... 2463
- Nucofed 2051
- Phenergan with Codeine................... 2777
- Phenergan VC with Codeine 2781
- Robitussin A-C Syrup 2073
- Robitussin-DAC Syrup 2074
- Ryna .... ▣ 841
- Soma Compound w/Codeine Tablets 2676
- Tussi-Organidin NR Liquid and S NR Liquid 2677
- Tylenol with Codeine 1583

Desflurane (Enhanced effect of CNS depressants). Products include:
- Suprane 1813

Dezocine (Enhanced effect of CNS depressants). Products include:
- Dalgan Injection 538

Diazepam (Enhanced effect of CNS depressants). Products include:
- Dizac 1809
- Valium Injectable 2182
- Valium Tablets 2183
- Valrelease Capsules 2169

Dicyclomine Hydrochloride (Use cyclobenzaprine with caution). Products include:
- Bentyl 1501

Droperidol (Enhanced effect of CNS depressants). Products include:
- Inapsine Injection............................. 1296

Enflurane (Enhanced effect of CNS depressants).
- No products indexed under this heading.

Estazolam (Enhanced effect of CNS depressants). Products include:
- ProSom Tablets 449

Ethchlorvynol (Enhanced effect of CNS depressants). Products include:
- Placidyl Capsules.............................. 448

Ethinamate (Enhanced effect of CNS depressants).
- No products indexed under this heading.

Fentanyl (Enhanced effect of CNS depressants). Products include:
- Duragesic Transdermal System........ 1288

Fentanyl Citrate (Enhanced effect of CNS depressants). Products include:
- Sublimaze Injection.......................... 1307

Fluphenazine Decanoate (Enhanced effect of CNS depressants). Products include:
- Prolixin Decanoate 509

Fluphenazine Enanthate (Enhanced effect of CNS depressants). Products include:
- Prolixin Enanthate 509

Fluphenazine Hydrochloride (Enhanced effect of CNS depressants). Products include:
- Prolixin 509

Flurazepam Hydrochloride (Enhanced effect of CNS depressants). Products include:
- Dalmane Capsules............................. 2173

Furazolidone (Contraindication; hyperpyretic crisis; severe convulsions; death). Products include:
- Furoxone 2046

Glutethimide (Enhanced effect of CNS depressants).
- No products indexed under this heading.

Glycopyrrolate (Use cyclobenzaprine with caution). Products include:
- Robinul Forte Tablets........................ 2072
- Robinul Injectable 2072
- Robinul Tablets................................. 2072

Guanethidine Monosulfate (Antihypertensive action of guanethidine blocked). Products include:
- Esimil Tablets 822
- Ismelin Tablets 827

Haloperidol (Enhanced effect of CNS depressants). Products include:
- Haldol Injection, Tablets and Concentrate 1575

Haloperidol Decanoate (Enhanced effect of CNS depressants). Products include:
- Haldol Decanoate.............................. 1577

Hydrocodone Bitartrate (Enhanced effect of CNS depressants). Products include:
- Anexsia 5/500 Elixir 1781
- Anexia Tablets.................................. 1782
- Codiclear DH Syrup 791
- Deconamine CX Cough and Cold Liquid and Tablets.......................... 1319
- Duratuss HD Elixir............................ 2565
- Hycodan Tablets and Syrup 930
- Hycomine Compound Tablets 932
- Hycomine 931

IMPORTANT NOTE: Always consult each drug listing in the patient's regimen for possible interactions.

Flexeril **Interactions Index** **420**

Hycotuss Expectorant Syrup 933
Hydrocet Capsules 782
Lorcet 10/650 1018
Lortab 2566
Tussend 1783
Tussend Expectorant 1785
Vicodin Tablets 1356
Vicodin ES Tablets 1357
Vicodin Tuss Expectorant 1358
Zydone Capsules 949

Hydrocodone Polistirex (Enhanced effect of CNS depressants). Products include:
Tussionex Pennkinetic Extended-Release Suspension 998

Hydroxyzine Hydrochloride (Enhanced effect of CNS depressants). Products include:
Atarax Tablets & Syrup 2185
Marax Tablets & DF Syrup 2200
Vistaril Intramuscular Solution 2216

Hyoscyamine (Use cyclobenzaprine with caution). Products include:
Cystospaz Tablets 1963
Urised Tablets 1964

Hyoscyamine Sulfate (Use cyclobenzaprine with caution). Products include:
Arco-Lase Plus Tablets 512
Atrohist Plus Tablets 454
Cystospaz-M Capsules 1963
Donnatal 2060
Donnatal Extentabs 2061
Donnatal Tablets 2060
Kutrase Capsules 2402
Levsin/Levsinex/Levbid 2405

Ipratropium Bromide (Use cyclobenzaprine with caution). Products include:
Atrovent Inhalation Aerosol 671
Atrovent Inhalation Solution 673

Isocarboxazid (Contraindication; hyperpyretic crisis; severe convulsions; death).
No products indexed under this heading.

Isoflurane (Enhanced effect of CNS depressants).
No products indexed under this heading.

Ketamine Hydrochloride (Enhanced effect of CNS depressants).
No products indexed under this heading.

Levomethadyl Acetate Hydrochloride (Enhanced effect of CNS depressants). Products include:
Orlamm 2239

Levorphanol Tartrate (Enhanced effect of CNS depressants). Products include:
Levo-Dromoran 2129

Lorazepam (Enhanced effect of CNS depressants). Products include:
Ativan Injection 2698
Ativan Tablets 2700

Loxapine Hydrochloride (Enhanced effect of CNS depressants). Products include:
Loxitane 1378

Loxapine Succinate (Enhanced effect of CNS depressants). Products include:
Loxitane Capsules 1378

Mepenzolate Bromide (Use cyclobenzaprine with caution).
No products indexed under this heading.

Meperidine Hydrochloride (Enhanced effect of CNS depressants). Products include:
Demerol 2308
Mepergan Injection 2753

Mephobarbital (Enhanced effect of barbiturates). Products include:
Mebaral Tablets 2322

Meprobamate (Enhanced effect of CNS depressants). Products include:
Miltown Tablets 2672

PMB 200 and PMB 400 2783

Mesoridazine Besylate (Enhanced effect of CNS depressants). Products include:
Serentil 684

Methadone Hydrochloride (Enhanced effect of CNS depressants). Products include:
Methadone Hydrochloride Oral Concentrate 2233
Methadone Hydrochloride Oral Solution & Tablets 2235

Methohexital Sodium (Enhanced effect of CNS depressants). Products include:
Brevital Sodium Vials 1429

Methotrimeprazine (Enhanced effect of CNS depressants). Products include:
Levoprome 1274

Methoxyflurane (Enhanced effect of CNS depressants).
No products indexed under this heading.

Midazolam Hydrochloride (Enhanced effect of CNS depressants). Products include:
Versed Injection 2170

Molindone Hydrochloride (Enhanced effect of CNS depressants). Products include:
Moban Tablets and Concentrate 1048

Morphine Sulfate (Enhanced effect of CNS depressants). Products include:
Astramorph/PF Injection, USP (Preservative-Free) 535
Duramorph 962
Infumorph 200 and Infumorph 500 Sterile Solutions 965
MS Contin Tablets 1994
MSIR 1997
Oramorph SR (Morphine Sulfate Sustained Release Tablets) 2236
RMS Suppositories 2657
Roxanol 2243

Opium Alkaloids (Enhanced effect of CNS depressants).
No products indexed under this heading.

Oxazepam (Enhanced effect of CNS depressants). Products include:
Serax Capsules 2810
Serax Tablets 2810

Oxybutynin Chloride (Use cyclobenzaprine with caution). Products include:
Ditropan 1516

Oxycodone Hydrochloride (Enhanced effect of CNS depressants). Products include:
Percocet Tablets 938
Percodan Tablets 939
Percodan-Demi Tablets 940
Roxicodone Tablets, Oral Solution & Intensol (Oxycodone) 2244
Tylox Capsules 1584

Oxyphenonium Bromide (Use cyclobenzaprine with caution).

Pentobarbital Sodium (Enhanced effect of barbiturates). Products include:
Nembutal Sodium Capsules 436
Nembutal Sodium Solution 438
Nembutal Sodium Suppositories 440

Perphenazine (Enhanced effect of CNS depressants). Products include:
Etrafon 2355
Triavil Tablets 1757
Trilafon 2389

Phenelzine Sulfate (Contraindication; hyperpyretic crisis; severe convulsions; death). Products include:
Nardil 1920

Phenobarbital (Enhanced effect of barbiturates). Products include:
Arco-Lase Plus Tablets 512
Bellergal-S Tablets 2250
Donnatal 2060
Donnatal Extentabs 2061
Donnatal Tablets 2060
Phenobarbital Elixir and Tablets 1469
Quadrinal Tablets 1350

Prazepam (Enhanced effect of CNS depressants).
No products indexed under this heading.

Prochlorperazine (Enhanced effects of CNS depressants). Products include:
Compazine 2470

Procyclidine Hydrochloride (Use cyclobenzaprine with caution). Products include:
Kemadrin Tablets 1112

Promethazine Hydrochloride (Enhanced effect of CNS depressants). Products include:
Mepergan Injection 2753
Phenergan with Codeine 2777
Phenergan with Dextromethorphan 2778
Phenergan Injection 2773
Phenergan Suppositories 2775
Phenergan Syrup 2774
Phenergan Tablets 2775
Phenergan VC 2779
Phenergan VC with Codeine 2781

Propantheline Bromide (Use cyclobenzaprine with caution). Products include:
Pro-Banthīne Tablets 2052

Propofol (Enhanced effect of CNS depressants). Products include:
Diprivan Injection 2833

Propoxyphene Hydrochloride (Enhanced effect of CNS depressants). Products include:
Darvon 1435
Wygesic Tablets 2827

Propoxyphene Napsylate (Enhanced effect of CNS depressants). Products include:
Darvon-N/Darvocet-N 1433

Quazepam (Enhanced effect of CNS depressants). Products include:
Doral Tablets 2664

Risperidone (Enhanced effect of CNS depressants). Products include:
Risperdal 1301

Scopolamine (Use cyclobenzaprine with caution). Products include:
Transderm Scōp Transdermal Therapeutic System 869

Scopolamine Hydrobromide (Use cyclobenzaprine with caution). Products include:
Atrohist Plus Tablets 454
Donnatal 2060
Donnatal Extentabs 2061
Donnatal Tablets 2060

Secobarbital Sodium (Enhanced effect of barbiturates). Products include:
Seconal Sodium Pulvules 1474

Selegiline Hydrochloride (Contraindication; hyperpyretic crisis; severe convulsions; death). Products include:
Eldepryl Tablets 2550

Sufentanil Citrate (Enhanced effect of CNS depressants). Products include:
Sufenta Injection 1309

Temazepam (Enhanced effect of CNS depressants). Products include:
Restoril Capsules 2284

Thiamylal Sodium (Enhanced effect of barbiturates).
No products indexed under this heading.

Thioridazine Hydrochloride (Enhanced effect of CNS depressants). Products include:
Mellaril 2269

Thiothixene (Enhanced effect of CNS depressants). Products include:
Navane Capsules and Concentrate 2201
Navane Intramuscular 2202

Tranylcypromine Sulfate (Contraindication; hyperpyretic crisis; severe convulsions; death). Products include:
Parnate Tablets 2503

Triazolam (Enhanced effect of CNS depressants). Products include:
Halcion Tablets 2611

Tridihexethyl Chloride (Use cyclobenzaprine with caution).
No products indexed under this heading.

Trifluoperazine Hydrochloride (Enhanced effect of CNS depressants). Products include:
Stelazine 2514

Trihexyphenidyl Hydrochloride (Use cyclobenzaprine with caution). Products include:
Artane 1368

Zolpidem Tartrate (Enhanced effect of CNS depressants). Products include:
Ambien Tablets 2416

Food Interactions

Alcohol (Enhanced effect of alcohol).

FLINTSTONES CHILDREN'S CHEWABLE VITAMINS
(Vitamins with Minerals) .... ▣ 718
None cited in PDR database.

FLINTSTONES CHILDREN'S CHEWABLE VITAMINS PLUS EXTRA C
(Vitamins with Minerals) .... ▣ 722
None cited in PDR database.

FLINTSTONES CHILDREN'S CHEWABLE VITAMINS PLUS IRON
(Vitamins with Iron) .... ▣ 718
None cited in PDR database.

FLINTSTONES COMPLETE WITH CALCIUM, IRON & MINERALS CHILDREN'S CHEWABLE VITAMINS
(Vitamins with Minerals) .... ▣ 721
None cited in PDR database.

FLINTSTONES PLUS CALCIUM CHILDREN'S CHEWABLE VITAMINS
(Vitamins with Minerals) .... ▣ 721
None cited in PDR database.

FLONASE NASAL SPRAY
(Fluticasone Propionate) 1098
None cited in PDR database.

FLORINEF ACETATE TABLETS
(Fludrocortisone Acetate) 505
May interact with barbiturates, estrogens, androgens, potassium-depleting diuretics, loop diuretics, cardiac glycosides, oral anticoagulants, oral hypoglycemic agents, insulin, and certain other agents. Compounds in these categories include:

Acarbose (Diminished antidiabetic effect; monitor symptoms of hyperglycemia).
No products indexed under this heading.

Amphotericin B (Potential for enhanced hypokalemia; serum potassium levels should be monitored frequently). Products include:
Fungizone Intravenous 506

Florinef Acetate

Aprobarbital (Increased metabolic clearance of fludrocortisone acetate because of the induction of hepatic enzymes).

No products indexed under this heading.

Aspirin (Increased ulcerogenic effect; decreased pharmacologic effect of aspirin). Products include:

Alka-Seltzer Effervescent Antacid and Pain Reliever .... ⊕ 701
Alka-Seltzer Extra Strength Effervescent Antacid and Pain Reliever .... ⊕ 703
Alka-Seltzer Lemon Lime Effervescent Antacid and Pain Reliever .... ⊕ 703
Alka-Seltzer Plus Cold Medicine .... ⊕ 705
Alka-Seltzer Plus Cold & Cough Medicine .... ⊕ 708
Alka-Seltzer Plus Night-Time Cold Medicine .... ⊕ 707
Alka Seltzer Plus Sinus Medicine .. ⊕ 707
Arthritis Foundation Safety Coated Aspirin Tablets .... ⊕ 675
Arthritis Pain Ascriptin .... ⊕ 631
Maximum Strength Ascriptin .... ⊕ 630
Regular Strength Ascriptin Tablets .... ⊕ 629
Arthritis Strength BC Powder .... ⊕ 609
BC Cold Powder Multi-Symptom Formula (Cold-Sinus-Allergy) ...... ⊕ 609
BC Cold Powder Non-Drowsy Formula (Cold-Sinus) .... ⊕ 609
BC Powder .... ⊕ 609
Bayer Children's Chewable Aspirin .... ⊕ 711
Genuine Bayer Aspirin Tablets & Caplets .... ⊕ 713
Extra Strength Bayer Arthritis Pain Regimen Formula .... ⊕ 711
Extra Strength Bayer Aspirin Caplets & Tablets .... ⊕ 712
Extended-Release Bayer 8-Hour Aspirin .... ⊕ 712
Extra Strength Bayer Plus Aspirin Caplets .... ⊕ 713
Extra Strength Bayer PM Aspirin .. ⊕ 713
Bayer Enteric Aspirin .... ⊕ 709
Bufferin Analgesic Tablets and Caplets .... ⊕ 613
Arthritis Strength Bufferin Analgesic Caplets .... ⊕ 614
Extra Strength Bufferin Analgesic Tablets .... ⊕ 615
Cama Arthritis Pain Reliever .... ⊕ 785
Darvon Compound-65 Pulvules 1435
Easprin 1914
Ecotrin 2455
Ecotrin Enteric Coated Aspirin Maximum Strength Tablets and Caplets .... ⊕ 816
Ecotrin Enteric Coated Aspirin Regular Strength Tablets 2455
Empirin Aspirin Tablets .... ⊕ 854
Empirin with Codeine Tablets........... 1093
Excedrin Extra-Strength Analgesic Tablets & Caplets 732
Fiorinal Capsules 2261
Fiorinal with Codeine Capsules 2262
Fiorinal Tablets 2261
Halfprin 1362
Healthprin Aspirin 2455
Norgesic.. 1496
Percodan Tablets.................................. 939
Percodan-Demi Tablets........................ 940
Robaxisal Tablets.................................. 2071
Soma Compound w/Codeine Tablets 2676
Soma Compound Tablets 2675
St. Joseph Adult Chewable Aspirin (81 mg.) .... ⊕ 808
Talwin Compound 2335
Ursinus Inlay-Tabs................................ ⊕ 794
Vanquish Analgesic Caplets .... ⊕ 731

Bendroflumethiazide (Potential for enhanced hypokalemia; serum potassium levels should be monitored frequently).

No products indexed under this heading.

Bumetanide (Potential for enhanced hypokalemia; serum potassium levels should be monitored frequently). Products include:

Bumex 2093

Butabarbital (Increased metabolic clearance of fludrocortisone acetate because of the induction of hepatic enzymes).

No products indexed under this heading.

Butalbital (Increased metabolic clearance of fludrocortisone acetate because of the induction of hepatic enzymes). Products include:

Esgic-plus Tablets 1013
Fioricet Tablets 2258
Fioricet with Codeine Capsules 2260
Fiorinal Capsules 2261
Fiorinal with Codeine Capsules 2262
Fiorinal Tablets 2261
Phenrelin 785
Sedapap Tablets 50 mg/650 mg .. 1543

Chlorothiazide (Potential for enhanced hypokalemia; serum potassium levels should be monitored frequently). Products include:

Aldoclor Tablets 1598
Diupres Tablets 1650
Diuril Oral 1653

Chlorothiazide Sodium (Potential for enhanced hypokalemia; serum potassium levels should be monitored frequently). Products include:

Diuril Sodium Intravenous 1652

Chlorotrianisene (Increased levels of corticosteroid-binding globulin, thereby increasing the bound (inactive) fraction).

No products indexed under this heading.

Chlorpropamide (Diminished antidiabetic effect; monitor symptoms of hyperglycemia). Products include:

Diabinese Tablets 1935

Deslanoside (Enhanced possibility of arrhythmias or digitalis toxicity associated with hypokalemia).

No products indexed under this heading.

Dicumarol (Decreased prothrombin time response).

No products indexed under this heading.

Dienestrol (Increased levels of corticosteroid-binding globulin, thereby increasing the bound (inactive) fraction). Products include:

Ortho Dienestrol Cream 1866

Diethylstilbestrol (Increased levels of corticosteroid-binding globulin, thereby increasing the bound (inactive) fraction). Products include:

Diethylstilbestrol Tablets 1437

Digitoxin (Enhanced possibility of arrhythmias or digitalis toxicity associated with hypokalemia). Products include:

Crystodigin Tablets 1433

Digoxin (Enhanced possibility of arrhythmias or digitalis toxicity associated with hypokalemia). Products include:

Lanoxicaps 1117
Lanoxin Elixir Pediatric 1120
Lanoxin Injection 1123
Lanoxin Injection Pediatric.................. 1126
Lanoxin Tablets 1128

Estradiol (Increased levels of corticosteroid-binding globulin, thereby increasing the bound (inactive) fraction). Products include:

Climara Transdermal System 645
Estrace Cream and Tablets 749
Estraderm Transdermal System 824

Estrogens, Conjugated (Increased levels of corticosteroid-binding globulin, thereby increasing the bound (inactive) fraction). Products include:

PMB 200 and PMB 400 2783
Premarin Intravenous 2787
Premarin with Methyltestosterone.. 2794
Premarin Tablets 2789
Premarin Vaginal Cream.................... 2791
Premphase 2797
Prempro.. 2801

Estrogens, Esterified (Increased levels of corticosteroid-binding globulin, thereby increasing the bound (inactive) fraction). Products include:

ESTRATAB Tablets (0.3, 0.625, 1.25, 2.5 mg) 2536
Estratest 2539
Menest Tablets 2494

Estropipate (Increased levels of corticosteroid-binding globulin, thereby increasing the bound (inactive) fraction). Products include:

Ogen Tablets 2627
Ogen Vaginal Cream............................ 2630
Ortho-Est.. 1869

Ethacrynic Acid (Potential for enhanced hypokalemia; serum potassium levels should be monitored frequently). Products include:

Edecrin Tablets.. 1657

Ethinyl Estradiol (Increased levels of corticosteroid-binding globulin, thereby increasing the bound (inactive) fraction). Products include:

Brevicon.. 2088
Demulen 2428
Desogen Tablets.................................... 1817
Levlen/Tri-Levlen 651
Lo/Ovral Tablets 2746
Lo/Ovral-28 Tablets.............................. 2751
Modicon.. 1872
Nordette-21 Tablets.............................. 2755
Nordette-28 Tablets.............................. 2758
Norinyl 2088
Ortho-Cept 1851
Ortho-Cyclen/Ortho-Tri-Cyclen 1858
Ortho-Novum.. 1872
Ortho-Cyclen/Ortho Tri-Cyclen 1858
Ovcon 760
Ovral Tablets 2770
Ovral-28 Tablets 2770
Levlen/Tri-Levlen 651
Tri-Norinyl.. 2164
Triphasil-21 Tablets 2814
Triphasil-28 Tablets 2819

Fluoxymesterone (Enhanced tendency toward edema). Products include:

Halotestin Tablets 2614

Furosemide (Potential for enhanced hypokalemia; serum potassium levels should be monitored frequently). Products include:

Lasix Injection, Oral Solution and Tablets 1240

Glipizide (Diminished antidiabetic effect; monitor symptoms of hyperglycemia). Products include:

Glucotrol Tablets 1967
Glucotrol XL Extended Release Tablets 1968

Glyburide (Diminished antidiabetic effect; monitor symptoms of hyperglycemia). Products include:

DiaBeta Tablets 1239
Glynase PresTab Tablets 2609
Micronase Tablets 2623

Hydrochlorothiazide (Potential for enhanced hypokalemia; serum potassium levels should be monitored frequently). Products include:

Aldactazide.. 2413
Aldoril Tablets 1604
Apresazide Capsules 808
Capozide 742
Dyazide 2479
Esidrix Tablets 821
Esimil Tablets 822
HydroDIURIL Tablets 1674
Hydropres Tablets.................................. 1675
Hyzaar Tablets 1677
Inderide Tablets 2732
Inderide LA Long Acting Capsules .. 2734
Lopressor HCT Tablets 832
Lotensin HCT 837
Maxzide 1380
Moduretic Tablets 1705
Oretic Tablets 443
Prinzide Tablets 1737
Ser-Ap-Es Tablets 849
Timolide Tablets...................................... 1748
Vaseretic Tablets 1765
Zestoretic 2850
Ziac 1415

Hydroflumethiazide (Potential for enhanced hypokalemia; serum potassium levels should be monitored frequently). Products include:

Diucardin Tablets.................................... 2718

Insulin, Human (Diminished antidiabetic effect; monitor symptoms of hyperglycemia).

No products indexed under this heading.

Insulin, Human Isophane Suspension (Diminished antidiabetic effect; monitor symptoms of hyperglycemia). Products include:

Novolin N Human Insulin 10 ml Vials.. 1795

Insulin, Human NPH (Diminished antidiabetic effect; monitor symptoms of hyperglycemia). Products include:

Humulin N, 100 Units 1448
Novolin N PenFill Cartridges Durable Insulin Delivery System 1798
Novolin N Prefilled Syringe Disposable Insulin Delivery System 1798

Insulin, Human Regular (Diminished antidiabetic effect; monitor symptoms of hyperglycemia). Products include:

Humulin R, 100 Units 1449
Novolin R Human Insulin 10 ml Vials.. 1795
Novolin R PenFill Cartridges Durable Insulin Delivery System 1798
Novolin R Prefilled Syringe Disposable Insulin Delivery System 1798
Velosulin BR Human Insulin 10 ml Vials.. 1795

Insulin, Human, Zinc Suspension (Diminished antidiabetic effect; monitor symptoms of hyperglycemia). Products include:

Humulin L, 100 Units 1446
Humulin U, 100 Units 1450
Novolin L Human Insulin 10 ml Vials.. 1795

Insulin, NPH (Diminished antidiabetic effect; monitor symptoms of hyperglycemia). Products include:

NPH, 100 Units 1450
Pork NPH, 100 Units.......................... 1452
Purified Pork NPH Isophane Insulin 1801

Insulin, Regular (Diminished antidiabetic effect; monitor symptoms of hyperglycemia). Products include:

Regular, 100 Units 1450
Pork Regular, 100 Units 1452
Pork Regular (Concentrated), 500 Units 1453
Purified Pork Regular Insulin 1801

Insulin, Zinc Crystals (Diminished antidiabetic effect; monitor symptoms of hyperglycemia). Products include:

NPH, 100 Units 1450

Insulin, Zinc Suspension (Diminished antidiabetic effect; monitor symptoms of hyperglycemia). Products include:

Iletin I 1450
Lente, 100 Units 1450
Iletin II 1452
Pork Lente, 100 Units.......................... 1452
Purified Pork Lente Insulin 1801

Mephobarbital (Increased metabolic clearance of fludrocortisone acetate because of the induction of hepatic enzymes). Products include:

Mebaral Tablets 2322

Metformin Hydrochloride (Diminished antidiabetic effect; monitor symptoms of hyperglycemia). Products include:

Glucophage 752

Methandrostinolone (Enhanced tendency toward edema).

IMPORTANT NOTE: Always consult each drug listing in the patient's regimen for possible interactions.

Methyclothiazide (Potential for enhanced hypokalemia; serum potassium levels should be monitored frequently). Products include:
- Enduron Tablets 420

Methyltestosterone (Enhanced tendency toward edema). Products include:
- Android Capsules, 10 mg 1250
- Android 1251
- Estratest 2539
- Oreton Methyl 1255
- Premarin with Methyltestosterone .. 2794
- Testred Capsules 1262

Norethandrolone (Enhanced tendency toward edema).

Oxandrolone (Enhanced tendency toward edema). Products include:
- Oxandrin 2862

Oxymetholone (Enhanced tendency toward edema).
- No products indexed under this heading.

Pentobarbital Sodium (Increased metabolic clearance of fludrocortisone acetate because of the induction of hepatic enzymes). Products include:
- Nembutal Sodium Capsules 436
- Nembutal Sodium Solution 438
- Nembutal Sodium Suppositories 440

Phenobarbital (Increased metabolic clearance of fludrocortisone acetate because of the induction of hepatic enzymes). Products include:
- Arco-Lase Plus Tablets 512
- Bellergal-S Tablets 2250
- Donnatal 2060
- Donnatal Extentabs 2061
- Donnatal Tablets 2060
- Phenobarbital Elixir and Tablets 1469
- Quadrinal Tablets 1350

Phenytoin (Increased metabolic clearance of fludrocortisone acetate because of the induction of hepatic enzymes). Products include:
- Dilantin Infatabs 1908
- Dilantin-125 Suspension 1911

Phenytoin Sodium (Increased metabolic clearance of fludrocortisone acetate because of the induction of hepatic enzymes). Products include:
- Dilantin Kapseals 1906
- Dilantin Parenteral 1910

Polyestradiol Phosphate (Increased levels of corticosteroid-binding globulin, thereby increasing the bound (inactive) fraction).
- No products indexed under this heading.

Polythiazide (Potential for enhanced hypokalemia; serum potassium levels should be monitored frequently). Products include:
- Minizide Capsules 1938

Quinestrol (Increased levels of corticosteroid-binding globulin, thereby increasing the bound (inactive) fraction).
- No products indexed under this heading.

Rifampin (Increased metabolic clearance of fludrocortisone acetate because of the induction of hepatic enzymes). Products include:
- Rifadin 1528
- Rifamate Capsules 1530
- Rifater 1532
- Rimactane Capsules 847

Secobarbital Sodium (Increased metabolic clearance of fludrocortisone acetate because of the induction of hepatic enzymes). Products include:
- Seconal Sodium Pulvules 1474

Stanozolol (Enhanced tendency toward edema). Products include:
- Winstrol Tablets 2337

Thiamylal Sodium (Increased metabolic clearance of fludrocortisone acetate because of the induction of hepatic enzymes).
- No products indexed under this heading.

Tolazamide (Diminished antidiabetic effect; monitor symptoms of hyperglycemia).
- No products indexed under this heading.

Tolbutamide (Diminished antidiabetic effect; monitor symptoms of hyperglycemia).
- No products indexed under this heading.

Torsemide (Potential for enhanced hypokalemia; serum potassium levels should be monitored frequently). Products include:
- Demadex Tablets and Injection 686

Warfarin Sodium (Decreased prothrombin time response). Products include:
- Coumadin 926

FLORONE CREAM 0.05%
(Diflorasone Diacetate) 906
None cited in PDR database.

FLORONE E EMOLLIENT CREAM 0.05%
(Diflorasone Diacetate) 906
None cited in PDR database.

FLORONE OINTMENT 0.05%
(Diflorasone Diacetate) 906
None cited in PDR database.

FLOROPRYL STERILE OPHTHALMIC OINTMENT
(Isoflurophate) 1662
May interact with cholinergic agents and certain other agents. Compounds in these categories include:

Edrophonium Chloride (Additive adverse effects). Products include:
- Tensilon Injectable 1261

Neostigmine Bromide (Additive adverse effects). Products include:
- Prostigmin Tablets 1261

Neostigmine Methylsulfate (Additive adverse effects). Products include:
- Prostigmin Injectable 1260

Pyridostigmine Bromide (Additive adverse effects). Products include:
- Mestinon Injectable 1253
- Mestinon 1254

Succinylcholine Chloride (Possible respiratory and cardiovascular collapse). Products include:
- Anectine 1073

FLOXIN I.V.
(Ofloxacin) 1571
May interact with oral anticoagulants, xanthine bronchodilators, nonsteroidal anti-inflammatory agents, insulin, oral hypoglycemic agents, drugs which undergo biotransformation by cytochrome p-450 mixed function oxidase, and certain other agents. Compounds in these categories include:

Acarbose (Potentiation of hypoglycemic action).
- No products indexed under this heading.

Aminophylline (Increased steady-state theophylline levels; concurrent therapy may prolong the half-life of theophylline, elevate serum theophylline levels, and increase the risk of theophylline-related adverse reactions).
- No products indexed under this heading.

Chlorpropamide (Potentiation of hypoglycemic action). Products include:
- Diabinese Tablets 1935

Cimetidine (May interfere with the elimination of quinolones resulting in significant increase in half-life and AUC of some quinolones; this interaction has not been studied with ofloxacin). Products include:
- Tagamet Tablets 2516

Cimetidine Hydrochloride (May interfere with the elimination of quinolones resulting in significant increase in half-life and AUC of some quinolones; this interaction has not been studied with ofloxacin). Products include:
- Tagamet 2516

Cyclosporine (Potential for prolonged half-life and elevated serum levels of cyclosporine). Products include:
- Neoral 2276
- Sandimmune 2286

Diclofenac Potassium (Increased risk of CNS stimulation and convulsive seizures). Products include:
- Cataflam 816

Diclofenac Sodium (Increased risk of CNS stimulation and convulsive seizures). Products include:
- Voltaren Ophthalmic Sterile Ophthalmic Solution .... ◉ 272
- Voltaren Tablets 861

Dicumarol (Potential for enhanced effects of the oral anticoagulant).
- No products indexed under this heading.

Drugs which undergo biotransformation by cytochrome P-450 mixed function oxidase (Quinolone antibacterials inhibit cytochrome P450 enzyme activity resulting in prolonged half-life for some drugs that are also metabolized by this system).

Dyphylline (Increased steady-state theophylline levels; concurrent therapy may prolong the half-life of theophylline, elevate serum theophylline levels, and increase the risk of theophylline-related adverse reactions). Products include:
- Lufyllin & Lufyllin-400 Tablets 2670
- Lufyllin-GG Elixir & Tablets 2671

Etodolac (Increased risk of CNS stimulation and convulsive seizures). Products include:
- Lodine Capsules and Tablets 2743

Fenbufen (Increased risk of CNS stimulation convulsive seizures).

Fenoprofen Calcium (Increased risk of CNS stimulation and convulsive seizures). Products include:
- Nalfon 200 Pulvules & Nalfon Tablets 917

Flurbiprofen (Increased risk of CNS stimulation and convulsive seizures). Products include:
- Ansaid Tablets 2579

Glipizide (Potentiation of hypoglycemic action). Products include:
- Glucotrol Tablets 1967
- Glucotrol XL Extended Release Tablets 1968

Glyburide (Potentiation of hypoglycemic action). Products include:
- DiaBeta Tablets 1239
- Glynase PresTab Tablets 2609
- Micronase Tablets 2623

Ibuprofen (Increased risk of CNS stimulation and convulsive seizures). Products include:
- Advil Cold and Sinus Caplets and Tablets (formerly CoAdvil) .... ▣ 870
- Advil Ibuprofen Tablets and Caplets .... ▣ 870
- Children's Advil Suspension 2692
- Arthritis Foundation Ibuprofen Tablets .... ▣ 674
- Bayer Select Ibuprofen Pain Relief Formula .... ▣ 715
- Cramp End Tablets .... ▣ 735
- Dimetapp Sinus Caplets .... ▣ 775
- Haltran Tablets .... ▣ 771
- IBU Tablets 1342
- Ibuprohm .... ▣ 735
- Children's Motrin Ibuprofen Oral Suspension 1546
- Motrin Tablets 2625
- Motrin IB Caplets, Tablets, and Geltabs .... ▣ 838
- Motrin IB Sinus .... ▣ 838
- Motrin Ibuprofen Suspension, Oral Drops, Chewable Tablets, Caplets 1546
- Nuprin Ibuprofen/Analgesic Tablets & Caplets .... ▣ 622
- Sine-Aid IB Caplets 1554
- Vicks DayQuil SINUS Pressure & PAIN Relief with IBUPROFEN .... ▣ 762

Indomethacin (Increased risk of CNS stimulation and convulsive seizures). Products include:
- Indocin 1680

Indomethacin Sodium Trihydrate (Increased risk of CNS stimulation and convulsive seizures). Products include:
- Indocin I.V. 1684

Insulin, Human (Potentiation of hypoglycemic action).
- No products indexed under this heading.

Insulin, Human Isophane Suspension (Potentiation of hypoglycemic action). Products include:
- Novolin N Human Insulin 10 ml Vials 1795

Insulin, Human NPH (Potentiation of hypoglycemic action). Products include:
- Humulin N, 100 Units 1448
- Novolin N PenFill Cartridges Durable Insulin Delivery System 1798
- Novolin N Prefilled Syringe Disposable Insulin Delivery System 1798

Insulin, Human Regular (Potentiation of hypoglycemic action). Products include:
- Humulin R, 100 Units 1449
- Novolin R Human Insulin 10 ml Vials 1795
- Novolin R PenFill Cartridges Durable Insulin Delivery System 1798
- Novolin R Prefilled Syringe Disposable Insulin Delivery System 1798
- Velosulin BR Human Insulin 10 ml Vials 1795

Insulin, Human, Zinc Suspension (Potentiation of hypoglycemic action). Products include:
- Humulin L, 100 Units 1446
- Humulin U, 100 Units 1450
- Novolin L Human Insulin 10 ml Vials 1795

Insulin, NPH (Potentiation of hypoglycemic action). Products include:
- NPH, 100 Units 1450
- Pork NPH, 100 Units 1452
- Purified Pork NPH Isophane Insulin 1801

Insulin, Regular (Potentiation of hypoglycemic action). Products include:
- Regular, 100 Units 1450
- Pork Regular, 100 Units 1452
- Pork Regular (Concentrated), 500 Units 1453
- Purified Pork Regular Insulin 1801

(▣ Described in PDR For Nonprescription Drugs) (◉ Described in PDR For Ophthalmology)

423 **Interactions Index** **Floxin**

Insulin, Zinc Crystals (Potentiation of hypoglycemic action). Products include:

NPH, 100 Units ... 1450

Insulin, Zinc Suspension (Potentiation of hypoglycemic action). Products include:

Iletin I ... 1450
Lente, 100 Units ... 1450
Iletin II ... 1452
Pork Lente, 100 Units ... 1452
Purified Pork Lente Insulin ... 1801

Ketoprofen (Increased risk of CNS stimulation and convulsive seizures). Products include:

Orudis Capsules ... 2766
Oruvail Capsules ... 2766

Ketorolac Tromethamine (Increased risk of CNS stimulation and convulsive seizures). Products include:

Acular ... 474
Acular ... ⊙ 277
Toradol ... 2159

Meclofenamate Sodium (Increased risk of CNS stimulation and convulsive seizures).

No products indexed under this heading.

Mefenamic Acid (Increased risk of CNS stimulation and convulsive seizures). Products include:

Ponstel ... 1925

Metformin Hydrochloride (Potentiation of hypoglycemic action). Products include:

Glucophage ... 752

Nabumetone (Increased risk of CNS stimulation and convulsive seizures). Products include:

Relafen Tablets ... 2510

Naproxen (Increased risk of CNS stimulation and convulsive seizures). Products include:

Anaprox/Naprosyn ... 2117

Naproxen Sodium (Increased risk of CNS stimulation and convulsive seizures). Products include:

Aleve ... 1975
Anaprox/Naprosyn ... 2117

Oxaprozin (Increased risk of CNS stimulation and convulsive seizures). Products include:

Daypro Caplets ... 2426

Phenylbutazone (Increased risk of CNS stimulation and convulsive seizures).

No products indexed under this heading.

Piroxicam (Increased risk of CNS stimulation and convulsive seizures). Products include:

Feldene Capsules ... 1965

Probenecid (Potential to affect renal tubular secretion; this interaction has not been studied with ofloxacin). Products include:

Benemid Tablets ... 1611
ColBENEMID Tablets ... 1622

Sulindac (Increased risk of CNS stimulation and convulsive seizures). Products include:

Clinoril Tablets ... 1618

Theophylline (Increased steady-state theophylline levels; concurrent therapy may prolong the half-life of theophylline, elevate serum theophylline levels, and increase the risk of theophylline-related adverse reactions). Products include:

Marax Tablets & DF Syrup ... 2200
Quibron ... 2053

Theophylline Anhydrous (Increased steady-state theophylline levels; concurrent therapy may prolong the half-life of theophylline, elevate serum theophylline levels, and increase the risk of theophylline-related adverse reactions). Products include:

Aerolate ... 1004
Primatene Dual Action Formula ... ■D 872
Primatene Tablets ... ■D 873
Respbid Tablets ... 682
Slo-bid Gyrocaps ... 2033
Theo-24 Extended Release Capsules ... 2568
Theo-Dur Extended-Release Tablets ... 1327
Theo-X Extended-Release Tablets ... 788
Uni-Dur Extended-Release Tablets ... 1331
Uniphyl 400 mg Tablets ... 2001

Theophylline Calcium Salicylate (Increased steady-state theophylline levels; concurrent therapy may prolong the half-life of theophylline, elevate serum theophylline levels, and increase the risk of theophylline-related adverse reactions). Products include:

Quadrinal Tablets ... 1350

Theophylline Sodium Glycinate (Increased steady-state theophylline levels; concurrent therapy may prolong the half-life of theophylline, elevate serum theophylline levels, and increase the risk of theophylline-related adverse reactions).

No products indexed under this heading.

Tolazamide (Potentiation of hypoglycemic action).

No products indexed under this heading.

Tolbutamide (Potentiation of hypoglycemic action).

No products indexed under this heading.

Tolmetin Sodium (Increased risk of CNS stimulation and convulsive seizures). Products include:

Tolectin (200, 400 and 600 mg) ... 1581

Warfarin Sodium (Potential for enhanced effects of the oral anticoagulant). Products include:

Coumadin ... 926

FLOXIN TABLETS (200 MG, 300 MG, 400 MG)

(Ofloxacin) ... 1567

May interact with xanthine bronchodilators, antacids containing aluminium, calcium and magnesium, oral anticoagulants, non-steroidal anti-inflammatory agents, insulin, oral hypoglycemic agents, drugs which undergo biotransformation by cytochrome p-450 mixed function oxidase, and certain other agents. Compounds in these categories include:

Acarbose (Potentiation of hypoglycemic action).

No products indexed under this heading.

Aluminum Carbonate Gel (May substantially interfere with the absorption of quinolones). Products include:

Basaljel ... 2703

Aluminum Hydroxide (May substantially interfere with the absorption of quinolones). Products include:

ALternaGEL Liquid ... 1316
Maximum Strength Ascriptin ... ■D 630
Cama Arthritis Pain Reliever ... ■D 785
Gaviscon Extra Strength Relief Formula Antacid Tablets ... ■D 819
Gaviscon Extra Strength Relief Formula Liquid Antacid ... ■D 819
Gaviscon Liquid Antacid ... ■D 820
Gelusil Liquid & Tablets ... ■D 855
Maalox Heartburn Relief Suspension ... ■D 642
Maalox Heartburn Relief Tablets ... ■D 641
Maalox Magnesia and Alumina Oral Suspension ... ■D 642
Maalox Plus Tablets ... ■D 643
Extra Strength Maalox Antacid Plus Antigas Liquid and Tablets ■D 638
Tempo Soft Antacid ... ■D 835

Aluminum Hydroxide Gel (May substantially interfere with the absorption of quinolones). Products include:

ALternaGEL Liquid ... ■D 659
Aludrox Oral Suspension ... 2695
Amphojel Suspension ... 2695
Amphojel Suspension without Flavor ... 2695
Amphojel Tablets ... 2695
Arthritis Pain Ascriptin ... ■D 631
Regular Strength Ascriptin Tablets ... ■D 629
Gaviscon Antacid Tablets ... ■D 819
Gaviscon-2 Antacid Tablets ... ■D 820
Mylanta Liquid ... 1317
Mylanta Tablets ... ■D 660
Mylanta Double Strength Liquid ... 1317
Mylanta Double Strength Tablets ... ■D 660
Nephrox Suspension ... ■D 655

Aluminum Hydroxide Gel, Dried (May substantially interfere with the absorption of quinolones).

Aminophylline (Increased steady-state theophylline levels; concurrent therapy may prolong the half-life of theophylline, elevate serum theophylline levels, and increase the risk of theophylline-related adverse reactions).

No products indexed under this heading.

Chlorpropamide (Potentiation of hypoglycemic action). Products include:

Diabinese Tablets ... 1935

Cimetidine (May interfere with the elimination of quinolones resulting in significant increase in half-life and AUC of some quinolones; this interaction has not been studied with ofloxacin). Products include:

Tagamet Tablets ... 2516

Cimetidine Hydrochloride (May interfere with the elimination of quinolones resulting in significant increase in half-life and AUC of some quinolones; this interaction has not been studied with ofloxacin). Products include:

Tagamet ... 2516

Cyclosporine (Potential for prolonged half-life and elevated serum levels of cyclosporine). Products include:

Neoral ... 2276
Sandimmune ... 2286

Diclofenac Potassium (Increased risk of CNS stimulation and convulsive seizures). Products include:

Cataflam ... 816

Diclofenac Sodium (Increased risk of CNS stimulation and convulsive seizures). Products include:

Voltaren Ophthalmic Sterile Ophthalmic Solution ... ⊙ 272
Voltaren Tablets ... 861

Dicumarol (Potential for enhanced effects of the oral anticoagulant).

No products indexed under this heading.

Drugs which undergo biotransformation by cytochrome P-450 mixed function oxidase (Quinolone antibacterials inhibit cytochrome P450 enzyme activity resulting in prolonged half-life for some drugs that are also metabolized by this system).

Dyphylline (Increased steady-state theophylline levels; concurrent therapy may prolong the half-life of theophylline, elevate serum theophylline levels, and increase the risk of theophylline-related adverse reactions). Products include:

Lufyllin & Lufyllin-400 Tablets ... 2670
Lufyllin-GG Elixir & Tablets ... 2671

Etodolac (Increased risk of CNS stimulation and convulsive seizures). Products include:

Lodine Capsules and Tablets ... 2743

Fenoprofen Calcium (Increased risk of CNS stimulation and convulsive seizures). Products include:

Nalfon 200 Pulvules & Nalfon Tablets ... 917

Flurbiprofen (Increased risk of CNS stimulation and convulsive seizures). Products include:

Ansaid Tablets ... 2579

Glipizide (Potentiation of hypoglycemic action). Products include:

Glucotrol Tablets ... 1967
Glucotrol XL Extended Release Tablets ... 1968

Glyburide (Potentiation of hypoglycemic action). Products include:

DiaBeta Tablets ... 1239
Glynase PresTab Tablets ... 2609
Micronase Tablets ... 2623

Ibuprofen (Increased risk of CNS stimulation and convulsive seizures). Products include:

Advil Cold and Sinus Caplets and Tablets (formerly CoAdvil) ... ■D 870
Advil Ibuprofen Tablets and Caplets ... ■D 870
Children's Advil Suspension ... 2692
Arthritis Foundation Ibuprofen Tablets ... ■D 674
Bayer Select Ibuprofen Pain Relief Formula ... ■D 715
Cramp End Tablets ... ■D 735
Dimetapp Sinus Caplets ... ■D 775
Haltran Tablets ... ■D 771
IBU Tablets ... 1342
Ibuprohm ... ■D 735
Children's Motrin Ibuprofen Oral Suspension ... 1546
Motrin Tablets ... 2625
Motrin IB Caplets, Tablets, and Geltabs ... ■D 838
Motrin IB Sinus ... ■D 838
Motrin Ibuprofen Suspension, Oral Drops, Chewable Tablets, Caplets ... 1546
Nuprin Ibuprofen/Analgesic Tablets & Caplets ... ■D 622
Sine-Aid IB Caplets ... 1554
Vicks DayQuil SINUS Pressure & PAIN Relief with IBUPROFEN ... ■D 762

Indomethacin (Increased risk of CNS stimulation and convulsive seizures). Products include:

Indocin ... 1680

Indomethacin Sodium Trihydrate (Increased risk of CNS stimulation and convulsive seizures). Products include:

Indocin I.V. ... 1684

Insulin, Human (Potentiation of hypoglycemic action).

No products indexed under this heading.

Insulin, Human Isophane Suspension (Potentiation of hypoglycemic action). Products include:

Novolin N Human Insulin 10 ml Vials ... 1795

Insulin, Human NPH (Potentiation of hypoglycemic action). Products include:

Humulin N, 100 Units ... 1448
Novolin N PenFill Cartridges Durable Insulin Delivery System ... 1798
Novolin N Prefilled Syringe Disposable Insulin Delivery System ... 1798

IMPORTANT NOTE: Always consult each drug listing in the patient's regimen for possible interactions.

Insulin, Human Regular (Potentiation of hypoglycemic action). Products include:
- Humulin R, 100 Units 1449
- Novolin R Human Insulin 10 ml Vials 1795
- Novolin R PenFill Cartridges Durable Insulin Delivery System 1798
- Novolin R Prefilled Syringe Disposable Insulin Delivery System 1798
- Velosulin BR Human Insulin 10 ml Vials 1795

Insulin, Human, Zinc Suspension (Potentiation of hypoglycemic action). Products include:
- Humulin L, 100 Units 1446
- Humulin U, 100 Units 1450
- Novolin L Human Insulin 10 ml Vials 1795

Insulin, NPH (Potentiation of hypoglycemic action). Products include:
- NPH, 100 Units 1450
- Pork NPH, 100 Units 1452
- Purified Pork NPH Isophane Insulin 1801

Insulin, Regular (Potentiation of hypoglycemic action). Products include:
- Regular, 100 Units 1450
- Pork Regular, 100 Units 1452
- Pork Regular (Concentrated), 500 Units 1453
- Purified Pork Regular Insulin 1801

Insulin, Zinc Crystals (Potentiation of hypoglycemic action). Products include:
- NPH, 100 Units 1450

Insulin, Zinc Suspension (Potentiation of hypoglycemic action). Products include:
- Iletin I 1450
- Lente, 100 Units 1450
- Iletin II 1452
- Pork Lente, 100 Units 1452
- Purified Pork Lente Insulin 1801

Ketoprofen (Increased risk of CNS stimulation and convulsive seizures). Products include:
- Orudis Capsules 2766
- Oruvail Capsules 2766

Ketorolac Tromethamine (Increased risk of CNS stimulation and convulsive seizures). Products include:
- Acular 474
- Acular .... ⊙ 277
- Toradol 2159

Magaldrate (May substantially interfere with the absorption of quinolones).
- No products indexed under this heading.

Magnesium Hydroxide (May substantially interfere with the absorption of quinolones). Products include:
- Aludrox Oral Suspension 2695
- Arthritis Pain Ascriptin .... ▣ 631
- Maximum Strength Ascriptin .... ▣ 630
- Regular Strength Ascriptin Tablets .... ▣ 629
- Di-Gel Antacid/Anti-Gas .... ▣ 801
- Gelusil Liquid & Tablets .... ▣ 855
- Maalox Magnesia and Alumina Oral Suspension .... ▣ 642
- Maalox Plus Tablets .... ▣ 643
- Extra Strength Maalox Antacid Plus Antigas Liquid and Tablets ▣ 638
- Mylanta Calcium Carbonate and Magnesium Hydroxide Tablets 1318
- Mylanta Liquid 1317
- Mylanta Tablets .... ▣ 660
- Mylanta Double Strength Liquid 1317
- Mylanta Double Strength Tablets .... ▣ 660
- Phillips' Milk of Magnesia Liquid .... ▣ 729
- Rolaids Tablets .... ▣ 843
- Tempo Soft Antacid .... ▣ 835

Magnesium Oxide (May substantially interfere with the absorption of quinolones). Products include:
- Beelith Tablets 639
- Bufferin Analgesic Tablets and Caplets .... ▣ 613
- Caltrate PLUS .... ▣ 665
- Cama Arthritis Pain Reliever .... ▣ 785
- Mag-Ox 400 668
- Uro-Mag 668

Meclofenamate Sodium (Increased risk of CNS stimulation and convulsive seizures).
- No products indexed under this heading.

Mefenamic Acid (Increased risk of CNS stimulation and convulsive seizures). Products include:
- Ponstel 1925

Metformin Hydrochloride (Potentiation of hypoglycemic action). Products include:
- Glucophage 752

Nabumetone (Increased risk of CNS stimulation and convulsive seizures). Products include:
- Relafen Tablets 2510

Naproxen (Increased risk of CNS stimulation and convulsive seizures). Products include:
- Anaprox/Naprosyn 2117

Naproxen Sodium (Increased risk of CNS stimulation and convulsive seizures). Products include:
- Aleve 1975
- Anaprox/Naprosyn 2117

Oxaprozin (Increased risk of CNS stimulation and convulsive seizures). Products include:
- Daypro Caplets 2426

Phenylbutazone (Increased risk of CNS stimulation and convulsive seizures).
- No products indexed under this heading.

Piroxicam (Increased risk of CNS stimulation and convulsive seizures). Products include:
- Feldene Capsules 1965

Probenecid (Potential to affect renal tubular secretion; this interaction has not been studied with ofloxacin). Products include:
- Benemid Tablets 1611
- ColBENEMID Tablets 1622

Sucralfate (May substantially interfere with the absorption of quinolones). Products include:
- Carafate Suspension 1505
- Carafate Tablets 1504

Sulindac (Increased risk of CNS stimulation and convulsive seizures). Products include:
- Clinoril Tablets 1618

Theophylline (Increased steady-state theophylline levels; concurrent therapy may prolong the half-life of theophylline, elevate serum theophylline levels, and increase the risk of theophylline-related adverse reactions). Products include:
- Marax Tablets & DF Syrup 2200
- Quibron 2053

Theophylline Anhydrous (Increased steady-state theophylline levels; concurrent therapy may prolong the half-life of theophylline, elevate serum theophylline levels, and increase the risk of theophylline-related adverse reactions). Products include:
- Aerolate 1004
- Primatene Dual Action Formula .... ▣ 872
- Primatene Tablets .... ▣ 873
- Respbid Tablets 682
- Slo-bid Gyrocaps 2033
- Theo-24 Extended Release Capsules 2568
- Theo-Dur Extended-Release Tablets 1327
- Theo-X Extended-Release Tablets 788
- Uni-Dur Extended-Release Tablets 1331
- Uniphyl 400 mg Tablets 2001

Theophylline Calcium Salicylate (Increased steady-state theophylline levels; concurrent therapy may prolong the half-life of theophylline, elevate serum theophylline levels, and increase the risk of theophylline-related adverse reactions). Products include:
- Quadrinal Tablets 1350

Theophylline Sodium Glycinate (Increased steady-state theophylline levels; concurrent therapy may prolong the half-life of theophylline, elevate serum theophylline levels, and increase the risk of theophylline-related adverse reactions).
- No products indexed under this heading.

Tolazamide (Potentiation of hypoglycemic action).
- No products indexed under this heading.

Tolbutamide (Potentiation of hypoglycemic action).
- No products indexed under this heading.

Tolmetin Sodium (Increased risk of CNS stimulation and convulsive seizures). Products include:
- Tolectin (200, 400 and 600 mg) .. 1581

Warfarin Sodium (Potential for enhanced effects of the oral anticoagulant). Products include:
- Coumadin 926

Zinc Sulfate (May substantially interfere with the absorption of quinolones). Products include:
- Clear Eyes ACR Astringent/Lubricant Eye Redness Reliever Eye Drops .... ⊙ 316
- Visine Maximum Strength Allergy Relief .... ⊙ 313

Food Interactions

Food, unspecified (Food does not affect the C_{max} and AUC_{∞} of the drug, but T_{max} is prolonged).

FLUDARA FOR INJECTION

(Fludarabine Phosphate) 663

May interact with:

Pentostatin (Co-administration may produce severe pulmonary toxicity; the use of Fludara in combination with pentostatin is not recommended).
- No products indexed under this heading.

FLUMADINE TABLETS & SYRUP

(Rimantadine Hydrochloride) 1015

May interact with:

Acetaminophen (Coadministration reduces the peak concentration and AUC values for rimantadine). Products include:
- Actifed Plus Caplets .... ▣ 845
- Actifed Plus Tablets .... ▣ 845
- Actifed Sinus Daytime/Nighttime Tablets and Caplets .... ▣ 846
- Alka-Seltzer Plus Cold Medicine Liqui-Gels .... ▣ 706
- Alka-Seltzer Plus Cold & Cough Medicine Liqui-Gels .... ▣ 705
- Alka-Seltzer Plus Night-Time Cold Medicine Liqui-Gels .... ▣ 706
- Allerest Headache Strength Tablets .... ▣ 627
- Allerest No Drowsiness Tablets .... ▣ 627
- Allerest Sinus Pain Formula .... ▣ 627
- Anexsia 5/500 Elixir 1781
- Anexia Tablets 1782
- Arthritis Foundation Aspirin Free Caplets .... ▣ 673
- Arthritis Foundation NightTime Caplets .... ▣ 674
- Bayer Select Headache Pain Relief Formula .... ▣ 716
- Bayer Select Menstrual Multi-Symptom Formula .... ▣ 716
- Bayer Select Night Time Pain Relief Formula .... ▣ 716
- Bayer Select Sinus Pain Relief Formula .... ▣ 717
- Benadryl Allergy Sinus Headache Formula Caplets .... ▣ 849
- Comtrex Multi-Symptom Cold Reliever Tablets/Caplets/Liqui-Gels/Liquid .... ▣ 615
- Allergy-Sinus Comtrex Multi-Symptom Allergy-Sinus Formula Tablets .... ▣ 617
- Comtrex Non-Drowsy .... ▣ 618
- Contac Day Allergy/Sinus Caplets ▣ 812
- Contac Day & Night .... ▣ 812
- Contac Night Allergy/Sinus Caplets .... ▣ 812
- Contac Severe Cold and Flu Formula Caplets .... ▣ 814
- Contac Severe Cold & Flu Non-Drowsy .... ▣ 815
- Coricidin 'D' Decongestant Tablets .... ▣ 800
- Coricidin Tablets .... ▣ 800
- DHCplus Capsules 1993
- Darvon-N/Darvocet-N 1433
- Drixoral Cold and Flu Extended-Release Tablets .... ▣ 803
- Drixoral Cough + Sore Throat Liquid Caps .... ▣ 802
- Drixoral Allergy/Sinus Extended Release Tablets .... ▣ 804
- Esgic-plus Tablets 1013
- Aspirin Free Excedrin Analgesic Caplets and Geltabs 732
- Excedrin Extra-Strength Analgesic Tablets & Caplets 732
- Excedrin P.M. Analgesic/Sleeping Aid Tablets, Caplets, Liquigels 733
- Fioricet Tablets 2258
- Fioricet with Codeine Capsules 2260
- Hycomine Compound Tablets 932
- Hydrocet Capsules 782
- Legatrin PM .... ▣ 651
- Lorcet 10/650 1018
- Lortab 2566
- Lurline PMS Tablets 982
- Maximum Strength Multi-Symptom Formula Midol .... ▣ 722
- PMS Multi-Symptom Formula Midol .... ▣ 723
- Teen Multi-Symptom Formula Midol .... ▣ 722
- Midrin Capsules 783
- Migralam Capsules 2038
- Panodol Tablets and Caplets .... ▣ 824
- Children's Panadol Chewable Tablets, Liquid, Infant's Drops .... ▣ 824
- Percocet Tablets 938
- Percogesic Analgesic Tablets .... ▣ 754
- Phrenilin 785
- Pyrroxate Caplets .... ▣ 772
- Sedapap Tablets 50 mg/650 mg .. 1543
- Sinarest Tablets .... ▣ 648
- Sinarest Extra Strength Tablets .... ▣ 648
- Sinarest No Drowsiness Tablets .... ▣ 648
- Sine-Aid Maximum Strength Sinus Medication Gelcaps, Caplets and Tablets 1554
- Sine-Off No Drowsiness Formula Caplets .... ▣ 824
- Sine-Off Sinus Medicine .... ▣ 825
- Singlet Tablets .... ▣ 825
- Sinulin Tablets 787
- Sinutab Sinus Allergy Medication, Maximum Strength Tablets and Caplets .... ▣ 860
- Sinutab Sinus Medication, Maximum Strength Without Drowsiness Formula, Tablets & Caplets .... ▣ 860
- Sinutab Sinus Medication, Regular Strength Without Drowsiness Formula .... ▣ 859
- Sudafed Cold and Cough Liquidcaps .... ▣ 862
- Sudafed Severe Cold Formula Caplets .... ▣ 863
- Sudafed Severe Cold Formula Tablets .... ▣ 864
- Sudafed Sinus Caplets .... ▣ 864
- Sudafed Sinus Tablets .... ▣ 864
- Talacen 2333
- TheraFlu .... ▣ 787
- TheraFlu Maximum Strength Nighttime Flu, Cold & Cough Medicine .... ▣ 788

(▣ Described in PDR For Nonprescription Drugs) (⊙ Described in PDR For Ophthalmology)

TheraFlu Maximum Strength Non-Drowsy Formula Flu, Cold & Cough Medicine .... ✦D 788

Thera Flu Maximum Strength, Non-Drowsy Formula Flu, Cold and Cough Caplets .... ✦D 789

Triaminic Sore Throat Formula ...... ✦D 791

Triaminicin Tablets .... ✦D 793

Children's TYLENOL acetaminophen Chewable Tablets, Elixir, Suspension Liquid 1555

Children's TYLENOL Cold Multi-Symptom Liquid Formula and Chewable Tablets................................ 1561

Children's TYLENOL Cold Plus Cough Multi Symptom Tablets and Liquid .... ✦D 681

Infants' TYLENOL acetaminophen Drops and Suspension Drops........ 1555

Infants' TYLENOL Cold Decongestant & Fever-Reducer Drops 1556

TYLENOL Extended Relief Caplets.. 1558

TYLENOL, Extra Strength, Acetaminophen Adult Liquid Pain Reliever 1560

TYLENOL, Extra Strength, acetaminophen Gelcaps, Geltabs, Caplets, Tablets 1559

TYLENOL, Extra Strength, Headache Plus Pain Reliever with Antacid Caplets 1559

TYLENOL, Junior Strength, acetaminophen Coated Caplets, Grape and Fruit Chewable Tablets 1557

TYLENOL Maximum Strength Allergy Sinus Medication Gelcaps and Caplets 1563

TYLENOL Maximum Strength Allergy Sinus NightTime Medication Caplets 1555

TYLENOL Flu Maximum Strength Gelcaps 1565

TYLENOL Flu NightTime, Maximum Strength, Gelcaps 1566

TYLENOL Maximum Strength Flu NightTime Hot Medication Packets 1562

TYLENOL, Maximum Strength, Sinus Medication Geltabs, Gelcaps, Caplets and Tablets 1566

TYLENOL Cold Multi-Symptom Formula Medication Tablets and Caplets 1561

TYLENOL Cold Medication No Drowsiness Formula Gelcaps and Caplets 1562

TYLENOL Cold Multi-Symptom Hot Medication Liquid Packets.............. 1557

TYLENOL Cough Multi-Symptom Medication 1564

TYLENOL Cough Multi-Symptom Medication with Decongestant...... 1565

TYLENOL, Regular Strength, acetaminophen Caplets and Tablets .. 1558

TYLENOL PM, Extra Strength Pain Reliever/Sleep Aid Caplets, Geltabs, Gelcaps 1560

TYLENOL Severe Allergy Medication Caplets 1564

Tylenol with Codeine 1583

Tylox Capsules 1584

Unisom With Pain Relief-Nighttime Sleep Aid and Pain Reliever............ 1934

Vanquish Analgesic Caplets .... ✦D 731

Vicks 44 LiquiCaps Cough, Cold & Flu Relief... ✦D 755

Vicks 44M Cough, Cold & Flu Relief.. ✦D 756

Vicks DayQuil .... ✦D 761

Vicks Nyquil Hot Therapy.................. ✦D 762

Vicks NyQuil LiquiCaps Multi-Symptom Cold/Flu Relief .... ✦D 763

Vicks NyQuil Multi-Symptom Cold/Flu Relief - (Original & Cherry Flavor)....................................... ✦D 763

Vicodin Tablets... 1356

Vicodin ES Tablets 1357

Wygesic Tablets 2827

Zydone Capsules 949

Aspirin (Coadministration reduces the peak concentration and AUC values for rimantadine). Products include:

Alka-Seltzer Effervescent Antacid and Pain Reliever .... ✦D 701

Alka-Seltzer Extra Strength Effervescent Antacid and Pain Reliever .... ✦D 703

Alka-Seltzer Lemon Lime Effervescent Antacid and Pain Reliever .... ✦D 703

Alka-Seltzer Plus Cold Medicine .... ✦D 705

Alka-Seltzer Plus Cold & Cough Medicine .... ✦D 708

Alka-Seltzer Plus Night-Time Cold Medicine .... ✦D 707

Alka Seltzer Plus Sinus Medicine .. ✦D 707

Arthritis Foundation Safety Coated Aspirin Tablets .... ✦D 675

Arthritis Pain Ascriptin .... ✦D 631

Maximum Strength Ascriptin .... ✦D 630

Regular Strength Ascriptin Tablets .... ✦D 629

Arthritis Strength BC Powder.... ✦D 609

BC Cold Powder Multi-Symptom Formula (Cold-Sinus-Allergy) ...... ✦D 609

BC Cold Powder Non-Drowsy Formula (Cold-Sinus).......................... ✦D 609

BC Powder .... ✦D 609

Bayer Children's Chewable Aspirin .... ✦D 711

Genuine Bayer Aspirin Tablets & Caplets .... ✦D 713

Extra Strength Bayer Arthritis Pain Regimen Formula .... ✦D 711

Extra Strength Bayer Aspirin Caplets & Tablets .... ✦D 712

Extended-Release Bayer 8-Hour Aspirin .... ✦D 712

Extra Strength Bayer Plus Aspirin Caplets .... ✦D 713

Extra Strength Bayer PM Aspirin .. ✦D 713

Bayer Enteric Aspirin .... ✦D 709

Bufferin Analgesic Tablets and Caplets .... ✦D 613

Arthritis Strength Bufferin Analgesic Caplets .... ✦D 614

Extra Strength Bufferin Analgesic Tablets .... ✦D 615

Cama Arthritis Pain Reliever............ ✦D 785

Darvon Compound-65 Pulvules 1435

Easprin 1914

Ecotrin 2455

Ecotrin Enteric Coated Aspirin Maximum Strength Tablets and Caplets .... ✦D 816

Ecotrin Enteric Coated Aspirin Regular Strength Tablets 2455

Empirin Aspirin Tablets .... ✦D 854

Empirin with Codeine Tablets............ 1093

Excedrin Extra-Strength Analgesic Tablets & Caplets 732

Fiorinal Capsules 2261

Fiorinal with Codeine Capsules 2262

Fiorinal Tablets... 2261

Halfprin 1362

Healthprin Aspirin 2455

Norgesic... 1496

Percodan Tablets....................................... 939

Percodan-Demi Tablets.......................... 940

Robaxisal Tablets...................................... 2071

Soma Compound w/Codeine Tablets 2676

Soma Compound Tablets...................... 2675

St. Joseph Adult Chewable Aspirin (81 mg.) .... ✦D 808

Talwin Compound 2335

Ursinus Inlay-Tabs.................................. ✦D 794

Vanquish Analgesic Caplets .... ✦D 731

Cimetidine (Potential for reduced clearance of total rimantadine). Products include:

Tagamet Tablets 2516

Cimetidine Hydrochloride (Potential for reduced clearance of total rimantadine). Products include:

Tagamet... 2516

FLUORACAINE

(Fluorescein Sodium, Proparacaine Hydrochloride).. ◎ 206

None cited in PDR database.

FLUORESCITE INJECTION

(Fluorescein Sodium) .... ◎ 219

None cited in PDR database.

FLUORESCITE SYRINGE

(Fluorescein Sodium) .... ◎ 219

None cited in PDR database.

FLUORI-METHANE

(Dichlorodifluoromethane, Trichloromonofluoromethane) 1053

None cited in PDR database.

FLUOR-I-STRIP

(Fluorescein Sodium) .... ◎ 326

None cited in PDR database.

FLUOR-I-STRIP A.T.

(Fluorescein Sodium) .... ◎ 326

None cited in PDR database.

FLUOR-OP OPHTHALMIC SUSPENSION

(Fluorometholone)................................... ◎ 264

None cited in PDR database.

FLUOROPLEX TOPICAL SOLUTION & CREAM 1%

(Fluorouracil) 479

None cited in PDR database.

FLUOROURACIL INJECTION

(Fluorouracil) 2116

May interact with alkylating agents and certain other agents. Compounds in these categories include:

Busulfan (Fluorouracil should be used with extreme caution in patients with previous use of alkylating agents). Products include:

Myleran Tablets 1143

Carmustine (BCNU) (Fluorouracil should be used with extreme caution in patients with previous use of alkylating agents; use with caution in patients with previous use of alkylating agents). Products include:

BiCNU 691

Chlorambucil (Fluorouracil should be used with extreme caution in patients with previous use of alkylating agents; use with caution in patients with previous use of alkylating agents). Products include:

Leukeran Tablets 1133

Cyclophosphamide (Fluorouracil should be used with extreme caution in patients with previous use of alkylating agents; use with caution in patients with previous use of alkylating agents). Products include:

Cytoxan 694

NEOSAR Lyophilized/Neosar 1959

Dacarbazine (Fluorouracil should be used with extreme caution in patients with previous use of alkylating agents; use with caution in patients with previous use of alkylating agents). Products include:

DTIC-Dome 600

Leucovorin Calcium (Increased toxicity of fluorouracil). Products include:

Leucovorin Calcium for Injection, Wellcovorin Brand 1132

Leucovorin Calcium for Injection 1268

Leucovorin Calcium Tablets, Wellcovorin Brand 1132

Leucovorin Calcium Tablets 1270

Lomustine (CCNU) (Fluorouracil should be used with extreme caution in patients with previous use of alkylating agents; use with caution in patients with previous use of alkylating agents). Products include:

CeeNU 693

Mechlorethamine Hydrochloride (Fluorouracil should be used with extreme caution in patients with previous use of alkylating agents; use with caution in patients with previous use of alkylating agents). Products include:

Mustargen... 1709

Melphalan (Fluorouracil should be used with extreme caution in patients with previous use of alkylating agents; use with caution in patients with previous use of alkylating agents). Products include:

Alkeran Tablets.. 1071

Thiotepa (Fluorouracil should be used with extreme caution in patients with previous use of alkylating agents; use with caution in patients with previous use of alkylating agents). Products include:

Thioplex (Thiotepa For Injection) 1281

FLUOTHANE

(Halothane)..2724

May interact with nondepolarizing neuromuscular blocking agents, ganglionic blocking agents, and certain other agents. Compounds in these categories include:

Atracurium Besylate (Actions augmented by Fluothane). Products include:

Tracrium Injection 1183

Epinephrine Hydrochloride (Simultaneous use may induce ventricular tachycardia or fibrillation). Products include:

Ana-Kit Anaphylaxis Emergency Treatment Kit 617

Guanethidine Monosulfate (Actions augmented by Fluothane). Products include:

Esimil Tablets 822

Ismelin Tablets 827

Mecamylamine Hydrochloride (Actions augmented by Fluothane). Products include:

Inversine Tablets 1686

Metocurine Iodide (Actions augmented by Fluothane). Products include:

Metubine Iodide Vials............................ 916

Mivacurium Chloride (Actions augmented by Fluothane). Products include:

Mivacron 1138

Norepinephrine Bitartrate (Simultaneous use may induce ventricular tachycardia or fibrillation). Products include:

Levophed Bitartrate Injection 2315

Pancuronium Bromide Injection (Actions augmented by Fluothane).

No products indexed under this heading.

Rocuronium Bromide (Actions augmented by Fluothane). Products include:

Zemuron 1830

Trimethaphan Camsylate (Actions augmented by Fluothane). Products include:

Arfonad Ampuls 2080

Vecuronium Bromide (Actions augmented by Fluothane). Products include:

Norcuron 1826

FLURESS

(Fluorescein Sodium, Benoxinate Hydrochloride).. ◎ 207

None cited in PDR database.

FLURO-ETHYL

(Dichlorotetrafluoroethane, Ethyl Chloride) 1053

None cited in PDR database.

FLUVIRIN

(Influenza Virus Vaccine) 460

May interact with xanthine bronchodilators, corticosteroids, antineoplastics, cytotoxic drugs, alkylating agents, and certain other agents.

IMPORTANT NOTE: Always consult each drug listing in the patient's regimen for possible interactions.

Fluvirin Interactions Index 426

Compounds in these categories include:

Altretamine (Potential for reduced antibody response in active immunization procedures). Products include:
Hexalen Capsules 2571

Aminophylline (Influenza immunization can inhibit the clearance of theophylline).
No products indexed under this heading.

Asparaginase (Potential for reduced antibody response in active immunization procedures). Products include:
Elspar 1659

Betamethasone Acetate (Potential for reduced antibody response in active immunization procedures). Products include:
Celestone Soluspan Suspension 2347

Betamethasone Sodium Phosphate (Potential for reduced antibody response in active immunization procedures). Products include:
Celestone Soluspan Suspension 2347

Bleomycin Sulfate (Potential for reduced antibody response in active immunization procedures). Products include:
Blenoxane 692

Busulfan (Potential for reduced antibody response in active immunization procedures). Products include:
Myleran Tablets 1143

Carboplatin (Potential for reduced antibody response in active immunization procedures). Products include:
Paraplatin for Injection 705

Carmustine (BCNU) (Potential for reduced antibody response in active immunization procedures). Products include:
BiCNU 691

Chlorambucil (Potential for reduced antibody response in active immunization procedures). Products include:
Leukeran Tablets 1133

Cisplatin (Potential for reduced antibody response in active immunization procedures). Products include:
Platinol 708
Platinol-AQ Injection 710

Cortisone Acetate (Potential for reduced antibody response in active immunization procedures). Products include:
Cortone Acetate Sterile Suspension 1623
Cortone Acetate Tablets 1624

Cyclophosphamide (Potential for reduced antibody response in active immunization procedures). Products include:
Cytoxan 694
NEOSAR Lyophilized/Neosar 1959

Dacarbazine (Potential for reduced antibody response in active immunization procedures). Products include:
DTIC-Dome 600

Daunorubicin Hydrochloride (Potential for reduced antibody response in active immunization procedures). Products include:
Cerubidine 795

Dexamethasone (Potential for reduced antibody response in active immunization procedures). Products include:
AK-Trol Ointment & Suspension .... ⊙ 205
Decadron Elixir 1633
Decadron Tablets 1635
Decaspray Topical Aerosol 1648
Dexacidin Ointment .... ⊙ 263
Maxitrol Ophthalmic Ointment and Suspension .... ⊙ 224
TobraDex Ophthalmic Suspension and Ointment 473

Dexamethasone Acetate (Potential for reduced antibody response in active immunization procedures). Products include:
Dalalone D.P. Injectable 1011
Decadron-LA Sterile Suspension 1646

Dexamethasone Sodium Phosphate (Potential for reduced antibody response in active immunization procedures). Products include:
Decadron Phosphate Injection 1637
Decadron Phosphate Respihaler 1642
Decadron Phosphate Sterile Ophthalmic Ointment 1641
Decadron Phosphate Sterile Ophthalmic Solution 1642
Decadron Phosphate Topical Cream 1644
Decadron Phosphate Turbinaire 1645
Decadron Phosphate with Xylocaine Injection, Sterile 1639
Dexacort Phosphate in Respihaler 458
Dexacort Phosphate in Turbinaire 459
NeoDecadron Sterile Ophthalmic Ointment 1712
NeoDecadron Sterile Ophthalmic Solution 1713
NeoDecadron Topical Cream 1714

Doxorubicin Hydrochloride (Potential for reduced antibody response in active immunization procedures). Products include:
Adriamycin PFS 1947
Adriamycin RDF 1947
Doxorubicin Astra 540
Rubex 712

Dyphylline (Influenza immunization can inhibit the clearance of theophylline). Products include:
Lufyllin & Lufyllin-400 Tablets 2670
Lufyllin-GG Elixir & Tablets 2671

Estramustine Phosphate Sodium (Potential for reduced antibody response in active immunization procedures). Products include:
Emcyt Capsules 1953

Etoposide (Potential for reduced antibody response in active immunization procedures). Products include:
VePesid Capsules and Injection 718

Floxuridine (Potential for reduced antibody response in active immunization procedures). Products include:
Sterile FUDR 2118

Fludrocortisone Acetate (Potential for reduced antibody response in active immunization procedures). Products include:
Florinef Acetate Tablets 505

Fluorouracil (Potential for reduced antibody response in active immunization procedures). Products include:
Efudex 2113
Fluoroplex Topical Solution & Cream 1% 479
Fluorouracil Injection 2116

Flutamide (Potential for reduced antibody response in active immunization procedures). Products include:
Eulexin Capsules 2358

Hydrocortisone (Potential for reduced antibody response in active immunization procedures). Products include:
Anusol-HC Cream 2.5% 1896
Aquanil HC Lotion 1931
Bactine Hydrocortisone Anti-Itch Cream .... ⊞ 709
Caldecort Anti-Itch Hydrocortisone Spray .... ⊞ 631
Cortaid .... ⊞ 836
CORTENEMA 2535
Cortisporin Ointment 1085
Cortisporin Ophthalmic Ointment Sterile 1085
Cortisporin Ophthalmic Suspension Sterile 1086
Cortisporin Otic Solution Sterile 1087
Cortisporin Otic Suspension Sterile 1088
Cortizone-5 .... ⊞ 831
Cortizone-10 .... ⊞ 831
Hydrocortone Tablets 1672
Hytone 907
Massengill Medicated Soft Cloth Towelettes 2458
PediOtic Suspension Sterile 1153
Preparation H Hydrocortisone 1% Cream .... ⊞ 872
ProctoCream-HC 2.5% 2408
VōSoL HC Otic Solution 2678

Hydrocortisone Acetate (Potential for reduced antibody response in active immunization procedures). Products include:
Analpram-HC Rectal Cream 1% and 2.5% 977
Anusol HC-1 Anti-Itch Hydrocortisone Ointment .... ⊞ 847
Anusol-HC Suppositories 1897
Caldecort .... ⊞ 631
Carmol HC 924
Coly-Mycin S Otic w/Neomycin & Hydrocortisone 1906
Cortaid .... ⊞ 836
Cortifoam 2396
Cortisporin Cream 1084
Epifoam 2399
Hydrocortone Acetate Sterile Suspension 1669
Mantadil Cream 1135
Nupercainal Hydrocortisone 1% Cream .... ⊞ 645
Ophthocort .... ⊙ 311
Pramosone Cream, Lotion & Ointment 978
ProctoCream-HC 2408
ProctoFoam-HC 2409
Terra-Cortril Ophthalmic Suspension 2210

Hydrocortisone Sodium Phosphate (Potential for reduced antibody response in active immunization procedures). Products include:
Hydrocortone Phosphate Injection, Sterile 1670

Hydrocortisone Sodium Succinate (Potential for reduced antibody response in active immunization procedures). Products include:
Solu-Cortef Sterile Powder 2641

Hydroxyurea (Potential for reduced antibody response in active immunization procedures). Products include:
Hydrea Capsules 696

Idarubicin Hydrochloride (Potential for reduced antibody response in active immunization procedures). Products include:
Idamycin 1955

Ifosfamide (Potential for reduced antibody response in active immunization procedures). Products include:
IFEX 697

Interferon alfa-2A, Recombinant (Potential for reduced antibody response in active immunization procedures). Products include:
Roferon-A Injection 2145

Interferon alfa-2B, Recombinant (Potential for reduced antibody response in active immunization procedures). Products include:
Intron A 2364

Levamisole Hydrochloride (Potential for reduced antibody response in active immunization procedures). Products include:
Ergamisol Tablets 1292

Lomustine (CCNU) (Potential for reduced antibody response in active immunization procedures). Products include:
CeeNU 693

Mechlorethamine Hydrochloride (Potential for reduced antibody response in active immunization procedures). Products include:
Mustargen 1709

Megestrol Acetate (Potential for reduced antibody response in active immunization procedures). Products include:
Megace Oral Suspension 699
Megace Tablets 701

Melphalan (Potential for reduced antibody response in active immunization procedures). Products include:
Alkeran Tablets 1071

Mercaptopurine (Potential for reduced antibody response in active immunization procedures). Products include:
Purinethol Tablets 1156

Methotrexate Sodium (Potential for reduced antibody response in active immunization procedures). Products include:
Methotrexate Sodium Tablets, Injection, for Injection and LPF Injection 1275

Methylprednisolone Acetate (Potential for reduced antibody response in active immunization procedures). Products include:
Depo-Medrol Single-Dose Vial 2600
Depo-Medrol Sterile Aqueous Suspension 2597

Methylprednisolone Sodium Succinate (Potential for reduced antibody response in active immunization procedures). Products include:
Solu-Medrol Sterile Powder 2643

Mitomycin (Mitomycin-C) (Potential for reduced antibody response in active immunization procedures). Products include:
Mutamycin 703

Mitotane (Potential for reduced antibody response in active immunization procedures). Products include:
Lysodren 698

Mitoxantrone Hydrochloride (Potential for reduced antibody response in active immunization procedures). Products include:
Novantrone 1279

Paclitaxel (Potential for reduced antibody response in active immunization procedures). Products include:
Taxol 714

Prednisolone Acetate (Potential for reduced antibody response in active immunization procedures). Products include:
AK-CIDE .... ⊙ 202
AK-CIDE Ointment .... ⊙ 202
Blephamide Liquifilm Sterile Ophthalmic Suspension 476
Blephamide Ointment .... ⊙ 237
Econopred & Econopred Plus Ophthalmic Suspensions .... ⊙ 217
Poly-Pred Liquifilm .... ⊙ 248
Pred Forte .... ⊙ 250
Pred Mild .... ⊙ 253
Pred-G Liquifilm Sterile Ophthalmic Suspension .... ⊙ 251
Pred-G S.O.P. Sterile Ophthalmic Ointment .... ⊙ 252
Vasocidin Ointment .... ⊙ 268

Prednisolone Sodium Phosphate (Potential for reduced antibody response in active immunization procedures). Products include:
AK-Pred .... ⊙ 204

(⊞ Described in PDR For Nonprescription Drugs) (⊙ Described in PDR For Ophthalmology)

427 **Interactions Index** **Foscavir**

Hydeltrasol Injection, Sterile 1665
Inflamase ⊙ 265
Pediapred Oral Liquid 995
Vasocidin Ophthalmic Solution ⊙ 270

Prednisolone Tebutate (Potential for reduced antibody response in active immunization procedures). Products include:
Hydeltra-T.B.A. Sterile Suspension 1667

Prednisone (Potential for reduced antibody response in active immunization procedures). Products include:
Deltasone Tablets 2595

Procarbazine Hydrochloride (Potential for reduced antibody response in active immunization procedures). Products include:
Matulane Capsules 2131

Streptozocin (Potential for reduced antibody response in active immunization procedures). Products include:
Zanosar Sterile Powder 2653

Tamoxifen Citrate (Potential for reduced antibody response in active immunization procedures). Products include:
Nolvadex Tablets 2841

Teniposide (Potential for reduced antibody response in active immunization procedures). Products include:
Vumon 727

Theophylline (Influenza immunization can inhibit the clearance of theophylline). Products include:
Marax Tablets & DF Syrup 2200
Quibron 2053

Theophylline Anhydrous (Influenza immunization can inhibit the clearance of theophylline). Products include:
Aerolate 1004
Primatene Dual Action Formula ■ 872
Primatene Tablets ■ 873
Respbid Tablets 682
Slo-bid Gyrocaps 2033
Theo-24 Extended Release Capsules 2568
Theo-Dur Extended-Release Tablets 1327
Theo-X Extended-Release Tablets 788
Uni-Dur Extended-Release Tablets 1331
Uniphyl 400 mg Tablets 2001

Theophylline Calcium Salicylate (Influenza immunization can inhibit the clearance of theophylline). Products include:
Quadrinal Tablets 1350

Theophylline Sodium Glycinate (Influenza immunization can inhibit the clearance of theophylline).
No products indexed under this heading.

Thioguanine (Potential for reduced antibody response in active immunization procedures). Products include:
Thioguanine Tablets, Tabloid Brand 1181

Thiotepa (Potential for reduced antibody response in active immunization procedures). Products include:
Thioplex (Thiotepa For Injection) 1281

Triamcinolone (Potential for reduced antibody response in active immunization procedures). Products include:
Aristocort Tablets 1022

Triamcinolone Acetonide (Potential for reduced antibody response in active immunization procedures). Products include:
Aristocort A 0.025% Cream 1027
Aristocort A 0.5% Cream 1031
Aristocort A 0.1% Cream 1029
Aristocort A 0.1% Ointment 1030
Azmacort Oral Inhaler 2011
Nasacort Nasal Inhaler 2024

Triamcinolone Diacetate (Potential for reduced antibody response in active immunization procedures). Products include:
Aristocort Suspension (Forte Parenteral) 1027
Aristocort Suspension (Intralesional) 1025

Triamcinolone Hexacetonide (Potential for reduced antibody response in active immunization procedures). Products include:
Aristospan Suspension (Intra-articular) 1033
Aristospan Suspension (Intralesional) 1032

Vincristine Sulfate (Potential for reduced antibody response in active immunization procedures). Products include:
Oncovin Solution Vials & Hyporets 1466

Vinorelbine Tartrate (Potential for reduced antibody response in active immunization procedures). Products include:
Navelbine Injection 1145

Warfarin Sodium (Influenza immunization can inhibit the clearance of warfarin). Products include:
Coumadin 926

FOOD FOR THOUGHT
(Nutritional Beverage) ■ 867
May interact with:

Aluminum Carbonate Gel (Concomitant use with aluminum-containing antacids should be avoided). Products include:
Basaljel 2703

Aluminum Hydroxide (Concomitant use with aluminum-containing antacids should be avoided). Products include:
ALternaGEL Liquid 1316
Maximum Strength Ascriptin ■ 630
Cama Arthritis Pain Reliever ■ 785
Gaviscon Extra Strength Relief Formula Antacid Tablets ■ 819
Gaviscon Extra Strength Relief Formula Liquid Antacid ■ 819
Gaviscon Liquid Antacid ■ 820
Gelusil Liquid & Tablets ■ 855
Maalox Heartburn Relief Suspension ■ 642
Maalox Heartburn Relief Tablets ■ 641
Maalox Magnesia and Alumina Oral Suspension ■ 642
Maalox Plus Tablets ■ 643
Extra Strength Maalox Antacid Plus Antigas Liquid and Tablets ■ 638
Tempo Soft Antacid ■ 835

Aluminum Hydroxide Gel (Concomitant use with aluminum-containing antacids should be avoided). Products include:
ALternaGEL Liquid ■ 659
Aludrox Oral Suspension 2695
Amphojel Suspension 2695
Amphojel Suspension without Flavor 2695
Amphojel Tablets 2695
Arthritis Pain Ascriptin ■ 631
Regular Strength Ascriptin Tablets ■ 629
Gaviscon Antacid Tablets ■ 819
Gaviscon-2 Antacid Tablets ■ 820
Mylanta Liquid 1317
Mylanta Tablets ■ 660
Mylanta Double Strength Liquid 1317
Mylanta Double Strength Tablets ■ 660
Nephrox Suspension ■ 655

FORMULA MAGIC ANTIBACTERIAL POWDER
(Benzethonium Chloride) ■ 625
None cited in PDR database.

FORTAZ
(Ceftazidime) 1100
May interact with aminoglycosides and certain other agents. Compounds in these categories include:

Amikacin Sulfate (Potential for nephrotoxicity following concomitant administration). Products include:
Amikacin Sulfate Injection, USP 960
Amikin Injectable 501

Chloramphenicol (Possibility of antagonism *in vivo*, particularly when bactericidal activity is desired; avoid this combination). Products include:
Chloromycetin Ophthalmic Ointment, 1% ⊙ 310
Chloromycetin Ophthalmic Solution ⊙ 310
Chloroptic S.O.P. ⊙ 239
Chloroptic Sterile Ophthalmic Solution ⊙ 239
Elase-Chloromycetin Ointment 1040
Ophthocort ⊙ 311

Chloramphenicol Palmitate (Possibility of antagonism *in vivo*, particularly when bactericidal activity is desired; avoid this combination).
No products indexed under this heading.

Chloramphenicol Sodium Succinate (Possibility of antagonism *in vivo*, particularly when bactericidal activity is desired; avoid this combination). Products include:
Chloromycetin Sodium Succinate 1900

Furosemide (Potential for nephrotoxicity following concomitant administration). Products include:
Lasix Injection, Oral Solution and Tablets 1240

Gentamicin Sulfate (Potential for nephrotoxicity following concomitant administration). Products include:
Garamycin Injectable 2360
Genoptic Sterile Ophthalmic Solution ⊙ 243
Genoptic Sterile Ophthalmic Ointment ⊙ 243
Gentacidin Ointment ⊙ 264
Gentacidin Solution ⊙ 264
Gentak ⊙ 208
Pred-G Liquifilm Sterile Ophthalmic Suspension ⊙ 251
Pred-G S.O.P. Sterile Ophthalmic Ointment ⊙ 252

Kanamycin Sulfate (Potential for nephrotoxicity following concomitant administration).
No products indexed under this heading.

Streptomycin Sulfate (Potential for nephrotoxicity following concomitant administration). Products include:
Streptomycin Sulfate Injection 2208

Tobramycin (Potential for nephrotoxicity following concomitant administration). Products include:
AKTOB ⊙ 206
TobraDex Ophthalmic Suspension and Ointment 473
Tobrex Ophthalmic Ointment and Solution ⊙ 229

Tobramycin Sulfate (Potential for nephrotoxicity following concomitant administration). Products include:
Nebcin Vials, Hyporets & ADD-Vantage 1464
Tobramycin Sulfate Injection 968

FOSCAVIR INJECTION
(Foscarnet Sodium) 547
May interact with aminoglycosides, drugs known to influence serum calcium levels (selected), inhibitors of renal tubular secretion or resorption, and certain other agents. Compounds in these categories include:

Amikacin Sulfate (Concurrent administration should be avoided because of foscarnet's tendency to cause renal impairment). Products include:
Amikacin Sulfate Injection, USP 960
Amikin Injectable 501

Amphotericin B (Concurrent administration should be avoided because of foscarnet's tendency to cause renal impairment). Products include:
Fungizone Intravenous 506

Carboplatin (Potential for increased hypocalcemia). Products include:
Paraplatin for Injection 705

Cisplatin (Potential for increased hypocalcemia). Products include:
Platinol 708
Platinol-AQ Injection 710

Gallium Nitrate (Potential for increased hypocalcemia). Products include:
Ganite 2533

Gentamicin Sulfate (Concurrent administration should be avoided because of foscarnet's tendency to cause renal impairment). Products include:
Garamycin Injectable 2360
Genoptic Sterile Ophthalmic Solution ⊙ 243
Genoptic Sterile Ophthalmic Ointment ⊙ 243
Gentacidin Ointment ⊙ 264
Gentacidin Solution ⊙ 264
Gentak ⊙ 208
Pred-G Liquifilm Sterile Ophthalmic Suspension ⊙ 251
Pred-G S.O.P. Sterile Ophthalmic Ointment ⊙ 252

Kanamycin Sulfate (Concurrent administration should be avoided because of foscarnet's tendency to cause renal impairment).
No products indexed under this heading.

Pentamidine Isethionate (Concomitant administration with intravenous pentamidine may cause hypocalcemia). Products include:
NebuPent for Inhalation Solution 1040
Pentam 300 Injection 1041

Probenecid (Elimination of foscarnet may be impaired). Products include:
Benemid Tablets 1611
ColBENEMID Tablets 1622

Sodium Polystyrene Sulfonate (Potential for increased hypocalcemia). Products include:
Kayexalate 2314
Sodium Polystyrene Sulfonate Suspension 2244

Streptomycin Sulfate (Concurrent administration should be avoided because of foscarnet's tendency to cause renal impairment). Products include:
Streptomycin Sulfate Injection 2208

Sulfinpyrazone (Elimination of foscarnet may be impaired). Products include:
Anturane 807

Tobramycin (Concurrent administration should be avoided because of foscarnet's tendency to cause renal impairment). Products include:
AKTOB ⊙ 206
TobraDex Ophthalmic Suspension and Ointment 473
Tobrex Ophthalmic Ointment and Solution ⊙ 229

IMPORTANT NOTE: Always consult each drug listing in the patient's regimen for possible interactions.

Foscavir **Interactions Index** 428

Tobramycin Sulfate (Concurrent administration should be avoided because of foscarnet's tendency to cause renal impairment). Products include:
- Nebcin Vials, Hyporets & ADD-Vantage ... 1464
- Tobramycin Sulfate Injection ... 968

Zidovudine (Potential for additive effects on anemia). Products include:
- Retrovir Capsules ... 1158
- Retrovir I.V. Infusion ... 1163
- Retrovir Syrup ... 1158

FOTOTAR CREAM
(Coal Tar) ... 1253
None cited in PDR database.

FRAGMIN
(Dalteparin Sodium) ... 1954
May interact with oral anticoagulants and platelet inhibitors. Compounds in these categories include:

Aspirin (Potential for increased risk of bleeding). Products include:
- Alka-Seltzer Effervescent Antacid and Pain Reliever ... ▣ 701
- Alka-Seltzer Extra Strength Effervescent Antacid and Pain Reliever ... ▣ 703
- Alka-Seltzer Lemon Lime Effervescent Antacid and Pain Reliever ... ▣ 703
- Alka-Seltzer Plus Cold Medicine ... ▣ 705
- Alka-Seltzer Plus Cold & Cough Medicine ... ▣ 708
- Alka-Seltzer Plus Night-Time Cold Medicine ... ▣ 707
- Alka Seltzer Plus Sinus Medicine .. ▣ 707
- Arthritis Foundation Safety Coated Aspirin Tablets ... ▣ 675
- Arthritis Pain Ascriptin ... ▣ 631
- Maximum Strength Ascriptin ... ▣ 630
- Regular Strength Ascriptin Tablets ... ▣ 629
- Arthritis Strength BC Powder ... ▣ 609
- BC Cold Powder Multi-Symptom Formula (Cold-Sinus-Allergy) ... ▣ 609
- BC Cold Powder Non-Drowsy Formula (Cold-Sinus) ... ▣ 609
- BC Powder ... ▣ 609
- Bayer Children's Chewable Aspirin ... ▣ 711
- Genuine Bayer Aspirin Tablets & Caplets ... ▣ 713
- Extra Strength Bayer Arthritis Pain Regimen Formula ... ▣ 711
- Extra Strength Bayer Aspirin Caplets & Tablets ... ▣ 712
- Extended-Release Bayer 8-Hour Aspirin ... ▣ 712
- Extra Strength Bayer Plus Aspirin Caplets ... ▣ 713
- Extra Strength Bayer PM Aspirin .. ▣ 713
- Bayer Enteric Aspirin ... ▣ 709
- Bufferin Analgesic Tablets and Caplets ... ▣ 613
- Arthritis Strength Bufferin Analgesic Caplets ... ▣ 614
- Extra Strength Bufferin Analgesic Tablets ... ▣ 615
- Cama Arthritis Pain Reliever ... ▣ 785
- Darvon Compound-65 Pulvules ... 1435
- Easprin ... 1914
- Ecotrin ... 2455
- Ecotrin Enteric Coated Aspirin Maximum Strength Tablets and Caplets ... ▣ 816
- Ecotrin Enteric Coated Aspirin Regular Strength Tablets ... 2455
- Empirin Aspirin Tablets ... ▣ 854
- Empirin with Codeine Tablets ... 1093
- Excedrin Extra-Strength Analgesic Tablets & Caplets ... 732
- Fiorinal Capsules ... 2261
- Fiorinal with Codeine Capsules ... 2262
- Fiorinal Tablets ... 2261
- Halfprin ... 1362
- Healthprin Aspirin ... 2455
- Norgesic ... 1496
- Percodan Tablets ... 939
- Percodan-Demi Tablets ... 940
- Robaxisal Tablets ... 2071
- Soma Compound w/Codeine Tablets ... 2676
- Soma Compound Tablets ... 2675
- St. Joseph Adult Chewable Aspirin (81 mg.) ... ▣ 808
- Talwin Compound ... 2335
- Ursinus Inlay-Tabs ... ▣ 794
- Vanquish Analgesic Caplets ... ▣ 731

Azlocillin Sodium (Potential for increased risk of bleeding).
- No products indexed under this heading.

Carbenicillin Indanyl Sodium (Potential for increased risk of bleeding). Products include:
- Geocillin Tablets ... 2199

Choline Magnesium Trisalicylate (Potential for increased risk of bleeding). Products include:
- Trilisate ... 2000

Diclofenac Potassium (Potential for increased risk of bleeding). Products include:
- Cataflam ... 816

Diclofenac Sodium (Potential for increased risk of bleeding). Products include:
- Voltaren Ophthalmic Sterile Ophthalmic Solution ... ◉ 272
- Voltaren Tablets ... 861

Dicumarol (Potential for increased risk of bleeding).
- No products indexed under this heading.

Diflunisal (Potential for increased risk of bleeding). Products include:
- Dolobid Tablets ... 1654

Dipyridamole (Potential for increased risk of bleeding). Products include:
- Persantine Tablets ... 681

Fenoprofen Calcium (Potential for increased risk of bleeding). Products include:
- Nalfon 200 Pulvules & Nalfon Tablets ... 917

Flurbiprofen (Potential for increased risk of bleeding). Products include:
- Ansaid Tablets ... 2579

Ibuprofen (Potential for increased risk of bleeding). Products include:
- Advil Cold and Sinus Caplets and Tablets (formerly CoAdvil) ... ▣ 870
- Advil Ibuprofen Tablets and Caplets ... ▣ 870
- Children's Advil Suspension ... 2692
- Arthritis Foundation Ibuprofen Tablets ... ▣ 674
- Bayer Select Ibuprofen Pain Relief Formula ... ▣ 715
- Cramp End Tablets ... ▣ 735
- Dimetapp Sinus Caplets ... ▣ 775
- Haltran Tablets ... ▣ 771
- IBU Tablets ... 1342
- Ibuprohm ... ▣ 735
- Children's Motrin Ibuprofen Oral Suspension ... 1546
- Motrin Tablets ... 2625
- Motrin IB Caplets, Tablets, and Geltabs ... ▣ 838
- Motrin IB Sinus ... ▣ 838
- Motrin Ibuprofen Suspension, Oral Drops, Chewable Tablets, Caplets ... 1546
- Nuprin Ibuprofen/Analgesic Tablets & Caplets ... ▣ 622
- Sine-Aid IB Caplets ... 1554
- Vicks DayQuil SINUS Pressure & PAIN Relief with IBUPROFEN ... ▣ 762

Indomethacin (Potential for increased risk of bleeding). Products include:
- Indocin ... 1680

Indomethacin Sodium Trihydrate (Potential for increased risk of bleeding). Products include:
- Indocin I.V. ... 1684

Ketoprofen (Potential for increased risk of bleeding). Products include:
- Orudis Capsules ... 2766
- Oruvail Capsules ... 2766

Magnesium Salicylate (Potential for increased risk of bleeding). Products include:
- Backache Caplets ... ▣ 613
- Bayer Select Backache Pain Relief Formula ... ▣ 715
- Doan's Extra-Strength Analgesic ... ▣ 633
- Extra Strength Doan's P.M. ... ▣ 633
- Doan's Regular Strength Analgesic ... ▣ 634
- Mobigesic Tablets ... ▣ 602

Meclofenamate Sodium (Potential for increased risk of bleeding).
- No products indexed under this heading.

Mefenamic Acid (Potential for increased risk of bleeding). Products include:
- Ponstel ... 1925

Mezlocillin Sodium (Potential for increased risk of bleeding). Products include:
- Mezlin ... 601
- Mezlin Pharmacy Bulk Package ... 604

Nafcillin Sodium (Potential for increased risk of bleeding).
- No products indexed under this heading.

Naproxen (Potential for increased risk of bleeding). Products include:
- Anaprox/Naprosyn ... 2117

Naproxen Sodium (Potential for increased risk of bleeding). Products include:
- Aleve ... 1975
- Anaprox/Naprosyn ... 2117

Penicillin G Benzathine (Potential for increased risk of bleeding). Products include:
- Bicillin C-R Injection ... 2704
- Bicillin C-R 900/300 Injection ... 2706
- Bicillin L-A Injection ... 2707

Penicillin G Procaine (Potential for increased risk of bleeding). Products include:
- Bicillin C-R Injection ... 2704
- Bicillin C-R 900/300 Injection ... 2706

Phenylbutazone (Potential for increased risk of bleeding).
- No products indexed under this heading.

Piroxicam (Potential for increased risk of bleeding). Products include:
- Feldene Capsules ... 1965

Salsalate (Potential for increased risk of bleeding). Products include:
- Mono-Gesic Tablets ... 792
- Salflex Tablets ... 786

Sulindac (Potential for increased risk of bleeding). Products include:
- Clinoril Tablets ... 1618

Ticarcillin Disodium (Potential for increased risk of bleeding). Products include:
- Ticar for Injection ... 2526
- Timentin for Injection ... 2528

Ticlopidine Hydrochloride (Potential for increased risk of bleeding). Products include:
- Ticlid Tablets ... 2156

Tolmetin Sodium (Potential for increased risk of bleeding). Products include:
- Tolectin (200, 400 and 600 mg) .. 1581

Warfarin Sodium (Potential for increased risk of bleeding). Products include:
- Coumadin ... 926

STERILE FUDR
(Floxuridine) ... 2118
May interact with alkylating agents. Compounds in this category include:

Bone Marrow Depressants, unspecified (Increased toxicity of FUDR).

Busulfan (FUDR should be used with extreme caution in patients with previous use of alkylating agents). Products include:
- Myleran Tablets ... 1143

Carmustine (BCNU) (FUDR should be used with extreme caution in patients with previous use of alkylating agents). Products include:
- BiCNU ... 691

Chlorambucil (FUDR should be used with extreme caution in patients with previous use of alkylating agents). Products include:
- Leukeran Tablets ... 1133

Cyclophosphamide (FUDR should be used with extreme caution in patients with previous use of alkylating agents). Products include:
- Cytoxan ... 694
- NEOSAR Lyophilized/Neosar ... 1959

Dacarbazine (FUDR should be used with extreme caution in patients with previous use of alkylating agents). Products include:
- DTIC-Dome ... 600

Lomustine (CCNU) (FUDR should be used with extreme caution in patients with previous use of alkylating agents). Products include:
- CeeNU ... 693

Mechlorethamine Hydrochloride (FUDR should be used with extreme caution in patients with previous use of alkylating agents). Products include:
- Mustargen ... 1709

Melphalan (FUDR should be used with extreme caution in patients with previous use of alkylating agents). Products include:
- Alkeran Tablets ... 1071

Thiotepa (FUDR should be used with extreme caution in patients with previous use of alkylating agents). Products include:
- Thioplex (Thiotepa For Injection) ... 1281

FULVICIN P/G TABLETS
(Griseofulvin) ... 2359
May interact with barbiturates, oral anticoagulants, oral contraceptives, and certain other agents. Compounds in these categories include:

Aprobarbital (Depresses griseofulvin activity).
- No products indexed under this heading.

Butabarbital (Depresses griseofulvin activity).
- No products indexed under this heading.

Butalbital (Depresses griseofulvin activity). Products include:
- Esgic-plus Tablets ... 1013
- Fioricet Tablets ... 2258
- Fioricet with Codeine Capsules ... 2260
- Fiorinal Capsules ... 2261
- Fiorinal with Codeine Capsules ... 2262
- Fiorinal Tablets ... 2261
- Phrenilin ... 785
- Sedapap Tablets 50 mg/650 mg .. 1543

Desogestrel (Decreased contraceptive effects; possible menstrual irregularities). Products include:
- Desogen Tablets ... 1817
- Ortho-Cept ... 1851

Dicumarol (Decreased anticoagulant effects).
- No products indexed under this heading.

Ethinyl Estradiol (Decreased contraceptive effects; possible menstrual irregularities). Products include:
- Brevicon ... 2088
- Demulen ... 2428
- Desogen Tablets ... 1817

(▣ Described in PDR For Nonprescription Drugs) (◉ Described in PDR For Ophthalmology)

429 **Interactions Index** **Fungizone I.V.**

Levlen/Tri-Levlen 651
Lo/Ovral Tablets 2746
Lo/Ovral-28 Tablets 2751
Modicon 1872
Nordette-21 Tablets 2755
Nordette-28 Tablets 2758
Norinyl 2088
Ortho-Cept 1851
Ortho-Cyclen/Ortho-Tri-Cyclen 1858
Ortho-Novum 1872
Ortho-Cyclen/Ortho Tri-Cyclen 1858
Ovcon 760
Ovral Tablets 2770
Ovral-28 Tablets 2770
Levlen/Tri-Levlen 651
Tri-Norinyl 2164
Triphasil-21 Tablets 2814
Triphasil-28 Tablets 2819

Ethynodiol Diacetate (Decreased contraceptive effects; possible menstrual irregularities). Products include:
Demulen 2428

Levonorgestrel (Decreased contraceptive effects; possible menstrual irregularities). Products include:
Levlen/Tri-Levlen 651
Nordette-21 Tablets 2755
Nordette-28 Tablets 2758
Norplant System 2759
Levlen/Tri-Levlen 651
Triphasil-21 Tablets 2814
Triphasil-28 Tablets 2819

Mephobarbital (Depresses griseofulvin activity). Products include:
Mebaral Tablets 2322

Mestranol (Decreased contraceptive effects; possible menstrual irregularities). Products include:
Norinyl 2088
Ortho-Novum 1872

Norethindrone (Decreased contraceptive effects; possible menstrual irregularities). Products include:
Brevicon 2088
Micronor Tablets 1872
Modicon 1872
Norinyl 2088
Nor-Q D Tablets 2135
Ortho-Novum 1872
Ovcon 760
Tri-Norinyl 2164

Norethynodrel (Decreased contraceptive effects; possible menstrual irregularities).
No products indexed under this heading.

Norgestimate (Decreased contraceptive effects; possible menstrual irregularities). Products include:
Ortho-Cyclen/Ortho-Tri-Cyclen 1858
Ortho-Cyclen/Ortho Tri-Cyclen 1858

Norgestrel (Decreased contraceptive effects; possible menstrual irregularities). Products include:
Lo/Ovral Tablets 2746
Lo/Ovral-28 Tablets 2751
Ovral Tablets 2770
Ovral-28 Tablets 2770
Ovrette Tablets 2771

Pentobarbital Sodium (Depresses griseofulvin activity). Products include:
Nembutal Sodium Capsules 436
Nembutal Sodium Solution 438
Nembutal Sodium Suppositories 440

Phenobarbital (Depresses griseofulvin activity). Products include:
Arco-Lase Plus Tablets 512
Bellergal-S Tablets 2250
Donnatal 2060
Donnatal Extentabs 2061
Donnatal Tablets 2060
Phenobarbital Elixir and Tablets 1469
Quadrinal Tablets 1350

Secobarbital Sodium (Depresses griseofulvin activity). Products include:
Seconal Sodium Pulvules 1474

Thiamylal Sodium (Depresses griseofulvin activity).
No products indexed under this heading.

Warfarin Sodium (Depresses anticoagulant effects). Products include:
Coumadin 926

Food Interactions

Alcohol (Potentiation of effects of alcohol).

FULVICIN P/G 165 & 330 TABLETS
(Griseofulvin) 2359
May interact with oral anticoagulants, barbiturates, oral contraceptives, and certain other agents. Compounds in these categories include:

Aprobarbital (Depresses griseofulvin activity).
No products indexed under this heading.

Butabarbital (Depresses griseofulvin activity).
No products indexed under this heading.

Butalbital (Depresses griseofulvin activity). Products include:
Esgic-plus Tablets 1013
Fioricet Tablets 2258
Fioricet with Codeine Capsules 2260
Fiorinal Capsules 2261
Fiorinal with Codeine Capsules 2262
Fiorinal Tablets 2261
Phrenilin 785
Sedapap Tablets 50 mg/650 mg 1543

Desogestrel (Decreased contraceptive effects; possible menstrual irregularities). Products include:
Desogen Tablets 1817
Ortho-Cept 1851

Dicumarol (Decreased anticoagulant effect).
No products indexed under this heading.

Ethinyl Estradiol (Decreased contraceptive effects; possible menstrual irregularities). Products include:
Brevicon 2088
Demulen 2428
Desogen Tablets 1817
Levlen/Tri-Levlen 651
Lo/Ovral Tablets 2746
Lo/Ovral-28 Tablets 2751
Modicon 1872
Nordette-21 Tablets 2755
Nordette-28 Tablets 2758
Norinyl 2088
Ortho-Cept 1851
Ortho-Cyclen/Ortho-Tri-Cyclen 1858
Ortho-Novum 1872
Ortho-Cyclen/Ortho Tri-Cyclen 1858
Ovcon 760
Ovral Tablets 2770
Ovral-28 Tablets 2770
Levlen/Tri-Levlen 651
Tri-Norinyl 2164
Triphasil-21 Tablets 2814
Triphasil-28 Tablets 2819

Ethynodiol Diacetate (Decreased contraceptive effects; possible menstrual irregularities). Products include:
Demulen 2428

Levonorgestrel (Decreased contraceptive effects; possible menstrual irregularities). Products include:
Levlen/Tri-Levlen 651
Nordette-21 Tablets 2755
Nordette-28 Tablets 2758
Norplant System 2759
Levlen/Tri-Levlen 651
Triphasil-21 Tablets 2814
Triphasil-28 Tablets 2819

Mephobarbital (Depresses griseofulvin activity). Products include:
Mebaral Tablets 2322

Mestranol (Decreased contraceptive effects; possible menstrual irregularities). Products include:
Norinyl 2088
Ortho-Novum 1872

Norethindrone (Decreased contraceptive effects; possible menstrual irregularities). Products include:
Brevicon 2088
Micronor Tablets 1872
Modicon 1872
Norinyl 2088
Nor-Q D Tablets 2135
Ortho-Novum 1872
Ovcon 760
Tri-Norinyl 2164

Norethynodrel (Decreased contraceptive effects; possible menstrual irregularities).
No products indexed under this heading.

Norgestimate (Decreased contraceptive effects; possible menstrual irregularities). Products include:
Ortho-Cyclen/Ortho-Tri-Cyclen 1858
Ortho-Cyclen/Ortho Tri-Cyclen 1858

Norgestrel (Decreased contraceptive effects; possible menstrual irregularities). Products include:
Lo/Ovral Tablets 2746
Lo/Ovral-28 Tablets 2751
Ovral Tablets 2770
Ovral-28 Tablets 2770
Ovrette Tablets 2771

Pentobarbital Sodium (Depresses griseofulvin activity). Products include:
Nembutal Sodium Capsules 436
Nembutal Sodium Solution 438
Nembutal Sodium Suppositories 440

Phenobarbital (Depresses griseofulvin activity). Products include:
Arco-Lase Plus Tablets 512
Bellergal-S Tablets 2250
Donnatal 2060
Donnatal Extentabs 2061
Donnatal Tablets 2060
Phenobarbital Elixir and Tablets 1469
Quadrinal Tablets 1350

Secobarbital Sodium (Depresses griseofulvin activity). Products include:
Seconal Sodium Pulvules 1474

Thiamylal Sodium (Depresses griseofulvin activity).
No products indexed under this heading.

Warfarin Sodium (Decreased anticoagulant effect). Products include:
Coumadin 926

Food Interactions

Alcohol (Potentiation of effects of alcohol).

FUNGIZONE INTRAVENOUS
(Amphotericin B) 506
May interact with antineoplastics, nitrogen-mustard-type alkylating agents, corticosteroids, cardiac glycosides, aminoglycosides, imidazoles, muscle relaxants, and certain other agents. Compounds in these categories include:

ACTH (May potentiate amphotericin B-induced hypokalemia which may predispose the patient to cardiac dysfunction; avoid concomitant use).
No products indexed under this heading.

Altretamine (May enhance the potential for renal toxicity, bronchospasm and hypotension). Products include:
Hexalen Capsules 2571

Amikacin Sulfate (May enhance the potential for drug-induced renal toxicity, and should be used concomitantly only with great caution). Products include:
Amikacin Sulfate Injection, USP 960
Amikin Injectable 501

Asparaginase (May enhance the potential for renal toxicity, bronchospasm and hypotension). Products include:
Elspar 1659

Atracurium Besylate (Amphotericin B-induced hypokalemia may enhance the curariform effect of skeletal muscle relaxants). Products include:
Tracrium Injection 1183

Baclofen (Amphotericin B-induced hypokalemia may enhance the curariform effect of skeletal muscle relaxants). Products include:
Lioresal Intrathecal 1596
Lioresal Tablets 829

Betamethasone Acetate (May potentiate amphotericin B-induced hypokalemia which may predispose the patient to cardiac dysfunction; avoid concomitant use). Products include:
Celestone Soluspan Suspension 2347

Betamethasone Sodium Phosphate (May potentiate amphotericin B-induced hypokalemia which may predispose the patient to cardiac dysfunction; avoid concomitant use). Products include:
Celestone Soluspan Suspension 2347

Bleomycin Sulfate (May enhance the potential for renal toxicity, bronchospasm and hypotension). Products include:
Blenoxane 692

Busulfan (May enhance the potential for renal toxicity, bronchospasm and hypotension). Products include:
Myleran Tablets 1143

Carboplatin (May enhance the potential for renal toxicity, bronchospasm and hypotension). Products include:
Paraplatin for Injection 705

Carisoprodol (Amphotericin B-induced hypokalemia may enhance the curariform effect of skeletal muscle relaxants). Products include:
Soma Compound w/Codeine Tablets 2676
Soma Compound Tablets 2675
Soma Tablets 2674

Carmustine (BCNU) (May enhance the potential for renal toxicity, bronchospasm and hypotension). Products include:
BiCNU 691

Chlorambucil (May enhance the potential for renal toxicity, bronchospasm and hypotension). Products include:
Leukeran Tablets 1133

Chlorzoxazone (Amphotericin B-induced hypokalemia may enhance the curariform effect of skeletal muscle relaxants). Products include:
Paraflex Caplets 1580
Parafon Forte DSC Caplets 1581

Cisplatin (May enhance the potential for renal toxicity, bronchospasm and hypotension). Products include:
Platinol 708
Platinol-AQ Injection 710

Clotrimazole (*In vitro* studies with combination therapy suggest that imidazoles may induce fungal resistance to amphotericin-B). Products include:
Prescription Strength Desenex Cream ◘ 633

IMPORTANT NOTE: Always consult each drug listing in the patient's regimen for possible interactions.

Gyne-Lotrimin .... ■ 805
Gyne-Lotrimin Pack .... ■ 806
Lotrimin 2371
Lotrimin AF Antifungal Cream, Lotion and Solution .... ■ 806
Lotrisone Cream 2372
Mycelex OTC Cream Antifungal .... ■ 724
Mycelex OTC Solution Antifungal .... ■ 724
Mycelex Troches 608
Mycelex-7 Vaginal Cream Antifungal .... ■ 724
Mycelex-7 Vaginal Antifungal Cream with 7 Disposable Applicators .... ■ 724
Mycelex-7 Vaginal Inserts Antifungal .... ■ 725
Mycelex-7 Combination-Pack Vaginal Inserts & External Vulvar Cream .... ■ 725
Mycelex-G 500 mg Vaginal Tablets 609

Cortisone Acetate (May potentiate amphotericin B-induced hypokalemia which may predispose the patient to cardiac dysfunction; avoid concomitant use). Products include:
Cortone Acetate Sterile Suspension 1623
Cortone Acetate Tablets 1624

Cyclobenzaprine Hydrochloride (Amphotericin B-induced hypokalemia may enhance the curariform effect of skeletal muscle relaxants). Products include:
Flexeril Tablets 1661

Cyclophosphamide (May enhance the potential for renal toxicity, bronchospasm and hypotension). Products include:
Cytoxan 694
NEOSAR Lyophilized/Neosar 1959

Cyclosporine (May enhance the potential for drug-induced renal toxicity, and should be used concomitantly only with great caution). Products include:
Neoral 2276
Sandimmune 2286

Dacarbazine (May enhance the potential for renal toxicity, bronchospasm and hypotension). Products include:
DTIC-Dome 600

Dantrolene Sodium (Amphotericin B-induced hypokalemia may enhance the curariform effect of skeletal muscle relaxants). Products include:
Dantrium Capsules 1982
Dantrium Intravenous 1983

Daunorubicin Hydrochloride (May enhance the potential for renal toxicity, bronchospasm and hypotension). Products include:
Cerubidine 795

Deslanoside (Amphotericin B-induced hypokalemia may potentiate digitalis toxicity).
No products indexed under this heading.

Dexamethasone (May potentiate amphotericin B-induced hypokalemia which may predispose the patient to cardiac dysfunction; avoid concomitant use). Products include:
AK-Trol Ointment & Suspension .... ◎ 205
Decadron Elixir 1633
Decadron Tablets 1635
Decaspray Topical Aerosol 1648
Dexacidin Ointment .... ◎ 263
Maxitrol Ophthalmic Ointment and Suspension .... ◎ 224
TobraDex Ophthalmic Suspension and Ointment 473

Dexamethasone Acetate (May potentiate amphotericin B-induced hypokalemia which may predispose the patient to cardiac dysfunction; avoid concomitant use). Products include:
Dalalone D.P. Injectable 1011
Decadron-LA Sterile Suspension 1646

Dexamethasone Sodium Phosphate (May potentiate amphotericin B-induced hypokalemia which may predispose the patient to cardiac dysfunction; avoid concomitant use). Products include:
Decadron Phosphate Injection 1637
Decadron Phosphate Respihaler 1642
Decadron Phosphate Sterile Ophthalmic Ointment 1641
Decadron Phosphate Sterile Ophthalmic Solution 1642
Decadron Phosphate Topical Cream 1644
Decadron Phosphate Turbinaire 1645
Decadron Phosphate with Xylocaine Injection, Sterile 1639
Dexacort Phosphate in Respihaler .. 458
Dexacort Phosphate in Turbinaire .. 459
NeoDecadron Sterile Ophthalmic Ointment 1712
NeoDecadron Sterile Ophthalmic Solution 1713
NeoDecadron Topical Cream 1714

Digitoxin (Amphotericin B-induced hypokalemia may potentiate digitalis toxicity). Products include:
Crystodigin Tablets 1433

Digoxin (Amphotericin B-induced hypokalemia may potentiate digitalis toxicity). Products include:
Lanoxicaps 1117
Lanoxin Elixir Pediatric 1120
Lanoxin Injection 1123
Lanoxin Injection Pediatric 1126
Lanoxin Tablets 1128

Doxacurium Chloride (Amphotericin B-induced hypokalemia may enhance the curariform effect of skeletal muscle relaxants). Products include:
Nuromax Injection 1149

Doxorubicin Hydrochloride (May enhance the potential for renal toxicity, bronchospasm and hypotension). Products include:
Adriamycin PFS 1947
Adriamycin RDF 1947
Doxorubicin Astra 540
Rubex 712

Estramustine Phosphate Sodium (May enhance the potential for renal toxicity, bronchospasm and hypotension). Products include:
Emcyt Capsules 1953

Etoposide (May enhance the potential for renal toxicity, bronchospasm and hypotension). Products include:
VePesid Capsules and Injection 718

Floxuridine (May enhance the potential for renal toxicity, bronchospasm and hypotension). Products include:
Sterile FUDR 2118

Fluconazole (*In vitro* studies with combination therapy suggest that imidazoles may induce fungal resistance to amphotericin-B). Products include:
Diflucan Injection, Tablets, and Oral Suspension 2194

Flucytosine (Concomitant use may increase the toxicity of flucytosine by possibly increasing its cellular uptake and/or impairing its renal excretion). Products include:
Ancobon Capsules 2079

Fludrocortisone Acetate (May potentiate amphotericin B-induced hypokalemia which may predispose the patient to cardiac dysfunction; avoid concomitant use). Products include:
Florinef Acetate Tablets 505

Fluorouracil (May enhance the potential for renal toxicity, bronchospasm and hypotension). Products include:
Efudex 2113
Fluoroplex Topical Solution & Cream 1% 479
Fluorouracil Injection 2116

Flutamide (May enhance the potential for renal toxicity, bronchospasm and hypotension). Products include:
Eulexin Capsules 2358

Gentamicin Sulfate (May enhance the potential for drug-induced renal toxicity, and should be used concomitantly only with great caution). Products include:
Garamycin Injectable 2360
Genoptic Sterile Ophthalmic Solution .... ◎ 243
Genoptic Sterile Ophthalmic Ointment .... ◎ 243
Gentacidin Ointment .... ◎ 264
Gentacidin Solution .... ◎ 264
Gentak .... ◎ 208
Pred-G Liquifilm Sterile Ophthalmic Suspension .... ◎ 251
Pred-G S.O.P. Sterile Ophthalmic Ointment .... ◎ 252

Hydrocortisone (May potentiate amphotericin B-induced hypokalemia which may predispose the patient to cardiac dysfunction; avoid concomitant use). Products include:
Anusol-HC Cream 2.5% 1896
Aquanil HC Lotion 1931
Bactine Hydrocortisone Anti-Itch Cream .... ■ 709
Caldecort Anti-Itch Hydrocortisone Spray .... ■ 631
Cortaid .... ■ 836
CORTENEMA 2535
Cortisporin Ointment 1085
Cortisporin Ophthalmic Ointment Sterile 1085
Cortisporin Ophthalmic Suspension Sterile 1086
Cortisporin Otic Solution Sterile 1087
Cortisporin Otic Suspension Sterile 1088
Cortizone-5 .... ■ 831
Cortizone-10 .... ■ 831
Hydrocortone Tablets 1672
Hytone 907
Massengill Medicated Soft Cloth Towelettes 2458
PediOtic Suspension Sterile 1153
Preparation H Hydrocortisone 1% Cream .... ■ 872
ProctoCream-HC 2.5% 2408
VōSoL HC Otic Solution 2678

Hydrocortisone Acetate (May potentiate amphotericin B-induced hypokalemia which may predispose the patient to cardiac dysfunction; avoid concomitant use). Products include:
Analpram-HC Rectal Cream 1% and 2.5% 977
Anusol HC-1 Anti-Itch Hydrocortisone Ointment .... ■ 847
Anusol-HC Suppositories 1897
Caldecort .... ■ 631
Carmol HC 924
Coly-Mycin S Otic w/Neomycin & Hydrocortisone 1906
Cortaid .... ■ 836
Cortifoam 2396
Cortisporin Cream 1084
Epifoam 2399
Hydrocortone Acetate Sterile Suspension 1669
Mantadil Cream 1135
Nupercainal Hydrocortisone 1% Cream .... ■ 645
Ophthocort .... ◎ 311
Pramosone Cream, Lotion & Ointment 978
ProctoCream-HC 2408
ProctoFoam-HC 2409
Terra-Cortril Ophthalmic Suspension 2210

Hydrocortisone Sodium Phosphate (May potentiate amphotericin B-induced hypokalemia which may predispose the patient to cardiac dysfunction; avoid concomitant use). Products include:
Hydrocortone Phosphate Injection, Sterile 1670

Hydrocortisone Sodium Succinate (May potentiate amphotericin B-induced hypokalemia which may predispose the patient to cardiac dysfunction; avoid concomitant use). Products include:
Solu-Cortef Sterile Powder 2641

Hydroxyurea (May enhance the potential for renal toxicity, bronchospasm and hypotension). Products include:
Hydrea Capsules 696

Idarubicin Hydrochloride (May enhance the potential for renal toxicity, bronchospasm and hypotension). Products include:
Idamycin 1955

Ifosfamide (May enhance the potential for renal toxicity, bronchospasm and hypotension). Products include:
IFEX 697

Interferon alfa-2A, Recombinant (May enhance the potential for renal toxicity, bronchospasm and hypotension). Products include:
Roferon-A Injection 2145

Interferon alfa-2B, Recombinant (May enhance the potential for renal toxicity, bronchospasm and hypotension). Products include:
Intron A 2364

Kanamycin Sulfate (May enhance the potential for drug-induced renal toxicity, and should be used concomitantly only with great caution).
No products indexed under this heading.

Ketoconazole (*In vitro* studies with combination therapy suggest that imidazoles may induce fungal resistance to amphotericin-B). Products include:
Nizoral 2% Cream 1297
Nizoral 2% Shampoo 1298
Nizoral Tablets 1298

Leukocyte transfusions (Potential for acute pulmonary toxicity with concomitant administration).

Levamisole Hydrochloride (May enhance the potential for renal toxicity, bronchospasm and hypotension). Products include:
Ergamisol Tablets 1292

Lomustine (CCNU) (May enhance the potential for renal toxicity, bronchospasm and hypotension). Products include:
CeeNU 693

Mechlorethamine Hydrochloride (May enhance the potential for renal toxicity, bronchospasm and hypotension). Products include:
Mustargen 1709

Megestrol Acetate (May enhance the potential for renal toxicity, bronchospasm and hypotension). Products include:
Megace Oral Suspension 699
Megace Tablets 701

Melphalan (May enhance the potential for renal toxicity, bronchospasm and hypotension). Products include:
Alkeran Tablets 1071

Mercaptopurine (May enhance the potential for renal toxicity, bronchospasm and hypotension). Products include:
Purinethol Tablets 1156

Metaxalone (Amphotericin B-induced hypokalemia may enhance the curariform effect of skeletal muscle relaxants). Products include:
Skelaxin Tablets 788

(■ Described in PDR For Nonprescription Drugs) (◎ Described in PDR For Ophthalmology)

431 Interactions Index Furoxone

Methocarbamol (Amphotericin B-induced hypokalemia may enhance the curariform effect of skeletal muscle relaxants). Products include:

Robaxin Injectable 2070
Robaxin Tablets 2071
Robaxisal Tablets 2071

Methotrexate Sodium (May enhance the potential for renal toxicity, bronchospasm and hypotension). Products include:

Methotrexate Sodium Tablets, Injection, for Injection and LPF Injection 1275

Methylprednisolone Acetate (May potentiate amphotericin B-induced hypokalemia which may predispose the patient to cardiac dysfunction; avoid concomitant use). Products include:

Depo-Medrol Single-Dose Vial 2600
Depo-Medrol Sterile Aqueous Suspension 2597

Methylprednisolone Sodium Succinate (May potentiate amphotericin B-induced hypokalemia which may predispose the patient to cardiac dysfunction; avoid concomitant use). Products include:

Solu-Medrol Sterile Powder 2643

Metocurine Iodide (Amphotericin B-induced hypokalemia may enhance the curariform effect of skeletal muscle relaxants). Products include:

Metubine Iodide Vials 916

Miconazole (*In vitro* studies with combination therapy suggest that imidazoles may induce fungal resistance to amphotericin-B).

No products indexed under this heading.

Miconazole Nitrate (*In vitro* studies with combination therapy suggest that imidazoles may induce fungal resistance to amphotericin-B). Products include:

Prescription Strength Desenex Spray Powder and Spray Liquid ▣ 633
Lotrimin AF Antifungal Spray Liquid, Spray Powder, Powder and Jock Itch Spray Powder .... ▣ 807
Monistat Dual-Pak 1850
Monistat 3 Vaginal Suppositories 1850
Monistat-Derm (miconazole nitrate 2%) Cream 1889

Mitomycin (Mitomycin-C) (May enhance the potential for renal toxicity, bronchospasm and hypotension). Products include:

Mutamycin 703

Mitotane (May enhance the potential for renal toxicity, bronchospasm and hypotension). Products include:

Lysodren 698

Mitoxantrone Hydrochloride (May enhance the potential for renal toxicity, bronchospasm and hypotension). Products include:

Novantrone 1279

Mivacurium Chloride (Amphotericin B-induced hypokalemia may enhance the curariform effect of skeletal muscle relaxants). Products include:

Mivacron 1138

Orphenadrine Citrate (Amphotericin B-induced hypokalemia may enhance the curariform effect of skeletal muscle relaxants). Products include:

Norflex 1496
Norgesic 1496

Paclitaxel (May enhance the potential for renal toxicity, bronchospasm and hypotension). Products include:

Taxol 714

Pancuronium Bromide Injection (Amphotericin B-induced hypokalemia may enhance the curariform effect of skeletal muscle relaxants).

No products indexed under this heading.

Pentamidine Isethionate (May enhance the potential for drug-induced renal toxicity, and should be used concomitantly only with great caution). Products include:

NebuPent for Inhalation Solution 1040
Pentam 300 Injection 1041

Prednisolone Acetate (May potentiate amphotericin B-induced hypokalemia which may predispose the patient to cardiac dysfunction; avoid concomitant use). Products include:

AK-CIDE .... ◉ 202
AK-CIDE Ointment .... ◉ 202
Blephamide Liquifilm Sterile Ophthalmic Suspension 476
Blephamide Ointment .... ◉ 237
Econopred & Econopred Plus Ophthalmic Suspensions .... ◉ 217
Poly-Pred Liquifilm .... ◉ 248
Pred Forte .... ◉ 250
Pred Mild .... ◉ 253
Pred-G Liquifilm Sterile Ophthalmic Suspension .... ◉ 251
Pred-G S.O.P. Sterile Ophthalmic Ointment .... ◉ 252
Vasocidin Ointment .... ◉ 268

Prednisolone Sodium Phosphate (May potentiate amphotericin B-induced hypokalemia which may predispose the patient to cardiac dysfunction; avoid concomitant use). Products include:

AK-Pred .... ◉ 204
Hydeltrasol Injection, Sterile 1665
Inflamase .... ◉ 265
Pediapred Oral Liquid 995
Vasocidin Ophthalmic Solution .... ◉ 270

Prednisolone Tebutate (May potentiate amphotericin B-induced hypokalemia which may predispose the patient to cardiac dysfunction; avoid concomitant use). Products include:

Hydeltra-T.B.A. Sterile Suspension 1667

Prednisone (May potentiate amphotericin B-induced hypokalemia which may predispose the patient to cardiac dysfunction; avoid concomitant use). Products include:

Deltasone Tablets 2595

Procarbazine Hydrochloride (May enhance the potential for renal toxicity, bronchospasm and hypotension). Products include:

Matulane Capsules 2131

Rocuronium Bromide (Amphotericin B-induced hypokalemia may enhance the curariform effect of skeletal muscle relaxants). Products include:

Zemuron 1830

Streptomycin Sulfate (May enhance the potential for drug-induced renal toxicity, and should be used concomitantly only with great caution). Products include:

Streptomycin Sulfate Injection 2208

Streptozocin (May enhance the potential for renal toxicity, bronchospasm and hypotension). Products include:

Zanosar Sterile Powder 2653

Succinylcholine Chloride (Amphotericin B-induced hypokalemia may enhance the curariform effect of skeletal muscle relaxants). Products include:

Anectine 1073

Tamoxifen Citrate (May enhance the potential for renal toxicity, bronchospasm and hypotension). Products include:

Nolvadex Tablets 2841

Teniposide (May enhance the potential for renal toxicity, bronchospasm and hypotension). Products include:

Vumon 727

Thioguanine (May enhance the potential for renal toxicity, bronchospasm and hypotension). Products include:

Thioguanine Tablets, Tabloid Brand 1181

Thiotepa (May enhance the potential for renal toxicity, bronchospasm and hypotension). Products include:

Thioplex (Thiotepa For Injection) 1281

Tobramycin (May enhance the potential for drug-induced renal toxicity, and should be used concomitantly only with great caution). Products include:

AKTOB .... ◉ 206
TobraDex Ophthalmic Suspension and Ointment 473
Tobrex Ophthalmic Ointment and Solution .... ◉ 229

Tobramycin Sulfate (May enhance the potential for drug-induced renal toxicity, and should be used concomitantly only with great caution). Products include:

Nebcin Vials, Hyporets & ADD-Vantage 1464
Tobramycin Sulfate Injection 968

Triamcinolone (May potentiate amphotericin B-induced hypokalemia which may predispose the patient to cardiac dysfunction; avoid concomitant use). Products include:

Aristocort Tablets 1022

Triamcinolone Acetonide (May potentiate amphotericin B-induced hypokalemia which may predispose the patient to cardiac dysfunction; avoid concomitant use). Products include:

Aristocort A 0.025% Cream 1027
Aristocort A 0.5% Cream 1031
Aristocort A 0.1% Cream 1029
Aristocort A 0.1% Ointment 1030
Azmacort Oral Inhaler 2011
Nasacort Nasal Inhaler 2024

Triamcinolone Diacetate (May potentiate amphotericin B-induced hypokalemia which may predispose the patient to cardiac dysfunction; avoid concomitant use). Products include:

Aristocort Suspension (Forte Parenteral) 1027
Aristocort Suspension (Intralesional) 1025

Triamcinolone Hexacetonide (May potentiate amphotericin B-induced hypokalemia which may predispose the patient to cardiac dysfunction; avoid concomitant use). Products include:

Aristospan Suspension (Intra-articular) 1033
Aristospan Suspension (Intralesional) 1032

Tubocurarine Chloride (Amphotericin B-induced hypokalemia may enhance the curariform effect of skeletal muscle relaxants).

No products indexed under this heading.

Vecuronium Bromide (Amphotericin B-induced hypokalemia may enhance the curariform effect of skeletal muscle relaxants). Products include:

Norcuron 1826

Vincristine Sulfate (May enhance the potential for renal toxicity, bronchospasm and hypotension). Products include:

Oncovin Solution Vials & Hyporets 1466

Vinorelbine Tartrate (May enhance the potential for renal toxicity, bronchospasm and hypotension). Products include:

Navelbine Injection 1145

FURACIN SOLUBLE DRESSING
(Nitrofurazone) 2045
None cited in PDR database.

FURACIN TOPICAL CREAM
(Nitrofurazone) 2045
None cited in PDR database.

FUROXONE LIQUID
(Furazolidone) 2046
May interact with anorexiants, monoamine oxidase inhibitors, antihistamines, hypnotics and sedatives, narcotic analgesics, tranquilizers, indirect-acting sympathomimetic amines, and certain other agents. Compounds in these categories include:

Acrivastine (Predisposition to hypertensive crises; use with caution at reduced dosages). Products include:

Semprex-D Capsules 463
Semprex-D Capsules 1167

Alfentanil Hydrochloride (Predisposition to hypertensive crises; use with caution at reduced dosages). Products include:

Alfenta Injection 1286

Alprazolam (Predisposition to hypertensive crises; use with caution at reduced dosages). Products include:

Xanax Tablets 2649

Amphetamine Resins (Predisposition to hypertensive crises; concurrent administration is contraindicated). Products include:

Biphetamine Capsules 983

Astemizole (Predisposition to hypertensive crises; use with caution at reduced dosages). Products include:

Hismanal Tablets 1293

Azatadine Maleate (Predisposition to hypertensive crises; use with caution at reduced dosages). Products include:

Trinalin Repetabs Tablets 1330

Benzphetamine Hydrochloride (Predisposition to hypertensive crises; concurrent administration is contraindicated). Products include:

Didrex Tablets 2607

Bromodiphenhydramine Hydrochloride (Predisposition to hypertensive crises; use with caution at reduced dosages).

No products indexed under this heading.

Brompheniramine Maleate (Predisposition to hypertensive crises; use with caution at reduced dosages). Products include:

Alka Seltzer Plus Sinus Medicine .. ▣ 707
Bromfed Capsules (Extended-Release) 1785
Bromfed Syrup .... ▣ 733
Bromfed Tablets 1785
Bromfed-DM Cough Syrup 1786
Bromfed-PD Capsules (Extended-Release) 1785
Dimetane-DC Cough Syrup 2059
Dimetane-DX Cough Syrup 2059
Dimetapp Elixir .... ▣ 773
Dimetapp Extentabs .... ▣ 774
Dimetapp Tablets/Liqui-Gels .... ▣ 775

IMPORTANT NOTE: Always consult each drug listing in the patient's regimen for possible interactions.

Furoxone Interactions Index 432

Dimetapp Cold & Allergy Chewable Tablets ▣ 773
Dimetapp DM Elixir ▣ 774
Vicks DayQuil Allergy Relief 12-Hour Extended Release Tablets ▣ 760
Vicks DayQuil Allergy Relief 4-Hour Tablets ▣ 760

Buprenorphine (Predisposition to hypertensive crises; use with caution at reduced dosages). Products include:
Buprenex Injectable 2006

Buspirone Hydrochloride (Predisposition to hypertensive crises; use with caution at reduced dosages). Products include:
BuSpar 737

Chlordiazepoxide (Predisposition to hypertensive crises; use with caution at reduced dosages). Products include:
Libritabs Tablets 2177
Limbitrol 2180

Chlordiazepoxide Hydrochloride (Predisposition to hypertensive crises; use with caution at reduced dosages). Products include:
Librax Capsules 2176
Librium Capsules 2178
Librium Injectable 2179

Chlorpheniramine Maleate (Predisposition to hypertensive crises; use with caution at reduced dosages). Products include:
Alka-Seltzer Plus Cold Medicine ▣ 705
Alka-Seltzer Plus Cold Medicine Liqui-Gels ▣ 706
Alka-Seltzer Plus Cold & Cough Medicine ▣ 708
Alka-Seltzer Plus Cold & Cough Medicine Liqui-Gels ▣ 705
Allerest Children's Chewable Tablets ▣ 627
Allerest Headache Strength Tablets ▣ 627
Allerest Maximum Strength Tablets ▣ 627
Allerest Sinus Pain Formula ▣ 627
Allerest 12 Hour Caplets ▣ 627
Ana-Kit Anaphylaxis Emergency Treatment Kit 617
Atrohist Pediatric Capsules 453
Atrohist Plus Tablets 454
BC Cold Powder Multi-Symptom Formula (Cold-Sinus-Allergy) ▣ 609
Cerose DM ▣ 878
Cheracol Plus Head Cold/Cough Formula ▣ 769
Children's Vicks DayQuil Allergy Relief ▣ 757
Children's Vicks NyQuil Cold/Cough Relief ▣ 758
Chlor-Trimeton Allergy Decongestant Tablets ▣ 799
Chlor-Trimeton Allergy Tablets ▣ 798
Comhist 2038
Comtrex Multi-Symptom Cold Reliever Tablets/Caplets/Liqui-Gels/Liquid ▣ 615
Allergy-Sinus Comtrex Multi-Symptom Allergy-Sinus Formula Tablets ▣ 617
Contac Continuous Action Nasal Decongestant/Antihistamine 12 Hour Capsules ▣ 813
Contac Maximum Strength Continuous Action Decongestant/Antihistamine 12 Hour Caplets ▣ 813
Contac Severe Cold and Flu Formula Caplets ▣ 814
Coricidin 'D' Decongestant Tablets ▣ 800
Coricidin Tablets ▣ 800
D.A. Chewable Tablets 951
Deconamine 1320
Dura-Tap/PD Capsules 2867
Dura-Vent/DA Tablets 953
Extendryl 1005
Fedahist Gyrocaps 2401
Fedahist Timecaps 2401
Hycomine Compound Tablets 932
Isoclor Timesule Capsules ▣ 637
Kronofed-A 977
Nolamine Timed-Release Tablets 785
Novahistine DH 2462
Novahistine Elixir ▣ 823
Ornade Spansule Capsules 2502
PediaCare Cold Allergy Chewable Tablets ▣ 677
PediaCare Cough-Cold Chewable Tablets 1553
PediaCare Cough-Cold Liquid 1553
PediaCare NightRest Cough-Cold Liquid 1553
Pediatric Vicks 44m Cough & Cold Relief ▣ 764
Pyrroxate Caplets ▣ 772
Ryna ▣ 841
Sinarest Tablets ▣ 648
Sinarest Extra Strength Tablets ▣ 648
Sine-Off Sinus Medicine ▣ 825
Singlet Tablets ▣ 825
Sinulin Tablets 787
Sinutab Sinus Allergy Medication, Maximum Strength Tablets and Caplets ▣ 860
Sudafed Plus Liquid ▣ 862
Sudafed Plus Tablets ▣ 863
Teldrin 12 Hour Antihistamine/Nasal Decongestant Allergy Relief Capsules ▣ 826
TheraFlu ▣ 787
TheraFlu Maximum Strength Nighttime Flu, Cold & Cough Medicine ▣ 788
Triaminic Allergy Tablets ▣ 789
Triaminic Cold Tablets ▣ 790
Triaminic Nite Light ▣ 791
Triaminic Syrup ▣ 792
Triaminic-12 Tablets ▣ 792
Triaminicin Tablets ▣ 793
Triaminicol Multi-Symptom Cold Tablets ▣ 793
Triaminicol Multi-Symptom Relief ▣ 794
Tussend 1783
Children's TYLENOL Cold Multi-Symptom Liquid Formula and Chewable Tablets 1561
Children's TYLENOL Cold Plus Cough Multi Symptom Tablets and Liquid ▣ 681
TYLENOL Maximum Strength Allergy Sinus Medication Gelcaps and Caplets 1563
TYLENOL Cold Multi-Symptom Formula Medication Tablets and Caplets 1561
TYLENOL Cold Multi-Symptom Hot Medication Liquid Packets 1557
Vicks 44 LiquiCaps Cough, Cold & Flu Relief ▣ 755
Vicks 44M Cough, Cold & Flu Relief ▣ 756

Chlorpheniramine Polistirex (Predisposition to hypertensive crises; use with caution at reduced dosages). Products include:
Tussionex Pennkinetic Extended-Release Suspension 998

Chlorpheniramine Tannate (Predisposition to hypertensive crises; use with caution at reduced dosages). Products include:
Atrohist Pediatric Suspension 454
Ricobid Tablets and Pediatric Suspension 2038
Rynatan 2673
Rynatuss 2673

Chlorpromazine (Predisposition to hypertensive crises; use with caution at reduced dosages). Products include:
Thorazine Suppositories 2523

Chlorprothixene (Predisposition to hypertensive crises; use with caution at reduced dosages).
No products indexed under this heading.

Chlorprothixene Hydrochloride (Predisposition to hypertensive crises; use with caution at reduced dosages).
No products indexed under this heading.

Clemastine Fumarate (Predisposition to hypertensive crises; use with caution at reduced dosages). Products include:
Tavist Syrup 2297
Tavist Tablets 2298
Tavist-1 12 Hour Relief Tablets ▣ 787
Tavist-D 12 Hour Relief Tablets ▣ 787

Clorazepate Dipotassium (Predisposition to hypertensive crises; use with caution at reduced dosages). Products include:
Tranxene 451

Codeine Phosphate (Predisposition to hypertensive crises; use with caution at reduced dosages). Products include:
Actifed with Codeine Cough Syrup 1067
Brontex 1981
Deconsal C Expectorant Syrup 456
Deconsal Pediatric Syrup 457
Dimetane-DC Cough Syrup 2059
Empirin with Codeine Tablets 1093
Fioricet with Codeine Capsules 2260
Fiorinal with Codeine Capsules 2262
Isoclor Expectorant 990
Novahistine DH 2462
Novahistine Expectorant 2463
Nucofed 2051
Phenergan with Codeine 2777
Phenergan VC with Codeine 2781
Robitussin A-C Syrup 2073
Robitussin-DAC Syrup 2074
Ryna ▣ 841
Soma Compound w/Codeine Tablets 2676
Tussi-Organidin NR Liquid and S NR Liquid 2677
Tylenol with Codeine 1583

Cyproheptadine Hydrochloride (Predisposition to hypertensive crises; use with caution at reduced dosages). Products include:
Periactin 1724

Dexchlorpheniramine Maleate (Predisposition to hypertensive crises; use with caution at reduced dosages).
No products indexed under this heading.

Dextroamphetamine Sulfate (Predisposition to hypertensive crises; concurrent administration is contraindicated). Products include:
Dexedrine 2474
DextroStat Dextroamphetamine Tablets 2036

Dezocine (Predisposition to hypertensive crises; use with caution at reduced dosages). Products include:
Dalgan Injection 538

Diazepam (Predisposition to hypertensive crises; use with caution at reduced dosages). Products include:
Dizac 1809
Valium Injectable 2182
Valium Tablets 2183
Valrelease Capsules 2169

Diethylpropion Hydrochloride (Predisposition to hypertensive crises; use with caution at reduced dosages).
No products indexed under this heading.

Diphenhydramine Citrate (Predisposition to hypertensive crises; use with caution at reduced dosages). Products include:
Excedrin P.M. Analgesic/Sleeping Aid Tablets, Caplets, Liquigels 733

Diphenhydramine Hydrochloride (Predisposition to hypertensive crises; use with caution at reduced dosages). Products include:
Actifed Allergy Daytime/Nighttime Caplets ▣ 844
Actifed Sinus Daytime/Nighttime Tablets and Caplets ▣ 846
Arthritis Foundation NightTime Caplets ▣ 674
Extra Strength Bayer PM Aspirin ▣ 713
Bayer Select Night Time Pain Relief Formula ▣ 716
Benadryl Allergy Decongestant Liquid Medication ▣ 848
Benadryl Allergy Decongestant Tablets ▣ 848
Benadryl Allergy Liquid Medication ▣ 849
Benadryl Allergy ▣ 848
Benadryl Allergy Sinus Headache Formula Caplets ▣ 849
Benadryl Capsules 1898
Benadryl Dye-Free Allergy Liqui-gel Softgels ▣ 850
Benadryl Dye-Free Allergy Liquid Medication ▣ 850
Benadryl Itch Relief Cream, Children's Formula and Maximum Strength 2% ▣ 851
Benadryl Itch Relief Spray, Children's Formula and Maximum Strength 2% ▣ 851
Benadryl Itch Relief Stick Maximum Strength 2% ▣ 850
Benadryl Itch Stopping Gel, Children's Formula and Maximum Strength 2% ▣ 851
Benadryl Kapseals 1898
Benadryl Injection 1898
Contac Day & Night Cold/Flu Night Caplets ▣ 812
Contac Night Allergy/Sinus Caplets ▣ 812
Extra Strength Doan's P.M. ▣ 633
Legatrin PM ▣ 651
Miles Nervine Nighttime Sleep-Aid ▣ 723
Nytol QuickCaps Caplets ▣ 610
Sleepinal Night-time Sleep Aid Capsules and Softgels ▣ 834
TYLENOL Maximum Strength Allergy Sinus NightTime Medication Caplets 1555
TYLENOL Flu NightTime, Maximum Strength, Gelcaps 1566
TYLENOL Maximum Strength Flu NightTime Hot Medication Packets 1562
TYLENOL PM, Extra Strength Pain Reliever/Sleep Aid Caplets, Geltabs, Gelcaps 1560
TYLENOL Severe Allergy Medication Caplets 1564
Maximum Strength Unisom Sleepgels 1934
Unisom With Pain Relief-Nighttime Sleep Aid and Pain Reliever 1934

Diphenylpyraline Hydrochloride (Predisposition to hypertensive crises; use with caution at reduced dosages).
No products indexed under this heading.

Droperidol (Predisposition to hypertensive crises; use with caution at reduced dosages). Products include:
Inapsine Injection 1296

Ephedrine Hydrochloride (Predisposition to hypertensive crises; concurrent administration is contraindicated). Products include:
Primatene Dual Action Formula ▣ 872
Primatene Tablets ▣ 873
Quadrinal Tablets 1350

Ephedrine Sulfate (Predisposition to hypertensive crises; concurrent administration is contraindicated). Products include:
Bronkaid Caplets ▣ 717
Marax Tablets & DF Syrup 2200

Ephedrine Tannate (Predisposition to hypertensive crises; concurrent administration is contraindicated). Products include:
Rynatuss 2673

Estazolam (Predisposition to hypertensive crises; use with caution at reduced dosages). Products include:
ProSom Tablets 449

Ethchlorvynol (Predisposition to hypertensive crises; use with caution at reduced dosages). Products include:
Placidyl Capsules 448

Ethinamate (Predisposition to hypertensive crises; use with caution at reduced dosages).
No products indexed under this heading.

Fenfluramine Hydrochloride (Predisposition to hypertensive crises; concurrent administration is contraindicated). Products include:
Pondimin Tablets 2066

(▣ Described in PDR For Nonprescription Drugs) (◉ Described in PDR For Ophthalmology)

433 **Interactions Index** **Furoxone**

Fentanyl (Predisposition to hypertensive crises; use with caution at reduced dosages). Products include:
- Duragesic Transdermal System 1288

Fentanyl Citrate (Predisposition to hypertensive crises; use with caution at reduced dosages). Products include:
- Sublimaze Injection 1307

Fluphenazine Decanoate (Predisposition to hypertensive crises; use with caution at reduced dosages). Products include:
- Prolixin Decanoate 509

Fluphenazine Enanthate (Predisposition to hypertensive crises; use with caution at reduced dosages). Products include:
- Prolixin Enanthate 509

Fluphenazine Hydrochloride (Predisposition to hypertensive crises; use with caution at reduced dosages). Products include:
- Prolixin 509

Flurazepam Hydrochloride (Predisposition to hypertensive crises; use with caution at reduced dosages). Products include:
- Dalmane Capsules 2173

Glutethimide (Predisposition to hypertensive crises; use with caution at reduced dosages).
- No products indexed under this heading.

Haloperidol (Predisposition to hypertensive crises; use with caution at reduced dosages). Products include:
- Haldol Injection, Tablets and Concentrate 1575

Haloperidol Decanoate (Predisposition to hypertensive crises; use with caution at reduced dosages). Products include:
- Haldol Decanoate 1577

Hydrocodone Bitartrate (Predisposition to hypertensive crises; use with caution at reduced dosages). Products include:
- Anexsia 5/500 Elixir 1781
- Anexia Tablets 1782
- Codiclear DH Syrup 791
- Deconamine CX Cough and Cold Liquid and Tablets 1319
- Duratuss HD Elixir 2565
- Hycodan Tablets and Syrup 930
- Hycomine Compound Tablets 932
- Hycomine 931
- Hycotuss Expectorant Syrup 933
- Hydrocet Capsules 782
- Lorcet 10/650 1018
- Lortab 2566
- Tussend 1783
- Tussend Expectorant 1785
- Vicodin Tablets 1356
- Vicodin ES Tablets 1357
- Vicodin Tuss Expectorant 1358
- Zydone Capsules 949

Hydrocodone Polistirex (Predisposition to hypertensive crises; use with caution at reduced dosages). Products include:
- Tussionex Pennkinetic Extended-Release Suspension 998

Hydroxyzine Hydrochloride (Predisposition to hypertensive crises; use with caution at reduced dosages). Products include:
- Atarax Tablets & Syrup 2185
- Marax Tablets & DF Syrup 2200
- Vistaril Intramuscular Solution 2216

Isocarboxazid (Predisposition to hypertensive crises; concurrent administration is contraindicated).
- No products indexed under this heading.

Levorphanol Tartrate (Predisposition to hypertensive crises; use with caution at reduced dosages). Products include:
- Levo-Dromoran 2129

Loratadine (Predisposition to hypertensive crises; use with caution at reduced dosages). Products include:
- Claritin 2349
- Claritin-D 2350

Lorazepam (Predisposition to hypertensive crises; use with caution at reduced dosages). Products include:
- Ativan Injection 2698
- Ativan Tablets 2700

Loxapine Hydrochloride (Predisposition to hypertensive crises; use with caution at reduced dosages). Products include:
- Loxitane 1378

Loxapine Succinate (Predisposition to hypertensive crises; use with caution at reduced dosages). Products include:
- Loxitane Capsules 1378

Mazindol (Predisposition to hypertensive crises; concurrent administration is contraindicated). Products include:
- Sanorex Tablets 2294

Meperidine Hydrochloride (Predisposition to hypertensive crises; use with caution at reduced dosages). Products include:
- Demerol 2308
- Mepergan Injection 2753

Meprobamate (Predisposition to hypertensive crises; use with caution at reduced dosages). Products include:
- Miltown Tablets 2672
- PMB 200 and PMB 400 2783

Mesoridazine Besylate (Predisposition to hypertensive crises; use with caution at reduced dosages). Products include:
- Serentil 684

Methadone Hydrochloride (Predisposition to hypertensive crises; use with caution at reduced dosages). Products include:
- Methadone Hydrochloride Oral Concentrate 2233
- Methadone Hydrochloride Oral Solution & Tablets 2235

Methamphetamine Hydrochloride (Predisposition to hypertensive crises; concurrent administration is contraindicated). Products include:
- Desoxyn Gradumet Tablets 419

Methdilazine Hydrochloride (Predisposition to hypertensive crises; use with caution at reduced dosages).
- No products indexed under this heading.

Midazolam Hydrochloride (Predisposition to hypertensive crises; use with caution at reduced dosages). Products include:
- Versed Injection 2170

Molindone Hydrochloride (Predisposition to hypertensive crises; use with caution at reduced dosages). Products include:
- Moban Tablets and Concentrate 1048

Morphine Sulfate (Predisposition to hypertensive crises; use with caution at reduced dosages). Products include:
- Astramorph/PF Injection, USP (Preservative-Free) 535
- Duramorph 962
- Infumorph 200 and Infumorph 500 Sterile Solutions 965
- MS Contin Tablets 1994
- MSIR 1997
- Oramorph SR (Morphine Sulfate Sustained Release Tablets) 2236
- RMS Suppositories 2657
- Roxanol 2243

Naphazoline Hydrochloride (Predisposition to hypertensive crises; concurrent administration is contraindicated). Products include:
- Albalon Solution with Liquifilm .... ⊙ 231
- Clear Eyes ACR Astringent/Lubricant Eye Redness Reliever Eye Drops .... ⊙ 316
- Clear Eyes Lubricant Eye Redness Reliever .... ⊙ 316
- 4-Way Fast Acting Nasal Spray (regular & mentholated) .... ▣ 621
- Naphcon-A Ophthalmic Solution 473
- Privine .... ▣ 647
- Vasocon-A .... ⊙ 271

Opium Alkaloids (Predisposition to hypertensive crises; use with caution at reduced dosages).
- No products indexed under this heading.

Oxazepam (Predisposition to hypertensive crises; use with caution at reduced dosages). Products include:
- Serax Capsules 2810
- Serax Tablets 2810

Oxycodone Hydrochloride (Predisposition to hypertensive crises; use with caution at reduced dosages). Products include:
- Percocet Tablets 938
- Percodan Tablets 939
- Percodan-Demi Tablets 940
- Roxicodone Tablets, Oral Solution & Intensol (Oxycodone) 2244
- Tylox Capsules 1584

Oxymetazoline Hydrochloride (Predisposition to hypertensive crises; concurrent administration is contraindicated). Products include:
- Afrin .... ▣ 797
- Cheracol Nasal Spray Pump .... ▣ 768
- Duration 12 Hour Nasal Spray .... ▣ 805
- 4-Way Long Lasting Nasal Spray .... ▣ 621
- NTZ Long Acting Nasal Spray & Drops 0.05% .... ▣ 727
- Neo-Synephrine Maximum Strength 12 Hour Nasal Spray .... ▣ 726
- Neo-Synephrine 12 Hour .... ▣ 726
- Nōstrilla Long Acting Nasal Decongestant .... ▣ 644
- Vicks Sinex 12-Hour Nasal Decongestant Spray and Ultra Fine Mist .... ▣ 765
- Visine L.R. Eye Drops .... ▣ 746
- Visine L.R. Eye Drops .... ⊙ 313

Perphenazine (Predisposition to hypertensive crises; use with caution at reduced dosages). Products include:
- Etrafon 2355
- Triavil Tablets 1757
- Trilafon 2389

Phendimetrazine Tartrate (Predisposition to hypertensive crises; concurrent administration is contraindicated). Products include:
- Bontril Slow-Release Capsules 781
- Prelu-2 Timed Release Capsules 681

Phenelzine Sulfate (Predisposition to hypertensive crises; concurrent administration is contraindicated). Products include:
- Nardil 1920

Phenmetrazine Hydrochloride (Predisposition to hypertensive crises; concurrent administration is contraindicated).
- No products indexed under this heading.

Phenylephrine Hydrochloride (Predisposition to hypertensive crises; concurrent administration is contraindicated). Products include:
- Atrohist Plus Tablets 454
- Cerose DM .... ▣ 878
- Comhist 2038
- D.A. Chewable Tablets 951
- Deconsal Pediatric Capsules 454
- Dura-Vent/DA Tablets 953
- Entex Capsules 1986
- Entex Liquid 1986
- Extendryl 1005
- 4-Way Fast Acting Nasal Spray (regular & mentholated) .... ▣ 621
- Hemorid For Women .... ▣ 834
- Hycomine Compound Tablets 932
- Neo-Synephrine Hydrochloride 1% Carpuject 2324
- Neo-Synephrine Hydrochloride 1% Injection 2324
- Neo-Synephrine Hydrochloride (Ophthalmic) 2325
- Neo-Synephrine .... ▣ 726
- Nōstril .... ▣ 644
- Novahistine Elixir .... ▣ 823
- Phenergan VC 2779
- Phenergan VC with Codeine 2781
- Preparation H .... ▣ 871
- Tympagesic Ear Drops 2342
- Vasosulf .... ⊙ 271
- Vicks Sinex Nasal Spray and Ultra Fine Mist .... ▣ 765

Phenylpropanolamine Hydrochloride (Predisposition to hypertensive crises; concurrent administration is contraindicated). Products include:
- Acutrim .... ▣ 628
- Allerest Children's Chewable Tablets .... ▣ 627
- Allerest 12 Hour Caplets .... ▣ 627
- Atrohist Plus Tablets 454
- BC Cold Powder Multi-Symptom Formula (Cold-Sinus-Allergy) .... ▣ 609
- BC Cold Powder Non-Drowsy Formula (Cold-Sinus) .... ▣ 609
- Cheracol Plus Head Cold/Cough Formula .... ▣ 769
- Comtrex Multi-Symptom Non-Drowsy Liqui-gels .... ▣ 618
- Contac Continuous Action Nasal Decongestant/Antihistamine 12 Hour Capsules .... ▣ 813
- Contac Maximum Strength Continuous Action Decongestant/Antihistamine 12 Hour Caplets .... ▣ 813
- Contac Severe Cold and Flu Formula Caplets .... ▣ 814
- Coricidin 'D' Decongestant Tablets .... ▣ 800
- Dexatrim .... ▣ 832
- Dexatrim Plus Vitamins Caplets .... ▣ 832
- Dimetane-DC Cough Syrup 2059
- Dimetapp Elixir .... ▣ 773
- Dimetapp Extentabs .... ▣ 774
- Dimetapp Tablets/Liqui-Gels .... ▣ 775
- Dimetapp Cold & Allergy Chewable Tablets .... ▣ 773
- Dimetapp DM Elixir .... ▣ 774
- Dura-Vent Tablets 952
- Entex Capsules 1986
- Entex LA Tablets 1987
- Entex Liquid 1986
- Exgest LA Tablets 782
- Hycomine 931
- Isoclor Timesule Capsules .... ▣ 637
- Nolamine Timed-Release Tablets 785
- Ornade Spansule Capsules 2502
- Propagest Tablets 786
- Pyrroxate Caplets .... ▣ 772
- Robitussin-CF .... ▣ 777
- Sinulin Tablets 787
- Tavist-D 12 Hour Relief Tablets .... ▣ 787
- Teldrin 12 Hour Antihistamine/Nasal Decongestant Allergy Relief Capsules .... ▣ 826
- Triaminic Allergy Tablets .... ▣ 789
- Triaminic Cold Tablets .... ▣ 790
- Triaminic Expectorant .... ▣ 790
- Triaminic Syrup .... ▣ 792
- Triaminic-12 Tablets .... ▣ 792
- Triaminic-DM Syrup .... ▣ 792
- Triaminicin Tablets .... ▣ 793
- Triaminicol Multi-Symptom Cold Tablets .... ▣ 793
- Triaminicol Multi-Symptom Relief .... ▣ 794
- Vicks DayQuil Allergy Relief 12-Hour Extended Release Tablets .... ▣ 760
- Vicks DayQuil Allergy Relief 4-Hour Tablets .... ▣ 760
- Vicks DayQuil SINUS Pressure & CONGESTION Relief .... ▣ 761

Prazepam (Predisposition to hypertensive crises; use with caution at reduced dosages).
- No products indexed under this heading.

IMPORTANT NOTE: Always consult each drug listing in the patient's regimen for possible interactions.

Furoxone Interactions Index 434

Prochlorperazine (Predisposition to hypertensive crises; use with caution at reduced dosages). Products include:
- Compazine ... 2470

Promethazine Hydrochloride (Predisposition to hypertensive crises; use with caution at reduced dosages). Products include:
- Mepergan Injection ... 2753
- Phenergan with Codeine ... 2777
- Phenergan with Dextromethorphan 2778
- Phenergan Injection ... 2773
- Phenergan Suppositories ... 2775
- Phenergan Syrup ... 2774
- Phenergan Tablets ... 2775
- Phenergan VC ... 2779
- Phenergan VC with Codeine ... 2781

Propofol (Predisposition to hypertensive crises; use with caution at reduced dosages). Products include:
- Diprivan Injection ... 2833

Propoxyphene Hydrochloride (Predisposition to hypertensive crises; use with caution at reduced dosages). Products include:
- Darvon ... 1435
- Wygesic Tablets ... 2827

Propoxyphene Napsylate (Predisposition to hypertensive crises; use with caution at reduced dosages). Products include:
- Darvon-N/Darvocet-N ... 1433

Pseudoephedrine Hydrochloride (Predisposition to hypertensive crises; concurrent administration is contraindicated). Products include:
- Actifed Allergy Daytime/Nighttime Caplets ... ▣ 844
- Actifed Plus Caplets ... ▣ 845
- Actifed Plus Tablets ... ▣ 845
- Actifed with Codeine Cough Syrup.. 1067
- Actifed Sinus Daytime/Nighttime Tablets and Caplets ... ▣ 846
- Actifed Syrup ... ▣ 846
- Actifed Tablets ... ▣ 844
- Advil Cold and Sinus Caplets and Tablets (formerly CoAdvil) ... ▣ 870
- Alka-Seltzer Plus Cold Medicine Liqui-Gels ... ▣ 706
- Alka-Seltzer Plus Cold & Cough Medicine Liqui-Gels ... ▣ 705
- Alka-Seltzer Plus Night-Time Cold Medicine Liqui-Gels ... ▣ 706
- Allerest Headache Strength Tablets ... ▣ 627
- Allerest Maximum Strength Tablets ... ▣ 627
- Allerest No Drowsiness Tablets ... ▣ 627
- Allerest Sinus Pain Formula ... ▣ 627
- Anatuss LA Tablets ... 1542
- Atrohist Pediatric Capsules ... 453
- Bayer Select Sinus Pain Relief Formula ... ▣ 717
- Benadryl Allergy Decongestant Liquid Medication ... ▣ 848
- Benadryl Allergy Decongestant Tablets ... ▣ 848
- Benadryl Allergy Sinus Headache Formula Caplets ... ▣ 849
- Benylin Multisymptom ... ▣ 852
- Bromfed Capsules (Extended-Release) ... 1785
- Bromfed Syrup ... ▣ 733
- Bromfed Tablets ... 1785
- Bromfed-DM Cough Syrup ... 1786
- Bromfed-PD Capsules (Extended-Release) ... 1785
- Children's Vicks DayQuil Allergy Relief ... ▣ 757
- Children's Vicks NyQuil Cold/Cough Relief ... ▣ 758
- Comtrex Multi-Symptom Cold Reliever Tablets/Caplets/Liqui-Gels/Liquid ... ▣ 615
- Allergy-Sinus Comtrex Multi-Symptom Allergy-Sinus Formula Tablets ... ▣ 617
- Comtrex Multi-Symptom Non-Drowsy Caplets ... ▣ 618
- Congess ... 1004
- Contac Day Allergy/Sinus Caplets ▣ 812
- Contac Day & Night ... ▣ 812
- Contac Night Allergy/Sinus Caplets ... ▣ 812
- Contac Severe Cold & Flu Non-Drowsy ... ▣ 815
- Deconamine Chewable Tablets ... 1320
- Deconamine CX Cough and Cold Liquid and Tablets ... 1319
- Deconamine ... 1320
- Deconsal C Expectorant Syrup ... 456
- Deconsal Pediatric Syrup ... 457
- Deconsal II Tablets ... 454
- Dimetane-DX Cough Syrup ... 2059
- Dimetapp Sinus Caplets ... ▣ 775
- Dorcol Children's Cough Syrup ... ▣ 785
- Drixoral Cough + Congestion Liquid Caps ... ▣ 802
- Dura-Tap/PD Capsules ... 2867
- Duratuss Tablets ... 2565
- Duratuss HD Elixir ... 2565
- Efidac/24 ... ▣ 635
- Entex PSE Tablets ... 1987
- Fedahist Gyrocaps ... 2401
- Fedahist Timecaps ... 2401
- Guaifed ... 1787
- Guaifed Syrup ... ▣ 734
- Guaimax-D Tablets ... 792
- Guaitab Tablets ... ▣ 734
- Isoclor Expectorant ... 990
- Kronofed-A ... 977
- Motrin IB Sinus ... ▣ 838
- Novahistine DH ... 2462
- Novahistine DMX ... ▣ 822
- Novahistine Expectorant ... 2463
- Nucofed ... 2051
- PediaCare Cold Allergy Chewable Tablets ... ▣ 677
- PediaCare Cough-Cold Chewable Tablets ... 1553
- PediaCare ... 1553
- PediaCare Infants' Decongestant Drops ... ▣ 677
- PediCare Infant's Drops Decongestant Plus Cough ... 1553
- PediaCare NightRest Cough-Cold Liquid ... 1553
- Pediatric Vicks 44d Dry Hacking Cough & Head Congestion ... ▣ 763
- Pediatric Vicks 44m Cough & Cold Relief ... ▣ 764
- Robitussin Cold & Cough Liqui-Gels ... ▣ 776
- Robitussin Maximum Strength Cough & Cold ... ▣ 778
- Robitussin Pediatric Cough & Cold Formula ... ▣ 779
- Robitussin Severe Congestion Liqui-Gels ... ▣ 776
- Robitussin-DAC Syrup ... 2074
- Robitussin-PE ... ▣ 778
- Rondec Oral Drops ... 953
- Rondec Syrup ... 953
- Rondec Tablet ... 953
- Rondec-DM Oral Drops ... 954
- Rondec-DM Syrup ... 954
- Rondec-TR Tablet ... 953
- Ryna ... ▣ 841
- Seldane-D Extended-Release Tablets ... 1538
- Semprex-D Capsules ... 463
- Semprex-D Capsules ... 1167
- Sinarest Tablets ... ▣ 648
- Sinarest Extra Strength Tablets ... ▣ 648
- Sinarest No Drowsiness Tablets ... ▣ 648
- Sine-Aid IB Caplets ... 1554
- Sine-Aid Maximum Strength Sinus Medication Gelcaps, Caplets and Tablets ... 1554
- Sine-Off No Drowsiness Formula Caplets ... ▣ 824
- Sine-Off Sinus Medicine ... ▣ 825
- Singlet Tablets ... ▣ 825
- Sinutab Non-Drying Liquid Caps ... ▣ 859
- Sinutab Sinus Allergy Medication, Maximum Strength Tablets and Caplets ... ▣ 860
- Sinutab Sinus Medication, Maximum Strength Without Drowsiness Formula, Tablets & Caplets ... ▣ 860
- Sinutab Sinus Medication, Regular Strength Without Drowsiness Formula ... ▣ 859
- Sudafed Children's Liquid ... ▣ 861
- Sudafed Cold and Cough Liquidcaps ... ▣ 862
- Sudafed Cough Syrup ... ▣ 862
- Sudafed Plus Liquid ... ▣ 862
- Sudafed Plus Tablets ... ▣ 863
- Sudafed Severe Cold Formula Caplets ... ▣ 863
- Sudafed Severe Cold Formula Tablets ... ▣ 864
- Sudafed Sinus Caplets ... ▣ 864
- Sudafed Sinus Tablets ... ▣ 864
- Sudafed Tablets, 30 mg ... ▣ 861
- Sudafed Tablets, 60 mg ... ▣ 861
- Sudafed 12 Hour Caplets ... ▣ 861
- Syn-Rx Tablets ... 465
- Syn-Rx DM Tablets ... 466
- TheraFlu ... ▣ 787
- TheraFlu Maximum Strength Nighttime Flu, Cold & Cough Medicine ... ▣ 788
- TheraFlu Maximum Strength Non-Drowsy Formula Flu, Cold & Cough Medicine ... ▣ 788
- Thera Flu Maximum Strength, Non-Drowsy Formula Flu, Cold and Cough Caplets ... ▣ 789
- Triaminic AM Cough and Decongestant Formula ... ▣ 789
- Triaminic AM Decongestant Formula ... ▣ 790
- Triaminic Nite Light ... ▣ 791
- Triaminic Sore Throat Formula ... ▣ 791
- Tussend ... 1783
- Tussend Expectorant ... 1785
- Children's TYLENOL Cold Multi-Symptom Liquid Formula and Chewable Tablets ... 1561
- Children's TYLENOL Cold Plus Cough Multi Symptom Tablets and Liquid ... ▣ 681
- Infants' TYLENOL Cold Decongestant & Fever-Reducer Drops ... 1556
- TYLENOL Maximum Strength Allergy Sinus Medication Gelcaps and Caplets ... 1563
- TYLENOL Maximum Strength Allergy Sinus NightTime Medication Caplets ... 1555
- TYLENOL Flu Maximum Strength Gelcaps ... 1565
- TYLENOL Flu NightTime, Maximum Strength, Gelcaps ... 1566
- TYLENOL Maximum Strength Flu NightTime Hot Medication Packets ... 1562
- TYLENOL, Maximum Strength, Sinus Medication Geltabs, Gelcaps, Caplets and Tablets ... 1566
- TYLENOL Cold Multi-Symptom Formula Medication Tablets and Caplets ... 1561
- TYLENOL Cold Medication No Drowsiness Formula Gelcaps and Caplets ... 1562
- TYLENOL Cold Multi-Symptom Hot Medication Liquid Packets ... 1557
- TYLENOL Cough Multi-Symptom Medication with Decongestant ... 1565
- Ursinus Inlay-Tabs ... ▣ 794
- Vicks 44 LiquiCaps Cough, Cold & Flu Relief ... ▣ 755
- Vicks 44 LiquiCaps Non-Drowsy Cough & Cold Relief ... ▣ 756
- Vicks 44D Dry Hacking Cough & Head Congestion ... ▣ 755
- Vicks 44M Cough, Cold & Flu Relief ... ▣ 756
- Vicks DayQuil ... ▣ 761
- Vicks DayQuil SINUS Pressure & PAIN Relief with IBUPROFEN ... ▣ 762
- Vicks Nyquil Hot Therapy ... ▣ 762
- Vicks NyQuil LiquiCaps Multi-Symptom Cold/Flu Relief ... ▣ 763
- Vicks NyQuil Multi-Symptom Cold/Flu Relief - (Original & Cherry Flavor) ... ▣ 763

Pyrilamine Maleate (Predisposition to hypertensive crises; use with caution at reduced dosages). Products include:
- 4-Way Fast Acting Nasal Spray (regular & mentholated) ... ▣ 621
- Maximum Strength Multi-Symptom Formula Midol ... ▣ 722
- PMS Multi-Symptom Formula Midol ... ▣ 723

Pyrilamine Tannate (Predisposition to hypertensive crises; use with caution at reduced dosages). Products include:
- Atrohist Pediatric Suspension ... 454
- Rynatan ... 2673

Quazepam (Predisposition to hypertensive crises; use with caution at reduced dosages). Products include:
- Doral Tablets ... 2664

Secobarbital Sodium (Predisposition to hypertensive crises; use with caution at reduced dosages). Products include:
- Seconal Sodium Pulvules ... 1474

Selegiline Hydrochloride (Predisposition to hypertensive crises; concurrent administration is contraindicated). Products include:
- Eldepryl Tablets ... 2550

Sufentanil Citrate (Predisposition to hypertensive crises; use with caution at reduced dosages). Products include:
- Sufenta Injection ... 1309

Temazepam (Predisposition to hypertensive crises; use with caution at reduced dosages). Products include:
- Restoril Capsules ... 2284

Terfenadine (Predisposition to hypertensive crises; use with caution at reduced dosages). Products include:
- Seldane Tablets ... 1536
- Seldane-D Extended-Release Tablets ... 1538

Tetrahydrozoline Hydrochloride (Predisposition to hypertensive crises; concurrent administration is contraindicated). Products include:
- Collyrium Fresh ... ⊙ 325
- Murine Plus Lubricant Redness Reliever Eye Drops ... ▣ 781
- Murine Tears Plus Lubricant Redness Reliever Eye Drops ... ⊙ 316
- Visine Maximum Strength Allergy Relief ... ⊙ 313
- Visine Moisturizing Eye Drops ... ⊙ 313
- Visine Original Eye Drops ... ⊙ 314

Thioridazine Hydrochloride (Predisposition to hypertensive crises; use with caution at reduced dosages). Products include:
- Mellaril ... 2269

Thiothixene (Predisposition to hypertensive crises; use with caution at reduced dosages). Products include:
- Navane Capsules and Concentrate 2201
- Navane Intramuscular ... 2202

Tranylcypromine Sulfate (Predisposition to hypertensive crises; concurrent administration is contraindicated). Products include:
- Parnate Tablets ... 2503

Triazolam (Predisposition to hypertensive crises; use with caution at reduced dosages). Products include:
- Halcion Tablets ... 2611

Trifluoperazine Hydrochloride (Predisposition to hypertensive crises; use with caution at reduced dosages). Products include:
- Stelazine ... 2514

Trimeprazine Tartrate (Predisposition to hypertensive crises; use with caution at reduced dosages). Products include:
- Temaril Tablets, Syrup and Spansule Extended-Release Capsules.. 483

Tripelennamine Hydrochloride (Predisposition to hypertensive crises; use with caution at reduced dosages). Products include:
- PBZ Tablets ... 845
- PBZ-SR Tablets ... 844

Triprolidine Hydrochloride (Predisposition to hypertensive crises; use with caution at reduced dosages). Products include:
- Actifed Plus Caplets ... ▣ 845
- Actifed Plus Tablets ... ▣ 845
- Actifed with Codeine Cough Syrup.. 1067
- Actifed Syrup ... ▣ 846
- Actifed Tablets ... ▣ 844

Tyramine (Predisposition to hypertensive crises; concurrent administration is contraindicated).

(▣ Described in PDR For Nonprescription Drugs) (⊙ Described in PDR For Ophthalmology)

Zolpidem Tartrate (Predisposition to hypertensive crises; use with caution at reduced dosages). Products include:

Ambien Tablets....................................... 2416

Food Interactions

Alcohol (Possible disulfiram-like reaction may occur; alcohol intake should be avoided during or within four days after Furoxone therapy).

Beans, broad (Concurrent and/or sequential intake must be avoided).

Beer, unspecified (Concurrent and/or sequential intake must be avoided).

Cheese, strong, unpasteurized (Concurrent and/or sequential intake must be avoided).

Food with high concentration of tyramine (Concurrent and/or sequential intake must be avoided).

Herring, pickled (Concurrent and/or sequential intake must be avoided).

Liver, chicken (Concurrent and/or sequential intake must be avoided).

Wine, unspecified (Concurrent and/or sequential intake must be avoided).

Yeast extract (Concurrent and/or sequential intake must be avoided).

FUROXONE TABLETS

(Furazolidone) 2046

See Furoxone Liquid

GAMIMUNE N, 5% IMMUNE GLOBULIN INTRAVENOUS (HUMAN), 5%

(Globulin, Immune (Human)) 619

May interact with:

Measles, Mumps & Rubella Virus Vaccine Live (Antibodies in Gamimune N, 5% may interfere with the response to live virus vaccine; use of such vaccines should be deferred until approximately 6 months after Gamimune N, 10% administration). Products include:

M-M-R II 1687

GAMIMUNE N, 10% IMMUNE GLOBULIN INTRAVENOUS (HUMAN), 10%

(Globulin, Immune (Human)) 621

May interact with:

Measles, Mumps & Rubella Virus Vaccine Live (Antibodies in Gamimune N, 10% may interfere with the response to live virus vaccine; use of such vaccines should be deferred until approximately 6 months after Gamimune N., 10% administration). Products include:

M-M-R II 1687

GAMMAGARD S/D, IMMUNE GLOBULIN, INTRAVENOUS (HUMAN)

(Globulin, Immune (Human)) 585

May interact with:

Measles, Mumps & Rubella Virus Vaccine Live (Antibodies in immune globulin may interfere with patient response to vaccine). Products include:

M-M-R II 1687

GAMMAR, IMMUNE GLOBULIN (HUMAN) U.S.P.

(Globulin, Immune (Human)) 515

May interact with:

Measles Virus Vaccine Live (Interference with the response to live viral vaccines). Products include:

Attenuvax 1610

Measles & Rubella Virus Vaccine Live (Interference with the response to live viral vaccines). Products include:

M-R-VAX II 1689

Measles, Mumps & Rubella Virus Vaccine Live (Interference with the response to live viral vaccines). Products include:

M-M-R II 1687

GAMMAR I.V., IMMUNE GLOBULIN INTRAVENOUS (HUMAN), LYOPHILIZED

(Globulin, Immune (Human)) 516

May interact with:

Measles Virus Vaccine Live (Antibodies in immune globulin preparations may interfere with the response by pediatric patients to live viral vaccines). Products include:

Attenuvax 1610

Measles & Rubella Virus Vaccine Live (Antibodies in immune globulin preparations may interfere with the response by pediatric patients to live viral vaccines). Products include:

M-R-VAX II 1689

Measles, Mumps & Rubella Virus Vaccine Live (Antibodies in immune globulin preparations may interfere with the response by pediatric patients to live viral vaccines). Products include:

M-M-R II 1687

GAMULIN RH, Rh_0(D) IMMUNE GLOBULIN (HUMAN)

(Rh_0(D) Immune Globulin (Human)) .. 517

None cited in PDR database.

GANITE

(Gallium Nitrate) 2533

May interact with aminoglycosides and certain other agents. Compounds in these categories include:

Amikacin Sulfate (Concomitant administration increases the risk for developing severe renal insufficiency). Products include:

Amikacin Sulfate Injection, USP 960
Amikin Injectable 501

Amphotericin B (Concomitant administration increases the risk for developing severe renal insufficiency). Products include:

Fungizone Intravenous 506

Gentamicin Sulfate (Concomitant administration increases the risk for developing severe renal insufficiency). Products include:

Garamycin Injectable 2360
Genoptic Sterile Ophthalmic Solution .... ⊙ 243
Genoptic Sterile Ophthalmic Ointment .... ⊙ 243
Gentacidin Ointment .... ⊙ 264
Gentacidin Solution............................... ⊙ 264
Gentak .... ⊙ 208
Pred-G Liquifilm Sterile Ophthalmic Suspension .... ⊙ 251
Pred-G S.O.P. Sterile Ophthalmic Ointment .... ⊙ 252

Kanamycin Sulfate (Concomitant administration increases the risk for developing severe renal insufficiency).

No products indexed under this heading.

Nephrotoxic Drugs (Concomitant administration may increase the risk for development of renal insufficiency).

Streptomycin Sulfate (Concomitant administration increases the risk for developing severe renal insufficiency). Products include:

Streptomycin Sulfate Injection......... 2208

Tobramycin (Concomitant administration increases the risk for developing severe renal insufficiency). Products include:

AKTOB .... ⊙ 206
TobraDex Ophthalmic Suspension and Ointment.. 473
Tobrex Ophthalmic Ointment and Solution .... ⊙ 229

Tobramycin Sulfate (Concomitant administration increases the risk for developing severe renal insufficiency). Products include:

Nebcin Vials, Hyporets & ADD-Vantage 1464
Tobramycin Sulfate Injection 968

GANTANOL TABLETS

(Sulfamethoxazole) 2119

May interact with thiazides, oral anticoagulants, and certain other agents. Compounds in these categories include:

Bendroflumethiazide (Increased incidence of thrombopenia with purpura in elderly).

No products indexed under this heading.

Chlorothiazide (Increased incidence of thrombopenia with purpura in elderly). Products include:

Aldoclor Tablets 1598
Diupres Tablets 1650
Diuril Oral 1653

Chlorothiazide Sodium (Increased incidence of thrombopenia with purpura in elderly). Products include:

Diuril Sodium Intravenous 1652

Dicumarol (Increased prothrombin time).

No products indexed under this heading.

Hydrochlorothiazide (Increased incidence of thrombopenia with purpura in elderly). Products include:

Aldactazide... 2413
Aldoril Tablets... 1604
Apresazide Capsules 808
Capozide 742
Dyazide.. 2479
Esidrix Tablets 821
Esimil Tablets 822
HydroDIURIL Tablets 1674
Hydropres Tablets.................................. 1675
Hyzaar Tablets 1677
Inderide Tablets 2732
Inderide LA Long Acting Capsules.. 2734
Lopressor HCT Tablets 832
Lotensin HCT... 837
Maxzide.. 1380
Moduretic Tablets 1705
Oretic Tablets 443
Prinzide Tablets 1737
Ser-Ap-Es Tablets 849
Timolide Tablets...................................... 1748
Vaseretic Tablets 1765
Zestoretic 2850
Ziac 1415

Hydroflumethiazide (Increased incidence of thrombopenia with purpura in elderly). Products include:

Diucardin Tablets................................... 2718

Methotrexate Sodium (May be displaced from protein-binding sites, thus increasing free methotrexate concentrations). Products include:

Methotrexate Sodium Tablets, Injection, for Injection and LPF Injection 1275

Methyclothiazide (Increased incidence of thrombopenia with purpura in elderly). Products include:

Enduron Tablets...................................... 420

Phenytoin (May inhibit hepatic metabolism; possible excessive phenytoin effect). Products include:

Dilantin Infatabs 1908
Dilantin-125 Suspension 1911

Phenytoin Sodium (May inhibit hepatic metabolism; possible excessive phenytoin effect). Products include:

Dilantin Kapseals 1906
Dilantin Parenteral 1910

Polythiazide (Increased incidence of thrombopenia with purpura in elderly). Products include:

Minizide Capsules 1938

Warfarin Sodium (Increased prothrombin time). Products include:

Coumadin 926

GANTRISIN PEDIATRIC SUSPENSION

(Acetyl Sulfisoxazole) 2120

May interact with oral anticoagulants, sulfonylureas, and certain other agents. Compounds in these categories include:

Chlorpropamide (Sulfisoxazole can potentiate the hypoglycemic activity of sulfonylurea). Products include:

Diabinese Tablets 1935

Dicumarol (Prolonged prothrombin time).

No products indexed under this heading.

Glipizide (Sulfisoxazole can potentiate the hypoglycemic activity of sulfonylurea). Products include:

Glucotrol Tablets 1967
Glucotrol XL Extended Release Tablets 1968

Glyburide (Sulfisoxazole can potentiate the hypoglycemic activity of sulfonylurea). Products include:

DiaBeta Tablets 1239
Glynase PresTab Tablets 2609
Micronase Tablets 2623

Methotrexate Sodium (Displaced from plasma protein-binding sites). Products include:

Methotrexate Sodium Tablets, Injection, for Injection and LPF Injection 1275

Sodium Thiopental (Potential for decrease in the amount of thiopental required for anesthesia and in a shortening of the awakening time when concomitantly administered with I.V. sulfisoxazole).

No products indexed under this heading.

Tolazamide (Sulfisoxazole can potentiate the hypoglycemic activity of sulfonylurea).

No products indexed under this heading.

Tolbutamide (Sulfisoxazole can potentiate the hypoglycemic activity of sulfonylurea).

No products indexed under this heading.

Warfarin Sodium (Prolonged prothrombin time). Products include:

Coumadin 926

IMPORTANT NOTE: Always consult each drug listing in the patient's regimen for possible interactions.

GANTRISIN SYRUP
(Acetyl Sulfisoxazole) 2120
See **Gantrisin Pediatric Suspension**

GANTRISIN TABLETS
(Sulfisoxazole) 2120
See **Gantrisin Pediatric Suspension**

GARAMYCIN INJECTABLE
(Gentamicin Sulfate) 2360
May interact with aminoglycosides, cephalosporins, anesthetics, neuromuscular blocking agents, and certain other agents. Compounds in these categories include:

Alfentanil Hydrochloride (Increased potential for neuromuscular blockade and respiratory paralysis). Products include:
Alfenta Injection 1286

Amikacin Sulfate (Concurrent and/or sequential use increases the risk of neurotoxicity and/or nephrotoxicity). Products include:
Amikacin Sulfate Injection, USP 960
Amikin Injectable 501

Atracurium Besylate (Increased potential for neuromuscular blockade and respiratory paralysis). Products include:
Tracrium Injection 1183

Carbenicillin Indanyl Sodium (Potential for reduction in gentamicin serum half-life in patients with severe renal impairment receiving concomitant carbenicillin and gentamicin). Products include:
Geocillin Tablets 2199

Cefaclor (Potential for increased nephrotoxicity). Products include:
Ceclor Pulvules & Suspension 1431

Cefadroxil Monohydrate (Potential for increased nephrotoxicity). Products include:
Duricef 748

Cefamandole Nafate (Potential for increased nephrotoxicity). Products include:
Mandol Vials, Faspak & ADD-Vantage 1461

Cefazolin Sodium (Potential for increased nephrotoxicity). Products include:
Ancef Injection 2465
Kefzol Vials, Faspak & ADD-Vantage 1456

Cefixime (Potential for increased nephrotoxicity). Products include:
Suprax 1399

Cefmetazole Sodium (Potential for increased nephrotoxicity). Products include:
Zefazone 2654

Cefonicid Sodium (Potential for increased nephrotoxicity). Products include:
Monocid Injection 2497

Cefoperazone Sodium (Potential for increased nephrotoxicity). Products include:
Cefobid Intravenous/Intramuscular 2189
Cefobid Pharmacy Bulk Package - Not for Direct Infusion 2192

Ceforanide (Potential for increased nephrotoxicity).
No products indexed under this heading.

Cefotaxime Sodium (Potential for increased nephrotoxicity). Products include:
Claforan Sterile and Injection 1235

Cefotetan (Potential for increased nephrotoxicity). Products include:
Cefotan 2829

Cefoxitin Sodium (Potential for increased nephrotoxicity). Products include:
Mefoxin 1691
Mefoxin Premixed Intravenous Solution 1694

Cefpodoxime Proxetil (Potential for increased nephrotoxicity). Products include:
Vantin for Oral Suspension and Vantin Tablets 2646

Cefprozil (Potential for increased nephrotoxicity). Products include:
Cefzil Tablets and Oral Suspension 746

Ceftazidime (Potential for increased nephrotoxicity). Products include:
Ceptaz 1081
Fortaz 1100
Tazicef for Injection 2519
Tazidime Vials, Faspak & ADD-Vantage 1478

Ceftizoxime Sodium (Potential for increased nephrotoxicity). Products include:
Cefizox for Intramuscular or Intravenous Use 1034

Ceftriaxone Sodium (Potential for increased nephrotoxicity). Products include:
Rocephin Injectable Vials, ADD-Vantage, Galaxy Container 2142

Cefuroxime Axetil (Potential for increased nephrotoxicity). Products include:
Ceftin 1078

Cefuroxime Sodium (Potential for increased nephrotoxicity). Products include:
Kefurox Vials, Faspak & ADD-Vantage 1454
Zinacef 1211

Cephalexin (Potential for increased nephrotoxicity). Products include:
Keflex Pulvules & Oral Suspension 914

Cephaloridine (Concurrent and/or sequential use increases the risk of neurotoxicity and/or nephrotoxicity).

Cephalothin Sodium (Potential for increased nephrotoxicity).

Cephapirin Sodium (Potential for increased nephrotoxicity).
No products indexed under this heading.

Cephradine (Potential for increased nephrotoxicity).
No products indexed under this heading.

Cisplatin (Concurrent and/or sequential use increases the risk of neurotoxicity and/or nephrotoxicity). Products include:
Platinol 708
Platinol-AQ Injection 710

Colistin Sulfate (Concurrent and/or sequential use increases the risk of neurotoxicity and/or nephrotoxicity). Products include:
Coly-Mycin S Otic w/Neomycin & Hydrocortisone 1906

Doxacurium Chloride (Increased potential for neuromuscular blockade and respiratory paralysis). Products include:
Nuromax Injection 1149

Enflurane (Increased potential for neuromuscular blockade and respiratory paralysis).
No products indexed under this heading.

Ethacrynic Acid (Potential for increased ototoxicity; concurrent use should be avoided). Products include:
Edecrin Tablets 1657

Fentanyl Citrate (Increased potential for neuromuscular blockade and respiratory paralysis). Products include:
Sublimaze Injection 1307

Furosemide (Potential for increased ototoxicity; concurrent use should be avoided). Products include:
Lasix Injection, Oral Solution and Tablets 1240

Halothane (Increased potential for neuromuscular blockade and respiratory paralysis). Products include:
Fluothane 2724

Isoflurane (Increased potential for neuromuscular blockade and respiratory paralysis).
No products indexed under this heading.

Kanamycin Sulfate (Concurrent and/or sequential use increases the risk of neurotoxicity and/or nephrotoxicity).
No products indexed under this heading.

Ketamine Hydrochloride (Increased potential for neuromuscular blockade and respiratory paralysis).
No products indexed under this heading.

Lithium Carbonate (Increased potential for neuromuscular blockade and respiratory paralysis). Products include:
Eskalith 2485
Lithium Carbonate Capsules & Tablets 2230
Lithonate/Lithotabs/Lithobid 2543

Lithium Citrate (Increased potential for neuromuscular blockade and respiratory paralysis).
No products indexed under this heading.

Loracarbef (Potential for increased nephrotoxicity). Products include:
Lorabid Suspension and Pulvules 1459

Methohexital Sodium (Increased potential for neuromuscular blockade and respiratory paralysis). Products include:
Brevital Sodium Vials 1429

Metocurine Iodide (Increased potential for neuromuscular blockade and respiratory paralysis). Products include:
Metubine Iodide Vials 916

Midazolam Hydrochloride (Increased potential for neuromuscular blockade and respiratory paralysis). Products include:
Versed Injection 2170

Mivacurium Chloride (Increased potential for neuromuscular blockade and respiratory paralysis). Products include:
Mivacron 1138

Neomycin Sulfate (Concurrent and/or sequential use increases the risk of neurotoxicity and/or nephrotoxicity). Products include:
AK-Spore .... ⊙ 204
AK-Trol Ointment & Suspension .... ⊙ 205
Bactine First Aid Antibiotic Plus Anesthetic Ointment .... ▣ 708
Campho-Phenique Maximum Strength First Aid Antibiotic Plus Pain Reliever Ointment .... ▣ 719
Coly-Mycin S Otic w/Neomycin & Hydrocortisone 1906
Cortisporin Cream 1084
Cortisporin Ointment 1085
Cortisporin Ophthalmic Ointment Sterile 1085
Cortisporin Ophthalmic Suspension Sterile 1086
Cortisporin Otic Solution Sterile 1087
Cortisporin Otic Suspension Sterile 1088
Dexacidin Ointment .... ⊙ 263
Maxitrol Ophthalmic Ointment and Suspension .... ⊙ 224
Mycitracin .... ▣ 839
NeoDecadron Sterile Ophthalmic Ointment 1712
NeoDecadron Sterile Ophthalmic Solution 1713
NeoDecadron Topical Cream 1714
Neosporin G.U. Irrigant Sterile 1148
Neosporin Ointment .... ▣ 857
Neosporin Plus Maximum Strength Cream .... ▣ 858
Neosporin Plus Maximum Strength Ointment .... ▣ 858
Neosporin Ophthalmic Ointment Sterile 1148
Neosporin Ophthalmic Solution Sterile 1149
PediOtic Suspension Sterile 1153
Poly-Pred Liquifilm .... ⊙ 248

Neomycin, oral (Concurrent and/or sequential use increases the risk of neurotoxicity and/or nephrotoxicity).

Pancuronium Bromide Injection (Increased potential for neuromuscular blockade and respiratory paralysis).
No products indexed under this heading.

Paromomycin Sulfate (Concurrent and/or sequential use increases the risk of neurotoxicity and/or nephrotoxicity).
No products indexed under this heading.

Polymyxin B Sulfate (Concurrent and/or sequential use increases the risk of neurotoxicity and/or nephrotoxicity). Products include:
AK-Spore .... ⊙ 204
AK-Trol Ointment & Suspension .... ⊙ 205
Bactine First Aid Antibiotic Plus Anesthetic Ointment .... ▣ 708
Betadine Brand First Aid Antibiotics & Moisturizer Ointment 1991
Campho-Phenique Maximum Strength First Aid Antibiotic Plus Pain Reliever Ointment .... ▣ 719
Cortisporin Cream 1084
Cortisporin Ointment 1085
Cortisporin Ophthalmic Ointment Sterile 1085
Cortisporin Ophthalmic Suspension Sterile 1086
Cortisporin Otic Solution Sterile 1087
Cortisporin Otic Suspension Sterile 1088
Dexacidin Ointment .... ⊙ 263
Maxitrol Ophthalmic Ointment and Suspension .... ⊙ 224
Mycitracin .... ▣ 839
Neosporin G.U. Irrigant Sterile 1148
Neosporin Ointment .... ▣ 857
Neosporin Plus Maximum Strength Cream .... ▣ 858
Neosporin Plus Maximum Strength Ointment .... ▣ 858
Neosporin Ophthalmic Ointment Sterile 1148
Neosporin Ophthalmic Solution Sterile 1149
Ophthocort .... ⊙ 311
PediOtic Suspension Sterile 1153
Polymyxin B Sulfate, Aerosporin Brand Sterile Powder 1154
Poly-Pred Liquifilm .... ⊙ 248
Polysporin Ointment .... ▣ 858
Polysporin Ophthalmic Ointment Sterile 1154
Polysporin Powder .... ▣ 859
Polytrim Ophthalmic Solution Sterile 482
TERAK Ointment .... ⊙ 209
Terramycin with Polymyxin B Sulfate Ophthalmic Ointment 2211

Propofol (Increased potential for neuromuscular blockade and respiratory paralysis). Products include:
Diprivan Injection 2833

Rocuronium Bromide (Increased potential for neuromuscular blockade and respiratory paralysis). Products include:
Zemuron 1830

(▣ Described in PDR For Nonprescription Drugs) (⊙ Described in PDR For Ophthalmology)

Streptomycin Sulfate (Concurrent and/or sequential use increases the risk of neurotoxicity and/or nephrotoxicity). Products include:
Streptomycin Sulfate Injection......... 2208

Succinylcholine Chloride (Increased potential for neuromuscular blockade and respiratory paralysis). Products include:
Anectine.. 1073

Sufentanil Citrate (Increased potential for neuromuscular blockade and respiratory paralysis). Products include:
Sufenta Injection 1309

Thiamylal Sodium (Increased potential for neuromuscular blockade and respiratory paralysis).
No products indexed under this heading.

Tobramycin (Concurrent and/or sequential use increases the risk of neurotoxicity and/or nephrotoxicity). Products include:
AKTOB .... ◉ 206
TobraDex Ophthalmic Suspension and Ointment...................................... 473
Tobrex Ophthalmic Ointment and Solution .... ◉ 229

Tobramycin Sulfate (Concurrent and/or sequential use increases the risk of neurotoxicity and/or nephrotoxicity). Products include:
Nebcin Vials, Hyporets & ADD-Vantage 1464
Tobramycin Sulfate Injection 968

Tubocurarine Chloride (Increased potential for neuromuscular blockade and respiratory paralysis).
No products indexed under this heading.

Vancomycin Hydrochloride (Concurrent and/or sequential use increases the risk of neurotoxicity and/or nephrotoxicity). Products include:
Vancocin HCl, Oral Solution & Pulvules 1483
Vancocin HCl, Vials & ADD-Vantage 1481

Vecuronium Bromide (Increased potential for neuromuscular blockade and respiratory paralysis). Products include:
Norcuron 1826

Viomycin (Concurrent and/or sequential use increases the risk of neurotoxicity and/or nephrotoxicity).

GAS-X CHEWABLE TABLETS

(Simethicone) .... ◘ 786
None cited in PDR database.

EXTRA STRENGTH GAS-X CHEWABLE TABLETS

(Simethicone) .... ◘ 786
None cited in PDR database.

GASTROCROM CAPSULES

(Cromolyn Sodium) 984
May interact with:

Isoproterenol Hydrochloride (Concurrent use at extremely high doses of both drugs appears to have increased resorptions and malformations in animal studies). Products include:
Isuprel Hydrochloride Injection 1:5000 2311
Isuprel Hydrochloride Solution 1:200 & 1:100 2313
Isuprel Mistometer 2312

GAVISCON ANTACID TABLETS

(Aluminum Hydroxide Gel, Magnesium Trisilicate) .... ◘ 819
May interact with:

Prescription Drugs, unspecified (Concurrent use with certain unspecified drugs is not recommended; consult your physicians).

GAVISCON-2 ANTACID TABLETS

(Aluminum Hydroxide Gel, Magnesium Trisilicate) .... ◘ 820
May interact with:

Prescription Drugs, unspecified (Concurrent use with certain unspecified drugs is not recommended; consult your physicians).

GAVISCON EXTRA STRENGTH RELIEF FORMULA ANTACID TABLETS

(Aluminum Hydroxide, Magnesium Carbonate) .... ◘ 819
May interact with:

Prescription Drugs, unspecified (Concurrent use with certain unspecified drugs is not recommended; consult your physicians).

GAVISCON EXTRA STRENGTH RELIEF FORMULA LIQUID ANTACID

(Aluminum Hydroxide, Magnesium Carbonate) .... ◘ 819
May interact with:

Prescription Drugs, unspecified (Concurrent use with certain unspecified drugs is not recommended; consult your physicians).

GAVISCON LIQUID ANTACID

(Aluminum Hydroxide, Magnesium Carbonate) .... ◘ 820
May interact with:

Prescription Drugs, unspecified (Concurrent use with certain unspecified drugs is not recommended; consult your physicians).

GELFOAM STERILE SPONGE

(Gelatin Preparations) 2608
May interact with:

Thrombin (The safety and efficacy of the combined use has not been evaluated and therefore cannot be recommended). Products include:
THROMBOGEN* Topical Thrombin, USP with Diluent and Transfer Needle 1315
THROMBOGEN* Topical Thrombin, USP, Spray Kit 1315

GELUSIL LIQUID & TABLETS

(Aluminum Hydroxide, Magnesium Hydroxide, Simethicone) .... ◘ 855
May interact with:

Prescription Drugs, unspecified (Concurrent use is not recommended; consult your doctor).

GENOPTIC STERILE OPHTHALMIC SOLUTION

(Gentamicin Sulfate)............................ ◉ 243
None cited in PDR database.

GENOPTIC STERILE OPHTHALMIC OINTMENT

(Gentamicin Sulfate)............................ ◉ 243
None cited in PDR database.

GENOTROPIN

(Somatropin) 006
May interact with glucocorticoids. Compounds in this category include:

Betamethasone Acetate (Concomitant glucocorticoid therapy may inhibit human growth promoting effect). Products include:
Celestone Soluspan Suspension 2347

Betamethasone Sodium Phosphate (Concomitant glucocorticoid therapy may inhibit human growth promoting effect). Products include:
Celestone Soluspan Suspension 2347

Cortisone Acetate (Concomitant glucocorticoid therapy may inhibit human growth promoting effect). Products include:
Cortone Acetate Sterile Suspension 1623
Cortone Acetate Tablets..................... 1624

Dexamethasone (Concomitant glucocorticoid therapy may inhibit human growth promoting effect). Products include:
AK-Trol Ointment & Suspension .... ◉ 205
Decadron Elixir 1633
Decadron Tablets................................. 1635
Decaspray Topical Aerosol 1648
Dexacidin Ointment .... ◉ 263
Maxitrol Ophthalmic Ointment and Suspension .... ◉ 224
TobraDex Ophthalmic Suspension and Ointment...................................... 473

Dexamethasone Acetate (Concomitant glucocorticoid therapy may inhibit human growth promoting effect). Products include:
Dalalone D.P. Injectable 1011
Decadron-LA Sterile Suspension...... 1646

Dexamethasone Sodium Phosphate (Concomitant glucocorticoid therapy may inhibit human growth promoting effect). Products include:
Decadron Phosphate Injection 1637
Decadron Phosphate Respihaler 1642
Decadron Phosphate Sterile Ophthalmic Ointment 1641
Decadron Phosphate Sterile Ophthalmic Solution 1642
Decadron Phosphate Topical Cream.. 1644
Decadron Phosphate Turbinaire 1645
Decadron Phosphate with Xylocaine Injection, Sterile 1639
Dexacort Phosphate in Respihaler .. 458
Dexacort Phosphate in Turbinaire .. 459
NeoDecadron Sterile Ophthalmic Ointment 1712
NeoDecadron Sterile Ophthalmic Solution 1713
NeoDecadron Topical Cream 1714

Fludrocortisone Acetate (Concomitant glucocorticoid therapy may inhibit human growth promoting effect). Products include:
Florinef Acetate Tablets 505

Hydrocortisone (Concomitant glucocorticoid therapy may inhibit human growth promoting effect). Products include:
Anusol-HC Cream 2.5% 1896
Aquanil HC Lotion 1931
Bactine Hydrocortisone Anti-Itch Cream... ◘ 709
Caldecort Anti-Itch Hydrocortisone Spray .... ◘ 631
Cortaid .... ◘ 836
CORTENEMA.. 2535
Cortisporin Ointment 1085
Cortisporin Ophthalmic Ointment Sterile 1085
Cortisporin Ophthalmic Suspension Sterile 1086
Cortisporin Otic Solution Sterile 1087
Cortisporin Otic Suspension Sterile 1088
Cortizone-5 .... ◘ 831
Cortizone-10 .... ◘ 831
Hydrocortone Tablets 1672
Hytone 907
Massengill Medicated Soft Cloth Towelettes... 2458
PediOtic Suspension Sterile 1153
Preparation H Hydrocortisone 1% Cream .... ◘ 872
ProctoCream-HC 2.5% 2408
VōSoL HC Otic Solution...................... 2678

Hydrocortisone Acetate (Concomitant glucocorticoid therapy may inhibit human growth promoting effect). Products include:
Analpram-HC Rectal Cream 1% and 2.5% 977
Anusol HC-1 Anti-Itch Hydrocortisone Ointment...................................... ◘ 847
Anusol-HC Suppositories 1897
Caldecort.. ◘ 631
Carmol HC 924
Coly-Mycin S Otic w/Neomycin & Hydrocortisone 1906
Cortaid .... ◘ 836
Cortifoam 2396
Cortisporin Cream................................ 1084
Epifoam 2399
Hydrocortone Acetate Sterile Suspension... 1669
Mantadil Cream 1135
Nupercainal Hydrocortisone 1% Cream... ◘ 645
Ophthocort .... ◉ 311
Pramosone Cream, Lotion & Ointment 978
ProctoCream-HC 2408
ProctoFoam-HC 2409
Terra-Cortril Ophthalmic Suspension 2210

Hydrocortisone Sodium Phosphate (Concomitant glucocorticoid therapy may inhibit human growth promoting effect). Products include:
Hydrocortone Phosphate Injection, Sterile 1670

Hydrocortisone Sodium Succinate (Concomitant glucocorticoid therapy may inhibit human growth promoting effect). Products include:
Solu-Cortef Sterile Powder................. 2641

Methylprednisolone Acetate (Concomitant glucocorticoid therapy may inhibit human growth promoting effect). Products include:
Depo-Medrol Single-Dose Vial 2600
Depo-Medrol Sterile Aqueous Suspension... 2597

Methylprednisolone Sodium Succinate (Concomitant glucocorticoid therapy may inhibit human growth promoting effect). Products include:
Solu-Medrol Sterile Powder............... 2643

Prednisolone Acetate (Concomitant glucocorticoid therapy may inhibit human growth promoting effect). Products include:
AK-CIDE .... ◉ 202
AK-CIDE Ointment............................... ◉ 202
Blephamide Liquifilm Sterile Ophthalmic Suspension............................. 476
Blephamide Ointment .... ◉ 237
Econopred & Econopred Plus Ophthalmic Suspensions .... ◉ 217
Poly-Pred Liquifilm .... ◉ 248
Pred Forte .... ◉ 250
Pred Mild.. ◉ 253
Pred-G Liquifilm Sterile Ophthalmic Suspension .... ◉ 251
Pred-G S.O.P. Sterile Ophthalmic Ointment .... ◉ 252
Vasocidin Ointment .... ◉ 268

Prednisolone Sodium Phosphate (Concomitant glucocorticoid therapy may inhibit human growth promoting effect). Products include:
AK-Pred .... ◉ 204
Hydeltrasol Injection, Sterile.............. 1665
Inflamase... ◉ 265
Pediapred Oral Liquid 995
Vasocidin Ophthalmic Solution ...... ◉ 270

Prednisolone Tebutate (Concomitant glucocorticoid therapy may inhibit human growth promoting effect). Products include:
Hydeltra-T.B.A. Sterile Suspension 1667

IMPORTANT NOTE: Always consult each drug listing in the patient's regimen for possible interactions.

Prednisone (Concomitant glucocorticoid therapy may inhibit human growth promoting effect). Products include:
- Deltasone Tablets ... 2595

Triamcinolone (Concomitant glucocorticoid therapy may inhibit human growth promoting effect). Products include:
- Aristocort Tablets ... 1022

Triamcinolone Acetonide (Concomitant glucocorticoid therapy may inhibit human growth promoting effect). Products include:
- Aristocort A 0.025% Cream ... 1027
- Aristocort A 0.5% Cream ... 1031
- Aristocort A 0.1% Cream ... 1029
- Aristocort A 0.1% Ointment ... 1030
- Azmacort Oral Inhaler ... 2011
- Nasacort Nasal Inhaler ... 2024

Triamcinolone Diacetate (Concomitant glucocorticoid therapy may inhibit human growth promoting effect). Products include:
- Aristocort Suspension (Forte Parenteral) ... 1027
- Aristocort Suspension (Intralesional) ... 1025

Triamcinolone Hexacetonide (Concomitant glucocorticoid therapy may inhibit human growth promoting effect). Products include:
- Aristospan Suspension (Intra-articular) ... 1033
- Aristospan Suspension (Intralesional) ... 1032

GENTACIDIN OINTMENT
(Gentamicin Sulfate) ... ⊙ 264
None cited in PDR database.

GENTACIDIN SOLUTION
(Gentamicin Sulfate) ... ⊙ 264
None cited in PDR database.

GENTAK
(Gentamicin Sulfate) ... ⊙ 208
None cited in PDR database.

GENTAK OPHTHALMIC OINTMENT
(Gentamicin Sulfate) ... ⊙ 208
None cited in PDR database.

GEOCILLIN TABLETS
(Carbenicillin Indanyl Sodium) ... 2199
May interact with:

Probenecid (Geocillin blood levels may be increased and prolonged). Products include:
- Benemid Tablets ... 1611
- ColBENEMID Tablets ... 1622

GEREF (SERMORELIN ACETATE FOR INJECTION)
(Sermorelin Acetate) ... 2876
May interact with drugs directly affecting the pituitary secretion of somatotropin, cyclo-oxygenase inhibitors, antimuscarinic drugs, antithyroid agents, and certain other agents. Compounds in these categories include:

Aspirin (The Geref test should not be conducted in the presence of this drug). Products include:
- Alka-Seltzer Effervescent Antacid and Pain Reliever ... ▣ 701
- Alka-Seltzer Extra Strength Effervescent Antacid and Pain Reliever ... ▣ 703
- Alka-Seltzer Lemon Lime Effervescent Antacid and Pain Reliever ... ▣ 703
- Alka-Seltzer Plus Cold Medicine ... ▣ 705
- Alka-Seltzer Plus Cold & Cough Medicine ... ▣ 708
- Alka-Seltzer Plus Night-Time Cold Medicine ... ▣ 707
- Alka Seltzer Plus Sinus Medicine ... ▣ 707
- Arthritis Foundation Safety Coated Aspirin Tablets ... ▣ 675
- Arthritis Pain Ascriptin ... ▣ 631
- Maximum Strength Ascriptin ... ▣ 630
- Regular Strength Ascriptin Tablets ... ▣ 629
- Arthritis Strength BC Powder ... ▣ 609
- BC Cold Powder Multi-Symptom Formula (Cold-Sinus-Allergy) ... ▣ 609
- BC Cold Powder Non-Drowsy Formula (Cold-Sinus) ... ▣ 609
- BC Powder ... ▣ 609
- Bayer Children's Chewable Aspirin ... ▣ 711
- Genuine Bayer Aspirin Tablets & Caplets ... ▣ 713
- Extra Strength Bayer Arthritis Pain Regimen Formula ... ▣ 711
- Extra Strength Bayer Aspirin Caplets & Tablets ... ▣ 712
- Extended-Release Bayer 8-Hour Aspirin ... ▣ 712
- Extra Strength Bayer Plus Aspirin Caplets ... ▣ 713
- Extra Strength Bayer PM Aspirin ... ▣ 713
- Bayer Enteric Aspirin ... ▣ 709
- Bufferin Analgesic Tablets and Caplets ... ▣ 613
- Arthritis Strength Bufferin Analgesic Caplets ... ▣ 614
- Extra Strength Bufferin Analgesic Tablets ... ▣ 615
- Cama Arthritis Pain Reliever ... ▣ 785
- Darvon Compound-65 Pulvules ... 1435
- Easprin ... 1914
- Ecotrin ... 2455
- Ecotrin Enteric Coated Aspirin Maximum Strength Tablets and Caplets ... ▣ 816
- Ecotrin Enteric Coated Aspirin Regular Strength Tablets ... 2455
- Empirin Aspirin Tablets ... ▣ 854
- Empirin with Codeine Tablets ... 1093
- Excedrin Extra-Strength Analgesic Tablets & Caplets ... 732
- Fiorinal Capsules ... 2261
- Fiorinal with Codeine Capsules ... 2262
- Fiorinal Tablets ... 2261
- Halfprin ... 1362
- Healthprin Aspirin ... 2455
- Norgesic ... 1496
- Percodan Tablets ... 939
- Percodan-Demi Tablets ... 940
- Robaxisal Tablets ... 2071
- Soma Compound w/Codeine Tablets ... 2676
- Soma Compound Tablets ... 2675
- St. Joseph Adult Chewable Aspirin (81 mg.) ... ▣ 808
- Talwin Compound ... 2335
- Ursinus Inlay-Tabs ... ▣ 794
- Vanquish Analgesic Caplets ... ▣ 731

Atropine Sulfate (Response to Geref may be blunted). Products include:
- Arco-Lase Plus Tablets ... 512
- Atrohist Plus Tablets ... 454
- Atropine Sulfate Sterile Ophthalmic Solution ... ⊙ 233
- Donnatal ... 2060
- Donnatal Extentabs ... 2061
- Donnatal Tablets ... 2060
- Lomotil ... 2439
- Motofen Tablets ... 784
- Urised Tablets ... 1964

Belladonna Alkaloids (Response to Geref may be blunted). Products include:
- Bellergal-S Tablets ... 2250
- Hyland's Bed Wetting Tablets ... ▣ 828
- Hyland's EnurAid Tablets ... ▣ 829
- Hyland's Teething Tablets ... ▣ 830

Betamethasone Acetate (The Geref test should not be conducted in the presence of this drug). Products include:
- Celestone Soluspan Suspension ... 2347

Betamethasone Sodium Phosphate (The Geref test should not be conducted in the presence of this drug). Products include:
- Celestone Soluspan Suspension ... 2347

Clidinium Bromide (Response to Geref may be blunted). Products include:
- Librax Capsules ... 2176
- Quarzan Capsules ... 2181

Cortisone Acetate (The Geref test should not be conducted in the presence of this drug). Products include:
- Cortone Acetate Sterile Suspension ... 1623
- Cortone Acetate Tablets ... 1624

Dexamethasone (The Geref test should not be conducted in the presence of this drug). Products include:
- AK-Trol Ointment & Suspension ... ⊙ 205
- Decadron Elixir ... 1633
- Decadron Tablets ... 1635
- Decaspray Topical Aerosol ... 1648
- Dexacidin Ointment ... ⊙ 263
- Maxitrol Ophthalmic Ointment and Suspension ... ⊙ 224
- TobraDex Ophthalmic Suspension and Ointment ... 473

Dexamethasone Acetate (The Geref test should not be conducted in the presence of this drug). Products include:
- Dalalone D.P. Injectable ... 1011
- Decadron-LA Sterile Suspension ... 1646

Dexamethasone Sodium Phosphate (The Geref test should not be conducted in the presence of this drug). Products include:
- Decadron Phosphate Injection ... 1637
- Decadron Phosphate Respihaler ... 1642
- Decadron Phosphate Sterile Ophthalmic Ointment ... 1641
- Decadron Phosphate Sterile Ophthalmic Solution ... 1642
- Decadron Phosphate Topical Cream ... 1644
- Decadron Phosphate Turbinaire ... 1645
- Decadron Phosphate with Xylocaine Injection, Sterile ... 1639
- Dexacort Phosphate in Respihaler ... 458
- Dexacort Phosphate in Turbinaire ... 459
- NeoDecadron Sterile Ophthalmic Ointment ... 1712
- NeoDecadron Sterile Ophthalmic Solution ... 1713
- NeoDecadron Topical Cream ... 1714

Dicyclomine Hydrochloride (Response to Geref may be blunted). Products include:
- Bentyl ... 1501

Glycopyrrolate (Response to Geref may be blunted). Products include:
- Robinul Forte Tablets ... 2072
- Robinul Injectable ... 2072
- Robinul Tablets ... 2072

Hydrocortisone (The Geref test should not be conducted in the presence of this drug). Products include:
- Anusol-HC Cream 2.5% ... 1896
- Aquanil HC Lotion ... 1931
- Bactine Hydrocortisone Anti-Itch Cream ... ▣ 709
- Caldecort Anti-Itch Hydrocortisone Spray ... ▣ 631
- Cortaid ... ▣ 836
- CORTENEMA ... 2535
- Cortisporin Ointment ... 1085
- Cortisporin Ophthalmic Ointment Sterile ... 1085
- Cortisporin Ophthalmic Suspension Sterile ... 1086
- Cortisporin Otic Solution Sterile ... 1087
- Cortisporin Otic Suspension Sterile ... 1088
- Cortizone-5 ... ▣ 831
- Cortizone-10 ... ▣ 831
- Hydrocortone Tablets ... 1672
- Hytone ... 907
- Massengill Medicated Soft Cloth Towelettes ... 2458
- PediOtic Suspension Sterile ... 1153
- Preparation H Hydrocortisone 1% Cream ... ▣ 872
- ProctoCream-HC 2.5% ... 2408
- VōSoL HC Otic Solution ... 2678

Hydrocortisone Acetate (The Geref test should not be conducted in the presence of this drug). Products include:
- Analpram-HC Rectal Cream 1% and 2.5% ... 977
- Anusol HC-1 Anti-Itch Hydrocortisone Ointment ... ▣ 847
- Anusol-HC Suppositories ... 1897
- Caldecort ... ▣ 631
- Carmol HC ... 924
- Coly-Mycin S Otic w/Neomycin & Hydrocortisone ... 1906
- Cortaid ... ▣ 836
- Cortifoam ... 2396
- Cortisporin Cream ... 1084
- Epifoam ... 2399
- Hydrocortone Acetate Sterile Suspension ... 1669
- Mantadil Cream ... 1135
- Nupercainal Hydrocortisone 1% Cream ... ▣ 645
- Ophthocort ... ⊙ 311
- Pramosone Cream, Lotion & Ointment ... 978
- ProctoCream-HC ... 2408
- ProctoFoam-HC ... 2409
- Terra-Cortril Ophthalmic Suspension ... 2210

Hydrocortisone Sodium Phosphate (The Geref test should not be conducted in the presence of this drug). Products include:
- Hydrocortone Phosphate Injection, Sterile ... 1670

Hydrocortisone Sodium Succinate (The Geref test should not be conducted in the presence of this drug). Products include:
- Solu-Cortef Sterile Powder ... 2641

Hyoscyamine (Response to Geref may be blunted). Products include:
- Cystospaz Tablets ... 1963
- Urised Tablets ... 1964

Hyoscyamine Sulfate (Response to Geref may be blunted). Products include:
- Arco-Lase Plus Tablets ... 512
- Atrohist Plus Tablets ... 454
- Cystospaz-M Capsules ... 1963
- Donnatal ... 2060
- Donnatal Extentabs ... 2061
- Donnatal Tablets ... 2060
- Kutrase Capsules ... 2402
- Levsin/Levsinex/Levbid ... 2405

Indomethacin (The Geref test should not be conducted in the presence of this drug). Products include:
- Indocin ... 1680

Indomethacin Sodium Trihydrate (The Geref test should not be conducted in the presence of this drug). Products include:
- Indocin I.V. ... 1684

Insulin, Human (The Geref test should not be conducted in the presence of this drug).
- No products indexed under this heading.

Insulin, Human Isophane Suspension (The Geref test should not be conducted in the presence of this drug). Products include:
- Novolin N Human Insulin 10 ml Vials ... 1795

Insulin, Human NPH (The Geref test should not be conducted in the presence of this drug). Products include:
- Humulin N, 100 Units ... 1448
- Novolin N PenFill Cartridges Durable Insulin Delivery System ... 1798
- Novolin N Prefilled Syringe Disposable Insulin Delivery System ... 1798

Insulin, Human Regular (The Geref test should not be conducted in the presence of this drug). Products include:
- Humulin R, 100 Units ... 1449
- Novolin R Human Insulin 10 ml Vials ... 1795
- Novolin R PenFill Cartridges Durable Insulin Delivery System ... 1798
- Novolin R Prefilled Syringe Disposable Insulin Delivery System ... 1798
- Velosulin BR Human Insulin 10 ml Vials ... 1795

Insulin, Human, Zinc Suspension (The Geref test should not be conducted in the presence of this drug). Products include:
- Humulin L, 100 Units ... 1446

(▣ Described in PDR For Nonprescription Drugs) (⊙ Described in PDR For Ophthalmology)

439 **Interactions Index** **Glauctabs**

- Humulin U, 100 Units ... 1450
- Novolin L Human Insulin 10 ml Vials ... 1795

Insulin, NPH (The Geref test should not be conducted in the presence of this drug). Products include:
- NPH, 100 Units ... 1450
- Pork NPH, 100 Units ... 1452
- Purified Pork NPH Isophane Insulin ... 1801

Insulin, Regular (The Geref test should not be conducted in the presence of this drug). Products include:
- Regular, 100 Units ... 1450
- Pork Regular, 100 Units ... 1452
- Pork Regular (Concentrated), 500 Units ... 1453
- Purified Pork Regular Insulin ... 1801

Insulin, Zinc Crystals (The Geref test should not be conducted in the presence of this drug). Products include:
- NPH, 100 Units ... 1450

Insulin, Zinc Suspension (The Geref test should not be conducted in the presence of this drug). Products include:
- Iletin I ... 1450
- Lente, 100 Units ... 1450
- Iletin II ... 1452
- Pork Lente, 100 Units ... 1452
- Purified Pork Lente Insulin ... 1801

Ipratropium Bromide (Response to Geref may be blunted). Products include:
- Atrovent Inhalation Aerosol ... 671
- Atrovent Inhalation Solution ... 673

Levodopa (Somatropin levels may be transiently elevated by levodopa). Products include:
- Atamet ... 572
- Larodopa Tablets ... 2129
- Sinemet Tablets ... 943
- Sinemet CR Tablets ... 944

Mepenzolate Bromide (Response to Geref may be blunted).
- No products indexed under this heading.

Methimazole (Response to Geref may be blunted). Products include:
- Tapazole Tablets ... 1477

Methylprednisolone Acetate (The Geref test should not be conducted in the presence of this drug). Products include:
- Depo-Medrol Single-Dose Vial ... 2600
- Depo-Medrol Sterile Aqueous Suspension ... 2597

Methylprednisolone Sodium Succinate (The Geref test should not be conducted in the presence of this drug). Products include:
- Solu-Medrol Sterile Powder ... 2643

Oxyphenonium Bromide (Response to Geref may be blunted).

Prednisolone Acetate (The Geref test should not be conducted in the presence of this drug). Products include:
- AK-CIDE ... ⊙ 202
- AK-CIDE Ointment ... ⊙ 202
- Blephamide Liquifilm Sterile Ophthalmic Suspension ... 476
- Blephamide Ointment ... ⊙ 237
- Econopred & Econopred Plus Ophthalmic Suspensions ... ⊙ 217
- Poly-Pred Liquifilm ... ⊙ 248
- Pred Forte ... ⊙ 250
- Pred Mild ... ⊙ 253
- Pred-G Liquifilm Sterile Ophthalmic Suspension ... ⊙ 251
- Pred-G S.O.P. Sterile Ophthalmic Ointment ... ⊙ 252
- Vasocidin Ointment ... ⊙ 268

Prednisolone Sodium Phosphate (The Geref test should not be conducted in the presence of this drug). Products include:
- AK-Pred ... ⊙ 204
- Hydeltrasol Injection, Sterile ... 1665
- Inflamase ... ⊙ 265
- Pediapred Oral Liquid ... 995
- Vasocidin Ophthalmic Solution ... ⊙ 270

Prednisolone Tebutate (The Geref test should not be conducted in the presence of this drug). Products include:
- Hydeltra-T.B.A. Sterile Suspension 1667

Prednisone (The Geref test should not be conducted in the presence of this drug). Products include:
- Deltasone Tablets ... 2595

Propantheline Bromide (Response to Geref may be blunted). Products include:
- Pro-Banthine Tablets ... 2052

Propylthiouracil (Response to Geref may be blunted).
- No products indexed under this heading.

Scopolamine (Response to Geref may be blunted). Products include:
- Transderm Scōp Transdermal Therapeutic System ... 869

Scopolamine Hydrobromide (Response to Geref may be blunted). Products include:
- Atrohist Plus Tablets ... 454
- Donnatal ... 2060
- Donnatal Extentabs ... 2061
- Donnatal Tablets ... 2060

Triamcinolone (The Geref test should not be conducted in the presence of this drug). Products include:
- Aristocort Tablets ... 1022

Triamcinolone Acetonide (The Geref test should not be conducted in the presence of this drug). Products include:
- Aristocort A 0.025% Cream ... 1027
- Aristocort A 0.5% Cream ... 1031
- Aristocort A 0.1% Cream ... 1029
- Aristocort A 0.1% Ointment ... 1030
- Azmacort Oral Inhaler ... 2011
- Nasacort Nasal Inhaler ... 2024

Triamcinolone Diacetate (The Geref test should not be conducted in the presence of this drug). Products include:
- Aristocort Suspension (Forte Parenteral) ... 1027
- Aristocort Suspension (Intralesional) ... 1025

Triamcinolone Hexacetonide (The Geref test should not be conducted in the presence of this drug). Products include:
- Aristospan Suspension (Intra-articular) ... 1033
- Aristospan Suspension (Intralesional) ... 1032

Tridihexethyl Chloride (Response to Geref may be blunted).
- No products indexed under this heading.

GERIMED TABLETS
(Vitamins with Minerals) ... 982
None cited in PDR database.

GEVRABON LIQUID
(Vitamins with Minerals) ... ▣ 670
None cited in PDR database.

GLAUCTABS 25 MG
(Methazolamide) ... ⊙ 208
May interact with corticosteroids and certain other agents. Compounds in these categories include:

Aspirin (Concomitant use with high-dose aspirin may result in anorexia, tachypnea, lethargy, coma, and death). Products include:
- Alka-Seltzer Effervescent Antacid and Pain Reliever ... ▣ 701
- Alka-Seltzer Extra Strength Effervescent Antacid and Pain Reliever ... ▣ 703
- Alka-Seltzer Lemon Lime Effervescent Antacid and Pain Reliever ... ▣ 703
- Alka-Seltzer Plus Cold Medicine ... ▣ 705
- Alka-Seltzer Plus Cold & Cough Medicine ... ▣ 708
- Alka-Seltzer Plus Night-Time Cold Medicine ... ▣ 707
- Alka Seltzer Plus Sinus Medicine .. ▣ 707
- Arthritis Foundation Safety Coated Aspirin Tablets ... ▣ 675
- Arthritis Pain Ascriptin ... ▣ 631
- Maximum Strength Ascriptin ... ▣ 630
- Regular Strength Ascriptin Tablets ... ▣ 629
- Arthritis Strength BC Powder ... ▣ 609
- BC Cold Powder Multi-Symptom Formula (Cold-Sinus-Allergy) ... ▣ 609
- BC Cold Powder Non-Drowsy Formula (Cold-Sinus) ... ▣ 609
- BC Powder ... ▣ 609
- Bayer Children's Chewable Aspirin ... ▣ 711
- Genuine Bayer Aspirin Tablets & Caplets ... ▣ 713
- Extra Strength Bayer Arthritis Pain Regimen Formula ... ▣ 711
- Extra Strength Bayer Aspirin Caplets & Tablets ... ▣ 712
- Extended-Release Bayer 8-Hour Aspirin ... ▣ 712
- Extra Strength Bayer Plus Aspirin Caplets ... ▣ 713
- Extra Strength Bayer PM Aspirin .. ▣ 713
- Bayer Enteric Aspirin ... ▣ 709
- Bufferin Analgesic Tablets and Caplets ... ▣ 613
- Arthritis Strength Bufferin Analgesic Caplets ... ▣ 614
- Extra Strength Bufferin Analgesic Tablets ... ▣ 615
- Cama Arthritis Pain Reliever ... ▣ 785
- Darvon Compound-65 Pulvules ... 1435
- Easprin ... 1914
- Ecotrin ... 2455
- Ecotrin Enteric Coated Aspirin Maximum Strength Tablets and Caplets ... ▣ 816
- Ecotrin Enteric Coated Aspirin Regular Strength Tablets ... 2455
- Empirin Aspirin Tablets ... ▣ 854
- Empirin with Codeine Tablets ... 1093
- Excedrin Extra-Strength Analgesic Tablets & Caplets ... 732
- Fiorinal Capsules ... 2261
- Fiorinal with Codeine Capsules ... 2262
- Fiorinal Tablets ... 2261
- Halfprin ... 1362
- Healthprin Aspirin ... 2455
- Norgesic ... 1496
- Percodan Tablets ... 939
- Percodan-Demi Tablets ... 940
- Robaxisal Tablets ... 2071
- Soma Compound w/Codeine Tablets ... 2676
- Soma Compound Tablets ... 2675
- St. Joseph Adult Chewable Aspirin (81 mg.) ... ▣ 808
- Talwin Compound ... 2335
- Ursinus Inlay-Tabs ... ▣ 794
- Vanquish Analgesic Caplets ... ▣ 731

Betamethasone Acetate (Potential for developing hypokalemia). Products include:
- Celestone Soluspan Suspension ... 2347

Betamethasone Sodium Phosphate (Potential for developing hypokalemia). Products include:
- Celestone Soluspan Suspension ... 2347

Cortisone Acetate (Potential for developing hypokalemia). Products include:
- Cortone Acetate Sterile Suspension ... 1623
- Cortone Acetate Tablets ... 1624

Dexamethasone (Potential for developing hypokalemia). Products include:
- AK-Trol Ointment & Suspension ... ⊙ 205
- Decadron Elixir ... 1633
- Decadron Tablets ... 1635
- Decaspray Topical Aerosol ... 1648
- Dexacidin Ointment ... ⊙ 263
- Maxitrol Ophthalmic Ointment and Suspension ... ⊙ 224
- TobraDex Ophthalmic Suspension and Ointment ... 473

Dexamethasone Acetate (Potential for developing hypokalemia). Products include:
- Dalalone D.P. Injectable ... 1011
- Decadron-LA Sterile Suspension ... 1646

Dexamethasone Sodium Phosphate (Potential for developing hypokalemia). Products include:
- Decadron Phosphate Injection ... 1637
- Decadron Phosphate Respihaler ... 1642
- Decadron Phosphate Sterile Ophthalmic Ointment ... 1641
- Decadron Phosphate Sterile Ophthalmic Solution ... 1642
- Decadron Phosphate Topical Cream ... 1644
- Decadron Phosphate Turbinaire ... 1645
- Decadron Phosphate with Xylocaine Injection, Sterile ... 1639
- Dexacort Phosphate in Respihaler .. 458
- Dexacort Phosphate in Turbinaire .. 459
- NeoDecadron Sterile Ophthalmic Ointment ... 1712
- NeoDecadron Sterile Ophthalmic Solution ... 1713
- NeoDecadron Topical Cream ... 1714

Fludrocortisone Acetate (Potential for developing hypokalemia). Products include:
- Florinef Acetate Tablets ... 505

Hydrocortisone (Potential for developing hypokalemia). Products include:
- Anusol-HC Cream 2.5% ... 1896
- Aquanil HC Lotion ... 1931
- Bactine Hydrocortisone Anti-Itch Cream ... ▣ 709
- Caldecort Anti-Itch Hydrocortisone Spray ... ▣ 631
- Cortaid ... ▣ 836
- CORTENEMA ... 2535
- Cortisporin Ointment ... 1085
- Cortisporin Ophthalmic Ointment Sterile ... 1085
- Cortisporin Ophthalmic Suspension Sterile ... 1086
- Cortisporin Otic Solution Sterile ... 1087
- Cortisporin Otic Suspension Sterile 1088
- Cortizone-5 ... ▣ 831
- Cortizone-10 ... ▣ 831
- Hydrocortone Tablets ... 1672
- Hytone ... 907
- Massengill Medicated Soft Cloth Towelettes ... 2458
- PediOtic Suspension Sterile ... 1153
- Preparation H Hydrocortisone 1% Cream ... ▣ 872
- ProctoCream-HC 2.5% ... 2408
- VōSoL HC Otic Solution ... 2678

Hydrocortisone Acetate (Potential for developing hypokalemia). Products include:
- Analpram-HC Rectal Cream 1% and 2.5% ... 977
- Anusol HC-1 Anti-Itch Hydrocortisone Ointment ... ▣ 847
- Anusol-HC Suppositories ... 1897
- Caldecort ... ▣ 631
- Carmol HC ... 924
- Coly-Mycin S Otic w/Neomycin & Hydrocortisone ... 1906
- Cortaid ... ▣ 836
- Cortifoam ... 2396
- Cortisporin Cream ... 1084
- Epifoam ... 2399
- Hydrocortone Acetate Sterile Suspension ... 1669
- Mantadil Cream ... 1135
- Nupercainal Hydrocortisone 1% Cream ... ▣ 645
- Ophthocort ... ⊙ 311
- Pramosone Cream, Lotion & Ointment ... 978
- ProctoCream-HC ... 2408
- ProctoFoam-HC ... 2409
- Terra-Cortril Ophthalmic Suspension ... 2210

Hydrocortisone Sodium Phosphate (Potential for developing hypokalemia). Products include:
- Hydrocortone Phosphate Injection, Sterile ... 1670

Hydrocortisone Sodium Succinate (Potential for developing hypokalemia). Products include:
- Solu-Cortef Sterile Powder ... 2641

Methylprednisolone Acetate (Potential for developing hypokalemia). Products include:
- Depo-Medrol Single-Dose Vial ... 2600
- Depo-Medrol Sterile Aqueous Suspension ... 2597

IMPORTANT NOTE: Always consult each drug listing in the patient's regimen for possible interactions.

Methylprednisolone Sodium Succinate (Potential for developing hypokalemia). Products include:
- Solu-Medrol Sterile Powder ... 2643

Prednisolone Acetate (Potential for developing hypokalemia). Products include:
- AK-CIDE ... ◉ 202
- AK-CIDE Ointment ... ◉ 202
- Blephamide Liquifilm Sterile Ophthalmic Suspension ... 476
- Blephamide Ointment ... ◉ 237
- Econopred & Econopred Plus Ophthalmic Suspensions ... ◉ 217
- Poly-Pred Liquifilm ... ◉ 248
- Pred Forte ... ◉ 250
- Pred Mild ... ◉ 253
- Pred-G Liquifilm Sterile Ophthalmic Suspension ... ◉ 251
- Pred-G S.O.P. Sterile Ophthalmic Ointment ... ◉ 252
- Vasocidin Ointment ... ◉ 268

Prednisolone Sodium Phosphate (Potential for developing hypokalemia). Products include:
- AK-Pred ... ◉ 204
- Hydeltrasol Injection, Sterile ... 1665
- Inflamase ... ◉ 265
- Pediapred Oral Liquid ... 995
- Vasocidin Ophthalmic Solution ... ◉ 270

Prednisolone Tebutate (Potential for developing hypokalemia). Products include:
- Hydeltra-T.B.A. Sterile Suspension 1667

Prednisone (Potential for developing hypokalemia). Products include:
- Deltasone Tablets ... 2595

Triamcinolone (Potential for developing hypokalemia). Products include:
- Aristocort Tablets ... 1022

Triamcinolone Acetonide (Potential for developing hypokalemia). Products include:
- Aristocort A 0.025% Cream ... 1027
- Aristocort A 0.5% Cream ... 1031
- Aristocort A 0.1% Cream ... 1029
- Aristocort A 0.1% Ointment ... 1030
- Azmacort Oral Inhaler ... 2011
- Nasacort Nasal Inhaler ... 2024

Triamcinolone Diacetate (Potential for developing hypokalemia). Products include:
- Aristocort Suspension (Forte Parenteral) ... 1027
- Aristocort Suspension (Intralesional) ... 1025

Triamcinolone Hexacetonide (Potential for developing hypokalemia). Products include:
- Aristospan Suspension (Intra-articular) ... 1033
- Aristospan Suspension (Intralesional) ... 1032

GLAUCTABS 50 MG
(Methazolamide) ... ◉ 208
See **Glauctabs 25 mg**

GLUCAGON FOR INJECTION VIALS AND EMERGENCY KIT
(Glucagon) ... 1440
None cited in PDR database.

GLUCERNA SPECIALIZED NUTRITION WITH FIBER FOR PATIENTS WITH ABNORMAL GLUCOSE TOLERANCE
(Nutritional Supplement) ... 2221
None cited in PDR database.

GLUCOPHAGE
(Metformin Hydrochloride) ... 752
May interact with radiographic iodinated contrast media, cationic drugs that are eliminated by renal tubular secretion, diuretics, corticosteroids, phenothiazines, thyroid preparations, estrogens, oral contraceptives, calcium channel blockers, sympathomimetics, and certain other agents. Compounds in these categories include:

Albuterol (Potential for loss of glycemic control). Products include:
- Proventil Inhalation Aerosol ... 2382
- Ventolin Inhalation Aerosol and Refill ... 1197

Albuterol Sulfate (Potential for loss of glycemic control). Products include:
- Airet Solution for Inhalation ... 452
- Proventil Inhalation Solution 0.083% ... 2384
- Proventil Repetabs Tablets ... 2386
- Proventil Solution for Inhalation 0.5% ... 2383
- Proventil Syrup ... 2385
- Proventil Tablets ... 2386
- Ventolin Inhalation Solution ... 1198
- Ventolin Nebules Inhalation Solution ... 1199
- Ventolin Rotacaps for Inhalation ... 1200
- Ventolin Syrup ... 1202
- Ventolin Tablets ... 1203
- Volmax Extended-Release Tablets .. 1788

Amiloride Hydrochloride (Potential for loss of glycemic control; theoretical potential for interaction with metformin by competing for common renal tubular transport system). Products include:
- Midamor Tablets ... 1703
- Moduretic Tablets ... 1705

Amlodipine Besylate (Potential for loss of glycemic control). Products include:
- Lotrel Capsules ... 840
- Norvasc Tablets ... 1940

Bendroflumethiazide (Potential for loss of glycemic control).
- No products indexed under this heading.

Bepridil Hydrochloride (Potential for loss of glycemic control). Products include:
- Vascor (200, 300 and 400 mg) Tablets ... 1587

Betamethasone Acetate (Potential for loss of glycemic control). Products include:
- Celestone Soluspan Suspension ... 2347

Betamethasone Sodium Phosphate (Potential for loss of glycemic control). Products include:
- Celestone Soluspan Suspension ... 2347

Bumetanide (Potential for loss of glycemic control). Products include:
- Bumex ... 2093

Chlorothiazide (Potential for loss of glycemic control). Products include:
- Aldoclor Tablets ... 1598
- Diupres Tablets ... 1650
- Diuril Oral ... 1653

Chlorothiazide Sodium (Potential for loss of glycemic control). Products include:
- Diuril Sodium Intravenous ... 1652

Chlorotrianisene (Potential for loss of glycemic control).
- No products indexed under this heading.

Chlorpromazine (Potential for loss of glycemic control). Products include:
- Thorazine Suppositories ... 2523

Chlorpromazine Hydrochloride (Potential for loss of glycemic control). Products include:
- Thorazine ... 2523

Chlorthalidone (Potential for loss of glycemic control). Products include:
- Combipres Tablets ... 677
- Tenoretic Tablets ... 2845
- Thalitone ... 1245

Cimetidine (Co-administered with oral cimetidine may increase peak metformin plasma and whole blood concentrations by 60% and a 40% increase in plasma and whole blood metformin AUC). Products include:
- Tagamet Tablets ... 2516

Cortisone Acetate (Potential for loss of glycemic control). Products include:
- Cortone Acetate Sterile Suspension ... 1623
- Cortone Acetate Tablets ... 1624

Desogestrel (Potential for loss of glycemic control). Products include:
- Desogen Tablets ... 1817
- Ortho-Cept ... 1851

Dexamethasone (Potential for loss of glycemic control). Products include:
- AK-Trol Ointment & Suspension ... ◉ 205
- Decadron Elixir ... 1633
- Decadron Tablets ... 1635
- Decaspray Topical Aerosol ... 1648
- Dexacidin Ointment ... ◉ 263
- Maxitrol Ophthalmic Ointment and Suspension ... ◉ 224
- TobraDex Ophthalmic Suspension and Ointment ... 473

Dexamethasone Acetate (Potential for loss of glycemic control). Products include:
- Dalalone D.P. Injectable ... 1011
- Decadron-LA Sterile Suspension ... 1646

Dexamethasone Sodium Phosphate (Potential for loss of glycemic control). Products include:
- Decadron Phosphate Injection ... 1637
- Decadron Phosphate Respihaler ... 1642
- Decadron Phosphate Sterile Ophthalmic Ointment ... 1641
- Decadron Phosphate Sterile Ophthalmic Solution ... 1642
- Decadron Phosphate Topical Cream ... 1644
- Decadron Phosphate Turbinaire ... 1645
- Decadron Phosphate with Xylocaine Injection, Sterile ... 1639
- Dexacort Phosphate in Respihaler .. 458
- Dexacort Phosphate in Turbinaire .. 459
- NeoDecadron Sterile Ophthalmic Ointment ... 1712
- NeoDecadron Sterile Ophthalmic Solution ... 1713
- NeoDecadron Topical Cream ... 1714

Diatrizoate Meglumine (Potential for acute alteration of renal function; metformin should be temporarily withheld in patients undergoing radiologic studies involving parenteral iodinated contrast material).

Diatrizoate Sodium (Potential for acute alteration of renal function; metformin should be temporarily withheld in patients undergoing radiologic studies involving parenteral iodinated contrast material).

Dienestrol (Potential for loss of glycemic control). Products include:
- Ortho Dienestrol Cream ... 1866

Diethylstilbestrol (Potential for loss of glycemic control). Products include:
- Diethylstilbestrol Tablets ... 1437

Digoxin (Theoretical potential for interaction with metformin by competing for common renal tubular transport system). Products include:
- Lanoxicaps ... 1117
- Lanoxin Elixir Pediatric ... 1120
- Lanoxin Injection ... 1123
- Lanoxin Injection Pediatric ... 1126
- Lanoxin Tablets ... 1128

Diltiazem Hydrochloride (Potential for loss of glycemic control). Products include:
- Cardizem CD Capsules ... 1506
- Cardizem SR Capsules ... 1510
- Cardizem Injectable ... 1508
- Cardizem Tablets ... 1512
- Dilacor XR Extended-release Capsules ... 2018

Dobutamine Hydrochloride (Potential for loss of glycemic control). Products include:
- Dobutrex Solution Vials ... 1439

Dopamine Hydrochloride (Potential for loss of glycemic control).
- No products indexed under this heading.

Ephedrine Hydrochloride (Potential for loss of glycemic control). Products include:
- Primatene Dual Action Formula ... 📖 872
- Primatene Tablets ... 📖 873
- Quadrinal Tablets ... 1350

Ephedrine Sulfate (Potential for loss of glycemic control). Products include:
- Bronkaid Caplets ... 📖 717
- Marax Tablets & DF Syrup ... 2200

Ephedrine Tannate (Potential for loss of glycemic control). Products include:
- Rynatuss ... 2673

Epinephrine (Potential for loss of glycemic control). Products include:
- Bronkaid Mist ... 📖 717
- EPIFRIN ... ◉ 239
- EpiPen ... 790
- Marcaine Hydrochloride with Epinephrine 1:200,000 ... 2316
- Primatene Mist ... 📖 873
- Sensorcaine with Epinephrine Injection ... 559
- Sus-Phrine Injection ... 1019
- Xylocaine with Epinephrine Injections ... 567

Epinephrine Bitartrate (Potential for loss of glycemic control). Products include:
- Bronkaid Mist Suspension ... 📖 718
- Sensorcaine-MPF with Epinephrine Injection ... 559

Epinephrine Hydrochloride (Potential for loss of glycemic control). Products include:
- Ana-Kit Anaphylaxis Emergency Treatment Kit ... 617

Estradiol (Potential for loss of glycemic control). Products include:
- Climara Transdermal System ... 645
- Estrace Cream and Tablets ... 749
- Estraderm Transdermal System ... 824

Estrogens, Conjugated (Potential for loss of glycemic control). Products include:
- PMB 200 and PMB 400 ... 2783
- Premarin Intravenous ... 2787
- Premarin with Methyltestosterone .. 2794
- Premarin Tablets ... 2789
- Premarin Vaginal Cream ... 2791
- Premphase ... 2797
- Prempro ... 2801

Estrogens, Esterified (Potential for loss of glycemic control). Products include:
- ESTRATAB Tablets (0.3, 0.625, 1.25, 2.5 mg) ... 2536
- Estratest ... 2539
- Menest Tablets ... 2494

Estropipate (Potential for loss of glycemic control). Products include:
- Ogen Tablets ... 2627
- Ogen Vaginal Cream ... 2630
- Ortho-Est ... 1869

Ethacrynic Acid (Potential for loss of glycemic control). Products include:
- Edecrin Tablets ... 1657

Ethinyl Estradiol (Potential for loss of glycemic control). Products include:
- Brevicon ... 2088
- Demulen ... 2428
- Desogen Tablets ... 1817
- Levlen/Tri-Levlen ... 651
- Lo/Ovral Tablets ... 2746
- Lo/Ovral-28 Tablets ... 2751
- Modicon ... 1872
- Nordette-21 Tablets ... 2755
- Nordette-28 Tablets ... 2758
- Norinyl ... 2088
- Ortho-Cept ... 1851

441 **Interactions Index** **Glucophage**

Ortho-Cyclen/Ortho-Tri-Cyclen 1858
Ortho-Novum 1872
Ortho-Cyclen/Ortho Tri-Cyclen 1858
Ovcon 760
Ovral Tablets 2770
Ovral-28 Tablets 2770
Levlen/Tri-Levlen 651
Tri-Norinyl 2164
Triphasil-21 Tablets 2814
Triphasil-28 Tablets 2819

Ethiodized Oil (Potential for acute alteration of renal function; metformin should be temporarily withheld in patients undergoing radiologic studies involving parenteral iodinated contrast material).
No products indexed under this heading.

Ethynodiol Diacetate (Potential for loss of glycemic control). Products include:
Demulen 2428

Felodipine (Potential for loss of glycemic control). Products include:
Plendil Extended-Release Tablets 527

Fludrocortisone Acetate (Potential for loss of glycemic control). Products include:
Florinef Acetate Tablets 505

Fluphenazine Decanoate (Potential for loss of glycemic control). Products include:
Prolixin Decanoate 509

Fluphenazine Enanthate (Potential for loss of glycemic control). Products include:
Prolixin Enanthate 509

Fluphenazine Hydrochloride (Potential for loss of glycemic control). Products include:
Prolixin 509

Furosemide (Increases metformin plasma and blood C_{max} by 22% and blood AUC by 15%; the C_{max} and AUC of furosemide were 31% and 12% smaller when co-administered; potential for loss of glycemic control). Products include:
Lasix Injection, Oral Solution and Tablets 1240

Gadopentetate Dimeglumine (Potential for acute alteration of renal function; metformin should be temporarily withheld in patients undergoing radiologic studies involving parenteral iodinated contrast material).
No products indexed under this heading.

Glyburide (Decrease in glyburide AUC and C_{max} have been observed, but were highly variable). Products include:
DiaBeta Tablets 1239
Glynase PresTab Tablets 2609
Micronase Tablets 2623

Hydrochlorothiazide (Potential for loss of glycemic control). Products include:
Aldactazide 2413
Aldoril Tablets 1604
Apresazide Capsules 808
Capozide 742
Dyazide 2479
Esidrix Tablets 821
Esimil Tablets 822
HydroDIURIL Tablets 1674
Hydropres Tablets 1675
Hyzaar Tablets 1677
Inderide Tablets 2732
Inderide LA Long Acting Capsules 2734
Lopressor HCT Tablets 832
Lotensin HCT 837
Maxzide 1380
Moduretic Tablets 1705
Oretic Tablets 443
Prinzide Tablets 1737
Ser-Ap-Es Tablets 849
Timolide Tablets 1748
Vaseretic Tablets 1765
Zestoretic 2850
Ziac 1415

Hydrocortisone (Potential for loss of glycemic control). Products include:
Anusol-HC Cream 2.5% 1896
Aquanil HC Lotion 1931
Bactine Hydrocortisone Anti-Itch Cream 709
Caldecort Anti-Itch Hydrocortisone Spray 631
Cortaid 836
CORTENEMA 2535
Cortisporin Ointment 1085
Cortisporin Ophthalmic Ointment Sterile 1085
Cortisporin Ophthalmic Suspension Sterile 1086
Cortisporin Otic Solution Sterile 1087
Cortisporin Otic Suspension Sterile 1088
Cortizone-5 831
Cortizone-10 831
Hydrocortone Tablets 1672
Hytone 907
Massengill Medicated Soft Cloth Towelettes 2458
PediOtic Suspension Sterile 1153
Preparation H Hydrocortisone 1% Cream 872
ProctoCream-HC 2.5% 2408
VōSoL HC Otic Solution 2678

Hydrocortisone Acetate (Potential for loss of glycemic control). Products include:
Analpram-HC Rectal Cream 1% and 2.5% 977
Anusol HC-1 Anti-Itch Hydrocortisone Ointment 847
Anusol-HC Suppositories 1897
Caldecort 631
Carmol HC 924
Coly-Mycin S Otic w/Neomycin & Hydrocortisone 1906
Cortaid 836
Cortifoam 2396
Cortisporin Cream 1084
Epifoam 2399
Hydrocortone Acetate Sterile Suspension 1669
Mantadil Cream 1135
Nupercainal Hydrocortisone 1% Cream 645
Ophthocort .... ⊙ 311
Pramosone Cream, Lotion & Ointment 978
ProctoCream-HC 2408
ProctoFoam-HC 2409
Terra-Cortril Ophthalmic Suspension 2210

Hydrocortisone Sodium Phosphate (Potential for loss of glycemic control). Products include:
Hydrocortone Phosphate Injection, Sterile 1670

Hydrocortisone Sodium Succinate (Potential for loss of glycemic control). Products include:
Solu-Cortef Sterile Powder 2641

Hydroflumethiazide (Potential for loss of glycemic control). Products include:
Diucardin Tablets 2718

Indapamide (Potential for loss of glycemic control). Products include:
Lozol Tablets 2022

Iodamide Meglumine (Potential for acute alteration of renal function; metformin should be temporarily withheld in patients undergoing radiologic studies involving parenteral iodinated contrast material).
No products indexed under this heading.

Iohexol (Potential for acute alteration of renal function; metformin should be temporarily withheld in patients undergoing radiologic studies involving parenteral iodinated contrast material).
No products indexed under this heading.

Iopamidol (Potential for acute alteration of renal function; metformin should be temporarily withheld in patients undergoing radiologic studies involving parenteral iodinated contrast material).
No products indexed under this heading.

Iothalamate Meglumine (Potential for acute alteration of renal function; metformin should be temporarily withheld in patients undergoing radiologic studies involving parenteral iodinated contrast material).
No products indexed under this heading.

Iopanoic Acid (Potential for acute alteration of renal function; metformin should be temporarily withheld in patients undergoing radiologic studies involving parenteral iodinated contrast material).

Ioxaglate Meglumine (Potential for acute alteration of renal function; metformin should be temporarily withheld in patients undergoing radiologic studies involving parenteral iodinated contrast material).
No products indexed under this heading.

Ioxaglate Sodium (Potential for acute alteration of renal function; metformin should be temporarily withheld in patients undergoing radiologic studies involving parenteral iodinated contrast material).
No products indexed under this heading.

Isoniazid (Potential for loss of glycemic control). Products include:
Nydrazid Injection 508
Rifamate Capsules 1530
Rifater 1532

Isoproterenol Hydrochloride (Potential for loss of glycemic control). Products include:
Isuprel Hydrochloride Injection 1:5000 2311
Isuprel Hydrochloride Solution 1:200 & 1:100 2313
Isuprel Mistometer 2312

Isoproterenol Sulfate (Potential for loss of glycemic control). Products include:
Norisodrine with Calcium Iodide Syrup 442

Isradipine (Potential for loss of glycemic control). Products include:
DynaCirc Capsules 2256

Levonorgestrel (Potential for loss of glycemic control). Products include:
Levlen/Tri-Levlen 651
Nordette-21 Tablets 2755
Nordette-28 Tablets 2758
Norplant System 2759
Levlen/Tri-Levlen 651
Triphasil-21 Tablets 2814
Triphasil-28 Tablets 2819

Levothyroxine Sodium (Potential for loss of glycemic control). Products include:
Levothroid Tablets 1016
Levoxyl Tablets 903
Synthroid 1359

Liothyronine Sodium (Potential for loss of glycemic control). Products include:
Cytomel Tablets 2473
Triostat Injection 2530

Liotrix (Potential for loss of glycemic control).
No products indexed under this heading.

Mesoridazine Besylate (Potential for loss of glycemic control). Products include:
Serentil 684

Mestranol (Potential for loss of glycemic control). Products include:
Norinyl 2088
Ortho-Novum 1872

Metaproterenol Sulfate (Potential for loss of glycemic control). Products include:
Alupent 669
Metaproterenol Sulfate Inhalation Solution, USP, Arm-a-Med 552

Metaraminol Bitartrate (Potential for loss of glycemic control). Products include:
Aramine Injection 1609

Methotrimeprazine (Potential for loss of glycemic control). Products include:
Levoprome 1274

Methoxamine Hydrochloride (Potential for loss of glycemic control). Products include:
Vasoxyl Injection 1196

Methyclothiazide (Potential for loss of glycemic control). Products include:
Enduron Tablets 420

Methylprednisolone Acetate (Potential for loss of glycemic control). Products include:
Depo-Medrol Single-Dose Vial 2600
Depo-Medrol Sterile Aqueous Suspension 2597

Methylprednisolone Sodium Succinate (Potential for loss of glycemic control). Products include:
Solu-Medrol Sterile Powder 2643

Metolazone (Potential for loss of glycemic control). Products include:
Mykrox Tablets 993
Zaroxolyn Tablets 1000

Morphine Sulfate (Theoretical potential for interaction with metformin by competing for common renal tubular transport system). Products include:
Astramorph/PF Injection, USP (Preservative-Free) 535
Duramorph 962
Infumorph 200 and Infumorph 500 Sterile Solutions 965
MS Contin Tablets 1994
MSIR 1997
Oramorph SR (Morphine Sulfate Sustained Release Tablets) 2236
RMS Suppositories 2657
Roxanol 2243

Nicardipine Hydrochloride (Potential for loss of glycemic control). Products include:
Cardene Capsules 2095
Cardene I.V. 2709
Cardene SR Capsules 2097

Nicotinic Acid (Potential for loss of glycemic control).
No products indexed under this heading.

Nifedipine (Enhances the absorption of metformin by increasing plasma metformin C_{max} and AUC; potential for loss of glycemic control). Products include:
Adalat Capsules (10 mg and 20 mg) 587
Adalat CC 589
Procardia Capsules 1971
Procardia XL Extended Release Tablets 1972

Nimodipine (Potential for loss of glycemic control). Products include:
Nimotop Capsules 610

Nisoldipine (Potential for loss of glycemic control).
No products indexed under this heading.

Norepinephrine Bitartrate (Potential for loss of glycemic control). Products include:
Levophed Bitartrate Injection 2315

IMPORTANT NOTE: Always consult each drug listing in the patient's regimen for possible interactions.

Glucophage | Interactions Index | 442

Norethindrone (Potential for loss of glycemic control). Products include:
- Brevicon 2088
- Micronor Tablets 1872
- Modicon 1872
- Norinyl 2088
- Nor-Q D Tablets 2135
- Ortho-Novum 1872
- Ovcon 760
- Tri-Norinyl 2164

Norethynodrel (Potential for loss of glycemic control).
- No products indexed under this heading.

Norgestimate (Potential for loss of glycemic control). Products include:
- Ortho-Cyclen/Ortho-Tri-Cyclen 1858
- Ortho-Cyclen/Ortho Tri-Cyclen 1858

Norgestrel (Potential for loss of glycemic control). Products include:
- Lo/Ovral Tablets 2746
- Lo/Ovral-28 Tablets 2751
- Ovral Tablets 2770
- Ovral-28 Tablets 2770
- Ovrette Tablets 2771

Perphenazine (Potential for loss of glycemic control). Products include:
- Etrafon 2355
- Triavil Tablets 1757
- Trilafon 2389

Phenylephrine Bitartrate (Potential for loss of glycemic control).
- No products indexed under this heading.

Phenylephrine Hydrochloride (Potential for loss of glycemic control). Products include:
- Atrohist Plus Tablets 454
- Cerose DM ▣ 878
- Comhist 2038
- D.A. Chewable Tablets 951
- Deconsal Pediatric Capsules 454
- Dura-Vent/DA Tablets 953
- Entex Capsules 1986
- Entex Liquid 1986
- Extendryl 1005
- 4-Way Fast Acting Nasal Spray (regular & mentholated) ▣ 621
- Hemorid For Women ▣ 834
- Hycomine Compound Tablets 932
- Neo-Synephrine Hydrochloride 1% Carpuject 2324
- Neo-Synephrine Hydrochloride 1% Injection 2324
- Neo-Synephrine Hydrochloride (Ophthalmic) 2325
- Neo-Synephrine ▣ 726
- Nōstril ▣ 644
- Novahistine Elixir ▣ 823
- Phenergan VC 2779
- Phenergan VC with Codeine 2781
- Preparation H ▣ 871
- Tympagesic Ear Drops 2342
- Vasosulf ⊙ 271
- Vicks Sinex Nasal Spray and Ultra Fine Mist ▣ 765

Phenylephrine Tannate (Potential for loss of glycemic control). Products include:
- Atrohist Pediatric Suspension 454
- Ricobid-D Pediatric Suspension 2038
- Ricobid Tablets and Pediatric Suspension 2038
- Rynatan 2673
- Rynatuss 2673

Phenylpropanolamine Hydrochloride (Potential for loss of glycemic control). Products include:
- Acutrim ▣ 628
- Allerest Children's Chewable Tablets ▣ 627
- Allerest 12 Hour Caplets ▣ 627
- Atrohist Plus Tablets 454
- BC Cold Powder Multi-Symptom Formula (Cold-Sinus-Allergy) ▣ 609
- BC Cold Powder Non-Drowsy Formula (Cold-Sinus) ▣ 609
- Cheracol Plus Head Cold/Cough Formula ▣ 769
- Comtrex Multi-Symptom Non-Drowsy Liqui-gels ▣ 618
- Contac Continuous Action Nasal Decongestant/Antihistamine 12 Hour Capsules ▣ 813
- Contac Maximum Strength Continuous Action Decongestant/Antihistamine 12 Hour Caplets ▣ 813
- Contac Severe Cold and Flu Formula Caplets ▣ 814
- Coricidin 'D' Decongestant Tablets ▣ 800
- Dexatrim ▣ 832
- Dexatrim Plus Vitamins Caplets ▣ 832
- Dimetane-DC Cough Syrup 2059
- Dimetapp Elixir ▣ 773
- Dimetapp Extentabs ▣ 774
- Dimetapp Tablets/Liqui-Gels ▣ 775
- Dimetapp Cold & Allergy Chewable Tablets ▣ 773
- Dimetapp DM Elixir ▣ 774
- Dura-Vent Tablets 952
- Entex Capsules 1986
- Entex LA Tablets 1987
- Entex Liquid 1986
- Exgest LA Tablets 782
- Hycomine 931
- Isoclor Timesule Capsules ▣ 637
- Nolamine Timed-Release Tablets 785
- Ornade Spansule Capsules 2502
- Propagest Tablets 786
- Pyrroxate Caplets ▣ 772
- Robitussin-CF ▣ 777
- Sinulin Tablets 787
- Tavist-D 12 Hour Relief Tablets ▣ 787
- Teldrin 12 Hour Antihistamine/Nasal Decongestant Allergy Relief Capsules ▣ 826
- Triaminic Allergy Tablets ▣ 789
- Triaminic Cold Tablets ▣ 790
- Triaminic Expectorant ▣ 790
- Triaminic Syrup ▣ 792
- Triaminic-12 Tablets ▣ 792
- Triaminic-DM Syrup ▣ 792
- Triaminicin Tablets ▣ 793
- Triaminicol Multi-Symptom Cold Tablets ▣ 793
- Triaminicol Multi-Symptom Relief ▣ 794
- Vicks DayQuil Allergy Relief 12-Hour Extended Release Tablets ▣ 760
- Vicks DayQuil Allergy Relief 4-Hour Tablets ▣ 760
- Vicks DayQuil SINUS Pressure & CONGESTION Relief ▣ 761

Phenytoin (Potential for loss of glycemic control). Products include:
- Dilantin Infatabs 1908
- Dilantin-125 Suspension 1911

Phenytoin Sodium (Potential for loss of glycemic control). Products include:
- Dilantin Kapseals 1906
- Dilantin Parenteral 1910

Pirbuterol Acetate (Potential for loss of glycemic control). Products include:
- Maxair Autohaler 1492
- Maxair Inhaler 1494

Polyestradiol Phosphate (Potential for loss of glycemic control).
- No products indexed under this heading.

Polythiazide (Potential for loss of glycemic control). Products include:
- Minizide Capsules 1938

Prednisolone Acetate (Potential for loss of glycemic control). Products include:
- AK-CIDE ⊙ 202
- AK-CIDE Ointment ⊙ 202
- Blephamide Liquifilm Sterile Ophthalmic Suspension 476
- Blephamide Ointment ⊙ 237
- Econopred & Econopred Plus Ophthalmic Suspensions ⊙ 217
- Poly-Pred Liquifilm ⊙ 248
- Pred Forte ⊙ 250
- Pred Mild ⊙ 253
- Pred-G Liquifilm Sterile Ophthalmic Suspension ⊙ 251
- Pred-G S.O.P. Sterile Ophthalmic Ointment ⊙ 252
- Vasocidin Ointment ⊙ 268

Prednisolone Sodium Phosphate (Potential for loss of glycemic control). Products include:
- AK-Pred ⊙ 204
- Hydeltrasol Injection, Sterile 1665
- Inflamase ⊙ 265
- Pediapred Oral Liquid 995
- Vasocidin Ophthalmic Solution ⊙ 270

Prednisolone Tebutate (Potential for loss of glycemic control). Products include:
- Hydeltra-T.B.A. Sterile Suspension 1667

Prednisone (Potential for loss of glycemic control). Products include:
- Deltasone Tablets 2595

Procainamide Hydrochloride (Theoretical potential for interaction with metformin by competing for common renal tubular transport system). Products include:
- Procan SR Tablets 1926

Prochlorperazine (Potential for loss of glycemic control). Products include:
- Compazine 2470

Promethazine Hydrochloride (Potential for loss of glycemic control). Products include:
- Mepergan Injection 2753
- Phenergan with Codeine 2777
- Phenergan with Dextromethorphan 2778
- Phenergan Injection 2773
- Phenergan Suppositories 2775
- Phenergan Syrup 2774
- Phenergan Tablets 2775
- Phenergan VC 2779
- Phenergan VC with Codeine 2781

Pseudoephedrine Hydrochloride (Potential for loss of glycemic control). Products include:
- Actifed Allergy Daytime/Nighttime Caplets ▣ 844
- Actifed Plus Caplets ▣ 845
- Actifed Plus Tablets ▣ 845
- Actifed with Codeine Cough Syrup 1067
- Actifed Sinus Daytime/Nighttime Tablets and Caplets ▣ 846
- Actifed Syrup ▣ 846
- Actifed Tablets ▣ 844
- Advil Cold and Sinus Caplets and Tablets (formerly CoAdvil) ▣ 870
- Alka-Seltzer Plus Cold Medicine Liqui-Gels ▣ 706
- Alka-Seltzer Plus Cold & Cough Medicine Liqui-Gels ▣ 705
- Alka-Seltzer Plus Night-Time Cold Medicine Liqui-Gels ▣ 706
- Allerest Headache Strength Tablets ▣ 627
- Allerest Maximum Strength Tablets ▣ 627
- Allerest No Drowsiness Tablets ▣ 627
- Allerest Sinus Pain Formula ▣ 627
- Anatuss LA Tablets 1542
- Atrohist Pediatric Capsules 453
- Bayer Select Sinus Pain Relief Formula ▣ 717
- Benadryl Allergy Decongestant Liquid Medication ▣ 848
- Benadryl Allergy Decongestant Tablets ▣ 848
- Benadryl Allergy Sinus Headache Formula Caplets ▣ 849
- Benylin Multisymptom ▣ 852
- Bromfed Capsules (Extended-Release) 1785
- Bromfed Syrup ▣ 733
- Bromfed Tablets 1785
- Bromfed-DM Cough Syrup 1786
- Bromfed-PD Capsules (Extended-Release) 1785
- Children's Vicks DayQuil Allergy Relief ▣ 757
- Children's Vicks NyQuil Cold/Cough Relief ▣ 758
- Comtrex Multi-Symptom Cold Reliever Tablets/Caplets/Liqui-Gels/Liquid ▣ 615
- Allergy-Sinus Comtrex Multi-Symptom Allergy-Sinus Formula Tablets ▣ 617
- Comtrex Multi-Symptom Non-Drowsy Caplets ▣ 618
- Congess 1004
- Contac Day Allergy/Sinus Caplets ▣ 812
- Contac Day & Night ▣ 812
- Contac Night Allergy/Sinus Caplets ▣ 812
- Contac Severe Cold & Flu Non-Drowsy ▣ 815
- Deconamine Chewable Tablets 1320
- Deconamine CX Cough and Cold Liquid and Tablets 1319
- Deconamine 1320
- Deconsal C Expectorant Syrup 456
- Deconsal Pediatric Syrup 457
- Deconsal II Tablets 454
- Dimetane-DX Cough Syrup 2059
- Dimetapp Sinus Caplets ▣ 775
- Dorcol Children's Cough Syrup ▣ 785
- Drixoral Cough + Congestion Liquid Caps ▣ 802
- Dura-Tap/PD Capsules 2867
- Duratuss Tablets 2565
- Duratuss HD Elixir 2565
- Efidac/24 ▣ 635
- Entex PSE Tablets 1987
- Fedahist Gyrocaps 2401
- Fedahist Timecaps 2401
- Guaifed 1787
- Guaifed Syrup ▣ 734
- Guaimax-D Tablets 792
- Guaitab Tablets ▣ 734
- Isoclor Expectorant 990
- Kronofed-A 977
- Motrin IB Sinus ▣ 838
- Novahistine DH 2462
- Novahistine DMX ▣ 822
- Novahistine Expectorant 2463
- Nucofed 2051
- PediaCare Cold Allergy Chewable Tablets ▣ 677
- PediaCare Cough-Cold Chewable Tablets 1553
- PediaCare 1553
- PediaCare Infants' Decongestant Drops ▣ 677
- PediCare Infant's Drops Decongestant Plus Cough 1553
- PediaCare NightRest Cough-Cold Liquid 1553
- Pediatric Vicks 44d Dry Hacking Cough & Head Congestion ▣ 763
- Pediatric Vicks 44m Cough & Cold Relief ▣ 764
- Robitussin Cold & Cough Liqui-Gels ▣ 776
- Robitussin Maximum Strength Cough & Cold ▣ 778
- Robitussin Pediatric Cough & Cold Formula ▣ 779
- Robitussin Severe Congestion Liqui-Gels ▣ 776
- Robitussin-DAC Syrup 2074
- Robitussin-PE ▣ 778
- Rondec Oral Drops 953
- Rondec Syrup 953
- Rondec Tablet 953
- Rondec-DM Oral Drops 954
- Rondec-DM Syrup 954
- Rondec-TR Tablet 953
- Ryna ▣ 841
- Seldane-D Extended-Release Tablets 1538
- Semprex-D Capsules 463
- Semprex-D Capsules 1167
- Sinarest Tablets ▣ 648
- Sinarest Extra Strength Tablets ▣ 648
- Sinarest No Drowsiness Tablets ▣ 648
- Sine-Aid IB Caplets 1554
- Sine-Aid Maximum Strength Sinus Medication Gelcaps, Caplets and Tablets 1554
- Sine-Off No Drowsiness Formula Caplets ▣ 824
- Sine-Off Sinus Medicine ▣ 825
- Singlet Tablets ▣ 825
- Sinutab Non-Drying Liquid Caps ▣ 859
- Sinutab Sinus Allergy Medication, Maximum Strength Tablets and Caplets ▣ 860
- Sinutab Sinus Medication, Maximum Strength Without Drowsiness Formula, Tablets & Caplets ▣ 860
- Sinutab Sinus Medication, Regular Strength Without Drowsiness Formula ▣ 859
- Sudafed Children's Liquid ▣ 861
- Sudafed Cold and Cough Liquidcaps ▣ 862
- Sudafed Cough Syrup ▣ 862
- Sudafed Plus Liquid ▣ 862
- Sudafed Plus Tablets ▣ 863
- Sudafed Severe Cold Formula Caplets ▣ 863
- Sudafed Severe Cold Formula Tablets ▣ 864
- Sudafed Sinus Caplets ▣ 864
- Sudafed Sinus Tablets ▣ 864
- Sudafed Tablets, 30 mg ▣ 861
- Sudafed Tablets, 60 mg ▣ 861
- Sudafed 12 Hour Caplets ▣ 861
- Syn-Rx Tablets 465

(▣ Described in PDR For Nonprescription Drugs) (⊙ Described in PDR For Ophthalmology)

Interactions Index — Glucotrol

Syn-Rx DM Tablets 466
TheraFlu .... **⊕** 787
TheraFlu Maximum Strength Nighttime Flu, Cold & Cough Medicine .... **⊕** 788
TheraFlu Maximum Strength Non-Drowsy Formula Flu, Cold & Cough Medicine .... **⊕** 788
Thera Flu Maximum Strength, Non-Drowsy Formula Flu, Cold and Cough Caplets .... **⊕** 789
Triaminic AM Cough and Decongestant Formula .... **⊕** 789
Triaminic AM Decongestant Formula .... **⊕** 790
Triaminic Nite Light .... **⊕** 791
Triaminic Sore Throat Formula ..... **⊕** 791
Tussend 1783
Tussend Expectorant 1785
Children's TYLENOL Cold Multi-Symptom Liquid Formula and Chewable Tablets 1561
Children's TYLENOL Cold Plus Cough Multi Symptom Tablets and Liquid .... **⊕** 681
Infants' TYLENOL Cold Decongestant & Fever-Reducer Drops 1556
TYLENOL Maximum Strength Allergy Sinus Medication Gelcaps and Caplets 1563
TYLENOL Maximum Strength Allergy Sinus NightTime Medication Caplets 1555
TYLENOL Flu Maximum Strength Gelcaps 1565
TYLENOL Flu NightTime, Maximum Strength, Gelcaps 1566
TYLENOL Maximum Strength Flu NightTime Hot Medication Packets 1562
TYLENOL, Maximum Strength, Sinus Medication Geltabs, Gelcaps, Caplets and Tablets 1566
TYLENOL Cold Multi-Symptom Formula Medication Tablets and Caplets 1561
TYLENOL Cold Medication No Drowsiness Formula Gelcaps and Caplets 1562
TYLENOL Cold Multi-Symptom Hot Medication Liquid Packets 1557
TYLENOL Cough Multi-Symptom Medication with Decongestant 1565
Ursinus Inlay-Tabs .... **⊕** 794
Vicks 44 LiquiCaps Cough, Cold & Flu Relief .... **⊕** 755
Vicks 44 LiquiCaps Non-Drowsy Cough & Cold Relief .... **⊕** 756
Vicks 44D Dry Hacking Cough & Head Congestion .... **⊕** 755
Vicks 44M Cough, Cold & Flu Relief .... **⊕** 756
Vicks DayQuil .... **⊕** 761
Vicks DayQuil SINUS Pressure & PAIN Relief with IBUPROFEN ...... **⊕** 762
Vicks Nyquil Hot Therapy .... **⊕** 762
Vicks NyQuil LiquiCaps Multi-Symptom Cold/Flu Relief .... **⊕** 763
Vicks NyQuil Multi-Symptom Cold/Flu Relief - (Original & Cherry Flavor) .... **⊕** 763

Pseudoephedrine Sulfate (Potential for loss of glycemic control). Products include:

Cheracol Sinus .... **⊕** 768
Chlor-Trimeton Allergy Decongestant Tablets .... **⊕** 799
Claritin-D 2350
Drixoral Cold and Allergy Sustained-Action Tablets .... **⊕** 802
Drixoral Cold and Flu Extended-Release Tablets .... **⊕** 803
Drixoral Non-Drowsy Formula Extended-Release Tablets .... **⊕** 803
Drixoral Allergy/Sinus Extended Release Tablets .... **⊕** 804
Trinalin Repetabs Tablets 1330

Quinestrol (Potential for loss of glycemic control).

No products indexed under this heading.

Quinidine Gluconate (Theoretical potential for interaction with metformin by competing for common renal tubular transport system). Products include:

Quinaglute Dura-Tabs Tablets 649

Quinidine Polygalacturonate (Theoretical potential for interaction with metformin by competing for common renal tubular transport system).

No products indexed under this heading.

Quinidine Sulfate (Theoretical potential for interaction with metformin by competing for common renal tubular transport system). Products include:

Quinidex Extentabs 2067

Quinine Sulfate (Theoretical potential for interaction with metformin by competing for common renal tubular transport system).

No products indexed under this heading.

Ranitidine Hydrochloride (Theoretical potential for interaction with metformin by competing for common renal tubular transport system). Products include:

Zantac 1209
Zantac Injection 1207
Zantac Syrup 1209

Salmeterol Xinafoate (Potential for loss of glycemic control). Products include:

Serevent Inhalation Aerosol 1176

Spironolactone (Potential for loss of glycemic control). Products include:

Aldactazide 2413
Aldactone 2414

Terbutaline Sulfate (Potential for loss of glycemic control). Products include:

Brethaire Inhaler 813
Brethine Ampuls 815
Brethine Tablets 814
Bricanyl Subcutaneous Injection 1502
Bricanyl Tablets 1503

Thioridazine Hydrochloride (Potential for loss of glycemic control). Products include:

Mellaril 2269

Thyroglobulin (Potential for loss of glycemic control).

No products indexed under this heading.

Thyroid (Potential for loss of glycemic control).

No products indexed under this heading.

Thyroxine (Potential for loss of glycemic control).

No products indexed under this heading.

Thyroxine Sodium (Potential for loss of glycemic control).

No products indexed under this heading.

Torsemide (Potential for loss of glycemic control). Products include:

Demadex Tablets and Injection 686

Triamcinolone (Potential for loss of glycemic control). Products include:

Aristocort Tablets 1022

Triamcinolone Acetonide (Potential for loss of glycemic control). Products include:

Aristocort A 0.025% Cream 1027
Aristocort A 0.5% Cream 1031
Aristocort A 0.1% Cream 1029
Aristocort A 0.1% Ointment 1030
Azmacort Oral Inhaler 2011
Nasacort Nasal Inhaler 2024

Triamcinolone Diacetate (Potential for loss of glycemic control). Products include:

Aristocort Suspension (Forte Parenteral) 1027
Aristocort Suspension (Intralesional) 1025

Triamcinolone Hexacetonide (Potential for loss of glycemic control). Products include:

Aristospan Suspension (Intra-articular) 1033
Aristospan Suspension (Intralesional) 1032

Triamterene (Potential for loss of glycemic control; theoretical potential for interaction with metformin by competing for common renal tubular transport system). Products include:

Dyazide 2479
Dyrenium Capsules 2481
Maxzide 1380

Trifluoperazine Hydrochloride (Potential for loss of glycemic control). Products include:

Stelazine 2514

Trimethoprim (Theoretical potential for interaction with metformin by competing for common renal tubular transport system). Products include:

Bactrim DS Tablets 2084
Bactrim I.V. Infusion 2082
Bactrim 2084
Proloprim Tablets 1155
Septra 1174
Septra I.V. Infusion 1169
Septra I.V. Infusion ADD-Vantage Vials 1171
Septra 1174
Trimpex Tablets 2163

Trimethoprim Sulfate (Theoretical potential for interaction with metformin by competing for common renal tubular transport system). Products include:

Polytrim Ophthalmic Solution Sterile 482

Tyropanoate Sodium (Potential for acute alteration of renal function; metformin should be temporarily withheld in patients undergoing radiologic studies involving parenteral iodinated contrast material).

No products indexed under this heading.

Vancomycin Hydrochloride (Theoretical potential for interaction with metformin by competing for common renal tubular transport system). Products include:

Vancocin HCl, Oral Solution & Pulvules 1483
Vancocin HCl, Vials & ADD-Vantage 1481

Verapamil Hydrochloride (Potential for loss of glycemic control). Products include:

Calan SR Caplets 2422
Calan Tablets 2419
Isoptin Injectable 1344
Isoptin Oral Tablets 1346
Isoptin SR Tablets 1348
Verelan Capsules 1410
Verelan Capsules 2824

Food Interactions

Alcohol (Alcohol potentiates the effect of metformin on lactate metabolism; patients should be warned against excessive alcohol intake, acute or chronic).

Food, unspecified (Food decreases the extent and slightly delays the absorption of metformin).

GLUCOTROL TABLETS

(Glipizide) 1967

May interact with non-steroidal anti-inflammatory agents, salicylates, sulfonamides, beta blockers, oral anticoagulants, highly protein bound drugs (selected), monoamine oxidase inhibitors, thiazides, diuretics, corticosteroids, phenothiazines, thyroid preparations, estrogens, sympathomimetics, calcium channel blockers, oral contraceptives, and certain other agents. Compounds in these categories include:

Acebutolol Hydrochloride (Potentiates the hypoglycemic action; patients should be observed for hypoglycemia or loss of control). Products include:

Sectral Capsules 2807

Albuterol (Potential for hyperglycemia leading to loss of control). Products include:

Proventil Inhalation Aerosol 2382
Ventolin Inhalation Aerosol and Refill 1197

Albuterol Sulfate (Potential for hyperglycemia leading to loss of control). Products include:

Airet Solution for Inhalation 452
Proventil Inhalation Solution 0.083% 2384
Proventil Repetabs Tablets 2386
Proventil Solution for Inhalation 0.5% 2383
Proventil Syrup 2385
Proventil Tablets 2386
Ventolin Inhalation Solution 1198
Ventolin Nebules Inhalation Solution 1199
Ventolin Rotacaps for Inhalation 1200
Ventolin Syrup 1202
Ventolin Tablets 1203
Volmax Extended-Release Tablets .. 1788

Amiloride Hydrochloride (Potential for hyperglycemia leading to loss of control). Products include:

Midamor Tablets 1703
Moduretic Tablets 1705

Amiodarone Hydrochloride (Potentiates the hypoglycemic action; patients should be observed for hypoglycemia or loss of control). Products include:

Cordarone Intravenous 2715
Cordarone Tablets 2712

Amitriptyline Hydrochloride (Potentiates the hypoglycemic action; patients should be observed for hypoglycemia or loss of control). Products include:

Elavil 2838
Endep Tablets 2174
Etrafon 2355
Limbitrol 2180
Triavil Tablets 1757

Amlodipine Besylate (Potential for hyperglycemia leading to loss of control). Products include:

Lotrel Capsules 840
Norvasc Tablets 1940

Aspirin (Potentiates the hypoglycemic action; patients should be observed for hypoglycemia or loss of control). Products include:

Alka-Seltzer Effervescent Antacid and Pain Reliever .... **⊕** 701
Alka-Seltzer Extra Strength Effervescent Antacid and Pain Reliever .... **⊕** 703
Alka-Seltzer Lemon Lime Effervescent Antacid and Pain Reliever .... **⊕** 703
Alka-Seltzer Plus Cold Medicine .... **⊕** 705
Alka-Seltzer Plus Cold & Cough Medicine .... **⊕** 708
Alka-Seltzer Plus Night-Time Cold Medicine .... **⊕** 707
Alka Seltzer Plus Sinus Medicine .. **⊕** 707
Arthritis Foundation Safety Coated Aspirin Tablets .... **⊕** 675
Arthritis Pain Ascriptin .... **⊕** 631
Maximum Strength Ascriptin .... **⊕** 630
Regular Strength Ascriptin Tablets .... **⊕** 629
Arthritis Strength BC Powder .... **⊕** 609
BC Cold Powder Multi-Symptom Formula (Cold-Sinus-Allergy) ...... **⊕** 609
BC Cold Powder Non-Drowsy Formula (Cold-Sinus) .... **⊕** 609
BC Powder .... **⊕** 609
Bayer Children's Chewable Aspirin .... **⊕** 711
Genuine Bayer Aspirin Tablets & Caplets .... **⊕** 713

IMPORTANT NOTE: Always consult each drug listing in the patient's regimen for possible interactions.

Glucotrol | Interactions Index | 444

Extra Strength Bayer Arthritis Pain Regimen Formula ▣ 711
Extra Strength Bayer Aspirin Caplets & Tablets ▣ 712
Extended-Release Bayer 8-Hour Aspirin ▣ 712
Extra Strength Bayer Plus Aspirin Caplets ▣ 713
Extra Strength Bayer PM Aspirin .. ▣ 713
Bayer Enteric Aspirin ▣ 709
Bufferin Analgesic Tablets and Caplets ▣ 613
Arthritis Strength Bufferin Analgesic Caplets ▣ 614
Extra Strength Bufferin Analgesic Tablets ▣ 615
Cama Arthritis Pain Reliever ▣ 785
Darvon Compound-65 Pulvules 1435
Easprin 1914
Ecotrin 2455
Ecotrin Enteric Coated Aspirin Maximum Strength Tablets and Caplets ▣ 816
Ecotrin Enteric Coated Aspirin Regular Strength Tablets 2455
Empirin Aspirin Tablets ▣ 854
Empirin with Codeine Tablets 1093
Excedrin Extra-Strength Analgesic Tablets & Caplets 732
Fiorinal Capsules 2261
Fiorinal with Codeine Capsules 2262
Fiorinal Tablets 2261
Halfprin 1362
Healthprin Aspirin 2455
Norgesic 1496
Percodan Tablets 939
Percodan-Demi Tablets 940
Robaxisal Tablets 2071
Soma Compound w/Codeine Tablets 2676
Soma Compound Tablets 2675
St. Joseph Adult Chewable Aspirin (81 mg.) ▣ 808
Talwin Compound 2335
Ursinus Inlay-Tabs ▣ 794
Vanquish Analgesic Caplets ▣ 731

Atenolol (Potentiates the hypoglycemic action; patients should be observed for hypoglycemia or loss of control). Products include:
Tenoretic Tablets 2845
Tenormin Tablets and I.V. Injection 2847

Atovaquone (Potentiates the hypoglycemic action; patients should be observed for hypoglycemia or loss of control). Products include:
Mepron Suspension 1135

Bendroflumethiazide (Potential for hyperglycemia leading to loss of control).
No products indexed under this heading.

Bepridil Hydrochloride (Potential for hyperglycemia leading to loss of control). Products include:
Vascor (200, 300 and 400 mg) Tablets 1587

Betamethasone Acetate (Potential for hyperglycemia leading to loss of control). Products include:
Celestone Soluspan Suspension 2347

Betamethasone Sodium Phosphate (Potential for hyperglycemia leading to loss of control). Products include:
Celestone Soluspan Suspension 2347

Betaxolol Hydrochloride (Potentiates the hypoglycemic action; patients should be observed for hypoglycemia or loss of control). Products include:
Betoptic Ophthalmic Solution 469
Betoptic S Ophthalmic Suspension 471
Kerlone Tablets 2436

Bisoprolol Fumarate (Potentiates the hypoglycemic action; patients should be observed for hypoglycemia or loss of control). Products include:
Zebeta Tablets 1413
Ziac 1415

Bumetanide (Potential for hyperglycemia leading to loss of control). Products include:
Bumex 2093

Carteolol Hydrochloride (Potentiates the hypoglycemic action; patients should be observed for hypoglycemia or loss of control). Products include:
Cartrol Tablets 410
Ocupress Ophthalmic Solution, 1% Sterile ⊙ 309

Cefonicid Sodium (Potentiates the hypoglycemic action; patients should be observed for hypoglycemia or loss of control). Products include:
Monocid Injection 2497

Chloramphenicol (Potentiates the hypoglycemic action; patients should be observed for hypoglycemia or loss of control). Products include:
Chloromycetin Ophthalmic Ointment, 1% ⊙ 310
Chloromycetin Ophthalmic Solution ⊙ 310
Chloroptic S.O.P. ⊙ 239
Chloroptic Sterile Ophthalmic Solution ⊙ 239
Elase-Chloromycetin Ointment 1040
Ophthocort ⊙ 311

Chloramphenicol Palmitate (Potentiates the hypoglycemic action; patients should be observed for hypoglycemia or loss of control).
No products indexed under this heading.

Chloramphenicol Sodium Succinate (Potentiates the hypoglycemic action; patients should be observed for hypoglycemia or loss of control). Products include:
Chloromycetin Sodium Succinate 1900

Chlordiazepoxide (Potentiates the hypoglycemic action; patients should be observed for hypoglycemia or loss of control). Products include:
Libritabs Tablets 2177
Limbitrol 2180

Chlordiazepoxide Hydrochloride (Potentiates the hypoglycemic action; patients should be observed for hypoglycemia or loss of control). Products include:
Librax Capsules 2176
Librium Capsules 2178
Librium Injectable 2179

Chlorothiazide (Potential for hyperglycemia leading to loss of control). Products include:
Aldoclor Tablets 1598
Diupres Tablets 1650
Diuril Oral 1653

Chlorothiazide Sodium (Potential for hyperglycemia leading to loss of control). Products include:
Diuril Sodium Intravenous 1652

Chlorotrianisene (Potential for hyperglycemia leading to loss of control).
No products indexed under this heading.

Chlorpromazine (Potential for hyperglycemia leading to loss of control). Products include:
Thorazine Suppositories 2523

Chlorpromazine Hydrochloride (Potential for hyperglycemia leading to loss of control). Products include:
Thorazine 2523

Chlorpropamide (Potentiates the hypoglycemic action; patients should be observed for hypoglycemia or loss of control). Products include:
Diabinese Tablets 1935

Chlorthalidone (Potential for hyperglycemia leading to loss of control). Products include:
Combipres Tablets 677
Tenoretic Tablets 2845
Thalitone 1245

Choline Magnesium Trisalicylate (Potentiates the hypoglycemic action; patients should be observed for hypoglycemia or loss of control). Products include:
Trilisate 2000

Clomipramine Hydrochloride (Potentiates the hypoglycemic action; patients should be observed for hypoglycemia or loss of control). Products include:
Anafranil Capsules 803

Clozapine (Potentiates the hypoglycemic action; patients should be observed for hypoglycemia or loss of control). Products include:
Clozaril Tablets 2252

Cortisone Acetate (Potential for hyperglycemia leading to loss of control). Products include:
Cortone Acetate Sterile Suspension 1623
Cortone Acetate Tablets 1624

Cyclosporine (Potentiates the hypoglycemic action; patients should be observed for hypoglycemia or loss of control). Products include:
Neoral 2276
Sandimmune 2286

Desogestrel (Potential for hyperglycemia leading to loss of control). Products include:
Desogen Tablets 1817
Ortho-Cept 1851

Dexamethasone (Potential for hyperglycemia leading to loss of control). Products include:
AK-Trol Ointment & Suspension ⊙ 205
Decadron Elixir 1633
Decadron Tablets 1635
Decaspray Topical Aerosol 1648
Dexacidin Ointment ⊙ 263
Maxitrol Ophthalmic Ointment and Suspension ⊙ 224
TobraDex Ophthalmic Suspension and Ointment 473

Dexamethasone Acetate (Potential for hyperglycemia leading to loss of control). Products include:
Dalalone D.P. Injectable 1011
Decadron-LA Sterile Suspension 1646

Dexamethasone Sodium Phosphate (Potential for hyperglycemia leading to loss of control). Products include:
Decadron Phosphate Injection 1637
Decadron Phosphate Respihaler 1642
Decadron Phosphate Sterile Ophthalmic Ointment 1641
Decadron Phosphate Sterile Ophthalmic Solution 1642
Decadron Phosphate Topical Cream 1644
Decadron Phosphate Turbinaire 1645
Decadron Phosphate with Xylocaine Injection, Sterile 1639
Dexacort Phosphate in Respihaler .. 458
Dexacort Phosphate in Turbinaire .. 459
NeoDecadron Sterile Ophthalmic Ointment 1712
NeoDecadron Sterile Ophthalmic Solution 1713
NeoDecadron Topical Cream 1714

Diazepam (Potentiates the hypoglycemic action; patients should be observed for hypoglycemia or loss of control). Products include:
Dizac 1809
Valium Injectable 2182
Valium Tablets 2183
Valrelease Capsules 2169

Diclofenac Potassium (Potentiates the hypoglycemic action; patients should be observed for hypoglycemia or loss of control). Products include:
Cataflam 816

Diclofenac Sodium (Potentiates the hypoglycemic action; patients should be observed for hypoglycemia or loss of control). Products include:
Voltaren Ophthalmic Sterile Ophthalmic Solution ⊙ 272
Voltaren Tablets 861

Dicumarol (Potentiates the hypoglycemic action; patients should be observed for hypoglycemia or loss of control).
No products indexed under this heading.

Dienestrol (Potential for hyperglycemia leading to loss of control). Products include:
Ortho Dienestrol Cream 1866

Diethylstilbestrol (Potential for hyperglycemia leading to loss of control). Products include:
Diethylstilbestrol Tablets 1437

Diflunisal (Potentiates the hypoglycemic action; patients should be observed for hypoglycemia or loss of control). Products include:
Dolobid Tablets 1654

Diltiazem Hydrochloride (Potential for hyperglycemia leading to loss of control). Products include:
Cardizem CD Capsules 1506
Cardizem SR Capsules 1510
Cardizem Injectable 1508
Cardizem Tablets 1512
Dilacor XR Extended-release Capsules 2018

Dipyridamole (Potentiates the hypoglycemic action; patients should be observed for hypoglycemia or loss of control). Products include:
Persantine Tablets 681

Dobutamine Hydrochloride (Potential for hyperglycemia leading to loss of control). Products include:
Dobutrex Solution Vials 1439

Dopamine Hydrochloride (Potential for hyperglycemia leading to loss of control).
No products indexed under this heading.

Ephedrine Hydrochloride (Potential for hyperglycemia leading to loss of control). Products include:
Primatene Dual Action Formula ▣ 872
Primatene Tablets ▣ 873
Quadrinal Tablets 1350

Ephedrine Sulfate (Potential for hyperglycemia leading to loss of control). Products include:
Bronkaid Caplets ▣ 717
Marax Tablets & DF Syrup 2200

Ephedrine Tannate (Potential for hyperglycemia leading to loss of control). Products include:
Rynatuss 2673

Epinephrine (Potential for hyperglycemia leading to loss of control). Products include:
Bronkaid Mist ▣ 717
EPIFRIN ⊙ 239
EpiPen 790
Marcaine Hydrochloride with Epinephrine 1:200,000 2316
Primatene Mist ▣ 873
Sensorcaine with Epinephrine Injection 559
Sus-Phrine Injection 1019
Xylocaine with Epinephrine Injections 567

Epinephrine Bitartrate (Potential for hyperglycemia leading to loss of control). Products include:
Bronkaid Mist Suspension ▣ 718

(▣ Described in PDR For Nonprescription Drugs) (⊙ Described in PDR For Ophthalmology)

445 **Interactions Index** **Glucotrol**

Sensorcaine-MPF with Epinephrine Injection ... 559

Epinephrine Hydrochloride (Potential for hyperglycemia leading to loss of control). Products include:
Ana-Kit Anaphylaxis Emergency Treatment Kit ... 617

Esmolol Hydrochloride (Potentiates the hypoglycemic action; patients should be observed for hypoglycemia or loss of control). Products include:
Brevibloc Injection ... 1808

Estradiol (Potential for hyperglycemia leading to loss of control). Products include:
Climara Transdermal System ... 645
Estrace Cream and Tablets ... 749
Estraderm Transdermal System ... 824

Estrogens, Conjugated (Potential for hyperglycemia leading to loss of control). Products include:
PMB 200 and PMB 400 ... 2783
Premarin Intravenous ... 2787
Premarin with Methyltestosterone .. 2794
Premarin Tablets ... 2789
Premarin Vaginal Cream ... 2791
Premphase ... 2797
Prempro ... 2801

Estrogens, Esterified (Potential for hyperglycemia leading to loss of control). Products include:
ESTRATAB Tablets (0.3, 0.625, 1.25, 2.5 mg) ... 2536
Estratest ... 2539
Menest Tablets ... 2494

Estropipate (Potential for hyperglycemia leading to loss of control). Products include:
Ogen Tablets ... 2627
Ogen Vaginal Cream ... 2630
Ortho-Est ... 1869

Ethacrynic Acid (Potential for hyperglycemia leading to loss of control). Products include:
Edecrin Tablets ... 1657

Ethinyl Estradiol (Potential for hyperglycemia leading to loss of control). Products include:
Brevicon ... 2088
Demulen ... 2428
Desogen Tablets ... 1817
Levlen/Tri-Levlen ... 651
Lo/Ovral Tablets ... 2746
Lo/Ovral-28 Tablets ... 2751
Modicon ... 1872
Nordette-21 Tablets ... 2755
Nordette-28 Tablets ... 2758
Norinyl ... 2088
Ortho-Cept ... 1851
Ortho-Cyclen/Ortho-Tri-Cyclen ... 1858
Ortho-Novum ... 1872
Ortho-Cyclen/Ortho Tri-Cyclen ... 1858
Ovcon ... 760
Ovral Tablets ... 2770
Ovral-28 Tablets ... 2770
Levlen/Tri-Levlen ... 651
Tri-Norinyl ... 2164
Triphasil-21 Tablets ... 2814
Triphasil-28 Tablets ... 2819

Ethynodiol Diacetate (Potential for hyperglycemia leading to loss of control). Products include:
Demulen ... 2428

Etodolac (Potentiates the hypoglycemic action; patients should be observed for hypoglycemia or loss of control). Products include:
Lodine Capsules and Tablets ... 2743

Felodipine (Potential for hyperglycemia leading to loss of control). Products include:
Plendil Extended-Release Tablets ... 527

Fenoprofen Calcium (Potentiates the hypoglycemic action; patients should be observed for hypoglycemia or loss of control). Products include:
Nalfon 200 Pulvules & Nalfon Tablets ... 917

Fluconazole (Potential for severe hypoglycemia when co-administered with fluconazole; increased in the Glucotrol AUC after fluconazole administration was 56.9%). Products include:
Diflucan Injection, Tablets, and Oral Suspension ... 2194

Fludrocortisone Acetate (Potential for hyperglycemia leading to loss of control). Products include:
Florinef Acetate Tablets ... 505

Fluphenazine Decanoate (Potential for hyperglycemia leading to loss of control). Products include:
Prolixin Decanoate ... 509

Fluphenazine Enanthate (Potential for hyperglycemia leading to loss of control). Products include:
Prolixin Enanthate ... 509

Fluphenazine Hydrochloride (Potential for hyperglycemia leading to loss of control). Products include:
Prolixin ... 509

Flurazepam Hydrochloride (Potentiates the hypoglycemic action; patients should be observed for hypoglycemia or loss of control). Products include:
Dalmane Capsules ... 2173

Flurbiprofen (Potentiates the hypoglycemic action; patients should be observed for hypoglycemia or loss of control). Products include:
Ansaid Tablets ... 2579

Furazolidone (Potentiates the hypoglycemic action; patients should be observed for hypoglycemia or loss of control). Products include:
Furoxone ... 2046

Furosemide (Potential for hyperglycemia leading to loss of control). Products include:
Lasix Injection, Oral Solution and Tablets ... 1240

Glyburide (Potentiates the hypoglycemic action; patients should be observed for hypoglycemia or loss of control). Products include:
DiaBeta Tablets ... 1239
Glynase PresTab Tablets ... 2609
Micronase Tablets ... 2623

Hydrochlorothiazide (Potential for hyperglycemia leading to loss of control). Products include:
Aldactazide ... 2413
Aldoril Tablets ... 1604
Apresazide Capsules ... 808
Capozide ... 742
Dyazide ... 2479
Esidrix Tablets ... 821
Esimil Tablets ... 822
HydroDIURIL Tablets ... 1674
Hydropres Tablets ... 1675
Hyzaar Tablets ... 1677
Inderide Tablets ... 2732
Inderide LA Long Acting Capsules .. 2734
Lopressor HCT Tablets ... 832
Lotensin HCT ... 837
Maxzide ... 1380
Moduretic Tablets ... 1705
Oretic Tablets ... 443
Prinzide Tablets ... 1737
Ser-Ap-Es Tablets ... 849
Timolide Tablets ... 1748
Vaseretic Tablets ... 1765
Zestoretic ... 2850
Ziac ... 1415

Hydrocortisone (Potential for hyperglycemia leading to loss of control). Products include:
Anusol-HC Cream 2.5% ... 1896
Aquanil HC Lotion ... 1931
Bactine Hydrocortisone Anti-Itch Cream ... ▣ 709
Caldecort Anti-Itch Hydrocortisone Spray ... ▣ 631
Cortaid ... ▣ 836
CORTENEMA ... 2535
Cortisporin Ointment ... 1085
Cortisporin Ophthalmic Ointment Sterile ... 1085
Cortisporin Ophthalmic Suspension Sterile ... 1086
Cortisporin Otic Solution Sterile ... 1087
Cortisporin Otic Suspension Sterile 1088
Cortizone-5 ... ▣ 831
Cortizone-10 ... ▣ 831
Hydrocortone Tablets ... 1672
Hytone ... 907
Massengill Medicated Soft Cloth Towelettes ... 2458
PediOtic Suspension Sterile ... 1153
Preparation H Hydrocortisone 1% Cream ... ▣ 872
ProctoCream-HC 2.5% ... 2408
VōSoL HC Otic Solution ... 2678

Hydrocortisone Acetate (Potential for hyperglycemia leading to loss of control). Products include:
Analpram-HC Rectal Cream 1% and 2.5% ... 977
Anusol HC-1 Anti-Itch Hydrocortisone Ointment ... ▣ 847
Anusol-HC Suppositories ... 1897
Caldecort ... ▣ 631
Carmol HC ... 924
Coly-Mycin S Otic w/Neomycin & Hydrocortisone ... 1906
Cortaid ... ▣ 836
Cortifoam ... 2396
Cortisporin Cream ... 1084
Epifoam ... 2399
Hydrocortone Acetate Sterile Suspension ... 1669
Mantadil Cream ... 1135
Nupercainal Hydrocortisone 1% Cream ... ▣ 645
Ophthocort ... ⊙ 311
Pramosone Cream, Lotion & Ointment ... 978
ProctoCream-HC ... 2408
ProctoFoam-HC ... 2409
Terra-Cortril Ophthalmic Suspension ... 2210

Hydrocortisone Sodium Phosphate (Potential for hyperglycemia leading to loss of control). Products include:
Hydrocortone Phosphate Injection, Sterile ... 1670

Hydrocortisone Sodium Succinate (Potential for hyperglycemia leading to loss of control). Products include:
Solu-Cortef Sterile Powder ... 2641

Hydroflumethiazide (Potential for hyperglycemia leading to loss of control). Products include:
Diucardin Tablets ... 2718

Ibuprofen (Potentiates the hypoglycemic action; patients should be observed for hypoglycemia or loss of control). Products include:
Advil Cold and Sinus Caplets and Tablets (formerly CoAdvil) ... ▣ 870
Advil Ibuprofen Tablets and Caplets ... ▣ 870
Children's Advil Suspension ... 2692
Arthritis Foundation Ibuprofen Tablets ... ▣ 674
Bayer Select Ibuprofen Pain Relief Formula ... ▣ 715
Cramp End Tablets ... ▣ 735
Dimetapp Sinus Caplets ... ▣ 775
Haltran Tablets ... ▣ 771
IBU Tablets ... 1342
Ibuprohm ... ▣ 735
Children's Motrin Ibuprofen Oral Suspension ... 1546
Motrin Tablets ... 2625
Motrin IB Caplets, Tablets, and Geltabs ... ▣ 838
Motrin IB Sinus ... ▣ 838
Motrin Ibuprofen Suspension, Oral Drops, Chewable Tablets, Caplets ... 1546
Nuprin Ibuprofen/Analgesic Tablets & Caplets ... ▣ 622
Sine-Aid IB Caplets ... 1554
Vicks DayQuil SINUS Pressure & PAIN Relief with IBUPROFEN ... ▣ 762

Imipramine Hydrochloride (Potentiates the hypoglycemic action; patients should be observed for hypoglycemia or loss of control). Products include:
Tofranil Ampuls ... 854
Tofranil Tablets ... 856

Imipramine Pamoate (Potentiates the hypoglycemic action; patients should be observed for hypoglycemia or loss of control). Products include:
Tofranil-PM Capsules ... 857

Indapamide (Potential for hyperglycemia leading to loss of control). Products include:
Lozol Tablets ... 2022

Indomethacin (Potentiates the hypoglycemic action; patients should be observed for hypoglycemia or loss of control). Products include:
Indocin ... 1680

Indomethacin Sodium Trihydrate (Potentiates the hypoglycemic action; patients should be observed for hypoglycemia or loss of control). Products include:
Indocin I.V. ... 1684

Isocarboxazid (Potentiates the hypoglycemic action; patients should be observed for hypoglycemia or loss of control).
No products indexed under this heading.

Isoniazid (Potential for hyperglycemia leading to loss of control). Products include:
Nydrazid Injection ... 508
Rifamate Capsules ... 1530
Rifater ... 1532

Isoproterenol Hydrochloride (Potential for hyperglycemia leading to loss of control). Products include:
Isuprel Hydrochloride Injection 1:5000 ... 2311
Isuprel Hydrochloride Solution 1:200 & 1:100 ... 2313
Isuprel Mistometer ... 2312

Isoproterenol Sulfate (Potential for hyperglycemia leading to loss of control). Products include:
Norisodrine with Calcium Iodide Syrup ... 442

Isradipine (Potential for hyperglycemia leading to loss of control). Products include:
DynaCirc Capsules ... 2256

Ketoprofen (Potentiates the hypoglycemic action; patients should be observed for hypoglycemia or loss of control). Products include:
Orudis Capsules ... 2766
Oruvail Capsules ... 2766

Ketorolac Tromethamine (Potentiates the hypoglycemic action; patients should be observed for hypoglycemia or loss of control). Products include:
Acular ... 474
Acular ... ⊙ 277
Toradol ... 2159

Labetalol Hydrochloride (Potentiates the hypoglycemic action; patients should be observed for hypoglycemia or loss of control). Products include:
Normodyne Injection ... 2377
Normodyne Tablets ... 2379
Trandate ... 1185

Levobunolol Hydrochloride (Potentiates the hypoglycemic action; patients should be observed for hypoglycemia or loss of control). Products include:
Betagan ... ⊙ 233

Levonorgestrel (Potential for hyperglycemia leading to loss of control). Products include:
Levlen/Tri-Levlen ... 651
Nordette-21 Tablets ... 2755
Nordette-28 Tablets ... 2758
Norplant System ... 2759
Levlen/Tri-Levlen ... 651
Triphasil-21 Tablets ... 2814
Triphasil-28 Tablets ... 2819

IMPORTANT NOTE: Always consult each drug listing in the patient's regimen for possible interactions.

Glucotrol

Interactions Index

Levothyroxine Sodium (Potential for hyperglycemia leading to loss of control). Products include:

Levothroid Tablets 1016
Levoxyl Tablets 903
Synthroid 1359

Liothyronine Sodium (Potential for hyperglycemia leading to loss of control). Products include:

Cytomel Tablets 2473
Triostat Injection 2530

Liotrix (Potential for hyperglycemia leading to loss of control).

No products indexed under this heading.

Magnesium Salicylate (Potentiates the hypoglycemic action; patients should be observed for hypoglycemia or loss of control). Products include:

Backache Caplets .... ⊕D 613
Bayer Select Backache Pain Relief Formula .... ⊕D 715
Doan's Extra-Strength Analgesic.... ⊕D 633
Extra Strength Doan's P.M. .... ⊕D 633
Doan's Regular Strength Analgesic .... ⊕D 634
Mobigesic Tablets .... ⊕D 602

Meclofenamate Sodium (Potentiates the hypoglycemic action; patients should be observed for hypoglycemia or loss of control).

No products indexed under this heading.

Mefenamic Acid (Potentiates the hypoglycemic action; patients should be observed for hypoglycemia or loss of control). Products include:

Ponstel 1925

Mesoridazine Besylate (Potential for hyperglycemia leading to loss of control). Products include:

Serentil 684

Mestranol (Potential for hyperglycemia leading to loss of control). Products include:

Norinyl 2088
Ortho-Novum 1872

Metaproterenol Sulfate (Potential for hyperglycemia leading to loss of control). Products include:

Alupent 669
Metaproterenol Sulfate Inhalation Solution, USP, Arm-a-Med 552

Metaraminol Bitartrate (Potential for hyperglycemia leading to loss of control). Products include:

Aramine Injection 1609

Methotrimeprazine (Potential for hyperglycemia leading to loss of control). Products include:

Levoprome 1274

Methoxamine Hydrochloride (Potential for hyperglycemia leading to loss of control). Products include:

Vasoxyl Injection 1196

Methylclothiazide (Potential for hyperglycemia leading to loss of control). Products include:

Enduron Tablets 420

Methylprednisolone Acetate (Potential for hyperglycemia leading to loss of control). Products include:

Depo-Medrol Single-Dose Vial 2600
Depo-Medrol Sterile Aqueous Suspension 2597

Methylprednisolone Sodium Succinate (Potential for hyperglycemia leading to loss of control). Products include:

Solu-Medrol Sterile Powder 2643

Metipranolol Hydrochloride (Potentiates the hypoglycemic action; patients should be observed for hypoglycemia or loss of control). Products include:

OptiPranolol (Metipranolol 0.3%) Sterile Ophthalmic Solution.......... ◎ 258

Metolazone (Potential for hyperglycemia leading to loss of control). Products include:

Mykrox Tablets 993
Zaroxolyn Tablets 1000

Metoprolol Succinate (Potentiates the hypoglycemic action; patients should be observed for hypoglycemia or loss of control). Products include:

Toprol-XL Tablets 565

Metoprolol Tartrate (Potentiates the hypoglycemic action; patients should be observed for hypoglycemia or loss of control). Products include:

Lopressor Ampuls 830
Lopressor HCT Tablets 832
Lopressor Tablets 830

Miconazole (Potential for severe hypoglycemia when co-administered with oral miconazole).

No products indexed under this heading.

Midazolam Hydrochloride (Potentiates the hypoglycemic action; patients should be observed for hypoglycemia or loss of control). Products include:

Versed Injection 2170

Nabumetone (Potentiates the hypoglycemic action; patients should be observed for hypoglycemia or loss of control). Products include:

Relafen Tablets 2510

Nadolol (Potentiates the hypoglycemic action; patients should be observed for hypoglycemia or loss of control).

No products indexed under this heading.

Naproxen (Potentiates the hypoglycemic action; patients should be observed for hypoglycemia or loss of control). Products include:

Anaprox/Naprosyn 2117

Naproxen Sodium (Potentiates the hypoglycemic action; patients should be observed for hypoglycemia or loss of control). Products include:

Aleve 1975
Anaprox/Naprosyn 2117

Niacin (Potential for hyperglycemia leading to loss of control). Products include:

Nicobid 2026
Nicolar Tablets 2026
Nicotinex Elixir .... ⊕D 655
Sigtab Tablets .... ⊕D 772
Slo-Niacin Tablets 2659
Stuart Prenatal Tablets .... ⊕D 881
The Stuart Formula Tablets .... ⊕D 663
Zymacap Capsules .... ⊕D 772

Nicardipine Hydrochloride (Potential for hyperglycemia leading to loss of control). Products include:

Cardene Capsules 2095
Cardene I.V. 2709
Cardene SR Capsules 2097

Nifedipine (Potential for hyperglycemia leading to loss of control). Products include:

Adalat Capsules (10 mg and 20 mg) 587
Adalat CC 589
Procardia Capsules 1971
Procardia XL Extended Release Tablets 1972

Nimodipine (Potential for hyperglycemia leading to loss of control). Products include:

Nimotop Capsules 610

Nisoldipine (Potential for hyperglycemia leading to loss of control).

No products indexed under this heading.

Norepinephrine Bitartrate (Potential for hyperglycemia leading to loss of control). Products include:

Levophed Bitartrate Injection 2315

Norethindrone (Potential for hyperglycemia leading to loss of control). Products include:

Brevicon 2088
Micronor Tablets 1872
Modicon 1872
Norinyl 2088
Nor-Q D Tablets 2135
Ortho-Novum 1872
Ovcon 760
Tri-Norinyl 2164

Norethynodrel (Potential for hyperglycemia leading to loss of control).

No products indexed under this heading.

Norgestimate (Potential for hyperglycemia leading to loss of control). Products include:

Ortho-Cyclen/Ortho-Tri-Cyclen 1858
Ortho-Cyclen/Ortho Tri-Cyclen 1858

Norgestrel (Potential for hyperglycemia leading to loss of control). Products include:

Lo/Ovral Tablets 2746
Lo/Ovral-28 Tablets 2751
Ovral Tablets 2770
Ovral-28 Tablets 2770
Ovrette Tablets 2771

Nortriptyline Hydrochloride (Potentiates the hypoglycemic action; patients should be observed for hypoglycemia or loss of control). Products include:

Pamelor 2280

Oxaprozin (Potentiates the hypoglycemic action; patients should be observed for hypoglycemia or loss of control). Products include:

Daypro Caplets 2426

Oxazepam (Potentiates the hypoglycemic action; patients should be observed for hypoglycemia or loss of control). Products include:

Serax Capsules 2810
Serax Tablets 2810

Penbutolol Sulfate (Potentiates the hypoglycemic action; patients should be observed for hypoglycemia or loss of control). Products include:

Levatol 2403

Perphenazine (Potential for hyperglycemia leading to loss of control). Products include:

Etrafon 2355
Triavil Tablets 1757
Trilafon 2389

Phenelzine Sulfate (Potentiates the hypoglycemic action; patients should be observed for hypoglycemia or loss of control). Products include:

Nardil 1920

Phenylbutazone (Potentiates the hypoglycemic action; patients should be observed for hypoglycemia or loss of control).

No products indexed under this heading.

Phenylephrine Bitartrate (Potential for hyperglycemia leading to loss of control).

No products indexed under this heading.

Phenylephrine Hydrochloride (Potential for hyperglycemia leading to loss of control). Products include:

Atrohist Plus Tablets 454
Cerose DM .... ⊕D 878
Comhist 2038
D.A. Chewable Tablets 951
Deconsal Pediatric Capsules 454
Dura-Vent/DA Tablets 953
Entex Capsules 1986
Entex Liquid 1986
Extendryl 1005
4-Way Fast Acting Nasal Spray (regular & mentholated) .... ⊕D 621
Hemorid For Women .... ⊕D 834
Hycomine Compound Tablets 932
Neo-Synephrine Hydrochloride 1% Carpuject 2324
Neo-Synephrine Hydrochloride 1% Injection 2324
Neo-Synephrine Hydrochloride (Ophthalmic) 2325
Neo-Synephrine .... ⊕D 726
Nostril .... ⊕D 644
Novahistine Elixir .... ⊕D 823
Phenergan VC 2779
Phenergan VC with Codeine 2781
Preparation H .... ⊕D 871
Tympagesic Ear Drops 2342
Vasosulf .... ◎ 271
Vicks Sinex Nasal Spray and Ultra Fine Mist .... ⊕D 765

Phenylephrine Tannate (Potential for hyperglycemia leading to loss of control). Products include:

Atrohist Pediatric Suspension 454
Ricobid-D Pediatric Suspension 2038
Ricobid Tablets and Pediatric Suspension 2038
Rynatan 2673
Rynatuss 2673

Phenylpropanolamine Hydrochloride (Potential for hyperglycemia leading to loss of control). Products include:

Acutrim .... ⊕D 628
Allerest Children's Chewable Tablets .... ⊕D 627
Allerest 12 Hour Caplets .... ⊕D 627
Atrohist Plus Tablets 454
BC Cold Powder Multi-Symptom Formula (Cold-Sinus-Allergy) ...... ⊕D 609
BC Cold Powder Non-Drowsy Formula (Cold-Sinus) .... ⊕D 609
Cheracol Plus Head Cold/Cough Formula .... ⊕D 769
Comtrex Multi-Symptom Non-Drowsy Liqui-gels .... ⊕D 618
Contac Continuous Action Nasal Decongestant/Antihistamine 12 Hour Capsules .... ⊕D 813
Contac Maximum Strength Continuous Action Decongestant/Antihistamine 12 Hour Caplets.. ⊕D 813
Contac Severe Cold and Flu Formula Caplets .... ⊕D 814
Coricidin 'D' Decongestant Tablets .... ⊕D 800
Dexatrim .... ⊕D 832
Dexatrim Plus Vitamins Caplets .... ⊕D 832
Dimetane-DC Cough Syrup 2059
Dimetapp Elixir .... ⊕D 773
Dimetapp Extentabs .... ⊕D 774
Dimetapp Tablets/Liqui-Gels .... ⊕D 775
Dimetapp Cold & Allergy Chewable Tablets .... ⊕D 773
Dimetapp DM Elixir .... ⊕D 774
Dura-Vent Tablets 952
Entex Capsules 1986
Entex LA Tablets 1987
Entex Liquid 1986
Exgest LA Tablets 782
Hycomine 931
Isoclor Timesule Capsules .... ⊕D 637
Nolamine Timed-Release Tablets 785
Ornade Spansule Capsules 2502
Propagest Tablets 786
Pyrroxate Caplets .... ⊕D 772
Robitussin-CF .... ⊕D 777
Sinulin Tablets 787
Tavist-D 12 Hour Relief Tablets .... ⊕D 787
Teldrin 12 Hour Antihistamine/Nasal Decongestant Allergy Relief Capsules .... ⊕D 826
Triaminic Allergy Tablets .... ⊕D 789
Triaminic Cold Tablets .... ⊕D 790
Triaminic Expectorant .... ⊕D 790
Triaminic Syrup .... ⊕D 792
Triaminic-12 Tablets .... ⊕D 792
Triaminic-DM Syrup .... ⊕D 792
Triaminicin Tablets .... ⊕D 793
Triaminicol Multi-Symptom Cold Tablets .... ⊕D 793
Triaminicol Multi-Symptom Relief ⊕D 794
Vicks DayQuil Allergy Relief 12-Hour Extended Release Tablets.. ⊕D 760
Vicks DayQuil Allergy Relief 4-Hour Tablets .... ⊕D 760
Vicks DayQuil SINUS Pressure & CONGESTION Relief .... ⊕D 761

(⊕D Described in PDR For Nonprescription Drugs) (◎ Described in PDR For Ophthalmology)

Phenytoin (Potential for hyperglycemia leading to loss of control). Products include:

Dilantin Infatabs 1908
Dilantin-125 Suspension 1911

Phenytoin Sodium (Potential for hyperglycemia leading to loss of control). Products include:

Dilantin Kapseals 1906
Dilantin Parenteral 1910

Pindolol (Potentiates the hypoglycemic action; patients should be observed for hypoglycemia or loss of control). Products include:

Visken Tablets... 2299

Pirbuterol Acetate (Potential for hyperglycemia leading to loss of control). Products include:

Maxair Autohaler 1492
Maxair Inhaler 1494

Piroxicam (Potentiates the hypoglycemic action; patients should be observed for hypoglycemia or loss of control). Products include:

Feldene Capsules...................................... 1965

Polyestradiol Phosphate (Potential for hyperglycemia leading to loss of control).

No products indexed under this heading.

Polythiazide (Potential for hyperglycemia leading to loss of control). Products include:

Minizide Capsules 1938

Prednisolone Acetate (Potential for hyperglycemia leading to loss of control). Products include:

AK-CIDE .... ◉ 202
AK-CIDE Ointment................................... ◉ 202
Blephamide Liquifilm Sterile Ophthalmic Suspension 476
Blephamide Ointment .... ◉ 237
Econopred & Econopred Plus Ophthalmic Suspensions .... ◉ 217
Poly-Pred Liquifilm .... ◉ 248
Pred Forte.. ◉ 250
Pred Mild.. ◉ 253
Pred-G Liquifilm Sterile Ophthalmic Suspension .... ◉ 251
Pred-G S.O.P. Sterile Ophthalmic Ointment .... ◉ 252
Vasocidin Ointment .... ◉ 268

Prednisolone Sodium Phosphate (Potential for hyperglycemia leading to loss of control). Products include:

AK-Pred .... ◉ 204
Hydeltrasol Injection, Sterile................ 1665
Inflamase... ◉ 265
Pediapred Oral Liquid 995
Vasocidin Ophthalmic Solution .... ◉ 270

Prednisolone Tebutate (Potential for hyperglycemia leading to loss of control). Products include:

Hydeltra-T.B.A. Sterile Suspension 1667

Prednisone (Potential for hyperglycemia leading to loss of control). Products include:

Deltasone Tablets 2595

Probenecid (Potentiates the hypoglycemic action; patients should be observed for hypoglycemia or loss of control). Products include:

Benemid Tablets 1611
ColBENEMID Tablets 1622

Prochlorperazine (Potential for hyperglycemia leading to loss of control). Products include:

Compazine 2470

Promethazine Hydrochloride (Potential for hyperglycemia leading to loss of control). Products include:

Mepergan Injection 2753
Phenergan with Codeine.......................... 2777
Phenergan with Dextromethorphan 2778
Phenergan Injection 2773
Phenergan Suppositories 2775
Phenergan Syrup 2774
Phenergan Tablets 2775
Phenergan VC.. 2779
Phenergan VC with Codeine 2781

Propranolol Hydrochloride (Potentiates the hypoglycemic action; patients should be observed for hypoglycemia or loss of control). Products include:

Inderal 2728
Inderal LA Long Acting Capsules 2730
Inderide Tablets 2732
Inderide LA Long Acting Capsules .. 2734

Pseudoephedrine Hydrochloride (Potential for hyperglycemia leading to loss of control). Products include:

Actifed Allergy Daytime/Nighttime Caplets... ⊕ 844
Actifed Plus Caplets .... ⊕ 845
Actifed Plus Tablets .... ⊕ 845
Actifed with Codeine Cough Syrup.. 1067
Actifed Sinus Daytime/Nighttime Tablets and Caplets .... ⊕ 846
Actifed Syrup... ⊕ 846
Actifed Tablets .... ⊕ 844
Advil Cold and Sinus Caplets and Tablets (formerly CoAdvil) .... ⊕ 870
Alka-Seltzer Plus Cold Medicine Liqui-Gels .... ⊕ 706
Alka-Seltzer Plus Cold & Cough Medicine Liqui-Gels.......................... ⊕ 705
Alka-Seltzer Plus Night-Time Cold Medicine Liqui-Gels.......................... ⊕ 706
Allerest Headache Strength Tablets .... ⊕ 627
Allerest Maximum Strength Tablets .... ⊕ 627
Allerest No Drowsiness Tablets ...... ⊕ 627
Allerest Sinus Pain Formula .... ⊕ 627
Anatuss LA Tablets................................... 1542
Atrohist Pediatric Capsules 453
Bayer Select Sinus Pain Relief Formula .... ⊕ 717
Benadryl Allergy Decongestant Liquid Medication .... ⊕ 848
Benadryl Allergy Decongestant Tablets .... ⊕ 848
Benadryl Allergy Sinus Headache Formula Caplets.................................... ⊕ 849
Benylin Multisymptom............................ ⊕ 852
Bromfed Capsules (Extended-Release) 1785
Bromfed Syrup .... ⊕ 733
Bromfed Tablets 1785
Bromfed-DM Cough Syrup..................... 1786
Bromfed-PD Capsules (Extended-Release) 1785
Children's Vicks DayQuil Allergy Relief.. ⊕ 757
Children's Vicks NyQuil Cold/ Cough Relief... ⊕ 758
Comtrex Multi-Symptom Cold Reliever Tablets/Caplets/Liqui-Gels/Liquid.. ⊕ 615
Allergy-Sinus Comtrex Multi-Symptom Allergy-Sinus Formula Tablets .... ⊕ 617
Comtrex Multi-Symptom Non-Drowsy Caplets..................................... ⊕ 618
Congess 1004
Contac Day Allergy/Sinus Caplets ⊕ 812
Contac Day & Night .... ⊕ 812
Contac Night Allergy/Sinus Caplets .... ⊕ 812
Contac Severe Cold & Flu Non-Drowsy .... ⊕ 815
Deconamine Chewable Tablets 1320
Deconamine CX Cough and Cold Liquid and Tablets............................... 1319
Deconamine 1320
Deconsal C Expectorant Syrup 456
Deconsal Pediatric Syrup..................... 457
Deconsal II Tablets 454
Dimetane-DX Cough Syrup 2059
Dimetapp Sinus Caplets .... ⊕ 775
Dorcol Children's Cough Syrup .... ⊕ 785
Drixoral Cough + Congestion Liquid Caps .... ⊕ 802
Dura-Tap/PD Capsules........................... 2867
Duratuss Tablets 2565
Duratuss HD Elixir.................................... 2565
Efidac/24 .... ⊕ 635
Entex PSE Tablets 1987
Fedahist Gyrocaps.................................... 2401
Fedahist Timecaps 2401
Guaifed.. 1787
Guaifed Syrup .... ⊕ 734
Guaimax-D Tablets 792
Guaitab Tablets .... ⊕ 734
Isoclor Expectorant.................................. 990
Kronofed-A 977
Motrin IB Sinus .... ⊕ 838
Novahistine DH... 2462
Novahistine DMX .... ⊕ 822
Novahistine Expectorant......................... 2463
Nucofed 2051
PediaCare Cold Allergy Chewable Tablets .... ⊕ 677
PediaCare Cough-Cold Chewable Tablets 1553
PediaCare 1553
PediaCare Infants' Decongestant Drops .... ⊕ 677
PediCare Infant's Drops Decongestant Plus Cough 1553
PediaCare NightRest Cough-Cold Liquid 1553
Pediatric Vicks 44d Dry Hacking Cough & Head Congestion.............. ⊕ 763
Pediatric Vicks 44m Cough & Cold Relief .... ⊕ 764
Robitussin Cold & Cough Liqui-Gels .... ⊕ 776
Robitussin Maximum Strength Cough & Cold .... ⊕ 778
Robitussin Pediatric Cough & Cold Formula... ⊕ 779
Robitussin Severe Congestion Liqui-Gels .... ⊕ 776
Robitussin-DAC Syrup 2074
Robitussin-PE .... ⊕ 778
Rondec Oral Drops 953
Rondec Syrup 953
Rondec Tablet.. 953
Rondec-DM Oral Drops 954
Rondec-DM Syrup 954
Rondec-TR Tablet 953
Ryna .... ⊕ 841
Seldane-D Extended-Release Tablets 1538
Semprex-D Capsules 463
Semprex-D Capsules 1167
Sinarest Tablets .... ⊕ 648
Sinarest Extra Strength Tablets....... ⊕ 648
Sinarest No Drowsiness Tablets .... ⊕ 648
Sine-Aid IB Caplets 1554
Sine-Aid Maximum Strength Sinus Medication Gelcaps, Caplets and Tablets 1554
Sine-Off No Drowsiness Formula Caplets.. ⊕ 824
Sine-Off Sinus Medicine .... ⊕ 825
Singlet Tablets .... ⊕ 825
Sinutab Non-Drying Liquid Caps .... ⊕ 859
Sinutab Sinus Allergy Medication, Maximum Strength Tablets and Caplets.. ⊕ 860
Sinutab Sinus Medication, Maximum Strength Without Drowsiness Formula, Tablets & Caplets .... ⊕ 860
Sinutab Sinus Medication, Regular Strength Without Drowsiness Formula .... ⊕ 859
Sudafed Children's Liquid .... ⊕ 861
Sudafed Cold and Cough Liquidcaps .... ⊕ 862
Sudafed Cough Syrup .... ⊕ 862
Sudafed Plus Liquid .... ⊕ 862
Sudafed Plus Tablets................................ ⊕ 863
Sudafed Severe Cold Formula Caplets.. ⊕ 863
Sudafed Severe Cold Formula Tablets .... ⊕ 864
Sudafed Sinus Caplets............................ ⊕ 864
Sudafed Sinus Tablets............................. ⊕ 864
Sudafed Tablets, 30 mg........................... ⊕ 861
Sudafed Tablets, 60 mg........................... ⊕ 861
Sudafed 12 Hour Caplets .... ⊕ 861
Syn-Rx Tablets 465
Syn-Rx DM Tablets 466
TheraFlu.. ⊕ 787
TheraFlu Maximum Strength Nighttime Flu, Cold & Cough Medicine .... ⊕ 788
TheraFlu Maximum Strength Non-Drowsy Formula Flu, Cold & Cough Medicine .... ⊕ 788
Thera Flu Maximum Strength, Non-Drowsy Formula Flu, Cold and Cough Caplets .... ⊕ 789
Triaminic AM Cough and Decongestant Formula .... ⊕ 789
Triaminic AM Decongestant Formula .... ⊕ 790
Triaminic Nite Light .... ⊕ 791
Triaminic Sore Throat Formula ...... ⊕ 791
Tussend 1783
Tussend Expectorant 1785
Children's TYLENOL Cold Multi-Symptom Liquid Formula and Chewable Tablets................................... 1561
Children's TYLENOL Cold Plus Cough Multi Symptom Tablets and Liquid... ⊕ 681
Infants' TYLENOL Cold Decongestant & Fever-Reducer Drops 1556
TYLENOL Maximum Strength Allergy Sinus Medication Gelcaps and Caplets 1563
TYLENOL Maximum Strength Allergy Sinus NightTime Medication Caplets 1555
TYLENOL Flu Maximum Strength Gelcaps 1565
TYLENOL Flu NightTime, Maximum Strength, Gelcaps 1566
TYLENOL Maximum Strength Flu NightTime Hot Medication Packets 1562
TYLENOL, Maximum Strength, Sinus Medication Geltabs, Gelcaps, Caplets and Tablets 1566
TYLENOL Cold Multi-Symptom Formula Medication Tablets and Caplets.. 1561
TYLENOL Cold Medication No Drowsiness Formula Gelcaps and Caplets.. 1562
TYLENOL Cold Multi-Symptom Hot Medication Liquid Packets.............. 1557
TYLENOL Cough Multi-Symptom Medication with Decongestant...... 1565
Ursinus Inlay-Tabs................................... ⊕ 794
Vicks 44 LiquiCaps Cough, Cold & Flu Relief... ⊕ 755
Vicks 44 LiquiCaps Non-Drowsy Cough & Cold Relief .... ⊕ 756
Vicks 44D Dry Hacking Cough & Head Congestion .... ⊕ 755
Vicks 44M Cough, Cold & Flu Relief.. ⊕ 756
Vicks DayQuil .... ⊕ 761
Vicks DayQuil SINUS Pressure & PAIN Relief with IBUPROFEN ...... ⊕ 762
Vicks Nyquil Hot Therapy.................... ⊕ 762
Vicks NyQuil LiquiCaps Multi-Symptom Cold/Flu Relief .... ⊕ 763
Vicks NyQuil Multi-Symptom Cold/Flu Relief · (Original & Cherry Flavor) .... ⊕ 763

Pseudoephedrine Sulfate (Potential for hyperglycemia leading to loss of control). Products include:

Cheracol Sinus .... ⊕ 768
Chlor-Trimeton Allergy Decongestant Tablets .... ⊕ 799
Claritin-D... 2350
Drixoral Cold and Allergy Sustained-Action Tablets.......................... ⊕ 802
Drixoral Cold and Flu Extended-Release Tablets.................................... ⊕ 803
Drixoral Non-Drowsy Formula Extended-Release Tablets .... ⊕ 803
Drixoral Allergy/Sinus Extended Release Tablets.................................... ⊕ 804
Trinalin Repetabs Tablets 1330

Quinestrol (Potential for hyperglycemia leading to loss of control).

No products indexed under this heading.

Salmeterol Xinafoate (Potential for hyperglycemia leading to loss of control). Products include:

Serevent Inhalation Aerosol................. 1176

Salsalate (Potentiates the hypoglycemic action; patients should be observed for hypoglycemia or loss of control). Products include:

Mono-Gesic Tablets 792
Salflex Tablets... 786

Selegiline Hydrochloride (Potentiates the hypoglycemic action; patients should be observed for hypoglycemia or loss of control). Products include:

Eldepryl Tablets 2550

Sotalol Hydrochloride (Potentiates the hypoglycemic action; patients should be observed for hypoglycemia or loss of control). Products include:

Betapace Tablets 641

Spironolactone (Potential for hyperglycemia leading to loss of control). Products include:

Aldactazide... 2413
Aldactone 2414

IMPORTANT NOTE: Always consult each drug listing in the patient's regimen for possible interactions.

Sulfacytine (Potentiates the hypoglycemic action; patients should be observed for hypoglycemia or loss of control).

Sulfamethizole (Potentiates the hypoglycemic action; patients should be observed for hypoglycemia or loss of control). Products include:

Urobiotic-250 Capsules 2214

Sulfamethoxazole (Potentiates the hypoglycemic action; patients should be observed for hypoglycemia or loss of control). Products include:

Azo Gantanol Tablets 2080
Bactrim DS Tablets 2084
Bactrim I.V. Infusion 2082
Bactrim 2084
Gantanol Tablets 2119
Septra 1174
Septra I.V. Infusion 1169
Septra I.V. Infusion ADD-Vantage Vials 1171
Septra 1174

Sulfasalazine (Potentiates the hypoglycemic action; patients should be observed for hypoglycemia or loss of control). Products include:

Azulfidine 1949

Sulfinpyrazone (Potentiates the hypoglycemic action; patients should be observed for hypoglycemia or loss of control). Products include:

Anturane 807

Sulfisoxazole (Potentiates the hypoglycemic action; patients should be observed for hypoglycemia or loss of control). Products include:

Azo Gantrisin Tablets 2081
Gantrisin Tablets 2120

Sulfisoxazole Diolamine (Potentiates the hypoglycemic action; patients should be observed for hypoglycemia or loss of control).

No products indexed under this heading.

Sulindac (Potentiates the hypoglycemic action; patients should be observed for hypoglycemia or loss of control). Products include:

Clinoril Tablets 1618

Temazepam (Potentiates the hypoglycemic action; patients should be observed for hypoglycemia or loss of control). Products include:

Restoril Capsules 2284

Terbutaline Sulfate (Potential for hyperglycemia leading to loss of control). Products include:

Brethaire Inhaler 813
Brethine Ampuls 815
Brethine Tablets 814
Bricanyl Subcutaneous Injection 1502
Bricanyl Tablets 1503

Thioridazine Hydrochloride (Potential for hyperglycemia leading to loss of control). Products include:

Mellaril 2269

Thyroglobulin (Potential for hyperglycemia leading to loss of control).

No products indexed under this heading.

Thyroid (Potential for hyperglycemia leading to loss of control).

No products indexed under this heading.

Thyroxine (Potential for hyperglycemia leading to loss of control).

No products indexed under this heading.

Thyroxine Sodium (Potential for hyperglycemia leading to loss of control).

No products indexed under this heading.

Timolol Hemihydrate (Potentiates the hypoglycemic action; patients should be observed for hypoglycemia or loss of control). Products include:

Betimol 0.25%, 0.5% ..... ⊚ 261

Timolol Maleate (Potentiates the hypoglycemic action; patients should be observed for hypoglycemia or loss of control). Products include:

Blocadren Tablets 1614
Timolide Tablets 1748
Timoptic in Ocudose 1753
Timoptic Sterile Ophthalmic Solution 1751
Timoptic-XE 1755

Tolazamide (Potentiates the hypoglycemic action; patients should be observed for hypoglycemia or loss of control).

No products indexed under this heading.

Tolbutamide (Potentiates the hypoglycemic action; patients should be observed for hypoglycemia or loss of control).

No products indexed under this heading.

Tolmetin Sodium (Potentiates the hypoglycemic action; patients should be observed for hypoglycemia or loss of control). Products include:

Tolectin (200, 400 and 600 mg) .. 1581

Torsemide (Potential for hyperglycemia leading to loss of control). Products include:

Demadex Tablets and Injection 686

Tranylcypromine Sulfate (Potentiates the hypoglycemic action; patients should be observed for hypoglycemia or loss of control). Products include:

Parnate Tablets 2503

Triamcinolone (Potential for hyperglycemia leading to loss of control). Products include:

Aristocort Tablets 1022

Triamcinolone Acetonide (Potential for hyperglycemia leading to loss of control). Products include:

Aristocort A 0.025% Cream 1027
Aristocort A 0.5% Cream 1031
Aristocort A 0.1% Cream 1029
Aristocort A 0.1% Ointment 1030
Azmacort Oral Inhaler 2011
Nasacort Nasal Inhaler 2024

Triamcinolone Diacetate (Potential for hyperglycemia leading to loss of control). Products include:

Aristocort Suspension (Forte Parenteral) 1027
Aristocort Suspension (Intralesional) 1025

Triamcinolone Hexacetonide (Potential for hyperglycemia leading to loss of control). Products include:

Aristospan Suspension (Intra-articular) 1033
Aristospan Suspension (Intralesional) 1032

Triamterene (Potential for hyperglycemia leading to loss of control). Products include:

Dyazide 2479
Dyrenium Capsules 2481
Maxzide 1380

Trifluoperazine Hydrochloride (Potential for hyperglycemia leading to loss of control). Products include:

Stelazine 2514

Trimipramine Maleate (Potentiates the hypoglycemic action; patients should be observed for hypoglycemia or loss of control). Products include:

Surmontil Capsules 2811

Verapamil Hydrochloride (Potential for hyperglycemia leading to loss of control). Products include:

Calan SR Caplets 2422
Calan Tablets 2419
Isoptin Injectable 1344
Isoptin Oral Tablets 1346
Isoptin SR Tablets 1348
Verelan Capsules 1410
Verelan Capsules 2824

Warfarin Sodium (Potentiates the hypoglycemic action; patients should be observed for hypoglycemia or loss of control). Products include:

Coumadin 926

Food Interactions

Alcohol (Potential for hypoglycemia).

Food, unspecified (Delays the absorption by 40 minutes; total absorption and disposition is unaffected; Glucotrol is more effective when administered about 30 minutes before, rather than with, a meal).

GLUCOTROL XL EXTENDED RELEASE TABLETS

(Glipizide) **1968**

May interact with non-steroidal anti-inflammatory agents, salicylates, sulfonamides, beta blockers, monoamine oxidase inhibitors, oral anticoagulants, highly protein bound drugs (selected), thiazides, diuretics, corticosteroids, phenothiazines, thyroid preparations, estrogens, oral contraceptives, sympathomimetics, calcium channel blockers, and certain other agents. Compounds in these categories include:

Acebutolol Hydrochloride (Potentiates the hypoglycemic action; patient should be observed for hypoglycemia or loss of control). Products include:

Sectral Capsules 2807

Albuterol (Potential for hyperglycemia leading to loss of control). Products include:

Proventil Inhalation Aerosol 2382
Ventolin Inhalation Aerosol and Refill 1197

Albuterol Sulfate (Potential for hyperglycemia leading to loss of control). Products include:

Airet Solution for Inhalation 452
Proventil Inhalation Solution 0.083% 2384
Proventil Repetabs Tablets 2386
Proventil Solution for Inhalation 0.5% 2383
Proventil Syrup 2385
Proventil Tablets 2386
Ventolin Inhalation Solution 1198
Ventolin Nebules Inhalation Solution 1199
Ventolin Rotacaps for Inhalation 1200
Ventolin Syrup 1202
Ventolin Tablets 1203
Volmax Extended-Release Tablets .. 1788

Amiloride Hydrochloride (Potential for hyperglycemia leading to loss of control). Products include:

Midamor Tablets 1703
Moduretic Tablets 1705

Amiodarone Hydrochloride (Potentiates the hypoglycemic action; patient should be observed for hypoglycemia or loss of control). Products include:

Cordarone Intravenous 2715
Cordarone Tablets 2712

Amitriptyline Hydrochloride (Potentiates the hypoglycemic action; patient should be observed for hypoglycemia or loss of control). Products include:

Elavil 2838
Endep Tablets 2174
Etrafon 2355
Limbitrol 2180
Triavil Tablets 1757

Amlodipine Besylate (Potential for hyperglycemia leading to loss of control). Products include:

Lotrel Capsules 840
Norvasc Tablets 1940

Aspirin (Potentiates the hypoglycemic action; patient should be observed for hypoglycemia or loss of control). Products include:

Alka-Seltzer Effervescent Antacid and Pain Reliever ..... ▣ 701
Alka-Seltzer Extra Strength Effervescent Antacid and Pain Reliever ..... ▣ 703
Alka-Seltzer Lemon Lime Effervescent Antacid and Pain Reliever ..... ▣ 703
Alka-Seltzer Plus Cold Medicine ..... ▣ 705
Alka-Seltzer Plus Cold & Cough Medicine ..... ▣ 708
Alka-Seltzer Plus Night-Time Cold Medicine ..... ▣ 707
Alka Seltzer Plus Sinus Medicine .. ▣ 707
Arthritis Foundation Safety Coated Aspirin Tablets ..... ▣ 675
Arthritis Pain Ascriptin ..... ▣ 631
Maximum Strength Ascriptin ..... ▣ 630
Regular Strength Ascriptin Tablets ..... ▣ 629
Arthritis Strength BC Powder ..... ▣ 609
BC Cold Powder Multi-Symptom Formula (Cold-Sinus-Allergy) ..... ▣ 609
BC Cold Powder Non-Drowsy Formula (Cold-Sinus) ..... ▣ 609
BC Powder ..... ▣ 609
Bayer Children's Chewable Aspirin ..... ▣ 711
Genuine Bayer Aspirin Tablets & Caplets ..... ▣ 713
Extra Strength Bayer Arthritis Pain Regimen Formula ..... ▣ 711
Extra Strength Bayer Aspirin Caplets & Tablets ..... ▣ 712
Extended-Release Bayer 8-Hour Aspirin ..... ▣ 712
Extra Strength Bayer Plus Aspirin Caplets ..... ▣ 713
Extra Strength Bayer PM Aspirin .. ▣ 713
Bayer Enteric Aspirin ..... ▣ 709
Bufferin Analgesic Tablets and Caplets ..... ▣ 613
Arthritis Strength Bufferin Analgesic Caplets ..... ▣ 614
Extra Strength Bufferin Analgesic Tablets ..... ▣ 615
Cama Arthritis Pain Reliever ..... ▣ 785
Darvon Compound-65 Pulvules 1435
Easprin 1914
Ecotrin 2455
Ecotrin Enteric Coated Aspirin Maximum Strength Tablets and Caplets ..... ▣ 816
Ecotrin Enteric Coated Aspirin Regular Strength Tablets 2455
Empirin Aspirin Tablets ..... ▣ 854
Empirin with Codeine Tablets 1093
Excedrin Extra-Strength Analgesic Tablets & Caplets 732
Fiorinal Capsules 2261
Fiorinal with Codeine Capsules 2262
Fiorinal Tablets 2261
Halfprin 1362
Healthprin Aspirin 2455
Norgesic 1496
Percodan Tablets 939
Percodan-Demi Tablets 940
Robaxisal Tablets 2071
Soma Compound w/Codeine Tablets 2676
Soma Compound Tablets 2675
St. Joseph Adult Chewable Aspirin (81 mg.) ..... ▣ 808
Talwin Compound 2335
Ursinus Inlay-Tabs ..... ▣ 794
Vanquish Analgesic Caplets ..... ▣ 731

Atenolol (Potentiates the hypoglycemic action; patient should be observed for hypoglycemia or loss of control). Products include:

Tenoretic Tablets 2845
Tenormin Tablets and I.V. Injection 2847

Atovaquone (Potentiates the hypoglycemic action; patient should be observed for hypoglycemia or loss of control). Products include:

Mepron Suspension 1135

Bendroflumethiazide (Potential for hyperglycemia leading to loss of control).

No products indexed under this heading.

(▣ Described in PDR For Nonprescription Drugs) (⊚ Described in PDR For Ophthalmology)

Interactions Index — Glucotrol XL

Bepridil Hydrochloride (Potential for hyperglycemia leading to loss of control). Products include:

Vascor (200, 300 and 400 mg) Tablets 1587

Betamethasone Acetate (Potential for hyperglycemia leading to loss of control). Products include:

Celestone Soluspan Suspension 2347

Betamethasone Sodium Phosphate (Potential for hyperglycemia leading to loss of control). Products include:

Celestone Soluspan Suspension 2347

Betaxolol Hydrochloride (Potentiates the hypoglycemic action; patient should be observed for hypoglycemia or loss of control). Products include:

Betoptic Ophthalmic Solution........... 469
Betoptic S Ophthalmic Suspension 471
Kerlone Tablets................................... 2436

Bisoprolol Fumarate (Potentiates the hypoglycemic action; patient should be observed for hypoglycemia or loss of control). Products include:

Zebeta Tablets 1413
Ziac 1415

Bumetanide (Potential for hyperglycemia leading to loss of control). Products include:

Bumex 2093

Carteolol Hydrochloride (Potentiates the hypoglycemic action; patient should be observed for hypoglycemia or loss of control). Products include:

Cartrol Tablets 410
Ocupress Ophthalmic Solution, 1% Sterile....................................... ⊕ 309

Cefonicid Sodium (Potentiates the hypoglycemic action; patient should be observed for hypoglycemia or loss of control). Products include:

Monocid Injection 2497

Chloramphenicol (Potentiates the hypoglycemic action; patient should be observed for hypoglycemia or loss of control). Products include:

Chloromycetin Ophthalmic Ointment, 1% .... ⊕ 310
Chloromycetin Ophthalmic Solution .... ⊕ 310
Chloroptic S.O.P. .... ⊕ 239
Chloroptic Sterile Ophthalmic Solution .... ⊕ 239
Elase-Chloromycetin Ointment 1040
Ophthocort .... ⊕ 311

Chloramphenicol Palmitate (Potentiates the hypoglycemic action; patient should be observed for hypoglycemia or loss of control).

No products indexed under this heading.

Chloramphenicol Sodium Succinate (Potentiates the hypoglycemic action; patient should be observed for hypoglycemia or loss of control). Products include:

Chloromycetin Sodium Succinate.... 1900

Chlordiazepoxide (Potentiates the hypoglycemic action; patient should be observed for hypoglycemia or loss of control). Products include:

Libritabs Tablets 2177
Limbitrol 2180

Chlordiazepoxide Hydrochloride (Potentiates the hypoglycemic action; patient should be observed for hypoglycemia or loss of control). Products include:

Librax Capsules 2176
Librium Capsules................................. 2178
Librium Injectable 2179

Chlorothiazide (Potential for hyperglycemia leading to loss of control). Products include:

Aldoclor Tablets................................... 1598
Diupres Tablets 1650
Diuril Oral 1653

Chlorothiazide Sodium (Potential for hyperglycemia leading to loss of control). Products include:

Diuril Sodium Intravenous 1652

Chlorotrianisene (Potential for hyperglycemia leading to loss of control).

No products indexed under this heading.

Chlorpromazine (Potential for hyperglycemia leading to loss of control). Products include:

Thorazine Suppositories 2523

Chlorpromazine Hydrochloride (Potential for hyperglycemia leading to loss of control). Products include:

Thorazine 2523

Chlorpropamide (Potentiates the hypoglycemic action; patient should be observed for hypoglycemia or loss of control). Products include:

Diabinese Tablets 1935

Chlorthalidone (Potential for hyperglycemia leading to loss of control). Products include:

Combipres Tablets 677
Tenoretic Tablets................................. 2845
Thalitone 1245

Choline Magnesium Trisalicylate (Potentiates the hypoglycemic action; patient should be observed for hypoglycemia or loss of control). Products include:

Trilisate 2000

Clomipramine Hydrochloride (Potentiates the hypoglycemic action; patient should be observed for hypoglycemia or loss of control). Products include:

Anafranil Capsules 803

Clozapine (Potentiates the hypoglycemic action; patient should be observed for hypoglycemia or loss of control). Products include:

Clozaril Tablets.................................... 2252

Cortisone Acetate (Potential for hyperglycemia leading to loss of control). Products include:

Cortone Acetate Sterile Suspension 1623
Cortone Acetate Tablets.................... 1624

Cyclosporine (Potentiates the hypoglycemic action; patient should be observed for hypoglycemia or loss of control). Products include:

Neoral... 2276
Sandimmune 2286

Desogestrel (Potential for hyperglycemia leading to loss of control). Products include:

Desogen Tablets.................................. 1817
Ortho-Cept 1851

Dexamethasone (Potential for hyperglycemia leading to loss of control). Products include:

AK-Trol Ointment & Suspension .... ⊕ 205
Decadron Elixir 1633
Decadron Tablets................................ 1635
Decaspray Topical Aerosol 1648
Dexacidin Ointment .... ⊕ 263
Maxitrol Ophthalmic Ointment and Suspension .... ⊕ 224
TobraDex Ophthalmic Suspension and Ointment....................................... 473

Dexamethasone Acetate (Potential for hyperglycemia leading to loss of control). Products include:

Dalalone D.P. Injectable 1011
Decadron-LA Sterile Suspension 1646

Dexamethasone Sodium Phosphate (Potential for hyperglycemia leading to loss of control). Products include:

Decadron Phosphate Injection 1637
Decadron Phosphate Respihaler 1642
Decadron Phosphate Sterile Ophthalmic Ointment 1641
Decadron Phosphate Sterile Ophthalmic Solution 1642
Decadron Phosphate Topical Cream.. 1644
Decadron Phosphate Turbinaire 1645
Decadron Phosphate with Xylocaine Injection, Sterile 1639
Dexacort Phosphate in Respihaler .. 458
Dexacort Phosphate in Turbinaire .. 459
NeoDecadron Sterile Ophthalmic Ointment 1712
NeoDecadron Sterile Ophthalmic Solution 1713
NeoDecadron Topical Cream 1714

Diazepam (Potentiates the hypoglycemic action; patient should be observed for hypoglycemia or loss of control). Products include:

Dizac 1809
Valium Injectable 2182
Valium Tablets 2183
Valrelease Capsules 2169

Diclofenac Potassium (Potentiates the hypoglycemic action; patient should be observed for hypoglycemia or loss of control). Products include:

Cataflam 816

Diclofenac Sodium (Potentiates the hypoglycemic action; patient should be observed for hypoglycemia or loss of control). Products include:

Voltaren Ophthalmic Sterile Ophthalmic Solution .... ⊕ 272
Voltaren Tablets.................................. 861

Dicumarol (Potentiates the hypoglycemic action; patient should be observed for hypoglycemia or loss of control).

No products indexed under this heading.

Dienestrol (Potential for hyperglycemia leading to loss of control). Products include:

Ortho Dienestrol Cream 1866

Diethylstilbestrol (Potential for hyperglycemia leading to loss of control). Products include:

Diethylstilbestrol Tablets 1437

Diflunisal (Potentiates the hypoglycemic action; patient should be observed for hypoglycemia or loss of control). Products include:

Dolobid Tablets.................................... 1654

Diltiazem Hydrochloride (Potential for hyperglycemia leading to loss of control). Products include:

Cardizem CD Capsules 1506
Cardizem SR Capsules 1510
Cardizem Injectable 1508
Cardizem Tablets................................. 1512
Dilacor XR Extended-release Capsules 2018

Dipyridamole (Potentiates the hypoglycemic action; patient should be observed for hypoglycemia or loss of control). Products include:

Persantine Tablets 681

Dobutamine Hydrochloride (Potential for hyperglycemia leading to loss of control). Products include:

Dobutrex Solution Vials...................... 1439

Dopamine Hydrochloride (Potential for hyperglycemia leading to loss of control).

No products indexed under this heading.

Ephedrine Hydrochloride (Potential for hyperglycemia leading to loss of control). Products include:

Primatene Dual Action Formula...... ⊕D 872
Primatene Tablets .... ⊕D 873

Quadrinal Tablets 1350

Ephedrine Sulfate (Potential for hyperglycemia leading to loss of control). Products include:

Bronkaid Caplets .... ⊕D 717
Marax Tablets & DF Syrup................. 2200

Ephedrine Tannate (Potential for hyperglycemia leading to loss of control). Products include:

Rynatuss 2673

Epinephrine (Potential for hyperglycemia leading to loss of control). Products include:

Bronkaid Mist .... ⊕D 717
EPIFRIN .... ⊕ 239
EpiPen 790
Marcaine Hydrochloride with Epinephrine 1:200,000 2316
Primatene Mist.................................... ⊕D 873
Sensorcaine with Epinephrine Injection.. 559
Sus-Phrine Injection 1019
Xylocaine with Epinephrine Injections.. 567

Epinephrine Bitartrate (Potential for hyperglycemia leading to loss of control). Products include:

Bronkaid Mist Suspension .... ⊕D 718
Sensorcaine-MPF with Epinephrine Injection 559

Epinephrine Hydrochloride (Potential for hyperglycemia leading to loss of control). Products include:

Ana-Kit Anaphylaxis Emergency Treatment Kit 617

Esmolol Hydrochloride (Potentiates the hypoglycemic action; patient should be observed for hypoglycemia or loss of control). Products include:

Brevibloc Injection............................... 1808

Estradiol (Potential for hyperglycemia leading to loss of control). Products include:

Climara Transdermal System............ 645
Estrace Cream and Tablets 749
Estraderm Transdermal System 824

Estrogens, Conjugated (Potential for hyperglycemia leading to loss of control). Products include:

PMB 200 and PMB 400 2783
Premarin Intravenous 2787
Premarin with Methyltestosterone .. 2794
Premarin Tablets 2789
Premarin Vaginal Cream.................... 2791
Premphase 2797
Prempro... 2801

Estrogens, Esterified (Potential for hyperglycemia leading to loss of control). Products include:

ESTRATAB Tablets (0.3, 0.625, 1.25, 2.5 mg)...................................... 2536
Estratest 2539
Menest Tablets 2494

Estropipate (Potential for hyperglycemia leading to loss of control). Products include:

Ogen Tablets 2627
Ogen Vaginal Cream........................... 2630
Ortho-Est... 1869

Ethacrynic Acid (Potential for hyperglycemia leading to loss of control). Products include:

Edecrin Tablets..................................... 1657

Ethinyl Estradiol (Potential for hyperglycemia leading to loss of control). Products include:

Brevicon... 2088
Demulen 2428
Desogen Tablets................................... 1817
Levlen/Tri-Levlen................................. 651
Lo/Ovral Tablets 2746
Lo/Ovral-28 Tablets............................. 2751
Modicon 1872
Nordette-21 Tablets............................. 2755
Nordette-28 Tablets............................. 2758
Norinyl 2088
Ortho-Cept 1851
Ortho-Cyclen/Ortho-Tri-Cyclen 1858
Ortho-Novum... 1872
Ortho-Cyclen/Ortho Tri-Cyclen 1858
Ovcon 760
Ovral Tablets 2770

IMPORTANT NOTE: Always consult each drug listing in the patient's regimen for possible interactions.

Glucotrol XL

Interactions Index

Ovral-28 Tablets 2770
Levlen/Tri-Levlen 651
Tri-Norinyl 2164
Triphasil-21 Tablets 2814
Triphasil-28 Tablets 2819

Ethynodiol Diacetate (Potential for hyperglycemia leading to loss of control). Products include:

Demulen 2428

Etodolac (Potentiates the hypoglycemic action; patient should be observed for hypoglycemia or loss of control). Products include:

Lodine Capsules and Tablets 2743

Felodipine (Potential for hyperglycemia leading to loss of control). Products include:

Plendil Extended-Release Tablets 527

Fenoprofen Calcium (Potentiates the hypoglycemic action; patient should be observed for hypoglycemia or loss of control). Products include:

Nalfon 200 Pulvules & Nalfon Tablets 917

Fluconazole (Increase in the Glucotrol AUC by 56.9%). Products include:

Diflucan Injection, Tablets, and Oral Suspension 2194

Fludrocortisone Acetate (Potential for hyperglycemia leading to loss of control). Products include:

Florinef Acetate Tablets 505

Fluphenazine Decanoate (Potential for hyperglycemia leading to loss of control). Products include:

Prolixin Decanoate 509

Fluphenazine Enanthate (Potential for hyperglycemia leading to loss of control). Products include:

Prolixin Enanthate 509

Fluphenazine Hydrochloride (Potential for hyperglycemia leading to loss of control). Products include:

Prolixin 509

Flurazepam Hydrochloride (Potentiates the hypoglycemic action; patient should be observed for hypoglycemia or loss of control). Products include:

Dalmane Capsules 2173

Flurbiprofen (Potentiates the hypoglycemic action; patient should be observed for hypoglycemia or loss of control). Products include:

Ansaid Tablets 2579

Furazolidone (Potentiates the hypoglycemic action; patient should be observed for hypoglycemia or loss of control). Products include:

Furoxone 2046

Furosemide (Potential for hyperglycemia leading to loss of control). Products include:

Lasix Injection, Oral Solution and Tablets 1240

Glyburide (Potentiates the hypoglycemic action; patient should be observed for hypoglycemia or loss of control). Products include:

DiaBeta Tablets 1239
Glynase PresTab Tablets 2609
Micronase Tablets 2623

Hydrochlorothiazide (Potential for hyperglycemia leading to loss of control). Products include:

Aldactazide 2413
Aldoril Tablets 1604
Apresazide Capsules 808
Capozide 742
Dyazide 2479
Esidrix Tablets 821
Esimil Tablets 822
HydroDIURIL Tablets 1674
Hydropres Tablets 1675
Hyzaar Tablets 1677
Inderide Tablets 2732
Inderide LA Long Acting Capsules .. 2734

Lopressor HCT Tablets 832
Lotensin HCT 837
Maxzide 1380
Moduretic Tablets 1705
Oretic Tablets 443
Prinzide Tablets 1737
Ser-Ap-Es Tablets 849
Timolide Tablets 1748
Vaseretic Tablets 1765
Zestoretic 2850
Ziac 1415

Hydrocortisone (Potential for hyperglycemia leading to loss of control). Products include:

Anusol-HC Cream 2.5% 1896
Aquanil HC Lotion 1931
Bactine Hydrocortisone Anti-Itch Cream .... ᴹᴰ 709
Caldecort Anti-Itch Hydrocortisone Spray .... ᴹᴰ 631
Cortaid .... ᴹᴰ 836
CORTENEMA 2535
Cortisporin Ointment 1085
Cortisporin Ophthalmic Ointment Sterile 1085
Cortisporin Ophthalmic Suspension Sterile 1086
Cortisporin Otic Solution Sterile 1087
Cortisporin Otic Suspension Sterile 1088
Cortizone-5 .... ᴹᴰ 831
Cortizone-10 .... ᴹᴰ 831
Hydrocortone Tablets 1672
Hytone 907
Massengill Medicated Soft Cloth Towelettes 2458
PediOtic Suspension Sterile 1153
Preparation H Hydrocortisone 1% Cream .... ᴹᴰ 872
ProctoCream-HC 2.5% 2408
V6Sol HC Otic Solution 2678

Hydrocortisone Acetate (Potential for hyperglycemia leading to loss of control). Products include:

Analpram-HC Rectal Cream 1% and 2.5% 977
Anusol HC-1 Anti-Itch Hydrocortisone Ointment .... ᴹᴰ 847
Anusol-HC Suppositories 1897
Caldecort .... ᴹᴰ 631
Carmol HC 924
Coly-Mycin S Otic w/Neomycin & Hydrocortisone 1906
Cortaid .... ᴹᴰ 836
Cortifoam 2396
Cortisporin Cream 1084
Epifoam 2399
Hydrocortone Acetate Sterile Suspension 1669
Mantadil Cream 1135
Nupercainal Hydrocortisone 1% Cream .... ᴹᴰ 645
Ophthocort .... ◎ 311
Pramosone Cream, Lotion & Ointment 978
ProctoCream-HC 2408
ProctoFoam-HC 2409
Terra-Cortril Ophthalmic Suspension 2210

Hydrocortisone Sodium Phosphate (Potential for hyperglycemia leading to loss of control). Products include:

Hydrocortone Phosphate Injection, Sterile 1670

Hydrocortisone Sodium Succinate (Potential for hyperglycemia leading to loss of control). Products include:

Solu-Cortef Sterile Powder 2641

Hydroflumethiazide (Potential for hyperglycemia leading to loss of control). Products include:

Diucardin Tablets 2718

Ibuprofen (Potentiates the hypoglycemic action; patient should be observed for hypoglycemia or loss of control). Products include:

Advil Cold and Sinus Caplets and Tablets (formerly CoAdvil) .... ᴹᴰ 870
Advil Ibuprofen Tablets and Caplets .... ᴹᴰ 870
Children's Advil Suspension 2692
Arthritis Foundation Ibuprofen Tablets .... ᴹᴰ 674
Bayer Select Ibuprofen Pain Relief Formula .... ᴹᴰ 715

Cramp End Tablets .... ᴹᴰ 735
Dimetapp Sinus Caplets .... ᴹᴰ 775
Haltran Tablets .... ᴹᴰ 771
IBU Tablets 1342
Ibuprohm .... ᴹᴰ 735
Children's Motrin Ibuprofen Oral Suspension 1546
Motrin Tablets 2625
Motrin IB Caplets, Tablets, and Geltabs .... ᴹᴰ 838
Motrin IB Sinus .... ᴹᴰ 838
Motrin Ibuprofen Suspension, Oral Drops, Chewable Tablets, Caplets 1546
Nuprin Ibuprofen/Analgesic Tablets & Caplets .... ᴹᴰ 622
Sine-Aid IB Caplets 1554
Vicks DayQuil SINUS Pressure & PAIN Relief with IBUPROFEN ...... ᴹᴰ 762

Imipramine Hydrochloride (Potentiates the hypoglycemic action; patient should be observed for hypoglycemia or loss of control). Products include:

Tofranil Ampuls 854
Tofranil Tablets 856

Imipramine Pamoate (Potentiates the hypoglycemic action; patient should be observed for hypoglycemia or loss of control). Products include:

Tofranil-PM Capsules 857

Indapamide (Potential for hyperglycemia leading to loss of control). Products include:

Lozol Tablets 2022

Indomethacin (Potentiates the hypoglycemic action; patient should be observed for hypoglycemia or loss of control). Products include:

Indocin 1680

Indomethacin Sodium Trihydrate (Potentiates the hypoglycemic action; patient should be observed for hypoglycemia or loss of control). Products include:

Indocin I.V. 1684

Isocarboxazid (Potentiates the hypoglycemic action; patient should be observed for hypoglycemia or loss of control).

No products indexed under this heading.

Isoniazid (Potential for hyperglycemia leading to loss of control). Products include:

Nydrazid Injection 508
Rifamate Capsules 1530
Rifater 1532

Isoproterenol Hydrochloride (Potential for hyperglycemia leading to loss of control). Products include:

Isuprel Hydrochloride Injection 1:5000 2311
Isuprel Hydrochloride Solution 1:200 & 1:100 2313
Isuprel Mistometer 2312

Isoproterenol Sulfate (Potential for hyperglycemia leading to loss of control). Products include:

Norisodrine with Calcium Iodide Syrup 442

Isradipine (Potential for hyperglycemia leading to loss of control). Products include:

DynaCirc Capsules 2256

Ketoprofen (Potentiates the hypoglycemic action; patient should be observed for hypoglycemia or loss of control). Products include:

Orudis Capsules 2766
Oruvail Capsules 2766

Ketorolac Tromethamine (Potentiates the hypoglycemic action; patient should be observed for hypoglycemia or loss of control). Products include:

Acular 474
Acular .... ◎ 277
Toradol 2159

Labetalol Hydrochloride (Potentiates the hypoglycemic action; patient should be observed for hypoglycemia or loss of control). Products include:

Normodyne Injection 2377
Normodyne Tablets 2379
Trandate 1185

Levobunolol Hydrochloride (Potentiates the hypoglycemic action; patient should be observed for hypoglycemia or loss of control). Products include:

Betagan .... ◎ 233

Levonorgestrel (Potential for hyperglycemia leading to loss of control). Products include:

Levlen/Tri-Levlen 651
Nordette-21 Tablets 2755
Nordette-28 Tablets 2758
Norplant System 2759
Levlen/Tri-Levlen 651
Triphasil-21 Tablets 2814
Triphasil-28 Tablets 2819

Levothyroxine Sodium (Potential for hyperglycemia leading to loss of control). Products include:

Levothroid Tablets 1016
Levoxyl Tablets 903
Synthroid 1359

Liothyronine Sodium (Potential for hyperglycemia leading to loss of control). Products include:

Cytomel Tablets 2473
Triostat Injection 2530

Liotrix (Potential for hyperglycemia leading to loss of control).

No products indexed under this heading.

Magnesium Salicylate (Potentiates the hypoglycemic action; patient should be observed for hypoglycemia or loss of control). Products include:

Backache Caplets .... ᴹᴰ 613
Bayer Select Backache Pain Relief Formula .... ᴹᴰ 715
Doan's Extra-Strength Analgesic .... ᴹᴰ 633
Extra Strength Doan's P.M. .... ᴹᴰ 633
Doan's Regular Strength Analgesic .... ᴹᴰ 634
Mobigesic Tablets .... ᴹᴰ 602

Meclofenamate Sodium (Potentiates the hypoglycemic action; patient should be observed for hypoglycemia or loss of control).

No products indexed under this heading.

Mefenamic Acid (Potentiates the hypoglycemic action; patient should be observed for hypoglycemia or loss of control). Products include:

Ponstel 1925

Mesoridazine Besylate (Potential for hyperglycemia leading to loss of control). Products include:

Serentil 684

Mestranol (Potential for hyperglycemia leading to loss of control). Products include:

Norinyl 2088
Ortho-Novum 1872

Metaproterenol Sulfate (Potential for hyperglycemia leading to loss of control). Products include:

Alupent 669
Metaproterenol Sulfate Inhalation Solution, USP, Arm-a-Med 552

Metaraminol Bitartrate (Potential for hyperglycemia leading to loss of control). Products include:

Aramine Injection 1609

Methotrimeprazine (Potential for hyperglycemia leading to loss of control). Products include:

Levoprome 1274

Methoxamine Hydrochloride (Potential for hyperglycemia leading to loss of control). Products include:

Vasoxyl Injection 1196

(ᴹᴰ Described in PDR For Nonprescription Drugs) (◎ Described in PDR For Ophthalmology)

Methyclothiazide (Potential for hyperglycemia leading to loss of control). Products include:
Enduron Tablets ... 420

Methylprednisolone Acetate (Potential for hyperglycemia leading to loss of control). Products include:
Depo-Medrol Single-Dose Vial ... 2600
Depo-Medrol Sterile Aqueous Suspension ... 2597

Methylprednisolone Sodium Succinate (Potential for hyperglycemia leading to loss of control). Products include:
Solu-Medrol Sterile Powder ... 2643

Metipranolol Hydrochloride (Potentiates the hypoglycemic action; patient should be observed for hypoglycemia or loss of control). Products include:
OptiPranolol (Metipranolol 0.3%) Sterile Ophthalmic Solution ... ◉ 258

Metolazone (Potential for hyperglycemia leading to loss of control). Products include:
Mykrox Tablets ... 993
Zaroxolyn Tablets ... 1000

Metoprolol Succinate (Potentiates the hypoglycemic action; patient should be observed for hypoglycemia or loss of control). Products include:
Toprol-XL Tablets ... 565

Metoprolol Tartrate (Potentiates the hypoglycemic action; patient should be observed for hypoglycemia or loss of control). Products include:
Lopressor Ampuls ... 830
Lopressor HCT Tablets ... 832
Lopressor Tablets ... 830

Miconazole (Potential for severe hypoglycemia when co-administered with oral miconazole).
No products indexed under this heading.

Midazolam Hydrochloride (Potentiates the hypoglycemic action; patient should be observed for hypoglycemia or loss of control). Products include:
Versed Injection ... 2170

Nabumetone (Potentiates the hypoglycemic action; patient should be observed for hypoglycemia or loss of control). Products include:
Relafen Tablets ... 2510

Nadolol (Potentiates the hypoglycemic action; patient should be observed for hypoglycemia or loss of control).
No products indexed under this heading.

Naproxen (Potentiates the hypoglycemic action; patient should be observed for hypoglycemia or loss of control). Products include:
Anaprox/Naprosyn ... 2117

Naproxen Sodium (Potentiates the hypoglycemic action; patient should be observed for hypoglycemia or loss of control). Products include:
Aleve ... 1975
Anaprox/Naprosyn ... 2117

Niacin (Potential for hyperglycemia leading to loss of control). Products include:
Nicobid ... 2026
Nicolar Tablets ... 2026
Nicotinex Elixir ... ▣ 655
Sigtab Tablets ... ▣ 772
Slo-Niacin Tablets ... 2659
Stuart Prenatal Tablets ... ▣ 881
The Stuart Formula Tablets ... ▣ 663
Zymacap Capsules ... ▣ 772

Nicardipine Hydrochloride (Potential for hyperglycemia leading to loss of control). Products include:
Cardene Capsules ... 2095
Cardene I.V. ... 2709
Cardene SR Capsules ... 2097

Nicotinic Acid (Potential for hyperglycemia leading to loss of control).
No products indexed under this heading.

Nifedipine (Potential for hyperglycemia leading to loss of control). Products include:
Adalat Capsules (10 mg and 20 mg) ... 587
Adalat CC ... 589
Procardia Capsules ... 1971
Procardia XL Extended Release Tablets ... 1972

Nimodipine (Potential for hyperglycemia leading to loss of control). Products include:
Nimotop Capsules ... 610

Nisoldipine (Potential for hyperglycemia leading to loss of control).
No products indexed under this heading.

Norepinephrine Bitartrate (Potential for hyperglycemia leading to loss of control). Products include:
Levophed Bitartrate Injection ... 2315

Norethindrone (Potential for hyperglycemia leading to loss of control). Products include:
Brevicon ... 2088
Micronor Tablets ... 1872
Modicon ... 1872
Norinyl ... 2088
Nor-Q D Tablets ... 2135
Ortho-Novum ... 1872
Ovcon ... 760
Tri-Norinyl ... 2164

Norethynodrel (Potential for hyperglycemia leading to loss of control).
No products indexed under this heading.

Norgestimate (Potential for hyperglycemia leading to loss of control). Products include:
Ortho-Cyclen/Ortho-Tri-Cyclen ... 1858
Ortho-Cyclen/Ortho Tri-Cyclen ... 1858

Norgestrel (Potential for hyperglycemia leading to loss of control). Products include:
Lo/Ovral Tablets ... 2746
Lo/Ovral-28 Tablets ... 2751
Ovral Tablets ... 2770
Ovral-28 Tablets ... 2770
Ovrette Tablets ... 2771

Nortriptyline Hydrochloride (Potentiates the hypoglycemic action; patient should be observed for hypoglycemia or loss of control). Products include:
Pamelor ... 2280

Oxaprozin (Potentiates the hypoglycemic action; patient should be observed for hypoglycemia or loss of control). Products include:
Daypro Caplets ... 2426

Oxazepam (Potentiates the hypoglycemic action; patient should be observed for hypoglycemia or loss of control). Products include:
Serax Capsules ... 2810
Serax Tablets ... 2810

Penbutolol Sulfate (Potentiates the hypoglycemic action; patient should be observed for hypoglycemia or loss of control). Products include:
Levatol ... 2403

Perphenazine (Potential for hyperglycemia leading to loss of control). Products include:
Etrafon ... 2355
Triavil Tablets ... 1757
Trilafon ... 2389

Phenelzine Sulfate (Potentiates the hypoglycemic action; patient should be observed for hypoglycemia or loss of control). Products include:
Nardil ... 1920

Phenylbutazone (Potentiates the hypoglycemic action; patient should be observed for hypoglycemia or loss of control).
No products indexed under this heading.

Phenylephrine Bitartrate (Potential for hyperglycemia leading to loss of control).
No products indexed under this heading.

Phenylephrine Hydrochloride (Potential for hyperglycemia leading to loss of control). Products include:
Atrohist Plus Tablets ... 454
Cerose DM ... ▣ 878
Comhist ... 2038
D.A. Chewable Tablets ... 951
Deconsal Pediatric Capsules ... 454
Dura-Vent/DA Tablets ... 953
Entex Capsules ... 1986
Entex Liquid ... 1986
Extendryl ... 1005
4-Way Fast Acting Nasal Spray (regular & mentholated) ... ▣ 621
Hemorid For Women ... ▣ 834
Hycomine Compound Tablets ... 932
Neo-Synephrine Hydrochloride 1% Carpuject ... 2324
Neo-Synephrine Hydrochloride 1% Injection ... 2324
Neo-Synephrine Hydrochloride (Ophthalmic) ... 2325
Neo-Synephrine ... ▣ 726
Nōstril ... ▣ 644
Novahistine Elixir ... ▣ 823
Phenergan VC ... 2779
Phenergan VC with Codeine ... 2781
Preparation H ... ▣ 871
Tympagesic Ear Drops ... 2342
Vasosulf ... ◉ 271
Vicks Sinex Nasal Spray and Ultra Fine Mist ... ▣ 765

Phenylephrine Tannate (Potential for hyperglycemia leading to loss of control). Products include:
Atrohist Pediatric Suspension ... 454
Ricobid-D Pediatric Suspension ... 2038
Ricobid Tablets and Pediatric Suspension ... 2038
Rynatan ... 2673
Rynatuss ... 2673

Phenylpropanolamine Hydrochloride (Potential for hyperglycemia leading to loss of control). Products include:
Acutrim ... ▣ 628
Allerest Children's Chewable Tablets ... ▣ 627
Allerest 12 Hour Caplets ... ▣ 627
Atrohist Plus Tablets ... 454
BC Cold Powder Multi-Symptom Formula (Cold-Sinus-Allergy) ... ▣ 609
BC Cold Powder Non-Drowsy Formula (Cold-Sinus) ... ▣ 609
Cheracol Plus Head Cold/Cough Formula ... ▣ 769
Comtrex Multi-Symptom Non-Drowsy Liqui-gels ... ▣ 618
Contac Continuous Action Nasal Decongestant/Antihistamine 12 Hour Capsules ... ▣ 813
Contac Maximum Strength Continuous Action Decongestant/Antihistamine 12 Hour Caplets ... ▣ 813
Contac Severe Cold and Flu Formula Caplets ... ▣ 814
Coricidin 'D' Decongestant Tablets ... ▣ 800
Dexatrim ... ▣ 832
Dexatrim Plus Vitamins Caplets ... ▣ 832
Dimetane-DC Cough Syrup ... 2059
Dimetapp Elixir ... ▣ 773
Dimetapp Extentabs ... ▣ 774
Dimetapp Tablets/Liqui-Gels ... ▣ 775
Dimetapp Cold & Allergy Chewable Tablets ... ▣ 773
Dimetapp DM Elixir ... ▣ 774
Dura-Vent Tablets ... 952
Entex Capsules ... 1986
Entex LA Tablets ... 1987
Entex Liquid ... 1986
Exgest LA Tablets ... 782
Hycomine ... 931
Isoclor Timesule Capsules ... ▣ 637
Nolamine Timed-Release Tablets ... 785
Ornade Spansule Capsules ... 2502
Propagest Tablets ... 786
Pyrroxate Caplets ... ▣ 772
Robitussin-CF ... ▣ 777
Sinulin Tablets ... 787
Tavist-D 12 Hour Relief Tablets ... ▣ 787
Teldrin 12 Hour Antihistamine/Nasal Decongestant Allergy Relief Capsules ... ▣ 826
Triaminic Allergy Tablets ... ▣ 789
Triaminic Cold Tablets ... ▣ 790
Triaminic Expectorant ... ▣ 790
Triaminic Syrup ... ▣ 792
Triaminic-12 Tablets ... ▣ 792
Triaminic-DM Syrup ... ▣ 792
Triaminicin Tablets ... ▣ 793
Triaminicol Multi-Symptom Cold Tablets ... ▣ 793
Triaminicol Multi-Symptom Relief ... ▣ 794
Vicks DayQuil Allergy Relief 12-Hour Extended Release Tablets ... ▣ 760
Vicks DayQuil Allergy Relief 4-Hour Tablets ... ▣ 760
Vicks DayQuil SINUS Pressure & CONGESTION Relief ... ▣ 761

Phenytoin (Potential for hyperglycemia leading to loss of control). Products include:
Dilantin Infatabs ... 1908
Dilantin-125 Suspension ... 1911

Phenytoin Sodium (Potential for hyperglycemia leading to loss of control). Products include:
Dilantin Kapseals ... 1906
Dilantin Parenteral ... 1910

Pindolol (Potentiates the hypoglycemic action; patient should be observed for hypoglycemia or loss of control). Products include:
Visken Tablets ... 2299

Pirbuterol Acetate (Potential for hyperglycemia leading to loss of control). Products include:
Maxair Autohaler ... 1492
Maxair Inhaler ... 1494

Piroxicam (Potentiates the hypoglycemic action; patient should be observed for hypoglycemia or loss of control). Products include:
Feldene Capsules ... 1965

Polyestradiol Phosphate (Potential for hyperglycemia leading to loss of control).
No products indexed under this heading.

Polythiazide (Potential for hyperglycemia leading to loss of control). Products include:
Minizide Capsules ... 1938

Prednisolone Acetate (Potential for hyperglycemia leading to loss of control). Products include:
AK-CIDE ... ◉ 202
AK-CIDE Ointment ... ◉ 202
Blephamide Liquifilm Sterile Ophthalmic Suspension ... 476
Blephamide Ointment ... ◉ 237
Econopred & Econopred Plus Ophthalmic Suspensions ... ◉ 217
Poly-Pred Liquifilm ... ◉ 248
Pred Forte ... ◉ 250
Pred Mild ... ◉ 253
Pred-G Liquifilm Sterile Ophthalmic Suspension ... ◉ 251
Pred-G S.O.P. Sterile Ophthalmic Ointment ... ◉ 252
Vasocidin Ointment ... ◉ 268

Prednisolone Sodium Phosphate (Potential for hyperglycemia leading to loss of control). Products include:
AK-Pred ... ◉ 204
Hydeltrasol Injection, Sterile ... 1665
Inflamase ... ◉ 265
Pediapred Oral Liquid ... 995
Vasocidin Ophthalmic Solution ... ◉ 270

IMPORTANT NOTE: Always consult each drug listing in the patient's regimen for possible interactions.

Glucotrol XL

Prednisolone Tebutate (Potential for hyperglycemia leading to loss of control). Products include:

Hydeltra-T.B.A. Sterile Suspension 1667

Prednisone (Potential for hyperglycemia leading to loss of control). Products include:

Deltasone Tablets 2595

Probenecid (Potentiates the hypoglycemic action; patient should be observed for hypoglycemia or loss of control). Products include:

Benemid Tablets 1611
ColBENEMID Tablets 1622

Prochlorperazine (Potential for hyperglycemia leading to loss of control). Products include:

Compazine 2470

Promethazine Hydrochloride (Potential for hyperglycemia leading to loss of control). Products include:

Mepergan Injection 2753
Phenergan with Codeine 2777
Phenergan with Dextromethorphan 2778
Phenergan Injection 2773
Phenergan Suppositories 2775
Phenergan Syrup 2774
Phenergan Tablets 2775
Phenergan VC 2779
Phenergan VC with Codeine 2781

Propranolol Hydrochloride (Potentiates the hypoglycemic action; patient should be observed for hypoglycemia or loss of control). Products include:

Inderal 2728
Inderal LA Long Acting Capsules 2730
Inderide Tablets 2732
Inderide LA Long Acting Capsules .. 2734

Pseudoephedrine Hydrochloride (Potential for hyperglycemia leading to loss of control). Products include:

Actifed Allergy Daytime/Nighttime Caplets .... ◆D 844
Actifed Plus Caplets .... ◆D 845
Actifed Plus Tablets .... ◆D 845
Actifed with Codeine Cough Syrup.. 1067
Actifed Sinus Daytime/Nighttime Tablets and Caplets .... ◆D 846
Actifed Syrup .... ◆D 846
Actifed Tablets .... ◆D 844
Advil Cold and Sinus Caplets and Tablets (formerly CoAdvil) .... ◆D 870
Alka-Seltzer Plus Cold Medicine Liqui-Gels .... ◆D 706
Alka-Seltzer Plus Cold & Cough Medicine Liqui-Gels .... ◆D 705
Alka-Seltzer Plus Night-Time Cold Medicine Liqui-Gels .... ◆D 706
Allerest Headache Strength Tablets .... ◆D 627
Allerest Maximum Strength Tablets .... ◆D 627
Allerest No Drowsiness Tablets ..... ◆D 627
Allerest Sinus Pain Formula .... ◆D 627
Anatuss LA Tablets 1542
Atrohist Pediatric Capsules 453
Bayer Select Sinus Pain Relief Formula .... ◆D 717
Benadryl Allergy Decongestant Liquid Medication .... ◆D 848
Benadryl Allergy Decongestant Tablets .... ◆D 848
Benadryl Allergy Sinus Headache Formula Caplets .... ◆D 849
Benylin Multisymptom .... ◆D 852
Bromfed Capsules (Extended-Release) 1785
Bromfed Syrup .... ◆D 733
Bromfed Tablets 1785
Bromfed-DM Cough Syrup 1786
Bromfed-PD Capsules (Extended-Release) 1785
Children's Vicks DayQuil Allergy Relief .... ◆D 757
Children's Vicks NyQuil Cold/Cough Relief .... ◆D 758
Comtrex Multi-Symptom Cold Reliever Tablets/Caplets/Liqui-Gels/Liquid .... ◆D 615
Allergy-Sinus Comtrex Multi-Symptom Allergy-Sinus Formula Tablets .... ◆D 617
Comtrex Multi-Symptom Non-Drowsy Caplets .... ◆D 618
Congess 1004
Contac Day Allergy/Sinus Caplets ◆D 812
Contac Day & Night .... ◆D 812
Contac Night Allergy/Sinus Caplets .... ◆D 812
Contac Severe Cold & Flu Non-Drowsy .... ◆D 815
Deconamine Chewable Tablets 1320
Deconamine CX Cough and Cold Liquid and Tablets 1319
Deconamine 1320
Deconsal C Expectorant Syrup 456
Deconsal Pediatric Syrup 457
Deconsal II Tablets 454
Dimetane-DX Cough Syrup 2059
Dimetapp Sinus Caplets .... ◆D 775
Dorcol Children's Cough Syrup ...... ◆D 785
Drixoral Cough + Congestion Liquid Caps .... ◆D 802
Dura-Tap/PD Capsules 2867
Duratuss Tablets 2565
Duratuss HD Elixir 2565
Efidac/24 .... ◆D 635
Entex PSE Tablets 1987
Fedahist Gyrocaps 2401
Fedahist Timecaps 2401
Guaifed 1787
Guaifed Syrup .... ◆D 734
Guaimax-D Tablets 792
Guaitab Tablets .... ◆D 734
Isoclor Expectorant 990
Kronofed-A 977
Motrin IB Sinus .... ◆D 838
Novahistine DH 2462
Novahistine DMX .... ◆D 822
Novahistine Expectorant 2463
Nucofed 2051
PediaCare Cold Allergy Chewable Tablets .... ◆D 677
PediaCare Cough-Cold Chewable Tablets 1553
PediaCare 1553
PediaCare Infants' Decongestant Drops .... ◆D 677
PediCare Infant's Drops Decongestant Plus Cough 1553
PediaCare NightRest Cough-Cold Liquid 1553
Pediatric Vicks 44d Dry Hacking Cough & Head Congestion .... ◆D 763
Pediatric Vicks 44m Cough & Cold Relief .... ◆D 764
Robitussin Cold & Cough Liqui-Gels .... ◆D 776
Robitussin Maximum Strength Cough & Cold .... ◆D 778
Robitussin Pediatric Cough & Cold Formula .... ◆D 779
Robitussin Severe Congestion Liqui-Gels .... ◆D 776
Robitussin-DAC Syrup 2074
Robitussin-PE .... ◆D 778
Rondec Oral Drops 953
Rondec Syrup 953
Rondec Tablet 953
Rondec-DM Oral Drops 954
Rondec-DM Syrup 954
Rondec-TR Tablet 953
Ryna .... ◆D 841
Seldane-D Extended-Release Tablets 1538
Semprex-D Capsules 463
Semprex-D Capsules 1167
Sinarest Tablets .... ◆D 648
Sinarest Extra Strength Tablets ...... ◆D 648
Sinarest No Drowsiness Tablets .... ◆D 648
Sine-Aid IB Caplets 1554
Sine-Aid Maximum Strength Sinus Medication Gelcaps, Caplets and Tablets 1554
Sine-Off No Drowsiness Formula Caplets .... ◆D 824
Sine-Off Sinus Medicine .... ◆D 825
Singlet Tablets .... ◆D 825
Sinutab Non-Drying Liquid Caps .... ◆D 859
Sinutab Sinus Allergy Medication, Maximum Strength Tablets and Caplets .... ◆D 860
Sinutab Sinus Medication, Maximum Strength Without Drowsiness Formula, Tablets & Caplets .... ◆D 860
Sinutab Sinus Medication, Regular Strength Without Drowsiness Formula .... ◆D 859
Sudafed Children's Liquid .... ◆D 861
Sudafed Cold and Cough Liquidcaps .... ◆D 862
Sudafed Cough Syrup .... ◆D 862
Sudafed Plus Liquid .... ◆D 862
Sudafed Plus Tablets .... ◆D 863
Sudafed Severe Cold Formula Caplets .... ◆D 863
Sudafed Severe Cold Formula Tablets .... ◆D 864
Sudafed Sinus Caplets .... ◆D 864
Sudafed Sinus Tablets .... ◆D 864
Sudafed Tablets, 30 mg .... ◆D 861
Sudafed Tablets, 60 mg .... ◆D 861
Sudafed 12 Hour Caplets .... ◆D 861
Syn-Rx Tablets 465
Syn-Rx DM Tablets 466
TheraFlu .... ◆D 787
TheraFlu Maximum Strength Nighttime Flu, Cold & Cough Medicine .... ◆D 788
TheraFlu Maximum Strength Non-Drowsy Formula Flu, Cold & Cough Medicine .... ◆D 788
Thera Flu Maximum Strength, Non-Drowsy Formula Flu, Cold and Cough Caplets .... ◆D 789
Triaminic AM Cough and Decongestant Formula .... ◆D 789
Triaminic AM Decongestant Formula .... ◆D 790
Triaminic Nite Light .... ◆D 791
Triaminic Sore Throat Formula ...... ◆D 791
Tussend 1783
Tussend Expectorant 1785
Children's TYLENOL Cold Multi-Symptom Liquid Formula and Chewable Tablets 1561
Children's TYLENOL Cold Plus Cough Multi Symptom Tablets and Liquid .... ◆D 681
Infants' TYLENOL Cold Decongestant & Fever-Reducer Drops 1556
TYLENOL Maximum Strength Allergy Sinus Medication Gelcaps and Caplets 1563
TYLENOL Maximum Strength Allergy Sinus NightTime Medication Caplets 1555
TYLENOL Flu Maximum Strength Gelcaps 1565
TYLENOL Flu NightTime, Maximum Strength, Gelcaps 1566
TYLENOL Maximum Strength Flu NightTime Hot Medication Packets 1562
TYLENOL, Maximum Strength, Sinus Medication Geltabs, Gelcaps, Caplets and Tablets 1566
TYLENOL Cold Multi-Symptom Formula Medication Tablets and Caplets 1561
TYLENOL Cold Medication No Drowsiness Formula Gelcaps and Caplets 1562
TYLENOL Cold Multi-Symptom Hot Medication Liquid Packets 1557
TYLENOL Cough Multi-Symptom Medication with Decongestant 1565
Ursinus Inlay-Tabs .... ◆D 794
Vicks 44 LiquiCaps Cough, Cold & Flu Relief .... ◆D 755
Vicks 44 LiquiCaps Non-Drowsy Cough & Cold Relief .... ◆D 756
Vicks 44D Dry Hacking Cough & Head Congestion .... ◆D 755
Vicks 44M, Cough, Cold & Flu Relief .... ◆D 756
Vicks DayQuil .... ◆D 761
Vicks DayQuil SINUS Pressure & PAIN Relief with IBUPROFEN ...... ◆D 762
Vicks Nyquil Hot Therapy .... ◆D 762
Vicks NyQuil LiquiCaps Multi-Symptom Cold/Flu Relief .... ◆D 763
Vicks NyQuil Multi-Symptom Cold/Flu Relief - (Original & Cherry Flavor) .... ◆D 763

Pseudoephedrine Sulfate (Potential for hyperglycemia leading to loss of control). Products include:

Cheracol Sinus .... ◆D 768
Chlor-Trimeton Allergy Decongestant Tablets .... ◆D 799
Claritin-D 2350
Drixoral Cold and Allergy Sustained-Action Tablets .... ◆D 802
Drixoral Cold and Flu Extended-Release Tablets .... ◆D 803
Drixoral Non-Drowsy Formula Extended-Release Tablets .... ◆D 803
Drixoral Allergy/Sinus Extended Release Tablets .... ◆D 804
Trinalin Repetabs Tablets 1330

Quinestrol (Potential for hyperglycemia leading to loss of control).

No products indexed under this heading.

Salmeterol Xinafoate (Potential for hyperglycemia leading to loss of control). Products include:

Serevent Inhalation Aerosol 1176

Salsalate (Potentiates the hypoglycemic action; patient should be observed for hypoglycemia or loss of control). Products include:

Mono-Gesic Tablets 792
Salflex Tablets 786

Selegiline Hydrochloride (Potentiates the hypoglycemic action; patient should be observed for hypoglycemia or loss of control). Products include:

Eldepryl Tablets 2550

Sotalol Hydrochloride (Potentiates the hypoglycemic action; patient should be observed for hypoglycemia or loss of control). Products include:

Betapace Tablets 641

Spironolactone (Potential for hyperglycemia leading to loss of control). Products include:

Aldactazide 2413
Aldactone 2414

Sulfacytine (Potentiates the hypoglycemic action; patient should be observed for hypoglycemia or loss of control).

Sulfamethizole (Potentiates the hypoglycemic action; patient should be observed for hypoglycemia or loss of control). Products include:

Urobiotic-250 Capsules 2214

Sulfamethoxazole (Potentiates the hypoglycemic action; patient should be observed for hypoglycemia or loss of control). Products include:

Azo Gantanol Tablets 2080
Bactrim DS Tablets 2084
Bactrim I.V. Infusion 2082
Bactrim 2084
Gantanol Tablets 2119
Septra 1174
Septra I.V. Infusion 1169
Septra I.V. Infusion ADD-Vantage Vials 1171
Septra 1174

Sulfasalazine (Potentiates the hypoglycemic action; patient should be observed for hypoglycemia or loss of control). Products include:

Azulfidine 1949

Sulfinpyrazone (Potentiates the hypoglycemic action; patient should be observed for hypoglycemia or loss of control). Products include:

Anturane 807

Sulfisoxazole (Potentiates the hypoglycemic action; patient should be observed for hypoglycemia or loss of control). Products include:

Azo Gantrisin Tablets 2081
Gantrisin Tablets 2120

Sulfisoxazole Diolamine (Potentiates the hypoglycemic action; patient should be observed for hypoglycemia or loss of control).

No products indexed under this heading.

Sulindac (Potentiates the hypoglycemic action; patient should be observed for hypoglycemia or loss of control). Products include:

Clinoril Tablets 1618

Temazepam (Potentiates the hypoglycemic action; patient should be observed for hypoglycemia or loss of control). Products include:

Restoril Capsules 2284

(◆D Described in PDR For Nonprescription Drugs) (⊙ Described in PDR For Ophthalmology)

Terbutaline Sulfate (Potential for hyperglycemia leading to loss of control). Products include:

Brethaire Inhaler 813
Brethine Ampuls 815
Brethine Tablets 814
Bricanyl Subcutaneous Injection 1502
Bricanyl Tablets 1503

Thioridazine Hydrochloride (Potential for hyperglycemia leading to loss of control). Products include:

Mellaril 2269

Thyroglobulin (Potential for hyperglycemia leading to loss of control).

No products indexed under this heading.

Thyroid (Potential for hyperglycemia leading to loss of control).

No products indexed under this heading.

Thyroxine (Potential for hyperglycemia leading to loss of control).

No products indexed under this heading.

Thyroxine Sodium (Potential for hyperglycemia leading to loss of control).

No products indexed under this heading.

Timolol Hemihydrate (Potentiates the hypoglycemic action; patient should be observed for hypoglycemia or loss of control). Products include:

Betimol 0.25%, 0.5% .... ⊙ 261

Timolol Maleate (Potentiates the hypoglycemic action; patient should be observed for hypoglycemia or loss of control). Products include:

Blocadren Tablets 1614
Timolide Tablets................................... 1748
Timoptic in Ocudose 1753
Timoptic Sterile Ophthalmic Solution 1751
Timoptic-XE 1755

Tolazamide (Potentiates the hypoglycemic action; patient should be observed for hypoglycemia or loss of control).

No products indexed under this heading.

Tolbutamide (Potentiates the hypoglycemic action; patient should be observed for hypoglycemia or loss of control).

No products indexed under this heading.

Tolmetin Sodium (Potentiates the hypoglycemic action; patient should be observed for hypoglycemia or loss of control). Products include:

Tolectin (200, 400 and 600 mg) .. 1581

Torsemide (Potential for hyperglycemia leading to loss of control). Products include:

Demadex Tablets and Injection 686

Tranylcypromine Sulfate (Potentiates the hypoglycemic action; patient should be observed for hypoglycemia or loss of control). Products include:

Parnate Tablets 2503

Triamcinolone (Potential for hyperglycemia leading to loss of control). Products include:

Aristocort Tablets 1022

Triamcinolone Acetonide (Potential for hyperglycemia leading to loss of control). Products include:

Aristocort A 0.025% Cream 1027
Aristocort A 0.5% Cream 1031
Aristocort A 0.1% Cream 1029
Aristocort A 0.1% Ointment 1030
Azmacort Oral Inhaler 2011
Nasacort Nasal Inhaler 2024

Triamcinolone Diacetate (Potential for hyperglycemia leading to loss of control). Products include:

Aristocort Suspension (Forte Parenteral)... 1027
Aristocort Suspension (Intralesional)... 1025

Triamcinolone Hexacetonide (Potential for hyperglycemia leading to loss of control). Products include:

Aristospan Suspension (Intra-articular)... 1033
Aristospan Suspension (Intralesional)... 1032

Triamterene (Potential for hyperglycemia leading to loss of control). Products include:

Dyazide 2479
Dyrenium Capsules 2481
Maxzide 1380

Trifluoperazine Hydrochloride (Potential for hyperglycemia leading to loss of control). Products include:

Stelazine 2514

Trimipramine Maleate (Potentiates the hypoglycemic action; patient should be observed for hypoglycemia or loss of control). Products include:

Surmontil Capsules.............................. 2811

Verapamil Hydrochloride (Potential for hyperglycemia leading to loss of control). Products include:

Calan SR Caplets 2422
Calan Tablets.. 2419
Isoptin Injectable 1344
Isoptin Oral Tablets 1346
Isoptin SR Tablets 1348
Verelan Capsules 1410
Verelan Capsules 2824

Warfarin Sodium (Potentiates the hypoglycemic action; patient should be observed for hypoglycemia or loss of control). Products include:

Coumadin 926

Food Interactions

Diet, high-lipid (Administration of Glucotrol XL immediately before a high fat breakfast resulted in a 40% increase in the glipizide mean Cmax value; the effect on the AUC was not significant).

GLYNASE PRESTAB TABLETS

(Glyburide) 2609

May interact with beta blockers, thiazides, calcium channel blockers, non-steroidal anti-inflammatory agents, salicylates, sulfonamides, oral anticoagulants, monoamine oxidase inhibitors, sympathomimetics, oral contraceptives, diuretics, corticosteroids, phenothiazines, thyroid preparations, estrogens, and certain other agents. Compounds in these categories include:

Acebutolol Hydrochloride (Potentiates hypoglycemic action). Products include:

Sectral Capsules 2807

Albuterol (Concurrent administration may lead to loss of control due to hyperglycemia). Products include:

Proventil Inhalation Aerosol 2382
Ventolin Inhalation Aerosol and Refill 1197

Albuterol Sulfate (Concurrent administration may lead to loss of control due to hyperglycemia). Products include:

Airet Solution for Inhalation 452
Proventil Inhalation Solution 0.083% 2384
Proventil Repetabs Tablets 2386
Proventil Solution for Inhalation 0.5% 2383
Proventil Syrup 2385
Proventil Tablets 2386
Ventolin Inhalation Solution................ 1198
Ventolin Nebules Inhalation Solution 1199

Ventolin Rotacaps for Inhalation 1200
Ventolin Syrup...................................... 1202
Ventolin Tablets 1203
Volmax Extended-Release Tablets .. 1788

Amiloride Hydrochloride (Concurrent administration may lead to loss of control due to hyperglycemia). Products include:

Midamor Tablets 1703
Moduretic Tablets 1705

Amlodipine Besylate (Concurrent administration may lead to loss of control due to hyperglycemia). Products include:

Lotrel Capsules.................................... 840
Norvasc Tablets 1940

Aspirin (Potentiates hypoglycemic action). Products include:

Alka-Seltzer Effervescent Antacid and Pain Reliever .... ⊞ 701
Alka-Seltzer Extra Strength Effervescent Antacid and Pain Reliever .... ⊞ 703
Alka-Seltzer Lemon Lime Effervescent Antacid and Pain Reliever .... ⊞ 703
Alka-Seltzer Plus Cold Medicine .... ⊞ 705
Alka-Seltzer Plus Cold & Cough Medicine .... ⊞ 708
Alka-Seltzer Plus Night-Time Cold Medicine .... ⊞ 707
Alka Seltzer Plus Sinus Medicine .. ⊞ 707
Arthritis Foundation Safety Coated Aspirin Tablets .... ⊞ 675
Arthritis Pain Ascriptin .... ⊞ 631
Maximum Strength Ascriptin .... ⊞ 630
Regular Strength Ascriptin Tablets .... ⊞ 629
Arthritis Strength BC Powder.......... ⊞ 609
BC Cold Powder Multi-Symptom Formula (Cold-Sinus-Allergy) ...... ⊞ 609
BC Cold Powder Non-Drowsy Formula (Cold-Sinus) .... ⊞ 609
BC Powder .... ⊞ 609
Bayer Children's Chewable Aspirin .... ⊞ 711
Genuine Bayer Aspirin Tablets & Caplets .... ⊞ 713
Extra Strength Bayer Arthritis Pain Regimen Formula .... ⊞ 711
Extra Strength Bayer Aspirin Caplets & Tablets .... ⊞ 712
Extended-Release Bayer 8-Hour Aspirin .... ⊞ 712
Extra Strength Bayer Plus Aspirin Caplets .... ⊞ 713
Extra Strength Bayer PM Aspirin .. ⊞ 713
Bayer Enteric Aspirin .... ⊞ 709
Bufferin Analgesic Tablets and Caplets .... ⊞ 613
Arthritis Strength Bufferin Analgesic Caplets .... ⊞ 614
Extra Strength Bufferin Analgesic Tablets .... ⊞ 615
Cama Arthritis Pain Reliever........... ⊞ 785
Darvon Compound-65 Pulvules 1435
Easprin... 1914
Ecotrin 2455
Ecotrin Enteric Coated Aspirin Maximum Strength Tablets and Caplets .... ⊞ 816
Ecotrin Enteric Coated Aspirin Regular Strength Tablets 2455
Empirin Aspirin Tablets .... ⊞ 854
Empirin with Codeine Tablets........... 1093
Excedrin Extra-Strength Analgesic Tablets & Caplets 732
Fiorinal Capsules 2261
Fiorinal with Codeine Capsules 2262
Fiorinal Tablets 2261
Halfprin 1362
Healthprin Aspirin 2455
Norgesic... 1496
Percodan Tablets.................................. 939
Percodan-Demi Tablets....................... 940
Robaxisal Tablets................................. 2071
Soma Compound w/Codeine Tablets 2676
Soma Compound Tablets.................... 2675
St. Joseph Adult Chewable Aspirin (81 mg.) .... ⊞ 808
Talwin Compound 2335
Ursinus Inlay-Tabs............................... ⊞ 794
Vanquish Analgesic Caplets .... ⊞ 731

Atenolol (Potentiates hypoglycemic action). Products include:

Tenoretic Tablets.................................. 2845

Tenormin Tablets and I.V. Injection 2847

Bendroflumethiazide (Concurrent administration may lead to loss of control due to hyperglycemia; potentiates hypoglycemic action).

No products indexed under this heading.

Bepridil Hydrochloride (Concurrent administration may lead to loss of control due to hyperglycemia). Products include:

Vascor (200, 300 and 400 mg) Tablets 1587

Betamethasone Acetate (Concurrent administration may lead to loss of control due to hyperglycemia). Products include:

Celestone Soluspan Suspension 2347

Betamethasone Sodium Phosphate (Concurrent administration may lead to loss of control due to hyperglycemia). Products include:

Celestone Soluspan Suspension 2347

Betaxolol Hydrochloride (Potentiates hypoglycemic action). Products include:

Betoptic Ophthalmic Solution............ 469
Betoptic S Ophthalmic Suspension 471
Kerlone Tablets..................................... 2436

Bisoprolol Fumarate (Potentiates hypoglycemic action). Products include:

Zebeta Tablets 1413
Ziac 1415

Bumetanide (Concurrent administration may lead to loss of control due to hyperglycemia). Products include:

Bumex 2093

Carteolol Hydrochloride (Potentiates hypoglycemic action). Products include:

Cartrol Tablets 410
Ocupress Ophthalmic Solution, 1% Sterile... ⊙ 309

Chloramphenicol (Potentiates hypoglycemic action). Products include:

Chloromycetin Ophthalmic Ointment, 1% .... ⊙ 310
Chloromycetin Ophthalmic Solution .... ⊙ 310
Chloroptic S.O.P. .... ⊙ 239
Chloroptic Sterile Ophthalmic Solution .... ⊙ 239
Elase-Chloromycetin Ointment 1040
Ophthocort .... ⊙ 311

Chloramphenicol Palmitate (Potentiates hypoglycemic action).

No products indexed under this heading.

Chloramphenicol Sodium Succinate (Potentiates hypoglycemic action). Products include:

Chloromycetin Sodium Succinate 1900

Chlorothiazide (Concurrent administration may lead to loss of control due to hyperglycemia). Products include:

Aldoclor Tablets 1598
Diupres Tablets 1650
Diuril Oral 1653

Chlorothiazide Sodium (Concurrent administration may lead to loss of control due to hyperglycemia). Products include:

Diuril Sodium Intravenous 1652

Chlorotrianisene (Concurrent administration may lead to loss of control due to hyperglycemia).

No products indexed under this heading.

Chlorpromazine (Concurrent administration may lead to loss of control due to hyperglycemia). Products include:

Thorazine Suppositories 2523

IMPORTANT NOTE: Always consult each drug listing in the patient's regimen for possible interactions.

Glynase

Interactions Index

454

Chlorpromazine Hydrochloride (Concurrent administration may lead to loss of control due to hyperglycemia). Products include:

Thorazine 2523

Chlorthalidone (Concurrent administration may lead to loss of control due to hyperglycemia). Products include:

Combipres Tablets 677
Tenoretic Tablets 2845
Thalitone 1245

Choline Magnesium Trisalicylate (Potentiates hypoglycemic action). Products include:

Trilisate 2000

Ciprofloxacin (Potentiation of the hypoglycemic action). Products include:

Cipro I.V. 595
Cipro I.V. Pharmacy Bulk Package.. 597

Ciprofloxacin Hydrochloride (Potentiation of the hypoglycemic action). Products include:

Ciloxan Ophthalmic Solution 472
Cipro Tablets 592

Cortisone Acetate (Concurrent administration may lead to loss of control due to hyperglycemia). Products include:

Cortone Acetate Sterile Suspension 1623
Cortone Acetate Tablets 1624

Desogestrel (Concurrent administration may lead to loss of control due to hyperglycemia). Products include:

Desogen Tablets 1817
Ortho-Cept 1851

Dexamethasone (Concurrent administration may lead to loss of control due to hyperglycemia). Products include:

AK-Trol Ointment & Suspension .... ⊙ 205
Decadron Elixir 1633
Decadron Tablets 1635
Decaspray Topical Aerosol 1648
Dexacidin Ointment .... ⊙ 263
Maxitrol Ophthalmic Ointment and Suspension .... ⊙ 224
TobraDex Ophthalmic Suspension and Ointment 473

Dexamethasone Acetate (Concurrent administration may lead to loss of control due to hyperglycemia). Products include:

Dalalone D.P. Injectable 1011
Decadron-LA Sterile Suspension 1646

Dexamethasone Sodium Phosphate (Concurrent administration may lead to loss of control due to hyperglycemia). Products include:

Decadron Phosphate Injection 1637
Decadron Phosphate Respihaler 1642
Decadron Phosphate Sterile Ophthalmic Ointment 1641
Decadron Phosphate Sterile Ophthalmic Solution 1642
Decadron Phosphate Topical Cream 1644
Decadron Phosphate Turbinaire 1645
Decadron Phosphate with Xylocaine Injection, Sterile 1639
Dexacort Phosphate in Respihaler .. 458
Dexacort Phosphate in Turbinaire .. 459
NeoDecadron Sterile Ophthalmic Ointment 1712
NeoDecadron Sterile Ophthalmic Solution 1713
NeoDecadron Topical Cream 1714

Diclofenac Potassium (Potentiates hypoglycemic action). Products include:

Cataflam 816

Diclofenac Sodium (Potentiates hypoglycemic action). Products include:

Voltaren Ophthalmic Sterile Ophthalmic Solution .... ⊙ 272
Voltaren Tablets 861

Dicumarol (Potentiates hypoglycemic action).

No products indexed under this heading.

Dienestrol (Concurrent administration may lead to loss of control due to hyperglycemia). Products include:

Ortho Dienestrol Cream 1866

Diethylstilbestrol (Concurrent administration may lead to loss of control due to hyperglycemia). Products include:

Diethylstilbestrol Tablets 1437

Diflunisal (Potentiates hypoglycemic action). Products include:

Dolobid Tablets 1654

Diltiazem Hydrochloride (Concurrent administration may lead to loss of control due to hyperglycemia). Products include:

Cardizem CD Capsules 1506
Cardizem SR Capsules 1510
Cardizem Injectable 1508
Cardizem Tablets 1512
Dilacor XR Extended-release Capsules 2018

Dobutamine Hydrochloride (Concurrent administration may lead to loss of control due to hyperglycemia). Products include:

Dobutrex Solution Vials 1439

Dopamine Hydrochloride (Concurrent administration may lead to loss of control due to hyperglycemia).

No products indexed under this heading.

Ephedrine Hydrochloride (Concurrent administration may lead to loss of control due to hyperglycemia). Products include:

Primatene Dual Action Formula .... ▣ 872
Primatene Tablets .... ▣ 873
Quadrinal Tablets 1350

Ephedrine Sulfate (Concurrent administration may lead to loss of control due to hyperglycemia). Products include:

Bronkaid Caplets .... ▣ 717
Marax Tablets & DF Syrup 2200

Ephedrine Tannate (Concurrent administration may lead to loss of control due to hyperglycemia). Products include:

Rynatuss 2673

Epinephrine (Concurrent administration may lead to loss of control due to hyperglycemia). Products include:

Bronkaid Mist .... ▣ 717
EPIFRIN .... ⊙ 239
EpiPen 790
Marcaine Hydrochloride with Epinephrine 1:200,000 2316
Primatene Mist .... ▣ 873
Sensorcaine with Epinephrine Injection 559
Sus-Phrine Injection 1019
Xylocaine with Epinephrine Injections 567

Epinephrine Bitartrate (Concurrent administration may lead to loss of control due to hyperglycemia). Products include:

Bronkaid Mist Suspension .... ▣ 718
Sensorcaine-MPF with Epinephrine Injection 559

Epinephrine Hydrochloride (Concurrent administration may lead to loss of control due to hyperglycemia). Products include:

Ana-Kit Anaphylaxis Emergency Treatment Kit 617

Esmolol Hydrochloride (Potentiates hypoglycemic action). Products include:

Brevibloc Injection 1808

Estradiol (Concurrent administration may lead to loss of control due to hyperglycemia). Products include:

Climara Transdermal System 645
Estrace Cream and Tablets 749
Estraderm Transdermal System 824

Estrogens, Conjugated (Concurrent administration may lead to loss of control due to hyperglycemia). Products include:

PMB 200 and PMB 400 2783
Premarin Intravenous 2787
Premarin with Methyltestosterone .. 2794
Premarin Tablets 2789
Premarin Vaginal Cream 2791
Premphase 2797
Prempro 2801

Estrogens, Esterified (Concurrent administration may lead to loss of control due to hyperglycemia). Products include:

ESTRATAB Tablets (0.3, 0.625, 1.25, 2.5 mg) 2536
Estratest 2539
Menest Tablets 2494

Estropipate (Concurrent administration may lead to loss of control due to hyperglycemia). Products include:

Ogen Tablets 2627
Ogen Vaginal Cream 2630
Ortho-Est 1869

Ethacrynic Acid (Concurrent administration may lead to loss of control due to hyperglycemia). Products include:

Edecrin Tablets 1657

Ethinyl Estradiol (Concurrent administration may lead to loss of control due to hyperglycemia). Products include:

Brevicon 2088
Demulen 2428
Desogen Tablets 1817
Levlen/Tri-Levlen 651
Lo/Ovral Tablets 2746
Lo/Ovral-28 Tablets 2751
Modicon 1872
Nordette-21 Tablets 2755
Nordette-28 Tablets 2758
Norinyl 2088
Ortho-Cept 1851
Ortho-Cyclen/Ortho-Tri-Cyclen 1858
Ortho-Novum 1872
Ortho-Cyclen/Ortho Tri-Cyclen 1858
Ovcon 760
Ovral Tablets 2770
Ovral-28 Tablets 2770
Levlen/Tri-Levlen 651
Tri-Norinyl 2164
Triphasil-21 Tablets 2814
Triphasil-28 Tablets 2819

Ethynodiol Diacetate (Concurrent administration may lead to loss of control due to hyperglycemia). Products include:

Demulen 2428

Etodolac (Potentiates hypoglycemic action). Products include:

Lodine Capsules and Tablets 2743

Felodipine (Concurrent administration may lead to loss of control due to hyperglycemia). Products include:

Plendil Extended-Release Tablets 527

Fenoprofen Calcium (Potentiates hypoglycemic action). Products include:

Nalfon 200 Pulvules & Nalfon Tablets 917

Fludrocortisone Acetate (Concurrent administration may lead to loss of control due to hyperglycemia). Products include:

Florinef Acetate Tablets 505

Fluphenazine Decanoate (Concurrent administration may lead to loss of control due to hyperglycemia). Products include:

Prolixin Decanoate 509

Fluphenazine Enanthate (Concurrent administration may lead to loss of control due to hyperglycemia). Products include:

Prolixin Enanthate 509

Fluphenazine Hydrochloride (Concurrent administration may lead to loss of control due to hyperglycemia). Products include:

Prolixin 509

Flurbiprofen (Potentiates hypoglycemic action). Products include:

Ansaid Tablets 2579

Furazolidone (Potentiates hypoglycemic action). Products include:

Furoxone 2046

Furosemide (Concurrent administration may lead to loss of control due to hyperglycemia). Products include:

Lasix Injection, Oral Solution and Tablets 1240

Glipizide (Potentiates hypoglycemic action). Products include:

Glucotrol Tablets 1967
Glucotrol XL Extended Release Tablets 1968

Hydrochlorothiazide (Concurrent administration may lead to loss of control due to hyperglycemia). Products include:

Aldactazide 2413
Aldoril Tablets 1604
Apresazide Capsules 808
Capozide 742
Dyazide 2479
Esidrix Tablets 821
Esimil Tablets 822
HydroDIURIL Tablets 1674
Hydropres Tablets 1675
Hyzaar Tablets 1677
Inderide Tablets 2732
Inderide LA Long Acting Capsules .. 2734
Lopressor HCT Tablets 832
Lotensin HCT 837
Maxzide 1380
Moduretic Tablets 1705
Oretic Tablets 443
Prinzide Tablets 1737
Ser-Ap-Es Tablets 849
Timolide Tablets 1748
Vaseretic Tablets 1765
Zestoretic 2850
Ziac 1415

Hydrocortisone (Concurrent administration may lead to loss of control due to hyperglycemia). Products include:

Anusol-HC Cream 2.5% 1896
Aquanil HC Lotion 1931
Bactine Hydrocortisone Anti-Itch Cream .... ▣ 709
Caldecort Anti-Itch Hydrocortisone Spray .... ▣ 631
Cortaid .... ▣ 836
CORTENEMA 2535
Cortisporin Ointment 1085
Cortisporin Ophthalmic Ointment Sterile 1085
Cortisporin Ophthalmic Suspension Sterile 1086
Cortisporin Otic Solution Sterile 1087
Cortisporin Otic Suspension Sterile 1088
Cortizone-5 .... ▣ 831
Cortizone-10 .... ▣ 831
Hydrocortone Tablets 1672
Hytone 907
Massengill Medicated Soft Cloth Towelettes 2458
PediOtic Suspension Sterile 1153
Preparation H Hydrocortisone 1% Cream .... ▣ 872
ProctoCream-HC 2.5% 2408
VōSoL HC Otic Solution 2678

Hydrocortisone Acetate (Concurrent administration may lead to loss of control due to hyperglycemia). Products include:

Analpram-HC Rectal Cream 1% and 2.5% 977
Anusol HC-1 Anti-Itch Hydrocortisone Ointment .... ▣ 847
Anusol-HC Suppositories 1897
Caldecort .... ▣ 631
Carmol HC 924

(▣ Described in PDR For Nonprescription Drugs)

(⊙ Described in PDR For Ophthalmology)

455 **Interactions Index** **Glynase**

Coly-Mycin S Otic w/Neomycin & Hydrocortisone 1906
Cortaid .... ⊞ 836
Cortifoam 2396
Cortisporin Cream 1084
Epifoam 2399
Hydrocortone Acetate Sterile Suspension 1669
Mantadil Cream 1135
Nupercainal Hydrocortisone 1% Cream .... ⊞ 645
Ophthocort .... ◉ 311
Pramosone Cream, Lotion & Ointment 978
ProctoCream-HC 2408
ProctoFoam-HC 2409
Terra-Cortril Ophthalmic Suspension 2210

Hydrocortisone Sodium Phosphate (Concurrent administration may lead to loss of control due to hyperglycemia). Products include:
Hydrocortone Phosphate Injection, Sterile 1670

Hydrocortisone Sodium Succinate (Concurrent administration may lead to loss of control due to hyperglycemia). Products include:
Solu-Cortef Sterile Powder 2641

Hydroflumethiazide (Concurrent administration may lead to loss of control due to hyperglycemia). Products include:
Diucardin Tablets 2718

Ibuprofen (Potentiates hypoglycemic action). Products include:
Advil Cold and Sinus Caplets and Tablets (formerly CoAdvil) .... ⊞ 870
Advil Ibuprofen Tablets and Caplets .... ⊞ 870
Children's Advil Suspension 2692
Arthritis Foundation Ibuprofen Tablets .... ⊞ 674
Bayer Select Ibuprofen Pain Relief Formula .... ⊞ 715
Cramp End Tablets .... ⊞ 735
Dimetapp Sinus Caplets .... ⊞ 775
Haltran Tablets .... ⊞ 771
IBU Tablets 1342
Ibuprohm .... ⊞ 735
Children's Motrin Ibuprofen Oral Suspension 1546
Motrin Tablets 2625
Motrin IB Caplets, Tablets, and Geltabs .... ⊞ 838
Motrin IB Sinus .... ⊞ 838
Motrin Ibuprofen Suspension, Oral Drops, Chewable Tablets, Caplets 1546
Nuprin Ibuprofen/Analgesic Tablets & Caplets .... ⊞ 622
Sine-Aid IB Caplets 1554
Vicks DayQuil SINUS Pressure & PAIN Relief with IBUPROFEN .... ⊞ 762

Indapamide (Concurrent administration may lead to loss of control due to hyperglycemia). Products include:
Lozol Tablets 2022

Indomethacin (Potentiates hypoglycemic action). Products include:
Indocin 1680

Indomethacin Sodium Trihydrate (Potentiates hypoglycemic action). Products include:
Indocin I.V. 1684

Isocarboxazid (Potentiates hypoglycemic action).
No products indexed under this heading.

Isoniazid (Concurrent administration may lead to loss of control due to hyperglycemia). Products include:
Nydrazid Injection 508
Rifamate Capsules 1530
Rifater 1532

Isoproterenol Hydrochloride (Concurrent administration may lead to loss of control due to hyperglycemia). Products include:
Isuprel Hydrochloride Injection 1:5000 2311
Isuprel Hydrochloride Solution 1:200 & 1:100 2313
Isuprel Mistometer 2312

Isoproterenol Sulfate (Concurrent administration may lead to loss of control due to hyperglycemia). Products include:
Norisodrine with Calcium Iodide Syrup 442

Isradipine (Concurrent administration may lead to loss of control due to hyperglycemia). Products include:
DynaCirc Capsules 2256

Ketoprofen (Potentiates hypoglycemic action). Products include:
Orudis Capsules 2766
Oruvail Capsules 2766

Ketorolac Tromethamine (Potentiates hypoglycemic action). Products include:
Acular 474
Acular .... ◉ 277
Toradol 2159

Labetalol Hydrochloride (Potentiates hypoglycemic action). Products include:
Normodyne Injection 2377
Normodyne Tablets 2379
Trandate 1185

Levobunolol Hydrochloride (Potentiates hypoglycemic action). Products include:
Betagan .... ◉ 233

Levonorgestrel (Concurrent administration may lead to loss of control due to hyperglycemia). Products include:
Levlen/Tri-Levlen 651
Nordette-21 Tablets 2755
Nordette-28 Tablets 2758
Norplant System 2759
Levlen/Tri-Levlen 651
Triphasil-21 Tablets 2814
Triphasil-28 Tablets 2819

Levothyroxine Sodium (Concurrent administration may lead to loss of control due to hyperglycemia). Products include:
Levothroid Tablets 1016
Levoxyl Tablets 903
Synthroid 1359

Liothyronine Sodium (Concurrent administration may lead to loss of control due to hyperglycemia). Products include:
Cytomel Tablets 2473
Triostat Injection 2530

Liotrix (Concurrent administration may lead to loss of control due to hyperglycemia).
No products indexed under this heading.

Magnesium Salicylate (Potentiates hypoglycemic action). Products include:
Backache Caplets .... ⊞ 613
Bayer Select Backache Pain Relief Formula .... ⊞ 715
Doan's Extra-Strength Analgesic .... ⊞ 633
Extra Strength Doan's P.M. .... ⊞ 633
Doan's Regular Strength Analgesic .... ⊞ 634
Mobigesic Tablets .... ⊞ 602

Meclofenamate Sodium (Potentiates hypoglycemic action).
No products indexed under this heading.

Mefenamic Acid (Potentiates hypoglycemic action). Products include:
Ponstel 1925

Mesoridazine Besylate (Concurrent administration may lead to loss of control due to hyperglycemia). Products include:
Serentil 684

Mestranol (Concurrent administration may lead to loss of control due to hyperglycemia). Products include:
Norinyl 2088
Ortho-Novum 1872

Metaproterenol Sulfate (Concurrent administration may lead to loss of control due to hyperglycemia). Products include:
Alupent 669
Metaproterenol Sulfate Inhalation Solution, USP, Arm-a-Med 552

Metaraminol Bitartrate (Concurrent administration may lead to loss of control due to hyperglycemia). Products include:
Aramine Injection 1609

Methotrimeprazine (Concurrent administration may lead to loss of control due to hyperglycemia). Products include:
Levoprome 1274

Methoxamine Hydrochloride (Concurrent administration may lead to loss of control due to hyperglycemia). Products include:
Vasoxyl Injection 1196

Methyclothiazide (Concurrent administration may lead to loss of control due to hyperglycemia). Products include:
Enduron Tablets 420

Methylprednisolone Acetate (Concurrent administration may lead to loss of control due to hyperglycemia). Products include:
Depo-Medrol Single-Dose Vial 2600
Depo-Medrol Sterile Aqueous Suspension 2597

Methylprednisolone Sodium Succinate (Concurrent administration may lead to loss of control due to hyperglycemia). Products include:
Solu-Medrol Sterile Powder 2643

Metipranolol Hydrochloride (Potentiates hypoglycemic action). Products include:
OptiPranolol (Metipranolol 0.3%) Sterile Ophthalmic Solution .... ◉ 258

Metolazone (Concurrent administration may lead to loss of control due to hyperglycemia). Products include:
Mykrox Tablets 993
Zaroxolyn Tablets 1000

Metoprolol Succinate (Potentiates hypoglycemic action). Products include:
Toprol-XL Tablets 565

Metoprolol Tartrate (Potentiates hypoglycemic action). Products include:
Lopressor Ampuls 830
Lopressor HCT Tablets 832
Lopressor Tablets 830

Miconazole (Potential for severe hypoglycemia with concurrent administration of oral miconazole).
No products indexed under this heading.

Nabumetone (Potentiates hypoglycemic action). Products include:
Relafen Tablets 2510

Nadolol (Potentiates hypoglycemic action).
No products indexed under this heading.

Naproxen (Potentiates hypoglycemic action). Products include:
Anaprox/Naprosyn 2117

Naproxen Sodium (Potentiates hypoglycemic action). Products include:
Aleve 1975
Anaprox/Naprosyn 2117

Nicardipine Hydrochloride (Concurrent administration may lead to loss of control due to hyperglycemia). Products include:
Cardene Capsules 2095
Cardene I.V. 2709
Cardene SR Capsules 2097

Nicotinic Acid (Concurrent administration may lead to loss of control due to hyperglycemia).
No products indexed under this heading.

Nifedipine (Concurrent administration may lead to loss of control due to hyperglycemia). Products include:
Adalat Capsules (10 mg and 20 mg) 587
Adalat CC 589
Procardia Capsules 1971
Procardia XL Extended Release Tablets 1972

Nimodipine (Concurrent administration may lead to loss of control due to hyperglycemia). Products include:
Nimotop Capsules 610

Nisoldipine (Concurrent administration may lead to loss of control due to hyperglycemia).
No products indexed under this heading.

Norepinephrine Bitartrate (Concurrent administration may lead to loss of control due to hyperglycemia). Products include:
Levophed Bitartrate Injection 2315

Norethindrone (Concurrent administration may lead to loss of control due to hyperglycemia). Products include:
Brevicon 2088
Micronor Tablets 1872
Modicon 1872
Norinyl 2088
Nor-Q D Tablets 2135
Ortho-Novum 1872
Ovcon 760
Tri-Norinyl 2164

Norethynodrel (Concurrent administration may lead to loss of control due to hyperglycemia).
No products indexed under this heading.

Norgestimate (Concurrent administration may lead to loss of control due to hyperglycemia). Products include:
Ortho-Cyclen/Ortho-Tri-Cyclen 1858
Ortho-Cyclen/Ortho Tri-Cyclen 1858

Norgestrel (Concurrent administration may lead to loss of control due to hyperglycemia). Products include:
Lo/Ovral Tablets 2746
Lo/Ovral-28 Tablets 2751
Ovral Tablets 2770
Ovral-28 Tablets 2770
Ovrette Tablets 2771

Oxaprozin (Potentiates hypoglycemic action). Products include:
Daypro Caplets 2426

Penbutolol Sulfate (Potentiates hypoglycemic action). Products include:
Levatol 2403

Perphenazine (Concurrent administration may lead to loss of control due to hyperglycemia). Products include:
Etrafon 2355
Triavil Tablets 1757
Trilafon 2389

Phenelzine Sulfate (Potentiates hypoglycemic action). Products include:
Nardil 1920

Phenylbutazone (Potentiates hypoglycemic action).
No products indexed under this heading.

Phenylephrine Bitartrate (Concurrent administration may lead to loss of control due to hyperglycemia).
No products indexed under this heading.

IMPORTANT NOTE: Always consult each drug listing in the patient's regimen for possible interactions.

Glynase | Interactions Index | 456

Phenylephrine Hydrochloride (Concurrent administration may lead to loss of control due to hyperglycemia). Products include:

- Atrohist Plus Tablets ... 454
- Cerose DM ... ▣ 878
- Comhist ... 2038
- D.A. Chewable Tablets ... 951
- Deconsal Pediatric Capsules ... 454
- Dura-Vent/DA Tablets ... 953
- Entex Capsules ... 1986
- Entex Liquid ... 1986
- Extendryl ... 1005
- 4-Way Fast Acting Nasal Spray (regular & mentholated) ... ▣ 621
- Hemorid For Women ... ▣ 834
- Hycomine Compound Tablets ... 932
- Neo-Synephrine Hydrochloride 1% Carpuject ... 2324
- Neo-Synephrine Hydrochloride 1% Injection ... 2324
- Neo-Synephrine Hydrochloride (Ophthalmic) ... 2325
- Neo-Synephrine ... ▣ 726
- Nōstril ... ▣ 644
- Novahistine Elixir ... ▣ 823
- Phenergan VC ... 2779
- Phenergan VC with Codeine ... 2781
- Preparation H ... ▣ 871
- Tympagesic Ear Drops ... 2342
- Vasosulf ... ⊙ 271
- Vicks Sinex Nasal Spray and Ultra Fine Mist ... ▣ 765

Phenylephrine Tannate (Concurrent administration may lead to loss of control due to hyperglycemia). Products include:

- Atrohist Pediatric Suspension ... 454
- Ricobid-D Pediatric Suspension ... 2038
- Ricobid Tablets and Pediatric Suspension ... 2038
- Rynatan ... 2673
- Rynatuss ... 2673

Phenylpropanolamine Hydrochloride (Concurrent administration may lead to loss of control due to hyperglycemia). Products include:

- Acutrim ... ▣ 628
- Allerest Children's Chewable Tablets ... ▣ 627
- Allerest 12 Hour Caplets ... ▣ 627
- Atrohist Plus Tablets ... 454
- BC Cold Powder Multi-Symptom Formula (Cold-Sinus-Allergy) ... ▣ 609
- BC Cold Powder Non-Drowsy Formula (Cold-Sinus) ... ▣ 609
- Cheracol Plus Head Cold/Cough Formula ... ▣ 769
- Comtrex Multi-Symptom Non-Drowsy Liqui-gels ... ▣ 618
- Contac Continuous Action Nasal Decongestant/Antihistamine 12 Hour Capsules ... ▣ 813
- Contac Maximum Strength Continuous Action Decongestant/Antihistamine 12 Hour Caplets ... ▣ 813
- Contac Severe Cold and Flu Formula Caplets ... ▣ 814
- Coricidin 'D' Decongestant Tablets ... ▣ 800
- Dexatrim ... ▣ 832
- Dexatrim Plus Vitamins Caplets ... ▣ 832
- Dimetane-DC Cough Syrup ... 2059
- Dimetapp Elixir ... ▣ 773
- Dimetapp Extentabs ... ▣ 774
- Dimetapp Tablets/Liqui-Gels ... ▣ 775
- Dimetapp Cold & Allergy Chewable Tablets ... ▣ 773
- Dimetapp DM Elixir ... ▣ 774
- Dura-Vent Tablets ... 952
- Entex Capsules ... 1986
- Entex LA Tablets ... 1987
- Entex Liquid ... 1986
- Exgest LA Tablets ... 782
- Hycomine ... 931
- Isoclor Timesule Capsules ... ▣ 637
- Nolamine Timed-Release Tablets ... 785
- Ornade Spansule Capsules ... 2502
- Propagest Tablets ... 786
- Pyrroxate Caplets ... ▣ 772
- Robitussin-CF ... ▣ 777
- Sinulin Tablets ... 787
- Tavist-D 12 Hour Relief Tablets ... ▣ 787
- Teldrin 12 Hour Antihistamine/Nasal Decongestant Allergy Relief Capsules ... ▣ 826
- Triaminic Allergy Tablets ... ▣ 789
- Triaminic Cold Tablets ... ▣ 790
- Triaminic Expectorant ... ▣ 790
- Triaminic Syrup ... ▣ 792
- Triaminic-12 Tablets ... ▣ 792
- Triaminic-DM Syrup ... ▣ 792
- Triaminicin Tablets ... ▣ 793
- Triaminicol Multi-Symptom Cold Tablets ... ▣ 793
- Triaminicol Multi-Symptom Relief ... ▣ 794
- Vicks DayQuil Allergy Relief 12-Hour Extended Release Tablets ... ▣ 760
- Vicks DayQuil Allergy Relief 4-Hour Tablets ... ▣ 760
- Vicks DayQuil SINUS Pressure & CONGESTION Relief ... ▣ 761

Phenytoin (Concurrent administration may lead to loss of control due to hyperglycemia). Products include:

- Dilantin Infatabs ... 1908
- Dilantin-125 Suspension ... 1911

Phenytoin Sodium (Concurrent administration may lead to loss of control due to hyperglycemia). Products include:

- Dilantin Kapseals ... 1906
- Dilantin Parenteral ... 1910

Pindolol (Potentiates hypoglycemic action). Products include:

- Visken Tablets ... 2299

Pirbuterol Acetate (Concurrent administration may lead to loss of control due to hyperglycemia). Products include:

- Maxair Autohaler ... 1492
- Maxair Inhaler ... 1494

Piroxicam (Potentiates hypoglycemic action). Products include:

- Feldene Capsules ... 1965

Polyestradiol Phosphate (Concurrent administration may lead to loss of control due to hyperglycemia).

- No products indexed under this heading.

Polythiazide (Concurrent administration may lead to loss of control due to hyperglycemia). Products include:

- Minizide Capsules ... 1938

Prednisolone Acetate (Concurrent administration may lead to loss of control due to hyperglycemia). Products include:

- AK-CIDE ... ⊙ 202
- AK-CIDE Ointment ... ⊙ 202
- Blephamide Liquifilm Sterile Ophthalmic Suspension ... 476
- Blephamide Ointment ... ⊙ 237
- Econopred & Econopred Plus Ophthalmic Suspensions ... ⊙ 217
- Poly-Pred Liquifilm ... ⊙ 248
- Pred Forte ... ⊙ 250
- Pred Mild ... ⊙ 253
- Pred-G Liquifilm Sterile Ophthalmic Suspension ... ⊙ 251
- Pred-G S.O.P. Sterile Ophthalmic Ointment ... ⊙ 252
- Vasocidin Ointment ... ⊙ 268

Prednisolone Sodium Phosphate (Concurrent administration may lead to loss of control due to hyperglycemia). Products include:

- AK-Pred ... ⊙ 204
- Hydeltrasol Injection, Sterile ... 1665
- Inflamase ... ⊙ 265
- Pediapred Oral Liquid ... 995
- Vasocidin Ophthalmic Solution ... ⊙ 270

Prednisolone Tebutate (Concurrent administration may lead to loss of control due to hyperglycemia). Products include:

- Hydeltra-T.B.A. Sterile Suspension ... 1667

Prednisone (Concurrent administration may lead to loss of control due to hyperglycemia). Products include:

- Deltasone Tablets ... 2595

Probenecid (Potentiates hypoglycemic action). Products include:

- Benemid Tablets ... 1611
- ColBENEMID Tablets ... 1622

Prochlorperazine (Concurrent administration may lead to loss of control due to hyperglycemia). Products include:

- Compazine ... 2470

Promethazine Hydrochloride (Concurrent administration may lead to loss of control due to hyperglycemia). Products include:

- Mepergan Injection ... 2753
- Phenergan with Codeine ... 2777
- Phenergan with Dextromethorphan ... 2778
- Phenergan Injection ... 2773
- Phenergan Suppositories ... 2775
- Phenergan Syrup ... 2774
- Phenergan Tablets ... 2775
- Phenergan VC ... 2779
- Phenergan VC with Codeine ... 2781

Propranolol Hydrochloride (Potentiates hypoglycemic action). Products include:

- Inderal ... 2728
- Inderal LA Long Acting Capsules ... 2730
- Inderide Tablets ... 2732
- Inderide LA Long Acting Capsules ... 2734

Pseudoephedrine Hydrochloride (Concurrent administration may lead to loss of control due to hyperglycemia). Products include:

- Actifed Allergy Daytime/Nighttime Caplets ... ▣ 844
- Actifed Plus Caplets ... ▣ 845
- Actifed Plus Tablets ... ▣ 845
- Actifed with Codeine Cough Syrup ... 1067
- Actifed Sinus Daytime/Nighttime Tablets and Caplets ... ▣ 846
- Actifed Syrup ... ▣ 846
- Actifed Tablets ... ▣ 844
- Advil Cold and Sinus Caplets and Tablets (formerly CoAdvil) ... ▣ 870
- Alka-Seltzer Plus Cold Medicine Liqui-Gels ... ▣ 706
- Alka-Seltzer Plus Cold & Cough Medicine Liqui-Gels ... ▣ 705
- Alka-Seltzer Plus Night-Time Cold Medicine Liqui-Gels ... ▣ 706
- Allerest Headache Strength Tablets ... ▣ 627
- Allerest Maximum Strength Tablets ... ▣ 627
- Allerest No Drowsiness Tablets ... ▣ 627
- Allerest Sinus Pain Formula ... ▣ 627
- Anatuss LA Tablets ... 1542
- Atrohist Pediatric Capsules ... 453
- Bayer Select Sinus Pain Relief Formula ... ▣ 717
- Benadryl Allergy Decongestant Liquid Medication ... ▣ 848
- Benadryl Allergy Decongestant Tablets ... ▣ 848
- Benadryl Allergy Sinus Headache Formula Caplets ... ▣ 849
- Benylin Multisymptom ... ▣ 852
- Bromfed Capsules (Extended-Release) ... 1785
- Bromfed Syrup ... ▣ 733
- Bromfed Tablets ... 1785
- Bromfed-DM Cough Syrup ... 1786
- Bromfed-PD Capsules (Extended-Release) ... 1785
- Children's Vicks DayQuil Allergy Relief ... ▣ 757
- Children's Vicks NyQuil Cold/Cough Relief ... ▣ 758
- Comtrex Multi-Symptom Cold Reliever Tablets/Caplets/Liqui-Gels/Liquid ... ▣ 615
- Allergy-Sinus Comtrex Multi-Symptom Allergy-Sinus Formula Tablets ... ▣ 617
- Comtrex Multi-Symptom Non-Drowsy Caplets ... ▣ 618
- Congess ... 1004
- Contac Day Allergy/Sinus Caplets ... ▣ 812
- Contac Day & Night ... ▣ 812
- Contac Night Allergy/Sinus Caplets ... ▣ 812
- Contac Severe Cold & Flu Non-Drowsy ... ▣ 815
- Deconamine Chewable Tablets ... 1320
- Deconamine CX Cough and Cold Liquid and Tablets ... 1319
- Deconamine ... 1320
- Deconsal C Expectorant Syrup ... 456
- Deconsal Pediatric Syrup ... 457
- Deconsal II Tablets ... 454
- Dimetane-DX Cough Syrup ... 2059
- Dimetapp Sinus Caplets ... ▣ 775
- Dorcol Children's Cough Syrup ... ▣ 785
- Drixoral Cough + Congestion Liquid Caps ... ▣ 802
- Dura-Tap/PD Capsules ... 2867
- Duratuss Tablets ... 2565
- Duratuss HD Elixir ... 2565
- Efidac/24 ... ▣ 635
- Entex PSE Tablets ... 1987
- Fedahist Gyrocaps ... 2401
- Fedahist Timecaps ... 2401
- Guaifed ... 1787
- Guaifed Syrup ... ▣ 734
- Guaimax-D Tablets ... 792
- Guaitab Tablets ... ▣ 734
- Isoclor Expectorant ... 990
- Kronofed-A ... 977
- Motrin IB Sinus ... ▣ 838
- Novahistine DH ... 2462
- Novahistine DMX ... ▣ 822
- Novahistine Expectorant ... 2463
- Nucofed ... 2051
- PediaCare Cold Allergy Chewable Tablets ... ▣ 677
- PediaCare Cough-Cold Chewable Tablets ... 1553
- PediaCare ... 1553
- PediaCare Infants' Decongestant Drops ... ▣ 677
- PediCare Infant's Drops Decongestant Plus Cough ... 1553
- PediaCare NightRest Cough-Cold Liquid ... 1553
- Pediatric Vicks 44d Dry Hacking Cough & Head Congestion ... ▣ 763
- Pediatric Vicks 44m Cough & Cold Relief ... ▣ 764
- Robitussin Cold & Cough Liqui-Gels ... ▣ 776
- Robitussin Maximum Strength Cough & Cold ... ▣ 778
- Robitussin Pediatric Cough & Cold Formula ... ▣ 779
- Robitussin Severe Congestion Liqui-Gels ... ▣ 776
- Robitussin-DAC Syrup ... 2074
- Robitussin-PE ... ▣ 778
- Rondec Oral Drops ... 953
- Rondec Syrup ... 953
- Rondec Tablet ... 953
- Rondec-DM Oral Drops ... 954
- Rondec-DM Syrup ... 954
- Rondec-TR Tablet ... 953
- Ryna ... ▣ 841
- Seldane-D Extended-Release Tablets ... 1538
- Semprex-D Capsules ... 463
- Semprex-D Capsules ... 1167
- Sinarest Tablets ... ▣ 648
- Sinarest Extra Strength Tablets ... ▣ 648
- Sinarest No Drowsiness Tablets ... ▣ 648
- Sine-Aid IB Caplets ... 1554
- Sine-Aid Maximum Strength Sinus Medication Gelcaps, Caplets and Tablets ... 1554
- Sine-Off No Drowsiness Formula Caplets ... ▣ 824
- Sine-Off Sinus Medicine ... ▣ 825
- Singlet Tablets ... ▣ 825
- Sinutab Non-Drying Liquid Caps ... ▣ 859
- Sinutab Sinus Allergy Medication, Maximum Strength Tablets and Caplets ... ▣ 860
- Sinutab Sinus Medication, Maximum Strength Without Drowsiness Formula, Tablets & Caplets ... ▣ 860
- Sinutab Sinus Medication, Regular Strength Without Drowsiness Formula ... ▣ 859
- Sudafed Children's Liquid ... ▣ 861
- Sudafed Cold and Cough Liquidcaps ... ▣ 862
- Sudafed Cough Syrup ... ▣ 862
- Sudafed Plus Liquid ... ▣ 862
- Sudafed Plus Tablets ... ▣ 863
- Sudafed Severe Cold Formula Caplets ... ▣ 863
- Sudafed Severe Cold Formula Tablets ... ▣ 864
- Sudafed Sinus Caplets ... ▣ 864
- Sudafed Sinus Tablets ... ▣ 864
- Sudafed Tablets, 30 mg ... ▣ 861
- Sudafed Tablets, 60 mg ... ▣ 861
- Sudafed 12 Hour Caplets ... ▣ 861
- Syn-Rx Tablets ... 465
- Syn-Rx DM Tablets ... 466
- TheraFlu ... ▣ 787
- TheraFlu Maximum Strength Nighttime Flu, Cold & Cough Medicine ... ▣ 788

(▣ Described in PDR For Nonprescription Drugs) (⊙ Described in PDR For Ophthalmology)

Interactions Index

TheraFlu Maximum Strength Non-Drowsy Formula Flu, Cold & Cough Medicine .... ✦ 788

Thera Flu Maximum Strength, Non-Drowsy Formula Flu, Cold and Cough Caplets .... ✦ 789

Triaminic AM Cough and Decongestant Formula .... ✦ 789

Triaminic AM Decongestant Formula .... ✦ 790

Triaminic Nite Light .... ✦ 791

Triaminic Sore Throat Formula ..... ✦ 791

Tussend 1783

Tussend Expectorant 1785

Children's TYLENOL Cold Multi-Symptom Liquid Formula and Chewable Tablets................................ 1561

Children's TYLENOL Cold Plus Cough Multi Symptom Tablets and Liquid .... ✦ 681

Infants' TYLENOL Cold Decongestant & Fever-Reducer Drops 1556

TYLENOL Maximum Strength Allergy Sinus Medication Gelcaps and Caplets 1563

TYLENOL Maximum Strength Allergy Sinus NightTime Medication Caplets 1555

TYLENOL Flu Maximum Strength Gelcaps 1565

TYLENOL Flu NightTime, Maximum Strength, Gelcaps 1566

TYLENOL Maximum Strength Flu NightTime Hot Medication Packets 1562

TYLENOL, Maximum Strength, Sinus Medication Geltabs, Gelcaps, Caplets and Tablets 1566

TYLENOL Cold Multi-Symptom Formula Medication Tablets and Caplets 1561

TYLENOL Cold Medication No Drowsiness Formula Gelcaps and Caplets 1562

TYLENOL Cold Multi-Symptom Hot Medication Liquid Packets 1557

TYLENOL Cough Multi-Symptom Medication with Decongestant 1565

Ursinus Inlay-Tabs .... ✦ 794

Vicks 44 LiquiCaps Cough, Cold & Flu Relief .... ✦ 755

Vicks 44 LiquiCaps Non-Drowsy Cough & Cold Relief .... ✦ 756

Vicks 44D Dry Hacking Cough & Head Congestion .... ✦ 755

Vicks 44M Cough, Cold & Flu Relief .... ✦ 756

Vicks DayQuil .... ✦ 761

Vicks DayQuil SINUS Pressure & PAIN Relief with IBUPROFEN ...... ✦ 762

Vicks Nyquil Hot Therapy .... ✦ 762

Vicks NyQuil LiquiCaps Multi-Symptom Cold/Flu Relief .... ✦ 763

Vicks NyQuil Multi-Symptom Cold/Flu Relief - (Original & Cherry Flavor) .... ✦ 763

Pseudoephedrine Sulfate (Concurrent administration may lead to loss of control due to hyperglycemia). Products include:

Cheracol Sinus .... ✦ 768

Chlor-Trimeton Allergy Decongestant Tablets .... ✦ 799

Claritin-D 2350

Drixoral Cold and Allergy Sustained-Action Tablets .... ✦ 802

Drixoral Cold and Flu Extended-Release Tablets .... ✦ 803

Drixoral Non-Drowsy Formula Extended-Release Tablets .... ✦ 803

Drixoral Allergy/Sinus Extended Release Tablets .... ✦ 804

Trinalin Repetabs Tablets 1330

Quinestrol (Concurrent administration may lead to loss of control due to hyperglycemia).

No products indexed under this heading.

Salmeterol Xinafoate (Concurrent administration may lead to loss of control due to hyperglycemia). Products include:

Serevent Inhalation Aerosol 1176

Salsalate (Potentiates hypoglycemic action). Products include:

Mono-Gesic Tablets 792

Salflex Tablets 786

Selegiline Hydrochloride (Potentiates hypoglycemic action). Products include:

Eldepryl Tablets 2550

Sotalol Hydrochloride (Potentiates hypoglycemic action). Products include:

Betapace Tablets 641

Spironolactone (Concurrent administration may lead to loss of control due to hyperglycemia). Products include:

Aldactazide 2413

Aldactone 2414

Sulfacytine (Potentiates hypoglycemic action).

Sulfamethizole (Potentiates hypoglycemic action). Products include:

Urobiotic-250 Capsules 2214

Sulfamethoxazole (Potentiates hypoglycemic action). Products include:

Azo Gantanol Tablets 2080

Bactrim DS Tablets 2084

Bactrim I.V. Infusion 2082

Bactrim 2084

Gantanol Tablets 2119

Septra 1174

Septra I.V. Infusion 1169

Septra I.V. Infusion ADD-Vantage Vials 1171

Septra 1174

Sulfasalazine (Potentiates hypoglycemic action). Products include:

Azulfidine 1949

Sulfinpyrazone (Potentiates hypoglycemic action). Products include:

Anturane 807

Sulfisoxazole (Potentiates hypoglycemic action). Products include:

Azo Gantrisin Tablets 2081

Gantrisin Tablets 2120

Sulfisoxazole Diolamine (Potentiates hypoglycemic action).

No products indexed under this heading.

Sulindac (Potentiates hypoglycemic action). Products include:

Clinoril Tablets 1618

Terbutaline Sulfate (Concurrent administration may lead to loss of control due to hyperglycemia). Products include:

Brethaire Inhaler 813

Brethine Ampuls 815

Brethine Tablets 814

Bricanyl Subcutaneous Injection 1502

Bricanyl Tablets 1503

Thioridazine Hydrochloride (Concurrent administration may lead to loss of control due to hyperglycemia). Products include:

Mellaril 2269

Thyroglobulin (Concurrent administration may lead to loss of control due to hyperglycemia).

No products indexed under this heading.

Thyroid (Concurrent administration may lead to loss of control due to hyperglycemia).

No products indexed under this heading.

Thyroxine (Concurrent administration may lead to loss of control due to hyperglycemia).

No products indexed under this heading.

Thyroxine Sodium (Concurrent administration may lead to loss of control due to hyperglycemia).

No products indexed under this heading.

Timolol Hemihydrate (Potentiates hypoglycemic action). Products include:

Betimol 0.25%, 0.5% .... © 261

Timolol Maleate (Potentiates hypoglycemic action). Products include:

Blocadren Tablets 1614

Timolide Tablets 1748

Timoptic in Ocudose 1753

Timoptic Sterile Ophthalmic Solution 1751

Timoptic-XE 1755

Tolazamide (Potentiates hypoglycemic action).

No products indexed under this heading.

Tolbutamide (Potentiates hypoglycemic action).

No products indexed under this heading.

Tolmetin Sodium (Potentiates hypoglycemic action). Products include:

Tolectin (200, 400 and 600 mg) .. 1581

Torsemide (Concurrent administration may lead to loss of control due to hyperglycemia). Products include:

Demadex Tablets and Injection 686

Tranylcypromine Sulfate (Potentiates hypoglycemic action). Products include:

Parnate Tablets 2503

Triamcinolone (Concurrent administration may lead to loss of control due to hyperglycemia). Products include:

Aristocort Tablets 1022

Triamcinolone Acetonide (Concurrent administration may lead to loss of control due to hyperglycemia). Products include:

Aristocort A 0.025% Cream 1027

Aristocort A 0.5% Cream 1031

Aristocort A 0.1% Cream 1029

Aristocort A 0.1% Ointment 1030

Azmacort Oral Inhaler 2011

Nasacort Nasal Inhaler 2024

Triamcinolone Diacetate (Concurrent administration may lead to loss of control due to hyperglycemia). Products include:

Aristocort Suspension (Forte Parenteral) 1027

Aristocort Suspension (Intralesional) 1025

Triamcinolone Hexacetonide (Concurrent administration may lead to loss of control due to hyperglycemia). Products include:

Aristospan Suspension (Intra-articular) 1033

Aristospan Suspension (Intralesional) 1032

Triamterene (Concurrent administration may lead to loss of control due to hyperglycemia). Products include:

Dyazide 2479

Dyrenium Capsules 2481

Maxzide 1380

Trifluoperazine Hydrochloride (Concurrent administration may lead to loss of control due to hyperglycemia). Products include:

Stelazine 2514

Verapamil Hydrochloride (Concurrent administration may lead to loss of control due to hyperglycemia). Products include:

Calan SR Caplets 2422

Calan Tablets 2419

Isoptin Injectable 1344

Isoptin Oral Tablets 1346

Isoptin SR Tablets 1348

Verelan Capsules 1410

Verelan Capsules 2824

Warfarin Sodium (Potentiates hypoglycemic action). Products include:

Coumadin 926

GLY-OXIDE LIQUID

(Carbamide Peroxide) .... ✦ 820

None cited in PDR database.

GOLYTELY

(Polyethylene Glycol) 688

May interact with:

Oral Medications, unspecified

(Those administered within one hour of GoLYTELY usage may be flushed from the gastrointestinal tract and not absorbed).

Food Interactions

Food, unspecified (For best results, no solid food should be consumed during 3 to 4 hour period before drinking solution).

GRANULEX

(Trypsin, Balsam Peru, Castor Oil) 925

None cited in PDR database.

GRIFULVIN V (GRISEOFULVIN TABLETS) MICROSIZE (GRISEOFULVIN ORAL SUSPENSION) MICROSIZE

(Griseofulvin) 1888

May interact with oral anticoagulants, barbiturates, and oral contraceptives. Compounds in these categories include:

Aprobarbital (Usually depresses griseofulvin activity; may necessitate dosage increase).

No products indexed under this heading.

Butabarbital (Usually depresses griseofulvin activity; may necessitate dosage increase).

No products indexed under this heading.

Butalbital (Usually depresses griseofulvin activity; may necessitate dosage increase). Products include:

Esgic-plus Tablets 1013

Fioricet Tablets 2258

Fioricet with Codeine Capsules 2260

Fiorinal Capsules 2261

Fiorinal with Codeine Capsules 2262

Fiorinal Tablets 2261

Phrenilin 785

Sedapap Tablets 50 mg/650 mg .. 1543

Desogestrel (Reduced contraceptive efficacy; increased incidence of breakthrough bleeding). Products include:

Desogen Tablets 1817

Ortho-Cept 1851

Dicumarol (Dosage adjustment of anticoagulant may be necessary).

No products indexed under this heading.

Ethinyl Estradiol (Reduced contraceptive efficacy; increased incidence of breakthrough bleeding). Products include:

Brevicon 2088

Demulen 2428

Desogen Tablets 1817

Levlen/Tri-Levlen 651

Lo/Ovral Tablets 2746

Lo/Ovral-28 Tablets 2751

Modicon 1872

Nordette-21 Tablets 2755

Nordette-28 Tablets 2758

Norinyl 2088

Ortho-Cept 1851

Ortho-Cyclen/Ortho-Tri-Cyclen 1858

Ortho-Novum 1872

Ortho-Cyclen/Ortho Tri-Cyclen 1858

Ovcon 760

Ovral Tablets 2770

Ovral-28 Tablets 2770

Levlen/Tri-Levlen 651

Tri-Norinyl 2164

Triphasil-21 Tablets 2814

Triphasil-28 Tablets 2819

IMPORTANT NOTE: Always consult each drug listing in the patient's regimen for possible interactions.

Ethynodiol Diacetate (Reduced contraceptive efficacy; increased incidence of breakthrough bleeding). Products include:
- Demulen ... 2428

Levonorgestrel (Reduced contraceptive efficacy; increased incidence of breakthrough bleeding). Products include:
- Levlen/Tri-Levlen ... 651
- Nordette-21 Tablets ... 2755
- Nordette-28 Tablets ... 2758
- Norplant System ... 2759
- Levlen/Tri-Levlen ... 651
- Triphasil-21 Tablets ... 2814
- Triphasil-28 Tablets ... 2819

Mephobarbital (Usually depresses griseofulvin activity; may necessitate dosage increase). Products include:
- Mebaral Tablets ... 2322

Mestranol (Reduced contraceptive efficacy; increased incidence of breakthrough bleeding). Products include:
- Norinyl ... 2088
- Ortho-Novum ... 1872

Norethindrone (Reduced contraceptive efficacy; increased incidence of breakthrough bleeding). Products include:
- Brevicon ... 2088
- Micronor Tablets ... 1872
- Modicon ... 1872
- Norinyl ... 2088
- Nor-Q D Tablets ... 2135
- Ortho-Novum ... 1872
- Ovcon ... 760
- Tri-Norinyl ... 2164

Norethynodrel (Reduced contraceptive efficacy; increased incidence of breakthrough bleeding).
- No products indexed under this heading.

Norgestimate (Reduced contraceptive efficacy; increased incidence of breakthrough bleeding). Products include:
- Ortho-Cyclen/Ortho-Tri-Cyclen ... 1858
- Ortho-Cyclen/Ortho Tri-Cyclen ... 1858

Norgestrel (Reduced contraceptive efficacy; increased incidence of breakthrough bleeding). Products include:
- Lo/Ovral Tablets ... 2746
- Lo/Ovral-28 Tablets ... 2751
- Ovral Tablets ... 2770
- Ovral-28 Tablets ... 2770
- Ovrette Tablets ... 2771

Pentobarbital Sodium (Usually depresses griseofulvin activity; may necessitate dosage increase). Products include:
- Nembutal Sodium Capsules ... 436
- Nembutal Sodium Solution ... 438
- Nembutal Sodium Suppositories ... 440

Phenobarbital (Usually depresses griseofulvin activity; may necessitate dosage increase). Products include:
- Arco-Lase Plus Tablets ... 512
- Bellergal-S Tablets ... 2250
- Donnatal ... 2060
- Donnatal Extentabs ... 2061
- Donnatal Tablets ... 2060
- Phenobarbital Elixir and Tablets ... 1469
- Quadrinal Tablets ... 1350

Secobarbital Sodium (Usually depresses griseofulvin activity; may necessitate dosage increase). Products include:
- Seconal Sodium Pulvules ... 1474

Thiamylal Sodium (Usually depresses griseofulvin activity; may necessitate dosage increase).
- No products indexed under this heading.

Warfarin Sodium (Dosage adjustment of anticoagulant may be necessary). Products include:
- Coumadin ... 926

GRIS-PEG TABLETS, 125 MG & 250 MG

(Griseofulvin) ... 479

May interact with oral anticoagulants, barbiturates, oral contraceptives, and certain other agents. Compounds in these categories include:

Aprobarbital (Depresses griseofulvin activity).
- No products indexed under this heading.

Butabarbital (Depresses griseofulvin activity).
- No products indexed under this heading.

Butalbital (Depresses griseofulvin activity). Products include:
- Esgic-plus Tablets ... 1013
- Fioricet Tablets ... 2258
- Fioricet with Codeine Capsules ... 2260
- Fiorinal Capsules ... 2261
- Fiorinal with Codeine Capsules ... 2262
- Fiorinal Tablets ... 2261
- Phrenilin ... 785
- Sedapap Tablets 50 mg/650 mg .. 1543

Desogestrel (Effects not specified). Products include:
- Desogen Tablets ... 1817
- Ortho-Cept ... 1851

Dicumarol (Decreased activity of anticoagulants; dosage adjustment may be required).
- No products indexed under this heading.

Ethinyl Estradiol (Effects not specified). Products include:
- Brevicon ... 2088
- Demulen ... 2428
- Desogen Tablets ... 1817
- Levlen/Tri-Levlen ... 651
- Lo/Ovral Tablets ... 2746
- Lo/Ovral-28 Tablets ... 2751
- Modicon ... 1872
- Nordette-21 Tablets ... 2755
- Nordette-28 Tablets ... 2758
- Norinyl ... 2088
- Ortho-Cept ... 1851
- Ortho-Cyclen/Ortho-Tri-Cyclen ... 1858
- Ortho-Novum ... 1872
- Ortho-Cyclen/Ortho Tri-Cyclen ... 1858
- Ovcon ... 760
- Ovral Tablets ... 2770
- Ovral-28 Tablets ... 2770
- Levlen/Tri-Levlen ... 651
- Tri-Norinyl ... 2164
- Triphasil-21 Tablets ... 2814
- Triphasil-28 Tablets ... 2819

Ethynodiol Diacetate (Effects not specified). Products include:
- Demulen ... 2428

Levonorgestrel (Effects not specified). Products include:
- Levlen/Tri-Levlen ... 651
- Nordette-21 Tablets ... 2755
- Nordette-28 Tablets ... 2758
- Norplant System ... 2759
- Levlen/Tri-Levlen ... 651
- Triphasil-21 Tablets ... 2814
- Triphasil-28 Tablets ... 2819

Mephobarbital (Depresses griseofulvin activity). Products include:
- Mebaral Tablets ... 2322

Mestranol (Effects not specified). Products include:
- Norinyl ... 2088
- Ortho-Novum ... 1872

Norethindrone (Effects not specified). Products include:
- Brevicon ... 2088
- Micronor Tablets ... 1872
- Modicon ... 1872
- Norinyl ... 2088
- Nor-Q D Tablets ... 2135
- Ortho-Novum ... 1872
- Ovcon ... 760
- Tri-Norinyl ... 2164

Norethynodrel (Effects not specified).
- No products indexed under this heading.

Norgestimate (Effects not specified). Products include:
- Ortho-Cyclen/Ortho-Tri-Cyclen ... 1858
- Ortho-Cyclen/Ortho Tri-Cyclen ... 1858

Norgestrel (Effects not specified). Products include:
- Lo/Ovral Tablets ... 2746
- Lo/Ovral-28 Tablets ... 2751
- Ovral Tablets ... 2770
- Ovral-28 Tablets ... 2770
- Ovrette Tablets ... 2771

Pentobarbital Sodium (Depresses griseofulvin activity). Products include:
- Nembutal Sodium Capsules ... 436
- Nembutal Sodium Solution ... 438
- Nembutal Sodium Suppositories ... 440

Phenobarbital (Depresses griseofulvin activity). Products include:
- Arco-Lase Plus Tablets ... 512
- Bellergal-S Tablets ... 2250
- Donnatal ... 2060
- Donnatal Extentabs ... 2061
- Donnatal Tablets ... 2060
- Phenobarbital Elixir and Tablets ... 1469
- Quadrinal Tablets ... 1350

Secobarbital Sodium (Depresses griseofulvin activity). Products include:
- Seconal Sodium Pulvules ... 1474

Thiamylal Sodium (Depresses griseofulvin activity).
- No products indexed under this heading.

Warfarin Sodium (Decreased activity of anticoagulants; dosage adjustment may be required). Products include:
- Coumadin ... 926

Food Interactions

Alcohol (The effect of alcohol may be potentiated).

GUAIFED CAPSULES (EXTENDED-RELEASE)

(Guaifenesin, Pseudoephedrine Hydrochloride) ... 1787

May interact with monoamine oxidase inhibitors, beta blockers, veratrum alkaloids, cardiac glycosides, and certain other agents. Compounds in these categories include:

Acebutolol Hydrochloride (Increased effect of sympathomimetic). Products include:
- Sectral Capsules ... 2807

Antidepressant Medications, unspecified (Effect not specified).

Atenolol (Increased effect of sympathomimetic). Products include:
- Tenoretic Tablets ... 2845
- Tenormin Tablets and I.V. Injection 2847

Betaxolol Hydrochloride (Increased effect of sympathomimetic). Products include:
- Betoptic Ophthalmic Solution ... 469
- Betoptic S Ophthalmic Suspension 471
- Kerlone Tablets ... 2436

Bisoprolol Fumarate (Increased effect of sympathomimetic). Products include:
- Zebeta Tablets ... 1413
- Ziac ... 1415

Blood Pressure Medications, unspecified (Effect not specified).
- No products indexed under this heading.

Carteolol Hydrochloride (Increased effect of sympathomimetic). Products include:
- Cartrol Tablets ... 410
- Ocupress Ophthalmic Solution, 1% Sterile ... ◉ 309

Cryptenamine Preparations (Reduced antihypertensive effects).

Deslanoside (Increased possibility of cardiac arrhythmias).
- No products indexed under this heading.

Digitoxin (Increased possibility of cardiac arrhythmias). Products include:
- Crystodigin Tablets ... 1433

Digoxin (Increased possibility of cardiac arrhythmias). Products include:
- Lanoxicaps ... 1117
- Lanoxin Elixir Pediatric ... 1120
- Lanoxin Injection ... 1123
- Lanoxin Injection Pediatric ... 1126
- Lanoxin Tablets ... 1128

Esmolol Hydrochloride (Increased effect of sympathomimetic). Products include:
- Brevibloc Injection ... 1808

Furazolidone (Increased effect of sympathomimetic; concurrent therapy is contraindicated). Products include:
- Furoxone ... 2046

Isocarboxazid (Increased effect of sympathomimetic; concurrent therapy is contraindicated).
- No products indexed under this heading.

Labetalol Hydrochloride (Increased effect of sympathomimetic). Products include:
- Normodyne Injection ... 2377
- Normodyne Tablets ... 2379
- Trandate ... 1185

Levobunolol Hydrochloride (Increased effect of sympathomimetic). Products include:
- Betagan ... ◉ 233

Mecamylamine Hydrochloride (Reduced antihypertensive effects). Products include:
- Inversine Tablets ... 1686

Methyldopa (Reduced antihypertensive effects). Products include:
- Aldoclor Tablets ... 1598
- Aldomet Oral ... 1600
- Aldoril Tablets ... 1604

Methyldopate Hydrochloride (Reduced antihypertensive effects). Products include:
- Aldomet Ester HCl Injection ... 1602

Metipranolol Hydrochloride (Increased effect of sympathomimetic). Products include:
- OptiPranolol (Metipranolol 0.3%) Sterile Ophthalmic Solution ... ◉ 258

Metoprolol Succinate (Increased effect of sympathomimetic). Products include:
- Toprol-XL Tablets ... 565

Metoprolol Tartrate (Increased effect of sympathomimetic). Products include:
- Lopressor Ampuls ... 830
- Lopressor HCT Tablets ... 832
- Lopressor Tablets ... 830

Nadolol (Increased effect of sympathomimetic).
- No products indexed under this heading.

Penbutolol Sulfate (Increased effect of sympathomimetic). Products include:
- Levatol ... 2403

Phenelzine Sulfate (Increased effect of sympathomimetic; concurrent therapy is contraindicated). Products include:
- Nardil ... 1920

Pindolol (Increased effect of sympathomimetic). Products include:
- Visken Tablets ... 2299

Propranolol Hydrochloride (Increased effect of sympathomimetic). Products include:
- Inderal ... 2728
- Inderal LA Long Acting Capsules ... 2730

(▣ Described in PDR For Nonprescription Drugs) (◉ Described in PDR For Ophthalmology)

459 Interactions Index Habitrol

Inderide Tablets ... 2732
Inderide LA Long Acting Capsules .. 2734

Reserpine (Reduced antihypertensive effects). Products include:
Diupres Tablets ... 1650
Hydropres Tablets ... 1675
Ser-Ap-Es Tablets ... 849

Selegiline Hydrochloride (Increased effect of sympathomimetic; concurrent therapy is contraindicated). Products include:
Eldepryl Tablets ... 2550

Sotalol Hydrochloride (Increased effect of sympathomimetic). Products include:
Betapace Tablets ... 641

Timolol Hemihydrate (Increased effect of sympathomimetic). Products include:
Betimol 0.25%, 0.5% ... ◉ 261

Timolol Maleate (Increased effect of sympathomimetic). Products include:
Blocadren Tablets ... 1614
Timolide Tablets ... 1748
Timoptic in Ocudose ... 1753
Timoptic Sterile Ophthalmic Solution ... 1751
Timoptic-XE ... 1755

Tranylcypromine Sulfate (Increased effect of sympathomimetic; concurrent therapy is contraindicated). Products include:
Parnate Tablets ... 2503

GUAIFED-PD CAPSULES (EXTENDED-RELEASE)
(Guaifenesin, Pseudoephedrine Hydrochloride) ... 1787
See **Guaifed Capsules (Extended-Release)**

GUAIFED SYRUP
(Guaifenesin, Pseudoephedrine Hydrochloride) ... ▣ 734
May interact with monoamine oxidase inhibitors. Compounds in this category include:

Furazolidone (Concurrent use is contraindicated). Products include:
Furoxone ... 2046

Isocarboxazid (Concurrent use is contraindicated).
No products indexed under this heading.

Phenelzine Sulfate (Concurrent use is contraindicated). Products include:
Nardil ... 1920

Selegiline Hydrochloride (Concurrent use is contraindicated). Products include:
Eldepryl Tablets ... 2550

Tranylcypromine Sulfate (Concurrent use is contraindicated). Products include:
Parnate Tablets ... 2503

GUAIMAX-D TABLETS
(Pseudoephedrine Hydrochloride, Guaifenesin) ... 792
May interact with monoamine oxidase inhibitors, beta blockers, veratrum alkaloids, catecholamine depleting drugs, and certain other agents. Compounds in these categories include:

Acebutolol Hydrochloride (Increases effects of sympathomimetics). Products include:
Sectral Capsules ... 2807

Atenolol (Increases effects of sympathomimetics). Products include:
Tenoretic Tablets ... 2845
Tenormin Tablets and I.V. Injection 2847

Betaxolol Hydrochloride (Increases effects of sympathomimetics). Products include:
Betoptic Ophthalmic Solution ... 469
Betoptic S Ophthalmic Suspension 471
Kerlone Tablets ... 2436

Bisoprolol Fumarate (Increases effects of sympathomimetics). Products include:
Zebeta Tablets ... 1413
Ziac ... 1415

Carteolol Hydrochloride (Increases effects of sympathomimetics). Products include:
Cartrol Tablets ... 410
Ocupress Ophthalmic Solution, 1% Sterile ... ◉ 309

Cryptenamine Preparations (Reduced antihypertensive effects).

Deserpidine (Reduced antihypertensive effects).
No products indexed under this heading.

Esmolol Hydrochloride (Increases effects of sympathomimetics). Products include:
Brevibloc Injection ... 1808

Furazolidone (Increases effects of sympathomimetics; concurrent use is contraindicated). Products include:
Furoxone ... 2046

Guanethidine Monosulfate (Reduced antihypertensive effects). Products include:
Esimil Tablets ... 822
Ismelin Tablets ... 827

Isocarboxazid (Increases effects of sympathomimetics; concurrent use is contraindicated).
No products indexed under this heading.

Labetalol Hydrochloride (Increases effects of sympathomimetics). Products include:
Normodyne Injection ... 2377
Normodyne Tablets ... 2379
Trandate ... 1185

Levobunolol Hydrochloride (Increases effects of sympathomimetics). Products include:
Betagan ... ◉ 233

Mecamylamine Hydrochloride (Reduced antihypertensive effects). Products include:
Inversine Tablets ... 1686

Methyldopa (Reduced antihypertensive effects). Products include:
Aldoclor Tablets ... 1598
Aldomet Oral ... 1600
Aldoril Tablets ... 1604

Metipranolol Hydrochloride (Increases effects of sympathomimetics). Products include:
OptiPranolol (Metipranolol 0.3%) Sterile Ophthalmic Solution ... ◉ 258

Metoprolol Succinate (Increases effects of sympathomimetics). Products include:
Toprol-XL Tablets ... 565

Metoprolol Tartrate (Increases effects of sympathomimetics). Products include:
Lopressor Ampuls ... 830
Lopressor HCT Tablets ... 832
Lopressor Tablets ... 830

Nadolol (Increases effects of sympathomimetics).
No products indexed under this heading.

Penbutolol Sulfate (Increases effects of sympathomimetics). Products include:
Levatol ... 2403

Phenelzine Sulfate (Increases effects of sympathomimetics; concurrent use is contraindicated). Products include:
Nardil ... 1920

Pindolol (Increases effects of sympathomimetics). Products include:
Visken Tablets ... 2299

Propranolol Hydrochloride (Increases effects of sympathomimetics). Products include:
Inderal ... 2728
Inderal LA Long Acting Capsules ... 2730
Inderide Tablets ... 2732
Inderide LA Long Acting Capsules .. 2734

Rauwolfia Serpentina (Reduced antihypertensive effects).
No products indexed under this heading.

Rescinnamine (Reduced antihypertensive effects).
No products indexed under this heading.

Reserpine (Reduced antihypertensive effects). Products include:
Diupres Tablets ... 1650
Hydropres Tablets ... 1675
Ser-Ap-Es Tablets ... 849

Selegiline Hydrochloride (Increases effects of sympathomimetics; concurrent use is contraindicated). Products include:
Eldepryl Tablets ... 2550

Sotalol Hydrochloride (Increases effects of sympathomimetics). Products include:
Betapace Tablets ... 641

Timolol Hemihydrate (Increases effects of sympathomimetics). Products include:
Betimol 0.25%, 0.5% ... ◉ 261

Timolol Maleate (Increases effects of sympathomimetics). Products include:
Blocadren Tablets ... 1614
Timolide Tablets ... 1748
Timoptic in Ocudose ... 1753
Timoptic Sterile Ophthalmic Solution ... 1751
Timoptic-XE ... 1755

Tranylcypromine Sulfate (Increases effects of sympathomimetics; concurrent use is contraindicated). Products include:
Parnate Tablets ... 2503

GUAITAB TABLETS
(Pseudoephedrine Hydrochloride, Guaifenesin) ... ▣ 734
See **Guaifed Syrup**

GYNE-LOTRIMIN VAGINAL CREAM
(Clotrimazole) ... ▣ 805
None cited in PDR database.

GYNE-LOTRIMIN VAGINAL CREAM WITH 7 DISPOSABLE APPLICATORS
(Clotrimazole) ... ▣ 805
None cited in PDR database.

GYNE-LOTRIMIN VAGINAL CREAM IN PREFILLED APPLICATORS
(Clotrimazole) ... ▣ 805
None cited in PDR database.

GYNE-LOTRIMIN VAGINAL INSERTS
(Clotrimazole) ... ▣ 806
None cited in PDR database.

GYNE-LOTRIMIN COMBINATION PACK
(Clotrimazole) ... ▣ 806
None cited in PDR database.

GYNE-MOISTRIN VAGINAL MOISTURIZING GEL
(Lubricant, Polyglycerylmethacrylate) ... ▣ 806
None cited in PDR database.

GYNOL II EXTRA STRENGTH CONTRACEPTIVE JELLY
(Nonoxynol-9) ... ▣ 739
None cited in PDR database.

GYNOL II ORIGINAL FORMULA CONTRACEPTIVE JELLY
(Nonoxynol-9) ... ▣ 738
None cited in PDR database.

HMS LIQUIFILM
(Medrysone) ... ◉ 244
None cited in PDR database.

HABITROL NICOTINE TRANSDERMAL SYSTEM
(Nicotine) ... 865
May interact with insulin and certain other agents. Compounds in these categories include:

Acetaminophen (Deinduction of hepatic enzymes on smoking cessation; may require a decrease in dose at cessation of smoking). Products include:
Actifed Plus Caplets ... ▣ 845
Actifed Plus Tablets ... ▣ 845
Actifed Sinus Daytime/Nighttime Tablets and Caplets ... ▣ 846
Alka-Seltzer Plus Cold Medicine Liqui-Gels ... ▣ 706
Alka-Seltzer Plus Cold & Cough Medicine Liqui-Gels ... ▣ 705
Alka-Seltzer Plus Night-Time Cold Medicine Liqui-Gels ... ▣ 706
Allerest Headache Strength Tablets ... ▣ 627
Allerest No Drowsiness Tablets ... ▣ 627
Allerest Sinus Pain Formula ... ▣ 627
Anexsia 5/500 Elixir ... 1781
Anexia Tablets ... 1782
Arthritis Foundation Aspirin Free Caplets ... ▣ 673
Arthritis Foundation NightTime Caplets ... ▣ 674
Bayer Select Headache Pain Relief Formula ... ▣ 716
Bayer Select Menstrual Multi-Symptom Formula ... ▣ 716
Bayer Select Night Time Pain Relief Formula ... ▣ 716
Bayer Select Sinus Pain Relief Formula ... ▣ 717
Benadryl Allergy Sinus Headache Formula Caplets ... ▣ 849
Comtrex Multi-Symptom Cold Reliever Tablets/Caplets/Liqui-Gels/Liquid ... ▣ 615
Allergy-Sinus Comtrex Multi-Symptom Allergy-Sinus Formula Tablets ... ▣ 617
Comtrex Non-Drowsy ... ▣ 618
Contac Day Allergy/Sinus Caplets ▣ 812
Contac Day & Night ... ▣ 812
Contac Night Allergy/Sinus Caplets ... ▣ 812
Contac Severe Cold and Flu Formula Caplets ... ▣ 814
Contac Severe Cold & Flu Non-Drowsy ... ▣ 815
Coricidin 'D' Decongestant Tablets ... ▣ 800
Coricidin Tablets ... ▣ 800
DHCplus Capsules ... 1993
Darvon-N/Darvocet-N ... 1433
Drixoral Cold and Flu Extended-Release Tablets ... ▣ 803
Drixoral Cough + Sore Throat Liquid Caps ... ▣ 802
Drixoral Allergy/Sinus Extended Release Tablets ... ▣ 804
Esgic-plus Tablets ... 1013
Aspirin Free Excedrin Analgesic Caplets and Geltabs ... 732
Excedrin Extra-Strength Analgesic Tablets & Caplets ... 732
Excedrin P.M. Analgesic/Sleeping Aid Tablets, Caplets, Liquigels ... 733
Fioricet Tablets ... 2258
Fioricet with Codeine Capsules ... 2260
Hycomine Compound Tablets ... 932
Hydrocet Capsules ... 782

IMPORTANT NOTE: Always consult each drug listing in the patient's regimen for possible interactions.

Habitrol Interactions Index 460

Legatrin PM ◘ 651
Lorcet 10/650 1018
Lortab 2566
Lurline PMS Tablets 982
Maximum Strength Multi-Symptom Formula Midol ◘ 722
PMS Multi-Symptom Formula Midol ◘ 723
Teen Multi-Symptom Formula Midol ◘ 722
Midrin Capsules 783
Migralam Capsules 2038
Panodol Tablets and Caplets ◘ 824
Children's Panadol Chewable Tablets, Liquid, Infant's Drops ◘ 824
Percocet Tablets 938
Percogesic Analgesic Tablets ◘ 754
Phrenilin 785
Pyrroxate Caplets ◘ 772
Sedapap Tablets 50 mg/650 mg 1543
Sinarest Tablets ◘ 648
Sinarest Extra Strength Tablets ◘ 648
Sinarest No Drowsiness Tablets ◘ 648
Sine-Aid Maximum Strength Sinus Medication Gelcaps, Caplets and Tablets 1554
Sine-Off No Drowsiness Formula Caplets ◘ 824
Sine-Off Sinus Medicine ◘ 825
Singlet Tablets ◘ 825
Sinulin Tablets 787
Sinutab Sinus Allergy Medication, Maximum Strength Tablets and Caplets ◘ 860
Sinutab Sinus Medication, Maximum Strength Without Drowsiness Formula, Tablets & Caplets ◘ 860
Sinutab Sinus Medication, Regular Strength Without Drowsiness Formula ◘ 859
Sudafed Cold and Cough Liquidcaps ◘ 862
Sudafed Severe Cold Formula Caplets ◘ 863
Sudafed Severe Cold Formula Tablets ◘ 864
Sudafed Sinus Caplets ◘ 864
Sudafed Sinus Tablets ◘ 864
Talacen 2333
TheraFlu ◘ 787
TheraFlu Maximum Strength Nighttime Flu, Cold & Cough Medicine ◘ 788
TheraFlu Maximum Strength Non-Drowsy Formula Flu, Cold & Cough Medicine ◘ 788
Thera Flu Maximum Strength, Non-Drowsy Formula Flu, Cold and Cough Caplets ◘ 789
Triaminic Sore Throat Formula ◘ 791
Triaminicin Tablets ◘ 793
Children's TYLENOL acetaminophen Chewable Tablets, Elixir, Suspension Liquid 1555
Children's TYLENOL Cold Multi-Symptom Liquid Formula and Chewable Tablets 1561
Children's TYLENOL Cold Plus Cough Multi Symptom Tablets and Liquid ◘ 681
Infants' TYLENOL acetaminophen Drops and Suspension Drops 1555
Infants' TYLENOL Cold Decongestant & Fever-Reducer Drops 1556
TYLENOL Extended Relief Caplets 1558
TYLENOL, Extra Strength, Acetaminophen Adult Liquid Pain Reliever 1560
TYLENOL, Extra Strength, acetaminophen Gelcaps, Geltabs, Caplets, Tablets 1559
TYLENOL, Extra Strength, Headache Plus Pain Reliever with Antacid Caplets 1559
TYLENOL, Junior Strength, acetaminophen Coated Caplets, Grape and Fruit Chewable Tablets 1557
TYLENOL Maximum Strength Allergy Sinus Medication Gelcaps and Caplets 1563
TYLENOL Maximum Strength Allergy Sinus NightTime Medication Caplets 1555
TYLENOL Flu Maximum Strength Gelcaps 1565
TYLENOL Flu NightTime, Maximum Strength, Gelcaps 1566
TYLENOL Maximum Strength Flu NightTime Hot Medication Packets 1562
TYLENOL, Maximum Strength, Sinus Medication Geltabs, Gelcaps, Caplets and Tablets 1566
TYLENOL Cold Multi-Symptom Formula Medication Tablets and Caplets 1561
TYLENOL Cold Medication No Drowsiness Formula Gelcaps and Caplets 1562
TYLENOL Cold Multi-Symptom Hot Medication Liquid Packets 1557
TYLENOL Cough Multi-Symptom Medication 1564
TYLENOL Cough Multi-Symptom Medication with Decongestant 1565
TYLENOL, Regular Strength, acetaminophen Caplets and Tablets 1558
TYLENOL PM, Extra Strength Pain Reliever/Sleep Aid Caplets, Geltabs, Gelcaps 1560
TYLENOL Severe Allergy Medication Caplets 1564
Tylenol with Codeine 1583
Tylox Capsules 1584
Unisom With Pain Relief-Nighttime Sleep Aid and Pain Reliever 1934
Vanquish Analgesic Caplets ◘ 731
Vicks 44 LiquiCaps Cough, Cold & Flu Relief ◘ 755
Vicks 44M Cough, Cold & Flu Relief ◘ 756
Vicks DayQuil ◘ 761
Vicks Nyquil Hot Therapy ◘ 762
Vicks NyQuil LiquiCaps Multi-Symptom Cold/Flu Relief ◘ 763
Vicks NyQuil Multi-Symptom Cold/Flu Relief - (Original & Cherry Flavor) ◘ 763
Vicodin Tablets 1356
Vicodin ES Tablets 1357
Wygesic Tablets 2827
Zydone Capsules 949

Aminophylline (Deinduction of hepatic enzymes on smoking cessation; may require a decrease in dose at cessation of smoking).
No products indexed under this heading.

Caffeine (Deinduction of hepatic enzymes on smoking cessation; may require a decrease in dose at cessation of smoking). Products include:
Arthritis Strength BC Powder ◘ 609
BC Powder ◘ 609
Bayer Select Headache Pain Relief Formula ◘ 716
Cafergot 2251
DHCplus Capsules 1993
Darvon Compound-65 Pulvules 1435
Esgic-plus Tablets 1013
Aspirin Free Excedrin Analgesic Caplets and Geltabs 732
Excedrin Extra-Strength Analgesic Tablets & Caplets 732
Fioricet Tablets 2258
Fioricet with Codeine Capsules 2260
Fiorinal Capsules 2261
Fiorinal with Codeine Capsules 2262
Fiorinal Tablets 2261
Maximum Strength Multi-Symptom Formula Midol ◘ 722
Migralam Capsules 2038
No Doz Maximum Strength Caplets ◘ 622
Norgesic 1496
Vanquish Analgesic Caplets ◘ 731
Wigraine Tablets & Suppositories 1829

Caffeine Anhydrous (Deinduction of hepatic enzymes on smoking cessation; may require a decrease in dose at cessation of smoking).
No products indexed under this heading.

Caffeine Citrate (Deinduction of hepatic enzymes on smoking cessation; may require a decrease in dose at cessation of smoking).
No products indexed under this heading.

Caffeine Sodium Benzoate (Deinduction of hepatic enzymes on smoking cessation; may require a decrease in dose at cessation of smoking).
No products indexed under this heading.

Dyphylline (Deinduction of hepatic enzymes on smoking cessation; may require a decrease in dose at cessation of smoking). Products include:
Lufyllin & Lufyllin-400 Tablets 2670
Lufyllin-GG Elixir & Tablets 2671

Imipramine Hydrochloride (Deinduction of hepatic enzymes on smoking cessation; may require a decrease in dose at cessation of smoking). Products include:
Tofranil Ampuls 854
Tofranil Tablets 856

Imipramine Pamoate (Deinduction of hepatic enzymes on smoking cessation; may require a decrease in dose at cessation of smoking). Products include:
Tofranil-PM Capsules 857

Insulin, Human (Increased subcutaneous insulin absorption with smoking cessation).
No products indexed under this heading.

Insulin, Human Isophane Suspension (Increased subcutaneous insulin absorption with smoking cessation). Products include:
Novolin N Human Insulin 10 ml Vials 1795

Insulin, Human NPH (Increased subcutaneous insulin absorption with smoking cessation). Products include:
Humulin N, 100 Units 1448
Novolin N PenFill Cartridges Durable Insulin Delivery System 1798
Novolin N Prefilled Syringe Disposable Insulin Delivery System 1798

Insulin, Human Regular (Increased subcutaneous insulin absorption with smoking cessation). Products include:
Humulin R, 100 Units 1449
Novolin R Human Insulin 10 ml Vials 1795
Novolin R PenFill Cartridges Durable Insulin Delivery System 1798
Novolin R Prefilled Syringe Disposable Insulin Delivery System 1798
Velosulin BR Human Insulin 10 ml Vials 1795

Insulin, Human, Zinc Suspension (Increased subcutaneous insulin absorption with smoking cessation). Products include:
Humulin L, 100 Units 1446
Humulin U, 100 Units 1450
Novolin L Human Insulin 10 ml Vials 1795

Insulin, NPH (Increased subcutaneous insulin absorption with smoking cessation). Products include:
NPH, 100 Units 1450
Pork NPH, 100 Units 1452
Purified Pork NPH Isophane Insulin 1801

Insulin, Regular (Increased subcutaneous insulin absorption with smoking cessation). Products include:
Regular, 100 Units 1450
Pork Regular, 100 Units 1452
Pork Regular (Concentrated), 500 Units 1453
Purified Pork Regular Insulin 1801

Insulin, Zinc Crystals (Increased subcutaneous insulin absorption with smoking cessation). Products include:
NPH, 100 Units 1450

Insulin, Zinc Suspension (Increased subcutaneous insulin absorption with smoking cessation). Products include:
Iletin I 1450
Lente, 100 Units 1450
Iletin II 1452
Pork Lente, 100 Units 1452
Purified Pork Lente Insulin 1801

Isoproterenol Hydrochloride (Decrease in circulating catecholamines with smoking cessation). Products include:
Isuprel Hydrochloride Injection 1:5000 2311
Isuprel Hydrochloride Solution 1:200 & 1:100 2313
Isuprel Mistometer 2312

Labetalol Hydrochloride (Decrease in circulating catecholamines with smoking cessation). Products include:
Normodyne Injection 2377
Normodyne Tablets 2379
Trandate 1185

Oxazepam (Deinduction of hepatic enzymes on smoking cessation; may require a decrease in dose at cessation of smoking). Products include:
Serax Capsules 2810
Serax Tablets 2810

Pentazocine Hydrochloride (Deinduction of hepatic enzymes on smoking cessation; may require a decrease in dose at cessation of smoking). Products include:
Talacen 2333
Talwin Compound 2335
Talwin Nx 2336

Pentazocine Lactate (Deinduction of hepatic enzymes on smoking cessation; may require a decrease in dose at cessation of smoking). Products include:
Talwin Injection 2334

Phenylephrine Hydrochloride (Decrease in circulating catecholamines with smoking cessation). Products include:
Atrohist Plus Tablets 454
Cerose DM ◘ 878
Comhist 2038
D.A. Chewable Tablets 951
Deconsal Pediatric Capsules 454
Dura-Vent/DA Tablets 953
Entex Capsules 1986
Entex Liquid 1986
Extendryl 1005
4-Way Fast Acting Nasal Spray (regular & mentholated) ◘ 621
Hemorid For Women ◘ 834
Hycomine Compound Tablets 932
Neo-Synephrine Hydrochloride 1% Carpuject 2324
Neo-Synephrine Hydrochloride 1% Injection 2324
Neo-Synephrine Hydrochloride (Ophthalmic) 2325
Neo-Synephrine ◘ 726
Nōstril ◘ 644
Novahistine Elixir ◘ 823
Phenergan VC 2779
Phenergan VC with Codeine 2781
Preparation H ◘ 871
Tympagesic Ear Drops 2342
Vasosulf ⊙ 271
Vicks Sinex Nasal Spray and Ultra Fine Mist ◘ 765

Prazosin Hydrochloride (Decrease in circulating catecholamines with smoking cessation). Products include:
Minipress Capsules 1937
Minizide Capsules 1938

Propranolol Hydrochloride (Deinduction of hepatic enzymes on smoking cessation; may require a decrease in dose at cessation of smoking). Products include:
Inderal 2728
Inderal LA Long Acting Capsules 2730
Inderide Tablets 2732
Inderide LA Long Acting Capsules 2734

(◘ Described in PDR For Nonprescription Drugs) (⊙ Described in PDR For Ophthalmology)

Interactions Index

Theophylline (Deinduction of hepatic enzymes on smoking cessation; may require a decrease in dose at cessation of smoking). Products include:

Marax Tablets & DF Syrup.................. 2200
Quibron 2053

Theophylline Anhydrous (Deinduction of hepatic enzymes on smoking cessation; may require a decrease in dose at cessation of smoking). Products include:

Aerolate 1004
Primatene Dual Action Formula...... ⊕ 872
Primatene Tablets................................ ⊕ 873
Respbid Tablets................................... 682
Slo-bid Gyrocaps................................. 2033
Theo-24 Extended Release Capsules.. 2568
Theo-Dur Extended-Release Tablets... 1327
Theo-X Extended-Release Tablets.. 788
Uni-Dur Extended-Release Tablets.. 1331
Uniphyl 400 mg Tablets...................... 2001

Theophylline Calcium Salicylate (Deinduction of hepatic enzymes on smoking cessation; may require a decrease in dose at cessation of smoking). Products include:

Quadrinal Tablets................................ 1350

Theophylline Sodium Glycinate (Deinduction of hepatic enzymes on smoking cessation; may require a decrease in dose at cessation of smoking).

No products indexed under this heading.

HALCION TABLETS

(Triazolam) 2611

May interact with benzodiazepines, psychotropics, anticonvulsants, antihistamines, central nervous system depressants, and certain other agents. Compounds in these categories include:

Acrivastine (Additive CNS depressant effects). Products include:

Semprex-D Capsules.......................... 463
Semprex-D Capsules.......................... 1167

Alfentanil Hydrochloride (Additive CNS depressant effects). Products include:

Alfenta Injection.................................. 1286

Alprazolam (Additive CNS depressant effects). Products include:

Xanax Tablets...................................... 2649

Amitriptyline Hydrochloride (Additive CNS depressant effects). Products include:

Elavil... 2838
Endep Tablets...................................... 2174
Etrafon.. 2355
Limbitrol... 2180
Triavil Tablets...................................... 1757

Amoxapine (Additive CNS depressant effects). Products include:

Asendin Tablets................................... 1369

Aprobarbital (Additive CNS depressant effects).

No products indexed under this heading.

Astemizole (Additive CNS depressant effects). Products include:

Hismanal Tablets................................. 1293

Azatadine Maleate (Additive CNS depressant effects). Products include:

Trinalin Repetabs Tablets.................. 1330

Bromodiphenhydramine Hydrochloride (Additive CNS depressant effects).

No products indexed under this heading.

Brompheniramine Maleate (Additive CNS depressant effects). Products include:

Alka Seltzer Plus Sinus Medicine.. ⊕ 707

Bromfed Capsules (Extended-Release).. 1785
Bromfed Syrup.................................... ⊕ 733
Bromfed Tablets.................................. 1785
Bromfed-DM Cough Syrup................ 1786
Bromfed-PD Capsules (Extended-Release).. 1785
Dimetane-DC Cough Syrup............... 2059
Dimetane-DX Cough Syrup............... 2059
Dimetapp Elixir................................... ⊕ 773
Dimetapp Extentabs........................... ⊕ 774
Dimetapp Tablets/Liqui-Gels.......... ⊕ 775
Dimetapp Cold & Allergy Chewable Tablets...................................... ⊕ 773
Dimetapp DM Elixir............................ ⊕ 774
Vicks DayQuil Allergy Relief 12-Hour Extended Release Tablets.. ⊕ 760
Vicks DayQuil Allergy Relief 4-Hour Tablets...................................... ⊕ 760

Buprenorphine (Additive CNS depressant effects). Products include:

Buprenex Injectable........................... 2006

Buspirone Hydrochloride (Additive CNS depressant effects). Products include:

BuSpar.. 737

Butabarbital (Additive CNS depressant effects).

No products indexed under this heading.

Butalbital (Additive CNS depressant effects). Products include:

Esgic-plus Tablets............................... 1013
Fioricet Tablets.................................... 2258
Fioricet with Codeine Capsules........ 2260
Fiorinal Capsules................................ 2261
Fiorinal with Codeine Capsules........ 2262
Fiorinal Tablets.................................... 2261
Phrenilin.. 785
Sedapap Tablets 50 mg/650 mg.. 1543

Carbamazepine (Additive CNS depressant effects). Products include:

Atretol Tablets..................................... 573
Tegretol Chewable Tablets................ 852
Tegretol Suspension........................... 852
Tegretol Tablets................................... 852

Chlordiazepoxide (Additive CNS depressant effects). Products include:

Libritabs Tablets.................................. 2177
Limbitrol... 2180

Chlordiazepoxide Hydrochloride (Additive CNS depressant effects). Products include:

Librax Capsules................................... 2176
Librium Capsules................................. 2178
Librium Injectable............................... 2179

Chlorpheniramine Maleate (Additive CNS depressant effects). Products include:

Alka-Seltzer Plus Cold Medicine.... ⊕ 705
Alka-Seltzer Plus Cold Medicine Liqui-Gels... ⊕ 706
Alka-Seltzer Plus Cold & Cough Medicine.. ⊕ 708
Alka-Seltzer Plus Cold & Cough Medicine Liqui-Gels........................... ⊕ 705
Allerest Children's Chewable Tablets... ⊕ 627
Allerest Headache Strength Tablets... ⊕ 627
Allerest Maximum Strength Tablets... ⊕ 627
Allerest Sinus Pain Formula............ ⊕ 627
Allerest 12 Hour Caplets.................. ⊕ 627
Ana-Kit Anaphylaxis Emergency Treatment Kit...................................... 617
Atrohist Pediatric Capsules.............. 453
Atrohist Plus Tablets.......................... 454
BC Cold Powder Multi-Symptom Formula (Cold-Sinus-Allergy)...... ⊕ 609
Cerose DM... ⊕ 878
Cheracol Plus Head Cold/Cough Formula... ⊕ 769
Children's Vicks DayQuil Allergy Relief.. ⊕ 757
Children's Vicks NyQuil Cold/Cough Relief.. ⊕ 758
Chlor-Trimeton Allergy Decongestant Tablets.. ⊕ 799
Chlor-Trimeton Allergy Tablets...... ⊕ 798
Comhist.. 2038

Comtrex Multi-Symptom Cold Reliever Tablets/Caplets/Liqui-Gels/Liquid.. ⊕ 615
Allergy-Sinus Comtrex Multi-Symptom Allergy-Sinus Formula Tablets.. ⊕ 617
Contac Continuous Action Nasal Decongestant/Antihistamine 12 Hour Capsules..................................... ⊕ 813
Contac Maximum Strength Continuous Action Decongestant/Antihistamine 12 Hour Caplets.. ⊕ 813
Contac Severe Cold and Flu Formula Caplets................................... ⊕ 814
Coricidin 'D' Decongestant Tablets... ⊕ 800
Coricidin Tablets................................. ⊕ 800
D.A. Chewable Tablets....................... 951
Deconamine... 1320
Dura-Tap/PD Capsules...................... 2867
Dura-Vent/DA Tablets........................ 953
Extendryl.. 1005
Fedahist Gyrocaps.............................. 2401
Fedahist Timecaps.............................. 2401
Hycomine Compound Tablets.......... 932
Isoclor Timesule Capsules................ ⊕ 637
Kronofed-A... 977
Nolamine Timed-Release Tablets.... 785
Novahistine DH................................... 2462
Novahistine Elixir............................... ⊕ 823
Ornade Spansule Capsules............... 2502
PediaCare Cold Allergy Chewable Tablets.. ⊕ 677
PediaCare Cough-Cold Chewable Tablets.. 1553
PediaCare Cough-Cold Liquid........... 1553
PediaCare NightRest Cough-Cold Liquid... 1553
Pediatric Vicks 44m Cough & Cold Relief... ⊕ 764
Pyrroxate Caplets............................... ⊕ 772
Ryna.. ⊕ 841
Sinarest Tablets................................... ⊕ 648
Sinarest Extra Strength Tablets...... ⊕ 648
Sine-Off Sinus Medicine.................... ⊕ 825
Singlet Tablets..................................... ⊕ 825
Sinulin Tablets..................................... 787
Sinutab Sinus Allergy Medication, Maximum Strength Tablets and Caplets.. ⊕ 860
Sudafed Plus Liquid............................ ⊕ 862
Sudafed Plus Tablets.......................... ⊕ 863
Teldrin 12 Hour Antihistamine/Nasal Decongestant Allergy Relief Capsules................................... ⊕ 826
TheraFlu... ⊕ 787
TheraFlu Maximum Strength Nighttime Flu, Cold & Cough Medicine.. ⊕ 788
Triaminic Allergy Tablets.................. ⊕ 789
Triaminic Cold Tablets....................... ⊕ 790
Triaminic Nite Light........................... ⊕ 791
Triaminic Syrup................................... ⊕ 792
Triaminic-12 Tablets........................... ⊕ 792
Triaminicin Tablets............................. ⊕ 793
Triaminicol Multi-Symptom Cold Tablets.. ⊕ 793
Triaminicol Multi-Symptom Relief ⊕ 794
Tussend... 1783
Children's TYLENOL Cold Multi-Symptom Liquid Formula and Chewable Tablets............................. 1561
Children's TYLENOL Cold Plus Cough Multi Symptom Tablets and Liquid... ⊕ 681
TYLENOL Maximum Strength Allergy Sinus Medication Gelcaps and Caplets... 1563
TYLENOL Cold Multi-Symptom Formula Medication Tablets and Caplets.. 1561
TYLENOL Cold Multi-Symptom Hot Medication Liquid Packets.............. 1557
Vicks 44 LiquiCaps Cough, Cold & Flu Relief... ⊕ 755
Vicks 44M Cough, Cold & Flu Relief.. ⊕ 756

Chlorpheniramine Polistirex (Additive CNS depressant effects). Products include:

Tussionex Pennkinetic Extended-Release Suspension.......................... 998

Chlorpheniramine Tannate (Additive CNS depressant effects). Products include:

Atrohist Pediatric Suspension......... 454
Ricobid Tablets and Pediatric Suspension.. 2038

Rynatan... 2673
Rynatuss... 2673

Chlorpromazine (Additive CNS depressant effects). Products include:

Thorazine Suppositories.................... 2523

Chlorpromazine Hydrochloride (Additive CNS depressant effects). Products include:

Thorazine.. 2523

Chlorprothixene (Additive CNS depressant effects).

No products indexed under this heading.

Chlorprothixene Hydrochloride (Additive CNS depressant effects).

No products indexed under this heading.

Cimetidine (Plasma levels and elimination half-life of triazolam doubled). Products include:

Tagamet Tablets.................................. 2516

Cimetidine Hydrochloride (Plasma levels and elimination half-life of triazolam doubled). Products include:

Tagamet... 2516

Clemastine Fumarate (Additive CNS depressant effects). Products include:

Tavist Syrup... 2297
Tavist Tablets....................................... 2298
Tavist-1 12 Hour Relief Tablets.... ⊕ 787
Tavist-D 12 Hour Relief Tablets.... ⊕ 787

Clorazepate Dipotassium (Additive CNS depressant effects). Products include:

Tranxene... 451

Clozapine (Additive CNS depressant effects). Products include:

Clozaril Tablets.................................... 2252

Codeine Phosphate (Additive CNS depressant effects). Products include:

Actifed with Codeine Cough Syrup.. 1067
Brontex.. 1981
Deconsal C Expectorant Syrup........ 456
Deconsal Pediatric Syrup.................. 457
Dimetane-DC Cough Syrup............... 2059
Empirin with Codeine Tablets........... 1093
Fioricet with Codeine Capsules........ 2260
Fiorinal with Codeine Capsules........ 2262
Isoclor Expectorant............................ 990
Novahistine DH................................... 2462
Novahistine Expectorant.................... 2463
Nucofed... 2051
Phenergan with Codeine.................... 2777
Phenergan VC with Codeine.............. 2781
Robitussin A-C Syrup.......................... 2073
Robitussin-DAC Syrup........................ 2074
Ryna.. ⊕ 841
Soma Compound w/Codeine Tablets... 2676
Tussi-Organidin NR Liquid and S NR Liquid.. 2677
Tylenol with Codeine.......................... 1583

Cyproheptadine Hydrochloride (Additive CNS depressant effects). Products include:

Periactin... 1724

Desflurane (Additive CNS depressant effects). Products include:

Suprane... 1813

Desipramine Hydrochloride (Additive CNS depressant effects). Products include:

Norpramin Tablets.............................. 1526

Dexchlorpheniramine Maleate (Additive CNS depressant effects).

No products indexed under this heading.

Dezocine (Additive CNS depressant effects). Products include:

Dalgan Injection.................................. 538

Diazepam (Additive CNS depressant effects). Products include:

Dizac.. 1809
Valium Injectable................................. 2182
Valium Tablets..................................... 2183
Valrelease Capsules............................ 2169

IMPORTANT NOTE: Always consult each drug listing in the patient's regimen for possible interactions.

Halcion

Interactions Index

Diphenhydramine Citrate (Additive CNS depressant effects). Products include:

Excedrin P.M. Analgesic/Sleeping Aid Tablets, Caplets, Liquigels...... 733

Diphenhydramine Hydrochloride (Additive CNS depressant effects). Products include:

Actifed Allergy Daytime/Nighttime Caplets................................. ⊞ 844
Actifed Sinus Daytime/Nighttime Tablets and Caplets..................... ⊞ 846
Arthritis Foundation NightTime Caplets.. ⊞ 674
Extra Strength Bayer PM Aspirin.. ⊞ 713
Bayer Select Night Time Pain Relief Formula................................. ⊞ 716
Benadryl Allergy Decongestant Liquid Medication.......................... ⊞ 848
Benadryl Allergy Decongestant Tablets.. ⊞ 848
Benadryl Allergy Liquid Medication.. ⊞ 849
Benadryl Allergy.............................. ⊞ 848
Benadryl Allergy Sinus Headache Formula Caplets......................... ⊞ 849
Benadryl Capsules........................... 1898
Benadryl Dye-Free Allergy Liquigel Softgels................................... ⊞ 850
Benadryl Dye-Free Allergy Liquid Medication.................................. ⊞ 850
Benadryl Itch Relief Cream, Children's Formula and Maximum Strength 2%................................... ⊞ 851
Benadryl Itch Relief Spray, Children's Formula and Maximum Strength 2%................................... ⊞ 851
Benadryl Itch Relief Stick Maximum Strength 2%........................... ⊞ 850
Benadryl Itch Stopping Gel, Children's Formula and Maximum Strength 2%................................... ⊞ 851
Benadryl Kapseals........................... 1898
Benadryl Injection........................... 1898
Contac Day & Night Cold/Flu Night Caplets................................... ⊞ 812
Contac Night Allergy/Sinus Caplets.. ⊞ 812
Extra Strength Doan's P.M............. ⊞ 633
Legatrin PM..................................... ⊞ 651
Miles Nervine Nighttime Sleep-Aid ⊞ 723
Nytol QuickCaps Caplets................ ⊞ 610
Sleepinal Night-time Sleep Aid Capsules and Softgels.................... ⊞ 834
TYLENOL Maximum Strength Allergy Sinus NightTime Medication Caplets.. 1555
TYLENOL Flu NightTime, Maximum Strength, Gelcaps................. 1566
TYLENOL Maximum Strength Flu NightTime Hot Medication Packets.. 1562
TYLENOL PM, Extra Strength Pain Reliever/Sleep Aid Caplets, Geltabs, Gelcaps.................................. 1560
TYLENOL Severe Allergy Medication Caplets.................................. 1564
Maximum Strength Unisom Sleepgels.. 1934
Unisom With Pain Relief-Nighttime Sleep Aid and Pain Reliever........... 1934

Diphenylpyraline Hydrochloride (Additive CNS depressant effects).

No products indexed under this heading.

Divalproex Sodium (Additive CNS depressant effects). Products include:

Depakote Tablets.............................. 415

Doxepin Hydrochloride (Additive CNS depressant effects). Products include:

Sinequan.. 2205
Zonalon Cream................................ 1055

Droperidol (Additive CNS depressant effects). Products include:

Inapsine Injection............................ 1296

Enflurane (Additive CNS depressant effects).

No products indexed under this heading.

Erythromycin (Plasma levels and elimination half-life of triazolam doubled). Products include:

A/T/S 2% Acne Topical Gel and Solution.. 1234
Benzamycin Topical Gel.................. 905
E-Mycin Tablets............................... 1341
Emgel 2% Topical Gel..................... 1093
ERYC.. 1915
Erycette (erythromycin 2%) Topical Solution.. 1888
Ery-Tab Tablets................................ 422
Erythromycin Base Filmtab.............. 426
Erythromycin Delayed-Release Capsules, USP.................................. 427
Ilotycin Ophthalmic Ointment......... 912
PCE Dispertab Tablets..................... 444
T-Stat 2.0% Topical Solution and Pads... 2688
Theramycin Z Topical Solution 2% 1592

Erythromycin Estolate (Plasma levels and elimination half-life of triazolam doubled). Products include:

Ilosone.. 911

Erythromycin Ethylsuccinate (Plasma levels and elimination half-life of triazolam doubled). Products include:

E.E.S... 424
EryPed.. 421

Erythromycin Gluceptate (Plasma levels and elimination half-life of triazolam doubled). Products include:

Ilotycin Gluceptate, IV, Vials.......... 913

Erythromycin Stearate (Plasma levels and elimination half-life of triazolam doubled). Products include:

Erythrocin Stearate Filmtab............. 425

Estazolam (Additive CNS depressant effects). Products include:

ProSom Tablets................................ 449

Ethchlorvynol (Additive CNS depressant effects). Products include:

Placidyl Capsules............................. 448

Ethinamate (Additive CNS depressant effects).

No products indexed under this heading.

Ethosuximide (Additive CNS depressant effects). Products include:

Zarontin Capsules............................ 1928
Zarontin Syrup................................. 1929

Ethotoin (Additive CNS depressant effects). Products include:

Peganone Tablets............................. 446

Felbamate (Additive CNS depressant effects). Products include:

Felbatol... 2666

Fentanyl (Additive CNS depressant effects). Products include:

Duragesic Transdermal System....... 1288

Fentanyl Citrate (Additive CNS depressant effects). Products include:

Sublimaze Injection.......................... 1307

Fluphenazine Decanoate (Additive CNS depressant effects). Products include:

Prolixin Decanoate........................... 509

Fluphenazine Enanthate (Additive CNS depressant effects). Products include:

Prolixin Enanthate........................... 509

Fluphenazine Hydrochloride (Additive CNS depressant effects). Products include:

Prolixin... 509

Flurazepam Hydrochloride (Additive CNS depressant effects). Products include:

Dalmane Capsules............................ 2173

Glutethimide (Additive CNS depressant effects).

No products indexed under this heading.

Halazepam (Additive CNS depressant effects).

No products indexed under this heading.

Haloperidol (Additive CNS depressant effects). Products include:

Haldol Injection, Tablets and Concentrate.. 1575

Haloperidol Decanoate (Additive CNS depressant effects). Products include:

Haldol Decanoate............................. 1577

Hydrocodone Bitartrate (Additive CNS depressant effects). Products include:

Anexsia 5/500 Elixir........................ 1781
Anexia Tablets.................................. 1782
Codiclear DH Syrup........................ 791
Deconamine CX Cough and Cold Liquid and Tablets............................ 1319
Duratuss HD Elixir.......................... 2565
Hycodan Tablets and Syrup............ 930
Hycomine Compound Tablets......... 932
Hycomine.. 931
Hycotuss Expectorant Syrup........... 933
Hydrocet Capsules........................... 782
Lorcet 10/650................................... 1018
Lortab... 2566
Tussend... 1783
Tussend Expectorant....................... 1785
Vicodin Tablets................................. 1356
Vicodin ES Tablets........................... 1357
Vicodin Tuss Expectorant............... 1358
Zydone Capsules.............................. 949

Hydrocodone Polistirex (Additive CNS depressant effects). Products include:

Tussionex Pennkinetic Extended-Release Suspension.......................... 998

Hydroxyzine Hydrochloride (Additive CNS depressant effects). Products include:

Atarax Tablets & Syrup................... 2185
Marax Tablets & DF Syrup.............. 2200
Vistaril Intramuscular Solution........ 2216

Imipramine Hydrochloride (Additive CNS depressant effects). Products include:

Tofranil Ampuls............................... 854
Tofranil Tablets................................ 856

Imipramine Pamoate (Additive CNS depressant effects). Products include:

Tofranil-PM Capsules...................... 857

Isocarboxazid (Additive CNS depressant effects).

No products indexed under this heading.

Isoflurane (Additive CNS depressant effects).

No products indexed under this heading.

Ketamine Hydrochloride (Additive CNS depressant effects).

No products indexed under this heading.

Lamotrigine (Additive CNS depressant effects). Products include:

Lamictal Tablets............................... 1112

Levomethadyl Acetate Hydrochloride (Additive CNS depressant effects). Products include:

Orlaam.. 2239

Levorphanol Tartrate (Additive CNS depressant effects). Products include:

Levo-Dromoran................................ 2129

Lithium Carbonate (Additive CNS depressant effects). Products include:

Eskalith.. 2485
Lithium Carbonate Capsules & Tablets... 2230
Lithonate/Lithotabs/Lithobid.......... 2543

Lithium Citrate (Additive CNS depressant effects).

No products indexed under this heading.

Loratadine (Additive CNS depressant effects). Products include:

Claritin.. 2349

Claritin-D.. 2350

Lorazepam (Additive CNS depressant effects). Products include:

Ativan Injection................................ 2698
Ativan Tablets.................................. 2700

Loxapine Hydrochloride (Additive CNS depressant effects). Products include:

Loxitane.. 1378

Loxapine Succinate (Additive CNS depressant effects). Products include:

Loxitane Capsules............................ 1378

Maprotiline Hydrochloride (Additive CNS depressant effects). Products include:

Ludiomil Tablets............................... 843

Meperidine Hydrochloride (Additive CNS depressant effects). Products include:

Demerol... 2308
Mepergan Injection.......................... 2753

Mephenytoin (Additive CNS depressant effects). Products include:

Mesantoin Tablets............................ 2272

Mephobarbital (Additive CNS depressant effects). Products include:

Mebaral Tablets............................... 2322

Meprobamate (Additive CNS depressant effects). Products include:

Miltown Tablets................................ 2672
PMB 200 and PMB 400.................. 2783

Mesoridazine Besylate (Additive CNS depressant effects). Products include:

Serentil... 684

Methadone Hydrochloride (Additive CNS depressant effects). Products include:

Methadone Hydrochloride Oral Concentrate...................................... 2233
Methadone Hydrochloride Oral Solution & Tablets............................ 2235

Methdilazine Hydrochloride (Additive CNS depressant effects).

No products indexed under this heading.

Methohexital Sodium (Additive CNS depressant effects). Products include:

Brevital Sodium Vials...................... 1429

Methotrimeprazine (Additive CNS depressant effects). Products include:

Levoprome....................................... 1274

Methoxyflurane (Additive CNS depressant effects).

No products indexed under this heading.

Methsuximide (Additive CNS depressant effects). Products include:

Celontin Kapseals............................ 1899

Midazolam Hydrochloride (Additive CNS depressant effects). Products include:

Versed Injection............................... 2170

Molindone Hydrochloride (Additive CNS depressant effects). Products include:

Moban Tablets and Concentrate...... 1048

Morphine Sulfate (Additive CNS depressant effects). Products include:

Astramorph/PF Injection, USP (Preservative-Free)........................... 535
Duramorph.. 962
Infumorph 200 and Infumorph 500 Sterile Solutions........................ 965
MS Contin Tablets............................ 1994
MSIR... 1997
Oramorph SR (Morphine Sulfate Sustained Release Tablets)............ 2236
RMS Suppositories.......................... 2657
Roxanol... 2243

Nortriptyline Hydrochloride (Additive CNS depressant effects). Products include:

Pamelor... 2280

(⊞ Described in PDR For Nonprescription Drugs) (◉ Described in PDR For Ophthalmology)

Interactions Index — Haldol Decanoate

Opium Alkaloids (Additive CNS depressant effects).

No products indexed under this heading.

Oxazepam (Additive CNS depressant effects). Products include:

Serax Capsules 2810
Serax Tablets... 2810

Oxycodone Hydrochloride (Additive CNS depressant effects). Products include:

Percocet Tablets 938
Percodan Tablets..................................... 939
Percodan-Demi Tablets........................... 940
Roxicodone Tablets, Oral Solution & Intensol (Oxycodone) 2244
Tylox Capsules 1584

Paramethadione (Additive CNS depressant effects).

No products indexed under this heading.

Pentobarbital Sodium (Additive CNS depressant effects). Products include:

Nembutal Sodium Capsules 436
Nembutal Sodium Solution 438
Nembutal Sodium Suppositories...... 440

Perphenazine (Additive CNS depressant effects). Products include:

Etrafon 2355
Triavil Tablets 1757
Trilafon... 2389

Phenacemide (Additive CNS depressant effects). Products include:

Phenurone Tablets 447

Phenelzine Sulfate (Additive CNS depressant effects). Products include:

Nardil 1920

Phenobarbital (Additive CNS depressant effects). Products include:

Arco-Lase Plus Tablets 512
Bellergal-S Tablets 2250
Donnatal 2060
Donnatal Extentabs................................ 2061
Donnatal Tablets 2060
Phenobarbital Elixir and Tablets 1469
Quadrinal Tablets 1350

Phensuximide (Additive CNS depressant effects). Products include:

Milontin Kapseals................................... 1920

Phenytoin (Additive CNS depressant effects). Products include:

Dilantin Infatabs..................................... 1908
Dilantin-125 Suspension 1911

Phenytoin Sodium (Additive CNS depressant effects). Products include:

Dilantin Kapseals 1906
Dilantin Parenteral 1910

Prazepam (Additive CNS depressant effects).

No products indexed under this heading.

Primidone (Additive CNS depressant effects). Products include:

Mysoline... 2754

Prochlorperazine (Additive CNS depressant effects). Products include:

Compazine 2470

Promethazine Hydrochloride (Additive CNS depressant effects). Products include:

Mepergan Injection 2753
Phenergan with Codeine....................... 2777
Phenergan with Dextromethorphan 2778
Phenergan Injection 2773
Phenergan Suppositories 2775
Phenergan Syrup 2774
Phenergan Tablets 2775
Phenergan VC 2779
Phenergan VC with Codeine 2781

Propofol (Additive CNS depressant effects). Products include:

Diprivan Injection................................... 2833

Propoxyphene Hydrochloride (Additive CNS depressant effects). Products include:

Darvon 1435

Wygesic Tablets 2827

Propoxyphene Napsylate (Additive CNS depressant effects). Products include:

Darvon-N/Darvocet-N 1433

Protriptyline Hydrochloride (Additive CNS depressant effects). Products include:

Vivactil Tablets 1774

Pyrilamine Maleate (Additive CNS depressant effects). Products include:

4-Way Fast Acting Nasal Spray (regular & mentholated) .... ⊕ 621
Maximum Strength Multi-Symptom Formula Midol .... ⊕ 722
PMS Multi-Symptom Formula Midol .... ⊕ 723

Pyrilamine Tannate (Additive CNS depressant effects). Products include:

Atrohist Pediatric Suspension 454
Rynatan 2673

Quazepam (Additive CNS depressant effects). Products include:

Doral Tablets 2664

Risperidone (Additive CNS depressant effects). Products include:

Risperdal 1301

Secobarbital Sodium (Additive CNS depressant effects). Products include:

Seconal Sodium Pulvules 1474

Sufentanil Citrate (Additive CNS depressant effects). Products include:

Sufenta Injection 1309

Temazepam (Additive CNS depressant effects). Products include:

Restoril Capsules................................... 2284

Terfenadine (Additive CNS depressant effects). Products include:

Seldane Tablets 1536
Seldane-D Extended-Release Tablets 1538

Thiamylal Sodium (Additive CNS depressant effects).

No products indexed under this heading.

Thioridazine Hydrochloride (Additive CNS depressant effects). Products include:

Mellaril 2269

Thiothixene (Additive CNS depressant effects). Products include:

Navane Capsules and Concentrate 2201
Navane Intramuscular........................... 2202

Tranylcypromine Sulfate (Additive CNS depressant effects). Products include:

Parnate Tablets 2503

Trifluoperazine Hydrochloride (Additive CNS depressant effects). Products include:

Stelazine 2514

Trimeprazine Tartrate (Additive CNS depressant effects). Products include:

Temaril Tablets, Syrup and Spansule Extended-Release Capsules.. 483

Trimethadione (Additive CNS depressant effects).

No products indexed under this heading.

Trimipramine Maleate (Additive CNS depressant effects). Products include:

Surmontil Capsules................................ 2811

Tripelennamine Hydrochloride (Additive CNS depressant effects). Products include:

PBZ Tablets... 845
PBZ-SR Tablets....................................... 844

Triprolidine Hydrochloride (Additive CNS depressant effects). Products include:

Actifed Plus Caplets .... ⊕ 845
Actifed Plus Tablets .... ⊕ 845

Actifed with Codeine Cough Syrup.. 1067
Actifed Syrup.. ⊕ 846
Actifed Tablets .... ⊕ 844

Valproic Acid (Additive CNS depressant effects). Products include:

Depakene 413

Zolpidem Tartrate (Additive CNS depressant effects). Products include:

Ambien Tablets....................................... 2416

Food Interactions

Alcohol (Additive CNS depressant effects).

HALDOL DECANOATE 50 (50 MG/ML) INJECTION

(Haloperidol Decanoate) 1577

May interact with narcotic analgesics, general anesthetics, oral anticoagulants, lithium preparations, central nervous system depressants, anticonvulsants, anticholinergics, anticholinergic-type antiparkinsonism drugs, and certain other agents. Compounds in these categories include:

Alfentanil Hydrochloride (CNS depressant potentiated). Products include:

Alfenta Injection 1286

Alprazolam (CNS depressant potentiated). Products include:

Xanax Tablets 2649

Aprobarbital (CNS depressant potentiated).

No products indexed under this heading.

Atropine Sulfate (Possible increase in intraocular pressure when anticholinergic drugs including antiparkinson agents are administered concomitantly with haloperidol). Products include:

Arco-Lase Plus Tablets 512
Atrohist Plus Tablets.............................. 454
Atropine Sulfate Sterile Ophthalmic Solution .... © 233
Donnatal 2060
Donnatal Extentabs............................... 2061
Donnatal Tablets 2060
Lomotil 2439
Motofen Tablets 784
Urised Tablets... 1964

Belladonna Alkaloids (Possible increase in intraocular pressure when anticholinergic drugs including antiparkinson agents are administered concomitantly with haloperidol). Products include:

Bellergal-S Tablets 2250
Hyland's Bed Wetting Tablets .... ⊕ 828
Hyland's EnurAid Tablets.................. ⊕ 829
Hyland's Teething Tablets .... ⊕ 830

Benztropine Mesylate (Possible increase in intraocular pressure when anticholinergic drugs including antiparkinson agents are administered concomitantly with haloperidol). Products include:

Cogentin 1621

Biperiden Hydrochloride (Possible increase in intraocular pressure when anticholinergic drugs including antiparkinson agents are administered concomitantly with haloperidol). Products include:

Akineton 1333

Buprenorphine (CNS depressant potentiated). Products include:

Buprenex Injectable 2006

Buspirone Hydrochloride (CNS depressant potentiated). Products include:

BuSpar 737

Butabarbital (CNS depressant potentiated).

No products indexed under this heading.

Butalbital (CNS depressant potentiated). Products include:

Esgic-plus Tablets 1013
Fioricet Tablets....................................... 2258
Fioricet with Codeine Capsules 2260
Fiorinal Capsules 2261
Fiorinal with Codeine Capsules 2262
Fiorinal Tablets....................................... 2261
Phrenilin 785
Sedapap Tablets 50 mg/650 mg .. 1543

Carbamazepine (Haldol lowers the convulsive threshold). Products include:

Atretol Tablets 573
Tegretol Chewable Tablets 852
Tegretol Suspension............................... 852
Tegretol Tablets 852

Chlordiazepoxide (CNS depressant potentiated). Products include:

Libritabs Tablets 2177
Limbitrol 2180

Chlordiazepoxide Hydrochloride (CNS depressant potentiated). Products include:

Librax Capsules 2176
Librium Capsules 2178
Librium Injectable 2179

Chlorpromazine (CNS depressant potentiated). Products include:

Thorazine Suppositories 2523

Chlorprothixene (CNS depressant potentiated).

No products indexed under this heading.

Chlorprothixene Hydrochloride (CNS depressant potentiated).

No products indexed under this heading.

Clidinium Bromide (Possible increase in intraocular pressure when anticholinergic drugs including antiparkinson agents are administered concomitantly with haloperidol). Products include:

Librax Capsules 2176
Quarzan Capsules 2181

Clorazepate Dipotassium (CNS depressant potentiated). Products include:

Tranxene 451

Clozapine (CNS depressant potentiated). Products include:

Clozaril Tablets....................................... 2252

Codeine Phosphate (CNS depressant potentiated). Products include:

Actifed with Codeine Cough Syrup.. 1067
Brontex 1981
Deconsal C Expectorant Syrup 456
Deconsal Pediatric Syrup 457
Dimetane-DC Cough Syrup 2059
Empirin with Codeine Tablets............ 1093
Fioricet with Codeine Capsules 2260
Fiorinal with Codeine Capsules 2262
Isoclor Expectorant................................ 990
Novahistine DH...................................... 2462
Novahistine Expectorant...................... 2463
Nucofed 2051
Phenergan with Codeine 2777
Phenergan VC with Codeine 2781
Robitussin A-C Syrup 2073
Robitussin-DAC Syrup 2074
Ryna .... ⊕ 841
Soma Compound w/Codeine Tablets 2676
Tussi-Organidin NR Liquid and S NR Liquid 2677
Tylenol with Codeine 1583

Desflurane (CNS depressant potentiated). Products include:

Suprane 1813

Dezocine (CNS depressant potentiated). Products include:

Dalgan Injection 538

Diazepam (CNS depressant potentiated). Products include:

Dizac 1809
Valium Injectable 2182
Valium Tablets 2183
Valrelease Capsules 2169

IMPORTANT NOTE: Always consult each drug listing in the patient's regimen for possible interactions.

Dicumarol (Potential interference with anticoagulant activity).
No products indexed under this heading.

Dicyclomine Hydrochloride (Possible increase in intraocular pressure when anticholinergic drugs including antiparkinson agents are administered concomitantly with haloperidol). Products include:
Bentyl ... 1501

Diphenhydramine Hydrochloride (Possible increase in intraocular pressure when antiparkinson agents are administered concomitantly with haloperidol). Products include:
Actifed Allergy Daytime/Nighttime Caplets ... ▣ 844
Actifed Sinus Daytime/Nighttime Tablets and Caplets ... ▣ 846
Arthritis Foundation NightTime Caplets ... ▣ 674
Extra Strength Bayer PM Aspirin .. ▣ 713
Bayer Select Night Time Pain Relief Formula ... ▣ 716
Benadryl Allergy Decongestant Liquid Medication ... ▣ 848
Benadryl Allergy Decongestant Tablets ... ▣ 848
Benadryl Allergy Liquid Medication ... ▣ 849
Benadryl Allergy ... ▣ 848
Benadryl Allergy Sinus Headache Formula Caplets ... ▣ 849
Benadryl Capsules ... 1898
Benadryl Dye-Free Allergy Liquigel Softgels ... ▣ 850
Benadryl Dye-Free Allergy Liquid Medication ... ▣ 850
Benadryl Itch Relief Cream, Children's Formula and Maximum Strength 2% ... ▣ 851
Benadryl Itch Relief Spray, Children's Formula and Maximum Strength 2% ... ▣ 851
Benadryl Itch Relief Stick Maximum Strength 2% ... ▣ 850
Benadryl Itch Stopping Gel, Children's Formula and Maximum Strength 2% ... ▣ 851
Benadryl Kapseals ... 1898
Benadryl Injection ... 1898
Contac Day & Night Cold/Flu Night Caplets ... ▣ 812
Contac Night Allergy/Sinus Caplets ... ▣ 812
Extra Strength Doan's P.M. ... ▣ 633
Legatrin PM ... ▣ 651
Miles Nervine Nighttime Sleep-Aid ▣ 723
Nytol QuickCaps Caplets ... ▣ 610
Sleepinal Night-time Sleep Aid Capsules and Softgels ... ▣ 834
TYLENOL Maximum Strength Allergy Sinus NightTime Medication Caplets ... 1555
TYLENOL Flu NightTime, Maximum Strength, Gelcaps ... 1566
TYLENOL Maximum Strength Flu NightTime Hot Medication Packets ... 1562
TYLENOL PM, Extra Strength Pain Reliever/Sleep Aid Caplets, Geltabs, Gelcaps ... 1560
TYLENOL Severe Allergy Medication Caplets ... 1564
Maximum Strength Unisom Sleepgels ... 1934
Unisom With Pain Relief-Nighttime Sleep Aid and Pain Reliever ... 1934

Divalproex Sodium (Haldol lowers the convulsive threshold). Products include:
Depakote Tablets ... 415

Droperidol (CNS depressant potentiated). Products include:
Inapsine Injection ... 1296

Enflurane (CNS depressant potentiated).
No products indexed under this heading.

Epinephrine Hydrochloride (Haloperidol may block vasopressor activity of epinephrine). Products include:
Ana-Kit Anaphylaxis Emergency Treatment Kit ... 617

Estazolam (CNS depressant potentiated). Products include:
ProSom Tablets ... 449

Ethchlorvynol (CNS depressant potentiated). Products include:
Placidyl Capsules ... 448

Ethinamate (CNS depressant potentiated).
No products indexed under this heading.

Ethosuximide (Haldol lowers the convulsive threshold). Products include:
Zarontin Capsules ... 1928
Zarontin Syrup ... 1929

Ethotoin (Haldol lowers the convulsive threshold). Products include:
Peganone Tablets ... 446

Felbamate (Haldol lowers the convulsive threshold). Products include:
Felbatol ... 2666

Fentanyl (CNS depressant potentiated). Products include:
Duragesic Transdermal System ... 1288

Fentanyl Citrate (CNS depressant potentiated). Products include:
Sublimaze Injection ... 1307

Fluphenazine Decanoate (CNS depressant potentiated). Products include:
Prolixin Decanoate ... 509

Fluphenazine Enanthate (CNS depressant potentiated). Products include:
Prolixin Enanthate ... 509

Fluphenazine Hydrochloride (CNS depressant potentiated). Products include:
Prolixin ... 509

Flurazepam Hydrochloride (CNS depressant potentiated). Products include:
Dalmane Capsules ... 2173

Glutethimide (CNS depressant potentiated).
No products indexed under this heading.

Glycopyrrolate (Possible increase in intraocular pressure when anticholinergic drugs including antiparkinson agents are administered concomitantly with haloperidol). Products include:
Robinul Forte Tablets ... 2072
Robinul Injectable ... 2072
Robinul Tablets ... 2072

Haloperidol (CNS depressant potentiated). Products include:
Haldol Injection, Tablets and Concentrate ... 1575

Hydrocodone Bitartrate (CNS depressant potentiated). Products include:
Anexsia 5/500 Elixir ... 1781
Anexia Tablets ... 1782
Codiclear DH Syrup ... 791
Deconamine CX Cough and Cold Liquid and Tablets ... 1319
Duratuss HD Elixir ... 2565
Hycodan Tablets and Syrup ... 930
Hycomine Compound Tablets ... 932
Hycomine ... 931
Hycotuss Expectorant Syrup ... 933
Hydrocet Capsules ... 782
Lorcet 10/650 ... 1018
Lortab ... 2566
Tussend ... 1783
Tussend Expectorant ... 1785
Vicodin Tablets ... 1356
Vicodin ES Tablets ... 1357
Vicodin Tuss Expectorant ... 1358
Zydone Capsules ... 949

Hydrocodone Polistirex (CNS depressant potentiated). Products include:
Tussionex Pennkinetic Extended-Release Suspension ... 998

Hydroxyzine Hydrochloride (CNS depressant potentiated). Products include:
Atarax Tablets & Syrup ... 2185
Marax Tablets & DF Syrup ... 2200
Vistaril Intramuscular Solution ... 2216

Hyoscyamine (Possible increase in intraocular pressure when anticholinergic drugs including antiparkinson agents are administered concomitantly with haloperidol). Products include:
Cystospaz Tablets ... 1963
Urised Tablets ... 1964

Hyoscyamine Sulfate (Possible increase in intraocular pressure when anticholinergic drugs including antiparkinson agents are administered concomitantly with haloperidol). Products include:
Arco-Lase Plus Tablets ... 512
Atrohist Plus Tablets ... 454
Cystospaz-M Capsules ... 1963
Donnatal ... 2060
Donnatal Extentabs ... 2061
Donnatal Tablets ... 2060
Kutrase Capsules ... 2402
Levsin/Levsinex/Levbid ... 2405

Ipratropium Bromide (Possible increase in intraocular pressure when anticholinergic drugs including antiparkinson agents are administered concomitantly with haloperidol). Products include:
Atrovent Inhalation Aerosol ... 671
Atrovent Inhalation Solution ... 673

Isoflurane (CNS depressant potentiated).
No products indexed under this heading.

Ketamine Hydrochloride (CNS depressant potentiated).
No products indexed under this heading.

Lamotrigine (Haldol lowers the convulsive threshold). Products include:
Lamictal Tablets ... 1112

Levomethadyl Acetate Hydrochloride (CNS depressant potentiated). Products include:
Orlamm ... 2239

Levorphanol Tartrate (CNS depressant potentiated). Products include:
Levo-Dromoran ... 2129

Lithium Carbonate (Potential for an encephalopathic syndrome followed by irreversible brain damage). Products include:
Eskalith ... 2485
Lithium Carbonate Capsules & Tablets ... 2230
Lithonate/Lithotabs/Lithobid ... 2543

Lithium Citrate (Potential for an encephalopathic syndrome followed by irreversible brain damage).
No products indexed under this heading.

Lorazepam (CNS depressant potentiated). Products include:
Ativan Injection ... 2698
Ativan Tablets ... 2700

Loxapine Hydrochloride (CNS depressant potentiated). Products include:
Loxitane ... 1378

Loxapine Succinate (CNS depressant potentiated). Products include:
Loxitane Capsules ... 1378

Mepenzolate Bromide (Possible increase in intraocular pressure when anticholinergic drugs including antiparkinson agents are administered concomitantly with haloperidol).
No products indexed under this heading.

Meperidine Hydrochloride (CNS depressant potentiated). Products include:
Demerol ... 2308
Mepergan Injection ... 2753

Mephenytoin (Haldol lowers the convulsive threshold). Products include:
Mesantoin Tablets ... 2272

Mephobarbital (CNS depressant potentiated). Products include:
Mebaral Tablets ... 2322

Meprobamate (CNS depressant potentiated). Products include:
Miltown Tablets ... 2672
PMB 200 and PMB 400 ... 2783

Mesoridazine Besylate (CNS depressant potentiated). Products include:
Serentil ... 684

Methadone Hydrochloride (CNS depressant potentiated). Products include:
Methadone Hydrochloride Oral Concentrate ... 2233
Methadone Hydrochloride Oral Solution & Tablets ... 2235

Methohexital Sodium (CNS depressant potentiated). Products include:
Brevital Sodium Vials ... 1429

Methotrimeprazine (CNS depressant potentiated). Products include:
Levoprome ... 1274

Methoxyflurane (CNS depressant potentiated).
No products indexed under this heading.

Methsuximide (Haldol lowers the convulsive threshold). Products include:
Celontin Kapseals ... 1899

Midazolam Hydrochloride (CNS depressant potentiated). Products include:
Versed Injection ... 2170

Molindone Hydrochloride (CNS depressant potentiated). Products include:
Moban Tablets and Concentrate ... 1048

Morphine Sulfate (CNS depressant potentiated). Products include:
Astramorph/PF Injection, USP (Preservative-Free) ... 535
Duramorph ... 962
Infumorph 200 and Infumorph 500 Sterile Solutions ... 965
MS Contin Tablets ... 1994
MSIR ... 1997
Oramorph SR (Morphine Sulfate Sustained Release Tablets) ... 2236
RMS Suppositories ... 2657
Roxanol ... 2243

Opium Alkaloids (CNS depressant potentiated).
No products indexed under this heading.

Oxazepam (CNS depressant potentiated). Products include:
Serax Capsules ... 2810
Serax Tablets ... 2810

Oxybutynin Chloride (Possible increase in intraocular pressure when anticholinergic drugs including antiparkinson agents are administered concomitantly with haloperidol). Products include:
Ditropan ... 1516

(▣ Described in PDR For Nonprescription Drugs)   (◉ Described in PDR For Ophthalmology)

Oxycodone Hydrochloride (CNS depressant potentiated). Products include:
Percocet Tablets ... 938
Percodan Tablets ... 939
Percodan-Demi Tablets ... 940
Roxicodone Tablets, Oral Solution & Intensol (Oxycodone) ... 2244
Tylox Capsules ... 1584
Paramethadione (Haldol lowers the convulsive threshold).
No products indexed under this heading.
Pentobarbital Sodium (CNS depressant potentiated). Products include:
Nembutal Sodium Capsules ... 436
Nembutal Sodium Solution ... 438
Nembutal Sodium Suppositories ... 440
Perphenazine (CNS depressant potentiated). Products include:
Etrafon ... 2355
Triavil Tablets ... 1757
Trilafon ... 2389
Phenacemide (Haldol lowers the convulsive threshold). Products include:
Phenurone Tablets ... 447
Phenobarbital (Haldol lowers the convulsive threshold). Products include:
Arco-Lase Plus Tablets ... 512
Bellergal-S Tablets ... 2250
Donnatal ... 2060
Donnatal Extentabs ... 2061
Donnatal Tablets ... 2060
Phenobarbital Elixir and Tablets ... 1469
Quadrinal Tablets ... 1350
Phensuximide (Haldol lowers the convulsive threshold). Products include:
Milontin Kapseals ... 1920
Phenytoin (Haldol lowers the convulsive threshold). Products include:
Dilantin Infatabs ... 1908
Dilantin-125 Suspension ... 1911
Phenytoin Sodium (Haldol lowers the convulsive threshold). Products include:
Dilantin Kapseals ... 1906
Dilantin Parenteral ... 1910
Prazepam (CNS depressant potentiated).
No products indexed under this heading.
Primidone (Haldol lowers the convulsive threshold). Products include:
Mysoline ... 2754
Prochlorperazine (CNS depressant potentiated). Products include:
Compazine ... 2470
Procyclidine Hydrochloride (Possible increase in intraocular pressure when anticholinergic drugs including antiparkinson agents are administered concomitantly with haloperidol). Products include:
Kemadrin Tablets ... 1112
Promethazine Hydrochloride (CNS depressant potentiated). Products include:
Mepergan Injection ... 2753
Phenergan with Codeine ... 2777
Phenergan with Dextromethorphan ... 2778
Phenergan Injection ... 2773
Phenergan Suppositories ... 2775
Phenergan Syrup ... 2774
Phenergan Tablets ... 2775
Phenergan VC ... 2779
Phenergan VC with Codeine ... 2781
Propantheline Bromide (Possible increase in intraocular pressure when anticholinergic drugs including antiparkinson agents are administered concomitantly with haloperidol). Products include:
Pro-Banthīne Tablets ... 2052
Propofol (CNS depressant potentiated). Products include:
Diprivan Injection ... 2833
Propoxyphene Hydrochloride (CNS depressant potentiated). Products include:
Darvon ... 1435
Wygesic Tablets ... 2827
Propoxyphene Napsylate (CNS depressant potentiated). Products include:
Darvon-N/Darvocet-N ... 1433
Quazepam (CNS depressant potentiated). Products include:
Doral Tablets ... 2664
Risperidone (CNS depressant potentiated). Products include:
Risperdal ... 1301
Scopolamine (Possible increase in intraocular pressure when anticholinergic drugs including antiparkinson agents are administered concomitantly with haloperidol). Products include:
Transderm Scōp Transdermal Therapeutic System ... 869
Scopolamine Hydrobromide (Possible increase in intraocular pressure when anticholinergic drugs including antiparkinson agents are administered concomitantly with haloperidol). Products include:
Atrohist Plus Tablets ... 454
Donnatal ... 2060
Donnatal Extentabs ... 2061
Donnatal Tablets ... 2060
Secobarbital Sodium (CNS depressant potentiated). Products include:
Seconal Sodium Pulvules ... 1474
Sufentanil Citrate (CNS depressant potentiated). Products include:
Sufenta Injection ... 1309
Temazepam (CNS depressant potentiated). Products include:
Restoril Capsules ... 2284
Thiamylal Sodium (CNS depressant potentiated).
No products indexed under this heading.
Thioridazine Hydrochloride (CNS depressant potentiated). Products include:
Mellaril ... 2269
Thiothixene (CNS depressant potentiated). Products include:
Navane Capsules and Concentrate ... 2201
Navane Intramuscular ... 2202
Triazolam (CNS depressant potentiated). Products include:
Halcion Tablets ... 2611
Tridihexethyl Chloride (Possible increase in intraocular pressure when anticholinergic drugs including antiparkinson agents are administered concomitantly with haloperidol).
No products indexed under this heading.
Trifluoperazine Hydrochloride (CNS depressant potentiated). Products include:
Stelazine ... 2514
Trihexyphenidyl Hydrochloride (Possible increase in intraocular pressure when anticholinergic drugs including antiparkinson agents are administered concomitantly with haloperidol). Products include:
Artane ... 1368
Trimethadione (Haldol lowers the convulsive threshold).
No products indexed under this heading.
Valproic Acid (Haldol lowers the convulsive threshold). Products include:
Depakene ... 413
Warfarin Sodium (Potential interference with anticoagulant activity). Products include:
Coumadin ... 926
Zolpidem Tartrate (CNS depressant potentiated). Products include:
Ambien Tablets ... 2416

Food Interactions

Alcohol (CNS depressant potentiated).

HALDOL DECANOATE 100 (100 MG/ML) INJECTION

(Haloperidol Decanoate) ... 1577
See **Haldol Decanoate 50 (50 mg/mL) Injection**

HALDOL INJECTION, TABLETS AND CONCENTRATE

(Haloperidol) ... 1575
May interact with general anesthetics, narcotic analgesics, anticholinergics, lithium preparations, and certain other agents. Compounds in these categories include:

Alfentanil Hydrochloride (CNS depressant potentiated). Products include:
Alfenta Injection ... 1286
Atropine Sulfate (Possible increase in intraocular pressure). Products include:
Arco-Lase Plus Tablets ... 512
Atrohist Plus Tablets ... 454
Atropine Sulfate Sterile Ophthalmic Solution ... ◉ 233
Donnatal ... 2060
Donnatal Extentabs ... 2061
Donnatal Tablets ... 2060
Lomotil ... 2439
Motofen Tablets ... 784
Urised Tablets ... 1964
Belladonna Alkaloids (Possible increase in intraocular pressure). Products include:
Bellergal-S Tablets ... 2250
Hyland's Bed Wetting Tablets ... ▣ 828
Hyland's EnurAid Tablets ... ▣ 829
Hyland's Teething Tablets ... ▣ 830
Benztropine Mesylate (Possible increase in intraocular pressure). Products include:
Cogentin ... 1621
Biperiden Hydrochloride (Possible increase in intraocular pressure). Products include:
Akineton ... 1333
Buprenorphine (CNS depressant potentiated). Products include:
Buprenex Injectable ... 2006
Clidinium Bromide (Possible increase in intraocular pressure). Products include:
Librax Capsules ... 2176
Quarzan Capsules ... 2181
Codeine Phosphate (CNS depressant potentiated). Products include:
Actifed with Codeine Cough Syrup ... 1067
Brontex ... 1981
Deconsal C Expectorant Syrup ... 456
Deconsal Pediatric Syrup ... 457
Dimetane-DC Cough Syrup ... 2059
Empirin with Codeine Tablets ... 1093
Fioricet with Codeine Capsules ... 2260
Fiorinal with Codeine Capsules ... 2262
Isoclor Expectorant ... 990
Novahistine DH ... 2462
Novahistine Expectorant ... 2463
Nucofed ... 2051
Phenergan with Codeine ... 2777
Phenergan VC with Codeine ... 2781
Robitussin A-C Syrup ... 2073
Robitussin-DAC Syrup ... 2074
Ryna ... ▣ 841
Soma Compound w/Codeine Tablets ... 2676
Tussi-Organidin NR Liquid and S NR Liquid ... 2677
Tylenol with Codeine ... 1583
Dezocine (CNS depressant potentiated). Products include:
Dalgan Injection ... 538
Dicyclomine Hydrochloride (Possible increase in intraocular pressure). Products include:
Bentyl ... 1501
Enflurane (CNS depressant potentiated).
No products indexed under this heading.
Epinephrine Hydrochloride (Haloperidol may block vasopressor activity of epinephrine). Products include:
Ana-Kit Anaphylaxis Emergency Treatment Kit ... 617
Ethopropazine Hydrochloride (Possible increase in intraocular pressure).
Fentanyl (CNS depressant potentiated). Products include:
Duragesic Transdermal System ... 1288
Fentanyl Citrate (CNS depressant potentiated). Products include:
Sublimaze Injection ... 1307
Glycopyrrolate (Possible increase in intraocular pressure). Products include:
Robinul Forte Tablets ... 2072
Robinul Injectable ... 2072
Robinul Tablets ... 2072
Hydrocodone Bitartrate (CNS depressant potentiated). Products include:
Anexsia 5/500 Elixir ... 1781
Anexia Tablets ... 1782
Codiclear DH Syrup ... 791
Deconamine CX Cough and Cold Liquid and Tablets ... 1319
Duratuss HD Elixir ... 2565
Hycodan Tablets and Syrup ... 930
Hycomine Compound Tablets ... 932
Hycomine ... 931
Hycotuss Expectorant Syrup ... 933
Hydrocet Capsules ... 782
Lorcet 10/650 ... 1018
Lortab ... 2566
Tussend ... 1783
Tussend Expectorant ... 1785
Vicodin Tablets ... 1356
Vicodin ES Tablets ... 1357
Vicodin Tuss Expectorant ... 1358
Zydone Capsules ... 949
Hydrocodone Polistirex (CNS depressant potentiated). Products include:
Tussionex Pennkinetic Extended-Release Suspension ... 998
Hyoscyamine (Possible increase in intraocular pressure). Products include:
Cystospaz Tablets ... 1963
Urised Tablets ... 1964
Hyoscyamine Sulfate (Possible increase in intraocular pressure). Products include:
Arco-Lase Plus Tablets ... 512
Atrohist Plus Tablets ... 454
Cystospaz-M Capsules ... 1963
Donnatal ... 2060
Donnatal Extentabs ... 2061
Donnatal Tablets ... 2060
Kutrase Capsules ... 2402
Levsin/Levsinex/Levbid ... 2405
Ipratropium Bromide (Possible increase in intraocular pressure). Products include:
Atrovent Inhalation Aerosol ... 671
Atrovent Inhalation Solution ... 673
Isoflurane (CNS depressant potentiated).
No products indexed under this heading.
Levorphanol Tartrate (CNS depressant potentiated). Products include:
Levo-Dromoran ... 2129

IMPORTANT NOTE: Always consult each drug listing in the patient's regimen for possible interactions.

Lithium Carbonate (Potential for an encephalopathic syndrome followed by irreversible brain damage). Products include:
- Eskalith ... 2485
- Lithium Carbonate Capsules & Tablets ... 2230
- Lithonate/Lithotabs/Lithobid ... 2543

Lithium Citrate (Potential for an encephalopathic syndrome followed by irreversible brain damage).
- No products indexed under this heading.

Mepenzolate Bromide (Possible increase in intraocular pressure).
- No products indexed under this heading.

Meperidine Hydrochloride (CNS depressant potentiated). Products include:
- Demerol ... 2308
- Mepergan Injection ... 2753

Methadone Hydrochloride (CNS depressant potentiated). Products include:
- Methadone Hydrochloride Oral Concentrate ... 2233
- Methadone Hydrochloride Oral Solution & Tablets ... 2235

Methohexital Sodium (CNS depressant potentiated). Products include:
- Brevital Sodium Vials ... 1429

Methoxyflurane (CNS depressant potentiated).
- No products indexed under this heading.

Morphine Sulfate (CNS depressant potentiated). Products include:
- Astramorph/PF Injection, USP (Preservative-Free) ... 535
- Duramorph ... 962
- Infumorph 200 and Infumorph 500 Sterile Solutions ... 965
- MS Contin Tablets ... 1994
- MSIR ... 1997
- Oramorph SR (Morphine Sulfate Sustained Release Tablets) ... 2236
- RMS Suppositories ... 2657
- Roxanol ... 2243

Opium Alkaloids (CNS depressant potentiated).
- No products indexed under this heading.

Oxybutynin Chloride (Possible increase in intraocular pressure). Products include:
- Ditropan ... 1516

Oxycodone Hydrochloride (CNS depressant potentiated). Products include:
- Percocet Tablets ... 938
- Percodan Tablets ... 939
- Percodan-Demi Tablets ... 940
- Roxicodone Tablets, Oral Solution & Intensol (Oxycodone) ... 2244
- Tylox Capsules ... 1584

Oxyphenonium Bromide (Possible increase in intraocular pressure).

Procyclidine Hydrochloride (Possible increase in intraocular pressure). Products include:
- Kemadrin Tablets ... 1112

Propantheline Bromide (Possible increase in intraocular pressure). Products include:
- Pro-Banthīne Tablets ... 2052

Propofol (CNS depressant potentiated). Products include:
- Diprivan Injection ... 2833

Propoxyphene Hydrochloride (CNS depressant potentiated). Products include:
- Darvon ... 1435
- Wygesic Tablets ... 2827

Propoxyphene Napsylate (CNS depressant potentiated). Products include:
- Darvon-N/Darvocet-N ... 1433

Scopolamine (Possible increase in intraocular pressure). Products include:
- Transderm Scōp Transdermal Therapeutic System ... 869

Scopolamine Hydrobromide (Possible increase in intraocular pressure). Products include:
- Atrohist Plus Tablets ... 454
- Donnatal ... 2060
- Donnatal Extentabs ... 2061
- Donnatal Tablets ... 2060

Sufentanil Citrate (CNS depressant potentiated). Products include:
- Sufenta Injection ... 1309

Tridihexethyl Chloride (Possible increase in intraocular pressure).
- No products indexed under this heading.

Trihexyphenidyl Hydrochloride (Possible increase in intraocular pressure). Products include:
- Artane ... 1368

Food Interactions

Alcohol (CNS depressant potentiated).

HALFPRIN
(Aspirin) ... 1362
None cited in PDR database.

HALLS MENTHO-LYPTUS COUGH SUPPRESSANT TABLETS
(Eucalyptus, Oil of, Menthol) ... ▣ 842
None cited in PDR database.

MAXIMUM STRENGTH HALLS PLUS COUGH SUPPRESSANT TABLETS
(Menthol) ... ▣ 843
None cited in PDR database.

HALLS SUGAR FREE COUGH SUPPRESSANT TABLETS
(Menthol, Eucalyptus, Oil of) ... ▣ 842
None cited in PDR database.

HALLS VITAMIN C DROPS
(Vitamin C) ... ▣ 843
None cited in PDR database.

HALOG CREAM, OINTMENT & SOLUTION
(Halcinonide) ... 2686
None cited in PDR database.

HALOG-E CREAM
(Halcinonide) ... 2686
None cited in PDR database.

HALOTESTIN TABLETS
(Fluoxymesterone) ... 2614
May interact with oral anticoagulants, insulin, and certain other agents. Compounds in these categories include:

Dicumarol (Increased sensitivity to dicumarol).
- No products indexed under this heading.

Insulin, Human (Insulin requirements may be decreased).
- No products indexed under this heading.

Insulin, Human Isophane Suspension (Insulin requirements may be decreased). Products include:
- Novolin N Human Insulin 10 ml Vials ... 1795

Insulin, Human NPH (Insulin requirements may be decreased). Products include:
- Humulin N, 100 Units ... 1448
- Novolin N PenFill Cartridges Durable Insulin Delivery System ... 1798
- Novolin N Prefilled Syringe Disposable Insulin Delivery System ... 1798

Insulin, Human Regular (Insulin requirements may be decreased). Products include:
- Humulin R, 100 Units ... 1449
- Novolin R Human Insulin 10 ml Vials ... 1795
- Novolin R PenFill Cartridges Durable Insulin Delivery System ... 1798
- Novolin R Prefilled Syringe Disposable Insulin Delivery System ... 1798
- Velosulin BR Human Insulin 10 ml Vials ... 1795

Insulin, Human, Zinc Suspension (Insulin requirements may be decreased). Products include:
- Humulin L, 100 Units ... 1446
- Humulin U, 100 Units ... 1450
- Novolin L Human Insulin 10 ml Vials ... 1795

Insulin, NPH (Insulin requirements may be decreased). Products include:
- NPH, 100 Units ... 1450
- Pork NPH, 100 Units ... 1452
- Purified Pork NPH Isophane Insulin ... 1801

Insulin, Regular (Insulin requirements may be decreased). Products include:
- Regular, 100 Units ... 1450
- Pork Regular, 100 Units ... 1452
- Pork Regular (Concentrated), 500 Units ... 1453
- Purified Pork Regular Insulin ... 1801

Insulin, Zinc Crystals (Insulin requirements may be decreased). Products include:
- NPH, 100 Units ... 1450

Insulin, Zinc Suspension (Insulin requirements may be decreased). Products include:
- Iletin I ... 1450
- Lente, 100 Units ... 1450
- Iletin II ... 1452
- Pork Lente, 100 Units ... 1452
- Purified Pork Lente Insulin ... 1801

Oxyphenbutazone (Elevated serum levels of oxyphenbutazone).

Warfarin Sodium (Increased sensitivity to warfarin). Products include:
- Coumadin ... 926

HALTRAN TABLETS
(Ibuprofen) ... ▣ 771
May interact with aspirin and acetaminophen containing products. Compounds in this category include:

Acetaminophen (Effect not specified). Products include:
- Actifed Plus Caplets ... ▣ 845
- Actifed Plus Tablets ... ▣ 845
- Actifed Sinus Daytime/Nighttime Tablets and Caplets ... ▣ 846
- Alka-Seltzer Plus Cold Medicine Liqui-Gels ... ▣ 706
- Alka-Seltzer Plus Cold & Cough Medicine Liqui-Gels ... ▣ 705
- Alka-Seltzer Plus Night-Time Cold Medicine Liqui-Gels ... ▣ 706
- Allerest Headache Strength Tablets ... ▣ 627
- Allerest No Drowsiness Tablets ... ▣ 627
- Allerest Sinus Pain Formula ... ▣ 627
- Anexsia 5/500 Elixir ... 1781
- Anexia Tablets ... 1782
- Arthritis Foundation Aspirin Free Caplets ... ▣ 673
- Arthritis Foundation NightTime Caplets ... ▣ 674
- Bayer Select Headache Pain Relief Formula ... ▣ 716
- Bayer Select Menstrual Multi-Symptom Formula ... ▣ 716
- Bayer Select Night Time Pain Relief Formula ... ▣ 716
- Bayer Select Sinus Pain Relief Formula ... ▣ 717
- Benadryl Allergy Sinus Headache Formula Caplets ... ▣ 849
- Comtrex Multi-Symptom Cold Reliever Tablets/Caplets/Liqui-Gels/Liquid ... ▣ 615
- Allergy-Sinus Comtrex Multi-Symptom Allergy-Sinus Formula Tablets ... ▣ 617
- Comtrex Non-Drowsy ... ▣ 618
- Contac Day Allergy/Sinus Caplets ▣ 812
- Contac Day & Night ... ▣ 812
- Contac Night Allergy/Sinus Caplets ... ▣ 812
- Contac Severe Cold and Flu Formula Caplets ... ▣ 814
- Contac Severe Cold & Flu Non-Drowsy ... ▣ 815
- Coricidin 'D' Decongestant Tablets ... ▣ 800
- Coricidin Tablets ... ▣ 800
- DHCplus Capsules ... 1993
- Darvon-N/Darvocet-N ... 1433
- Drixoral Cold and Flu Extended-Release Tablets ... ▣ 803
- Drixoral Cough + Sore Throat Liquid Caps ... ▣ 802
- Drixoral Allergy/Sinus Extended Release Tablets ... ▣ 804
- Esgic-plus Tablets ... 1013
- Aspirin Free Excedrin Analgesic Caplets and Geltabs ... 732
- Excedrin Extra-Strength Analgesic Tablets & Caplets ... 732
- Excedrin P.M. Analgesic/Sleeping Aid Tablets, Caplets, Liquigels ... 733
- Fioricet Tablets ... 2258
- Fioricet with Codeine Capsules ... 2260
- Hycomine Compound Tablets ... 932
- Hydrocet Capsules ... 782
- Legatrin PM ... ▣ 651
- Lorcet 10/650 ... 1018
- Lortab ... 2566
- Lurline PMS Tablets ... 982
- Maximum Strength Multi-Symptom Formula Midol ... ▣ 722
- PMS Multi-Symptom Formula Midol ... ▣ 723
- Teen Multi-Symptom Formula Midol ... ▣ 722
- Midrin Capsules ... 783
- Migralam Capsules ... 2038
- Panodol Tablets and Caplets ... ▣ 824
- Children's Panadol Chewable Tablets, Liquid, Infant's Drops ... ▣ 824
- Percocet Tablets ... 938
- Percogesic Analgesic Tablets ... ▣ 754
- Phrenilin ... 785
- Pyrroxate Caplets ... ▣ 772
- Sedapap Tablets 50 mg/650 mg .. 1543
- Sinarest Tablets ... ▣ 648
- Sinarest Extra Strength Tablets ... ▣ 648
- Sinarest No Drowsiness Tablets ... ▣ 648
- Sine-Aid Maximum Strength Sinus Medication Gelcaps, Caplets and Tablets ... 1554
- Sine-Off No Drowsiness Formula Caplets ... ▣ 824
- Sine-Off Sinus Medicine ... ▣ 825
- Singlet Tablets ... ▣ 825
- Sinulin Tablets ... 787
- Sinutab Sinus Allergy Medication, Maximum Strength Tablets and Caplets ... ▣ 860
- Sinutab Sinus Medication, Maximum Strength Without Drowsiness Formula, Tablets & Caplets ... ▣ 860
- Sinutab Sinus Medication, Regular Strength Without Drowsiness Formula ... ▣ 859
- Sudafed Cold and Cough Liquidcaps ... ▣ 862
- Sudafed Severe Cold Formula Caplets ... ▣ 863
- Sudafed Severe Cold Formula Tablets ... ▣ 864
- Sudafed Sinus Caplets ... ▣ 864
- Sudafed Sinus Tablets ... ▣ 864
- Talacen ... 2333
- TheraFlu ... ▣ 787
- TheraFlu Maximum Strength Nighttime Flu, Cold & Cough Medicine ... ▣ 788
- TheraFlu Maximum Strength Non-Drowsy Formula Flu, Cold & Cough Medicine ... ▣ 788
- Thera Flu Maximum Strength, Non-Drowsy Formula Flu, Cold and Cough Caplets ... ▣ 789
- Triaminic Sore Throat Formula ... ▣ 791
- Triaminicin Tablets ... ▣ 793

(▣ Described in PDR For Nonprescription Drugs) (◉ Described in PDR For Ophthalmology)

Children's TYLENOL acetaminophen Chewable Tablets, Elixir, Suspension Liquid 1555
Children's TYLENOL Cold Multi-Symptom Liquid Formula and Chewable Tablets.............................. 1561
Children's TYLENOL Cold Plus Cough Multi Symptom Tablets and Liquid .... ⊞ 681
Infants' TYLENOL acetaminophen Drops and Suspension Drops 1555
Infants' TYLENOL Cold Decongestant & Fever-Reducer Drops 1556
TYLENOL Extended Relief Caplets.. 1558
TYLENOL, Extra Strength, Acetaminophen Adult Liquid Pain Reliever 1560
TYLENOL, Extra Strength, acetaminophen Gelcaps, Geltabs, Caplets, Tablets 1559
TYLENOL, Extra Strength, Headache Plus Pain Reliever with Antacid Caplets 1559
TYLENOL, Junior Strength, acetaminophen Coated Caplets, Grape and Fruit Chewable Tablets 1557
TYLENOL Maximum Strength Allergy Sinus Medication Gelcaps and Caplets 1563
TYLENOL Maximum Strength Allergy Sinus NightTime Medication Caplets 1555
TYLENOL Flu Maximum Strength Gelcaps 1565
TYLENOL Flu NightTime, Maximum Strength, Gelcaps 1566
TYLENOL Maximum Strength Flu NightTime Hot Medication Packets 1562
TYLENOL, Maximum Strength, Sinus Medication Geltabs, Gelcaps, Caplets and Tablets 1566
TYLENOL Cold Multi-Symptom Formula Medication Tablets and Caplets 1561
TYLENOL Cold Medication No Drowsiness Formula Gelcaps and Caplets 1562
TYLENOL Cold Multi-Symptom Hot Medication Liquid Packets............... 1557
TYLENOL Cough Multi-Symptom Medication 1564
TYLENOL Cough Multi-Symptom Medication with Decongestant 1565
TYLENOL, Regular Strength, acetaminophen Caplets and Tablets .. 1558
TYLENOL PM, Extra Strength Pain Reliever/Sleep Aid Caplets, Geltabs, Gelcaps 1560
TYLENOL Severe Allergy Medication Caplets 1564
Tylenol with Codeine 1583
Tylox Capsules 1584
Unisom With Pain Relief-Nighttime Sleep Aid and Pain Reliever............. 1934
Vanquish Analgesic Caplets .... ⊞ 731
Vicks 44 LiquiCaps Cough, Cold & Flu Relief.. ⊞ 755
Vicks 44M Cough, Cold & Flu Relief... ⊞ 756
Vicks DayQuil .... ⊞ 761
Vicks Nyquil Hot Therapy................. ⊞ 762
Vicks NyQuil LiquiCaps Multi-Symptom Cold/Flu Relief .... ⊞ 763
Vicks NyQuil Multi-Symptom Cold/Flu Relief - (Original & Cherry Flavor) .... ⊞ 763
Vicodin Tablets................................... 1356
Vicodin ES Tablets 1357
Wygesic Tablets 2827
Zydone Capsules 949

Aspirin (Effect not specified). Products include:

Alka-Seltzer Effervescent Antacid and Pain Reliever.............................. ⊞ 701
Alka-Seltzer Extra Strength Effervescent Antacid and Pain Reliever .... ⊞ 703
Alka-Seltzer Lemon Lime Effervescent Antacid and Pain Reliever .... ⊞ 703
Alka-Seltzer Plus Cold Medicine .... ⊞ 705
Alka-Seltzer Plus Cold & Cough Medicine .... ⊞ 708
Alka-Seltzer Plus Night-Time Cold Medicine .... ⊞ 707
Alka Seltzer Plus Sinus Medicine .. ⊞ 707
Arthritis Foundation Safety Coated Aspirin Tablets .... ⊞ 675

Arthritis Pain Ascriptin .... ⊞ 631
Maximum Strength Ascriptin .... ⊞ 630
Regular Strength Ascriptin Tablets .... ⊞ 629
Arthritis Strength BC Powder.......... ⊞ 609
BC Cold Powder Multi-Symptom Formula (Cold-Sinus-Allergy) ...... ⊞ 609
BC Cold Powder Non-Drowsy Formula (Cold-Sinus) .... ⊞ 609
BC Powder .... ⊞ 609
Bayer Children's Chewable Aspirin .... ⊞ 711
Genuine Bayer Aspirin Tablets & Caplets .... ⊞ 713
Extra Strength Bayer Arthritis Pain Regimen Formula .... ⊞ 711
Extra Strength Bayer Aspirin Caplets & Tablets .... ⊞ 712
Extended-Release Bayer 8-Hour Aspirin .... ⊞ 712
Extra Strength Bayer Plus Aspirin Caplets .... ⊞ 713
Extra Strength Bayer PM Aspirin .. ⊞ 713
Bayer Enteric Aspirin .... ⊞ 709
Bufferin Analgesic Tablets and Caplets .... ⊞ 613
Arthritis Strength Bufferin Analgesic Caplets .... ⊞ 614
Extra Strength Bufferin Analgesic Tablets .... ⊞ 615
Cama Arthritis Pain Reliever............ ⊞ 785
Darvon Compound-65 Pulvules 1435
Easprin 1914
Ecotrin 2455
Ecotrin Enteric Coated Aspirin Maximum Strength Tablets and Caplets .... ⊞ 816
Ecotrin Enteric Coated Aspirin Regular Strength Tablets 2455
Empirin Aspirin Tablets .... ⊞ 854
Empirin with Codeine Tablets.......... 1093
Excedrin Extra-Strength Analgesic Tablets & Caplets 732
Fiorinal Capsules 2261
Fiorinal with Codeine Capsules 2262
Fiorinal Tablets 2261
Halfprin 1362
Healthprin Aspirin 2455
Norgesic... 1496
Percodan Tablets.................................. 939
Percodan-Demi Tablets....................... 940
Robaxisal Tablets................................. 2071
Soma Compound w/Codeine Tablets 2676
Soma Compound Tablets.................... 2675
St. Joseph Adult Chewable Aspirin (81 mg.) .... ⊞ 808
Talwin Compound 2335
Ursinus Inlay-Tabs.............................. ⊞ 794
Vanquish Analgesic Caplets .... ⊞ 731

HAVRIX

(Hepatitis A Vaccine, Inactivated) 2489
May interact with anticoagulants. Compounds in this category include:

Dalteparin Sodium (Havrix should be given with caution to individuals on anticoagulant therapy). Products include:

Fragmin 1954

Dicumarol (Havrix should be given with caution to individuals on anticoagulant therapy).

No products indexed under this heading.

Enoxaparin (Havrix should be given with caution to individuals on anticoagulant therapy). Products include:

Lovenox Injection.. 2020

Heparin Calcium (Havrix should be given with caution to individuals on anticoagulant therapy).

No products indexed under this heading.

Heparin Sodium (Havrix should be given with caution to individuals on anticoagulant therapy). Products include:

Heparin Lock Flush Solution 2725
Heparin Sodium Injection..................... 2726
Heparin Sodium Injection, USP, Sterile Solution 2615
Heparin Sodium Vials............................ 1441

Warfarin Sodium (Havrix should be given with caution to individuals on anticoagulant therapy). Products include:

Coumadin 926

HEAD & SHOULDERS INTENSIVE TREATMENT DANDRUFF SHAMPOO

(Selenium Sulfide)................................ ⊞ 750
None cited in PDR database.

HEAD & SHOULDERS INTENSIVE TREATMENT DANDRUFF SHAMPOO 2-IN-1 PLUS CONDITIONER

(Selenium Sulfide)................................ ⊞ 750
None cited in PDR database.

HEALON

(Sodium Hyaluronate) .... ◎ 314
None cited in PDR database.

HEALON GV

(Sodium Hyaluronate) .... ◎ 315
None cited in PDR database.

HEALTHPRIN ASPIRIN

(Aspirin) 2455
May interact with oral anticoagulants. Compounds in this category include:

Antiarthritic Drugs, unspecified (Concurrent use not recommended unless directed by a doctor).

Antidiabetic Drugs, unspecified (Concurrent use not recommended unless directed by a doctor).

Antigout Drugs, unspecified (Concurrent use not recommended unless directed by a doctor).

Dicumarol (Concurrent use not recommended unless directed by a doctor).

No products indexed under this heading.

Warfarin Sodium (Concurrent use not recommended unless directed by a doctor). Products include:

Coumadin 926

HEMORID FOR WOMEN CLEANSER

(Cleanser)... ⊞ 834
None cited in PDR database.

HEMORID FOR WOMEN CREME

(Petrolatum, White, Mineral Oil, Pramoxine Hydrochloride, Phenylephrine Hydrochloride).......... ⊞ 834
None cited in PDR database.

HEMORID FOR WOMEN SUPPOSITORIES

(Zinc Oxide, Phenylephrine Hydrochloride, Fat, Hard) .... ⊞ 834
None cited in PDR database.

HEPARIN LOCK FLUSH SOLUTION

(Heparin Sodium) 2725
May interact with cardiac glycosides, antihistamines, tetracyclines, nonsteroidal anti-inflammatory agents, platelet inhibitors, and certain other agents. Compounds in these categories include:

Acrivastine (Anticoagulant action partially counteracted). Products include:

Semprex-D Capsules 463
Semprex-D Capsules 1167

Aspirin (Interferes with platelet-aggregation reactions and may induce bleeding). Products include:

Alka-Seltzer Effervescent Antacid and Pain Reliever.............................. ⊞ 701
Alka-Seltzer Extra Strength Effervescent Antacid and Pain Reliever .... ⊞ 703
Alka-Seltzer Lemon Lime Effervescent Antacid and Pain Reliever .... ⊞ 703
Alka-Seltzer Plus Cold Medicine .... ⊞ 705
Alka-Seltzer Plus Cold & Cough Medicine .... ⊞ 708
Alka-Seltzer Plus Night-Time Cold Medicine .... ⊞ 707
Alka Seltzer Plus Sinus Medicine .. ⊞ 707
Arthritis Foundation Safety Coated Aspirin Tablets .... ⊞ 675
Arthritis Pain Ascriptin .... ⊞ 631
Maximum Strength Ascriptin .... ⊞ 630
Regular Strength Ascriptin Tablets .... ⊞ 629
Arthritis Strength BC Powder.......... ⊞ 609
BC Cold Powder Multi-Symptom Formula (Cold-Sinus-Allergy) ...... ⊞ 609
BC Cold Powder Non-Drowsy Formula (Cold-Sinus) .... ⊞ 609
BC Powder .... ⊞ 609
Bayer Children's Chewable Aspirin .... ⊞ 711
Genuine Bayer Aspirin Tablets & Caplets .... ⊞ 713
Extra Strength Bayer Arthritis Pain Regimen Formula .... ⊞ 711
Extra Strength Bayer Aspirin Caplets & Tablets .... ⊞ 712
Extended-Release Bayer 8-Hour Aspirin .... ⊞ 712
Extra Strength Bayer Plus Aspirin Caplets .... ⊞ 713
Extra Strength Bayer PM Aspirin .. ⊞ 713
Bayer Enteric Aspirin .... ⊞ 709
Bufferin Analgesic Tablets and Caplets .... ⊞ 613
Arthritis Strength Bufferin Analgesic Caplets .... ⊞ 614
Extra Strength Bufferin Analgesic Tablets .... ⊞ 615
Cama Arthritis Pain Reliever............ ⊞ 785
Darvon Compound-65 Pulvules 1435
Easprin 1914
Ecotrin 2455
Ecotrin Enteric Coated Aspirin Maximum Strength Tablets and Caplets .... ⊞ 816
Ecotrin Enteric Coated Aspirin Regular Strength Tablets 2455
Empirin Aspirin Tablets .... ⊞ 854
Empirin with Codeine Tablets.......... 1093
Excedrin Extra-Strength Analgesic Tablets & Caplets 732
Fiorinal Capsules 2261
Fiorinal with Codeine Capsules 2262
Fiorinal Tablets 2261
Halfprin 1362
Healthprin Aspirin 2455
Norgesic... 1496
Percodan Tablets.................................. 939
Percodan-Demi Tablets....................... 940
Robaxisal Tablets................................. 2071
Soma Compound w/Codeine Tablets 2676
Soma Compound Tablets.................... 2675
St. Joseph Adult Chewable Aspirin (81 mg.) .... ⊞ 808
Talwin Compound 2335
Ursinus Inlay-Tabs.............................. ⊞ 794
Vanquish Analgesic Caplets .... ⊞ 731

Astemizole (Anticoagulant action partially counteracted). Products include:

Hismanal Tablets................................... 1293

Azatadine Maleate (Anticoagulant action partially counteracted). Products include:

Trinalin Repetabs Tablets 1330

Azlocillin Sodium (Interferes with platelet-aggregation reactions and may induce bleeding).

No products indexed under this heading.

Bromodiphenhydramine Hydrochloride (Anticoagulant action partially counteracted).

No products indexed under this heading.

IMPORTANT NOTE: Always consult each drug listing in the patient's regimen for possible interactions.

Heparin Lock Flush | Interactions Index | 468

Brompheniramine Maleate (Anticoagulant action partially counteracted). Products include:

- Alka Seltzer Plus Sinus Medicine .. ▣ 707
- Bromfed Capsules (Extended-Release) 1785
- Bromfed Syrup .... ▣ 733
- Bromfed Tablets 1785
- Bromfed-DM Cough Syrup 1786
- Bromfed-PD Capsules (Extended-Release) 1785
- Dimetane-DC Cough Syrup 2059
- Dimetane-DX Cough Syrup 2059
- Dimetapp Elixir .... ▣ 773
- Dimetapp Extentabs .... ▣ 774
- Dimetapp Tablets/Liqui-Gels .... ▣ 775
- Dimetapp Cold & Allergy Chewable Tablets .... ▣ 773
- Dimetapp DM Elixir .... ▣ 774
- Vicks DayQuil Allergy Relief 12-Hour Extended Release Tablets .. ▣ 760
- Vicks DayQuil Allergy Relief 4-Hour Tablets .... ▣ 760

Carbenicillin Indanyl Sodium (Interferes with platelet-aggregation reactions and may induce bleeding). Products include:

- Geocillin Tablets 2199

Chlorpheniramine Maleate (Anticoagulant action partially counteracted). Products include:

- Alka-Seltzer Plus Cold Medicine .... ▣ 705
- Alka-Seltzer Plus Cold Medicine Liqui-Gels .... ▣ 706
- Alka-Seltzer Plus Cold & Cough Medicine .... ▣ 708
- Alka-Seltzer Plus Cold & Cough Medicine Liqui-Gels .... ▣ 705
- Allerest Children's Chewable Tablets .... ▣ 627
- Allerest Headache Strength Tablets .... ▣ 627
- Allerest Maximum Strength Tablets .... ▣ 627
- Allerest Sinus Pain Formula .... ▣ 627
- Allerest 12 Hour Caplets .... ▣ 627
- Ana-Kit Anaphylaxis Emergency Treatment Kit 617
- Atrohist Pediatric Capsules 453
- Atrohist Plus Tablets 454
- BC Cold Powder Multi-Symptom Formula (Cold-Sinus-Allergy) .... ▣ 609
- Cerose DM .... ▣ 878
- Cheracol Plus Head Cold/Cough Formula .... ▣ 769
- Children's Vicks DayQuil Allergy Relief .... ▣ 757
- Children's Vicks NyQuil Cold/Cough Relief .... ▣ 758
- Chlor-Trimeton Allergy Decongestant Tablets .... ▣ 799
- Chlor-Trimeton Allergy Tablets .... ▣ 798
- Comhist 2038
- Comtrex Multi-Symptom Cold Reliever Tablets/Caplets/Liqui-Gels/Liquid .... ▣ 615
- Allergy-Sinus Comtrex Multi-Symptom Allergy-Sinus Formula Tablets .... ▣ 617
- Contac Continuous Action Nasal Decongestant/Antihistamine 12 Hour Capsules .... ▣ 813
- Contac Maximum Strength Continuous Action Decongestant/Antihistamine 12 Hour Caplets .. ▣ 813
- Contac Severe Cold and Flu Formula Caplets .... ▣ 814
- Coricidin 'D' Decongestant Tablets .... ▣ 800
- Coricidin Tablets .... ▣ 800
- D.A. Chewable Tablets 951
- Deconamine 1320
- Dura-Tap/PD Capsules 2867
- Dura-Vent/DA Tablets 953
- Extendryl 1005
- Fedahist Gyrocaps 2401
- Fedahist Timecaps 2401
- Hycomine Compound Tablets 932
- Isoclor Timesule Capsules .... ▣ 637
- Kronofed-A 977
- Nolamine Timed-Release Tablets 785
- Novahistine DH 2462
- Novahistine Elixir .... ▣ 823
- Ornade Spansule Capsules 2502
- PediaCare Cold Allergy Chewable Tablets .... ▣ 677
- PediaCare Cough-Cold Chewable Tablets 1553
- PediaCare Cough-Cold Liquid 1553
- PediaCare NightRest Cough-Cold Liquid 1553
- Pediatric Vicks 44m Cough & Cold Relief .... ▣ 764
- Pyrroxate Caplets .... ▣ 772
- Ryna .... ▣ 841
- Sinarest Tablets .... ▣ 648
- Sinarest Extra Strength Tablets .... ▣ 648
- Sine-Off Sinus Medicine .... ▣ 825
- Singlet Tablets .... ▣ 825
- Sinulin Tablets 787
- Sinutab Sinus Allergy Medication, Maximum Strength Tablets and Caplets .... ▣ 860
- Sudafed Plus Liquid .... ▣ 862
- Sudafed Plus Tablets .... ▣ 863
- Teldrin 12 Hour Antihistamine/Nasal Decongestant Allergy Relief Capsules .... ▣ 826
- TheraFlu .... ▣ 787
- TheraFlu Maximum Strength Nighttime Flu, Cold & Cough Medicine .... ▣ 788
- Triaminic Allergy Tablets .... ▣ 789
- Triaminic Cold Tablets .... ▣ 790
- Triaminic Nite Light .... ▣ 791
- Triaminic Syrup .... ▣ 792
- Triaminic-12 Tablets .... ▣ 792
- Triaminicin Tablets .... ▣ 793
- Triaminicol Multi-Symptom Cold Tablets .... ▣ 793
- Triaminicol Multi-Symptom Relief ▣ 794
- Tussend 1783
- Children's TYLENOL Cold Multi-Symptom Liquid Formula and Chewable Tablets 1561
- Children's TYLENOL Cold Plus Cough Multi Symptom Tablets and Liquid .... ▣ 681
- TYLENOL Maximum Strength Allergy Sinus Medication Gelcaps and Caplets 1563
- TYLENOL Cold Multi-Symptom Formula Medication Tablets and Caplets 1561
- TYLENOL Cold Multi-Symptom Hot Medication Liquid Packets 1557
- Vicks 44 LiquiCaps Cough, Cold & Flu Relief .... ▣ 755
- Vicks 44M Cough, Cold & Flu Relief .... ▣ 756

Chlorpheniramine Polistirex (Anticoagulant action partially counteracted). Products include:

- Tussionex Pennkinetic Extended-Release Suspension 998

Chlorpheniramine Tannate (Anticoagulant action partially counteracted). Products include:

- Atrohist Pediatric Suspension 454
- Ricobid Tablets and Pediatric Suspension 2038
- Rynatan 2673
- Rynatuss 2673

Choline Magnesium Trisalicylate (Interferes with platelet-aggregation reactions and may induce bleeding). Products include:

- Trilisate 2000

Clemastine Fumarate (Anticoagulant action partially counteracted). Products include:

- Tavist Syrup 2297
- Tavist Tablets 2298
- Tavist-1 12 Hour Relief Tablets .... ▣ 787
- Tavist-D 12 Hour Relief Tablets .... ▣ 787

Cyproheptadine Hydrochloride (Anticoagulant action partially counteracted). Products include:

- Periactin 1724

Demeclocycline Hydrochloride (Anticoagulant action partially counteracted). Products include:

- Declomycin Tablets 1371

Deslanoside (Anticoagulant action partially counteracted).

- No products indexed under this heading.

Dexchlorpheniramine Maleate (Anticoagulant action partially counteracted).

- No products indexed under this heading.

Dextran 40 (Interferes with platelet-aggregation reactions and may induce bleeding).

- No products indexed under this heading.

Diclofenac Potassium (Interferes with platelet-aggregation reactions and may induce bleeding). Products include:

- Cataflam 816

Diclofenac Sodium (Interferes with platelet-aggregation reactions and may induce bleeding). Products include:

- Voltaren Ophthalmic Sterile Ophthalmic Solution .... ⊙ 272
- Voltaren Tablets 861

Diflunisal (Interferes with platelet-aggregation reactions and may induce bleeding). Products include:

- Dolobid Tablets 1654

Digitoxin (Anticoagulant action partially counteracted). Products include:

- Crystodigin Tablets 1433

Digoxin (Anticoagulant action partially counteracted). Products include:

- Lanoxicaps 1117
- Lanoxin Elixir Pediatric 1120
- Lanoxin Injection 1123
- Lanoxin Injection Pediatric 1126
- Lanoxin Tablets 1128

Diphenhydramine Citrate (Anticoagulant action partially counteracted). Products include:

- Excedrin P.M. Analgesic/Sleeping Aid Tablets, Caplets, Liquigels 733

Diphenylpyraline Hydrochloride (Anticoagulant action partially counteracted).

- No products indexed under this heading.

Dipyridamole (Interferes with platelet-aggregation reactions and may induce bleeding). Products include:

- Persantine Tablets 681

Doxycycline Calcium (Anticoagulant action partially counteracted). Products include:

- Vibramycin Calcium Oral Suspension Syrup 1941

Doxycycline Hyclate (Anticoagulant action partially counteracted). Products include:

- Doryx Capsules 1913
- Vibramycin Hyclate Capsules 1941
- Vibramycin Hyclate Intravenous 2215
- Vibra-Tabs Film Coated Tablets 1941

Doxycycline Monohydrate (Anticoagulant action partially counteracted). Products include:

- Monodox Capsules 1805
- Vibramycin Monohydrate for Oral Suspension 1941

Etodolac (Interferes with platelet-aggregation reactions and may induce bleeding). Products include:

- Lodine Capsules and Tablets 2743

Fenoprofen Calcium (Interferes with platelet-aggregation ractions and may induce bleeding). Products include:

- Nalfon 200 Pulvules & Nalfon Tablets 917

Flurbiprofen (Interferes with platelet-aggregation reactions and may induce bleeding). Products include:

- Ansaid Tablets 2579

Hydroxychloroquine Sulfate (Interferes with platelet-aggregation reactions and may induce bleeding). Products include:

- Plaquenil Sulfate Tablets 2328

Ibuprofen (Interferes with platelet-aggregation reactions and may induce bleeding). Products include:

- Advil Cold and Sinus Caplets and Tablets (formerly CoAdvil) .... ▣ 870
- Advil Ibuprofen Tablets and Caplets .... ▣ 870
- Children's Advil Suspension 2692
- Arthritis Foundation Ibuprofen Tablets .... ▣ 674
- Bayer Select Ibuprofen Pain Relief Formula .... ▣ 715
- Cramp End Tablets .... ▣ 735
- Dimetapp Sinus Caplets .... ▣ 775
- Haltran Tablets .... ▣ 771
- IBU Tablets 1342
- Ibuprohm .... ▣ 735
- Children's Motrin Ibuprofen Oral Suspension 1546
- Motrin Tablets 2625
- Motrin IB Caplets, Tablets, and Geltabs .... ▣ 838
- Motrin IB Sinus .... ▣ 838
- Motrin Ibuprofen Suspension, Oral Drops, Chewable Tablets, Caplets 1546
- Nuprin Ibuprofen/Analgesic Tablets & Caplets .... ▣ 622
- Sine-Aid IB Caplets 1554
- Vicks DayQuil SINUS Pressure & PAIN Relief with IBUPROFEN .... ▣ 762

Indomethacin (Interferes with platelet-aggregation reactions and may induce bleeding). Products include:

- Indocin 1680

Indomethacin Sodium Trihydrate (Interferes with platelet-aggregation reactions and may induce bleeding). Products include:

- Indocin I.V. 1684

Ketoprofen (Interferes with platelet-aggregation reactions and may induce bleeding). Products include:

- Orudis Capsules 2766
- Oruvail Capsules 2766

Ketorolac Tromethamine (Interferes with platelet-aggregation reactions and may induce bleeding). Products include:

- Acular 474
- Acular .... ⊙ 277
- Toradol 2159

Loratadine (Anticoagulant action partially counteracted). Products include:

- Claritin 2349
- Claritin-D 2350

Magnesium Salicylate (Interferes with platelet-aggregation reactions and may induce bleeding). Products include:

- Backache Caplets .... ▣ 613
- Bayer Select Backache Pain Relief Formula .... ▣ 715
- Doan's Extra-Strength Analgesic .... ▣ 633
- Extra Strength Doan's P.M. .... ▣ 633
- Doan's Regular Strength Analgesic .... ▣ 634
- Mobigesic Tablets .... ▣ 602

Meclofenamate Sodium (Interferes with platelet-aggregation reactions and may induce bleeding).

- No products indexed under this heading.

Mefenamic Acid (Interferes with platelet-aggregation reactions and may induce bleeding). Products include:

- Ponstel 1925

Methacycline Hydrochloride (Anticoagulant action partially counteracted).

- No products indexed under this heading.

Methdilazine Hydrochloride (Anticoagulant action partially counteracted).

- No products indexed under this heading.

(▣ Described in PDR For Nonprescription Drugs) (⊙ Described in PDR For Ophthalmology)

Interactions Index

Heparin Sodium Injection

Mezlocillin Sodium (Interferes with platelet-aggregation reactions and may induce bleeding). Products include:

Mezlin 601
Mezlin Pharmacy Bulk Package....... 604

Minocycline Hydrochloride (Anticoagulant action partially counteracted). Products include:

Dynacin Capsules 1590
Minocin Intravenous 1382
Minocin Oral Suspension 1385
Minocin Pellet-Filled Capsules 1383

Nabumetone (Interferes with platelet-aggregation reactions and may induce bleeding). Products include:

Relafen Tablets 2510

Nafcillin Sodium (Interferes with platelet-aggregation reactions and may induce bleeding).

No products indexed under this heading.

Naproxen (Interferes with platelet-aggregation reactions and may induce bleeding). Products include:

Anaprox/Naprosyn 2117

Naproxen Sodium (Interferes with platelet-aggregation reactions and may induce bleeding). Products include:

Aleve 1975
Anaprox/Naprosyn 2117

Nicotine Polacrilex (Anticoagulant action partially counteracted). Products include:

Nicorette 2458

Oxaprozin (Interferes with platelet-aggregation reactions and may induce bleeding). Products include:

Daypro Caplets 2426

Oxytetracycline (Anticoagulant action partially counteracted). Products include:

Terramycin Intramuscular Solution 2210

Oxytetracycline Hydrochloride (Anticoagulant action partially counteracted). Products include:

TERAK Ointment .... ⓒ 209
Terra-Cortril Ophthalmic Suspension 2210
Terramycin with Polymyxin B Sulfate Ophthalmic Ointment 2211
Urobiotic-250 Capsules 2214

Penicillin G Benzathine (Interferes with platelet-aggregation reactions and may induce bleeding). Products include:

Bicillin C-R Injection 2704
Bicillin C-R 900/300 Injection 2706
Bicillin L-A Injection 2707

Penicillin G Procaine (Interferes with platelet-aggregation reactions and may induce bleeding). Products include:

Bicillin C-R Injection 2704
Bicillin C-R 900/300 Injection 2706

Phenylbutazone (Interferes with platelet-aggregation reactions and may induce bleeding).

No products indexed under this heading.

Piroxicam (Interferes with platelet-aggregation reactions and may induce bleeding). Products include:

Feldene Capsules 1965

Promethazine Hydrochloride (Anticoagulant action partially counteracted). Products include:

Mepergan Injection 2753
Phenergan with Codeine 2777
Phenergan with Dextromethorphan 2778
Phenergan Injection 2773
Phenergan Suppositories 2775
Phenergan Syrup 2774
Phenergan Tablets 2775
Phenergan VC 2779
Phenergan VC with Codeine 2781

Pyrilamine Maleate (Anticoagulant action partially counteracted). Products include:

4-Way Fast Acting Nasal Spray (regular & mentholated) .... ⊕ 621
Maximum Strength Multi-Symptom Formula Midol .... ⊕ 722
PMS Multi-Symptom Formula Midol .... ⊕ 723

Pyrilamine Tannate (Anticoagulant action partially counteracted). Products include:

Atrohist Pediatric Suspension 454
Rynatan 2673

Salsalate (Interferes with platelet-aggregation reactions and may induce bleeding). Products include:

Mono-Gesic Tablets 792
Salflex Tablets 786

Sulindac (Interferes with platelet-aggregation reactions and may induce bleeding). Products include:

Clinoril Tablets 1618

Terfenadine (Anticoagulant action partially counteracted). Products include:

Seldane Tablets 1536
Seldane-D Extended-Release Tablets 1538

Tetracycline Hydrochloride (Anticoagulant action partially counteracted). Products include:

Achromycin V Capsules 1367

Ticarcillin Disodium (Interferes with platelet-aggregation reactions and may induce bleeding). Products include:

Ticar for Injection 2526
Timentin for Injection 2528

Ticlopidine Hydrochloride (Interferes with platelet-aggregation reactions and may induce bleeding). Products include:

Ticlid Tablets 2156

Tolmetin Sodium (Interferes with platelet-aggregation reactions and may induce bleeding). Products include:

Tolectin (200, 400 and 600 mg) .. 1581

Trimeprazine Tartrate (Anticoagulant action partially counteracted). Products include:

Temaril Tablets, Syrup and Spansule Extended-Release Capsules .. 483

Tripelennamine Hydrochloride (Anticoagulant action partially counteracted). Products include:

PBZ Tablets 845
PBZ-SR Tablets 844

Triprolidine Hydrochloride (Anticoagulant action partially counteracted). Products include:

Actifed Plus Caplets .... ⊕ 845
Actifed Plus Tablets .... ⊕ 845
Actifed with Codeine Cough Syrup.. 1067
Actifed Syrup .... ⊕ 846
Actifed Tablets .... ⊕ 844

HEPARIN SODIUM INJECTION

(Heparin Sodium) 2726

May interact with cardiac glycosides, antihistamines, oral anticoagulants, tetracyclines, non-steroidal anti-inflammatory agents, platelet inhibitors, and certain other agents. Compounds in these categories include:

Acrivastine (Anticoagulant action partially counteracted). Products include:

Semprex-D Capsules 463
Semprex-D Capsules 1167

Aspirin (Interferes with platelet-aggregation reactions and may induce bleeding). Products include:

Alka-Seltzer Effervescent Antacid and Pain Reliever .... ⊕ 701
Alka-Seltzer Extra Strength Effervescent Antacid and Pain Reliever .... ⊕ 703
Alka-Seltzer Lemon Lime Effervescent Antacid and Pain Reliever .... ⊕ 703
Alka-Seltzer Plus Cold Medicine .... ⊕ 705
Alka-Seltzer Plus Cold & Cough Medicine .... ⊕ 708
Alka-Seltzer Plus Night-Time Cold Medicine .... ⊕ 707
Alka Seltzer Plus Sinus Medicine .. ⊕ 707
Arthritis Foundation Safety Coated Aspirin Tablets .... ⊕ 675
Arthritis Pain Ascriptin .... ⊕ 631
Maximum Strength Ascriptin .... ⊕ 630
Regular Strength Ascriptin Tablets .... ⊕ 629
Arthritis Strength BC Powder .... ⊕ 609
BC Cold Powder Multi-Symptom Formula (Cold-Sinus-Allergy) ...... ⊕ 609
BC Cold Powder Non-Drowsy Formula (Cold-Sinus) .... ⊕ 609
BC Powder .... ⊕ 609
Bayer Children's Chewable Aspirin .... ⊕ 711
Genuine Bayer Aspirin Tablets & Caplets .... ⊕ 713
Extra Strength Bayer Arthritis Pain Regimen Formula .... ⊕ 711
Extra Strength Bayer Aspirin Caplets & Tablets .... ⊕ 712
Extended-Release Bayer 8-Hour Aspirin .... ⊕ 712
Extra Strength Bayer Plus Aspirin Caplets .... ⊕ 713
Extra Strength Bayer PM Aspirin .. ⊕ 713
Bayer Enteric Aspirin .... ⊕ 709
Bufferin Analgesic Tablets and Caplets .... ⊕ 613
Arthritis Strength Bufferin Analgesic Caplets .... ⊕ 614
Extra Strength Bufferin Analgesic Tablets .... ⊕ 615
Cama Arthritis Pain Reliever .... ⊕ 785
Darvon Compound-65 Pulvules 1435
Easprin 1914
Ecotrin 2455
Ecotrin Enteric Coated Aspirin Maximum Strength Tablets and Caplets .... ⊕ 816
Ecotrin Enteric Coated Aspirin Regular Strength Tablets 2455
Empirin Aspirin Tablets .... ⊕ 854
Empirin with Codeine Tablets 1093
Excedrin Extra-Strength Analgesic Tablets & Caplets 732
Fiorinal Capsules 2261
Fiorinal with Codeine Capsules 2262
Fiorinal Tablets 2261
Halfprin 1362
Healthprin Aspirin 2455
Norgesic 1496
Percodan Tablets 939
Percodan-Demi Tablets 940
Robaxisal Tablets 2071
Soma Compound w/Codeine Tablets 2676
Soma Compound Tablets 2675
St. Joseph Adult Chewable Aspirin (81 mg.) .... ⊕ 808
Talwin Compound 2335
Ursinus Inlay-Tabs .... ⊕ 794
Vanquish Analgesic Caplets .... ⊕ 731

Astemizole (Anticoagulant action partially counteracted). Products include:

Hismanal Tablets 1293

Azatadine Maleate (Anticoagulant action partially counteracted). Products include:

Trinalin Repetabs Tablets 1330

Azlocillin Sodium (Interferes with platelet-aggregation reactions and may induce bleeding).

No products indexed under this heading.

Bromodiphenhydramine Hydrochloride (Anticoagulant action partially counteracted).

No products indexed under this heading.

Brompheniramine Maleate (Anticoagulant action partially counteracted). Products include:

Alka Seltzer Plus Sinus Medicine .. ⊕ 707
Bromfed Capsules (Extended-Release) 1785
Bromfed Syrup .... ⊕ 733
Bromfed Tablets 1785
Bromfed-DM Cough Syrup 1786
Bromfed-PD Capsules (Extended-Release) 1785
Dimetane-DC Cough Syrup 2059
Dimetane-DX Cough Syrup 2059
Dimetapp Elixir .... ⊕ 773
Dimetapp Extentabs .... ⊕ 774
Dimetapp Tablets/Liqui-Gels .... ⊕ 775
Dimetapp Cold & Allergy Chewable Tablets .... ⊕ 773
Dimetapp DM Elixir .... ⊕ 774
Vicks DayQuil Allergy Relief 12-Hour Extended Release Tablets .. ⊕ 760
Vicks DayQuil Allergy Relief 4-Hour Tablets .... ⊕ 760

Carbenicillin Indanyl Sodium (Interferes with platelet-aggregation reactions and may induce bleeding). Products include:

Geocillin Tablets 2199

Chlorpheniramine Maleate (Anticoagulant action partially counteracted). Products include:

Alka-Seltzer Plus Cold Medicine ... ⊕ 705
Alka-Seltzer Plus Cold Medicine Liqui-Gels .... ⊕ 706
Alka-Seltzer Plus Cold & Cough Medicine .... ⊕ 708
Alka-Seltzer Plus Cold & Cough Medicine Liqui-Gels .... ⊕ 705
Allerest Children's Chewable Tablets .... ⊕ 627
Allerest Headache Strength Tablets .... ⊕ 627
Allerest Maximum Strength Tablets .... ⊕ 627
Allerest Sinus Pain Formula .... ⊕ 627
Allerest 12 Hour Caplets .... ⊕ 627
Ana-Kit Anaphylaxis Emergency Treatment Kit 617
Atrohist Pediatric Capsules 453
Atrohist Plus Tablets 454
BC Cold Powder Multi-Symptom Formula (Cold-Sinus-Allergy) ...... ⊕ 609
Cerose DM .... ⊕ 878
Cheracol Plus Head Cold/Cough Formula .... ⊕ 769
Children's Vicks DayQuil Allergy Relief .... ⊕ 757
Children's Vicks NyQuil Cold/Cough Relief .... ⊕ 758
Chlor-Trimeton Allergy Decongestant Tablets .... ⊕ 799
Chlor-Trimeton Allergy Tablets ...... ⊕ 798
Comhist 2038
Comtrex Multi-Symptom Cold Reliever Tablets/Caplets/Liqui-Gels/Liquid .... ⊕ 615
Allergy-Sinus Comtrex Multi-Symptom Allergy-Sinus Formula Tablets .... ⊕ 617
Contac Continuous Action Nasal Decongestant/Antihistamine 12 Hour Capsules .... ⊕ 813
Contac Maximum Strength Continuous Action Decongestant/Antihistamine 12 Hour Caplets .. ⊕ 813
Contac Severe Cold and Flu Formula Caplets .... ⊕ 814
Coricidin 'D' Decongestant Tablets .... ⊕ 800
Coricidin Tablets .... ⊕ 800
D.A. Chewable Tablets 951
Deconamine 1320
Dura-Tap/PD Capsules 2867
Dura-Vent/DA Tablets 953
Extendryl 1005
Fedahist Gyrocaps 2401
Fedahist Timecaps 2401
Hycomine Compound Tablets 932
Isoclor Timesule Capsules .... ⊕ 637
Kronofed-A 977
Nolamine Timed-Release Tablets 785
Novahistine DH 2462
Novahistine Elixir .... ⊕ 823
Ornade Spansule Capsules 2502
PediaCare Cold Allergy Chewable Tablets .... ⊕ 677
PediaCare Cough-Cold Chewable Tablets 1553
PediaCare Cough-Cold Liquid 1553
PediaCare NightRest Cough-Cold Liquid 1553
Pediatric Vicks 44m Cough & Cold Relief .... ⊕ 764
Pyrroxate Caplets .... ⊕ 772
Ryna .... ⊕ 841
Sinarest Tablets .... ⊕ 648
Sinarest Extra Strength Tablets ...... ⊕ 648
Sine-Off Sinus Medicine .... ⊕ 825
Singlet Tablets .... ⊕ 825

IMPORTANT NOTE: Always consult each drug listing in the patient's regimen for possible interactions.

Heparin Sodium Injection **Interactions Index** **470**

Sinulin Tablets 787
Sinutab Sinus Allergy Medication, Maximum Strength Tablets and Caplets .... ▣ 860
Sudafed Plus Liquid .... ▣ 862
Sudafed Plus Tablets .... ▣ 863
Teldrin 12 Hour Antihistamine/ Nasal Decongestant Allergy Relief Capsules .... ▣ 826
TheraFlu .... ▣ 787
TheraFlu Maximum Strength Nighttime Flu, Cold & Cough Medicine .... ▣ 788
Triaminic Allergy Tablets .... ▣ 789
Triaminic Cold Tablets .... ▣ 790
Triaminic Nite Light .... ▣ 791
Triaminic Syrup .... ▣ 792
Triaminic-12 Tablets .... ▣ 792
Triaminicin Tablets .... ▣ 793
Triaminicol Multi-Symptom Cold Tablets .... ▣ 793
Triaminicol Multi-Symptom Relief ▣ 794
Tussend 1783
Children's TYLENOL Cold Multi-Symptom Liquid Formula and Chewable Tablets 1561
Children's TYLENOL Cold Plus Cough Multi Symptom Tablets and Liquid .... ▣ 681
TYLENOL Maximum Strength Allergy Sinus Medication Gelcaps and Caplets 1563
TYLENOL Cold Multi-Symptom Formula Medication Tablets and Caplets 1561
TYLENOL Cold Multi-Symptom Hot Medication Liquid Packets 1557
Vicks 44 LiquiCaps Cough, Cold & Flu Relief .... ▣ 755
Vicks 44M Cough, Cold & Flu Relief .... ▣ 756

Chlorpheniramine Polistirex (Anticoagulant action partially counteracted). Products include:
Tussionex Pennkinetic Extended-Release Suspension 998

Chlorpheniramine Tannate (Anticoagulant action partially counteracted). Products include:
Atrohist Pediatric Suspension 454
Ricobid Tablets and Pediatric Suspension 2038
Rynatan 2673
Rynatuss 2673

Choline Magnesium Trisalicylate (Interferes with platelet-aggregation reactions and may induce bleeding). Products include:
Trilisate 2000

Clemastine Fumarate (Anticoagulant action partially counteracted). Products include:
Tavist Syrup 2297
Tavist Tablets 2298
Tavist-1 12 Hour Relief Tablets .... ▣ 787
Tavist-D 12 Hour Relief Tablets .... ▣ 787

Cyproheptadine Hydrochloride (Anticoagulant action partially counteracted). Products include:
Periactin 1724

Demeclocycline Hydrochloride (Anticoagulant action partially counteracted). Products include:
Declomycin Tablets 1371

Deslanoside (Anticoagulant action partially counteracted).
No products indexed under this heading.

Dexchlorpheniramine Maleate (Anticoagulant action partially counteracted).
No products indexed under this heading.

Dextran 40 (Interferes with platelet-aggregation reactions and may induce bleeding).
No products indexed under this heading.

Diclofenac Potassium (Interferes with platelet-aggregation reactions and may induce bleeding). Products include:
Cataflam 816

Diclofenac Sodium (Interferes with platelet-aggregation reactions and may induce bleeding). Products include:
Voltaren Ophthalmic Sterile Ophthalmic Solution .... ◉ 272
Voltaren Tablets 861

Dicumarol (Prolonged prothrombin time).
No products indexed under this heading.

Diflunisal (Interferes with platelet-aggregation reactions and may induce bleeding). Products include:
Dolobid Tablets 1654

Digitoxin (Anticoagulant action partially counteracted). Products include:
Crystodigin Tablets 1433

Digoxin (Anticoagulant action partially counteracted). Products include:
Lanoxicaps 1117
Lanoxin Elixir Pediatric 1120
Lanoxin Injection 1123
Lanoxin Injection Pediatric 1126
Lanoxin Tablets 1128

Diphenhydramine Citrate (Anticoagulant action partially counteracted). Products include:
Excedrin P.M. Analgesic/Sleeping Aid Tablets, Caplets, Liquigels 733

Diphenhydramine Hydrochloride (Anticoagulant action partially counteracted). Products include:
Actifed Allergy Daytime/Nighttime Caplets .... ▣ 844
Actifed Sinus Daytime/Nighttime Tablets and Caplets .... ▣ 846
Arthritis Foundation NightTime Caplets .... ▣ 674
Extra Strength Bayer PM Aspirin .... ▣ 713
Bayer Select Night Time Pain Relief Formula .... ▣ 716
Benadryl Allergy Decongestant Liquid Medication .... ▣ 848
Benadryl Allergy Decongestant Tablets .... ▣ 848
Benadryl Allergy Liquid Medication .... ▣ 849
Benadryl Allergy .... ▣ 848
Benadryl Allergy Sinus Headache Formula Caplets .... ▣ 849
Benadryl Capsules 1898
Benadryl Dye-Free Allergy Liquigel Softgels .... ▣ 850
Benadryl Dye-Free Allergy Liquid Medication .... ▣ 850
Benadryl Itch Relief Cream, Children's Formula and Maximum Strength 2% .... ▣ 851
Benadryl Itch Relief Spray, Children's Formula and Maximum Strength 2% .... ▣ 851
Benadryl Itch Relief Stick Maximum Strength 2% .... ▣ 850
Benadryl Itch Stopping Gel, Children's Formula and Maximum Strength 2% .... ▣ 851
Benadryl Kapseals 1898
Benadryl Injection 1898
Contac Day & Night Cold/Flu Night Caplets .... ▣ 812
Contac Night Allergy/Sinus Caplets .... ▣ 812
Extra Strength Doan's P.M. .... ▣ 633
Legatrin PM .... ▣ 651
Miles Nervine Nighttime Sleep-Aid ▣ 723
Nytol QuickCaps Caplets .... ▣ 610
Sleepinal Night-time Sleep Aid Capsules and Softgels .... ▣ 834
TYLENOL Maximum Strength Allergy Sinus NightTime Medication Caplets 1555
TYLENOL Flu NightTime, Maximum Strength, Gelcaps 1566
TYLENOL Maximum Strength Flu NightTime Hot Medication Packets 1562
TYLENOL PM, Extra Strength Pain Reliever/Sleep Aid Caplets, Geltabs, Gelcaps 1560
TYLENOL Severe Allergy Medication Caplets 1564
Maximum Strength Unisom Sleepgels 1934
Unisom With Pain Relief-Nighttime Sleep Aid and Pain Reliever 1934

Diphenylpyraline Hydrochloride (Anticoagulant action partially counteracted).
No products indexed under this heading.

Dipyridamole (Interferes with platelet-aggregation reactions and may induce bleeding). Products include:
Persantine Tablets 681

Doxycycline Calcium (Anticoagulant action partially counteracted). Products include:
Vibramycin Calcium Oral Suspension Syrup 1941

Doxycycline Hyclate (Anticoagulant action partially counteracted). Products include:
Doryx Capsules 1913
Vibramycin Hyclate Capsules 1941
Vibramycin Hyclate Intravenous 2215
Vibra-Tabs Film Coated Tablets 1941

Doxycycline Monohydrate (Anticoagulant action partially counteracted). Products include:
Monodox Capsules 1805
Vibramycin Monohydrate for Oral Suspension 1941

Etodolac (Interferes with platelet-aggregation reactions and may induce bleeding). Products include:
Lodine Capsules and Tablets 2743

Fenoprofen Calcium (Interferes with platelet-aggregation reactions and may induce bleeding). Products include:
Nalfon 200 Pulvules & Nalfon Tablets 917

Flurbiprofen (Interferes with platelet-aggregation reactions and may induce bleeding). Products include:
Ansaid Tablets 2579

Hydroxychloroquine Sulfate (Interferes with platelet-aggregation reactions and may induce bleeding). Products include:
Plaquenil Sulfate Tablets 2328

Ibuprofen (Interferes with platelet-aggregation reactions and may induce bleeding). Products include:
Advil Cold and Sinus Caplets and Tablets (formerly CoAdvil) .... ▣ 870
Advil Ibuprofen Tablets and Caplets .... ▣ 870
Children's Advil Suspension 2692
Arthritis Foundation Ibuprofen Tablets .... ▣ 674
Bayer Select Ibuprofen Pain Relief Formula .... ▣ 715
Cramp End Tablets .... ▣ 735
Dimetapp Sinus Caplets .... ▣ 775
Haltran Tablets .... ▣ 771
IBU Tablets 1342
Ibuprohm .... ▣ 735
Children's Motrin Ibuprofen Oral Suspension 1546
Motrin Tablets 2625
Motrin IB Caplets, Tablets, and Geltabs .... ▣ 838
Motrin IB Sinus .... ▣ 838
Motrin Ibuprofen Suspension, Oral Drops, Chewable Tablets, Caplets 1546
Nuprin Ibuprofen/Analgesic Tablets & Caplets .... ▣ 622
Sine-Aid IB Caplets 1554
Vicks DayQuil SINUS Pressure & PAIN Relief with IBUPROFEN .... ▣ 762

Indomethacin (Interferes with platelet-aggregation reactions and may induce bleeding). Products include:
Indocin 1680

Indomethacin Sodium Trihydrate (Interferes with platelet-aggregation reactions and may induce bleeding). Products include:
Indocin I.V. 1684

Ketoprofen (Interferes with platelet-aggregation reactions and may induce bleeding). Products include:
Orudis Capsules 2766
Oruvail Capsules 2766

Ketorolac Tromethamine (Interferes with platelet-aggregation reactions and may induce bleeding). Products include:
Acular 474
Acular .... ◉ 277
Toradol 2159

Loratadine (Anticoagulant action partially counteracted). Products include:
Claritin 2349
Claritin-D 2350

Magnesium Salicylate (Interferes with platelet-aggregation reactions and may induce bleeding). Products include:
Backache Caplets .... ▣ 613
Bayer Select Backache Pain Relief Formula .... ▣ 715
Doan's Extra-Strength Analgesic .... ▣ 633
Extra Strength Doan's P.M. .... ▣ 633
Doan's Regular Strength Analgesic .... ▣ 634
Mobigesic Tablets .... ▣ 602

Meclofenamate Sodium (Interferes with platelet-aggregation reactions and may induce bleeding).
No products indexed under this heading.

Mefenamic Acid (Interferes with platelet-aggregation reactions and may induce bleeding). Products include:
Ponstel 1925

Methacycline Hydrochloride (Anticoagulant action partially counteracted).
No products indexed under this heading.

Methdilazine Hydrochloride (Anticoagulant action partially counteracted).
No products indexed under this heading.

Mezlocillin Sodium (Interferes with platelet-aggregation reactions and may induce bleeding). Products include:
Mezlin 601
Mezlin Pharmacy Bulk Package 604

Minocycline Hydrochloride (Anticoagulant action partially counteracted). Products include:
Dynacin Capsules 1590
Minocin Intravenous 1382
Minocin Oral Suspension 1385
Minocin Pellet-Filled Capsules 1383

Nabumetone (Interferes with platelet-aggregation reactions and may induce bleeding). Products include:
Relafen Tablets 2510

Nafcillin Sodium (Interferes with platelet-aggregation reactions and may induce bleeding).
No products indexed under this heading.

Naproxen (Interferes with platelet-aggregation reactions and may induce bleeding). Products include:
Anaprox/Naprosyn 2117

Naproxen Sodium (Interferes with platelet-aggregation reactions and may induce bleeding). Products include:
Aleve 1975
Anaprox/Naprosyn 2117

Nicotine Polacrilex (Anticoagulant action partially counteracted). Products include:
Nicorette 2458

Oxaprozin (Interferes with platelet-aggregation reactions and may induce bleeding). Products include:
Daypro Caplets 2426

(▣ Described in PDR For Nonprescription Drugs) (◉ Described in PDR For Ophthalmology)

Oxytetracycline (Anticoagulant action partially counteracted). Products include:
- Terramycin Intramuscular Solution 2210

Oxytetracycline Hydrochloride (Anticoagulant action partially counteracted). Products include:
- TERAK Ointment 209
- Terra-Cortril Ophthalmic Suspension 2210
- Terramycin with Polymyxin B Sulfate Ophthalmic Ointment 2211
- Urobiotic-250 Capsules 2214

Penicillin G Benzathine (Interferes with platelet-aggregation reactions and may induce bleeding). Products include:
- Bicillin C-R Injection 2704
- Bicillin C-R 900/300 Injection 2706
- Bicillin L-A Injection 2707

Penicillin G Procaine (Interferes with platelet-aggregation reactions and may induce bleeding). Products include:
- Bicillin C-R Injection 2704
- Bicillin C-R 900/300 Injection 2706

Phenylbutazone (Interferes with platelet-aggregation reactions and may induce bleeding).
- No products indexed under this heading.

Piroxicam (Interferes with platelet-aggregation reactions and may induce bleeding). Products include:
- Feldene Capsules 1965

Promethazine Hydrochloride (Anticoagulant action partially counteracted). Products include:
- Mepergan Injection 2753
- Phenergan with Codeine 2777
- Phenergan with Dextromethorphan 2778
- Phenergan Injection 2773
- Phenergan Suppositories 2775
- Phenergan Syrup 2774
- Phenergan Tablets 2775
- Phenergan VC 2779
- Phenergan VC with Codeine 2781

Pyrilamine Maleate (Anticoagulant action partially counteracted). Products include:
- 4-Way Fast Acting Nasal Spray (regular & mentholated) 621
- Maximum Strength Multi-Symptom Formula Midol 722
- PMS Multi-Symptom Formula Midol 723

Pyrilamine Tannate (Anticoagulant action partially counteracted). Products include:
- Atrohist Pediatric Suspension 454
- Rynatan 2673

Salsalate (Interferes with platelet-aggregation reactions and may induce bleeding). Products include:
- Mono-Gesic Tablets 792
- Salflex Tablets 786

Sulindac (Interferes with platelet-aggregation reactions and may induce bleeding). Products include:
- Clinoril Tablets 1618

Terfenadine (Anticoagulant action partially counteracted). Products include:
- Seldane Tablets 1536
- Seldane-D Extended-Release Tablets 1538

Tetracycline Hydrochloride (Anticoagulant action partially counteracted). Products include:
- Achromycin V Capsules 1367

Ticarcillin Disodium (Interferes with platelet-aggregation reactions and may induce bleeding). Products include:
- Ticar for Injection 2526
- Timentin for Injection 2528

Ticlopidine Hydrochloride (Interferes with platelet-aggregation reactions and may induce bleeding). Products include:
- Ticlid Tablets 2156

Tolmetin Sodium (Interferes with platelet-aggregation reactions and may induce bleeding). Products include:
- Tolectin (200, 400 and 600 mg) 1581

Trimeprazine Tartrate (Anticoagulant action partially counteracted). Products include:
- Temaril Tablets, Syrup and Spansule Extended-Release Capsules 483

Tripelennamine Hydrochloride (Anticoagulant action partially counteracted). Products include:
- PBZ Tablets 845
- PBZ-SR Tablets 844

Triprolidine Hydrochloride (Anticoagulant action partially counteracted). Products include:
- Actifed Plus Caplets 845
- Actifed Plus Tablets 845
- Actifed with Codeine Cough Syrup 1067
- Actifed Syrup 846
- Actifed Tablets 844

Warfarin Sodium (Prolonged prothrombin time). Products include:
- Coumadin 926

HEPARIN SODIUM INJECTION, USP, STERILE SOLUTION

(Heparin Sodium) 2615

May interact with oral anticoagulants, antihistamines, salicylates, cardiac glycosides, tetracyclines, non-steroidal anti-inflammatory agents, and certain other agents. Compounds in these categories include:

Acrivastine (May partially counteract anticoagulant effect of Heparin). Products include:
- Semprex-D Capsules 463
- Semprex-D Capsules 1167

Aspirin (May induce bleeding). Products include:
- Alka-Seltzer Effervescent Antacid and Pain Reliever 701
- Alka-Seltzer Extra Strength Effervescent Antacid and Pain Reliever 703
- Alka-Seltzer Lemon Lime Effervescent Antacid and Pain Reliever 703
- Alka-Seltzer Plus Cold Medicine 705
- Alka-Seltzer Plus Cold & Cough Medicine 708
- Alka-Seltzer Plus Night-Time Cold Medicine 707
- Alka Seltzer Plus Sinus Medicine 707
- Arthritis Foundation Safety Coated Aspirin Tablets 675
- Arthritis Pain Ascriptin 631
- Maximum Strength Ascriptin 630
- Regular Strength Ascriptin Tablets 629
- Arthritis Strength BC Powder 609
- BC Cold Powder Multi-Symptom Formula (Cold-Sinus-Allergy) 609
- BC Cold Powder Non-Drowsy Formula (Cold-Sinus) 609
- BC Powder 609
- Bayer Children's Chewable Aspirin 711
- Genuine Bayer Aspirin Tablets & Caplets 713
- Extra Strength Bayer Arthritis Pain Regimen Formula 711
- Extra Strength Bayer Aspirin Caplets & Tablets 712
- Extended-Release Bayer 8-Hour Aspirin 712
- Extra Strength Bayer Plus Aspirin Caplets 713
- Extra Strength Bayer PM Aspirin 713
- Bayer Enteric Aspirin 709
- Bufferin Analgesic Tablets and Caplets 613
- Arthritis Strength Bufferin Analgesic Caplets 614
- Extra Strength Bufferin Analgesic Tablets 615
- Cama Arthritis Pain Reliever 785
- Darvon Compound-65 Pulvules 1435
- Easprin 1914
- Ecotrin 2455
- Ecotrin Enteric Coated Aspirin Maximum Strength Tablets and Caplets 816
- Ecotrin Enteric Coated Aspirin Regular Strength Tablets 2455
- Empirin Aspirin Tablets 854
- Empirin with Codeine Tablets 1093
- Excedrin Extra-Strength Analgesic Tablets & Caplets 732
- Fiorinal Capsules 2261
- Fiorinal with Codeine Capsules 2262
- Fiorinal Tablets 2261
- Halfprin 1362
- Healthprin Aspirin 2455
- Norgesic 1496
- Percodan Tablets 939
- Percodan-Demi Tablets 940
- Robaxisal Tablets 2071
- Soma Compound w/Codeine Tablets 2676
- Soma Compound Tablets 2675
- St. Joseph Adult Chewable Aspirin (81 mg.) 808
- Talwin Compound 2335
- Ursinus Inlay-Tabs 794
- Vanquish Analgesic Caplets 731

Astemizole (May partially counteract anticoagulant effect of Heparin). Products include:
- Hismanal Tablets 1293

Azatadine Maleate (May partially counteract anticoagulant effect of Heparin). Products include:
- Trinalin Repetabs Tablets 1330

Bromodiphenhydramine Hydrochloride (May partially counteract anticoagulant effect of Heparin).
- No products indexed under this heading.

Brompheniramine Maleate (May partially counteract anticoagulant effect of Heparin). Products include:
- Alka Seltzer Plus Sinus Medicine 707
- Bromfed Capsules (Extended-Release) 1785
- Bromfed Syrup 733
- Bromfed Tablets 1785
- Bromfed-DM Cough Syrup 1786
- Bromfed-PD Capsules (Extended-Release) 1785
- Dimetane-DC Cough Syrup 2059
- Dimetane-DX Cough Syrup 2059
- Dimetapp Elixir 773
- Dimetapp Extentabs 774
- Dimetapp Tablets/Liqui-Gels 775
- Dimetapp Cold & Allergy Chewable Tablets 773
- Dimetapp DM Elixir 774
- Vicks DayQuil Allergy Relief 12-Hour Extended Release Tablets 760
- Vicks DayQuil Allergy Relief 4-Hour Tablets 760

Chlorpheniramine Maleate (May partially counteract anticoagulant effect of Heparin). Products include:
- Alka-Seltzer Plus Cold Medicine 705
- Alka-Seltzer Plus Cold Medicine Liqui-Gels 706
- Alka-Seltzer Plus Cold & Cough Medicine 708
- Alka-Seltzer Plus Cold & Cough Medicine Liqui-Gels 705
- Allerest Children's Chewable Tablets 627
- Allerest Headache Strength Tablets 627
- Allerest Maximum Strength Tablets 627
- Allerest Sinus Pain Formula 627
- Allerest 12 Hour Caplets 627
- Ana-Kit Anaphylaxis Emergency Treatment Kit 617
- Atrohist Pediatric Capsules 453
- Atrohist Plus Tablets 454
- BC Cold Powder Multi-Symptom Formula (Cold-Sinus-Allergy) 609
- Cerose DM 878
- Cheracol Plus Head Cold/Cough Formula 769
- Children's Vicks DayQuil Allergy Relief 757
- Children's Vicks NyQuil Cold/Cough Relief 758
- Chlor-Trimeton Allergy Decongestant Tablets 799
- Chlor-Trimeton Allergy Tablets 798
- Comhist 2038
- Comtrex Multi-Symptom Cold Reliever Tablets/Caplets/Liqui-Gels/Liquid 615
- Allergy-Sinus Comtrex Multi-Symptom Allergy-Sinus Formula Tablets 617
- Contac Continuous Action Nasal Decongestant/Antihistamine 12 Hour Capsules 813
- Contac Maximum Strength Continuous Action Decongestant/Antihistamine 12 Hour Caplets 813
- Contac Severe Cold and Flu Formula Caplets 814
- Coricidin 'D' Decongestant Tablets 800
- Coricidin Tablets 800
- D.A. Chewable Tablets 951
- Deconamine 1320
- Dura-Tap/PD Capsules 2867
- Dura-Vent/DA Tablets 953
- Extendryl 1005
- Fedahist Gyrocaps 2401
- Fedahist Timecaps 2401
- Hycomine Compound Tablets 932
- Isoclor Timesule Capsules 637
- Kronofed-A 977
- Nolamine Timed-Release Tablets 785
- Novahistine DH 2462
- Novahistine Elixir 823
- Ornade Spansule Capsules 2502
- PediaCare Cold Allergy Chewable Tablets 677
- PediaCare Cough-Cold Chewable Tablets 1553
- PediaCare Cough-Cold Liquid 1553
- PediaCare NightRest Cough-Cold Liquid 1553
- Pediatric Vicks 44m Cough & Cold Relief 764
- Pyrroxate Caplets 772
- Ryna 841
- Sinarest Tablets 648
- Sinarest Extra Strength Tablets 648
- Sine-Off Sinus Medicine 825
- Singlet Tablets 825
- Sinulin Tablets 787
- Sinutab Sinus Allergy Medication, Maximum Strength Tablets and Caplets 860
- Sudafed Plus Liquid 862
- Sudafed Plus Tablets 863
- Teldrin 12 Hour Antihistamine/Nasal Decongestant Allergy Relief Capsules 826
- TheraFlu 787
- TheraFlu Maximum Strength Nighttime Flu, Cold & Cough Medicine 788
- Triaminic Allergy Tablets 789
- Triaminic Cold Tablets 790
- Triaminic Nite Light 791
- Triaminic Syrup 792
- Triaminic-12 Tablets 792
- Triaminicin Tablets 793
- Triaminicol Multi-Symptom Cold Tablets 793
- Triaminicol Multi-Symptom Relief 794
- Tussend 1783
- Children's TYLENOL Cold Multi-Symptom Liquid Formula and Chewable Tablets 1561
- Children's TYLENOL Cold Plus Cough Multi Symptom Tablets and Liquid 681
- TYLENOL Maximum Strength Allergy Sinus Medication Gelcaps and Caplets 1563
- TYLENOL Cold Multi-Symptom Formula Medication Tablets and Caplets 1561
- TYLENOL Cold Multi-Symptom Hot Medication Liquid Packets 1557
- Vicks 44 LiquiCaps Cough, Cold & Flu Relief 755
- Vicks 44M Cough, Cold & Flu Relief 756

Chlorpheniramine Polistirex (May partially counteract anticoagulant effect of Heparin). Products include:
- Tussionex Pennkinetic Extended-Release Suspension 998

Chlorpheniramine Tannate (May partially counteract anticoagulant effect of Heparin). Products include:
- Atrohist Pediatric Suspension 454

IMPORTANT NOTE: Always consult each drug listing in the patient's regimen for possible interactions.

Heparin Sodium Injection **Interactions Index** **472**

Ricobid Tablets and Pediatric Suspension ... 2038
Rynatan ... 2673
Rynatuss ... 2673

Choline Magnesium Trisalicylate (May induce bleeding). Products include:
Trilisate ... 2000

Clemastine Fumarate (May partially counteract anticoagulant effect of Heparin). Products include:
Tavist Syrup ... 2297
Tavist Tablets ... 2298
Tavist-1 12 Hour Relief Tablets ... ▣ 787
Tavist-D 12 Hour Relief Tablets ... ▣ 787

Cyproheptadine Hydrochloride (May partially counteract anticoagulant effect of Heparin). Products include:
Periactin ... 1724

Demeclocycline Hydrochloride (May partially counteract anticoagulant effect of Heparin). Products include:
Declomycin Tablets ... 1371

Deslanoside (May partially counteract anticoagulant effect of Heparin).
No products indexed under this heading.

Dexchlorpheniramine Maleate (May partially counteract anticoagulant effect of Heparin).
No products indexed under this heading.

Dextrans (Low Molecular Weight) (May induce bleeding).
No products indexed under this heading.

Diclofenac Potassium (May induce bleeding). Products include:
Cataflam ... 816

Diclofenac Sodium (May induce bleeding). Products include:
Voltaren Ophthalmic Sterile Ophthalmic Solution ... ⊙ 272
Voltaren Tablets ... 861

Dicumarol (Prolonged one-state prothrombin time).
No products indexed under this heading.

Diflunisal (May induce bleeding). Products include:
Dolobid Tablets ... 1654

Digitoxin (May partially counteract anticoagulant effect of Heparin). Products include:
Crystodigin Tablets ... 1433

Digoxin (May partially counteract anticoagulant effect of Heparin). Products include:
Lanoxicaps ... 1117
Lanoxin Elixir Pediatric ... 1120
Lanoxin Injection ... 1123
Lanoxin Injection Pediatric ... 1126
Lanoxin Tablets ... 1128

Diphenhydramine Citrate (May partially counteract anticoagulant effect of Heparin). Products include:
Excedrin P.M. Analgesic/Sleeping Aid Tablets, Caplets, Liquigels ... 733

Diphenhydramine Hydrochloride (May partially counteract anticoagulant effect of Heparin). Products include:
Actifed Allergy Daytime/Nighttime Caplets ... ▣ 844
Actifed Sinus Daytime/Nighttime Tablets and Caplets ... ▣ 846
Arthritis Foundation NightTime Caplets ... ▣ 674
Extra Strength Bayer PM Aspirin ... ▣ 713
Bayer Select Night Time Pain Relief Formula ... ▣ 716
Benadryl Allergy Decongestant Liquid Medication ... ▣ 848
Benadryl Allergy Decongestant Tablets ... ▣ 848
Benadryl Allergy Liquid Medication ... ▣ 849
Benadryl Allergy ... ▣ 848
Benadryl Allergy Sinus Headache Formula Caplets ... ▣ 849
Benadryl Capsules ... 1898
Benadryl Dye-Free Allergy Liqui-gel Softgels ... ▣ 850
Benadryl Dye-Free Allergy Liquid Medication ... ▣ 850
Benadryl Itch Relief Cream, Children's Formula and Maximum Strength 2% ... ▣ 851
Benadryl Itch Relief Spray, Children's Formula and Maximum Strength 2% ... ▣ 851
Benadryl Itch Relief Stick Maximum Strength 2% ... ▣ 850
Benadryl Itch Stopping Gel, Children's Formula and Maximum Strength 2% ... ▣ 851
Benadryl Kapseals ... 1898
Benadryl Injection ... 1898
Contac Day & Night Cold/Flu Night Caplets ... ▣ 812
Contac Night Allergy/Sinus Caplets ... ▣ 812
Extra Strength Doan's P.M. ... ▣ 633
Legatrin PM ... ▣ 651
Miles Nervine Nighttime Sleep-Aid ▣ 723
Nytol QuickCaps Caplets ... ▣ 610
Sleepinal Night-time Sleep Aid Capsules and Softgels ... ▣ 834
TYLENOL Maximum Strength Allergy Sinus NightTime Medication Caplets ... 1555
TYLENOL Flu NightTime, Maximum Strength, Gelcaps ... 1566
TYLENOL Maximum Strength Flu NightTime Hot Medication Packets ... 1562
TYLENOL PM, Extra Strength Pain Reliever/Sleep Aid Caplets, Geltabs, Gelcaps ... 1560
TYLENOL Severe Allergy Medication Caplets ... 1564
Maximum Strength Unisom Sleepgels ... 1934
Unisom With Pain Relief-Nighttime Sleep Aid and Pain Reliever ... 1934

Diphenylpyraline Hydrochloride (May partially counteract anticoagulant effect of Heparin).
No products indexed under this heading.

Dipyridamole (May induce bleeding). Products include:
Persantine Tablets ... 681

Doxycycline Calcium (May partially counteract anticoagulant effect of Heparin). Products include:
Vibramycin Calcium Oral Suspension Syrup ... 1941

Doxycycline Hyclate (May partially counteract anticoagulant effect of Heparin). Products include:
Doryx Capsules ... 1913
Vibramycin Hyclate Capsules ... 1941
Vibramycin Hyclate Intravenous ... 2215
Vibra-Tabs Film Coated Tablets ... 1941

Doxycycline Monohydrate (May partially counteract anticoagulant effect of Heparin). Products include:
Monodox Capsules ... 1805
Vibramycin Monohydrate for Oral Suspension ... 1941

Etodolac (May induce bleeding). Products include:
Lodine Capsules and Tablets ... 2743

Fenoprofen Calcium (May induce bleeding). Products include:
Nalfon 200 Pulvules & Nalfon Tablets ... 917

Flurbiprofen (May induce bleeding). Products include:
Ansaid Tablets ... 2579

Hydroxychloroquine Sulfate (May induce bleeding). Products include:
Plaquenil Sulfate Tablets ... 2328

Ibuprofen (May induce bleeding). Products include:
Advil Cold and Sinus Caplets and Tablets (formerly CoAdvil) ... ▣ 870
Advil Ibuprofen Tablets and Caplets ... ▣ 870
Children's Advil Suspension ... 2692
Arthritis Foundation Ibuprofen Tablets ... ▣ 674
Bayer Select Ibuprofen Pain Relief Formula ... ▣ 715
Cramp End Tablets ... ▣ 735
Dimetapp Sinus Caplets ... ▣ 775
Haltran Tablets ... ▣ 771
IBU Tablets ... 1342
Ibuprohm ... ▣ 735
Children's Motrin Ibuprofen Oral Suspension ... 1546
Motrin Tablets ... 2625
Motrin IB Caplets, Tablets, and Geltabs ... ▣ 838
Motrin IB Sinus ... ▣ 838
Motrin Ibuprofen Suspension, Oral Drops, Chewable Tablets, Caplets ... 1546
Nuprin Ibuprofen/Analgesic Tablets & Caplets ... ▣ 622
Sine-Aid IB Caplets ... 1554
Vicks DayQuil SINUS Pressure & PAIN Relief with IBUPROFEN ... ▣ 762

Indomethacin (May induce bleeding). Products include:
Indocin ... 1680

Indomethacin Sodium Trihydrate (May induce bleeding). Products include:
Indocin I.V. ... 1684

Ketoprofen (May induce bleeding). Products include:
Orudis Capsules ... 2766
Oruvail Capsules ... 2766

Ketorolac Tromethamine (May induce bleeding). Products include:
Acular ... 474
Acular ... ⊙ 277
Toradol ... 2159

Loratadine (May partially counteract anticoagulant effect of Heparin). Products include:
Claritin ... 2349
Claritin-D ... 2350

Magnesium Salicylate (May induce bleeding). Products include:
Backache Caplets ... ▣ 613
Bayer Select Backache Pain Relief Formula ... ▣ 715
Doan's Extra-Strength Analgesic ... ▣ 633
Extra Strength Doan's P.M. ... ▣ 633
Doan's Regular Strength Analgesic ... ▣ 634
Mobigesic Tablets ... ▣ 602

Meclofenamate Sodium (May induce bleeding).
No products indexed under this heading.

Mefenamic Acid (May induce bleeding). Products include:
Ponstel ... 1925

Methacycline Hydrochloride (May partially counteract anticoagulant effect of Heparin).
No products indexed under this heading.

Methdilazine Hydrochloride (May partially counteract anticoagulant effect of Heparin).
No products indexed under this heading.

Minocycline Hydrochloride (May partially counteract anticoagulant effect of Heparin). Products include:
Dynacin Capsules ... 1590
Minocin Intravenous ... 1382
Minocin Oral Suspension ... 1385
Minocin Pellet-Filled Capsules ... 1383

Nabumetone (May induce bleeding). Products include:
Relafen Tablets ... 2510

Naproxen (May induce bleeding). Products include:
Anaprox/Naprosyn ... 2117

Naproxen Sodium (May induce bleeding). Products include:
Aleve ... 1975
Anaprox/Naprosyn ... 2117

Nicotine Polacrilex (May partially counteract anticoagulant effect of Heparin). Products include:
Nicorette ... 2458

Oxaprozin (May induce bleeding). Products include:
Daypro Caplets ... 2426

Oxytetracycline (May partially counteract anticoagulant effect of Heparin). Products include:
Terramycin Intramuscular Solution 2210

Oxytetracycline Hydrochloride (May partially counteract anticoagulant effect of Heparin). Products include:
TERAK Ointment ... ⊙ 209
Terra-Cortril Ophthalmic Suspension ... 2210
Terramycin with Polymyxin B Sulfate Ophthalmic Ointment ... 2211
Urobiotic-250 Capsules ... 2214

Phenylbutazone (May induce bleeding).
No products indexed under this heading.

Piroxicam (May induce bleeding). Products include:
Feldene Capsules ... 1965

Promethazine Hydrochloride (May partially counteract anticoagulant effect of Heparin). Products include:
Mepergan Injection ... 2753
Phenergan with Codeine ... 2777
Phenergan with Dextromethorphan 2778
Phenergan Injection ... 2773
Phenergan Suppositories ... 2775
Phenergan Syrup ... 2774
Phenergan Tablets ... 2775
Phenergan VC ... 2779
Phenergan VC with Codeine ... 2781

Pyrilamine Maleate (May partially counteract anticoagulant effect of Heparin). Products include:
4-Way Fast Acting Nasal Spray (regular & mentholated) ... ▣ 621
Maximum Strength Multi-Symptom Formula Midol ... ▣ 722
PMS Multi-Symptom Formula Midol ... ▣ 723

Pyrilamine Tannate (May partially counteract anticoagulant effect of Heparin). Products include:
Atrohist Pediatric Suspension ... 454
Rynatan ... 2673

Salsalate (May induce bleeding). Products include:
Mono-Gesic Tablets ... 792
Salflex Tablets ... 786

Sulindac (May induce bleeding). Products include:
Clinoril Tablets ... 1618

Terfenadine (May partially counteract anticoagulant effect of Heparin). Products include:
Seldane Tablets ... 1536
Seldane-D Extended-Release Tablets ... 1538

Tetracycline Hydrochloride (May partially counteract anticoagulant effect of Heparin). Products include:
Achromycin V Capsules ... 1367

Tolmetin Sodium (May induce bleeding). Products include:
Tolectin (200, 400 and 600 mg) .. 1581

Trimeprazine Tartrate (May partially counteract anticoagulant effect of Heparin). Products include:
Temaril Tablets, Syrup and Spansule Extended-Release Capsules .. 483

Tripelennamine Hydrochloride (May partially counteract anticoagulant effect of Heparin). Products include:
PBZ Tablets ... 845
PBZ-SR Tablets ... 844

(▣ Described in PDR For Nonprescription Drugs) (⊙ Described in PDR For Ophthalmology)

473 Interactions Index Heparin Sodium

Triprolidine Hydrochloride (May partially counteract anticoagulant effect of Heparin). Products include:
Actifed Plus Caplets ... 845
Actifed Plus Tablets ... 845
Actifed with Codeine Cough Syrup .. 1067
Actifed Syrup ... 846
Actifed Tablets ... 844

Warfarin Sodium (Prolonged one-statge prothrombin time). Products include:
Coumadin ... 926

HEPARIN SODIUM VIALS
(Heparin Sodium) ... 1441
May interact with oral anticoagulants, non-steroidal anti-inflammatory agents, salicylates, cardiac glycosides, high doses of parenteral penicillins, phenothiazines, tetracyclines, antihistamines, platelet inhibitors, cephalosporins with methylthiotetrazole side chains, macrolide antibiotics, and certain other agents. Compounds in these categories include:

Acrivastine (Antagonizes the antithrombotic activity of heparin). Products include:
Semprex-D Capsules ... 463
Semprex-D Capsules ... 1167

Aspirin (Coadministration may result in an additive or synergistic activity and can result in an increased risk of bleeding). Products include:
Alka-Seltzer Effervescent Antacid and Pain Reliever ... 701
Alka-Seltzer Extra Strength Effervescent Antacid and Pain Reliever ... 703
Alka-Seltzer Lemon Lime Effervescent Antacid and Pain Reliever ... 703
Alka-Seltzer Plus Cold Medicine ... 705
Alka-Seltzer Plus Cold & Cough Medicine ... 708
Alka-Seltzer Plus Night-Time Cold Medicine ... 707
Alka Seltzer Plus Sinus Medicine .. 707
Arthritis Foundation Safety Coated Aspirin Tablets ... 675
Arthritis Pain Ascriptin ... 631
Maximum Strength Ascriptin ... 630
Regular Strength Ascriptin Tablets ... 629
Arthritis Strength BC Powder ... 609
BC Cold Powder Multi-Symptom Formula (Cold-Sinus-Allergy) ... 609
BC Cold Powder Non-Drowsy Formula (Cold-Sinus) ... 609
BC Powder ... 609
Bayer Children's Chewable Aspirin ... 711
Genuine Bayer Aspirin Tablets & Caplets ... 713
Extra Strength Bayer Arthritis Pain Regimen Formula ... 711
Extra Strength Bayer Aspirin Caplets & Tablets ... 712
Extended-Release Bayer 8-Hour Aspirin ... 712
Extra Strength Bayer Plus Aspirin Caplets ... 713
Extra Strength Bayer PM Aspirin .. 713
Bayer Enteric Aspirin ... 709
Bufferin Analgesic Tablets and Caplets ... 613
Arthritis Strength Bufferin Analgesic Caplets ... 614
Extra Strength Bufferin Analgesic Tablets ... 615
Cama Arthritis Pain Reliever ... 785
Darvon Compound-65 Pulvules ... 1435
Easprin ... 1914
Ecotrin ... 2455
Ecotrin Enteric Coated Aspirin Maximum Strength Tablets and Caplets ... 816
Ecotrin Enteric Coated Aspirin Regular Strength Tablets ... 2455
Empirin Aspirin Tablets ... 854
Empirin with Codeine Tablets ... 1093
Excedrin Extra-Strength Analgesic Tablets & Caplets ... 732
Fiorinal Capsules ... 2261
Fiorinal with Codeine Capsules ... 2262
Fiorinal Tablets ... 2261
Halfprin ... 1362
Healthprin Aspirin ... 2455
Norgesic ... 1496
Percodan Tablets ... 939
Percodan-Demi Tablets ... 940
Robaxisal Tablets ... 2071
Soma Compound w/Codeine Tablets ... 2676
Soma Compound Tablets ... 2675
St. Joseph Adult Chewable Aspirin (81 mg.) ... 808
Talwin Compound ... 2335
Ursinus Inlay-Tabs ... 794
Vanquish Analgesic Caplets ... 731

Astemizole (Antagonizes the antithrombotic activity of heparin). Products include:
Hismanal Tablets ... 1293

Azatadine Maleate (Antagonizes the antithrombotic activity of heparin). Products include:
Trinalin Repetabs Tablets ... 1330

Azithromycin (Loss of pharmacological activity of either or both drugs). Products include:
Zithromax ... 1944

Azlocillin Sodium (Coadministration may result in an additive or synergistic activity and can result in an increased risk of bleeding).
No products indexed under this heading.

Bromodiphenhydramine Hydrochloride (Antagonizes the antithrombotic activity of heparin).
No products indexed under this heading.

Brompheniramine Maleate (Antagonizes the antithrombotic activity of heparin). Products include:
Alka Seltzer Plus Sinus Medicine .. 707
Bromfed Capsules (Extended-Release) ... 1785
Bromfed Syrup ... 733
Bromfed Tablets ... 1785
Bromfed-DM Cough Syrup ... 1786
Bromfed-PD Capsules (Extended-Release) ... 1785
Dimetane-DC Cough Syrup ... 2059
Dimetane-DX Cough Syrup ... 2059
Dimetapp Elixir ... 773
Dimetapp Extentabs ... 774
Dimetapp Tablets/Liqui-Gels ... 775
Dimetapp Cold & Allergy Chewable Tablets ... 773
Dimetapp DM Elixir ... 774
Vicks DayQuil Allergy Relief 12-Hour Extended Release Tablets .. 760
Vicks DayQuil Allergy Relief 4-Hour Tablets ... 760

Carbenicillin Indanyl Sodium (Coadministration may result in an additive or synergistic activity and can result in an increased risk of bleeding). Products include:
Geocillin Tablets ... 2199

Cefamandole Nafate (Coadministration may result in an additive or synergistic activity and can result in an increased risk of bleeding). Products include:
Mandol Vials, Faspak & ADD-Vantage ... 1461

Cefmetazole Sodium (Coadministration may result in an additive or synergistic activity and can result in an increased risk of bleeding). Products include:
Zefazone ... 2654

Cefoperazone Sodium (Coadministration may result in an additive or synergistic activity and can result in an increased risk of bleeding). Products include:
Cefobid Intravenous/Intramuscular 2189
Cefobid Pharmacy Bulk Package - Not for Direct Infusion ... 2192

Cefotetan (Coadministration may result in an additive or synergistic activity and can result in an increased risk of bleeding). Products include:
Cefotan ... 2829

Chlorpheniramine Maleate (Antagonizes the antithrombotic activity of heparin). Products include:
Alka-Seltzer Plus Cold Medicine ... 705
Alka-Seltzer Plus Cold Medicine Liqui-Gels ... 706
Alka-Seltzer Plus Cold & Cough Medicine ... 708
Alka-Seltzer Plus Cold & Cough Medicine Liqui-Gels ... 705
Allerest Children's Chewable Tablets ... 627
Allerest Headache Strength Tablets ... 627
Allerest Maximum Strength Tablets ... 627
Allerest Sinus Pain Formula ... 627
Allerest 12 Hour Caplets ... 627
Ana-Kit Anaphylaxis Emergency Treatment Kit ... 617
Atrohist Pediatric Capsules ... 453
Atrohist Plus Tablets ... 454
BC Cold Powder Multi-Symptom Formula (Cold-Sinus-Allergy) ... 609
Cerose DM ... 878
Cheracol Plus Head Cold/Cough Formula ... 769
Children's Vicks DayQuil Allergy Relief ... 757
Children's Vicks NyQuil Cold/Cough Relief ... 758
Chlor-Trimeton Allergy Decongestant Tablets ... 799
Chlor-Trimeton Allergy Tablets ... 798
Comhist ... 2038
Comtrex Multi-Symptom Cold Reliever Tablets/Caplets/Liqui-Gels/Liquid ... 615
Allergy-Sinus Comtrex Multi-Symptom Allergy-Sinus Formula Tablets ... 617
Contac Continuous Action Nasal Decongestant/Antihistamine 12 Hour Capsules ... 813
Contac Maximum Strength Continuous Action Decongestant/Antihistamine 12 Hour Caplets .. 813
Contac Severe Cold and Flu Formula Caplets ... 814
Coricidin 'D' Decongestant Tablets ... 800
Coricidin Tablets ... 800
D.A. Chewable Tablets ... 951
Deconamine ... 1320
Dura-Tap/PD Capsules ... 2867
Dura-Vent/DA Tablets ... 953
Extendryl ... 1005
Fedahist Gyrocaps ... 2401
Fedahist Timecaps ... 2401
Hycomine Compound Tablets ... 932
Isoclor Timesule Capsules ... 637
Kronofed-A ... 977
Nolamine Timed-Release Tablets ... 785
Novahistine DH ... 2462
Novahistine Elixir ... 823
Ornade Spansule Capsules ... 2502
PediaCare Cold Allergy Chewable Tablets ... 677
PediaCare Cough-Cold Chewable Tablets ... 1553
PediaCare Cough-Cold Liquid ... 1553
PediaCare NightRest Cough-Cold Liquid ... 1553
Pediatric Vicks 44m Cough & Cold Relief ... 764
Pyrroxate Caplets ... 772
Ryna ... 841
Sinarest Tablets ... 648
Sinarest Extra Strength Tablets ... 648
Sine-Off Sinus Medicine ... 825
Singlet Tablets ... 825
Sinulin Tablets ... 787
Sinutab Sinus Allergy Medication, Maximum Strength Tablets and Caplets ... 860
Sudafed Plus Liquid ... 862
Sudafed Plus Tablets ... 863
Teldrin 12 Hour Antihistamine/Nasal Decongestant Allergy Relief Capsules ... 826
TheraFlu ... 787
TheraFlu Maximum Strength Nighttime Flu, Cold & Cough Medicine ... 788
Triaminic Allergy Tablets ... 789
Triaminic Cold Tablets ... 790
Triaminic Nite Light ... 791
Triaminic Syrup ... 792
Triaminic-12 Tablets ... 792
Triaminicin Tablets ... 793
Triaminicol Multi-Symptom Cold Tablets ... 793
Triaminicol Multi-Symptom Relief 794
Tussend ... 1783
Children's TYLENOL Cold Multi-Symptom Liquid Formula and Chewable Tablets ... 1561
Children's TYLENOL Cold Plus Cough Multi Symptom Tablets and Liquid ... 681
TYLENOL Maximum Strength Allergy Sinus Medication Gelcaps and Caplets ... 1563
TYLENOL Cold Multi-Symptom Formula Medication Tablets and Caplets ... 1561
TYLENOL Cold Multi-Symptom Hot Medication Liquid Packets ... 1557
Vicks 44 LiquiCaps Cough, Cold & Flu Relief ... 755
Vicks 44M Cough, Cold & Flu Relief ... 756

Chlorpheniramine Polistirex (Antagonizes the antithrombotic activity of heparin). Products include:
Tussionex Pennkinetic Extended-Release Suspension ... 998

Chlorpheniramine Tannate (Antagonizes the antithrombotic activity of heparin). Products include:
Atrohist Pediatric Suspension ... 454
Ricobid Tablets and Pediatric Suspension ... 2038
Rynatan ... 2673
Rynatuss ... 2673

Chlorpromazine (Antagonizes the antithrombotic activity of heparin). Products include:
Thorazine Suppositories ... 2523

Choline Magnesium Trisalicylate (Coadministration may result in an additive or synergistic activity and can result in an increased risk of bleeding). Products include:
Trilisate ... 2000

Clarithromycin (Loss of pharmacological activity of either or both drugs). Products include:
Biaxin ... 405

Clemastine Fumarate (Antagonizes the antithrombotic activity of heparin). Products include:
Tavist Syrup ... 2297
Tavist Tablets ... 2298
Tavist-1 12 Hour Relief Tablets ... 787
Tavist-D 12 Hour Relief Tablets ... 787

Cyproheptadine Hydrochloride (Antagonizes the antithrombotic activity of heparin). Products include:
Periactin ... 1724

Demeclocycline Hydrochloride (Loss of pharmacological activity of either or both drugs). Products include:
Declomycin Tablets ... 1371

Deslanoside (Antagonizes the antithrombotic activity of heparin).
No products indexed under this heading.

Dexchlorpheniramine Maleate (Antagonizes the antithrombotic activity of heparin).
No products indexed under this heading.

Dextran 40 (Interferes with platelet aggregation reactions).
No products indexed under this heading.

IMPORTANT NOTE: Always consult each drug listing in the patient's regimen for possible interactions.

Dextran 70 (Interferes with platelet aggregation reactions). Products include:

AquaSite Eye Drops ◉ 261
Hyskon Hysteroscopy Fluid 1595
Ocucoat and Ocucoat PF Eye Drops ◉ 322
Tears Naturale II Lubricant Eye Drops 473
Tears Naturale Free 473

Diclofenac Potassium (Coadministration may result in an additive or synergistic activity and can result in an increased risk of bleeding). Products include:

Cataflam 816

Diclofenac Sodium (Coadministration may result in an additive or synergistic activity and can result in an increased risk of bleeding). Products include:

Voltaren Ophthalmic Sterile Ophthalmic Solution ◉ 272
Voltaren Tablets 861

Dicumarol (One-stage prothrombin time prolonged).

No products indexed under this heading.

Diflunisal (Coadministration may result in an additive or synergistic activity and can result in an increased risk of bleeding). Products include:

Dolobid Tablets 1654

Digitoxin (Antagonizes the antithrombotic activity of heparin). Products include:

Crystodigin Tablets 1433

Digoxin (Antagonizes the antithrombotic activity of heparin). Products include:

Lanoxicaps 1117
Lanoxin Elixir Pediatric 1120
Lanoxin Injection 1123
Lanoxin Injection Pediatric 1126
Lanoxin Tablets 1128

Diphenhydramine Citrate (Antagonizes the antithrombotic activity of heparin). Products include:

Excedrin P.M. Analgesic/Sleeping Aid Tablets, Caplets, Liquigels 733

Diphenhydramine Hydrochloride (Antagonizes the antithrombotic activity of heparin). Products include:

Actifed Allergy Daytime/Nighttime Caplets ■ 844
Actifed Sinus Daytime/Nighttime Tablets and Caplets ■ 846
Arthritis Foundation NightTime Caplets ■ 674
Extra Strength Bayer PM Aspirin ■ 713
Bayer Select Night Time Pain Relief Formula ■ 716
Benadryl Allergy Decongestant Liquid Medication ■ 848
Benadryl Allergy Decongestant Tablets ■ 848
Benadryl Allergy Liquid Medication ■ 849
Benadryl Allergy ■ 848
Benadryl Allergy Sinus Headache Formula Caplets ■ 849
Benadryl Capsules 1898
Benadryl Dye-Free Allergy Liquigel Softgels ■ 850
Benadryl Dye-Free Allergy Liquid Medication ■ 850
Benadryl Itch Relief Cream, Children's Formula and Maximum Strength 2% ■ 851
Benadryl Itch Relief Spray, Children's Formula and Maximum Strength 2% ■ 851
Benadryl Itch Relief Stick Maximum Strength 2% ■ 850
Benadryl Itch Stopping Gel, Children's Formula and Maximum Strength 2% ■ 851
Benadryl Kapseals 1898
Benadryl Injection 1898
Contac Day & Night Cold/Flu Night Caplets ■ 812
Contac Night Allergy/Sinus Caplets ■ 812
Extra Strength Doan's P.M. ■ 633
Legatrin PM ■ 651
Miles Nervine Nighttime Sleep-Aid ■ 723
Nytol QuickCaps Caplets ■ 610
Sleepinal Night-time Sleep Aid Capsules and Softgels ■ 834
TYLENOL Maximum Strength Allergy Sinus NightTime Medication Caplets 1555
TYLENOL Flu NightTime, Maximum Strength, Gelcaps 1566
TYLENOL Maximum Strength Flu NightTime Hot Medication Packets 1562
TYLENOL PM, Extra Strength Pain Reliever/Sleep Aid Caplets, Geltabs, Gelcaps 1560
TYLENOL Severe Allergy Medication Caplets 1564
Maximum Strength Unisom Sleepgels 1934
Unisom With Pain Relief-Nighttime Sleep Aid and Pain Reliever 1934

Diphenylpyraline Hydrochloride (Antagonizes the antithrombotic activity of heparin).

No products indexed under this heading.

Dipyridamole (Coadministration may result in an additive or synergistic activity and can result in an increased risk of bleeding). Products include:

Persantine Tablets 681

Doxycycline Calcium (Loss of pharmacological activity of either or both drugs). Products include:

Vibramycin Calcium Oral Suspension Syrup 1941

Doxycycline Hyclate (Loss of pharmacological activity of either or both drugs). Products include:

Doryx Capsules 1913
Vibramycin Hyclate Capsules 1941
Vibramycin Hyclate Intravenous 2215
Vibra-Tabs Film Coated Tablets 1941

Doxycycline Monohydrate (Loss of pharmacological activity of either or both drugs). Products include:

Monodox Capsules 1805
Vibramycin Monohydrate for Oral Suspension 1941

Erythromycin (Loss of pharmacological activity of either or both drugs). Products include:

A/T/S 2% Acne Topical Gel and Solution 1234
Benzamycin Topical Gel 905
E-Mycin Tablets 1341
Emgel 2% Topical Gel 1093
ERYC 1915
Erycette (erythromycin 2%) Topical Solution 1888
Ery-Tab Tablets 422
Erythromycin Base Filmtab 426
Erythromycin Delayed-Release Capsules, USP 427
Ilotycin Ophthalmic Ointment 912
PCE Dispertab Tablets 444
T-Stat 2.0% Topical Solution and Pads 2688
Theramycin Z Topical Solution 2% 1592

Erythromycin Estolate (Loss of pharmacological activity of either or both drugs). Products include:

Ilosone 911

Erythromycin Ethylsuccinate (Loss of pharmacological activity of either or both drugs). Products include:

E.E.S. 424
EryPed 421

Erythromycin Gluceptate (Loss of pharmacological activity of either or both drugs). Products include:

Ilotycin Gluceptate, IV, Vials 913

Erythromycin Stearate (Loss of pharmacological activity of either or both drugs). Products include:

Erythrocin Stearate Filmtab 425

Etodolac (Coadministration may result in an additive or synergistic activity and can result in an increased risk of bleeding). Products include:

Lodine Capsules and Tablets 2743

Fenoprofen Calcium (Coadministration may result in an additive or synergistic activity and can result in an increased risk of bleeding). Products include:

Nalfon 200 Pulvules & Nalfon Tablets 917

Fluphenazine Decanoate (Antagonizes the antithrombotic activity of heparin). Products include:

Prolixin Decanoate 509

Fluphenazine Enanthate (Antagonizes the antithrombotic activity of heparin). Products include:

Prolixin Enanthate 509

Fluphenazine Hydrochloride (Antagonizes the antithrombotic activity of heparin). Products include:

Prolixin 509

Flurbiprofen (Coadministration may result in an additive or synergistic activity and can result in an increased risk of bleeding). Products include:

Ansaid Tablets 2579

Gentamicin Sulfate (Loss of pharmacological activity of either or both drugs). Products include:

Garamycin Injectable 2360
Genoptic Sterile Ophthalmic Solution ◉ 243
Genoptic Sterile Ophthalmic Ointment ◉ 243
Gentacidin Ointment ◉ 264
Gentacidin Solution ◉ 264
Gentak ◉ 208
Pred-G Liquifilm Sterile Ophthalmic Suspension ◉ 251
Pred-G S.O.P. Sterile Ophthalmic Ointment ◉ 252

Ibuprofen (Coadministration may result in an additive or synergistic activity and can result in an increased risk of bleeding). Products include:

Advil Cold and Sinus Caplets and Tablets (formerly CoAdvil) ■ 870
Advil Ibuprofen Tablets and Caplets ■ 870
Children's Advil Suspension 2692
Arthritis Foundation Ibuprofen Tablets ■ 674
Bayer Select Ibuprofen Pain Relief Formula ■ 715
Cramp End Tablets ■ 735
Dimetapp Sinus Caplets ■ 775
Haltran Tablets ■ 771
IBU Tablets 1342
Ibuprohm ■ 735
Children's Motrin Ibuprofen Oral Suspension 1546
Motrin Tablets 2625
Motrin IB Caplets, Tablets, and Geltabs ■ 838
Motrin IB Sinus ■ 838
Motrin Ibuprofen Suspension, Oral Drops, Chewable Tablets, Caplets 1546
Nuprin Ibuprofen/Analgesic Tablets & Caplets ■ 622
Sine-Aid IB Caplets 1554
Vicks DayQuil SINUS Pressure & PAIN Relief with IBUPROFEN ■ 762

Indomethacin (Coadministration may result in an additive or synergistic activity and can result in an increased risk of bleeding). Products include:

Indocin 1680

Indomethacin Sodium Trihydrate (Coadministration may result in an additive or synergistic activity and can result in an increased risk of bleeding). Products include:

Indocin I.V. 1684

Ketoprofen (Coadministration may result in an additive or synergistic activity and can result in an increased risk of bleeding). Products include:

Orudis Capsules 2766
Oruvail Capsules 2766

Ketorolac Tromethamine (Coadministration may result in an additive or synergistic activity and can result in an increased risk of bleeding). Products include:

Acular 474
Acular ◉ 277
Toradol 2159

Loratadine (Antagonizes the antithrombotic activity of heparin). Products include:

Claritin 2349
Claritin-D 2350

Magnesium Salicylate (Coadministration may result in an additive or synergistic activity and can result in an increased risk of bleeding). Products include:

Backache Caplets ■ 613
Bayer Select Backache Pain Relief Formula ■ 715
Doan's Extra-Strength Analgesic ■ 633
Extra Strength Doan's P.M. ■ 633
Doan's Regular Strength Analgesic ■ 634
Mobigesic Tablets ■ 602

Meclofenamate Sodium (Coadministration may result in an additive or synergistic activity and can result in an increased risk of bleeding).

No products indexed under this heading.

Mefenamic Acid (Coadministration may result in an additive or synergistic activity and can result in an increased risk of bleeding). Products include:

Ponstel 1925

Mesoridazine Besylate (Antagonizes the antithrombotic activity of heparin). Products include:

Serentil 684

Methacycline Hydrochloride (Loss of pharmacological activity of either or both drugs).

No products indexed under this heading.

Methdilazine Hydrochloride (Antagonizes the antithrombotic activity of heparin).

No products indexed under this heading.

Methotrimeprazine (Antagonizes the antithrombotic activity of heparin). Products include:

Levoprome 1274

Mezlocillin Sodium (Coadministration may result in an additive or synergistic activity and can result in an increased risk of bleeding). Products include:

Mezlin 601
Mezlin Pharmacy Bulk Package 604

Minocycline Hydrochloride (Loss of pharmacological activity of either or both drugs). Products include:

Dynacin Capsules 1590
Minocin Intravenous 1382
Minocin Oral Suspension 1385
Minocin Pellet-Filled Capsules 1383

Moxalactam Disodium (Coadministration may result in an additive or synergistic activity and can result in an increased risk of bleeding).

475 **Interactions Index** **Hexalen**

Nabumetone (Coadministration may result in an additive or synergistic activity and can result in an increased risk of bleeding). Products include:
- Relafen Tablets ... 2510

Nafcillin Sodium (Coadministration may result in an additive or synergistic activity and can result in an increased risk of bleeding).
- No products indexed under this heading.

Naproxen (Coadministration may result in an additive or synergistic activity and can result in an increased risk of bleeding). Products include:
- Anaprox/Naprosyn ... 2117

Naproxen Sodium (Coadministration may result in an additive or synergistic activity and can result in an increased risk of bleeding). Products include:
- Aleve ... 1975
- Anaprox/Naprosyn ... 2117

Neomycin, oral (Loss of pharmacological activity of either or both drugs).

Nicotine Polacrilex (Antagonizes the antithrombotic activity of heparin). Products include:
- Nicorette ... 2458

Nitroglycerin Intravenous (May require higher doses of heparin; close monitoring of the partial thromboplastin time is required).

Oxaprozin (Coadministration may result in an additive or synergistic activity and can result in an increased risk of bleeding). Products include:
- Daypro Caplets ... 2426

Oxytetracycline Hydrochloride (Loss of pharmacological activity of either or both drugs). Products include:
- TERAK Ointment ... ⊙ 209
- Terra-Cortril Ophthalmic Suspension ... 2210
- Terramycin with Polymyxin B Sulfate Ophthalmic Ointment ... 2211
- Urobiotic-250 Capsules ... 2214

Penicillin G Benzathine (Coadministration may result in an additive or synergistic activity and can result in an increased risk of bleeding). Products include:
- Bicillin C-R Injection ... 2704
- Bicillin C-R 900/300 Injection ... 2706
- Bicillin L-A Injection ... 2707

Penicillin G Procaine (Coadministration may result in an additive or synergistic activity and can result in an increased risk of bleeding). Products include:
- Bicillin C-R Injection ... 2704
- Bicillin C-R 900/300 Injection ... 2706

Perphenazine (Antagonizes the antithrombotic activity of heparin). Products include:
- Etrafon ... 2355
- Triavil Tablets ... 1757
- Trilafon ... 2389

Phenylbutazone (Coadministration may result in an additive or synergistic activity and can result in an increased risk of bleeding).
- No products indexed under this heading.

Piroxicam (Coadministration may result in an additive or synergistic activity and can result in an increased risk of bleeding). Products include:
- Feldene Capsules ... 1965

Polymyxin B Sulfate (Loss of pharmacological activity of either or both drugs). Products include:
- AK-Spore ... ⊙ 204
- AK-Trol Ointment & Suspension ... ⊙ 205
- Bactine First Aid Antibiotic Plus Anesthetic Ointment ... ▣ 708
- Betadine Brand First Aid Antibiotics & Moisturizer Ointment ... 1991
- Campho-Phenique Maximum Strength First Aid Antibiotic Plus Pain Reliever Ointment ... ▣ 719
- Cortisporin Cream ... 1084
- Cortisporin Ointment ... 1085
- Cortisporin Ophthalmic Ointment Sterile ... 1085
- Cortisporin Ophthalmic Suspension Sterile ... 1086
- Cortisporin Otic Solution Sterile ... 1087
- Cortisporin Otic Suspension Sterile 1088
- Dexacidin Ointment ... ⊙ 263
- Maxitrol Ophthalmic Ointment and Suspension ... ⊙ 224
- Mycitracin ... ▣ 839
- Neosporin G.U. Irrigant Sterile ... 1148
- Neosporin Ointment ... ▣ 857
- Neosporin Plus Maximum Strength Cream ... ▣ 858
- Neosporin Plus Maximum Strength Ointment ... ▣ 858
- Neosporin Ophthalmic Ointment Sterile ... 1148
- Neosporin Ophthalmic Solution Sterile ... 1149
- Ophthocort ... ⊙ 311
- PediOtic Suspension Sterile ... 1153
- Polymyxin B Sulfate, Aerosporin Brand Sterile Powder ... 1154
- Poly-Pred Liquifilm ... ⊙ 248
- Polysporin Ointment ... ▣ 858
- Polysporin Ophthalmic Ointment Sterile ... 1154
- Polysporin Powder ... ▣ 859
- Polytrim Ophthalmic Solution Sterile ... 482
- TERAK Ointment ... ⊙ 209
- Terramycin with Polymyxin B Sulfate Ophthalmic Ointment ... 2211

Prochlorperazine (Antagonizes the antithrombotic activity of heparin). Products include:
- Compazine ... 2470

Promethazine Hydrochloride (Antagonizes the antithrombotic activity of heparin). Products include:
- Mepergan Injection ... 2753
- Phenergan with Codeine ... 2777
- Phenergan with Dextromethorphan 2778
- Phenergan Injection ... 2773
- Phenergan Suppositories ... 2775
- Phenergan Syrup ... 2774
- Phenergan Tablets ... 2775
- Phenergan VC ... 2779
- Phenergan VC with Codeine ... 2781

Pyrilamine Maleate (Antagonizes the antithrombotic activity of heparin). Products include:
- 4-Way Fast Acting Nasal Spray (regular & mentholated) ... ▣ 621
- Maximum Strength Multi-Symptom Formula Midol ... ▣ 722
- PMS Multi-Symptom Formula Midol ... ▣ 723

Pyrilamine Tannate (Antagonizes the antithrombotic activity of heparin). Products include:
- Atrohist Pediatric Suspension ... 454
- Rynatan ... 2673

Salsalate (Coadministration may result in an additive or synergistic activity and can result in an increased risk of bleeding). Products include:
- Mono-Gesic Tablets ... 792
- Salflex Tablets ... 786

Streptomycin Sulfate (Loss of pharmacological activity of either or both drugs). Products include:
- Streptomycin Sulfate Injection ... 2208

Sulindac (Coadministration may result in an additive or synergistic activity and can result in an increased risk of bleeding). Products include:
- Clinoril Tablets ... 1618

Terfenadine (Antagonizes the antithrombotic activity of heparin). Products include:
- Seldane Tablets ... 1536
- Seldane-D Extended-Release Tablets ... 1538

Tetracycline Hydrochloride (Loss of pharmacological activity of either or both drugs). Products include:
- Achromycin V Capsules ... 1367

Thioridazine Hydrochloride (Antagonizes the antithrombotic activity of heparin). Products include:
- Mellaril ... 2269

Ticarcillin Disodium (Coadministration may result in an additive or synergistic activity and can result in an increased risk of bleeding). Products include:
- Ticar for Injection ... 2526
- Timentin for Injection ... 2528

Ticlopidine Hydrochloride (Coadministration may result in an additive or synergistic activity and can result in an increased risk of bleeding). Products include:
- Ticlid Tablets ... 2156

Tolmetin Sodium (Coadministration may result in an additive or synergistic activity and can result in an increased risk of bleeding). Products include:
- Tolectin (200, 400 and 600 mg) .. 1581

Trifluoperazine Hydrochloride (Antagonizes the antithrombotic activity of heparin). Products include:
- Stelazine ... 2514

Trimeprazine Tartrate (Antagonizes the antithrombotic activity of heparin). Products include:
- Temaril Tablets, Syrup and Spansule Extended-Release Capsules .. 483

Tripelennamine Hydrochloride (Antagonizes the antithrombotic activity of heparin). Products include:
- PBZ Tablets ... 845
- PBZ-SR Tablets ... 844

Triprolidine Hydrochloride (Antagonizes the antithrombotic activity of heparin). Products include:
- Actifed Plus Caplets ... ▣ 845
- Actifed Plus Tablets ... ▣ 845
- Actifed with Codeine Cough Syrup .. 1067
- Actifed Syrup ... ▣ 846
- Actifed Tablets ... ▣ 844

Troleandomycin (Loss of pharmacological activity of either or both drugs). Products include:
- Tao Capsules ... 2209

Vitamin C (Antagonizes the antithrombotic activity of heparin). Products include:
- ANTIOX Capsules ... 1543
- C-Buff ... 667
- Centrum Singles Vitamin C ... ▣ 669
- Chromagen Capsules ... 2339
- Dexatrim Maximum Strength Plus Vitamin C/Caffeine-free Caplets ▣ 832
- Ester-C Mineral Ascorbates Powder ... ▣ 658
- Fero-Folic-500 Filmtab ... 429
- Fero-Grad-500 Filmtab ... 429
- Halls Vitamin C Drops ... ▣ 843
- Hyland's Vitamin C for Children ... ▣ 830
- Irospan ... 982
- Materna Tablets ... 1379
- Nature Made Antioxidant Formula ▣ 748
- Niferex w/Vitamin C Tablets ... 793
- One-A-Day Extras Antioxidant ... ▣ 728
- One-A-Day Extras Vitamin C ... ▣ 728
- Protegra Antioxidant Vitamin & Mineral Supplement ... ▣ 670
- Stuart Prenatal Tablets ... ▣ 881
- The Stuart Formula Tablets ... ▣ 663
- Sunkist Children's Chewable Multivitamins - Plus Extra C ... ▣ 649
- Sunkist Vitamin C ... ▣ 649
- Theragran Antioxidant ... ▣ 623
- Trinsicon Capsules ... 2570
- Vitron-C Tablets ... ▣ 650

Warfarin Sodium (One-stage prothrombin time prolonged). Products include:
- Coumadin ... 926

HEP-B-GAMMAGEE
(Hepatitis B Immune Globulin (Human)) ... 1663
May interact with:

Measles Virus Vaccine Live (Interference with immune response to live virus vaccines). Products include:
- Attenuvax ... 1610

Measles & Rubella Virus Vaccine Live (Interference with immune response to live virus vaccines). Products include:
- M-R-VAX II ... 1689

Measles, Mumps & Rubella Virus Vaccine Live (Interference with immune response to live virus vaccines). Products include:
- M-M-R II ... 1687

Rubella Virus Vaccine Live (Interference with immune response to live virus vaccines). Products include:
- Meruvax II ... 1697

Rubella & Mumps Virus Vaccine Live (Interference with immune response to live virus vaccines). Products include:
- Biavax II ... 1613

HEP-FORTE CAPSULES
(Vitamins with Minerals) ... 1541
None cited in PDR database.

HERPECIN-L COLD SORE LIP BALM STICK
(Allantoin) ... 779
None cited in PDR database.

HERPLEX LIQUIFILM
(Idoxuridine) ... ⊙ 244
May interact with:

Boric Acid (Concurrent administration is not recommended). Products include:
- Collyrium for Fresh Eyes ... ⊙ 325
- Collyrium Fresh ... ▣ 879
- Lens Plus Rewetting Drops ... ⊙ 336
- Star-Otic Ear Solution ... ▣ 830

HERRICK LACRIMAL PLUGS
(Collagen) ... ⊙ 285
None cited in PDR database.

HESPAN INJECTION
(Hetastarch) ... 929
None cited in PDR database.

HEXALEN CAPSULES
(Altretamine) ... 2571
May interact with monoamine oxidase inhibitors and certain other agents. Compounds in these categories include:

Cimetidine (Increases altretamine's half-life and toxicity in a rat model). Products include:
- Tagamet Tablets ... 2516

IMPORTANT NOTE: Always consult each drug listing in the patient's regimen for possible interactions.

Hexalen Interactions Index 476

Cimetidine Hydrochloride (Increases altretamine's half-life and toxicity in a rat model). Products include:
- Tagamet ... 2516

Furazolidone (Potential for severe orthostatic hypotension). Products include:
- Furoxone ... 2046

Isocarboxazid (Potential for severe orthostatic hypotension).
- No products indexed under this heading.

Phenelzine Sulfate (Potential for severe orthostatic hypotension). Products include:
- Nardil ... 1920

Pyridoxine Hydrochloride (May adversely affect response duration; should not be administered with Hexalen and/or Cisplatin).
- No products indexed under this heading.

Selegiline Hydrochloride (Potential for severe orthostatic hypotension). Products include:
- Eldepryl Tablets ... 2550

Tranylcypromine Sulfate (Potential for severe orthostatic hypotension). Products include:
- Parnate Tablets ... 2503

HELIXATE, ANTIHEMOPHILIC FACTOR (RECOMBINANT)
(Antihemophilic Factor (Recombinant)) ... 518
None cited in PDR database.

HIBICLENS ANTIMICROBIAL SKIN CLEANSER
(Chlorhexidine Gluconate) ... 2840
None cited in PDR database.

HIBISTAT GERMICIDAL HAND RINSE
(Chlorhexidine Gluconate) ... 2841
None cited in PDR database.

HIBISTAT TOWELETTE
(Chlorhexidine Gluconate) ... 2841
None cited in PDR database.

HIBTITER
(Haemophilus B Conjugate Vaccine) .. 1375
May interact with immunosuppressive agents, corticosteroids, cytotoxic drugs, alkylating agents, and anticoagulants. Compounds in these categories include:

Azathioprine (Reduces antibody response to active immunization procedures). Products include:
- Imuran ... 1110

Betamethasone Acetate (Reduces antibody response to active immunization procedures). Products include:
- Celestone Soluspan Suspension ... 2347

Betamethasone Sodium Phosphate (Reduces antibody response to active immunization procedures). Products include:
- Celestone Soluspan Suspension ... 2347

Bleomycin Sulfate (Reduces antibody response to active immunization procedures). Products include:
- Blenoxane ... 692

Busulfan (Reduces antibody response to active immunization procedures). Products include:
- Myleran Tablets ... 1143

Carmustine (BCNU) (Reduces antibody response to active immunization procedures). Products include:
- BiCNU ... 691

Chlorambucil (Reduces antibody response to active immunization procedures). Products include:
- Leukeran Tablets ... 1133

Cortisone Acetate (Reduces antibody response to active immunization procedures). Products include:
- Cortone Acetate Sterile Suspension ... 1623
- Cortone Acetate Tablets ... 1624

Cyclophosphamide (Reduces antibody response to active immunization). Products include:
- Cytoxan ... 694
- NEOSAR Lyophilized/Neosar ... 1959

Cyclosporine (Reduces antibody response to active immunization procedures). Products include:
- Neoral ... 2276
- Sandimmune ... 2286

Dacarbazine (Reduces antibody response to active immunization procedures). Products include:
- DTIC-Dome ... 600

Dalteparin Sodium (HibTITER should be given with caution to children on anticoagulant therapy). Products include:
- Fragmin ... 1954

Daunorubicin Hydrochloride (Reduces antibody response to active immunization procedures). Products include:
- Cerubidine ... 795

Dexamethasone (Reduces antibody response to active immunization procedures). Products include:
- AK-Trol Ointment & Suspension ... ◉ 205
- Decadron Elixir ... 1633
- Decadron Tablets ... 1635
- Decaspray Topical Aerosol ... 1648
- Dexacidin Ointment ... ◉ 263
- Maxitrol Ophthalmic Ointment and Suspension ... ◉ 224
- TobraDex Ophthalmic Suspension and Ointment ... 473

Dexamethasone Acetate (Reduces antibody response to active immunization procedures). Products include:
- Dalalone D.P. Injectable ... 1011
- Decadron-LA Sterile Suspension ... 1646

Dexamethasone Sodium Phosphate (Reduces antibody response to active immunization procedures). Products include:
- Decadron Phosphate Injection ... 1637
- Decadron Phosphate Respihaler ... 1642
- Decadron Phosphate Sterile Ophthalmic Ointment ... 1641
- Decadron Phosphate Sterile Ophthalmic Solution ... 1642
- Decadron Phosphate Topical Cream ... 1644
- Decadron Phosphate Turbinaire ... 1645
- Decadron Phosphate with Xylocaine Injection, Sterile ... 1639
- Dexacort Phosphate in Respihaler .. 458
- Dexacort Phosphate in Turbinaire .. 459
- NeoDecadron Sterile Ophthalmic Ointment ... 1712
- NeoDecadron Sterile Ophthalmic Solution ... 1713
- NeoDecadron Topical Cream ... 1714

Dicumarol (HibTITER should be given with caution to children on anticoagulant therapy).
- No products indexed under this heading.

Doxorubicin Hydrochloride (Reduces antibody response to active immunization procedures). Products include:
- Adriamycin PFS ... 1947
- Adriamycin RDF ... 1947
- Doxorubicin Astra ... 540
- Rubex ... 712

Enoxaparin (HibTITER should be given with caution to children on anticoagulant therapy). Products include:
- Lovenox Injection ... 2020

Fludrocortisone Acetate (Reduces antibody response to active immunization procedures). Products include:
- Florinef Acetate Tablets ... 505

Fluorouracil (Reduces antibody response to active immunization procedures). Products include:
- Efudex ... 2113
- Fluoroplex Topical Solution & Cream 1% ... 479
- Fluorouracil Injection ... 2116

Heparin Calcium (HibTITER should be given with caution to children on anticoagulant therapy).
- No products indexed under this heading.

Heparin Sodium (HibTITER should be given with caution to children on anticoagulant therapy). Products include:
- Heparin Lock Flush Solution ... 2725
- Heparin Sodium Injection ... 2726
- Heparin Sodium Injection, USP, Sterile Solution ... 2615
- Heparin Sodium Vials ... 1441

Hydrocortisone (Reduces antibody response to active immunization procedures). Products include:
- Anusol-HC Cream 2.5% ... 1896
- Aquanil HC Lotion ... 1931
- Bactine Hydrocortisone Anti-Itch Cream ... ▣ 709
- Caldecort Anti-Itch Hydrocortisone Spray ... ▣ 631
- Cortaid ... ▣ 836
- CORTENEMA ... 2535
- Cortisporin Ointment ... 1085
- Cortisporin Ophthalmic Ointment Sterile ... 1085
- Cortisporin Ophthalmic Suspension Sterile ... 1086
- Cortisporin Otic Solution Sterile ... 1087
- Cortisporin Otic Suspension Sterile 1088
- Cortizone-5 ... ▣ 831
- Cortizone-10 ... ▣ 831
- Hydrocortone Tablets ... 1672
- Hytone ... 907
- Massengill Medicated Soft Cloth Towelettes ... 2458
- PediOtic Suspension Sterile ... 1153
- Preparation H Hydrocortisone 1% Cream ... ▣ 872
- ProctoCream-HC 2.5% ... 2408
- VōSoL HC Otic Solution ... 2678

Hydrocortisone Acetate (Reduces antibody response to active immunization procedures). Products include:
- Analpram-HC Rectal Cream 1% and 2.5% ... 977
- Anusol HC-1 Anti-Itch Hydrocortisone Ointment ... ▣ 847
- Anusol-HC Suppositories ... 1897
- Caldecort ... ▣ 631
- Carmol HC ... 924
- Coly-Mycin S Otic w/Neomycin & Hydrocortisone ... 1906
- Cortaid ... ▣ 836
- Cortifoam ... 2396
- Cortisporin Cream ... 1084
- Epifoam ... 2399
- Hydrocortone Acetate Sterile Suspension ... 1669
- Mantadil Cream ... 1135
- Nupercainal Hydrocortisone 1% Cream ... ▣ 645
- Ophthocort ... ◉ 311
- Pramosone Cream, Lotion & Ointment ... 978
- ProctoCream-HC ... 2408
- ProctoFoam-HC ... 2409
- Terra-Cortril Ophthalmic Suspension ... 2210

Hydrocortisone Sodium Phosphate (Reduces antibody response to active immunization procedures). Products include:
- Hydrocortone Phosphate Injection, Sterile ... 1670

Hydrocortisone Sodium Succinate (Reduces antibody response to active immunization procedures). Products include:
- Solu-Cortef Sterile Powder ... 2641

Hydroxyurea (Reduces antibody response to active immunization procedures). Products include:
- Hydrea Capsules ... 696

Immune Globulin (Human) (Reduces antibody response to active immunization procedures).
- No products indexed under this heading.

Immune Globulin Intravenous (Human) (Reduces antibody response to active immunization procedures).

Lomustine (CCNU) (Reduces antibody response to active immunization procedures). Products include:
- CeeNU ... 693

Mechlorethamine Hydrochloride (Reduces antibody response to active immunization procedures). Products include:
- Mustargen ... 1709

Melphalan (Reduces antibody response to active immunization procedures). Products include:
- Alkeran Tablets ... 1071

Methotrexate Sodium (Reduces antibody response to active immunization procedures). Products include:
- Methotrexate Sodium Tablets, Injection, for Injection and LPF Injection ... 1275

Methylprednisolone Acetate (Reduces antibody response to active immunization procedures). Products include:
- Depo-Medrol Single-Dose Vial ... 2600
- Depo-Medrol Sterile Aqueous Suspension ... 2597

Methylprednisolone Sodium Succinate (Reduces antibody response to active immunization procedures). Products include:
- Solu-Medrol Sterile Powder ... 2643

Mitotane (Reduces antibody response to active immunization procedures). Products include:
- Lysodren ... 698

Mitoxantrone Hydrochloride (Reduces antibody response to active immunization procedures). Products include:
- Novantrone ... 1279

Muromonab-CD3 (Reduces antibody response to active immunization procedures). Products include:
- Orthoclone OKT3 Sterile Solution .. 1837

Mycophenolate Mofetil (Reduces antibody response to active immunization procedures). Products include:
- CellCept Capsules ... 2099

Prednisolone Acetate (Reduces antibody response to active immunization procedures). Products include:
- AK-CIDE ... ◉ 202
- AK-CIDE Ointment ... ◉ 202
- Blephamide Liquifilm Sterile Ophthalmic Suspension ... 476
- Blephamide Ointment ... ◉ 237
- Econopred & Econopred Plus Ophthalmic Suspensions ... ◉ 217
- Poly-Pred Liquifilm ... ◉ 248
- Pred Forte ... ◉ 250
- Pred Mild ... ◉ 253

(▣ Described in PDR For Nonprescription Drugs) (◉ Described in PDR For Ophthalmology)

Pred-G Liquifilm Sterile Ophthalmic Suspension .... ◉ 251
Pred-G S.O.P. Sterile Ophthalmic Ointment .... ◉ 252
Vasocidin Ointment .... ◉ 268

Prednisolone Sodium Phosphate (Reduces antibody response to active immunization procedures). Products include:

AK-Pred .... ◉ 204
Hydeltrasol Injection, Sterile 1665
Inflamase .... ◉ 265
Pediapred Oral Liquid 995
Vasocidin Ophthalmic Solution .... ◉ 270

Prednisolone Tebutate (Reduces antibody response to active immunization procedures). Products include:

Hydeltra-T.B.A. Sterile Suspension 1667

Prednisone (Reduces antibody response to active immunization procedures). Products include:

Deltasone Tablets 2595

Procarbazine Hydrochloride (Reduces antibody response to active immunization procedures). Products include:

Matulane Capsules 2131

Tacrolimus (Reduces antibody response to active immunization procedures). Products include:

Prograf 1042

Tamoxifen Citrate (Reduces antibody response to active immunization procedures). Products include:

Nolvadex Tablets 2841

Thiotepa (Reduces antibody response to active immunization procedures). Products include:

Thioplex (Thiotepa For Injection) 1281

Triamcinolone (Reduces antibody response to active immunization procedures). Products include:

Aristocort Tablets 1022

Triamcinolone Acetonide (Reduces antibody response to active immunization procedures). Products include:

Aristocort A 0.025% Cream 1027
Aristocort A 0.5% Cream 1031
Aristocort A 0.1% Cream 1029
Aristocort A 0.1% Ointment 1030
Azmacort Oral Inhaler 2011
Nasacort Nasal Inhaler 2024

Triamcinolone Diacetate (Reduces antibody response to active immunization procedures). Products include:

Aristocort Suspension (Forte Parenteral) 1027
Aristocort Suspension (Intralesional) 1025

Triamcinolone Hexacetonide (Reduces antibody response to active immunization procedures). Products include:

Aristospan Suspension (Intra-articular) 1033
Aristospan Suspension (Intralesional) 1032

Vincristine Sulfate (Reduces antibody response to active immunization procedures). Products include:

Oncovin Solution Vials & Hyporets 1466

Warfarin Sodium (HibTITER should be given with caution to children on anticoagulant therapy). Products include:

Coumadin 926

HISMANAL TABLETS

(Astemizole) 1293

May interact with macrolide antibiotics and certain other agents. Compounds in these categories include:

Azithromycin (Concomitant administration is contraindicated; potential for syncope with Torsades de Pointes). Products include:

Zithromax 1944

Clarithromycin (Concomitant administration is contraindicated; potential for syncope with Torsades de Pointes). Products include:

Biaxin 405

Erythromycin (Concomitant administration is contraindicated; potential for syncope with Torsades de Pointes). Products include:

A/T/S 2% Acne Topical Gel and Solution 1234
Benzamycin Topical Gel 905
E-Mycin Tablets 1341
Emgel 2% Topical Gel 1093
ERYC 1915
Erycette (erythromycin 2%) Topical Solution 1888
Ery-Tab Tablets 422
Erythromycin Base Filmtab 426
Erythromycin Delayed-Release Capsules, USP 427
Ilotycin Ophthalmic Ointment 912
PCE Dispertab Tablets 444
T-Stat 2.0% Topical Solution and Pads 2688
Theramycin Z Topical Solution 2% 1592

Erythromycin Estolate (Concomitant administration is contraindicated; potential for syncope with Torsades de Pointes). Products include:

Ilosone 911

Erythromycin Ethylsuccinate (Concomitant administration is contraindicated; potential for syncope with Torsades de Pointes). Products include:

E.E.S. 424
EryPed 421

Erythromycin Gluceptate (Concomitant administration is contraindicated; potential for syncope with Torsades de Pointes). Products include:

Ilotycin Gluceptate, IV, Vials 913

Erythromycin Stearate (Concomitant administration is contraindicated; potential for syncope with Torsades de Pointes). Products include:

Erythrocin Stearate Filmtab 425

Fluconazole (Concomitant use with astemizole is not recommended due to chemical similarity of fluconazole to ketoconazole). Products include:

Diflucan Injection, Tablets, and Oral Suspension 2194

Itraconazole (Concomitant administration with astemizole is contraindicated based on the chemical resemblance of itraconazole and ketoconazole). Products include:

Sporanox Capsules 1305

Ketoconazole (Concomitant administration with ketoconazole tablets is contraindicated; potential for cardiovascular events including electrographic QT prolongation). Products include:

Nizoral 2% Cream 1297
Nizoral 2% Shampoo 1298
Nizoral Tablets 1298

Metronidazole (Concomitant use with astemizole is not recommended due to chemical similarity of metronidazole to ketoconazole). Products include:

Flagyl 375 Capsules 2434
Flagyl I.V. RTU 2247
MetroGel 1047
MetroGel-Vaginal 902
Protostat Tablets 1883

Metronidazole Hydrochloride (Concomitant use with astemizole is not recommended due to chemical similarity of metronidazole to ketoconazole). Products include:

Flagyl I.V. 2247

Miconazole (Concomitant use with astemizole is not recommended due to chemical similarity of intravenous form of miconazole to ketoconazole).

No products indexed under this heading.

Troleandomycin (Concomitant administration is contraindicated; potential for syncope with Torsades de Pointes). Products include:

Tao Capsules 2209

Food Interactions

Meal, unspecified (Reduces the absorption by 60%; patients should be instructed to take Hismanal on an empty stomach, e.g. at least 2 hours after a meal).

HIVID TABLETS

(Zalcitabine) 2121

May interact with aminoglycosides, drugs that are known to cause peripheral neuropathy and pancreatitis (selected), antacids containing aluminium, calcium and magnesium, and certain other agents. Compounds in these categories include:

Altretamine (Potential for increased peripheral neuropathy; concomitant use should be avoided). Products include:

Hexalen Capsules 2571

Aluminum Carbonate Gel (Absorption of zalcitabine is moderately reduced (approximately 25%) when coadministered with magnesium/aluminum containing antacids). Products include:

Basaljel 2703

Aluminum Hydroxide (Absorption of zalcitabine is moderately reduced (approximately 25%) when coadministered with magnesium/aluminum containing antacids). Products include:

ALternaGEL Liquid 1316
Maximum Strength Ascriptin .... ▣ 630
Cama Arthritis Pain Reliever .... ▣ 785
Gaviscon Extra Strength Relief Formula Antacid Tablets .... ▣ 819
Gaviscon Extra Strength Relief Formula Liquid Antacid .... ▣ 819
Gaviscon Liquid Antacid .... ▣ 820
Gelusil Liquid & Tablets .... ▣ 855
Maalox Heartburn Relief Suspension .... ▣ 642
Maalox Heartburn Relief Tablets .... ▣ 641
Maalox Magnesia and Alumina Oral Suspension .... ▣ 642
Maalox Plus Tablets .... ▣ 643
Extra Strength Maalox Antacid Plus Antigas Liquid and Tablets ▣ 638
Tempo Soft Antacid .... ▣ 835

Aluminum Hydroxide Gel (Absorption of zalcitabine is moderately reduced (approximately 25%) when coadministered with magnesium/aluminum containing antacids). Products include:

ALternaGEL Liquid .... ▣ 659
Aludrox Oral Suspension 2695
Amphojel Suspension 2695
Amphojel Suspension without Flavor 2695
Amphojel Tablets 2695
Arthritis Pain Ascriptin .... ▣ 631
Regular Strength Ascriptin Tablets .... ▣ 629
Gaviscon Antacid Tablets .... ▣ 819
Gaviscon-2 Antacid Tablets .... ▣ 820
Mylanta Liquid 1317
Mylanta Tablets .... ▣ 660
Mylanta Double Strength Liquid 1317
Mylanta Double Strength Tablets .... ▣ 660
Nephrox Suspension .... ▣ 655

Amikacin Sulfate (Increases the risk of developing peripheral neuropathy or other Hivid-associated toxicities by interfering with the renal clearance of zalcitabine). Products include:

Amikacin Sulfate Injection, USP 960
Amikin Injectable 501

Amphotericin B (Increases the risk of developing peripheral neuropathy or other Hivid-associated toxicities by interfering with the renal clearance of zalcitabine). Products include:

Fungizone Intravenous 506

Auranofin (Potential for increased peripheral neuropathy; concomitant use should be avoided). Products include:

Ridaura Capsules 2513

Carboplatin (Potential for increased peripheral neuropathy; concomitant use should be avoided). Products include:

Paraplatin for Injection 705

Chloramphenicol (Potential for increased peripheral neuropathy; concomitant use should be avoided). Products include:

Chloromycetin Ophthalmic Ointment, 1% .... ◉ 310
Chloromycetin Ophthalmic Solution .... ◉ 310
Chloroptic S.O.P. .... ◉ 239
Chloroptic Sterile Ophthalmic Solution .... ◉ 239
Elase-Chloromycetin Ointment 1040
Ophthocort .... ◉ 311

Chloramphenicol Palmitate (Potential for increased peripheral neuropathy; concomitant use should be avoided).

No products indexed under this heading.

Chloramphenicol Sodium Succinate (Potential for increased peripheral neuropathy; concomitant use should be avoided). Products include:

Chloromycetin Sodium Succinate 1900

Cimetidine (Concomitant administration decreases the elimination of zalcitabine, most likely by inhibition of renal tubular secretion of zalcitabine). Products include:

Tagamet Tablets 2516

Cimetidine Hydrochloride (Concomitant administration decreases the elimination of zalcitabine, most likely by inhibition of renal tubular secretion of zalcitabine). Products include:

Tagamet 2516

Cisplatin (Potential for increased peripheral neuropathy; concomitant use should be avoided). Products include:

Platinol 708
Platinol-AQ Injection 710

Dapsone (Potential for increased peripheral neuropathy; concomitant use should be avoided). Products include:

Dapsone Tablets USP 1284

Didanosine (Concomitant use is not recommended). Products include:

Videx Tablets, Powder for Oral Solution, & Pediatric Powder for Oral Solution 720

Dihydroxyaluminum Sodium Carbonate (Absorption of zalcitabine is moderately reduced (approximately 25%) when coadministered with magnesium/aluminum containing antacids).

No products indexed under this heading.

IMPORTANT NOTE: Always consult each drug listing in the patient's regimen for possible interactions.

Disulfiram (Potential for increased peripheral neuropathy; concomitant use should be avoided). Products include:

Antabuse Tablets 2695

Ethionamide (Potential for increased peripheral neuropathy; concomitant use should be avoided). Products include:

Trecator-SC Tablets 2814

Foscarnet Sodium (Increases the risk of developing peripheral neuropathy or other Hivid-associated toxicities by interfering with the renal clearance of zalcitabine). Products include:

Foscavir Injection 547

Gentamicin Sulfate (Increases the risk of developing peripheral neuropathy or other Hivid-associated toxicities by interfering with the renal clearance of zalcitabine). Products include:

Garamycin Injectable 2360
Genoptic Sterile Ophthalmic Solution ..... ◉ 243
Genoptic Sterile Ophthalmic Ointment ..... ◉ 243
Gentacidin Ointment ..... ◉ 264
Gentacidin Solution ..... ◉ 264
Gentak ..... ◉ 208
Pred-G Liquifilm Sterile Ophthalmic Suspension ..... ◉ 251
Pred-G S.O.P. Sterile Ophthalmic Ointment ..... ◉ 252

Glutethimide (Potential for increased peripheral neuropathy; concomitant use should be avoided).

No products indexed under this heading.

Gold Sodium Thiomalate (Potential for increased peripheral neuropathy; concomitant use should be avoided). Products include:

Myochrysine Injection 1711

Hydralazine Hydrochloride (Potential for increased peripheral neuropathy; concomitant use should be avoided). Products include:

Apresazide Capsules 808
Apresoline Hydrochloride Tablets .. 809
Ser-Ap-Es Tablets 849

Iodoquinol (Potential for increased peripheral neuropathy; concomitant use should be avoided). Products include:

Yodoxin 1230

Isoniazid (Potential for increased peripheral neuropathy; concomitant use should be avoided). Products include:

Nydrazid Injection 508
Rifamate Capsules 1530
Rifater 1532

Kanamycin Sulfate (Increases the risk of developing peripheral neuropathy or other Hivid-associated toxicities by interfering with the renal clearance of zalcitabine).

No products indexed under this heading.

Leuprolide Acetate (Potential for increased peripheral neuropathy; concomitant use should be avoided). Products include:

Lupron Depot 3.75 mg 2556
Lupron Depot 7.5 mg 2559
Lupron Depot-PED 7.5 mg, 11.25 mg and 15 mg 2560
Lupron Injection 2555

Magaldrate (Absorption of zalcitabine is moderately reduced (approximately 25%) when coadministered with magnesium/aluminum containing antacids).

No products indexed under this heading.

Magnesium Hydroxide (Absorption of zalcitabine is moderately reduced (approximately 25%) when coadministered with magnesium/aluminum containing antacids). Products include:

Aludrox Oral Suspension 2695
Arthritis Pain Ascriptin ..... ▣ 631
Maximum Strength Ascriptin ..... ▣ 630
Regular Strength Ascriptin Tablets ..... ▣ 629
Di-Gel Antacid/Anti-Gas ..... ▣ 801
Gelusil Liquid & Tablets ..... ▣ 855
Maalox Magnesia and Alumina Oral Suspension ..... ▣ 642
Maalox Plus Tablets ..... ▣ 643
Extra Strength Maalox Antacid Plus Antigas Liquid and Tablets ▣ 638
Mylanta Calcium Carbonate and Magnesium Hydroxide Tablets 1318
Mylanta Liquid 1317
Mylanta Tablets ..... ▣ 660
Mylanta Double Strength Liquid 1317
Mylanta Double Strength Tablets .. ▣ 660
Phillips' Milk of Magnesia Liquid ..... ▣ 729
Rolaids Tablets ..... ▣ 843
Tempo Soft Antacid ..... ▣ 835

Magnesium Oxide (Absorption of zalcitabine is moderately reduced (approximately 25%) when coadministered with magnesium/aluminum containing antacids). Products include:

Beelith Tablets 639
Bufferin Analgesic Tablets and Caplets ..... ▣ 613
Caltrate PLUS ..... ▣ 665
Cama Arthritis Pain Reliever ..... ▣ 785
Mag-Ox 400 668
Uro-Mag 668

Metoclopramide Hydrochloride (Co-administration may reduce bioavailability (approximately 10%)). Products include:

Reglan 2068

Metronidazole (Potential for increased peripheral neuropathy; concomitant use should be avoided). Products include:

Flagyl 375 Capsules 2434
Flagyl I.V. RTU 2247
MetroGel 1047
MetroGel-Vaginal 902
Protostat Tablets 1883

Nitrofurantoin (Potential for increased peripheral neuropathy; concomitant use should be avoided). Products include:

Macrodantin Capsules 1989

Pentamidine Isethionate (Death due to fulminant pancreatitis possibly related to intravenous pentamidine and Hivid has been reported; treatment with Hivid should be interrupted if intravenous pentamidine is required to treat Pneumocystis carinii pneumonia). Products include:

NebuPent for Inhalation Solution 1040
Pentam 300 Injection 1041

Phenytoin (Potential for increased peripheral neuropathy; concomitant use should be avoided). Products include:

Dilantin Infatabs 1908
Dilantin-125 Suspension 1911

Phenytoin Sodium (Potential for increased peripheral neuropathy; concomitant use should be avoided). Products include:

Dilantin Kapseals 1906
Dilantin Parenteral 1910

Probenecid (Concomitant administration decreases the elimination of zalcitabine, most likely by inhibition of renal tubular secretion of zalcitabine). Products include:

Benemid Tablets 1611
ColBENEMID Tablets 1622

Ribavirin (Potential for increased peripheral neuropathy; concomitant use should be avoided). Products include:

Virazole 1264

Streptomycin Sulfate (Increases the risk of developing peripheral neuropathy or other Hivid-associated toxicities by interfering with the renal clearance of zalcitabine). Products include:

Streptomycin Sulfate Injection 2208

Sulfamethoxazole (Potential for increased peripheral neuropathy; concomitant use should be avoided). Products include:

Azo Gantanol Tablets 2080
Bactrim DS Tablets 2084
Bactrim I.V. Infusion 2082
Bactrim 2084
Gantanol Tablets 2119
Septra 1174
Septra I.V. Infusion 1169
Septra I.V. Infusion ADD-Vantage Vials 1171
Septra 1174

Tobramycin (Increases the risk of developing peripheral neuropathy or other Hivid-associated toxicities by interfering with the renal clearance of zalcitabine). Products include:

AKTOB ..... ◉ 206
TobraDex Ophthalmic Suspension and Ointment 473
Tobrex Ophthalmic Ointment and Solution ..... ◉ 229

Tobramycin Sulfate (Increases the risk of developing peripheral neuropathy or other Hivid-associated toxicities by interfering with the renal clearance of zalcitabine). Products include:

Nebcin Vials, Hyporets & ADD-Vantage 1464
Tobramycin Sulfate Injection 968

Vincristine Sulfate (Potential for increased peripheral neuropathy; concomitant use should be avoided). Products include:

Oncovin Solution Vials & Hyporets 1466

HUMATE-P, ANTIHEMOPHILIC FACTOR (HUMAN), PASTEURIZED

(Antihemophilic Factor (Human)) **520**
None cited in PDR database.

HUMATROPE VIALS

(Somatropin) **1443**
May interact with glucocorticoids. Compounds in this category include:

Betamethasone Acetate (Excessive glucocorticoid therapy will inhibit the growth promoting effect of somatropin). Products include:

Celestone Soluspan Suspension 2347

Betamethasone Sodium Phosphate (Excessive glucocorticoid therapy will inhibit the growth promoting effect of somatropin). Products include:

Celestone Soluspan Suspension 2347

Cortisone Acetate (Excessive glucocorticoid therapy will inhibit the growth promoting effect of somatropin). Products include:

Cortone Acetate Sterile Suspension 1623
Cortone Acetate Tablets 1624

Dexamethasone (Excessive glucocorticoid therapy will inhibit the growth promoting effect of somatropin). Products include:

AK-Trol Ointment & Suspension ..... ◉ 205
Decadron Elixir 1633
Decadron Tablets 1635
Decaspray Topical Aerosol 1648
Dexacidin Ointment ..... ◉ 263
Maxitrol Ophthalmic Ointment and Suspension ..... ◉ 224
TobraDex Ophthalmic Suspension and Ointment 473

Dexamethasone Acetate (Excessive glucocorticoid therapy will inhibit the growth promoting effect of somatropin). Products include:

Dalalone D.P. Injectable 1011
Decadron-LA Sterile Suspension 1646

Dexamethasone Sodium Phosphate (Excessive glucocorticoid therapy will inhibit the growth promoting effect of somatropin). Products include:

Decadron Phosphate Injection 1637
Decadron Phosphate Respihaler 1642
Decadron Phosphate Sterile Ophthalmic Ointment 1641
Decadron Phosphate Sterile Ophthalmic Solution 1642
Decadron Phosphate Topical Cream 1644
Decadron Phosphate Turbinaire 1645
Decadron Phosphate with Xylocaine Injection, Sterile 1639
Dexacort Phosphate in Respihaler .. 458
Dexacort Phosphate in Turbinaire .. 459
NeoDecadron Sterile Ophthalmic Ointment 1712
NeoDecadron Sterile Ophthalmic Solution 1713
NeoDecadron Topical Cream 1714

Fludrocortisone Acetate (Excessive glucocorticoid therapy will inhibit the growth promoting effect of somatropin). Products include:

Florinef Acetate Tablets 505

Hydrocortisone (Excessive glucocorticoid therapy will inhibit the growth promoting effect of somatropin). Products include:

Anusol-HC Cream 2.5% 1896
Aquanil HC Lotion 1931
Bactine Hydrocortisone Anti-Itch Cream ..... ▣ 709
Caldecort Anti-Itch Hydrocortisone Spray ..... ▣ 631
Cortaid ..... ▣ 836
CORTENEMA 2535
Cortisporin Ointment 1085
Cortisporin Ophthalmic Ointment Sterile 1085
Cortisporin Ophthalmic Suspension Sterile 1086
Cortisporin Otic Solution Sterile 1087
Cortisporin Otic Suspension Sterile 1088
Cortizone-5 ..... ▣ 831
Cortizone-10 ..... ▣ 831
Hydrocortone Tablets 1672
Hytone 907
Massengill Medicated Soft Cloth Towelettes 2458
PediOtic Suspension Sterile 1153
Preparation H Hydrocortisone 1% Cream ..... ▣ 872
ProctoCream-HC 2.5% 2408
VōSoL HC Otic Solution 2678

Hydrocortisone Acetate (Excessive glucocorticoid therapy will inhibit the growth promoting effect of somatropin). Products include:

Analpram-HC Rectal Cream 1% and 2.5% 977
Anusol HC-1 Anti-Itch Hydrocortisone Ointment ..... ▣ 847
Anusol-HC Suppositories 1897
Caldecort ..... ▣ 631
Carmol HC 924
Coly-Mycin S Otic w/Neomycin & Hydrocortisone 1906
Cortaid ..... ▣ 836
Cortifoam 2396
Cortisporin Cream 1084
Epifoam 2399
Hydrocortone Acetate Sterile Suspension 1669
Mantadil Cream 1135
Nupercainal Hydrocortisone 1% Cream ..... ▣ 645
Ophthocort ..... ◉ 311
Pramosone Cream, Lotion & Ointment 978
ProctoCream-HC 2408
ProctoFoam-HC 2409
Terra-Cortril Ophthalmic Suspension 2210

(▣ Described in PDR For Nonprescription Drugs) (◉ Described in PDR For Ophthalmology)

479 **Interactions Index** **Hycodan**

Hydrocortisone Sodium Phosphate (Excessive glucocorticoid therapy will inhibit the growth promoting effect of somatropin). Products include:
- Hydrocortone Phosphate Injection, Sterile ... 1670

Hydrocortisone Sodium Succinate (Excessive glucocorticoid therapy will inhibit the growth promoting effect of somatropin). Products include:
- Solu-Cortef Sterile Powder ... 2641

Methylprednisolone Acetate (Excessive glucocorticoid therapy will inhibit the growth promoting effect of somatropin). Products include:
- Depo-Medrol Single-Dose Vial ... 2600
- Depo-Medrol Sterile Aqueous Suspension ... 2597

Methylprednisolone Sodium Succinate (Excessive glucocorticoid therapy will inhibit the growth promoting effect of somatropin). Products include:
- Solu-Medrol Sterile Powder ... 2643

Prednisolone Acetate (Excessive glucocorticoid therapy will inhibit the growth promoting effect of somatropin). Products include:
- AK-CIDE ... ◉ 202
- AK-CIDE Ointment ... ◉ 202
- Blephamide Liquifilm Sterile Ophthalmic Suspension ... 476
- Blephamide Ointment ... ◉ 237
- Econopred & Econopred Plus Ophthalmic Suspensions ... ◉ 217
- Poly-Pred Liquifilm ... ◉ 248
- Pred Forte ... ◉ 250
- Pred Mild ... ◉ 253
- Pred-G Liquifilm Sterile Ophthalmic Suspension ... ◉ 251
- Pred-G S.O.P. Sterile Ophthalmic Ointment ... ◉ 252
- Vasocidin Ointment ... ◉ 268

Prednisolone Sodium Phosphate (Excessive glucocorticoid therapy will inhibit the growth promoting effect of somatropin). Products include:
- AK-Pred ... ◉ 204
- Hydeltrasol Injection, Sterile ... 1665
- Inflamase ... ◉ 265
- Pediapred Oral Liquid ... 995
- Vasocidin Ophthalmic Solution ... ◉ 270

Prednisolone Tebutate (Excessive glucocorticoid therapy will inhibit the growth promoting effect of somatropin). Products include:
- Hydeltra-T.B.A. Sterile Suspension 1667

Prednisone (Excessive glucocorticoid therapy will inhibit the growth promoting effect of somatropin). Products include:
- Deltasone Tablets ... 2595

Triamcinolone (Excessive glucocorticoid therapy will inhibit the growth promoting effect of somatropin). Products include:
- Aristocort Tablets ... 1022

Triamcinolone Acetonide (Excessive glucocorticoid therapy will inhibit the growth promoting effect of somatropin). Products include:
- Aristocort A 0.025% Cream ... 1027
- Aristocort A 0.5% Cream ... 1031
- Aristocort A 0.1% Cream ... 1029
- Aristocort A 0.1% Ointment ... 1030
- Azmacort Oral Inhaler ... 2011
- Nasacort Nasal Inhaler ... 2024

Triamcinolone Diacetate (Excessive glucocorticoid therapy will inhibit the growth promoting effect of somatropin). Products include:
- Aristocort Suspension (Forte Parenteral) ... 1027
- Aristocort Suspension (Intralesional) ... 1025

Triamcinolone Hexacetonide (Excessive glucocorticoid therapy will inhibit the growth promoting effect of somatropin). Products include:
- Aristospan Suspension (Intra-articular) ... 1033
- Aristospan Suspension (Intralesional) ... 1032

HUMEGON
(Menotropins) ... 1824
None cited in PDR database.

HUMIBID DM PEDIATRIC CAPSULES
(Dextromethorphan Hydrobromide, Guaifenesin) ... 462
See **Humibid DM Tablets**

HUMIBID DM TABLETS
(Guaifenesin, Dextromethorphan Hydrobromide) ... 462
May interact with monoamine oxidase inhibitors. Compounds in this category include:

Furazolidone (Concurrent and/or sequential use is contraindicated). Products include:
- Furoxone ... 2046

Isocarboxazid (Concurrent and/or sequential use is contraindicated).
- No products indexed under this heading.

Phenelzine Sulfate (Concurrent and/or sequential use is contraindicated). Products include:
- Nardil ... 1920

Selegiline Hydrochloride (Concurrent and/or sequential use is contraindicated). Products include:
- Eldepryl Tablets ... 2550

Tranylcypromine Sulfate (Concurrent and/or sequential use is contraindicated). Products include:
- Parnate Tablets ... 2503

HUMIBID L.A. TABLETS
(Guaifenesin) ... 462
None cited in PDR database.

HUMIBID PEDIATRIC CAPSULES
(Guaifenesin) ... 462
None cited in PDR database.

HUMORSOL STERILE OPHTHALMIC SOLUTION
(Demecarium Bromide) ... 1664
May interact with cholinergic agents and certain other agents. Compounds in these categories include:

Edrophonium Chloride (Additive adverse effects). Products include:
- Tensilon Injectable ... 1261

Neostigmine Bromide (Additive adverse effects). Products include:
- Prostigmin Tablets ... 1261

Neostigmine Methylsulfate (Additive adverse effects). Products include:
- Prostigmin Injectable ... 1260

Pyridostigmine Bromide (Additive adverse effects). Products include:
- Mestinon Injectable ... 1253
- Mestinon ... 1254

Succinylcholine Chloride (Possible respiratory and cardiovascular collapse). Products include:
- Anectine ... 1073

HUMULIN 50/50, 100 UNITS
(Insulin, Human Isophane Suspension, Insulin, Human) ... 1444
None cited in PDR database.

HUMULIN 70/30, 100 UNITS
(Insulin, Human Regular and Human NPH Mixture) ... 1445
None cited in PDR database.

HUMULIN L, 100 UNITS
(Insulin, Human, Zinc Suspension) ... 1446
None cited in PDR database.

HUMULIN N, 100 UNITS
(Insulin, Human NPH) ... 1448
None cited in PDR database.

HUMULIN R, 100 UNITS
(Insulin, Human Regular) ... 1449
None cited in PDR database.

HUMULIN U, 100 UNITS
(Insulin, Human, Zinc Suspension) ... 1450
None cited in PDR database.

HURRICAINE TOPICAL ANESTHETIC AEROSOL SPRAY, 2 OZ (WILD CHERRY FLAVOR)
(Benzocaine) ... 666
None cited in PDR database.

HURRICAINE TOPICAL ANESTHETIC SPRAY KIT
(Benzocaine) ... 666
None cited in PDR database.

HURRICAINE TOPICAL ANESTHETIC GEL, 1 OZ WILD CHERRY, PINA COLADA, WATERMELON, 1/6 OZ WILD CHERRY, WATERMELON
(Benzocaine) ... 666
None cited in PDR database.

HURRICAINE TOPICAL ANESTHETIC LIQUID, .25 GM, 1 OZ WILD CHERRY AND PINA COLADA .25 ML DRY HANDLE SWAB WILD CHERRY, 1/6 OZ WILD CHERRY
(Benzocaine) ... 666
None cited in PDR database.

HYCODAN TABLETS AND SYRUP
(Hydrocodone Bitartrate, Homatropine Methylbromide) ... 930
May interact with central nervous system depressants, narcotic analgesics, antihistamines, antipsychotic agents, tranquilizers, monoamine oxidase inhibitors, tricyclic antidepressants, and certain other agents. Compounds in these categories include:

Acrivastine (Exhibits an additive CNS depression). Products include:
- Semprex-D Capsules ... 463
- Semprex-D Capsules ... 1167

Alfentanil Hydrochloride (Exhibits an additive CNS depression). Products include:
- Alfenta Injection ... 1286

Alprazolam (Exhibits an additive CNS depression). Products include:
- Xanax Tablets ... 2649

Amitriptyline Hydrochloride (Increased effect of either the antidepressant or hydrocodone). Products include:
- Elavil ... 2838
- Endep Tablets ... 2174
- Etrafon ... 2355
- Limbitrol ... 2180
- Triavil Tablets ... 1757

Amoxapine (Increased effect of either the antidepressant or hydrocodone). Products include:
- Asendin Tablets ... 1369

Aprobarbital (Exhibits an additive CNS depression).
- No products indexed under this heading.

Astemizole (Exhibits an additive CNS depression). Products include:
- Hismanal Tablets ... 1293

Azatadine Maleate (Exhibits an additive CNS depression). Products include:
- Trinalin Repetabs Tablets ... 1330

Bromodiphenhydramine Hydrochloride (Exhibits an additive CNS depression).
- No products indexed under this heading.

Brompheniramine Maleate (Exhibits an additive CNS depression). Products include:
- Alka Seltzer Plus Sinus Medicine ... ■ 707
- Bromfed Capsules (Extended-Release) ... 1785
- Bromfed Syrup ... ■ 733
- Bromfed Tablets ... 1785
- Bromfed-DM Cough Syrup ... 1786
- Bromfed-PD Capsules (Extended-Release) ... 1785
- Dimetane-DC Cough Syrup ... 2059
- Dimetane-DX Cough Syrup ... 2059
- Dimetapp Elixir ... ■ 773
- Dimetapp Extentabs ... ■ 774
- Dimetapp Tablets/Liqui-Gels ... ■ 775
- Dimetapp Cold & Allergy Chewable Tablets ... ■ 773
- Dimetapp DM Elixir ... ■ 774
- Vicks DayQuil Allergy Relief 12-Hour Extended Release Tablets ... ■ 760
- Vicks DayQuil Allergy Relief 4-Hour Tablets ... ■ 760

Buprenorphine (Exhibits an additive CNS depression). Products include:
- Buprenex Injectable ... 2006

Buspirone Hydrochloride (Exhibits an additive CNS depression). Products include:
- BuSpar ... 737

Butabarbital (Exhibits an additive CNS depression).
- No products indexed under this heading.

Butalbital (Exhibits an additive CNS depression). Products include:
- Esgic-plus Tablets ... 1013
- Fioricet Tablets ... 2258
- Fioricet with Codeine Capsules ... 2260
- Fiorinal Capsules ... 2261
- Fiorinal with Codeine Capsules ... 2262
- Fiorinal Tablets ... 2261
- Phrenilin ... 785
- Sedapap Tablets 50 mg/650 mg ... 1543

Chlordiazepoxide (Exhibits an additive CNS depression). Products include:
- Libritabs Tablets ... 2177
- Limbitrol ... 2180

Chlordiazepoxide Hydrochloride (Exhibits an additive CNS depression). Products include:
- Librax Capsules ... 2176
- Librium Capsules ... 2178
- Librium Injectable ... 2179

Chlorpheniramine Maleate (Exhibits an additive CNS depression). Products include:
- Alka-Seltzer Plus Cold Medicine ... ■ 705
- Alka-Seltzer Plus Cold Medicine Liqui-Gels ... ■ 706
- Alka-Seltzer Plus Cold & Cough Medicine ... ■ 708
- Alka-Seltzer Plus Cold & Cough Medicine Liqui-Gels ... ■ 705
- Allerest Children's Chewable Tablets ... ■ 627
- Allerest Headache Strength Tablets ... ■ 627
- Allerest Maximum Strength Tablets ... ■ 627
- Allerest Sinus Pain Formula ... ■ 627

IMPORTANT NOTE: Always consult each drug listing in the patient's regimen for possible interactions.

Hycodan Interactions Index 480

Allerest 12 Hour Caplets ■ 627
Ana-Kit Anaphylaxis Emergency Treatment Kit 617
Atrohist Pediatric Capsules 453
Atrohist Plus Tablets 454
BC Cold Powder Multi-Symptom Formula (Cold-Sinus-Allergy) ■ 609
Cerose DM ■ 878
Cheracol Plus Head Cold/Cough Formula ■ 769
Children's Vicks DayQuil Allergy Relief ■ 757
Children's Vicks NyQuil Cold/Cough Relief ■ 758
Chlor-Trimeton Allergy Decongestant Tablets ■ 799
Chlor-Trimeton Allergy Tablets ■ 798
Comhist 2038
Comtrex Multi-Symptom Cold Reliever Tablets/Caplets/Liqui-Gels/Liquid ■ 615
Allergy-Sinus Comtrex Multi-Symptom Allergy-Sinus Formula Tablets ■ 617
Contac Continuous Action Nasal Decongestant/Antihistamine 12 Hour Capsules ■ 813
Contac Maximum Strength Continuous Action Decongestant/Antihistamine 12 Hour Caplets ■ 813
Contac Severe Cold and Flu Formula Caplets ■ 814
Coricidin 'D' Decongestant Tablets ■ 800
Coricidin Tablets ■ 800
D.A. Chewable Tablets 951
Deconamine 1320
Dura-Tap/PD Capsules 2867
Dura-Vent/DA Tablets 953
Extendryl 1005
Fedahist Gyrocaps 2401
Fedahist Timecaps 2401
Hycomine Compound Tablets 932
Isoclor Timesule Capsules ■ 637
Kronofed-A 977
Nolamine Timed-Release Tablets 785
Novahistine DH 2462
Novahistine Elixir ■ 823
Ornade Spansule Capsules 2502
PediaCare Cold Allergy Chewable Tablets ■ 677
PediaCare Cough-Cold Chewable Tablets 1553
PediaCare Cough-Cold Liquid 1553
PediaCare NightRest Cough-Cold Liquid 1553
Pediatric Vicks 44m Cough & Cold Relief ■ 764
Pyrroxate Caplets ■ 772
Ryna ■ 841
Sinarest Tablets ■ 648
Sinarest Extra Strength Tablets ■ 648
Sine-Off Sinus Medicine ■ 825
Singlet Tablets ■ 825
Sinulin Tablets 787
Sinutab Sinus Allergy Medication, Maximum Strength Tablets and Caplets ■ 860
Sudafed Plus Liquid ■ 862
Sudafed Plus Tablets ■ 863
Teldrin 12 Hour Antihistamine/Nasal Decongestant Allergy Relief Capsules ■ 826
TheraFlu ■ 787
TheraFlu Maximum Strength Nighttime Flu, Cold & Cough Medicine ■ 788
Triaminic Allergy Tablets ■ 789
Triaminic Cold Tablets ■ 790
Triaminic Nite Light ■ 791
Triaminic Syrup ■ 792
Triaminic-12 Tablets ■ 792
Triaminicin Tablets ■ 793
Triaminicol Multi-Symptom Cold Tablets ■ 793
Triaminicol Multi-Symptom Relief ■ 794
Tussend 1783
Children's TYLENOL Cold Multi-Symptom Liquid Formula and Chewable Tablets 1561
Children's TYLENOL Cold Plus Cough Multi Symptom Tablets and Liquid ■ 681
TYLENOL Maximum Strength Allergy Sinus Medication Gelcaps and Caplets 1563
TYLENOL Cold Multi-Symptom Formula Medication Tablets and Caplets 1561
TYLENOL Cold Multi-Symptom Hot Medication Liquid Packets 1557
Vicks 44 LiquiCaps Cough, Cold & Flu Relief ■ 755
Vicks 44M Cough, Cold & Flu Relief ■ 756

Chlorpheniramine Polistirex (Exhibits an additive CNS depression). Products include:
Tussionex Pennkinetic Extended-Release Suspension 998

Chlorpheniramine Tannate (Exhibits an additive CNS depression). Products include:
Atrohist Pediatric Suspension 454
Ricobid Tablets and Pediatric Suspension 2038
Rynatan 2673
Rynatuss 2673

Chlorpromazine (Exhibits an additive CNS depression). Products include:
Thorazine Suppositories 2523

Chlorpromazine Hydrochloride (Exhibits an additive CNS depression). Products include:
Thorazine 2523

Chlorprothixene (Exhibits an additive CNS depression).
No products indexed under this heading.

Chlorprothixene Hydrochloride (Exhibits an additive CNS depression).
No products indexed under this heading.

Clemastine Fumarate (Exhibits an additive CNS depression). Products include:
Tavist Syrup 2297
Tavist Tablets 2298
Tavist-1 12 Hour Relief Tablets ■ 787
Tavist-D 12 Hour Relief Tablets ■ 787

Clomipramine Hydrochloride (Increased effect of either the antidepressant or hydrocodone). Products include:
Anafranil Capsules 803

Clorazepate Dipotassium (Exhibits an additive CNS depression). Products include:
Tranxene 451

Clozapine (Exhibits an additive CNS depression). Products include:
Clozaril Tablets 2252

Codeine Phosphate (Exhibits an additive CNS depression). Products include:
Actifed with Codeine Cough Syrup 1067
Brontex 1981
Deconsal C Expectorant Syrup 456
Deconsal Pediatric Syrup 457
Dimetane-DC Cough Syrup 2059
Empirin with Codeine Tablets 1093
Fioricet with Codeine Capsules 2260
Fiorinal with Codeine Capsules 2262
Isoclor Expectorant 990
Novahistine DH 2462
Novahistine Expectorant 2463
Nucofed 2051
Phenergan with Codeine 2777
Phenergan VC with Codeine 2781
Robitussin A-C Syrup 2073
Robitussin-DAC Syrup 2074
Ryna ■ 841
Soma Compound w/Codeine Tablets 2676
Tussi-Organidin NR Liquid and S NR Liquid 2677
Tylenol with Codeine 1583

Cyproheptadine Hydrochloride (Exhibits an additive CNS depression). Products include:
Periactin 1724

Desflurane (Exhibits an additive CNS depression). Products include:
Suprane 1813

Desipramine Hydrochloride (Increased effect of either the antidepressant or hydrocodone). Products include:
Norpramin Tablets 1526

Dexchlorpheniramine Maleate (Exhibits an additive CNS depression).
No products indexed under this heading.

Dezocine (Exhibits an additive CNS depression). Products include:
Dalgan Injection 538

Diazepam (Exhibits an additive CNS depression). Products include:
Dizac 1809
Valium Injectable 2182
Valium Tablets 2183
Valrelease Capsules 2169

Diphenhydramine Citrate (Exhibits an additive CNS depression). Products include:
Excedrin P.M. Analgesic/Sleeping Aid Tablets, Caplets, Liquigels 733

Diphenhydramine Hydrochloride (Exhibits an additive CNS depression). Products include:
Actifed Allergy Daytime/Nighttime Caplets ■ 844
Actifed Sinus Daytime/Nighttime Tablets and Caplets ■ 846
Arthritis Foundation NightTime Caplets ■ 674
Extra Strength Bayer PM Aspirin ■ 713
Bayer Select Night Time Pain Relief Formula ■ 716
Benadryl Allergy Decongestant Liquid Medication ■ 848
Benadryl Allergy Decongestant Tablets ■ 848
Benadryl Allergy Liquid Medication ■ 849
Benadryl Allergy ■ 848
Benadryl Allergy Sinus Headache Formula Caplets ■ 849
Benadryl Capsules 1898
Benadryl Dye-Free Allergy Liqui-gel Softgels ■ 850
Benadryl Dye-Free Allergy Liquid Medication ■ 850
Benadryl Itch Relief Cream, Children's Formula and Maximum Strength 2% ■ 851
Benadryl Itch Relief Spray, Children's Formula and Maximum Strength 2% ■ 851
Benadryl Itch Relief Stick Maximum Strength 2% ■ 850
Benadryl Itch Stopping Gel, Children's Formula and Maximum Strength 2% ■ 851
Benadryl Kapseals 1898
Benadryl Injection 1898
Contac Day & Night Cold/Flu Night Caplets ■ 812
Contac Night Allergy/Sinus Caplets ■ 812
Extra Strength Doan's P.M. ■ 633
Legatrin PM ■ 651
Miles Nervine Nighttime Sleep-Aid ■ 723
Nytol QuickCaps Caplets ■ 610
Sleepinal Night-time Sleep Aid Capsules and Softgels ■ 834
TYLENOL Maximum Strength Allergy Sinus NightTime Medication Caplets 1555
TYLENOL Flu NightTime, Maximum Strength, Gelcaps 1566
TYLENOL Maximum Strength Flu NightTime Hot Medication Packets 1562
TYLENOL PM, Extra Strength Pain Reliever/Sleep Aid Caplets, Geltabs, Gelcaps 1560
TYLENOL Severe Allergy Medication Caplets 1564
Maximum Strength Unisom Sleepgels 1934
Unisom With Pain Relief-Nighttime Sleep Aid and Pain Reliever 1934

Diphenylpyraline Hydrochloride (Exhibits an additive CNS depression).
No products indexed under this heading.

Doxepin Hydrochloride (Increased effect of either the antidepressant or hydrocodone). Products include:
Sinequan 2205
Zonalon Cream 1055

Droperidol (Exhibits an additive CNS depression). Products include:
Inapsine Injection 1296

Enflurane (Exhibits an additive CNS depression).
No products indexed under this heading.

Estazolam (Exhibits an additive CNS depression). Products include:
ProSom Tablets 449

Ethchlorvynol (Exhibits an additive CNS depression). Products include:
Placidyl Capsules 448

Ethinamate (Exhibits an additive CNS depression).
No products indexed under this heading.

Fentanyl (Exhibits an additive CNS depression). Products include:
Duragesic Transdermal System 1288

Fentanyl Citrate (Exhibits an additive CNS depression). Products include:
Sublimaze Injection 1307

Fluphenazine Decanoate (Exhibits an additive CNS depression). Products include:
Prolixin Decanoate 509

Fluphenazine Enanthate (Exhibits an additive CNS depression). Products include:
Prolixin Enanthate 509

Fluphenazine Hydrochloride (Exhibits an additive CNS depression). Products include:
Prolixin 509

Flurazepam Hydrochloride (Exhibits an additive CNS depression). Products include:
Dalmane Capsules 2173

Furazolidone (May increase the effect of either MAO inhibitor or hydrocodone). Products include:
Furoxone 2046

Glutethimide (Exhibits an additive CNS depression).
No products indexed under this heading.

Haloperidol (Exhibits an additive CNS depression). Products include:
Haldol Injection, Tablets and Concentrate 1575

Haloperidol Decanoate (Exhibits an additive CNS depression). Products include:
Haldol Decanoate 1577

Hydrocodone Polistirex (Exhibits an additive CNS depression). Products include:
Tussionex Pennkinetic Extended-Release Suspension 998

Hydroxyzine Hydrochloride (Exhibits an additive CNS depression). Products include:
Atarax Tablets & Syrup 2185
Marax Tablets & DF Syrup 2200
Vistaril Intramuscular Solution 2216

Imipramine Hydrochloride (Increased effect of either the antidepressant or hydrocodone). Products include:
Tofranil Ampuls 854
Tofranil Tablets 856

Imipramine Pamoate (Increased effect of either the antidepressant or hydrocodone). Products include:
Tofranil-PM Capsules 857

Isocarboxazid (May increase the effect of either MAO inhibitor or hydrocodone).
No products indexed under this heading.

Isoflurane (Exhibits an additive CNS depression).
No products indexed under this heading.

(■ Described in PDR For Nonprescription Drugs) (◉ Described in PDR For Ophthalmology)

Interactions Index

Ketamine Hydrochloride (Exhibits an additive CNS depression).

No products indexed under this heading.

Levomethadyl Acetate Hydrochloride (Exhibits an additive CNS depression). Products include:

Orlamm 2239

Levorphanol Tartrate (Exhibits an additive CNS depression). Products include:

Levo-Dromoran 2129

Lithium Carbonate (Exhibits an additive CNS depression). Products include:

Eskalith 2485
Lithium Carbonate Capsules & Tablets 2230
Lithonate/Lithotabs/Lithobid 2543

Lithium Citrate (Exhibits an additive CNS depression).

No products indexed under this heading.

Loratadine (Exhibits an additive CNS depression). Products include:

Claritin 2349
Claritin-D 2350

Lorazepam (Exhibits an additive CNS depression). Products include:

Ativan Injection 2698
Ativan Tablets 2700

Loxapine Hydrochloride (Exhibits an additive CNS depression). Products include:

Loxitane 1378

Loxapine Succinate (Exhibits an additive CNS depression). Products include:

Loxitane Capsules 1378

Maprotiline Hydrochloride (Increased effect of either the antidepressant or hydrocodone). Products include:

Ludiomil Tablets 843

Meperidine Hydrochloride (Exhibits an additive CNS depression). Products include:

Demerol 2308
Mepergan Injection 2753

Mephobarbital (Exhibits an additive CNS depression). Products include:

Mebaral Tablets 2322

Meprobamate (Exhibits an additive CNS depression). Products include:

Miltown Tablets 2672
PMB 200 and PMB 400 2783

Mesoridazine Besylate (Exhibits an additive CNS depression). Products include:

Serentil 684

Methadone Hydrochloride (Exhibits an additive CNS depression). Products include:

Methadone Hydrochloride Oral Concentrate 2233
Methadone Hydrochloride Oral Solution & Tablets 2235

Methdilazine Hydrochloride (Exhibits an additive CNS depression).

No products indexed under this heading.

Methohexital Sodium (Exhibits an additive CNS depression). Products include:

Brevital Sodium Vials 1429

Methotrimeprazine (Exhibits an additive CNS depression). Products include:

Levoprome 1274

Methoxyflurane (Exhibits an additive CNS depression).

No products indexed under this heading.

Midazolam Hydrochloride (Exhibits an additive CNS depression). Products include:

Versed Injection 2170

Molindone Hydrochloride (Exhibits an additive CNS depression). Products include:

Moban Tablets and Concentrate 1048

Morphine Sulfate (Exhibits an additive CNS depression). Products include:

Astramorph/PF Injection, USP (Preservative-Free) 535
Duramorph 962
Infumorph 200 and Infumorph 500 Sterile Solutions 965
MS Contin Tablets 1994
MSIR 1997
Oramorph SR (Morphine Sulfate Sustained Release Tablets) 2236
RMS Suppositories 2657
Roxanol 2243

Nortriptyline Hydrochloride (Increased effect of either the antidepressant or hydrocodone). Products include:

Pamelor 2280

Opium Alkaloids (Exhibits an additive CNS depression).

No products indexed under this heading.

Oxazepam (Exhibits an additive CNS depression). Products include:

Serax Capsules 2810
Serax Tablets 2810

Oxycodone Hydrochloride (Exhibits an additive CNS depression). Products include:

Percocet Tablets 938
Percodan Tablets 939
Percodan-Demi Tablets 940
Roxicodone Tablets, Oral Solution & Intensol (Oxycodone) 2244
Tylox Capsules 1584

Pentobarbital Sodium (Exhibits an additive CNS depression). Products include:

Nembutal Sodium Capsules 436
Nembutal Sodium Solution 438
Nembutal Sodium Suppositories 440

Perphenazine (Exhibits an additive CNS depression). Products include:

Etrafon 2355
Triavil Tablets 1757
Trilafon 2389

Phenelzine Sulfate (May increase the effect of either MAO inhibitor or hydrocodone). Products include:

Nardil 1920

Phenobarbital (Exhibits an additive CNS depression). Products include:

Arco-Lase Plus Tablets 512
Bellergal-S Tablets 2250
Donnatal 2060
Donnatal Extentabs 2061
Donnatal Tablets 2060
Phenobarbital Elixir and Tablets 1469
Quadrinal Tablets 1350

Pimozide (Exhibits an additive CNS depression). Products include:

Orap Tablets 1050

Prazepam (Exhibits an additive CNS depression).

No products indexed under this heading.

Prochlorperazine (Exhibits an additive CNS depression). Products include:

Compazine 2470

Promethazine Hydrochloride (Exhibits an additive CNS depression). Products include:

Mepergan Injection 2753
Phenergan with Codeine 2777
Phenergan with Dextromethorphan 2778
Phenergan Injection 2773
Phenergan Suppositories 2775
Phenergan Syrup 2774
Phenergan Tablets 2775
Phenergan VC 2779
Phenergan VC with Codeine 2781

Propofol (Exhibits an additive CNS depression). Products include:

Diprivan Injection 2833

Propoxyphene Hydrochloride (Exhibits an additive CNS depression). Products include:

Darvon 1435
Wygesic Tablets 2827

Propoxyphene Napsylate (Exhibits an additive CNS depression). Products include:

Darvon-N/Darvocet-N 1433

Protriptyline Hydrochloride (Increased effect of either the antidepressant or hydrocodone). Products include:

Vivactil Tablets 1774

Pyrilamine Maleate (Exhibits an additive CNS depression). Products include:

4-Way Fast Acting Nasal Spray (regular & mentholated) .... ⊞ 621
Maximum Strength Multi-Symptom Formula Midol .... ⊞ 722
PMS Multi-Symptom Formula Midol .... ⊞ 723

Pyrilamine Tannate (Exhibits an additive CNS depression). Products include:

Atrohist Pediatric Suspension 454
Rynatan 2673

Quazepam (Exhibits an additive CNS depression). Products include:

Doral Tablets 2664

Risperidone (Exhibits an additive CNS depression). Products include:

Risperdal 1301

Secobarbital Sodium (Exhibits an additive CNS depression). Products include:

Seconal Sodium Pulvules 1474

Selegiline Hydrochloride (May increase the effect of either MAO inhibitor or hydrocodone). Products include:

Eldepryl Tablets 2550

Sufentanil Citrate (Exhibits an additive CNS depression). Products include:

Sufenta Injection 1309

Temazepam (Exhibits an additive CNS depression). Products include:

Restoril Capsules 2284

Terfenadine (Exhibits an additive CNS depression). Products include:

Seldane Tablets 1536
Seldane-D Extended-Release Tablets 1538

Thiamylal Sodium (Exhibits an additive CNS depression).

No products indexed under this heading.

Thioridazine Hydrochloride (Exhibits an additive CNS depression). Products include:

Mellaril 2269

Thiothixene (Exhibits an additive CNS depression). Products include:

Navane Capsules and Concentrate 2201
Navane Intramuscular 2202

Tranylcypromine Sulfate (May increase the effect of either MAO inhibitor or hydrocodone). Products include:

Parnate Tablets 2503

Triazolam (Exhibits an additive CNS depression). Products include:

Halcion Tablets 2611

Trifluoperazine Hydrochloride (Exhibits an additive CNS depression). Products include:

Stelazine 2514

Trimeprazine Tartrate (Exhibits an additive CNS depression). Products include:

Temaril Tablets, Syrup and Spansule Extended-Release Capsules .. 483

Trimipramine Maleate (Increased effect of either the antidepressant or hydrocodone). Products include:

Surmontil Capsules 2811

Tripelennamine Hydrochloride (Exhibits an additive CNS depression). Products include:

PBZ Tablets 845
PBZ-SR Tablets 844

Triprolidine Hydrochloride (Exhibits an additive CNS depression). Products include:

Actifed Plus Caplets .... ⊞ 845
Actifed Plus Tablets .... ⊞ 845
Actifed with Codeine Cough Syrup.. 1067
Actifed Syrup .... ⊞ 846
Actifed Tablets .... ⊞ 844

Zolpidem Tartrate (Exhibits an additive CNS depression). Products include:

Ambien Tablets 2416

Food Interactions

Alcohol (Exhibits an additive CNS depression).

HYCOMINE COMPOUND TABLETS

(Hydrocodone Bitartrate, Chlorpheniramine Maleate, Acetaminophen, Phenylephrine Hydrochloride) 932

May interact with monoamine oxidase inhibitors, narcotic analgesics, general anesthetics, central nervous system depressants, phenothiazines, tranquilizers, hypnotics and sedatives, sympathomimetics, beta blockers, and certain other agents. Compounds in these categories include:

Acebutolol Hydrochloride (Potential for hypertensive crises). Products include:

Sectral Capsules 2807

Albuterol (Additive elevation of blood pressure). Products include:

Proventil Inhalation Aerosol 2382
Ventolin Inhalation Aerosol and Refill 1197

Albuterol Sulfate (Additive elevation of blood pressure). Products include:

Airet Solution for Inhalation 452
Proventil Inhalation Solution 0.083% 2384
Proventil Repetabs Tablets 2386
Proventil Solution for Inhalation 0.5% 2383
Proventil Syrup 2385
Proventil Tablets 2386
Ventolin Inhalation Solution 1198
Ventolin Nebules Inhalation Solution 1199
Ventolin Rotacaps for Inhalation 1200
Ventolin Syrup 1202
Ventolin Tablets 1203
Volmax Extended-Release Tablets .. 1788

Alfentanil Hydrochloride (Exhibits an additive CNS depression). Products include:

Alfenta Injection 1286

Alprazolam (Exhibits an additive CNS depression). Products include:

Xanax Tablets 2649

Aprobarbital (Exhibits an additive CNS depression).

No products indexed under this heading.

Atenolol (Potential for hypertensive crises). Products include:

Tenoretic Tablets 2845
Tenormin Tablets and I.V. Injection 2847

IMPORTANT NOTE: Always consult each drug listing in the patient's regimen for possible interactions.

Hycomine Compound

Betaxolol Hydrochloride (Potential for hypertensive crises). Products include:

Betoptic Ophthalmic Solution............. 469
Betoptic S Ophthalmic Suspension 471
Kerlone Tablets.. 2436

Bisoprolol Fumarate (Potential for hypertensive crises). Products include:

Zebeta Tablets 1413
Ziac 1415

Buprenorphine (Exhibits an additive CNS depression). Products include:

Buprenex Injectable 2006

Buspirone Hydrochloride (Exhibits an additive CNS depression). Products include:

BuSpar 737

Butabarbital (Exhibits an additive CNS depression).

No products indexed under this heading.

Butalbital (Exhibits an additive CNS depression). Products include:

Esgic-plus Tablets 1013
Fioricet Tablets.. 2258
Fioricet with Codeine Capsules 2260
Fiorinal Capsules 2261
Fiorinal with Codeine Capsules 2262
Fiorinal Tablets.. 2261
Phrenilin 785
Sedapap Tablets 50 mg/650 mg .. 1543

Carteolol Hydrochloride (Potential for hypertensive crises). Products include:

Cartrol Tablets 410
Ocupress Ophthalmic Solution, 1% Sterile... ◉ 309

Chlordiazepoxide (Exhibits an additive CNS depression). Products include:

Libritabs Tablets 2177
Limbitrol 2180

Chlordiazepoxide Hydrochloride (Exhibits an additive CNS depression). Products include:

Librax Capsules 2176
Librium Capsules..................................... 2178
Librium Injectable 2179

Chlorpromazine (Exhibits an additive CNS depression). Products include:

Thorazine Suppositories........................ 2523

Chlorpromazine Hydrochloride (Exhibits an additive CNS depression). Products include:

Thorazine 2523

Chlorprothixene (Exhibits an additive CNS depression).

No products indexed under this heading.

Chlorprothixene Hydrochloride (Exhibits an additive CNS depression).

No products indexed under this heading.

Clorazepate Dipotassium (Exhibits an additive CNS depression). Products include:

Tranxene 451

Clozapine (Exhibits an additive CNS depression). Products include:

Clozaril Tablets... 2252

Codeine Phosphate (Exhibits an additive CNS depression). Products include:

Actifed with Codeine Cough Syrup.. 1067
Brontex 1981
Deconsal C Expectorant Syrup 456
Deconsal Pediatric Syrup 457
Dimetane-DC Cough Syrup 2059
Empirin with Codeine Tablets............ 1093
Fioricet with Codeine Capsules 2260
Fiorinal with Codeine Capsules 2262
Isoclor Expectorant................................. 990
Novahistine DH.. 2462
Novahistine Expectorant....................... 2463
Nucofed 2051
Phenergan with Codeine....................... 2777

Phenergan VC with Codeine 2781
Robitussin A-C Syrup............................. 2073
Robitussin-DAC Syrup 2074
Ryna .... ⊞ 841
Soma Compound w/Codeine Tablets 2676
Tussi-Organidin NR Liquid and S NR Liquid 2677
Tylenol with Codeine 1583

Desflurane (Exhibits an additive CNS depression). Products include:

Suprane 1813

Dezocine (Exhibits an additive CNS depression). Products include:

Dalgan Injection 538

Diazepam (Exhibits an additive CNS depression). Products include:

Dizac 1809
Valium Injectable 2182
Valium Tablets 2183
Valrelease Capsules 2169

Dobutamine Hydrochloride (Additive elevation of blood pressure). Products include:

Dobutrex Solution Vials......................... 1439

Dopamine Hydrochloride (Additive elevation of blood pressure).

No products indexed under this heading.

Droperidol (Exhibits an additive CNS depression). Products include:

Inapsine Injection.................................... 1296

Enflurane (Exhibits an additive CNS depression).

No products indexed under this heading.

Ephedrine Hydrochloride (Additive elevation of blood pressure). Products include:

Primatene Dual Action Formula....... ⊞ 872
Primatene Tablets .... ⊞ 873
Quadrinal Tablets 1350

Ephedrine Sulfate (Additive elevation of blood pressure). Products include:

Bronkaid Caplets .... ⊞ 717
Marax Tablets & DF Syrup.................... 2200

Ephedrine Tannate (Additive elevation of blood pressure). Products include:

Rynatuss 2673

Epinephrine (Additive elevation of blood pressure). Products include:

Bronkaid Mist .... ⊞ 717
EPIFRIN .... ◉ 239
EpiPen 790
Marcaine Hydrochloride with Epinephrine 1:200,000 2316
Primatene Mist .... ⊞ 873
Sensorcaine with Epinephrine Injection... 559
Sus-Phrine Injection 1019
Xylocaine with Epinephrine Injections... 567

Epinephrine Bitartrate (Additive elevation of blood pressure). Products include:

Bronkaid Mist Suspension .... ⊞ 718
Sensorcaine-MPF with Epinephrine Injection... 559

Epinephrine Hydrochloride (Additive elevation of blood pressure). Products include:

Ana-Kit Anaphylaxis Emergency Treatment Kit 617

Esmolol Hydrochloride (Potential for hypertensive crises). Products include:

Brevibloc Injection................................... 1808

Estazolam (Exhibits an additive CNS depression). Products include:

ProSom Tablets 449

Ethchlorvynol (Exhibits an additive CNS depression). Products include:

Placidyl Capsules..................................... 448

Ethinamate (Exhibits an additive CNS depression).

No products indexed under this heading.

Fentanyl (Exhibits an additive CNS depression). Products include:

Duragesic Transdermal System......... 1288

Fentanyl Citrate (Exhibits an additive CNS depression). Products include:

Sublimaze Injection................................. 1307

Fluphenazine Decanoate (Exhibits an additive CNS depression). Products include:

Prolixin Decanoate 509

Fluphenazine Enanthate (Exhibits an additive CNS depression). Products include:

Prolixin Enanthate 509

Fluphenazine Hydrochloride (Exhibits an additive CNS depression). Products include:

Prolixin 509

Flurazepam Hydrochloride (Exhibits an additive CNS depression). Products include:

Dalmane Capsules 2173

Furazolidone (Additive elevation of blood pressure; concurrent use is contraindicated; prolongs the anticholinergic effects of antihistamines). Products include:

Furoxone 2046

Glutethimide (Exhibits an additive CNS depression).

No products indexed under this heading.

Haloperidol (Exhibits an additive CNS depression). Products include:

Haldol Injection, Tablets and Concentrate 1575

Haloperidol Decanoate (Exhibits an additive CNS depression). Products include:

Haldol Decanoate..................................... 1577

Hydrocodone Polistirex (Exhibits an additive CNS depression). Products include:

Tussionex Pennkinetic Extended-Release Suspension 998

Hydroxyzine Hydrochloride (Exhibits an additive CNS depression). Products include:

Atarax Tablets & Syrup.......................... 2185
Marax Tablets & DF Syrup.................... 2200
Vistaril Intramuscular Solution.......... 2216

Indomethacin (Potential for hypertensive crises). Products include:

Indocin 1680

Indomethacin Sodium Trihydrate (Potential for hypertensive crises). Products include:

Indocin I.V. 1684

Isocarboxazid (Additive elevation of blood pressure; concurrent use is contraindicated; prolongs the anticholinergic effects of antihistamines).

No products indexed under this heading.

Isoflurane (Exhibits an additive CNS depression).

No products indexed under this heading.

Isoproterenol Hydrochloride (Additive elevation of blood pressure). Products include:

Isuprel Hydrochloride Injection 1:5000 2311
Isuprel Hydrochloride Solution 1:200 & 1:100 2313
Isuprel Mistometer 2312

Isoproterenol Sulfate (Additive elevation of blood pressure). Products include:

Norisodrine with Calcium Iodide Syrup... 442

Ketamine Hydrochloride (Exhibits an additive CNS depression).

No products indexed under this heading.

Labetalol Hydrochloride (Potential for hypertensive crises). Products include:

Normodyne Injection 2377
Normodyne Tablets 2379
Trandate 1185

Levobunolol Hydrochloride (Potential for hypertensive crises). Products include:

Betagan .... ◉ 233

Levomethadyl Acetate Hydrochloride (Exhibits an additive CNS depression). Products include:

Orlaam 2239

Levorphanol Tartrate (Exhibits an additive CNS depression). Products include:

Levo-Dromoran.. 2129

Lorazepam (Exhibits an additive CNS depression). Products include:

Ativan Injection... 2698
Ativan Tablets 2700

Loxapine Hydrochloride (Exhibits an additive CNS depression). Products include:

Loxitane 1378

Loxapine Succinate (Exhibits an additive CNS depression). Products include:

Loxitane Capsules 1378

Meperidine Hydrochloride (Exhibits an additive CNS depression). Products include:

Demerol 2308
Mepergan Injection 2753

Mephobarbital (Exhibits an additive CNS depression). Products include:

Mebaral Tablets 2322

Meprobamate (Exhibits an additive CNS depression). Products include:

Miltown Tablets 2672
PMB 200 and PMB 400 2783

Mesoridazine (Exhibits an additive CNS depression).

Metaproterenol Sulfate (Additive elevation of blood pressure). Products include:

Alupent.. 669
Metaproterenol Sulfate Inhalation Solution, USP, Arm-a-Med 552

Metaraminol Bitartrate (Additive elevation of blood pressure). Products include:

Aramine Injection..................................... 1609

Methadone Hydrochloride (Exhibits an additive CNS depression). Products include:

Methadone Hydrochloride Oral Concentrate 2233
Methadone Hydrochloride Oral Solution & Tablets..................................... 2235

Methohexital Sodium (Exhibits an additive CNS depression). Products include:

Brevital Sodium Vials.............................. 1429

Methotrimeprazine (Exhibits an additive CNS depression). Products include:

Levoprome 1274

Methoxamine Hydrochloride (Additive elevation of blood pressure). Products include:

Vasoxyl Injection 1196

Methoxyflurane (Exhibits an additive CNS depression).

No products indexed under this heading.

Methyldopa (Potential for hypertensive crises). Products include:

Aldoclor Tablets 1598
Aldomet Oral 1600
Aldoril Tablets.. 1604

(⊞ Described in PDR For Nonprescription Drugs) (◉ Described in PDR For Ophthalmology)

Metipranolol Hydrochloride (Potential for hypertensive crises). Products include:

OptiPranolol (Metipranolol 0.3%) Sterile Ophthalmic Solution.......... ◆ 258

Metoprolol Succinate (Potential for hypertensive crises). Products include:

Toprol-XL Tablets 565

Metoprolol Tartrate (Potential for hypertensive crises). Products include:

Lopressor Ampuls 830
Lopressor HCT Tablets 832
Lopressor Tablets 830

Midazolam Hydrochloride (Exhibits an additive CNS depression). Products include:

Versed Injection 2170

Molindone Hydrochloride (Exhibits an additive CNS depression). Products include:

Moban Tablets and Concentrate 1048

Morphine Sulfate (Exhibits an additive CNS depression). Products include:

Astramorph/PF Injection, USP (Preservative-Free) 535
Duramorph 962
Infumorph 200 and Infumorph 500 Sterile Solutions 965
MS Contin Tablets 1994
MSIR 1997
Oramorph SR (Morphine Sulfate Sustained Release Tablets) 2236
RMS Suppositories 2657
Roxanol 2243

Nadolol (Potential for hypertensive crises).

No products indexed under this heading.

Norepinephrine Bitartrate (Additive elevation of blood pressure). Products include:

Levophed Bitartrate Injection 2315

Opium Alkaloids (Exhibits an additive CNS depression).

No products indexed under this heading.

Oxazepam (Exhibits an additive CNS depression). Products include:

Serax Capsules 2810
Serax Tablets 2810

Oxycodone Hydrochloride (Exhibits an additive CNS depression). Products include:

Percocet Tablets 938
Percodan Tablets 939
Percodan-Demi Tablets 940
Roxicodone Tablets, Oral Solution & Intensol (Oxycodone) 2244
Tylox Capsules 1584

Penbutolol Sulfate (Potential for hypertensive crises). Products include:

Levatol 2403

Pentobarbital Sodium (Exhibits an additive CNS depression). Products include:

Nembutal Sodium Capsules 436
Nembutal Sodium Solution 438
Nembutal Sodium Suppositories 440

Perphenazine (Exhibits an additive CNS depression). Products include:

Etrafon 2355
Triavil Tablets 1757
Trilafon 2389

Phenelzine Sulfate (Additive elevation of blood pressure; concurrent use is contraindicated; prolongs the anticholinergic effects of antihistamines). Products include:

Nardil 1920

Phenobarbital (Exhibits an additive CNS depression). Products include:

Arco-Lase Plus Tablets 512
Bellergal-S Tablets 2250
Donnatal 2060
Donnatal Extentabs 2061
Donnatal Tablets 2060
Phenobarbital Elixir and Tablets 1469
Quadrinal Tablets 1350

Phenylephrine Bitartrate (Additive elevation of blood pressure).

No products indexed under this heading.

Phenylephrine Tannate (Additive elevation of blood pressure). Products include:

Atrohist Pediatric Suspension 454
Ricobid-D Pediatric Suspension 2038
Ricobid Tablets and Pediatric Suspension 2038
Rynatan 2673
Rynatuss 2673

Phenylpropanolamine Hydrochloride (Additive elevation of blood pressure). Products include:

Acutrim .... ⊕ 628
Allerest Children's Chewable Tablets .... ⊕ 627
Allerest 12 Hour Caplets .... ⊕ 627
Atrohist Plus Tablets 454
BC Cold Powder Multi-Symptom Formula (Cold-Sinus-Allergy) ...... ⊕ 609
BC Cold Powder Non-Drowsy Formula (Cold-Sinus) .... ⊕ 609
Cheracol Plus Head Cold/Cough Formula .... ⊕ 769
Comtrex Multi-Symptom Non-Drowsy Liqui-gels .... ⊕ 618
Contac Continuous Action Nasal Decongestant/Antihistamine 12 Hour Capsules .... ⊕ 813
Contac Maximum Strength Continuous Action Decongestant/Antihistamine 12 Hour Caplets .. ⊕ 813
Contac Severe Cold and Flu Formula Caplets .... ⊕ 814
Coricidin 'D' Decongestant Tablets .... ⊕ 800
Dexatrim .... ⊕ 832
Dexatrim Plus Vitamins Caplets .... ⊕ 832
Dimetane-DC Cough Syrup 2059
Dimetapp Elixir .... ⊕ 773
Dimetapp Extentabs .... ⊕ 774
Dimetapp Tablets/Liqui-Gels .... ⊕ 775
Dimetapp Cold & Allergy Chewable Tablets .... ⊕ 773
Dimetapp DM Elixir .... ⊕ 774
Dura-Vent Tablets 952
Entex Capsules 1986
Entex LA Tablets 1987
Entex Liquid 1986
Exgest LA Tablets 782
Hycomine 931
Isoclor Timesule Capsules .... ⊕ 637
Nolamine Timed-Release Tablets 785
Ornade Spansule Capsules 2502
Propagest Tablets 786
Pyrroxate Caplets .... ⊕ 772
Robitussin-CF .... ⊕ 777
Sinulin Tablets 787
Tavist-D 12 Hour Relief Tablets .... ⊕ 787
Teldrin 12 Hour Antihistamine/Nasal Decongestant Allergy Relief Capsules .... ⊕ 826
Triaminic Allergy Tablets .... ⊕ 789
Triaminic Cold Tablets .... ⊕ 790
Triaminic Expectorant .... ⊕ 790
Triaminic Syrup .... ⊕ 792
Triaminic-12 Tablets .... ⊕ 792
Triaminic-DM Syrup .... ⊕ 792
Triaminicin Tablets .... ⊕ 793
Triaminicol Multi-Symptom Cold Tablets .... ⊕ 793
Triaminicol Multi-Symptom Relief ⊕ 794
Vicks DayQuil Allergy Relief 12-Hour Extended Release Tablets .. ⊕ 760
Vicks DayQuil Allergy Relief 4-Hour Tablets .... ⊕ 760
Vicks DayQuil SINUS Pressure & CONGESTION Relief .... ⊕ 761

Pindolol (Potential for hypertensive crises). Products include:

Visken Tablets 2299

Pirbuterol Acetate (Additive elevation of blood pressure). Products include:

Maxair Autohaler 1492
Maxair Inhaler 1494

Prazepam (Exhibits an additive CNS depression).

No products indexed under this heading.

Prochlorperazine (Exhibits an additive CNS depression). Products include:

Compazine 2470

Promethazine Hydrochloride (Exhibits an additive CNS depression). Products include:

Mepergan Injection 2753
Phenergan with Codeine 2777
Phenergan with Dextromethorphan 2778
Phenergan Injection 2773
Phenergan Suppositories 2775
Phenergan Syrup 2774
Phenergan Tablets 2775
Phenergan VC 2779
Phenergan VC with Codeine 2781

Propofol (Exhibits an additive CNS depression). Products include:

Diprivan Injection 2833

Propoxyphene Hydrochloride (Exhibits an additive CNS depression). Products include:

Darvon 1435
Wygesic Tablets 2827

Propoxyphene Napsylate (Exhibits an additive CNS depression). Products include:

Darvon-N/Darvocet-N 1433

Propranolol Hydrochloride (Potential for hypertensive crises). Products include:

Inderal 2728
Inderal LA Long Acting Capsules 2730
Inderide Tablets 2732
Inderide LA Long Acting Capsules .. 2734

Pseudoephedrine Hydrochloride (Additive elevation of blood pressure). Products include:

Actifed Allergy Daytime/Nighttime Caplets .... ⊕ 844
Actifed Plus Caplets .... ⊕ 845
Actifed Plus Tablets .... ⊕ 845
Actifed with Codeine Cough Syrup .. 1067
Actifed Sinus Daytime/Nighttime Tablets and Caplets .... ⊕ 846
Actifed Syrup .... ⊕ 846
Actifed Tablets .... ⊕ 844
Advil Cold and Sinus Caplets and Tablets (formerly CoAdvil) .... ⊕ 870
Alka-Seltzer Plus Cold Medicine Liqui-Gels .... ⊕ 706
Alka-Seltzer Plus Cold & Cough Medicine Liqui-Gels .... ⊕ 705
Alka-Seltzer Plus Night-Time Cold Medicine Liqui-Gels .... ⊕ 706
Allerest Headache Strength Tablets .... ⊕ 627
Allerest Maximum Strength Tablets .... ⊕ 627
Allerest No Drowsiness Tablets ...... ⊕ 627
Allerest Sinus Pain Formula .... ⊕ 627
Anatuss LA Tablets 1542
Atrohist Pediatric Capsules 453
Bayer Select Sinus Pain Relief Formula .... ⊕ 717
Benadryl Allergy Decongestant Liquid Medication .... ⊕ 848
Benadryl Allergy Decongestant Tablets .... ⊕ 848
Benadryl Allergy Sinus Headache Formula Caplets .... ⊕ 849
Benylin Multisymptom .... ⊕ 852
Bromfed Capsules (Extended-Release) 1785
Bromfed Syrup .... ⊕ 733
Bromfed Tablets 1785
Bromfed-DM Cough Syrup 1786
Bromfed-PD Capsules (Extended-Release) 1785
Children's Vicks DayQuil Allergy Relief .... ⊕ 757
Children's Vicks NyQuil Cold/Cough Relief .... ⊕ 758
Comtrex Multi-Symptom Cold Reliever Tablets/Caplets/Liqui-Gels/Liquid .... ⊕ 615
Allergy-Sinus Comtrex Multi-Symptom Allergy-Sinus Formula Tablets .... ⊕ 617
Comtrex Multi-Symptom Non-Drowsy Caplets .... ⊕ 618
Congess 1004
Contac Day Allergy/Sinus Caplets ⊕ 812
Contac Day & Night .... ⊕ 812
Contac Night Allergy/Sinus Caplets .... ⊕ 812
Contac Severe Cold & Flu Non-Drowsy .... ⊕ 815
Deconamine Chewable Tablets 1320
Deconamine CX Cough and Cold Liquid and Tablets 1319
Deconamine 1320
Deconsal C Expectorant Syrup 456
Deconsal Pediatric Syrup 457
Deconsal II Tablets 454
Dimetane-DX Cough Syrup 2059
Dimetapp Sinus Caplets .... ⊕ 775
Dorcol Children's Cough Syrup ...... ⊕ 785
Drixoral Cough + Congestion Liquid Caps .... ⊕ 802
Dura-Tap/PD Capsules 2867
Duratuss Tablets 2565
Duratuss HD Elixir 2565
Efidac/24 .... ⊕ 635
Entex PSE Tablets 1987
Fedahist Gyrocaps 2401
Fedahist Timecaps 2401
Guaifed 1787
Guaifed Syrup .... ⊕ 734
Guaimax-D Tablets 792
Guaitab Tablets .... ⊕ 734
Isoclor Expectorant 990
Kronofed-A 977
Motrin IB Sinus .... ⊕ 838
Novahistine DH 2462
Novahistine DMX .... ⊕ 822
Novahistine Expectorant 2463
Nucofed 2051
PediaCare Cold Allergy Chewable Tablets .... ⊕ 677
PediaCare Cough-Cold Chewable Tablets 1553
PediaCare 1553
PediaCare Infants' Decongestant Drops .... ⊕ 677
PediCare Infant's Drops Decongestant Plus Cough 1553
PediaCare NightRest Cough-Cold Liquid 1553
Pediatric Vicks 44d Dry Hacking Cough & Head Congestion .... ⊕ 763
Pediatric Vicks 44m Cough & Cold Relief .... ⊕ 764
Robitussin Cold & Cough Liqui-Gels .... ⊕ 776
Robitussin Maximum Strength Cough & Cold .... ⊕ 778
Robitussin Pediatric Cough & Cold Formula .... ⊕ 779
Robitussin Severe Congestion Liqui-Gels .... ⊕ 776
Robitussin-DAC Syrup 2074
Robitussin-PE .... ⊕ 778
Rondec Oral Drops 953
Rondec Syrup 953
Rondec Tablet 953
Rondec-DM Oral Drops 954
Rondec-DM Syrup 954
Rondec-TR Tablet 953
Ryna .... ⊕ 841
Seldane-D Extended-Release Tablets 1538
Semprex-D Capsules 463
Semprex-D Capsules 1167
Sinarest Tablets .... ⊕ 648
Sinarest Extra Strength Tablets ...... ⊕ 648
Sinarest No Drowsiness Tablets ..... ⊕ 648
Sine-Aid IB Caplets 1554
Sine-Aid Maximum Strength Sinus Medication Gelcaps, Caplets and Tablets 1554
Sine-Off No Drowsiness Formula Caplets .... ⊕ 824
Sine-Off Sinus Medicine .... ⊕ 825
Singlet Tablets .... ⊕ 825
Sinutab Non-Drying Liquid Caps .... ⊕ 859
Sinutab Sinus Allergy Medication, Maximum Strength Tablets and Caplets .... ⊕ 860
Sinutab Sinus Medication, Maximum Strength Without Drowsiness Formula, Tablets & Caplets .... ⊕ 860
Sinutab Sinus Medication, Regular Strength Without Drowsiness Formula .... ⊕ 859
Sudafed Children's Liquid .... ⊕ 861
Sudafed Cold and Cough Liquidcaps .... ⊕ 862
Sudafed Cough Syrup .... ⊕ 862
Sudafed Plus Liquid .... ⊕ 862
Sudafed Plus Tablets .... ⊕ 863
Sudafed Severe Cold Formula Caplets .... ⊕ 863
Sudafed Severe Cold Formula Tablets .... ⊕ 864
Sudafed Sinus Caplets .... ⊕ 864

IMPORTANT NOTE: Always consult each drug listing in the patient's regimen for possible interactions.

Sudafed Sinus Tablets ▣ 864
Sudafed Tablets, 30 mg ▣ 861
Sudafed Tablets, 60 mg ▣ 861
Sudafed 12 Hour Caplets ▣ 861
Syn-Rx Tablets 465
Syn-Rx DM Tablets 466
TheraFlu ▣ 787
TheraFlu Maximum Strength Nighttime Flu, Cold & Cough Medicine ▣ 788
TheraFlu Maximum Strength Non-Drowsy Formula Flu, Cold & Cough Medicine ▣ 788
Thera Flu Maximum Strength, Non-Drowsy Formula Flu, Cold and Cough Caplets ▣ 789
Triaminic AM Cough and Decongestant Formula ▣ 789
Triaminic AM Decongestant Formula ▣ 790
Triaminic Nite Light ▣ 791
Triaminic Sore Throat Formula ▣ 791
Tussend 1783
Tussend Expectorant 1785
Children's TYLENOL Cold Multi-Symptom Liquid Formula and Chewable Tablets 1561
Children's TYLENOL Cold Plus Cough Multi Symptom Tablets and Liquid ▣ 681
Infants' TYLENOL Cold Decongestant & Fever-Reducer Drops 1556
TYLENOL Maximum Strength Allergy Sinus Medication Gelcaps and Caplets 1563
TYLENOL Maximum Strength Allergy Sinus NightTime Medication Caplets 1555
TYLENOL Flu Maximum Strength Gelcaps 1565
TYLENOL Flu NightTime, Maximum Strength, Gelcaps 1566
TYLENOL Maximum Strength Flu NightTime Hot Medication Packets 1562
TYLENOL, Maximum Strength, Sinus Medication Geltabs, Gelcaps, Caplets and Tablets 1566
TYLENOL Cold Multi-Symptom Formula Medication Tablets and Caplets 1561
TYLENOL Cold Medication No Drowsiness Formula Gelcaps and Caplets 1562
TYLENOL Cold Multi-Symptom Hot Medication Liquid Packets 1557
TYLENOL Cough Multi-Symptom Medication with Decongestant 1565
Ursinus Inlay-Tabs ▣ 794
Vicks 44 LiquiCaps Cough, Cold & Flu Relief ▣ 755
Vicks 44 LiquiCaps Non-Drowsy Cough & Cold Relief ▣ 756
Vicks 44D Dry Hacking Cough & Head Congestion ▣ 755
Vicks 44M Cough, Cold & Flu Relief ▣ 756
Vicks DayQuil ▣ 761
Vicks DayQuil SINUS Pressure & PAIN Relief with IBUPROFEN ▣ 762
Vicks Nyquil Hot Therapy ▣ 762
Vicks NyQuil LiquiCaps Multi-Symptom Cold/Flu Relief ▣ 763
Vicks NyQuil Multi-Symptom Cold/Flu Relief - (Original & Cherry Flavor) ▣ 763

Pseudoephedrine Sulfate (Additive elevation of blood pressure). Products include:
Cheracol Sinus ▣ 768
Chlor-Trimeton Allergy Decongestant Tablets ▣ 799
Claritin-D 2350
Drixoral Cold and Allergy Sustained-Action Tablets ▣ 802
Drixoral Cold and Flu Extended-Release Tablets ▣ 803
Drixoral Non-Drowsy Formula Extended-Release Tablets ▣ 803
Drixoral Allergy/Sinus Extended Release Tablets ▣ 804
Trinalin Repetabs Tablets 1330

Quazepam (Exhibits an additive CNS depression). Products include:
Doral Tablets 2664

Risperidone (Exhibits an additive CNS depression). Products include:
Risperdal 1301

Salmeterol Xinafoate (Additive elevation of blood pressure). Products include:
Serevent Inhalation Aerosol 1176

Secobarbital Sodium (Exhibits an additive CNS depression). Products include:
Seconal Sodium Pulvules 1474

Selegiline Hydrochloride (Additive elevation of blood pressure; concurrent use is contraindicated; prolongs the anticholinergic effects of antihistamines). Products include:
Eldepryl Tablets 2550

Sotalol Hydrochloride (Potential for hypertensive crises). Products include:
Betapace Tablets 641

Sufentanil Citrate (Exhibits an additive CNS depression). Products include:
Sufenta Injection 1309

Temazepam (Exhibits an additive CNS depression). Products include:
Restoril Capsules 2284

Terbutaline Sulfate (Additive elevation of blood pressure). Products include:
Brethaire Inhaler 813
Brethine Ampuls 815
Brethine Tablets 814
Bricanyl Subcutaneous Injection 1502
Bricanyl Tablets 1503

Thiamylal Sodium (Exhibits an additive CNS depression).
No products indexed under this heading.

Thioridazine Hydrochloride (Exhibits an additive CNS depression). Products include:
Mellaril 2269

Thiothixene (Exhibits an additive CNS depression). Products include:
Navane Capsules and Concentrate 2201
Navane Intramuscular 2202

Timolol Hemihydrate (Potential for hypertensive crises). Products include:
Betimol 0.25%, 0.5% ⊙ 261

Timolol Maleate (Potential for hypertensive crises). Products include:
Blocadren Tablets 1614
Timolide Tablets 1748
Timoptic in Ocudose 1753
Timoptic Sterile Ophthalmic Solution 1751
Timoptic-XE 1755

Tranylcypromine Sulfate (Additive elevation of blood pressure; concurrent use is contraindicated; prolongs the anticholinergic effects of antihistamines). Products include:
Parnate Tablets 2503

Triazolam (Exhibits an additive CNS depression). Products include:
Halcion Tablets 2611

Trifluoperazine Hydrochloride (Exhibits an additive CNS depression). Products include:
Stelazine 2514

Zolpidem Tartrate (Exhibits an additive CNS depression). Products include:
Ambien Tablets 2416

Food Interactions

Alcohol (Exhibits an additive CNS depression).

HYCOMINE PEDIATRIC SYRUP

(Hydrocodone Bitartrate, Phenylpropanolamine Hydrochloride) 931

May interact with sympathomimetics, monoamine oxidase inhibitors, beta blockers, central nervous system depressants, narcotic analgesics, hypnotics and sedatives, general anesthetics, phenothiazines, tranquilizers, and certain other agents. Compounds in these categories include:

Acebutolol Hydrochloride (Concurrent use may produce additive elevation in blood pressure). Products include:
Sectral Capsules 2807

Albuterol (Concurrent use may produce additive elevation of blood pressure). Products include:
Proventil Inhalation Aerosol 2382
Ventolin Inhalation Aerosol and Refill 1197

Albuterol Sulfate (Concurrent use may produce additive elevation of blood pressure). Products include:
Airet Solution for Inhalation 452
Proventil Inhalation Solution 0.083% 2384
Proventil Repetabs Tablets 2386
Proventil Solution for Inhalation 0.5% 2383
Proventil Syrup 2385
Proventil Tablets 2386
Ventolin Inhalation Solution 1198
Ventolin Nebules Inhalation Solution 1199
Ventolin Rotacaps for Inhalation 1200
Ventolin Syrup 1202
Ventolin Tablets 1203
Volmax Extended-Release Tablets 1788

Alfentanil Hydrochloride (Additive CNS depression). Products include:
Alfenta Injection 1286

Alprazolam (Additive CNS depression). Products include:
Xanax Tablets 2649

Aprobarbital (Additive CNS depression).
No products indexed under this heading.

Atenolol (Concurrent use may produce additive elevation in blood pressure). Products include:
Tenoretic Tablets 2845
Tenormin Tablets and I.V. Injection 2847

Betaxolol Hydrochloride (Concurrent use may produce additive elevation in blood pressure). Products include:
Betoptic Ophthalmic Solution 469
Betoptic S Ophthalmic Suspension 471
Kerlone Tablets 2436

Bisoprolol Fumarate (Concurrent use may produce additive elevation in blood pressure). Products include:
Zebeta Tablets 1413
Ziac 1415

Buprenorphine (Additive CNS depression). Products include:
Buprenex Injectable 2006

Buspirone Hydrochloride (Additive CNS depression). Products include:
BuSpar 737

Butabarbital (Additive CNS depression).
No products indexed under this heading.

Butalbital (Additive CNS depression). Products include:
Esgic-plus Tablets 1013
Fioricet Tablets 2258
Fioricet with Codeine Capsules 2260
Fiorinal Capsules 2261
Fiorinal with Codeine Capsules 2262
Fiorinal Tablets 2261
Phrenilin 785
Sedapap Tablets 50 mg/650 mg 1543

Carteolol Hydrochloride (Concurrent use may produce additive elevation in blood pressure). Products include:
Cartrol Tablets 410
Ocupress Ophthalmic Solution, 1% Sterile ⊙ 309

Chlordiazepoxide (Additive CNS depression). Products include:
Libritabs Tablets 2177
Limbitrol 2180

Chlordiazepoxide Hydrochloride (Additive CNS depression). Products include:
Librax Capsules 2176
Librium Capsules 2178
Librium Injectable 2179

Chlorpromazine (Additive CNS depression). Products include:
Thorazine Suppositories 2523

Chlorpromazine Hydrochloride (Additive CNS depression). Products include:
Thorazine 2523

Chlorprothixene (Additive CNS depression).
No products indexed under this heading.

Chlorprothixene Hydrochloride (Additive CNS depression).
No products indexed under this heading.

Clorazepate Dipotassium (Additive CNS depression). Products include:
Tranxene 451

Clozapine (Additive CNS depression). Products include:
Clozaril Tablets 2252

Codeine Phosphate (Additive CNS depression). Products include:
Actifed with Codeine Cough Syrup 1067
Brontex 1981
Deconsal C Expectorant Syrup 456
Deconsal Pediatric Syrup 457
Dimetane-DC Cough Syrup 2059
Empirin with Codeine Tablets 1093
Fioricet with Codeine Capsules 2260
Fiorinal with Codeine Capsules 2262
Isoclor Expectorant 990
Novahistine DH 2462
Novahistine Expectorant 2463
Nucofed 2051
Phenergan with Codeine 2777
Phenergan VC with Codeine 2781
Robitussin A-C Syrup 2073
Robitussin-DAC Syrup 2074
Ryna ▣ 841
Soma Compound w/Codeine Tablets 2676
Tussi-Organidin NR Liquid and S NR Liquid 2677
Tylenol with Codeine 1583

Desflurane (Additive CNS depression). Products include:
Suprane 1813

Dezocine (Additive CNS depression). Products include:
Dalgan Injection 538

Diazepam (Additive CNS depression). Products include:
Dizac 1809
Valium Injectable 2182
Valium Tablets 2183
Valrelease Capsules 2169

Dobutamine Hydrochloride (Concurrent use may produce additive elevation of blood pressure). Products include:
Dobutrex Solution Vials 1439

Dopamine Hydrochloride (Concurrent use may produce additive elevation of blood pressure).
No products indexed under this heading.

Droperidol (Additive CNS depression). Products include:
Inapsine Injection 1296

Enflurane (Additive CNS depression).
No products indexed under this heading.

Ephedrine Hydrochloride (Concurrent use may produce additive elevation of blood pressure). Products include:
Primatene Dual Action Formula ▣ 872
Primatene Tablets ▣ 873

(▣ Described in PDR For Nonprescription Drugs) (⊙ Described in PDR For Ophthalmology)

485 **Interactions Index** **Hycomine**

Quadrinal Tablets 1350

Ephedrine Sulfate (Concurrent use may produce additive elevation of blood pressure). Products include:
Bronkaid Caplets ..... ▣ 717
Marax Tablets & DF Syrup 2200

Ephedrine Tannate (Concurrent use may produce additive elevation of blood pressure). Products include:
Rynatuss 2673

Epinephrine (Concurrent use may produce additive elevation of blood pressure). Products include:
Bronkaid Mist ..... ▣ 717
EPIFRIN ..... ◉ 239
EpiPen 790
Marcaine Hydrochloride with Epinephrine 1:200,000 2316
Primatene Mist ..... ▣ 873
Sensorcaine with Epinephrine Injection 559
Sus-Phrine Injection 1019
Xylocaine with Epinephrine Injections 567

Epinephrine Bitartrate (Concurrent use may produce additive elevation of blood pressure). Products include:
Bronkaid Mist Suspension ..... ▣ 718
Sensorcaine-MPF with Epinephrine Injection 559

Epinephrine Hydrochloride (Concurrent use may produce additive elevation of blood pressure). Products include:
Ana-Kit Anaphylaxis Emergency Treatment Kit 617

Esmolol Hydrochloride (Concurrent use may produce additive elevation in blood pressure). Products include:
Brevibloc Injection 1808

Estazolam (Additive CNS depression). Products include:
ProSom Tablets 449

Ethchlorvynol (Additive CNS depression). Products include:
Placidyl Capsules 448

Ethinamate (Additive CNS depression).
No products indexed under this heading.

Fentanyl (Additive CNS depression). Products include:
Duragesic Transdermal System 1288

Fentanyl Citrate (Additive CNS depression). Products include:
Sublimaze Injection 1307

Fluphenazine Decanoate (Additive CNS depression). Products include:
Prolixin Decanoate 509

Fluphenazine Enanthate (Additive CNS depression). Products include:
Prolixin Enanthate 509

Fluphenazine Hydrochloride (Additive CNS depression). Products include:
Prolixin 509

Flurazepam Hydrochloride (Additive CNS depression). Products include:
Dalmane Capsules 2173

Furazolidone (Potential for hypertensive crises; concurrent use is contraindicated). Products include:
Furoxone 2046

Glutethimide (Additive CNS depression).
No products indexed under this heading.

Haloperidol (Additive CNS depression). Products include:
Haldol Injection, Tablets and Concentrate 1575

Haloperidol Decanoate (Additive CNS depression). Products include:
Haldol Decanoate 1577

Hydrocodone Polistirex (Additive CNS depression). Products include:
Tussionex Pennkinetic Extended-Release Suspension 998

Hydroxyzine Hydrochloride (Additive CNS depression). Products include:
Atarax Tablets & Syrup 2185
Marax Tablets & DF Syrup 2200
Vistaril Intramuscular Solution 2216

Indomethacin (Hypertensive crisis can occur with concurrent use). Products include:
Indocin 1680

Indomethacin Sodium Trihydrate (Hypertensive crisis can occur with concurrent use). Products include:
Indocin I.V. 1684

Isocarboxazid (Potential for hypertensive crises; concurrent use is contraindicated).
No products indexed under this heading.

Isoflurane (Additive CNS depression).
No products indexed under this heading.

Isoproterenol Hydrochloride (Concurrent use may produce additive elevation of blood pressure). Products include:
Isuprel Hydrochloride Injection 1:5000 2311
Isuprel Hydrochloride Solution 1:200 & 1:100 2313
Isuprel Mistometer 2312

Isoproterenol Sulfate (Concurrent use may produce additive elevation of blood pressure). Products include:
Norisodrine with Calcium Iodide Syrup 442

Ketamine Hydrochloride (Additive CNS depression).
No products indexed under this heading.

Labetalol Hydrochloride (Concurrent use may produce additive elevation in blood pressure). Products include:
Normodyne Injection 2377
Normodyne Tablets 2379
Trandate 1185

Levobunolol Hydrochloride (Concurrent use may produce additive elevation in blood pressure). Products include:
Betagan ..... ◉ 233

Levomethadyl Acetate Hydrochloride (Additive CNS depression). Products include:
Orlamm 2239

Levorphanol Tartrate (Additive CNS depression). Products include:
Levo-Dromoran 2129

Lorazepam (Additive CNS depression). Products include:
Ativan Injection 2698
Ativan Tablets 2700

Loxapine Hydrochloride (Additive CNS depression). Products include:
Loxitane 1378

Loxapine Succinate (Additive CNS depression). Products include:
Loxitane Capsules 1378

Meperidine Hydrochloride (Additive CNS depression). Products include:
Demerol 2308
Mepergan Injection 2753

Mephobarbital (Additive CNS depression). Products include:
Mebaral Tablets 2322

Meprobamate (Additive CNS depression). Products include:
Miltown Tablets 2672
PMB 200 and PMB 400 2783

Mesoridazine (Additive CNS depression).

Mesoridazine Besylate (Additive CNS depression). Products include:
Serentil 684

Metaproterenol Sulfate (Concurrent use may produce additive elevation of blood pressure). Products include:
Alupent 669
Metaproterenol Sulfate Inhalation Solution, USP, Arm-a-Med 552

Metaraminol Bitartrate (Concurrent use may produce additive elevation of blood pressure). Products include:
Aramine Injection 1609

Methadone Hydrochloride (Additive CNS depression). Products include:
Methadone Hydrochloride Oral Concentrate 2233
Methadone Hydrochloride Oral Solution & Tablets 2235

Methohexital Sodium (Additive CNS depression). Products include:
Brevital Sodium Vials 1429

Methotrimeprazine (Additive CNS depression). Products include:
Levoprome 1274

Methoxamine Hydrochloride (Concurrent use may produce additive elevation of blood pressure). Products include:
Vasoxyl Injection 1196

Methoxyflurane (Additive CNS depression).
No products indexed under this heading.

Methyldopa (Hypertensive crisis can occur with concurrent use). Products include:
Aldoclor Tablets 1598
Aldomet Oral 1600
Aldoril Tablets 1604

Methyldopate Hydrochloride (Hypertensive crisis can occur with concurrent use). Products include:
Aldomet Ester HCl Injection 1602

Metipranolol Hydrochloride (Concurrent use may produce additive elevation in blood pressure). Products include:
OptiPranolol (Metipranolol 0.3%) Sterile Ophthalmic Solution ..... ◉ 258

Metoprolol Succinate (Concurrent use may produce additive elevation in blood pressure). Products include:
Toprol-XL Tablets 565

Metoprolol Tartrate (Concurrent use may produce additive elevation in blood pressure). Products include:
Lopressor Ampuls 830
Lopressor HCT Tablets 832
Lopressor Tablets 830

Midazolam Hydrochloride (Additive CNS depression). Products include:
Versed Injection 2170

Molindone Hydrochloride (Additive CNS depression). Products include:
Moban Tablets and Concentrate 1048

Morphine Sulfate (Additive CNS depression). Products include:
Astramorph/PF Injection, USP (Preservative-Free) 535
Duramorph 962
Infumorph 200 and Infumorph 500 Sterile Solutions 965
MS Contin Tablets 1994
MSIR 1997
Oramorph SR (Morphine Sulfate Sustained Release Tablets) 2236
RMS Suppositories 2657
Roxanol 2243

Nadolol (Concurrent use may produce additive elevation in blood pressure).
No products indexed under this heading.

Norepinephrine Bitartrate (Concurrent use may produce additive elevation of blood pressure). Products include:
Levophed Bitartrate Injection 2315

Opium Alkaloids (Additive CNS depression).
No products indexed under this heading.

Oxazepam (Additive CNS depression). Products include:
Serax Capsules 2810
Serax Tablets 2810

Oxycodone Hydrochloride (Additive CNS depression). Products include:
Percocet Tablets 938
Percodan Tablets 939
Percodan-Demi Tablets 940
Roxicodone Tablets, Oral Solution & Intensol (Oxycodone) 2244
Tylox Capsules 1584

Penbutolol Sulfate (Concurrent use may produce additive elevation in blood pressure). Products include:
Levatol 2403

Pentobarbital Sodium (Additive CNS depression). Products include:
Nembutal Sodium Capsules 436
Nembutal Sodium Solution 438
Nembutal Sodium Suppositories 440

Perphenazine (Additive CNS depression). Products include:
Etrafon 2355
Triavil Tablets 1757
Trilafon 2389

Phenelzine Sulfate (Potential for hypertensive crises; concurrent use is contraindicated). Products include:
Nardil 1920

Phenobarbital (Additive CNS depression). Products include:
Arco-Lase Plus Tablets 512
Bellergal-S Tablets 2250
Donnatal 2060
Donnatal Extentabs 2061
Donnatal Tablets 2060
Phenobarbital Elixir and Tablets 1469
Quadrinal Tablets 1350

Phenylephrine Bitartrate (Concurrent use may produce additive elevation of blood pressure).
No products indexed under this heading.

Phenylephrine Hydrochloride (Concurrent use may produce additive elevation of blood pressure). Products include:
Atrohist Plus Tablets 454
Cerose DM ..... ▣ 878
Comhist 2038
D.A. Chewable Tablets 951
Deconsal Pediatric Capsules 454
Dura-Vent/DA Tablets 953
Entex Capsules 1986
Entex Liquid 1986
Extendryl 1005
4-Way Fast Acting Nasal Spray (regular & mentholated) ..... ▣ 621
Hemorid For Women ..... ▣ 834
Hycomine Compound Tablets 932
Neo-Synephrine Hydrochloride 1% Carpuject 2324
Neo-Synephrine Hydrochloride 1% Injection 2324
Neo-Synephrine Hydrochloride (Ophthalmic) 2325
Neo-Synephrine ..... ▣ 726
Nōstril ..... ▣ 644
Novahistine Elixir ..... ▣ 823
Phenergan VC 2779
Phenergan VC with Codeine 2781
Preparation H ..... ▣ 871
Tympagesic Ear Drops 2342
Vasosulf ..... ◉ 271
Vicks Sinex Nasal Spray and Ultra Fine Mist ..... ▣ 765

IMPORTANT NOTE: Always consult each drug listing in the patient's regimen for possible interactions.

Hycomine

Interactions Index

Phenylephrine Tannate (Concurrent use may produce additive elevation of blood pressure). Products include:

Atrohist Pediatric Suspension 454
Ricobid-D Pediatric Suspension........ 2038
Ricobid Tablets and Pediatric Suspension.. 2038
Rynatan 2673
Rynatuss 2673

Pindolol (Concurrent use may produce additive elevation in blood pressure). Products include:

Visken Tablets... 2299

Pirbuterol Acetate (Concurrent use may produce additive elevation of blood pressure). Products include:

Maxair Autohaler 1492
Maxair Inhaler 1494

Prazepam (Additive CNS depression).

No products indexed under this heading.

Prochlorperazine (Additive CNS depression). Products include:

Compazine 2470

Promethazine Hydrochloride (Additive CNS depression). Products include:

Mepergan Injection 2753
Phenergan with Codeine 2777
Phenergan with Dextromethorphan 2778
Phenergan Injection 2773
Phenergan Suppositories 2775
Phenergan Syrup 2774
Phenergan Tablets 2775
Phenergan VC 2779
Phenergan VC with Codeine 2781

Propofol (Additive CNS depression). Products include:

Diprivan Injection..................................... 2833

Propoxyphene Hydrochloride (Additive CNS depression). Products include:

Darvon 1435
Wygesic Tablets 2827

Propoxyphene Napsylate (Additive CNS depression). Products include:

Darvon-N/Darvocet-N 1433

Propranolol Hydrochloride (Concurrent use may produce additive elevation in blood pressure). Products include:

Inderal 2728
Inderal LA Long Acting Capsules 2730
Inderide Tablets 2732
Inderide LA Long Acting Capsules .. 2734

Pseudoephedrine Hydrochloride (Concurrent use may produce additive elevation of blood pressure). Products include:

Actifed Allergy Daytime/Nighttime Caplets... ᴮᴰ 844
Actifed Plus Caplets .... ᴮᴰ 845
Actifed Plus Tablets .... ᴮᴰ 845
Actifed with Codeine Cough Syrup.. 1067
Actifed Sinus Daytime/Nighttime Tablets and Caplets .... ᴮᴰ 846
Actifed Syrup... ᴮᴰ 846
Actifed Tablets .... ᴮᴰ 844
Advil Cold and Sinus Caplets and Tablets (formerly CoAdvil) .... ᴮᴰ 870
Alka-Seltzer Plus Cold Medicine Liqui-Gels .... ᴮᴰ 706
Alka-Seltzer Plus Cold & Cough Medicine Liqui-Gels............................ ᴮᴰ 705
Alka-Seltzer Plus Night-Time Cold Medicine Liqui-Gels............................ ᴮᴰ 706
Allerest Headache Strength Tablets .... ᴮᴰ 627
Allerest Maximum Strength Tablets .... ᴮᴰ 627
Allerest No Drowsiness Tablets ...... ᴮᴰ 627
Allerest Sinus Pain Formula .... ᴮᴰ 627
Anatuss LA Tablets................................. 1542
Atrohist Pediatric Capsules.................. 453
Bayer Select Sinus Pain Relief Formula .... ᴮᴰ 717
Benadryl Allergy Decongestant Liquid Medication .... ᴮᴰ 848
Benadryl Allergy Decongestant Tablets .... ᴮᴰ 848
Benadryl Allergy Sinus Headache Formula Caplets................................. ᴮᴰ 849
Benylin Multisymptom........................ ᴮᴰ 852
Bromfed Capsules (Extended-Release) 1785
Bromfed Syrup .... ᴮᴰ 733
Bromfed Tablets....................................... 1785
Bromfed-DM Cough Syrup................... 1786
Bromfed-PD Capsules (Extended-Release) 1785
Children's Vicks DayQuil Allergy Relief .... ᴮᴰ 757
Children's Vicks NyQuil Cold/ Cough Relief.. ᴮᴰ 758
Comtrex Multi-Symptom Cold Reliever Tablets/Caplets/Liqui-Gels/Liquid.. ᴮᴰ 615
Allergy-Sinus Comtrex Multi-Symptom Allergy-Sinus Formula Tablets .... ᴮᴰ 617
Comtrex Multi-Symptom Non-Drowsy Caplets................................... ᴮᴰ 618
Congess... 1004
Contac Day Allergy/Sinus Caplets ᴮᴰ 812
Contac Day & Night .... ᴮᴰ 812
Contac Night Allergy/Sinus Caplets .... ᴮᴰ 812
Contac Severe Cold & Flu Non-Drowsy .... ᴮᴰ 815
Deconamine Chewable Tablets 1320
Deconamine CX Cough and Cold Liquid and Tablets............................... 1319
Deconamine 1320
Deconsal C Expectorant Syrup 456
Deconsal Pediatric Syrup..................... 457
Deconsal II Tablets.................................. 454
Dimetane-DX Cough Syrup 2059
Dimetapp Sinus Caplets .... ᴮᴰ 775
Dorcol Children's Cough Syrup ..... ᴮᴰ 785
Drixoral Cough + Congestion Liquid Caps .... ᴮᴰ 802
Dura-Tap/PD Capsules 2867
Duratuss Tablets...................................... 2565
Duratuss HD Elixir................................... 2565
Efidac/24 .... ᴮᴰ 635
Entex PSE Tablets................................... 1987
Fedahist Gyrocaps.................................. 2401
Fedahist Timecaps 2401
Guaifed... 1787
Guaifed Syrup .... ᴮᴰ 734
Guaimax-D Tablets.................................. 792
Guaitab Tablets .... ᴮᴰ 734
Isoclor Expectorant................................ 990
Kronofed-A 977
Motrin IB Sinus... ᴮᴰ 838
Novahistine DH... 2462
Novahistine DMX .... ᴮᴰ 822
Novahistine Expectorant....................... 2463
Nucofed 2051
PediaCare Cold Allergy Chewable Tablets .... ᴮᴰ 677
PediaCare Cough-Cold Chewable Tablets 1553
PediaCare 1553
PediaCare Infants' Decongestant Drops .... ᴮᴰ 677
PediCare Infant's Drops Decongestant Plus Cough 1553
PediaCare NightRest Cough-Cold Liquid 1553
Pediatric Vicks 44d Dry Hacking Cough & Head Congestion............ ᴮᴰ 763
Pediatric Vicks 44m Cough & Cold Relief .... ᴮᴰ 764
Robitussin Cold & Cough Liqui-Gels .... ᴮᴰ 776
Robitussin Maximum Strength Cough & Cold .... ᴮᴰ 778
Robitussin Pediatric Cough & Cold Formula.. ᴮᴰ 779
Robitussin Severe Congestion Liqui-Gels .... ᴮᴰ 776
Robitussin-DAC Syrup 2074
Robitussin-PE .... ᴮᴰ 778
Rondec Oral Drops 953
Rondec Syrup 953
Rondec Tablet 953
Rondec-DM Oral Drops 954
Rondec-DM Syrup 954
Rondec-TR Tablet 953
Ryna .... ᴮᴰ 841
Seldane-D Extended-Release Tablets 1538
Semprex-D Capsules 463
Semprex-D Capsules 1167
Sinarest Tablets .... ᴮᴰ 648
Sinarest Extra Strength Tablets...... ᴮᴰ 648
Sinarest No Drowsiness Tablets .... ᴮᴰ 648
Sine-Aid IB Caplets 1554
Sine-Aid Maximum Strength Sinus Medication Gelcaps, Caplets and Tablets 1554
Sine-Off No Drowsiness Formula Caplets .... ᴮᴰ 824
Sine-Off Sinus Medicine .... ᴮᴰ 825
Singlet Tablets .... ᴮᴰ 825
Sinutab Non-Drying Liquid Caps .... ᴮᴰ 859
Sinutab Sinus Allergy Medication, Maximum Strength Tablets and Caplets .... ᴮᴰ 860
Sinutab Sinus Medication, Maximum Strength Without Drowsiness Formula, Tablets & Caplets .... ᴮᴰ 860
Sinutab Sinus Medication, Regular Strength Without Drowsiness Formula .... ᴮᴰ 859
Sudafed Children's Liquid .... ᴮᴰ 861
Sudafed Cold and Cough Liquidcaps .... ᴮᴰ 862
Sudafed Cough Syrup .... ᴮᴰ 862
Sudafed Plus Liquid .... ᴮᴰ 862
Sudafed Plus Tablets............................. ᴮᴰ 863
Sudafed Severe Cold Formula Caplets .... ᴮᴰ 863
Sudafed Severe Cold Formula Tablets .... ᴮᴰ 864
Sudafed Sinus Caplets.......................... ᴮᴰ 864
Sudafed Sinus Tablets.......................... ᴮᴰ 864
Sudafed Tablets, 30 mg........................ ᴮᴰ 861
Sudafed Tablets, 60 mg........................ ᴮᴰ 861
Sudafed 12 Hour Caplets .... ᴮᴰ 861
Syn-Rx Tablets 465
Syn-Rx DM Tablets 466
TheraFlu... ᴮᴰ 787
TheraFlu Maximum Strength Nighttime Flu, Cold & Cough Medicine .... ᴮᴰ 788
TheraFlu Maximum Strength Non-Drowsy Formula Flu, Cold & Cough Medicine .... ᴮᴰ 788
Thera Flu Maximum Strength, Non-Drowsy Formula Flu, Cold and Cough Caplets .... ᴮᴰ 789
Triaminic AM Cough and Decongestant Formula .... ᴮᴰ 789
Triaminic AM Decongestant Formula .... ᴮᴰ 790
Triaminic Nite Light .... ᴮᴰ 791
Triaminic Sore Throat Formula ...... ᴮᴰ 791
Tussend 1783
Tussend Expectorant 1785
Children's TYLENOL Cold Multi-Symptom Liquid Formula and Chewable Tablets................................. 1561
Children's TYLENOL Cold Plus Cough Multi Symptom Tablets and Liquid .... ᴮᴰ 681
Infants' TYLENOL Cold Decongestant & Fever-Reducer Drops 1556
TYLENOL Maximum Strength Allergy Sinus Medication Gelcaps and Caplets 1563
TYLENOL Maximum Strength Allergy Sinus NightTime Medication Caplets 1555
TYLENOL Flu Maximum Strength Gelcaps 1565
TYLENOL Flu NightTime, Maximum Strength, Gelcaps 1566
TYLENOL Maximum Strength Flu NightTime Hot Medication Packets 1562
TYLENOL, Maximum Strength, Sinus Medication Geltabs, Gelcaps, Caplets and Tablets 1566
TYLENOL Cold Multi-Symptom Formula Medication Tablets and Caplets 1561
TYLENOL Cold Medication No Drowsiness Formula Gelcaps and Caplets 1562
TYLENOL Cold Multi-Symptom Hot Medication Liquid Packets............... 1557
TYLENOL Cough Multi-Symptom Medication with Decongestant...... 1565
Ursinus Inlay-Tabs.................................. ᴮᴰ 794
Vicks 44 LiquiCaps Cough, Cold & Flu Relief... ᴮᴰ 755
Vicks 44 LiquiCaps Non-Drowsy Cough & Cold Relief .... ᴮᴰ 756
Vicks 44D Dry Hacking Cough & Head Congestion .... ᴮᴰ 755
Vicks 44M Cough, Cold & Flu Relief.. ᴮᴰ 756
Vicks DayQuil .... ᴮᴰ 761
Vicks DayQuil SINUS Pressure & PAIN Relief with IBUPROFEN ...... ᴮᴰ 762
Vicks Nyquil Hot Therapy................... ᴮᴰ 762
Vicks NyQuil LiquiCaps Multi-Symptom Cold/Flu Relief .... ᴮᴰ 763
Vicks NyQuil Multi-Symptom Cold/Flu Relief - (Original & Cherry Flavor).................................... ᴮᴰ 763

Pseudoephedrine Sulfate (Concurrent use may produce additive elevation of blood pressure). Products include:

Cheracol Sinus .... ᴮᴰ 768
Chlor-Trimeton Allergy Decongestant Tablets .... ᴮᴰ 799
Claritin-D 2350
Drixoral Cold and Allergy Sustained-Action Tablets .... ᴮᴰ 802
Drixoral Cold and Flu Extended-Release Tablets................................... ᴮᴰ 803
Drixoral Non-Drowsy Formula Extended-Release Tablets .... ᴮᴰ 803
Drixoral Allergy/Sinus Extended Release Tablets................................... ᴮᴰ 804
Trinalin Repetabs Tablets 1330

Quazepam (Additive CNS depression). Products include:

Doral Tablets 2664

Risperidone (Additive CNS depression). Products include:

Risperdal 1301

Salmeterol Xinafoate (Concurrent use may produce additive elevation of blood pressure). Products include:

Serevent Inhalation Aerosol................ 1176

Secobarbital Sodium (Additive CNS depression). Products include:

Seconal Sodium Pulvules 1474

Selegiline Hydrochloride (Potential for hypertensive crises; concurrent use is contraindicated). Products include:

Eldepryl Tablets 2550

Sotalol Hydrochloride (Concurrent use may produce additive elevation in blood pressure). Products include:

Betapace Tablets 641

Sufentanil Citrate (Additive CNS depression). Products include:

Sufenta Injection 1309

Temazepam (Additive CNS depression). Products include:

Restoril Capsules..................................... 2284

Terbutaline Sulfate (Concurrent use may produce additive elevation of blood pressure). Products include:

Brethaire Inhaler 813
Brethine Ampuls 815
Brethine Tablets....................................... 814
Bricanyl Subcutaneous Injection...... 1502
Bricanyl Tablets 1503

Thiamylal Sodium (Additive CNS depression).

No products indexed under this heading.

Thioridazine Hydrochloride (Additive CNS depression). Products include:

Mellaril 2269

Thiothixene (Additive CNS depression). Products include:

Navane Capsules and Concentrate 2201
Navane Intramuscular 2202

Timolol Hemihydrate (Concurrent use may produce additive elevation in blood pressure). Products include:

Betimol 0.25%, 0.5% .... ◉ 261

Timolol Maleate (Concurrent use may produce additive elevation in blood pressure). Products include:

Blocadren Tablets 1614
Timolide Tablets....................................... 1748
Timoptic in Ocudose 1753
Timoptic Sterile Ophthalmic Solution.. 1751
Timoptic-XE 1755

(ᴮᴰ Described in PDR For Nonprescription Drugs) (◉ Described in PDR For Ophthalmology)

Tranylcypromine Sulfate (Potential for hypertensive crises; concurrent use is contraindicated). Products include:

Parnate Tablets 2503

Triazolam (Additive CNS depression). Products include:

Halcion Tablets 2611

Trifluoperazine Hydrochloride (Additive CNS depression). Products include:

Stelazine 2514

Zolpidem Tartrate (Additive CNS depression). Products include:

Ambien Tablets 2416

HYCOMINE SYRUP

(Hydrocodone Bitartrate, Phenylpropanolamine Hydrochloride) 931

See Hycomine Pediatric Syrup

HYCOTUSS EXPECTORANT SYRUP

(Hydrocodone Bitartrate, Guaifenesin) 933

May interact with central nervous system depressants, narcotic analgesics, antipsychotic agents, tranquilizers, and certain other agents. Compounds in these categories include:

Alfentanil Hydrochloride (Exhibits an additive CNS depression). Products include:

Alfenta Injection 1286

Alprazolam (Exhibits an additive CNS depression). Products include:

Xanax Tablets 2649

Aprobarbital (Exhibits an additive CNS depression).

No products indexed under this heading.

Buprenorphine (Exhibits an additive CNS depression). Products include:

Buprenex Injectable 2006

Buspirone Hydrochloride (Exhibits an additive CNS depression). Products include:

BuSpar 737

Butabarbital (Exhibits an additive CNS depression).

No products indexed under this heading.

Butalbital (Exhibits an additive CNS depression). Products include:

Esgic-plus Tablets 1013
Fioricet Tablets 2258
Fioricet with Codeine Capsules 2260
Fiorinal Capsules 2261
Fiorinal with Codeine Capsules 2262
Fiorinal Tablets 2261
Phrenilin 785
Sedapap Tablets 50 mg/650 mg .. 1543

Chlordiazepoxide (Exhibits an additive CNS depression). Products include:

Libritabs Tablets 2177
Limbitrol 2180

Chlordiazepoxide Hydrochloride (Exhibits an additive CNS depression). Products include:

Librax Capsules 2176
Librium Capsules 2178
Librium Injectable 2179

Chlorpromazine (Exhibits an additive CNS depression). Products include:

Thorazine Suppositories 2523

Chlorpromazine Hydrochloride (Exhibits an additive CNS depression). Products include:

Thorazine 2523

Chlorprothixene (Exhibits an additive CNS depression).

No products indexed under this heading.

Chlorprothixene Hydrochloride (Exhibits an additive CNS depression).

No products indexed under this heading.

Clorazepate Dipotassium (Exhibits an additive CNS depression). Products include:

Tranxene 451

Clozapine (Exhibits an additive CNS depression). Products include:

Clozaril Tablets 2252

Codeine Phosphate (Exhibits an additive CNS depression). Products include:

Actifed with Codeine Cough Syrup.. 1067
Brontex 1981
Deconsal C Expectorant Syrup 456
Deconsal Pediatric Syrup 457
Dimetane-DC Cough Syrup 2059
Empirin with Codeine Tablets 1093
Fioricet with Codeine Capsules 2260
Fiorinal with Codeine Capsules 2262
Isoclor Expectorant 990
Novahistine DH 2462
Novahistine Expectorant 2463
Nucofed 2051
Phenergan with Codeine 2777
Phenergan VC with Codeine 2781
Robitussin A-C Syrup 2073
Robitussin-DAC Syrup 2074
Ryna .... ◻ 841
Soma Compound w/Codeine Tablets 2676
Tussi-Organidin NR Liquid and S NR Liquid 2677
Tylenol with Codeine 1583

Desflurane (Exhibits an additive CNS depression). Products include:

Suprane 1813

Dezocine (Exhibits an additive CNS depression). Products include:

Dalgan Injection 538

Diazepam (Exhibits an additive CNS depression). Products include:

Dizac 1809
Valium Injectable 2182
Valium Tablets 2183
Valrelease Capsules 2169

Droperidol (Exhibits an additive CNS depression). Products include:

Inapsine Injection 1296

Enflurane (Exhibits an additive CNS depression).

No products indexed under this heading.

Estazolam (Exhibits an additive CNS depression). Products include:

ProSom Tablets 449

Ethchlorvynol (Exhibits an additive CNS depression). Products include:

Placidyl Capsules 448

Ethinamate (Exhibits an additive CNS depression).

No products indexed under this heading.

Fentanyl (Exhibits an additive CNS depression). Products include:

Duragesic Transdermal System 1288

Fentanyl Citrate (Exhibits an additive CNS depression). Products include:

Sublimaze Injection 1307

Fluphenazine Decanoate (Exhibits an additive CNS depression). Products include:

Prolixin Decanoate 509

Fluphenazine Enanthate (Exhibits an additive CNS depression). Products include:

Prolixin Enanthate 509

Fluphenazine Hydrochloride (Exhibits an additive CNS depression). Products include:

Prolixin 509

Flurazepam Hydrochloride (Exhibits an additive CNS depression). Products include:

Dalmane Capsules 2173

Glutethimide (Exhibits an additive CNS depression).

No products indexed under this heading.

Haloperidol (Exhibits an additive CNS depression). Products include:

Haldol Injection, Tablets and Concentrate 1575

Haloperidol Decanoate (Exhibits an additive CNS depression). Products include:

Haldol Decanoate 1577

Hydrocodone Polistirex (Exhibits an additive CNS depression). Products include:

Tussionex Pennkinetic Extended-Release Suspension 998

Hydroxyzine Hydrochloride (Exhibits an additive CNS depression). Products include:

Atarax Tablets & Syrup 2185
Marax Tablets & DF Syrup 2200
Vistaril Intramuscular Solution 2216

Isoflurane (Exhibits an additive CNS depression).

No products indexed under this heading.

Ketamine Hydrochloride (Exhibits an additive CNS depression).

No products indexed under this heading.

Levomethadyl Acetate Hydrochloride (Exhibits an additive CNS depression). Products include:

Orlaam 2239

Levorphanol Tartrate (Exhibits an additive CNS depression). Products include:

Levo-Dromoran 2129

Lithium Carbonate (Exhibits an additive CNS depression). Products include:

Eskalith 2485
Lithium Carbonate Capsules & Tablets 2230
Lithonate/Lithotabs/Lithobid 2543

Lithium Citrate (Exhibits an additive CNS depression).

No products indexed under this heading.

Lorazepam (Exhibits an additive CNS depression). Products include:

Ativan Injection 2698
Ativan Tablets 2700

Loxapine Hydrochloride (Exhibits an additive CNS depression). Products include:

Loxitane 1378

Loxapine Succinate (Exhibits an additive CNS depression). Products include:

Loxitane Capsules 1378

Meperidine Hydrochloride (Exhibits an additive CNS depression). Products include:

Demerol 2308
Mepergan Injection 2753

Mephobarbital (Exhibits an additive CNS depression). Products include:

Mebaral Tablets 2322

Meprobamate (Exhibits an additive CNS depression). Products include:

Miltown Tablets 2672
PMB 200 and PMB 400 2783

Mesoridazine (Exhibits an additive CNS depression).

Mesoridazine Besylate (Exhibits an additive CNS depression). Products include:

Serentil 684

Methadone Hydrochloride (Exhibits an additive CNS depression). Products include:

Methadone Hydrochloride Oral Concentrate 2233

Methadone Hydrochloride Oral Solution & Tablets 2235

Methohexital Sodium (Exhibits an additive CNS depression). Products include:

Brevital Sodium Vials 1429

Methotrimeprazine (Exhibits an additive CNS depression). Products include:

Levoprome 1274

Methoxyflurane (Exhibits an additive CNS depression).

No products indexed under this heading.

Midazolam Hydrochloride (Exhibits an additive CNS depression). Products include:

Versed Injection 2170

Molindone Hydrochloride (Exhibits an additive CNS depression). Products include:

Moban Tablets and Concentrate 1048

Morphine Sulfate (Exhibits an additive CNS depression). Products include:

Astramorph/PF Injection, USP (Preservative-Free) 535
Duramorph 962
Infumorph 200 and Infumorph 500 Sterile Solutions 965
MS Contin Tablets 1994
MSIR 1997
Oramorph SR (Morphine Sulfate Sustained Release Tablets) 2236
RMS Suppositories 2657
Roxanol 2243

Opium Alkaloids (Exhibits an additive CNS depression).

No products indexed under this heading.

Oxazepam (Exhibits an additive CNS depression). Products include:

Serax Capsules 2810
Serax Tablets 2810

Oxycodone Hydrochloride (Exhibits an additive CNS depression). Products include:

Percocet Tablets 938
Percodan Tablets 939
Percodan-Demi Tablets 940
Roxicodone Tablets, Oral Solution & Intensol (Oxycodone) 2244
Tylox Capsules 1584

Pentobarbital Sodium (Exhibits an additive CNS depression). Products include:

Nembutal Sodium Capsules 436
Nembutal Sodium Solution 438
Nembutal Sodium Suppositories 440

Perphenazine (Exhibits an additive CNS depression). Products include:

Etrafon 2355
Triavil Tablets 1757
Trilafon 2389

Phenobarbital (Exhibits an additive CNS depression). Products include:

Arco-Lase Plus Tablets 512
Bellergal-S Tablets 2250
Donnatal 2060
Donnatal Extentabs 2061
Donnatal Tablets 2060
Phenobarbital Elixir and Tablets 1469
Quadrinal Tablets 1350

Pimozide (Exhibits an additive CNS depression). Products include:

Orap Tablets 1050

Prazepam (Exhibits an additive CNS depression).

No products indexed under this heading.

Prochlorperazine (Exhibits an additive CNS depression). Products include:

Compazine 2470

Promethazine Hydrochloride (Exhibits an additive CNS depression). Products include:

Mepergan Injection 2753
Phenergan with Codeine 2777

IMPORTANT NOTE: Always consult each drug listing in the patient's regimen for possible interactions.

Phenergan with Dextromethorphan 2778
Phenergan Injection 2773
Phenergan Suppositories 2775
Phenergan Syrup 2774
Phenergan Tablets 2775
Phenergan VC 2779
Phenergan VC with Codeine 2781

Propofol (Exhibits an additive CNS depression). Products include:
Diprivan Injection 2833

Propoxyphene Hydrochloride (Exhibits an additive CNS depression). Products include:
Darvon 1435
Wygesic Tablets 2827

Propoxyphene Napsylate (Exhibits an additive CNS depression). Products include:
Darvon-N/Darvocet-N 1433

Quazepam (Exhibits an additive CNS depression). Products include:
Doral Tablets 2664

Risperidone (Exhibits an additive CNS depression). Products include:
Risperdal 1301

Secobarbital Sodium (Exhibits an additive CNS depression). Products include:
Seconal Sodium Pulvules 1474

Sufentanil Citrate (Exhibits an additive CNS depression). Products include:
Sufenta Injection 1309

Temazepam (Exhibits an additive CNS depression). Products include:
Restoril Capsules 2284

Thiamylal Sodium (Exhibits an additive CNS depression).
No products indexed under this heading.

Thioridazine Hydrochloride (Exhibits an additive CNS depression). Products include:
Mellaril 2269

Thiothixene (Exhibits an additive CNS depression). Products include:
Navane Capsules and Concentrate 2201
Navane Intramuscular 2202

Triazolam (Exhibits an additive CNS depression). Products include:
Halcion Tablets 2611

Trifluoperazine Hydrochloride (Exhibits an additive CNS depression). Products include:
Stelazine 2514

Zolpidem Tartrate (Exhibits an additive CNS depression). Products include:
Ambien Tablets 2416

Food Interactions

Alcohol (Exhibits an additive CNS depression).

HYDELTRASOL INJECTION, STERILE

(Prednisolone Sodium Phosphate) 1665
May interact with oral anticoagulants, potassium sparing diuretics, and certain other agents. Compounds in these categories include:

Amiloride Hydrochloride (Hypokalemia). Products include:
Midamor Tablets 1703
Moduretic Tablets 1705

Aspirin (Aspirin should be used cautiously in conjunction with corticosteroids in hypoprothrombinemia). Products include:
Alka-Seltzer Effervescent Antacid and Pain Reliever ◘ 701
Alka-Seltzer Extra Strength Effervescent Antacid and Pain Reliever ◘ 703
Alka-Seltzer Lemon Lime Effervescent Antacid and Pain Reliever ◘ 703
Alka-Seltzer Plus Cold Medicine ◘ 705
Alka-Seltzer Plus Cold & Cough Medicine ◘ 708
Alka-Seltzer Plus Night-Time Cold Medicine ◘ 707
Alka Seltzer Plus Sinus Medicine ◘ 707
Arthritis Foundation Safety Coated Aspirin Tablets ◘ 675
Arthritis Pain Ascriptin ◘ 631
Maximum Strength Ascriptin ◘ 630
Regular Strength Ascriptin Tablets ◘ 629
Arthritis Strength BC Powder ◘ 609
BC Cold Powder Multi-Symptom Formula (Cold-Sinus-Allergy) ◘ 609
BC Cold Powder Non-Drowsy Formula (Cold-Sinus) ◘ 609
BC Powder ◘ 609
Bayer Children's Chewable Aspirin ◘ 711
Genuine Bayer Aspirin Tablets & Caplets ◘ 713
Extra Strength Bayer Arthritis Pain Regimen Formula ◘ 711
Extra Strength Bayer Aspirin Caplets & Tablets ◘ 712
Extended-Release Bayer 8-Hour Aspirin ◘ 712
Extra Strength Bayer Plus Aspirin Caplets ◘ 713
Extra Strength Bayer PM Aspirin ◘ 713
Bayer Enteric Aspirin ◘ 709
Bufferin Analgesic Tablets and Caplets ◘ 613
Arthritis Strength Bufferin Analgesic Caplets ◘ 614
Extra Strength Bufferin Analgesic Tablets ◘ 615
Cama Arthritis Pain Reliever ◘ 785
Darvon Compound-65 Pulvules 1435
Easprin 1914
Ecotrin 2455
Ecotrin Enteric Coated Aspirin Maximum Strength Tablets and Caplets ◘ 816
Ecotrin Enteric Coated Aspirin Regular Strength Tablets 2455
Empirin Aspirin Tablets ◘ 854
Empirin with Codeine Tablets 1093
Excedrin Extra-Strength Analgesic Tablets & Caplets 732
Fiorinal Capsules 2261
Fiorinal with Codeine Capsules 2262
Fiorinal Tablets 2261
Halfprin 1362
Healthprin Aspirin 2455
Norgesic 1496
Percodan Tablets 939
Percodan-Demi Tablets 940
Robaxisal Tablets 2071
Soma Compound w/Codeine Tablets 2676
Soma Compound Tablets 2675
St. Joseph Adult Chewable Aspirin (81 mg.) ◘ 808
Talwin Compound 2335
Ursinus Inlay-Tabs ◘ 794
Vanquish Analgesic Caplets ◘ 731

Dicumarol (Inhibited response to coumarins).
No products indexed under this heading.

Ephedrine Hydrochloride (Lessened physiologic activity of corticosteroids). Products include:
Primatene Dual Action Formula ◘ 872
Primatene Tablets ◘ 873
Quadrinal Tablets 1350

Ephedrine Sulfate (Lessened physiologic activity of corticosteroids). Products include:
Bronkaid Caplets ◘ 717
Marax Tablets & DF Syrup 2200

Ephedrine Tannate (Lessened physiologic activity to corticosteroids). Products include:
Rynatuss 2673

Live virus vaccines; smallpox (Contraindicated).

Phenobarbital (Lessened physiologic activity of corticosteroids). Products include:
Arco-Lase Plus Tablets 512
Bellergal-S Tablets 2250
Donnatal 2060
Donnatal Extentabs 2061
Donnatal Tablets 2060
Phenobarbital Elixir and Tablets 1469
Quadrinal Tablets 1350

Phenytoin (Lessened physiologic activity of corticosteroids). Products include:
Dilantin Infatabs 1908
Dilantin-125 Suspension 1911

Phenytoin Sodium (Lessened physiologic activity of corticosteroids). Products include:
Dilantin Kapseals 1906
Dilantin Parenteral 1910

Rifampin (Lessened physiologic activity of corticosteroids). Products include:
Rifadin 1528
Rifamate Capsules 1530
Rifater 1532
Rimactane Capsules 847

Spironolactone (Hypokalemia). Products include:
Aldactazide 2413
Aldactone 2414

Triamterene (Hypokalemia). Products include:
Dyazide 2479
Dyrenium Capsules 2481
Maxzide 1380

Warfarin Sodium (Inhibited response to coumarins). Products include:
Coumadin 926

HYDELTRA-T.B.A. STERILE SUSPENSION

(Prednisolone Tebutate) 1667
May interact with oral anticoagulants, potassium sparing diuretics, and certain other agents. Compounds in these categories include:

Amiloride Hydrochloride (Hypokalemia). Products include:
Midamor Tablets 1703
Moduretic Tablets 1705

Aspirin (Aspirin should be used cautiously in conjunction with corticosteroids in hypoprothrombinemia). Products include:
Alka-Seltzer Effervescent Antacid and Pain Reliever ◘ 701
Alka-Seltzer Extra Strength Effervescent Antacid and Pain Reliever ◘ 703
Alka-Seltzer Lemon Lime Effervescent Antacid and Pain Reliever ◘ 703
Alka-Seltzer Plus Cold Medicine ◘ 705
Alka-Seltzer Plus Cold & Cough Medicine ◘ 708
Alka-Seltzer Plus Night-Time Cold Medicine ◘ 707
Alka Seltzer Plus Sinus Medicine ◘ 707
Arthritis Foundation Safety Coated Aspirin Tablets ◘ 675
Arthritis Pain Ascriptin ◘ 631
Maximum Strength Ascriptin ◘ 630
Regular Strength Ascriptin Tablets ◘ 629
Arthritis Strength BC Powder ◘ 609
BC Cold Powder Multi-Symptom Formula (Cold-Sinus-Allergy) ◘ 609
BC Cold Powder Non-Drowsy Formula (Cold-Sinus) ◘ 609
BC Powder ◘ 609
Bayer Children's Chewable Aspirin ◘ 711
Genuine Bayer Aspirin Tablets & Caplets ◘ 713
Extra Strength Bayer Arthritis Pain Regimen Formula ◘ 711
Extra Strength Bayer Aspirin Caplets & Tablets ◘ 712
Extended-Release Bayer 8-Hour Aspirin ◘ 712
Extra Strength Bayer Plus Aspirin Caplets ◘ 713
Extra Strength Bayer PM Aspirin ◘ 713
Bayer Enteric Aspirin ◘ 709
Bufferin Analgesic Tablets and Caplets ◘ 613
Arthritis Strength Bufferin Analgesic Caplets ◘ 614
Extra Strength Bufferin Analgesic Tablets ◘ 615
Cama Arthritis Pain Reliever ◘ 785
Darvon Compound-65 Pulvules 1435
Easprin 1914
Ecotrin 2455
Ecotrin Enteric Coated Aspirin Maximum Strength Tablets and Caplets ◘ 816
Ecotrin Enteric Coated Aspirin Regular Strength Tablets 2455
Empirin Aspirin Tablets ◘ 854
Empirin with Codeine Tablets 1093
Excedrin Extra-Strength Analgesic Tablets & Caplets 732
Fiorinal Capsules 2261
Fiorinal with Codeine Capsules 2262
Fiorinal Tablets 2261
Halfprin 1362
Healthprin Aspirin 2455
Norgesic 1496
Percodan Tablets 939
Percodan-Demi Tablets 940
Robaxisal Tablets 2071
Soma Compound w/Codeine Tablets 2676
Soma Compound Tablets 2675
St. Joseph Adult Chewable Aspirin (81 mg.) ◘ 808
Talwin Compound 2335
Ursinus Inlay-Tabs ◘ 794
Vanquish Analgesic Caplets ◘ 731

Dicumarol (Inhibited response to coumarins).
No products indexed under this heading.

Ephedrine Hydrochloride (Lessened physiologic activity of corticosteroids). Products include:
Primatene Dual Action Formula ◘ 872
Primatene Tablets ◘ 873
Quadrinal Tablets 1350

Ephedrine Sulfate (Lessened physiologic activity of corticosteroids). Products include:
Bronkaid Caplets ◘ 717
Marax Tablets & DF Syrup 2200

Ephedrine Tannate (Lessened physiologic activity of corticosteroids). Products include:
Rynatuss 2673

Phenobarbital (Lessened physiologic activity of corticosteroids). Products include:
Arco-Lase Plus Tablets 512
Bellergal-S Tablets 2250
Donnatal 2060
Donnatal Extentabs 2061
Donnatal Tablets 2060
Phenobarbital Elixir and Tablets 1469
Quadrinal Tablets 1350

Phenytoin (Lessened physiologic activity of corticosteroids). Products include:
Dilantin Infatabs 1908
Dilantin-125 Suspension 1911

Phenytoin Sodium (Lessened physiologic activity of corticosteroids). Products include:
Dilantin Kapseals 1906
Dilantin Parenteral 1910

Rifampin (Lessened physiologic activity of corticosteroids). Products include:
Rifadin 1528
Rifamate Capsules 1530
Rifater 1532
Rimactane Capsules 847

Spironolactone (Hypokalemia). Products include:
Aldactazide 2413
Aldactone 2414

Triamterene (Hypokalemia). Products include:
Dyazide 2479
Dyrenium Capsules 2481
Maxzide 1380

Warfarin Sodium (Inhibited response to coumarins). Products include:
Coumadin 926

HYDERGINE LC LIQUID CAPSULES

(Ergoloid Mesylates) 2265
None cited in PDR database.

(◘ Described in PDR For Nonprescription Drugs) (⊙ Described in PDR For Ophthalmology)

HYDERGINE LIQUID
(Ergoloid Mesylates) 2265
None cited in PDR database.

HYDERGINE ORAL TABLETS
(Ergoloid Mesylates) 2265
None cited in PDR database.

HYDERGINE SUBLINGUAL TABLETS
(Ergoloid Mesylates) 2265
None cited in PDR database.

HYDRASORB STERILE DRESSINGS
(Dressings, sterile)..................................2865
None cited in PDR database.

HYDREA CAPSULES
(Hydroxyurea) 696
None cited in PDR database.

HYDROCET CAPSULES
(Acetaminophen, Hydrocodone Bitartrate) 782

May interact with monoamine oxidase inhibitors, tricyclic antidepressants, central nervous system depressants, antipsychotic agents, narcotic analgesics, antihistamines, and certain other agents. Compounds in these categories include:

Acrivastine (Additive CNS depression). Products include:

Semprex-D Capsules 463
Semprex-D Capsules 1167

Alfentanil Hydrochloride (Additive CNS depression). Products include:

Alfenta Injection 1286

Alprazolam (Additive CNS depression). Products include:

Xanax Tablets 2649

Amitriptyline Hydrochloride (Enhanced effect of either/both drugs). Products include:

Elavil 2838
Endep Tablets 2174
Etrafon 2355
Limbitrol 2180
Triavil Tablets 1757

Amoxapine (Enhanced effect of either/both drugs). Products include:

Asendin Tablets 1369

Aprobarbital (Additive CNS depression).

No products indexed under this heading.

Astemizole (Additive CNS depression). Products include:

Hismanal Tablets 1293

Azatadine Maleate (Additive CNS depression). Products include:

Trinalin Repetabs Tablets 1330

Bromodiphenhydramine Hydrochloride (Additive CNS depression).

No products indexed under this heading.

Brompheniramine Maleate (Additive CNS depression). Products include:

Alka Seltzer Plus Sinus Medicine .. ⊞ 707
Bromfed Capsules (Extended-Release) 1785
Bromfed Syrup .... ⊞ 733
Bromfed Tablets 1785
Bromfed-DM Cough Syrup................... 1786
Bromfed-PD Capsules (Extended-Release).. 1785
Dimetane-DC Cough Syrup 2059
Dimetane-DX Cough Syrup 2059
Dimetapp Elixir .... ⊞ 773
Dimetapp Extentabs .... ⊞ 774
Dimetapp Tablets/Liqui-Gels .... ⊞ 775
Dimetapp Cold & Allergy Chewable Tablets .... ⊞ 773
Dimetapp DM Elixir .... ⊞ 774

Vicks DayQuil Allergy Relief 12-Hour Extended Release Tablets.. ⊞ 760
Vicks DayQuil Allergy Relief 4-Hour Tablets .... ⊞ 760

Buprenorphine (Additive CNS depression). Products include:

Buprenex Injectable 2006

Buspirone Hydrochloride (Additive CNS depression). Products include:

BuSpar 737

Butabarbital (Additive CNS depression).

No products indexed under this heading.

Butalbital (Additive CNS depression). Products include:

Esgic-plus Tablets 1013
Fioricet Tablets 2258
Fioricet with Codeine Capsules 2260
Fiorinal Capsules 2261
Fiorinal with Codeine Capsules 2262
Fiorinal Tablets 2261
Phrenilin 785
Sedapap Tablets 50 mg/650 mg .. 1543

Chlordiazepoxide (Additive CNS depression). Products include:

Libritabs Tablets 2177
Limbitrol 2180

Chlordiazepoxide Hydrochloride (Additive CNS depression). Products include:

Librax Capsules 2176
Librium Capsules 2178
Librium Injectable 2179

Chlorpheniramine Maleate (Additive CNS depression). Products include:

Alka-Seltzer Plus Cold Medicine .... ⊞ 705
Alka-Seltzer Plus Cold Medicine Liqui-Gels .... ⊞ 706
Alka-Seltzer Plus Cold & Cough Medicine .... ⊞ 708
Alka-Seltzer Plus Cold & Cough Medicine Liqui-Gels.......................... ⊞ 705
Allerest Children's Chewable Tablets .... ⊞ 627
Allerest Headache Strength Tablets .... ⊞ 627
Allerest Maximum Strength Tablets .... ⊞ 627
Allerest Sinus Pain Formula .... ⊞ 627
Allerest 12 Hour Caplets .... ⊞ 627
Ana-Kit Anaphylaxis Emergency Treatment Kit 617
Atrohist Pediatric Capsules.................. 453
Atrohist Plus Tablets 454
BC Cold Powder Multi-Symptom Formula (Cold-Sinus-Allergy) ...... ⊞ 609
Cerose DM .... ⊞ 878
Cheracol Plus Head Cold/Cough Formula .... ⊞ 769
Children's Vicks DayQuil Allergy Relief.. ⊞ 757
Children's Vicks NyQuil Cold/Cough Relief.. ⊞ 758
Chlor-Trimeton Allergy Decongestant Tablets .... ⊞ 799
Chlor-Trimeton Allergy Tablets ...... ⊞ 798
Comhist 2038
Comtrex Multi-Symptom Cold Reliever Tablets/Caplets/Liqui-Gels/Liquid.. ⊞ 615
Allergy-Sinus Comtrex Multi-Symptom Allergy-Sinus Formula Tablets .... ⊞ 617
Contac Continuous Action Nasal Decongestant/Antihistamine 12 Hour Capsules..................................... ⊞ 813
Contac Maximum Strength Continuous Action Decongestant/Antihistamine 12 Hour Caplets.. ⊞ 813
Contac Severe Cold and Flu Formula Caplets .... ⊞ 814
Coricidin 'D' Decongestant Tablets .... ⊞ 800
Coricidin Tablets .... ⊞ 800
D.A. Chewable Tablets........................... 951
Deconamine 1320
Dura-Tap/PD Capsules 2867
Dura-Vent/DA Tablets 953
Extendryl 1005
Fedahist Gyrocaps................................. 2401
Fedahist Timecaps 2401
Hycomine Compound Tablets 932
Isoclor Timesule Capsules .... ⊞ 637
Kronofed-A 977

Nolamine Timed-Release Tablets 785
Novahistine DH..................................... 2462
Novahistine Elixir .... ⊞ 823
Ornade Spansule Capsules 2502
PediaCare Cold Allergy Chewable Tablets .... ⊞ 677
PediaCare Cough-Cold Chewable Tablets 1553
PediaCare Cough-Cold Liquid.............. 1553
PediaCare NightRest Cough-Cold Liquid 1553
Pediatric Vicks 44m Cough & Cold Relief .... ⊞ 764
Pyrroxate Caplets .... ⊞ 772
Ryna .... ⊞ 841
Sinarest Tablets .... ⊞ 648
Sinarest Extra Strength Tablets...... ⊞ 648
Sine-Off Sinus Medicine .... ⊞ 825
Singlet Tablets .... ⊞ 825
Sinulin Tablets 787
Sinutab Sinus Allergy Medication, Maximum Strength Tablets and Caplets .... ⊞ 860
Sudafed Plus Liquid .... ⊞ 862
Sudafed Plus Tablets............................. ⊞ 863
Teldrin 12 Hour Antihistamine/Nasal Decongestant Allergy Relief Capsules .... ⊞ 826
TheraFlu.. ⊞ 787
TheraFlu Maximum Strength Nighttime Flu, Cold & Cough Medicine .... ⊞ 788
Triaminic Allergy Tablets .... ⊞ 789
Triaminic Cold Tablets .... ⊞ 790
Triaminic Nite Light .... ⊞ 791
Triaminic Syrup .... ⊞ 792
Triaminic-12 Tablets .... ⊞ 792
Triaminicin Tablets .... ⊞ 793
Triaminicol Multi-Symptom Cold Tablets .... ⊞ 793
Triaminicol Multi-Symptom Relief ⊞ 794
Tussend 1783
Children's TYLENOL Cold Multi-Symptom Liquid Formula and Chewable Tablets................................... 1561
Children's TYLENOL Cold Plus Cough Multi Symptom Tablets and Liquid .... ⊞ 681
TYLENOL Maximum Strength Allergy Sinus Medication Gelcaps and Caplets 1563
TYLENOL Cold Multi-Symptom Formula Medication Tablets and Caplets 1561
TYLENOL Cold Multi-Symptom Hot Medication Liquid Packets.............. 1557
Vicks 44 LiquiCaps Cough, Cold & Flu Relief .... ⊞ 755
Vicks 44M Cough, Cold & Flu Relief.. ⊞ 756

Chlorpheniramine Polistirex (Additive CNS depression). Products include:

Tussionex Pennkinetic Extended-Release Suspension 998

Chlorpheniramine Tannate (Additive CNS depression). Products include:

Atrohist Pediatric Suspension 454
Ricobid Tablets and Pediatric Suspension... 2038
Rynatan 2673
Rynatuss 2673

Chlorpromazine (Additive CNS depression). Products include:

Thorazine Suppositories....................... 2523

Chlorpromazine Hydrochloride (Additive CNS depression). Products include:

Thorazine 2523

Chlorprothixene (Additive CNS depression).

No products indexed under this heading.

Chlorprothixene Hydrochloride (Additive CNS depression).

No products indexed under this heading.

Chlorprothixene Lactate (Additive CNS depression).

No products indexed under this heading.

Clemastine Fumarate (Additive CNS depression). Products include:

Tavist Syrup... 2297
Tavist Tablets 2298
Tavist-1 12 Hour Relief Tablets .... ⊞ 787

Tavist-D 12 Hour Relief Tablets .... ⊞ 787

Clomipramine Hydrochloride (Enhanced effect of either/both drugs). Products include:

Anafranil Capsules 803

Clorazepate Dipotassium (Additive CNS depression). Products include:

Tranxene 451

Clozapine (Additive CNS depression). Products include:

Clozaril Tablets...................................... 2252

Codeine Phosphate (Additive CNS depression). Products include:

Actifed with Codeine Cough Syrup.. 1067
Brontex 1981
Deconsal C Expectorant Syrup 456
Deconsal Pediatric Syrup..................... 457
Dimetane-DC Cough Syrup 2059
Empirin with Codeine Tablets........... 1093
Fioricet with Codeine Capsules 2260
Fiorinal with Codeine Capsules 2262
Isoclor Expectorant................................ 990
Novahistine DH..................................... 2462
Novahistine Expectorant....................... 2463
Nucofed 2051
Phenergan with Codeine 2777
Phenergan VC with Codeine 2781
Robitussin A-C Syrup............................. 2073
Robitussin-DAC Syrup 2074
Ryna .... ⊞ 841
Soma Compound w/Codeine Tablets 2676
Tussi-Organidin NR Liquid and S NR Liquid 2677
Tylenol with Codeine 1583

Cyproheptadine Hydrochloride (Additive CNS depression). Products include:

Periactin 1724

Desflurane (Additive CNS depression). Products include:

Suprane 1813

Desipramine Hydrochloride (Enhanced effect of either/both drugs). Products include:

Norpramin Tablets 1526

Dexchlorpheniramine Maleate (Additive CNS depression).

No products indexed under this heading.

Dezocine (Additive CNS depression). Products include:

Dalgan Injection 538

Diazepam (Additive CNS depression). Products include:

Dizac 1809
Valium Injectable 2182
Valium Tablets 2183
Valrelease Capsules 2169

Diphenhydramine Citrate (Additive CNS depression). Products include:

Excedrin P.M. Analgesic/Sleeping Aid Tablets, Caplets, Liquigels 733

Diphenhydramine Hydrochloride (Additive CNS depression). Products include:

Actifed Allergy Daytime/Nighttime Caplets .... ⊞ 844
Actifed Sinus Daytime/Nighttime Tablets and Caplets .... ⊞ 846
Arthritis Foundation NightTime Caplets .... ⊞ 674
Extra Strength Bayer PM Aspirin .. ⊞ 713
Bayer Select Night Time Pain Relief Formula....................................... ⊞ 716
Benadryl Allergy Decongestant Liquid Medication .... ⊞ 848
Benadryl Allergy Decongestant Tablets .... ⊞ 848
Benadryl Allergy Liquid Medication.. ⊞ 849
Benadryl Allergy .... ⊞ 848
Benadryl Allergy Sinus Headache Formula Caplets .... ⊞ 849
Benadryl Capsules................................. 1898
Benadryl Dye-Free Allergy Liquigel Softgels.. ⊞ 850
Benadryl Dye-Free Allergy Liquid Medication .... ⊞ 850
Benadryl Itch Relief Cream, Children's Formula and Maximum Strength 2% .... ⊞ 851

IMPORTANT NOTE: Always consult each drug listing in the patient's regimen for possible interactions.

Hydrocet **Interactions Index** 490

Benadryl Itch Relief Spray, Children's Formula and Maximum Strength 2% ◘ 851
Benadryl Itch Relief Stick Maximum Strength 2% ◘ 850
Benadryl Itch Stopping Gel, Children's Formula and Maximum Strength 2% ◘ 851
Benadryl Kapseals 1898
Benadryl Injection 1898
Contac Day & Night Cold/Flu Night Caplets ◘ 812
Contac Night Allergy/Sinus Caplets ◘ 812
Extra Strength Doan's P.M. ◘ 633
Legatrin PM ◘ 651
Miles Nervine Nighttime Sleep-Aid ◘ 723
Nytol QuickCaps Caplets ◘ 610
Sleepinal Night-time Sleep Aid Capsules and Softgels ◘ 834
TYLENOL Maximum Strength Allergy Sinus NightTime Medication Caplets 1555
TYLENOL Flu NightTime, Maximum Strength, Gelcaps 1566
TYLENOL Maximum Strength Flu NightTime Hot Medication Packets 1562
TYLENOL PM, Extra Strength Pain Reliever/Sleep Aid Caplets, Geltabs, Gelcaps 1560
TYLENOL Severe Allergy Medication Caplets 1564
Maximum Strength Unisom Sleepgels 1934
Unisom With Pain Relief-Nighttime Sleep Aid and Pain Reliever 1934

Diphenylpyraline Hydrochloride (Additive CNS depression).
No products indexed under this heading.

Doxepin Hydrochloride (Enhanced effect of either/both drugs). Products include:
Sinequan 2205
Zonalon Cream 1055

Droperidol (Additive CNS depression). Products include:
Inapsine Injection 1296

Enflurane (Additive CNS depression).
No products indexed under this heading.

Estazolam (Additive CNS depression). Products include:
ProSom Tablets 449

Ethchlorvynol (Additive CNS depression). Products include:
Placidyl Capsules 448

Ethinamate (Additive CNS depression).
No products indexed under this heading.

Fentanyl (Additive CNS depression). Products include:
Duragesic Transdermal System 1288

Fentanyl Citrate (Additive CNS depression). Products include:
Sublimaze Injection 1307

Fluphenazine Decanoate (Additive CNS depression). Products include:
Prolixin Decanoate 509

Fluphenazine Enanthate (Additive CNS depression). Products include:
Prolixin Enanthate 509

Fluphenazine Hydrochloride (Additive CNS depression). Products include:
Prolixin 509

Flurazepam Hydrochloride (Additive CNS depression). Products include:
Dalmane Capsules 2173

Furazolidone (Enhanced effect of either/both drugs). Products include:
Furoxone 2046

Glutethimide (Additive CNS depression).
No products indexed under this heading.

Haloperidol (Additive CNS depression). Products include:
Haldol Injection, Tablets and Concentrate 1575

Haloperidol Decanoate (Additive CNS depression). Products include:
Haldol Decanoate 1577

Hydrocodone Polistirex (Additive CNS depression). Products include:
Tussionex Pennkinetic Extended-Release Suspension 998

Hydroxyzine Hydrochloride (Additive CNS depression). Products include:
Atarax Tablets & Syrup 2185
Marax Tablets & DF Syrup 2200
Vistaril Intramuscular Solution 2216

Imipramine Hydrochloride (Enhanced effect of either/both drugs). Products include:
Tofranil Ampuls 854
Tofranil Tablets 856

Imipramine Pamoate (Enhanced effect of either/both drugs). Products include:
Tofranil-PM Capsules 857

Isocarboxazid (Enhanced effect of either/both drugs).
No products indexed under this heading.

Isoflurane (Additive CNS depression).
No products indexed under this heading.

Ketamine Hydrochloride (Additive CNS depression).
No products indexed under this heading.

Levomethadyl Acetate Hydrochloride (Additive CNS depression). Products include:
Orlamm 2239

Levorphanol Tartrate (Additive CNS depression). Products include:
Levo-Dromoran 2129

Lithium Carbonate (Additive CNS depression). Products include:
Eskalith 2485
Lithium Carbonate Capsules & Tablets 2230
Lithonate/Lithotabs/Lithobid 2543

Lithium Citrate (Additive CNS depression).
No products indexed under this heading.

Loratadine (Additive CNS depression). Products include:
Claritin 2349
Claritin-D 2350

Lorazepam (Additive CNS depression). Products include:
Ativan Injection 2698
Ativan Tablets 2700

Loxapine Hydrochloride (Additive CNS depression). Products include:
Loxitane 1378

Loxapine Succinate (Additive CNS depression). Products include:
Loxitane Capsules 1378

Maprotiline Hydrochloride (Enhanced effect of either/both drugs). Products include:
Ludiomil Tablets 843

Meperidine Hydrochloride (Additive CNS depression). Products include:
Demerol 2308
Mepergan Injection 2753

Mephobarbital (Additive CNS depression). Products include:
Mebaral Tablets 2322

Meprobamate (Additive CNS depression). Products include:
Miltown Tablets 2672
PMB 200 and PMB 400 2783

Mesoridazine Besylate (Additive CNS depression). Products include:
Serentil 684

Methadone Hydrochloride (Additive CNS depression). Products include:
Methadone Hydrochloride Oral Concentrate 2233
Methadone Hydrochloride Oral Solution & Tablets 2235

Methdilazine Hydrochloride (Additive CNS depression).
No products indexed under this heading.

Methohexital Sodium (Additive CNS depression). Products include:
Brevital Sodium Vials 1429

Methotrimeprazine (Additive CNS depression). Products include:
Levoprome 1274

Methoxyflurane (Additive CNS depression).
No products indexed under this heading.

Midazolam Hydrochloride (Additive CNS depression). Products include:
Versed Injection 2170

Molindone Hydrochloride (Additive CNS depression). Products include:
Moban Tablets and Concentrate 1048

Morphine Sulfate (Additive CNS depression). Products include:
Astramorph/PF Injection, USP (Preservative-Free) 535
Duramorph 962
Infumorph 200 and Infumorph 500 Sterile Solutions 965
MS Contin Tablets 1994
MSIR 1997
Oramorph SR (Morphine Sulfate Sustained Release Tablets) 2236
RMS Suppositories 2657
Roxanol 2243

Nortriptyline Hydrochloride (Enhanced effect of either/both drugs). Products include:
Pamelor 2280

Opium Alkaloids (Additive CNS depression).
No products indexed under this heading.

Oxazepam (Additive CNS depression). Products include:
Serax Capsules 2810
Serax Tablets 2810

Oxycodone Hydrochloride (Additive CNS depression). Products include:
Percocet Tablets 938
Percodan Tablets 939
Percodan-Demi Tablets 940
Roxicodone Tablets, Oral Solution & Intensol (Oxycodone) 2244
Tylox Capsules 1584

Pentobarbital Sodium (Additive CNS depression). Products include:
Nembutal Sodium Capsules 436
Nembutal Sodium Solution 438
Nembutal Sodium Suppositories 440

Perphenazine (Additive CNS depression). Products include:
Etrafon 2355
Triavil Tablets 1757
Trilafon 2389

Phenelzine Sulfate (Enhanced effect of either/both drugs). Products include:
Nardil 1920

Phenobarbital (Additive CNS depression). Products include:
Arco-Lase Plus Tablets 512
Bellergal-S Tablets 2250
Donnatal 2060
Donnatal Extentabs 2061
Donnatal Tablets 2060
Phenobarbital Elixir and Tablets 1469
Quadrinal Tablets 1350

Pimozide (Additive CNS depression). Products include:
Orap Tablets 1050

Prazepam (Additive CNS depression).
No products indexed under this heading.

Prochlorperazine (Additive CNS depression). Products include:
Compazine 2470

Promethazine Hydrochloride (Additive CNS depression). Products include:
Mepergan Injection 2753
Phenergan with Codeine 2777
Phenergan with Dextromethorphan 2778
Phenergan Injection 2773
Phenergan Suppositories 2775
Phenergan Syrup 2774
Phenergan Tablets 2775
Phenergan VC 2779
Phenergan VC with Codeine 2781

Propofol (Additive CNS depression). Products include:
Diprivan Injection 2833

Propoxyphene Hydrochloride (Additive CNS depression). Products include:
Darvon 1435
Wygesic Tablets 2827

Propoxyphene Napsylate (Additive CNS depression). Products include:
Darvon-N/Darvocet-N 1433

Protriptyline Hydrochloride (Enhanced effect of either/both drugs). Products include:
Vivactil Tablets 1774

Pyrilamine Maleate (Additive CNS depression). Products include:
4-Way Fast Acting Nasal Spray (regular & mentholated) ◘ 621
Maximum Strength Multi-Symptom Formula Midol ◘ 722
PMS Multi-Symptom Formula Midol ◘ 723

Pyrilamine Tannate (Additive CNS depression). Products include:
Atrohist Pediatric Suspension 454
Rynatan 2673

Quazepam (Additive CNS depression). Products include:
Doral Tablets 2664

Risperidone (Additive CNS depression). Products include:
Risperdal 1301

Secobarbital Sodium (Additive CNS depression). Products include:
Seconal Sodium Pulvules 1474

Selegiline Hydrochloride (Enhanced effect of either/both drugs). Products include:
Eldepryl Tablets 2550

Sufentanil Citrate (Additive CNS depression). Products include:
Sufenta Injection 1309

Temazepam (Additive CNS depression). Products include:
Restoril Capsules 2284

Terfenadine (Additive CNS depression). Products include:
Seldane Tablets 1536
Seldane-D Extended-Release Tablets 1538

Thiamylal Sodium (Additive CNS depression).
No products indexed under this heading.

Thioridazine Hydrochloride (Additive CNS depression). Products include:
Mellaril 2269

Thiothixene (Additive CNS depression). Products include:
Navane Capsules and Concentrate 2201
Navane Intramuscular 2202

(◘ Described in PDR For Nonprescription Drugs) (⊙ Described in PDR For Ophthalmology)

Interactions Index

Hydrocortone Tablets

Tranylcypromine Sulfate (Enhanced effect of either/both drugs). Products include:

Parnate Tablets 2503

Triazolam (Additive CNS depression). Products include:

Halcion Tablets 2611

Tridihexethyl Chloride (Paralytic ileus).

No products indexed under this heading.

Trifluoperazine Hydrochloride (Additive CNS depression). Products include:

Stelazine 2514

Trihexyphenidyl Hydrochloride (Paralytic ileus). Products include:

Artane 1368

Trimeprazine Tartrate (Additive CNS depression). Products include:

Temaril Tablets, Syrup and Spansule Extended-Release Capsules .. 483

Trimipramine Maleate (Enhanced effect of either/both drugs). Products include:

Surmontil Capsules 2811

Tripelennamine Hydrochloride (Additive CNS depression). Products include:

PBZ Tablets 845
PBZ-SR Tablets 844

Triprolidine Hydrochloride (Additive CNS depression). Products include:

Actifed Plus Caplets .... ◉ 845
Actifed Plus Tablets .... ◉ 845
Actifed with Codeine Cough Syrup.. 1067
Actifed Syrup .... ◉ 846
Actifed Tablets .... ◉ 844

Zolpidem Tartrate (Additive CNS depression). Products include:

Ambien Tablets 2416

Food Interactions

Alcohol (Additive CNS depression).

HYDROCORTONE ACETATE STERILE SUSPENSION

(Hydrocortisone Acetate) 1669

May interact with oral anticoagulants, potassium sparing diuretics, and certain other agents. Compounds in these categories include:

Amiloride Hydrochloride (Hypokalemia). Products include:

Midamor Tablets 1703
Moduretic Tablets 1705

Aspirin (Aspirin should be used cautiously in conjunction with corticosteroids in hypoprothrombinemia). Products include:

Alka-Seltzer Effervescent Antacid and Pain Reliever .... ◉ 701
Alka-Seltzer Extra Strength Effervescent Antacid and Pain Reliever .... ◉ 703
Alka-Seltzer Lemon Lime Effervescent Antacid and Pain Reliever .... ◉ 703
Alka-Seltzer Plus Cold Medicine .... ◉ 705
Alka-Seltzer Plus Cold & Cough Medicine .... ◉ 708
Alka-Seltzer Plus Night-Time Cold Medicine .... ◉ 707
Alka Seltzer Plus Sinus Medicine .. ◉ 707
Arthritis Foundation Safety Coated Aspirin Tablets .... ◉ 675
Arthritis Pain Ascriptin .... ◉ 631
Maximum Strength Ascriptin .... ◉ 630
Regular Strength Ascriptin Tablets .... ◉ 629
Arthritis Strength BC Powder .... ◉ 609
BC Cold Powder Multi-Symptom Formula (Cold-Sinus-Allergy) ...... ◉ 609
BC Cold Powder Non-Drowsy Formula (Cold-Sinus) .... ◉ 609
BC Powder .... ◉ 609
Bayer Children's Chewable Aspirin .... ◉ 711
Genuine Bayer Aspirin Tablets & Caplets .... ◉ 713
Extra Strength Bayer Arthritis Pain Regimen Formula .... ◉ 711
Extra Strength Bayer Aspirin Caplets & Tablets .... ◉ 712
Extended-Release Bayer 8-Hour Aspirin .... ◉ 712
Extra Strength Bayer Plus Aspirin Caplets .... ◉ 713
Extra Strength Bayer PM Aspirin .. ◉ 713
Bayer Enteric Aspirin .... ◉ 709
Bufferin Analgesic Tablets and Caplets .... ◉ 613
Arthritis Strength Bufferin Analgesic Caplets .... ◉ 614
Extra Strength Bufferin Analgesic Tablets .... ◉ 615
Cama Arthritis Pain Reliever .... ◉ 785
Darvon Compound-65 Pulvules 1435
Easprin 1914
Ecotrin 2455
Ecotrin Enteric Coated Aspirin Maximum Strength Tablets and Caplets .... ◉ 816
Ecotrin Enteric Coated Aspirin Regular Strength Tablets 2455
Empirin Aspirin Tablets .... ◉ 854
Empirin with Codeine Tablets 1093
Excedrin Extra-Strength Analgesic Tablets & Caplets 732
Fiorinal Capsules 2261
Fiorinal with Codeine Capsules 2262
Fiorinal Tablets 2261
Halfprin 1362
Healthprin Aspirin 2455
Norgesic 1496
Percodan Tablets 939
Percodan-Demi Tablets 940
Robaxisal Tablets 2071
Soma Compound w/Codeine Tablets 2676
Soma Compound Tablets 2675
St. Joseph Adult Chewable Aspirin (81 mg.) .... ◉ 808
Talwin Compound 2335
Ursinus Inlay-Tabs .... ◉ 794
Vanquish Analgesic Caplets .... ◉ 731

Dicumarol (Inhibited response to coumarins).

No products indexed under this heading.

Ephedrine Hydrochloride (Lessened physiologic activity of corticosteroids). Products include:

Primatene Dual Action Formula ...... ◉ 872
Primatene Tablets .... ◉ 873
Quadrinal Tablets 1350

Ephedrine Sulfate (Lessened physiologic activity of corticosteroids). Products include:

Bronkaid Caplets .... ◉ 717
Marax Tablets & DF Syrup 2200

Ephedrine Tannate (Lessened physiologic activity of corticosteroids). Products include:

Rynatuss 2673

Live virus vaccines; smallpox (Contraindicated).

Phenobarbital (Lessened physiologic activity of corticosteroids). Products include:

Arco-Lase Plus Tablets 512
Bellergal-S Tablets 2250
Donnatal 2060
Donnatal Extentabs 2061
Donnatal Tablets 2060
Phenobarbital Elixir and Tablets 1469
Quadrinal Tablets 1350

Phenytoin (Lessened physiologic activity of corticosteroids). Products include:

Dilantin Infatabs 1908
Dilantin-125 Suspension 1911

Phenytoin Sodium (Lessened physiologic activity of corticosteroids). Products include:

Dilantin Kapseals 1906
Dilantin Parenteral 1910

Rifampin (Lessened physiologic activity of corticosteroids). Products include:

Rifadin 1528
Rifamate Capsules 1530
Rifater 1532
Rimactane Capsules 847

Spironolactone (Hypokalemia). Products include:

Aldactazide 2413
Aldactone 2414

Triamterene (Hypokalemia). Products include:

Dyazide 2479
Dyrenium Capsules 2481
Maxzide 1380

Warfarin Sodium (Inhibited response to coumarins). Products include:

Coumadin 926

HYDROCORTONE PHOSPHATE INJECTION, STERILE

(Hydrocortisone Sodium Phosphate) 1670

May interact with oral anticoagulants, potassium sparing diuretics, and certain other agents. Compounds in these categories include:

Amiloride Hydrochloride (Hypokalemia). Products include:

Midamor Tablets 1703
Moduretic Tablets 1705

Amphotericin B (Cardiac enlargement and congestive failure). Products include:

Fungizone Intravenous 506

Aspirin (Aspirin should be used cautiously in conjunction with corticosteroids in hypoprothrombinemia). Products include:

Alka-Seltzer Effervescent Antacid and Pain Reliever .... ◉ 701
Alka-Seltzer Extra Strength Effervescent Antacid and Pain Reliever .... ◉ 703
Alka-Seltzer Lemon Lime Effervescent Antacid and Pain Reliever .... ◉ 703
Alka-Seltzer Plus Cold Medicine .... ◉ 705
Alka-Seltzer Plus Cold & Cough Medicine .... ◉ 708
Alka-Seltzer Plus Night-Time Cold Medicine .... ◉ 707
Alka Seltzer Plus Sinus Medicine .. ◉ 707
Arthritis Foundation Safety Coated Aspirin Tablets .... ◉ 675
Arthritis Pain Ascriptin .... ◉ 631
Maximum Strength Ascriptin .... ◉ 630
Regular Strength Ascriptin Tablets .... ◉ 629
Arthritis Strength BC Powder .... ◉ 609
BC Cold Powder Multi-Symptom Formula (Cold-Sinus-Allergy) ...... ◉ 609
BC Cold Powder Non-Drowsy Formula (Cold-Sinus) .... ◉ 609
BC Powder .... ◉ 609
Bayer Children's Chewable Aspirin .... ◉ 711
Genuine Bayer Aspirin Tablets & Caplets .... ◉ 713
Extra Strength Bayer Arthritis Pain Regimen Formula .... ◉ 711
Extra Strength Bayer Aspirin Caplets & Tablets .... ◉ 712
Extended-Release Bayer 8-Hour Aspirin .... ◉ 712
Extra Strength Bayer Plus Aspirin Caplets .... ◉ 713
Extra Strength Bayer PM Aspirin .. ◉ 713
Bayer Enteric Aspirin .... ◉ 709
Bufferin Analgesic Tablets and Caplets .... ◉ 613
Arthritis Strength Bufferin Analgesic Caplets .... ◉ 614
Extra Strength Bufferin Analgesic Tablets .... ◉ 615
Cama Arthritis Pain Reliever .... ◉ 785
Darvon Compound-65 Pulvules 1435
Easprin 1914
Ecotrin 2455
Ecotrin Enteric Coated Aspirin Maximum Strength Tablets and Caplets .... ◉ 816
Ecotrin Enteric Coated Aspirin Regular Strength Tablets 2455
Empirin Aspirin Tablets .... ◉ 854
Empirin with Codeine Tablets 1093
Excedrin Extra-Strength Analgesic Tablets & Caplets 732
Fiorinal Capsules 2261
Fiorinal with Codeine Capsules 2262
Fiorinal Tablets 2261
Halfprin 1362
Healthprin Aspirin 2455
Norgesic 1496
Percodan Tablets 939
Percodan-Demi Tablets 940
Robaxisal Tablets 2071
Soma Compound w/Codeine Tablets 2676
Soma Compound Tablets 2675
St. Joseph Adult Chewable Aspirin (81 mg.) .... ◉ 808
Talwin Compound 2335
Ursinus Inlay-Tabs .... ◉ 794
Vanquish Analgesic Caplets .... ◉ 731

Dicumarol (Inhibited response to coumarins).

No products indexed under this heading.

Ephedrine Hydrochloride (Lessened physiologic activity of corticosteroids). Products include:

Primatene Dual Action Formula ...... ◉ 872
Primatene Tablets .... ◉ 873
Quadrinal Tablets 1350

Ephedrine Sulfate (Lessened physiologic activity of corticosteroids). Products include:

Bronkaid Caplets .... ◉ 717
Marax Tablets & DF Syrup 2200

Ephedrine Tannate (Lessened physiologic activity of corticosteroids). Products include:

Rynatuss 2673

Live Virus Vaccines (Contraindicated).

Phenobarbital (Lessened physiologic activity of corticosteroids). Products include:

Arco-Lase Plus Tablets 512
Bellergal-S Tablets 2250
Donnatal 2060
Donnatal Extentabs 2061
Donnatal Tablets 2060
Phenobarbital Elixir and Tablets 1469
Quadrinal Tablets 1350

Phenytoin (Lessened physiologic activity of corticosteroids). Products include:

Dilantin Infatabs 1908
Dilantin-125 Suspension 1911

Phenytoin Sodium (Lessened physiologic activity of corticosteroids). Products include:

Dilantin Kapseals 1906
Dilantin Parenteral 1910

Rifampin (Lessened physiologic activity of corticosteroids). Products include:

Rifadin 1528
Rifamate Capsules 1530
Rifater 1532
Rimactane Capsules 847

Spironolactone (Hypokalemia). Products include:

Aldactazide 2413
Aldactone 2414

Triamterene (Hypokalemia). Products include:

Dyazide 2479
Dyrenium Capsules 2481
Maxzide 1380

Warfarin Sodium (Inhibited response to coumarins). Products include:

Coumadin 926

HYDROCORTONE TABLETS

(Hydrocortisone) 1672

May interact with oral anticoagulants, potassium sparing diuretics, oral hypoglycemic agents, insulin, and certain other agents. Compounds in these categories include:

Acarbose (Increased requirements for hypoglycemic agents in diabetics).

No products indexed under this heading.

IMPORTANT NOTE: Always consult each drug listing in the patient's regimen for possible interactions.

Amiloride Hydrochloride (Hypokalemia). Products include:
- Midamor Tablets ... 1703
- Moduretic Tablets ... 1705

Aspirin (Aspirin should be used cautiously in conjunction with corticosteroids in hypoprothrombinemia). Products include:
- Alka-Seltzer Effervescent Antacid and Pain Reliever ... ▣ 701
- Alka-Seltzer Extra Strength Effervescent Antacid and Pain Reliever ... ▣ 703
- Alka-Seltzer Lemon Lime Effervescent Antacid and Pain Reliever ... ▣ 703
- Alka-Seltzer Plus Cold Medicine ... ▣ 705
- Alka-Seltzer Plus Cold & Cough Medicine ... ▣ 708
- Alka-Seltzer Plus Night-Time Cold Medicine ... ▣ 707
- Alka Seltzer Plus Sinus Medicine .. ▣ 707
- Arthritis Foundation Safety Coated Aspirin Tablets ... ▣ 675
- Arthritis Pain Ascriptin ... ▣ 631
- Maximum Strength Ascriptin ... ▣ 630
- Regular Strength Ascriptin Tablets ... ▣ 629
- Arthritis Strength BC Powder ... ▣ 609
- BC Cold Powder Multi-Symptom Formula (Cold-Sinus-Allergy) ... ▣ 609
- BC Cold Powder Non-Drowsy Formula (Cold-Sinus) ... ▣ 609
- BC Powder ... ▣ 609
- Bayer Children's Chewable Aspirin ... ▣ 711
- Genuine Bayer Aspirin Tablets & Caplets ... ▣ 713
- Extra Strength Bayer Arthritis Pain Regimen Formula ... ▣ 711
- Extra Strength Bayer Aspirin Caplets & Tablets ... ▣ 712
- Extended-Release Bayer 8-Hour Aspirin ... ▣ 712
- Extra Strength Bayer Plus Aspirin Caplets ... ▣ 713
- Extra Strength Bayer PM Aspirin .. ▣ 713
- Bayer Enteric Aspirin ... ▣ 709
- Bufferin Analgesic Tablets and Caplets ... ▣ 613
- Arthritis Strength Bufferin Analgesic Caplets ... ▣ 614
- Extra Strength Bufferin Analgesic Tablets ... ▣ 615
- Cama Arthritis Pain Reliever ... ▣ 785
- Darvon Compound-65 Pulvules ... 1435
- Easprin ... 1914
- Ecotrin ... 2455
- Ecotrin Enteric Coated Aspirin Maximum Strength Tablets and Caplets ... ▣ 816
- Ecotrin Enteric Coated Aspirin Regular Strength Tablets ... 2455
- Empirin Aspirin Tablets ... ▣ 854
- Empirin with Codeine Tablets ... 1093
- Excedrin Extra-Strength Analgesic Tablets & Caplets ... 732
- Fiorinal Capsules ... 2261
- Fiorinal with Codeine Capsules ... 2262
- Fiorinal Tablets ... 2261
- Halfprin ... 1362
- Healthprin Aspirin ... 2455
- Norgesic ... 1496
- Percodan Tablets ... 939
- Percodan-Demi Tablets ... 940
- Robaxisal Tablets ... 2071
- Soma Compound w/Codeine Tablets ... 2676
- Soma Compound Tablets ... 2675
- St. Joseph Adult Chewable Aspirin (81 mg.) ... ▣ 808
- Talwin Compound ... 2335
- Ursinus Inlay-Tabs ... ▣ 794
- Vanquish Analgesic Caplets ... ▣ 731

Chlorpropamide (Increased requirements for hypoglycemic agents in diabetics). Products include:
- Diabinese Tablets ... 1935

Dicumarol (Inhibited response to coumarins).
- No products indexed under this heading.

Ephedrine Hydrochloride (Reduces physiologic activity of corticosteroids). Products include:
- Primatene Dual Action Formula ... ▣ 872
- Primatene Tablets ... ▣ 873
- Quadrinal Tablets ... 1350

Glipizide (Increased requirements for hypoglycemic agents in diabetics). Products include:
- Glucotrol Tablets ... 1967
- Glucotrol XL Extended Release Tablets ... 1968

Glyburide (Increased requirements for hypoglycemic agents in diabetics). Products include:
- DiaBeta Tablets ... 1239
- Glynase PresTab Tablets ... 2609
- Micronase Tablets ... 2623

Insulin, Human (Increased requirements for insulin in diabetics).
- No products indexed under this heading.

Insulin, Human Isophane Suspension (Increased requirements for insulin in diabetics). Products include:
- Novolin N Human Insulin 10 ml Vials ... 1795

Insulin, Human NPH (Increased requirements for insulin in diabetics). Products include:
- Humulin N, 100 Units ... 1448
- Novolin N PenFill Cartridges Durable Insulin Delivery System ... 1798
- Novolin N Prefilled Syringe Disposable Insulin Delivery System ... 1798

Insulin, Human Regular (Increased requirements for insulin in diabetics). Products include:
- Humulin R, 100 Units ... 1449
- Novolin R Human Insulin 10 ml Vials ... 1795
- Novolin R PenFill Cartridges Durable Insulin Delivery System ... 1798
- Novolin R Prefilled Syringe Disposable Insulin Delivery System ... 1798
- Velosulin BR Human Insulin 10 ml Vials ... 1795

Insulin, Human, Zinc Suspension (Increased requirements for insulin in diabetics). Products include:
- Humulin L, 100 Units ... 1446
- Humulin U, 100 Units ... 1450
- Novolin L Human Insulin 10 ml Vials ... 1795

Insulin, NPH (Increased requirements for insulin in diabetics). Products include:
- NPH, 100 Units ... 1450
- Pork NPH, 100 Units ... 1452
- Purified Pork NPH Isophane Insulin ... 1801

Insulin, Regular (Increased requirements for insulin in diabetics). Products include:
- Regular, 100 Units ... 1450
- Pork Regular, 100 Units ... 1452
- Pork Regular (Concentrated), 500 Units ... 1453
- Purified Pork Regular Insulin ... 1801

Insulin, Zinc Crystals (Increased requirements for insulin in diabetics). Products include:
- NPH, 100 Units ... 1450

Insulin, Zinc Suspension (Increased requirements for insulin in diabetics). Products include:
- Iletin I ... 1450
- Lente, 100 Units ... 1450
- Iletin II ... 1452
- Pork Lente, 100 Units ... 1452
- Purified Pork Lente Insulin ... 1801

Metformin Hydrochloride (Increased requirements for hypoglycemic agents in diabetics). Products include:
- Glucophage ... 752

Phenobarbital (Lessened physiologic activity of corticosteroids). Products include:
- Arco-Lase Plus Tablets ... 512
- Bellergal-S Tablets ... 2250
- Donnatal ... 2060
- Donnatal Extentabs ... 2061
- Donnatal Tablets ... 2060
- Phenobarbital Elixir and Tablets ... 1469
- Quadrinal Tablets ... 1350

Phenytoin (Lessened physiologic activity of corticosteroids). Products include:
- Dilantin Infatabs ... 1908
- Dilantin-125 Suspension ... 1911

Phenytoin Sodium (Lessened physiologic activity of corticosteroids). Products include:
- Dilantin Kapseals ... 1906
- Dilantin Parenteral ... 1910

Rifampin (Lessened physiologic activity of corticosteroids). Products include:
- Rifadin ... 1528
- Rifamate Capsules ... 1530
- Rifater ... 1532
- Rimactane Capsules ... 847

Spironolactone (Hypokalemia). Products include:
- Aldactazide ... 2413
- Aldactone ... 2414

Tolazamide (Increased requirements for hypoglycemic agents in diabetics).
- No products indexed under this heading.

Tolbutamide (Increased requirements for hypoglycemic agents in diabetics).
- No products indexed under this heading.

Triamterene (Hypokalemia). Products include:
- Dyazide ... 2479
- Dyrenium Capsules ... 2481
- Maxzide ... 1380

Warfarin Sodium (Inhibited response to coumarins). Products include:
- Coumadin ... 926

HYDRODIURIL TABLETS

(Hydrochlorothiazide) ... **1674**

May interact with antihypertensives, lithium preparations, corticosteroids, cardiac glycosides, insulin, non-steroidal anti-inflammatory agents, barbiturates, narcotic analgesics, oral hypoglycemic agents, bile acid sequestering agents, and certain other agents. Compounds in these categories include:

Acarbose (Dosage adjustment of oral hypoglycemic may be necessary).
- No products indexed under this heading.

Acebutolol Hydrochloride (Potentiation of antihypertensive drugs). Products include:
- Sectral Capsules ... 2807

ACTH (Hypokalemia).
- No products indexed under this heading.

Alfentanil Hydrochloride (Potentiation of orthostatic hypotension). Products include:
- Alfenta Injection ... 1286

Amlodipine Besylate (Potentiation of antihypertensive drugs). Products include:
- Lotrel Capsules ... 840
- Norvasc Tablets ... 1940

Aprobarbital (Potentiation of orthostatic hypotension).
- No products indexed under this heading.

Atenolol (Potentiation of antihypertensive drugs). Products include:
- Tenoretic Tablets ... 2845
- Tenormin Tablets and I.V. Injection 2847

Benazepril Hydrochloride (Potentiation of antihypertensive drugs). Products include:
- Lotensin Tablets ... 834
- Lotensin HCT ... 837
- Lotrel Capsules ... 840

Bendroflumethiazide (Potentiation of antihypertensive drugs).
- No products indexed under this heading.

Betamethasone Acetate (Hypokalemia). Products include:
- Celestone Soluspan Suspension ... 2347

Betamethasone Sodium Phosphate (Hypokalemia). Products include:
- Celestone Soluspan Suspension ... 2347

Betaxolol Hydrochloride (Potentiation of antihypertensive drugs). Products include:
- Betoptic Ophthalmic Solution ... 469
- Betoptic S Ophthalmic Suspension 471
- Kerlone Tablets ... 2436

Bisoprolol Fumarate (Potentiation of antihypertensive drugs). Products include:
- Zebeta Tablets ... 1413
- Ziac ... 1415

Buprenorphine (Potentiation of orthostatic hypotension). Products include:
- Buprenex Injectable ... 2006

Butabarbital (Potentiation of orthostatic hypotension).
- No products indexed under this heading.

Butalbital (Potentiation of orthostatic hypotension). Products include:
- Esgic-plus Tablets ... 1013
- Fioricet Tablets ... 2258
- Fioricet with Codeine Capsules ... 2260
- Fiorinal Capsules ... 2261
- Fiorinal with Codeine Capsules ... 2262
- Fiorinal Tablets ... 2261
- Phrenilin ... 785
- Sedapap Tablets 50 mg/650 mg .. 1543

Captopril (Potentiation of antihypertensive drugs). Products include:
- Capoten ... 739
- Capozide ... 742

Carteolol Hydrochloride (Potentiation of antihypertensive drugs). Products include:
- Cartrol Tablets ... 410
- Ocupress Ophthalmic Solution, 1% Sterile ... ⊙ 309

Chlorothiazide (Potentiation of antihypertensive drugs). Products include:
- Aldoclor Tablets ... 1598
- Diupres Tablets ... 1650
- Diuril Oral ... 1653

Chlorothiazide Sodium (Potentiation of antihypertensive drugs). Products include:
- Diuril Sodium Intravenous ... 1652

Chlorpropamide (Dosage adjustment of oral hypoglycemic may be necessary). Products include:
- Diabinese Tablets ... 1935

Chlorthalidone (Potentiation of antihypertensive drugs). Products include:
- Combipres Tablets ... 677
- Tenoretic Tablets ... 2845
- Thalitone ... 1245

Cholestyramine (Cholestyramine resin has potential of binding hydrochlorothiazide and reducing its absorption from the GI tract by up to 85%). Products include:
- Questran Light ... 769
- Questran Powder ... 770

Clonidine (Potentiation of antihypertensive drugs). Products include:
- Catapres-TTS ... 675

Clonidine Hydrochloride (Potentiation of antihypertensive drugs). Products include:
- Catapres Tablets ... 674
- Combipres Tablets ... 677

(▣ Described in PDR For Nonprescription Drugs) (⊙ Described in PDR For Ophthalmology)

493 **Interactions Index** **HydroDIURIL**

Codeine Phosphate (Potentiation of orthostatic hypotension). Products include:
- Actifed with Codeine Cough Syrup.. 1067
- Brontex 1981
- Deconsal C Expectorant Syrup 456
- Deconsal Pediatric Syrup 457
- Dimetane-DC Cough Syrup 2059
- Empirin with Codeine Tablets........ 1093
- Fioricet with Codeine Capsules 2260
- Fiorinal with Codeine Capsules 2262
- Isoclor Expectorant........ 990
- Novahistine DH........ 2462
- Novahistine Expectorant........ 2463
- Nucofed 2051
- Phenergan with Codeine........ 2777
- Phenergan VC with Codeine 2781
- Robitussin A-C Syrup........ 2073
- Robitussin-DAC Syrup........ 2074
- Ryna .... ▣ 841
- Soma Compound w/Codeine Tablets 2676
- Tussi-Organidin NR Liquid and S NR Liquid 2677
- Tylenol with Codeine 1583

Colestipol Hydrochloride (Colestipol resin has potential of binding hydrochlorothiazide and reducing its absorption from the GI tract by up to 43%). Products include:
- Colestid Tablets 2591

Cortisone Acetate (Hypokalemia). Products include:
- Cortone Acetate Sterile Suspension 1623
- Cortone Acetate Tablets........ 1624

Deserpidine (Potentiation of antihypertensive drugs).
- No products indexed under this heading.

Deslanoside (Resultant hypokalemia may exaggerate cardiac toxicity of digitalis).
- No products indexed under this heading.

Dexamethasone (Hypokalemia). Products include:
- AK-Trol Ointment & Suspension .... ◉ 205
- Decadron Elixir 1633
- Decadron Tablets........ 1635
- Decaspray Topical Aerosol 1648
- Dexacidin Ointment .... ◉ 263
- Maxitrol Ophthalmic Ointment and Suspension .... ◉ 224
- TobraDex Ophthalmic Suspension and Ointment........ 473

Dexamethasone Acetate (Hypokalemia). Products include:
- Dalalone D.P. Injectable 1011
- Decadron-LA Sterile Suspension........ 1646

Dexamethasone Sodium Phosphate (Hypokalemia). Products include:
- Decadron Phosphate Injection 1637
- Decadron Phosphate Respihaler........ 1642
- Decadron Phosphate Sterile Ophthalmic Ointment........ 1641
- Decadron Phosphate Sterile Ophthalmic Solution 1642
- Decadron Phosphate Topical Cream........ 1644
- Decadron Phosphate Turbinaire 1645
- Decadron Phosphate with Xylocaine Injection, Sterile 1639
- Dexacort Phosphate in Respihaler .. 458
- Dexacort Phosphate in Turbinaire .. 459
- NeoDecadron Sterile Ophthalmic Ointment 1712
- NeoDecadron Sterile Ophthalmic Solution 1713
- NeoDecadron Topical Cream 1714

Dezocine (Potentiation of orthostatic hypotension). Products include:
- Dalgan Injection 538

Diazoxide (Potentiation of antihypertensive drugs). Products include:
- Hyperstat I.V. Injection 2363
- Proglycem........ 580

Diclofenac Potassium (Reduced diuretic, natriuretic, and antihypertensive effects). Products include:
- Cataflam 816

Diclofenac Sodium (Reduced diuretic, natriuretic, and antihypertensive effects). Products include:
- Voltaren Ophthalmic Sterile Ophthalmic Solution .... ◉ 272
- Voltaren Tablets........ 861

Digitoxin (Resultant hypokalemia may exaggerate cardiac toxicity of digitalis). Products include:
- Crystodigin Tablets........ 1433

Digoxin (Resultant hypokalemia may exaggerate cardiac toxicity of digitalis). Products include:
- Lanoxicaps 1117
- Lanoxin Elixir Pediatric 1120
- Lanoxin Injection 1123
- Lanoxin Injection Pediatric........ 1126
- Lanoxin Tablets 1128

Diltiazem Hydrochloride (Potentiation of antihypertensive drugs). Products include:
- Cardizem CD Capsules 1506
- Cardizem SR Capsules 1510
- Cardizem Injectable 1508
- Cardizem Tablets........ 1512
- Dilacor XR Extended-release Capsules 2018

Doxazosin Mesylate (Potentiation of antihypertensive drugs). Products include:
- Cardura Tablets 2186

Enalapril Maleate (Potentiation of antihypertensive drugs). Products include:
- Vaseretic Tablets 1765
- Vasotec Tablets 1771

Enalaprilat (Potentiation of antihypertensive drugs). Products include:
- Vasotec I.V........ 1768

Esmolol Hydrochloride (Potentiation of antihypertensive drugs). Products include:
- Brevibloc Injection........ 1808

Etodolac (Reduced diuretic, natriuretic, and antihypertensive effects). Products include:
- Lodine Capsules and Tablets 2743

Felodipine (Potentiation of antihypertensive drugs). Products include:
- Plendil Extended-Release Tablets.... 527

Fenoprofen Calcium (Reduced diuretic, natriuretic, and antihypertensive effects). Products include:
- Nalfon 200 Pulvules & Nalfon Tablets 917

Fentanyl (Potentiation of orthostatic hypotension). Products include:
- Duragesic Transdermal System........ 1288

Fentanyl Citrate (Potentiation of orthostatic hypotension). Products include:
- Sublimaze Injection........ 1307

Fludrocortisone Acetate (Hypokalemia). Products include:
- Florinef Acetate Tablets 505

Flurbiprofen (Reduced diuretic, natriuretic, and antihypertensive effects). Products include:
- Ansaid Tablets 2579

Fosinopril Sodium (Potentiation of antihypertensive drugs). Products include:
- Monopril Tablets 757

Furosemide (Potentiation of antihypertensive drugs). Products include:
- Lasix Injection, Oral Solution and Tablets 1240

Glipizide (Dosage adjustment of oral hypoglycemic may be necessary). Products include:
- Glucotrol Tablets 1967
- Glucotrol XL Extended Release Tablets 1968

Glyburide (Dosage adjustment of oral hypoglycemic may be necessary). Products include:
- DiaBeta Tablets 1239
- Glynase PresTab Tablets 2609
- Micronase Tablets 2623

Guanabenz Acetate (Potentiation of antihypertensive drugs).
- No products indexed under this heading.

Guanethidine Monosulfate (Potentiation of antihypertensive drugs). Products include:
- Esimil Tablets 822
- Ismelin Tablets 827

Hydralazine Hydrochloride (Potentiation of antihypertensive drugs). Products include:
- Apresazide Capsules 808
- Apresoline Hydrochloride Tablets .. 809
- Ser-Ap-Es Tablets 849

Hydrocodone Bitartrate (Potentiation of orthostatic hypotension). Products include:
- Anexsia 5/500 Elixir 1781
- Anexia Tablets........ 1782
- Codiclear DH Syrup 791
- Deconamine CX Cough and Cold Liquid and Tablets........ 1319
- Duratuss HD Elixir........ 2565
- Hycodan Tablets and Syrup 930
- Hycomine Compound Tablets 932
- Hycomine 931
- Hycotuss Expectorant Syrup 933
- Hydrocet Capsules 782
- Lorcet 10/650........ 1018
- Lortab 2566
- Tussend 1783
- Tussend Expectorant 1785
- Vicodin Tablets 1356
- Vicodin ES Tablets 1357
- Vicodin Tuss Expectorant 1358
- Zydone Capsules 949

Hydrocodone Polistirex (Potentiation of orthostatic hypotension). Products include:
- Tussionex Pennkinetic Extended-Release Suspension 998

Hydrocortisone (Hypokalemia). Products include:
- Anusol-HC Cream 2.5%........ 1896
- Aquanil HC Lotion 1931
- Bactine Hydrocortisone Anti-Itch Cream........ ▣ 709
- Caldecort Anti-Itch Hydrocortisone Spray .... ▣ 631
- Cortaid .... ▣ 836
- CORTENEMA........ 2535
- Cortisporin Ointment........ 1085
- Cortisporin Ophthalmic Ointment Sterile 1085
- Cortisporin Ophthalmic Suspension Sterile 1086
- Cortisporin Otic Solution Sterile 1087
- Cortisporin Otic Suspension Sterile 1088
- Cortizone-5 .... ▣ 831
- Cortizone-10........ ▣ 831
- Hydrocortone Tablets 1672
- Hytone 907
- Massengill Medicated Soft Cloth Towelettes........ 2458
- PediOtic Suspension Sterile 1153
- Preparation H Hydrocortisone 1% Cream .... ▣ 872
- ProctoCream-HC 2.5%........ 2408
- VōSoL HC Otic Solution........ 2678

Hydrocortisone Acetate (Hypokalemia). Products include:
- Analpram-HC Rectal Cream 1% and 2.5% 977
- Anusol HC-1 Anti-Itch Hydrocortisone Ointment........ ▣ 847
- Anusol-HC Suppositories 1897
- Caldecort........ ▣ 631
- Carmol HC 924
- Coly-Mycin S Otic w/Neomycin & Hydrocortisone........ 1906
- Cortaid .... ▣ 836
- Cortifoam 2396
- Cortisporin Cream........ 1084
- Epifoam 2399
- Hydrocortone Acetate Sterile Suspension........ 1669
- Mantadil Cream 1135
- Nupercainal Hydrocortisone 1% Cream........ ▣ 645
- Ophthocort........ ◉ 311
- Pramosone Cream, Lotion & Ointment 978
- ProctoCream-HC 2408
- ProctoFoam-HC 2409
- Terra-Cortril Ophthalmic Suspension 2210

Hydrocortisone Sodium Phosphate (Hypokalemia). Products include:
- Hydrocortone Phosphate Injection, Sterile 1670

Hydrocortisone Sodium Succinate (Hypokalemia). Products include:
- Solu-Cortef Sterile Powder........ 2641

Hydroflumethiazide (Potentiation of antihypertensive drugs). Products include:
- Diucardin Tablets........ 2718

Ibuprofen (Reduced diuretic, natriuretic, and antihypertensive effects). Products include:
- Advil Cold and Sinus Caplets and Tablets (formerly CoAdvil) .... ▣ 870
- Advil Ibuprofen Tablets and Caplets .... ▣ 870
- Children's Advil Suspension 2692
- Arthritis Foundation Ibuprofen Tablets .... ▣ 674
- Bayer Select Ibuprofen Pain Relief Formula .... ▣ 715
- Cramp End Tablets .... ▣ 735
- Dimetapp Sinus Caplets .... ▣ 775
- Haltran Tablets........ ▣ 771
- IBU Tablets........ 1342
- Ibuprohm........ ▣ 735
- Children's Motrin Ibuprofen Oral Suspension 1546
- Motrin Tablets........ 2625
- Motrin IB Caplets, Tablets, and Geltabs........ ▣ 838
- Motrin IB Sinus........ ▣ 838
- Motrin Ibuprofen Suspension, Oral Drops, Chewable Tablets, Caplets 1546
- Nuprin Ibuprofen/Analgesic Tablets & Caplets .... ▣ 622
- Sine-Aid IB Caplets 1554
- Vicks DayQuil SINUS Pressure & PAIN Relief with IBUPROFEN ...... ▣ 762

Indapamide (Potentiation of antihypertensive drugs). Products include:
- Lozol Tablets 2022

Indomethacin (Reducted diuretic, natriuretic, and antihypertensive effects). Products include:
- Indocin 1680

Indomethacin Sodium Trihydrate (Reduced diuretic, natriuretic, and antihypertensive effects). Products include:
- Indocin I.V. 1684

Insulin, Human (Altered insulin requirements).
- No products indexed under this heading.

Insulin, Human Isophane Suspension (Altered insulin requirements). Products include:
- Novolin N Human Insulin 10 ml Vials........ 1795

Insulin, Human NPH (Altered insulin requirements). Products include:
- Humulin N, 100 Units........ 1448
- Novolin N PenFill Cartridges Durable Insulin Delivery System 1798
- Novolin N Prefilled Syringe Disposable Insulin Delivery System 1798

Insulin, Human Regular (Altered insulin requirements). Products include:
- Humulin R, 100 Units 1449
- Novolin R Human Insulin 10 ml Vials........ 1795
- Novolin R PenFill Cartridges Durable Insulin Delivery System 1798
- Novolin R Prefilled Syringe Disposable Insulin Delivery System 1798
- Velosulin BR Human Insulin 10 ml Vials........ 1795

IMPORTANT NOTE: Always consult each drug listing in the patient's regimen for possible interactions.

HydroDIURIL | Interactions Index | 494

Insulin, Human, Zinc Suspension (Altered insulin requirements). Products include:
Humulin L, 100 Units 1446
Humulin U, 100 Units 1450
Novolin L Human Insulin 10 ml Vials 1795
Insulin, NPH (Altered insulin requirements). Products include:
NPH, 100 Units 1450
Pork NPH, 100 Units 1452
Purified Pork NPH Isophane Insulin 1801
Insulin, Regular (Altered insulin requirements). Products include:
Regular, 100 Units 1450
Pork Regular, 100 Units 1452
Pork Regular (Concentrated), 500 Units 1453
Purified Pork Regular Insulin 1801
Insulin, Zinc Crystals (Altered insulin requirements). Products include:
NPH, 100 Units 1450
Insulin, Zinc Suspension (Altered insulin requirements). Products include:
Iletin I 1450
Lente, 100 Units 1450
Iletin II 1452
Pork Lente, 100 Units 1452
Purified Pork Lente Insulin 1801
Isradipine (Potentiation of antihypertensive drugs). Products include:
DynaCirc Capsules 2256
Ketoprofen (Reduced diuretic, natriuretic, antihypertensive effects). Products include:
Orudis Capsules 2766
Oruvail Capsules 2766
Ketorolac Tromethamine (Reduced diuretic, natriuretic, and antihypertensive effects). Products include:
Acular 474
Acular .... ⊙ 277
Toradol 2159
Labetalol Hydrochloride (Potentiation of antihypertensive drugs). Products include:
Normodyne Injection 2377
Normodyne Tablets 2379
Trandate 1185
Levorphanol Tartrate (Potentiation of orthostatic hypotension). Products include:
Levo-Dromoran 2129
Lisinopril (Potentiation of antihypertensive drugs). Products include:
Prinivil Tablets 1733
Prinzide Tablets 1737
Zestoretic 2850
Zestril Tablets 2854
Lithium Carbonate (High risk of lithium toxicity). Products include:
Eskalith 2485
Lithium Carbonate Capsules & Tablets 2230
Lithonate/Lithotabs/Lithobid 2543
Lithium Citrate (High risk of lithium toxicity).
No products indexed under this heading.
Losartan Potassium (Potentiation of antihypertensive drugs). Products include:
Cozaar Tablets 1628
Hyzaar Tablets 1677
Mecamylamine Hydrochloride (Potentiation of antihypertensive drugs). Products include:
Inversine Tablets 1686
Meclofenamate Sodium (Reduced diuretic, natriuretic, and antihypertensive effects).
No products indexed under this heading.
Mefenamic Acid (Reduced diuretic, natriuretic, and antihypertensive effects). Products include:
Ponstel 1925
Meperidine Hydrochloride (Potentiation of orthostatic hypotension). Products include:
Demerol 2308
Mepergan Injection 2753
Mephobarbital (Potentiation of orthostatic hypotension). Products include:
Mebaral Tablets 2322
Metformin Hydrochloride (Dosage adjustment of oral hypoglycemic may be necessary). Products include:
Glucophage 752
Methadone Hydrochloride (Potentiation of orthostatic hypotension). Products include:
Methadone Hydrochloride Oral Concentrate 2233
Methadone Hydrochloride Oral Solution & Tablets 2235
Methyclothiazide (Potentiation of antihypertensive drugs). Products include:
Enduron Tablets 420
Methyldopa (Potentiation of antihypertensive drugs). Products include:
Aldoclor Tablets 1598
Aldomet Oral 1600
Aldoril Tablets 1604
Methyldopate Hydrochloride (Potentiation of antihypertensive drugs). Products include:
Aldomet Ester HCl Injection 1602
Methylprednisolone (Hypokalemia). Products include:
Medrol 2621
Methylprednisolone Acetate (Hypokalemia). Products include:
Depo-Medrol Single-Dose Vial 2600
Depo-Medrol Sterile Aqueous Suspension 2597
Methylprednisolone Sodium Succinate (Hypokalemia). Products include:
Solu-Medrol Sterile Powder 2643
Metolazone (Potentiation of antihypertensive drugs). Products include:
Mykrox Tablets 993
Zaroxolyn Tablets 1000
Metoprolol Succinate (Potentiation of antihypertensive drugs). Products include:
Toprol-XL Tablets 565
Metoprolol Tartrate (Potentiation of antihypertensive drugs). Products include:
Lopressor Ampuls 830
Lopressor HCT Tablets 832
Lopressor Tablets 830
Metyrosine (Potentiation of antihypertensive drugs). Products include:
Demser Capsules 1649
Minoxidil (Potentiation of antihypertensive drugs). Products include:
Loniten Tablets 2618
Rogaine Topical Solution 2637
Moexipril Hydrochloride (Potentiation of antihypertensive drugs). Products include:
Univasc Tablets 2410
Morphine Sulfate (Potentiation of orthostatic hypotension). Products include:
Astramorph/PF Injection, USP (Preservative-Free) 535
Duramorph 962
Infumorph 200 and Infumorph 500 Sterile Solutions 965
MS Contin Tablets 1994
MSIR 1997
Oramorph SR (Morphine Sulfate Sustained Release Tablets) 2236
RMS Suppositories 2657
Roxanol 2243
Nabumetone (Reduced diuretic, natriuretic, and antihypertensive effects). Products include:
Relafen Tablets 2510
Nadolol (Potentiation of antihypertensive drugs).
No products indexed under this heading.
Naproxen (Reduced diuretic, natriuretic, and antihypertensive effects). Products include:
Anaprox/Naprosyn 2117
Naproxen Sodium (Reduced diuretic, natriuretic, and antihypertensive effects). Products include:
Aleve 1975
Anaprox/Naprosyn 2117
Nicardipine Hydrochloride (Potentiation of ahtihypertensive drugs). Products include:
Cardene Capsules 2095
Cardene I.V. 2709
Cardene SR Capsules 2097
Nifedipine (Potentiation of antihypertensive drugs). Products include:
Adalat Capsules (10 mg and 20 mg) 587
Adalat CC 589
Procardia Capsules 1971
Procardia XL Extended Release Tablets 1972
Nisoldipine (Potentiation of antihypertensive drugs).
No products indexed under this heading.
Nitroglycerin (Potentiation of antihypertensive drugs). Products include:
Deponit NTG Transdermal Delivery System 2397
Nitro-Bid IV 1523
Nitro-Bid Ointment 1524
Nitrodisc 2047
Nitro-Dur (nitroglycerin) Transdermal Infusion System 1326
Nitrolingual Spray 2027
Nitrostat Tablets 1925
Transderm-Nitro Transdermal Therapeutic System 859
Norepinephrine Bitartrate (Decreased arterial responsiveness to norepinephrine). Products include:
Levophed Bitartrate Injection 2315
Opium Alkaloids (Potentiation of orthostatic hypotension).
No products indexed under this heading.
Oxaprozin (Reduced diuretic, natriuretic, and antihypertensive effects). Products include:
Daypro Caplets 2426
Oxycodone Hydrochloride (Potentiation of orthostatic hypotension). Products include:
Percocet Tablets 938
Percodan Tablets 939
Percodan-Demi Tablets 940
Roxicodone Tablets, Oral Solution & Intensol (Oxycodone) 2244
Tylox Capsules 1584
Penbutolol Sulfate (Potentiation of antihypertensive drugs). Products include:
Levatol 2403
Pentobarbital Sodium (Potentiation of orthostatic hypotension). Products include:
Nembutal Sodium Capsules 436
Nembutal Sodium Solution 438
Nembutal Sodium Suppositories 440
Phenobarbital (Potentiation of orthostatic hypotension). Products include:
Arco-Lase Plus Tablets 512
Bellergal-S Tablets 2250
Donnatal 2060
Donnatal Extentabs 2061
Donnatal Tablets 2060
Phenobarbital Elixir and Tablets 1469
Quadrinal Tablets 1350
Phenoxybenzamine Hydrochloride (Potentiation of antihypertensive drugs). Products include:
Dibenzyline Capsules 2476
Phentolamine Mesylate (Potentiation of antihypertensive drugs). Products include:
Regitine 846
Phenylbutazone (Reduced diuretic, natriuretic, and antihypertensive effects).
No products indexed under this heading.
Pindolol (Potentiation of antihypertensive drugs). Products include:
Visken Tablets 2299
Piroxicam (Reduced diuretic, natriuretic, and antihypertensive effects). Products include:
Feldene Capsules 1965
Polythiazide (Potentiation of antihypertensive drugs). Products include:
Minizide Capsules 1938
Prazosin Hydrochloride (Potentiation of antihypertensive drugs). Products include:
Minipress Capsules 1937
Minizide Capsules 1938
Prednisolone Acetate (Hypokalemia). Products include:
AK-CIDE .... ⊙ 202
AK-CIDE Ointment .... ⊙ 202
Blephamide Liquifilm Sterile Ophthalmic Suspension 476
Blephamide Ointment .... ⊙ 237
Econopred & Econopred Plus Ophthalmic Suspensions .... ⊙ 217
Poly-Pred Liquifilm .... ⊙ 248
Pred Forte .... ⊙ 250
Pred Mild .... ⊙ 253
Pred-G Liquifilm Sterile Ophthalmic Suspension .... ⊙ 251
Pred-G S.O.P. Sterile Ophthalmic Ointment .... ⊙ 252
Vasocidin Ointment .... ⊙ 268
Prednisolone Sodium Phosphate (Hypokalemia). Products include:
AK-Pred .... ⊙ 204
Hydeltrasol Injection, Sterile 1665
Inflamase .... ⊙ 265
Pediapred Oral Liquid 995
Vasocidin Ophthalmic Solution .... ⊙ 270
Prednisolone Tebutate (Hypokalemia). Products include:
Hydeltra-T.B.A. Sterile Suspension 1667
Prednisone (Hypokalemia). Products include:
Deltasone Tablets 2595
Propoxyphene Hydrochloride (Potentiation of orthostatic hypotension). Products include:
Darvon 1435
Wygesic Tablets 2827
Propoxyphene Napsylate (Potentiation of orthostatic hypotension). Products include:
Darvon-N/Darvocet-N 1433
Propranolol Hydrochloride (Potentiation of antihypertensive drugs). Products include:
Inderal 2728
Inderal LA Long Acting Capsules 2730
Inderide Tablets 2732
Inderide LA Long Acting Capsules 2734
Quinapril Hydrochloride (Potentiation of antihypertensive drugs). Products include:
Accupril Tablets 1893
Ramipril (Potentiation of antihypertensive drugs). Products include:
Altace Capsules 1232
Rauwolfia Serpentina (Potentiation of antihypertensive drugs).
No products indexed under this heading.

(▭ Described in PDR For Nonprescription Drugs) (⊙ Described in PDR For Ophthalmology)

Rescinnamine (Potentiation of antihypertensive drugs).
No products indexed under this heading.

Reserpine (Potentiation of antihypertensive drugs). Products include:
Diupres Tablets ... 1650
Hydropres Tablets ... 1675
Ser-Ap-Es Tablets ... 849

Secobarbital Sodium (Potentiation of orthostatic hypotension). Products include:
Seconal Sodium Pulvules ... 1474

Sodium Nitroprusside (Potentiation of antihypertensive drugs).
No products indexed under this heading.

Sotalol Hydrochloride (Potentiation of antihypertensive drugs). Products include:
Betapace Tablets ... 641

Spirapril Hydrochloride (Potentiation of antihypertensive drugs).
No products indexed under this heading.

Sufentanil Citrate (Potentiation of orthostatic hypotension). Products include:
Sufenta Injection ... 1309

Sulindac (Reduced diuretic, natriuretic, and antihypertensive effects). Products include:
Clinoril Tablets ... 1618

Terazosin Hydrochloride (Potentiation of antihypertensive drugs). Products include:
Hytrin Capsules ... 430

Thiamylal Sodium (Potentiation of orthostatic hypotension).
No products indexed under this heading.

Timolol Maleate (Potentiation of antihypertensive drugs). Products include:
Blocadren Tablets ... 1614
Timolide Tablets ... 1748
Timoptic in Ocudose ... 1753
Timoptic Sterile Ophthalmic Solution ... 1751
Timoptic-XE ... 1755

Tolazamide (Dosage adjustment of oral hypoglycemic may be necessary).
No products indexed under this heading.

Tolbutamide (Dosage adjustment of oral hypoglycemic may be necessary).
No products indexed under this heading.

Tolmetin Sodium (Reduced diuretic, natriuretic, and antihypertensive effects). Products include:
Tolectin (200, 400 and 600 mg) .. 1581

Torsemide (Potentiation of antihypertensive drugs). Products include:
Demadex Tablets and Injection ... 686

Triamcinolone (Hypokalemia). Products include:
Aristocort Tablets ... 1022

Triamcinolone Acetonide (Hypokalemia). Products include:
Aristocort A 0.025% Cream ... 1027
Aristocort A 0.5% Cream ... 1031
Aristocort A 0.1% Cream ... 1029
Aristocort A 0.1% Ointment ... 1030
Azmacort Oral Inhaler ... 2011
Nasacort Nasal Inhaler ... 2024

Triamcinolone Diacetate (Hypokalemia). Products include:
Aristocort Suspension (Forte Parenteral) ... 1027
Aristocort Suspension (Intralesional) ... 1025

Triamcinolone Hexacetonide (Hypokalemia). Products include:
Aristospan Suspension (Intra-articular) ... 1033
Aristospan Suspension (Intralesional) ... 1032

Trimethaphan Camsylate (Potentiation of antihypertensive drugs). Products include:
Arfonad Ampuls ... 2080

Tubocurarine Chloride (Increased responsiveness to tubocurarine).
No products indexed under this heading.

Verapamil Hydrochloride (Potentiation of antihypertensive drugs). Products include:
Calan SR Caplets ... 2422
Calan Tablets ... 2419
Isoptin Injectable ... 1344
Isoptin Oral Tablets ... 1346
Isoptin SR Tablets ... 1348
Verelan Capsules ... 1410
Verelan Capsules ... 2824

Food Interactions

Alcohol (Potentiation of orthostatic hypotension).

HYDROPRES TABLETS

(Reserpine, Hydrochlorothiazide) 1675
May interact with antihypertensives, lithium preparations, corticosteroids, insulin, non-steroidal anti-inflammatory agents, barbiturates, narcotic analgesics, monoamine oxidase inhibitors, oral hypoglycemic agents, cardiac glycosides, bile acid sequestering agents, and certain other agents. Compounds in these categories include:

Acarbose (Dosage adjustment of the antidiabetic drug may be required).
No products indexed under this heading.

Acebutolol Hydrochloride (Potentiation of antihypertensive drugs). Products include:
Sectral Capsules ... 2807

ACTH (Hypokalemia).
No products indexed under this heading.

Alfentanil Hydrochloride (Potentiation of orthostatic hypotension; enhanced CNS depressant effects of reserpine). Products include:
Alfenta Injection ... 1286

Amlodipine Besylate (Potentiation of antihypertensive drugs). Products include:
Lotrel Capsules ... 840
Norvasc Tablets ... 1940

Aprobarbital (Potentiation of orthostatic hypotension; enhanced CNS depressant effects of reserpine).
No products indexed under this heading.

Atenolol (Potentiation of antihypertensive drugs). Products include:
Tenoretic Tablets ... 2845
Tenormin Tablets and I.V. Injection 2847

Benazepril Hydrochloride (Potentiation of antihypertensive drugs). Products include:
Lotensin Tablets ... 834
Lotensin HCT ... 837
Lotrel Capsules ... 840

Bendroflumethiazide (Potentiation of antihypertensive drugs).
No products indexed under this heading.

Betamethasone Acetate (Hypokalemia). Products include:
Celestone Soluspan Suspension ... 2347

Betamethasone Sodium Phosphate (Hypokalemia). Products include:
Celestone Soluspan Suspension ... 2347

Betaxolol Hydrochloride (Potentiation of antihypertensive drugs). Products include:
Betoptic Ophthalmic Solution ... 469
Betoptic S Ophthalmic Suspension 471
Kerlone Tablets ... 2436

Bisoprolol Fumarate (Potentiation of antihypertensive drugs). Products include:
Zebeta Tablets ... 1413
Ziac ... 1415

Buprenorphine (Potentiation of orthostatic hypotension; enhanced CNS depressant effects of reserpine). Products include:
Buprenex Injectable ... 2006

Butabarbital (Potentiation of orthostatic hypotension; enhanced CNS depressant effects of reserpine).
No products indexed under this heading.

Butalbital (Potentiation of orthostatic hypotension; enhanced CNS depressant effects of reserpine). Products include:
Esgic-plus Tablets ... 1013
Fioricet Tablets ... 2258
Fioricet with Codeine Capsules ... 2260
Fiorinal Capsules ... 2261
Fiorinal with Codeine Capsules ... 2262
Fiorinal Tablets ... 2261
Phrenilin ... 785
Sedapap Tablets 50 mg/650 mg .. 1543

Captopril (Potentiation of antihypertensive drugs). Products include:
Capoten ... 739
Capozide ... 742

Carteolol Hydrochloride (Potentiation of antihypertensive drugs). Products include:
Cartrol Tablets ... 410
Ocupress Ophthalmic Solution, 1% Sterile ... ◉ 309

Chlorothiazide (Potentiation of antihypertensive drugs). Products include:
Aldoclor Tablets ... 1598
Diupres Tablets ... 1650
Diuril Oral ... 1653

Chlorothiazide Sodium (Potentiation of antihypertensive drugs). Products include:
Diuril Sodium Intravenous ... 1652

Chlorpropamide (Dosage adjustment of the antidiabetic drug may be required). Products include:
Diabinese Tablets ... 1935

Chlorthalidone (Potentiation of antihypertensive drugs). Products include:
Combipres Tablets ... 677
Tenoretic Tablets ... 2845
Thalitone ... 1245

Cholestyramine (Cholestyramine resin has potential of binding hydrochlorothiazide and reducing its absorption from the GI tract by up to 85%). Products include:
Questran Light ... 769
Questran Powder ... 770

Clobetasol Propionate (Hypokalemia). Products include:
Temovate ... 1179

Clonidine (Potentiation of antihypertensive drugs). Products include:
Catapres-TTS ... 675

Clonidine Hydrochloride (Potentiation of antihypertensive drugs). Products include:
Catapres Tablets ... 674
Combipres Tablets ... 677

Codeine Phosphate (Potentiation of orthostatic hypotension; enhanced CNS depressant effects of reserpine). Products include:
Actifed with Codeine Cough Syrup.. 1067
Brontex ... 1981
Deconsal C Expectorant Syrup ... 456
Deconsal Pediatric Syrup ... 457
Dimetane-DC Cough Syrup ... 2059
Empirin with Codeine Tablets ... 1093
Fioricet with Codeine Capsules ... 2260
Fiorinal with Codeine Capsules ... 2262
Isoclor Expectorant ... 990
Novahistine DH ... 2462
Novahistine Expectorant ... 2463
Nucofed ... 2051
Phenergan with Codeine ... 2777
Phenergan VC with Codeine ... 2781
Robitussin A-C Syrup ... 2073
Robitussin-DAC Syrup ... 2074
Ryna ... ⊞ 841
Soma Compound w/Codeine Tablets ... 2676
Tussi-Organidin NR Liquid and S NR Liquid ... 2677
Tylenol with Codeine ... 1583

Colestipol Hydrochloride (Colestipol resin has potential of binding hydrochlorothiazide and reducing its absorption from the GI tract by up to 43%). Products include:
Colestid Tablets ... 2591

Cortisone Acetate (Hypokalemia). Products include:
Cortone Acetate Sterile Suspension ... 1623
Cortone Acetate Tablets ... 1624

Deserpidine (Potentiation of antihypertensive drugs).
No products indexed under this heading.

Deslanoside (Use cautiously; cardiac arrhythmias have occurred with reserpine).
No products indexed under this heading.

Dexamethasone (Hypokalemia). Products include:
AK-Trol Ointment & Suspension ... ◉ 205
Decadron Elixir ... 1633
Decadron Tablets ... 1635
Decaspray Topical Aerosol ... 1648
Dexacidin Ointment ... ◉ 263
Maxitrol Ophthalmic Ointment and Suspension ... ◉ 224
TobraDex Ophthalmic Suspension and Ointment ... 473

Dexamethasone Acetate (Hypokalemia). Products include:
Dalalone D.P. Injectable ... 1011
Decadron-LA Sterile Suspension ... 1646

Dexamethasone Sodium Phosphate (Hypokalemia). Products include:
Decadron Phosphate Injection ... 1637
Decadron Phosphate Respihaler ... 1642
Decadron Phosphate Sterile Ophthalmic Ointment ... 1641
Decadron Phosphate Sterile Ophthalmic Solution ... 1642
Decadron Phosphate Topical Cream ... 1644
Decadron Phosphate Turbinaire ... 1645
Decadron Phosphate with Xylocaine Injection, Sterile ... 1639
Dexacort Phosphate in Respihaler .. 458
Dexacort Phosphate in Turbinaire .. 459
NeoDecadron Sterile Ophthalmic Ointment ... 1712
NeoDecadron Sterile Ophthalmic Solution ... 1713
NeoDecadron Topical Cream ... 1714

Dezocine (Potentiation of orthostatic hypotension; enhanced CNS depressant effects of reserpine). Products include:
Dalgan Injection ... 538

Diazoxide (Potentiation of antihypertensive drugs). Products include:
Hyperstat I.V. Injection ... 2363
Proglycem ... 580

Diclofenac Potassium (Reduced diuretic, natriuretic, and antihypertensive effects). Products include:
Cataflam ... 816

Diclofenac Sodium (Reduced diuretic, natriuretic, and antihypertensive effects). Products include:
Voltaren Ophthalmic Sterile Ophthalmic Solution ... ◉ 272
Voltaren Tablets ... 861

IMPORTANT NOTE: Always consult each drug listing in the patient's regimen for possible interactions.

Hydropres **Interactions Index** 496

Digitoxin (Use cautiously; cardiac arrhythmias have occurred with reserpine). Products include:
Crystodigin Tablets 1433

Digoxin (Use cautiously; cardiac arrhythmias have occurred with reserpine). Products include:
Lanoxicaps 1117
Lanoxin Elixir Pediatric 1120
Lanoxin Injection 1123
Lanoxin Injection Pediatric 1126
Lanoxin Tablets 1128

Diltiazem Hydrochloride (Potentiation of antihypertensive drugs). Products include:
Cardizem CD Capsules 1506
Cardizem SR Capsules 1510
Cardizem Injectable 1508
Cardizem Tablets 1512
Dilacor XR Extended-release Capsules 2018

Doxazosin Mesylate (Potentiation of antihypertensive drugs). Products include:
Cardura Tablets 2186

Enalapril Maleate (Potentiation of antihypertensive drugs). Products include:
Vaseretic Tablets 1765
Vasotec Tablets 1771

Enalaprilat (Potentiation of antihypertensive drugs). Products include:
Vasotec I.V. 1768

Esmolol Hydrochloride (Potentiation of antihypertensive drugs). Products include:
Brevibloc Injection 1808

Etodolac (Reduced diuretic, natriuretic, and antihypertensive effects). Products include:
Lodine Capsules and Tablets 2743

Felodipine (Potentiation of antihypertensive drugs). Products include:
Plendil Extended-Release Tablets 527

Fenoprofen Calcium (Reduced diuretic, natriuretic, and antihypertensive effects). Products include:
Nalfon 200 Pulvules & Nalfon Tablets 917

Fentanyl (Potentiation of orthostatic hypotension; enhanced CNS depressant effects of reserpine). Products include:
Duragesic Transdermal System 1288

Fentanyl Citrate (Potentiation of orthostatic hypotension; enhanced CNS depressant effects of reserpine). Products include:
Sublimaze Injection 1307

Fludrocortisone Acetate (Hypokalemia). Products include:
Florinef Acetate Tablets 505

Flurbiprofen (Reduced diuretic, natriuretic, and antihypertensive effects). Products include:
Ansaid Tablets 2579

Fosinopril Sodium (Potentiation of antihypertensive drugs). Products include:
Monopril Tablets 757

Furazolidone (Concurrent use is contraindicated). Products include:
Furoxone 2046

Furosemide (Potentiation of antihypertensive drugs). Products include:
Lasix Injection, Oral Solution and Tablets 1240

Glipizide (Dosage adjustment of the antidiabetic drug may be required). Products include:
Glucotrol Tablets 1967
Glucotrol XL Extended Release Tablets 1968

Glyburide (Dosage adjustment of the antidiabetic drug may be required). Products include:
DiaBeta Tablets 1239
Glynase PresTab Tablets 2609
Micronase Tablets 2623

Guanabenz Acetate (Potentiation of antihypertensive drugs).
No products indexed under this heading.

Guanethidine Monosulfate (Potentiation of antihypertensive drugs). Products include:
Esimil Tablets 822
Ismelin Tablets 827

Hydralazine Hydrochloride (Potentiation of antihypertensive drugs). Products include:
Apresazide Capsules 808
Apresoline Hydrochloride Tablets 809
Ser-Ap-Es Tablets 849

Hydrocodone Bitartrate (Potentiation of orthostatic hypotension; enhanced CNS depressant effects of reserpine). Products include:
Anexsia 5/500 Elixir 1781
Anexia Tablets 1782
Codiclear DH Syrup 791
Deconamine CX Cough and Cold Liquid and Tablets 1319
Duratuss HD Elixir 2565
Hycodan Tablets and Syrup 930
Hycomine Compound Tablets 932
Hycomine 931
Hycotuss Expectorant Syrup 933
Hydrocet Capsules 782
Lorcet 10/650 1018
Lortab 2566
Tussend 1783
Tussend Expectorant 1785
Vicodin Tablets 1356
Vicodin ES Tablets 1357
Vicodin Tuss Expectorant 1358
Zydone Capsules 949

Hydrocodone Polistirex (Potentiation of orthostatic hypotension; enhanced CNS depressant effects of reserpine). Products include:
Tussionex Pennkinetic Extended-Release Suspension 998

Hydrocortisone (Hypokalemia). Products include:
Anusol-HC Cream 2.5% 1896
Aquanil HC Lotion 1931
Bactine Hydrocortisone Anti-Itch Cream .... ▣ 709
Caldecort Anti-Itch Hydrocortisone Spray .... ▣ 631
Cortaid .... ▣ 836
CORTENEMA 2535
Cortisporin Ointment 1085
Cortisporin Ophthalmic Ointment Sterile 1085
Cortisporin Ophthalmic Suspension Sterile 1086
Cortisporin Otic Solution Sterile 1087
Cortisporin Otic Suspension Sterile 1088
Cortizone-5 .... ▣ 831
Cortizone-10 .... ▣ 831
Hydrocortone Tablets 1672
Hytone 907
Massengill Medicated Soft Cloth Towelettes 2458
PediOtic Suspension Sterile 1153
Preparation H Hydrocortisone 1% Cream .... ▣ 872
ProctoCream-HC 2.5% 2408
VōSoL HC Otic Solution 2678

Hydrocortisone Acetate (Hypokalemia). Products include:
Analpram-HC Rectal Cream 1% and 2.5% 977
Anusol HC-1 Anti-Itch Hydrocortisone Ointment .... ▣ 847
Anusol-HC Suppositories 1897
Caldecort .... ▣ 631
Carmol HC 924
Coly-Mycin S Otic w/Neomycin & Hydrocortisone 1906
Cortaid .... ▣ 836
Cortifoam 2396
Cortisporin Cream 1084
Epifoam 2399
Hydrocortone Acetate Sterile Suspension 1669
Mantadil Cream 1135
Nupercainal Hydrocortisone 1% Cream .... ▣ 645
Ophthocort .... ⊙ 311
Pramosone Cream, Lotion & Ointment 978
ProctoCream-HC 2408
ProctoFoam-HC 2409
Terra-Cortril Ophthalmic Suspension 2210

Hydrocortisone Sodium Phosphate (Hypokalemia). Products include:
Hydrocortone Phosphate Injection, Sterile 1670

Hydrocortisone Sodium Succinate (Hypokalemia). Products include:
Solu-Cortef Sterile Powder 2641

Hydroflumethiazide (Potentiation of antihypertensive drugs). Products include:
Diucardin Tablets 2718

Ibuprofen (Reduced diuretic, natriuretic, and antihypertensive effects). Products include:
Advil Cold and Sinus Caplets and Tablets (formerly CoAdvil) .... ▣ 870
Advil Ibuprofen Tablets and Caplets .... ▣ 870
Children's Advil Suspension 2692
Arthritis Foundation Ibuprofen Tablets .... ▣ 674
Bayer Select Ibuprofen Pain Relief Formula .... ▣ 715
Cramp End Tablets .... ▣ 735
Dimetapp Sinus Caplets .... ▣ 775
Haltran Tablets .... ▣ 771
IBU Tablets 1342
Ibuprohm .... ▣ 735
Children's Motrin Ibuprofen Oral Suspension 1546
Motrin Tablets 2625
Motrin IB Caplets, Tablets, and Geltabs .... ▣ 838
Motrin IB Sinus .... ▣ 838
Motrin Ibuprofen Suspension, Oral Drops, Chewable Tablets, Caplets 1546
Nuprin Ibuprofen/Analgesic Tablets & Caplets .... ▣ 622
Sine-Aid IB Caplets 1554
Vicks DayQuil SINUS Pressure & PAIN Relief with IBUPROFEN .... ▣ 762

Indapamide (Potentiation of antihypertensive drugs). Products include:
Lozol Tablets 2022

Indomethacin (Reduced diuretic, natriuretic, and antihypertensive effects). Products include:
Indocin 1680

Indomethacin Sodium Trihydrate (Reduced diuretic, natriuretic, and antihypertensive effects). Products include:
Indocin I.V. 1684

Insulin, Human (Altered insulin requirements).
No products indexed under this heading.

Insulin, Human Isophane Suspension (Altered insulin requirements). Products include:
Novolin N Human Insulin 10 ml Vials 1795

Insulin, Human NPH (Altered insulin requirements). Products include:
Humulin N, 100 Units 1448
Novolin N PenFill Cartridges Durable Insulin Delivery System 1798
Novolin N Prefilled Syringe Disposable Insulin Delivery System 1798

Insulin, Human Regular (Altered insulin requirements). Products include:
Humulin R, 100 Units 1449
Novolin R Human Insulin 10 ml Vials 1795
Novolin R PenFill Cartridges Durable Insulin Delivery System 1798
Novolin R Prefilled Syringe Disposable Insulin Delivery System 1798
Velosulin BR Human Insulin 10 ml Vials 1795

Insulin, Human, Zinc Suspension (Altered insulin requirements). Products include:
Humulin L, 100 Units 1446
Humulin U, 100 Units 1450
Novolin L Human Insulin 10 ml Vials 1795

Insulin, NPH (Altered insulin requirements). Products include:
NPH, 100 Units 1450
Pork NPH, 100 Units 1452
Purified Pork NPH Isophane Insulin 1801

Insulin, Regular (Altered insulin requirements). Products include:
Regular, 100 Units 1450
Pork Regular, 100 Units 1452
Pork Regular (Concentrated), 500 Units 1453
Purified Pork Regular Insulin 1801

Insulin, Zinc Crystals (Altered insulin requirements). Products include:
NPH, 100 Units 1450

Insulin, Zinc Suspension (Altered insulin requirements). Products include:
Iletin I 1450
Lente, 100 Units 1450
Iletin II 1452
Pork Lente, 100 Units 1452
Purified Pork Lente Insulin 1801

Isocarboxazid (Concurrent use is contraindicated).
No products indexed under this heading.

Isradipine (Potentiation of antihypertensive drugs). Products include:
DynaCirc Capsules 2256

Ketoprofen (Reduced diuretic, natriuretic, and antihypertensive effects). Products include:
Orudis Capsules 2766
Oruvail Capsules 2766

Ketorolac Tromethamine (Reduced diuretic, natriuretic, and antihypertensive effects). Products include:
Acular 474
Acular .... ⊙ 277
Toradol 2159

Labetalol Hydrochloride (Potentiation of antihypertensive drugs). Products include:
Normodyne Injection 2377
Normodyne Tablets 2379
Trandate 1185

Levorphanol Tartrate (Potentiation of orthostatic hypotension; enhanced CNS depressant effects of reserpine). Products include:
Levo-Dromoran 2129

Lisinopril (Potentiation of antihypertensive drugs). Products include:
Prinivil Tablets 1733
Prinzide Tablets 1737
Zestoretic 2850
Zestril Tablets 2854

Lithium Carbonate (High risk of lithium toxicity). Products include:
Eskalith 2485
Lithium Carbonate Capsules & Tablets 2230
Lithonate/Lithotabs/Lithobid 2543

Lithium Citrate (High risk of lithium toxicity).
No products indexed under this heading.

Losartan Potassium (Potentiation of antihypertensive drugs). Products include:
Cozaar Tablets 1628
Hyzaar Tablets 1677

Mecamylamine Hydrochloride (Potentiation of antihypertensive drugs). Products include:
Inversine Tablets 1686

(▣ Described in PDR For Nonprescription Drugs) (⊙ Described in PDR For Ophthalmology)

497 **Interactions Index** **Hydropres**

Meclofenamate Sodium (Reduced diuretic, natriuretic, and antihypertensive effects).
No products indexed under this heading.

Mefenamic Acid (Reduced diuretic, natriuretic, and antihypertensive effects). Products include:
Ponstel 1925

Meperidine Hydrochloride (Potentiation of orthostatic hypotension; enhanced CNS depressant effects of reserpine). Products include:
Demerol 2308
Mepergan Injection 2753

Mephobarbital (Potentiation of orthostatic hypotension; enhanced CNS depressant effects of reserpine). Products include:
Mebaral Tablets 2322

Metformin Hydrochloride (Dosage adjustment of the antidiabetic drug may be required). Products include:
Glucophage 752

Methadone Hydrochloride (Potentiation of orthostatic hypotension; enhanced CNS depressant effects of reserpine). Products include:
Methadone Hydrochloride Oral Concentrate 2233
Methadone Hydrochloride Oral Solution & Tablets 2235

Methyclothiazide (Potentiation of antihypertensive drugs). Products include:
Enduron Tablets 420

Methyldopa (Potentiation of antihypertensive drugs). Products include:
Aldoclor Tablets 1598
Aldomet Oral 1600
Aldoril Tablets 1604

Methyldopate Hydrochloride (Potentiation of antihypertensive drugs). Products include:
Aldomet Ester HCl Injection 1602

Methylprednisolone Acetate (Hypokalemia). Products include:
Depo-Medrol Single-Dose Vial 2600
Depo-Medrol Sterile Aqueous Suspension 2597

Methylprednisolone Sodium Succinate (Hypokalemia). Products include:
Solu-Medrol Sterile Powder 2643

Metolazone (Potentiation of antihypertensive drugs). Products include:
Mykrox Tablets 993
Zaroxolyn Tablets 1000

Metoprolol Succinate (Potentiation of antihypertensive drugs). Products include:
Toprol-XL Tablets 565

Metoprolol Tartrate (Potentiation of antihypertensive drugs). Products include:
Lopressor Ampuls 830
Lopressor HCT Tablets 832
Lopressor Tablets 830

Metyrosine (Potentiation of antihypertensive drugs). Products include:
Demser Capsules 1649

Minoxidil (Potentiation of antihypertensive drugs). Products include:
Loniten Tablets 2618
Rogaine Topical Solution 2637

Moexipril Hydrochloride (Potentiation of antihypertensive drugs). Products include:
Univasc Tablets 2410

Morphine Sulfate (Potentiation of orthostatic hypotension; enhanced CNS depressant effects of reserpine). Products include:
Astramorph/PF Injection, USP (Preservative-Free) 535
Duramorph 962
Infumorph 200 and Infumorph 500 Sterile Solutions 965
MS Contin Tablets 1994
MSIR 1997
Oramorph SR (Morphine Sulfate Sustained Release Tablets) 2236
RMS Suppositories 2657
Roxanol 2243

Nabumetone (Reduced diuretic, natriuretic, and antihypertensive effects). Products include:
Relafen Tablets 2510

Nadolol (Potentiation of antihypertensive drugs).
No products indexed under this heading.

Naproxen (Reduced diuretic, natriuretic, and antihypertensive effects). Products include:
Anaprox/Naprosyn 2117

Naproxen Sodium (Reduced diuretic, natriuretic, and antihypertensive effects). Products include:
Aleve 1975
Anaprox/Naprosyn 2117

Nicardipine Hydrochloride (Potentiation of antihypertensive drugs). Products include:
Cardene Capsules 2095
Cardene I.V. 2709
Cardene SR Capsules 2097

Nifedipine (Potentiation of antihypertensive drugs). Products include:
Adalat Capsules (10 mg and 20 mg) 587
Adalat CC 589
Procardia Capsules 1971
Procardia XL Extended Release Tablets 1972

Nisoldipine (Potentiation of antihypertensive drugs).
No products indexed under this heading.

Nitroglycerin (Potentiation of antihypertensive drugs). Products include:
Deponit NTG Transdermal Delivery System 2397
Nitro-Bid IV 1523
Nitro-Bid Ointment 1524
Nitrodisc 2047
Nitro-Dur (nitroglycerin) Transdermal Infusion System 1326
Nitrolingual Spray 2027
Nitrostat Tablets 1925
Transderm-Nitro Transdermal Therapeutic System 859

Norepinephrine Bitartrate (Decreased arterial responsiveness to norepinephrine). Products include:
Levophed Bitartrate Injection 2315

Opium Alkaloids (Potentiation of orthostatic hypotension; enhanced CNS depressant effects of reserpine).
No products indexed under this heading.

Oxaprozin (Reduced diuretic, natriuretic, and antihypertensive effects). Products include:
Daypro Caplets 2426

Oxycodone Hydrochloride (Potentiation of orthostatic hypotension; enhanced CNS depressant effects of reserpine). Products include:
Percocet Tablets 938
Percodan Tablets 939
Percodan-Demi Tablets 940
Roxicodone Tablets, Oral Solution & Intensol (Oxycodone) 2244
Tylox Capsules 1584

Penbutolol Sulfate (Potentiation of antihypertensive drugs). Products include:
Levatol 2403

Pentobarbital Sodium (Potentiation of orthostatic hypotension; enhanced CNS depressant effects of reserpine). Products include:
Nembutal Sodium Capsules 436
Nembutal Sodium Solution 438
Nembutal Sodium Suppositories 440

Phenelzine Sulfate (Concurrent use is contraindicated). Products include:
Nardil 1920

Phenobarbital (Potentiation of orthostatic hypotension; enhanced CNS depressant effects of reserpine). Products include:
Arco-Lase Plus Tablets 512
Bellergal-S Tablets 2250
Donnatal 2060
Donnatal Extentabs 2061
Donnatal Tablets 2060
Phenobarbital Elixir and Tablets 1469
Quadrinal Tablets 1350

Phenoxybenzamine Hydrochloride (Potentiation of antihypertensive drugs). Products include:
Dibenzyline Capsules 2476

Phentolamine Mesylate (Potentiation of antihypertensive drugs). Products include:
Regitine 846

Phenylbutazone (Reduced diuretic, natriuretic, and antihypertensive effects).
No products indexed under this heading.

Pindolol (Potentiation of antihypertensive drugs). Products include:
Visken Tablets 2299

Piroxicam (Reduced diuretic, natriuretic, and antihypertensive effects). Products include:
Feldene Capsules 1965

Polythiazide (Potentiation of antihypertensive drugs). Products include:
Minizide Capsules 1938

Prazosin Hydrochloride (Potentiation of antihypertensive drugs). Products include:
Minipress Capsules 1937
Minizide Capsules 1938

Prednisolone Acetate (Hypokalemia). Products include:
AK-CIDE ..... ⊙ 202
AK-CIDE Ointment ..... ⊙ 202
Blephamide Liquifilm Sterile Ophthalmic Suspension 476
Blephamide Ointment ..... ⊙ 237
Econopred & Econopred Plus Ophthalmic Suspensions ..... ⊙ 217
Poly-Pred Liquifilm ..... ⊙ 248
Pred Forte ..... ⊙ 250
Pred Mild ..... ⊙ 253
Pred-G Liquifilm Sterile Ophthalmic Suspension ..... ⊙ 251
Pred-G S.O.P. Sterile Ophthalmic Ointment ..... ⊙ 252
Vasocidin Ointment ..... ⊙ 268

Prednisolone Sodium Phosphate (Hypokalemia). Products include:
AK-Pred ..... ⊙ 204
Hydeltrasol Injection, Sterile 1665
Inflamase ..... ⊙ 265
Pediapred Oral Liquid 995
Vasocidin Ophthalmic Solution ..... ⊙ 270

Prednisolone Tebutate (Hypokalemia). Products include:
Hydeltra-T.B.A. Sterile Suspension 1667

Prednisone (Hypokalemia). Products include:
Deltasone Tablets 2595

Propoxyphene Hydrochloride (Potentiation of orthostatic hypotension; enhanced CNS depressant effects of reserpine). Products include:
Darvon 1435
Wygesic Tablets 2827

Propoxyphene Napsylate (Potentiation of orthostatic hypotension; enhanced CNS depressant effects of reserpine). Products include:
Darvon-N/Darvocet-N 1433

Propranolol Hydrochloride (Potentiation of antihypertensive drugs). Products include:
Inderal 2728
Inderal LA Long Acting Capsules 2730
Inderide Tablets 2732
Inderide LA Long Acting Capsules 2734

Quinapril Hydrochloride (Potentiation of antihypertensive drugs). Products include:
Accupril Tablets 1893

Quinidine Gluconate (Use cautiously; cardiac arrhythmias have occurred with reserpine). Products include:
Quinaglute Dura-Tabs Tablets 649

Quinidine Polygalacturonate (Use cautiously; cardiac arrhythmias have occurred with reserpine).
No products indexed under this heading.

Quinidine Sulfate (Use cautiously; cardiac arrhythmias have occurred with reserpine). Products include:
Quinidex Extentabs 2067

Ramipril (Potentiation of antihypertensive drugs). Products include:
Altace Capsules 1232

Rauwolfia Serpentina (Potentiation of antihypertensive drugs).
No products indexed under this heading.

Rescinnamine (Potentiation of antihypertensive drugs).
No products indexed under this heading.

Secobarbital Sodium (Potentiation of orthostatic hypotension; enhanced CNS depressant effects of reserpine). Products include:
Seconal Sodium Pulvules 1474

Selegiline Hydrochloride (Concurrent use is contraindicated). Products include:
Eldepryl Tablets 2550

Sodium Nitroprusside (Potentiation of antihypertensive drugs).
No products indexed under this heading.

Sotalol Hydrochloride (Potentiation of antihypertensive drugs). Products include:
Betapace Tablets 641

Spirapril Hydrochloride (Potentiation of antihypertensive drugs).
No products indexed under this heading.

Sufentanil Citrate (Potentiation of orthostatic hypotension; enhanced CNS depressant effects of reserpine). Products include:
Sufenta Injection 1309

Sulindac (Reduced diuretic, natriuretic, and antihypertensive effects). Products include:
Clinoril Tablets 1618

Terazosin Hydrochloride (Potentiation of antihypertensive drugs). Products include:
Hytrin Capsules 430

Thiamylal Sodium (Potentiation of orthostatic hypotension; enhanced CNS depressant effects of reserpine).
No products indexed under this heading.

Timolol Maleate (Potentiation of antihypertensive drugs). Products include:
Blocadren Tablets 1614
Timolide Tablets 1748
Timoptic in Ocudose 1753
Timoptic Sterile Ophthalmic Solution 1751
Timoptic-XE 1755

IMPORTANT NOTE: Always consult each drug listing in the patient's regimen for possible interactions.

Tolazamide (Dosage adjustment of the antidiabetic drug may be required).
No products indexed under this heading.

Tolbutamide (Dosage adjustment of the antidiabetic drug may be required).
No products indexed under this heading.

Tolmetin Sodium (Reduced diuretic, natriuretic, and antihypertensive effects). Products include:
Tolectin (200, 400 and 600 mg) .. 1581

Torsemide (Potentiation of antihypertensive drugs). Products include:
Demadex Tablets and Injection 686

Tranylcypromine Sulfate (Concurrent use is contraindicated). Products include:
Parnate Tablets 2503

Triamcinolone (Hypokalemia). Products include:
Aristocort Tablets 1022

Triamcinolone Acetonide (Hypokalemia). Products include:
Aristocort A 0.025% Cream 1027
Aristocort A 0.5% Cream 1031
Aristocort A 0.1% Cream 1029
Aristocort A 0.1% Ointment 1030
Azmacort Oral Inhaler 2011
Nasacort Nasal Inhaler 2024

Triamcinolone Diacetate (Hypokalemia). Products include:
Aristocort Suspension (Forte Parenteral) 1027
Aristocort Suspension (Intralesional) 1025

Triamcinolone Hexacetonide (Hypokalemia). Products include:
Aristospan Suspension (Intra-articular) 1033
Aristospan Suspension (Intralesional) 1032

Trimethaphan Camsylate (Potentiation of antihypertensive drugs). Products include:
Arfonad Ampuls 2080

Tubocurarine Chloride (Increased responsiveness to tubocurarine).
No products indexed under this heading.

Verapamil Hydrochloride (Potentiation of antihypertensive drugs). Products include:
Calan SR Caplets 2422
Calan Tablets 2419
Isoptin Injectable 1344
Isoptin Oral Tablets 1346
Isoptin SR Tablets 1348
Verelan Capsules 1410
Verelan Capsules 2824

Food Interactions

Alcohol (Potentiation of orthostatic hypotension).

HYLAND'S ARNICAID TABLETS
(Homeopathic Medications) .... ▣ 828
None cited in PDR database.

HYLAND'S BED WETTING TABLETS
(Homeopathic Medications) .... ▣ 828
None cited in PDR database.

HYLAND'S CALMS FORTé TABLETS
(Homeopathic Medications) .... ▣ 828
None cited in PDR database.

HYLAND'S CLEARAC
(Homeopathic Medications) .... ▣ 828
None cited in PDR database.

HYLAND'S COLIC TABLETS
(Homeopathic Medications) .... ▣ 829
None cited in PDR database.

HYLAND'S COUGH SYRUP WITH HONEY
(Ipecac) .... ▣ 829
None cited in PDR database.

HYLAND'S C-PLUS COLD TABLETS
(Homeopathic Medications) .... ▣ 829
None cited in PDR database.

HYLAND'S DIARREX TABLETS
(Homeopathic Medications) .... ▣ 829
None cited in PDR database.

HYLAND'S ENURAID TABLETS
(Homeopathic Medications) .... ▣ 829
None cited in PDR database.

HYLAND'S TEETHING TABLETS
(Calcium Phosphate, Homeopathic Medications) .... ▣ 830
None cited in PDR database.

HYLAND'S VITAMIN C FOR CHILDREN
(Vitamin C) .... ▣ 830
None cited in PDR database.

HYLOREL TABLETS
(Guanadrel Sulfate) 985

May interact with monoamine oxidase inhibitors, phenothiazines, tricyclic antidepressants, vasodilators, sympathomimetic bronchodilators, alpha adrenergic blockers, direct-acting sympathomimetic amines, indirect-acting sympathomimetic amines, beta blockers, catecholamine depleting drugs, and certain other agents. Compounds in these categories include:

Acebutolol Hydrochloride (May cause excessive postural hypotension and bradycardia). Products include:
Sectral Capsules 2807

Albuterol (May interfere with the hypotensive effect). Products include:
Proventil Inhalation Aerosol 2382
Ventolin Inhalation Aerosol and Refill 1197

Albuterol Sulfate (May interfere with the hypotensive effect). Products include:
Airet Solution for Inhalation 452
Proventil Inhalation Solution 0.083% 2384
Proventil Repetabs Tablets 2386
Proventil Solution for Inhalation 0.5% 2383
Proventil Syrup 2385
Proventil Tablets 2386
Ventolin Inhalation Solution 1198
Ventolin Nebules Inhalation Solution 1199
Ventolin Rotacaps for Inhalation 1200
Ventolin Syrup 1202
Ventolin Tablets 1203
Volmax Extended-Release Tablets .. 1788

Amitriptyline Hydrochloride (Possible reversal of the effects of guanadrel; tricyclic antidepressant, if discontinued abruptly, may enhance effect of guanadrel). Products include:
Elavil 2838
Endep Tablets 2174
Etrafon 2355
Limbitrol 2180
Triavil Tablets 1757

Amoxapine (Possible reversal of the effects of guanadrel; tricyclic antidepressant, if discontinued abruptly, may enhance effect of guanadrel). Products include:
Asendin Tablets 1369

Amphetamine Resins (May reverse the effects of neuronal blocking agents). Products include:
Biphetamine Capsules 983

Atenolol (May cause excessive postural hypotension and bradycardia). Products include:
Tenoretic Tablets 2845
Tenormin Tablets and I.V. Injection 2847

Betaxolol Hydrochloride (May cause excessive postural hypotension and bradycardia). Products include:
Betoptic Ophthalmic Solution 469
Betoptic S Ophthalmic Suspension 471
Kerlone Tablets 2436

Bisoprolol Fumarate (May cause excessive postural hypotension and bradycardia). Products include:
Zebeta Tablets 1413
Ziac 1415

Bitolterol Mesylate (May interfere with the hypotensive effect). Products include:
Tornalate Solution for Inhalation, 0.2% 956
Tornalate Metered Dose Inhaler 957

Carteolol Hydrochloride (May cause excessive postural hypotension and bradycardia). Products include:
Cartrol Tablets 410
Ocupress Ophthalmic Solution, 1% Sterile .... ⊙ 309

Chlorpromazine (Possible reversal of the effects of guanadrel). Products include:
Thorazine Suppositories 2523

Chlorpromazine Hydrochloride (Possible reversal of the effects of guanadrel). Products include:
Thorazine 2523

Clomipramine Hydrochloride (Possible reversal of the effects of guanadrel; tricyclic antidepressant, if discontinued abruptly, may enhance effect of guanadrel). Products include:
Anafranil Capsules 803

Deserpidine (May cause excessive postural hypotension and bradycardia).
No products indexed under this heading.

Desipramine Hydrochloride (Possible reversal of the effects of guanadrel; tricyclic antidepressant, if discontinued abruptly, may enhance effect of guanadrel). Products include:
Norpramin Tablets 1526

Dextroamphetamine Sulfate (May reverse the effects of neuronal blocking agents). Products include:
Dexedrine 2474
DextroStat Dextroamphetamine Tablets 2036

Diazoxide (Comcomitant use may increase the potential for symptomatic or orthostatic hypotension). Products include:
Hyperstat I.V. Injection 2363
Proglycem 580

Doxazosin Mesylate (May cause excessive postural hypotension and bradycardia). Products include:
Cardura Tablets 2186

Doxepin Hydrochloride (Possible reversal of the effects of guanadrel; tricyclic antidepressant, if discontinued abruptly, may enhance effect of guanadrel). Products include:
Sinequan 2205
Zonalon Cream 1055

Ephedrine Hydrochloride (May interfere with the hypotensive effect; may reverse the effects of neuronal blocking agents). Products include:
Primatene Dual Action Formula .... ▣ 872
Primatene Tablets .... ▣ 873
Quadrinal Tablets 1350

Ephedrine Sulfate (May interfere with the hypotensive effect; may reverse the effects of neuronal blocking agents). Products include:
Bronkaid Caplets .... ▣ 717
Marax Tablets & DF Syrup 2200

Ephedrine Tannate (May interfere with the hypotensive effect; may reverse the effects of neuronal blocking agents). Products include:
Rynatuss 2673

Epinephrine (May interfere with the hypotensive effect). Products include:
Bronkaid Mist .... ▣ 717
EPIFRIN .... ⊙ 239
EpiPen 790
Marcaine Hydrochloride with Epinephrine 1:200,000 2316
Primatene Mist .... ▣ 873
Sensorcaine with Epinephrine Injection 559
Sus-Phrine Injection 1019
Xylocaine with Epinephrine Injections 567

Epinephrine Hydrochloride (May interfere with the hypotensive effect; enhances the activity of direct acting sympathomimetic amines). Products include:
Ana-Kit Anaphylaxis Emergency Treatment Kit 617

Esmolol Hydrochloride (May cause excessive postural hypotension and bradycardia). Products include:
Brevibloc Injection 1808

Ethylnorepinephrine Hydrochloride (May interfere with the hypotensive effect).
No products indexed under this heading.

Fluphenazine Decanoate (Possible reversal of the effects of guanadrel). Products include:
Prolixin Decanoate 509

Fluphenazine Enanthate (Possible reversal of the effects of guanadrel). Products include:
Prolixin Enanthate 509

Fluphenazine Hydrochloride (Possible reversal of the effects of guanadrel). Products include:
Prolixin 509

Furazolidone (Concurrent or sequential use with MAO inhibitor is contraindicated). Products include:
Furoxone 2046

Guanethidine Monosulfate (May cause excessive postural hypotension and bradycardia). Products include:
Esimil Tablets 822
Ismelin Tablets 827

Hydralazine Hydrochloride (Comcomitant use may increase the potential for symptomatic or orthostatic hypotension). Products include:
Apresazide Capsules 808
Apresoline Hydrochloride Tablets .. 809
Ser-Ap-Es Tablets 849

(▣ Described in PDR For Nonprescription Drugs) (⊙ Described in PDR For Ophthalmology)

499 **Interactions Index** **Hylorel**

Imipramine Hydrochloride (Possible reversal of the effects of guanadrel; tricyclic antidepressant, if discontinued abruptly, may enhance effect of guanadrel). Products include:

Tofranil Ampuls ... 854
Tofranil Tablets ... 856

Imipramine Pamoate (Possible reversal of the effects of guanadrel; tricyclic antidepressant, if discontinued abruptly, may enhance effect of guanadrel). Products include:

Tofranil-PM Capsules ... 857

Isocarboxazid (Concurrent or sequential use with MAO inhibitor is contraindicated).

No products indexed under this heading.

Isoetharine (May interfere with the hypotensive effect). Products include:

Bronkometer Aerosol ... 2302
Bronkosol Solution ... 2302
Isoetharine Inhalation Solution, USP, Arm-a-Med ... 551

Isoproterenol Hydrochloride (May interfere with the hypotensive effect; enhances the activity of direct acting sympathomimetic amines). Products include:

Isuprel Hydrochloride Injection 1:5000 ... 2311
Isuprel Hydrochloride Solution 1:200 & 1:100 ... 2313
Isuprel Mistometer ... 2312

Isoproterenol Sulfate (May interfere with the hypotensive effect; enhances the activity of direct acting sympathomimetic amines). Products include:

Norisodrine with Calcium Iodide Syrup ... 442

Labetalol Hydrochloride (May cause excessive postural hypotension and bradycardia). Products include:

Normodyne Injection ... 2377
Normodyne Tablets ... 2379
Trandate ... 1185

Levobunolol Hydrochloride (May cause excessive postural hypotension and bradycardia). Products include:

Betagan ... ◉ 233

Maprotiline Hydrochloride (Possible reversal of the effects of guanadrel; tricyclic antidepressant, if discontinued abruptly, may enhance effect of guanadrel). Products include:

Ludiomil Tablets ... 843

Mesoridazine Besylate (Possible reversal of the effects of guanadrel). Products include:

Serentil ... 684

Metaproterenol Sulfate (May interfere with the hypotensive effect). Products include:

Alupent ... 669
Metaproterenol Sulfate Inhalation Solution, USP, Arm-a-Med ... 552

Metaraminol Bitartrate (Enhances the activity of direct acting sympathomimetic amines). Products include:

Aramine Injection ... 1609

Methotrimeprazine (Possible reversal of the effects of guanadrel). Products include:

Levoprome ... 1274

Metipranolol Hydrochloride (May cause excessive postural hypotension and bradycardia). Products include:

OptiPranolol (Metipranolol 0.3%) Sterile Ophthalmic Solution ... ◉ 258

Metoprolol Succinate (May cause excessive postural hypotension and bradycardia). Products include:

Toprol-XL Tablets ... 565

Metoprolol Tartrate (May cause excessive postural hypotension and bradycardia). Products include:

Lopressor Ampuls ... 830
Lopressor HCT Tablets ... 832
Lopressor Tablets ... 830

Minoxidil (Comcomitant use may increase the potential for symptomatic or orthostatic hypotension). Products include:

Loniten Tablets ... 2618
Rogaine Topical Solution ... 2637

Nadolol (May cause excessive postural hypotension and bradycardia).

No products indexed under this heading.

Norepinephrine Bitartrate (Enhanced effect of norepinephrine). Products include:

Levophed Bitartrate Injection ... 2315

Norepinephrine Hydrochloride (Enhances the activity of direct acting sympathomimetic amines).

Nortriptyline Hydrochloride (Possible reversal of the effects of guanadrel; tricyclic antidepressant, if discontinued abruptly, may enhance effect of guanadrel). Products include:

Pamelor ... 2280

Penbutolol Sulfate (May cause excessive postural hypotension and bradycardia). Products include:

Levatol ... 2403

Perphenazine (Possible reversal of the effects of guanadrel). Products include:

Etrafon ... 2355
Triavil Tablets ... 1757
Trilafon ... 2389

Phenelzine Sulfate (Concurrent or sequential use with MAO inhibitor is contraindicated). Products include:

Nardil ... 1920

Phenylephrine Hydrochloride (Enhances the activity of direct acting sympathomimetic amines). Products include:

Atrohist Plus Tablets ... 454
Cerose DM ... 🕮 878
Comhist ... 2038
D.A. Chewable Tablets ... 951
Deconsal Pediatric Capsules ... 454
Dura-Vent/DA Tablets ... 953
Entex Capsules ... 1986
Entex Liquid ... 1986
Extendryl ... 1005
4-Way Fast Acting Nasal Spray (regular & mentholated) ... 🕮 621
Hemorid For Women ... 🕮 834
Hycomine Compound Tablets ... 932
Neo-Synephrine Hydrochloride 1% Carpuject ... 2324
Neo-Synephrine Hydrochloride 1% Injection ... 2324
Neo-Synephrine Hydrochloride (Ophthalmic) ... 2325
Neo-Synephrine ... 🕮 726
Nōstril ... 🕮 644
Novahistine Elixir ... 🕮 823
Phenergan VC ... 2779
Phenergan VC with Codeine ... 2781
Preparation H ... 🕮 871
Tympagesic Ear Drops ... 2342
Vasosulf ... ◉ 271
Vicks Sinex Nasal Spray and Ultra Fine Mist ... 🕮 765

Phenylephrine Tannate (Enhances the activity of direct acting sympathomimetic amines). Products include:

Atrohist Pediatric Suspension ... 454
Ricobid-D Pediatric Suspension ... 2038
Ricobid Tablets and Pediatric Suspension ... 2038
Rynatan ... 2673
Rynatuss ... 2673

Phenylpropanolamine Hydrochloride (May reverse the effects of neuronal blocking agents). Products include:

Acutrim ... 🕮 628
Allerest Children's Chewable Tablets ... 🕮 627
Allerest 12 Hour Caplets ... 🕮 627
Atrohist Plus Tablets ... 454
BC Cold Powder Multi-Symptom Formula (Cold-Sinus-Allergy) ... 🕮 609
BC Cold Powder Non-Drowsy Formula (Cold-Sinus) ... 🕮 609
Cheracol Plus Head Cold/Cough Formula ... 🕮 769
Comtrex Multi-Symptom Non-Drowsy Liqui-gels ... 🕮 618
Contac Continuous Action Nasal Decongestant/Antihistamine 12 Hour Capsules ... 🕮 813
Contac Maximum Strength Continuous Action Decongestant/Antihistamine 12 Hour Caplets ... 🕮 813
Contac Severe Cold and Flu Formula Caplets ... 🕮 814
Coricidin 'D' Decongestant Tablets ... 🕮 800
Dexatrim ... 🕮 832
Dexatrim Plus Vitamins Caplets ... 🕮 832
Dimetane-DC Cough Syrup ... 2059
Dimetapp Elixir ... 🕮 773
Dimetapp Extentabs ... 🕮 774
Dimetapp Tablets/Liqui-Gels ... 🕮 775
Dimetapp Cold & Allergy Chewable Tablets ... 🕮 773
Dimetapp DM Elixir ... 🕮 774
Dura-Vent Tablets ... 952
Entex Capsules ... 1986
Entex LA Tablets ... 1987
Entex Liquid ... 1986
Exgest LA Tablets ... 782
Hycomine ... 931
Isoclor Timesule Capsules ... 🕮 637
Nolamine Timed-Release Tablets ... 785
Ornade Spansule Capsules ... 2502
Propagest Tablets ... 786
Pyrroxate Caplets ... 🕮 772
Robitussin-CF ... 🕮 777
Sinulin Tablets ... 787
Tavist-D 12 Hour Relief Tablets ... 🕮 787
Teldrin 12 Hour Antihistamine/Nasal Decongestant Allergy Relief Capsules ... 🕮 826
Triaminic Allergy Tablets ... 🕮 789
Triaminic Cold Tablets ... 🕮 790
Triaminic Expectorant ... 🕮 790
Triaminic Syrup ... 🕮 792
Triaminic-12 Tablets ... 🕮 792
Triaminic-DM Syrup ... 🕮 792
Triaminicin Tablets ... 🕮 793
Triaminicol Multi-Symptom Cold Tablets ... 🕮 793
Triaminicol Multi-Symptom Relief ... 🕮 794
Vicks DayQuil Allergy Relief 12-Hour Extended Release Tablets ... 🕮 760
Vicks DayQuil Allergy Relief 4-Hour Tablets ... 🕮 760
Vicks DayQuil SINUS Pressure & CONGESTION Relief ... 🕮 761

Pindolol (May cause excessive postural hypotension and bradycardia). Products include:

Visken Tablets ... 2299

Pirbuterol Acetate (May interfere with the hypotensive effect). Products include:

Maxair Autohaler ... 1492
Maxair Inhaler ... 1494

Prazosin Hydrochloride (May cause excessive postural hypotension and bradycardia). Products include:

Minipress Capsules ... 1937
Minizide Capsules ... 1938

Prochlorperazine (Possible reversal of the effects of guanadrel). Products include:

Compazine ... 2470

Promethazine Hydrochloride (Possible reversal of the effects of guanadrel). Products include:

Mepergan Injection ... 2753
Phenergan with Codeine ... 2777
Phenergan with Dextromethorphan ... 2778
Phenergan Injection ... 2773
Phenergan Suppositories ... 2775
Phenergan Syrup ... 2774
Phenergan Tablets ... 2775
Phenergan VC ... 2779
Phenergan VC with Codeine ... 2781

Propranolol Hydrochloride (May cause excessive postural hypotension and bradycardia). Products include:

Inderal ... 2728
Inderal LA Long Acting Capsules ... 2730
Inderide Tablets ... 2732
Inderide LA Long Acting Capsules ... 2734

Protriptyline Hydrochloride (Possible reversal of the effects of guanadrel; tricyclic antidepressant, if discontinued abruptly, may enhance effect of guanadrel). Products include:

Vivactil Tablets ... 1774

Rauwolfia Serpentina (May cause excessive postural hypotension and bradycardia).

No products indexed under this heading.

Rescinnamine (May cause excessive postural hypotension and bradycardia).

No products indexed under this heading.

Reserpine (May cause excessive postural hypotension and bradycardia). Products include:

Diupres Tablets ... 1650
Hydropres Tablets ... 1675
Ser-Ap-Es Tablets ... 849

Salmeterol Xinafoate (May interfere with the hypotensive effect). Products include:

Serevent Inhalation Aerosol ... 1176

Selegiline Hydrochloride (Concurrent or sequential use with MAO inhibitor is contraindicated). Products include:

Eldepryl Tablets ... 2550

Sotalol Hydrochloride (May cause excessive postural hypotension and bradycardia). Products include:

Betapace Tablets ... 641

Terazosin Hydrochloride (May cause excessive postural hypotension and bradycardia). Products include:

Hytrin Capsules ... 430

Terbutaline Sulfate (May interfere with the hypotensive effect). Products include:

Brethaire Inhaler ... 813
Brethine Ampuls ... 815
Brethine Tablets ... 814
Bricanyl Subcutaneous Injection ... 1502
Bricanyl Tablets ... 1503

Thioridazine Hydrochloride (Possible reversal of the effects of guanadrel). Products include:

Mellaril ... 2269

Timolol Hemihydrate (May cause excessive postural hypotension and bradycardia). Products include:

Betimol 0.25%, 0.5% ... ◉ 261

Timolol Maleate (May cause excessive postural hypotension and bradycardia). Products include:

Blocadren Tablets ... 1614
Timolide Tablets ... 1748
Timoptic in Ocudose ... 1753
Timoptic Sterile Ophthalmic Solution ... 1751
Timoptic-XE ... 1755

Tranylcypromine Sulfate (Concurrent or sequential use with MAO inhibitor is contraindicated). Products include:

Parnate Tablets ... 2503

Trifluoperazine Hydrochloride (Possible reversal of the effects of guanadrel). Products include:

Stelazine ... 2514

IMPORTANT NOTE: Always consult each drug listing in the patient's regimen for possible interactions.

Hylorel **Interactions Index** 500

Trimipramine Maleate (Possible reversal of the effects of guanadrel; tricyclic antidepressant, if discontinued abruptly, may enhance effect of guanadrel). Products include:
- Surmontil Capsules ... 2811

Food Interactions

Alcohol (Exaggerates postural hypotension).

HYPERAB RABIES IMMUNE GLOBULIN (HUMAN)

(Rabies Immune Globulin (Human)) .. 624
May interact with:

Measles Virus Vaccine Live (Interference with the response to live viral vaccines). Products include:
- Attenuvax ... 1610

Measles & Rubella Virus Vaccine Live (Interference with the response to live viral vaccines). Products include:
- M-R-VAX II ... 1689

Measles, Mumps & Rubella Virus Vaccine Live (Interference with the response to live viral vaccines). Products include:
- M-M-R II ... 1687

Mumps Virus Vaccine, Live (Interference with the response to live viral vaccines). Products include:
- Mumpsvax ... 1708

Poliovirus Vaccine, Live, Oral, Trivalent, Types 1,2,3 (Sabin) (Interference with the response to live viral vaccines). Products include:
- Orimune ... 1388

Rubella Virus Vaccine Live (Interference with the response to live viral vaccines). Products include:
- Meruvax II ... 1697

Rubella & Mumps Virus Vaccine Live (Interference with the response to live viral vaccines). Products include:
- Biavax II ... 1613

HYPERHEP HEPATITIS B IMMUNE GLOBULIN (HUMAN)

(Hepatitis B Immune Globulin (Human)) ... 626
May interact with:

Vaccines (Live) (May interfere with response. Use should be deferred for 3 months after administration of HyperHep).

HYPERSTAT I.V. INJECTION

(Diazoxide) ... 2363
May interact with oral anticoagulants, antihypertensives, beta blockers, thiazides, diuretics, and certain other agents. Compounds in these categories include:

Acebutolol Hydrochloride (Potentiation of effects of diazoxide; hypotension). Products include:
- Sectral Capsules ... 2807

Alphaprodine Hydrochloride (Potentiation of effects of diazoxide).

Amlodipine Besylate (Hypotension). Products include:
- Lotrel Capsules ... 840
- Norvasc Tablets ... 1940

Atenolol (Potentiation of effects of diazoxide; hypotension). Products include:
- Tenoretic Tablets ... 2845
- Tenormin Tablets and I.V. Injection 2847

Benazepril Hydrochloride (Hypotension). Products include:
- Lotensin Tablets ... 834
- Lotensin HCT ... 837
- Lotrel Capsules ... 840

Bendroflumethiazide (Potentiation of effects of diazoxide; hypotension).
No products indexed under this heading.

Betaxolol Hydrochloride (Hypotension). Products include:
- Betoptic Ophthalmic Solution ... 469
- Betoptic S Ophthalmic Suspension 471
- Kerlone Tablets ... 2436

Bisoprolol Fumarate (Potentiation of effects of diazoxide; hypotension). Products include:
- Zebeta Tablets ... 1413
- Ziac ... 1415

Captopril (Hypotension). Products include:
- Capoten ... 739
- Capozide ... 742

Carteolol Hydrochloride (Potentiation of effects of diazoxide; hypotension). Products include:
- Cartrol Tablets ... 410
- Ocupress Ophthalmic Solution, 1% Sterile ... ◉ 309

Chlorothiazide (Potentiation of effects of diazoxide; hypotension). Products include:
- Aldoclor Tablets ... 1598
- Diupres Tablets ... 1650
- Diuril Oral ... 1653

Chlorothiazide Sodium (Potentiation of effects of diazoxide; hypotension). Products include:
- Diuril Sodium Intravenous ... 1652

Chlorthalidone (Potentiation of effects of diazoxide; hypotension). Products include:
- Combipres Tablets ... 677
- Tenoretic Tablets ... 2845
- Thalitone ... 1245

Clonidine (Hypotension). Products include:
- Catapres-TTS ... 675

Clonidine Hydrochloride (Hypotension; potentiation of effects of diazoxide). Products include:
- Catapres Tablets ... 674
- Combipres Tablets ... 677

Deserpidine (Hypotension).
No products indexed under this heading.

Dicumarol (Increased blood levels).
No products indexed under this heading.

Diltiazem Hydrochloride (Hypotension). Products include:
- Cardizem CD Capsules ... 1506
- Cardizem SR Capsules ... 1510
- Cardizem Injectable ... 1508
- Cardizem Tablets ... 1512
- Dilacor XR Extended-release Capsules ... 2018

Doxazosin Mesylate (Hypotension). Products include:
- Cardura Tablets ... 2186

Enalapril Maleate (Hypotension). Products include:
- Vaseretic Tablets ... 1765
- Vasotec Tablets ... 1771

Enalaprilat (Potentiation of effects of diazoxide; hypotension). Products include:
- Vasotec I.V. ... 1768

Esmolol Hydrochloride (Potentiation of effects of diazoxide; hypotension). Products include:
- Brevibloc Injection ... 1808

Felodipine (Hypotension). Products include:
- Plendil Extended-Release Tablets ... 527

Fosinopril Sodium (Hypotension). Products include:
- Monopril Tablets ... 757

Furosemide (Hypotension). Products include:
- Lasix Injection, Oral Solution and Tablets ... 1240

Guanabenz Acetate (Hypotension).
No products indexed under this heading.

Guanethidine Monosulfate (Hypotension). Products include:
- Esimil Tablets ... 822
- Ismelin Tablets ... 827

Hydralazine Hydrochloride (Potentiation of effects of diazoxide; hypotension). Products include:
- Apresazide Capsules ... 808
- Apresoline Hydrochloride Tablets .. 809
- Ser-Ap-Es Tablets ... 849

Hydrochlorothiazide (Potentiation of effects of diazoxide; hypotension). Products include:
- Aldactazide ... 2413
- Aldoril Tablets ... 1604
- Apresazide Capsules ... 808
- Capozide ... 742
- Dyazide ... 2479
- Esidrix Tablets ... 821
- Esimil Tablets ... 822
- HydroDIURIL Tablets ... 1674
- Hydropres Tablets ... 1675
- Hyzaar Tablets ... 1677
- Inderide Tablets ... 2732
- Inderide LA Long Acting Capsules .. 2734
- Lopressor HCT Tablets ... 832
- Lotensin HCT ... 837
- Maxzide ... 1380
- Moduretic Tablets ... 1705
- Oretic Tablets ... 443
- Prinzide Tablets ... 1737
- Ser-Ap-Es Tablets ... 849
- Timolide Tablets ... 1748
- Vaseretic Tablets ... 1765
- Zestoretic ... 2850
- Ziac ... 1415

Hydroflumethiazide (Potentiation of effects of diazoxide; hypotension). Products include:
- Diucardin Tablets ... 2718

Indapamide (Hypotension). Products include:
- Lozol Tablets ... 2022

Isradipine (Hypotension). Products include:
- DynaCirc Capsules ... 2256

Labetalol Hydrochloride (Potentiation of effects of diazoxide; hypotension). Products include:
- Normodyne Injection ... 2377
- Normodyne Tablets ... 2379
- Trandate ... 1185

Levobunolol Hydrochloride (Potentiation of effects of diazoxide; hypotension). Products include:
- Betagan ... ◉ 233

Lisinopril (Potentiation of effects of diazoxide; hypotension). Products include:
- Prinivil Tablets ... 1733
- Prinzide Tablets ... 1737
- Zestoretic ... 2850
- Zestril Tablets ... 2854

Losartan Potassium (Hypotension). Products include:
- Cozaar Tablets ... 1628
- Hyzaar Tablets ... 1677

Mecamylamine Hydrochloride (Hypotension). Products include:
- Inversine Tablets ... 1686

Methyclothiazide (Potentiation of effects of diazoxide; hypotension). Products include:
- Enduron Tablets ... 420

Methyldopa (Hypotension). Products include:
- Aldoclor Tablets ... 1598
- Aldomet Oral ... 1600
- Aldoril Tablets ... 1604

Methyldopate Hydrochloride (Hypotension). Products include:
- Aldomet Ester HCl Injection ... 1602

Metipranolol Hydrochloride (Potentiation of effects of diazoxide; hypotension). Products include:
- OptiPranolol (Metipranolol 0.3%) Sterile Ophthalmic Solution ... ◉ 258

Metolazone (Hypotension). Products include:
- Mykrox Tablets ... 993
- Zaroxolyn Tablets ... 1000

Metoprolol Succinate (Hypotension). Products include:
- Toprol-XL Tablets ... 565

Metoprolol Tartrate (Potentiation of effects of diazoxide; hypotension). Products include:
- Lopressor Ampuls ... 830
- Lopressor HCT Tablets ... 832
- Lopressor Tablets ... 830

Metyrosine (Hypotension). Products include:
- Demser Capsules ... 1649

Minoxidil (Potentiation of effects of diazoxide; hypotension). Products include:
- Loniten Tablets ... 2618
- Rogaine Topical Solution ... 2637

Moexipril Hydrochloride (Hypotension). Products include:
- Univasc Tablets ... 2410

Nadolol (Potentiation of effects of diazoxide; hypotension).
No products indexed under this heading.

Nicardipine Hydrochloride (Potentiation of effects of diazoxide; hypotension). Products include:
- Cardene Capsules ... 2095
- Cardene I.V. ... 2709
- Cardene SR Capsules ... 2097

Nifedipine (Hypotension). Products include:
- Adalat Capsules (10 mg and 20 mg) ... 587
- Adalat CC ... 589
- Procardia Capsules ... 1971
- Procardia XL Extended Release Tablets ... 1972

Nisoldipine (Hypotension).
No products indexed under this heading.

Nitroglycerin (Hypotension). Products include:
- Deponit NTG Transdermal Delivery System ... 2397
- Nitro-Bid IV ... 1523
- Nitro-Bid Ointment ... 1524
- Nitrodisc ... 2047
- Nitro-Dur (nitroglycerin) Transdermal Infusion System ... 1326
- Nitrolingual Spray ... 2027
- Nitrostat Tablets ... 1925
- Transderm-Nitro Transdermal Therapeutic System ... 859

Papaverine Hydrochloride (Potentiation of effects of diazoxide). Products include:
- Papaverine Hydrochloride Vials and Ampoules ... 1468

Penbutolol Sulfate (Potentiation of effects of diazoxide; hypotension). Products include:
- Levatol ... 2403

Phenoxybenzamine Hydrochloride (Hypotension). Products include:
- Dibenzyline Capsules ... 2476

Phentolamine Mesylate (Hypotension). Products include:
- Regitine ... 846

Pindolol (Potentiation of effects of diazoxide; hypotension). Products include:
- Visken Tablets ... 2299

Polythiazide (Potentiation of effects of diazoxide; hypotension). Products include:
- Minizide Capsules ... 1938

(▣ Described in PDR For Nonprescription Drugs) (◉ Described in PDR For Ophthalmology)

501 Interactions Index Hytrin

Prazosin Hydrochloride (Potentiation of effects of diazoxide; hypotension). Products include:
- Minipress Capsules ... 1937
- Minizide Capsules ... 1938

Propranolol Hydrochloride (Potentiation of effects of diazoxide; hypotension). Products include:
- Inderal ... 2728
- Inderal LA Long Acting Capsules ... 2730
- Inderide Tablets ... 2732
- Inderide LA Long Acting Capsules .. 2734

Quinapril Hydrochloride (Hypotension). Products include:
- Accupril Tablets ... 1893

Ramipril (Hypotension). Products include:
- Altace Capsules ... 1232

Rauwolfia Serpentina (Hypotension).
- No products indexed under this heading.

Rescinnamine (Hypotension).
- No products indexed under this heading.

Reserpine (Hypotension). Products include:
- Diupres Tablets ... 1650
- Hydropres Tablets ... 1675
- Ser-Ap-Es Tablets ... 849

Sodium Nitroprusside (Hypotension).
- No products indexed under this heading.

Sotalol Hydrochloride (Potentiation of effects of diazoxide; hypotension). Products include:
- Betapace Tablets ... 641

Spirapril Hydrochloride (Hypotension).
- No products indexed under this heading.

Terazosin Hydrochloride (Hypotension). Products include:
- Hytrin Capsules ... 430

Timolol Hemihydrate (Potentiation of effects of diazoxide; hypotension). Products include:
- Betimol 0.25%, 0.5% ... ◎ 261

Timolol Maleate (Potentiation of effects of diazoxide; hypotension). Products include:
- Blocadren Tablets ... 1614
- Timolide Tablets ... 1748
- Timoptic in Ocudose ... 1753
- Timoptic Sterile Ophthalmic Solution ... 1751
- Timoptic-XE ... 1755

Torsemide (Hypotension). Products include:
- Demadex Tablets and Injection ... 686

Trimethaphan Camsylate (Hypotension). Products include:
- Arfonad Ampuls ... 2080

Verapamil Hydrochloride (Hypotension). Products include:
- Calan SR Caplets ... 2422
- Calan Tablets ... 2419
- Isoptin Injectable ... 1344
- Isoptin Oral Tablets ... 1346
- Isoptin SR Tablets ... 1348
- Verelan Capsules ... 1410
- Verelan Capsules ... 2824

Warfarin Sodium (Increased blood levels). Products include:
- Coumadin ... 926

HYPER-TET TETANUS IMMUNE GLOBULIN (HUMAN)
(Tetanus Immune Globulin (Human)) 627
May interact with:

Vaccines (Live) (May interfere with response. Use should be deferred for 3 months).

HYPOTEARS LUBRICANT EYE DROPS
(Polyvinyl Alcohol) ... ◎ 265
None cited in PDR database.

HYPOTEARS OINTMENT
(Petrolatum, White) ... ◎ 265
None cited in PDR database.

HYPOTEARS PF LUBRICANT EYE DROPS
(Polyvinyl Alcohol) ... ◎ 265
None cited in PDR database.

HYPRHO-D FULL DOSE RHO (D) IMMUNE GLOBULIN (HUMAN)
(Immune Globulin (Human)) ... 629
May interact with:

Measles Virus Vaccine Live (Interference with response to live vaccines). Products include:
- Attenuvax ... 1610

Measles & Rubella Virus Vaccine Live (Interference with response to live vaccines). Products include:
- M-R-VAX II ... 1689

Measles, Mumps & Rubella Virus Vaccine Live (Interference with response to live vaccines). Products include:
- M-M-R II ... 1687

Rubella Virus Vaccine Live (Interference with response to live vaccines). Products include:
- Meruvax II ... 1697

Rubella & Mumps Virus Vaccine Live (Interference with response to live vaccines). Products include:
- Biavax II ... 1613

HYPRHO-D MINI-DOSE RHO (D) IMMUNE GLOBULIN (HUMAN)
(Immune Globulin (Human)) ... 628
May interact with:

Measles Virus Vaccine Live (Interference with response to live vaccines). Products include:
- Attenuvax ... 1610

Measles & Rubella Virus Vaccine Live (Interference with response to live vaccines). Products include:
- M-R-VAX II ... 1689

Measles, Mumps & Rubella Virus Vaccine Live (Interference with response to live vaccines). Products include:
- M-M-R II ... 1687

Rubella Virus Vaccine Live (Interference with response to live vaccines). Products include:
- Meruvax II ... 1697

Rubella & Mumps Virus Vaccine Live (Interference with response to live vaccines). Products include:
- Biavax II ... 1613

HYSKON HYSTEROSCOPY FLUID
(Dextran 70) ... 1595
None cited in PDR database.

HYTONE CREAM 2 ½%
(Hydrocortisone) ... 907
None cited in PDR database.

HYTONE LOTION 2 ½%
(Hydrocortisone) ... 907
None cited in PDR database.

HYTONE OINTMENT 2 ½%
(Hydrocortisone) ... 907
None cited in PDR database.

HYTRIN CAPSULES
(Terazosin Hydrochloride) ... 430
May interact with antihypertensives and certain other agents. Compounds in these categories include:

Acebutolol Hydrochloride (Possibility of significant hypotension; dosage adjustment may be necessary). Products include:
- Sectral Capsules ... 2807

Amlodipine Besylate (Possibility of significant hypotension; dosage adjustment may be necessary). Products include:
- Lotrel Capsules ... 840
- Norvasc Tablets ... 1940

Atenolol (Possibility of significant hypotension; dosage adjustment may be necessary). Products include:
- Tenoretic Tablets ... 2845
- Tenormin Tablets and I.V. Injection 2847

Benazepril Hydrochloride (Possibility of significant hypotension; dosage adjustment may be necessary). Products include:
- Lotensin Tablets ... 834
- Lotensin HCT ... 837
- Lotrel Capsules ... 840

Bendroflumethiazide (Possibility of significant hypotension; dosage adjustment may be necessary).
- No products indexed under this heading.

Betaxolol Hydrochloride (Possibility of significant hypotension; dosage adjustment may be necessary). Products include:
- Betoptic Ophthalmic Solution ... 469
- Betoptic S Ophthalmic Suspension 471
- Kerlone Tablets ... 2436

Bisoprolol Fumarate (Possibility of significant hypotension; dosage adjustment may be necessary). Products include:
- Zebeta Tablets ... 1413
- Ziac ... 1415

Captopril (Co-administration increases terazosine's maximum plasma concentrations linearly with dose at steady-state after administration of terazosine plus captopril). Products include:
- Capoten ... 739
- Capozide ... 742

Carteolol Hydrochloride (Possibility of significant hypotension; dosage adjustment may be necessary). Products include:
- Cartrol Tablets ... 410
- Ocupress Ophthalmic Solution, 1% Sterile ... ◎ 309

Chlorothiazide (Possibility of significant hypotension; dosage adjustment may be necessary). Products include:
- Aldoclor Tablets ... 1598
- Diupres Tablets ... 1650
- Diuril Oral ... 1653

Chlorothiazide Sodium (Possibility of significant hypotension; dosage adjustment may be necessary). Products include:
- Diuril Sodium Intravenous ... 1652

Chlorthalidone (Possibility of significant hypotension; dosage adjustment may be necessary). Products include:
- Combipres Tablets ... 677
- Tenoretic Tablets ... 2845
- Thalitone ... 1245

Clonidine (Possibility of significant hypotension; dosage adjustment may be necessary). Products include:
- Catapres-TTS ... 675

Clonidine Hydrochloride (Possibility of significant hypotension; dosage adjustment may be necessary). Products include:
- Catapres Tablets ... 674
- Combipres Tablets ... 677

Deserpidine (Possibility of significant hypotension; dosage adjustment may be necessary).
- No products indexed under this heading.

Diazoxide (Possibility of significant hypotension; dosage adjustment may be necessary). Products include:
- Hyperstat I.V. Injection ... 2363
- Proglycem ... 580

Diltiazem Hydrochloride (Possibility of significant hypotension; dosage adjustment may be necessary). Products include:
- Cardizem CD Capsules ... 1506
- Cardizem SR Capsules ... 1510
- Cardizem Injectable ... 1508
- Cardizem Tablets ... 1512
- Dilacor XR Extended-release Capsules ... 2018

Doxazosin Mesylate (Possibility of significant hypotension; dosage adjustment may be necessary). Products include:
- Cardura Tablets ... 2186

Enalapril Maleate (Possibility of significant hypotension; dosage adjustment may be necessary). Products include:
- Vaseretic Tablets ... 1765
- Vasotec Tablets ... 1771

Enalaprilat (Possibility of significant hypotension; dosage adjustment may be necessary). Products include:
- Vasotec I.V. ... 1768

Esmolol Hydrochloride (Possibility of significant hypotension; dosage adjustment may be necessary). Products include:
- Brevibloc Injection ... 1808

Felodipine (Possibility of significant hypotension; dosage adjustment may be necessary). Products include:
- Plendil Extended-Release Tablets ... 527

Fosinopril Sodium (Possibility of significant hypotension; dosage adjustment may be necessary). Products include:
- Monopril Tablets ... 757

Furosemide (Possibility of significant hypotension; dosage adjustment may be necessary). Products include:
- Lasix Injection, Oral Solution and Tablets ... 1240

Guanabenz Acetate (Possibility of significant hypotension; dosage adjustment may be necessary).
- No products indexed under this heading.

Guanethidine Monosulfate (Possibility of significant hypotension; dosage adjustment may be necessary). Products include:
- Esimil Tablets ... 822
- Ismelin Tablets ... 827

Hydralazine Hydrochloride (Possibility of significant hypotension; dosage adjustment may be necessary). Products include:
- Apresazide Capsules ... 808
- Apresoline Hydrochloride Tablets .. 809
- Ser-Ap-Es Tablets ... 849

IMPORTANT NOTE: Always consult each drug listing in the patient's regimen for possible interactions.

Hytrin | Interactions Index | 502

Hydrochlorothiazide (Possibility of significant hypotension; dosage adjustment may be necessary). Products include:
- Aldactazide 2413
- Aldoril Tablets 1604
- Apresazide Capsules 808
- Capozide 742
- Dyazide 2479
- Esidrix Tablets 821
- Esimil Tablets 822
- HydroDIURIL Tablets 1674
- Hydropres Tablets 1675
- Hyzaar Tablets 1677
- Inderide Tablets 2732
- Inderide LA Long Acting Capsules .. 2734
- Lopressor HCT Tablets 832
- Lotensin HCT 837
- Maxzide 1380
- Moduretic Tablets 1705
- Oretic Tablets 443
- Prinzide Tablets 1737
- Ser-Ap-Es Tablets 849
- Timolide Tablets 1748
- Vaseretic Tablets 1765
- Zestoretic 2850
- Ziac 1415

Hydroflumethiazide (Possibility of significant hypotension; dosage adjustment may be necessary). Products include:
- Diucardin Tablets 2718

Indapamide (Possibility of significant hypotension; dosage adjustment may be necessary). Products include:
- Lozol Tablets 2022

Isradipine (Possibility of significant hypotension; dosage adjustment may be necessary). Products include:
- DynaCirc Capsules 2256

Labetalol Hydrochloride (Possibility of significant hypotension; dosage adjustment may be necessary). Products include:
- Normodyne Injection 2377
- Normodyne Tablets 2379
- Trandate 1185

Levobunolol Hydrochloride (Possibility of significant hypotension; dosage adjustment may be necessary). Products include:
- Betagan .... ⊙ 233

Lisinopril (Possibility of significant hypotension; dosage adjustment may be necessary). Products include:
- Prinivil Tablets 1733
- Prinzide Tablets 1737
- Zestoretic 2850
- Zestril Tablets 2854

Losartan Potassium (Possibility of significant hypotension; dosage adjustment may be necessary). Products include:
- Cozaar Tablets 1628
- Hyzaar Tablets 1677

Mecamylamine Hydrochloride (Possibility of significant hypotension; dosage adjustment may be necessary). Products include:
- Inversine Tablets 1686

Methyclothiazide (Possibility of significant hypotension; dosage adjustment may be necessary). Products include:
- Enduron Tablets 420

Methyldopa (Possibility of significant hypotension; dosage adjustment may be necessary). Products include:
- Aldoclor Tablets 1598
- Aldomet Oral 1600
- Aldoril Tablets 1604

Methyldopate Hydrochloride (Possibility of significant hypotension; dosage adjustment may be necessary). Products include:
- Aldomet Ester HCl Injection 1602

Metipranolol Hydrochloride (Possibility of significant hypotension; dosage adjustment may be necessary). Products include:
- OptiPranolol (Metipranolol 0.3%) Sterile Ophthalmic Solution .... ⊙ 258

Metolazone (Possibility of significant hypotension; dosage adjustment may be necessary). Products include:
- Mykrox Tablets 993
- Zaroxolyn Tablets 1000

Metoprolol Succinate (Possibility of significant hypotension; dosage adjustment may be necessary). Products include:
- Toprol-XL Tablets 565

Metoprolol Tartrate (Possibility of significant hypotension; dosage adjustment may be necessary). Products include:
- Lopressor Ampuls 830
- Lopressor HCT Tablets 832
- Lopressor Tablets 830

Metyrosine (Possibility of significant hypotension; dosage adjustment may be necessary). Products include:
- Demser Capsules 1649

Minoxidil (Possibility of significant hypotension; dosage adjustment may be necessary). Products include:
- Loniten Tablets 2618
- Rogaine Topical Solution 2637

Moexipril Hydrochloride (Possibility of significant hypotension; dosage adjustment may be necessary). Products include:
- Univasc Tablets 2410

Nadolol (Possibility of significant hypotension; dosage adjustment may be necessary).
- No products indexed under this heading.

Nicardipine Hydrochloride (Possibility of significant hypotension; dosage adjustment may be necessary). Products include:
- Cardene Capsules 2095
- Cardene I.V. 2709
- Cardene SR Capsules 2097

Nifedipine (Possibility of significant hypotension; dosage adjustment may be necessary). Products include:
- Adalat Capsules (10 mg and 20 mg) 587
- Adalat CC 589
- Procardia Capsules 1971
- Procardia XL Extended Release Tablets 1972

Nisoldipine (Possibility of significant hypotension; dosage adjustment may be necessary).
- No products indexed under this heading.

Nitroglycerin (Possibility of significant hypotension; dosage adjustment may be necessary). Products include:
- Deponit NTG Transdermal Delivery System 2397
- Nitro-Bid IV 1523
- Nitro-Bid Ointment 1524
- Nitrodisc 2047
- Nitro-Dur (nitroglycerin) Transdermal Infusion System 1326
- Nitrolingual Spray 2027
- Nitrostat Tablets 1925
- Transderm-Nitro Transdermal Therapeutic System 859

Penbutolol Sulfate (Possibility of significant hypotension; dosage adjustment may be necessary). Products include:
- Levatol 2403

Phenoxybenzamine Hydrochloride (Possibility of significant hypotension; dosage adjustment may be necessary). Products include:
- Dibenzyline Capsules 2476

Phentolamine Mesylate (Possibility of significant hypotension; dosage adjustment may be necessary). Products include:
- Regitine 846

Pindolol (Possibility of significant hypotension; dosage adjustment may be necessary). Products include:
- Visken Tablets 2299

Polythiazide (Possibility of significant hypotension; dosage adjustment may be necessary). Products include:
- Minizide Capsules 1938

Prazosin Hydrochloride (Possibility of significant hypotension; dosage adjustment may be necessary). Products include:
- Minipress Capsules 1937
- Minizide Capsules 1938

Propranolol Hydrochloride (Possibility of significant hypotension; dosage adjustment may be necessary). Products include:
- Inderal 2728
- Inderal LA Long Acting Capsules 2730
- Inderide Tablets 2732
- Inderide LA Long Acting Capsules .. 2734

Quinapril Hydrochloride (Possibility of significant hypotension; dosage adjustment may be necessary). Products include:
- Accupril Tablets 1893

Ramipril (Possibility of significant hypotension; dosage adjustment may be necessary). Products include:
- Altace Capsules 1232

Rauwolfia Serpentina (Possibility of significant hypotension; dosage adjustment may be necessary).
- No products indexed under this heading.

Rescinnamine (Possibility of significant hypotension; dosage adjustment may be necessary).
- No products indexed under this heading.

Reserpine (Possibility of significant hypotension; dosage adjustment may be necessary). Products include:
- Diupres Tablets 1650
- Hydropres Tablets 1675
- Ser-Ap-Es Tablets 849

Sodium Nitroprusside (Possibility of significant hypotension; dosage adjustment may be necessary).
- No products indexed under this heading.

Sotalol Hydrochloride (Possibility of significant hypotension; dosage adjustment may be necessary). Products include:
- Betapace Tablets 641

Spirapril Hydrochloride (Possibility of significant hypotension; dosage adjustment may be necessary).
- No products indexed under this heading.

Timolol Hemihydrate (Possibility of significant hypotension; dosage adjustment may be necessary). Products include:
- Betimol 0.25%, 0.5% .... ⊙ 261

Timolol Maleate (Possibility of significant hypotension; dosage adjustment may be necessary). Products include:
- Blocadren Tablets 1614
- Timolide Tablets 1748
- Timoptic in Ocudose 1753
- Timoptic Sterile Ophthalmic Solution 1751
- Timoptic-XE 1755

Torsemide (Possibility of significant hypotension; dosage adjustment may be necessary). Products include:
- Demadex Tablets and Injection 686

Trimethaphan Camsylate (Possibility of significant hypotension; dosage adjustment may be necessary). Products include:
- Arfonad Ampuls 2080

Verapamil Hydrochloride (Co-administration increases terazosine's mean AUC_{0-24} by 11% to 24% with associated increase in C_{max} (25%) and C_{min} (32%)). Products include:
- Calan SR Caplets 2422
- Calan Tablets 2419
- Isoptin Injectable 1344
- Isoptin Oral Tablets 1346
- Isoptin SR Tablets 1348
- Verelan Capsules 1410
- Verelan Capsules 2824

Food Interactions

Food, unspecified (Delays the time to peak concentration by about 40 minutes).

HYZAAR TABLETS

(Losartan Potassium, Hydrochlorothiazide) 1677

May interact with barbiturates, narcotic analgesics, oral hypoglycemic agents, insulin, antihypertensives, corticosteroids, lithium preparations, non-steroidal anti-inflammatory agents, nondepolarizing neuromuscular blocking agents, and certain other agents. Compounds in these categories include:

Acarbose (Hyperglycemia may occur with thiazide diuretics; dosage adjustment of the antidiabetic drug may be required).
- No products indexed under this heading.

Acebutolol Hydrochloride (Additive effect or potentiation of other antihypertensives). Products include:
- Sectral Capsules 2807

ACTH (Potential for intensified electrolyte depletion particularly hypokalemia).
- No products indexed under this heading.

Alfentanil Hydrochloride (Potentiation of orthostatic hypotension). Products include:
- Alfenta Injection 1286

Amlodipine Besylate (Additive effect or potentiation of other antihypertensives). Products include:
- Lotrel Capsules 840
- Norvasc Tablets 1940

Aprobarbital (Potentiation of orthostatic hypotension).
- No products indexed under this heading.

Atenolol (Additive effect or potentiation of other antihypertensives). Products include:
- Tenoretic Tablets 2845
- Tenormin Tablets and I.V. Injection 2847

Atracurium Besylate (Possible increased responsiveness to the muscle relaxant). Products include:
- Tracrium Injection 1183

Benazepril Hydrochloride (Additive effect or potentiation of other antihypertensives). Products include:
- Lotensin Tablets 834
- Lotensin HCT 837
- Lotrel Capsules 840

503 **Interactions Index** **Hyzaar**

Bendroflumethiazide (Additive effect or potentiation of other antihypertensives).
- No products indexed under this heading.

Betamethasone Acetate (Potential for intensified electrolyte depletion particularly hypokalemia). Products include:
- Celestone Soluspan Suspension 2347

Betamethasone Sodium Phosphate (Potential for intensified electrolyte depletion particularly hypokalemia). Products include:
- Celestone Soluspan Suspension 2347

Betaxolol Hydrochloride (Additive effect or potentiation of other antihypertensives). Products include:
- Betoptic Ophthalmic Solution 469
- Betoptic S Ophthalmic Suspension 471
- Kerlone Tablets 2436

Bisoprolol Fumarate (Additive effect or potentiation of other antihypertensives). Products include:
- Zebeta Tablets 1413
- Ziac 1415

Buprenorphine (Potentiation of orthostatic hypotension). Products include:
- Buprenex Injectable 2006

Butabarbital (Potentiation of orthostatic hypotension).
- No products indexed under this heading.

Butalbital (Potentiation of orthostatic hypotension). Products include:
- Esgic-plus Tablets 1013
- Fioricet Tablets 2258
- Fioricet with Codeine Capsules 2260
- Fiorinal Capsules 2261
- Fiorinal with Codeine Capsules 2262
- Fiorinal Tablets 2261
- Phrenilin 785
- Sedapap Tablets 50 mg/650 mg .. 1543

Captopril (Additive effect or potentiation of other antihypertensives). Products include:
- Capoten 739
- Capozide 742

Carteolol Hydrochloride (Additive effect or potentiation of other antihypertensives). Products include:
- Cartrol Tablets 410
- Ocupress Ophthalmic Solution, 1% Sterile ...... ◉ 309

Chlorothiazide (Additive effect or potentiation of other antihypertensives). Products include:
- Aldoclor Tablets 1598
- Diupres Tablets 1650
- Diuril Oral 1653

Chlorothiazide Sodium (Additive effect or potentiation of other antihypertensives). Products include:
- Diuril Sodium Intravenous 1652

Chlorpropamide (Hyperglycemia may occur with thiazide diuretics; dosage adjustment of the antidiabetic drug may be required). Products include:
- Diabinese Tablets 1935

Chlorthalidone (Additive effect or potentiation of other antihypertensives). Products include:
- Combipres Tablets 677
- Tenoretic Tablets 2845
- Thalitone 1245

Cholestyramine (Absorption of hydrochlorothiazide is impaired in the presence of anionic exchange resins; cholestyramine binds hydrochlorothiazide and reduces its absorption from GI tract by up to 85%). Products include:
- Questran Light 769
- Questran Powder 770

Cimetidine (Co-administration may lead to an increase of about 18% in AUC of losartan but did not affect the pharmacokinetics of its active metabolite). Products include:
- Tagamet Tablets 2516

Cimetidine Hydrochloride (Co-administration may lead to an increase of about 18% in AUC of losartan but did not affect the pharmacokinetics of its active metabolite). Products include:
- Tagamet 2516

Clonidine (Additive effect or potentiation of other antihypertensives). Products include:
- Catapres-TTS 675

Clonidine Hydrochloride (Additive effect or potentiation of other antihypertensives). Products include:
- Catapres Tablets 674
- Combipres Tablets 677

Codeine Phosphate (Potentiation of orthostatic hypotension). Products include:
- Actifed with Codeine Cough Syrup.. 1067
- Brontex 1981
- Deconsal C Expectorant Syrup 456
- Deconsal Pediatric Syrup 457
- Dimetane-DC Cough Syrup 2059
- Empirin with Codeine Tablets 1093
- Fioricet with Codeine Capsules 2260
- Fiorinal with Codeine Capsules 2262
- Isoclor Expectorant 990
- Novahistine DH 2462
- Novahistine Expectorant 2463
- Nucofed 2051
- Phenergan with Codeine 2777
- Phenergan VC with Codeine 2781
- Robitussin A-C Syrup 2073
- Robitussin-DAC Syrup 2074
- Ryna ...... ▣ 841
- Soma Compound w/Codeine Tablets 2676
- Tussi-Organidin NR Liquid and S NR Liquid 2677
- Tylenol with Codeine 1583

Colestipol Hydrochloride (Absorption of hydrochlorothiazide is impaired in the presence of anionic exchange resins; cholestyramine binds hydrochlorothiazide and reduces its absorption from GI tract by up to 85%). Products include:
- Colestid Tablets 2591

Cortisone Acetate (Potential for intensified electrolyte depletion particularly hypokalemia). Products include:
- Cortone Acetate Sterile Suspension 1623
- Cortone Acetate Tablets 1624

Deserpidine (Additive effect or potentiation of other antihypertensives).
- No products indexed under this heading.

Dexamethasone (Potential for intensified electrolyte depletion particularly hypokalemia). Products include:
- AK-Trol Ointment & Suspension .... ◉ 205
- Decadron Elixir 1633
- Decadron Tablets 1635
- Decaspray Topical Aerosol 1648
- Dexacidin Ointment ...... ◉ 263
- Maxitrol Ophthalmic Ointment and Suspension ...... ◉ 224
- TobraDex Ophthalmic Suspension and Ointment 473

Dexamethasone Acetate (Potential for intensified electrolyte depletion particularly hypokalemia). Products include:
- Dalalone D.P. Injectable 1011
- Decadron-LA Sterile Suspension 1646

Dexamethasone Sodium Phosphate (Potential for intensified electrolyte depletion particularly hypokalemia). Products include:
- Decadron Phosphate Injection 1637
- Decadron Phosphate Respihaler 1642
- Decadron Phosphate Sterile Ophthalmic Ointment 1641
- Decadron Phosphate Sterile Ophthalmic Solution 1642
- Decadron Phosphate Topical Cream 1644
- Decadron Phosphate Turbinaire 1645
- Decadron Phosphate with Xylocaine Injection, Sterile 1639
- Dexacort Phosphate in Respihaler .. 458
- Dexacort Phosphate in Turbinaire .. 459
- NeoDecadron Sterile Ophthalmic Ointment 1712
- NeoDecadron Sterile Ophthalmic Solution 1713
- NeoDecadron Topical Cream 1714

Dezocine (Potentiation of orthostatic hypotension). Products include:
- Dalgan Injection 538

Diazoxide (Additive effect or potentiation of other antihypertensives). Products include:
- Hyperstat I.V. Injection 2363
- Proglycem 580

Diclofenac Potassium (Potential reduced diuretic, natriuretic, and antihypertensive effects). Products include:
- Cataflam 816

Diclofenac Sodium (Potential reduced diuretic, natriuretic, and antihypertensive effects). Products include:
- Voltaren Ophthalmic Sterile Ophthalmic Solution ...... ◉ 272
- Voltaren Tablets 861

Diltiazem Hydrochloride (Additive effect or potentiation of other antihypertensives). Products include:
- Cardizem CD Capsules 1506
- Cardizem SR Capsules 1510
- Cardizem Injectable 1508
- Cardizem Tablets 1512
- Dilacor XR Extended-release Capsules 2018

Doxazosin Mesylate (Additive effect or potentiation of other antihypertensives). Products include:
- Cardura Tablets 2186

Enalapril Maleate (Additive effect or potentiation of other antihypertensives). Products include:
- Vaseretic Tablets 1765
- Vasotec Tablets 1771

Enalaprilat (Additive effect or potentiation of other antihypertensives). Products include:
- Vasotec I.V. 1768

Esmolol Hydrochloride (Additive effect or potentiation of other antihypertensives). Products include:
- Brevibloc Injection 1808

Etodolac (Potential reduced diuretic, natriuretic, and antihypertensive effects). Products include:
- Lodine Capsules and Tablets 2743

Felodipine (Additive effect or potentiation of other antihypertensives). Products include:
- Plendil Extended-Release Tablets 527

Fenoprofen Calcium (Potential reduced diuretic, natriuretic, and antihypertensive effects). Products include:
- Nalfon 200 Pulvules & Nalfon Tablets 917

Fentanyl (Potentiation of orthostatic hypotension). Products include:
- Duragesic Transdermal System 1288

Fentanyl Citrate (Potentiation of orthostatic hypotension). Products include:
- Sublimaze Injection 1307

Fludrocortisone Acetate (Potential for intensified electrolyte depletion particularly hypokalemia). Products include:
- Florinef Acetate Tablets 505

Flurbiprofen (Potential reduced diuretic, natriuretic, and antihypertensive effects). Products include:
- Ansaid Tablets 2579

Fosinopril Sodium (Additive effect or potentiation of other antihypertensives). Products include:
- Monopril Tablets 757

Furosemide (Additive effect or potentiation of other antihypertensives). Products include:
- Lasix Injection, Oral Solution and Tablets 1240

Gestodene (*In Vitro* studies show significant inhibition of the formation of the active metabolite by inhibitors of P450 3A4 such as gestodene; pharmacodynamic consequences of concomitant use is undefined).
- No products indexed under this heading.

Glipizide (Hyperglycemia may occur with thiazide diuretics; dosage adjustment of the antidiabetic drug may be required). Products include:
- Glucotrol Tablets 1967
- Glucotrol XL Extended Release Tablets 1968

Glyburide (Hyperglycemia may occur with thiazide diuretics; dosage adjustment of the antidiabetic drug may be required). Products include:
- DiaBeta Tablets 1239
- Glynase PresTab Tablets 2609
- Micronase Tablets 2623

Guanabenz Acetate (Additive effect or potentiation of other antihypertensives).
- No products indexed under this heading.

Guanethidine Monosulfate (Additive effect or potentiation of other antihypertensives). Products include:
- Esimil Tablets 822
- Ismelin Tablets 827

Hydralazine Hydrochloride (Additive effect or potentiation of other antihypertensives). Products include:
- Apresazide Capsules 808
- Apresoline Hydrochloride Tablets .. 809
- Ser-Ap-Es Tablets 849

Hydrocodone Bitartrate (Potentiation of orthostatic hypotension). Products include:
- Anexsia 5/500 Elixir 1781
- Anexia Tablets 1782
- Codiclear DH Syrup 791
- Deconamine CX Cough and Cold Liquid and Tablets 1319
- Duratuss HD Elixir 2565
- Hycodan Tablets and Syrup 930
- Hycomine Compound Tablets 932
- Hycomine 931
- Hycotuss Expectorant Syrup 933
- Hydrocet Capsules 782
- Lorcet 10/650 1018
- Lortab 2566
- Tussend 1783
- Tussend Expectorant 1785
- Vicodin Tablets 1356
- Vicodin ES Tablets 1357
- Vicodin Tuss Expectorant 1358
- Zydone Capsules 949

Hydrocodone Polistirex (Potentiation of orthostatic hypotension). Products include:
- Tussionex Pennkinetic Extended-Release Suspension 998

Hydrocortisone (Potential for intensified electrolyte depletion particularly hypokalemia). Products include:
- Anusol-HC Cream 2.5% 1896
- Aquanil HC Lotion 1931
- Bactine Hydrocortisone Anti-Itch Cream ...... ▣ 709
- Caldecort Anti-Itch Hydrocortisone Spray ...... ▣ 631
- Cortaid ...... ▣ 836
- CORTENEMA 2535
- Cortisporin Ointment 1085

IMPORTANT NOTE: Always consult each drug listing in the patient's regimen for possible interactions.

Hyzaar **Interactions Index** 504

Cortisporin Ophthalmic Ointment Sterile 1085
Cortisporin Ophthalmic Suspension Sterile 1086
Cortisporin Otic Solution Sterile 1087
Cortisporin Otic Suspension Sterile 1088
Cortizone-5 .... ◘ 831
Cortizone-10 .... ◘ 831
Hydrocortone Tablets 1672
Hytone 907
Massengill Medicated Soft Cloth Towelettes 2458
PediOtic Suspension Sterile 1153
Preparation H Hydrocortisone 1% Cream .... ◘ 872
ProctoCream-HC 2.5% 2408
VōSoL HC Otic Solution 2678

Hydrocortisone Acetate (Potential for intensified electrolyte depletion particularly hypokalemia). Products include:
Analpram-HC Rectal Cream 1% and 2.5% 977
Anusol HC-1 Anti-Itch Hydrocortisone Ointment .... ◘ 847
Anusol-HC Suppositories 1897
Caldecort .... ◘ 631
Carmol HC 924
Coly-Mycin S Otic w/Neomycin & Hydrocortisone 1906
Cortaid .... ◘ 836
Cortifoam 2396
Cortisporin Cream 1084
Epifoam 2399
Hydrocortone Acetate Sterile Suspension 1669
Mantadil Cream 1135
Nupercainal Hydrocortisone 1% Cream .... ◘ 645
Ophthocort .... ⊙ 311
Pramosone Cream, Lotion & Ointment 978
ProctoCream-HC 2408
ProctoFoam-HC 2409
Terra-Cortril Ophthalmic Suspension 2210

Hydrocortisone Sodium Phosphate (Potential for intensified electrolyte depletion particularly hypokalemia). Products include:
Hydrocortone Phosphate Injection, Sterile 1670

Hydrocortisone Sodium Succinate (Potential for intensified electrolyte depletion particularly hypokalemia). Products include:
Solu-Cortef Sterile Powder 2641

Hydroflumethiazide (Additive effect or potentiation of other antihypertensives). Products include:
Diucardin Tablets 2718

Ibuprofen (Potential reduced diuretic, natriuretic, and antihypertensive effects). Products include:
Advil Cold and Sinus Caplets and Tablets (formerly CoAdvil) .... ◘ 870
Advil Ibuprofen Tablets and Caplets .... ◘ 870
Children's Advil Suspension 2692
Arthritis Foundation Ibuprofen Tablets .... ◘ 674
Bayer Select Ibuprofen Pain Relief Formula .... ◘ 715
Cramp End Tablets .... ◘ 735
Dimetapp Sinus Caplets .... ◘ 775
Haltran Tablets .... ◘ 771
IBU Tablets 1342
Ibuprohm .... ◘ 735
Children's Motrin Ibuprofen Oral Suspension 1546
Motrin Tablets 2625
Motrin IB Caplets, Tablets, and Geltabs .... ◘ 838
Motrin IB Sinus .... ◘ 838
Motrin Ibuprofen Suspension, Oral Drops, Chewable Tablets, Caplets 1546
Nuprin Ibuprofen/Analgesic Tablets & Caplets .... ◘ 622
Sine-Aid IB Caplets 1554
Vicks DayQuil SINUS Pressure & PAIN Relief with IBUPROFEN .... ◘ 762

Indapamide (Additive effect or potentiation of other antihypertensives). Products include:
Lozol Tablets 2022

Indomethacin (Potential reduced diuretic, natriuretic, and antihypertensive effects). Products include:
Indocin 1680

Indomethacin Sodium Trihydrate (Potential reduced diuretic, natriuretic, and antihypertensive effects). Products include:
Indocin I.V. 1684

Insulin, Human (Hyperglycemia may occur with thiazide diuretics; dosage adjustment of the antidiabetic drug may be required).
No products indexed under this heading.

Insulin, Human Isophane Suspension (Hyperglycemia may occur with thiazide diuretics; dosage adjustment of the antidiabetic drug may be required). Products include:
Novolin N Human Insulin 10 ml Vials 1795

Insulin, Human NPH (Hyperglycemia may occur with thiazide diuretics; dosage adjustment of the antidiabetic drug may be required). Products include:
Humulin N, 100 Units 1448
Novolin N PenFill Cartridges Durable Insulin Delivery System 1798
Novolin N Prefilled Syringe Disposable Insulin Delivery System 1798

Insulin, Human Regular (Hyperglycemia may occur with thiazide diuretics; dosage adjustment of the antidiabetic drug may be required). Products include:
Humulin R, 100 Units 1449
Novolin R Human Insulin 10 ml Vials 1795
Novolin R PenFill Cartridges Durable Insulin Delivery System 1798
Novolin R Prefilled Syringe Disposable Insulin Delivery System 1798
Velosulin BR Human Insulin 10 ml Vials 1795

Insulin, Human, Zinc Suspension (Hyperglycemia may occur with thiazide diuretics; dosage adjustment of the antidiabetic drug may be required). Products include:
Humulin L, 100 Units 1446
Humulin U, 100 Units 1450
Novolin L Human Insulin 10 ml Vials 1795

Insulin, NPH (Hyperglycemia may occur with thiazide diuretics; dosage adjustment of the antidiabetic drug may be required). Products include:
NPH, 100 Units 1450
Pork NPH, 100 Units 1452
Purified Pork NPH Isophane Insulin 1801

Insulin, Regular (Hyperglycemia may occur with thiazide diuretics; dosage adjustment of the antidiabetic drug may be required). Products include:
Regular, 100 Units 1450
Pork Regular, 100 Units 1452
Pork Regular (Concentrated), 500 Units 1453
Purified Pork Regular Insulin 1801

Insulin, Zinc Crystals (Hyperglycemia may occur with thiazide diuretics; dosage adjustment of the antidiabetic drug may be required). Products include:
NPH, 100 Units 1450

Insulin, Zinc Suspension (Hyperglycemia may occur with thiazide diuretics; dosage adjustment of the antidiabetic drug may be required). Products include:
Iletin I 1450
Lente, 100 Units 1450
Iletin II 1452
Pork Lente, 100 Units 1452
Purified Pork Lente Insulin 1801

Isradipine (Additive effect or potentiation of other antihypertensives). Products include:
DynaCirc Capsules 2256

Ketoconazole (*In Vitro* studies show significant inhibition of the formation of the active metabolite by inhibitors of P450 3A4 such as ketoconazole or complete inhibition by the combination of ketoconazole and sulfaphenazole; pharmacodynamic consequences of concomitant use is undefined). Products include:
Nizoral 2% Cream 1297
Nizoral 2% Shampoo 1298
Nizoral Tablets 1298

Ketoprofen (Potential reduced diuretic, natriuretic, and antihypertensive effects). Products include:
Orudis Capsules 2766
Oruvail Capsules 2766

Ketorolac Tromethamine (Potential reduced diuretic, natriuretic, and antihypertensive effects). Products include:
Acular 474
Acular .... ⊙ 277
Toradol 2159

Labetalol Hydrochloride (Additive effect or potentiation of other antihypertensives). Products include:
Normodyne Injection 2377
Normodyne Tablets 2379
Trandate 1185

Levobunolol Hydrochloride (Additive effect or potentiation of other antihypertensives). Products include:
Betagan .... ⊙ 233

Levorphanol Tartrate (Potentiation of orthostatic hypotension). Products include:
Levo-Dromoran 2129

Lisinopril (Additive effect or potentiation of other antihypertensives). Products include:
Prinivil Tablets 1733
Prinzide Tablets 1737
Zestoretic 2850
Zestril Tablets 2854

Lithium Carbonate (Diuretics reduce the renal clearance of lithium and add a high risk of lithium toxicity; concurrent use should be avoided). Products include:
Eskalith 2485
Lithium Carbonate Capsules & Tablets 2230
Lithonate/Lithotabs/Lithobid 2543

Lithium Citrate (Diuretics reduce the renal clearance of lithium and add a high risk of lithium toxicity; concurrent use should be avoided).
No products indexed under this heading.

Mecamylamine Hydrochloride (Additive effect or potentiation of other antihypertensives). Products include:
Inversine Tablets 1686

Meclofenamate Sodium (Potential reduced diuretic, natriuretic, and antihypertensive effects).
No products indexed under this heading.

Mefenamic Acid (Potential reduced diuretic, natriuretic, and antihypertensive effects). Products include:
Ponstel 1925

Meperidine Hydrochloride (Potentiation of orthostatic hypotension). Products include:
Demerol 2308
Mepergan Injection 2753

Mephobarbital (Potentiation of orthostatic hypotension). Products include:
Mebaral Tablets 2322

Metformin Hydrochloride (Hyperglycemia may occur with thiazide diuretics; dosage adjustment of the antidiabetic drug may be required). Products include:
Glucophage 752

Methadone Hydrochloride (Potentiation of orthostatic hypotension). Products include:
Methadone Hydrochloride Oral Concentrate 2233
Methadone Hydrochloride Oral Solution & Tablets 2235

Methyclothiazide (Additive effect or potentiation of other antihypertensives). Products include:
Enduron Tablets 420

Methyldopa (Additive effect or potentiation of other antihypertensives). Products include:
Aldoclor Tablets 1598
Aldomet Oral 1600
Aldoril Tablets 1604

Methyldopate Hydrochloride (Additive effect or potentiation of other antihypertensives). Products include:
Aldomet Ester HCl Injection 1602

Methylprednisolone Acetate (Potential for intensified electrolyte depletion particularly hypokalemia). Products include:
Depo-Medrol Single-Dose Vial 2600
Depo-Medrol Sterile Aqueous Suspension 2597

Methylprednisolone Sodium Succinate (Potential for intensified electrolyte depletion particularly hypokalemia). Products include:
Solu-Medrol Sterile Powder 2643

Metipranolol Hydrochloride (Additive effect or potentiation of other antihypertensives). Products include:
OptiPranolol (Metipranolol 0.3%) Sterile Ophthalmic Solution .... ⊙ 258

Metocurine Iodide (Possible increased responsiveness to the muscle relaxant). Products include:
Metubine Iodide Vials 916

Metolazone (Additive effect or potentiation of other antihypertensives). Products include:
Mykrox Tablets 993
Zaroxolyn Tablets 1000

Metoprolol Succinate (Additive effect or potentiation of other antihypertensives). Products include:
Toprol-XL Tablets 565

Metoprolol Tartrate (Additive effect or potentiation of other antihypertensives). Products include:
Lopressor Ampuls 830
Lopressor HCT Tablets 832
Lopressor Tablets 830

Metyrosine (Additive effect or potentiation of other antihypertensives). Products include:
Demser Capsules 1649

Minoxidil (Additive effect or potentiation of other antihypertensives). Products include:
Loniten Tablets 2618
Rogaine Topical Solution 2637

Mivacurium Chloride (Possible increased responsiveness to the muscle relaxant). Products include:
Mivacron 1138

Moexipril Hydrochloride (Additive effect or potentiation of other antihypertensives). Products include:
Univasc Tablets 2410

Morphine Sulfate (Potentiation of orthostatic hypotension). Products include:
Astramorph/PF Injection, USP (Preservative-Free) 535
Duramorph 962

(◘ Described in PDR For Nonprescription Drugs) (⊙ Described in PDR For Ophthalmology)

505 Interactions Index Hyzaar

Infumorph 200 and Infumorph 500 Sterile Solutions ... 965
MS Contin Tablets ... 1994
MSIR ... 1997
Oramorph SR (Morphine Sulfate Sustained Release Tablets) ... 2236
RMS Suppositories ... 2657
Roxanol ... 2243

Nabumetone (Potential reduced diuretic, natriuretic, and antihypertensive effects). Products include:
Relafen Tablets ... 2510

Nadolol (Additive effect or potentiation of other antihypertensives).
No products indexed under this heading.

Naproxen (Potential reduced diuretic, natriuretic, and antihypertensive effects). Products include:
Anaprox/Naprosyn ... 2117

Naproxen Sodium (Potential reduced diuretic, natriuretic, and antihypertensive effects). Products include:
Aleve ... 1975
Anaprox/Naprosyn ... 2117

Nicardipine Hydrochloride (Additive effect or potentiation of other antihypertensives). Products include:
Cardene Capsules ... 2095
Cardene I.V. ... 2709
Cardene SR Capsules ... 2097

Nifedipine (Additive effect or potentiation of other antihypertensives). Products include:
Adalat Capsules (10 mg and 20 mg) ... 587
Adalat CC ... 589
Procardia Capsules ... 1971
Procardia XL Extended Release Tablets ... 1972

Nisoldipine (Additive effect or potentiation of other antihypertensives).
No products indexed under this heading.

Nitroglycerin (Additive effect or potentiation of other antihypertensives). Products include:
Deponit NTG Transdermal Delivery System ... 2397
Nitro-Bid IV ... 1523
Nitro-Bid Ointment ... 1524
Nitrodisc ... 2047
Nitro-Dur (nitroglycerin) Transdermal Infusion System ... 1326
Nitrolingual Spray ... 2027
Nitrostat Tablets ... 1925
Transderm-Nitro Transdermal Therapeutic System ... 859

Norepinephrine Bitartrate (Possible decreased response to pressor amines). Products include:
Levophed Bitartrate Injection ... 2315

Opium Alkaloids (Potentiation of orthostatic hypotension).
No products indexed under this heading.

Oxaprozin (Potential reduced diuretic, natriuretic, and antihypertensive effects). Products include:
Daypro Caplets ... 2426

Oxycodone Hydrochloride (Potentiation of orthostatic hypotension). Products include:
Percocet Tablets ... 938
Percodan Tablets ... 939
Percodan-Demi Tablets ... 940
Roxicodone Tablets, Oral Solution & Intensol (Oxycodone) ... 2244
Tylox Capsules ... 1584

Pancuronium Bromide Injection (Possible increased responsiveness to the muscle relaxant).
No products indexed under this heading.

Penbutolol Sulfate (Additive effect or potentiation of other antihypertensives). Products include:
Levatol ... 2403

Pentobarbital Sodium (Potentiation of orthostatic hypotension). Products include:
Nembutal Sodium Capsules ... 436
Nembutal Sodium Solution ... 438
Nembutal Sodium Suppositories ... 440

Phenobarbital (Co-administration may lead to a reduction of about 20% in AUC of losartan and its active metabolite; potentiation of orthostatic hypotension). Products include:
Arco-Lase Plus Tablets ... 512
Bellergal-S Tablets ... 2250
Donnatal ... 2060
Donnatal Extentabs ... 2061
Donnatal Tablets ... 2060
Phenobarbital Elixir and Tablets ... 1469
Quadrinal Tablets ... 1350

Phenoxybenzamine Hydrochloride (Additive effect or potentiation of other antihypertensives). Products include:
Dibenzyline Capsules ... 2476

Phentolamine Mesylate (Additive effect or potentiation of other antihypertensives). Products include:
Regitine ... 846

Phenylbutazone (Potential reduced diuretic, natriuretic, and antihypertensive effects).
No products indexed under this heading.

Pindolol (Additive effect or potentiation of other antihypertensives). Products include:
Visken Tablets ... 2299

Piroxicam (Potential reduced diuretic, natriuretic, and antihypertensive effects). Products include:
Feldene Capsules ... 1965

Polythiazide (Additive effect or potentiation of other antihypertensives). Products include:
Minizide Capsules ... 1938

Prazosin Hydrochloride (Additive effect or potentiation of other antihypertensives). Products include:
Minipress Capsules ... 1937
Minizide Capsules ... 1938

Prednisolone Acetate (Potential for intensified electrolyte depletion particularly hypokalemia). Products include:
AK-CIDE ... ◉ 202
AK-CIDE Ointment ... ◉ 202
Blephamide Liquifilm Sterile Ophthalmic Suspension ... 476
Blephamide Ointment ... ◉ 237
Econopred & Econopred Plus Ophthalmic Suspensions ... ◉ 217
Poly-Pred Liquifilm ... ◉ 248
Pred Forte ... ◉ 250
Pred Mild ... ◉ 253
Pred-G Liquifilm Sterile Ophthalmic Suspension ... ◉ 251
Pred-G S.O.P. Sterile Ophthalmic Ointment ... ◉ 252
Vasocidin Ointment ... ◉ 268

Prednisolone Sodium Phosphate (Potential for intensified electrolyte depletion particularly hypokalemia). Products include:
AK-Pred ... ◉ 204
Hydeltrasol Injection, Sterile ... 1665
Inflamase ... ◉ 265
Pediapred Oral Liquid ... 995
Vasocidin Ophthalmic Solution ... ◉ 270

Prednisolone Tebutate (Potential for intensified electrolyte depletion particularly hypokalemia). Products include:
Hydeltra-T.B.A. Sterile Suspension 1667

Prednisone (Potential for intensified electrolyte depletion particularly hypokalemia). Products include:
Deltasone Tablets ... 2595

Propoxyphene Hydrochloride (Potentiation of orthostatic hypotension). Products include:
Darvon ... 1435
Wygesic Tablets ... 2827

Propoxyphene Napsylate (Potentiation of orthostatic hypotension). Products include:
Darvon-N/Darvocet-N ... 1433

Propranolol Hydrochloride (Additive effect or potentiation of other antihypertensives). Products include:
Inderal ... 2728
Inderal LA Long Acting Capsules ... 2730
Inderide Tablets ... 2732
Inderide LA Long Acting Capsules .. 2734

Quinapril Hydrochloride (Additive effect or potentiation of other antihypertensives). Products include:
Accupril Tablets ... 1893

Ramipril (Additive effect or potentiation of other antihypertensives). Products include:
Altace Capsules ... 1232

Rauwolfia Serpentina (Additive effect or potentiation of other antihypertensives).
No products indexed under this heading.

Rescinnamine (Additive effect or potentiation of other antihypertensives).
No products indexed under this heading.

Reserpine (Additive effect or potentiation of other antihypertensives). Products include:
Diupres Tablets ... 1650
Hydropres Tablets ... 1675
Ser-Ap-Es Tablets ... 849

Rocuronium Bromide (Possible increased responsiveness to the muscle relaxant). Products include:
Zemuron ... 1830

Secobarbital Sodium (Potentiation of orthostatic hypotension). Products include:
Seconal Sodium Pulvules ... 1474

Sodium Nitroprusside (Additive effect or potentiation of other antihypertensives).
No products indexed under this heading.

Sotalol Hydrochloride (Additive effect or potentiation of other antihypertensives). Products include:
Betapace Tablets ... 641

Spirapril Hydrochloride (Additive effect or potentiation of other antihypertensives).
No products indexed under this heading.

Sufentanil Citrate (Potentiation of orthostatic hypotension). Products include:
Sufenta Injection ... 1309

Sulfaphenazole (*In Vitro* studies show significant inhibition of the formation of the active metabolite by inhibitors of P450 3A4 such as sulfaphenazole; pharmacodynamic consequences of concomitant use is undefined).
No products indexed under this heading.

Sulindac (Potential reduced diuretic, natriuretic, and antihypertensive effects). Products include:
Clinoril Tablets ... 1618

Terazosin Hydrochloride (Additive effect or potentiation of other antihypertensives). Products include:
Hytrin Capsules ... 430

Thiamylal Sodium (Potentiation of orthostatic hypotension).
No products indexed under this heading.

Timolol Maleate (Additive effect or potentiation of other antihypertensives). Products include:
Blocadren Tablets ... 1614
Timolide Tablets ... 1748
Timoptic in Ocudose ... 1753
Timoptic Sterile Ophthalmic Solution ... 1751
Timoptic-XE ... 1755

Tolazamide (Hyperglycemia may occur with thiazide diuretics; dosage adjustment of the antidiabetic drug may be required).
No products indexed under this heading.

Tolbutamide (Hyperglycemia may occur with thiazide diuretics; dosage adjustment of the antidiabetic drug may be required).
No products indexed under this heading.

Tolmetin Sodium (Potential reduced diuretic, natriuretic, and antihypertensive effects). Products include:
Tolectin (200, 400 and 600 mg) .. 1581

Torsemide (Additive effect or potentiation of other antihypertensives). Products include:
Demadex Tablets and Injection ... 686

Triamcinolone (Potential for intensified electrolyte depletion particularly hypokalemia). Products include:
Aristocort Tablets ... 1022

Triamcinolone Acetonide (Potential for intensified electrolyte depletion particularly hypokalemia). Products include:
Aristocort A 0.025% Cream ... 1027
Aristocort A 0.5% Cream ... 1031
Aristocort A 0.1% Cream ... 1029
Aristocort A 0.1% Ointment ... 1030
Azmacort Oral Inhaler ... 2011
Nasacort Nasal Inhaler ... 2024

Triamcinolone Diacetate (Potential for intensified electrolyte depletion particularly hypokalemia). Products include:
Aristocort Suspension (Forte Parenteral) ... 1027
Aristocort Suspension (Intralesional) ... 1025

Triamcinolone Hexacetonide (Potential for intensified electrolyte depletion particularly hypokalemia). Products include:
Aristospan Suspension (Intra-articular) ... 1033
Aristospan Suspension (Intralesional) ... 1032

Trimethaphan Camsylate (Additive effect or potentiation of other antihypertensives). Products include:
Arfonad Ampuls ... 2080

Troleandomycin (*In Vitro* studies show significant inhibition of the formation of the active metabolite by inhibitors of P450 3A4 such as troleandomycin; pharmacodynamic consequences of concomitant use is undefined). Products include:
Tao Capsules ... 2209

Vecuronium Bromide (Possible increased responsiveness to the muscle relaxant). Products include:
Norcuron ... 1826

Verapamil Hydrochloride (Additive effect or potentiation of other antihypertensives). Products include:
Calan SR Caplets ... 2422
Calan Tablets ... 2419
Isoptin Injectable ... 1344
Isoptin Oral Tablets ... 1346
Isoptin SR Tablets ... 1348
Verelan Capsules ... 1410
Verelan Capsules ... 2824

Food Interactions

Alcohol (Potentiation of orthostatic hypotension).

Meal, unspecified (Meal slows absorption and decreases C_{max} but has minor

IMPORTANT NOTE: Always consult each drug listing in the patient's regimen for possible interactions.

effects on losartan AUC or on the AUC of the metabolite).

IBU TABLETS

(Ibuprofen) 1342

May interact with oral anticoagulants, thiazides, lithium preparations, and certain other agents. Compounds in these categories include:

Aspirin (Yields a net decrease in anti-inflammatory activity with lowered blood levels of non-aspirin drug in animal studies). Products include:

- Alka-Seltzer Effervescent Antacid and Pain Reliever .... ▣ 701
- Alka-Seltzer Extra Strength Effervescent Antacid and Pain Reliever .... ▣ 703
- Alka-Seltzer Lemon Lime Effervescent Antacid and Pain Reliever .... ▣ 703
- Alka-Seltzer Plus Cold Medicine .... ▣ 705
- Alka-Seltzer Plus Cold & Cough Medicine .... ▣ 708
- Alka-Seltzer Plus Night-Time Cold Medicine .... ▣ 707
- Alka Seltzer Plus Sinus Medicine .. ▣ 707
- Arthritis Foundation Safety Coated Aspirin Tablets .... ▣ 675
- Arthritis Pain Ascriptin .... ▣ 631
- Maximum Strength Ascriptin .... ▣ 630
- Regular Strength Ascriptin Tablets .... ▣ 629
- Arthritis Strength BC Powder .... ▣ 609
- BC Cold Powder Multi-Symptom Formula (Cold-Sinus-Allergy) ...... ▣ 609
- BC Cold Powder Non-Drowsy Formula (Cold-Sinus) .... ▣ 609
- BC Powder .... ▣ 609
- Bayer Children's Chewable Aspirin .... ▣ 711
- Genuine Bayer Aspirin Tablets & Caplets .... ▣ 713
- Extra Strength Bayer Arthritis Pain Regimen Formula .... ▣ 711
- Extra Strength Bayer Aspirin Caplets & Tablets .... ▣ 712
- Extended-Release Bayer 8-Hour Aspirin .... ▣ 712
- Extra Strength Bayer Plus Aspirin Caplets .... ▣ 713
- Extra Strength Bayer PM Aspirin .. ▣ 713
- Bayer Enteric Aspirin .... ▣ 709
- Bufferin Analgesic Tablets and Caplets .... ▣ 613
- Arthritis Strength Bufferin Analgesic Caplets .... ▣ 614
- Extra Strength Bufferin Analgesic Tablets .... ▣ 615
- Cama Arthritis Pain Reliever .... ▣ 785
- Darvon Compound-65 Pulvules 1435
- Easprin 1914
- Ecotrin 2455
- Ecotrin Enteric Coated Aspirin Maximum Strength Tablets and Caplets .... ▣ 816
- Ecotrin Enteric Coated Aspirin Regular Strength Tablets 2455
- Empirin Aspirin Tablets .... ▣ 854
- Empirin with Codeine Tablets 1093
- Excedrin Extra-Strength Analgesic Tablets & Caplets 732
- Fiorinal Capsules 2261
- Fiorinal with Codeine Capsules 2262
- Fiorinal Tablets 2261
- Halfprin 1362
- Healthprin Aspirin 2455
- Norgesic 1496
- Percodan Tablets 939
- Percodan-Demi Tablets 940
- Robaxisal Tablets 2071
- Soma Compound w/Codeine Tablets 2676
- Soma Compound Tablets 2675
- St. Joseph Adult Chewable Aspirin (81 mg.) .... ▣ 808
- Talwin Compound 2335
- Ursinus Inlay-Tabs .... ▣ 794
- Vanquish Analgesic Caplets .... ▣ 731

Bendroflumethiazide (Ibuprofen can reduce the natriuretic effect of thiazide diuretics in some patients).

No products indexed under this heading.

Chlorothiazide (Ibuprofen can reduce the natriuretic effect of thiazide diuretics in some patients). Products include:

- Aldoclor Tablets 1598
- Diupres Tablets 1650
- Diuril Oral 1653

Chlorothiazide Sodium (Ibuprofen can reduce the natriuretic effect of thiazide diuretics in some patients). Products include:

- Diuril Sodium Intravenous 1652

Dicumarol (Concurrent use may result in bleeding).

No products indexed under this heading.

Furosemide (Ibuprofen can reduce the natriurectic effect furosemide). Products include:

- Lasix Injection, Oral Solution and Tablets 1240

Hydrochlorothiazide (Ibuprofen can reduce the natriuretic effect of thiazide diuretics in some patients). Products include:

- Aldactazide 2413
- Aldoril Tablets 1604
- Apresazide Capsules 808
- Capozide 742
- Dyazide 2479
- Esidrix Tablets 821
- Esimil Tablets 822
- HydroDIURIL Tablets 1674
- Hydropres Tablets 1675
- Hyzaar Tablets 1677
- Inderide Tablets 2732
- Inderide LA Long Acting Capsules .. 2734
- Lopressor HCT Tablets 832
- Lotensin HCT 837
- Maxzide 1380
- Moduretic Tablets 1705
- Oretic Tablets 443
- Prinzide Tablets 1737
- Ser-Ap-Es Tablets 849
- Timolide Tablets 1748
- Vaseretic Tablets 1765
- Zestoretic 2850
- Ziac 1415

Hydroflumethiazide (Ibuprofen can reduce the natriuretic effect of thiazide diuretics in some patients). Products include:

- Diucardin Tablets 2718

Lithium Carbonate (Ibuprofen can produce an elevation of plasma lithium levels and a reduction in renal lithium clearance). Products include:

- Eskalith 2485
- Lithium Carbonate Capsules & Tablets 2230
- Lithonate/Lithotabs/Lithobid 2543

Lithium Citrate (Ibuprofen can produce an elevation of plasma lithium levels and a reduction in renal lithium clearance).

No products indexed under this heading.

Methotrexate Sodium (Potential for enhanced methotrexate toxicity possibly resulting from competitively inhibiting methotrexate accumulation). Products include:

- Methotrexate Sodium Tablets, Injection, for Injection and LPF Injection 1275

Methyclothiazide (Ibuprofen can reduce the natriuretic effect of thiazide diuretics in some patients). Products include:

- Enduron Tablets 420

Polythiazide (Ibuprofen can reduce the natriuretic effect of thiazide diuretics in some patients). Products include:

- Minizide Capsules 1938

Warfarin Sodium (Concurrent use may result in bleeding). Products include:

- Coumadin 926

Food Interactions

Food, unspecified (Food affects the rate but not the extent of absorption).

IBERET FILMTAB

(Vitamin B Complex With Vitamin C, Ferrous Sulfate) 433

None cited in PDR database.

IBERET-500 FILMTAB

(Vitamin B Complex With Vitamin C, Ferrous Sulfate) 433

None cited in PDR database.

IBERET-500 LIQUID

(Vitamin B Complex With Vitamin C, Ferrous Sulfate) 433

None cited in PDR database.

IBERET-FOLIC-500 FILMTAB

(Vitamin B Complex With Vitamin C, Ferrous Sulfate) 429

See **Fero-Folic-500 Filmtab**

IBERET-LIQUID

(Vitamin B Complex With Vitamin C, Ferrous Sulfate) 433

None cited in PDR database.

IBUPROHM (IBUPROFEN) CAPLETS, 200 MG

(Ibuprofen) .... ▣ 735

May interact with aspirin and acetaminophen containing products. Compounds in this category include:

Acetaminophen (Concurrent use not recommended). Products include:

- Actifed Plus Caplets .... ▣ 845
- Actifed Plus Tablets .... ▣ 845
- Actifed Sinus Daytime/Nighttime Tablets and Caplets .... ▣ 846
- Alka-Seltzer Plus Cold Medicine Liqui-Gels .... ▣ 706
- Alka-Seltzer Plus Cold & Cough Medicine Liqui-Gels .... ▣ 705
- Alka-Seltzer Plus Night-Time Cold Medicine Liqui-Gels .... ▣ 706
- Allerest Headache Strength Tablets .... ▣ 627
- Allerest No Drowsiness Tablets .... ▣ 627
- Allerest Sinus Pain Formula .... ▣ 627
- Anexsia 5/500 Elixir 1781
- Anexia Tablets 1782
- Arthritis Foundation Aspirin Free Caplets .... ▣ 673
- Arthritis Foundation NightTime Caplets .... ▣ 674
- Bayer Select Headache Pain Relief Formula .... ▣ 716
- Bayer Select Menstrual Multi-Symptom Formula .... ▣ 716
- Bayer Select Night Time Pain Relief Formula .... ▣ 716
- Bayer Select Sinus Pain Relief Formula .... ▣ 717
- Benadryl Allergy Sinus Headache Formula Caplets .... ▣ 849
- Comtrex Multi-Symptom Cold Reliever Tablets/Caplets/Liqui-Gels/Liquid .... ▣ 615
- Allergy-Sinus Comtrex Multi-Symptom Allergy-Sinus Formula Tablets .... ▣ 617
- Comtrex Non-Drowsy .... ▣ 618
- Contac Day Allergy/Sinus Caplets ▣ 812
- Contac Day & Night .... ▣ 812
- Contac Night Allergy/Sinus Caplets .... ▣ 812
- Contac Severe Cold and Flu Formula Caplets .... ▣ 814
- Contac Severe Cold & Flu Non-Drowsy .... ▣ 815
- Coricidin 'D' Decongestant Tablets .... ▣ 800
- Coricidin Tablets .... ▣ 800
- DHCplus Capsules 1993
- Darvon-N/Darvocet-N 1433
- Drixoral Cold and Flu Extended-Release Tablets .... ▣ 803
- Drixoral Cough + Sore Throat Liquid Caps .... ▣ 802
- Drixoral Allergy/Sinus Extended Release Tablets .... ▣ 804
- Esgic-plus Tablets 1013
- Aspirin Free Excedrin Analgesic Caplets and Geltabs 732
- Excedrin Extra-Strength Analgesic Tablets & Caplets 732
- Excedrin P.M. Analgesic/Sleeping Aid Tablets, Caplets, Liquigels 733
- Fioricet Tablets 2258
- Fioricet with Codeine Capsules 2260
- Hycomine Compound Tablets 932
- Hydrocet Capsules 782
- Legatrin PM .... ▣ 651
- Lorcet 10/650 1018
- Lortab 2566
- Lurline PMS Tablets 982
- Maximum Strength Multi-Symptom Formula Midol .... ▣ 722
- PMS Multi-Symptom Formula Midol .... ▣ 723
- Teen Multi-Symptom Formula Midol .... ▣ 722
- Midrin Capsules 783
- Migralam Capsules 2038
- Panodol Tablets and Caplets .... ▣ 824
- Children's Panadol Chewable Tablets, Liquid, Infant's Drops .... ▣ 824
- Percocet Tablets 938
- Percogesic Analgesic Tablets .... ▣ 754
- Phrenilin 785
- Pyrroxate Caplets .... ▣ 772
- Sedapap Tablets 50 mg/650 mg .. 1543
- Sinarest Tablets .... ▣ 648
- Sinarest Extra Strength Tablets .... ▣ 648
- Sinarest No Drowsiness Tablets .... ▣ 648
- Sine-Aid Maximum Strength Sinus Medication Gelcaps, Caplets and Tablets 1554
- Sine-Off No Drowsiness Formula Caplets .... ▣ 824
- Sine-Off Sinus Medicine .... ▣ 825
- Singlet Tablets .... ▣ 825
- Sinulin Tablets 787
- Sinutab Sinus Allergy Medication, Maximum Strength Tablets and Caplets .... ▣ 860
- Sinutab Sinus Medication, Maximum Strength Without Drowsiness Formula, Tablets & Caplets .... ▣ 860
- Sinutab Sinus Medication, Regular Strength Without Drowsiness Formula .... ▣ 859
- Sudafed Cold and Cough Liquidcaps .... ▣ 862
- Sudafed Severe Cold Formula Caplets .... ▣ 863
- Sudafed Severe Cold Formula Tablets .... ▣ 864
- Sudafed Sinus Caplets .... ▣ 864
- Sudafed Sinus Tablets .... ▣ 864
- Talacen 2333
- TheraFlu .... ▣ 787
- TheraFlu Maximum Strength Nighttime Flu, Cold & Cough Medicine .... ▣ 788
- TheraFlu Maximum Strength Non-Drowsy Formula Flu, Cold & Cough Medicine .... ▣ 788
- Thera Flu Maximum Strength, Non-Drowsy Formula Flu, Cold and Cough Caplets .... ▣ 789
- Triaminic Sore Throat Formula .... ▣ 791
- Triaminicin Tablets .... ▣ 793
- Children's TYLENOL acetaminophen Chewable Tablets, Elixir, Suspension Liquid 1555
- Children's TYLENOL Cold Multi-Symptom Liquid Formula and Chewable Tablets 1561
- Children's TYLENOL Cold Plus Cough Multi Symptom Tablets and Liquid .... ▣ 681
- Infants' TYLENOL acetaminophen Drops and Suspension Drops 1555
- Infants' TYLENOL Cold Decongestant & Fever-Reducer Drops 1556
- TYLENOL Extended Relief Caplets .. 1558
- TYLENOL, Extra Strength, Acetaminophen Adult Liquid Pain Reliever 1560
- TYLENOL, Extra Strength, acetaminophen Gelcaps, Geltabs, Caplets, Tablets 1559
- TYLENOL, Extra Strength, Headache Plus Pain Reliever with Antacid Caplets 1559
- TYLENOL, Junior Strength, acetaminophen Coated Caplets, Grape and Fruit Chewable Tablets 1557

(▣ Described in PDR For Nonprescription Drugs) (◉ Described in PDR For Ophthalmology)

TYLENOL Maximum Strength Allergy Sinus Medication Gelcaps and Caplets 1563
TYLENOL Maximum Strength Allergy Sinus NightTime Medication Caplets 1555
TYLENOL Flu Maximum Strength Gelcaps 1565
TYLENOL Flu NightTime, Maximum Strength, Gelcaps 1566
TYLENOL Maximum Strength Flu NightTime Hot Medication Packets 1562
TYLENOL, Maximum Strength, Sinus Medication Geltabs, Gelcaps, Caplets and Tablets 1566
TYLENOL Cold Multi-Symptom Formula Medication Tablets and Caplets 1561
TYLENOL Cold Medication No Drowsiness Formula Gelcaps and Caplets 1562
TYLENOL Cold Multi-Symptom Hot Medication Liquid Packets............ 1557
TYLENOL Cough Multi-Symptom Medication 1564
TYLENOL Cough Multi-Symptom Medication with Decongestant...... 1565
TYLENOL, Regular Strength, acetaminophen Caplets and Tablets .. 1558
TYLENOL PM, Extra Strength Pain Reliever/Sleep Aid Caplets, Geltabs, Gelcaps.............................. 1560
TYLENOL Severe Allergy Medication Caplets 1564
Tylenol with Codeine 1583
Tylox Capsules 1584
Unisom With Pain Relief-Nighttime Sleep Aid and Pain Reliever............ 1934
Vanquish Analgesic Caplets .... ✹ 731
Vicks 44 LiquiCaps Cough, Cold & Flu Relief...................................... ✹ 755
Vicks 44M Cough, Cold & Flu Relief .... ✹ 756
Vicks DayQuil .... ✹ 761
Vicks Nyquil Hot Therapy................. ✹ 762
Vicks NyQuil LiquiCaps Multi-Symptom Cold/Flu Relief .... ✹ 763
Vicks NyQuil Multi-Symptom Cold/Flu Relief - (Original & Cherry Flavor)................................... ✹ 763
Vicodin Tablets.................................. 1356
Vicodin ES Tablets 1357
Wygesic Tablets 2827
Zydone Capsules 949

Aspirin (Concurrent use not recommended). Products include:

Alka-Seltzer Effervescent Antacid and Pain Reliever............................ ✹ 701
Alka-Seltzer Extra Strength Effervescent Antacid and Pain Reliever .... ✹ 703
Alka-Seltzer Lemon Lime Effervescent Antacid and Pain Reliever .... ✹ 703
Alka-Seltzer Plus Cold Medicine .... ✹ 705
Alka-Seltzer Plus Cold & Cough Medicine .... ✹ 708
Alka-Seltzer Plus Night-Time Cold Medicine .... ✹ 707
Alka Seltzer Plus Sinus Medicine .. ✹ 707
Arthritis Foundation Safety Coated Aspirin Tablets .... ✹ 675
Arthritis Pain Ascriptin .... ✹ 631
Maximum Strength Ascriptin .... ✹ 630
Regular Strength Ascriptin Tablets .... ✹ 629
Arthritis Strength BC Powder......... ✹ 609
BC Cold Powder Multi-Symptom Formula (Cold-Sinus-Allergy) ...... ✹ 609
BC Cold Powder Non-Drowsy Formula (Cold-Sinus) .... ✹ 609
BC Powder .... ✹ 609
Bayer Children's Chewable Aspirin .... ✹ 711
Genuine Bayer Aspirin Tablets & Caplets .... ✹ 713
Extra Strength Bayer Arthritis Pain Regimen Formula .... ✹ 711
Extra Strength Bayer Aspirin Caplets & Tablets .... ✹ 712
Extended-Release Bayer 8-Hour Aspirin .... ✹ 712
Extra Strength Bayer Plus Aspirin Caplets .... ✹ 713
Extra Strength Bayer PM Aspirin .. ✹ 713
Bayer Enteric Aspirin .... ✹ 709
Bufferin Analgesic Tablets and Caplets .... ✹ 613
Arthritis Strength Bufferin Analgesic Caplets .... ✹ 614

Extra Strength Bufferin Analgesic Tablets .... ✹ 615
Cama Arthritis Pain Reliever........... ✹ 785
Darvon Compound-65 Pulvules 1435
Easprin 1914
Ecotrin 2455
Ecotrin Enteric Coated Aspirin Maximum Strength Tablets and Caplets .... ✹ 816
Ecotrin Enteric Coated Aspirin Regular Strength Tablets 2455
Empirin Aspirin Tablets .... ✹ 854
Empirin with Codeine Tablets........... 1093
Excedrin Extra-Strength Analgesic Tablets & Caplets 732
Fiorinal Capsules 2261
Fiorinal with Codeine Capsules 2262
Fiorinal Tablets 2261
Halfprin 1362
Healthprin Aspirin 2455
Norgesic... 1496
Percodan Tablets................................ 939
Percodan-Demi Tablets...................... 940
Robaxisal Tablets............................... 2071
Soma Compound w/Codeine Tablets 2676
Soma Compound Tablets.................. 2675
St. Joseph Adult Chewable Aspirin (81 mg.) .... ✹ 808
Talwin Compound 2335
Ursinus Inlay-Tabs............................. ✹ 794
Vanquish Analgesic Caplets .... ✹ 731

IBUPROHM (IBUPROFEN) TABLETS, 200 MG

(Ibuprofen) .... ✹ 735
See Ibuprohm (Ibuprofen) Caplets, 200 mg

IDAMYCIN

(Idarubicin Hydrochloride) 1955
May interact with anthracyclines. Compounds in this category include:

Daunorubicin Hydrochloride (Previous therapy with anthracyclines is co-factor for increased cardiac toxicity). Products include:

Cerubidine 795

Doxorubicin Hydrochloride (Previous therapy with anthracyclines is co-factor for increased cardiac toxicity). Products include:

Adriamycin PFS 1947
Adriamycin RDF 1947
Doxorubicin Astra 540
Rubex 712

IFEX

(Ifosfamide) 697
May interact with:

Bone Marrow Depressants, unspecified (Adjustments in dosing may be necessary).

ILETIN I

(Insulin, Zinc Suspension)....................1450
None cited in PDR database.

LENTE, 100 UNITS

(Insulin, Zinc Suspension)....................1450
None cited in PDR database.

NPH, 100 UNITS

(Insulin, NPH) 1450
None cited in PDR database.

REGULAR, 100 UNITS

(Insulin, Regular) 1450
None cited in PDR database.

ILETIN II

(Insulin, Zinc Suspension)....................1452
None cited in PDR database.

PORK LENTE, 100 UNITS

(Insulin, Zinc Suspension)....................1452
None cited in PDR database.

PORK NPH, 100 UNITS

(Insulin, NPH) 1452
None cited in PDR database.

PORK REGULAR, 100 UNITS

(Insulin, Regular) 1452
None cited in PDR database.

PORK REGULAR (CONCENTRATED), 500 UNITS

(Insulin, Regular) 1453
None cited in PDR database.

ILOSONE LIQUID, ORAL SUSPENSIONS

(Erythromycin Estolate) 911
See Ilosone Pulvules & Tablets

ILOSONE PULVULES & TABLETS

(Erythromycin Estolate) 911
May interact with drugs which undergo biotransformation by cytochrome p-450 mixed function oxidase, oral anticoagulants, xanthine bronchodilators, and certain other agents. Compounds in these categories include:

Alfentanil Hydrochloride (Concurrent use may be associated with elevation in serum level of alfentanil; monitor serum levels closely). Products include:

Alfenta Injection 1286

Aminophylline (Co-administration with high doses of theophylline may be associated with increased serum theophylline levels and potential theophylline toxicity).

No products indexed under this heading.

Astemizole (Concomitant use may significantly alter the metabolism of astemizole; rare cases of serious cardiovascular adverse events, including electrocardiographic QT/QTc interval prolongation, death, cardiac arrest, torsades de pointes and other ventricular arrhythmias have been reported; concurrent use is contraindicated). Products include:

Hismanal Tablets 1293

Bromocriptine Mesylate (Concurrent use may be associated with elevation in serum level of bromocriptine; monitor serum levels closely). Products include:

Parlodel 2281

Carbamazepine (Concurrent use may be associated with elevation in serum level of carbamazepine; monitor serum levels closely). Products include:

Atretol Tablets 573
Tegretol Chewable Tablets 852
Tegretol Suspension.......................... 852
Tegretol Tablets.................................. 852

Clindamycin Hydrochloride (Antagonistic under some conditions).

No products indexed under this heading.

Clindamycin Palmitate Hydrochloride (Antagonistic under some conditions).

No products indexed under this heading.

Cyclosporine (Concurrent use may be associated with elevation in serum level of cyclosporine; monitor serum levels closely). Products include:

Neoral 2276
Sandimmune 2286

Dicumarol (Concomitant therapy may result in increased anticoagulant effects).

No products indexed under this heading.

Digoxin (Co-administration may result in elevated digoxin serum levels). Products include:

Lanoxicaps 1117
Lanoxin Elixir Pediatric 1120
Lanoxin Injection 1123
Lanoxin Injection Pediatric............... 1126
Lanoxin Tablets 1128

Dihydroergotamine Mesylate (Concurrent use has been associated with acute ergot toxicity characterized by severe peripheral vasospasm and dysesthesia). Products include:

D.H.E. 45 Injection 2255

Disopyramide Phosphate (Concurrent use may be associated with elevation in serum level of disopyramide; monitor serum levels closely). Products include:

Norpace 2444

Divalproex Sodium (Concurrent use may be associated with elevation in serum level of valproate; monitor serum levels closely). Products include:

Depakote Tablets................................ 415

Drugs which undergo biotransformation by cytochrome P-450 mixed function oxidase (Concurrent use may be associated with elevation in serum level of drugs metabolized by the cytochrome P-450 system).

Dyphylline (Co-administration with high doses of theophylline may be associated with increased serum theophylline levels and potential theophylline toxicity). Products include:

Lufyllin & Lufyllin-400 Tablets 2670
Lufyllin-GG Elixir & Tablets 2671

Ergotamine Tartrate (Concurrent use has been associated with acute ergot toxicity characterized by severe peripheral vasospasm and dysesthesia). Products include:

Bellergal-S Tablets 2250
Cafergot... 2251
Ergomar.. 1486
Wigraine Tablets & Suppositories .. 1829

Hexobarbital (Concurrent use may be associated with elevation in serum level of hexobarbital; monitor serum levels closely).

Lincomycin Hydrochloride Monohydrate (Antagonistic under some conditions).

No products indexed under this heading.

Lovastatin (Potential for rhabdomyolysis with or without renal impairment in seriously ill patients; concurrent use may be associated with elevation in serum level of lovastatin; monitor serum levels closely). Products include:

Mevacor Tablets................................. 1699

Midazolam Hydrochloride (Decreased clearance of midazolam; potential for increased pharmacologic effect of midazolam). Products include:

Versed Injection 2170

Phenytoin (Concurrent use may be associated with elevation in serum level of phenytoin; monitor serum levels closely). Products include:

Dilantin Infatabs................................. 1908
Dilantin-125 Suspension 1911

Phenytoin Sodium (Concurrent use may be associated with elevation in serum level of phenytoin; monitor serum levels closely). Products include:

Dilantin Kapseals 1906
Dilantin Parenteral 1910

IMPORTANT NOTE: Always consult each drug listing in the patient's regimen for possible interactions.

Probenecid (Inhibits tubular reabsorption of erythromycin). Products include:

- Benemid Tablets ... 1611
- ColBENEMID Tablets ... 1622

Terfenadine (Concomitant use may significantly alter the metabolism of terfenadine; rare cases of serious cardiovascular adverse events, including electrocardiographic QT/QTc interval prolongation, death, cardiac arrest, torsades de pointes and other ventricular arrhythmias have been reported; concurrent use is contraindicated). Products include:

- Seldane Tablets ... 1536
- Seldane-D Extended-Release Tablets ... 1538

Theophylline (Co-administration with high doses of theophylline may be associated with increased serum theophylline levels and potential theophylline toxicity). Products include:

- Marax Tablets & DF Syrup ... 2200
- Quibron ... 2053

Theophylline Anhydrous (Co-administration with high doses of theophylline may be associated with increased serum theophylline levels and potential theophylline toxicity). Products include:

- Aerolate ... 1004
- Primatene Dual Action Formula ... ▣ 872
- Primatene Tablets ... ▣ 873
- Respbid Tablets ... 682
- Slo-bid Gyrocaps ... 2033
- Theo-24 Extended Release Capsules ... 2568
- Theo-Dur Extended-Release Tablets ... 1327
- Theo-X Extended-Release Tablets .. 788
- Uni-Dur Extended-Release Tablets .. 1331
- Uniphyl 400 mg Tablets ... 2001

Theophylline Calcium Salicylate (Co-administration with high doses of theophylline may be associated with increased serum theophylline levels and potential theophylline toxicity). Products include:

- Quadrinal Tablets ... 1350

Theophylline Sodium Glycinate (Co-administration with high doses of theophylline may be associated with increased serum theophylline levels and potential theophylline toxicity).

No products indexed under this heading.

Triazolam (Decreased clearance of triazolam; potential for increased pharmacologic effect of triazolam). Products include:

- Halcion Tablets ... 2611

Valproic Acid (Concurrent use may be associated with elevation in serum level of valproate; monitor serum levels closely). Products include:

- Depakene ... 413

Warfarin Sodium (Concomitant therapy may result in increased anticoagulant effects). Products include:

- Coumadin ... 926

ILOTYCIN GLUCEPTATE, IV, VIALS

(Erythromycin Gluceptate) ... 913

May interact with oral anticoagulants, drugs which undergo biotransformation by cytochrome p-450 mixed function oxidase, xanthine bronchodilators, and certain other agents. Compounds in these categories include:

Alfentanil Hydrochloride (Concurrent use may be associated with elevation in serum level of alfentanil; monitor serum levels closely). Products include:

- Alfenta Injection ... 1286

Aminophylline (Co-administration with high doses of theophylline may be associated with increased serum theophylline levels and potential theophylline toxicity).

No products indexed under this heading.

Astemizole (Concomitant use may significantly alter the metabolism of astemizole; rare cases of serious cardiovascular adverse events, including electrocardiographic QT/QTc interval prolongation, death, cardiac arrest, torsades de pointes and other ventricular arrhythmias have been reported; concurrent use is contraindicated). Products include:

- Hismanal Tablets ... 1293

Bromocriptine Mesylate (Concurrent use may be associated with elevation in serum level of bromocriptine; monitor serum levels closely). Products include:

- Parlodel ... 2281

Carbamazepine (Concurrent use may be associated with elevation in serum level of carbamazepine; monitor serum levels closely). Products include:

- Atretol Tablets ... 573
- Tegretol Chewable Tablets ... 852
- Tegretol Suspension ... 852
- Tegretol Tablets ... 852

Cyclosporine (Concurrent use may be associated with elevation in serum level of cyclosporine; monitor serum levels closely). Products include:

- Neoral ... 2276
- Sandimmune ... 2286

Dicumarol (Concomitant therapy may result in increased anticoagulant effects).

No products indexed under this heading.

Digoxin (Co-administration may result in elevated digoxin serum levels). Products include:

- Lanoxicaps ... 1117
- Lanoxin Elixir Pediatric ... 1120
- Lanoxin Injection ... 1123
- Lanoxin Injection Pediatric ... 1126
- Lanoxin Tablets ... 1128

Dihydroergotamine Mesylate (Concurrent use has been associated with acute ergot toxicity characterized by severe peripheral vasospasm and dysesthesia). Products include:

- D.H.E. 45 Injection ... 2255

Disopyramide Phosphate (Concurrent use may be associated with elevation in serum level of disopyramide; monitor serum levels closely). Products include:

- Norpace ... 2444

Drugs which undergo biotransformation by cytochrome P-450 mixed function oxidase (Concurrent use may be associated with elevation in serum level of drugs metabolized by the cytochrome P-450 system).

Dyphylline (Co-administration with high doses of theophylline may be associated with increased serum theophylline levels and potential theophylline toxicity). Products include:

- Lufyllin & Lufyllin-400 Tablets ... 2670
- Lufyllin-GG Elixir & Tablets ... 2671

Ergotamine Tartrate (Concurrent use has been associated with acute ergot toxicity characterized by severe peripheral vasospasm and dysesthesia). Products include:

- Bellergal-S Tablets ... 2250
- Cafergot ... 2251
- Ergomar ... 1486
- Wigraine Tablets & Suppositories .. 1829

Hexobarbital (Concurrent use may be associated with elevation in serum level of hexobarbital; monitor serum levels closely).

Lovastatin (Potential for rhabdomyolysis with or without renal impairment in seriously ill patients; concurrent use may be associated with elevation in serum level of lovastatin; monitor serum levels closely). Products include:

- Mevacor Tablets ... 1699

Midazolam Hydrochloride (Decreased clearance of midazolam; potential for increased pharmacologic effect of midazolam). Products include:

- Versed Injection ... 2170

Phenytoin (Concurrent use may be associated with elevation in serum level of phenytoin; monitor serum levels closely). Products include:

- Dilantin Infatabs ... 1908
- Dilantin-125 Suspension ... 1911

Phenytoin Sodium (Concurrent use may be associated with elevation in serum level of phenytoin; monitor serum levels closely). Products include:

- Dilantin Kapseals ... 1906
- Dilantin Parenteral ... 1910

Terfenadine (Concomitant use may significantly alter the metabolism of terfenadine; rare cases of serious cardiovascular adverse events, including electrocardiographic QT/QTc interval prolongation, death, cardiac arrest, torsades de pointes and other ventricular arrhythmias have been reported; concurrent use is contraindicated). Products include:

- Seldane Tablets ... 1536
- Seldane-D Extended-Release Tablets ... 1538

Theophylline (Co-administration with high doses of theophylline may be associated with increased serum theophylline levels and potential theophylline toxicity). Products include:

- Marax Tablets & DF Syrup ... 2200
- Quibron ... 2053

Theophylline Anhydrous (Co-administration with high doses of theophylline may be associated with increased serum theophylline levels and potential theophylline toxicity). Products include:

- Aerolate ... 1004
- Primatene Dual Action Formula ... ▣ 872
- Primatene Tablets ... ▣ 873
- Respbid Tablets ... 682
- Slo-bid Gyrocaps ... 2033
- Theo-24 Extended Release Capsules ... 2568
- Theo-Dur Extended-Release Tablets ... 1327
- Theo-X Extended-Release Tablets .. 788
- Uni-Dur Extended-Release Tablets .. 1331
- Uniphyl 400 mg Tablets ... 2001

Theophylline Calcium Salicylate (Co-administration with high doses of theophylline may be associated with increased serum theophylline levels and potential theophylline toxicity). Products include:

- Quadrinal Tablets ... 1350

Theophylline Sodium Glycinate (Co-administration with high doses of theophylline may be associated with increased serum theophylline levels and potential theophylline toxicity).

No products indexed under this heading.

Triazolam (Decreased clearance of triazolam; potential for increased pharmacologic effect of triazolam). Products include:

- Halcion Tablets ... 2611

Warfarin Sodium (Concomitant therapy may result in increased anticoagulant effects). Products include:

- Coumadin ... 926

ILOTYCIN OPHTHALMIC OINTMENT

(Erythromycin) ... 912

None cited in PDR database.

IMDUR

(Isosorbide Mononitrate) ... 1323

May interact with calcium channel blockers, vasodilators, and certain other agents. Compounds in these categories include:

Amlodipine Besylate (Potential for marked symptomatic orthostatic hypotension; dosage adjustments may be necessary). Products include:

- Lotrel Capsules ... 840
- Norvasc Tablets ... 1940

Bepridil Hydrochloride (Potential for marked symptomatic orthostatic hypotension; dosage adjustments may be necessary). Products include:

- Vascor (200, 300 and 400 mg) Tablets ... 1587

Diazoxide (Additive vasodilating effects). Products include:

- Hyperstat I.V. Injection ... 2363
- Proglycem ... 580

Diltiazem Hydrochloride (Potential for marked symptomatic orthostatic hypotension; dosage adjustments may be necessary). Products include:

- Cardizem CD Capsules ... 1506
- Cardizem SR Capsules ... 1510
- Cardizem Injectable ... 1508
- Cardizem Tablets ... 1512
- Dilacor XR Extended-release Capsules ... 2018

Felodipine (Potential for marked symptomatic orthostatic hypotension; dosage adjustments may be necessary). Products include:

- Plendil Extended-Release Tablets ... 527

Hydralazine Hydrochloride (Additive vasodilating effects). Products include:

- Apresazide Capsules ... 808
- Apresoline Hydrochloride Tablets .. 809
- Ser-Ap-Es Tablets ... 849

Isradipine (Potential for marked symptomatic orthostatic hypotension; dosage adjustments may be necessary). Products include:

- DynaCirc Capsules ... 2256

Minoxidil (Additive vasodilating effects). Products include:

- Loniten Tablets ... 2618
- Rogaine Topical Solution ... 2637

Nicardipine Hydrochloride (Potential for marked symptomatic orthostatic hypotension; dosage adjustments may be necessary). Products include:

- Cardene Capsules ... 2095
- Cardene I.V. ... 2709
- Cardene SR Capsules ... 2097

Nifedipine (Potential for marked symptomatic orthostatic hypotension; dosage adjustments may be necessary). Products include:

Adalat Capsules (10 mg and 20 mg) 587
Adalat CC 589
Procardia Capsules 1971
Procardia XL Extended Release Tablets 1972

Nimodipine (Potential for marked symptomatic orthostatic hypotension; dosage adjustments may be necessary). Products include:

Nimotop Capsules 610

Nisoldipine (Potential for marked symptomatic orthostatic hypotension; dosage adjustments may be necessary).

No products indexed under this heading.

Verapamil Hydrochloride (Potential for marked symptomatic orthostatic hypotension; dosage adjustments may be necessary). Products include:

Calan SR Caplets 2422
Calan Tablets 2419
Isoptin Injectable 1344
Isoptin Oral Tablets 1346
Isoptin SR Tablets 1348
Verelan Capsules 1410
Verelan Capsules 2824

Food Interactions

Alcohol (Additive vasodilating effects).

Food, unspecified (May decrease the rate (increase in T_{max}) but not the extent (AUC) of absorption).

IMITREX INJECTION

(Sumatriptan Succinate) 1103

May interact with ergot-containing drugs and monoamine oxidase inhibitors. Compounds in these categories include:

Dihydroergotamine Mesylate (Concomitant use is contraindicated; potential for prolonged vasospastic reactions). Products include:

D.H.E. 45 Injection 2255

Ergotamine Tartrate (Concomitant use is contraindicated; potential for prolonged vasospastic reactions). Products include:

Bellergal-S Tablets 2250
Cafergot 2251
Ergomar 1486
Wigraine Tablets & Suppositories .. 1829

Furazolidone (Potential for MAO inhibitors to alter sumatriptan pharmacokinetics, increased systemic exposure, reduce sumatriptan dose). Products include:

Furoxone 2046

Isocarboxazid (Potential for MAO inhibitors to alter sumatriptan pharmacokinetics, increased systemic exposure, reduce sumatriptan dose).

No products indexed under this heading.

Methylergonovine Maleate (Concomitant use is contraindicated; potential for prolonged vasospastic reactions). Products include:

Methergine 2272

Methysergide Maleate (Concomitant use is contraindicated; potential for prolonged vasospastic reactions). Products include:

Sansert Tablets 2295

Phenelzine Sulfate (Potential for MAO inhibitors to alter sumatriptan pharmacokinetics, increased systemic exposure, reduce sumatriptan dose). Products include:

Nardil 1920

Selegiline Hydrochloride (Potential for MAO inhibitors to alter sumatripatan pharmacokinetics, increased systemic exposure, reduce sumatriptan dose). Products include:

Eldepryl Tablets 2550

Tranylcypromine Sulfate (Potential for MAO inhibitors to alter sumatripatan pharmacokinetics, increased systemic exposure, reduce sumatriptan dose). Products include:

Parnate Tablets 2503

IMITREX TABLETS

(Sumatriptan Succinate) 1106

May interact with monoamine oxidase inhibitors, ergot-containing drugs, and certain other agents. Compounds in these categories include:

Dihydroergotamine Mesylate (Ergot-containing drugs have been reported to cause prolonged vasospastic reactions which may result in additive effects; concurrent use within 24 hours of each other should be avoided). Products include:

D.H.E. 45 Injection 2255

Ergotamine Tartrate (Ergot-containing drugs have been reported to cause prolonged vasospastic reactions which may result in additive effects; concurrent use within 24 hours of each other should be avoided). Products include:

Bellergal-S Tablets 2250
Cafergot 2251
Ergomar 1486
Wigraine Tablets & Suppositories .. 1829

Furazolidone (Concurrent and/or sequential use is contraindicated; MAOI can markedly increase sumatriptan systemic exposure; potential for marked increase in sumatriptan AUC and half-life and marked decrease in Cl_p/F). Products include:

Furoxone 2046

Isocarboxazid (Concurrent and/or sequential use is contraindicated; MAOI can markedly increase sumatriptan systemic exposure; potential for marked increase in sumatriptan AUC and half-life and marked decrease in Cl_p/F).

No products indexed under this heading.

Methylergonovine Maleate (Ergot-containing drugs have been reported to cause prolonged vasospastic reactions which may result in additive effects; concurrent use within 24 hours of each other should be avoided). Products include:

Methergine 2272

Methysergide Maleate (Ergot-containing drugs have been reported to cause prolonged vasospastic reactions which may result in additive effects; concurrent use within 24 hours of each other should be avoided). Products include:

Sansert Tablets 2295

Phenelzine Sulfate (Concurrent and/or sequential use is contraindicated; MAOI can markedly increase sumatriptan systemic exposure; potential for marked increase in sumatriptan AUC and half-life and marked decrease in Cl_p/F). Products include:

Nardil 1920

Selegiline Hydrochloride (Concurrent and/or sequential use is contraindicated; MAOI can markedly increase sumatriptan systemic exposure; potential for marked increase in sumatriptan AUC and half-life and marked decrease in Cl_p/F). Products include:

Eldepryl Tablets 2550

Tranylcypromine Sulfate (Concurrent and/or sequential use is contraindicated; MAOI can markedly increase sumatriptan systemic exposure; potential for marked increase in sumatriptan AUC and half-life and marked decrease in Cl_p/F). Products include:

Parnate Tablets 2503

Food Interactions

Food, unspecified (Delays the T_{max} slightly by about 0.5 hour with no significant effect on the bioavailability).

IMODIUM A-D CAPLETS AND LIQUID

(Loperamide Hydrochloride) 1549

None cited in PDR database.

IMODIUM CAPSULES

(Loperamide Hydrochloride) 1295

None cited in PDR database.

IMOGAM RABIES IMMUNE GLOBULIN (HUMAN)

(Rabies Immune Globulin (Human)) .. 880

May interact with:

Measles Virus Vaccine Live (Antibodies may interfere with the immune response to the vaccine). Products include:

Attenuvax 1610

IMOVAX RABIES VACCINE

(Rabies Vaccine) 881

May interact with corticosteroids and immunosuppressive agents. Compounds in these categories include:

Azathioprine (Can interfere with the development of active immunity and predispose the patient to develop rabies). Products include:

Imuran 1110

Betamethasone Acetate (Can interfere with the development of active immunity and predispose the patient to develop rabies). Products include:

Celestone Soluspan Suspension 2347

Betamethasone Sodium Phosphate (Can interfere with the development of active immunity and predispose the patient to develop rabies). Products include:

Celestone Soluspan Suspension 2347

Cortisone Acetate (Can interfere with the development of active immunity and predispose the patient to develop rabies). Products include:

Cortone Acetate Sterile Suspension 1623
Cortone Acetate Tablets 1624

Cyclosporine (Can interfere with the development of active immunity and predispose the patient to develop rabies). Products include:

Neoral 2276
Sandimmune 2286

Dexamethasone (Can interfere with the development of active immunity and predispose the patient to develop rabies). Products include:

AK-Trol Ointment & Suspension .... ◉ 205
Decadron Elixir 1633
Decadron Tablets 1635
Decaspray Topical Aerosol 1648
Dexacidin Ointment .... ◉ 263

Maxitrol Ophthalmic Ointment and Suspension .... ◉ 224
TobraDex Ophthalmic Suspension and Ointment 473

Dexamethasone Acetate (Can interfere with the development of active immunity and predispose the patient to develop rabies). Products include:

Dalalone D.P. Injectable 1011
Decadron-LA Sterile Suspension 1646

Dexamethasone Sodium Phosphate (Can interfere with the development of active immunity and predispose the patient to develop rabies). Products include:

Decadron Phosphate Injection 1637
Decadron Phosphate Respihaler 1642
Decadron Phosphate Sterile Ophthalmic Ointment 1641
Decadron Phosphate Sterile Ophthalmic Solution 1642
Decadron Phosphate Topical Cream 1644
Decadron Phosphate Turbinaire 1645
Decadron Phosphate with Xylocaine Injection, Sterile 1639
Dexacort Phosphate in Respihaler .. 458
Dexacort Phosphate in Turbinaire .. 459
NeoDecadron Sterile Ophthalmic Ointment 1712
NeoDecadron Sterile Ophthalmic Solution 1713
NeoDecadron Topical Cream 1714

Fludrocortisone Acetate (Can interfere with the development of active immunity and predispose the patient to develop rabies). Products include:

Florinef Acetate Tablets 505

Hydrocortisone (Can interfere with the development of active immunity and predispose the patient to develop rabies). Products include:

Anusol-HC Cream 2.5% 1896
Aquanil HC Lotion 1931
Bactine Hydrocortisone Anti-Itch Cream .... ᴴᴰ 709
Caldecort Anti-Itch Hydrocortisone Spray .... ᴴᴰ 631
Cortaid .... ᴴᴰ 836
CORTENEMA 2535
Cortisporin Ointment 1085
Cortisporin Ophthalmic Ointment Sterile 1085
Cortisporin Ophthalmic Suspension Sterile 1086
Cortisporin Otic Solution Sterile 1087
Cortisporin Otic Suspension Sterile 1088
Cortizone-5 .... ᴴᴰ 831
Cortizone-10 .... ᴴᴰ 831
Hydrocortone Tablets 1672
Hytone 907
Massengill Medicated Soft Cloth Towelettes 2458
PediOtic Suspension Sterile 1153
Preparation H Hydrocortisone 1% Cream .... ᴴᴰ 872
ProctoCream-HC 2.5% 2408
VōSoL HC Otic Solution 2678

Hydrocortisone Acetate (Can interfere with the development of active immunity and predispose the patient to develop rabies). Products include:

Analpram-HC Rectal Cream 1% and 2.5% 977
Anusol HC-1 Anti-Itch Hydrocortisone Ointment .... ᴴᴰ 847
Anusol-HC Suppositories 1897
Caldecort .... ᴴᴰ 631
Carmol HC 924
Coly-Mycin S Otic w/Neomycin & Hydrocortisone 1906
Cortaid .... ᴴᴰ 836
Cortifoam 2396
Cortisporin Cream 1084
Epifoam 2399
Hydrocortone Acetate Sterile Suspension 1669
Mantadil Cream 1135
Nupercainal Hydrocortisone 1% Cream .... ᴴᴰ 645
Ophthocort .... ◉ 311
Pramosone Cream, Lotion & Ointment 978
ProctoCream-HC 2408

IMPORTANT NOTE: Always consult each drug listing in the patient's regimen for possible interactions.

ProctoFoam-HC 2409
Terra-Cortril Ophthalmic Suspension 2210

Hydrocortisone Sodium Phosphate (Can interfere with the development of active immunity and predispose the patient to develop rabies). Products include:
Hydrocortone Phosphate Injection, Sterile 1670

Hydrocortisone Sodium Succinate (Can interfere with the development of active immunity and predispose the patient to develop rabies). Products include:
Solu-Cortef Sterile Powder 2641

Immune Globulin (Human) (Can interfere with the development of active immunity and predispose the patient to develop rabies).
No products indexed under this heading.

Immune Globulin Intravenous (Human) (Can interfere with the development of active immunity and predispose the patient to develop rabies).

Methylprednisolone Acetate (Can interfere with the development of active immunity and predispose the patient to develop rabies). Products include:
Depo-Medrol Single-Dose Vial 2600
Depo-Medrol Sterile Aqueous Suspension 2597

Methylprednisolone Sodium Succinate (Can interfere with the development of active immunity and predispose the patient to develop rabies). Products include:
Solu-Medrol Sterile Powder 2643

Muromonab-CD3 (Can interfere with the development of active immunity and predispose the patient to develop rabies). Products include:
Orthoclone OKT3 Sterile Solution 1837

Mycophenolate Mofetil (Can interfere with the development of active immunity and predispose the patient to develop rabies). Products include:
CellCept Capsules 2099

Prednisolone Acetate (Can interfere with the development of active immunity and predispose the patient to develop rabies). Products include:
AK-CIDE ◉ 202
AK-CIDE Ointment ◉ 202
Blephamide Liquifilm Sterile Ophthalmic Suspension 476
Blephamide Ointment ◉ 237
Econopred & Econopred Plus Ophthalmic Suspensions ◉ 217
Poly-Pred Liquifilm ◉ 248
Pred Forte ◉ 250
Pred Mild ◉ 253
Pred-G Liquifilm Sterile Ophthalmic Suspension ◉ 251
Pred-G S.O.P. Sterile Ophthalmic Ointment ◉ 252
Vasocidin Ointment ◉ 268

Prednisolone Sodium Phosphate (Can interfere with the development of active immunity and predispose the patient to develop rabies). Products include:
AK-Pred ◉ 204
Hydeltrasol Injection, Sterile 1665
Inflamase ◉ 265
Pediapred Oral Liquid 995
Vasocidin Ophthalmic Solution ◉ 270

Prednisolone Tebutate (Can interfere with the development of active immunity and predispose the patient to develop rabies). Products include:
Hydeltra-T.B.A. Sterile Suspension 1667

Prednisone (Can interfere with the development of active immunity and predispose the patient to develop rabies). Products include:
Deltasone Tablets 2595

Tacrolimus (Can interfere with the development of active immunity and predispose the patient to develop rabies). Products include:
Prograf 1042

Triamcinolone (Can interfere with the development of active immunity and predispose the patient to develop rabies). Products include:
Aristocort Tablets 1022

Triamcinolone Acetonide (Can interfere with the development of active immunity and predispose the patient to develop rabies). Products include:
Aristocort A 0.025% Cream 1027
Aristocort A 0.5% Cream 1031
Aristocort A 0.1% Cream 1029
Aristocort A 0.1% Ointment 1030
Azmacort Oral Inhaler 2011
Nasacort Nasal Inhaler 2024

Triamcinolone Diacetate (Can interfere with the development of active immunity and predispose the patient to develop rabies). Products include:
Aristocort Suspension (Forte Parenteral) 1027
Aristocort Suspension (Intralesional) 1025

Triamcinolone Hexacetonide (Can interfere with the development of active immunity and predispose the patient to develop rabies). Products include:
Aristospan Suspension (Intra-articular) 1033
Aristospan Suspension (Intralesional) 1032

IMPREGON CONCENTRATE

(Tetrachlorosalicylanilide) 1005
None cited in PDR database.

IMURAN INJECTION

(Azathioprine) 1110
See **Imuran Tablets**

IMURAN TABLETS

(Azathioprine) 1110
May interact with ACE inhibitors and certain other agents. Compounds in these categories include:

Allopurinol (Inhibition of degradative pathway of azathioprine; reduce Imuran dosage by 1/3 to 1/4 the usual dose). Products include:
Zyloprim Tablets 1226

Benazepril Hydrochloride (Potential for severe leukopenia). Products include:
Lotensin Tablets 834
Lotensin HCT 837
Lotrel Capsules 840

Captopril (Potential for severe leukopenia). Products include:
Capoten 739
Capozide 742

Enalapril Maleate (Potential for severe leukopenia). Products include:
Vaseretic Tablets 1765
Vasotec Tablets 1771

Enalaprilat (Potential for severe leukopenia). Products include:
Vasotec I.V. 1768

Fosinopril Sodium (Potential for severe leukopenia). Products include:
Monopril Tablets 757

Lisinopril (Potential for severe leukopenia). Products include:
Prinivil Tablets 1733
Prinzide Tablets 1737
Zestoretic 2850
Zestril Tablets 2854

Moexipril Hydrochloride (Potential for severe leukopenia). Products include:
Univasc Tablets 2410

Quinapril Hydrochloride (Potential for severe leukopenia). Products include:
Accupril Tablets 1893

Ramipril (Potential for severe leukopenia). Products include:
Altace Capsules 1232

Spirapril Hydrochloride (Potential for severe leukopenia).
No products indexed under this heading.

Sulfamethoxazole (Potential for exaggerated leukopenia). Products include:
Azo Gantanol Tablets 2080
Bactrim DS Tablets 2084
Bactrim I.V. Infusion 2082
Bactrim 2084
Gantanol Tablets 2119
Septra 1174
Septra I.V. Infusion 1169
Septra I.V. Infusion ADD-Vantage Vials 1171
Septra 1174

Trimethoprim (Potential for exaggerated leukopenia). Products include:
Bactrim DS Tablets 2084
Bactrim I.V. Infusion 2082
Bactrim 2084
Proloprim Tablets 1155
Septra 1174
Septra I.V. Infusion 1169
Septra I.V. Infusion ADD-Vantage Vials 1171
Septra 1174
Trimpex Tablets 2163

INAPSINE INJECTION

(Droperidol) 1296
May interact with central nervous system depressants, barbiturates, tranquilizers, narcotic analgesics, general anesthetics, and certain other agents. Compounds in these categories include:

Alfentanil Hydrochloride (Additive or potentiating effects). Products include:
Alfenta Injection 1286

Alprazolam (Additive or potentiating effects). Products include:
Xanax Tablets 2649

Aprobarbital (Additive or potentiating effects).
No products indexed under this heading.

Buprenorphine (Additive or potentiating effects). Products include:
Buprenex Injectable 2006

Buspirone Hydrochloride (Additive or potentiating effects). Products include:
BuSpar 737

Butabarbital (Additive or potentiating effects).
No products indexed under this heading.

Butalbital (Additive or potentiating effects). Products include:
Esgic-plus Tablets 1013
Fioricet Tablets 2258
Fioricet with Codeine Capsules 2260
Fiorinal Capsules 2261
Fiorinal with Codeine Capsules 2262
Fiorinal Tablets 2261
Phrenilin 785
Sedapap Tablets 50 mg/650 mg 1543

Chlordiazepoxide (Additive or potentiating effects). Products include:
Libritabs Tablets 2177
Limbitrol 2180

Chlordiazepoxide Hydrochloride (Additive or potentiating effects). Products include:
Librax Capsules 2176
Librium Capsules 2178
Librium Injectable 2179

Chlorpromazine (Additive or potentiating effects). Products include:
Thorazine Suppositories 2523

Chlorpromazine Hydrochloride (Additive or potentiating effects). Products include:
Thorazine 2523

Chlorprothixene (Additive or potentiating effects).
No products indexed under this heading.

Chlorprothixene Hydrochloride (Additive or potentiating effects).
No products indexed under this heading.

Clorazepate Dipotassium (Additive or potentiating effects). Products include:
Tranxene 451

Clozapine (Additive or potentiating effects). Products include:
Clozaril Tablets 2252

Codeine Phosphate (Additive or potentiating effects). Products include:
Actifed with Codeine Cough Syrup 1067
Brontex 1981
Deconsal C Expectorant Syrup 456
Deconsal Pediatric Syrup 457
Dimetane-DC Cough Syrup 2059
Empirin with Codeine Tablets 1093
Fioricet with Codeine Capsules 2260
Fiorinal with Codeine Capsules 2262
Isoclor Expectorant 990
Novahistine DH 2462
Novahistine Expectorant 2463
Nucofed 2051
Phenergan with Codeine 2777
Phenergan VC with Codeine 2781
Robitussin A-C Syrup 2073
Robitussin-DAC Syrup 2074
Ryna ▣ 841
Soma Compound w/Codeine Tablets 2676
Tussi-Organidin NR Liquid and S NR Liquid 2677
Tylenol with Codeine 1583

Desflurane (Additive or potentiating effects). Products include:
Suprane 1813

Dezocine (Additive or potentiating effects). Products include:
Dalgan Injection 538

Diazepam (Additive or potentiating effects). Products include:
Dizac 1809
Valium Injectable 2182
Valium Tablets 2183
Valrelease Capsules 2169

Enflurane (Additive or potentiating effects).
No products indexed under this heading.

Epinephrine (Epinephrine may cause paradoxical hypotension due to alpha blockade produced by Inapsine). Products include:
Bronkaid Mist ▣ 717
EPIFRIN ◉ 239
EpiPen 790
Marcaine Hydrochloride with Epinephrine 1:200,000 2316
Primatene Mist ▣ 873
Sensorcaine with Epinephrine Injection 559
Sus-Phrine Injection 1019
Xylocaine with Epinephrine Injections 567

Estazolam (Additive or potentiating effects). Products include:
ProSom Tablets 449

Ethchlorvynol (Additive or potentiating effects). Products include:
Placidyl Capsules 448

(▣ Described in PDR For Nonprescription Drugs) (◉ Described in PDR For Ophthalmology)

Interactions Index

Inderal

Ethinamate (Additive or potentiating effects).

No products indexed under this heading.

Fentanyl (Additive or potentiating effects). Products include:

Duragesic Transdermal System........ 1288

Fentanyl Citrate (Additive or potentiating effects). Products include:

Sublimaze Injection................................. 1307

Fluphenazine Decanoate (Additive or potentiating effects). Products include:

Prolixin Decanoate 509

Fluphenazine Enanthate (Additive or potentiating effects). Products include:

Prolixin Enanthate 509

Fluphenazine Hydrochloride (Additive or potentiating effects). Products include:

Prolixin 509

Flurazepam Hydrochloride (Additive or potentiating effects). Products include:

Dalmane Capsules 2173

Glutethimide (Additive or potentiating effects).

No products indexed under this heading.

Haloperidol (Additive or potentiating effects). Products include:

Haldol Injection, Tablets and Concentrate 1575

Haloperidol Decanoate (Additive or potentiating effects). Products include:

Haldol Decanoate..................................... 1577

Hydrocodone Bitartrate (Additive or potentiating effects). Products include:

Anexsia 5/500 Elixir 1781
Anexia Tablets.. 1782
Codiclear DH Syrup 791
Deconamine CX Cough and Cold Liquid and Tablets................................. 1319
Duratuss HD Elixir 2565
Hycodan Tablets and Syrup 930
Hycomine Compound Tablets 932
Hycomine 931
Hycotuss Expectorant Syrup 933
Hydrocet Capsules 782
Lorcet 10/650.. 1018
Lortab.. 2566
Tussend 1783
Tussend Expectorant 1785
Vicodin Tablets 1356
Vicodin ES Tablets 1357
Vicodin Tuss Expectorant 1358
Zydone Capsules 949

Hydrocodone Polistirex (Additive or potentiating effects). Products include:

Tussionex Pennkinetic Extended-Release Suspension 998

Hydroxyzine Hydrochloride (Additive or potentiating effects). Products include:

Atarax Tablets & Syrup.......................... 2185
Marax Tablets & DF Syrup.................... 2200
Vistaril Intramuscular Solution.......... 2216

Isoflurane (Additive or potentiating effects).

No products indexed under this heading.

Ketamine Hydrochloride (Additive or potentiating effects).

No products indexed under this heading.

Levomethadyl Acetate Hydrochloride (Additive or potentiating effects). Products include:

Orlamm 2239

Levorphanol Tartrate (Additive or potentiating effects). Products include:

Levo-Dromoran... 2129

Lorazepam (Additive or potentiating effects). Products include:

Ativan Injection.. 2698

Ativan Tablets 2700

Loxapine Hydrochloride (Additive or potentiating effects). Products include:

Loxitane 1378

Loxapine Succinate (Additive or potentiating effects). Products include:

Loxitane Capsules 1378

Meperidine Hydrochloride (Additive or potentiating effects). Products include:

Demerol 2308
Mepergan Injection 2753

Mephobarbital (Additive or potentiating effects). Products include:

Mebaral Tablets 2322

Meprobamate (Additive or potentiating effects). Products include:

Miltown Tablets 2672
PMB 200 and PMB 400 2783

Mesoridazine Besylate (Additive or potentiating effects). Products include:

Serentil.. 684

Methadone Hydrochloride (Additive or potentiating effects). Products include:

Methadone Hydrochloride Oral Concentrate 2233
Methadone Hydrochloride Oral Solution & Tablets................................ 2235

Methohexital Sodium (Additive or potentiating effects). Products include:

Brevital Sodium Vials 1429

Methotrimeprazine (Additive or potentiating effects). Products include:

Levoprome 1274

Methoxyflurane (Additive or potentiating effects).

No products indexed under this heading.

Midazolam Hydrochloride (Additive or potentiating effects). Products include:

Versed Injection 2170

Molindone Hydrochloride (Additive or potentiating effects). Products include:

Moban Tablets and Concentrate...... 1048

Morphine Sulfate (Additive or potentiating effects). Products include:

Astramorph/PF Injection, USP (Preservative-Free) 535
Duramorph 962
Infumorph 200 and Infumorph 500 Sterile Solutions.............................. 965
MS Contin Tablets................................... 1994
MSIR 1997
Oramorph SR (Morphine Sulfate Sustained Release Tablets) 2236
RMS Suppositories 2657
Roxanol 2243

Opium Alkaloids (Additive or potentiating effects).

No products indexed under this heading.

Oxazepam (Additive or potentiating effects). Products include:

Serax Capsules... 2810
Serax Tablets.. 2810

Oxycodone Hydrochloride (Additive or potentiating effects). Products include:

Percocet Tablets 938
Percodan Tablets...................................... 939
Percodan-Demi Tablets........................... 940
Roxicodone Tablets, Oral Solution & Intensol (Oxycodone) 2244
Tylox Capsules 1584

Pentobarbital Sodium (Additive or potentiating effects). Products include:

Nembutal Sodium Capsules 436
Nembutal Sodium Solution 438

Nembutal Sodium Suppositories...... 440

Perphenazine (Additive or potentiating effects). Products include:

Etrafon... 2355
Triavil Tablets 1757
Trilafon... 2389

Phenobarbital (Additive or potentiating effects). Products include:

Arco-Lase Plus Tablets 512
Bellergal-S Tablets 2250
Donnatal 2060
Donnatal Extentabs................................. 2061
Donnatal Tablets 2060
Phenobarbital Elixir and Tablets 1469
Quadrinal Tablets 1350

Prazepam (Additive or potentiating effects).

No products indexed under this heading.

Prochlorperazine (Additive or potentiating effects). Products include:

Compazine 2470

Promethazine Hydrochloride (Additive or potentiating effects). Products include:

Mepergan Injection 2753
Phenergan with Codeine......................... 2777
Phenergan with Dextromethorphan 2778
Phenergan Injection 2773
Phenergan Suppositories 2775
Phenergan Syrup 2774
Phenergan Tablets 2775
Phenergan VC 2779
Phenergan VC with Codeine 2781

Propofol (Additive or potentiating effects). Products include:

Diprivan Injection.................................... 2833

Propoxyphene Hydrochloride (Additive or potentiating effects). Products include:

Darvon 1435
Wygesic Tablets 2827

Propoxyphene Napsylate (Additive or potentiating effects). Products include:

Darvon-N/Darvocet-N 1433

Quazepam (Additive or potentiating effects). Products include:

Doral Tablets 2664

Risperidone (Additive or potentiating effects). Products include:

Risperdal.. 1301

Secobarbital Sodium (Additive or potentiating effects). Products include:

Seconal Sodium Pulvules 1474

Sufentanil Citrate (Additive or potentiating effects). Products include:

Sufenta Injection 1309

Temazepam (Additive or potentiating effects). Products include:

Restoril Capsules 2284

Thiamylal Sodium (Additive or potentiating effects).

No products indexed under this heading.

Thioridazine Hydrochloride (Additive or potentiating effects). Products include:

Mellaril 2269

Thiothixene (Additive or potentiating effects). Products include:

Navane Capsules and Concentrate 2201
Navane Intramuscular 2202

Triazolam (Additive or potentiating effects). Products include:

Halcion Tablets... 2611

Trifluoperazine Hydrochloride (Additive or potentiating effects). Products include:

Stelazine 2514

Zolpidem Tartrate (Additive or potentiating effects). Products include:

Ambien Tablets... 2416

INCHES AWAY

(Aminophylline) ....ᴿᴰ 867

None cited in PDR database.

INDERAL INJECTABLE

(Propranolol Hydrochloride)................2728

May interact with insulin, catecholamine depleting drugs, calcium channel blockers, non-steroidal anti-inflammatory agents, beta-adrenergic stimulating agents, oral hypoglycemic agents, and certain other agents. Compounds in these categories include:

Acarbose (Delay in the recovery of blood glucose to normal levels following insulin-induced hypoglycemia).

No products indexed under this heading.

Albuterol (Propranolol may block bronchodilation produced by exogenous catecholamine stimulation of beta receptors). Products include:

Proventil Inhalation Aerosol 2382
Ventolin Inhalation Aerosol and Refill 1197

Albuterol Sulfate (Propranolol may block bronchodilation produced by exogenous catecholamine stimulation of beta receptors). Products include:

Airet Solution for Inhalation 452
Proventil Inhalation Solution 0.083% 2384
Proventil Repetabs Tablets 2386
Proventil Solution for Inhalation 0.5% 2383
Proventil Syrup 2385
Proventil Tablets 2386
Ventolin Inhalation Solution................. 1198
Ventolin Nebules Inhalation Solution... 1199
Ventolin Rotacaps for Inhalation...... 1200
Ventolin Syrup.. 1202
Ventolin Tablets 1203
Volmax Extended-Release Tablets .. 1788

Aluminum Hydroxide (Greatly reduces intestinal absorption of propranolol). Products include:

ALternaGEL Liquid 1316
Maximum Strength Ascriptin ....ᴿᴰ 630
Cama Arthritis Pain Reliever............ᴿᴰ 785
Gaviscon Extra Strength Relief Formula Antacid Tablets.................ᴿᴰ 819
Gaviscon Extra Strength Relief Formula Liquid Antacid...................ᴿᴰ 819
Gaviscon Liquid Antacid ....ᴿᴰ 820
Gelusil Liquid & Tablets ....ᴿᴰ 855
Maalox Heartburn Relief Suspension ....ᴿᴰ 642
Maalox Heartburn Relief Tablets....ᴿᴰ 641
Maalox Magnesia and Alumina Oral Suspension ....ᴿᴰ 642
Maalox Plus Tablets ....ᴿᴰ 643
Extra Strength Maalox Antacid Plus Antigas Liquid and Tablets ᴿᴰ 638
Tempo Soft Antacid ....ᴿᴰ 835

Aluminum Hydroxide Gel (Greatly reduces intestinal absorption of propranolol). Products include:

ALternaGEL Liquid ....ᴿᴰ 659
Aludrox Oral Suspension 2695
Amphojel Suspension 2695
Amphojel Suspension without Flavor 2695
Amphojel Tablets..................................... 2695
Arthritis Pain Ascriptin ....ᴿᴰ 631
Regular Strength Ascriptin Tablets ....ᴿᴰ 629
Gaviscon Antacid Tablets...................ᴿᴰ 819
Gaviscon-2 Antacid Tablets ....ᴿᴰ 820
Mylanta Liquid 1317
Mylanta Tablets ....ᴿᴰ 660
Mylanta Double Strength Liquid 1317
Mylanta Double Strength Tablets ..ᴿᴰ 660
Nephrox Suspension ....ᴿᴰ 655

Aluminum Hydroxide Gel, Dried (Greatly reduces intestinal absorption of propranolol).

IMPORTANT NOTE: Always consult each drug listing in the patient's regimen for possible interactions.

Inderal — Interactions Index — 512

Aminophylline (Reduced theophylline clearance).
No products indexed under this heading.

Amlodipine Besylate (Both agents may depress myocardial contractility or AV conduction resulting in increased adverse reactions). Products include:
- Lotrel Capsules 840
- Norvasc Tablets 1940

Antipyrine (Reduced clearance of antipyrine). Products include:
- Auralgan Otic Solution 2703
- Tympagesic Ear Drops 2342

Bepridil Hydrochloride (Both agents may depress myocardial contractility or AV conduction resulting in increased adverse reactions). Products include:
- Vascor (200, 300 and 400 mg) Tablets 1587

Bitolterol Mesylate (Propranolol may block bronchodilation produced by exogenous catecholamine stimulation of beta receptors). Products include:
- Tornalate Solution for Inhalation, 0.2% 956
- Tornalate Metered Dose Inhaler 957

Chlorpromazine (Increased plasma levels of both drugs). Products include:
- Thorazine Suppositories 2523

Chlorpromazine Hydrochloride (Increased plasma levels of both drugs). Products include:
- Thorazine 2523

Chlorpropamide (Delay in the recovery of blood glucose to normal levels following insulin-induced hypoglycemia). Products include:
- Diabinese Tablets 1935

Cimetidine (Decreases hepatic metabolism of propranolol resulting in increased blood levels). Products include:
- Tagamet Tablets 2516

Cimetidine Hydrochloride (Decreases hepatic metabolism of propranolol resulting in increased blood levels). Products include:
- Tagamet 2516

Deserpidine (May produce an excessive hypotension with bradycardia and orthostatic effects).
No products indexed under this heading.

Diclofenac Potassium (Blunts antihypertensive effect of beta blocker). Products include:
- Cataflam 816

Diclofenac Sodium (Blunts antihypertensive effect of beta blocker). Products include:
- Voltaren Ophthalmic Sterile Ophthalmic Solution .... ◉ 272
- Voltaren Tablets 861

Diltiazem Hydrochloride (Both agents may depress myocardial contractility or AV conduction resulting in increased adverse reactions). Products include:
- Cardizem CD Capsules 1506
- Cardizem SR Capsules 1510
- Cardizem Injectable 1508
- Cardizem Tablets 1512
- Dilacor XR Extended-release Capsules 2018

Dobutamine Hydrochloride (Reversed effects of propranolol). Products include:
- Dobutrex Solution Vials 1439

Dyphylline (Reduced theophylline clearance). Products include:
- Lufyllin & Lufyllin-400 Tablets 2670
- Lufyllin-GG Elixir & Tablets 2671

Ephedrine Hydrochloride (Propranolol may block bronchodilation produced by exogenous catecholamine stimulation of beta receptors). Products include:
- Primatene Dual Action Formula .... ▣ 872
- Primatene Tablets .... ▣ 873
- Quadrinal Tablets 1350

Ephedrine Sulfate (Propranolol may block bronchodilation produced by exogenous catecholamine stimulation of beta receptors). Products include:
- Bronkaid Caplets .... ▣ 717
- Marax Tablets & DF Syrup 2200

Ephedrine Tannate (Propranolol may block bronchodilation produced by exogenous catecholamine stimulation of beta receptors). Products include:
- Rynatuss 2673

Epinephrine (Propranolol may block bronchodilation produced by exogenous catecholamine stimulation of beta receptors). Products include:
- Bronkaid Mist .... ▣ 717
- EPIFRIN .... ◉ 239
- EpiPen 790
- Marcaine Hydrochloride with Epinephrine 1:200,000 2316
- Primatene Mist .... ▣ 873
- Sensorcaine with Epinephrine Injection 559
- Sus-Phrine Injection 1019
- Xylocaine with Epinephrine Injections 567

Epinephrine Hydrochloride (Propranolol may block bronchodilation produced by exogenous catecholamine stimulation of beta receptors). Products include:
- Ana-Kit Anaphylaxis Emergency Treatment Kit 617

Ethylnorepinephrine Hydrochloride (Propranolol may block bronchodilation produced by exogenous catecholamine stimulation of beta receptors).
No products indexed under this heading.

Etodolac (Blunts antihypertensive effect of beta blocker). Products include:
- Lodine Capsules and Tablets 2743

Felodipine (Both agents may depress myocardial contractility or AV conduction resulting in increased adverse reactions). Products include:
- Plendil Extended-Release Tablets 527

Fenoprofen Calcium (Blunts antihypertensive effect of beta blocker). Products include:
- Nalfon 200 Pulvules & Nalfon Tablets 917

Flurbiprofen (Blunts antihypertensive effect of beta blocker). Products include:
- Ansaid Tablets 2579

Glipizide (Delay in the recovery of blood glucose to normal levels following insulin-induced hypoglycemia). Products include:
- Glucotrol Tablets 1967
- Glucotrol XL Extended Release Tablets 1968

Glyburide (Delay in the recovery of blood glucose to normal levels following insulin-induced hypoglycemia). Products include:
- DiaBeta Tablets 1239
- Glynase PresTab Tablets 2609
- Micronase Tablets 2623

Guanethidine Monosulfate (May produce an excessive hypotension with bradycardia and orthostatic effects). Products include:
- Esimil Tablets 822
- Ismelin Tablets 827

Haloperidol (Hypotension and cardiac arrest have been reported with the concomitant use of propranolol and haloperidol). Products include:
- Haldol Injection, Tablets and Concentrate 1575

Haloperidol Decanoate (Hypotension and cardiac arrest have been reported with the concomitant use of propranolol and haloperidol). Products include:
- Haldol Decanoate 1577

Ibuprofen (Blunts antihypertensive effect of beta blocker). Products include:
- Advil Cold and Sinus Caplets and Tablets (formerly CoAdvil) .... ▣ 870
- Advil Ibuprofen Tablets and Caplets .... ▣ 870
- Children's Advil Suspension 2692
- Arthritis Foundation Ibuprofen Tablets .... ▣ 674
- Bayer Select Ibuprofen Pain Relief Formula .... ▣ 715
- Cramp End Tablets .... ▣ 735
- Dimetapp Sinus Caplets .... ▣ 775
- Haltran Tablets .... ▣ 771
- IBU Tablets 1342
- Ibuprohm .... ▣ 735
- Children's Motrin Ibuprofen Oral Suspension 1546
- Motrin Tablets 2625
- Motrin IB Caplets, Tablets, and Geltabs .... ▣ 838
- Motrin IB Sinus .... ▣ 838
- Motrin Ibuprofen Suspension, Oral Drops, Chewable Tablets, Caplets 1546
- Nuprin Ibuprofen/Analgesic Tablets & Caplets .... ▣ 622
- Sine-Aid IB Caplets 1554
- Vicks DayQuil SINUS Pressure & PAIN Relief with IBUPROFEN .... ▣ 762

Indomethacin (Blunts antihypertensive effect of beta blocker). Products include:
- Indocin 1680

Indomethacin Sodium Trihydrate (Blunts antihypertensive effect of beta blocker). Products include:
- Indocin I.V. 1684

Insulin, Human (Delayed recovery of blood glucose to normal levels following insulin-induced hypoglycemia).
No products indexed under this heading.

Insulin, Human Isophane Suspension (Delayed recovery of blood glucose to normal levels following insulin-induced hypoglycemia). Products include:
- Novolin N Human Insulin 10 ml Vials 1795

Insulin, Human NPH (Delayed recovery of blood glucose to normal levels following insulin-induced hypoglycemia). Products include:
- Humulin N, 100 Units 1448
- Novolin N PenFill Cartridges Durable Insulin Delivery System 1798
- Novolin N Prefilled Syringe Disposable Insulin Delivery System 1798

Insulin, Human Regular (Delayed recovery of blood glucose to normal levels following insulin-induced hypoglycemia). Products include:
- Humulin R, 100 Units 1449
- Novolin R Human Insulin 10 ml Vials 1795
- Novolin R PenFill Cartridges Durable Insulin Delivery System 1798
- Novolin R Prefilled Syringe Disposable Insulin Delivery System 1798
- Velosulin BR Human Insulin 10 ml Vials 1795

Insulin, Human, Zinc Suspension (Delayed recovery of blood glucose to normal levels following insulin-induced hypoglycemia). Products include:
- Humulin L, 100 Units 1446
- Humulin U, 100 Units 1450
- Novolin L Human Insulin 10 ml Vials 1795

Insulin, NPH (Delayed recovery of blood glucose to normal levels following insulin-induced hypoglycemia). Products include:
- NPH, 100 Units 1450
- Pork NPH, 100 Units 1452
- Purified Pork NPH Isophane Insulin 1801

Insulin, Regular (Delayed recovery of blood glucose to normal levels following insulin-induced hypoglycemia). Products include:
- Regular, 100 Units 1450
- Pork Regular, 100 Units 1452
- Pork Regular (Concentrated), 500 Units 1453
- Purified Pork Regular Insulin 1801

Insulin, Zinc Crystals (Delayed recovery of blood glucose to normal levels following insulin-induced hypoglycemia). Products include:
- NPH, 100 Units 1450

Insulin, Zinc Suspension (Delayed recovery of blood glucose to normal levels following insulin-induced hypoglycemia). Products include:
- Iletin I 1450
- Lente, 100 Units 1450
- Iletin II 1452
- Pork Lente, 100 Units 1452
- Purified Pork Lente Insulin 1801

Isoetharine (Propranolol may block bronchodilation produced by exogenous catecholamine stimulation of beta receptors). Products include:
- Bronkometer Aerosol 2302
- Bronkosol Solution 2302
- Isoetharine Inhalation Solution, USP, Arm-a-Med 551

Isoproterenol Hydrochloride (Propranolol may block bronchodilation produced by exogenous catecholamine stimulation of beta receptors). Products include:
- Isuprel Hydrochloride Injection 1:5000 2311
- Isuprel Hydrochloride Solution 1:200 & 1:100 2313
- Isuprel Mistometer 2312

Isoproterenol Sulfate (Propranolol may block bronchodilation produced by exogenous catecholamine stimulation of beta receptors). Products include:
- Norisodrine with Calcium Iodide Syrup 442

Isradipine (Both agents may depress myocardial contractility or AV conduction resulting in increased adverse reactions). Products include:
- DynaCirc Capsules 2256

Ketoprofen (Blunts antihypertensive effect of beta blocker). Products include:
- Orudis Capsules 2766
- Oruvail Capsules 2766

Ketorolac Tromethamine (Blunts antihypertensive effect of beta blocker). Products include:
- Acular 474
- Acular .... ◉ 277
- Toradol 2159

Lidocaine Hydrochloride (Reduced clearance of lidocaine). Products include:
- Bactine Antiseptic/Anesthetic First Aid Liquid .... ▣ 708
- Campho-Phenique Maximum Strength First Aid Antibiotic Plus Pain Reliever Ointment .... ▣ 719

(▣ Described in PDR For Nonprescription Drugs) (◉ Described in PDR For Ophthalmology)

Decadron Phosphate with Xylocaine Injection, Sterile 1639
Xylocaine Injections 567

Meclofenamate Sodium (Blunts antihypertensive effect of beta blocker).

No products indexed under this heading.

Mefenamic Acid (Blunts antihypertensive effect of beta blocker). Products include:

Ponstel 1925

Metaproterenol Sulfate (Propranolol may block bronchodilation produced by exogenous catecholamine stimulation of beta receptors). Products include:

Alupent... 669
Metaproterenol Sulfate Inhalation Solution, USP, Arm-a-Med 552

Metformin Hydrochloride (Delay in the recovery of blood glucose to normal levels following insulin-induced hypoglycemia). Products include:

Glucophage 752

Nabumetone (Blunts antihypertensive effect of beta blocker). Products include:

Relafen Tablets... 2510

Naproxen (Blunts antihypertensive effect of beta blocker). Products include:

Anaprox/Naprosyn 2117

Naproxen Sodium (Blunts antihypertensive effect of beta blocker). Products include:

Aleve 1975
Anaprox/Naprosyn 2117

Nicardipine Hydrochloride (Both agents may depress myocardial contractility or AV conduction resulting in increased adverse reactions). Products include:

Cardene Capsules 2095
Cardene I.V. 2709
Cardene SR Capsules................................ 2097

Nifedipine (Both agents may depress myocardial contractility or AV conduction resulting in increased adverse reactions). Products include:

Adalat Capsules (10 mg and 20 mg) 587
Adalat CC 589
Procardia Capsules 1971
Procardia XL Extended Release Tablets 1972

Nimodipine (Both agents may depress myocardial contractility or AV conduction resulting in increased adverse reactions). Products include:

Nimotop Capsules 610

Nisoldipine (Both agents may depress myocardial contractility or AV conduction resulting in increased adverse reactions).

No products indexed under this heading.

Oxaprozin (Blunts antihypertensive effect of beta blocker). Products include:

Daypro Caplets 2426

Phenobarbital (Accelerates propranolol clearance). Products include:

Arco-Lase Plus Tablets 512
Bellergal-S Tablets 2250
Donnatal 2060
Donnatal Extentabs................................... 2061
Donnatal Tablets 2060
Phenobarbital Elixir and Tablets 1469
Quadrinal Tablets 1350

Phenylbutazone (Blunts antihypertensive effect of beta blocker).

No products indexed under this heading.

Phenytoin (Accelerates propranolol clearance). Products include:

Dilantin Infatabs.. 1908
Dilantin-125 Suspension 1911

Phenytoin Sodium (Accelerates propranolol clearance). Products include:

Dilantin Kapseals 1906
Dilantin Parenteral 1910

Pirbuterol Acetate (Propranolol may block bronchodilation produced by exogenous catecholamine stimulation of beta receptors). Products include:

Maxair Autohaler 1492
Maxair Inhaler 1494

Piroxicam (Blunts antihypertensive effect of beta blocker). Products include:

Feldene Capsules 1965

Rauwolfia Serpentina (May produce an excessive hypotension with bradycardia and orthostatic effects).

No products indexed under this heading.

Rescinnamine (May produce an excessive hypotension with bradycardia and orthostatic effects).

No products indexed under this heading.

Reserpine (May produce an excessive hypotension with bradycardia and orthostatic effects). Products include:

Diupres Tablets 1650
Hydropres Tablets..................................... 1675
Ser-Ap-Es Tablets 849

Rifampin (Accelerates propranolol clearance). Products include:

Rifadin 1528
Rifamate Capsules 1530
Rifater... 1532
Rimactane Capsules 847

Salmeterol Xinafoate (Propranolol may block bronchodilation produced by exogenous catecholamine stimulation of beta receptors). Products include:

Serevent Inhalation Aerosol.................. 1176

Sulindac (Blunts antihypertensive effect of beta blocker). Products include:

Clinoril Tablets 1618

Terbutaline Sulfate (Propranolol may block bronchodilation produced by exogenous catecholamine stimulation of beta receptors). Products include:

Brethaire Inhaler 813
Brethine Ampuls 815
Brethine Tablets... 814
Bricanyl Subcutaneous Injection 1502
Bricanyl Tablets 1503

Theophylline (Reduced theophylline clearance). Products include:

Marax Tablets & DF Syrup..................... 2200
Quibron 2053

Theophylline Anhydrous (Reduced theophylline clearance). Products include:

Aerolate 1004
Primatene Dual Action Formula...... ⊕ 872
Primatene Tablets .... ⊕ 873
Respbid Tablets 682
Slo-bid Gyrocaps 2033
Theo-24 Extended Release Capsules 2568
Theo-Dur Extended-Release Tablets 1327
Theo-X Extended-Release Tablets .. 788
Uni-Dur Extended-Release Tablets.. 1331
Uniphyl 400 mg Tablets.......................... 2001

Theophylline Calcium Salicylate (Reduced theophylline clearance). Products include:

Quadrinal Tablets 1350

Theophylline Sodium Glycinate (Reduced theophylline clearance).

No products indexed under this heading.

Thyroxine (Lower than expected T3 concentration).

No products indexed under this heading.

Thyroxine Sodium (Lower than expected T3 concentration).

No products indexed under this heading.

Tolazamide (Delay in the recovery of blood glucose to normal levels following insulin-induced hypoglycemia).

No products indexed under this heading.

Tolbutamide (Delay in the recovery of blood glucose to normal levels following insulin-induced hypoglycemia).

No products indexed under this heading.

Tolmetin Sodium (Blunts antihypertensive effect of beta blocker). Products include:

Tolectin (200, 400 and 600 mg) .. 1581

Verapamil Hydrochloride (Both agents may depress myocardial contractility or AV conduction resulting in increased adverse reactions). Products include:

Calan SR Caplets 2422
Calan Tablets... 2419
Isoptin Injectable 1344
Isoptin Oral Tablets 1346
Isoptin SR Tablets 1348
Verelan Capsules 1410
Verelan Capsules 2824

Food Interactions

Alcohol (Slows the rate of absorption of propranolol).

INDERAL TABLETS

(Propranolol Hydrochloride)....................2728

See Inderal Injectable

INDERAL LA LONG ACTING CAPSULES

(Propranolol Hydrochloride)....................2730

May interact with catecholamine depleting drugs, calcium channel blockers, insulin, beta-adrenergic stimulating agents, oral hypoglycemic agents, non-steroidal anti-inflammatory agents, and certain other agents. Compounds in these categories include:

Acarbose (Delay in the recovery of blood glucose to normal levels following insulin-induced hypoglycemia).

No products indexed under this heading.

Albuterol (Propranolol may block bronchodilation produced by exogenous catecholamine stimulation of beta receptors). Products include:

Proventil Inhalation Aerosol 2382
Ventolin Inhalation Aerosol and Refill 1197

Albuterol Sulfate (Propranolol may block bronchodilation produced by exogenous catecholamine stimulation of beta receptors). Products include:

Airet Solution for Inhalation 452
Proventil Inhalation Solution 0.083% 2384
Proventil Repetabs Tablets 2386
Proventil Solution for Inhalation 0.5% 2383
Proventil Syrup 2385
Proventil Tablets 2386
Ventolin Inhalation Solution.................. 1198
Ventolin Nebules Inhalation Solution 1199
Ventolin Rotacaps for Inhalation 1200
Ventolin Syrup.. 1202
Ventolin Tablets 1203
Volmax Extended-Release Tablets .. 1788

Aluminum Hydroxide Gel (Intestinal absorption of propranolol greatly reduced). Products include:

ALternaGEL Liquid .... ⊕ 659
Aludrox Oral Suspension 2695
Amphojel Suspension 2695

Amphojel Suspension without Flavor 2695
Amphojel Tablets....................................... 2695
Arthritis Pain Ascriptin .... ⊕ 631
Regular Strength Ascriptin Tablets .... ⊕ 629
Gaviscon Antacid Tablets.................... ⊕ 819
Gaviscon-2 Antacid Tablets .... ⊕ 820
Mylanta Liquid 1317
Mylanta Tablets .... ⊕ 660
Mylanta Double Strength Liquid 1317
Mylanta Double Strength Tablets .. ⊕ 660
Nephrox Suspension .... ⊕ 655

Amlodipine Besylate (Caution should be exercised when administered concomitantly). Products include:

Lotrel Capsules 840
Norvasc Tablets 1940

Antipyrine (Reduced clearance of antipyrine). Products include:

Auralgan Otic Solution............................ 2703
Tympagesic Ear Drops 2342

Bepridil Hydrochloride (Caution should be exercised when administered concomitantly). Products include:

Vascor (200, 300 and 400 mg) Tablets 1587

Bitolterol Mesylate (Propranolol may block bronchodilation produced by exogenous catecholamine stimulation of beta receptors). Products include:

Tornalate Solution for Inhalation, 0.2% 956
Tornalate Metered Dose Inhaler 957

Chlorpromazine (Increased plasma levels of both drugs). Products include:

Thorazine Suppositories 2523

Chlorpromazine Hydrochloride (Increased plasma levels of both drugs). Products include:

Thorazine 2523

Chlorpropamide (Delay in the recovery of blood glucose to normal levels following insulin-induced hypoglycemia). Products include:

Diabinese Tablets 1935

Cimetidine (Delayed elimination and increased blood levels of propranolol). Products include:

Tagamet Tablets 2516

Cimetidine Hydrochloride (Delayed elimination and increased blood levels of propranolol). Products include:

Tagamet... 2516

Deserpidine (May produce excessive hypotension with bradycardia and orthostatic effects).

No products indexed under this heading.

Diclofenac Potassium (Blunts antihypertensive effect of beta blocker). Products include:

Cataflam 816

Diclofenac Sodium (Blunts antihypertensive effect of beta blocker). Products include:

Voltaren Ophthalmic Sterile Ophthalmic Solution .... ◉ 272
Voltaren Tablets 861

Diltiazem Hydrochloride (Caution should be exercised when administered concomitantly). Products include:

Cardizem CD Capsules 1506
Cardizem SR Capsules 1510
Cardizem Injectable 1508
Cardizem Tablets....................................... 1512
Dilacor XR Extended-release Capsules 2018

Ephedrine Hydrochloride (Propranolol may block bronchodilation produced by exogenous catecholamine stimulation of beta receptors). Products include:

Primatene Dual Action Formula...... ⊕ 872

IMPORTANT NOTE: Always consult each drug listing in the patient's regimen for possible interactions.

Inderal LA **Interactions Index** **514**

Primatene Tablets ▣ 873
Quadrinal Tablets 1350

Ephedrine Sulfate (Propranolol may block bronchodilation produced by exogenous catecholamine stimulation of beta receptors). Products include:
Bronkaid Caplets ▣ 717
Marax Tablets & DF Syrup 2200

Ephedrine Tannate (Propranolol may block bronchodilation produced by exogenous catecholamine stimulation of beta receptors). Products include:
Rynatuss 2673

Epinephrine (Propranolol may block bronchodilation produced by exogenous catecholamine stimulation of beta receptors). Products include:
Bronkaid Mist ▣ 717
EPIFRIN ◉ 239
EpiPen 790
Marcaine Hydrochloride with Epinephrine 1:200,000 2316
Primatene Mist ▣ 873
Sensorcaine with Epinephrine Injection 559
Sus-Phrine Injection 1019
Xylocaine with Epinephrine Injections 567

Epinephrine Hydrochloride (Propranolol may block bronchodilation produced by exogenous catecholamine stimulation of beta receptors). Products include:
Ana-Kit Anaphylaxis Emergency Treatment Kit 617

Ethylnorepinephrine Hydrochloride (Propranolol may block bronchodilation produced by exogenous catecholamine stimulation of beta receptors).
No products indexed under this heading.

Etodolac (Blunts antihypertensive effect of beta blocker). Products include:
Lodine Capsules and Tablets 2743

Felodipine (Caution should be exercised when administered concomitantly). Products include:
Plendil Extended-Release Tablets 527

Fenoprofen Calcium (Blunts antihypertensive effect of beta blocker). Products include:
Nalfon 200 Pulvules & Nalfon Tablets 917

Flurbiprofen (Blunts antihypertensive effect of beta blocker). Products include:
Ansaid Tablets 2579

Glipizide (Delay in the recovery of blood glucose to normal levels following insulin-induced hypoglycemia). Products include:
Glucotrol Tablets 1967
Glucotrol XL Extended Release Tablets 1968

Glyburide (Delay in the recovery of blood glucose to normal levels following insulin-induced hypoglycemia). Products include:
DiaBeta Tablets 1239
Glynase PresTab Tablets 2609
Micronase Tablets 2623

Guanethidine Monosulfate (May produce excessive hypotension with bradycardia and orthostatic effects). Products include:
Esimil Tablets 822
Ismelin Tablets 827

Haloperidol (Hypotension and cardiac arrest have been reported with the concomitant use of propranolol and haloperidol). Products include:
Haldol Injection, Tablets and Concentrate 1575

Haloperidol Decanoate (Hypotension and cardiac arrest have been reported with the concomitant use of propranolol and haloperidol). Products include:
Haldol Decanoate 1577

Ibuprofen (Blunts antihypertensive effect of beta blocker). Products include:
Advil Cold and Sinus Caplets and Tablets (formerly CoAdvil) ▣ 870
Advil Ibuprofen Tablets and Caplets ▣ 870
Children's Advil Suspension 2692
Arthritis Foundation Ibuprofen Tablets ▣ 674
Bayer Select Ibuprofen Pain Relief Formula ▣ 715
Cramp End Tablets ▣ 735
Dimetapp Sinus Caplets ▣ 775
Haltran Tablets ▣ 771
IBU Tablets 1342
Ibuprohm ▣ 735
Children's Motrin Ibuprofen Oral Suspension 1546
Motrin Tablets 2625
Motrin IB Caplets, Tablets, and Geltabs ▣ 838
Motrin IB Sinus ▣ 838
Motrin Ibuprofen Suspension, Oral Drops, Chewable Tablets, Caplets 1546
Nuprin Ibuprofen/Analgesic Tablets & Caplets ▣ 622
Sine-Aid IB Caplets 1554
Vicks DayQuil SINUS Pressure & PAIN Relief with IBUPROFEN ▣ 762

Indomethacin (Blunts antihypertensive effect of beta blocker). Products include:
Indocin 1680

Indomethacin Sodium Trihydrate (Blunts antihypertensive effect of beta blocker). Products include:
Indocin I.V. 1684

Insulin, Human (Delayed recovery of blood glucose to normal levels following insulin-induced hypoglycemia).
No products indexed under this heading.

Insulin, Human Isophane Suspension (Delayed recovery of blood glucose to normal levels following insulin-induced hypoglycemia). Products include:
Novolin N Human Insulin 10 ml Vials 1795

Insulin, Human NPH (Delayed recovery of blood glucose to normal levels following insulin-induced hypoglycemia). Products include:
Humulin N, 100 Units 1448
Novolin N PenFill Cartridges Durable Insulin Delivery System 1798
Novolin N Prefilled Syringe Disposable Insulin Delivery System 1798

Insulin, Human Regular (Delayed recovery of blood glucose to normal levels following insulin-induced hypoglycemia). Products include:
Humulin R, 100 Units 1449
Novolin R Human Insulin 10 ml Vials 1795
Novolin R PenFill Cartridges Durable Insulin Delivery System 1798
Novolin R Prefilled Syringe Disposable Insulin Delivery System 1798
Velosulin BR Human Insulin 10 ml Vials 1795

Insulin, Human, Zinc Suspension (Delayed recovery of blood glucose to normal levels following insulin-induced hypoglycemia). Products include:
Humulin L, 100 Units 1446
Humulin U, 100 Units 1450
Novolin L Human Insulin 10 ml Vials 1795

Insulin, NPH (Delayed recovery of blood glucose to normal levels following insulin-induced hypoglycemia). Products include:
NPH, 100 Units 1450
Pork NPH, 100 Units 1452
Purified Pork NPH Isophane Insulin 1801

Insulin, Regular (Delayed recovery of blood glucose to normal levels following insulin-induced hypoglycemia). Products include:
Regular, 100 Units 1450
Pork Regular, 100 Units 1452
Pork Regular (Concentrated), 500 Units 1453
Purified Pork Regular Insulin 1801

Insulin, Zinc Crystals (Delayed recovery of blood glucose to normal levels following insulin-induced hypoglycemia). Products include:
NPH, 100 Units 1450

Insulin, Zinc Suspension (Delayed recovery of blood glucose to normal levels following insulin-induced hypoglycemia). Products include:
Iletin I 1450
Lente, 100 Units 1450
Iletin II 1452
Pork Lente, 100 Units 1452
Purified Pork Lente Insulin 1801

Isoetharine (Propranolol may block bronchodilation produced by exogenous catecholamine stimulation of beta receptors). Products include:
Bronkometer Aerosol 2302
Bronkosol Solution 2302
Isoetharine Inhalation Solution, USP, Arm-a-Med 551

Isoproterenol Hydrochloride (Propranolol may block bronchodilation produced by exogenous catecholamine stimulation of beta receptors). Products include:
Isuprel Hydrochloride Injection 1:5000 2311
Isuprel Hydrochloride Solution 1:200 & 1:100 2313
Isuprel Mistometer 2312

Isoproterenol Sulfate (Propranolol may block bronchodilation produced by exogenous catecholamine stimulation of beta receptors). Products include:
Norisodrine with Calcium Iodide Syrup 442

Isradipine (Caution should be exercised when administered concomitantly). Products include:
DynaCirc Capsules 2256

Ketoprofen (Blunts antihypertensive effect of beta blocker). Products include:
Orudis Capsules 2766
Oruvail Capsules 2766

Ketorolac Tromethamine (Blunts antihypertensive effect of beta blocker). Products include:
Acular 474
Acular ◉ 277
Toradol 2159

Levothyroxine Sodium (Concurrent use may result in lower than expected T_3 concentration). Products include:
Levothroid Tablets 1016
Levoxyl Tablets 903
Synthroid 1359

Lidocaine Hydrochloride (Reduced clearance of lidocaine). Products include:
Bactine Antiseptic/Anesthetic First Aid Liquid ▣ 708
Campho-Phenique Maximum Strength First Aid Antibiotic Plus Pain Reliever Ointment ▣ 719
Decadron Phosphate with Xylocaine Injection, Sterile 1639
Xylocaine Injections 567

Meclofenamate Sodium (Blunts antihypertensive effect of beta blocker).
No products indexed under this heading.

Mefenamic Acid (Blunts antihypertensive effect of beta blocker). Products include:
Ponstel 1925

Metaproterenol Sulfate (Propranolol may block bronchodilation produced by exogenous catecholamine stimulation of beta receptors). Products include:
Alupent 669
Metaproterenol Sulfate Inhalation Solution, USP, Arm-a-Med 552

Metformin Hydrochloride (Delay in the recovery of blood glucose to normal levels following insulin-induced hypoglycemia). Products include:
Glucophage 752

Nabumetone (Blunts antihypertensive effect of beta blocker). Products include:
Relafen Tablets 2510

Naproxen (Blunts antihypertensive effect of beta blocker). Products include:
Anaprox/Naprosyn 2117

Naproxen Sodium (Blunts antihypertensive effect of beta blocker). Products include:
Aleve 1975
Anaprox/Naprosyn 2117

Nicardipine Hydrochloride (Caution should be exercised when administered concomitantly). Products include:
Cardene Capsules 2095
Cardene I.V. 2709
Cardene SR Capsules 2097

Nifedipine (Caution should be exercised when administered concomitantly). Products include:
Adalat Capsules (10 mg and 20 mg) 587
Adalat CC 589
Procardia Capsules 1971
Procardia XL Extended Release Tablets 1972

Nimodipine (Caution should be exercised when administered concomitantly). Products include:
Nimotop Capsules 610

Nisoldipine (Caution should be exercised when administered concomitantly).
No products indexed under this heading.

Oxaprozin (Blunts antihypertensive effect of beta blocker). Products include:
Daypro Caplets 2426

Phenobarbital (Propranolol clearance accelerated). Products include:
Arco-Lase Plus Tablets 512
Bellergal-S Tablets 2250
Donnatal 2060
Donnatal Extentabs 2061
Donnatal Tablets 2060
Phenobarbital Elixir and Tablets 1469
Quadrinal Tablets 1350

Phenylbutazone (Blunts antihypertensive effect of beta blocker).
No products indexed under this heading.

Phenytoin (Propranolol clearance accelerated). Products include:
Dilantin Infatabs 1908
Dilantin-125 Suspension 1911

Phenytoin Sodium (Propranolol clearance accelerated). Products include:
Dilantin Kapseals 1906
Dilantin Parenteral 1910

(▣ Described in PDR For Nonprescription Drugs) (◉ Described in PDR For Ophthalmology)

Pirbuterol Acetate (Propranolol may block bronchodilation produced by exogenous catecholamine stimulation of beta receptors). Products include:

Maxair Autohaler 1492
Maxair Inhaler 1494

Piroxicam (Blunts antihypertensive effect of beta blocker). Products include:

Feldene Capsules 1965

Rauwolfia Serpentina (May produce excessive hypotension with bradycardia and orthostatic effects).

No products indexed under this heading.

Rescinnamine (May produce excessive hypotension with bradycardia and orthostatic effects).

No products indexed under this heading.

Reserpine (May produce excessive hypotension with bradycardia and orthostatic effects). Products include:

Diupres Tablets 1650
Hydropres Tablets 1675
Ser-Ap-Es Tablets 849

Rifampin (Propranolol clearance accelerated). Products include:

Rifadin 1528
Rifamate Capsules 1530
Rifater 1532
Rimactane Capsules 847

Salmeterol Xinafoate (Propranolol may block bronchodilation produced by exogenous catecholamine stimulation of beta receptors). Products include:

Serevent Inhalation Aerosol 1176

Sulindac (Blunts antihypertensive effect of beta blocker). Products include:

Clinoril Tablets 1618

Terbutaline Sulfate (Propranolol may block bronchodilation produced by exogenous catecholamine stimulation of beta receptors). Products include:

Brethaire Inhaler 813
Brethine Ampuls 815
Brethine Tablets 814
Bricanyl Subcutaneous Injection 1502
Bricanyl Tablets 1503

Theophylline (Reduced theophylline clearance). Products include:

Marax Tablets & DF Syrup 2200
Quibron 2053

Theophylline Anhydrous (Reduced theophylline clearance). Products include:

Aerolate 1004
Primatene Dual Action Formula .... ▣ 872
Primatene Tablets .... ▣ 873
Respbid Tablets 682
Slo-bid Gyrocaps 2033
Theo-24 Extended Release Capsules 2568
Theo-Dur Extended-Release Tablets 1327
Theo-X Extended-Release Tablets 788
Uni-Dur Extended-Release Tablets 1331
Uniphyl 400 mg Tablets 2001

Theophylline Calcium Salicylate (Reduced theophylline clearance). Products include:

Quadrinal Tablets 1350

Theophylline Sodium Glycinate (Reduced theophylline clearance).

No products indexed under this heading.

Thyroxine (Lower-than-expected T3 concentration may result).

No products indexed under this heading.

Tolazamide (Delay in the recovery of blood glucose to normal levels following insulin-induced hypoglycemia).

No products indexed under this heading.

Tolbutamide (Delay in the recovery of blood glucose to normal levels following insulin-induced hypoglycemia).

No products indexed under this heading.

Tolmetin Sodium (Blunts antihypertensive effect of beta blocker). Products include:

Tolectin (200, 400 and 600 mg) 1581

Verapamil Hydrochloride (Intravenous use of beta blocker and verapamil has resulted in serious adverse reactions in patients with severe cardiomyopathy, CHF or recent MI). Products include:

Calan SR Caplets 2422
Calan Tablets 2419
Isoptin Injectable 1344
Isoptin Oral Tablets 1346
Isoptin SR Tablets 1348
Verelan Capsules 1410
Verelan Capsules 2824

Food Interactions

Alcohol (Absorption rate of propranolol slowed).

INDERIDE TABLETS

(Propranolol Hydrochloride, Hydrochlorothiazide) 2732

May interact with antihypertensives, peripheral adrenergic blockers, catecholamine depleting drugs, cardiac glycosides, corticosteroids, calcium channel blockers, ganglionic blocking agents, insulin, non-steroidal anti-inflammatory agents, barbiturates, narcotic analgesics, xanthine bronchodilators, and certain other agents. Compounds in these categories include:

Acebutolol Hydrochloride (Potentiated or additive action). Products include:

Sectral Capsules 2807

ACTH (Hypokalemia).

No products indexed under this heading.

Alfentanil Hydrochloride (Aggravates orthostatic hypotension). Products include:

Alfenta Injection 1286

Aluminum Hydroxide (Greatly reduces intestinal absorption of propranolol). Products include:

ALternaGEL Liquid 1316
Maximum Strength Ascriptin .... ▣ 630
Cama Arthritis Pain Reliever .... ▣ 785
Gaviscon Extra Strength Relief Formula Antacid Tablets .... ▣ 819
Gaviscon Extra Strength Relief Formula Liquid Antacid .... ▣ 819
Gaviscon Liquid Antacid .... ▣ 820
Gelusil Liquid & Tablets .... ▣ 855
Maalox Heartburn Relief Suspension .... ▣ 642
Maalox Heartburn Relief Tablets .... ▣ 641
Maalox Magnesia and Alumina Oral Suspension .... ▣ 642
Maalox Plus Tablets .... ▣ 643
Extra Strength Maalox Antacid Plus Antigas Liquid and Tablets ▣ 638
Tempo Soft Antacid .... ▣ 835

Aluminum Hydroxide Gel (Greatly reduces intestinal absorption of propranolol). Products include:

ALternaGEL Liquid .... ▣ 659
Aludrox Oral Suspension 2695
Amphojel Suspension 2695
Amphojel Suspension without Flavor 2695
Amphojel Tablets 2695
Arthritis Pain Ascriptin .... ▣ 631
Regular Strength Ascriptin Tablets .... ▣ 629
Gaviscon Antacid Tablets .... ▣ 819
Gaviscon-2 Antacid Tablets .... ▣ 820
Mylanta Liquid 1317
Mylanta Tablets .... ▣ 660
Mylanta Double Strength Liquid 1317
Mylanta Double Strength Tablets .... ▣ 660
Nephrox Suspension .... ▣ 655

Aluminum Hydroxide Gel, Dried (Greatly reduces intestinal absorption of propranolol).

Aminophylline (Reduced theophylline clearance).

No products indexed under this heading.

Amlodipine Besylate (Potentiated or additive action). Products include:

Lotrel Capsules 840
Norvasc Tablets 1940

Antipyrine (Reduced clearance of antipyrine). Products include:

Auralgan Otic Solution 2703
Tympagesic Ear Drops 2342

Aprobarbital (Aggravates orthostatic hypotension).

No products indexed under this heading.

Atenolol (Potentiated or additive action). Products include:

Tenoretic Tablets 2845
Tenormin Tablets and I.V. Injection 2847

Benazepril Hydrochloride (Potentiated or additive action). Products include:

Lotensin Tablets 834
Lotensin HCT 837
Lotrel Capsules 840

Bendroflumethiazide (Potentiated or additive action).

No products indexed under this heading.

Bepridil Hydrochloride (Both agents may depress myocardial contractility or AV conduction resulting in increased adverse reactions). Products include:

Vascor (200, 300 and 400 mg) Tablets 1587

Betamethasone Acetate (Hypokalemia). Products include:

Celestone Soluspan Suspension 2347

Betamethasone Sodium Phosphate (Hypokalemia). Products include:

Celestone Soluspan Suspension 2347

Betaxolol Hydrochloride (Potentiated or additive action). Products include:

Betoptic Ophthalmic Solution 469
Betoptic S Ophthalmic Suspension 471
Kerlone Tablets 2436

Bisoprolol Fumarate (Potentiated or additive action). Products include:

Zebeta Tablets 1413
Ziac 1415

Buprenorphine (Aggravates orthostatic hypotension). Products include:

Buprenex Injectable 2006

Butabarbital (Aggravates orthostatic hypotension).

No products indexed under this heading.

Butalbital (Aggravates orthostatic hypotension). Products include:

Esgic-plus Tablets 1013
Fioricet Tablets 2258
Fioricet with Codeine Capsules 2260
Fiorinal Capsules 2261
Fiorinal with Codeine Capsules 2262
Fiorinal Tablets 2261
Phrenilin 785
Sedapap Tablets 50 mg/650 mg 1543

Captopril (Potentiated or additive action). Products include:

Capoten 739
Capozide 742

Carteolol Hydrochloride (Potentiated or additive action). Products include:

Cartrol Tablets 410
Ocupress Ophthalmic Solution, 1% Sterile .... ⊙ 309

Chlorothiazide (Potentiated or additive action). Products include:

Aldoclor Tablets 1598
Diupres Tablets 1650
Diuril Oral 1653

Chlorothiazide Sodium (Potentiated or additive action). Products include:

Diuril Sodium Intravenous 1652

Chlorpromazine (Increased plasma levels of both drugs). Products include:

Thorazine Suppositories 2523

Chlorthalidone (Potentiated or additive action). Products include:

Combipres Tablets 677
Tenoretic Tablets 2845
Thalitone 1245

Cimetidine (Decreases hepatic metabolism of propranolol resulting in increased blood levels). Products include:

Tagamet Tablets 2516

Cimetidine Hydrochloride (Decreases hepatic metabolism of propranolol resulting in increased blood levels). Products include:

Tagamet 2516

Clonidine (Potentiated or additive action). Products include:

Catapres-TTS 675

Clonidine Hydrochloride (Potentiated or additive action). Products include:

Catapres Tablets 674
Combipres Tablets 677

Codeine Phosphate (Aggravates orthostatic hypotension). Products include:

Actifed with Codeine Cough Syrup 1067
Brontex 1981
Deconsal C Expectorant Syrup 456
Deconsal Pediatric Syrup 457
Dimetane-DC Cough Syrup 2059
Empirin with Codeine Tablets 1093
Fioricet with Codeine Capsules 2260
Fiorinal with Codeine Capsules 2262
Isoclor Expectorant 990
Novahistine DH 2462
Novahistine Expectorant 2463
Nucofed 2051
Phenergan with Codeine 2777
Phenergan VC with Codeine 2781
Robitussin A-C Syrup 2073
Robitussin-DAC Syrup 2074
Ryna .... ▣ 841
Soma Compound w/Codeine Tablets 2676
Tussi-Organidin NR Liquid and S NR Liquid 2677
Tylenol with Codeine 1583

Cortisone Acetate (Hypokalemia). Products include:

Cortone Acetate Sterile Suspension 1623
Cortone Acetate Tablets 1624

Deserpidine (May produce an excessive hypotension with bradycardia and orthostatic effects).

No products indexed under this heading.

Deslanoside (Hypokalemia can sensitize or exaggerate the response of the heart to digitalis toxicity).

No products indexed under this heading.

Dexamethasone (Hypokalemia). Products include:

AK-Trol Ointment & Suspension .... ⊙ 205
Decadron Elixir 1633
Decadron Tablets 1635
Decaspray Topical Aerosol 1648
Dexacidin Ointment .... ⊙ 263
Maxitrol Ophthalmic Ointment and Suspension .... ⊙ 224

IMPORTANT NOTE: Always consult each drug listing in the patient's regimen for possible interactions.

Inderide **Interactions Index** **516**

TobraDex Ophthalmic Suspension and Ointment.... 473

Dexamethasone Acetate (Hypokalemia). Products include:

Dalalone D.P. Injectable 1011
Decadron-LA Sterile Suspension.... 1646

Dexamethasone Sodium Phosphate (Hypokalemia). Products include:

Decadron Phosphate Injection 1637
Decadron Phosphate Respihaler.... 1642
Decadron Phosphate Sterile Ophthalmic Ointment 1641
Decadron Phosphate Sterile Ophthalmic Solution 1642
Decadron Phosphate Topical Cream 1644
Decadron Phosphate Turbinaire 1645
Decadron Phosphate with Xylocaine Injection, Sterile 1639
Dexacort Phosphate in Respihaler .. 458
Dexacort Phosphate in Turbinaire .. 459
NeoDecadron Sterile Ophthalmic Ointment 1712
NeoDecadron Sterile Ophthalmic Solution 1713
NeoDecadron Topical Cream 1714

Dezocine (Aggravates orthostatic hypotension). Products include:

Dalgan Injection 538

Diazoxide (Potentiated or additive action). Products include:

Hyperstat I.V. Injection 2363
Proglycem.... 580

Diclofenac Potassium (Blunting of the antihypertensive effect). Products include:

Cataflam 816

Diclofenac Sodium (Blunting of the antihypertensive effect). Products include:

Voltaren Ophthalmic Sterile Ophthalmic Solution .... ◉ 272
Voltaren Tablets 861

Digitoxin (Hypokalemia can sensitize or exaggerate the response of the heart to digitalis toxicity). Products include:

Crystodigin Tablets.... 1433

Digoxin (Hypokalemia can sensitize or exaggerate the response of the heart to digitalis toxicity). Products include:

Lanoxicaps 1117
Lanoxin Elixir Pediatric 1120
Lanoxin Injection 1123
Lanoxin Injection Pediatric.... 1126
Lanoxin Tablets 1128

Diltiazem Hydrochloride (Both agents may depress myocardial contractility or AV conduction resulting in increased adverse reactions). Products include:

Cardizem CD Capsules 1506
Cardizem SR Capsules 1510
Cardizem Injectable 1508
Cardizem Tablets.... 1512
Dilacor XR Extended-release Capsules 2018

Doxazosin Mesylate (Potentiated or additive action). Products include:

Cardura Tablets 2186

Dyphylline (Reduced theophylline clearance). Products include:

Lufyllin & Lufyllin-400 Tablets 2670
Lufyllin-GG Elixir & Tablets 2671

Enalapril Maleate (Potentiated or additive action). Products include:

Vaseretic Tablets.... 1765
Vasotec Tablets 1771

Enalaprilat (Potentiated or additive action). Products include:

Vasotec I.V..... 1768

Esmolol Hydrochloride (Potentiated or additive action). Products include:

Brevibloc Injection.... 1808

Etodolac (Blunting of the antihypertensive effect). Products include:

Lodine Capsules and Tablets 2743

Felodipine (Potentiated or additive action). Products include:

Plendil Extended-Release Tablets.... 527

Fenoprofen Calcium (Blunting of the antihypertensive effect). Products include:

Nalfon 200 Pulvules & Nalfon Tablets 917

Fentanyl (Aggravates orthostatic hypotension). Products include:

Duragesic Transdermal System.... 1288

Fentanyl Citrate (Aggravates orthostatic hypotension). Products include:

Sublimaze Injection.... 1307

Fludrocortisone Acetate (Hypokalemia). Products include:

Florinef Acetate Tablets 505

Flurbiprofen (Blunting of the antihypertensive effect). Products include:

Ansaid Tablets 2579

Fosinopril Sodium (Potentiated or additive action). Products include:

Monopril Tablets 757

Furosemide (Potentiated or additive action). Products include:

Lasix Injection, Oral Solution and Tablets 1240

Guanabenz Acetate (Potentiated or additive action).

No products indexed under this heading.

Guanethidine Monosulfate (Potentiation). Products include:

Esimil Tablets 822
Ismelin Tablets 827

Haloperidol (Concomitant use may result in hypotension and coronary arrest). Products include:

Haldol Injection, Tablets and Concentrate 1575

Haloperidol Decanoate (Concomitant use may result in hypotension and coronary arrest). Products include:

Haldol Decanoate.... 1577

Hydralazine Hydrochloride (Potentiated or additive action). Products include:

Apresazide Capsules 808
Apresoline Hydrochloride Tablets .. 809
Ser-Ap-Es Tablets 849

Hydrocodone Bitartrate (Aggravates orthostatic hypotension). Products include:

Anexsia 5/500 Elixir 1781
Anexia Tablets.... 1782
Codiclear DH Syrup 791
Deconamine CX Cough and Cold Liquid and Tablets.... 1319
Duratuss HD Elixir.... 2565
Hycodan Tablets and Syrup 930
Hycomine Compound Tablets 932
Hycomine 931
Hycotuss Expectorant Syrup 933
Hydrocet Capsules 782
Lorcet 10/650.... 1018
Lortab.... 2566
Tussend 1783
Tussend Expectorant 1785
Vicodin Tablets 1356
Vicodin ES Tablets 1357
Vicodin Tuss Expectorant 1358
Zydone Capsules 949

Hydrocodone Polistirex (Aggravates orthostatic hypotension). Products include:

Tussionex Pennkinetic Extended-Release Suspension 998

Hydrocortisone (Hypokalemia). Products include:

Anusol-HC Cream 2.5% 1896
Aquanil HC Lotion 1931
Bactine Hydrocortisone Anti-Itch Cream.... ▣ 709
Caldecort Anti-Itch Hydrocortisone Spray .... ▣ 631
Cortaid .... ▣ 836
CORTENEMA.... 2535
Cortisporin Ointment 1085
Cortisporin Ophthalmic Ointment Sterile 1085
Cortisporin Ophthalmic Suspension Sterile 1086
Cortisporin Otic Solution Sterile 1087
Cortisporin Otic Suspension Sterile 1088
Cortizone-5 .... ▣ 831
Cortizone-10 .... ▣ 831
Hydrocortone Tablets 1672
Hytone 907
Massengill Medicated Soft Cloth Towelettes.... 2458
PediOtic Suspension Sterile 1153
Preparation H Hydrocortisone 1% Cream .... ▣ 872
ProctoCream-HC 2.5%.... 2408
VōSoL HC Otic Solution.... 2678

Hydrocortisone Acetate (Hypokalemia). Products include:

Analpram-HC Rectal Cream 1% and 2.5% 977
Anusol HC-1 Anti-Itch Hydrocortisone Ointment.... ▣ 847
Anusol-HC Suppositories 1897
Caldecort.... ▣ 631
Carmol HC 924
Coly-Mycin S Otic w/Neomycin & Hydrocortisone.... 1906
Cortaid .... ▣ 836
Cortifoam 2396
Cortisporin Cream.... 1084
Epifoam 2399
Hydrocortone Acetate Sterile Suspension.... 1669
Mantadil Cream 1135
Nupercainal Hydrocortisone 1% Cream .... ▣ 645
Ophthocort .... ◉ 311
Pramosone Cream, Lotion & Ointment 978
ProctoCream-HC 2408
ProctoFoam-HC 2409
Terra-Cortril Ophthalmic Suspension 2210

Hydrocortisone Sodium Phosphate (Hypokalemia). Products include:

Hydrocortone Phosphate Injection, Sterile 1670

Hydrocortisone Sodium Succinate (Hypokalemia). Products include:

Solu-Cortef Sterile Powder.... 2641

Hydroflumethiazide (Potentiated or additive action). Products include:

Diucardin Tablets.... 2718

Ibuprofen (Blunting of the antihypertensive effect). Products include:

Advil Cold and Sinus Caplets and Tablets (formerly CoAdvil) .... ▣ 870
Advil Ibuprofen Tablets and Caplets .... ▣ 870
Children's Advil Suspension 2692
Arthritis Foundation Ibuprofen Tablets .... ▣ 674
Bayer Select Ibuprofen Pain Relief Formula .... ▣ 715
Cramp End Tablets .... ▣ 735
Dimetapp Sinus Caplets .... ▣ 775
Haltran Tablets .... ▣ 771
IBU Tablets.... 1342
Ibuprohm.... ▣ 735
Children's Motrin Ibuprofen Oral Suspension 1546
Motrin Tablets.... 2625
Motrin IB Caplets, Tablets, and Geltabs.... ▣ 838
Motrin IB Sinus.... ▣ 838
Motrin Ibuprofen Suspension, Oral Drops, Chewable Tablets, Caplets 1546
Nuprin Ibuprofen/Analgesic Tablets & Caplets .... ▣ 622
Sine-Aid IB Caplets 1554
Vicks DayQuil SINUS Pressure & PAIN Relief with IBUPROFEN .... ▣ 762

Indapamide (Potentiated or additive action). Products include:

Lozol Tablets 2022

Indomethacin (Blunting of the antihypertensive effect). Products include:

Indocin 1680

Indomethacin Sodium Trihydrate (Blunting of the antihypertensive effect). Products include:

Indocin I.V. 1684

Insulin, Human (Insulin requirements may be altered).

No products indexed under this heading.

Insulin, Human Isophane Suspension (Insulin requirements may be altered). Products include:

Novolin N Human Insulin 10 ml Vials.... 1795

Insulin, Human NPH (Insulin requirements may be altered). Products include:

Humulin N, 100 Units.... 1448
Novolin N PenFill Cartridges Durable Insulin Delivery System 1798
Novolin N Prefilled Syringe Disposable Insulin Delivery System 1798

Insulin, Human Regular (Insulin requirements may be altered). Products include:

Humulin R, 100 Units 1449
Novolin R Human Insulin 10 ml Vials.... 1795
Novolin R PenFill Cartridges Durable Insulin Delivery System 1798
Novolin R Prefilled Syringe Disposable Insulin Delivery System 1798
Velosulin BR Human Insulin 10 ml Vials.... 1795

Insulin, Human, Zinc Suspension (Insulin requirements may be altered). Products include:

Humulin L, 100 Units 1446
Humulin U, 100 Units.... 1450
Novolin L Human Insulin 10 ml Vials.... 1795

Insulin, NPH (Insulin requirements may be altered). Products include:

NPH, 100 Units 1450
Pork NPH, 100 Units.... 1452
Purified Pork NPH Isophane Insulin 1801

Insulin, Regular (Insulin requirements may be altered). Products include:

Regular, 100 Units.... 1450
Pork Regular, 100 Units 1452
Pork Regular (Concentrated), 500 Units 1453
Purified Pork Regular Insulin 1801

Insulin, Zinc Crystals (Insulin requirements may be altered). Products include:

NPH, 100 Units 1450

Insulin, Zinc Suspension (Insulin requirements may be altered). Products include:

Iletin I 1450
Lente, 100 Units 1450
Iletin II.... 1452
Pork Lente, 100 Units.... 1452
Purified Pork Lente Insulin 1801

Isoproterenol Hydrochloride (Effects of propranolol reversed). Products include:

Isuprel Hydrochloride Injection 1:5000 2311
Isuprel Hydrochloride Solution 1:200 & 1:100 2313
Isuprel Mistometer 2312

Isoproterenol Sulfate (Effects of propranolol reversed). Products include:

Norisodrine with Calcium Iodide Syrup.... 442

Isradipine (Potentiated or additive action). Products include:

DynaCirc Capsules 2256

Ketoprofen (Blunting of the antihypertensive effect). Products include:

Orudis Capsules.... 2766
Oruvail Capsules 2766

Ketorolac Tromethamine (Blunting of the antihypertensive effect). Products include:

Acular 474
Acular .... ◉ 277
Toradol.... 2159

(▣ Described in PDR For Nonprescription Drugs) (◉ Described in PDR For Ophthalmology)

517 **Interactions Index** **Inderide**

Labetalol Hydrochloride (Potentiated or additive action). Products include:
- Normodyne Injection ... 2377
- Normodyne Tablets ... 2379
- Trandate ... 1185

Levorphanol Tartrate (Aggravates orthostatic hypotension). Products include:
- Levo-Dromoran ... 2129

Lidocaine Hydrochloride (Reduced clearance of lidocaine). Products include:
- Bactine Antiseptic/Anesthetic First Aid Liquid ... ▣ 708
- Campho-Phenique Maximum Strength First Aid Antibiotic Plus Pain Reliever Ointment ... ▣ 719
- Decadron Phosphate with Xylocaine Injection, Sterile ... 1639
- Xylocaine Injections ... 567

Lisinopril (Potentiated or additive action). Products include:
- Prinivil Tablets ... 1733
- Prinzide Tablets ... 1737
- Zestoretic ... 2850
- Zestril Tablets ... 2854

Losartan Potassium (Potentiated or additive action). Products include:
- Cozaar Tablets ... 1628
- Hyzaar Tablets ... 1677

Mecamylamine Hydrochloride (Potentiated or additive action). Products include:
- Inversine Tablets ... 1686

Meclofenamate Sodium (Blunting of the antihypertensive effect).
- No products indexed under this heading.

Mefenamic Acid (Blunting of the antihypertensive effect). Products include:
- Ponstel ... 1925

Meperidine Hydrochloride (Aggravates orthostatic hypotension). Products include:
- Demerol ... 2308
- Mepergan Injection ... 2753

Mephobarbital (Aggravates orthostatic hypotension). Products include:
- Mebaral Tablets ... 2322

Methadone Hydrochloride (Aggravates orthostatic hypotension). Products include:
- Methadone Hydrochloride Oral Concentrate ... 2233
- Methadone Hydrochloride Oral Solution & Tablets ... 2235

Methyclothiazide (Potentiated or additive action). Products include:
- Enduron Tablets ... 420

Methyldopa (Potentiated or additive action). Products include:
- Aldoclor Tablets ... 1598
- Aldomet Oral ... 1600
- Aldoril Tablets ... 1604

Methyldopate Hydrochloride (Potentiated or additive action). Products include:
- Aldomet Ester HCl Injection ... 1602

Methylprednisolone Acetate (Hypokalemia). Products include:
- Depo-Medrol Single-Dose Vial ... 2600
- Depo-Medrol Sterile Aqueous Suspension ... 2597

Methylprednisolone Sodium Succinate (Hypokalemia). Products include:
- Solu-Medrol Sterile Powder ... 2643

Metolazone (Potentiated or additive action). Products include:
- Mykrox Tablets ... 993
- Zaroxolyn Tablets ... 1000

Metoprolol Succinate (Potentiated or additive action). Products include:
- Toprol-XL Tablets ... 565

Metoprolol Tartrate (Potentiated or additive action). Products include:
- Lopressor Ampuls ... 830
- Lopressor HCT Tablets ... 832
- Lopressor Tablets ... 830

Metyrosine (Potentiated or additive action). Products include:
- Demser Capsules ... 1649

Minoxidil (Potentiated or additive action). Products include:
- Loniten Tablets ... 2618
- Rogaine Topical Solution ... 2637

Moexipril Hydrochloride (Potentiated or additive action). Products include:
- Univasc Tablets ... 2410

Morphine Sulfate (Aggravates orthostatic hypotension). Products include:
- Astramorph/PF Injection, USP (Preservative-Free) ... 535
- Duramorph ... 962
- Infumorph 200 and Infumorph 500 Sterile Solutions ... 965
- MS Contin Tablets ... 1994
- MSIR ... 1997
- Oramorph SR (Morphine Sulfate Sustained Release Tablets) ... 2236
- RMS Suppositories ... 2657
- Roxanol ... 2243

Nabumetone (Blunting of the antihypertensive effect). Products include:
- Relafen Tablets ... 2510

Nadolol (Potentiated or additive action).
- No products indexed under this heading.

Naproxen (Blunting of the antihypertensive effect). Products include:
- Anaprox/Naprosyn ... 2117

Naproxen Sodium (Blunting of the antihypertensive effect). Products include:
- Aleve ... 1975
- Anaprox/Naprosyn ... 2117

Nicardipine Hydrochloride (Both agents may depress myocardial contractility or AV conduction resulting in increased adverse reactions). Products include:
- Cardene Capsules ... 2095
- Cardene I.V. ... 2709
- Cardene SR Capsules ... 2097

Nifedipine (Both agents may depress myocardial contractility or AV conduction resulting in increased adverse reactions). Products include:
- Adalat Capsules (10 mg and 20 mg) ... 587
- Adalat CC ... 589
- Procardia Capsules ... 1971
- Procardia XL Extended Release Tablets ... 1972

Nimodipine (Both agents may depress myocardial contractility or AV conduction resulting in increased adverse reactions). Products include:
- Nimotop Capsules ... 610

Nisoldipine (Potentiated or additive action).
- No products indexed under this heading.

Nitroglycerin (Potentiated or additive action). Products include:
- Deponit NTG Transdermal Delivery System ... 2397
- Nitro-Bid IV ... 1523
- Nitro-Bid Ointment ... 1524
- Nitrodisc ... 2047
- Nitro-Dur (nitroglycerin) Transdermal Infusion System ... 1326
- Nitrolingual Spray ... 2027
- Nitrostat Tablets ... 1925
- Transderm-Nitro Transdermal Therapeutic System ... 859

Norepinephrine Bitartrate (Decreased arterial responsiveness to norepinephrine). Products include:
- Levophed Bitartrate Injection ... 2315

Opium Alkaloids (Aggravates orthostatic hypotension).
- No products indexed under this heading.

Oxaprozin (Blunting of the antihypertensive effect). Products include:
- Daypro Caplets ... 2426

Oxycodone Hydrochloride (Aggravates orthostatic hypotension). Products include:
- Percocet Tablets ... 938
- Percodan Tablets ... 939
- Percodan-Demi Tablets ... 940
- Roxicodone Tablets, Oral Solution & Intensol (Oxycodone) ... 2244
- Tylox Capsules ... 1584

Penbutolol Sulfate (Potentiated or additive action). Products include:
- Levatol ... 2403

Pentobarbital Sodium (Aggravates orthostatic hypotension). Products include:
- Nembutal Sodium Capsules ... 436
- Nembutal Sodium Solution ... 438
- Nembutal Sodium Suppositories ... 440

Phenobarbital (Accelerates propranolol clearance). Products include:
- Arco-Lase Plus Tablets ... 512
- Bellergal-S Tablets ... 2250
- Donnatal ... 2060
- Donnatal Extentabs ... 2061
- Donnatal Tablets ... 2060
- Phenobarbital Elixir and Tablets ... 1469
- Quadrinal Tablets ... 1350

Phenoxybenzamine Hydrochloride (Potentiated or additive action). Products include:
- Dibenzyline Capsules ... 2476

Phentolamine Mesylate (Potentiated or additive action). Products include:
- Regitine ... 846

Phenylbutazone (Blunting of the antihypertensive effect).
- No products indexed under this heading.

Phenytoin (Accelerates propranolol clearance). Products include:
- Dilantin Infatabs ... 1908
- Dilantin-125 Suspension ... 1911

Phenytoin Sodium (Accelerates propranolol clearance). Products include:
- Dilantin Kapseals ... 1906
- Dilantin Parenteral ... 1910

Pindolol (Potentiated or additive action). Products include:
- Visken Tablets ... 2299

Piroxicam (Blunting of the antihypertensive effect). Products include:
- Feldene Capsules ... 1965

Polythiazide (Potentiated or additive action). Products include:
- Minizide Capsules ... 1938

Prazosin Hydrochloride (Potentiated or additive action). Products include:
- Minipress Capsules ... 1937
- Minizide Capsules ... 1938

Prednisolone Acetate (Hypokalemia). Products include:
- AK-CIDE ... ◉ 202
- AK-CIDE Ointment ... ◉ 202
- Blephamide Liquifilm Sterile Ophthalmic Suspension ... 476
- Blephamide Ointment ... ◉ 237
- Econopred & Econopred Plus Ophthalmic Suspensions ... ◉ 217
- Poly-Pred Liquifilm ... ◉ 248
- Pred Forte ... ◉ 250
- Pred Mild ... ◉ 253
- Pred-G Liquifilm Sterile Ophthalmic Suspension ... ◉ 251
- Pred-G S.O.P. Sterile Ophthalmic Ointment ... ◉ 252
- Vasocidin Ointment ... ◉ 268

Prednisolone Sodium Phosphate (Hypokalemia). Products include:
- AK-Pred ... ◉ 204
- Hydeltrasol Injection, Sterile ... 1665
- Inflamase ... ◉ 265
- Pediapred Oral Liquid ... 995
- Vasocidin Ophthalmic Solution ... ◉ 270

Prednisolone Tebutate (Hypokalemia). Products include:
- Hydeltra-T.B.A. Sterile Suspension 1667

Prednisone (Hypokalemia). Products include:
- Deltasone Tablets ... 2595

Propoxyphene Hydrochloride (Aggravates orthostatic hypotension). Products include:
- Darvon ... 1435
- Wygesic Tablets ... 2827

Propoxyphene Napsylate (Aggravates orthostatic hypotension). Products include:
- Darvon-N/Darvocet-N ... 1433

Quinapril Hydrochloride (Potentiated or additive action). Products include:
- Accupril Tablets ... 1893

Ramipril (Potentiated or additive action). Products include:
- Altace Capsules ... 1232

Rauwolfia Serpentina (May produce an excessive hypotension with bradycardia and orthostatic effects).
- No products indexed under this heading.

Rescinnamine (May produce an excessive hypotension with bradycardia and orthostatic effects).
- No products indexed under this heading.

Reserpine (May produce an excessive hypotension with bradycardia and orthostatic effects). Products include:
- Diupres Tablets ... 1650
- Hydropres Tablets ... 1675
- Ser-Ap-Es Tablets ... 849

Rifampin (Accelerates propranolol clearance). Products include:
- Rifadin ... 1528
- Rifamate Capsules ... 1530
- Rifater ... 1532
- Rimactane Capsules ... 847

Secobarbital Sodium (Aggravates orthostatic hypotension). Products include:
- Seconal Sodium Pulvules ... 1474

Sodium Nitroprusside (Potentiated or additive action).
- No products indexed under this heading.

Sotalol Hydrochloride (Potentiated or additive action). Products include:
- Betapace Tablets ... 641

Spirapril Hydrochloride (Potentiated or additive action).
- No products indexed under this heading.

Sufentanil Citrate (Aggravates orthostatic hypotension). Products include:
- Sufenta Injection ... 1309

Sulindac (Blunting of the antihypertensive effect). Products include:
- Clinoril Tablets ... 1618

Terazosin Hydrochloride (Potentiated or additive action). Products include:
- Hytrin Capsules ... 430

Theophylline (Reduced theophylline clearance). Products include:
- Marax Tablets & DF Syrup ... 2200
- Quibron ... 2053

Theophylline Anhydrous (Reduced theophylline clearance). Products include:
- Aerolate ... 1004
- Primatene Dual Action Formula ... ▣ 872
- Primatene Tablets ... ▣ 873
- Respbid Tablets ... 682
- Slo-bid Gyrocaps ... 2033

IMPORTANT NOTE: Always consult each drug listing in the patient's regimen for possible interactions.

Inderide Interactions Index 518

Theo-24 Extended Release Capsules ... 2568
Theo-Dur Extended-Release Tablets ... 1327
Theo-X Extended-Release Tablets .. 788
Uni-Dur Extended-Release Tablets .. 1331
Uniphyl 400 mg Tablets ... 2001

Theophylline Calcium Salicylate (Reduced theophylline clearance). Products include:
Quadrinal Tablets ... 1350

Theophylline Sodium Glycinate (Reduced theophylline clearance).
No products indexed under this heading.

Thiamylal Sodium (Aggravates orthostatic hypotension).
No products indexed under this heading.

Thyroxine (Lower than expected T3 concentration).
No products indexed under this heading.

Thyroxine Sodium (Lower than expected T3 concentration).
No products indexed under this heading.

Timolol Maleate (Potentiated or additive action). Products include:
Blocadren Tablets ... 1614
Timolide Tablets ... 1748
Timoptic in Ocudose ... 1753
Timoptic Sterile Ophthalmic Solution ... 1751
Timoptic-XE ... 1755

Tolmetin Sodium (Blunting of the antihypertensive effect). Products include:
Tolectin (200, 400 and 600 mg) .. 1581

Torsemide (Potentiated or additive action). Products include:
Demadex Tablets and Injection ... 686

Triamcinolone (Hypokalemia). Products include:
Aristocort Tablets ... 1022

Triamcinolone Acetonide (Hypokalemia). Products include:
Aristocort A 0.025% Cream ... 1027
Aristocort A 0.5% Cream ... 1031
Aristocort A 0.1% Cream ... 1029
Aristocort A 0.1% Ointment ... 1030
Azmacort Oral Inhaler ... 2011
Nasacort Nasal Inhaler ... 2024

Triamcinolone Diacetate (Hypokalemia). Products include:
Aristocort Suspension (Forte Parenteral) ... 1027
Aristocort Suspension (Intralesional) ... 1025

Triamcinolone Hexacetonide (Hypokalemia). Products include:
Aristospan Suspension (Intra-articular) ... 1033
Aristospan Suspension (Intralesional) ... 1032

Trimethaphan Camsylate (Potentiated or additive action). Products include:
Arfonad Ampuls ... 2080

Tubocurarine Chloride (Increased responsiveness to tubocurarine).
No products indexed under this heading.

Verapamil Hydrochloride (Both agents may depress myocardial contractility or AV conduction resulting in increased adverse reactions). Products include:
Calan SR Caplets ... 2422
Calan Tablets ... 2419
Isoptin Injectable ... 1344
Isoptin Oral Tablets ... 1346
Isoptin SR Tablets ... 1348
Verelan Capsules ... 1410
Verelan Capsules ... 2824

Food Interactions

Alcohol (Slows the rate of absorption of propranolol).

INDERIDE LA LONG ACTING CAPSULES

(Propranolol Hydrochloride, Hydrochlorothiazide) ... 2734
May interact with antihypertensives, peripheral adrenergic blockers, catecholamine depleting drugs, cardiac glycosides, corticosteroids, insulin, ganglionic blocking agents, barbiturates, non-steroidal anti-inflammatory agents, narcotic analgesics, and certain other agents. Compounds in these categories include:

Acebutolol Hydrochloride (Potentiated or additive action). Products include:
Sectral Capsules ... 2807

ACTH (Hypokalemia).
No products indexed under this heading.

Alfentanil Hydrochloride (May aggravate orthostatic hypotension). Products include:
Alfenta Injection ... 1286

Amlodipine Besylate (Potentiated or additive action). Products include:
Lotrel Capsules ... 840
Norvasc Tablets ... 1940

Aprobarbital (May aggravate orthostatic hypotension).
No products indexed under this heading.

Atenolol (Potentiated or additive action). Products include:
Tenoretic Tablets ... 2845
Tenormin Tablets and I.V. Injection 2847

Benazepril Hydrochloride (Potentiated or additive action). Products include:
Lotensin Tablets ... 834
Lotensin HCT ... 837
Lotrel Capsules ... 840

Bendroflumethiazide (Potentiated or additive action).
No products indexed under this heading.

Betamethasone Acetate (Hypokalemia). Products include:
Celestone Soluspan Suspension ... 2347

Betamethasone Sodium Phosphate (Hypokalemia). Products include:
Celestone Soluspan Suspension ... 2347

Betaxolol Hydrochloride (Potentiated or additive action). Products include:
Betoptic Ophthalmic Solution ... 469
Betoptic S Ophthalmic Suspension ... 471
Kerlone Tablets ... 2436

Bisoprolol Fumarate (Potentiated or additive action). Products include:
Zebeta Tablets ... 1413
Ziac ... 1415

Buprenorphine (May aggravate orthostatic hypotension). Products include:
Buprenex Injectable ... 2006

Butabarbital (May aggravate orthostatic hypotension).
No products indexed under this heading.

Butalbital (May aggravate orthostatic hypotension). Products include:
Esgic-plus Tablets ... 1013
Fioricet Tablets ... 2258
Fioricet with Codeine Capsules ... 2260
Fiorinal Capsules ... 2261
Fiorinal with Codeine Capsules ... 2262
Fiorinal Tablets ... 2261
Phrenilin ... 785
Sedapap Tablets 50 mg/650 mg .. 1543

Captopril (Potentiated or additive action). Products include:
Capoten ... 739
Capozide ... 742

Carteolol Hydrochloride (Potentiated or additive action). Products include:
Cartrol Tablets ... 410
Ocupress Ophthalmic Solution, 1% Sterile ... ⊙ 309

Chlorothiazide (Potentiated or additive action). Products include:
Aldoclor Tablets ... 1598
Diupres Tablets ... 1650
Diuril Oral ... 1653

Chlorothiazide Sodium (Potentiated or additive action). Products include:
Diuril Sodium Intravenous ... 1652

Chlorthalidone (Potentiated or additive action). Products include:
Combipres Tablets ... 677
Tenoretic Tablets ... 2845
Thalitone ... 1245

Clonidine (Potentiated or additive action). Products include:
Catapres-TTS ... 675

Clonidine Hydrochloride (Potentiated or additive action). Products include:
Catapres Tablets ... 674
Combipres Tablets ... 677

Codeine Phosphate (May aggravate orthostatic hypotension). Products include:
Actifed with Codeine Cough Syrup.. 1067
Brontex ... 1981
Deconsal C Expectorant Syrup ... 456
Deconsal Pediatric Syrup ... 457
Dimetane-DC Cough Syrup ... 2059
Empirin with Codeine Tablets ... 1093
Fioricet with Codeine Capsules ... 2260
Fiorinal with Codeine Capsules ... 2262
Isoclor Expectorant ... 990
Novahistine DH ... 2462
Novahistine Expectorant ... 2463
Nucofed ... 2051
Phenergan with Codeine ... 2777
Phenergan VC with Codeine ... 2781
Robitussin A-C Syrup ... 2073
Robitussin-DAC Syrup ... 2074
Ryna ... ▣ 841
Soma Compound w/Codeine Tablets ... 2676
Tussi-Organidin NR Liquid and S NR Liquid ... 2677
Tylenol with Codeine ... 1583

Cortisone Acetate (Hypokalemia). Products include:
Cortone Acetate Sterile Suspension ... 1623
Cortone Acetate Tablets ... 1624

Deserpidine (May produce an excessive hypotension with bradycardia and orthostatic effects).
No products indexed under this heading.

Deslanoside (Hypokalemia produced by thiazides can exaggerate cardiotoxicity of digitalis).
No products indexed under this heading.

Dexamethasone Acetate (Hypokalemia). Products include:
Dalalone D.P. Injectable ... 1011
Decadron-LA Sterile Suspension ... 1646

Dexamethasone Sodium Phosphate (Hypokalemia). Products include:
Decadron Phosphate Injection ... 1637
Decadron Phosphate Respihaler ... 1642
Decadron Phosphate Sterile Ophthalmic Ointment ... 1641
Decadron Phosphate Sterile Ophthalmic Solution ... 1642
Decadron Phosphate Topical Cream ... 1644
Decadron Phosphate Turbinaire ... 1645
Decadron Phosphate with Xylocaine Injection, Sterile ... 1639
Dexacort Phosphate in Respihaler .. 458
Dexacort Phosphate in Turbinaire .. 459
NeoDecadron Sterile Ophthalmic Ointment ... 1712
NeoDecadron Sterile Ophthalmic Solution ... 1713
NeoDecadron Topical Cream ... 1714

Dezocine (May aggravate orthostatic hypotension). Products include:
Dalgan Injection ... 538

Diazoxide (Potentiated or additive action). Products include:
Hyperstat I.V. Injection ... 2363
Proglycem ... 580

Diclofenac Potassium (Blunts antihypertensive effect of beta blocker). Products include:
Cataflam ... 816

Diclofenac Sodium (Blunts antihypertensive effect of beta blocker). Products include:
Voltaren Ophthalmic Sterile Ophthalmic Solution ... ⊙ 272
Voltaren Tablets ... 861

Digitoxin (Hypokalemia produced by thiazides can exaggerate cardiotoxicity of digitalis). Products include:
Crystodigin Tablets ... 1433

Digoxin (Hypokalemia produced by thiazides can exaggerate cardiotoxicity of digitalis). Products include:
Lanoxicaps ... 1117
Lanoxin Elixir Pediatric ... 1120
Lanoxin Injection ... 1123
Lanoxin Injection Pediatric ... 1126
Lanoxin Tablets ... 1128

Diltiazem Hydrochloride (Potentiated or additive action). Products include:
Cardizem CD Capsules ... 1506
Cardizem SR Capsules ... 1510
Cardizem Injectable ... 1508
Cardizem Tablets ... 1512
Dilacor XR Extended-release Capsules ... 2018

Doxazosin Mesylate (Potentiated or additive action). Products include:
Cardura Tablets ... 2186

Enalapril Maleate (Potentiated or additive action). Products include:
Vaseretic Tablets ... 1765
Vasotec Tablets ... 1771

Enalaprilat (Potentiated or additive action). Products include:
Vasotec I.V. ... 1768

Esmolol Hydrochloride (Potentiated or additive action). Products include:
Brevibloc Injection ... 1808

Etodolac (Blunts antihypertensive effect of beta blocker). Products include:
Lodine Capsules and Tablets ... 2743

Felodipine (Potentiated or additive action). Products include:
Plendil Extended-Release Tablets ... 527

Fenoprofen Calcium (Blunts antihypertensive effect of beta blocker). Products include:
Nalfon 200 Pulvules & Nalfon Tablets ... 917

Fentanyl (May aggravate orthostatic hypotension). Products include:
Duragesic Transdermal System ... 1288

Fentanyl Citrate (May aggravate orthostatic hypotension). Products include:
Sublimaze Injection ... 1307

Fludrocortisone Acetate (Hypokalemia). Products include:
Florinef Acetate Tablets ... 505

Flurbiprofen (Blunts antihypertensive effect of beta blocker). Products include:
Ansaid Tablets ... 2579

Fosinopril Sodium (Potentiated or additive action). Products include:
Monopril Tablets ... 757

Furosemide (Potentiated or additive action). Products include:
Lasix Injection, Oral Solution and Tablets ... 1240

(▣ Described in PDR For Nonprescription Drugs) (⊙ Described in PDR For Ophthalmology)

519 **Interactions Index** **Inderide LA**

Guanabenz Acetate (Potentiated or additive action).
- No products indexed under this heading.

Guanethidine Monosulfate (Potentiated). Products include:
- Esimil Tablets ... 822
- Ismelin Tablets ... 827

Haloperidol (Hypotension and cardiac arrest have been reported with the concomitant use of propranolol and haloperidol). Products include:
- Haldol Injection, Tablets and Concentrate ... 1575

Haloperidol Decanoate (Hypotension and cardiac arrest have been reported with the concomitant use of propranolol and haloperidol). Products include:
- Haldol Decanoate ... 1577

Hydralazine Hydrochloride (Potentiated or additive action). Products include:
- Apresazide Capsules ... 808
- Apresoline Hydrochloride Tablets .. 809
- Ser-Ap-Es Tablets ... 849

Hydrocodone Bitartrate (May aggravate orthostatic hypotension). Products include:
- Anexsia 5/500 Elixir ... 1781
- Anexia Tablets ... 1782
- Codiclear DH Syrup ... 791
- Deconamine CX Cough and Cold Liquid and Tablets ... 1319
- Duratuss HD Elixir ... 2565
- Hycodan Tablets and Syrup ... 930
- Hycomine Compound Tablets ... 932
- Hycomine ... 931
- Hycotuss Expectorant Syrup ... 933
- Hydrocet Capsules ... 782
- Lorcet 10/650 ... 1018
- Lortab ... 2566
- Tussend ... 1783
- Tussend Expectorant ... 1785
- Vicodin Tablets ... 1356
- Vicodin ES Tablets ... 1357
- Vicodin Tuss Expectorant ... 1358
- Zydone Capsules ... 949

Hydrocodone Polistirex (May aggravate orthostatic hypotension). Products include:
- Tussionex Pennkinetic Extended-Release Suspension ... 998

Hydrocortisone (Hypokalemia). Products include:
- Anusol-HC Cream 2.5% ... 1896
- Aquanil HC Lotion ... 1931
- Bactine Hydrocortisone Anti-Itch Cream ... ▣ 709
- Caldecort Anti-Itch Hydrocortisone Spray ... ▣ 631
- Cortaid ... ▣ 836
- CORTENEMA ... 2535
- Cortisporin Ointment ... 1085
- Cortisporin Ophthalmic Ointment Sterile ... 1085
- Cortisporin Ophthalmic Suspension Sterile ... 1086
- Cortisporin Otic Solution Sterile ... 1087
- Cortisporin Otic Suspension Sterile 1088
- Cortizone-5 ... ▣ 831
- Cortizone-10 ... ▣ 831
- Hydrocortone Tablets ... 1672
- Hytone ... 907
- Massengill Medicated Soft Cloth Towelettes ... 2458
- PediOtic Suspension Sterile ... 1153
- Preparation H Hydrocortisone 1% Cream ... ▣ 872
- ProctoCream-HC 2.5% ... 2408
- VōSoL HC Otic Solution ... 2678

Hydrocortisone Acetate (Hypokalemia). Products include:
- Analpram-HC Rectal Cream 1% and 2.5% ... 977
- Anusol HC-1 Anti-Itch Hydrocortisone Ointment ... ▣ 847
- Anusol-HC Suppositories ... 1897
- Caldecort ... ▣ 631
- Carmol HC ... 924
- Coly-Mycin S Otic w/Neomycin & Hydrocortisone ... 1906
- Cortaid ... ▣ 836
- Cortifoam ... 2396
- Cortisporin Cream ... 1084
- Epifoam ... 2399
- Hydrocortone Acetate Sterile Suspension ... 1669
- Mantadil Cream ... 1135
- Nupercainal Hydrocortisone 1% Cream ... ▣ 645
- Ophthocort ... ◉ 311
- Pramosone Cream, Lotion & Ointment ... 978
- ProctoCream-HC ... 2408
- ProctoFoam-HC ... 2409
- Terra-Cortril Ophthalmic Suspension ... 2210

Hydrocortisone Sodium Phosphate (Hypokalemia). Products include:
- Hydrocortone Phosphate Injection, Sterile ... 1670

Hydrocortisone Sodium Succinate (Hypokalemia). Products include:
- Solu-Cortef Sterile Powder ... 2641

Hydroflumethiazide (Potentiated or additive action). Products include:
- Diucardin Tablets ... 2718

Ibuprofen (Blunts antihypertensive effect of beta blocker). Products include:
- Advil Cold and Sinus Caplets and Tablets (formerly CoAdvil) ... ▣ 870
- Advil Ibuprofen Tablets and Caplets ... ▣ 870
- Children's Advil Suspension ... 2692
- Arthritis Foundation Ibuprofen Tablets ... ▣ 674
- Bayer Select Ibuprofen Pain Relief Formula ... ▣ 715
- Cramp End Tablets ... ▣ 735
- Dimetapp Sinus Caplets ... ▣ 775
- Haltran Tablets ... ▣ 771
- IBU Tablets ... 1342
- Ibuprohm ... ▣ 735
- Children's Motrin Ibuprofen Oral Suspension ... 1546
- Motrin Tablets ... 2625
- Motrin IB Caplets, Tablets, and Geltabs ... ▣ 838
- Motrin IB Sinus ... ▣ 838
- Motrin Ibuprofen Suspension, Oral Drops, Chewable Tablets, Caplets ... 1546
- Nuprin Ibuprofen/Analgesic Tablets & Caplets ... ▣ 622
- Sine-Aid IB Caplets ... 1554
- Vicks DayQuil SINUS Pressure & PAIN Relief with IBUPROFEN ... ▣ 762

Indapamide (Potentiated or additive action). Products include:
- Lozol Tablets ... 2022

Indomethacin (Blunts antihypertensive effect of beta blocker). Products include:
- Indocin ... 1680

Indomethacin Sodium Trihydrate (Blunts antihypertensive effect of beta blocker). Products include:
- Indocin I.V. ... 1684

Insulin, Human (Insulin requirements may be increased, decreased, or unchanged).
- No products indexed under this heading.

Insulin, Human Isophane Suspension (Insulin requirements may be increased, decreased, or unchanged). Products include:
- Novolin N Human Insulin 10 ml Vials ... 1795

Insulin, Human NPH (Insulin requirements may be increased, decreased, or unchanged). Products include:
- Humulin N, 100 Units ... 1448
- Novolin N PenFill Cartridges Durable Insulin Delivery System ... 1798
- Novolin N Prefilled Syringe Disposable Insulin Delivery System ... 1798

Insulin, Human Regular (Insulin requirements may be increased, decreased, or unchanged). Products include:
- Humulin R, 100 Units ... 1449
- Novolin R Human Insulin 10 ml Vials ... 1795
- Novolin R PenFill Cartridges Durable Insulin Delivery System ... 1798
- Novolin R Prefilled Syringe Disposable Insulin Delivery System ... 1798
- Velosulin BR Human Insulin 10 ml Vials ... 1795

Insulin, Human, Zinc Suspension (Insulin requirements may be increased, decreased, or unchanged). Products include:
- Humulin L, 100 Units ... 1446
- Humulin U, 100 Units ... 1450
- Novolin L Human Insulin 10 ml Vials ... 1795

Insulin, NPH (Insulin requirements may be increased, decreased, or unchanged). Products include:
- NPH, 100 Units ... 1450
- Pork NPH, 100 Units ... 1452
- Purified Pork NPH Isophane Insulin ... 1801

Insulin, Regular (Insulin requirements may be increased, decreased, or unchanged). Products include:
- Regular, 100 Units ... 1450
- Pork Regular, 100 Units ... 1452
- Pork Regular (Concentrated), 500 Units ... 1453
- Purified Pork Regular Insulin ... 1801

Insulin, Zinc Crystals (Insulin requirements may be increased, decreased, or unchanged). Products include:
- NPH, 100 Units ... 1450

Insulin, Zinc Suspension (Insulin requirements may be increased, decreased, or unchanged). Products include:
- Iletin I ... 1450
- Lente, 100 Units ... 1450
- Iletin II ... 1452
- Pork Lente, 100 Units ... 1452
- Purified Pork Lente Insulin ... 1801

Isradipine (Potentiated or additive action). Products include:
- DynaCirc Capsules ... 2256

Ketoprofen (Blunts antihypertensive effect of beta blocker). Products include:
- Orudis Capsules ... 2766
- Oruvail Capsules ... 2766

Ketorolac Tromethamine (Blunts antihypertensive effect of beta blocker). Products include:
- Acular ... 474
- Acular ... ◉ 277
- Toradol ... 2159

Labetalol Hydrochloride (Potentiated or additive action). Products include:
- Normodyne Injection ... 2377
- Normodyne Tablets ... 2379
- Trandate ... 1185

Levorphanol Tartrate (May aggravate orthostatic hypotension). Products include:
- Levo-Dromoran ... 2129

Lisinopril (Potentiated or additive action). Products include:
- Prinivil Tablets ... 1733
- Prinzide Tablets ... 1737
- Zestoretic ... 2850
- Zestril Tablets ... 2854

Losartan Potassium (Potentiated or additive action). Products include:
- Cozaar Tablets ... 1628
- Hyzaar Tablets ... 1677

Mecamylamine Hydrochloride (Potentiated or additive action). Products include:
- Inversine Tablets ... 1686

Meclofenamate Sodium (Blunts antihypertensive effect of beta blocker).
- No products indexed under this heading.

Mefenamic Acid (Blunts antihypertensive effect of beta blocker). Products include:
- Ponstel ... 1925

Meperidine Hydrochloride (May aggravate orthostatic hypotension). Products include:
- Demerol ... 2308
- Mepergan Injection ... 2753

Mephobarbital (May aggravate orthostatic hypotension). Products include:
- Mebaral Tablets ... 2322

Methadone Hydrochloride (May aggravate orthostatic hypotension). Products include:
- Methadone Hydrochloride Oral Concentrate ... 2233
- Methadone Hydrochloride Oral Solution & Tablets ... 2235

Methyclothiazide (Potentiated or additive action). Products include:
- Enduron Tablets ... 420

Methyldopa (Potentiated or additive action). Products include:
- Aldoclor Tablets ... 1598
- Aldomet Oral ... 1600
- Aldoril Tablets ... 1604

Methyldopate Hydrochloride (Potentiated or additive action). Products include:
- Aldomet Ester HCl Injection ... 1602

Methylprednisolone Acetate (Hypokalemia). Products include:
- Depo-Medrol Single-Dose Vial ... 2600
- Depo-Medrol Sterile Aqueous Suspension ... 2597

Methylprednisolone Sodium Succinate (Hypokalemia). Products include:
- Solu-Medrol Sterile Powder ... 2643

Metolazone (Potentiated or additive action). Products include:
- Mykrox Tablets ... 993
- Zaroxolyn Tablets ... 1000

Metoprolol Succinate (Potentiated or additive action). Products include:
- Toprol-XL Tablets ... 565

Metoprolol Tartrate (Potentiated or additive action). Products include:
- Lopressor Ampuls ... 830
- Lopressor HCT Tablets ... 832
- Lopressor Tablets ... 830

Metyrosine (Potentiated or additive action). Products include:
- Demser Capsules ... 1649

Minoxidil (Potentiated or additive action). Products include:
- Loniten Tablets ... 2618
- Rogaine Topical Solution ... 2637

Moexipril Hydrochloride (Potentiated or additive action). Products include:
- Univasc Tablets ... 2410

Morphine Sulfate (May aggravate orthostatic hypotension). Products include:
- Astramorph/PF Injection, USP (Preservative-Free) ... 535
- Duramorph ... 962
- Infumorph 200 and Infumorph 500 Sterile Solutions ... 965
- MS Contin Tablets ... 1994
- MSIR ... 1997
- Oramorph SR (Morphine Sulfate Sustained Release Tablets) ... 2236
- RMS Suppositories ... 2657
- Roxanol ... 2243

Nabumetone (Blunts antihypertensive effect of beta blocker). Products include:
- Relafen Tablets ... 2510

IMPORTANT NOTE: Always consult each drug listing in the patient's regimen for possible interactions.

Nadolol (Potentiated or additive action).
- No products indexed under this heading.

Naproxen (Blunts antihypertensive effect of beta blocker). Products include:
- Anaprox/Naprosyn 2117

Naproxen Sodium (Blunts antihypertensive effect of beta blocker). Products include:
- Aleve 1975
- Anaprox/Naprosyn 2117

Nicardipine Hydrochloride (Potentiated or additive action). Products include:
- Cardene Capsules 2095
- Cardene I.V. 2709
- Cardene SR Capsules 2097

Nifedipine (Potentiated or additive action). Products include:
- Adalat Capsules (10 mg and 20 mg) 587
- Adalat CC 589
- Procardia Capsules 1971
- Procardia XL Extended Release Tablets 1972

Nisoldipine (Potentiated or additive action).
- No products indexed under this heading.

Nitroglycerin (Potentiated or additive action). Products include:
- Deponit NTG Transdermal Delivery System 2397
- Nitro-Bid IV 1523
- Nitro-Bid Ointment 1524
- Nitrodisc 2047
- Nitro-Dur (nitroglycerin) Transdermal Infusion System 1326
- Nitrolingual Spray 2027
- Nitrostat Tablets 1925
- Transderm-Nitro Transdermal Therapeutic System 859

Norepinephrine Bitartrate (Decreased arterial responsiveness to norepinephrine). Products include:
- Levophed Bitartrate Injection 2315

Opium Alkaloids (May aggravate orthostatic hypotension).
- No products indexed under this heading.

Oxaprozin (Blunts antihypertensive effect of beta blocker). Products include:
- Daypro Caplets 2426

Oxycodone Hydrochloride (May aggravate orthostatic hypotension). Products include:
- Percocet Tablets 938
- Percodan Tablets 939
- Percodan-Demi Tablets 940
- Roxicodone Tablets, Oral Solution & Intensol (Oxycodone) 2244
- Tylox Capsules 1584

Penbutolol Sulfate (Potentiated or additive action). Products include:
- Levatol 2403

Pentobarbital Sodium (May aggravate orthostatic hypotension). Products include:
- Nembutal Sodium Capsules 436
- Nembutal Sodium Solution 438
- Nembutal Sodium Suppositories 440

Phenobarbital (May aggravate orthostatic hypotension). Products include:
- Arco-Lase Plus Tablets 512
- Bellergal-S Tablets 2250
- Donnatal 2060
- Donnatal Extentabs 2061
- Donnatal Tablets 2060
- Phenobarbital Elixir and Tablets 1469
- Quadrinal Tablets 1350

Phenoxybenzamine Hydrochloride (Potentiated or additive action). Products include:
- Dibenzyline Capsules 2476

Phentolamine Mesylate (Potentiated or additive action). Products include:
- Regitine 846

Phenylbutazone (Blunts antihypertensive effect of beta blocker).
- No products indexed under this heading.

Pindolol (Potentiated or additive action). Products include:
- Visken Tablets 2299

Piroxicam (Blunts antihypertensive effect of beta blocker). Products include:
- Feldene Capsules 1965

Polythiazide (Potentiated or additive action). Products include:
- Minizide Capsules 1938

Prazosin Hydrochloride (Potentiated). Products include:
- Minipress Capsules 1937
- Minizide Capsules 1938

Prednisolone Acetate (Hypokalemia). Products include:
- AK-CIDE ⊙ 202
- AK-CIDE Ointment ⊙ 202
- Blephamide Liquifilm Sterile Ophthalmic Suspension 476
- Blephamide Ointment ⊙ 237
- Econopred & Econopred Plus Ophthalmic Suspensions ⊙ 217
- Poly-Pred Liquifilm ⊙ 248
- Pred Forte ⊙ 250
- Pred Mild ⊙ 253
- Pred-G Liquifilm Sterile Ophthalmic Suspension ⊙ 251
- Pred-G S.O.P. Sterile Ophthalmic Ointment ⊙ 252
- Vasocidin Ointment ⊙ 268

Prednisolone Sodium Phosphate (Hypokalemia). Products include:
- AK-Pred ⊙ 204
- Hydeltrasol Injection, Sterile 1665
- Inflamase ⊙ 265
- Pediapred Oral Liquid 995
- Vasocidin Ophthalmic Solution ⊙ 270

Prednisolone Tebutate (Hypokalemia). Products include:
- Hydeltra-T.B.A. Sterile Suspension 1667

Prednisone (Hypokalemia). Products include:
- Deltasone Tablets 2595

Propoxyphene Hydrochloride (May aggravate orthostatic hypotension). Products include:
- Darvon 1435
- Wygesic Tablets 2827

Propoxyphene Napsylate (May aggravate orthostatic hypotension). Products include:
- Darvon-N/Darvocet-N 1433

Quinapril Hydrochloride (Potentiated or additive action). Products include:
- Accupril Tablets 1893

Ramipril (Potentiated or additive action). Products include:
- Altace Capsules 1232

Rauwolfia Serpentina (May produce an excessive hypotension with bradycardia and orthostatic effects).
- No products indexed under this heading.

Rescinnamine (May produce an excessive hypotension with bradycardia and orthostatic effects).
- No products indexed under this heading.

Reserpine (May produce an excessive hypotension with bradycardia and orthostatic effects). Products include:
- Diupres Tablets 1650
- Hydropres Tablets 1675
- Ser-Ap-Es Tablets 849

Secobarbital Sodium (May aggravate orthostatic hypotension). Products include:
- Seconal Sodium Pulvules 1474

Sodium Nitroprusside (Potentiated or additive action).
- No products indexed under this heading.

Sotalol Hydrochloride (Potentiated or additive action). Products include:
- Betapace Tablets 641

Spirapril Hydrochloride (Potentiated or additive action).
- No products indexed under this heading.

Sufentanil Citrate (May aggravate orthostatic hypotension). Products include:
- Sufenta Injection 1309

Sulindac (Blunts antihypertensive effect of beta blocker). Products include:
- Clinoril Tablets 1618

Terazosin Hydrochloride (Potentiated or additive action). Products include:
- Hytrin Capsules 430

Thiamylal Sodium (May aggravate orthostatic hypotension).
- No products indexed under this heading.

Timolol Maleate (Potentiated or additive action). Products include:
- Blocadren Tablets 1614
- Timolide Tablets 1748
- Timoptic in Ocudose 1753
- Timoptic Sterile Ophthalmic Solution 1751
- Timoptic-XE 1755

Tolmetin Sodium (Blunts antihypertensive effect of beta blocker). Products include:
- Tolectin (200, 400 and 600 mg) 1581

Torsemide (Potentiated or additive action). Products include:
- Demadex Tablets and Injection 686

Triamcinolone (Hypokalemia). Products include:
- Aristocort Tablets 1022

Triamcinolone Acetonide (Hypokalemia). Products include:
- Aristocort A 0.025% Cream 1027
- Aristocort A 0.5% Cream 1031
- Aristocort A 0.1% Cream 1029
- Aristocort A 0.1% Ointment 1030
- Azmacort Oral Inhaler 2011
- Nasacort Nasal Inhaler 2024

Triamcinolone Diacetate (Hypokalemia). Products include:
- Aristocort Suspension (Forte Parenteral) 1027
- Aristocort Suspension (Intralesional) 1025

Triamcinolone Hexacetonide (Hypokalemia). Products include:
- Aristospan Suspension (Intra-articular) 1033
- Aristospan Suspension (Intralesional) 1032

Trimethaphan Camsylate (Potentiated). Products include:
- Arfonad Ampuls 2080

Tubocurarine Chloride (Increased responsiveness to tubocurarine).
- No products indexed under this heading.

Verapamil Hydrochloride (Potentiated or additive action). Products include:
- Calan SR Caplets 2422
- Calan Tablets 2419
- Isoptin Injectable 1344
- Isoptin Oral Tablets 1346
- Isoptin SR Tablets 1348
- Verelan Capsules 1410
- Verelan Capsules 2824

Food Interactions

Alcohol (May aggravate orthostatic hypotension).

INDOCIN CAPSULES

(Indomethacin) 1680

May interact with loop diuretics, oral anticoagulants, thiazides, potassium sparing diuretics, beta blockers, and certain other agents. Compounds in these categories include:

Acebutolol Hydrochloride (Blunting of antihypertensive effect of beta blockers). Products include:
- Sectral Capsules 2807

Amiloride Hydrochloride (Reduced diuretic, natriuretic, and antihypertensive effects and increased serum potassium levels). Products include:
- Midamor Tablets 1703
- Moduretic Tablets 1705

Aspirin (Decreases indomethacin blood levels). Products include:
- Alka-Seltzer Effervescent Antacid and Pain Reliever ▣ 701
- Alka-Seltzer Extra Strength Effervescent Antacid and Pain Reliever ▣ 703
- Alka-Seltzer Lemon Lime Effervescent Antacid and Pain Reliever ▣ 703
- Alka-Seltzer Plus Cold Medicine ▣ 705
- Alka-Seltzer Plus Cold & Cough Medicine ▣ 708
- Alka-Seltzer Plus Night-Time Cold Medicine ▣ 707
- Alka Seltzer Plus Sinus Medicine ▣ 707
- Arthritis Foundation Safety Coated Aspirin Tablets ▣ 675
- Arthritis Pain Ascriptin ▣ 631
- Maximum Strength Ascriptin ▣ 630
- Regular Strength Ascriptin Tablets ▣ 629
- Arthritis Strength BC Powder ▣ 609
- BC Cold Powder Multi-Symptom Formula (Cold-Sinus-Allergy) ▣ 609
- BC Cold Powder Non-Drowsy Formula (Cold-Sinus) ▣ 609
- BC Powder ▣ 609
- Bayer Children's Chewable Aspirin ▣ 711
- Genuine Bayer Aspirin Tablets & Caplets ▣ 713
- Extra Strength Bayer Arthritis Pain Regimen Formula ▣ 711
- Extra Strength Bayer Aspirin Caplets & Tablets ▣ 712
- Extended-Release Bayer 8-Hour Aspirin ▣ 712
- Extra Strength Bayer Plus Aspirin Caplets ▣ 713
- Extra Strength Bayer PM Aspirin ▣ 713
- Bayer Enteric Aspirin ▣ 709
- Bufferin Analgesic Tablets and Caplets ▣ 613
- Arthritis Strength Bufferin Analgesic Caplets ▣ 614
- Extra Strength Bufferin Analgesic Tablets ▣ 615
- Cama Arthritis Pain Reliever ▣ 785
- Darvon Compound-65 Pulvules 1435
- Easprin 1914
- Ecotrin 2455
- Ecotrin Enteric Coated Aspirin Maximum Strength Tablets and Caplets ▣ 816
- Ecotrin Enteric Coated Aspirin Regular Strength Tablets 2455
- Empirin Aspirin Tablets ▣ 854
- Empirin with Codeine Tablets 1093
- Excedrin Extra-Strength Analgesic Tablets & Caplets 732
- Fiorinal Capsules 2261
- Fiorinal with Codeine Capsules 2262
- Fiorinal Tablets 2261
- Halfprin 1362
- Healthprin Aspirin 2455
- Norgesic 1496
- Percodan Tablets 939
- Percodan-Demi Tablets 940
- Robaxisal Tablets 2071
- Soma Compound w/Codeine Tablets 2676
- Soma Compound Tablets 2675
- St. Joseph Adult Chewable Aspirin (81 mg.) ▣ 808
- Talwin Compound 2335
- Ursinus Inlay-Tabs ▣ 794
- Vanquish Analgesic Caplets ▣ 731

(▣ Described in PDR For Nonprescription Drugs) (⊙ Described in PDR For Ophthalmology)

Atenolol (Blunting of antihypertensive effect of beta blockers). Products include:
- Tenoretic Tablets 2845
- Tenormin Tablets and I.V. Injection 2847

Bendroflumethiazide (Reduced diuretic, natriuretic, and antihypertensive effects of thiazide diuretics).
- No products indexed under this heading.

Betaxolol Hydrochloride (Blunting of antihypertensive effect of beta blockers). Products include:
- Betoptic Ophthalmic Solution 469
- Betoptic S Ophthalmic Suspension 471
- Kerlone Tablets 2436

Bisoprolol Fumarate (Blunting of antihypertensive effect of beta blockers). Products include:
- Zebeta Tablets 1413
- Ziac 1415

Bumetanide (Reduced diuretic, natriuretic, and antihypertensive effects of loop diuretics). Products include:
- Bumex 2093

Captopril (Reduced antihypertensive effect of captopril). Products include:
- Capoten 739
- Capozide 742

Carteolol Hydrochloride (Blunting of antihypertensive effect of beta blockers). Products include:
- Cartrol Tablets 410
- Ocupress Ophthalmic Solution, 1% Sterile ◉ 309

Chlorothiazide (Reduced diuretic, natriuretic, and antihypertensive effects of thiazide diuretics). Products include:
- Aldoclor Tablets 1598
- Diupres Tablets 1650
- Diuril Oral 1653

Chlorothiazide Sodium (Reduced diuretic, natriuretic, and antihypertensive effects of thiazide diuretics). Products include:
- Diuril Sodium Intravenous 1652

Cyclosporine (Increase in cyclosporine-induced toxicity). Products include:
- Neoral 2276
- Sandimmune 2286

Dexamethasone (False-negative results in dexamethasone suppression test). Products include:
- AK-Trol Ointment & Suspension ◉ 205
- Decadron Elixir 1633
- Decadron Tablets 1635
- Decaspray Topical Aerosol 1648
- Dexacidin Ointment ◉ 263
- Maxitrol Ophthalmic Ointment and Suspension ◉ 224
- TobraDex Ophthalmic Suspension and Ointment 473

Dexamethasone Acetate (False-negative results in dexamethasone suppression test). Products include:
- Dalalone D.P. Injectable 1011
- Decadron-LA Sterile Suspension 1646

Dexamethasone Sodium Phosphate (False-negative results in dexamethasone suppression test). Products include:
- Decadron Phosphate Injection 1637
- Decadron Phosphate Respihaler 1642
- Decadron Phosphate Sterile Ophthalmic Ointment 1641
- Decadron Phosphate Sterile Ophthalmic Solution 1642
- Decadron Phosphate Topical Cream 1644
- Decadron Phosphate Turbinaire 1645
- Decadron Phosphate with Xylocaine Injection, Sterile 1639
- Dexacort Phosphate in Respihaler 458
- Dexacort Phosphate in Turbinaire 459
- NeoDecadron Sterile Ophthalmic Ointment 1712
- NeoDecadron Sterile Ophthalmic Solution 1713
- NeoDecadron Topical Cream 1714

Dicumarol (Altered prothrombin time).
- No products indexed under this heading.

Diflunisal (Do not use concomitantly; fatal gastrointestinal hemorrhage). Products include:
- Dolobid Tablets 1654

Digoxin (Increased serum digoxin concentration and prolonged half-life). Products include:
- Lanoxicaps 1117
- Lanoxin Elixir Pediatric 1120
- Lanoxin Injection 1123
- Lanoxin Injection Pediatric 1126
- Lanoxin Tablets 1128

Esmolol Hydrochloride (Blunting of antihypertensive effect of beta blockers). Products include:
- Brevibloc Injection 1808

Ethacrynic Acid (Reduced diuretic, natriuretic, and antihypertensive effects of loop diuretics). Products include:
- Edecrin Tablets 1657

Furosemide (Reduced diuretic, natriuretic, and antihypertensive effects of loop diuretics). Products include:
- Lasix Injection, Oral Solution and Tablets 1240

Hydrochlorothiazide (Reduced diuretic, natriuretic, and antihypertensive effects of thiazide diuretics). Products include:
- Aldactazide 2413
- Aldoril Tablets 1604
- Apresazide Capsules 808
- Capozide 742
- Dyazide 2479
- Esidrix Tablets 821
- Esimil Tablets 822
- HydroDIURIL Tablets 1674
- Hydropres Tablets 1675
- Hyzaar Tablets 1677
- Inderide Tablets 2732
- Inderide LA Long Acting Capsules 2734
- Lopressor HCT Tablets 832
- Lotensin HCT 837
- Maxzide 1380
- Moduretic Tablets 1705
- Oretic Tablets 443
- Prinzide Tablets 1737
- Ser-Ap-Es Tablets 849
- Timolide Tablets 1748
- Vaseretic Tablets 1765
- Zestoretic 2850
- Ziac 1415

Hydroflumethiazide (Reduced diuretic, natriuretic, and antihypertensive effects of thiazide diuretics). Products include:
- Diucardin Tablets 2718

Labetalol Hydrochloride (Blunting of antihypertensive effect of beta blockers). Products include:
- Normodyne Injection 2377
- Normodyne Tablets 2379
- Trandate 1185

Levobunolol Hydrochloride (Blunting of antihypertensive effect of beta blockers). Products include:
- Betagan ◉ 233

Lithium Carbonate (Elevated plasma lithium levels; toxicity). Products include:
- Eskalith 2485
- Lithium Carbonate Capsules & Tablets 2230
- Lithonate/Lithotabs/Lithobid 2543

Lithium Citrate (Elevated plasma lithium levels; toxicity).
- No products indexed under this heading.

Methotrexate Sodium (Potentiation of methotrexate toxicity). Products include:
- Methotrexate Sodium Tablets, Injection, for Injection and LPF Injection 1275

Methyclothiazide (Reduced diuretic, natriuretic, and antihypertensive effects of thiazide diuretics). Products include:
- Enduron Tablets 420

Metipranolol Hydrochloride (Blunting of antihypertensive effect of beta blockers). Products include:
- OptiPranolol (Metipranolol 0.3%) Sterile Ophthalmic Solution ◉ 258

Metoprolol Succinate (Blunting of antihypertensive effect of beta blockers). Products include:
- Toprol-XL Tablets 565

Metoprolol Tartrate (Blunting of antihypertensive effect of beta blockers). Products include:
- Lopressor Ampuls 830
- Lopressor HCT Tablets 832
- Lopressor Tablets 830

Nadolol (Blunting of antihypertensive effect of beta blockers).
- No products indexed under this heading.

Nephrotoxic Drugs (Overt renal decompensation).

Penbutolol Sulfate (Blunting of antihypertensive effect of beta blockers). Products include:
- Levatol 2403

Pindolol (Blunting of antihypertensive effect of beta blockers). Products include:
- Visken Tablets 2299

Polythiazide (Reduced diuretic, natriuretic, and antihypertensive effects of thiazide diuretics). Products include:
- Minizide Capsules 1938

Probenecid (Increased plasma levels of indomethacin). Products include:
- Benemid Tablets 1611
- ColBENEMID Tablets 1622

Propranolol Hydrochloride (Blunting of antihypertensive effect of beta blockers). Products include:
- Inderal 2728
- Inderal LA Long Acting Capsules 2730
- Inderide Tablets 2732
- Inderide LA Long Acting Capsules 2734

Sotalol Hydrochloride (Blunting of antihypertensive effect of beta blockers). Products include:
- Betapace Tablets 641

Spironolactone (Reduced diuretic, natriuretic, and antihypertensive effects and increased serum potassium levels). Products include:
- Aldactazide 2413
- Aldactone 2414

Timolol Hemihydrate (Blunting of antihypertensive effect of beta blockers). Products include:
- Betimol 0.25%, 0.5% ◉ 261

Timolol Maleate (Blunting of antihypertensive effect of beta blockers). Products include:
- Blocadren Tablets 1614
- Timolide Tablets 1748
- Timoptic in Ocudose 1753
- Timoptic Sterile Ophthalmic Solution 1751
- Timoptic-XE 1755

Torsemide (Reduced diuretic, natriuretic, and antihypertensive effects of loop diuretics). Products include:
- Demadex Tablets and Injection 686

Triamterene (Potential for reversible acute renal failure and hyperkalemia). Products include:
- Dyazide 2479
- Dyrenium Capsules 2481
- Maxzide 1380

Warfarin Sodium (Altered prothrombin time). Products include:
- Coumadin 926

INDOCIN I.V.
(Indomethacin Sodium Trihydrate) 1684
May interact with cardiac glycosides and certain other agents. Compounds in these categories include:

Amikacin Sulfate (Serum levels of amikacin significantly elevated). Products include:
- Amikacin Sulfate Injection, USP 960
- Amikin Injectable 501

Deslanoside (Half-life of digitalis may be prolonged when given concomitantly).
- No products indexed under this heading.

Digitoxin (Half-life of digitalis may be prolonged when given concomitantly). Products include:
- Crystodigin Tablets 1433

Digoxin (Half-life of digitalis may be prolonged when given concomitantly). Products include:
- Lanoxicaps 1117
- Lanoxin Elixir Pediatric 1120
- Lanoxin Injection 1123
- Lanoxin Injection Pediatric 1126
- Lanoxin Tablets 1128

Furosemide (Blunted natriuretic effect of furosemide). Products include:
- Lasix Injection, Oral Solution and Tablets 1240

Gentamicin Sulfate (Serum levels of gentamicin significantly elevated). Products include:
- Garamycin Injectable 2360
- Genoptic Sterile Ophthalmic Solution ◉ 243
- Genoptic Sterile Ophthalmic Ointment ◉ 243
- Gentacidin Ointment ◉ 264
- Gentacidin Solution ◉ 264
- Gentak ◉ 208
- Pred-G Liquifilm Sterile Ophthalmic Suspension ◉ 251
- Pred-G S.O.P. Sterile Ophthalmic Ointment ◉ 252

INDOCIN ORAL SUSPENSION
(Indomethacin) 1680
See **Indocin Capsules**

INDOCIN SR CAPSULES
(Indomethacin) 1680
See **Indocin Capsules**

INDOCIN SUPPOSITORIES
(Indomethacin) 1680
See **Indocin Capsules**

INFED (IRON DEXTRAN INJECTION, USP)
(Iron Dextran) 2345
None cited in PDR database.

INFLAMASE FORTE 1%
(Prednisolone Sodium Phosphate) ◉ 265
None cited in PDR database.

INFLAMASE MILD ⅛%
(Prednisolone Sodium Phosphate) ◉ 265
None cited in PDR database.

INFLUENZA VIRUS VACCINE, TRIVALENT, TYPES A AND B (CHROMATOGRAPH- AND FILTER-PURIFIED SUBVIRON ANTIGEN) FLUSHIELD, 1995-1996 FORMULA
(Influenza Virus Vaccine) 2736
May interact with corticosteroids, alkylating agents, cytotoxic drugs, xanthine bronchodilators, and certain other agents. Compounds in these categories include:

Aminophylline (Potential for ele-

IMPORTANT NOTE: Always consult each drug listing in the patient's regimen for possible interactions.

FluShield **Interactions Index** 522

vated theophylline serum concentrations resulting in possible enhanced effects or toxicity).
No products indexed under this heading.

Betamethasone Acetate (Individual receiving large amount of corticosteroids as immunosuppressive agents may not respond optimally to active immunization procedures). Products include:
Celestone Soluspan Suspension 2347

Betamethasone Sodium Phosphate (Individual receiving large amount of corticosteroids as immunosuppressive agents may not respond optimally to active immunization procedures). Products include:
Celestone Soluspan Suspension 2347

Bleomycin Sulfate (Individual receiving large amount of cytotoxic agents may not respond optimally to active immunization procedures). Products include:
Blenoxane 692

Busulfan (Individual receiving large amount of alkylating agents may not respond optimally to active immunization procedures). Products include:
Myleran Tablets 1143

Carmustine (BCNU) (Individual receiving large amount of alkylating agents may not respond optimally to active immunization procedures). Products include:
BiCNU 691

Chlorambucil (Individual receiving large amount of alkylating agents may not respond optimally to active immunization procedures). Products include:
Leukeran Tablets 1133

Cortisone Acetate (Individual receiving large amount of corticosteroids as immunosuppressive agents may not respond optimally to active immunization procedures). Products include:
Cortone Acetate Sterile Suspension 1623
Cortone Acetate Tablets 1624

Cyclophosphamide (Individual receiving large amount of alkylating agents may not respond optimally to active immunization procedures). Products include:
Cytoxan 694
NEOSAR Lyophilized/Neosar 1959

Dacarbazine (Individual receiving large amount of alkylating agents may not respond optimally to active immunization procedures). Products include:
DTIC-Dome 600

Daunorubicin Hydrochloride (Individual receiving large amount of cytotoxic agents may not respond optimally to active immunization procedures). Products include:
Cerubidine 795

Dexamethasone (Individual receiving large amount of corticosteroids as immunosuppressive agents may not respond optimally to active immunization procedures). Products include:
AK-Trol Ointment & Suspension ...... ⊙ 205
Decadron Elixir 1633
Decadron Tablets 1635
Decaspray Topical Aerosol 1648
Dexacidin Ointment ...... ⊙ 263
Maxitrol Ophthalmic Ointment and Suspension ...... ⊙ 224
TobraDex Ophthalmic Suspension and Ointment 473

Dexamethasone Acetate (Individual receiving large amount of corticosteroids as immunosuppressive agents may not respond optimally to active immunization procedures). Products include:
Dalalone D.P. Injectable 1011
Decadron-LA Sterile Suspension 1646

Dexamethasone Sodium Phosphate (Individual receiving large amount of corticosteroids as immunosuppressive agents may not respond optimally to active immunization procedures). Products include:
Decadron Phosphate Injection 1637
Decadron Phosphate Respihaler 1642
Decadron Phosphate Sterile Ophthalmic Ointment 1641
Decadron Phosphate Sterile Ophthalmic Solution 1642
Decadron Phosphate Topical Cream 1644
Decadron Phosphate Turbinaire 1645
Decadron Phosphate with Xylocaine Injection, Sterile 1639
Dexacort Phosphate in Respihaler 458
Dexacort Phosphate in Turbinaire 459
NeoDecadron Sterile Ophthalmic Ointment 1712
NeoDecadron Sterile Ophthalmic Solution 1713
NeoDecadron Topical Cream 1714

Doxorubicin Hydrochloride (Individual receiving large amount of cytotoxic agents may not respond optimally to active immunization procedures). Products include:
Adriamycin PFS 1947
Adriamycin RDF 1947
Doxorubicin Astra 540
Rubex 712

Dyphylline (Potential for elevated theophylline serum concentrations resulting in possible enhanced effects or toxicity). Products include:
Lufyllin & Lufyllin-400 Tablets 2670
Lufyllin-GG Elixir & Tablets 2671

Fludrocortisone Acetate (Individual receiving large amount of corticosteroids as immunosuppressive agents may not respond optimally to active immunization procedures). Products include:
Florinef Acetate Tablets 505

Fluorouracil (Individual receiving large amount of cytotoxic agents may not respond optimally to active immunization procedures). Products include:
Efudex 2113
Fluoroplex Topical Solution & Cream 1% 479
Fluorouracil Injection 2116

Hydrocortisone (Individual receiving large amount of corticosteroids as immunosuppressive agents may not respond optimally to active immunization procedures). Products include:
Anusol-HC Cream 2.5% 1896
Aquanil HC Lotion 1931
Bactine Hydrocortisone Anti-Itch Cream ...... ▭ 709
Caldecort Anti-Itch Hydrocortisone Spray ...... ▭ 631
Cortaid ...... ▭ 836
CORTENEMA 2535
Cortisporin Ointment 1085
Cortisporin Ophthalmic Ointment Sterile 1085
Cortisporin Ophthalmic Suspension Sterile 1086
Cortisporin Otic Solution Sterile 1087
Cortisporin Otic Suspension Sterile 1088
Cortizone-5 ...... ▭ 831
Cortizone-10 ...... ▭ 831
Hydrocortone Tablets 1672
Hytone 907
Massengill Medicated Soft Cloth Towelettes 2458
PediOtic Suspension Sterile 1153
Preparation H Hydrocortisone 1% Cream ...... ▭ 872
ProctoCream-HC 2.5% 2408
VōSoL HC Otic Solution 2678

Hydrocortisone Acetate (Individual receiving large amount of corticosteroids as immunosuppressive agents may not respond optimally to active immunization procedures). Products include:
Analpram-HC Rectal Cream 1% and 2.5% 977
Anusol HC-1 Anti-Itch Hydrocortisone Ointment ...... ▭ 847
Anusol-HC Suppositories 1897
Caldecort ...... ▭ 631
Carmol HC 924
Coly-Mycin S Otic w/Neomycin & Hydrocortisone 1906
Cortaid ...... ▭ 836
Cortifoam 2396
Cortisporin Cream 1084
Epifoam 2399
Hydrocortone Acetate Sterile Suspension 1669
Mantadil Cream 1135
Nupercainal Hydrocortisone 1% Cream ...... ▭ 645
Ophthocort ...... ⊙ 311
Pramosone Cream, Lotion & Ointment 978
ProctoCream-HC 2408
ProctoFoam-HC 2409
Terra-Cortril Ophthalmic Suspension 2210

Hydrocortisone Sodium Phosphate (Individual receiving large amount of corticosteroids as immunosuppressive agents may not respond optimally to active immunization procedures). Products include:
Hydrocortone Phosphate Injection, Sterile 1670

Hydrocortisone Sodium Succinate (Individual receiving large amount of corticosteroids as immunosuppressive agents may not respond optimally to active immunization procedures). Products include:
Solu-Cortef Sterile Powder 2641

Hydroxyurea (Individual receiving large amount of cytotoxic agents may not respond optimally to active immunization procedures). Products include:
Hydrea Capsules 696

Lomustine (CCNU) (Individual receiving large amount of alkylating agents may not respond optimally to active immunization procedures). Products include:
CeeNU 693

Mechlorethamine Hydrochloride (Individual receiving large amount of alkylating agents may not respond optimally to active immunization procedures). Products include:
Mustargen 1709

Melphalan (Individual receiving large amount of alkylating agents may not respond optimally to active immunization procedures). Products include:
Alkeran Tablets 1071

Methotrexate Sodium (Individual receiving large amount of cytotoxic agents may not respond optimally to active immunization procedures). Products include:
Methotrexate Sodium Tablets, Injection, for Injection and LPF Injection 1275

Methylprednisolone Acetate (Individual receiving large amount of corticosteroids as immunosuppressive agents may not respond optimally to active immunization procedures). Products include:
Depo-Medrol Single-Dose Vial 2600
Depo-Medrol Sterile Aqueous Suspension 2597

Methylprednisolone Sodium Succinate (Individual receiving large amount of corticosteriods as immunosuppressive agents may not respond optimally to active immunization procedures). Products include:
Solu-Medrol Sterile Powder 2643

Mitotane (Individual receiving large amount of cytotoxic agents may not respond optimally to active immunization procedures). Products include:
Lysodren 698

Mitoxantrone Hydrochloride (Individual receiving large amount of cytotoxic agents may not respond optimally to active immunization procedures). Products include:
Novantrone 1279

Prednisolone Acetate (Individual receiving large amount of corticosteroids as immunosuppressive agents may not respond optimally to active immunization procedures). Products include:
AK-CIDE ...... ⊙ 202
AK-CIDE Ointment ...... ⊙ 202
Blephamide Liquifilm Sterile Ophthalmic Suspension 476
Blephamide Ointment ...... ⊙ 237
Econopred & Econopred Plus Ophthalmic Suspensions ...... ⊙ 217
Poly-Pred Liquifilm ...... ⊙ 248
Pred Forte ...... ⊙ 250
Pred Mild ...... ⊙ 253
Pred-G Liquifilm Sterile Ophthalmic Suspension ...... ⊙ 251
Pred-G S.O.P. Sterile Ophthalmic Ointment ...... ⊙ 252
Vasocidin Ointment ...... ⊙ 268

Prednisolone Sodium Phosphate (Individual receiving large amount of corticosteroids as immunosuppressive agents may not respond optimally to active immunization procedures). Products include:
AK-Pred ...... ⊙ 204
Hydeltrasol Injection, Sterile 1665
Inflamase ...... ⊙ 265
Pediapred Oral Liquid 995
Vasocidin Ophthalmic Solution ...... ⊙ 270

Prednisolone Tebutate (Individual receiving large amount of corticosteroids as immunosuppressive agents may not respond optimally to active immunization procedures). Products include:
Hydeltra-T.B.A. Sterile Suspension 1667

Prednisone (Individual receiving large amount of corticosteriods as immunosuppressive agents may not respond optimally to active immunization procedures). Products include:
Deltasone Tablets 2595

Procarbazine Hydrochloride (Individual receiving large amount of cytotoxic agents may not respond optimally to active immunization procedures). Products include:
Matulane Capsules 2131

Tamoxifen Citrate (Individual receiving large amount of cytotoxic agents may not respond optimally to active immunization procedures). Products include:
Nolvadex Tablets 2841

Theophylline (Potential for elevated theophylline serum concentrations resulting in possible enhanced effects or toxicity). Products include:
Marax Tablets & DF Syrup 2200
Quibron 2053

Theophylline Anhydrous (Potential for elevated theophylline serum concentrations resulting in possible enhanced effects or toxicity). Products include:
Aerolate 1004

(▭ Described in PDR For Nonprescription Drugs) (⊙ Described in PDR For Ophthalmology)

Primatene Dual Action Formula...... ✦D 872
Primatene Tablets .... ✦D 873
Respbid Tablets 682
Slo-bid Gyrocaps 2033
Theo-24 Extended Release Capsules 2568
Theo-Dur Extended-Release Tablets 1327
Theo-X Extended-Release Tablets .. 788
Uni-Dur Extended-Release Tablets.. 1331
Uniphyl 400 mg Tablets........................ 2001

Theophylline Calcium Salicylate (Potential for elevated theophylline serum concentrations resulting in possible enhanced effects or toxicity). Products include:

Quadrinal Tablets 1350

Theophylline Sodium Glycinate (Potential for elevated theophylline serum concentrations resulting in possible enhanced effects or toxicity).

No products indexed under this heading.

Thiotepa (Individual receiving large amount of alkylating agents may not respond optimally to active immunization procedures). Products include:

Thioplex (Thiotepa For Injection) 1281

Triamcinolone (Individual receiving large amount of corticosteriods as immunosuppressive agents may not respond optimally to active immunization procedures). Products include:

Aristocort Tablets 1022

Triamcinolone Acetonide (Individual receiving large amount of corticosteriods as immunosuppressive agents may not respond optimally to active immunization procedures). Products include:

Aristocort A 0.025% Cream 1027
Aristocort A 0.5% Cream 1031
Aristocort A 0.1% Cream 1029
Aristocort A 0.1% Ointment 1030
Azmacort Oral Inhaler 2011
Nasacort Nasal Inhaler 2024

Triamcinolone Diacetate (Individual receiving large amount of corticosteriods as immunosuppressive agents may not respond optimally to active immunization procedures). Products include:

Aristocort Suspension (Forte Parenteral).. 1027
Aristocort Suspension (Intralesional) 1025

Triamcinolone Hexacetonide (Individual receiving large amount of corticosteriods as immunosuppressive agents may not respond optimally to active immunization procedures). Products include:

Aristospan Suspension (Intra-articular) 1033
Aristospan Suspension (Intralesional) 1032

Vincristine Sulfate (Individual receiving large amount of cytotoxic agents may not respond optimally to active immunization procedures). Products include:

Oncovin Solution Vials & Hyporets 1466

Warfarin Sodium (Potential for hypoprothrombinemia resulting in possible enhanced effects or toxicity). Products include:

Coumadin 926

INFUMORPH 200 AND INFUMORPH 500 STERILE SOLUTIONS

(Morphine Sulfate).................................... 965

May interact with central nervous system depressants, antihistamines, antipsychotic agents, and certain other agents. Compounds in these categories include:

Acrivastine (Potentiates CNS depressant effects). Products include:

Semprex-D Capsules 463
Semprex-D Capsules 1167

Alfentanil Hydrochloride (Potentiates CNS depressant effects). Products include:

Alfenta Injection 1286

Alprazolam (Potentiates CNS depressant effects). Products include:

Xanax Tablets 2649

Aprobarbital (Potentiates CNS depressant effects).

No products indexed under this heading.

Astemizole (Potentiates CNS depressant effects). Products include:

Hismanal Tablets 1293

Azatadine Maleate (Potentiates CNS depressant effects). Products include:

Trinalin Repetabs Tablets 1330

Bromodiphenhydramine Hydrochloride (Potentiates CNS depressant effects).

No products indexed under this heading.

Brompheniramine Maleate (Potentiates CNS depressant effects). Products include:

Alka Seltzer Plus Sinus Medicine .. ✦D 707
Bromfed Capsules (Extended-Release) 1785
Bromfed Syrup .... ✦D 733
Bromfed Tablets 1785
Bromfed-DM Cough Syrup.................. 1786
Bromfed-PD Capsules (Extended-Release).. 1785
Dimetane-DC Cough Syrup 2059
Dimetane-DX Cough Syrup 2059
Dimetapp Elixir .... ✦D 773
Dimetapp Extentabs .... ✦D 774
Dimetapp Tablets/Liqui-Gels .... ✦D 775
Dimetapp Cold & Allergy Chewable Tablets .... ✦D 773
Dimetapp DM Elixir .... ✦D 774
Vicks DayQuil Allergy Relief 12-Hour Extended Release Tablets.. ✦D 760
Vicks DayQuil Allergy Relief 4-Hour Tablets .... ✦D 760

Buprenorphine (Potentiates CNS depressant effects). Products include:

Buprenex Injectable 2006

Buspirone Hydrochloride (Potentiates CNS depressant effects). Products include:

BuSpar 737

Butabarbital (Potentiates CNS depressant effects).

No products indexed under this heading.

Butalbital (Potentiates CNS depressant effects). Products include:

Esgic-plus Tablets 1013
Fioricet Tablets.. 2258
Fioricet with Codeine Capsules 2260
Fiorinal Capsules 2261
Fiorinal with Codeine Capsules 2262
Fiorinal Tablets.. 2261
Phrenilin 785
Sedapap Tablets 50 mg/650 mg .. 1543

Chlordiazepoxide (Potentiates CNS depressant effects). Products include:

Libritabs Tablets 2177
Limbitrol 2180

Chlordiazepoxide Hydrochloride (Potentiates CNS depressant effects). Products include:

Librax Capsules 2176
Librium Capsules.................................... 2178
Librium Injectable 2179

Chlorpheniramine Maleate (Potentiates CNS depressant effects). Products include:

Alka-Seltzer Plus Cold Medicine .... ✦D 705
Alka-Seltzer Plus Cold Medicine Liqui-Gels .... ✦D 706
Alka-Seltzer Plus Cold & Cough Medicine .... ✦D 708
Alka-Seltzer Plus Cold & Cough Medicine Liqui-Gels......................... ✦D 705
Allerest Children's Chewable Tablets .... ✦D 627
Allerest Headache Strength Tablets .... ✦D 627
Allerest Maximum Strength Tablets .... ✦D 627
Allerest Sinus Pain Formula .... ✦D 627
Allerest 12 Hour Caplets .... ✦D 627
Ana-Kit Anaphylaxis Emergency Treatment Kit 617
Atrohist Pediatric Capsules.................. 453
Atrohist Plus Tablets 454
BC Cold Powder Multi-Symptom Formula (Cold-Sinus-Allergy) ...... ✦D 609
Cerose DM .... ✦D 878
Cheracol Plus Head Cold/Cough Formula .... ✦D 769
Children's Vicks DayQuil Allergy Relief.. ✦D 757
Children's Vicks NyQuil Cold/Cough Relief.. ✦D 758
Chlor-Trimeton Allergy Decongestant Tablets .... ✦D 799
Chlor-Trimeton Allergy Tablets ...... ✦D 798
Combist 2038
Comtrex Multi-Symptom Cold Reliever Tablets/Caplets/Liqui-Gels/Liquid .... ✦D 615
Allergy-Sinus Comtrex Multi-Symptom Allergy-Sinus Formula Tablets .... ✦D 617
Contac Continuous Action Nasal Decongestant/Antihistamine 12 Hour Capsules.................................... ✦D 813
Contac Maximum Strength Continuous Action Decongestant/Antihistamine 12 Hour Caplets.. ✦D 813
Contac Severe Cold and Flu Formula Caplets .... ✦D 814
Coricidin 'D' Decongestant Tablets .... ✦D 800
Coricidin Tablets .... ✦D 800
D.A. Chewable Tablets.......................... 951
Deconamine 1320
Dura-Tap/PD Capsules 2867
Dura-Vent/DA Tablets 953
Extendryl 1005
Fedahist Gyrocaps.................................. 2401
Fedahist Timecaps 2401
Hycomine Compound Tablets 932
Isoclor Timesule Capsules .... ✦D 637
Kronofed-A 977
Nolamine Timed-Release Tablets 785
Novahistine DH.. 2462
Novahistine Elixir .... ✦D 823
Ornade Spansule Capsules 2502
PediaCare Cold Allergy Chewable Tablets .... ✦D 677
PediaCare Cough-Cold Chewable Tablets 1553
PediaCare Cough-Cold Liquid............ 1553
PediaCare NightRest Cough-Cold Liquid 1553
Pediatric Vicks 44m Cough & Cold Relief .... ✦D 764
Pyrroxate Caplets .... ✦D 772
Ryna .... ✦D 841
Sinarest Tablets .... ✦D 648
Sinarest Extra Strength Tablets...... ✦D 648
Sine-Off Sinus Medicine .... ✦D 825
Singlet Tablets .... ✦D 825
Sinulin Tablets 787
Sinutab Sinus Allergy Medication, Maximum Strength Tablets and Caplets .... ✦D 860
Sudafed Plus Liquid .... ✦D 862
Sudafed Plus Tablets .... ✦D 863
Teldrin 12 Hour Antihistamine/Nasal Decongestant Allergy Relief Capsules .... ✦D 826
TheraFlu... ✦D 787
TheraFlu Maximum Strength Nighttime Flu, Cold & Cough Medicine .... ✦D 788
Triaminic Allergy Tablets .... ✦D 789
Triaminic Cold Tablets .... ✦D 790
Triaminic Nite Light .... ✦D 791
Triaminic Syrup .... ✦D 792
Triaminic-12 Tablets .... ✦D 792
Triaminicin Tablets .... ✦D 793
Triaminicol Multi-Symptom Cold Tablets .... ✦D 793
Triaminicol Multi-Symptom Relief ✦D 794
Tussend 1783
Children's TYLENOL Cold Multi-Symptom Liquid Formula and Chewable Tablets............................. 1561

Children's TYLENOL Cold Plus Cough Multi Symptom Tablets and Liquid .... ✦D 681
TYLENOL Maximum Strength Allergy Sinus Medication Gelcaps and Caplets 1563
TYLENOL Cold Multi-Symptom Formula Medication Tablets and Caplets 1561
TYLENOL Cold Multi-Symptom Hot Medication Liquid Packets.............. 1557
Vicks 44 LiquiCaps Cough, Cold & Flu Relief.. ✦D 755
Vicks 44M Cough, Cold & Flu Relief... ✦D 756

Chlorpheniramine Polistirex (Potentiates CNS depressant effects). Products include:

Tussionex Pennkinetic Extended-Release Suspension 998

Chlorpheniramine Tannate (Potentiates CNS depressant effects). Products include:

Atrohist Pediatric Suspension 454
Ricobid Tablets and Pediatric Suspension.. 2038
Rynatan 2673
Rynatuss 2673

Chlorpromazine (Potentiates CNS depressant effects; increases the risk of respiratory depression). Products include:

Thorazine Suppositories 2523

Chlorprothixene (Potentiates CNS depressant effects; increases the risk of respiratory depression).

No products indexed under this heading.

Chlorprothixene Hydrochloride (Potentiates CNS depressant effects; increases the risk of respiratory depression).

No products indexed under this heading.

Clemastine Fumarate (Potentiates CNS depressant effects). Products include:

Tavist Syrup.. 2297
Tavist Tablets 2298
Tavist-1 12 Hour Relief Tablets .... ✦D 787
Tavist-D 12 Hour Relief Tablets .... ✦D 787

Clorazepate Dipotassium (Potentiates CNS depressant effects). Products include:

Tranxene 451

Clozapine (Potentiates CNS depressant effects; increases the risk of respiratory depression). Products include:

Clozaril Tablets.. 2252

Codeine Phosphate (Potentiates CNS depressant effects). Products include:

Actifed with Codeine Cough Syrup.. 1067
Brontex 1981
Deconsal C Expectorant Syrup 456
Deconsal Pediatric Syrup.................... 457
Dimetane-DC Cough Syrup 2059
Empirin with Codeine Tablets............ 1093
Fioricet with Codeine Capsules 2260
Fiorinal with Codeine Capsules 2262
Isoclor Expectorant................................ 990
Novahistine DH.. 2462
Novahistine Expectorant...................... 2463
Nucofed 2051
Phenergan with Codeine 2777
Phenergan VC with Codeine 2781
Robitussin A-C Syrup............................ 2073
Robitussin-DAC Syrup........................... 2074
Ryna .... ✦D 841
Soma Compound w/Codeine Tablets 2676
Tussi-Organidin NR Liquid and S NR Liquid 2677
Tylenol with Codeine 1583

Cyproheptadine Hydrochloride (Potentiates CNS depressant effects). Products include:

Periactin 1724

Desflurane (Potentiates CNS depressant effects). Products include:

Suprane 1813

IMPORTANT NOTE: Always consult each drug listing in the patient's regimen for possible interactions.

Dexchlorpheniramine Maleate (Potentiates CNS depressant effects).
No products indexed under this heading.

Dezocine (Potentiates CNS depressant effects). Products include:
Dalgan Injection 538

Diazepam (Potentiates CNS depressant effects). Products include:
Dizac 1809
Valium Injectable 2182
Valium Tablets 2183
Valrelease Capsules 2169

Diphenhydramine Citrate (Potentiates CNS depressant effects). Products include:
Excedrin P.M. Analgesic/Sleeping Aid Tablets, Caplets, Liquigels 733

Diphenhydramine Hydrochloride (Potentiates CNS depressant effects). Products include:
Actifed Allergy Daytime/Nighttime Caplets .... ▣ 844
Actifed Sinus Daytime/Nighttime Tablets and Caplets .... ▣ 846
Arthritis Foundation NightTime Caplets .... ▣ 674
Extra Strength Bayer PM Aspirin .. ▣ 713
Bayer Select Night Time Pain Relief Formula .... ▣ 716
Benadryl Allergy Decongestant Liquid Medication .... ▣ 848
Benadryl Allergy Decongestant Tablets .... ▣ 848
Benadryl Allergy Liquid Medication .... ▣ 849
Benadryl Allergy .... ▣ 848
Benadryl Allergy Sinus Headache Formula Caplets .... ▣ 849
Benadryl Capsules 1898
Benadryl Dye-Free Allergy Liquigel Softgels .... ▣ 850
Benadryl Dye-Free Allergy Liquid Medication .... ▣ 850
Benadryl Itch Relief Cream, Children's Formula and Maximum Strength 2% .... ▣ 851
Benadryl Itch Relief Spray, Children's Formula and Maximum Strength 2% .... ▣ 851
Benadryl Itch Relief Stick Maximum Strength 2% .... ▣ 850
Benadryl Itch Stopping Gel, Children's Formula and Maximum Strength 2% .... ▣ 851
Benadryl Kapseals 1898
Benadryl Injection 1898
Contac Day & Night Cold/Flu Night Caplets .... ▣ 812
Contac Night Allergy/Sinus Caplets .... ▣ 812
Extra Strength Doan's P.M. .... ▣ 633
Legatrin PM .... ▣ 651
Miles Nervine Nighttime Sleep-Aid ▣ 723
Nytol QuickCaps Caplets .... ▣ 610
Sleepinal Night-time Sleep Aid Capsules and Softgels .... ▣ 834
TYLENOL Maximum Strength Allergy Sinus NightTime Medication Caplets 1555
TYLENOL Flu NightTime, Maximum Strength, Gelcaps 1566
TYLENOL Maximum Strength Flu NightTime Hot Medication Packets 1562
TYLENOL PM, Extra Strength Pain Reliever/Sleep Aid Caplets, Geltabs, Gelcaps 1560
TYLENOL Severe Allergy Medication Caplets 1564
Maximum Strength Unisom Sleepgels 1934
Unisom With Pain Relief-Nighttime Sleep Aid and Pain Reliever 1934

Diphenylpyraline Hydrochloride (Potentiates CNS depressant effects).
No products indexed under this heading.

Droperidol (Potentiates CNS depressant effects). Products include:
Inapsine Injection 1296

Enflurane (Potentiates CNS depressant effects).
No products indexed under this heading.

Estazolam (Potentiates CNS depressant effects). Products include:
ProSom Tablets 449

Ethchlorvynol (Potentiates CNS depressant effects). Products include:
Placidyl Capsules 448

Ethinamate (Potentiates CNS depressant effects).
No products indexed under this heading.

Fentanyl (Potentiates CNS depressant effects). Products include:
Duragesic Transdermal System 1288

Fentanyl Citrate (Potentiates CNS depressant effects). Products include:
Sublimaze Injection 1307

Fluphenazine Decanoate (Potentiates CNS depressant effects; increases the risk of respiratory depression). Products include:
Prolixin Decanoate 509

Fluphenazine Enanthate (Potentiates CNS depressant effects; increases the risk of respiratory depression). Products include:
Prolixin Enanthate 509

Fluphenazine Hydrochloride (Potentiates CNS depressant effects; increases the risk of respiratory depression). Products include:
Prolixin 509

Flurazepam Hydrochloride (Potentiates CNS depressant effects). Products include:
Dalmane Capsules 2173

Glutethimide (Potentiates CNS depressant effects).
No products indexed under this heading.

Haloperidol (Potentiates CNS depressant effects; increases the risk of respiratory depression). Products include:
Haldol Injection, Tablets and Concentrate 1575

Haloperidol Decanoate (Potentiates CNS depressant effects; increases the risk of respiratory depression). Products include:
Haldol Decanoate 1577

Hydrocodone Bitartrate (Potentiates CNS depressant effects). Products include:
Anexsia 5/500 Elixir 1781
Anexia Tablets 1782
Codiclear DH Syrup 791
Deconamine CX Cough and Cold Liquid and Tablets 1319
Duratuss HD Elixir 2565
Hycodan Tablets and Syrup 930
Hycomine Compound Tablets 932
Hycomine 931
Hycotuss Expectorant Syrup 933
Hydrocet Capsules 782
Lorcet 10/650 1018
Lortab 2566
Tussend 1783
Tussend Expectorant 1785
Vicodin Tablets 1356
Vicodin ES Tablets 1357
Vicodin Tuss Expectorant 1358
Zydone Capsules 949

Hydrocodone Polistirex (Potentiates CNS depressant effects). Products include:
Tussionex Pennkinetic Extended-Release Suspension 998

Hydroxyzine Hydrochloride (Potentiates CNS depressant effects). Products include:
Atarax Tablets & Syrup 2185
Marax Tablets & DF Syrup 2200
Vistaril Intramuscular Solution 2216

Isoflurane (Potentiates CNS depressant effects).
No products indexed under this heading.

Ketamine Hydrochloride (Potentiates CNS depressant effects).
No products indexed under this heading.

Levomethadyl Acetate Hydrochloride (Potentiates CNS depressant effects). Products include:
Orlamm 2239

Levorphanol Tartrate (Potentiates CNS depressant effects). Products include:
Levo-Dromoran 2129

Lithium Carbonate (Potentiates CNS depressant effects; increases the risk of respiratory depression). Products include:
Eskalith 2485
Lithium Carbonate Capsules & Tablets 2230
Lithonate/Lithotabs/Lithobid 2543

Lithium Citrate (Potentiates CNS depressant effects; increases the risk of respiratory depression).
No products indexed under this heading.

Loratadine (Potentiates CNS depressant effects). Products include:
Claritin 2349
Claritin-D 2350

Lorazepam (Potentiates CNS depressant effects). Products include:
Ativan Injection 2698
Ativan Tablets 2700

Loxapine Hydrochloride (Potentiates CNS depressant effects; increases the risk of respiratory depression). Products include:
Loxitane 1378

Loxapine Succinate (Potentiates CNS depressant effects; increases the risk of respiratory depression). Products include:
Loxitane Capsules 1378

Meperidine Hydrochloride (Potentiates CNS depressant effects). Products include:
Demerol 2308
Mepergan Injection 2753

Mephobarbital (Potentiates CNS depressant effects). Products include:
Mebaral Tablets 2322

Meprobamate (Potentiates CNS depressant effects). Products include:
Miltown Tablets 2672
PMB 200 and PMB 400 2783

Mesoridazine Besylate (Potentiates CNS depressant effects; increases the risk of respiratory depression). Products include:
Serentil 684

Methadone Hydrochloride (Potentiates CNS depressant effects). Products include:
Methadone Hydrochloride Oral Concentrate 2233
Methadone Hydrochloride Oral Solution & Tablets 2235

Methdilazine Hydrochloride (Potentiates CNS depressant effects).
No products indexed under this heading.

Methohexital Sodium (Potentiates CNS depressant effects). Products include:
Brevital Sodium Vials 1429

Methotrimeprazine (Potentiates CNS depressant effects). Products include:
Levoprome 1274

Methoxyflurane (Potentiates CNS depressant effects).
No products indexed under this heading.

Midazolam Hydrochloride (Potentiates CNS depressant effects). Products include:
Versed Injection 2170

Molindone Hydrochloride (Potentiates CNS depressant effects; increases the risk of respiratory depression). Products include:
Moban Tablets and Concentrate 1048

Opium Alkaloids (Potentiates CNS depressant effects).
No products indexed under this heading.

Oxazepam (Potentiates CNS depressant effects). Products include:
Serax Capsules 2810
Serax Tablets 2810

Oxycodone Hydrochloride (Potentiates CNS depressant effects). Products include:
Percocet Tablets 938
Percodan Tablets 939
Percodan-Demi Tablets 940
Roxicodone Tablets, Oral Solution & Intensol (Oxycodone) 2244
Tylox Capsules 1584

Pentobarbital Sodium (Potentiates CNS depressant effects). Products include:
Nembutal Sodium Capsules 436
Nembutal Sodium Solution 438
Nembutal Sodium Suppositories 440

Perphenazine (Potentiates CNS depressant effects; increases the risk of respiratory depression). Products include:
Etrafon 2355
Triavil Tablets 1757
Trilafon 2389

Phenobarbital (Potentiates CNS depressant effects). Products include:
Arco-Lase Plus Tablets 512
Bellergal-S Tablets 2250
Donnatal 2060
Donnatal Extentabs 2061
Donnatal Tablets 2060
Phenobarbital Elixir and Tablets 1469
Quadrinal Tablets 1350

Pimozide (Potentiates CNS depressant effects; increases the risk of respiratory depression). Products include:
Orap Tablets 1050

Prazepam (Potentiates CNS depressant effects).
No products indexed under this heading.

Prochlorperazine (Potentiates CNS depressant effects; increases the risk of respiratory depression). Products include:
Compazine 2470

Promethazine Hydrochloride (Potentiates CNS depressant effects; increases the risk of respiratory depression). Products include:
Mepergan Injection 2753
Phenergan with Codeine 2777
Phenergan with Dextromethorphan 2778
Phenergan Injection 2773
Phenergan Suppositories 2775
Phenergan Syrup 2774
Phenergan Tablets 2775
Phenergan VC 2779
Phenergan VC with Codeine 2781

Propofol (Potentiates CNS depressant effects). Products include:
Diprivan Injection 2833

Propoxyphene Hydrochloride (Potentiates CNS depressant effects). Products include:
Darvon 1435
Wygesic Tablets 2827

(▣ Described in PDR For Nonprescription Drugs) (◉ Described in PDR For Ophthalmology)

Propoxyphene Napsylate (Potentiates CNS depressant effects). Products include:

Darvon-N/Darvocet-N 1433

Pyrilamine Maleate (Potentiates CNS depressant effects). Products include:

4-Way Fast Acting Nasal Spray (regular & mentholated) .... ⊕ 621
Maximum Strength Multi-Symptom Formula Midol .... ⊕ 722
PMS Multi-Symptom Formula Midol .... ⊕ 723

Pyrilamine Tannate (Potentiates CNS depressant effects). Products include:

Atrohist Pediatric Suspension 454
Rynatan 2673

Quazepam (Potentiates CNS depressant effects). Products include:

Doral Tablets 2664

Risperidone (Potentiates CNS depressant effects). Products include:

Risperdal 1301

Secobarbital Sodium (Potentiates CNS depressant effects). Products include:

Seconal Sodium Pulvules 1474

Sufentanil Citrate (Potentiates CNS depressant effects). Products include:

Sufenta Injection 1309

Temazepam (Potentiates CNS depressant effects). Products include:

Restoril Capsules 2284

Terfenadine (Potentiates CNS depressant effects). Products include:

Seldane Tablets 1536
Seldane-D Extended-Release Tablets 1538

Thiamylal Sodium (Potentiates CNS depressant effects).

No products indexed under this heading.

Thioridazine Hydrochloride (Potentiates CNS depressant effects; increases the risk of respiratory depression). Products include:

Mellaril 2269

Thiothixene (Potentiates CNS depressant effects; increases the risk of respiratory depression). Products include:

Navane Capsules and Concentrate 2201
Navane Intramuscular 2202

Triazolam (Potentiates CNS depressant effects). Products include:

Halcion Tablets 2611

Trifluoperazine Hydrochloride (Potentiates CNS depressant effects; increases the risk of respiratory depression). Products include:

Stelazine 2514

Trimeprazine Tartrate (Potentiates CNS depressant effects). Products include:

Temaril Tablets, Syrup and Spansule Extended-Release Capsules.. 483

Tripelennamine Hydrochloride (Potentiates CNS depressant effects). Products include:

PBZ Tablets 845
PBZ-SR Tablets 844

Triprolidine Hydrochloride (Potentiates CNS depressant effects). Products include:

Actifed Plus Caplets .... ⊕ 845
Actifed Plus Tablets .... ⊕ 845
Actifed with Codeine Cough Syrup.. 1067
Actifed Syrup .... ⊕ 846
Actifed Tablets .... ⊕ 844

Zolpidem Tartrate (Potentiates CNS depressant effects). Products include:

Ambien Tablets 2416

Food Interactions

Alcohol (Potentiates CNS depressant effects).

INNOGEL PLUS
(Pyrethrum Extract, Piperonyl Butoxide) .... ⊕ 657
None cited in PDR database.

INOCOR LACTATE INJECTION
(Amrinone Lactate) 2309
May interact with:

Disopyramide Phosphate (Excessive hypotension; concurrent administration should be undertaken with caution). Products include:

Norpace 2444

INSTAT* COLLAGEN ABSORBABLE HEMOSTAT
(Collagen) 1312
None cited in PDR database.

INSTAT* MCH MICROFIBRILLAR COLLAGEN HEMOSTAT
(Collagen, bovine) 1313
None cited in PDR database.

INTAL CAPSULES
(Cromolyn Sodium) 987
May interact with:

Isoproterenol Hydrochloride (The addition of cromolyn sodium increases resorptions and malformations in animal studies). Products include:

Isuprel Hydrochloride Injection 1:5000 2311
Isuprel Hydrochloride Solution 1:200 & 1:100 2313
Isuprel Mistometer 2312

INTAL INHALER
(Cromolyn Sodium) 988
May interact with:

Isoproterenol Hydrochloride (The addition of cromolyn sodium increases incidence of both resorptions and malformations in animal studies). Products include:

Isuprel Hydrochloride Injection 1:5000 2311
Isuprel Hydrochloride Solution 1:200 & 1:100 2313
Isuprel Mistometer 2312

INTAL NEBULIZER SOLUTION
(Cromolyn Sodium) 989
May interact with:

Isoproterenol Hydrochloride (The addition of cromolyn sodium increases the incidence of both resorption and malformations in animal studies). Products include:

Isuprel Hydrochloride Injection 1:5000 2311
Isuprel Hydrochloride Solution 1:200 & 1:100 2313
Isuprel Mistometer 2312

INTERCEED* (TC7) ABSORBABLE ADHESION BARRIER
(Cellulose, Oxidized Regenerated)......1313
None cited in PDR database.

INTRON A
(Interferon alfa-2B, Recombinant) 2364
May interact with:

Bone Marrow Depressants, unspecified (Careful monitoring of the WBC count is indicated).

Zidovudine (Concomitant administration may result in a higher incidence of neutropenia). Products include:

Retrovir Capsules 1158
Retrovir I.V. Infusion 1163
Retrovir Syrup 1158

INVERSINE TABLETS

(Mecamylamine Hydrochloride)..........1686
May interact with sulfonamides, general anesthetics, antihypertensives, and certain other agents. Compounds in these categories include:

Acebutolol Hydrochloride (Potentiation of Inversine). Products include:

Sectral Capsules 2807

Amlodipine Besylate (Potentiation of Inversine). Products include:

Lotrel Capsules 840
Norvasc Tablets 1940

Antibiotics, unspecified (Patients receiving antibiotics generally should not be treated with ganglionic blockers).

Atenolol (Potentiation of Inversine). Products include:

Tenoretic Tablets 2845
Tenormin Tablets and I.V. Injection 2847

Benazepril Hydrochloride (Potentiation of Inversine). Products include:

Lotensin Tablets 834
Lotensin HCT 837
Lotrel Capsules 840

Bendroflumethiazide (Potentiation of Inversine; patients receiving sulfonamides generally should not be treated with ganglion blockers).

No products indexed under this heading.

Betaxolol Hydrochloride (Potentiation of Inversine). Products include:

Betoptic Ophthalmic Solution........... 469
Betoptic S Ophthalmic Suspension 471
Kerlone Tablets 2436

Bisoprolol Fumarate (Potentiation of Inversine). Products include:

Zebeta Tablets 1413
Ziac 1415

Captopril (Potentiation of Inversine). Products include:

Capoten 739
Capozide 742

Carteolol Hydrochloride (Potentiation of Inversine). Products include:

Cartrol Tablets 410
Ocupress Ophthalmic Solution, 1% Sterile .... ⊙ 309

Chlorothiazide (Potentiation of Inversine; patients receiving sulfonamides generally should not be treated with ganglion blockers). Products include:

Aldoclor Tablets 1598
Diupres Tablets 1650
Diuril Oral 1653

Chlorothiazide Sodium (Potentiation of Inversine; patients receiving sulfonamides generally should not be treated with ganglion blockers). Products include:

Diuril Sodium Intravenous 1652

Chlorpropamide (Patients receiving sulfonamides generally should not be treated with ganglionic blockers). Products include:

Diabinese Tablets 1935

Chlorthalidone (Potentiation of Inversine). Products include:

Combipres Tablets 677
Tenoretic Tablets 2845
Thalitone 1245

Clonidine (Potentiation of Inversine). Products include:

Catapres-TTS 675

Clonidine Hydrochloride (Potentiation of Inversine). Products include:

Catapres Tablets 674
Combipres Tablets 677

Deserpidine (Potentiation of Inversine).

No products indexed under this heading.

Diazoxide (Potentiation of Inversine). Products include:

Hyperstat I.V. Injection 2363
Proglycem 580

Diltiazem Hydrochloride (Potentiation of Inversine). Products include:

Cardizem CD Capsules 1506
Cardizem SR Capsules 1510
Cardizem Injectable 1508
Cardizem Tablets 1512
Dilacor XR Extended-release Capsules 2018

Doxazosin Mesylate (Potentiation of Inversine). Products include:

Cardura Tablets 2186

Enalapril Maleate (Potentiation of Inversine). Products include:

Vaseretic Tablets 1765
Vasotec Tablets 1771

Enalaprilat (Potentiation of Inversine). Products include:

Vasotec I.V. 1768

Enflurane (Potentiation of Inversine).

No products indexed under this heading.

Esmolol Hydrochloride (Potentiation of Inversine). Products include:

Brevibloc Injection 1808

Felodipine (Potentiation of Inversine). Products include:

Plendil Extended-Release Tablets.... 527

Fosinopril Sodium (Potentiation of Inversine). Products include:

Monopril Tablets 757

Furosemide (Potentiation of Inversine). Products include:

Lasix Injection, Oral Solution and Tablets 1240

Glipizide (Patients receiving sulfonamides generally should not be treated with ganglionic blockers). Products include:

Glucotrol Tablets 1967
Glucotrol XL Extended Release Tablets 1968

Glyburide (Patients receiving sulfonamides generally should not be treated with ganglionic blockers). Products include:

DiaBeta Tablets 1239
Glynase PresTab Tablets 2609
Micronase Tablets 2623

Guanabenz Acetate (Potentiation of Inversine).

No products indexed under this heading.

Guanethidine Monosulfate (Potentiation of Inversine). Products include:

Esimil Tablets 822
Ismelin Tablets 827

Hydralazine Hydrochloride (Potentiation of Inversine). Products include:

Apresazide Capsules 808
Apresoline Hydrochloride Tablets .. 809
Ser-Ap-Es Tablets 849

Hydrochlorothiazide (Potentiation of Inversine; patients receiving sulfonamides generally should not receive ganglion blockers). Products include:

Aldactazide 2413
Aldoril Tablets 1604
Apresazide Capsules 808

IMPORTANT NOTE: Always consult each drug listing in the patient's regimen for possible interactions.

Inversine Interactions Index 526

Capozide 742
Dyazide 2479
Esidrix Tablets 821
Esimil Tablets 822
HydroDIURIL Tablets 1674
Hydropres Tablets 1675
Hyzaar Tablets 1677
Inderide Tablets 2732
Inderide LA Long Acting Capsules .. 2734
Lopressor HCT Tablets 832
Lotensin HCT 837
Maxzide 1380
Moduretic Tablets 1705
Oretic Tablets 443
Prinzide Tablets 1737
Ser-Ap-Es Tablets 849
Timolide Tablets 1748
Vaseretic Tablets 1765
Zestoretic 2850
Ziac 1415

Hydroflumethiazide (Potentiation of Inversine; patients receiving sulfonamides generally should not be treated with ganglion blockers). Products include:
Diucardin Tablets 2718

Indapamide (Potentiation of Inversine). Products include:
Lozol Tablets 2022

Isoflurane (Potentiation of Inversine).
No products indexed under this heading.

Isradipine (Potentiation of Inversine). Products include:
DynaCirc Capsules 2256

Labetalol Hydrochloride (Potentiation of Inversine). Products include:
Normodyne Injection 2377
Normodyne Tablets 2379
Trandate 1185

Lisinopril (Potentiation of Inversine). Products include:
Prinivil Tablets 1733
Prinzide Tablets 1737
Zestoretic 2850
Zestril Tablets 2854

Losartan Potassium (Potentiation of Inversine). Products include:
Cozaar Tablets 1628
Hyzaar Tablets 1677

Methohexital Sodium (Potentiation of Inversine). Products include:
Brevital Sodium Vials 1429

Methoxyflurane (Potentiation of Inversine).
No products indexed under this heading.

Methyclothiazide (Potentiation of Inversine; patients receiving sulfonamides generally should not be treated with ganglion blockers). Products include:
Enduron Tablets 420

Methyldopa (Potentiation of Inversine). Products include:
Aldoclor Tablets 1598
Aldomet Oral 1600
Aldoril Tablets 1604

Methyldopate Hydrochloride (Potentiation of Inversine). Products include:
Aldomet Ester HCl Injection 1602

Metolazone (Potentiation of Inversine). Products include:
Mykrox Tablets 993
Zaroxolyn Tablets 1000

Metoprolol Succinate (Potentiation of Inversine). Products include:
Toprol-XL Tablets 565

Metoprolol Tartrate (Potentiation of Inversine). Products include:
Lopressor Ampuls 830
Lopressor HCT Tablets 832
Lopressor Tablets 830

Metyrosine (Potentiation of Inversine). Products include:
Demser Capsules 1649

Minoxidil (Potentiation of Inversine). Products include:
Loniten Tablets 2618
Rogaine Topical Solution 2637

Moexipril Hydrochloride (Potentiation of Inversine). Products include:
Univasc Tablets 2410

Nadolol (Potentiation of Inversine).
No products indexed under this heading.

Nicardipine Hydrochloride (Potentiation of Inversine). Products include:
Cardene Capsules 2095
Cardene I.V. 2709
Cardene SR Capsules 2097

Nifedipine (Potentiation of Inversine). Products include:
Adalat Capsules (10 mg and 20 mg) 587
Adalat CC 589
Procardia Capsules 1971
Procardia XL Extended Release Tablets 1972

Nisoldipine (Potentiation of Inversine).
No products indexed under this heading.

Nitroglycerin (Potentiation of Inversine). Products include:
Deponit NTG Transdermal Delivery System 2397
Nitro-Bid IV 1523
Nitro-Bid Ointment 1524
Nitrodisc 2047
Nitro-Dur (nitroglycerin) Transdermal Infusion System 1326
Nitrolingual Spray 2027
Nitrostat Tablets 1925
Transderm-Nitro Transdermal Therapeutic System 859

Penbutolol Sulfate (Potentiation of Inversine). Products include:
Levatol 2403

Phenoxybenzamine Hydrochloride (Potentiation of Inversine). Products include:
Dibenzyline Capsules 2476

Phentolamine Mesylate (Potentiation of Inversine). Products include:
Regitine 846

Pindolol (Potentiation of Inversine). Products include:
Visken Tablets 2299

Polythiazide (Potentiation of Inversine; patients receiving sulfonamides generally should not be treated with ganglion blockers). Products include:
Minizide Capsules 1938

Prazosin Hydrochloride (Potentiation of Inversine). Products include:
Minipress Capsules 1937
Minizide Capsules 1938

Propofol (Potentiation of Inversine). Products include:
Diprivan Injection 2833

Propranolol Hydrochloride (Potentiation of Inversine). Products include:
Inderal 2728
Inderal LA Long Acting Capsules 2730
Inderide Tablets 2732
Inderide LA Long Acting Capsules .. 2734

Quinapril Hydrochloride (Potentiation of Inversine). Products include:
Accupril Tablets 1893

Ramipril (Potentiation of Inversine). Products include:
Altace Capsules 1232

Rauwolfia Serpentina (Potentiation of Inversine).
No products indexed under this heading.

Rescinnamine (Potentiation of Inversine).
No products indexed under this heading.

Reserpine (Potentiation of Inversine). Products include:
Diupres Tablets 1650
Hydropres Tablets 1675
Ser-Ap-Es Tablets 849

Sodium Nitroprusside (Potentiation of Inversine).
No products indexed under this heading.

Sotalol Hydrochloride (Potentiation of Inversine). Products include:
Betapace Tablets 641

Spirapril Hydrochloride (Potentiation of Inversine).
No products indexed under this heading.

Sulfamethizole (Patients receiving sulfonamides generally should not be treated with ganglionic blockers). Products include:
Urobiotic-250 Capsules 2214

Sulfamethoxazole (Patients receiving sulfonamides generally should not be treated with ganglionic blockers). Products include:
Azo Gantanol Tablets 2080
Bactrim DS Tablets 2084
Bactrim I.V. Infusion 2082
Bactrim 2084
Gantanol Tablets 2119
Septra 1174
Septra I.V. Infusion 1169
Septra I.V. Infusion ADD-Vantage Vials 1171
Septra 1174

Sulfasalazine (Patients receiving sulfonamides generally should not be treated with ganglionic blockers). Products include:
Azulfidine 1949

Sulfinpyrazone (Patients receiving sulfonamides generally should not be treated with ganglionic blockers). Products include:
Anturane 807

Sulfisoxazole (Patients receiving sulfonamides generally should not be treated with ganglionic blockers). Products include:
Azo Gantrisin Tablets 2081
Gantrisin Tablets 2120

Sulfisoxazole Diolamine (Patients receiving sulfonamides generally should not be treated with ganglionic blockers).
No products indexed under this heading.

Terazosin Hydrochloride (Potentiation of Inversine). Products include:
Hytrin Capsules 430

Timolol Maleate (Potentiation of Inversine). Products include:
Blocadren Tablets 1614
Timolide Tablets 1748
Timoptic in Ocudose 1753
Timoptic Sterile Ophthalmic Solution 1751
Timoptic-XE 1755

Tolazamide (Patients receiving sulfonamides generally should not be treated with ganglionic blockers).
No products indexed under this heading.

Tolbutamide (Patients receiving sulfonamides generally should not be treated with ganglionic blockers).
No products indexed under this heading.

Torsemide (Potentiation of Inversine). Products include:
Demadex Tablets and Injection 686

Trimethaphan Camsylate (Potentiation of Inversine). Products include:
Arfonad Ampuls 2080

Verapamil Hydrochloride (Potentiation of Inversine). Products include:
Calan SR Caplets 2422
Calan Tablets 2419
Isoptin Injectable 1344
Isoptin Oral Tablets 1346
Isoptin SR Tablets 1348
Verelan Capsules 1410
Verelan Capsules 2824

Food Interactions

Alcohol (Potentiation of Inversine).

IONAMIN CAPSULES
(Phentermine Resin) 990
May interact with monoamine oxidase inhibitors, insulin, and certain other agents. Compounds in these categories include:

Furazolidone (Concurrent use is contraindicated). Products include:
Furoxone 2046

Guanethidine Monosulfate (Decreased hypotensive effect of guanethidine). Products include:
Esimil Tablets 822
Ismelin Tablets 827

Insulin, Human (Insulin requirement may be altered in diabetics).
No products indexed under this heading.

Insulin, Human Isophane Suspension (Insulin requirement may be altered in diabetics). Products include:
Novolin N Human Insulin 10 ml Vials 1795

Insulin, Human NPH (Insulin requirement may be altered in diabetics). Products include:
Humulin N, 100 Units 1448
Novolin N PenFill Cartridges Durable Insulin Delivery System 1798
Novolin N Prefilled Syringe Disposable Insulin Delivery System 1798

Insulin, Human Regular (Insulin requirement may be altered in diabetics). Products include:
Humulin R, 100 Units 1449
Novolin R Human Insulin 10 ml Vials 1795
Novolin R PenFill Cartridges Durable Insulin Delivery System 1798
Novolin R Prefilled Syringe Disposable Insulin Delivery System 1798
Velosulin BR Human Insulin 10 ml Vials 1795

Insulin, Human, Zinc Suspension (Insulin requirement may be altered in diabetics). Products include:
Humulin L, 100 Units 1446
Humulin U, 100 Units 1450
Novolin L Human Insulin 10 ml Vials 1795

Insulin, NPH (Insulin requirement may be altered in diabetics). Products include:
NPH, 100 Units 1450
Pork NPH, 100 Units 1452
Purified Pork NPH Isophane Insulin 1801

Insulin, Regular (Insulin requirement may be altered in diabetics). Products include:
Regular, 100 Units 1450
Pork Regular, 100 Units 1452
Pork Regular (Concentrated), 500 Units 1453
Purified Pork Regular Insulin 1801

Insulin, Zinc Crystals (Insulin requirement may be altered in diabetics). Products include:
NPH, 100 Units 1450

(▣ Described in PDR For Nonprescription Drugs) (◉ Described in PDR For Ophthalmology)

Insulin, Zinc Suspension (Insulin requirement may be altered in diabetics). Products include:

Iletin I 1450
Lente, 100 Units 1450
Iletin II... 1452
Pork Lente, 100 Units........................... 1452
Purified Pork Lente Insulin 1801

Isocarboxazid (Concurrent use is contraindicated).

No products indexed under this heading.

Phenelzine Sulfate (Concurrent use is contraindicated). Products include:

Nardil 1920

Selegiline Hydrochloride (Concurrent use is contraindicated). Products include:

Eldepryl Tablets 2550

Tranylcypromine Sulfate (Concurrent use is contraindicated). Products include:

Parnate Tablets 2503

Food Interactions

Alcohol (Possibility of adverse interactions).

IOPIDINE STERILE OPHTHALMIC SOLUTION

(Apraclonidine Hydrochloride) .... ⊛ 219

May interact with monoamine oxidase inhibitors. Compounds in this category include:

Furazolidone (Concurrent therapy is contraindicated). Products include:

Furoxone 2046

Isocarboxazid (Concurrent therapy is contraindicated).

No products indexed under this heading.

Phenelzine Sulfate (Concurrent therapy is contraindicated). Products include:

Nardil 1920

Selegiline Hydrochloride (Concurrent therapy is contraindicated). Products include:

Eldepryl Tablets 2550

Tranylcypromine Sulfate (Concurrent therapy is contraindicated). Products include:

Parnate Tablets 2503

IOPIDINE 0.5%

(Apraclonidine Hydrochloride) .... ⊛ 221

May interact with monoamine oxidase inhibitors, central nervous system depressants, barbiturates, narcotic analgesics, general anesthetics, hypnotics and sedatives, tricyclic antidepressants, antipsychotic agents, insulin, beta blockers, antihypertensives, and cardiac glycosides. Compounds in these categories include:

Acebutolol Hydrochloride (Apraclonidine reduces pulse and blood pressure, caution is advised when used concurrently). Products include:

Sectral Capsules 2807

Alfentanil Hydrochloride (Possible additive or potentiating effect with CNS depressant). Products include:

Alfenta Injection 1286

Alprazolam (Possible additive or potentiating effect with CNS depressant). Products include:

Xanax Tablets 2649

Amitriptyline Hydrochloride (Tricyclic antidepressants have been reported to blunt the hypotensive effect of clonidine; it is not known whether the concurrent use with apraclonidine can lead to reduction in IOP lowering effect). Products include:

Elavil 2838
Endep Tablets 2174
Etrafon 2355
Limbitrol 2180
Triavil Tablets 1757

Amlodipine Besylate (Apraclonidine reduces pulse and blood pressure, caution is advised when used concurrently). Products include:

Lotrel Capsules 840
Norvasc Tablets 1940

Amoxapine (Tricyclic antidepressants have been reported to blunt the hypotensive effect of clonidine; it is not known whether the concurrent use with apraclonidine can lead to reduction in IOP lowering effect). Products include:

Asendin Tablets 1369

Aprobarbital (Possible additive or potentiating effect with CNS depressant).

No products indexed under this heading.

Atenolol (Apraclonidine reduces pulse and blood pressure, caution is advised when used concurrently). Products include:

Tenoretic Tablets....................................... 2845
Tenormin Tablets and I.V. Injection 2847

Benazepril Hydrochloride (Apraclonidine reduces pulse and blood pressure, caution is advised when used concurrently). Products include:

Lotensin Tablets... 834
Lotensin HCT.. 837
Lotrel Capsules... 840

Bendroflumethiazide (Apraclonidine reduces pulse and blood pressure, caution is advised when used concurrently).

No products indexed under this heading.

Betaxolol Hydrochloride (Apraclonidine reduces pulse and blood pressure, caution is advised when used concurrently). Products include:

Betoptic Ophthalmic Solution............. 469
Betoptic S Ophthalmic Suspension 471
Kerlone Tablets.. 2436

Bisoprolol Fumarate (Apraclonidine reduces pulse and blood pressure, caution is advised when used concurrently). Products include:

Zebeta Tablets 1413
Ziac 1415

Buprenorphine (Possible additive or potentiating effect with CNS depressant). Products include:

Buprenex Injectable 2006

Buspirone Hydrochloride (Possible additive or potentiating effect with CNS depressant). Products include:

BuSpar 737

Butabarbital (Possible additive or potentiating effect with CNS depressant).

No products indexed under this heading.

Butalbital (Possible additive or potentiating effect with CNS depressant). Products include:

Esgic-plus Tablets 1013
Fioricet Tablets 2258
Fioricet with Codeine Capsules 2260
Fiorinal Capsules 2261
Fiorinal with Codeine Capsules 2262
Fiorinal Tablets... 2261
Phrenilin 785

Sedapap Tablets 50 mg/650 mg .. 1543

Captopril (Apraclonidine reduces pulse and blood pressure, caution is advised when used concurrently). Products include:

Capoten 739
Capozide 742

Carteolol Hydrochloride (Apraclonidine reduces pulse and blood pressure, caution is advised when used concurrently). Products include:

Cartrol Tablets 410
Ocupress Ophthalmic Solution, 1% Sterile.. ⊛ 309

Chlordiazepoxide (Possible additive or potentiating effect with CNS depressant). Products include:

Libritabs Tablets 2177
Limbitrol 2180

Chlordiazepoxide Hydrochloride (Possible additive or potentiating effect with CNS depressant). Products include:

Librax Capsules 2176
Librium Capsules....................................... 2178
Librium Injectable 2179

Chlorothiazide (Apraclonidine reduces pulse and blood pressure, caution is advised when used concurrently). Products include:

Aldoclor Tablets... 1598
Diupres Tablets 1650
Diuril Oral 1653

Chlorothiazide Sodium (Apraclonidine reduces pulse and blood pressure, caution is advised when used concurrently). Products include:

Diuril Sodium Intravenous 1652

Chlorpromazine (An additive hypotensive effect has been reported with the combination of systemic clonidine and neuroleptic therapy; possible additive or potentiating effect with CNS depressant). Products include:

Thorazine Suppositories........................ 2523

Chlorpromazine Hydrochloride (An additive hypotensive effect has been reported with the combination of systemic clonidine and neuroleptic therapy; possible additive or potentiating effect with CNS depressant). Products include:

Thorazine 2523

Chlorprothixene (An additive hypotensive effect has been reported with the combination of systemic clonidine and neuroleptic therapy; possible additive or potentiating effect with CNS depressant).

No products indexed under this heading.

Chlorprothixene Hydrochloride (An additive hypotensive effect has been reported with the combination of systemic clonidine and neuroleptic therapy; possible additive or potentiating effect with CNS depressant).

No products indexed under this heading.

Chlorthalidone (Apraclonidine reduces pulse and blood pressure, caution is advised when used concurrently). Products include:

Combipres Tablets 677
Tenoretic Tablets....................................... 2845
Thalitone 1245

Clomipramine Hydrochloride (Tricyclic antidepressants have been reported to blunt the hypotensive effect of clonidine; it is not known whether the concurrent use with apraclonidine can lead to reduction in IOP lowering effect). Products include:

Anafranil Capsules 803

Clonidine (Apraclonidine reduces pulse and blood pressure, caution is advised when used concurrently). Products include:

Catapres-TTS.. 675

Clonidine Hydrochloride (Apraclonidine reduces pulse and blood pressure, caution is advised when used concurrently). Products include:

Catapres Tablets 674
Combipres Tablets 677

Clorazepate Dipotassium (Possible additive or potentiating effect with CNS depressant). Products include:

Tranxene 451

Clozapine (An additive hypotensive effect has been reported with the combination of systemic clonidine and neuroleptic therapy; possible additive or potentiating effect with CNS depressant). Products include:

Clozaril Tablets... 2252

Codeine Phosphate (Possible additive or potentiating effect with CNS depressant). Products include:

Actifed with Codeine Cough Syrup.. 1067
Brontex 1981
Deconsal C Expectorant Syrup 456
Deconsal Pediatric Syrup 457
Dimetane-DC Cough Syrup 2059
Empirin with Codeine Tablets............ 1093
Fioricet with Codeine Capsules 2260
Fiorinal with Codeine Capsules 2262
Isoclor Expectorant.................................. 990
Novahistine DH.. 2462
Novahistine Expectorant........................ 2463
Nucofed 2051
Phenergan with Codeine....................... 2777
Phenergan VC with Codeine 2781
Robitussin A-C Syrup............................... 2073
Robitussin-DAC Syrup 2074
Ryna .... ⊕D 841
Soma Compound w/Codeine Tablets 2676
Tussi-Organidin NR Liquid and S NR Liquid 2677
Tylenol with Codeine 1583

Deserpidine (Apraclonidine reduces pulse and blood pressure, caution is advised when used concurrently).

No products indexed under this heading.

Desflurane (Possible additive or potentiating effect with CNS depressant). Products include:

Suprane 1813

Desipramine Hydrochloride (Tricyclic antidepressants have been reported to blunt the hypotensive effect of clonidine; it is not known whether the concurrent use with apraclonidine can lead to reduction in IOP lowering effect). Products include:

Norpramin Tablets 1526

Deslanoside (Apraclonidine reduces pulse and blood pressure, caution is advised when used concurrently).

No products indexed under this heading.

Dezocine (Possible additive or potentiating effect with CNS depressant). Products include:

Dalgan Injection 538

Diazepam (Possible additive or potentiating effect with CNS depressant). Products include:

Dizac 1809
Valium Injectable 2182
Valium Tablets 2183
Valrelease Capsules 2169

Diazoxide (Apraclonidine reduces pulse and blood pressure, caution is advised when used concurrently). Products include:

Hyperstat I.V. Injection 2363
Proglycem... 580

IMPORTANT NOTE: Always consult each drug listing in the patient's regimen for possible interactions.

Digitoxin (Apraclonidine reduces pulse and blood pressure, caution is advised when used concurrently). Products include:
- Crystodigin Tablets ... 1433

Digoxin (Apraclonidine reduces pulse and blood pressure, caution is advised when used concurrently). Products include:
- Lanoxicaps ... 1117
- Lanoxin Elixir Pediatric ... 1120
- Lanoxin Injection ... 1123
- Lanoxin Injection Pediatric ... 1126
- Lanoxin Tablets ... 1128

Diltiazem Hydrochloride (Apraclonidine reduces pulse and blood pressure, caution is advised when used concurrently). Products include:
- Cardizem CD Capsules ... 1506
- Cardizem SR Capsules ... 1510
- Cardizem Injectable ... 1508
- Cardizem Tablets ... 1512
- Dilacor XR Extended-release Capsules ... 2018

Doxazosin Mesylate (Apraclonidine reduces pulse and blood pressure, caution is advised when used concurrently). Products include:
- Cardura Tablets ... 2186

Doxepin Hydrochloride (Tricyclic antidepressants have been reported to blunt the hypotensive effect of clonidine; it is not known whether the concurrent use with apraclonidine can lead to reduction in IOP lowering effect). Products include:
- Sinequan ... 2205
- Zonalon Cream ... 1055

Droperidol (Possible additive or potentiating effect with CNS depressant). Products include:
- Inapsine Injection ... 1296

Enalapril Maleate (Apraclonidine reduces pulse and blood pressure, caution is advised when used concurrently). Products include:
- Vaseretic Tablets ... 1765
- Vasotec Tablets ... 1771

Enalaprilat (Apraclonidine reduces pulse and blood pressure, caution is advised when used concurrently). Products include:
- Vasotec I.V. ... 1768

Enflurane (Possible additive or potentiating effect with CNS depressant).
- No products indexed under this heading.

Esmolol Hydrochloride (Apraclonidine reduces pulse and blood pressure, caution is advised when used concurrently). Products include:
- Brevibloc Injection ... 1808

Estazolam (Possible additive or potentiating effect with CNS depressant). Products include:
- ProSom Tablets ... 449

Ethchlorvynol (Possible additive or potentiating effect with CNS depressant). Products include:
- Placidyl Capsules ... 448

Ethinamate (Possible additive or potentiating effect with CNS depressant).
- No products indexed under this heading.

Felodipine (Apraclonidine reduces pulse and blood pressure, caution is advised when used concurrently). Products include:
- Plendil Extended-Release Tablets ... 527

Fentanyl (Possible additive or potentiating effect with CNS depressant). Products include:
- Duragesic Transdermal System ... 1288

Fentanyl Citrate (Possible additive or potentiating effect with CNS depressant). Products include:
- Sublimaze Injection ... 1307

Fluphenazine Decanoate (An additive hypotensive effect has been reported with the combination of systemic clonidine and neuroleptic therapy; possible additive or potentiating effect with CNS depressant). Products include:
- Prolixin Decanoate ... 509

Fluphenazine Enanthate (An additive hypotensive effect has been reported with the combination of systemic clonidine and neuroleptic therapy; possible additive or potentiating effect with CNS depressant). Products include:
- Prolixin Enanthate ... 509

Fluphenazine Hydrochloride (An additive hypotensive effect has been reported with the combination of systemic clonidine and neuroleptic therapy; possible additive or potentiating effect with CNS depressant). Products include:
- Prolixin ... 509

Flurazepam Hydrochloride (Possible additive or potentiating effect with CNS depressant). Products include:
- Dalmane Capsules ... 2173

Fosinopril Sodium (Apraclonidine reduces pulse and blood pressure, caution is advised when used concurrently). Products include:
- Monopril Tablets ... 757

Furazolidone (Concurrent use is contraindicated). Products include:
- Furoxone ... 2046

Furosemide (Apraclonidine reduces pulse and blood pressure, caution is advised when used concurrently). Products include:
- Lasix Injection, Oral Solution and Tablets ... 1240

Glutethimide (Possible additive or potentiating effect with CNS depressant).
- No products indexed under this heading.

Guanabenz Acetate (Apraclonidine reduces pulse and blood pressure, caution is advised when used concurrently).
- No products indexed under this heading.

Guanethidine Monosulfate (Apraclonidine reduces pulse and blood pressure, caution is advised when used concurrently). Products include:
- Esimil Tablets ... 822
- Ismelin Tablets ... 827

Haloperidol (An additive hypotensive effect has been reported with the combination of systemic clonidine and neuroleptic therapy; possible additive or potentiating effect with CNS depressant). Products include:
- Haldol Injection, Tablets and Concentrate ... 1575

Haloperidol Decanoate (An additive hypotensive effect has been reported with the combination of systemic clonidine and neuroleptic therapy; possible additive or potentiating effect with CNS depressant). Products include:
- Haldol Decanoate ... 1577

Hydralazine Hydrochloride (Apraclonidine reduces pulse and blood pressure, caution is advised when used concurrently). Products include:
- Apresazide Capsules ... 808
- Apresoline Hydrochloride Tablets ... 809
- Ser-Ap-Es Tablets ... 849

Hydrochlorothiazide (Apraclonidine reduces pulse and blood pressure, caution is advised when used concurrently). Products include:
- Aldactazide ... 2413
- Aldoril Tablets ... 1604
- Apresazide Capsules ... 808
- Capozide ... 742
- Dyazide ... 2479
- Esidrix Tablets ... 821
- Esimil Tablets ... 822
- HydroDIURIL Tablets ... 1674
- Hydropres Tablets ... 1675
- Hyzaar Tablets ... 1677
- Inderide Tablets ... 2732
- Inderide LA Long Acting Capsules ... 2734
- Lopressor HCT Tablets ... 832
- Lotensin HCT ... 837
- Maxzide ... 1380
- Moduretic Tablets ... 1705
- Oretic Tablets ... 443
- Prinzide Tablets ... 1737
- Ser-Ap-Es Tablets ... 849
- Timolide Tablets ... 1748
- Vaseretic Tablets ... 1765
- Zestoretic ... 2850
- Ziac ... 1415

Hydrocodone Bitartrate (Possible additive or potentiating effect with CNS depressant). Products include:
- Anexsia 5/500 Elixir ... 1781
- Anexia Tablets ... 1782
- Codiclear DH Syrup ... 791
- Deconamine CX Cough and Cold Liquid and Tablets ... 1319
- Duratuss HD Elixir ... 2565
- Hycodan Tablets and Syrup ... 930
- Hycomine Compound Tablets ... 932
- Hycomine ... 931
- Hycotuss Expectorant Syrup ... 933
- Hydrocet Capsules ... 782
- Lorcet 10/650 ... 1018
- Lortab ... 2566
- Tussend ... 1783
- Tussend Expectorant ... 1785
- Vicodin Tablets ... 1356
- Vicodin ES Tablets ... 1357
- Vicodin Tuss Expectorant ... 1358
- Zydone Capsules ... 949

Hydrocodone Polistirex (Possible additive or potentiating effect with CNS depressant). Products include:
- Tussionex Pennkinetic Extended-Release Suspension ... 998

Hydroflumethiazide (Apraclonidine reduces pulse and blood pressure, caution is advised when used concurrently). Products include:
- Diucardin Tablets ... 2718

Hydroxyzine Hydrochloride (Possible additive or potentiating effect with CNS depressant). Products include:
- Atarax Tablets & Syrup ... 2185
- Marax Tablets & DF Syrup ... 2200
- Vistaril Intramuscular Solution ... 2216

Imipramine Hydrochloride (Tricyclic antidepressants have been reported to blunt the hypotensive effect of clonidine; it is not known whether the concurrent use with apraclonidine can lead to reduction in IOP lowering effect). Products include:
- Tofranil Ampuls ... 854
- Tofranil Tablets ... 856

Imipramine Pamoate (Tricyclic antidepressants have been reported to blunt the hypotensive effect of clonidine; it is not known whether the concurrent use with apraclonidine can lead to reduction in IOP lowering effect). Products include:
- Tofranil-PM Capsules ... 857

Indapamide (Apraclonidine reduces pulse and blood pressure, caution is advised when used concurrently). Products include:
- Lozol Tablets ... 2022

Insulin, Human (Systemic clonidine may inhibit the production of catecholamines in response to insulin-induced hypoglycemia and mask the signs and symptoms of hypoglycemia).
- No products indexed under this heading.

Insulin, Human Isophane Suspension (Systemic clonidine may inhibit the production of catecholamines in response to insulin-induced hypoglycemia and mask the signs and symptoms of hypoglycemia). Products include:
- Novolin N Human Insulin 10 ml Vials ... 1795

Insulin, Human NPH (Systemic clonidine may inhibit the production of catecholamines in response to insulin-induced hypoglycemia and mask the signs and symptoms of hypoglycemia). Products include:
- Humulin N, 100 Units ... 1448
- Novolin N PenFill Cartridges Durable Insulin Delivery System ... 1798
- Novolin N Prefilled Syringe Disposable Insulin Delivery System ... 1798

Insulin, Human Regular (Systemic clonidine may inhibit the production of catecholamines in response to insulin-induced hypoglycemia and mask the signs and symptoms of hypoglycemia). Products include:
- Humulin R, 100 Units ... 1449
- Novolin R Human Insulin 10 ml Vials ... 1795
- Novolin R PenFill Cartridges Durable Insulin Delivery System ... 1798
- Novolin R Prefilled Syringe Disposable Insulin Delivery System ... 1798
- Velosulin BR Human Insulin 10 ml Vials ... 1795

Insulin, Human, Zinc Suspension (Systemic clonidine may inhibit the production of catecholamines in response to insulin-induced hypoglycemia and mask the signs and symptoms of hypoglycemia). Products include:
- Humulin L, 100 Units ... 1446
- Humulin U, 100 Units ... 1450
- Novolin L Human Insulin 10 ml Vials ... 1795

Insulin, NPH (Systemic clonidine may inhibit the production of catecholamines in response to insulin-induced hypoglycemia and mask the signs and symptoms of hypoglycemia). Products include:
- NPH, 100 Units ... 1450
- Pork NPH, 100 Units ... 1452
- Purified Pork NPH Isophane Insulin ... 1801

Insulin, Regular (Systemic clonidine may inhibit the production of catecholamines in response to insulin-induced hypoglycemia and mask the signs and symptoms of hypoglycemia). Products include:
- Regular, 100 Units ... 1450
- Pork Regular, 100 Units ... 1452
- Pork Regular (Concentrated), 500 Units ... 1453
- Purified Pork Regular Insulin ... 1801

Insulin, Zinc Crystals (Systemic clonidine may inhibit the production of catecholamines in response to insulin-induced hypoglycemia and mask the signs and symptoms of hypoglycemia). Products include:
- NPH, 100 Units ... 1450

Insulin, Zinc Suspension (Systemic clonidine may inhibit the production of catecholamines in response to insulin-induced hypoglycemia and mask the signs and symptoms of hypoglycemia). Products include:
- Iletin I ... 1450

529 **Interactions Index** **Iopidine**

Lente, 100 Units ... 1450
Iletin II ... 1452
Pork Lente, 100 Units ... 1452
Purified Pork Lente Insulin ... 1801

Isocarboxazid (Concurrent use is contraindicated).
No products indexed under this heading.

Isoflurane (Possible additive or potentiating effect with CNS depressant).
No products indexed under this heading.

Isradipine (Apraclonidine reduces pulse and blood pressure, caution is advised when used concurrently). Products include:
DynaCirc Capsules ... 2256

Ketamine Hydrochloride (Possible additive or potentiating effect with CNS depressant).
No products indexed under this heading.

Labetalol Hydrochloride (Apraclonidine reduces pulse and blood pressure, caution is advised when used concurrently). Products include:
Normodyne Injection ... 2377
Normodyne Tablets ... 2379
Trandate ... 1185

Levobunolol Hydrochloride (Apraclonidine reduces pulse and blood pressure, caution is advised when used concurrently). Products include:
Betagan ... ⊙ 233

Levomethadyl Acetate Hydrochloride (Possible additive or potentiating effect with CNS depressant). Products include:
Orlamm ... 2239

Levorphanol Tartrate (Possible additive or potentiating effect with CNS depressant). Products include:
Levo-Dromoran ... 2129

Lisinopril (Apraclonidine reduces pulse and blood pressure, caution is advised when used concurrently). Products include:
Prinivil Tablets ... 1733
Prinzide Tablets ... 1737
Zestoretic ... 2850
Zestril Tablets ... 2854

Lithium Carbonate (An additive hypotensive effect has been reported with the combination of systemic clonidine and neuroleptic therapy). Products include:
Eskalith ... 2485
Lithium Carbonate Capsules & Tablets ... 2230
Lithonate/Lithotabs/Lithobid ... 2543

Lithium Citrate (An additive hypotensive effect has been reported with the combination of systemic clonidine and neuroleptic therapy).
No products indexed under this heading.

Lorazepam (Possible additive or potentiating effect with CNS depressant). Products include:
Ativan Injection ... 2698
Ativan Tablets ... 2700

Losartan Potassium (Apraclonidine reduces pulse and blood pressure, caution is advised when used concurrently). Products include:
Cozaar Tablets ... 1628
Hyzaar Tablets ... 1677

Loxapine Hydrochloride (An additive hypotensive effect has been reported with the combination of systemic clonidine and neuroleptic therapy; possible additive or potentiating effect with CNS depressant). Products include:
Loxitane ... 1378

Loxapine Succinate (An additive hypotensive effect has been reported with the combination of systemic clonidine and neuroleptic therapy; possible additive or potentiating effect with CNS depressant). Products include:
Loxitane Capsules ... 1378

Maprotiline Hydrochloride (Tricyclic antidepressants have been reported to blunt the hypotensive effect of clonidine; it is not known whether the concurrent use with apraclonidine can lead to reduction in IOP lowering effect). Products include:
Ludiomil Tablets ... 843

Mecamylamine Hydrochloride (Apraclonidine reduces pulse and blood pressure, caution is advised when used concurrently). Products include:
Inversine Tablets ... 1686

Meperidine Hydrochloride (Possible additive or potentiating effect with CNS depressant). Products include:
Demerol ... 2308
Mepergan Injection ... 2753

Mephobarbital (Possible additive or potentiating effect with CNS depressant). Products include:
Mebaral Tablets ... 2322

Meprobamate (Possible additive or potentiating effect with CNS depressant). Products include:
Miltown Tablets ... 2672
PMB 200 and PMB 400 ... 2783

Mesoridazine (Possible additive or potentiating effect with CNS depressant).

Mesoridazine Besylate (An additive hypotensive effect has been reported with the combination of systemic clonidine and neuroleptic therapy). Products include:
Serentil ... 684

Methadone Hydrochloride (Possible additive or potentiating effect with CNS depressant). Products include:
Methadone Hydrochloride Oral Concentrate ... 2233
Methadone Hydrochloride Oral Solution & Tablets ... 2235

Methohexital Sodium (Possible additive or potentiating effect with CNS depressant). Products include:
Brevital Sodium Vials ... 1429

Methotrimeprazine (An additive hypotensive effect has been reported with the combination of systemic clonidine and neuroleptic therapy; possible additive or potentiating effect with CNS depressant). Products include:
Levoprome ... 1274

Methoxyflurane (Possible additive or potentiating effect with CNS depressant).
No products indexed under this heading.

Methyclothiazide (Apraclonidine reduces pulse and blood pressure, caution is advised when used concurrently). Products include:
Enduron Tablets ... 420

Methyldopa (Apraclonidine reduces pulse and blood pressure, caution is advised when used concurrently). Products include:
Aldoclor Tablets ... 1598
Aldomet Oral ... 1600
Aldoril Tablets ... 1604

Methyldopate Hydrochloride (Apraclonidine reduces pulse and blood pressure, caution is advised when used concurrently). Products include:
Aldomet Ester HCl Injection ... 1602

Metipranolol Hydrochloride (Apraclonidine reduces pulse and blood pressure, caution is advised when used concurrently). Products include:
OptiPranolol (Metipranolol 0.3%) Sterile Ophthalmic Solution ... ⊙ 258

Metolazone (Apraclonidine reduces pulse and blood pressure, caution is advised when used concurrently). Products include:
Mykrox Tablets ... 993
Zaroxolyn Tablets ... 1000

Metoprolol Succinate (Apraclonidine reduces pulse and blood pressure, caution is advised when used concurrently). Products include:
Toprol-XL Tablets ... 565

Metoprolol Tartrate (Apraclonidine reduces pulse and blood pressure, caution is advised when used concurrently). Products include:
Lopressor Ampuls ... 830
Lopressor HCT Tablets ... 832
Lopressor Tablets ... 830

Metyrosine (Apraclonidine reduces pulse and blood pressure, caution is advised when used concurrently). Products include:
Demser Capsules ... 1649

Midazolam Hydrochloride (Possible additive or potentiating effect with CNS depressant). Products include:
Versed Injection ... 2170

Minoxidil (Apraclonidine reduces pulse and blood pressure, caution is advised when used concurrently). Products include:
Loniten Tablets ... 2618
Rogaine Topical Solution ... 2637

Moexipril Hydrochloride (Apraclonidine reduces pulse and blood pressure, caution is advised when used concurrently). Products include:
Univasc Tablets ... 2410

Molindone Hydrochloride (An additive hypotensive effect has been reported with the combination of systemic clonidine and neuroleptic therapy; possible additive or potentiating effect with CNS depressant). Products include:
Moban Tablets and Concentrate ... 1048

Morphine Sulfate (Possible additive or potentiating effect with CNS depressant). Products include:
Astramorph/PF Injection, USP (Preservative-Free) ... 535
Duramorph ... 962
Infumorph 200 and Infumorph 500 Sterile Solutions ... 965
MS Contin Tablets ... 1994
MSIR ... 1997
Oramorph SR (Morphine Sulfate Sustained Release Tablets) ... 2236
RMS Suppositories ... 2657
Roxanol ... 2243

Nadolol (Apraclonidine reduces pulse and blood pressure, caution is advised when used concurrently).
No products indexed under this heading.

Nicardipine Hydrochloride (Apraclonidine reduces pulse and blood pressure, caution is advised when used concurrently). Products include:
Cardene Capsules ... 2095
Cardene I.V. ... 2709
Cardene SR Capsules ... 2097

Nifedipine (Apraclonidine reduces pulse and blood pressure, caution is advised when used concurrently). Products include:
Adalat Capsules (10 mg and 20 mg) ... 587
Adalat CC ... 589
Procardia Capsules ... 1971
Procardia XL Extended Release Tablets ... 1972

Nisoldipine (Apraclonidine reduces pulse and blood pressure, caution is advised when used concurrently).
No products indexed under this heading.

Nitroglycerin (Apraclonidine reduces pulse and blood pressure, caution is advised when used concurrently). Products include:
Deponit NTG Transdermal Delivery System ... 2397
Nitro-Bid IV ... 1523
Nitro-Bid Ointment ... 1524
Nitrodisc ... 2047
Nitro-Dur (nitroglycerin) Transdermal Infusion System ... 1326
Nitrolingual Spray ... 2027
Nitrostat Tablets ... 1925
Transderm-Nitro Transdermal Therapeutic System ... 859

Nortriptyline Hydrochloride (Tricyclic antidepressants have been reported to blunt the hypotensive effect of clonidine; it is not known whether the concurrent use with apraclonidine can lead to reduction in IOP lowering effect). Products include:
Pamelor ... 2280

Opium Alkaloids (Possible additive or potentiating effect with CNS depressant).
No products indexed under this heading.

Oxazepam (Possible additive or potentiating effect with CNS depressant). Products include:
Serax Capsules ... 2810
Serax Tablets ... 2810

Oxycodone Hydrochloride (Possible additive or potentiating effect with CNS depressant). Products include:
Percocet Tablets ... 938
Percodan Tablets ... 939
Percodan-Demi Tablets ... 940
Roxicodone Tablets, Oral Solution & Intensol (Oxycodone) ... 2244
Tylox Capsules ... 1584

Penbutolol Sulfate (Apraclonidine reduces pulse and blood pressure, caution is advised when used concurrently). Products include:
Levatol ... 2403

Pentobarbital Sodium (Possible additive or potentiating effect with CNS depressant). Products include:
Nembutal Sodium Capsules ... 436
Nembutal Sodium Solution ... 438
Nembutal Sodium Suppositories ... 440

Perphenazine (An additive hypotensive effect has been reported with the combination of systemic clonidine and neuroleptic therapy; possible additive or potentiating effect with CNS depressant). Products include:
Etrafon ... 2355
Triavil Tablets ... 1757
Trilafon ... 2389

Phenelzine Sulfate (Concurrent use is contraindicated). Products include:
Nardil ... 1920

Phenobarbital (Possible additive or potentiating effect with CNS depressant). Products include:
Arco-Lase Plus Tablets ... 512
Bellergal-S Tablets ... 2250
Donnatal ... 2060

IMPORTANT NOTE: Always consult each drug listing in the patient's regimen for possible interactions.

Donnatal Extentabs ... 2061
Donnatal Tablets ... 2060
Phenobarbital Elixir and Tablets ... 1469
Quadrinal Tablets ... 1350

Phenoxybenzamine Hydrochloride (Apraclonidine reduces pulse and blood pressure, caution is advised when used concurrently). Products include:
Dibenzyline Capsules ... 2476

Phentolamine Mesylate (Apraclonidine reduces pulse and blood pressure, caution is advised when used concurrently). Products include:
Regitine ... 846

Pimozide (An additive hypotensive effect has been reported with the combination of systemic clonidine and neuroleptic therapy). Products include:
Orap Tablets ... 1050

Pindolol (Apraclonidine reduces pulse and blood pressure, caution is advised when used concurrently). Products include:
Visken Tablets ... 2299

Polythiazide (Apraclonidine reduces pulse and blood pressure, caution is advised when used concurrently). Products include:
Minizide Capsules ... 1938

Prazepam (Possible additive or potentiating effect with CNS depressant).
No products indexed under this heading.

Prazosin Hydrochloride (Apraclonidine reduces pulse and blood pressure, caution is advised when used concurrently). Products include:
Minipress Capsules ... 1937
Minizide Capsules ... 1938

Prochlorperazine (An additive hypotensive effect has been reported with the combination of systemic clonidine and neuroleptic therapy; possible additive or potentiating effect with CNS depressant). Products include:
Compazine ... 2470

Promethazine Hydrochloride (An additive hypotensive effect has been reported with the combination of systemic clonidine and neuroleptic therapy; possible additive or potentiating effect with CNS depressant). Products include:
Mepergan Injection ... 2753
Phenergan with Codeine ... 2777
Phenergan with Dextromethorphan 2778
Phenergan Injection ... 2773
Phenergan Suppositories ... 2775
Phenergan Syrup ... 2774
Phenergan Tablets ... 2775
Phenergan VC ... 2779
Phenergan VC with Codeine ... 2781

Propofol (Possible additive or potentiating effect with CNS depressant). Products include:
Diprivan Injection ... 2833

Propoxyphene Hydrochloride (Possible additive or potentiating effect with CNS depressant). Products include:
Darvon ... 1435
Wygesic Tablets ... 2827

Propoxyphene Napsylate (Possible additive or potentiating effect with CNS depressant). Products include:
Darvon-N/Darvocet-N ... 1433

Propranolol Hydrochloride (Apraclonidine reduces pulse and blood pressure, caution is advised when used concurrently). Products include:
Inderal ... 2728
Inderal LA Long Acting Capsules ... 2730
Inderide Tablets ... 2732
Inderide LA Long Acting Capsules .. 2734

Protriptyline Hydrochloride (Tricyclic antidepressants have been reported to blunt the hypotensive effect of clonidine; it is not known whether the concurrent use with apraclonidine can lead to reduction in IOP lowering effect). Products include:
Vivactil Tablets ... 1774

Quazepam (Possible additive or potentiating effect with CNS depressant). Products include:
Doral Tablets ... 2664

Quinapril Hydrochloride (Apraclonidine reduces pulse and blood pressure, caution is advised when used concurrently). Products include.
Accupril Tablets ... 1893

Ramipril (Apraclonidine reduces pulse and blood pressure, caution is advised when used concurrently). Products include:
Altace Capsules ... 1232

Rauwolfia Serpentina (Apraclonidine reduces pulse and blood pressure, caution is advised when used concurrently).
No products indexed under this heading.

Rescinnamine (Apraclonidine reduces pulse and blood pressure, caution is advised when used concurrently).
No products indexed under this heading.

Reserpine (Apraclonidine reduces pulse and blood pressure, caution is advised when used concurrently). Products include:
Diupres Tablets ... 1650
Hydropres Tablets ... 1675
Ser-Ap-Es Tablets ... 849

Risperidone (An additive hypotensive effect has been reported with the combination of systemic clonidine and neuroleptic therapy; possible additive or potentiating effect with CNS depressant). Products include:
Risperdal ... 1301

Secobarbital Sodium (Possible additive or potentiating effect with CNS depressant). Products include:
Seconal Sodium Pulvules ... 1474

Selegiline Hydrochloride (Concurrent use is contraindicated). Products include:
Eldepryl Tablets ... 2550

Sodium Nitroprusside (Apraclonidine reduces pulse and blood pressure, caution is advised when used concurrently).
No products indexed under this heading.

Sotalol Hydrochloride (Apraclonidine reduces pulse and blood pressure, caution is advised when used concurrently). Products include:
Betapace Tablets ... 641

Spirapril Hydrochloride (Apraclonidine reduces pulse and blood pressure, caution is advised when used concurrently).
No products indexed under this heading.

Sufentanil Citrate (Possible additive or potentiating effect with CNS depressant). Products include:
Sufenta Injection ... 1309

Temazepam (Possible additive or potentiating effect with CNS depressant). Products include:
Restoril Capsules ... 2284

Terazosin Hydrochloride (Apraclonidine reduces pulse and blood pressure, caution is advised when used concurrently). Products include:
Hytrin Capsules ... 430

Thiamylal Sodium (Possible additive or potentiating effect with CNS depressant).
No products indexed under this heading.

Thioridazine Hydrochloride (An additive hypotensive effect has been reported with the combination of systemic clonidine and neuroleptic therapy; possible additive or potentiating effect with CNS depressant). Products include:
Mellaril ... 2269

Thiothixene (An additive hypotensive effect has been reported with the combination of systemic clonidine and neuroleptic therapy; possible additive or potentiating effect with CNS depressant). Products include:
Navane Capsules and Concentrate 2201
Navane Intramuscular 2202

Timolol Hemihydrate (Apraclonidine reduces pulse and blood pressure, caution is advised when used concurrently). Products include:
Betimol 0.25%, 0.5% ... ⊙ 261

Timolol Maleate (Apraclonidine reduces pulse and blood pressure, caution is advised when used concurrently). Products include:
Blocadren Tablets ... 1614
Timolide Tablets ... 1748
Timoptic in Ocudose ... 1753
Timoptic Sterile Ophthalmic Solution ... 1751
Timoptic-XE ... 1755

Torsemide (Apraclonidine reduces pulse and blood pressure, caution is advised when used concurrently). Products include:
Demadex Tablets and Injection ... 686

Tranylcypromine Sulfate (Concurrent use is contraindicated). Products include:
Parnate Tablets ... 2503

Triazolam (Possible additive or potentiating effect with CNS depressant). Products include:
Halcion Tablets ... 2611

Trifluoperazine Hydrochloride (An additive hypotensive effect has been reported with the combination of systemic clonidine and neuroleptic therapy; possible additive or potentiating effect with CNS depressant). Products include:
Stelazine ... 2514

Trimethaphan Camsylate (Apraclonidine reduces pulse and blood pressure, caution is advised when used concurrently). Products include:
Arfonad Ampuls ... 2080

Trimipramine Maleate (Tricyclic antidepressants have been reported to blunt the hypotensive effect of clonidine; it is not known whether the concurrent use with apraclonidine can lead to reduction in IOP lowering effect). Products include:
Surmontil Capsules ... 2811

Verapamil Hydrochloride (Apraclonidine reduces pulse and blood pressure, caution is advised when used concurrently). Products include:
Calan SR Caplets ... 2422
Calan Tablets ... 2419
Isoptin Injectable ... 1344
Isoptin Oral Tablets ... 1346
Isoptin SR Tablets ... 1348
Verelan Capsules ... 1410
Verelan Capsules ... 2824

Zolpidem Tartrate (Possible additive or potentiating effect with CNS depressant). Products include:
Ambien Tablets ... 2416

IPOL POLIOVIRUS VACCINE INACTIVATED

(Poliovirus Vaccine Inactivated, Trivalent Types 1,2,3) ... 885
None cited in PDR database.

IROSPAN CAPSULES

(Ferrous Sulfate, Vitamin C) ... 982
None cited in PDR database.

IROSPAN TABLETS

(Ferrous Sulfate, Vitamin C) ... 982
None cited in PDR database.

ISMELIN TABLETS

(Guanethidine Monosulfate) ... 827
May interact with monoamine oxidase inhibitors, tricyclic antidepressants, phenothiazines, estrogens, thiazides, oral contraceptives, cardiac glycosides, and certain other agents. Compounds in these categories include:

Amitriptyline Hydrochloride (Reduces hypotensive effect). Products include:
Elavil ... 2838
Endep Tablets ... 2174
Etrafon ... 2355
Limbitrol ... 2180
Triavil Tablets ... 1757

Amoxapine (Reduces hypotensive effect). Products include:
Asendin Tablets ... 1369

Bendroflumethiazide (Enhances antihypertensive action of Ismelin).
No products indexed under this heading.

Chlorothiazide (Enhances antihypertensive action of Ismelin). Products include:
Aldoclor Tablets ... 1598
Diupres Tablets ... 1650
Diuril Oral ... 1653

Chlorothiazide Sodium (Enhances antihypertensive action of Ismelin). Products include:
Diuril Sodium Intravenous ... 1652

Chlorotrianisene (Reduces hypotensive effect).
No products indexed under this heading.

Chlorpromazine (Reduces hypotensive effect). Products include:
Thorazine Suppositories ... 2523

Clomipramine Hydrochloride (Reduces hypotensive effect). Products include:
Anafranil Capsules ... 803

Deserpidine (May result in excessive postural hypotension, bradycardia, and mental depression).
No products indexed under this heading.

Desipramine Hydrochloride (Reduces hypotensive effect). Products include:
Norpramin Tablets ... 1526

Deslanoside (Slow heart rate).
No products indexed under this heading.

Desogestrel (Reduces hypotensive effect). Products include:
Desogen Tablets ... 1817
Ortho-Cept ... 1851

Dienestrol (Reduces hypotensive effect). Products include:
Ortho Dienestrol Cream ... 1866

Diethylstilbestrol (Reduces hypotensive effect). Products include:
Diethylstilbestrol Tablets ... 1437

(▣ Described in PDR For Nonprescription Drugs) (⊙ Described in PDR For Ophthalmology)

Interactions Index

Digitoxin (Slow heart rate). Products include:

Crystodigin Tablets 1433

Digoxin (Slow heart rate). Products include:

Lanoxicaps 1117
Lanoxin Elixir Pediatric 1120
Lanoxin Injection 1123
Lanoxin Injection Pediatric..................... 1126
Lanoxin Tablets 1128

Doxepin Hydrochloride (Reduces hypotensive effect). Products include:

Sinequan 2205
Zonalon Cream 1055

Ephedrine Hydrochloride (Reduces hypotensive effect). Products include:

Primatene Dual Action Formula....◆ 872
Primatene Tablets ....◆ 873
Quadrinal Tablets 1350

Ephedrine Sulfate (Reduces hypotensive effect). Products include:

Bronkaid Caplets ....◆ 717
Marax Tablets & DF Syrup.................... 2200

Ephedrine Tannate (Reduces hypotensive effect). Products include:

Rynatuss 2673

Estradiol (Reduces hypotensive effect). Products include:

Climara Transdermal System 645
Estrace Cream and Tablets 749
Estraderm Transdermal System 824

Estrogens, Conjugated (Reduces hypotensive effect). Products include:

PMB 200 and PMB 400 2783
Premarin Intravenous 2787
Premarin with Methyltestosterone.. 2794
Premarin Tablets 2789
Premarin Vaginal Cream........................ 2791
Premphase 2797
Prempro... 2801

Estrogens, Esterified (Reduces hypotensive effect). Products include:

ESTRATAB Tablets (0.3, 0.625, 1.25, 2.5 mg) 2536
Estratest 2539
Menest Tablets 2494

Estropipate (Reduces hypotensive effect). Products include:

Ogen Tablets 2627
Ogen Vaginal Cream............................... 2630
Ortho-Est... 1869

Ethinyl Estradiol (Reduces hypotensive effect). Products include:

Brevicon... 2088
Demulen 2428
Desogen Tablets....................................... 1817
Levlen/Tri-Levlen.................................... 651
Lo/Ovral Tablets 2746
Lo/Ovral-28 Tablets................................. 2751
Modicon.. 1872
Nordette-21 Tablets................................. 2755
Nordette-28 Tablets................................. 2758
Norinyl 2088
Ortho-Cept 1851
Ortho-Cyclen/Ortho-Tri-Cyclen 1858
Ortho-Novum.. 1872
Ortho-Cyclen/Ortho Tri-Cyclen 1858
Ovcon 760
Ovral Tablets... 2770
Ovral-28 Tablets 2770
Levlen/Tri-Levlen.................................... 651
Tri-Norinyl... 2164
Triphasil-21 Tablets 2814
Triphasil-28 Tablets 2819

Ethynodiol Diacetate (Reduces hypotensive effect). Products include:

Demulen 2428

Fluphenazine Decanoate (Reduces hypotensive effect). Products include:

Prolixin Decanoate 509

Fluphenazine Enanthate (Reduces hypotensive effect). Products include:

Prolixin Enanthate 509

Fluphenazine Hydrochloride (Reduces hypotensive effect). Products include:

Prolixin 509

Furazolidone (Concurrent use contraindicated). Products include:

Furoxone 2046

Hydrochlorothiazide (Enhances antihypertensive action of Ismelin). Products include:

Aldactazide.. 2413
Aldoril Tablets.. 1604
Apresazide Capsules 808
Capozide 742
Dyazide 2479
Esidrix Tablets 821
Esimil Tablets 822
HydroDIURIL Tablets 1674
Hydropres Tablets.................................... 1675
Hyzaar Tablets 1677
Inderide Tablets 2732
Inderide LA Long Acting Capsules .. 2734
Lopressor HCT Tablets 832
Lotensin HCT... 837
Maxzide 1380
Moduretic Tablets 1705
Oretic Tablets 443
Prinzide Tablets 1737
Ser-Ap-Es Tablets 849
Timolide Tablets....................................... 1748
Vaseretic Tablets 1765
Zestoretic 2850
Ziac 1415

Hydroflumethiazide (Enhances antihypertensive action of Ismelin). Products include:

Diucardin Tablets..................................... 2718

Imipramine Hydrochloride (Reduces hypotensive effect). Products include:

Tofranil Ampuls 854
Tofranil Tablets 856

Imipramine Pamoate (Reduces hypotensive effect). Products include:

Tofranil-PM Capsules............................. 857

Isocarboxazid (Concurrent use contraindicated).

No products indexed under this heading.

Levonorgestrel (Reduces hypotensive effect). Products include:

Levlen/Tri-Levlen.................................... 651
Nordette-21 Tablets................................. 2755
Nordette-28 Tablets................................. 2758
Norplant System 2759
Levlen/Tri-Levlen.................................... 651
Triphasil-21 Tablets 2814
Triphasil-28 Tablets 2819

Maprotiline Hydrochloride (Reduces hypotensive effect). Products include:

Ludiomil Tablets...................................... 843

Mesoridazine Besylate (Reduces hypotensive effect). Products include:

Serentil... 684

Mestranol (Reduces hypotensive effect). Products include:

Norinyl 2088
Ortho-Novum.. 1872

Methotrimeprazine (Reduces hypotensive effect). Products include:

Levoprome 1274

Methyclothiazide (Reduces hypotensive effect). Products include:

Enduron Tablets....................................... 420

Methylphenidate Hydrochloride (Reduces hypotensive effect). Products include:

Ritalin 848

Norethindrone (Reduces hypotensive effect). Products include:

Brevicon... 2088
Micronor Tablets 1872
Modicon.. 1872
Norinyl 2088
Nor-Q D Tablets 2135
Ortho-Novum.. 1872
Ovcon 760

Tri-Norinyl... 2164

Norethynodrel (Reduces hypotensive effect).

No products indexed under this heading.

Norgestimate (Reduces hypotensive effect). Products include:

Ortho-Cyclen/Ortho-Tri-Cyclen 1858
Ortho-Cyclen/Ortho Tri-Cyclen 1858

Norgestrel (Reduces hypotensive effect). Products include:

Lo/Ovral Tablets 2746
Lo/Ovral-28 Tablets................................. 2751
Ovral Tablets... 2770
Ovral-28 Tablets 2770
Ovrette Tablets... 2771

Nortriptyline Hydrochloride (Reduces hypotensive effect). Products include:

Pamelor 2280

Perphenazine (Reduces hypotensive effect). Products include:

Etrafon 2355
Triavil Tablets 1757
Trilafon... 2389

Phenelzine Sulfate (Concurrent use contraindicated). Products include:

Nardil 1920

Polyestradiol Phosphate (Reduces hypotensive effect).

No products indexed under this heading.

Polythiazide (Enhances antihypertensive action of Ismelin). Products include:

Minizide Capsules 1938

Prochlorperazine (Reduces hypotensive effect). Products include:

Compazine 2470

Promethazine Hydrochloride (Reduces hypotensive effect). Products include:

Mepergan Injection 2753
Phenergan with Codeine........................ 2777
Phenergan with Dextromethorphan 2778
Phenergan Injection 2773
Phenergan Suppositories 2775
Phenergan Syrup 2774
Phenergan Tablets 2775
Phenergan VC 2779
Phenergan VC with Codeine 2781

Protriptyline Hydrochloride (Reduces hypotensive effect). Products include:

Vivactil Tablets 1774

Quinestrol (Reduces hypotensive effect).

No products indexed under this heading.

Rauwolfia Serpentina (May result in excessive postural hypotension, bradycardia, and mental depression).

No products indexed under this heading.

Rescinnamine (May result in excessive postural hypotension, bradycardia, and mental depression).

No products indexed under this heading.

Reserpine (May result in excessive postural hypotension, bradycardia, and mental depression). Products include:

Diupres Tablets 1650
Hydropres Tablets.................................... 1675
Ser-Ap-Es Tablets 849

Selegiline Hydrochloride (Concurrent use contraindicated). Products include:

Eldepryl Tablets 2550

Thioridazine Hydrochloride (Reduces hypotensive effect). Products include:

Mellaril 2269

Tranylcypromine Sulfate (Concurrent use contraindicated). Products include:

Parnate Tablets 2503

Trifluoperazine Hydrochloride (Reduces hypotensive effect). Products include:

Stelazine 2514

Trimipramine Maleate (Reduces hypotensive effect). Products include:

Surmontil Capsules................................. 2811

Food Interactions

Alcohol (Aggravates orthostatic hypotensive effects).

ISMO TABLETS

(Isosorbide Mononitrate) **2738**

May interact with vasodilators, calcium channel blockers, and certain other agents. Compounds in these categories include:

Amlodipine Besylate (Potential for marked symptomatic orthostatic hypotension). Products include:

Lotrel Capsules... 840
Norvasc Tablets 1940

Bepridil Hydrochloride (Potential for marked symptomatic orthostatic hypotension). Products include:

Vascor (200, 300 and 400 mg) Tablets 1587

Diazoxide (Additive vasodilating effects). Products include:

Hyperstat I.V. Injection 2363
Proglycem.. 580

Diltiazem Hydrochloride (Potential for marked symptomatic orthostatic hypotension). Products include:

Cardizem CD Capsules 1506
Cardizem SR Capsules 1510
Cardizem Injectable 1508
Cardizem Tablets..................................... 1512
Dilacor XR Extended-release Capsules 2018

Felodipine (Potential for marked symptomatic orthostatic hypotension). Products include:

Plendil Extended-Release Tablets.... 527

Hydralazine Hydrochloride (Additive vasodilating effects). Products include:

Apresazide Capsules 808
Apresoline Hydrochloride Tablets .. 809
Ser-Ap-Es Tablets 849

Isradipine (Potential for marked symptomatic orthostatic hypotension). Products include:

DynaCirc Capsules 2256

Minoxidil (Additive vasodilating effects). Products include:

Loniten Tablets... 2618
Rogaine Topical Solution 2637

Nicardipine Hydrochloride (Potential for marked symptomatic orthostatic hypotension). Products include:

Cardene Capsules 2095
Cardene I.V. 2709
Cardene SR Capsules.............................. 2097

Nifedipine (Potential for marked symptomatic orthostatic hypotension). Products include:

Adalat Capsules (10 mg and 20 mg) 587
Adalat CC 589
Procardia Capsules.................................. 1971
Procardia XL Extended Release Tablets 1972

Nimodipine (Potential for marked symptomatic orthostatic hypotension). Products include:

Nimotop Capsules 610

Nisoldipine (Potential for marked symptomatic orthostatic hypotension).

No products indexed under this heading.

IMPORTANT NOTE: Always consult each drug listing in the patient's regimen for possible interactions.

Verapamil Hydrochloride (Potential for marked symptomatic orthostatic hypotension). Products include:

- Calan SR Caplets 2422
- Calan Tablets 2419
- Isoptin Injectable 1344
- Isoptin Oral Tablets 1346
- Isoptin SR Tablets 1348
- Verelan Capsules 1410
- Verelan Capsules 2824

Food Interactions

Alcohol (Additive vasodilating effects).

ISMOTIC 45% W/V SOLUTION

(Isosorbide) .... ⊙ 222
None cited in PDR database.

ISOCLOR EXPECTORANT

(Codeine Phosphate, Guaifenesin, Pseudoephedrine Hydrochloride) 990
None cited in PDR database.

ISOCLOR TIMESULE CAPSULES

(Phenylpropanolamine Hydrochloride, Chlorpheniramine Maleate) .... ▣ 637
May interact with monoamine oxidase inhibitors and certain other agents. Compounds in these categories include:

Furazolidone (Concurrent use is not recommended). Products include:

- Furoxone 2046

Isocarboxazid (Concurrent use is not recommended).

- No products indexed under this heading.

Phenelzine Sulfate (Concurrent use is not recommended). Products include:

- Nardil 1920

Phenylpropanolamine Containing Anorectics (Concurrent use is not recommended).

Selegiline Hydrochloride (Concurrent use is not recommended). Products include:

- Eldepryl Tablets 2550

Tranylcypromine Sulfate (Concurrent use is not recommended). Products include:

- Parnate Tablets 2503

Food Interactions

Alcohol (Concurrent use is not recommended).

ISOETHARINE INHALATION SOLUTION, USP, ARM-A-MED

(Isoetharine) 551
May interact with sympathomimetics. Compounds in this category include:

Albuterol (May cause excessive tachycardia). Products include:

- Proventil Inhalation Aerosol 2382
- Ventolin Inhalation Aerosol and Refill 1197

Albuterol Sulfate (May cause excessive tachycardia). Products include:

- Airet Solution for Inhalation 452
- Proventil Inhalation Solution 0.083% 2384
- Proventil Repetabs Tablets 2386
- Proventil Solution for Inhalation 0.5% 2383
- Proventil Syrup 2385
- Proventil Tablets 2386
- Ventolin Inhalation Solution 1198
- Ventolin Nebules Inhalation Solution 1199
- Ventolin Rotacaps for Inhalation 1200
- Ventolin Syrup 1202
- Ventolin Tablets 1203
- Volmax Extended-Release Tablets 1788

Dobutamine Hydrochloride (May cause excessive tachycardia). Products include:

- Dobutrex Solution Vials 1439

Dopamine Hydrochloride (May cause excessive tachycardia).

- No products indexed under this heading.

Ephedrine Hydrochloride (May cause excessive tachycardia). Products include:

- Primatene Dual Action Formula .... ▣ 872
- Primatene Tablets .... ▣ 873
- Quadrinal Tablets 1350

Ephedrine Sulfate (May cause excessive tachycardia). Products include:

- Bronkaid Caplets .... ▣ 717
- Marax Tablets & DF Syrup 2200

Ephedrine Tannate (May cause excessive tachycardia). Products include:

- Rynatuss 2673

Epinephrine (May cause excessive tachycardia). Products include:

- Bronkaid Mist .... ▣ 717
- EPIFRIN .... ⊙ 239
- EpiPen 790
- Marcaine Hydrochloride with Epinephrine 1:200,000 2316
- Primatene Mist .... ▣ 873
- Sensorcaine with Epinephrine Injection 559
- Sus-Phrine Injection 1019
- Xylocaine with Epinephrine Injections 567

Epinephrine Bitartrate (May cause excessive tachycardia). Products include:

- Bronkaid Mist Suspension .... ▣ 718
- Sensorcaine-MPF with Epinephrine Injection 559

Epinephrine Hydrochloride (May cause excessive tachycardia). Products include:

- Ana-Kit Anaphylaxis Emergency Treatment Kit 617

Isoproterenol Hydrochloride (May cause excessive tachycardia). Products include:

- Isuprel Hydrochloride Injection 1:5000 2311
- Isuprel Hydrochloride Solution 1:200 & 1:100 2313
- Isuprel Mistometer 2312

Isoproterenol Sulfate (May cause excessive tachycardia). Products include:

- Norisodrine with Calcium Iodide Syrup 442

Metaproterenol Sulfate (May cause excessive tachycardia). Products include:

- Alupent 669
- Metaproterenol Sulfate Inhalation Solution, USP, Arm-a-Med 552

Metaraminol Bitartrate (May cause excessive tachycardia). Products include:

- Aramine Injection 1609

Methoxamine Hydrochloride (May cause excessive tachycardia). Products include:

- Vasoxyl Injection 1196

Norepinephrine Bitartrate (May cause excessive tachycardia). Products include:

- Levophed Bitartrate Injection 2315

Phenylephrine Bitartrate (May cause excessive tachycardia).

- No products indexed under this heading.

Phenylephrine Hydrochloride (May cause excessive tachycardia). Products include:

- Atrohist Plus Tablets 454
- Cerose DM .... ▣ 878
- Comhist 2038
- D.A. Chewable Tablets 951
- Deconsal Pediatric Capsules 454
- Dura-Vent/DA Tablets 953
- Entex Capsules 1986
- Entex Liquid 1986
- Extendryl 1005
- 4-Way Fast Acting Nasal Spray (regular & mentholated) .... ▣ 621
- Hemorid For Women .... ▣ 834
- Hycomine Compound Tablets 932
- Neo-Synephrine Hydrochloride 1% Carpuject 2324
- Neo-Synephrine Hydrochloride 1% Injection 2324
- Neo-Synephrine Hydrochloride (Ophthalmic) 2325
- Neo-Synephrine .... ▣ 726
- Nōstril .... ▣ 644
- Novahistine Elixir .... ▣ 823
- Phenergan VC 2779
- Phenergan VC with Codeine 2781
- Preparation H .... ▣ 871
- Tympagesic Ear Drops 2342
- Vasosulf .... ⊙ 271
- Vicks Sinex Nasal Spray and Ultra Fine Mist .... ▣ 765

Phenylephrine Tannate (May cause excessive tachycardia). Products include:

- Atrohist Pediatric Suspension 454
- Ricobid-D Pediatric Suspension 2038
- Ricobid Tablets and Pediatric Suspension 2038
- Rynatan 2673
- Rynatuss 2673

Phenylpropanolamine Hydrochloride (May cause excessive tachycardia). Products include:

- Acutrim .... ▣ 628
- Allerest Children's Chewable Tablets .... ▣ 627
- Allerest 12 Hour Caplets .... ▣ 627
- Atrohist Plus Tablets 454
- BC Cold Powder Multi-Symptom Formula (Cold-Sinus-Allergy) .... ▣ 609
- BC Cold Powder Non-Drowsy Formula (Cold-Sinus) .... ▣ 609
- Cheracol Plus Head Cold/Cough Formula .... ▣ 769
- Comtrex Multi-Symptom Non-Drowsy Liqui-gels .... ▣ 618
- Contac Continuous Action Nasal Decongestant/Antihistamine 12 Hour Capsules .... ▣ 813
- Contac Maximum Strength Continuous Action Decongestant/Antihistamine 12 Hour Caplets .... ▣ 813
- Contac Severe Cold and Flu Formula Caplets .... ▣ 814
- Coricidin 'D' Decongestant Tablets .... ▣ 800
- Dexatrim .... ▣ 832
- Dexatrim Plus Vitamins Caplets .... ▣ 832
- Dimetane-DC Cough Syrup 2059
- Dimetapp Elixir .... ▣ 773
- Dimetapp Extentabs .... ▣ 774
- Dimetapp Tablets/Liqui-Gels .... ▣ 775
- Dimetapp Cold & Allergy Chewable Tablets .... ▣ 773
- Dimetapp DM Elixir .... ▣ 774
- Dura-Vent Tablets 952
- Entex Capsules 1986
- Entex LA Tablets 1987
- Entex Liquid 1986
- Exgest LA Tablets 782
- Hycomine 931
- Isoclor Timesule Capsules .... ▣ 637
- Nolamine Timed-Release Tablets 785
- Ornade Spansule Capsules 2502
- Propagest Tablets 786
- Pyrroxate Caplets .... ▣ 772
- Robitussin-CF .... ▣ 777
- Sinulin Tablets 787
- Tavist-D 12 Hour Relief Tablets .... ▣ 787
- Teldrin 12 Hour Antihistamine/Nasal Decongestant Allergy Relief Capsules .... ▣ 826
- Triaminic Allergy Tablets .... ▣ 789
- Triaminic Cold Tablets .... ▣ 790
- Triaminic Expectorant .... ▣ 790
- Triaminic Syrup .... ▣ 792
- Triaminic-12 Tablets .... ▣ 792
- Triaminic-DM Syrup .... ▣ 792
- Triaminicin Tablets .... ▣ 793
- Triaminicol Multi-Symptom Cold Tablets .... ▣ 793
- Triaminicol Multi-Symptom Relief ▣ 794
- Vicks DayQuil Allergy Relief 12-Hour Extended Release Tablets .... ▣ 760
- Vicks DayQuil Allergy Relief 4-Hour Tablets .... ▣ 760
- Vicks DayQuil SINUS Pressure & CONGESTION Relief .... ▣ 761

Pirbuterol Acetate (May cause excessive tachycardia). Products include:

- Maxair Autohaler 1492
- Maxair Inhaler 1494

Pseudoephedrine Hydrochloride (May cause excessive tachycardia). Products include:

- Actifed Allergy Daytime/Nighttime Caplets .... ▣ 844
- Actifed Plus Caplets .... ▣ 845
- Actifed Plus Tablets .... ▣ 845
- Actifed with Codeine Cough Syrup 1067
- Actifed Sinus Daytime/Nighttime Tablets and Caplets .... ▣ 846
- Actifed Syrup .... ▣ 846
- Actifed Tablets .... ▣ 844
- Advil Cold and Sinus Caplets and Tablets (formerly CoAdvil) .... ▣ 870
- Alka-Seltzer Plus Cold Medicine Liqui-Gels .... ▣ 706
- Alka-Seltzer Plus Cold & Cough Medicine Liqui-Gels .... ▣ 705
- Alka-Seltzer Plus Night-Time Cold Medicine Liqui-Gels .... ▣ 706
- Allerest Headache Strength Tablets .... ▣ 627
- Allerest Maximum Strength Tablets .... ▣ 627
- Allerest No Drowsiness Tablets .... ▣ 627
- Allerest Sinus Pain Formula .... ▣ 627
- Anatuss LA Tablets 1542
- Atrohist Pediatric Capsules 453
- Bayer Select Sinus Pain Relief Formula .... ▣ 717
- Benadryl Allergy Decongestant Liquid Medication .... ▣ 848
- Benadryl Allergy Decongestant Tablets .... ▣ 848
- Benadryl Allergy Sinus Headache Formula Caplets .... ▣ 849
- Benylin Multisymptom .... ▣ 852
- Bromfed Capsules (Extended-Release) 1785
- Bromfed Syrup .... ▣ 733
- Bromfed Tablets 1785
- Bromfed-DM Cough Syrup 1786
- Bromfed-PD Capsules (Extended-Release) 1785
- Children's Vicks DayQuil Allergy Relief .... ▣ 757
- Children's Vicks NyQuil Cold/Cough Relief .... ▣ 758
- Comtrex Multi-Symptom Cold Reliever Tablets/Caplets/Liqui-Gels/Liquid .... ▣ 615
- Allergy-Sinus Comtrex Multi-Symptom Allergy-Sinus Formula Tablets .... ▣ 617
- Comtrex Multi-Symptom Non-Drowsy Caplets .... ▣ 618
- Congess 1004
- Contac Day Allergy/Sinus Caplets ▣ 812
- Contac Day & Night .... ▣ 812
- Contac Night Allergy/Sinus Caplets .... ▣ 812
- Contac Severe Cold & Flu Non-Drowsy .... ▣ 815
- Deconamine Chewable Tablets 1320
- Deconamine CX Cough and Cold Liquid and Tablets 1319
- Deconamine 1320
- Deconsal C Expectorant Syrup 456
- Deconsal Pediatric Syrup 457
- Deconsal II Tablets 454
- Dimetane-DX Cough Syrup 2059
- Dimetapp Sinus Caplets .... ▣ 775
- Dorcol Children's Cough Syrup .... ▣ 785
- Drixoral Cough + Congestion Liquid Caps .... ▣ 802
- Dura-Tap/PD Capsules 2867
- Duratuss Tablets 2565
- Duratuss HD Elixir 2565
- Efidac/24 .... ▣ 635
- Entex PSE Tablets 1987
- Fedahist Gyrocaps 2401
- Fedahist Timecaps 2401
- Guaifed 1787
- Guaifed Syrup .... ▣ 734
- Guaimax-D Tablets 792
- Guaitab Tablets .... ▣ 734
- Isoclor Expectorant 990
- Kronofed-A 977
- Motrin IB Sinus .... ▣ 838
- Novahistine DH 2462
- Novahistine DMX .... ▣ 822
- Novahistine Expectorant 2463
- Nucofed 2051

(▣ Described in PDR For Nonprescription Drugs) (⊙ Described in PDR For Ophthalmology)

533 **Interactions Index** **Isoptin Injectable**

PediaCare Cold Allergy Chewable Tablets ▣ 677
PediaCare Cough-Cold Chewable Tablets 1553
PediaCare 1553
PediaCare Infants' Decongestant Drops ▣ 677
PediCare Infant's Drops Decongestant Plus Cough 1553
PediaCare NightRest Cough-Cold Liquid 1553
Pediatric Vicks 44d Dry Hacking Cough & Head Congestion ▣ 763
Pediatric Vicks 44m Cough & Cold Relief ▣ 764
Robitussin Cold & Cough Liqui-Gels ▣ 776
Robitussin Maximum Strength Cough & Cold ▣ 778
Robitussin Pediatric Cough & Cold Formula ▣ 779
Robitussin Severe Congestion Liqui-Gels ▣ 776
Robitussin-DAC Syrup 2074
Robitussin-PE ▣ 778
Rondec Oral Drops 953
Rondec Syrup 953
Rondec Tablet 953
Rondec-DM Oral Drops 954
Rondec-DM Syrup 954
Rondec-TR Tablet 953
Ryna ▣ 841
Seldane-D Extended-Release Tablets 1538
Semprex-D Capsules 463
Semprex-D Capsules 1167
Sinarest Tablets ▣ 648
Sinarest Extra Strength Tablets ▣ 648
Sinarest No Drowsiness Tablets ▣ 648
Sine-Aid IB Caplets 1554
Sine-Aid Maximum Strength Sinus Medication Gelcaps, Caplets and Tablets 1554
Sine-Off No Drowsiness Formula Caplets ▣ 824
Sine-Off Sinus Medicine ▣ 825
Singlet Tablets ▣ 825
Sinutab Non-Drying Liquid Caps ▣ 859
Sinutab Sinus Allergy Medication, Maximum Strength Tablets and Caplets ▣ 860
Sinutab Sinus Medication, Maximum Strength Without Drowsiness Formula, Tablets & Caplets ▣ 860
Sinutab Sinus Medication, Regular Strength Without Drowsiness Formula ▣ 859
Sudafed Children's Liquid ▣ 861
Sudafed Cold and Cough Liquidcaps ▣ 862
Sudafed Cough Syrup ▣ 862
Sudafed Plus Liquid ▣ 862
Sudafed Plus Tablets ▣ 863
Sudafed Severe Cold Formula Caplets ▣ 863
Sudafed Severe Cold Formula Tablets ▣ 864
Sudafed Sinus Caplets ▣ 864
Sudafed Sinus Tablets ▣ 864
Sudafed Tablets, 30 mg ▣ 861
Sudafed Tablets, 60 mg ▣ 861
Sudafed 12 Hour Caplets ▣ 861
Syn-Rx Tablets 465
Syn-Rx DM Tablets 466
TheraFlu ▣ 787
TheraFlu Maximum Strength Nighttime Flu, Cold & Cough Medicine ▣ 788
TheraFlu Maximum Strength Non-Drowsy Formula Flu, Cold & Cough Medicine ▣ 788
Thera Flu Maximum Strength, Non-Drowsy Formula Flu, Cold and Cough Caplets ▣ 789
Triaminic AM Cough and Decongestant Formula ▣ 789
Triaminic AM Decongestant Formula ▣ 790
Triaminic Nite Light ▣ 791
Triaminic Sore Throat Formula ▣ 791
Tussend 1783
Tussend Expectorant 1785
Children's TYLENOL Cold Multi-Symptom Liquid Formula and Chewable Tablets 1561
Children's TYLENOL Cold Plus Cough Multi Symptom Tablets and Liquid ▣ 681
Infants' TYLENOL Cold Decongestant & Fever-Reducer Drops 1556
TYLENOL Maximum Strength Allergy Sinus Medication Gelcaps and Caplets 1563
TYLENOL Maximum Strength Allergy Sinus NightTime Medication Caplets 1555
TYLENOL Flu Maximum Strength Gelcaps 1565
TYLENOL Flu NightTime, Maximum Strength, Gelcaps 1566
TYLENOL Maximum Strength Flu NightTime Hot Medication Packets 1562
TYLENOL, Maximum Strength, Sinus Medication Geltabs, Gelcaps, Caplets and Tablets 1566
TYLENOL Cold Multi-Symptom Formula Medication Tablets and Caplets 1561
TYLENOL Cold Medication No Drowsiness Formula Gelcaps and Caplets 1562
TYLENOL Cold Multi-Symptom Hot Medication Liquid Packets 1557
TYLENOL Cough Multi-Symptom Medication with Decongestant 1565
Ursinus Inlay-Tabs ▣ 794
Vicks 44 LiquiCaps Cough, Cold & Flu Relief ▣ 755
Vicks 44 LiquiCaps Non-Drowsy Cough & Cold Relief ▣ 756
Vicks 44D Dry Hacking Cough & Head Congestion ▣ 755
Vicks 44M Cough, Cold & Flu Relief ▣ 756
Vicks DayQuil ▣ 761
Vicks DayQuil SINUS Pressure & PAIN Relief with IBUPROFEN ▣ 762
Vicks Nyquil Hot Therapy ▣ 762
Vicks NyQuil LiquiCaps Multi-Symptom Cold/Flu Relief ▣ 763
Vicks NyQuil Multi-Symptom Cold/Flu Relief - (Original & Cherry Flavor) ▣ 763

Pseudoephedrine Sulfate (May cause excessive tachycardia). Products include:
Cheracol Sinus ▣ 768
Chlor-Trimeton Allergy Decongestant Tablets ▣ 799
Claritin-D 2350
Drixoral Cold and Allergy Sustained-Action Tablets ▣ 802
Drixoral Cold and Flu Extended-Release Tablets ▣ 803
Drixoral Non-Drowsy Formula Extended-Release Tablets ▣ 803
Drixoral Allergy/Sinus Extended Release Tablets ▣ 804
Trinalin Repetabs Tablets 1330

Salmeterol Xinafoate (May cause excessive tachycardia). Products include:
Serevent Inhalation Aerosol 1176

Terbutaline Sulfate (May cause excessive tachycardia). Products include:
Brethaire Inhaler 813
Brethine Ampuls 815
Brethine Tablets 814
Bricanyl Subcutaneous Injection 1502
Bricanyl Tablets 1503

ISOPTIN AMPULES 5MG/2ML
(Verapamil Hydrochloride) 1344
May interact with beta blockers, alpha adrenergic blockers, inhalant anesthetics, nondepolarizing neuromuscular blocking agents, cardiac glycosides, lithium preparations, highly protein bound drugs (selected), and certain other agents. Compounds in these categories include:

Acebutolol Hydrochloride (Concomitant intravenous beta blocker therapy results in serious toxicity in patients with CHF, recent MI or severe cardiomyopathy). Products include:
Sectral Capsules 2807

Amiodarone Hydrochloride (Administer with caution to patients receiving other highly protein bound drugs). Products include:
Cordarone Intravenous 2715
Cordarone Tablets 2712

Amitriptyline Hydrochloride (Administer with caution to patients receiving other highly protein bound drugs). Products include:
Elavil 2838
Endep Tablets 2174
Etrafon 2355
Limbitrol 2180
Triavil Tablets 1757

Atenolol (Concomitant intravenous beta blocker therapy results in serious toxicity in patients with CHF, recent MI or severe cardiomyopathy). Products include:
Tenoretic Tablets 2845
Tenormin Tablets and I.V. Injection 2847

Atovaquone (Administer with caution to patients receiving other highly protein bound drugs). Products include:
Mepron Suspension 1135

Atracurium Besylate (Verapamil may potentiate the activity of neuromuscular blocking agents). Products include:
Tracrium Injection 1183

Betaxolol Hydrochloride (Concomitant intravenous beta blocker therapy results in serious toxicity in patients with CHF, recent MI or severe cardiomyopathy). Products include:
Betoptic Ophthalmic Solution 469
Betoptic S Ophthalmic Suspension 471
Kerlone Tablets 2436

Bisoprolol Fumarate (Concomitant intravenous beta blocker therapy results in serious toxicity in patients with CHF, recent MI or severe cardiomyopathy). Products include:
Zebeta Tablets 1413
Ziac 1415

Carbamazepine (Increased carbamazepine concentrations resulting in increased side effects of carbamazepine). Products include:
Atretol Tablets 573
Tegretol Chewable Tablets 852
Tegretol Suspension 852
Tegretol Tablets 852

Carteolol Hydrochloride (Concomitant intravenous beta blocker therapy results in serious toxicity in patients with CHF, recent MI or severe cardiomyopathy). Products include:
Cartrol Tablets 410
Ocupress Ophthalmic Solution, 1% Sterile ⊙ 309

Cefonicid Sodium (Administer with caution to patients receiving other highly protein bound drugs). Products include:
Monocid Injection 2497

Chlordiazepoxide (Administer with caution to patients receiving other highly protein bound drugs). Products include:
Libritabs Tablets 2177
Limbitrol 2180

Chlordiazepoxide Hydrochloride (Administer with caution to patients receiving other highly protein bound drugs). Products include:
Librax Capsules 2176
Librium Capsules 2178
Librium Injectable 2179

Chlorpromazine (Administer with caution to patients receiving other highly protein bound drugs). Products include:
Thorazine Suppositories 2523

Chlorpromazine Hydrochloride (Administer with caution to patients receiving other highly protein bound drugs). Products include:
Thorazine 2523

Cimetidine (Variable results on verapamil clearance). Products include:
Tagamet Tablets 2516

Cimetidine Hydrochloride (Variable results on verapamil clearance). Products include:
Tagamet 2516

Clomipramine Hydrochloride (Administer with caution to patients receiving other highly protein bound drugs). Products include:
Anafranil Capsules 803

Clozapine (Administer with caution to patients receiving other highly protein bound drugs). Products include:
Clozaril Tablets 2252

Cyclosporine (Increased serum levels of cyclosporin; administer with caution to patients receiving other highly protein bound drugs). Products include:
Neoral 2276
Sandimmune 2286

Dantrolene Sodium (Concomitant use of both drugs by intravenous route may result in cardiovascular collapse). Products include:
Dantrium Capsules 1982
Dantrium Intravenous 1983

Desflurane (Excessive cardiovascular depression). Products include:
Suprane 1813

Deslanoside (Both drugs slow AV conduction resulting in possible AV block or excessive bradycardia).
No products indexed under this heading.

Diazepam (Administer with caution to patients receiving other highly protein bound drugs). Products include:
Dizac 1809
Valium Injectable 2182
Valium Tablets 2183
Valrelease Capsules 2169

Diclofenac Potassium (Administer with caution to patients receiving other highly protein bound drugs). Products include:
Cataflam 816

Diclofenac Sodium (Administer with caution to patients receiving other highly protein bound drugs). Products include:
Voltaren Ophthalmic Sterile Ophthalmic Solution ⊙ 272
Voltaren Tablets 861

Digitoxin (Both drugs slow AV conduction resulting in possible AV block or excessive bradycardia). Products include:
Crystodigin Tablets 1433

Digoxin (Both drugs slow AV conduction resulting in possible AV block or excessive bradycardia). Products include:
Lanoxicaps 1117
Lanoxin Elixir Pediatric 1120
Lanoxin Injection 1123
Lanoxin Injection Pediatric 1126
Lanoxin Tablets 1128

Dipyridamole (Administer with caution to patients receiving other highly protein bound drugs). Products include:
Persantine Tablets 681

Disopyramide Phosphate (Do not administer within 48 hours before or 24 hours after verapamil). Products include:
Norpace 2444

IMPORTANT NOTE: Always consult each drug listing in the patient's regimen for possible interactions.

Isoptin Injectable | Interactions Index | 534

Doxazosin Mesylate (Exaggerated hypotensive response). Products include:
- Cardura Tablets 2186

Enflurane (Excessive cardiovascular depression).
- No products indexed under this heading.

Esmolol Hydrochloride (Concomitant intravenous beta blocker therapy results in serious toxicity in patients with CHF, recent MI or severe cardiomyopathy). Products include:
- Brevibloc Injection 1808

Fenoprofen Calcium (Administer with caution to patients receiving other highly protein bound drugs). Products include:
- Nalfon 200 Pulvules & Nalfon Tablets 917

Flecainide Acetate (Additive effects on myocardial contractility, AV conduction, and repolarization). Products include:
- Tambocor Tablets 1497

Flurazepam Hydrochloride (Administer with caution to patients receiving other highly protein bound drugs). Products include:
- Dalmane Capsules 2173

Flurbiprofen (Administer with caution to patients receiving other highly protein bound drugs). Products include:
- Ansaid Tablets 2579

Glipizide (Administer with caution to patients receiving other highly protein bound drugs). Products include:
- Glucotrol Tablets 1967
- Glucotrol XL Extended Release Tablets 1968

Halothane (Excessive cardiovascular depression). Products include:
- Fluothane 2724

Ibuprofen (Administer with caution to patients receiving other highly protein bound drugs). Products include:
- Advil Cold and Sinus Caplets and Tablets (formerly CoAdvil) ..... ▣ 870
- Advil Ibuprofen Tablets and Caplets ..... ▣ 870
- Children's Advil Suspension 2692
- Arthritis Foundation Ibuprofen Tablets ..... ▣ 674
- Bayer Select Ibuprofen Pain Relief Formula ..... ▣ 715
- Cramp End Tablets ..... ▣ 735
- Dimetapp Sinus Caplets ..... ▣ 775
- Haltran Tablets ..... ▣ 771
- IBU Tablets 1342
- Ibuprohm ..... ▣ 735
- Children's Motrin Ibuprofen Oral Suspension 1546
- Motrin Tablets 2625
- Motrin IB Caplets, Tablets, and Geltabs ..... ▣ 838
- Motrin IB Sinus ..... ▣ 838
- Motrin Ibuprofen Suspension, Oral Drops, Chewable Tablets, Caplets 1546
- Nuprin Ibuprofen/Analgesic Tablets & Caplets ..... ▣ 622
- Sine-Aid IB Caplets 1554
- Vicks DayQuil SINUS Pressure & PAIN Relief with IBUPROFEN ..... ▣ 762

Imipramine Hydrochloride (Administer with caution to patients receiving other highly protein bound drugs). Products include:
- Tofranil Ampuls 854
- Tofranil Tablets 856

Imipramine Pamoate (Administer with caution to patients receiving other highly protein bound drugs). Products include:
- Tofranil-PM Capsules 857

Indomethacin (Administer with caution to patients receiving other highly protein bound drugs). Products include:
- Indocin 1680

Indomethacin Sodium Trihydrate (Administer with caution to patients receiving other highly protein bound drugs). Products include:
- Indocin I.V. 1684

Isoflurane (Excessive cardiovascular depression).
- No products indexed under this heading.

Ketoprofen (Administer with caution to patients receiving other highly protein bound drugs). Products include:
- Orudis Capsules 2766
- Oruvail Capsules 2766

Ketorolac Tromethamine (Administer with caution to patients receiving other highly protein bound drugs). Products include:
- Acular 474
- Acular ..... ⊙ 277
- Toradol 2159

Labetalol Hydrochloride (Concomitant intravenous beta blocker therapy results in serious toxicity in patients with CHF, recent MI or severe cardiomyopathy). Products include:
- Normodyne Injection 2377
- Normodyne Tablets 2379
- Trandate 1185

Levobunolol Hydrochloride (Concomitant intravenous beta blocker therapy results in serious toxicity in patients with CHF, recent MI or severe cardiomyopathy). Products include:
- Betagan ..... ⊙ 233

Lithium Carbonate (Increased sensitivity to effects of lithium). Products include:
- Eskalith 2485
- Lithium Carbonate Capsules & Tablets 2230
- Lithonate/Lithotabs/Lithobid 2543

Lithium Citrate (Increased sensitivity to effects of lithium).
- No products indexed under this heading.

Meclofenamate Sodium (Administer with caution to patients receiving other highly protein bound drugs).
- No products indexed under this heading.

Mefenamic Acid (Administer with caution to patients receiving other highly protein bound drugs). Products include:
- Ponstel 1925

Methoxyflurane (Excessive cardiovascular depression).
- No products indexed under this heading.

Metipranolol Hydrochloride (Concomitant intravenous beta blocker therapy results in serious toxicity in patients with CHF, recent MI or severe cardiomyopathy). Products include:
- OptiPranolol (Metipranolol 0.3%) Sterile Ophthalmic Solution ..... ⊙ 258

Metocurine Iodide (Verapamil may potentiate the activity of neuromuscular blocking agents). Products include:
- Metubine Iodide Vials 916

Metoprolol Succinate (Concomitant intravenous beta blocker therapy results in serious toxicity in patients with CHF, recent MI or severe cardiomyopathy). Products include:
- Toprol-XL Tablets 565

Metoprolol Tartrate (Concomitant intravenous beta blocker therapy results in serious toxicity in patients with CHF, recent MI or severe cardiomyopathy). Products include:
- Lopressor Ampuls 830
- Lopressor HCT Tablets 832
- Lopressor Tablets 830

Midazolam Hydrochloride (Administer with caution to patients receiving other highly protein bound drugs). Products include:
- Versed Injection 2170

Mivacurium Chloride (Verapamil may potentiate the activity of neuromuscular blocking agents). Products include:
- Mivacron 1138

Nadolol (Concomitant intravenous beta blocker therapy results in serious toxicity in patients with CHF, recent MI or severe cardiomyopathy).
- No products indexed under this heading.

Naproxen (Administer with caution to patients receiving other highly protein bound drugs). Products include:
- Anaprox/Naprosyn 2117

Naproxen Sodium (Administer with caution to patients receiving other highly protein bound drugs). Products include:
- Aleve 1975
- Anaprox/Naprosyn 2117

Nortriptyline Hydrochloride (Administer with caution to patients receiving other highly protein bound drugs). Products include:
- Pamelor 2280

Oxaprozin (Administer with caution to patients receiving other highly protein bound drugs). Products include:
- Daypro Caplets 2426

Oxazepam (Administer with caution to patients receiving other highly protein bound drugs). Products include:
- Serax Capsules 2810
- Serax Tablets 2810

Pancuronium Bromide Injection (Verapamil may potentiate the activity of neuromuscular blocking agents).
- No products indexed under this heading.

Penbutolol Sulfate (Concomitant intravenous beta blocker therapy results in serious toxicity in patients with CHF, recent MI or severe cardiomyopathy). Products include:
- Levatol 2403

Phenobarbital (Increases verapamil serum levels). Products include:
- Arco-Lase Plus Tablets 512
- Bellergal-S Tablets 2250
- Donnatal 2060
- Donnatal Extentabs 2061
- Donnatal Tablets 2060
- Phenobarbital Elixir and Tablets 1469
- Quadrinal Tablets 1350

Phenylbutazone (Administer with caution to patients receiving other highly protein bound drugs).
- No products indexed under this heading.

Pindolol (Concomitant intravenous beta blocker therapy results in serious toxicity in patients with CHF, recent MI or severe cardiomyopathy). Products include:
- Visken Tablets 2299

Piroxicam (Administer with caution to patients receiving other highly protein bound drugs). Products include:
- Feldene Capsules 1965

Prazosin Hydrochloride (Exaggerated hypotensive response). Products include:
- Minipress Capsules 1937
- Minizide Capsules 1938

Propranolol Hydrochloride (Concomitant intravenous beta blocker therapy results in serious toxicity in patients with CHF, recent MI or severe cardiomyopathy). Products include:
- Inderal 2728
- Inderal LA Long Acting Capsules 2730
- Inderide Tablets 2732
- Inderide LA Long Acting Capsules 2734

Quinidine Gluconate (Exaggerated hypotensive response). Products include:
- Quinaglute Dura-Tabs Tablets 649

Quinidine Polygalacturonate (Exaggerated hypotensive response).
- No products indexed under this heading.

Quinidine Sulfate (Exaggerated hypotensive response). Products include:
- Quinidex Extentabs 2067

Rifampin (Markedly reduces oral verapamil bioavailability). Products include:
- Rifadin 1528
- Rifamate Capsules 1530
- Rifater 1532
- Rimactane Capsules 847

Rocuronium Bromide (Verapamil may potentiate the activity of neuromuscular blocking agents). Products include:
- Zemuron 1830

Sotalol Hydrochloride (Concomitant intravenous beta blocker therapy results in serious toxicity in patients with CHF, recent MI or severe cardiomyopathy). Products include:
- Betapace Tablets 641

Sulindac (Administer with caution to patients receiving other highly protein bound drugs). Products include:
- Clinoril Tablets 1618

Temazepam (Administer with caution to patients receiving other highly protein bound drugs). Products include:
- Restoril Capsules 2284

Terazosin Hydrochloride (Exaggerated hypotensive response). Products include:
- Hytrin Capsules 430

Timolol Hemihydrate (Concomitant intravenous beta blocker therapy results in serious toxicity in patients with CHF, recent MI or severe cardiomyopathy). Products include:
- Betimol 0.25%, 0.5% ..... ⊙ 261

Timolol Maleate (Concomitant intravenous beta blocker therapy results in serious toxicity in patients with CHF, recent MI or severe cardiomyopathy). Products include:
- Blocadren Tablets 1614
- Timolide Tablets 1748
- Timoptic in Ocudose 1753
- Timoptic Sterile Ophthalmic Solution 1751
- Timoptic-XE 1755

Tolbutamide (Administer with caution to patients receiving other highly protein bound drugs).
- No products indexed under this heading.

Tolmetin Sodium (Administer with caution to patients receiving other highly protein bound drugs). Products include:
- Tolectin (200, 400 and 600 mg) 1581

(▣ Described in PDR For Nonprescription Drugs) (⊙ Described in PDR For Ophthalmology)

535 **Interactions Index** **Isoptin Oral**

Trimipramine Maleate (Administer with caution to patients receiving other highly protein bound drugs). Products include:
Surmontil Capsules 2811

Vecuronium Bromide (Verapamil may potentiate the activity of neuromuscular blocking agents). Products include:
Norcuron 1826

Warfarin Sodium (Administer with caution to patients receiving other highly protein bound drugs). Products include:
Coumadin 926

ISOPTIN FOR INTRAVENOUS INJECTION 5MG/2ML
(Verapamil Hydrochloride) 1344
See **Isoptin Ampules 5mg/2mL**

ISOPTIN ORAL TABLETS
(Verapamil Hydrochloride) 1346
May interact with antihypertensives, beta blockers, diuretics, inhalant anesthetics, nondepolarizing neuromuscular blocking agents, vasodilators, cardiac glycosides, lithium preparations, and ACE inhibitors. Compounds in these categories include:

Acebutolol Hydrochloride (Additive negative effects on heart rate, AV conduction and/or cardiac contractility). Products include:
Sectral Capsules 2807

Amiloride Hydrochloride (Additive effect on lowering blood pressure). Products include:
Midamor Tablets 1703
Moduretic Tablets 1705

Amlodipine Besylate (Additive effect on lowering blood pressure). Products include:
Lotrel Capsules 840
Norvasc Tablets 1940

Atenolol (Additive negative effects on heart rate, AV conduction and/or cardiac contractility). Products include:
Tenoretic Tablets 2845
Tenormin Tablets and I.V. Injection 2847

Atracurium Besylate (Potentiated). Products include:
Tracrium Injection 1183

Benazepril Hydrochloride (Additive effect on lowering blood pressure). Products include:
Lotensin Tablets 834
Lotensin HCT 837
Lotrel Capsules 840

Bendroflumethiazide (Additive effect on lowering blood pressure).
No products indexed under this heading.

Betaxolol Hydrochloride (Additive effect on lowering blood pressure). Products include:
Betoptic Ophthalmic Solution 469
Betoptic S Ophthalmic Suspension 471
Kerlone Tablets 2436

Bisoprolol Fumarate (Additive negative effects on heart rate, AV conduction and/or cardiac contractility). Products include:
Zebeta Tablets 1413
Ziac 1415

Bumetanide (Additive effect on lowering blood pressure). Products include:
Bumex 2093

Captopril (Additive effect on lowering blood pressure). Products include:
Capoten 739
Capozide 742

Carbamazepine (Increased carbamazepine concentrations). Products include:
Atretol Tablets 573
Tegretol Chewable Tablets 852
Tegretol Suspension 852
Tegretol Tablets 852

Carteolol Hydrochloride (Additive negative effects on heart rate, AV conduction and/or cardiac contractility). Products include:
Cartrol Tablets 410
Ocupress Ophthalmic Solution, 1% Sterile .... ◉ 309

Chlorothiazide (Additive effect on lowering blood pressure). Products include:
Aldoclor Tablets 1598
Diupres Tablets 1650
Diuril Oral 1653

Chlorothiazide Sodium (Additive effect on lowering blood pressure). Products include:
Diuril Sodium Intravenous 1652

Chlorthalidone (Adverse effects on cardiac function; additive effect on lowering blood pressure). Products include:
Combipres Tablets 677
Tenoretic Tablets 2845
Thalitone 1245

Cimetidine (Possible reduced verapamil clearance). Products include:
Tagamet Tablets 2516

Cimetidine Hydrochloride (Possible reduced verapamil clearance). Products include:
Tagamet 2516

Clonidine (Additive effect on lowering blood pressure). Products include:
Catapres-TTS 675

Clonidine Hydrochloride (Additive effect on lowering blood pressure; adverse effects on cardiac function). Products include:
Catapres Tablets 674
Combipres Tablets 677

Cyclosporine (Increased serum levels of cyclosporin). Products include:
Neoral 2276
Sandimmune 2286

Deserpidine (Additive effect on lowering blood pressure).
No products indexed under this heading.

Desflurane (Potential for excessive cardiovascular depression). Products include:
Suprane 1813

Deslanoside (Chronic verapamil treatment can increase serum digoxin levels and this can result in digitalis toxicity).
No products indexed under this heading.

Diazoxide (Additive negative effects on heart rate, AV conduction and/or cardiac contractility). Products include:
Hyperstat I.V. Injection 2363
Proglycem 580

Digitoxin (Chronic verapamil treatment can increase serum digoxin levels and this can result in digitalis toxicity). Products include:
Crystodigin Tablets 1433

Digoxin (Chronic verapamil treatment can increase serum digoxin levels and this can result in digitalis toxicity). Products include:
Lanoxicaps 1117
Lanoxin Elixir Pediatric 1120
Lanoxin Injection 1123
Lanoxin Injection Pediatric 1126
Lanoxin Tablets 1128

Diltiazem Hydrochloride (Additive effect on lowering blood pressure). Products include:
Cardizem CD Capsules 1506
Cardizem SR Capsules 1510
Cardizem Injectable 1508
Cardizem Tablets 1512
Dilacor XR Extended-release Capsules 2018

Disopyramide Phosphate (Should not be administered within 48 hours before or 24 hours after verapamil administration). Products include:
Norpace 2444

Doxazosin Mesylate (Additive effect on lowering blood pressure). Products include:
Cardura Tablets 2186

Enalapril Maleate (Additive effect on lowering blood pressure). Products include:
Vaseretic Tablets 1765
Vasotec Tablets 1771

Enalaprilat (Additive effect on lowering blood pressure). Products include:
Vasotec I.V. 1768

Enflurane (Potential for excessive cardiovascular depression).
No products indexed under this heading.

Esmolol Hydrochloride (Additive negative effects on heart rate, AV conduction and/or cardiac contractility). Products include:
Brevibloc Injection 1808

Ethacrynic Acid (Additive effect on lowering blood pressure). Products include:
Edecrin Tablets 1657

Felodipine (Additive effect on lowering blood pressure). Products include:
Plendil Extended-Release Tablets 527

Flecainide Acetate (Additive effects on myocardial contractility, AV conduction, and repolarization; concomitant therapy may result in negative inotropic effect and prolongation of atrioventricular conduction). Products include:
Tambocor Tablets 1497

Fosinopril Sodium (Additive effect on lowering blood pressure). Products include:
Monopril Tablets 757

Furosemide (Additive effect on lowering blood pressure). Products include:
Lasix Injection, Oral Solution and Tablets 1240

Guanabenz Acetate (Additive effect on lowering blood pressure).
No products indexed under this heading.

Guanethidine Monosulfate (Additive effect on lowering blood pressure). Products include:
Esimil Tablets 822
Ismelin Tablets 827

Halothane (Potential for excessive cardiovascular depression). Products include:
Fluothane 2724

Hydralazine Hydrochloride (Additive effect on lowering blood pressure; adverse effects on cardiac function). Products include:
Apresazide Capsules 808
Apresoline Hydrochloride Tablets .. 809
Ser-Ap-Es Tablets 849

Hydrochlorothiazide (Additive effect on lowering blood pressure). Products include:
Aldactazide 2413
Aldoril Tablets 1604
Apresazide Capsules 808
Capozide 742
Dyazide 2479
Esidrix Tablets 821
Esimil Tablets 822
HydroDIURIL Tablets 1674
Hydropres Tablets 1675
Hyzaar Tablets 1677
Inderide Tablets 2732
Inderide LA Long Acting Capsules .. 2734
Lopressor HCT Tablets 832
Lotensin HCT 837
Maxzide 1380
Moduretic Tablets 1705
Oretic Tablets 443
Prinzide Tablets 1737
Ser-Ap-Es Tablets 849
Timolide Tablets 1748
Vaseretic Tablets 1765
Zestoretic 2850
Ziac 1415

Hydroflumethiazide (Additive effect on lowering blood pressure). Products include:
Diucardin Tablets 2718

Indapamide (Additive effect on lowering blood pressure). Products include:
Lozol Tablets 2022

Isoflurane (Potential for excessive cardiovascular depression).
No products indexed under this heading.

Isradipine (Additive effect on lowering blood pressure). Products include:
DynaCirc Capsules 2256

Labetalol Hydrochloride (Additive negative effects on heart rate, AV conduction and/or cardiac contractility). Products include:
Normodyne Injection 2377
Normodyne Tablets 2379
Trandate 1185

Levobunolol Hydrochloride (Additive negative effects on heart rate, AV conduction and/or cardiac contractility). Products include:
Betagan .... ◉ 233

Lisinopril (Additive effect on lowering blood pressure). Products include:
Prinivil Tablets 1733
Prinzide Tablets 1737
Zestoretic 2850
Zestril Tablets 2854

Lithium Carbonate (May result in lowering of serum lithium levels and increased sensitivity to the effects of lithium). Products include:
Eskalith 2485
Lithium Carbonate Capsules & Tablets 2230
Lithonate/Lithotabs/Lithobid 2543

Lithium Citrate (May result in lowering of serum lithium levels and increased sensitivity to the effects of lithium).
No products indexed under this heading.

Losartan Potassium (Additive effect on lowering blood pressure). Products include:
Cozaar Tablets 1628
Hyzaar Tablets 1677

Mecamylamine Hydrochloride (Additive effect on lowering blood pressure). Products include:
Inversine Tablets 1686

Methoxyflurane (Potential for excessive cardiovascular depression).
No products indexed under this heading.

Methyclothiazide (Additive effect on lowering blood pressure). Products include:
Enduron Tablets 420

Methyldopa (Additive effect on lowering blood pressure). Products include:
Aldoclor Tablets 1598
Aldomet Oral 1600

IMPORTANT NOTE: Always consult each drug listing in the patient's regimen for possible interactions.

Aldoril Tablets ... **1604**

Methyldopate Hydrochloride (Additive effect on lowering blood pressure). Products include:

Aldomet Ester HCl Injection ... **1602**

Metipranolol Hydrochloride (Additive negative effects on heart rate, AV conduction and/or cardiac contractility). Products include:

OptiPranolol (Metipranolol 0.3%) Sterile Ophthalmic Solution ... ⊙ **258**

Metocurine Iodide (Potentiated). Products include:

Metubine Iodide Vials ... **916**

Metolazone (Additive effect on lowering blood pressure). Products include:

Mykrox Tablets ... **993**
Zaroxolyn Tablets ... **1000**

Metoprolol Succinate (Additive effect on lowering blood pressure). Products include:

Toprol-XL Tablets ... **565**

Metoprolol Tartrate (Additive negative effects on heart rate, AV conduction and/or cardiac contractility). Products include:

Lopressor Ampuls ... **830**
Lopressor HCT Tablets ... **832**
Lopressor Tablets ... **830**

Metyrosine (Additive effect on lowering blood pressure). Products include:

Demser Capsules ... **1649**

Minoxidil (Additive effect on lowering blood pressure). Products include:

Loniten Tablets ... **2618**
Rogaine Topical Solution ... **2637**

Mivacurium Chloride (Potentiated). Products include:

Mivacron ... **1138**

Moexipril Hydrochloride (Additive effect on lowering blood pressure). Products include:

Univasc Tablets ... **2410**

Nadolol (Additive negative effects on heart rate, AV conduction and/or cardiac contractility).

No products indexed under this heading.

Nicardipine Hydrochloride (Additive negative effects on heart rate, AV conduction and/or cardiac contractility). Products include:

Cardene Capsules ... **2095**
Cardene I.V. ... **2709**
Cardene SR Capsules ... **2097**

Nifedipine (Additive effect on lowering blood pressure). Products include:

Adalat Capsules (10 mg and 20 mg) ... **587**
Adalat CC ... **589**
Procardia Capsules ... **1971**
Procardia XL Extended Release Tablets ... **1972**

Nisoldipine (Additive effect on lowering blood pressure).

No products indexed under this heading.

Nitroglycerin (Additive effect on lowering blood pressure). Products include:

Deponit NTG Transdermal Delivery System ... **2397**
Nitro-Bid IV ... **1523**
Nitro-Bid Ointment ... **1524**
Nitrodisc ... **2047**
Nitro-Dur (nitroglycerin) Transdermal Infusion System ... **1326**
Nitrolingual Spray ... **2027**
Nitrostat Tablets ... **1925**
Transderm-Nitro Transdermal Therapeutic System ... **859**

Pancuronium Bromide Injection (Potentiated).

No products indexed under this heading.

Penbutolol Sulfate (Additive negative effects on heart rate, AV conduction and/or cardiac contractility). Products include:

Levatol ... **2403**

Phenoxybenzamine Hydrochloride (Additive effect on lowering blood pressure). Products include:

Dibenzyline Capsules ... **2476**

Phentolamine Mesylate (Additive effect on lowering blood pressure). Products include:

Regitine ... **846**

Pindolol (Additive negative effects on heart rate, AV conduction and/or cardiac contractility). Products include:

Visken Tablets ... **2299**

Polythiazide (Additive effect on lowering blood pressure). Products include:

Minizide Capsules ... **1938**

Prazosin Hydrochloride (May result in a reduction in blood pressure that is excessive in some patients). Products include:

Minipress Capsules ... **1937**
Minizide Capsules ... **1938**

Propranolol Hydrochloride (Additive negative effects on heart rate, AV conduction and/or cardiac contractility). Products include:

Inderal ... **2728**
Inderal LA Long Acting Capsules ... **2730**
Inderide Tablets ... **2732**
Inderide LA Long Acting Capsules ... **2734**

Quinapril Hydrochloride (Additive effect on lowering blood pressure). Products include:

Accupril Tablets ... **1893**

Quinidine Gluconate (Hypotension in patients with hypertrophic cardiomyopathy; increased quinidine levels). Products include:

Quinaglute Dura-Tabs Tablets ... **649**

Quinidine Polygalacturonate (Hypotension in patients with hypertrophic cardiomyopathy; increased quinidine levels).

No products indexed under this heading.

Quinidine Sulfate (Hypotension in patients with hypertrophic cardiomyopathy; increased quinidine levels). Products include:

Quinidex Extentabs ... **2067**

Ramipril (Additive effect on lowering blood pressure). Products include:

Altace Capsules ... **1232**

Rauwolfia Serpentina (Additive effect on lowering blood pressure).

No products indexed under this heading.

Rescinnamine (Additive effect on lowering blood pressure).

No products indexed under this heading.

Reserpine (Additive effect on lowering blood pressure). Products include:

Diupres Tablets ... **1650**
Hydropres Tablets ... **1675**
Ser-Ap-Es Tablets ... **849**

Rifampin (Reduced verapamil bioavailability). Products include:

Rifadin ... **1528**
Rifamate Capsules ... **1530**
Rifater ... **1532**
Rimactane Capsules ... **847**

Rocuronium Bromide (Potentiated). Products include:

Zemuron ... **1830**

Sodium Nitroprusside (Additive effect on lowering blood pressure).

No products indexed under this heading.

Sotalol Hydrochloride (Additive negative effects on heart rate, AV conduction and/or cardiac contractility). Products include:

Betapace Tablets ... **641**

Spirapril Hydrochloride (Additive effect on lowering blood pressure).

No products indexed under this heading.

Spironolactone (Additive effect on lowering blood pressure). Products include:

Aldactazide ... **2413**
Aldactone ... **2414**

Terazosin Hydrochloride (May result in a reduction in blood pressure that is excessive in some patients). Products include:

Hytrin Capsules ... **430**

Timolol Hemihydrate (Additive negative effects on heart rate, AV conduction and/or cardiac contractility). Products include:

Betimol 0.25%, 0.5% ... ⊙ **261**

Timolol Maleate (Additive negative effects on heart rate, AV conduction and/or cardiac contractility). Products include:

Blocadren Tablets ... **1614**
Timolide Tablets ... **1748**
Timoptic in Ocudose ... **1753**
Timoptic Sterile Ophthalmic Solution ... **1751**
Timoptic-XE ... **1755**

Torsemide (Additive effect on lowering blood pressure). Products include:

Demadex Tablets and Injection ... **686**

Triamterene (Additive effect on lowering blood pressure). Products include:

Dyazide ... **2479**
Dyrenium Capsules ... **2481**
Maxzide ... **1380**

Trimethaphan Camsylate (Additive effect on lowering blood pressure). Products include:

Arfonad Ampuls ... **2080**

Vecuronium Bromide (Verapamil prolongs recovery from the neuromuscular blockade produced by vecuronium). Products include:

Norcuron ... **1826**

ISOPTIN SR TABLETS

(Verapamil Hydrochloride) ... **1348**

May interact with antihypertensives, beta blockers, diuretics, inhalant anesthetics, neuromuscular blocking agents, vasodilators, ACE inhibitors, xanthine bronchodilators, lithium preparations, alpha adrenergic blockers, cardiac glycosides, and certain other agents. Compounds in these categories include:

Acebutolol Hydrochloride (Additive negative effects on heart rate, AV conduction and/or cardiac contractility; additive effect on lowering blood pressure). Products include:

Sectral Capsules ... **2807**

Amiloride Hydrochloride (Additive effect on lowering blood pressure). Products include:

Midamor Tablets ... **1703**
Moduretic Tablets ... **1705**

Aminophylline (Inhibition of theophylline clearance and increased plasma levels of theophylline).

No products indexed under this heading.

Amlodipine Besylate (Additive effect on lowering blood pressure). Products include:

Lotrel Capsules ... **840**
Norvasc Tablets ... **1940**

Atenolol (Additive negative effects on heart rate, AV conduction and/or cardiac contractility; potential for a variable effect on atenolol clearance; additive effect on lowering blood pressure). Products include:

Tenoretic Tablets ... **2845**
Tenormin Tablets and I.V. Injection **2847**

Atracurium Besylate (Verapamil may potentiate the activity of neuromuscular blocking agents). Products include:

Tracrium Injection ... **1183**

Benazepril Hydrochloride (Additive effect on lowering blood pressure). Products include:

Lotensin Tablets ... **834**
Lotensin HCT ... **837**
Lotrel Capsules ... **840**

Bendroflumethiazide (Additive effect on lowering blood pressure).

No products indexed under this heading.

Betaxolol Hydrochloride (Additive effect on lowering blood pressure). Products include:

Betoptic Ophthalmic Solution ... **469**
Betoptic S Ophthalmic Suspension **471**
Kerlone Tablets ... **2436**

Bisoprolol Fumarate (Additive negative effects on heart rate, AV conduction and/or cardiac contractility; additive effect on lowering blood pressure). Products include:

Zebeta Tablets ... **1413**
Ziac ... **1415**

Bumetanide (Additive effect on lowering blood pressure). Products include:

Bumex ... **2093**

Captopril (Additive effect on lowering blood pressure). Products include:

Capoten ... **739**
Capozide ... **742**

Carbamazepine (Increased carbamazepine concentrations; potential for diplopia, headache, ataxia, or dizziness). Products include:

Atretol Tablets ... **573**
Tegretol Chewable Tablets ... **852**
Tegretol Suspension ... **852**
Tegretol Tablets ... **852**

Carteolol Hydrochloride (Additive negative effects on heart rate, AV conduction and/or cardiac contractility; additive effect on lowering blood pressure). Products include:

Cartrol Tablets ... **410**
Ocupress Ophthalmic Solution, 1% Sterile ... ⊙ **309**

Chlorothiazide (Additive effect on lowering blood pressure). Products include:

Aldoclor Tablets ... **1598**
Diupres Tablets ... **1650**
Diuril Oral ... **1653**

Chlorothiazide Sodium (Additive effect on lowering blood pressure). Products include:

Diuril Sodium Intravenous ... **1652**

Chlorthalidone (Adverse effects on cardiac function; additive effect on lowering blood pressure). Products include:

Combipres Tablets ... **677**
Tenoretic Tablets ... **2845**
Thalitone ... **1245**

Cimetidine (Possible reduced verapamil clearance). Products include:

Tagamet Tablets ... **2516**

Cimetidine Hydrochloride (Possible reduced verapamil clearance). Products include:

Tagamet ... **2516**

537 Interactions Index Isoptin SR

Clonidine (Additive effect on lowering blood pressure). Products include:
Catapres-TTS ... 675

Clonidine Hydrochloride (Additive effect on lowering blood pressure; adverse effects on cardiac function). Products include:
Catapres Tablets ... 674
Combipres Tablets ... 677

Cyclosporine (Increased serum levels of cyclosporin). Products include:
Neoral ... 2276
Sandimmune ... 2286

Deserpidine (Additive effect on lowering blood pressure).
No products indexed under this heading.

Desflurane (Potential for excessive cardiovascular depression). Products include:
Suprane ... 1813

Deslanoside (Chronic verapamil treatment can increase serum digoxin levels and this can result in digitalis toxicity).
No products indexed under this heading.

Diazoxide (Additive negative effects on heart rate, AV conduction and/or cardiac contractility). Products include:
Hyperstat I.V. Injection ... 2363
Proglycem ... 580

Digitoxin (Chronic verapamil treatment can increase serum digoxin levels and this can result in digitalis toxicity). Products include:
Crystodigin Tablets ... 1433

Digoxin (Chronic verapamil treatment can increase serum digoxin levels and this can result in digitalis toxicity). Products include:
Lanoxicaps ... 1117
Lanoxin Elixir Pediatric ... 1120
Lanoxin Injection ... 1123
Lanoxin Injection Pediatric ... 1126
Lanoxin Tablets ... 1128

Diltiazem Hydrochloride (Additive effect on lowering blood pressure). Products include:
Cardizem CD Capsules ... 1506
Cardizem SR Capsules ... 1510
Cardizem Injectable ... 1508
Cardizem Tablets ... 1512
Dilacor XR Extended-release Capsules ... 2018

Disopyramide Phosphate (Should not be administered within 48 hours before or 24 hours after verapamil administration). Products include:
Norpace ... 2444

Doxacurium Chloride (Verapamil may potentiate the activity of neuromuscular blocking agents). Products include:
Nuromax Injection ... 1149

Doxazosin Mesylate (May result in a reduction in blood pressure that is excessive in some patients). Products include:
Cardura Tablets ... 2186

Dyphylline (Inhibition of theophylline clearance and increased plasma levels of theophylline). Products include:
Lufyllin & Lufyllin-400 Tablets ... 2670
Lufyllin-GG Elixir & Tablets ... 2671

Enalapril Maleate (Additive effect on lowering blood pressure). Products include:
Vaseretic Tablets ... 1765
Vasotec Tablets ... 1771

Enalaprilat (Additive effect on lowering blood pressure). Products include:
Vasotec I.V. ... 1768

Enflurane (Potential for excessive cardiovascular depression).
No products indexed under this heading.

Esmolol Hydrochloride (Additive negative effects on heart rate, AV conduction and/or cardiac contractility; additive effect on lowering blood pressure cardiac contractility; additive effect on lowering blood pressure). Products include:
Brevibloc Injection ... 1808

Ethacrynic Acid (Additive effect on lowering blood pressure). Products include:
Edecrin Tablets ... 1657

Felodipine (Additive effect on lowering blood pressure). Products include:
Plendil Extended-Release Tablets ... 527

Flecainide Acetate (Additive effects on myocardial contractility, AV conduction, and repolarization; additive negative inotropic effect). Products include:
Tambocor Tablets ... 1497

Fosinopril Sodium (Additive effect on lowering blood pressure). Products include:
Monopril Tablets ... 757

Furosemide (Additive effect on lowering blood pressure). Products include:
Lasix Injection, Oral Solution and Tablets ... 1240

Guanabenz Acetate (Additive effect on lowering blood pressure).
No products indexed under this heading.

Guanethidine Monosulfate (Additive effect on lowering blood pressure). Products include:
Esimil Tablets ... 822
Ismelin Tablets ... 827

Halothane (Potential for excessive cardiovascular depression). Products include:
Fluothane ... 2724

Hydralazine Hydrochloride (Additive effect on lowering blood pressure; adverse effects on cardiac function). Products include:
Apresazide Capsules ... 808
Apresoline Hydrochloride Tablets ... 809
Ser-Ap-Es Tablets ... 849

Hydrochlorothiazide (Additive effect on lowering blood pressure). Products include:
Aldactazide ... 2413
Aldoril Tablets ... 1604
Apresazide Capsules ... 808
Capozide ... 742
Dyazide ... 2479
Esidrix Tablets ... 821
Esimil Tablets ... 822
HydroDIURIL Tablets ... 1674
Hydropres Tablets ... 1675
Hyzaar Tablets ... 1677
Inderide Tablets ... 2732
Inderide LA Long Acting Capsules ... 2734
Lopressor HCT Tablets ... 832
Lotensin HCT ... 837
Maxzide ... 1380
Moduretic Tablets ... 1705
Oretic Tablets ... 443
Prinzide Tablets ... 1737
Ser-Ap-Es Tablets ... 849
Timolide Tablets ... 1748
Vaseretic Tablets ... 1765
Zestoretic ... 2850
Ziac ... 1415

Hydroflumethiazide (Additive effect on lowering blood pressure). Products include:
Diucardin Tablets ... 2718

Indapamide (Additive effect on lowering blood pressure). Products include:
Lozol Tablets ... 2022

Isoflurane (Potential for excessive cardiovascular depression).
No products indexed under this heading.

Isradipine (Additive effect on lowering blood pressure). Products include:
DynaCirc Capsules ... 2256

Labetalol Hydrochloride (Additive negative effects on heart rate, AV conduction and/or cardiac contractility; additive effect on lowering blood pressure). Products include:
Normodyne Injection ... 2377
Normodyne Tablets ... 2379
Trandate ... 1185

Levobunolol Hydrochloride (Additive negative effects on heart rate, AV conduction and/or cardiac contractility; additive effect on lowering blood pressure). Products include:
Betagan ... ◉ 233

Lisinopril (Additive effect on lowering blood pressure). Products include:
Prinivil Tablets ... 1733
Prinzide Tablets ... 1737
Zestoretic ... 2850
Zestril Tablets ... 2854

Lithium Carbonate (May result in lowering of serum lithium levels and increased sensitivity to the effects of lithium). Products include:
Eskalith ... 2485
Lithium Carbonate Capsules & Tablets ... 2230
Lithonate/Lithotabs/Lithobid ... 2543

Lithium Citrate (May result in lowering of serum lithium levels and increased sensitivity to the effects of lithium).
No products indexed under this heading.

Losartan Potassium (Additive effect on lowering blood pressure). Products include:
Cozaar Tablets ... 1628
Hyzaar Tablets ... 1677

Mecamylamine Hydrochloride (Additive effect on lowering blood pressure). Products include:
Inversine Tablets ... 1686

Methoxyflurane (Potential for excessive cardiovascular depression).
No products indexed under this heading.

Methyclothiazide (Additive effect on lowering blood pressure). Products include:
Enduron Tablets ... 420

Methyldopa (Additive effect on lowering blood pressure). Products include:
Aldoclor Tablets ... 1598
Aldomet Oral ... 1600
Aldoril Tablets ... 1604

Methyldopate Hydrochloride (Additive effect on lowering blood pressure). Products include:
Aldomet Ester HCl Injection ... 1602

Metipranolol Hydrochloride (Additive negative effects on heart rate, AV conduction and/or cardiac contractility; additive effect on lowering blood pressure). Products include:
OptiPranolol (Metipranolol 0.3%) Sterile Ophthalmic Solution ... ◉ 258

Metocurine Iodide (Verapamil may potentiate the activity of neuromuscular blocking agents). Products include:
Metubine Iodide Vials ... 916

Metolazone (Additive effect on lowering blood pressure). Products include:
Mykrox Tablets ... 993
Zaroxolyn Tablets ... 1000

Metoprolol Succinate (Additive negative effects on heart rate, AV conduction and/or cardiac contractility; a decrease in metoprolol clearance; additive effect on lowering blood pressure). Products include:
Toprol-XL Tablets ... 565

Metoprolol Tartrate (Additive negative effects on heart rate, AV conduction and/or cardiac contractility; a decrease in metoprolol clearance; additive effect on lowering blood pressure). Products include:
Lopressor Ampuls ... 830
Lopressor HCT Tablets ... 832
Lopressor Tablets ... 830

Metyrosine (Additive effect on lowering blood pressure). Products include:
Demser Capsules ... 1649

Minoxidil (Additive effect on lowering blood pressure). Products include:
Loniten Tablets ... 2618
Rogaine Topical Solution ... 2637

Mivacurium Chloride (Verapamil may potentiate the activity of neuromuscular blocking agents). Products include:
Mivacron ... 1138

Moexipril Hydrochloride (Additive effect on lowering blood pressure). Products include:
Univasc Tablets ... 2410

Nadolol (Additive negative effects on heart rate, AV conduction and/or cardiac contractility; additive effect on lowering blood pressure).
No products indexed under this heading.

Nicardipine Hydrochloride (Additive effect on lowering blood pressure). Products include:
Cardene Capsules ... 2095
Cardene I.V. ... 2709
Cardene SR Capsules ... 2097

Nifedipine (Additive effect on lowering blood pressure). Products include:
Adalat Capsules (10 mg and 20 mg) ... 587
Adalat CC ... 589
Procardia Capsules ... 1971
Procardia XL Extended Release Tablets ... 1972

Nisoldipine (Additive effect on lowering blood pressure).
No products indexed under this heading.

Pancuronium Bromide Injection (Verapamil may potentiate the activity of neuromuscular blocking agents).
No products indexed under this heading.

Penbutolol Sulfate (Additive negative effects on heart rate, AV conduction and/or cardiac contractility; additive effect on lowering blood pressure). Products include:
Levatol ... 2403

Phenobarbital (Increases verapamil clearance). Products include:
Arco-Lase Plus Tablets ... 512
Bellergal-S Tablets ... 2250
Donnatal ... 2060
Donnatal Extentabs ... 2061
Donnatal Tablets ... 2060
Phenobarbital Elixir and Tablets ... 1469
Quadrinal Tablets ... 1350

Phenoxybenzamine Hydrochloride (Additive effect on lowering blood pressure). Products include:
Dibenzyline Capsules ... 2476

Phentolamine Mesylate (Additive effect on lowering blood pressure). Products include:
Regitine ... 846

IMPORTANT NOTE: Always consult each drug listing in the patient's regimen for possible interactions.

Isoptin SR

Pindolol (Additive negative effects on heart rate, AV conduction and/or cardiac contractility; additive effect on lowering blood pressure). Products include:

Visken Tablets....................................... 2299

Polythiazide (Additive effect on lowering blood pressure). Products include:

Minizide Capsules 1938

Prazosin Hydrochloride (May result in a reduction in blood pressure that is excessive in some patients). Products include:

Minipress Capsules................................ 1937
Minizide Capsules 1938

Propranolol Hydrochloride (Additive negative effects on heart rate, AV conduction and/or cardiac contractility; potential for a decrease in propranolol clearance; additive effect on lowering blood pressure). Products include:

Inderal 2728
Inderal LA Long Acting Capsules 2730
Inderide Tablets 2732
Inderide LA Long Acting Capsules .. 2734

Quinapril Hydrochloride (Additive effect on lowering blood pressure). Products include:

Accupril Tablets 1893

Quinidine Gluconate (Hypotension (in patients with hypertrophic cardiomyopathy); increased quinidine levels). Products include:

Quinaglute Dura-Tabs Tablets 649

Quinidine Polygalacturonate (Hypotension (in patients with hypertrophic cardiomyopathy); increased quinidine levels).

No products indexed under this heading.

Quinidine Sulfate (Hypotension (in patients with hypertrophic cardiomyopathy); increased quinidine levels). Products include:

Quinidex Extentabs 2067

Ramipril (Additive effect on lowering blood pressure). Products include:

Altace Capsules 1232

Rauwolfia Serpentina (Additive effect on lowering blood pressure).

No products indexed under this heading.

Rescinnamine (Additive effect on lowering blood pressure).

No products indexed under this heading.

Reserpine (Additive effect on lowering blood pressure). Products include:

Diupres Tablets 1650
Hydropres Tablets................................. 1675
Ser-Ap-Es Tablets 849

Rifampin (Reduces oral verapamil bioavailability). Products include:

Rifadin 1528
Rifamate Capsules 1530
Rifater.. 1532
Rimactane Capsules.............................. 847

Rocuronium Bromide (Verapamil may potentiate the activity of neuromuscular blocking agents). Products include:

Zemuron 1830

Sodium Nitroprusside (Additive effect on lowering blood pressure).

No products indexed under this heading.

Sotalol Hydrochloride (Additive negative effects on heart rate, AV conduction and/or cardiac contractility; additive effect on lowering blood pressure). Products include:

Betapace Tablets 641

Spirapril Hydrochloride (Additive effect on lowering blood pressure).

No products indexed under this heading.

Spironolactone (Additive effect on lowering blood pressure). Products include:

Aldactazide... 2413
Aldactone 2414

Succinylcholine Chloride (Verapamil may potentiate the activity of neuromuscular blocking agents). Products include:

Anectine... 1073

Terazosin Hydrochloride (May result in a reduction in blood pressure that is excessive in some patients). Products include:

Hytrin Capsules 430

Theophylline (Inhibition of theophylline clearance and increased plasma levels of theophylline). Products include:

Marax Tablets & DF Syrup.................. 2200
Quibron 2053

Theophylline Anhydrous (Inhibition of theophylline clearance and increased plasma levels of theophylline). Products include:

Aerolate 1004
Primatene Dual Action Formula...... ⊕ 872
Primatene Tablets .... ⊕ 873
Respbid Tablets 682
Slo-bid Gyrocaps 2033
Theo-24 Extended Release Capsules 2568
Theo-Dur Extended-Release Tablets 1327
Theo-X Extended-Release Tablets .. 788
Uni-Dur Extended-Release Tablets.. 1331
Uniphyl 400 mg Tablets....................... 2001

Theophylline Calcium Salicylate (Inhibition of theophylline clearance and increased plasma levels of theophylline). Products include:

Quadrinal Tablets 1350

Theophylline Sodium Glycinate (Inhibition of theophylline clearance and increased plasma levels of theophylline).

No products indexed under this heading.

Timolol Hemihydrate (Additive negative effects on heart rate, AV conduction and/or cardiac contractility; additive effect on lowering blood pressure). Products include:

Betimol 0.25%, 0.5% .... ◎ 261

Timolol Maleate (Additive negative effects on heart rate, AV conduction and/or cardiac contractility; asymptomatic bradycardia has been reported with ophthalmic timolol and oral verapamil; additive effect on lowering blood pressure). Products include:

Blocadren Tablets 1614
Timolide Tablets.................................... 1748
Timoptic in Ocudose 1753
Timoptic Sterile Ophthalmic Solution... 1751
Timoptic-XE 1755

Torsemide (Additive effect on lowering blood pressure). Products include:

Demadex Tablets and Injection 686

Triamterene (Additive effect on lowering blood pressure). Products include:

Dyazide 2479
Dyrenium Capsules............................... 2481
Maxzide 1380

Trimethaphan Camsylate (Additive effect on lowering blood pressure). Products include:

Arfonad Ampuls 2080

Vecuronium Bromide (Verapamil prolongs recovery from the neuromuscular blockade; may potentiate the activity of neuromuscular blocking agents). Products include:

Norcuron 1826

Food Interactions

Food, unspecified (Produces decreased bioavailability (AUC) but a narrower peak to trough ratio).

ISOPTO CARBACHOL OPHTHALMIC SOLUTION

(Carbachol) .... ◎ 223
None cited in PDR database.

ISOPTO CARPINE OPHTHALMIC SOLUTION

(Pilocarpine Hydrochloride)............... ◎ 223
None cited in PDR database.

ISORDIL SUBLINGUAL TABLETS

(Isosorbide Dinitrate) 2739
May interact with vasodilators and certain other agents. Compounds in these categories include:

Diazoxide (The vasodilating effects of isosorbide dinitrate may be additive with those of other vasodilators). Products include:

Hyperstat I.V. Injection 2363
Proglycem.. 580

Hydralazine Hydrochloride (The vasodilating effects of isosorbide dinitrate may be additive with those of other vasodilators). Products include:

Apresazide Capsules 808
Apresoline Hydrochloride Tablets .. 809
Ser-Ap-Es Tablets 849

Minoxidil (The vasodilating effects of isosorbide dinitrate may be additive with those of other vasodilators). Products include:

Loniten Tablets...................................... 2618
Rogaine Topical Solution 2637

Food Interactions

Alcohol (Alcohol exhibits additive vasodilating effects).

ISORDIL TEMBIDS CAPSULES

(Isosorbide Dinitrate) 2741
May interact with vasodilators and certain other agents. Compounds in these categories include:

Diazoxide (The vasodilating effects of isosorbide dinitrate may be additive with those of other vasodilators). Products include:

Hyperstat I.V. Injection 2363
Proglycem.. 580

Hydralazine Hydrochloride (The vasodilating effects of isosorbide dinitrate may be additive with those of other vasodilators). Products include:

Apresazide Capsules 808
Apresoline Hydrochloride Tablets .. 809
Ser-Ap-Es Tablets 849

Minoxidil (The vasodilating effects of isosorbide dinitrate may be additive with those of other vasodilators). Products include:

Loniten Tablets...................................... 2618
Rogaine Topical Solution 2637

Food Interactions

Alcohol (Alcohol exhibits additive vasodilating effects).

ISORDIL TEMBIDS CONTROLLED-RELEASE TABLETS

(Isosorbide Dinitrate) 2741
See Isordil Tembids Capsules

ISORDIL TITRADOSE TABLETS

(Isosorbide Dinitrate) 2742
May interact with vasodilators and certain other agents. Compounds in these categories include:

Diazoxide (The vasodilating effects of isosorbide dinitrate may be additive with those of other vasodilators). Products include:

Hyperstat I.V. Injection 2363
Proglycem.. 580

Hydralazine Hydrochloride (The vasodilating effects of isosorbide dinitrate may be additive with those of other vasodilators). Products include:

Apresazide Capsules 808
Apresoline Hydrochloride Tablets .. 809
Ser-Ap-Es Tablets 849

Minoxidil (The vasodilating effects of isosorbide dinitrate may be additive with those of other vasodilators). Products include:

Loniten Tablets...................................... 2618
Rogaine Topical Solution 2637

Food Interactions

Alcohol (Alcohol exhibits additive vasodilating effects).

ISPAN PERFLUOROPROPANE

(Perfluoropropane) .... ◎ 276
None cited in PDR database.

ISPAN SULFUR HEXAFLUORIDE

(Sulfur Hexafluoride) .... ◎ 275
None cited in PDR database.

ISUPREL HYDROCHLORIDE INJECTION 1:5000

(Isoproterenol Hydrochloride) 2311
May interact with inhalant anesthetics and certain other agents. Compounds in these categories include:

Desflurane (Myocardium sensitized to sympathomimetic amines). Products include:

Suprane 1813

Enflurane (Myocardium sensitized to sympathomimetic amines).

No products indexed under this heading.

Epinephrine Hydrochloride (May induce serious arrhythmias). Products include:

Ana-Kit Anaphylaxis Emergency Treatment Kit 617

Halothane (Myocardium sensitized to sympathomimetic amines). Products include:

Fluothane 2724

Isoflurane (Myocardium sensitized to sympathomimetic amines).

No products indexed under this heading.

Methoxyflurane (Myocardium sensitized to sympathomimetic amines).

No products indexed under this heading.

ISUPREL HYDROCHLORIDE SOLUTION 1:200 & 1:100

(Isoproterenol Hydrochloride) 2313
May interact with beta blockers, monoamine oxidase inhibitors, tricy-

clic antidepressants, sympathomimetic bronchodilators, and sympathomimetic aerosol bronchodilators. Compounds in these categories include:

Acebutolol Hydrochloride (Inhibition of the effects of each other). Products include:

Sectral Capsules 2807

Albuterol (Potential for deleterious cardiovascular effects; should not be used concomitantly). Products include:

Proventil Inhalation Aerosol 2382
Ventolin Inhalation Aerosol and Refill 1197

Albuterol Sulfate (Potential for deleterious cardiovascular effects). Products include:

Airet Solution for Inhalation 452
Proventil Inhalation Solution 0.083% 2384
Proventil Repetabs Tablets 2386
Proventil Solution for Inhalation 0.5% 2383
Proventil Syrup 2385
Proventil Tablets 2386
Ventolin Inhalation Solution................ 1198
Ventolin Nebules Inhalation Solution 1199
Ventolin Rotacaps for Inhalation 1200
Ventolin Syrup... 1202
Ventolin Tablets....................................... 1203
Volmax Extended-Release Tablets .. 1788

Amitriptyline Hydrochloride (The action of beta adrenergic agonists on the vascular system may be potentiated). Products include:

Elavil 2838
Endep Tablets 2174
Etrafon 2355
Limbitrol 2180
Triavil Tablets 1757

Amoxapine (The action of beta adrenergic agonists on the vascular system may be potentiated). Products include:

Asendin Tablets 1369

Atenolol (Inhibition of the effects of each other). Products include:

Tenoretic Tablets.................................... 2845
Tenormin Tablets and I.V. Injection 2847

Betaxolol Hydrochloride (Inhibition of the effects of each other). Products include:

Betoptic Ophthalmic Solution........... 469
Betoptic S Ophthalmic Suspension 471
Kerlone Tablets....................................... 2436

Bisoprolol Fumarate (Inhibition of the effects of each other). Products include:

Zebeta Tablets 1413
Ziac 1415

Bitolterol Mesylate (Potential for deleterious cardiovascular effects; should not be used concomitantly). Products include:

Tornalate Solution for Inhalation, 0.2% 956
Tornalate Metered Dose Inhaler 957

Carteolol Hydrochloride (Inhibition of the effects of each other). Products include:

Cartrol Tablets 410
Ocupress Ophthalmic Solution, 1% Sterile... ◎ 309

Clomipramine Hydrochloride (The action of beta adrenergic agonists on the vascular system may be potentiated). Products include:

Anafranil Capsules 803

Desipramine Hydrochloride (The action of beta adrenergic agonists on the vascular system may be potentiated). Products include:

Norpramin Tablets 1526

Doxepin Hydrochloride (The action of beta adrenergic agonists on the vascular system may be potentiated). Products include:

Sinequan 2205

Zonalon Cream 1055

Ephedrine Hydrochloride (Potential for deleterious cardiovascular effects). Products include:

Primatene Dual Action Formula...... 🔲 872
Primatene Tablets .... 🔲 873
Quadrinal Tablets 1350

Ephedrine Sulfate (Potential for deleterious cardiovascular effects). Products include:

Bronkaid Caplets .... 🔲 717
Marax Tablets & DF Syrup.................. 2200

Ephedrine Tannate (Potential for deleterious cardiovascular effects). Products include:

Rynatuss 2673

Epinephrine (Potential for deleterious cardiovascular effects). Products include:

Bronkaid Mist .... 🔲 717
EPIFRIN .... ◎ 239
EpiPen 790
Marcaine Hydrochloride with Epinephrine 1:200,000 2316
Primatene Mist .... 🔲 873
Sensorcaine with Epinephrine Injection 559
Sus-Phrine Injection 1019
Xylocaine with Epinephrine Injections... 567

Epinephrine Hydrochloride (Potential for deleterious cardiovascular effects). Products include:

Ana-Kit Anaphylaxis Emergency Treatment Kit 617

Esmolol Hydrochloride (Inhibition of the effects of each other). Products include:

Brevibloc Injection................................. 1808

Ethylnorepinephrine Hydrochloride (Potential for deleterious cardiovascular effects).

No products indexed under this heading.

Furazolidone (The action of beta adrenergic agonists on the vascular system may be potentiated). Products include:

Furoxone 2046

Imipramine Hydrochloride (The action of beta adrenergic agonists on the vascular system may be potentiated). Products include:

Tofranil Ampuls 854
Tofranil Tablets 856

Imipramine Pamoate (The action of beta adrenergic agonists on the vascular system may be potentiated). Products include:

Tofranil-PM Capsules............................ 857

Isocarboxazid (The action of beta adrenergic agonists on the vascular system may be potentiated).

No products indexed under this heading.

Isoetharine (Potential for deleterious cardiovascular effects; should not be used concomitantly). Products include:

Bronkometer Aerosol............................ 2302
Bronkosol Solution 2302
Isoetharine Inhalation Solution, USP, Arm-a-Med................................... 551

Isoproterenol Sulfate (Potential for deleterious cardiovascular effects; should not be used concomitantly). Products include:

Norisodrine with Calcium Iodide Syrup... 442

Labetalol Hydrochloride (Inhibition of the effects of each other). Products include:

Normodyne Injection 2377
Normodyne Tablets 2379
Trandate 1185

Levobunolol Hydrochloride (Inhibition of the effects of each other). Products include:

Betagan .... ◎ 233

Maprotiline Hydrochloride (The action of beta adrenergic agonists on the vascular system may be potentiated). Products include:

Ludiomil Tablets..................................... 843

Metaproterenol Sulfate (Potential for deleterious cardiovascular effects; should not be used concomitantly). Products include:

Alupent... 669
Metaproterenol Sulfate Inhalation Solution, USP, Arm-a-Med 552

Metipranolol Hydrochloride (Inhibition of the effects of each other). Products include:

OptiPranolol (Metipranolol 0.3%) Sterile Ophthalmic Solution.......... ◎ 258

Metoprolol Succinate (Inhibition of the effects of each other). Products include:

Toprol-XL Tablets 565

Metoprolol Tartrate (Inhibition of the effects of each other). Products include:

Lopressor Ampuls 830
Lopressor HCT Tablets 832
Lopressor Tablets 830

Nadolol (Inhibition of the effects of each other).

No products indexed under this heading.

Nortriptyline Hydrochloride (The action of beta adrenergic agonists on the vascular system may be potentiated). Products include:

Pamelor 2280

Penbutolol Sulfate (Inhibition of the effects of each other). Products include:

Levatol 2403

Phenelzine Sulfate (The action of beta adrenergic agonists on the vascular system may be potentiated). Products include:

Nardil 1920

Pindolol (Inhibition of the effects of each other). Products include:

Visken Tablets... 2299

Pirbuterol Acetate (Potential for deleterious cardiovascular effects; should not be used concomitantly). Products include:

Maxair Autohaler 1492
Maxair Inhaler 1494

Propranolol Hydrochloride (Inhibition of the effects of each other). Products include:

Inderal 2728
Inderal LA Long Acting Capsules 2730
Inderide Tablets 2732
Inderide LA Long Acting Capsules .. 2734

Protriptyline Hydrochloride (The action of beta adrenergic agonists on the vascular system may be potentiated). Products include:

Vivactil Tablets 1774

Salmeterol Xinafoate (Potential for deleterious cardiovascular effects; should not be used concomitantly). Products include:

Serevent Inhalation Aerosol............... 1176

Selegiline Hydrochloride (The action of beta adrenergic agonists on the vascular system may be potentiated). Products include:

Eldepryl Tablets 2550

Sotalol Hydrochloride (Inhibition of the effects of each other). Products include:

Betapace Tablets 641

Terbutaline Sulfate (Potential for deleterious cardiovascular effects; should not be used concomitantly). Products include:

Brethaire Inhaler 813
Brethine Ampuls 815
Brethine Tablets...................................... 814
Bricanyl Subcutaneous Injection...... 1502

Bricanyl Tablets 1503

Timolol Hemihydrate (Inhibition of the effects of each other). Products include:

Betimol 0.25%, 0.5% .... ◎ 261

Timolol Maleate (Inhibition of the effects of each other). Products include:

Blocadren Tablets 1614
Timolide Tablets..................................... 1748
Timoptic in Ocudose 1753
Timoptic Sterile Ophthalmic Solution 1751
Timoptic-XE 1755

Tranylcypromine Sulfate (The action of beta adrenergic agonists on the vascular system may be potentiated). Products include:

Parnate Tablets 2503

Trimipramine Maleate (The action of beta adrenergic agonists on the vascular system may be potentiated). Products include:

Surmontil Capsules................................ 2811

ISUPREL MISTOMETER (Isoproterenol Hydrochloride) ....2312 May interact with:

Epinephrine Hydrochloride (May induce serious arrhythmias). Products include:

Ana-Kit Anaphylaxis Emergency Treatment Kit 617

ITCH-X GEL (Pramoxine Hydrochloride, Benzyl Alcohol) .... 🔲 602 None cited in PDR database.

ITCH-X SPRAY (Pramoxine Hydrochloride, Benzyl Alcohol) .... 🔲 602 None cited in PDR database.

JE-VAX (Japanese Encephalitis Vaccine Inactivated)... 886 None cited in PDR database.

JEVITY ISOTONIC LIQUID NUTRITION WITH FIBER (Nutritional Supplement) ....2221 None cited in PDR database.

K-DUR MICROBURST RELEASE SYSTEM (POTASSIUM CHLORIDE, USP) E.R. TABLETS (Potassium Chloride)..............................1325 May interact with potassium sparing diuretics and ACE inhibitors. Compounds in these categories include:

Amiloride Hydrochloride (Severe hyperkalemia). Products include:

Midamor Tablets 1703
Moduretic Tablets 1705

Benazepril Hydrochloride (Potential for increased potassium retention). Products include:

Lotensin Tablets 834
Lotensin HCT.. 837
Lotrel Capsules....................................... 840

Captopril (Potential for increased potassium retention). Products include:

Capoten 739
Capozide 742

Enalapril Maleate (Potential for increased potassium retention). Products include:

Vaseretic Tablets 1765
Vasotec Tablets 1771

Enalaprilat (Potential for increased potassium retention). Products include:

Vasotec I.V. 1768

IMPORTANT NOTE: Always consult each drug listing in the patient's regimen for possible interactions.

K-Dur Interactions Index 540

Fosinopril Sodium (Potential for increased potassium retention). Products include:

- Monopril Tablets 757

Lisinopril (Potential for increased potassium retention). Products include:

- Prinivil Tablets 1733
- Prinzide Tablets 1737
- Zestoretic 2850
- Zestril Tablets 2854

Moexipril Hydrochloride (Potential for increased potassium retention). Products include:

- Univasc Tablets 2410

Quinapril Hydrochloride (Potential for increased potassium retention). Products include:

- Accupril Tablets 1893

Ramipril (Potential for increased potassium retention). Products include:

- Altace Capsules 1232

Spirapril Hydrochloride (Potential for increased potassium retention).

No products indexed under this heading.

Spironolactone (Severe hyperkalemia). Products include:

- Aldactazide........ 2413
- Aldactone 2414

Triamterene (Severe hyperkalemia). Products include:

- Dyazide 2479
- Dyrenium Capsules........ 2481
- Maxzide 1380

K-LOR POWDER PACKETS

(Potassium Chloride)........ 434

May interact with potassium sparing diuretics and ACE inhibitors. Compounds in these categories include:

Amiloride Hydrochloride (Potential for severe hyperkalemia). Products include:

- Midamor Tablets 1703
- Moduretic Tablets 1705

Benazepril Hydrochloride (Potential for hyperkalemia). Products include:

- Lotensin Tablets........ 834
- Lotensin HCT........ 837
- Lotrel Capsules........ 840

Captopril (Potential for hyperkalemia). Products include:

- Capoten 739
- Capozide 742

Enalapril Maleate (Potential for hyperkalemia). Products include:

- Vaseretic Tablets 1765
- Vasotec Tablets 1771

Enalaprilat (Potential for hyperkalemia). Products include:

- Vasotec I.V........ 1768

Fosinopril Sodium (Potential for hyperkalemia). Products include:

- Monopril Tablets 757

Lisinopril (Potential for hyperkalemia). Products include:

- Prinivil Tablets 1733
- Prinzide Tablets 1737
- Zestoretic 2850
- Zestril Tablets 2854

Moexipril Hydrochloride (Potential for hyperkalemia). Products include:

- Univasc Tablets 2410

Quinapril Hydrochloride (Potential for hyperkalemia). Products include:

- Accupril Tablets 1893

Ramipril (Potential for hyperkalemia). Products include:

- Altace Capsules 1232

Spirapril Hydrochloride (Potential for hyperkalemia).

No products indexed under this heading.

Spironolactone (Potential for severe hyperkalemia). Products include:

- Aldactazide........ 2413
- Aldactone 2414

Triamterene (Potential for severe hyperkalemia). Products include:

- Dyazide 2479
- Dyrenium Capsules........ 2481
- Maxzide 1380

K-NORM EXTENDED-RELEASE CAPSULES

(Potassium Chloride)........ 991

May interact with potassium sparing diuretics, ACE inhibitors, and anticholinergics. Compounds in these categories include:

Amiloride Hydrochloride (Concurrent administration can produce severe hyperkalemia). Products include:

- Midamor Tablets 1703
- Moduretic Tablets 1705

Atropine Sulfate (Anticholinergic drugs can be cause for delay or arrest in tablet passage through the gastrointestinal tract; concomitant administration of drugs capable of decreasing GI motility should be avoided). Products include:

- Arco-Lase Plus Tablets 512
- Atrohist Plus Tablets 454
- Atropine Sulfate Sterile Ophthalmic Solution .... ◉ 233
- Donnatal 2060
- Donnatal Extentabs........ 2061
- Donnatal Tablets 2060
- Lomotil 2439
- Motofen Tablets 784
- Urised Tablets........ 1964

Belladonna Alkaloids (Anticholinergic drugs can be cause for delay or arrest in tablet passage through the gastrointestinal tract; concomitant administration of drugs capable of decreasing GI motility should be avoided). Products include:

- Bellergal-S Tablets 2250
- Hyland's Bed Wetting Tablets .... ▣ 828
- Hyland's EnurAid Tablets........ ▣ 829
- Hyland's Teething Tablets .... ▣ 830

Benazepril Hydrochloride (Potential for severe hyperkalemia). Products include:

- Lotensin Tablets........ 834
- Lotensin HCT........ 837
- Lotrel Capsules........ 840

Benztropine Mesylate (Anticholinergic drugs can be cause for delay or arrest in tablet passage through the gastrointestinal tract; concomitant administration of drugs capable of decreasing GI motility should be avoided). Products include:

- Cogentin 1621

Biperiden Hydrochloride (Anticholinergic drugs can be cause for delay or arrest in tablet passage through the gastrointestinal tract; concomitant administration of drugs capable of decreasing GI motility should be avoided). Products include:

- Akineton 1333

Captopril (Potential for severe hyperkalemia). Products include:

- Capoten 739
- Capozide 742

Clidinium Bromide (Anticholinergic drugs can be cause for delay or arrest in tablet passage through the gastrointestinal tract; concomitant administration of drugs capable of decreasing GI motility should be avoided). Products include:

- Librax Capsules 2176
- Quarzan Capsules 2181

Dicyclomine Hydrochloride (Anticholinergic drugs can be cause for delay or arrest in tablet passage through the gastrointestinal tract; concomitant administration of drugs capable of decreasing GI motility should be avoided). Products include:

- Bentyl 1501

Enalapril Maleate (Potential for severe hyperkalemia). Products include:

- Vaseretic Tablets 1765
- Vasotec Tablets 1771

Enalaprilat (Potential for severe hyperkalemia). Products include:

- Vasotec I.V........ 1768

Fosinopril Sodium (Potential for severe hyperkalemia). Products include:

- Monopril Tablets 757

Glycopyrrolate (Anticholinergic drugs can be cause for delay or arrest in tablet passage through the gastrointestinal tract; concomitant administration of drugs capable of decreasing GI motility should be avoided). Products include:

- Robinul Forte Tablets........ 2072
- Robinul Injectable 2072
- Robinul Tablets........ 2072

Hyoscyamine (Anticholinergic drugs can be cause for delay or arrest in tablet passage through the gastrointestinal tract; concomitant administration of drugs capable of decreasing GI motility should be avoided). Products include:

- Cystospaz Tablets 1963
- Urised Tablets........ 1964

Hyoscyamine Sulfate (Anticholinergic drugs can be cause for delay or arrest in tablet passage through the gastrointestinal tract; concomitant administration of drugs capable of decreasing GI motility should be avoided). Products include:

- Arco-Lase Plus Tablets 512
- Atrohist Plus Tablets 454
- Cystospaz-M Capsules 1963
- Donnatal 2060
- Donnatal Extentabs........ 2061
- Donnatal Tablets 2060
- Kutrase Capsules........ 2402
- Levsin/Levsinex/Levbid 2405

Ipratropium Bromide (Anticholinergic drugs can be cause for delay or arrest in tablet passage through the gastrointestinal tract; concomitant administration of drugs capable of decreasing GI motility should be avoided). Products include:

- Atrovent Inhalation Aerosol........ 671
- Atrovent Inhalation Solution 673

Lisinopril (Potential for severe hyperkalemia). Products include:

- Prinivil Tablets 1733
- Prinzide Tablets........ 1737
- Zestoretic 2850
- Zestril Tablets........ 2854

Mepenzolate Bromide (Anticholinergic drugs can be cause for delay or arrest in tablet passage through the gastrointestinal tract; concomitant administration of drugs capable of decreasing GI motility should be avoided).

No products indexed under this heading.

Moexipril Hydrochloride (Potential for severe hyperkalemia). Products include:

- Univasc Tablets 2410

Oxybutynin Chloride (Anticholinergic drugs can be cause for delay or arrest in tablet passage through the gastrointestinal tract; concomitant administration of drugs capable of decreasing GI motility should be avoided). Products include:

- Ditropan........ 1516

Procyclidine Hydrochloride (Anticholinergic drugs can be cause for delay or arrest in tablet passage through the gastrointestinal tract; concomitant administration of drugs capable of decreasing GI motility should be avoided). Products include:

- Kemadrin Tablets 1112

Propantheline Bromide (Anticholinergic drugs can be cause for delay or arrest in tablet passage through the gastrointestinal tract; concomitant administration of drugs capable of decreasing GI motility should be avoided). Products include:

- Pro-Banthīne Tablets........ 2052

Quinapril Hydrochloride (Potential for severe hyperkalemia). Products include:

- Accupril Tablets 1893

Ramipril (Potential for severe hyperkalemia). Products include:

- Altace Capsules 1232

Scopolamine (Anticholinergic drugs can be cause for delay or arrest in tablet passage through the gastrointestinal tract; concomitant administration of drugs capable of decreasing GI motility should be avoided). Products include:

- Transderm Scōp Transdermal Therapeutic System 869

Scopolamine Hydrobromide (Anticholinergic drugs can be cause for delay or arrest in tablet passage through the gastrointestinal tract; concomitant administration of drugs capable of decreasing GI motility should be avoided). Products include:

- Atrohist Plus Tablets 454
- Donnatal 2060
- Donnatal Extentabs........ 2061
- Donnatal Tablets 2060

Spirapril Hydrochloride (Potential for severe hyperkalemia).

No products indexed under this heading.

Spironolactone (Concurrent administration can produce severe hyperkalemia). Products include:

- Aldactazide........ 2413
- Aldactone 2414

Triamterene (Concurrent administration can produce severe hyperkalemia). Products include:

- Dyazide 2479
- Dyrenium Capsules........ 2481
- Maxzide 1380

Tridihexethyl Chloride (Anticholinergic drugs can be cause for delay or arrest in tablet passage through the gastrointestinal tract; concomitant administration of drugs capable of decreasing GI motility should be avoided).

No products indexed under this heading.

(▣ Described in PDR For Nonprescription Drugs) (◉ Described in PDR For Ophthalmology)

Trihexyphenidyl Hydrochloride

(Anticholinergic drugs can be cause for delay or arrest in tablet passage through the gastrointestinal tract; concomitant administration of drugs capable of decreasing GI motility should be avoided). Products include:

Artane 1368

K-PHOS NEUTRAL TABLETS

(Potassium Phosphate, Monobasic, Sodium Phosphate, Monobasic, Sodium Phosphate, Dibasic) **639**

May interact with antacids, catecholamine depleting drugs, calcium preparations, salicylates, potassium preparations, corticosteroids, potassium sparing diuretics, and certain other agents. Compounds in these categories include:

ACTH (Hypernatremia).

No products indexed under this heading.

Aluminum Carbonate Gel (May bind phosphate and prevent its absorption). Products include:

Basaljel 2703

Aluminum Hydroxide (May bind phosphate and prevent its absorption). Products include:

ALternaGEL Liquid 1316
Maximum Strength Ascriptin .... ⊕ 630
Cama Arthritis Pain Reliever .... ⊕ 785
Gaviscon Extra Strength Relief Formula Antacid Tablets .... ⊕ 819
Gaviscon Extra Strength Relief Formula Liquid Antacid .... ⊕ 819
Gaviscon Liquid Antacid .... ⊕ 820
Gelusil Liquid & Tablets .... ⊕ 855
Maalox Heartburn Relief Suspension .... ⊕ 642
Maalox Heartburn Relief Tablets .... ⊕ 641
Maalox Magnesia and Alumina Oral Suspension .... ⊕ 642
Maalox Plus Tablets .... ⊕ 643
Extra Strength Maalox Antacid Plus Antigas Liquid and Tablets ⊕ 638
Tempo Soft Antacid .... ⊕ 835

Aluminum Hydroxide Gel (May bind phosphate and prevent its absorption). Products include:

ALternaGEL Liquid .... ⊕ 659
Aludrox Oral Suspension 2695
Amphojel Suspension 2695
Amphojel Suspension without Flavor 2695
Amphojel Tablets 2695
Arthritis Pain Ascriptin .... ⊕ 631
Regular Strength Ascriptin Tablets .... ⊕ 629
Gaviscon Antacid Tablets .... ⊕ 819
Gaviscon-2 Antacid Tablets .... ⊕ 820
Mylanta Liquid 1317
Mylanta Tablets .... ⊕ 660
Mylanta Double Strength Liquid 1317
Mylanta Double Strength Tablets .. ⊕ 660
Nephrox Suspension .... ⊕ 655

Aluminum Hydroxide Gel, Dried (May bind phosphate and prevent its absorption).

Amiloride Hydrochloride (Hyperkalemia; monitor potassium levels periodically). Products include:

Midamor Tablets 1703
Moduretic Tablets 1705

Betamethasone Acetate (Hypernatremia). Products include:

Celestone Soluspan Suspension 2347

Betamethasone Sodium Phosphate (Hypernatremia). Products include:

Celestone Soluspan Suspension 2347

Calcium Carbonate (May antagonize effects of phosphates in treatment of hypercalcemia). Products include:

Alka-Mints Chewable Antacid .... ⊕ 701
Arthritis Pain Ascriptin .... ⊕ 631
Maximum Strength Ascriptin .... ⊕ 630
Regular Strength Ascriptin Tablets .... ⊕ 629
Extra Strength Bayer Plus Aspirin Caplets .... ⊕ 713
Bufferin Analgesic Tablets and Caplets .... ⊕ 613
Calci-Chew Tablets 2004
Calci-Mix Capsules 2004
Caltrate 600 .... ⊕ 665
Caltrate PLUS .... ⊕ 665
Caltrate 600 + D .... ⊕ 665
Centrum Singles Calcium .... ⊕ 669
Chooz Antacid Gum .... ⊕ 799
Di-Gel Antacid/Anti-Gas .... ⊕ 801
Gerimed Tablets 982
Maalox Antacid Caplets .... ⊕ 638
Marblen .... ⊕ 655
Materna Tablets 1379
Mylanta Calcium Carbonate and Magnesium Hydroxide Tablets 1318
Mylanta Gelcaps Antacid .... ⊕ 662
Mylanta Soothing Lozenges 1319
Nephro-Calci Tablets 2004
Rolaids Tablets .... ⊕ 843
Rolaids (Calcium Rich/Sodium Free) Tablets .... ⊕ 843
Tempo Soft Antacid .... ⊕ 835
Titralac .... ⊕ 672
Titralac Plus .... ⊕ 672
Tums Antacid Tablets .... ⊕ 827
Tums Anti-gas/Antacid Formula Tablets, Assorted Fruit .... ⊕ 827
Tums E-X Antacid Tablets .... ⊕ 827
Tums 500 Calcium Supplement .... ⊕ 828
Tums ULTRA Antacid Tablets .... ⊕ 827
TYLENOL, Extra Strength, Headache Plus Pain Reliever with Antacid Caplets 1559

Calcium Chloride (May antagonize effects of phosphates in treatment of hypercalcemia).

No products indexed under this heading.

Calcium Citrate (May antagonize effects of phosphates in treatment of hypercalcemia). Products include:

Citracal 1779
Citracal Caplets + D 1780
Citracal Liquitab 1780

Calcium Glubionate (May antagonize effects of phosphates in treatment of hypercalcemia).

No products indexed under this heading.

Cortisone Acetate (Hypernatremia). Products include:

Cortone Acetate Sterile Suspension 1623
Cortone Acetate Tablets 1624

Deserpidine (Hypernatremia).

No products indexed under this heading.

Desoxycorticosterone Acetate (Hypernatremia).

Dexamethasone (Hypernatremia). Products include:

AK-Trol Ointment & Suspension .... ◎ 205
Decadron Elixir 1633
Decadron Tablets 1635
Decaspray Topical Aerosol 1648
Dexacidin Ointment .... ◎ 263
Maxitrol Ophthalmic Ointment and Suspension .... ◎ 224
TobraDex Ophthalmic Suspension and Ointment 473

Dexamethasone Acetate (Hypernatremia). Products include:

Dalalone D.P. Injectable 1011
Decadron-LA Sterile Suspension 1646

Dexamethasone Sodium Phosphate (Hypernatremia). Products include:

Decadron Phosphate Injection 1637
Decadron Phosphate Respihaler 1642
Decadron Phosphate Sterile Ophthalmic Ointment 1641
Decadron Phosphate Sterile Ophthalmic Solution 1642
Decadron Phosphate Topical Cream 1644
Decadron Phosphate Turbinaire 1645
Decadron Phosphate with Xylocaine Injection, Sterile 1639
Dexacort Phosphate in Respihaler .. 458
Dexacort Phosphate in Turbinaire .. 459

NeoDecadron Sterile Ophthalmic Ointment 1712
NeoDecadron Sterile Ophthalmic Solution 1713
NeoDecadron Topical Cream 1714

Diazoxide (Hypernatremia). Products include:

Hyperstat I.V. Injection 2363
Proglycem 580

Dihydroxyaluminum Sodium Carbonate (May bind phosphate and prevent its absorption).

No products indexed under this heading.

Fludrocortisone Acetate (Hypernatremia). Products include:

Florinef Acetate Tablets 505

Guanethidine Monosulfate (Hypernatremia). Products include:

Esimil Tablets 822
Ismelin Tablets 827

Hydralazine Hydrochloride (Hypernatremia). Products include:

Apresazide Capsules 808
Apresoline Hydrochloride Tablets .. 809
Ser-Ap-Es Tablets 849

Hydrocortisone (Hypernatremia). Products include:

Anusol-HC Cream 2.5% 1896
Aquanil HC Lotion 1931
Bactine Hydrocortisone Anti-Itch Cream .... ⊕ 709
Caldecort Anti-Itch Hydrocortisone Spray .... ⊕ 631
Cortaid .... ⊕ 836
CORTENEMA 2535
Cortisporin Ointment 1085
Cortisporin Ophthalmic Ointment Sterile 1085
Cortisporin Ophthalmic Suspension Sterile 1086
Cortisporin Otic Solution Sterile 1087
Cortisporin Otic Suspension Sterile 1088
Cortizone-5 .... ⊕ 831
Cortizone-10 .... ⊕ 831
Hydrocortone Tablets 1672
Hytone 907
Massengill Medicated Soft Cloth Towelettes 2458
PediOtic Suspension Sterile 1153
Preparation H Hydrocortisone 1% Cream .... ⊕ 872
ProctoCream-HC 2.5% 2408
VōSoL HC Otic Solution 2678

Hydrocortisone Acetate (Hypernatremia). Products include:

Analpram-HC Rectal Cream 1% and 2.5% 977
Anusol HC-1 Anti-Itch Hydrocortisone Ointment .... ⊕ 847
Anusol-HC Suppositories 1897
Caldecort .... ⊕ 631
Carmol HC 924
Coly-Mycin S Otic w/Neomycin & Hydrocortisone 1906
Cortaid .... ⊕ 836
Cortifoam 2396
Cortisporin Cream 1084
Epifoam 2399
Hydrocortone Acetate Sterile Suspension 1669
Mantadil Cream 1135
Nupercainal Hydrocortisone 1% Cream .... ⊕ 645
Ophthocort .... ◎ 311
Pramosone Cream, Lotion & Ointment 978
ProctoCream-HC 2408
ProctoFoam-HC 2409
Terra-Cortril Ophthalmic Suspension 2210

Hydrocortisone Sodium Phosphate (Hypernatremia). Products include:

Hydrocortone Phosphate Injection, Sterile 1670

Hydrocortisone Sodium Succinate (Hypernatremia). Products include:

Solu-Cortef Sterile Powder 2641

Magaldrate (May bind phosphate and prevent its absorption).

No products indexed under this heading.

Magnesium Hydroxide (May bind phosphate and prevent its absorption). Products include:

Aludrox Oral Suspension 2695
Arthritis Pain Ascriptin .... ⊕ 631
Maximum Strength Ascriptin .... ⊕ 630
Regular Strength Ascriptin Tablets .... ⊕ 629
Di-Gel Antacid/Anti-Gas .... ⊕ 801
Gelusil Liquid & Tablets .... ⊕ 855
Maalox Magnesia and Alumina Oral Suspension .... ⊕ 642
Maalox Plus Tablets .... ⊕ 643
Extra Strength Maalox Antacid Plus Antigas Liquid and Tablets ⊕ 638
Mylanta Calcium Carbonate and Magnesium Hydroxide Tablets 1318
Mylanta Liquid 1317
Mylanta Tablets .... ⊕ 660
Mylanta Double Strength Liquid 1317
Mylanta Double Strength Tablets .. ⊕ 660
Phillips' Milk of Magnesia Liquid .... ⊕ 729
Rolaids Tablets .... ⊕ 843
Tempo Soft Antacid .... ⊕ 835

Magnesium Oxide (May bind phosphate and prevent its absorption). Products include:

Beelith Tablets 639
Bufferin Analgesic Tablets and Caplets .... ⊕ 613
Caltrate PLUS .... ⊕ 665
Cama Arthritis Pain Reliever .... ⊕ 785
Mag-Ox 400 668
Uro-Mag 668

Methyldopa (Hypernatremia). Products include:

Aldoclor Tablets 1598
Aldomet Oral 1600
Aldoril Tablets 1604

Methyldopate Hydrochloride (Hypernatremia). Products include:

Aldomet Ester HCl Injection 1602

Methylprednisolone Acetate (Hypernatremia). Products include:

Depo-Medrol Single-Dose Vial 2600
Depo-Medrol Sterile Aqueous Suspension 2597

Methylprednisolone Sodium Succinate (Hypernatremia). Products include:

Solu-Medrol Sterile Powder 2643

Potassium Acid Phosphate (Hyperkalemia; monitor potassium levels periodically). Products include:

K-Phos Original Formula 'Sodium Free' Tablets 639

Potassium Bicarbonate (Hyperkalemia; monitor potassium levels periodically). Products include:

Alka-Seltzer Gold Effervescent Antacid .... ⊕ 703

Potassium Chloride (Hyperkalemia; monitor potassium levels periodically). Products include:

Chlor-3 Condiment 1004
K-Dur Microburst Release System (potassium chloride, USP) E.R. Tablets 1325
K-Lor Powder Packets 434
K-Norm Extended-Release Capsules 991
K-Tab Filmtab 434
Kolyum Liquid 992
Micro-K 2063
Micro-K LS Packets 2064
NuLYTELY 689
Cherry Flavor NuLYTELY 689
Rum-K Syrup 1005
Slow-K Extended-Release Tablets 851

Potassium Citrate (Hyperkalemia; monitor potassium levels periodically). Products include:

Polycitra Syrup 578
Polycitra-K Crystals 579
Polycitra-K Oral Solution 579
Polycitra-LC 578

Potassium Gluconate (Hyperkalemia; monitor potassium levels periodically). Products include:

Kolyum Liquid 992

IMPORTANT NOTE: Always consult each drug listing in the patient's regimen for possible interactions.

Potassium Phosphate, Dibasic (Hyperkalemia; monitor potassium levels periodically).
No products indexed under this heading.

Prednisolone Acetate (Hypernatremia). Products include:
AK-CIDE ... ⊙ 202
AK-CIDE Ointment ... ⊙ 202
Blephamide Liquifilm Sterile Ophthalmic Suspension ... 476
Blephamide Ointment ... ⊙ 237
Econopred & Econopred Plus Ophthalmic Suspensions ... ⊙ 217
Poly-Pred Liquifilm ... ⊙ 248
Pred Forte ... ⊙ 250
Pred Mild ... ⊙ 253
Pred-G Liquifilm Sterile Ophthalmic Suspension ... ⊙ 251
Pred-G S.O.P. Sterile Ophthalmic Ointment ... ⊙ 252
Vasocidin Ointment ... ⊙ 268

Prednisolone Sodium Phosphate (Hypernatremia). Products include:
AK-Pred ... ⊙ 204
Hydeltrasol Injection, Sterile ... 1665
Inflamase ... ⊙ 265
Pediapred Oral Liquid ... 995
Vasocidin Ophthalmic Solution ... ⊙ 270

Prednisolone Tebutate (Hypernatremia). Products include:
Hydeltra-T.B.A. Sterile Suspension 1667

Prednisone (Hypernatremia). Products include:
Deltasone Tablets ... 2595

Rauwolfia Serpentina (Hypernatremia).
No products indexed under this heading.

Rescinnamine (Hypernatremia).
No products indexed under this heading.

Reserpine (Hypernatremia). Products include:
Diupres Tablets ... 1650
Hydropres Tablets ... 1675
Ser-Ap-Es Tablets ... 849

Spironolactone (Hyperkalemia; monitor potassium levels periodically). Products include:
Aldactazide ... 2413
Aldactone ... 2414

Triamcinolone (Hypernatremia). Products include:
Aristocort Tablets ... 1022

Triamcinolone Acetonide (Hypernatremia). Products include:
Aristocort A 0.025% Cream ... 1027
Aristocort A 0.5% Cream ... 1031
Aristocort A 0.1% Cream ... 1029
Aristocort A 0.1% Ointment ... 1030
Azmacort Oral Inhaler ... 2011
Nasacort Nasal Inhaler ... 2024

Triamcinolone Diacetate (Hypernatremia). Products include:
Aristocort Suspension (Forte Parenteral) ... 1027
Aristocort Suspension (Intralesional) ... 1025

Triamcinolone Hexacetonide (Hypernatremia). Products include:
Aristospan Suspension (Intra-articular) ... 1033
Aristospan Suspension (Intralesional) ... 1032

Triamterene (Hyperkalemia; monitor potassium levels periodically). Products include:
Dyazide ... 2479
Dyrenium Capsules ... 2481
Maxzide ... 1380

Trichlormethiazide (Hypernatremia).
No products indexed under this heading.

Vitamin D (May antagonize effects of phosphates in treatment of hypercalcemia). Products include:
Caltrate PLUS ... ▣ 665
Caltrate 600 + D ... ▣ 665
Citracal Caplets + D ... 1780
Dical-D Tablets & Wafers ... 420
Drisdol ... ▣ 794
Materna Tablets ... 1379
Megadose ... 512
Zymacap Capsules ... ▣ 772

K-PHOS ORIGINAL FORMULA 'SODIUM FREE' TABLETS

(Potassium Acid Phosphate) ... 639
May interact with antacids, potassium sparing diuretics, salicylates, potassium preparations, and certain other agents. Compounds in these categories include:

Aluminum Carbonate Gel (May bind phosphate and prevent its absorption). Products include:
Basaljel ... 2703

Aluminum Hydroxide (May bind phosphate and prevent its absorption). Products include:
ALternaGEL Liquid ... 1316
Maximum Strength Ascriptin ... ▣ 630
Cama Arthritis Pain Reliever ... ▣ 785
Gaviscon Extra Strength Relief Formula Antacid Tablets ... ▣ 819
Gaviscon Extra Strength Relief Formula Liquid Antacid ... ▣ 819
Gaviscon Liquid Antacid ... ▣ 820
Gelusil Liquid & Tablets ... ▣ 855
Maalox Heartburn Relief Suspension ... ▣ 642
Maalox Heartburn Relief Tablets ... ▣ 641
Maalox Magnesia and Alumina Oral Suspension ... ▣ 642
Maalox Plus Tablets ... ▣ 643
Extra Strength Maalox Antacid Plus Antigas Liquid and Tablets ▣ 638
Tempo Soft Antacid ... ▣ 835

Aluminum Hydroxide Gel (May bind phosphate and prevent its absorption). Products include:
ALternaGEL Liquid ... ▣ 659
Aludrox Oral Suspension ... 2695
Amphojel Suspension ... 2695
Amphojel Suspension without Flavor ... 2695
Amphojel Tablets ... 2695
Arthritis Pain Ascriptin ... ▣ 631
Regular Strength Ascriptin Tablets ... ▣ 629
Gaviscon Antacid Tablets ... ▣ 819
Gaviscon-2 Antacid Tablets ... ▣ 820
Mylanta Liquid ... 1317
Mylanta Tablets ... ▣ 660
Mylanta Double Strength Liquid ... 1317
Mylanta Double Strength Tablets .. ▣ 660
Nephrox Suspension ... ▣ 655

Aluminum Hydroxide Gel, Dried (May bind phosphate and prevent its absorption).

Amiloride Hydrochloride (Hyperkalemia). Products include:
Midamor Tablets ... 1703
Moduretic Tablets ... 1705

Aspirin (Increased serum salicylate levels; possible toxicity). Products include:
Alka-Seltzer Effervescent Antacid and Pain Reliever ... ▣ 701
Alka-Seltzer Extra Strength Effervescent Antacid and Pain Reliever ... ▣ 703
Alka-Seltzer Lemon Lime Effervescent Antacid and Pain Reliever ... ▣ 703
Alka-Seltzer Plus Cold Medicine ... ▣ 705
Alka-Seltzer Plus Cold & Cough Medicine ... ▣ 708
Alka-Seltzer Plus Night-Time Cold Medicine ... ▣ 707
Alka Seltzer Plus Sinus Medicine .. ▣ 707
Arthritis Foundation Safety Coated Aspirin Tablets ... ▣ 675
Arthritis Pain Ascriptin ... ▣ 631
Maximum Strength Ascriptin ... ▣ 630
Regular Strength Ascriptin Tablets ... ▣ 629
Arthritis Strength BC Powder ... ▣ 609
BC Cold Powder Multi-Symptom Formula (Cold-Sinus-Allergy) ... ▣ 609
BC Cold Powder Non-Drowsy Formula (Cold-Sinus) ... ▣ 609
BC Powder ... ▣ 609
Bayer Children's Chewable Aspirin ... ▣ 711
Genuine Bayer Aspirin Tablets & Caplets ... ▣ 713
Extra Strength Bayer Arthritis Pain Regimen Formula ... ▣ 711
Extra Strength Bayer Aspirin Caplets & Tablets ... ▣ 712
Extended-Release Bayer 8-Hour Aspirin ... ▣ 712
Extra Strength Bayer Plus Aspirin Caplets ... ▣ 713
Extra Strength Bayer PM Aspirin .. ▣ 713
Bayer Enteric Aspirin ... ▣ 709
Bufferin Analgesic Tablets and Caplets ... ▣ 613
Arthritis Strength Bufferin Analgesic Caplets ... ▣ 614
Extra Strength Bufferin Analgesic Tablets ... ▣ 615
Cama Arthritis Pain Reliever ... ▣ 785
Darvon Compound-65 Pulvules ... 1435
Easprin ... 1914
Ecotrin ... 2455
Ecotrin Enteric Coated Aspirin Maximum Strength Tablets and Caplets ... ▣ 816
Ecotrin Enteric Coated Aspirin Regular Strength Tablets ... 2455
Empirin Aspirin Tablets ... ▣ 854
Empirin with Codeine Tablets ... 1093
Excedrin Extra-Strength Analgesic Tablets & Caplets ... 732
Fiorinal Capsules ... 2261
Fiorinal with Codeine Capsules ... 2262
Fiorinal Tablets ... 2261
Halfprin ... 1362
Healthprin Aspirin ... 2455
Norgesic ... 1496
Percodan Tablets ... 939
Percodan-Demi Tablets ... 940
Robaxisal Tablets ... 2071
Soma Compound w/Codeine Tablets ... 2676
Soma Compound Tablets ... 2675
St. Joseph Adult Chewable Aspirin (81 mg.) ... ▣ 808
Talwin Compound ... 2335
Ursinus Inlay-Tabs ... ▣ 794
Vanquish Analgesic Caplets ... ▣ 731

Choline Magnesium Trisalicylate (Increased serum salicylate levels; possible toxicity). Products include:
Trilisate ... 2000

Diflunisal (Increased serum salicylate levels; possible toxicity). Products include:
Dolobid Tablets ... 1654

Dihydroxyaluminum Sodium Carbonate (May bind phosphate and prevent its absorption).
No products indexed under this heading.

Magaldrate (May bind phosphate and prevent its absorption).
No products indexed under this heading.

Magnesium Hydroxide (May bind phosphate and prevent its absorption). Products include:
Aludrox Oral Suspension ... 2695
Arthritis Pain Ascriptin ... ▣ 631
Maximum Strength Ascriptin ... ▣ 630
Regular Strength Ascriptin Tablets ... ▣ 629
Di-Gel Antacid/Anti-Gas ... ▣ 801
Gelusil Liquid & Tablets ... ▣ 855
Maalox Magnesia and Alumina Oral Suspension ... ▣ 642
Maalox Plus Tablets ... ▣ 643
Extra Strength Maalox Antacid Plus Antigas Liquid and Tablets ▣ 638
Mylanta Calcium Carbonate and Magnesium Hydroxide Tablets ... 1318
Mylanta Liquid ... 1317
Mylanta Tablets ... ▣ 660
Mylanta Double Strength Liquid ... 1317
Mylanta Double Strength Tablets .. ▣ 660
Phillips' Milk of Magnesia Liquid ... ▣ 729
Rolaids Tablets ... ▣ 843
Tempo Soft Antacid ... ▣ 835

Magnesium Oxide (May bind phosphate and prevent its absorption). Products include:
Beelith Tablets ... 639
Bufferin Analgesic Tablets and Caplets ... ▣ 613
Caltrate PLUS ... ▣ 665
Cama Arthritis Pain Reliever ... ▣ 785
Mag-Ox 400 ... 668
Uro-Mag ... 668

Magnesium Salicylate (Increased serum salicylate levels; possible toxicity). Products include:
Backache Caplets ... ▣ 613
Bayer Select Backache Pain Relief Formula ... ▣ 715
Doan's Extra-Strength Analgesic ... ▣ 633
Extra Strength Doan's P.M. ... ▣ 633
Doan's Regular Strength Analgesic ... ▣ 634
Mobigesic Tablets ... ▣ 602

Potassium Bicarbonate (Potential for hyperkalemia). Products include:
Alka-Seltzer Gold Effervescent Antacid ... ▣ 703

Potassium Chloride (Potential for hyperkalemia). Products include:
Chlor-3 Condiment ... 1004
K-Dur Microburst Release System (potassium chloride, USP) E.R. Tablets ... 1325
K-Lor Powder Packets ... 434
K-Norm Extended-Release Capsules ... 991
K-Tab Filmtab ... 434
Kolyum Liquid ... 992
Micro-K ... 2063
Micro-K LS Packets ... 2064
NuLYTELY ... 689
Cherry Flavor NuLYTELY ... 689
Rum-K Syrup ... 1005
Slow-K Extended-Release Tablets ... 851

Potassium Citrate (Potential for hyperkalemia). Products include:
Polycitra Syrup ... 578
Polycitra-K Crystals ... 579
Polycitra-K Oral Solution ... 579
Polycitra-LC ... 578

Potassium Gluconate (Potential for hyperkalemia). Products include:
Kolyum Liquid ... 992

Potassium Phosphate, Dibasic (Potential for hyperkalemia).
No products indexed under this heading.

Potassium Phosphate, Monobasic (Potential for hyperkalemia). Products include:
K-Phos Neutral Tablets ... 639
K-Phos Original Formula 'Sodium Free' Tablets ... 639

Salsalate (Increased serum salicylate levels; possible toxicity). Products include:
Mono-Gesic Tablets ... 792
Salflex Tablets ... 786

Spironolactone (Hyperkalemia). Products include:
Aldactazide ... 2413
Aldactone ... 2414

Triamterene (Hyperkalemia). Products include:
Dyazide ... 2479
Dyrenium Capsules ... 2481
Maxzide ... 1380

K-TAB FILMTAB

(Potassium Chloride) ... 434
May interact with potassium sparing diuretics, ACE inhibitors, and anticholinergics. Compounds in these categories include:

Amiloride Hydrochloride (Potential for severe hyperkalemia). Products include:
Midamor Tablets ... 1703
Moduretic Tablets ... 1705

Atropine Sulfate (Anticholinergic drugs can be cause for delay or arrest in tablet passage through the gastrointestinal tract; concomitant administration of drugs capable of decreasing GI motility should be avoided). Products include:
Arco-Lase Plus Tablets ... 512

(▣ Described in PDR For Nonprescription Drugs) (⊙ Described in PDR For Ophthalmology)

Atrohist Plus Tablets 454
Atropine Sulfate Sterile Ophthalmic Solution .... ◉ 233
Donnatal 2060
Donnatal Extentabs 2061
Donnatal Tablets 2060
Lomotil 2439
Motofen Tablets 784
Urised Tablets 1964

Belladonna Alkaloids (Anticholinergic drugs can be cause for delay or arrest in tablet passage through the gastrointestinal tract; concomitant administration of drugs capable of decreasing GI motility should be avoided). Products include:
Bellergal-S Tablets 2250
Hyland's Bed Wetting Tablets .... ▣ 828
Hyland's EnurAid Tablets .... ▣ 829
Hyland's Teething Tablets .... ▣ 830

Benazepril Hydrochloride (Concomitant therapy may result in hyperkalemia; close monitoring is advised). Products include:
Lotensin Tablets 834
Lotensin HCT 837
Lotrel Capsules 840

Benztropine Mesylate (Anticholinergic drugs can be cause for delay or arrest in tablet passage through the gastrointestinal tract; concomitant administration of drugs capable of decreasing GI motility should be avoided). Products include:
Cogentin 1621

Biperiden Hydrochloride (Anticholinergic drugs can be cause for delay or arrest in tablet passage through the gastrointestinal tract; concomitant administration of drugs capable of decreasing GI motility should be avoided). Products include:
Akineton 1333

Captopril (Concomitant therapy may result in hyperkalemia; close monitoring is advised). Products include:
Capoten 739
Capozide 742

Clidinium Bromide (Anticholinergic drugs can be cause for delay or arrest in tablet passage through the gastrointestinal tract; concomitant administration of drugs capable of decreasing GI motility should be avoided). Products include:
Librax Capsules 2176
Quarzan Capsules 2181

Dicyclomine Hydrochloride (Anticholinergic drugs can be cause for delay or arrest in tablet passage through the gastrointestinal tract; concomitant administration of drugs capable of decreasing GI motility should be avoided). Products include:
Bentyl 1501

Enalapril Maleate (Concomitant therapy may result in hyperkalemia; close monitoring is advised). Products include:
Vaseretic Tablets 1765
Vasotec Tablets 1771

Enalaprilat (Concomitant therapy may result in hyperkalemia; close monitoring is advised). Products include:
Vasotec I.V. 1768

Fosinopril Sodium (Concomitant therapy may result in hyperkalemia; close monitoring is advised). Products include:
Monopril Tablets 757

Glycopyrrolate (Anticholinergic drugs can be cause for delay or arrest in tablet passage through the gastrointestinal tract; concomitant administration of drugs capable of decreasing GI motility should be avoided). Products include:
Robinul Forte Tablets 2072
Robinul Injectable 2072
Robinul Tablets 2072

Hyoscyamine (Anticholinergic drugs can be cause for delay or arrest in tablet passage through the gastrointestinal tract; concomitant administration of drugs capable of decreasing GI motility should be avoided). Products include:
Cystospaz Tablets 1963
Urised Tablets 1964

Hyoscyamine Sulfate (Anticholinergic drugs can be cause for delay or arrest in tablet passage through the gastrointestinal tract; concomitant administration of drugs capable of decreasing GI motility should be avoided). Products include:
Arco-Lase Plus Tablets 512
Atrohist Plus Tablets 454
Cystospaz-M Capsules 1963
Donnatal 2060
Donnatal Extentabs 2061
Donnatal Tablets 2060
Kutrase Capsules 2402
Levsin/Levsinex/Levbid 2405

Ipratropium Bromide (Anticholinergic drugs can be cause for delay or arrest in tablet passage through the gastrointestinal tract; concomitant administration of drugs capable of decreasing GI motility should be avoided). Products include:
Atrovent Inhalation Aerosol 671
Atrovent Inhalation Solution 673

Lisinopril (Concomitant therapy may result in hyperkalemia; close monitoring is advised). Products include:
Prinivil Tablets 1733
Prinzide Tablets 1737
Zestoretic 2850
Zestril Tablets 2854

Mepenzolate Bromide (Anticholinergic drugs can be cause for delay or arrest in tablet passage through the gastrointestinal tract; concomitant administration of drugs capable of decreasing GI motility should be avoided).
No products indexed under this heading.

Moexipril Hydrochloride (Concomitant therapy may result in hyperkalemia; close monitoring is advised). Products include:
Univasc Tablets 2410

Oxybutynin Chloride (Anticholinergic drugs can be cause for delay or arrest in tablet passage through the gastrointestinal tract; concomitant administration of drugs capable of decreasing GI motility should be avoided). Products include:
Ditropan 1516

Procyclidine Hydrochloride (Anticholinergic drugs can be cause for delay or arrest in tablet passage through the gastrointestinal tract; concomitant administration of drugs capable of decreasing GI motility should be avoided). Products include:
Kemadrin Tablets 1112

Propantheline Bromide (Anticholinergic drugs can be cause for delay or arrest in tablet passage through the gastrointestinal tract; concomitant administration of drugs capable of decreasing GI motility should be avoided). Products include:
Pro-Banthīne Tablets 2052

Quinapril Hydrochloride (Concomitant therapy may result in hyperkalemia; close monitoring is advised). Products include:
Accupril Tablets 1893

Ramipril (Concomitant therapy may result in hyperkalemia; close monitoring is advised). Products include:
Altace Capsules 1232

Scopolamine (Anticholinergic drugs can be cause for delay or arrest in tablet passage through the gastrointestinal tract; concomitant administration of drugs capable of decreasing GI motility should be avoided). Products include:
Transderm Scōp Transdermal Therapeutic System 869

Scopolamine Hydrobromide (Anticholinergic drugs can be cause for delay or arrest in tablet passage through the gastrointestinal tract; concomitant administration of drugs capable of decreasing GI motility should be avoided). Products include:
Atrohist Plus Tablets 454
Donnatal 2060
Donnatal Extentabs 2061
Donnatal Tablets 2060

Spirapril Hydrochloride (Concomitant therapy may result in hyperkalemia; close monitoring is advised).
No products indexed under this heading.

Spironolactone (Potential for severe hyperkalemia). Products include:
Aldactazide 2413
Aldactone 2414

Triamterene (Potential for severe hyperkalemia). Products include:
Dyazide 2479
Dyrenium Capsules 2481
Maxzide 1380

Tridihexethyl Chloride (Anticholinergic drugs can be cause for delay or arrest in tablet passage through the gastrointestinal tract; concomitant administration of drugs capable of decreasing GI motility should be avoided).
No products indexed under this heading.

Trihexyphenidyl Hydrochloride (Anticholinergic drugs can be cause for delay or arrest in tablet passage through the gastrointestinal tract; concomitant administration of drugs capable of decreasing GI motility should be avoided). Products include:
Artane 1368

K-Y JELLY PERSONAL LUBRICANT
(Chlorhexidine Gluconate) .... ▣ 658
None cited in PDR database.

K-Y PLUS VAGINAL CONTRACEPTIVE AND PERSONAL LUBRICANT
(Nonoxynol-9) .... ▣ 659
None cited in PDR database.

KALTOSTAT WOUND DRESSING
(Calcium Sodium Alginate Fiber) 2866
None cited in PDR database.

KAOPECTATE CONCENTRATED ANTI-DIARRHEAL, PEPPERMINT FLAVOR
(Attapulgite) .... ▣ 837
None cited in PDR database.

KAOPECTATE CONCENTRATED ANTI-DIARRHEAL, REGULAR FLAVOR
(Attapulgite) .... ▣ 837
None cited in PDR database.

KAOPECTATE CHILDREN'S LIQUID
(Attapulgite) .... ▣ 837
None cited in PDR database.

KAOPECTATE MAXIMUM STRENGTH CAPLETS
(Attapulgite) .... ▣ 837
None cited in PDR database.

KAOPECTATE 1-D
(Loperamide Hydrochloride) .... ▣ 838
None cited in PDR database.

KAYEXALATE
(Sodium Polystyrene Sulfonate) 2314
May interact with antacids, cardiac glycosides, and certain other agents. Compounds in these categories include:

Aluminum Carbonate Gel (May reduce potassium exchange capability). Products include:
Basaljel 2703

Aluminum Hydroxide (May reduce potassium exchange capability; potential for intestinal obstruction). Products include:
ALternaGEL Liquid 1316
Maximum Strength Ascriptin .... ▣ 630
Cama Arthritis Pain Reliever .... ▣ 785
Gaviscon Extra Strength Relief Formula Antacid Tablets .... ▣ 819
Gaviscon Extra Strength Relief Formula Liquid Antacid .... ▣ 819
Gaviscon Liquid Antacid .... ▣ 820
Gelusil Liquid & Tablets .... ▣ 855
Maalox Heartburn Relief Suspension .... ▣ 642
Maalox Heartburn Relief Tablets .... ▣ 641
Maalox Magnesia and Alumina Oral Suspension .... ▣ 642
Maalox Plus Tablets .... ▣ 643
Extra Strength Maalox Antacid Plus Antigas Liquid and Tablets ▣ 638
Tempo Soft Antacid .... ▣ 835

Aluminum Hydroxide Gel (May reduce potassium exchange capability; potential for intestinal obstruction). Products include:
ALternaGEL Liquid .... ▣ 659
Aludrox Oral Suspension 2695
Amphojel Suspension 2695
Amphojel Suspension without Flavor 2695
Amphojel Tablets 2695
Arthritis Pain Ascriptin .... ▣ 631
Regular Strength Ascriptin Tablets .... ▣ 629
Gaviscon Antacid Tablets .... ▣ 819
Gaviscon-2 Antacid Tablets .... ▣ 820
Mylanta Liquid 1317
Mylanta Tablets .... ▣ 660
Mylanta Double Strength Liquid 1317
Mylanta Double Strength Tablets .... ▣ 660
Nephrox Suspension .... ▣ 655

Aluminum Hydroxide Gel, Dried (May reduce potassium exchange capability; potential for intestinal obstruction).

IMPORTANT NOTE: Always consult each drug listing in the patient's regimen for possible interactions.

Deslanoside (Cardiac toxicity of digitalis may be exaggerated).
No products indexed under this heading.

Digitoxin (Cardiac toxicity of digitalis may be exaggerated). Products include:
- Crystodigin Tablets ... 1433

Digoxin (Cardiac toxicity of digitalis may be exaggerated). Products include:
- Lanoxicaps ... 1117
- Lanoxin Elixir Pediatric ... 1120
- Lanoxin Injection ... 1123
- Lanoxin Injection Pediatric ... 1126
- Lanoxin Tablets ... 1128

Dihydroxyaluminum Sodium Carbonate (May reduce potassium exchange capability).
No products indexed under this heading.

Magaldrate (May reduce potassium exchange capability).
No products indexed under this heading.

Magnesium Hydroxide (May reduce potassium exchange capability; potential for grand mal seizure). Products include:
- Aludrox Oral Suspension ... 2695
- Arthritis Pain Ascriptin ... ▣ 631
- Maximum Strength Ascriptin ... ▣ 630
- Regular Strength Ascriptin Tablets ... ▣ 629
- Di-Gel Antacid/Anti-Gas ... ▣ 801
- Gelusil Liquid & Tablets ... ▣ 855
- Maalox Magnesia and Alumina Oral Suspension ... ▣ 642
- Maalox Plus Tablets ... ▣ 643
- Extra Strength Maalox Antacid Plus Antigas Liquid and Tablets ▣ 638
- Mylanta Calcium Carbonate and Magnesium Hydroxide Tablets ... 1318
- Mylanta Liquid ... 1317
- Mylanta Tablets ... ▣ 660
- Mylanta Double Strength Liquid ... 1317
- Mylanta Double Strength Tablets .. ▣ 660
- Phillips' Milk of Magnesia Liquid ... ▣ 729
- Rolaids Tablets ... ▣ 843
- Tempo Soft Antacid ... ▣ 835

Magnesium Oxide (May reduce potassium exchange capability). Products include:
- Beelith Tablets ... 639
- Bufferin Analgesic Tablets and Caplets ... ▣ 613
- Caltrate PLUS ... ▣ 665
- Cama Arthritis Pain Reliever ... ▣ 785
- Mag-Ox 400 ... 668
- Uro-Mag ... 668

KEFLEX PULVULES & ORAL SUSPENSION
(Cephalexin) ... 914
None cited in PDR database.

KEFTAB TABLETS
(Cephalexin Hydrochloride) ... 915
None cited in PDR database.

KEFUROX VIALS, FASPAK & ADD-VANTAGE
(Cefuroxime Sodium) ... 1454
May interact with aminoglycosides and diuretics. Compounds in these categories include:

Amikacin Sulfate (Nephrotoxicity). Products include:
- Amikacin Sulfate Injection, USP ... 960
- Amikin Injectable ... 501

Amiloride Hydrochloride (Possible adverse effects on renal function). Products include:
- Midamor Tablets ... 1703
- Moduretic Tablets ... 1705

Bendroflumethiazide (Possible adverse effects on renal function).
No products indexed under this heading.

Bumetanide (Possible adverse effects on renal function). Products include:
- Bumex ... 2093

Chlorothiazide (Possible adverse effects on renal function). Products include:
- Aldoclor Tablets ... 1598
- Diupres Tablets ... 1650
- Diuril Oral ... 1653

Chlorothiazide Sodium (Possible adverse effects on renal function). Products include:
- Diuril Sodium Intravenous ... 1652

Chlorthalidone (Possible adverse effects on renal function). Products include:
- Combipres Tablets ... 677
- Tenoretic Tablets ... 2845
- Thalitone ... 1245

Ethacrynic Acid (Possible adverse effects on renal function). Products include:
- Edecrin Tablets ... 1657

Furosemide (Possible adverse effects on renal function). Products include:
- Lasix Injection, Oral Solution and Tablets ... 1240

Gentamicin Sulfate (Nephrotoxicity). Products include:
- Garamycin Injectable ... 2360
- Genoptic Sterile Ophthalmic Solution ... ◉ 243
- Genoptic Sterile Ophthalmic Ointment ... ◉ 243
- Gentacidin Ointment ... ◉ 264
- Gentacidin Solution ... ◉ 264
- Gentak ... ◉ 208
- Pred-G Liquifilm Sterile Ophthalmic Suspension ... ◉ 251
- Pred-G S.O.P. Sterile Ophthalmic Ointment ... ◉ 252

Hydrochlorothiazide (Possible adverse effects on renal function). Products include:
- Aldactazide ... 2413
- Aldoril Tablets ... 1604
- Apresazide Capsules ... 808
- Capozide ... 742
- Dyazide ... 2479
- Esidrix Tablets ... 821
- Esimil Tablets ... 822
- HydroDIURIL Tablets ... 1674
- Hydropres Tablets ... 1675
- Hyzaar Tablets ... 1677
- Inderide Tablets ... 2732
- Inderide LA Long Acting Capsules .. 2734
- Lopressor HCT Tablets ... 832
- Lotensin HCT ... 837
- Maxzide ... 1380
- Moduretic Tablets ... 1705
- Oretic Tablets ... 443
- Prinzide Tablets ... 1737
- Ser-Ap-Es Tablets ... 849
- Timolide Tablets ... 1748
- Vaseretic Tablets ... 1765
- Zestoretic ... 2850
- Ziac ... 1415

Hydroflumethiazide (Possible adverse effects on renal function). Products include:
- Diucardin Tablets ... 2718

Indapamide (Possible adverse effects on renal function). Products include:
- Lozol Tablets ... 2022

Kanamycin Sulfate (Nephrotoxicity).
No products indexed under this heading.

Methyclothiazide (Possible adverse effects on renal function). Products include:
- Enduron Tablets ... 420

Metolazone (Possible adverse effects on renal function). Products include:
- Mykrox Tablets ... 993
- Zaroxolyn Tablets ... 1000

Polythiazide (Possible adverse effects on renal function). Products include:
- Minizide Capsules ... 1938

Spironolactone (Possible adverse effects on renal function). Products include:
- Aldactazide ... 2413
- Aldactone ... 2414

Streptomycin Sulfate (Nephrotoxicity). Products include:
- Streptomycin Sulfate Injection ... 2208

Tobramycin (Nephrotoxicity). Products include:
- AKTOB ... ◉ 206
- TobraDex Ophthalmic Suspension and Ointment ... 473
- Tobrex Ophthalmic Ointment and Solution ... ◉ 229

Tobramycin Sulfate (Nephrotoxicity). Products include:
- Nebcin Vials, Hyporets & ADD-Vantage ... 1464
- Tobramycin Sulfate Injection ... 968

Torsemide (Possible adverse effects on renal function). Products include:
- Demadex Tablets and Injection ... 686

Triamterene (Possible adverse effects on renal function). Products include:
- Dyazide ... 2479
- Dyrenium Capsules ... 2481
- Maxzide ... 1380

KEFZOL VIALS, FASPAK & ADD-VANTAGE
(Cefazolin Sodium) ... 1456
May interact with:

Probenecid (Increases and prolongs cephalosporin blood levels). Products include:
- Benemid Tablets ... 1611
- ColBENEMID Tablets ... 1622

KEMADRIN TABLETS
(Procyclidine Hydrochloride) ... 1112
None cited in PDR database.

KERI LOTION - ORIGINAL FORMULA
(Mineral Oil) ... ▣ 622
None cited in PDR database.

KERI LOTION - SILKY SMOOTH
(Petrolatum) ... ▣ 622
None cited in PDR database.

KERI LOTION - SENSITIVE SKIN
(Petrolatum) ... ▣ 622
None cited in PDR database.

KERLONE TABLETS
(Betaxolol Hydrochloride) ... 2436
May interact with catecholamine depleting drugs, calcium channel blockers, and certain other agents. Compounds in these categories include:

Amlodipine Besylate (Potential for hypotension, AV conduction disturbances, and LVF in patients with impaired cardiac function). Products include:
- Lotrel Capsules ... 840
- Norvasc Tablets ... 1940

Bepridil Hydrochloride (Potential for hypotension, AV conduction disturbances, and LVF in patients with impaired cardiac function). Products include:
- Vascor (200, 300 and 400 mg) Tablets ... 1587

Clonidine (Potential for withdrawal reactions). Products include:
- Catapres-TTS ... 675

Clonidine Hydrochloride (Potential for withdrawal). Products include:
- Catapres Tablets ... 674
- Combipres Tablets ... 677

Deserpidine (Additive effect resulting in marked bradycardia, vertigo, syncope or postural hypotension).
No products indexed under this heading.

Diltiazem Hydrochloride (Potential for hypotension, AV conduction disturbances, and LVF in patients with impaired cardiac function). Products include:
- Cardizem CD Capsules ... 1506
- Cardizem SR Capsules ... 1510
- Cardizem Injectable ... 1508
- Cardizem Tablets ... 1512
- Dilacor XR Extended-release Capsules ... 2018

Felodipine (Potential for hypotension, AV conduction disturbances, and LVF in patients with impaired cardiac function). Products include:
- Plendil Extended-Release Tablets ... 527

Guanethidine Monosulfate (Additive effect resulting in marked bradycardia, vertigo, syncope or postural hypotension). Products include:
- Esimil Tablets ... 822
- Ismelin Tablets ... 827

Isradipine (Potential for hypotension, AV conduction disturbances, and LVF in patients with impaired cardiac function). Products include:
- DynaCirc Capsules ... 2256

Nicardipine Hydrochloride (Potential for hypotension, AV conduction disturbances, and LVF in patients with impaired cardiac function). Products include:
- Cardene Capsules ... 2095
- Cardene I.V. ... 2709
- Cardene SR Capsules ... 2097

Nifedipine (Potential for hypotension, AV conduction disturbances, and LVF in patients with impaired cardiac function). Products include:
- Adalat Capsules (10 mg and 20 mg) ... 587
- Adalat CC ... 589
- Procardia Capsules ... 1971
- Procardia XL Extended Release Tablets ... 1972

Nimodipine (Potential for hypotension, AV conduction disturbances, and LVF in patients with impaired cardiac function). Products include:
- Nimotop Capsules ... 610

Nisoldipine (Potential for hypotension, AV conduction disturbances, and LVF in patients with impaired cardiac function).
No products indexed under this heading.

Rauwolfia Serpentina (Additive effect resulting in marked bradycardia, vertigo, syncope or postural hypotension).
No products indexed under this heading.

Rescinnamine (Additive effect resulting in marked bradycardia, vertigo, syncope or postural hypotension).
No products indexed under this heading.

Reserpine (Additive effect resulting in marked bradycardia, vertigo, syncope or postural hypotension). Products include:
- Diupres Tablets ... 1650
- Hydropres Tablets ... 1675
- Ser-Ap-Es Tablets ... 849

Verapamil Hydrochloride (Potential for hypotension, AV conduction disturbances, and LVF in patients with impaired cardiac function). Products include:

Calan SR Caplets 2422
Calan Tablets 2419
Isoptin Injectable 1344
Isoptin Oral Tablets 1346
Isoptin SR Tablets 1348
Verelan Capsules 1410
Verelan Capsules 2824

KLONOPIN TABLETS

(Clonazepam) 2126

May interact with narcotic analgesics, barbiturates, hypnotics and sedatives, tranquilizers, phenothiazines, monoamine oxidase inhibitors, tricyclic antidepressants, anticonvulsants, and certain other agents. Compounds in these categories include:

Alfentanil Hydrochloride (Potentiates CNS-depressant action). Products include:

Alfenta Injection 1286

Alprazolam (Potentiates CNS-depressant action). Products include:

Xanax Tablets 2649

Amitriptyline Hydrochloride (Potentiates CNS-depressant action). Products include:

Elavil 2838
Endep Tablets 2174
Etrafon 2355
Limbitrol 2180
Triavil Tablets 1757

Amoxapine (Potentiates CNS-depressant action). Products include:

Asendin Tablets 1369

Aprobarbital (Potentiates CNS-depressant action).

No products indexed under this heading.

Buprenorphine (Potentiates CNS-depressant action). Products include:

Buprenex Injectable 2006

Buspirone Hydrochloride (Potentiates CNS-depressant action). Products include:

BuSpar 737

Butabarbital (Potentiates CNS-depressant action).

No products indexed under this heading.

Butalbital (Potentiates CNS-depressant action). Products include:

Esgic-plus Tablets 1013
Fioricet Tablets 2258
Fioricet with Codeine Capsules 2260
Fiorinal Capsules 2261
Fiorinal with Codeine Capsules 2262
Fiorinal Tablets 2261
Phrenilin 785
Sedapap Tablets 50 mg/650 mg .. 1543

Carbamazepine (Potentiates CNS-depressant action). Products include:

Atretol Tablets 573
Tegretol Chewable Tablets 852
Tegretol Suspension 852
Tegretol Tablets 852

Chlordiazepoxide (Potentiates CNS-depressant action). Products include:

Libritabs Tablets 2177
Limbitrol 2180

Chlordiazepoxide Hydrochloride (Potentiates CNS-depressant action). Products include:

Librax Capsules 2176
Librium Capsules 2178
Librium Injectable 2179

Chlorpromazine (Potentiates CNS-depressant action). Products include:

Thorazine Suppositories 2523

Chlorprothixene (Potentiates CNS-depressant action).

No products indexed under this heading.

Chlorprothixene Hydrochloride (Potentiates CNS-depressant action).

No products indexed under this heading.

Clomipramine Hydrochloride (Potentiates CNS-depressant action). Products include:

Anafranil Capsules 803

Clorazepate Dipotassium (Potentiates CNS-depressant action). Products include:

Tranxene 451

Codeine Phosphate (Potentiates CNS-depressant action). Products include:

Actifed with Codeine Cough Syrup.. 1067
Brontex 1981
Deconsal C Expectorant Syrup 456
Deconsal Pediatric Syrup 457
Dimetane-DC Cough Syrup 2059
Empirin with Codeine Tablets............ 1093
Fioricet with Codeine Capsules 2260
Fiorinal with Codeine Capsules 2262
Isoclor Expectorant 990
Novahistine DH 2462
Novahistine Expectorant 2463
Nucofed 2051
Phenergan with Codeine 2777
Phenergan VC with Codeine 2781
Robitussin A-C Syrup 2073
Robitussin-DAC Syrup 2074
Ryna .... ◻◻ 841
Soma Compound w/Codeine Tablets 2676
Tussi-Organidin NR Liquid and S NR Liquid 2677
Tylenol with Codeine 1583

Desipramine Hydrochloride (Potentiates CNS-depressant action). Products include:

Norpramin Tablets 1526

Dezocine (Potentiates CNS-depressant action). Products include:

Dalgan Injection 538

Diazepam (Potentiates CNS-depressant action). Products include:

Dizac 1809
Valium Injectable 2182
Valium Tablets 2183
Valrelease Capsules 2169

Divalproex Sodium (Potentiates CNS-depressant action). Products include:

Depakote Tablets 415

Doxepin Hydrochloride (Potentiates CNS-depressant action). Products include:

Sinequan 2205
Zonalon Cream 1055

Droperidol (Potentiates CNS-depressant action). Products include:

Inapsine Injection 1296

Estazolam (Potentiates CNS-depressant action). Products include:

ProSom Tablets 449

Ethchlorvynol (Potentiates CNS-depressant action). Products include:

Placidyl Capsules 448

Ethinamate (Potentiates CNS-depressant action).

No products indexed under this heading.

Ethosuximide (Potentiates CNS-depressant action). Products include:

Zarontin Capsules 1928
Zarontin Syrup 1929

Ethotoin (Potentiates CNS-depressant action). Products include:

Peganone Tablets 446

Felbamate (Potentiates CNS-depressant action). Products include:

Felbatol 2666

Fentanyl (Potentiates CNS-depressant action). Products include:

Duragesic Transdermal System......... 1288

Fentanyl Citrate (Potentiates CNS-depressant action). Products include:

Sublimaze Injection 1307

Fluphenazine Decanoate (Potentiates CNS-depressant action). Products include:

Prolixin Decanoate 509

Fluphenazine Enanthate (Potentiates CNS-depressant action). Products include:

Prolixin Enanthate 509

Fluphenazine Hydrochloride (Potentiates CNS-depressant action). Products include:

Prolixin 509

Flurazepam Hydrochloride (Potentiates CNS-depressant action). Products include:

Dalmane Capsules 2173

Furazolidone (Potentiates CNS-depressant action). Products include:

Furoxone 2046

Glutethimide (Potentiates CNS-depressant action).

No products indexed under this heading.

Haloperidol (Potentiates CNS-depressant action). Products include:

Haldol Injection, Tablets and Concentrate 1575

Haloperidol Decanoate (Potentiates CNS-depressant action). Products include:

Haldol Decanoate 1577

Hydrocodone Bitartrate (Potentiates CNS-depressant action). Products include:

Anexsia 5/500 Elixir 1781
Anexia Tablets 1782
Codiclear DH Syrup 791
Deconamine CX Cough and Cold Liquid and Tablets 1319
Duratuss HD Elixir 2565
Hycodan Tablets and Syrup 930
Hycomine Compound Tablets 932
Hycomine 931
Hycotuss Expectorant Syrup 933
Hydrocet Capsules 782
Lorcet 10/650 1018
Lortab 2566
Tussend 1783
Tussend Expectorant 1785
Vicodin Tablets 1356
Vicodin ES Tablets 1357
Vicodin Tuss Expectorant 1358
Zydone Capsules 949

Hydrocodone Polistirex (Potentiates CNS-depressant action). Products include:

Tussionex Pennkinetic Extended-Release Suspension 998

Hydroxyzine Hydrochloride (Potentiates CNS-depressant action). Products include:

Atarax Tablets & Syrup 2185
Marax Tablets & DF Syrup 2200
Vistaril Intramuscular Solution 2216

Imipramine Hydrochloride (Potentiates CNS-depressant action). Products include:

Tofranil Ampuls 854
Tofranil Tablets 856

Imipramine Pamoate (Potentiates CNS-depressant action). Products include:

Tofranil-PM Capsules 857

Isocarboxazid (Potentiates CNS-depressant action).

No products indexed under this heading.

Lamotrigine (Potentiates CNS-depressant action). Products include:

Lamictal Tablets 1112

Levorphanol Tartrate (Potentiates CNS-depressant action). Products include:

Levo-Dromoran 2129

Lorazepam (Potentiates CNS-depressant action). Products include:

Ativan Injection 2698
Ativan Tablets 2700

Loxapine Hydrochloride (Potentiates CNS-depressant action). Products include:

Loxitane 1378

Maprotiline Hydrochloride (Potentiates CNS-depressant action). Products include:

Ludiomil Tablets 843

Meperidine Hydrochloride (Potentiates CNS-depressant action). Products include:

Demerol 2308
Mepergan Injection 2753

Mephenytoin (Potentiates CNS-depressant action). Products include:

Mesantoin Tablets 2272

Mephobarbital (Potentiates CNS-depressant action). Products include:

Mebaral Tablets 2322

Meprobamate (Potentiates CNS-depressant action). Products include:

Miltown Tablets 2672
PMB 200 and PMB 400 2783

Mesoridazine Besylate (Potentiates CNS-depressant action). Products include:

Serentil 684

Methadone Hydrochloride (Potentiates CNS-depressant action). Products include:

Methadone Hydrochloride Oral Concentrate 2233
Methadone Hydrochloride Oral Solution & Tablets 2235

Methotrimeprazine (Potentiates CNS-depressant action). Products include:

Levoprome 1274

Methsuximide (Potentiates CNS-depressant action). Products include:

Celontin Kapseals 1899

Midazolam Hydrochloride (Potentiates CNS-depressant action). Products include:

Versed Injection 2170

Molindone Hydrochloride (Potentiates CNS-depressant action). Products include:

Moban Tablets and Concentrate 1048

Morphine Sulfate (Potentiates CNS-depressant action). Products include:

Astramorph/PF Injection, USP (Preservative-Free) 535
Duramorph 962
Infumorph 200 and Infumorph 500 Sterile Solutions 965
MS Contin Tablets 1994
MSIR 1997
Oramorph SR (Morphine Sulfate Sustained Release Tablets) 2236
RMS Suppositories 2657
Roxanol 2243

Nortriptyline Hydrochloride (Potentiates CNS-depressant action). Products include:

Pamelor 2280

Opium Alkaloids (Potentiates CNS-depressant action).

No products indexed under this heading.

Oxazepam (Potentiates CNS-depressant action). Products include:

Serax Capsules 2810
Serax Tablets 2810

IMPORTANT NOTE: Always consult each drug listing in the patient's regimen for possible interactions.

Oxycodone Hydrochloride (Potentiates CNS-depressant action). Products include:
- Percocet Tablets ... 938
- Percodan Tablets ... 939
- Percodan-Demi Tablets ... 940
- Roxicodone Tablets, Oral Solution & Intensol (Oxycodone) ... 2244
- Tylox Capsules ... 1584

Paramethadione (Potentiates CNS-depressant action).
- No products indexed under this heading.

Pentobarbital Sodium (Potentiates CNS-depressant action). Products include:
- Nembutal Sodium Capsules ... 436
- Nembutal Sodium Solution ... 438
- Nembutal Sodium Suppositories ... 440

Perphenazine (Potentiates CNS-depressant action). Products include:
- Etrafon ... 2355
- Triavil Tablets ... 1757
- Trilafon ... 2389

Phenacemide (Potentiates CNS-depressant action). Products include:
- Phenurone Tablets ... 447

Phenelzine Sulfate (Potentiates CNS-depressant action). Products include:
- Nardil ... 1920

Phenobarbital (Potentiates CNS-depressant action). Products include:
- Arco-Lase Plus Tablets ... 512
- Bellergal-S Tablets ... 2250
- Donnatal ... 2060
- Donnatal Extentabs ... 2061
- Donnatal Tablets ... 2060
- Phenobarbital Elixir and Tablets ... 1469
- Quadrinal Tablets ... 1350

Phenothiazine Derivatives (Potentiates CNS-depressant action).

Phensuximide (Potentiates CNS-depressant action). Products include:
- Milontin Kapseals ... 1920

Phenytoin (Potentiates CNS-depressant action). Products include:
- Dilantin Infatabs ... 1908
- Dilantin-125 Suspension ... 1911

Phenytoin Sodium (Potentiates CNS-depressant action). Products include:
- Dilantin Kapseals ... 1906
- Dilantin Parenteral ... 1910

Prazepam (Potentiates CNS-depressant action).
- No products indexed under this heading.

Primidone (Potentiates CNS-depressant action). Products include:
- Mysoline ... 2754

Prochlorperazine (Potentiates CNS-depressant action). Products include:
- Compazine ... 2470

Promethazine Hydrochloride (Potentiates CNS-depressant action). Products include:
- Mepergan Injection ... 2753
- Phenergan with Codeine ... 2777
- Phenergan with Dextromethorphan 2778
- Phenergan Injection ... 2773
- Phenergan Suppositories ... 2775
- Phenergan Syrup ... 2774
- Phenergan Tablets ... 2775
- Phenergan VC ... 2779
- Phenergan VC with Codeine ... 2781

Propofol (Potentiates CNS-depressant action). Products include:
- Diprivan Injection ... 2833

Propoxyphene Hydrochloride (Potentiates CNS-depressant action). Products include:
- Darvon ... 1435
- Wygesic Tablets ... 2827

Propoxyphene Napsylate (Potentiates CNS-depressant action). Products include:
- Darvon-N/Darvocet-N ... 1433

Protriptyline Hydrochloride (Potentiates CNS-depressant action). Products include:
- Vivactil Tablets ... 1774

Quazepam (Potentiates CNS-depressant action). Products include:
- Doral Tablets ... 2664

Secobarbital Sodium (Potentiates CNS-depressant action). Products include:
- Seconal Sodium Pulvules ... 1474

Selegiline Hydrochloride (Potentiates CNS-depressant action). Products include:
- Eldepryl Tablets ... 2550

Sufentanil Citrate (Potentiates CNS-depressant action). Products include:
- Sufenta Injection ... 1309

Temazepam (Potentiates CNS-depressant action). Products include:
- Restoril Capsules ... 2284

Thiamylal Sodium (Potentiates CNS-depressant action).
- No products indexed under this heading.

Thioridazine Hydrochloride (Potentiates CNS-depressant action). Products include:
- Mellaril ... 2269

Thiothixene (Potentiates CNS-depressant action). Products include:
- Navane Capsules and Concentrate 2201
- Navane Intramuscular ... 2202

Tranylcypromine Sulfate (Potentiates CNS-depressant action). Products include:
- Parnate Tablets ... 2503

Triazolam (Potentiates CNS-depressant action). Products include:
- Halcion Tablets ... 2611

Trifluoperazine Hydrochloride (Potentiates CNS-depressant action). Products include:
- Stelazine ... 2514

Trimethadione (Potentiates CNS-depressant action).
- No products indexed under this heading.

Trimipramine Maleate (Potentiates CNS-depressant action). Products include:
- Surmontil Capsules ... 2811

Valproic Acid (Potentiates CNS-depressant action). Products include:
- Depakene ... 413

Zolpidem Tartrate (Potentiates CNS-depressant action). Products include:
- Ambien Tablets ... 2416

Food Interactions

Alcohol (Potentiates CNS-depressant action).

KOāTE-HP ANTIHEMOPHILIC FACTOR (HUMAN)

(Antihemophilic Factor (Human)) ... 630

None cited in PDR database.

KOGENATE ANTIHEMOPHILIC FACTOR (RECOMBINANT)

(Antihemophilic Factor (Recombinant)) ... 632

None cited in PDR database.

KOLYUM LIQUID

(Potassium Gluconate, Potassium Chloride) ... 992

May interact with potassium sparing diuretics and ACE inhibitors. Compounds in these categories include:

Amiloride Hydrochloride (Potential for severe hyperkalemia). Products include:
- Midamor Tablets ... 1703
- Moduretic Tablets ... 1705

Benazepril Hydrochloride (Potential for increased potassium retention; potassium supplements should be given to patients on ACE inhibitors only with close monitoring). Products include:
- Lotensin Tablets ... 834
- Lotensin HCT ... 837
- Lotrel Capsules ... 840

Captopril (Potential for increased potassium retention; potassium supplements should be given to patients on ACE inhibitors only with close monitoring). Products include:
- Capoten ... 739
- Capozide ... 742

Enalapril Maleate (Potential for increased potassium retention; potassium supplements should be given to patients on ACE inhibitors only with close monitoring). Products include:
- Vaseretic Tablets ... 1765
- Vasotec Tablets ... 1771

Enalaprilat (Potential for increased potassium retention; potassium supplements should be given to patients on ACE inhibitors only with close monitoring). Products include:
- Vasotec I.V. ... 1768

Fosinopril Sodium (Potential for increased potassium retention; potassium supplements should be given to patients on ACE inhibitors only with close monitoring). Products include:
- Monopril Tablets ... 757

Lisinopril (Potential for increased potassium retention; potassium supplements should be given to patients on ACE inhibitors only with close monitoring). Products include:
- Prinivil Tablets ... 1733
- Prinzide Tablets ... 1737
- Zestoretic ... 2850
- Zestril Tablets ... 2854

Moexipril Hydrochloride (Potential for increased potassium retention; potassium supplements should be given to patients on ACE inhibitors only with close monitoring). Products include:
- Univasc Tablets ... 2410

Quinapril Hydrochloride (Potential for increased potassium retention; potassium supplements should be given to patients on ACE inhibitors only with close monitoring). Products include:
- Accupril Tablets ... 1893

Ramipril (Potential for increased potassium retention; potassium supplements should be given to patients on ACE inhibitors only with close monitoring). Products include:
- Altace Capsules ... 1232

Spirapril Hydrochloride (Potential for increased potassium retention; potassium supplements should be given to patients on ACE inhibitors only with close monitoring).
- No products indexed under this heading.

Spironolactone (Potential for severe hyperkalemia). Products include:
- Aldactazide ... 2413
- Aldactone ... 2414

Triamterene (Potential for severe hyperkalemia). Products include:
- Dyazide ... 2479
- Dyrenium Capsules ... 2481
- Maxzide ... 1380

KONAKION INJECTION

(Phytonadione) ... 2127

May interact with oral anticoagulants. Compounds in this category include:

Dicumarol (Concomitant use is not recommended except for excessive hypoprothrombinemia).
- No products indexed under this heading.

Warfarin Sodium (Concomitant use is not recommended except for excessive hypoprothrombinemia). Products include:
- Coumadin ... 926

KONDREMUL

(Mineral Oil) ... ▣ 637

May interact with stool softener laxatives. Compounds in this category include:

Docusate Calcium (Concurrent use is not recommended). Products include:
- Doxidan Liqui-Gels ... ▣ 836
- Surfak Liqui-Gels ... ▣ 839

Docusate Potassium (Concurrent use is not recommended).
- No products indexed under this heading.

Docusate Sodium (Concurrent use is not recommended). Products include:
- Colace ... 2044
- Correctol Extra Gentle Stool Softener ... ▣ 801
- Correctol Laxative Tablets & Caplets ... ▣ 801
- Dialose Tablets ... 1317
- Dialose Plus Tablets ... 1317
- Extra Gentle Ex-Lax Laxative Pills ... ▣ 786
- Feen-A-Mint Laxative Pills ... ▣ 805
- Ferro-Sequels ... ▣ 669
- Fleet Sof-Lax ... 1004
- Fleet Sof-Lax Overnight ... 1004
- Peri-Colace ... 2052
- Phillips' Gelcaps ... ▣ 729
- Senokot-S Tablets ... 1999

KONSYL FIBER TABLETS

(Calcium Polycarbophil) ... ▣ 663

May interact with tetracyclines. Compounds in this category include:

Demeclocycline Hydrochloride (Take KONSYL at least one hour before or two hours after taking the antibiotic). Products include:
- Declomycin Tablets ... 1371

Doxycycline Calcium (Take KONSYL at least one hour before or two hours after taking the antibiotic). Products include:
- Vibramycin Calcium Oral Suspension Syrup ... 1941

Doxycycline Hyclate (Take KONSYL at least one hour before or two hours after taking the antibiotic). Products include:
- Doryx Capsules ... 1913
- Vibramycin Hyclate Capsules ... 1941
- Vibramycin Hyclate Intravenous ... 2215
- Vibra-Tabs Film Coated Tablets ... 1941

Doxycycline Monohydrate (Take KONSYL at least one hour before or two hours after taking the antibiotic). Products include:
- Monodox Capsules ... 1805
- Vibramycin Monohydrate for Oral Suspension ... 1941

(▣ Described in PDR For Nonprescription Drugs) (⊙ Described in PDR For Ophthalmology)

Methacycline Hydrochloride (Take KONSYL at least one hour before or two hours after taking the antibiotic).

No products indexed under this heading.

Minocycline Hydrochloride (Take KONSYL at least one hour before or two hours after taking the antibiotic). Products include:

Dynacin Capsules 1590
Minocin Intravenous 1382
Minocin Oral Suspension 1385
Minocin Pellet-Filled Capsules 1383

Oxytetracycline Hydrochloride (Take KONSYL at least one hour before or two hours after taking the antibiotic). Products include:

TERAK Ointment .... ⓒ 209
Terra-Cortril Ophthalmic Suspension 2210
Terramycin with Polymyxin B Sulfate Ophthalmic Ointment 2211
Urobiotic-250 Capsules 2214

Tetracycline Hydrochloride (Take KONSYL at least one hour before or two hours after taking the antibiotic). Products include:

Achromycin V Capsules 1367

KONSYL POWDER SUGAR FREE UNFLAVORED

(Psyllium Preparations) .... ⊕ 664
None cited in PDR database.

KONSYL-D POWDER UNFLAVORED

(Psyllium Preparations) .... ⊕ 664
None cited in PDR database.

KONSYL-ORANGE ULTRA FINE POWDER

(Psyllium Preparations) .... ⊕ 664
None cited in PDR database.

KONINE 80 FACTOR IX COMPLEX

(Factor IX Complex)................................ 634
None cited in PDR database.

KRONOFED-A KRONOCAPS

(Chlorpheniramine Maleate, Pseudoephedrine Hydrochloride) 977
None cited in PDR database.

KRONOFED-A-JR. KRONOCAPS

(Pseudoephedrine Hydrochloride, Chlorpheniramine Maleate) 977
None cited in PDR database.

KUTRASE CAPSULES

(Hyoscyamine Sulfate, Phenyltoloxamine Citrate, Enzymes, Digestive) 2402
None cited in PDR database.

KU-ZYME CAPSULES

(Enzymes, Digestive) 2402
None cited in PDR database.

KU-ZYME HP CAPSULES

(Pancrelipase) 2402
May interact with:

Ferrous Fumarate (Decreased serum response to oral iron). Products include:

Chromagen Capsules 2339
Ferro-Sequels .... ⊕ 669
Nephro-Fer Tablets 2004
Nephro-Fer Rx Tablets........................... 2005
Nephro-Vite + Fe Tablets 2006
Sigtab-M Tablets .... ⊕ 772
Stresstabs + Iron .... ⊕ 671
The Stuart Formula Tablets............... ⊕ 663
Theragran-M Tablets with Beta Carotene .... ⊕ 623

Trinsicon Capsules 2570
Vitron-C Tablets .... ⊕ 650

Ferrous Gluconate (Decreased serum response to oral iron). Products include:

Fergon Iron Supplement Tablets.... ⊕ 721
Megadose 512

Ferrous Sulfate (Decreased serum response to oral iron). Products include:

Feosol Capsules 2456
Feosol Elixir 2456
Feosol Tablets 2457
Fero-Folic-500 Filmtab 429
Fero-Grad-500 Filmtab.......................... 429
Fero-Gradumet Filmtab......................... 429
Iberet Tablets 433
Iberet-500 Liquid 433
Iberet-Folic-500 Filmtab....................... 429
Iberet-Liquid... 433
Irospan 982
Slow Fe Tablets.. 869
Slow Fe with Folic Acid 869

KWELL CREAM & LOTION

(Lindane) 2008
May interact with:

Oil Based Products (May enhance absorption; avoid concomitant use).

KWELL SHAMPOO

(Lindane) 2009
May interact with:

Oil Based Products (Oils may enhance absorption; avoid using immediately before or after using Kwell Shampoo).

Oils, unspecified (Oils may enhance absorption; avoid using immediately before or after using Kwell Shampoo).

KYOLIC

(Garlic Extract) .... ⊕ 839
None cited in PDR database.

KYTRIL INJECTION

(Granisetron Hydrochloride) 2490
May interact with drugs affecting hepatic drug metabolizing enzyme systems and certain other agents. Compounds in these categories include:

Carbamazepine (May change the clearance and, hence, the half-life of granisetron). Products include:

Atretol Tablets 573
Tegretol Chewable Tablets 852
Tegretol Suspension............................... 852
Tegretol Tablets 852

Cimetidine (May change the clearance and hence, the half-life of granisetron). Products include:

Tagamet Tablets 2516

Cimetidine Hydrochloride (May change the clearance and hence, the half-life of granisetron). Products include:

Tagamet.. 2516

Phenobarbital (May change the clearance and, hence, the half-life of granisetron). Products include:

Arco-Lase Plus Tablets 512
Bellergal-S Tablets 2250
Donnatal 2060
Donnatal Extentabs................................ 2061
Donnatal Tablets 2060
Phenobarbital Elixir and Tablets 1469
Quadrinal Tablets 1350

Phenytoin (May change the clearance and, hence, the half-life of granisetron). Products include:

Dilantin Infatabs..................................... 1908
Dilantin-125 Suspension 1911

Phenytoin Sodium (May change the clearance and, hence, the half-life of granisetron). Products include:

Dilantin Kapseals 1906
Dilantin Parenteral 1910

Rifampin (May change the clearance and, hence, the half-life of granisetron). Products include:

Rifadin 1528
Rifamate Capsules 1530
Rifater.. 1532
Rimactane Capsules................................ 847

KYTRIL TABLETS

(Granisetron Hydrochloride) 2492
May interact with drugs affecting hepatic drug metabolizing enzyme systems. Compounds in this category include:

Carbamazepine (May change the clearance and, hence, the half-life of granisetron). Products include:

Atretol Tablets 573
Tegretol Chewable Tablets 852
Tegretol Suspension............................... 852
Tegretol Tablets 852

Cimetidine (May change the clearance and, hence, the half-life of granisetron). Products include:

Tagamet Tablets 2516

Cimetidine Hydrochloride (May change the clearance and, hence the half-life of granisetron). Products include:

Tagamet.. 2516

Phenobarbital (May change the clearance and, hence the half-life of granisetron). Products include:

Arco-Lase Plus Tablets 512
Bellergal-S Tablets 2250
Donnatal 2060
Donnatal Extentabs................................ 2061
Donnatal Tablets 2060
Phenobarbital Elixir and Tablets 1469
Quadrinal Tablets 1350

Phenytoin (May change the clearance and, hence, the half-life of granisetron). Products include:

Dilantin Infatabs..................................... 1908
Dilantin-125 Suspension 1911

Phenytoin Sodium (May change the clearance and, hence the half-life of granisetron). Products include:

Dilantin Kapseals 1906
Dilantin Parenteral 1910

Food Interactions

Food, unspecified (When oral granisetron was administered with food, AUC was decreased by 5% and C_{max} increased by 30% in non-fasted individuals).

LAC-HYDRIN 12% LOTION

(Ammonium Lactate).............................2687
None cited in PDR database.

LACRISERT STERILE OPHTHALMIC INSERT

(Hydroxypropyl Cellulose) 1686
None cited in PDR database.

LACTAID CAPLETS

(Lactase (beta-d-Galactosidase)).........1550
None cited in PDR database.

LACTAID DROPS

(Lactase (beta-d-Galactosidase)).........1550
None cited in PDR database.

LAMICTAL TABLETS

(Lamotrigine) 1112
May interact with dihydrofolate reductase inhibitors and certain other agents. Compounds in these categories include:

Carbamazepine (Potential for higher incidence of dizziness, diplopia, ataxia, and blurred vision; decreases lamotrigine steady-state concentrations by approximately 40%). Products include:

Atretol Tablets 573
Tegretol Chewable Tablets 852
Tegretol Suspension............................... 852
Tegretol Tablets 852

Divalproex Sodium (Decreases the clearance of lamotrigine, i.e., more than doubles the elimination t½ of lamotrigine, whether given with or without hepatic enzyme inducing antiepileptic drugs; the steady-state valproic acid concentrations in plasma may be decreased by an average of 25%). Products include:

Depakote Tablets..................................... 415

Methotrexate Sodium (Lamotrigine is an inhibitor of dihydrofolate reductase; prescribers should be aware of this action when used concurrently with agents which inhibit folate metabolism). Products include:

Methotrexate Sodium Tablets, Injection, for Injection and LPF Injection 1275

Phenobarbital (Decreases lamotrigine steady-state concentrations by approximately 40%). Products include:

Arco-Lase Plus Tablets 512
Bellergal-S Tablets 2250
Donnatal 2060
Donnatal Extentabs................................ 2061
Donnatal Tablets 2060
Phenobarbital Elixir and Tablets 1469
Quadrinal Tablets 1350

Phenytoin (Decreases lamotrigine steady-state concentrations by approximately 45% to 54%). Products include:

Dilantin Infatabs..................................... 1908
Dilantin-125 Suspension 1911

Phenytoin Sodium (Decreases lamotrigine steady-state concentrations by approximately 45% to 54%). Products include:

Dilantin Kapseals 1906
Dilantin Parenteral 1910

Primidone (Decreases lamotrigine steady-state concentrations by approximately 40%). Products include:

Mysoline... 2754

Sodium Valproate (Decreases the clearance of lamotrigine, i.e., more than doubles the elimination t½ of lamotrigine, whether given with or without hepatic enzyme-inducing antiepileptic drugs; the steady-state valproic acid concentrations in plasma may be decreased by an average of 25%).

Trimethoprim (Lamotrigine is an inhibitor of dihydrofolate reductase; prescribers should be aware of this action when used concurrently with agents which inhibit folate metabolism). Products include:

Bactrim DS Tablets................................. 2084
Bactrim I.V. Infusion 2082
Bactrim 2084
Proloprim Tablets 1155
Septra 1174
Septra I.V. Infusion 1169
Septra I.V. Infusion ADD-Vantage Vials.. 1171
Septra 1174
Trimpex Tablets 2163

Trimetrexate Glucuronate (Lamotrigine is an inhibitor of dihydrofolate reductase; prescribers should be aware of this action when used concurrently with agents which inhibit folate metabolism). Products include:

Neutrexin.. 2572

IMPORTANT NOTE: Always consult each drug listing in the patient's regimen for possible interactions.

Lamictal Interactions Index 548

Valproic Acid (Decreases the clearance of lamotrigine, i.e., more than doubles the elimination t½ of lamotrigine, whether given with or without hepatic enzyme-inducing antiepileptic drugs; the steady-state valproic acid concentrations in plasma may be decreased by an average of 25%). Products include:
- Depakene 413

LAMISIL CREAM 1%
(Terbinafine Hydrochloride) 2265
None cited in PDR database.

LAMPRENE CAPSULES
(Clofazimine) 828
None cited in PDR database.

LANOXICAPS
(Digoxin) 1117
May interact with potassium-depleting diuretics, potassium-depleting corticosteroids, mineralocorticoids, thyroid preparations, diuretics, antacids, sympathomimetics, beta blockers, calcium channel blockers, tetracyclines, macrolide antibiotics, and certain other agents. Compounds in these categories include:

Acebutolol Hydrochloride (Additive effects on AV node conduction). Products include:
- Sectral Capsules 2807

Albuterol (Increased risk of cardiac arrhythmias). Products include:
- Proventil Inhalation Aerosol 2382
- Ventolin Inhalation Aerosol and Refill 1197

Albuterol Sulfate (Increased risk of cardiac arrhythmias). Products include:
- Airet Solution for Inhalation 452
- Proventil Inhalation Solution 0.083% 2384
- Proventil Repetabs Tablets 2386
- Proventil Solution for Inhalation 0.5% 2383
- Proventil Syrup 2385
- Proventil Tablets 2386
- Ventolin Inhalation Solution 1198
- Ventolin Nebules Inhalation Solution 1199
- Ventolin Rotacaps for Inhalation 1200
- Ventolin Syrup 1202
- Ventolin Tablets 1203
- Volmax Extended-Release Tablets .. 1788

Alprazolam (Causes a rise in serum digoxin concentration, with the implication that digitalis intoxication may result). Products include:
- Xanax Tablets 2649

Aluminum Carbonate Gel (Interferes with intestinal digoxin absorption). Products include:
- Basaljel 2703

Aluminum Hydroxide (Interferes with intestinal digoxin absorption). Products include:
- ALternaGEL Liquid 1316
- Maximum Strength Ascriptin .... ▣ 630
- Cama Arthritis Pain Reliever .... ▣ 785
- Gaviscon Extra Strength Relief Formula Antacid Tablets .... ▣ 819
- Gaviscon Extra Strength Relief Formula Liquid Antacid .... ▣ 819
- Gaviscon Liquid Antacid .... ▣ 820
- Gelusil Liquid & Tablets .... ▣ 855
- Maalox Heartburn Relief Suspension .... ▣ 642
- Maalox Heartburn Relief Tablets .... ▣ 641
- Maalox Magnesia and Alumina Oral Suspension .... ▣ 642
- Maalox Plus Tablets .... ▣ 643
- Extra Strength Maalox Antacid Plus Antigas Liquid and Tablets ▣ 638
- Tempo Soft Antacid .... ▣ 835

Aluminum Hydroxide Gel (Interferes with intestinal digoxin absorption). Products include:
- ALternaGEL Liquid .... ▣ 659
- Aludrox Oral Suspension 2695
- Amphojel Suspension 2695
- Amphojel Suspension without Flavor 2695
- Amphojel Tablets 2695
- Arthritis Pain Ascriptin .... ▣ 631
- Regular Strength Ascriptin Tablets .... ▣ 629
- Gaviscon Antacid Tablets .... ▣ 819
- Gaviscon-2 Antacid Tablets .... ▣ 820
- Mylanta Liquid 1317
- Mylanta Tablets .... ▣ 660
- Mylanta Double Strength Liquid 1317
- Mylanta Double Strength Tablets .. ▣ 660
- Nephrox Suspension .... ▣ 655

Aluminum Hydroxide Gel, Dried (Interferes with intestinal digoxin absorption).

Amiodarone Hydrochloride (Causes a rise in serum digoxin concentration, with the implication that digitalis intoxication may result). Products include:
- Cordarone Intravenous 2715
- Cordarone Tablets 2712

Amlodipine Besylate (Additive effects on AV node conduction). Products include:
- Lotrel Capsules 840
- Norvasc Tablets 1940

Amphotericin B (Amphotericin B-induced hypokalemia sensitizes the myocardium to digitalis resulting in possible digitalis toxicity). Products include:
- Fungizone Intravenous 506

Anticancer Drugs, unspecified (Interferes with intestinal digoxin absorption).

Atenolol (Additive effects on AV node conduction). Products include:
- Tenoretic Tablets 2845
- Tenormin Tablets and I.V. Injection 2847

Azithromycin (May increase digoxin absorption in patients who convert digoxin to inactive metabolites in the gut resulting in increased serum levels of digoxin). Products include:
- Zithromax 1944

Bendroflumethiazide (Diuretic-induced hypokalemia sensitizes the myocardium to digitalis resulting in possible digitalis toxicity).
- No products indexed under this heading.

Bepridil Hydrochloride (Additive effects on AV node conduction). Products include:
- Vascor (200, 300 and 400 mg) Tablets 1587

Betamethasone Acetate (Corticosteroid-induced hypokalemia sensitizes the myocardium to digitalis resulting in possible digitalis toxicity). Products include:
- Celestone Soluspan Suspension 2347

Betamethasone Sodium Phosphate (Corticosteroid-induced hypokalemia sensitizes the myocardium to digitalis resulting in possible digitalis toxicity). Products include:
- Celestone Soluspan Suspension 2347

Betaxolol Hydrochloride (Additive effects on AV node conduction). Products include:
- Betoptic Ophthalmic Solution 469
- Betoptic S Ophthalmic Suspension 471
- Kerlone Tablets 2436

Bisoprolol Fumarate (Additive effects on AV node conduction). Products include:
- Zebeta Tablets 1413
- Ziac 1415

Calcium, intravenous (May produce serious arrhythmias in digitalized patients).
- No products indexed under this heading.

Carteolol Hydrochloride (Additive effects on Av node conduction). Products include:
- Cartrol Tablets 410
- Ocupress Ophthalmic Solution, 1% Sterile .... ⊙ 309

Chlorothiazide (Diuretic-induced hypokalemia sensitizes the myocardium to digitalis resulting in possible digitalis toxicity). Products include:
- Aldoclor Tablets 1598
- Diupres Tablets 1650
- Diuril Oral 1653

Chlorothiazide Sodium (Diuretic-induced hypokalemia sensitizes the myocardium to digitalis resulting in possible digitalis toxicity). Products include:
- Diuril Sodium Intravenous 1652

Chlorthalidone (Diuretic-induced hypokalemia sensitizes the myocardium to digitalis resulting in possible digitalis toxicity). Products include:
- Combipres Tablets 677
- Tenoretic Tablets 2845
- Thalitone 1245

Cholestyramine (Interferes with intestinal digoxin absorption). Products include:
- Questran Light 769
- Questran Powder 770

Clarithromycin (May increase digoxin absorption in patients who convert digoxin to inactive metabolites in the gut resulting in increased serum levels of digoxin). Products include:
- Biaxin 405

Cortisone Acetate (Corticosteroid-induced hypokalemia sensitizes the myocardium to digitalis resulting in possible digitalis toxicity). Products include:
- Cortone Acetate Sterile Suspension 1623
- Cortone Acetate Tablets 1624

Demeclocycline Hydrochloride (May increase digoxin absorption in patients who convert digoxin to inactive metabolites in the gut resulting in increased serum levels of digoxin). Products include:
- Declomycin Tablets 1371

Desoxycorticosterone Acetate (Contributing factor to digitalis toxicity).

Dexamethasone (Corticosteroid-induced hypokalemia sensitizes the myocardium to digitalis resulting in possible digitalis toxicity). Products include:
- AK-Trol Ointment & Suspension .... ⊙ 205
- Decadron Elixir 1633
- Decadron Tablets 1635
- Decaspray Topical Aerosol 1648
- Dexacidin Ointment .... ⊙ 263
- Maxitrol Ophthalmic Ointment and Suspension .... ⊙ 224
- TobraDex Ophthalmic Suspension and Ointment 473

Dexamethasone Acetate (Corticosteroid-induced hypokalemia sensitizes the myocardium to digitalis resulting in possible digitalis toxicity). Products include:
- Dalalone D.P. Injectable 1011
- Decadron-LA Sterile Suspension 1646

Dexamethasone Sodium Phosphate (Corticosteroid-induced hypokalemia sensitizes the myocardium to digitalis resulting in possible digitalis toxicity). Products include:
- Decadron Phosphate Injection 1637
- Decadron Phosphate Respihaler 1642
- Decadron Phosphate Sterile Ophthalmic Ointment 1641
- Decadron Phosphate Sterile Ophthalmic Solution 1642
- Decadron Phosphate Topical Cream 1644
- Decadron Phosphate Turbinaire 1645
- Decadron Phosphate with Xylocaine Injection, Sterile 1639
- Dexacort Phosphate in Respihaler .. 458
- Dexacort Phosphate in Turbinaire .. 459
- NeoDecadron Sterile Ophthalmic Ointment 1712
- NeoDecadron Sterile Ophthalmic Solution 1713
- NeoDecadron Topical Cream 1714

Dihydroxyaluminum Sodium Carbonate (Interferes with intestinal digoxin absorption).
- No products indexed under this heading.

Diltiazem Hydrochloride (Additive effects on AV node conduction). Products include:
- Cardizem CD Capsules 1506
- Cardizem SR Capsules 1510
- Cardizem Injectable 1508
- Cardizem Tablets 1512
- Dilacor XR Extended-release Capsules 2018

Diphenoxylate Hydrochloride (Increases digoxin absorption). Products include:
- Lomotil 2439

Dobutamine Hydrochloride (Increased risk of cardiac arrhythmias). Products include:
- Dobutrex Solution Vials 1439

Dopamine Hydrochloride (Increased risk of cardiac arrhythmias).
- No products indexed under this heading.

Doxycycline Calcium (May increase digoxin absorption in patients who convert digoxin to inactive metabolites in the gut resulting in increased serum levels of digoxin). Products include:
- Vibramycin Calcium Oral Suspension Syrup 1941

Doxycycline Hyclate (May increase digoxin absorption in patients who convert digoxin to inactive metabolites in the gut resulting in increased serum levels of digoxin). Products include:
- Doryx Capsules 1913
- Vibramycin Hyclate Capsules 1941
- Vibramycin Hyclate Intravenous 2215
- Vibra-Tabs Film Coated Tablets 1941

Doxycycline Monohydrate (May increase digoxin absorption in patients who convert digoxin to inactive metabolites in the gut resulting in increased serum levels of digoxin). Products include:
- Monodox Capsules 1805
- Vibramycin Monohydrate for Oral Suspension 1941

Ephedrine Hydrochloride (Increased risk of cardiac arrhythmias). Products include:
- Primatene Dual Action Formula .... ▣ 872
- Primatene Tablets .... ▣ 873
- Quadrinal Tablets 1350

Ephedrine Sulfate (Increased risk of cardiac arrhythmias). Products include:
- Bronkaid Caplets .... ▣ 717
- Marax Tablets & DF Syrup 2200

Ephedrine Tannate (Increased risk of cardiac arrhythmias). Products include:
- Rynatuss 2673

Epinephrine (Increased risk of cardiac arrhythmias). Products include:
- Bronkaid Mist .... ▣ 717
- EPIFRIN .... ⊙ 239
- EpiPen 790
- Marcaine Hydrochloride with Epinephrine 1:200,000 2316
- Primatene Mist .... ▣ 873
- Sensorcaine with Epinephrine Injection 559
- Sus-Phrine Injection 1019
- Xylocaine with Epinephrine Injections 567

(▣ Described in PDR For Nonprescription Drugs) (⊙ Described in PDR For Ophthalmology)

549 Interactions Index Lanoxicaps

Epinephrine Bitartrate (Increased risk of cardiac arrhythmias). Products include:
Bronkaid Mist Suspension ⊞ 718
Sensorcaine-MPF with Epinephrine Injection 559

Epinephrine Hydrochloride (Increased risk of cardiac arrhythmias). Products include:
Ana-Kit Anaphylaxis Emergency Treatment Kit 617

Erythromycin (May increase digoxin absorption in patients who convert digoxin to inactive metabolites in the gut resulting in increased serum levels of digoxin). Products include:
A/T/S 2% Acne Topical Gel and Solution 1234
Benzamycin Topical Gel 905
E-Mycin Tablets 1341
Emgel 2% Topical Gel 1093
ERYC 1915
Erycette (erythromycin 2%) Topical Solution 1888
Ery-Tab Tablets 422
Erythromycin Base Filmtab 426
Erythromycin Delayed-Release Capsules, USP 427
Ilotycin Ophthalmic Ointment 912
PCE Dispertab Tablets 444
T-Stat 2.0% Topical Solution and Pads 2688
Theramycin Z Topical Solution 2% 1592

Erythromycin Estolate (May increase digoxin absorption in patients who convert digoxin to inactive metabolites in the gut resulting in increased serum levels of digoxin). Products include:
Ilosone 911

Erythromycin Ethylsuccinate (May increase digoxin absorption in patients who convert digoxin to inactive metabolites in the gut resulting in increased serum levels of digoxin). Products include:
E.E.S. 424
EryPed 421

Erythromycin Gluceptate (May increase digoxin absorption in patients who convert digoxin to inactive metabolites in the gut resulting in increased serum levels of digoxin). Products include:
Ilotycin Gluceptate, IV, Vials 913

Erythromycin Stearate (May increase digoxin absorption in patients who convert digoxin to inactive metabolites in the gut resulting in increased serum levels of digoxin). Products include:
Erythrocin Stearate Filmtab 425

Esmolol Hydrochloride (Additive effects on AV node conduction). Products include:
Brevibloc Injection 1808

Felodipine (Additive effects on AV node conduction). Products include:
Plendil Extended-Release Tablets 527

Furosemide (Diuretic-induced hypokalemia sensitizes the myocardium to digitalis resulting in possible digitalis toxicity). Products include:
Lasix Injection, Oral Solution and Tablets 1240

Hydrochlorothiazide (Diuretic-induced hypokalemia sensitizes the myocardium to digitalis resulting in possible digitalis toxicity). Products include:
Aldactazide 2413
Aldoril Tablets 1604
Apresazide Capsules 808
Capozide 742
Dyazide 2479
Esidrix Tablets 821
Esimil Tablets 822
HydroDIURIL Tablets 1674
Hydropres Tablets 1675
Hyzaar Tablets 1677
Inderide Tablets 2732
Inderide LA Long Acting Capsules 2734
Lopressor HCT Tablets 832
Lotensin HCT 837
Maxzide 1380
Moduretic Tablets 1705
Oretic Tablets 443
Prinzide Tablets 1737
Ser-Ap-Es Tablets 849
Timolide Tablets 1748
Vaseretic Tablets 1765
Zestoretic 2850
Ziac 1415

Hydrocortisone (Corticosteroid-induced hypokalemia sensitizes the myocardium to digitalis resulting in possible digitalis toxicity). Products include:
Anusol-HC Cream 2.5% 1896
Aquanil HC Lotion 1931
Bactine Hydrocortisone Anti-Itch Cream ⊞ 709
Caldecort Anti-Itch Hydrocortisone Spray ⊞ 631
Cortaid ⊞ 836
CORTENEMA 2535
Cortisporin Ointment 1085
Cortisporin Ophthalmic Ointment Sterile 1085
Cortisporin Ophthalmic Suspension Sterile 1086
Cortisporin Otic Solution Sterile 1087
Cortisporin Otic Suspension Sterile 1088
Cortizone-5 ⊞ 831
Cortizone-10 ⊞ 831
Hydrocortone Tablets 1672
Hytone 907
Massengill Medicated Soft Cloth Towelettes 2458
PediOtic Suspension Sterile 1153
Preparation H Hydrocortisone 1% Cream ⊞ 872
ProctoCream-HC 2.5% 2408
VōSoL HC Otic Solution 2678

Hydrocortisone Acetate (Corticosteroid-induced hypokalemia sensitizes the myocardium to digitalis resulting in possible digitalis toxicity). Products include:
Analpram-HC Rectal Cream 1% and 2.5% 977
Anusol HC-1 Anti-Itch Hydrocortisone Ointment ⊞ 847
Anusol-HC Suppositories 1897
Caldecort ⊞ 631
Carmol HC 924
Coly-Mycin S Otic w/Neomycin & Hydrocortisone 1906
Cortaid ⊞ 836
Cortifoam 2396
Cortisporin Cream 1084
Epifoam 2399
Hydrocortone Acetate Sterile Suspension 1669
Mantadil Cream 1135
Nupercainal Hydrocortisone 1% Cream ⊞ 645
Ophthocort ◉ 311
Pramosone Cream, Lotion & Ointment 978
ProctoCream-HC 2408
ProctoFoam-HC 2409
Terra-Cortril Ophthalmic Suspension 2210

Hydrocortisone Sodium Phosphate (Corticosteroid-induced hypokalemia sensitizes the myocardium to digitalis resulting in possible digitalis toxicity). Products include:
Hydrocortone Phosphate Injection, Sterile 1670

Hydrocortisone Sodium Succinate (Corticosteroid-induced hypokalemia sensitizes the myocardium to digitalis resulting in possible digitalis toxicity). Products include:
Solu-Cortef Sterile Powder 2641

Hydroflumethiazide (Diuretic-induced hypokalemia sensitizes the myocardium to digitalis resulting in possible digitalis toxicity). Products include:
Diucardin Tablets 2718

Indapamide (Diuretic-induced hypokalemia sensitizes the myocardium to digitalis resulting in possible digitalis toxicity). Products include:
Lozol Tablets 2022

Indomethacin (Causes a rise in serum digoxin concentration, with the implication that digitalis intoxication may result). Products include:
Indocin 1680

Indomethacin Sodium Trihydrate (Causes a rise in serum digoxin concentration, with the implication that digitalis intoxication may result). Products include:
Indocin I.V. 1684

Isoproterenol Hydrochloride (Increased risk of cardiac arrhythmias). Products include:
Isuprel Hydrochloride Injection 1:5000 2311
Isuprel Hydrochloride Solution 1:200 & 1:100 2313
Isuprel Mistometer 2312

Isoproterenol Sulfate (Increased risk of cardiac arrhythmias). Products include:
Norisodrine with Calcium Iodide Syrup 442

Isradipine (Additive effects on AV node conduction). Products include:
DynaCirc Capsules 2256

Itraconazole (Causes a rise in serum digoxin concentration, with the implication that digitalis intoxication may result). Products include:
Sporanox Capsules 1305

Kaolin (Interferes with intestinal digoxin absorption).
No products indexed under this heading.

Labetalol Hydrochloride (Additive effects on AV node conduction). Products include:
Normodyne Injection 2377
Normodyne Tablets 2379
Trandate 1185

Levobunolol Hydrochloride (Additive effects on AV node conduction). Products include:
Betagan ◉ 233

Liothyronine Sodium (Hypothyroid patients may require increased digoxin dose). Products include:
Cytomel Tablets 2473
Triostat Injection 2530

Magaldrate (Interferes with intestinal digoxin absorption).
No products indexed under this heading.

Magnesium Hydroxide (Interferes with intestinal digoxin absorption). Products include:
Aludrox Oral Suspension 2695
Arthritis Pain Ascriptin ⊞ 631
Maximum Strength Ascriptin ⊞ 630
Regular Strength Ascriptin Tablets ⊞ 629
Di-Gel Antacid/Anti-Gas ⊞ 801
Gelusil Liquid & Tablets ⊞ 855
Maalox Magnesia and Alumina Oral Suspension ⊞ 642
Maalox Plus Tablets ⊞ 643
Extra Strength Maalox Antacid Plus Antigas Liquid and Tablets ⊞ 638
Mylanta Calcium Carbonate and Magnesium Hydroxide Tablets 1318
Mylanta Liquid 1317
Mylanta Tablets ⊞ 660
Mylanta Double Strength Liquid 1317
Mylanta Double Strength Tablets ⊞ 660
Phillips' Milk of Magnesia Liquid ⊞ 729
Rolaids Tablets ⊞ 843
Tempo Soft Antacid ⊞ 835

Magnesium Oxide (Interferes with intestinal digoxin absorption). Products include:
Beelith Tablets 639
Bufferin Analgesic Tablets and Caplets ⊞ 613
Caltrate PLUS ⊞ 665
Cama Arthritis Pain Reliever ⊞ 785
Mag-Ox 400 668
Uro-Mag 668

Metaproterenol Sulfate (Increased risk of cardiac arrhythmias). Products include:
Alupent 669
Metaproterenol Sulfate Inhalation Solution, USP, Arm-a-Med 552

Metaraminol Bitartrate (Increased risk of cardiac arrhythmias). Products include:
Aramine Injection 1609

Methacycline Hydrochloride (May increase digoxin absorption in patients who convert digoxin to inactive metabolites in the gut resulting in increased serum levels of digoxin).
No products indexed under this heading.

Methoxamine Hydrochloride (Increased risk of cardiac arrhythmias). Products include:
Vasoxyl Injection 1196

Methyclothiazide (Diuretic-induced hypokalemia sensitizes the myocardium to digitalis resulting in possible digitalis toxicity). Products include:
Enduron Tablets 420

Methylprednisolone Acetate (Corticosteroid-induced hypokalemia sensitizes the myocardium to digitalis resulting in possible digitalis toxicity). Products include:
Depo-Medrol Single-Dose Vial 2600
Depo-Medrol Sterile Aqueous Suspension 2597

Methylprednisolone Sodium Succinate (Corticosteroid-induced hypokalemia sensitizes the myocardium to digitalis resulting in possible digitalis toxicity). Products include:
Solu-Medrol Sterile Powder 2643

Metipranolol Hydrochloride (Additive effects on AV node conduction). Products include:
OptiPranolol (Metipranolol 0.3%) Sterile Ophthalmic Solution ◉ 258

Metolazone (Diuretic-induced hypokalemia sensitizes the myocardium to digitalis resulting in possible digitalis toxicity). Products include:
Mykrox Tablets 993
Zaroxolyn Tablets 1000

Metoprolol Succinate (Additive effects on AV node conduction). Products include:
Toprol-XL Tablets 565

Metoprolol Tartrate (Additive effects on AV node conduction). Products include:
Lopressor Ampuls 830
Lopressor HCT Tablets 832
Lopressor Tablets 830

Minocycline Hydrochloride (May increase digoxin absorption in patients who convert digoxin to inactive metabolites in the gut resulting in increased serum levels of digoxin). Products include:
Dynacin Capsules 1590
Minocin Intravenous 1382
Minocin Oral Suspension 1385
Minocin Pellet-Filled Capsules 1383

Nadolol (Additive effects on AV node conduction).
No products indexed under this heading.

Neomycin, oral (Interferes with intestinal digoxin absorption).

Nephrotoxic Drugs (May impair the excretion of digoxin).

Nicardipine Hydrochloride (Additive effects on AV node conduction). Products include:
Cardene Capsules 2095
Cardene I.V. 2709
Cardene SR Capsules 2097

IMPORTANT NOTE: Always consult each drug listing in the patient's regimen for possible interactions.

Lanoxicaps

Interactions Index

Nifedipine (Additive effects on AV node conduction). Products include:

Adalat Capsules (10 mg and 20 mg) 587
Adalat CC 589
Procardia Capsules 1971
Procardia XL Extended Release Tablets 1972

Nimodipine (Additive effects on AV node conduction). Products include:

Nimotop Capsules 610

Nisoldipine (Additive effects on AV node conduction).

No products indexed under this heading.

Norepinephrine Bitartrate (Increased risk of cardiac arrhythmias). Products include:

Levophed Bitartrate Injection 2315

Oxytetracycline Hydrochloride (May increase digoxin absorption in patients who convert digoxin to inactive metabolites in the gut resulting in increased serum levels of digoxin). Products include:

TERAK Ointment .... ⊙ 209
Terra-Cortril Ophthalmic Suspension 2210
Terramycin with Polymyxin B Sulfate Ophthalmic Ointment 2211
Urobiotic-250 Capsules 2214

Pectin (Interferes with intestinal digoxin absorption). Products include:

Celestial Seasonings Soothers Throat Drops .... ®D 842

Penbutolol Sulfate (Additive effects on AV node conduction). Products include:

Levatol 2403

Phenylephrine Bitartrate (Increased risk of cardiac arrhythmias).

No products indexed under this heading.

Phenylephrine Hydrochloride (Increased risk of cardiac arrhythmias). Products include:

Atrohist Plus Tablets 454
Cerose DM .... ®D 878
Comhist 2038
D.A. Chewable Tablets 951
Deconsal Pediatric Capsules 454
Dura-Vent/DA Tablets 953
Entex Capsules 1986
Entex Liquid 1986
Extendryl 1005
4-Way Fast Acting Nasal Spray (regular & mentholated) .... ®D 621
Hemorid For Women .... ®D 834
Hycomine Compound Tablets 932
Neo-Synephrine Hydrochloride 1% Carpuject 2324
Neo-Synephrine Hydrochloride 1% Injection 2324
Neo-Synephrine Hydrochloride (Ophthalmic) 2325
Neo-Synephrine .... ®D 726
Nōstril .... ®D 644
Novahistine Elixir .... ®D 823
Phenergan VC 2779
Phenergan VC with Codeine 2781
Preparation H .... ®D 871
Tympagesic Ear Drops 2342
Vasosulf .... ⊙ 271
Vicks Sinex Nasal Spray and Ultra Fine Mist .... ®D 765

Phenylephrine Tannate (Increased risk of cardiac arrhythmias). Products include:

Atrohist Pediatric Suspension 454
Ricobid-D Pediatric Suspension 2038
Ricobid Tablets and Pediatric Suspension 2038
Rynatan 2673
Rynatuss 2673

Phenylpropanolamine Hydrochloride (Increased risk of cardiac arrhythmias). Products include:

Acutrim .... ®D 628
Allerest Children's Chewable Tablets .... ®D 627
Allerest 12 Hour Caplets .... ®D 627
Atrohist Plus Tablets 454

BC Cold Powder Multi-Symptom Formula (Cold-Sinus-Allergy) ...... ®D 609
BC Cold Powder Non-Drowsy Formula (Cold-Sinus) .... ®D 609
Cheracol Plus Head Cold/Cough Formula .... ®D 769
Comtrex Multi-Symptom Non-Drowsy Liqui-gels .... ®D 618
Contac Continuous Action Nasal Decongestant/Antihistamine 12 Hour Capsules .... ®D 813
Contac Maximum Strength Continuous Action Decongestant/ Antihistamine 12 Hour Caplets .. ®D 813
Contac Severe Cold and Flu Formula Caplets .... ®D 814
Coricidin 'D' Decongestant Tablets .... ®D 800
Dexatrim .... ®D 832
Dexatrim Plus Vitamins Caplets .... ®D 832
Dimetane-DC Cough Syrup 2059
Dimetapp Elixir .... ®D 773
Dimetapp Extentabs .... ®D 774
Dimetapp Tablets/Liqui-Gels .... ®D 775
Dimetapp Cold & Allergy Chewable Tablets .... ®D 773
Dimetapp DM Elixir .... ®D 774
Dura-Vent Tablets 952
Entex Capsules 1986
Entex LA Tablets 1987
Entex Liquid 1986
Exgest LA Tablets 782
Hycomine 931
Isoclor Timesule Capsules .... ®D 637
Nolamine Timed-Release Tablets 785
Ornade Spansule Capsules 2502
Propagest Tablets 786
Pyrroxate Caplets .... ®D 772
Robitussin-CF .... ®D 777
Sinulin Tablets 787
Tavist-D 12 Hour Relief Tablets .... ®D 787
Teldrin 12 Hour Antihistamine/ Nasal Decongestant Allergy Relief Capsules .... ®D 826
Triaminic Allergy Tablets .... ®D 789
Triaminic Cold Tablets .... ®D 790
Triaminic Expectorant .... ®D 790
Triaminic Syrup .... ®D 792
Triaminic-12 Tablets .... ®D 792
Triaminic-DM Syrup .... ®D 792
Triaminicin Tablets .... ®D 793
Triaminicol Multi-Symptom Cold Tablets .... ®D 793
Triaminicol Multi-Symptom Relief ®D 794
Vicks DayQuil Allergy Relief 12-Hour Extended Release Tablets .. ®D 760
Vicks DayQuil Allergy Relief 4-Hour Tablets .... ®D 760
Vicks DayQuil SINUS Pressure & CONGESTION Relief .... ®D 761

Pindolol (Additive effects on AV node conduction). Products include:

Visken Tablets 2299

Pirbuterol Acetate (Increased risk of cardiac arrhythmias). Products include:

Maxair Autohaler 1492
Maxair Inhaler 1494

Polythiazide (Diuretic-induced hypokalemia sensitizes the myocardium to digitalis resulting in possible digitalis toxicity). Products include:

Minizide Capsules 1938

Prednisolone Acetate (Corticosteroid-induced hypokalemia sensitizes the myocardium to digitalis resulting in possible digitalis toxicity). Products include:

AK-CIDE .... ⊙ 202
AK-CIDE Ointment .... ⊙ 202
Blephamide Liquifilm Sterile Ophthalmic Suspension 476
Blephamide Ointment .... ⊙ 237
Econopred & Econopred Plus Ophthalmic Suspensions .... ⊙ 217
Poly-Pred Liquifilm .... ⊙ 248
Pred Forte .... ⊙ 250
Pred Mild .... ⊙ 253
Pred-G Liquifilm Sterile Ophthalmic Suspension .... ⊙ 251
Pred-G S.O.P. Sterile Ophthalmic Ointment .... ⊙ 252
Vasocidin Ointment .... ⊙ 268

Prednisolone Sodium Phosphate (Corticosteroid-induced hypokalemia sensitizes the myocardium to digitalis resulting in possible digitalis toxicity). Products include:

AK-Pred .... ⊙ 204
Hydeltrasol Injection, Sterile 1665
Inflamase .... ⊙ 265
Pediapred Oral Liquid 995
Vasocidin Ophthalmic Solution ...... ⊙ 270

Prednisolone Tebutate (Corticosteroid-induced hypokalemia sensitizes the myocardium to digitalis resulting in possible digitalis toxicity). Products include:

Hydeltra-T.B.A. Sterile Suspension 1667

Prednisone (Corticosteroid-induced hypokalemia sensitizes the myocardium to digitalis resulting in possible digitalis toxicity). Products include:

Deltasone Tablets 2595

Propafenone Hydrochloride (Causes a rise in serum digoxin concentration, with the implication that digitalis intoxication may result). Products include:

Rythmol Tablets–150mg, 225mg, 300mg 1352

Propantheline Bromide (Increases digoxin absorption). Products include:

Pro-Banthine Tablets 2052

Propranolol Hydrochloride (Additive effects on AV node conduction). Products include:

Inderal 2728
Inderal LA Long Acting Capsules 2730
Inderide Tablets 2732
Inderide LA Long Acting Capsules .. 2734

Pseudoephedrine Hydrochloride (Increased risk of cardiac arrhythmias). Products include:

Actifed Allergy Daytime/Nighttime Caplets .... ®D 844
Actifed Plus Caplets .... ®D 845
Actifed Plus Tablets .... ®D 845
Actifed with Codeine Cough Syrup.. 1067
Actifed Sinus Daytime/Nighttime Tablets and Caplets .... ®D 846
Actifed Syrup .... ®D 846
Actifed Tablets .... ®D 844
Advil Cold and Sinus Caplets and Tablets (formerly CoAdvil) .... ®D 870
Alka-Seltzer Plus Cold Medicine Liqui-Gels .... ®D 706
Alka-Seltzer Plus Cold & Cough Medicine Liqui-Gels .... ®D 705
Alka-Seltzer Plus Night-Time Cold Medicine Liqui-Gels .... ®D 706
Allerest Headache Strength Tablets .... ®D 627
Allerest Maximum Strength Tablets .... ®D 627
Allerest No Drowsiness Tablets ...... ®D 627
Allerest Sinus Pain Formula .... ®D 627
Anatuss LA Tablets 1542
Atrohist Pediatric Capsules 453
Bayer Select Sinus Pain Relief Formula .... ®D 717
Benadryl Allergy Decongestant Liquid Medication .... ®D 848
Benadryl Allergy Decongestant Tablets .... ®D 848
Benadryl Allergy Sinus Headache Formula Caplets .... ®D 849
Benylin Multisymptom .... ®D 852
Bromfed Capsules (Extended-Release) 1785
Bromfed Syrup .... ®D 733
Bromfed Tablets 1785
Bromfed-DM Cough Syrup 1786
Bromfed-PD Capsules (Extended-Release) 1785
Children's Vicks DayQuil Allergy Relief .... ®D 757
Children's Vicks NyQuil Cold/ Cough Relief .... ®D 758
Comtrex Multi-Symptom Cold Reliever Tablets/Caplets/Liqui-Gels/Liquid .... ®D 615
Allergy-Sinus Comtrex Multi-Symptom Allergy-Sinus Formula Tablets .... ®D 617
Comtrex Multi-Symptom Non-Drowsy Caplets .... ®D 618

Congess 1004
Contac Day Allergy/Sinus Caplets ®D 812
Contac Day & Night .... ®D 812
Contac Night Allergy/Sinus Caplets .... ®D 812
Contac Severe Cold & Flu Non-Drowsy .... ®D 815
Deconamine Chewable Tablets 1320
Deconamine CX Cough and Cold Liquid and Tablets 1319
Deconamine 1320
Deconsal C Expectorant Syrup 456
Deconsal Pediatric Syrup 457
Deconsal II Tablets 454
Dimetane-DX Cough Syrup 2059
Dimetapp Sinus Caplets .... ®D 775
Dorcol Children's Cough Syrup ...... ®D 785
Drixoral Cough + Congestion Liquid Caps .... ®D 802
Dura-Tap/PD Capsules 2867
Duratuss Tablets 2565
Duratuss HD Elixir 2565
Efidac/24 .... ®D 635
Entex PSE Tablets 1987
Fedahist Gyrocaps 2401
Fedahist Timecaps 2401
Guaifed 1787
Guaifed Syrup .... ®D 734
Guaimax-D Tablets 792
Guaitab Tablets .... ®D 734
Isoclor Expectorant 990
Kronofed-A 977
Motrin IB Sinus .... ®D 838
Novahistine DH 2462
Novahistine DMX .... ®D 822
Novahistine Expectorant 2463
Nucofed 2051
PediaCare Cold Allergy Chewable Tablets .... ®D 677
PediaCare Cough-Cold Chewable Tablets 1553
PediaCare 1553
PediaCare Infants' Decongestant Drops .... ®D 677
PediCare Infant's Drops Decongestant Plus Cough 1553
PediaCare NightRest Cough-Cold Liquid 1553
Pediatric Vicks 44d Dry Hacking Cough & Head Congestion .... ®D 763
Pediatric Vicks 44m Cough & Cold Relief .... ®D 764
Robitussin Cold & Cough Liqui-Gels .... ®D 776
Robitussin Maximum Strength Cough & Cold .... ®D 778
Robitussin Pediatric Cough & Cold Formula .... ®D 779
Robitussin Severe Congestion Liqui-Gels .... ®D 776
Robitussin-DAC Syrup 2074
Robitussin-PE .... ®D 778
Rondec Oral Drops 953
Rondec Syrup 953
Rondec Tablet 953
Rondec-DM Oral Drops 954
Rondec-DM Syrup 954
Rondec-TR Tablet 953
Ryna .... ®D 841
Seldane-D Extended-Release Tablets 1538
Semprex-D Capsules 463
Semprex-D Capsules 1167
Sinarest Tablets .... ®D 648
Sinarest Extra Strength Tablets ...... ®D 648
Sinarest No Drowsiness Tablets .... ®D 648
Sine-Aid IB Caplets 1554
Sine-Aid Maximum Strength Sinus Medication Gelcaps, Caplets and Tablets 1554
Sine-Off No Drowsiness Formula Caplets .... ®D 824
Sine-Off Sinus Medicine .... ®D 825
Singlet Tablets .... ®D 825
Sinutab Non-Drying Liquid Caps .... ®D 859
Sinutab Sinus Allergy Medication, Maximum Strength Tablets and Caplets .... ®D 860
Sinutab Sinus Medication, Maximum Strength Without Drowsiness Formula, Tablets & Caplets .... ®D 860
Sinutab Sinus Medication, Regular Strength Without Drowsiness Formula .... ®D 859
Sudafed Children's Liquid .... ®D 861
Sudafed Cold and Cough Liquidcaps .... ®D 862
Sudafed Cough Syrup .... ®D 862
Sudafed Plus Liquid .... ®D 862
Sudafed Plus Tablets .... ®D 863

(®D Described in PDR For Nonprescription Drugs) (⊙ Described in PDR For Ophthalmology)

Interactions Index

Lanoxin Elixir

Sudafed Severe Cold Formula Caplets .... ⓢⓓ 863
Sudafed Severe Cold Formula Tablets .... ⓢⓓ 864
Sudafed Sinus Caplets........................... ⓢⓓ 864
Sudafed Sinus Tablets........................... ⓢⓓ 864
Sudafed Tablets, 30 mg .... ⓢⓓ 861
Sudafed Tablets, 60 mg .... ⓢⓓ 861
Sudafed 12 Hour Caplets .... ⓢⓓ 861
Syn-Rx Tablets 465
Syn-Rx DM Tablets 466
TheraFlu.. ⓢⓓ 787
TheraFlu Maximum Strength Nighttime Flu, Cold & Cough Medicine .... ⓢⓓ 788
TheraFlu Maximum Strength Non-Drowsy Formula Flu, Cold & Cough Medicine .... ⓢⓓ 788
Thera Flu Maximum Strength, Non-Drowsy Formula Flu, Cold and Cough Caplets .... ⓢⓓ 789
Triaminic AM Cough and Decongestant Formula .... ⓢⓓ 789
Triaminic AM Decongestant Formula .... ⓢⓓ 799
Triaminic Nite Light .... ⓢⓓ 791
Triaminic Sore Throat Formula ...... ⓢⓓ 791
Tussend 1783
Tussend Expectorant 1785
Children's TYLENOL Cold Multi-Symptom Liquid Formula and Chewable Tablets................................ 1561
Children's TYLENOL Cold Plus Cough Multi Symptom Tablets and Liquid .... ⓢⓓ 681
Infants' TYLENOL Cold Decongestant & Fever-Reducer Drops 1556
TYLENOL Maximum Strength Allergy Sinus Medication Gelcaps and Caplets 1563
TYLENOL Maximum Strength Allergy Sinus NightTime Medication Caplets 1555
TYLENOL Flu Maximum Strength Gelcaps 1565
TYLENOL Flu NightTime, Maximum Strength, Gelcaps 1566
TYLENOL Maximum Strength Flu NightTime Hot Medication Packets 1562
TYLENOL, Maximum Strength, Sinus Medication Geltabs, Gelcaps, Caplets and Tablets 1566
TYLENOL Cold Multi-Symptom Formula Medication Tablets and Caplets 1561
TYLENOL Cold Medication No Drowsiness Formula Gelcaps and Caplets 1562
TYLENOL Cold Multi-Symptom Hot Medication Liquid Packets............ 1557
TYLENOL Cough Multi-Symptom Medication with Decongestant 1565
Ursinus Inlay-Tabs................................. ⓢⓓ 794
Vicks 44 LiquiCaps Cough, Cold & Flu Relief.. ⓢⓓ 755
Vicks 44 LiquiCaps Non-Drowsy Cough & Cold Relief .... ⓢⓓ 756
Vicks 44D Dry Hacking Cough & Head Congestion .... ⓢⓓ 755
Vicks 44M Cough, Cold & Flu Relief.. ⓢⓓ 756
Vicks DayQuil .... ⓢⓓ 761
Vicks DayQuil SINUS Pressure & PAIN Relief with IBUPROFEN ...... ⓢⓓ 762
Vicks Nyquil Hot Therapy................... ⓢⓓ 762
Vicks NyQuil LiquiCaps Multi-Symptom Cold/Flu Relief .... ⓢⓓ 763
Vicks NyQuil Multi-Symptom Cold/Flu Relief - (Original & Cherry Flavor) .... ⓢⓓ 763

Pseudoephedrine Sulfate (Increased risk of cardiac arrhythmias). Products include:

Cheracol Sinus .... ⓢⓓ 768
Chlor-Trimeton Allergy Decongestant Tablets .... ⓢⓓ 799
Claritin-D 2350
Drixoral Cold and Allergy Sustained-Action Tablets .... ⓢⓓ 802
Drixoral Cold and Flu Extended-Release Tablets.................................... ⓢⓓ 803
Drixoral Non-Drowsy Formula Extended-Release Tablets .... ⓢⓓ 803
Drixoral Allergy/Sinus Extended Release Tablets.................................... ⓢⓓ 804
Trinalin Repetabs Tablets 1330

Quinidine Gluconate (Causes a rise in serum digoxin concentration, with the implication that digitalis intoxication may result). Products include:

Quinaglute Dura-Tabs Tablets 649

Quinidine Polygalacturonate (Causes a rise in serum digoxin concentration, with the implication that digitalis intoxication may result).

No products indexed under this heading.

Quinidine Sulfate (Causes a rise in serum digoxin concentration, with the implication that digitalis intoxication may result). Products include:

Quinidex Extentabs 2067

Salmeterol Xinafoate (Increased risk of cardiac arrhythmias). Products include:

Serevent Inhalation Aerosol................ 1176

Sotalol Hydrochloride (Additive effects on AV node conduction). Products include:

Betapace Tablets 641

Succinylcholine Chloride (May cause arrhythmias). Products include:

Anectine.. 1073

Sulfasalazine (Interferes with intestinal digoxin absorption). Products include:

Azulfidine 1949

Terbutaline Sulfate (Increased risk of cardiac arrhythmias). Products include:

Brethaire Inhaler 813
Brethine Ampuls 815
Brethine Tablets....................................... 814
Bricanyl Subcutaneous Injection 1502
Bricanyl Tablets 1503

Tetracycline Hydrochloride (May increase digoxin absorption in patients who convert digoxin to inactive metabolites in the gut resulting in increased serum levels of digoxin). Products include:

Achromycin V Capsules 1367

Thyroid (Hypothyroid patients may require increased digoxin dose).

No products indexed under this heading.

Thyroxine (Hypothyroid patients may require increased digoxin dose).

No products indexed under this heading.

Timolol Hemihydrate (Additive effects on AV node conduction). Products include:

Betimol 0.25%, 0.5% .... © 261

Timolol Maleate (Additive effects on AV node conduction). Products include:

Blocadren Tablets 1614
Timolide Tablets...................................... 1748
Timoptic in Ocudose 1753
Timoptic Sterile Ophthalmic Solution.. 1751
Timoptic-XE 1755

Torsemide (Diuretic-induced hypokalemia sensitizes the myocardium to digitalis resulting in possible digitalis toxicity). Products include:

Demadex Tablets and Injection 686

Triamcinolone (Corticosteroid-induced hypokalemia sensitizes the myocardium to digitalis resulting in possible digitalis toxicity). Products include:

Aristocort Tablets 1022

Triamcinolone Acetonide (Corticosteroid-induced hypokalemia sensitizes the myocardium to digitalis resulting in possible digitalis toxicity). Products include:

Aristocort A 0.025% Cream 1027
Aristocort A 0.5% Cream 1031
Aristocort A 0.1% Cream 1029

Aristocort A 0.1% Ointment 1030
Azmacort Oral Inhaler 2011
Nasacort Nasal Inhaler 2024

Triamcinolone Diacetate (Corticosteroid-induced hypokalemia sensitizes the myocardium to digitalis resulting in possible digitalis toxicity). Products include:

Aristocort Suspension (Forte Parenteral).. 1027
Aristocort Suspension (Intralesional) 1025

Triamcinolone Hexacetonide (Corticosteroid-induced hypokalemia sensitizes the myocardium to digitalis resulting in possible digitalis toxicity). Products include:

Aristospan Suspension (Intra-articular)... 1033
Aristospan Suspension (Intralesional)... 1032

Troleandomycin (May increase digoxin absorption in patients who convert digoxin to inactive metabolites in the gut resulting in increased serum levels of digoxin). Products include:

Tao Capsules 2209

Verapamil Hydrochloride (Causes a rise in serum digoxin concentration, with the implication that digitalis intoxication may result). Products include:

Calan SR Caplets 2422
Calan Tablets... 2419
Isoptin Injectable 1344
Isoptin Oral Tablets 1346
Isoptin SR Tablets 1348
Verelan Capsules 1410
Verelan Capsules 2824

Food Interactions

Meal, high in bran fiber (Reduces the amount of digoxin from an oral dose).

Meal, unspecified (The rate of absorption is slowed).

LANOXIN ELIXIR PEDIATRIC

(Digoxin) 1120

May interact with potassium-depleting corticosteroids, potassium-depleting diuretics, antacids, sympathomimetics, beta blockers, calcium channel blockers, thyroid preparations, mineralocorticoids, tetracyclines, macrolide antibiotics, and certain other agents. Compounds in these categories include:

Acebutolol Hydrochloride (Additive effects on AV node conduction). Products include:

Sectral Capsules 2807

Albuterol (Increased risk of cardiac arrhythmias). Products include:

Proventil Inhalation Aerosol 2382
Ventolin Inhalation Aerosol and Refill 1197

Albuterol Sulfate (Increased risk of cardiac arrhythmias). Products include:

Airet Solution for Inhalation 452
Proventil Inhalation Solution 0.083% 2384
Proventil Repetabs Tablets 2386
Proventil Solution for Inhalation 0.5% 2383
Proventil Syrup... 2385
Proventil Tablets 2386
Ventolin Inhalation Solution................ 1198
Ventolin Nebules Inhalation Solution.. 1199
Ventolin Rotacaps for Inhalation 1200
Ventolin Syrup... 1202
Ventolin Tablets 1203
Volmax Extended-Release Tablets .. 1788

Alprazolam (Causes a rise in serum digoxin concentration, with the implication that digitalis intoxication may result). Products include:

Xanax Tablets 2649

Aluminum Carbonate Gel (Interferes with intestinal digoxin absorption). Products include:

Basaljel... 2703

Aluminum Hydroxide (Interferes with intestinal digoxin absorption). Products include:

ALternaGEL Liquid 1316
Maximum Strength Ascriptin .... ⓢⓓ 630
Cama Arthritis Pain Reliever............. ⓢⓓ 785
Gaviscon Extra Strength Relief Formula Antacid Tablets.................. ⓢⓓ 819
Gaviscon Extra Strength Relief Formula Liquid Antacid .... ⓢⓓ 819
Gaviscon Liquid Antacid .... ⓢⓓ 820
Gelusil Liquid & Tablets .... ⓢⓓ 855
Maalox Heartburn Relief Suspension .... ⓢⓓ 642
Maalox Heartburn Relief Tablets.... ⓢⓓ 641
Maalox Magnesia and Alumina Oral Suspension................................... ⓢⓓ 642
Maalox Plus Tablets .... ⓢⓓ 643
Extra Strength Maalox Antacid Plus Antigas Liquid and Tablets ⓢⓓ 638
Tempo Soft Antacid .... ⓢⓓ 835

Aluminum Hydroxide Gel (Interferes with intestinal digoxin absorption). Products include:

ALternaGEL Liquid .... ⓢⓓ 659
Aludrox Oral Suspension 2695
Amphojel Suspension 2695
Amphojel Suspension without Flavor 2695
Amphojel Tablets...................................... 2695
Arthritis Pain Ascriptin .... ⓢⓓ 631
Regular Strength Ascriptin Tablets .... ⓢⓓ 629
Gaviscon Antacid Tablets.................... ⓢⓓ 819
Gaviscon-2 Antacid Tablets .... ⓢⓓ 820
Mylanta Liquid 1317
Mylanta Tablets .... ⓢⓓ 660
Mylanta Double Strength Liquid 1317
Mylanta Double Strength Tablets .. ⓢⓓ 660
Nephrox Suspension .... ⓢⓓ 655

Aluminum Hydroxide Gel, Dried (Interferes with intestinal digoxin absorption).

Amiodarone Hydrochloride (Causes a rise in serum digoxin concentration, with the implication that digitalis intoxication may result). Products include:

Cordarone Intravenous 2715
Cordarone Tablets.................................... 2712

Amlodipine Besylate (Additive effects on AV node conduction). Products include:

Lotrel Capsules.. 840
Norvasc Tablets 1940

Amphotericin B (Amphotericin B-induced hypokalemia sensitizes the myocardium to digitalis resulting in possible digitalis toxicity). Products include:

Fungizone Intravenous 506

Anticancer Drugs, unspecified (Interferes with intestinal digoxin absorption).

Atenolol (Additive effects on AV node conduction). Products include:

Tenoretic Tablets....................................... 2845
Tenormin Tablets and I.V. Injection 2847

Azithromycin (May increase digoxin absorption in patients who convert digoxin to inactive metabolites in the gut resulting in increased serum levels of digoxin). Products include:

Zithromax 1944

Bendroflumethiazide (Diuretic-induced hypokalemia sensitizes the myocardium to digitalis resulting in possible digitalis toxicity).

No products indexed under this heading.

Bepridil Hydrochloride (Additive effects on AV node conduction). Products include:

Vascor (200, 300 and 400 mg) Tablets 1587

IMPORTANT NOTE: Always consult each drug listing in the patient's regimen for possible interactions.

Betamethasone Acetate (Corticosteroid-induced hypokalemia sensitizes the myocardium to digitalis resulting in possible digitalis toxicity). Products include:
- Celestone Soluspan Suspension 2347

Betamethasone Sodium Phosphate (Corticosteroid-induced hypokalemia sensitizes the myocardium to digitalis resulting in possible digitalis toxicity). Products include:
- Celestone Soluspan Suspension 2347

Betaxolol Hydrochloride (Additive effects on AV node conduction). Products include:
- Betoptic Ophthalmic Solution 469
- Betoptic S Ophthalmic Suspension 471
- Kerlone Tablets 2436

Bisoprolol Fumarate (Additive effects on AV node conduction). Products include:
- Zebeta Tablets 1413
- Ziac 1415

Calcium, intravenous (May produce serious arrhythmias in digitalized patients).
- No products indexed under this heading.

Carteolol Hydrochloride (Additive effects on AV node conduction). Products include:
- Cartrol Tablets 410
- Ocupress Ophthalmic Solution, 1% Sterile ...... ⊙ 309

Chlorothiazide (Diuretic-induced hypokalemia sensitizes the myocardium to digitalis resulting in possible digitalis toxicity). Products include:
- Aldoclor Tablets 1598
- Diupres Tablets 1650
- Diuril Oral 1653

Chlorothiazide Sodium (Diuretic-induced hypokalemia sensitizes the myocardium to digitalis resulting in possible digitalis toxicity). Products include:
- Diuril Sodium Intravenous 1652

Chlorthalidone (Diuretic-induced hypokalemia sensitizes the myocardium to digitalis resulting in possible digitalis toxicity). Products include:
- Combipres Tablets 677
- Tenoretic Tablets 2845
- Thalitone 1245

Cholestyramine (Interferes with intestinal digoxin absorption). Products include:
- Questran Light 769
- Questran Powder 770

Clarithromycin (May increase digoxin absorption in patients who convert digoxin to inactive metabolites in the gut resulting in increased serum levels of digoxin). Products include:
- Biaxin 405

Cortisone Acetate (Corticosteroid-induced hypokalemia sensitizes the myocardium to digitalis resulting in possible digitalis toxicity). Products include:
- Cortone Acetate Sterile Suspension 1623
- Cortone Acetate Tablets 1624

Demeclocycline Hydrochloride (May increase digoxin absorption in patients who convert digoxin to inactive metabolites in the gut resulting in increased serum levels of digoxin). Products include:
- Declomycin Tablets 1371

Dexamethasone (Corticosteroid-induced hypokalemia sensitizes the myocardium to digitalis resulting in possible digitalis toxicity). Products include:
- AK-Trol Ointment & Suspension ...... ⊙ 205
- Decadron Elixir 1633
- Decadron Tablets 1635
- Decaspray Topical Aerosol 1648
- Dexacidin Ointment ...... ⊙ 263
- Maxitrol Ophthalmic Ointment and Suspension ...... ⊙ 224
- TobraDex Ophthalmic Suspension and Ointment 473

Dexamethasone Acetate (Corticosteroid-induced hypokalemia sensitizes the myocardium to digitalis resulting in possible digitalis toxicity). Products include:
- Dalalone D.P. Injectable 1011
- Decadron-LA Sterile Suspension 1646

Dexamethasone Sodium Phosphate (Corticosteroid-induced hypokalemia sensitizes the myocardium to digitalis resulting in possible digitalis toxicity). Products include:
- Decadron Phosphate Injection 1637
- Decadron Phosphate Respihaler 1642
- Decadron Phosphate Sterile Ophthalmic Ointment 1641
- Decadron Phosphate Sterile Ophthalmic Solution 1642
- Decadron Phosphate Topical Cream 1644
- Decadron Phosphate Turbinaire 1645
- Decadron Phosphate with Xylocaine Injection, Sterile 1639
- Dexacort Phosphate in Respihaler .. 458
- Dexacort Phosphate in Turbinaire .. 459
- NeoDecadron Sterile Ophthalmic Ointment 1712
- NeoDecadron Sterile Ophthalmic Solution 1713
- NeoDecadron Topical Cream 1714

Dihydroxyaluminum Sodium Carbonate (Interferes with intestinal digoxin absorption).
- No products indexed under this heading.

Diltiazem Hydrochloride (Additive effects on AV node conduction). Products include:
- Cardizem CD Capsules 1506
- Cardizem SR Capsules 1510
- Cardizem Injectable 1508
- Cardizem Tablets 1512
- Dilacor XR Extended-release Capsules 2018

Diphenoxylate Hydrochloride (Increases digoxin absorption). Products include:
- Lomotil 2439

Dobutamine Hydrochloride (Increased risk of cardiac arrhythmias). Products include:
- Dobutrex Solution Vials 1439

Dopamine Hydrochloride (Increased risk of cardiac arrhythmias).
- No products indexed under this heading.

Doxycycline Calcium (May increase digoxin absorption in patients who convert digoxin to inactive metabolites in the gut resulting in increased serum levels of digoxin). Products include:
- Vibramycin Calcium Oral Suspension Syrup 1941

Doxycycline Hyclate (May increase digoxin absorption in patients who convert digoxin to inactive metabolites in the gut resulting in increased serum levels of digoxin). Products include:
- Doryx Capsules 1913
- Vibramycin Hyclate Capsules 1941
- Vibramycin Hyclate Intravenous 2215
- Vibra-Tabs Film Coated Tablets 1941

Doxycycline Monohydrate (May increase digoxin absorption in patients who convert digoxin to inactive metabolites in the gut resulting in increased serum levels of digoxin). Products include:
- Monodox Capsules 1805
- Vibramycin Monohydrate for Oral Suspension 1941

Ephedrine Hydrochloride (Increased risk of cardiac arrhythmias). Products include:
- Primatene Dual Action Formula ...... ▣ 872
- Primatene Tablets ...... ▣ 873
- Quadrinal Tablets 1350

Ephedrine Sulfate (Increased risk of cardiac arrhythmias). Products include:
- Bronkaid Caplets ...... ▣ 717
- Marax Tablets & DF Syrup 2200

Ephedrine Tannate (Increased risk of cardiac arrhythmias). Products include:
- Rynatuss 2673

Epinephrine (Increased risk of cardiac arrhythmias). Products include:
- Bronkaid Mist ...... ▣ 717
- EPIFRIN ...... ⊙ 239
- EpiPen 790
- Marcaine Hydrochloride with Epinephrine 1:200,000 2316
- Primatene Mist ...... ▣ 873
- Sensorcaine with Epinephrine Injection 559
- Sus-Phrine Injection 1019
- Xylocaine with Epinephrine Injections 567

Epinephrine Bitartrate (Increased risk of cardiac arrhythmias). Products include:
- Bronkaid Mist Suspension ...... ▣ 718
- Sensorcaine-MPF with Epinephrine Injection 559

Epinephrine Hydrochloride (Increased risk of cardiac arrhythmias). Products include:
- Ana-Kit Anaphylaxis Emergency Treatment Kit 617

Erythromycin (May increase digoxin absorption in patients who convert digoxin to inactive metabolites in the gut resulting in increased serum levels of digoxin). Products include:
- A/T/S 2% Acne Topical Gel and Solution 1234
- Benzamycin Topical Gel 905
- E-Mycin Tablets 1341
- Emgel 2% Topical Gel 1093
- ERYC 1915
- Erycette (erythromycin 2%) Topical Solution 1888
- Ery-Tab Tablets 422
- Erythromycin Base Filmtab 426
- Erythromycin Delayed-Release Capsules, USP 427
- Ilotycin Ophthalmic Ointment 912
- PCE Dispertab Tablets 444
- T-Stat 2.0% Topical Solution and Pads 2688
- Theramycin Z Topical Solution 2% 1592

Erythromycin Estolate (May increase digoxin absorption in patients who convert digoxin to inactive metabolites in the gut resulting in increased serum levels of digoxin). Products include:
- Ilosone 911

Erythromycin Ethylsuccinate (May increase digoxin absorption in patients who convert digoxin to inactive metabolites in the gut resulting in increased serum levels of digoxin). Products include:
- E.E.S. 424
- EryPed 421

Erythromycin Gluceptate (May increase digoxin absorption in patients who convert digoxin to inactive metabolites in the gut resulting in increased serum levels of digoxin). Products include:
- Ilotycin Gluceptate, IV, Vials 913

Erythromycin Stearate (May increase digoxin absorption in patients who convert digoxin to inactive metabolites in the gut resulting in increased serum levels of digoxin). Products include:
- Erythrocin Stearate Filmtab 425

Esmolol Hydrochloride (Additive effects on AV node conduction). Products include:
- Brevibloc Injection 1808

Felodipine (Additive effects on AV node conduction). Products include:
- Plendil Extended-Release Tablets 527

Furosemide (Diuretic-induced hypokalemia sensitizes the myocardium to digitalis resulting in possible digitalis toxicity). Products include:
- Lasix Injection, Oral Solution and Tablets 1240

Hydrochlorothiazide (Diuretic-induced hypokalemia sensitizes the myocardium to digitalis resulting in possible digitalis toxicity). Products include:
- Aldactazide 2413
- Aldoril Tablets 1604
- Apresazide Capsules 808
- Capozide 742
- Dyazide 2479
- Esidrix Tablets 821
- Esimil Tablets 822
- HydroDIURIL Tablets 1674
- Hydropres Tablets 1675
- Hyzaar Tablets 1677
- Inderide Tablets 2732
- Inderide LA Long Acting Capsules .. 2734
- Lopressor HCT Tablets 832
- Lotensin HCT 837
- Maxzide 1380
- Moduretic Tablets 1705
- Oretic Tablets 443
- Prinzide Tablets 1737
- Ser-Ap-Es Tablets 849
- Timolide Tablets 1748
- Vaseretic Tablets 1765
- Zestoretic 2850
- Ziac 1415

Hydrocortisone (Corticosteroid-induced hypokalemia sensitizes the myocardium to digitalis resulting in possible digitalis toxicity). Products include:
- Anusol-HC Cream 2.5% 1896
- Aquanil HC Lotion 1931
- Bactine Hydrocortisone Anti-Itch Cream ...... ▣ 709
- Caldecort Anti-Itch Hydrocortisone Spray ...... ▣ 631
- Cortaid ...... ▣ 836
- CORTENEMA 2535
- Cortisporin Ointment 1085
- Cortisporin Ophthalmic Ointment Sterile 1085
- Cortisporin Ophthalmic Suspension Sterile 1086
- Cortisporin Otic Solution Sterile 1087
- Cortisporin Otic Suspension Sterile 1088
- Cortizone-5 ...... ▣ 831
- Cortizone-10 ...... ▣ 831
- Hydrocortone Tablets 1672
- Hytone 907
- Massengill Medicated Soft Cloth Towelettes 2458
- PediOtic Suspension Sterile 1153
- Preparation H Hydrocortisone 1% Cream ...... ▣ 872
- ProctoCream-HC 2.5% 2408
- VōSoL HC Otic Solution 2678

Hydrocortisone Acetate (Corticosteroid-induced hypokalemia sensitizes the myocardium to digitalis resulting in possible digitalis toxicity). Products include:
- Analpram-HC Rectal Cream 1% and 2.5% 977
- Anusol HC-1 Anti-Itch Hydrocortisone Ointment ...... ▣ 847
- Anusol-HC Suppositories 1897
- Caldecort ...... ▣ 631
- Carmol HC 924
- Coly-Mycin S Otic w/Neomycin & Hydrocortisone 1906
- Cortaid ...... ▣ 836
- Cortifoam 2396
- Cortisporin Cream 1084
- Epifoam 2399
- Hydrocortone Acetate Sterile Suspension 1669
- Mantadil Cream 1135
- Nupercainal Hydrocortisone 1% Cream ...... ▣ 645
- Ophthocort ...... ⊙ 311

(▣ Described in PDR For Nonprescription Drugs) (⊙ Described in PDR For Ophthalmology)

Pramosone Cream, Lotion & Ointment 978
ProctoCream-HC 2408
ProctoFoam-HC 2409
Terra-Cortril Ophthalmic Suspension 2210

Hydrocortisone Sodium Phosphate (Corticosteroid-induced hypokalemia sensitizes the myocardium to digitalis resulting in possible digitalis toxicity). Products include:

Hydrocortone Phosphate Injection, Sterile 1670

Hydrocortisone Sodium Succinate (Corticosteroid-induced hypokalemia sensitizes the myocardium to digitalis resulting in possible digitalis toxicity). Products include:

Solu-Cortef Sterile Powder................. 2641

Hydroflumethiazide (Diuretic-induced hypokalemia sensitizes the myocardium to digitalis resulting in possible digitalis toxicity). Products include:

Diucardin Tablets................................ 2718

Indapamide (Diuretic-induced hypokalemia sensitizes the myocardium to digitalis resulting in possible digitalis toxicity). Products include:

Lozol Tablets 2022

Indomethacin (Causes a rise in serum digoxin concentration, with the implication that digitalis intoxication may result). Products include:

Indocin 1680

Indomethacin Sodium Trihydrate (Causes a rise in serum digoxin concentration, with the implication that digitalis intoxication may result). Products include:

Indocin I.V. 1684

Isoproterenol Hydrochloride (Increased risk of cardiac arrhythmias). Products include:

Isuprel Hydrochloride Injection 1:5000 2311
Isuprel Hydrochloride Solution 1:200 & 1:100 2313
Isuprel Mistometer 2312

Isoproterenol Sulfate (Increased risk of cardiac arrhythmias). Products include:

Norisodrine with Calcium Iodide Syrup.. 442

Isradipine (Additive effects on AV node conduction). Products include:

DynaCirc Capsules 2256

Itraconazole (Causes a rise in serum digoxin concentration, with the implication that digitalis intoxication may result). Products include:

Sporanox Capsules 1305

Labetalol Hydrochloride (Additive effects on AV node conduction). Products include:

Normodyne Injection 2377
Normodyne Tablets 2379
Trandate 1185

Levobunolol Hydrochloride (Additive effects on AV node conduction). Products include:

Betagan .... ⊛ 233

Levothyroxine Sodium (Hypothyroid patients may require increased digoxin dose). Products include:

Levothroid Tablets 1016
Levoxyl Tablets.................................... 903
Synthroid.. 1359

Liothyronine Sodium (Hypothyroid patients may require increased digoxin dose). Products include:

Cytomel Tablets 2473
Triostat Injection 2530

Liotrix (Hypothyroid patients may require increased digoxin dose).

No products indexed under this heading.

Magaldrate (Interferes with intestinal digoxin absorption).

No products indexed under this heading.

Magnesium Hydroxide (Interferes with intestinal digoxin absorption). Products include:

Aludrox Oral Suspension 2695
Arthritis Pain Ascriptin .... ᵍᵈ 631
Maximum Strength Ascriptin .... ᵍᵈ 630
Regular Strength Ascriptin Tablets .... ᵍᵈ 629
Di-Gel Antacid/Anti-Gas .... ᵍᵈ 801
Gelusil Liquid & Tablets .... ᵍᵈ 855
Maalox Magnesia and Alumina Oral Suspension .... ᵍᵈ 642
Maalox Plus Tablets .... ᵍᵈ 643
Extra Strength Maalox Antacid Plus Antigas Liquid and Tablets ᵍᵈ 638
Mylanta Calcium Carbonate and Magnesium Hydroxide Tablets...... 1318
Mylanta Liquid 1317
Mylanta Tablets .... ᵍᵈ 660
Mylanta Double Strength Liquid 1317
Mylanta Double Strength Tablets .. ᵍᵈ 660
Phillips' Milk of Magnesia Liquid.... ᵍᵈ 729
Rolaids Tablets .... ᵍᵈ 843
Tempo Soft Antacid .... ᵍᵈ 835

Magnesium Oxide (Interferes with intestinal digoxin absorption). Products include:

Beelith Tablets 639
Bufferin Analgesic Tablets and Caplets .... ᵍᵈ 613
Caltrate PLUS .... ᵍᵈ 665
Cama Arthritis Pain Reliever.............. ᵍᵈ 785
Mag-Ox 400 668
Uro-Mag... 668

Metaproterenol Sulfate (Increased risk of cardiac arrhythmias). Products include:

Alupent... 669
Metaproterenol Sulfate Inhalation Solution, USP, Arm-a-Med 552

Metaraminol Bitartrate (Increased risk of cardiac arrhythmias). Products include:

Aramine Injection................................ 1609

Methacycline Hydrochloride (May increase digoxin absorption in patients who convert digoxin to inactive metabolites in the gut resulting in increased serum levels of digoxin).

No products indexed under this heading.

Methoxamine Hydrochloride (Increased risk of cardiac arrhythmias). Products include:

Vasoxyl Injection 1196

Methyclothiazide (Diuretic-induced hypokalemia sensitizes the myocardium to digitalis resulting in possible digitalis toxicity). Products include:

Enduron Tablets................................... 420

Methylprednisolone Acetate (Corticosteroid-induced hypokalemia sensitizes the myocardium to digitalis resulting in possible digitalis toxicity). Products include:

Depo-Medrol Single-Dose Vial 2600
Depo-Medrol Sterile Aqueous Suspension... 2597

Methylprednisolone Sodium Succinate (Corticosteroid-induced hypokalemia sensitizes the myocardium to digitalis resulting in possible digitalis toxicity). Products include:

Solu-Medrol Sterile Powder................ 2643

Metipranolol Hydrochloride (Additive effects on AV node conduction). Products include:

OptiPranolol (Metipranolol 0.3%) Sterile Ophthalmic Solution........... ⊛ 258

Metolazone (Diuretic-induced hypokalemia sensitizes the myocardium to digitalis resulting in possible digitalis toxicity). Products include:

Mykrox Tablets 993
Zaroxolyn Tablets 1000

Metoprolol Succinate (Additive effects on AV node conduction). Products include:

Toprol-XL Tablets 565

Metoprolol Tartrate (Additive effects on AV node conduction). Products include:

Lopressor Ampuls 830
Lopressor HCT Tablets 832
Lopressor Tablets 830

Minocycline Hydrochloride (May increase digoxin absorption in patients who convert digoxin to inactive metabolites in the gut resulting in increased serum levels of digoxin). Products include:

Dynacin Capsules 1590
Minocin Intravenous 1382
Minocin Oral Suspension 1385
Minocin Pellet-Filled Capsules 1383

Nadolol (Additive effects on AV node conduction).

No products indexed under this heading.

Neomycin, oral (Interferes with intestinal digoxin absorption).

Nephrotoxic Drugs (May impair the excretion of digoxin).

Nicardipine Hydrochloride (Additive effects on AV node conduction). Products include:

Cardene Capsules 2095
Cardene I.V. 2709
Cardene SR Capsules........................... 2097

Nifedipine (Additive effects on AV node conduction). Products include:

Adalat Capsules (10 mg and 20 mg) 587
Adalat CC 589
Procardia Capsules............................... 1971
Procardia XL Extended Release Tablets 1972

Nimodipine (Additive effects on AV node conduction). Products include:

Nimotop Capsules 610

Nisoldipine (Additive effects on AV node conduction).

No products indexed under this heading.

Norepinephrine Bitartrate (Increased risk of cardiac arrhythmias). Products include:

Levophed Bitartrate Injection 2315

Oxytetracycline Hydrochloride (May increase digoxin absorption in patients who convert digoxin to inactive metabolites in the gut resulting in increased serum levels of digoxin). Products include:

TERAK Ointment .... ⊛ 209
Terra-Cortril Ophthalmic Suspension 2210
Terramycin with Polymyxin B Sulfate Ophthalmic Ointment 2211
Urobiotic-250 Capsules 2214

Pectin (Low digoxin serum concentration; interferes with intestinal digoxin absorption). Products include:

Celestial Seasonings Soothers Throat Drops .... ᵍᵈ 842

Penbutolol Sulfate (Additive effects on AV node conduction). Products include:

Levatol 2403

Phenylephrine Bitartrate (Increased risk of cardiac arrhythmias).

No products indexed under this heading.

Phenylephrine Hydrochloride (Increased risk of cardiac arrhythmias). Products include:

Atrohist Plus Tablets 454
Cerose DM .... ᵍᵈ 878
Comhist 2038
D.A. Chewable Tablets........................ 951
Deconsal Pediatric Capsules............... 454
Dura-Vent/DA Tablets 953
Entex Capsules 1986
Entex Liquid 1986
Extendryl 1005
4-Way Fast Acting Nasal Spray (regular & mentholated) .... ᵍᵈ 621
Hemorid For Women .... ᵍᵈ 834
Hycomine Compound Tablets 932
Neo-Synephrine Hydrochloride 1% Carpuject.. 2324
Neo-Synephrine Hydrochloride 1% Injection 2324
Neo-Synephrine Hydrochloride (Ophthalmic) 2325
Neo-Synephrine .... ᵍᵈ 726
Nöstril .... ᵍᵈ 644
Novahistine Elixir .... ᵍᵈ 823
Phenergan VC 2779
Phenergan VC with Codeine 2781
Preparation H .... ᵍᵈ 871
Tympagesic Ear Drops 2342
Vasosulf .... ⊛ 271
Vicks Sinex Nasal Spray and Ultra Fine Mist .... ᵍᵈ 765

Phenylephrine Tannate (Increased risk of cardiac arrhythmias). Products include:

Atrohist Pediatric Suspension 454
Ricobid-D Pediatric Suspension........ 2038
Ricobid Tablets and Pediatric Suspension.. 2038
Rynatan 2673
Rynatuss 2673

Phenylpropanolamine Hydrochloride (Increased risk of cardiac arrhythmias). Products include:

Acutrim .... ᵍᵈ 628
Allerest Children's Chewable Tablets .... ᵍᵈ 627
Allerest 12 Hour Caplets .... ᵍᵈ 627
Atrohist Plus Tablets 454
BC Cold Powder Multi-Symptom Formula (Cold-Sinus-Allergy) ...... ᵍᵈ 609
BC Cold Powder Non-Drowsy Formula (Cold-Sinus) .... ᵍᵈ 609
Cheracol Plus Head Cold/Cough Formula .... ᵍᵈ 769
Comtrex Multi-Symptom Non-Drowsy Liqui-gels................................ ᵍᵈ 618
Contac Continuous Action Nasal Decongestant/Antihistamine 12 Hour Capsules..................................... ᵍᵈ 813
Contac Maximum Strength Continuous Action Decongestant/ Antihistamine 12 Hour Caplets.. ᵍᵈ 813
Contac Severe Cold and Flu Formula Caplets .... ᵍᵈ 814
Coricidin 'D' Decongestant Tablets .... ᵍᵈ 800
Dexatrim .... ᵍᵈ 832
Dexatrim Plus Vitamins Caplets .... ᵍᵈ 832
Dimetane-DC Cough Syrup 2059
Dimetapp Elixir.................................... ᵍᵈ 773
Dimetapp Extentabs............................ ᵍᵈ 774
Dimetapp Tablets/Liqui-Gels .... ᵍᵈ 775
Dimetapp Cold & Allergy Chewable Tablets .... ᵍᵈ 773
Dimetapp DM Elixir............................. ᵍᵈ 774
Dura-Vent Tablets 952
Entex Capsules 1986
Entex LA Tablets 1987
Entex Liquid 1986
Exgest LA Tablets 782
Hycomine 931
Isoclor Timesule Capsules .... ᵍᵈ 637
Nolamine Timed-Release Tablets 785
Ornade Spansule Capsules 2502
Propagest Tablets 786
Pyrroxate Caplets .... ᵍᵈ 772
Robitussin-CF .... ᵍᵈ 777
Sinulin Tablets 787
Tavist-D 12 Hour Relief Tablets .... ᵍᵈ 787
Teldrin 12 Hour Antihistamine/ Nasal Decongestant Allergy Relief Capsules .... ᵍᵈ 826
Triaminic Allergy Tablets .... ᵍᵈ 789
Triaminic Cold Tablets .... ᵍᵈ 790
Triaminic Expectorant .... ᵍᵈ 790
Triaminic Syrup .... ᵍᵈ 792
Triaminic-12 Tablets .... ᵍᵈ 792
Triaminic-DM Syrup .... ᵍᵈ 792
Triaminicin Tablets .... ᵍᵈ 793
Triaminicol Multi-Symptom Cold Tablets .... ᵍᵈ 793
Triaminicol Multi-Symptom Relief ᵍᵈ 794
Vicks DayQuil Allergy Relief 12-Hour Extended Release Tablets.. ᵍᵈ 760
Vicks DayQuil Allergy Relief 4-Hour Tablets .... ᵍᵈ 760
Vicks DayQuil SINUS Pressure & CONGESTION Relief........................ ᵍᵈ 761

IMPORTANT NOTE: Always consult each drug listing in the patient's regimen for possible interactions.

Lanoxin Elixir — Interactions Index — 554

Pindolol (Additive effects on AV node conduction). Products include:
Visken Tablets 2299

Pirbuterol Acetate (Increased risk of cardiac arrhythmias). Products include:
Maxair Autohaler 1492
Maxair Inhaler 1494

Polythiazide (Diuretic-induced hypokalemia sensitizes the myocardium to digitalis resulting in possible digitalis toxicity). Products include:
Minizide Capsules 1938

Prednisolone Acetate (Corticosteroid-induced hypokalemia sensitizes the myocardium to digitalis resulting in possible digitalis toxicity). Products include:
AK-CIDE ⊙ 202
AK-CIDE Ointment ⊙ 202
Blephamide Liquifilm Sterile Ophthalmic Suspension 476
Blephamide Ointment ⊙ 237
Econopred & Econopred Plus Ophthalmic Suspensions ⊙ 217
Poly-Pred Liquifilm ⊙ 248
Pred Forte ⊙ 250
Pred Mild ⊙ 253
Pred-G Liquifilm Sterile Ophthalmic Suspension ⊙ 251
Pred-G S.O.P. Sterile Ophthalmic Ointment ⊙ 252
Vasocidin Ointment ⊙ 268

Prednisolone Sodium Phosphate (Corticosteroid-induced hypokalemia sensitizes the myocardium to digitalis resulting in possible digitalis toxicity). Products include:
AK-Pred ⊙ 204
Hydeltrasol Injection, Sterile 1665
Inflamase ⊙ 265
Pediapred Oral Liquid 995
Vasocidin Ophthalmic Solution ⊙ 270

Prednisolone Tebutate (Corticosteroid-induced hypokalemia sensitizes the myocardium to digitalis resulting in possible digitalis toxicity). Products include:
Hydeltra-T.B.A. Sterile Suspension 1667

Prednisone (Corticosteroid-induced hypokalemia sensitizes the myocardium to digitalis resulting in possible digitalis toxicity). Products include:
Deltasone Tablets 2595

Propafenone Hydrochloride (Causes a rise in serum digoxin concentration, with the implication that digitalis intoxication may result). Products include:
Rythmol Tablets–150mg, 225mg, 300mg 1352

Propantheline Bromide (Increases digoxin absorption). Products include:
Pro-Banthīne Tablets 2052

Propranolol Hydrochloride (Additive effects on AV node conduction). Products include:
Inderal 2728
Inderal LA Long Acting Capsules 2730
Inderide Tablets 2732
Inderide LA Long Acting Capsules 2734

Pseudoephedrine Hydrochloride (Increased risk of cardiac arrhythmias). Products include:
Actifed Allergy Daytime/Nighttime Caplets ◘ 844
Actifed Plus Caplets ◘ 845
Actifed Plus Tablets ◘ 845
Actifed with Codeine Cough Syrup 1067
Actifed Sinus Daytime/Nighttime Tablets and Caplets ◘ 846
Actifed Syrup ◘ 846
Actifed Tablets ◘ 844
Advil Cold and Sinus Caplets and Tablets (formerly CoAdvil) ◘ 870
Alka-Seltzer Plus Cold Medicine Liqui-Gels ◘ 706
Alka-Seltzer Plus Cold & Cough Medicine Liqui-Gels ◘ 705
Alka-Seltzer Plus Night-Time Cold Medicine Liqui-Gels ◘ 706
Allerest Headache Strength Tablets ◘ 627
Allerest Maximum Strength Tablets ◘ 627
Allerest No Drowsiness Tablets ◘ 627
Allerest Sinus Pain Formula ◘ 627
Anatuss LA Tablets 1542
Atrohist Pediatric Capsules 453
Bayer Select Sinus Pain Relief Formula ◘ 717
Benadryl Allergy Decongestant Liquid Medication ◘ 848
Benadryl Allergy Decongestant Tablets ◘ 848
Benadryl Allergy Sinus Headache Formula Caplets ◘ 849
Benylin Multisymptom ◘ 852
Bromfed Capsules (Extended-Release) 1785
Bromfed Syrup ◘ 733
Bromfed Tablets 1785
Bromfed-DM Cough Syrup 1786
Bromfed-PD Capsules (Extended-Release) 1785
Children's Vicks DayQuil Allergy Relief ◘ 757
Children's Vicks NyQuil Cold/Cough Relief ◘ 758
Comtrex Multi-Symptom Cold Reliever Tablets/Caplets/Liqui-Gels/Liquid ◘ 615
Allergy-Sinus Comtrex Multi-Symptom Allergy-Sinus Formula Tablets ◘ 617
Comtrex Multi-Symptom Non-Drowsy Caplets ◘ 618
Congess 1004
Contac Day Allergy/Sinus Caplets ◘ 812
Contac Day & Night ◘ 812
Contac Night Allergy/Sinus Caplets ◘ 812
Contac Severe Cold & Flu Non-Drowsy ◘ 815
Deconamine Chewable Tablets 1320
Deconamine CX Cough and Cold Liquid and Tablets 1319
Deconamine 1320
Deconsal C Expectorant Syrup 456
Deconsal Pediatric Syrup 457
Deconsal II Tablets 454
Dimetane-DX Cough Syrup 2059
Dimetapp Sinus Caplets ◘ 775
Dorcol Children's Cough Syrup ◘ 785
Drixoral Cough + Congestion Liquid Caps ◘ 802
Dura-Tap/PD Capsules 2867
Duratuss Tablets 2565
Duratuss HD Elixir 2565
Efidac/24 ◘ 635
Entex PSE Tablets 1987
Fedahist Gyrocaps 2401
Fedahist Timecaps 2401
Guaifed 1787
Guaifed Syrup ◘ 734
Guaimax-D Tablets 792
Guaitab Tablets ◘ 734
Isoclor Expectorant 990
Kronofed-A 977
Motrin IB Sinus ◘ 838
Novahistine DH 2462
Novahistine DMX ◘ 822
Novahistine Expectorant 2463
Nucofed 2051
PediaCare Cold Allergy Chewable Tablets ◘ 677
PediaCare Cough-Cold Chewable Tablets 1553
PediaCare 1553
PediaCare Infants' Decongestant Drops ◘ 677
PediCare Infant's Drops Decongestant Plus Cough 1553
PediaCare NightRest Cough-Cold Liquid 1553
Pediatric Vicks 44d Dry Hacking Cough & Head Congestion ◘ 763
Pediatric Vicks 44m Cough & Cold Relief ◘ 764
Robitussin Cold & Cough Liqui-Gels ◘ 776
Robitussin Maximum Strength Cough & Cold ◘ 778
Robitussin Pediatric Cough & Cold Formula ◘ 779
Robitussin Severe Congestion Liqui-Gels ◘ 776
Robitussin-DAC Syrup 2074
Robitussin-PE ◘ 778
Rondec Oral Drops 953
Rondec Syrup 953
Rondec Tablet 953
Rondec-DM Oral Drops 954
Rondec-DM Syrup 954
Rondec-TR Tablet 953
Ryna ◘ 841
Seldane-D Extended-Release Tablets 1538
Semprex-D Capsules 463
Semprex-D Capsules 1167
Sinarest Tablets ◘ 648
Sinarest Extra Strength Tablets ◘ 648
Sinarest No Drowsiness Tablets ◘ 648
Sine-Aid IB Caplets 1554
Sine-Aid Maximum Strength Sinus Medication Gelcaps, Caplets and Tablets 1554
Sine-Off No Drowsiness Formula Caplets ◘ 824
Sine-Off Sinus Medicine ◘ 825
Singlet Tablets ◘ 825
Sinutab Non-Drying Liquid Caps ◘ 859
Sinutab Sinus Allergy Medication, Maximum Strength Tablets and Caplets ◘ 860
Sinutab Sinus Medication, Maximum Strength Without Drowsiness Formula, Tablets & Caplets ◘ 860
Sinutab Sinus Medication, Regular Strength Without Drowsiness Formula ◘ 859
Sudafed Children's Liquid ◘ 861
Sudafed Cold and Cough Liquidcaps ◘ 862
Sudafed Cough Syrup ◘ 862
Sudafed Plus Liquid ◘ 862
Sudafed Plus Tablets ◘ 863
Sudafed Severe Cold Formula Caplets ◘ 863
Sudafed Severe Cold Formula Tablets ◘ 864
Sudafed Sinus Caplets ◘ 864
Sudafed Sinus Tablets ◘ 864
Sudafed Tablets, 30 mg ◘ 861
Sudafed Tablets, 60 mg ◘ 861
Sudafed 12 Hour Caplets ◘ 861
Syn-Rx Tablets 465
Syn-Rx DM Tablets 466
TheraFlu ◘ 787
TheraFlu Maximum Strength Nighttime Flu, Cold & Cough Medicine ◘ 788
TheraFlu Maximum Strength Non-Drowsy Formula Flu, Cold & Cough Medicine ◘ 788
Thera Flu Maximum Strength, Non-Drowsy Formula Flu, Cold and Cough Caplets ◘ 789
Triaminic AM Cough and Decongestant Formula ◘ 789
Triaminic AM Decongestant Formula ◘ 790
Triaminic Nite Light ◘ 791
Triaminic Sore Throat Formula ◘ 791
Tussend 1783
Tussend Expectorant 1785
Children's TYLENOL Cold Multi-Symptom Liquid Formula and Chewable Tablets 1561
Children's TYLENOL Cold Plus Cough Multi Symptom Tablets and Liquid ◘ 681
Infants' TYLENOL Cold Decongestant & Fever-Reducer Drops 1556
TYLENOL Maximum Strength Allergy Sinus Medication Gelcaps and Caplets 1563
TYLENOL Maximum Strength Allergy Sinus NightTime Medication Caplets 1555
TYLENOL Flu Maximum Strength Gelcaps 1565
TYLENOL Flu NightTime, Maximum Strength, Gelcaps 1566
TYLENOL Maximum Strength Flu NightTime Hot Medication Packets 1562
TYLENOL, Maximum Strength, Sinus Medication Geltabs, Gelcaps, Caplets and Tablets 1566
TYLENOL Cold Multi-Symptom Formula Medication Tablets and Caplets 1561
TYLENOL Cold Medication No Drowsiness Formula Gelcaps and Caplets 1562
TYLENOL Cold Multi-Symptom Hot Medication Liquid Packets 1557
TYLENOL Cough Multi-Symptom Medication with Decongestant 1565
Ursinus Inlay-Tabs ◘ 794
Vicks 44 LiquiCaps Cough, Cold & Flu Relief ◘ 755
Vicks 44 LiquiCaps Non-Drowsy Cough & Cold Relief ◘ 756
Vicks 44D Dry Hacking Cough & Head Congestion ◘ 755
Vicks 44M Cough, Cold & Flu Relief ◘ 756
Vicks DayQuil ◘ 761
Vicks DayQuil SINUS Pressure & PAIN Relief with IBUPROFEN ◘ 762
Vicks Nyquil Hot Therapy ◘ 762
Vicks NyQuil LiquiCaps Multi-Symptom Cold/Flu Relief ◘ 763
Vicks NyQuil Multi-Symptom Cold/Flu Relief - (Original & Cherry Flavor) ◘ 763

Pseudoephedrine Sulfate (Increased risk of cardiac arrhythmias). Products include:
Cheracol Sinus ◘ 768
Chlor-Trimeton Allergy Decongestant Tablets ◘ 799
Claritin-D 2350
Drixoral Cold and Allergy Sustained-Action Tablets ◘ 802
Drixoral Cold and Flu Extended-Release Tablets ◘ 803
Drixoral Non-Drowsy Formula Extended-Release Tablets ◘ 803
Drixoral Allergy/Sinus Extended Release Tablets ◘ 804
Trinalin Repetabs Tablets 1330

Quinidine Gluconate (Causes a rise in serum digoxin concentration, with the implication that digitalis intoxication may result). Products include:
Quinaglute Dura-Tabs Tablets 649

Quinidine Polygalacturonate (Causes a rise in serum digoxin concentration, with the implication that digitalis intoxication may result).
No products indexed under this heading.

Quinidine Sulfate (Causes a rise in serum digoxin concentration, with the implication that digitalis intoxication may result). Products include:
Quinidex Extentabs 2067

Salmeterol Xinafoate (Increased risk of cardiac arrhythmias). Products include:
Serevent Inhalation Aerosol 1176

Sodium Bicarbonate (Interferes with intestinal digoxin absorption). Products include:
Alka-Seltzer Effervescent Antacid and Pain Reliever ◘ 701
Alka-Seltzer Extra Strength Effervescent Antacid and Pain Reliever ◘ 703
Alka-Seltzer Gold Effervescent Antacid ◘ 703
Alka-Seltzer Lemon Lime Effervescent Antacid and Pain Reliever ◘ 703
Arm & Hammer Pure Baking Soda ◘ 627
Ceo-Two Rectal Suppositories 666
Citrocarbonate Antacid ◘ 770
Massengill Disposable Douches ◘ 820
Massengill Liquid Concentrate ◘ 820
NuLYTELY 689
Cherry Flavor NuLYTELY 689

Sotalol Hydrochloride (Additive effects on AV node conduction). Products include:
Betapace Tablets 641

Succinylcholine Chloride (May cause arrhythmias). Products include:
Anectine 1073

Sulfasalazine (Low digoxin serum concentration; interferes with intestinal digoxin absorption). Products include:
Azulfidine 1949

Terbutaline Sulfate (Increased risk of cardiac arrhythmias). Products include:
Brethaire Inhaler 813
Brethine Ampuls 815

(◘ Described in PDR For Nonprescription Drugs) (⊙ Described in PDR For Ophthalmology)

555 Interactions Index Lanoxin Injection

Brethine Tablets 814
Bricanyl Subcutaneous Injection 1502
Bricanyl Tablets 1503

Tetracycline Hydrochloride (May increase digoxin absorption in patients who convert digoxin to inactive metabolites in the gut resulting in increased serum levels of digoxin). Products include:
Achromycin V Capsules 1367

Thyroglobulin (Hypothyroid patients may require increased digoxin dose).
No products indexed under this heading.

Thyroid (Hypothyroid patients may require increased digoxin dose).
No products indexed under this heading.

Thyroxine (Hypothyroid patients may require increased digoxin dose).
No products indexed under this heading.

Thyroxine Sodium (Hypothyroid patients may require increased digoxin dose).
No products indexed under this heading.

Timolol Hemihydrate (Additive effects on AV node conduction). Products include:
Betimol 0.25%, 0.5% .... ◉ 261

Timolol Maleate (Additive effects on AV node conduction). Products include:
Blocadren Tablets 1614
Timolide Tablets 1748
Timoptic in Ocudose 1753
Timoptic Sterile Ophthalmic Solution 1751
Timoptic-XE 1755

Triamcinolone (Corticosteroid-induced hypokalemia sensitizes the myocardium to digitalis resulting in possible digitalis toxicity). Products include:
Aristocort Tablets 1022

Triamcinolone Acetonide (Corticosteroid-induced hypokalemia sensitizes the myocardium to digitalis resulting in possible digitalis toxicity). Products include:
Aristocort A 0.025% Cream 1027
Aristocort A 0.5% Cream 1031
Aristocort A 0.1% Cream 1029
Aristocort A 0.1% Ointment 1030
Azmacort Oral Inhaler 2011
Nasacort Nasal Inhaler 2024

Triamcinolone Diacetate (Corticosteroid-induced hypokalemia sensitizes the myocardium to digitalis resulting in possible digitalis toxicity). Products include:
Aristocort Suspension (Forte Parenteral) 1027
Aristocort Suspension (Intralesional) 1025

Triamcinolone Hexacetonide (Corticosteroid-induced hypokalemia sensitizes the myocardium to digitalis resulting in possible digitalis toxicity). Products include:
Aristospan Suspension (Intra-articular) 1033
Aristospan Suspension (Intralesional) 1032

Troleandomycin (May increase digoxin absorption in patients who convert digoxin to inactive metabolites in the gut resulting in increased serum levels of digoxin). Products include:
Tao Capsules 2209

Verapamil Hydrochloride (Causes a rise in serum digoxin concentration, with the implication that digitalis intoxication may result). Products include:
Calan SR Caplets 2422
Calan Tablets 2419
Isoptin Injectable 1344
Isoptin Oral Tablets 1346
Isoptin SR Tablets 1348
Verelan Capsules 1410
Verelan Capsules 2824

LANOXIN INJECTION

(Digoxin) 1123

May interact with potassium-depleting corticosteroids, potassium-depleting diuretics, antacids, sympathomimetics, beta blockers, calcium channel blockers, thyroid preparations, mineralocorticoids, tetracyclines, macrolide antibiotics, and certain other agents. Compounds in these categories include:

Acebutolol Hydrochloride (Additive effects on AV node conduction). Products include:
Sectral Capsules 2807

Albuterol (Increased risk of cardiac arrhythmias). Products include:
Proventil Inhalation Aerosol 2382
Ventolin Inhalation Aerosol and Refill 1197

Albuterol Sulfate (Increased risk of cardiac arrhythmias). Products include:
Airet Solution for Inhalation 452
Proventil Inhalation Solution 0.083% 2384
Proventil Repetabs Tablets 2386
Proventil Solution for Inhalation 0.5% 2383
Proventil Syrup 2385
Proventil Tablets 2386
Ventolin Inhalation Solution 1198
Ventolin Nebules Inhalation Solution 1199
Ventolin Rotacaps for Inhalation 1200
Ventolin Syrup 1202
Ventolin Tablets 1203
Volmax Extended-Release Tablets 1788

Alprazolam (Causes a rise in serum digoxin concentration, with the implication that digitalis intoxication may result). Products include:
Xanax Tablets 2649

Aluminum Carbonate Gel (Interferes with intestinal digoxin absorption). Products include:
Basaljel 2703

Aluminum Hydroxide (Interferes with intestinal digoxin absorption). Products include:
ALternaGEL Liquid 1316
Maximum Strength Ascriptin .... ▣ 630
Cama Arthritis Pain Reliever .... ▣ 785
Gaviscon Extra Strength Relief Formula Antacid Tablets .... ▣ 819
Gaviscon Extra Strength Relief Formula Liquid Antacid .... ▣ 819
Gaviscon Liquid Antacid .... ▣ 820
Gelusil Liquid & Tablets .... ▣ 855
Maalox Heartburn Relief Suspension .... ▣ 642
Maalox Heartburn Relief Tablets .... ▣ 641
Maalox Magnesia and Alumina Oral Suspension .... ▣ 642
Maalox Plus Tablets .... ▣ 643
Extra Strength Maalox Antacid Plus Antigas Liquid and Tablets .... ▣ 638
Tempo Soft Antacid .... ▣ 835

Aluminum Hydroxide Gel (Interferes with intestinal digoxin absorption). Products include:
ALternaGEL Liquid .... ▣ 659
Aludrox Oral Suspension 2695
Amphojel Suspension 2695
Amphojel Suspension without Flavor 2695
Amphojel Tablets 2695
Arthritis Pain Ascriptin .... ▣ 631
Regular Strength Ascriptin Tablets .... ▣ 629
Gaviscon Antacid Tablets .... ▣ 819
Gaviscon-2 Antacid Tablets .... ▣ 820
Mylanta Liquid 1317
Mylanta Tablets .... ▣ 660
Mylanta Double Strength Liquid 1317
Mylanta Double Strength Tablets .... ▣ 660
Nephrox Suspension .... ▣ 655

Aluminum Hydroxide Gel, Dried (Interferes with intestinal digoxin absorption).

Amiodarone Hydrochloride (Causes a rise in serum digoxin concentration, with the implication that digitalis intoxication may result). Products include:
Cordarone Intravenous 2715
Cordarone Tablets 2712

Amlodipine Besylate (Additive effects on AV node conduction). Products include:
Lotrel Capsules 840
Norvasc Tablets 1940

Amphotericin B (Amphotericin B-induced hypokalemia sensitizes the myocardium to digitalis resulting in possible digitalis toxicity). Products include:
Fungizone Intravenous 506

Antibiotics, unspecified (Increases digoxin absorption in patients who inactivate digoxin by bacterial metabolism).

Anticancer Drugs, unspecified (Interferes with intestinal digoxin absorption).

Atenolol (Additive effects on AV node conduction). Products include:
Tenoretic Tablets 2845
Tenormin Tablets and I.V. Injection 2847

Azithromycin (May increase digoxin absorption in patients who convert digoxin to inactive metabolites in the gut resulting in increased serum levels of digoxin). Products include:
Zithromax 1944

Bendroflumethiazide (Diuretic-induced hypokalemia sensitizes the myocardium to digitalis resulting in possible digitalis toxicity).
No products indexed under this heading.

Bepridil Hydrochloride (Additive effects on AV node conduction). Products include:
Vascor (200, 300 and 400 mg) Tablets 1587

Betamethasone Acetate (Corticosteroid-induced hypokalemia sensitizes the myocardium to digitalis resulting in possible digitalis toxicity). Products include:
Celestone Soluspan Suspension 2347

Betamethasone Sodium Phosphate (Corticosteroid-induced hypokalemia sensitizes the myocardium to digitalis resulting in possible digitalis toxicity). Products include:
Celestone Soluspan Suspension 2347

Betaxolol Hydrochloride (Additive effects on AV node conduction). Products include:
Betoptic Ophthalmic Solution 469
Betoptic S Ophthalmic Suspension 471
Kerlone Tablets 2436

Bisoprolol Fumarate (Additive effects on AV node conduction). Products include:
Zebeta Tablets 1413
Ziac 1415

Calcium, intravenous (May produce serious arrhythmias in digitalized patients).
No products indexed under this heading.

Carteolol Hydrochloride (Additive effects on AV node conduction). Products include:
Cartrol Tablets 410
Ocupress Ophthalmic Solution, 1% Sterile .... ◉ 309

Chlorothiazide (Diuretic-induced hypokalemia sensitizes the myocardium to digitalis resulting in possible digitalis toxicity). Products include:
Aldoclor Tablets 1598
Diupres Tablets 1650
Diuril Oral 1653

Chlorothiazide Sodium (Diuretic-induced hypokalemia sensitizes the myocardium to digitalis resulting in possible digitalis toxicity). Products include:
Diuril Sodium Intravenous 1652

Chlorthalidone (Diuretic-induced hypokalemia sensitizes the myocardium to digitalis resulting in possible digitalis toxicity). Products include:
Combipres Tablets 677
Tenoretic Tablets 2845
Thalitone 1245

Cholestyramine (Interferes with intestinal digoxin absorption). Products include:
Questran Light 769
Questran Powder 770

Clarithromycin (May increase digoxin absorption in patients who convert digoxin to inactive metabolites in the gut resulting in increased serum levels of digoxin). Products include:
Biaxin 405

Cortisone Acetate (Corticosteroid-induced hypokalemia sensitizes the myocardium to digitalis resulting in possible digitalis toxicity). Products include:
Cortone Acetate Sterile Suspension 1623
Cortone Acetate Tablets 1624

Demeclocycline Hydrochloride (May increase digoxin absorption in patients who convert digoxin to inactive metabolites in the gut resulting in increased serum levels of digoxin). Products include:
Declomycin Tablets 1371

Dexamethasone (Corticosteroid-induced hypokalemia sensitizes the myocardium to digitalis resulting in possible digitalis toxicity). Products include:
AK-Trol Ointment & Suspension .... ◉ 205
Decadron Elixir 1633
Decadron Tablets 1635
Decaspray Topical Aerosol 1648
Dexacidin Ointment .... ◉ 263
Maxitrol Ophthalmic Ointment and Suspension .... ◉ 224
TobraDex Ophthalmic Suspension and Ointment 473

Dexamethasone Acetate (Corticosteroid-induced hypokalemia sensitizes the myocardium to digitalis resulting in possible digitalis toxicity). Products include:
Dalalone D.P. Injectable 1011
Decadron-LA Sterile Suspension 1646

Dexamethasone Sodium Phosphate (Corticosteroid-induced hypokalemia sensitizes the myocardium to digitalis resulting in possible digitalis toxicity). Products include:
Decadron Phosphate Injection 1637
Decadron Phosphate Respihaler 1642
Decadron Phosphate Sterile Ophthalmic Ointment 1641
Decadron Phosphate Sterile Ophthalmic Solution 1642
Decadron Phosphate Topical Cream 1644
Decadron Phosphate Turbinaire 1645
Decadron Phosphate with Xylocaine Injection, Sterile 1639
Dexacort Phosphate in Respihaler 458
Dexacort Phosphate in Turbinaire 459
NeoDecadron Sterile Ophthalmic Ointment 1712
NeoDecadron Sterile Ophthalmic Solution 1713
NeoDecadron Topical Cream 1714

Dihydroxyaluminum Sodium Carbonate (Interferes with intestinal digoxin absorption).
No products indexed under this heading.

IMPORTANT NOTE: Always consult each drug listing in the patient's regimen for possible interactions.

Lanoxin Injection — Interactions Index — 556

Diltiazem Hydrochloride (Additive effects on AV node conduction). Products include:
- Cardizem CD Capsules ... 1506
- Cardizem SR Capsules ... 1510
- Cardizem Injectable ... 1508
- Cardizem Tablets ... 1512
- Dilacor XR Extended-release Capsules ... 2018

Diphenoxylate Hydrochloride (Increases digoxin absorption). Products include:
- Lomotil ... 2439

Dobutamine Hydrochloride (Increased risk of cardiac arrhythmias). Products include:
- Dobutrex Solution Vials ... 1439

Dopamine Hydrochloride (Increased risk of cardiac arrhythmias).
- No products indexed under this heading.

Doxycycline Calcium (May increase digoxin absorption in patients who convert digoxin to inactive metabolites in the gut resulting in increased serum levels of digoxin). Products include:
- Vibramycin Calcium Oral Suspension Syrup ... 1941

Doxycycline Hyclate (May increase digoxin absorption in patients who convert digoxin to inactive metabolites in the gut resulting in increased serum levels of digoxin). Products include:
- Doryx Capsules ... 1913
- Vibramycin Hyclate Capsules ... 1941
- Vibramycin Hyclate Intravenous ... 2215
- Vibra-Tabs Film Coated Tablets ... 1941

Doxycycline Monohydrate (May increase digoxin absorption in patients who convert digoxin to inactive metabolites in the gut resulting in increased serum levels of digoxin). Products include:
- Monodox Capsules ... 1805
- Vibramycin Monohydrate for Oral Suspension ... 1941

Ephedrine Hydrochloride (Increased risk of cardiac arrhythmias). Products include:
- Primatene Dual Action Formula ... ◘ 872
- Primatene Tablets ... ◘ 873
- Quadrinal Tablets ... 1350

Ephedrine Sulfate (Increased risk of cardiac arrhythmias). Products include:
- Bronkaid Caplets ... ◘ 717
- Marax Tablets & DF Syrup ... 2200

Ephedrine Tannate (Increased risk of cardiac arrhythmias). Products include:
- Rynatuss ... 2673

Epinephrine (Increased risk of cardiac arrhythmias). Products include:
- Bronkaid Mist ... ◘ 717
- EPIFRIN ... ⊙ 239
- EpiPen ... 790
- Marcaine Hydrochloride with Epinephrine 1:200,000 ... 2316
- Primatene Mist ... ◘ 873
- Sensorcaine with Epinephrine Injection ... 559
- Sus-Phrine Injection ... 1019
- Xylocaine with Epinephrine Injections ... 567

Epinephrine Bitartrate (Increased risk of cardiac arrhythmias). Products include:
- Bronkaid Mist Suspension ... ◘ 718
- Sensorcaine-MPF with Epinephrine Injection ... 559

Epinephrine Hydrochloride (Increased risk of cardiac arrhythmias). Products include:
- Ana-Kit Anaphylaxis Emergency Treatment Kit ... 617

Erythromycin (May increase digoxin absorption in patients who convert digoxin to inactive metabolites in the gut resulting in increased serum levels of digoxin). Products include:
- A/T/S 2% Acne Topical Gel and Solution ... 1234
- Benzamycin Topical Gel ... 905
- E-Mycin Tablets ... 1341
- Emgel 2% Topical Gel ... 1093
- ERYC ... 1915
- Erycette (erythromycin 2%) Topical Solution ... 1888
- Ery-Tab Tablets ... 422
- Erythromycin Base Filmtab ... 426
- Erythromycin Delayed-Release Capsules, USP ... 427
- Ilotycin Ophthalmic Ointment ... 912
- PCE Dispertab Tablets ... 444
- T-Stat 2.0% Topical Solution and Pads ... 2688
- Theramycin Z Topical Solution 2% ... 1592

Erythromycin Estolate (May increase digoxin absorption in patients who convert digoxin to inactive metabolites in the gut resulting in increased serum levels of digoxin). Products include:
- Ilosone ... 911

Erythromycin Ethylsuccinate (May increase digoxin absorption in patients who convert digoxin to inactive metabolites in the gut resulting in increased serum levels of digoxin). Products include:
- E.E.S. ... 424
- EryPed ... 421

Erythromycin Gluceptate (May increase digoxin absorption in patients who convert digoxin to inactive metabolites in the gut resulting in increased serum levels of digoxin). Products include:
- Ilotycin Gluceptate, IV, Vials ... 913

Erythromycin Stearate (May increase digoxin absorption in patients who convert digoxin to inactive metabolites in the gut resulting in increased serum levels of digoxin). Products include:
- Erythrocin Stearate Filmtab ... 425

Esmolol Hydrochloride (Additive effects on AV node conduction). Products include:
- Brevibloc Injection ... 1808

Felodipine (Additive effects on AV node conduction). Products include:
- Plendil Extended-Release Tablets ... 527

Furosemide (Diuretic-induced hypokalemia sensitizes the myocardium to digitalis resulting in possible digitalis toxicity). Products include:
- Lasix Injection, Oral Solution and Tablets ... 1240

Hydrochlorothiazide (Diuretic-induced hypokalemia sensitizes the myocardium to digitalis resulting in possible digitalis toxicity). Products include:
- Aldactazide ... 2413
- Aldoril Tablets ... 1604
- Apresazide Capsules ... 808
- Capozide ... 742
- Dyazide ... 2479
- Esidrix Tablets ... 821
- Esimil Tablets ... 822
- HydroDIURIL Tablets ... 1674
- Hydropres Tablets ... 1675
- Hyzaar Tablets ... 1677
- Inderide Tablets ... 2732
- Inderide LA Long Acting Capsules ... 2734
- Lopressor HCT Tablets ... 832
- Lotensin HCT ... 837
- Maxzide ... 1380
- Moduretic Tablets ... 1705
- Oretic Tablets ... 443
- Prinzide Tablets ... 1737
- Ser-Ap-Es Tablets ... 849
- Timolide Tablets ... 1748
- Vaseretic Tablets ... 1765
- Zestoretic ... 2850
- Ziac ... 1415

Hydrocortisone (Corticosteroid-induced hypokalemia sensitizes the myocardium to digitalis resulting in possible digitalis toxicity). Products include:
- Anusol-HC Cream 2.5% ... 1896
- Aquanil HC Lotion ... 1931
- Bactine Hydrocortisone Anti-Itch Cream ... ◘ 709
- Caldecort Anti-Itch Hydrocortisone Spray ... ◘ 631
- Cortaid ... ◘ 836
- CORTENEMA ... 2535
- Cortisporin Ointment ... 1085
- Cortisporin Ophthalmic Ointment Sterile ... 1085
- Cortisporin Ophthalmic Suspension Sterile ... 1086
- Cortisporin Otic Solution Sterile ... 1087
- Cortisporin Otic Suspension Sterile ... 1088
- Cortizone-5 ... ◘ 831
- Cortizone-10 ... ◘ 831
- Hydrocortone Tablets ... 1672
- Hytone ... 907
- Massengill Medicated Soft Cloth Towelettes ... 2458
- PediOtic Suspension Sterile ... 1153
- Preparation H Hydrocortisone 1% Cream ... ◘ 872
- ProctoCream-HC 2.5% ... 2408
- VōSoL HC Otic Solution ... 2678

Hydrocortisone Acetate (Corticosteroid-induced hypokalemia sensitizes the myocardium to digitalis resulting in possible digitalis toxicity). Products include:
- Analpram-HC Rectal Cream 1% and 2.5% ... 977
- Anusol HC-1 Anti-Itch Hydrocortisone Ointment ... ◘ 847
- Anusol-HC Suppositories ... 1897
- Caldecort ... ◘ 631
- Carmol HC ... 924
- Coly-Mycin S Otic w/Neomycin & Hydrocortisone ... 1906
- Cortaid ... ◘ 836
- Cortifoam ... 2396
- Cortisporin Cream ... 1084
- Epifoam ... 2399
- Hydrocortone Acetate Sterile Suspension ... 1669
- Mantadil Cream ... 1135
- Nupercainal Hydrocortisone 1% Cream ... ◘ 645
- Ophthocort ... ⊙ 311
- Pramosone Cream, Lotion & Ointment ... 978
- ProctoCream-HC ... 2408
- ProctoFoam-HC ... 2409
- Terra-Cortril Ophthalmic Suspension ... 2210

Hydrocortisone Sodium Phosphate (Corticosteroid-induced hypokalemia sensitizes the myocardium to digitalis resulting in possible digitalis toxicity). Products include:
- Hydrocortone Phosphate Injection, Sterile ... 1670

Hydrocortisone Sodium Succinate (Corticosteroid-induced hypokalemia sensitizes the myocardium to digitalis resulting in possible digitalis toxicity). Products include:
- Solu-Cortef Sterile Powder ... 2641

Hydroflumethiazide (Diuretic-induced hypokalemia sensitizes the myocardium to digitalis resulting in possible digitalis toxicity). Products include:
- Diucardin Tablets ... 2718

Indapamide (Diuretic-induced hypokalemia sensitizes the myocardium to digitalis resulting in possible digitalis toxicity). Products include:
- Lozol Tablets ... 2022

Indomethacin (Causes a rise in serum digoxin concentration, with the implication that digitalis intoxication may result). Products include:
- Indocin ... 1680

Indomethacin Sodium Trihydrate (Causes a rise in serum digoxin concentration, with the implication that digitalis intoxication may result). Products include:
- Indocin I.V. ... 1684

Isoproterenol Hydrochloride (Increased risk of cardiac arrhythmias). Products include:
- Isuprel Hydrochloride Injection 1:5000 ... 2311
- Isuprel Hydrochloride Solution 1:200 & 1:100 ... 2313
- Isuprel Mistometer ... 2312

Isoproterenol Sulfate (Increased risk of cardiac arrhythmias). Products include:
- Norisodrine with Calcium Iodide Syrup ... 442

Isradipine (Additive effects on AV node conduction). Products include:
- DynaCirc Capsules ... 2256

Itraconazole (Causes a rise in serum digoxin concentration, with the implication that digitalis intoxication may result). Products include:
- Sporanox Capsules ... 1305

Labetalol Hydrochloride (Additive effects on AV node conduction). Products include:
- Normodyne Injection ... 2377
- Normodyne Tablets ... 2379
- Trandate ... 1185

Levobunolol Hydrochloride (Additive effects on AV node conduction). Products include:
- Betagan ... ⊙ 233

Levothyroxine Sodium (Hypothyroid patients may require increased digoxin dose). Products include:
- Levothroid Tablets ... 1016
- Levoxyl Tablets ... 903
- Synthroid ... 1359

Liothyronine Sodium (Hypothyroid patients may require increased digoxin dose). Products include:
- Cytomel Tablets ... 2473
- Triostat Injection ... 2530

Liotrix (Hypothyroid patients may require increased digoxin dose).
- No products indexed under this heading.

Magaldrate (Interferes with intestinal digoxin absorption).
- No products indexed under this heading.

Magnesium Hydroxide (Interferes with intestinal digoxin absorption). Products include:
- Aludrox Oral Suspension ... 2695
- Arthritis Pain Ascriptin ... ◘ 631
- Maximum Strength Ascriptin ... ◘ 630
- Regular Strength Ascriptin Tablets ... ◘ 629
- Di-Gel Antacid/Anti-Gas ... ◘ 801
- Gelusil Liquid & Tablets ... ◘ 855
- Maalox Magnesia and Alumina Oral Suspension ... ◘ 642
- Maalox Plus Tablets ... ◘ 643
- Extra Strength Maalox Antacid Plus Antigas Liquid and Tablets ◘ 638
- Mylanta Calcium Carbonate and Magnesium Hydroxide Tablets ... 1318
- Mylanta Liquid ... 1317
- Mylanta Tablets ... ◘ 660
- Mylanta Double Strength Liquid ... 1317
- Mylanta Double Strength Tablets .. ◘ 660
- Phillips' Milk of Magnesia Liquid ... ◘ 729
- Rolaids Tablets ... ◘ 843
- Tempo Soft Antacid ... ◘ 835

Magnesium Oxide (Interferes with intestinal digoxin absorption). Products include:
- Beelith Tablets ... 639
- Bufferin Analgesic Tablets and Caplets ... ◘ 613
- Caltrate PLUS ... ◘ 665
- Cama Arthritis Pain Reliever ... ◘ 785
- Mag-Ox 400 ... 668
- Uro-Mag ... 668

(◘ Described in PDR For Nonprescription Drugs) (⊙ Described in PDR For Ophthalmology)

557 **Interactions Index** **Lanoxin Injection**

Metaproterenol Sulfate (Increased risk of cardiac arrhythmias). Products include:
- Alupent 669
- Metaproterenol Sulfate Inhalation Solution, USP, Arm-a-Med 552

Metaraminol Bitartrate (Increased risk of cardiac arrhythmias). Products include:
- Aramine Injection 1609

Methacycline Hydrochloride (May increase digoxin absorption in patients who convert digoxin to inactive metabolites in the gut resulting in increased serum levels of digoxin).
- No products indexed under this heading.

Methoxamine Hydrochloride (Increased risk of cardiac arrhythmias). Products include:
- Vasoxyl Injection 1196

Methyclothiazide (Diuretic-induced hypokalemia sensitizes the myocardium to digitalis resulting in possible digitalis toxicity). Products include:
- Enduron Tablets 420

Methylprednisolone Acetate (Corticosteroid-induced hypokalemia sensitizes the myocardium to digitalis resulting in possible digitalis toxicity). Products include:
- Depo-Medrol Single-Dose Vial 2600
- Depo-Medrol Sterile Aqueous Suspension 2597

Methylprednisolone Sodium Succinate (Corticosteroid-induced hypokalemia sensitizes the myocardium to digitalis resulting in possible digitalis toxicity). Products include:
- Solu-Medrol Sterile Powder 2643

Metipranolol Hydrochloride (Additive effects on AV node conduction). Products include:
- OptiPranolol (Metipranolol 0.3%) Sterile Ophthalmic Solution .... ◉ 258

Metolazone (Diuretic-induced hypokalemia sensitizes the myocardium to digitalis resulting in possible digitalis toxicity). Products include:
- Mykrox Tablets 993
- Zaroxolyn Tablets 1000

Metoprolol Succinate (Additive effects on AV node conduction). Products include:
- Toprol-XL Tablets 565

Metoprolol Tartrate (Additive effects on AV node conduction). Products include:
- Lopressor Ampuls 830
- Lopressor HCT Tablets 832
- Lopressor Tablets 830

Minocycline Hydrochloride (May increase digoxin absorption in patients who convert digoxin to inactive metabolites in the gut resulting in increased serum levels of digoxin). Products include:
- Dynacin Capsules 1590
- Minocin Intravenous 1382
- Minocin Oral Suspension 1385
- Minocin Pellet-Filled Capsules 1383

Nadolol (Additive effects on AV node conduction).
- No products indexed under this heading.

Neomycin, oral (Interferes with intestinal digoxin absorption).

Nephrotoxic Drugs (May impair the excretion of digoxin).

Nicardipine Hydrochloride (Additive effects on AV node conduction). Products include:
- Cardene Capsules 2095
- Cardene I.V. 2709
- Cardene SR Capsules 2097

Nifedipine (Additive effects on AV node conduction). Products include:
- Adalat Capsules (10 mg and 20 mg) 587
- Adalat CC 589
- Procardia Capsules 1971
- Procardia XL Extended Release Tablets 1972

Nimodipine (Additive effects on AV node conduction). Products include:
- Nimotop Capsules 610

Nisoldipine (Additive effects on AV node conduction).
- No products indexed under this heading.

Norepinephrine Bitartrate (Increased risk of cardiac arrhythmias). Products include:
- Levophed Bitartrate Injection 2315

Oxytetracycline Hydrochloride (May increase digoxin absorption in patients who convert digoxin to inactive metabolites in the gut resulting in increased serum levels of digoxin). Products include:
- TERAK Ointment .... ◉ 209
- Terra-Cortril Ophthalmic Suspension 2210
- Terramycin with Polymyxin B Sulfate Ophthalmic Ointment 2211
- Urobiotic-250 Capsules 2214

Pectin (Low digoxin serum concentration; interferes with intestinal digoxin absorption). Products include:
- Celestial Seasonings Soothers Throat Drops .... ▣ 842

Penbutolol Sulfate (Additive effects on AV node conduction). Products include:
- Levatol 2403

Phenylephrine Bitartrate (Increased risk of cardiac arrhythmias).
- No products indexed under this heading.

Phenylephrine Hydrochloride (Increased risk of cardiac arrhythmias). Products include:
- Atrohist Plus Tablets 454
- Cerose DM .... ▣ 878
- Comhist 2038
- D.A. Chewable Tablets 951
- Deconsal Pediatric Capsules 454
- Dura-Vent/DA Tablets 953
- Entex Capsules 1986
- Entex Liquid 1986
- Extendryl 1005
- 4-Way Fast Acting Nasal Spray (regular & mentholated) .... ▣ 621
- Hemorid For Women .... ▣ 834
- Hycomine Compound Tablets 932
- Neo-Synephrine Hydrochloride 1% Carpuject 2324
- Neo-Synephrine Hydrochloride 1% Injection 2324
- Neo-Synephrine Hydrochloride (Ophthalmic) 2325
- Neo-Synephrine .... ▣ 726
- Nōstril .... ▣ 644
- Novahistine Elixir .... ▣ 823
- Phenergan VC 2779
- Phenergan VC with Codeine 2781
- Preparation H .... ▣ 871
- Tympagesic Ear Drops 2342
- Vasosulf .... ◉ 271
- Vicks Sinex Nasal Spray and Ultra Fine Mist .... ▣ 765

Phenylephrine Tannate (Increased risk of cardiac arrhythmias). Products include:
- Atrohist Pediatric Suspension 454
- Ricobid-D Pediatric Suspension 2038
- Ricobid Tablets and Pediatric Suspension 2038
- Rynatan 2673
- Rynatuss 2673

Phenylpropanolamine Hydrochloride (Increased risk of cardiac arrhythmias). Products include:
- Acutrim .... ▣ 628
- Allerest Children's Chewable Tablets .... ▣ 627
- Allerest 12 Hour Caplets .... ▣ 627
- Atrohist Plus Tablets 454
- BC Cold Powder Multi-Symptom Formula (Cold-Sinus-Allergy) .... ▣ 609
- BC Cold Powder Non-Drowsy Formula (Cold-Sinus) .... ▣ 609
- Cheracol Plus Head Cold/Cough Formula .... ▣ 769
- Comtrex Multi-Symptom Non-Drowsy Liqui-gels .... ▣ 618
- Contac Continuous Action Nasal Decongestant/Antihistamine 12 Hour Capsules .... ▣ 813
- Contac Maximum Strength Continuous Action Decongestant/Antihistamine 12 Hour Caplets .... ▣ 813
- Contac Severe Cold and Flu Formula Caplets .... ▣ 814
- Coricidin 'D' Decongestant Tablets .... ▣ 800
- Dexatrim .... ▣ 832
- Dexatrim Plus Vitamins Caplets .... ▣ 832
- Dimetane-DC Cough Syrup 2059
- Dimetapp Elixir .... ▣ 773
- Dimetapp Extentabs .... ▣ 774
- Dimetapp Tablets/Liqui-Gels .... ▣ 775
- Dimetapp Cold & Allergy Chewable Tablets .... ▣ 773
- Dimetapp DM Elixir .... ▣ 774
- Dura-Vent Tablets 952
- Entex Capsules 1986
- Entex LA Tablets 1987
- Entex Liquid 1986
- Exgest LA Tablets 782
- Hycomine 931
- Isoclor Timesule Capsules .... ▣ 637
- Nolamine Timed-Release Tablets 785
- Ornade Spansule Capsules 2502
- Propagest Tablets 786
- Pyrroxate Caplets .... ▣ 772
- Robitussin-CF .... ▣ 777
- Sinulin Tablets 787
- Tavist-D 12 Hour Relief Tablets .... ▣ 787
- Teldrin 12 Hour Antihistamine/Nasal Decongestant Allergy Relief Capsules .... ▣ 826
- Triaminic Allergy Tablets .... ▣ 789
- Triaminic Cold Tablets .... ▣ 790
- Triaminic Expectorant .... ▣ 790
- Triaminic Syrup .... ▣ 792
- Triaminic-12 Tablets .... ▣ 792
- Triaminic-DM Syrup .... ▣ 792
- Triaminicin Tablets .... ▣ 793
- Triaminicol Multi-Symptom Cold Tablets .... ▣ 793
- Triaminicol Multi-Symptom Relief .... ▣ 794
- Vicks DayQuil Allergy Relief 12-Hour Extended Release Tablets .... ▣ 760
- Vicks DayQuil Allergy Relief 4-Hour Tablets .... ▣ 760
- Vicks DayQuil SINUS Pressure & CONGESTION Relief .... ▣ 761

Pindolol (Additive effects on AV node conduction). Products include:
- Visken Tablets 2299

Pirbuterol Acetate (Increased risk of cardiac arrhythmias). Products include:
- Maxair Autohaler 1492
- Maxair Inhaler 1494

Polythiazide (Diuretic-induced hypokalemia sensitizes the myocardium to digitalis resulting in possible digitalis toxicity). Products include:
- Minizide Capsules 1938

Prednisolone Acetate (Corticosteroid-induced hypokalemia sensitizes the myocardium to digitalis resulting in possible digitalis toxicity). Products include:
- AK-CIDE .... ◉ 202
- AK-CIDE Ointment .... ◉ 202
- Blephamide Liquifilm Sterile Ophthalmic Suspension 476
- Blephamide Ointment .... ◉ 237
- Econopred & Econopred Plus Ophthalmic Suspensions .... ◉ 217
- Poly-Pred Liquifilm .... ◉ 248
- Pred Forte .... ◉ 250
- Pred Mild .... ◉ 253
- Pred-G Liquifilm Sterile Ophthalmic Suspension .... ◉ 251
- Pred-G S.O.P. Sterile Ophthalmic Ointment .... ◉ 252
- Vasocidin Ointment .... ◉ 268

Prednisolone Sodium Phosphate (Corticosteroid-induced hypokalemia sensitizes the myocardium to digitalis resulting in possible digitalis toxicity). Products include:
- AK-Pred .... ◉ 204
- Hydeltrasol Injection, Sterile 1665
- Inflamase .... ◉ 265
- Pediapred Oral Liquid 995
- Vasocidin Ophthalmic Solution .... ◉ 270

Prednisolone Tebutate (Corticosteroid-induced hypokalemia sensitizes the myocardium to digitalis resulting in possible digitalis toxicity). Products include:
- Hydeltra-T.B.A. Sterile Suspension 1667

Prednisone (Corticosteroid-induced hypokalemia sensitizes the myocardium to digitalis resulting in possible digitalis toxicity). Products include:
- Deltasone Tablets 2595

Propafenone Hydrochloride (Causes a rise in serum digoxin concentration, with the implication that digitalis intoxication may result). Products include:
- Rythmol Tablets–150mg, 225mg, 300mg 1352

Propantheline Bromide (Increases digoxin absorption). Products include:
- Pro-Banthīne Tablets 2052

Propranolol Hydrochloride (Additive effects on AV node conduction). Products include:
- Inderal 2728
- Inderal LA Long Acting Capsules 2730
- Inderide Tablets 2732
- Inderide LA Long Acting Capsules 2734

Pseudoephedrine Hydrochloride (Increased risk of cardiac arrhythmias). Products include:
- Actifed Allergy Daytime/Nighttime Caplets .... ▣ 844
- Actifed Plus Caplets .... ▣ 845
- Actifed Plus Tablets .... ▣ 845
- Actifed with Codeine Cough Syrup 1067
- Actifed Sinus Daytime/Nighttime Tablets and Caplets .... ▣ 846
- Actifed Syrup .... ▣ 846
- Actifed Tablets .... ▣ 844
- Advil Cold and Sinus Caplets and Tablets (formerly CoAdvil) .... ▣ 870
- Alka-Seltzer Plus Cold Medicine Liqui-Gels .... ▣ 706
- Alka-Seltzer Plus Cold & Cough Medicine Liqui-Gels .... ▣ 705
- Alka-Seltzer Plus Night-Time Cold Medicine Liqui-Gels .... ▣ 706
- Allerest Headache Strength Tablets .... ▣ 627
- Allerest Maximum Strength Tablets .... ▣ 627
- Allerest No Drowsiness Tablets .... ▣ 627
- Allerest Sinus Pain Formula .... ▣ 627
- Anatuss LA Tablets 1542
- Atrohist Pediatric Capsules 453
- Bayer Select Sinus Pain Relief Formula .... ▣ 717
- Benadryl Allergy Decongestant Liquid Medication .... ▣ 848
- Benadryl Allergy Decongestant Tablets .... ▣ 848
- Benadryl Allergy Sinus Headache Formula Caplets .... ▣ 849
- Benylin Multisymptom .... ▣ 852
- Bromfed Capsules (Extended-Release) 1785
- Bromfed Syrup .... ▣ 733
- Bromfed Tablets 1785
- Bromfed-DM Cough Syrup 1786
- Bromfed-PD Capsules (Extended-Release) 1785
- Children's Vicks DayQuil Allergy Relief .... ▣ 757
- Children's Vicks NyQuil Cold/Cough Relief .... ▣ 758
- Comtrex Multi-Symptom Cold Reliever Tablets/Caplets/Liqui-Gels/Liquid .... ▣ 615
- Allergy-Sinus Comtrex Multi-Symptom Allergy-Sinus Formula Tablets .... ▣ 617
- Comtrex Multi-Symptom Non-Drowsy Caplets .... ▣ 618

IMPORTANT NOTE: Always consult each drug listing in the patient's regimen for possible interactions.

Congess ... 1004
Contac Day Allergy/Sinus Caplets ■ 812
Contac Day & Night ■ 812
Contac Night Allergy/Sinus Caplets ■ 812
Contac Severe Cold & Flu Non-Drowsy ■ 815
Deconamine Chewable Tablets ... 1320
Deconamine CX Cough and Cold Liquid and Tablets ... 1319
Deconamine ... 1320
Deconsal C Expectorant Syrup ... 456
Deconsal Pediatric Syrup ... 457
Deconsal II Tablets ... 454
Dimetane-DX Cough Syrup ... 2059
Dimetapp Sinus Caplets ■ 775
Dorcol Children's Cough Syrup ■ 785
Drixoral Cough + Congestion Liquid Caps ■ 802
Dura-Tap/PD Capsules ... 2867
Duratuss Tablets ... 2565
Duratuss HD Elixir ... 2565
Efidac/24 ■ 635
Entex PSE Tablets ... 1987
Fedahist Gyrocaps ... 2401
Fedahist Timecaps ... 2401
Guaifed ... 1787
Guaifed Syrup ■ 734
Guaimax-D Tablets ... 792
Guaitab Tablets ■ 734
Isoclor Expectorant ... 990
Kronofed-A ... 977
Motrin IB Sinus ■ 838
Novahistine DH ... 2462
Novahistine DMX ■ 822
Novahistine Expectorant ... 2463
Nucofed ... 2051
PediaCare Cold Allergy Chewable Tablets ■ 677
PediaCare Cough-Cold Chewable Tablets ... 1553
PediaCare ... 1553
PediaCare Infants' Decongestant Drops ■ 677
PediCare Infant's Drops Decongestant Plus Cough ... 1553
PediaCare NightRest Cough-Cold Liquid ... 1553
Pediatric Vicks 44d Dry Hacking Cough & Head Congestion ■ 763
Pediatric Vicks 44m Cough & Cold Relief ■ 764
Robitussin Cold & Cough Liqui-Gels ■ 776
Robitussin Maximum Strength Cough & Cold ■ 778
Robitussin Pediatric Cough & Cold Formula ■ 779
Robitussin Severe Congestion Liqui-Gels ■ 776
Robitussin-DAC Syrup ... 2074
Robitussin-PE ■ 778
Rondec Oral Drops ... 953
Rondec Syrup ... 953
Rondec Tablet ... 953
Rondec-DM Oral Drops ... 954
Rondec-DM Syrup ... 954
Rondec-TR Tablet ... 953
Ryna ■ 841
Seldane-D Extended-Release Tablets ... 1538
Semprex-D Capsules ... 463
Semprex-D Capsules ... 1167
Sinarest Tablets ■ 648
Sinarest Extra Strength Tablets ■ 648
Sinarest No Drowsiness Tablets ■ 648
Sine-Aid IB Caplets ... 1554
Sine-Aid Maximum Strength Sinus Medication Gelcaps, Caplets and Tablets ... 1554
Sine-Off No Drowsiness Formula Caplets ■ 824
Sine-Off Sinus Medicine ■ 825
Singlet Tablets ■ 825
Sinutab Non-Drying Liquid Caps ■ 859
Sinutab Sinus Allergy Medication, Maximum Strength Tablets and Caplets ■ 860
Sinutab Sinus Medication, Maximum Strength Without Drowsiness Formula, Tablets & Caplets ■ 860
Sinutab Sinus Medication, Regular Strength Without Drowsiness Formula ■ 859
Sudafed Children's Liquid ■ 861
Sudafed Cold and Cough Liquidcaps ■ 862
Sudafed Cough Syrup ■ 862
Sudafed Plus Liquid ■ 862
Sudafed Plus Tablets ■ 863
Sudafed Severe Cold Formula Caplets ■ 863
Sudafed Severe Cold Formula Tablets ■ 864
Sudafed Sinus Caplets ■ 864
Sudafed Sinus Tablets ■ 864
Sudafed Tablets, 30 mg ■ 861
Sudafed Tablets, 60 mg ■ 861
Sudafed 12 Hour Caplets ■ 861
Syn-Rx Tablets ... 465
Syn-Rx DM Tablets ... 466
TheraFlu ■ 787
TheraFlu Maximum Strength Nighttime Flu, Cold & Cough Medicine ■ 788
TheraFlu Maximum Strength Non-Drowsy Formula Flu, Cold & Cough Medicine ■ 788
Thera Flu Maximum Strength, Non-Drowsy Formula Flu, Cold and Cough Caplets ■ 789
Triaminic AM Cough and Decongestant Formula ■ 789
Triaminic AM Decongestant Formula ■ 790
Triaminic Nite Light ■ 791
Triaminic Sore Throat Formula ■ 791
Tussend ... 1783
Tussend Expectorant ... 1785
Children's TYLENOL Cold Multi-Symptom Liquid Formula and Chewable Tablets ... 1561
Children's TYLENOL Cold Plus Cough Multi Symptom Tablets and Liquid ■ 681
Infants' TYLENOL Cold Decongestant & Fever-Reducer Drops ... 1556
TYLENOL Maximum Strength Allergy Sinus Medication Gelcaps and Caplets ... 1563
TYLENOL Maximum Strength Allergy Sinus NightTime Medication Caplets ... 1555
TYLENOL Flu Maximum Strength Gelcaps ... 1565
TYLENOL Flu NightTime, Maximum Strength, Gelcaps ... 1566
TYLENOL Maximum Strength Flu NightTime Hot Medication Packets ... 1562
TYLENOL, Maximum Strength, Sinus Medication Geltabs, Gelcaps, Caplets and Tablets ... 1566
TYLENOL Cold Multi-Symptom Formula Medication Tablets and Caplets ... 1561
TYLENOL Cold Medication No Drowsiness Formula Gelcaps and Caplets ... 1562
TYLENOL Cold Multi-Symptom Hot Medication Liquid Packets ... 1557
TYLENOL Cough Multi-Symptom Medication with Decongestant ... 1565
Ursinus Inlay-Tabs ■ 794
Vicks 44 LiquiCaps Cough, Cold & Flu Relief ■ 755
Vicks 44 LiquiCaps Non-Drowsy Cough & Cold Relief ■ 756
Vicks 44D Dry Hacking Cough & Head Congestion ■ 755
Vicks 44M Cough, Cold & Flu Relief ■ 756
Vicks DayQuil ■ 761
Vicks DayQuil SINUS Pressure & PAIN Relief with IBUPROFEN ■ 762
Vicks Nyquil Hot Therapy ■ 762
Vicks NyQuil LiquiCaps Multi-Symptom Cold/Flu Relief ■ 763
Vicks NyQuil Multi-Symptom Cold/Flu Relief - (Original & Cherry Flavor) ■ 763

Pseudoephedrine Sulfate (Increased risk of cardiac arrhythmias). Products include:
Cheracol Sinus ■ 768
Chlor-Trimeton Allergy Decongestant Tablets ■ 799
Claritin-D ... 2350
Drixoral Cold and Allergy Sustained-Action Tablets ■ 802
Drixoral Cold and Flu Extended-Release Tablets ■ 803
Drixoral Non-Drowsy Formula Extended-Release Tablets ■ 803
Drixoral Allergy/Sinus Extended Release Tablets ■ 804
Trinalin Repetabs Tablets ... 1330

Quinidine Gluconate (Causes a rise in serum digoxin concentration, with the implication that digitalis intoxication may result). Products include:
Quinaglute Dura-Tabs Tablets ... 649

Quinidine Polygalacturonate (Causes a rise in serum digoxin concentration, with the implication that digitalis intoxication may result).
No products indexed under this heading.

Quinidine Sulfate (Causes a rise in serum digoxin concentration, with the implication that digitalis intoxication may result). Products include:
Quinidex Extentabs ... 2067

Salmeterol Xinafoate (Increased risk of cardiac arrhythmias). Products include:
Serevent Inhalation Aerosol ... 1176

Sodium Bicarbonate (Interferes with intestinal digoxin absorption). Products include:
Alka-Seltzer Effervescent Antacid and Pain Reliever ■ 701
Alka-Seltzer Extra Strength Effervescent Antacid and Pain Reliever ■ 703
Alka-Seltzer Gold Effervescent Antacid ■ 703
Alka-Seltzer Lemon Lime Effervescent Antacid and Pain Reliever ■ 703
Arm & Hammer Pure Baking Soda ■ 627
Ceo-Two Rectal Suppositories ... 666
Citrocarbonate Antacid ■ 770
Massengill Disposable Douches ■ 820
Massengill Liquid Concentrate ■ 820
NuLYTELY ... 689
Cherry Flavor NuLYTELY ... 689

Sotalol Hydrochloride (Additive effects on AV node conduction). Products include:
Betapace Tablets ... 641

Succinylcholine Chloride (May cause arrhythmias). Products include:
Anectine ... 1073

Sulfasalazine (Low digoxin serum concentration; interferes with intestinal digoxin absorption). Products include:
Azulfidine ... 1949

Terbutaline Sulfate (Increased risk of cardiac arrhythmias). Products include:
Brethaire Inhaler ... 813
Brethine Ampuls ... 815
Brethine Tablets ... 814
Bricanyl Subcutaneous Injection ... 1502
Bricanyl Tablets ... 1503

Tetracycline Hydrochloride (May increase digoxin absorption in patients who convert digoxin to inactive metabolites in the gut resulting in increased serum levels of digoxin). Products include:
Achromycin V Capsules ... 1367

Thyroglobulin (Hypothyroid patients may require increased digoxin dose).
No products indexed under this heading.

Thyroid (Hypothyroid patients may require increased digoxin dose).
No products indexed under this heading.

Thyroxine (Hypothyroid patients may require increased digoxin dose).
No products indexed under this heading.

Thyroxine Sodium (Hypothyroid patients may require increased digoxin dose).
No products indexed under this heading.

Timolol Hemihydrate (Additive effects on AV node conduction). Products include:
Betimol 0.25%, 0.5% ◉ 261

Timolol Maleate (Additive effects on AV node conduction). Products include:
Blocadren Tablets ... 1614
Timolide Tablets ... 1748
Timoptic in Ocudose ... 1753
Timoptic Sterile Ophthalmic Solution ... 1751
Timoptic-XE ... 1755

Triamcinolone (Corticosteroid-induced hypokalemia sensitizes the myocardium to digitalis resulting in possible digitalis toxicity). Products include:
Aristocort Tablets ... 1022

Triamcinolone Acetonide (Corticosteroid-induced hypokalemia sensitizes the myocardium to digitalis resulting in possible digitalis toxicity). Products include:
Aristocort A 0.025% Cream ... 1027
Aristocort A 0.5% Cream ... 1031
Aristocort A 0.1% Cream ... 1029
Aristocort A 0.1% Ointment ... 1030
Azmacort Oral Inhaler ... 2011
Nasacort Nasal Inhaler ... 2024

Triamcinolone Diacetate (Corticosteroid-induced hypokalemia sensitizes the myocardium to digitalis resulting in possible digitalis toxicity). Products include:
Aristocort Suspension (Forte Parenteral) ... 1027
Aristocort Suspension (Intralesional) ... 1025

Triamcinolone Hexacetonide (Corticosteroid-induced hypokalemia sensitizes the myocardium to digitalis resulting in possible digitalis toxicity). Products include:
Aristospan Suspension (Intra-articular) ... 1033
Aristospan Suspension (Intralesional) ... 1032

Troleandomycin (May increase digoxin absorption in patients who convert digoxin to inactive metabolites in the gut resulting in increased serum levels of digoxin). Products include:
Tao Capsules ... 2209

Verapamil Hydrochloride (Causes a rise in serum digoxin concentration, with the implication that digitalis intoxication may result). Products include:
Calan SR Caplets ... 2422
Calan Tablets ... 2419
Isoptin Injectable ... 1344
Isoptin Oral Tablets ... 1346
Isoptin SR Tablets ... 1348
Verelan Capsules ... 1410
Verelan Capsules ... 2824

LANOXIN INJECTION PEDIATRIC

(Digoxin) ... 1126

May interact with potassium-depleting corticosteroids, potassium-depleting diuretics, antacids, sympathomimetics, beta blockers, calcium channel blockers, thyroid preparations, mineralocorticoids, tetracyclines, macrolide antibiotics, and certain other agents. Compounds in these categories include:

Acebutolol Hydrochloride (Additive effects on AV node conduction). Products include:
Sectral Capsules ... 2807

Albuterol (Increased risk of cardiac arrhythmias). Products include:
Proventil Inhalation Aerosol ... 2382
Ventolin Inhalation Aerosol and Refill ... 1197

(■ Described in PDR For Nonprescription Drugs) (◉ Described in PDR For Ophthalmology)

559 **Interactions Index** **Lanoxin Injection Pediatric**

Albuterol Sulfate (Increased risk of cardiac arrhythmias). Products include:
- Airet Solution for Inhalation ... 452
- Proventil Inhalation Solution 0.083% ... 2384
- Proventil Repetabs Tablets ... 2386
- Proventil Solution for Inhalation 0.5% ... 2383
- Proventil Syrup ... 2385
- Proventil Tablets ... 2386
- Ventolin Inhalation Solution ... 1198
- Ventolin Nebules Inhalation Solution ... 1199
- Ventolin Rotacaps for Inhalation ... 1200
- Ventolin Syrup ... 1202
- Ventolin Tablets ... 1203
- Volmax Extended-Release Tablets .. 1788

Alprazolam (Causes a rise in serum digoxin concentration, with the implication that digitalis intoxication may result). Products include:
- Xanax Tablets ... 2649

Aluminum Carbonate Gel (Interferes with intestinal digoxin absorption). Products include:
- Basaljel ... 2703

Aluminum Hydroxide (Interferes with intestinal digoxin absorption). Products include:
- ALternaGEL Liquid ... 1316
- Maximum Strength Ascriptin ... ▣ 630
- Cama Arthritis Pain Reliever ... ▣ 785
- Gaviscon Extra Strength Relief Formula Antacid Tablets ... ▣ 819
- Gaviscon Extra Strength Relief Formula Liquid Antacid ... ▣ 819
- Gaviscon Liquid Antacid ... ▣ 820
- Gelusil Liquid & Tablets ... ▣ 855
- Maalox Heartburn Relief Suspension ... ▣ 642
- Maalox Heartburn Relief Tablets ... ▣ 641
- Maalox Magnesia and Alumina Oral Suspension ... ▣ 642
- Maalox Plus Tablets ... ▣ 643
- Extra Strength Maalox Antacid Plus Antigas Liquid and Tablets ▣ 638
- Tempo Soft Antacid ... ▣ 835

Aluminum Hydroxide Gel (Interferes with intestinal digoxin absorption). Products include:
- ALternaGEL Liquid ... ▣ 659
- Aludrox Oral Suspension ... 2695
- Amphojel Suspension ... 2695
- Amphojel Suspension without Flavor ... 2695
- Amphojel Tablets ... 2695
- Arthritis Pain Ascriptin ... ▣ 631
- Regular Strength Ascriptin Tablets ... ▣ 629
- Gaviscon Antacid Tablets ... ▣ 819
- Gaviscon-2 Antacid Tablets ... ▣ 820
- Mylanta Liquid ... 1317
- Mylanta Tablets ... ▣ 660
- Mylanta Double Strength Liquid ... 1317
- Mylanta Double Strength Tablets .. ▣ 660
- Nephrox Suspension ... ▣ 655

Aluminum Hydroxide Gel, Dried (Interferes with intestinal digoxin absorption).

Amiodarone Hydrochloride (Causes a rise in serum digoxin concentration, with the implication that digitalis intoxication may result). Products include:
- Cordarone Intravenous ... 2715
- Cordarone Tablets ... 2712

Amlodipine Besylate (Additive effects on AV node conduction). Products include:
- Lotrel Capsules ... 840
- Norvasc Tablets ... 1940

Amphotericin B (Amphotericin B-induced hypokalemia sensitizes the myocardium to digitalis resulting in possible digitalis toxicity). Products include:
- Fungizone Intravenous ... 506

Anticancer Drugs, unspecified (Interferes with intestinal digoxin absorption).

Atenolol (Additive effects on AV node conduction). Products include:
- Tenoretic Tablets ... 2845
- Tenormin Tablets and I.V. Injection 2847

Azithromycin (May increase digoxin absorption in patients who convert digoxin to inactive metabolites in the gut resulting in increased serum levels of digoxin). Products include:
- Zithromax ... 1944

Bendroflumethiazide (Diuretic-induced hypokalemia sensitizes the myocardium to digitalis resulting in possible digitalis toxicity).
- No products indexed under this heading.

Bepridil Hydrochloride (Additive effects on AV node conduction). Products include:
- Vascor (200, 300 and 400 mg) Tablets ... 1587

Betamethasone Acetate (Corticosteroid-induced hypokalemia sensitizes the myocardium to digitalis resulting in possible digitalis toxicity). Products include:
- Celestone Soluspan Suspension ... 2347

Betamethasone Sodium Phosphate (Corticosteroid-induced hypokalemia sensitizes the myocardium to digitalis resulting in possible digitalis toxicity). Products include:
- Celestone Soluspan Suspension ... 2347

Betaxolol Hydrochloride (Additive effects on AV node conduction). Products include:
- Betoptic Ophthalmic Solution ... 469
- Betoptic S Ophthalmic Suspension 471
- Kerlone Tablets ... 2436

Bisoprolol Fumarate (Additive effects on AV node conduction). Products include:
- Zebeta Tablets ... 1413
- Ziac ... 1415

Calcium, intravenous (May produce serious arrhythmias in digitalized patients).
- No products indexed under this heading.

Carteolol Hydrochloride (Additive effects on AV node conduction). Products include:
- Cartrol Tablets ... 410
- Ocupress Ophthalmic Solution, 1% Sterile ... ◉ 309

Chlorothiazide (Diuretic-induced hypokalemia sensitizes the myocardium to digitalis resulting in possible digitalis toxicity). Products include:
- Aldoclor Tablets ... 1598
- Diupres Tablets ... 1650
- Diuril Oral ... 1653

Chlorothiazide Sodium (Diuretic-induced hypokalemia sensitizes the myocardium to digitalis resulting in possible digitalis toxicity). Products include:
- Diuril Sodium Intravenous ... 1652

Chlorthalidone (Diuretic-induced hypokalemia sensitizes the myocardium to digitalis resulting in possible digitalis toxicity). Products include:
- Combipres Tablets ... 677
- Tenoretic Tablets ... 2845
- Thalitone ... 1245

Cholestyramine (Interferes with intestinal digoxin absorption). Products include:
- Questran Light ... 769
- Questran Powder ... 770

Clarithromycin (May increase digoxin absorption in patients who convert digoxin to inactive metabolites in the gut resulting in increased serum levels of digoxin). Products include:
- Biaxin ... 405

Cortisone Acetate (Corticosteroid-induced hypokalemia sensitizes the myocardium to digitalis resulting in possible digitalis toxicity). Products include:
- Cortone Acetate Sterile Suspension ... 1623
- Cortone Acetate Tablets ... 1624

Demeclocycline Hydrochloride (May increase digoxin absorption in patients who convert digoxin to inactive metabolites in the gut resulting in increased serum levels of digoxin). Products include:
- Declomycin Tablets ... 1371

Dexamethasone (Corticosteroid-induced hypokalemia sensitizes the myocardium to digitalis resulting in possible digitalis toxicity). Products include:
- AK-Trol Ointment & Suspension ... ◉ 205
- Decadron Elixir ... 1633
- Decadron Tablets ... 1635
- Decaspray Topical Aerosol ... 1648
- Dexacidin Ointment ... ◉ 263
- Maxitrol Ophthalmic Ointment and Suspension ... ◉ 224
- TobraDex Ophthalmic Suspension and Ointment ... 473

Dexamethasone Acetate (Corticosteroid-induced hypokalemia sensitizes the myocardium to digitalis resulting in possible digitalis toxicity). Products include:
- Dalalone D.P. Injectable ... 1011
- Decadron-LA Sterile Suspension ... 1646

Dexamethasone Sodium Phosphate (Corticosteroid-induced hypokalemia sensitizes the myocardium to digitalis resulting in possible digitalis toxicity). Products include:
- Decadron Phosphate Injection ... 1637
- Decadron Phosphate Respihaler ... 1642
- Decadron Phosphate Sterile Ophthalmic Ointment ... 1641
- Decadron Phosphate Sterile Ophthalmic Solution ... 1642
- Decadron Phosphate Topical Cream ... 1644
- Decadron Phosphate Turbinaire ... 1645
- Decadron Phosphate with Xylocaine Injection, Sterile ... 1639
- Dexacort Phosphate in Respihaler .. 458
- Dexacort Phosphate in Turbinaire .. 459
- NeoDecadron Sterile Ophthalmic Ointment ... 1712
- NeoDecadron Sterile Ophthalmic Solution ... 1713
- NeoDecadron Topical Cream ... 1714

Dihydroxyaluminum Sodium Carbonate (Interferes with intestinal digoxin absorption).
- No products indexed under this heading.

Diltiazem Hydrochloride (Additive effects on AV node conduction). Products include:
- Cardizem CD Capsules ... 1506
- Cardizem SR Capsules ... 1510
- Cardizem Injectable ... 1508
- Cardizem Tablets ... 1512
- Dilacor XR Extended-release Capsules ... 2018

Diphenoxylate Hydrochloride (Increases digoxin absorption). Products include:
- Lomotil ... 2439

Dobutamine Hydrochloride (Increased risk of cardiac arrhythmias). Products include:
- Dobutrex Solution Vials ... 1439

Dopamine Hydrochloride (Increased risk of cardiac arrhythmias).
- No products indexed under this heading.

Doxycycline Calcium (May increase digoxin absorption in patients who convert digoxin to inactive metabolites in the gut resulting in increased serum levels of digoxin). Products include:
- Vibramycin Calcium Oral Suspension Syrup ... 1941

Doxycycline Hyclate (May increase digoxin absorption in patients who convert digoxin to inactive metabolites in the gut resulting in increased serum levels of digoxin). Products include:
- Doryx Capsules ... 1913
- Vibramycin Hyclate Capsules ... 1941
- Vibramycin Hyclate Intravenous ... 2215
- Vibra-Tabs Film Coated Tablets ... 1941

Doxycycline Monohydrate (May increase digoxin absorption in patients who convert digoxin to inactive metabolites in the gut resulting in increased serum levels of digoxin). Products include:
- Monodox Capsules ... 1805
- Vibramycin Monohydrate for Oral Suspension ... 1941

Ephedrine Hydrochloride (Increased risk of cardiac arrhythmias). Products include:
- Primatene Dual Action Formula ... ▣ 872
- Primatene Tablets ... ▣ 873
- Quadrinal Tablets ... 1350

Ephedrine Sulfate (Increased risk of cardiac arrhythmias). Products include:
- Bronkaid Caplets ... ▣ 717
- Marax Tablets & DF Syrup ... 2200

Ephedrine Tannate (Increased risk of cardiac arrhythmias). Products include:
- Rynatuss ... 2673

Epinephrine (Increased risk of cardiac arrhythmias). Products include:
- Bronkaid Mist ... ▣ 717
- EPIFRIN ... ◉ 239
- EpiPen ... 790
- Marcaine Hydrochloride with Epinephrine 1:200,000 ... 2316
- Primatene Mist ... ▣ 873
- Sensorcaine with Epinephrine Injection ... 559
- Sus-Phrine Injection ... 1019
- Xylocaine with Epinephrine Injections ... 567

Epinephrine Bitartrate (Increased risk of cardiac arrhythmias). Products include:
- Bronkaid Mist Suspension ... ▣ 718
- Sensorcaine-MPF with Epinephrine Injection ... 559

Epinephrine Hydrochloride (Increased risk of cardiac arrhythmias). Products include:
- Ana-Kit Anaphylaxis Emergency Treatment Kit ... 617

Erythromycin (May increase digoxin absorption in patients who convert digoxin to inactive metabolites in the gut resulting in increased serum levels of digoxin). Products include:
- A/T/S 2% Acne Topical Gel and Solution ... 1234
- Benzamycin Topical Gel ... 905
- E-Mycin Tablets ... 1341
- Emgel 2% Topical Gel ... 1093
- ERYC ... 1915
- Erycette (erythromycin 2%) Topical Solution ... 1888
- Ery-Tab Tablets ... 422
- Erythromycin Base Filmtab ... 426
- Erythromycin Delayed-Release Capsules, USP ... 427
- Ilotycin Ophthalmic Ointment ... 912
- PCE Dispertab Tablets ... 444
- T-Stat 2.0% Topical Solution and Pads ... 2688
- Theramycin Z Topical Solution 2% 1592

IMPORTANT NOTE: Always consult each drug listing in the patient's regimen for possible interactions.

Lanoxin Injection Pediatric **Interactions Index** **560**

Erythromycin Estolate (May increase digoxin absorption in patients who convert digoxin to inactive metabolites in the gut resulting in increased serum levels of digoxin). Products include:
- Ilosone 911

Erythromycin Ethylsuccinate (May increase digoxin absorption in patients who convert digoxin to inactive metabolites in the gut resulting in increased serum levels of digoxin). Products include:
- E.E.S. 424
- EryPed 421

Erythromycin Gluceptate (May increase digoxin absorption in patients who convert digoxin to inactive metabolites in the gut resulting in increased serum levels of digoxin). Products include:
- Ilotycin Gluceptate, IV, Vials 913

Erythromycin Stearate (May increase digoxin absorption in patients who convert digoxin to inactive metabolites in the gut resulting in increased serum levels of digoxin). Products include:
- Erythrocin Stearate Filmtab 425

Esmolol Hydrochloride (Additive effects on AV node conduction). Products include:
- Brevibloc Injection 1808

Felodipine (Additive effects on AV node conduction). Products include:
- Plendil Extended-Release Tablets 527

Furosemide (Diuretic-induced hypokalemia sensitizes the myocardium to digitalis resulting in possible digitalis toxicity). Products include:
- Lasix Injection, Oral Solution and Tablets 1240

Hydrochlorothiazide (Diuretic-induced hypokalemia sensitizes the myocardium to digitalis resulting in possible digitalis toxicity). Products include:
- Aldactazide 2413
- Aldoril Tablets 1604
- Apresazide Capsules 808
- Capozide 742
- Dyazide 2479
- Esidrix Tablets 821
- Esimil Tablets 822
- HydroDIURIL Tablets 1674
- Hydropres Tablets 1675
- Hyzaar Tablets 1677
- Inderide Tablets 2732
- Inderide LA Long Acting Capsules .. 2734
- Lopressor HCT Tablets 832
- Lotensin HCT 837
- Maxzide 1380
- Moduretic Tablets 1705
- Oretic Tablets 443
- Prinzide Tablets 1737
- Ser-Ap-Es Tablets 849
- Timolide Tablets 1748
- Vaseretic Tablets 1765
- Zestoretic 2850
- Ziac 1415

Hydrocortisone (Corticosteroid-induced hypokalemia sensitizes the myocardium to digitalis resulting in possible digitalis toxicity). Products include:
- Anusol-HC Cream 2.5% 1896
- Aquanil HC Lotion 1931
- Bactine Hydrocortisone Anti-Itch Cream .... ◙ 709
- Caldecort Anti-Itch Hydrocortisone Spray .... ◙ 631
- Cortaid .... ◙ 836
- CORTENEMA 2535
- Cortisporin Ointment 1085
- Cortisporin Ophthalmic Ointment Sterile 1085
- Cortisporin Ophthalmic Suspension Sterile 1086
- Cortisporin Otic Solution Sterile 1087
- Cortisporin Otic Suspension Sterile 1088
- Cortizone-5 .... ◙ 831
- Cortizone-10 .... ◙ 831
- Hydrocortone Tablets 1672
- Hytone 907
- Massengill Medicated Soft Cloth Towelettes 2458
- PediOtic Suspension Sterile 1153
- Preparation H Hydrocortisone 1% Cream .... ◙ 872
- ProctoCream-HC 2.5% 2408
- VōSoL HC Otic Solution 2678

Hydrocortisone Acetate (Corticosteroid-induced hypokalemia sensitizes the myocardium to digitalis resulting in possible digitalis toxicity). Products include:
- Analpram-HC Rectal Cream 1% and 2.5% 977
- Anusol HC-1 Anti-Itch Hydrocortisone Ointment .... ◙ 847
- Anusol-HC Suppositories 1897
- Caldecort .... ◙ 631
- Carmol HC 924
- Coly-Mycin S Otic w/Neomycin & Hydrocortisone 1906
- Cortaid .... ◙ 836
- Cortifoam 2396
- Cortisporin Cream 1084
- Epifoam 2399
- Hydrocortone Acetate Sterile Suspension 1669
- Mantadil Cream 1135
- Nupercainal Hydrocortisone 1% Cream .... ◙ 645
- Ophthocort .... ◉ 311
- Pramosone Cream, Lotion & Ointment 978
- ProctoCream-HC 2408
- ProctoFoam-HC 2409
- Terra-Cortril Ophthalmic Suspension 2210

Hydrocortisone Sodium Phosphate (Corticosteroid-induced hypokalemia sensitizes the myocardium to digitalis resulting in possible digitalis toxicity). Products include:
- Hydrocortone Phosphate Injection, Sterile 1670

Hydrocortisone Sodium Succinate (Corticosteroid-induced hypokalemia sensitizes the myocardium to digitalis resulting in possible digitalis toxicity). Products include:
- Solu-Cortef Sterile Powder 2641

Hydroflumethiazide (Diuretic-induced hypokalemia sensitizes the myocardium to digitalis resulting in possible digitalis toxicity). Products include:
- Diucardin Tablets 2718

Indapamide (Diuretic-induced hypokalemia sensitizes the myocardium to digitalis resulting in possible digitalis toxicity). Products include:
- Lozol Tablets 2022

Indomethacin (Causes a rise in serum digoxin concentration, with the implication that digitalis intoxication may result). Products include:
- Indocin 1680

Indomethacin Sodium Trihydrate (Causes a rise in serum digoxin concentration, with the implication that digitalis intoxication may result). Products include:
- Indocin I.V. 1684

Isoproterenol Hydrochloride (Increased risk of cardiac arrhythmias). Products include:
- Isuprel Hydrochloride Injection 1:5000 2311
- Isuprel Hydrochloride Solution 1:200 & 1:100 2313
- Isuprel Mistometer 2312

Isoproterenol Sulfate (Increased risk of cardiac arrhythmias). Products include:
- Norisodrine with Calcium Iodide Syrup 442

Isradipine (Additive effects on AV node conduction). Products include:
- DynaCirc Capsules 2256

Itraconazole (Causes a rise in serum digoxin concentration, with the implication that digitalis intoxication may result). Products include:
- Sporanox Capsules 1305

Labetalol Hydrochloride (Additive effects on AV node conduction). Products include:
- Normodyne Injection 2377
- Normodyne Tablets 2379
- Trandate 1185

Levobunolol Hydrochloride (Additive effects on AV node conduction). Products include:
- Betagan .... ◉ 233

Levothyroxine Sodium (Hypothyroid patients may require increased digoxin dose). Products include:
- Levothroid Tablets 1016
- Levoxyl Tablets 903
- Synthroid 1359

Liothyronine Sodium (Hypothyroid patients may require increased digoxin dose). Products include:
- Cytomel Tablets 2473
- Triostat Injection 2530

Liotrix (Hypothyroid patients may require increased digoxin dose).
- No products indexed under this heading.

Magaldrate (Interferes with intestinal digoxin absorption).
- No products indexed under this heading.

Magnesium Hydroxide (Interferes with intestinal digoxin absorption). Products include:
- Aludrox Oral Suspension 2695
- Arthritis Pain Ascriptin .... ◙ 631
- Maximum Strength Ascriptin .... ◙ 630
- Regular Strength Ascriptin Tablets .... ◙ 629
- Di-Gel Antacid/Anti-Gas .... ◙ 801
- Gelusil Liquid & Tablets .... ◙ 855
- Maalox Magnesia and Alumina Oral Suspension .... ◙ 642
- Maalox Plus Tablets .... ◙ 643
- Extra Strength Maalox Antacid Plus Antigas Liquid and Tablets ◙ 638
- Mylanta Calcium Carbonate and Magnesium Hydroxide Tablets...... 1318
- Mylanta Liquid 1317
- Mylanta Tablets .... ◙ 660
- Mylanta Double Strength Liquid 1317
- Mylanta Double Strength Tablets .. ◙ 660
- Phillips' Milk of Magnesia Liquid.... ◙ 729
- Rolaids Tablets .... ◙ 843
- Tempo Soft Antacid .... ◙ 835

Magnesium Oxide (Interferes with intestinal digoxin absorption). Products include:
- Beelith Tablets 639
- Bufferin Analgesic Tablets and Caplets .... ◙ 613
- Caltrate PLUS .... ◙ 665
- Cama Arthritis Pain Reliever .... ◙ 785
- Mag-Ox 400 668
- Uro-Mag 668

Metaproterenol Sulfate (Increased risk of cardiac arrhythmias). Products include:
- Alupent 669
- Metaproterenol Sulfate Inhalation Solution, USP, Arm-a-Med 552

Metaraminol Bitartrate (Increased risk of cardiac arrhythmias). Products include:
- Aramine Injection 1609

Methacycline Hydrochloride (May increase digoxin absorption in patients who convert digoxin to inactive metabolites in the gut resulting in increased serum levels of digoxin).
- No products indexed under this heading.

Methoxamine Hydrochloride (Increased risk of cardiac arrhythmias). Products include:
- Vasoxyl Injection 1196

Methyclothiazide (Diuretic-induced hypokalemia sensitizes the myocardium to digitalis resulting in possible digitalis toxicity). Products include:
- Enduron Tablets 420

Methylprednisolone Acetate (Corticosteroid-induced hypokalemia sensitizes the myocardium to digitalis resulting in possible digitalis toxicity). Products include:
- Depo-Medrol Single-Dose Vial 2600
- Depo-Medrol Sterile Aqueous Suspension 2597

Methylprednisolone Sodium Succinate (Corticosteroid-induced hypokalemia sensitizes the myocardium to digitalis resulting in possible digitalis toxicity). Products include:
- Solu-Medrol Sterile Powder 2643

Metipranolol Hydrochloride (Additive effects on AV node conduction). Products include:
- OptiPranolol (Metipranolol 0.3%) Sterile Ophthalmic Solution.......... ◉ 258

Metolazone (Diuretic-induced hypokalemia sensitizes the myocardium to digitalis resulting in possible digitalis toxicity). Products include:
- Mykrox Tablets 993
- Zaroxolyn Tablets 1000

Metoprolol Succinate (Additive effects on AV node conduction). Products include:
- Toprol-XL Tablets 565

Metoprolol Tartrate (Additive effects on AV node conduction). Products include:
- Lopressor Ampuls 830
- Lopressor HCT Tablets 832
- Lopressor Tablets 830

Minocycline Hydrochloride (May increase digoxin absorption in patients who convert digoxin to inactive metabolites in the gut resulting in increased serum levels of digoxin). Products include:
- Dynacin Capsules 1590
- Minocin Intravenous 1382
- Minocin Oral Suspension 1385
- Minocin Pellet-Filled Capsules 1383

Nadolol (Additive effects on AV node conduction).
- No products indexed under this heading.

Neomycin, oral (Interferes with intestinal digoxin absorption).

Nephrotoxic Drugs (May impair the excretion of digoxin).

Nicardipine Hydrochloride (Additive effects on AV node conduction). Products include:
- Cardene Capsules 2095
- Cardene I.V. 2709
- Cardene SR Capsules 2097

Nifedipine (Additive effects on AV node conduction). Products include:
- Adalat Capsules (10 mg and 20 mg) 587
- Adalat CC 589
- Procardia Capsules 1971
- Procardia XL Extended Release Tablets 1972

Nimodipine (Additive effects on AV node conduction). Products include:
- Nimotop Capsules 610

Nisoldipine (Additive effects on AV node conduction).
- No products indexed under this heading.

Norepinephrine Bitartrate (Increased risk of cardiac arrhythmias). Products include:
- Levophed Bitartrate Injection 2315

561 Interactions Index Lanoxin Injection Pediatric

Oxytetracycline Hydrochloride (May increase digoxin absorption in patients who convert digoxin to inactive metabolites in the gut resulting in increased serum levels of digoxin). Products include:

- TERAK Ointment ◉ 209
- Terra-Cortril Ophthalmic Suspension 2210
- Terramycin with Polymyxin B Sulfate Ophthalmic Ointment 2211
- Urobiotic-250 Capsules 2214

Pectin (Low digoxin serum concentration; interferes with intestinal digoxin absorption). Products include:

- Celestial Seasonings Soothers Throat Drops ▣ 842

Penbutolol Sulfate (Additive effects on AV node conduction). Products include:

- Levatol 2403

Phenylephrine Bitartrate (Increased risk of cardiac arrhythmias).

- No products indexed under this heading.

Phenylephrine Hydrochloride (Increased risk of cardiac arrhythmias). Products include:

- Atrohist Plus Tablets 454
- Cerose DM ▣ 878
- Comhist 2038
- D.A. Chewable Tablets 951
- Deconsal Pediatric Capsules 454
- Dura-Vent/DA Tablets 953
- Entex Capsules 1986
- Entex Liquid 1986
- Extendryl 1005
- 4-Way Fast Acting Nasal Spray (regular & mentholated) ▣ 621
- Hemorid For Women ▣ 834
- Hycomine Compound Tablets 932
- Neo-Synephrine Hydrochloride 1% Carpuject 2324
- Neo-Synephrine Hydrochloride 1% Injection 2324
- Neo-Synephrine Hydrochloride (Ophthalmic) 2325
- Neo-Synephrine ▣ 726
- Nōstril ▣ 644
- Novahistine Elixir ▣ 823
- Phenergan VC 2779
- Phenergan VC with Codeine 2781
- Preparation H ▣ 871
- Tympagesic Ear Drops 2342
- Vasosulf ◉ 271
- Vicks Sinex Nasal Spray and Ultra Fine Mist ▣ 765

Phenylephrine Tannate (Increased risk of cardiac arrhythmias). Products include:

- Atrohist Pediatric Suspension 454
- Ricobid-D Pediatric Suspension 2038
- Ricobid Tablets and Pediatric Suspension 2038
- Rynatan 2673
- Rynatuss 2673

Phenylpropanolamine Hydrochloride (Increased risk of cardiac arrhythmias). Products include:

- Acutrim ▣ 628
- Allerest Children's Chewable Tablets ▣ 627
- Allerest 12 Hour Caplets ▣ 627
- Atrohist Plus Tablets 454
- BC Cold Powder Multi-Symptom Formula (Cold-Sinus-Allergy) ▣ 609
- BC Cold Powder Non-Drowsy Formula (Cold-Sinus) ▣ 609
- Cheracol Plus Head Cold/Cough Formula ▣ 769
- Comtrex Multi-Symptom Non-Drowsy Liqui-gels ▣ 618
- Contac Continuous Action Nasal Decongestant/Antihistamine 12 Hour Capsules ▣ 813
- Contac Maximum Strength Continuous Action Decongestant/Antihistamine 12 Hour Caplets ▣ 813
- Contac Severe Cold and Flu Formula Caplets ▣ 814
- Coricidin 'D' Decongestant Tablets ▣ 800
- Dexatrim ▣ 832
- Dexatrim Plus Vitamins Caplets ▣ 832
- Dimetane-DC Cough Syrup 2059
- Dimetapp Elixir ▣ 773
- Dimetapp Extentabs ▣ 774
- Dimetapp Tablets/Liqui-Gels ▣ 775
- Dimetapp Cold & Allergy Chewable Tablets ▣ 773
- Dimetapp DM Elixir ▣ 774
- Dura-Vent Tablets 952
- Entex Capsules 1986
- Entex LA Tablets 1987
- Entex Liquid 1986
- Exgest LA Tablets 782
- Hycomine 931
- Isoclor Timesule Capsules ▣ 637
- Nolamine Timed-Release Tablets 785
- Ornade Spansule Capsules 2502
- Propagest Tablets 786
- Pyrroxate Caplets ▣ 772
- Robitussin-CF ▣ 777
- Sinulin Tablets 787
- Tavist-D 12 Hour Relief Tablets ▣ 787
- Teldrin 12 Hour Antihistamine/Nasal Decongestant Allergy Relief Capsules ▣ 826
- Triaminic Allergy Tablets ▣ 789
- Triaminic Cold Tablets ▣ 790
- Triaminic Expectorant ▣ 790
- Triaminic Syrup ▣ 792
- Triaminic-12 Tablets ▣ 792
- Triaminic-DM Syrup ▣ 792
- Triaminicin Tablets ▣ 793
- Triaminicol Multi-Symptom Cold Tablets ▣ 793
- Triaminicol Multi-Symptom Relief ▣ 794
- Vicks DayQuil Allergy Relief 12-Hour Extended Release Tablets ▣ 760
- Vicks DayQuil Allergy Relief 4-Hour Tablets ▣ 760
- Vicks DayQuil SINUS Pressure & CONGESTION Relief ▣ 761

Pindolol (Additive effects on AV node conduction). Products include:

- Visken Tablets 2299

Pirbuterol Acetate (Increased risk of cardiac arrhythmias). Products include:

- Maxair Autohaler 1492
- Maxair Inhaler 1494

Polythiazide (Diuretic-induced hypokalemia sensitizes the myocardium to digitalis resulting in possible digitalis toxicity). Products include:

- Minizide Capsules 1938

Prednisolone Acetate (Corticosteroid-induced hypokalemia sensitizes the myocardium to digitalis resulting in possible digitalis toxicity). Products include:

- AK-CIDE ◉ 202
- AK-CIDE Ointment ◉ 202
- Blephamide Liquifilm Sterile Ophthalmic Suspension 476
- Blephamide Ointment ◉ 237
- Econopred & Econopred Plus Ophthalmic Suspensions ◉ 217
- Poly-Pred Liquifilm ◉ 248
- Pred Forte ◉ 250
- Pred Mild ◉ 253
- Pred-G Liquifilm Sterile Ophthalmic Suspension ◉ 251
- Pred-G S.O.P. Sterile Ophthalmic Ointment ◉ 252
- Vasocidin Ointment ◉ 268

Prednisolone Sodium Phosphate (Corticosteroid-induced hypokalemia sensitizes the myocardium to digitalis resulting in possible digitalis toxicity). Products include:

- AK-Pred ◉ 204
- Hydeltrasol Injection, Sterile 1665
- Inflamase ◉ 265
- Pediapred Oral Liquid 995
- Vasocidin Ophthalmic Solution ◉ 270

Prednisolone Tebutate (Corticosteroid-induced hypokalemia sensitizes the myocardium to digitalis resulting in possible digitalis toxicity). Products include:

- Hydeltra-T.B.A. Sterile Suspension 1667

Prednisone (Corticosteroid-induced hypokalemia sensitizes the myocardium to digitalis resulting in possible digitalis toxicity). Products include:

- Deltasone Tablets 2595

Propafenone Hydrochloride (Causes a rise in serum digoxin concentration, with the implication that digitalis intoxication may result). Products include:

- Rythmol Tablets–150mg, 225mg, 300mg 1352

Propantheline Bromide (Increases digoxin absorption). Products include:

- Pro-Banthine Tablets 2052

Propranolol Hydrochloride (Additive effects on AV node conduction). Products include:

- Inderal 2728
- Inderal LA Long Acting Capsules 2730
- Inderide Tablets 2732
- Inderide LA Long Acting Capsules 2734

Pseudoephedrine Hydrochloride (Increased risk of cardiac arrhythmias). Products include:

- Actifed Allergy Daytime/Nighttime Caplets ▣ 844
- Actifed Plus Caplets ▣ 845
- Actifed Plus Tablets ▣ 845
- Actifed with Codeine Cough Syrup 1067
- Actifed Sinus Daytime/Nighttime Tablets and Caplets ▣ 846
- Actifed Syrup ▣ 846
- Actifed Tablets ▣ 844
- Advil Cold and Sinus Caplets and Tablets (formerly CoAdvil) ▣ 870
- Alka-Seltzer Plus Cold Medicine Liqui-Gels ▣ 706
- Alka-Seltzer Plus Cold & Cough Medicine Liqui-Gels ▣ 705
- Alka-Seltzer Plus Night-Time Cold Medicine Liqui-Gels ▣ 706
- Allerest Headache Strength Tablets ▣ 627
- Allerest Maximum Strength Tablets ▣ 627
- Allerest No Drowsiness Tablets ▣ 627
- Allerest Sinus Pain Formula ▣ 627
- Anatuss LA Tablets 1542
- Atrohist Pediatric Capsules 453
- Bayer Select Sinus Pain Relief Formula ▣ 717
- Benadryl Allergy Decongestant Liquid Medication ▣ 848
- Benadryl Allergy Decongestant Tablets ▣ 848
- Benadryl Allergy Sinus Headache Formula Caplets ▣ 849
- Benylin Multisymptom ▣ 852
- Bromfed Capsules (Extended-Release) 1785
- Bromfed Syrup ▣ 733
- Bromfed Tablets 1785
- Bromfed-DM Cough Syrup 1786
- Bromfed-PD Capsules (Extended-Release) 1785
- Children's Vicks DayQuil Allergy Relief ▣ 757
- Children's Vicks NyQuil Cold/Cough Relief ▣ 758
- Comtrex Multi-Symptom Cold Reliever Tablets/Caplets/Liqui-Gels/Liquid ▣ 615
- Allergy-Sinus Comtrex Multi-Symptom Allergy-Sinus Formula Tablets ▣ 617
- Comtrex Multi-Symptom Non-Drowsy Caplets ▣ 618
- Congess 1004
- Contac Day Allergy/Sinus Caplets ▣ 812
- Contac Day & Night ▣ 812
- Contac Night Allergy/Sinus Caplets ▣ 812
- Contac Severe Cold & Flu Non-Drowsy ▣ 815
- Deconamine Chewable Tablets 1320
- Deconamine CX Cough and Cold Liquid and Tablets 1319
- Deconamine 1320
- Deconsal C Expectorant Syrup 456
- Deconsal Pediatric Syrup 457
- Deconsal II Tablets 454
- Dimetane-DX Cough Syrup 2059
- Dimetapp Sinus Caplets ▣ 775
- Dorcol Children's Cough Syrup ▣ 785
- Drixoral Cough + Congestion Liquid Caps ▣ 802
- Dura-Tap/PD Capsules 2867
- Duratuss Tablets 2565
- Duratuss HD Elixir 2565
- Efidac/24 ▣ 635
- Entex PSE Tablets 1987
- Fedahist Gyrocaps 2401
- Fedahist Timecaps 2401
- Guaifed 1787
- Guaifed Syrup ▣ 734
- Guaimax-D Tablets 792
- Guaitab Tablets ▣ 734
- Isoclor Expectorant 990
- Kronofed-A 977
- Motrin IB Sinus ▣ 838
- Novahistine DH 2462
- Novahistine DMX ▣ 822
- Novahistine Expectorant 2463
- Nucofed 2051
- PediaCare Cold Allergy Chewable Tablets ▣ 677
- PediaCare Cough-Cold Chewable Tablets 1553
- PediaCare 1553
- PediaCare Infants' Decongestant Drops ▣ 677
- PediCare Infant's Drops Decongestant Plus Cough 1553
- PediaCare NightRest Cough-Cold Liquid 1553
- Pediatric Vicks 44d Dry Hacking Cough & Head Congestion ▣ 763
- Pediatric Vicks 44m Cough & Cold Relief ▣ 764
- Robitussin Cold & Cough Liqui-Gels ▣ 776
- Robitussin Maximum Strength Cough & Cold ▣ 778
- Robitussin Pediatric Cough & Cold Formula ▣ 779
- Robitussin Severe Congestion Liqui-Gels ▣ 776
- Robitussin-DAC Syrup 2074
- Robitussin-PE ▣ 778
- Rondec Oral Drops 953
- Rondec Syrup 953
- Rondec Tablet 953
- Rondec-DM Oral Drops 954
- Rondec-DM Syrup 954
- Rondec-TR Tablet 953
- Ryna ▣ 841
- Seldane-D Extended-Release Tablets 1538
- Semprex-D Capsules 463
- Semprex-D Capsules 1167
- Sinarest Tablets ▣ 648
- Sinarest Extra Strength Tablets ▣ 648
- Sinarest No Drowsiness Tablets ▣ 648
- Sine-Aid IB Caplets 1554
- Sine-Aid Maximum Strength Sinus Medication Gelcaps, Caplets and Tablets 1554
- Sine-Off No Drowsiness Formula Caplets ▣ 824
- Sine-Off Sinus Medicine ▣ 825
- Singlet Tablets ▣ 825
- Sinutab Non-Drying Liquid Caps ▣ 859
- Sinutab Sinus Allergy Medication, Maximum Strength Tablets and Caplets ▣ 860
- Sinutab Sinus Medication, Maximum Strength Without Drowsiness Formula, Tablets & Caplets ▣ 860
- Sinutab Sinus Medication, Regular Strength Without Drowsiness Formula ▣ 859
- Sudafed Children's Liquid ▣ 861
- Sudafed Cold and Cough Liquidcaps ▣ 862
- Sudafed Cough Syrup ▣ 862
- Sudafed Plus Liquid ▣ 862
- Sudafed Plus Tablets ▣ 863
- Sudafed Severe Cold Formula Caplets ▣ 863
- Sudafed Severe Cold Formula Tablets ▣ 864
- Sudafed Sinus Caplets ▣ 864
- Sudafed Sinus Tablets ▣ 864
- Sudafed Tablets, 30 mg ▣ 861
- Sudafed Tablets, 60 mg ▣ 861
- Sudafed 12 Hour Caplets ▣ 861
- Syn-Rx Tablets 465
- Syn-Rx DM Tablets 466
- TheraFlu ▣ 787
- TheraFlu Maximum Strength Nighttime Flu, Cold & Cough Medicine ▣ 788
- TheraFlu Maximum Strength Non-Drowsy Formula Flu, Cold & Cough Medicine ▣ 788
- Thera Flu Maximum Strength, Non-Drowsy Formula Flu, Cold and Cough Caplets ▣ 789
- Triaminic AM Cough and Decongestant Formula ▣ 789
- Triaminic AM Decongestant Formula ▣ 790

IMPORTANT NOTE: Always consult each drug listing in the patient's regimen for possible interactions.

- Triaminic Nite Light ▣ 791
- Triaminic Sore Throat Formula ▣ 791
- Tussend 1783
- Tussend Expectorant 1785
- Children's TYLENOL Cold Multi-Symptom Liquid Formula and Chewable Tablets 1561
- Children's TYLENOL Cold Plus Cough Multi Symptom Tablets and Liquid ▣ 681
- Infants' TYLENOL Cold Decongestant & Fever-Reducer Drops 1556
- TYLENOL Maximum Strength Allergy Sinus Medication Gelcaps and Caplets 1563
- TYLENOL Maximum Strength Allergy Sinus NightTime Medication Caplets 1555
- TYLENOL Flu Maximum Strength Gelcaps 1565
- TYLENOL Flu NightTime, Maximum Strength, Gelcaps 1566
- TYLENOL Maximum Strength Flu NightTime Hot Medication Packets 1562
- TYLENOL, Maximum Strength, Sinus Medication Geltabs, Gelcaps, Caplets and Tablets 1566
- TYLENOL Cold Multi-Symptom Formula Medication Tablets and Caplets 1561
- TYLENOL Cold Medication No Drowsiness Formula Gelcaps and Caplets 1562
- TYLENOL Cold Multi-Symptom Hot Medication Liquid Packets 1557
- TYLENOL Cough Multi-Symptom Medication with Decongestant 1565
- Ursinus Inlay-Tabs ▣ 794
- Vicks 44 LiquiCaps Cough, Cold & Flu Relief ▣ 755
- Vicks 44 LiquiCaps Non-Drowsy Cough & Cold Relief ▣ 756
- Vicks 44D Dry Hacking Cough & Head Congestion ▣ 755
- Vicks 44M Cough, Cold & Flu Relief ▣ 756
- Vicks DayQuil ▣ 761
- Vicks DayQuil SINUS Pressure & PAIN Relief with IBUPROFEN ▣ 762
- Vicks Nyquil Hot Therapy ▣ 762
- Vicks NyQuil LiquiCaps Multi-Symptom Cold/Flu Relief ▣ 763
- Vicks NyQuil Multi-Symptom Cold/Flu Relief - (Original & Cherry Flavor) ▣ 763

Pseudoephedrine Sulfate (Increased risk of cardiac arrhythmias). Products include:
- Cheracol Sinus ▣ 768
- Chlor-Trimeton Allergy Decongestant Tablets ▣ 799
- Claritin-D 2350
- Drixoral Cold and Allergy Sustained-Action Tablets ▣ 802
- Drixoral Cold and Flu Extended-Release Tablets ▣ 803
- Drixoral Non-Drowsy Formula Extended-Release Tablets ▣ 803
- Drixoral Allergy/Sinus Extended Release Tablets ▣ 804
- Trinalin Repetabs Tablets 1330

Quinidine Gluconate (Causes a rise in serum digoxin concentration, with the implication that digitalis intoxication may result). Products include:
- Quinaglute Dura-Tabs Tablets 649

Quinidine Polygalacturonate (Causes a rise in serum digoxin concentration, with the implication that digitalis intoxication may result).
- No products indexed under this heading.

Quinidine Sulfate (Causes a rise in serum digoxin concentration, with the implication that digitalis intoxication may result). Products include:
- Quinidex Extentabs 2067

Salmeterol Xinafoate (Increased risk of cardiac arrhythmias). Products include:
- Serevent Inhalation Aerosol 1176

Sodium Bicarbonate (Interferes with intestinal digoxin absorption). Products include:
- Alka-Seltzer Effervescent Antacid and Pain Reliever ▣ 701
- Alka-Seltzer Extra Strength Effervescent Antacid and Pain Reliever ▣ 703
- Alka-Seltzer Gold Effervescent Antacid ▣ 703
- Alka-Seltzer Lemon Lime Effervescent Antacid and Pain Reliever ▣ 703
- Arm & Hammer Pure Baking Soda ▣ 627
- Ceo-Two Rectal Suppositories 666
- Citrocarbonate Antacid ▣ 770
- Massengill Disposable Douches ▣ 820
- Massengill Liquid Concentrate ▣ 820
- NuLYTELY 689
- Cherry Flavor NuLYTELY 689

Sotalol Hydrochloride (Additive effects on AV node conduction). Products include:
- Betapace Tablets 641

Succinylcholine Chloride (May cause arrhythmias). Products include:
- Anectine 1073

Sulfasalazine (Low digoxin serum concentration; interferes with intestinal digoxin absorption). Products include:
- Azulfidine 1949

Terbutaline Sulfate (Increased risk of cardiac arrhythmias). Products include:
- Brethaire Inhaler 813
- Brethine Ampuls 815
- Brethine Tablets 814
- Bricanyl Subcutaneous Injection 1502
- Bricanyl Tablets 1503

Tetracycline Hydrochloride (May increase digoxin absorption in patients who convert digoxin to inactive metabolites in the gut resulting in increased serum levels of digoxin). Products include:
- Achromycin V Capsules 1367

Thyroglobulin (Hypothyroid patients may require increased digoxin dose).
- No products indexed under this heading.

Thyroid (Hypothyroid patients may require increased digoxin dose).
- No products indexed under this heading.

Thyroxine (Hypothyroid patients may require increased digoxin dose).
- No products indexed under this heading.

Thyroxine Sodium (Hypothyroid patients may require increased digoxin dose).
- No products indexed under this heading.

Timolol Hemihydrate (Additive effects on AV node conduction). Products include:
- Betimol 0.25%, 0.5% ◉ 261

Timolol Maleate (Additive effects on AV node conduction). Products include:
- Blocadren Tablets 1614
- Timolide Tablets 1748
- Timoptic in Ocudose 1753
- Timoptic Sterile Ophthalmic Solution 1751
- Timoptic-XE 1755

Triamcinolone (Corticosteroid-induced hypokalemia sensitizes the myocardium to digitalis resulting in possible digitalis toxicity). Products include:
- Aristocort Tablets 1022

Triamcinolone Acetonide (Corticosteroid-induced hypokalemia sensitizes the myocardium to digitalis resulting in possible digitalis toxicity). Products include:
- Aristocort A 0.025% Cream 1027
- Aristocort A 0.5% Cream 1031
- Aristocort A 0.1% Cream 1029
- Aristocort A 0.1% Ointment 1030
- Azmacort Oral Inhaler 2011
- Nasacort Nasal Inhaler 2024

Triamcinolone Diacetate (Corticosteroid-induced hypokalemia sensitizes the myocardium to digitalis resulting in possible digitalis toxicity). Products include:
- Aristocort Suspension (Forte Parenteral) 1027
- Aristocort Suspension (Intralesional) 1025

Triamcinolone Hexacetonide (Corticosteroid-induced hypokalemia sensitizes the myocardium to digitalis resulting in possible digitalis toxicity). Products include:
- Aristospan Suspension (Intra-articular) 1033
- Aristospan Suspension (Intralesional) 1032

Troleandomycin (May increase digoxin absorption in patients who convert digoxin to inactive metabolites in the gut resulting in increased serum levels of digoxin). Products include:
- Tao Capsules 2209

Verapamil Hydrochloride (Causes a rise in serum digoxin concentration, with the implication that digitalis intoxication may result). Products include:
- Calan SR Caplets 2422
- Calan Tablets 2419
- Isoptin Injectable 1344
- Isoptin Oral Tablets 1346
- Isoptin SR Tablets 1348
- Verelan Capsules 1410
- Verelan Capsules 2824

LANOXIN TABLETS

(Digoxin) 1128

May interact with potassium-depleting corticosteroids, potassium-depleting diuretics, antacids, sympathomimetics, beta blockers, calcium channel blockers, thyroid preparations, mineralocorticoids, tetracyclines, macrolide antibiotics, and certain other agents. Compounds in these categories include:

Acebutolol Hydrochloride (Additive effects on AV node conduction). Products include:
- Sectral Capsules 2807

Albuterol (Increased risk of cardiac arrhythmias). Products include:
- Proventil Inhalation Aerosol 2382
- Ventolin Inhalation Aerosol and Refill 1197

Albuterol Sulfate (Increased risk of cardiac arrhythmias). Products include:
- Airet Solution for Inhalation 452
- Proventil Inhalation Solution 0.083% 2384
- Proventil Repetabs Tablets 2386
- Proventil Solution for Inhalation 0.5% 2383
- Proventil Syrup 2385
- Proventil Tablets 2386
- Ventolin Inhalation Solution 1198
- Ventolin Nebules Inhalation Solution 1199
- Ventolin Rotacaps for Inhalation 1200
- Ventolin Syrup 1202
- Ventolin Tablets 1203
- Volmax Extended-Release Tablets 1788

Alprazolam (Causes a rise in serum digoxin concentration, with the implication that digitalis intoxication may result). Products include:
- Xanax Tablets 2649

Aluminum Carbonate Gel (Interferes with intestinal digoxin absorption). Products include:
- Basaljel 2703

Aluminum Hydroxide (Interferes with intestinal digoxin absorption). Products include:
- ALternaGEL Liquid 1316
- Maximum Strength Ascriptin ▣ 630
- Cama Arthritis Pain Reliever ▣ 785
- Gaviscon Extra Strength Relief Formula Antacid Tablets ▣ 819
- Gaviscon Extra Strength Relief Formula Liquid Antacid ▣ 819
- Gaviscon Liquid Antacid ▣ 820
- Gelusil Liquid & Tablets ▣ 855
- Maalox Heartburn Relief Suspension ▣ 642
- Maalox Heartburn Relief Tablets ▣ 641
- Maalox Magnesia and Alumina Oral Suspension ▣ 642
- Maalox Plus Tablets ▣ 643
- Extra Strength Maalox Antacid Plus Antigas Liquid and Tablets ▣ 638
- Tempo Soft Antacid ▣ 835

Aluminum Hydroxide Gel (Interferes with intestinal digoxin absorption). Products include:
- ALternaGEL Liquid ▣ 659
- Aludrox Oral Suspension 2695
- Amphojel Suspension 2695
- Amphojel Suspension without Flavor 2695
- Amphojel Tablets 2695
- Arthritis Pain Ascriptin ▣ 631
- Regular Strength Ascriptin Tablets ▣ 629
- Gaviscon Antacid Tablets ▣ 819
- Gaviscon-2 Antacid Tablets ▣ 820
- Mylanta Liquid 1317
- Mylanta Tablets ▣ 660
- Mylanta Double Strength Liquid 1317
- Mylanta Double Strength Tablets ▣ 660
- Nephrox Suspension ▣ 655

Aluminum Hydroxide Gel, Dried (Interferes with intestinal digoxin absorption).

Amiodarone Hydrochloride (Causes a rise in serum digoxin concentration, with the implication that digitalis intoxication may result). Products include:
- Cordarone Intravenous 2715
- Cordarone Tablets 2712

Amlodipine Besylate (Additive effects on AV node conduction). Products include:
- Lotrel Capsules 840
- Norvasc Tablets 1940

Amphotericin B (Amphotericin B-induced hypokalemia sensitizes the myocardium to digitalis resulting in possible digitalis toxicity). Products include:
- Fungizone Intravenous 506

Anticancer Drugs, unspecified (Interferes with intestinal digoxin absorption).

Atenolol (Additive effects on AV node conduction). Products include:
- Tenoretic Tablets 2845
- Tenormin Tablets and I.V. Injection 2847

Azithromycin (May increase digoxin absorption in patients who convert digoxin to inactive metabolites in the gut resulting in increased serum levels of digoxin). Products include:
- Zithromax 1944

Bendroflumethiazide (Diuretic-induced hypokalemia sensitizes the myocardium to digitalis resulting in possible digitalis toxicity).
- No products indexed under this heading.

Bepridil Hydrochloride (Additive effects on AV node conduction). Products include:
- Vascor (200, 300 and 400 mg) Tablets 1587

Interactions Index — Lanoxin Tablets

Betamethasone Acetate (Corticosteroid-induced hypokalemia sensitizes the myocardium to digitalis resulting in possible digitalis toxicity). Products include:

Celestone Soluspan Suspension 2347

Betamethasone Sodium Phosphate (Corticosteroid-induced hypokalemia sensitizes the myocardium to digitalis resulting in possible digitalis toxicity). Products include:

Celestone Soluspan Suspension 2347

Betaxolol Hydrochloride (Additive effects on AV node conduction). Products include:

Betoptic Ophthalmic Solution............ 469
Betoptic S Ophthalmic Suspension 471
Kerlone Tablets................................... 2436

Bisoprolol Fumarate (Additive effects on AV node conduction). Products include:

Zebeta Tablets 1413
Ziac 1415

Calcium, intravenous (May produce serious arrhythmias in digitalized patients).

No products indexed under this heading.

Carteolol Hydrochloride (Additive effects on AV node conduction). Products include:

Cartrol Tablets 410
Ocupress Ophthalmic Solution, 1% Sterile... ◊ 309

Chlorothiazide (Diuretic-induced hypokalemia sensitizes the myocardium to digitalis resulting in possible digitalis toxicity). Products include:

Aldoclor Tablets 1598
Diupres Tablets 1650
Diuril Oral 1653

Chlorothiazide Sodium (Diuretic-induced hypokalemia sensitizes the myocardium to digitalis resulting in possible digitalis toxicity). Products include:

Diuril Sodium Intravenous 1652

Chlorthalidone (Diuretic-induced hypokalemia sensitizes the myocardium to digitalis resulting in possible digitalis toxicity). Products include:

Combipres Tablets 677
Tenoretic Tablets................................. 2845
Thalitone 1245

Cholestyramine (Interferes with intestinal digoxin absorption). Products include:

Questran Light 769
Questran Powder 770

Clarithromycin (May increase digoxin absorption in patients who convert digoxin to inactive metabolites in the gut resulting in increased serum levels of digoxin). Products include:

Biaxin 405

Cortisone Acetate (Corticosteroid-induced hypokalemia sensitizes the myocardium to digitalis resulting in possible digitalis toxicity). Products include:

Cortone Acetate Sterile Suspension 1623
Cortone Acetate Tablets...................... 1624

Demeclocycline Hydrochloride (May increase digoxin absorption in patients who convert digoxin to inactive metabolites in the gut resulting in increased serum levels of digoxin). Products include:

Declomycin Tablets............................. 1371

Dexamethasone (Corticosteroid-induced hypokalemia sensitizes the myocardium to digitalis resulting in possible digitalis toxicity). Products include:

AK-Trol Ointment & Suspension .... ◊ 205
Decadron Elixir 1633
Decadron Tablets................................. 1635
Decaspray Topical Aerosol 1648
Dexacidin Ointment .... ◊ 263
Maxitrol Ophthalmic Ointment and Suspension .... ◊ 224
TobraDex Ophthalmic Suspension and Ointment... 473

Dexamethasone Acetate (Corticosteroid-induced hypokalemia sensitizes the myocardium to digitalis resulting in possible digitalis toxicity). Products include:

Dalalone D.P. Injectable 1011
Decadron-LA Sterile Suspension...... 1646

Dexamethasone Sodium Phosphate (Corticosteroid-induced hypokalemia sensitizes the myocardium to digitalis resulting in possible digitalis toxicity). Products include:

Decadron Phosphate Injection 1637
Decadron Phosphate Respihaler 1642
Decadron Phosphate Sterile Ophthalmic Ointment 1641
Decadron Phosphate Sterile Ophthalmic Solution 1642
Decadron Phosphate Topical Cream... 1644
Decadron Phosphate Turbinaire 1645
Decadron Phosphate with Xylocaine Injection, Sterile 1639
Dexacort Phosphate in Respihaler .. 458
Dexacort Phosphate in Turbinaire .. 459
NeoDecadron Sterile Ophthalmic Ointment 1712
NeoDecadron Sterile Ophthalmic Solution 1713
NeoDecadron Topical Cream 1714

Dihydroxyaluminum Sodium Carbonate (Interfers with intestinal digoxin absorption).

No products indexed under this heading.

Diltiazem Hydrochloride (Additive effects on AV node conduction). Products include:

Cardizem CD Capsules 1506
Cardizem SR Capsules 1510
Cardizem Injectable 1508
Cardizem Tablets................................. 1512
Dilacor XR Extended-release Capsules 2018

Diphenoxylate Hydrochloride (Increases digoxin absorption). Products include:

Lomotil... 2439

Dobutamine Hydrochloride (Increased risk of cardiac arrhythmias). Products include:

Dobutrex Solution Vials...................... 1439

Dopamine Hydrochloride (Increased risk of cardiac arrhythmias).

No products indexed under this heading.

Doxycycline Calcium (May increase digoxin absorption in patients who convert digoxin to inactive metabolites in the gut resulting in increased serum levels of digoxin). Products include:

Vibramycin Calcium Oral Suspension Syrup... 1941

Doxycycline Hyclate (May increase digoxin absorption in patients who convert digoxin to inactive metabolites in the gut resulting in increased serum levels of digoxin). Products include:

Doryx Capsules.................................... 1913
Vibramycin Hyclate Capsules 1941
Vibramycin Hyclate Intravenous 2215
Vibra-Tabs Film Coated Tablets 1941

Doxycycline Monohydrate (May increase digoxin absorption in patients who convert digoxin to inactive metabolites in the gut resulting in increased serum levels of digoxin). Products include:

Monodox Capsules 1805
Vibramycin Monohydrate for Oral Suspension 1941

Ephedrine Hydrochloride (Increased risk of cardiac arrhythmias). Products include:

Primatene Dual Action Formula...... ⊕D 872
Primatene Tablets .... ⊕D 873
Quadrinal Tablets 1350

Ephedrine Sulfate (Increased risk of cardiac arrhythmias). Products include:

Bronkaid Caplets .... ⊕D 717
Marax Tablets & DF Syrup................. 2200

Ephedrine Tannate (Increased risk of cardiac arrhythmias). Products include:

Rynatuss 2673

Epinephrine (Increased risk of cardiac arrhythmias). Products include:

Bronkaid Mist .... ⊕D 717
EPIFRIN .... ◊ 239
EpiPen 790
Marcaine Hydrochloride with Epinephrine 1:200,000 2316
Primatene Mist .... ⊕D 873
Sensorcaine with Epinephrine Injection 559
Sus-Phrine Injection 1019
Xylocaine with Epinephrine Injections... 567

Epinephrine Bitartrate (Increased risk of cardiac arrhythmias). Products include:

Bronkaid Mist Suspension .... ⊕D 718
Sensorcaine-MPF with Epinephrine Injection 559

Epinephrine Hydrochloride (Increased risk of cardiac arrhythmias). Products include:

Ana-Kit Anaphylaxis Emergency Treatment Kit 617

Erythromycin (May increase digoxin absorption in patients who convert digoxin to inactive metabolites in the gut resulting in increased serum levels of digoxin). Products include:

A/T/S 2% Acne Topical Gel and Solution 1234
Benzamycin Topical Gel 905
E-Mycin Tablets 1341
Emgel 2% Topical Gel......................... 1093
ERYC... 1915
Erycette (erythromycin 2%) Topical Solution... 1888
Ery-Tab Tablets 422
Erythromycin Base Filmtab 426
Erythromycin Delayed-Release Capsules, USP...................................... 427
Ilotycin Ophthalmic Ointment............ 912
PCE Dispertab Tablets 444
T-Stat 2.0% Topical Solution and Pads 2688
Theramycin Z Topical Solution 2% 1592

Erythromycin Estolate (May increase digoxin absorption in patients who convert digoxin to inactive metabolites in the gut resulting in increased serum levels of digoxin). Products include:

Ilosone 911

Erythromycin Ethylsuccinate (May increase digoxin absorption in patients who convert digoxin to inactive metabolites in the gut resulting in increased serum levels of digoxin). Products include:

E.E.S.. 424
EryPed 421

Erythromycin Gluceptate (May increase digoxin absorption in patients who convert digoxin to inactive metabolites in the gut resulting in increased serum levels of digoxin). Products include:

Ilotycin Gluceptate, IV, Vials 913

Erythromycin Stearate (May increase digoxin absorption in patients who convert digoxin to inactive metabolites in the gut resulting in increased serum levels of digoxin). Products include:

Erythrocin Stearate Filmtab 425

Esmolol Hydrochloride (Additive effects on AV node conduction). Products include:

Brevibloc Injection............................... 1808

Felodipine (Additive effects on AV node conduction). Products include:

Plendil Extended-Release Tablets..... 527

Furosemide (Diuretic-induced hypokalemia sensitizes the myocardium to digitalis resulting in possible digitalis toxicity). Products include:

Lasix Injection, Oral Solution and Tablets 1240

Hydrochlorothiazide (Diuretic-induced hypokalemia sensitizes the myocardium to digitalis resulting in possible digitalis toxicity). Products include:

Aldactazide... 2413
Aldoril Tablets...................................... 1604
Apresazide Capsules 808
Capozide 742
Dyazide 2479
Esidrix Tablets 821
Esimil Tablets 822
HydroDIURIL Tablets 1674
Hydropres Tablets................................ 1675
Hyzaar Tablets 1677
Inderide Tablets 2732
Inderide LA Long Acting Capsules .. 2734
Lopressor HCT Tablets 832
Lotensin HCT....................................... 837
Maxzide 1380
Moduretic Tablets 1705
Oretic Tablets 443
Prinzide Tablets................................... 1737
Ser-Ap-Es Tablets 849
Timolide Tablets................................... 1748
Vaseretic Tablets 1765
Zestoretic 2850
Ziac 1415

Hydrocortisone (Corticosteroid-induced hypokalemia sensitizes the myocardium to digitalis resulting in possible digitalis toxicity). Products include:

Anusol-HC Cream 2.5% 1896
Aquanil HC Lotion 1931
Bactine Hydrocortisone Anti-Itch Cream... ⊕D 709
Caldecort Anti-Itch Hydrocortisone Spray .... ⊕D 631
Cortaid .... ⊕D 836
CORTENEMA.. 2535
Cortisporin Ointment 1085
Cortisporin Ophthalmic Ointment Sterile 1085
Cortisporin Ophthalmic Suspension Sterile 1086
Cortisporin Otic Solution Sterile 1087
Cortisporin Otic Suspension Sterile 1088
Cortizone-5 .... ⊕D 831
Cortizone-10 .... ⊕D 831
Hydrocortone Tablets 1672
Hytone 907
Massengill Medicated Soft Cloth Towelettes.. 2458
PediOtic Suspension Sterile 1153
Preparation H Hydrocortisone 1% Cream .... ⊕D 872
ProctoCream-HC 2.5%........................ 2408
VōSoL HC Otic Solution...................... 2678

Hydrocortisone Acetate (Corticosteroid-induced hypokalemia sensitizes the myocardium to digitalis resulting in possible digitalis toxicity). Products include:

Analpram-HC Rectal Cream 1% and 2.5% 977
Anusol HC-1 Anti-Itch Hydrocortisone Ointment.................................... ⊕D 847
Anusol-HC Suppositories 1897
Caldecort.. ⊕D 631
Carmol HC 924
Coly-Mycin S Otic w/Neomycin & Hydrocortisone 1906
Cortaid .... ⊕D 836
Cortifoam 2396
Cortisporin Cream............................... 1084
Epifoam 2399
Hydrocortone Acetate Sterile Suspension.. 1669
Mantadil Cream 1135
Nupercainal Hydrocortisone 1% Cream... ⊕D 645
Ophthocort .... ◊ 311

IMPORTANT NOTE: Always consult each drug listing in the patient's regimen for possible interactions.

Lanoxin Tablets | Interactions Index | 564

Pramosone Cream, Lotion & Ointment ... 978
ProctoCream-HC ... 2408
ProctoFoam-HC ... 2409
Terra-Cortril Ophthalmic Suspension ... 2210

Hydrocortisone Sodium Phosphate (Corticosteroid-induced hypokalemia sensitizes the myocardium to digitalis resulting in possible digitalis toxicity). Products include:
Hydrocortone Phosphate Injection, Sterile ... 1670

Hydrocortisone Sodium Succinate (Corticosteroid-induced hypokalemia sensitizes the myocardium to digitalis resulting in possible digitalis toxicity). Products include:
Solu-Cortef Sterile Powder ... 2641

Hydroflumethiazide (Diuretic-induced hypokalemia sensitizes the myocardium to digitalis resulting in possible digitalis toxicity). Products include:
Diucardin Tablets ... 2718

Indapamide (Diuretic-induced hypokalemia sensitizes the myocardium to digitalis resulting in possible digitalis toxicity). Products include:
Lozol Tablets ... 2022

Indomethacin (Causes a rise in serum digoxin concentration, with the implication that digitalis intoxication may result). Products include:
Indocin ... 1680

Indomethacin Sodium Trihydrate (Causes a rise in serum digoxin concentration, with the implication that digitalis intoxication may result). Products include:
Indocin I.V. ... 1684

Isoproterenol Hydrochloride (Increased risk of cardiac arrhythmias). Products include:
Isuprel Hydrochloride Injection 1:5000 ... 2311
Isuprel Hydrochloride Solution 1:200 & 1:100 ... 2313
Isuprel Mistometer ... 2312

Isoproterenol Sulfate (Increased risk of cardiac arrhythmias). Products include:
Norisodrine with Calcium Iodide Syrup ... 442

Isradipine (Additive effects on AV node conduction). Products include:
DynaCirc Capsules ... 2256

Itraconazole (Causes a rise in serum digoxin concentration, with the implication that digitalis intoxication may result). Products include:
Sporanox Capsules ... 1305

Kaolin (Low digoxin serum concentration; interferes with intestinal digoxin absorption).
No products indexed under this heading.

Labetalol Hydrochloride (Additive effects on AV node conduction). Products include:
Normodyne Injection ... 2377
Normodyne Tablets ... 2379
Trandate ... 1185

Levobunolol Hydrochloride (Additive effects on AV node conduction). Products include:
Betagan ... ⊙ 233

Liothyronine Sodium (Hypothyroid patients may require increased digoxin dose). Products include:
Cytomel Tablets ... 2473
Triostat Injection ... 2530

Magaldrate (Interferes with intestinal digoxin absorption).
No products indexed under this heading.

Magnesium Hydroxide (Interferes with intestinal digoxin absorption). Products include:
Aludrox Oral Suspension ... 2695
Arthritis Pain Ascriptin ... ◘ 631
Maximum Strength Ascriptin ... ◘ 630
Regular Strength Ascriptin Tablets ... ◘ 629
Di-Gel Antacid/Anti-Gas ... ◘ 801
Gelusil Liquid & Tablets ... ◘ 855
Maalox Magnesia and Alumina Oral Suspension ... ◘ 642
Maalox Plus Tablets ... ◘ 643
Extra Strength Maalox Antacid Plus Antigas Liquid and Tablets ◘ 638
Mylanta Calcium Carbonate and Magnesium Hydroxide Tablets ... 1318
Mylanta Liquid ... 1317
Mylanta Tablets ... ◘ 660
Mylanta Double Strength Liquid ... 1317
Mylanta Double Strength Tablets ... ◘ 660
Phillips' Milk of Magnesia Liquid ... ◘ 729
Rolaids Tablets ... ◘ 843
Tempo Soft Antacid ... ◘ 835

Magnesium Oxide (Interferes with intestinal digoxin absorption). Products include:
Beelith Tablets ... 639
Bufferin Analgesic Tablets and Caplets ... ◘ 613
Caltrate PLUS ... ◘ 665
Cama Arthritis Pain Reliever ... ◘ 785
Mag-Ox 400 ... 668
Uro-Mag ... 668

Metaproterenol Sulfate (Increased risk of cardiac arrhythmias). Products include:
Alupent ... 669
Metaproterenol Sulfate Inhalation Solution, USP, Arm-a-Med ... 552

Metaraminol Bitartrate (Increased risk of cardiac arrhythmias). Products include:
Aramine Injection ... 1609

Methacycline Hydrochloride (May increase digoxin absorption in patients who convert digoxin to inactive metabolites in the gut resulting in increased serum levels of digoxin).
No products indexed under this heading.

Methoxamine Hydrochloride (Increased risk of cardiac arrhythmias). Products include:
Vasoxyl Injection ... 1196

Methyclothiazide (Diuretic-induced hypokalemia sensitizes the myocardium to digitalis resulting in possible digitalis toxicity). Products include:
Enduron Tablets ... 420

Methylprednisolone Acetate (Corticosteroid-induced hypokalemia sensitizes the myocardium to digitalis resulting in possible digitalis toxicity). Products include:
Depo-Medrol Single-Dose Vial ... 2600
Depo-Medrol Sterile Aqueous Suspension ... 2597

Methylprednisolone Sodium Succinate (Corticosteroid-induced hypokalemia sensitizes the myocardium to digitalis resulting in possible digitalis toxicity). Products include:
Solu-Medrol Sterile Powder ... 2643

Metipranolol Hydrochloride (Additive effects on AV node conduction). Products include:
OptiPranolol (Metipranolol 0.3%) Sterile Ophthalmic Solution ... ⊙ 258

Metoclopramide Hydrochloride (Reduces intestinal digoxin absorption, resulting in unexpectedly low serum concentration). Products include:
Reglan ... 2068

Metolazone (Diuretic-induced hypokalemia sensitizes the myocardium to digitalis resulting in possible digitalis toxicity). Products include:
Mykrox Tablets ... 993
Zaroxolyn Tablets ... 1000

Metoprolol Succinate (Additive effects on AV node conduction). Products include:
Toprol-XL Tablets ... 565

Metoprolol Tartrate (Additive effects on AV node conduction). Products include:
Lopressor Ampuls ... 830
Lopressor HCT Tablets ... 832
Lopressor Tablets ... 830

Minocycline Hydrochloride (May increase digoxin absorption in patients who convert digoxin to inactive metabolites in the gut resulting in increased serum levels of digoxin). Products include:
Dynacin Capsules ... 1590
Minocin Intravenous ... 1382
Minocin Oral Suspension ... 1385
Minocin Pellet-Filled Capsules ... 1383

Nadolol (Additive effects on AV node conduction).
No products indexed under this heading.

Neomycin, oral (Interferes with intestinal digoxin absorption).

Nephrotoxic Drugs (May impair the excretion of digoxin).

Nicardipine Hydrochloride (Additive effects on AV node conduction). Products include:
Cardene Capsules ... 2095
Cardene I.V. ... 2709
Cardene SR Capsules ... 2097

Nifedipine (Additive effects on AV node conduction). Products include:
Adalat Capsules (10 mg and 20 mg) ... 587
Adalat CC ... 589
Procardia Capsules ... 1971
Procardia XL Extended Release Tablets ... 1972

Nimodipine (Additive effects on AV node conduction). Products include:
Nimotop Capsules ... 610

Nisoldipine (Additive effects on AV node conduction).
No products indexed under this heading.

Norepinephrine Bitartrate (Increase risk of cardiac arrhythmias). Products include:
Levophed Bitartrate Injection ... 2315

Oxytetracycline Hydrochloride (May increase digoxin absorption in patients who convert digoxin to inactive metabolites in the gut resulting in increased serum levels of digoxin). Products include:
TERAK Ointment ... ⊙ 209
Terra-Cortril Ophthalmic Suspension ... 2210
Terramycin with Polymyxin B Sulfate Ophthalmic Ointment ... 2211
Urobiotic-250 Capsules ... 2214

Pectin (Low digoxin serum concentration; interferes with intestinal digoxin absorption). Products include:
Celestial Seasonings Soothers Throat Drops ... ◘ 842

Penbutolol Sulfate (Additive effects on AV node conduction). Products include:
Levatol ... 2403

Phenylephrine Bitartrate (Increased risk of cardiac arrhythmias).
No products indexed under this heading.

Phenylephrine Hydrochloride (Increased risk of cardiac arrhythmias). Products include:
Atrohist Plus Tablets ... 454
Cerose DM ... ◘ 878
Comhist ... 2038
D.A. Chewable Tablets ... 951
Deconsal Pediatric Capsules ... 454
Dura-Vent/DA Tablets ... 953
Entex Capsules ... 1986
Entex Liquid ... 1986
Extendryl ... 1005
4-Way Fast Acting Nasal Spray (regular & mentholated) ... ◘ 621
Hemorid For Women ... ◘ 834
Hycomine Compound Tablets ... 932
Neo-Synephrine Hydrochloride 1% Carpuject ... 2324
Neo-Synephrine Hydrochloride 1% Injection ... 2324
Neo-Synephrine Hydrochloride (Ophthalmic) ... 2325
Neo-Synephrine ... ◘ 726
Nōstril ... ◘ 644
Novahistine Elixir ... ◘ 823
Phenergan VC ... 2779
Phenergan VC with Codeine ... 2781
Preparation H ... ◘ 871
Tympagesic Ear Drops ... 2342
Vasosulf ... ⊙ 271
Vicks Sinex Nasal Spray and Ultra Fine Mist ... ◘ 765

Phenylephrine Tannate (Increased risk of cardiac arrhythmias). Products include:
Atrohist Pediatric Suspension ... 454
Ricobid-D Pediatric Suspension ... 2038
Ricobid Tablets and Pediatric Suspension ... 2038
Rynatan ... 2673
Rynatuss ... 2673

Phenylpropanolamine Hydrochloride (Increased risk of cardiac arrhythmias). Products include:
Acutrim ... ◘ 628
Allerest Children's Chewable Tablets ... ◘ 627
Allerest 12 Hour Caplets ... ◘ 627
Atrohist Plus Tablets ... 454
BC Cold Powder Multi-Symptom Formula (Cold-Sinus-Allergy) ... ◘ 609
BC Cold Powder Non-Drowsy Formula (Cold-Sinus) ... ◘ 609
Cheracol Plus Head Cold/Cough Formula ... ◘ 769
Comtrex Multi-Symptom Non-Drowsy Liqui-gels ... ◘ 618
Contac Continuous Action Nasal Decongestant/Antihistamine 12 Hour Capsules ... ◘ 813
Contac Maximum Strength Continuous Action Decongestant/Antihistamine 12 Hour Caplets ... ◘ 813
Contac Severe Cold and Flu Formula Caplets ... ◘ 814
Coricidin 'D' Decongestant Tablets ... ◘ 800
Dexatrim ... ◘ 832
Dexatrim Plus Vitamins Caplets ... ◘ 832
Dimetane-DC Cough Syrup ... 2059
Dimetapp Elixir ... ◘ 773
Dimetapp Extentabs ... ◘ 774
Dimetapp Tablets/Liqui-Gels ... ◘ 775
Dimetapp Cold & Allergy Chewable Tablets ... ◘ 773
Dimetapp DM Elixir ... ◘ 774
Dura-Vent Tablets ... 952
Entex Capsules ... 1986
Entex LA Tablets ... 1987
Entex Liquid ... 1986
Exgest LA Tablets ... 782
Hycomine ... 931
Isoclor Timesule Capsules ... ◘ 637
Nolamine Timed-Release Tablets ... 785
Ornade Spansule Capsules ... 2502
Propagest Tablets ... 786
Pyrroxate Caplets ... ◘ 772
Robitussin-CF ... ◘ 777
Sinulin Tablets ... 787
Tavist-D 12 Hour Relief Tablets ... ◘ 787
Teldrin 12 Hour Antihistamine/Nasal Decongestant Allergy Relief Capsules ... ◘ 826
Triaminic Allergy Tablets ... ◘ 789
Triaminic Cold Tablets ... ◘ 790
Triaminic Expectorant ... ◘ 790
Triaminic Syrup ... ◘ 792
Triaminic-12 Tablets ... ◘ 792
Triaminic-DM Syrup ... ◘ 792
Triaminicin Tablets ... ◘ 793
Triaminicol Multi-Symptom Cold Tablets ... ◘ 793
Triaminicol Multi-Symptom Relief ◘ 794
Vicks DayQuil Allergy Relief 12-Hour Extended Release Tablets ... ◘ 760
Vicks DayQuil Allergy Relief 4-Hour Tablets ... ◘ 760
Vicks DayQuil SINUS Pressure & CONGESTION Relief ... ◘ 761

(◘ Described in PDR For Nonprescription Drugs) (⊙ Described in PDR For Ophthalmology)

Pindolol (Additive effects on AV node conduction). Products include:
Visken Tablets ... 2299

Pirbuterol Acetate (Increased risk of cardiac arrhythmias). Products include:
Maxair Autohaler ... 1492
Maxair Inhaler ... 1494

Polythiazide (Diuretic-induced hypokalemia sensitizes the myocardium to digitalis resulting in possible digitalis toxicity). Products include:
Minizide Capsules ... 1938

Prednisolone Acetate (Corticosteroid-induced hypokalemia sensitizes the myocardium to digitalis resulting in possible digitalis toxicity). Products include:
AK-CIDE ... ◉ 202
AK-CIDE Ointment ... ◉ 202
Blephamide Liquifilm Sterile Ophthalmic Suspension ... 476
Blephamide Ointment ... ◉ 237
Econopred & Econopred Plus Ophthalmic Suspensions ... ◉ 217
Poly-Pred Liquifilm ... ◉ 248
Pred Forte ... ◉ 250
Pred Mild ... ◉ 253
Pred-G Liquifilm Sterile Ophthalmic Suspension ... ◉ 251
Pred-G S.O.P. Sterile Ophthalmic Ointment ... ◉ 252
Vasocidin Ointment ... ◉ 268

Prednisolone Sodium Phosphate (Corticosteroid-induced hypokalemia sensitizes the myocardium to digitalis resulting in possible digitalis toxicity). Products include:
AK-Pred ... ◉ 204
Hydeltrasol Injection, Sterile ... 1665
Inflamase ... ◉ 265
Pediapred Oral Liquid ... 995
Vasocidin Ophthalmic Solution ... ◉ 270

Prednisolone Tebutate (Corticosteroid-induced hypokalemia sensitizes the myocardium to digitalis resulting in possible digitalis toxicity). Products include:
Hydeltra-T.B.A. Sterile Suspension 1667

Prednisone (Corticosteroid-induced hypokalemia sensitizes the myocardium to digitalis resulting in possible digitalis toxicity). Products include:
Deltasone Tablets ... 2595

Propafenone Hydrochloride (Causes a rise in serum digoxin concentration, with the implication that digitalis intoxication may result). Products include:
Rythmol Tablets–150mg, 225mg, 300mg ... 1352

Propantheline Bromide (Increases digoxin absorption). Products include:
Pro-Banthīne Tablets ... 2052

Propranolol Hydrochloride (Additive effects on AV node conduction). Products include:
Inderal ... 2728
Inderal LA Long Acting Capsules ... 2730
Inderide Tablets ... 2732
Inderide LA Long Acting Capsules .. 2734

Pseudoephedrine Hydrochloride (Increased risk of cardiac arrhythmias). Products include:
Actifed Allergy Daytime/Nighttime Caplets ... ▣ 844
Actifed Plus Caplets ... ▣ 845
Actifed Plus Tablets ... ▣ 845
Actifed with Codeine Cough Syrup.. 1067
Actifed Sinus Daytime/Nighttime Tablets and Caplets ... ▣ 846
Actifed Syrup ... ▣ 846
Actifed Tablets ... ▣ 844
Advil Cold and Sinus Caplets and Tablets (formerly CoAdvil) ... ▣ 870
Alka-Seltzer Plus Cold Medicine Liqui-Gels ... ▣ 706
Alka-Seltzer Plus Cold & Cough Medicine Liqui-Gels ... ▣ 705
Alka-Seltzer Plus Night-Time Cold Medicine Liqui-Gels ... ▣ 706
Allerest Headache Strength Tablets ... ▣ 627
Allerest Maximum Strength Tablets ... ▣ 627
Allerest No Drowsiness Tablets ... ▣ 627
Allerest Sinus Pain Formula ... ▣ 627
Anatuss LA Tablets ... 1542
Atrohist Pediatric Capsules ... 453
Bayer Select Sinus Pain Relief Formula ... ▣ 717
Benadryl Allergy Decongestant Liquid Medication ... ▣ 848
Benadryl Allergy Decongestant Tablets ... ▣ 848
Benadryl Allergy Sinus Headache Formula Caplets ... ▣ 849
Benylin Multisymptom ... ▣ 852
Bromfed Capsules (Extended-Release) ... 1785
Bromfed Syrup ... ▣ 733
Bromfed Tablets ... 1785
Bromfed-DM Cough Syrup ... 1786
Bromfed-PD Capsules (Extended-Release) ... 1785
Children's Vicks DayQuil Allergy Relief ... ▣ 757
Children's Vicks NyQuil Cold/Cough Relief ... ▣ 758
Comtrex Multi-Symptom Cold Reliever Tablets/Caplets/Liqui-Gels/Liquid ... ▣ 615
Allergy-Sinus Comtrex Multi-Symptom Allergy-Sinus Formula Tablets ... ▣ 617
Comtrex Multi-Symptom Non-Drowsy Caplets ... ▣ 618
Congess ... 1004
Contac Day Allergy/Sinus Caplets ▣ 812
Contac Day & Night ... ▣ 812
Contac Night Allergy/Sinus Caplets ... ▣ 812
Contac Severe Cold & Flu Non-Drowsy ... ▣ 815
Deconamine Chewable Tablets ... 1320
Deconamine CX Cough and Cold Liquid and Tablets ... 1319
Deconamine ... 1320
Deconsal C Expectorant Syrup ... 456
Deconsal Pediatric Syrup ... 457
Deconsal II Tablets ... 454
Dimetane-DX Cough Syrup ... 2059
Dimetapp Sinus Caplets ... ▣ 775
Dorcol Children's Cough Syrup ... ▣ 785
Drixoral Cough + Congestion Liquid Caps ... ▣ 802
Dura-Tap/PD Capsules ... 2867
Duratuss Tablets ... 2565
Duratuss HD Elixir ... 2565
Efidac/24 ... ▣ 635
Entex PSE Tablets ... 1987
Fedahist Gyrocaps ... 2401
Fedahist Timecaps ... 2401
Guaifed ... 1787
Guaifed Syrup ... ▣ 734
Guaimax-D Tablets ... 792
Guaitab Tablets ... ▣ 734
Isoclor Expectorant ... 990
Kronofed-A ... 977
Motrin IB Sinus ... ▣ 838
Novahistine DH ... 2462
Novahistine DMX ... ▣ 822
Novahistine Expectorant ... 2463
Nucofed ... 2051
PediaCare Cold Allergy Chewable Tablets ... ▣ 677
PediaCare Cough-Cold Chewable Tablets ... 1553
PediaCare ... 1553
PediaCare Infants' Decongestant Drops ... ▣ 677
PediCare Infant's Drops Decongestant Plus Cough ... 1553
PediaCare NightRest Cough-Cold Liquid ... 1553
Pediatric Vicks 44d Dry Hacking Cough & Head Congestion ... ▣ 763
Pediatric Vicks 44m Cough & Cold Relief ... ▣ 764
Robitussin Cold & Cough Liqui-Gels ... ▣ 776
Robitussin Maximum Strength Cough & Cold ... ▣ 778
Robitussin Pediatric Cough & Cold Formula ... ▣ 779
Robitussin Severe Congestion Liqui-Gels ... ▣ 776
Robitussin-DAC Syrup ... 2074
Robitussin-PE ... ▣ 778
Rondec Oral Drops ... 953
Rondec Syrup ... 953
Rondec Tablet ... 953
Rondec-DM Oral Drops ... 954
Rondec-DM Syrup ... 954
Rondec-TR Tablet ... 953
Ryna ... ▣ 841
Seldane-D Extended-Release Tablets ... 1538
Semprex-D Capsules ... 463
Semprex-D Capsules ... 1167
Sinarest Tablets ... ▣ 648
Sinarest Extra Strength Tablets ... ▣ 648
Sinarest No Drowsiness Tablets ... ▣ 648
Sine-Aid IB Caplets ... 1554
Sine-Aid Maximum Strength Sinus Medication Gelcaps, Caplets and Tablets ... 1554
Sine-Off No Drowsiness Formula Caplets ... ▣ 824
Sine-Off Sinus Medicine ... ▣ 825
Singlet Tablets ... ▣ 825
Sinutab Non-Drying Liquid Caps ... ▣ 859
Sinutab Sinus Allergy Medication, Maximum Strength Tablets and Caplets ... ▣ 860
Sinutab Sinus Medication, Maximum Strength Without Drowsiness Formula, Tablets & Caplets ... ▣ 860
Sinutab Sinus Medication, Regular Strength Without Drowsiness Formula ... ▣ 859
Sudafed Children's Liquid ... ▣ 861
Sudafed Cold and Cough Liquidcaps ... ▣ 862
Sudafed Cough Syrup ... ▣ 862
Sudafed Plus Liquid ... ▣ 862
Sudafed Plus Tablets ... ▣ 863
Sudafed Severe Cold Formula Caplets ... ▣ 863
Sudafed Severe Cold Formula Tablets ... ▣ 864
Sudafed Sinus Caplets ... ▣ 864
Sudafed Sinus Tablets ... ▣ 864
Sudafed Tablets, 30 mg ... ▣ 861
Sudafed Tablets, 60 mg ... ▣ 861
Sudafed 12 Hour Caplets ... ▣ 861
Syn-Rx Tablets ... 465
Syn-Rx DM Tablets ... 466
TheraFlu ... ▣ 787
TheraFlu Maximum Strength Nighttime Flu, Cold & Cough Medicine ... ▣ 788
TheraFlu Maximum Strength Non-Drowsy Formula Flu, Cold & Cough Medicine ... ▣ 788
Thera Flu Maximum Strength, Non-Drowsy Formula Flu, Cold and Cough Caplets ... ▣ 789
Triaminic AM Cough and Decongestant Formula ... ▣ 789
Triaminic AM Decongestant Formula ... ▣ 790
Triaminic Nite Light ... ▣ 791
Triaminic Sore Throat Formula ... ▣ 791
Tussend ... 1783
Tussend Expectorant ... 1785
Children's TYLENOL Cold Multi-Symptom Liquid Formula and Chewable Tablets ... 1561
Children's TYLENOL Cold Plus Cough Multi Symptom Tablets and Liquid ... ▣ 681
Infants' TYLENOL Cold Decongestant & Fever-Reducer Drops ... 1556
TYLENOL Maximum Strength Allergy Sinus Medication Gelcaps and Caplets ... 1563
TYLENOL Maximum Strength Allergy Sinus NightTime Medication Caplets ... 1555
TYLENOL Flu Maximum Strength Gelcaps ... 1565
TYLENOL Flu NightTime, Maximum Strength, Gelcaps ... 1566
TYLENOL Maximum Strength Flu NightTime Hot Medication Packets ... 1562
TYLENOL, Maximum Strength, Sinus Medication Geltabs, Gelcaps, Caplets and Tablets ... 1566
TYLENOL Cold Multi-Symptom Formula Medication Tablets and Caplets ... 1561
TYLENOL Cold Medication No Drowsiness Formula Gelcaps and Caplets ... 1562
TYLENOL Cold Multi-Symptom Hot Medication Liquid Packets ... 1557
TYLENOL Cough Multi-Symptom Medication with Decongestant ... 1565
Ursinus Inlay-Tabs ... ▣ 794
Vicks 44 LiquiCaps Cough, Cold & Flu Relief ... ▣ 755
Vicks 44 LiquiCaps Non-Drowsy Cough & Cold Relief ... ▣ 756
Vicks 44D Dry Hacking Cough & Head Congestion ... ▣ 755
Vicks 44M Cough, Cold & Flu Relief ... ▣ 756
Vicks DayQuil ... ▣ 761
Vicks DayQuil SINUS Pressure & PAIN Relief with IBUPROFEN ... ▣ 762
Vicks Nyquil Hot Therapy ... ▣ 762
Vicks NyQuil LiquiCaps Multi-Symptom Cold/Flu Relief ... ▣ 763
Vicks NyQuil Multi-Symptom Cold/Flu Relief - (Original & Cherry Flavor) ... ▣ 763

Pseudoephedrine Sulfate (Increased risk of cardiac arrhythmias). Products include:
Cheracol Sinus ... ▣ 768
Chlor-Trimeton Allergy Decongestant Tablets ... ▣ 799
Claritin-D ... 2350
Drixoral Cold and Allergy Sustained-Action Tablets ... ▣ 802
Drixoral Cold and Flu Extended-Release Tablets ... ▣ 803
Drixoral Non-Drowsy Formula Extended-Release Tablets ... ▣ 803
Drixoral Allergy/Sinus Extended Release Tablets ... ▣ 804
Trinalin Repetabs Tablets ... 1330

Quinidine Gluconate (Causes a rise in serum digoxin concentration, with the implication that digitalis intoxication may result). Products include:
Quinaglute Dura-Tabs Tablets ... 649

Quinidine Polygalacturonate (Causes a rise in serum digoxin concentration, with the implication that digitalis intoxication may result).
No products indexed under this heading.

Quinidine Sulfate (Causes a rise in serum digoxin concentration, with the implication that digitalis intoxication may result). Products include:
Quinidex Extentabs ... 2067

Salmeterol Xinafoate (Increased risk of cardiac arrhythmias). Products include:
Serevent Inhalation Aerosol ... 1176

Sotalol Hydrochloride (Additive effects on AV node conduction). Products include:
Betapace Tablets ... 641

Succinylcholine Chloride (May cause arrhythmias). Products include:
Anectine ... 1073

Sulfasalazine (Low serum digoxin; interferes with intestinal digoxin absorption). Products include:
Azulfidine ... 1949

Terbutaline Sulfate (Increased risk of cardiac arrhythmias). Products include:
Brethaire Inhaler ... 813
Brethine Ampuls ... 815
Brethine Tablets ... 814
Bricanyl Subcutaneous Injection ... 1502
Bricanyl Tablets ... 1503

Tetracycline Hydrochloride (May increase digoxin absorption in patients who convert digoxin to inactive metabolites in the gut resulting in increased serum levels of digoxin). Products include:
Achromycin V Capsules ... 1367

Thyroid (Hypothyroid patients may require increased digoxin dose).
No products indexed under this heading.

Thyroxine (Hypothyroid patients may require increased digoxin dose).
No products indexed under this heading.

IMPORTANT NOTE: Always consult each drug listing in the patient's regimen for possible interactions.

Lanoxin Tablets | Interactions Index | 566

Timolol Hemihydrate (Additive effects on AV node conduction). Products include:
Betimol 0.25%, 0.5% ⊙ 261
Timolol Maleate (Additive effects on AV node conduction). Products include:
Blocadren Tablets 1614
Timolide Tablets 1748
Timoptic in Ocudose 1753
Timoptic Sterile Ophthalmic Solution 1751
Timoptic-XE 1755
Triamcinolone (Corticosteroid-induced hypokalemia sensitizes the myocardium to digitalis resulting in possible digitalis toxicity). Products include:
Aristocort Tablets 1022
Triamcinolone Acetonide (Corticosteroid-induced hypokalemia sensitizes the myocardium to digitalis resulting in possible digitalis toxicity). Products include:
Aristocort A 0.025% Cream 1027
Aristocort A 0.5% Cream 1031
Aristocort A 0.1% Cream 1029
Aristocort A 0.1% Ointment 1030
Azmacort Oral Inhaler 2011
Nasacort Nasal Inhaler 2024
Triamcinolone Diacetate (Corticosteroid-induced hypokalemia sensitizes the myocardium to digitalis resulting in possible digitalis toxicity). Products include:
Aristocort Suspension (Forte Parenteral) 1027
Aristocort Suspension (Intralesional) 1025
Triamcinolone Hexacetonide (Corticosteroid-induced hypokalemia sensitizes the myocardium to digitalis resulting in possible digitalis toxicity). Products include:
Aristospan Suspension (Intra-articular) 1033
Aristospan Suspension (Intralesional) 1032
Troleandomycin (May increase digoxin absorption in patients who convert digoxin to inactive metabolites in the gut resulting in increased serum levels of digoxin). Products include:
Tao Capsules 2209
Verapamil Hydrochloride (Causes a rise in serum digoxin concentration, with the implication that digitalis intoxication may result). Products include:
Calan SR Caplets 2422
Calan Tablets 2419
Isoptin Injectable 1344
Isoptin Oral Tablets 1346
Isoptin SR Tablets 1348
Verelan Capsules 1410
Verelan Capsules 2824

Food Interactions

Meal, high in bran fiber (The amount of digoxin from an oral dose may be reduced).
Meal, unspecified (Slows the rate of absorption).

LARIAM TABLETS

(Mefloquine Hydrochloride) 2128
May interact with beta blockers, anticonvulsants, and certain other agents. Compounds in these categories include:

Acebutolol Hydrochloride (May produce electrocardiographic abnormalities or cardiac arrest). Products include:
Sectral Capsules 2807
Atenolol (May produce electrocardiographic abnormalities or cardiac arrest). Products include:
Tenoretic Tablets 2845
Tenormin Tablets and I.V. Injection 2847
Betaxolol Hydrochloride (May produce electrocardiographic abnormalities or cardiac arrest). Products include:
Betoptic Ophthalmic Solution 469
Betoptic S Ophthalmic Suspension 471
Kerlone Tablets 2436
Bisoprolol Fumarate (May produce electrocardiographic abnormalities or cardiac arrest). Products include:
Zebeta Tablets 1413
Ziac 1415
Carbamazepine (Potential for loss of seizure control and lower than expected serum levels). Products include:
Atretol Tablets 573
Tegretol Chewable Tablets 852
Tegretol Suspension 852
Tegretol Tablets 852
Carteolol Hydrochloride (May produce electrocardiographic abnormalities or cardiac arrest). Products include:
Cartrol Tablets 410
Ocupress Ophthalmic Solution, 1% Sterile ⊙ 309
Chloroquine Hydrochloride (Increased risk of convulsions). Products include:
Aralen Hydrochloride Injection 2301
Chloroquine Phosphate (Increased risk of convulsions). Products include:
Aralen Phosphate Tablets 2301
Divalproex Sodium (Potential for loss of seizure control and lower than expected serum levels). Products include:
Depakote Tablets 415
Esmolol Hydrochloride (May produce electrocardiographic abnormalities or cardiac arrest). Products include:
Brevibloc Injection 1808
Ethosuximide (Potential for loss of seizure control and lower than expected serum levels). Products include:
Zarontin Capsules 1928
Zarontin Syrup 1929
Ethotoin (Potential for loss of seizure control and lower than expected serum levels). Products include:
Peganone Tablets 446
Felbamate (Potential for loss of seizure control and lower than expected serum levels). Products include:
Felbatol 2666
Halofantrine (Concurrent use may result in potentially fatal prolongation of Qtc interval; concurrent and/or sequential use is not recommended).
No products indexed under this heading.
Labetalol Hydrochloride (May produce electrocardiographic abnormalities or cardiac arrest). Products include:
Normodyne Injection 2377
Normodyne Tablets 2379
Trandate 1185
Lamotrigine (Potential for loss of seizure control and lower than expected serum levels). Products include:
Lamictal Tablets 1112
Levobunolol Hydrochloride (May produce electrocardiographic abnormalities or cardiac arrest). Products include:
Betagan ⊙ 233
Mephenytoin (Potential for loss of seizure control and lower than expected serum levels). Products include:
Mesantoin Tablets 2272
Methsuximide (Potential for loss of seizure control and lower than expected serum levels). Products include:
Celontin Kapseals 1899
Metipranolol Hydrochloride (May produce electrocardiographic abnormalities or cardiac arrest). Products include:
OptiPranolol (Metipranolol 0.3%) Sterile Ophthalmic Solution ⊙ 258
Metoprolol Succinate (May produce electrocardiographic abnormalities or cardiac arrest). Products include:
Toprol-XL Tablets 565
Metoprolol Tartrate (May produce electrocardiographic abnormalities or cardiac arrest). Products include:
Lopressor Ampuls 830
Lopressor HCT Tablets 832
Lopressor Tablets 830
Nadolol (May produce electrocardiographic abnormalities or cardiac arrest).
No products indexed under this heading.
Paramethadione (Potential for loss of seizure control and lower than expected serum levels).
No products indexed under this heading.
Penbutolol Sulfate (May produce electrocardiographic abnormalities or cardiac arrest). Products include:
Levatol 2403
Phenacemide (Potential for loss of seizure control and lower than expected serum levels). Products include:
Phenurone Tablets 447
Phenobarbital (Potential for loss of seizure control and lower than expected serum levels). Products include:
Arco-Lase Plus Tablets 512
Bellergal-S Tablets 2250
Donnatal 2060
Donnatal Extentabs 2061
Donnatal Tablets 2060
Phenobarbital Elixir and Tablets 1469
Quadrinal Tablets 1350
Phensuximide (Potential for loss of seizure control and lower than expected serum levels). Products include:
Milontin Kapseals 1920
Phenytoin (Potential for loss of seizure control and lower than expected serum levels). Products include:
Dilantin Infatabs 1908
Dilantin-125 Suspension 1911
Phenytoin Sodium (Potential for loss of seizure control and lower than expected serum levels). Products include:
Dilantin Kapseals 1906
Dilantin Parenteral 1910
Pindolol (May produce electrocardiographic abnormalities or cardiac arrest). Products include:
Visken Tablets 2299
Primidone (Potential for loss of seizure control and lower than expected serum levels). Products include:
Mysoline 2754
Propranolol Hydrochloride (May produce electrocardiographic abnormalities or cardiac arrest). Products include:
Inderal 2728
Inderal LA Long Acting Capsules 2730
Inderide Tablets 2732
Inderide LA Long Acting Capsules 2734
Quinidine Gluconate (May produce electrocardiographic abnormalities or cardiac arrest). Products include:
Quinaglute Dura-Tabs Tablets 649
Quinidine Polygalacturonate (May produce electrocardiographic abnormalities or cardiac arrest).
No products indexed under this heading.
Quinidine Sulfate (May produce electrocardiographic abnormalities or cardiac arrest). Products include:
Quinidex Extentabs 2067
Quinine Sulfate (Increased risk of convulsions; potential for electrocardiographic abnormalities or cardiac arrest).
No products indexed under this heading.
Sotalol Hydrochloride (May produce electrocardiographic abnormalities or cardiac arrest). Products include:
Betapace Tablets 641
Timolol Hemihydrate (May produce electrocardiographic abnormalities or cardiac arrest). Products include:
Betimol 0.25%, 0.5% ⊙ 261
Timolol Maleate (May produce electrocardiographic abnormalities or cardiac arrest). Products include:
Blocadren Tablets 1614
Timolide Tablets 1748
Timoptic in Ocudose 1753
Timoptic Sterile Ophthalmic Solution 1751
Timoptic-XE 1755
Trimethadione (Potential for loss of seizure control and lower than expected serum levels).
No products indexed under this heading.
Valproic Acid (Potential for loss of seizure control and lower than expected serum levels). Products include:
Depakene 413

LARODOPA TABLETS

(Levodopa) 2129
May interact with monoamine oxidase inhibitors and antihypertensives. Compounds in these categories include:

Acebutolol Hydrochloride (Postural hypotensive episodes have been reported). Products include:
Sectral Capsules 2807
Amlodipine Besylate (Postural hypotensive episodes have been reported). Products include:
Lotrel Capsules 840
Norvasc Tablets 1940
Atenolol (Postural hypotensive episodes have been reported). Products include:
Tenoretic Tablets 2845
Tenormin Tablets and I.V. Injection 2847
Benazepril Hydrochloride (Postural hypotensive episodes have been reported). Products include:
Lotensin Tablets 834
Lotensin HCT 837
Lotrel Capsules 840
Bendroflumethiazide (Postural hypotensive episodes have been reported).
No products indexed under this heading.
Betaxolol Hydrochloride (Postural hypotensive episodes have been reported). Products include:
Betoptic Ophthalmic Solution 469
Betoptic S Ophthalmic Suspension 471

567 Interactions Index Larodopa

Kerlone Tablets ... 2436

Bisoprolol Fumarate (Postural hypotensive episodes have been reported). Products include:
Zebeta Tablets ... 1413
Ziac ... 1415

Captopril (Postural hypotensive episodes have been reported). Products include:
Capoten ... 739
Capozide ... 742

Carteolol Hydrochloride (Postural hypotensive episodes have been reported). Products include:
Cartrol Tablets ... 410
Ocupress Ophthalmic Solution, 1% Sterile ... ◉ 309

Chlorothiazide (Postural hypotensive episodes have been reported). Products include:
Aldoclor Tablets ... 1598
Diupres Tablets ... 1650
Diuril Oral ... 1653

Chlorothiazide Sodium (Postural hypotensive episodes have been reported). Products include:
Diuril Sodium Intravenous ... 1652

Chlorthalidone (Postural hypotensive episodes have been reported). Products include:
Combipres Tablets ... 677
Tenoretic Tablets ... 2845
Thalitone ... 1245

Clonidine (Postural hypotensive episodes have been reported). Products include:
Catapres-TTS ... 675

Clonidine Hydrochloride (Postural hypotensive episodes have been reported). Products include:
Catapres Tablets ... 674
Combipres Tablets ... 677

Deserpidine (Postural hypotensive episodes have been reported).
No products indexed under this heading.

Diazoxide (Postural hypotensive episodes have been reported). Products include:
Hyperstat I.V. Injection ... 2363
Proglycem ... 580

Diltiazem Hydrochloride (Postural hypotensive episodes have been reported). Products include:
Cardizem CD Capsules ... 1506
Cardizem SR Capsules ... 1510
Cardizem Injectable ... 1508
Cardizem Tablets ... 1512
Dilacor XR Extended-release Capsules ... 2018

Doxazosin Mesylate (Postural hypotensive episodes have been reported). Products include:
Cardura Tablets ... 2186

Enalapril Maleate (Postural hypotensive episodes have been reported). Products include:
Vaseretic Tablets ... 1765
Vasotec Tablets ... 1771

Enalaprilat (Postural hypotensive episodes have been reported). Products include:
Vasotec I.V. ... 1768

Esmolol Hydrochloride (Postural hypotensive episodes have been reported). Products include:
Brevibloc Injection ... 1808

Felodipine (Postural hypotensive episodes have been reported). Products include:
Plendil Extended-Release Tablets ... 527

Fosinopril Sodium (Postural hypotensive episodes have been reported). Products include:
Monopril Tablets ... 757

Furazolidone (Concurrent administration is contraindicated). Products include:
Furoxone ... 2046

Furosemide (Postural hypotensive episodes have been reported). Products include:
Lasix Injection, Oral Solution and Tablets ... 1240

Guanabenz Acetate (Postural hypotensive episodes have been reported).
No products indexed under this heading.

Guanethidine Monosulfate (Postural hypotensive episodes have been reported). Products include:
Esimil Tablets ... 822
Ismelin Tablets ... 827

Hydralazine Hydrochloride (Postural hypotensive episodes have been reported). Products include:
Apresazide Capsules ... 808
Apresoline Hydrochloride Tablets ... 809
Ser-Ap-Es Tablets ... 849

Hydrochlorothiazide (Postural hypotensive episodes have been reported). Products include:
Aldactazide ... 2413
Aldoril Tablets ... 1604
Apresazide Capsules ... 808
Capozide ... 742
Dyazide ... 2479
Esidrix Tablets ... 821
Esimil Tablets ... 822
HydroDIURIL Tablets ... 1674
Hydropres Tablets ... 1675
Hyzaar Tablets ... 1677
Inderide Tablets ... 2732
Inderide LA Long Acting Capsules ... 2734
Lopressor HCT Tablets ... 832
Lotensin HCT ... 837
Maxzide ... 1380
Moduretic Tablets ... 1705
Oretic Tablets ... 443
Prinzide Tablets ... 1737
Ser-Ap-Es Tablets ... 849
Timolide Tablets ... 1748
Vaseretic Tablets ... 1765
Zestoretic ... 2850
Ziac ... 1415

Hydroflumethiazide (Postural hypotensive episodes have been reported). Products include:
Diucardin Tablets ... 2718

Indapamide (Postural hypotensive episodes have been reported). Products include:
Lozol Tablets ... 2022

Isocarboxazid (Concurrent administration is contraindicated).
No products indexed under this heading.

Isradipine (Postural hypotensive episodes have been reported). Products include:
DynaCirc Capsules ... 2256

Labetalol Hydrochloride (Postural hypotensive episodes have been reported). Products include:
Normodyne Injection ... 2377
Normodyne Tablets ... 2379
Trandate ... 1185

Lisinopril (Postural hypotensive episodes have been reported). Products include:
Prinivil Tablets ... 1733
Prinzide Tablets ... 1737
Zestoretic ... 2850
Zestril Tablets ... 2854

Losartan Potassium (Postural hypotensive episodes have been reported). Products include:
Cozaar Tablets ... 1628
Hyzaar Tablets ... 1677

Mecamylamine Hydrochloride (Postural hypotensive episodes have been reported). Products include:
Inversine Tablets ... 1686

Methyclothiazide (Postural hypotensive episodes have been reported). Products include:
Enduron Tablets ... 420

Methyldopa (Postural hypotensive episodes have been reported). Products include:
Aldoclor Tablets ... 1598
Aldomet Oral ... 1600
Aldoril Tablets ... 1604

Methyldopate Hydrochloride (Postural hypotensive episodes have been reported). Products include:
Aldomet Ester HCl Injection ... 1602

Metolazone (Postural hypotensive episodes have been reported). Products include:
Mykrox Tablets ... 993
Zaroxolyn Tablets ... 1000

Metoprolol Succinate (Postural hypotensive episodes have been reported). Products include:
Toprol-XL Tablets ... 565

Metoprolol Tartrate (Postural hypotensive episodes have been reported). Products include:
Lopressor Ampuls ... 830
Lopressor HCT Tablets ... 832
Lopressor Tablets ... 830

Metyrosine (Postural hypotensive episodes have been reported). Products include:
Demser Capsules ... 1649

Minoxidil (Postural hypotensive episodes have been reported). Products include:
Loniten Tablets ... 2618
Rogaine Topical Solution ... 2637

Moexipril Hydrochloride (Postural hypotensive episodes have been reported). Products include:
Univasc Tablets ... 2410

Nadolol (Postural hypotensive episodes have been reported).
No products indexed under this heading.

Nicardipine Hydrochloride (Postural hypotensive episodes have been reported). Products include:
Cardene Capsules ... 2095
Cardene I.V. ... 2709
Cardene SR Capsules ... 2097

Nifedipine (Postural hypotensive episodes have been reported). Products include:
Adalat Capsules (10 mg and 20 mg) ... 587
Adalat CC ... 589
Procardia Capsules ... 1971
Procardia XL Extended Release Tablets ... 1972

Nisoldipine (Postural hypotensive episodes have been reported).
No products indexed under this heading.

Nitroglycerin (Postural hypotensive episodes have been reported). Products include:
Deponit NTG Transdermal Delivery System ... 2397
Nitro-Bid IV ... 1523
Nitro-Bid Ointment ... 1524
Nitrodisc ... 2047
Nitro-Dur (nitroglycerin) Transdermal Infusion System ... 1326
Nitrolingual Spray ... 2027
Nitrostat Tablets ... 1925
Transderm-Nitro Transdermal Therapeutic System ... 859

Penbutolol Sulfate (Postural hypotensive episodes have been reported). Products include:
Levatol ... 2403

Phenelzine Sulfate (Concurrent administration is contraindicated). Products include:
Nardil ... 1920

Phenoxybenzamine Hydrochloride (Postural hypotensive episodes have been reported). Products include:
Dibenzyline Capsules ... 2476

Phentolamine Mesylate (Postural hypotensive episodes have been reported). Products include:
Regitine ... 846

Pindolol (Postural hypotensive episodes have been reported). Products include:
Visken Tablets ... 2299

Polythiazide (Postural hypotensive episodes have been reported). Products include:
Minizide Capsules ... 1938

Prazosin Hydrochloride (Postural hypotensive episodes have been reported). Products include:
Minipress Capsules ... 1937
Minizide Capsules ... 1938

Propranolol Hydrochloride (Postural hypotensive episodes have been reported). Products include:
Inderal ... 2728
Inderal LA Long Acting Capsules ... 2730
Inderide Tablets ... 2732
Inderide LA Long Acting Capsules ... 2734

Quinapril Hydrochloride (Postural hypotensive episodes have been reported). Products include:
Accupril Tablets ... 1893

Ramipril (Postural hypotensive episodes have been reported). Products include:
Altace Capsules ... 1232

Rauwolfia Serpentina (Postural hypotensive episodes have been reported).
No products indexed under this heading.

Rescinnamine (Postural hypotensive episodes have been reported).
No products indexed under this heading.

Reserpine (Postural hypotensive episodes have been reported). Products include:
Diupres Tablets ... 1650
Hydropres Tablets ... 1675
Ser-Ap-Es Tablets ... 849

Selegiline Hydrochloride (Concurrent administration is contraindicated). Products include:
Eldepryl Tablets ... 2550

Sodium Nitroprusside (Postural hypotensive episodes have been reported).
No products indexed under this heading.

Sotalol Hydrochloride (Postural hypotensive episodes have been reported). Products include:
Betapace Tablets ... 641

Spirapril Hydrochloride (Postural hypotensive episodes have been reported).
No products indexed under this heading.

Terazosin Hydrochloride (Postural hypotensive episodes have been reported). Products include:
Hytrin Capsules ... 430

Timolol Maleate (Postural hypotensive episodes have been reported). Products include:
Blocadren Tablets ... 1614
Timolide Tablets ... 1748
Timoptic in Ocudose ... 1753
Timoptic Sterile Ophthalmic Solution ... 1751
Timoptic-XE ... 1755

Torsemide (Postural hypotensive episodes have been reported). Products include:
Demadex Tablets and Injection ... 686

Tranylcypromine Sulfate (Concurrent administration is contraindicated). Products include:
Parnate Tablets ... 2503

IMPORTANT NOTE: Always consult each drug listing in the patient's regimen for possible interactions.

Larodopa Interactions Index 568

Trimethaphan Camsylate (Postural hypotensive episodes have been reported). Products include:
Arfonad Ampuls ... 2080
Verapamil Hydrochloride (Postural hypotensive episodes have been reported). Products include:
Calan SR Caplets ... 2422
Calan Tablets ... 2419
Isoptin Injectable ... 1344
Isoptin Oral Tablets ... 1346
Isoptin SR Tablets ... 1348
Verelan Capsules ... 1410
Verelan Capsules ... 2824

LASIX INJECTION, ORAL SOLUTION AND TABLETS
(Furosemide) ... 1240
May interact with aminoglycosides, salicylates, lithium preparations, antihypertensives, ganglionic blocking agents, peripheral adrenergic blockers, cardiac glycosides, corticosteroids, and certain other agents. Compounds in these categories include:

Acebutolol Hydrochloride (Added therapeutic effect). Products include:
Sectral Capsules ... 2807
ACTH (Concomitant therapy may exaggerate metabolic effects of hypokalemia, especially myocardial effects).
No products indexed under this heading.
Amikacin Sulfate (Increased ototoxic potential). Products include:
Amikacin Sulfate Injection, USP ... 960
Amikin Injectable ... 501
Amlodipine Besylate (Added therapeutic effect). Products include:
Lotrel Capsules ... 840
Norvasc Tablets ... 1940
Aspirin (Salicylate toxicity at lower doses; reduced creatinine clearance in patients with chronic renal insufficiency). Products include:
Alka-Seltzer Effervescent Antacid and Pain Reliever ... ▣ 701
Alka-Seltzer Extra Strength Effervescent Antacid and Pain Reliever ... ▣ 703
Alka-Seltzer Lemon Lime Effervescent Antacid and Pain Reliever ... ▣ 703
Alka-Seltzer Plus Cold Medicine ... ▣ 705
Alka-Seltzer Plus Cold & Cough Medicine ... ▣ 708
Alka-Seltzer Plus Night-Time Cold Medicine ... ▣ 707
Alka Seltzer Plus Sinus Medicine ... ▣ 707
Arthritis Foundation Safety Coated Aspirin Tablets ... ▣ 675
Arthritis Pain Ascriptin ... ▣ 631
Maximum Strength Ascriptin ... ▣ 630
Regular Strength Ascriptin Tablets ... ▣ 629
Arthritis Strength BC Powder ... ▣ 609
BC Cold Powder Multi-Symptom Formula (Cold-Sinus-Allergy) ... ▣ 609
BC Cold Powder Non-Drowsy Formula (Cold-Sinus) ... ▣ 609
BC Powder ... ▣ 609
Bayer Children's Chewable Aspirin ... ▣ 711
Genuine Bayer Aspirin Tablets & Caplets ... ▣ 713
Extra Strength Bayer Arthritis Pain Regimen Formula ... ▣ 711
Extra Strength Bayer Aspirin Caplets & Tablets ... ▣ 712
Extended-Release Bayer 8-Hour Aspirin ... ▣ 712
Extra Strength Bayer Plus Aspirin Caplets ... ▣ 713
Extra Strength Bayer PM Aspirin ... ▣ 713
Bayer Enteric Aspirin ... ▣ 709
Bufferin Analgesic Tablets and Caplets ... ▣ 613
Arthritis Strength Bufferin Analgesic Caplets ... ▣ 614
Extra Strength Bufferin Analgesic Tablets ... ▣ 615
Cama Arthritis Pain Reliever ... ▣ 785
Darvon Compound-65 Pulvules ... 1435
Easprin ... 1914
Ecotrin ... 2455
Ecotrin Enteric Coated Aspirin Maximum Strength Tablets and Caplets ... ▣ 816
Ecotrin Enteric Coated Aspirin Regular Strength Tablets ... 2455
Empirin Aspirin Tablets ... ▣ 854
Empirin with Codeine Tablets ... 1093
Excedrin Extra-Strength Analgesic Tablets & Caplets ... 732
Fiorinal Capsules ... 2261
Fiorinal with Codeine Capsules ... 2262
Fiorinal Tablets ... 2261
Halfprin ... 1362
Healthprin Aspirin ... 2455
Norgesic ... 1496
Percodan Tablets ... 939
Percodan-Demi Tablets ... 940
Robaxisal Tablets ... 2071
Soma Compound w/Codeine Tablets ... 2676
Soma Compound Tablets ... 2675
St. Joseph Adult Chewable Aspirin (81 mg.) ... ▣ 808
Talwin Compound ... 2335
Ursinus Inlay-Tabs ... ▣ 794
Vanquish Analgesic Caplets ... ▣ 731
Atenolol (Added therapeutic effect). Products include:
Tenoretic Tablets ... 2845
Tenormin Tablets and I.V. Injection 2847
Benazepril Hydrochloride (Added therapeutic effect). Products include:
Lotensin Tablets ... 834
Lotensin HCT ... 837
Lotrel Capsules ... 840
Bendroflumethiazide (Added therapeutic effect).
No products indexed under this heading.
Betamethasone Acetate (Concomitant therapy may exaggerate metabolic effects of hypokalemia, especially myocardial effects). Products include:
Celestone Soluspan Suspension ... 2347
Betamethasone Sodium Phosphate (Concomitant therapy may exaggerate metabolic effects of hypokalemia, especially myocardial effects). Products include:
Celestone Soluspan Suspension ... 2347
Betaxolol Hydrochloride (Added therapeutic effect). Products include:
Betoptic Ophthalmic Solution ... 469
Betoptic S Ophthalmic Suspension ... 471
Kerlone Tablets ... 2436
Bisoprolol Fumarate (Added therapeutic effect). Products include:
Zebeta Tablets ... 1413
Ziac ... 1415
Captopril (Added therapeutic effect). Products include:
Capoten ... 739
Capozide ... 742
Carteolol Hydrochloride (Added therapeutic effect). Products include:
Cartrol Tablets ... 410
Ocupress Ophthalmic Solution, 1% Sterile ... ⊙ 309
Chlorothiazide (Added therapeutic effect). Products include:
Aldoclor Tablets ... 1598
Diupres Tablets ... 1650
Diuril Oral ... 1653
Chlorothiazide Sodium (Added therapeutic effect). Products include:
Diuril Sodium Intravenous ... 1652
Chlorthalidone (Added therapeutic effect). Products include:
Combipres Tablets ... 677
Tenoretic Tablets ... 2845
Thalitone ... 1245
Choline Magnesium Trisalicylate (Salicylate toxicity at lower doses). Products include:
Trilisate ... 2000
Clonidine (Added therapeutic effect). Products include:
Catapres-TTS ... 675
Clonidine Hydrochloride (Added therapeutic effect). Products include:
Catapres Tablets ... 674
Combipres Tablets ... 677
Cortisone Acetate (Concomitant therapy may exaggerate metabolic effects of hypokalemia, especially myocardial effects). Products include:
Cortone Acetate Sterile Suspension ... 1623
Cortone Acetate Tablets ... 1624
Deserpidine (Potentiated therapeutic effect).
No products indexed under this heading.
Deslanoside (Concomitant therapy may exaggerate metabolic effects of hypokalemia, especially myocardial effects).
No products indexed under this heading.
Dexamethasone (Concomitant therapy may exaggerate metabolic effects of hypokalemia, especially myocardial effects). Products include:
AK-Trol Ointment & Suspension ... ⊙ 205
Decadron Elixir ... 1633
Decadron Tablets ... 1635
Decaspray Topical Aerosol ... 1648
Dexacidin Ointment ... ⊙ 263
Maxitrol Ophthalmic Ointment and Suspension ... ⊙ 224
TobraDex Ophthalmic Suspension and Ointment ... 473
Dexamethasone Acetate (Concomitant therapy may exaggerate metabolic effects of hypokalemia, especially myocardial effects). Products include:
Dalalone D.P. Injectable ... 1011
Decadron-LA Sterile Suspension ... 1646
Dexamethasone Sodium Phosphate (Concomitant therapy may exaggerate metabolic effects of hypokalemia, especially myocardial effects). Products include:
Decadron Phosphate Injection ... 1637
Decadron Phosphate Respihaler ... 1642
Decadron Phosphate Sterile Ophthalmic Ointment ... 1641
Decadron Phosphate Sterile Ophthalmic Solution ... 1642
Decadron Phosphate Topical Cream ... 1644
Decadron Phosphate Turbinaire ... 1645
Decadron Phosphate with Xylocaine Injection, Sterile ... 1639
Dexacort Phosphate in Respihaler ... 458
Dexacort Phosphate in Turbinaire ... 459
NeoDecadron Sterile Ophthalmic Ointment ... 1712
NeoDecadron Sterile Ophthalmic Solution ... 1713
NeoDecadron Topical Cream ... 1714
Diazoxide (Added therapeutic effect). Products include:
Hyperstat I.V. Injection ... 2363
Proglycem ... 580
Diflunisal (Salicylate toxicity at lower doses). Products include:
Dolobid Tablets ... 1654
Digitoxin (Concomitant therapy may exaggerate metabolic effects of hypokalemia, especially myocardial effects). Products include:
Crystodigin Tablets ... 1433
Digoxin (Concomitant therapy may exaggerate metabolic effects of hypokalemia, especially myocardial effects). Products include:
Lanoxicaps ... 1117
Lanoxin Elixir Pediatric ... 1120
Lanoxin Injection ... 1123
Lanoxin Injection Pediatric ... 1126
Lanoxin Tablets ... 1128
Diltiazem Hydrochloride (Added therapeutic effect). Products include:
Cardizem CD Capsules ... 1506
Cardizem SR Capsules ... 1510
Cardizem Injectable ... 1508
Cardizem Tablets ... 1512
Dilacor XR Extended-release Capsules ... 2018
Doxazosin Mesylate (Added therapeutic effect). Products include:
Cardura Tablets ... 2186
Enalapril Maleate (Added therapeutic effect). Products include:
Vaseretic Tablets ... 1765
Vasotec Tablets ... 1771
Enalaprilat (Added therapeutic effect). Products include:
Vasotec I.V. ... 1768
Esmolol Hydrochloride (Added therapeutic effect). Products include:
Brevibloc Injection ... 1808
Ethacrynic Acid (Increased possibility of otoxicity). Products include:
Edecrin Tablets ... 1657
Felodipine (Added therapeutic effect). Products include:
Plendil Extended-Release Tablets ... 527
Fludrocortisone Acetate (Concomitant therapy may exaggerate metabolic effects of hypokalemia, especially myocardial effects). Products include:
Florinef Acetate Tablets ... 505
Fosinopril Sodium (Added therapeutic effect). Products include:
Monopril Tablets ... 757
Gentamicin Sulfate (Increased ototoxic potential). Products include:
Garamycin Injectable ... 2360
Genoptic Sterile Ophthalmic Solution ... ⊙ 243
Genoptic Sterile Ophthalmic Ointment ... ⊙ 243
Gentacidin Ointment ... ⊙ 264
Gentacidin Solution ... ⊙ 264
Gentak ... ⊙ 208
Pred-G Liquifilm Sterile Ophthalmic Suspension ... ⊙ 251
Pred-G S.O.P. Sterile Ophthalmic Ointment ... ⊙ 252
Guanabenz Acetate (Added therapeutic effect).
No products indexed under this heading.
Guanethidine Monosulfate (Potentiated therapeutic effect). Products include:
Esimil Tablets ... 822
Ismelin Tablets ... 827
Hydralazine Hydrochloride (Added therapeutic effect). Products include:
Apresazide Capsules ... 808
Apresoline Hydrochloride Tablets ... 809
Ser-Ap-Es Tablets ... 849
Hydrochlorothiazide (Added therapeutic effect). Products include:
Aldactazide ... 2413
Aldoril Tablets ... 1604
Apresazide Capsules ... 808
Capozide ... 742
Dyazide ... 2479
Esidrix Tablets ... 821
Esimil Tablets ... 822
HydroDIURIL Tablets ... 1674
Hydropres Tablets ... 1675
Hyzaar Tablets ... 1677
Inderide Tablets ... 2732
Inderide LA Long Acting Capsules ... 2734
Lopressor HCT Tablets ... 832
Lotensin HCT ... 837
Maxzide ... 1380
Moduretic Tablets ... 1705
Oretic Tablets ... 443
Prinzide Tablets ... 1737
Ser-Ap-Es Tablets ... 849
Timolide Tablets ... 1748
Vaseretic Tablets ... 1765
Zestoretic ... 2850
Ziac ... 1415

(▣ Described in PDR For Nonprescription Drugs) (⊙ Described in PDR For Ophthalmology)

Hydrocortisone (Concomitant therapy may exaggerate metabolic effects of hypokalemia, especially myocardial effects). Products include:
- Anusol-HC Cream 2.5% 1896
- Aquanil HC Lotion 1931
- Bactine Hydrocortisone Anti-Itch Cream 709
- Caldecort Anti-Itch Hydrocortisone Spray 631
- Cortaid 836
- CORTENEMA 2535
- Cortisporin Ointment 1085
- Cortisporin Ophthalmic Ointment Sterile 1085
- Cortisporin Ophthalmic Suspension Sterile 1086
- Cortisporin Otic Solution Sterile 1087
- Cortisporin Otic Suspension Sterile 1088
- Cortizone-5 831
- Cortizone-10 831
- Hydrocortone Tablets 1672
- Hytone 907
- Massengill Medicated Soft Cloth Towelettes 2458
- PediOtic Suspension Sterile 1153
- Preparation H Hydrocortisone 1% Cream 872
- ProctoCream-HC 2.5% 2408
- VōSoL HC Otic Solution 2678

Hydrocortisone Acetate (Concomitant therapy may exaggerate metabolic effects of hypokalemia, especially myocardial effects). Products include:
- Analpram-HC Rectal Cream 1% and 2.5% 977
- Anusol HC-1 Anti-Itch Hydrocortisone Ointment 847
- Anusol-HC Suppositories 1897
- Caldecort 631
- Carmol HC 924
- Coly-Mycin S Otic w/Neomycin & Hydrocortisone 1906
- Cortaid 836
- Cortifoam 2396
- Cortisporin Cream 1084
- Epifoam 2399
- Hydrocortone Acetate Sterile Suspension 1669
- Mantadil Cream 1135
- Nupercainal Hydrocortisone 1% Cream 645
- Ophthocort .... ◉ 311
- Pramosone Cream, Lotion & Ointment 978
- ProctoCream-HC 2408
- ProctoFoam-HC 2409
- Terra-Cortril Ophthalmic Suspension 2210

Hydrocortisone Sodium Phosphate (Concomitant therapy may exaggerate metabolic effects of hypokalemia, especially myocardial effects). Products include:
- Hydrocortone Phosphate Injection, Sterile 1670

Hydrocortisone Sodium Succinate (Concomitant therapy may exaggerate metabolic effects of hypokalemia, especially myocardial effects). Products include:
- Solu-Cortef Sterile Powder 2641

Hydroflumethiazide (Added therapeutic effect). Products include:
- Diucardin Tablets 2718

Indapamide (Added therapeutic effect). Products include:
- Lozol Tablets 2022

Indomethacin (Reduced natriuretic and antihypertensive effects of Lasix). Products include:
- Indocin 1680

Indomethacin Sodium Trihydrate (Reduced natriuretic and antihypertensive effects of Lasix). Products include:
- Indocin I.V. 1684

Isradipine (Added therapeutic effect). Products include:
- DynaCirc Capsules 2256

Kanamycin Sulfate (Increased ototoxic potential).
- No products indexed under this heading.

Labetalol Hydrochloride (Added therapeutic effect). Products include:
- Normodyne Injection 2377
- Normodyne Tablets 2379
- Trandate 1185

Lisinopril (Added therapeutic effect). Products include:
- Prinivil Tablets 1733
- Prinzide Tablets 1737
- Zestoretic 2850
- Zestril Tablets 2854

Lithium Carbonate (Reduced renal clearance of lithium; lithium toxicity). Products include:
- Eskalith 2485
- Lithium Carbonate Capsules & Tablets 2230
- Lithonate/Lithotabs/Lithobid 2543

Lithium Citrate (Reduced renal clearance of lithium; lithium toxicity).
- No products indexed under this heading.

Losartan Potassium (Added therapeutic effect). Products include:
- Cozaar Tablets 1628
- Hyzaar Tablets 1677

Magnesium Salicylate (Salicylate toxicity at lower doses). Products include:
- Backache Caplets 613
- Bayer Select Backache Pain Relief Formula 715
- Doan's Extra-Strength Analgesic 633
- Extra Strength Doan's P.M. 633
- Doan's Regular Strength Analgesic 634
- Mobigesic Tablets 602

Mecamylamine Hydrochloride (Potentiated therapeutic effect). Products include:
- Inversine Tablets 1686

Methyclothiazide (Added therapeutic effect). Products include:
- Enduron Tablets 420

Methyldopa (Added therapeutic effect). Products include:
- Aldoclor Tablets 1598
- Aldomet Oral 1600
- Aldoril Tablets 1604

Methyldopate Hydrochloride (Added therapeutic effect). Products include:
- Aldomet Ester HCl Injection 1602

Methylprednisolone Acetate (Concomitant therapy may exaggerate metabolic effects of hypokalemia, especially myocardial effects). Products include:
- Depo-Medrol Single-Dose Vial 2600
- Depo-Medrol Sterile Aqueous Suspension 2597

Methylprednisolone Sodium Succinate (Concomitant therapy may exaggerate metabolic effects of hypokalemia, especially myocardial effects). Products include:
- Solu-Medrol Sterile Powder 2643

Metolazone (Added therapeutic effect). Products include:
- Mykrox Tablets 993
- Zaroxolyn Tablets 1000

Metoprolol Succinate (Added therapeutic effect). Products include:
- Toprol-XL Tablets 565

Metoprolol Tartrate (Added therapeutic effect). Products include:
- Lopressor Ampuls 830
- Lopressor HCT Tablets 832
- Lopressor Tablets 830

Metyrosine (Added therapeutic effect). Products include:
- Demser Capsules 1649

Minoxidil (Added therapeutic effect). Products include:
- Loniten Tablets 2618
- Rogaine Topical Solution 2637

Moexipril Hydrochloride (Added therapeutic effect). Products include:
- Univasc Tablets 2410

Nadolol (Added therapeutic effect).
- No products indexed under this heading.

Nicardipine Hydrochloride (Added therapeutic effect). Products include:
- Cardene Capsules 2095
- Cardene I.V. 2709
- Cardene SR Capsules 2097

Nifedipine (Added therapeutic effect). Products include:
- Adalat Capsules (10 mg and 20 mg) 587
- Adalat CC 589
- Procardia Capsules 1971
- Procardia XL Extended Release Tablets 1972

Nisoldipine (Added therapeutic effect).
- No products indexed under this heading.

Nitroglycerin (Added therapeutic effect). Products include:
- Deponit NTG Transdermal Delivery System 2397
- Nitro-Bid IV 1523
- Nitro-Bid Ointment 1524
- Nitrodisc 2047
- Nitro-Dur (nitroglycerin) Transdermal Infusion System 1326
- Nitrolingual Spray 2027
- Nitrostat Tablets 1925
- Transderm-Nitro Transdermal Therapeutic System 859

Norepinephrine Bitartrate (Decreased arterial response to norepinephrine). Products include:
- Levophed Bitartrate Injection 2315

Penbutolol Sulfate (Added therapeutic effect). Products include:
- Levatol 2403

Phenoxybenzamine Hydrochloride (Added therapeutic effect). Products include:
- Dibenzyline Capsules 2476

Phentolamine Mesylate (Added therapeutic effect). Products include:
- Regitine 846

Pindolol (Added therapeutic effect). Products include:
- Visken Tablets 2299

Polythiazide (Added therapeutic effect). Products include:
- Minizide Capsules 1938

Prazosin Hydrochloride (Potentiated therapeutic effect). Products include:
- Minipress Capsules 1937
- Minizide Capsules 1938

Prednisolone Acetate (Concomitant therapy may exaggerate metabolic effects of hypokalemia, especially myocardial effects). Products include:
- AK-CIDE .... ◉ 202
- AK-CIDE Ointment .... ◉ 202
- Blephamide Liquifilm Sterile Ophthalmic Suspension 476
- Blephamide Ointment .... ◉ 237
- Econopred & Econopred Plus Ophthalmic Suspensions .... ◉ 217
- Poly-Pred Liquifilm .... ◉ 248
- Pred Forte .... ◉ 250
- Pred Mild .... ◉ 253
- Pred-G Liquifilm Sterile Ophthalmic Suspension .... ◉ 251
- Pred-G S.O.P. Sterile Ophthalmic Ointment .... ◉ 252
- Vasocidin Ointment .... ◉ 268

Prednisolone Sodium Phosphate (Concomitant therapy may exaggerate metabolic effects of hypokalemia, especially myocardial effects). Products include:
- AK-Pred .... ◉ 204
- Hydeltrasol Injection, Sterile 1665
- Inflamase .... ◉ 265
- Pediapred Oral Liquid 995
- Vasocidin Ophthalmic Solution .... ◉ 270

Prednisolone Tebutate (Concomitant therapy may exaggerate metabolic effects of hypokalemia, especially myocardial effects). Products include:
- Hydeltra-T.B.A. Sterile Suspension 1667

Prednisone (Concomitant therapy may exaggerate metabolic effects of hypokalemia, especially myocardial effects). Products include:
- Deltasone Tablets 2595

Propranolol Hydrochloride (Added therapeutic effect). Products include:
- Inderal 2728
- Inderal LA Long Acting Capsules 2730
- Inderide Tablets 2732
- Inderide LA Long Acting Capsules .. 2734

Quinapril Hydrochloride (Added therapeutic effect). Products include:
- Accupril Tablets 1893

Ramipril (Added therapeutic effect). Products include:
- Altace Capsules 1232

Rauwolfia Serpentina (Potentiated therapeutic effect).
- No products indexed under this heading.

Rescinnamine (Potentiated therapeutic effect).
- No products indexed under this heading.

Reserpine (Potentiated therapeutic effect). Products include:
- Diupres Tablets 1650
- Hydropres Tablets 1675
- Ser-Ap-Es Tablets 849

Salsalate (Salicylate toxicity at lower doses). Products include:
- Mono-Gesic Tablets 792
- Salflex Tablets 786

Sodium Nitroprusside (Added therapeutic effect).
- No products indexed under this heading.

Sotalol Hydrochloride (Added therapeutic effect). Products include:
- Betapace Tablets 641

Spirapril Hydrochloride (Added therapeutic effect).
- No products indexed under this heading.

Streptomycin Sulfate (Increased ototoxic potential). Products include:
- Streptomycin Sulfate Injection 2208

Succinylcholine Chloride (Potentiated action of succinylcholine). Products include:
- Anectine 1073

Sucralfate (Co-administration may reduce the natriuretic and antihypertensive effects of furosemide; the intake of these two drugs should be separated by at least two hours). Products include:
- Carafate Suspension 1505
- Carafate Tablets 1504

Terazosin Hydrochloride (Added therapeutic effect). Products include:
- Hytrin Capsules 430

Timolol Maleate (Added therapeutic effect). Products include:
- Blocadren Tablets 1614
- Timolide Tablets 1748
- Timoptic in Ocudose 1753
- Timoptic Sterile Ophthalmic Solution 1751
- Timoptic-XE 1755

Tobramycin Sulfate (Increased ototoxic potential). Products include:
- Nebcin Vials, Hyporets & ADD-Vantage 1464
- Tobramycin Sulfate Injection 968

Torsemide (Added therapeutic effect). Products include:
- Demadex Tablets and Injection 686

IMPORTANT NOTE: Always consult each drug listing in the patient's regimen for possible interactions.

Lasix

Triamcinolone (Concomitant therapy may exaggerate metabolic effects of hypokalemia, especially myocardial effects). Products include:

Aristocort Tablets 1022

Triamcinolone Acetonide (Concomitant therapy may exaggerate metabolic effects of hypokalemia, especially myocardial effects). Products include:

Aristocort A 0.025% Cream 1027
Aristocort A 0.5% Cream 1031
Aristocort A 0.1% Cream 1029
Aristocort A 0.1% Ointment 1030
Azmacort Oral Inhaler 2011
Nasacort Nasal Inhaler 2024

Triamcinolone Diacetate (Concomitant therapy may exaggerate metabolic effects of hypokalemia, especially myocardial effects). Products include:

Aristocort Suspension (Forte Parenteral).. 1027
Aristocort Suspension (Intralesional) 1025

Triamcinolone Hexacetonide (Concomitant therapy may exaggerate metabolic effects of hypokalemia, especially myocardial effects). Products include:

Aristospan Suspension (Intra-articular) 1033
Aristospan Suspension (Intralesional) 1032

Trimethaphan Camsylate (Potentiated therapeutic effect). Products include:

Arfonad Ampuls 2080

Tubocurarine Chloride (Antagonized skeletal muscle relaxing effect).

No products indexed under this heading.

Verapamil Hydrochloride (Added therapeutic effect). Products include:

Calan SR Caplets 2422
Calan Tablets.. 2419
Isoptin Injectable 1344
Isoptin Oral Tablets 1346
Isoptin SR Tablets 1348
Verelan Capsules 1410
Verelan Capsules 2824

LAVOPTIK EYE WASH (Isotonic Solution) ....◆◻ 665
None cited in PDR database.

LEGATRIN PM (Acetaminophen, Diphenhydramine Hydrochloride)......................................◆◻ 651
May interact with hypnotics and sedatives, tranquilizers, and certain other agents. Compounds in these categories include:

Alprazolam (Concurrent use not recommended; consult your doctor). Products include:

Xanax Tablets 2649

Buspirone Hydrochloride (Concurrent use not recommended; consult your doctor). Products include:

BuSpar 737

Chlordiazepoxide (Concurrent use not recommended; consult your doctor). Products include:

Libritabs Tablets 2177
Limbitrol 2180

Chlordiazepoxide Hydrochloride (Concurrent use not recommended; consult your doctor). Products include:

Librax Capsules 2176
Librium Capsules 2178
Librium Injectable 2179

Chlorpromazine (Concurrent use not recommended; consult your doctor). Products include:

Thorazine Suppositories 2523

Chlorpromazine Hydrochloride (Concurrent use not recommended; consult your doctor). Products include:

Thorazine 2523

Chlorprothixene (Concurrent use not recommended; consult your doctor).

No products indexed under this heading.

Chlorprothixene Hydrochloride (Concurrent use not recommended; consult your doctor).

No products indexed under this heading.

Clorazepate Dipotassium (Concurrent use not recommended; consult your doctor). Products include:

Tranxene 451

Diazepam (Concurrent use not recommended; consult your doctor). Products include:

Dizac 1809
Valium Injectable 2182
Valium Tablets 2183
Valrelease Capsules 2169

Droperidol (Concurrent use not recommended; consult your doctor). Products include:

Inapsine Injection.................................... 1296

Estazolam (Concurrent use not recommended; consult your doctor). Products include:

ProSom Tablets 449

Ethchlorvynol (Concurrent use not recommended; consult your doctor). Products include:

Placidyl Capsules..................................... 448

Ethinamate (Concurrent use not recommended; consult your doctor).

No products indexed under this heading.

Fluphenazine Decanoate (Concurrent use not recommended; consult your doctor). Products include:

Prolixin Decanoate 509

Fluphenazine Enanthate (Concurrent use not recommended; consult your doctor). Products include:

Prolixin Enanthate 509

Fluphenazine Hydrochloride (Concurrent use not recommended; consult your doctor). Products include:

Prolixin 509

Flurazepam Hydrochloride (Concurrent use not recommended; consult your doctor). Products include:

Dalmane Capsules.................................... 2173

Glutethimide (Concurrent use not recommended; consult your doctor).

No products indexed under this heading.

Haloperidol (Concurrent use not recommended; consult your doctor). Products include:

Haldol Injection, Tablets and Concentrate 1575

Haloperidol Decanoate (Concurrent use not recommended; consult your doctor). Products include:

Haldol Decanoate 1577

Hydroxyzine Hydrochloride (Concurrent use not recommended; consult your doctor). Products include:

Atarax Tablets & Syrup.......................... 2185
Marax Tablets & DF Syrup.................... 2200
Vistaril Intramuscular Solution.......... 2216

Lorazepam (Concurrent use not recommended; consult your doctor). Products include:

Ativan Injection... 2698

Ativan Tablets 2700

Loxapine Hydrochloride (Concurrent use not recommended; consult your doctor). Products include:

Loxitane 1378

Loxapine Succinate (Concurrent use not recommended; consult your doctor). Products include:

Loxitane Capsules 1378

Meprobamate (Concurrent use not recommended; consult your doctor). Products include:

Miltown Tablets 2672
PMB 200 and PMB 400 2783

Mesoridazine Besylate (Concurrent use not recommended; consult your doctor). Products include:

Serentil... 684

Midazolam Hydrochloride (Concurrent use not recommended; consult your doctor). Products include:

Versed Injection 2170

Molindone Hydrochloride (Concurrent use not recommended; consult your doctor). Products include:

Moban Tablets and Concentrate...... 1048

Oxazepam (Concurrent use not recommended; consult your doctor). Products include:

Serax Capsules... 2810
Serax Tablets... 2810

Perphenazine (Concurrent use not recommended; consult your doctor). Products include:

Etrafon 2355
Triavil Tablets 1757
Trilafon... 2389

Prazepam (Concurrent use not recommended; consult your doctor).

No products indexed under this heading.

Prochlorperazine (Concurrent use not recommended; consult your doctor). Products include:

Compazine 2470

Promethazine Hydrochloride (Concurrent use not recommended; consult your doctor). Products include:

Mepergan Injection 2753
Phenergan with Codeine........................ 2777
Phenergan with Dextromethorphan 2778
Phenergan Injection 2773
Phenergan Suppositories 2775
Phenergan Syrup 2774
Phenergan Tablets 2775
Phenergan VC 2779
Phenergan VC with Codeine 2781

Propofol (Concurrent use not recommended; consult your doctor). Products include:

Diprivan Injection..................................... 2833

Quazepam (Concurrent use not recommended; consult your doctor). Products include:

Doral Tablets 2664

Secobarbital Sodium (Concurrent use not recommended; consult your doctor). Products include:

Seconal Sodium Pulvules 1474

Temazepam (Concurrent use not recommended; consult your doctor). Products include:

Restoril Capsules 2284

Thioridazine Hydrochloride (Concurrent use not recommended; consult your doctor). Products include:

Mellaril 2269

Thiothixene (Concurrent use not recommended; consult your doctor). Products include:

Navane Capsules and Concentrate 2201
Navane Intramuscular 2202

Triazolam (Concurrent use not recommended; consult your doctor). Products include:

Halcion Tablets... 2611

Trifluoperazine Hydrochloride (Concurrent use not recommended; consult your doctor). Products include:

Stelazine 2514

Zolpidem Tartrate (Concurrent use not recommended; consult your doctor). Products include:

Ambien Tablets... 2416

Food Interactions

Alcohol (Concurrent use not recommended; consult your doctor).

LESCOL CAPSULES

(Fluvastatin Sodium) 2267

May interact with immunosuppressive agents, fibrates, and certain other agents. Compounds in these categories include:

Azathioprine (Potential for increased risk of myopathy resulted with immunosuppressive drug cyclosporine). Products include:

Imuran 1110

Cholestyramine (Coadministration with or up to 4 hours after the resin decreases fluvastatin AUC by 50% and C_{max} by 50%-80%; additive effects if administered 4 hours after cholestyramine). Products include:

Questran Light 769
Questran Powder 770

Cimetidine (A significant increase in the fluvastatin C_{max} 43% and AUC (24%-33%) with an 18%-23% decrease in plasma clearance). Products include:

Tagamet Tablets 2516

Cimetidine Hydrochloride (A significant increase in the fluvastatin C_{max} 43% and AUC (24%-33%) with an 18%-23% decrease in plasma clearance). Products include:

Tagamet.. 2516

Clofibrate (Potential for increased risk of myopathy; combined use should be avoided). Products include:

Atromid-S Capsules 2701

Cyclosporine (Potential for increased risk of myopathy resulted with immunosuppressive drug cyclosporine). Products include:

Neoral 2276
Sandimmune 2286

Digoxin (Coadministration results in an 11% increase in digoxin C_{max} and small increase in digoxin urinary clearance). Products include:

Lanoxicaps 1117
Lanoxin Elixir Pediatric 1120
Lanoxin Injection 1123
Lanoxin Injection Pediatric.................. 1126
Lanoxin Tablets 1128

Erythromycin (Potential for increased risk of myopathy). Products include:

A/T/S 2% Acne Topical Gel and Solution 1234
Benzamycin Topical Gel 905
E-Mycin Tablets 1341
Emgel 2% Topical Gel............................. 1093
ERYC.. 1915
Erycette (erythromycin 2%) Topical Solution.. 1888
Ery-Tab Tablets 422
Erythromycin Base Filmtab 426
Erythromycin Delayed-Release Capsules, USP... 427
Ilotycin Ophthalmic Ointment........... 912
PCE Dispertab Tablets 444
T-Stat 2.0% Topical Solution and Pads 2688
Theramycin Z Topical Solution 2% 1592

Erythromycin Estolate (Potential for increased risk of myopathy). Products include:

Ilosone 911

Erythromycin Ethylsuccinate (Potential for increased risk of myopathy). Products include:
- E.E.S. ... 424
- EryPed ... 421

Erythromycin Gluceptate (Potential for increased risk of myopathy). Products include:
- Ilotycin Gluceptate, IV, Vials ... 913

Erythromycin Stearate (Potential for increased risk of myopathy). Products include:
- Erythrocin Stearate Filmtab ... 425

Gemfibrozil (Potential for increased risk of myopathy; combined use should be avoided). Products include:
- Lopid Tablets ... 1917

Ketoconazole (Caution should be exercised if used concurrently with drugs that may decrease the levels of endogenous steroid hormones; increase potential for endocrine dysfunction). Products include:
- Nizoral 2% Cream ... 1297
- Nizoral 2% Shampoo ... 1298
- Nizoral Tablets ... 1298

Muromonab-CD3 (Potential for increased risk of myopathy resulted with immunosuppressive drug cyclosporine). Products include:
- Orthoclone OKT3 Sterile Solution .. 1837

Mycophenolate Mofetil (Potential for increased risk of myopathy resulted with immunosuppressive drug cyclosporine). Products include:
- CellCept Capsules ... 2099

Nicotinic Acid (Potential for increased risk of myopathy with lipid lowering doses of nicotinic acid).
- No products indexed under this heading.

Omeprazole (A significant increase in the fluvastatin C_{max} 50% and AUC (24%-33%) with an 18%-23% decrease in plasma clearance). Products include:
- Prilosec Delayed-Release Capsules 529

Ranitidine Hydrochloride (A significant increase in the fluvastatin C_{max} 70% and AUC (24%-33%) with an 18%-23% decrease in plasma clearance). Products include:
- Zantac ... 1209
- Zantac Injection ... 1207
- Zantac Syrup ... 1209

Rifampin (Administration of fluvastatin to subjects pretreated with rifampin results in significant reduction in C_{max} (59%) and AUC (51%), with a large increase (95%) in plasma clearance). Products include:
- Rifadin ... 1528
- Rifamate Capsules ... 1530
- Rifater ... 1532
- Rimactane Capsules ... 847

Spironolactone (Caution should be exercised if used concurrently with drugs that may decrease the levels of endogenous steroid hormones; increase potential for endocrine dysfunction). Products include:
- Aldactazide ... 2413
- Aldactone ... 2414

Tacrolimus (Potential for increased risk of myopathy resulted with immunosuppressive drug cyclosporine). Products include:
- Prograf ... 1042

Warfarin Sodium (Bleeding and/or increased prothrombin time has been reported with other HMG-CoA reductase inhibitors when used concurrently; no interactions at therapeutic concentrations have been demonstrated with fluvastatin and warfarin). Products include:
- Coumadin ... 926

Food Interactions

Meal, unspecified (Administration of fluvastatin with the evening meal results in a two-fold decrease in C_{max} and more than two-fold increase in t_{max} as compared to patients receiving the drug 4 hours after evening meal).

LEUCOVORIN CALCIUM FOR INJECTION, WELLCOVORIN BRAND

(Leucovorin Calcium) ... 1132
May interact with:

Fluorouracil (Concomitant administration results in enhanced toxicity of fluorouracil). Products include:
- Efudex ... 2113
- Fluoroplex Topical Solution & Cream 1% ... 479
- Fluorouracil Injection ... 2116

Phenobarbital (May counteract antiepileptic effects and increases frequency of seizures in susceptible children). Products include:
- Arco-Lase Plus Tablets ... 512
- Bellergal-S Tablets ... 2250
- Donnatal ... 2060
- Donnatal Extentabs ... 2061
- Donnatal Tablets ... 2060
- Phenobarbital Elixir and Tablets ... 1469
- Quadrinal Tablets ... 1350

Phenytoin (May counteract antiepileptic effects and increases frequency of seizures in susceptible children). Products include:
- Dilantin Infatabs ... 1908
- Dilantin-125 Suspension ... 1911

Phenytoin Sodium (May counteract antiepileptic effects and increases frequency of seizures in susceptible children). Products include:
- Dilantin Kapseals ... 1906
- Dilantin Parenteral ... 1910

Primidone (May counteract antiepileptic effects and increases frequency of seizures in susceptible children). Products include:
- Mysoline ... 2754

LEUCOVORIN CALCIUM FOR INJECTION

(Leucovorin Calcium) ... 1268
May interact with:

Fluorouracil (Enhanced toxicity of fluorouracil). Products include:
- Efudex ... 2113
- Fluoroplex Topical Solution & Cream 1% ... 479
- Fluorouracil Injection ... 2116

Methotrexate Sodium (High doses of leucovorin may reduce the efficacy of intrathecally administered methotrexate). Products include:
- Methotrexate Sodium Tablets, Injection, for Injection and LPF Injection ... 1275

Phenobarbital (Antiepileptic effect counteracted by large amount of folic acid; increased frequency of seizures in susceptible children). Products include:
- Arco-Lase Plus Tablets ... 512
- Bellergal-S Tablets ... 2250
- Donnatal ... 2060
- Donnatal Extentabs ... 2061
- Donnatal Tablets ... 2060
- Phenobarbital Elixir and Tablets ... 1469
- Quadrinal Tablets ... 1350

Phenytoin (Antiepileptic effect counteracted by large amount of folic acid; increased frequency of seizures in susceptible children). Products include:
- Dilantin Infatabs ... 1908
- Dilantin-125 Suspension ... 1911

Phenytoin Sodium (Antiepileptic effect counteracted by large amount of folic acid; increased frequency of seizures in susceptible children). Products include:
- Dilantin Kapseals ... 1906
- Dilantin Parenteral ... 1910

Primidone (Antiepileptic effect counteracted by large amount of folic acid; increased frequency of seizures in susceptible children). Products include:
- Mysoline ... 2754

LEUCOVORIN CALCIUM TABLETS, WELLCOVORIN BRAND

(Leucovorin Calcium) ... 1132
May interact with:

Fluorouracil (Enhanced toxicity of fluorouracil). Products include:
- Efudex ... 2113
- Fluoroplex Topical Solution & Cream 1% ... 479
- Fluorouracil Injection ... 2116

Phenobarbital (Increased frequency of seizures in children). Products include:
- Arco-Lase Plus Tablets ... 512
- Bellergal-S Tablets ... 2250
- Donnatal ... 2060
- Donnatal Extentabs ... 2061
- Donnatal Tablets ... 2060
- Phenobarbital Elixir and Tablets ... 1469
- Quadrinal Tablets ... 1350

Phenytoin (Increased frequency of seizures in children). Products include:
- Dilantin Infatabs ... 1908
- Dilantin-125 Suspension ... 1911

Phenytoin Sodium (Increased frequency of seizures in children). Products include:
- Dilantin Kapseals ... 1906
- Dilantin Parenteral ... 1910

Primidone (Increased frequency of seizures in children). Products include:
- Mysoline ... 2754

LEUCOVORIN CALCIUM TABLETS

(Leucovorin Calcium) ... 1270
May interact with:

Fluorouracil (Enhanced toxicity of fluorouracil). Products include:
- Efudex ... 2113
- Fluoroplex Topical Solution & Cream 1% ... 479
- Fluorouracil Injection ... 2116

Methotrexate Sodium (High doses of leucovorin may reduce the efficacy of intrathecally administered methotrexate). Products include:
- Methotrexate Sodium Tablets, Injection, for Injection and LPF Injection ... 1275

Phenobarbital (Antiepileptic effect counteracted by large amount of folic acid). Products include:
- Arco-Lase Plus Tablets ... 512
- Bellergal-S Tablets ... 2250
- Donnatal ... 2060
- Donnatal Extentabs ... 2061
- Donnatal Tablets ... 2060
- Phenobarbital Elixir and Tablets ... 1469
- Quadrinal Tablets ... 1350

Phenytoin (Antiepileptic effect counteracted by large amount of folic acid). Products include:
- Dilantin Infatabs ... 1908
- Dilantin-125 Suspension ... 1911

Phenytoin Sodium (Antiepileptic effect counteracted by large amount of folic acid). Products include:
- Dilantin Kapseals ... 1906
- Dilantin Parenteral ... 1910

Primidone (Antiepileptic effect counteracted by large amount of folic acid). Products include:
- Mysoline ... 2754

LEUKERAN TABLETS

(Chlorambucil) ... 1133
None cited in PDR database.

LEUKINE FOR IV INFUSION

(Sargramostim) ... 1271
May interact with drugs with myeloproliferative effects and cytotoxic drugs. Compounds in these categories include:

Betamethasone Acetate (May potentiate the myeloproliferative effect). Products include:
- Celestone Soluspan Suspension ... 2347

Betamethasone Sodium Phosphate (May potentiate the myeloproliferative effect). Products include:
- Celestone Soluspan Suspension ... 2347

Bleomycin Sulfate (Coadministration within 24 hours preceding or following chemotherapy is not recommended because of potential sensitivity of rapidly dividing hematopoietic progenitor cells to cytotoxic therapy). Products include:
- Blenoxane ... 692

Cortisone Acetate (May potentiate the myeloproliferative effect). Products include:
- Cortone Acetate Sterile Suspension ... 1623
- Cortone Acetate Tablets ... 1624

Daunorubicin Hydrochloride (Coadministration within 24 hours preceding or following chemotherapy is not recommended because of potential sensitivity of rapidly dividing hematopoietic progenitor cells to cytotoxic therapy). Products include:
- Cerubidine ... 795

Dexamethasone (May potentiate the myeloproliferative effect). Products include:
- AK-Trol Ointment & Suspension ... ◉ 205
- Decadron Elixir ... 1633
- Decadron Tablets ... 1635
- Decaspray Topical Aerosol ... 1648
- Dexacidin Ointment ... ◉ 263
- Maxitrol Ophthalmic Ointment and Suspension ... ◉ 224
- TobraDex Ophthalmic Suspension and Ointment ... 473

Dexamethasone Acetate (May potentiate the myeloproliferative effect). Products include:
- Dalalone D.P. Injectable ... 1011
- Decadron-LA Sterile Suspension ... 1646

Dexamethasone Sodium Phosphate (May potentiate the myeloproliferative effect). Products include:
- Decadron Phosphate Injection ... 1637
- Decadron Phosphate Respihaler ... 1642
- Decadron Phosphate Sterile Ophthalmic Ointment ... 1641
- Decadron Phosphate Sterile Ophthalmic Solution ... 1642
- Decadron Phosphate Topical Cream ... 1644
- Decadron Phosphate Turbinaire ... 1645
- Decadron Phosphate with Xylocaine Injection, Sterile ... 1639
- Dexacort Phosphate in Respihaler .. 458
- Dexacort Phosphate in Turbinaire .. 459
- NeoDecadron Sterile Ophthalmic Ointment ... 1712
- NeoDecadron Sterile Ophthalmic Solution ... 1713
- NeoDecadron Topical Cream ... 1714

IMPORTANT NOTE: Always consult each drug listing in the patient's regimen for possible interactions.

Doxorubicin Hydrochloride (Coadministration within 24 hours preceding or following chemotherapy is not recommended because of potential sensitivity of rapidly dividing hematopoietic progenitor cells to cytotoxic therapy). Products include:
- Adriamycin PFS ... **1947**
- Adriamycin RDF ... **1947**
- Doxorubicin Astra ... **540**
- Rubex ... **712**

Fluorouracil (Coadministration within 24 hours preceding or following chemotherapy is not recommended because of potential sensitivity of rapidly dividing hematopoietic progenitor cells to cytotoxic therapy). Products include:
- Efudex ... **2113**
- Fluoroplex Topical Solution & Cream 1% ... **479**
- Fluorouracil Injection ... **2116**

Hydrocortisone (May potentiate the myeloproliferative effect). Products include:
- Anusol-HC Cream 2.5% ... **1896**
- Aquanil HC Lotion ... **1931**
- Bactine Hydrocortisone Anti-Itch Cream ... ⊞ **709**
- Caldecort Anti-Itch Hydrocortisone Spray ... ⊞ **631**
- Cortaid ... ⊞ **836**
- CORTENEMA ... **2535**
- Cortisporin Ointment ... **1085**
- Cortisporin Ophthalmic Ointment Sterile ... **1085**
- Cortisporin Ophthalmic Suspension Sterile ... **1086**
- Cortisporin Otic Solution Sterile ... **1087**
- Cortisporin Otic Suspension Sterile **1088**
- Cortizone-5 ... ⊞ **831**
- Cortizone-10 ... ⊞ **831**
- Hydrocortone Tablets ... **1672**
- Hytone ... **907**
- Massengill Medicated Soft Cloth Towelettes ... **2458**
- PediOtic Suspension Sterile ... **1153**
- Preparation H Hydrocortisone 1% Cream ... ⊞ **872**
- ProctoCream-HC 2.5% ... **2408**
- VōSoL HC Otic Solution ... **2678**

Hydrocortisone Acetate (May potentiate the myeloproliferative effect). Products include:
- Analpram-HC Rectal Cream 1% and 2.5% ... **977**
- Anusol HC-1 Anti-Itch Hydrocortisone Ointment ... ⊞ **847**
- Anusol-HC Suppositories ... **1897**
- Caldecort ... ⊞ **631**
- Carmol HC ... **924**
- Coly-Mycin S Otic w/Neomycin & Hydrocortisone ... **1906**
- Cortaid ... ⊞ **836**
- Cortifoam ... **2396**
- Cortisporin Cream ... **1084**
- Epifoam ... **2399**
- Hydrocortone Acetate Sterile Suspension ... **1669**
- Mantadil Cream ... **1135**
- Nupercainal Hydrocortisone 1% Cream ... ⊞ **645**
- Ophthocort ... ◉ **311**
- Pramosone Cream, Lotion & Ointment ... **978**
- ProctoCream-HC ... **2408**
- ProctoFoam-HC ... **2409**
- Terra-Cortril Ophthalmic Suspension ... **2210**

Hydrocortisone Sodium Phosphate (May potentiate the myeloproliferative effect). Products include:
- Hydrocortone Phosphate Injection, Sterile ... **1670**

Hydrocortisone Sodium Succinate (May potentiate the myeloproliferative effect). Products include:
- Solu-Cortef Sterile Powder ... **2641**

Hydroxyurea (Coadministration within 24 hours preceding or following chemotherapy is not recommended because of potential sensitivity of rapidly dividing hematopoietic progenitor cells to cytotoxic therapy). Products include:
- Hydrea Capsules ... **696**

Lithium Carbonate (May potentiate the myeloproliferative effect). Products include:
- Eskalith ... **2485**
- Lithium Carbonate Capsules & Tablets ... **2230**
- Lithonate/Lithotabs/Lithobid ... **2543**

Lithium Citrate (May potentiate the myeloproliferative effect).
- No products indexed under this heading.

Methotrexate Sodium (Coadministration within 24 hours preceding or following chemotherapy is not recommended because of potential sensitivity of rapidly dividing hematopoietic progenitor cells to cytotoxic therapy). Products include:
- Methotrexate Sodium Tablets, Injection, for Injection and LPF Injection ... **1275**

Methylprednisolone Acetate (May potentiate the myeloproliferative effect). Products include:
- Depo-Medrol Single-Dose Vial ... **2600**
- Depo-Medrol Sterile Aqueous Suspension ... **2597**

Methylprednisolone Sodium Succinate (May potentiate the myeloproliferative effect). Products include:
- Solu-Medrol Sterile Powder ... **2643**

Mitotane (Coadministration within 24 hours preceding or following chemotherapy is not recommended because of potential sensitivity of rapidly dividing hematopoietic progenitor cells to cytotoxic therapy). Products include:
- Lysodren ... **698**

Mitoxantrone Hydrochloride (Coadministration within 24 hours preceding or following chemotherapy is not recommended because of potential sensitivity of rapidly dividing hematopoietic progenitor cells to cytotoxic therapy). Products include:
- Novantrone ... **1279**

Prednisolone Acetate (May potentiate the myeloproliferative effect). Products include:
- AK-CIDE ... ◉ **202**
- AK-CIDE Ointment ... ◉ **202**
- Blephamide Liquifilm Sterile Ophthalmic Suspension ... **476**
- Blephamide Ointment ... ◉ **237**
- Econopred & Econopred Plus Ophthalmic Suspensions ... ◉ **217**
- Poly-Pred Liquifilm ... ◉ **248**
- Pred Forte ... ◉ **250**
- Pred Mild ... ◉ **253**
- Pred-G Liquifilm Sterile Ophthalmic Suspension ... ◉ **251**
- Pred-G S.O.P. Sterile Ophthalmic Ointment ... ◉ **252**
- Vasocidin Ointment ... ◉ **268**

Prednisolone Sodium Phosphate (May potentiate the myeloproliferative effect). Products include:
- AK-Pred ... ◉ **204**
- Hydeltrasol Injection, Sterile ... **1665**
- Inflamase ... ◉ **265**
- Pediapred Oral Liquid ... **995**
- Vasocidin Ophthalmic Solution ... ◉ **270**

Prednisolone Tebutate (May potentiate the myeloproliferative effect). Products include:
- Hydeltra-T.B.A. Sterile Suspension **1667**

Prednisone (May potentiate the myeloproliferative effect). Products include:
- Deltasone Tablets ... **2595**

Procarbazine Hydrochloride (Coadministration within 24 hours preceding or following chemotherapy is not recommended because of potential sensitivity of rapidly dividing hematopoietic progenitor cells to cytotoxic therapy). Products include:
- Matulane Capsules ... **2131**

Tamoxifen Citrate (Coadministration within 24 hours preceding or following chemotherapy is not recommended because of potential sensitivity of rapidly dividing hematopoietic progenitor cells to cytotoxic therapy). Products include:
- Nolvadex Tablets ... **2841**

Triamcinolone (May potentiate the myeloproliferative effect). Products include:
- Aristocort Tablets ... **1022**

Triamcinolone Acetonide (May potentiate the myeloproliferative effect). Products include:
- Aristocort A 0.025% Cream ... **1027**
- Aristocort A 0.5% Cream ... **1031**
- Aristocort A 0.1% Cream ... **1029**
- Aristocort A 0.1% Ointment ... **1030**
- Azmacort Oral Inhaler ... **2011**
- Nasacort Nasal Inhaler ... **2024**

Triamcinolone Diacetate (May potentiate the myeloproliferative effect). Products include:
- Aristocort Suspension (Forte Parenteral) ... **1027**
- Aristocort Suspension (Intralesional) ... **1025**

Triamcinolone Hexacetonide (May potentiate the myeloproliferative effect). Products include:
- Aristospan Suspension (Intra-articular) ... **1033**
- Aristospan Suspension (Intralesional) ... **1032**

Vincristine Sulfate (Coadministration within 24 hours preceding or following chemotherapy is not recommended because of potential sensitivity of rapidly dividing hematopoietic progenitor cells to cytotoxic therapy). Products include:
- Oncovin Solution Vials & Hyporets **1466**

LEUSTATIN
(Cladribine) ... **1834**
May interact with:

Bone Marrow Depressants, unspecified (Caution should be exercised if co-administered with other drugs known to cause myelosuppression).

LEVATOL
(Penbutolol Sulfate) ... **2403**
May interact with calcium channel blockers, catecholamine depleting drugs, insulin, and certain other agents. Compounds in these categories include:

Amlodipine Besylate (Potential for synergistic hypotensive effects, bradycardia, and arrhythmias). Products include:
- Lotrel Capsules ... **840**
- Norvasc Tablets ... **1940**

Bepridil Hydrochloride (Potential for synergistic hypotensive effects, bradycardia, and arrhythmias). Products include:
- Vascor (200, 300 and 400 mg) Tablets ... **1587**

Cyclopropane (Potential for excessive myocardial depression).

Deserpidine (Concurrent use is not recommended).
- No products indexed under this heading.

Diltiazem Hydrochloride (Potential for synergistic hypotensive effects, bradycardia, and arrhythmias). Products include:
- Cardizem CD Capsules ... **1506**
- Cardizem SR Capsules ... **1510**
- Cardizem Injectable ... **1508**
- Cardizem Tablets ... **1512**
- Dilacor XR Extended-release Capsules ... **2018**

Ether (Potential for excessive myocardial depression).

Felodipine (Potential for synergistic hypotensive effects, bradycardia, and arrhythmias). Products include:
- Plendil Extended-Release Tablets ... **527**

Guanethidine Monosulfate (Concurrent use is not recommended). Products include:
- Esimil Tablets ... **822**
- Ismelin Tablets ... **827**

Insulin, Human (Beta-blockade reduces the release of insulin in response to hyperglycemia).
- No products indexed under this heading.

Insulin, Human Isophane Suspension (Beta-blockade reduces the release of insulin in response to hyperglycemia). Products include:
- Novolin N Human Insulin 10 ml Vials ... **1795**

Insulin, Human NPH (Beta-blockade reduces the release of insulin in response to hyperglycemia). Products include:
- Humulin N, 100 Units ... **1448**
- Novolin N PenFill Cartridges Durable Insulin Delivery System ... **1798**
- Novolin N Prefilled Syringe Disposable Insulin Delivery System ... **1798**

Insulin, Human Regular (Beta-blockade reduces the release of insulin in response to hyperglycemia). Products include:
- Humulin R, 100 Units ... **1449**
- Novolin R Human Insulin 10 ml Vials ... **1795**
- Novolin R PenFill Cartridges Durable Insulin Delivery System ... **1798**
- Novolin R Prefilled Syringe Disposable Insulin Delivery System ... **1798**
- Velosulin BR Human Insulin 10 ml Vials ... **1795**

Insulin, Human, Zinc Suspension (Beta-blockade reduces the release of insulin in response to hyperglycemia). Products include:
- Humulin L, 100 Units ... **1446**
- Humulin U, 100 Units ... **1450**
- Novolin L Human Insulin 10 ml Vials ... **1795**

Insulin, NPH (Beta-blockade reduces the release of insulin in response to hyperglycemia). Products include:
- NPH, 100 Units ... **1450**
- Pork NPH, 100 Units ... **1452**
- Purified Pork NPH Isophane Insulin ... **1801**

Insulin, Regular (Beta-blockade reduces the release of insulin in response to hyperglycemia). Products include:
- Regular, 100 Units ... **1450**
- Pork Regular, 100 Units ... **1452**
- Pork Regular (Concentrated), 500 Units ... **1453**
- Purified Pork Regular Insulin ... **1801**

Insulin, Zinc Crystals (Beta-blockade reduces the release of insulin in response to hyperglycemia). Products include:
- NPH, 100 Units ... **1450**

Insulin, Zinc Suspension (Beta-blockade reduces the release of insulin in response to hyperglycemia). Products include:
- Iletin I ... **1450**
- Lente, 100 Units ... **1450**
- Iletin II ... **1452**

(⊞ Described in PDR For Nonprescription Drugs) (◉ Described in PDR For Ophthalmology)

Pork Lente, 100 Units........................ 1452
Purified Pork Lente Insulin 1801

Isradipine (Potential for synergistic hypotensive effects, bradycardia, and arrhythmias). Products include:

DynaCirc Capsules 2256

Lidocaine Hydrochloride (Increased volume of distribution of lidocaine). Products include:

Bactine Antiseptic/Anesthetic First Aid Liquid .... ✦D 708
Campho-Phenique Maximum Strength First Aid Antibiotic Plus Pain Reliever Ointment .... ✦D 719
Decadron Phosphate with Xylocaine Injection, Sterile 1639
Xylocaine Injections 567

Nicardipine Hydrochloride (Potential for synergistic hypotensive effects, bradycardia, and arrhythmias). Products include:

Cardene Capsules 2095
Cardene I.V. 2709
Cardene SR Capsules............................ 2097

Nifedipine (Potential for synergistic hypotensive effects, bradycardia, and arrhythmias). Products include:

Adalat Capsules (10 mg and 20 mg) 587
Adalat CC 589
Procardia Capsules................................ 1971
Procardia XL Extended Release Tablets 1972

Nimodipine (Potential for synergistic hypotensive effects, bradycardia, and arrhythmias). Products include:

Nimotop Capsules 610

Nisoldipine (Potential for synergistic hypotensive effects, bradycardia, and arrhythmias).

No products indexed under this heading.

Rauwolfia Serpentina (Concurrent use is not recommended).

No products indexed under this heading.

Rescinnamine (Concurrent use is not recommended).

No products indexed under this heading.

Reserpine (Concurrent use is not recommended). Products include:

Diupres Tablets 1650
Hydropres Tablets.................................. 1675
Ser-Ap-Es Tablets 849

Verapamil Hydrochloride (Potential for synergistic hypotensive effects, bradycardia, and arrhythmias). Products include:

Calan SR Caplets 2422
Calan Tablets.. 2419
Isoptin Injectable 1344
Isoptin Oral Tablets 1346
Isoptin SR Tablets 1348
Verelan Capsules 1410
Verelan Capsules 2824

Food Interactions

Alcohol (Increased number of errors in the eye-hand psychomotor function test).

LEVBID EXTENDED-RELEASE TABLETS

(Hyoscyamine Sulfate) 2405

See Levsin Drops

LEVER 2000

(Triclosan) .... ✦D 672
None cited in PDR database.

LIQUID LEVER 2000

(Triclosan) .... ✦D 672
None cited in PDR database.

UNSCENTED LEVER 2000

(Triclosan) .... ✦D 672
None cited in PDR database.

LEVLEN 21 TABLETS

(Levonorgestrel, Ethinyl Estradiol) 651
May interact with barbiturates, tetracyclines, and certain other agents. Compounds in these categories include:

Ampicillin Sodium (Reduced efficacy; breakthrough bleeding). Products include:

Unasyn 2212

Aprobarbital (Reduced efficacy; breakthrough bleeding).

No products indexed under this heading.

Butabarbital (Reduced efficacy; breakthrough bleeding).

No products indexed under this heading.

Butalbital (Reduced efficacy; breakthrough bleeding). Products include:

Esgic-plus Tablets 1013
Fioricet Tablets 2258
Fioricet with Codeine Capsules 2260
Fiorinal Capsules 2261
Fiorinal with Codeine Capsules 2262
Fiorinal Tablets....................................... 2261
Phrenilin.. 785
Sedapap Tablets 50 mg/650 mg .. 1543

Demeclocycline Hydrochloride (Reduced efficacy; breakthrough bleeding). Products include:

Declomycin Tablets................................ 1371

Doxycycline Calcium (Reduced efficacy; breakthrough bleeding). Products include:

Vibramycin Calcium Oral Suspension Syrup 1941

Doxycycline Hyclate (Reduced efficacy; breakthrough bleeding). Products include:

Doryx Capsules....................................... 1913
Vibramycin Hyclate Capsules 1941
Vibramycin Hyclate Intravenous 2215
Vibra-Tabs Film Coated Tablets 1941

Doxycycline Monohydrate (Reduced efficacy; breakthrough bleeding). Products include:

Monodox Capsules 1805
Vibramycin Monohydrate for Oral Suspension 1941

Griseofulvin (Reduced efficacy; breakthrough bleeding). Products include:

Fulvicin P/G Tablets.............................. 2359
Fulvicin P/G 165 & 330 Tablets 2359
Grifulvin V (griseofulvin tablets) Microsize (griseofulvin oral suspension) Microsize 1888
Gris-PEG Tablets, 125 mg & 250 mg 479

Mephobarbital (Reduced efficacy; breakthrough bleeding). Products include:

Mebaral Tablets 2322

Methacycline Hydrochloride (Reduced efficacy; breakthrough bleeding).

No products indexed under this heading.

Minocycline Hydrochloride (Reduced efficacy; breakthrough bleeding). Products include:

Dynacin Capsules 1590
Minocin Intravenous 1382
Minocin Oral Suspension 1385
Minocin Pellet-Filled Capsules 1383

Oxytetracycline (Reduced efficacy; breakthrough bleeding). Products include:

Terramycin Intramuscular Solution 2210

Oxytetracycline Hydrochloride (Reduced efficacy; breakthrough bleeding). Products include:

TERAK Ointment .... © 209
Terra-Cortril Ophthalmic Suspension 2210
Terramycin with Polymyxin B Sulfate Ophthalmic Ointment 2211
Urobiotic-250 Capsules 2214

Pentobarbital Sodium (Reduced efficacy; breakthrough bleeding). Products include:

Nembutal Sodium Capsules 436
Nembutal Sodium Solution 438
Nembutal Sodium Suppositories...... 440

Phenobarbital (Reduced efficacy; breakthrough bleeding). Products include:

Arco-Lase Plus Tablets 512
Bellergal-S Tablets 2250
Donnatal 2060
Donnatal Extentabs............................... 2061
Donnatal Tablets 2060
Phenobarbital Elixir and Tablets 1469
Quadrinal Tablets 1350

Phenylbutazone (Reduced efficacy; breakthrough bleeding).

No products indexed under this heading.

Phenytoin Sodium (Reduced efficacy; breakthrough bleeding). Products include:

Dilantin Kapseals 1906
Dilantin Parenteral 1910

Rifampin (Reduced efficacy; breakthrough bleeding). Products include:

Rifadin 1528
Rifamate Capsules 1530
Rifater... 1532
Rimactane Capsules 847

Secobarbital Sodium (Reduced efficacy; breakthrough bleeding). Products include:

Seconal Sodium Pulvules 1474

Tetracycline Hydrochloride (Reduced efficacy; breakthrough bleeding). Products include:

Achromycin V Capsules 1367

Thiamylal Sodium (Reduced efficacy; breakthrough bleeding).

No products indexed under this heading.

LEVLEN 28 TABLETS

(Levonorgestrel, Ethinyl Estradiol) 651

See Levlen 21 Tablets

LEVO-DROMORAN INJECTABLE

(Levorphanol Tartrate) 2129
None cited in PDR database.

LEVO-DROMORAN TABLETS

(Levorphanol Tartrate) 2129
None cited in PDR database.

LEVOPHED BITARTRATE INJECTION

(Norepinephrine Bitartrate) 2315
May interact with monoamine oxidase inhibitors, tricyclic antidepressants, and certain other agents. Compounds in these categories include:

Amitriptyline Hydrochloride (Severe prolonged hypertension). Products include:

Elavil 2838
Endep Tablets 2174
Etrafon 2355
Limbitrol 2180
Triavil Tablets 1757

Amoxapine (Severe prolonged hypertension). Products include:

Asendin Tablets 1369

Clomipramine Hydrochloride (Severe prolonged hypertension). Products include:

Anafranil Capsules 803

Cyclopropane (Increases cardiac autonomic irritability).

Desipramine Hydrochloride (Severe prolonged hypertension). Products include:

Norpramin Tablets 1526

Doxepin Hydrochloride (Severe prolonged hypertension). Products include:

Sinequan 2205
Zonalon Cream....................................... 1055

Furazolidone (Severe prolonged hypertension). Products include:

Furoxone 2046

Halothane (Increases cardiac autonomic irritability). Products include:

Fluothane 2724

Imipramine Hydrochloride (Severe prolonged hypertension). Products include:

Tofranil Ampuls 854
Tofranil Tablets 856

Imipramine Pamoate (Severe prolonged hypertension). Products include:

Tofranil-PM Capsules............................ 857

Isocarboxazid (Severe prolonged hypertension).

No products indexed under this heading.

Maprotiline Hydrochloride (Severe prolonged hypertension). Products include:

Ludiomil Tablets..................................... 843

Nortriptyline Hydrochloride (Severe prolonged hypertension). Products include:

Pamelor 2280

Phenelzine Sulfate (Severe prolonged hypertension). Products include:

Nardil 1920

Protriptyline Hydrochloride (Severe prolonged hypertension). Products include:

Vivactil Tablets 1774

Selegiline Hydrochloride (Severe prolonged hypertension). Products include:

Eldepryl Tablets 2550

Tranylcypromine Sulfate (Severe prolonged hypertension). Products include:

Parnate Tablets 2503

Trimipramine Maleate (Severe prolonged hypertension). Products include:

Surmontil Capsules................................ 2811

LEVOPROME

(Methotrimeprazine) 1274
May interact with monoamine oxidase inhibitors, antihypertensives, central nervous system depressants, narcotic analgesics, barbiturates, general anesthetics, antihistamines, and certain other agents. Compounds in these categories include:

Acebutolol Hydrochloride (Concurrent use is contraindicated). Products include:

Sectral Capsules 2807

Acrivastine (Potentiation of CNS depression). Products include:

Semprex-D Capsules 463
Semprex-D Capsules 1167

Alfentanil Hydrochloride (Potential for additive effects; the dosage of either drug should be reduced and critically adjusted when used concomitantly or in sequence). Products include:

Alfenta Injection 1286

Alprazolam (Potential for additive effects; the dosage of either drug should be reduced and critically adjusted when used concomitantly or in sequence). Products include:

Xanax Tablets 2649

Amlodipine Besylate (Concurrent use is contraindicated). Products include:

Lotrel Capsules....................................... 840

IMPORTANT NOTE: Always consult each drug listing in the patient's regimen for possible interactions.

Levoprome **Interactions Index** **574**

Norvasc Tablets 1940

Analgesics, unspecified (Potentiation of CNS depression).

Aprobarbital (Potential for additive effects; the dosage of either drug should be reduced and critically adjusted when used concomitantly or in sequence).

No products indexed under this heading.

Aspirin (Potential for additive effects; the dosage of either drug should be reduced and critically adjusted when used concomitantly or in sequence). Products include:

Alka-Seltzer Effervescent Antacid and Pain Reliever .... ▣ 701
Alka-Seltzer Extra Strength Effervescent Antacid and Pain Reliever .... ▣ 703
Alka-Seltzer Lemon Lime Effervescent Antacid and Pain Reliever .... ▣ 703
Alka-Seltzer Plus Cold Medicine .... ▣ 705
Alka-Seltzer Plus Cold & Cough Medicine .... ▣ 708
Alka-Seltzer Plus Night-Time Cold Medicine .... ▣ 707
Alka Seltzer Plus Sinus Medicine .... ▣ 707
Arthritis Foundation Safety Coated Aspirin Tablets .... ▣ 675
Arthritis Pain Ascriptin .... ▣ 631
Maximum Strength Ascriptin .... ▣ 630
Regular Strength Ascriptin Tablets .... ▣ 629
Arthritis Strength BC Powder .... ▣ 609
BC Cold Powder Multi-Symptom Formula (Cold-Sinus-Allergy) .... ▣ 609
BC Cold Powder Non-Drowsy Formula (Cold-Sinus) .... ▣ 609
BC Powder .... ▣ 609
Bayer Children's Chewable Aspirin .... ▣ 711
Genuine Bayer Aspirin Tablets & Caplets .... ▣ 713
Extra Strength Bayer Arthritis Pain Regimen Formula .... ▣ 711
Extra Strength Bayer Aspirin Caplets & Tablets .... ▣ 712
Extended-Release Bayer 8-Hour Aspirin .... ▣ 712
Extra Strength Bayer Plus Aspirin Caplets .... ▣ 713
Extra Strength Bayer PM Aspirin .... ▣ 713
Bayer Enteric Aspirin .... ▣ 709
Bufferin Analgesic Tablets and Caplets .... ▣ 613
Arthritis Strength Bufferin Analgesic Caplets .... ▣ 614
Extra Strength Bufferin Analgesic Tablets .... ▣ 615
Cama Arthritis Pain Reliever .... ▣ 785
Darvon Compound-65 Pulvules 1435
Easprin 1914
Ecotrin 2455
Ecotrin Enteric Coated Aspirin Maximum Strength Tablets and Caplets .... ▣ 816
Ecotrin Enteric Coated Aspirin Regular Strength Tablets 2455
Empirin Aspirin Tablets .... ▣ 854
Empirin with Codeine Tablets 1093
Excedrin Extra-Strength Analgesic Tablets & Caplets 732
Fiorinal Capsules 2261
Fiorinal with Codeine Capsules 2262
Fiorinal Tablets 2261
Halfprin 1362
Healthprin Aspirin 2455
Norgesic 1496
Percodan Tablets 939
Percodan-Demi Tablets 940
Robaxisal Tablets 2071
Soma Compound w/Codeine Tablets 2676
Soma Compound Tablets 2675
St. Joseph Adult Chewable Aspirin (81 mg.) .... ▣ 808
Talwin Compound 2335
Ursinus Inlay-Tabs .... ▣ 794
Vanquish Analgesic Caplets .... ▣ 731

Astemizole (Potentiation of CNS depression). Products include:

Hismanal Tablets 1293

Atenolol (Concurrent use is contraindicated). Products include:

Tenoretic Tablets 2845
Tenormin Tablets and I.V. Injection 2847

Atropine Sulfate (Potential for tachycardia, hypotension, undesirable CNS effects such as stimulation, delirium, and extrapyramidal symptoms may be aggravated). Products include:

Arco-Lase Plus Tablets 512
Atrohist Plus Tablets 454
Atropine Sulfate Sterile Ophthalmic Solution .... ⊙ 233
Donnatal 2060
Donnatal Extentabs 2061
Donnatal Tablets 2060
Lomotil 2439
Motofen Tablets 784
Urised Tablets 1964

Azatadine Maleate (Potentiation of CNS depression). Products include:

Trinalin Repetabs Tablets 1330

Benazepril Hydrochloride (Concurrent use is contraindicated). Products include:

Lotensin Tablets 834
Lotensin HCT 837
Lotrel Capsules 840

Bendroflumethiazide (Concurrent use is contraindicated).

No products indexed under this heading.

Betaxolol Hydrochloride (Concurrent use is contraindicated). Products include:

Betoptic Ophthalmic Solution 469
Betoptic S Ophthalmic Suspension 471
Kerlone Tablets 2436

Bisoprolol Fumarate (Concurrent use is contraindicated). Products include:

Zebeta Tablets 1413
Ziac 1415

Bromodiphenhydramine Hydrochloride (Potentiation of CNS depression).

No products indexed under this heading.

Brompheniramine Maleate (Potentiation of CNS depression). Products include:

Alka Seltzer Plus Sinus Medicine .. ▣ 707
Bromfed Capsules (Extended-Release) 1785
Bromfed Syrup .... ▣ 733
Bromfed Tablets 1785
Bromfed-DM Cough Syrup 1786
Bromfed-PD Capsules (Extended-Release) 1785
Dimetane-DC Cough Syrup 2059
Dimetane-DX Cough Syrup 2059
Dimetapp Elixir .... ▣ 773
Dimetapp Extentabs .... ▣ 774
Dimetapp Tablets/Liqui-Gels .... ▣ 775
Dimetapp Cold & Allergy Chewable Tablets .... ▣ 773
Dimetapp DM Elixir .... ▣ 774
Vicks DayQuil Allergy Relief 12-Hour Extended Release Tablets .... ▣ 760
Vicks DayQuil Allergy Relief 4-Hour Tablets .... ▣ 760

Buprenorphine (Potential for additive effects; the dosage of either drug should be reduced and critically adjusted when used concomitantly or in sequence). Products include:

Buprenex Injectable 2006

Buspirone Hydrochloride (Potential for additive effects; the dosage of either drug should be reduced and critically adjusted when used concomitantly or in sequence). Products include:

BuSpar 737

Butabarbital (Potential for additive effects; the dosage of either drug should be reduced and critically adjusted when used concomitantly or in sequence).

No products indexed under this heading.

Butalbital (Potential for additive effects; the dosage of either drug should be reduced and critically adjusted when used concomitantly or in sequence). Products include:

Esgic-plus Tablets 1013
Fioricet Tablets 2258
Fioricet with Codeine Capsules 2260
Fiorinal Capsules 2261
Fiorinal with Codeine Capsules 2262
Fiorinal Tablets 2261
Phrenilin 785
Sedapap Tablets 50 mg/650 mg .. 1543

Captopril (Concurrent use is contraindicated). Products include:

Capoten 739
Capozide 742

Carteolol Hydrochloride (Concurrent use is contraindicated). Products include:

Cartrol Tablets 410
Ocupress Ophthalmic Solution, 1% Sterile .... ⊙ 309

Chlordiazepoxide (Potential for additive effects; the dosage of either drug should be reduced and critically adjusted when used concomitantly or in sequence). Products include:

Libritabs Tablets 2177
Limbitrol 2180

Chlordiazepoxide Hydrochloride (Potential for additive effects; the dosage of either drug should be reduced and critically adjusted when used concomitantly or in sequence). Products include:

Librax Capsules 2176
Librium Capsules 2178
Librium Injectable 2179

Chlorothiazide (Concurrent use is contraindicated). Products include:

Aldoclor Tablets 1598
Diupres Tablets 1650
Diuril Oral 1653

Chlorothiazide Sodium (Concurrent use is contraindicated). Products include:

Diuril Sodium Intravenous 1652

Chlorpheniramine Maleate (Potentiation of CNS depression). Products include:

Alka-Seltzer Plus Cold Medicine .... ▣ 705
Alka-Seltzer Plus Cold Medicine Liqui-Gels .... ▣ 706
Alka-Seltzer Plus Cold & Cough Medicine .... ▣ 708
Alka-Seltzer Plus Cold & Cough Medicine Liqui-Gels .... ▣ 705
Allerest Children's Chewable Tablets .... ▣ 627
Allerest Headache Strength Tablets .... ▣ 627
Allerest Maximum Strength Tablets .... ▣ 627
Allerest Sinus Pain Formula .... ▣ 627
Allerest 12 Hour Caplets .... ▣ 627
Ana-Kit Anaphylaxis Emergency Treatment Kit 617
Atrohist Pediatric Capsules 453
Atrohist Plus Tablets 454
BC Cold Powder Multi-Symptom Formula (Cold-Sinus-Allergy) .... ▣ 609
Cerose DM .... ▣ 878
Cheracol Plus Head Cold/Cough Formula .... ▣ 769
Children's Vicks DayQuil Allergy Relief .... ▣ 757
Children's Vicks NyQuil Cold/Cough Relief .... ▣ 758
Chlor-Trimeton Allergy Decongestant Tablets .... ▣ 799
Chlor-Trimeton Allergy Tablets .... ▣ 798
Comhist 2038
Comtrex Multi-Symptom Cold Reliever Tablets/Caplets/Liqui-Gels/Liquid .... ▣ 615
Allergy-Sinus Comtrex Multi-Symptom Allergy-Sinus Formula Tablets .... ▣ 617
Contac Continuous Action Nasal Decongestant/Antihistamine 12 Hour Capsules .... ▣ 813
Contac Maximum Strength Continuous Action Decongestant/Antihistamine 12 Hour Caplets .... ▣ 813
Contac Severe Cold and Flu Formula Caplets .... ▣ 814
Coricidin 'D' Decongestant Tablets .... ▣ 800
Coricidin Tablets .... ▣ 800
D.A. Chewable Tablets 951
Deconamine 1320
Dura-Tap/PD Capsules 2867
Dura-Vent/DA Tablets 953
Extendryl 1005
Fedahist Gyrocaps 2401
Fedahist Timecaps 2401
Hycomine Compound Tablets 932
Isoclor Timesule Capsules .... ▣ 637
Kronofed-A 977
Nolamine Timed-Release Tablets 785
Novahistine DH 2462
Novahistine Elixir .... ▣ 823
Ornade Spansule Capsules 2502
PediaCare Cold Allergy Chewable Tablets .... ▣ 677
PediaCare Cough-Cold Chewable Tablets 1553
PediaCare Cough-Cold Liquid 1553
PediaCare NightRest Cough-Cold Liquid 1553
Pediatric Vicks 44m Cough & Cold Relief .... ▣ 764
Pyrroxate Caplets .... ▣ 772
Ryna .... ▣ 841
Sinarest Tablets .... ▣ 648
Sinarest Extra Strength Tablets .... ▣ 648
Sine-Off Sinus Medicine .... ▣ 825
Singlet Tablets .... ▣ 825
Sinulin Tablets 787
Sinutab Sinus Allergy Medication, Maximum Strength Tablets and Caplets .... ▣ 860
Sudafed Plus Liquid .... ▣ 862
Sudafed Plus Tablets .... ▣ 863
Teldrin 12 Hour Antihistamine/Nasal Decongestant Allergy Relief Capsules .... ▣ 826
TheraFlu .... ▣ 787
TheraFlu Maximum Strength Nighttime Flu, Cold & Cough Medicine .... ▣ 788
Triaminic Allergy Tablets .... ▣ 789
Triaminic Cold Tablets .... ▣ 790
Triaminic Nite Light .... ▣ 791
Triaminic Syrup .... ▣ 792
Triaminic-12 Tablets .... ▣ 792
Triaminicin Tablets .... ▣ 793
Triaminicol Multi-Symptom Cold Tablets .... ▣ 793
Triaminicol Multi-Symptom Relief ▣ 794
Tussend 1783
Children's TYLENOL Cold Multi-Symptom Liquid Formula and Chewable Tablets 1561
Children's TYLENOL Cold Plus Cough Multi Symptom Tablets and Liquid .... ▣ 681
TYLENOL Maximum Strength Allergy Sinus Medication Gelcaps and Caplets 1563
TYLENOL Cold Multi-Symptom Formula Medication Tablets and Caplets 1561
TYLENOL Cold Multi-Symptom Hot Medication Liquid Packets 1557
Vicks 44 LiquiCaps Cough, Cold & Flu Relief .... ▣ 755
Vicks 44M Cough, Cold & Flu Relief .... ▣ 756

Chlorpheniramine Polistirex (Potentiation of CNS depression). Products include:

Tussionex Pennkinetic Extended-Release Suspension 998

Chlorpheniramine Tannate (Potentiation of CNS depression). Products include:

Atrohist Pediatric Suspension 454
Ricobid Tablets and Pediatric Suspension 2038
Rynatan 2673
Rynatuss 2673

Chlorpromazine (Potential for additive effects; the dosage of either drug should be reduced and critically adjusted when used concomitantly or in sequence). Products include:

Thorazine Suppositories 2523

(▣ Described in PDR For Nonprescription Drugs) (⊙ Described in PDR For Ophthalmology)

Interactions Index

Chlorpromazine Hydrochloride (Potential for additive effects; the dosage of either drug should be reduced and critically adjusted when used concomitantly or in sequence). Products include:

Thorazine 2523

Chlorprothixene (Potential for additive effects; the dosage of either drug should be reduced and critically adjusted when used concomitantly or in sequence).

No products indexed under this heading.

Chlorprothixene Hydrochloride (Potential for additive effects; the dosage of either drug should be reduced and critically adjusted when used concomitantly or in sequence).

No products indexed under this heading.

Chlorthalidone (Concurrent use is contraindicated). Products include:

Combipres Tablets 677
Tenoretic Tablets 2845
Thalitone 1245

Clemastine Fumarate (Potentiation of CNS depression). Products include:

Tavist Syrup 2297
Tavist Tablets 2298
Tavist-1 12 Hour Relief Tablets ....ⓐ 787
Tavist-D 12 Hour Relief Tablets ....ⓐ 787

Clonidine (Concurrent use is contraindicated). Products include:

Catapres-TTS 675

Clonidine Hydrochloride (Concurrent use is contraindicated). Products include:

Catapres Tablets 674
Combipres Tablets 677

Clorazepate Dipotassium (Potential for additive effects; the dosage of either drug should be reduced and critically adjusted when used concomitantly or in sequence). Products include:

Tranxene 451

Clozapine (Potential for additive effects; the dosage of either drug should be reduced and critically adjusted when used concomitantly or in sequence). Products include:

Clozaril Tablets 2252

Codeine Phosphate (Potential for additive effects; the dosage of either drug should be reduced and critically adjusted when used concomitantly or in sequence). Products include:

Actifed with Codeine Cough Syrup.. 1067
Brontex 1981
Deconsal C Expectorant Syrup 456
Deconsal Pediatric Syrup 457
Dimetane-DC Cough Syrup 2059
Empirin with Codeine Tablets........... 1093
Fioricet with Codeine Capsules 2260
Fiorinal with Codeine Capsules 2262
Isoclor Expectorant 990
Novahistine DH 2462
Novahistine Expectorant 2463
Nucofed 2051
Phenergan with Codeine 2777
Phenergan VC with Codeine 2781
Robitussin A-C Syrup 2073
Robitussin-DAC Syrup 2074
Ryna .... ⓐ 841
Soma Compound w/Codeine Tablets 2676
Tussi-Organidin NR Liquid and S NR Liquid 2677
Tylenol with Codeine 1583

Cyproheptadine Hydrochloride (Potentiation of CNS depression). Products include:

Periactin 1724

Deserpidine (Concurrent use is contraindicated).

No products indexed under this heading.

Desflurane (Potential for additive effects; the dosage of either drug should be reduced and critically adjusted when used concomitantly or in sequence). Products include:

Suprane 1813

Dexchlorpheniramine Maleate (Potentiation of CNS depression).

No products indexed under this heading.

Dezocine (Potential for additive effects; the dosage of either drug should be reduced and critically adjusted when used concomitantly or in sequence). Products include:

Dalgan Injection 538

Diazepam (Potential for additive effects; the dosage of either drug should be reduced and critically adjusted when used concomitantly or in sequence). Products include:

Dizac 1809
Valium Injectable 2182
Valium Tablets 2183
Valrelease Capsules 2169

Diazoxide (Concurrent use is contraindicated). Products include:

Hyperstat I.V. Injection 2363
Proglycem 580

Diltiazem Hydrochloride (Concurrent use is contraindicated). Products include:

Cardizem CD Capsules 1506
Cardizem SR Capsules 1510
Cardizem Injectable 1508
Cardizem Tablets 1512
Dilacor XR Extended-release Capsules 2018

Diphenhydramine Citrate (Potentiation of CNS depression). Products include:

Excedrin P.M. Analgesic/Sleeping Aid Tablets, Caplets, Liquigels 733

Diphenhydramine Hydrochloride (Potentiation of CNS depression). Products include:

Actifed Allergy Daytime/Nighttime Caplets .... ⓐ 844
Actifed Sinus Daytime/Nighttime Tablets and Caplets .... ⓐ 846
Arthritis Foundation NightTime Caplets .... ⓐ 674
Extra Strength Bayer PM Aspirin ..ⓐ 713
Bayer Select Night Time Pain Relief Formula .... ⓐ 716
Benadryl Allergy Decongestant Liquid Medication .... ⓐ 848
Benadryl Allergy Decongestant Tablets .... ⓐ 848
Benadryl Allergy Liquid Medication .... ⓐ 849
Benadryl Allergy .... ⓐ 848
Benadryl Allergy Sinus Headache Formula Caplets .... ⓐ 849
Benadryl Capsules 1898
Benadryl Dye-Free Allergy Liquigel Softgels .... ⓐ 850
Benadryl Dye-Free Allergy Liquid Medication .... ⓐ 850
Benadryl Itch Relief Cream, Children's Formula and Maximum Strength 2% .... ⓐ 851
Benadryl Itch Relief Spray, Children's Formula and Maximum Strength 2% .... ⓐ 851
Benadryl Itch Relief Stick Maximum Strength 2% .... ⓐ 850
Benadryl Itch Stopping Gel, Children's Formula and Maximum Strength 2% .... ⓐ 851
Benadryl Kapseals 1898
Benadryl Injection 1898
Contac Day & Night Cold/Flu Night Caplets .... ⓐ 812
Contac Night Allergy/Sinus Caplets .... ⓐ 812
Extra Strength Doan's P.M. .... ⓐ 633
Legatrin PM .... ⓐ 651
Miles Nervine Nighttime Sleep-Aid ⓐ 723
Nytol QuickCaps Caplets .... ⓐ 610
Sleepinal Night-time Sleep Aid Capsules and Softgels .... ⓐ 834
TYLENOL Maximum Strength Allergy Sinus NightTime Medication Caplets 1555

TYLENOL Flu NightTime, Maximum Strength, Gelcaps 1566
TYLENOL Maximum Strength Flu NightTime Hot Medication Packets 1562
TYLENOL PM, Extra Strength Pain Reliever/Sleep Aid Caplets, Geltabs, Gelcaps 1560
TYLENOL Severe Allergy Medication Caplets 1564
Maximum Strength Unisom Sleepgels 1934
Unisom With Pain Relief-Nighttime Sleep Aid and Pain Reliever............ 1934

Diphenylpyraline Hydrochloride (Potentiation of CNS depression).

No products indexed under this heading.

Doxazosin Mesylate (Concurrent use is contraindicated). Products include:

Cardura Tablets 2186

Droperidol (Potential for additive effects; the dosage of either drug should be reduced and critically adjusted when used concomitantly or in sequence). Products include:

Inapsine Injection 1296

Enalapril Maleate (Concurrent use is contraindicated). Products include:

Vaseretic Tablets 1765
Vasotec Tablets 1771

Enalaprilat (Concurrent use is contraindicated). Products include:

Vasotec I.V. 1768

Enflurane (Potential for additive effects; the dosage of either drug should be reduced and critically adjusted when used concomitantly or in sequence).

No products indexed under this heading.

Epinephrine Hydrochloride (Potential for paradoxical decrease in blood pressure). Products include:

Ana-Kit Anaphylaxis Emergency Treatment Kit 617

Esmolol Hydrochloride (Concurrent use is contraindicated). Products include:

Brevibloc Injection 1808

Estazolam (Potential for additive effects; the dosage of either drug should be reduced and critically adjusted when used concomitantly or in sequence). Products include:

ProSom Tablets 449

Ethchlorvynol (Potential for additive effects; the dosage of either drug should be reduced and critically adjusted when used concomitantly or in sequence). Products include:

Placidyl Capsules 448

Ethinamate (Potential for additive effects; the dosage of either drug should be reduced and critically adjusted when used concomitantly or in sequence).

No products indexed under this heading.

Felodipine (Concurrent use is contraindicated). Products include:

Plendil Extended-Release Tablets..... 527

Fentanyl (Potential for additive effects; the dosage of either drug should be reduced and critically adjusted when used concomitantly or in sequence). Products include:

Duragesic Transdermal System......... 1288

Fentanyl Citrate (Potential for additive effects; the dosage of either drug should be reduced and critically adjusted when used concomitantly or in sequence). Products include:

Sublimaze Injection 1307

Fluphenazine Decanoate (Potential for additive effects; the dosage of either drug should be reduced and critically adjusted when used concomitantly or in sequence). Products include:

Prolixin Decanoate 509

Fluphenazine Enanthate (Potential for additive effects; the dosage of either drug should be reduced and critically adjusted when used concomitantly or in sequence). Products include:

Prolixin Enanthate 509

Fluphenazine Hydrochloride (Potential for additive effects; the dosage of either drug should be reduced and critically adjusted when used concomitantly or in sequence). Products include:

Prolixin 509

Flurazepam Hydrochloride (Potential for additive effects; the dosage of either drug should be reduced and critically adjusted when used concomitantly or in sequence). Products include:

Dalmane Capsules 2173

Fosinopril Sodium (Concurrent use is contraindicated). Products include:

Monopril Tablets 757

Furazolidone (Concurrent use is contraindicated). Products include:

Furoxone 2046

Furosemide (Concurrent use is contraindicated). Products include:

Lasix Injection, Oral Solution and Tablets 1240

Glutethimide (Potential for additive effects; the dosage of either drug should be reduced and critically adjusted when used concomitantly or in sequence).

No products indexed under this heading.

Guanabenz Acetate (Concurrent use is contraindicated).

No products indexed under this heading.

Guanethidine Monosulfate (Concurrent use is contraindicated). Products include:

Esimil Tablets 822
Ismelin Tablets 827

Haloperidol (Potential for additive effects; the dosage of either drug should be reduced and critically adjusted when used concomitantly or in sequence). Products include:

Haldol Injection, Tablets and Concentrate 1575

Haloperidol Decanoate (Potential for additive effects; the dosage of either drug should be reduced and critically adjusted when used concomitantly or in sequence). Products include:

Haldol Decanoate 1577

Hydralazine Hydrochloride (Concurrent use is contraindicated). Products include:

Apresazide Capsules 808
Apresoline Hydrochloride Tablets .. 809
Ser-Ap-Es Tablets 849

Hydrochlorothiazide (Concurrent use is contraindicated). Products include:

Aldactazide 2413
Aldoril Tablets 1604
Apresazide Capsules 808
Capozide 742
Dyazide 2479
Esidrix Tablets 821
Esimil Tablets 822
HydroDIURIL Tablets 1674
Hydropres Tablets 1675
Hyzaar Tablets 1677
Inderide Tablets 2732
Inderide LA Long Acting Capsules .. 2734

IMPORTANT NOTE: Always consult each drug listing in the patient's regimen for possible interactions.

Levoprome Interactions Index 576

Lopressor HCT Tablets 832
Lotensin HCT........ 837
Maxzide 1380
Moduretic Tablets 1705
Oretic Tablets 443
Prinzide Tablets 1737
Ser-Ap-Es Tablets 849
Timolide Tablets........ 1748
Vaseretic Tablets 1765
Zestoretic 2850
Ziac 1415

Hydrocodone Bitartrate (Potential for additive effects; the dosage of either drug should be reduced and critically adjusted when used concomitantly or in sequence). Products include:

Anexsia 5/500 Elixir 1781
Anexia Tablets........ 1782
Codiclear DH Syrup 791
Deconamine CX Cough and Cold Liquid and Tablets........ 1319
Duratuss HD Elixir........ 2565
Hycodan Tablets and Syrup 930
Hycomine Compound Tablets 932
Hycomine 931
Hycotuss Expectorant Syrup 933
Hydrocet Capsules 782
Lorcet 10/650........ 1018
Lortab 2566
Tussend 1783
Tussend Expectorant 1785
Vicodin Tablets........ 1356
Vicodin ES Tablets 1357
Vicodin Tuss Expectorant 1358
Zydone Capsules 949

Hydrocodone Polistirex (Potential for additive effects; the dosage of either drug should be reduced and critically adjusted when used concomitantly or in sequence). Products include:

Tussionex Pennkinetic Extended-Release Suspension 998

Hydroflumethiazide (Concurrent use is contraindicated). Products include:

Diucardin Tablets........ 2718

Hydroxyzine Hydrochloride (Potential for additive effects; the dosage of either drug should be reduced and critically adjusted when used concomitantly or in sequence). Products include:

Atarax Tablets & Syrup........ 2185
Marax Tablets & DF Syrup........ 2200
Vistaril Intramuscular Solution........ 2216

Indapamide (Concurrent use is contraindicated). Products include:

Lozol Tablets 2022

Isocarboxazid (Concurrent use is contraindicated).

No products indexed under this heading.

Isoflurane (Potential for additive effects; the dosage of either drug should be reduced and critically adjusted when used concomitantly or in sequence).

No products indexed under this heading.

Isradipine (Concurrent use is contraindicated). Products include:

DynaCirc Capsules 2256

Ketamine Hydrochloride (Potential for additive effects; the dosage of either drug should be reduced and critically adjusted when used concomitantly or in sequence).

No products indexed under this heading.

Labetalol Hydrochloride (Concurrent use is contraindicated). Products include:

Normodyne Injection 2377
Normodyne Tablets 2379
Trandate 1185

Levomethadyl Acetate Hydrochloride (Potential for additive effects; the dosage of either drug should be reduced and critically adjusted when used concomitantly or in sequence). Products include:

Orlamm 2239

Levorphanol Tartrate (Potential for additive effects; the dosage of either drug should be reduced and critically adjusted when used concomitantly or in sequence). Products include:

Levo-Dromoran........ 2129

Lisinopril (Concurrent use is contraindicated). Products include:

Prinivil Tablets 1733
Prinzide Tablets 1737
Zestoretic 2850
Zestril Tablets 2854

Loratadine (Potentiation of CNS depression). Products include:

Claritin 2349
Claritin-D 2350

Lorazepam (Potential for additive effects; the dosage of either drug should be reduced and critically adjusted when used concomitantly or in sequence). Products include:

Ativan Injection........ 2698
Ativan Tablets 2700

Losartan Potassium (Concurrent use is contraindicated). Products include:

Cozaar Tablets 1628
Hyzaar Tablets 1677

Loxapine Hydrochloride (Potential for additive effects; the dosage of either drug should be reduced and critically adjusted when used concomitantly or in sequence). Products include:

Loxitane 1378

Loxapine Succinate (Potential for additive effects; the dosage of either drug should be reduced and critically adjusted when used concomitantly or in sequence). Products include:

Loxitane Capsules 1378

Mecamylamine Hydrochloride (Concurrent use is contraindicated). Products include:

Inversine Tablets 1686

Meperidine Hydrochloride (Potential for additive effects; the dosage of either drug should be reduced and critically adjusted when used concomitantly or in sequence). Products include:

Demerol 2308
Mepergan Injection 2753

Mephobarbital (Potential for additive effects; the dosage of either drug should be reduced and critically adjusted when used concomitantly or in sequence). Products include:

Mebaral Tablets 2322

Meprobamate (Potential for additive effects; the dosage of either drug should be reduced and critically adjusted when used concomitantly or in sequence). Products include:

Miltown Tablets 2672
PMB 200 and PMB 400 2783

Mesoridazine (Potential for additive effects; the dosage of either drug should be reduced and critically adjusted when used concomitantly or in sequence).

Methadone Hydrochloride (Potential for additive effects; the dosage of either drug should be reduced and critically adjusted when used concomitantly or in sequence). Products include:

Methadone Hydrochloride Oral Concentrate 2233
Methadone Hydrochloride Oral Solution & Tablets........ 2235

Methdilazine Hydrochloride (Potentiation of CNS depression).

No products indexed under this heading.

Methohexital Sodium (Potential for additive effects; the dosage of either drug should be reduced and critically adjusted when used concomitantly or in sequence). Products include:

Brevital Sodium Vials........ 1429

Methoxyflurane (Potential for additive effects; the dosage of either drug should be reduced and critically adjusted when used concomitantly or in sequence).

No products indexed under this heading.

Methyclothiazide (Concurrent use is contraindicated). Products include:

Enduron Tablets........ 420

Methyldopa (Concurrent use is contraindicated). Products include:

Aldoclor Tablets 1598
Aldomet Oral 1600
Aldoril Tablets........ 1604

Methyldopate Hydrochloride (Concurrent use is contraindicated). Products include:

Aldomet Ester HCl Injection 1602

Metolazone (Concurrent use is contraindicated). Products include:

Mykrox Tablets........ 993
Zaroxolyn Tablets 1000

Metoprolol Succinate (Concurrent use is contraindicated). Products include:

Toprol-XL Tablets 565

Metoprolol Tartrate (Concurrent use is contraindicated). Products include:

Lopressor Ampuls........ 830
Lopressor HCT Tablets........ 832
Lopressor Tablets 830

Metyrosine (Concurrent use is contraindicated). Products include:

Demser Capsules........ 1649

Midazolam Hydrochloride (Potential for additive effects; the dosage of either drug should be reduced and critically adjusted when used concomitantly or in sequence). Products include:

Versed Injection 2170

Minoxidil (Concurrent use is contraindicated). Products include:

Loniten Tablets........ 2618
Rogaine Topical Solution 2637

Moexipril Hydrochloride (Concurrent use is contraindicated). Products include:

Univasc Tablets 2410

Molindone Hydrochloride (Potential for additive effects; the dosage of either drug should be reduced and critically adjusted when used concomitantly or in sequence). Products include:

Moban Tablets and Concentrate........ 1048

Morphine Sulfate (Potential for additive effects; the dosage of either drug should be reduced and critically adjusted when used concomitantly or in sequence). Products include:

Astramorph/PF Injection, USP (Preservative-Free) 535
Duramorph........ 962
Infumorph 200 and Infumorph 500 Sterile Solutions........ 965
MS Contin Tablets........ 1994
MSIR 1997
Oramorph SR (Morphine Sulfate Sustained Release Tablets)........ 2236
RMS Suppositories 2657
Roxanol 2243

Nadolol (Concurrent use is contraindicated).

No products indexed under this heading.

Nicardipine Hydrochloride (Concurrent use is contraindicated). Products include:

Cardene Capsules 2095
Cardene I.V. 2709
Cardene SR Capsules........ 2097

Nifedipine (Concurrent use is contraindicated). Products include:

Adalat Capsules (10 mg and 20 mg) 587
Adalat CC 589
Procardia Capsules........ 1971
Procardia XL Extended Release Tablets 1972

Nisoldipine (Concurrent use is contraindicated).

No products indexed under this heading.

Nitroglycerin (Concurrent use is contraindicated). Products include:

Deponit NTG Transdermal Delivery System 2397
Nitro-Bid IV........ 1523
Nitro-Bid Ointment 1524
Nitrodisc 2047
Nitro-Dur (nitroglycerin) Transdermal Infusion System 1326
Nitrolingual Spray 2027
Nitrostat Tablets 1925
Transderm-Nitro Transdermal Therapeutic System 859

Opium Alkaloids (Potential for additive effects; the dosage of either drug should be reduced and critically adjusted when used concomitantly or in sequence).

No products indexed under this heading.

Oxazepam (Potential for additive effects; the dosage of either drug should be reduced and critically adjusted when used concomitantly or in sequence). Products include:

Serax Capsules 2810
Serax Tablets........ 2810

Oxycodone Hydrochloride (Potential for additive effects; the dosage of either drug should be reduced and critically adjusted when used concomitantly or in sequence). Products include:

Percocet Tablets 938
Percodan Tablets........ 939
Percodan-Demi Tablets........ 940
Roxicodone Tablets, Oral Solution & Intensol (Oxycodone) 2244
Tylox Capsules 1584

Penbutolol Sulfate (Concurrent use is contraindicated). Products include:

Levatol 2403

Pentobarbital Sodium (Potential for additive effects; the dosage of either drug should be reduced and critically adjusted when used concomitantly or in sequence). Products include:

Nembutal Sodium Capsules 436
Nembutal Sodium Solution 438
Nembutal Sodium Suppositories........ 440

Perphenazine (Potential for additive effects; the dosage of either drug should be reduced and critically adjusted when used concomitantly or in sequence). Products include:

Etrafon 2355
Triavil Tablets 1757
Trilafon........ 2389

Phenelzine Sulfate (Concurrent use is contraindicated). Products include:

Nardil 1920

(▭ Described in PDR For Nonprescription Drugs) (⊙ Described in PDR For Ophthalmology)

Phenobarbital (Potential for additive effects; the dosage of either drug should be reduced and critically adjusted when used concomitantly or in sequence). Products include:

Arco-Lase Plus Tablets 512
Bellergal-S Tablets 2250
Donnatal 2060
Donnatal Extentabs................................. 2061
Donnatal Tablets 2060
Phenobarbital Elixir and Tablets 1469
Quadrinal Tablets 1350

Phenoxybenzamine Hydrochloride (Concurrent use is contraindicated). Products include:

Dibenzyline Capsules 2476

Phentolamine Mesylate (Concurrent use is contraindicated). Products include:

Regitine 846

Pindolol (Concurrent use is contraindicated). Products include:

Visken Tablets.. 2299

Polythiazide (Concurrent use is contraindicated). Products include:

Minizide Capsules 1938

Prazepam (Potential for additive effects; the dosage of either drug should be reduced and critically adjusted when used concomitantly or in sequence).

No products indexed under this heading.

Prazosin Hydrochloride (Concurrent use is contraindicated). Products include:

Minipress Capsules................................. 1937
Minizide Capsules 1938

Prochlorperazine (Potential for additive effects; the dosage of either drug should be reduced and critically adjusted when used concomitantly or in sequence). Products include:

Compazine 2470

Promethazine Hydrochloride (Potential for additive effects; the dosage of either drug should be reduced and critically adjusted when used concomitantly or in sequence; potentiation of CNS depression). Products include:

Mepergan Injection 2753
Phenergan with Codeine........................ 2777
Phenergan with Dextromethorphan 2778
Phenergan Injection 2773
Phenergan Suppositories 2775
Phenergan Syrup 2774
Phenergan Tablets 2775
Phenergan VC 2779
Phenergan VC with Codeine 2781

Propofol (Potential for additive effects; the dosage of either drug should be reduced and critically adjusted when used concomitantly or in sequence). Products include:

Diprivan Injection.................................... 2833

Propoxyphene Hydrochloride (Potential for additive effects; the dosage of either drug should be reduced and critically adjusted when used concomitantly or in sequence). Products include:

Darvon 1435
Wygesic Tablets 2827

Propoxyphene Napsylate (Potential for additive effects; the dosage of either drug should be reduced and critically adjusted when used concomitantly or in sequence). Products include:

Darvon-N/Darvocet-N 1433

Propranolol Hydrochloride (Concurrent use is contraindicated). Products include:

Inderal 2728
Inderal LA Long Acting Capsules 2730
Inderide Tablets 2732
Inderide LA Long Acting Capsules .. 2734

Pyrilamine Maleate (Potentiation of CNS depression). Products include:

4-Way Fast Acting Nasal Spray (regular & mentholated) .... ◆◻ 621
Maximum Strength Multi-Symptom Formula Midol .... ◆◻ 722
PMS Multi-Symptom Formula Midol .... ◆◻ 723

Pyrilamine Tannate (Potentiation of CNS depression). Products include:

Atrohist Pediatric Suspension 454
Rynatan 2673

Quazepam (Potential for additive effects; the dosage of either drug should be reduced and critically adjusted when used concomitantly or in sequence). Products include:

Doral Tablets 2664

Quinapril Hydrochloride (Concurrent use is contraindicated). Products include:

Accupril Tablets 1893

Ramipril (Concurrent use is contraindicated). Products include:

Altace Capsules 1232

Rauwolfia Serpentina (Concurrent use is contraindicated).

No products indexed under this heading.

Rescinnamine (Concurrent use is contraindicated).

No products indexed under this heading.

Reserpine (Potential for additive effects; the dosage of either drug should be reduced and critically adjusted when used concomitantly or in sequence; concurrent use is contraindicated). Products include:

Diupres Tablets 1650
Hydropres Tablets................................... 1675
Ser-Ap-Es Tablets 849

Risperidone (Potential for additive effects; the dosage of either drug should be reduced and critically adjusted when used concomitantly or in sequence). Products include:

Risperdal 1301

Scopolamine (Potential for tachycardia, hypotension, undesirable CNS effects such as stimulation, delirium, and extrapyramidal symptoms may be aggravated). Products include:

Transderm Scōp Transdermal Therapeutic System 869

Scopolamine Hydrobromide (Potential for tachycardia, hypotension, undesirable CNS effects such as stimulation, delirium, and extrapyramidal symptoms may be aggravated). Products include:

Atrohist Plus Tablets 454
Donnatal 2060
Donnatal Extentabs................................ 2061
Donnatal Tablets 2060

Secobarbital Sodium (Potential for additive effects; the dosage of either drug should be reduced and critically adjusted when used concomitantly or in sequence). Products include:

Seconal Sodium Pulvules 1474

Selegiline Hydrochloride (Concurrent use is contraindicated). Products include:

Eldepryl Tablets 2550

Sodium Nitroprusside (Concurrent use is contraindicated).

No products indexed under this heading.

Sotalol Hydrochloride (Concurrent use is contraindicated). Products include:

Betapace Tablets 641

Spirapril Hydrochloride (Concurrent use is contraindicated).

No products indexed under this heading.

Succinylcholine Chloride (Potential for tachycardia, hypotension, undesirable CNS effects such as stimulation, delirium, and extrapyramidal symptoms may be aggravated). Products include:

Anectine.. 1073

Sufentanil Citrate (Potential for additive effects; the dosage of either drug should be reduced and critically adjusted when used concomitantly or in sequence). Products include:

Sufenta Injection 1309

Temazepam (Potential for additive effects; the dosage of either drug should be reduced and critically adjusted when used concomitantly or in sequence). Products include:

Restoril Capsules 2284

Terazosin Hydrochloride (Concurrent use is contraindicated). Products include:

Hytrin Capsules 430

Terfenadine (Potentiation of CNS depression). Products include:

Seldane Tablets 1536
Seldane-D Extended-Release Tablets 1538

Thiamylal Sodium (Potential for additive effects; the dosage of either drug should be reduced and critically adjusted when used concomitantly or in sequence).

No products indexed under this heading.

Thioridazine Hydrochloride (Potential for additive effects; the dosage of either drug should be reduced and critically adjusted when used concomitantly or in sequence). Products include:

Mellaril 2269

Thiothixene (Potential for additive effects; the dosage of either drug should be reduced and critically adjusted when used concomitantly or in sequence). Products include:

Navane Capsules and Concentrate 2201
Navane Intramuscular 2202

Timolol Maleate (Concurrent use is contraindicated). Products include:

Blocadren Tablets 1614
Timolide Tablets...................................... 1748
Timoptic in Ocudose 1753
Timoptic Sterile Ophthalmic Solution.. 1751
Timoptic-XE 1755

Torsemide (Concurrent use is contraindicated). Products include:

Demadex Tablets and Injection 686

Tranylcypromine Sulfate (Concurrent use is contraindicated). Products include:

Parnate Tablets 2503

Triazolam (Potential for additive effects; the dosage of either drug should be reduced and critically adjusted when used concomitantly or in sequence). Products include:

Halcion Tablets.. 2611

Trifluoperazine Hydrochloride (Potential for additive effects; the dosage of either drug should be reduced and critically adjusted when used concomitantly or in sequence). Products include:

Stelazine 2514

Trimeprazine Tartrate (Potentiation of CNS depression). Products include:

Temaril Tablets, Syrup and Spansule Extended-Release Capsules.. 483

Trimethaphan Camsylate (Concurrent use is contraindicated). Products include:

Arfonad Ampuls 2080

Tripelennamine Hydrochloride (Potentiation of CNS depression). Products include:

PBZ Tablets 845
PBZ-SR Tablets.. 844

Triprolidine Hydrochloride (Potentiation of CNS depression). Products include:

Actifed Plus Caplets .... ◆◻ 845
Actifed Plus Tablets .... ◆◻ 845
Actifed with Codeine Cough Syrup.. 1067
Actifed Syrup... ◆◻ 846
Actifed Tablets .... ◆◻ 844

Verapamil Hydrochloride (Concurrent use is contraindicated). Products include:

Calan SR Caplets 2422
Calan Tablets.. 2419
Isoptin Injectable 1344
Isoptin Oral Tablets 1346
Isoptin SR Tablets 1348
Verelan Capsules 1410
Verelan Capsules 2824

Zolpidem Tartrate (Potential for additive effects; the dosage of either drug should be reduced and critically adjusted when used concomitantly or in sequence). Products include:

Ambien Tablets... 2416

Food Interactions

Alcohol (Potentiation of CNS depression).

LEVOTHROID TABLETS

(Levothyroxine Sodium) 1016

May interact with oral hypoglycemic agents, insulin, oral anticoagulants, oral contraceptives, estrogens, and certain other agents. Compounds in these categories include:

Acarbose (Dosage of hypoglycemic agent may need to be adjusted).

No products indexed under this heading.

Chlorotrianisene (Estrogens tend to increase serum thyroxine-binding globulin; patients with non-functioning thyroid may need to adjust thyroid dosage).

No products indexed under this heading.

Chlorpropamide (Dosage of hypoglycemic agent may need to be adjusted). Products include:

Diabinese Tablets 1935

Cholestyramine (Binds both T_4 and T_3 in the intestine, thus impairing absorption of thyroid hormone; four to five hours should elapse between administration of cholestyramine and thyroid hormone). Products include:

Questran Light 769
Questran Powder 770

Colestipol Hydrochloride (Binds both T_4 and T_3 in the intestine, thus impairing absorption of thyroid hormone; four to five hours should elapse between administration of cholestyramine and thyroid hormone). Products include:

Colestid Tablets 2591

Desogestrel (Estrogens tend to increase serum thyroxine-binding globulin; patients with non-functioning thyroid may need to adjust thyroid dosage). Products include:

Desogen Tablets....................................... 1817
Ortho-Cept 1851

Dicumarol (Anticoagulant effects may be potentiated; dosage adjustment should be made).

No products indexed under this heading.

IMPORTANT NOTE: Always consult each drug listing in the patient's regimen for possible interactions.

Levothroid Tablets

Dienestrol (Estrogens tend to increase serum thyroxine-binding globulin; patients with non-functioning thyroid may need to adjust thyroid dosage). Products include:

Ortho Dienestrol Cream 1866

Diethylstilbestrol (Estrogens tend to increase serum thyroxine-binding globulin; patients with non-functioning thyroid may need to adjust thyroid dosage). Products include:

Diethylstilbestrol Tablets 1437

Epinephrine Hydrochloride (Enhanced coronary insufficiency). Products include:

Ana-Kit Anaphylaxis Emergency Treatment Kit 617

Estradiol (Estrogens tend to increase serum thyroxine-binding globulin; patients with non-functioning thyroid may need to adjust thyroid dosage). Products include:

Climara Transdermal System 645
Estrace Cream and Tablets 749
Estraderm Transdermal System 824

Estrogens, Conjugated (Estrogens tend to increase serum thyroxine-binding globulin; patients with non-functioning thyroid may need to adjust thyroid dosage). Products include:

PMB 200 and PMB 400 2783
Premarin Intravenous 2787
Premarin with Methyltestosterone .. 2794
Premarin Tablets 2789
Premarin Vaginal Cream.................... 2791
Premphase 2797
Prempro.. 2801

Estrogens, Esterified (Estrogens tend to increase serum thyroxine-binding globulin; patients with non-functioning thyroid may need to adjust thyroid dosage). Products include:

ESTRATAB Tablets (0.3, 0.625, 1.25, 2.5 mg) 2536
Estratest 2539
Menest Tablets 2494

Estropipate (Estrogens tend to increase serum thyroxine-binding globulin; patients with non-functioning thyroid may need to adjust thyroid dosage). Products include:

Ogen Tablets 2627
Ogen Vaginal Cream............................ 2630
Ortho-Est.. 1869

Ethinyl Estradiol (Estrogens tend to increase serum thyroxine-binding globulin; patients with non-functioning thyroid may need to adjust thyroid dosage). Products include:

Brevicon.. 2088
Demulen 2428
Desogen Tablets.................................... 1817
Levlen/Tri-Levlen.................................. 651
Lo/Ovral Tablets 2746
Lo/Ovral-28 Tablets............................. 2751
Modicon 1872
Nordette-21 Tablets............................. 2755
Nordette-28 Tablets............................. 2758
Norinyl 2088
Ortho-Cept 1851
Ortho-Cyclen/Ortho-Tri-Cyclen 1858
Ortho-Novum.. 1872
Ortho-Cyclen/Ortho Tri-Cyclen 1858
Ovcon 760
Ovral Tablets 2770
Ovral-28 Tablets 2770
Levlen/Tri-Levlen.................................. 651
Tri-Norinyl.. 2164
Triphasil-21 Tablets 2814
Triphasil-28 Tablets 2819

Ethynodiol Diacetate (Estrogens tend to increase serum thyroxine-binding globulin; patients with non-functioning thyroid may need to adjust thyroid dosage). Products include:

Demulen 2428

Glipizide (Dosage of hypoglycemic agent may need to be adjusted). Products include:

Glucotrol Tablets 1967
Glucotrol XL Extended Release Tablets 1968

Glyburide (Dosage of hypoglycemic agent may need to be adjusted). Products include:

DiaBeta Tablets 1239
Glynase PresTab Tablets 2609
Micronase Tablets 2623

Insulin, Human (Dosage of insulin may need to be adjusted).

No products indexed under this heading.

Insulin, Human Isophane Suspension (Dosage of insulin may need to be adjusted). Products include:

Novolin N Human Insulin 10 ml Vials.. 1795

Insulin, Human NPH (Dosage of insulin may need to be adjusted). Products include:

Humulin N, 100 Units 1448
Novolin N PenFill Cartridges Durable Insulin Delivery System 1798
Novolin N Prefilled Syringe Disposable Insulin Delivery System 1798

Insulin, Human Regular (Dosage of insulin may need to be adjusted). Products include:

Humulin R, 100 Units 1449
Novolin R Human Insulin 10 ml Vials.. 1795
Novolin R PenFill Cartridges Durable Insulin Delivery System 1798
Novolin R Prefilled Syringe Disposable Insulin Delivery System 1798
Velosulin BR Human Insulin 10 ml Vials.. 1795

Insulin, Human, Zinc Suspension (Dosage of insulin may need to be adjusted). Products include:

Humulin L, 100 Units 1446
Humulin U, 100 Units 1450
Novolin L Human Insulin 10 ml Vials.. 1795

Insulin, NPH (Dosage of insulin may need to be adjusted). Products include:

NPH, 100 Units 1450
Pork NPH, 100 Units.......................... 1452
Purified Pork NPH Isophane Insulin 1801

Insulin, Regular (Dosage of insulin may need to be adjusted). Products include:

Regular, 100 Units 1450
Pork Regular, 100 Units 1452
Pork Regular (Concentrated), 500 Units 1453
Purified Pork Regular Insulin 1801

Insulin, Zinc Crystals (Dosage of insulin may need to be adjusted). Products include:

NPH, 100 Units 1450

Insulin, Zinc Suspension (Dosage of insulin may need to be adjusted). Products include:

Iletin I 1450
Lente, 100 Units 1450
Iletin II.. 1452
Pork Lente, 100 Units.......................... 1452
Purified Pork Lente Insulin 1801

Levonorgestrel (Estrogens tend to increase serum thyroxine-binding globulin; patients with non-functioning thyroid may need to adjust thyroid dosage). Products include:

Levlen/Tri-Levlen.................................. 651
Nordette-21 Tablets............................. 2755
Nordette-28 Tablets............................. 2758
Norplant System 2759
Levlen/Tri-Levlen.................................. 651
Triphasil-21 Tablets 2814
Triphasil-28 Tablets 2819

Mestranol (Estrogens tend to increase serum thyroxine-binding globulin; patients with non-functioning thyroid may need to adjust thyroid dosage). Products include:

Norinyl 2088
Ortho-Novum.. 1872

Metformin Hydrochloride (Dosage of hypoglycemic agent may need to be adjusted). Products include:

Glucophage 752

Norethindrone (Estrogens tend to increase serum thyroxine-binding globulin; patients with non-functioning thyroid may need to adjust thyroid dosage). Products include:

Brevicon.. 2088
Micronor Tablets 1872
Modicon 1872
Norinyl 2088
Nor-Q D Tablets 2135
Ortho-Novum.. 1872
Ovcon 760
Tri-Norinyl.. 2164

Norethynodrel (Estrogens tend to increase serum thyroxine-binding globulin; patients with non-functioning thyroid may need to adjust thyroid dosage).

No products indexed under this heading.

Norgestimate (Estrogens tend to increase serum thyroxine-binding globulin; patients with non-functioning thyroid may need to adjust thyroid dosage). Products include:

Ortho-Cyclen/Ortho-Tri-Cyclen 1858
Ortho-Cyclen/Ortho Tri-Cyclen 1858

Norgestrel (Estrogens tend to increase serum thyroxine-binding globulin; patients with non-functioning thyroid may need to adjust thyroid dosage). Products include:

Lo/Ovral Tablets 2746
Lo/Ovral-28 Tablets............................. 2751
Ovral Tablets 2770
Ovral-28 Tablets 2770
Ovrette Tablets...................................... 2771

Polyestradiol Phosphate (Estrogens tend to increase serum thyroxine-binding globulin; patients with non-functioning thyroid may need to adjust thyroid dosage).

No products indexed under this heading.

Quinestrol (Estrogens tend to increase serum thyroxine-binding globulin; patients with non-functioning thyroid may need to adjust thyroid dosage).

No products indexed under this heading.

Tolazamide (Dosage of hypoglycemic agent may need to be adjusted).

No products indexed under this heading.

Tolbutamide (Dosage of hypoglycemic agent may need to be adjusted).

No products indexed under this heading.

Warfarin Sodium (Anticoagulant effects may be potentiated; dosage adjustment should be made). Products include:

Coumadin 926

LEVOXYL TABLETS

(Levothyroxine Sodium) 903

May interact with insulin, oral hypoglycemic agents, oral anticoagulants, estrogens, and certain other agents. Compounds in these categories include:

Acarbose (May cause an increase in the required dosage of oral hypoglycemics).

No products indexed under this heading.

Chlorotrianisene (Increases serum thyroxine-binding globulin (TBG) in patients with a non-functioning thyroid gland who are receiving thyroid replacement therapy thus decreasing thyroxine and increasing thyroid requirements in patients who are on estrogens or estrogen containing oral contraceptives).

No products indexed under this heading.

Chlorpropamide (May cause an increase in the required dosage of oral hypoglycemics). Products include:

Diabinese Tablets 1935

Cholestyramine (Impairs absorption; 4 to 5 hours should elapse between administration of cholestyramine and thyroid hormones). Products include:

Questran Light 769
Questran Powder 770

Dicumarol (Close supervision is advised; possible reduction in anticoagulant dosage).

No products indexed under this heading.

Dienestrol (Increases serum thyroxine-binding globulin (TBG) in patients with a non-functioning thyroid gland who are receiving thyroid replacement therapy thus decreasing thyroxine and increasing thyroid requirements in patients who are on estrogens or estrogen containing oral contraceptives). Products include:

Ortho Dienestrol Cream 1866

Diethylstilbestrol (Increases serum thyroxine-binding globulin (TBG) in patients with a non-functioning thyroid gland who are receiving thyroid replacement therapy thus decreasing thyroxine and increasing thyroid requirements in patients who are on estrogens or estrogen containing oral contraceptives). Products include:

Diethylstilbestrol Tablets 1437

Estradiol (Increases serum thyroxine-binding globulin (TBG) in patients with a non-functioning thyroid gland who are receiving thyroid replacement therapy thus decreasing thyroxine and increasing thyroid requirements in patients who are on estrogens or estrogen containing oral contraceptives). Products include:

Climara Transdermal System 645
Estrace Cream and Tablets 749
Estraderm Transdermal System 824

Estrogens, Conjugated (Increases serum thyroxine-binding globulin (TBG) in patients with a non-functioning thyroid gland who are receiving thyroid replacement therapy thus decreasing thyroxine and increasing thyroid requirements in patients who are on estrogens or estrogen containing oral contraceptives). Products include:

PMB 200 and PMB 400 2783
Premarin Intravenous 2787
Premarin with Methyltestosterone .. 2794
Premarin Tablets 2789
Premarin Vaginal Cream.................... 2791
Premphase 2797
Prempro.. 2801

(◻ Described in PDR For Nonprescription Drugs) (◉ Described in PDR For Ophthalmology)

Estrogens, Esterified (Increases serum thyroxine-binding globulin (TBG) in patients with a non-functioning thyroid gland who are receiving thyroid replacement therapy thus decreasing thyroxine and increasing thyroid requirements in patients who are on estrogens or estrogen containing oral contraceptives). Products include:

ESTRATAB Tablets (0.3, 0.625, 1.25, 2.5 mg) 2536
Estratest 2539
Menest Tablets 2494

Estropipate (Increases serum thyroxine-binding globulin (TBG) in patients with a non-functioning thyroid gland who are receiving thyroid replacement therapy thus decreasing thyroxine and increasing thyroid requirements in patients who are on estrogens or estrogen containing oral contraceptives). Products include:

Ogen Tablets 2627
Ogen Vaginal Cream 2630
Ortho-Est 1869

Ethinyl Estradiol (Increases serum thyroxine-binding globulin (TBG) in patients with a non-functioning thyroid gland who are receiving thyroid replacement therapy thus decreasing thyroxine and increasing thyroid requirements in patients who are on estrogens or estrogen containing oral contraceptives). Products include:

Brevicon 2088
Demulen 2428
Desogen Tablets 1817
Levlen/Tri-Levlen 651
Lo/Ovral Tablets 2746
Lo/Ovral-28 Tablets 2751
Modicon 1872
Nordette-21 Tablets 2755
Nordette-28 Tablets 2758
Norinyl 2088
Ortho-Cept 1851
Ortho-Cyclen/Ortho-Tri-Cyclen 1858
Ortho-Novum 1872
Ortho-Cyclen/Ortho Tri-Cyclen 1858
Ovcon 760
Ovral Tablets 2770
Ovral-28 Tablets 2770
Levlen/Tri-Levlen 651
Tri-Norinyl 2164
Triphasil-21 Tablets 2814
Triphasil-28 Tablets 2819

Glipizide (May cause an increase in the required dosage of oral hypoglycemics). Products include:

Glucotrol Tablets 1967
Glucotrol XL Extended Release Tablets 1968

Glyburide (May cause an increase in the required dosage of oral hypoglycemics). Products include:

DiaBeta Tablets 1239
Glynase PresTab Tablets 2609
Micronase Tablets 2623

Insulin, Human (May cause an increase in the required dosage of insulin).

No products indexed under this heading.

Insulin, Human Isophane Suspension (May cause an increase in the required dosage of insulin). Products include:

Novolin N Human Insulin 10 ml Vials 1795

Insulin, Human NPH (May cause an increase in the required dosage of insulin). Products include:

Humulin N, 100 Units 1448
Novolin N PenFill Cartridges Durable Insulin Delivery System 1798
Novolin N Prefilled Syringe Disposable Insulin Delivery System 1798

Insulin, Human Regular (May cause an increase in the required dosage of insulin). Products include:

Humulin R, 100 Units 1449
Novolin R Human Insulin 10 ml Vials 1795
Novolin R PenFill Cartridges Durable Insulin Delivery System 1798
Novolin R Prefilled Syringe Disposable Insulin Delivery System 1798
Velosulin BR Human Insulin 10 ml Vials 1795

Insulin, Human, Zinc Suspension (May cause an increase in the required dosage of insulin). Products include:

Humulin L, 100 Units 1446
Humulin U, 100 Units 1450
Novolin L Human Insulin 10 ml Vials 1795

Insulin, NPH (May cause an increase in the required dosage of insulin). Products include:

NPH, 100 Units 1450
Pork NPH, 100 Units 1452
Purified Pork NPH Isophane Insulin 1801

Insulin, Regular (May cause an increase in the required dosage of insulin). Products include:

Regular, 100 Units 1450
Pork Regular, 100 Units 1452
Pork Regular (Concentrated), 500 Units 1453
Purified Pork Regular Insulin 1801

Insulin, Zinc Crystals (May cause an increase in the required dosage of insulin). Products include:

NPH, 100 Units 1450

Insulin, Zinc Suspension (May cause an increase in the required dosage of insulin). Products include:

Iletin I 1450
Lente, 100 Units 1450
Iletin II 1452
Pork Lente, 100 Units 1452
Purified Pork Lente Insulin 1801

Metformin Hydrochloride (May cause an increase in the required dosage of oral hypoglycemics). Products include:

Glucophage 752

Polyestradiol Phosphate (Increases serum thyroxine-binding globulin (TBG) in patients with a non-functioning thyroid gland who are receiving thyroid replacement therapy thus decreasing thyroxine and increasing thyroid requirements in patients who are on estrogens or estrogen containing oral contraceptives).

No products indexed under this heading.

Quinestrol (Increases serum thyroxine-binding globulin (TBG) in patients with a non-functioning thyroid gland who are receiving thyroid replacement therapy thus decreasing thyroxine and increasing thyroid requirements in patients who are on estrogens or estrogen containing oral contraceptives).

No products indexed under this heading.

Tolazamide (May cause an increase in the required dosage of oral hypoglycemics).

No products indexed under this heading.

Tolbutamide (May cause an increase in the required dosage of oral hypoglycemics).

No products indexed under this heading.

Warfarin Sodium (Close supervision is advised; possible reduction in anticoagulant dosage). Products include:

Coumadin 926

LEVSIN DROPS

(Hyoscyamine Sulfate) ....2405 May interact with antimuscarinic drugs, phenothiazines, monoamine oxidase inhibitors, tricyclic antidepressants, antihistamines, antacids, and certain other agents. Compounds in these categories include:

Acrivastine (Additive adverse effects). Products include:

Semprex-D Capsules 463
Semprex-D Capsules 1167

Aluminum Carbonate Gel (Interferes with absorption of Levsin). Products include:

Basaljel 2703

Aluminum Hydroxide (Interferes with absorption of Levsin). Products include:

ALternaGEL Liquid 1316
Maximum Strength Ascriptin .... ⊕ 630
Cama Arthritis Pain Reliever .... ⊕ 785
Gaviscon Extra Strength Relief Formula Antacid Tablets .... ⊕ 819
Gaviscon Extra Strength Relief Formula Liquid Antacid .... ⊕ 819
Gaviscon Liquid Antacid .... ⊕ 820
Gelusil Liquid & Tablets .... ⊕ 855
Maalox Heartburn Relief Suspension .... ⊕ 642
Maalox Heartburn Relief Tablets .... ⊕ 641
Maalox Magnesia and Alumina Oral Suspension .... ⊕ 642
Maalox Plus Tablets .... ⊕ 643
Extra Strength Maalox Antacid Plus Antigas Liquid and Tablets ⊕ 638
Tempo Soft Antacid .... ⊕ 835

Aluminum Hydroxide Gel (Interferes with absorption of Levsin). Products include:

ALternaGEL Liquid .... ⊕ 659
Aludrox Oral Suspension 2695
Amphojel Suspension 2695
Amphojel Suspension without Flavor 2695
Amphojel Tablets 2695
Arthritis Pain Ascriptin .... ⊕ 631
Regular Strength Ascriptin Tablets .... ⊕ 629
Gaviscon Antacid Tablets .... ⊕ 819
Gaviscon-2 Antacid Tablets .... ⊕ 820
Mylanta Liquid 1317
Mylanta Tablets .... ⊕ 660
Mylanta Double Strength Liquid 1317
Mylanta Double Strength Tablets .. ⊕ 660
Nephrox Suspension .... ⊕ 655

Amantadine Hydrochloride (Additive adverse effects). Products include:

Symmetrel Capsules and Syrup 946

Amitriptyline Hydrochloride (Additive adverse effects). Products include:

Elavil 2838
Endep Tablets 2174
Etrafon 2355
Limbitrol 2180
Triavil Tablets 1757

Amoxapine (Additive adverse effects). Products include:

Asendin Tablets 1369

Astemizole (Additive adverse effects). Products include:

Hismanal Tablets 1293

Atropine Sulfate (Additive adverse effects). Products include:

Arco-Lase Plus Tablets 512
Atrohist Plus Tablets 454
Atropine Sulfate Sterile Ophthalmic Solution .... © 233
Donnatal 2060
Donnatal Extentabs 2061
Donnatal Tablets 2060
Lomotil 2439
Motofen Tablets 784
Urised Tablets 1964

Azatadine Maleate (Additive adverse effects). Products include:

Trinalin Repetabs Tablets 1330

Belladonna Alkaloids (Additive adverse effects). Products include:

Bellergal-S Tablets 2250
Hyland's Bed Wetting Tablets .... ⊕ 828
Hyland's EnurAid Tablets .... ⊕ 829

Hyland's Teething Tablets .... ⊕ 830

Bromodiphenhydramine Hydrochloride (Additive adverse effects).

No products indexed under this heading.

Brompheniramine Maleate (Additive adverse effects). Products include:

Alka Seltzer Plus Sinus Medicine .. ⊕ 707
Bromfed Capsules (Extended-Release) 1785
Bromfed Syrup .... ⊕ 733
Bromfed Tablets 1785
Bromfed-DM Cough Syrup 1786
Bromfed-PD Capsules (Extended-Release) 1785
Dimetane-DC Cough Syrup 2059
Dimetane-DX Cough Syrup 2059
Dimetapp Elixir .... ⊕ 773
Dimetapp Extentabs .... ⊕ 774
Dimetapp Tablets/Liqui-Gels .... ⊕ 775
Dimetapp Cold & Allergy Chewable Tablets .... ⊕ 773
Dimetapp DM Elixir .... ⊕ 774
Vicks DayQuil Allergy Relief 12-Hour Extended Release Tablets .. ⊕ 760
Vicks DayQuil Allergy Relief 4-Hour Tablets .... ⊕ 760

Chlorpheniramine Maleate (Additive adverse effects). Products include:

Alka-Seltzer Plus Cold Medicine .... ⊕ 705
Alka-Seltzer Plus Cold Medicine Liqui-Gels .... ⊕ 706
Alka-Seltzer Plus Cold & Cough Medicine .... ⊕ 708
Alka-Seltzer Plus Cold & Cough Medicine Liqui-Gels .... ⊕ 705
Allerest Children's Chewable Tablets .... ⊕ 627
Allerest Headache Strength Tablets .... ⊕ 627
Allerest Maximum Strength Tablets .... ⊕ 627
Allerest Sinus Pain Formula .... ⊕ 627
Allerest 12 Hour Caplets .... ⊕ 627
Ana-Kit Anaphylaxis Emergency Treatment Kit 617
Atrohist Pediatric Capsules 453
Atrohist Plus Tablets 454
BC Cold Powder Multi-Symptom Formula (Cold-Sinus-Allergy) ...... ⊕ 609
Cerose DM .... ⊕ 878
Cheracol Plus Head Cold/Cough Formula .... ⊕ 769
Children's Vicks DayQuil Allergy Relief .... ⊕ 757
Children's Vicks NyQuil Cold/Cough Relief .... ⊕ 758
Chlor-Trimeton Allergy Decongestant Tablets .... ⊕ 799
Chlor-Trimeton Allergy Tablets ...... ⊕ 798
Combist 2038
Comtrex Multi-Symptom Cold Reliever Tablets/Caplets/Liqui-Gels/Liquid .... ⊕ 615
Allergy-Sinus Comtrex Multi-Symptom Allergy-Sinus Formula Tablets .... ⊕ 617
Contac Continuous Action Nasal Decongestant/Antihistamine 12 Hour Capsules .... ⊕ 813
Contac Maximum Strength Continuous Action Decongestant/Antihistamine 12 Hour Caplets .. ⊕ 813
Contac Severe Cold and Flu Formula Caplets .... ⊕ 814
Coricidin 'D' Decongestant Tablets .... ⊕ 800
Coricidin Tablets .... ⊕ 800
D.A. Chewable Tablets 951
Deconamine 1320
Dura-Tap/PD Capsules 2867
Dura-Vent/DA Tablets 953
Extendryl 1005
Fedahist Gyrocaps 2401
Fedahist Timecaps 2401
Hycomine Compound Tablets 932
Isoclor Timesule Capsules .... ⊕ 637
Kronofed-A 977
Nolamine Timed-Release Tablets 785
Novahistine DH 2462
Novahistine Elixir .... ⊕ 823
Ornade Spansule Capsules 2502
PediaCare Cold Allergy Chewable Tablets .... ⊕ 677
PediaCare Cough-Cold Chewable Tablets 1553
PediaCare Cough-Cold Liquid 1553

IMPORTANT NOTE: Always consult each drug listing in the patient's regimen for possible interactions.

Levsin/Levsinex/Levbid | Interactions Index | 580

PediaCare NightRest Cough-Cold Liquid ... 1553
Pediatric Vicks 44m Cough & Cold Relief ... ▣ 764
Pyrroxate Caplets ... ▣ 772
Ryna ... ▣ 841
Sinarest Tablets ... ▣ 648
Sinarest Extra Strength Tablets ... ▣ 648
Sine-Off Sinus Medicine ... ▣ 825
Singlet Tablets ... ▣ 825
Sinulin Tablets ... 787
Sinutab Sinus Allergy Medication, Maximum Strength Tablets and Caplets ... ▣ 860
Sudafed Plus Liquid ... ▣ 862
Sudafed Plus Tablets ... ▣ 863
Teldrin 12 Hour Antihistamine/Nasal Decongestant Allergy Relief Capsules ... ▣ 826
TheraFlu ... ▣ 787
TheraFlu Maximum Strength Nighttime Flu, Cold & Cough Medicine ... ▣ 788
Triaminic Allergy Tablets ... ▣ 789
Triaminic Cold Tablets ... ▣ 790
Triaminic Nite Light ... ▣ 791
Triaminic Syrup ... ▣ 792
Triaminic-12 Tablets ... ▣ 792
Triaminicin Tablets ... ▣ 793
Triaminicol Multi-Symptom Cold Tablets ... ▣ 793
Triaminicol Multi-Symptom Relief ▣ 794
Tussend ... 1783
Children's TYLENOL Cold Multi-Symptom Liquid Formula and Chewable Tablets ... 1561
Children's TYLENOL Cold Plus Cough Multi Symptom Tablets and Liquid ... ▣ 681
TYLENOL Maximum Strength Allergy Sinus Medication Gelcaps and Caplets ... 1563
TYLENOL Cold Multi-Symptom Formula Medication Tablets and Caplets ... 1561
TYLENOL Cold Multi-Symptom Hot Medication Liquid Packets ... 1557
Vicks 44 LiquiCaps Cough, Cold & Flu Relief ... ▣ 755
Vicks 44M Cough, Cold & Flu Relief ... ▣ 756

Chlorpheniramine Polistirex (Additive adverse effects). Products include:
Tussionex Pennkinetic Extended-Release Suspension ... 998

Chlorpheniramine Tannate (Additive adverse effects). Products include:
Atrohist Pediatric Suspension ... 454
Ricobid Tablets and Pediatric Suspension ... 2038
Rynatan ... 2673
Rynatuss ... 2673

Chlorpromazine (Additive adverse effects). Products include:
Thorazine Suppositories ... 2523

Chlorpromazine Hydrochloride (Additive adverse effects). Products include:
Thorazine ... 2523

Clemastine Fumarate (Additive adverse effects). Products include:
Tavist Syrup ... 2297
Tavist Tablets ... 2298
Tavist-1 12 Hour Relief Tablets ... ▣ 787
Tavist-D 12 Hour Relief Tablets ... ▣ 787

Clidinium Bromide (Additive adverse effects). Products include:
Librax Capsules ... 2176
Quarzan Capsules ... 2181

Clomipramine Hydrochloride (Additive adverse effects). Products include:
Anafranil Capsules ... 803

Cyproheptadine Hydrochloride (Additive adverse effects). Products include:
Periactin ... 1724

Desipramine Hydrochloride (Additive adverse effects). Products include:
Norpramin Tablets ... 1526

Dexchlorpheniramine Maleate (Additive adverse effects).
No products indexed under this heading.

Dicyclomine Hydrochloride (Additive adverse effects). Products include:
Bentyl ... 1501

Dihydroxyaluminum Sodium Carbonate (Interferes with absorption of Levsin).
No products indexed under this heading.

Diphenhydramine Citrate (Additive adverse effects). Products include:
Excedrin P.M. Analgesic/Sleeping Aid Tablets, Caplets, Liquigels ... 733

Diphenhydramine Hydrochloride (Additive adverse effects). Products include:
Actifed Allergy Daytime/Nighttime Caplets ... ▣ 844
Actifed Sinus Daytime/Nighttime Tablets and Caplets ... ▣ 846
Arthritis Foundation NightTime Caplets ... ▣ 674
Extra Strength Bayer PM Aspirin .. ▣ 713
Bayer Select Night Time Pain Relief Formula ... ▣ 716
Benadryl Allergy Decongestant Liquid Medication ... ▣ 848
Benadryl Allergy Decongestant Tablets ... ▣ 848
Benadryl Allergy Liquid Medication ... ▣ 849
Benadryl Allergy ... ▣ 848
Benadryl Allergy Sinus Headache Formula Caplets ... ▣ 849
Benadryl Capsules ... 1898
Benadryl Dye-Free Allergy Liquigel Softgels ... ▣ 850
Benadryl Dye-Free Allergy Liquid Medication ... ▣ 850
Benadryl Itch Relief Cream, Children's Formula and Maximum Strength 2% ... ▣ 851
Benadryl Itch Relief Spray, Children's Formula and Maximum Strength 2% ... ▣ 851
Benadryl Itch Relief Stick Maximum Strength 2% ... ▣ 850
Benadryl Itch Stopping Gel, Children's Formula and Maximum Strength 2% ... ▣ 851
Benadryl Kapseals ... 1898
Benadryl Injection ... 1898
Contac Day & Night Cold/Flu Night Caplets ... ▣ 812
Contac Night Allergy/Sinus Caplets ... ▣ 812
Extra Strength Doan's P.M. ... ▣ 633
Legatrin PM ... ▣ 651
Miles Nervine Nighttime Sleep-Aid ▣ 723
Nytol QuickCaps Caplets ... ▣ 610
Sleepinal Night-time Sleep Aid Capsules and Softgels ... ▣ 834
TYLENOL Maximum Strength Allergy Sinus NightTime Medication Caplets ... 1555
TYLENOL Flu NightTime, Maximum Strength, Gelcaps ... 1566
TYLENOL Maximum Strength Flu NightTime Hot Medication Packets ... 1562
TYLENOL PM, Extra Strength Pain Reliever/Sleep Aid Caplets, Geltabs, Gelcaps ... 1560
TYLENOL Severe Allergy Medication Caplets ... 1564
Maximum Strength Unisom Sleepgels ... 1934
Unisom With Pain Relief-Nighttime Sleep Aid and Pain Reliever ... 1934

Diphenylpyraline Hydrochloride (Additive adverse effects).
No products indexed under this heading.

Doxepin Hydrochloride (Additive adverse effects). Products include:
Sinequan ... 2205
Zonalon Cream ... 1055

Fluphenazine Decanoate (Additive adverse effects). Products include:
Prolixin Decanoate ... 509

Fluphenazine Enanthate (Additive adverse effects). Products include:
Prolixin Enanthate ... 509

Fluphenazine Hydrochloride (Additive adverse effects). Products include:
Prolixin ... 509

Furazolidone (Additive adverse effects). Products include:
Furoxone ... 2046

Glycopyrrolate (Additive adverse effects). Products include:
Robinul Forte Tablets ... 2072
Robinul Injectable ... 2072
Robinul Tablets ... 2072

Haloperidol (Additive adverse effects). Products include:
Haldol Injection, Tablets and Concentrate ... 1575

Haloperidol Decanoate (Additive adverse effects). Products include:
Haldol Decanoate ... 1577

Hyoscyamine (Additive adverse effects). Products include:
Cystospaz Tablets ... 1963
Urised Tablets ... 1964

Imipramine Hydrochloride (Additive adverse effects). Products include:
Tofranil Ampuls ... 854
Tofranil Tablets ... 856

Imipramine Pamoate (Additive adverse effects). Products include:
Tofranil-PM Capsules ... 857

Ipratropium Bromide (Additive adverse effects). Products include:
Atrovent Inhalation Aerosol ... 671
Atrovent Inhalation Solution ... 673

Isocarboxazid (Additive adverse effects).
No products indexed under this heading.

Loratadine (Additive adverse effects). Products include:
Claritin ... 2349
Claritin-D ... 2350

Magaldrate (Interferes with absorption of Levsin).
No products indexed under this heading.

Magnesium Hydroxide (Interferes with absorption of Levsin). Products include:
Aludrox Oral Suspension ... 2695
Arthritis Pain Ascriptin ... ▣ 631
Maximum Strength Ascriptin ... ▣ 630
Regular Strength Ascriptin Tablets ... ▣ 629
Di-Gel Antacid/Anti-Gas ... ▣ 801
Gelusil Liquid & Tablets ... ▣ 855
Maalox Magnesia and Alumina Oral Suspension ... ▣ 642
Maalox Plus Tablets ... ▣ 643
Extra Strength Maalox Antacid Plus Antigas Liquid and Tablets ▣ 638
Mylanta Calcium Carbonate and Magnesium Hydroxide Tablets ... 1318
Mylanta Liquid ... 1317
Mylanta Tablets ... ▣ 660
Mylanta Double Strength Liquid ... 1317
Mylanta Double Strength Tablets .. ▣ 660
Phillips' Milk of Magnesia Liquid ... ▣ 729
Rolaids Tablets ... ▣ 843
Tempo Soft Antacid ... ▣ 835

Magnesium Oxide (Interferes with absorption of Levsin). Products include:
Beelith Tablets ... 639
Bufferin Analgesic Tablets and Caplets ... ▣ 613
Caltrate PLUS ... ▣ 665
Cama Arthritis Pain Reliever ... ▣ 785
Mag-Ox 400 ... 668
Uro-Mag ... 668

Maprotiline Hydrochloride (Additive adverse effects). Products include:
Ludiomil Tablets ... 843

Mepenzolate Bromide (Additive adverse effects).
No products indexed under this heading.

Mesoridazine Besylate (Additive adverse effects). Products include:
Serentil ... 684

Methdilazine Hydrochloride (Additive adverse effects).
No products indexed under this heading.

Methotrimeprazine (Additive adverse effects). Products include:
Levoprome ... 1274

Nortriptyline Hydrochloride (Additive adverse effects). Products include:
Pamelor ... 2280

Oxyphenonium Bromide (Additive adverse effects).

Perphenazine (Additive adverse effects). Products include:
Etrafon ... 2355
Triavil Tablets ... 1757
Trilafon ... 2389

Phenelzine Sulfate (Additive adverse effects). Products include:
Nardil ... 1920

Prochlorperazine (Additive adverse effect). Products include:
Compazine ... 2470

Promethazine Hydrochloride (Additive adverse effects). Products include:
Mepergan Injection ... 2753
Phenergan with Codeine ... 2777
Phenergan with Dextromethorphan 2778
Phenergan Injection ... 2773
Phenergan Suppositories ... 2775
Phenergan Syrup ... 2774
Phenergan Tablets ... 2775
Phenergan VC ... 2779
Phenergan VC with Codeine ... 2781

Propantheline Bromide (Additive adverse effects). Products include:
Pro-Banthine Tablets ... 2052

Protriptyline Hydrochloride (Additive adverse effects). Products include:
Vivactil Tablets ... 1774

Pyrilamine Maleate (Additive adverse effects). Products include:
4-Way Fast Acting Nasal Spray (regular & mentholated) ... ▣ 621
Maximum Strength Multi-Symptom Formula Midol ... ▣ 722
PMS Multi-Symptom Formula Midol ... ▣ 723

Pyrilamine Tannate (Additive adverse effects). Products include:
Atrohist Pediatric Suspension ... 454
Rynatan ... 2673

Scopolamine (Additive adverse effects). Products include:
Transderm Scōp Transdermal Therapeutic System ... 869

Scopolamine Hydrobromide (Additive adverse effects). Products include:
Atrohist Plus Tablets ... 454
Donnatal ... 2060
Donnatal Extentabs ... 2061
Donnatal Tablets ... 2060

Selegiline Hydrochloride (Additive adverse effects). Products include:
Eldepryl Tablets ... 2550

Terfenadine (Additive adverse effects). Products include:
Seldane Tablets ... 1536
Seldane-D Extended-Release Tablets ... 1538

Thioridazine Hydrochloride (Additive adverse effects). Products include:
Mellaril ... 2269

(▣ Described in PDR For Nonprescription Drugs) (⊙ Described in PDR For Ophthalmology)

Interactions Index

Librax

Tranylcypromine Sulfate (Additive adverse effects). Products include:

Parnate Tablets 2503

Tridihexethyl Chloride (Additive adverse effects).

No products indexed under this heading.

Trifluoperazine Hydrochloride (Additive adverse effects). Products include:

Stelazine 2514

Trimeprazine Tartrate (Additive adverse effects). Products include:

Temaril Tablets, Syrup and Spansule Extended-Release Capsules... 483

Trimipramine Maleate (Additive adverse effects). Products include:

Surmontil Capsules.................................. 2811

Tripelennamine Hydrochloride (Additive adverse effects). Products include:

PBZ Tablets 845
PBZ-SR Tablets.. 844

Triprolidine Hydrochloride (Additive adverse effects). Products include:

Actifed Plus Caplets .... ⊕ 845
Actifed Plus Tablets .... ⊕ 845
Actifed with Codeine Cough Syrup.. 1067
Actifed Syrup... ⊕ 846
Actifed Tablets .... ⊕ 844

LEVSIN ELIXIR

(Hyoscyamine Sulfate) 2405
See **Levsin Drops**

LEVSIN INJECTION

(Hyoscyamine Sulfate) 2405
See **Levsin Drops**

LEVSIN TABLETS

(Hyoscyamine Sulfate) 2405
See **Levsin Drops**

LEVSIN/SL TABLETS

(Hyoscyamine Sulfate) 2405
See **Levsin Drops**

LEVSINEX TIMECAPS

(Hyoscyamine Sulfate) 2405
See **Levsin Drops**

LIBRAX CAPSULES

(Chlordiazepoxide Hydrochloride, Clidinium Bromide) 2176

May interact with monoamine oxidase inhibitors, phenothiazines, psychotropics, central nervous system depressants, and certain other agents. Compounds in these categories include:

Alfentanil Hydrochloride (Additive effects). Products include:

Alfenta Injection 1286

Alprazolam (Additive effects; concomitant use not recommended). Products include:

Xanax Tablets 2649

Amitriptyline Hydrochloride (Additive effects; concomitant use not recommended). Products include:

Elavil 2838
Endep Tablets 2174
Etrafon 2355
Limbitrol 2180
Triavil Tablets 1757

Amoxapine (Concomitant use not recommended). Products include:

Asendin Tablets 1369

Aprobarbital (Additive effects).

No products indexed under this heading.

Buprenorphine (Additive effects). Products include:

Buprenex Injectable 2006

Buspirone Hydrochloride (Additive effects; concomitant use not recommended). Products include:

BuSpar 737

Butabarbital (Additive effects).

No products indexed under this heading.

Butalbital (Additive effects). Products include:

Esgic-plus Tablets 1013
Fioricet Tablets... 2258
Fioricet with Codeine Capsules 2260
Fiorinal Capsules 2261
Fiorinal with Codeine Capsules 2262
Fiorinal Tablets 2261
Phrenilin 785
Sedapap Tablets 50 mg/650 mg .. 1543

Chlordiazepoxide (Additive effects). Products include:

Libritabs Tablets 2177
Limbitrol 2180

Chlorpromazine (Additive effects; concomitant use not recommended; potentiates Librax). Products include:

Thorazine Suppositories 2523

Chlorprothixene (Additive effects; concomitant use not recommended).

No products indexed under this heading.

Chlorprothixene Hydrochloride (Additive effects; concomitant use not recommended).

No products indexed under this heading.

Clorazepate Dipotassium (Additive effects; concomitant use not recommended). Products include:

Tranxene 451

Clozapine (Additive effects). Products include:

Clozaril Tablets.. 2252

Codeine Phosphate (Additive effects). Products include:

Actifed with Codeine Cough Syrup.. 1067
Brontex 1981
Deconsal C Expectorant Syrup 456
Deconsal Pediatric Syrup 457
Dimetane-DC Cough Syrup 2059
Empirin with Codeine Tablets........... 1093
Fioricet with Codeine Capsules 2260
Fiorinal with Codeine Capsules 2262
Isoclor Expectorant.................................. 990
Novahistine DH....................................... 2462
Novahistine Expectorant.......................... 2463
Nucofed 2051
Phenergan with Codeine.......................... 2777
Phenergan VC with Codeine 2781
Robitussin A-C Syrup.............................. 2073
Robitussin-DAC Syrup 2074
Ryna .... ⊕ 841
Soma Compound w/Codeine Tablets 2676
Tussi-Organidin NR Liquid and S NR Liquid 2677
Tylenol with Codeine 1583

Desflurane (Additive effects). Products include:

Suprane 1813

Desipramine Hydrochloride (Concomitant use not recommended). Products include:

Norpramin Tablets 1526

Dezocine (Additive effects). Products include:

Dalgan Injection 538

Diazepam (Additive effects; concomitant use not recommended). Products include:

Dizac 1809
Valium Injectable 2182
Valium Tablets 2183
Valrelease Capsules 2169

Doxepin Hydrochloride (Concomitant use not recommended). Products include:

Sinequan 2205
Zonalon Cream 1055

Droperidol (Additive effects; concomitant use not recommended). Products include:

Inapsine Injection..................................... 1296

Enflurane (Additive effects).

No products indexed under this heading.

Estazolam (Additive effects). Products include:

ProSom Tablets 449

Ethchlorvynol (Additive effects). Products include:

Placidyl Capsules..................................... 448

Ethinamate (Additive effects).

No products indexed under this heading.

Fentanyl (Additive effects). Products include:

Duragesic Transdermal System........ 1288

Fentanyl Citrate (Additive effects). Products include:

Sublimaze Injection.................................. 1307

Fluphenazine Decanoate (Additive effects; concomitant use not recommended; potentiates Librax). Products include:

Prolixin Decanoate 509

Fluphenazine Enanthate (Additive effects; concomitant use not recommended; potentiates Librax). Products include:

Prolixin Enanthate 509

Fluphenazine Hydrochloride (Additive effects; concomitant use not recommended; potentiates Librax). Products include:

Prolixin 509

Flurazepam Hydrochloride (Additive effects). Products include:

Dalmane Capsules.................................... 2173

Furazolidone (Potentiates Librax; concomitant use not recommended). Products include:

Furoxone 2046

Glutethimide (Additive effects).

No products indexed under this heading.

Haloperidol (Additive effects; concomitant use not recommended). Products include:

Haldol Injection, Tablets and Concentrate 1575

Haloperidol Decanoate (Additive effects; concomitant use not recommended). Products include:

Haldol Decanoate..................................... 1577

Hydrocodone Bitartrate (Additive effects). Products include:

Anexsia 5/500 Elixir 1781
Anexia Tablets.. 1782
Codiclear DH Syrup 791
Deconamine CX Cough and Cold Liquid and Tablets.................................... 1319
Duratuss HD Elixir................................... 2565
Hycodan Tablets and Syrup 930
Hycomine Compound Tablets 932
Hycomine 931
Hycotuss Expectorant Syrup 933
Hydrocet Capsules 782
Lorcet 10/650.. 1018
Lortab 2566
Tussend 1783
Tussend Expectorant 1785
Vicodin Tablets 1356
Vicodin ES Tablets 1357
Vicodin Tuss Expectorant 1358
Zydone Capsules 949

Hydrocodone Polistirex (Additive effects). Products include:

Tussionex Pennkinetic Extended-Release Suspension 998

Hydroxyzine Hydrochloride (Additive effects; concomitant use not recommended). Products include:

Atarax Tablets & Syrup........................... 2185
Marax Tablets & DF Syrup...................... 2200
Vistaril Intramuscular Solution......... 2216

Imipramine Hydrochloride (Concomitant use not recommended). Products include:

Tofranil Ampuls 854
Tofranil Tablets 856

Imipramine Pamoate (Concomitant use not recommended). Products include:

Tofranil-PM Capsules.............................. 857

Isocarboxazid (Potentiates Librax; concomitant use not recommended).

No products indexed under this heading.

Isoflurane (Additive effects).

No products indexed under this heading.

Ketamine Hydrochloride (Additive effects).

No products indexed under this heading.

Levomethadyl Acetate Hydrochloride (Additive effects). Products include:

Orlaam 2239

Levorphanol Tartrate (Additive effects). Products include:

Levo-Dromoran 2129

Lithium Carbonate (Concomitant use not recommended). Products include:

Eskalith 2485
Lithium Carbonate Capsules & Tablets 2230
Lithonate/Lithotabs/Lithobid 2543

Lithium Citrate (Concomitant use not recommended).

No products indexed under this heading.

Lorazepam (Additive effects; concomitant use not recommended). Products include:

Ativan Injection.. 2698
Ativan Tablets 2700

Loxapine Hydrochloride (Additive effects; concomitant use not recommended). Products include:

Loxitane 1378

Loxapine Succinate (Additive effects). Products include:

Loxitane Capsules 1378

Maprotiline Hydrochloride (Concomitant use not recommended). Products include:

Ludiomil Tablets...................................... 843

Meperidine Hydrochloride (Additive effects). Products include:

Demerol 2308
Mepergan Injection 2753

Mephobarbital (Additive effects). Products include:

Mebaral Tablets 2322

Meprobamate (Additive effects; concomitant use not recommended). Products include:

Miltown Tablets 2672
PMB 200 and PMB 400 2783

Mesoridazine Besylate (Additive effects; concomitant use not recommended; potentiates Librax). Products include:

Serentil... 684

Methadone Hydrochloride (Additive effects). Products include:

Methadone Hydrochloride Oral Concentrate 2233
Methadone Hydrochloride Oral Solution & Tablets................................... 2235

Methohexital Sodium (Additive effects). Products include:

Brevital Sodium Vials.............................. 1429

Methotrimeprazine (Additive effects). Products include:

Levoprome 1274

Methoxyflurane (Additive effects).

No products indexed under this heading.

IMPORTANT NOTE: Always consult each drug listing in the patient's regimen for possible interactions.

Midazolam Hydrochloride (Additive effects; concomitant use not recommended). Products include:
- Versed Injection ... 2170

Molindone Hydrochloride (Additive effects; concomitant use not recommended). Products include:
- Moban Tablets and Concentrate ... 1048

Morphine Sulfate (Additive effects). Products include:
- Astramorph/PF Injection, USP (Preservative-Free) ... 535
- Duramorph ... 962
- Infumorph 200 and Infumorph 500 Sterile Solutions ... 965
- MS Contin Tablets ... 1994
- MSIR ... 1997
- Oramorph SR (Morphine Sulfate Sustained Release Tablets) ... 2236
- RMS Suppositories ... 2657
- Roxanol ... 2243

Nortriptyline Hydrochloride (Concomitant use not recommended). Products include:
- Pamelor ... 2280

Opium Alkaloids (Additive effects).
- No products indexed under this heading.

Oxazepam (Additive effects; concomitant use not recommended). Products include:
- Serax Capsules ... 2810
- Serax Tablets ... 2810

Oxycodone Hydrochloride (Additive effects). Products include:
- Percocet Tablets ... 938
- Percodan Tablets ... 939
- Percodan-Demi Tablets ... 940
- Roxicodone Tablets, Oral Solution & Intensol (Oxycodone) ... 2244
- Tylox Capsules ... 1584

Pentobarbital Sodium (Additive effects). Products include:
- Nembutal Sodium Capsules ... 436
- Nembutal Sodium Solution ... 438
- Nembutal Sodium Suppositories ... 440

Perphenazine (Additive effects; concomitant use not recommended; potentiates Librax). Products include:
- Etrafon ... 2355
- Triavil Tablets ... 1757
- Trilafon ... 2389

Phenelzine Sulfate (Potentiates Librax; concomitant use not recommended). Products include:
- Nardil ... 1920

Phenobarbital (Additive effects). Products include:
- Arco-Lase Plus Tablets ... 512
- Bellergal-S Tablets ... 2250
- Donnatal ... 2060
- Donnatal Extentabs ... 2061
- Donnatal Tablets ... 2060
- Phenobarbital Elixir and Tablets ... 1469
- Quadrinal Tablets ... 1350

Prazepam (Additive effects; concomitant use not recommended).
- No products indexed under this heading.

Prochlorperazine (Additive effects; concomitant use not recommended). Products include:
- Compazine ... 2470

Promethazine Hydrochloride (Additive effects; concomitant use not recommended; potentiates Librax). Products include:
- Mepergan Injection ... 2753
- Phenergan with Codeine ... 2777
- Phenergan with Dextromethorphan ... 2778
- Phenergan Injection ... 2773
- Phenergan Suppositories ... 2775
- Phenergan Syrup ... 2774
- Phenergan Tablets ... 2775
- Phenergan VC ... 2779
- Phenergan VC with Codeine ... 2781

Propofol (Additive effects). Products include:
- Diprivan Injection ... 2833

Propoxyphene Hydrochloride (Additive effects). Products include:
- Darvon ... 1435
- Wygesic Tablets ... 2827

Propoxyphene Napsylate (Additive effects). Products include:
- Darvon-N/Darvocet-N ... 1433

Protriptyline Hydrochloride (Concomitant use not recommended). Products include:
- Vivactil Tablets ... 1774

Quazepam (Additive effects). Products include:
- Doral Tablets ... 2664

Risperidone (Additive effects). Products include:
- Risperdal ... 1301

Secobarbital Sodium (Additive effects). Products include:
- Seconal Sodium Pulvules ... 1474

Selegiline Hydrochloride (Potentiates Librax; concomitant use not recommended). Products include:
- Eldepryl Tablets ... 2550

Sufentanil Citrate (Additive effects). Products include:
- Sufenta Injection ... 1309

Temazepam (Additive effects). Products include:
- Restoril Capsules ... 2284

Thiamylal Sodium (Additive effects).
- No products indexed under this heading.

Thioridazine Hydrochloride (Additive effects; concomitant use not recommended; potentiates Librax). Products include:
- Mellaril ... 2269

Thiothixene (Additive effects; concomitant use not recommended). Products include:
- Navane Capsules and Concentrate ... 2201
- Navane Intramuscular ... 2202

Tranylcypromine Sulfate (Potentiates Librax; concomitant use not recommended). Products include:
- Parnate Tablets ... 2503

Triazolam (Additive effects). Products include:
- Halcion Tablets ... 2611

Trifluoperazine Hydrochloride (Additive effects; concomitant use not recommended; potentiates Librax). Products include:
- Stelazine ... 2514

Trimipramine Maleate (Concomitant use not recommended). Products include:
- Surmontil Capsules ... 2811

Zolpidem Tartrate (Additive effects). Products include:
- Ambien Tablets ... 2416

Food Interactions

Alcohol (Additive effects).

LIBRITABS TABLETS

(Chlordiazepoxide) ... 2177

May interact with central nervous system depressants, monoamine oxidase inhibitors, phenothiazines, oral anticoagulants, and certain other agents. Compounds in these categories include:

Alfentanil Hydrochloride (Additive effect). Products include:
- Alfenta Injection ... 1286

Alprazolam (Additive effect). Products include:
- Xanax Tablets ... 2649

Aprobarbital (Additive effect).
- No products indexed under this heading.

Buprenorphine (Additive effect). Products include:
- Buprenex Injectable ... 2006

Buspirone Hydrochloride (Additive effect). Products include:
- BuSpar ... 737

Butabarbital (Additive effect).
- No products indexed under this heading.

Butalbital (Additive effect). Products include:
- Esgic-plus Tablets ... 1013
- Fioricet Tablets ... 2258
- Fioricet with Codeine Capsules ... 2260
- Fiorinal Capsules ... 2261
- Fiorinal with Codeine Capsules ... 2262
- Fiorinal Tablets ... 2261
- Phrenilin ... 785
- Sedapap Tablets 50 mg/650 mg ... 1543

Chlordiazepoxide Hydrochloride (Additive effect). Products include:
- Librax Capsules ... 2176
- Librium Capsules ... 2178
- Librium Injectable ... 2179

Chlorpromazine (Additive effect; potentiates Librium). Products include:
- Thorazine Suppositories ... 2523

Chlorprothixene (Additive effects).
- No products indexed under this heading.

Chlorprothixene Hydrochloride (Additive effect).
- No products indexed under this heading.

Clorazepate Dipotassium (Additive effect). Products include:
- Tranxene ... 451

Clozapine (Additive effect). Products include:
- Clozaril Tablets ... 2252

Codeine Phosphate (Additive effect). Products include:
- Actifed with Codeine Cough Syrup ... 1067
- Brontex ... 1981
- Deconsal C Expectorant Syrup ... 456
- Deconsal Pediatric Syrup ... 457
- Dimetane-DC Cough Syrup ... 2059
- Empirin with Codeine Tablets ... 1093
- Fioricet with Codeine Capsules ... 2260
- Fiorinal with Codeine Capsules ... 2262
- Isoclor Expectorant ... 990
- Novahistine DH ... 2462
- Novahistine Expectorant ... 2463
- Nucofed ... 2051
- Phenergan with Codeine ... 2777
- Phenergan VC with Codeine ... 2781
- Robitussin A-C Syrup ... 2073
- Robitussin-DAC Syrup ... 2074
- Ryna ... ▣ 841
- Soma Compound w/Codeine Tablets ... 2676
- Tussi-Organidin NR Liquid and S NR Liquid ... 2677
- Tylenol with Codeine ... 1583

Desflurane (Additive effect). Products include:
- Suprane ... 1813

Dezocine (Additive effect). Products include:
- Dalgan Injection ... 538

Diazepam (Additive effect). Products include:
- Dizac ... 1809
- Valium Injectable ... 2182
- Valium Tablets ... 2183
- Valrelease Capsules ... 2169

Dicumarol (Potential for variable effects on blood coagulation).
- No products indexed under this heading.

Droperidol (Additive effect). Products include:
- Inapsine Injection ... 1296

Enflurane (Additive effect).
- No products indexed under this heading.

Estazolam (Additive effect). Products include:
- ProSom Tablets ... 449

Ethchlorvynol (Additive effect). Products include:
- Placidyl Capsules ... 448

Ethinamate (Additive effect).
- No products indexed under this heading.

Fentanyl (Additive effect). Products include:
- Duragesic Transdermal System ... 1288

Fentanyl Citrate (Additive effect). Products include:
- Sublimaze Injection ... 1307

Fluphenazine Decanoate (Additive effect; potentiates Librium). Products include:
- Prolixin Decanoate ... 509

Fluphenazine Enanthate (Additive effect; potentiates Librium). Products include:
- Prolixin Enanthate ... 509

Fluphenazine Hydrochloride (Additive effect; potentiates Librium). Products include:
- Prolixin ... 509

Flurazepam Hydrochloride (Additive effect). Products include:
- Dalmane Capsules ... 2173

Furazolidone (Potentiates Librium). Products include:
- Furoxone ... 2046

Glutethimide (Additive effect).
- No products indexed under this heading.

Haloperidol (Additive effect). Products include:
- Haldol Injection, Tablets and Concentrate ... 1575

Haloperidol Decanoate (Additive effect). Products include:
- Haldol Decanoate ... 1577

Hydrocodone Bitartrate (Additive effect). Products include:
- Anexsia 5/500 Elixir ... 1781
- Anexia Tablets ... 1782
- Codiclear DH Syrup ... 791
- Deconamine CX Cough and Cold Liquid and Tablets ... 1319
- Duratuss HD Elixir ... 2565
- Hycodan Tablets and Syrup ... 930
- Hycomine Compound Tablets ... 932
- Hycomine ... 931
- Hycotuss Expectorant Syrup ... 933
- Hydrocet Capsules ... 782
- Lorcet 10/650 ... 1018
- Lortab ... 2566
- Tussend ... 1783
- Tussend Expectorant ... 1785
- Vicodin Tablets ... 1356
- Vicodin ES Tablets ... 1357
- Vicodin Tuss Expectorant ... 1358
- Zydone Capsules ... 949

Hydrocodone Polistirex (Additive effect). Products include:
- Tussionex Pennkinetic Extended-Release Suspension ... 998

Hydroxyzine Hydrochloride (Additive effect). Products include:
- Atarax Tablets & Syrup ... 2185
- Marax Tablets & DF Syrup ... 2200
- Vistaril Intramuscular Solution ... 2216

Isocarboxazid (Potentiates Librium).
- No products indexed under this heading.

Isoflurane (Additive effect).
- No products indexed under this heading.

Ketamine Hydrochloride (Additive effect).
- No products indexed under this heading.

Levomethadyl Acetate Hydrochloride (Additive effect). Products include:
- Orlamm ... 2239

Levorphanol Tartrate (Additive effect). Products include:
- Levo-Dromoran ... 2129

(▣ Described in PDR For Nonprescription Drugs) (◉ Described in PDR For Ophthalmology)

583 Interactions Index Librium Injectable

Lorazepam (Additive effect). Products include:
Ativan Injection 2698
Ativan Tablets 2700
Loxapine Hydrochloride (Additive effect). Products include:
Loxitane 1378
Loxapine Succinate (Additive effect). Products include:
Loxitane Capsules 1378
Meperidine Hydrochloride (Additive effect). Products include:
Demerol 2308
Mepergan Injection 2753
Mephobarbital (Additive effect). Products include:
Mebaral Tablets 2322
Meprobamate (Additive effect). Products include:
Miltown Tablets 2672
PMB 200 and PMB 400 2783
Mesoridazine Besylate (Additive effect; potentiates Librium). Products include:
Serentil 684
Methadone Hydrochloride (Additive effect). Products include:
Methadone Hydrochloride Oral Concentrate 2233
Methadone Hydrochloride Oral Solution & Tablets 2235
Methohexital Sodium (Additive effect). Products include:
Brevital Sodium Vials 1429
Methotrimeprazine (Additive effect). Products include:
Levoprome 1274
Methoxyflurane (Additive effect).
No products indexed under this heading.
Midazolam Hydrochloride (Additive effect). Products include:
Versed Injection 2170
Molindone Hydrochloride (Additive effect). Products include:
Moban Tablets and Concentrate 1048
Morphine Sulfate (Additive effect). Products include:
Astramorph/PF Injection, USP (Preservative-Free) 535
Duramorph 962
Infumorph 200 and Infumorph 500 Sterile Solutions 965
MS Contin Tablets 1994
MSIR 1997
Oramorph SR (Morphine Sulfate Sustained Release Tablets) 2236
RMS Suppositories 2657
Roxanol 2243
Opium Alkaloids (Additive effect).
No products indexed under this heading.
Oxazepam (Additive effect). Products include:
Serax Capsules 2810
Serax Tablets 2810
Oxycodone Hydrochloride (Additive effect). Products include:
Percocet Tablets 938
Percodan Tablets 939
Percodan-Demi Tablets 940
Roxicodone Tablets, Oral Solution & Intensol (Oxycodone) 2244
Tylox Capsules 1584
Pentobarbital Sodium (Additive effect). Products include:
Nembutal Sodium Capsules 436
Nembutal Sodium Solution 438
Nembutal Sodium Suppositories 440
Perphenazine (Additive effect; potentiates Librium). Products include:
Etrafon 2355
Triavil Tablets 1757
Trilafon 2389
Phenelzine Sulfate (Potentiates Librium). Products include:
Nardil 1920
Phenobarbital (Additive effect). Products include:
Arco-Lase Plus Tablets 512
Bellergal-S Tablets 2250
Donnatal 2060
Donnatal Extentabs 2061
Donnatal Tablets 2060
Phenobarbital Elixir and Tablets 1469
Quadrinal Tablets 1350
Prazepam (Additive effect).
No products indexed under this heading.
Prochlorperazine (Additive effect; potentiates Librium). Products include:
Compazine 2470
Promethazine Hydrochloride (Additive effect; potentiates Librium). Products include:
Mepergan Injection 2753
Phenergan with Codeine 2777
Phenergan with Dextromethorphan 2778
Phenergan Injection 2773
Phenergan Suppositories 2775
Phenergan Syrup 2774
Phenergan Tablets 2775
Phenergan VC 2779
Phenergan VC with Codeine 2781
Propofol (Additive effect). Products include:
Diprivan Injection 2833
Propoxyphene Hydrochloride (Additive effect). Products include:
Darvon 1435
Wygesic Tablets 2827
Propoxyphene Napsylate (Additive effect). Products include:
Darvon-N/Darvocet-N 1433
Quazepam (Additive effect). Products include:
Doral Tablets 2664
Risperidone (Additive effect). Products include:
Risperdal 1301
Secobarbital Sodium (Additive effect). Products include:
Seconal Sodium Pulvules 1474
Selegiline Hydrochloride (Potentiates Librium). Products include:
Eldepryl Tablets 2550
Sufentanil Citrate (Additive effect). Products include:
Sufenta Injection 1309
Temazepam (Additive effect). Products include:
Restoril Capsules 2284
Thiamylal Sodium (Additive effect).
No products indexed under this heading.
Thioridazine Hydrochloride (Additive effect; potentiates Librium). Products include:
Mellaril 2269
Thiothixene (Additive effect). Products include:
Navane Capsules and Concentrate 2201
Navane Intramuscular 2202
Tranylcypromine Sulfate (Potentiates Librium). Products include:
Parnate Tablets 2503
Triazolam (Additive effect). Products include:
Halcion Tablets 2611
Trifluoperazine Hydrochloride (Additive effect; potentiates Librium). Products include:
Stelazine 2514
Warfarin Sodium (Potential for variable effects on blood coagulation). Products include:
Coumadin 926
Zolpidem Tartrate (Additive effect). Products include:
Ambien Tablets 2416

Food Interactions

Alcohol (Additive effect).

LIBRIUM CAPSULES
(Chlordiazepoxide Hydrochloride) 2178
May interact with monoamine oxidase inhibitors, phenothiazines, and oral anticoagulants. Compounds in these categories include:

Chlorpromazine (Combination therapy requires careful monitoring from pharmacological point of view). Products include:
Thorazine Suppositories 2523
Dicumarol (Variable effects on blood coagulation).
No products indexed under this heading.
Fluphenazine Decanoate (Combination therapy requires careful monitoring from pharmacological point of view). Products include:
Prolixin Decanoate 509
Fluphenazine Enanthate (Combination therapy requires careful monitoring from pharmacological point of view). Products include:
Prolixin Enanthate 509
Fluphenazine Hydrochloride (Combination therapy requires careful monitoring from pharmacological point of view). Products include:
Prolixin 509
Furazolidone (Combination therapy requires careful monitoring from pharmacological point of view). Products include:
Furoxone 2046
Isocarboxazid (Combination therapy requires careful monitoring from pharmacological point of view).
No products indexed under this heading.
Mesoridazine Besylate (Combination therapy requires careful monitoring from pharmacological point of view). Products include:
Serentil 684
Methotrimeprazine (Combination therapy requires careful monitoring from pharmacological point of view). Products include:
Levoprome 1274
Perphenazine (Combination therapy requires careful monitoring from pharmacological point of view). Products include:
Etrafon 2355
Triavil Tablets 1757
Trilafon 2389
Phenelzine Sulfate (Combination therapy requires careful monitoring from pharmacological point of view). Products include:
Nardil 1920
Prochlorperazine (Combination therapy requires careful monitoring from pharmacological point of view). Products include:
Compazine 2470
Promethazine Hydrochloride (Combination therapy requires careful monitoring from pharmacological point of view). Products include:
Mepergan Injection 2753
Phenergan with Codeine 2777
Phenergan with Dextromethorphan 2778
Phenergan Injection 2773
Phenergan Suppositories 2775
Phenergan Syrup 2774
Phenergan Tablets 2775
Phenergan VC 2779
Phenergan VC with Codeine 2781
Selegiline Hydrochloride (Combination therapy requires careful monitoring from pharmacological point of view). Products include:
Eldepryl Tablets 2550
Thioridazine Hydrochloride (Combination therapy requires careful monitoring from pharmacological point of view). Products include:
Mellaril 2269
Tranylcypromine Sulfate (Combination therapy requires careful monitoring from pharmacological point of view). Products include:
Parnate Tablets 2503
Trifluoperazine Hydrochloride (Combination therapy requires careful monitoring from pharmacological point of view). Products include:
Stelazine 2514
Warfarin Sodium (Variable effects on blood coagulation). Products include:
Coumadin 926

LIBRIUM INJECTABLE
(Chlordiazepoxide Hydrochloride) 2179
May interact with central nervous system depressants, monoamine oxidase inhibitors, phenothiazines, and certain other agents. Compounds in these categories include:

Alfentanil Hydrochloride (Additive effect). Products include:
Alfenta Injection 1286
Alprazolam (Additive effect). Products include:
Xanax Tablets 2649
Aprobarbital (Additive effect).
No products indexed under this heading.
Buprenorphine (Additive effect). Products include:
Buprenex Injectable 2006
Buspirone Hydrochloride (Additive effect). Products include:
BuSpar 737
Butabarbital (Additive effect).
No products indexed under this heading.
Butalbital (Additive effect). Products include:
Esgic-plus Tablets 1013
Fioricet Tablets 2258
Fioricet with Codeine Capsules 2260
Fiorinal Capsules 2261
Fiorinal with Codeine Capsules 2262
Fiorinal Tablets 2261
Phrenilin 785
Sedapap Tablets 50 mg/650 mg 1543
Chlordiazepoxide (Additive effect). Products include:
Libritabs Tablets 2177
Limbitrol 2180
Chlorpromazine (Additive effect; potentiates Librium). Products include:
Thorazine Suppositories 2523
Chlorprothixene (Additive effect).
No products indexed under this heading.
Chlorprothixene Hydrochloride (Additive effect).
No products indexed under this heading.
Clorazepate Dipotassium (Additive effect). Products include:
Tranxene 451
Clozapine (Additive effect). Products include:
Clozaril Tablets 2252
Codeine Phosphate (Additive effect). Products include:
Actifed with Codeine Cough Syrup 1067
Brontex 1981
Deconsal C Expectorant Syrup 456
Deconsal Pediatric Syrup 457
Dimetane-DC Cough Syrup 2059
Empirin with Codeine Tablets 1093
Fioricet with Codeine Capsules 2260
Fiorinal with Codeine Capsules 2262
Isoclor Expectorant 990
Novahistine DH 2462
Novahistine Expectorant 2463
Nucofed 2051

IMPORTANT NOTE: Always consult each drug listing in the patient's regimen for possible interactions.

Phenergan with Codeine 2777
Phenergan VC with Codeine 2781
Robitussin A-C Syrup 2073
Robitussin-DAC Syrup 2074
Ryna .... ▣ 841
Soma Compound w/Codeine Tablets 2676
Tussi-Organidin NR Liquid and S NR Liquid 2677
Tylenol with Codeine 1583

Desflurane (Additive effect). Products include:
Suprane 1813

Dezocine (Additive effect). Products include:
Dalgan Injection 538

Diazepam (Additive effect). Products include:
Dizac 1809
Valium Injectable 2182
Valium Tablets 2183
Valrelease Capsules 2169

Droperidol (Additive effect). Products include:
Inapsine Injection 1296

Enflurane (Additive effect).
No products indexed under this heading.

Estazolam (Additive effect). Products include:
ProSom Tablets 449

Ethchlorvynol (Additive effect). Products include:
Placidyl Capsules 448

Ethinamate (Additive effect).
No products indexed under this heading.

Fentanyl (Additive effect). Products include:
Duragesic Transdermal System 1288

Fentanyl Citrate (Additive effect). Products include:
Sublimaze Injection 1307

Fluphenazine Decanoate (Additive effect; potentiates Librium). Products include:
Prolixin Decanoate 509

Fluphenazine Enanthate (Additive effect; potentiates Librium). Products include:
Prolixin Enanthate 509

Fluphenazine Hydrochloride (Additive effect; potentiates Librium). Products include:
Prolixin 509

Flurazepam Hydrochloride (Additive effect). Products include:
Dalmane Capsules 2173

Furazolidone (Potentiates Librium). Products include:
Furoxone 2046

Glutethimide (Additive effect).
No products indexed under this heading.

Haloperidol (Additive effect). Products include:
Haldol Injection, Tablets and Concentrate 1575

Haloperidol Decanoate (Additive effect). Products include:
Haldol Decanoate 1577

Hydrocodone Bitartrate (Additive effect). Products include:
Anexsia 5/500 Elixir 1781
Anexia Tablets 1782
Codiclear DH Syrup 791
Deconamine CX Cough and Cold Liquid and Tablets 1319
Duratuss HD Elixir 2565
Hycodan Tablets and Syrup 930
Hycomine Compound Tablets 932
Hycomine 931
Hycotuss Expectorant Syrup 933
Hydrocet Capsules 782
Lorcet 10/650 1018
Lortab 2566
Tussend 1783
Tussend Expectorant 1785
Vicodin Tablets 1356
Vicodin ES Tablets 1357
Vicodin Tuss Expectorant 1358
Zydone Capsules 949

Hydrocodone Polistirex (Additive effect). Products include:
Tussionex Pennkinetic Extended-Release Suspension 998

Hydroxyzine Hydrochloride (Additive effect). Products include:
Atarax Tablets & Syrup 2185
Marax Tablets & DF Syrup 2200
Vistaril Intramuscular Solution 2216

Isocarboxazid (Potentiates Librium).
No products indexed under this heading.

Isoflurane (Additive effect).
No products indexed under this heading.

Ketamine Hydrochloride (Additive effect).
No products indexed under this heading.

Levomethadyl Acetate Hydrochloride (Additive effect). Products include:
Orlamm 2239

Levorphanol Tartrate (Additive effect). Products include:
Levo-Dromoran 2129

Lorazepam (Additive effect). Products include:
Ativan Injection 2698
Ativan Tablets 2700

Loxapine Hydrochloride (Additive effect). Products include:
Loxitane 1378

Loxapine Succinate (Additive effect). Products include:
Loxitane Capsules 1378

Meperidine Hydrochloride (Additive effect). Products include:
Demerol 2308
Mepergan Injection 2753

Mephobarbital (Additive effect). Products include:
Mebaral Tablets 2322

Meprobamate (Additive effect). Products include:
Miltown Tablets 2672
PMB 200 and PMB 400 2783

Mesoridazine Besylate (Additive effect; potentiates Librium). Products include:
Serentil 684

Methadone Hydrochloride (Additive effect). Products include:
Methadone Hydrochloride Oral Concentrate 2233
Methadone Hydrochloride Oral Solution & Tablets 2235

Methohexital Sodium (Additive effect). Products include:
Brevital Sodium Vials 1429

Methotrimeprazine (Additive effect). Products include:
Levoprome 1274

Methoxyflurane (Additive effect).
No products indexed under this heading.

Midazolam Hydrochloride (Additive effect). Products include:
Versed Injection 2170

Molindone Hydrochloride (Additive effect). Products include:
Moban Tablets and Concentrate 1048

Morphine Sulfate (Additive effect). Products include:
Astramorph/PF Injection, USP (Preservative-Free) 535
Duramorph 962
Infumorph 200 and Infumorph 500 Sterile Solutions 965
MS Contin Tablets 1994
MSIR 1997
Oramorph SR (Morphine Sulfate Sustained Release Tablets) 2236
RMS Suppositories 2657
Roxanol 2243

Opium Alkaloids (Additive effect).
No products indexed under this heading.

Oxazepam (Additive effect). Products include:
Serax Capsules 2810
Serax Tablets 2810

Oxycodone Hydrochloride (Additive effect). Products include:
Percocet Tablets 938
Percodan Tablets 939
Percodan-Demi Tablets 940
Roxicodone Tablets, Oral Solution & Intensol (Oxycodone) 2244
Tylox Capsules 1584

Pentobarbital Sodium (Additive effect). Products include:
Nembutal Sodium Capsules 436
Nembutal Sodium Solution 438
Nembutal Sodium Suppositories 440

Perphenazine (Additive effect; potentiates Librium). Products include:
Etrafon 2355
Triavil Tablets 1757
Trilafon 2389

Phenelzine Sulfate (Potentiates Librium). Products include:
Nardil 1920

Phenobarbital (Additive effect). Products include:
Arco-Lase Plus Tablets 512
Bellergal-S Tablets 2250
Donnatal 2060
Donnatal Extentabs 2061
Donnatal Tablets 2060
Phenobarbital Elixir and Tablets 1469
Quadrinal Tablets 1350

Prazepam (Additive effect).
No products indexed under this heading.

Prochlorperazine (Additive effect; potentiates Librium). Products include:
Compazine 2470

Promethazine Hydrochloride (Additive effect; potentiates Librium). Products include:
Mepergan Injection 2753
Phenergan with Codeine 2777
Phenergan with Dextromethorphan 2778
Phenergan Injection 2773
Phenergan Suppositories 2775
Phenergan Syrup 2774
Phenergan Tablets 2775
Phenergan VC 2779
Phenergan VC with Codeine 2781

Propofol (Additive effect). Products include:
Diprivan Injection 2833

Propoxyphene Hydrochloride (Additive effect). Products include:
Darvon 1435
Wygesic Tablets 2827

Propoxyphene Napsylate (Additive effect). Products include:
Darvon-N/Darvocet-N 1433

Quazepam (Additive effect). Products include:
Doral Tablets 2664

Risperidone (Additive effect). Products include:
Risperdal 1301

Secobarbital Sodium (Additive effect). Products include:
Seconal Sodium Pulvules 1474

Selegiline Hydrochloride (Potentiates Librium). Products include:
Eldepryl Tablets 2550

Sufentanil Citrate (Additive effect). Products include:
Sufenta Injection 1309

Temazepam (Additive effect). Products include:
Restoril Capsules 2284

Thiamylal Sodium (Additive effect).
No products indexed under this heading.

Thioridazine Hydrochloride (Additive effect; potentiates Librium). Products include:
Mellaril 2269

Thiothixene (Additive effect). Products include:
Navane Capsules and Concentrate 2201
Navane Intramuscular 2202

Tranylcypromine Sulfate (Potentiates Librium). Products include:
Parnate Tablets 2503

Triazolam (Additive effect). Products include:
Halcion Tablets 2611

Trifluoperazine Hydrochloride (Additive effect). Products include:
Stelazine 2514

Zolpidem Tartrate (Additive effect). Products include:
Ambien Tablets 2416

Food Interactions

Alcohol (Additive effect).

LID WIPES-SPF
(Peg-200 Glyceryl Monotallowate).. ⊙ 209
None cited in PDR database.

LIDEX CREAM 0.05%
(Fluocinonide) 2130
None cited in PDR database.

LIDEX GEL 0.05%
(Fluocinonide) 2130
None cited in PDR database.

LIDEX OINTMENT 0.05%
(Fluocinonide) 2130
None cited in PDR database.

LIDEX TOPICAL SOLUTION 0.05%
(Fluocinonide) 2130
None cited in PDR database.

LIDEX-E CREAM 0.05%
(Fluocinonide) 2130
None cited in PDR database.

LIMBITROL DS TABLETS
(Chlordiazepoxide, Amitriptyline Hydrochloride) 2180
See **Limbitrol Tablets**

LIMBITROL TABLETS
(Chlordiazepoxide, Amitriptyline Hydrochloride) 2180
May interact with monoamine oxidase inhibitors, anticholinergics, central nervous system depressants, antidepressant drugs, selective serotonin reuptake inhibitors, phenothiazines, drugs that inhibit cytochrome p450iid6, and certain other agents. Compounds in these categories include:

Alfentanil Hydrochloride (Potential for additive effects leading to harmful level of sedation and CNS depression). Products include:
Alfenta Injection 1286

Alprazolam (Potential for additive effects leading to harmful level of sedation and CNS depression). Products include:
Xanax Tablets 2649

Amoxapine (Concurrent use with drugs that are substrate for cytochrome $P_{450}IID_6$ may make normal metabolizer resemble poor metabolizer leading to higher than expected plasma concentrations of TCA with resultant toxicity). Products include:
Asendin Tablets 1369

Aprobarbital (Potential for additive effects leading to harmful level of sedation and CNS depression).
No products indexed under this heading.

(▣ Described in PDR For Nonprescription Drugs) (⊙ Described in PDR For Ophthalmology)

585 **Interactions Index** **Limbitrol**

Atropine Sulfate (Concurrent use may result in additive anticholinergic effects including severe constipation). Products include:
Arco-Lase Plus Tablets ... 512
Atrohist Plus Tablets ... 454
Atropine Sulfate Sterile Ophthalmic Solution ... ⊙ 233
Donnatal ... 2060
Donnatal Extentabs ... 2061
Donnatal Tablets ... 2060
Lomotil ... 2439
Motofen Tablets ... 784
Urised Tablets ... 1964

Belladonna Alkaloids (Concurrent use may result in additive anticholinergic effects including severe constipation). Products include:
Bellergal-S Tablets ... 2250
Hyland's Bed Wetting Tablets ... ▣ 828
Hyland's EnurAid Tablets ... ▣ 829
Hyland's Teething Tablets ... ▣ 830

Benztropine Mesylate (Concurrent use may result in additive anticholinergic effects including severe constipation). Products include:
Cogentin ... 1621

Biperiden Hydrochloride (Concurrent use may result in additive anticholinergic effects including severe constipation). Products include:
Akineton ... 1333

Buprenorphine (Potential for additive effects leading to harmful level of sedation and CNS depression). Products include:
Buprenex Injectable ... 2006

Bupropion Hydrochloride (Concurrent use with drugs that are substrate for cytochrome $P_{450}IID_6$ may make normal metabolizer resemble poor metabolizer leading to higher than expected plasma concentrations of TCA with resultant toxicity). Products include:
Wellbutrin Tablets ... 1204

Buspirone Hydrochloride (Potential for additive effects leading to harmful level of sedation and CNS depression). Products include:
BuSpar ... 737

Butabarbital (Potential for additive effects leading to harmful level of sedation and CNS depression).
No products indexed under this heading.

Butalbital (Potential for additive effects leading to harmful level of sedation and CNS depression). Products include:
Esgic-plus Tablets ... 1013
Fioricet Tablets ... 2258
Fioricet with Codeine Capsules ... 2260
Fiorinal Capsules ... 2261
Fiorinal with Codeine Capsules ... 2262
Fiorinal Tablets ... 2261
Phrenilin ... 785
Sedapap Tablets 50 mg/650 mg .. 1543

Chlordiazepoxide Hydrochloride (Potential for additive effects leading to harmful level of sedation and CNS depression). Products include:
Librax Capsules ... 2176
Librium Capsules ... 2178
Librium Injectable ... 2179

Chlorpromazine (Concurrent use with drugs that are substrate for cytochrome $P_{450}IID_6$ may make normal metabolizer resemble poor metabolizer leading to higher than expected plasma concentrations of TCA with resultant toxicity; potential for additive effects leading to harmful level of sedation and CNS depression). Products include:
Thorazine Suppositories ... 2523

Chlorpromazine Hydrochloride (Concurrent use with drugs that are substrate for cytochrome $P_{450}IID_6$ may make normal metabolizer resemble poor metabolizer leading to higher than expected plasma concentrations of TCA with resultant toxicity; potential for additive effects leading to harmful level of sedation and CNS depression). Products include:
Thorazine ... 2523

Chlorprothixene (Potential for additive effects leading to harmful level of sedation and CNS depression).
No products indexed under this heading.

Chlorprothixene Hydrochloride (Potential for additive effects leading to harmful level of sedation and CNS depression).
No products indexed under this heading.

Cimetidine (Reduces hepatic metabolism of certain tricyclic antidepressants and benzodiazepines, thereby delaying elimination and increasing steady state concentrations of these drugs resulting in clinically significant effects). Products include:
Tagamet Tablets ... 2516

Cimetidine Hydrochloride (Reduces hepatic metabolism of certain tricyclic antidepressants and benzodiazepines, thereby delaying elimination and increasing steady state concentrations of these drugs resulting in clinically significant effects). Products include:
Tagamet ... 2516

Clidinium Bromide (Concurrent use may result in additive anticholinergic effects including severe constipation). Products include:
Librax Capsules ... 2176
Quarzan Capsules ... 2181

Clonidine (Amitriptyline may block the antihypertensive effect). Products include:
Catapres-TTS ... 675

Clonidine Hydrochloride (Amitriptyline may block the antihypertensive effect). Products include:
Catapres Tablets ... 674
Combipres Tablets ... 677

Clorazepate Dipotassium (Potential for additive effects leading to harmful level of sedation and CNS depression). Products include:
Tranxene ... 451

Clozapine (Potential for additive effects leading to harmful level of sedation and CNS depression). Products include:
Clozaril Tablets ... 2252

Codeine Phosphate (Potential for additive effects leading to harmful level of sedation and CNS depression). Products include:
Actifed with Codeine Cough Syrup.. 1067
Brontex ... 1981
Deconsal C Expectorant Syrup ... 456
Deconsal Pediatric Syrup ... 457
Dimetane-DC Cough Syrup ... 2059
Empirin with Codeine Tablets ... 1093
Fioricet with Codeine Capsules ... 2260
Fiorinal with Codeine Capsules ... 2262
Isoclor Expectorant ... 990
Novahistine DH ... 2462
Novahistine Expectorant ... 2463
Nucofed ... 2051
Phenergan with Codeine ... 2777
Phenergan VC with Codeine ... 2781
Robitussin A-C Syrup ... 2073
Robitussin-DAC Syrup ... 2074
Ryna ... ▣ 841
Soma Compound w/Codeine Tablets ... 2676
Tussi-Organidin NR Liquid and S NR Liquid ... 2677
Tylenol with Codeine ... 1583

Desflurane (Potential for additive effects leading to harmful level of sedation and CNS depression). Products include:
Suprane ... 1813

Desipramine Hydrochloride (Concurrent use with drugs that are substrate for cytochrome $P_{450}IID_6$ may make normal metabolizer resemble poor metabolizer leading to higher than expected plasma concentrations of TCA with resultant toxicity). Products include:
Norpramin Tablets ... 1526

Dezocine (Potential for additive effects leading to harmful level of sedation and CNS depression). Products include:
Dalgan Injection ... 538

Diazepam (Potential for additive effects leading to harmful level of sedation and CNS depression). Products include:
Dizac ... 1809
Valium Injectable ... 2182
Valium Tablets ... 2183
Valrelease Capsules ... 2169

Dicyclomine Hydrochloride (Concurrent use may result in additive anticholinergic effects including severe constipation). Products include:
Bentyl ... 1501

Doxepin Hydrochloride (Concurrent use with drugs that are substrate for cytochrome $P_{450}IID_6$ may make normal metabolizer resemble poor metabolizer leading to higher than expected plasma concentrations of TCA with resultant toxicity). Products include:
Sinequan ... 2205
Zonalon Cream ... 1055

Droperidol (Potential for additive effects leading to harmful level of sedation and CNS depression). Products include:
Inapsine Injection ... 1296

Enflurane (Potential for additive effects leading to harmful level of sedation and CNS depression).
No products indexed under this heading.

Estazolam (Potential for additive effects leading to harmful level of sedation and CNS depression). Products include:
ProSom Tablets ... 449

Ethchlorvynol (Potential for additive effects leading to harmful level of sedation and CNS depression). Products include:
Placidyl Capsules ... 448

Ethinamate (Potential for additive effects leading to harmful level of sedation and CNS depression).
No products indexed under this heading.

Fentanyl (Potential for additive effects leading to harmful level of sedation and CNS depression). Products include:
Duragesic Transdermal System ... 1288

Fentanyl Citrate (Potential for additive effects leading to harmful level of sedation and CNS depression). Products include:
Sublimaze Injection ... 1307

Flecainide Acetate (Concurrent use with drugs that are substrate for cytochrome $P_{450}IID_6$ may make normal metabolizer resemble poor metabolizer leading to higher than expected plasma concentrations of TCA with resultant toxicity). Products include:
Tambocor Tablets ... 1497

Fluoxetine Hydrochloride (Concurrent use with drugs that are substrate for cytochrome $P_{450}IID_6$ may make normal metabolizer resemble poor metabolizer leading to higher than expected plasma concentrations of TCA with resultant toxicity; due to variation in the extent of inhibition of $P_{450}IID_6$ and long half-life of the parent (fluoxetine) and active metabolite sufficient time must elapse, at least 5 weeks before switching to TCA). Products include:
Prozac Pulvules & Liquid, Oral Solution ... 919

Fluphenazine Decanoate (Concurrent use with drugs that are substrate for cytochrome $P_{450}IID_6$ may make normal metabolizer resemble poor metabolizer leading to higher than expected plasma concentrations of TCA with resultant toxicity; potential for additive effects leading to harmful level of sedation and CNS depression). Products include:
Prolixin Decanoate ... 509

Fluphenazine Enanthate (Concurrent use with drugs that are substrate for cytochrome $P_{450}IID_6$ may make normal metabolizer resemble poor metabolizer leading to higher than expected plasma concentrations of TCA with resultant toxicity; potential for additive effects leading to harmful level of sedation and CNS depression). Products include:
Prolixin Enanthate ... 509

Fluphenazine Hydrochloride (Concurrent use with drugs that are substrate for cytochrome $P_{450}IID_6$ may make normal metabolizer resemble poor metabolizer leading to higher than expected plasma concentrations of TCA with resultant toxicity; potential for additive effects leading to harmful level of sedation and CNS depression). Products include:
Prolixin ... 509

Flurazepam Hydrochloride (Potential for additive effects leading to harmful level of sedation and CNS depression). Products include:
Dalmane Capsules ... 2173

Fluvoxamine Maleate (Concurrent use with drugs that are substrate for cytochrome $P_{450}IID_6$ may make normal metabolizer resemble poor metabolizer leading to higher than expected plasma concentrations of TCA with resultant toxicity; due to variation in the extent of inhibition of $P_{450}IID_6$ caution is indicated if co-administered sufficient time must elapse). Products include:
Luvox Tablets ... 2544

Furazolidone (Potential for hyperpyretic crises, severe convulsions, and deaths; concurrent and/or sequential use is contraindicated). Products include:
Furoxone ... 2046

Glutethimide (Potential for additive effects leading to harmful level of sedation and CNS depression).
No products indexed under this heading.

IMPORTANT NOTE: Always consult each drug listing in the patient's regimen for possible interactions.

Limbitrol Interactions Index 586

Glycopyrrolate (Concurrent use may result in additive anticholinergic effects including severe constipation). Products include:
- Robinul Forte Tablets ... 2072
- Robinul Injectable ... 2072
- Robinul Tablets ... 2072

Guanadrel Sulfate (Amitriptyline may block the antihypertensive effect). Products include:
- Hylorel Tablets ... 985

Guanethidine Monosulfate (Amitriptyline may block the antihypertensive effect of guanethidine or similarly acting compounds). Products include:
- Esimil Tablets ... 822
- Ismelin Tablets ... 827

Haloperidol (Potential for additive effects leading to harmful level of sedation and CNS depression). Products include:
- Haldol Injection, Tablets and Concentrate ... 1575

Haloperidol Decanoate (Potential for additive effects leading to harmful level of sedation and CNS depression). Products include:
- Haldol Decanoate ... 1577

Hydrocodone Bitartrate (Potential for additive effects leading to harmful level of sedation and CNS depression). Products include:
- Anexsia 5/500 Elixir ... 1781
- Anexia Tablets ... 1782
- Codiclear DH Syrup ... 791
- Deconamine CX Cough and Cold Liquid and Tablets ... 1319
- Duratuss HD Elixir ... 2565
- Hycodan Tablets and Syrup ... 930
- Hycomine Compound Tablets ... 932
- Hycomine ... 931
- Hycotuss Expectorant Syrup ... 933
- Hydrocet Capsules ... 782
- Lorcet 10/650 ... 1018
- Lortab ... 2566
- Tussend ... 1783
- Tussend Expectorant ... 1785
- Vicodin Tablets ... 1356
- Vicodin ES Tablets ... 1357
- Vicodin Tuss Expectorant ... 1358
- Zydone Capsules ... 949

Hydrocodone Polistirex (Potential for additive effects leading to harmful level of sedation and CNS depression). Products include:
- Tussionex Pennkinetic Extended-Release Suspension ... 998

Hydroxyzine Hydrochloride (Potential for additive effects leading to harmful level of sedation and CNS depression). Products include:
- Atarax Tablets & Syrup ... 2185
- Marax Tablets & DF Syrup ... 2200
- Vistaril Intramuscular Solution ... 2216

Hyoscyamine (Concurrent use may result in additive anticholinergic effects including severe constipation). Products include:
- Cystospaz Tablets ... 1963
- Urised Tablets ... 1964

Hyoscyamine Sulfate (Concurrent use may result in additive anticholinergic effects including severe constipation). Products include:
- Arco-Lase Plus Tablets ... 512
- Atrohist Plus Tablets ... 454
- Cystospaz-M Capsules ... 1963
- Donnatal ... 2060
- Donnatal Extentabs ... 2061
- Donnatal Tablets ... 2060
- Kutrase Capsules ... 2402
- Levsin/Levsinex/Levbid ... 2405

Imipramine Hydrochloride (Concurrent use with drugs that are substrate for cytochrome $P_{450}IID_6$ may make normal metabolizer resemble poor metabolizer leading to higher than expected plasma concentrations of TCA with resultant toxicity). Products include:
- Tofranil Ampuls ... 854
- Tofranil Tablets ... 856

Imipramine Pamoate (Concurrent use with drugs that are substrate for cytochrome $P_{450}IID_6$ may make normal metabolizer resemble poor metabolizer leading to higher than expected plasma concentrations of TCA with resultant toxicity). Products include:
- Tofranil-PM Capsules ... 857

Ipratropium Bromide (Concurrent use may result in additive anticholinergic effects including severe constipation). Products include:
- Atrovent Inhalation Aerosol ... 671
- Atrovent Inhalation Solution ... 673

Isocarboxazid (Potential for hyperpyretic crises, severe convulsions, and deaths; concurrent and/or sequential use is contraindicated).
- No products indexed under this heading.

Isoflurane (Potential for additive effects leading to harmful level of sedation and CNS depression).
- No products indexed under this heading.

Ketamine Hydrochloride (Potential for additive effects leading to harmful level of sedation and CNS depression).
- No products indexed under this heading.

Levomethadyl Acetate Hydrochloride (Potential for additive effects leading to harmful level of sedation and CNS depression). Products include:
- Orlamm ... 2239

Levorphanol Tartrate (Potential for additive effects leading to harmful level of sedation and CNS depression). Products include:
- Levo-Dromoran ... 2129

Lorazepam (Potential for additive effects leading to harmful level of sedation and CNS depression). Products include:
- Ativan Injection ... 2698
- Ativan Tablets ... 2700

Loxapine Hydrochloride (Potential for additive effects leading to harmful level of sedation and CNS depression). Products include:
- Loxitane ... 1378

Loxapine Succinate (Potential for additive effects leading to harmful level of sedation and CNS depression). Products include:
- Loxitane Capsules ... 1378

Maprotiline Hydrochloride (Concurrent use with drugs that are substrate for cytochrome $P_{450}IID_6$ may make normal metabolizer resemble poor metabolizer leading to higher than expected plasma concentrations of TCA with resultant toxicity). Products include:
- Ludiomil Tablets ... 843

Mepenzolate Bromide (Concurrent use may result in additive anticholinergic effects including severe constipation).
- No products indexed under this heading.

Meperidine Hydrochloride (Potential for additive effects leading to harmful level of sedation and CNS depression). Products include:
- Demerol ... 2308
- Mepergan Injection ... 2753

Mephobarbital (Potential for additive effects leading to harmful level of sedation and CNS depression). Products include:
- Mebaral Tablets ... 2322

Meprobamate (Potential for additive effects leading to harmful level of sedation and CNS depression). Products include:
- Miltown Tablets ... 2672
- PMB 200 and PMB 400 ... 2783

Mesoridazine Besylate (Concurrent use with drugs that are substrate for cytochrome $P_{450}IID_6$ may make normal metabolizer resemble poor metabolizer leading to higher than expected plasma concentrations of TCA with resultant toxicity; potential for additive effects leading to harmful level of sedation and CNS depression). Products include:
- Serentil ... 684

Methadone Hydrochloride (Potential for additive effects leading to harmful level of sedation and CNS depression). Products include:
- Methadone Hydrochloride Oral Concentrate ... 2233
- Methadone Hydrochloride Oral Solution & Tablets ... 2235

Methohexital Sodium (Potential for additive effects leading to harmful level of sedation and CNS depression). Products include:
- Brevital Sodium Vials ... 1429

Methotrimeprazine (Concurrent use with drugs that are substrate for cytochrome $P_{450}IID_6$ may make normal metabolizer resemble poor metabolizer leading to higher than expected plasma concentrations of TCA with resultant toxicity; potential for additive effects leading to harmful level of sedation and CNS depression). Products include:
- Levoprome ... 1274

Methoxyflurane (Potential for additive effects leading to harmful level of sedation and CNS depression).
- No products indexed under this heading.

Midazolam Hydrochloride (Potential for additive effects leading to harmful level of sedation and CNS depression). Products include:
- Versed Injection ... 2170

Molindone Hydrochloride (Potential for additive effects leading to harmful level of sedation and CNS depression). Products include:
- Moban Tablets and Concentrate ... 1048

Morphine Sulfate (Potential for additive effects leading to harmful level of sedation and CNS depression). Products include:
- Astramorph/PF Injection, USP (Preservative-Free) ... 535
- Duramorph ... 962
- Infumorph 200 and Infumorph 500 Sterile Solutions ... 965
- MS Contin Tablets ... 1994
- MSIR ... 1997
- Oramorph SR (Morphine Sulfate Sustained Release Tablets) ... 2236
- RMS Suppositories ... 2657
- Roxanol ... 2243

Nefazodone Hydrochloride (Concurrent use with drugs that are substrate for cytochrome $P_{450}IID_6$ may make normal metabolizer resemble poor metabolizer leading to higher than expected plasma concentrations of TCA with resultant toxicity). Products include:
- Serzone Tablets ... 771

Nortriptyline Hydrochloride (Concurrent use with drugs that are substrate for cytochrome $P_{450}IID_6$ may make normal metabolizer resemble poor metabolizer leading to higher than expected plasma concentrations of TCA with resultant toxicity). Products include:
- Pamelor ... 2280

Opium Alkaloids (Potential for additive effects leading to harmful level of sedation and CNS depression).
- No products indexed under this heading.

Oxazepam (Potential for additive effects leading to harmful level of sedation and CNS depression). Products include:
- Serax Capsules ... 2810
- Serax Tablets ... 2810

Oxybutynin Chloride (Concurrent use may result in additive anticholinergic effects including severe constipation). Products include:
- Ditropan ... 1516

Oxycodone Hydrochloride (Potential for additive effects leading to harmful level of sedation and CNS depression). Products include:
- Percocet Tablets ... 938
- Percodan Tablets ... 939
- Percodan-Demi Tablets ... 940
- Roxicodone Tablets, Oral Solution & Intensol (Oxycodone) ... 2244
- Tylox Capsules ... 1584

Paroxetine Hydrochloride (Concurrent use with drugs that are substrate for cytochrome $P_{450}IID_6$ may make normal metabolizer resemble poor metabolizer leading to higher than expected plasma concentrations of TCA with resultant toxicity; due to variation in the extent of inhibition of $P_{450}IID_6$ caution is indicated if co-administered sufficient time must elapse). Products include:
- Paxil Tablets ... 2505

Pentobarbital Sodium (Potential for additive effects leading to harmful level of sedation and CNS depression). Products include:
- Nembutal Sodium Capsules ... 436
- Nembutal Sodium Solution ... 438
- Nembutal Sodium Suppositories ... 440

Perphenazine (Concurrent use with drugs that are substrate for cytochrome $P_{450}IID_6$ may make normal metabolizer resemble poor metabolizer leading to higher than expected plasma concentrations of TCA with resultant toxicity; potential for additive effects leading to harmful level of sedation and CNS depression). Products include:
- Etrafon ... 2355
- Triavil Tablets ... 1757
- Trilafon ... 2389

Phenelzine Sulfate (Potential for hyperpyretic crises, severe convulsions, and deaths; concurrent and/or sequential use is contraindicated). Products include:
- Nardil ... 1920

Phenobarbital (Potential for additive effects leading to harmful level of sedation and CNS depression). Products include:
- Arco-Lase Plus Tablets ... 512
- Bellergal-S Tablets ... 2250
- Donnatal ... 2060
- Donnatal Extentabs ... 2061
- Donnatal Tablets ... 2060
- Phenobarbital Elixir and Tablets ... 1469
- Quadrinal Tablets ... 1350

Prazepam (Potential for additive effects leading to harmful level of sedation and CNS depression).
- No products indexed under this heading.

Interactions Index

Lioresal Intrathecal

Prochlorperazine (Concurrent use with drugs that are substrate for cytochrome $P_{450}IID_6$ may make normal metabolizer resemble poor metabolizer leading to higher than expected plasma concentrations of TCA with resultant toxicity; potential for additive effects leading to harmful level of sedation and CNS depression). Products include:

Compazine 2470

Procyclidine Hydrochloride (Concurrent use may result in additive anticholinergic effects including severe constipation). Products include:

Kemadrin Tablets 1112

Promethazine Hydrochloride (Concurrent use with drugs that are substrate for cytochrome $P_{450}IID_6$ may make normal metabolizer resemble poor metabolizer leading to higher than expected plasma concentrations of TCA with resultant toxicity; potential for additive effects leading to harmful level of sedation and CNS depression). Products include:

Mepergan Injection 2753
Phenergan with Codeine 2777
Phenergan with Dextromethorphan 2778
Phenergan Injection 2773
Phenergan Suppositories 2775
Phenergan Syrup 2774
Phenergan Tablets 2775
Phenergan VC 2779
Phenergan VC with Codeine 2781

Propafenone Hydrochloride (Concurrent use with drugs that are substrate for cytochrome $P_{450}IID_6$ may make normal metabolizer resemble poor metabolizer leading to higher than expected plasma concentrations of TCA with resultant toxicity). Products include:

Rythmol Tablets–150mg, 225mg, 300mg 1352

Propantheline Bromide (Concurrent use may result in additive anticholinergic effects including severe constipation). Products include:

Pro-Banthine Tablets 2052

Propofol (Potential for additive effects leading to harmful level of sedation and CNS depression). Products include:

Diprivan Injection 2833

Propoxyphene Hydrochloride (Potential for additive effects leading to harmful level of sedation and CNS depression). Products include:

Darvon 1435
Wygesic Tablets 2827

Propoxyphene Napsylate (Potential for additive effects leading to harmful level of sedation and CNS depression). Products include:

Darvon-N/Darvocet-N 1433

Protriptyline Hydrochloride (Concurrent use with drugs that are substrate for cytochrome $P_{450}IID_6$ may make normal metabolizer resemble poor metabolizer leading to higher than expected plasma concentrations of TCA with resultant toxicity). Products include:

Vivactil Tablets 1774

Quazepam (Potential for additive effects leading to harmful level of sedation and CNS depression). Products include:

Doral Tablets 2664

Quinidine Gluconate (Concurrent use with drugs that inhibit cytochrome $P_{450}IID_6$ may make normal metabolizer resemble poor metabolizer leading to higher than expected plasma concentrations of TCA with resultant toxicity). Products include:

Quinaglute Dura-Tabs Tablets 649

Quinidine Polygalacturonate (Concurrent use with drugs that inhibit cytochrome $P_{450}IID_6$ may make normal metabolizer resemble poor metabolizer leading to higher than expected plasma concentrations of TCA with resultant toxicity).

No products indexed under this heading.

Quinidine Sulfate (Concurrent use with drugs that inhibit cytochrome $P_{450}IID_6$ may make normal metabolizer resemble poor metabolizer leading to higher than expected plasma concentrations of TCA with resultant toxicity). Products include:

Quinidex Extentabs 2067

Risperidone (Potential for additive effects leading to harmful level of sedation and CNS depression). Products include:

Risperdal 1301

Scopolamine (Concurrent use may result in additive anticholinergic effects including severe constipation). Products include:

Transderm Scōp Transdermal Therapeutic System 869

Scopolamine Hydrobromide (Concurrent use may result in additive anticholinergic effects including severe constipation). Products include:

Atrohist Plus Tablets 454
Donnatal 2060
Donnatal Extentabs 2061
Donnatal Tablets 2060

Secobarbital Sodium (Potential for additive effects leading to harmful level of sedation and CNS depression). Products include:

Seconal Sodium Pulvules 1474

Selegiline Hydrochloride (Potential for hyperpyretic crises, severe convulsions, and deaths; concurrent and/or sequential use is contraindicated). Products include:

Eldepryl Tablets 2550

Sertraline Hydrochloride (Concurrent use with drugs that are substrate for cytochrome $P_{450}IID_6$ may make normal metaoblizer resemble poor metabolizer leading to higher than expected plasma concentrations of TCA with resultant toxicity; due to variation in the extent of inhibition of $P_{450}IID_6$ caution is indicated if co-administered sufficient time must elapse). Products include:

Zoloft Tablets 2217

Sufentanil Citrate (Potential for additive effects leading to harmful level of sedation and CNS depression). Products include:

Sufenta Injection 1309

Temazepam (Potential for additive effects leading to harmful level of sedation and CNS depression). Products include:

Restoril Capsules 2284

Thiamylal Sodium (Potential for additive effects leading to harmful level of sedation and CNS depression).

No products indexed under this heading.

Thioridazine Hydrochloride (Concurrent use with drugs that are substrate for cytochrome $P_{450}IID_6$ may make normal metabolizer resemble poor metabolizer leading to higher than expected plasma concentrations of TCA with resultant toxicity; potential for additive effects leading to harmful level of sedation and CNS depression). Products include:

Mellaril 2269

Thiothixene (Potential for additive effects leading to harmful level of sedation and CNS depression). Products include:

Navane Capsules and Concentrate 2201
Navane Intramuscular 2202

Tranylcypromine Sulfate (Potential for hyperpyretic crises, severe convulsions, and deaths; concurrent and/or sequential use is contraindicated). Products include:

Parnate Tablets 2503

Trazodone Hydrochloride (Concurrent use with drugs that are substrate for cytochrome $P_{450}IID_6$ may make normal metabolizer resemble poor metabolizer leading to higher than expected plasma concentrations of TCA with resultant toxicity). Products include:

Desyrel and Desyrel Dividose 503

Triazolam (Potential for additive effects leading to harmful level of sedation and CNS depression). Products include:

Halcion Tablets 2611

Tridihexethyl Chloride (Concurrent use may result in additive anticholinergic effects including severe constipation).

No products indexed under this heading.

Trifluoperazine Hydrochloride (Concurrent use with drugs that are substrate for cytochrome $P_{450}IID_6$ may make normal metabolizer resemble poor metabolizer leading to higher than expected plasma concentrations of TCA with resultant toxicity; potential for additive effects leading to harmful level of sedation and CNS depression). Products include:

Stelazine 2514

Trihexyphenidyl Hydrochloride (Concurrent use may result in additive anticholinergic effects including severe constipation). Products include:

Artane 1368

Trimipramine Maleate (Concurrent use with drugs that are substrate for cytochrome $P_{450}IID_6$ may make normal metabolizer resemble poor metabolizer leading to higher than expected plasma concentrations of TCA with resultant toxicity). Products include:

Surmontil Capsules 2811

Venlafaxine Hydrochloride (Concurrent use with drugs that are substrate for cytochrome $P_{450}IID_6$ may make normal metaoblizer resemble poor metabolizer leading to higher than expected plasma concentrations of TCA with resultant toxicity; due to variation in the extent of inhibition of $P_{450}IID_6$ caution is indicated if co-administered sufficient time must elapse). Products include:

Effexor 2719

Zolpidem Tartrate (Potential for additive effects leading to harmful level of sedation and CNS depression). Products include:

Ambien Tablets 2416

Food Interactions

Alcohol (Potential for additive effects leading to harmful level of sedation and CNS depression).

LINCOCIN CAPSULES

(Lincomycin Hydrochloride) 2617
May interact with nondepolarizing neuromuscular blocking agents and certain other agents. Compounds in these categories include:

Atracurium Besylate (Enhanced neuromuscular blocking activity). Products include:

Tracrium Injection 1183

Diphenoxylate Hydrochloride (May prolong and/or worsen colitis). Products include:

Lomotil 2439

Metocurine Iodide (Enhanced neuromuscular blocking activity). Products include:

Metubine Iodide Vials 916

Mivacurium Chloride (Enhanced neuromuscular blocking activity). Products include:

Mivacron 1138

Pancuronium Bromide Injection (Enhanced neuromuscular blocking activity).

No products indexed under this heading.

Paregoric (May prolong and/or worsen colitis).

No products indexed under this heading.

Rocuronium Bromide (Enhanced neuromuscular blocking activity). Products include:

Zemuron 1830

Vecuronium Bromide (Enhanced neuromuscular blocking activity). Products include:

Norcuron 1826

LINCOCIN PEDIATRIC CAPSULES

(Lincomycin Hydrochloride) 2617
See Lincocin Capsules

LINCOCIN STERILE SOLUTION

(Lincomycin Hydrochloride) 2617
See Lincocin Capsules

LINDANE LOTION USP 1%

(Lindane) 582
May interact with:

Oils, unspecified (May enhance absorption; avoid concurrent use).

LINDANE SHAMPOO USP 1%

(Lindane) 583
May interact with:

Oils, unspecified (May enhance absorption; avoid concurrent use).

LIORESAL INTRATHECAL

(Baclofen) 1596
May interact with central nervous system depressants and certain other agents. Compounds in these categories include:

Alfentanil Hydrochloride (CNS depressant effect of Lioresal Intrathecal may be additive to those of other CNS depressants). Products include:

Alfenta Injection 1286

IMPORTANT NOTE: Always consult each drug listing in the patient's regimen for possible interactions.

Alprazolam (CNS depressant effect of Lioresal Intrathecal may be additive to those of other CNS depressants). Products include:

Xanax Tablets 2649

Aprobarbital (CNS depressant effect of Lioresal Intrathecal may be additive to those of other CNS depressants).

No products indexed under this heading.

Buprenorphine (CNS depressant effect of Lioresal Intrathecal may be additive to those of other CNS depressants). Products include:

Buprenex Injectable 2006

Buspirone Hydrochloride (CNS depressant effect of Lioresal Intrathecal may be additive to those of other CNS depressants). Products include:

BuSpar 737

Butabarbital (CNS depressant effect of Lioresal Intrathecal may be additive to those of other CNS depressants).

No products indexed under this heading.

Butalbital (CNS depressant effect of Lioresal Intrathecal may be additive to those of other CNS depressants). Products include:

Esgic-plus Tablets 1013
Fioricet Tablets 2258
Fioricet with Codeine Capsules 2260
Fiorinal Capsules 2261
Fiorinal with Codeine Capsules 2262
Fiorinal Tablets 2261
Phrenilin 785
Sedapap Tablets 50 mg/650 mg .. 1543

Chlordiazepoxide (CNS depressant effect of Lioresal Intrathecal may be additive to those of other CNS depressants). Products include:

Libritabs Tablets 2177
Limbitrol 2180

Chlordiazepoxide Hydrochloride (CNS depressant effect of Lioresal Intrathecal may be additive to those of other CNS depressants). Products include:

Librax Capsules 2176
Librium Capsules 2178
Librium Injectable 2179

Chlorpromazine (CNS depressant effect of Lioresal Intrathecal may be additive to those of other CNS depressants). Products include:

Thorazine Suppositories 2523

Chlorpromazine Hydrochloride (CNS depressant effect of Lioresal Intrathecal may be additive to those of other CNS depressants). Products include:

Thorazine 2523

Chlorprothixene (CNS depressant effect of Lioresal Intrathecal may be additive to those of other CNS depressants).

No products indexed under this heading.

Chlorprothixene Hydrochloride (CNS depressant effect of Lioresal Intrathecal may be additive to those of other CNS depressants).

No products indexed under this heading.

Clorazepate Dipotassium (CNS depressant effect of Lioresal Intrathecal may be additive to those of other CNS depressants). Products include:

Tranxene 451

Clozapine (CNS depressant effect of Lioresal Intrathecal may be additive to those of other CNS depressants). Products include:

Clozaril Tablets 2252

Codeine Phosphate (CNS depressant effect of Lioresal Intrathecal may be additive to those of other CNS depressants). Products include:

Actifed with Codeine Cough Syrup.. 1067
Brontex 1981
Deconsal C Expectorant Syrup 456
Deconsal Pediatric Syrup 457
Dimetane-DC Cough Syrup 2059
Empirin with Codeine Tablets 1093
Fioricet with Codeine Capsules 2260
Fiorinal with Codeine Capsules 2262
Isoclor Expectorant 990
Novahistine DH 2462
Novahistine Expectorant 2463
Nucofed 2051
Phenergan with Codeine 2777
Phenergan VC with Codeine 2781
Robitussin A-C Syrup 2073
Robitussin-DAC Syrup 2074
Ryna .... ■ 841
Soma Compound w/Codeine Tablets 2676
Tussi-Organidin NR Liquid and S NR Liquid 2677
Tylenol with Codeine 1583

Desflurane (CNS depressant effect of Lioresal Intrathecal may be additive to those of other CNS depressants). Products include:

Suprane 1813

Dezocine (CNS depressant effect of Lioresal Intrathecal may be additive to those of other CNS depressants). Products include:

Dalgan Injection 538

Diazepam (CNS depressant effect of Lioresal Intrathecal may be additive to those of other CNS depressants). Products include:

Dizac 1809
Valium Injectable 2182
Valium Tablets 2183
Valrelease Capsules 2169

Droperidol (CNS depressant effect of Lioresal Intrathecal may be additive to those of other CNS depressants). Products include:

Inapsine Injection 1296

Enflurane (CNS depressant effect of Lioresal Intrathecal may be additive to those of other CNS depressants).

No products indexed under this heading.

Estazolam (CNS depressant effect of Lioresal Intrathecal may be additive to those of other CNS depressants). Products include:

ProSom Tablets 449

Ethchlorvynol (CNS depressant effect of Lioresal Intrathecal may be additive to those of other CNS depressants). Products include:

Placidyl Capsules 448

Ethinamate (CNS depressant effect of Lioresal Intrathecal may be additive to those of other CNS depressants).

No products indexed under this heading.

Fentanyl (CNS depressant effect of Lioresal Intrathecal may be additive to those of other CNS depressants). Products include:

Duragesic Transdermal System 1288

Fentanyl Citrate (CNS depressant effect of Lioresal Intrathecal may be additive to those of other CNS depressants). Products include:

Sublimaze Injection 1307

Fluphenazine Decanoate (CNS depressant effect of Lioresal Intrathecal may be additive to those of other CNS depressants). Products include:

Prolixin Decanoate 509

Fluphenazine Enanthate (CNS depressant effect of Lioresal Intrathecal may be additive to those of other CNS depressants). Products include:

Prolixin Enanthate 509

Fluphenazine Hydrochloride (CNS depressant effect of Lioresal Intrathecal may be additive to those of other CNS depressants). Products include:

Prolixin 509

Flurazepam Hydrochloride (CNS depressant effect of Lioresal Intrathecal may be additive to those of other CNS depressants). Products include:

Dalmane Capsules 2173

Glutethimide (CNS depressant effect of Lioresal Intrathecal may be additive to those of other CNS depressants).

No products indexed under this heading.

Haloperidol (CNS depressant effect of Lioresal Intrathecal may be additive to those of other CNS depressants). Products include:

Haldol Injection, Tablets and Concentrate 1575

Haloperidol Decanoate (CNS depressant effect of Lioresal Intrathecal may be additive to those of other CNS depressants). Products include:

Haldol Decanoate 1577

Hydrocodone Bitartrate (CNS depressant effect of Lioresal Intrathecal may be additive to those of other CNS depressants). Products include:

Anexsia 5/500 Elixir 1781
Anexia Tablets 1782
Codiclear DH Syrup 791
Deconamine CX Cough and Cold Liquid and Tablets 1319
Duratuss HD Elixir 2565
Hycodan Tablets and Syrup 930
Hycomine Compound Tablets 932
Hycomine 931
Hycotuss Expectorant Syrup 933
Hydrocet Capsules 782
Lorcet 10/650 1018
Lortab 2566
Tussend 1783
Tussend Expectorant 1785
Vicodin Tablets 1356
Vicodin ES Tablets 1357
Vicodin Tuss Expectorant 1358
Zydone Capsules 949

Hydrocodone Polistirex (CNS depressant effect of Lioresal Intrathecal may be additive to those of other CNS depressants). Products include:

Tussionex Pennkinetic Extended-Release Suspension 998

Hydroxyzine Hydrochloride (CNS depressant effect of Lioresal Intrathecal may be additive to those of other CNS depressants). Products include:

Atarax Tablets & Syrup 2185
Marax Tablets & DF Syrup 2200
Vistaril Intramuscular Solution 2216

Isoflurane (CNS depressant effect of Lioresal Intrathecal may be additive to those of other CNS depressants).

No products indexed under this heading.

Ketamine Hydrochloride (CNS depressant effect of Lioresal Intrathecal may be additive to those of other CNS depressants).

No products indexed under this heading.

Levomethadyl Acetate Hydrochloride (CNS depressant effect of Lioresal Intrathecal may be additive to those of other CNS depressants). Products include:

Orlamm 2239

Levorphanol Tartrate (CNS depressant effect of Lioresal Intrathecal may be additive to those of other CNS depressants). Products include:

Levo-Dromoran 2129

Lorazepam (CNS depressant effect of Lioresal Intrathecal may be additive to those of other CNS depressants). Products include:

Ativan Injection 2698
Ativan Tablets 2700

Loxapine Hydrochloride (CNS depressant effect of Lioresal Intrathecal may be additive to those of other CNS depressants). Products include:

Loxitane 1378

Loxapine Succinate (CNS depressant effect of Lioresal Intrathecal may be additive to those of other CNS depressants). Products include:

Loxitane Capsules 1378

Meperidine Hydrochloride (CNS depressant effect of Lioresal Intrathecal may be additive to those of other CNS depressants). Products include:

Demerol 2308
Mepergan Injection 2753

Mephobarbital (CNS depressant effect of Lioresal Intrathecal may be additive to those of other CNS depressants). Products include:

Mebaral Tablets 2322

Meprobamate (CNS depressant effect of Lioresal Intrathecal may be additive to those of other CNS depressants). Products include:

Miltown Tablets 2672
PMB 200 and PMB 400 2783

Mesoridazine (CNS depressant effect of Lioresal Intrathecal may be additive to those of other CNS depressants).

Methadone Hydrochloride (CNS depressant effect of Lioresal Intrathecal may be additive to those of other CNS depressants). Products include:

Methadone Hydrochloride Oral Concentrate 2233
Methadone Hydrochloride Oral Solution & Tablets 2235

Methohexital Sodium (CNS depressant effect of Lioresal Intrathecal may be additive to those of other CNS depressants). Products include:

Brevital Sodium Vials 1429

Methotrimeprazine (CNS depressant effect of Lioresal Intrathecal may be additive to those of other CNS depressants). Products include:

Levoprome 1274

Methoxyflurane (CNS depressant effect of Lioresal Intrathecal may be additive to those of other CNS depressants).

No products indexed under this heading.

Midazolam Hydrochloride (CNS depressant effect of Lioresal Intrathecal may be additive to those of other CNS depressants). Products include:

Versed Injection 2170

Molindone Hydrochloride (CNS depressant effect of Lioresal Intrathecal may be additive to those of other CNS depressants). Products include:

Moban Tablets and Concentrate 1048

589 **Interactions Index** **Lioresal**

Morphine Sulfate (CNS depressant effect of Lioresal Intrathecal may be additive to those of other CNS depressants; potential for hypotension and dyspnea with concurrent administration of Lioresal Intrathecal and epidural morphine). Products include:

Astramorph/PF Injection, USP (Preservative-Free) 535
Duramorph 962
Infumorph 200 and Infumorph 500 Sterile Solutions 965
MS Contin Tablets 1994
MSIR 1997
Oramorph SR (Morphine Sulfate Sustained Release Tablets) 2236
RMS Suppositories 2657
Roxanol 2243

Opium Alkaloids (CNS depressant effect of Lioresal Intrathecal may be additive to those of other CNS depressants).

No products indexed under this heading.

Oxazepam (CNS depressant effect of Lioresal Intrathecal may be additive to those of other CNS depressants). Products include:

Serax Capsules 2810
Serax Tablets 2810

Oxycodone Hydrochloride (CNS depressant effect of Lioresal Intrathecal may be additive to those of other CNS depressants). Products include:

Percocet Tablets 938
Percodan Tablets 939
Percodan-Demi Tablets 940
Roxicodone Tablets, Oral Solution & Intensol (Oxycodone) 2244
Tylox Capsules 1584

Pentobarbital Sodium (CNS depressant effect of Lioresal Intrathecal may be additive to those of other CNS depressants). Products include:

Nembutal Sodium Capsules 436
Nembutal Sodium Solution 438
Nembutal Sodium Suppositories 440

Perphenazine (CNS depressant effect of Lioresal Intrathecal may be additive to those of other CNS depressants). Products include:

Etrafon 2355
Triavil Tablets 1757
Trilafon 2389

Phenobarbital (CNS depressant effect of Lioresal Intrathecal may be additive to those of other CNS depressants). Products include:

Arco-Lase Plus Tablets 512
Bellergal-S Tablets 2250
Donnatal 2060
Donnatal Extentabs 2061
Donnatal Tablets 2060
Phenobarbital Elixir and Tablets 1469
Quadrinal Tablets 1350

Prazepam (CNS depressant effect of Lioresal Intrathecal may be additive to those of other CNS depressants).

No products indexed under this heading.

Prochlorperazine (CNS depressant effect of Lioresal Intrathecal may be additive to those of other CNS depressants). Products include:

Compazine 2470

Promethazine Hydrochloride (CNS depressant effect of Lioresal Intrathecal may be additive to those of other CNS depressants). Products include:

Mepergan Injection 2753
Phenergan with Codeine 2777
Phenergan with Dextromethorphan 2778
Phenergan Injection 2773
Phenergan Suppositories 2775
Phenergan Syrup 2774
Phenergan Tablets 2775
Phenergan VC 2779
Phenergan VC with Codeine 2781

Propofol (CNS depressant effect of Lioresal Intrathecal may be additive to those of other CNS depressants). Products include:

Diprivan Injection 2833

Propoxyphene Hydrochloride (CNS depressant effect of Lioresal Intrathecal may be additive to those of other CNS depressants). Products include:

Darvon 1435
Wygesic Tablets 2827

Propoxyphene Napsylate (CNS depressant effect of Lioresal Intrathecal may be additive to those of other CNS depressants). Products include:

Darvon-N/Darvocet-N 1433

Quazepam (CNS depressant effect of Lioresal Intrathecal may be additive to those of other CNS depressants). Products include:

Doral Tablets 2664

Risperidone (CNS depressant effect of Lioresal Intrathecal may be additive to those of other CNS depressants). Products include:

Risperdal 1301

Secobarbital Sodium (CNS depressant effect of Lioresal Intrathecal may be additive to those of other CNS depressants). Products include:

Seconal Sodium Pulvules 1474

Sufentanil Citrate (CNS depressant effect of Lioresal Intrathecal may be additive to those of other CNS depressants). Products include:

Sufenta Injection 1309

Temazepam (CNS depressant effect of Lioresal Intrathecal may be additive to those of other CNS depressants). Products include:

Restoril Capsules 2284

Thiamylal Sodium (CNS depressant effect of Lioresal Intrathecal may be additive to those of other CNS depressants).

No products indexed under this heading.

Thioridazine Hydrochloride (CNS depressant effect of Lioresal Intrathecal may be additive to those of other CNS depressants). Products include:

Mellaril 2269

Thiothixene (CNS depressant effect of Lioresal Intrathecal may be additive to those of other CNS depressants). Products include:

Navane Capsules and Concentrate 2201
Navane Intramuscular 2202

Triazolam (CNS depressant effect of Lioresal Intrathecal may be additive to those of other CNS depressants). Products include:

Halcion Tablets 2611

Trifluoperazine Hydrochloride (CNS depressant effect of Lioresal Intrathecal may be additive to those of other CNS depressants). Products include:

Stelazine 2514

Zolpidem Tartrate (CNS depressant effect of Lioresal Intrathecal may be additive to those of other CNS depressants). Products include:

Ambien Tablets 2416

Food Interactions

Alcohol (CNS depressant effect of Lioresal Intrathecal may be additive to those of alcohol).

LIORESAL TABLETS
(Baclofen) 829

May interact with central nervous system depressants and certain other agents. Compounds in these categories include:

Alfentanil Hydrochloride (Additive depressant effect). Products include:

Alfenta Injection 1286

Alprazolam (Additive depressant effect). Products include:

Xanax Tablets 2649

Aprobarbital (Additive depressant effect).

No products indexed under this heading.

Buprenorphine (Additive depressant effect). Products include:

Buprenex Injectable 2006

Buspirone Hydrochloride (Additive depressant effect). Products include:

BuSpar 737

Butabarbital (Additive depressant effect).

No products indexed under this heading.

Butalbital (Additive depressant effect). Products include:

Esgic-plus Tablets 1013
Fioricet Tablets 2258
Fioricet with Codeine Capsules 2260
Fiorinal Capsules 2261
Fiorinal with Codeine Capsules 2262
Fiorinal Tablets 2261
Phrenilin 785
Sedapap Tablets 50 mg/650 mg .. 1543

Chlordiazepoxide (Additive depressant effect). Products include:

Libritabs Tablets 2177
Limbitrol 2180

Chlordiazepoxide Hydrochloride (Additive depressant effect). Products include:

Librax Capsules 2176
Librium Capsules 2178
Librium Injectable 2179

Chlorpromazine (Additive depressant effect). Products include:

Thorazine Suppositories 2523

Chlorprothixene (Additive depressant effect).

No products indexed under this heading.

Chlorprothixene Hydrochloride (Additive depressant effect).

No products indexed under this heading.

Chlorprothixene Lactate (Additive depressant effect).

No products indexed under this heading.

Clorazepate Dipotassium (Additive depressant effect). Products include:

Tranxene 451

Clozapine (Additive depressant effect). Products include:

Clozaril Tablets 2252

Codeine Phosphate (Additive depressant effect). Products include:

Actifed with Codeine Cough Syrup.. 1067
Brontex 1981
Deconsal C Expectorant Syrup 456
Deconsal Pediatric Syrup 457
Dimetane-DC Cough Syrup 2059
Empirin with Codeine Tablets 1093
Fioricet with Codeine Capsules 2260
Fiorinal with Codeine Capsules 2262
Isoclor Expectorant 990
Novahistine DH 2462
Novahistine Expectorant 2463
Nucofed 2051
Phenergan with Codeine 2777
Phenergan VC with Codeine 2781
Robitussin A-C Syrup 2073
Robitussin-DAC Syrup 2074
Ryna .... ⊞ 841
Soma Compound w/Codeine Tablets 2676
Tussi-Organidin NR Liquid and S NR Liquid 2677
Tylenol with Codeine 1583

Desflurane (Additive depressant effect). Products include:

Suprane 1813

Dezocine (Additive depressant effect). Products include:

Dalgan Injection 538

Diazepam (Additive depressant effect). Products include:

Dizac 1809
Valium Injectable 2182
Valium Tablets 2183
Valrelease Capsules 2169

Droperidol (Additive depressant effect). Products include:

Inapsine Injection 1296

Enflurane (Additive depressant effect).

No products indexed under this heading.

Estazolam (Additive depressant effect). Products include:

ProSom Tablets 449

Ethchlorvynol (Additive depressant effect). Products include:

Placidyl Capsules 448

Ethinamate (Additive depressant effect).

No products indexed under this heading.

Fentanyl (Additive depressant effect). Products include:

Duragesic Transdermal System 1288

Fentanyl Citrate (Additive depressant effect). Products include:

Sublimaze Injection 1307

Fluphenazine Decanoate (Additive depressant effect). Products include:

Prolixin Decanoate 509

Fluphenazine Enanthate (Additive depressant effect). Products include:

Prolixin Enanthate 509

Fluphenazine Hydrochloride (Additive depressant effect). Products include:

Prolixin 509

Flurazepam Hydrochloride (Additive depressant effect). Products include:

Dalmane Capsules 2173

Glutethimide (Additive depressant effect).

No products indexed under this heading.

Haloperidol (Additive depressant effect). Products include:

Haldol Injection, Tablets and Concentrate 1575

Haloperidol Decanoate (Additive depressant effect). Products include:

Haldol Decanoate 1577

Hydrocodone Bitartrate (Additive depressant effect). Products include:

Anexsia 5/500 Elixir 1781
Anexia Tablets 1782
Codiclear DH Syrup 791
Deconamine CX Cough and Cold Liquid and Tablets 1319
Duratuss HD Elixir 2565
Hycodan Tablets and Syrup 930
Hycomine Compound Tablets 932
Hycomine 931
Hycotuss Expectorant Syrup 933
Hydrocet Capsules 782
Lorcet 10/650 1018
Lortab 2566
Tussend 1783
Tussend Expectorant 1785
Vicodin Tablets 1356
Vicodin ES Tablets 1357
Vicodin Tuss Expectorant 1358
Zydone Capsules 949

Hydrocodone Polistirex (Additive depressant effect). Products include:

Tussionex Pennkinetic Extended-Release Suspension 998

IMPORTANT NOTE: Always consult each drug listing in the patient's regimen for possible interactions.

Hydroxyzine Hydrochloride (Additive depressant effect). Products include:
- Atarax Tablets & Syrup ... 2185
- Marax Tablets & DF Syrup ... 2200
- Vistaril Intramuscular Solution ... 2216

Isoflurane (Additive depressant effect).
- No products indexed under this heading.

Ketamine Hydrochloride (Additive depressant effect).
- No products indexed under this heading.

Levomethadyl Acetate Hydrochloride (Additive depressant effect). Products include:
- Orlamm ... 2239

Levorphanol Tartrate (Additive depressant effect). Products include:
- Levo-Dromoran ... 2129

Lorazepam (Additive depressant effect). Products include:
- Ativan Injection ... 2698
- Ativan Tablets ... 2700

Loxapine Hydrochloride (Additive depressant effect). Products include:
- Loxitane ... 1378

Loxapine Succinate (Additive depressant effect). Products include:
- Loxitane Capsules ... 1378

Meperidine Hydrochloride (Additive depressant effect). Products include:
- Demerol ... 2308
- Mepergan Injection ... 2753

Mephobarbital (Additive depressant effect). Products include:
- Mebaral Tablets ... 2322

Meprobamate (Additive depressant effect). Products include:
- Miltown Tablets ... 2672
- PMB 200 and PMB 400 ... 2783

Mesoridazine Besylate (Additive depressant effect). Products include:
- Serentil ... 684

Methadone Hydrochloride (Additive depressant effect). Products include:
- Methadone Hydrochloride Oral Concentrate ... 2233
- Methadone Hydrochloride Oral Solution & Tablets ... 2235

Methohexital Sodium (Additive depressant effect). Products include:
- Brevital Sodium Vials ... 1429

Methotrimeprazine (Additive depressant effect). Products include:
- Levoprome ... 1274

Methoxyflurane (Additive depressant effect).
- No products indexed under this heading.

Midazolam Hydrochloride (Additive depressant effect). Products include:
- Versed Injection ... 2170

Molindone Hydrochloride (Additive depressant effect). Products include:
- Moban Tablets and Concentrate ... 1048

Morphine Sulfate (Additive depressant effect). Products include:
- Astramorph/PF Injection, USP (Preservative-Free) ... 535
- Duramorph ... 962
- Infumorph 200 and Infumorph 500 Sterile Solutions ... 965
- MS Contin Tablets ... 1994
- MSIR ... 1997
- Oramorph SR (Morphine Sulfate Sustained Release Tablets) ... 2236
- RMS Suppositories ... 2657
- Roxanol ... 2243

Opium Alkaloids (Additive depressant effect).
- No products indexed under this heading.

Oxazepam (Additive depressant effect). Products include:
- Serax Capsules ... 2810
- Serax Tablets ... 2810

Oxycodone Hydrochloride (Additive depressant effect). Products include:
- Percocet Tablets ... 938
- Percodan Tablets ... 939
- Percodan-Demi Tablets ... 940
- Roxicodone Tablets, Oral Solution & Intensol (Oxycodone) ... 2244
- Tylox Capsules ... 1584

Pentobarbital Sodium (Additive depressant effects). Products include:
- Nembutal Sodium Capsules ... 436
- Nembutal Sodium Solution ... 438
- Nembutal Sodium Suppositories ... 440

Perphenazine (Additive depressant effect). Products include:
- Etrafon ... 2355
- Triavil Tablets ... 1757
- Trilafon ... 2389

Phenobarbital (Additive depressant effect). Products include:
- Arco-Lase Plus Tablets ... 512
- Bellergal-S Tablets ... 2250
- Donnatal ... 2060
- Donnatal Extentabs ... 2061
- Donnatal Tablets ... 2060
- Phenobarbital Elixir and Tablets ... 1469
- Quadrinal Tablets ... 1350

Prazepam (Additive depressant effect).
- No products indexed under this heading.

Prochlorperazine (Additive depressant effect). Products include:
- Compazine ... 2470

Promethazine Hydrochloride (Additive depressant effect). Products include:
- Mepergan Injection ... 2753
- Phenergan with Codeine ... 2777
- Phenergan with Dextromethorphan ... 2778
- Phenergan Injection ... 2773
- Phenergan Suppositories ... 2775
- Phenergan Syrup ... 2774
- Phenergan Tablets ... 2775
- Phenergan VC ... 2779
- Phenergan VC with Codeine ... 2781

Propofol (Additive depressant effect). Products include:
- Diprivan Injection ... 2833

Propoxyphene Hydrochloride (Additive depressant effect). Products include:
- Darvon ... 1435
- Wygesic Tablets ... 2827

Propoxyphene Napsylate (Additive depressant effect). Products include:
- Darvon-N/Darvocet-N ... 1433

Quazepam (Additive depressant effect). Products include:
- Doral Tablets ... 2664

Risperidone (Additive depressant effect). Products include:
- Risperdal ... 1301

Secobarbital Sodium (Additive depressant effect). Products include:
- Seconal Sodium Pulvules ... 1474

Sufentanil Citrate (Additive depressant effect). Products include:
- Sufenta Injection ... 1309

Temazepam (Additive depressant effect). Products include:
- Restoril Capsules ... 2284

Thiamylal Sodium (Additive depressant effect).
- No products indexed under this heading.

Thioridazine Hydrochloride (Additive depressant effect). Products include:
- Mellaril ... 2269

Thiothixene (Additive depressant effect). Products include:
- Navane Capsules and Concentrate ... 2201
- Navane Intramuscular ... 2202

Triazolam (Additive depressant effect). Products include:
- Halcion Tablets ... 2611

Trifluoperazine Hydrochloride (Additive depressant effect). Products include:
- Stelazine ... 2514

Zolpidem Tartrate (Additive depressant effect). Products include:
- Ambien Tablets ... 2416

Food Interactions

Alcohol (Additive depressant effect).

LIPPES LOOP INTRAUTERINE DOUBLE-S

(Intrauterine device) ... 1848

None cited in PDR database.

LISTERINE ANTISEPTIC

(Eucalyptol, Menthol, Methyl Salicylate) ... ◘ 855

None cited in PDR database.

COOL MINT LISTERINE

(Thymol, Eucalyptol, Methyl Salicylate, Menthol) ... ◘ 856

None cited in PDR database.

FRESHBURST LISTERINE

(Thymol, Eucalyptol, Methyl Salicylate, Menthol) ... ◘ 856

None cited in PDR database.

LISTERMINT ALCOHOL-FREE MOUTHWASH

(Sodium Fluoride) ... ◘ 855

None cited in PDR database.

LITHIUM CARBONATE CAPSULES & TABLETS

(Lithium Carbonate) ... 2230

May interact with antipsychotic agents, nondepolarizing neuromuscular blocking agents, non-steroidal anti-inflammatory agents, diuretics, ACE inhibitors, and certain other agents. Compounds in these categories include:

Amiloride Hydrochloride (High risk of lithium toxicity). Products include:
- Midamor Tablets ... 1703
- Moduretic Tablets ... 1705

Atracurium Besylate (Prolonged effects of neuromuscular blockers). Products include:
- Tracrium Injection ... 1183

Benazepril Hydrochloride (Reduces lithium clearance and increases serum lithium levels resulting in risk of lithium toxicity). Products include:
- Lotensin Tablets ... 834
- Lotensin HCT ... 837
- Lotrel Capsules ... 840

Bendroflumethiazide (High risk of lithium toxicity).
- No products indexed under this heading.

Bumetanide (High risk of lithium toxicity). Products include:
- Bumex ... 2093

Captopril (Reduces lithium clearance and increases serum lithium levels resulting in risk of lithium toxicity). Products include:
- Capoten ... 739
- Capozide ... 742

Chlorothiazide (High risk of lithium toxicity). Products include:
- Aldoclor Tablets ... 1598
- Diupres Tablets ... 1650
- Diuril Oral ... 1653

Chlorothiazide Sodium (High risk of lithium toxicity). Products include:
- Diuril Sodium Intravenous ... 1652

Chlorpromazine (Neurological toxicity has occurred; encephalopathic syndrome followed by irreversible brain damage). Products include:
- Thorazine Suppositories ... 2523

Chlorprothixene (Neurological toxicity has occurred; encephalopathic syndrome followed by irreversible brain damage).
- No products indexed under this heading.

Chlorprothixene Hydrochloride (Neurological toxicity has occurred; encephalopathic syndrome followed by irreversible brain damage).
- No products indexed under this heading.

Chlorthalidone (High risk of lithium toxicity). Products include:
- Combipres Tablets ... 677
- Tenoretic Tablets ... 2845
- Thalitone ... 1245

Clozapine (Neurological toxicity has occurred; encephalopathic syndrome followed by irreversible brain damage). Products include:
- Clozaril Tablets ... 2252

Diclofenac Potassium (Significant increase in steady state plasma lithium levels; possible lithium toxicity). Products include:
- Cataflam ... 816

Diclofenac Sodium (Significant increase in steady state plasma lithium levels; possible lithium toxicity). Products include:
- Voltaren Ophthalmic Sterile Ophthalmic Solution ... ⊙ 272
- Voltaren Tablets ... 861

Enalapril Maleate (Reduces lithium clearance and increases serum lithium levels resulting in risk of lithium toxicity). Products include:
- Vaseretic Tablets ... 1765
- Vasotec Tablets ... 1771

Enalaprilat (Reduces lithium clearance and increases serum lithium levels resulting in risk of lithium toxicity). Products include:
- Vasotec I.V. ... 1768

Ethacrynic Acid (High risk of lithium toxicity). Products include:
- Edecrin Tablets ... 1657

Etodolac (Significant increase in steady state plasma lithium levels; possible lithium toxicity). Products include:
- Lodine Capsules and Tablets ... 2743

Fenoprofen Calcium (Significant increase in steady state plasma lithium levels; possible lithium toxicity). Products include:
- Nalfon 200 Pulvules & Nalfon Tablets ... 917

Fluphenazine Decanoate (Neurological toxicity has occurred; encephalopathic syndrome followed by irreversible brain damage). Products include:
- Prolixin Decanoate ... 509

Fluphenazine Enanthate (Neurological toxicity has occurred; encephalopathic syndrome followed by irreversible brain damage). Products include:
- Prolixin Enanthate ... 509

Fluphenazine Hydrochloride (Neurological toxicity has occurred; encephalopathic syndrome followed by irreversible brain damage). Products include:
- Prolixin ... 509

(◘ Described in PDR For Nonprescription Drugs) (⊙ Described in PDR For Ophthalmology)

Interactions Index

Lithonate/Lithotabs/Lithobid

Flurbiprofen (Significant increase in steady state plasma lithium levels; possible lithium toxicity). Products include:

Ansaid Tablets 2579

Fosinopril Sodium (Reduces lithium clearance and increases serum lithium levels resulting in risk of lithium toxicity). Products include:

Monopril Tablets 757

Furosemide (High risk of lithium toxicity). Products include:

Lasix Injection, Oral Solution and Tablets 1240

Haloperidol (Neurological toxicity has occurred; encephalopathic syndrome followed by irreversible brain damage). Products include:

Haldol Injection, Tablets and Concentrate 1575

Haloperidol Decanoate (Neurological toxicity has occurred; encephalopathic syndrome followed by irreversible brain damage). Products include:

Haldol Decanoate................................... 1577

Hydrochlorothiazide (High risk of lithium toxicity). Products include:

Aldactazide.. 2413
Aldoril Tablets... 1604
Apresazide Capsules 808
Capozide 742
Dyazide 2479
Esidrix Tablets 821
Esimil Tablets.. 822
HydroDIURIL Tablets 1674
Hydropres Tablets................................... 1675
Hyzaar Tablets 1677
Inderide Tablets 2732
Inderide LA Long Acting Capsules .. 2734
Lopressor HCT Tablets 832
Lotensin HCT.. 837
Maxzide 1380
Moduretic Tablets 1705
Oretic Tablets 443
Prinzide Tablets 1737
Ser-Ap-Es Tablets................................... 849
Timolide Tablets...................................... 1748
Vaseretic Tablets 1765
Zestoretic 2850
Ziac 1415

Hydroflumethiazide (High risk of lithium toxicity). Products include:

Diucardin Tablets.................................... 2718

Ibuprofen (Significant increase in steady state plasma lithium levels; possible lithium toxicity). Products include:

Advil Cold and Sinus Caplets and Tablets (formerly CoAdvil) .... ®D 870
Advil Ibuprofen Tablets and Caplets .... ®D 870
Children's Advil Suspension 2692
Arthritis Foundation Ibuprofen Tablets .... ®D 674
Bayer Select Ibuprofen Pain Relief Formula .... ®D 715
Cramp End Tablets .... ®D 735
Dimetapp Sinus Caplets .... ®D 775
Haltran Tablets.. ®D 771
IBU Tablets.. 1342
Ibuprohm... ®D 735
Children's Motrin Ibuprofen Oral Suspension 1546
Motrin Tablets.. 2625
Motrin IB Caplets, Tablets, and Geltabs .... ®D 838
Motrin IB Sinus .... ®D 838
Motrin Ibuprofen Suspension, Oral Drops, Chewable Tablets, Caplets 1546
Nuprin Ibuprofen/Analgesic Tablets & Caplets .... ®D 622
Sine-Aid IB Caplets 1554
Vicks DayQuil SINUS Pressure & PAIN Relief with IBUPROFEN ...... ®D 762

Indapamide (High risk of lithium toxicity). Products include:

Lozol Tablets 2022

Indomethacin (Significant increase in steady state plasma lithium levels; possible lithium toxicity). Products include:

Indocin 1680

Indomethacin Sodium Trihydrate (Significant increase in steady state plasma lithium levels; possible lithium toxicity). Products include:

Indocin I.V. 1684

Ketoprofen (Significant increase in steady state plasma lithium levels; possible lithium toxicity). Products include:

Orudis Capsules 2766
Oruvail Capsules 2766

Ketorolac Tromethamine (Significant increase in steady state plasma lithium levels; possible lithium toxicity). Products include:

Acular 474
Acular .... © 277
Toradol... 2159

Lisinopril (Reduces lithium clearance and increases serum lithium levels resulting in risk of lithium toxicity). Products include:

Prinivil Tablets 1733
Prinzide Tablets 1737
Zestoretic 2850
Zestril Tablets 2854

Loxapine Hydrochloride (Neurological toxicity has occurred; encephalopathic syndrome followed by irreversible brain damage). Products include:

Loxitane 1378

Meclofenamate Sodium (Significant increase in steady state plasma lithium levels; possible lithium toxicity).

No products indexed under this heading.

Mefenamic Acid (Significant increase in steady state plasma lithium levels; possible lithium toxicity). Products include:

Ponstel 1925

Mesoridazine Besylate (Neurological toxicity has occurred; encephalopathic syndrome followed by irreversible brain damage). Products include:

Serentil... 684

Methyclothiazide (High risk of lithium toxicity). Products include:

Enduron Tablets...................................... 420

Metocurine Iodide (Prolonged effects of neuromuscular blockers). Products include:

Metubine Iodide Vials............................ 916

Metolazone (High risk of lithium toxicity). Products include:

Mykrox Tablets.. 993
Zaroxolyn Tablets 1000

Mivacurium Chloride (Prolonged effects of neuromuscular blockers). Products include:

Mivacron 1138

Moexipril Hydrochloride (Reduces lithium clearance and increases serum lithium levels resulting in risk of lithium toxicity). Products include:

Univasc Tablets 2410

Molindone Hydrochloride (Neurological toxicity has occurred; encephalopathic syndrome followed by irreversible brain damage). Products include:

Moban Tablets and Concentrate...... 1048

Nabumetone (Significant increase in steady state plasma lithium levels; possible lithium toxicity). Products include:

Relafen Tablets....................................... 2510

Naproxen (Significant increase in steady state plasma lithium levels; possible lithium toxicity). Products include:

Anaprox/Naprosyn 2117

Naproxen Sodium (Significant increase in steady state plasma lithium levels; possible lithium toxicity). Products include:

Aleve 1975
Anaprox/Naprosyn 2117

Oxaprozin (Significant increase in steady state plasma lithium levels; possible lithium toxicity). Products include:

Daypro Caplets 2426

Pancuronium Bromide Injection (Prolonged effects of neuromuscular blockers).

No products indexed under this heading.

Perphenazine (Neurological toxicity has occurred; encephalopathic syndrome followed by irreversible brain damage). Products include:

Etrafon 2355
Triavil Tablets.. 1757
Trilafon... 2389

Phenylbutazone (Significant increase in steady state plasma lithium levels; possible lithium toxicity).

No products indexed under this heading.

Pimozide (Neurological toxicity has occurred; encephalopathic syndrome followed by irreversible brain damage). Products include:

Orap Tablets 1050

Piroxicam (Significant increase in steady state plasma lithium levels; possible lithium toxicity). Products include:

Feldene Capsules 1965

Polythiazide (High risk of lithium toxicity). Products include:

Minizide Capsules 1938

Prochlorperazine (Neurological toxicity has occurred; encephalopathic syndrome followed by irreversible brain damage). Products include:

Compazine 2470

Promethazine Hydrochloride (Neurological toxicity has occurred; encephalopathic syndrome followed by irreversible brain damage). Products include:

Mepergan Injection 2753
Phenergan with Codeine....................... 2777
Phenergan with Dextromethorphan 2778
Phenergan Injection 2773
Phenergan Suppositories 2775
Phenergan Syrup 2774
Phenergan Tablets 2775
Phenergan VC 2779
Phenergan VC with Codeine 2781

Quinapril Hydrochloride (Reduces lithium clearance and increases serum lithium levels resulting in risk of lithium toxicity). Products include:

Accupril Tablets 1893

Ramipril (Reduces lithium clearance and increases serum lithium levels resulting in risk of lithium toxicity). Products include:

Altace Capsules 1232

Risperidone (Neurological toxicity has occurred; encephalopathic syndrome followed by irreversible brain damage). Products include:

Risperdal.. 1301

Rocuronium Bromide (Prolonged effects of neuromuscular blockers). Products include:

Zemuron 1830

Spirapril Hydrochloride (Reduces lithium clearance and increases serum lithium levels resulting in risk of lithium toxicity).

No products indexed under this heading.

Spironolactone (High risk of lithium toxicity). Products include:

Aldactazide.. 2413
Aldactone 2414

Sulindac (Significant increase in steady state plasma lithium levels; possible lithium toxicity). Products include:

Clinoril Tablets 1618

Thioridazine Hydrochloride (Neurological toxicity has occurred; encephalopathic syndrome followed by irreversible brain damage). Products include:

Mellaril 2269

Thiothixene (Neurological toxicity has occurred; encephalopathic syndrome followed by irreversible brain damage). Products include:

Navane Capsules and Concentrate 2201
Navane Intramuscular 2202

Tolmetin Sodium (Significant increase in steady state plasma lithium levels; possible lithium toxicity). Products include:

Tolectin (200, 400 and 600 mg) .. 1581

Torsemide (High risk of lithium toxicity). Products include:

Demadex Tablets and Injection 686

Triamterene (High risk of lithium toxicity). Products include:

Dyazide 2479
Dyrenium Capsules................................ 2481
Maxzide 1380

Trifluoperazine Hydrochloride (Neurological toxicity has occurred; encephalopathic syndrome followed by irreversible brain damage). Products include:

Stelazine 2514

Vecuronium Bromide (Prolonged effects of neuromuscular blockers). Products include:

Norcuron 1826

LITHOBID SLOW-RELEASE TABLETS

(Lithium Carbonate) 2543

See **LITHONATE Capsules**

LITHONATE CAPSULES

(Lithium Carbonate) 2543

May interact with ACE inhibitors, diuretics, calcium channel blockers, antipsychotic agents, thiazides, neuromuscular blocking agents, xanthine bronchodilators, non-steroidal anti-inflammatory agents, and certain other agents. Compounds in these categories include:

Acetazolamide (Lowers serum lithium concentrations by increasing urinary lithium excretions). Products include:

Diamox Sequels (Sustained Release) 1373
Diamox Sequels (Sustained Release) .... © 319
Diamox Tablets.. 1372
Diamox Tablets.. © 317

Amiloride Hydrochloride (Concomitant use should be avoided; potential for lithium toxicity). Products include:

Midamor Tablets 1703
Moduretic Tablets 1705

Aminophylline (Lowers serum lithium concentrations by increasing urinary lithium excretions).

No products indexed under this heading.

Amlodipine Besylate (Concurrent use may increase the risk of neurotoxicity in the form of ataxia, tremors, nausea, vomiting, diarrhea, and/or tinnitus). Products include:

Lotrel Capsules....................................... 840
Norvasc Tablets 1940

IMPORTANT NOTE: Always consult each drug listing in the patient's regimen for possible interactions.

Lithonate/Lithotabs/Lithobid | Interactions Index | 592

Atracurium Besylate (Prolonged effects of neuromuscular blocking agents). Products include:

Tracrium Injection 1183

Benazepril Hydrochloride (Concomitant use should be avoided; potential for lithium toxicity). Products include:

Lotensin Tablets 834
Lotensin HCT 837
Lotrel Capsules 840

Bendroflumethiazide (Concomitant use should be avoided; potential for lithium toxicity).

No products indexed under this heading.

Bepridil Hydrochloride (Concurrent use may increase the risk of neurotoxicity in the form of ataxia, tremors, nausea, vomiting, diarrhea, and/or tinnitus). Products include:

Vascor (200, 300 and 400 mg) Tablets 1587

Bumetanide (Concomitant use should be avoided; potential for lithium toxicity). Products include:

Bumex 2093

Captopril (Concomitant use should be avoided; potential for lithium toxicity). Products include:

Capoten 739
Capozide 742

Carbamazepine (Increased risk of neurotoxic side effects). Products include:

Atretol Tablets 573
Tegretol Chewable Tablets 852
Tegretol Suspension 852
Tegretol Tablets 852

Chlorothiazide (Concomitant use should be avoided; potential for lithium toxicity). Products include:

Aldoclor Tablets 1598
Diupres Tablets 1650
Diuril Oral 1653

Chlorothiazide Sodium (Concomitant use should be avoided; potential for lithium toxicity). Products include:

Diuril Sodium Intravenous 1652

Chlorpromazine (Possible haloperidol-type interaction has been extended to other antipsychotics). Products include:

Thorazine Suppositories 2523

Chlorprothixene (Possible haloperidol-type interaction has been extended to other antipsychotics).

No products indexed under this heading.

Chlorprothixene Hydrochloride (Possible haloperidol-type interaction has been extended to other antipsychotics).

No products indexed under this heading.

Chlorthalidone (Concomitant use should be avoided; potential for lithium toxicity). Products include:

Combipres Tablets 677
Tenoretic Tablets 2845
Thalitone 1245

Clozapine (Possible haloperidol-type interaction has been extended to other antipsychotics). Products include:

Clozaril Tablets 2252

Decamethonium (Prolonged effects of neuromuscular blocking agents).

Diclofenac Potassium (Potential for increased steady-state plasma lithium levels resulting in lithium toxicity). Products include:

Cataflam 816

Diclofenac Sodium (Potential for increased steady-state plasma lithium levels resulting in lithium toxicity). Products include:

Voltaren Ophthalmic Sterile Ophthalmic Solution .... ⊙ 272
Voltaren Tablets 861

Diltiazem Hydrochloride (Concurrent use may increase the risk of neurotoxicity in the form of ataxia, tremors, nausea, vomiting, diarrhea, and/or tinnitus). Products include:

Cardizem CD Capsules 1506
Cardizem SR Capsules 1510
Cardizem Injectable 1508
Cardizem Tablets 1512
Dilacor XR Extended-release Capsules 2018

Doxacurium Chloride (Prolonged effects of neuromuscular blocking agents). Products include:

Nuromax Injection 1149

Dyphylline (Lowers serum lithium concentrations by increasing urinary lithium excretions). Products include:

Lufyllin & Lufyllin-400 Tablets 2670
Lufyllin-GG Elixir & Tablets 2671

Enalapril Maleate (Concomitant use should be avoided; potential for lithium toxicity). Products include:

Vaseretic Tablets 1765
Vasotec Tablets 1771

Enalaprilat (Concomitant use should be avoided; potential for lithium toxicity). Products include:

Vasotec I.V. 1768

Ethacrynic Acid (Concomitant use should be avoided; potential for lithium toxicity). Products include:

Edecrin Tablets 1657

Etodolac (Potential for increased steady-state plasma lithium levels resulting in lithium toxicity). Products include:

Lodine Capsules and Tablets 2743

Felodipine (Concurrent use may increase the risk of neurotoxicity in the form of ataxia, tremors, nausea, vomiting, diarrhea, and/or tinnitus). Products include:

Plendil Extended-Release Tablets 527

Fenoprofen Calcium (Potential for increased steady-state plasma lithium levels resulting in lithium toxicity). Products include:

Nalfon 200 Pulvules & Nalfon Tablets 917

Fluoxetine Hydrochloride (Concurrent use has resulted in both increased and decreased lithium levels). Products include:

Prozac Pulvules & Liquid, Oral Solution 919

Fluphenazine Decanoate (Possible haloperidol-type interaction has been extended to other antipsychotics). Products include:

Prolixin Decanoate 509

Fluphenazine Enanthate (Possible haloperidol-type interaction has been extended to other antipsychotics). Products include:

Prolixin Enanthate 509

Fluphenazine Hydrochloride (Possible haloperidol-type interaction has been extended to other antipsychotics). Products include:

Prolixin 509

Flurbiprofen (Potential for increased steady-state plasma lithium levels resulting in lithium toxicity). Products include:

Ansaid Tablets 2579

Fosinopril Sodium (Concomitant use should be avoided; potential for lithium toxicity). Products include:

Monopril Tablets 757

Furosemide (Concomitant use should be avoided; potential for lithium toxicity). Products include:

Lasix Injection, Oral Solution and Tablets 1240

Haloperidol (Concomitant use may lead to encephalopathic syndrome followed by irreversible brain damage; possible haloperidol-type interaction has been extended to other antipsychotic). Products include:

Haldol Injection, Tablets and Concentrate 1575

Haloperidol Decanoate (Concomitant use may lead to encephalopathic syndrome followed by irreversible brain damage; possible haloperidol-type interaction has been extended to other antipsychotic). Products include:

Haldol Decanoate 1577

Hydrochlorothiazide (Concomitant use should be avoided; potential for lithium toxicity). Products include:

Aldactazide 2413
Aldoril Tablets 1604
Apresazide Capsules 808
Capozide 742
Dyazide 2479
Esidrix Tablets 821
Esimil Tablets 822
HydroDIURIL Tablets 1674
Hydropres Tablets 1675
Hyzaar Tablets 1677
Inderide Tablets 2732
Inderide LA Long Acting Capsules .. 2734
Lopressor HCT Tablets 832
Lotensin HCT 837
Maxzide 1380
Moduretic Tablets 1705
Oretic Tablets 443
Prinzide Tablets 1737
Ser-Ap-Es Tablets 849
Timolide Tablets 1748
Vaseretic Tablets 1765
Zestoretic 2850
Ziac 1415

Hydroflumethiazide (Concomitant use should be avoided; potential for lithium toxicity). Products include:

Diucardin Tablets 2718

Ibuprofen (Potential for increased steady-state plasma lithium levels resulting in lithium toxicity). Products include:

Advil Cold and Sinus Caplets and Tablets (formerly CoAdvil) .... ▣ 870
Advil Ibuprofen Tablets and Caplets .... ▣ 870
Children's Advil Suspension 2692
Arthritis Foundation Ibuprofen Tablets .... ▣ 674
Bayer Select Ibuprofen Pain Relief Formula .... ▣ 715
Cramp End Tablets .... ▣ 735
Dimetapp Sinus Caplets .... ▣ 775
Haltran Tablets .... ▣ 771
IBU Tablets 1342
Ibuprohm .... ▣ 735
Children's Motrin Ibuprofen Oral Suspension 1546
Motrin Tablets 2625
Motrin IB Caplets, Tablets, and Geltabs .... ▣ 838
Motrin IB Sinus .... ▣ 838
Motrin Ibuprofen Suspension, Oral Drops, Chewable Tablets, Caplets 1546
Nuprin Ibuprofen/Analgesic Tablets & Caplets .... ▣ 622
Sine-Aid IB Caplets 1554
Vicks DayQuil SINUS Pressure & PAIN Relief with IBUPROFEN .... ▣ 762

Indapamide (Concomitant use should be avoided; potential for lithium toxicity). Products include:

Lozol Tablets 2022

Indomethacin (Potential for increased steady-state plasma lithium levels resulting in lithium toxicity). Products include:

Indocin 1680

Indomethacin Sodium Trihydrate (Potential for increased steady-state plasma lithium levels resulting in lithium toxicity). Products include:

Indocin I.V. 1684

Isradipine (Concurrent use may increase the risk of neurotoxicity in the form of ataxia, tremors, nausea, vomiting, diarrhea, and/or tinnitus). Products include:

DynaCirc Capsules 2256

Ketoprofen (Potential for increased steady-state plasma lithium levels resulting in lithium toxicity). Products include:

Orudis Capsules 2766
Oruvail Capsules 2766

Ketorolac Tromethamine (Potential for increased steady-state plasma lithium levels resulting in lithium toxicity). Products include:

Acular 474
Acular .... ⊙ 277
Toradol 2159

Lisinopril (Concomitant use should be avoided; potential for lithium toxicity). Products include:

Prinivil Tablets 1733
Prinzide Tablets 1737
Zestoretic 2850
Zestril Tablets 2854

Loxapine Hydrochloride (Possible haloperidol-type interaction has been extended to other antipsychotics). Products include:

Loxitane 1378

Loxapine Succinate (Possible haloperidol-type interaction has been extended to other antipsychotics). Products include:

Loxitane Capsules 1378

Meclofenamate Sodium (Potential for increased steady-state plasma lithium levels resulting in lithium toxicity).

No products indexed under this heading.

Mefenamic Acid (Potential for increased steady-state plasma lithium levels resulting in lithium toxicity). Products include:

Ponstel 1925

Mesoridazine Besylate (Possible haloperidol-type interaction has been extended to other antipsychotics). Products include:

Serentil 684

Methyclothiazide (Concomitant use should be avoided; potential for lithium toxicity). Products include:

Enduron Tablets 420

Metocurine Iodide (Prolonged effects of neuromuscular blocking agents). Products include:

Metubine Iodide Vials 916

Metolazone (Concomitant use should be avoided; potential for lithium toxicity). Products include:

Mykrox Tablets 993
Zaroxolyn Tablets 1000

Metronidazole (Concurrent use may provoke lithium toxicity due to reduced renal clearance). Products include:

Flagyl 375 Capsules 2434
Flagyl I.V. RTU 2247
MetroGel 1047
MetroGel-Vaginal 902
Protostat Tablets 1883

Mivacurium Chloride (Prolonged effects of neuromuscular blocking agents). Products include:

Mivacron 1138

(▣ Described in PDR For Nonprescription Drugs) (⊙ Described in PDR For Ophthalmology)

Moexipril Hydrochloride (Concomitant use should be avoided; potential for lithium toxicity). Products include:

Univasc Tablets 2410

Molindone Hydrochloride (Possible haloperidol-type interaction has been extended to other antipsychotics). Products include:

Moban Tablets and Concentrate 1048

Nabumetone (Potential for increased steady-state plasma lithium levels resulting in lithium toxicity). Products include:

Relafen Tablets................................... 2510

Naproxen (Potential for increased steady-state plasma lithium levels resulting in lithium toxicity). Products include:

Anaprox/Naprosyn 2117

Naproxen Sodium (Potential for increased steady-state plasma lithium levels resulting in lithium toxicity). Products include:

Aleve 1975
Anaprox/Naprosyn 2117

Nicardipine Hydrochloride (Concurrent use may increase the risk of neurotoxicity in the form of ataxia, tremors, nausea, vomiting, diarrhea, and/or tinnitus). Products include:

Cardene Capsules 2095
Cardene I.V. 2709
Cardene SR Capsules.......................... 2097

Nifedipine (Concurrent use may increase the risk of neurotoxicity in the form of ataxia, tremors, nausea, vomiting, diarrhea, and/or tinnitus). Products include:

Adalat Capsules (10 mg and 20 mg) 587
Adalat CC 589
Procardia Capsules............................. 1971
Procardia XL Extended Release Tablets 1972

Nimodipine (Concurrent use may increase the risk of neurotoxicity in the form of ataxia, tremors, nausea, vomiting, diarrhea, and/or tinnitus). Products include:

Nimotop Capsules 610

Nisoldipine (Concurrent use may increase the risk of neurotoxicity in the form of ataxia, tremors, nausea, vomiting, diarrhea, and/or tinnitus).

No products indexed under this heading.

Oxaprozin (Potential for increased steady-state plasma lithium levels resulting in lithium toxicity). Products include:

Daypro Caplets 2426

Pancuronium Bromide Injection (Prolonged effects of neuromuscular blocking agents).

No products indexed under this heading.

Perphenazine (Possible haloperidol-type interaction has been extended to other antipsychotics). Products include:

Etrafon 2355
Triavil Tablets 1757
Trilafon... 2389

Phenylbutazone (Potential for increased steady-state plasma lithium levels resulting in lithium toxicity).

No products indexed under this heading.

Pimozide (Possible haloperidol-type interaction has been extended to other antipsychotics). Products include:

Orap Tablets 1050

Piroxicam (Potential for increased steady-state plasma lithium levels resulting in lithium toxicity). Products include:

Feldene Capsules................................. 1965

Polythiazide (Concomitant use should be avoided; potential for lithium toxicity). Products include:

Minizide Capsules 1938

Potassium Iodide (Concomitant extended use of iodide preparation may produce hypothyroidism). Products include:

Hyland's C-Plus Cold Tablets .... ⊞ 829
Pima Syrup.. 1005
Quadrinal Tablets 1350
SSKI Solution 2658

Prochlorperazine (Possible haloperidol-type interaction has been extended to other antipsychotics). Products include:

Compazine 2470

Promethazine Hydrochloride (Possible haloperidol-type interaction has been extended to other antipsychotics). Products include:

Mepergan Injection 2753
Phenergan with Codeine.................... 2777
Phenergan with Dextromethorphan 2778
Phenergan Injection 2773
Phenergan Suppositories.................... 2775
Phenergan Syrup 2774
Phenergan Tablets 2775
Phenergan VC 2779
Phenergan VC with Codeine 2781

Quinapril Hydrochloride (Concomitant use should be avoided; potential for lithium toxicity). Products include:

Accupril Tablets 1893

Ramipril (Concomitant use should be avoided; potential for lithium toxicity). Products include:

Altace Capsules 1232

Risperidone (Possible haloperidol-type interaction has been extended to other antipsychotics). Products include:

Risperdal 1301

Rocuronium Bromide (Prolonged effects of neuromuscular blocking agents). Products include:

Zemuron 1830

Sodium Bicarbonate (Lowers serum lithium concentrations by increasing urinary lithium excretions). Products include:

Alka-Seltzer Effervescent Antacid and Pain Reliever............................ ⊞ 701
Alka-Seltzer Extra Strength Effervescent Antacid and Pain Reliever .... ⊞ 703
Alka-Seltzer Gold Effervescent Antacid... ⊞ 703
Alka-Seltzer Lemon Lime Effervescent Antacid and Pain Reliever .... ⊞ 703
Arm & Hammer Pure Baking Soda .... ⊞ 627
Ceo-Two Rectal Suppositories 666
Citrocarbonate Antacid...................... ⊞ 770
Massengill Disposable Douches....... ⊞ 820
Massengill Liquid Concentrate........ ⊞ 820
NuLYTELY... 689
Cherry Flavor NuLYTELY 689

Spirapril Hydrochloride (Concomitant use should be avoided; potential for lithium toxicity).

No products indexed under this heading.

Spironolactone (Concomitant use should be avoided; potential for lithium toxicity). Products include:

Aldactazide... 2413
Aldactone 2414

Succinylcholine Chloride (Prolonged effects of neuromuscular blocking agents). Products include:

Anectine... 1073

Sulindac (Potential for increased steady-state plasma lithium levels resulting in lithium toxicity). Products include:

Clinoril Tablets 1618

Theophylline (Lowers serum lithium concentrations by increasing urinary lithium excretions). Products include:

Marax Tablets & DF Syrup................. 2200
Quibron 2053

Theophylline Anhydrous (Lowers serum lithium concentrations by increasing urinary lithium excretions). Products include:

Aerolate 1004
Primatene Dual Action Formula...... ⊞ 872
Primatene Tablets............................... ⊞ 873
Respbid Tablets 682
Slo-bid Gyrocaps 2033
Theo-24 Extended Release Capsules 2568
Theo-Dur Extended-Release Tablets 1327
Theo-X Extended-Release Tablets .. 788
Uni-Dur Extended-Release Tablets.. 1331
Uniphyl 400 mg Tablets..................... 2001

Theophylline Calcium Salicylate (Lowers serum lithium concentrations by increasing urinary lithium excretions). Products include:

Quadrinal Tablets 1350

Theophylline Sodium Glycinate (Lowers serum lithium concentrations by increasing urinary lithium excretions).

No products indexed under this heading.

Thioridazine Hydrochloride (Possible haloperidol-type interaction has been extended to other antipsychotics). Products include:

Mellaril 2269

Thiothixene (Possible haloperidol-type interaction has been extended to other antipsychotics). Products include:

Navane Capsules and Concentrate 2201
Navane Intramuscular 2202

Tolmetin Sodium (Potential for increased steady-state plasma lithium levels resulting in lithium toxicity). Products include:

Tolectin (200, 400 and 600 mg) .. 1581

Torsemide (Concomitant use should be avoided; potential for lithium toxicity). Products include:

Demadex Tablets and Injection 686

Triamterene (Concomitant use should be avoided; potential for lithium toxicity). Products include:

Dyazide 2479
Dyrenium Capsules............................. 2481
Maxzide 1380

Trifluoperazine Hydrochloride (Possible haloperidol-type interaction has been extended to other antipsychotics). Products include:

Stelazine 2514

Vecuronium Bromide (Prolonged effects of neuromuscular blocking agents). Products include:

Norcuron 1826

Verapamil Hydrochloride (Concurrent use may increase the risk of neurotoxicity in the form of ataxia, tremors, nausea, vomiting, diarrhea, and/or tinnitus). Products include:

Calan SR Caplets 2422
Calan Tablets....................................... 2419
Isoptin Injectable 1344
Isoptin Oral Tablets 1346
Isoptin SR Tablets 1348
Verelan Capsules 1410
Verelan Capsules 2824

LITHOTABS TABLETS
(Lithium Carbonate) 2543

See LITHONATE Capsules

LIVOSTIN
(Levocabastine Hydrochloride) .... ◆ 266
None cited in PDR database.

LOCOID CREAM, OINTMENT AND TOPICAL SOLUTION
(Hydrocortisone Butyrate) 978
None cited in PDR database.

LODINE CAPSULES AND TABLETS
(Etodolac) 2743
May interact with lithium preparations, diuretics, antacids, and certain other agents. Compounds in these categories include:

Aluminum Carbonate Gel (Coadministration decreases the peak concentration reached by about 15 to 20%). Products include:

Basaljel... 2703

Aluminum Hydroxide (Coadministration decreases the peak concentration reached by about 15 to 20%). Products include:

ALternaGEL Liquid 1316
Maximum Strength Ascriptin .... ⊞ 630
Cama Arthritis Pain Reliever............ ⊞ 785
Gaviscon Extra Strength Relief Formula Antacid Tablets.................. ⊞ 819
Gaviscon Extra Strength Relief Formula Liquid Antacid................... ⊞ 819
Gaviscon Liquid Antacid .... ⊞ 820
Gelusil Liquid & Tablets .... ⊞ 855
Maalox Heartburn Relief Suspension .... ⊞ 642
Maalox Heartburn Relief Tablets.... ⊞ 641
Maalox Magnesia and Alumina Oral Suspension................................. ⊞ 642
Maalox Plus Tablets .... ⊞ 643
Extra Strength Maalox Antacid Plus Antigas Liquid and Tablets ⊞ 638
Tempo Soft Antacid .... ⊞ 835

Aluminum Hydroxide Gel (Coadministration decreases the peak concentration reached by about 15 to 20%). Products include:

ALternaGEL Liquid .... ⊞ 659
Aludrox Oral Suspension 2695
Amphojel Suspension 2695
Amphojel Suspension without Flavor 2695
Amphojel Tablets................................. 2695
Arthritis Pain Ascriptin .... ⊞ 631
Regular Strength Ascriptin Tablets .... ⊞ 629
Gaviscon Antacid Tablets................... ⊞ 819
Gaviscon-2 Antacid Tablets .... ⊞ 820
Mylanta Liquid 1317
Mylanta Tablets .... ⊞ 660
Mylanta Double Strength Liquid 1317
Mylanta Double Strength Tablets .. ⊞ 660
Nephrox Suspension .... ⊞ 655

Aluminum Hydroxide Gel, Dried (Coadministration decreases the peak concentration reached by about 15 to 20%).

Amiloride Hydrochloride (Caution is recommended if coadministered to patients with cardiac, renal or hepatic failure). Products include:

Midamor Tablets 1703
Moduretic Tablets 1705

Aspirin (Potential for increased adverse effects). Products include:

Alka-Seltzer Effervescent Antacid and Pain Reliever............................ ⊞ 701
Alka-Seltzer Extra Strength Effervescent Antacid and Pain Reliever .... ⊞ 703
Alka-Seltzer Lemon Lime Effervescent Antacid and Pain Reliever .... ⊞ 703
Alka-Seltzer Plus Cold Medicine .... ⊞ 705
Alka-Seltzer Plus Cold & Cough Medicine .... ⊞ 708
Alka-Seltzer Plus Night-Time Cold Medicine .... ⊞ 707
Alka Seltzer Plus Sinus Medicine .. ⊞ 707
Arthritis Foundation Safety Coated Aspirin Tablets .... ⊞ 675

IMPORTANT NOTE: Always consult each drug listing in the patient's regimen for possible interactions.

Lodine Interactions Index 594

Arthritis Pain Ascriptin ▣ 631
Maximum Strength Ascriptin ▣ 630
Regular Strength Ascriptin Tablets ▣ 629
Arthritis Strength BC Powder ▣ 609
BC Cold Powder Multi-Symptom Formula (Cold-Sinus-Allergy) ▣ 609
BC Cold Powder Non-Drowsy Formula (Cold-Sinus) ▣ 609
BC Powder ▣ 609
Bayer Children's Chewable Aspirin ▣ 711
Genuine Bayer Aspirin Tablets & Caplets ▣ 713
Extra Strength Bayer Arthritis Pain Regimen Formula ▣ 711
Extra Strength Bayer Aspirin Caplets & Tablets ▣ 712
Extended-Release Bayer 8-Hour Aspirin ▣ 712
Extra Strength Bayer Plus Aspirin Caplets ▣ 713
Extra Strength Bayer PM Aspirin ▣ 713
Bayer Enteric Aspirin ▣ 709
Bufferin Analgesic Tablets and Caplets ▣ 613
Arthritis Strength Bufferin Analgesic Caplets ▣ 614
Extra Strength Bufferin Analgesic Tablets ▣ 615
Cama Arthritis Pain Reliever ▣ 785
Darvon Compound-65 Pulvules 1435
Easprin 1914
Ecotrin 2455
Ecotrin Enteric Coated Aspirin Maximum Strength Tablets and Caplets ▣ 816
Ecotrin Enteric Coated Aspirin Regular Strength Tablets 2455
Empirin Aspirin Tablets ▣ 854
Empirin with Codeine Tablets 1093
Excedrin Extra-Strength Analgesic Tablets & Caplets 732
Fiorinal Capsules 2261
Fiorinal with Codeine Capsules 2262
Fiorinal Tablets 2261
Halfprin 1362
Healthprin Aspirin 2455
Norgesic 1496
Percodan Tablets 939
Percodan-Demi Tablets 940
Robaxisal Tablets 2071
Soma Compound w/Codeine Tablets 2676
Soma Compound Tablets 2675
St. Joseph Adult Chewable Aspirin (81 mg.) ▣ 808
Talwin Compound 2335
Ursinus Inlay-Tabs ▣ 794
Vanquish Analgesic Caplets ▣ 731

Bendroflumethiazide (Caution is recommended if coadministered to patients with cardiac, renal or hepatic failure).
No products indexed under this heading.

Bumetanide (Caution is recommended if coadministered to patients with cardiac, renal or hepatic failure). Products include:
Bumex 2093

Chlorothiazide (Caution is recommended if coadministered to patients with cardiac, renal or hepatic failure). Products include:
Aldoclor Tablets 1598
Diupres Tablets 1650
Diuril Oral 1653

Chlorothiazide Sodium (Caution is recommended if coadministered to patients with cardiac, renal or hepatic failure). Products include:
Diuril Sodium Intravenous 1652

Chlorthalidone (Caution is recommended if coadministered to patients with cardiac, renal or hepatic failure). Products include:
Combipres Tablets 677
Tenoretic Tablets 2845
Thalitone 1245

Cyclosporine (Potential for elevated serum levels of cyclosporine and increased nephrotoxicity). Products include:
Neoral 2276
Sandimmune 2286

Digoxin (Potential for elevated serum levels of digoxin and increased toxicity). Products include:
Lanoxicaps 1117
Lanoxin Elixir Pediatric 1120
Lanoxin Injection 1123
Lanoxin Injection Pediatric 1126
Lanoxin Tablets 1128

Dihydroxyaluminum Sodium Carbonate (Coadministration decreases the peak concentration reached by about 15 to 20%).
No products indexed under this heading.

Ethacrynic Acid (Caution is recommended if coadministered to patients with cardiac, renal or hepatic failure). Products include:
Edecrin Tablets 1657

Furosemide (Caution is recommended if coadministered to patients with cardiac, renal or hepatic failure). Products include:
Lasix Injection, Oral Solution and Tablets 1240

Hydrochlorothiazide (Caution is recommended if coadministered to patients with cardiac, renal or hepatic failure). Products include:
Aldactazide 2413
Aldoril Tablets 1604
Apresazide Capsules 808
Capozide 742
Dyazide 2479
Esidrix Tablets 821
Esimil Tablets 822
HydroDIURIL Tablets 1674
Hydropres Tablets 1675
Hyzaar Tablets 1677
Inderide Tablets 2732
Inderide LA Long Acting Capsules 2734
Lopressor HCT Tablets 832
Lotensin HCT 837
Maxzide 1380
Moduretic Tablets 1705
Oretic Tablets 443
Prinzide Tablets 1737
Ser-Ap-Es Tablets 849
Timolide Tablets 1748
Vaseretic Tablets 1765
Zestoretic 2850
Ziac 1415

Hydroflumethiazide (Caution is recommended if coadministered to patients with cardiac, renal or hepatic failure). Products include:
Diucardin Tablets 2718

Indapamide (Caution is recommended if coadministered to patients with cardiac, renal or hepatic failure). Products include:
Lozol Tablets 2022

Lithium Carbonate (Potential for elevated serum levels of lithium and increased toxicity). Products include:
Eskalith 2485
Lithium Carbonate Capsules & Tablets 2230
Lithonate/Lithotabs/Lithobid 2543

Lithium Citrate (Potential for elevated serum levels of lithium and increased toxicity).
No products indexed under this heading.

Magaldrate (Coadministration decreases the peak concentration reached by about 15 to 20%).
No products indexed under this heading.

Magnesium Hydroxide (Coadministration decreases the peak concentration reached by about 15 to 20%). Products include:
Aludrox Oral Suspension 2695
Arthritis Pain Ascriptin ▣ 631
Maximum Strength Ascriptin ▣ 630
Regular Strength Ascriptin Tablets ▣ 629
Di-Gel Antacid/Anti-Gas ▣ 801
Gelusil Liquid & Tablets ▣ 855
Maalox Magnesia and Alumina Oral Suspension ▣ 642
Maalox Plus Tablets ▣ 643
Extra Strength Maalox Antacid Plus Antigas Liquid and Tablets ▣ 638
Mylanta Calcium Carbonate and Magnesium Hydroxide Tablets 1318
Mylanta Liquid 1317
Mylanta Tablets ▣ 660
Mylanta Double Strength Liquid 1317
Mylanta Double Strength Tablets ▣ 660
Phillips' Milk of Magnesia Liquid ▣ 729
Rolaids Tablets ▣ 843
Tempo Soft Antacid ▣ 835

Magnesium Oxide (Coadministration decreases the peak concentration reached by about 15 to 20%). Products include:
Beelith Tablets 639
Bufferin Analgesic Tablets and Caplets ▣ 613
Caltrate PLUS ▣ 665
Cama Arthritis Pain Reliever ▣ 785
Mag-Ox 400 668
Uro-Mag 668

Methotrexate Sodium (Potential for elevated serum levels of methotrexate and increased toxicity). Products include:
Methotrexate Sodium Tablets, Injection, for Injection and LPF Injection 1275

Methyclothiazide (Caution is recommended if coadministered to patients with cardiac, renal or hepatic failure). Products include:
Enduron Tablets 420

Metolazone (Caution is recommended if coadministered to patients with cardiac, renal or hepatic failure). Products include:
Mykrox Tablets 993
Zaroxolyn Tablets 1000

Phenylbutazone (Increases (by about 80%) in the free fraction of etodolac in vitro studies).
No products indexed under this heading.

Polythiazide (Caution is recommended if coadministered to patients with cardiac, renal or hepatic failure). Products include:
Minizide Capsules 1938

Sodium Bicarbonate (Coadministration decreases the peak concentration reached by about 15 to 20%). Products include:
Alka-Seltzer Effervescent Antacid and Pain Reliever ▣ 701
Alka-Seltzer Extra Strength Effervescent Antacid and Pain Reliever ▣ 703
Alka-Seltzer Gold Effervescent Antacid ▣ 703
Alka-Seltzer Lemon Lime Effervescent Antacid and Pain Reliever ▣ 703
Arm & Hammer Pure Baking Soda ▣ 627
Ceo-Two Rectal Suppositories 666
Citrocarbonate Antacid ▣ 770
Massengill Disposable Douches ▣ 820
Massengill Liquid Concentrate ▣ 820
NuLYTELY 689
Cherry Flavor NuLYTELY 689

Spironolactone (Caution is recommended if coadministered to patients with cardiac, renal or hepatic failure). Products include:
Aldactazide 2413
Aldactone 2414

Torsemide (Caution is recommended if coadministered to patients with cardiac, renal or hepatic failure). Products include:
Demadex Tablets and Injection 686

Triamterene (Caution is recommended if coadministered to patients with cardiac, renal or hepatic failure). Products include:
Dyazide 2479
Dyrenium Capsules 2481
Maxzide 1380

Warfarin Sodium (Reduced protein binding of warfarin; few spontaneous reports of prolonged prothrombin times with concomitant therapy). Products include:
Coumadin 926

Food Interactions

Food, unspecified (Reduces the peak concentration reached by approximately one-half and increases the time-to-peak concentration by 1.4 to 3.8 hours).

LOMOTIL LIQUID
(Diphenoxylate Hydrochloride, Atropine Sulfate) 2439
May interact with monoamine oxidase inhibitors, barbiturates, tranquilizers, and certain other agents. Compounds in these categories include:

Alprazolam (Potentiation of tranquilizers). Products include:
Xanax Tablets 2649

Aprobarbital (Potentiation of barbiturates).
No products indexed under this heading.

Buspirone Hydrochloride (Potentiation of tranquilizers). Products include:
BuSpar 737

Butabarbital (Potentiation of barbiturates).
No products indexed under this heading.

Butalbital (Potentiation of barbiturates). Products include:
Esgic-plus Tablets 1013
Fioricet Tablets 2258
Fioricet with Codeine Capsules 2260
Fiorinal Capsules 2261
Fiorinal with Codeine Capsules 2262
Fiorinal Tablets 2261
Phrenilin 785
Sedapap Tablets 50 mg/650 mg 1543

Chlordiazepoxide (Potentiation of tranquilizers). Products include:
Libritabs Tablets 2177
Limbitrol 2180

Chlordiazepoxide Hydrochloride (Potentiation of tranquilizers). Products include:
Librax Capsules 2176
Librium Capsules 2178
Librium Injectable 2179

Chlorpromazine (Potentiation of tranquilizers). Products include:
Thorazine Suppositories 2523

Chlorprothixene (Potentiation of tranquilizers).
No products indexed under this heading.

Chlorprothixene Lactate (Potentiation of tranquilizers).
No products indexed under this heading.

Clorazepate Dipotassium (Potentiation of tranquilizers). Products include:
Tranxene 451

Diazepam (Potentiation of tranquilizers). Products include:
Dizac 1809
Valium Injectable 2182
Valium Tablets 2183
Valrelease Capsules 2169

Droperidol (Potentiation of tranquilizers). Products include:
Inapsine Injection 1296

Fluphenazine Decanoate (Potentiation of tranquilizers). Products include:
Prolixin Decanoate 509

Fluphenazine Enanthate (Potentiation of tranquilizers). Products include:
Prolixin Enanthate 509

(▣ Described in PDR For Nonprescription Drugs) (◉ Described in PDR For Ophthalmology)

Interactions Index — Lopressor HCT

Fluphenazine Hydrochloride (Potentiation of tranquilizers). Products include:

Prolixin 509

Furazolidone (Hypertensive crisis). Products include:

Furoxone 2046

Haloperidol (Potentiation of tranquilizers). Products include:

Haldol Injection, Tablets and Concentrate 1575

Haloperidol Decanoate (Potentiation of tranquilizers). Products include:

Haldol Decanoate................................. 1577

Hydroxyzine Hydrochloride (Potentiation of tranquilizers). Products include:

Atarax Tablets & Syrup........................ 2185
Marax Tablets & DF Syrup................... 2200
Vistaril Intramuscular Solution........... 2216

Isocarboxazid (Hypertensive crisis).

No products indexed under this heading.

Lorazepam (Potentiation of tranquilizers). Products include:

Ativan Injection.................................... 2698
Ativan Tablets 2700

Loxapine Hydrochloride (Potentiation of tranquilizers). Products include:

Loxitane 1378

Mephobarbital (Potentiation of barbiturates). Products include:

Mebaral Tablets 2322

Meprobamate (Potentiation of tranquilizers). Products include:

Miltown Tablets 2672
PMB 200 and PMB 400 2783

Mesoridazine Besylate (Potentiation of tranquilizers). Products include:

Serentil 684

Molindone Hydrochloride (Potentiation of tranquilizers). Products include:

Moban Tablets and Concentrate 1048

Oxazepam (Potentiation of tranquilizers). Products include:

Serax Capsules 2810
Serax Tablets.. 2810

Pentobarbital Sodium (Potentiation of barbiturates). Products include:

Nembutal Sodium Capsules 436
Nembutal Sodium Solution 438
Nembutal Sodium Suppositories........ 440

Perphenazine (Potentiation of tranquilizers). Products include:

Etrafon 2355
Triavil Tablets 1757
Trilafon.. 2389

Phenelzine Sulfate (Hypertensive crisis). Products include:

Nardil 1920

Phenobarbital (Potentiation of barbiturates). Products include:

Arco-Lase Plus Tablets 512
Bellergal-S Tablets 2250
Donnatal 2060
Donnatal Extentabs.............................. 2061
Donnatal Tablets 2060
Phenobarbital Elixir and Tablets 1469
Quadrinal Tablets 1350

Prazepam (Potentiation of tranquilizers).

No products indexed under this heading.

Prochlorperazine (Potentiation of tranquilizers). Products include:

Compazine 2470

Promethazine Hydrochloride (Potentiation of tranquilizers). Products include:

Mepergan Injection 2753
Phenergan with Codeine 2777
Phenergan with Dextromethorphan 2778
Phenergan Injection 2773
Phenergan Suppositories 2775
Phenergan Syrup 2774
Phenergan Tablets 2775
Phenergan VC 2779
Phenergan VC with Codeine 2781

Secobarbital Sodium (Potentiation of barbiturates). Products include:

Seconal Sodium Pulvules 1474

Selegiline Hydrochloride (Hypertensive crisis). Products include:

Eldepryl Tablets 2550

Thiamylal Sodium (Potentiation of barbiturates).

No products indexed under this heading.

Thioridazine Hydrochloride (Potentiation of tranquilizers). Products include:

Mellaril 2269

Thiothixene (Potentiation of tranquilizers). Products include:

Navane Capsules and Concentrate 2201
Navane Intramuscular 2202

Tranylcypromine Sulfate (Hypertensive crisis). Products include:

Parnate Tablets 2503

Trifluoperazine Hydrochloride (Potentiation of tranquilizers). Products include:

Stelazine 2514

Food Interactions

Alcohol (Potentiation of alcohol).

LOMOTIL TABLETS

(Diphenoxylate Hydrochloride, Atropine Sulfate) 2439

See **Lomotil Liquid**

LONITEN TABLETS

(Minoxidil) 2618

May interact with:

Guanethidine Monosulfate (Profound orthostatic effects). Products include:

Esimil Tablets 822
Ismelin Tablets 827

LO/OVRAL TABLETS

(Norgestrel, Ethinyl Estradiol) 2746

May interact with barbiturates and certain other agents. Compounds in these categories include:

Ampicillin Sodium (Reduced efficacy; increased incidence of breakthrough bleeding). Products include:

Unasyn 2212

Aprobarbital (Reduced efficacy; increased incidence of breakthrough bleeding).

No products indexed under this heading.

Butabarbital (Reduced efficacy; increased incidence of breakthrough bleeding).

No products indexed under this heading.

Butalbital (Reduced efficacy; increased incidence of breakthrough bleeding). Products include:

Esgic-plus Tablets 1013
Fioricet Tablets..................................... 2258
Fioricet with Codeine Capsules 2260
Fiorinal Capsules 2261
Fiorinal with Codeine Capsules 2262
Fiorinal Tablets 2261
Phrenilin 785
Sedapap Tablets 50 mg/650 mg .. 1543

Mephobarbital (Reduced efficacy; increased incidence of breakthrough bleeding). Products include:

Mebaral Tablets 2322

Oxytetracycline (Reduced efficacy; increased incidence of breakthrough bleeding). Products include:

Terramycin Intramuscular Solution 2210

Oxytetracycline Hydrochloride (Reduced efficacy; increased incidence of breakthrough bleeding). Products include:

TERAK Ointment .... ⊙ 209
Terra-Cortril Ophthalmic Suspension 2210
Terramycin with Polymyxin B Sulfate Ophthalmic Ointment 2211
Urobiotic-250 Capsules 2214

Pentobarbital Sodium (Reduced efficacy; increased incidence of breakthrough bleeding). Products include:

Nembutal Sodium Capsules 436
Nembutal Sodium Solution 438
Nembutal Sodium Suppositories........ 440

Phenobarbital (Reduced efficacy; increased incidence of breakthrough bleeding). Products include:

Arco-Lase Plus Tablets 512
Bellergal-S Tablets 2250
Donnatal 2060
Donnatal Extentabs.............................. 2061
Donnatal Tablets 2060
Phenobarbital Elixir and Tablets 1469
Quadrinal Tablets 1350

Phenylbutazone (Reduced efficacy; increased incidence of breakthrough bleeding).

No products indexed under this heading.

Phenytoin Sodium (Reduced efficacy; increased incidence of breakthrough bleeding). Products include:

Dilantin Kapseals 1906
Dilantin Parenteral 1910

Rifampin (Reduced efficacy; increased incidence of breakthrough bleeding). Products include:

Rifadin 1528
Rifamate Capsules 1530
Rifater.. 1532
Rimactane Capsules 847

Secobarbital Sodium (Reduced efficacy; increased incidence of breakthrough bleeding). Products include:

Seconal Sodium Pulvules 1474

Tetracycline Hydrochloride (Reduced efficacy; increased incidence of breakthrough bleeding). Products include:

Achromycin V Capsules 1367

Thiamylal Sodium (Reduced efficacy; increased incidence of breakthrough bleeding).

No products indexed under this heading.

LO/OVRAL-28 TABLETS

(Norgestrel, Ethinyl Estradiol) 2751

See **Lo/Ovral Tablets**

LOPERAMIDE HYDROCHLORIDE CAPLETS, 2 MG

(Loperamide Hydrochloride) ....ⓂⒹ 736

May interact with:

Antibiotics, unspecified (Effect not specified).

LOPID TABLETS

(Gemfibrozil) 1917

May interact with anticoagulants, hmg-coa reductase inhibitors, and certain other agents. Compounds in these categories include:

Dalteparin Sodium (May affect prothrombin time resulting in bleeding complication). Products include:

Fragmin 1954

Dicumarol (May affect prothrombin time resulting in bleeding complication).

No products indexed under this heading.

Enoxaparin (May affect prothrombin time resulting in bleeding complication). Products include:

Lovenox Injection 2020

Fluvastatin Sodium (Potential for severe myopathy, rhabdomyolysis, and acute renal failure). Products include:

Lescol Capsules 2267

Heparin Calcium (May affect prothrombin time resulting in bleeding complication).

No products indexed under this heading.

Heparin Sodium (May affect prothrombin time resulting in bleeding complication). Products include:

Heparin Lock Flush Solution 2725
Heparin Sodium Injection.................... 2726
Heparin Sodium Injection, USP, Sterile Solution 2615
Heparin Sodium Vials........................... 1441

Lovastatin (Potential for severe myopathy, rhabdomyolysis, and acute renal failure). Products include:

Mevacor Tablets................................... 1699

Pravastatin Sodium (Potential for severe myopathy, rhabdomyolysis, and acute renal failure). Products include:

Pravachol 765

Simvastatin (Potential for severe myopathy, rhabdomyolysis, and acute renal failure). Products include:

Zocor Tablets 1775

Warfarin Sodium (May affect prothrombin time resulting in bleeding complication). Products include:

Coumadin 926

LOPRESSOR AMPULS

(Metoprolol Tartrate)............................ 830

May interact with catecholamine depleting drugs and certain other agents. Compounds in these categories include:

Deserpidine (Potential for additive effect).

No products indexed under this heading.

Epinephrine Hydrochloride (Potential for unresponsiveness to epinephrine to treat allergic reactions in certain patients). Products include:

Ana-Kit Anaphylaxis Emergency Treatment Kit 617

Guanethidine Monosulfate (Potential for additive effect). Products include:

Esimil Tablets 822
Ismelin Tablets 827

Rauwolfia Serpentina (Potential for additive effect).

No products indexed under this heading.

Rescinnamine (Potential for additive effect).

No products indexed under this heading.

Reserpine (Potential for additive effect). Products include:

Diupres Tablets 1650
Hydropres Tablets................................. 1675
Ser-Ap-Es Tablets 849

LOPRESSOR HCT TABLETS

(Metoprolol Tartrate, Hydrochlorothiazide) 832

May interact with catecholamine depleting drugs, cardiac glycosides, corticosteroids, peripheral adrenergic blockers, ganglionic blocking agents, antihypertensives, non-steroidal anti-inflammatory agents, barbiturates, narcotic analgesics,

IMPORTANT NOTE: Always consult each drug listing in the patient's regimen for possible interactions.

and certain other agents. Compounds in these categories include:

Acebutolol Hydrochloride (Potentiation of antihypertensive action). Products include:
- Sectral Capsules ... 2807

ACTH (Hypokalemia may develop during concomitant use).
- No products indexed under this heading.

Alfentanil Hydrochloride (Orthostatic hypotension may be potentiated). Products include:
- Alfenta Injection ... 1286

Amlodipine Besylate (Potentiation of antihypertensive action). Products include:
- Lotrel Capsules ... 840
- Norvasc Tablets ... 1940

Aprobarbital (Orthostatic hypotension may be potentiated).
- No products indexed under this heading.

Atenolol (Potentiation of antihypertensive action). Products include:
- Tenoretic Tablets ... 2845
- Tenormin Tablets and I.V. Injection 2847

Benazepril Hydrochloride (Potentiation of antihypertensive action). Products include:
- Lotensin Tablets ... 834
- Lotensin HCT ... 837
- Lotrel Capsules ... 840

Bendroflumethiazide (Potentiation of antihypertensive action).
- No products indexed under this heading.

Betamethasone Acetate (Hypokalemia may develop during concomitant use). Products include:
- Celestone Soluspan Suspension ... 2347

Betamethasone Sodium Phosphate (Hypokalemia may develop during concomitant use). Products include:
- Celestone Soluspan Suspension ... 2347

Betaxolol Hydrochloride (Potentiation of antihypertensive action). Products include:
- Betoptic Ophthalmic Solution ... 469
- Betoptic S Ophthalmic Suspension 471
- Kerlone Tablets ... 2436

Bisoprolol Fumarate (Potentiation of antihypertensive action). Products include:
- Zebeta Tablets ... 1413
- Ziac ... 1415

Buprenorphine (Orthostatic hypotension may be potentiated). Products include:
- Buprenex Injectable ... 2006

Butabarbital (Orthostatic hypotension may be potentiated).
- No products indexed under this heading.

Butalbital (Orthostatic hypotension may be potentiated). Products include:
- Esgic-plus Tablets ... 1013
- Fioricet Tablets ... 2258
- Fioricet with Codeine Capsules ... 2260
- Fiorinal Capsules ... 2261
- Fiorinal with Codeine Capsules ... 2262
- Fiorinal Tablets ... 2261
- Phrenilin ... 785
- Sedapap Tablets 50 mg/650 mg .. 1543

Captopril (Potentiation of antihypertensive action). Products include:
- Capoten ... 739
- Capozide ... 742

Carteolol Hydrochloride (Potentiation of antihypertensive action). Products include:
- Cartrol Tablets ... 410
- Ocupress Ophthalmic Solution, 1% Sterile ... ◉ 309

Chlorothiazide (Potentiation of antihypertensive action). Products include:
- Aldoclor Tablets ... 1598
- Diupres Tablets ... 1650
- Diuril Oral ... 1653

Chlorothiazide Sodium (Potentiation of antihypertensive action). Products include:
- Diuril Sodium Intravenous ... 1652

Chlorthalidone (Potentiation of antihypertensive action). Products include:
- Combipres Tablets ... 677
- Tenoretic Tablets ... 2845
- Thalitone ... 1245

Cholestyramine (Impairs the oral absorption of hydrochlorothiazide from gastrointestinal tract by up to 85%). Products include:
- Questran Light ... 769
- Questran Powder ... 770

Clonidine (Potentiation of antihypertensive action). Products include:
- Catapres-TTS ... 675

Clonidine Hydrochloride (Potentiation of antihypertensive action). Products include:
- Catapres Tablets ... 674
- Combipres Tablets ... 677

Codeine Phosphate (Orthostatic hypotension may be potentiated). Products include:
- Actifed with Codeine Cough Syrup.. 1067
- Brontex ... 1981
- Deconsal C Expectorant Syrup ... 456
- Deconsal Pediatric Syrup ... 457
- Dimetane-DC Cough Syrup ... 2059
- Empirin with Codeine Tablets ... 1093
- Fioricet with Codeine Capsules ... 2260
- Fiorinal with Codeine Capsules ... 2262
- Isoclor Expectorant ... 990
- Novahistine DH ... 2462
- Novahistine Expectorant ... 2463
- Nucofed ... 2051
- Phenergan with Codeine ... 2777
- Phenergan VC with Codeine ... 2781
- Robitussin A-C Syrup ... 2073
- Robitussin-DAC Syrup ... 2074
- Ryna ... ▣ 841
- Soma Compound w/Codeine Tablets ... 2676
- Tussi-Organidin NR Liquid and S NR Liquid ... 2677
- Tylenol with Codeine ... 1583

Colestipol Hydrochloride (Impairs the oral absorption of hydrochlorothiazide from gastrointestinal tract by up to 43%). Products include:
- Colestid Tablets ... 2591

Cortisone Acetate (Hypokalemia may develop during concomitant use). Products include:
- Cortone Acetate Sterile Suspension ... 1623
- Cortone Acetate Tablets ... 1624

Deserpidine (Potentiation of antihypertensive action; potential for additive effects).
- No products indexed under this heading.

Deslanoside (Potential for toxic effects of deslanoside on heart).
- No products indexed under this heading.

Dexamethasone (Hypokalemia may develop during concomitant use). Products include:
- AK-Trol Ointment & Suspension ... ◉ 205
- Decadron Elixir ... 1633
- Decadron Tablets ... 1635
- Decaspray Topical Aerosol ... 1648
- Dexacidin Ointment ... ◉ 263
- Maxitrol Ophthalmic Ointment and Suspension ... ◉ 224
- TobraDex Ophthalmic Suspension and Ointment ... 473

Dexamethasone Acetate (Hypokalemia may develop during concomitant use). Products include:
- Dalalone D.P. Injectable ... 1011
- Decadron-LA Sterile Suspension ... 1646

Dexamethasone Sodium Phosphate (Hypokalemia may develop during concomitant use). Products include:
- Decadron Phosphate Injection ... 1637
- Decadron Phosphate Respihaler ... 1642
- Decadron Phosphate Sterile Ophthalmic Ointment ... 1641
- Decadron Phosphate Sterile Ophthalmic Solution ... 1642
- Decadron Phosphate Topical Cream ... 1644
- Decadron Phosphate Turbinaire ... 1645
- Decadron Phosphate with Xylocaine Injection, Sterile ... 1639
- Dexacort Phosphate in Respihaler .. 458
- Dexacort Phosphate in Turbinaire .. 459
- NeoDecadron Sterile Ophthalmic Ointment ... 1712
- NeoDecadron Sterile Ophthalmic Solution ... 1713
- NeoDecadron Topical Cream ... 1714

Dezocine (Orthostatic hypotension may be potentiated). Products include:
- Dalgan Injection ... 538

Diazoxide (Potentiation of antihypertensive action). Products include:
- Hyperstat I.V. Injection ... 2363
- Proglycem ... 580

Diclofenac Potassium (Reduces diuretic, natriuretic and antihypertensive effects of thiazides). Products include:
- Cataflam ... 816

Diclofenac Sodium (Reduces diuretic, natriuretic and antihypertensive effects of thiazides). Products include:
- Voltaren Ophthalmic Sterile Ophthalmic Solution ... ◉ 272
- Voltaren Tablets ... 861

Digitoxin (Potential for toxic effects of digitalis on heart). Products include:
- Crystodigin Tablets ... 1433

Digoxin (Potential for toxic effects of digitalis on heart). Products include:
- Lanoxicaps ... 1117
- Lanoxin Elixir Pediatric ... 1120
- Lanoxin Injection ... 1123
- Lanoxin Injection Pediatric ... 1126
- Lanoxin Tablets ... 1128

Diltiazem Hydrochloride (Potentiation of antihypertensive action). Products include:
- Cardizem CD Capsules ... 1506
- Cardizem SR Capsules ... 1510
- Cardizem Injectable ... 1508
- Cardizem Tablets ... 1512
- Dilacor XR Extended-release Capsules ... 2018

Doxazosin Mesylate (Potentiation of antihypertensive action). Products include:
- Cardura Tablets ... 2186

Enalapril Maleate (Potentiation of antihypertensive action). Products include:
- Vaseretic Tablets ... 1765
- Vasotec Tablets ... 1771

Enalaprilat (Potentiation of antihypertensive effects). Products include:
- Vasotec I.V. ... 1768

Epinephrine Hydrochloride (Potential for unresponsiveness to epinephrine to treat allergic reactions in certain patients). Products include:
- Ana-Kit Anaphylaxis Emergency Treatment Kit ... 617

Esmolol Hydrochloride (Potentiation of antihypertensive action). Products include:
- Brevibloc Injection ... 1808

Etodolac (Reduces diuretic, natriuretic and antihypertensive effects of thiazides). Products include:
- Lodine Capsules and Tablets ... 2743

Felodipine (Potentiation of antihypertensive action). Products include:
- Plendil Extended-Release Tablets ... 527

Fenoprofen Calcium (Reduces diuretic, natriuretic and antihypertensive effects of thiazides). Products include:
- Nalfon 200 Pulvules & Nalfon Tablets ... 917

Fentanyl (Orthostatic hypotension may be potentiated). Products include:
- Duragesic Transdermal System ... 1288

Fentanyl Citrate (Orthostatic hypotension may be potentiated). Products include:
- Sublimaze Injection ... 1307

Fludrocortisone Acetate (Hypokalemia may develop during concomitant use). Products include:
- Florinef Acetate Tablets ... 505

Flurbiprofen (Reduces diuretic, natriuretic and antihypertensive effects of thiazides). Products include:
- Ansaid Tablets ... 2579

Fosinopril Sodium (Potentiation of antihypertensive action). Products include:
- Monopril Tablets ... 757

Furosemide (Potentiation of antihypertensive action). Products include:
- Lasix Injection, Oral Solution and Tablets ... 1240

Guanabenz Acetate (Potentiation of antihypertensive action).
- No products indexed under this heading.

Guanethidine Monosulfate (Potentiation of antihypertensive action). Products include:
- Esimil Tablets ... 822
- Ismelin Tablets ... 827

Hydralazine Hydrochloride (Potentiation of antihypertensive action). Products include:
- Apresazide Capsules ... 808
- Apresoline Hydrochloride Tablets .. 809
- Ser-Ap-Es Tablets ... 849

Hydrocodone Bitartrate (Orthostatic hypotension may be potentiated). Products include:
- Anexsia 5/500 Elixir ... 1781
- Anexia Tablets ... 1782
- Codiclear DH Syrup ... 791
- Deconamine CX Cough and Cold Liquid and Tablets ... 1319
- Duratuss HD Elixir ... 2565
- Hycodan Tablets and Syrup ... 930
- Hycomine Compound Tablets ... 932
- Hycomine ... 931
- Hycotuss Expectorant Syrup ... 933
- Hydrocet Capsules ... 782
- Lorcet 10/650 ... 1018
- Lortab ... 2566
- Tussend ... 1783
- Tussend Expectorant ... 1785
- Vicodin Tablets ... 1356
- Vicodin ES Tablets ... 1357
- Vicodin Tuss Expectorant ... 1358
- Zydone Capsules ... 949

Hydrocodone Polistirex (Orthostatic hypotension may be potentiated). Products include:
- Tussionex Pennkinetic Extended-Release Suspension ... 998

Hydrocortisone (Hypokalemia may develop during concomitant use). Products include:
- Anusol-HC Cream 2.5% ... 1896
- Aquanil HC Lotion ... 1931
- Bactine Hydrocortisone Anti-Itch Cream ... ▣ 709
- Caldecort Anti-Itch Hydrocortisone Spray ... ▣ 631
- Cortaid ... ▣ 836

(▣ Described in PDR For Nonprescription Drugs) (◉ Described in PDR For Ophthalmology)

Interactions Index — Lopressor HCT

CORTENEMA 2535
Cortisporin Ointment 1085
Cortisporin Ophthalmic Ointment Sterile 1085
Cortisporin Ophthalmic Suspension Sterile 1086
Cortisporin Otic Solution Sterile 1087
Cortisporin Otic Suspension Sterile 1088
Cortizone-5 .... ⓑⓓ 831
Cortizone-10 .... ⓑⓓ 831
Hydrocortone Tablets 1672
Hytone 907
Massengill Medicated Soft Cloth Towelettes 2458
PediOtic Suspension Sterile 1153
Preparation H Hydrocortisone 1% Cream .... ⓑⓓ 872
ProctoCream-HC 2.5% 2408
VōSoL HC Otic Solution 2678

Hydrocortisone Acetate (Hypokalemia may develop during concomitant use). Products include:

Analpram-HC Rectal Cream 1% and 2.5% 977
Anusol HC-1 Anti-Itch Hydrocortisone Ointment .... ⓑⓓ 847
Anusol-HC Suppositories 1897
Caldecort .... ⓑⓓ 631
Carmol HC 924
Coly-Mycin S Otic w/Neomycin & Hydrocortisone 1906
Cortaid .... ⓑⓓ 836
Cortifoam 2396
Cortisporin Cream 1084
Epifoam 2399
Hydrocortone Acetate Sterile Suspension 1669
Mantadil Cream 1135
Nupercainal Hydrocortisone 1% Cream .... ⓑⓓ 645
Ophthocort .... ⓒ 311
Pramosone Cream, Lotion & Ointment 978
ProctoCream-HC 2408
ProctoFoam-HC 2409
Terra-Cortril Ophthalmic Suspension 2210

Hydrocortisone Sodium Phosphate (Hypokalemia may develop during concomitant use). Products include:

Hydrocortone Phosphate Injection, Sterile 1670

Hydrocortisone Sodium Succinate (Hypokalemia may develop during concomitant use). Products include:

Solu-Cortef Sterile Powder 2641

Hydroflumethiazide (Potentiation of antihypertensive action). Products include:

Diucardin Tablets 2718

Ibuprofen (Reduces diuretic, natriuretic and antihypertensive effects of thiazides). Products include:

Advil Cold and Sinus Caplets and Tablets (formerly CoAdvil) .... ⓑⓓ 870
Advil Ibuprofen Tablets and Caplets .... ⓑⓓ 870
Children's Advil Suspension 2692
Arthritis Foundation Ibuprofen Tablets .... ⓑⓓ 674
Bayer Select Ibuprofen Pain Relief Formula .... ⓑⓓ 715
Cramp End Tablets .... ⓑⓓ 735
Dimetapp Sinus Caplets .... ⓑⓓ 775
Haltran Tablets .... ⓑⓓ 771
IBU Tablets 1342
Ibuprohm .... ⓑⓓ 735
Children's Motrin Ibuprofen Oral Suspension 1546
Motrin Tablets 2625
Motrin IB Caplets, Tablets, and Geltabs .... ⓑⓓ 838
Motrin IB Sinus .... ⓑⓓ 838
Motrin Ibuprofen Suspension, Oral Drops, Chewable Tablets, Caplets 1546
Nuprin Ibuprofen/Analgesic Tablets & Caplets .... ⓑⓓ 622
Sine-Aid IB Caplets 1554
Vicks DayQuil SINUS Pressure & PAIN Relief with IBUPROFEN ...... ⓑⓓ 762

Indapamide (Potentiation of antihypertensive action). Products include:

Lozol Tablets 2022

Indomethacin (Reduces diuretic, natriuretic and antihypertensive effects of thiazides). Products include:

Indocin 1680

Indomethacin Sodium Trihydrate (Reduces diuretic, natriuretic and antihypertensive effects of thiazides). Products include:

Indocin I.V. 1684

Isradipine (Potentiation of antihypertensive action). Products include:

DynaCirc Capsules 2256

Ketoprofen (Reduces diuretic, natriuretic and antihypertensive effects of thiazides). Products include:

Orudis Capsules 2766
Oruvail Capsules 2766

Ketorolac Tromethamine (Reduces diuretic, natriuretic and antihypertensive effects of thiazides). Products include:

Acular 474
Acular .... ⓒ 277
Toradol 2159

Labetalol Hydrochloride (Potentiation of antihypertensive action). Products include:

Normodyne Injection 2377
Normodyne Tablets 2379
Trandate 1185

Levorphanol Tartrate (Orthostatic hypotension may be potentiated). Products include:

Levo-Dromoran 2129

Lisinopril (Potentiation of antihypertensive effects). Products include:

Prinivil Tablets 1733
Prinzide Tablets 1737
Zestoretic 2850
Zestril Tablets 2854

Lithium Carbonate (Lithium renal clearance is reduced, increasing risk of lithium toxicity). Products include:

Eskalith 2485
Lithium Carbonate Capsules & Tablets 2230
Lithonate/Lithotabs/Lithobid 2543

Lithium Citrate (Lithium renal clearance is reduced, increasing risk of lithium toxicity).

No products indexed under this heading.

Losartan Potassium (Potentiation of antihypertensive action). Products include:

Cozaar Tablets 1628
Hyzaar Tablets 1677

Mecamylamine Hydrochloride (Potentiation of antihypertensive action). Products include:

Inversine Tablets 1686

Meclofenamate Sodium (Reduces diuretic, natriuretic and antihypertensive effects of thiazides).

No products indexed under this heading.

Mefenamic Acid (Reduces diuretic, natriuretic and antihypertensive effects of thiazides). Products include:

Ponstel 1925

Meperidine Hydrochloride (Orthostatic hypotension may be potentiated). Products include:

Demerol 2308
Mepergan Injection 2753

Mephobarbital (Orthostatic hypotension may be potentiated). Products include:

Mebaral Tablets 2322

Methadone Hydrochloride (Orthostatic hypotension may be potentiated). Products include:

Methadone Hydrochloride Oral Concentrate 2233

Methadone Hydrochloride Oral Solution & Tablets 2235

Methyclothiazide (Potentiation of antihypertensive action). Products include:

Enduron Tablets 420

Methyldopa (Potentiation of antihypertensive action; hemolytic anemia). Products include:

Aldoclor Tablets 1598
Aldomet Oral 1600
Aldoril Tablets 1604

Methyldopate Hydrochloride (Potentiation of antihypertensive action; hemolytic anemia). Products include:

Aldomet Ester HCl Injection 1602

Methylprednisolone Acetate (Hypokalemia may develop during concomitant use). Products include:

Depo-Medrol Single-Dose Vial 2600
Depo-Medrol Sterile Aqueous Suspension 2597

Methylprednisolone Sodium Succinate (Hypokalemia may develop during concomitant use). Products include:

Solu-Medrol Sterile Powder 2643

Metolazone (Potentiation of antihypertensive action). Products include:

Mykrox Tablets 993
Zaroxolyn Tablets 1000

Metoprolol Succinate (Potentiation of antihypertensive action). Products include:

Toprol-XL Tablets 565

Metyrosine (Potentiation of antihypertensive action). Products include:

Demser Capsules 1649

Minoxidil (Potentiation of antihypertensive action). Products include:

Loniten Tablets 2618
Rogaine Topical Solution 2637

Moexipril Hydrochloride (Potentiation of antihypertensive action). Products include:

Univasc Tablets 2410

Morphine Sulfate (Orthostatic hypotension may be potentiated). Products include:

Astramorph/PF Injection, USP (Preservative-Free) 535
Duramorph 962
Infumorph 200 and Infumorph 500 Sterile Solutions 965
MS Contin Tablets 1994
MSIR 1997
Oramorph SR (Morphine Sulfate Sustained Release Tablets) 2236
RMS Suppositories 2657
Roxanol 2243

Nabumetone (Reduces diuretic, natriuretic and antihypertensive effects of thiazides). Products include:

Relafen Tablets 2510

Nadolol (Potentiation of antihypertensive action).

No products indexed under this heading.

Naproxen (Reduces diuretic, natriuretic and antihypertensive effects of thiazides). Products include:

Anaprox/Naprosyn 2117

Naproxen Sodium (Reduces diuretic, natriuretic and antihypertensive effects of thiazides). Products include:

Aleve 1975
Anaprox/Naprosyn 2117

Nicardipine Hydrochloride (Potentiation of antihypertensive action). Products include:

Cardene Capsules 2095
Cardene I.V. 2709
Cardene SR Capsules 2097

Nifedipine (Potentiation of antihypertensive action). Products include:

Adalat Capsules (10 mg and 20 mg) 587
Adalat CC 589
Procardia Capsules 1971
Procardia XL Extended Release Tablets 1972

Nisoldipine (Potentiation of antihypertensive action).

No products indexed under this heading.

Nitroglycerin (Potentiation of antihypertensive action). Products include:

Deponit NTG Transdermal Delivery System 2397
Nitro-Bid IV 1523
Nitro-Bid Ointment 1524
Nitrodisc 2047
Nitro-Dur (nitroglycerin) Transdermal Infusion System 1326
Nitrolingual Spray 2027
Nitrostat Tablets 1925
Transderm-Nitro Transdermal Therapeutic System 859

Norepinephrine Bitartrate (Arterial responsiveness may be decreased, but not enough to preclude effectiveness of pressor agent). Products include:

Levophed Bitartrate Injection 2315

Opium Alkaloids (Orthostatic hypotension may be potentiated).

No products indexed under this heading.

Oxaprozin (Reduces diuretic, natriuretic and antihypertensive effects of thiazides). Products include:

Daypro Caplets 2426

Oxycodone Hydrochloride (Orthostatic hypotension may be potentiated). Products include:

Percocet Tablets 938
Percodan Tablets 939
Percodan-Demi Tablets 940
Roxicodone Tablets, Oral Solution & Intensol (Oxycodone) 2244
Tylox Capsules 1584

Penbutolol Sulfate (Potentiation of antihypertensive action). Products include:

Levatol 2403

Pentobarbital Sodium (Orthostatic hypotension may be potentiated). Products include:

Nembutal Sodium Capsules 436
Nembutal Sodium Solution 438
Nembutal Sodium Suppositories 440

Phenobarbital (Orthostatic hypotension may be potentiated). Products include:

Arco-Lase Plus Tablets 512
Bellergal-S Tablets 2250
Donnatal 2060
Donnatal Extentabs 2061
Donnatal Tablets 2060
Phenobarbital Elixir and Tablets 1469
Quadrinal Tablets 1350

Phenoxybenzamine Hydrochloride (Potentiation of antihypertensive action). Products include:

Dibenzyline Capsules 2476

Phentolamine Mesylate (Potentiation of antihypertensive action). Products include:

Regitine 846

Phenylbutazone (Reduces diuretic, natriuretic and antihypertensive effects of thiazides).

No products indexed under this heading.

Pindolol (Potentiation of antihypertensive action). Products include:

Visken Tablets 2299

Piroxicam (Reduces diuretic, natriuretic and antihypertensive effects of thiazides). Products include:

Feldene Capsules 1965

IMPORTANT NOTE: Always consult each drug listing in the patient's regimen for possible interactions.

Polythiazide (Potentiation of antihypertensive action). Products include:
Minizide Capsules 1938

Prazosin Hydrochloride (Potentiation of antihypertensive action). Products include:
Minipress Capsules 1937
Minizide Capsules 1938

Prednisolone Acetate (Hypokalemia may develop during concomitant use). Products include:
AK-CIDE .... ⊙ 202
AK-CIDE Ointment .... ⊙ 202
Blephamide Liquifilm Sterile Ophthalmic Suspension 476
Blephamide Ointment .... ⊙ 237
Econopred & Econopred Plus Ophthalmic Suspensions .... ⊙ 217
Poly-Pred Liquifilm .... ⊙ 248
Pred Forte .... ⊙ 250
Pred Mild .... ⊙ 253
Pred-G Liquifilm Sterile Ophthalmic Suspension .... ⊙ 251
Pred-G S.O.P. Sterile Ophthalmic Ointment .... ⊙ 252
Vasocidin Ointment .... ⊙ 268

Prednisolone Sodium Phosphate (Hypokalemia may develop during concomitant use). Products include:
AK-Pred .... ⊙ 204
Hydeltrasol Injection, Sterile 1665
Inflamase .... ⊙ 265
Pediapred Oral Liquid 995
Vasocidin Ophthalmic Solution .... ⊙ 270

Prednisolone Tebutate (Hypokalemia may develop during concomitant use). Products include:
Hydeltra-T.B.A. Sterile Suspension 1667

Prednisone (Hypokalemia may develop during concomitant use). Products include:
Deltasone Tablets 2595

Propoxyphene Hydrochloride (Orthostatic hypotension may be potentiated). Products include:
Darvon 1435
Wygesic Tablets 2827

Propoxyphene Napsylate (Orthostatic hypotension may be potentiated). Products include:
Darvon-N/Darvocet-N 1433

Propranolol Hydrochloride (Potentiation of antihypertensive action). Products include:
Inderal 2728
Inderal LA Long Acting Capsules 2730
Inderide Tablets 2732
Inderide LA Long Acting Capsules 2734

Quinapril Hydrochloride (Potentiation of antihypertensive action). Products include:
Accupril Tablets 1893

Ramipril (Potentiation of antihypertensive action). Products include:
Altace Capsules 1232

Rauwolfia Serpentina (Potentiation of antihypertensive action; potential for additive effects).
No products indexed under this heading.

Rescinnamine (Potentiation of antihypertensive action; potential for additive effects).
No products indexed under this heading.

Reserpine (Potentiation of antihypertensive action; potential for additive effects). Products include:
Diupres Tablets 1650
Hydropres Tablets 1675
Ser-Ap-Es Tablets 849

Secobarbital Sodium (Orthostatic hypotension may be potentiated). Products include:
Seconal Sodium Pulvules 1474

Sodium Nitroprusside (Potentiation of antihypertensive action).
No products indexed under this heading.

Sotalol Hydrochloride (Potentiation of antihypertensive action). Products include:
Betapace Tablets 641

Spirapril Hydrochloride (Potentiation of antihypertensive action).
No products indexed under this heading.

Sufentanil Citrate (Orthostatic hypotension may be potentiated). Products include:
Sufenta Injection 1309

Sulindac (Reduces diuretic, natriuretic and antihypertensive effects of thiazides). Products include:
Clinoril Tablets 1618

Terazosin Hydrochloride (Potentiation of antihypertensive action). Products include:
Hytrin Capsules 430

Thiamylal Sodium (Orthostatic hypotension may be potentiated).
No products indexed under this heading.

Timolol Maleate (Potentiation of antihypertensive action). Products include:
Blocadren Tablets 1614
Timolide Tablets 1748
Timoptic in Ocudose 1753
Timoptic Sterile Ophthalmic Solution 1751
Timoptic-XE 1755

Tolmetin Sodium (Reduces diuretic, natriuretic and antihypertensive effects of thiazides). Products include:
Tolectin (200, 400 and 600 mg) .. 1581

Torsemide (Potentiation of antihypertensive action). Products include:
Demadex Tablets and Injection 686

Triamcinolone (Hypokalemia may develop during concomitant use). Products include:
Aristocort Tablets 1022

Triamcinolone Acetonide (Hypokalemia may develop during concomitant use). Products include:
Aristocort A 0.025% Cream 1027
Aristocort A 0.5% Cream 1031
Aristocort A 0.1% Cream 1029
Aristocort A 0.1% Ointment 1030
Azmacort Oral Inhaler 2011
Nasacort Nasal Inhaler 2024

Triamcinolone Diacetate (Hypokalemia may develop during concomitant use). Products include:
Aristocort Suspension (Forte Parenteral) 1027
Aristocort Suspension (Intralesional) 1025

Triamcinolone Hexacetonide (Hypokalemia may develop during concomitant use). Products include:
Aristospan Suspension (Intra-articular) 1033
Aristospan Suspension (Intralesional) 1032

Trimethaphan Camsylate (Potentiation of antihypertensive action). Products include:
Arfonad Ampuls 2080

Tubocurarine Chloride (Increase responsiveness to tubocurarine).
No products indexed under this heading.

Verapamil Hydrochloride (Potentiation of antihypertensive action). Products include:
Calan SR Caplets 2422
Calan Tablets 2419
Isoptin Injectable 1344
Isoptin Oral Tablets 1346
Isoptin SR Tablets 1348
Verelan Capsules 1410
Verelan Capsules 2824

Food Interactions

Alcohol (Orthostatic hypotension may be potentiated).

LOPRESSOR TABLETS
(Metoprolol Tartrate) 830
See **Lopressor Ampuls**

LOPROX 1% CREAM AND LOTION
(Ciclopirox Olamine) 1242
None cited in PDR database.

LORABID SUSPENSION AND PULVULES
(Loracarbef) 1459
May interact with:

Probenecid (Inhibits renal excretion resulting in an approximately 80% increase in the AUC for loracarbef). Products include:
Benemid Tablets 1611
ColBENEMID Tablets 1622

Food Interactions

Food, unspecified (Delays the peak plasma concentration with no change in the total absorption).

LORCET 10/650
(Hydrocodone Bitartrate, Acetaminophen) 1018
May interact with narcotic analgesics, tricyclic antidepressants, monoamine oxidase inhibitors, tranquilizers, central nervous system depressants, anticholinergics, and certain other agents. Compounds in these categories include:

Alfentanil Hydrochloride (Potential for additive CNS depression). Products include:
Alfenta Injection 1286

Alprazolam (Potential for additive CNS depression). Products include:
Xanax Tablets 2649

Amitriptyline Hydrochloride (Increased effect of either the antidepressant or hydrocodone). Products include:
Elavil 2838
Endep Tablets 2174
Etrafon 2355
Limbitrol 2180
Triavil Tablets 1757

Amoxapine (Increased effect of either the antidepressant or hydrocodone). Products include:
Asendin Tablets 1369

Aprobarbital (Potential for additive CNS depression).
No products indexed under this heading.

Atropine Sulfate (Concurrent use may produce paralytic ileus). Products include:
Arco-Lase Plus Tablets 512
Atrohist Plus Tablets 454
Atropine Sulfate Sterile Ophthalmic Solution .... ⊙ 233
Donnatal 2060
Donnatal Extentabs 2061
Donnatal Tablets 2060
Lomotil 2439
Motofen Tablets 784
Urised Tablets 1964

Belladonna Alkaloids (Concurrent use may produce paralytic ileus). Products include:
Bellergal-S Tablets 2250
Hyland's Bed Wetting Tablets .... ▣ 828
Hyland's EnurAid Tablets .... ▣ 829
Hyland's Teething Tablets .... ▣ 830

Benztropine Mesylate (Concurrent use may produce paralytic ileus). Products include:
Cogentin 1621

Biperiden Hydrochloride (Concurrent use may produce paralytic ileus). Products include:
Akineton 1333

Buprenorphine (Potential for additive CNS depression). Products include:
Buprenex Injectable 2006

Buspirone Hydrochloride (Potential for additive CNS depression). Products include:
BuSpar 737

Butabarbital (Potential for additive CNS depression).
No products indexed under this heading.

Butalbital (Potential for additive CNS depression). Products include:
Esgic-plus Tablets 1013
Fioricet Tablets 2258
Fioricet with Codeine Capsules 2260
Fiorinal Capsules 2261
Fiorinal with Codeine Capsules 2262
Fiorinal Tablets 2261
Phrenilin 785
Sedapap Tablets 50 mg/650 mg .. 1543

Chlordiazepoxide (Potential for additive CNS depression). Products include:
Libritabs Tablets 2177
Limbitrol 2180

Chlordiazepoxide Hydrochloride (Potential for additive CNS depression). Products include:
Librax Capsules 2176
Librium Capsules 2178
Librium Injectable 2179

Chlorpromazine (Potential for additive CNS depression). Products include:
Thorazine Suppositories 2523

Chlorpromazine Hydrochloride (Potential for additive CNS depression). Products include:
Thorazine 2523

Chlorprothixene (Potential for additive CNS depression).
No products indexed under this heading.

Chlorprothixene Hydrochloride (Potential for additive CNS depression).
No products indexed under this heading.

Clidinium Bromide (Concurrent use may produce paralytic ileus). Products include:
Librax Capsules 2176
Quarzan Capsules 2181

Clomipramine Hydrochloride (Increased effect of either the antidepressant or hydrocodone). Products include:
Anafranil Capsules 803

Clorazepate Dipotassium (Potential for additive CNS depression). Products include:
Tranxene 451

Clozapine (Potential for additive CNS depression). Products include:
Clozaril Tablets 2252

Codeine Phosphate (Potential for additive CNS depression). Products include:
Actifed with Codeine Cough Syrup.. 1067
Brontex 1981
Deconsal C Expectorant Syrup 456
Deconsal Pediatric Syrup 457
Dimetane-DC Cough Syrup 2059
Empirin with Codeine Tablets 1093
Fioricet with Codeine Capsules 2260
Fiorinal with Codeine Capsules 2262
Isoclor Expectorant 990
Novahistine DH 2462
Novahistine Expectorant 2463
Nucofed 2051
Phenergan with Codeine 2777
Phenergan VC with Codeine 2781
Robitussin A-C Syrup 2073
Robitussin-DAC Syrup 2074
Ryna .... ▣ 841

(▣ Described in PDR For Nonprescription Drugs) (⊙ Described in PDR For Ophthalmology)

599 Interactions Index Lorcet 10/650

Soma Compound w/Codeine Tablets 2676
Tussi-Organidin NR Liquid and S NR Liquid 2677
Tylenol with Codeine 1583

Desflurane (Potential for additive CNS depression). Products include:
Suprane 1813

Desipramine Hydrochloride (Increased effect of either the antidepressant or hydrocodone). Products include:
Norpramin Tablets 1526

Dezocine (Potential for additive CNS depression). Products include:
Dalgan Injection 538

Diazepam (Potential for additive CNS depression). Products include:
Dizac 1809
Valium Injectable 2182
Valium Tablets 2183
Valrelease Capsules 2169

Dicyclomine Hydrochloride (Concurrent use may produce paralytic ileus). Products include:
Bentyl 1501

Doxepin Hydrochloride (Increased effect of either the antidepressant or hydrocodone). Products include:
Sinequan 2205
Zonalon Cream 1055

Droperidol (Potential for additive CNS depression). Products include:
Inapsine Injection 1296

Enflurane (Potential for additive CNS depression).
No products indexed under this heading.

Estazolam (Potential for additive CNS depression). Products include:
ProSom Tablets 449

Ethchlorvynol (Potential for additive CNS depression). Products include:
Placidyl Capsules 448

Ethinamate (Potential for additive CNS depression).
No products indexed under this heading.

Fentanyl (Potential for additive CNS depression). Products include:
Duragesic Transdermal System 1288

Fentanyl Citrate (Potential for additive CNS depression). Products include:
Sublimaze Injection 1307

Fluphenazine Decanoate (Potential for additive CNS depression). Products include:
Prolixin Decanoate 509

Fluphenazine Enanthate (Potential for additive CNS depression). Products include:
Prolixin Enanthate 509

Fluphenazine Hydrochloride (Potential for additive CNS depression). Products include:
Prolixin 509

Flurazepam Hydrochloride (Potential for additive CNS depression). Products include:
Dalmane Capsules 2173

Furazolidone (Increased effect of either the antidepressant or hydrocodone). Products include:
Furoxone 2046

Glutethimide (Potential for additive CNS depression).
No products indexed under this heading.

Glycopyrrolate (Concurrent use may produce paralytic ileus). Products include:
Robinul Forte Tablets 2072
Robinul Injectable 2072
Robinul Tablets 2072

Haloperidol (Potential for additive CNS depression). Products include:
Haldol Injection, Tablets and Concentrate 1575

Haloperidol Decanoate (Potential for additive CNS depression). Products include:
Haldol Decanoate 1577

Hydrocodone Polistirex (Potential for additive CNS depression). Products include:
Tussionex Pennkinetic Extended-Release Suspension 998

Hydroxyzine Hydrochloride (Potential for additive CNS depression). Products include:
Atarax Tablets & Syrup 2185
Marax Tablets & DF Syrup 2200
Vistaril Intramuscular Solution 2216

Hyoscyamine (Concurrent use may produce paralytic ileus). Products include:
Cystospaz Tablets 1963
Urised Tablets 1964

Hyoscyamine Sulfate (Concurrent use may produce paralytic ileus). Products include:
Arco-Lase Plus Tablets 512
Atrohist Plus Tablets 454
Cystospaz-M Capsules 1963
Donnatal 2060
Donnatal Extentabs 2061
Donnatal Tablets 2060
Kutrase Capsules 2402
Levsin/Levsinex/Levbid 2405

Imipramine Hydrochloride (Increased effect of either the antidepressant or hydrocodone). Products include:
Tofranil Ampuls 854
Tofranil Tablets 856

Imipramine Pamoate (Increased effect of either the antidepressant or hydrocodone). Products include:
Tofranil-PM Capsules 857

Ipratropium Bromide (Concurrent use may produce paralytic ileus). Products include:
Atrovent Inhalation Aerosol 671
Atrovent Inhalation Solution 673

Isocarboxazid (Increased effect of either the antidepressant or hydrocodone).
No products indexed under this heading.

Isoflurane (Potential for additive CNS depression).
No products indexed under this heading.

Ketamine Hydrochloride (Potential for additive CNS depression).
No products indexed under this heading.

Levomethadyl Acetate Hydrochloride (Potential for additive CNS depression). Products include:
Orlamm 2239

Levorphanol Tartrate (Potential for additive CNS depression). Products include:
Levo-Dromoran 2129

Lorazepam (Potential for additive CNS depression). Products include:
Ativan Injection 2698
Ativan Tablets 2700

Loxapine Hydrochloride (Potential for additive CNS depression). Products include:
Loxitane 1378

Loxapine Succinate (Potential for additive CNS depression). Products include:
Loxitane Capsules 1378

Maprotiline Hydrochloride (Increased effect of either the antidepressant or hydrocodone). Products include:
Ludiomil Tablets 843

Mepenzolate Bromide (Concurrent use may produce paralytic ileus).
No products indexed under this heading.

Meperidine Hydrochloride (Potential for additive CNS depression). Products include:
Demerol 2308
Mepergan Injection 2753

Mephobarbital (Potential for additive CNS depression). Products include:
Mebaral Tablets 2322

Meprobamate (Potential for additive CNS depression). Products include:
Miltown Tablets 2672
PMB 200 and PMB 400 2783

Mesoridazine (Potential for additive CNS depression).

Methadone Hydrochloride (Potential for additive CNS depression). Products include:
Methadone Hydrochloride Oral Concentrate 2233
Methadone Hydrochloride Oral Solution & Tablets 2235

Methohexital Sodium (Potential for additive CNS depression). Products include:
Brevital Sodium Vials 1429

Methotrimeprazine (Potential for additive CNS depression). Products include:
Levoprome 1274

Methoxyflurane (Potential for additive CNS depression).
No products indexed under this heading.

Midazolam Hydrochloride (Potential for additive CNS depression). Products include:
Versed Injection 2170

Molindone Hydrochloride (Potential for additive CNS depression). Products include:
Moban Tablets and Concentrate 1048

Morphine Sulfate (Potential for additive CNS depression). Products include:
Astramorph/PF Injection, USP (Preservative-Free) 535
Duramorph 962
Infumorph 200 and Infumorph 500 Sterile Solutions 965
MS Contin Tablets 1994
MSIR 1997
Oramorph SR (Morphine Sulfate Sustained Release Tablets) 2236
RMS Suppositories 2657
Roxanol 2243

Nortriptyline Hydrochloride (Increased effect of either the antidepressant or hydrocodone). Products include:
Pamelor 2280

Opium Alkaloids (Potential for additive CNS depression).
No products indexed under this heading.

Oxazepam (Potential for additive CNS depression). Products include:
Serax Capsules 2810
Serax Tablets 2810

Oxybutynin Chloride (Concurrent use may produce paralytic ileus). Products include:
Ditropan 1516

Oxycodone Hydrochloride (Potential for additive CNS depression). Products include:
Percocet Tablets 938
Percodan Tablets 939
Percodan-Demi Tablets 940
Roxicodone Tablets, Oral Solution & Intensol (Oxycodone) 2244
Tylox Capsules 1584

Pentobarbital Sodium (Potential for additive CNS depression). Products include:
Nembutal Sodium Capsules 436
Nembutal Sodium Solution 438
Nembutal Sodium Suppositories 440

Perphenazine (Potential for additive CNS depression). Products include:
Etrafon 2355
Triavil Tablets 1757
Trilafon 2389

Phenelzine Sulfate (Increased effect of either the antidepressant or hydrocodone). Products include:
Nardil 1920

Phenobarbital (Potential for additive CNS depression). Products include:
Arco-Lase Plus Tablets 512
Bellergal-S Tablets 2250
Donnatal 2060
Donnatal Extentabs 2061
Donnatal Tablets 2060
Phenobarbital Elixir and Tablets 1469
Quadrinal Tablets 1350

Prazepam (Potential for additive CNS depression).
No products indexed under this heading.

Prochlorperazine (Potential for additive CNS depression). Products include:
Compazine 2470

Procyclidine Hydrochloride (Concurrent use may produce paralytic ileus). Products include:
Kemadrin Tablets 1112

Promethazine Hydrochloride (Potential for additive CNS depression). Products include:
Mepergan Injection 2753
Phenergan with Codeine 2777
Phenergan with Dextromethorphan 2778
Phenergan Injection 2773
Phenergan Suppositories 2775
Phenergan Syrup 2774
Phenergan Tablets 2775
Phenergan VC 2779
Phenergan VC with Codeine 2781

Propantheline Bromide (Concurrent use may produce paralytic ileus). Products include:
Pro-Banthīne Tablets 2052

Propofol (Potential for additive CNS depression). Products include:
Diprivan Injection 2833

Propoxyphene Hydrochloride (Potential for additive CNS depression). Products include:
Darvon 1435
Wygesic Tablets 2827

Propoxyphene Napsylate (Potential for additive CNS depression). Products include:
Darvon-N/Darvocet-N 1433

Protriptyline Hydrochloride (Increased effect of either the antidepressant or hydrocodone). Products include:
Vivactil Tablets 1774

Quazepam (Potential for additive CNS depression). Products include:
Doral Tablets 2664

Risperidone (Potential for additive CNS depression). Products include:
Risperdal 1301

Scopolamine (Concurrent use may produce paralytic ileus). Products include:
Transderm Scōp Transdermal Therapeutic System 869

Scopolamine Hydrobromide (Concurrent use may produce paralytic ileus). Products include:
Atrohist Plus Tablets 454
Donnatal 2060
Donnatal Extentabs 2061
Donnatal Tablets 2060

IMPORTANT NOTE: Always consult each drug listing in the patient's regimen for possible interactions.

Secobarbital Sodium (Potential for additive CNS depression). Products include:
- Seconal Sodium Pulvules ... 1474

Selegiline Hydrochloride (Increased effect of either the antidepressant or hydrocodone). Products include:
- Eldepryl Tablets ... 2550

Sufentanil Citrate (Potential for additive CNS depression). Products include:
- Sufenta Injection ... 1309

Temazepam (Potential for additive CNS depression). Products include:
- Restoril Capsules ... 2284

Thiamylal Sodium (Potential for additive CNS depression).
- No products indexed under this heading.

Thioridazine Hydrochloride (Potential for additive CNS depression). Products include:
- Mellaril ... 2269

Thiothixene (Potential for additive CNS depression). Products include:
- Navane Capsules and Concentrate 2201
- Navane Intramuscular ... 2202

Tranylcypromine Sulfate (Increased effect of either the antidepressant or hydrocodone). Products include:
- Parnate Tablets ... 2503

Triazolam (Potential for additive CNS depression). Products include:
- Halcion Tablets ... 2611

Tridihexethyl Chloride (Concurrent use may produce paralytic ileus).
- No products indexed under this heading.

Trifluoperazine Hydrochloride (Potential for additive CNS depression). Products include:
- Stelazine ... 2514

Trihexyphenidyl Hydrochloride (Concurrent use may produce paralytic ileus). Products include:
- Artane ... 1368

Trimipramine Maleate (Increased effect of either the antidepressant or hydrocodone). Products include:
- Surmontil Capsules ... 2811

Zolpidem Tartrate (Potential for additive CNS depression). Products include:
- Ambien Tablets ... 2416

Food Interactions

Alcohol (Potential for additive CNS depression).

LORELCO TABLETS

(Probucol) ... 1517

May interact with drugs that prolong the qt interval and certain other agents. Compounds in these categories include:

Amiodarone Hydrochloride (Increases the risk of serious arrhythmia). Products include:
- Cordarone Intravenous ... 2715
- Cordarone Tablets ... 2712

Amitriptyline Hydrochloride (Increases the risk of serious arrhythmia). Products include:
- Elavil ... 2838
- Endep Tablets ... 2174
- Etrafon ... 2355
- Limbitrol ... 2180
- Triavil Tablets ... 1757

Amoxapine (Increases the risk of serious arrhythmia). Products include:
- Asendin Tablets ... 1369

Astemizole (Increases the risk of serious arrhythmia). Products include:
- Hismanal Tablets ... 1293

Bretylium Tosylate (Increases the risk of serious arrhythmia).
- No products indexed under this heading.

Chlorpromazine (Increases the risk of serious arrhythmia). Products include:
- Thorazine Suppositories ... 2523

Clofibrate (Pronounced lowering of HDL-cholesterol). Products include:
- Atromid-S Capsules ... 2701

Clomipramine Hydrochloride (Increases the risk of serious arrhythmia). Products include:
- Anafranil Capsules ... 803

Desipramine Hydrochloride (Increases the risk of serious arrhythmia). Products include:
- Norpramin Tablets ... 1526

Disopyramide Phosphate (Increases the risk of serious arrhythmia). Products include:
- Norpace ... 2444

Doxepin Hydrochloride (Increases the risk of serious arrhythmia). Products include:
- Sinequan ... 2205
- Zonalon Cream ... 1055

Flecainide Acetate (Increases the risk of serious arrhythmia). Products include:
- Tambocor Tablets ... 1497

Fluphenazine Decanoate (Increases the risk of serious arrhythmia). Products include:
- Prolixin Decanoate ... 509

Fluphenazine Enanthate (Increases the risk of serious arrhythmia). Products include:
- Prolixin Enanthate ... 509

Fluphenazine Hydrochloride (Increases the risk of serious arrhythmia). Products include:
- Prolixin ... 509

Imipramine Hydrochloride (Increases the risk of serious arrhythmia). Products include:
- Tofranil Ampuls ... 854
- Tofranil Tablets ... 856

Imipramine Pamoate (Increases the risk of serious arrhythmia). Products include:
- Tofranil-PM Capsules ... 857

Lidocaine Hydrochloride (Increases the risk of serious arrhythmia). Products include:
- Bactine Antiseptic/Anesthetic First Aid Liquid ... ▣ 708
- Campho-Phenique Maximum Strength First Aid Antibiotic Plus Pain Reliever Ointment ... ▣ 719
- Decadron Phosphate with Xylocaine Injection, Sterile ... 1639
- Xylocaine Injections ... 567

Maprotiline Hydrochloride (Increases the risk of serious arrhythmia). Products include:
- Ludiomil Tablets ... 843

Mesoridazine Besylate (Increases the risk of serious arrhythmia). Products include:
- Serentil ... 684

Mexiletine Hydrochloride (Increases the risk of serious arrhythmia). Products include:
- Mexitil Capsules ... 678

Nortriptyline Hydrochloride (Increases the risk of serious arrhythmia). Products include:
- Pamelor ... 2280

Perphenazine (Increases the risk of serious arrhythmia). Products include:
- Etrafon ... 2355
- Triavil Tablets ... 1757
- Trilafon ... 2389

Procainamide Hydrochloride (Increases the risk of serious arrhythmia). Products include:
- Procan SR Tablets ... 1926

Prochlorperazine (Increases the risk of serious arrhythmia). Products include:
- Compazine ... 2470

Promethazine Hydrochloride (Increases the risk of serious arrhythmia). Products include:
- Mepergan Injection ... 2753
- Phenergan with Codeine ... 2777
- Phenergan with Dextromethorphan 2778
- Phenergan Injection ... 2773
- Phenergan Suppositories ... 2775
- Phenergan Syrup ... 2774
- Phenergan Tablets ... 2775
- Phenergan VC ... 2779
- Phenergan VC with Codeine ... 2781

Propafenone Hydrochloride (Increases the risk of serious arrhythmia). Products include:
- Rythmol Tablets–150mg, 225mg, 300mg ... 1352

Protriptyline Hydrochloride (Increases the risk of serious arrhythmia). Products include:
- Vivactil Tablets ... 1774

Quinidine Gluconate (Increases the risk of serious arrhythmia). Products include:
- Quinaglute Dura-Tabs Tablets ... 649

Quinidine Polygalacturonate (Increases the risk of serious arrhythmia).
- No products indexed under this heading.

Quinidine Sulfate (Increases the risk of serious arrhythmia). Products include:
- Quinidex Extentabs ... 2067

Terfenadine (Increases the risk of serious arrhythmia). Products include:
- Seldane Tablets ... 1536
- Seldane-D Extended-Release Tablets ... 1538

Thioridazine Hydrochloride (Increases the risk of serious arrhythmia). Products include:
- Mellaril ... 2269

Tocainide Hydrochloride (Increases the risk of serious arrhythmia). Products include:
- Tonocard Tablets ... 531

Trifluoperazine Hydrochloride (Increases the risk of serious arrhythmia). Products include:
- Stelazine ... 2514

Trimipramine Maleate (Increases the risk of serious arrhythmia). Products include:
- Surmontil Capsules ... 2811

LORTAB 2.5/500 TABLETS

(Hydrocodone Bitartrate, Acetaminophen) ... 2566

May interact with central nervous system depressants, narcotic analgesics, psychotropics, tranquilizers, antihistamines, tricyclic antidepressants, monoamine oxidase inhibitors, and certain other agents. Compounds in these categories include:

Acrivastine (Additive CNS depression; the dose of one or both agents should be reduced). Products include:
- Semprex-D Capsules ... 463
- Semprex-D Capsules ... 1167

Alfentanil Hydrochloride (Additive CNS depression; the dose of one or both agents should be reduced). Products include:
- Alfenta Injection ... 1286

Alprazolam (Additive CNS depression; the dose of one or both agents should be reduced). Products include:
- Xanax Tablets ... 2649

Amitriptyline Hydrochloride (Increased effect of either hydrocodone or antidepressant; additive CNS depression; the dose of one or both agents should be reduced). Products include:
- Elavil ... 2838
- Endep Tablets ... 2174
- Etrafon ... 2355
- Limbitrol ... 2180
- Triavil Tablets ... 1757

Amoxapine (Increased effect of either hydrocodone or antidepressant; additive CNS depression; the dose of one or both agents should be reduced). Products include:
- Asendin Tablets ... 1369

Aprobarbital (Additive CNS depression; the dose of one or both agents should be reduced).
- No products indexed under this heading.

Astemizole (Additive CNS depression; the dose of one or both agents should be reduced). Products include:
- Hismanal Tablets ... 1293

Azatadine Maleate (Additive CNS depression; the dose of one or both agents should be reduced). Products include:
- Trinalin Repetabs Tablets ... 1330

Bromodiphenhydramine Hydrochloride (Additive CNS depression; the dose of one or both agents should be reduced).
- No products indexed under this heading.

Brompheniramine Maleate (Additive CNS depression; the dose of one or both agents should be reduced). Products include:
- Alka Seltzer Plus Sinus Medicine .. ▣ 707
- Bromfed Capsules (Extended-Release) ... 1785
- Bromfed Syrup ... ▣ 733
- Bromfed Tablets ... 1785
- Bromfed-DM Cough Syrup ... 1786
- Bromfed-PD Capsules (Extended-Release) ... 1785
- Dimetane-DC Cough Syrup ... 2059
- Dimetane-DX Cough Syrup ... 2059
- Dimetapp Elixir ... ▣ 773
- Dimetapp Extentabs ... ▣ 774
- Dimetapp Tablets/Liqui-Gels ... ▣ 775
- Dimetapp Cold & Allergy Chewable Tablets ... ▣ 773
- Dimetapp DM Elixir ... ▣ 774
- Vicks DayQuil Allergy Relief 12-Hour Extended Release Tablets.. ▣ 760
- Vicks DayQuil Allergy Relief 4-Hour Tablets ... ▣ 760

Buprenorphine (Additive CNS depression; the dose of one or both agents should be reduced). Products include:
- Buprenex Injectable ... 2006

Buspirone Hydrochloride (Additive CNS depression; the dose of one or both agents should be reduced). Products include:
- BuSpar ... 737

Butabarbital (Additive CNS depression; the dose of one or both agents should be reduced).
- No products indexed under this heading.

Butalbital (Additive CNS depression; the dose of one or both agents should be reduced). Products include:
- Esgic-plus Tablets ... 1013
- Fioricet Tablets ... 2258
- Fioricet with Codeine Capsules ... 2260
- Fiorinal Capsules ... 2261
- Fiorinal with Codeine Capsules ... 2262

(▣ Described in PDR For Nonprescription Drugs) (◉ Described in PDR For Ophthalmology)

601 Interactions Index Lortab

Fiorinal Tablets 2261
Phrenilin 785
Sedapap Tablets 50 mg/650 mg .. 1543

Chlordiazepoxide (Additive CNS depression; the dose of one or both agents should be reduced). Products include:
Libritabs Tablets 2177
Limbitrol 2180

Chlordiazepoxide Hydrochloride (Additive CNS depression; the dose of one or both agents should be reduced). Products include:
Librax Capsules 2176
Librium Capsules 2178
Librium Injectable 2179

Chlorpheniramine Maleate (Additive CNS depression; the dose of one or both agents should be reduced). Products include:
Alka-Seltzer Plus Cold Medicine 705
Alka-Seltzer Plus Cold Medicine Liqui-Gels 706
Alka-Seltzer Plus Cold & Cough Medicine 708
Alka-Seltzer Plus Cold & Cough Medicine Liqui-Gels 705
Allerest Children's Chewable Tablets 627
Allerest Headache Strength Tablets 627
Allerest Maximum Strength Tablets 627
Allerest Sinus Pain Formula 627
Allerest 12 Hour Caplets 627
Ana-Kit Anaphylaxis Emergency Treatment Kit 617
Atrohist Pediatric Capsules 453
Atrohist Plus Tablets 454
BC Cold Powder Multi-Symptom Formula (Cold-Sinus-Allergy) 609
Cerose DM 878
Cheracol Plus Head Cold/Cough Formula 769
Children's Vicks DayQuil Allergy Relief 757
Children's Vicks NyQuil Cold/Cough Relief 758
Chlor-Trimeton Allergy Decongestant Tablets 799
Chlor-Trimeton Allergy Tablets 798
Comhist 2038
Comtrex Multi-Symptom Cold Reliever Tablets/Caplets/Liqui-Gels/Liquid 615
Allergy-Sinus Comtrex Multi-Symptom Allergy-Sinus Formula Tablets 617
Contac Continuous Action Nasal Decongestant/Antihistamine 12 Hour Capsules 813
Contac Maximum Strength Continuous Action Decongestant/Antihistamine 12 Hour Caplets .. 813
Contac Severe Cold and Flu Formula Caplets 814
Coricidin 'D' Decongestant Tablets 800
Coricidin Tablets 800
D.A. Chewable Tablets 951
Deconamine 1320
Dura-Tap/PD Capsules 2867
Dura-Vent/DA Tablets 953
Extendryl 1005
Fedahist Gyrocaps 2401
Fedahist Timecaps 2401
Hycomine Compound Tablets 932
Isoclor Timesule Capsules 637
Kronofed-A 977
Nolamine Timed-Release Tablets 785
Novahistine DH 2462
Novahistine Elixir 823
Ornade Spansule Capsules 2502
PediaCare Cold Allergy Chewable Tablets 677
PediaCare Cough-Cold Chewable Tablets 1553
PediaCare Cough-Cold Liquid 1553
PediaCare NightRest Cough-Cold Liquid 1553
Pediatric Vicks 44m Cough & Cold Relief 764
Pyrroxate Caplets 772
Ryna 841
Sinarest Tablets 648
Sinarest Extra Strength Tablets 648
Sine-Off Sinus Medicine 825
Singlet Tablets 825
Sinulin Tablets 787
Sinutab Sinus Allergy Medication, Maximum Strength Tablets and Caplets 860
Sudafed Plus Liquid 862
Sudafed Plus Tablets 863
Teldrin 12 Hour Antihistamine/Nasal Decongestant Allergy Relief Capsules 826
TheraFlu 787
TheraFlu Maximum Strength Nighttime Flu, Cold & Cough Medicine 788
Triaminic Allergy Tablets 789
Triaminic Cold Tablets 790
Triaminic Nite Light 791
Triaminic Syrup 792
Triaminic-12 Tablets 792
Triaminicin Tablets 793
Triaminicol Multi-Symptom Cold Tablets 793
Triaminicol Multi-Symptom Relief 794
Tussend 1783
Children's TYLENOL Cold Multi-Symptom Liquid Formula and Chewable Tablets 1561
Children's TYLENOL Cold Plus Cough Multi Symptom Tablets and Liquid 681
TYLENOL Maximum Strength Allergy Sinus Medication Gelcaps and Caplets 1563
TYLENOL Cold Multi-Symptom Formula Medication Tablets and Caplets 1561
TYLENOL Cold Multi-Symptom Hot Medication Liquid Packets 1557
Vicks 44 LiquiCaps Cough, Cold & Flu Relief 755
Vicks 44M Cough, Cold & Flu Relief 756

Chlorpheniramine Polistirex (Additive CNS depression; the dose of one or both agents should be reduced). Products include:
Tussionex Pennkinetic Extended-Release Suspension 998

Chlorpheniramine Tannate (Additive CNS depression; the dose of one or both agents should be reduced). Products include:
Atrohist Pediatric Suspension 454
Ricobid Tablets and Pediatric Suspension 2038
Rynatan 2673
Rynatuss 2673

Chlorpromazine (Additive CNS depression; the dose of one or both agents should be reduced). Products include:
Thorazine Suppositories 2523

Chlorpromazine Hydrochloride (Additive CNS depression; the dose of one or both agents should be reduced). Products include:
Thorazine 2523

Chlorprothixene (Additive CNS depression; the dose of one or both agents should be reduced).
No products indexed under this heading.

Chlorprothixene Hydrochloride (Additive CNS depression; the dose of one or both agents should be reduced).
No products indexed under this heading.

Clemastine Fumarate (Additive CNS depression; the dose of one or both agents should be reduced). Products include:
Tavist Syrup 2297
Tavist Tablets 2298
Tavist-1 12 Hour Relief Tablets 787
Tavist-D 12 Hour Relief Tablets 787

Clomipramine Hydrochloride (Increased effect of either hydrocodone or antidepressant). Products include:
Anafranil Capsules 803

Clorazepate Dipotassium (Additive CNS depression; the dose of one or both agents should be reduced). Products include:
Tranxene 451

Clozapine (Additive CNS depression; the dose of one or both agents should be reduced). Products include:
Clozaril Tablets 2252

Codeine Phosphate (Additive CNS depression; the dose of one or both agents should be reduced). Products include:
Actifed with Codeine Cough Syrup.. 1067
Brontex 1981
Deconsal C Expectorant Syrup 456
Deconsal Pediatric Syrup 457
Dimetane-DC Cough Syrup 2059
Empirin with Codeine Tablets 1093
Fioricet with Codeine Capsules 2260
Fiorinal with Codeine Capsules 2262
Isoclor Expectorant 990
Novahistine DH 2462
Novahistine Expectorant 2463
Nucofed 2051
Phenergan with Codeine 2777
Phenergan VC with Codeine 2781
Robitussin A-C Syrup 2073
Robitussin-DAC Syrup 2074
Ryna 841
Soma Compound w/Codeine Tablets 2676
Tussi-Organidin NR Liquid and S NR Liquid 2677
Tylenol with Codeine 1583

Cyproheptadine Hydrochloride (Additive CNS depression; the dose of one or both agents should be reduced). Products include:
Periactin 1724

Desflurane (Additive CNS depression; the dose of one or both agents should be reduced). Products include:
Suprane 1813

Desipramine Hydrochloride (Increased effect of either hydrocodone or antidepressant; additive CNS depression; the dose of one or both agents should be reduced). Products include:
Norpramin Tablets 1526

Dexchlorpheniramine Maleate (Additive CNS depression; the dose of one or both agents should be reduced).
No products indexed under this heading.

Dezocine (Additive CNS depression; the dose of one or both agents should be reduced). Products include:
Dalgan Injection 538

Diazepam (Additive CNS depression; the dose of one or both agents should be reduced). Products include:
Dizac 1809
Valium Injectable 2182
Valium Tablets 2183
Valrelease Capsules 2169

Diphenhydramine Citrate (Additive CNS depression; the dose of one or both agents should be reduced). Products include:
Excedrin P.M. Analgesic/Sleeping Aid Tablets, Caplets, Liquigels 733

Diphenhydramine Hydrochloride (Additive CNS depression; the dose of one or both agents should be reduced). Products include:
Actifed Allergy Daytime/Nighttime Caplets 844
Actifed Sinus Daytime/Nighttime Tablets and Caplets 846
Arthritis Foundation NightTime Caplets 674
Extra Strength Bayer PM Aspirin .. 713
Bayer Select Night Time Pain Relief Formula 716
Benadryl Allergy Decongestant Liquid Medication 848
Benadryl Allergy Decongestant Tablets 848
Benadryl Allergy Liquid Medication 849
Benadryl Allergy 848
Benadryl Allergy Sinus Headache Formula Caplets 849
Benadryl Capsules 1898
Benadryl Dye-Free Allergy Liqui-gel Softgels 850
Benadryl Dye-Free Allergy Liquid Medication 850
Benadryl Itch Relief Cream, Children's Formula and Maximum Strength 2% 851
Benadryl Itch Relief Spray, Children's Formula and Maximum Strength 2% 851
Benadryl Itch Relief Stick Maximum Strength 2% 850
Benadryl Itch Stopping Gel, Children's Formula and Maximum Strength 2% 851
Benadryl Kapseals 1898
Benadryl Injection 1898
Contac Day & Night Cold/Flu Night Caplets 812
Contac Night Allergy/Sinus Caplets 812
Extra Strength Doan's P.M. 633
Legatrin PM 651
Miles Nervine Nighttime Sleep-Aid 723
Nytol QuickCaps Caplets 610
Sleepinal Night-time Sleep Aid Capsules and Softgels 834
TYLENOL Maximum Strength Allergy Sinus NightTime Medication Caplets 1555
TYLENOL Flu NightTime, Maximum Strength, Gelcaps 1566
TYLENOL Maximum Strength Flu NightTime Hot Medication Packets 1562
TYLENOL PM, Extra Strength Pain Reliever/Sleep Aid Caplets, Geltabs, Gelcaps 1560
TYLENOL Severe Allergy Medication Caplets 1564
Maximum Strength Unisom Sleepgels 1934
Unisom With Pain Relief-Nighttime Sleep Aid and Pain Reliever 1934

Diphenylpyraline Hydrochloride (Additive CNS depression; the dose of one or both agents should be reduced).
No products indexed under this heading.

Doxepin Hydrochloride (Increased effect of either hydrocodone or antidepressant; additive CNS depression; the dose of one or both agents should be reduced). Products include:
Sinequan 2205
Zonalon Cream 1055

Droperidol (Additive CNS depression; the dose of one or both agents should be reduced). Products include:
Inapsine Injection 1296

Enflurane (Additive CNS depression; the dose of one or both agents should be reduced).
No products indexed under this heading.

Estazolam (Additive CNS depression; the dose of one or both agents should be reduced). Products include:
ProSom Tablets 449

Ethchlorvynol (Additive CNS depression; the dose of one or both agents should be reduced). Products include:
Placidyl Capsules 448

Ethinamate (Additive CNS depression; the dose of one or both agents should be reduced).
No products indexed under this heading.

Fentanyl (Additive CNS depression; the dose of one or both agents should be reduced). Products include:
Duragesic Transdermal System 1288

IMPORTANT NOTE: Always consult each drug listing in the patient's regimen for possible interactions.

Lortab Interactions Index 602

Fentanyl Citrate (Additive CNS depression; the dose of one or both agents should be reduced). Products include:
- Sublimaze Injection 1307

Fluphenazine Decanoate (Additive CNS depression; the dose of one or both agents should be reduced). Products include:
- Prolixin Decanoate 509

Fluphenazine Enanthate (Additive CNS depression; the dose of one or both agents should be reduced). Products include:
- Prolixin Enanthate 509

Fluphenazine Hydrochloride (Additive CNS depression; the dose of one or both agents should be reduced). Products include:
- Prolixin 509

Flurazepam Hydrochloride (Additive CNS depression; the dose of one or both agents should be reduced). Products include:
- Dalmane Capsules 2173

Furazolidone (Increased effect of either hydrocodone or MAOI inhibitor). Products include:
- Furoxone 2046

Glutethimide (Additive CNS depression; the dose of one or both agents should be reduced).
- No products indexed under this heading.

Haloperidol (Additive CNS depression; the dose of one or both agents should be reduced). Products include:
- Haldol Injection, Tablets and Concentrate 1575

Haloperidol Decanoate (Additive CNS depression; the dose of one or both agents should be reduced). Products include:
- Haldol Decanoate 1577

Hydrocodone Polistirex (Additive CNS depression; the dose of one or both agents should be reduced). Products include:
- Tussionex Pennkinetic Extended-Release Suspension 998

Hydroxyzine Hydrochloride (Additive CNS depression; the dose of one or both agents should be reduced). Products include:
- Atarax Tablets & Syrup 2185
- Marax Tablets & DF Syrup 2200
- Vistaril Intramuscular Solution 2216

Imipramine Hydrochloride (Increased effect of either hydrocodone or antidepressant; additive CNS depression; the dose of one or both agents should be reduced). Products include:
- Tofranil Ampuls 854
- Tofranil Tablets 856

Imipramine Pamoate (Increased effect of either hydrocodone or antidepressant; additive CNS depression; the dose of one or both agents should be reduced). Products include:
- Tofranil-PM Capsules 857

Isocarboxazid (Increased effect of either hydrocodone or MAOI inhibitor; additive CNS depression; the dose of one or both agents should be reduced).
- No products indexed under this heading.

Isoflurane (Additive CNS depression; the dose of one or both agents should be reduced).
- No products indexed under this heading.

Ketamine Hydrochloride (Additive CNS depression; the dose of one or both agents should be reduced).
- No products indexed under this heading.

Levomethadyl Acetate Hydrochloride (Additive CNS depression; the dose of one or both agents should be reduced). Products include:
- Orlamm 2239

Levorphanol Tartrate (Additive CNS depression; the dose of one or both agents should be reduced). Products include:
- Levo-Dromoran 2129

Lithium Carbonate (Additive CNS depression; the dose of one or both agents should be reduced). Products include:
- Eskalith 2485
- Lithium Carbonate Capsules & Tablets 2230
- Lithonate/Lithotabs/Lithobid 2543

Lithium Citrate (Additive CNS depression; the dose of one or both agents should be reduced).
- No products indexed under this heading.

Loratadine (Additive CNS depression; the dose of one or both agents should be reduced). Products include:
- Claritin 2349
- Claritin-D 2350

Lorazepam (Additive CNS depression; the dose of one or both agents should be reduced). Products include:
- Ativan Injection 2698
- Ativan Tablets 2700

Loxapine Hydrochloride (Additive CNS depression; the dose of one or both agents should be reduced). Products include:
- Loxitane 1378

Loxapine Succinate (Additive CNS depression; the dose of one or both agents should be reduced). Products include:
- Loxitane Capsules 1378

Maprotiline Hydrochloride (Increased effect of either hydrocodone or antidepressant; additive CNS depression; the dose of one or both agents should be reduced). Products include:
- Ludiomil Tablets 843

Meperidine Hydrochloride (Additive CNS depression; the dose of one or both agents should be reduced). Products include:
- Demerol 2308
- Mepergan Injection 2753

Mephobarbital (Additive CNS depression; the dose of one or both agents should be reduced). Products include:
- Mebaral Tablets 2322

Meprobamate (Additive CNS depression; the dose of one or both agents should be reduced). Products include:
- Miltown Tablets 2672
- PMB 200 and PMB 400 2783

Mesoridazine Besylate (Additive CNS depression; the dose of one or both agents should be reduced). Products include:
- Serentil 684

Methadone Hydrochloride (Additive CNS depression; the dose of one or both agents should be reduced). Products include:
- Methadone Hydrochloride Oral Concentrate 2233
- Methadone Hydrochloride Oral Solution & Tablets 2235

Methdilazine Hydrochloride (Additive CNS depression; the dose of one or both agents should be reduced).
- No products indexed under this heading.

Methohexital Sodium (Additive CNS depression; the dose of one or both agents should be reduced). Products include:
- Brevital Sodium Vials 1429

Methotrimeprazine (Additive CNS depression; the dose of one or both agents should be reduced). Products include:
- Levoprome 1274

Methoxyflurane (Additive CNS depression; the dose of one or both agents should be reduced).
- No products indexed under this heading.

Midazolam Hydrochloride (Additive CNS depression; the dose of one or both agents should be reduced). Products include:
- Versed Injection 2170

Molindone Hydrochloride (Additive CNS depression; the dose of one or both agents should be reduced). Products include:
- Moban Tablets and Concentrate 1048

Morphine Sulfate (Additive CNS depression; the dose of one or both agents should be reduced). Products include:
- Astramorph/PF Injection, USP (Preservative-Free) 535
- Duramorph 962
- Infumorph 200 and Infumorph 500 Sterile Solutions 965
- MS Contin Tablets 1994
- MSIR 1997
- Oramorph SR (Morphine Sulfate Sustained Release Tablets) 2236
- RMS Suppositories 2657
- Roxanol 2243

Nortriptyline Hydrochloride (Increased effect of either hydrocodone or antidepressant; additive CNS depression; the dose of one or both agents should be reduced). Products include:
- Pamelor 2280

Opium Alkaloids (Additive CNS depression; the dose of one or both agents should be reduced).
- No products indexed under this heading.

Oxazepam (Additive CNS depression; the dose of one or both agents should be reduced). Products include:
- Serax Capsules 2810
- Serax Tablets 2810

Oxycodone Hydrochloride (Additive CNS depression; the dose of one or both agents should be reduced). Products include:
- Percocet Tablets 938
- Percodan Tablets 939
- Percodan-Demi Tablets 940
- Roxicodone Tablets, Oral Solution & Intensol (Oxycodone) 2244
- Tylox Capsules 1584

Pentobarbital Sodium (Additive CNS depression; the dose of one or both agents should be reduced). Products include:
- Nembutal Sodium Capsules 436
- Nembutal Sodium Solution 438
- Nembutal Sodium Suppositories 440

Perphenazine (Additive CNS depression; the dose of one or both agents should be reduced). Products include:
- Etrafon 2355
- Triavil Tablets 1757
- Trilafon 2389

Phenelzine Sulfate (Increased effect of either hydrocodone or MAOI inhibitor). Products include:
- Nardil 1920

Phenobarbital (Additive CNS depression; the dose of one or both agents should be reduced). Products include:
- Arco-Lase Plus Tablets 512
- Bellergal-S Tablets 2250
- Donnatal 2060
- Donnatal Extentabs 2061
- Donnatal Tablets 2060
- Phenobarbital Elixir and Tablets 1469
- Quadrinal Tablets 1350

Prazepam (Additive CNS depression; the dose of one or both agents should be reduced).
- No products indexed under this heading.

Prochlorperazine (Additive CNS depression; the dose of one or both agents should be reduced). Products include:
- Compazine 2470

Promethazine Hydrochloride (Additive CNS depression; the dose of one or both agents should be reduced). Products include:
- Mepergan Injection 2753
- Phenergan with Codeine 2777
- Phenergan with Dextromethorphan 2778
- Phenergan Injection 2773
- Phenergan Suppositories 2775
- Phenergan Syrup 2774
- Phenergan Tablets 2775
- Phenergan VC 2779
- Phenergan VC with Codeine 2781

Propofol (Additive CNS depression; the dose of one or both agents should be reduced). Products include:
- Diprivan Injection 2833

Propoxyphene Hydrochloride (Additive CNS depression; the dose of one or both agents should be reduced). Products include:
- Darvon 1435
- Wygesic Tablets 2827

Propoxyphene Napsylate (Additive CNS depression; the dose of one or both agents should be reduced). Products include:
- Darvon-N/Darvocet-N 1433

Protriptyline Hydrochloride (Increased effect of either hydrocodone or antidepressant; additive CNS depression; the dose of one or both agents should be reduced). Products include:
- Vivactil Tablets 1774

Pyrilamine Maleate (Additive CNS depression; the dose of one or both agents should be reduced). Products include:
- 4-Way Fast Acting Nasal Spray (regular & mentholated) .... ▣ 621
- Maximum Strength Multi-Symptom Formula Midol .... ▣ 722
- PMS Multi-Symptom Formula Midol .... ▣ 723

Pyrilamine Tannate (Additive CNS depression; the dose of one or both agents should be reduced). Products include:
- Atrohist Pediatric Suspension 454
- Rynatan 2673

Quazepam (Additive CNS depression; the dose of one or both agents should be reduced). Products include:
- Doral Tablets 2664

Risperidone (Additive CNS depression; the dose of one or both agents should be reduced). Products include:
- Risperdal 1301

(▣ Described in PDR For Nonprescription Drugs) (◉ Described in PDR For Ophthalmology)

Interactions Index

Secobarbital Sodium (Additive CNS depression; the dose of one or both agents should be reduced). Products include:

Seconal Sodium Pulvules 1474

Selegiline Hydrochloride (Increased effect of either hydrocodone or MAOI inhibitor). Products include:

Eldepryl Tablets 2550

Sufentanil Citrate (Additive CNS depression; the dose of one or both agents should be reduced). Products include:

Sufenta Injection 1309

Temazepam (Additive CNS depression; the dose of one or both agents should be reduced). Products include:

Restoril Capsules 2284

Terfenadine (Additive CNS depression; the dose of one or both agents should be reduced). Products include:

Seldane Tablets 1536
Seldane-D Extended-Release Tablets 1538

Thiamylal Sodium (Additive CNS depression; the dose of one or both agents should be reduced).

No products indexed under this heading.

Thioridazine Hydrochloride (Additive CNS depression; the dose of one or both agents should be reduced). Products include:

Mellaril 2269

Thiothixene (Additive CNS depression; the dose of one or both agents should be reduced). Products include:

Navane Capsules and Concentrate 2201
Navane Intramuscular 2202

Tranylcypromine Sulfate (Increased effect of either hydrocodone or MAOI inhibitor; additive CNS depression; the dose of one or both agents should be reduced). Products include:

Parnate Tablets 2503

Triazolam (Additive CNS depression; the dose of one or both agents should be reduced). Products include:

Halcion Tablets.................................... 2611

Trifluoperazine Hydrochloride (Additive CNS depression; the dose of one or both agents should be reduced). Products include:

Stelazine 2514

Trimeprazine Tartrate (Additive CNS depression; the dose of one or both agents should be reduced). Products include:

Temaril Tablets, Syrup and Spansule Extended-Release Capsules.. 483

Trimipramine Maleate (Increased effect of either hydrocodone or antidepressant; additive CNS depression; the dose of one or both agents should be reduced). Products include:

Surmontil Capsules.............................. 2811

Tripelennamine Hydrochloride (Additive CNS depression; the dose of one or both agents should be reduced). Products include:

PBZ Tablets 845
PBZ-SR Tablets.................................... 844

Triprolidine Hydrochloride (Additive CNS depression; the dose of one or both agents should be reduced). Products include:

Actifed Plus Caplets .... ◻️ 845
Actifed Plus Tablets .... ◻️ 845
Actifed with Codeine Cough Syrup.. 1067
Actifed Syrup.. ◻️ 846
Actifed Tablets .... ◻️ 844

Zolpidem Tartrate (Additive CNS depression; the dose of one or both agents should be reduced). Products include:

Ambien Tablets.................................... 2416

Food Interactions

Alcohol (Additive CNS depression).

LORTAB 5/500 TABLETS

(Hydrocodone Bitartrate, Acetaminophen).....................................2566
See Lortab 2.5/500 Tablets

LORTAB 7.5/500 TABLETS

(Hydrocodone Bitartrate, Acetaminophen).....................................2566
See Lortab 2.5/500 Tablets

LORTAB ELIXIR

(Hydrocodone Bitartrate, Acetaminophen).....................................2566
See Lortab 2.5/500 Tablets

LOTENSIN TABLETS

(Benazepril Hydrochloride) 834
May interact with diuretics, potassium sparing diuretics, potassium preparations, lithium preparations, and certain other agents. Compounds in these categories include:

Amiloride Hydrochloride (Potential for excessive reduction of blood pressure; potential for hyperkalemia). Products include:

Midamor Tablets 1703
Moduretic Tablets 1705

Bendroflumethiazide (Potential for excessive reduction of blood pressure).

No products indexed under this heading.

Bumetanide (Potential for excessive reduction of blood pressure). Products include:

Bumex 2093

Chlorothiazide (Potential for excessive reduction of blood pressure). Products include:

Aldoclor Tablets 1598
Diupres Tablets 1650
Diuril Oral 1653

Chlorothiazide Sodium (Potential for excessive reduction of blood pressure). Products include:

Diuril Sodium Intravenous 1652

Chlorthalidone (Potential for excessive reduction of blood pressure). Products include:

Combipres Tablets 677
Tenoretic Tablets.................................. 2845
Thalitone 1245

Ethacrynic Acid (Potential for excessive reduction of blood pressure). Products include:

Edecrin Tablets..................................... 1657

Furosemide (Potential for excessive reduction of blood pressure). Products include:

Lasix Injection, Oral Solution and Tablets 1240

Hydrochlorothiazide (Potential for excessive reduction of blood pressure). Products include:

Aldactazide.. 2413
Aldoril Tablets....................................... 1604
Apresazide Capsules 808
Capozide 742
Dyazide 2479
Esidrix Tablets 821
Esimil Tablets 822
HydroDIURIL Tablets 1674
Hydropres Tablets................................. 1675
Hyzaar Tablets 1677
Inderide Tablets 2732
Inderide LA Long Acting Capsules .. 2734
Lopressor HCT Tablets 832
Lotensin HCT.. 837
Maxzide 1380
Moduretic Tablets 1705

Oretic Tablets 443
Prinzide Tablets 1737
Ser-Ap-Es Tablets 849
Timolide Tablets................................... 1748
Vaseretic Tablets 1765
Zestoretic 2850
Ziac 1415

Hydroflumethiazide (Potential for excessive reduction of blood pressure). Products include:

Diucardin Tablets................................. 2718

Indapamide (Potential for excessive reduction of blood pressure). Products include:

Lozol Tablets 2022

Lithium Carbonate (Increased serum lithium levels and symptoms of lithium toxicity). Products include:

Eskalith 2485
Lithium Carbonate Capsules & Tablets 2230
Lithonate/Lithotabs/Lithobid 2543

Lithium Citrate (Increased serum lithium levels and symptoms of lithium toxicity).

No products indexed under this heading.

Methyclothiazide (Potential for excessive reduction of blood pressure). Products include:

Enduron Tablets................................... 420

Metolazone (Potential for excessive reduction of blood pressure). Products include:

Mykrox Tablets 993
Zaroxolyn Tablets 1000

Polythiazide (Potential for excessive reduction of blood pressure). Products include:

Minizide Capsules 1938

Potassium Acid Phosphate (Potential for hyperkalemia). Products include:

K-Phos Original Formula 'Sodium Free' Tablets 639

Potassium Bicarbonate (Potential for hyperkalemia). Products include:

Alka-Seltzer Gold Effervescent Antacid .... ◻️ 703

Potassium Chloride (Potential for hyperkalemia). Products include:

Chlor-3 Condiment 1004
K-Dur Microburst Release System (potassium chloride, USP) E.R. Tablets 1325
K-Lor Powder Packets 434
K-Norm Extended-Release Capsules 991
K-Tab Filmtab 434
Kolyum Liquid 992
Micro-K.. 2063
Micro-K LS Packets.............................. 2064
NuLYTELY... 689
Cherry Flavor NuLYTELY 689
Rum-K Syrup 1005
Slow-K Extended-Release Tablets..... 851

Potassium Citrate (Potential for hyperkalemia). Products include:

Polycitra Syrup 578
Polycitra-K Crystals 579
Polycitra-K Oral Solution 579
Polycitra-LC 578

Potassium Gluconate (Potential for hyperkalemia). Products include:

Kolyum Liquid 992

Potassium Phosphate, Dibasic (Potential for hyperkalemia).

No products indexed under this heading.

Potassium Phosphate, Monobasic (Potential for hyperkalemia). Products include:

K-Phos Neutral Tablets 639
K-Phos Original Formula 'Sodium Free' Tablets 639

Spironolactone (Potential for excessive reduction of blood pressure; potential for hyperkalemia). Products include:

Aldactazide.. 2413
Aldactone 2414

Torsemide (Potential for excessive reduction of blood pressure). Products include:

Demadex Tablets and Injection 686

Triamterene (Potential for excessive reduction of blood pressure; potential for hyperkalemia). Products include:

Dyazide 2479
Dyrenium Capsules.............................. 2481
Maxzide 1380

LOTENSIN HCT

(Benazepril Hydrochloride, Hydrochlorothiazide)............................ 837
May interact with potassium sparing diuretics, potassium preparations, lithium preparations, insulin, non-steroidal anti-inflammatory agents, barbiturates, narcotic analgesics, and certain other agents. Compounds in these categories include:

Alfentanil Hydrochloride (Thiazide-induced orthostatic hypotension potentiated by narcotics). Products include:

Alfenta Injection 1286

Amiloride Hydrochloride (Increases the risk of hyperkalemia). Products include:

Midamor Tablets 1703
Moduretic Tablets 1705

Aprobarbital (Thiazide-induced orthostatic hypotension potentiated by barbiturates).

No products indexed under this heading.

Buprenorphine (Thiazide-induced orthostatic hypotension potentiated by narcotics). Products include:

Buprenex Injectable 2006

Butabarbital (Thiazide-induced orthostatic hypotension potentiated by barbiturates).

No products indexed under this heading.

Butalbital (Thiazide-induced orthostatic hypotension potentiated by barbiturates). Products include:

Esgic-plus Tablets 1013
Fioricet Tablets..................................... 2258
Fioricet with Codeine Capsules 2260
Fiorinal Capsules 2261
Fiorinal with Codeine Capsules 2262
Fiorinal Tablets..................................... 2261
Phrenilin 785
Sedapap Tablets 50 mg/650 mg .. 1543

Cholestyramine (Cholestyramine resin has potential of binding hydrochlorothiazide and reducing its absorption from the GI tract by up to 85%). Products include:

Questran Light 769
Questran Powder 770

Codeine Phosphate (Thiazide-induced orthostatic hypotension potentiated by narcotics). Products include:

Actifed with Codeine Cough Syrup.. 1067
Brontex 1981
Deconsal C Expectorant Syrup 456
Deconsal Pediatric Syrup 457
Dimetane-DC Cough Syrup 2059
Empirin with Codeine Tablets............ 1093
Fioricet with Codeine Capsules 2260
Fiorinal with Codeine Capsules 2262
Isoclor Expectorant 990
Novahistine DH.................................... 2462
Novahistine Expectorant..................... 2463
Nucofed 2051
Phenergan with Codeine..................... 2777
Phenergan VC with Codeine 2781
Robitussin A-C Syrup.......................... 2073
Robitussin-DAC Syrup 2074
Ryna .... ◻️ 841
Soma Compound w/Codeine Tablets 2676
Tussi-Organidin NR Liquid and S NR Liquid 2677
Tylenol with Codeine 1583

IMPORTANT NOTE: Always consult each drug listing in the patient's regimen for possible interactions.

Lotensin HCT | Interactions Index | 604

Colestipol Hydrochloride (Colestipol resin has potential of binding hydrochlorothiazide and reducing its absorption from the GI tract by up to 43%). Products include:

Colestid Tablets ... 2591

Dezocine (Thiazide-induced orthostatic hypotension potentiated by narcotics). Products include:

Dalgan Injection ... 538

Diclofenac Potassium (Reduces diuretic, natriuretic, and antihypertensive effects). Products include:

Cataflam ... 816

Diclofenac Sodium (Reduces diuretic, natriuretic, and antihypertensive effects). Products include:

Voltaren Ophthalmic Sterile Ophthalmic Solution ... ⊙ 272
Voltaren Tablets ... 861

Etodolac (Reduces diuretic, natriuretic, and antihypertensive effects). Products include:

Lodine Capsules and Tablets ... 2743

Fenoprofen Calcium (Reduces diuretic, natriuretic, and antihypertensive effects). Products include:

Nalfon 200 Pulvules & Nalfon Tablets ... 917

Fentanyl (Thiazide-induced orthostatic hypotension potentiated by narcotics). Products include:

Duragesic Transdermal System ... 1288

Fentanyl Citrate (Thiazide-induced orthostatic hypotension potentiated by narcotics). Products include:

Sublimaze Injection ... 1307

Flurbiprofen (Reduces diuretic, natriuretic, and antihypertensive effects). Products include:

Ansaid Tablets ... 2579

Hydrocodone Bitartrate (Thiazide-induced orthostatic hypotension potentiated by narcotics). Products include:

Anexsia 5/500 Elixir ... 1781
Anexia Tablets ... 1782
Codiclear DH Syrup ... 791
Deconamine CX Cough and Cold Liquid and Tablets ... 1319
Duratuss HD Elixir ... 2565
Hycodan Tablets and Syrup ... 930
Hycomine Compound Tablets ... 932
Hycomine ... 931
Hycotuss Expectorant Syrup ... 933
Hydrocet Capsules ... 782
Lorcet 10/650 ... 1018
Lortab ... 2566
Tussend ... 1783
Tussend Expectorant ... 1785
Vicodin Tablets ... 1356
Vicodin ES Tablets ... 1357
Vicodin Tuss Expectorant ... 1358
Zydone Capsules ... 949

Hydrocodone Polistirex (Thiazide-induced orthostatic hypotension potentiated by narcotics). Products include:

Tussionex Pennkinetic Extended-Release Suspension ... 998

Ibuprofen (Reduces diuretic, natriuretic, and antihypertensive effects). Products include:

Advil Cold and Sinus Caplets and Tablets (formerly CoAdvil) ... ■ 870
Advil Ibuprofen Tablets and Caplets ... ■ 870
Children's Advil Suspension ... 2692
Arthritis Foundation Ibuprofen Tablets ... ■ 674
Bayer Select Ibuprofen Pain Relief Formula ... ■ 715
Cramp End Tablets ... ■ 735
Dimetapp Sinus Caplets ... ■ 775
Haltran Tablets ... ■ 771
IBU Tablets ... 1342
Ibuprohm ... ■ 735
Children's Motrin Ibuprofen Oral Suspension ... 1546
Motrin Tablets ... 2625
Motrin IB Caplets, Tablets, and Geltabs ... ■ 838
Motrin IB Sinus ... ■ 838
Motrin Ibuprofen Suspension, Oral Drops, Chewable Tablets, Caplets ... 1546
Nuprin Ibuprofen/Analgesic Tablets & Caplets ... ■ 622
Sine-Aid IB Caplets ... 1554
Vicks DayQuil SINUS Pressure & PAIN Relief with IBUPROFEN ... ■ 762

Indomethacin (Reduces diuretic, natriuretic, and antihypertensive effects). Products include:

Indocin ... 1680

Indomethacin Sodium Trihydrate (Reduces diuretic, natriuretic, and antihypertensive effects). Products include:

Indocin I.V. ... 1684

Insulin, Human (Insulin requirements may be increased, decreased, or unchanged).

No products indexed under this heading.

Insulin, Human Isophane Suspension (Insulin requirements may be increased, decreased, or unchanged). Products include:

Novolin N Human Insulin 10 ml Vials ... 1795

Insulin, Human NPH (Insulin requirements may be increased, decreased, or unchanged). Products include:

Humulin N, 100 Units ... 1448
Novolin N PenFill Cartridges Durable Insulin Delivery System ... 1798
Novolin N Prefilled Syringe Disposable Insulin Delivery System ... 1798

Insulin, Human Regular (Insulin requirements may be increased, decreased, or unchanged). Products include:

Humulin R, 100 Units ... 1449
Novolin R Human Insulin 10 ml Vials ... 1795
Novolin R PenFill Cartridges Durable Insulin Delivery System ... 1798
Novolin R Prefilled Syringe Disposable Insulin Delivery System ... 1798
Velosulin BR Human Insulin 10 ml Vials ... 1795

Insulin, Human, Zinc Suspension (Insulin requirements may be increased, decreased, or unchanged). Products include:

Humulin L, 100 Units ... 1446
Humulin U, 100 Units ... 1450
Novolin L Human Insulin 10 ml Vials ... 1795

Insulin, NPH (Insulin requirements may be increased, decreased, or unchanged). Products include:

NPH, 100 Units ... 1450
Pork NPH, 100 Units ... 1452
Purified Pork NPH Isophane Insulin ... 1801

Insulin, Regular (Insulin requirements may be increased, decreased, or unchanged). Products include:

Regular, 100 Units ... 1450
Pork Regular, 100 Units ... 1452
Pork Regular (Concentrated), 500 Units ... 1453
Purified Pork Regular Insulin ... 1801

Insulin, Zinc Crystals (Insulin requirements may be increased, decreased, or unchanged). Products include:

NPH, 100 Units ... 1450

Insulin, Zinc Suspension (Insulin requirements may be increased, decreased, or unchanged). Products include:

Iletin I ... 1450
Lente, 100 Units ... 1450
Iletin II ... 1452
Pork Lente, 100 Units ... 1452
Purified Pork Lente Insulin ... 1801

Ketoprofen (Reduces diuretic, natriuretic, and antihypertensive effects). Products include:

Orudis Capsules ... 2766
Oruvail Capsules ... 2766

Ketorolac Tromethamine (Reduces diuretic, natriuretic, and antihypertensive effects). Products include:

Acular ... 474
Acular ... ⊙ 277
Toradol ... 2159

Levorphanol Tartrate (Thiazide-induced orthostatic hypotension potentiated by narcotics). Products include:

Levo-Dromoran ... 2129

Lithium Carbonate (Increased serum lithium levels and symptoms of lithium toxicity; potential for reduced lithium renal clearance). Products include:

Eskalith ... 2485
Lithium Carbonate Capsules & Tablets ... 2230
Lithonate/Lithotabs/Lithobid ... 2543

Lithium Citrate (Increased serum lithium levels and symptoms of lithium toxicity; potential for reduced lithium renal clearance).

No products indexed under this heading.

Meclofenamate Sodium (Reduces diuretic, natriuretic, and antihypertensive effects).

No products indexed under this heading.

Mefenamic Acid (Reduces diuretic, natriuretic, and antihypertensive effects). Products include:

Ponstel ... 1925

Meperidine Hydrochloride (Thiazide-induced orthostatic hypotension potentiated by narcotics). Products include:

Demerol ... 2308
Mepergan Injection ... 2753

Mephobarbital (Thiazide-induced orthostatic hypotension potentiated by barbiturates). Products include:

Mebaral Tablets ... 2322

Methadone Hydrochloride (Thiazide-induced orthostatic hypotension potentiated by narcotics). Products include:

Methadone Hydrochloride Oral Concentrate ... 2233
Methadone Hydrochloride Oral Solution & Tablets ... 2235

Morphine Sulfate (Thiazide-induced orthostatic hypotension potentiated by narcotics). Products include:

Astramorph/PF Injection, USP (Preservative-Free) ... 535
Duramorph ... 962
Infumorph 200 and Infumorph 500 Sterile Solutions ... 965
MS Contin Tablets ... 1994
MSIR ... 1997
Oramorph SR (Morphine Sulfate Sustained Release Tablets) ... 2236
RMS Suppositories ... 2657
Roxanol ... 2243

Nabumetone (Reduces diuretic, natriuretic, and antihypertensive effects). Products include:

Relafen Tablets ... 2510

Naproxen (Reduces diuretic, natriuretic, and antihypertensive effects). Products include:

Anaprox/Naprosyn ... 2117

Naproxen Sodium (Reduces diuretic, natriuretic, and antihypertensive effects). Products include:

Aleve ... 1975
Anaprox/Naprosyn ... 2117

Norepinephrine Bitartrate (Thiazides may decrease arterial responsiveness to norepinephrine). Products include:

Levophed Bitartrate Injection ... 2315

Opium Alkaloids (Thiazide-induced orthostatic hypotension potentiated by narcotics).

No products indexed under this heading.

Oxaprozin (Reduces diuretic, natriuretic, and antihypertensive effects). Products include:

Daypro Caplets ... 2426

Oxycodone Hydrochloride (Thiazide-induced orthostatic hypotension potentiated by narcotics). Products include:

Percocet Tablets ... 938
Percodan Tablets ... 939
Percodan-Demi Tablets ... 940
Roxicodone Tablets, Oral Solution & Intensol (Oxycodone) ... 2244
Tylox Capsules ... 1584

Pentobarbital Sodium (Thiazide-induced orthostatic hypotension potentiated by barbiturates). Products include:

Nembutal Sodium Capsules ... 436
Nembutal Sodium Solution ... 438
Nembutal Sodium Suppositories ... 440

Phenobarbital (Thiazide-induced orthostatic hypotension potentiated by barbiturates). Products include:

Arco-Lase Plus Tablets ... 512
Bellergal-S Tablets ... 2250
Donnatal ... 2060
Donnatal Extentabs ... 2061
Donnatal Tablets ... 2060
Phenobarbital Elixir and Tablets ... 1469
Quadrinal Tablets ... 1350

Phenylbutazone (Reduces diuretic, natriuretic, and antihypertensive effects).

No products indexed under this heading.

Piroxicam (Reduces diuretic, natriuretic, and antihypertensive effects). Products include:

Feldene Capsules ... 1965

Potassium Acid Phosphate (Increases the risk of hyperkalemia). Products include:

K-Phos Original Formula 'Sodium Free' Tablets ... 639

Potassium Bicarbonate (Increases the risk of hyperkalemia). Products include:

Alka-Seltzer Gold Effervescent Antacid ... ■ 703

Potassium Chloride (Increases the risk of hyperkalemia). Products include:

Chlor-3 Condiment ... 1004
K-Dur Microburst Release System (potassium chloride, USP) E.R. Tablets ... 1325
K-Lor Powder Packets ... 434
K-Norm Extended-Release Capsules ... 991
K-Tab Filmtab ... 434
Kolyum Liquid ... 992
Micro-K ... 2063
Micro-K LS Packets ... 2064
NuLYTELY ... 689
Cherry Flavor NuLYTELY ... 689
Rum-K Syrup ... 1005
Slow-K Extended-Release Tablets ... 851

Potassium Citrate (Increases the risk of hyperkalemia). Products include:

Polycitra Syrup ... 578
Polycitra-K Crystals ... 579
Polycitra-K Oral Solution ... 579
Polycitra-LC ... 578

Potassium Gluconate (Increases the risk of hyperkalemia). Products include:

Kolyum Liquid ... 992

(■ Described in PDR For Nonprescription Drugs) (⊙ Described in PDR For Ophthalmology)

Potassium Phosphate, Dibasic (Increases the risk of hyperkalemia).

No products indexed under this heading.

Potassium Phosphate, Monobasic (Increases the risk of hyperkalemia). Products include:

K-Phos Neutral Tablets 639
K-Phos Original Formula 'Sodium Free' Tablets 639

Propoxyphene Hydrochloride (Thiazide-induced orthostatic hypotension potentiated by narcotics). Products include:

Darvon 1435
Wygesic Tablets 2827

Propoxyphene Napsylate (Thiazide-induced orthostatic hypotension potentiated by narcotics). Products include:

Darvon-N/Darvocet-N 1433

Secobarbital Sodium (Thiazide-induced orthostatic hypotension potentiated by barbiturates). Products include:

Seconal Sodium Pulvules 1474

Spironolactone (Increases the risk of hyperkalemia). Products include:

Aldactazide 2413
Aldactone 2414

Sufentanil Citrate (Thiazide-induced orthostatic hypotension potentiated by narcotics). Products include:

Sufenta Injection 1309

Sulindac (Reduces diuretic, natriuretic, and antihypertensive effects). Products include:

Clinoril Tablets 1618

Thiamylal Sodium (Thiazide-induced orthostatic hypotension potentiated by barbiturates).

No products indexed under this heading.

Tolmetin Sodium (Reduces diuretic, natriuretic, and antihypertensive effects). Products include:

Tolectin (200, 400 and 600 mg) .. 1581

Triamterene (Increases the risk of hyperkalemia). Products include:

Dyazide 2479
Dyrenium Capsules 2481
Maxzide 1380

Tubocurarine Chloride (Thiazides may increase the responsiveness to tubocurarine).

No products indexed under this heading.

Food Interactions

Alcohol (Thiazide-induced orthostatic hypotension potentiated by alcohol).

LOTREL CAPSULES

(Amlodipine Besylate, Benazepril Hydrochloride) 840

May interact with potassium sparing diuretics, potassium preparations, lithium preparations, and diuretics. Compounds in these categories include:

Amiloride Hydrochloride (Potential for the increased risk of hyperkalemia; patients on diuretics, especially those in whom diuretic therapy was recently instituted, may experience an excessive reduction in blood pressure). Products include:

Midamor Tablets 1703
Moduretic Tablets 1705

Bendroflumethiazide (Patients on diuretics, especially those in whom diuretic therapy was recently instituted, may experience an excessive reduction in blood pressure).

No products indexed under this heading.

Bumetanide (Patients on diuretics, especially those in whom diuretic therapy was recently instituted, may experience an excessive reduction in blood pressure). Products include:

Bumex 2093

Chlorothiazide (Patients on diuretics, especially those in whom diuretic therapy was recently instituted, may experience an excessive reduction in blood pressure). Products include:

Aldoclor Tablets 1598
Diupres Tablets 1650
Diuril Oral 1653

Chlorothiazide Sodium (Patients on diuretics, especially those in whom diuretic therapy was recently instituted, may experience an excessive reduction in blood pressure). Products include:

Diuril Sodium Intravenous 1652

Chlorthalidone (Patients on diuretics, especially those in whom diuretic therapy was recently instituted, may experience an excessive reduction in blood pressure). Products include:

Combipres Tablets 677
Tenoretic Tablets 2845
Thalitone 1245

Ethacrynic Acid (Patients on diuretics, especially those in whom diuretic therapy was recently instituted, may experience an excessive reduction in blood pressure). Products include:

Edecrin Tablets....................................... 1657

Furosemide (Patients on diuretics, especially those in whom diuretic therapy was recently instituted, may experience an excessive reduction in blood pressure). Products include:

Lasix Injection, Oral Solution and Tablets 1240

Hydrochlorothiazide (Patients on diuretics, especially those in whom diuretic therapy was recently instituted, may experience an excessive reduction in blood pressure). Products include:

Aldactazide... 2413
Aldoril Tablets.. 1604
Apresazide Capsules 808
Capozide 742
Dyazide 2479
Esidrix Tablets 821
Esimil Tablets 822
HydroDIURIL Tablets 1674
Hydropres Tablets.................................. 1675
Hyzaar Tablets 1677
Inderide Tablets 2732
Inderide LA Long Acting Capsules .. 2734
Lopressor HCT Tablets 832
Lotensin HCT... 837
Maxzide 1380
Moduretic Tablets 1705
Oretic Tablets 443
Prinzide Tablets 1737
Ser-Ap-Es Tablets 849
Timolide Tablets..................................... 1748
Vaseretic Tablets 1765
Zestoretic 2850
Ziac 1415

Hydroflumethiazide (Patients on diuretics, especially those in whom diuretic therapy was recently instituted, may experience an excessive reduction in blood pressure). Products include:

Diucardin Tablets................................... 2718

Indapamide (Patients on diuretics, especially those in whom diuretic therapy was recently instituted, may experience an excessive reduction in blood pressure). Products include:

Lozol Tablets 2022

Lithium Carbonate (Potential for increased serum lithium levels and symptoms of lithium toxicity). Products include:

Eskalith 2485
Lithium Carbonate Capsules & Tablets 2230
Lithonate/Lithotabs/Lithobid 2543

Lithium Citrate (Potential for increased serum lithium levels and symptoms of lithium toxicity).

No products indexed under this heading.

Methyclothiazide (Patients on diuretics, especially those in whom diuretic therapy was recently instituted, may experience an excessive reduction in blood pressure). Products include:

Enduron Tablets..................................... 420

Metolazone (Patients on diuretics, especially those in whom diuretic therapy was recently instituted, may experience an excessive reduction in blood pressure). Products include:

Mykrox Tablets 993
Zaroxolyn Tablets 1000

Polythiazide (Patients on diuretics, especially those in whom diuretic therapy was recently instituted, may experience an excessive reduction in blood pressure). Products include:

Minizide Capsules 1938

Potassium Acid Phosphate (Potential for the increased risk of hyperkalemia). Products include:

K-Phos Original Formula 'Sodium Free' Tablets 639

Potassium Bicarbonate (Potential for the increased risk of hyperkalemia). Products include:

Alka-Seltzer Gold+ Effervescent Antacid .... ⊞ 703

Potassium Chloride (Potential for the increased risk of hyperkalemia). Products include:

Chlor-3 Condiment 1004
K-Dur Microburst Release System (potassium chloride, USP) E.R. Tablets 1325
K-Lor Powder Packets 434
K-Norm Extended-Release Capsules 991
K-Tab Filmtab 434
Kolyum Liquid 992
Micro-K... 2063
Micro-K LS Packets............................... 2064
NuLYTELY... 689
Cherry Flavor NuLYTELY 689
Rum-K Syrup 1005
Slow-K Extended-Release Tablets..... 851

Potassium Citrate (Potential for the increased risk of hyperkalemia). Products include:

Polycitra Syrup 578
Polycitra-K Crystals 579
Polycitra-K Oral Solution 579
Polycitra-LC 578

Potassium Gluconate (Potential for the increased risk of hyperkalemia). Products include:

Kolyum Liquid 992

Potassium Phosphate, Dibasic (Potential for the increased risk of hyperkalemia).

No products indexed under this heading.

Potassium Phosphate, Monobasic (Potential for the increased risk of hyperkalemia). Products include:

K-Phos Neutral Tablets 639
K-Phos Original Formula 'Sodium Free' Tablets 639

Spironolactone (Potential for the increased risk of hyperkalemia; patients on diuretics, especially those in whom diuretic therapy was recently instituted, may experience an excessive reduction in blood pressure). Products include:

Aldactazide 2413
Aldactone 2414

Torsemide (Patients on diuretics, especially those in whom diuretic therapy was recently instituted, may experience an excessive reduction in blood pressure). Products include:

Demadex Tablets and Injection 686

Triamterene (Potential for the increased risk of hyperkalemia; patients on diuretics, especially those in whom diuretic therapy was recently instituted, may experience an excessive reduction in blood pressure). Products include:

Dyazide 2479
Dyrenium Capsules 2481
Maxzide 1380

LOTRIMIN CREAM 1%

(Clotrimazole)..2371

None cited in PDR database.

LOTRIMIN LOTION 1%

(Clotrimazole)..2371

None cited in PDR database.

LOTRIMIN SOLUTION 1%

(Clotrimazole)..2371

None cited in PDR database.

LOTRIMIN AF ANTIFUNGAL CREAM, LOTION AND SOLUTION

(Clotrimazole) ....⊞ 806

None cited in PDR database.

LOTRIMIN AF ANTIFUNGAL SPRAY LIQUID, SPRAY POWDER, POWDER AND JOCK ITCH SPRAY POWDER

(Miconazole Nitrate) ....⊞ 807

None cited in PDR database.

LOTRISONE CREAM

(Clotrimazole, Betamethasone Dipropionate) 2372

None cited in PDR database.

LOVENOX INJECTION

(Enoxaparin)...2020

May interact with oral anticoagulants, platelet inhibitors, non-steroidal anti-inflammatory agents, salicylates, and certain other agents. Compounds in these categories include:

Aspirin (May enhance the risk of hemorrhage). Products include:

Alka-Seltzer Effervescent Antacid and Pain Reliever .... ⊞ 701
Alka-Seltzer Extra Strength Effervescent Antacid and Pain Reliever .... ⊞ 703
Alka-Seltzer Lemon Lime Effervescent Antacid and Pain Reliever .... ⊞ 703
Alka-Seltzer Plus Cold Medicine .... ⊞ 705
Alka-Seltzer Plus Cold & Cough Medicine .... ⊞ 708
Alka-Seltzer Plus Night-Time Cold Medicine .... ⊞ 707
Alka Seltzer Plus Sinus Medicine .. ⊞ 707
Arthritis Foundation Safety Coated Aspirin Tablets .... ⊞ 675
Arthritis Pain Ascriptin .... ⊞ 631
Maximum Strength Ascriptin .... ⊞ 630
Regular Strength Ascriptin Tablets .... ⊞ 629
Arthritis Strength BC Powder.......... ⊞ 609
BC Cold Powder Multi-Symptom Formula (Cold-Sinus-Allergy) ...... ⊞ 609

IMPORTANT NOTE: Always consult each drug listing in the patient's regimen for possible interactions.

BC Cold Powder Non-Drowsy Formula (Cold-Sinus) ▣ 609
BC Powder ▣ 609
Bayer Children's Chewable Aspirin ▣ 711
Genuine Bayer Aspirin Tablets & Caplets ▣ 713
Extra Strength Bayer Arthritis Pain Regimen Formula ▣ 711
Extra Strength Bayer Aspirin Caplets & Tablets ▣ 712
Extended-Release Bayer 8-Hour Aspirin ▣ 712
Extra Strength Bayer Plus Aspirin Caplets ▣ 713
Extra Strength Bayer PM Aspirin .. ▣ 713
Bayer Enteric Aspirin ▣ 709
Bufferin Analgesic Tablets and Caplets ▣ 613
Arthritis Strength Bufferin Analgesic Caplets ▣ 614
Extra Strength Bufferin Analgesic Tablets ▣ 615
Cama Arthritis Pain Reliever ▣ 785
Darvon Compound-65 Pulvules 1435
Easprin 1914
Ecotrin 2455
Ecotrin Enteric Coated Aspirin Maximum Strength Tablets and Caplets ▣ 816
Ecotrin Enteric Coated Aspirin Regular Strength Tablets 2455
Empirin Aspirin Tablets ▣ 854
Empirin with Codeine Tablets 1093
Excedrin Extra-Strength Analgesic Tablets & Caplets 732
Fiorinal Capsules 2261
Fiorinal with Codeine Capsules 2262
Fiorinal Tablets 2261
Halfprin 1362
Healthprin Aspirin 2455
Norgesic 1496
Percodan Tablets 939
Percodan-Demi Tablets 940
Robaxisal Tablets 2071
Soma Compound w/Codeine Tablets 2676
Soma Compound Tablets 2675
St. Joseph Adult Chewable Aspirin (81 mg.) ▣ 808
Talwin Compound 2335
Ursinus Inlay-Tabs ▣ 794
Vanquish Analgesic Caplets ▣ 731

Azlocillin Sodium (May enhance the risk of hemorrhage).
No products indexed under this heading.

Carbenicillin Indanyl Sodium (May enhance the risk of hemorrhage). Products include:
Geocillin Tablets 2199

Choline Magnesium Trisalicylate (May enhance the risk of hemorrhage). Products include:
Trilisate 2000

Diclofenac Potassium (May enhance the risk of hemorrhage). Products include:
Cataflam 816

Diclofenac Sodium (May enhance the risk of hemorrhage). Products include:
Voltaren Ophthalmic Sterile Ophthalmic Solution ◉ 272
Voltaren Tablets 861

Dicumarol (May enhance the risk of hemorrhage).
No products indexed under this heading.

Diflunisal (May enhance the risk of hemorrhage). Products include:
Dolobid Tablets 1654

Dipyridamole (May enhance the risk of hemorrhage). Products include:
Persantine Tablets 681

Etodolac (May enhance the risk of hemorrhage). Products include:
Lodine Capsules and Tablets 2743

Fenoprofen Calcium (May enhance the risk of hemorrhage). Products include:
Nalfon 200 Pulvules & Nalfon Tablets 917

Flurbiprofen (May enhance the risk of hemorrhage). Products include:
Ansaid Tablets 2579

Ibuprofen (May enhance the risk of hemorrhage). Products include:
Advil Cold and Sinus Caplets and Tablets (formerly CoAdvil) ▣ 870
Advil Ibuprofen Tablets and Caplets ▣ 870
Children's Advil Suspension 2692
Arthritis Foundation Ibuprofen Tablets ▣ 674
Bayer Select Ibuprofen Pain Relief Formula ▣ 715
Cramp End Tablets ▣ 735
Dimetapp Sinus Caplets ▣ 775
Haltran Tablets ▣ 771
IBU Tablets 1342
Ibuprohm ▣ 735
Children's Motrin Ibuprofen Oral Suspension 1546
Motrin Tablets 2625
Motrin IB Caplets, Tablets, and Geltabs ▣ 838
Motrin IB Sinus ▣ 838
Motrin Ibuprofen Suspension, Oral Drops, Chewable Tablets, Caplets 1546
Nuprin Ibuprofen/Analgesic Tablets & Caplets ▣ 622
Sine-Aid IB Caplets 1554
Vicks DayQuil SINUS Pressure & PAIN Relief with IBUPROFEN ▣ 762

Indomethacin (May enhance the risk of hemorrhage). Products include:
Indocin 1680

Indomethacin Sodium Trihydrate (May enhance the risk of hemorrhage). Products include:
Indocin I.V. 1684

Ketoprofen (May enhance the risk of hemorrhage). Products include:
Orudis Capsules 2766
Oruvail Capsules 2766

Ketorolac Tromethamine (May enhance the risk of hemorrhage). Products include:
Acular 474
Acular ◉ 277
Toradol 2159

Magnesium Salicylate (May enhance the risk of hemorrhage). Products include:
Backache Caplets ▣ 613
Bayer Select Backache Pain Relief Formula ▣ 715
Doan's Extra-Strength Analgesic ▣ 633
Extra Strength Doan's P.M. ▣ 633
Doan's Regular Strength Analgesic ▣ 634
Mobigesic Tablets ▣ 602

Meclofenamate Sodium (May enhance the risk of hemorrhage).
No products indexed under this heading.

Mefenamic Acid (May enhance the risk of hemorrhage). Products include:
Ponstel 1925

Mezlocillin Sodium (May enhance the risk of hemorrhage). Products include:
Mezlin 601
Mezlin Pharmacy Bulk Package 604

Nabumetone (May enhance the risk of hemorrhage). Products include:
Relafen Tablets 2510

Nafcillin Sodium (May enhance the risk of hemorrhage).
No products indexed under this heading.

Naproxen (May enhance the risk of hemorrhage). Products include:
Anaprox/Naprosyn 2117

Naproxen Sodium (May enhance the risk of hemorrhage). Products include:
Aleve 1975
Anaprox/Naprosyn 2117

Oxaprozin (May enhance the risk of hemorrhage). Products include:
Daypro Caplets 2426

Penicillin G Benzathine (May enhance the risk of hemorrhage). Products include:
Bicillin C-R Injection 2704
Bicillin C-R 900/300 Injection 2706
Bicillin L-A Injection 2707

Penicillin G Procaine (May enhance the risk of hemorrhage). Products include:
Bicillin C-R Injection 2704
Bicillin C-R 900/300 Injection 2706

Phenylbutazone (May enhance the risk of hemorrhage).
No products indexed under this heading.

Piroxicam (May enhance the risk of hemorrhage). Products include:
Feldene Capsules 1965

Salsalate (May enhance the risk of hemorrhage). Products include:
Mono-Gesic Tablets 792
Salflex Tablets 786

Sulfinpyrazone (May enhance the risk of hemorrhage). Products include:
Anturane 807

Sulindac (May enhance the risk of hemorrhage). Products include:
Clinoril Tablets 1618

Ticarcillin Disodium (May enhance the risk of hemorrhage). Products include:
Ticar for Injection 2526
Timentin for Injection 2528

Ticlopidine Hydrochloride (May enhance the risk of hemorrhage). Products include:
Ticlid Tablets 2156

Tolmetin Sodium (May enhance the risk of hemorrhage). Products include:
Tolectin (200, 400 and 600 mg) .. 1581

Warfarin Sodium (May enhance the risk of hemorrhage). Products include:
Coumadin 926

LOXITANE C ORAL CONCENTRATE

(Loxapine Hydrochloride) 1378
See **Loxitane Capsules**

LOXITANE CAPSULES

(Loxapine Succinate) 1378
May interact with anticholinergic-type anitparkinsonism drugs, barbiturates, narcotic analgesics, general anesthetics, and certain other agents. Compounds in these categories include:

Alfentanil Hydrochloride (Loxitane is contraindicated in severe narcotic-induced depressed state). Products include:
Alfenta Injection 1286

Aprobarbital (Loxitane is contraindicated in severe barbiturate-induced depressed state).
No products indexed under this heading.

Benztropine Mesylate (Use Loxitane cautiously). Products include:
Cogentin 1621

Biperiden Hydrochloride (Use Loxitane cautiously). Products include:
Akineton 1333

Buprenorphine (Loxitane is contraindicated in severe narcotic-induced depressed state). Products include:
Buprenex Injectable 2006

Butabarbital (Loxitane is contraindicated in severe barbiturate-induced depressed state).
No products indexed under this heading.

Butalbital (Loxitane is contraindicated in severe barbiturate-induced depressed state). Products include:
Esgic-plus Tablets 1013
Fioricet Tablets 2258
Fioricet with Codeine Capsules 2260
Fiorinal Capsules 2261
Fiorinal with Codeine Capsules 2262
Fiorinal Tablets 2261
Phrenilin 785
Sedapap Tablets 50 mg/650 mg .. 1543

Codeine Phosphate (Loxitane is contraindicated in severe narcotic-induced depressed state). Products include:
Actifed with Codeine Cough Syrup.. 1067
Brontex 1981
Deconsal C Expectorant Syrup 456
Deconsal Pediatric Syrup 457
Dimetane-DC Cough Syrup 2059
Empirin with Codeine Tablets 1093
Fioricet with Codeine Capsules 2260
Fiorinal with Codeine Capsules 2262
Isoclor Expectorant 990
Novahistine DH 2462
Novahistine Expectorant 2463
Nucofed 2051
Phenergan with Codeine 2777
Phenergan VC with Codeine 2781
Robitussin A-C Syrup 2073
Robitussin-DAC Syrup 2074
Ryna ▣ 841
Soma Compound w/Codeine Tablets 2676
Tussi-Organidin NR Liquid and S NR Liquid 2677
Tylenol with Codeine 1583

Dezocine (Loxitane is contraindicated in severe narcotic-induced depressed state). Products include:
Dalgan Injection 538

Diphenhydramine Hydrochloride (Use Loxitane cautiously). Products include:
Actifed Allergy Daytime/Nighttime Caplets ▣ 844
Actifed Sinus Daytime/Nighttime Tablets and Caplets ▣ 846
Arthritis Foundation NightTime Caplets ▣ 674
Extra Strength Bayer PM Aspirin .. ▣ 713
Bayer Select Night Time Pain Relief Formula ▣ 716
Benadryl Allergy Decongestant Liquid Medication ▣ 848
Benadryl Allergy Decongestant Tablets ▣ 848
Benadryl Allergy Liquid Medication ▣ 849
Benadryl Allergy ▣ 848
Benadryl Allergy Sinus Headache Formula Caplets ▣ 849
Benadryl Capsules 1898
Benadryl Dye-Free Allergy Liquigel Softgels ▣ 850
Benadryl Dye-Free Allergy Liquid Medication ▣ 850
Benadryl Itch Relief Cream, Children's Formula and Maximum Strength 2% ▣ 851
Benadryl Itch Relief Spray, Children's Formula and Maximum Strength 2% ▣ 851
Benadryl Itch Relief Stick Maximum Strength 2% ▣ 850
Benadryl Itch Stopping Gel, Children's Formula and Maximum Strength 2% ▣ 851
Benadryl Kapseals 1898
Benadryl Injection 1898
Contac Day & Night Cold/Flu Night Caplets ▣ 812
Contac Night Allergy/Sinus Caplets ▣ 812
Extra Strength Doan's P.M. ▣ 633
Legatrin PM ▣ 651
Miles Nervine Nighttime Sleep-Aid ▣ 723
Nytol QuickCaps Caplets ▣ 610
Sleepinal Night-time Sleep Aid Capsules and Softgels ▣ 834
TYLENOL Maximum Strength Allergy Sinus NightTime Medication Caplets 1555

(▣ Described in PDR For Nonprescription Drugs) (◉ Described in PDR For Ophthalmology)

607 **Interactions Index** **Lozol**

TYLENOL Flu NightTime, Maximum Strength, Gelcaps ... 1566
TYLENOL Maximum Strength Flu NightTime Hot Medication Packets ... 1562
TYLENOL PM, Extra Strength Pain Reliever/Sleep Aid Caplets, Geltabs, Gelcaps ... 1560
TYLENOL Severe Allergy Medication Caplets ... 1564
Maximum Strength Unisom Sleepgels ... 1934
Unisom With Pain Relief-Nighttime Sleep Aid and Pain Reliever ... 1934

Enflurane (Loxitane is contraindicated in severe anesthetic-induced depressed state).
No products indexed under this heading.

Epinephrine (Inhibition of vasopressor effect by Loxitane). Products include:
Bronkaid Mist ... 717
EPIFRIN ... ⊙ 239
EpiPen ... 790
Marcaine Hydrochloride with Epinephrine 1:200,000 ... 2316
Primatene Mist ... 873
Sensorcaine with Epinephrine Injection ... 559
Sus-Phrine Injection ... 1019
Xylocaine with Epinephrine Injections ... 567

Fentanyl (Loxitane is contraindicated in severe narcotic-induced depressed state). Products include:
Duragesic Transdermal System ... 1288

Fentanyl Citrate (Loxitane is contraindicated in severe narcotic-induced depressed state). Products include:
Sublimaze Injection ... 1307

Hydrocodone Bitartrate (Loxitane is contraindicated in severe narcotic-induced depressed state). Products include:
Anexsia 5/500 Elixir ... 1781
Anexia Tablets ... 1782
Codiclear DH Syrup ... 791
Deconamine CX Cough and Cold Liquid and Tablets ... 1319
Duratuss HD Elixir ... 2565
Hycodan Tablets and Syrup ... 930
Hycomine Compound Tablets ... 932
Hycomine ... 931
Hycotuss Expectorant Syrup ... 933
Hydrocet Capsules ... 782
Lorcet 10/650 ... 1018
Lortab ... 2566
Tussend ... 1783
Tussend Expectorant ... 1785
Vicodin Tablets ... 1356
Vicodin ES Tablets ... 1357
Vicodin Tuss Expectorant ... 1358
Zydone Capsules ... 949

Hydrocodone Polistirex (Loxitane is contraindicated in severe narcotic-induced depressed state). Products include:
Tussionex Pennkinetic Extended-Release Suspension ... 998

Isoflurane (Loxitane is contraindicated in severe anesthetic-induced depressed state).
No products indexed under this heading.

Ketamine Hydrochloride (Loxitane is contraindicated in severe anesthetic-induced depressed state).
No products indexed under this heading.

Levorphanol Tartrate (Loxitane is contraindicated in severe narcotic-induced depressed state). Products include:
Levo-Dromoran ... 2129

Meperidine Hydrochloride (Loxitane is contraindicated in severe narcotic-induced depressed state). Products include:
Demerol ... 2308
Mepergan Injection ... 2753

Mephobarbital (Loxitane is contraindicated in severe barbiturate-induced depressed state). Products include:
Mebaral Tablets ... 2322

Methadone Hydrochloride (Loxitane is contraindicated in severe narcotic-induced depressed state). Products include:
Methadone Hydrochloride Oral Concentrate ... 2233
Methadone Hydrochloride Oral Solution & Tablets ... 2235

Methohexital Sodium (Loxitane is contraindicated in severe anesthetic-induced depressed state). Products include:
Brevital Sodium Vials ... 1429

Methoxyflurane (Loxitane is contraindicated in severe anesthetic-induced depressed state).
No products indexed under this heading.

Morphine Sulfate (Loxitane is contraindicated in severe narcotic-induced depressed state). Products include:
Astramorph/PF Injection, USP (Preservative-Free) ... 535
Duramorph ... 962
Infumorph 200 and Infumorph 500 Sterile Solutions ... 965
MS Contin Tablets ... 1994
MSIR ... 1997
Oramorph SR (Morphine Sulfate Sustained Release Tablets) ... 2236
RMS Suppositories ... 2657
Roxanol ... 2243

Opium Alkaloids (Loxitane is contraindicated in severe narcotic-induced depressed state).
No products indexed under this heading.

Oxycodone Hydrochloride (Loxitane is contraindicated in severe narcotic-induced depressed state). Products include:
Percocet Tablets ... 938
Percodan Tablets ... 939
Percodan-Demi Tablets ... 940
Roxicodone Tablets, Oral Solution & Intensol (Oxycodone) ... 2244
Tylox Capsules ... 1584

Pentobarbital Sodium (Loxitane is contraindicated in severe barbiturate-induced depressed state). Products include:
Nembutal Sodium Capsules ... 436
Nembutal Sodium Solution ... 438
Nembutal Sodium Suppositories ... 440

Phenobarbital (Loxitane is contraindicated in severe barbiturate-induced depressed state). Products include:
Arco-Lase Plus Tablets ... 512
Bellergal-S Tablets ... 2250
Donnatal ... 2060
Donnatal Extentabs ... 2061
Donnatal Tablets ... 2060
Phenobarbital Elixir and Tablets ... 1469
Quadrinal Tablets ... 1350

Procyclidine Hydrochloride (Use Loxitane cautiously). Products include:
Kemadrin Tablets ... 1112

Propofol (Loxitane is contraindicated in severe anesthetic-induced depressed state). Products include:
Diprivan Injection ... 2833

Propoxyphene Hydrochloride (Loxitane is contraindicated in severe narcotic-induced depressed state). Products include:
Darvon ... 1435
Wygesic Tablets ... 2827

Propoxyphene Napsylate (Loxitane is contraindicated in severe narcotic-induced depressed state). Products include:
Darvon-N/Darvocet-N ... 1433

Secobarbital Sodium (Loxitane is contraindicated in severe barbiturate-induced depressed state). Products include:
Seconal Sodium Pulvules ... 1474

Sufentanil Citrate (Loxitane is contraindicated in severe narcotic-induced depressed state). Products include:
Sufenta Injection ... 1309

Thiamylal Sodium (Loxitane is contraindicated in severe barbiturate-induced depressed state).
No products indexed under this heading.

Tridihexethyl Chloride (Use Loxitane cautiously).
No products indexed under this heading.

Trihexyphenidyl Hydrochloride (Use Loxitane cautiously). Products include:
Artane ... 1368

LOXITANE IM
(Loxapine Hydrochloride) ... 1378
See **Loxitane Capsules**

LOZOL TABLETS
(Indapamide) ... 2022
May interact with antihypertensives, lithium preparations, corticosteroids, insulin, cardiac glycosides, and certain other agents. Compounds in these categories include:

Acebutolol Hydrochloride (Additive or potentiated antihypertensive action). Products include:
Sectral Capsules ... 2807

ACTH (Increased potential for hypokalemia).
No products indexed under this heading.

Amlodipine Besylate (Additive or potentiated antihypertensive action). Products include:
Lotrel Capsules ... 840
Norvasc Tablets ... 1940

Atenolol (Additive or potentiated antihypertensive action). Products include:
Tenoretic Tablets ... 2845
Tenormin Tablets and I.V. Injection ... 2847

Benazepril Hydrochloride (Additive or potentiated antihypertensive action). Products include:
Lotensin Tablets ... 834
Lotensin HCT ... 837
Lotrel Capsules ... 840

Bendroflumethiazide (Additive or potentiated antihypertensive action).
No products indexed under this heading.

Betamethasone Acetate (Concomitant use increases the risk of hypokalemia). Products include:
Celestone Soluspan Suspension ... 2347

Betamethasone Sodium Phosphate (Concomitant use increases the risk of hypokalemia). Products include:
Celestone Soluspan Suspension ... 2347

Betaxolol Hydrochloride (Additive or potentiated antihypertensive action). Products include:
Betoptic Ophthalmic Solution ... 469
Betoptic S Ophthalmic Suspension ... 471
Kerlone Tablets ... 2436

Bisoprolol Fumarate (Additive or potentiated antihypertensive action). Products include:
Zebeta Tablets ... 1413
Ziac ... 1415

Captopril (Additive or potentiated antihypertensive action). Products include:
Capoten ... 739
Capozide ... 742

Carteolol Hydrochloride (Additive or potentiated antihypertensive action). Products include:
Cartrol Tablets ... 410
Ocupress Ophthalmic Solution, 1% Sterile ... ⊙ 309

Chlorothiazide (Additive or potentiated antihypertensive action). Products include:
Aldoclor Tablets ... 1598
Diupres Tablets ... 1650
Diuril Oral ... 1653

Chlorothiazide Sodium (Additive or potentiated antihypertensive action). Products include:
Diuril Sodium Intravenous ... 1652

Chlorthalidone (Possible additive or potentiated antihypertensive action). Products include:
Combipres Tablets ... 677
Tenoretic Tablets ... 2845
Thalitone ... 1245

Clonidine (Additive or potentiated antihypertensive action). Products include:
Catapres-TTS ... 675

Clonidine Hydrochloride (Additive or potentiated antihypertensive action). Products include:
Catapres Tablets ... 674
Combipres Tablets ... 677

Cortisone Acetate (Concomitant use increases the risk of hypokalemia). Products include:
Cortone Acetate Sterile Suspension ... 1623
Cortone Acetate Tablets ... 1624

Deserpidine (Additive or potentiated antihypertensive action).
No products indexed under this heading.

Deslanoside (Hypokalemia can sensitize or exaggerate digitalis toxicity).
No products indexed under this heading.

Dexamethasone (Concomitant use increases the risk of hypokalemia). Products include:
AK-Trol Ointment & Suspension ... ⊙ 205
Decadron Elixir ... 1633
Decadron Tablets ... 1635
Decaspray Topical Aerosol ... 1648
Dexacidin Ointment ... ⊙ 263
Maxitrol Ophthalmic Ointment and Suspension ... ⊙ 224
TobraDex Ophthalmic Suspension and Ointment ... 473

Dexamethasone Acetate (Concomitant use increases the risk of hypokalemia). Products include:
Dalalone D.P. Injectable ... 1011
Decadron-LA Sterile Suspension ... 1646

Dexamethasone Sodium Phosphate (Concomitant use increases the risk of hypokalemia). Products include:
Decadron Phosphate Injection ... 1637
Decadron Phosphate Respihaler ... 1642
Decadron Phosphate Sterile Ophthalmic Ointment ... 1641
Decadron Phosphate Sterile Ophthalmic Solution ... 1642
Decadron Phosphate Topical Cream ... 1644
Decadron Phosphate Turbinaire ... 1645
Decadron Phosphate with Xylocaine Injection, Sterile ... 1639
Dexacort Phosphate in Respihaler ... 458
Dexacort Phosphate in Turbinaire ... 459
NeoDecadron Sterile Ophthalmic Ointment ... 1712
NeoDecadron Sterile Ophthalmic Solution ... 1713
NeoDecadron Topical Cream ... 1714

Diazoxide (Additive or potentiated antihypertensive action). Products include:
Hyperstat I.V. Injection ... 2363
Proglycem ... 580

IMPORTANT NOTE: Always consult each drug listing in the patient's regimen for possible interactions.

Lozol

Digitoxin (Hypokalemia can sensitize or exaggerate digitalis toxicity). Products include:

Crystodigin Tablets 1433

Digoxin (Hypokalemia can sensitize or exaggerate digitalis toxicity). Products include:

Lanoxicaps 1117
Lanoxin Elixir Pediatric 1120
Lanoxin Injection 1123
Lanoxin Injection Pediatric.................... 1126
Lanoxin Tablets 1128

Diltiazem Hydrochloride (Additive or potentiated antihypertensive action). Products include:

Cardizem CD Capsules 1506
Cardizem SR Capsules 1510
Cardizem Injectable 1508
Cardizem Tablets...................................... 1512
Dilacor XR Extended-release Capsules 2018

Doxazosin Mesylate (Additive or potentiated antihypertensive action). Products include:

Cardura Tablets 2186

Enalapril Maleate (Additive or potentiated antihypertensive action). Products include:

Vaseretic Tablets 1765
Vasotec Tablets 1771

Enalaprilat (Additive or potentiated antihypertensive action). Products include:

Vasotec I.V... 1768

Esmolol Hydrochloride (Additive or potentiated antihypertensive action). Products include:

Brevibloc Injection................................... 1808

Felodipine (Additive or potentiated antihypertensive action). Products include:

Plendil Extended-Release Tablets.... 527

Fludrocortisone Acetate (Concomitant use increases the risk of hypokalemia). Products include:

Florinef Acetate Tablets 505

Fosinopril Sodium (Additive or potentiated antihypertensive action). Products include:

Monopril Tablets 757

Furosemide (Additive or potentiated antihypertensive action). Products include:

Lasix Injection, Oral Solution and Tablets 1240

Guanabenz Acetate (Additive or potentiated antihypertensive action).

No products indexed under this heading.

Guanethidine Monosulfate (Additive or potentiated antihypertensive action). Products include:

Esimil Tablets 822
Ismelin Tablets 827

Hydralazine Hydrochloride (Possible additive or potentiated antihypertensive action). Products include:

Apresazide Capsules 808
Apresoline Hydrochloride Tablets .. 809
Ser-Ap-Es Tablets 849

Hydrochlorothiazide (Additive or potentiated antihypertensive action). Products include:

Aldactazide... 2413
Aldoril Tablets... 1604
Apresazide Capsules 808
Capozide 742
Dyazide 2479
Esidrix Tablets 821
Esimil Tablets 822
HydroDIURIL Tablets 1674
Hydropres Tablets.................................... 1675
Hyzaar Tablets 1677
Inderide Tablets 2732
Inderide LA Long Acting Capsules .. 2734
Lopressor HCT Tablets 832
Lotensin HCT.. 837
Maxzide 1380
Moduretic Tablets 1705
Oretic Tablets 443

Prinzide Tablets 1737
Ser-Ap-Es Tablets 849
Timolide Tablets....................................... 1748
Vaseretic Tablets 1765
Zestoretic 2850
Ziac 1415

Hydrocortisone (Concomitant use increases the risk of hypokalemia). Products include:

Anusol-HC Cream 2.5% 1896
Aquanil HC Lotion 1931
Bactine Hydrocortisone Anti-Itch Cream.. ᴾᴰ 709
Caldecort Anti-Itch Hydrocortisone Spray .... ᴾᴰ 631
Cortaid .... ᴾᴰ 836
CORTENEMA... 2535
Cortisporin Ointment 1085
Cortisporin Ophthalmic Ointment Sterile 1085
Cortisporin Ophthalmic Suspension Sterile 1086
Cortisporin Otic Solution Sterile 1087
Cortisporin Otic Suspension Sterile 1088
Cortizone-5 .... ᴾᴰ 831
Cortizone-10 .... ᴾᴰ 831
Hydrocortone Tablets 1672
Hytone 907
Massengill Medicated Soft Cloth Towelettes.. 2458
PediOtic Suspension Sterile 1153
Preparation H Hydrocortisone 1% Cream .... ᴾᴰ 872
ProctoCream-HC 2.5% 2408
VōSoL HC Otic Solution.......................... 2678

Hydrocortisone Acetate (Concomitant use increases the risk of hypokalemia). Products include:

Analpram-HC Rectal Cream 1% and 2.5% 977
Anusol HC-1 Anti-Itch Hydrocortisone Ointment... ᴾᴰ 847
Anusol-HC Suppositories 1897
Caldecort.. ᴾᴰ 631
Carmol HC 924
Coly-Mycin S Otic w/Neomycin & Hydrocortisone 1906
Cortaid .... ᴾᴰ 836
Cortifoam 2396
Cortisporin Cream.................................... 1084
Epifoam 2399
Hydrocortone Acetate Sterile Suspension... 1669
Mantadil Cream 1135
Nupercainal Hydrocortisone 1% Cream... ᴾᴰ 645
Ophthocort .... ⊙ 311
Pramosone Cream, Lotion & Ointment 978
ProctoCream-HC 2408
ProctoFoam-HC 2409
Terra-Cortril Ophthalmic Suspension 2210

Hydrocortisone Sodium Phosphate (Concomitant use increases the risk of hypokalemia). Products include:

Hydrocortone Phosphate Injection, Sterile 1670

Hydrocortisone Sodium Succinate (Concomitant use increases the risk of hypokalemia). Products include:

Solu-Cortef Sterile Powder................... 2641

Hydroflumethiazide (Additive or potentiated antihypertensive action). Products include:

Diucardin Tablets..................................... 2718

Insulin, Human (Insulin requirements may be altered).

No products indexed under this heading.

Insulin, Human Isophane Suspension (Insulin requirements may be altered). Products include:

Novolin N Human Insulin 10 ml Vials... 1795

Insulin, Human NPH (Insulin requirements may be altered). Products include:

Humulin N, 100 Units............................ 1448
Novolin N PenFill Cartridges Durable Insulin Delivery System 1798
Novolin N Prefilled Syringe Disposable Insulin Delivery System 1798

Insulin, Human Regular (Insulin requirements may be altered). Products include:

Humulin R, 100 Units 1449
Novolin R Human Insulin 10 ml Vials... 1795
Novolin R PenFill Cartridges Durable Insulin Delivery System 1798
Novolin R Prefilled Syringe Disposable Insulin Delivery System 1798
Velosulin BR Human Insulin 10 ml Vials... 1795

Insulin, Human, Zinc Suspension (Insulin requirements may be altered). Products include:

Humulin L, 100 Units 1446
Humulin U, 100 Units 1450
Novolin L Human Insulin 10 ml Vials... 1795

Insulin, NPH (Insulin requirements may be altered). Products include:

NPH, 100 Units 1450
Pork NPH, 100 Units.............................. 1452
Purified Pork NPH Isophane Insulin 1801

Insulin, Regular (Insulin requirements may be altered). Products include:

Regular, 100 Units 1450
Pork Regular, 100 Units 1452
Pork Regular (Concentrated), 500 Units 1453
Purified Pork Regular Insulin 1801

Insulin, Zinc Crystals (Insulin requirements may be altered). Products include:

NPH, 100 Units 1450

Insulin, Zinc Suspension (Insulin requirements may be altered). Products include:

Iletin I 1450
Lente, 100 Units 1450
Iletin II... 1452
Pork Lente, 100 Units............................. 1452
Purified Pork Lente Insulin 1801

Isradipine (Additive or potentiated antihypertensive action). Products include:

DynaCirc Capsules 2256

Labetalol Hydrochloride (Additive or potentiated antihypertensive action). Products include:

Normodyne Injection 2377
Normodyne Tablets 2379
Trandate 1185

Lisinopril (Additive or potentiated antihypertensive action). Products include:

Prinivil Tablets 1733
Prinzide Tablets 1737
Zestoretic 2850
Zestril Tablets 2854

Lithium Carbonate (Reduced renal clearance; high risk of lithium toxicity). Products include:

Eskalith 2485
Lithium Carbonate Capsules & Tablets.. 2230
Lithonate/Lithotabs/Lithobid 2543

Lithium Citrate (Reduced renal clearance; high risk of lithium toxicity).

No products indexed under this heading.

Losartan Potassium (Additive or potentiated antihypertensive action). Products include:

Cozaar Tablets 1628
Hyzaar Tablets 1677

Mecamylamine Hydrochloride (Additive or potentiated antihypertensive action). Products include:

Inversine Tablets 1686

Methyclothiazide (Additive or potentiated antihypertensive action). Products include:

Enduron Tablets.. 420

Methyldopa (Additive or potentiated antihypertensive action). Products include:

Aldoclor Tablets 1598

Aldomet Oral 1600
Aldoril Tablets... 1604

Methyldopate Hydrochloride (Additive or potentiated antihypertensive action). Products include:

Aldomet Ester HCl Injection 1602

Methylprednisolone Acetate (Concomitant use increases the risk of hypokalemia). Products include:

Depo-Medrol Single-Dose Vial 2600
Depo-Medrol Sterile Aqueous Suspension... 2597

Methylprednisolone Sodium Succinate (Concomitant use increases the risk of hypokalemia). Products include:

Solu-Medrol Sterile Powder 2643

Metolazone (Additive or potentiated antihypertensive action). Products include:

Mykrox Tablets 993
Zaroxolyn Tablets 1000

Metoprolol Succinate (Additive or potentiated antihypertensive action). Products include:

Toprol-XL Tablets 565

Metoprolol Tartrate (Additive or potentiated antihypertensive action). Products include:

Lopressor Ampuls 830
Lopressor HCT Tablets 832
Lopressor Tablets 830

Metyrosine (Additive or potentiated antihypertensive action). Products include:

Demser Capsules 1649

Minoxidil (Additive or potentiated antihypertensive action). Products include:

Loniten Tablets 2618
Rogaine Topical Solution 2637

Moexipril Hydrochloride (Additive or potentiated antihypertensive action). Products include:

Univasc Tablets 2410

Nadolol (Additive or potentiated antihypertensive action).

No products indexed under this heading.

Nicardipine Hydrochloride (Additive or potentiated antihypertensive action). Products include:

Cardene Capsules 2095
Cardene I.V. 2709
Cardene SR Capsules............................... 2097

Nifedipine (Additive or potentiated antihypertensive action). Products include:

Adalat Capsules (10 mg and 20 mg) 587
Adalat CC 589
Procardia Capsules 1971
Procardia XL Extended Release Tablets 1972

Nisoldipine (Additive or potentiated antihypertensive action).

No products indexed under this heading.

Nitroglycerin (Additive or potentiated antihypertensive action). Products include:

Deponit NTG Transdermal Delivery System 2397
Nitro-Bid IV 1523
Nitro-Bid Ointment 1524
Nitrodisc 2047
Nitro-Dur (nitroglycerin) Transdermal Infusion System 1326
Nitrolingual Spray 2027
Nitrostat Tablets 1925
Transderm-Nitro Transdermal Therapeutic System 859

Norepinephrine Bitartrate (Decreased arterial responsiveness to norepinephrine). Products include:

Levophed Bitartrate Injection.............. 2315

Penbutolol Sulfate (Additive or potentiated antihypertensive action). Products include:

Levatol 2403

Phenoxybenzamine Hydrochloride (Additive or potentiated antihypertensive action). Products include:

Dibenzyline Capsules 2476

Phentolamine Mesylate (Additive or potentiated antihypertensive action). Products include:

Regitine 846

Pindolol (Additive or potentiated antihypertensive action). Products include:

Visken Tablets 2299

Polythiazide (Additive or potentiated antihypertensive action). Products include:

Minizide Capsules 1938

Prazosin Hydrochloride (Additive or potentiated antihypertensive action). Products include:

Minipress Capsules 1937
Minizide Capsules 1938

Prednisolone Acetate (Concomitant use increases the risk of hypokalemia). Products include:

AK-CIDE .... ⊙ 202
AK-CIDE Ointment .... ⊙ 202
Blephamide Liquifilm Sterile Ophthalmic Suspension 476
Blephamide Ointment .... ⊙ 237
Econopred & Econopred Plus Ophthalmic Suspensions .... ⊙ 217
Poly-Pred Liquifilm .... ⊙ 248
Pred Forte .... ⊙ 250
Pred Mild .... ⊙ 253
Pred-G Liquifilm Sterile Ophthalmic Suspension .... ⊙ 251
Pred-G S.O.P. Sterile Ophthalmic Ointment .... ⊙ 252
Vasocidin Ointment .... ⊙ 268

Prednisolone Sodium Phosphate (Concomitant use increases the risk of hypokalemia). Products include:

AK-Pred .... ⊙ 204
Hydeltrasol Injection, Sterile 1665
Inflamase .... ⊙ 265
Pediapred Oral Liquid 995
Vasocidin Ophthalmic Solution .... ⊙ 270

Prednisolone Tebutate (Concomitant use increases the risk of hypokalemia). Products include:

Hydeltra-T.B.A. Sterile Suspension 1667

Prednisone (Concomitant use increases the risk of hypokalemia). Products include:

Deltasone Tablets 2595

Propranolol Hydrochloride (Additive or potentiated antihypertensive action). Products include:

Inderal 2728
Inderal LA Long Acting Capsules 2730
Inderide Tablets 2732
Inderide LA Long Acting Capsules .. 2734

Quinapril Hydrochloride (Additive or potentiated antihypertensive action). Products include:

Accupril Tablets 1893

Ramipril (Additive or potentiated antihypertensive action). Products include:

Altace Capsules 1232

Rauwolfia Serpentina (Additive or potentiated antihypertensive action).

No products indexed under this heading.

Rescinnamine (Additive or potentiated antihypertensive action).

No products indexed under this heading.

Reserpine (Additive or potentiated antihypertensive action). Products include:

Diupres Tablets 1650
Hydropres Tablets 1675
Ser-Ap-Es Tablets 849

Sodium Nitroprusside (Additive or potentiated antihypertensive action).

No products indexed under this heading.

Sotalol Hydrochloride (Additive or potentiated antihypertensive action). Products include:

Betapace Tablets 641

Spirapril Hydrochloride (Additive or potentiated antihypertensive action).

No products indexed under this heading.

Terazosin Hydrochloride (Additive or potentiated antihypertensive action). Products include:

Hytrin Capsules 430

Timolol Maleate (Additive or potentiated antihypertensive action). Products include:

Blocadren Tablets 1614
Timolide Tablets 1748
Timoptic in Ocudose 1753
Timoptic Sterile Ophthalmic Solution 1751
Timoptic-XE 1755

Torsemide (Additive or potentiated antihypertensive action). Products include:

Demadex Tablets and Injection 686

Triamcinolone (Concomitant use increases the risk of hypokalemia). Products include:

Aristocort Tablets 1022

Triamcinolone Acetonide (Concomitant use increases the risk of hypokalemia). Products include:

Aristocort A 0.025% Cream 1027
Aristocort A 0.5% Cream 1031
Aristocort A 0.1% Cream 1029
Aristocort A 0.1% Ointment 1030
Azmacort Oral Inhaler 2011
Nasacort Nasal Inhaler 2024

Triamcinolone Diacetate (Concomitant use increases the risk of hypokalemia). Products include:

Aristocort Suspension (Forte Parenteral) 1027
Aristocort Suspension (Intralesional) 1025

Triamcinolone Hexacetonide (Concomitant use increases the risk of hypokalemia). Products include:

Aristospan Suspension (Intra-articular) 1033
Aristospan Suspension (Intralesional) 1032

Trimethaphan Camsylate (Additive or potentiated antihypertensive action). Products include:

Arfonad Ampuls 2080

Verapamil Hydrochloride (Additive or potentiated antihypertensive action). Products include:

Calan SR Caplets 2422
Calan Tablets 2419
Isoptin Injectable 1344
Isoptin Oral Tablets 1346
Isoptin SR Tablets 1348
Verelan Capsules 1410
Verelan Capsules 2824

LUBRIDERM BATH AND SHOWER OIL

(Emollient, Mineral Oil) .... ▣ 856
None cited in PDR database.

LUBRIDERM CARE LOTION

(Emollient) .... ▣ 856
None cited in PDR database.

LUBRIDERM MOISTURE RECOVERY ALPHA HYDROXY FORMULA CREAM AND LOTION

(Moisturizing formula) .... ▣ 856
None cited in PDR database.

LUBRIDERM MOISTURE RECOVERY GELCREME

(Cetyl Alcohol, Glycerin, Mineral Oil) .... ▣ 857
None cited in PDR database.

LUBRIDERM SERIOUSLY SENSITIVE LOTION

(Glycerin, Mineral Oil, Petrolatum) .. ▣ 857
None cited in PDR database.

LUDIOMIL TABLETS

(Maprotiline Hydrochloride) 843
May interact with monoamine oxidase inhibitors, benzodiazepines, phenothiazines, barbiturates, anticholinergics, sympathomimetics, thyroid preparations, central nervous system depressants, and certain other agents. Compounds in these categories include:

Albuterol (Possible additive atropine-like effects; careful adjustment of dosage and close supervision are required). Products include:

Proventil Inhalation Aerosol 2382
Ventolin Inhalation Aerosol and Refill 1197

Albuterol Sulfate (Possible additive atropine-like effects; careful adjustment of dosage and close supervision are required). Products include:

Airet Solution for Inhalation 452
Proventil Inhalation Solution 0.083% 2384
Proventil Repetabs Tablets 2386
Proventil Solution for Inhalation 0.5% 2383
Proventil Syrup 2385
Proventil Tablets 2386
Ventolin Inhalation Solution 1198
Ventolin Nebules Inhalation Solution 1199
Ventolin Rotacaps for Inhalation 1200
Ventolin Syrup 1202
Ventolin Tablets 1203
Volmax Extended-Release Tablets .. 1788

Alfentanil Hydrochloride (Ludiomil may enhance the response to CNS depressants). Products include:

Alfenta Injection 1286

Alprazolam (The risk of seizures may be increased when the dosage of benzodiazepines is rapidly tapered in patients receiving Ludiomil or when the recommended dosage of Ludiomil is exceeded; Ludiomol may enhance the response to CNS depressants). Products include:

Xanax Tablets 2649

Aprobarbital (Ludiomil may enhance the response to barbiturates; certain barbiturates may decrease the plasma levels of malprotiliine due to hepatic enzyme induction).

No products indexed under this heading.

Atropine Sulfate (Possible additive atropine-like effects; careful adjustment of dosage and close supervision are required). Products include:

Arco-Lase Plus Tablets 512
Atrohist Plus Tablets 454
Atropine Sulfate Sterile Ophthalmic Solution .... ⊙ 233
Donnatal 2060
Donnatal Extentabs 2061
Donnatal Tablets 2060
Lomotil 2439
Motofen Tablets 784
Urised Tablets 1964

Belladonna Alkaloids (Possible additive atropine-like effects; careful adjustment of dosage and close supervision are required). Products include:

Bellergal-S Tablets 2250
Hyland's Bed Wetting Tablets .... ▣ 828
Hyland's EnurAid Tablets .... ▣ 829
Hyland's Teething Tablets .... ▣ 830

Benztropine Mesylate (Possible additive atropine-like effects; careful adjustment of dosage and close supervision are required). Products include:

Cogentin 1621

Biperiden Hydrochloride (Possible additive atropine-like effects; careful adjustment of dosage and close supervision are required). Products include:

Akineton 1333

Buprenorphine (Ludiomil may enhance the response to CNS depressants). Products include:

Buprenex Injectable 2006

Buspirone Hydrochloride (Ludiomil may enhance the response to CNS depressants). Products include:

BuSpar 737

Butabarbital (Ludiomil may enhance the response to barbiturates; certain barbiturates may decrease the plasma levels of maprotiline due to hepatic enzyme induction).

No products indexed under this heading.

Butalbital (Ludiomil may enhance the response to barbiturates; certain barbiturates may decrease the plasma levels of maprotiline due to hepatic enzyme induction). Products include:

Esgic-plus Tablets 1013
Fioricet Tablets 2258
Fioricet with Codeine Capsules 2260
Fiorinal Capsules 2261
Fiorinal with Codeine Capsules 2262
Fiorinal Tablets 2261
Phrenilin 785
Sedapap Tablets 50 mg/650 mg .. 1543

Chlordiazepoxide (The risk of seizures may be increased when the dosage of benzodiazepines is rapidly tapered in patients receiving Ludiomil or when the recommended dosage of Ludiomil is exceeded; Ludiomol may enhance the response to CNS depressants). Products include:

Libritabs Tablets 2177
Limbitrol 2180

Chlordiazepoxide Hydrochloride (The risk of seizures may be increased when the dosage of benzodiazepines is rapidly tapered in patients receiving Ludiomil or when the recommended dosage of Ludiomil is exceeded; Ludiomol may enhance the response to CNS depressants). Products include:

Librax Capsules 2176
Librium Capsules 2178
Librium Injectable 2179

Chlorpromazine (The risk of seizures may be increased when used concomitantly; Ludiomil may enhance the response to CNS depressants). Products include:

Thorazine Suppositories 2523

Chlorpromazine Hydrochloride (The risk of seizures may be increased when used concomitantly; Ludiomil may enhance the response to CNS depressants). Products include:

Thorazine 2523

Chlorprothixene (Ludiomil may enhance the response to CNS depressants).

No products indexed under this heading.

Chlorprothixene Hydrochloride (Ludiomil may enhance the response to CNS depressants).

No products indexed under this heading.

IMPORTANT NOTE: Always consult each drug listing in the patient's regimen for possible interactions.

Cimetidine (May increase the plasma levels of maprotiline due to hepatic enzyme inhibition). Products include:

Tagamet Tablets ... 2516

Cimetidine Hydrochloride (May increase the plasma levels of maprotiline due to hepatic enzyme inhibition). Products include:

Tagamet ... 2516

Clidinium Bromide (Possible additive atropine-like effects; careful adjustment of dosage and close supervision are required). Products include:

Librax Capsules ... 2176
Quarzan Capsules ... 2181

Clonidine (Maprotiline may block the pharmacological effect). Products include:

Catapres-TTS ... 675

Clonidine Hydrochloride (Maprotiline may block the pharmacological effect). Products include:

Catapres Tablets ... 674
Combipres Tablets ... 677

Clorazepate Dipotassium (The risk of seizures may be increased when the dosage of benzodiazepines is rapidly tapered in patients receiving Ludiomil or when the recommended dosage of Ludiomil is exceeded; Ludiomol may enhance the response to CNS depressants). Products include:

Tranxene ... 451

Clozapine (Ludiomil may enhance the response to CNS depressants). Products include:

Clozaril Tablets ... 2252

Codeine Phosphate (Ludiomil may enhance the response to CNS depressants). Products include:

Actifed with Codeine Cough Syrup.. 1067
Brontex ... 1981
Deconsal C Expectorant Syrup ... 456
Deconsal Pediatric Syrup ... 457
Dimetane-DC Cough Syrup ... 2059
Empirin with Codeine Tablets ... 1093
Fioricet with Codeine Capsules ... 2260
Fiorinal with Codeine Capsules ... 2262
Isoclor Expectorant ... 990
Novahistine DH ... 2462
Novahistine Expectorant ... 2463
Nucofed ... 2051
Phenergan with Codeine ... 2777
Phenergan VC with Codeine ... 2781
Robitussin A-C Syrup ... 2073
Robitussin-DAC Syrup ... 2074
Ryna ... ▣ 841
Soma Compound w/Codeine Tablets ... 2676
Tussi-Organidin NR Liquid and S NR Liquid ... 2677
Tylenol with Codeine ... 1583

Desflurane (Ludiomil may enhance the response to CNS depressants). Products include:

Suprane ... 1813

Dezocine (Ludiomil may enhance the response to CNS depressants). Products include:

Dalgan Injection ... 538

Diazepam (The risk of seizures may be increased when the dosage of benzodiazepines is rapidly tapered in patients receiving Ludiomil or when the recommended dosage of Ludiomil is exceeded; Ludiomol may enhance the response to CNS depressants). Products include:

Dizac ... 1809
Valium Injectable ... 2182
Valium Tablets ... 2183
Valrelease Capsules ... 2169

Dicyclomine Hydrochloride (Possible additive atropine-like effects; careful adjustment of dosage and close supervision are required). Products include:

Bentyl ... 1501

Dobutamine Hydrochloride (Possible additive atropiine-like effects; careful adjustment of dosage and close supervision are required). Products include:

Dobutrex Solution Vials ... 1439

Dopamine Hydrochloride (Possible additive atropine-like effects; careful adjustment of dosage and close supervision are required).

No products indexed under this heading.

Droperidol (Ludiomil may enhance the response to CNS depressants). Products include:

Inapsine Injection ... 1296

Enflurane (Ludiomil may enhance the response to CNS depressants).

No products indexed under this heading.

Ephedrine Hydrochloride (Possible additive atropine-like effects; careful adjustment of dosage and close supervision are required). Products include:

Primatene Dual Action Formula ... ▣ 872
Primatene Tablets ... ▣ 873
Quadrinal Tablets ... 1350

Ephedrine Sulfate (Possible additive atropine-like effects; careful adjustment of dosage and close supervision are required). Products include:

Bronkaid Caplets ... ▣ 717
Marax Tablets & DF Syrup ... 2200

Ephedrine Tannate (Possible additive atropine-like effects; careful adjustment of dosage and close supervision are required). Products include:

Rynatuss ... 2673

Epinephrine (Possible additive atropine-like effects; careful adjustment of dosage and close supervision are required). Products include:

Bronkaid Mist ... ▣ 717
EPIFRIN ... ⊙ 239
EpiPen ... 790
Marcaine Hydrochloride with Epinephrine 1:200,000 ... 2316
Primatene Mist ... ▣ 873
Sensorcaine with Epinephrine Injection ... 559
Sus-Phrine Injection ... 1019
Xylocaine with Epinephrine Injections ... 567

Epinephrine Bitartrate (Possible additive atropine-like effects; careful adjustment of dosage and close supervision are required). Products include:

Bronkaid Mist Suspension ... ▣ 718
Sensorcaine-MPF with Epinephrine Injection ... 559

Epinephrine Hydrochloride (Possible additive atropine-like effects; careful adjustment of dosage and close supervision are required). Products include:

Ana-Kit Anaphylaxis Emergency Treatment Kit ... 617

Estazolam (The risk of seizures may be increased when the dosage of benzodiazepines is rapidly tapered in patients receiving Ludiomil or when the recommended dosage of Ludiomil is exceeded; Ludiomol may enhance the response to CNS depressants). Products include:

ProSom Tablets ... 449

Ethchlorvynol (Ludiomil may enhance the response to CNS depressants). Products include:

Placidyl Capsules ... 448

Ethinamate (Ludiomil may enhance the response to CNS depressants).

No products indexed under this heading.

Fentanyl (Ludiomil may enhance the response to CNS depressants). Products include:

Duragesic Transdermal System ... 1288

Fentanyl Citrate (Ludiomil may enhance the response to CNS depressants). Products include:

Sublimaze Injection ... 1307

Fluoxetine Hydrochloride (May increase the plasma levels of maprotiline due to hepatic enzyme inhibition). Products include:

Prozac Pulvules & Liquid, Oral Solution ... 919

Fluphenazine Decanoate (The risk of seizures may be increased when used concomitantly; Ludiomil may enhance the response to CNS depressants). Products include:

Prolixin Decanoate ... 509

Fluphenazine Enanthate (The risk of seizures may be increased when used concomitantly; Ludiomil may enhance the response to CNS depressants). Products include:

Prolixin Enanthate ... 509

Fluphenazine Hydrochloride (The risk of seizures may be increased when used concomitantly; Ludiomil may enhance the response to CNS depressants). Products include:

Prolixin ... 509

Flurazepam Hydrochloride (The risk of seizures may be increased when the dosage of benzodiazepines is rapidly tapered in patients receiving Ludiomil or when the recommended dosage of Ludiomil is exceeded; Ludiomol may enhance the response to CNS depressants). Products include:

Dalmane Capsules ... 2173

Furazolidone (Concurrent and/or sequential use is contraindicated). Products include:

Furoxone ... 2046

Glutethimide (Ludiomil may enhance the response to CNS depressants).

No products indexed under this heading.

Glycopyrrolate (Possible additive atropine-like effects; careful adjustment of dosage and close supervision are required). Products include:

Robinul Forte Tablets ... 2072
Robinul Injectable ... 2072
Robinul Tablets ... 2072

Guanethidine Monosulfate (Maprotiline may block the pharmacological effect of guanethidine or similar agents). Products include:

Esimil Tablets ... 822
Ismelin Tablets ... 827

Halazepam (The risk of seizures may be increased when the dosage of benzodiazepines is rapidly tapered in patients receiving Ludiomil or when the recommended dosage of Ludiomil is exceeded; Ludiomol may enhance the response to CNS depressants).

No products indexed under this heading.

Haloperidol (Ludiomil may enhance the response to CNS depressants). Products include:

Haldol Injection, Tablets and Concentrate ... 1575

Haloperidol Decanoate (Ludiomil may enhance the response to CNS depressants). Products include:

Haldol Decanoate ... 1577

Hydrocodone Bitartrate (Ludiomil may enhance the response to CNS depressants). Products include:

Anexsia 5/500 Elixir ... 1781
Anexia Tablets ... 1782
Codiclear DH Syrup ... 791
Deconamine CX Cough and Cold Liquid and Tablets ... 1319
Duratuss HD Elixir ... 2565
Hycodan Tablets and Syrup ... 930
Hycomine Compound Tablets ... 932
Hycomine ... 931
Hycotuss Expectorant Syrup ... 933
Hydrocet Capsules ... 782
Lorcet 10/650 ... 1018
Lortab ... 2566
Tussend ... 1783
Tussend Expectorant ... 1785
Vicodin Tablets ... 1356
Vicodin ES Tablets ... 1357
Vicodin Tuss Expectorant ... 1358
Zydone Capsules ... 949

Hydrocodone Polistirex (Ludiomil may enhance the response to CNS depressants). Products include:

Tussionex Pennkinetic Extended-Release Suspension ... 998

Hydroxyzine Hydrochloride (Ludiomil may enhance the response to CNS depressants). Products include:

Atarax Tablets & Syrup ... 2185
Marax Tablets & DF Syrup ... 2200
Vistaril Intramuscular Solution ... 2216

Hyoscyamine (Possible additive atropine-like effects; careful adjustment of dosage and close supervision are required). Products include:

Cystospaz Tablets ... 1963
Urised Tablets ... 1964

Hyoscyamine Sulfate (Possible additive atropine-like effects; careful adjustment of dosage and close supervision are required). Products include:

Arco-Lase Plus Tablets ... 512
Atrohist Plus Tablets ... 454
Cystospaz-M Capsules ... 1963
Donnatal ... 2060
Donnatal Extentabs ... 2061
Donnatal Tablets ... 2060
Kutrase Capsules ... 2402
Levsin/Levsinex/Levbid ... 2405

Ipratropium Bromide (Possible additive atropine-like effects; careful adjustment of dosage and close supervision are required). Products include:

Atrovent Inhalation Aerosol ... 671
Atrovent Inhalation Solution ... 673

Isocarboxazid (Concurrent and/or sequential use is contraindicated).

No products indexed under this heading.

Isoflurane (Ludiomil may enhance the response to CNS depressants).

No products indexed under this heading.

Isoproterenol Hydrochloride (Possible additive atropine-like effects; careful adjustment of dosage and close supervision are required). Products include:

Isuprel Hydrochloride Injection 1:5000 ... 2311
Isuprel Hydrochloride Solution 1:200 & 1:100 ... 2313
Isuprel Mistometer ... 2312

Isoproterenol Sulfate (Possible additive atropine-like effects; careful adjustment of dosage and close supervision are required). Products include:

Norisodrine with Calcium Iodide Syrup ... 442

Ketamine Hydrochloride (Ludiomil may enhance the response to CNS depressants).

No products indexed under this heading.

Levomethadyl Acetate Hydrochloride (Ludiomil may enhance the response to CNS depressants). Products include:

Orlamm ... 2239

(▣ Described in PDR For Nonprescription Drugs) (⊙ Described in PDR For Ophthalmology)

Interactions Index — Ludiomil

Levorphanol Tartrate (Ludiomil may enhance the response to CNS depressants). Products include:

Levo-Dromoran 2129

Levothyroxine Sodium (Possibility of enhanced potential for cardiovascular toxicity of Ludiomil). Products include:

Levothroid Tablets 1016
Levoxyl Tablets 903
Synthroid 1359

Liothyronine Sodium (Possibility of enhanced potential for cardiovascular toxicity of Ludiomil). Products include:

Cytomel Tablets 2473
Triostat Injection 2530

Liotrix (Possibility of enhanced potential for cardiovascular toxicity of Ludiomil).

No products indexed under this heading.

Lorazepam (The risk of seizures may be increased when the dosage of benzodiazepines is rapidly tapered in patients receiving Ludiomil or when the recommended dosage of Ludiomil is exceeded; Ludiomol may enhance the response to CNS depressants). Products include:

Ativan Injection 2698
Ativan Tablets 2700

Loxapine Hydrochloride (Ludiomil may enhance the response to CNS depressants). Products include:

Loxitane 1378

Loxapine Succinate (Ludiomil may enhance the response to CNS depressants). Products include:

Loxitane Capsules 1378

Mepenzolate Bromide (Possible additive atropine-like effects; careful adjustment of dosage and close supervision are required).

No products indexed under this heading.

Meperidine Hydrochloride (Ludiomil may enhance the response to CNS depressants). Products include:

Demerol 2308
Mepergan Injection 2753

Mephobarbital (Ludiomil may enhance the response to barbiturates; certain barbiturates may decrease the plasma levels of maprotiline due to hepatic enzyme induction). Products include:

Mebaral Tablets 2322

Meprobamate (Ludiomil may enhance the response to CNS depressants). Products include:

Miltown Tablets 2672
PMB 200 and PMB 400 2783

Mesoridazine (Ludiomil may enhance the response to CNS depressants).

Mesoridazine Besylate (The risk of seizures may be increased when used concomitantly; Ludiomil may enhance the response to CNS depressants). Products include:

Serentil 684

Metaproterenol Sulfate (Possible additive atropiine-like effects; careful adjustment of dosage and close supervision are required). Products include:

Alupent 669
Metaproterenol Sulfate Inhalation Solution, USP, Arm-a-Med 552

Metaraminol Bitartrate (Possible additive atropiine-like effects; careful adjustment of dosage and close supervision are required). Products include:

Aramine Injection 1609

Methadone Hydrochloride (Ludiomil may enhance the response to CNS depressants). Products include:

Methadone Hydrochloride Oral Concentrate 2233
Methadone Hydrochloride Oral Solution & Tablets 2235

Methohexital Sodium (Ludiomil may enhance the response to CNS depressants). Products include:

Brevital Sodium Vials 1429

Methotrimeprazine (The risk of seizures may be increased when used concomitantly; Ludiomil may enhance the response to CNS depressants). Products include:

Levoprome 1274

Methoxamine Hydrochloride (Possible additive atropine-like effects; careful adjustment of dosage and close supervision are required). Products include:

Vasoxyl Injection 1196

Methoxyflurane (Ludiomil may enhance the response to CNS depressants).

No products indexed under this heading.

Midazolam Hydrochloride (The risk of seizures may be increased when the dosage of benzodiazepines is rapidly tapered in patients receiving Ludiomil or when the recommended dosage of Ludiomil is exceeded; Ludiomol may enhance the response to CNS depressants). Products include:

Versed Injection 2170

Molindone Hydrochloride (Ludiomil may enhance the response to CNS depressants). Products include:

Moban Tablets and Concentrate 1048

Morphine Sulfate (Ludiomil may enhance the response to CNS depressants). Products include:

Astramorph/PF Injection, USP (Preservative-Free) 535
Duramorph 962
Infumorph 200 and Infumorph 500 Sterile Solutions 965
MS Contin Tablets 1994
MSIR 1997
Oramorph SR (Morphine Sulfate Sustained Release Tablets) 2236
RMS Suppositories 2657
Roxanol 2243

Norepinephrine Bitartrate (Possible additive atropiine-like effects; careful adjustment of dosage and close supervision are required). Products include:

Levophed Bitartrate Injection 2315

Opium Alkaloids (Ludiomil may enhance the response to CNS depressants).

No products indexed under this heading.

Oxazepam (The risk of seizures may be increased when the dosage of benzodiazepines is rapidly tapered in patients receiving Ludiomil or when the recommended dosage of Ludiomil is exceeded; Ludiomol may enhance the response to CNS depressants). Products include:

Serax Capsules 2810
Serax Tablets 2810

Oxybutynin Chloride (Possible additive atropine-like effects; careful adjustment of dosage and close supervision are required). Products include:

Ditropan 1516

Oxycodone Hydrochloride (Ludiomil may enhance the response to CNS depressants). Products include:

Percocet Tablets 938
Percodan Tablets 939
Percodan-Demi Tablets 940
Roxicodone Tablets, Oral Solution & Intensol (Oxycodone) 2244
Tylox Capsules 1584

Pentobarbital Sodium (Ludiomil may enhance the response to barbiturates; certain barbiturates may decrease the plasma levels of maprotiline due to hepatic enzyme induction). Products include:

Nembutal Sodium Capsules 436
Nembutal Sodium Solution 438
Nembutal Sodium Suppositories 440

Perphenazine (The risk of seizures may be increased when used concomitantly; Ludiomil may enhance the response to CNS depressants). Products include:

Etrafon 2355
Triavil Tablets 1757
Trilafon 2389

Phenelzine Sulfate (Concurrent and/or sequential use is contraindicated). Products include:

Nardil 1920

Phenobarbital (Ludiomil may enhance the response to barbiturates; certain barbiturates may decrease the plasma levels of maprotiline due to hepatic enzyme induction). Products include:

Arco-Lase Plus Tablets 512
Bellergal-S Tablets 2250
Donnatal 2060
Donnatal Extentabs 2061
Donnatal Tablets 2060
Phenobarbital Elixir and Tablets 1469
Quadrinal Tablets 1350

Phenylephrine Bitartrate (Possible additive atropine-like effects; careful adjustment of dosage and close supervision are required).

No products indexed under this heading.

Phenylephrine Hydrochloride (Possible additive atropine-like effects; careful adjustment of dosage and close supervision are required). Products include:

Atrohist Plus Tablets 454
Cerose DM .... ◆□ 878
Comhist 2038
D.A. Chewable Tablets 951
Deconsal Pediatric Capsules 454
Dura-Vent/DA Tablets 953
Entex Capsules 1986
Entex Liquid 1986
Extendryl 1005
4-Way Fast Acting Nasal Spray (regular & mentholated) .... ◆□ 621
Hemorid For Women .... ◆□ 834
Hycomine Compound Tablets 932
Neo-Synephrine Hydrochloride 1% Carpuject 2324
Neo-Synephrine Hydrochloride 1% Injection 2324
Neo-Synephrine Hydrochloride (Ophthalmic) 2325
Neo-Synephrine .... ◆□ 726
Nōstril .... ◆□ 644
Novahistine Elixir .... ◆□ 823
Phenergan VC 2779
Phenergan VC with Codeine 2781
Preparation H .... ◆□ 871
Tympagesic Ear Drops 2342
Vasosulf .... ◎ 271
Vicks Sinex Nasal Spray and Ultra Fine Mist .... ◆□ 765

Phenylephrine Tannate (Possible additive atropine-like effects; careful adjustment of dosage and close supervision are required). Products include:

Atrohist Pediatric Suspension 454

Ricobid-D Pediatric Suspension 2038
Ricobid Tablets and Pediatric Suspension 2038
Rynatan 2673
Rynatuss 2673

Phenylpropanolamine Hydrochloride (Possible additive atropine-like effects; careful adjustment of dosage and close supervision are required). Products include:

Acutrim .... ◆□ 628
Allerest Children's Chewable Tablets .... ◆□ 627
Allerest 12 Hour Caplets .... ◆□ 627
Atrohist Plus Tablets 454
BC Cold Powder Multi-Symptom Formula (Cold-Sinus-Allergy) ...... ◆□ 609
BC Cold Powder Non-Drowsy Formula (Cold-Sinus) .... ◆□ 609
Cheracol Plus Head Cold/Cough Formula .... ◆□ 769
Comtrex Multi-Symptom Non-Drowsy Liqui-gels .... ◆□ 618
Contac Continuous Action Nasal Decongestant/Antihistamine 12 Hour Capsules .... ◆□ 813
Contac Maximum Strength Continuous Action Decongestant/ Antihistamine 12 Hour Caplets .. ◆□ 813
Contac Severe Cold and Flu Formula Caplets .... ◆□ 814
Coricidin 'D' Decongestant Tablets .... ◆□ 800
Dexatrim .... ◆□ 832
Dexatrim Plus Vitamins Caplets .... ◆□ 832
Dimetane-DC Cough Syrup 2059
Dimetapp Elixir .... ◆□ 773
Dimetapp Extentabs .... ◆□ 774
Dimetapp Tablets/Liqui-Gels .... ◆□ 775
Dimetapp Cold & Allergy Chewable Tablets .... ◆□ 773
Dimetapp DM Elixir .... ◆□ 774
Dura-Vent Tablets 952
Entex Capsules 1986
Entex LA Tablets 1987
Entex Liquid 1986
Exgest LA Tablets 782
Hycomine 931
Isoclor Timesule Capsules .... ◆□ 637
Nolamine Timed-Release Tablets 785
Ornade Spansule Capsules 2502
Propagest Tablets 786
Pyrroxate Caplets .... ◆□ 772
Robitussin-CF .... ◆□ 777
Sinulin Tablets 787
Tavist-D 12 Hour Relief Tablets .... ◆□ 787
Teldrin 12 Hour Antihistamine/ Nasal Decongestant Allergy Relief Capsules .... ◆□ 826
Triaminic Allergy Tablets .... ◆□ 789
Triaminic Cold Tablets .... ◆□ 790
Triaminic Expectorant .... ◆□ 790
Triaminic Syrup .... ◆□ 792
Triaminic-12 Tablets .... ◆□ 792
Triaminic-DM Syrup .... ◆□ 792
Triaminicin Tablets .... ◆□ 793
Triaminicol Multi-Symptom Cold Tablets .... ◆□ 793
Triaminicol Multi-Symptom Relief ◆□ 794
Vicks DayQuil Allergy Relief 12-Hour Extended Release Tablets .. ◆□ 760
Vicks DayQuil Allergy Relief 4-Hour Tablets .... ◆□ 760
Vicks DayQuil SINUS Pressure & CONGESTION Relief .... ◆□ 761

Phenytoin (May decrease the plasma levels of maprotiline due to hepatic enzyme induction). Products include:

Dilantin Infatabs 1908
Dilantin-125 Suspension 1911

Phenytoin Sodium (May decrease the plasma levels of maprotiline due to hepatic enzyme induction). Products include:

Dilantin Kapseals 1906
Dilantin Parenteral 1910

Pirbuterol Acetate (Possible additive atropine-like effects; careful adjustment of dosage and close supervision are required). Products include:

Maxair Autohaler 1492
Maxair Inhaler 1494

IMPORTANT NOTE: Always consult each drug listing in the patient's regimen for possible interactions.

Prazepam (The risk of seizures may be increased when the dosage of benzodiazepines is rapidly tapered in patients receiving Ludiomil or when the recommended dosage of Ludiomil is exceeded; Ludiomol may enhance the response to CNS depressants).

No products indexed under this heading.

Prochlorperazine (The risk of seizures may be increased when used concomitantly; Ludiomil may enhance the response to CNS depressants). Products include:

Compazine ... 2470

Procyclidine Hydrochloride (Possible additive atropine-like effects; careful adjustment of dosage and close supervision are required). Products include:

Kemadrin Tablets ... 1112

Promethazine Hydrochloride (The risk of seizures may be increased when used concomitantly; Ludiomil may enhance the response to CNS depressants). Products include:

Mepergan Injection ... 2753
Phenergan with Codeine ... 2777
Phenergan with Dextromethorphan 2778
Phenergan Injection ... 2773
Phenergan Suppositories ... 2775
Phenergan Syrup ... 2774
Phenergan Tablets ... 2775
Phenergan VC ... 2779
Phenergan VC with Codeine ... 2781

Propantheline Bromide (Possible additive atropine-like effects; careful adjustment of dosage and close supervision are required). Products include:

Pro-Banthīne Tablets ... 2052

Propofol (Ludiomil may enhance the response to CNS depressants). Products include:

Diprivan Injection ... 2833

Propoxyphene Hydrochloride (Ludiomil may enhance the response to CNS depressants). Products include:

Darvon ... 1435
Wygesic Tablets ... 2827

Propoxyphene Napsylate (Ludiomil may enhance the response to CNS depressants). Products include:

Darvon-N/Darvocet-N ... 1433

Pseudoephedrine Hydrochloride (Possible additive atropiine-like effects; careful adjustment of dosage and close supervision are required). Products include:

Actifed Allergy Daytime/Nighttime Caplets ... ◘ 844
Actifed Plus Caplets ... ◘ 845
Actifed Plus Tablets ... ◘ 845
Actifed with Codeine Cough Syrup.. 1067
Actifed Sinus Daytime/Nighttime Tablets and Caplets ... ◘ 846
Actifed Syrup ... ◘ 846
Actifed Tablets ... ◘ 844
Advil Cold and Sinus Caplets and Tablets (formerly CoAdvil) ... ◘ 870
Alka-Seltzer Plus Cold Medicine Liqui-Gels ... ◘ 706
Alka-Seltzer Plus Cold & Cough Medicine Liqui-Gels ... ◘ 705
Alka-Seltzer Plus Night-Time Cold Medicine Liqui-Gels ... ◘ 706
Allerest Headache Strength Tablets ... ◘ 627
Allerest Maximum Strength Tablets ... ◘ 627
Allerest No Drowsiness Tablets ... ◘ 627
Allerest Sinus Pain Formula ... ◘ 627
Anatuss LA Tablets ... 1542
Atrohist Pediatric Capsules ... 453
Bayer Select Sinus Pain Relief Formula ... ◘ 717
Benadryl Allergy Decongestant Liquid Medication ... ◘ 848
Benadryl Allergy Decongestant Tablets ... ◘ 848
Benadryl Allergy Sinus Headache Formula Caplets ... ◘ 849
Benylin Multisymptom ... ◘ 852
Bromfed Capsules (Extended-Release) ... 1785
Bromfed Syrup ... ◘ 733
Bromfed Tablets ... 1785
Bromfed-DM Cough Syrup ... 1786
Bromfed-PD Capsules (Extended-Release) ... 1785
Children's Vicks DayQuil Allergy Relief ... ◘ 757
Children's Vicks NyQuil Cold/Cough Relief ... ◘ 758
Comtrex Multi-Symptom Cold Reliever Tablets/Caplets/Liqui-Gels/Liquid ... ◘ 615
Allergy-Sinus Comtrex Multi-Symptom Allergy-Sinus Formula Tablets ... ◘ 617
Comtrex Multi-Symptom Non-Drowsy Caplets ... ◘ 618
Congess ... 1004
Contac Day Allergy/Sinus Caplets ◘ 812
Contac Day & Night ... ◘ 812
Contac Night Allergy/Sinus Caplets ... ◘ 812
Contac Severe Cold & Flu Non-Drowsy ... ◘ 815
Deconamine Chewable Tablets ... 1320
Deconamine CX Cough and Cold Liquid and Tablets ... 1319
Deconamine ... 1320
Deconsal C Expectorant Syrup ... 456
Deconsal Pediatric Syrup ... 457
Deconsal II Tablets ... 454
Dimetane-DX Cough Syrup ... 2059
Dimetapp Sinus Caplets ... ◘ 775
Dorcol Children's Cough Syrup ... ◘ 785
Drixoral Cough + Congestion Liquid Caps ... ◘ 802
Dura-Tap/PD Capsules ... 2867
Duratuss Tablets ... 2565
Duratuss HD Elixir ... 2565
Efidac/24 ... ◘ 635
Entex PSE Tablets ... 1987
Fedahist Gyrocaps ... 2401
Fedahist Timecaps ... 2401
Guaifed ... 1787
Guaifed Syrup ... ◘ 734
Guaimax-D Tablets ... 792
Guaitab Tablets ... ◘ 734
Isoclor Expectorant ... 990
Kronofed-A ... 977
Motrin IB Sinus ... ◘ 838
Novahistine DH ... 2462
Novahistine DMX ... ◘ 822
Novahistine Expectorant ... 2463
Nucofed ... 2051
PediaCare Cold Allergy Chewable Tablets ... ◘ 677
PediaCare Cough-Cold Chewable Tablets ... 1553
PediaCare ... 1553
PediaCare Infants' Decongestant Drops ... ◘ 677
PediCare Infant's Drops Decongestant Plus Cough ... 1553
PediaCare NightRest Cough-Cold Liquid ... 1553
Pediatric Vicks 44d Dry Hacking Cough & Head Congestion ... ◘ 763
Pediatric Vicks 44m Cough & Cold Relief ... ◘ 764
Robitussin Cold & Cough Liqui-Gels ... ◘ 776
Robitussin Maximum Strength Cough & Cold ... ◘ 778
Robitussin Pediatric Cough & Cold Formula ... ◘ 779
Robitussin Severe Congestion Liqui-Gels ... ◘ 776
Robitussin-DAC Syrup ... 2074
Robitussin-PE ... ◘ 778
Rondec Oral Drops ... 953
Rondec Syrup ... 953
Rondec Tablet ... 953
Rondec-DM Oral Drops ... 954
Rondec-DM Syrup ... 954
Rondec-TR Tablet ... 953
Ryna ... ◘ 841
Seldane-D Extended-Release Tablets ... 1538
Semprex-D Capsules ... 463
Semprex-D Capsules ... 1167
Sinarest Tablets ... ◘ 648
Sinarest Extra Strength Tablets ... ◘ 648
Sinarest No Drowsiness Tablets ... ◘ 648
Sine-Aid IB Caplets ... 1554
Sine-Aid Maximum Strength Sinus Medication Gelcaps, Caplets and Tablets ... 1554
Sine-Off No Drowsiness Formula Caplets ... ◘ 824
Sine-Off Sinus Medicine ... ◘ 825
Singlet Tablets ... ◘ 825
Sinutab Non-Drying Liquid Caps ... ◘ 859
Sinutab Sinus Allergy Medication, Maximum Strength Tablets and Caplets ... ◘ 860
Sinutab Sinus Medication, Maximum Strength Without Drowsiness Formula, Tablets & Caplets ... ◘ 860
Sinutab Sinus Medication, Regular Strength Without Drowsiness Formula ... ◘ 859
Sudafed Children's Liquid ... ◘ 861
Sudafed Cold and Cough Liquidcaps ... ◘ 862
Sudafed Cough Syrup ... ◘ 862
Sudafed Plus Liquid ... ◘ 862
Sudafed Plus Tablets ... ◘ 863
Sudafed Severe Cold Formula Caplets ... ◘ 863
Sudafed Severe Cold Formula Tablets ... ◘ 864
Sudafed Sinus Caplets ... ◘ 864
Sudafed Sinus Tablets ... ◘ 864
Sudafed Tablets, 30 mg ... ◘ 861
Sudafed Tablets, 60 mg ... ◘ 861
Sudafed 12 Hour Caplets ... ◘ 861
Syn-Rx Tablets ... 465
Syn-Rx DM Tablets ... 466
TheraFlu ... ◘ 787
TheraFlu Maximum Strength Nighttime Flu, Cold & Cough Medicine ... ◘ 788
TheraFlu Maximum Strength Non-Drowsy Formula Flu, Cold & Cough Medicine ... ◘ 788
Thera Flu Maximum Strength, Non-Drowsy Formula Flu, Cold and Cough Caplets ... ◘ 789
Triaminic AM Cough and Decongestant Formula ... ◘ 789
Triaminic AM Decongestant Formula ... ◘ 790
Triaminic Nite Light ... ◘ 791
Triaminic Sore Throat Formula ... ◘ 791
Tussend ... 1783
Tussend Expectorant ... 1785
Children's TYLENOL Cold Multi-Symptom Liquid Formula and Chewable Tablets ... 1561
Children's TYLENOL Cold Plus Cough Multi Symptom Tablets and Liquid ... ◘ 681
Infants' TYLENOL Cold Decongestant & Fever-Reducer Drops ... 1556
TYLENOL Maximum Strength Allergy Sinus Medication Gelcaps and Caplets ... 1563
TYLENOL Maximum Strength Allergy Sinus NightTime Medication Caplets ... 1555
TYLENOL Flu Maximum Strength Gelcaps ... 1565
TYLENOL Flu NightTime, Maximum Strength, Gelcaps ... 1566
TYLENOL Maximum Strength Flu NightTime Hot Medication Packets ... 1562
TYLENOL, Maximum Strength, Sinus Medication Geltabs, Gelcaps, Caplets and Tablets ... 1566
TYLENOL Cold Multi-Symptom Formula Medication Tablets and Caplets ... 1561
TYLENOL Cold Medication No Drowsiness Formula Gelcaps and Caplets ... 1562
TYLENOL Cold Multi-Symptom Hot Medication Liquid Packets ... 1557
TYLENOL Cough Multi-Symptom Medication with Decongestant ... 1565
Ursinus Inlay-Tabs ... ◘ 794
Vicks 44 LiquiCaps Cough, Cold & Flu Relief ... ◘ 755
Vicks 44 LiquiCaps Non-Drowsy Cough & Cold Relief ... ◘ 756
Vicks 44D Dry Hacking Cough & Head Congestion ... ◘ 755
Vicks 44M Cough, Cold & Flu Relief ... ◘ 756
Vicks DayQuil ... ◘ 761
Vicks DayQuil SINUS Pressure & PAIN Relief with IBUPROFEN ... ◘ 762
Vicks Nyquil Hot Therapy ... ◘ 762
Vicks NyQuil LiquiCaps Multi-Symptom Cold/Flu Relief ... ◘ 763
Vicks NyQuil Multi-Symptom Cold/Flu Relief - (Original & Cherry Flavor) ... ◘ 763

Pseudoephedrine Sulfate (Possible additive atropine-like effects; careful adjustment of dosage and close supervision are required). Products include:

Cheracol Sinus ... ◘ 768
Chlor-Trimeton Allergy Decongestant Tablets ... ◘ 799
Claritin-D ... 2350
Drixoral Cold and Allergy Sustained-Action Tablets ... ◘ 802
Drixoral Cold and Flu Extended-Release Tablets ... ◘ 803
Drixoral Non-Drowsy Formula Extended-Release Tablets ... ◘ 803
Drixoral Allergy/Sinus Extended Release Tablets ... ◘ 804
Trinalin Repetabs Tablets ... 1330

Quazepam (The risk of seizures may be increased when the dosage of benzodiazepines is rapidly tapered in patients receiving Ludiomil or when the recommended dosage of Ludiomil is exceeded; Ludiomol may enhance the response to CNS depressants). Products include:

Doral Tablets ... 2664

Risperidone (Ludiomil may enhance the response to CNS depressants). Products include:

Risperdal ... 1301

Salmeterol Xinafoate (Possible additive atropiine-like effects; careful adjustment of dosage and close supervision are required). Products include:

Serevent Inhalation Aerosol ... 1176

Scopolamine (Possible additive atropine-like effects; careful adjustment of dosage and close supervision are required). Products include:

Transderm Scōp Transdermal Therapeutic System ... 869

Scopolamine Hydrobromide (Possible additive atropine-like effects; careful adjustment of dosage and close supervision are required). Products include:

Atrohist Plus Tablets ... 454
Donnatal ... 2060
Donnatal Extentabs ... 2061
Donnatal Tablets ... 2060

Secobarbital Sodium (Ludiomil may enhance the response to barbiturates; certain barbiturates may decrease the plasma levels of malprotiliine due to hepatic enzyme induction). Products include:

Seconal Sodium Pulvules ... 1474

Selegiline Hydrochloride (Concurrent and/or sequential use is contraindicated). Products include:

Eldepryl Tablets ... 2550

Sufentanil Citrate (Ludiomil may enhance the response to CNS depressants). Products include:

Sufenta Injection ... 1309

Temazepam (The risk of seizures may be increased when the dosage of benzodiazepines is rapidly tapered in patients receiving Ludiomil or when the recommended dosage of Ludiomil is exceeded; Ludiomil may enhance the response to CNS depressants). Products include:

Restoril Capsules ... 2284

Terbutaline Sulfate (Possible additive atropine-like effects; careful adjustment of dosage and close supervision are required). Products include:

Brethaire Inhaler ... 813
Brethine Ampuls ... 815
Brethine Tablets ... 814
Bricanyl Subcutaneous Injection ... 1502
Bricanyl Tablets ... 1503

Thiamylal Sodium (Ludiomil may enhance the response to barbiturates; certain barbiturates may decrease the plasma levels of maprotiline due to hepatic enzyme induction).

No products indexed under this heading.

Thioridazine Hydrochloride (The risk of seizures may be increased when used concomitantly; Ludiomil may enhance the response to CNS depressants). Products include:

Mellaril 2269

Thiothixene (Ludiomil may enhance the response to CNS depressants). Products include:

Navane Capsules and Concentrate **2201**
Navane Intramuscular **2202**

Thyroglobulin (Possibility of enhanced potential for cardiovascular toxicity of Ludiomil).

No products indexed under this heading.

Thyroid (Possibility of enhanced potential for cardiovascular toxicity of Ludiomil).

No products indexed under this heading.

Thyroxine (Possibility of enhanced potential for cardiovascular toxicity of Ludiomil).

No products indexed under this heading.

Thyroxine Sodium (Possibility of enhanced potential for cardiovascular toxicity of Ludiomil).

No products indexed under this heading.

Tranylcypromine Sulfate (Concurrent and/or sequential use is contraindicated). Products include:

Parnate Tablets 2503

Triazolam (The risk of seizures may be increased when the dosage of benzodiazepines is rapidly tapered in patients receiving Ludiomil or when the recommended dosage of Ludiomil is exceeded; Ludiomol may enhance the response to CNS depressants). Products include:

Halcion Tablets.. 2611

Tridihexethyl Chloride (Possible additive atropine-like effects; careful adjustment of dosage and close supervision are required).

No products indexed under this heading.

Trifluoperazine Hydrochloride (The risk of seizures may be increased when used concomitantly; Ludiomil may enhance the response to CNS depressants). Products include:

Stelazine 2514

Trihexyphenidyl Hydrochloride (Possible additive atropine-like effects; careful adjustment of dosage and close supervision are required). Products include:

Artane... 1368

Zolpidem Tartrate (Ludiomil may enhance the response to CNS depressants). Products include:

Ambien Tablets.. 2416

Food Interactions

Alcohol (Enhanced response to alcohol).

LUFYLLIN & LUFYLLIN-400 TABLETS

(Dyphylline)...2670

May interact with sympathomimetic bronchodilators and certain other agents. Compounds in these categories include:

Albuterol (Synergism). Products include:

Proventil Inhalation Aerosol 2382
Ventolin Inhalation Aerosol and Refill 1197

Albuterol Sulfate (Synergism). Products include:

Airet Solution for Inhalation 452
Proventil Inhalation Solution 0.083% 2384
Proventil Repetabs Tablets 2386
Proventil Solution for Inhalation 0.5% 2383
Proventil Syrup....................................... 2385
Proventil Tablets 2386
Ventolin Inhalation Solution................. 1198
Ventolin Nebules Inhalation Solution... 1199
Ventolin Rotacaps for Inhalation 1200
Ventolin Syrup... 1202
Ventolin Tablets 1203
Volmax Extended-Release Tablets .. 1788

Bitolterol Mesylate (Synergism). Products include:

Tornalate Solution for Inhalation, 0.2% 956
Tornalate Metered Dose Inhaler 957

Ephedrine Hydrochloride (Synergism). Products include:

Primatene Dual Action Formula...... ⊕ 872
Primatene Tablets .... ⊕ 873
Quadrinal Tablets 1350

Ephedrine Sulfate (Synergism). Products include:

Bronkaid Caplets .... ⊕ 717
Marax Tablets & DF Syrup.................. 2200

Ephedrine Tannate (Synergism). Products include:

Rynatuss 2673

Epinephrine (Synergism). Products include:

Bronkaid Mist .... ⊕ 717
EPIFRIN .... © 239
EpiPen 790
Marcaine Hydrochloride with Epinephrine 1:200,000 2316
Primatene Mist .... ⊕ 873
Sensorcaine with Epinephrine Injection... 559
Sus-Phrine Injection 1019
Xylocaine with Epinephrine Injections... 567

Epinephrine Bitartrate (Synergism). Products include:

Bronkaid Mist Suspension .... ⊕ 718
Sensorcaine-MPF with Epinephrine Injection 559

Ethylnorepinephrine Hydrochloride (Synergism).

No products indexed under this heading.

Isoetharine (Synergism). Products include:

Bronkometer Aerosol............................ 2302
Bronkosol Solution 2302
Isoetharine Inhalation Solution, USP, Arm-a-Med................................... 551

Isoproterenol Hydrochloride (Synergism). Products include:

Isuprel Hydrochloride Injection 1:5000 2311
Isuprel Hydrochloride Solution 1:200 & 1:100 2313
Isuprel Mistometer 2312

Isoproterenol Sulfate (Synergism). Products include:

Norisodrine with Calcium Iodide Syrup... 442

Metaproterenol Sulfate (Synergism). Products include:

Alupent... 669
Metaproterenol Sulfate Inhalation Solution, USP, Arm-a-Med 552

Pirbuterol Acetate (Synergism). Products include:

Maxair Autohaler 1492
Maxair Inhaler 1494

Probenecid (Increased plasma half-life of dyphylline). Products include:

Benemid Tablets 1611
ColBENEMID Tablets 1622

Salmeterol Xinafoate (Synergism). Products include:

Serevent Inhalation Aerosol................ 1176

Terbutaline Sulfate (Synergism). Products include:

Brethaire Inhaler 813
Brethine Ampuls 815
Brethine Tablets...................................... 814
Bricanyl Subcutaneous Injection 1502
Bricanyl Tablets 1503

LUFYLLIN-GG ELIXIR & TABLETS

(Dyphylline, Guaifenesin) 2671

May interact with sympathomimetic bronchodilators and certain other agents. Compounds in these categories include:

Albuterol (Synergism). Products include:

Proventil Inhalation Aerosol 2382
Ventolin Inhalation Aerosol and Refill 1197

Albuterol Sulfate (Synergism). Products include:

Airet Solution for Inhalation 452
Proventil Inhalation Solution 0.083% 2384
Proventil Repetabs Tablets 2386
Proventil Solution for Inhalation 0.5% 2383
Proventil Syrup....................................... 2385
Proventil Tablets 2386
Ventolin Inhalation Solution................. 1198
Ventolin Nebules Inhalation Solution... 1199
Ventolin Rotacaps for Inhalation 1200
Ventolin Syrup... 1202
Ventolin Tablets 1203
Volmax Extended-Release Tablets .. 1788

Ephedrine Hydrochloride (Synergism). Products include:

Primatene Dual Action Formula...... ⊕ 872
Primatene Tablets .... ⊕ 873
Quadrinal Tablets 1350

Ephedrine Sulfate (Synergism). Products include:

Bronkaid Caplets .... ⊕ 717
Marax Tablets & DF Syrup.................. 2200

Ephedrine Tannate (Synergism). Products include:

Rynatuss 2673

Epinephrine (Synergism). Products include:

Bronkaid Mist .... ⊕ 717
EPIFRIN .... © 239
EpiPen 790
Marcaine Hydrochloride with Epinephrine 1:200,000 2316
Primatene Mist .... ⊕ 873
Sensorcaine with Epinephrine Injection... 559
Sus-Phrine Injection 1019
Xylocaine with Epinephrine Injections... 567

Epinephrine Hydrochloride (Synergism). Products include:

Ana-Kit Anaphylaxis Emergency Treatment Kit 617

Ethylnorepinephrine Hydrochloride (Synergism).

No products indexed under this heading.

Isoetharine (Synergism). Products include:

Bronkometer Aerosol............................ 2302
Bronkosol Solution 2302
Isoetharine Inhalation Solution, USP, Arm-a-Med................................... 551

Isoproterenol Hydrochloride (Synergism). Products include:

Isuprel Hydrochloride Injection 1:5000 2311
Isuprel Hydrochloride Solution 1:200 & 1:100 2313

Isuprel Mistometer 2312

Isoproterenol Sulfate (Synergism). Products include:

Norisodrine with Calcium Iodide Syrup... 442

Metaproterenol Sulfate (Synergism). Products include:

Alupent... 669
Metaproterenol Sulfate Inhalation Solution, USP, Arm-a-Med 552

Pirbuterol Acetate (Synergism). Products include:

Maxair Autohaler 1492
Maxair Inhaler 1494

Probenecid (Increased plasma half-life of dyphylline). Products include:

Benemid Tablets 1611
ColBENEMID Tablets 1622

Salmeterol Xinafoate (Synergism). Products include:

Serevent Inhalation Aerosol................ 1176

Terbutaline Sulfate (Synergism). Products include:

Brethaire Inhaler 813
Brethine Ampuls 815
Brethine Tablets...................................... 814
Bricanyl Subcutaneous Injection 1502
Bricanyl Tablets 1503

LUPRON DEPOT 3.75 MG

(Leuprolide Acetate) 2556

None cited in PDR database.

LUPRON DEPOT 7.5 MG

(Leuprolide Acetate) 2559

None cited in PDR database.

LUPRON DEPOT-PED 7.5 MG, 11.25 MG AND 15 MG

(Leuprolide Acetate) 2560

None cited in PDR database.

LUPRON INJECTION

(Leuprolide Acetate) 2555

None cited in PDR database.

LURIDE DROPS 50 ML

(Sodium Fluoride) 871

Food Interactions

Dairy products (Incompatibility of fluoride with dairy).

LURIDE LOZI-TABS TABLETS

(Sodium Fluoride) 871

Food Interactions

Dairy products (Incompatibility of fluoride with dairy foods results in the formation of poorly absorbed calcium fluoride).

LURLINE PMS TABLETS

(Acetaminophen, Pamabrom) 982

None cited in PDR database.

LUTREPULSE FOR INJECTION

(Gonadorelin Acetate) 980

May interact with ovulation stimulators. Compounds in this category include:

Chorionic Gonadotropin (Lutrepulse should not be used concomitantly with other ovulation stimulators). Products include:

Pregnyl 1828
Profasi (chorionic gonadotropin for injection, USP) 2450

Clomiphene Citrate (Lutrepulse should not be used concomitantly with other ovulation stimulators). Products include:

Clomid 1514
Serophene (clomiphene citrate tablets, USP) 2451

Menotropins (Lutrepulse should not be used concomitantly with other ovulation stimulators). Products include:

Humegon ... 1824
Pergonal (menotropins for injection, USP) ... 2448

Urofollitropin (Lutrepulse should not be used concomitantly with other ovulation stimulators). Products include:

Metrodin (urofollitropin for injection) ... 2446

LUVOX TABLETS

(Fluvoxamine Maleate) ... **2544**

May interact with monoamine oxidase inhibitors, benzodiazepines metabolized by hepatic oxidation, benzodiazepines metabolized by glucuronidation, xanthine bronchodilators, lithium preparations, tricyclic antidepressants, and certain other agents. Compounds in these categories include:

Alprazolam (Co-administration may result in reduced alprazolam clearance, pharmacokinetic parameters (AUC, C_{max}, T½) and steady state plasma concentrations of alprazolam are twice those observed when alprazolam was used alone). Products include:

Xanax Tablets ... 2649

Aminophylline (Decreased clearance of theophylline by approximately 3-fold; dose of theophylline should be reduced to one-third of the usual daily dose).

No products indexed under this heading.

Amitriptyline Hydrochloride (Potential for increased plasma tricyclic antidepressants levels). Products include:

Elavil ... 2838
Endep Tablets ... 2174
Etrafon ... 2355
Limbitrol ... 2180
Triavil Tablets ... 1757

Amoxapine (Potential for increased plasma tricyclic antidepressants levels). Products include:

Asendin Tablets ... 1369

Astemizole (Concurrent use is contraindicated; fluvoxamine may be a potent inhibitor of IIIA4 leading to the potential for QT prolongation and torsades de pointes-type ventricular tachycardia). Products include:

Hismanal Tablets ... 1293

Carbamazepine (Elevated plasma carbamazepine levels and symptoms of toxicity). Products include:

Atretol Tablets ... 573
Tegretol Chewable Tablets ... 852
Tegretol Suspension ... 852
Tegretol Tablets ... 852

Chlordiazepoxide (Potential for reduced clearance of benzodiazepines metabolized by hepatic oxidation). Products include:

Libritabs Tablets ... 2177
Limbitrol ... 2180

Chlordiazepoxide Hydrochloride (Potential for reduced clearance of benzodiazepines metabolized by hepatic oxidation). Products include:

Librax Capsules ... 2176
Librium Capsules ... 2178
Librium Injectable ... 2179

Clomipramine Hydrochloride (Potential for increased plasma tricyclic antidepressants levels). Products include:

Anafranil Capsules ... 803

Clozapine (Elevated serum levels of clozapine). Products include:

Clozaril Tablets ... 2252

Desipramine Hydrochloride (Potential for increased plasma tricyclic antidepressants levels). Products include:

Norpramin Tablets ... 1526

Diazepam (Reduced clearance of both diazepam and its active metabolite; co-administration is not advisable). Products include:

Dizac ... 1809
Valium Injectable ... 2182
Valium Tablets ... 2183
Valrelease Capsules ... 2169

Diltiazem Hydrochloride (Co-administration may produce bradycardia). Products include:

Cardizem CD Capsules ... 1506
Cardizem SR Capsules ... 1510
Cardizem Injectable ... 1508
Cardizem Tablets ... 1512
Dilacor XR Extended-release Capsules ... 2018

Doxepin Hydrochloride (Potential for increased plasma tricyclic antidepressants levels). Products include:

Sinequan ... 2205
Zonalon Cream ... 1055

Dyphylline (Decreased clearance of theophylline by approximately 3-fold; dose of theophylline should be reduced to one-third of the usual daily dose). Products include:

Lufyllin & Lufyllin-400 Tablets ... 2670
Lufyllin-GG Elixir & Tablets ... 2671

Estazolam (Potential for reduced clearance of benzodiazepines metabolized by hepatic oxidation). Products include:

ProSom Tablets ... 449

Flurazepam Hydrochloride (Potential for reduced clearance of benzodiazepines metabolized by hepatic oxidation). Products include:

Dalmane Capsules ... 2173

Furazolidone (Potential exists for serious, sometimes fatal, reactions including hyperthermia, rigidity, myoclonus, autonomic instability with possible fluctuations of vital signs, extreme agitation, and coma; concurrent and/sequential use is not recommended). Products include:

Furoxone ... 2046

Halazepam (Potential for reduced clearance of benzodiazepines metabolized by hepatic oxidation).

No products indexed under this heading.

Imipramine Hydrochloride (Potential for increased plasma tricyclic antidepressants levels). Products include:

Tofranil Ampuls ... 854
Tofranil Tablets ... 856

Imipramine Pamoate (Potential for increased plasma tricyclic antidepressants levels). Products include:

Tofranil-PM Capsules ... 857

Isocarboxazid (Potential exists for serious, sometimes fatal, reactions including hyperthermia, rigidity, myoclonus, autonomic instability with possible fluctuations of vital signs, extreme agitation, and coma; concurrent and/sequential use is not recommended).

No products indexed under this heading.

Lithium Carbonate (Potential for seizures; enhanced serotogenic effects). Products include:

Eskalith ... 2485
Lithium Carbonate Capsules & Tablets ... 2230
Lithonate/Lithotabs/Lithobid ... 2543

Lithium Citrate (Potential for seizures; enhanced serotogenic effects).

No products indexed under this heading.

Lorazepam (Possible substantial decrements in cognitive functioning; the clearance of benzodiazepines metabolized by glucuronidation is unlikely to be affected). Products include:

Ativan Injection ... 2698
Ativan Tablets ... 2700

Maprotiline Hydrochloride (Potential for increased plasma tricyclic antidepressants levels). Products include:

Ludiomil Tablets ... 843

Methadone Hydrochloride (Significantly increased methadone (plasma level:dose) ratios). Products include:

Methadone Hydrochloride Oral Concentrate ... 2233
Methadone Hydrochloride Oral Solution & Tablets ... 2235

Metoprolol Succinate (Potential for bradycardia, hypotension and orthostatic hypotension). Products include:

Toprol-XL Tablets ... 565

Metoprolol Tartrate (Potential for bradycardia, hypotension and orthostatic hypotension). Products include:

Lopressor Ampuls ... 830
Lopressor HCT Tablets ... 832
Lopressor Tablets ... 830

Midazolam Hydrochloride (Potential for reduced clearance of benzodiazepines metabolized by hepatic oxidation). Products include:

Versed Injection ... 2170

Nortriptyline Hydrochloride (Potential for increased plasma tricyclic antidepressants levels). Products include:

Pamelor ... 2280

Oxazepam (The clearance of benzodiazepines metabolized by glucuronidation is unlikely to be affected). Products include:

Serax Capsules ... 2810
Serax Tablets ... 2810

Phenelzine Sulfate (Potential exists for serious, sometimes fatal, reactions including hyperthermia, rigidity, myoclonus, autonomic instability with possible fluctuations of vital signs, extreme agitation, and coma; concurrent and/sequential use is not recommended). Products include:

Nardil ... 1920

Propranolol Hydrochloride (Potential for five-fold increase in minimum propranolol plasma concentrations; slight potentiation of the propranolol-induced reduction in heart rate and reduction in the exercise diastolic pressure). Products include:

Inderal ... 2728
Inderal LA Long Acting Capsules ... 2730
Inderide Tablets ... 2732
Inderide LA Long Acting Capsules ... 2734

Protriptyline Hydrochloride (Potential for increased plasma tricyclic antidepressants levels). Products include:

Vivactil Tablets ... 1774

Quazepam (Potential for reduced clearance of benzodiazepines metabolized by hepatic oxidation). Products include:

Doral Tablets ... 2664

Selegiline Hydrochloride (Potential exists for serious, sometimes fatal, reactions including hyperthermia, rigidity, myoclonus, autonomic instability with possible fluctuations of vital signs, extreme agitation, and coma; concurrent and/sequential use is not recommended). Products include:

Eldepryl Tablets ... 2550

Temazepam (The clearance of benzodiazepines metabolized by glucuronidation is unlikely to be affected). Products include:

Restoril Capsules ... 2284

Terfenadine (Concurrent use is contraindicated; fluvoxamine may be a potent inhibitor of IIIA4 leading to the potential for QT prolongation and torsades de pointes-type ventricular tachycardia). Products include:

Seldane Tablets ... 1536
Seldane-D Extended-Release Tablets ... 1538

Theophylline (Decreased clearance of theophylline by approximately 3-fold; dose of theophylline should be reduced to one-third of the usual daily dose). Products include:

Marax Tablets & DF Syrup ... 2200
Quibron ... 2053

Theophylline Anhydrous (Decreased clearance of theophylline by approximately 3-fold; dose of theophylline should be reduced to one-third of the usual daily dose). Products include:

Aerolate ... 1004
Primatene Dual Action Formula ... ▣ 872
Primatene Tablets ... ▣ 873
Respbid Tablets ... 682
Slo-bid Gyrocaps ... 2033
Theo-24 Extended Release Capsules ... 2568
Theo-Dur Extended-Release Tablets ... 1327
Theo-X Extended-Release Tablets ... 788
Uni-Dur Extended-Release Tablets ... 1331
Uniphyl 400 mg Tablets ... 2001

Theophylline Calcium Salicylate (Decreased clearance of theophylline by approximately 3-fold; dose of theophylline should be reduced to one-third of the usual daily dose). Products include:

Quadrinal Tablets ... 1350

Theophylline Sodium Glycinate (Decreased clearance of theophylline by approximately 3-fold; dose of theophylline should be reduced to one-third of the usual daily dose).

No products indexed under this heading.

Tranylcypromine Sulfate (Potential exists for serious, sometimes fatal, reactions including hyperthermia, rigidity, myoclonus, autonomic instability with possible fluctuations of vital signs, extreme agitation, and coma; concurrent and/sequential use is not recommended). Products include:

Parnate Tablets ... 2503

Triazolam (The clearance of benzodiazepines metabolized by glucuronidation is unlikely to be affected). Products include:

Halcion Tablets ... 2611

Trimipramine Maleate (Potential for increased plasma tricyclic antidepressants levels). Products include:

Surmontil Capsules ... 2811

L-Tryptophan (Enhances serotogenic effects; potential for severe vomiting).

No products indexed under this heading.

(▣ Described in PDR For Nonprescription Drugs) (◉ Described in PDR For Ophthalmology)

615 Interactions Index MS Contin

Warfarin Sodium (Potential for increased plasma concentrations of warfarin and prolonged prothrombin time). Products include:

Coumadin ... 926

Food Interactions

Alcohol (Concurrent use should be avoided).

LYSODREN
(Mitotane) ... 698
May interact with oral anticoagulants. Compounds in this category include:

Dicumarol (Accelerated metabolism of dicumarol).

No products indexed under this heading.

Warfarin Sodium (Accelerated metabolism of warfarin). Products include:

Coumadin ... 926

MDR FITNESS TABS FOR MEN AND WOMEN
(Vitamins with Minerals) ... 1487
None cited in PDR database.

MG 217 MEDICATED TAR SHAMPOO
(Coal Tar) ... 835
None cited in PDR database.

MG 217 MEDICATED TAR-FREE SHAMPOO
(Sulfur, Salicylic Acid) ... 835
None cited in PDR database.

MG 217 PSORIASIS OINTMENT AND LOTION
(Coal Tar) ... 835
None cited in PDR database.

MICRHOGAM RH$_O$(D) IMMUNE GLOBULIN (HUMAN)
(Immune Globulin (Human)) ... 1847
None cited in PDR database.

M-M-R II
(Measles, Mumps & Rubella Virus Vaccine Live) ... 1687
May interact with immunosuppressive agents. Compounds in this category include:

Azathioprine (Concurrent administration is contraindicated). Products include:

Imuran ... 1110

Cyclosporine (Concurrent administration is contraindicated). Products include:

Neoral ... 2276
Sandimmune ... 2286

Immune Globulin (Human) (Concurrent administration is contraindicated).

No products indexed under this heading.

Immune Globulin Intravenous (Human) (Concurrent administration is contraindicated).

Muromonab-CD3 (Concurrent administration is contraindicated). Products include:

Orthoclone OKT3 Sterile Solution .. 1837

Mycophenolate Mofetil (Concurrent administration is contraindicated). Products include:

CellCept Capsules ... 2099

Tacrolimus (Concurrent administration is contraindicated). Products include:

Prograf ... 1042

M-R-VAX II
(Measles & Rubella Virus Vaccine Live) ... 1689
May interact with immunosuppressive agents. Compounds in this category include:

Azathioprine (Concurrent administration is containdicated). Products include:

Imuran ... 1110

Cyclosporine (Concurrent administration is containdicated). Products include:

Neoral ... 2276
Sandimmune ... 2286

Immune Globulin (Human) (Concurrent administration is containdicated).

No products indexed under this heading.

Immune Globulin Intravenous (Human) (Concurrent administration is containdicated).

Muromonab-CD3 (Concurrent administration is containdicated). Products include:

Orthoclone OKT3 Sterile Solution .. 1837

Mycophenolate Mofetil (Concurrent administration is containdicated). Products include:

CellCept Capsules ... 2099

Tacrolimus (Concurrent administration is containdicated). Products include:

Prograf ... 1042

MS CONTIN TABLETS
(Morphine Sulfate) ... 1994
May interact with phenothiazines, general anesthetics, hypnotics and sedatives, tranquilizers, neuromuscular blocking agents, mixed agonist/antagonist opioid analgesics, central nervous system depressants, and certain other agents. Compounds in these categories include:

Alfentanil Hydrochloride (Profound sedation; coma; severe hypotension; respiratory depression). Products include:

Alfenta Injection ... 1286

Alprazolam (Profound sedation; coma; severe hypotension; respiratory depression). Products include:

Xanax Tablets ... 2649

Aprobarbital (Profound sedation; coma; severe hypotension; respiratory depression).

No products indexed under this heading.

Atracurium Besylate (Increased respiratory depression). Products include:

Tracrium Injection ... 1183

Buprenorphine (Mixed agonist/antagonist analgesics may reduce the analgesic effect or may precipitate withdrawal symptoms). Products include:

Buprenex Injectable ... 2006

Buspirone Hydrochloride (Profound sedation; coma; severe hypotension; respiratory depression). Products include:

BuSpar ... 737

Butabarbital (Profound sedation; coma; severe hypotension; respiratory depression).

No products indexed under this heading.

Butalbital (Profound sedation; coma; severe hypotension; respiratory depression). Products include:

Esgic-plus Tablets ... 1013
Fioricet Tablets ... 2258
Fioricet with Codeine Capsules ... 2260
Fiorinal Capsules ... 2261
Fiorinal with Codeine Capsules ... 2262
Fiorinal Tablets ... 2261
Phrenilin ... 785
Sedapap Tablets 50 mg/650 mg .. 1543

Butorphanol Tartrate (Mixed agonist/antagonist analgesics may reduce the analgesic effect or may precipitate withdrawal symptoms). Products include:

Stadol ... 775

Chlordiazepoxide (Profound sedation; coma; severe hypotension; respiratory depression). Products include:

Libritabs Tablets ... 2177
Limbitrol ... 2180

Chlordiazepoxide Hydrochloride (Profound sedation; coma; severe hypotension; respiratory depression). Products include:

Librax Capsules ... 2176
Librium Capsules ... 2178
Librium Injectable ... 2179

Chlorpromazine (Profound sedation; coma; severe hypotension; respiratory depression). Products include:

Thorazine Suppositories ... 2523

Chlorpromazine Hydrochloride (Profound sedation; coma; severe hypotension; respiratory depression). Products include:

Thorazine ... 2523

Chlorprothixene (Profound sedation; coma; severe hypotension; respiratory depression).

No products indexed under this heading.

Chlorprothixene Hydrochloride (Profound sedation; coma; severe hypotension; respiratory depression).

No products indexed under this heading.

Clorazepate Dipotassium (Profound sedation; coma; severe hypotension; respiratory depression). Products include:

Tranxene ... 451

Clozapine (Profound sedation; coma; severe hypotension; respiratory depression). Products include:

Clozaril Tablets ... 2252

Codeine Phosphate (Profound sedation; coma; severe hypotension; respiratory depression). Products include:

Actifed with Codeine Cough Syrup.. 1067
Brontex ... 1981
Deconsal C Expectorant Syrup ... 456
Deconsal Pediatric Syrup ... 457
Dimetane-DC Cough Syrup ... 2059
Empirin with Codeine Tablets ... 1093
Fioricet with Codeine Capsules ... 2260
Fiorinal with Codeine Capsules ... 2262
Isoclor Expectorant ... 990
Novahistine DH ... 2462
Novahistine Expectorant ... 2463
Nucofed ... 2051
Phenergan with Codeine ... 2777
Phenergan VC with Codeine ... 2781
Robitussin A-C Syrup ... 2073
Robitussin-DAC Syrup ... 2074
Ryna ... 841
Soma Compound w/Codeine Tablets ... 2676
Tussi-Organidin NR Liquid and S NR Liquid ... 2677
Tylenol with Codeine ... 1583

Desflurane (Profound sedation; coma; severe hypotension; respiratory depression). Products include:

Suprane ... 1813

Dezocine (Profound sedation; coma; severe hypotension; respiratory depression). Products include:

Dalgan Injection ... 538

Diazepam (Profound sedation; coma; severe hypotension; respiratory depression). Products include:

Dizac ... 1809
Valium Injectable ... 2182
Valium Tablets ... 2183
Valrelease Capsules ... 2169

Doxacurium Chloride (Increased respiratory depression). Products include:

Nuromax Injection ... 1149

Droperidol (Profound sedation; coma; severe hypotension; respiratory depression). Products include:

Inapsine Injection ... 1296

Enflurane (Profound sedation; coma; severe hypotension; respiratory depression).

No products indexed under this heading.

Estazolam (Profound sedation; coma; severe hypotension; respiratory depression). Products include:

ProSom Tablets ... 449

Ethchlorvynol (Profound sedation; coma; severe hypotension; respiratory depression). Products include:

Placidyl Capsules ... 448

Ethinamate (Profound sedation; coma; severe hypotension; respiratory depression).

No products indexed under this heading.

Fentanyl (Profound sedation; coma; severe hypotension; respiratory depression). Products include:

Duragesic Transdermal System ... 1288

Fentanyl Citrate (Profound sedation; coma; severe hypotension; respiratory depression). Products include:

Sublimaze Injection ... 1307

Fluphenazine Decanoate (Profound sedation; coma; severe hypotension; respiratory depression). Products include:

Prolixin Decanoate ... 509

Fluphenazine Enanthate (Profound sedation; coma; severe hypotension; respiratory depression). Products include:

Prolixin Enanthate ... 509

Fluphenazine Hydrochloride (Profound sedation; coma; severe hypotension; respiratory depression). Products include:

Prolixin ... 509

Flurazepam Hydrochloride (Profound sedation; coma; severe hypotension; respiratory depression). Products include:

Dalmane Capsules ... 2173

Glutethimide (Profound sedation; coma; severe hypotension; respiratory depression).

No products indexed under this heading.

Haloperidol (Profound sedation; coma; severe hypotension; respiratory depression). Products include:

Haldol Injection, Tablets and Concentrate ... 1575

Haloperidol Decanoate (Profound sedation; coma; severe hypotension; respiratory depression). Products include:

Haldol Decanoate ... 1577

Hydrocodone Bitartrate (Profound sedation; coma; severe hypotension; respiratory depression). Products include:

Anexsia 5/500 Elixir ... 1781
Anexia Tablets ... 1782
Codiclear DH Syrup ... 791
Deconamine CX Cough and Cold Liquid and Tablets ... 1319
Duratuss HD Elixir ... 2565
Hycodan Tablets and Syrup ... 930
Hycomine Compound Tablets ... 932
Hycomine ... 931
Hycotuss Expectorant Syrup ... 933
Hydrocet Capsules ... 782
Lorcet 10/650 ... 1018
Lortab ... 2566

IMPORTANT NOTE: Always consult each drug listing in the patient's regimen for possible interactions.

Tussend 1783
Tussend Expectorant 1785
Vicodin Tablets 1356
Vicodin ES Tablets 1357
Vicodin Tuss Expectorant 1358
Zydone Capsules 949

Hydrocodone Polistirex (Profound sedation; coma; severe hypotension; respiratory depression). Products include:
Tussionex Pennkinetic Extended-Release Suspension 998

Hydroxyzine Hydrochloride (Profound sedation; coma; severe hypotension; respiratory depression). Products include:
Atarax Tablets & Syrup 2185
Marax Tablets & DF Syrup 2200
Vistaril Intramuscular Solution 2216

Isoflurane (Profound sedation; coma; severe hypotension; respiratory depression).
No products indexed under this heading.

Ketamine Hydrochloride (Profound sedation; coma; severe hypotension; respiratory depression).
No products indexed under this heading.

Levomethadyl Acetate Hydrochloride (Profound sedation; coma; severe hypotension; respiratory depression). Products include:
Orlamm 2239

Levorphanol Tartrate (Profound sedation; coma; severe hypotension; respiratory depression). Products include:
Levo-Dromoran 2129

Lorazepam (Profound sedation; coma; severe hypotension; respiratory depression). Products include:
Ativan Injection 2698
Ativan Tablets 2700

Loxapine Hydrochloride (Profound sedation; coma; severe hypotension; respiratory depression). Products include:
Loxitane 1378

Loxapine Succinate (Profound sedation; coma; severe hypotension; respiratory depression). Products include:
Loxitane Capsules 1378

Meperidine Hydrochloride (Profound sedation; coma; severe hypotension; respiratory depression). Products include:
Demerol 2308
Mepergan Injection 2753

Mephobarbital (Profound sedation; coma; severe hypotension; respiratory depression). Products include:
Mebaral Tablets 2322

Meprobamate (Profound sedation; coma; severe hypotension; respiratory depression). Products include:
Miltown Tablets 2672
PMB 200 and PMB 400 2783

Mesoridazine Besylate (Profound sedation; coma; severe hypotension; respiratory depression). Products include:
Serentil 684

Methadone Hydrochloride (Profound sedation; coma; severe hypotension; respiratory depression). Products include:
Methadone Hydrochloride Oral Concentrate 2233
Methadone Hydrochloride Oral Solution & Tablets 2235

Methohexital Sodium (Profound sedation; coma; severe hypotension; respiratory depression). Products include:
Brevital Sodium Vials 1429

Methotrimeprazine (Profound sedation; coma; severe hypotension; respiratory depression). Products include:
Levoprome 1274

Methoxyflurane (Profound sedation; coma; severe hypotension; respiratory depression).
No products indexed under this heading.

Metocurine Iodide (Increased respiratory depression). Products include:
Metubine Iodide Vials 916

Midazolam Hydrochloride (Profound sedation; coma; severe hypotension; respiratory depression). Products include:
Versed Injection 2170

Mivacurium Chloride (Increased respiratory depression). Products include:
Mivacron 1138

Molindone Hydrochloride (Profound sedation; coma; severe hypotension; respiratory depression). Products include:
Moban Tablets and Concentrate 1048

Nalbuphine Hydrochloride (Mixed agonist/antagonist analgesics may reduce the analgesic effect or may precipitate withdrawal symptoms). Products include:
Nubain Injection 935

Opium Alkaloids (Profound sedation; coma; severe hypotension; respiratory depression).
No products indexed under this heading.

Oxazepam (Profound sedation; coma; severe hypotension; respiratory depression). Products include:
Serax Capsules 2810
Serax Tablets 2810

Oxycodone Hydrochloride (Profound sedation; coma; severe hypotension; respiratory depression). Products include:
Percocet Tablets 938
Percodan Tablets 939
Percodan-Demi Tablets 940
Roxicodone Tablets, Oral Solution & Intensol (Oxycodone) 2244
Tylox Capsules 1584

Pancuronium Bromide Injection (Increased respiratory depression).
No products indexed under this heading.

Pentazocine Hydrochloride (Mixed agonist/antagonist analgesics may reduce the analgesic effect or may precipitate withdrawal symptoms). Products include:
Talacen 2333
Talwin Compound 2335
Talwin Nx 2336

Pentazocine Lactate (Mixed agonist/antagonist analgesics may reduce the analgesic effect or may precipitate withdrawal symptoms). Products include:
Talwin Injection 2334

Pentobarbital Sodium (Profound sedation; coma; severe hypotension; respiratory depression). Products include:
Nembutal Sodium Capsules 436
Nembutal Sodium Solution 438
Nembutal Sodium Suppositories 440

Perphenazine (Profound sedation; coma; severe hypotension; respiratory depression). Products include:
Etrafon 2355
Triavil Tablets 1757
Trilafon 2389

Phenobarbital (Profound sedation; coma; severe hypotension; respiratory depression). Products include:
Arco-Lase Plus Tablets 512
Bellergal-S Tablets 2250
Donnatal 2060
Donnatal Extentabs 2061
Donnatal Tablets 2060
Phenobarbital Elixir and Tablets 1469
Quadrinal Tablets 1350

Prazepam (Profound sedation; coma; severe hypotension; respiratory depression).
No products indexed under this heading.

Prochlorperazine (Profound sedation; coma; severe hypotension; respiratory depression). Products include:
Compazine 2470

Promethazine Hydrochloride (Profound sedation; coma; severe hypotension; respiratory depression). Products include:
Mepergan Injection 2753
Phenergan with Codeine 2777
Phenergan with Dextromethorphan 2778
Phenergan Injection 2773
Phenergan Suppositories 2775
Phenergan Syrup 2774
Phenergan Tablets 2775
Phenergan VC 2779
Phenergan VC with Codeine 2781

Propofol (Profound sedation; coma; severe hypotension; respiratory depression). Products include:
Diprivan Injection 2833

Propoxyphene Hydrochloride (Profound sedation; coma; severe hypotension; respiratory depression). Products include:
Darvon 1435
Wygesic Tablets 2827

Propoxyphene Napsylate (Profound sedation; coma; severe hypotension; respiratory depression). Products include:
Darvon-N/Darvocet-N 1433

Quazepam (Profound sedation; coma; severe hypotension; respiratory depression). Products include:
Doral Tablets 2664

Risperidone (Profound sedation; coma; severe hypotension; respiratory depression). Products include:
Risperdal 1301

Rocuronium Bromide (Increased respiratory depression). Products include:
Zemuron 1830

Secobarbital Sodium (Profound sedation; coma; severe hypotension; respiratory depression). Products include:
Seconal Sodium Pulvules 1474

Succinylcholine Chloride (Increased respiratory depression). Products include:
Anectine 1073

Sufentanil Citrate (Profound sedation; coma; severe hypotension; respiratory depression). Products include:
Sufenta Injection 1309

Temazepam (Profound sedation; coma; severe hypotension; respiratory depression). Products include:
Restoril Capsules 2284

Thiamylal Sodium (Profound sedation; coma; severe hypotension; respiratory depression).
No products indexed under this heading.

Thioridazine Hydrochloride (Profound sedation; coma; severe hypotension; respiratory depression). Products include:
Mellaril 2269

Thiothixene (Profound sedation; coma; severe hypotension; respiratory depression). Products include:
Navane Capsules and Concentrate 2201
Navane Intramuscular 2202

Triazolam (Profound sedation; coma; severe hypotension; respiratory depression). Products include:
Halcion Tablets 2611

Trifluoperazine Hydrochloride (Profound sedation; coma; severe hypotension; respiratory depression). Products include:
Stelazine 2514

Vecuronium Bromide (Increased respiratory depression). Products include:
Norcuron 1826

Zolpidem Tartrate (Profound sedation; coma; severe hypotension; respiratory depression). Products include:
Ambien Tablets 2416

Food Interactions

Alcohol (Respiratory depression, hypotension and profound sedation or coma may result).

MSIR ORAL CAPSULES

(Morphine Sulfate) 1997
See **MSIR Oral Solution**

MSIR ORAL SOLUTION

(Morphine Sulfate) 1997
May interact with hypnotics and sedatives, general anesthetics, phenothiazines, tranquilizers, muscle relaxants, central nervous system depressants, and certain other agents. Compounds in these categories include:

Alfentanil Hydrochloride (Additive depressant effects; potential for respiratory depression, hypotension and profound sedation or coma; the dose of one or both agents should be reduced). Products include:
Alfenta Injection 1286

Alprazolam (Additive depressant effects; potential for respiratory depression, hypotension and profound sedation or coma; the dose of one or both agents should be reduced). Products include:
Xanax Tablets 2649

Aprobarbital (Additive depressant effects; potential for respiratory depression, hypotension and profound sedation or coma; the dose of one or both agents should be reduced).
No products indexed under this heading.

Atracurium Besylate (Increased respiratory depression). Products include:
Tracrium Injection 1183

Baclofen (Increased respiratory depression). Products include:
Lioresal Intrathecal 1596
Lioresal Tablets 829

Buprenorphine (Additive depressant effects; potential for respiratory depression, hypotension and profound sedation or coma; the dose of one or both agents should be reduced). Products include:
Buprenex Injectable 2006

Buspirone Hydrochloride (Additive depressant effects; potential for respiratory depression, hypotension and profound sedation or coma; the dose of one or both agents should be reduced). Products include:
BuSpar 737

Butabarbital (Additive depressant effects; potential for respiratory depression, hypotension and profound sedation or coma; the dose of one or both agents should be reduced).

No products indexed under this heading.

Butalbital (Additive depressant effects; potential for respiratory depression, hypotension and profound sedation or coma; the dose of one or both agents should be reduced). Products include:

Esgic-plus Tablets 1013
Fioricet Tablets 2258
Fioricet with Codeine Capsules 2260
Fiorinal Capsules 2261
Fiorinal with Codeine Capsules 2262
Fiorinal Tablets 2261
Phrenilin 785
Sedapap Tablets 50 mg/650 mg .. 1543

Carisoprodol (Increased respiratory depression). Products include:

Soma Compound w/Codeine Tablets 2676
Soma Compound Tablets 2675
Soma Tablets 2674

Chlordiazepoxide (Additive depressant effects; potential for respiratory depression, hypotension and profound sedation or coma; the dose of one or both agents should be reduced). Products include:

Libritabs Tablets 2177
Limbitrol 2180

Chlordiazepoxide Hydrochloride (Additive depressant effects; potential for respiratory depression, hypotension and profound sedation or coma; the dose of one or both agents should be reduced). Products include:

Librax Capsules 2176
Librium Capsules 2178
Librium Injectable 2179

Chlorpromazine (Additive depressant effects; potential for respiratory depression, hypotension and profound sedation or coma; the dose of one or both agents should be reduced). Products include:

Thorazine Suppositories 2523

Chlorpromazine Hydrochloride (Additive depressant effects; potential for respiratory depression, hypotension and profound sedation or coma; the dose of one or both agents should be reduced). Products include:

Thorazine 2523

Chlorprothixene (Additive depressant effects; potential for respiratory depression, hypotension and profound sedation or coma; the dose of one or both agents should be reduced).

No products indexed under this heading.

Chlorprothixene Hydrochloride (Additive depressant effects; potential for respiratory depression, hypotension and profound sedation or coma; the dose of one or both agents should be reduced).

No products indexed under this heading.

Chlorzoxazone (Increased respiratory depression). Products include:

Paraflex Caplets 1580
Parafon Forte DSC Caplets 1581

Clorazepate Dipotassium (Additive depressant effects; potential for respiratory depression, hypotension and profound sedation or coma; the dose of one or both agents should be reduced). Products include:

Tranxene 451

Clozapine (Additive depressant effects; potential for respiratory depression, hypotension and profound sedation or coma; the dose of one or both agents should be reduced). Products include:

Clozaril Tablets 2252

Codeine Phosphate (Additive depressant effects; potential for respiratory depression, hypotension and profound sedation or coma; the dose of one or both agents should be reduced). Products include:

Actifed with Codeine Cough Syrup.. 1067
Brontex 1981
Deconsal C Expectorant Syrup 456
Deconsal Pediatric Syrup 457
Dimetane-DC Cough Syrup 2059
Empirin with Codeine Tablets........... 1093
Fioricet with Codeine Capsules 2260
Fiorinal with Codeine Capsules 2262
Isoclor Expectorant 990
Novahistine DH 2462
Novahistine Expectorant 2463
Nucofed 2051
Phenergan with Codeine 2777
Phenergan VC with Codeine 2781
Robitussin A-C Syrup 2073
Robitussin-DAC Syrup 2074
Ryna .... ⊕ 841
Soma Compound w/Codeine Tablets 2676
Tussi-Organidin NR Liquid and S NR Liquid 2677
Tylenol with Codeine 1583

Cyclobenzaprine Hydrochloride (Increased respiratory depression). Products include:

Flexeril Tablets 1661

Dantrolene Sodium (Increased respiratory depression). Products include:

Dantrium Capsules 1982
Dantrium Intravenous 1983

Desflurane (Additive depressant effects; potential for respiratory depression, hypotension and profound sedation or coma; the dose of one or both agents should be reduced). Products include:

Suprane 1813

Dezocine (Additive depressant effects; potential for respiratory depression, hypotension and profound sedation or coma; the dose of one or both agents should be reduced). Products include:

Dalgan Injection 538

Diazepam (Additive depressant effects; potential for respiratory depression, hypotension and profound sedation or coma; the dose of one or both agents should be reduced). Products include:

Dizac 1809
Valium Injectable 2182
Valium Tablets 2183
Valrelease Capsules 2169

Doxacurium Chloride (Increased respiratory depression). Products include:

Nuromax Injection 1149

Droperidol (Additive depressant effects; potential for respiratory depression, hypotension and profound sedation or coma; the dose of one or both agents should be reduced). Products include:

Inapsine Injection 1296

Enflurane (Additive depressant effects; potential for respiratory depression, hypotension and profound sedation or coma; the dose of one or both agents should be reduced).

No products indexed under this heading.

Estazolam (Additive depressant effects; potential for respiratory depression, hypotension and profound sedation or coma; the dose of one or both agents should be reduced). Products include:

ProSom Tablets 449

Ethchlorvynol (Additive depressant effects; potential for respiratory depression, hypotension and profound sedation or coma; the dose of one or both agents should be reduced). Products include:

Placidyl Capsules 448

Ethinamate (Additive depressant effects; potential for respiratory depression, hypotension and profound sedation or coma; the dose of one or both agents should be reduced).

No products indexed under this heading.

Fentanyl (Additive depressant effects; potential for respiratory depression, hypotension and profound sedation or coma; the dose of one or both agents should be reduced). Products include:

Duragesic Transdermal System......... 1288

Fentanyl Citrate (Additive depressant effects; potential for respiratory depression, hypotension and profound sedation or coma; the dose of one or both agents should be reduced). Products include:

Sublimaze Injection 1307

Fluphenazine Decanoate (Additive depressant effects; potential for respiratory depression, hypotension and profound sedation or coma; the dose of one or both agents should be reduced). Products include:

Prolixin Decanoate 509

Fluphenazine Enanthate (Additive depressant effects; potential for respiratory depression, hypotension and profound sedation or coma; the dose of one or both agents should be reduced). Products include:

Prolixin Enanthate 509

Fluphenazine Hydrochloride (Additive depressant effects; potential for respiratory depression, hypotension and profound sedation or coma; the dose of one or both agents should be reduced). Products include:

Prolixin 509

Flurazepam Hydrochloride (Additive depressant effects; potential for respiratory depression, hypotension and profound sedation or coma; the dose of one or both agents should be reduced). Products include:

Dalmane Capsules 2173

Glutethimide (Additive depressant effects; potential for respiratory depression, hypotension and profound sedation or coma; the dose of one or both agents should be reduced).

No products indexed under this heading.

Haloperidol (Additive depressant effects; potential for respiratory depression, hypotension and profound sedation or coma; the dose of one or both agents should be reduced). Products include:

Haldol Injection, Tablets and Concentrate 1575

Haloperidol Decanoate (Additive depressant effects; potential for respiratory depression, hypotension and profound sedation or coma; the dose of one or both agents should be reduced). Products include:

Haldol Decanoate 1577

Hydrocodone Bitartrate (Additive depressant effects; potential for respiratory depression, hypotension and profound sedation or coma; the dose of one or both agents should be reduced). Products include:

Anexsia 5/500 Elixir 1781
Anexia Tablets 1782
Codiclear DH Syrup 791
Deconamine CX Cough and Cold Liquid and Tablets 1319
Duratuss HD Elixir 2565
Hycodan Tablets and Syrup 930
Hycomine Compound Tablets 932
Hycomine 931
Hycotuss Expectorant Syrup 933
Hydrocet Capsules 782
Lorcet 10/650 1018
Lortab 2566
Tussend 1783
Tussend Expectorant 1785
Vicodin Tablets 1356
Vicodin ES Tablets 1357
Vicodin Tuss Expectorant 1358
Zydone Capsules 949

Hydrocodone Polistirex (Additive depressant effects; potential for respiratory depression, hypotension and profound sedation or coma; the dose of one or both agents should be reduced). Products include:

Tussionex Pennkinetic Extended-Release Suspension 998

Hydroxyzine Hydrochloride (Additive depressant effects; potential for respiratory depression, hypotension and profound sedation or coma; the dose of one or both agents should be reduced). Products include:

Atarax Tablets & Syrup 2185
Marax Tablets & DF Syrup 2200
Vistaril Intramuscular Solution 2216

Isoflurane (Additive depressant effects; potential for respiratory depression, hypotension and profound sedation or coma; the dose of one or both agents should be reduced).

No products indexed under this heading.

Ketamine Hydrochloride (Additive depressant effects; potential for respiratory depression, hypotension and profound sedation or coma; the dose of one or both agents should be reduced).

No products indexed under this heading.

Levomethadyl Acetate Hydrochloride (Additive depressant effects; potential for respiratory depression, hypotension and profound sedation or coma; the dose of one or both agents should be reduced). Products include:

Orlamm 2239

Levorphanol Tartrate (Additive depressant effects; potential for respiratory depression, hypotension and profound sedation or coma; the dose of one or both agents should be reduced). Products include:

Levo-Dromoran 2129

Lorazepam (Additive depressant effects; potential for respiratory depression, hypotension and profound sedation or coma; the dose of one or both agents should be reduced). Products include:

Ativan Injection 2698
Ativan Tablets 2700

IMPORTANT NOTE: Always consult each drug listing in the patient's regimen for possible interactions.

MSIR Interactions Index 618

Loxapine Hydrochloride (Additive depressant effects; potential for respiratory depression, hypotension and profound sedation or coma; the dose of one or both agents should be reduced). Products include:
Loxitane 1378
Loxapine Succinate (Additive depressant effects; potential for respiratory depression, hypotension and profound sedation or coma; the dose of one or both agents should be reduced). Products include:
Loxitane Capsules 1378
Meperidine Hydrochloride (Additive depressant effects; potential for respiratory depression, hypotension and profound sedation or coma; the dose of one or both agents should be reduced). Products include:
Demerol 2308
Mepergan Injection 2753
Mephobarbital (Additive depressant effects; potential for respiratory depression, hypotension and profound sedation or coma; the dose of one or both agents should be reduced). Products include:
Mebaral Tablets 2322
Meprobamate (Additive depressant effects; potential for respiratory depression, hypotension and profound sedation or coma; the dose of one or both agents should be reduced). Products include:
Miltown Tablets 2672
PMB 200 and PMB 400 2783
Mesoridazine (Additive depressant effects; potential for respiratory depression, hypotension and profound sedation or coma; the dose of one or both agents should be reduced).
Mesoridazine Besylate (Additive depressant effects; potential for respiratory depression, hypotension and profound sedation or coma; the dose of one or both agents should be reduced). Products include:
Serentil 684
Metaxalone (Increased respiratory depression). Products include:
Skelaxin Tablets 788
Methadone Hydrochloride (Additive depressant effects; potential for respiratory depression, hypotension and profound sedation or coma; the dose of one or both agents should be reduced). Products include:
Methadone Hydrochloride Oral Concentrate 2233
Methadone Hydrochloride Oral Solution & Tablets 2235
Methocarbamol (Increased respiratory depression). Products include:
Robaxin Injectable 2070
Robaxin Tablets 2071
Robaxisal Tablets 2071
Methohexital Sodium (Additive depressant effects; potential for respiratory depression, hypotension and profound sedation or coma; the dose of one or both agents should be reduced). Products include:
Brevital Sodium Vials 1429
Methotrimeprazine (Additive depressant effects; potential for respiratory depression, hypotension and profound sedation or coma; the dose of one or both agents should be reduced). Products include:
Levoprome 1274
Methoxyflurane (Additive depressant effects; potential for respiratory depression, hypotension and profound sedation or coma; the dose of one or both agents should be reduced).
No products indexed under this heading.
Metocurine Iodide (Increased respiratory depression). Products include:
Metubine Iodide Vials 916
Midazolam Hydrochloride (Additive depressant effects; potential for respiratory depression, hypotension and profound sedation or coma; the dose of one or both agents should be reduced). Products include:
Versed Injection 2170
Mivacurium Chloride (Increased respiratory depression). Products include:
Mivacron 1138
Molindone Hydrochloride (Additive depressant effects; potential for respiratory depression, hypotension and profound sedation or coma; the dose of one or both agents should be reduced). Products include:
Moban Tablets and Concentrate 1048
Opium Alkaloids (Additive depressant effects; potential for respiratory depression, hypotension and profound sedation or coma; the dose of one or both agents should be reduced).
No products indexed under this heading.
Orphenadrine Citrate (Increased respiratory depression). Products include:
Norflex 1496
Norgesic 1496
Oxazepam (Additive depressant effects; potential for respiratory depression, hypotension and profound sedation or coma; the dose of one or both agents should be reduced). Products include:
Serax Capsules 2810
Serax Tablets 2810
Oxycodone Hydrochloride (Additive depressant effects; potential for respiratory depression, hypotension and profound sedation or coma; the dose of one or both agents should be reduced). Products include:
Percocet Tablets 938
Percodan Tablets 939
Percodan-Demi Tablets 940
Roxicodone Tablets, Oral Solution & Intensol (Oxycodone) 2244
Tylox Capsules 1584
Pancuronium Bromide Injection (Increased respiratory depression).
No products indexed under this heading.
Pentazocine Hydrochloride (Reduced analgesic effect; precipitation of withdrawal). Products include:
Talacen 2333
Talwin Compound 2335
Talwin Nx 2336
Pentazocine Lactate (Reduced analgesic effect; precipitation of withdrawal). Products include:
Talwin Injection 2334
Pentobarbital Sodium (Additive depressant effects; potential for respiratory depression, hypotension and profound sedation or coma; the dose of one or both agents should be reduced). Products include:
Nembutal Sodium Capsules 436
Nembutal Sodium Solution 438
Nembutal Sodium Suppositories 440
Perphenazine (Additive depressant effects; potential for respiratory depression, hypotension and profound sedation or coma; the dose of one or both agents should be reduced). Products include:
Etrafon 2355
Triavil Tablets 1757
Trilafon 2389
Phenobarbital (Additive depressant effects; potential for respiratory depression, hypotension and profound sedation or coma; the dose of one or both agents should be reduced). Products include:
Arco-Lase Plus Tablets 512
Bellergal-S Tablets 2250
Donnatal 2060
Donnatal Extentabs 2061
Donnatal Tablets 2060
Phenobarbital Elixir and Tablets 1469
Quadrinal Tablets 1350
Prazepam (Additive depressant effects; potential for respiratory depression, hypotension and profound sedation or coma; the dose of one or both agents should be reduced).
No products indexed under this heading.
Prochlorperazine (Additive depressant effects; potential for respiratory depression, hypotension and profound sedation or coma; the dose of one or both agents should be reduced). Products include:
Compazine 2470
Promethazine Hydrochloride (Additive depressant effects; potential for respiratory depression, hypotension and profound sedation or coma; the dose of one or both agents should be reduced). Products include:
Mepergan Injection 2753
Phenergan with Codeine 2777
Phenergan with Dextromethorphan 2778
Phenergan Injection 2773
Phenergan Suppositories 2775
Phenergan Syrup 2774
Phenergan Tablets 2775
Phenergan VC 2779
Phenergan VC with Codeine 2781
Propofol (Additive depressant effects; potential for respiratory depression, hypotension and profound sedation or coma; the dose of one or both agents should be reduced). Products include:
Diprivan Injection 2833
Propoxyphene Hydrochloride (Additive depressant effects; potential for respiratory depression, hypotension and profound sedation or coma; the dose of one or both agents should be reduced). Products include:
Darvon 1435
Wygesic Tablets 2827
Propoxyphene Napsylate (Additive depressant effects; potential for respiratory depression, hypotension and profound sedation or coma; the dose of one or both agents should be reduced). Products include:
Darvon-N/Darvocet-N 1433
Quazepam (Additive depressant effects; potential for respiratory depression, hypotension and profound sedation or coma; the dose of one or both agents should be reduced). Products include:
Doral Tablets 2664
Risperidone (Additive depressant effects; potential for respiratory depression, hypotension and profound sedation or coma; the dose of one or both agents should be reduced). Products include:
Risperdal 1301
Rocuronium Bromide (Increased respiratory depression). Products include:
Zemuron 1830
Secobarbital Sodium (Additive depressant effects; potential for respiratory depression, hypotension and profound sedation or coma; the dose of one or both agents should be reduced). Products include:
Seconal Sodium Pulvules 1474
Succinylcholine Chloride (Increased respiratory depression). Products include:
Anectine 1073
Sufentanil Citrate (Additive depressant effects; potential for respiratory depression, hypotension and profound sedation or coma; the dose of one or both agents should be reduced). Products include:
Sufenta Injection 1309
Temazepam (Additive depressant effects; potential for respiratory depression, hypotension and profound sedation or coma; the dose of one or both agents should be reduced). Products include:
Restoril Capsules 2284
Thiamylal Sodium (Additive depressant effects; potential for respiratory depression, hypotension and profound sedation or coma; the dose of one or both agents should be reduced).
No products indexed under this heading.
Thioridazine Hydrochloride (Additive depressant effects; potential for respiratory depression, hypotension and profound sedation or coma; the dose of one or both agents should be reduced). Products include:
Mellaril 2269
Thiothixene (Additive depressant effects; potential for respiratory depression, hypotension and profound sedation or coma; the dose of one or both agents should be reduced). Products include:
Navane Capsules and Concentrate 2201
Navane Intramuscular 2202
Triazolam (Additive depressant effects; potential for respiratory depression, hypotension and profound sedation or coma; the dose of one or both agents should be reduced). Products include:
Halcion Tablets 2611
Trifluoperazine Hydrochloride (Additive depressant effects; potential for respiratory depression, hypotension and profound sedation or coma; the dose of one or both agents should be reduced). Products include:
Stelazine 2514
Vecuronium Bromide (Increased respiratory depression). Products include:
Norcuron 1826
Zolpidem Tartrate (Additive depressant effects; potential for respiratory depression, hypotension and profound sedation or coma; the dose of one or both agents should be reduced). Products include:
Ambien Tablets 2416

(▭ Described in PDR For Nonprescription Drugs) (◉ Described in PDR For Ophthalmology)

619 Interactions Index Maalox Antacid Caplets

Food Interactions

Alcohol (Additive depressant effects; potential for respiratory depression, hypotension and profound sedation or coma).

MSIR ORAL SOLUTION CONCENTRATE
(Morphine Sulfate) 1997
See **MSIR Oral Solution**

MSIR TABLETS
(Morphine Sulfate) 1997
See **MSIR Oral Solution**

MZM
(Methazolamide) .... ⊙ 267
May interact with corticosteroids and certain other agents. Compounds in these categories include:

Aspirin (Concurrent use with high dose aspirin may result in anorexia, tachypnea, lethargy, coma and death). Products include:
- Alka-Seltzer Effervescent Antacid and Pain Reliever .... ▣ 701
- Alka-Seltzer Extra Strength Effervescent Antacid and Pain Reliever .... ▣ 703
- Alka-Seltzer Lemon Lime Effervescent Antacid and Pain Reliever .... ▣ 703
- Alka-Seltzer Plus Cold Medicine .... ▣ 705
- Alka-Seltzer Plus Cold & Cough Medicine .... ▣ 708
- Alka-Seltzer Plus Night-Time Cold Medicine .... ▣ 707
- Alka Seltzer Plus Sinus Medicine .... ▣ 707
- Arthritis Foundation Safety Coated Aspirin Tablets .... ▣ 675
- Arthritis Pain Ascriptin .... ▣ 631
- Maximum Strength Ascriptin .... ▣ 630
- Regular Strength Ascriptin Tablets .... ▣ 629
- Arthritis Strength BC Powder .... ▣ 609
- BC Cold Powder Multi-Symptom Formula (Cold-Sinus-Allergy) .... ▣ 609
- BC Cold Powder Non-Drowsy Formula (Cold-Sinus) .... ▣ 609
- BC Powder .... ▣ 609
- Bayer Children's Chewable Aspirin .... ▣ 711
- Genuine Bayer Aspirin Tablets & Caplets .... ▣ 713
- Extra Strength Bayer Arthritis Pain Regimen Formula .... ▣ 711
- Extra Strength Bayer Aspirin Caplets & Tablets .... ▣ 712
- Extended-Release Bayer 8-Hour Aspirin .... ▣ 712
- Extra Strength Bayer Plus Aspirin Caplets .... ▣ 713
- Extra Strength Bayer PM Aspirin .... ▣ 713
- Bayer Enteric Aspirin .... ▣ 709
- Bufferin Analgesic Tablets and Caplets .... ▣ 613
- Arthritis Strength Bufferin Analgesic Caplets .... ▣ 614
- Extra Strength Bufferin Analgesic Tablets .... ▣ 615
- Cama Arthritis Pain Reliever .... ▣ 785
- Darvon Compound-65 Pulvules 1435
- Easprin 1914
- Ecotrin 2455
- Ecotrin Enteric Coated Aspirin Maximum Strength Tablets and Caplets .... ▣ 816
- Ecotrin Enteric Coated Aspirin Regular Strength Tablets 2455
- Empirin Aspirin Tablets .... ▣ 854
- Empirin with Codeine Tablets 1093
- Excedrin Extra-Strength Analgesic Tablets & Caplets 732
- Fiorinal Capsules 2261
- Fiorinal with Codeine Capsules 2262
- Fiorinal Tablets 2261
- Halfprin 1362
- Healthprin Aspirin 2455
- Norgesic 1496
- Percodan Tablets 939
- Percodan-Demi Tablets 940
- Robaxisal Tablets 2071
- Soma Compound w/Codeine Tablets 2676
- Soma Compound Tablets 2675
- St. Joseph Adult Chewable Aspirin (81 mg.) .... ▣ 808
- Talwin Compound 2335
- Ursinus Inlay-Tabs .... ▣ 794
- Vanquish Analgesic Caplets .... ▣ 731

Betamethasone Acetate (Potential for developing hypokalemia). Products include:
- Celestone Soluspan Suspension 2347

Betamethasone Sodium Phosphate (Potential for developing hypokalemia). Products include:
- Celestone Soluspan Suspension 2347

Cortisone Acetate (Potential for developing hypokalemia). Products include:
- Cortone Acetate Sterile Suspension 1623
- Cortone Acetate Tablets 1624

Dexamethasone (Potential for developing hypokalemia). Products include:
- AK-Trol Ointment & Suspension .... ⊙ 205
- Decadron Elixir 1633
- Decadron Tablets 1635
- Decaspray Topical Aerosol 1648
- Dexacidin Ointment .... ⊙ 263
- Maxitrol Ophthalmic Ointment and Suspension .... ⊙ 224
- TobraDex Ophthalmic Suspension and Ointment 473

Dexamethasone Acetate (Potential for developing hypokalemia). Products include:
- Dalalone D.P. Injectable 1011
- Decadron-LA Sterile Suspension 1646

Dexamethasone Sodium Phosphate (Potential for developing hypokalemia). Products include:
- Decadron Phosphate Injection 1637
- Decadron Phosphate Respihaler 1642
- Decadron Phosphate Sterile Ophthalmic Ointment 1641
- Decadron Phosphate Sterile Ophthalmic Solution 1642
- Decadron Phosphate Topical Cream 1644
- Decadron Phosphate Turbinaire 1645
- Decadron Phosphate with Xylocaine Injection, Sterile 1639
- Dexacort Phosphate in Respihaler .. 458
- Dexacort Phosphate in Turbinaire .. 459
- NeoDecadron Sterile Ophthalmic Ointment 1712
- NeoDecadron Sterile Ophthalmic Solution 1713
- NeoDecadron Topical Cream 1714

Fludrocortisone Acetate (Potential for developing hypokalemia). Products include:
- Florinef Acetate Tablets 505

Hydrocortisone (Potential for developing hypokalemia). Products include:
- Anusol-HC Cream 2.5% 1896
- Aquanil HC Lotion 1931
- Bactine Hydrocortisone Anti-Itch Cream .... ▣ 709
- Caldecort Anti-Itch Hydrocortisone Spray .... ▣ 631
- Cortaid .... ▣ 836
- CORTENEMA 2535
- Cortisporin Ointment 1085
- Cortisporin Ophthalmic Ointment Sterile 1085
- Cortisporin Ophthalmic Suspension Sterile 1086
- Cortisporin Otic Solution Sterile 1087
- Cortisporin Otic Suspension Sterile 1088
- Cortizone-5 .... ▣ 831
- Cortizone-10 .... ▣ 831
- Hydrocortone Tablets 1672
- Hytone 907
- Massengill Medicated Soft Cloth Towelettes 2458
- PediOtic Suspension Sterile 1153
- Preparation H Hydrocortisone 1% Cream .... ▣ 872
- ProctoCream-HC 2.5% 2408
- VōSoL HC Otic Solution 2678

Hydrocortisone Acetate (Potential for developing hypokalemia). Products include:
- Analpram-HC Rectal Cream 1% and 2.5% 977
- Anusol HC-1 Anti-Itch Hydrocortisone Ointment .... ▣ 847
- Anusol-HC Suppositories 1897
- Caldecort .... ▣ 631
- Carmol HC 924
- Coly-Mycin S Otic w/Neomycin & Hydrocortisone 1906
- Cortaid .... ▣ 836
- Cortifoam 2396
- Cortisporin Cream 1084
- Epifoam 2399
- Hydrocortone Acetate Sterile Suspension 1669
- Mantadil Cream 1135
- Nupercainal Hydrocortisone 1% Cream .... ▣ 645
- Ophthocort .... ⊙ 311
- Pramosone Cream, Lotion & Ointment 978
- ProctoCream-HC 2408
- ProctoFoam-HC 2409
- Terra-Cortril Ophthalmic Suspension 2210

Hydrocortisone Sodium Phosphate (Potential for developing hypokalemia). Products include:
- Hydrocortone Phosphate Injection, Sterile 1670

Hydrocortisone Sodium Succinate (Potential for developing hypokalemia). Products include:
- Solu-Cortef Sterile Powder 2641

Methylprednisolone Acetate (Potential for developing hypokalemia). Products include:
- Depo-Medrol Single-Dose Vial 2600
- Depo-Medrol Sterile Aqueous Suspension 2597

Methylprednisolone Sodium Succinate (Potential for developing hypokalemia). Products include:
- Solu-Medrol Sterile Powder 2643

Prednisolone Acetate (Potential for developing hypokalemia). Products include:
- AK-CIDE .... ⊙ 202
- AK-CIDE Ointment .... ⊙ 202
- Blephamide Liquifilm Sterile Ophthalmic Suspension 476
- Blephamide Ointment .... ⊙ 237
- Econopred & Econopred Plus Ophthalmic Suspensions .... ⊙ 217
- Poly-Pred Liquifilm .... ⊙ 248
- Pred Forte .... ⊙ 250
- Pred Mild .... ⊙ 253
- Pred-G Liquifilm Sterile Ophthalmic Suspension .... ⊙ 251
- Pred-G S.O.P. Sterile Ophthalmic Ointment .... ⊙ 252
- Vasocidin Ointment .... ⊙ 268

Prednisolone Sodium Phosphate (Potential for developing hypokalemia). Products include:
- AK-Pred .... ⊙ 204
- Hydeltrasol Injection, Sterile 1665
- Inflamase .... ⊙ 265
- Pediapred Oral Liquid 995
- Vasocidin Ophthalmic Solution .... ⊙ 270

Prednisolone Tebutate (Potential for developing hypokalemia). Products include:
- Hydeltra-T.B.A. Sterile Suspension 1667

Prednisone (Potential for developing hypokalemia). Products include:
- Deltasone Tablets 2595

Triamcinolone (Potential for developing hypokalemia). Products include:
- Aristocort Tablets 1022

Triamcinolone Acetonide (Potential for developing hypokalemia). Products include:
- Aristocort A 0.025% Cream 1027
- Aristocort A 0.5% Cream 1031
- Aristocort A 0.1% Cream 1029
- Aristocort A 0.1% Ointment 1030
- Azmacort Oral Inhaler 2011
- Nasacort Nasal Inhaler 2024

Triamcinolone Diacetate (Potential for developing hypokalemia). Products include:
- Aristocort Suspension (Forte Parenteral) 1027
- Aristocort Suspension (Intralesional) 1025

Triamcinolone Hexacetonide (Potential for developing hypokalemia). Products include:
- Aristospan Suspension (Intra-articular) 1033
- Aristospan Suspension (Intralesional) 1032

MAALOX ANTACID CAPLETS
(Calcium Carbonate) .... ▣ 638
May interact with beta blockers, thiazides, and certain other agents. Compounds in these categories include:

Acebutolol Hydrochloride (Decreased absorption of beta blockers). Products include:
- Sectral Capsules 2807

Atenolol (Decreased absorption of beta blockers). Products include:
- Tenoretic Tablets 2845
- Tenormin Tablets and I.V. Injection 2847

Bendroflumethiazide (Can cause hypercalcemia).
- No products indexed under this heading.

Betaxolol Hydrochloride (Decreased absorption of beta blockers). Products include:
- Betoptic Ophthalmic Solution 469
- Betoptic S Ophthalmic Suspension 471
- Kerlone Tablets 2436

Bisoprolol Fumarate (Decreased absorption of beta blockers). Products include:
- Zebeta Tablets 1413
- Ziac 1415

Carteolol Hydrochloride (Decreased absorption of beta blockers). Products include:
- Cartrol Tablets 410
- Ocupress Ophthalmic Solution, 1% Sterile .... ⊙ 309

Chlorothiazide (Can cause hypercalcemia). Products include:
- Aldoclor Tablets 1598
- Diupres Tablets 1650
- Diuril Oral 1653

Chlorothiazide Sodium (Can cause hypercalcemia). Products include:
- Diuril Sodium Intravenous 1652

Esmolol Hydrochloride (Decreased absorption of beta blockers). Products include:
- Brevibloc Injection 1808

Hydrochlorothiazide (Can cause hypercalcemia). Products include:
- Aldactazide 2413
- Aldoril Tablets 1604
- Apresazide Capsules 808
- Capozide 742
- Dyazide 2479
- Esidrix Tablets 821
- Esimil Tablets 822
- HydroDIURIL Tablets 1674
- Hydropres Tablets 1675
- Hyzaar Tablets 1677
- Inderide Tablets 2732
- Inderide LA Long Acting Capsules .. 2734
- Lopressor HCT Tablets 832
- Lotensin HCT 837
- Maxzide 1380
- Moduretic Tablets 1705
- Oretic Tablets 443
- Prinzide Tablets 1737
- Ser-Ap-Es Tablets 849
- Timolide Tablets 1748
- Vaseretic Tablets 1765
- Zestoretic 2850
- Ziac 1415

Hydroflumethiazide (Can cause hypercalcemia). Products include:
- Diucardin Tablets 2718

Labetalol Hydrochloride (Decreased absorption of beta blockers). Products include:
- Normodyne Injection 2377
- Normodyne Tablets 2379
- Trandate 1185

IMPORTANT NOTE: Always consult each drug listing in the patient's regimen for possible interactions.

Maalox Antacid Caplets

Levobunolol Hydrochloride (Decreased absorption of beta blockers). Products include:

Betagan .... ◉ 233

Methylclothiazide (Can cause hypercalcemia). Products include:

Enduron Tablets...................................... 420

Metipranolol Hydrochloride (Decreased absorption of beta blockers). Products include:

OptiPranolol (Metipranolol 0.3%) Sterile Ophthalmic Solution......... ◉ 258

Metoprolol Succinate (Decreased absorption of beta blockers). Products include:

Toprol-XL Tablets 565

Metoprolol Tartrate (Decreased absorption of beta blockers). Products include:

Lopressor Ampuls 830
Lopressor HCT Tablets 832
Lopressor Tablets 830

Nadolol (Decreased absorption of beta blockers).

No products indexed under this heading.

Penbutolol Sulfate (Decreased absorption of beta blockers). Products include:

Levatol 2403

Phenytoin (Decreased absorption of phenytoin). Products include:

Dilantin Infatabs 1908
Dilantin-125 Suspension 1911

Phenytoin Sodium (Decreased absorption of phenytoin). Products include:

Dilantin Kapseals 1906
Dilantin Parenteral 1910

Pindolol (Decreased absorption of beta blockers). Products include:

Visken Tablets.. 2299

Polythiazide (Can cause hypercalcemia). Products include:

Minizide Capsules 1938

Prescription Drugs, unspecified (Antacids may interact with certain unspecified prescription drugs).

Propranolol Hydrochloride (Decreased absorption of beta blockers). Products include:

Inderal 2728
Inderal LA Long Acting Capsules 2730
Inderide Tablets 2732
Inderide LA Long Acting Capsules .. 2734

Sotalol Hydrochloride (Decreased absorption of beta blockers). Products include:

Betapace Tablets 641

Timolol Hemihydrate (Decreased absorption of beta blockers). Products include:

Betimol 0.25%, 0.5% .... ◉ 261

Timolol Maleate (Decreased absorption of beta blockers). Products include:

Blocadren Tablets 1614
Timolide Tablets..................................... 1748
Timoptic in Ocudose 1753
Timoptic Sterile Ophthalmic Solution... 1751
Timoptic-XE 1755

Food Interactions

Dairy products (Concurrent prolonged use with homogenized milk containing Vitamin D may result in the milk-alkali syndrome).

MAALOX ANTI-DIARRHEAL CAPLETS

(Loperamide Hydrochloride) ....ⓂⒹ 640

May interact with:

Antibiotics, unspecified (Effect not specified; consult your doctor).

MAALOX ANTI-DIARRHEAL ORAL SOLUTION

(Loperamide Hydrochloride) ....ⓂⒹ 639

May interact with:

Antibiotics, unspecified (Effect not specified; consult your doctor).

MAALOX ANTI-GAS TABLETS, REGULAR STRENGTH

(Simethicone) ....ⓂⒹ 640

None cited in PDR database.

MAALOX ANTI-GAS TABLETS, EXTRA STRENGTH

(Simethicone) ....ⓂⒹ 640

None cited in PDR database.

MAALOX DAILY FIBER THERAPY

(Psyllium Preparations) ....ⓂⒹ 641

None cited in PDR database.

MAALOX HEARTBURN RELIEF SUSPENSION

(Aluminum Hydroxide, Magnesium Carbonate) ....ⓂⒹ 642

May interact with:

Prescription Drugs, unspecified (Effect of concurrent use with unspecified prescription drugs not cited).

MAALOX HEARTBURN RELIEF TABLETS

(Aluminum Hydroxide, Magnesium Carbonate) ....ⓂⒹ 641

May interact with:

Prescription Drugs, unspecified (Effect of concurrent use with unspecified prescription drugs not cited).

MAALOX MAGNESIA AND ALUMINA ORAL SUSPENSION

(Magnesium Hydroxide, Aluminum Hydroxide) ....ⓂⒹ 642

May interact with:

Prescription Drugs, unspecified (Antacids may interact with certain unspecified prescription drugs).

MAALOX PLUS TABLETS

(Aluminum Hydroxide, Magnesium Hydroxide, Simethicone) ....ⓂⒹ 643

May interact with tetracyclines and certain other agents. Compounds in these categories include:

Demeclocycline Hydrochloride (Concurrent use with any form of tetracycline should be avoided). Products include:

Declomycin Tablets................................ 1371

Doxycycline Calcium (Concurrent use with any form of tetracycline should be avoided). Products include:

Vibramycin Calcium Oral Suspension Syrup... 1941

Doxycycline Hyclate (Concurrent use with any form of tetracycline should be avoided). Products include:

Doryx Capsules....................................... 1913
Vibramycin Hyclate Capsules 1941
Vibramycin Hyclate Intravenous 2215
Vibra-Tabs Film Coated Tablets 1941

Doxycycline Monohydrate (Concurrent use with any form of tetracycline should be avoided). Products include:

Monodox Capsules 1805
Vibramycin Monohydrate for Oral Suspension 1941

Methacycline Hydrochloride (Concurrent use with any form of tetracycline should be avoided).

No products indexed under this heading.

Minocycline Hydrochloride (Concurrent use with any form of tetracycline should be avoided). Products include:

Dynacin Capsules 1590
Minocin Intravenous 1382
Minocin Oral Suspension 1385
Minocin Pellet-Filled Capsules 1383

Oxytetracycline Hydrochloride (Concurrent use with any form of tetracycline should be avoided). Products include:

TERAK Ointment .... ◉ 209
Terra-Cortril Ophthalmic Suspension 2210
Terramycin with Polymyxin B Sulfate Ophthalmic Ointment 2211
Urobiotic-250 Capsules 2214

Prescription Drugs, unspecified (Antacids may interfere with certain unspecified prescription drugs; resulting effect not specified).

Tetracycline Hydrochloride (Concurrent use with any form of tetracycline should be avoided). Products include:

Achromycin V Capsules 1367

EXTRA STRENGTH MAALOX ANTACID PLUS ANTIGAS LIQUID AND TABLETS

(Aluminum Hydroxide, Magnesium Hydroxide, Simethicone) ....ⓂⒹ 638

May interact with tetracyclines and certain other agents. Compounds in these categories include:

Demeclocycline Hydrochloride (Concurrent use with any form of tetracycline should be avoided). Products include:

Declomycin Tablets................................ 1371

Doxycycline Calcium (Concurrent use with any form of tetracycline should be avoided). Products include:

Vibramycin Calcium Oral Suspension Syrup... 1941

Doxycycline Hyclate (Concurrent use with any form of tetracycline should be avoided). Products include:

Doryx Capsules....................................... 1913
Vibramycin Hyclate Capsules 1941
Vibramycin Hyclate Intravenous 2215
Vibra-Tabs Film Coated Tablets 1941

Doxycycline Monohydrate (Concurrent use with any form of tetracycline should be avoided). Products include:

Monodox Capsules 1805
Vibramycin Monohydrate for Oral Suspension 1941

Methacycline Hydrochloride (Concurrent use with any form of tetracycline should be avoided).

No products indexed under this heading.

Minocycline Hydrochloride (Concurrent use with any form of tetracycline should be avoided). Products include:

Dynacin Capsules 1590
Minocin Intravenous 1382
Minocin Oral Suspension 1385
Minocin Pellet-Filled Capsules 1383

Oxytetracycline Hydrochloride (Concurrent use with any form of tetracycline should be avoided). Products include:

TERAK Ointment .... ◉ 209
Terra-Cortril Ophthalmic Suspension 2210
Terramycin with Polymyxin B Sulfate Ophthalmic Ointment 2211
Urobiotic-250 Capsules 2214

Prescription Drugs, unspecified (Antacids may interfere with certain unspecified prescription drugs; resulting effect not specified).

Tetracycline Hydrochloride (Concurrent use with any form of tetracycline should be avoided). Products include:

Achromycin V Capsules 1367

MACROBID CAPSULES

(Nitrofurantoin Monohydrate) 1988

May interact with:

Magnesium Trisilicate (Concomitant administration reduces both the rate and extent of absorption). Products include:

Gaviscon Antacid Tablets...................ⓂⒹ 819
Gaviscon-2 Antacid Tablets ....ⓂⒹ 820

Probenecid (Inhibition of renal tubular secretion of nitrofurantoin; increases toxicity and could lessen its efficacy as a urinary tract antibacterial). Products include:

Benemid Tablets 1611
ColBENEMID Tablets 1622

Sulfinpyrazone (Inhibition of renal tubular secretion of nitrofurantoin; increases toxicity and could lessen its efficacy as a urinary tract antibacterial). Products include:

Anturane 807

Food Interactions

Food, unspecified (Increases bioavailability by approximately 40%).

MACRODANTIN CAPSULES

(Nitrofurantoin) 1989

May interact with:

Magnesium Trisilicate (Rate and extent of Macrodantin absorption reduced). Products include:

Gaviscon Antacid Tablets...................ⓂⒹ 819
Gaviscon-2 Antacid Tablets ....ⓂⒹ 820

Probenecid (Possible toxicity and decreased efficacy of Macrodantin). Products include:

Benemid Tablets 1611
ColBENEMID Tablets 1622

Sulfinpyrazone (Possible toxicity and decreased efficacy of Macrodantin). Products include:

Anturane 807

Food Interactions

Food, unspecified (Increases bioavailability of Macrodantin).

MAG-L-100

(Magnesium Chloride).......................... 668

None cited in PDR database.

MAGONATE TABLETS AND LIQUID

(Magnesium Gluconate) 1005

None cited in PDR database.

MAG-OX 400

(Magnesium Oxide) 668

None cited in PDR database.

MAGTAB SR CAPLETS

(Magnesium Lactate).............................1793

None cited in PDR database.

621 **Interactions Index** **Marax**

MALTSUPEX LIQUID, POWDER & TABLES
(Malt Soup Extract) ▣ 840
None cited in PDR database.

MANDOL VIALS, FASPAK & ADD-VANTAGE
(Cefamandole Nafate) 1461
May interact with aminoglycosides and certain other agents. Compounds in these categories include:

Amikacin Sulfate (Nephrotoxicity). Products include:
- Amikacin Sulfate Injection, USP 960
- Amikin Injectable 501

Gentamicin Sulfate (Nephrotoxicity). Products include:
- Garamycin Injectable 2360
- Genoptic Sterile Ophthalmic Solution ⊙ 243
- Genoptic Sterile Ophthalmic Ointment ⊙ 243
- Gentacidin Ointment ⊙ 264
- Gentacidin Solution ⊙ 264
- Gentak ⊙ 208
- Pred-G Liquifilm Sterile Ophthalmic Suspension ⊙ 251
- Pred-G S.O.P. Sterile Ophthalmic Ointment ⊙ 252

Kanamycin Sulfate (Nephrotoxicity).
No products indexed under this heading.

Probenecid (Slows tubular excretion and doubles the peak serum levels). Products include:
- Benemid Tablets 1611
- ColBENEMID Tablets 1622

Streptomycin Sulfate (Nephrotoxicity). Products include:
- Streptomycin Sulfate Injection 2208

Tobramycin Sulfate (Nephrotoxicity). Products include:
- Nebcin Vials, Hyporets & ADD-Vantage 1464
- Tobramycin Sulfate Injection 968

Food Interactions

Alcohol (Concurrent ingestion of ethanol may result in nausea, vomiting, vasomotor instability with hypotension and peripheral vasodilation).

MANTADIL CREAM
(Chlorcyclizine Hydrochloride) 1135
None cited in PDR database.

MARAX TABLETS & DF SYRUP
(Ephedrine Sulfate, Theophylline, Hydroxyzine Hydrochloride) 2200
May interact with central nervous system depressants and certain other agents. Compounds in these categories include:

Alfentanil Hydrochloride (Potentiated). Products include:
- Alfenta Injection 1286

Alprazolam (Potentiated). Products include:
- Xanax Tablets 2649

Aprobarbital (Potentiated).
No products indexed under this heading.

Buprenorphine (Potentiated). Products include:
- Buprenex Injectable 2006

Buspirone Hydrochloride (Potentiated). Products include:
- BuSpar 737

Butabarbital (Potentiated).
No products indexed under this heading.

Butalbital (Potentiated). Products include:
- Esgic-plus Tablets 1013
- Fioricet Tablets 2258
- Fioricet with Codeine Capsules 2260
- Fiorinal Capsules 2261
- Fiorinal with Codeine Capsules 2262
- Fiorinal Tablets 2261
- Phrenilin 785
- Sedapap Tablets 50 mg/650 mg 1543

Chlordiazepoxide (Potentiated). Products include:
- Libritabs Tablets 2177
- Limbitrol 2180

Chlordiazepoxide Hydrochloride (Potentiated). Products include:
- Librax Capsules 2176
- Librium Capsules 2178
- Librium Injectable 2179

Chlorpromazine (Potentiated). Products include:
- Thorazine Suppositories 2523

Chlorprothixene (Potentiated).
No products indexed under this heading.

Chlorprothixene Hydrochloride (Potentiated).
No products indexed under this heading.

Chlorprothixene Lactate (Potentiated).
No products indexed under this heading.

Clorazepate Dipotassium (Potentiated). Products include:
- Tranxene 451

Clozapine (Potentiated). Products include:
- Clozaril Tablets 2252

Codeine Phosphate (Potentiated). Products include:
- Actifed with Codeine Cough Syrup 1067
- Brontex 1981
- Deconsal C Expectorant Syrup 456
- Deconsal Pediatric Syrup 457
- Dimetane-DC Cough Syrup 2059
- Empirin with Codeine Tablets 1093
- Fioricet with Codeine Capsules 2260
- Fiorinal with Codeine Capsules 2262
- Isoclor Expectorant 990
- Novahistine DH 2462
- Novahistine Expectorant 2463
- Nucofed 2051
- Phenergan with Codeine 2777
- Phenergan VC with Codeine 2781
- Robitussin A-C Syrup 2073
- Robitussin-DAC Syrup 2074
- Ryna ▣ 841
- Soma Compound w/Codeine Tablets 2676
- Tussi-Organidin NR Liquid and S NR Liquid 2677
- Tylenol with Codeine 1583

Desflurane (Potentiated). Products include:
- Suprane 1813

Dezocine (Potentiated). Products include:
- Dalgan Injection 538

Diazepam (Potentiated). Products include:
- Dizac 1809
- Valium Injectable 2182
- Valium Tablets 2183
- Valrelease Capsules 2169

Droperidol (Potentiated). Products include:
- Inapsine Injection 1296

Enflurane (Potentiated).
No products indexed under this heading.

Estazolam (Potentiated). Products include:
- ProSom Tablets 449

Ethchlorvynol (Potentiated). Products include:
- Placidyl Capsules 448

Ethinamate (Potentiated).
No products indexed under this heading.

Fentanyl (Potentiated). Products include:
- Duragesic Transdermal System 1288

Fentanyl Citrate (Potentiated). Products include:
- Sublimaze Injection 1307

Fluphenazine Decanoate (Potentiated). Products include:
- Prolixin Decanoate 509

Fluphenazine Enanthate (Potentiated). Products include:
- Prolixin Enanthate 509

Fluphenazine Hydrochloride (Potentiated). Products include:
- Prolixin 509

Flurazepam Hydrochloride (Potentiated). Products include:
- Dalmane Capsules 2173

Glutethimide (Potentiated).
No products indexed under this heading.

Haloperidol (Potentiated). Products include:
- Haldol Injection, Tablets and Concentrate 1575

Haloperidol Decanoate (Potentiated). Products include:
- Haldol Decanoate 1577

Hydrocodone Bitartrate (Potentiated). Products include:
- Anexsia 5/500 Elixir 1781
- Anexia Tablets 1782
- Codiclear DH Syrup 791
- Deconamine CX Cough and Cold Liquid and Tablets 1319
- Duratuss HD Elixir 2565
- Hycodan Tablets and Syrup 930
- Hycomine Compound Tablets 932
- Hycomine 931
- Hycotuss Expectorant Syrup 933
- Hydrocet Capsules 782
- Lorcet 10/650 1018
- Lortab 2566
- Tussend 1783
- Tussend Expectorant 1785
- Vicodin Tablets 1356
- Vicodin ES Tablets 1357
- Vicodin Tuss Expectorant 1358
- Zydone Capsules 949

Hydrocodone Polistirex (Potentiated). Products include:
- Tussionex Pennkinetic Extended-Release Suspension 998

Isoflurane (Potentiated).
No products indexed under this heading.

Ketamine Hydrochloride (Potentiated).
No products indexed under this heading.

Levomethadyl Acetate Hydrochloride (Potentiated). Products include:
- Orlamm 2239

Levorphanol Tartrate (Potentiated). Products include:
- Levo-Dromoran 2129

Lorazepam (Potentiated). Products include:
- Ativan Injection 2698
- Ativan Tablets 2700

Loxapine Hydrochloride (Potentiated). Products include:
- Loxitane 1378

Loxapine Succinate (Potentiated). Products include:
- Loxitane Capsules 1378

Meperidine Hydrochloride (Potentiated). Products include:
- Demerol 2308
- Mepergan Injection 2753

Mephobarbital (Potentiated). Products include:
- Mebaral Tablets 2322

Meprobamate (Potentiated). Products include:
- Miltown Tablets 2672
- PMB 200 and PMB 400 2783

Mesoridazine Besylate (Potentiated). Products include:
- Serentil 684

Methadone Hydrochloride (Potentiated). Products include:
- Methadone Hydrochloride Oral Concentrate 2233
- Methadone Hydrochloride Oral Solution & Tablets 2235

Methohexital Sodium (Potentiated). Products include:
- Brevital Sodium Vials 1429

Methotrimeprazine (Potentiated). Products include:
- Levoprome 1274

Methoxyflurane (Potentiated).
No products indexed under this heading.

Midazolam Hydrochloride (Potentiated). Products include:
- Versed Injection 2170

Molindone Hydrochloride (Potentiated). Products include:
- Moban Tablets and Concentrate 1048

Morphine Sulfate (Potentiated). Products include:
- Astramorph/PF Injection, USP (Preservative-Free) 535
- Duramorph 962
- Infumorph 200 and Infumorph 500 Sterile Solutions 965
- MS Contin Tablets 1994
- MSIR 1997
- Oramorph SR (Morphine Sulfate Sustained Release Tablets) 2236
- RMS Suppositories 2657
- Roxanol 2243

Opium Alkaloids (Potentiated).
No products indexed under this heading.

Oxazepam (Potentiated). Products include:
- Serax Capsules 2810
- Serax Tablets 2810

Oxycodone Hydrochloride (Potentiated). Products include:
- Percocet Tablets 938
- Percodan Tablets 939
- Percodan-Demi Tablets 940
- Roxicodone Tablets, Oral Solution & Intensol (Oxycodone) 2244
- Tylox Capsules 1584

Pentobarbital Sodium (Potentiated). Products include:
- Nembutal Sodium Capsules 436
- Nembutal Sodium Solution 438
- Nembutal Sodium Suppositories 440

Perphenazine (Potentiated). Products include:
- Etrafon 2355
- Triavil Tablets 1757
- Trilafon 2389

Phenobarbital (Potentiated). Products include:
- Arco-Lase Plus Tablets 512
- Bellergal-S Tablets 2250
- Donnatal 2060
- Donnatal Extentabs 2061
- Donnatal Tablets 2060
- Phenobarbital Elixir and Tablets 1469
- Quadrinal Tablets 1350

Prazepam (Potentiated).
No products indexed under this heading.

Prochlorperazine (Potentiated). Products include:
- Compazine 2470

Promethazine Hydrochloride (Potentiated). Products include:
- Mepergan Injection 2753
- Phenergan with Codeine 2777
- Phenergan with Dextromethorphan 2778
- Phenergan Injection 2773
- Phenergan Suppositories 2775
- Phenergan Syrup 2774
- Phenergan Tablets 2775
- Phenergan VC 2779
- Phenergan VC with Codeine 2781

Propofol (Potentiated). Products include:
- Diprivan Injection 2833

Propoxyphene Hydrochloride (Potentiated). Products include:
- Darvon 1435
- Wygesic Tablets 2827

Propoxyphene Napsylate (Potentiated). Products include:
- Darvon-N/Darvocet-N 1433

IMPORTANT NOTE: Always consult each drug listing in the patient's regimen for possible interactions.

Quazepam (Potentiated). Products include:
Doral Tablets ... 2664
Risperidone (Potentiated). Products include:
Risperdal ... 1301
Secobarbital Sodium (Potentiated). Products include:
Seconal Sodium Pulvules ... 1474
Sufentanil Citrate (Potentiated). Products include:
Sufenta Injection ... 1309
Temazepam (Potentiated). Products include:
Restoril Capsules ... 2284
Thiamylal Sodium (Potentiated).
No products indexed under this heading.
Thioridazine Hydrochloride (Potentiated). Products include:
Mellaril ... 2269
Thiothixene (Potentiated). Products include:
Navane Capsules and Concentrate 2201
Navane Intramuscular ... 2202
Triazolam (Potentiated). Products include:
Halcion Tablets ... 2611
Trifluoperazine Hydrochloride (Potentiated). Products include:
Stelazine ... 2514
Zolpidem Tartrate (Potentiated). Products include:
Ambien Tablets ... 2416

Food Interactions

Alcohol (Potentiated).

MARBLEN SUSPENSION PEACH/APRICOT
(Calcium Carbonate, Magnesium Carbonate) ... ■ 655
None cited in PDR database.

MARBLEN TABLETS
(Calcium Carbonate, Magnesium Carbonate) ... ■ 655
None cited in PDR database.

MARCAINE HYDROCHLORIDE WITH EPINEPHRINE 1:200,000
(Bupivacaine Hydrochloride, Epinephrine) ... 2316
May interact with monoamine oxidase inhibitors, tricyclic antidepressants, vasopressors, phenothiazines, butyrophenones, and certain other agents. Compounds in these categories include:

Amitriptyline Hydrochloride (Severe, persistent hypertension). Products include:
Elavil ... 2838
Endep Tablets ... 2174
Etrafon ... 2355
Limbitrol ... 2180
Triavil Tablets ... 1757
Amoxapine (Severe, persistent hypertension). Products include:
Asendin Tablets ... 1369
Chlorpromazine (May reduce or reverse the pressor effect of epinephrine). Products include:
Thorazine Suppositories ... 2523
Clomipramine Hydrochloride (Severe, persistent hypertension). Products include:
Anafranil Capsules ... 803
Desipramine Hydrochloride (Severe, persistent hypertension). Products include:
Norpramin Tablets ... 1526
Dopamine Hydrochloride (Severe, persistent hypertension).
No products indexed under this heading.
Doxepin Hydrochloride (Severe, persistent hypertension). Products include:
Sinequan ... 2205
Zonalon Cream ... 1055
Epinephrine Hydrochloride (Severe, persistent hypertension). Products include:
Ana-Kit Anaphylaxis Emergency Treatment Kit ... 617
Fluphenazine Decanoate (May reduce or reverse the pressor effect of epinephrine). Products include:
Prolixin Decanoate ... 509
Fluphenazine Enanthate (May reduce or reverse the pressor effect of epinephrine). Products include:
Prolixin Enanthate ... 509
Fluphenazine Hydrochloride (May reduce or reverse the pressor effect of epinephrine). Products include:
Prolixin ... 509
Furazolidone (Severe, persistent hypertension). Products include:
Furoxone ... 2046
Haloperidol (May reduce or reverse the pressor effect of epinephrine). Products include:
Haldol Injection, Tablets and Concentrate ... 1575
Haloperidol Decanoate (May reduce or reverse the pressor effect of epinephrine). Products include:
Haldol Decanoate ... 1577
Imipramine Hydrochloride (Severe, persistent hypertension). Products include:
Tofranil Ampuls ... 854
Tofranil Tablets ... 856
Imipramine Pamoate (Severe, persistent hypertension). Products include:
Tofranil-PM Capsules ... 857
Isocarboxazid (Severe, persistent hypertension).
No products indexed under this heading.
Maprotiline Hydrochloride (Severe, persistent hypertension). Products include:
Ludiomil Tablets ... 843
Mesoridazine Besylate (May reduce or reverse the pressor effect of epinephrine). Products include:
Serentil ... 684
Metaraminol Bitartrate (Severe, persistent hypertension). Products include:
Aramine Injection ... 1609
Methotrimeprazine (May reduce or reverse the pressor effect of epinephrine). Products include:
Levoprome ... 1274
Methoxamine Hydrochloride (Severe, persistent hypertension). Products include:
Vasoxyl Injection ... 1196
Norepinephrine Bitartrate (Severe, persistent hypertension). Products include:
Levophed Bitartrate Injection ... 2315
Nortriptyline Hydrochloride (Severe, persistent hypertension). Products include:
Pamelor ... 2280
Oxytocin (Severe, persistent hypertension). Products include:
Oxytocin Injection ... 2771
Syntocinon Injection ... 2296
Oxytocin (Nasal Spray) (Severe, persistent hypertension).
Perphenazine (May reduce or reverse the pressor effect of epinephrine). Products include:
Etrafon ... 2355
Triavil Tablets ... 1757
Trilafon ... 2389
Phenelzine Sulfate (Severe, persistent hypertension). Products include:
Nardil ... 1920
Phenylephrine Hydrochloride (Severe, persistent hypertension). Products include:
Atrohist Plus Tablets ... 454
Cerose DM ... ■ 878
Comhist ... 2038
D.A. Chewable Tablets ... 951
Deconsal Pediatric Capsules ... 454
Dura-Vent/DA Tablets ... 953
Entex Capsules ... 1986
Entex Liquid ... 1986
Extendryl ... 1005
4-Way Fast Acting Nasal Spray (regular & mentholated) ... ■ 621
Hemorid For Women ... ■ 834
Hycomine Compound Tablets ... 932
Neo-Synephrine Hydrochloride 1% Carpuject ... 2324
Neo-Synephrine Hydrochloride 1% Injection ... 2324
Neo-Synephrine Hydrochloride (Ophthalmic) ... 2325
Neo-Synephrine ... ■ 726
Nōstril ... ■ 644
Novahistine Elixir ... ■ 823
Phenergan VC ... 2779
Phenergan VC with Codeine ... 2781
Preparation H ... ■ 871
Tympagesic Ear Drops ... 2342
Vasosulf ... ◉ 271
Vicks Sinex Nasal Spray and Ultra Fine Mist ... ■ 765
Prochlorperazine (May reduce or reverse the pressor effect of epinephrine). Products include:
Compazine ... 2470
Promethazine Hydrochloride (May reduce or reverse the pressor effect of epinephrine). Products include:
Mepergan Injection ... 2753
Phenergan with Codeine ... 2777
Phenergan with Dextromethorphan 2778
Phenergan Injection ... 2773
Phenergan Suppositories ... 2775
Phenergan Syrup ... 2774
Phenergan Tablets ... 2775
Phenergan VC ... 2779
Phenergan VC with Codeine ... 2781
Protriptyline Hydrochloride (Severe, persistent hypertension). Products include:
Vivactil Tablets ... 1774
Selegiline Hydrochloride (Severe, persistent hypertension). Products include:
Eldepryl Tablets ... 2550
Thioridazine Hydrochloride (May reduce or reverse the pressor effect of epinephrine). Products include:
Mellaril ... 2269
Tranylcypromine Sulfate (Severe, persistent hypertension). Products include:
Parnate Tablets ... 2503
Trifluoperazine Hydrochloride (May reduce or reverse the pressor effect of epinephrine). Products include:
Stelazine ... 2514
Trimipramine Maleate (Severe, persistent hypertension). Products include:
Surmontil Capsules ... 2811

MARCAINE HYDROCHLORIDE INJECTION
(Bupivacaine Hydrochloride) ... 2316
See **Marcaine Hydrochloride with Epinephrine 1:200,000**

MARCAINE SPINAL
(Bupivacaine Hydrochloride) ... 2319
May interact with monoamine oxidase inhibitors, tricyclic antidepressants, vasopressors, and certain other agents. Compounds in these categories include:

Amitriptyline Hydrochloride (Severe, persistent hypertension). Products include:
Elavil ... 2838
Endep Tablets ... 2174
Etrafon ... 2355
Limbitrol ... 2180
Triavil Tablets ... 1757
Amoxapine (Severe, persistent hypertension). Products include:
Asendin Tablets ... 1369
Clomipramine Hydrochloride (Severe, persistent hypertension). Products include:
Anafranil Capsules ... 803
Desipramine Hydrochloride (Severe, persistent hypertension). Products include:
Norpramin Tablets ... 1526
Dopamine Hydrochloride (Severe, persistent hypertension).
No products indexed under this heading.
Doxepin Hydrochloride (Severe, persistent hypertension). Products include:
Sinequan ... 2205
Zonalon Cream ... 1055
Epinephrine Hydrochloride (Severe, persistent hypertension). Products include:
Ana-Kit Anaphylaxis Emergency Treatment Kit ... 617
Furazolidone (Severe, persistent hypertension). Products include:
Furoxone ... 2046
Imipramine Hydrochloride (Severe, persistent hypertension). Products include:
Tofranil Ampuls ... 854
Tofranil Tablets ... 856
Imipramine Pamoate (Severe, persistent hypertension). Products include:
Tofranil-PM Capsules ... 857
Isocarboxazid (Severe, persistent hypertension).
No products indexed under this heading.
Maprotiline Hydrochloride (Severe, persistent hypertension). Products include:
Ludiomil Tablets ... 843
Metaraminol Bitartrate (Severe, persistent hypertension). Products include:
Aramine Injection ... 1609
Methoxamine Hydrochloride (Severe, persistent hypertension). Products include:
Vasoxyl Injection ... 1196
Norepinephrine Bitartrate (Severe, persistent hypertension). Products include:
Levophed Bitartrate Injection ... 2315
Nortriptyline Hydrochloride (Severe, persistent hypertension). Products include:
Pamelor ... 2280
Oxytocin (Severe, persistent hypertension). Products include:
Oxytocin Injection ... 2771
Syntocinon Injection ... 2296
Oxytocin (Nasal Spray) (Severe, persistent hypertension).
Phenelzine Sulfate (Severe, persistent hypertension). Products include:
Nardil ... 1920
Phenylephrine Hydrochloride (Severe, persistent hypertension). Products include:
Atrohist Plus Tablets ... 454
Cerose DM ... ■ 878
Comhist ... 2038
D.A. Chewable Tablets ... 951

(■ Described in PDR For Nonprescription Drugs) (◉ Described in PDR For Ophthalmology)

Deconsal Pediatric Capsules ... 454
Dura-Vent/DA Tablets ... 953
Entex Capsules ... 1986
Entex Liquid ... 1986
Extendryl ... 1005
4-Way Fast Acting Nasal Spray (regular & mentholated) ... ◘ 621
Hemorid For Women ... ◘ 834
Hycomine Compound Tablets ... 932
Neo-Synephrine Hydrochloride 1% Carpuject ... 2324
Neo-Synephrine Hydrochloride 1% Injection ... 2324
Neo-Synephrine Hydrochloride (Oohthalmic) ... 2325
Neo-Synephrine ... ◘ 726
Nōstril ... ◘ 644
Novahistine Elixir ... ◘ 823
Phenergan VC ... 2779
Phenergan VC with Codeine ... 2781
Preparation H ... ◘ 871
Tympagesic Ear Drops ... 2342
Vasosulf ... ◉ 271
Vicks Sinex Nasal Spray and Ultra Fine Mist ... ◘ 765

Protriptyline Hydrochloride (Severe, persistent hypertension). Products include:
Vivactil Tablets ... 1774

Selegiline Hydrochloride (Severe, persistent hypertension). Products include:
Eldepryl Tablets ... 2550

Tranylcypromine Sulfate (Severe, persistent hypertension). Products include:
Parnate Tablets ... 2503

Trimipramine Maleate (Severe, persistent hypertension). Products include:
Surmontil Capsules ... 2811

MARINOL (DRONABINOL) CAPSULES

(Dronabinol) ... 2231
May interact with central nervous system depressants, hypnotics and sedatives, benzodiazepines, barbiturates, antipsychotic agents, sympathomimetics, antihistamines, anticholinergics, tricyclic antidepressants, lithium preparations, muscle relaxants, narcotic analgesics, xanthine bronchodilators, and certain other agents. Compounds in these categories include:

Acrivastine (Potential for additive or super-additive tachycardia and drowsiness). Products include:
Semprex-D Capsules ... 463
Semprex-D Capsules ... 1167

Albuterol (Potential for additive hypertension, tachycardia and possibly cardiotoxicity). Products include:
Proventil Inhalation Aerosol ... 2382
Ventolin Inhalation Aerosol and Refill ... 1197

Albuterol Sulfate (Potential for additive hypertension, tachycardia and possibly cardiotoxicity). Products include:
Airet Solution for Inhalation ... 452
Proventil Inhalation Solution 0.083% ... 2384
Proventil Repetabs Tablets ... 2386
Proventil Solution for Inhalation 0.5% ... 2383
Proventil Syrup ... 2385
Proventil Tablets ... 2386
Ventolin Inhalation Solution ... 1198
Ventolin Nebules Inhalation Solution ... 1199
Ventolin Rotacaps for Inhalation ... 1200
Ventolin Syrup ... 1202
Ventolin Tablets ... 1203
Volmax Extended-Release Tablets .. 1788

Alfentanil Hydrochloride (Potential for additive drowsiness and CNS depression; potential for additive or synergistic CNS effects). Products include:
Alfenta Injection ... 1286

Alprazolam (Potential for additive or synergistic CNS effects). Products include:
Xanax Tablets ... 2649

Aminophylline (Potential for increased theophylline metabolism).
No products indexed under this heading.

Amitriptyline Hydrochloride (Potential for additive tachycardia, hypertension and drowsiness). Products include:
Elavil ... 2838
Endep Tablets ... 2174
Etrafon ... 2355
Limbitrol ... 2180
Triavil Tablets ... 1757

Amoxapine (Potential for additive tachycardia, hypertension and drowsiness). Products include:
Asendin Tablets ... 1369

Amphetamine Resins (Potential for additive hypertension, tachycardia and possibly cardiotoxicity). Products include:
Biphetamine Capsules ... 983

Antipyrine (Potential for decreased antipyrine clearance). Products include:
Auralgan Otic Solution ... 2703
Tympagesic Ear Drops ... 2342

Aprobarbital (Potential for additive or synergistic CNS effects; potential for decreased barbiturate clearance).
No products indexed under this heading.

Astemizole (Potential for additive or super-additive tachycardia and drowsiness). Products include:
Hismanal Tablets ... 1293

Atracurium Besylate (Potential for additive drowsiness and CNS depression). Products include:
Tracrium Injection ... 1183

Atropine Sulfate (Potential for additive or super-additive tachycardia and drowsiness). Products include:
Arco-Lase Plus Tablets ... 512
Atrohist Plus Tablets ... 454
Atropine Sulfate Sterile Ophthalmic Solution ... ◉ 233
Donnatal ... 2060
Donnatal Extentabs ... 2061
Donnatal Tablets ... 2060
Lomotil ... 2439
Motofen Tablets ... 784
Urised Tablets ... 1964

Azatadine Maleate (Potential for additive or super-additive tachycardia and drowsiness). Products include:
Trinalin Repetabs Tablets ... 1330

Baclofen (Potential for additive drowsiness and CNSD depression). Products include:
Lioresal Intrathecal ... 1596
Lioresal Tablets ... 829

Belladonna Alkaloids (Potential for additive or super-additive tachycardia and drowsiness). Products include:
Bellergal-S Tablets ... 2250
Hyland's Bed Wetting Tablets ... ◘ 828
Hyland's EnurAid Tablets ... ◘ 829
Hyland's Teething Tablets ... ◘ 830

Benztropine Mesylate (Potential for additive or super-additive tachycardia and drowsiness). Products include:
Cogentin ... 1621

Biperiden Hydrochloride (Potential for additive or super-additive tachycardia and drowsiness). Products include:
Akineton ... 1333

Bromodiphenhydramine Hydrochloride (Potential for additive or super-additive tachycardia and drowsiness).
No products indexed under this heading.

Brompheniramine Maleate (Potential for additive or super-additive tachycardia and drowsiness). Products include:
Alka Seltzer Plus Sinus Medicine .. ◘ 707
Bromfed Capsules (Extended-Release) ... 1785
Bromfed Syrup ... ◘ 733
Bromfed Tablets ... 1785
Bromfed-DM Cough Syrup ... 1786
Bromfed-PD Capsules (Extended-Release) ... 1785
Dimetane-DC Cough Syrup ... 2059
Dimetane-DX Cough Syrup ... 2059
Dimetapp Elixir ... ◘ 773
Dimetapp Extentabs ... ◘ 774
Dimetapp Tablets/Liqui-Gels ... ◘ 775
Dimetapp Cold & Allergy Chewable Tablets ... ◘ 773
Dimetapp DM Elixir ... ◘ 774
Vicks DayQuil Allergy Relief 12-Hour Extended Release Tablets.. ◘ 760
Vicks DayQuil Allergy Relief 4-Hour Tablets ... ◘ 760

Buprenorphine (Potential for additive drowsiness and CNS depression; potential for additive or synergistic CNS effects). Products include:
Buprenex Injectable ... 2006

Buspirone Hydrochloride (Potential for additive or synergistic CNS effects). Products include:
BuSpar ... 737

Butabarbital (Potential for additive or synergistic CNS effects; potential for decreased barbiturate clearance).
No products indexed under this heading.

Butalbital (Potential for additive or synergistic CNS effects; potential for decreased barbiturate clearance). Products include:
Esgic-plus Tablets ... 1013
Fioricet Tablets ... 2258
Fioricet with Codeine Capsules ... 2260
Fiorinal Capsules ... 2261
Fiorinal with Codeine Capsules ... 2262
Fiorinal Tablets ... 2261
Phrenilin ... 785
Sedapap Tablets 50 mg/650 mg .. 1543

Carisoprodol (Potential for additive drowsiness and CNS depression). Products include:
Soma Compound w/Codeine Tablets ... 2676
Soma Compound Tablets ... 2675
Soma Tablets ... 2674

Chlordiazepoxide (Potential for additive or synergistic CNS effects). Products include:
Libritabs Tablets ... 2177
Limbitrol ... 2180

Chlordiazepoxide Hydrochloride (Potential for additive or synergistic CNS effects). Products include:
Librax Capsules ... 2176
Librium Capsules ... 2178
Librium Injectable ... 2179

Chlorpheniramine Maleate (Potential for additive or super-additive tachycardia and drowsiness). Products include:
Alka-Seltzer Plus Cold Medicine ... ◘ 705
Alka-Seltzer Plus Cold Medicine Liqui-Gels ... ◘ 706
Alka-Seltzer Plus Cold & Cough Medicine ... ◘ 708
Alka-Seltzer Plus Cold & Cough Medicine Liqui-Gels ... ◘ 705
Allerest Children's Chewable Tablets ... ◘ 627
Allerest Headache Strength Tablets ... ◘ 627
Allerest Maximum Strength Tablets ... ◘ 627
Allerest Sinus Pain Formula ... ◘ 627
Allerest 12 Hour Caplets ... ◘ 627
Ana-Kit Anaphylaxis Emergency Treatment Kit ... 617
Atrohist Pediatric Capsules ... 453
Atrohist Plus Tablets ... 454
BC Cold Powder Multi-Symptom Formula (Cold-Sinus-Allergy) ... ◘ 609
Cerose DM ... ◘ 878
Cheracol Plus Head Cold/Cough Formula ... ◘ 769
Children's Vicks DayQuil Allergy Relief ... ◘ 757
Children's Vicks NyQuil Cold/Cough Relief ... ◘ 758
Chlor-Trimeton Allergy Decongestant Tablets ... ◘ 799
Chlor-Trimeton Allergy Tablets ... ◘ 798
Comhist ... 2038
Comtrex Multi-Symptom Cold Reliever Tablets/Caplets/Liqui-Gels/Liquid ... ◘ 615
Allergy-Sinus Comtrex Multi-Symptom Allergy-Sinus Formula Tablets ... ◘ 617
Contac Continuous Action Nasal Decongestant/Antihistamine 12 Hour Capsules ... ◘ 813
Contac Maximum Strength Continuous Action Decongestant/Antihistamine 12 Hour Caplets .. ◘ 813
Contac Severe Cold and Flu Formula Caplets ... ◘ 814
Coricidin 'D' Decongestant Tablets ... ◘ 800
Coricidin Tablets ... ◘ 800
D.A. Chewable Tablets ... 951
Deconamine ... 1320
Dura-Tap/PD Capsules ... 2867
Dura-Vent/DA Tablets ... 953
Extendryl ... 1005
Fedahist Gyrocaps ... 2401
Fedahist Timecaps ... 2401
Hycomine Compound Tablets ... 932
Isoclor Timesule Capsules ... ◘ 637
Kronofed-A ... 977
Nolamine Timed-Release Tablets ... 785
Novahistine DH ... 2462
Novahistine Elixir ... ◘ 823
Ornade Spansule Capsules ... 2502
PediaCare Cold Allergy Chewable Tablets ... ◘ 677
PediaCare Cough-Cold Chewable Tablets ... 1553
PediaCare Cough-Cold Liquid ... 1553
PediaCare NightRest Cough-Cold Liquid ... 1553
Pediatric Vicks 44m Cough & Cold Relief ... ◘ 764
Pyrroxate Caplets ... ◘ 772
Ryna ... ◘ 841
Sinarest Tablets ... ◘ 648
Sinarest Extra Strength Tablets ... ◘ 648
Sine-Off Sinus Medicine ... ◘ 825
Singlet Tablets ... ◘ 825
Sinulin Tablets ... 787
Sinutab Sinus Allergy Medication, Maximum Strength Tablets and Caplets ... ◘ 860
Sudafed Plus Liquid ... ◘ 862
Sudafed Plus Tablets ... ◘ 863
Teldrin 12 Hour Antihistamine/Nasal Decongestant Allergy Relief Capsules ... ◘ 826
TheraFlu ... ◘ 787
TheraFlu Maximum Strength Nighttime Flu, Cold & Cough Medicine ... ◘ 788
Triaminic Allergy Tablets ... ◘ 789
Triaminic Cold Tablets ... ◘ 790
Triaminic Nite Light ... ◘ 791
Triaminic Syrup ... ◘ 792
Triaminic-12 Tablets ... ◘ 792
Triaminicin Tablets ... ◘ 793
Triaminicol Multi-Symptom Cold Tablets ... ◘ 793
Triaminicol Multi-Symptom Relief ◘ 794
Tussend ... 1783
Children's TYLENOL Cold Multi-Symptom Liquid Formula and Chewable Tablets ... 1561
Children's TYLENOL Cold Plus Cough Multi Symptom Tablets and Liquid ... ◘ 681
TYLENOL Maximum Strength Allergy Sinus Medication Gelcaps and Caplets ... 1563
TYLENOL Cold Multi-Symptom Formula Medication Tablets and Caplets ... 1561
TYLENOL Cold Multi-Symptom Hot Medication Liquid Packets ... 1557

IMPORTANT NOTE: Always consult each drug listing in the patient's regimen for possible interactions.

Marinol **Interactions Index** **624**

Vicks 44 LiquiCaps Cough, Cold & Flu Relief ▣ 755
Vicks 44M Cough, Cold & Flu Relief ▣ 756

Chlorpheniramine Polistirex (Potential for additive or super-additive tachycardia and drowsiness). Products include:
Tussionex Pennkinetic Extended-Release Suspension 998

Chlorpheniramine Tannate (Potential for additive or super-additive tachycardia and drowsiness). Products include:
Atrohist Pediatric Suspension 454
Ricobid Tablets and Pediatric Suspension 2038
Rynatan 2673
Rynatuss 2673

Chlorpromazine (Potential for additive or synergistic CNS effects). Products include:
Thorazine Suppositories 2523

Chlorpromazine Hydrochloride (Potential for additive or synergistic CNS effects). Products include:
Thorazine 2523

Chlorprothixene (Potential for additive or synergistic CNS effects).
No products indexed under this heading.

Chlorprothixene Hydrochloride (Potential for additive or synergistic CNS effects).
No products indexed under this heading.

Chlorzoxazone (Potential for additive drowsiness and CNS depression). Products include:
Paraflex Caplets 1580
Parafon Forte DSC Caplets 1581

Clemastine Fumarate (Potential for additive or super-additive tachycardia and drowsiness). Products include:
Tavist Syrup 2297
Tavist Tablets 2298
Tavist-1 12 Hour Relief Tablets ▣ 787
Tavist-D 12 Hour Relief Tablets ▣ 787

Clidinium Bromide (Potential for additive or super-additive tachycardia and drowsiness). Products include:
Librax Capsules 2176
Quarzan Capsules 2181

Clomipramine Hydrochloride (Potential for additive tachycardia, hypertension and drowsiness). Products include:
Anafranil Capsules 803

Clorazepate Dipotassium (Potential for additive or synergistic CNS effects). Products include:
Tranxene 451

Clozapine (Potential for additive or synergistic CNS effects). Products include:
Clozaril Tablets 2252

Cocaine Hydrochloride (Potential for additive hypertension, tachycardia and possibly cardiotoxicity). Products include:
Cocaine Hydrochloride Topical Solution 537

Codeine Phosphate (Potential for additive drowsiness and CNS depression; potential for additive or synergistic CNS effects). Products include:
Actifed with Codeine Cough Syrup 1067
Brontex 1981
Deconsal C Expectorant Syrup 456
Deconsal Pediatric Syrup 457
Dimetane-DC Cough Syrup 2059
Empirin with Codeine Tablets 1093
Fioricet with Codeine Capsules 2260
Fiorinal with Codeine Capsules 2262
Isoclor Expectorant 990
Novahistine DH 2462
Novahistine Expectorant 2463
Nucofed 2051
Phenergan with Codeine 2777
Phenergan VC with Codeine 2781
Robitussin A-C Syrup 2073
Robitussin-DAC Syrup 2074
Ryna ▣ 841
Soma Compound w/Codeine Tablets 2676
Tussi-Organidin NR Liquid and S NR Liquid 2677
Tylenol with Codeine 1583

Cyclobenzaprine Hydrochloride (Potential for additive drowsiness and CNSD depression). Products include:
Flexeril Tablets 1661

Cyproheptadine Hydrochloride (Potential for additive or super-additive tachycardia and drowsiness). Products include:
Periactin 1724

Dantrolene Sodium (Potential for additive drowsiness and CNSD depression). Products include:
Dantrium Capsules 1982
Dantrium Intravenous 1983

Desflurane (Potential for additive drowsiness and CNS depression; potential for additive or synergistic CNS effects). Products include:
Suprane 1813

Desipramine Hydrochloride (Potential for additive tachycardia, hypertension and drowsiness). Products include:
Norpramin Tablets 1526

Dexchlorpheniramine Maleate (Potential for additive or super-additive tachycardia and drowsiness).
No products indexed under this heading.

Dextroamphetamine Sulfate (Potential for additive hypertension, tachycardia and possibly cardiotoxicity). Products include:
Dexedrine 2474
DextroStat Dextroamphetamine Tablets 2036

Dezocine (Potential for additive drowsiness and CNS depression; potential for additive or synergistic CNS effects). Products include:
Dalgan Injection 538

Diazepam (Potential for additive or synergistic CNS effects). Products include:
Dizac 1809
Valium Injectable 2182
Valium Tablets 2183
Valrelease Capsules 2169

Dicyclomine Hydrochloride (Potential for additive or super-additive tachycardia and drowsiness). Products include:
Bentyl 1501

Diphenhydramine Citrate (Potential for additive or super-additive tachycardia and drowsiness). Products include:
Excedrin P.M. Analgesic/Sleeping Aid Tablets, Caplets, Liquigels 733

Diphenhydramine Hydrochloride (Potential for additive or super-additive tachycardia and drowsiness). Products include:
Actifed Allergy Daytime/Nighttime Caplets ▣ 844
Actifed Sinus Daytime/Nighttime Tablets and Caplets ▣ 846
Arthritis Foundation NightTime Caplets ▣ 674
Extra Strength Bayer PM Aspirin ▣ 713
Bayer Select Night Time Pain Relief Formula ▣ 716
Benadryl Allergy Decongestant Liquid Medication ▣ 848
Benadryl Allergy Decongestant Tablets ▣ 848
Benadryl Allergy Liquid Medication ▣ 849
Benadryl Allergy ▣ 848
Benadryl Allergy Sinus Headache Formula Caplets ▣ 849
Benadryl Capsules 1898
Benadryl Dye-Free Allergy Liqui-gel Softgels ▣ 850
Benadryl Dye-Free Allergy Liquid Medication ▣ 850
Benadryl Itch Relief Cream, Children's Formula and Maximum Strength 2% ▣ 851
Benadryl Itch Relief Spray, Children's Formula and Maximum Strength 2% ▣ 851
Benadryl Itch Relief Stick Maximum Strength 2% ▣ 850
Benadryl Itch Stopping Gel, Children's Formula and Maximum Strength 2% ▣ 851
Benadryl Kapseals 1898
Benadryl Injection 1898
Contac Day & Night Cold/Flu Night Caplets ▣ 812
Contac Night Allergy/Sinus Caplets ▣ 812
Extra Strength Doan's P.M. ▣ 633
Legatrin PM ▣ 651
Miles Nervine Nighttime Sleep-Aid ▣ 723
Nytol QuickCaps Caplets ▣ 610
Sleepinal Night-time Sleep Aid Capsules and Softgels ▣ 834
TYLENOL Maximum Strength Allergy Sinus NightTime Medication Caplets 1555
TYLENOL Flu NightTime, Maximum Strength, Gelcaps 1566
TYLENOL Maximum Strength Flu NightTime Hot Medication Packets 1562
TYLENOL PM, Extra Strength Pain Reliever/Sleep Aid Caplets, Geltabs, Gelcaps 1560
TYLENOL Severe Allergy Medication Caplets 1564
Maximum Strength Unisom Sleepgels 1934
Unisom With Pain Relief-Nighttime Sleep Aid and Pain Reliever 1934

Diphenylpyraline Hydrochloride (Potential for additive or super-additive tachycardia and drowsiness).
No products indexed under this heading.

Disulfiram (Potential for reversible hypomanic reaction). Products include:
Antabuse Tablets 2695

Dobutamine Hydrochloride (Potential for additive hypertension, tachycardia and possibly cardiotoxicity). Products include:
Dobutrex Solution Vials 1439

Dopamine Hydrochloride (Potential for additive hypertension, tachycardia and possibly cardiotoxicity).
No products indexed under this heading.

Doxacurium Chloride (Potential for additive drowsiness and CNS depression). Products include:
Nuromax Injection 1149

Doxepin Hydrochloride (Potential for additive tachycardia, hypertension and drowsiness). Products include:
Sinequan 2205
Zonalon Cream 1055

Droperidol (Potential for additive or synergistic CNS effects). Products include:
Inapsine Injection 1296

Dyphylline (Potential for increased theophylline metabolism). Products include:
Lufyllin & Lufyllin-400 Tablets 2670
Lufyllin-GG Elixir & Tablets 2671

Enflurane (Potential for additive or synergistic CNS effects).
No products indexed under this heading.

Ephedrine Hydrochloride (Potential for additive hypertension, tachycardia and possibly cardiotoxicity). Products include:
Primatene Dual Action Formula ▣ 872
Primatene Tablets ▣ 873
Quadrinal Tablets 1350

Ephedrine Sulfate (Potential for additive hypertension, tachycardia and possibly cardiotoxicity). Products include:
Bronkaid Caplets ▣ 717
Marax Tablets & DF Syrup 2200

Ephedrine Tannate (Potential for additive hypertension, tachycardia and possibly cardiotoxicity). Products include:
Rynatuss 2673

Epinephrine (Potential for additive hypertension, tachycardia and possibly cardiotoxicity). Products include:
Bronkaid Mist ▣ 717
EPIFRIN ⊙ 239
EpiPen 790
Marcaine Hydrochloride with Epinephrine 1:200,000 2316
Primatene Mist ▣ 873
Sensorcaine with Epinephrine Injection 559
Sus-Phrine Injection 1019
Xylocaine with Epinephrine Injections 567

Epinephrine Bitartrate (Potential for additive hypertension, tachycardia and possibly cardiotoxicity). Products include:
Bronkaid Mist Suspension ▣ 718
Sensorcaine-MPF with Epinephrine Injection 559

Epinephrine Hydrochloride (Potential for additive hypertension, tachycardia and possibly cardiotoxicity). Products include:
Ana-Kit Anaphylaxis Emergency Treatment Kit 617

Estazolam (Potential for additive or synergistic CNS effects). Products include:
ProSom Tablets 449

Ethchlorvynol (Potential for additive or synergistic CNS effects). Products include:
Placidyl Capsules 448

Ethinamate (Potential for additive or synergistic CNS effects).
No products indexed under this heading.

Fentanyl (Potential for additive drowsiness and CNS depression). Products include:
Duragesic Transdermal System 1288

Fentanyl Citrate (Potential for additive drowsiness and CNS depression; potential for additive or synergistic CNS effects). Products include:
Sublimaze Injection 1307

Fluoxetine Hydrochloride (Potential for hypomanic reaction). Products include:
Prozac Pulvules & Liquid, Oral Solution 919

Fluphenazine Decanoate (Potential for additive or synergistic CNS effects). Products include:
Prolixin Decanoate 509

Fluphenazine Enanthate (Potential for additive or synergistic CNS effects). Products include:
Prolixin Enanthate 509

Fluphenazine Hydrochloride (Potential for additive or synergistic CNS effects). Products include:
Prolixin 509

Flurazepam Hydrochloride (Potential for additive or synergistic CNS effects). Products include:
Dalmane Capsules 2173

Glutethimide (Potential for additive or synergistic CNS effects).
No products indexed under this heading.

(▣ Described in PDR For Nonprescription Drugs) (⊙ Described in PDR For Ophthalmology)

Glycopyrrolate (Potential for additive or super-additive tachycardia and drowsiness). Products include:
- Robinul Forte Tablets ... 2072
- Robinul Injectable ... 2072
- Robinul Tablets ... 2072

Halazepam (Potential for additive or synergistic CNS effects).
- No products indexed under this heading.

Haloperidol (Potential for additive or synergistic CNS effects). Products include:
- Haldol Injection, Tablets and Concentrate ... 1575

Haloperidol Decanoate (Potential for additive or synergistic CNS effects). Products include:
- Haldol Decanoate ... 1577

Hydrocodone Bitartrate (Potential for additive drowsiness and CNS effects; potential for additive or synergistic CNS effects). Products include:
- Anexsia 5/500 Elixir ... 1781
- Anexia Tablets ... 1782
- Codiclear DH Syrup ... 791
- Deconamine CX Cough and Cold Liquid and Tablets ... 1319
- Duratuss HD Elixir ... 2565
- Hycodan Tablets and Syrup ... 930
- Hycomine Compound Tablets ... 932
- Hycomine ... 931
- Hycotuss Expectorant Syrup ... 933
- Hydrocet Capsules ... 782
- Lorcet 10/650 ... 1018
- Lortab ... 2566
- Tussend ... 1783
- Tussend Expectorant ... 1785
- Vicodin Tablets ... 1356
- Vicodin ES Tablets ... 1357
- Vicodin Tuss Expectorant ... 1358
- Zydone Capsules ... 949

Hydrocodone Polistirex (Potential for additive drowsiness and CNS depression; potential for additive or synergistic CNS effects). Products include:
- Tussionex Pennkinetic Extended-Release Suspension ... 998

Hydroxyzine Hydrochloride (Potential for additive or synergistic CNS effects). Products include:
- Atarax Tablets & Syrup ... 2185
- Marax Tablets & DF Syrup ... 2200
- Vistaril Intramuscular Solution ... 2216

Hyoscyamine (Potential for additive or super-additive tachycardia and drowsiness). Products include:
- Cystospaz Tablets ... 1963
- Urised Tablets ... 1964

Hyoscyamine Sulfate (Potential for additive or super-additive tachycardia and drowsiness). Products include:
- Arco-Lase Plus Tablets ... 512
- Atrohist Plus Tablets ... 454
- Cystospaz-M Capsules ... 1963
- Donnatal ... 2060
- Donnatal Extentabs ... 2061
- Donnatal Tablets ... 2060
- Kutrase Capsules ... 2402
- Levsin/Levsinex/Levbid ... 2405

Imipramine Hydrochloride (Potential for additive tachycardia, hypertension and drowsiness). Products include:
- Tofranil Ampuls ... 854
- Tofranil Tablets ... 856

Imipramine Pamoate (Potential for additive tachycardia, hypertension and drowsiness). Products include:
- Tofranil-PM Capsules ... 857

Ipratropium Bromide (Potential for additive or super-additive tachycardia and drowsiness). Products include:
- Atrovent Inhalation Aerosol ... 671
- Atrovent Inhalation Solution ... 673

Isoflurane (Potential for additive or synergistic CNS effects).
- No products indexed under this heading.

Isoproterenol Hydrochloride (Potential for additive hypertension, tachycardia and possibly cardiotoxicity). Products include:
- Isuprel Hydrochloride Injection 1:5000 ... 2311
- Isuprel Hydrochloride Solution 1:200 & 1:100 ... 2313
- Isuprel Mistometer ... 2312

Isoproterenol Sulfate (Potential for additive hypertension, tachycardia and possibly cardiotoxicity). Products include:
- Norisodrine with Calcium Iodide Syrup ... 442

Ketamine Hydrochloride (Potential for additive or synergistic CNS effects).
- No products indexed under this heading.

Levomethadyl Acetate Hydrochloride (Potential for additive drowsiness and CNS depression; potential for additive or synergistic CNS effects). Products include:
- Orlamm ... 2239

Levorphanol Tartrate (Potential for additive drowsiness and CNS depression; potential for additive or synergistic CNS effects). Products include:
- Levo-Dromoran ... 2129

Lithium Carbonate (Potential for additive drowsiness and CNS depression; potential for additive or synergistic CNS effects). Products include:
- Eskalith ... 2485
- Lithium Carbonate Capsules & Tablets ... 2230
- Lithonate/Lithotabs/Lithobid ... 2543

Lithium Citrate (Potential for additive drowsiness and CNS depression; potential for additive or synergistic CNS effects).
- No products indexed under this heading.

Loratadine (Potential for additive or super-additive tachycardia and drowsiness). Products include:
- Claritin ... 2349
- Claritin-D ... 2350

Lorazepam (Potential for additive or synergistic CNS effects). Products include:
- Ativan Injection ... 2698
- Ativan Tablets ... 2700

Loxapine Hydrochloride (Potential for additive or synergistic CNS effects). Products include:
- Loxitane ... 1378

Loxapine Succinate (Potential for additive or synergistic CNS effects). Products include:
- Loxitane Capsules ... 1378

Maprotiline Hydrochloride (Potential for additive tachycardia, hypertension and drowsiness). Products include:
- Ludiomil Tablets ... 843

Mepenzolate Bromide (Potential for additive or super-additive tachycardia and drowsiness).
- No products indexed under this heading.

Meperidine Hydrochloride (Potential for additive drowsiness and CNS depression; potential for additive or synergistic CNS effects). Products include:
- Demerol ... 2308
- Mepergan Injection ... 2753

Mephobarbital (Potential for additive or synergistic CNS effects; potential for decreased barbiturate clearance). Products include:
- Mebaral Tablets ... 2322

Meprobamate (Potential for additive or synergistic CNS effects). Products include:
- Miltown Tablets ... 2672
- PMB 200 and PMB 400 ... 2783

Mesoridazine (Potential for additive or synergistic CNS effects).

Mesoridazine Besylate (Potential for additive or synergistic CNS effects). Products include:
- Serentil ... 684

Metaproterenol Sulfate (Potential for additive hypertension, tachycardia and possibly cardiotoxicity). Products include:
- Alupent ... 669
- Metaproterenol Sulfate Inhalation Solution, USP, Arm-a-Med ... 552

Metaraminol Bitartrate (Potential for additive hypertension, tachycardia and possibly cardiotoxicity). Products include:
- Aramine Injection ... 1609

Metaxalone (Potential for additive drowsiness and CNS depression). Products include:
- Skelaxin Tablets ... 788

Methadone Hydrochloride (Potential for additive drowsiness and CNS depression; potential for additive or synergistic CNS effects). Products include:
- Methadone Hydrochloride Oral Concentrate ... 2233
- Methadone Hydrochloride Oral Solution & Tablets ... 2235

Methamphetamine Hydrochloride (Potential for additive hypertension, tachycardia and possibly cardiotoxicity). Products include:
- Desoxyn Gradumet Tablets ... 419

Methdilazine Hydrochloride (Potential for additive or super-additive tachycardia and drowsiness).
- No products indexed under this heading.

Methocarbamol (Potential for additive drowsiness and CNS depression). Products include:
- Robaxin Injectable ... 2070
- Robaxin Tablets ... 2071
- Robaxisal Tablets ... 2071

Methohexital Sodium (Potential for additive or synergistic CNS effects). Products include:
- Brevital Sodium Vials ... 1429

Methotrimeprazine (Potential for additive drowsiness and CNS depression; potential for additive or synergistic CNS effects). Products include:
- Levoprome ... 1274

Methoxamine Hydrochloride (Potential for additive hypertension, tachycardia and possibly cardiotoxicity). Products include:
- Vasoxyl Injection ... 1196

Methoxyflurane (Potential for additive or synergistic CNS effects).
- No products indexed under this heading.

Metocurine Iodide (Potential for additive drowsiness and CNS depression). Products include:
- Metubine Iodide Vials ... 916

Midazolam Hydrochloride (Potential for additive or synergistic CNS effects). Products include:
- Versed Injection ... 2170

Mivacurium Chloride (Potential for additive drowsiness and CNSD depression). Products include:
- Mivacron ... 1138

Molindone Hydrochloride (Potential for additive or synergistic CNS effects). Products include:
- Moban Tablets and Concentrate ... 1048

Morphine Sulfate (Potential for additive drowsiness and CNS depression; potential for additive or synergistic CNS effects). Products include:
- Astramorph/PF Injection, USP (Preservative-Free) ... 535
- Duramorph ... 962
- Infumorph 200 and Infumorph 500 Sterile Solutions ... 965
- MS Contin Tablets ... 1994
- MSIR ... 1997
- Oramorph SR (Morphine Sulfate Sustained Release Tablets) ... 2236
- RMS Suppositories ... 2657
- Roxanol ... 2243

Norepinephrine Bitartrate (Potential for additive hypertension, tachycardia and possibly cardiotoxicity). Products include:
- Levophed Bitartrate Injection ... 2315

Nortriptyline Hydrochloride (Potential for additive tachycardia, hypertension and drowsiness). Products include:
- Pamelor ... 2280

Opium Alkaloids (Potential for additive drowsiness and CNS depression; potential for additive or synergistic CNS effects).
- No products indexed under this heading.

Orphenadrine Citrate (Potential for additive drowsiness and CNS depression). Products include:
- Norflex ... 1496
- Norgesic ... 1496

Oxazepam (Potential for additive or synergistic CNS effects). Products include:
- Serax Capsules ... 2810
- Serax Tablets ... 2810

Oxybutynin Chloride (Potential for additive or super-additive tachycardia and drowsiness). Products include:
- Ditropan ... 1516

Oxycodone Hydrochloride (Potential for additive drowsiness and CNS depression; potential for additive or synergistic CNS effects). Products include:
- Percocet Tablets ... 938
- Percodan Tablets ... 939
- Percodan-Demi Tablets ... 940
- Roxicodone Tablets, Oral Solution & Intensol (Oxycodone) ... 2244
- Tylox Capsules ... 1584

Pancuronium Bromide Injection (Potential for additive drowsiness and CNSD depression).
- No products indexed under this heading.

Pentobarbital Sodium (Potential for additive or synergistic CNS effects; potential for decreased barbiturate clearance). Products include:
- Nembutal Sodium Capsules ... 436
- Nembutal Sodium Solution ... 438
- Nembutal Sodium Suppositories ... 440

Perphenazine (Potential for additive or synergistic CNS effects). Products include:
- Etrafon ... 2355
- Triavil Tablets ... 1757
- Trilafon ... 2389

Phenobarbital (Potential for additive or synergistic CNS effects; potential for decreased barbiturate clearance). Products include:
- Arco-Lase Plus Tablets ... 512
- Bellergal-S Tablets ... 2250
- Donnatal ... 2060
- Donnatal Extentabs ... 2061
- Donnatal Tablets ... 2060
- Phenobarbital Elixir and Tablets ... 1469
- Quadrinal Tablets ... 1350

IMPORTANT NOTE: Always consult each drug listing in the patient's regimen for possible interactions.

Marinol

Phenylephrine Bitartrate (Potential for additive hypertension, tachycardia and possibly cardiotoxicity).

No products indexed under this heading.

Phenylephrine Hydrochloride (Potential for additive hypertension, tachycardia and possibly cardiotoxicity). Products include:

Atrohist Plus Tablets 454
Cerose DM .... ⊕D 878
Comhist 2038
D.A. Chewable Tablets............................ 951
Deconsal Pediatric Capsules.................. 454
Dura-Vent/DA Tablets 953
Entex Capsules 1986
Entex Liquid 1986
Extendryl 1005
4-Way Fast Acting Nasal Spray (regular & mentholated).................. ⊕D 621
Hemorid For Women .... ⊕D 834
Hycomine Compound Tablets 932
Neo-Synephrine Hydrochloride 1% Carpuject.. 2324
Neo-Synephrine Hydrochloride 1% Injection 2324
Neo-Synephrine Hydrochloride (Ophthalmic) 2325
Neo-Synephrine .... ⊕D 726
Nöstril.. ⊕D 644
Novahistine Elixir .... ⊕D 823
Phenergan VC 2779
Phenergan VC with Codeine 2781
Preparation H .... ⊕D 871
Tympagesic Ear Drops 2342
Vasosulf .... ⊙ 271
Vicks Sinex Nasal Spray and Ultra Fine Mist .... ⊕D 765

Phenylephrine Tannate (Potential for additive hypertension, tachycardia and possibly cardiotoxicity). Products include:

Atrohist Pediatric Suspension 454
Ricobid-D Pediatric Suspension........ 2038
Ricobid Tablets and Pediatric Suspension.. 2038
Rynatan 2673
Rynatuss 2673

Phenylpropanolamine Hydrochloride (Potential for additive hypertension, tachycardia and possibly cardiotoxicity). Products include:

Acutrim .... ⊕D 628
Allerest Children's Chewable Tablets .... ⊕D 627
Allerest 12 Hour Caplets .... ⊕D 627
Atrohist Plus Tablets 454
BC Cold Powder Multi-Symptom Formula (Cold-Sinus-Allergy) ...... ⊕D 609
BC Cold Powder Non-Drowsy Formula (Cold-Sinus) .... ⊕D 609
Cheracol Plus Head Cold/Cough Formula .... ⊕D 769
Comtrex Multi-Symptom Non-Drowsy Liqui-gels............................... ⊕D 618
Contac Continuous Action Nasal Decongestant/Antihistamine 12 Hour Capsules.................................... ⊕D 813
Contac Maximum Strength Continuous Action Decongestant/ Antihistamine 12 Hour Caplets.. ⊕D 813
Contac Severe Cold and Flu Formula Caplets .... ⊕D 814
Coricidin 'D' Decongestant Tablets .... ⊕D 800
Dexatrim .... ⊕D 832
Dexatrim Plus Vitamins Caplets .... ⊕D 832
Dimetane-DC Cough Syrup 2059
Dimetapp Elixir .... ⊕D 773
Dimetapp Extentabs .... ⊕D 774
Dimetapp Tablets/Liqui-Gels .... ⊕D 775
Dimetapp Cold & Allergy Chewable Tablets .... ⊕D 773
Dimetapp DM Elixir.............................. ⊕D 774
Dura-Vent Tablets 952
Entex Capsules 1986
Entex LA Tablets 1987
Entex Liquid 1986
Exgest LA Tablets 782
Hycomine 931
Isoclor Timesule Capsules .... ⊕D 637
Nolamine Timed-Release Tablets 785
Ornade Spansule Capsules 2502
Propagest Tablets 786
Pyrroxate Caplets .... ⊕D 772
Robitussin-CF .... ⊕D 777
Sinulin Tablets 787

Tavist-D 12 Hour Relief Tablets .... ⊕D 787
Teldrin 12 Hour Antihistamine/ Nasal Decongestant Allergy Relief Capsules .... ⊕D 826
Triaminic Allergy Tablets .... ⊕D 789
Triaminic Cold Tablets .... ⊕D 790
Triaminic Expectorant........................ ⊕D 790
Triaminic Syrup .... ⊕D 792
Triaminic-12 Tablets .... ⊕D 792
Triaminic-DM Syrup .... ⊕D 792
Triaminicin Tablets............................... ⊕D 793
Triaminicol Multi-Symptom Cold Tablets .... ⊕D 793
Triaminicol Multi-Symptom Relief ⊕D 794
Vicks DayQuil Allergy Relief 12-Hour Extended Release Tablets.. ⊕D 760
Vicks DayQuil Allergy Relief 4-Hour Tablets .... ⊕D 760
Vicks DayQuil SINUS Pressure & CONGESTION Relief.......................... ⊕D 761

Pimozide (Potential for additive or synergistic CNS effects). Products include:

Orap Tablets 1050

Pirbuterol Acetate (Potential for additive hypertension, tachycardia and possibly cardiotoxicity). Products include:

Maxair Autohaler 1492
Maxair Inhaler 1494

Prazepam (Potential for additive or synergistic CNS effects).

No products indexed under this heading.

Prochlorperazine (Potential for additive or synergistic CNS effects). Products include:

Compazine 2470

Procyclidine Hydrochloride (Potential for additive or super-additive tachycardia and drowsiness). Products include:

Kemadrin Tablets 1112

Promethazine Hydrochloride (Potential for additive or super-additive tachycardia and drowsiness; potential for additive or synergistic CNS effects). Products include:

Mepergan Injection 2753
Phenergan with Codeine...................... 2777
Phenergan with Dextromethorphan 2778
Phenergan Injection 2773
Phenergan Suppositories 2775
Phenergan Syrup 2774
Phenergan Tablets 2775
Phenergan VC... 2779
Phenergan VC with Codeine 2781

Propantheline Bromide (Potential for additive or super-additive tachycardia and drowsiness). Products include:

Pro-Banthine Tablets.............................. 2052

Propofol (Potential for additive or synergistic CNS effects; potential for decreased barbiturate clearance). Products include:

Diprivan Injection................................... 2833

Propoxyphene Hydrochloride (Potential for additive drowsiness and CNS depression; potential for additive or synergistic CNS effects). Products include:

Darvon 1435
Wygesic Tablets 2827

Propoxyphene Napsylate (Potential for additive drowsiness and CNS depression; potential for additive or synergistic CNS effects). Products include:

Darvon-N/Darvocet-N 1433

Protriptyline Hydrochloride (Potential for additive tachycardia, hypertension and drowsiness). Products include:

Vivactil Tablets 1774

Pseudoephedrine Hydrochloride (Potential for additive hypertension, tachycardia and possibly cardiotoxicity). Products include:

Actifed Allergy Daytime/Nighttime Caplets .... ⊕D 844

Actifed Plus Caplets .... ⊕D 845
Actifed Plus Tablets .... ⊕D 845
Actifed with Codeine Cough Syrup.. 1067
Actifed Sinus Daytime/Nighttime Tablets and Caplets .... ⊕D 846
Actifed Syrup.. ⊕D 846
Actifed Tablets .... ⊕D 844
Advil Cold and Sinus Caplets and Tablets (formerly CoAdvil) .... ⊕D 870
Alka-Seltzer Plus Cold Medicine Liqui-Gels .... ⊕D 706
Alka-Seltzer Plus Cold & Cough Medicine Liqui-Gels........................... ⊕D 705
Alka-Seltzer Plus Night-Time Cold Medicine Liqui-Gels........................... ⊕D 706
Allerest Headache Strength Tablets .... ⊕D 627
Allerest Maximum Strength Tablets .... ⊕D 627
Allerest No Drowsiness Tablets ...... ⊕D 627
Allerest Sinus Pain Formula .... ⊕D 627
Anatuss LA Tablets.................................. 1542
Atrohist Pediatric Capsules.................. 453
Bayer Select Sinus Pain Relief Formula .... ⊕D 717
Benadryl Allergy Decongestant Liquid Medication .... ⊕D 848
Benadryl Allergy Decongestant Tablets .... ⊕D 848
Benadryl Allergy Sinus Headache Formula Caplets .... ⊕D 849
Benylin Multisymptom.......................... ⊕D 852
Bromfed Capsules (Extended-Release) 1785
Bromfed Syrup .... ⊕D 733
Bromfed Tablets 1785
Bromfed-DM Cough Syrup................... 1786
Bromfed-PD Capsules (Extended-Release) 1785
Children's Vicks DayQuil Allergy Relief .... ⊕D 757
Children's Vicks NyQuil Cold/ Cough Relief... ⊕D 758
Comtrex Multi-Symptom Cold Reliever Tablets/Caplets/Liqui-Gels/Liquid .... ⊕D 615
Allergy-Sinus Comtrex Multi-Symptom Allergy-Sinus Formula Tablets .... ⊕D 617
Comtrex Multi-Symptom Non-Drowsy Caplets..................................... ⊕D 618
Congess 1004
Contac Day Allergy/Sinus Caplets ⊕D 812
Contac Day & Night .... ⊕D 812
Contac Night Allergy/Sinus Caplets .... ⊕D 812
Contac Severe Cold & Flu Non-Drowsy .... ⊕D 815
Deconamine Chewable Tablets 1320
Deconamine CX Cough and Cold Liquid and Tablets................................ 1319
Deconamine 1320
Deconsal C Expectorant Syrup 456
Deconsal Pediatric Syrup 457
Deconsal II Tablets 454
Dimetane-DX Cough Syrup 2059
Dimetapp Sinus Caplets .... ⊕D 775
Dorcol Children's Cough Syrup ...... ⊕D 785
Drixoral Cough + Congestion Liquid Caps .... ⊕D 802
Dura-Tap/PD Capsules 2867
Duratuss Tablets 2565
Duratuss HD Elixir................................... 2565
Efidac/24 .... ⊕D 635
Entex PSE Tablets 1987
Fedahist Gyrocaps................................... 2401
Fedahist Timecaps 2401
Guaifed... 1787
Guaifed Syrup .... ⊕D 734
Guaimax-D Tablets 792
Guaitab Tablets .... ⊕D 734
Isoclor Expectorant................................. 990
Kronofed-A 977
Motrin IB Sinus .... ⊕D 838
Novahistine DH... 2462
Novahistine DMX .... ⊕D 822
Novahistine Expectorant....................... 2463
Nucofed 2051
PediaCare Cold Allergy Chewable Tablets .... ⊕D 677
PediaCare Cough-Cold Chewable Tablets 1553
PediaCare 1553
PediaCare Infants' Decongestant Drops .... ⊕D 677
PediCare Infant's Drops Decongestant Plus Cough 1553
PediaCare NightRest Cough-Cold Liquid 1553
Pediatric Vicks 44d Dry Hacking Cough & Head Congestion.............. ⊕D 763

Pediatric Vicks 44m Cough & Cold Relief .... ⊕D 764
Robitussin Cold & Cough Liqui-Gels .... ⊕D 776
Robitussin Maximum Strength Cough & Cold .... ⊕D 778
Robitussin Pediatric Cough & Cold Formula .... ⊕D 779
Robitussin Severe Congestion Liqui-Gels .... ⊕D 776
Robitussin-DAC Syrup 2074
Robitussin-PE .... ⊕D 778
Rondec Oral Drops 953
Rondec Syrup 953
Rondec Tablet.. 953
Rondec-DM Oral Drops 954
Rondec-DM Syrup.................................... 954
Rondec-TR Tablet 953
Ryna .... ⊕D 841
Seldane-D Extended-Release Tablets 1538
Semprex-D Capsules 463
Semprex-D Capsules 1167
Sinarest Tablets .... ⊕D 648
Sinarest Extra Strength Tablets...... ⊕D 648
Sinarest No Drowsiness Tablets .... ⊕D 648
Sine-Aid IB Caplets 1554
Sine-Aid Maximum Strength Sinus Medication Gelcaps, Caplets and Tablets 1554
Sine-Off No Drowsiness Formula Caplets .... ⊕D 824
Sine-Off Sinus Medicine .... ⊕D 825
Singlet Tablets .... ⊕D 825
Sinutab Non-Drying Liquid Caps .... ⊕D 859
Sinutab Sinus Allergy Medication, Maximum Strength Tablets and Caplets .... ⊕D 860
Sinutab Sinus Medication, Maximum Strength Without Drowsiness Formula, Tablets & Caplets .... ⊕D 860
Sinutab Sinus Medication, Regular Strength Without Drowsiness Formula .... ⊕D 859
Sudafed Children's Liquid .... ⊕D 861
Sudafed Cold and Cough Liquidcaps .... ⊕D 862
Sudafed Cough Syrup .... ⊕D 862
Sudafed Plus Liquid .... ⊕D 862
Sudafed Plus Tablets .... ⊕D 863
Sudafed Severe Cold Formula Caplets .... ⊕D 863
Sudafed Severe Cold Formula Tablets .... ⊕D 864
Sudafed Sinus Caplets.......................... ⊕D 864
Sudafed Sinus Tablets........................... ⊕D 864
Sudafed Tablets, 30 mg........................ ⊕D 861
Sudafed Tablets, 60 mg........................ ⊕D 861
Sudafed 12 Hour Caplets .... ⊕D 861
Syn-Rx Tablets 465
Syn-Rx DM Tablets 466
TheraFlu.. ⊕D 787
TheraFlu Maximum Strength Nighttime Flu, Cold & Cough Medicine .... ⊕D 788
TheraFlu Maximum Strength Non-Drowsy Formula Flu, Cold & Cough Medicine .... ⊕D 788
Thera Flu Maximum Strength, Non-Drowsy Formula Flu, Cold and Cough Caplets .... ⊕D 789
Triaminic AM Cough and Decongestant Formula .... ⊕D 789
Triaminic AM Decongestant Formula .... ⊕D 790
Triaminic Nite Light .... ⊕D 791
Triaminic Sore Throat Formula ...... ⊕D 791
Tussend 1783
Tussend Expectorant 1785
Children's TYLENOL Cold Multi-Symptom Liquid Formula and Chewable Tablets................................. 1561
Children's TYLENOL Cold Plus Cough Multi Symptom Tablets and Liquid... ⊕D 681
Infants' TYLENOL Cold Decongestant & Fever-Reducer Drops 1556
TYLENOL Maximum Strength Allergy Sinus Medication Gelcaps and Caplets 1563
TYLENOL Maximum Strength Allergy Sinus NightTime Medication Caplets 1555
TYLENOL Flu Maximum Strength Gelcaps 1565
TYLENOL Flu NightTime, Maximum Strength, Gelcaps 1566
TYLENOL Maximum Strength Flu NightTime Hot Medication Packets 1562

(⊕D Described in PDR For Nonprescription Drugs) (⊙ Described in PDR For Ophthalmology)

TYLENOL, Maximum Strength, Sinus Medication Geltabs, Gelcaps, Caplets and Tablets 1566
TYLENOL Cold Multi-Symptom Formula Medication Tablets and Caplets 1561
TYLENOL Cold Medication No Drowsiness Formula Gelcaps and Caplets 1562
TYLENOL Cold Multi-Symptom Hot Medication Liquid Packets.............. 1557
TYLENOL Cough Multi-Symptom Medication with Decongestant...... 1565
Ursinus Inlay-Tabs................................ⓢⓓ 794
Vicks 44 LiquiCaps Cough, Cold & Flu Relief... ⓢⓓ 755
Vicks 44 LiquiCaps Non-Drowsy Cough & Cold Relief........................ ⓢⓓ 756
Vicks 44D Dry Hacking Cough & Head Congestion .... ⓢⓓ 755
Vicks 44M Cough, Cold & Flu Relief.. ⓢⓓ 756
Vicks DayQuil .... ⓢⓓ 761
Vicks DayQuil SINUS Pressure & PAIN Relief with IBUPROFEN ...... ⓢⓓ 762
Vicks Nyquil Hot Therapy.................. ⓢⓓ 762
Vicks NyQuil LiquiCaps Multi-Symptom Cold/Flu Relief.............. ⓢⓓ 763
Vicks NyQuil Multi-Symptom Cold/Flu Relief - (Original & Cherry Flavor) .... ⓢⓓ 763

Pseudoephedrine Sulfate (Potential for additive hypertension, tachycardia and possibly cardiotoxicity). Products include:

Cheracol Sinus .... ⓢⓓ 768
Chlor-Trimeton Allergy Decongestant Tablets .... ⓢⓓ 799
Claritin-D 2350
Drixoral Cold and Allergy Sustained-Action Tablets .... ⓢⓓ 802
Drixoral Cold and Flu Extended-Release Tablets................................... ⓢⓓ 803
Drixoral Non-Drowsy Formula Extended-Release Tablets .... ⓢⓓ 803
Drixoral Allergy/Sinus Extended Release Tablets................................... ⓢⓓ 804
Trinalin Repetabs Tablets 1330

Pyrilamine Maleate (Potential for additive or super-additive tachycardia and drowsiness). Products include:

4-Way Fast Acting Nasal Spray (regular & mentholated) .... ⓢⓓ 621
Maximum Strength Multi-Symptom Formula Midol .... ⓢⓓ 722
PMS Multi-Symptom Formula Midol .... ⓢⓓ 723

Pyrilamine Tannate (Potential for additive or super-additive tachycardia and drowsiness). Products include:

Atrohist Pediatric Suspension 454
Rynatan 2673

Quazepam (Potential for additive or synergistic CNS effects). Products include:

Doral Tablets 2664

Risperidone (Potential for additive drowsiness and CNS depression; potential for additive or synergistic CNS effects). Products include:

Risperdal 1301

Rocuronium Bromide (Potential for additive drowsiness and CNSD depression). Products include:

Zemuron 1830

Salmeterol Xinafoate (Potential for additive hypertension, tachycardia and possibly cardiotoxicity). Products include:

Serevent Inhalation Aerosol................ 1176

Scopolamine (Potential for additive or super-additive tachycardia and drowsiness). Products include:

Transderm Scōp Transdermal Therapeutic System 869

Scopolamine Hydrobromide (Potential for additive or super-additive tachycardia and drowsiness). Products include:

Atrohist Plus Tablets 454
Donnatal 2060
Donnatal Extentabs................................ 2061

Donnatal Tablets 2060

Secobarbital Sodium (Potential for additive or synergistic CNS effects; potential for decreased barbiturate clearance). Products include:

Seconal Sodium Pulvules 1474

Succinylcholine Chloride (Potential for additive drowsiness and CNSD depression). Products include:

Anectine.. 1073

Sufentanil Citrate (Potential for additive drowsiness and CNS depression; potential for additive or synergistic CNS effects). Products include:

Sufenta Injection 1309

Temazepam (Potential for additive or synergistic CNS effects; potential for decreased barbiturate clearance). Products include:

Restoril Capsules.................................... 2284

Terbutaline Sulfate (Potential for additive hypertension, tachycardia and possibly cardiotoxicity). Products include:

Brethaire Inhaler 813
Brethine Ampuls 815
Brethine Tablets...................................... 814
Bricanyl Subcutaneous Injection...... 1502
Bricanyl Tablets 1503

Terfenadine (Potential for additive or super-additive tachycardia and drowsiness). Products include:

Seldane Tablets 1536
Seldane-D Extended-Release Tablets 1538

Theophylline (Potential for increased theophylline metabolism). Products include:

Marax Tablets & DF Syrup.................. 2200
Quibron 2053

Theophylline Anhydrous (Potential for increased theophylline metabolism). Products include:

Aerolate 1004
Primatene Dual Action Formula...... ⓢⓓ 872
Primatene Tablets .... ⓢⓓ 873
Respbid Tablets 682
Slo-bid Gyrocaps 2033
Theo-24 Extended Release Capsules 2568
Theo-Dur Extended-Release Tablets 1327
Theo-X Extended-Release Tablets .. 788
Uni-Dur Extended-Release Tablets.. 1331
Uniphyl 400 mg Tablets........................ 2001

Theophylline Calcium Salicylate (Potential for increased theophylline metabolism). Products include:

Quadrinal Tablets 1350

Theophylline Sodium Glycinate (Potential for increased theophylline metabolism).

No products indexed under this heading.

Thiamylal Sodium (Potential for additive or synergistic CNS effects; potential for decreased barbiturate clearance).

No products indexed under this heading.

Thioridazine Hydrochloride (Potential for additive or synergistic CNS effects). Products include:

Mellaril 2269

Thiothixene (Potential for additive or synergistic CNS effects). Products include:

Navane Capsules and Concentrate 2201
Navane Intramuscular 2202

Triazolam (Potential for additive or synergistic CNS effects; potential for decreased barbiturate clearance). Products include:

Halcion Tablets.. 2611

Tridihexethyl Chloride (Potential for additive or super-additive tachycardia and drowsiness).

No products indexed under this heading.

Trifluoperazine Hydrochloride (Potential for additive or synergistic CNS effects). Products include:

Stelazine 2514

Trihexyphenidyl Hydrochloride (Potential for additive or super-additive tachycardia and drowsiness). Products include:

Artane.. 1368

Trimeprazine Tartrate (Potential for additive or super-additive tachycardia and drowsiness). Products include:

Temaril Tablets, Syrup and Spansule Extended-Release Capsules.. 483

Trimipramine Maleate (Potential for additive tachycardia, hypertension and drowsiness). Products include:

Surmontil Capsules................................ 2811

Tripelennamine Hydrochloride (Potential for additive or super-additive tachycardia and drowsiness). Products include:

PBZ Tablets 845
PBZ-SR Tablets.. 844

Triprolidine Hydrochloride (Potential for additive or super-additive tachycardia and drowsiness). Products include:

Actifed Plus Caplets .... ⓢⓓ 845
Actifed Plus Tablets .... ⓢⓓ 845
Actifed with Codeine Cough Syrup.. 1067
Actifed Syrup...................................... ⓢⓓ 846
Actifed Tablets .... ⓢⓓ 844

Vecuronium Bromide (Potential for additive drowsiness and CNS depression). Products include:

Norcuron.. 1826

Zolpidem Tartrate (Potential for additive drowsiness and CNS depression; potential for additive or synergistic CNS effects). Products include:

Ambien Tablets.. 2416

Food Interactions

Alcohol (Additive drowsiness and CNS depression).

MARLYN FORMULA 50 CAPSULES

(Amino Acid Preparations, Vitamin B_6) 1541

None cited in PDR database.

MASSENGILL DISPOSABLE DOUCHE

(Vinegar) 2457

None cited in PDR database.

MASSENGILL FEMININE CLEANSING WASH

(Cleanser) 2458

None cited in PDR database.

MASSENGILL FRAGRANCE-FREE SOFT CLOTH TOWELETTE & BABY POWDER SCENT

(Lactic Acid, Potassium Sorbate, Sodium Lactate) 2458

None cited in PDR database.

MASSENGILL LIQUID CONCENTRATE

(Povidone Iodine) 2457

None cited in PDR database.

MASSENGILL MEDICATED DISPOSABLE DOUCHE

(Povidone Iodine) 2458

None cited in PDR database.

MASSENGILL MEDICATED LIQUID CONCENTRATE

(Povidone Iodine) ....ⓢⓓ 821

None cited in PDR database.

MASSENGILL MEDICATED SOFT CLOTH TOWELETTES

(Hydrocortisone) 2458

None cited in PDR database.

MASSENGILL POWDER

(Ammonium Alum, Sodium Chloride) 2457

None cited in PDR database.

MATERNA TABLETS

(Vitamins, Prenatal) 1379

None cited in PDR database.

MATULANE CAPSULES

(Procarbazine Hydrochloride) 2131

May interact with barbiturates, antihistamines, narcotic analgesics, phenothiazines, sympathomimetics, tricyclic antidepressants, antihypertensives, and certain other agents. Compounds in these categories include:

Acebutolol Hydrochloride (Possible potentiation and increased CNS depression). Products include:

Sectral Capsules 2807

Acrivastine (CNS depression). Products include:

Semprex-D Capsules 463
Semprex-D Capsules 1167

Albuterol (Avoided because of some maoi activity). Products include:

Proventil Inhalation Aerosol 2382
Ventolin Inhalation Aerosol and Refill 1197

Albuterol Sulfate (Avoided). Products include:

Airet Solution for Inhalation 452
Proventil Inhalation Solution 0.083%.. 2384
Proventil Repetabs Tablets 2386
Proventil Solution for Inhalation 0.5%.. 2383
Proventil Syrup...................................... 2385
Proventil Tablets 2386
Ventolin Inhalation Solution................ 1198
Ventolin Nebules Inhalation Solution.. 1199
Ventolin Rotacaps for Inhalation...... 1200
Ventolin Syrup.. 1202
Ventolin Tablets 1203
Volmax Extended-Release Tablets .. 1788

Alfentanil Hydrochloride (CNS depression). Products include:

Alfenta Injection 1286

Amitriptyline Hydrochloride (Avoid concurrent use). Products include:

Elavil 2838
Endep Tablets 2174
Etrafon 2355
Limbitrol 2180
Triavil Tablets 1757

Amlodipine Besylate (Possible potentiation and increased CNS depression). Products include:

Lotrel Capsules...................................... 840
Norvasc Tablets 1940

Amoxapine (Avoid concurrent use). Products include:

Asendin Tablets 1369

Aprobarbital (CNS depression).

No products indexed under this heading.

Astemizole (CNS depression). Products include:

Hismanal Tablets.................................... 1293

Atenolol (Possible potentiation and increased CNS depression). Products include:

Tenoretic Tablets.................................... 2845
Tenormin Tablets and I.V. Injection 2847

Azatadine Maleate (CNS depression). Products include:

Trinalin Repetabs Tablets 1330

IMPORTANT NOTE: Always consult each drug listing in the patient's regimen for possible interactions.

Matulane **Interactions Index** **628**

Benazepril Hydrochloride (Possible potentiation and increased CNS depression). Products include:
- Lotensin Tablets 834
- Lotensin HCT 837
- Lotrel Capsules 840

Bendroflumethiazide (Possible potentiation and increased CNS depression).
- No products indexed under this heading.

Betaxolol Hydrochloride (Possible potentiation and increased CNS depression). Products include:
- Betoptic Ophthalmic Solution 469
- Betoptic S Ophthalmic Suspension 471
- Kerlone Tablets 2436

Bisoprolol Fumarate (Possible potentiation and increased CNS depression). Products include:
- Zebeta Tablets 1413
- Ziac 1415

Bromodiphenhydramine Hydrochloride (CNS depression).
- No products indexed under this heading.

Brompheniramine Maleate (CNS depression). Products include:
- Alka Seltzer Plus Sinus Medicine .. ▣ 707
- Bromfed Capsules (Extended-Release) 1785
- Bromfed Syrup .... ▣ 733
- Bromfed Tablets 1785
- Bromfed-DM Cough Syrup 1786
- Bromfed-PD Capsules (Extended-Release) 1785
- Dimetane-DC Cough Syrup 2059
- Dimetane-DX Cough Syrup 2059
- Dimetapp Elixir .... ▣ 773
- Dimetapp Extentabs .... ▣ 774
- Dimetapp Tablets/Liqui-Gels .... ▣ 775
- Dimetapp Cold & Allergy Chewable Tablets .... ▣ 773
- Dimetapp DM Elixir .... ▣ 774
- Vicks DayQuil Allergy Relief 12-Hour Extended Release Tablets.. ▣ 760
- Vicks DayQuil Allergy Relief 4-Hour Tablets .... ▣ 760

Buprenorphine (CNS depression). Products include:
- Buprenex Injectable 2006

Butabarbital (CNS depression).
- No products indexed under this heading.

Butalbital (CNS depression). Products include:
- Esgic-plus Tablets 1013
- Fioricet Tablets 2258
- Fioricet with Codeine Capsules 2260
- Fiorinal Capsules 2261
- Fiorinal with Codeine Capsules 2262
- Fiorinal Tablets 2261
- Phrenilin 785
- Sedapap Tablets 50 mg/650 mg .. 1543

Captopril (Possible potentiation and increased CNS depression). Products include:
- Capoten 739
- Capozide 742

Carteolol Hydrochloride (Possible potentiation and increased CNS depression). Products include:
- Cartrol Tablets 410
- Ocupress Ophthalmic Solution, 1% Sterile .... ⊙ 309

Chlorothiazide (Possible potentiation and increased CNS depression). Products include:
- Aldoclor Tablets 1598
- Diupres Tablets 1650
- Diuril Oral 1653

Chlorothiazide Sodium (Possible potentiation and increased CNS depression). Products include:
- Diuril Sodium Intravenous 1652

Chlorpheniramine Maleate (CNS depression). Products include:
- Alka-Seltzer Plus Cold Medicine .... ▣ 705
- Alka-Seltzer Plus Cold Medicine Liqui-Gels .... ▣ 706
- Alka-Seltzer Plus Cold & Cough Medicine .... ▣ 708
- Alka-Seltzer Plus Cold & Cough Medicine Liqui-Gels .... ▣ 705
- Allerest Children's Chewable Tablets .... ▣ 627
- Allerest Headache Strength Tablets .... ▣ 627
- Allerest Maximum Strength Tablets .... ▣ 627
- Allerest Sinus Pain Formula .... ▣ 627
- Allerest 12 Hour Caplets .... ▣ 627
- Ana-Kit Anaphylaxis Emergency Treatment Kit 617
- Atrohist Pediatric Capsules 453
- Atrohist Plus Tablets 454
- BC Cold Powder Multi-Symptom Formula (Cold-Sinus-Allergy) ...... ▣ 609
- Cerose DM .... ▣ 878
- Cheracol Plus Head Cold/Cough Formula .... ▣ 769
- Children's Vicks DayQuil Allergy Relief .... ▣ 757
- Children's Vicks NyQuil Cold/Cough Relief .... ▣ 758
- Chlor-Trimeton Allergy Decongestant Tablets .... ▣ 799
- Chlor-Trimeton Allergy Tablets ...... ▣ 798
- Comhist 2038
- Comtrex Multi-Symptom Cold Reliever Tablets/Caplets/Liqui-Gels/Liquid .... ▣ 615
- Allergy-Sinus Comtrex Multi-Symptom Allergy-Sinus Formula Tablets .... ▣ 617
- Contac Continuous Action Nasal Decongestant/Antihistamine 12 Hour Capsules .... ▣ 813
- Contac Maximum Strength Continuous Action Decongestant/Antihistamine 12 Hour Caplets.. ▣ 813
- Contac Severe Cold and Flu Formula Caplets .... ▣ 814
- Coricidin 'D' Decongestant Tablets .... ▣ 800
- Coricidin Tablets .... ▣ 800
- D.A. Chewable Tablets 951
- Deconamine 1320
- Dura-Tap/PD Capsules 2867
- Dura-Vent/DA Tablets 953
- Extendryl 1005
- Fedahist Gyrocaps 2401
- Fedahist Timecaps 2401
- Hycomine Compound Tablets 932
- Isoclor Timesule Capsules .... ▣ 637
- Kronofed-A 977
- Nolamine Timed-Release Tablets 785
- Novahistine DH 2462
- Novahistine Elixir .... ▣ 823
- Ornade Spansule Capsules 2502
- PediaCare Cold Allergy Chewable Tablets .... ▣ 677
- PediaCare Cough-Cold Chewable Tablets 1553
- PediaCare Cough-Cold Liquid 1553
- PediaCare NightRest Cough-Cold Liquid 1553
- Pediatric Vicks 44m Cough & Cold Relief .... ▣ 764
- Pyrroxate Caplets .... ▣ 772
- Ryna .... ▣ 841
- Sinarest Tablets .... ▣ 648
- Sinarest Extra Strength Tablets .... ▣ 648
- Sine-Off Sinus Medicine .... ▣ 825
- Singlet Tablets .... ▣ 825
- Sinulin Tablets 787
- Sinutab Sinus Allergy Medication, Maximum Strength Tablets and Caplets .... ▣ 860
- Sudafed Plus Liquid .... ▣ 862
- Sudafed Plus Tablets .... ▣ 863
- Teldrin 12 Hour Antihistamine/Nasal Decongestant Allergy Relief Capsules .... ▣ 826
- TheraFlu .... ▣ 787
- TheraFlu Maximum Strength Nighttime Flu, Cold & Cough Medicine .... ▣ 788
- Triaminic Allergy Tablets .... ▣ 789
- Triaminic Cold Tablets .... ▣ 790
- Triaminic Nite Light .... ▣ 791
- Triaminic Syrup .... ▣ 792
- Triaminic-12 Tablets .... ▣ 792
- Triaminicin Tablets .... ▣ 793
- Triaminicol Multi-Symptom Cold Tablets .... ▣ 793
- Triaminicol Multi-Symptom Relief ▣ 794
- Tussend 1783
- Children's TYLENOL Cold Multi-Symptom Liquid Formula and Chewable Tablets 1561
- Children's TYLENOL Cold Plus Cough Multi Symptom Tablets and Liquid .... ▣ 681
- TYLENOL Maximum Strength Allergy Sinus Medication Gelcaps and Caplets 1563
- TYLENOL Cold Multi-Symptom Formula Medication Tablets and Caplets 1561
- TYLENOL Cold Multi-Symptom Hot Medication Liquid Packets 1557
- Vicks 44 LiquiCaps Cough, Cold & Flu Relief .... ▣ 755
- Vicks 44M Cough, Cold & Flu Relief .... ▣ 756

Chlorpheniramine Polistirex (CNS depression). Products include:
- Tussionex Pennkinetic Extended-Release Suspension 998

Chlorpheniramine Tannate (CNS depression). Products include:
- Atrohist Pediatric Suspension 454
- Ricobid Tablets and Pediatric Suspension 2038
- Rynatan 2673
- Rynatuss 2673

Chlorpromazine (CNS depression). Products include:
- Thorazine Suppositories 2523

Chlorthalidone (Possible potentiation and increased CNS depression). Products include:
- Combipres Tablets 677
- Tenoretic Tablets 2845
- Thalitone 1245

Clemastine Fumarate (CNS depression). Products include:
- Tavist Syrup 2297
- Tavist Tablets 2298
- Tavist-1 12 Hour Relief Tablets .... ▣ 787
- Tavist-D 12 Hour Relief Tablets .... ▣ 787

Clomipramine Hydrochloride (Avoid concurrent use). Products include:
- Anafranil Capsules 803

Clonidine (Possible potentiation and increased CNS depression). Products include:
- Catapres-TTS 675

Clonidine Hydrochloride (Possible potentiation and increased CNS depression). Products include:
- Catapres Tablets 674
- Combipres Tablets 677

Codeine Phosphate (CNS depression). Products include:
- Actifed with Codeine Cough Syrup.. 1067
- Brontex 1981
- Deconsal C Expectorant Syrup 456
- Deconsal Pediatric Syrup 457
- Dimetane-DC Cough Syrup 2059
- Empirin with Codeine Tablets 1093
- Fioricet with Codeine Capsules 2260
- Fiorinal with Codeine Capsules 2262
- Isoclor Expectorant 990
- Novahistine DH 2462
- Novahistine Expectorant 2463
- Nucofed 2051
- Phenergan with Codeine 2777
- Phenergan VC with Codeine 2781
- Robitussin A-C Syrup 2073
- Robitussin-DAC Syrup 2074
- Ryna .... ▣ 841
- Soma Compound w/Codeine Tablets 2676
- Tussi-Organidin NR Liquid and S NR Liquid 2677
- Tylenol with Codeine 1583

Cyproheptadine Hydrochloride (CNS depression). Products include:
- Periactin 1724

Deserpidine (Possible potentiation and increased CNS depression).
- No products indexed under this heading.

Desipramine Hydrochloride (Avoid concurrent use). Products include:
- Norpramin Tablets 1526

Dexchlorpheniramine Maleate (CNS depression).
- No products indexed under this heading.

Dezocine (CNS depression). Products include:
- Dalgan Injection 538

Diazoxide (Possible potentiation and increased CNS depression). Products include:
- Hyperstat I.V. Injection 2363
- Proglycem 580

Diltiazem Hydrochloride (Possible potentiation and increased CNS depression). Products include:
- Cardizem CD Capsules 1506
- Cardizem SR Capsules 1510
- Cardizem Injectable 1508
- Cardizem Tablets 1512
- Dilacor XR Extended-release Capsules 2018

Diphenhydramine Citrate (CNS depression). Products include:
- Excedrin P.M. Analgesic/Sleeping Aid Tablets, Caplets, Liquigels...... 733

Diphenhydramine Hydrochloride (CNS depression). Products include:
- Actifed Allergy Daytime/Nighttime Caplets .... ▣ 844
- Actifed Sinus Daytime/Nighttime Tablets and Caplets .... ▣ 846
- Arthritis Foundation NightTime Caplets .... ▣ 674
- Extra Strength Bayer PM Aspirin .. ▣ 713
- Bayer Select Night Time Pain Relief Formula .... ▣ 716
- Benadryl Allergy Decongestant Liquid Medication .... ▣ 848
- Benadryl Allergy Decongestant Tablets .... ▣ 848
- Benadryl Allergy Liquid Medication .... ▣ 849
- Benadryl Allergy .... ▣ 848
- Benadryl Allergy Sinus Headache Formula Caplets .... ▣ 849
- Benadryl Capsules 1898
- Benadryl Dye-Free Allergy Liqui-gel Softgels .... ▣ 850
- Benadryl Dye-Free Allergy Liquid Medication .... ▣ 850
- Benadryl Itch Relief Cream, Children's Formula and Maximum Strength 2% .... ▣ 851
- Benadryl Itch Relief Spray, Children's Formula and Maximum Strength 2% .... ▣ 851
- Benadryl Itch Relief Stick Maximum Strength 2% .... ▣ 850
- Benadryl Itch Stopping Gel, Children's Formula and Maximum Strength 2% .... ▣ 851
- Benadryl Kapseals 1898
- Benadryl Injection 1898
- Contac Day & Night Cold/Flu Night Caplets .... ▣ 812
- Contac Night Allergy/Sinus Caplets .... ▣ 812
- Extra Strength Doan's P.M. .... ▣ 633
- Legatrin PM .... ▣ 651
- Miles Nervine Nighttime Sleep-Aid ▣ 723
- Nytol QuickCaps Caplets .... ▣ 610
- Sleepinal Night-time Sleep Aid Capsules and Softgels .... ▣ 834
- TYLENOL Maximum Strength Allergy Sinus NightTime Medication Caplets 1555
- TYLENOL Flu NightTime, Maximum Strength, Gelcaps 1566
- TYLENOL Maximum Strength Flu NightTime Hot Medication Packets 1562
- TYLENOL PM, Extra Strength Pain Reliever/Sleep Aid Caplets, Geltabs, Gelcaps 1560
- TYLENOL Severe Allergy Medication Caplets 1564
- Maximum Strength Unisom Sleepgels 1934
- Unisom With Pain Relief-Nighttime Sleep Aid and Pain Reliever 1934

Diphenylpyraline Hydrochloride (CNS depression).
- No products indexed under this heading.

Dobutamine Hydrochloride (Avoid concurrent use). Products include:
- Dobutrex Solution Vials 1439

(▣ Described in PDR For Nonprescription Drugs) (⊙ Described in PDR For Ophthalmology)

Interactions Index

Dopamine Hydrochloride (Avoid concurrent use).

No products indexed under this heading.

Doxazosin Mesylate (Possible potentiation and increased CNS depression). Products include:

Cardura Tablets 2186

Doxepin Hydrochloride (Avoid concurrent use). Products include:

Sinequan 2205
Zonalon Cream 1055

Enalapril Maleate (Possible potentiation and increased CNS depression). Products include:

Vaseretic Tablets 1765
Vasotec Tablets 1771

Enalaprilat (Possible potentiation and increased CNS depression). Products include:

Vasotec I.V. 1768

Ephedrine Hydrochloride (Avoid concurrent use). Products include:

Primatene Dual Action Formula...... ◉□ 872
Primatene Tablets .... ◉□ 873
Quadrinal Tablets 1350

Ephedrine Sulfate (Avoid concurrent use). Products include:

Bronkaid Caplets .... ◉□ 717
Marax Tablets & DF Syrup.................... 2200

Ephedrine Tannate (Avoid concurrent use). Products include:

Rynatuss 2673

Epinephrine (Avoid concurrent use). Products include:

Bronkaid Mist .... ◉□ 717
EPIFRIN .... ⊙ 239
EpiPen 790
Marcaine Hydrochloride with Epinephrine 1:200,000 2316
Primatene Mist .... ◉□ 873
Sensorcaine with Epinephrine Injection 559
Sus-Phrine Injection 1019
Xylocaine with Epinephrine Injections 567

Epinephrine Bitartrate (Avoid concurrent use). Products include:

Bronkaid Mist Suspension .... ◉□ 718
Sensorcaine-MPF with Epinephrine Injection 559

Epinephrine Hydrochloride (Avoid concurrent use). Products include:

Ana-Kit Anaphylaxis Emergency Treatment Kit 617

Esmolol Hydrochloride (Possible potentiation and increased CNS depression). Products include:

Brevibloc Injection................................ 1808

Felodipine (Possible potentiation and increased CNS depression). Products include:

Plendil Extended-Release Tablets.... 527

Fentanyl (CNS depression). Products include:

Duragesic Transdermal System....... 1288

Fentanyl Citrate (CNS depression). Products include:

Sublimaze Injection............................... 1307

Fluphenazine Decanoate (CNS depression). Products include:

Prolixin Decanoate 509

Fluphenazine Enanthate (CNS depression). Products include:

Prolixin Enanthate 509

Fluphenazine Hydrochloride (CNS depression). Products include:

Prolixin 509

Fosinopril Sodium (Possible potentiation and increased CNS depression). Products include:

Monopril Tablets 757

Furosemide (Possible potentiation and increased CNS depression). Products include:

Lasix Injection, Oral Solution and Tablets 1240

Guanabenz Acetate (Possible potentiation and increased CNS depression).

No products indexed under this heading.

Guanethidine Monosulfate (Possible potentiation and increased CNS depression). Products include:

Esimil Tablets 822
Ismelin Tablets 827

Hydralazine Hydrochloride (Possible potentiation and increased CNS depression). Products include:

Apresazide Capsules 808
Apresoline Hydrochloride Tablets .. 809
Ser-Ap-Es Tablets 849

Hydrochlorothiazide (Possible potentiation and increased CNS depression). Products include:

Aldactazide... 2413
Aldoril Tablets....................................... 1604
Apresazide Capsules 808
Capozide 742
Dyazide 2479
Esidrix Tablets 821
Esimil Tablets 822
HydroDIURIL Tablets 1674
Hydropres Tablets................................. 1675
Hyzaar Tablets 1677
Inderide Tablets 2732
Inderide LA Long Acting Capsules .. 2734
Lopressor HCT Tablets 832
Lotensin HCT.. 837
Maxzide 1380
Moduretic Tablets 1705
Oretic Tablets 443
Prinzide Tablets 1737
Ser-Ap-Es Tablets 849
Timolide Tablets.................................... 1748
Vaseretic Tablets 1765
Zestoretic 2850
Ziac 1415

Hydrocodone Bitartrate (CNS depression). Products include:

Anexsia 5/500 Elixir 1781
Anexia Tablets....................................... 1782
Codiclear DH Syrup 791
Deconamine CX Cough and Cold Liquid and Tablets................................. 1319
Duratuss HD Elixir................................ 2565
Hycodan Tablets and Syrup 930
Hycomine Compound Tablets 932
Hycomine 931
Hycotuss Expectorant Syrup 933
Hydrocet Capsules 782
Lorcet 10/650....................................... 1018
Lortab 2566
Tussend 1783
Tussend Expectorant 1785
Vicodin Tablets..................................... 1356
Vicodin ES Tablets 1357
Vicodin Tuss Expectorant 1358
Zydone Capsules 949

Hydrocodone Polistirex (CNS depression). Products include:

Tussionex Pennkinetic Extended-Release Suspension 998

Hydroflumethiazide (Possible potentiation and increased CNS depression). Products include:

Diucardin Tablets.................................. 2718

Imipramine Hydrochloride (Avoid concurrent use). Products include:

Tofranil Ampuls 854
Tofranil Tablets 856

Imipramine Pamoate (Avoid concurrent use). Products include:

Tofranil-PM Capsules............................ 857

Indapamide (Possible potentiation and increased CNS depression). Products include:

Lozol Tablets 2022

Isoproterenol Hydrochloride (Avoid concurrent use). Products include:

Isuprel Hydrochloride Injection 1:5000 2311
Isuprel Hydrochloride Solution 1:200 & 1:100 2313
Isuprel Mistometer 2312

Isoproterenol Sulfate (Avoid concurrent use). Products include:

Norisodrine with Calcium Iodide Syrup... 442

Isradipine (Possible potentiation and increased CNS depression). Products include:

DynaCirc Capsules 2256

Labetalol Hydrochloride (Possible potentiation and increased CNS depression). Products include:

Normodyne Injection 2377
Normodyne Tablets 2379
Trandate 1185

Levorphanol Tartrate (CNS depression). Products include:

Levo-Dromoran..................................... 2129

Lisinopril (Possible potentiation and increased CNS depression). Products include:

Prinivil Tablets 1733
Prinzide Tablets 1737
Zestoretic 2850
Zestril Tablets 2854

Loratadine (CNS depression). Products include:

Claritin 2349
Claritin-D 2350

Losartan Potassium (Possible potentiation and increased CNS depression). Products include:

Cozaar Tablets 1628
Hyzaar Tablets 1677

Maprotiline Hydrochloride (Avoid concurrent use). Products include:

Ludiomil Tablets................................... 843

Mecamylamine Hydrochloride (Possible potentiation and increased CNS depression). Products include:

Inversine Tablets 1686

Meperidine Hydrochloride (CNS depression). Products include:

Demerol 2308
Mepergan Injection 2753

Mephobarbital (CNS depression). Products include:

Mebaral Tablets 2322

Mesoridazine Besylate (CNS depression). Products include:

Serentil.. 684

Metaproterenol Sulfate (Avoid concurrent use). Products include:

Alupent.. 669
Metaproterenol Sulfate Inhalation Solution, USP, Arm-a-Med 552

Metaraminol Bitartrate (Avoid concurrent use). Products include:

Aramine Injection.................................. 1609

Methadone Hydrochloride (CNS depression). Products include:

Methadone Hydrochloride Oral Concentrate 2233
Methadone Hydrochloride Oral Solution & Tablets................................ 2235

Methdilazine Hydrochloride (CNS depression).

No products indexed under this heading.

Methotrimeprazine (CNS depression). Products include:

Levoprome 1274

Methoxamine Hydrochloride (Avoid concurrent use). Products include:

Vasoxyl Injection 1196

Methylclothiazide (Possible potentiation and increased CNS depression). Products include:

Enduron Tablets.................................... 420

Methyldopa (Possible potentiation and increased CNS depression). Products include:

Aldoclor Tablets 1598
Aldomet Oral 1600
Aldoril Tablets....................................... 1604

Methyldopate Hydrochloride (Possible potentiation and increased CNS depression). Products include:

Aldomet Ester HCl Injection 1602

Metolazone (Possible potentiation and increased CNS depression). Products include:

Mykrox Tablets 993
Zaroxolyn Tablets 1000

Metoprolol Succinate (Possible potentiation and increased CNS depression). Products include:

Toprol-XL Tablets 565

Metoprolol Tartrate (Possible potentiation and increased CNS depression). Products include:

Lopressor Ampuls 830
Lopressor HCT Tablets 832
Lopressor Tablets 830

Metyrosine (Possible potentiation and increased CNS depression). Products include:

Demser Capsules.................................. 1649

Minoxidil (Possible potentiation and increased CNS depression). Products include:

Loniten Tablets 2618
Rogaine Topical Solution 2637

Moexipril Hydrochloride (Possible potentiation and increased CNS depression). Products include:

Univasc Tablets 2410

Morphine Sulfate (CNS depression). Products include:

Astramorph/PF Injection, USP (Preservative-Free) 535
Duramorph.. 962
Infumorph 200 and Infumorph 500 Sterile Solutions............................ 965
MS Contin Tablets................................. 1994
MSIR 1997
Oramorph SR (Morphine Sulfate Sustained Release Tablets) 2236
RMS Suppositories 2657
Roxanol 2243

Nadolol (Possible potentiation and increased CNS depression).

No products indexed under this heading.

Nicardipine Hydrochloride (Possible potentiation and increased CNS depression). Products include:

Cardene Capsules 2095
Cardene I.V. 2709
Cardene SR Capsules............................ 2097

Nifedipine (Possible potentiation and increased CNS depression). Products include:

Adalat Capsules (10 mg and 20 mg) 587
Adalat CC 589
Procardia Capsules............................... 1971
Procardia XL Extended Release Tablets 1972

Nisoldipine (Possible potentiation and increased CNS depression).

No products indexed under this heading.

Nitroglycerin (Possible potentiation and increased CNS depression). Products include:

Deponit NTG Transdermal Delivery System 2397
Nitro-Bid IV... 1523
Nitro-Bid Ointment 1524
Nitrodisc 2047
Nitro-Dur (nitroglycerin) Transdermal Infusion System 1326
Nitrolingual Spray 2027
Nitrostat Tablets 1925
Transderm-Nitro Transdermal Therapeutic System 859

Norepinephrine Bitartrate (Avoid concurrent use). Products include:

Levophed Bitartrate Injection........... 2315

Nortriptyline Hydrochloride (Avoid concurrent use). Products include:

Pamelor 2280

IMPORTANT NOTE: Always consult each drug listing in the patient's regimen for possible interactions.

Matulane Interactions Index 630

Opium Alkaloids (CNS depression).
- No products indexed under this heading.

Oxycodone Hydrochloride (CNS depression). Products include:
- Percocet Tablets ... 938
- Percodan Tablets ... 939
- Percodan-Demi Tablets ... 940
- Roxicodone Tablets, Oral Solution & Intensol (Oxycodone) ... 2244
- Tylox Capsules ... 1584

Penbutolol Sulfate (Possible potentiation and increased CNS depression). Products include:
- Levatol ... 2403

Pentobarbital Sodium (CNS depression). Products include:
- Nembutal Sodium Capsules ... 436
- Nembutal Sodium Solution ... 438
- Nembutal Sodium Suppositories ... 440

Perphenazine (CNS depression). Products include:
- Etrafon ... 2355
- Triavil Tablets ... 1757
- Trilafon ... 2389

Phenobarbital (CNS depression). Products include:
- Arco-Lase Plus Tablets ... 512
- Bellergal-S Tablets ... 2250
- Donnatal ... 2060
- Donnatal Extentabs ... 2061
- Donnatal Tablets ... 2060
- Phenobarbital Elixir and Tablets ... 1469
- Quadrinal Tablets ... 1350

Phenoxybenzamine Hydrochloride (Possible potentiation and increased CNS depression). Products include:
- Dibenzyline Capsules ... 2476

Phentolamine Mesylate (Possible potentiation and increased CNS depression). Products include:
- Regitine ... 846

Phenylephrine Bitartrate (Avoid concurrent use).
- No products indexed under this heading.

Phenylephrine Hydrochloride (Avoid concurrent use). Products include:
- Atrohist Plus Tablets ... 454
- Cerose DM ... ■ 878
- Comhist ... 2038
- D.A. Chewable Tablets ... 951
- Deconsal Pediatric Capsules ... 454
- Dura-Vent/DA Tablets ... 953
- Entex Capsules ... 1986
- Entex Liquid ... 1986
- Extendryl ... 1005
- 4-Way Fast Acting Nasal Spray (regular & mentholated) ... ■ 621
- Hemorid For Women ... ■ 834
- Hycomine Compound Tablets ... 932
- Neo-Synephrine Hydrochloride 1% Carpuject ... 2324
- Neo-Synephrine Hydrochloride 1% Injection ... 2324
- Neo-Synephrine Hydrochloride (Ophthalmic) ... 2325
- Neo-Synephrine ... ■ 726
- Nōstril ... ■ 644
- Novahistine Elixir ... ■ 823
- Phenergan VC ... 2779
- Phenergan VC with Codeine ... 2781
- Preparation H ... ■ 871
- Tympagesic Ear Drops ... 2342
- Vasosulf ... ⊙ 271
- Vicks Sinex Nasal Spray and Ultra Fine Mist ... ■ 765

Phenylephrine Tannate (Avoid concurrent use). Products include:
- Atrohist Pediatric Suspension ... 454
- Ricobid-D Pediatric Suspension ... 2038
- Ricobid Tablets and Pediatric Suspension ... 2038
- Rynatan ... 2673
- Rynatuss ... 2673

Phenylpropanolamine Hydrochloride (Avoid concurrent use). Products include:
- Acutrim ... ■ 628
- Allerest Children's Chewable Tablets ... ■ 627
- Allerest 12 Hour Caplets ... ■ 627
- Atrohist Plus Tablets ... 454
- BC Cold Powder Multi-Symptom Formula (Cold-Sinus-Allergy) ... ■ 609
- BC Cold Powder Non-Drowsy Formula (Cold-Sinus) ... ■ 609
- Cheracol Plus Head Cold/Cough Formula ... ■ 769
- Comtrex Multi-Symptom Non-Drowsy Liqui-gels ... ■ 618
- Contac Continuous Action Nasal Decongestant/Antihistamine 12 Hour Capsules ... ■ 813
- Contac Maximum Strength Continuous Action Decongestant/Antihistamine 12 Hour Caplets ... ■ 813
- Contac Severe Cold and Flu Formula Caplets ... ■ 814
- Coricidin 'D' Decongestant Tablets ... ■ 800
- Dexatrim ... ■ 832
- Dexatrim Plus Vitamins Caplets ... ■ 832
- Dimetane-DC Cough Syrup ... 2059
- Dimetapp Elixir ... ■ 773
- Dimetapp Extentabs ... ■ 774
- Dimetapp Tablets/Liqui-Gels ... ■ 775
- Dimetapp Cold & Allergy Chewable Tablets ... ■ 773
- Dimetapp DM Elixir ... ■ 774
- Dura-Vent Tablets ... 952
- Entex Capsules ... 1986
- Entex LA Tablets ... 1987
- Entex Liquid ... 1986
- Exgest LA Tablets ... 782
- Hycomine ... 931
- Isoclor Timesule Capsules ... ■ 637
- Nolamine Timed-Release Tablets ... 785
- Ornade Spansule Capsules ... 2502
- Propagest Tablets ... 786
- Pyrroxate Caplets ... ■ 772
- Robitussin-CF ... ■ 777
- Sinulin Tablets ... 787
- Tavist-D 12 Hour Relief Tablets ... ■ 787
- Teldrin 12 Hour Antihistamine/Nasal Decongestant Allergy Relief Capsules ... ■ 826
- Triaminic Allergy Tablets ... ■ 789
- Triaminic Cold Tablets ... ■ 790
- Triaminic Expectorant ... ■ 790
- Triaminic Syrup ... ■ 792
- Triaminic-12 Tablets ... ■ 792
- Triaminic-DM Syrup ... ■ 792
- Triaminicin Tablets ... ■ 793
- Triaminicol Multi-Symptom Cold Tablets ... ■ 793
- Triaminicol Multi-Symptom Relief ... ■ 794
- Vicks DayQuil Allergy Relief 12-Hour Extended Release Tablets ... ■ 760
- Vicks DayQuil Allergy Relief 4-Hour Tablets ... ■ 760
- Vicks DayQuil SINUS Pressure & CONGESTION Relief ... ■ 761

Pindolol (Possible potentiation and increased CNS depression). Products include:
- Visken Tablets ... 2299

Pirbuterol Acetate (Avoid concurrent use). Products include:
- Maxair Autohaler ... 1492
- Maxair Inhaler ... 1494

Polythiazide (Possible potentiation and increased CNS depression). Products include:
- Minizide Capsules ... 1938

Prazosin Hydrochloride (Possible potentiation and increased CNS depression). Products include:
- Minipress Capsules ... 1937
- Minizide Capsules ... 1938

Prochlorperazine (CNS depression). Products include:
- Compazine ... 2470

Promethazine Hydrochloride (CNS depression). Products include:
- Mepergan Injection ... 2753
- Phenergan with Codeine ... 2777
- Phenergan with Dextromethorphan ... 2778
- Phenergan Injection ... 2773
- Phenergan Suppositories ... 2775
- Phenergan Syrup ... 2774
- Phenergan Tablets ... 2775
- Phenergan VC ... 2779
- Phenergan VC with Codeine ... 2781

Propoxyphene Hydrochloride (CNS depression). Products include:
- Darvon ... 1435
- Wygesic Tablets ... 2827

Propoxyphene Napsylate (CNS depression). Products include:
- Darvon-N/Darvocet-N ... 1433

Propranolol Hydrochloride (Possible potentiation and increased CNS depression). Products include:
- Inderal ... 2728
- Inderal LA Long Acting Capsules ... 2730
- Inderide Tablets ... 2732
- Inderide LA Long Acting Capsules ... 2734

Protriptyline Hydrochloride (Avoid concurrent use). Products include:
- Vivactil Tablets ... 1774

Pseudoephedrine Hydrochloride (Avoid concurrent use). Products include:
- Actifed Allergy Daytime/Nighttime Caplets ... ■ 844
- Actifed Plus Caplets ... ■ 845
- Actifed Plus Tablets ... ■ 845
- Actifed with Codeine Cough Syrup ... 1067
- Actifed Sinus Daytime/Nighttime Tablets and Caplets ... ■ 846
- Actifed Syrup ... ■ 846
- Actifed Tablets ... ■ 844
- Advil Cold and Sinus Caplets and Tablets (formerly CoAdvil) ... ■ 870
- Alka-Seltzer Plus Cold Medicine Liqui-Gels ... ■ 706
- Alka-Seltzer Plus Cold & Cough Medicine Liqui-Gels ... ■ 705
- Alka-Seltzer Plus Night-Time Cold Medicine Liqui-Gels ... ■ 706
- Allerest Headache Strength Tablets ... ■ 627
- Allerest Maximum Strength Tablets ... ■ 627
- Allerest No Drowsiness Tablets ... ■ 627
- Allerest Sinus Pain Formula ... ■ 627
- Anatuss LA Tablets ... 1542
- Atrohist Pediatric Capsules ... 453
- Bayer Select Sinus Pain Relief Formula ... ■ 717
- Benadryl Allergy Decongestant Liquid Medication ... ■ 848
- Benadryl Allergy Decongestant Tablets ... ■ 848
- Benadryl Allergy Sinus Headache Formula Caplets ... ■ 849
- Benylin Multisymptom ... ■ 852
- Bromfed Capsules (Extended-Release) ... 1785
- Bromfed Syrup ... ■ 733
- Bromfed Tablets ... 1785
- Bromfed-DM Cough Syrup ... 1786
- Bromfed-PD Capsules (Extended-Release) ... 1785
- Children's Vicks DayQuil Allergy Relief ... ■ 757
- Children's Vicks NyQuil Cold/Cough Relief ... ■ 758
- Comtrex Multi-Symptom Cold Reliever Tablets/Caplets/Liqui-Gels/Liquid ... ■ 615
- Allergy-Sinus Comtrex Multi-Symptom Allergy-Sinus Formula Tablets ... ■ 617
- Comtrex Multi-Symptom Non-Drowsy Caplets ... ■ 618
- Congess ... 1004
- Contac Day Allergy/Sinus Caplets ... ■ 812
- Contac Day & Night ... ■ 812
- Contac Night Allergy/Sinus Caplets ... ■ 812
- Contac Severe Cold & Flu Non-Drowsy ... ■ 815
- Deconamine Chewable Tablets ... 1320
- Deconamine CX Cough and Cold Liquid and Tablets ... 1319
- Deconamine ... 1320
- Deconsal C Expectorant Syrup ... 456
- Deconsal Pediatric Syrup ... 457
- Deconsal II Tablets ... 454
- Dimetane-DX Cough Syrup ... 2059
- Dimetapp Sinus Caplets ... ■ 775
- Dorcol Children's Cough Syrup ... ■ 785
- Drixoral Cough + Congestion Liquid Caps ... ■ 802
- Dura-Tap/PD Capsules ... 2867
- Duratuss Tablets ... 2565
- Duratuss HD Elixir ... 2565
- Efidac/24 ... ■ 635
- Entex PSE Tablets ... 1987
- Fedahist Gyrocaps ... 2401
- Fedahist Timecaps ... 2401
- Guaifed ... 1787
- Guaifed Syrup ... ■ 734
- Guaimax-D Tablets ... 792
- Guaitab Tablets ... ■ 734
- Isoclor Expectorant ... 990
- Kronofed-A ... 977
- Motrin IB Sinus ... ■ 838
- Novahistine DH ... 2462
- Novahistine DMX ... ■ 822
- Novahistine Expectorant ... 2463
- Nucofed ... 2051
- PediaCare Cold Allergy Chewable Tablets ... ■ 677
- PediaCare Cough-Cold Chewable Tablets ... 1553
- PediaCare ... 1553
- PediaCare Infants' Decongestant Drops ... ■ 677
- PediCare Infant's Drops Decongestant Plus Cough ... 1553
- PediaCare NightRest Cough-Cold Liquid ... 1553
- Pediatric Vicks 44d Dry Hacking Cough & Head Congestion ... ■ 763
- Pediatric Vicks 44m Cough & Cold Relief ... ■ 764
- Robitussin Cold & Cough Liqui-Gels ... ■ 776
- Robitussin Maximum Strength Cough & Cold ... ■ 778
- Robitussin Pediatric Cough & Cold Formula ... ■ 779
- Robitussin Severe Congestion Liqui-Gels ... ■ 776
- Robitussin-DAC Syrup ... 2074
- Robitussin-PE ... ■ 778
- Rondec Oral Drops ... 953
- Rondec Syrup ... 953
- Rondec Tablet ... 953
- Rondec-DM Oral Drops ... 954
- Rondec-DM Syrup ... 954
- Rondec-TR Tablet ... 953
- Ryna ... ■ 841
- Seldane-D Extended-Release Tablets ... 1538
- Semprex-D Capsules ... 463
- Semprex-D Capsules ... 1167
- Sinarest Tablets ... ■ 648
- Sinarest Extra Strength Tablets ... ■ 648
- Sinarest No Drowsiness Tablets ... ■ 648
- Sine-Aid IB Caplets ... 1554
- Sine-Aid Maximum Strength Sinus Medication Gelcaps, Caplets and Tablets ... 1554
- Sine-Off No Drowsiness Formula Caplets ... ■ 824
- Sine-Off Sinus Medicine ... ■ 825
- Singlet Tablets ... ■ 825
- Sinutab Non-Drying Liquid Caps ... ■ 859
- Sinutab Sinus Allergy Medication, Maximum Strength Tablets and Caplets ... ■ 860
- Sinutab Sinus Medication, Maximum Strength Without Drowsiness Formula, Tablets & Caplets ... ■ 860
- Sinutab Sinus Medication, Regular Strength Without Drowsiness Formula ... ■ 859
- Sudafed Children's Liquid ... ■ 861
- Sudafed Cold and Cough Liquidcaps ... ■ 862
- Sudafed Cough Syrup ... ■ 862
- Sudafed Plus Liquid ... ■ 862
- Sudafed Plus Tablets ... ■ 863
- Sudafed Severe Cold Formula Caplets ... ■ 863
- Sudafed Severe Cold Formula Tablets ... ■ 864
- Sudafed Sinus Caplets ... ■ 864
- Sudafed Sinus Tablets ... ■ 864
- Sudafed Tablets, 30 mg ... ■ 861
- Sudafed Tablets, 60 mg ... ■ 861
- Sudafed 12 Hour Caplets ... ■ 861
- Syn-Rx Tablets ... 465
- Syn-Rx DM Tablets ... 466
- TheraFlu ... ■ 787
- TheraFlu Maximum Strength Nighttime Flu, Cold & Cough Medicine ... ■ 788
- TheraFlu Maximum Strength Non-Drowsy Formula Flu, Cold & Cough Medicine ... ■ 788
- Thera Flu Maximum Strength, Non-Drowsy Formula Flu, Cold and Cough Caplets ... ■ 789
- Triaminic AM Cough and Decongestant Formula ... ■ 789
- Triaminic AM Decongestant Formula ... ■ 790
- Triaminic Nite Light ... ■ 791
- Triaminic Sore Throat Formula ... ■ 791
- Tussend ... 1783
- Tussend Expectorant ... 1785

(■ Described in PDR For Nonprescription Drugs) (⊙ Described in PDR For Ophthalmology)

Interactions Index

Children's TYLENOL Cold Multi-Symptom Liquid Formula and Chewable Tablets 1561

Children's TYLENOL Cold Plus Cough Multi Symptom Tablets and Liquid .... ⊞ 681

Infants' TYLENOL Cold Decongestant & Fever-Reducer Drops 1556

TYLENOL Maximum Strength Allergy Sinus Medication Gelcaps and Caplets 1563

TYLENOL Maximum Strength Allergy Sinus NightTime Medication Caplets 1555

TYLENOL Flu Maximum Strength Gelcaps 1565

TYLENOL Flu NightTime, Maximum Strength, Gelcaps 1566

TYLENOL Maximum Strength Flu NightTime Hot Medication Packets 1562

TYLENOL, Maximum Strength, Sinus Medication Geltabs, Gelcaps, Caplets and Tablets 1566

TYLENOL Cold Multi-Symptom Formula Medication Tablets and Caplets 1561

TYLENOL Cold Medication No Drowsiness Formula Gelcaps and Caplets 1562

TYLENOL Cold Multi-Symptom Hot Medication Liquid Packets 1557

TYLENOL Cough Multi-Symptom Medication with Decongestant 1565

Ursinus Inlay-Tabs .... ⊞ 794

Vicks 44 LiquiCaps Cough, Cold & Flu Relief .... ⊞ 755

Vicks 44 LiquiCaps Non-Drowsy Cough & Cold Relief .... ⊞ 756

Vicks 44D Dry Hacking Cough & Head Congestion .... ⊞ 755

Vicks 44M Cough, Cold & Flu Relief .... ⊞ 756

Vicks DayQuil .... ⊞ 761

Vicks DayQuil SINUS Pressure & PAIN Relief with IBUPROFEN .... ⊞ 762

Vicks Nyquil Hot Therapy .... ⊞ 762

Vicks NyQuil LiquiCaps Multi-Symptom Cold/Flu Relief .... ⊞ 763

Vicks NyQuil Multi-Symptom Cold/Flu Relief - (Original & Cherry Flavor) .... ⊞ 763

Pseudoephedrine Sulfate (Avoid concurrent use). Products include:

Cheracol Sinus .... ⊞ 768

Chlor-Trimeton Allergy Decongestant Tablets .... ⊞ 799

Claritin-D 2350

Drixoral Cold and Allergy Sustained-Action Tablets .... ⊞ 802

Drixoral Cold and Flu Extended-Release Tablets..................................... ⊞ 803

Drixoral Non-Drowsy Formula Extended-Release Tablets .... ⊞ 803

Drixoral Allergy/Sinus Extended Release Tablets..................................... ⊞ 804

Trinalin Repetabs Tablets 1330

Pyrilamine Maleate (CNS depression). Products include:

4-Way Fast Acting Nasal Spray (regular & mentholated) .... ⊞ 621

Maximum Strength Multi-Symptom Formula Midol .... ⊞ 722

PMS Multi-Symptom Formula Midol .... ⊞ 723

Pyrilamine Tannate (CNS depression). Products include:

Atrohist Pediatric Suspension 454

Rynatan 2673

Quinapril Hydrochloride (Possible potentiation and increased CNS depression). Products include:

Accupril Tablets 1893

Ramipril (Possible potentiation and increased CNS depression). Products include:

Altace Capsules 1232

Rauwolfia Serpentina (Possible potentiation and increased CNS depression).

No products indexed under this heading.

Rescinnamine (Possible potentiation and increased CNS depression).

No products indexed under this heading.

Reserpine (Possible potentiation and increased CNS depression). Products include:

Diupres Tablets 1650

Hydropres Tablets 1675

Ser-Ap-Es Tablets 849

Salmeterol Xinafoate (Avoid concurrent use). Products include:

Serevent Inhalation Aerosol 1176

Secobarbital Sodium (CNS depression). Products include:

Seconal Sodium Pulvules 1474

Sodium Nitroprusside (Possible potentiation and increased CNS depression).

No products indexed under this heading.

Sotalol Hydrochloride (Possible potentiation and increased CNS depression). Products include:

Betapace Tablets 641

Spirapril Hydrochloride (Possible potentiation and increased CNS depression).

No products indexed under this heading.

Sufentanil Citrate (CNS depression). Products include:

Sufenta Injection 1309

Terazosin Hydrochloride (Possible potentiation and increased CNS depression). Products include:

Hytrin Capsules 430

Terbutaline Sulfate (Avoid concurrent use). Products include:

Brethaire Inhaler 813

Brethine Ampuls 815

Brethine Tablets 814

Bricanyl Subcutaneous Injection 1502

Bricanyl Tablets 1503

Terfenadine (CNS depression). Products include:

Seldane Tablets 1536

Seldane-D Extended-Release Tablets 1538

Thiamylal Sodium (CNS depression).

No products indexed under this heading.

Thioridazine Hydrochloride (CNS depression). Products include:

Mellaril 2269

Timolol Maleate (Possible potentiation and increased CNS depression). Products include:

Blocadren Tablets 1614

Timolide Tablets 1748

Timoptic in Ocudose 1753

Timoptic Sterile Ophthalmic Solution 1751

Timoptic-XE 1755

Torsemide (Possible potentiation and increased CNS depression). Products include:

Demadex Tablets and Injection 686

Trifluoperazine Hydrochloride (CNS depression). Products include:

Stelazine 2514

Trimeprazine Tartrate (CNS depression). Products include:

Temaril Tablets, Syrup and Spansule Extended-Release Capsules .. 483

Trimethaphan Camsylate (Possible potentiation and increased CNS depression). Products include:

Arfonad Ampuls 2080

Trimipramine Maleate (Avoid concurrent use). Products include:

Surmontil Capsules 2811

Tripelennamine Hydrochloride (CNS depression). Products include:

PBZ Tablets 845

PBZ-SR Tablets 844

Triprolidine Hydrochloride (CNS depression). Products include:

Actifed Plus Caplets .... ⊞ 845

Actifed Plus Tablets .... ⊞ 845

Actifed with Codeine Cough Syrup .. 1067

Actifed Syrup .... ⊞ 846

Actifed Tablets .... ⊞ 844

Verapamil Hydrochloride (Possible potentiation and increased CNS depression). Products include:

Calan SR Caplets 2422

Calan Tablets 2419

Isoptin Injectable 1344

Isoptin Oral Tablets 1346

Isoptin SR Tablets 1348

Verelan Capsules 1410

Verelan Capsules 2824

Food Interactions

Alcohol (May result in disulfiram-like reaction).

Bananas (Concurrent use should be avoided).

Cheese, aged (Concurrent use should be avoided).

Food with high concentration of tyramine (Concurrent use should be avoided).

Wine, unspecified (Concurrent use should be avoided).

Yogurt (Concurrent use should be avoided).

MAXAIR AUTOHALER

(Pirbuterol Acetate) 1492

May interact with sympathomimetic aerosol bronchodilators, monoamine oxidase inhibitors, and tricyclic antidepressants. Compounds in these categories include:

Albuterol (Potential for additive effects). Products include:

Proventil Inhalation Aerosol 2382

Ventolin Inhalation Aerosol and Refill 1197

Amitriptyline Hydrochloride (Potentiates the action of beta adrenergic agonists on the vascular system). Products include:

Elavil 2838

Endep Tablets 2174

Etrafon 2355

Limbitrol 2180

Triavil Tablets 1757

Amoxapine (Potentiates the action of beta adrenergic agonists on the vascular system). Products include:

Asendin Tablets 1369

Bitolterol Mesylate (Potential for additive effects). Products include:

Tornalate Solution for Inhalation, 0.2% 956

Tornalate Metered Dose Inhaler 957

Clomipramine Hydrochloride (Potentiates the action of beta adrenergic agonists on the vascular system). Products include:

Anafranil Capsules 803

Desipramine Hydrochloride (Potentiates the action of beta adrenergic agonists on the vascular system). Products include:

Norpramin Tablets 1526

Doxepin Hydrochloride (Potentiates the action of beta adrenergic agonists on the vascular system). Products include:

Sinequan 2205

Zonalon Cream 1055

Furazolidone (Potentiates the action of beta adrenergic agonists on the vascular system). Products include:

Furoxone 2046

Imipramine Hydrochloride (Potentiates the action of beta adrenergic agonists on the vascular system). Products include:

Tofranil Ampuls 854

Tofranil Tablets 856

Imipramine Pamoate (Potentiates the action of beta adrenergic agonists on the vascular system). Products include:

Tofranil-PM Capsules 857

Isocarboxazid (Potentiates the action of beta adrenergic agonists on the vascular system).

No products indexed under this heading.

Isoetharine (Potential for additive effects). Products include:

Bronkometer Aerosol 2302

Bronkosol Solution 2302

Isoetharine Inhalation Solution, USP, Arm-a-Med 551

Isoproterenol Hydrochloride (Potential for additive effects). Products include:

Isuprel Hydrochloride Injection 1:5000 2311

Isuprel Hydrochloride Solution 1:200 & 1:100 2313

Isuprel Mistometer 2312

Maprotiline Hydrochloride (Potentiates the action of beta adrenergic agonists on the vascular system). Products include:

Ludiomil Tablets 843

Metaproterenol Sulfate (Potential for additive effects). Products include:

Alupent 669

Metaproterenol Sulfate Inhalation Solution, USP, Arm-a-Med 552

Nortriptyline Hydrochloride (Potentiates the action of beta adrenergic agonists on the vascular system). Products include:

Pamelor 2280

Phenelzine Sulfate (Potentiates the action of beta adrenergic agonists on the vascular system). Products include:

Nardil 1920

Protriptyline Hydrochloride (Potentiates the action of beta adrenergic agonists on the vascular system). Products include:

Vivactil Tablets 1774

Salmeterol Xinafoate (Potential for additive effects). Products include:

Serevent Inhalation Aerosol 1176

Selegiline Hydrochloride (Potentiates the action of beta adrenergic agonists on the vascular system). Products include:

Eldepryl Tablets 2550

Terbutaline Sulfate (Potential for additive effects). Products include:

Brethaire Inhaler 813

Brethine Ampuls 815

Brethine Tablets 814

Bricanyl Subcutaneous Injection 1502

Bricanyl Tablets 1503

Tranylcypromine Sulfate (Potentiates the action of beta adrenergic agonists on the vascular system). Products include:

Parnate Tablets 2503

Trimipramine Maleate (Potentiates the action of beta adrenergic agonists on the vascular system). Products include:

Surmontil Capsules 2811

MAXAIR INHALER

(Pirbuterol Acetate) 1494

May interact with monoamine oxidase inhibitors, tricyclic antidepressants, and sympathomimetic aerosol bronchodilators. Compounds in these categories include:

Albuterol (Potential for additive effects). Products include:

Proventil Inhalation Aerosol 2382

Ventolin Inhalation Aerosol and Refill 1197

Amitriptyline Hydrochloride (Action of pirbuterol on vascular system may be potentiated). Products include:

Elavil 2838

IMPORTANT NOTE: Always consult each drug listing in the patient's regimen for possible interactions.

Maxair **Interactions Index** **632**

Endep Tablets ... 2174
Etrafon ... 2355
Limbitrol ... 2180
Triavil Tablets ... 1757

Amoxapine (Action of pirbuterol on vascular system may be potentiated). Products include:
Asendin Tablets ... 1369

Bitolterol Mesylate (Potential for additive effects). Products include:
Tornalate Solution for Inhalation, 0.2% ... 956
Tornalate Metered Dose Inhaler ... 957

Clomipramine Hydrochloride (Action of pirbuterol on vascular system may be potentiated). Products include:
Anafranil Capsules ... 803

Desipramine Hydrochloride (Action of pirbuterol on vascular system may be potentiated). Products include:
Norpramin Tablets ... 1526

Doxepin Hydrochloride (Action of pirbuterol on vascular system may be potentiated). Products include:
Sinequan ... 2205
Zonalon Cream ... 1055

Furazolidone (Action of pirbuterol on vascular system may be potentiated). Products include:
Furoxone ... 2046

Imipramine Hydrochloride (Action of pirbuterol on vascular system may be potentiated). Products include:
Tofranil Ampuls ... 854
Tofranil Tablets ... 856

Imipramine Pamoate (Action of pirbuterol on vascular system may be potentiated). Products include:
Tofranil-PM Capsules ... 857

Isocarboxazid (Action of pirbuterol on vascular system may be potentiated).
No products indexed under this heading.

Isoetharine (Potential for additive effects). Products include:
Bronkometer Aerosol ... 2302
Bronkosol Solution ... 2302
Isoetharine Inhalation Solution, USP, Arm-a-Med ... 551

Isoproterenol Hydrochloride (Potential for additive effects). Products include:
Isuprel Hydrochloride Injection 1:5000 ... 2311
Isuprel Hydrochloride Solution 1:200 & 1:100 ... 2313
Isuprel Mistometer ... 2312

Maprotiline Hydrochloride (Action of pirbuterol on vascular system may be potentiated). Products include:
Ludiomil Tablets ... 843

Metaproterenol Sulfate (Potential for additive effects). Products include:
Alupent ... 669
Metaproterenol Sulfate Inhalation Solution, USP, Arm-a-Med ... 552

Nortriptyline Hydrochloride (Action of pirbuterol on vascular system may be potentiated). Products include:
Pamelor ... 2280

Phenelzine Sulfate (Action of pirbuterol on vascular system may be potentiated). Products include:
Nardil ... 1920

Protriptyline Hydrochloride (Action of pirbuterol on vascular system may be potentiated). Products include:
Vivactil Tablets ... 1774

Salmeterol Xinafoate (Potential for additive effects). Products include:
Serevent Inhalation Aerosol ... 1176

Selegiline Hydrochloride (Action of pirbuterol on vascular system may be potentiated). Products include:
Eldepryl Tablets ... 2550

Terbutaline Sulfate (Potential for additive effects). Products include:
Brethaire Inhaler ... 813
Brethine Ampuls ... 815
Brethine Tablets ... 814
Bricanyl Subcutaneous Injection ... 1502
Bricanyl Tablets ... 1503

Tranylcypromine Sulfate (Action of pirbuterol on vascular system may be potentiated). Products include:
Parnate Tablets ... 2503

Trimipramine Maleate (Action of pirbuterol on vascular system may be potentiated). Products include:
Surmontil Capsules ... 2811

MAXAQUIN TABLETS
(Lomefloxacin Hydrochloride) ... 2440
May interact with xanthine bronchodilators, antacids containing aluminium, calcium and magnesium, oral anticoagulants, and certain other agents. Compounds in these categories include:

Aluminum Carbonate Gel (Interferes with the bioavailability of lomefloxacin). Products include:
Basaljel ... 2703

Aluminum Hydroxide (Interferes with the bioavailability of lomefloxacin). Products include:
ALternaGEL Liquid ... 1316
Maximum Strength Ascriptin ... ◙ 630
Cama Arthritis Pain Reliever ... ◙ 785
Gaviscon Extra Strength Relief Formula Antacid Tablets ... ◙ 819
Gaviscon Extra Strength Relief Formula Liquid Antacid ... ◙ 819
Gaviscon Liquid Antacid ... ◙ 820
Gelusil Liquid & Tablets ... ◙ 855
Maalox Heartburn Relief Suspension ... ◙ 642
Maalox Heartburn Relief Tablets ... ◙ 641
Maalox Magnesia and Alumina Oral Suspension ... ◙ 642
Maalox Plus Tablets ... ◙ 643
Extra Strength Maalox Antacid Plus Antigas Liquid and Tablets ◙ 638
Tempo Soft Antacid ... ◙ 835

Aluminum Hydroxide Gel (Interferes with the bioavailability of lomefloxacin). Products include:
ALternaGEL Liquid ... ◙ 659
Aludrox Oral Suspension ... 2695
Amphojel Suspension ... 2695
Amphojel Suspension without Flavor ... 2695
Amphojel Tablets ... 2695
Arthritis Pain Ascriptin ... ◙ 631
Regular Strength Ascriptin Tablets ... ◙ 629
Gaviscon Antacid Tablets ... ◙ 819
Gaviscon-2 Antacid Tablets ... ◙ 820
Mylanta Liquid ... 1317
Mylanta Tablets ... ◙ 660
Mylanta Double Strength Liquid ... 1317
Mylanta Double Strength Tablets .. ◙ 660
Nephrox Suspension ... ◙ 655

Aminophylline (Individual theophylline levels may fluctuate with no clinically significant symptoms of drug interactions).
No products indexed under this heading.

Caffeine-containing medications (May result in drug-induced central nervous system-related adverse effects in certain patient population at higher levels of caffeine).

Cimetidine (May interfere with the elimination of quinolones). Products include:
Tagamet Tablets ... 2516

Cimetidine Hydrochloride (May interfere with the elimination of quinolones). Products include:
Tagamet ... 2516

Cyclosporine (Elevated serum levels of cyclosporin have been reported with concomitant use of cyclosporin and quinolones). Products include:
Neoral ... 2276
Sandimmune ... 2286

Dicumarol (Quinolones may enhance the effects of oral anticoagulants).
No products indexed under this heading.

Dihydroxyaluminum Sodium Carbonate (Interferes with the bioavailability of lomefloxacin).
No products indexed under this heading.

Dyphylline (Individual theophylline levels may fluctuate with no clinically significant symptoms of drug interactions). Products include:
Lufyllin & Lufyllin-400 Tablets ... 2670
Lufyllin-GG Elixir & Tablets ... 2671

Fenbufen (Potential for increased risk of CNS stimulation and convulsive seizures).

Magaldrate (Interferes with the bioavailability of lomefloxacin).
No products indexed under this heading.

Magnesium Hydroxide (Interferes with the bioavailability of lomefloxacin). Products include:
Aludrox Oral Suspension ... 2695
Arthritis Pain Ascriptin ... ◙ 631
Maximum Strength Ascriptin ... ◙ 630
Regular Strength Ascriptin Tablets ... ◙ 629
Di-Gel Antacid/Anti-Gas ... ◙ 801
Gelusil Liquid & Tablets ... ◙ 855
Maalox Magnesia and Alumina Oral Suspension ... ◙ 642
Maalox Plus Tablets ... ◙ 643
Extra Strength Maalox Antacid Plus Antigas Liquid and Tablets ◙ 638
Mylanta Calcium Carbonate and Magnesium Hydroxide Tablets ... 1318
Mylanta Liquid ... 1317
Mylanta Tablets ... ◙ 660
Mylanta Double Strength Liquid ... 1317
Mylanta Double Strength Tablets .. ◙ 660
Phillips' Milk of Magnesia Liquid ... ◙ 729
Rolaids Tablets ... ◙ 843
Tempo Soft Antacid ... ◙ 835

Magnesium Oxide (Interferes with the bioavailability of lomefloxacin). Products include:
Beelith Tablets ... 639
Bufferin Analgesic Tablets and Caplets ... ◙ 613
Caltrate PLUS ... ◙ 665
Cama Arthritis Pain Reliever ... ◙ 785
Mag-Ox 400 ... 668
Uro-Mag ... 668

Probenecid (Slows the renal eliminaton of lomefloxacin). Products include:
Benemid Tablets ... 1611
ColBENEMID Tablets ... 1622

Sucralfate (Interferes with the bioavailability of lomefloxacin). Products include:
Carafate Suspension ... 1505
Carafate Tablets ... 1504

Theophylline (Individual theophylline levels may fluctuate with no clinically significant symptoms of drug interactions). Products include:
Marax Tablets & DF Syrup ... 2200
Quibron ... 2053

Theophylline Anhydrous (Individual theophylline levels may fluctuate with no clinically significant symptoms of drug interactions). Products include:
Aerolate ... 1004
Primatene Dual Action Formula ... ◙ 872
Primatene Tablets ... ◙ 873
Respbid Tablets ... 682
Slo-bid Gyrocaps ... 2033
Theo-24 Extended Release Capsules ... 2568
Theo-Dur Extended-Release Tablets ... 1327
Theo-X Extended-Release Tablets .. 788
Uni-Dur Extended-Release Tablets .. 1331
Uniphyl 400 mg Tablets ... 2001

Theophylline Calcium Salicylate (Individual theophylline levels may fluctuate with no clinically significant symptoms of drug interactions). Products include:
Quadrinal Tablets ... 1350

Theophylline Sodium Glycinate (Individual theophylline levels may fluctuate with no clinically significant symptoms of drug interactions).
No products indexed under this heading.

Warfarin Sodium (Quinolones may enhance the effects of oral anticoagulants). Products include:
Coumadin ... 926

Food Interactions

Food, unspecified (The rate of drug absorption may be delayed by 41%, however, the drug can be taken without regard to meal).

MAXITROL OPHTHALMIC OINTMENT AND SUSPENSION
(Dexamethasone, Neomycin Sulfate, Polymyxin B Sulfate) ... ⊙ 224
None cited in PDR database.

MAXZIDE TABLETS
(Triamterene, Hydrochlorothiazide) .. 1380
May interact with lithium preparations, antihypertensives, non-steroidal anti-inflammatory agents, barbiturates, narcotic analgesics, ACE inhibitors, insulin, potassium sparing diuretics, cardiac glycosides, potassium preparations, and certain other agents. Compounds in these categories include:

Acebutolol Hydrochloride (Potential for additive or augmentative effect). Products include:
Sectral Capsules ... 2807

Alfentanil Hydrochloride (May aggravate orthostatic hypotension). Products include:
Alfenta Injection ... 1286

Amiloride Hydrochloride (Concurrent use is contraindicated). Products include:
Midamor Tablets ... 1703
Moduretic Tablets ... 1705

Amlodipine Besylate (Antihypertensive effect potentiated). Products include:
Lotrel Capsules ... 840
Norvasc Tablets ... 1940

Aprobarbital (May aggravate orthostatic hypotension).
No products indexed under this heading.

Atenolol (Potential for additive or augmentative effect). Products include:
Tenoretic Tablets ... 2845
Tenormin Tablets and I.V. Injection 2847

Benazepril Hydrochloride (Increased risk of hyperkalemia and antihypertensive effect potentiated). Products include:
Lotensin Tablets ... 834
Lotensin HCT ... 837
Lotrel Capsules ... 840

Bendroflumethiazide (Potential for additive or augmentative effect).
No products indexed under this heading.

(◙ Described in PDR For Nonprescription Drugs) (⊙ Described in PDR For Ophthalmology)

Betaxolol Hydrochloride (Antihypertensive effect potentiated). Products include:
- Betoptic Ophthalmic Solution 469
- Betoptic S Ophthalmic Suspension 471
- Kerlone Tablets 2436

Bisoprolol Fumarate (Antihypertensive effect potentiated). Products include:
- Zebeta Tablets 1413
- Ziac 1415

Buprenorphine (May aggravate orthostatic hypotension). Products include:
- Buprenex Injectable 2006

Butabarbital (May aggravate orthostatic hypotension).
- No products indexed under this heading.

Butalbital (May aggravate orthostatic hypotension). Products include:
- Esgic-plus Tablets 1013
- Fioricet Tablets 2258
- Fioricet with Codeine Capsules 2260
- Fiorinal Capsules 2261
- Fiorinal with Codeine Capsules 2262
- Fiorinal Tablets 2261
- Phrenilin 785
- Sedapap Tablets 50 mg/650 mg .. 1543

Captopril (Increased risk of hyperkalemia and antihypertensive effect potentiated). Products include:
- Capoten 739
- Capozide 742

Carteolol Hydrochloride (Potential for additive or augmentative effect). Products include:
- Cartrol Tablets 410
- Ocupress Ophthalmic Solution, 1% Sterile .... ⊙ 309

Chlorothiazide (Potential for additive or augmentative effect). Products include:
- Aldoclor Tablets 1598
- Diupres Tablets 1650
- Diuril Oral 1653

Chlorothiazide Sodium (Potential for additive or augmentative effect). Products include:
- Diuril Sodium Intravenous 1652

Chlorthalidone (Potential for additive or augmentative effect). Products include:
- Combipres Tablets 677
- Tenoretic Tablets 2845
- Thalitone 1245

Clonidine (Potential for additive or augmentative effect). Products include:
- Catapres-TTS 675

Clonidine Hydrochloride (Potential for additive or augmentative effect). Products include:
- Catapres Tablets 674
- Combipres Tablets 677

Codeine Phosphate (May aggravate orthostatic hypotension). Products include:
- Actifed with Codeine Cough Syrup.. 1067
- Brontex 1981
- Deconsal C Expectorant Syrup 456
- Deconsal Pediatric Syrup 457
- Dimetane-DC Cough Syrup 2059
- Empirin with Codeine Tablets 1093
- Fioricet with Codeine Capsules 2260
- Fiorinal with Codeine Capsules 2262
- Isoclor Expectorant 990
- Novahistine DH 2462
- Novahistine Expectorant 2463
- Nucofed 2051
- Phenergan with Codeine 2777
- Phenergan VC with Codeine 2781
- Robitussin A-C Syrup 2073
- Robitussin-DAC Syrup 2074
- Ryna .... ▣ 841
- Soma Compound w/Codeine Tablets 2676
- Tussi-Organidin NR Liquid and S NR Liquid 2677
- Tylenol with Codeine 1583

Deserpidine (Potential for additive or augmentative effect).
- No products indexed under this heading.

Deslanoside (Potential for digitalis toxicity due to hypokalemia).
- No products indexed under this heading.

Dezocine (May aggravate orthostatic hypotension). Products include:
- Dalgan Injection 538

Diazoxide (Potential for additive or augmentative effect). Products include:
- Hyperstat I.V. Injection 2363
- Proglycem 580

Diclofenac Potassium (Potential for acute renal failure). Products include:
- Cataflam 816

Diclofenac Sodium (Potential for acute renal failure). Products include:
- Voltaren Ophthalmic Sterile Ophthalmic Solution .... ⊙ 272
- Voltaren Tablets 861

Digitoxin (Potential for digitalis toxicity due to hypokalemia). Products include:
- Crystodigin Tablets 1433

Digoxin (Potential for digitalis toxicity due to hypokalemia). Products include:
- Lanoxicaps 1117
- Lanoxin Elixir Pediatric 1120
- Lanoxin Injection 1123
- Lanoxin Injection Pediatric 1126
- Lanoxin Tablets 1128

Diltiazem Hydrochloride (Antihypertensive effect potentiated). Products include:
- Cardizem CD Capsules 1506
- Cardizem SR Capsules 1510
- Cardizem Injectable 1508
- Cardizem Tablets 1512
- Dilacor XR Extended-release Capsules 2018

Doxazosin Mesylate (Antihypertensive effect potentiated). Products include:
- Cardura Tablets 2186

Enalapril Maleate (Increased risk of hyperkalemia and antihypertensive effect potentiated). Products include:
- Vaseretic Tablets 1765
- Vasotec Tablets 1771

Enalaprilat (Increased risk of hyperkalemia and antihypertensive effect potentiated). Products include:
- Vasotec I.V. 1768

Esmolol Hydrochloride (Potential for additive or augmentative effect). Products include:
- Brevibloc Injection 1808

Etodolac (Potential for acute renal failure). Products include:
- Lodine Capsules and Tablets 2743

Felodipine (Antihypertensive effect potentiated). Products include:
- Plendil Extended-Release Tablets 527

Fenoprofen Calcium (Potential for acute renal failure). Products include:
- Nalfon 200 Pulvules & Nalfon Tablets 917

Fentanyl (May aggravate orthostatic hypotension). Products include:
- Duragesic Transdermal System 1288

Fentanyl Citrate (May aggravate orthostatic hypotension). Products include:
- Sublimaze Injection 1307

Flurbiprofen (Potential for acute renal failure). Products include:
- Ansaid Tablets 2579

Fosinopril Sodium (Increased risk of hyperkalemia and antihypertensive effect potentiated). Products include:
- Monopril Tablets 757

Furosemide (Potential for additive or augmentative effect). Products include:
- Lasix Injection, Oral Solution and Tablets 1240

Guanabenz Acetate (Potential for additive or augmentative effect).
- No products indexed under this heading.

Guanethidine Monosulfate (Potential for additive or augmentative effect). Products include:
- Esimil Tablets 822
- Ismelin Tablets 827

Hydralazine Hydrochloride (Potential for additive or augmentative effect). Products include:
- Apresazide Capsules 808
- Apresoline Hydrochloride Tablets .. 809
- Ser-Ap-Es Tablets 849

Hydrocodone Bitartrate (May aggravate orthostatic hypotension). Products include:
- Anexsia 5/500 Elixir 1781
- Anexia Tablets 1782
- Codiclear DH Syrup 791
- Deconamine CX Cough and Cold Liquid and Tablets 1319
- Duratuss HD Elixir 2565
- Hycodan Tablets and Syrup 930
- Hycomine Compound Tablets 932
- Hycomine 931
- Hycotuss Expectorant Syrup 933
- Hydrocet Capsules 782
- Lorcet 10/650 1018
- Lortab 2566
- Tussend 1783
- Tussend Expectorant 1785
- Vicodin Tablets 1356
- Vicodin ES Tablets 1357
- Vicodin Tuss Expectorant 1358
- Zydone Capsules 949

Hydrocodone Polistirex (May aggravate orthostatic hypotension). Products include:
- Tussionex Pennkinetic Extended-Release Suspension 998

Hydroflumethiazide (Potential for additive or augmentative effect). Products include:
- Diucardin Tablets 2718

Ibuprofen (Potential for acute renal failure). Products include:
- Advil Cold and Sinus Caplets and Tablets (formerly CoAdvil) .... ▣ 870
- Advil Ibuprofen Tablets and Caplets .... ▣ 870
- Children's Advil Suspension 2692
- Arthritis Foundation Ibuprofen Tablets .... ▣ 674
- Bayer Select Ibuprofen Pain Relief Formula .... ▣ 715
- Cramp End Tablets .... ▣ 735
- Dimetapp Sinus Caplets .... ▣ 775
- Haltran Tablets .... ▣ 771
- IBU Tablets 1342
- Ibuprohm .... ▣ 735
- Children's Motrin Ibuprofen Oral Suspension 1546
- Motrin Tablets 2625
- Motrin IB Caplets, Tablets, and Geltabs .... ▣ 838
- Motrin IB Sinus .... ▣ 838
- Motrin Ibuprofen Suspension, Oral Drops, Chewable Tablets, Caplets 1546
- Nuprin Ibuprofen/Analgesic Tablets & Caplets .... ▣ 622
- Sine-Aid IB Caplets 1554
- Vicks DayQuil SINUS Pressure & PAIN Relief with IBUPROFEN .... ▣ 762

Indapamide (Potential for additive or augmentative effect). Products include:
- Lozol Tablets 2022

Indomethacin (Potential for acute renal failure). Products include:
- Indocin 1680

Indomethacin Sodium Trihydrate (Potential for acute renal failure). Products include:
- Indocin I.V. 1684

Insulin, Human (Insulin requirements in diabetics may be altered).
- No products indexed under this heading.

Insulin, Human Isophane Suspension (Insulin requirements in diabetics may be altered). Products include:
- Novolin N Human Insulin 10 ml Vials 1795

Insulin, Human NPH (Insulin requirements in diabetics may be altered). Products include:
- Humulin N, 100 Units 1448
- Novolin N PenFill Cartridges Durable Insulin Delivery System 1798
- Novolin N Prefilled Syringe Disposable Insulin Delivery System 1798

Insulin, Human Regular (Insulin requirements in diabetics may be altered). Products include:
- Humulin R, 100 Units 1449
- Novolin R Human Insulin 10 ml Vials 1795
- Novolin R PenFill Cartridges Durable Insulin Delivery System 1798
- Novolin R Prefilled Syringe Disposable Insulin Delivery System 1798
- Velosulin BR Human Insulin 10 ml Vials 1795

Insulin, Human, Zinc Suspension (Insulin requirements in diabetics may be altered). Products include:
- Humulin L, 100 Units 1446
- Humulin U, 100 Units 1450
- Novolin L Human Insulin 10 ml Vials 1795

Insulin, NPH (Insulin requirements in diabetics may be altered). Products include:
- NPH, 100 Units 1450
- Pork NPH, 100 Units 1452
- Purified Pork NPH Isophane Insulin 1801

Insulin, Regular (Insulin requirements in diabetics may be altered). Products include:
- Regular, 100 Units 1450
- Pork Regular, 100 Units 1452
- Pork Regular (Concentrated), 500 Units 1453
- Purified Pork Regular Insulin 1801

Insulin, Zinc Crystals (Insulin requirements in diabetics may be altered). Products include:
- NPH, 100 Units 1450

Insulin, Zinc Suspension (Insulin requirements in diabetics may be altered). Products include:
- Iletin I 1450
- Lente, 100 Units 1450
- Iletin II 1452
- Pork Lente, 100 Units 1452
- Purified Pork Lente Insulin 1801

Isradipine (Antihypertensive effect potentiated). Products include:
- DynaCirc Capsules 2256

Ketoprofen (Potential for acute renal failure). Products include:
- Orudis Capsules 2766
- Oruvail Capsules 2766

Ketorolac Tromethamine (Potential for acute renal failure). Products include:
- Acular 474
- Acular .... ⊙ 277
- Toradol 2159

Labetalol Hydrochloride (Potential for additive or augmentative effect). Products include:
- Normodyne Injection 2377
- Normodyne Tablets 2379
- Trandate 1185

IMPORTANT NOTE: Always consult each drug listing in the patient's regimen for possible interactions.

Maxzide Interactions Index 634

Levorphanol Tartrate (May aggravate orthostatic hypotension). Products include:
Levo-Dromoran ... 2129

Lisinopril (Increased risk of hyperkalemia and antihypertensive effect potentiated). Products include:
Prinivil Tablets ... 1733
Prinzide Tablets ... 1737
Zestoretic ... 2850
Zestril Tablets ... 2854

Lithium Carbonate (High risk of lithium toxicity). Products include:
Eskalith ... 2485
Lithium Carbonate Capsules & Tablets ... 2230
Lithonate/Lithotabs/Lithobid ... 2543

Lithium Citrate (High risk of lithium toxicity).
No products indexed under this heading.

Losartan Potassium (Antihypertensive effect potentiated). Products include:
Cozaar Tablets ... 1628
Hyzaar Tablets ... 1677

Mecamylamine Hydrochloride (Potential for additive or augmentative effect). Products include:
Inversine Tablets ... 1686

Meclofenamate Sodium (Potential for acute renal failure).
No products indexed under this heading.

Mefenamic Acid (Potential for acute renal failure). Products include:
Ponstel ... 1925

Meperidine Hydrochloride (May aggravate orthostatic hypotension). Products include:
Demerol ... 2308
Mepergan Injection ... 2753

Mephobarbital (May aggravate orthostatic hypotension). Products include:
Mebaral Tablets ... 2322

Methadone Hydrochloride (May aggravate orthostatic hypotension). Products include:
Methadone Hydrochloride Oral Concentrate ... 2233
Methadone Hydrochloride Oral Solution & Tablets ... 2235

Methyclothiazide (Potential for additive or augmentative effect). Products include:
Enduron Tablets ... 420

Methyldopa (Potential for additive or augmentative effect). Products include:
Aldoclor Tablets ... 1598
Aldomet Oral ... 1600
Aldoril Tablets ... 1604

Methyldopate Hydrochloride (Potential for additive or augmentative effect). Products include:
Aldomet Ester HCl Injection ... 1602

Metolazone (Potential for additive or augmentative effect). Products include:
Mykrox Tablets ... 993
Zaroxolyn Tablets ... 1000

Metoprolol Succinate (Potential for additive or augmentative effect). Products include:
Toprol-XL Tablets ... 565

Metoprolol Tartrate (Potential for additive or augmentative effect). Products include:
Lopressor Ampuls ... 830
Lopressor HCT Tablets ... 832
Lopressor Tablets ... 830

Metyrosine (Potential for additive or augmentative effect). Products include:
Demser Capsules ... 1649

Minoxidil (Potential for additive or augmentative effect). Products include:
Loniten Tablets ... 2618
Rogaine Topical Solution ... 2637

Moexipril Hydrochloride (Increased risk of hyperkalemia and antihypertensive effect potentiated). Products include:
Univasc Tablets ... 2410

Morphine Sulfate (May aggravate orthostatic hypotension). Products include:
Astramorph/PF Injection, USP (Preservative-Free) ... 535
Duramorph ... 962
Infumorph 200 and Infumorph 500 Sterile Solutions ... 965
MS Contin Tablets ... 1994
MSIR ... 1997
Oramorph SR (Morphine Sulfate Sustained Release Tablets) ... 2236
RMS Suppositories ... 2657
Roxanol ... 2243

Nabumetone (Potential for acute renal failure). Products include:
Relafen Tablets ... 2510

Nadolol (Potential for additive or augmentative effect).
No products indexed under this heading.

Naproxen (Potential for acute renal failure). Products include:
Anaprox/Naprosyn ... 2117

Naproxen Sodium (Potential for acute renal failure). Products include:
Aleve ... 1975
Anaprox/Naprosyn ... 2117

Nicardipine Hydrochloride (Potential for additive or augmentative effect). Products include:
Cardene Capsules ... 2095
Cardene I.V. ... 2709
Cardene SR Capsules ... 2097

Nifedipine (Antihypertensive effect potentiated). Products include:
Adalat Capsules (10 mg and 20 mg) ... 587
Adalat CC ... 589
Procardia Capsules ... 1971
Procardia XL Extended Release Tablets ... 1972

Nisoldipine (Antihypertensive effect potentiated).
No products indexed under this heading.

Nitroglycerin (Potential for additive or augmentative effect). Products include:
Deponit NTG Transdermal Delivery System ... 2397
Nitro-Bid IV ... 1523
Nitro-Bid Ointment ... 1524
Nitrodisc ... 2047
Nitro-Dur (nitroglycerin) Transdermal Infusion System ... 1326
Nitrolingual Spray ... 2027
Nitrostat Tablets ... 1925
Transderm-Nitro Transdermal Therapeutic System ... 859

Norepinephrine Bitartrate (Decreased arterial responsiveness to norepinephrine). Products include:
Levophed Bitartrate Injection ... 2315

Opium Alkaloids (May aggravate orthostatic hypotension).
No products indexed under this heading.

Oxaprozin (Potential for acute renal failure). Products include:
Daypro Caplets ... 2426

Oxycodone Hydrochloride (May aggravate orthostatic hypotension). Products include:
Percocet Tablets ... 938
Percodan Tablets ... 939
Percodan-Demi Tablets ... 940
Roxicodone Tablets, Oral Solution & Intensol (Oxycodone) ... 2244
Tylox Capsules ... 1584

Penbutolol Sulfate (Potential for additive or augmentative effect). Products include:
Levatol ... 2403

Pentobarbital Sodium (May aggravate orthostatic hypotension). Products include:
Nembutal Sodium Capsules ... 436
Nembutal Sodium Solution ... 438
Nembutal Sodium Suppositories ... 440

Phenobarbital (May aggravate orthostatic hypotension). Products include:
Arco-Lase Plus Tablets ... 512
Bellergal-S Tablets ... 2250
Donnatal ... 2060
Donnatal Extentabs ... 2061
Donnatal Tablets ... 2060
Phenobarbital Elixir and Tablets ... 1469
Quadrinal Tablets ... 1350

Phenoxybenzamine Hydrochloride (Potential for additive or augmentative effect). Products include:
Dibenzyline Capsules ... 2476

Phentolamine Mesylate (Potential for additive or augmentative effect). Products include:
Regitine ... 846

Phenylbutazone (Potential for acute renal failure).
No products indexed under this heading.

Pindolol (Potential for additive or augmentative effect). Products include:
Visken Tablets ... 2299

Piroxicam (Potential for acute renal failure). Products include:
Feldene Capsules ... 1965

Polythiazide (Potential for additive or augmentative effect). Products include:
Minizide Capsules ... 1938

Potassium Acid Phosphate (Concomitant administration is contraindicated). Products include:
K-Phos Original Formula 'Sodium Free' Tablets ... 639

Potassium Bicarbonate (Concomitant administration is contraindicated). Products include:
Alka-Seltzer Gold Effervescent Antacid ... ▣ 703

Potassium Chloride (Concomitant administration is contraindicated). Products include:
Chlor-3 Condiment ... 1004
K-Dur Microburst Release System (potassium chloride, USP) E.R. Tablets ... 1325
K-Lor Powder Packets ... 434
K-Norm Extended-Release Capsules ... 991
K-Tab Filmtab ... 434
Kolyum Liquid ... 992
Micro-K ... 2063
Micro-K LS Packets ... 2064
NuLYTELY ... 689
Cherry Flavor NuLYTELY ... 689
Rum-K Syrup ... 1005
Slow-K Extended-Release Tablets ... 851

Potassium Citrate (Concomitant administration is contraindicated). Products include:
Polycitra Syrup ... 578
Polycitra-K Crystals ... 579
Polycitra-K Oral Solution ... 579
Polycitra-LC ... 578

Potassium Gluconate (Concomitant administration is contraindicated). Products include:
Kolyum Liquid ... 992

Potassium Phosphate, Dibasic (Concomitant administration is contraindicated).
No products indexed under this heading.

Potassium Phosphate, Monobasic (Concomitant administration is contraindicated). Products include:
K-Phos Neutral Tablets ... 639
K-Phos Original Formula 'Sodium Free' Tablets ... 639

Prazosin Hydrochloride (Potential for additive or augmentative effect). Products include:
Minipress Capsules ... 1937
Minizide Capsules ... 1938

Propoxyphene Hydrochloride (May aggravate orthostatic hypotension). Products include:
Darvon ... 1435
Wygesic Tablets ... 2827

Propoxyphene Napsylate (May aggravate orthostatic hypotension). Products include:
Darvon-N/Darvocet-N ... 1433

Propranolol Hydrochloride (Potential for additive or augmentative effect). Products include:
Inderal ... 2728
Inderal LA Long Acting Capsules ... 2730
Inderide Tablets ... 2732
Inderide LA Long Acting Capsules ... 2734

Quinapril Hydrochloride (Increased risk of hyperkalemia and antihypertensive effect potentiated). Products include:
Accupril Tablets ... 1893

Ramipril (Increased risk of hyperkalemia and antihypertensive effect potentiated). Products include:
Altace Capsules ... 1232

Rauwolfia Serpentina (Potential for additive or augmentative effect).
No products indexed under this heading.

Rescinnamine (Potential for additive or augmentative effect).
No products indexed under this heading.

Reserpine (Potential for additive or augmentative effect). Products include:
Diupres Tablets ... 1650
Hydropres Tablets ... 1675
Ser-Ap-Es Tablets ... 849

Secobarbital Sodium (May aggravate orthostatic hypotension). Products include:
Seconal Sodium Pulvules ... 1474

Sodium Nitroprusside (Potential for additive or augmentative effect).
No products indexed under this heading.

Sotalol Hydrochloride (Increased risk of hyperkalemia and antihypertensive effect potentiated). Products include:
Betapace Tablets ... 641

Spirapril Hydrochloride (Increased risk of hyperkalemia and antihypertensive effect potentiated).
No products indexed under this heading.

Spironolactone (Concurrent use is contraindicated). Products include:
Aldactazide ... 2413
Aldactone ... 2414

Sufentanil Citrate (May aggravate orthostatic hypotension). Products include:
Sufenta Injection ... 1309

Sulindac (Potential for acute renal failure). Products include:
Clinoril Tablets ... 1618

Terazosin Hydrochloride (Potential for additive or augmentative effect). Products include:
Hytrin Capsules ... 430

635 **Interactions Index** **Mebaral Tablets**

Thiamylal Sodium (May aggravate orthostatic hypotension).
- No products indexed under this heading.

Timolol Maleate (Potential for additive or augmentative effect). Products include:
- Blocadren Tablets ... 1614
- Timolide Tablets ... 1748
- Timoptic in Ocudose ... 1753
- Timoptic Sterile Ophthalmic Solution ... 1751
- Timoptic-XE ... 1755

Tolmetin Sodium (Potential for acute renal failure). Products include:
- Tolectin (200, 400 and 600 mg) .. 1581

Torsemide (Increased risk of hyperkalemia and antihypertensive effect potentiated). Products include:
- Demadex Tablets and Injection ... 686

Trimethaphan Camsylate (Potential for additive or augmentative effect). Products include:
- Arfonad Ampuls ... 2080

Tubocurarine Chloride (Increased responsiveness to tubocurarine).
- No products indexed under this heading.

Verapamil Hydrochloride (Increased risk of hyperkalemia and antihypertensive effect potentiated). Products include:
- Calan SR Caplets ... 2422
- Calan Tablets ... 2419
- Isoptin Injectable ... 1344
- Isoptin Oral Tablets ... 1346
- Isoptin SR Tablets ... 1348
- Verelan Capsules ... 1410
- Verelan Capsules ... 2824

Food Interactions

Alcohol (May aggravate orthostatic hypotension).

Diet, potassium-rich (Concurrent use is contraindicated).

MAXZIDE-25 MG TABLETS
(Triamterene, Hydrochlorothiazide) ..1380
See **Maxzide Tablets**

MAY-VITA ELIXIR
(Vitamins with Minerals) ...1543
None cited in PDR database.

MEBARAL TABLETS
(Mephobarbital) ...2322
May interact with corticosteroids, monoamine oxidase inhibitors, central nervous system depressants, oral anticoagulants, oral contraceptives, and certain other agents. Compounds in these categories include:

Alfentanil Hydrochloride (Additive depressant effects). Products include:
- Alfenta Injection ... 1286

Alprazolam (Additive depressant effects). Products include:
- Xanax Tablets ... 2649

Aprobarbital (Additive depressant effects).
- No products indexed under this heading.

Betamethasone Acetate (Enhanced metabolism of exogenous corticosteroids). Products include:
- Celestone Soluspan Suspension ... 2347

Betamethasone Sodium Phosphate (Enhanced metabolism of exogenous corticosteroids). Products include:
- Celestone Soluspan Suspension ... 2347

Buprenorphine (Additive depressant effects). Products include:
- Buprenex Injectable ... 2006

Buspirone Hydrochloride (Additive depressant effects). Products include:
- BuSpar ... 737

Butabarbital (Additive depressant effects).
- No products indexed under this heading.

Butalbital (Additive depressant effects). Products include:
- Esgic-plus Tablets ... 1013
- Fioricet Tablets ... 2258
- Fioricet with Codeine Capsules ... 2260
- Fiorinal Capsules ... 2261
- Fiorinal with Codeine Capsules ... 2262
- Fiorinal Tablets ... 2261
- Phrenilin ... 785
- Sedapap Tablets 50 mg/650 mg .. 1543

Chlordiazepoxide (Additive depressant effects). Products include:
- Libritabs Tablets ... 2177
- Limbitrol ... 2180

Chlordiazepoxide Hydrochloride (Additive depressant effects). Products include:
- Librax Capsules ... 2176
- Librium Capsules ... 2178
- Librium Injectable ... 2179

Chlorpromazine (Additive depressant effects). Products include:
- Thorazine Suppositories ... 2523

Chlorprothixene (Additive depressant effects).
- No products indexed under this heading.

Chlorprothixene Hydrochloride (Additive depressant effects).
- No products indexed under this heading.

Chlorprothixene Lactate (Additive depressant effects).
- No products indexed under this heading.

Clorazepate Dipotassium (Additive depressant effects). Products include:
- Tranxene ... 451

Clozapine (Additive depressant effects). Products include:
- Clozaril Tablets ... 2252

Codeine Phosphate (Additive depressant effects). Products include:
- Actifed with Codeine Cough Syrup.. 1067
- Brontex ... 1981
- Deconsal C Expectorant Syrup ... 456
- Deconsal Pediatric Syrup ... 457
- Dimetane-DC Cough Syrup ... 2059
- Empirin with Codeine Tablets ... 1093
- Fioricet with Codeine Capsules ... 2260
- Fiorinal with Codeine Capsules ... 2262
- Isoclor Expectorant ... 990
- Novahistine DH ... 2462
- Novahistine Expectorant ... 2463
- Nucofed ... 2051
- Phenergan with Codeine ... 2777
- Phenergan VC with Codeine ... 2781
- Robitussin A-C Syrup ... 2073
- Robitussin-DAC Syrup ... 2074
- Ryna ... 841
- Soma Compound w/Codeine Tablets ... 2676
- Tussi-Organidin NR Liquid and S NR Liquid ... 2677
- Tylenol with Codeine ... 1583

Cortisone Acetate (Enhanced metabolism of exogenous corticosteroids). Products include:
- Cortone Acetate Sterile Suspension ... 1623
- Cortone Acetate Tablets ... 1624

Desflurane (Additive depressant effects). Products include:
- Suprane ... 1813

Desogestrel (Decreased contraceptive effect). Products include:
- Desogen Tablets ... 1817
- Ortho-Cept ... 1851

Dexamethasone (Enhanced metabolism of exogenous corticosteroids). Products include:
- AK-Trol Ointment & Suspension ... ⊙ 205
- Decadron Elixir ... 1633
- Decadron Tablets ... 1635
- Decaspray Topical Aerosol ... 1648
- Dexacidin Ointment ... ⊙ 263
- Maxitrol Ophthalmic Ointment and Suspension ... ⊙ 224
- TobraDex Ophthalmic Suspension and Ointment ... 473

Dexamethasone Acetate (Enhanced metabolism of exogenous corticosteroids). Products include:
- Dalalone D.P. Injectable ... 1011
- Decadron-LA Sterile Suspension ... 1646

Dexamethasone Sodium Phosphate (Enhanced metabolism of exogenous corticosteroids). Products include:
- Decadron Phosphate Injection ... 1637
- Decadron Phosphate Respihaler ... 1642
- Decadron Phosphate Sterile Ophthalmic Ointment ... 1641
- Decadron Phosphate Sterile Ophthalmic Solution ... 1642
- Decadron Phosphate Topical Cream ... 1644
- Decadron Phosphate Turbinaire ... 1645
- Decadron Phosphate with Xylocaine Injection, Sterile ... 1639
- Dexacort Phosphate in Respihaler .. 458
- Dexacort Phosphate in Turbinaire .. 459
- NeoDecadron Sterile Ophthalmic Ointment ... 1712
- NeoDecadron Sterile Ophthalmic Solution ... 1713
- NeoDecadron Topical Cream ... 1714

Dezocine (Additive depressant effects). Products include:
- Dalgan Injection ... 538

Diazepam (Additive depressant effects). Products include:
- Dizac ... 1809
- Valium Injectable ... 2182
- Valium Tablets ... 2183
- Valrelease Capsules ... 2169

Dicumarol (Decreased anticoagulant response).
- No products indexed under this heading.

Doxycycline Calcium (Half-life of doxycycline shortened). Products include:
- Vibramycin Calcium Oral Suspension Syrup ... 1941

Doxycycline Hyclate (Half-life of doxycycline shortened). Products include:
- Doryx Capsules ... 1913
- Vibramycin Hyclate Capsules ... 1941
- Vibramycin Hyclate Intravenous ... 2215
- Vibra-Tabs Film Coated Tablets ... 1941

Doxycycline Monohydrate (Half-life of doxycycline shortened). Products include:
- Monodox Capsules ... 1805
- Vibramycin Monohydrate for Oral Suspension ... 1941

Droperidol (Additive depressant effects). Products include:
- Inapsine Injection ... 1296

Enflurane (Additive depressant effects).
- No products indexed under this heading.

Estazolam (Additive depressant effects). Products include:
- ProSom Tablets ... 449

Estradiol (Decreased effect of estradiol). Products include:
- Climara Transdermal System ... 645
- Estrace Cream and Tablets ... 749
- Estraderm Transdermal System ... 824

Estrone (Decreased effect of estrone).
- No products indexed under this heading.

Ethchlorvynol (Additive depressant effects). Products include:
- Placidyl Capsules ... 448

Ethinamate (Additive depressant effects).
- No products indexed under this heading.

Ethinyl Estradiol (Decreased contraceptive effect). Products include:
- Brevicon ... 2088
- Demulen ... 2428
- Desogen Tablets ... 1817
- Levlen/Tri-Levlen ... 651
- Lo/Ovral Tablets ... 2746
- Lo/Ovral-28 Tablets ... 2751
- Modicon ... 1872
- Nordette-21 Tablets ... 2755
- Nordette-28 Tablets ... 2758
- Norinyl ... 2088
- Ortho-Cept ... 1851
- Ortho-Cyclen/Ortho-Tri-Cyclen ... 1858
- Ortho-Novum ... 1872
- Ortho-Cyclen/Ortho Tri-Cyclen ... 1858
- Ovcon ... 760
- Ovral Tablets ... 2770
- Ovral-28 Tablets ... 2770
- Levlen/Tri-Levlen ... 651
- Tri-Norinyl ... 2164
- Triphasil-21 Tablets ... 2814
- Triphasil-28 Tablets ... 2819

Ethynodiol Diacetate (Decreased contraceptive effect). Products include:
- Demulen ... 2428

Fentanyl (Additive depressant effects). Products include:
- Duragesic Transdermal System ... 1288

Fentanyl Citrate (Additive depressant effects). Products include:
- Sublimaze Injection ... 1307

Fludrocortisone Acetate (Enhanced metabolism of exogenous corticosteroids). Products include:
- Florinef Acetate Tablets ... 505

Fluphenazine Decanoate (Additive depressant effects). Products include:
- Prolixin Decanoate ... 509

Fluphenazine Enanthate (Additive depressant effects). Products include:
- Prolixin Enanthate ... 509

Fluphenazine Hydrochloride (Additive depressant effects). Products include:
- Prolixin ... 509

Flurazepam Hydrochloride (Additive depressant effects). Products include:
- Dalmane Capsules ... 2173

Furazolidone (Prolongs effects of barbiturates). Products include:
- Furoxone ... 2046

Glutethimide (Additive depressant effects).
- No products indexed under this heading.

Griseofulvin (Decreased blood levels of griseofulvin). Products include:
- Fulvicin P/G Tablets ... 2359
- Fulvicin P/G 165 & 330 Tablets ... 2359
- Grifulvin V (griseofulvin tablets) Microsize (griseofulvin oral suspension) Microsize ... 1888
- Gris-PEG Tablets, 125 mg & 250 mg ... 479

Haloperidol (Additive depressant effects). Products include:
- Haldol Injection, Tablets and Concentrate ... 1575

Haloperidol Decanoate (Additive depressant effects). Products include:
- Haldol Decanoate ... 1577

Hydrocodone Bitartrate (Additive depressant effects). Products include:
- Anexsia 5/500 Elixir ... 1781
- Anexia Tablets ... 1782
- Codiclear DH Syrup ... 791
- Deconamine CX Cough and Cold Liquid and Tablets ... 1319
- Duratuss HD Elixir ... 2565
- Hycodan Tablets and Syrup ... 930
- Hycomine Compound Tablets ... 932
- Hycomine ... 931
- Hycotuss Expectorant Syrup ... 933
- Hydrocet Capsules ... 782

IMPORTANT NOTE: Always consult each drug listing in the patient's regimen for possible interactions.

Mebaral Tablets

Lorcet 10/650 1018
Lortab 2566
Tussend 1783
Tussend Expectorant 1785
Vicodin Tablets 1356
Vicodin ES Tablets 1357
Vicodin Tuss Expectorant 1358
Zydone Capsules 949

Hydrocodone Polistirex (Additive depressant effects). Products include:

Tussionex Pennkinetic Extended-Release Suspension 998

Hydrocortisone (Enhanced metabolism of exogenous corticosteroids). Products include:

Anusol-HC Cream 2.5% 1896
Aquanil HC Lotion 1931
Bactine Hydrocortisone Anti-Itch Cream .... ⊞ 709
Caldecort Anti-Itch Hydrocortisone Spray .... ⊞ 631
Cortaid .... ⊞ 836
CORTENEMA 2535
Cortisporin Ointment 1085
Cortisporin Ophthalmic Ointment Sterile 1085
Cortisporin Ophthalmic Suspension Sterile 1086
Cortisporin Otic Solution Sterile 1087
Cortisporin Otic Suspension Sterile 1088
Cortizone-5 .... ⊞ 831
Cortizone-10 .... ⊞ 831
Hydrocortone Tablets 1672
Hytone 907
Massengill Medicated Soft Cloth Towelettes 2458
PediOtic Suspension Sterile 1153
Preparation H Hydrocortisone 1% Cream .... ⊞ 872
ProctoCream-HC 2.5% 2408
VōSoL HC Otic Solution 2678

Hydrocortisone Acetate (Enhanced metabolism of exogenous corticosteroids). Products include:

Analpram-HC Rectal Cream 1% and 2.5% 977
Anusol HC-1 Anti-Itch Hydrocortisone Ointment .... ⊞ 847
Anusol-HC Suppositories 1897
Caldecort .... ⊞ 631
Carmol HC 924
Coly-Mycin S Otic w/Neomycin & Hydrocortisone 1906
Cortaid .... ⊞ 836
Cortifoam 2396
Cortisporin Cream 1084
Epifoam 2399
Hydrocortone Acetate Sterile Suspension 1669
Mantadil Cream 1135
Nupercainal Hydrocortisone 1% Cream .... ⊞ 645
Ophthocort .... ⊙ 311
Pramosone Cream, Lotion & Ointment 978
ProctoCream-HC 2408
ProctoFoam-HC 2409
Terra-Cortril Ophthalmic Suspension 2210

Hydrocortisone Sodium Phosphate (Enhanced metabolism of exogenous corticosteroids). Products include:

Hydrocortone Phosphate Injection, Sterile 1670

Hydrocortisone Sodium Succinate (Enhanced metabolism of exogenous corticosteroids). Products include:

Solu-Cortef Sterile Powder 2641

Hydroxyzine Hydrochloride (Additive depressant effects). Products include:

Atarax Tablets & Syrup 2185
Marax Tablets & DF Syrup 2200
Vistaril Intramuscular Solution 2216

Isocarboxazid (Prolongs effects of barbiturates).

No products indexed under this heading.

Isoflurane (Additive depressant effects).

No products indexed under this heading.

Ketamine Hydrochloride (Additive depressant effects).

No products indexed under this heading.

Levomethadyl Acetate Hydrochloride (Additive depressant effects). Products include:

Orlaam 2239

Levonorgestrel (Decreased contraceptive effect). Products include:

Levlen/Tri-Levlen 651
Nordette-21 Tablets 2755
Nordette-28 Tablets 2758
Norplant System 2759
Levlen/Tri-Levlen 651
Triphasil-21 Tablets 2814
Triphasil-28 Tablets 2819

Levorphanol Tartrate (Additive depressant effects). Products include:

Levo-Dromoran 2129

Lorazepam (Additive depressant effects). Products include:

Ativan Injection 2698
Ativan Tablets 2700

Loxapine Hydrochloride (Additive depressant effects). Products include:

Loxitane 1378

Loxapine Succinate (Additive depressant effects). Products include:

Loxitane Capsules 1378

Meperidine Hydrochloride (Additive depressant effects). Products include:

Demerol 2308
Mepergan Injection 2753

Meprobamate (Additive depressant effects). Products include:

Miltown Tablets 2672
PMB 200 and PMB 400 2783

Mesoridazine Besylate (Additive depressant effects). Products include:

Serentil 684

Mestranol (Decreased contraceptive effect). Products include:

Norinyl 2088
Ortho-Novum 1872

Methadone Hydrochloride (Additive depressant effects). Products include:

Methadone Hydrochloride Oral Concentrate 2233
Methadone Hydrochloride Oral Solution & Tablets 2235

Methohexital Sodium (Additive depressant effects). Products include:

Brevital Sodium Vials 1429

Methotrimeprazine (Additive depressant effects). Products include:

Levoprome 1274

Methoxyflurane (Additive depressant effects).

No products indexed under this heading.

Methylprednisolone Acetate (Enhanced metabolism of exogenous corticosteroids). Products include:

Depo-Medrol Single-Dose Vial 2600
Depo-Medrol Sterile Aqueous Suspension 2597

Methylprednisolone Sodium Succinate (Enhanced metabolism of exogenous corticosteroids). Products include:

Solu-Medrol Sterile Powder 2643

Midazolam Hydrochloride (Additive depressant effects). Products include:

Versed Injection 2170

Molindone Hydrochloride (Additive depressant effects). Products include:

Moban Tablets and Concentrate 1048

Morphine Sulfate (Additive depressant effects). Products include:

Astramorph/PF Injection, USP (Preservative-Free) 535
Duramorph 962
Infumorph 200 and Infumorph 500 Sterile Solutions 965
MS Contin Tablets 1994
MSIR 1997
Oramorph SR (Morphine Sulfate Sustained Release Tablets) 2236
RMS Suppositories 2657
Roxanol 2243

Norethindrone (Decreased contraceptive effect). Products include:

Brevicon 2088
Micronor Tablets 1872
Modicon 1872
Norinyl 2088
Nor-Q D Tablets 2135
Ortho-Novum 1872
Ovcon 760
Tri-Norinyl 2164

Norethynodrel (Decreased contraceptive effect).

No products indexed under this heading.

Norgestimate (Decreased contraceptive effect). Products include:

Ortho-Cyclen/Ortho-Tri-Cyclen 1858
Ortho-Cyclen/Ortho Tri-Cyclen 1858

Norgestrel (Decreased contraceptive effect). Products include:

Lo/Ovral Tablets 2746
Lo/Ovral-28 Tablets 2751
Ovral Tablets 2770
Ovral-28 Tablets 2770
Ovrette Tablets 2771

Opium Alkaloids (Additive depressant effects).

No products indexed under this heading.

Oxazepam (Additive depressant effects). Products include:

Serax Capsules 2810
Serax Tablets 2810

Oxycodone Hydrochloride (Additive depressant effects). Products include:

Percocet Tablets 938
Percodan Tablets 939
Percodan-Demi Tablets 940
Roxicodone Tablets, Oral Solution & Intensol (Oxycodone) 2244
Tylox Capsules 1584

Pentobarbital Sodium (Additive depressant effects). Products include:

Nembutal Sodium Capsules 436
Nembutal Sodium Solution 438
Nembutal Sodium Suppositories 440

Perphenazine (Additive depressant effects). Products include:

Etrafon 2355
Triavil Tablets 1757
Trilafon 2389

Phenelzine Sulfate (Prolongs effects of barbiturates). Products include:

Nardil 1920

Phenobarbital (Additive depressant effects). Products include:

Arco-Lase Plus Tablets 512
Bellergal-S Tablets 2250
Donnatal 2060
Donnatal Extentabs 2061
Donnatal Tablets 2060
Phenobarbital Elixir and Tablets 1469
Quadrinal Tablets 1350

Phenytoin (Unpredictable effects). Products include:

Dilantin Infatabs 1908
Dilantin-125 Suspension 1911

Phenytoin Sodium (Unpredictable effects). Products include:

Dilantin Kapseals 1906
Dilantin Parenteral 1910

Prazepam (Additive depressant effects).

No products indexed under this heading.

Prednisolone Acetate (Enhanced metabolism of exogenous corticosteroids). Products include:

AK-CIDE .... ⊙ 202
AK-CIDE Ointment .... ⊙ 202
Blephamide Liquifilm Sterile Ophthalmic Suspension 476
Blephamide Ointment .... ⊙ 237
Econopred & Econopred Plus Ophthalmic Suspensions .... ⊙ 217
Poly-Pred Liquifilm .... ⊙ 248
Pred Forte .... ⊙ 250
Pred Mild .... ⊙ 253
Pred-G Liquifilm Sterile Ophthalmic Suspension .... ⊙ 251
Pred-G S.O.P. Sterile Ophthalmic Ointment .... ⊙ 252
Vasocidin Ointment .... ⊙ 268

Prednisolone Sodium Phosphate (Enhanced metabolism of exogenous corticosteroids). Products include:

AK-Pred .... ⊙ 204
Hydeltrasol Injection, Sterile 1665
Inflamase .... ⊙ 265
Pediapred Oral Liquid 995
Vasocidin Ophthalmic Solution ...... ⊙ 270

Prednisolone Tebutate (Enhanced metabolism of exogenous corticosteroids). Products include:

Hydeltra-T.B.A. Sterile Suspension 1667

Prednisone (Enhanced metabolism of exogenous corticosteroids). Products include:

Deltasone Tablets 2595

Prochlorperazine (Additive depressant effects). Products include:

Compazine 2470

Progesterone (Decreased effect of progesterone).

No products indexed under this heading.

Promethazine Hydrochloride (Additive depressant effects). Products include:

Mepergan Injection 2753
Phenergan with Codeine 2777
Phenergan with Dextromethorphan 2778
Phenergan Injection 2773
Phenergan Suppositories 2775
Phenergan Syrup 2774
Phenergan Tablets 2775
Phenergan VC 2779
Phenergan VC with Codeine 2781

Propofol (Additive depressant effects). Products include:

Diprivan Injection 2833

Propoxyphene Hydrochloride (Additive depressant effects). Products include:

Darvon 1435
Wygesic Tablets 2827

Propoxyphene Napsylate (Additive depressant effects). Products include:

Darvon-N/Darvocet-N 1433

Quazepam (Additive depressant effects). Products include:

Doral Tablets 2664

Risperidone (Additive depressant effects). Products include:

Risperdal 1301

Secobarbital Sodium (Additive depressant effects). Products include:

Seconal Sodium Pulvules 1474

Selegiline Hydrochloride (Prolongs effects of barbiturates). Products include:

Eldepryl Tablets 2550

Sodium Valproate (Barbiturate metabolism decreased).

Sufentanil Citrate (Additive depressant effects). Products include:

Sufenta Injection 1309

Temazepam (Additive depressant effects). Products include:

Restoril Capsules 2284

(⊞ Described in PDR For Nonprescription Drugs) (⊙ Described in PDR For Ophthalmology)

Thiamylal Sodium (Additive depressant effects).

No products indexed under this heading.

Thioridazine Hydrochloride (Additive depressant effects). Products include:

Mellaril 2269

Thiothixene (Additive depressant effects). Products include:

Navane Capsules and Concentrate 2201
Navane Intramuscular 2202

Tranylcypromine Sulfate (Prolongs effects of barbiturates). Products include:

Parnate Tablets 2503

Triamcinolone (Enhanced metabolism of exogenous corticosteroids). Products include:

Aristocort Tablets 1022

Triamcinolone Acetonide (Enhanced metabolism of exogenous corticosteroids). Products include:

Aristocort A 0.025% Cream 1027
Aristocort A 0.5% Cream 1031
Aristocort A 0.1% Cream 1029
Aristocort A 0.1% Ointment 1030
Azmacort Oral Inhaler 2011
Nasacort Nasal Inhaler 2024

Triamcinolone Diacetate (Enhanced metabolism of exogenous corticosteroids). Products include:

Aristocort Suspension (Forte Parenteral)... 1027
Aristocort Suspension (Intralesional) 1025

Triamcinolone Hexacetonide (Enhanced metabolism of exogenous corticosteroids). Products include:

Aristospan Suspension (Intra-articular) 1033
Aristospan Suspension (Intralesional) 1032

Triazolam (Additive depressant effects). Products include:

Halcion Tablets.. 2611

Trifluoperazine Hydrochloride (Additive depressant effects). Products include:

Stelazine 2514

Valproic Acid (Decreased barbiturate metabolism). Products include:

Depakene 413

Warfarin Sodium (Decreased anticoagulant response). Products include:

Coumadin 926

Zolpidem Tartrate (Additive depressant effects). Products include:

Ambien Tablets.. 2416

MEDIFEN

(Fiber Supplement) 1807

None cited in PDR database.

MEDROL DOSEPAK UNIT OF USE

(Methylprednisolone) 2621

May interact with oral anticoagulants, certain other agents, oral hypoglycemic agents, and insulin. Compounds in these categories include:

Acarbose (Increased requirements for oral hypoglycemic agents in diabetes).

No products indexed under this heading.

Aspirin (Increased clearance of chronic high dose aspirin leading to decreased salicylate serum levels or increase the risk of salicylate toxicity when methylprednisolone is withdrawn). Products include:

Alka-Seltzer Effervescent Antacid and Pain Reliever .... ◆ 701
Alka-Seltzer Extra Strength Effervescent Antacid and Pain Reliever .... ◆ 703
Alka-Seltzer Lemon Lime Effervescent Antacid and Pain Reliever .... ◆ 703
Alka-Seltzer Plus Cold Medicine .... ◆ 705
Alka-Seltzer Plus Cold & Cough Medicine .... ◆ 708
Alka-Seltzer Plus Night-Time Cold Medicine .... ◆ 707
Alka Seltzer Plus Sinus Medicine .. ◆ 707
Arthritis Foundation Safety Coated Aspirin Tablets .... ◆ 675
Arthritis Pain Ascriptin .... ◆ 631
Maximum Strength Ascriptin .... ◆ 630
Regular Strength Ascriptin Tablets .... ◆ 629
Arthritis Strength BC Powder......... ◆ 609
BC Cold Powder Multi-Symptom Formula (Cold-Sinus-Allergy) ...... ◆ 609
BC Cold Powder Non-Drowsy Formula (Cold-Sinus) .... ◆ 609
BC Powder .... ◆ 609
Bayer Children's Chewable Aspirin .... ◆ 711
Genuine Bayer Aspirin Tablets & Caplets .... ◆ 713
Extra Strength Bayer Arthritis Pain Regimen Formula .... ◆ 711
Extra Strength Bayer Aspirin Caplets & Tablets .... ◆ 712
Extended-Release Bayer 8-Hour Aspirin .... ◆ 712
Extra Strength Bayer Plus Aspirin Caplets .... ◆ 713
Extra Strength Bayer PM Aspirin .. ◆ 713
Bayer Enteric Aspirin .... ◆ 709
Bufferin Analgesic Tablets and Caplets .... ◆ 613
Arthritis Strength Bufferin Analgesic Caplets .... ◆ 614
Extra Strength Bufferin Analgesic Tablets .... ◆ 615
Cama Arthritis Pain Reliever........... ◆ 785
Darvon Compound-65 Pulvules 1435
Easprin 1914
Ecotrin 2455
Ecotrin Enteric Coated Aspirin Maximum Strength Tablets and Caplets .... ◆ 816
Ecotrin Enteric Coated Aspirin Regular Strength Tablets 2455
Empirin Aspirin Tablets .... ◆ 854
Empirin with Codeine Tablets.......... 1093
Excedrin Extra-Strength Analgesic Tablets & Caplets 732
Fiorinal Capsules 2261
Fiorinal with Codeine Capsules 2262
Fiorinal Tablets 2261
Halfprin 1362
Healthprin Aspirin 2455
Norgesic... 1496
Percodan Tablets..................................... 939
Percodan-Demi Tablets........................ 940
Robaxisal Tablets.................................... 2071
Soma Compound w/Codeine Tablets 2676
Soma Compound Tablets..................... 2675
St. Joseph Adult Chewable Aspirin (81 mg.) .... ◆ 808
Talwin Compound 2335
Ursinus Inlay-Tabs................................ ◆ 794
Vanquish Analgesic Caplets .... ◆ 731

Chlorpropamide (Increased requirements for oral hypoglycemic agents in diabetes). Products include:

Diabinese Tablets 1935

Cyclosporine (Potential for convulsions; potential for mutual inhibition of metabolism). Products include:

Neoral 2276
Sandimmune 2286

Dicumarol (Potential for variable effect; concurrent use may result in enhanced as well as diminished effects of anticoagulant).

No products indexed under this heading.

Glipizide (Increased requirements for oral hypoglycemic agents in diabetes). Products include:

Glucotrol Tablets 1967
Glucotrol XL Extended Release Tablets 1968

Glyburide (Increased requirements for oral hypoglycemic agents in diabetes). Products include:

DiaBeta Tablets 1239
Glynase PresTab Tablets 2609
Micronase Tablets 2623

Immunization (Possible hazard of neurological complications and a lack of antibody response).

Insulin, Human (Increased requirements for insulin in diabetes).

No products indexed under this heading.

Insulin, Human Isophane Suspension (Increased requirements for insulin in diabetes). Products include:

Novolin N Human Insulin 10 ml Vials.. 1795

Insulin, Human NPH (Increased requirements for insulin in diabetes). Products include:

Humulin N, 100 Units 1448
Novolin N PenFill Cartridges Durable Insulin Delivery System 1798
Novolin N Prefilled Syringe Disposable Insulin Delivery System 1798

Insulin, Human Regular (Increased requirements for insulin in diabetes). Products include:

Humulin R, 100 Units.......................... 1449
Novolin R Human Insulin 10 ml Vials.. 1795
Novolin R PenFill Cartridges Durable Insulin Delivery System 1798
Novolin R Prefilled Syringe Disposable Insulin Delivery System 1798
Velosulin BR Human Insulin 10 ml Vials.. 1795

Insulin, Human, Zinc Suspension (Increased requirements for insulin in diabetes). Products include:

Humulin L, 100 Units 1446
Humulin U, 100 Units 1450
Novolin L Human Insulin 10 ml Vials.. 1795

Insulin, NPH (Increased requirements for insulin in diabetes). Products include:

NPH, 100 Units 1450
Pork NPH, 100 Units........................... 1452
Purified Pork NPH Isophane Insulin 1801

Insulin, Regular (Increased requirements for insulin in diabetes). Products include:

Regular, 100 Units 1450
Pork Regular, 100 Units 1452
Pork Regular (Concentrated), 500 Units 1453
Purified Pork Regular Insulin 1801

Insulin, Zinc Crystals (Increased requirements for insulin in diabetes). Products include:

NPH, 100 Units 1450

Insulin, Zinc Suspension (Increased requirements for insulin in diabetes). Products include:

Iletin I 1450
Lente, 100 Units 1450
Iletin II.. 1452
Pork Lente, 100 Units.......................... 1452
Purified Pork Lente Insulin 1801

Ketoconazole (May inhibit the metabolism of methylprednisolone and thus decrease its clearance; the dose of methylprednisolone should be titrated to avoid toxicity). Products include:

Nizoral 2% Cream.................................. 1297
Nizoral 2% Shampoo............................ 1298
Nizoral Tablets 1298

Metformin Hydrochloride (Increased requirements for oral hypoglycemic agents in diabetes). Products include:

Glucophage 752

Phenobarbital (Increases clearance of methylprednisolone and may require increase in dose of methylprednisolone to achieve the desired response). Products include:

Arco-Lase Plus Tablets 512
Bellergal-S Tablets 2250
Donnatal 2060
Donnatal Extentabs............................... 2061
Donnatal Tablets 2060
Phenobarbital Elixir and Tablets 1469
Quadrinal Tablets 1350

Phenytoin (Increases clearance of methylprednisolone and may require increase in dose of methylprednisolone to achieve the desired response). Products include:

Dilantin Infatabs 1908
Dilantin-125 Suspension 1911

Phenytoin Sodium (Increases clearance of methylprednisolone and may require increase in dose of methylprednisolone to achieve the desired response). Products include:

Dilantin Kapseals 1906
Dilantin Parenteral 1910

Rifampin (Increases clearance of methylprednisolone and may require increase in dose of methylprednisolone to achieve the desired response). Products include:

Rifadin 1528
Rifamate Capsules 1530
Rifater... 1532
Rimactane Capsules............................... 847

Smallpox Vaccine (Possible hazard of neurological complications and a lack of antibody response).

Tolazamide (Increased requirements for oral hypoglycemic agents in diabetes).

No products indexed under this heading.

Tolbutamide (Increased requirements for oral hypoglycemic agents in diabetes).

No products indexed under this heading.

Troleandomycin (May inhibit the metabolism of methylprednisolone and thus decrease its clearance; the dose of methylprednisolone should be titrated to avoid toxicity). Products include:

Tao Capsules 2209

Warfarin Sodium (Potential for variable effect; concurrent use may result in enhanced as well as diminished effects of anticoagulant). Products include:

Coumadin 926

MEDROL TABLETS

(Methylprednisolone) 2621

See **Medrol Dosepak Unit of Use**

MEFOXIN

(Cefoxitin Sodium).................................1691

May interact with aminoglycosides and certain other agents. Compounds in these categories include:

Amikacin Sulfate (Increased nephrotoxicity). Products include:

Amikacin Sulfate Injection, USP 960
Amikin Injectable 501

Gentamicin Sulfate (Increased nephrotoxicity). Products include:

Garamycin Injectable 2360
Genoptic Sterile Ophthalmic Solution.. ◎ 243
Genoptic Sterile Ophthalmic Ointment .... ◎ 243
Gentacidin Ointment .... ◎ 264
Gentacidin Solution............................... ◎ 264
Gentak .... ◎ 208
Pred-G Liquifilm Sterile Ophthalmic Suspension .... ◎ 251
Pred-G S.O.P. Sterile Ophthalmic Ointment .... ◎ 252

IMPORTANT NOTE: Always consult each drug listing in the patient's regimen for possible interactions.

Kanamycin Sulfate (Increased nephrotoxicity).
No products indexed under this heading.

Probenecid (Slows tubular excretion and produces higher serum levels of cefoxitin). Products include:
Benemid Tablets ... 1611
ColBENEMID Tablets ... 1622

Streptomycin Sulfate (Increased nephrotoxicity). Products include:
Streptomycin Sulfate Injection ... 2208

Tobramycin (Increased nephrotoxicity). Products include:
AKTOB ... ⊙ 206
TobraDex Ophthalmic Suspension and Ointment ... 473
Tobrex Ophthalmic Ointment and Solution ... ⊙ 229

Tobramycin Sulfate (Increased nephrotoxicity). Products include:
Nebcin Vials, Hyporets & ADD-Vantage ... 1464
Tobramycin Sulfate Injection ... 968

MEFOXIN PREMIXED INTRAVENOUS SOLUTION
(Cefoxitin Sodium) ... 1694
May interact with aminoglycosides and certain other agents. Compounds in these categories include:

Amikacin Sulfate (Increased nephrotoxicity). Products include:
Amikacin Sulfate Injection, USP ... 960
Amikin Injectable ... 501

Gentamicin Sulfate (Increased nephrotoxicity). Products include:
Garamycin Injectable ... 2360
Genoptic Sterile Ophthalmic Solution ... ⊙ 243
Genoptic Sterile Ophthalmic Ointment ... ⊙ 243
Gentacidin Ointment ... ⊙ 264
Gentacidin Solution ... ⊙ 264
Gentak ... ⊙ 208
Pred-G Liquifilm Sterile Ophthalmic Suspension ... ⊙ 251
Pred-G S.O.P. Sterile Ophthalmic Ointment ... ⊙ 252

Kanamycin Sulfate (Increased nephrotoxicity).
No products indexed under this heading.

Probenecid (Higher serum levels of cefoxitin). Products include:
Benemid Tablets ... 1611
ColBENEMID Tablets ... 1622

Streptomycin Sulfate (Increased nephrotoxicity). Products include:
Streptomycin Sulfate Injection ... 2208

Tobramycin Sulfate (Increased nephrotoxicity). Products include:
Nebcin Vials, Hyporets & ADD-Vantage ... 1464
Tobramycin Sulfate Injection ... 968

MEGA-B
(Vitamin B Complex) ... 512
None cited in PDR database.

MEGACE ORAL SUSPENSION
(Megestrol Acetate) ... 699
None cited in PDR database.

MEGACE TABLETS
(Megestrol Acetate) ... 701
None cited in PDR database.

MEGADOSE
(Vitamins with Minerals) ... 512
None cited in PDR database.

MELANEX TOPICAL SOLUTION
(Hydroquinone) ... 1793
May interact with:

Hydrogen Peroxide (May result in transient dark staining of skin areas so treated). Products include:
Oxysept Disinfection System ... ⊙ 340
Oxysept 1 Disinfecting Solution ... ⊙ 339
UltraCare System ... ⊙ 342

MELLARIL CONCENTRATE
(Thioridazine Hydrochloride) ... 2269
May interact with central nervous system depressants, narcotic analgesics, barbiturates, general anesthetics, and certain other agents. Compounds in these categories include:

Alfentanil Hydrochloride (Potentiation of central nervous system depressants). Products include:
Alfenta Injection ... 1286

Alprazolam (Potentiation of central nervous system depressants). Products include:
Xanax Tablets ... 2649

Aprobarbital (Potentiation of central nervous system depressants; severe respiratory depression and respiratory arrest have been reported when a patient was given a phenothiazine and a concomitant high dose of a barbiturate).
No products indexed under this heading.

Atropine Sulfate (Potentiation of central nervous system depressants). Products include:
Arco-Lase Plus Tablets ... 512
Atrohist Plus Tablets ... 454
Atropine Sulfate Sterile Ophthalmic Solution ... ⊙ 233
Donnatal ... 2060
Donnatal Extentabs ... 2061
Donnatal Tablets ... 2060
Lomotil ... 2439
Motofen Tablets ... 784
Urised Tablets ... 1964

Buprenorphine (Potentiation of central nervous system depressants). Products include:
Buprenex Injectable ... 2006

Buspirone Hydrochloride (Potentiation of central nervous system depressants). Products include:
BuSpar ... 737

Butabarbital (Potentiation of central nervous system depressants; severe respiratory depression and respiratory arrest have been reported when a patient was given a phenothiazine and a concomitant high dose of a barbiturate).
No products indexed under this heading.

Butalbital (Potentiation of central nervous system depressants; severe respiratory depression and respiratory arrest have been reported when a patient was given a phenothiazine and a concomitant high dose of a barbiturate). Products include:
Esgic-plus Tablets ... 1013
Fioricet Tablets ... 2258
Fioricet with Codeine Capsules ... 2260
Fiorinal Capsules ... 2261
Fiorinal with Codeine Capsules ... 2262
Fiorinal Tablets ... 2261
Phrenilin ... 785
Sedapap Tablets 50 mg/650 mg ... 1543

Chlordiazepoxide (Potentiation of central nervous system depressants). Products include:
Libritabs Tablets ... 2177
Limbitrol ... 2180

Chlordiazepoxide Hydrochloride (Potentiation of central nervous system depressants). Products include:
Librax Capsules ... 2176
Librium Capsules ... 2178
Librium Injectable ... 2179

Chlorpromazine (Potentiation of central nervous system depressants). Products include:
Thorazine Suppositories ... 2523

Chlorpromazine Hydrochloride (Potentiation of central nervous system depressants). Products include:
Thorazine ... 2523

Chlorprothixene (Potentiation of central nervous system depressants).
No products indexed under this heading.

Chlorprothixene Hydrochloride (Potentiation of central nervous system depressants).
No products indexed under this heading.

Clorazepate Dipotassium (Potentiation of central nervous system depressants). Products include:
Tranxene ... 451

Clozapine (Potentiation of central nervous system depressants). Products include:
Clozaril Tablets ... 2252

Codeine Phosphate (Potentiation of central nervous system depressants). Products include:
Actifed with Codeine Cough Syrup ... 1067
Brontex ... 1981
Deconsal C Expectorant Syrup ... 456
Deconsal Pediatric Syrup ... 457
Dimetane-DC Cough Syrup ... 2059
Empirin with Codeine Tablets ... 1093
Fioricet with Codeine Capsules ... 2260
Fiorinal with Codeine Capsules ... 2262
Isoclor Expectorant ... 990
Novahistine DH ... 2462
Novahistine Expectorant ... 2463
Nucofed ... 2051
Phenergan with Codeine ... 2777
Phenergan VC with Codeine ... 2781
Robitussin A-C Syrup ... 2073
Robitussin-DAC Syrup ... 2074
Ryna ... ▣ 841
Soma Compound w/Codeine Tablets ... 2676
Tussi-Organidin NR Liquid and S NR Liquid ... 2677
Tylenol with Codeine ... 1583

Desflurane (Potentiation of central nervous system depressants). Products include:
Suprane ... 1813

Dezocine (Potentiation of central nervous system depressants). Products include:
Dalgan Injection ... 538

Diazepam (Potentiation of central nervous system depressants). Products include:
Dizac ... 1809
Valium Injectable ... 2182
Valium Tablets ... 2183
Valrelease Capsules ... 2169

Droperidol (Potentiation of central nervous system depressants). Products include:
Inapsine Injection ... 1296

Enflurane (Potentiation of central nervous system depressants).
No products indexed under this heading.

Estazolam (Potentiation of central nervous system depressants). Products include:
ProSom Tablets ... 449

Ethchlorvynol (Potentiation of central nervous system depressants). Products include:
Placidyl Capsules ... 448

Ethinamate (Potentiation of central nervous system depressants).
No products indexed under this heading.

Fentanyl (Potentiation of central nervous system depressants). Products include:
Duragesic Transdermal System ... 1288

Fentanyl Citrate (Potentiation of central nervous system depressants). Products include:
Sublimaze Injection ... 1307

Fluphenazine Decanoate (Potentiation of central nervous system depressants). Products include:
Prolixin Decanoate ... 509

Fluphenazine Enanthate (Potentiation of central nervous system depressants). Products include:
Prolixin Enanthate ... 509

Fluphenazine Hydrochloride (Potentiation of central nervous system depressants). Products include:
Prolixin ... 509

Flurazepam Hydrochloride (Potentiation of central nervous system depressants). Products include:
Dalmane Capsules ... 2173

Glutethimide (Potentiation of central nervous system depressants).
No products indexed under this heading.

Haloperidol (Potentiation of central nervous system depressants). Products include:
Haldol Injection, Tablets and Concentrate ... 1575

Haloperidol Decanoate (Potentiation of central nervous system depressants). Products include:
Haldol Decanoate ... 1577

Hydrocodone Bitartrate (Potentiation of central nervous system depressants). Products include:
Anexsia 5/500 Elixir ... 1781
Anexia Tablets ... 1782
Codiclear DH Syrup ... 791
Deconamine CX Cough and Cold Liquid and Tablets ... 1319
Duratuss HD Elixir ... 2565
Hycodan Tablets and Syrup ... 930
Hycomine Compound Tablets ... 932
Hycomine ... 931
Hycotuss Expectorant Syrup ... 933
Hydrocet Capsules ... 782
Lorcet 10/650 ... 1018
Lortab ... 2566
Tussend ... 1783
Tussend Expectorant ... 1785
Vicodin Tablets ... 1356
Vicodin ES Tablets ... 1357
Vicodin Tuss Expectorant ... 1358
Zydone Capsules ... 949

Hydrocodone Polistirex (Potentiation of central nervous system depressants). Products include:
Tussionex Pennkinetic Extended-Release Suspension ... 998

Hydroxyzine Hydrochloride (Potentiation of central nervous system depressants). Products include:
Atarax Tablets & Syrup ... 2185
Marax Tablets & DF Syrup ... 2200
Vistaril Intramuscular Solution ... 2216

Isoflurane (Potentiation of central nervous system depressants).
No products indexed under this heading.

Ketamine Hydrochloride (Potentiation of central nervous system depressants).
No products indexed under this heading.

Levomethadyl Acetate Hydrochloride (Potentiation of central nervous system depressants). Products include:
Orlamm ... 2239

Levorphanol Tartrate (Potentiation of central nervous system depressants). Products include:
Levo-Dromoran ... 2129

Lorazepam (Potentiation of central nervous system depressants). Products include:
Ativan Injection ... 2698
Ativan Tablets ... 2700

639 Interactions Index Mepergan

Loxapine Hydrochloride (Potentiation of central nervous system depressants). Products include:
Loxitane ... 1378
Loxapine Succinate (Potentiation of central nervous system depressants). Products include:
Loxitane Capsules ... 1378
Meperidine Hydrochloride (Potentiation of central nervous system depressants). Products include:
Demerol ... 2308
Mepergan Injection ... 2753
Mephobarbital (Potentiation of central nervous system depressants; severe respiratory depression and respiratory arrest have been reported when a patient was given a phenothiazine and a concomitant high dose of a barbiturate). Products include:
Mebaral Tablets ... 2322
Meprobamate (Potentiation of central nervous system depressants). Products include:
Miltown Tablets ... 2672
PMB 200 and PMB 400 ... 2783
Mesoridazine Besylate (Potentiation of central nervous system depressants). Products include:
Serentil ... 684
Methadone Hydrochloride (Potentiation of central nervous system depressants). Products include:
Methadone Hydrochloride Oral Concentrate ... 2233
Methadone Hydrochloride Oral Solution & Tablets ... 2235
Methohexital Sodium (Potentiation of central nervous system depressants). Products include:
Brevital Sodium Vials ... 1429
Methotrimeprazine (Potentiation of central nervous system depressants). Products include:
Levoprome ... 1274
Methoxyflurane (Potentiation of central nervous system depressants).
No products indexed under this heading.
Midazolam Hydrochloride (Potentiation of central nervous system depressants). Products include:
Versed Injection ... 2170
Molindone Hydrochloride (Potentiation of central nervous system depressants). Products include:
Moban Tablets and Concentrate ... 1048
Morphine Sulfate (Potentiation of central nervous system depressants). Products include:
Astramorph/PF Injection, USP (Preservative-Free) ... 535
Duramorph ... 962
Infumorph 200 and Infumorph 500 Sterile Solutions ... 965
MS Contin Tablets ... 1994
MSIR ... 1997
Oramorph SR (Morphine Sulfate Sustained Release Tablets) ... 2236
RMS Suppositories ... 2657
Roxanol ... 2243
Opium Alkaloids (Potentiation of central nervous system depressants).
No products indexed under this heading.
Oxazepam (Potentiation of central nervous system depressants). Products include:
Serax Capsules ... 2810
Serax Tablets ... 2810
Oxycodone Hydrochloride (Potentiation of central nervous system depressants). Products include:
Percocet Tablets ... 938
Percodan Tablets ... 939
Percodan-Demi Tablets ... 940
Roxicodone Tablets, Oral Solution & Intensol (Oxycodone) ... 2244
Tylox Capsules ... 1584
Pentobarbital Sodium (Potentiation of central nervous system depressants; severe respiratory depression and respiratory arrest have been reported when a patient was given a phenothiazine and a concomitant high dose of a barbiturate). Products include:
Nembutal Sodium Capsules ... 436
Nembutal Sodium Solution ... 438
Nembutal Sodium Suppositories ... 440
Perphenazine (Potentiation of central nervous system depressants). Products include:
Etrafon ... 2355
Triavil Tablets ... 1757
Trilafon ... 2389
Phenobarbital (Potentiation of central nervous system depressants; severe respiratory depression and respiratory arrest have been reported when a patient was given a phenothiazine and a concomitant high dose of a barbiturate). Products include:
Arco-Lase Plus Tablets ... 512
Bellergal-S Tablets ... 2250
Donnatal ... 2060
Donnatal Extentabs ... 2061
Donnatal Tablets ... 2060
Phenobarbital Elixir and Tablets ... 1469
Quadrinal Tablets ... 1350
Pindolol (Concurrent administration of both drugs have resulted in higher serum levels of both). Products include:
Visken Tablets ... 2299
Prazepam (Potentiation of central nervous system depressants).
No products indexed under this heading.
Prochlorperazine (Potentiation of central nervous system depressants). Products include:
Compazine ... 2470
Promethazine Hydrochloride (Potentiation of central nervous system depressants). Products include:
Mepergan Injection ... 2753
Phenergan with Codeine ... 2777
Phenergan with Dextromethorphan 2778
Phenergan Injection ... 2773
Phenergan Suppositories ... 2775
Phenergan Syrup ... 2774
Phenergan Tablets ... 2775
Phenergan VC ... 2779
Phenergan VC with Codeine ... 2781
Propofol (Potentiation of central nervous system depressants). Products include:
Diprivan Injection ... 2833
Propoxyphene Hydrochloride (Potentiation of central nervous system depressants). Products include:
Darvon ... 1435
Wygesic Tablets ... 2827
Propoxyphene Napsylate (Potentiation of central nervous system depressants). Products include:
Darvon-N/Darvocet-N ... 1433
Propranolol Hydrochloride (Concurrent administration produces increases in plasma levels of thioridazine). Products include:
Inderal ... 2728
Inderal LA Long Acting Capsules ... 2730
Inderide Tablets ... 2732
Inderide LA Long Acting Capsules .. 2734
Quazepam (Potentiation of central nervous system depressants). Products include:
Doral Tablets ... 2664
Risperidone (Potentiation of central nervous system depressants). Products include:
Risperdal ... 1301
Secobarbital Sodium (Potentiation of central nervous system depressants; severe respiratory depression and respiratory arrest have been reported when a patient was given a phenothiazine and a concomitant high dose of a barbiturate). Products include:
Seconal Sodium Pulvules ... 1474
Sufentanil Citrate (Potentiation of central nervous system depressants). Products include:
Sufenta Injection ... 1309
Temazepam (Potentiation of central nervous system depressants). Products include:
Restoril Capsules ... 2284
Thiamylal Sodium (Potentiation of central nervous system depressants; severe respiratory depression and respiratory arrest have been reported when a patient was given a phenothiazine and a concomitant high dose of a barbiturate).
No products indexed under this heading.
Thiothixene (Potentiation of central nervous system depressants). Products include:
Navane Capsules and Concentrate 2201
Navane Intramuscular ... 2202
Triazolam (Potentiation of central nervous system depressants). Products include:
Halcion Tablets ... 2611
Trifluoperazine Hydrochloride (Potentiation of central nervous system depressants). Products include:
Stelazine ... 2514
Zolpidem Tartrate (Potentiation of central nervous system depressants). Products include:
Ambien Tablets ... 2416

Food Interactions

Alcohol (Potentiation of central nervous system depressants).

MELLARIL TABLETS
(Thioridazine Hydrochloride) ... 2269
See **Mellaril Concentrate**

MELLARIL-S SUSPENSION
(Thioridazine) ... 2269
See **Mellaril Concentrate**

MENEST TABLETS
(Estrogens, Esterified) ... 2494
None cited in PDR database.

MENOMUNE-A/C/Y/W-135-
(Meningococcal Polysaccharide Vaccine) ... 889
May interact with immunosuppressive agents. Compounds in this category include:

Azathioprine (The expected immune response may not be obtained). Products include:
Imuran ... 1110
Cyclosporine (The expected immune response may not be obtained). Products include:
Neoral ... 2276
Sandimmune ... 2286
Immune Globulin (Human) (The expected immune response may not be obtained).
No products indexed under this heading.
Immune Globulin Intravenous (Human) (The expected immune response may not be obtained).
Muromonab-CD3 (The expected immune response may not be obtained). Products include:
Orthoclone OKT3 Sterile Solution .. 1837
Mycophenolate Mofetil (The expected immune response may not be obtained). Products include:
CellCept Capsules ... 2099
Tacrolimus (The expected immune response may not be obtained). Products include:
Prograf ... 1042

MEPERGAN INJECTION
(Meperidine Hydrochloride, Promethazine Hydrochloride) ... 2753
May interact with narcotic analgesics, general anesthetics, phenothiazines, tranquilizers, hypnotics and sedatives, tricyclic antidepressants, barbiturates, central nervous system depressants, monoamine oxidase inhibitors, and certain other agents. Compounds in these categories include:

Alfentanil Hydrochloride (Respiratory depression, hypotension, profound sedation or coma). Products include:
Alfenta Injection ... 1286
Alprazolam (Respiratory depression, hypotension, profound sedation or coma). Products include:
Xanax Tablets ... 2649
Amitriptyline Hydrochloride (Respiratory depression, hypotension, profound sedation or coma). Products include:
Elavil ... 2838
Endep Tablets ... 2174
Etrafon ... 2355
Limbitrol ... 2180
Triavil Tablets ... 1757
Amoxapine (Respiratory depression, hypotension, profound sedation or coma). Products include:
Asendin Tablets ... 1369
Aprobarbital (Respiratory depression, hypotension, profound sedation or coma).
No products indexed under this heading.
Buprenorphine (Respiratory depression, hypotension, profound sedation or coma). Products include:
Buprenex Injectable ... 2006
Buspirone Hydrochloride (Respiratory depression, hypotension, profound sedation or coma). Products include:
BuSpar ... 737
Butabarbital (Respiratory depression, hypotension, profound sedation or coma).
No products indexed under this heading.
Butalbital (Respiratory depression, hypotension, profound sedation or coma). Products include:
Esgic-plus Tablets ... 1013
Fioricet Tablets ... 2258
Fioricet with Codeine Capsules ... 2260
Fiorinal Capsules ... 2261
Fiorinal with Codeine Capsules ... 2262
Fiorinal Tablets ... 2261
Phrenilin ... 785
Sedapap Tablets 50 mg/650 mg .. 1543
Chlordiazepoxide (Respiratory depression, hypotension, profound sedation or coma). Products include:
Libritabs Tablets ... 2177
Limbitrol ... 2180
Chlordiazepoxide Hydrochloride (Respiratory depression, hypotension, profound sedation or coma). Products include:
Librax Capsules ... 2176
Librium Capsules ... 2178
Librium Injectable ... 2179
Chlorpromazine (Respiratory depression, hypotension, profound sedation or coma). Products include:
Thorazine Suppositories ... 2523

IMPORTANT NOTE: Always consult each drug listing in the patient's regimen for possible interactions.

Mepergan

Interactions Index

Chlorprothixene (Respiratory depression, hypotension, profound sedation or coma).

No products indexed under this heading.

Chlorprothixene Hydrochloride (Respiratory depression, hypotension, profound sedation or coma).

No products indexed under this heading.

Clomipramine Hydrochloride (Respiratory depression, hypotension, profound sedation or coma). Products include:

Anafranil Capsules 803

Clorazepate Dipotassium (Respiratory depression, hypotension, profound sedation or coma). Products include:

Tranxene 451

Clozapine (Respiratory depression, hypotension, profound sedation or coma). Products include:

Clozaril Tablets.. 2252

Codeine Phosphate (Respiratory depression, hypotension, profound sedation or coma). Products include:

Actifed with Codeine Cough Syrup.. 1067
Brontex 1981
Deconsal C Expectorant Syrup 456
Deconsal Pediatric Syrup 457
Dimetane-DC Cough Syrup 2059
Empirin with Codeine Tablets............ 1093
Fioricet with Codeine Capsules 2260
Fiorinal with Codeine Capsules 2262
Isoclor Expectorant 990
Novahistine DH...................................... 2462
Novahistine Expectorant...................... 2463
Nucofed 2051
Phenergan with Codeine 2777
Phenergan VC with Codeine 2781
Robitussin A-C Syrup 2073
Robitussin-DAC Syrup 2074
Ryna .... ⊞ 841
Soma Compound w/Codeine Tablets 2676
Tussi-Organidin NR Liquid and S NR Liquid 2677
Tylenol with Codeine 1583

Desflurane (Respiratory depression, hypotension, profound sedation or coma). Products include:

Suprane 1813

Desipramine Hydrochloride (Respiratory depression, hypotension, profound sedation or coma). Products include:

Norpramin Tablets 1526

Dezocine (Respiratory depression, hypotension, profound sedation or coma). Products include:

Dalgan Injection 538

Diazepam (Respiratory depression, hypotension, profound sedation or coma). Products include:

Dizac 1809
Valium Injectable 2182
Valium Tablets 2183
Valrelease Capsules 2169

Doxepin Hydrochloride (Respiratory depression, hypotension, profound sedation or coma). Products include:

Sinequan 2205
Zonalon Cream 1055

Droperidol (Respiratory depression, hypotension, profound sedation or coma). Products include:

Inapsine Injection................................... 1296

Enflurane (Respiratory depression, hypotension, profound sedation or coma).

No products indexed under this heading.

Estazolam (Respiratory depression, hypotension, profound sedation or coma). Products include:

ProSom Tablets 449

Ethchlorvynol (Respiratory depression, hypotension, profound sedation or coma). Products include:

Placidyl Capsules................................... 448

Ethinamate (Respiratory depression, hypotension, profound sedation or coma).

No products indexed under this heading.

Fentanyl (Respiratory depression, hypotension, profound sedation or coma). Products include:

Duragesic Transdermal System........ 1288

Fentanyl Citrate (Respiratory depression, hypotension, profound sedation or coma). Products include:

Sublimaze Injection............................... 1307

Fluphenazine Decanoate (Respiratory depression, hypotension, profound sedation or coma). Products include:

Prolixin Decanoate 509

Fluphenazine Enanthate (Respiratory depression, hypotension, profound sedation or coma). Products include:

Prolixin Enanthate 509

Fluphenazine Hydrochloride (Respiratory depression, hypotension, profound sedation or coma). Products include:

Prolixin 509

Flurazepam Hydrochloride (Respiratory depression, hypotension, profound sedation or coma). Products include:

Dalmane Capsules.................................. 2173

Furazolidone (Concurrent administration is contraindicated). Products include:

Furoxone 2046

Glutethimide (Respiratory depression, hypotension, profound sedation or coma).

No products indexed under this heading.

Haloperidol (Respiratory depression, hypotension, profound sedation or coma). Products include:

Haldol Injection, Tablets and Concentrate 1575

Haloperidol Decanoate (Respiratory depression, hypotension, profound sedation or coma). Products include:

Haldol Decanoate................................... 1577

Hydrocodone Bitartrate (Respiratory depression, hypotension, profound sedation or coma). Products include:

Anexsia 5/500 Elixir 1781
Anexia Tablets... 1782
Codiclear DH Syrup 791
Deconamine CX Cough and Cold Liquid and Tablets................................... 1319
Duratuss HD Elixir................................. 2565
Hycodan Tablets and Syrup 930
Hycomine Compound Tablets 932
Hycomine 931
Hycotuss Expectorant Syrup 933
Hydrocet Capsules 782
Lorcet 10/650... 1018
Lortab 2566
Tussend 1783
Tussend Expectorant 1785
Vicodin Tablets 1356
Vicodin ES Tablets 1357
Vicodin Tuss Expectorant 1358
Zydone Capsules.................................... 949

Hydrocodone Polistirex (Respiratory depression, hypotension, profound sedation or coma). Products include:

Tussionex Pennkinetic Extended-Release Suspension 998

Hydroxyzine Hydrochloride (Respiratory depression, hypotension, profound sedation or coma). Products include:

Atarax Tablets & Syrup......................... 2185

Marax Tablets & DF Syrup................... 2200
Vistaril Intramuscular Solution.......... 2216

Imipramine Hydrochloride (Respiratory depression, hypotension, profound sedation or coma). Products include:

Tofranil Ampuls 854
Tofranil Tablets 856

Imipramine Pamoate (Respiratory depression, hypotension, profound sedation or coma). Products include:

Tofranil-PM Capsules............................ 857

Isocarboxazid (Concurrent administration is contraindicated).

No products indexed under this heading.

Isoflurane (Respiratory depression, hypotension, profound sedation or coma).

No products indexed under this heading.

Ketamine Hydrochloride (Respiratory depression, hypotension, profound sedation or coma).

No products indexed under this heading.

Levomethadyl Acetate Hydrochloride (Respiratory depression, hypotension, profound sedation or coma). Products include:

Orlamm 2239

Levorphanol Tartrate (Respiratory depression, hypotension, profound sedation or coma). Products include:

Levo-Dromoran....................................... 2129

Lorazepam (Respiratory depression, hypotension, profound sedation or coma). Products include:

Ativan Injection....................................... 2698
Ativan Tablets.. 2700

Loxapine Hydrochloride (Respiratory depression, hypotension, profound sedation or coma). Products include:

Loxitane 1378

Loxapine Succinate (Respiratory depression, hypotension, profound sedation or coma). Products include:

Loxitane Capsules 1378

Maprotiline Hydrochloride (Respiratory depression, hypotension, profound sedation or coma). Products include:

Ludiomil Tablets..................................... 843

Mephobarbital (Respiratory depression, hypotension, profound sedation or coma). Products include:

Mebaral Tablets 2322

Meprobamate (Respiratory depression, hypotension, profound sedation or coma). Products include:

Miltown Tablets 2672
PMB 200 and PMB 400 2783

Mesoridazine Besylate (Respiratory depression, hypotension, profound sedation or coma). Products include:

Serentil 684

Methadone Hydrochloride (Respiratory depression, hypotension, profound sedation or coma). Products include:

Methadone Hydrochloride Oral Concentrate 2233
Methadone Hydrochloride Oral Solution & Tablets.................................... 2235

Methohexital Sodium (Respiratory depression, hypotension, profound sedation or coma). Products include:

Brevital Sodium Vials 1429

Methotrimeprazine (Respiratory depression, hypotension, profound sedation or coma). Products include:

Levoprome 1274

Methoxyflurane (Respiratory depression, hypotension, profound sedation or coma).

No products indexed under this heading.

Midazolam Hydrochloride (Respiratory depression, hypotension, profound sedation or coma). Products include:

Versed Injection 2170

Molindone Hydrochloride (Respiratory depression, hypotension, profound sedation or coma). Products include:

Moban Tablets and Concentrate 1048

Morphine Sulfate (Respiratory depression, hypotension, profound sedation or coma). Products include:

Astramorph/PF Injection, USP (Preservative-Free) 535
Duramorph.. 962
Infumorph 200 and Infumorph 500 Sterile Solutions 965
MS Contin Tablets.................................. 1994
MSIR 1997
Oramorph SR (Morphine Sulfate Sustained Release Tablets) 2236
RMS Suppositories 2657
Roxanol 2243

Nortriptyline Hydrochloride (Respiratory depression, hypotension, profound sedation or coma). Products include:

Pamelor 2280

Opium Alkaloids (Respiratory depression, hypotension, profound sedation or coma).

No products indexed under this heading.

Oxazepam (Respiratory depression, hypotension, profound sedation or coma). Products include:

Serax Capsules 2810
Serax Tablets.. 2810

Oxycodone Hydrochloride (Respiratory depression, hypotension, profound sedation or coma). Products include:

Percocet Tablets 938
Percodan Tablets.................................... 939
Percodan-Demi Tablets......................... 940
Roxicodone Tablets, Oral Solution & Intensol (Oxycodone) 2244
Tylox Capsules 1584

Pentobarbital Sodium (Respiratory depression, hypotension, profound sedation or coma). Products include:

Nembutal Sodium Capsules 436
Nembutal Sodium Solution 438
Nembutal Sodium Suppositories...... 440

Perphenazine (Respiratory depression, hypotension, profound sedation or coma). Products include:

Etrafon 2355
Triavil Tablets 1757
Trilafon... 2389

Phenelzine Sulfate (Concurrent administration is contraindicated). Products include:

Nardil 1920

Phenobarbital (Respiratory depression, hypotension, profound sedation or coma). Products include:

Arco-Lase Plus Tablets 512
Bellergal-S Tablets 2250
Donnatal 2060
Donnatal Extentabs............................... 2061
Donnatal Tablets 2060
Phenobarbital Elixir and Tablets 1469
Quadrinal Tablets 1350

Prazepam (Respiratory depression, hypotension, profound sedation or coma).

No products indexed under this heading.

Prochlorperazine (Respiratory depression, hypotension, profound sedation or coma). Products include:

Compazine 2470

(⊞ Described in PDR For Nonprescription Drugs) (◉ Described in PDR For Ophthalmology)

Propofol (Respiratory depression, hypotension, profound sedation or coma). Products include:
- Diprivan Injection 2833

Propoxyphene Hydrochloride (Respiratory depression, hypotension, profound sedation or coma). Products include:
- Darvon 1435
- Wygesic Tablets 2827

Propoxyphene Napsylate (Respiratory depression, hypotension, profound sedation or coma). Products include:
- Darvon-N/Darvocet-N 1433

Protriptyline Hydrochloride (Respiratory depression, hypotension, profound sedation or coma). Products include:
- Vivactil Tablets 1774

Quazepam (Respiratory depression, hypotension, profound sedation or coma). Products include:
- Doral Tablets 2664

Risperidone (Respiratory depression, hypotension, profound sedation or coma). Products include:
- Risperdal 1301

Secobarbital Sodium (Respiratory depression, hypotension, profound sedation or coma). Products include:
- Seconal Sodium Pulvules 1474

Selegiline Hydrochloride (Concurrent administration is contraindicated). Products include:
- Eldepryl Tablets 2550

Sufentanil Citrate (Respiratory depression, hypotension, profound sedation or coma). Products include:
- Sufenta Injection 1309

Temazepam (Respiratory depression, hypotension, profound sedation or coma). Products include:
- Restoril Capsules 2284

Thiamylal Sodium (Respiratory depression, hypotension, profound sedation or coma).
- No products indexed under this heading.

Thioridazine Hydrochloride (Respiratory depression, hypotension, profound sedation or coma). Products include:
- Mellaril 2269

Thiothixene (Respiratory depression, hypotension, profound sedation or coma). Products include:
- Navane Capsules and Concentrate 2201
- Navane Intramuscular 2202

Tranylcypromine Sulfate (Concurrent administration is contraindicated). Products include:
- Parnate Tablets 2503

Triazolam (Respiratory depression, hypotension, profound sedation or coma). Products include:
- Halcion Tablets 2611

Trifluoperazine Hydrochloride (Respiratory depression, hypotension, profound sedation or coma). Products include:
- Stelazine 2514

Trimipramine Maleate (Respiratory depression, hypotension, profound sedation or coma). Products include:
- Surmontil Capsules 2811

Zolpidem Tartrate (Respiratory depression, hypotension, profound sedation or coma). Products include:
- Ambien Tablets 2416

Food Interactions

Alcohol (Respiratory depression, hypotension, profound sedation or coma).

MEPHYTON TABLETS

(Phytonadione) 1696

None cited in PDR database.

MEPRON SUSPENSION

(Atovaquone) 1135

May interact with highly protein bound drugs (selected) and certain other agents. Compounds in these categories include:

Amiodarone Hydrochloride (Atovaquone is highly bound to plasma protein (greater than 99.9%); caution is advised when co-administered with other highly protein bound drugs with narrow therapeutic indices). Products include:
- Cordarone Intravenous 2715
- Cordarone Tablets 2712

Amitriptyline Hydrochloride (Atovaquone is highly bound to plasma protein (greater than 99.9%); caution is advised when co-administered with other highly protein bound drugs with narrow therapeutic indices). Products include:
- Elavil 2838
- Endep Tablets 2174
- Etrafon 2355
- Limbitrol 2180
- Triavil Tablets 1757

Cefonicid Sodium (Atovaquone is highly bound to plasma protein (greater than 99.9%); caution is advised when co-administered with other highly protein bound drugs with narrow therapeutic indices). Products include:
- Monocid Injection 2497

Chlordiazepoxide (Atovaquone is highly bound to plasma protein (greater than 99.9%); caution is advised when co-administered with other highly protein bound drugs with narrow therapeutic indices). Products include:
- Libritabs Tablets 2177
- Limbitrol 2180

Chlordiazepoxide Hydrochloride (Atovaquone is highly bound to plasma protein (greater than 99.9%); caution is advised when co-administered with other highly protein bound drugs with narrow therapeutic indices). Products include:
- Librax Capsules 2176
- Librium Capsules 2178
- Librium Injectable 2179

Chlorpromazine (Atovaquone is highly bound to plasma protein (greater than 99.9%); caution is advised when co-administered with other highly protein bound drugs with narrow therapeutic indices). Products include:
- Thorazine Suppositories 2523

Chlorpromazine Hydrochloride (Atovaquone is highly bound to plasma protein (greater than 99.9%); caution is advised when co-administered with other highly protein bound drugs with narrow therapeutic indices). Products include:
- Thorazine 2523

Clomipramine Hydrochloride (Atovaquone is highly bound to plasma protein (greater than 99.9%); caution is advised when co-administered with other highly protein bound drugs with narrow therapeutic indices). Products include:
- Anafranil Capsules 803

Clozapine (Atovaquone is highly bound to plasma protein (greater than 99.9%); caution is advised when co-administered with other highly protein bound drugs with narrow therapeutic indices). Products include:
- Clozaril Tablets 2252

Cyclosporine (Atovaquone is highly bound to plasma protein (greater than 99.9%); caution is advised when co-administered with other highly protein bound drugs with narrow therapeutic indices). Products include:
- Neoral 2276
- Sandimmune 2286

Diazepam (Atovaquone is highly bound to plasma protein (greater than 99.9%); caution is advised when co-administered with other highly protein bound drugs with narrow therapeutic indices). Products include:
- Dizac 1809
- Valium Injectable 2182
- Valium Tablets 2183
- Valrelease Capsules 2169

Diclofenac Potassium (Atovaquone is highly bound to plasma protein (greater than 99.9%); caution is advised when co-administered with other highly protein bound drugs with narrow therapeutic indices). Products include:
- Cataflam 816

Diclofenac Sodium (Atovaquone is highly bound to plasma protein (greater than 99.9%); caution is advised when co-administered with other highly protein bound drugs with narrow therapeutic indices). Products include:
- Voltaren Ophthalmic Sterile Ophthalmic Solution .... ◉ 272
- Voltaren Tablets 861

Dipyridamole (Atovaquone is highly bound to plasma protein (greater than 99.9%); caution is advised when co-administered with other highly protein bound drugs with narrow therapeutic indices). Products include:
- Persantine Tablets 681

Fenoprofen Calcium (Atovaquone is highly bound to plasma protein (greater than 99.9%); caution is advised when co-administered with other highly protein bound drugs with narrow therapeutic indices). Products include:
- Nalfon 200 Pulvules & Nalfon Tablets 917

Flurazepam Hydrochloride (Atovaquone is highly bound to plasma protein (greater than 99.9%); caution is advised when co-administered with other highly protein bound drugs with narrow therapeutic indices). Products include:
- Dalmane Capsules 2173

Flurbiprofen (Atovaquone is highly bound to plasma protein (greater than 99.9%); caution is advised when co-administered with other highly protein bound drugs with narrow therapeutic indices). Products include:
- Ansaid Tablets 2579

Glipizide (Atovaquone is highly bound to plasma protein (greater than 99.9%); caution is advised when co-administered with other highly protein bound drugs with narrow therapeutic indices). Products include:
- Glucotrol Tablets 1967
- Glucotrol XL Extended Release Tablets 1968

Ibuprofen (Atovaquone is highly bound to plasma protein (greater than 99.9%); caution is advised when co-administered with other highly protein bound drugs with narrow therapeutic indices). Products include:
- Advil Cold and Sinus Caplets and Tablets (formerly CoAdvil) .... ▣ 870
- Advil Ibuprofen Tablets and Caplets .... ▣ 870
- Children's Advil Suspension 2692
- Arthritis Foundation Ibuprofen Tablets .... ▣ 674
- Bayer Select Ibuprofen Pain Relief Formula .... ▣ 715
- Cramp End Tablets .... ▣ 735
- Dimetapp Sinus Caplets .... ▣ 775
- Haltran Tablets .... ▣ 771
- IBU Tablets 1342
- Ibuprohm .... ▣ 735
- Children's Motrin Ibuprofen Oral Suspension 1546
- Motrin Tablets 2625
- Motrin IB Caplets, Tablets, and Geltabs .... ▣ 838
- Motrin IB Sinus .... ▣ 838
- Motrin Ibuprofen Suspension, Oral Drops, Chewable Tablets, Caplets 1546
- Nuprin Ibuprofen/Analgesic Tablets & Caplets .... ▣ 622
- Sine-Aid IB Caplets 1554
- Vicks DayQuil SINUS Pressure & PAIN Relief with IBUPROFEN .... ▣ 762

Imipramine Hydrochloride (Atovaquone is highly bound to plasma protein (greater than 99.9%); caution is advised when co-administered with other highly protein bound drugs with narrow therapeutic indices). Products include:
- Tofranil Ampuls 854
- Tofranil Tablets 856

Imipramine Pamoate (Atovaquone is highly bound to plasma protein (greater than 99.9%); caution is advised when co-administered with other highly protein bound drugs with narrow therapeutic indices). Products include:
- Tofranil-PM Capsules 857

Indomethacin (Atovaquone is highly bound to plasma protein (greater than 99.9%); caution is advised when co-administered with other highly protein bound drugs with narrow therapeutic indices). Products include:
- Indocin 1680

Indomethacin Sodium Trihydrate (Atovaquone is highly bound to plasma protein (greater than 99.9%); caution is advised when co-administered with other highly protein bound drugs with narrow therapeutic indices). Products include:
- Indocin I.V. 1684

Ketoprofen (Atovaquone is highly bound to plasma protein (greater than 99.9%); caution is advised when co-administered with other highly protein bound drugs with narrow therapeutic indices). Products include:
- Orudis Capsules 2766
- Oruvail Capsules 2766

Ketorolac Tromethamine (Atovaquone is highly bound to plasma protein (greater than 99.9%); caution is advised when co-administered with other highly protein bound drugs with narrow therapeutic indices). Products include:
- Acular 474
- Acular .... ◉ 277
- Toradol 2159

IMPORTANT NOTE: Always consult each drug listing in the patient's regimen for possible interactions.

Mepron suspension | Interactions Index | 642

Meclofenamate Sodium (Atovaquone is highly bound to plasma protein (greater than 99.9%); caution is advised when co-administered with other highly protein bound drugs with narrow therapeutic indices).

No products indexed under this heading.

Mefenamic Acid (Atovaquone is highly bound to plasma protein (greater than 99.9%); caution is advised when co-administered with other highly protein bound drugs with narrow therapeutic indices). Products include:

Ponstel 1925

Midazolam Hydrochloride (Atovaquone is highly bound to plasma protein (greater than 99.9%); caution is advised when co-administered with other highly protein bound drugs with narrow therapeutic indices). Products include:

Versed Injection 2170

Naproxen (Atovaquone is highly bound to plasma protein (greater than 99.9%); caution is advised when co-administered with other highly protein bound drugs with narrow therapeutic indices). Products include:

Anaprox/Naprosyn 2117

Naproxen Sodium (Atovaquone is highly bound to plasma protein (greater than 99.9%); caution is advised when co-administered with other highly protein bound drugs with narrow therapeutic indices). Products include:

Aleve 1975
Anaprox/Naprosyn 2117

Nortriptyline Hydrochloride (Atovaquone is highly bound to plasma protein (greater than 99.9%); caution is advised when co-administered with other highly protein bound drugs with narrow therapeutic indices). Products include:

Pamelor 2280

Oxaprozin (Atovaquone is highly bound to plasma protein (greater than 99.9%); caution is advised when co-administered with other highly protein bound drugs with narrow therapeutic indices). Products include:

Daypro Caplets 2426

Oxazepam (Atovaquone is highly bound to plasma protein (greater than 99.9%); caution is advised when co-administered with other highly protein bound drugs with narrow therapeutic indices). Products include:

Serax Capsules 2810
Serax Tablets 2810

Phenylbutazone (Atovaquone is highly bound to plasma protein (greater than 99.9%); caution is advised when co-administered with other highly protein bound drugs with narrow therapeutic indices).

No products indexed under this heading.

Piroxicam (Atovaquone is highly bound to plasma protein (greater than 99.9%); caution is advised when co-administered with other highly protein bound drugs with narrow therapeutic indices). Products include:

Feldene Capsules 1965

Propranolol Hydrochloride (Atovaquone is highly bound to plasma protein (greater than 99.9%); caution is advised when co-administered with other highly protein bound drugs with narrow therapeutic indices). Products include:

Inderal 2728
Inderal LA Long Acting Capsules 2730
Inderide Tablets 2732
Inderide LA Long Acting Capsules 2734

Rifabutin (Due to structural similarity to rifampin, rifabutin may decrease average steady-state plasma atovaquone concentration). Products include:

Mycobutin Capsules 1957

Rifampin (Co-administration with oral rifampin in HIV-infected individuals may result in a 52% +/− 13% decrease in the average steady-state plasma atovaquone concentration and a 37% 42% increase in the average steady-state plasma rifampin concentration). Products include:

Rifadin 1528
Rifamate Capsules 1530
Rifater 1532
Rimactane Capsules 847

Sulfamethoxazole (Co-administration with TMP-SMX may result in slight decrease in average steady-state concentrations of TMP-SMX; this effect is minor and would not expect to produce clinically significant events). Products include:

Azo Gantanol Tablets 2080
Bactrim DS Tablets 2084
Bactrim I.V. Infusion 2082
Bactrim 2084
Gantanol Tablets 2119
Septra 1174
Septra I.V. Infusion 1169
Septra I.V. Infusion ADD-Vantage Vials 1171
Septra 1174

Sulindac (Atovaquone is highly bound to plasma protein (greater than 99.9%); caution is advised when co-administered with other highly protein bound drugs with narrow therapeutic indices). Products include:

Clinoril Tablets 1618

Temazepam (Atovaquone is highly bound to plasma protein (greater than 99.9%); caution is advised when co-administered with other highly protein bound drugs with narrow therapeutic indices). Products include:

Restoril Capsules 2284

Tolbutamide (Atovaquone is highly bound to plasma protein (greater than 99.9%); caution is advised when co-administered with other highly protein bound drugs with narrow therapeutic indices).

No products indexed under this heading.

Tolmetin Sodium (Atovaquone is highly bound to plasma protein (greater than 99.9%); caution is advised when co-administered with other highly protein bound drugs with narrow therapeutic indices). Products include:

Tolectin (200, 400 and 600 mg) 1581

Trimethoprim (Co-administration with TMP-SMX may result in slight decrease in average steady-state concentrations of TMP-SMX; this effect is minor and would not expect to produce clinically significant events). Products include:

Bactrim DS Tablets 2084
Bactrim I.V. Infusion 2082
Bactrim 2084
Proloprim Tablets 1155
Septra 1174
Septra I.V. Infusion 1169
Septra I.V. Infusion ADD-Vantage Vials 1171
Septra 1174
Trimpex Tablets 2163

Trimipramine Maleate (Atovaquone is highly bound to plasma protein (greater than 99.9%); caution is advised when co-administered with other highly protein bound drugs with narrow therapeutic indices). Products include:

Surmontil Capsules 2811

Warfarin Sodium (Atovaquone is highly bound to plasma protein (greater than 99.9%); caution is advised when co-administered with other highly protein bound drugs with narrow therapeutic indices). Products include:

Coumadin 926

Zidovudine (Atovaquone tablets have shown to decrease zidovudine apparent oral clearance leading to an increase in plasma zidovudine AUC; this effect is minor and would not expect to produce clinically significant events). Products include:

Retrovir Capsules 1158
Retrovir I.V. Infusion 1163
Retrovir Syrup 1158

Food Interactions

Food, unspecified (Food enhances absorption by approximately two-fold).

MERUVAX II

(Rubella Virus Vaccine Live) 1697

May interact with immunosuppressive agents. Compounds in this category include:

Azathioprine (Concurrent administration is contraindicated). Products include:

Imuran 1110

Cyclosporine (Concurrent administration is contraindicated). Products include:

Neoral 2276
Sandimmune 2286

Immune Globulin (Human) (Concurrent administration is contraindicated).

No products indexed under this heading.

Immune Globulin Intravenous (Human) (Concurrent administration is contraindicated).

Muromonab-CD3 (Concurrent administration is contraindicated). Products include:

Orthoclone OKT3 Sterile Solution 1837

Mycophenolate Mofetil (Concurrent administration is contraindicated). Products include:

CellCept Capsules 2099

Tacrolimus (Concurrent administration is contraindicated). Products include:

Prograf 1042

MESANTOIN TABLETS

(Mephenytoin) 2272

May interact with central nervous system depressants and certain other agents. Compounds in these categories include:

Alfentanil Hydrochloride (Additive effects). Products include:

Alfenta Injection 1286

Alprazolam (Additive effects). Products include:

Xanax Tablets 2649

Aprobarbital (Additive effects).

No products indexed under this heading.

Buprenorphine (Additive effects). Products include:

Buprenex Injectable 2006

Buspirone Hydrochloride (Additive effects). Products include:

BuSpar 737

Butabarbital (Additive effects).

No products indexed under this heading.

Butalbital (Additive effects). Products include:

Esgic-plus Tablets 1013
Fioricet Tablets 2258
Fioricet with Codeine Capsules 2260
Fiorinal Capsules 2261
Fiorinal with Codeine Capsules 2262
Fiorinal Tablets 2261
Phrenilin 785
Sedapap Tablets 50 mg/650 mg 1543

Chlordiazepoxide (Additive effects). Products include:

Libritabs Tablets 2177
Limbitrol 2180

Chlordiazepoxide Hydrochloride (Additive effects). Products include:

Librax Capsules 2176
Librium Capsules 2178
Librium Injectable 2179

Chlorpromazine (Additive effects). Products include:

Thorazine Suppositories 2523

Chlorprothixene (Additive effects).

No products indexed under this heading.

Chlorprothixene Hydrochloride (Additive effects).

No products indexed under this heading.

Chlorprothixene Lactate (Additive effects).

No products indexed under this heading.

Clorazepate Dipotassium (Additive effects). Products include:

Tranxene 451

Clozapine (Additive effects). Products include:

Clozaril Tablets 2252

Codeine Phosphate (Additive effects). Products include:

Actifed with Codeine Cough Syrup 1067
Brontex 1981
Deconsal C Expectorant Syrup 456
Deconsal Pediatric Syrup 457
Dimetane-DC Cough Syrup 2059
Empirin with Codeine Tablets 1093
Fioricet with Codeine Capsules 2260
Fiorinal with Codeine Capsules 2262
Isoclor Expectorant 990
Novahistine DH 2462
Novahistine Expectorant 2463
Nucofed 2051
Phenergan with Codeine 2777
Phenergan VC with Codeine 2781
Robitussin A-C Syrup 2073
Robitussin-DAC Syrup 2074
Ryna .... ▭ 841
Soma Compound w/Codeine Tablets 2676
Tussi-Organidin NR Liquid and S NR Liquid 2677
Tylenol with Codeine 1583

Desflurane (Additive effects). Products include:

Suprane 1813

Dezocine (Additive effects). Products include:

Dalgan Injection 538

Diazepam (Additive effects). Products include:

Dizac 1809
Valium Injectable 2182
Valium Tablets 2183
Valrelease Capsules 2169

Droperidol (Additive effects). Products include:

Inapsine Injection 1296

Enflurane (Additive effects).
No products indexed under this heading.

Estazolam (Additive effects). Products include:
ProSom Tablets 449

Ethchlorvynol (Additive effects). Products include:
Placidyl Capsules 448

Ethinamate (Additive effects).
No products indexed under this heading.

Fentanyl (Additive effects). Products include:
Duragesic Transdermal System 1288

Fentanyl Citrate (Additive effects). Products include:
Sublimaze Injection 1307

Fluphenazine Decanoate (Additive effects). Products include:
Prolixin Decanoate 509

Fluphenazine Enanthate (Additive effects). Products include:
Prolixin Enanthate 509

Fluphenazine Hydrochloride (Additive effects). Products include:
Prolixin 509

Flurazepam Hydrochloride (Additive effects). Products include:
Dalmane Capsules 2173

Glutethimide (Additive effects).
No products indexed under this heading.

Haloperidol (Additive effects). Products include:
Haldol Injection, Tablets and Concentrate 1575

Haloperidol Decanoate (Additive effects). Products include:
Haldol Decanoate 1577

Hydrocodone Bitartrate (Additive effects). Products include:
Anexsia 5/500 Elixir 1781
Anexia Tablets 1782
Codiclear DH Syrup 791
Deconamine CX Cough and Cold Liquid and Tablets 1319
Duratuss HD Elixir 2565
Hycodan Tablets and Syrup 930
Hycomine Compound Tablets 932
Hycomine 931
Hycotuss Expectorant Syrup 933
Hydrocet Capsules 782
Lorcet 10/650 1018
Lortab 2566
Tussend 1783
Tussend Expectorant 1785
Vicodin Tablets 1356
Vicodin ES Tablets 1357
Vicodin Tuss Expectorant 1358
Zydone Capsules 949

Hydrocodone Polistirex (Additive effects). Products include:
Tussionex Pennkinetic Extended-Release Suspension 998

Hydroxyzine Hydrochloride (Additive effects). Products include:
Atarax Tablets & Syrup 2185
Marax Tablets & DF Syrup 2200
Vistaril Intramuscular Solution 2216

Isoflurane (Additive effects).
No products indexed under this heading.

Ketamine Hydrochloride (Additive effects).
No products indexed under this heading.

Levomethadyl Acetate Hydrochloride (Additive effects). Products include:
Orlamm 2239

Levorphanol Tartrate (Additive effects). Products include:
Levo-Dromoran 2129

Lorazepam (Additive effects). Products include:
Ativan Injection 2698
Ativan Tablets 2700

Loxapine Hydrochloride (Additive effects). Products include:
Loxitane 1378

Loxapine Succinate (Additive effects). Products include:
Loxitane Capsules 1378

Meperidine Hydrochloride (Additive effects). Products include:
Demerol 2308
Mepergan Injection 2753

Mephobarbital (Additive effects). Products include:
Mebaral Tablets 2322

Meprobamate (Additive effects). Products include:
Miltown Tablets 2672
PMB 200 and PMB 400 2783

Mesoridazine Besylate (Additive effects). Products include:
Serentil 684

Methadone Hydrochloride (Additive effects). Products include:
Methadone Hydrochloride Oral Concentrate 2233
Methadone Hydrochloride Oral Solution & Tablets 2235

Methohexital Sodium (Additive effects). Products include:
Brevital Sodium Vials 1429

Methotrimeprazine (Additive effects). Products include:
Levoprome 1274

Methoxyflurane (Additive effects).
No products indexed under this heading.

Midazolam Hydrochloride (Additive effects). Products include:
Versed Injection 2170

Molindone Hydrochloride (Additive effects). Products include:
Moban Tablets and Concentrate 1048

Morphine Sulfate (Additive effects). Products include:
Astramorph/PF Injection, USP (Preservative-Free) 535
Duramorph 962
Infumorph 200 and Infumorph 500 Sterile Solutions 965
MS Contin Tablets 1994
MSIR 1997
Oramorph SR (Morphine Sulfate Sustained Release Tablets) 2236
RMS Suppositories 2657
Roxanol 2243

Opium Alkaloids (Additive effects).
No products indexed under this heading.

Oxazepam (Additive effects). Products include:
Serax Capsules 2810
Serax Tablets 2810

Oxycodone Hydrochloride (Additive effects). Products include:
Percocet Tablets 938
Percodan Tablets 939
Percodan-Demi Tablets 940
Roxicodone Tablets, Oral Solution & Intensol (Oxycodone) 2244
Tylox Capsules 1584

Pentobarbital Sodium (Additive effects). Products include:
Nembutal Sodium Capsules 436
Nembutal Sodium Solution 438
Nembutal Sodium Suppositories 440

Perphenazine (Additive effects). Products include:
Etrafon 2355
Triavil Tablets 1757
Trilafon 2389

Phenobarbital (Additive effects). Products include:
Arco-Lase Plus Tablets 512
Bellergal-S Tablets 2250
Donnatal 2060
Donnatal Extentabs 2061
Donnatal Tablets 2060
Phenobarbital Elixir and Tablets 1469
Quadrinal Tablets 1350

Prazepam (Additive effects).
No products indexed under this heading.

Prochlorperazine (Additive effects). Products include:
Compazine 2470

Promethazine Hydrochloride (Additive effects). Products include:
Mepergan Injection 2753
Phenergan with Codeine 2777
Phenergan with Dextromethorphan 2778
Phenergan Injection 2773
Phenergan Suppositories 2775
Phenergan Syrup 2774
Phenergan Tablets 2775
Phenergan VC 2779
Phenergan VC with Codeine 2781

Propofol (Additive effects). Products include:
Diprivan Injection 2833

Propoxyphene Hydrochloride (Additive effects). Products include:
Darvon 1435
Wygesic Tablets 2827

Propoxyphene Napsylate (Additive effects). Products include:
Darvon-N/Darvocet-N 1433

Quazepam (Additive effects). Products include:
Doral Tablets 2664

Risperidone (Additive effects). Products include:
Risperdal 1301

Secobarbital Sodium (Additive effects). Products include:
Seconal Sodium Pulvules 1474

Sufentanil Citrate (Additive effects). Products include:
Sufenta Injection 1309

Temazepam (Additive effects). Products include:
Restoril Capsules 2284

Thiamylal Sodium (Additive effects).
No products indexed under this heading.

Thioridazine Hydrochloride (Additive effects). Products include:
Mellaril 2269

Thiothixene (Additive effects). Products include:
Navane Capsules and Concentrate 2201
Navane Intramuscular 2202

Triazolam (Additive effects). Products include:
Halcion Tablets 2611

Trifluoperazine Hydrochloride (Additive effects). Products include:
Stelazine 2514

Zolpidem Tartrate (Additive effects). Products include:
Ambien Tablets 2416

Food Interactions

Alcohol (Acute alcohol intoxication may increase the anticonvulsant effect; chronic alcohol abuse may decrease anticonvulsant effect).

MESNEX INJECTION
(Mesna) 702
None cited in PDR database.

MESTINON INJECTABLE
(Pyridostigmine Bromide) 1253
None cited in PDR database.

MESTINON SYRUP
(Pyridostigmine Bromide) 1254
None cited in PDR database.

MESTINON TABLETS
(Pyridostigmine Bromide) 1254
None cited in PDR database.

MESTINON TIMESPAN TABLETS
(Pyridostigmine Bromide) 1254
None cited in PDR database.

METAMUCIL EFFERVESCENT SUGAR-FREE, LEMON-LIME FLAVOR
(Psyllium Preparations) 1975
None cited in PDR database.

METAMUCIL EFFERVESCENT SUGAR-FREE, ORANGE FLAVOR
(Psyllium Preparations) 1975
None cited in PDR database.

METAMUCIL POWDER, ORANGE FLAVOR
(Psyllium Preparations) 1975
None cited in PDR database.

METAMUCIL ORIGINAL TEXTURE POWDER, REGULAR FLAVOR
(Psyllium Preparations) 1975
None cited in PDR database.

METAMUCIL SMOOTH TEXTURE, CITRUS FLAVOR
(Psyllium Preparations) 1975
None cited in PDR database.

METAMUCIL SMOOTH TEXTURE, SUGAR-FREE, CITRUS FLAVOR
(Psyllium Preparations) 1975
None cited in PDR database.

METAMUCIL SMOOTH TEXTURE POWDER, ORANGE FLAVOR
(Psyllium Preparations) 1975
None cited in PDR database.

METAMUCIL SMOOTH TEXTURE POWDER, SUGAR-FREE, ORANGE FLAVOR
(Psyllium Preparations) 1975
None cited in PDR database.

METAMUCIL SMOOTH TEXTURE, SUGAR-FREE, REGULAR FLAVOR
(Psyllium Preparations) 1975
None cited in PDR database.

METAMUCIL WAFERS, APPLE CRISP AND CINNAMON SPICE FLAVORS
(Psyllium Preparations) 1975
None cited in PDR database.

METAPROTERENOL SULFATE INHALATION SOLUTION, USP, ARM-A-MED
(Metaproterenol Sulfate) 552
May interact with sympathomimetics. Compounds in this category include:

Albuterol (Effect not specified). Products include:
Proventil Inhalation Aerosol 2382
Ventolin Inhalation Aerosol and Refill 1197

Albuterol Sulfate (Effect not specified). Products include:
Airet Solution for Inhalation 452
Proventil Inhalation Solution 0.083% 2384
Proventil Repetabs Tablets 2386
Proventil Solution for Inhalation 0.5% 2383
Proventil Syrup 2385
Proventil Tablets 2386

IMPORTANT NOTE: Always consult each drug listing in the patient's regimen for possible interactions.

Metaproterenol Arm-a-Med Interactions Index 644

Ventolin Inhalation Solution 1198
Ventolin Nebules Inhalation Solution 1199
Ventolin Rotacaps for Inhalation 1200
Ventolin Syrup 1202
Ventolin Tablets 1203
Volmax Extended-Release Tablets 1788

Dobutamine Hydrochloride (Effect not specified). Products include:
Dobutrex Solution Vials 1439

Dopamine Hydrochloride (Effect not specified).
No products indexed under this heading.

Ephedrine Hydrochloride (Effect not specified). Products include:
Primatene Dual Action Formula ⊡ 872
Primatene Tablets ⊡ 873
Quadrinal Tablets 1350

Ephedrine Sulfate (Effect not specified). Products include:
Bronkaid Caplets ⊡ 717
Marax Tablets & DF Syrup 2200

Ephedrine Tannate (Effect not specified). Products include:
Rynatuss 2673

Epinephrine (Effect not specified). Products include:
Bronkaid Mist ⊡ 717
EPIFRIN ⊙ 239
EpiPen 790
Marcaine Hydrochloride with Epinephrine 1:200,000 2316
Primatene Mist ⊡ 873
Sensorcaine with Epinephrine Injection 559
Sus-Phrine Injection 1019
Xylocaine with Epinephrine Injections 567

Epinephrine Bitartrate (Effect not specified). Products include:
Bronkaid Mist Suspension ⊡ 718
Sensorcaine-MPF with Epinephrine Injection 559

Epinephrine Hydrochloride (Effect not specified). Products include:
Ana-Kit Anaphylaxis Emergency Treatment Kit 617

Isoproterenol Hydrochloride (Effect not specified). Products include:
Isuprel Hydrochloride Injection 1:5000 2311
Isuprel Hydrochloride Solution 1:200 & 1:100 2313
Isuprel Mistometer 2312

Isoproterenol Sulfate (Effect not specified). Products include:
Norisodrine with Calcium Iodide Syrup 442

Metaraminol Bitartrate (Effect not specified). Products include:
Aramine Injection 1609

Methoxamine Hydrochloride (Effect not specified). Products include:
Vasoxyl Injection 1196

Norepinephrine Bitartrate (Effect not specified). Products include:
Levophed Bitartrate Injection 2315

Phenylephrine Bitartrate (Effect not specified).
No products indexed under this heading.

Phenylephrine Hydrochloride (Effect not specified). Products include:
Atrohist Plus Tablets 454
Cerose DM ⊡ 878
Comhist 2038
D.A. Chewable Tablets 951
Deconsal Pediatric Capsules 454
Dura-Vent/DA Tablets 953
Entex Capsules 1986
Entex Liquid 1986
Extendryl 1005
4-Way Fast Acting Nasal Spray (regular & mentholated) ⊡ 621
Hemorid For Women ⊡ 834
Hycomine Compound Tablets 932
Neo-Synephrine Hydrochloride 1% Carpuject 2324
Neo-Synephrine Hydrochloride 1% Injection 2324
Neo-Synephrine Hydrochloride (Ophthalmic) 2325
Neo-Synephrine ⊡ 726
Nōstril ⊡ 644
Novahistine Elixir ⊡ 823
Phenergan VC 2779
Phenergan VC with Codeine 2781
Preparation H ⊡ 871
Tympagesic Ear Drops 2342
Vasosulf ⊙ 271
Vicks Sinex Nasal Spray and Ultra Fine Mist ⊡ 765

Phenylephrine Tannate (Effect not specified). Products include:
Atrohist Pediatric Suspension 454
Ricobid-D Pediatric Suspension 2038
Ricobid Tablets and Pediatric Suspension 2038
Rynatan 2673
Rynatuss 2673

Phenylpropanolamine Hydrochloride (Effect not specified). Products include:
Acutrim ⊡ 628
Allerest Children's Chewable Tablets ⊡ 627
Allerest 12 Hour Caplets ⊡ 627
Atrohist Plus Tablets 454
BC Cold Powder Multi-Symptom Formula (Cold-Sinus-Allergy) ⊡ 609
BC Cold Powder Non-Drowsy Formula (Cold-Sinus) ⊡ 609
Cheracol Plus Head Cold/Cough Formula ⊡ 769
Comtrex Multi-Symptom Non-Drowsy Liqui-gels ⊡ 618
Contac Continuous Action Nasal Decongestant/Antihistamine 12 Hour Capsules ⊡ 813
Contac Maximum Strength Continuous Action Decongestant/Antihistamine 12 Hour Caplets ⊡ 813
Contac Severe Cold and Flu Formula Caplets ⊡ 814
Coricidin 'D' Decongestant Tablets ⊡ 800
Dexatrim ⊡ 832
Dexatrim Plus Vitamins Caplets ⊡ 832
Dimetane-DC Cough Syrup 2059
Dimetapp Elixir ⊡ 773
Dimetapp Extentabs ⊡ 774
Dimetapp Tablets/Liqui-Gels ⊡ 775
Dimetapp Cold & Allergy Chewable Tablets ⊡ 773
Dimetapp DM Elixir ⊡ 774
Dura-Vent Tablets 952
Entex Capsules 1986
Entex LA Tablets 1987
Entex Liquid 1986
Exgest LA Tablets 782
Hycomine 931
Isoclor Timesule Capsules ⊡ 637
Nolamine Timed-Release Tablets 785
Ornade Spansule Capsules 2502
Propagest Tablets 786
Pyrroxate Caplets ⊡ 772
Robitussin-CF ⊡ 777
Sinulin Tablets 787
Tavist-D 12 Hour Relief Tablets ⊡ 787
Teldrin 12 Hour Antihistamine/Nasal Decongestant Allergy Relief Capsules ⊡ 826
Triaminic Allergy Tablets ⊡ 789
Triaminic Cold Tablets ⊡ 790
Triaminic Expectorant ⊡ 790
Triaminic Syrup ⊡ 792
Triaminic-12 Tablets ⊡ 792
Triaminic-DM Syrup ⊡ 792
Triaminicin Tablets ⊡ 793
Triaminicol Multi-Symptom Cold Tablets ⊡ 793
Triaminicol Multi-Symptom Relief ⊡ 794
Vicks DayQuil Allergy Relief 12-Hour Extended Release Tablets ⊡ 760
Vicks DayQuil Allergy Relief 4-Hour Tablets ⊡ 760
Vicks DayQuil SINUS Pressure & CONGESTION Relief ⊡ 761

Pirbuterol Acetate (Effect not specified). Products include:
Maxair Autohaler 1492
Maxair Inhaler 1494

Pseudoephedrine Hydrochloride (Effect not specified). Products include:
Actifed Allergy Daytime/Nighttime Caplets ⊡ 844
Actifed Plus Caplets ⊡ 845
Actifed Plus Tablets ⊡ 845
Actifed with Codeine Cough Syrup 1067
Actifed Sinus Daytime/Nighttime Tablets and Caplets ⊡ 846
Actifed Syrup ⊡ 846
Actifed Tablets ⊡ 844
Advil Cold and Sinus Caplets and Tablets (formerly CoAdvil) ⊡ 870
Alka-Seltzer Plus Cold Medicine Liqui-Gels ⊡ 706
Alka-Seltzer Plus Cold & Cough Medicine Liqui-Gels ⊡ 705
Alka-Seltzer Plus Night-Time Cold Medicine Liqui-Gels ⊡ 706
Allerest Headache Strength Tablets ⊡ 627
Allerest Maximum Strength Tablets ⊡ 627
Allerest No Drowsiness Tablets ⊡ 627
Allerest Sinus Pain Formula ⊡ 627
Anatuss LA Tablets 1542
Atrohist Pediatric Capsules 453
Bayer Select Sinus Pain Relief Formula ⊡ 717
Benadryl Allergy Decongestant Liquid Medication ⊡ 848
Benadryl Allergy Decongestant Tablets ⊡ 848
Benadryl Allergy Sinus Headache Formula Caplets ⊡ 849
Benylin Multisymptom ⊡ 852
Bromfed Capsules (Extended-Release) 1785
Bromfed Syrup ⊡ 733
Bromfed Tablets 1785
Bromfed-DM Cough Syrup 1786
Bromfed-PD Capsules (Extended-Release) 1785
Children's Vicks DayQuil Allergy Relief ⊡ 757
Children's Vicks NyQuil Cold/Cough Relief ⊡ 758
Comtrex Multi-Symptom Cold Reliever Tablets/Caplets/Liqui-Gels/Liquid ⊡ 615
Allergy-Sinus Comtrex Multi-Symptom Allergy-Sinus Formula Tablets ⊡ 617
Comtrex Multi-Symptom Non-Drowsy Caplets ⊡ 618
Congess 1004
Contac Day Allergy/Sinus Caplets ⊡ 812
Contac Day & Night ⊡ 812
Contac Night Allergy/Sinus Caplets ⊡ 812
Contac Severe Cold & Flu Non-Drowsy ⊡ 815
Deconamine Chewable Tablets 1320
Deconamine CX Cough and Cold Liquid and Tablets 1319
Deconamine 1320
Deconsal C Expectorant Syrup 456
Deconsal Pediatric Syrup 457
Deconsal II Tablets 454
Dimetane-DX Cough Syrup 2059
Dimetapp Sinus Caplets ⊡ 775
Dorcol Children's Cough Syrup ⊡ 785
Drixoral Cough + Congestion Liquid Caps ⊡ 802
Dura-Tap/PD Capsules 2867
Duratuss Tablets 2565
Duratuss HD Elixir 2565
Efidac/24 ⊡ 635
Entex PSE Tablets 1987
Fedahist Gyrocaps 2401
Fedahist Timecaps 2401
Guaifed 1787
Guaifed Syrup ⊡ 734
Guaimax-D Tablets 792
Guaitab Tablets ⊡ 734
Isoclor Expectorant 990
Kronofed-A 977
Motrin IB Sinus ⊡ 838
Novahistine DH 2462
Novahistine DMX ⊡ 822
Novahistine Expectorant 2463
Nucofed 2051
PediaCare Cold Allergy Chewable Tablets ⊡ 677
PediaCare Cough-Cold Chewable Tablets 1553
PediaCare 1553
PediaCare Infants' Decongestant Drops ⊡ 677
PediCare Infant's Drops Decongestant Plus Cough 1553
PediaCare NightRest Cough-Cold Liquid 1553
Pediatric Vicks 44d Dry Hacking Cough & Head Congestion ⊡ 763
Pediatric Vicks 44m Cough & Cold Relief ⊡ 764
Robitussin Cold & Cough Liqui-Gels ⊡ 776
Robitussin Maximum Strength Cough & Cold ⊡ 778
Robitussin Pediatric Cough & Cold Formula ⊡ 779
Robitussin Severe Congestion Liqui-Gels ⊡ 776
Robitussin-DAC Syrup 2074
Robitussin-PE ⊡ 778
Rondec Oral Drops 953
Rondec Syrup 953
Rondec Tablet 953
Rondec-DM Oral Drops 954
Rondec-DM Syrup 954
Rondec-TR Tablet 953
Ryna ⊡ 841
Seldane-D Extended-Release Tablets 1538
Semprex-D Capsules 463
Semprex-D Capsules 1167
Sinarest Tablets ⊡ 648
Sinarest Extra Strength Tablets ⊡ 648
Sinarest No Drowsiness Tablets ⊡ 648
Sine-Aid IB Caplets 1554
Sine-Aid Maximum Strength Sinus Medication Gelcaps, Caplets and Tablets 1554
Sine-Off No Drowsiness Formula Caplets ⊡ 824
Sine-Off Sinus Medicine ⊡ 825
Singlet Tablets ⊡ 825
Sinutab Non-Drying Liquid Caps ⊡ 859
Sinutab Sinus Allergy Medication, Maximum Strength Tablets and Caplets ⊡ 860
Sinutab Sinus Medication, Maximum Strength Without Drowsiness Formula, Tablets & Caplets ⊡ 860
Sinutab Sinus Medication, Regular Strength Without Drowsiness Formula ⊡ 859
Sudafed Children's Liquid ⊡ 861
Sudafed Cold and Cough Liquidcaps ⊡ 862
Sudafed Cough Syrup ⊡ 862
Sudafed Plus Liquid ⊡ 862
Sudafed Plus Tablets ⊡ 863
Sudafed Severe Cold Formula Caplets ⊡ 863
Sudafed Severe Cold Formula Tablets ⊡ 864
Sudafed Sinus Caplets ⊡ 864
Sudafed Sinus Tablets ⊡ 864
Sudafed Tablets, 30 mg ⊡ 861
Sudafed Tablets, 60 mg ⊡ 861
Sudafed 12 Hour Caplets ⊡ 861
Syn-Rx Tablets 465
Syn-Rx DM Tablets 466
TheraFlu ⊡ 787
TheraFlu Maximum Strength Nighttime Flu, Cold & Cough Medicine ⊡ 788
TheraFlu Maximum Strength Non-Drowsy Formula Flu, Cold & Cough Medicine ⊡ 788
Thera Flu Maximum Strength, Non-Drowsy Formula Flu, Cold and Cough Caplets ⊡ 789
Triaminic AM Cough and Decongestant Formula ⊡ 789
Triaminic AM Decongestant Formula ⊡ 790
Triaminic Nite Light ⊡ 791
Triaminic Sore Throat Formula ⊡ 791
Tussend 1783
Tussend Expectorant 1785
Children's TYLENOL Cold Multi-Symptom Liquid Formula and Chewable Tablets 1561
Children's TYLENOL Cold Plus Cough Multi Symptom Tablets and Liquid ⊡ 681
Infants' TYLENOL Cold Decongestant & Fever-Reducer Drops 1556
TYLENOL Maximum Strength Allergy Sinus Medication Gelcaps and Caplets 1563
TYLENOL Maximum Strength Allergy Sinus NightTime Medication Caplets 1555

(⊡ Described in PDR For Nonprescription Drugs) (⊙ Described in PDR For Ophthalmology)

Interactions Index

Methadone Concentrate

TYLENOL Flu Maximum Strength Gelcaps 1565
TYLENOL Flu NightTime, Maximum Strength, Gelcaps 1566
TYLENOL Maximum Strength Flu NightTime Hot Medication Packets 1562
TYLENOL, Maximum Strength, Sinus Medication Geltabs, Gelcaps, Caplets and Tablets 1566
TYLENOL Cold Multi-Symptom Formula Medication Tablets and Caplets 1561
TYLENOL Cold Medication No Drowsiness Formula Gelcaps and Caplets 1562
TYLENOL Cold Multi-Symptom Hot Medication Liquid Packets.............. 1557
TYLENOL Cough Multi-Symptom Medication with Decongestant 1565
Ursinus Inlay-Tabs................................ ◻ 794
Vicks 44 LiquiCaps Cough, Cold & Flu Relief.. ◻ 755
Vicks 44 LiquiCaps Non-Drowsy Cough & Cold Relief .... ◻ 756
Vicks 44D Dry Hacking Cough & Head Congestion .... ◻ 755
Vicks 44M Cough, Cold & Flu Relief.. ◻ 756
Vicks DayQuil .... ◻ 761
Vicks DayQuil SINUS Pressure & PAIN Relief with IBUPROFEN ...... ◻ 762
Vicks Nyquil Hot Therapy.................... ◻ 762
Vicks NyQuil LiquiCaps Multi-Symptom Cold/Flu Relief.................. ◻ 763
Vicks NyQuil Multi-Symptom Cold/Flu Relief - (Original & Cherry Flavor) .... ◻ 763

Pseudoephedrine Sulfate (Effect not specified). Products include:

Cheracol Sinus .... ◻ 768
Chlor-Trimeton Allergy Decongestant Tablets .... ◻ 799
Claritin-D 2350
Drixoral Cold and Allergy Sustained-Action Tablets .... ◻ 802
Drixoral Cold and Flu Extended-Release Tablets...................................... ◻ 803
Drixoral Non-Drowsy Formula Extended-Release Tablets .... ◻ 803
Drixoral Allergy/Sinus Extended Release Tablets...................................... ◻ 804
Trinalin Repetabs Tablets 1330

Salmeterol Xinafoate (Effect not specified). Products include:

Serevent Inhalation Aerosol................ 1176

Terbutaline Sulfate (Effect not specified). Products include:

Brethaire Inhaler 813
Brethine Ampuls 815
Brethine Tablets.................................... 814
Bricanyl Subcutaneous Injection 1502
Bricanyl Tablets 1503

METASTRON

(Strontium Chloride) 1594
None cited in PDR database.

METHADONE HYDROCHLORIDE ORAL CONCENTRATE

(Methadone Hydrochloride) 2233
May interact with central nervous system depressants, narcotic analgesics, general anesthetics, phenothiazines, tranquilizers, hypnotics and sedatives, tricyclic antidepressants, monoamine oxidase inhibitors, and certain other agents. Compounds in these categories include:

Alfentanil Hydrochloride (Potential for respiratory depression, hypotension, and profound sedation or coma; use caution and reduced dosage in patients who are concurrently receiving these drugs). Products include:

Alfenta Injection 1286

Alprazolam (Potential for respiratory depression, hypotension, and profound sedation or coma; use caution and reduced dosage in patients who are concurrently receiving these drugs). Products include:

Xanax Tablets 2649

Amitriptyline Hydrochloride (Potential for respiratory depression, hypotension, and profound sedation or coma; use caution and reduced dosage in patients who are concurrently receiving these drugs). Products include:

Elavil 2838
Endep Tablets 2174
Etrafon 2355
Limbitrol 2180
Triavil Tablets 1757

Amoxapine (Potential for respiratory depression, hypotension, and profound sedation or coma; use caution and reduced dosage in patients who are concurrently receiving these drugs). Products include:

Asendin Tablets 1369

Aprobarbital (Potential for respiratory depression, hypotension, and profound sedation or coma; use caution and reduced dosage in patients who are concurrently receiving these drugs).

No products indexed under this heading.

Buprenorphine (Potential for respiratory depression, hypotension, and profound sedation or coma; use caution and reduced dosage in patients who are concurrently receiving these drugs). Products include:

Buprenex Injectable 2006

Buspirone Hydrochloride (Potential for respiratory depression, hypotension, and profound sedation or coma; use caution and reduced dosage in patients who are concurrently receiving these drugs). Products include:

BuSpar 737

Butabarbital (Potential for respiratory depression, hypotension, and profound sedation or coma; use caution and reduced dosage in patients who are concurrently receiving these drugs).

No products indexed under this heading.

Butalbital (Potential for respiratory depression, hypotension, and profound sedation or coma; use caution and reduced dosage in patients who are concurrently receiving these drugs). Products include:

Esgic-plus Tablets 1013
Fioricet Tablets.. 2258
Fioricet with Codeine Capsules 2260
Fiorinal Capsules 2261
Fiorinal with Codeine Capsules 2262
Fiorinal Tablets 2261
Phrenilin 785
Sedapap Tablets 50 mg/650 mg .. 1543

Chlordiazepoxide (Potential for respiratory depression, hypotension, and profound sedation or coma; use caution and reduced dosage in patients who are concurrently receiving these drugs). Products include:

Libritabs Tablets 2177
Limbitrol 2180

Chlordiazepoxide Hydrochloride (Potential for respiratory depression, hypotension, and profound sedation or coma; use caution and reduced dosage in patients who are concurrently receiving these drugs). Products include:

Librax Capsules 2176
Librium Capsules.................................... 2178
Librium Injectable 2179

Chlorpromazine (Potential for respiratory depression, hypotension, and profound sedation or coma; use caution and reduced dosage in patients who are concurrently receiving these drugs). Products include:

Thorazine Suppositories........................ 2523

Chlorpromazine Hydrochloride (Potential for respiratory depression, hypotension, and profound sedation or coma; use caution and reduced dosage in patients who are concurrently receiving these drugs). Products include:

Thorazine 2523

Chlorprothixene (Potential for respiratory depression, hypotension, and profound sedation or coma; use caution and reduced dosage in patients who are concurrently receiving these drugs).

No products indexed under this heading.

Chlorprothixene Hydrochloride (Potential for respiratory depression, hypotension, and profound sedation or coma; use caution and reduced dosage in patients who are concurrently receiving these drugs).

No products indexed under this heading.

Clomipramine Hydrochloride (Potential for respiratory depression, hypotension, and profound sedation or coma; use caution and reduced dosage in patients who are concurrently receiving these drugs). Products include:

Anafranil Capsules 803

Clorazepate Dipotassium (Potential for respiratory depression, hypotension, and profound sedation or coma; use caution and reduced dosage in patients who are concurrently receiving these drugs). Products include:

Tranxene 451

Clozapine (Potential for respiratory depression, hypotension, and profound sedation or coma; use caution and reduced dosage in patients who are concurrently receiving these drugs). Products include:

Clozaril Tablets.. 2252

Codeine Phosphate (Potential for respiratory depression, hypotension, and profound sedation or coma; use caution and reduced dosage in patients who are concurrently receiving these drugs). Products include:

Actifed with Codeine Cough Syrup.. 1067
Brontex 1981
Deconsal C Expectorant Syrup 456
Deconsal Pediatric Syrup.................... 457
Dimetane-DC Cough Syrup 2059
Empirin with Codeine Tablets............ 1093
Fioricet with Codeine Capsules 2260
Fiorinal with Codeine Capsules 2262
Isoclor Expectorant................................ 990
Novahistine DH...................................... 2462
Novahistine Expectorant...................... 2463
Nucofed 2051
Phenergan with Codeine 2777
Phenergan VC with Codeine 2781
Robitussin A-C Syrup............................ 2073
Robitussin-DAC Syrup 2074
Ryna .... ◻ 841
Soma Compound w/Codeine Tablets 2676
Tussi-Organidin NR Liquid and S NR Liquid 2677
Tylenol with Codeine 1583

Desflurane (Potential for respiratory depression, hypotension, and profound sedation or coma; use caution and reduced dosage in patients who are concurrently receiving these drugs). Products include:

Suprane 1813

Desipramine Hydrochloride (Potential for respiratory depression, hypotension, and profound sedation or coma; use caution and reduced dosage in patients who are concurrently receiving these drugs). Products include:

Norpramin Tablets 1526

Dezocine (Potential for respiratory depression, hypotension, and profound sedation or coma; use caution and reduced dosage in patients who are concurrently receiving these drugs). Products include:

Dalgan Injection 538

Diazepam (Potential for respiratory depression, hypotension, and profound sedation or coma; use caution and reduced dosage in patients who are concurrently receiving these drugs). Products include:

Dizac 1809
Valium Injectable 2182
Valium Tablets 2183
Valrelease Capsules 2169

Doxepin Hydrochloride (Potential for respiratory depression, hypotension, and profound sedation or coma; use caution and reduced dosage in patients who are concurrently receiving these drugs). Products include:

Sinequan 2205
Zonalon Cream 1055

Droperidol (Potential for respiratory depression, hypotension, and profound sedation or coma; use caution and reduced dosage in patients who are concurrently receiving these drugs). Products include:

Inapsine Injection.................................... 1296

Enflurane (Potential for respiratory depression, hypotension, and profound sedation or coma; use caution and reduced dosage in patients who are concurrently receiving these drugs).

No products indexed under this heading.

Estazolam (Potential for respiratory depression, hypotension, and profound sedation or coma; use caution and reduced dosage in patients who are concurrently receiving these drugs). Products include:

ProSom Tablets 449

Ethchlorvynol (Potential for respiratory depression, hypotension, and profound sedation or coma; use caution and reduced dosage in patients who are concurrently receiving these drugs). Products include:

Placidyl Capsules.................................... 448

Ethinamate (Potential for respiratory depression, hypotension, and profound sedation or coma; use caution and reduced dosage in patients who are concurrently receiving these drugs).

No products indexed under this heading.

Fentanyl (Potential for respiratory depression, hypotension, and profound sedation or coma; use caution and reduced dosage in patients who are concurrently receiving these drugs). Products include:

Duragesic Transdermal System........ 1288

Fentanyl Citrate (Potential for respiratory depression, hypotension, and profound sedation or coma; use caution and reduced dosage in patients who are concurrently receiving these drugs). Products include:

Sublimaze Injection................................ 1307

Fluphenazine Decanoate (Potential for respiratory depression, hypotension, and profound sedation or coma; use caution and reduced dosage in patients who are concurrently receiving these drugs). Products include:

Prolixin Decanoate 509

IMPORTANT NOTE: Always consult each drug listing in the patient's regimen for possible interactions.

Methadone Concentrate

Fluphenazine Enanthate (Potential for respiratory depression, hypotension, and profound sedation or coma; use caution and reduced dosage in patients who are concurrently receiving these drugs). Products include:

Prolixin Enanthate 509

Fluphenazine Hydrochloride (Potential for respiratory depression, hypotension, and profound sedation or coma; use caution and reduced dosage in patients who are concurrently receiving these drugs). Products include:

Prolixin 509

Flurazepam Hydrochloride (Potential for respiratory depression, hypotension, and profound sedation or coma; use caution and reduced dosage in patients who are concurrently receiving these drugs). Products include:

Dalmane Capsules 2173

Furazolidone (Potential for meperidine/MAOI-type reaction; sensitivity test should be performed). Products include:

Furoxone 2046

Glutethimide (Potential for respiratory depression, hypotension, and profound sedation or coma; use caution and reduced dosage in patients who are concurrently receiving these drugs).

No products indexed under this heading.

Haloperidol (Potential for respiratory depression, hypotension, and profound sedation or coma; use caution and reduced dosage in patients who are concurrently receiving these drugs). Products include:

Haldol Injection, Tablets and Concentrate 1575

Haloperidol Decanoate (Potential for respiratory depression, hypotension, and profound sedation or coma; use caution and reduced dosage in patients who are concurrently receiving these drugs). Products include:

Haldol Decanoate 1577

Hydrocodone Bitartrate (Potential for respiratory depression, hypotension, and profound sedation or coma; use caution and reduced dosage in patients who are concurrently receiving these drugs). Products include:

Anexsia 5/500 Elixir 1781
Anexia Tablets 1782
Codiclear DH Syrup 791
Deconamine CX Cough and Cold Liquid and Tablets 1319
Duratuss HD Elixir 2565
Hycodan Tablets and Syrup 930
Hycomine Compound Tablets 932
Hycomine 931
Hycotuss Expectorant Syrup 933
Hydrocet Capsules 782
Lorcet 10/650 1018
Lortab 2566
Tussend 1783
Tussend Expectorant 1785
Vicodin Tablets 1356
Vicodin ES Tablets 1357
Vicodin Tuss Expectorant 1358
Zydone Capsules 949

Hydrocodone Polistirex (Potential for respiratory depression, hypotension, and profound sedation or coma; use caution and reduced dosage in patients who are concurrently receiving these drugs). Products include:

Tussionex Pennkinetic Extended-Release Suspension 998

Hydroxyzine Hydrochloride (Potential for respiratory depression, hypotension, and profound sedation or coma; use caution and reduced dosage in patients who are concurrently receiving these drugs). Products include:

Atarax Tablets & Syrup 2185
Marax Tablets & DF Syrup 2200
Vistaril Intramuscular Solution 2216

Imipramine Hydrochloride (Potential for respiratory depression, hypotension, and profound sedation or coma; use caution and reduced dosage in patients who are concurrently receiving these drugs). Products include:

Tofranil Ampuls 854
Tofranil Tablets 856

Imipramine Pamoate (Potential for respiratory depression, hypotension, and profound sedation or coma; use caution and reduced dosage in patients who are concurrently receiving these drugs). Products include:

Tofranil-PM Capsules 857

Isocarboxazid (Potential for meperidine/MAOI-type reaction; sensitivity test should be performed).

No products indexed under this heading.

Isoflurane (Potential for respiratory depression, hypotension, and profound sedation or coma; use caution and reduced dosage in patients who are concurrently receiving these drugs).

No products indexed under this heading.

Ketamine Hydrochloride (Potential for respiratory depression, hypotension, and profound sedation or coma; use caution and reduced dosage in patients who are concurrently receiving these drugs).

No products indexed under this heading.

Levomethadyl Acetate Hydrochloride (Potential for respiratory depression, hypotension, and profound sedation or coma; use caution and reduced dosage in patients who are concurrently receiving these drugs). Products include:

Orlaam 2239

Levorphanol Tartrate (Potential for respiratory depression, hypotension, and profound sedation or coma; use caution and reduced dosage in patients who are concurrently receiving these drugs). Products include:

Levo-Dromoran 2129

Lorazepam (Potential for respiratory depression, hypotension, and profound sedation or coma; use caution and reduced dosage in patients who are concurrently receiving these drugs). Products include:

Ativan Injection 2698
Ativan Tablets 2700

Loxapine Hydrochloride (Potential for respiratory depression, hypotension, and profound sedation or coma; use caution and reduced dosage in patients who are concurrently receiving these drugs). Products include:

Loxitane 1378

Loxapine Succinate (Potential for respiratory depression, hypotension, and profound sedation or coma; use caution and reduced dosage in patients who are concurrently receiving these drugs). Products include:

Loxitane Capsules 1378

Maprotiline Hydrochloride (Potential for respiratory depression, hypotension, and profound sedation or coma; use caution and reduced dosage in patients who are concurrently receiving these drugs). Products include:

Ludiomil Tablets 843

Meperidine Hydrochloride (Potential for respiratory depression, hypotension, and profound sedation or coma; use caution and reduced dosage in patients who are concurrently receiving these drugs). Products include:

Demerol 2308
Mepergan Injection 2753

Mephobarbital (Potential for respiratory depression, hypotension, and profound sedation or coma; use caution and reduced dosage in patients who are concurrently receiving these drugs). Products include:

Mebaral Tablets 2322

Meprobamate (Potential for respiratory depression, hypotension, and profound sedation or coma; use caution and reduced dosage in patients who are concurrently receiving these drugs). Products include:

Miltown Tablets 2672
PMB 200 and PMB 400 2783

Mesoridazine (Potential for respiratory depression, hypotension, and profound sedation or coma; use caution and reduced dosage in patients who are concurrently receiving these drugs).

Mesoridazine Besylate (Potential for respiratory depression, hypotension, and profound sedation or coma; use caution and reduced dosage in patients who are concurrently receiving these drugs). Products include:

Serentil 684

Methohexital Sodium (Potential for respiratory depression, hypotension, and profound sedation or coma; use caution and reduced dosage in patients who are concurrently receiving these drugs). Products include:

Brevital Sodium Vials 1429

Methotrimeprazine (Potential for respiratory depression, hypotension, and profound sedation or coma; use caution and reduced dosage in patients who are concurrently receiving these drugs). Products include:

Levoprome 1274

Methoxyflurane (Potential for respiratory depression, hypotension, and profound sedation or coma; use caution and reduced dosage in patients who are concurrently receiving these drugs).

No products indexed under this heading.

Midazolam Hydrochloride (Potential for respiratory depression, hypotension, and profound sedation or coma; use caution and reduced dosage in patients who are concurrently receiving these drugs). Products include:

Versed Injection 2170

Molindone Hydrochloride (Potential for respiratory depression, hypotension, and profound sedation or coma; use caution and reduced dosage in patients who are concurrently receiving these drugs). Products include:

Moban Tablets and Concentrate 1048

Morphine Sulfate (Potential for respiratory depression, hypotension, and profound sedation or coma; use caution and reduced dosage in patients who are concurrently receiving these drugs). Products include:

Astramorph/PF Injection, USP (Preservative-Free) 535
Duramorph 962
Infumorph 200 and Infumorph 500 Sterile Solutions 965
MS Contin Tablets 1994
MSIR 1997
Oramorph SR (Morphine Sulfate Sustained Release Tablets) 2236
RMS Suppositories 2657
Roxanol 2243

Nortriptyline Hydrochloride (Potential for respiratory depression, hypotension, and profound sedation or coma; use caution and reduced dosage in patients who are concurrently receiving these drugs). Products include:

Pamelor 2280

Opium Alkaloids (Potential for respiratory depression, hypotension, and profound sedation or coma; use caution and reduced dosage in patients who are concurrently receiving these drugs).

No products indexed under this heading.

Oxazepam (Potential for respiratory depression, hypotension, and profound sedation or coma; use caution and reduced dosage in patients who are concurrently receiving these drugs). Products include:

Serax Capsules 2810
Serax Tablets 2810

Oxycodone Hydrochloride (Potential for respiratory depression, hypotension, and profound sedation or coma; use caution and reduced dosage in patients who are concurrently receiving these drugs). Products include:

Percocet Tablets 938
Percodan Tablets 939
Percodan-Demi Tablets 940
Roxicodone Tablets, Oral Solution & Intensol (Oxycodone) 2244
Tylox Capsules 1584

Pentazocine Hydrochloride (Potential for withdrawal symptoms in patients who are on the methadone maintenance program when given pentazocine). Products include:

Talacen 2333
Talwin Compound 2335
Talwin Nx 2336

Pentazocine Lactate (Potential for withdrawal symptoms in patients who are on the methadone maintenance program when given pentazocine). Products include:

Talwin Injection 2334

Pentobarbital Sodium (Potential for respiratory depression, hypotension, and profound sedation or coma; use caution and reduced dosage in patients who are concurrently receiving these drugs). Products include:

Nembutal Sodium Capsules 436
Nembutal Sodium Solution 438
Nembutal Sodium Suppositories 440

Perphenazine (Potential for respiratory depression, hypotension, and profound sedation or coma; use caution and reduced dosage in patients who are concurrently receiving these drugs). Products include:

Etrafon 2355
Triavil Tablets 1757
Trilafon 2389

647 Interactions Index Methadone Oral

Phenelzine Sulfate (Potential for meperidine/MAOI-type reaction; sensitivity test should be performed). Products include:
Nardil ... 1920

Phenobarbital (Potential for respiratory depression, hypotension, and profound sedation or coma; use caution and reduced dosage in patients who are concurrently receiving these drugs). Products include:
Arco-Lase Plus Tablets ... 512
Bellergal-S Tablets ... 2250
Donnatal ... 2060
Donnatal Extentabs ... 2061
Donnatal Tablets ... 2060
Phenobarbital Elixir and Tablets ... 1469
Quadrinal Tablets ... 1350

Prazepam (Potential for respiratory depression, hypotension, and profound sedation or coma; use caution and reduced dosage in patients who are concurrently receiving these drugs).
No products indexed under this heading.

Prochlorperazine (Potential for respiratory depression, hypotension, and profound sedation or coma; use caution and reduced dosage in patients who are concurrently receiving these drugs). Products include:
Compazine ... 2470

Promethazine Hydrochloride (Potential for respiratory depression, hypotension, and profound sedation or coma; use caution and reduced dosage in patients who are concurrently receiving these drugs). Products include:
Mepergan Injection ... 2753
Phenergan with Codeine ... 2777
Phenergan with Dextromethorphan 2778
Phenergan Injection ... 2773
Phenergan Suppositories ... 2775
Phenergan Syrup ... 2774
Phenergan Tablets ... 2775
Phenergan VC ... 2779
Phenergan VC with Codeine ... 2781

Propofol (Potential for respiratory depression, hypotension, and profound sedation or coma; use caution and reduced dosage in patients who are concurrently receiving these drugs). Products include:
Diprivan Injection ... 2833

Propoxyphene Hydrochloride (Potential for respiratory depression, hypotension, and profound sedation or coma; use caution and reduced dosage in patients who are concurrently receiving these drugs). Products include:
Darvon ... 1435
Wygesic Tablets ... 2827

Propoxyphene Napsylate (Potential for respiratory depression, hypotension, and profound sedation or coma; use caution and reduced dosage in patients who are concurrently receiving these drugs). Products include:
Darvon-N/Darvocet-N ... 1433

Protriptyline Hydrochloride (Potential for respiratory depression, hypotension, and profound sedation or coma; use caution and reduced dosage in patients who are concurrently receiving these drugs). Products include:
Vivactil Tablets ... 1774

Quazepam (Potential for respiratory depression, hypotension, and profound sedation or coma; use caution and reduced dosage in patients who are concurrently receiving these drugs). Products include:
Doral Tablets ... 2664

Rifampin (Concurrent administration may reduce the blood concentration of methadone to a degree sufficient to produce withdrawal symptoms). Products include:
Rifadin ... 1528
Rifamate Capsules ... 1530
Rifater ... 1532
Rimactane Capsules ... 847

Risperidone (Potential for respiratory depression, hypotension, and profound sedation or coma; use caution and reduced dosage in patients who are concurrently receiving these drugs). Products include:
Risperdal ... 1301

Secobarbital Sodium (Potential for respiratory depression, hypotension, and profound sedation or coma; use caution and reduced dosage in patients who are concurrently receiving these drugs). Products include:
Seconal Sodium Pulvules ... 1474

Selegiline Hydrochloride (Potential for meperidine/MAOI-type reaction; sensitivity test should be performed). Products include:
Eldepryl Tablets ... 2550

Sufentanil Citrate (Potential for respiratory depression, hypotension, and profound sedation or coma; use caution and reduced dosage in patients who are concurrently receiving these drugs). Products include:
Sufenta Injection ... 1309

Temazepam (Potential for respiratory depression, hypotension, and profound sedation or coma; use caution and reduced dosage in patients who are concurrently receiving these drugs). Products include:
Restoril Capsules ... 2284

Thiamylal Sodium (Potential for respiratory depression, hypotension, and profound sedation or coma; use caution and reduced dosage in patients who are concurrently receiving these drugs).
No products indexed under this heading.

Thioridazine Hydrochloride (Potential for respiratory depression, hypotension, and profound sedation or coma; use caution and reduced dosage in patients who are concurrently receiving these drugs). Products include:
Mellaril ... 2269

Thiothixene (Potential for respiratory depression, hypotension, and profound sedation or coma; use caution and reduced dosage in patients who are concurrently receiving these drugs). Products include:
Navane Capsules and Concentrate 2201
Navane Intramuscular ... 2202

Tranylcypromine Sulfate (Potential for meperidine/MAOI-type reaction; sensitivity test should be performed). Products include:
Parnate Tablets ... 2503

Triazolam (Potential for respiratory depression, hypotension, and profound sedation or coma; use caution and reduced dosage in patients who are concurrently receiving these drugs). Products include:
Halcion Tablets ... 2611

Trifluoperazine Hydrochloride (Potential for respiratory depression, hypotension, and profound sedation or coma; use caution and reduced dosage in patients who are concurrently receiving these drugs). Products include:
Stelazine ... 2514

Trimipramine Maleate (Potential for respiratory depression, hypotension, and profound sedation or coma; use caution and reduced dosage in patients who are concurrently receiving these drugs). Products include:
Surmontil Capsules ... 2811

Zolpidem Tartrate (Potential for respiratory depression, hypotension, and profound sedation or coma; use caution and reduced dosage in patients who are concurrently receiving these drugs). Products include:
Ambien Tablets ... 2416

Food Interactions

Alcohol (Potential for respiratory depression, hypotension, and profound sedation or coma; use caution and reduced dosage in patients who are concurrently receiving these drugs).

METHADONE HYDROCHLORIDE ORAL SOLUTION & TABLETS

(Methadone Hydrochloride) ... 2235

May interact with tricyclic antidepressants, central nervous system depressants, monoamine oxidase inhibitors, and certain other agents. Compounds in these categories include:

Alfentanil Hydrochloride (Respiratory depression, hypotension, and profound sedation or coma may result). Products include:
Alfenta Injection ... 1286

Alprazolam (Respiratory depression, hypotension, and profound sedation or coma may result). Products include:
Xanax Tablets ... 2649

Amitriptyline Hydrochloride (Respiratory depression, hypotension, and profound sedation or coma may result). Products include:
Elavil ... 2838
Endep Tablets ... 2174
Etrafon ... 2355
Limbitrol ... 2180
Triavil Tablets ... 1757

Amoxapine (Respiratory depression, hypotension, and profound sedation or coma may result). Products include:
Asendin Tablets ... 1369

Aprobarbital (Respiratory depression, hypotension, and profound sedation or coma may result).
No products indexed under this heading.

Buprenorphine (Respiratory depression, hypotension, and profound sedation or coma may result). Products include:
Buprenex Injectable ... 2006

Buspirone Hydrochloride (Respiratory depression, hypotension, and profound sedation or coma may result). Products include:
BuSpar ... 737

Butabarbital (Respiratory depression, hypotension, and profound sedation or coma may result).
No products indexed under this heading.

Butalbital (Respiratory depression, hypotension, and profound sedation or coma may result). Products include:
Esgic-plus Tablets ... 1013
Fioricet Tablets ... 2258
Fioricet with Codeine Capsules ... 2260
Fiorinal Capsules ... 2261
Fiorinal with Codeine Capsules ... 2262
Fiorinal Tablets ... 2261
Phrenilin ... 785
Sedapap Tablets 50 mg/650 mg .. 1543

Chlordiazepoxide (Respiratory depression, hypotension, and profound sedation or coma may result). Products include:
Libritabs Tablets ... 2177
Limbitrol ... 2180

Chlordiazepoxide Hydrochloride (Respiratory depression, hypotension, and profound sedation or coma may result). Products include:
Librax Capsules ... 2176
Librium Capsules ... 2178
Librium Injectable ... 2179

Chlorpromazine (Respiratory depression, hypotension, and profound sedation or coma may result). Products include:
Thorazine Suppositories ... 2523

Chlorprothixene (Respiratory depression, hypotension, and profound sedation or coma may result).
No products indexed under this heading.

Chlorprothixene Hydrochloride (Respiratory depression, hypotension, and profound sedation or coma may result).
No products indexed under this heading.

Chlorprothixene Lactate (Respiratory depression, hypotension, and profound sedation or coma may result).
No products indexed under this heading.

Clomipramine Hydrochloride (Respiratory depression, hypotension, and profound sedation or coma may result). Products include:
Anafranil Capsules ... 803

Clorazepate Dipotassium (Respiratory depression, hypotension, and profound sedation or coma may result). Products include:
Tranxene ... 451

Clozapine (Respiratory depression, hypotension, and profound sedation or coma may result). Products include:
Clozaril Tablets ... 2252

Codeine Phosphate (Respiratory depression, hypotension, and profound sedation or coma may result). Products include:
Actifed with Codeine Cough Syrup.. 1067
Brontex ... 1981
Deconsal C Expectorant Syrup ... 456
Deconsal Pediatric Syrup ... 457
Dimetane-DC Cough Syrup ... 2059
Empirin with Codeine Tablets ... 1093
Fioricet with Codeine Capsules ... 2260
Fiorinal with Codeine Capsules ... 2262
Isoclor Expectorant ... 990
Novahistine DH ... 2462
Novahistine Expectorant ... 2463
Nucofed ... 2051
Phenergan with Codeine ... 2777
Phenergan VC with Codeine ... 2781
Robitussin A-C Syrup ... 2073
Robitussin-DAC Syrup ... 2074
Ryna ... 841
Soma Compound w/Codeine Tablets ... 2676
Tussi-Organidin NR Liquid and S NR Liquid ... 2677
Tylenol with Codeine ... 1583

Desflurane (Respiratory depression, hypotension, and profound sedation or coma may result). Products include:
Suprane ... 1813

Desipramine Hydrochloride (Respiratory depression, hypotension, and profound sedation or coma may result). Products include:
Norpramin Tablets ... 1526

Dezocine (Respiratory depression, hypotension, and profound sedation or coma may result). Products include:
Dalgan Injection ... 538

IMPORTANT NOTE: Always consult each drug listing in the patient's regimen for possible interactions.

Diazepam (Respiratory depression, hypotension, and profound sedation or coma may result). Products include:
- Dizac ... **1809**
- Valium Injectable ... **2182**
- Valium Tablets ... **2183**
- Valrelease Capsules ... **2169**

Doxepin Hydrochloride (Respiratory depression, hypotension, and profound sedation or coma may result). Products include:
- Sinequan ... **2205**
- Zonalon Cream ... **1055**

Droperidol (Respiratory depression, hypotension, and profound sedation or coma may result). Products include:
- Inapsine Injection ... **1296**

Enflurane (Respiratory depression, hypotension, and profound sedation or coma may result).
- No products indexed under this heading.

Estazolam (Respiratory depression, hypotension, and profound sedation or coma may result). Products include:
- ProSom Tablets ... **449**

Ethchlorvynol (Respiratory depression, hypotension, and profound sedation or coma may result). Products include:
- Placidyl Capsules ... **448**

Ethinamate (Respiratory depression, hypotension, and profound sedation or coma may result).
- No products indexed under this heading.

Fentanyl (Respiratory depression, hypotension, and profound sedation or coma may result). Products include:
- Duragesic Transdermal System ... **1288**

Fentanyl Citrate (Respiratory depression, hypotension, and profound sedation or coma may result). Products include:
- Sublimaze Injection ... **1307**

Fluphenazine Decanoate (Respiratory depression, hypotension, and profound sedation or coma may result). Products include:
- Prolixin Decanoate ... **509**

Fluphenazine Enanthate (Respiratory depression, hypotension, and profound sedation or coma may result). Products include:
- Prolixin Enanthate ... **509**

Fluphenazine Hydrochloride (Respiratory depression, hypotension, and profound sedation or coma may result). Products include:
- Prolixin ... **509**

Flurazepam Hydrochloride (Respiratory depression, hypotension, and profound sedation or coma may result). Products include:
- Dalmane Capsules ... **2173**

Furazolidone (Severe reactions not reported, but a sensitivity test is advised). Products include:
- Furoxone ... **2046**

Glutethimide (Respiratory depression, hypotension, and profound sedation or coma may result).
- No products indexed under this heading.

Haloperidol (Respiratory depression, hypotension, and profound sedation or coma may result). Products include:
- Haldol Injection, Tablets and Concentrate ... **1575**

Haloperidol Decanoate (Respiratory depression, hypotension, and profound sedation or coma may result). Products include:
- Haldol Decanoate ... **1577**

Hydrocodone Bitartrate (Respiratory depression, hypotension, and profound sedation or coma may result). Products include:
- Anexsia 5/500 Elixir ... **1781**
- Anexia Tablets ... **1782**
- Codiclear DH Syrup ... **791**
- Deconamine CX Cough and Cold Liquid and Tablets ... **1319**
- Duratuss HD Elixir ... **2565**
- Hycodan Tablets and Syrup ... **930**
- Hycomine Compound Tablets ... **932**
- Hycomine ... **931**
- Hycotuss Expectorant Syrup ... **933**
- Hydrocet Capsules ... **782**
- Lorcet 10/650 ... **1018**
- Lortab ... **2566**
- Tussend ... **1783**
- Tussend Expectorant ... **1785**
- Vicodin Tablets ... **1356**
- Vicodin ES Tablets ... **1357**
- Vicodin Tuss Expectorant ... **1358**
- Zydone Capsules ... **949**

Hydrocodone Polistirex (Respiratory depression, hypotension, and profound sedation or coma may result). Products include:
- Tussionex Pennkinetic Extended-Release Suspension ... **998**

Hydroxyzine Hydrochloride (Respiratory depression, hypotension, and profound sedation or coma may result). Products include:
- Atarax Tablets & Syrup ... **2185**
- Marax Tablets & DF Syrup ... **2200**
- Vistaril Intramuscular Solution ... **2216**

Imipramine Hydrochloride (Respiratory depression, hypotension, and profound sedation or coma may result). Products include:
- Tofranil Ampuls ... **854**
- Tofranil Tablets ... **856**

Imipramine Pamoate (Respiratory depression, hypotension, and profound sedation or coma may result). Products include:
- Tofranil-PM Capsules ... **857**

Isocarboxazid (Severe reactions not reported, but a sensitivity test is advised).
- No products indexed under this heading.

Isoflurane (Respiratory depression, hypotension, and profound sedation or coma may result).
- No products indexed under this heading.

Ketamine Hydrochloride (Respiratory depression, hypotension, and profound sedation or coma may result).
- No products indexed under this heading.

Levomethadyl Acetate Hydrochloride (Respiratory depression, hypotension, and profound sedation or coma may result). Products include:
- Orlamm ... **2239**

Levorphanol Tartrate (Respiratory depression, hypotension, and profound sedation or coma may result). Products include:
- Levo-Dromoran ... **2129**

Lorazepam (Respiratory depression, hypotension, and profound sedation or coma may result). Products include:
- Ativan Injection ... **2698**
- Ativan Tablets ... **2700**

Loxapine Hydrochloride (Respiratory depression, hypotension, and profound sedation or coma may result). Products include:
- Loxitane ... **1378**

Loxapine Succinate (Respiratory depression, hypotension, and profound sedation or coma may result). Products include:
- Loxitane Capsules ... **1378**

Maprotiline Hydrochloride (Respiratory depression, hypotension, and profound sedation or coma may result). Products include:
- Ludiomil Tablets ... **843**

Meperidine Hydrochloride (Respiratory depression, hypotension, and profound sedation or coma may result). Products include:
- Demerol ... **2308**
- Mepergan Injection ... **2753**

Mephobarbital (Respiratory depression, hypotension, and profound sedation or coma may result). Products include:
- Mebaral Tablets ... **2322**

Meprobamate (Respiratory depression, hypotension, and profound sedation or coma may result). Products include:
- Miltown Tablets ... **2672**
- PMB 200 and PMB 400 ... **2783**

Mesoridazine Besylate (Respiratory depression, hypotension, and profound sedation or coma may result). Products include:
- Serentil ... **684**

Methohexital Sodium (Respiratory depression, hypotension, and profound sedation or coma may result). Products include:
- Brevital Sodium Vials ... **1429**

Methotrimeprazine (Respiratory depression, hypotension, and profound sedation or coma may result). Products include:
- Levoprome ... **1274**

Methoxyflurane (Respiratory depression, hypotension, and profound sedation or coma may result).
- No products indexed under this heading.

Methyldopate Hydrochloride (Respiratory depression, hypotension, and profound sedation or coma may result). Products include:
- Aldomet Ester HCl Injection ... **1602**

Midazolam Hydrochloride (Respiratory depression, hypotension, and profound sedation or coma may result). Products include:
- Versed Injection ... **2170**

Molindone Hydrochloride (Respiratory depression, hypotension, and profound sedation or coma may result). Products include:
- Moban Tablets and Concentrate ... **1048**

Morphine Sulfate (Respiratory depression, hypotension, and profound sedation or coma may result). Products include:
- Astramorph/PF Injection, USP (Preservative-Free) ... **535**
- Duramorph ... **962**
- Infumorph 200 and Infumorph 500 Sterile Solutions ... **965**
- MS Contin Tablets ... **1994**
- MSIR ... **1997**
- Oramorph SR (Morphine Sulfate Sustained Release Tablets) ... **2236**
- RMS Suppositories ... **2657**
- Roxanol ... **2243**

Nortriptyline Hydrochloride (Respiratory depression, hypotension, and profound sedation or coma may result). Products include:
- Pamelor ... **2280**

Opium Alkaloids (Respiratory depression, hypotension, and profound sedation or coma may result).
- No products indexed under this heading.

Oxazepam (Respiratory depression, hypotension, and profound sedation or coma may result). Products include:
- Serax Capsules ... **2810**
- Serax Tablets ... **2810**

Oxycodone Hydrochloride (Respiratory depression, hypotension, and profound sedation or coma may result). Products include:
- Percocet Tablets ... **938**
- Percodan Tablets ... **939**
- Percodan-Demi Tablets ... **940**
- Roxicodone Tablets, Oral Solution & Intensol (Oxycodone) ... **2244**
- Tylox Capsules ... **1584**

Pentazocine Hydrochloride (Possible withdrawal symptoms). Products include:
- Talacen ... **2333**
- Talwin Compound ... **2335**
- Talwin Nx ... **2336**

Pentazocine Lactate (Possible withdrawal symptoms). Products include:
- Talwin Injection ... **2334**

Pentobarbital Sodium (Respiratory depression, hypotension, and profound sedation or coma may result). Products include:
- Nembutal Sodium Capsules ... **436**
- Nembutal Sodium Solution ... **438**
- Nembutal Sodium Suppositories ... **440**

Perphenazine (Respiratory depression, hypotension, and profound sedation or coma may result). Products include:
- Etrafon ... **2355**
- Triavil Tablets ... **1757**
- Trilafon ... **2389**

Phenelzine Sulfate (Severe reactions not reported, but a sensitivity test is advised). Products include:
- Nardil ... **1920**

Phenobarbital (Respiratory depression, hypotension, and profound sedation or coma may result). Products include:
- Arco-Lase Plus Tablets ... **512**
- Bellergal-S Tablets ... **2250**
- Donnatal ... **2060**
- Donnatal Extentabs ... **2061**
- Donnatal Tablets ... **2060**
- Phenobarbital Elixir and Tablets ... **1469**
- Quadrinal Tablets ... **1350**

Prazepam (Respiratory depression, hypotension, and profound sedation or coma may result).
- No products indexed under this heading.

Prochlorperazine (Respiratory depression, hypotension, and profound sedation or coma may result). Products include:
- Compazine ... **2470**

Promethazine Hydrochloride (Respiratory depression, hypotension, and profound sedation or coma may result). Products include:
- Mepergan Injection ... **2753**
- Phenergan with Codeine ... **2777**
- Phenergan with Dextromethorphan **2778**
- Phenergan Injection ... **2773**
- Phenergan Suppositories ... **2775**
- Phenergan Syrup ... **2774**
- Phenergan Tablets ... **2775**
- Phenergan VC ... **2779**
- Phenergan VC with Codeine ... **2781**

Propofol (Respiratory depression, hypotension, and profound sedation or coma may result). Products include:
- Diprivan Injection ... **2833**

Propoxyphene Hydrochloride (Respiratory depression, hypotension, and profound sedation or coma may result). Products include:
- Darvon ... **1435**
- Wygesic Tablets ... **2827**

(Described in PDR For Nonprescription Drugs) (⊙ Described in PDR For Ophthalmology)

Interactions Index

Methotrexate/Rheumatrex

Propoxyphene Napsylate (Respiratory depression, hypotension, and profound sedation or coma may result). Products include:

Darvon-N/Darvocet-N 1433

Protriptyline Hydrochloride (Respiratory depression, hypotension, and profound sedation or coma may result). Products include:

Vivactil Tablets 1774

Quazepam (Respiratory depression, hypotension, and profound sedation or coma may result). Products include:

Doral Tablets 2664

Rifampin (Reduced blood concentration of methadone). Products include:

Rifadin 1528
Rifamate Capsules 1530
Rifater 1532
Rimactane Capsules 847

Risperidone (Respiratory depression, hypotension, and profound sedation or coma may result). Products include:

Risperdal 1301

Secobarbital Sodium (Respiratory depression, hypotension, and profound sedation or coma may result). Products include:

Seconal Sodium Pulvules 1474

Selegiline Hydrochloride (Severe reactions not reported, but a sensitivity test is advised). Products include:

Eldepryl Tablets 2550

Sufentanil Citrate (Respiratory depression, hypotension, and profound sedation or coma may result). Products include:

Sufenta Injection 1309

Temazepam (Respiratory depression, hypotension, and profound sedation or coma may result). Products include:

Restoril Capsules 2284

Thiamylal Sodium (Respiratory depression, hypotension, and profound sedation or coma may result).

No products indexed under this heading.

Thioridazine Hydrochloride (Respiratory depression, hypotension, and profound sedation or coma may result). Products include:

Mellaril 2269

Thiothixene (Respiratory depression, hypotension, and profound sedation or coma may result). Products include:

Navane Capsules and Concentrate 2201
Navane Intramuscular 2202

Tranylcypromine Sulfate (Severe reactions not reported, but a sensitivity test is advised). Products include:

Parnate Tablets 2503

Triazolam (Respiratory depression, hypotension, and profound sedation or coma may result). Products include:

Halcion Tablets.. 2611

Trifluoperazine Hydrochloride (Respiratory depression, hypotension, and profound sedation or coma may result). Products include:

Stelazine 2514

Trimipramine Maleate (Respiratory depression, hypotension, and profound sedation or coma may result). Products include:

Surmontil Capsules 2811

Zolpidem Tartrate (Respiratory depression, hypotension, and profound sedation or coma may result). Products include:

Ambien Tablets.. 2416

Food Interactions

Alcohol (Respiratory depression, hypotension, and profound sedation or coma may result).

METHERGINE INJECTION

(Methylergonovine Maleate)................2272

May interact with vasopressors and certain other agents. Compounds in these categories include:

Dopamine Hydrochloride (Use cautiously).

No products indexed under this heading.

Epinephrine Hydrochloride (Use cautiously). Products include:

Ana-Kit Anaphylaxis Emergency Treatment Kit 617

Ergoloid Mesylates (Use cautiously). Products include:

Hydergine 2265

Ergonovine Maleate (Use cautiously).

No products indexed under this heading.

Metaraminol Bitartrate (Use cautiously). Products include:

Aramine Injection.................................... 1609

Methoxamine Hydrochloride (Use cautiously). Products include:

Vasoxyl Injection 1196

Methysergide Maleate (Use cautiously). Products include:

Sansert Tablets.. 2295

Norepinephrine Bitartrate (Use cautiously). Products include:

Levophed Bitartrate Injection 2315

Phenylephrine Hydrochloride (Use cautiously). Products include:

Atrohist Plus Tablets 454
Cerose DM .... ⊕D 878
Comhist 2038
D.A. Chewable Tablets........................... 951
Deconsal Pediatric Capsules................ 454
Dura-Vent/DA Tablets 953
Entex Capsules 1986
Entex Liquid 1986
Extendryl 1005
4-Way Fast Acting Nasal Spray (regular & mentholated) .... ⊕D 621
Hemorid For Women .... ⊕D 834
Hycomine Compound Tablets 932
Neo-Synephrine Hydrochloride 1% Carpuject... 2324
Neo-Synephrine Hydrochloride 1% Injection 2324
Neo-Synephrine Hydrochloride (Ophthalmic) 2325
Neo-Synephrine .... ⊕D 726
Nöstril .... ⊕D 644
Novahistine Elixir .... ⊕D 823
Phenergan VC 2779
Phenergan VC with Codeine 2781
Preparation H .... ⊕D 871
Tympagesic Ear Drops 2342
Vasosulf .... © 271
Vicks Sinex Nasal Spray and Ultra Fine Mist .... ⊕D 765

METHERGINE TABLETS

(Methylergonovine Maleate)................2272

See Methergine Injection

METHOTREXATE SODIUM TABLETS, INJECTION, FOR INJECTION AND LPF INJECTION

(Methotrexate Sodium) 1275

May interact with salicylates, sulfonamides, tetracyclines, non-steroidal anti-inflammatory agents, cytotoxic drugs, and certain other agents. Compounds in these categories include:

Antibiotics, nonabsorbable broad spectrum, unspecified (Decreases intestinal absorption and interferes with enterohepatic circulation).

Aspirin (Increased toxicity). Products include:

Alka-Seltzer Effervescent Antacid and Pain Reliever .... ⊕D 701
Alka-Seltzer Extra Strength Effervescent Antacid and Pain Reliever .... ⊕D 703
Alka-Seltzer Lemon Lime Effervescent Antacid and Pain Reliever .... ⊕D 703
Alka-Seltzer Plus Cold Medicine .... ⊕D 705
Alka-Seltzer Plus Cold & Cough Medicine .... ⊕D 708
Alka-Seltzer Plus Night-Time Cold Medicine .... ⊕D 707
Alka Seltzer Plus Sinus Medicine .. ⊕D 707
Arthritis Foundation Safety Coated Aspirin Tablets .... ⊕D 675
Arthritis Pain Ascriptin .... ⊕D 631
Maximum Strength Ascriptin .... ⊕D 630
Regular Strength Ascriptin Tablets .... ⊕D 629
Arthritis Strength BC Powder.......... ⊕D 609
BC Cold Powder Multi-Symptom Formula (Cold-Sinus-Allergy) ...... ⊕D 609
BC Cold Powder Non-Drowsy Formula (Cold-Sinus) .... ⊕D 609
BC Powder .... ⊕D 609
Bayer Children's Chewable Aspirin .... ⊕D 711
Genuine Bayer Aspirin Tablets & Caplets .... ⊕D 713
Extra Strength Bayer Arthritis Pain Regimen Formula .... ⊕D 711
Extra Strength Bayer Aspirin Caplets & Tablets .... ⊕D 712
Extended-Release Bayer 8-Hour Aspirin .... ⊕D 712
Extra Strength Bayer Plus Aspirin Caplets .... ⊕D 713
Extra Strength Bayer PM Aspirin .. ⊕D 713
Bayer Enteric Aspirin .... ⊕D 709
Bufferin Analgesic Tablets and Caplets .... ⊕D 613
Arthritis Strength Bufferin Analgesic Caplets .... ⊕D 614
Extra Strength Bufferin Analgesic Tablets .... ⊕D 615
Cama Arthritis Pain Reliever........... ⊕D 785
Darvon Compound-65 Pulvules 1435
Easprin.. 1914
Ecotrin 2455
Ecotrin Enteric Coated Aspirin Maximum Strength Tablets and Caplets .... ⊕D 816
Ecotrin Enteric Coated Aspirin Regular Strength Tablets 2455
Empirin Aspirin Tablets .... ⊕D 854
Empirin with Codeine Tablets............ 1093
Excedrin Extra-Strength Analgesic Tablets & Caplets 732
Fiorinal Capsules 2261
Fiorinal with Codeine Capsules 2262
Fiorinal Tablets....................................... 2261
Halfprin 1362
Healthprin Aspirin 2455
Norgesic.. 1496
Percodan Tablets..................................... 939
Percodan-Demi Tablets.......................... 940
Robaxisal Tablets.................................... 2071
Soma Compound w/Codeine Tablets 2676
Soma Compound Tablets....................... 2675
St. Joseph Adult Chewable Aspirin (81 mg.) .... ⊕D 808
Talwin Compound 2335
Ursinus Inlay-Tabs............................. ⊕D 794
Vanquish Analgesic Caplets .... ⊕D 731

Auranofin (Combined use has not been studied and may increase the incidence of adverse effects). Products include:

Ridaura Capsules.................................... 2513

Aurothioglucose (Combined use has not been studied and may increase the incidence of adverse effects). Products include:

Solganal Suspension............................... 2388

Bleomycin Sulfate (Combined use has not been studied and may increase the incidence of adverse effects). Products include:

Blenoxane 692

Chloramphenicol (Decreases intestinal absorption and interferes with enterohepatic circulation). Products include:

Chloromycetin Ophthalmic Ointment, 1% .... © 310
Chloromycetin Ophthalmic Solution.. © 310
Chloroptic S.O.P. .... © 239
Chloroptic Sterile Ophthalmic Solution .... © 239
Elase-Chloromycetin Ointment 1040
Ophthocort .... © 311

Chloramphenicol Palmitate (Decreases intestinal absorption and interferes with enterohepatic circulation).

No products indexed under this heading.

Chloramphenicol Sodium Succinate (Increased toxicity). Products include:

Chloromycetin Sodium Succinate.... 1900

Choline Magnesium Trisalicylate (Increased toxicity). Products include:

Trilisate 2000

Cisplatin (Caution should be exercised if high-dose of methotrexate is used concurrently in the treatment of osteosarcoma). Products include:

Platinol 708
Platinol-AQ Injection.............................. 710

Daunorubicin Hydrochloride (Combined use has not been studied and may increase the incidence of adverse effects). Products include:

Cerubidine 795

Demeclocycline Hydrochloride (Decreases intestinal absorption and interferes with enterohepatic circulation). Products include:

Declomycin Tablets................................. 1371

Diclofenac Potassium (May elevate and prolong serum methotrexate levels; reduces the tubular secretion of methotrexate). Products include:

Cataflam 816

Diclofenac Sodium (May elevate and prolong serum methotrexate levels; reduces the tubular secretion of methotrexate). Products include:

Voltaren Ophthalmic Sterile Ophthalmic Solution .... © 272
Voltaren Tablets....................................... 861

Diflunisal (Increased toxicity). Products include:

Dolobid Tablets.. 1654

Doxorubicin Hydrochloride (Combined use has not been studied and may increase the incidence of adverse effects). Products include:

Adriamycin PFS 1947
Adriamycin RDF 1947
Doxorubicin Astra 540
Rubex 712

Doxycycline Calcium (Decreases intestinal absorption and interferes with enterohepatic circulation). Products include:

Vibramycin Calcium Oral Suspension Syrup.. 1941

Doxycycline Hyclate (Decreases intestinal absorption and interferes with enterohepatic circulation). Products include:

Doryx Capsules.. 1913
Vibramycin Hyclate Capsules 1941
Vibramycin Hyclate Intravenous 2215
Vibra-Tabs Film Coated Tablets 1941

Doxycycline Monohydrate (Decreases intestinal absorption and interferes with enterohepatic circulation). Products include:

Monodox Capsules 1805
Vibramycin Monohydrate for Oral Suspension 1941

IMPORTANT NOTE: Always consult each drug listing in the patient's regimen for possible interactions.

Etodolac (May elevate and prolong serum methotrexate levels; reduces the tubular secretion of methotrexate). Products include:
- Lodine Capsules and Tablets 2743

Fenoprofen Calcium (May elevate and prolong serum methotrexate levels; reduces the tubular secretion of methotrexate). Products include:
- Nalfon 200 Pulvules & Nalfon Tablets 917

Fluorouracil (Combined use has not been studied and may increase the incidence of adverse effects). Products include:
- Efudex 2113
- Fluoroplex Topical Solution & Cream 1% 479
- Fluorouracil Injection 2116

Flurbiprofen (May elevate and prolong serum methotrexate levels; reduces the tubular secretion of methotrexate). Products include:
- Ansaid Tablets 2579

Folic Acid (May decrease response to methotrexate). Products include:
- Cefol Filmtab 412
- Fero-Folic-500 Filmtab 429
- Iberet-Folic-500 Filmtab 429
- Materna Tablets 1379
- Mega-B 512
- Megadose 512
- Nephro-Fer Rx Tablets 2005
- Nephro-Vite + Fe Tablets 2006
- Nephro-Vite Rx Tablets 2006
- Niferex-150 Forte Capsules 794
- Niferex Forte Elixir 794
- Sigtab Tablets .... ▣ 772
- Slow Fe with Folic Acid 869
- Stuart Prenatal Tablets .... ▣ 881
- The Stuart Formula Tablets .... ▣ 663
- Trinsicon Capsules 2570
- Zymacap Capsules .... ▣ 772

Gold Sodium Thiomalate (Combined use has not been studied and may increase the incidence of adverse effects). Products include:
- Myochrysine Injection 1711

Hydroxychloroquine Sulfate (Combined use has not been studied and may increase the incidence of adverse effects). Products include:
- Plaquenil Sulfate Tablets 2328

Hydroxyurea (Combined use has not been studied and may increase the incidence of adverse effects). Products include:
- Hydrea Capsules 696

Ibuprofen (May elevate and prolong serum methotrexate levels; reduces the tubular secretion of methotrexate). Products include:
- Advil Cold and Sinus Caplets and Tablets (formerly CoAdvil) .... ▣ 870
- Advil Ibuprofen Tablets and Caplets .... ▣ 870
- Children's Advil Suspension 2692
- Arthritis Foundation Ibuprofen Tablets .... ▣ 674
- Bayer Select Ibuprofen Pain Relief Formula .... ▣ 715
- Cramp End Tablets .... ▣ 735
- Dimetapp Sinus Caplets .... ▣ 775
- Haltran Tablets .... ▣ 771
- IBU Tablets 1342
- Ibuprohm .... ▣ 735
- Children's Motrin Ibuprofen Oral Suspension 1546
- Motrin Tablets 2625
- Motrin IB Caplets, Tablets, and Geltabs .... ▣ 838
- Motrin IB Sinus .... ▣ 838
- Motrin Ibuprofen Suspension, Oral Drops, Chewable Tablets, Caplets 1546
- Nuprin Ibuprofen/Analgesic Tablets & Caplets .... ▣ 622
- Sine-Aid IB Caplets 1554
- Vicks DayQuil SINUS Pressure & PAIN Relief with IBUPROFEN .... ▣ 762

Indomethacin (May elevate and prolong serum methotrexate levels; reduces the tubular secretion of methotrexate). Products include:
- Indocin 1680

Indomethacin Sodium Trihydrate (May elevate and prolong serum methotrexate levels; reduces the tubular secretion of methotrexate). Products include:
- Indocin I.V. 1684

Ketoprofen (May elevate and prolong serum methotrexate levels; reduces the tubular secretion of methotrexate). Products include:
- Orudis Capsules 2766
- Oruvail Capsules 2766

Ketorolac Tromethamine (May elevate and prolong serum methotrexate levels; reduces the tubular secretion of methotrexate). Products include:
- Acular 474
- Acular .... ⊙ 277
- Toradol 2159

Leucovorin Calcium (High doses may reduce the efficacy of intrathecally administered methotrexate). Products include:
- Leucovorin Calcium for Injection, Wellcovorin Brand 1132
- Leucovorin Calcium for Injection 1268
- Leucovorin Calcium Tablets, Wellcovorin Brand 1132
- Leucovorin Calcium Tablets 1270

Magnesium Salicylate (Increased toxicity). Products include:
- Backache Caplets .... ▣ 613
- Bayer Select Backache Pain Relief Formula .... ▣ 715
- Doan's Extra-Strength Analgesic .... ▣ 633
- Extra Strength Doan's P.M. .... ▣ 633
- Doan's Regular Strength Analgesic .... ▣ 634
- Mobigesic Tablets .... ▣ 602

Meclofenamate Sodium (May elevate and prolong serum methotrexate levels; reduces the tubular secretion of methotrexate).
- No products indexed under this heading.

Mefenamic Acid (May elevate and prolong serum methotrexate levels; reduces the tubular secretion of methotrexate). Products include:
- Ponstel 1925

Methacycline Hydrochloride (Decreases intestinal absorption and interferes with enterohepatic circulation).
- No products indexed under this heading.

Minocycline Hydrochloride (Decreases intestinal absorption and interferes with enterohepatic circulation). Products include:
- Dynacin Capsules 1590
- Minocin Intravenous 1382
- Minocin Oral Suspension 1385
- Minocin Pellet-Filled Capsules 1383

Mitotane (Combined use has not been studied and may increase the incidence of adverse effects). Products include:
- Lysodren 698

Mitoxantrone Hydrochloride (Combined use has not been studied and may increase the incidence of adverse effects). Products include:
- Novantrone 1279

Nabumetone (May elevate and prolong serum methotrexate levels; reduces the tubular secretion of methotrexate). Products include:
- Relafen Tablets 2510

Naproxen (May elevate and prolong serum methotrexate levels; reduces the tubular secretion of methotrexate). Products include:
- Anaprox/Naprosyn 2117

Naproxen Sodium (May elevate and prolong serum methotrexate levels; reduces the tubular secretion of methotrexate). Products include:
- Aleve 1975
- Anaprox/Naprosyn 2117

Oxaprozin (May elevate and prolong serum methotrexate levels; reduces the tubular secretion of methotrexate). Products include:
- Daypro Caplets 2426

Oxytetracycline (Decreases intestinal absorption and interferes with enterohepatic circulation). Products include:
- Terramycin Intramuscular Solution 2210

Oxytetracycline Hydrochloride (Decreases intestinal absorption and interferes with enterohepatic circulation). Products include:
- TERAK Ointment .... ⊙ 209
- Terra-Cortril Ophthalmic Suspension 2210
- Terramycin with Polymyxin B Sulfate Ophthalmic Ointment 2211
- Urobiotic-250 Capsules 2214

Penicillamine (Combined use has not been studied and may increase the incidence of adverse effects). Products include:
- Cuprimine Capsules 1630
- Depen Titratable Tablets 2662

Phenylbutazone (Increased toxicity; may elevate and prolong serum methotrexate levels; reduces the tubular secretion of methotrexate).
- No products indexed under this heading.

Phenytoin (Increased toxicity). Products include:
- Dilantin Infatabs 1908
- Dilantin-125 Suspension 1911

Phenytoin Sodium (Increased toxicity). Products include:
- Dilantin Kapseals 1906
- Dilantin Parenteral 1910

Piroxicam (May elevate and prolong serum methotrexate levels; reduces the tubular secretion of methotrexate). Products include:
- Feldene Capsules 1965

Probenecid (Reduces renal tubular transport). Products include:
- Benemid Tablets 1611
- ColBENEMID Tablets 1622

Procarbazine Hydrochloride (Combined use has not been studied and may increase the incidence of adverse effects). Products include:
- Matulane Capsules 2131

Salsalate (Increased toxicity). Products include:
- Mono-Gesic Tablets 792
- Salflex Tablets 786

Sulfamethizole (Increased toxicity). Products include:
- Urobiotic-250 Capsules 2214

Sulfamethoxazole (Increased toxicity). Products include:
- Azo Gantanol Tablets 2080
- Bactrim DS Tablets 2084
- Bactrim I.V. Infusion 2082
- Bactrim 2084
- Gantanol Tablets 2119
- Septra 1174
- Septra I.V. Infusion 1169
- Septra I.V. Infusion ADD-Vantage Vials 1171
- Septra 1174

Sulfasalazine (Increased toxicity). Products include:
- Azulfidine 1949

Sulfinpyrazone (Increased toxicity). Products include:
- Anturane 807

Sulfisoxazole (Increased toxicity). Products include:
- Azo Gantrisin Tablets 2081
- Gantrisin Tablets 2120

Sulfisoxazole Diolamine (Increased toxicity).
- No products indexed under this heading.

Sulindac (May elevate and prolong serum methotrexate levels; reduces the tubular secretion of methotrexate). Products include:
- Clinoril Tablets 1618

Tamoxifen Citrate (Combined use has not been studied and may increase the incidence of adverse effects). Products include:
- Nolvadex Tablets 2841

Tetracycline Hydrochloride (Decreases intestinal absorption and interferes with enterohepatic circulation). Products include:
- Achromycin V Capsules 1367

Tolmetin Sodium (May elevate and prolong serum methotrexate levels; reduces the tubular secretion of methotrexate). Products include:
- Tolectin (200, 400 and 600 mg) .. 1581

Trimethoprim (May increase bone marrow suppression). Products include:
- Bactrim DS Tablets 2084
- Bactrim I.V. Infusion 2082
- Bactrim 2084
- Proloprim Tablets 1155
- Septra 1174
- Septra I.V. Infusion 1169
- Septra I.V. Infusion ADD-Vantage Vials 1171
- Septra 1174
- Trimpex Tablets 2163

Vincristine Sulfate (Combined use has not been studied and may increase the incidence of adverse effects). Products include:
- Oncovin Solution Vials & Hyporets 1466

Food Interactions

Food, unspecified (Delays absorption and reduces peak concentration).

METRODIN (UROFOLLITROPIN FOR INJECTION)

(Urofollitropin) 2446

None cited in PDR database.

METROGEL

(Metronidazole) 1047

May interact with oral anticoagulants. Compounds in this category include:

Dicumarol (Prolonged prothrombin time and potentiation of oral anticoagulant with systemic metronidazole; the effect of topical metronidazole on prothrombin is unknown).
- No products indexed under this heading.

Warfarin Sodium (Prolonged prothrombin time and potentiation of oral anticoagulant with systemic metronidazole; the effect of topical metronidazole on prothrombin is unknown). Products include:
- Coumadin 926

METROGEL-VAGINAL

(Metronidazole) 902

May interact with oral anticoagulants and certain other agents. Compounds in these categories include:

Dicumarol (Oral metronidazole potentiates the anticoagulant effect of warfarin).
- No products indexed under this heading.

(▣ Described in PDR For Nonprescription Drugs) (⊙ Described in PDR For Ophthalmology)

Disulfiram (Psychotic reactions to oral metronidazole have been reported in alcoholics who are using metronidazole and disulfiram concurrently). Products include:

Antabuse Tablets 2695

Warfarin Sodium (Oral metronidazole potentiates the anticoagulant effect of warfarin). Products include:

Coumadin 926

Food Interactions

Alcohol (Possibility of a disulfiram-like reaction).

METUBINE IODIDE VIALS

(Metocurine Iodide) 916

May interact with general anesthetics, muscle relaxants, tetracyclines, and certain other agents. Compounds in these categories include:

Atracurium Besylate (Synergistic or antagonistic effect). Products include:

Tracrium Injection 1183

Bacitracin (Intensified or similar neuroblocking action). Products include:

Mycitracin ▣ 839

Baclofen (Synergistic or antagonistic effect). Products include:

Lioresal Intrathecal 1596
Lioresal Tablets 829

Carisoprodol (Synergistic or antagonistic effect). Products include:

Soma Compound w/Codeine Tablets 2676
Soma Compound Tablets 2675
Soma Tablets 2674

Chlorzoxazone (Synergistic or antagonistic effect). Products include:

Paraflex Caplets 1580
Parafon Forte DSC Caplets 1581

Colistimethate Sodium (Intensified or similar neuroblocking action). Products include:

Coly-Mycin M Parenteral 1905

Colistin Sulfate (Intensified or similar neuroblocking action). Products include:

Coly-Mycin S Otic w/Neomycin & Hydrocortisone 1906

Cyclobenzaprine Hydrochloride (Synergistic or antagonistic effect). Products include:

Flexeril Tablets 1661

Dantrolene Sodium (Synergistic or antagonistic effect). Products include:

Dantrium Capsules 1982
Dantrium Intravenous 1983

Demeclocycline Hydrochloride (Intensified or similar neuroblocking action). Products include:

Declomycin Tablets 1371

Diethyl Ether (Potentiation of neuromuscular blocking action of metubine iodide).

Doxacurium Chloride (Synergistic or antagonistic effect). Products include:

Nuromax Injection 1149

Doxycycline Calcium (Intensified or similar neuroblocking action). Products include:

Vibramycin Calcium Oral Suspension Syrup 1941

Doxycycline Hyclate (Intensified or similar neuroblocking action). Products include:

Doryx Capsules 1913
Vibramycin Hyclate Capsules 1941
Vibramycin Hyclate Intravenous 2215
Vibra-Tabs Film Coated Tablets 1941

Doxycycline Monohydrate (Intensified or similar neuroblocking action). Products include:

Monodox Capsules 1805
Vibramycin Monohydrate for Oral Suspension 1941

Enflurane (Synergistic action).

No products indexed under this heading.

Gentamicin Sulfate (Intensified or similar neuroblocking action). Products include:

Garamycin Injectable 2360
Genoptic Sterile Ophthalmic Solution ◉ 243
Genoptic Sterile Ophthalmic Ointment ◉ 243
Gentacidin Ointment ◉ 264
Gentacidin Solution ◉ 264
Gentak ◉ 208
Pred-G Liquifilm Sterile Ophthalmic Suspension ◉ 251
Pred-G S.O.P. Sterile Ophthalmic Ointment ◉ 252

Halothane (Potentiation of neuromuscular blocking action of metubine iodide). Products include:

Fluothane 2724

Isoflurane (Potentiation of neuromuscular blocking action of metubine iodide; synergistic action).

No products indexed under this heading.

Kanamycin Sulfate (Intensified or similar neuroblocking action).

No products indexed under this heading.

Magnesium Sulfate (Potentiation of both depolarizing and nondepolarizing drugs).

No products indexed under this heading.

Metaxalone (Synergistic or antagonistic effect). Products include:

Skelaxin Tablets 788

Methacycline Hydrochloride (Intensified or similar neuroblocking action).

No products indexed under this heading.

Methocarbamol (Synegistic or antagonistic effect). Products include:

Robaxin Injectable 2070
Robaxin Tablets 2071
Robaxisal Tablets 2071

Methohexital Sodium (Potentiation of neuromuscular action of metubine iodide; synergistic action). Products include:

Brevital Sodium Vials 1429

Methoxyflurane (Potentiation of neuromuscular action of metubine iodide; synergistic action).

No products indexed under this heading.

Minocycline Hydrochloride (Intensified or similar neuroblocking action). Products include:

Dynacin Capsules 1590
Minocin Intravenous 1382
Minocin Oral Suspension 1385
Minocin Pellet-Filled Capsules 1383

Neomycin Sulfate (Intensified or similar neuroblocking action). Products include:

AK-Spore ◉ 204
AK-Trol Ointment & Suspension ◉ 205
Bactine First Aid Antibiotic Plus Anesthetic Ointment ▣ 708
Campho-Phenique Maximum Strength First Aid Antibiotic Plus Pain Reliever Ointment ▣ 719
Coly-Mycin S Otic w/Neomycin & Hydrocortisone 1906
Cortisporin Cream 1084
Cortisporin Ointment 1085
Cortisporin Ophthalmic Ointment Sterile 1085
Cortisporin Ophthalmic Suspension Sterile 1086
Cortisporin Otic Solution Sterile 1087
Cortisporin Otic Suspension Sterile 1088
Dexacidin Ointment ◉ 263
Maxitrol Ophthalmic Ointment and Suspension ◉ 224
Mycitracin ▣ 839
NeoDecadron Sterile Ophthalmic Ointment 1712
NeoDecadron Sterile Ophthalmic Solution 1713
NeoDecadron Topical Cream 1714
Neosporin G.U. Irrigant Sterile 1148
Neosporin Ointment ▣ 857
Neosporin Plus Maximum Strength Cream ▣ 858
Neosporin Plus Maximum Strength Ointment ▣ 858
Neosporin Ophthalmic Ointment Sterile 1148
Neosporin Ophthalmic Solution Sterile 1149
PediOtic Suspension Sterile 1153
Poly-Pred Liquifilm ◉ 248

Orphenadrine Citrate (Synergistic or antagonistic effect). Products include:

Norflex 1496
Norgesic 1496

Oxytetracycline (Intensified or similar neuroblocking action). Products include:

Terramycin Intramuscular Solution 2210

Oxytetracycline Hydrochloride (Intensified or similar neuroblocking action). Products include:

TERAK Ointment ◉ 209
Terra-Cortril Ophthalmic Suspension 2210
Terramycin with Polymyxin B Sulfate Ophthalmic Ointment 2211
Urobiotic-250 Capsules 2214

Pancuronium Bromide Injection (Synergistic or antagonistic effect).

No products indexed under this heading.

Polymyxin B Sulfate (Intensified or similar neuroblocking action). Products include:

AK-Spore ◉ 204
AK-Trol Ointment & Suspension ◉ 205
Bactine First Aid Antibiotic Plus Anesthetic Ointment ▣ 708
Betadine Brand First Aid Antibiotics & Moisturizer Ointment 1991
Campho-Phenique Maximum Strength First Aid Antibiotic Plus Pain Reliever Ointment ▣ 719
Cortisporin Cream 1084
Cortisporin Ointment 1085
Cortisporin Ophthalmic Ointment Sterile 1085
Cortisporin Ophthalmic Suspension Sterile 1086
Cortisporin Otic Solution Sterile 1087
Cortisporin Otic Suspension Sterile 1088
Dexacidin Ointment ◉ 263
Maxitrol Ophthalmic Ointment and Suspension ◉ 224
Mycitracin ▣ 839
Neosporin G.U. Irrigant Sterile 1148
Neosporin Ointment ▣ 857
Neosporin Plus Maximum Strength Cream ▣ 858
Neosporin Plus Maximum Strength Ointment ▣ 858
Neosporin Ophthalmic Ointment Sterile 1148
Neosporin Ophthalmic Solution Sterile 1149
Ophthocort ◉ 311
PediOtic Suspension Sterile 1153
Polymyxin B Sulfate, Aerosporin Brand Sterile Powder 1154
Poly-Pred Liquifilm ◉ 248
Polysporin Ointment ▣ 858
Polysporin Ophthalmic Ointment Sterile 1154
Polysporin Powder ▣ 859
Polytrim Ophthalmic Solution Sterile 482
TERAK Ointment ◉ 209
Terramycin with Polymyxin B Sulfate Ophthalmic Ointment 2211

Propofol (Synergistic action). Products include:

Diprivan Injection 2833

Quinidine Gluconate (Recurrent paralysis). Products include:

Quinaglute Dura-Tabs Tablets 649

Quinidine Polygalacturonate (Recurrent paralysis).

No products indexed under this heading.

Quinidine Sulfate (Recurrent paralysis). Products include:

Quinidex Extentabs 2067

Rocuronium Bromide (Synergistic or antagonistic effect). Products include:

Zemuron 1830

Streptomycin Sulfate (Intensified or similar neuroblocking action). Products include:

Streptomycin Sulfate Injection 2208

Succinylcholine Chloride (Synergistic or antagonistic effect). Products include:

Anectine 1073

Tetracycline Hydrochloride (Intensified or similar neuroblocking action). Products include:

Achromycin V Capsules 1367

Vecuronium Bromide (Synergistic or antagonistic effect). Products include:

Norcuron 1826

MEVACOR TABLETS

(Lovastatin) 1699

May interact with immunosuppressive agents, fibrates, oral anticoagulants, and certain other agents. Compounds in these categories include:

Azathioprine (Potential for myopathy and/or markedly elevated CPK levels). Products include:

Imuran 1110

Clofibrate (Potential for myopathy and/or markedly elevated CPK levels). Products include:

Atromid-S Capsules 2701

Cyclosporine (Potential for myopathy, markedly elevated CPK levels and/or acute renal failure from rhabdomyolysis). Products include:

Neoral 2276
Sandimmune 2286

Dicumarol (Potential for clinically evident bleeding and/or increased prothrombin time).

No products indexed under this heading.

Erythromycin (Concomitant therapy in seriously ill patients may result in rhabdomyolysis with or without renal impairment). Products include:

A/T/S 2% Acne Topical Gel and Solution 1234
Benzamycin Topical Gel 905
E-Mycin Tablets 1341
Emgel 2% Topical Gel 1093
ERYC 1915
Erycette (erythromycin 2%) Topical Solution 1888
Ery-Tab Tablets 422
Erythromycin Base Filmtab 426
Erythromycin Delayed-Release Capsules, USP 427
Ilotycin Ophthalmic Ointment 912
PCE Dispertab Tablets 444
T-Stat 2.0% Topical Solution and Pads 2688
Theramycin Z Topical Solution 2% 1592

Erythromycin Estolate (Concomitant therapy in seriously ill patients may result in rhabdomyolysis with or without renal impairment). Products include:

Ilosone 911

IMPORTANT NOTE: Always consult each drug listing in the patient's regimen for possible interactions.

Erythromycin Ethylsuccinate (Concomitant therapy in seriously ill patients may result in rhabdomyolysis with or without renal impairment). Products include:
- E.E.S. 424
- EryPed 421

Erythromycin Gluceptate (Concomitant therapy in seriously ill patients may result in rhabdomyolysis with or without renal impairment). Products include:
- Ilotycin Gluceptate, IV, Vials 913

Erythromycin Stearate (Concomitant therapy in seriously ill patients may result in rhabdomyolysis with or without renal impairment). Products include:
- Erythrocin Stearate Filmtab 425

Gemfibrozil (Potential for myopathy, markedly elevated CPK levels and/or acute renal failure from rhabdomyolysis). Products include:
- Lopid Tablets 1917

Itraconazole (The HMG Coa reductase inhibitors and the azole derivatives antifungal agents inhibit cholesterol biosynthesis at different points in the biosynthesis pathway; potential for muscle weakness accompanied by marked elevation of creatine phosphokinase). Products include:
- Sporanox Capsules 1305

Muromonab-CD3 (Potential for myopathy and/or markedly elevated CPK levels). Products include:
- Orthoclone OKT3 Sterile Solution .. 1837

Mycophenolate Mofetil (Potential for myopathy and/or markedly elevated CPK levels). Products include:
- CellCept Capsules 2099

Nicotinic Acid (Potential for myopathy and/or markedly elevated CPK levels with lipid-lowering doses of nicotinic acid).
- No products indexed under this heading.

Tacrolimus (Potential for myopathy and/or markedly elevated CPK levels). Products include:
- Prograf 1042

Warfarin Sodium (Potential for clinically evident bleeding and/or increased prothrombin time). Products include:
- Coumadin 926

Food Interactions

Alcohol (Increased potential for liver dysfunction in patients who consume substantial quantity of alcohol).

MEXITIL CAPSULES

(Mexiletine Hydrochloride) 678

May interact with narcotic analgesics and certain other agents. Compounds in these categories include:

Alfentanil Hydrochloride (Narcotics slow the absorption of Mexitil). Products include:
- Alfenta Injection 1286

Atropine Sulfate (Slows the absorption of Mexitil). Products include:
- Arco-Lase Plus Tablets 512
- Atrohist Plus Tablets 454
- Atropine Sulfate Sterile Ophthalmic Solution .... ⊙ 233
- Donnatal 2060
- Donnatal Extentabs 2061
- Donnatal Tablets 2060
- Lomotil 2439
- Motofen Tablets 784
- Urised Tablets 1964

Buprenorphine (Narcotics slow the absorption of Mexitil). Products include:
- Buprenex Injectable 2006

Caffeine-containing medications (Caffeine clearance decreased 50%).

Cimetidine (May alter Mexitil plasma levels). Products include:
- Tagamet Tablets 2516

Cimetidine Hydrochloride (May alter Mexitil plasma levels). Products include:
- Tagamet 2516

Codeine Phosphate (Narcotics slow the absorption of Mexitil). Products include:
- Actifed with Codeine Cough Syrup .. 1067
- Brontex 1981
- Deconsal C Expectorant Syrup 456
- Deconsal Pediatric Syrup 457
- Dimetane-DC Cough Syrup 2059
- Empirin with Codeine Tablets 1093
- Fioricet with Codeine Capsules 2260
- Fiorinal with Codeine Capsules 2262
- Isoclor Expectorant 990
- Novahistine DH 2462
- Novahistine Expectorant 2463
- Nucofed 2051
- Phenergan with Codeine 2777
- Phenergan VC with Codeine 2781
- Robitussin A-C Syrup 2073
- Robitussin-DAC Syrup 2074
- Ryna .... ⊡ 841
- Soma Compound w/Codeine Tablets 2676
- Tussi-Organidin NR Liquid and S NR Liquid 2677
- Tylenol with Codeine 1583

Dezocine (Narcotics slow the absorption of Mexitil). Products include:
- Dalgan Injection 538

Digoxin (Lowered serum digoxin levels in presence of magnesium-aluminum hydroxide). Products include:
- Lanoxicaps 1117
- Lanoxin Elixir Pediatric 1120
- Lanoxin Injection 1123
- Lanoxin Injection Pediatric 1126
- Lanoxin Tablets 1128

Fentanyl (Narcotics slow the absorption of Mexitil). Products include:
- Duragesic Transdermal System 1288

Fentanyl Citrate (Narcotics slow the absorption of Mexitil). Products include:
- Sublimaze Injection 1307

Hydrocodone Bitartrate (Narcotics slow the absorption of Mexitil). Products include:
- Anexsia 5/500 Elixir 1781
- Anexia Tablets 1782
- Codiclear DH Syrup 791
- Deconamine CX Cough and Cold Liquid and Tablets 1319
- Duratuss HD Elixir 2565
- Hycodan Tablets and Syrup 930
- Hycomine Compound Tablets 932
- Hycomine 931
- Hycotuss Expectorant Syrup 933
- Hydrocet Capsules 782
- Lorcet 10/650 1018
- Lortab 2566
- Tussend 1783
- Tussend Expectorant 1785
- Vicodin Tablets 1356
- Vicodin ES Tablets 1357
- Vicodin Tuss Expectorant 1358
- Zydone Capsules 949

Hydrocodone Polistirex (Narcotics slow the absorption of Mexitil). Products include:
- Tussionex Pennkinetic Extended-Release Suspension 998

Levorphanol Tartrate (Narcotics slow the absorption of Mexitil). Products include:
- Levo-Dromoran 2129

Magaldrate (Slows the absorption of Mexitil).
- No products indexed under this heading.

Meperidine Hydrochloride (Narcotics slow the absorption of Mexitil). Products include:
- Demerol 2308
- Mepergan Injection 2753

Methadone Hydrochloride (Narcotics slow the absorption of Mexitil). Products include:
- Methadone Hydrochloride Oral Concentrate 2233
- Methadone Hydrochloride Oral Solution & Tablets 2235

Metoclopramide Hydrochloride (Accelerates the absorption). Products include:
- Reglan 2068

Morphine Sulfate (Narcotics slow the absorption of Mexitil). Products include:
- Astramorph/PF Injection, USP (Preservative-Free) 535
- Duramorph 962
- Infumorph 200 and Infumorph 500 Sterile Solutions 965
- MS Contin Tablets 1994
- MSIR 1997
- Oramorph SR (Morphine Sulfate Sustained Release Tablets) 2236
- RMS Suppositories 2657
- Roxanol 2243

Opium Alkaloids (Narcotics slow the absorption of Mexitil).
- No products indexed under this heading.

Oxycodone Hydrochloride (Narcotics slow the absorption of Mexitil). Products include:
- Percocet Tablets 938
- Percodan Tablets 939
- Percodan-Demi Tablets 940
- Roxicodone Tablets, Oral Solution & Intensol (Oxycodone) 2244
- Tylox Capsules 1584

Phenobarbital (Lowers Mexitil plasma levels). Products include:
- Arco-Lase Plus Tablets 512
- Bellergal-S Tablets 2250
- Donnatal 2060
- Donnatal Extentabs 2061
- Donnatal Tablets 2060
- Phenobarbital Elixir and Tablets 1469
- Quadrinal Tablets 1350

Phenytoin (Lowers Mexitil plasma levels). Products include:
- Dilantin Infatabs 1908
- Dilantin-125 Suspension 1911

Phenytoin Sodium (Lowers Mexitil plasma levels). Products include:
- Dilantin Kapseals 1906
- Dilantin Parenteral 1910

Propoxyphene Hydrochloride (Narcotics slow the absorption of Mexitil). Products include:
- Darvon 1435
- Wygesic Tablets 2827

Propoxyphene Napsylate (Narcotics slow the absorption of Mexitil). Products include:
- Darvon-N/Darvocet-N 1433

Rifampin (Lowers Mexitil plasma levels). Products include:
- Rifadin 1528
- Rifamate Capsules 1530
- Rifater 1532
- Rimactane Capsules 847

Sufentanil Citrate (Narcotics slow the absorption of Mexitil). Products include:
- Sufenta Injection 1309

Theophylline (Potential for increased plasma theophylline levels). Products include:
- Marax Tablets & DF Syrup 2200
- Quibron 2053

Theophylline Anhydrous (Potential for increased plasma theophylline levels). Products include:
- Aerolate 1004
- Primatene Dual Action Formula .... ⊡ 872
- Primatene Tablets .... ⊡ 873
- Respbid Tablets 682
- Slo-bid Gyrocaps 2033
- Theo-24 Extended Release Capsules 2568
- Theo-Dur Extended-Release Tablets 1327
- Theo-X Extended-Release Tablets .. 788
- Uni-Dur Extended-Release Tablets .. 1331
- Uniphyl 400 mg Tablets 2001

Theophylline Calcium Salicylate (Potential for increased plasma theophylline levels). Products include:
- Quadrinal Tablets 1350

Theophylline Sodium Glycinate (Potential for increased plasma theophylline levels).
- No products indexed under this heading.

MEZLIN

(Mezlocillin Sodium) 601

May interact with aminoglycosides and certain other agents. Compounds in these categories include:

Amikacin Sulfate (Physical incompatibility resulting in substantial inactivation of the aminoglycoside). Products include:
- Amikacin Sulfate Injection, USP 960
- Amikin Injectable 501

Gentamicin Sulfate (Physical incompatibility resulting in substantial inactivation of the aminoglycoside). Products include:
- Garamycin Injectable 2360
- Genoptic Sterile Ophthalmic Solution .... ⊙ 243
- Genoptic Sterile Ophthalmic Ointment .... ⊙ 243
- Gentacidin Ointment .... ⊙ 264
- Gentacidin Solution .... ⊙ 264
- Gentak .... ⊙ 208
- Pred-G Liquifilm Sterile Ophthalmic Suspension .... ⊙ 251
- Pred-G S.O.P. Sterile Ophthalmic Ointment .... ⊙ 252

Kanamycin Sulfate (Physical incompatibility resulting in substantial inactivation of the aminoglycoside).
- No products indexed under this heading.

Probenecid (Increased serum concentrations and prolonged serum half-life of mezlocillin). Products include:
- Benemid Tablets 1611
- ColBENEMID Tablets 1622

Streptomycin Sulfate (Physical incompatibility resulting in substantial inactivation of the aminoglycoside). Products include:
- Streptomycin Sulfate Injection 2208

Tobramycin Sulfate (Physical incompatibility resulting in substantial inactivation of the aminoglycoside). Products include:
- Nebcin Vials, Hyporets & ADD-Vantage 1464
- Tobramycin Sulfate Injection 968

MEZLIN PHARMACY BULK PACKAGE

(Mezlocillin Sodium) 604

May interact with:

Probenecid (Prolongs serum half-life of antibiotic). Products include:
- Benemid Tablets 1611
- ColBENEMID Tablets 1622

MIACALCIN INJECTION

(Calcitonin, Synthetic) 2273

None cited in PDR database.

(⊡ Described in PDR For Nonprescription Drugs) (⊙ Described in PDR For Ophthalmology)

MIACALCIN NASAL SPRAY

(Calcitonin-Salmon) 2275

May interact with:

Etidronate Disodium (Diphosphonate) (Prior diphosphonate use may reduce the anti-resorptive response to calcitonin-salmon nasal spray).

Pamidronate Disodium (Prior diphosphonate use may reduce the anti-resorptive response to calcitonin-salmon nasal spray). Products include:

Aredia for Injection 810

MICRO-K EXTENCAPS

(Potassium Chloride) 2063

May interact with potassium sparing diuretics, ACE inhibitors, and anticholinergics. Compounds in these categories include:

Amiloride Hydrochloride (Simultaneous administration can produce severe hyperkalemia). Products include:

Midamor Tablets 1703
Moduretic Tablets 1705

Atropine Sulfate (Anticholinergic drugs can be cause for delay or arrest in tablet passage through the gastrointestinal tract; concomitant administration of drugs capable of decreasing GI motility should be avoided). Products include:

Arco-Lase Plus Tablets 512
Atrohist Plus Tablets 454
Atropine Sulfate Sterile Ophthalmic Solution .... ⊛ 233
Donnatal 2060
Donnatal Extentabs.................................. 2061
Donnatal Tablets 2060
Lomotil 2439
Motofen Tablets 784
Urised Tablets... 1964

Belladonna Alkaloids (Anticholinergic drugs can be cause for delay or arrest in tablet passage through the gastrointestinal tract; concomitant administration of drugs capable of decreasing GI motility should be avoided). Products include:

Bellergal-S Tablets 2250
Hyland's Bed Wetting Tablets ....ᴴᴰ 828
Hyland's EnurAid Tablets...................ᴴᴰ 829
Hyland's Teething Tablets ....ᴴᴰ 830

Benazepril Hydrochloride (Potential for hyperkalemia). Products include:

Lotensin Tablets....................................... 834
Lotensin HCT... 837
Lotrel Capsules 840

Benztropine Mesylate (Anticholinergic drugs can be cause for delay or arrest in tablet passage through the gastrointestinal tract; concomitant administration of drugs capable of decreasing GI motility should be avoided). Products include:

Cogentin 1621

Biperiden Hydrochloride (Anticholinergic drugs can be cause for delay or arrest in tablet passage through the gastrointestinal tract; concomitant administration of drugs capable of decreasing GI motility should be avoided). Products include:

Akineton 1333

Captopril (Potential for hyperkalemia). Products include:

Capoten 739
Capozide 742

Clidinium Bromide (Anticholinergic drugs can be cause for delay or arrest in tablet passage through the gastrointestinal tract; concomitant administration of drugs capable of decreasing GI motility should be avoided). Products include:

Librax Capsules 2176
Quarzan Capsules 2181

Dicyclomine Hydrochloride (Anticholinergic drugs can be cause for delay or arrest in tablet passage through the gastrointestinal tract; concomitant administration of drugs capable of decreasing GI motility should be avoided). Products include:

Bentyl 1501

Enalapril Maleate (Potential for hyperkalemia). Products include:

Vaseretic Tablets 1765
Vasotec Tablets 1771

Enalaprilat (Potential for hyperkalemia). Products include:

Vasotec I.V.. 1768

Fosinopril Sodium (Potential for hyperkalemia). Products include:

Monopril Tablets 757

Glycopyrrolate (Anticholinergic drugs can be cause for delay or arrest in tablet passage through the gastrointestinal tract; concomitant administration of drugs capable of decreasing GI motility should be avoided). Products include:

Robinul Forte Tablets............................... 2072
Robinul Injectable 2072
Robinul Tablets... 2072

Hyoscyamine (Anticholinergic drugs can be cause for delay or arrest in tablet passage through the gastrointestinal tract; concomitant administration of drugs capable of decreasing GI motility should be avoided). Products include:

Cystospaz Tablets..................................... 1963
Urised Tablets... 1964

Hyoscyamine Sulfate (Anticholinergic drugs can be cause for delay or arrest in tablet passage through the gastrointestinal tract; concomitant administration of drugs capable of decreasing GI motility should be avoided). Products include:

Arco-Lase Plus Tablets 512
Atrohist Plus Tablets 454
Cystospaz-M Capsules 1963
Donnatal 2060
Donnatal Extentabs.................................. 2061
Donnatal Tablets 2060
Kutrase Capsules...................................... 2402
Levsin/Levsinex/Levbid 2405

Ipratropium Bromide (Anticholinergic drugs can be cause for delay or arrest in tablet passage through the gastrointestinal tract; concomitant administration of drugs capable of decreasing GI motility should be avoided). Products include:

Atrovent Inhalation Aerosol.................... 671
Atrovent Inhalation Solution 673

Lisinopril (Potential for hyperkalemia). Products include:

Prinivil Tablets 1733
Prinzide Tablets 1737
Zestoretic 2850
Zestril Tablets 2854

Mepenzolate Bromide (Anticholinergic drugs can be cause for delay or arrest in tablet passage through the gastrointestinal tract; concomitant administration of drugs capable of decreasing GI motility should be avoided).

No products indexed under this heading.

Moexipril Hydrochloride (Potential for hyperkalemia). Products include:

Univasc Tablets 2410

Oxybutynin Chloride (Anticholinergic drugs can be cause for delay or arrest in tablet passage through the gastrointestinal tract; concomitant administration of drugs capable of decreasing GI motility should be avoided). Products include:

Ditropan... 1516

Procyclidine Hydrochloride (Anticholinergic drugs can be cause for delay or arrest in tablet passage through the gastrointestinal tract; concomitant administration of drugs capable of decreasing GI motility should be avoided). Products include:

Kemadrin Tablets 1112

Propantheline Bromide (Anticholinergic drugs can be cause for delay or arrest in tablet passage through the gastrointestinal tract; concomitant administration of drugs capable of decreasing GI motility should be avoided). Products include:

Pro-Banthine Tablets 2052

Quinapril Hydrochloride (Potential for hyperkalemia). Products include:

Accupril Tablets 1893

Ramipril (Potential for hyperkalemia). Products include:

Altace Capsules 1232

Scopolamine (Anticholinergic drugs can be cause for delay or arrest in tablet passage through the gastrointestinal tract; concomitant administration of drugs capable of decreasing GI motility should be avoided). Products include:

Transderm Scōp Transdermal Therapeutic System 869

Scopolamine Hydrobromide (Anticholinergic drugs can be cause for delay or arrest in tablet passage through the gastrointestinal tract; concomitant administration of drugs capable of decreasing GI motility should be avoided). Products include:

Atrohist Plus Tablets 454
Donnatal 2060
Donnatal Extentabs.................................. 2061
Donnatal Tablets 2060

Spirapril Hydrochloride (Potential for hyperkalemia).

No products indexed under this heading.

Spironolactone (Simultaneous administration can produce severe hyperkalemia). Products include:

Aldactazide.. 2413
Aldactone 2414

Triamterene (Simultaneous administration can produce severe hyperkalemia). Products include:

Dyazide 2479
Dyrenium Capsules.................................. 2481
Maxzide 1380

Tridihexethyl Chloride (Anticholinergic drugs can be cause for delay or arrest in tablet passage through the gastrointestinal tract; concomitant administration of drugs capable of decreasing GI motility should be avoided).

No products indexed under this heading.

Trihexyphenidyl Hydrochloride (Anticholinergic drugs can be cause for delay or arrest in tablet passage through the gastrointestinal tract; concomitant administration of drugs capable of decreasing GI motility should be avoided). Products include:

Artane.. 1368

MICRO-K 10 EXTENCAPS

(Potassium Chloride)...............................2063

See Micro-K Extencaps

MICRO-K LS PACKETS

(Potassium Chloride)...............................2064

May interact with potassium sparing diuretics and ACE inhibitors. Compounds in these categories include:

Amiloride Hydrochloride (Simultaneous administration can produce severe hyperkalemia). Products include:

Midamor Tablets 1703
Moduretic Tablets 1705

Benazepril Hydrochloride (Potential for hyperkalemia). Products include:

Lotensin Tablets....................................... 834
Lotensin HCT... 837
Lotrel Capsules 840

Captopril (Potential for hyperkalemia). Products include:

Capoten 739
Capozide 742

Enalapril Maleate (Potential for hyperkalemia). Products include:

Vaseretic Tablets 1765
Vasotec Tablets 1771

Enalaprilat (Potential for hyperkalemia). Products include:

Vasotec I.V.. 1768

Fosinopril Sodium (Potential for hyperkalemia). Products include:

Monopril Tablets 757

Lisinopril (Potential for hyperkalemia). Products include:

Prinivil Tablets 1733
Prinzide Tablets 1737
Zestoretic 2850
Zestril Tablets 2854

Moexipril Hydrochloride (Potential for hyperkalemia). Products include:

Univasc Tablets 2410

Quinapril Hydrochloride (Potential for hyperkalemia). Products include:

Accupril Tablets 1893

Ramipril (Potential for hyperkalemia). Products include:

Altace Capsules 1232

Spirapril Hydrochloride (Potential for hyperkalemia).

No products indexed under this heading.

Spironolactone (Simultaneous administration can produce severe hyperkalemia). Products include:

Aldactazide.. 2413
Aldactone 2414

Triamterene (Simultaneous administration can produce severe hyperkalemia). Products include:

Dyazide 2479
Dyrenium Capsules.................................. 2481
Maxzide 1380

MICRONASE TABLETS

(Glyburide) 2623

May interact with beta blockers, salicylates, non-steroidal anti-inflammatory agents, sulfonamides, oral anticoagulants, monoamine oxidase inhibitors, thiazides, potassium sparing diuretics, estrogens, phenothiazines, corticosteroids, oral contraceptives, sympathomimetics, calcium channel blockers, diuretics,

IMPORTANT NOTE: Always consult each drug listing in the patient's regimen for possible interactions.

Micronase Interactions Index 654

thyroid preparations, and certain other agents. Compounds in these categories include:

Acebutolol Hydrochloride (Hypoglycemic action potentiated). Products include:
Sectral Capsules 2807

Albuterol (Hyperglycemia). Products include:
Proventil Inhalation Aerosol 2382
Ventolin Inhalation Aerosol and Refill 1197

Albuterol Sulfate (Hyperglycemia). Products include:
Airet Solution for Inhalation 452
Proventil Inhalation Solution 0.083% 2384
Proventil Repetabs Tablets 2386
Proventil Solution for Inhalation 0.5% 2383
Proventil Syrup 2385
Proventil Tablets 2386
Ventolin Inhalation Solution 1198
Ventolin Nebules Inhalation Solution 1199
Ventolin Rotacaps for Inhalation 1200
Ventolin Syrup 1202
Ventolin Tablets 1203
Volmax Extended-Release Tablets 1788

Amiloride Hydrochloride (Hyperglycemia). Products include:
Midamor Tablets 1703
Moduretic Tablets 1705

Amlodipine Besylate (Hyperglycemia). Products include:
Lotrel Capsules 840
Norvasc Tablets 1940

Aspirin (Hypoglycemic action potentiated). Products include:
Alka-Seltzer Effervescent Antacid and Pain Reliever .... ▣ 701
Alka-Seltzer Extra Strength Effervescent Antacid and Pain Reliever .... ▣ 703
Alka-Seltzer Lemon Lime Effervescent Antacid and Pain Reliever .... ▣ 703
Alka-Seltzer Plus Cold Medicine .... ▣ 705
Alka-Seltzer Plus Cold & Cough Medicine .... ▣ 708
Alka-Seltzer Plus Night-Time Cold Medicine .... ▣ 707
Alka Seltzer Plus Sinus Medicine .... ▣ 707
Arthritis Foundation Safety Coated Aspirin Tablets .... ▣ 675
Arthritis Pain Ascriptin .... ▣ 631
Maximum Strength Ascriptin .... ▣ 630
Regular Strength Ascriptin Tablets .... ▣ 629
Arthritis Strength BC Powder .... ▣ 609
BC Cold Powder Multi-Symptom Formula (Cold-Sinus-Allergy) .... ▣ 609
BC Cold Powder Non-Drowsy Formula (Cold-Sinus) .... ▣ 609
BC Powder .... ▣ 609
Bayer Children's Chewable Aspirin .... ▣ 711
Genuine Bayer Aspirin Tablets & Caplets .... ▣ 713
Extra Strength Bayer Arthritis Pain Regimen Formula .... ▣ 711
Extra Strength Bayer Aspirin Caplets & Tablets .... ▣ 712
Extended-Release Bayer 8-Hour Aspirin .... ▣ 712
Extra Strength Bayer Plus Aspirin Caplets .... ▣ 713
Extra Strength Bayer PM Aspirin .... ▣ 713
Bayer Enteric Aspirin .... ▣ 709
Bufferin Analgesic Tablets and Caplets .... ▣ 613
Arthritis Strength Bufferin Analgesic Caplets .... ▣ 614
Extra Strength Bufferin Analgesic Tablets .... ▣ 615
Cama Arthritis Pain Reliever .... ▣ 785
Darvon Compound-65 Pulvules 1435
Easprin 1914
Ecotrin 2455
Ecotrin Enteric Coated Aspirin Maximum Strength Tablets and Caplets .... ▣ 816
Ecotrin Enteric Coated Aspirin Regular Strength Tablets 2455
Empirin Aspirin Tablets .... ▣ 854
Empirin with Codeine Tablets 1093
Excedrin Extra-Strength Analgesic Tablets & Caplets 732
Fiorinal Capsules 2261
Fiorinal with Codeine Capsules 2262
Fiorinal Tablets 2261
Halfprin 1362
Healthprin Aspirin 2455
Norgesic 1496
Percodan Tablets 939
Percodan-Demi Tablets 940
Robaxisal Tablets 2071
Soma Compound w/Codeine Tablets 2676
Soma Compound Tablets 2675
St. Joseph Adult Chewable Aspirin (81 mg.) .... ▣ 808
Talwin Compound 2335
Ursinus Inlay-Tabs .... ▣ 794
Vanquish Analgesic Caplets .... ▣ 731

Atenolol (Hypoglycemic action potentiated). Products include:
Tenoretic Tablets 2845
Tenormin Tablets and I.V. Injection 2847

Bendroflumethiazide (Thiazides tend to produce hyperglycemia and may lead to loss of control on concurrent use).
No products indexed under this heading.

Bepridil Hydrochloride (Hyperglycemia). Products include:
Vascor (200, 300 and 400 mg) Tablets 1587

Betamethasone Acetate (Hyperglycemia). Products include:
Celestone Soluspan Suspension 2347

Betamethasone Sodium Phosphate (Hyperglycemia). Products include:
Celestone Soluspan Suspension 2347

Betaxolol Hydrochloride (Hypoglycemic action potentiated). Products include:
Betoptic Ophthalmic Solution 469
Betoptic S Ophthalmic Suspension 471
Kerlone Tablets 2436

Bisoprolol Fumarate (Hypoglycemic action potentiated). Products include:
Zebeta Tablets 1413
Ziac 1415

Bumetanide (Hyperglycemia). Products include:
Bumex 2093

Carteolol Hydrochloride (Hypoglycemic action potentiated). Products include:
Cartrol Tablets 410
Ocupress Ophthalmic Solution, 1% Sterile .... ⊙ 309

Chloramphenicol (Hypoglycemic action potentiated). Products include:
Chloromycetin Ophthalmic Ointment, 1% .... ⊙ 310
Chloromycetin Ophthalmic Solution .... ⊙ 310
Chloroptic S.O.P. .... ⊙ 239
Chloroptic Sterile Ophthalmic Solution .... ⊙ 239
Elase-Chloromycetin Ointment 1040
Ophthocort .... ⊙ 311

Chloramphenicol Palmitate (Hypoglycemic action potentiated).
No products indexed under this heading.

Chloramphenicol Sodium Succinate (Hypoglycemic action potentiated). Products include:
Chloromycetin Sodium Succinate 1900

Chlorothiazide (Thiazides tend to produce hyperglycemia and may lead to loss of control on concurrent use). Products include:
Aldoclor Tablets 1598
Diupres Tablets 1650
Diuril Oral 1653

Chlorothiazide Sodium (Thiazides tend to produce hyperglycemia and may lead to loss of control on concurrent use). Products include:
Diuril Sodium Intravenous 1652

Chlorotrianisene (Hyperglycemia).
No products indexed under this heading.

Chlorpromazine (Hyperglycemia). Products include:
Thorazine Suppositories 2523

Chlorpromazine Hydrochloride (Hypoglycemic action potentiated). Products include:
Thorazine 2523

Chlorpropamide (Hypoglycemic action potentiated). Products include:
Diabinese Tablets 1935

Chlorthalidone (Hyperglycemia). Products include:
Combipres Tablets 677
Tenoretic Tablets 2845
Thalitone 1245

Choline Magnesium Trisalicylate (Hypoglycemic action potentiated). Products include:
Trilisate 2000

Ciprofloxacin (Potentiation of the hypoglycemic action). Products include:
Cipro I.V. 595
Cipro I.V. Pharmacy Bulk Package 597

Ciprofloxacin Hydrochloride (Potentiation of the hypoglycemic action). Products include:
Ciloxan Ophthalmic Solution 472
Cipro Tablets 592

Cortisone Acetate (Hyperglycemia). Products include:
Cortone Acetate Sterile Suspension 1623
Cortone Acetate Tablets 1624

Desogestrel (Hyperglycemia). Products include:
Desogen Tablets 1817
Ortho-Cept 1851

Dexamethasone (Hyperglycemia). Products include:
AK-Trol Ointment & Suspension .... ⊙ 205
Decadron Elixir 1633
Decadron Tablets 1635
Decaspray Topical Aerosol 1648
Dexacidin Ointment .... ⊙ 263
Maxitrol Ophthalmic Ointment and Suspension .... ⊙ 224
TobraDex Ophthalmic Suspension and Ointment 473

Dexamethasone Acetate (Hyperglycemia). Products include:
Dalalone D.P. Injectable 1011
Decadron-LA Sterile Suspension 1646

Dexamethasone Sodium Phosphate (Hyperglycemia). Products include:
Decadron Phosphate Injection 1637
Decadron Phosphate Respihaler 1642
Decadron Phosphate Sterile Ophthalmic Ointment 1641
Decadron Phosphate Sterile Ophthalmic Solution 1642
Decadron Phosphate Topical Cream 1644
Decadron Phosphate Turbinaire 1645
Decadron Phosphate with Xylocaine Injection, Sterile 1639
Dexacort Phosphate in Respihaler 458
Dexacort Phosphate in Turbinaire 459
NeoDecadron Sterile Ophthalmic Ointment 1712
NeoDecadron Sterile Ophthalmic Solution 1713
NeoDecadron Topical Cream 1714

Diclofenac Potassium (Hypoglycemic action potentiated; hyperglycemia). Products include:
Cataflam 816

Diclofenac Sodium (Hypoglycemic action potentiated; hyperglycemia). Products include:
Voltaren Ophthalmic Sterile Ophthalmic Solution .... ⊙ 272
Voltaren Tablets 861

Dicumarol (Hypoglycemic action potentiated).
No products indexed under this heading.

Dienestrol (Hyperglycemia). Products include:
Ortho Dienestrol Cream 1866

Diethylstilbestrol (Hyperglycemia). Products include:
Diethylstilbestrol Tablets 1437

Diflunisal (Hypoglycemic action potentiated). Products include:
Dolobid Tablets 1654

Diltiazem Hydrochloride (Hyperglycemia). Products include:
Cardizem CD Capsules 1506
Cardizem SR Capsules 1510
Cardizem Injectable 1508
Cardizem Tablets 1512
Dilacor XR Extended-release Capsules 2018

Dobutamine Hydrochloride (Hyperglycemia). Products include:
Dobutrex Solution Vials 1439

Dopamine Hydrochloride (Hyperglycemia).
No products indexed under this heading.

Ephedrine Hydrochloride (Hyperglycemia). Products include:
Primatene Dual Action Formula .... ▣ 872
Primatene Tablets .... ▣ 873
Quadrinal Tablets 1350

Ephedrine Sulfate (Hyperglycemia). Products include:
Bronkaid Caplets .... ▣ 717
Marax Tablets & DF Syrup 2200

Ephedrine Tannate (Hyperglycemia). Products include:
Rynatuss 2673

Epinephrine (Hyperglycemia). Products include:
Bronkaid Mist .... ▣ 717
EPIFRIN .... ⊙ 239
EpiPen 790
Marcaine Hydrochloride with Epinephrine 1:200,000 2316
Primatene Mist .... ▣ 873
Sensorcaine with Epinephrine Injection 559
Sus-Phrine Injection 1019
Xylocaine with Epinephrine Injections 567

Epinephrine Bitartrate (Hyperglycemia). Products include:
Bronkaid Mist Suspension .... ▣ 718
Sensorcaine-MPF with Epinephrine Injection 559

Epinephrine Hydrochloride (Hyperglycemia). Products include:
Ana-Kit Anaphylaxis Emergency Treatment Kit 617

Esmolol Hydrochloride (Hypoglycemic action potentiated). Products include:
Brevibloc Injection 1808

Estradiol (Hyperglycemia). Products include:
Climara Transdermal System 645
Estrace Cream and Tablets 749
Estraderm Transdermal System 824

Estrogens, Conjugated (Hyperglycemia). Products include:
PMB 200 and PMB 400 2783
Premarin Intravenous 2787
Premarin with Methyltestosterone 2794
Premarin Tablets 2789
Premarin Vaginal Cream 2791
Premphase 2797
Prempro 2801

Estrogens, Esterified (Hyperglycemia). Products include:
ESTRATAB Tablets (0.3, 0.625, 1.25, 2.5 mg) 2536
Estratest 2539
Menest Tablets 2494

Estropipate (Hyperglycemia). Products include:
Ogen Tablets 2627
Ogen Vaginal Cream 2630
Ortho-Est 1869

(▣ Described in PDR For Nonprescription Drugs) (⊙ Described in PDR For Ophthalmology)

Ethacrynic Acid (Hyperglycemia). Products include:
- Edecrin Tablets ... 1657

Ethinyl Estradiol (Hyperglycemia). Products include:
- Brevicon ... 2088
- Demulen ... 2428
- Desogen Tablets ... 1817
- Levlen/Tri-Levlen ... 651
- Lo/Ovral Tablets ... 2746
- Lo/Ovral-28 Tablets ... 2751
- Modicon ... 1872
- Nordette-21 Tablets ... 2755
- Nordette-28 Tablets ... 2758
- Norinyl ... 2088
- Ortho-Cept ... 1851
- Ortho-Cyclen/Ortho-Tri-Cyclen ... 1858
- Ortho-Novum ... 1872
- Ortho-Cyclen/Ortho Tri-Cyclen ... 1858
- Ovcon ... 760
- Ovral Tablets ... 2770
- Ovral-28 Tablets ... 2770
- Levlen/Tri-Levlen ... 651
- Tri-Norinyl ... 2164
- Triphasil-21 Tablets ... 2814
- Triphasil-28 Tablets ... 2819

Ethynodiol Diacetate (Hyperglycemia). Products include:
- Demulen ... 2428

Etodolac (Hypoglycemic action potentiated; hyperglycemia). Products include:
- Lodine Capsules and Tablets ... 2743

Felodipine (Hyperglycemia). Products include:
- Plendil Extended-Release Tablets ... 527

Fenoprofen Calcium (Hypoglycemic action potentiated). Products include:
- Nalfon 200 Pulvules & Nalfon Tablets ... 917

Fludrocortisone Acetate (Hyperglycemia). Products include:
- Florinef Acetate Tablets ... 505

Fluphenazine Decanoate (Hyperglycemia). Products include:
- Prolixin Decanoate ... 509

Fluphenazine Enanthate (Hyperglycemia). Products include:
- Prolixin Enanthate ... 509

Fluphenazine Hydrochloride (Hyperglycemia). Products include:
- Prolixin ... 509

Flurbiprofen (Hypoglycemic action potentiated). Products include:
- Ansaid Tablets ... 2579

Furazolidone (Hypoglycemic action potentiated). Products include:
- Furoxone ... 2046

Furosemide (Hyperglycemia). Products include:
- Lasix Injection, Oral Solution and Tablets ... 1240

Glipizide (Hypoglycemic action potentiated). Products include:
- Glucotrol Tablets ... 1967
- Glucotrol XL Extended Release Tablets ... 1968

Hydrochlorothiazide (Thiazides tend to produce hyperglycemia and may lead to loss of control on concurrent use). Products include:
- Aldactazide ... 2413
- Aldoril Tablets ... 1604
- Apresazide Capsules ... 808
- Capozide ... 742
- Dyazide ... 2479
- Esidrix Tablets ... 821
- Esimil Tablets ... 822
- HydroDIURIL Tablets ... 1674
- Hydropres Tablets ... 1675
- Hyzaar Tablets ... 1677
- Inderide Tablets ... 2732
- Inderide LA Long Acting Capsules ... 2734
- Lopressor HCT Tablets ... 832
- Lotensin HCT ... 837
- Maxzide ... 1380
- Moduretic Tablets ... 1705
- Oretic Tablets ... 443
- Prinzide Tablets ... 1737
- Ser-Ap-Es Tablets ... 849
- Timolide Tablets ... 1748
- Vaseretic Tablets ... 1765
- Zestoretic ... 2850
- Ziac ... 1415

Hydrocortisone (Hyperglycemia). Products include:
- Anusol-HC Cream 2.5% ... 1896
- Aquanil HC Lotion ... 1931
- Bactine Hydrocortisone Anti-Itch Cream ... ◘ 709
- Caldecort Anti-Itch Hydrocortisone Spray ... ◘ 631
- Cortaid ... ◘ 836
- CORTENEMA ... 2535
- Cortisporin Ointment ... 1085
- Cortisporin Ophthalmic Ointment Sterile ... 1085
- Cortisporin Ophthalmic Suspension Sterile ... 1086
- Cortisporin Otic Solution Sterile ... 1087
- Cortisporin Otic Suspension Sterile ... 1088
- Cortizone-5 ... ◘ 831
- Cortizone-10 ... ◘ 831
- Hydrocortone Tablets ... 1672
- Hytone ... 907
- Massengill Medicated Soft Cloth Towelettes ... 2458
- PediOtic Suspension Sterile ... 1153
- Preparation H Hydrocortisone 1% Cream ... ◘ 872
- ProctoCream-HC 2.5% ... 2408
- VõSoL HC Otic Solution ... 2678

Hydrocortisone Acetate (Hyperglycemia). Products include:
- Analpram-HC Rectal Cream 1% and 2.5% ... 977
- Anusol HC-1 Anti-Itch Hydrocortisone Ointment ... ◘ 847
- Anusol-HC Suppositories ... 1897
- Caldecort ... ◘ 631
- Carmol HC ... 924
- Coly-Mycin S Otic w/Neomycin & Hydrocortisone ... 1906
- Cortaid ... ◘ 836
- Cortifoam ... 2396
- Cortisporin Cream ... 1084
- Epifoam ... 2399
- Hydrocortone Acetate Sterile Suspension ... 1669
- Mantadil Cream ... 1135
- Nupercainal Hydrocortisone 1% Cream ... ◘ 645
- Ophthocort ... ⊙ 311
- Pramosone Cream, Lotion & Ointment ... 978
- ProctoCream-HC ... 2408
- ProctoFoam-HC ... 2409
- Terra-Cortril Ophthalmic Suspension ... 2210

Hydrocortisone Sodium Phosphate (Hyperglycemia). Products include:
- Hydrocortone Phosphate Injection, Sterile ... 1670

Hydrocortisone Sodium Succinate (Hyperglycemia). Products include:
- Solu-Cortef Sterile Powder ... 2641

Hydroflumethiazide (Thiazides tend to produce hyperglycemia and may lead to loss of control on concurrent use). Products include:
- Diucardin Tablets ... 2718

Ibuprofen (Hypoglycemic action potentiated). Products include:
- Advil Cold and Sinus Caplets and Tablets (formerly CoAdvil) ... ◘ 870
- Advil Ibuprofen Tablets and Caplets ... ◘ 870
- Children's Advil Suspension ... 2692
- Arthritis Foundation Ibuprofen Tablets ... ◘ 674
- Bayer Select Ibuprofen Pain Relief Formula ... ◘ 715
- Cramp End Tablets ... ◘ 735
- Dimetapp Sinus Caplets ... ◘ 775
- Haltran Tablets ... ◘ 771
- IBU Tablets ... 1342
- Ibuprohm ... ◘ 735
- Children's Motrin Ibuprofen Oral Suspension ... 1546
- Motrin Tablets ... 2625
- Motrin IB Caplets, Tablets, and Geltabs ... ◘ 838
- Motrin IB Sinus ... ◘ 838
- Motrin Ibuprofen Suspension, Oral Drops, Chewable Tablets, Caplets ... 1546
- Nuprin Ibuprofen/Analgesic Tablets & Caplets ... ◘ 622
- Sine-Aid IB Caplets ... 1554
- Vicks DayQuil SINUS Pressure & PAIN Relief with IBUPROFEN ... ◘ 762

Indapamide (Hyperglycemia). Products include:
- Lozol Tablets ... 2022

Indomethacin (Hypoglycemic action potentiated). Products include:
- Indocin ... 1680

Indomethacin Sodium Trihydrate (Hypoglycemic action potentiated). Products include:
- Indocin I.V. ... 1684

Isocarboxazid (Hypoglycemic action potentiated).
- No products indexed under this heading.

Isoniazid (Hyperglycemia). Products include:
- Nydrazid Injection ... 508
- Rifamate Capsules ... 1530
- Rifater ... 1532

Isoproterenol Hydrochloride (Hyperglycemia). Products include:
- Isuprel Hydrochloride Injection 1:5000 ... 2311
- Isuprel Hydrochloride Solution 1:200 & 1:100 ... 2313
- Isuprel Mistometer ... 2312

Isoproterenol Sulfate (Hyperglycemia). Products include:
- Norisodrine with Calcium Iodide Syrup ... 442

Isradipine (Hyperglycemia). Products include:
- DynaCirc Capsules ... 2256

Ketoprofen (Hypoglycemic action potentiated). Products include:
- Orudis Capsules ... 2766
- Oruvail Capsules ... 2766

Ketorolac Tromethamine (Hypoglycemic action potentiated). Products include:
- Acular ... 474
- Acular ... ⊙ 277
- Toradol ... 2159

Labetalol Hydrochloride (Hypoglycemic action potentiated). Products include:
- Normodyne Injection ... 2377
- Normodyne Tablets ... 2379
- Trandate ... 1185

Levobunolol Hydrochloride (Hypoglycemic action potentiated). Products include:
- Betagan ... ⊙ 233

Levonorgestrel (Hyperglycemia). Products include:
- Levlen/Tri-Levlen ... 651
- Nordette-21 Tablets ... 2755
- Nordette-28 Tablets ... 2758
- Norplant System ... 2759
- Levlen/Tri-Levlen ... 651
- Triphasil-21 Tablets ... 2814
- Triphasil-28 Tablets ... 2819

Levothyroxine Sodium (Hyperglycemia). Products include:
- Levothroid Tablets ... 1016
- Levoxyl Tablets ... 903
- Synthroid ... 1359

Liothyronine Sodium (Hyperglycemia). Products include:
- Cytomel Tablets ... 2473
- Triostat Injection ... 2530

Liotrix (Hyperglycemia).
- No products indexed under this heading.

Magnesium Salicylate (Hypoglycemic action potentiated). Products include:
- Backache Caplets ... ◘ 613
- Bayer Select Backache Pain Relief Formula ... ◘ 715
- Doan's Extra-Strength Analgesic ... ◘ 633
- Extra Strength Doan's P.M. ... ◘ 633
- Doan's Regular Strength Analgesic ... ◘ 634
- Mobigesic Tablets ... ◘ 602

Meclofenamate Sodium (Hypoglycemic action potentiated).
- No products indexed under this heading.

Mefenamic Acid (Hypoglycemic action potentiated). Products include:
- Ponstel ... 1925

Mesoridazine Besylate (Hyperglycemia). Products include:
- Serentil ... 684

Mestranol (Hyperglycemia). Products include:
- Norinyl ... 2088
- Ortho-Novum ... 1872

Metaproterenol Sulfate (Hyperglycemia). Products include:
- Alupent ... 669
- Metaproterenol Sulfate Inhalation Solution, USP, Arm-a-Med ... 552

Metaraminol Bitartrate (Hyperglycemia). Products include:
- Aramine Injection ... 1609

Methotrimeprazine (Hyperglycemia). Products include:
- Levoprome ... 1274

Methoxamine Hydrochloride (Hyperglycemia). Products include:
- Vasoxyl Injection ... 1196

Methyclothiazide (Thiazides tend to produce hyperglycemia and may lead to loss of control on concurrent use). Products include:
- Enduron Tablets ... 420

Methylprednisolone (Hyperglycemia). Products include:
- Medrol ... 2621

Methylprednisolone Acetate (Hyperglycemia). Products include:
- Depo-Medrol Single-Dose Vial ... 2600
- Depo-Medrol Sterile Aqueous Suspension ... 2597

Methylprednisolone Sodium Succinate (Hyperglycemia). Products include:
- Solu-Medrol Sterile Powder ... 2643

Metipranolol Hydrochloride (Hypoglycemic action potentiated). Products include:
- OptiPranolol (Metipranolol 0.3%) Sterile Ophthalmic Solution ... ⊙ 258

Metolazone (Hyperglycemia). Products include:
- Mykrox Tablets ... 993
- Zaroxolyn Tablets ... 1000

Metoprolol Succinate (Hypoglycemic action potentiated). Products include:
- Toprol-XL Tablets ... 565

Metoprolol Tartrate (Hypoglycemic action potentiated). Products include:
- Lopressor Ampuls ... 830
- Lopressor HCT Tablets ... 832
- Lopressor Tablets ... 830

Miconazole (Severe hypoglycemia).
- No products indexed under this heading.

Miconazole Nitrate (Severe hypoglycemia). Products include:
- Prescription Strength Desenex Spray Powder and Spray Liquid ... ◘ 633
- Lotrimin AF Antifungal Spray Liquid, Spray Powder, Powder and Jock Itch Spray Powder ... ◘ 807
- Monistat Dual-Pak ... 1850
- Monistat 3 Vaginal Suppositories ... 1850
- Monistat-Derm (miconazole nitrate 2%) Cream ... 1889

Nabumetone (Hypoglycemic action potentiated). Products include:
- Relafen Tablets ... 2510

Nadolol (Hypoglycemic action potentiated).
- No products indexed under this heading.

IMPORTANT NOTE: Always consult each drug listing in the patient's regimen for possible interactions.

Micronase

Interactions Index

Naproxen (Hypoglycemic action potentiated). Products include:

Anaprox/Naprosyn 2117

Naproxen Sodium (Hypoglycemic action potentiated). Products include:

Aleve 1975
Anaprox/Naprosyn 2117

Nicardipine Hydrochloride (Hyperglycemia). Products include:

Cardene Capsules 2095
Cardene I.V. 2709
Cardene SR Capsules.............................. 2097

Nicotinic Acid (Hyperglycemia).

No products indexed under this heading.

Nifedipine (Hyperglycemia). Products include:

Adalat Capsules (10 mg and 20 mg) 587
Adalat CC 589
Procardia Capsules................................. 1971
Procardia XL Extended Release Tablets 1972

Nimodipine (Hyperglycemia). Products include:

Nimotop Capsules................................... 610

Nisoldipine (Hyperglycemia).

No products indexed under this heading.

Norepinephrine Bitartrate (Hyperglycemia). Products include:

Levophed Bitartrate Injection 2315

Norethindrone (Hyperglycemia). Products include:

Brevicon.. 2088
Micronor Tablets 1872
Modicon 1872
Norinyl 2088
Nor-Q D Tablets 2135
Ortho-Novum... 1872
Ovcon 760
Tri-Norinyl.. 2164

Norethynodrel (Hyperglycemia).

No products indexed under this heading.

Norgestimate (Hyperglycemia). Products include:

Ortho-Cyclen/Ortho-Tri-Cyclen 1858
Ortho-Cyclen/Ortho Tri-Cyclen 1858

Norgestrel (Hyperglycemia). Products include:

Lo/Ovral Tablets 2746
Lo/Ovral-28 Tablets................................ 2751
Ovral Tablets 2770
Ovral-28 Tablets 2770
Ovrette Tablets.. 2771

Oxaprozin (Hypoglycemic action potentiated). Products include:

Daypro Caplets 2426

Penbutolol Sulfate (Hypoglycemic action potentiated). Products include:

Levatol 2403

Perphenazine (Hyperglycemia). Products include:

Etrafon 2355
Triavil Tablets 1757
Trilafon.. 2389

Phenelzine Sulfate (Hypoglycemic action potentiated). Products include:

Nardil 1920

Phenylbutazone (Hypoglycemic action potentiated).

No products indexed under this heading.

Phenylephrine Bitartrate (Hyperglycemia).

No products indexed under this heading.

Phenylephrine Hydrochloride (Hyperglycemia). Products include:

Atrohist Plus Tablets 454
Cerose DM .... ᴾᴰ 878
Comhist 2038
D.A. Chewable Tablets........................... 951
Deconsal Pediatric Capsules................. 454
Dura-Vent/DA Tablets 953
Entex Capsules 1986
Entex Liquid 1986
Extendryl 1005
4-Way Fast Acting Nasal Spray (regular & mentholated) .... ᴾᴰ 621
Hemorid For Women .... ᴾᴰ 834
Hycomine Compound Tablets 932
Neo-Synephrine Hydrochloride 1% Carpuject.. 2324
Neo-Synephrine Hydrochloride 1% Injection 2324
Neo-Synephrine Hydrochloride (Ophthalmic) 2325
Neo-Synephrine .... ᴾᴰ 726
Nōstril... ᴾᴰ 644
Novahistine Elixir .... ᴾᴰ 823
Phenergan VC.. 2779
Phenergan VC with Codeine 2781
Preparation H .... ᴾᴰ 871
Tympagesic Ear Drops 2342
Vasosulf .... © 271
Vicks Sinex Nasal Spray and Ultra Fine Mist .... ᴾᴰ 765

Phenylephrine Tannate (Hyperglycemia). Products include:

Atrohist Pediatric Suspension 454
Ricobid-D Pediatric Suspension........ 2038
Ricobid Tablets and Pediatric Suspension.. 2038
Rynatan 2673
Rynatuss 2673

Phenylpropanolamine Hydrochloride (Hyperglycemia). Products include:

Acutrim .... ᴾᴰ 628
Allerest Children's Chewable Tablets.. ᴾᴰ 627
Allerest 12 Hour Caplets .... ᴾᴰ 627
Atrohist Plus Tablets 454
BC Cold Powder Multi-Symptom Formula (Cold-Sinus-Allergy) ...... ᴾᴰ 609
BC Cold Powder Non-Drowsy Formula (Cold-Sinus)............................ ᴾᴰ 609
Cheracol Plus Head Cold/Cough Formula .... ᴾᴰ 769
Comtrex Multi-Symptom Non-Drowsy Liqui-gels................................... ᴾᴰ 618
Contac Continuous Action Nasal Decongestant/Antihistamine 12 Hour Capsules... ᴾᴰ 813
Contac Maximum Strength Continuous Action Decongestant/ Antihistamine 12 Hour Caplets.. ᴾᴰ 813
Contac Severe Cold and Flu Formula Caplets .... ᴾᴰ 814
Coricidin 'D' Decongestant Tablets.. ᴾᴰ 800
Dexatrim .... ᴾᴰ 832
Dexatrim Plus Vitamins Caplets .... ᴾᴰ 832
Dimetane-DC Cough Syrup 2059
Dimetapp Elixir .... ᴾᴰ 773
Dimetapp Extentabs............................... ᴾᴰ 774
Dimetapp Tablets/Liqui-Gels .... ᴾᴰ 775
Dimetapp Cold & Allergy Chewable Tablets .... ᴾᴰ 773
Dimetapp DM Elixir................................ ᴾᴰ 774
Dura-Vent Tablets................................... 952
Entex Capsules 1986
Entex LA Tablets 1987
Entex Liquid 1986
Exgest LA Tablets 782
Hycomine 931
Isoclor Timesule Capsules .... ᴾᴰ 637
Nalamine Timed-Release Tablets 785
Ornade Spansule Capsules 2502
Propagest Tablets.................................... 786
Pyrroxate Caplets .... ᴾᴰ 772
Robitussin-CF .... ᴾᴰ 777
Sinulin Tablets 787
Tavist-D 12 Hour Relief Tablets .... ᴾᴰ 787
Teldrin 12 Hour Antihistamine/ Nasal Decongestant Allergy Relief Capsules... ᴾᴰ 826
Triaminic Allergy Tablets .... ᴾᴰ 789
Triaminic Cold Tablets .... ᴾᴰ 790
Triaminic Expectorant .... ᴾᴰ 790
Triaminic Syrup .... ᴾᴰ 792
Triaminic-12 Tablets .... ᴾᴰ 792
Triaminic-DM Syrup .... ᴾᴰ 792
Triaminicin Tablets.................................. ᴾᴰ 793
Triaminicol Multi-Symptom Cold Tablets .... ᴾᴰ 793
Triaminicol Multi-Symptom Relief ᴾᴰ 794
Vicks DayQuil Allergy Relief 12-Hour Extended Release Tablets.. ᴾᴰ 760
Vicks DayQuil Allergy Relief 4-Hour Tablets .... ᴾᴰ 760
Vicks DayQuil SINUS Pressure & CONGESTION Relief............................ ᴾᴰ 761

Phenytoin (Hyperglycemia). Products include:

Dilantin Infatabs..................................... 1908
Dilantin-125 Suspension 1911

Phenytoin Sodium (Hyperglycemia). Products include:

Dilantin Kapseals 1906
Dilantin Parenteral 1910

Pindolol (Hypoglycemic action potentiated). Products include:

Visken Tablets.. 2299

Pirbuterol Acetate (Hyperglycemia). Products include:

Maxair Autohaler 1492
Maxair Inhaler 1494

Piroxicam (Hypoglycemic action potentiated). Products include:

Feldene Capsules..................................... 1965

Polyestradiol Phosphate (Hyperglycemia).

No products indexed under this heading.

Polythiazide (Thiazides tend to produce hyperglycemia and may lead to loss of control on concurrent use). Products include:

Minizide Capsules 1938

Prednisolone Acetate (Hyperglycemia). Products include:

AK-CIDE.. © 202
AK-CIDE Ointment.................................. © 202
Blephamide Liquifilm Sterile Ophthalmic Suspension................................ 476
Blephamide Ointment .... © 237
Econopred & Econopred Plus Ophthalmic Suspensions .... © 217
Poly-Pred Liquifilm .... © 248
Pred Forte... © 250
Pred Mild... © 253
Pred-G Liquifilm Sterile Ophthalmic Suspension .... © 251
Pred-G S.O.P. Sterile Ophthalmic Ointment .... © 252
Vasocidin Ointment .... © 268

Prednisolone Sodium Phosphate (Hyperglycemia). Products include:

AK-Pred .... © 204
Hydeltrasol Injection, Sterile 1665
Inflamase... © 265
Pediapred Oral Liquid 995
Vasocidin Ophthalmic Solution ...... © 270

Prednisolone Tebutate (Hyperglycemia). Products include:

Hydeltra-T.B.A. Sterile Suspension 1667

Prednisone (Hyperglycemia). Products include:

Deltasone Tablets.................................... 2595

Probenecid (Hypoglycemic action potentiated). Products include:

Benemid Tablets 1611
ColBENEMID Tablets................................ 1622

Prochlorperazine (Hyperglycemia). Products include:

Compazine 2470

Promethazine Hydrochloride (Hyperglycemia). Products include:

Mepergan Injection 2753
Phenergan with Codeine........................ 2777
Phenergan with Dextromethorphan 2778
Phenergan Injection 2773
Phenergan Suppositories 2775
Phenergan Syrup 2774
Phenergan Tablets 2775
Phenergan VC... 2779
Phenergan VC with Codeine 2781

Propranolol Hydrochloride (Hypoglycemic action potentiated). Products include:

Inderal 2728
Inderal LA Long Acting Capsules 2730
Inderide Tablets 2732
Inderide LA Long Acting Capsules.. 2734

Pseudoephedrine Hydrochloride (Hyperglycemia). Products include:

Actifed Allergy Daytime/Nighttime Caplets .... ᴾᴰ 844
Actifed Plus Caplets .... ᴾᴰ 845
Actifed Plus Tablets .... ᴾᴰ 845
Actifed with Codeine Cough Syrup.. 1067
Actifed Sinus Daytime/Nighttime Tablets and Caplets .... ᴾᴰ 846
Actifed Syrup.. ᴾᴰ 846
Actifed Tablets .... ᴾᴰ 844
Advil Cold and Sinus Caplets and Tablets (formerly CoAdvil) .... ᴾᴰ 870
Alka-Seltzer Plus Cold Medicine Liqui-Gels .... ᴾᴰ 706
Alka-Seltzer Plus Cold & Cough Medicine Liqui-Gels.............................. ᴾᴰ 705
Alka-Seltzer Plus Night-Time Cold Medicine Liqui-Gels.......................... ᴾᴰ 706
Allerest Headache Strength Tablets.. ᴾᴰ 627
Allerest Maximum Strength Tablets.. ᴾᴰ 627
Allerest No Drowsiness Tablets...... ᴾᴰ 627
Allerest Sinus Pain Formula .... ᴾᴰ 627
Anatuss LA Tablets.................................. 1542
Atrohist Pediatric Capsules.................. 453
Bayer Select Sinus Pain Relief Formula .... ᴾᴰ 717
Benadryl Allergy Decongestant Liquid Medication .... ᴾᴰ 848
Benadryl Allergy Decongestant Tablets .... ᴾᴰ 848
Benadryl Allergy Sinus Headache Formula Caplets .... ᴾᴰ 849
Benylin Multisymptom........................... ᴾᴰ 852
Bromfed Capsules (Extended-Release) 1785
Bromfed Syrup .... ᴾᴰ 733
Bromfed Tablets 1785
Bromfed-DM Cough Syrup................... 1786
Bromfed-PD Capsules (Extended-Release) 1785
Children's Vicks DayQuil Allergy Relief.. ᴾᴰ 757
Children's Vicks NyQuil Cold/ Cough Relief... ᴾᴰ 758
Comtrex Multi-Symptom Cold Reliever Tablets/Caplets/Liqui-Gels/Liquid.. ᴾᴰ 615
Allergy-Sinus Comtrex Multi-Symptom Allergy-Sinus Formula Tablets .... ᴾᴰ 617
Comtrex Multi-Symptom Non-Drowsy Caplets...................................... ᴾᴰ 618
Congess 1004
Contac Day Allergy/Sinus Caplets ᴾᴰ 812
Contac Day & Night .... ᴾᴰ 812
Contac Night Allergy/Sinus Caplets.. ᴾᴰ 812
Contac Severe Cold & Flu Non-Drowsy .... ᴾᴰ 815
Deconamine Chewable Tablets 1320
Deconamine CX Cough and Cold Liquid and Tablets.................................. 1319
Deconamine 1320
Deconsal C Expectorant Syrup 456
Deconsal Pediatric Syrup 457
Deconsal II Tablets 454
Dimetane-DX Cough Syrup 2059
Dimetapp Sinus Caplets .... ᴾᴰ 775
Dorcol Children's Cough Syrup ...... ᴾᴰ 785
Drixoral Cough + Congestion Liquid Caps .... ᴾᴰ 802
Dura-Tap/PD Capsules 2867
Duratuss Tablets 2565
Duratuss HD Elixir 2565
Efidac/24 .... ᴾᴰ 635
Entex PSE Tablets.................................... 1987
Fedahist Gyrocaps................................... 2401
Fedahist Timecaps 2401
Guaifed... 1787
Guaifed Syrup .... ᴾᴰ 734
Guaimax-D Tablets 792
Guaitab Tablets .... ᴾᴰ 734
Isoclor Expectorant 990
Kronofed-A 977
Motrin IB Sinus .... ᴾᴰ 838
Novahistine DH.. 2462
Novahistine DMX .... ᴾᴰ 822
Novahistine Expectorant....................... 2463
Nucofed 2051
PediaCare Cold Allergy Chewable Tablets .... ᴾᴰ 677
PediaCare Cough-Cold Chewable Tablets 1553
PediaCare 1553
PediaCare Infants' Decongestant Drops .... ᴾᴰ 677
PediCare Infant's Drops Decongestant Plus Cough 1553
PediaCare NightRest Cough-Cold Liquid 1553
Pediatric Vicks 44d Dry Hacking Cough & Head Congestion............ ᴾᴰ 763
Pediatric Vicks 44m Cough & Cold Relief .... ᴾᴰ 764
Robitussin Cold & Cough Liqui-Gels.. ᴾᴰ 776
Robitussin Maximum Strength Cough & Cold .... ᴾᴰ 778

(ᴾᴰ Described in PDR For Nonprescription Drugs)

(© Described in PDR For Ophthalmology)

Robitussin Pediatric Cough & Cold Formula .... ⓂⒹ 779
Robitussin Severe Congestion Liqui-Gels .... ⓂⒹ 776
Robitussin-DAC Syrup 2074
Robitussin-PE .... ⓂⒹ 778
Rondec Oral Drops 953
Rondec Syrup 953
Rondec Tablet 953
Rondec-DM Oral Drops 954
Rondec-DM Syrup 954
Rondec-TR Tablet 953
Ryna .... ⓂⒹ 841
Seldane-D Extended-Release Tablets 1538
Semprex-D Capsules 463
Semprex-D Capsules 1167
Sinarest Tablets .... ⓂⒹ 648
Sinarest Extra Strength Tablets...... ⓂⒹ 648
Sinarest No Drowsiness Tablets .... ⓂⒹ 648
Sine-Aid IB Caplets 1554
Sine-Aid Maximum Strength Sinus Medication Gelcaps, Caplets and Tablets 1554
Sine-Off No Drowsiness Formula Caplets .... ⓂⒹ 824
Sine-Off Sinus Medicine .... ⓂⒹ 825
Singlet Tablets .... ⓂⒹ 825
Sinutab Non-Drying Liquid Caps .... ⓂⒹ 859
Sinutab Sinus Allergy Medication, Maximum Strength Tablets and Caplets .... ⓂⒹ 860
Sinutab Sinus Medication, Maximum Strength Without Drowsiness Formula, Tablets & Caplets .... ⓂⒹ 860
Sinutab Sinus Medication, Regular Strength Without Drowsiness Formula .... ⓂⒹ 859
Sudafed Children's Liquid .... ⓂⒹ 861
Sudafed Cold and Cough Liquidcaps .... ⓂⒹ 862
Sudafed Cough Syrup .... ⓂⒹ 862
Sudafed Plus Liquid .... ⓂⒹ 862
Sudafed Plus Tablets .... ⓂⒹ 863
Sudafed Severe Cold Formula Caplets .... ⓂⒹ 863
Sudafed Severe Cold Formula Tablets .... ⓂⒹ 864
Sudafed Sinus Caplets......................... ⓂⒹ 864
Sudafed Sinus Tablets .... ⓂⒹ 864
Sudafed Tablets, 30 mg .... ⓂⒹ 861
Sudafed Tablets, 60 mg .... ⓂⒹ 861
Sudafed 12 Hour Caplets .... ⓂⒹ 861
Syn-Rx Tablets 465
Syn-Rx DM Tablets 466
TheraFlu .... ⓂⒹ 787
TheraFlu Maximum Strength Nighttime Flu, Cold & Cough Medicine .... ⓂⒹ 788
TheraFlu Maximum Strength Non-Drowsy Formula Flu, Cold & Cough Medicine .... ⓂⒹ 788
Thera Flu Maximum Strength, Non-Drowsy Formula Flu, Cold and Cough Caplets .... ⓂⒹ 789
Triaminic AM Cough and Decongestant Formula .... ⓂⒹ 789
Triaminic AM Decongestant Formula .... ⓂⒹ 790
Triaminic Nite Light .... ⓂⒹ 791
Triaminic Sore Throat Formula ...... ⓂⒹ 791
Tussend 1783
Tussend Expectorant 1785
Children's TYLENOL Cold Multi-Symptom Liquid Formula and Chewable Tablets................................ 1561
Children's TYLENOL Cold Plus Cough Multi Symptom Tablets and Liquid .... ⓂⒹ 681
Infants' TYLENOL Cold Decongestant & Fever-Reducer Drops 1556
TYLENOL Maximum Strength Allergy Sinus Medication Gelcaps and Caplets 1563
TYLENOL Maximum Strength Allergy Sinus NightTime Medication Caplets 1555
TYLENOL Flu Maximum Strength Gelcaps 1565
TYLENOL Flu NightTime, Maximum Strength, Gelcaps 1566
TYLENOL Maximum Strength Flu NightTime Hot Medication Packets 1562
TYLENOL, Maximum Strength, Sinus Medication Geltabs, Gelcaps, Caplets and Tablets 1566
TYLENOL Cold Multi-Symptom Formula Medication Tablets and Caplets 1561

TYLENOL Cold Medication No Drowsiness Formula Gelcaps and Caplets 1562
TYLENOL Cold Multi-Symptom Hot Medication Liquid Packets.............. 1557
TYLENOL Cough Multi-Symptom Medication with Decongestant...... 1565
Ursinus Inlay-Tabs................................ ⓂⒹ 794
Vicks 44 LiquiCaps Cough, Cold & Flu Relief .... ⓂⒹ 755
Vicks 44 LiquiCaps Non-Drowsy Cough & Cold Relief .... ⓂⒹ 756
Vicks 44D Dry Hacking Cough & Head Congestion .... ⓂⒹ 755
Vicks 44M Cough, Cold & Flu Relief .... ⓂⒹ 756
Vicks DayQuil .... ⓂⒹ 761
Vicks DayQuil SINUS Pressure & PAIN Relief with IBUPROFEN ...... ⓂⒹ 762
Vicks Nyquil Hot Therapy.................... ⓂⒹ 762
Vicks NyQuil LiquiCaps Multi-Symptom Cold/Flu Relief .... ⓂⒹ 763
Vicks NyQuil Multi-Symptom Cold/Flu Relief - (Original & Cherry Flavor) .... ⓂⒹ 763

Pseudoephedrine Sulfate (Hyperglycemia). Products include:

Cheracol Sinus .... ⓂⒹ 768
Chlor-Trimeton Allergy Decongestant Tablets .... ⓂⒹ 799
Claritin-D 2350
Drixoral Cold and Allergy Sustained-Action Tablets .... ⓂⒹ 802
Drixoral Cold and Flu Extended-Release Tablets................................... ⓂⒹ 803
Drixoral Non-Drowsy Formula Extended-Release Tablets .... ⓂⒹ 803
Drixoral Allergy/Sinus Extended Release Tablets................................... ⓂⒹ 804
Trinalin Repetabs Tablets 1330

Quinestrol (Hyperglycemia).

No products indexed under this heading.

Salmeterol Xinafoate (Hyperglycemia). Products include:

Serevent Inhalation Aerosol............... 1176

Salsalate (Hypoglycemic action potentiated). Products include:

Mono-Gesic Tablets 792
Salflex Tablets 786

Selegiline Hydrochloride (Hypoglycemic action potentiated). Products include:

Eldepryl Tablets 2550

Sotalol Hydrochloride (Hypoglycemic action potentiated). Products include:

Betapace Tablets 641

Spironolactone (Hyperglycemia). Products include:

Aldactazide 2413
Aldactone 2414

Sulfacytine (Hypoglycemic action potentiated).

Sulfamethizole (Hypoglycemic action potentiated). Products include:

Urobiotic-250 Capsules 2214

Sulfamethoxazole (Hypoglycemic action potentiated). Products include:

Azo Gantanol Tablets 2080
Bactrim DS Tablets 2084
Bactrim I.V. Infusion 2082
Bactrim 2084
Gantanol Tablets 2119
Septra 1174
Septra I.V. Infusion 1169
Septra I.V. Infusion ADD-Vantage Vials 1171
Septra 1174

Sulfasalazine (Hypoglycemic action potentiated). Products include:

Azulfidine 1949

Sulfinpyrazone (Hypoglycemic action potentiated). Products include:

Anturane 807

Sulfisoxazole (Hypoglycemic action potentiated). Products include:

Azo Gantrisin Tablets........................... 2081
Gantrisin Tablets 2120

Sulfisoxazole Diolamine (Hypoglycemic action potentiated).

No products indexed under this heading.

Sulindac (Hypoglycemic action potentiated). Products include:

Clinoril Tablets 1618

Terbutaline Sulfate (Hyperglycemia). Products include:

Brethaire Inhaler 813
Brethine Ampuls 815
Brethine Tablets 814
Bricanyl Subcutaneous Injection...... 1502
Bricanyl Tablets 1503

Thioridazine Hydrochloride (Hyperglycemia). Products include:

Mellaril 2269

Thyroglobulin (Hyperglycemia).

No products indexed under this heading.

Thyroid (Hyperglycemia).

No products indexed under this heading.

Thyroxine (Hyperglycemia).

No products indexed under this heading.

Thyroxine Sodium (Hyperglycemia).

No products indexed under this heading.

Timolol Hemihydrate (Hypoglycemic action potentiated). Products include:

Betimol 0.25%, 0.5% .... ⓒ 261

Timolol Maleate (Hypoglycemic action potentiated). Products include:

Blocadren Tablets 1614
Timolide Tablets 1748
Timoptic in Ocudose 1753
Timoptic Sterile Ophthalmic Solution 1751
Timoptic-XE 1755

Tolazamide (Hypoglycemic action potentiated).

No products indexed under this heading.

Tolbutamide (Hypoglycemic action potentiated).

No products indexed under this heading.

Tolmetin Sodium (Hypoglycemic action potentiated). Products include:

Tolectin (200, 400 and 600 mg) .. 1581

Torsemide (Hyperglycemia). Products include:

Demadex Tablets and Injection 686

Tranylcypromine Sulfate (Hypoglycemic action potentiated). Products include:

Parnate Tablets 2503

Triamcinolone (Hyperglycemia). Products include:

Aristocort Tablets 1022

Triamcinolone Acetonide (Hyperglycemia). Products include:

Aristocort A 0.025% Cream 1027
Aristocort A 0.5% Cream 1031
Aristocort A 0.1% Cream 1029
Aristocort A 0.1% Ointment 1030
Azmacort Oral Inhaler 2011
Nasacort Nasal Inhaler 2024

Triamcinolone Diacetate (Hyperglycemia). Products include:

Aristocort Suspension (Forte Parenteral) 1027
Aristocort Suspension (Intralesional) 1025

Triamcinolone Hexacetonide (Hyperglycemia). Products include:

Aristospan Suspension (Intra-articular) 1033
Aristospan Suspension (Intralesional) 1032

Triamterene (Hyperglycemia). Products include:

Dyazide 2479
Dyrenium Capsules 2481
Maxzide 1380

Trifluoperazine Hydrochloride (Hyperglycemia). Products include:

Stelazine 2514

Verapamil Hydrochloride (Hyperglycemia). Products include:

Calan SR Caplets 2422
Calan Tablets 2419
Isoptin Injectable 1344
Isoptin Oral Tablets 1346
Isoptin SR Tablets 1348
Verelan Capsules 1410
Verelan Capsules 2824

Warfarin Sodium (Hypoglycemic action potentiated). Products include:

Coumadin 926

MICRONOR TABLETS

(Norethindrone) 1872

See **Ortho-Novum 7/7/7** □21 **Tablets**

MIDAMOR TABLETS

(Amiloride Hydrochloride) 1703

May interact with diuretics, potassium sparing diuretics, lithium preparations, non-steroidal anti-inflammatory agents, potassium preparations, ACE inhibitors, and certain other agents. Compounds in these categories include:

Benazepril Hydrochloride (Increased risk of hyperkalemia). Products include:

Lotensin Tablets 834
Lotensin HCT 837
Lotrel Capsules 840

Bendroflumethiazide (Hyponatremia; hypochloremia; increases in BUN levels).

No products indexed under this heading.

Bumetanide (Hyponatremia; hypochloremia; increases in BUN levels). Products include:

Bumex 2093

Captopril (Increased risk of hyperkalemia). Products include:

Capoten 739
Capozide 742

Chlorothiazide (Hyponatremia; hypochloremia; increases in BUN levels). Products include:

Aldoclor Tablets 1598
Diupres Tablets 1650
Diuril Oral 1653

Chlorothiazide Sodium (Hyponatremia; hypochloremia; increases in BUN levels). Products include:

Diuril Sodium Intravenous 1652

Chlorthalidone (Hyponatremia; hypochloremia; increases in BUN levels). Products include:

Combipres Tablets 677
Tenoretic Tablets 2845
Thalitone 1245

Diclofenac Potassium (Reduced diuretic, natriuretic, and antihypertensive effects of Midamor). Products include:

Cataflam 816

Diclofenac Sodium (Reduced diuretic, natriuretic, and antihypertensive effects of Midamor). Products include:

Voltaren Ophthalmic Sterile Ophthalmic Solution .... ⓒ 272
Voltaren Tablets 861

Enalapril Maleate (Increased risk of hyperkalemia). Products include:

Vaseretic Tablets 1765
Vasotec Tablets 1771

Enalaprilat (Increased risk of hyperkalemia). Products include:

Vasotec I.V. 1768

Ethacrynic Acid (Hyponatremia; hypochloremia; increases in BUN levels). Products include:

Edecrin Tablets 1657

IMPORTANT NOTE: Always consult each drug listing in the patient's regimen for possible interactions.

Midamor **Interactions Index** 658

Etodolac (Reduced diuretic, natriuretic, and antihypertensive effects of Midamor). Products include:
Lodine Capsules and Tablets 2743
Fenoprofen Calcium (Reduced diuretic, natriuretic, and antihypertensive effects of Midamor). Products include:
Nalfon 200 Pulvules & Nalfon Tablets 917
Flurbiprofen (Reduced diuretic, natriuretic, and antihypertensive effects of Midamor). Products include:
Ansaid Tablets 2579
Fosinopril Sodium (Increased risk of hyperkalemia). Products include:
Monopril Tablets 757
Furosemide (Hyponatremia; hypochloremia; increases in BUN levels). Products include:
Lasix Injection, Oral Solution and Tablets 1240
Hydrochlorothiazide (Hyponatremia; hypochloremia; increases in BUN levels). Products include:
Aldactazide 2413
Aldoril Tablets 1604
Apresazide Capsules 808
Capozide 742
Dyazide 2479
Esidrix Tablets 821
Esimil Tablets 822
HydroDIURIL Tablets 1674
Hydropres Tablets 1675
Hyzaar Tablets 1677
Inderide Tablets 2732
Inderide LA Long Acting Capsules .. 2734
Lopressor HCT Tablets 832
Lotensin HCT 837
Maxzide 1380
Moduretic Tablets 1705
Oretic Tablets 443
Prinzide Tablets 1737
Ser-Ap-Es Tablets 849
Timolide Tablets 1748
Vaseretic Tablets 1765
Zestoretic 2850
Ziac 1415
Hydroflumethiazide (Hyponatremia; hypochloremia; increases in BUN levels). Products include:
Diucardin Tablets 2718
Ibuprofen (Reduced diuretic, natriuretic, and antihypertensive effects of Midamor). Products include:
Advil Cold and Sinus Caplets and Tablets (formerly CoAdvil) ◘ 870
Advil Ibuprofen Tablets and Caplets .... ◘ 870
Children's Advil Suspension 2692
Arthritis Foundation Ibuprofen Tablets .... ◘ 674
Bayer Select Ibuprofen Pain Relief Formula .... ◘ 715
Cramp End Tablets .... ◘ 735
Dimetapp Sinus Caplets .... ◘ 775
Haltran Tablets .... ◘ 771
IBU Tablets 1342
Ibuprohm .... ◘ 735
Children's Motrin Ibuprofen Oral Suspension 1546
Motrin Tablets 2625
Motrin IB Caplets, Tablets, and Geltabs .... ◘ 838
Motrin IB Sinus .... ◘ 838
Motrin Ibuprofen Suspension, Oral Drops, Chewable Tablets, Caplets 1546
Nuprin Ibuprofen/Analgesic Tablets & Caplets .... ◘ 622
Sine-Aid IB Caplets 1554
Vicks DayQuil SINUS Pressure & PAIN Relief with IBUPROFEN ...... ◘ 762
Indapamide (Hyponatremia; hypochloremia; increases in BUN levels). Products include:
Lozol Tablets 2022
Indomethacin (Reduced diuretic, natriuretic, and antihypertensive effects of Midamor; increased serum potassium levels of both drugs). Products include:
Indocin 1680
Indomethacin Sodium Trihydrate (Reduced diuretic, natriuretic, and antihypertensive effects of Midamor; increased serum potassium levels of both drugs). Products include:
Indocin I.V. 1684
Ketoprofen (Reduced diuretic, natriuretic, and antihypertensive effects of Midamor). Products include:
Orudis Capsules 2766
Oruvail Capsules 2766
Ketorolac Tromethamine (Reduced diuretic, natriuretic, and antihypertensive effects of Midamor). Products include:
Acular 474
Acular .... ⊙ 277
Toradol 2159
Lisinopril (Increased risk of hyperkalemia). Products include:
Prinivil Tablets 1733
Prinzide Tablets 1737
Zestoretic 2850
Zestril Tablets 2854
Lithium Carbonate (High risk of lithium toxicity). Products include:
Eskalith 2485
Lithium Carbonate Capsules & Tablets 2230
Lithonate/Lithotabs/Lithobid 2543
Lithium Citrate (High risk of lithium toxicity).
No products indexed under this heading.
Meclofenamate Sodium (Reduced diuretic, natiuretic, and antihypertensive effects of Midamor).
No products indexed under this heading.
Mefenamic Acid (Reduced diuretic, natriuretic, and antihypertensive effects of Midamor). Products include:
Ponstel 1925
Methyclothiazide (Hyponatremia; hypochloremia; increases in BUN levels). Products include:
Enduron Tablets 420
Metolazone (Hyponatremia; hypochloremia; increases in BUN levels). Products include:
Mykrox Tablets 993
Zaroxolyn Tablets 1000
Moexipril Hydrochloride (Increased risk of hyperkalemia). Products include:
Univasc Tablets 2410
Nabumetone (Reduced diuretic, natriuretic, and antihypertensive effects of Midamor). Products include:
Relafen Tablets 2510
Naproxen (Reduced diuretic, natriuretic, and antihypertensive effects of Midamor). Products include:
Anaprox/Naprosyn 2117
Naproxen Sodium (Reduced diuretic, natriuretic, and antihypertensive effects of Midamor). Products include:
Aleve 1975
Anaprox/Naprosyn 2117
Oxaprozin (Reduced diuretic, natriuretic, and antihypertensive effects of Midamor). Products include:
Daypro Caplets 2426
Phenylbutazone (Reduced diuretic, natriuretic, and antihypertensive effects of Midamor).
No products indexed under this heading.
Piroxicam (Reduced diuretic, natriuretic, and antihypertensive effects of Midamor). Products include:
Feldene Capsules 1965
Polythiazide (Hyponatremia; hypochloremia; increases in BUN levels). Products include:
Minizide Capsules 1938
Potassium Acid Phosphate (Concomitant therapy is contraindicated). Products include:
K-Phos Original Formula 'Sodium Free' Tablets 639
Potassium Bicarbonate (Concomitant therapy is contraindicated). Products include:
Alka-Seltzer Gold Effervescent Antacid .... ◘ 703
Potassium Chloride (Concomitant therapy is contraindicated). Products include:
Chlor-3 Condiment 1004
K-Dur Microburst Release System (potassium chloride, USP) E.R. Tablets 1325
K-Lor Powder Packets 434
K-Norm Extended-Release Capsules 991
K-Tab Filmtab 434
Kolyum Liquid 992
Micro-K 2063
Micro-K LS Packets 2064
NuLYTELY 689
Cherry Flavor NuLYTELY 689
Rum-K Syrup 1005
Slow-K Extended-Release Tablets.... 851
Potassium Citrate (Concomitant therapy is contraindicated). Products include:
Polycitra Syrup 578
Polycitra-K Crystals 579
Polycitra-K Oral Solution 579
Polycitra-LC 578
Potassium Gluconate (Concomitant therapy is contraindicated). Products include:
Kolyum Liquid 992
Potassium Phosphate, Dibasic (Concomitant therapy is contraindicated).
No products indexed under this heading.
Potassium Phosphate, Monobasic (Concomitant therapy is contraindicated). Products include:
K-Phos Neutral Tablets 639
K-Phos Original Formula 'Sodium Free' Tablets 639
Quinapril Hydrochloride (Increased risk of hyperkalemia). Products include:
Accupril Tablets 1893
Ramipril (Increased risk of hyperkalemia). Products include:
Altace Capsules 1232
Spirapril Hydrochloride (Increased risk of hyperkalemia).
No products indexed under this heading.
Spironolactone (Do not administer concomitantly; rapid increases in serum potassium). Products include:
Aldactazide 2413
Aldactone 2414
Sulindac (Reduced diuretic, natriuretic, and antihypertensive effects of Midamor). Products include:
Clinoril Tablets 1618
Tolmetin Sodium (Reduced diuretic, natriuretic, and antihypertensive effects of Midamor). Products include:
Tolectin (200, 400 and 600 mg) .. 1581
Torsemide (Hyponatremia; hypochloremia; increases in BUN levels). Products include:
Demadex Tablets and Injection 686
Triamterene (Do not administer concomitantly; rapid increases in serum potassium). Products include:
Dyazide 2479
Dyrenium Capsules 2481
Maxzide 1380

Food Interactions

Diet, potassium-rich (Potential for rapid increases in serum potassium levels).

MAXIMUM STRENGTH MULTI-SYMPTOM FORMULA MIDOL

(Acetaminophen, Caffeine, Pyrilamine Maleate) .... ◘ 722
May interact with hypnotics and sedatives, tranquilizers, and certain other agents. Compounds in these categories include:
Alprazolam (May increase drowsiness). Products include:
Xanax Tablets 2649
Buspirone Hydrochloride (May increase drowsiness). Products include:
BuSpar 737
Caffeine-containing medications (Concomitant use may cause nervousness, irritability, sleeplessness, and occasionally, rapid heartbeat).
Chlordiazepoxide (May increase drowsiness). Products include:
Libritabs Tablets 2177
Limbitrol 2180
Chlordiazepoxide Hydrochloride (May increase drowsiness). Products include:
Librax Capsules 2176
Librium Capsules 2178
Librium Injectable 2179
Chlorpromazine (May increase drowsiness). Products include:
Thorazine Suppositories 2523
Chlorprothixene (May increase drowsiness).
No products indexed under this heading.
Chlorprothixene Hydrochloride (May increase drowsiness).
No products indexed under this heading.
Clorazepate Dipotassium (May increase drowsiness). Products include:
Tranxene 451
Diazepam (May increase drowsiness). Products include:
Dizac 1809
Valium Injectable 2182
Valium Tablets 2183
Valrelease Capsules 2169
Droperidol (May increase drowsiness). Products include:
Inapsine Injection 1296
Estazolam (May increase drowsiness). Products include:
ProSom Tablets 449
Ethchlorvynol (May increase drowsiness). Products include:
Placidyl Capsules 448
Ethinamate (May increase drowsiness).
No products indexed under this heading.
Fluphenazine Decanoate (May increase drowsiness). Products include:
Prolixin Decanoate 509
Fluphenazine Enanthate (May increase drowsiness). Products include:
Prolixin Enanthate 509
Fluphenazine Hydrochloride (May increase drowsiness). Products include:
Prolixin 509
Flurazepam Hydrochloride (May increase drowsiness). Products include:
Dalmane Capsules 2173

(◘ Described in PDR For Nonprescription Drugs) (⊙ Described in PDR For Ophthalmology)

Glutethimide (May increase drowsiness).
No products indexed under this heading.

Haloperidol (May increase drowsiness). Products include:
Haldol Injection, Tablets and Concentrate 1575

Haloperidol Decanoate (May increase drowsiness). Products include:
Haldol Decanoate 1577

Hydroxyzine Hydrochloride (May increase drowsiness). Products include:
Atarax Tablets & Syrup 2185
Marax Tablets & DF Syrup 2200
Vistaril Intramuscular Solution 2216

Lorazepam (May increase drowsiness). Products include:
Ativan Injection 2698
Ativan Tablets 2700

Loxapine Hydrochloride (May increase drowsiness). Products include:
Loxitane 1378

Loxapine Succinate (May increase drowsiness). Products include:
Loxitane Capsules 1378

Meprobamate (May increase drowsiness). Products include:
Miltown Tablets 2672
PMB 200 and PMB 400 2783

Mesoridazine Besylate (May increase drowsiness). Products include:
Serentil 684

Midazolam Hydrochloride (May increase drowsiness). Products include:
Versed Injection 2170

Molindone Hydrochloride (May increase drowsiness). Products include:
Moban Tablets and Concentrate 1048

Oxazepam (May increase drowsiness). Products include:
Serax Capsules 2810
Serax Tablets 2810

Perphenazine (May increase drowsiness). Products include:
Etrafon 2355
Triavil Tablets 1757
Trilafon 2389

Prazepam (May increase drowsiness).
No products indexed under this heading.

Prochlorperazine (May increase drowsiness). Products include:
Compazine 2470

Promethazine Hydrochloride (May increase drowsiness). Products include:
Mepergan Injection 2753
Phenergan with Codeine 2777
Phenergan with Dextromethorphan 2778
Phenergan Injection 2773
Phenergan Suppositories 2775
Phenergan Syrup 2774
Phenergan Tablets 2775
Phenergan VC 2779
Phenergan VC with Codeine 2781

Propofol (May increase drowsiness). Products include:
Diprivan Injection 2833

Quazepam (May increase drowsiness). Products include:
Doral Tablets 2664

Secobarbital Sodium (May increase drowsiness). Products include:
Seconal Sodium Pulvules 1474

Temazepam (May increase drowsiness). Products include:
Restoril Capsules 2284

Thioridazine Hydrochloride (May increase drowsiness). Products include:
Mellaril 2269

Thiothixene (May increase drowsiness). Products include:
Navane Capsules and Concentrate 2201
Navane Intramuscular 2202

Triazolam (May increase drowsiness). Products include:
Halcion Tablets 2611

Trifluoperazine Hydrochloride (May increase drowsiness). Products include:
Stelazine 2514

Zolpidem Tartrate (May increase drowsiness). Products include:
Ambien Tablets 2416

Food Interactions

Alcohol (May increase drowsiness).

Beverages, caffeine-containing (Concomitant use may cause nervousness, irritability, sleeplessness, and occasionally, rapid heartbeat).

Food, caffeine-containing (Concomitant use may cause nervousness, irritability, sleeplessness, and occasionally, rapid heartbeat).

PMS MULTI-SYMPTOM FORMULA MIDOL

(Acetaminophen, Pamabrom, Pyrilamine Maleate) 723
May interact with hypnotics and sedatives, tranquilizers, and certain other agents. Compounds in these categories include:

Alprazolam (May increase drowsiness). Products include:
Xanax Tablets 2649

Buspirone Hydrochloride (May increase drowsiness). Products include:
BuSpar 737

Chlordiazepoxide (May increase drowsiness). Products include:
Libritabs Tablets 2177
Limbitrol 2180

Chlordiazepoxide Hydrochloride (May increase drowsiness). Products include:
Librax Capsules 2176
Librium Capsules 2178
Librium Injectable 2179

Chlorpromazine (May increase drowsiness). Products include:
Thorazine Suppositories 2523

Chlorprothixene (May increase drowsiness).
No products indexed under this heading.

Chlorprothixene Hydrochloride (May increase drowsiness).
No products indexed under this heading.

Clorazepate Dipotassium (May increase drowsiness). Products include:
Tranxene 451

Diazepam (May increase drowsiness). Products include:
Dizac 1809
Valium Injectable 2182
Valium Tablets 2183
Valrelease Capsules 2169

Droperidol (May increase drowsiness). Products include:
Inapsine Injection 1296

Estazolam (May increase drowsiness). Products include:
ProSom Tablets 449

Ethchlorvynol (May increase drowsiness). Products include:
Placidyl Capsules 448

Ethinamate (May increase drowsiness).
No products indexed under this heading.

Fluphenazine Decanoate (May increase drowsiness). Products include:
Prolixin Decanoate 509

Fluphenazine Enanthate (May increase drowsiness). Products include:
Prolixin Enanthate 509

Fluphenazine Hydrochloride (May increase drowsiness). Products include:
Prolixin 509

Flurazepam Hydrochloride (May increase drowsiness). Products include:
Dalmane Capsules 2173

Glutethimide (May increase drowsiness).
No products indexed under this heading.

Haloperidol (May increase drowsiness). Products include:
Haldol Injection, Tablets and Concentrate 1575

Haloperidol Decanoate (May increase drowsiness). Products include:
Haldol Decanoate 1577

Hydroxyzine Hydrochloride (May increase drowsiness). Products include:
Atarax Tablets & Syrup 2185
Marax Tablets & DF Syrup 2200
Vistaril Intramuscular Solution 2216

Lorazepam (May increase drowsiness). Products include:
Ativan Injection 2698
Ativan Tablets 2700

Loxapine Hydrochloride (May increase drowsiness). Products include:
Loxitane 1378

Loxapine Succinate (May increase drowsiness). Products include:
Loxitane Capsules 1378

Meprobamate (May increase drowsiness). Products include:
Miltown Tablets 2672
PMB 200 and PMB 400 2783

Mesoridazine Besylate (May increase drowsiness). Products include:
Serentil 684

Midazolam Hydrochloride (May increase drowsiness). Products include:
Versed Injection 2170

Molindone Hydrochloride (May increase drowsiness). Products include:
Moban Tablets and Concentrate 1048

Oxazepam (May increase drowsiness). Products include:
Serax Capsules 2810
Serax Tablets 2810

Perphenazine (May increase drowsiness). Products include:
Etrafon 2355
Triavil Tablets 1757
Trilafon 2389

Prazepam (May increase drowsiness).
No products indexed under this heading.

Prochlorperazine (May increase drowsiness). Products include:
Compazine 2470

Promethazine Hydrochloride (May increase drowsiness). Products include:
Mepergan Injection 2753
Phenergan with Codeine 2777
Phenergan with Dextromethorphan 2778
Phenergan Injection 2773
Phenergan Suppositories 2775
Phenergan Syrup 2774
Phenergan Tablets 2775
Phenergan VC 2779
Phenergan VC with Codeine 2781

Propofol (May increase drowsiness). Products include:
Diprivan Injection 2833

Quazepam (May increase drowsiness). Products include:
Doral Tablets 2664

Secobarbital Sodium (May increase drowsiness). Products include:
Seconal Sodium Pulvules 1474

Temazepam (May increase drowsiness). Products include:
Restoril Capsules 2284

Thioridazine Hydrochloride (May increase drowsiness). Products include:
Mellaril 2269

Thiothixene (May increase drowsiness). Products include:
Navane Capsules and Concentrate 2201
Navane Intramuscular 2202

Triazolam (May increase drowsiness). Products include:
Halcion Tablets 2611

Trifluoperazine Hydrochloride (May increase drowsiness). Products include:
Stelazine 2514

Zolpidem Tartrate (May increase drowsiness). Products include:
Ambien Tablets 2416

Food Interactions

Alcohol (May increase drowsiness).

TEEN MULTI-SYMPTOM FORMULA MIDOL

(Acetaminophen, Pamabrom) 722
None cited in PDR database.

MIDRIN CAPSULES

(Isometheptene Mucate, Dichloralphenazone, Acetaminophen) 783
May interact with monoamine oxidase inhibitors. Compounds in this category include:

Furazolidone (Concurrent therapy contraindicated). Products include:
Furoxone 2046

Isocarboxazid (Concurrent therapy contraindicated).
No products indexed under this heading.

Phenelzine Sulfate (Concurrent therapy contraindicated). Products include:
Nardil 1920

Selegiline Hydrochloride (Concurrent therapy contraindicated). Products include:
Eldepryl Tablets 2550

Tranylcypromine Sulfate (Concurrent therapy contraindicated). Products include:
Parnate Tablets 2503

MIGRALAM CAPSULES

(Isometheptene Mucate, Caffeine, Acetaminophen) 2038
May interact with monoamine oxidase inhibitors. Compounds in this category include:

Furazolidone (Concurrent use is contraindicated). Products include:
Furoxone 2046

Isocarboxazid (Concurrent use is contraindicated).
No products indexed under this heading.

IMPORTANT NOTE: Always consult each drug listing in the patient's regimen for possible interactions.

Phenelzine Sulfate (Concurrent use is contraindicated). Products include:
Nardil 1920

Selegiline Hydrochloride (Concurrent use is contraindicated). Products include:
Eldepryl Tablets 2550

Tranylcypromine Sulfate (Concurrent use is contraindicated). Products include:
Parnate Tablets 2503

MILES NERVINE NIGHTTIME SLEEP-AID
(Diphenhydramine Hydrochloride) .. ◘ 723
May interact with hypnotics and sedatives, tranquilizers, and certain other agents. Compounds in these categories include:

Alprazolam (Concurrent use not recommended). Products include:
Xanax Tablets 2649

Buspirone Hydrochloride (Concurrent use not recommended). Products include:
BuSpar 737

Chlordiazepoxide (Concurrent use not recommended). Products include:
Libritabs Tablets 2177
Limbitrol 2180

Chlordiazepoxide Hydrochloride (Concurrent use not recommended). Products include:
Librax Capsules 2176
Librium Capsules 2178
Librium Injectable 2179

Chlorpromazine (Concurrent use not recommended). Products include:
Thorazine Suppositories 2523

Chlorprothixene (Concurrent use not recommended).
No products indexed under this heading.

Chlorprothixene Hydrochloride (Concurrent use not recommended).
No products indexed under this heading.

Clorazepate Dipotassium (Concurrent use not recommended). Products include:
Tranxene 451

Diazepam (Concurrent use not recommended). Products include:
Dizac 1809
Valium Injectable 2182
Valium Tablets 2183
Valrelease Capsules 2169

Droperidol (Concurrent use not recommended). Products include:
Inapsine Injection 1296

Estazolam (Concurrent use not recommended). Products include:
ProSom Tablets 449

Ethchlorvynol (Concurrent use not recommended). Products include:
Placidyl Capsules 448

Ethinamate (Concurrent use not recommended).
No products indexed under this heading.

Fluphenazine Decanoate (Concurrent use not recommended). Products include:
Prolixin Decanoate 509

Fluphenazine Enanthate (Concurrent use not recommended). Products include:
Prolixin Enanthate 509

Fluphenazine Hydrochloride (Concurrent use not recommended). Products include:
Prolixin 509

Flurazepam Hydrochloride (Concurrent use not recommended). Products include:
Dalmane Capsules 2173

Glutethimide (Concurrent use not recommended).
No products indexed under this heading.

Haloperidol (Concurrent use not recommended). Products include:
Haldol Injection, Tablets and Concentrate 1575

Haloperidol Decanoate (Concurrent use not recommended). Products include:
Haldol Decanoate 1577

Hydroxyzine Hydrochloride (Concurrent use not recommended). Products include:
Atarax Tablets & Syrup 2185
Marax Tablets & DF Syrup 2200
Vistaril Intramuscular Solution 2216

Lorazepam (Concurrent use not recommended). Products include:
Ativan Injection 2698
Ativan Tablets 2700

Loxapine Hydrochloride (Concurrent use not recommended). Products include:
Loxitane 1378

Loxapine Succinate (Concurrent use not recommended). Products include:
Loxitane Capsules 1378

Meprobamate (Concurrent use not recommended). Products include:
Miltown Tablets 2672
PMB 200 and PMB 400 2783

Mesoridazine Besylate (Concurrent use not recommended). Products include:
Serentil 684

Midazolam Hydrochloride (Concurrent use not recommended). Products include:
Versed Injection 2170

Molindone Hydrochloride (Concurrent use not recommended). Products include:
Moban Tablets and Concentrate 1048

Oxazepam (Concurrent use not recommended). Products include:
Serax Capsules 2810
Serax Tablets 2810

Perphenazine (Concurrent use not recommended). Products include:
Etrafon 2355
Triavil Tablets 1757
Trilafon 2389

Prazepam (Concurrent use not recommended).
No products indexed under this heading.

Prochlorperazine (Concurrent use not recommended). Products include:
Compazine 2470

Promethazine Hydrochloride (Concurrent use not recommended). Products include:
Mepergan Injection 2753
Phenergan with Codeine 2777
Phenergan with Dextromethorphan 2778
Phenergan Injection 2773
Phenergan Suppositories 2775
Phenergan Syrup 2774
Phenergan Tablets 2775
Phenergan VC 2779
Phenergan VC with Codeine 2781

Propofol (Concurrent use not recommended). Products include:
Diprivan Injection 2833

Quazepam (Concurrent use not recommended). Products include:
Doral Tablets 2664

Secobarbital Sodium (Concurrent use not recommended). Products include:
Seconal Sodium Pulvules 1474

Temazepam (Concurrent use not recommended). Products include:
Restoril Capsules 2284

Thioridazine Hydrochloride (Concurrent use not recommended). Products include:
Mellaril 2269

Thiothixene (Concurrent use not recommended). Products include:
Navane Capsules and Concentrate 2201
Navane Intramuscular 2202

Triazolam (Concurrent use not recommended). Products include:
Halcion Tablets 2611

Trifluoperazine Hydrochloride (Concurrent use not recommended). Products include:
Stelazine 2514

Zolpidem Tartrate (Concurrent use not recommended). Products include:
Ambien Tablets 2416

Food Interactions

Alcohol (Concurrent use not recommended).

MILONTIN KAPSEALS
(Phensuximide) 1920
May interact with anticonvulsants. Compounds in this category include:

Carbamazepine (Effect not specified; periodic serum level determination may be necessary). Products include:
Atretol Tablets 573
Tegretol Chewable Tablets 852
Tegretol Suspension 852
Tegretol Tablets 852

Divalproex Sodium (Effect not specified; periodic serum level determination may be necessary). Products include:
Depakote Tablets 415

Ethosuximide (Effect not specified; periodic serum level determination may be necessary). Products include:
Zarontin Capsules 1928
Zarontin Syrup 1929

Ethotoin (Effect not specified; periodic serum level determination may be necessary). Products include:
Peganone Tablets 446

Felbamate (Effect not specified; periodic serum level determination may be necessary). Products include:
Felbatol 2666

Lamotrigine (Effect not specified; periodic serum level determination may be necessary). Products include:
Lamictal Tablets 1112

Mephenytoin (Effect not specified; periodic serum level determination may be necessary). Products include:
Mesantoin Tablets 2272

Methsuximide (Effect not specified; periodic serum level determination may be necessary). Products include:
Celontin Kapseals 1899

Paramethadione (Effect not specified; periodic serum level determination may be necessary).
No products indexed under this heading.

Phenacemide (Effect not specified; periodic serum level determination may be necessary). Products include:
Phenurone Tablets 447

Phenobarbital (Effect not specified; periodic serum level determination may be necessary). Products include:
Arco-Lase Plus Tablets 512
Bellergal-S Tablets 2250
Donnatal 2060
Donnatal Extentabs 2061
Donnatal Tablets 2060
Phenobarbital Elixir and Tablets 1469
Quadrinal Tablets 1350

Phenytoin (Effect not specified; periodic serum level determination may be necessary). Products include:
Dilantin Infatabs 1908
Dilantin-125 Suspension 1911

Phenytoin Sodium (Effect not specified; periodic serum level determination may be necessary). Products include:
Dilantin Kapseals 1906
Dilantin Parenteral 1910

Primidone (Effect not specified; periodic serum level determination may be necessary). Products include:
Mysoline 2754

Trimethadione (Effect not specified; periodic serum level determination may be necessary).
No products indexed under this heading.

Valproic Acid (Effect not specified; periodic serum level determination may be necessary). Products include:
Depakene 413

MILTOWN TABLETS
(Meprobamate) 2672
May interact with central nervous system depressants, psychotropics, and certain other agents. Compounds in these categories include:

Alfentanil Hydrochloride (Additive effects). Products include:
Alfenta Injection 1286

Alprazolam (Additive effects). Products include:
Xanax Tablets 2649

Amitriptyline Hydrochloride (Additive effects). Products include:
Elavil 2838
Endep Tablets 2174
Etrafon 2355
Limbitrol 2180
Triavil Tablets 1757

Amoxapine (Additive effects). Products include:
Asendin Tablets 1369

Aprobarbital (Additive effects).
No products indexed under this heading.

Buprenorphine (Additive effects). Products include:
Buprenex Injectable 2006

Buspirone Hydrochloride (Additive effects). Products include:
BuSpar 737

Butabarbital (Additive effects).
No products indexed under this heading.

Butalbital (Additive effects). Products include:
Esgic-plus Tablets 1013
Fioricet Tablets 2258
Fioricet with Codeine Capsules 2260
Fiorinal Capsules 2261
Fiorinal with Codeine Capsules 2262
Fiorinal Tablets 2261
Phrenilin 785
Sedapap Tablets 50 mg/650 mg .. 1543

(◘ Described in PDR For Nonprescription Drugs) (◉ Described in PDR For Ophthalmology)

661 **Interactions Index** **Mini-Gamulin Rh**

Chlordiazepoxide (Additive effects). Products include:
- Libritabs Tablets ... 2177
- Limbitrol ... 2180

Chlordiazepoxide Hydrochloride (Additive effects). Products include:
- Librax Capsules ... 2176
- Librium Capsules ... 2178
- Librium Injectable ... 2179

Chlorpromazine (Additive effects). Products include:
- Thorazine Suppositories ... 2523

Chlorpromazine Hydrochloride (Additive effects). Products include:
- Thorazine ... 2523

Chlorprothixene (Additive effects).
- No products indexed under this heading.

Chlorprothixene Hydrochloride (Additive effects).
- No products indexed under this heading.

Clorazepate Dipotassium (Additive effects). Products include:
- Tranxene ... 451

Clozapine (Additive effects). Products include:
- Clozaril Tablets ... 2252

Codeine Phosphate (Additive effects). Products include:
- Actifed with Codeine Cough Syrup.. 1067
- Brontex ... 1981
- Deconsal C Expectorant Syrup ... 456
- Deconsal Pediatric Syrup ... 457
- Dimetane-DC Cough Syrup ... 2059
- Empirin with Codeine Tablets ... 1093
- Fioricet with Codeine Capsules ... 2260
- Fiorinal with Codeine Capsules ... 2262
- Isoclor Expectorant ... 990
- Novahistine DH ... 2462
- Novahistine Expectorant ... 2463
- Nucofed ... 2051
- Phenergan with Codeine ... 2777
- Phenergan VC with Codeine ... 2781
- Robitussin A-C Syrup ... 2073
- Robitussin-DAC Syrup ... 2074
- Ryna ... 841
- Soma Compound w/Codeine Tablets ... 2676
- Tussi-Organidin NR Liquid and S NR Liquid ... 2677
- Tylenol with Codeine ... 1583

Desflurane (Additive effects). Products include:
- Suprane ... 1813

Desipramine Hydrochloride (Additive effects). Products include:
- Norpramin Tablets ... 1526

Dezocine (Additive effects). Products include:
- Dalgan Injection ... 538

Diazepam (Additive effects). Products include:
- Dizac ... 1809
- Valium Injectable ... 2182
- Valium Tablets ... 2183
- Valrelease Capsules ... 2169

Doxepin Hydrochloride (Additive effects). Products include:
- Sinequan ... 2205
- Zonalon Cream ... 1055

Droperidol (Additive effects). Products include:
- Inapsine Injection ... 1296

Enflurane (Additive effects).
- No products indexed under this heading.

Estazolam (Additive effects). Products include:
- ProSom Tablets ... 449

Ethchlorvynol (Additive effects). Products include:
- Placidyl Capsules ... 448

Ethinamate (Additive effects).
- No products indexed under this heading.

Fentanyl (Additive effects). Products include:
- Duragesic Transdermal System ... 1288

Fentanyl Citrate (Additive effects). Products include:
- Sublimaze Injection ... 1307

Fluphenazine Decanoate (Additive effects). Products include:
- Prolixin Decanoate ... 509

Fluphenazine Enanthate (Additive effects). Products include:
- Prolixin Enanthate ... 509

Fluphenazine Hydrochloride (Additive effects). Products include:
- Prolixin ... 509

Flurazepam Hydrochloride (Additive effects). Products include:
- Dalmane Capsules ... 2173

Glutethimide (Additive effects).
- No products indexed under this heading.

Haloperidol (Additive effects). Products include:
- Haldol Injection, Tablets and Concentrate ... 1575

Haloperidol Decanoate (Additive effects). Products include:
- Haldol Decanoate ... 1577

Hydrocodone Bitartrate (Additive effects). Products include:
- Anexsia 5/500 Elixir ... 1781
- Anexia Tablets ... 1782
- Codiclear DH Syrup ... 791
- Deconamine CX Cough and Cold Liquid and Tablets ... 1319
- Duratuss HD Elixir ... 2565
- Hycodan Tablets and Syrup ... 930
- Hycomine Compound Tablets ... 932
- Hycomine ... 931
- Hycotuss Expectorant Syrup ... 933
- Hydrocet Capsules ... 782
- Lorcet 10/650 ... 1018
- Lortab ... 2566
- Tussend ... 1783
- Tussend Expectorant ... 1785
- Vicodin Tablets ... 1356
- Vicodin ES Tablets ... 1357
- Vicodin Tuss Expectorant ... 1358
- Zydone Capsules ... 949

Hydrocodone Polistirex (Additive effects). Products include:
- Tussionex Pennkinetic Extended-Release Suspension ... 998

Hydroxyzine Hydrochloride (Additive effects). Products include:
- Atarax Tablets & Syrup ... 2185
- Marax Tablets & DF Syrup ... 2200
- Vistaril Intramuscular Solution ... 2216

Imipramine Hydrochloride (Additive effects). Products include:
- Tofranil Ampuls ... 854
- Tofranil Tablets ... 856

Imipramine Pamoate (Additive effects). Products include:
- Tofranil-PM Capsules ... 857

Isocarboxazid (Additive effects).
- No products indexed under this heading.

Isoflurane (Additive effects).
- No products indexed under this heading.

Ketamine Hydrochloride (Additive effects).
- No products indexed under this heading.

Levomethadyl Acetate Hydrochloride (Additive effects). Products include:
- Orlamm ... 2239

Levorphanol Tartrate (Additive effects). Products include:
- Levo-Dromoran ... 2129

Lithium Carbonate (Additive effects). Products include:
- Eskalith ... 2485
- Lithium Carbonate Capsules & Tablets ... 2230
- Lithonate/Lithotabs/Lithobid ... 2543

Lithium Citrate (Additive effects).
- No products indexed under this heading.

Lorazepam (Additive effects). Products include:
- Ativan Injection ... 2698
- Ativan Tablets ... 2700

Loxapine Hydrochloride (Additive effects). Products include:
- Loxitane ... 1378

Loxapine Succinate (Additive effects). Products include:
- Loxitane Capsules ... 1378

Maprotiline Hydrochloride (Additive effects). Products include:
- Ludiomil Tablets ... 843

Meperidine Hydrochloride (Additive effects). Products include:
- Demerol ... 2308
- Mepergan Injection ... 2753

Mephobarbital (Additive effects). Products include:
- Mebaral Tablets ... 2322

Mesoridazine Besylate (Additive effects). Products include:
- Serentil ... 684

Methadone Hydrochloride (Additive effects). Products include:
- Methadone Hydrochloride Oral Concentrate ... 2233
- Methadone Hydrochloride Oral Solution & Tablets ... 2235

Methohexital Sodium (Additive effects). Products include:
- Brevital Sodium Vials ... 1429

Methotrimeprazine (Additive effects). Products include:
- Levoprome ... 1274

Methoxyflurane (Additive effects).
- No products indexed under this heading.

Midazolam Hydrochloride (Additive effects). Products include:
- Versed Injection ... 2170

Molindone Hydrochloride (Additive effects). Products include:
- Moban Tablets and Concentrate ... 1048

Morphine Sulfate (Additive effects). Products include:
- Astramorph/PF Injection, USP (Preservative-Free) ... 535
- Duramorph ... 962
- Infumorph 200 and Infumorph 500 Sterile Solutions ... 965
- MS Contin Tablets ... 1994
- MSIR ... 1997
- Oramorph SR (Morphine Sulfate Sustained Release Tablets) ... 2236
- RMS Suppositories ... 2657
- Roxanol ... 2243

Nortriptyline Hydrochloride (Additive effects). Products include:
- Pamelor ... 2280

Opium Alkaloids (Additive effects).
- No products indexed under this heading.

Oxazepam (Additive effects). Products include:
- Serax Capsules ... 2810
- Serax Tablets ... 2810

Oxycodone Hydrochloride (Additive effects). Products include:
- Percocet Tablets ... 938
- Percodan Tablets ... 939
- Percodan-Demi Tablets ... 940
- Roxicodone Tablets, Oral Solution & Intensol (Oxycodone) ... 2244
- Tylox Capsules ... 1584

Pentobarbital Sodium (Additive effects). Products include:
- Nembutal Sodium Capsules ... 436
- Nembutal Sodium Solution ... 438
- Nembutal Sodium Suppositories ... 440

Perphenazine (Additive effects). Products include:
- Etrafon ... 2355
- Triavil Tablets ... 1757
- Trilafon ... 2389

Phenelzine Sulfate (Additive effects). Products include:
- Nardil ... 1920

Phenobarbital (Additive effects). Products include:
- Arco-Lase Plus Tablets ... 512
- Bellergal-S Tablets ... 2250
- Donnatal ... 2060
- Donnatal Extentabs ... 2061
- Donnatal Tablets ... 2060
- Phenobarbital Elixir and Tablets ... 1469
- Quadrinal Tablets ... 1350

Prazepam (Additive effects).
- No products indexed under this heading.

Prochlorperazine (Additive effects). Products include:
- Compazine ... 2470

Promethazine Hydrochloride (Additive effects). Products include:
- Mepergan Injection ... 2753
- Phenergan with Codeine ... 2777
- Phenergan with Dextromethorphan 2778
- Phenergan Injection ... 2773
- Phenergan Suppositories ... 2775
- Phenergan Syrup ... 2774
- Phenergan Tablets ... 2775
- Phenergan VC ... 2779
- Phenergan VC with Codeine ... 2781

Propofol (Additive effects). Products include:
- Diprivan Injection ... 2833

Propoxyphene Hydrochloride (Additive effects). Products include:
- Darvon ... 1435
- Wygesic Tablets ... 2827

Propoxyphene Napsylate (Additive effects). Products include:
- Darvon-N/Darvocet-N ... 1433

Protriptyline Hydrochloride (Additive effects). Products include:
- Vivactil Tablets ... 1774

Quazepam (Additive effects). Products include:
- Doral Tablets ... 2664

Risperidone (Additive effects). Products include:
- Risperdal ... 1301

Secobarbital Sodium (Additive effects). Products include:
- Seconal Sodium Pulvules ... 1474

Sufentanil Citrate (Additive effects). Products include:
- Sufenta Injection ... 1309

Temazepam (Additive effects). Products include:
- Restoril Capsules ... 2284

Thiamylal Sodium (Additive effects).
- No products indexed under this heading.

Thioridazine Hydrochloride (Additive effects). Products include:
- Mellaril ... 2269

Thiothixene (Additive effects). Products include:
- Navane Capsules and Concentrate 2201
- Navane Intramuscular ... 2202

Tranylcypromine Sulfate (Additive effects). Products include:
- Parnate Tablets ... 2503

Triazolam (Additive effects). Products include:
- Halcion Tablets ... 2611

Trifluoperazine Hydrochloride (Additive effects). Products include:
- Stelazine ... 2514

Trimipramine Maleate (Additive effects). Products include:
- Surmontil Capsules ... 2811

Zolpidem Tartrate (Additive effects). Products include:
- Ambien Tablets ... 2416

Food Interactions

Alcohol (Additive effects).

MINI-GAMULIN RH, RH_0(D) IMMUNE GLOBULIN (HUMAN)

(Rh_0(D) Immune Globulin (Human)) .. 520

None cited in PDR database.

IMPORTANT NOTE: Always consult each drug listing in the patient's regimen for possible interactions.

Minipress Interactions Index 662

MINIPRESS CAPSULES
(Prazosin Hydrochloride) 1937
May interact with beta blockers, diuretics, antihypertensives, and certain other agents. Compounds in these categories include:

Acebutolol Hydrochloride (Additive hypotensive effect; dosage retitration may be required). Products include:
- Sectral Capsules 2807

Amiloride Hydrochloride (Additive hypotensive effect). Products include:
- Midamor Tablets 1703
- Moduretic Tablets 1705

Amlodipine Besylate (Additive hypotensive effect; dosage retitration may be required). Products include:
- Lotrel Capsules 840
- Norvasc Tablets 1940

Atenolol (Additive hypotensive effect; dosage retitration may be required). Products include:
- Tenoretic Tablets 2845
- Tenormin Tablets and I.V. Injection 2847

Benazepril Hydrochloride (Additive hypotensive effect; dosage retitration may be required). Products include:
- Lotensin Tablets 834
- Lotensin HCT 837
- Lotrel Capsules 840

Bendroflumethiazide (Additive hypotensive effect; dosage retitration may be required).
- No products indexed under this heading.

Betaxolol Hydrochloride (Additive hypotensive effect; dosage retitration may be required). Products include:
- Betoptic Ophthalmic Solution 469
- Betoptic S Ophthalmic Suspension 471
- Kerlone Tablets 2436

Bisoprolol Fumarate (Additive hypotensive effect; dosage retitration may be required). Products include:
- Zebeta Tablets 1413
- Ziac 1415

Bumetanide (Additive hypotensive effect). Products include:
- Bumex 2093

Captopril (Additive hypotensive effect; dosage retitration may be required). Products include:
- Capoten 739
- Capozide 742

Carteolol Hydrochloride (Additive hypotensive effect; dosage retitration may be required). Products include:
- Cartrol Tablets 410
- Ocupress Ophthalmic Solution, 1% Sterile .... ◉ 309

Chlorothiazide (Additive hypotensive effect; dosage retitration may be required). Products include:
- Aldoclor Tablets 1598
- Diupres Tablets 1650
- Diuril Oral 1653

Chlorothiazide Sodium (Additive hypotensive effect; dosage retitration may be required). Products include:
- Diuril Sodium Intravenous 1652

Chlorthalidone (Additive hypotensive effect; dosage retitration may be required). Products include:
- Combipres Tablets 677
- Tenoretic Tablets 2845
- Thalitone 1245

Clonidine (Additive hypotensive effect; dosage retitration may be required). Products include:
- Catapres-TTS 675

Clonidine Hydrochloride (Additive hypotensive effect; dosage retitration may be required). Products include:
- Catapres Tablets 674
- Combipres Tablets 677

Deserpidine (Additive hypotensive effect; dosage retitration may be required).
- No products indexed under this heading.

Diazoxide (Additive hypotensive effect; dosage retitration may be required). Products include:
- Hyperstat I.V. Injection 2363
- Proglycem 580

Diltiazem Hydrochloride (Additive hypotensive effect; dosage retitration may be required). Products include:
- Cardizem CD Capsules 1506
- Cardizem SR Capsules 1510
- Cardizem Injectable 1508
- Cardizem Tablets 1512
- Dilacor XR Extended-release Capsules 2018

Doxazosin Mesylate (Additive hypotensive effect; dosage retitration may be required). Products include:
- Cardura Tablets 2186

Enalapril Maleate (Additive hypotensive effect; dosage retitration may be required). Products include:
- Vaseretic Tablets 1765
- Vasotec Tablets 1771

Enalaprilat (Additive hypotensive effect; dosage retitration may be required). Products include:
- Vasotec I.V. 1768

Esmolol Hydrochloride (Additive hypotensive effect; dosage retitration may be required). Products include:
- Brevibloc Injection 1808

Ethacrynic Acid (Additive hypotensive effect). Products include:
- Edecrin Tablets 1657

Felodipine (Additive hypotensive effect; dosage retitration may be required). Products include:
- Plendil Extended-Release Tablets 527

Fosinopril Sodium (Additive hypotensive effect; dosage retitration may be required). Products include:
- Monopril Tablets 757

Furosemide (Additive hypotensive effect; dosage retitration may be required). Products include:
- Lasix Injection, Oral Solution and Tablets 1240

Guanabenz Acetate (Additive hypotensive effect; dosage retitration may be required).
- No products indexed under this heading.

Guanethidine Monosulfate (Additive hypotensive effect; dosage retitration may be required). Products include:
- Esimil Tablets 822
- Ismelin Tablets 827

Hydralazine Hydrochloride (Additive hypotensive effect; dosage retitration may be required). Products include:
- Apresazide Capsules 808
- Apresoline Hydrochloride Tablets .. 809
- Ser-Ap-Es Tablets 849

Hydrochlorothiazide (Additive hypotensive effect; dosage retitration may be required). Products include:
- Aldactazide 2413
- Aldoril Tablets 1604
- Apresazide Capsules 808
- Capozide 742
- Dyazide 2479
- Esidrix Tablets 821
- Esimil Tablets 822
- HydroDIURIL Tablets 1674
- Hydropres Tablets 1675
- Hyzaar Tablets 1677
- Inderide Tablets 2732
- Inderide LA Long Acting Capsules .. 2734
- Lopressor HCT Tablets 832
- Lotensin HCT 837
- Maxzide 1380
- Moduretic Tablets 1705
- Oretic Tablets 443
- Prinzide Tablets 1737
- Ser-Ap-Es Tablets 849
- Timolide Tablets 1748
- Vaseretic Tablets 1765
- Zestoretic 2850
- Ziac 1415

Hydroflumethiazide (Additive hypotensive effect; dosage retitration may be required). Products include:
- Diucardin Tablets 2718

Indapamide (Additive hypotensive effect; dosage retitration may be required). Products include:
- Lozol Tablets 2022

Isradipine (Additive hypotensive effect; dosage retitration may be required). Products include:
- DynaCirc Capsules 2256

Labetalol Hydrochloride (Additive hypotensive effect; dosage retitration may be required). Products include:
- Normodyne Injection 2377
- Normodyne Tablets 2379
- Trandate 1185

Levobunolol Hydrochloride (Additive hypotensive effect; dosage retitration may be required). Products include:
- Betagan .... ◉ 233

Lisinopril (Additive hypotensive effect; dosage retitration may be required). Products include:
- Prinivil Tablets 1733
- Prinzide Tablets 1737
- Zestoretic 2850
- Zestril Tablets 2854

Losartan Potassium (Additive hypotensive effect; dosage retitration may be required). Products include:
- Cozaar Tablets 1628
- Hyzaar Tablets 1677

Mecamylamine Hydrochloride (Additive hypotensive effect; dosage retitration may be required). Products include:
- Inversine Tablets 1686

Methyclothiazide (Additive hypotensive effect; dosage retitration may be required). Products include:
- Enduron Tablets 420

Methyldopa (Additive hypotensive effect; dosage retitration may be required). Products include:
- Aldoclor Tablets 1598
- Aldomet Oral 1600
- Aldoril Tablets 1604

Methyldopate Hydrochloride (Additive hypotensive effect; dosage retitration may be required). Products include:
- Aldomet Ester HCl Injection 1602

Metipranolol Hydrochloride (Additive hypotensive effect; dosage retitration may be required). Products include:
- OptiPranolol (Metipranolol 0.3%) Sterile Ophthalmic Solution .... ◉ 258

Metolazone (Additive hypotensive effect; dosage retitration may be required). Products include:
- Mykrox Tablets 993
- Zaroxolyn Tablets 1000

Metoprolol Succinate (Additive hypotensive effect; dosage retitration may be required). Products include:
- Toprol-XL Tablets 565

Metoprolol Tartrate (Additive hypotensive effect; dosage retitration may be required). Products include:
- Lopressor Ampuls 830
- Lopressor HCT Tablets 832
- Lopressor Tablets 830

Metyrosine (Additive hypotensive effect; dosage retitration may be required). Products include:
- Demser Capsules 1649

Minoxidil (Additive hypotensive effect; dosage retitration may be required). Products include:
- Loniten Tablets 2618
- Rogaine Topical Solution 2637

Moexipril Hydrochloride (Additive hypotensive effect; dosage retitration may be required). Products include:
- Univasc Tablets 2410

Nadolol (Additive hypotensive effect; dosage retitration may be required).
- No products indexed under this heading.

Nicardipine Hydrochloride (Additive hypotensive effect; dosage retitration may be required). Products include:
- Cardene Capsules 2095
- Cardene I.V. 2709
- Cardene SR Capsules 2097

Nifedipine (Additive hypotensive effect; dosage retitration may be required). Products include:
- Adalat Capsules (10 mg and 20 mg) 587
- Adalat CC 589
- Procardia Capsules 1971
- Procardia XL Extended Release Tablets 1972

Nisoldipine (Additive hypotensive effect; dosage retitration may be required).
- No products indexed under this heading.

Nitroglycerin (Additive hypotensive effect; dosage retitration may be required). Products include:
- Deponit NTG Transdermal Delivery System 2397
- Nitro-Bid IV 1523
- Nitro-Bid Ointment 1524
- Nitrodisc 2047
- Nitro-Dur (nitroglycerin) Transdermal Infusion System 1326
- Nitrolingual Spray 2027
- Nitrostat Tablets 1925
- Transderm-Nitro Transdermal Therapeutic System 859

Penbutolol Sulfate (Additive hypotensive effect; dosage retitration may be required). Products include:
- Levatol 2403

Phenoxybenzamine Hydrochloride (Additive hypotensive effect; dosage retitration may be required). Products include:
- Dibenzyline Capsules 2476

Phentolamine Mesylate (Additive hypotensive effect; dosage retitration may be required). Products include:
- Regitine 846

Pindolol (Additive hypotensive effect; dosage retitration may be required). Products include:
- Visken Tablets 2299

Polythiazide (Additive hypotensive effect; dosage retitration may be required). Products include:
- Minizide Capsules 1938

Propranolol Hydrochloride (Additive hypotensive effect; dosage retitration may be required). Products include:
- Inderal 2728
- Inderal LA Long Acting Capsules 2730

(▣ Described in PDR For Nonprescription Drugs) (◉ Described in PDR For Ophthalmology)

663 **Interactions Index** **Minizide**

Inderide Tablets 2732
Inderide LA Long Acting Capsules .. 2734

Quinapril Hydrochloride (Additive hypotensive effect; dosage retitration may be required). Products include:
Accupril Tablets 1893

Ramipril (Additive hypotensive effect; dosage retitration may be required). Products include:
Altace Capsules 1232

Rauwolfia Serpentina (Additive hypotensive effect; dosage retitration may be required).
No products indexed under this heading.

Rescinnamine (Additive hypotensive effect; dosage retitration may be required).
No products indexed under this heading.

Reserpine (Additive hypotensive effect; dosage retitration may be required). Products include:
Diupres Tablets 1650
Hydropres Tablets 1675
Ser-Ap-Es Tablets 849

Sodium Nitroprusside (Additive hypotensive effect; dosage retitration may be required).
No products indexed under this heading.

Sotalol Hydrochloride (Additive hypotensive effect; dosage retitration may be required). Products include:
Betapace Tablets 641

Spirapril Hydrochloride (Additive hypotensive effect; dosage retitration may be required).
No products indexed under this heading.

Spironolactone (Additive hypotensive effect). Products include:
Aldactazide 2413
Aldactone 2414

Terazosin Hydrochloride (Additive hypotensive effect; dosage retitration may be required). Products include:
Hytrin Capsules 430

Timolol Hemihydrate (Additive hypotensive effect; dosage retitration may be required). Products include:
Betimol 0.25%, 0.5% .... ◉ 261

Timolol Maleate (Additive hypotensive effect; dosage retitration may be required). Products include:
Blocadren Tablets 1614
Timolide Tablets 1748
Timoptic in Ocudose 1753
Timoptic Sterile Ophthalmic Solution 1751
Timoptic-XE 1755

Torsemide (Additive hypotensive effect; dosage retitration may be required). Products include:
Demadex Tablets and Injection 686

Triamterene (Additive hypotensive effect). Products include:
Dyazide 2479
Dyrenium Capsules 2481
Maxzide 1380

Trimethaphan Camsylate (Additive hypotensive effect; dosage retitration may be required). Products include:
Arfonad Ampuls 2080

Verapamil Hydrochloride (Additive hypotensive effect; dosage retitration may be required). Products include:
Calan SR Caplets 2422
Calan Tablets 2419
Isoptin Injectable 1344
Isoptin Oral Tablets 1346
Isoptin SR Tablets 1348
Verelan Capsules 1410
Verelan Capsules 2824

MINIZIDE CAPSULES
(Prazosin Hydrochloride, Polythiazide) 1938
May interact with thiazides, ganglionic blocking agents, peripheral adrenergic blockers, insulin, barbiturates, narcotic analgesics, corticosteroids, cardiac glycosides, and certain other agents. Compounds in these categories include:

ACTH (Hypokalemia may be aggravated).
No products indexed under this heading.

Alfentanil Hydrochloride (Orthostatic hypotension). Products include:
Alfenta Injection 1286

Aprobarbital (Orthostatic hypotension).
No products indexed under this heading.

Bendroflumethiazide (Potentiation of antihypertensive action).
No products indexed under this heading.

Betamethasone Acetate (Hypokalemia may be aggravated). Products include:
Celestone Soluspan Suspension 2347

Betamethasone Sodium Phosphate (Hypokalemia may be aggravated). Products include:
Celestone Soluspan Suspension 2347

Buprenorphine (Orthostatic hypotension). Products include:
Buprenex Injectable 2006

Butabarbital (Orthostatic hypotension).
No products indexed under this heading.

Butalbital (Orthostatic hypotension). Products include:
Esgic-plus Tablets 1013
Fioricet Tablets 2258
Fioricet with Codeine Capsules 2260
Fiorinal Capsules 2261
Fiorinal with Codeine Capsules 2262
Fiorinal Tablets 2261
Phrenilin 785
Sedapap Tablets 50 mg/650 mg .. 1543

Chlorothiazide (Potentiation of antihypertensive action). Products include:
Aldoclor Tablets 1598
Diupres Tablets 1650
Diuril Oral 1653

Chlorothiazide Sodium (Potentiation of antihypertensive action). Products include:
Diuril Sodium Intravenous 1652

Codeine Phosphate (Orthostatic hypotension). Products include:
Actifed with Codeine Cough Syrup.. 1067
Brontex 1981
Deconsal C Expectorant Syrup 456
Deconsal Pediatric Syrup 457
Dimetane-DC Cough Syrup 2059
Empirin with Codeine Tablets 1093
Fioricet with Codeine Capsules 2260
Fiorinal with Codeine Capsules 2262
Isoclor Expectorant 990
Novahistine DH 2462
Novahistine Expectorant 2463
Nucofed 2051
Phenergan with Codeine 2777
Phenergan VC with Codeine 2781
Robitussin A-C Syrup 2073
Robitussin-DAC Syrup 2074
Ryna .... ▣ 841
Soma Compound w/Codeine Tablets 2676
Tussi-Organidin NR Liquid and S NR Liquid 2677
Tylenol with Codeine 1583

Cortisone Acetate (Hypokalemia may be aggravated). Products include:
Cortone Acetate Sterile Suspension 1623
Cortone Acetate Tablets 1624

Deserpidine (Potentiation of antihypertensive action of deserpidine).
No products indexed under this heading.

Deslanoside (May exaggerate the metabolic effects of hypokalemia).
No products indexed under this heading.

Dexamethasone (Hypokalemia may be aggravated). Products include:
AK-Trol Ointment & Suspension .... ◉ 205
Decadron Elixir 1633
Decadron Tablets 1635
Decaspray Topical Aerosol 1648
Dexacidin Ointment .... ◉ 263
Maxitrol Ophthalmic Ointment and Suspension .... ◉ 224
TobraDex Ophthalmic Suspension and Ointment 473

Dexamethasone Acetate (Hypokalemia may be aggravated). Products include:
Dalalone D.P. Injectable 1011
Decadron-LA Sterile Suspension 1646

Dexamethasone Sodium Phosphate (Hypokalemia may be aggravated). Products include:
Decadron Phosphate Injection 1637
Decadron Phosphate Respihaler 1642
Decadron Phosphate Sterile Ophthalmic Ointment 1641
Decadron Phosphate Sterile Ophthalmic Solution 1642
Decadron Phosphate Topical Cream 1644
Decadron Phosphate Turbinaire 1645
Decadron Phosphate with Xylocaine Injection, Sterile 1639
Dexacort Phosphate in Respihaler .. 458
Dexacort Phosphate in Turbinaire .. 459
NeoDecadron Sterile Ophthalmic Ointment 1712
NeoDecadron Sterile Ophthalmic Solution 1713
NeoDecadron Topical Cream 1714

Dezocine (Orthostatic hypotension). Products include:
Dalgan Injection 538

Digitoxin (May exaggerate the metabolic effects of hypokalemia). Products include:
Crystodigin Tablets 1433

Digoxin (May exaggerate the metabolic effects of hypokalemia). Products include:
Lanoxicaps 1117
Lanoxin Elixir Pediatric 1120
Lanoxin Injection 1123
Lanoxin Injection Pediatric 1126
Lanoxin Tablets 1128

Fentanyl (Orthostatic hypotension). Products include:
Duragesic Transdermal System 1288

Fentanyl Citrate (Orthostatic hypotension). Products include:
Sublimaze Injection 1307

Fludrocortisone Acetate (Hypokalemia may be aggravated). Products include:
Florinef Acetate Tablets 505

Guanethidine Monosulfate (Potentiation of antihypertensive action of guanethidine). Products include:
Esimil Tablets 822
Ismelin Tablets 827

Hydrochlorothiazide (Potentiation of antihypertensive action). Products include:
Aldactazide 2413
Aldoril Tablets 1604
Apresazide Capsules 808
Capozide 742
Dyazide 2479
Esidrix Tablets 821
Esimil Tablets 822
HydroDIURIL Tablets 1674
Hydropres Tablets 1675
Hyzaar Tablets 1677
Inderide Tablets 2732
Inderide LA Long Acting Capsules .. 2734
Lopressor HCT Tablets 832
Lotensin HCT 837
Maxzide 1380
Moduretic Tablets 1705
Oretic Tablets 443
Prinzide Tablets 1737
Ser-Ap-Es Tablets 849
Timolide Tablets 1748
Vaseretic Tablets 1765
Zestoretic 2850
Ziac 1415

Hydrocodone Bitartrate (Orthostatic hypotension). Products include:
Anexsia 5/500 Elixir 1781
Anexia Tablets 1782
Codiclear DH Syrup 791
Deconamine CX Cough and Cold Liquid and Tablets 1319
Duratuss HD Elixir 2565
Hycodan Tablets and Syrup 930
Hycomine Compound Tablets 932
Hycomine 931
Hycotuss Expectorant Syrup 933
Hydrocet Capsules 782
Lorcet 10/650 1018
Lortab 2566
Tussend 1783
Tussend Expectorant 1785
Vicodin Tablets 1356
Vicodin ES Tablets 1357
Vicodin Tuss Expectorant 1358
Zydone Capsules 949

Hydrocodone Polistirex (Orthostatic hypotension). Products include:
Tussionex Pennkinetic Extended-Release Suspension 998

Hydrocortisone (Hypokalemia may be aggravated). Products include:
Anusol-HC Cream 2.5% 1896
Aquanil HC Lotion 1931
Bactine Hydrocortisone Anti-Itch Cream .... ▣ 709
Caldecort Anti-Itch Hydrocortisone Spray .... ▣ 631
Cortaid .... ▣ 836
CORTENEMA 2535
Cortisporin Ointment 1085
Cortisporin Ophthalmic Ointment Sterile 1085
Cortisporin Ophthalmic Suspension Sterile 1086
Cortisporin Otic Solution Sterile 1087
Cortisporin Otic Suspension Sterile 1088
Cortizone-5 .... ▣ 831
Cortizone-10 .... ▣ 831
Hydrocortone Tablets 1672
Hytone 907
Massengill Medicated Soft Cloth Towelettes 2458
PediOtic Suspension Sterile 1153
Preparation H Hydrocortisone 1% Cream .... ▣ 872
ProctoCream-HC 2.5% 2408
VōSoL HC Otic Solution 2678

Hydrocortisone Acetate (Hypokalemia may be aggravated). Products include:
Analpram-HC Rectal Cream 1% and 2.5% 977
Anusol HC-1 Anti-Itch Hydrocortisone Ointment .... ▣ 847
Anusol-HC Suppositories 1897
Caldecort .... ▣ 631
Carmol HC 924
Coly-Mycin S Otic w/Neomycin & Hydrocortisone 1906
Cortaid .... ▣ 836
Cortifoam 2396
Cortisporin Cream 1084
Epifoam 2399
Hydrocortone Acetate Sterile Suspension 1669
Mantadil Cream 1135
Nupercainal Hydrocortisone 1% Cream .... ▣ 645
Ophthocort .... ◉ 311
Pramosone Cream, Lotion & Ointment 978
ProctoCream-HC 2408
ProctoFoam-HC 2409
Terra-Cortril Ophthalmic Suspension 2210

IMPORTANT NOTE: Always consult each drug listing in the patient's regimen for possible interactions.

Minizide **Interactions Index** 664

Hydrocortisone Sodium Phosphate (Hypokalemia may be aggravated). Products include:

Hydrocortone Phosphate Injection, Sterile 1670

Hydrocortisone Sodium Succinate (Hypokalemia may be aggravated). Products include:

Solu-Cortef Sterile Powder 2641

Hydroflumethiazide (Potentiation of antihypertensive action). Products include:

Diucardin Tablets 2718

Insulin, Human (Altered insulin requirements).

No products indexed under this heading.

Insulin, Human Isophane Suspension (Altered insulin requirements). Products include:

Novolin N Human Insulin 10 ml Vials 1795

Insulin, Human NPH (Altered insulin requirements). Products include:

Humulin N, 100 Units 1448
Novolin N PenFill Cartridges Durable Insulin Delivery System 1798
Novolin N Prefilled Syringe Disposable Insulin Delivery System 1798

Insulin, Human Regular (Altered insulin requirements). Products include:

Humulin R, 100 Units 1449
Novolin R Human Insulin 10 ml Vials 1795
Novolin R PenFill Cartridges Durable Insulin Delivery System 1798
Novolin R Prefilled Syringe Disposable Insulin Delivery System 1798
Velosulin BR Human Insulin 10 ml Vials 1795

Insulin, Human, Zinc Suspension (Altered insulin requirements). Products include:

Humulin L, 100 Units 1446
Humulin U, 100 Units 1450
Novolin L Human Insulin 10 ml Vials 1795

Insulin, NPH (Altered insulin requirements). Products include:

NPH, 100 Units 1450
Pork NPH, 100 Units 1452
Purified Pork NPH Isophane Insulin 1801

Insulin, Regular (Altered insulin requirements). Products include:

Regular, 100 Units 1450
Pork Regular, 100 Units 1452
Pork Regular (Concentrated), 500 Units 1453
Purified Pork Regular Insulin 1801

Insulin, Zinc Crystals (Altered insulin requirements). Products include:

NPH, 100 Units 1450

Insulin, Zinc Suspension (Altered insulin requirements). Products include:

Iletin I 1450
Lente, 100 Units 1450
Iletin II 1452
Pork Lente, 100 Units 1452
Purified Pork Lente Insulin 1801

Levorphanol Tartrate (Orthostatic hypotension). Products include:

Levo-Dromoran 2129

Mecamylamine Hydrochloride (Potentiation of antihypertensive action of mecamylamine). Products include:

Inversine Tablets 1686

Meperidine Hydrochloride (Orthostatic hypotension). Products include:

Demerol 2308
Mepergan Injection 2753

Mephobarbital (Orthostatic hypotension). Products include:

Mebaral Tablets 2322

Methadone Hydrochloride (Orthostatic hypotension). Products include:

Methadone Hydrochloride Oral Concentrate 2233
Methadone Hydrochloride Oral Solution & Tablets 2235

Methyclothiazide (Potentiation of antihypertensive action). Products include:

Enduron Tablets 420

Methylprednisolone Acetate (Hypokalemia may be aggravated). Products include:

Depo-Medrol Single-Dose Vial 2600
Depo-Medrol Sterile Aqueous Suspension 2597

Methylprednisolone Sodium Succinate (Hypokalemia may be aggravated). Products include:

Solu-Medrol Sterile Powder 2643

Morphine Sulfate (Orthostatic hypotension). Products include:

Astramorph/PF Injection, USP (Preservative-Free) 535
Duramorph 962
Infumorph 200 and Infumorph 500 Sterile Solutions 965
MS Contin Tablets 1994
MSIR 1997
Oramorph SR (Morphine Sulfate Sustained Release Tablets) 2236
RMS Suppositories 2657
Roxanol 2243

Norepinephrine Bitartrate (Decreased arterial responsiveness to norepinephrine). Products include:

Levophed Bitartrate Injection 2315

Opium Alkaloids (Orthostatic hypotension).

No products indexed under this heading.

Oxycodone Hydrochloride (Orthostatic hypotension). Products include:

Percocet Tablets 938
Percodan Tablets 939
Percodan-Demi Tablets 940
Roxicodone Tablets, Oral Solution & Intensol (Oxycodone) 2244
Tylox Capsules 1584

Pentobarbital Sodium (Orthostatic hypotension). Products include:

Nembutal Sodium Capsules 436
Nembutal Sodium Solution 438
Nembutal Sodium Suppositories 440

Phenobarbital (Orthostatic hypotension). Products include:

Arco-Lase Plus Tablets 512
Bellergal-S Tablets 2250
Donnatal 2060
Donnatal Extentabs 2061
Donnatal Tablets 2060
Phenobarbital Elixir and Tablets 1469
Quadrinal Tablets 1350

Prednisolone Acetate (Hypokalemia may be aggravated). Products include:

AK-CIDE .... ◉ 202
AK-CIDE Ointment .... ◉ 202
Blephamide Liquifilm Sterile Ophthalmic Suspension 476
Blephamide Ointment .... ◉ 237
Econopred & Econopred Plus Ophthalmic Suspensions .... ◉ 217
Poly-Pred Liquifilm .... ◉ 248
Pred Forte .... ◉ 250
Pred Mild .... ◉ 253
Pred-G Liquifilm Sterile Ophthalmic Suspension .... ◉ 251
Pred-G S.O.P. Sterile Ophthalmic Ointment .... ◉ 252
Vasocidin Ointment .... ◉ 268

Prednisolone Sodium Phosphate (Hypokalemia may be aggravated). Products include:

AK-Pred .... ◉ 204
Hydeltrasol Injection, Sterile 1665
Inflamase .... ◉ 265
Pediapred Oral Liquid 995
Vasocidin Ophthalmic Solution .... ◉ 270

Prednisolone Tebutate (Hypokalemia may be aggravated). Products include:

Hydeltra-T.B.A. Sterile Suspension 1667

Prednisone (Hypokalemia may be aggravated). Products include:

Deltasone Tablets 2595

Propoxyphene Hydrochloride (Orthostatic hypotension). Products include:

Darvon 1435
Wygesic Tablets 2827

Propoxyphene Napsylate (Orthostatic hypotension). Products include:

Darvon-N/Darvocet-N 1433

Rauwolfia Serpentina (Potentiation of antihypertensive action of rauwolfia alkaloids).

No products indexed under this heading.

Rescinnamine (Potentiation of antihypertensive action of rescinnamine).

No products indexed under this heading.

Reserpine (Potentiation of antihypertensive action of reserpine). Products include:

Diupres Tablets 1650
Hydropres Tablets 1675
Ser-Ap-Es Tablets 849

Secobarbital Sodium (Orthostatic hypotension). Products include:

Seconal Sodium Pulvules 1474

Sufentanil Citrate (Orthostatic hypotension). Products include:

Sufenta Injection 1309

Terazosin Hydrochloride (Potentiation of antihypertensive action of guanadrel). Products include:

Hytrin Capsules 430

Thiamylal Sodium (Orthostatic hypotension).

No products indexed under this heading.

Triamcinolone (Hypokalemia may be aggravated). Products include:

Aristocort Tablets 1022

Triamcinolone Acetonide (Hypokalemia may be aggravated). Products include:

Aristocort A 0.025% Cream 1027
Aristocort A 0.5% Cream 1031
Aristocort A 0.1% Cream 1029
Aristocort A 0.1% Ointment 1030
Azmacort Oral Inhaler 2011
Nasacort Nasal Inhaler 2024

Triamcinolone Diacetate (Hypokalemia may be aggravated). Products include:

Aristocort Suspension (Forte Parenteral) 1027
Aristocort Suspension (Intralesional) 1025

Triamcinolone Hexacetonide (Hypokalemia may be aggravated). Products include:

Aristospan Suspension (Intra-articular) 1033
Aristospan Suspension (Intralesional) 1032

Trimethaphan Camsylate (Potentiation of antihypertensive action of trimethaphan). Products include:

Arfonad Ampuls 2080

Tubocurarine Chloride (Increased responsiveness to tubocurarine).

No products indexed under this heading.

Food Interactions

Alcohol (Orthostatic hypotension).

MINOCIN INTRAVENOUS
(Minocycline Hydrochloride) 1382
May interact with penicillins, anticoagulants, oral contraceptives, and certain other agents. Compounds in these categories include:

Amoxicillin Trihydrate (Interference with bactericidal action of penicillins; avoid concurrent use). Products include:

Amoxil 2464
Augmentin 2468

Ampicillin (Interference with bactericidal action of penicillins; avoid concurrent use). Products include:

Omnipen Capsules 2764
Omnipen for Oral Suspension 2765

Ampicillin Sodium (Interference with bactericidal action of penicillins; avoid concurrent use). Products include:

Unasyn 2212

Ampicillin Trihydrate (Interference with bactericidal action of penicillins; avoid concurrent use).

No products indexed under this heading.

Azlocillin Sodium (Interference with bactericidal action of penicillins; avoid concurrent use).

No products indexed under this heading.

Bacampicillin Hydrochloride (Interference with bactericidal action of penicillins; avoid concurrent use). Products include:

Spectrobid Tablets 2206

Carbenicillin Disodium (Interference with bactericidal action of penicillins; avoid concurrent use).

No products indexed under this heading.

Carbenicillin Indanyl Sodium (Interference with bactericidal action of penicillins; avoid concurrent use). Products include:

Geocillin Tablets 2199

Dalteparin Sodium (Depressed plasma prothrombin activity). Products include:

Fragmin 1954

Desogestrel (Reduced efficacy and increased incidence of breakthrough bleeding). Products include:

Desogen Tablets 1817
Ortho-Cept 1851

Dicloxacillin Sodium (Interference with bactericidal action of penicillins; avoid concurrent use).

No products indexed under this heading.

Dicumarol (Depressed plasma prothrombin activity).

No products indexed under this heading.

Enoxaparin (Depressed plasma prothrombin activity). Products include:

Lovenox Injection 2020

Ethinyl Estradiol (Reduced efficacy and increased incidence of breakthrough bleeding). Products include:

Brevicon 2088
Demulen 2428
Desogen Tablets 1817
Levlen/Tri-Levlen 651
Lo/Ovral Tablets 2746
Lo/Ovral-28 Tablets 2751
Modicon 1872
Nordette-21 Tablets 2755
Nordette-28 Tablets 2758
Norinyl 2088
Ortho-Cept 1851
Ortho-Cyclen/Ortho-Tri-Cyclen 1858
Ortho-Novum 1872
Ortho-Cyclen/Ortho Tri-Cyclen 1858
Ovcon 760
Ovral Tablets 2770
Ovral-28 Tablets 2770
Levlen/Tri-Levlen 651
Tri-Norinyl 2164
Triphasil-21 Tablets 2814

(▣ Described in PDR For Nonprescription Drugs) (◉ Described in PDR For Ophthalmology)

Triphasil-28 Tablets 2819

Ethynodiol Diacetate (Reduced efficacy and increased incidence of breakthrough bleeding). Products include:

Demulen 2428

Heparin Calcium (Depressed plasma prothrombin activity).

No products indexed under this heading.

Heparin Sodium (Depressed plasma prothrombin activity). Products include:

Heparin Lock Flush Solution 2725
Heparin Sodium Injection.................... 2726
Heparin Sodium Injection, USP, Sterile Solution 2615
Heparin Sodium Vials............................ 1441

Levonorgestrel (Reduced efficacy and increased incidence of breakthrough bleeding). Products include:

Levlen/Tri-Levlen................................... 651
Nordette-21 Tablets............................... 2755
Nordette-28 Tablets............................... 2758
Norplant System 2759
Levlen/Tri-Levlen................................... 651
Triphasil-21 Tablets............................... 2814
Triphasil-28 Tablets............................... 2819

Mestranol (Reduced efficacy and increased incidence of breakthrough bleeding). Products include:

Norinyl 2088
Ortho-Novum... 1872

Mezlocillin Sodium (Interference with bactericidal action of penicillins; avoid concurrent use). Products include:

Mezlin 601
Mezlin Pharmacy Bulk Package......... 604

Nafcillin Sodium (Interference with bactericidal action of penicillins; avoid concurrent use).

No products indexed under this heading.

Norethindrone (Reduced efficacy and increased incidence of breakthrough bleeding). Products include:

Brevicon.. 2088
Micronor Tablets 1872
Modicon... 1872
Norinyl 2088
Nor-Q D Tablets...................................... 2135
Ortho-Novum... 1872
Ovcon 760
Tri-Norinyl.. 2164

Norethynodrel (Reduced efficacy and increased incidence of breakthrough bleeding).

No products indexed under this heading.

Norgestimate (Reduced efficacy and increased incidence of breakthrough bleeding). Products include:

Ortho-Cyclen/Ortho-Tri-Cyclen 1858
Ortho-Cyclen/Ortho Tri-Cyclen 1858

Norgestrel (Reduced efficacy and increased incidence of breakthrough bleeding). Products include:

Lo/Ovral Tablets 2746
Lo/Ovral-28 Tablets............................... 2751
Ovral Tablets 2770
Ovral-28 Tablets 2770
Ovrette Tablets.. 2771

Penicillin G Benzathine (Interference with bactericidal action of penicillins; avoid concurrent use). Products include:

Bicillin C-R Injection 2704
Bicillin C-R 900/300 Injection 2706
Bicillin L-A Injection 2707

Penicillin G Potassium (Interference with bactericidal action of penicillins; avoid concurrent use). Products include:

Pfizerpen for Injection 2203

Penicillin G Procaine (Interference with bactericidal action of penicillins; avoid concurrent use). Products include:

Bicillin C-R Injection 2704
Bicillin C-R 900/300 Injection 2706

Penicillin G Sodium (Interference with bactericidal action of penicillins; avoid concurrent use).

No products indexed under this heading.

Penicillin V Potassium (Interference with bactericidal action of penicillins; avoid concurrent use). Products include:

Pen•Vee K.. 2772

Ticarcillin Disodium (Interference with bactericidal action of penicillins; avoid concurrent use). Products include:

Ticar for Injection 2526
Timentin for Injection............................ 2528

Warfarin Sodium (Depressed plasma prothrombin activity). Products include:

Coumadin 926

MINOCIN ORAL SUSPENSION

(Minocycline Hydrochloride) 1385

May interact with anticoagulants, oral contraceptives, penicillins, antacids containing aluminium, calcium and magnesium, and certain other agents. Compounds in these categories include:

Aluminum Carbonate Gel (Absorption of tetracyclines is impaired). Products include:

Basaljel... 2703

Aluminum Hydroxide (Absorption of tetracyclines is impaired). Products include:

ALternaGEL Liquid 1316
Maximum Strength Ascriptin .... ᴹᴰ 630
Cama Arthritis Pain Reliever........... ᴹᴰ 785
Gaviscon Extra Strength Relief Formula Antacid Tablets................. ᴹᴰ 819
Gaviscon Extra Strength Relief Formula Liquid Antacid .... ᴹᴰ 819
Gaviscon Liquid Antacid .... ᴹᴰ 820
Gelusil Liquid & Tablets .... ᴹᴰ 855
Maalox Heartburn Relief Suspension .... ᴹᴰ 642
Maalox Heartburn Relief Tablets.... ᴹᴰ 641
Maalox Magnesia and Alumina Oral Suspension .... ᴹᴰ 642
Maalox Plus Tablets .... ᴹᴰ 643
Extra Strength Maalox Antacid Plus Antigas Liquid and Tablets ᴹᴰ 638
Tempo Soft Antacid .... ᴹᴰ 835

Aluminum Hydroxide Gel (Absorption of tetracyclines is impaired). Products include:

ALternaGEL Liquid .... ᴹᴰ 659
Aludrox Oral Suspension 2695
Amphojel Suspension 2695
Amphojel Suspension without Flavor 2695
Amphojel Tablets.................................... 2695
Arthritis Pain Ascriptin .... ᴹᴰ 631
Regular Strength Ascriptin Tablets .... ᴹᴰ 629
Gaviscon Antacid Tablets.................... ᴹᴰ 819
Gaviscon-2 Antacid Tablets .... ᴹᴰ 820
Mylanta Liquid 1317
Mylanta Tablets .... ᴹᴰ 660
Mylanta Double Strength Liquid 1317
Mylanta Double Strength Tablets .. ᴹᴰ 660
Nephrox Suspension .... ᴹᴰ 655

Amoxicillin Trihydrate (Interference with bactericidal action of penicillin; avoid concurrent use). Products include:

Amoxil.. 2464
Augmentin 2468

Ampicillin (Interference with bactericidal action of penicillin; avoid concurrent use). Products include:

Omnipen Capsules 2764
Omnipen for Oral Suspension 2765

Ampicillin Sodium (Interference with bactericidal action of penicillin; avoid concurrent use). Products include:

Unasyn 2212

Ampicillin Trihydrate (Interference with bactericidal action of penicillin; avoid concurrent use).

No products indexed under this heading.

Azlocillin Sodium (Interference with bactericidal action of penicillin; avoid concurrent use).

No products indexed under this heading.

Bacampicillin Hydrochloride (Interference with bactericidal action of penicillin; avoid concurrent use). Products include:

Spectrobid Tablets 2206

Carbenicillin Disodium (Interference with bactericidal action of penicillin; avoid concurrent use).

No products indexed under this heading.

Carbenicillin Indanyl Sodium (Interference with bactericidal action of penicillin; avoid concurrent use). Products include:

Geocillin Tablets..................................... 2199

Dalteparin Sodium (Depressed plasma prothrombin activity; may require downward adjustment of the anticoagulant dosage). Products include:

Fragmin 1954

Desogestrel (Concurrent use may render oral contraceptives less effective; potential for breakthrough bleeding). Products include:

Desogen Tablets...................................... 1817
Ortho-Cept 1851

Dicloxacillin Sodium (Interference with bactericidal action of penicillin; avoid concurrent use).

No products indexed under this heading.

Dicumarol (Depressed plasma prothrombin activity; may require downward adjustment of the anticoagulant dosage).

No products indexed under this heading.

Dihydroxyaluminum Sodium Carbonate (Absorption of tetracyclines is impaired).

No products indexed under this heading.

Enoxaparin (Depressed plasma prothrombin activity; may require downward adjustment of the anticoagulant dosage). Products include:

Lovenox Injection.................................... 2020

Ethinyl Estradiol (Concurrent use may render oral contraceptives less effective; potential for breakthrough bleeding). Products include:

Brevicon... 2088
Demulen 2428
Desogen Tablets...................................... 1817
Levlen/Tri-Levlen................................... 651
Lo/Ovral Tablets 2746
Lo/Ovral-28 Tablets............................... 2751
Modicon.. 1872
Nordette-21 Tablets............................... 2755
Nordette-28 Tablets............................... 2758
Norinyl 2088
Ortho-Cept 1851
Ortho-Cyclen/Ortho-Tri-Cyclen 1858
Ortho-Novum.. 1872
Ortho-Cyclen/Ortho Tri-Cyclen 1858
Ovcon 760
Ovral Tablets 2770
Ovral-28 Tablets 2770
Levlen/Tri-Levlen................................... 651
Tri-Norinyl... 2164
Triphasil-21 Tablets............................... 2814
Triphasil-28 Tablets............................... 2819

Ethynodiol Diacetate (Concurrent use may render oral contraceptives less effective; potential for breakthrough bleeding). Products include:

Demulen 2428

Ferrous Fumarate (Absorption of tetracyclines is impaired). Products include:

Chromagen Capsules 2339
Ferro-Sequels .... ᴹᴰ 669
Nephro-Fer Tablets................................ 2004
Nephro-Fer Rx Tablets.......................... 2005
Nephro-Vite + Fe Tablets 2006
Sigtab-M Tablets .... ᴹᴰ 772
Stresstabs + Iron .... ᴹᴰ 671
The Stuart Formula Tablets.............. ᴹᴰ 663
Theragran-M Tablets with Beta Carotene .... ᴹᴰ 623
Triniscon Capsules 2570
Vitron-C Tablets..................................... ᴹᴰ 650

Ferrous Gluconate (Absorption of tetracyclines is impaired). Products include:

Fergon Iron Supplement Tablets.... ᴹᴰ 721
Megadose 512

Ferrous Sulfate (Absorption of tetracyclines is impaired). Products include:

Feosol Capsules 2456
Feosol Elixir 2456
Feosol Tablets 2457
Fero-Folic-500 Filmtab 429
Fero-Grad-500 Filmtab......................... 429
Fero-Gradumet Filmtab........................ 429
Iberet Tablets 433
Iberet-500 Liquid 433
Iberet-Folic-500 Filmtab...................... 429
Iberet-Liquid.. 433
Irospan... 982
Slow Fe Tablets....................................... 869
Slow Fe with Folic Acid 869

Heparin Calcium (Depressed plasma prothrombin activity; may require downward adjustment of the anticoagulant dosage).

No products indexed under this heading.

Heparin Sodium (Depressed plasma prothrombin activity; may require downward adjustment of the anticoagulant dosage). Products include:

Heparin Lock Flush Solution.............. 2725
Heparin Sodium Injection.................... 2726
Heparin Sodium Injection, USP, Sterile Solution.................................... 2615
Heparin Sodium Vials............................ 1441

Levonorgestrel (Concurrent use may render oral contraceptives less effective; potential for breakthrough bleeding). Products include:

Levlen/Tri-Levlen................................... 651
Nordette-21 Tablets............................... 2755
Nordette-28 Tablets............................... 2758
Norplant System 2759
Levlen/Tri-Levlen................................... 651
Triphasil-21 Tablets............................... 2814
Triphasil-28 Tablets............................... 2819

Magaldrate (Absorption of tetracyclines is impaired).

No products indexed under this heading.

Magnesium Hydroxide (Absorption of tetracyclines is impaired). Products include:

Aludrox Oral Suspension 2695
Arthritis Pain Ascriptin .... ᴹᴰ 631
Maximum Strength Ascriptin .... ᴹᴰ 630
Regular Strength Ascriptin Tablets .... ᴹᴰ 629
Di-Gel Antacid/Anti-Gas .... ᴹᴰ 801
Gelusil Liquid & Tablets .... ᴹᴰ 855
Maalox Magnesia and Alumina Oral Suspension .... ᴹᴰ 642
Maalox Plus Tablets .... ᴹᴰ 643
Extra Strength Maalox Antacid Plus Antigas Liquid and Tablets ᴹᴰ 638
Mylanta Calcium Carbonate and Magnesium Hydroxide Tablets...... 1318
Mylanta Liquid 1317
Mylanta Tablets .... ᴹᴰ 660
Mylanta Double Strength Liquid 1317
Mylanta Double Strength Tablets .. ᴹᴰ 660
Phillips' Milk of Magnesia Liquid.... ᴹᴰ 729
Rolaids Tablets....................................... ᴹᴰ 843
Tempo Soft Antacid .... ᴹᴰ 835

Magnesium Oxide (Absorption of tetracyclines is impaired). Products include:

Beelith Tablets 639

IMPORTANT NOTE: Always consult each drug listing in the patient's regimen for possible interactions.

Minocin Oral Suspension Interactions Index 666

Bufferin Analgesic Tablets and Caplets ▣ 613
Caltrate PLUS ▣ 665
Cama Arthritis Pain Reliever ▣ 785
Mag-Ox 400 668
Uro-Mag 668

Mestranol (Concurrent use may render oral contraceptives less effective; potential for breakthrough bleeding). Products include:
Norinyl 2088
Ortho-Novum 1872

Methoxyflurane (Potential for fatal renal toxicity).
No products indexed under this heading.

Mezlocillin Sodium (Interference with bactericidal action of penicillin; avoid concurrent use). Products include:
Mezlin 601
Mezlin Pharmacy Bulk Package 604

Nafcillin Sodium (Interference with bactericidal action of penicillin; avoid concurrent use).
No products indexed under this heading.

Norethindrone (Concurrent use may render oral contraceptives less effective; potential for breakthrough bleeding). Products include:
Brevicon 2088
Micronor Tablets 1872
Modicon 1872
Norinyl 2088
Nor-Q D Tablets 2135
Ortho-Novum 1872
Ovcon 760
Tri-Norinyl 2164

Norethynodrel (Concurrent use may render oral contraceptives less effective; potential for breakthrough bleeding).
No products indexed under this heading.

Norgestimate (Concurrent use may render oral contraceptives less effective; potential for breakthrough bleeding). Products include:
Ortho-Cyclen/Ortho-Tri-Cyclen 1858
Ortho-Cyclen/Ortho Tri-Cyclen 1858

Norgestrel (Concurrent use may render oral contraceptives less effective; potential for breakthrough bleeding). Products include:
Lo/Ovral Tablets 2746
Lo/Ovral-28 Tablets 2751
Ovral Tablets 2770
Ovral-28 Tablets 2770
Ovrette Tablets 2771

Penicillin G Benzathine (Interference with bactericidal action of penicillin; avoid concurrent use). Products include:
Bicillin C-R Injection 2704
Bicillin C-R 900/300 Injection 2706
Bicillin L-A Injection 2707

Penicillin G Potassium (Interference with bactericidal action of penicillin; avoid concurrent use). Products include:
Pfizerpen for Injection 2203

Penicillin G Procaine (Interference with bactericidal action of penicillin; avoid concurrent use). Products include:
Bicillin C-R Injection 2704
Bicillin C-R 900/300 Injection 2706

Penicillin G Sodium (Interference with bactericidal action of penicillin; avoid concurrent use).
No products indexed under this heading.

Penicillin V Potassium (Interference with bactericidal action of penicillin; avoid concurrent use). Products include:
Pen•Vee K 2772

Ticarcillin Disodium (Interference with bactericidal action of penicillin; avoid concurrent use). Products include:
Ticar for Injection 2526
Timentin for Injection 2528

Warfarin Sodium (Depressed plasma prothrombin activity; may require downward adjustment of the anticoagulant dosage). Products include:
Coumadin 926

MINOCIN PELLET-FILLED CAPSULES

(Minocycline Hydrochloride) 1383
May interact with anticoagulants, oral contraceptives, penicillins, antacids containing aluminium, calcium and magnesium, iron containing oral preparations, and certain other agents. Compounds in these categories include:

Aluminum Carbonate Gel (Absorption of tetracyclines is impaired). Products include:
Basaljel 2703

Aluminum Hydroxide (Absorption of tetracyclines is impaired). Products include:
ALternaGEL Liquid 1316
Maximum Strength Ascriptin ▣ 630
Cama Arthritis Pain Reliever ▣ 785
Gaviscon Extra Strength Relief Formula Antacid Tablets ▣ 819
Gaviscon Extra Strength Relief Formula Liquid Antacid ▣ 819
Gaviscon Liquid Antacid ▣ 820
Gelusil Liquid & Tablets ▣ 855
Maalox Heartburn Relief Suspension ▣ 642
Maalox Heartburn Relief Tablets ▣ 641
Maalox Magnesia and Alumina Oral Suspension ▣ 642
Maalox Plus Tablets ▣ 643
Extra Strength Maalox Antacid Plus Antigas Liquid and Tablets ▣ 638
Tempo Soft Antacid ▣ 835

Aluminum Hydroxide Gel (Absorption of tetracyclines is impaired). Products include:
ALternaGEL Liquid ▣ 659
Aludrox Oral Suspension 2695
Amphojel Suspension 2695
Amphojel Suspension without Flavor 2695
Amphojel Tablets 2695
Arthritis Pain Ascriptin ▣ 631
Regular Strength Ascriptin Tablets ▣ 629
Gaviscon Antacid Tablets ▣ 819
Gaviscon-2 Antacid Tablets ▣ 820
Mylanta Liquid 1317
Mylanta Tablets ▣ 660
Mylanta Double Strength Liquid 1317
Mylanta Double Strength Tablets ▣ 660
Nephrox Suspension ▣ 655

Amoxicillin Trihydrate (Interference with bactericidal action of penicillin; avoid concurrent use). Products include:
Amoxil 2464
Augmentin 2468

Ampicillin (Interference with bactericidal action of penicillin; avoid concurrent use). Products include:
Omnipen Capsules 2764
Omnipen for Oral Suspension 2765

Ampicillin Sodium (Interference with bactericidal action of penicillin; avoid concurrent use). Products include:
Unasyn 2212

Ampicillin Trihydrate (Interference with bactericidal action of penicillin; avoid concurrent use).
No products indexed under this heading.

Azlocillin Sodium (Interference with bactericidal action of penicillin; avoid concurrent use).
No products indexed under this heading.

Bacampicillin Hydrochloride (Interference with bactericidal action of penicillin; avoid concurrent use). Products include:
Spectrobid Tablets 2206

Carbenicillin Disodium (Interference with bactericidal action of penicillin; avoid concurrent use).
No products indexed under this heading.

Carbenicillin Indanyl Sodium (Interference with bactericidal action of penicillin; avoid concurrent use). Products include:
Geocillin Tablets 2199

Dalteparin Sodium (Depressed plasma prothrombin activity; may require downward adjustment of the anticoagulant dosage). Products include:
Fragmin 1954

Desogestrel (Concurrent use may render oral contraceptives less effective; potential for breakthrough bleeding). Products include:
Desogen Tablets 1817
Ortho-Cept 1851

Dicloxacillin Sodium (Interference with bactericidal action of penicillin; avoid concurrent use).
No products indexed under this heading.

Dicumarol (Depressed plasma prothrombin activity; may require downward adjustment of the anticoagulant dosage).
No products indexed under this heading.

Dihydroxyaluminum Sodium Carbonate (Absorption of tetracyclines is impaired).
No products indexed under this heading.

Enoxaparin (Depressed plasma prothrombin activity; may require downward adjustment of the anticoagulant dosage). Products include:
Lovenox Injection 2020

Ethinyl Estradiol (Concurrent use may render oral contraceptives less effective; potential for breakthrough bleeding). Products include:
Brevicon 2088
Demulen 2428
Desogen Tablets 1817
Levlen/Tri-Levlen 651
Lo/Ovral Tablets 2746
Lo/Ovral-28 Tablets 2751
Modicon 1872
Nordette-21 Tablets 2755
Nordette-28 Tablets 2758
Norinyl 2088
Ortho-Cept 1851
Ortho-Cyclen/Ortho-Tri-Cyclen 1858
Ortho-Novum 1872
Ortho-Cyclen/Ortho Tri-Cyclen 1858
Ovcon 760
Ovral Tablets 2770
Ovral-28 Tablets 2770
Levlen/Tri-Levlen 651
Tri-Norinyl 2164
Triphasil-21 Tablets 2814
Triphasil-28 Tablets 2819

Ethynodiol Diacetate (Concurrent use may render oral contraceptives less effective; potential for breakthrough bleeding). Products include:
Demulen 2428

Ferrous Fumarate (Absorption of tetracyclines is impaired). Products include:
Chromagen Capsules 2339
Ferro-Sequels ▣ 669
Nephro-Fer Tablets 2004
Nephro-Fer Rx Tablets 2005
Nephro-Vite + Fe Tablets 2006
Sigtab-M Tablets ▣ 772
Stresstabs + Iron ▣ 671
The Stuart Formula Tablets ▣ 663
Theragran-M Tablets with Beta Carotene ▣ 623
Trinsicon Capsules 2570
Vitron-C Tablets ▣ 650

Ferrous Gluconate (Absorption of tetracyclines is impaired). Products include:
Fergon Iron Supplement Tablets ▣ 721
Megadose 512

Ferrous Sulfate (Absorption of tetracyclines is impaired). Products include:
Feosol Capsules 2456
Feosol Elixir 2456
Feosol Tablets 2457
Fero-Folic-500 Filmtab 429
Fero-Grad-500 Filmtab 429
Fero-Gradumet Filmtab 429
Iberet Tablets 433
Iberet-500 Liquid 433
Iberet-Folic-500 Filmtab 429
Iberet-Liquid 433
Irospan 982
Slow Fe Tablets 869
Slow Fe with Folic Acid 869

Heparin Calcium (Depressed plasma prothrombin activity; may require downward adjustment of the anticoagulant dosage).
No products indexed under this heading.

Heparin Sodium (Depressed plasma prothrombin activity; may require downward adjustment of the anticoagulant dosage). Products include:
Heparin Lock Flush Solution 2725
Heparin Sodium Injection 2726
Heparin Sodium Injection, USP, Sterile Solution 2615
Heparin Sodium Vials 1441

Levonorgestrel (Concurrent use may render oral contraceptives less effective; potential for breakthrough bleeding). Products include:
Levlen/Tri-Levlen 651
Nordette-21 Tablets 2755
Nordette-28 Tablets 2758
Norplant System 2759
Levlen/Tri-Levlen 651
Triphasil-21 Tablets 2814
Triphasil-28 Tablets 2819

Magaldrate (Absorption of tetracyclines is impaired).
No products indexed under this heading.

Magnesium Hydroxide (Absorption of tetracyclines is impaired). Products include:
Aludrox Oral Suspension 2695
Arthritis Pain Ascriptin ▣ 631
Maximum Strength Ascriptin ▣ 630
Regular Strength Ascriptin Tablets ▣ 629
Di-Gel Antacid/Anti-Gas ▣ 801
Gelusil Liquid & Tablets ▣ 855
Maalox Magnesia and Alumina Oral Suspension ▣ 642
Maalox Plus Tablets ▣ 643
Extra Strength Maalox Antacid Plus Antigas Liquid and Tablets ▣ 638
Mylanta Calcium Carbonate and Magnesium Hydroxide Tablets 1318
Mylanta Liquid 1317
Mylanta Tablets ▣ 660
Mylanta Double Strength Liquid 1317
Mylanta Double Strength Tablets ▣ 660
Phillips' Milk of Magnesia Liquid ▣ 729
Rolaids Tablets ▣ 843
Tempo Soft Antacid ▣ 835

Magnesium Oxide (Absorption of tetracyclines is impaired). Products include:
Beelith Tablets 639
Bufferin Analgesic Tablets and Caplets ▣ 613
Caltrate PLUS ▣ 665
Cama Arthritis Pain Reliever ▣ 785
Mag-Ox 400 668
Uro-Mag 668

(▣ Described in PDR For Nonprescription Drugs) (◉ Described in PDR For Ophthalmology)

Mestranol (Concurrent use may render oral contraceptives less effective; potential for breakthrough bleeding). Products include:

Norinyl 2088
Ortho-Novum 1872

Methoxyflurane (Potential for fatal renal toxicity).

No products indexed under this heading.

Mezlocillin Sodium (Interference with bactericidal action of penicillin; avoid concurrent use). Products include:

Mezlin 601
Mezlin Pharmacy Bulk Package 604

Nafcillin Sodium (Interference with bactericidal action of penicillin).

No products indexed under this heading.

Norethindrone (Concurrent use may render oral contraceptives less effective; potential for breakthrough bleeding). Products include:

Brevicon 2088
Micronor Tablets 1872
Modicon 1872
Norinyl 2088
Nor-Q D Tablets 2135
Ortho-Novum 1872
Ovcon 760
Tri-Norinyl 2164

Norethynodrel (Concurrent use may render oral contraceptives less effective; potential for breakthrough bleeding).

No products indexed under this heading.

Norgestimate (Concurrent use may render oral contraceptives less effective; potential for breakthrough bleeding). Products include:

Ortho-Cyclen/Ortho-Tri-Cyclen 1858
Ortho-Cyclen/Ortho Tri-Cyclen 1858

Norgestrel (Concurrent use may render oral contraceptives less effective; potential for breakthrough bleeding). Products include:

Lo/Ovral Tablets 2746
Lo/Ovral-28 Tablets 2751
Ovral Tablets 2770
Ovral-28 Tablets 2770
Ovrette Tablets 2771

Penicillin G Benzathine (Interference with bactericidal action of penicillin; avoid concurrent use). Products include:

Bicillin C-R Injection 2704
Bicillin C-R 900/300 Injection 2706
Bicillin L-A Injection 2707

Penicillin G Potassium (Interference with bactericidal action of penicillin; avoid concurrent use). Products include:

Pfizerpen for Injection 2203

Penicillin G Procaine (Interference with bactericidal action of penicillin; avoid concurrent use). Products include:

Bicillin C-R Injection 2704
Bicillin C-R 900/300 Injection 2706

Penicillin G Sodium (Interference with bactericidal action of penicillin; avoid concurrent use).

No products indexed under this heading.

Penicillin V Potassium (Interference with bactericidal action of penicillin; avoid concurrent use). Products include:

Pen•Vee K 2772

Polysaccharide-Iron Complex (Absorption of tetracyclines is impaired). Products include:

Niferex-150 Capsules 793
Niferex Elixir 793
Niferex-150 Forte Capsules 794
Niferex Forte Elixir 794
Niferex 793
Niferex-PN Tablets 794
Nu-Iron 150 Capsules 1543
Nu-Iron Elixir 1543
Sunkist Children's Chewable Multivitamins - Plus Iron .... ■ 649

Ticarcillin Disodium (Interference with bactericidal action of penicillin; avoid concurrent use). Products include:

Ticar for Injection 2526
Timentin for Injection 2528

Warfarin Sodium (Depressed plasma prothrombin activity; may require downward adjustment of the anticoagulant dosage). Products include:

Coumadin 926

Food Interactions

Dairy products (The peak plasma concentrations were slightly decreased (11.2%) and delayed by 1 hour).

Meal with dairy products (The peak plasma concentrations were slightly decreased (11.2%) and delayed by 1 hour).

MINTEZOL CHEWABLE TABLETS

(Thiabendazole) 1704

May interact with xanthine bronchodilators. Compounds in this category include:

Aminophylline (Xanthine toxicity).

No products indexed under this heading.

Dyphylline (Xanthine toxicity). Products include:

Lufyllin & Lufyllin-400 Tablets 2670
Lufyllin-GG Elixir & Tablets 2671

Theophylline (Xanthine toxicity). Products include:

Marax Tablets & DF Syrup 2200
Quibron 2053

Theophylline Anhydrous (Xanthine toxicity). Products include:

Aerolate 1004
Primatene Dual Action Formula .... ■ 872
Primatene Tablets .... ■ 873
Respbid Tablets 682
Slo-bid Gyrocaps 2033
Theo-24 Extended Release Capsules 2568
Theo-Dur Extended-Release Tablets 1327
Theo-X Extended-Release Tablets 788
Uni-Dur Extended-Release Tablets 1331
Uniphyl 400 mg Tablets 2001

Theophylline Calcium Salicylate (Xanthine toxicity). Products include:

Quadrinal Tablets 1350

Theophylline Sodium Glycinate (Xanthine toxicity).

No products indexed under this heading.

Xanthine Preparations (Xanthine toxicity).

MINTEZOL SUSPENSION

(Thiabendazole) 1704

See **Mintezol Chewable Tablets**

MIOCHOL-E WITH IOCARE STERI-TAGS AND MIOCHOL-E SYSTEM PAK

(Acetylcholine Chloride) .... ⊙ 273

May interact with topical nonsteroidal anti-inflammatory agents. Compounds in this category include:

Diclofenac Sodium (Acetylcholine and carbachol have been ineffective when used in patients with topical nonsteroidal anti-inflammatory agents). Products include:

Voltaren Ophthalmic Sterile Ophthalmic Solution .... ⊙ 272
Voltaren Tablets 861

Flurbiprofen Sodium (Acetylcholine and carbachol have been ineffective when used in patients with topical nonsteroidal anti-inflammatory agents). Products include:

Ocufen .... ⊙ 245

Suprofen (Acetylcholine and carbachol have been ineffective when used in patients with topical nonsteroidal anti-inflammatory agents). Products include:

Profenal 1% Sterile Ophthalmic Solution .... ⊙ 227

MIOSTAT INTRAOCULAR SOLUTION

(Carbachol) .... ⊙ 224

None cited in PDR database.

MITHRACIN

(Plicamycin) 607

None cited in PDR database.

MITRAFLEX WOUND DRESSING

(Polyurethane Film) 2866

None cited in PDR database.

MIVACRON INJECTION

(Mivacurium Chloride) 1138

May interact with aminoglycosides, tetracyclines, lithium preparations, local anesthetics, oral contraceptives, monoamine oxidase inhibitors, glucocorticoids, antineoplastics, and certain other agents. Compounds in these categories include:

Altretamine (Irreversible inhibition of plasma cholinesterase by certain unspecified antineoplastic drugs resulting in possible prolonged neuromuscular block). Products include:

Hexalen Capsules 2571

Amikacin Sulfate (Enhances the neuromuscular blocking action). Products include:

Amikacin Sulfate Injection, USP 960
Amikin Injectable 501

Asparaginase (Irreversible inhibition of plasma cholinesterase by certain unspecified antineoplastic drugs resulting in possible prolonged neuromuscular block). Products include:

Elspar 1659

Bacitracin (Enhances neuromuscular blocking action). Products include:

Mycitracin .... ■ 839

Betamethasone Acetate (Enhances the neuromuscular blocking effects by a reduction in plasma cholinesterase activity induced by chronic administration of glucocorticoids). Products include:

Celestone Soluspan Suspension 2347

Betamethasone Sodium Phosphate (Enhances the neuromuscular blocking effects by a reduction in plasma cholinesterase activity induced by chronic administration of glucocorticoids). Products include:

Celestone Soluspan Suspension 2347

Bleomycin Sulfate (Irreversible inhibition of plasma cholinesterase by certain unspecified antineoplastic drugs resulting in possible prolonged neuromuscular block). Products include:

Blenoxane 692

Bupivacaine Hydrochloride (Enhances neuromuscular blocking action). Products include:

Marcaine Hydrochloride with Epinephrine 1:200,000 2316
Marcaine Hydrochloride Injection 2316
Marcaine Spinal 2319
Sensorcaine 559

Busulfan (Irreversible inhibition of plasma cholinesterase by certain unspecified antineoplastic drugs resulting in possible prolonged neuromuscular block). Products include:

Myleran Tablets 1143

Carbamazepine (Potential for resistance to the neuromuscular blocking action in patients on chronic carbamazepine therapy). Products include:

Atretol Tablets 573
Tegretol Chewable Tablets 852
Tegretol Suspension 852
Tegretol Tablets 852

Carboplatin (Irreversible inhibition of plasma cholinesterase by certain unspecified antineoplastic drugs resulting in possible prolonged neuromuscular block). Products include:

Paraplatin for Injection 705

Carmustine (BCNU) (Irreversible inhibition of plasma cholinesterase by certain unspecified antineoplastic drugs resulting in possible prolonged neuromuscular block). Products include:

BiCNU 691

Chlorambucil (Irreversible inhibition of plasma cholinesterase by certain unspecified antineoplastic drugs resulting in possible prolonged neuromuscular block). Products include:

Leukeran Tablets 1133

Chloroprocaine Hydrochloride (Enhances neuromuscular blocking action). Products include:

Nescaine/Nescaine MPF 554

Cisplatin (Irreversible inhibition of plasma cholinesterase by certain unspecified antineoplastic drugs resulting in possible prolonged neuromuscular block). Products include:

Platinol 708
Platinol-AQ Injection 710

Clindamycin Hydrochloride (Enhances neuromuscular blocking action).

No products indexed under this heading.

Clindamycin Palmitate Hydrochloride (Enhances neuromuscular blocking action).

No products indexed under this heading.

Clindamycin Phosphate (Enhances neuromuscular blocking action). Products include:

Cleocin Phosphate Injection 2586
Cleocin T Topical 2590
Cleocin Vaginal Cream 2589

Colistimethate Sodium (Enhances neuromuscular blocking action). Products include:

Coly-Mycin M Parenteral 1905

Colistin Sulfate (Enhances neuromuscular blocking action). Products include:

Coly-Mycin S Otic w/Neomycin & Hydrocortisone 1906

Cortisone Acetate (Enhances the neuromuscular blocking effects by a reduction in plasma cholinesterase activity induced by chronic administration of glucocorticoids). Products include:

Cortone Acetate Sterile Suspension 1623
Cortone Acetate Tablets 1624

Cyclophosphamide (Irreversible inhibition of plasma cholinesterase by certain unspecified antineoplastic drugs resulting in possible prolonged neuromuscular block). Products include:

Cytoxan 694
NEOSAR Lyophilized/Neosar 1959

IMPORTANT NOTE: Always consult each drug listing in the patient's regimen for possible interactions.

Mivacron Interactions Index 668

Dacarbazine (Irreversible inhibition of plasma cholinesterase by certain unspecified antineoplastic drugs resulting in possible prolonged neuromuscular block). Products include:
DTIC-Dome 600

Daunorubicin Hydrochloride (Irreversible inhibition of plasma cholinesterase by certain unspecified antineoplastic drugs resulting in possible prolonged neuromuscular block). Products include:
Cerubidine 795

Demeclocycline Hydrochloride (Enhances neuromuscular blocking action). Products include:
Declomycin Tablets 1371

Desogestrel (Enhances the neuromuscular blocking effects by a reduction in plasma cholinesterase activity induced by chronic administration of oral contraceptives). Products include:
Desogen Tablets 1817
Ortho-Cept 1851

Dexamethasone (Enhances the neuromuscular blocking effects by a reduction in plasma cholinesterase activity induced by chronic administration of glucocorticoids). Products include:
AK-Trol Ointment & Suspension .... ◉ 205
Decadron Elixir 1633
Decadron Tablets 1635
Decaspray Topical Aerosol 1648
Dexacidin Ointment .... ◉ 263
Maxitrol Ophthalmic Ointment and Suspension .... ◉ 224
TobraDex Ophthalmic Suspension and Ointment 473

Dexamethasone Acetate (Enhances the neuromuscular blocking effects by a reduction in plasma cholinesterase activity induced by chronic administration of glucocorticoids). Products include:
Dalalone D.P. Injectable 1011
Decadron-LA Sterile Suspension 1646

Dexamethasone Sodium Phosphate (Enhances the neuromuscular blocking effects by a reduction in plasma cholinesterase activity induced by chronic administration of glucocorticoids). Products include:
Decadron Phosphate Injection 1637
Decadron Phosphate Respihaler 1642
Decadron Phosphate Sterile Ophthalmic Ointment 1641
Decadron Phosphate Sterile Ophthalmic Solution 1642
Decadron Phosphate Topical Cream 1644
Decadron Phosphate Turbinaire 1645
Decadron Phosphate with Xylocaine Injection, Sterile 1639
Dexacort Phosphate in Respihaler .. 458
Dexacort Phosphate in Turbinaire .. 459
NeoDecadron Sterile Ophthalmic Ointment 1712
NeoDecadron Sterile Ophthalmic Solution 1713
NeoDecadron Topical Cream 1714

Doxorubicin Hydrochloride (Irreversible inhibition of plasma cholinesterase by certain unspecified antineoplastic drugs resulting in possible prolonged neuromuscular block). Products include:
Adriamycin PFS 1947
Adriamycin RDF 1947
Doxorubicin Astra 540
Rubex 712

Doxycycline Calcium (Enhances neuromuscular blocking action). Products include:
Vibramycin Calcium Oral Suspension Syrup 1941

Doxycycline Hyclate (Enhances neuromuscular blocking action). Products include:
Doryx Capsules 1913
Vibramycin Hyclate Capsules 1941
Vibramycin Hyclate Intravenous 2215
Vibra-Tabs Film Coated Tablets 1941

Doxycycline Monohydrate (Enhances neuromuscular blocking action). Products include:
Monodox Capsules 1805
Vibramycin Monohydrate for Oral Suspension 1941

Echothiophate Iodide (Irreversible inhibition of plasma cholinesterase by echothiophate resulting in possible prolonged neuromuscular block). Products include:
Phospholine Iodide .... ◉ 326

Enflurane (Decreases ED_{50} of Mivacron by as much as 35% to 40%; prolongs the clinically effective duration of action).
No products indexed under this heading.

Estramustine Phosphate Sodium (Irreversible inhibition of plasma cholinesterase by certain unspecified antineoplastic drugs resulting in possible prolonged neuromuscular block). Products include:
Emcyt Capsules 1953

Ethinyl Estradiol (Enhances the neuromuscular blocking effects by a reduction in plasma cholinesterase activity induced by chronic administration of oral contraceptives). Products include:
Brevicon 2088
Demulen 2428
Desogen Tablets 1817
Levlen/Tri-Levlen 651
Lo/Ovral Tablets 2746
Lo/Ovral-28 Tablets 2751
Modicon 1872
Nordette-21 Tablets 2755
Nordette-28 Tablets 2758
Norinyl 2088
Ortho-Cept 1851
Ortho-Cyclen/Ortho-Tri-Cyclen 1858
Ortho-Novum 1872
Ortho-Cyclen/Ortho Tri-Cyclen 1858
Ovcon 760
Ovral Tablets 2770
Ovral-28 Tablets 2770
Levlen/Tri-Levlen 651
Tri-Norinyl 2164
Triphasil-21 Tablets 2814
Triphasil-28 Tablets 2819

Ethynodiol Diacetate (Enhances the neuromuscular blocking effects by a reduction in plasma cholinesterase activity induced by chronic administration of oral contraceptives). Products include:
Demulen 2428

Etidocaine Hydrochloride (Enhances neuromuscular blocking action). Products include:
Duranest Injections 542

Etoposide (Irreversible inhibition of plasma cholinesterase by certain unspecified antineoplastic drugs resulting in possible prolonged neuromuscular block). Products include:
VePesid Capsules and Injection 718

Floxuridine (Irreversible inhibition of plasma cholinesterase by certain unspecified antineoplastic drugs resulting in possible prolonged neuromuscular block). Products include:
Sterile FUDR 2118

Fludrocortisone Acetate (Enhances the neuromuscular blocking effects by a reduction in plasma cholinesterase activity induced by chronic administration of glucocorticoids). Products include:
Florinef Acetate Tablets 505

Fluorouracil (Irreversible inhibition of plasma cholinesterase by certain unspecified antineoplastic drugs resulting in possible prolonged neuromuscular block). Products include:
Efudex 2113
Fluoroplex Topical Solution & Cream 1% 479
Fluorouracil Injection 2116

Flutamide (Irreversible inhibition of plasma cholinesterase by certain unspecified antineoplastic drugs resulting in possible prolonged neuromuscular block). Products include:
Eulexin Capsules 2358

Furazolidone (Enhances the neuromuscular blocking effects by a reduction in plasma cholinesterase activity induced by chronic administration of certain unspecified monoamine oxidase inhibitors). Products include:
Furoxone 2046

Gentamicin Sulfate (Enhances the neuromuscular blocking action). Products include:
Garamycin Injectable 2360
Genoptic Sterile Ophthalmic Solution .... ◉ 243
Genoptic Sterile Ophthalmic Ointment .... ◉ 243
Gentacidin Ointment .... ◉ 264
Gentacidin Solution .... ◉ 264
Gentak .... ◉ 208
Pred-G Liquifilm Sterile Ophthalmic Suspension .... ◉ 251
Pred-G S.O.P. Sterile Ophthalmic Ointment .... ◉ 252

Halothane (Prolongs the duration of action). Products include:
Fluothane 2724

Hydrocortisone (Enhances the neuromuscular blocking effects by a reduction in plasma cholinesterase activity induced by chronic administration of glucocorticoids). Products include:
Anusol-HC Cream 2.5% 1896
Aquanil HC Lotion 1931
Bactine Hydrocortisone Anti-Itch Cream .... ▣ 709
Caldecort Anti-Itch Hydrocortisone Spray .... ▣ 631
Cortaid .... ▣ 836
CORTENEMA 2535
Cortisporin Ointment 1085
Cortisporin Ophthalmic Ointment Sterile 1085
Cortisporin Ophthalmic Suspension Sterile 1086
Cortisporin Otic Solution Sterile 1087
Cortisporin Otic Suspension Sterile 1088
Cortizone-5 .... ▣ 831
Cortizone-10 .... ▣ 831
Hydrocortone Tablets 1672
Hytone 907
Massengill Medicated Soft Cloth Towelettes 2458
PediOtic Suspension Sterile 1153
Preparation H Hydrocortisone 1% Cream .... ▣ 872
ProctoCream-HC 2.5% 2408
VōSoL HC Otic Solution 2678

Hydrocortisone Acetate (Enhances the neuromuscular blocking effects by a reduction in plasma cholinesterase activity induced by chronic administration of glucocorticoids). Products include:
Analpram-HC Rectal Cream 1% and 2.5% 977
Anusol HC-1 Anti-Itch Hydrocortisone Ointment .... ▣ 847
Anusol-HC Suppositories 1897
Caldecort .... ▣ 631
Carmol HC 924
Coly-Mycin S Otic w/Neomycin & Hydrocortisone 1906
Cortaid .... ▣ 836
Cortifoam 2396
Cortisporin Cream 1084
Epifoam 2399
Hydrocortone Acetate Sterile Suspension 1669
Mantadil Cream 1135
Nupercainal Hydrocortisone 1% Cream .... ▣ 645
Ophthocort .... ◉ 311
Pramosone Cream, Lotion & Ointment 978
ProctoCream-HC 2408
ProctoFoam-HC 2409
Terra-Cortril Ophthalmic Suspension 2210

Hydrocortisone Sodium Phosphate (Enhances the neuromuscular blocking effects by a reduction in plasma cholinesterase activity induced by chronic administration of glucocorticoids). Products include:
Hydrocortone Phosphate Injection, Sterile 1670

Hydrocortisone Sodium Succinate (Enhances the neuromuscular blocking effects by a reduction in plasma cholinesterase activity induced by chronic administration of glucocorticoids). Products include:
Solu-Cortef Sterile Powder 2641

Hydroxyurea (Irreversible inhibition of plasma cholinesterase by certain unspecified antineoplastic drugs resulting in possible prolonged neuromuscular block). Products include:
Hydrea Capsules 696

Idarubicin Hydrochloride (Irreversible inhibition of plasma cholinesterase by certain unspecified antineoplastic drugs resulting in possible prolonged neuromuscular block). Products include:
Idamycin 1955

Ifosfamide (Irreversible inhibition of plasma cholinesterase by certain unspecified antineoplastic drugs resulting in possible prolonged neuromuscular block). Products include:
IFEX 697

Interferon alfa-2A, Recombinant (Irreversible inhibition of plasma cholinesterase by certain unspecified antineoplastic drugs resulting in possible prolonged neuromuscular block). Products include:
Roferon-A Injection 2145

Interferon alfa-2B, Recombinant (Irreversible inhibition of plasma cholinesterase by certain unspecified antineoplastic drugs resulting in possible prolonged neuromuscular block). Products include:
Intron A 2364

Isocarboxazid (Enhances the neuromuscular blocking effects by a reduction in plasma cholinesterase activity induced by chronic administration of certain unspecified monoamine oxidase inhibitors).
No products indexed under this heading.

Isoflurane (Decreases ED_{50} of Mivacron by as much as 35% to 40%; prolongs the clinically effective duration of action).
No products indexed under this heading.

Kanamycin Sulfate (Enhances the neuromuscular blocking action).
No products indexed under this heading.

Levamisole Hydrochloride (Irreversible inhibition of plasma cholinesterase by certain unspecified antineoplastic drugs resulting in possible prolonged neuromuscular block). Products include:
Ergamisol Tablets 1292

Levonorgestrel (Enhances the neuromuscular blocking effects by a reduction in plasma cholinesterase activity induced by chronic administration of oral contraceptives). Products include:
Levlen/Tri-Levlen 651
Nordette-21 Tablets 2755
Nordette-28 Tablets 2758
Norplant System 2759
Levlen/Tri-Levlen 651
Triphasil-21 Tablets 2814
Triphasil-28 Tablets 2819

(▣ Described in PDR For Nonprescription Drugs) (◉ Described in PDR For Ophthalmology)

669 **Interactions Index** **Mivacron**

Lidocaine Hydrochloride (Enhances neuromuscular blocking action). Products include:
- Bactine Antiseptic/Anesthetic First Aid Liquid ... 708
- Campho-Phenique Maximum Strength First Aid Antibiotic Plus Pain Reliever Ointment ... 719
- Decadron Phosphate with Xylocaine Injection, Sterile ... 1639
- Xylocaine Injections ... 567

Lincomycin Hydrochloride (Enhances neuromuscular blocking action). Products include:
- Lincocin ... 2617

Lithium Carbonate (Enhances neuromuscular blocking action). Products include:
- Eskalith ... 2485
- Lithium Carbonate Capsules & Tablets ... 2230
- Lithonate/Lithotabs/Lithobid ... 2543

Lithium Citrate (Enhances neuromuscular blocking action).
- No products indexed under this heading.

Lomustine (CCNU) (Irreversible inhibition of plasma cholinesterase by certain unspecified antineoplastic drugs resulting in possible prolonged neuromuscular block). Products include:
- CeeNU ... 693

Magnesium Salts (Enhances neuromuscular blocking action).

Mechlorethamine Hydrochloride (Irreversible inhibition of plasma cholinesterase by certain unspecified antineoplastic drugs resulting in possible prolonged neuromuscular block). Products include:
- Mustargen ... 1709

Megestrol Acetate (Irreversible inhibition of plasma cholinesterase by certain unspecified antineoplastic drugs resulting in possible prolonged neuromuscular block). Products include:
- Megace Oral Suspension ... 699
- Megace Tablets ... 701

Melphalan (Irreversible inhibition of plasma cholinesterase by certain unspecified antineoplastic drugs resulting in possible prolonged neuromuscular block). Products include:
- Alkeran Tablets ... 1071

Mepivacaine Hydrochloride Injection (Enhances neuromuscular blocking action). Products include:
- Carbocaine Hydrochloride Injection 2303

Mercaptopurine (Irreversible inhibition of plasma cholinesterase by certain unspecified antineoplastic drugs resulting in possible prolonged neuromuscular block). Products include:
- Purinethol Tablets ... 1156

Mestranol (Enhances the neuromuscular blocking effects by a reduction in plasma cholinesterase activity induced by chronic administration of oral contraceptives). Products include:
- Norinyl ... 2088
- Ortho-Novum ... 1872

Methacycline Hydrochloride (Enhances neuromuscular blocking action).
- No products indexed under this heading.

Methotrexate Sodium (Irreversible inhibition of plasma cholinesterase by certain unspecified antineoplastic drugs resulting in possible prolonged neuromuscular block). Products include:
- Methotrexate Sodium Tablets, Injection, for Injection and LPF Injection ... 1275

Methylprednisolone Acetate (Enhances the neuromuscular blocking effects by a reduction in plasma cholinesterase activity induced by chronic administration of glucocorticoids). Products include:
- Depo-Medrol Single-Dose Vial ... 2600
- Depo-Medrol Sterile Aqueous Suspension ... 2597

Methylprednisolone Sodium Succinate (Enhances the neuromuscular blocking effects by a reduction in plasma cholinesterase activity induced by chronic administration of glucocorticoids). Products include:
- Solu-Medrol Sterile Powder ... 2643

Minocycline Hydrochloride (Enhances neuromuscular blocking action). Products include:
- Dynacin Capsules ... 1590
- Minocin Intravenous ... 1382
- Minocin Oral Suspension ... 1385
- Minocin Pellet-Filled Capsules ... 1383

Mitomycin (Mitomycin-C) (Irreversible inhibition of plasma cholinesterase by certain unspecified antineoplastic drugs resulting in possible prolonged neuromuscular block). Products include:
- Mutamycin ... 703

Mitotane (Irreversible inhibition of plasma cholinesterase by certain unspecified antineoplastic drugs resulting in possible prolonged neuromuscular block). Products include:
- Lysodren ... 698

Mitoxantrone Hydrochloride (Irreversible inhibition of plasma cholinesterase by certain unspecified antineoplastic drugs resulting in possible prolonged neuromuscular block). Products include:
- Novantrone ... 1279

Norethindrone (Enhances the neuromuscular blocking effects by a reduction in plasma cholinesterase activity induced by chronic administration of oral contraceptives). Products include:
- Brevicon ... 2088
- Micronor Tablets ... 1872
- Modicon ... 1872
- Norinyl ... 2088
- Nor-Q D Tablets ... 2135
- Ortho-Novum ... 1872
- Ovcon ... 760
- Tri-Norinyl ... 2164

Norethynodrel (Enhances the neuromuscular blocking effects by a reduction in plasma cholinesterase activity induced by chronic administration of oral contraceptives).
- No products indexed under this heading.

Norgestimate (Enhances the neuromuscular blocking effects by a reduction in plasma cholinesterase activity induced by chronic administration of oral contraceptives). Products include:
- Ortho-Cyclen/Ortho-Tri-Cyclen ... 1858
- Ortho-Cyclen/Ortho Tri-Cyclen ... 1858

Norgestrel (Enhances the neuromuscular blocking effects by a reduction in plasma cholinesterase activity induced by chronic administration of oral contraceptives). Products include:
- Lo/Ovral Tablets ... 2746
- Lo/Ovral-28 Tablets ... 2751
- Ovral Tablets ... 2770
- Ovral-28 Tablets ... 2770
- Ovrette Tablets ... 2771

Oxytetracycline Hydrochloride (Enhances neuromuscular blocking action). Products include:
- TERAK Ointment ... ◉ 209
- Terra-Cortril Ophthalmic Suspension ... 2210
- Terramycin with Polymyxin B Sulfate Ophthalmic Ointment ... 2211
- Urobiotic-250 Capsules ... 2214

Paclitaxel (Irreversible inhibition of plasma cholinesterase by certain unspecified antineoplastic drugs resulting in possible prolonged neuromuscular block). Products include:
- Taxol ... 714

Phenelzine Sulfate (Enhances the neuromuscular blocking effects by a reduction in plasma cholinesterase activity induced by chronic administration of certain unspecified monoamine oxidase inhibitors). Products include:
- Nardil ... 1920

Phenytoin (Potential for resistance to the neuromuscular blocking action in patients on chronic phenytoin therapy). Products include:
- Dilantin Infatabs ... 1908
- Dilantin-125 Suspension ... 1911

Phenytoin Sodium (Potential for resistance to the neuromuscular blocking action in patients on chronic phenytoin therapy). Products include:
- Dilantin Kapseals ... 1906
- Dilantin Parenteral ... 1910

Polymyxin Preparations (Enhances neuromuscular blocking action).

Prednisolone Acetate (Enhances the neuromuscular blocking effects by a reduction in plasma cholinesterase activity induced by chronic administration of glucocorticoids). Products include:
- AK-CIDE ... ◉ 202
- AK-CIDE Ointment ... ◉ 202
- Blephamide Liquifilm Sterile Ophthalmic Suspension ... 476
- Blephamide Ointment ... ◉ 237
- Econopred & Econopred Plus Ophthalmic Suspensions ... ◉ 217
- Poly-Pred Liquifilm ... ◉ 248
- Pred Forte ... ◉ 250
- Pred Mild ... ◉ 253
- Pred-G Liquifilm Sterile Ophthalmic Suspension ... ◉ 251
- Pred-G S.O.P. Sterile Ophthalmic Ointment ... ◉ 252
- Vasocidin Ointment ... ◉ 268

Prednisolone Sodium Phosphate (Enhances the neuromuscular blocking effects by a reduction in plasma cholinesterase activity induced by chronic administration of glucocorticoids). Products include:
- AK-Pred ... ◉ 204
- Hydeltrasol Injection, Sterile ... 1665
- Inflamase ... ◉ 265
- Pediapred Oral Liquid ... 995
- Vasocidin Ophthalmic Solution ... ◉ 270

Prednisolone Tebutate (Enhances the neuromuscular blocking effects by a reduction in plasma cholinesterase activity induced by chronic administration of glucocorticoids). Products include:
- Hydeltra-T.B.A. Sterile Suspension 1667

Prednisone (Enhances the neuromuscular blocking effects by a reduction in plasma cholinesterase activity induced by chronic administration of glucocorticoids). Products include:
- Deltasone Tablets ... 2595

Procainamide Hydrochloride (Enhances neuromuscular blocking action). Products include:
- Procan SR Tablets ... 1926

Procaine Hydrochloride (Enhances neuromuscular blocking action). Products include:
- Novocain Hydrochloride for Spinal Anesthesia ... 2326

Procarbazine Hydrochloride (Irreversible inhibition of plasma cholinesterase by certain unspecified antineoplastic drugs resulting in possible prolonged neuromuscular block). Products include:
- Matulane Capsules ... 2131

Quinidine Gluconate (Enhances neuromuscular blocking action). Products include:
- Quinaglute Dura-Tabs Tablets ... 649

Quinidine Polygalacturonate (Enhances neuromuscular blocking action).
- No products indexed under this heading.

Quinidine Sulfate (Enhances neuromuscular blocking action). Products include:
- Quinidex Extentabs ... 2067

Selegiline Hydrochloride (Enhances the neuromuscular blocking effects by a reduction in plasma cholinesterase activity induced by chronic administration of certain unspecified monoamine oxidase inhibitors). Products include:
- Eldepryl Tablets ... 2550

Streptomycin Sulfate (Enhances the neuromuscular blocking action). Products include:
- Streptomycin Sulfate Injection ... 2208

Streptozocin (Irreversible inhibition of plasma cholinesterase by certain unspecified antineoplastic drugs resulting in possible prolonged neuromuscular block). Products include:
- Zanosar Sterile Powder ... 2653

Succinylcholine Chloride (Prior administration of succinylcholine can potentiate neuromuscular blockade). Products include:
- Anectine ... 1073

Tamoxifen Citrate (Irreversible inhibition of plasma cholinesterase by certain unspecified antineoplastic drugs resulting in possible prolonged neuromuscular block). Products include:
- Nolvadex Tablets ... 2841

Teniposide (Irreversible inhibition of plasma cholinesterase by certain unspecified antineoplastic drugs resulting in possible prolonged neuromuscular block). Products include:
- Vumon ... 727

Tetracaine Hydrochloride (Enhances neuromuscular blocking action). Products include:
- Cetacaine Topical Anesthetic ... 794
- Pontocaine Hydrochloride for Spinal Anesthesia ... 2330

Tetracycline Hydrochloride (Enhances neuromuscular blocking action). Products include:
- Achromycin V Capsules ... 1367

Thioguanine (Irreversible inhibition of plasma cholinesterase by certain unspecified antineoplastic drugs resulting in possible prolonged neuromuscular block). Products include:
- Thioguanine Tablets, Tabloid Brand ... 1181

IMPORTANT NOTE: Always consult each drug listing in the patient's regimen for possible interactions.

Thiotepa (Irreversible inhibition of plasma cholinesterase by certain unspecified antineoplastic drugs resulting in possible prolonged neuromuscular block). Products include:
- Thioplex (Thiotepa For Injection) 1281

Tobramycin (Enhances the neuromuscular blocking action). Products include:
- AKTOB .... ⊙ 206
- TobraDex Ophthalmic Suspension and Ointment 473
- Tobrex Ophthalmic Ointment and Solution .... ⊙ 229

Tobramycin Sulfate (Enhances the neuromuscular blocking action). Products include:
- Nebcin Vials, Hyporets & ADD-Vantage 1464
- Tobramycin Sulfate Injection 968

Tranylcypromine Sulfate (Enhances the neuromuscular blocking effects by a reduction in plasma cholinesterase activity induced by chronic administration of certain unspecified monoamine oxidase inhibitors). Products include:
- Parnate Tablets 2503

Triamcinolone (Enhances the neuromuscular blocking effects by a reduction in plasma cholinesterase activity induced by chronic administration of glucocorticoids). Products include:
- Aristocort Tablets 1022

Triamcinolone Acetonide (Enhances the neuromuscular blocking effects by a reduction in plasma cholinesterase activity induced by chronic administration of glucocorticoids). Products include:
- Aristocort A 0.025% Cream 1027
- Aristocort A 0.5% Cream 1031
- Aristocort A 0.1% Cream 1029
- Aristocort A 0.1% Ointment 1030
- Azmacort Oral Inhaler 2011
- Nasacort Nasal Inhaler 2024

Triamcinolone Diacetate (Enhances the neuromuscular blocking effects by a reduction in plasma cholinesterase activity induced by chronic administration of glucocorticoids). Products include:
- Aristocort Suspension (Forte Parenteral) 1027
- Aristocort Suspension (Intralesional) 1025

Triamcinolone Hexacetonide (Enhances the neuromuscular blocking effects by a reduction in plasma cholinesterase activity induced by chronic administration of glucocorticoids). Products include:
- Aristospan Suspension (Intra-articular) 1033
- Aristospan Suspension (Intralesional) 1032

Vincristine Sulfate (Irreversible inhibition of plasma cholinesterase by certain unspecified antineoplastic drugs resulting in possible prolonged neuromuscular block). Products include:
- Oncovin Solution Vials & Hyporets 1466

Vinorelbine Tartrate (Irreversible inhibition of plasma cholinesterase by certain unspecified antineoplastic drugs resulting in possible prolonged neuromuscular block). Products include:
- Navelbine Injection 1145

MIVACRON PREMIXED INFUSION

(Mivacurium Chloride) 1138

See **Mivacron Injection**

MOBAN TABLETS AND CONCENTRATE

(Molindone Hydrochloride) 1048

May interact with tetracyclines and certain other agents. Compounds in these categories include:

Demeclocycline Hydrochloride (Calcium sulfate present as an excipient may interfere with the absorption of oral tetracyclines). Products include:
- Declomycin Tablets 1371

Doxycycline Calcium (Calcium sulfate present as an excipient may interfere with the absorption of oral tetracyclines). Products include:
- Vibramycin Calcium Oral Suspension Syrup 1941

Doxycycline Hyclate (Calcium sulfate present as an excipient may interfere with the absorption of oral tetracyclines). Products include:
- Doryx Capsules 1913
- Vibramycin Hyclate Capsules 1941
- Vibramycin Hyclate Intravenous 2215
- Vibra-Tabs Film Coated Tablets 1941

Doxycycline Monohydrate (Calcium sulfate present as an excipient may interfere with the absorption of oral tetracyclines). Products include:
- Monodox Capsules 1805
- Vibramycin Monohydrate for Oral Suspension 1941

Methacycline Hydrochloride (Calcium sulfate present as an excipient may interfere with the absorption of oral tetracyclines).
- No products indexed under this heading.

Minocycline Hydrochloride (Calcium sulfate present as an excipient may interfere with the absorption of oral tetracyclines). Products include:
- Dynacin Capsules 1590
- Minocin Intravenous 1382
- Minocin Oral Suspension 1385
- Minocin Pellet-Filled Capsules 1383

Oxytetracycline Hydrochloride (Calcium sulfate present as an excipient may interfere with the absorption of oral tetracyclines). Products include:
- TERAK Ointment .... ⊙ 209
- Terra-Cortril Ophthalmic Suspension 2210
- Terramycin with Polymyxin B Sulfate Ophthalmic Ointment 2211
- Urobiotic-250 Capsules 2214

Phenytoin Sodium (Calcium sulfate present as an excipient may interfere with the absorption of oral phenytoin sodium). Products include:
- Dilantin Kapseals 1906
- Dilantin Parenteral 1910

Tetracycline Hydrochloride (Calcium sulfate present as an excipient may interfere with the absorption of oral tetracyclines). Products include:
- Achromycin V Capsules 1367

MOBIGESIC TABLETS

(Magnesium Salicylate, Phenyltoloxamine Citrate) .... ▣ 602

May interact with hypnotics and sedatives, tranquilizers, and certain other agents. Compounds in these categories include:

Alprazolam (Concurrent use not recommended; consult your doctor). Products include:
- Xanax Tablets 2649

Buspirone Hydrochloride (Concurrent use not recommended; consult your doctor). Products include:
- BuSpar 737

Chlordiazepoxide (Concurrent use not recommended; consult your doctor). Products include:
- Libritabs Tablets 2177
- Limbitrol 2180

Chlordiazepoxide Hydrochloride (Concurrent use not recommended; consult your doctor). Products include:
- Librax Capsules 2176
- Librium Capsules 2178
- Librium Injectable 2179

Chlorpromazine (Concurrent use not recommended; consult your doctor). Products include:
- Thorazine Suppositories 2523

Chlorpromazine Hydrochloride (Concurrent use not recommended; consult your doctor). Products include:
- Thorazine 2523

Chlorprothixene (Concurrent use not recommended; consult your doctor).
- No products indexed under this heading.

Chlorprothixene Hydrochloride (Concurrent use not recommended; consult your doctor).
- No products indexed under this heading.

Clorazepate Dipotassium (Concurrent use not recommended; consult your doctor). Products include:
- Tranxene 451

Diazepam (Concurrent use not recommended; consult your doctor). Products include:
- Dizac 1809
- Valium Injectable 2182
- Valium Tablets 2183
- Valrelease Capsules 2169

Droperidol (Concurrent use not recommended; consult your doctor). Products include:
- Inapsine Injection 1296

Estazolam (Concurrent use not recommended; consult your doctor). Products include:
- ProSom Tablets 449

Ethchlorvynol (Concurrent use not recommended; consult your doctor). Products include:
- Placidyl Capsules 448

Ethinamate (Concurrent use not recommended; consult your doctor).
- No products indexed under this heading.

Fluphenazine Decanoate (Concurrent use not recommended; consult your doctor). Products include:
- Prolixin Decanoate 509

Fluphenazine Enanthate (Concurrent use not recommended; consult your doctor). Products include:
- Prolixin Enanthate 509

Fluphenazine Hydrochloride (Concurrent use not recommended; consult your doctor). Products include:
- Prolixin 509

Flurazepam Hydrochloride (Concurrent use not recommended; consult your doctor). Products include:
- Dalmane Capsules 2173

Glutethimide (Concurrent use not recommended; consult your doctor).
- No products indexed under this heading.

Haloperidol (Concurrent use not recommended; consult your doctor). Products include:
- Haldol Injection, Tablets and Concentrate 1575

Haloperidol Decanoate (Concurrent use not recommended; consult your doctor). Products include:
- Haldol Decanoate 1577

Hydroxyzine Hydrochloride (Concurrent use not recommended; consult your doctor). Products include:
- Atarax Tablets & Syrup 2185
- Marax Tablets & DF Syrup 2200
- Vistaril Intramuscular Solution 2216

Lorazepam (Concurrent use not recommended; consult your doctor). Products include:
- Ativan Injection 2698
- Ativan Tablets 2700

Loxapine Hydrochloride (Concurrent use not recommended; consult your doctor). Products include:
- Loxitane 1378

Loxapine Succinate (Concurrent use not recommended; consult your doctor). Products include:
- Loxitane Capsules 1378

Meprobamate (Concurrent use not recommended; consult your doctor). Products include:
- Miltown Tablets 2672
- PMB 200 and PMB 400 2783

Mesoridazine Besylate (Concurrent use not recommended; consult your doctor). Products include:
- Serentil 684

Midazolam Hydrochloride (Concurrent use not recommended; consult your doctor). Products include:
- Versed Injection 2170

Molindone Hydrochloride (Concurrent use not recommended; consult your doctor). Products include:
- Moban Tablets and Concentrate 1048

Oxazepam (Concurrent use not recommended; consult your doctor). Products include:
- Serax Capsules 2810
- Serax Tablets 2810

Perphenazine (Concurrent use not recommended; consult your doctor). Products include:
- Etrafon 2355
- Triavil Tablets 1757
- Trilafon 2389

Prazepam (Concurrent use not recommended; consult your doctor).
- No products indexed under this heading.

Prochlorperazine (Concurrent use not recommended; consult your doctor). Products include:
- Compazine 2470

Promethazine Hydrochloride (Concurrent use not recommended; consult your doctor). Products include:
- Mepergan Injection 2753
- Phenergan with Codeine 2777
- Phenergan with Dextromethorphan 2778
- Phenergan Injection 2773
- Phenergan Suppositories 2775
- Phenergan Syrup 2774
- Phenergan Tablets 2775
- Phenergan VC 2779
- Phenergan VC with Codeine 2781

Propofol (Concurrent use not recommended; consult your doctor). Products include:
- Diprivan Injection 2833

Quazepam (Concurrent use not recommended; consult your doctor). Products include:
- Doral Tablets 2664

Secobarbital Sodium (Concurrent use not recommended; consult your doctor). Products include:
- Seconal Sodium Pulvules 1474

Temazepam (Concurrent use not recommended; consult your doctor). Products include:
- Restoril Capsules 2284

Thioridazine Hydrochloride (Concurrent use not recommended; consult your doctor). Products include:

Mellaril 2269

Thiothixene (Concurrent use not recommended; consult your doctor). Products include:

Navane Capsules and Concentrate 2201
Navane Intramuscular 2202

Triazolam (Concurrent use not recommended; consult your doctor). Products include:

Halcion Tablets.. 2611

Trifluoperazine Hydrochloride (Concurrent use not recommended; consult your doctor). Products include:

Stelazine 2514

Zolpidem Tartrate (Concurrent use not recommended; consult your doctor). Products include:

Ambien Tablets... 2416

Food Interactions

Alcohol (Avoid concurrent use; may cause drowsiness).

MOBISYL ANALGESIC CREME

(Trolamine Salicylate)...........................◈ 603

None cited in PDR database.

MODICON 21 TABLETS

(Norethindrone, Ethinyl Estradiol)......1872
See **Ortho-Novum 7/7/7** ▢21 **Tablets**

MODICON 28 TABLETS

(Norethindrone, Ethinyl Estradiol)......1872
See **Ortho-Novum 7/7/7** ▢21 **Tablets**

MODURETIC TABLETS

(Amiloride Hydrochloride, Hydrochlorothiazide)............................1705

May interact with antihypertensives, lithium preparations, non-steroidal anti-inflammatory agents, insulin, cardiac glycosides, corticosteroids, potassium preparations, ACE inhibitors, oral hypoglycemic agents, barbiturates, narcotic analgesics, bile acid sequestering agents, and certain other agents. Compounds in these categories include:

Acarbose (Dosage adjustment of the antidiabetic drug may be required).

No products indexed under this heading.

Acebutolol Hydrochloride (Potentiated or additive action). Products include:

Sectral Capsules 2807

ACTH (Hypokalemia).

No products indexed under this heading.

Alfentanil Hydrochloride (Potentiation of orthostatic hypotension). Products include:

Alfenta Injection 1286

Amlodipine Besylate (Potentiated or additive action). Products include:

Lotrel Capsules... 840
Norvasc Tablets 1940

Aprobarbital (Potentiation of orthostatic hypotension).

No products indexed under this heading.

Atenolol (Potentiated or additive action). Products include:

Tenoretic Tablets..................................... 2845
Tenormin Tablets and I.V. Injection 2847

Benazepril Hydrochloride (Potentiated or additive action; increased risk of hyperkalemia). Products include:

Lotensin Tablets....................................... 834
Lotensin HCT.. 837
Lotrel Capsules... 840

Bendroflumethiazide (Potentiated or additive action).

No products indexed under this heading.

Betamethasone Acetate (Hypokalemia). Products include:

Celestone Soluspan Suspension 2347

Betamethasone Sodium Phosphate (Hypokalemia). Products include:

Celestone Soluspan Suspension 2347

Betaxolol Hydrochloride (Potentiated or additive action). Products include:

Betoptic Ophthalmic Solution............ 469
Betoptic S Ophthalmic Suspension 471
Kerlone Tablets.. 2436

Bisoprolol Fumarate (Potentiated or additive action). Products include:

Zebeta Tablets 1413
Ziac 1415

Buprenorphine (Potentiation of orthostatic hypotension). Products include:

Buprenex Injectable 2006

Butabarbital (Potentiation of orthostatic hypotension).

No products indexed under this heading.

Butalbital (Potentiation of orthostatic hypotension). Products include:

Esgic-plus Tablets 1013
Fioricet Tablets.. 2258
Fioricet with Codeine Capsules 2260
Fiorinal Capsules 2261
Fiorinal with Codeine Capsules 2262
Fiorinal Tablets 2261
Phrenilin 785
Sedapap Tablets 50 mg/650 mg .. 1543

Captopril (Potentiated or additive action; increased risk of hyperkalemia). Products include:

Capoten 739
Capozide 742

Carteolol Hydrochloride (Potentiated or additive action). Products include:

Cartrol Tablets 410
Ocupress Ophthalmic Solution, 1% Sterile... ⊙ 309

Chlorothiazide (Potentiated or additive action). Products include:

Aldoclor Tablets 1598
Diupres Tablets 1650
Diuril Oral 1653

Chlorothiazide Sodium (Potentiated or additive action). Products include:

Diuril Sodium Intravenous 1652

Chlorpropamide (Dosage adjustment of the antidiabetic drug may be required). Products include:

Diabinese Tablets 1935

Chlorthalidone (Potentiated or additive effects). Products include:

Combipres Tablets 677
Tenoretic Tablets..................................... 2845
Thalitone 1245

Cholestyramine (Cholestyramine resin has potential of binding hydrochlorothiazide and reducing its absorption from the GI tract by up to 85%). Products include:

Questran Light 769
Questran Powder 770

Clonidine (Potentiated or additive action). Products include:

Catapres-TTS.. 675

Clonidine Hydrochloride (Potentiated or additive action). Products include:

Catapres Tablets 674
Combipres Tablets 677

Codeine Phosphate (Potentiation of orthostatic hypotension). Products include:

Actifed with Codeine Cough Syrup.. 1067
Brontex 1981
Deconsal C Expectorant Syrup 456
Deconsal Pediatric Syrup 457
Dimetane-DC Cough Syrup 2059
Empirin with Codeine Tablets............ 1093
Fioricet with Codeine Capsules 2260
Fiorinal with Codeine Capsules 2262
Isoclor Expectorant................................ 990
Novahistine DH....................................... 2462
Novahistine Expectorant...................... 2463
Nucofed 2051
Phenergan with Codeine 2777
Phenergan VC with Codeine 2781
Robitussin A-C Syrup............................. 2073
Robitussin-DAC Syrup........................... 2074
Ryna .... ◈ 841
Soma Compound w/Codeine Tablets 2676
Tussi-Organidin NR Liquid and S NR Liquid 2677
Tylenol with Codeine 1583

Colestipol Hydrochloride (Colestipol resin has potential of binding hydrochlorothiazide and reducing its absorption from the GI tract by up to 43%). Products include:

Colestid Tablets 2591

Cortisone Acetate (Hypokalemia). Products include:

Cortone Acetate Sterile Suspension 1623
Cortone Acetate Tablets....................... 1624

Deserpidine (Potentiated or additive action).

No products indexed under this heading.

Deslanoside (Potential for exaggerated response of the heart to the toxic effects of digitalis).

No products indexed under this heading.

Dexamethasone (Hypokalemia). Products include:

AK-Trol Ointment & Suspension .... ⊙ 205
Decadron Elixir 1633
Decadron Tablets.................................... 1635
Decaspray Topical Aerosol 1648
Dexacidin Ointment .... ⊙ 263
Maxitrol Ophthalmic Ointment and Suspension .... ⊙ 224
TobraDex Ophthalmic Suspension and Ointment.. 473

Dexamethasone Acetate (Hypokalemia). Products include:

Dalalone D.P. Injectable 1011
Decadron-LA Sterile Suspension...... 1646

Dexamethasone Sodium Phosphate (Hypokalemia). Products include:

Decadron Phosphate Injection 1637
Decadron Phosphate Respihaler...... 1642
Decadron Phosphate Sterile Ophthalmic Ointment 1641
Decadron Phosphate Sterile Ophthalmic Solution 1642
Decadron Phosphate Topical Cream... 1644
Decadron Phosphate Turbinaire 1645
Decadron Phosphate with Xylocaine Injection, Sterile 1639
Dexacort Phosphate in Respihaler .. 458
Dexacort Phosphate in Turbinaire .. 459
NeoDecadron Sterile Ophthalmic Ointment 1712
NeoDecadron Sterile Ophthalmic Solution 1713
NeoDecadron Topical Cream 1714

Dezocine (Potentiation of orthostatic hypotension). Products include:

Dalgan Injection 538

Diazoxide (Potentiated or additive action). Products include:

Hyperstat I.V. Injection 2363
Proglycem... 580

Diclofenac Potassium (Reduced diuretic, natriuretic, and antihypertensive effects of Moduretic). Products include:

Cataflam 816

Diclofenac Sodium (Reduced diuretic, natriuretic, and antihypertensive effects of Moduretic). Products include:

Voltaren Ophthalmic Sterile Ophthalmic Solution .... ⊙ 272
Voltaren Tablets....................................... 861

Digitoxin (Potential for exaggerated response of the heart to the toxic effects of digitalis). Products include:

Crystodigin Tablets................................. 1433

Digoxin (Potential for exaggerated response of the heart to the toxic effects of digitalis). Products include:

Lanoxicaps 1117
Lanoxin Elixir Pediatric 1120
Lanoxin Injection 1123
Lanoxin Injection Pediatric................. 1126
Lanoxin Tablets 1128

Diltiazem Hydrochloride (Potentiated or additive action). Products include:

Cardizem CD Capsules 1506
Cardizem SR Capsules 1510
Cardizem Injectable 1508
Cardizem Tablets..................................... 1512
Dilacor XR Extended-release Capsules 2018

Doxazosin Mesylate (Potentiated or additive action). Products include:

Cardura Tablets 2186

Enalapril Maleate (Potentiated or additive action; increased risk of hyperkalemia). Products include:

Vaseretic Tablets 1765
Vasotec Tablets 1771

Enalaprilat (Potentiated or additive action; increased risk of hyperkalemia). Products include:

Vasotec I.V... 1768

Etodolac (Reduced diuretic, natriuretic, and antihypertensive effects of Moduretic). Products include:

Lodine Capsules and Tablets 2743

Felodipine (Potentiated or additive action). Products include:

Plendil Extended-Release Tablets.... 527

Fenoprofen Calcium (Reduced diuretic, natriuretic, and antihypertensive effects of Moduretic). Products include:

Nalfon 200 Pulvules & Nalfon Tablets 917

Fentanyl (Potentiation of orthostatic hypotension). Products include:

Duragesic Transdermal System........ 1288

Fentanyl Citrate (Potentiation of orthostatic hypotension). Products include:

Sublimaze Injection................................ 1307

Fludrocortisone Acetate (Hypokalemia). Products include:

Florinef Acetate Tablets 505

Flurbiprofen (Reduced diuretic, natriuretic, and antihypertensive effects of Moduretic). Products include:

Ansaid Tablets 2579

Fosinopril Sodium (Potentiated or additive action; increased risk of hyperkalemia). Products include:

Monopril Tablets 757

Furosemide (Potentiated or additive action). Products include:

Lasix Injection, Oral Solution and Tablets 1240

IMPORTANT NOTE: Always consult each drug listing in the patient's regimen for possible interactions.

Moduretic **Interactions Index** **672**

Glipizide (Dosage adjustment of the antidiabetic drug may be required). Products include:
Glucotrol Tablets ... 1967
Glucotrol XL Extended Release Tablets ... 1968

Glyburide (Dosage adjustment of the antidiabetic drug may be required). Products include:
DiaBeta Tablets ... 1239
Glynase PresTab Tablets ... 2609
Micronase Tablets ... 2623

Guanabenz Acetate (Potentiated or additive action).
No products indexed under this heading.

Guanethidine Monosulfate (Potentiated or additive action). Products include:
Esimil Tablets ... 822
Ismelin Tablets ... 827

Hydralazine Hydrochloride (Potentiated or additive effects). Products include:
Apresazide Capsules ... 808
Apresoline Hydrochloride Tablets .. 809
Ser-Ap-Es Tablets ... 849

Hydrocodone Bitartrate (Potentiation of orthostatic hypotension). Products include:
Anexsia 5/500 Elixir ... 1781
Anexia Tablets ... 1782
Codiclear DH Syrup ... 791
Deconamine CX Cough and Cold Liquid and Tablets ... 1319
Duratuss HD Elixir ... 2565
Hycodan Tablets and Syrup ... 930
Hycomine Compound Tablets ... 932
Hycomine ... 931
Hycotuss Expectorant Syrup ... 933
Hydrocet Capsules ... 782
Lorcet 10/650 ... 1018
Lortab ... 2566
Tussend ... 1783
Tussend Expectorant ... 1785
Vicodin Tablets ... 1356
Vicodin ES Tablets ... 1357
Vicodin Tuss Expectorant ... 1358
Zydone Capsules ... 949

Hydrocodone Polistirex (Potentiation of orthostatic hypotension). Products include:
Tussionex Pennkinetic Extended-Release Suspension ... 998

Hydrocortisone (Hypokalemia). Products include:
Anusol-HC Cream 2.5% ... 1896
Aquanil HC Lotion ... 1931
Bactine Hydrocortisone Anti-Itch Cream ... ◘ 709
Caldecort Anti-Itch Hydrocortisone Spray ... ◘ 631
Cortaid ... ◘ 836
CORTENEMA ... 2535
Cortisporin Ointment ... 1085
Cortisporin Ophthalmic Ointment Sterile ... 1085
Cortisporin Ophthalmic Suspension Sterile ... 1086
Cortisporin Otic Solution Sterile ... 1087
Cortisporin Otic Suspension Sterile 1088
Cortizone-5 ... ◘ 831
Cortizone-10 ... ◘ 831
Hydrocortone Tablets ... 1672
Hytone ... 907
Massengill Medicated Soft Cloth Towelettes ... 2458
PediOtic Suspension Sterile ... 1153
Preparation H Hydrocortisone 1% Cream ... ◘ 872
ProctoCream-HC 2.5% ... 2408
VōSoL HC Otic Solution ... 2678

Hydrocortisone Acetate (Hypokalemia). Products include:
Analpram-HC Rectal Cream 1% and 2.5% ... 977
Anusol HC-1 Anti-Itch Hydrocortisone Ointment ... ◘ 847
Anusol-HC Suppositories ... 1897
Caldecort ... ◘ 631
Carmol HC ... 924
Coly-Mycin S Otic w/Neomycin & Hydrocortisone ... 1906
Cortaid ... ◘ 836
Cortifoam ... 2396
Cortisporin Cream ... 1084
Epifoam ... 2399
Hydrocortone Acetate Sterile Suspension ... 1669
Mantadil Cream ... 1135
Nupercainal Hydrocortisone 1% Cream ... ◘ 645
Ophthocort ... ⊙ 311
Pramosone Cream, Lotion & Ointment ... 978
ProctoCream-HC ... 2408
ProctoFoam-HC ... 2409
Terra-Cortril Ophthalmic Suspension ... 2210

Hydrocortisone Sodium Phosphate (Hypokalemia). Products include:
Hydrocortone Phosphate Injection, Sterile ... 1670

Hydrocortisone Sodium Succinate (Hypokalemia). Products include:
Solu-Cortef Sterile Powder ... 2641

Hydroflumethiazide (Potentiated or additive action). Products include:
Diucardin Tablets ... 2718

Ibuprofen (Reduced diuretic, natriuretic, and antihypertensive effects of Moduretic). Products include:
Advil Cold and Sinus Caplets and Tablets (formerly CoAdvil) ... ◘ 870
Advil Ibuprofen Tablets and Caplets ... ◘ 870
Children's Advil Suspension ... 2692
Arthritis Foundation Ibuprofen Tablets ... ◘ 674
Bayer Select Ibuprofen Pain Relief Formula ... ◘ 715
Cramp End Tablets ... ◘ 735
Dimetapp Sinus Caplets ... ◘ 775
Haltran Tablets ... ◘ 771
IBU Tablets ... 1342
Ibuprohm ... ◘ 735
Children's Motrin Ibuprofen Oral Suspension ... 1546
Motrin Tablets ... 2625
Motrin IB Caplets, Tablets, and Geltabs ... ◘ 838
Motrin IB Sinus ... ◘ 838
Motrin Ibuprofen Suspension, Oral Drops, Chewable Tablets, Caplets ... 1546
Nuprin Ibuprofen/Analgesic Tablets & Caplets ... ◘ 622
Sine-Aid IB Caplets ... 1554
Vicks DayQuil SINUS Pressure & PAIN Relief with IBUPROFEN ... ◘ 762

Indapamide (Potentiated or additive action). Products include:
Lozol Tablets ... 2022

Indomethacin (Reduced diuretic, natriuretic, and antihypertensive effects of Moduretic; increased serum potassium levels of both drugs). Products include:
Indocin ... 1680

Indomethacin Sodium Trihydrate (Reduced diuretic, natriuretic, and antihypertensive effects of Moduretic; increased serum potassium levels of both drugs). Products include:
Indocin I.V. ... 1684

Insulin, Human (Altered insulin requirements).
No products indexed under this heading.

Insulin, Human Isophane Suspension (Altered insulin requirements). Products include:
Novolin N Human Insulin 10 ml Vials ... 1795

Insulin, Human NPH (Altered insulin requirements). Products include:
Humulin N, 100 Units ... 1448
Novolin N PenFill Cartridges Durable Insulin Delivery System ... 1798
Novolin N Prefilled Syringe Disposable Insulin Delivery System ... 1798

Insulin, Human Regular (Altered insulin requirements). Products include:
Humulin R, 100 Units ... 1449
Novolin R Human Insulin 10 ml Vials ... 1795
Novolin R PenFill Cartridges Durable Insulin Delivery System ... 1798
Novolin R Prefilled Syringe Disposable Insulin Delivery System ... 1798
Velosulin BR Human Insulin 10 ml Vials ... 1795

Insulin, Human, Zinc Suspension (Altered insulin requirements). Products include:
Humulin L, 100 Units ... 1446
Humulin U, 100 Units ... 1450
Novolin L Human Insulin 10 ml Vials ... 1795

Insulin, NPH (Altered insulin requirements). Products include:
NPH, 100 Units ... 1450
Pork NPH, 100 Units ... 1452
Purified Pork NPH Isophane Insulin ... 1801

Insulin, Regular (Altered insulin requirements). Products include:
Regular, 100 Units ... 1450
Pork Regular, 100 Units ... 1452
Pork Regular (Concentrated), 500 Units ... 1453
Purified Pork Regular Insulin ... 1801

Insulin, Zinc Crystals (Altered insulin requirements). Products include:
NPH, 100 Units ... 1450

Insulin, Zinc Suspension (Altered insulin requirements). Products include:
Iletin I ... 1450
Lente, 100 Units ... 1450
Iletin II ... 1452
Pork Lente, 100 Units ... 1452
Purified Pork Lente Insulin ... 1801

Isradipine (Potentiated or additive action). Products include:
DynaCirc Capsules ... 2256

Ketoprofen (Reduced diuretic, natriuretic, and antihypertensive effects of Moduretic). Products include:
Orudis Capsules ... 2766
Oruvail Capsules ... 2766

Ketorolac Tromethamine (Reduced diuretic, natriuretic, and antihypertensive effects of Moduretic). Products include:
Acular ... 474
Acular ... ⊙ 277
Toradol ... 2159

Labetalol Hydrochloride (Potentiated or additive action). Products include:
Normodyne Injection ... 2377
Normodyne Tablets ... 2379
Trandate ... 1185

Levorphanol Tartrate (Potentiation of orthostatic hypotension). Products include:
Levo-Dromoran ... 2129

Lisinopril (Potentiated or additive action; increased risk of hyperkalemia). Products include:
Prinivil Tablets ... 1733
Prinzide Tablets ... 1737
Zestoretic ... 2850
Zestril Tablets ... 2854

Lithium Carbonate (High risk of lithium toxicity). Products include:
Eskalith ... 2485
Lithium Carbonate Capsules & Tablets ... 2230
Lithonate/Lithotabs/Lithobid ... 2543

Lithium Citrate (High risk of lithium toxicity).
No products indexed under this heading.

Losartan Potassium (Potentiated or additive action). Products include:
Cozaar Tablets ... 1628
Hyzaar Tablets ... 1677

Mecamylamine Hydrochloride (Potentiated or additive action). Products include:
Inversine Tablets ... 1686

Meclofenamate Sodium (Reduced diuretic, natriuretic, and antihypertensive effects of Moduretic).
No products indexed under this heading.

Mefenamic Acid (Reduced diuretic, natriuretic, and antihypertensive effects of Modiuretic). Products include:
Ponstel ... 1925

Meperidine Hydrochloride (Potentiation of orthostatic hypotension). Products include:
Demerol ... 2308
Mepergan Injection ... 2753

Mephobarbital (Potentiation of orthostatic hypotension). Products include:
Mebaral Tablets ... 2322

Metformin Hydrochloride (Dosage adjustment of the antidiabetic drug may be required). Products include:
Glucophage ... 752

Methadone Hydrochloride (Potentiation of orthostatic hypotension). Products include:
Methadone Hydrochloride Oral Concentrate ... 2233
Methadone Hydrochloride Oral Solution & Tablets ... 2235

Methyclothiazide (Potentiated or additive action). Products include:
Enduron Tablets ... 420

Methyldopa (Potentiated or additive action). Products include:
Aldoclor Tablets ... 1598
Aldomet Oral ... 1600
Aldoril Tablets ... 1604

Methyldopate Hydrochloride (Potentiated or additive action). Products include:
Aldomet Ester HCl Injection ... 1602

Methylprednisolone Acetate (Hypokalemia). Products include:
Depo-Medrol Single-Dose Vial ... 2600
Depo-Medrol Sterile Aqueous Suspension ... 2597

Methylprednisolone Sodium Succinate (Hypokalemia). Products include:
Solu-Medrol Sterile Powder ... 2643

Metolazone (Potentiated or additive action). Products include:
Mykrox Tablets ... 993
Zaroxolyn Tablets ... 1000

Metoprolol Succinate (Potentiated or additive action). Products include:
Toprol-XL Tablets ... 565

Metoprolol Tartrate (Potentiated or additive action). Products include:
Lopressor Ampuls ... 830
Lopressor HCT Tablets ... 832
Lopressor Tablets ... 830

Metyrosine (Potentiated or additive action). Products include:
Demser Capsules ... 1649

Minoxidil (Potentiated or additive action). Products include:
Loniten Tablets ... 2618
Rogaine Topical Solution ... 2637

Moexipril Hydrochloride (Potentiated or additive action; increased risk of hyperkalemia). Products include:
Univasc Tablets ... 2410

Morphine Sulfate (Potentiation of orthostatic hypotension). Products include:
Astramorph/PF Injection, USP (Preservative-Free) ... 535
Duramorph ... 962
Infumorph 200 and Infumorph 500 Sterile Solutions ... 965
MS Contin Tablets ... 1994
MSIR ... 1997
Oramorph SR (Morphine Sulfate Sustained Release Tablets) ... 2236

(◘ Described in PDR For Nonprescription Drugs) (⊙ Described in PDR For Ophthalmology)

673 Interactions Index Moduretic

RMS Suppositories ... 2657
Roxanol ... 2243

Nabumetone (Reduced diuretic, natriuretic, and antihypertensive effects of Moduretic). Products include:
Relafen Tablets ... 2510

Nadolol (Potentiated or additive action).
No products indexed under this heading.

Naproxen (Reduced diuretic, natriuretic, and antihypertensive effects of Moduretic). Products include:
Anaprox/Naprosyn ... 2117

Naproxen Sodium (Reduced diuretic, natriuretic, and antihypertensive effects of Moduretic). Products include:
Aleve ... 1975
Anaprox/Naprosyn ... 2117

Nicardipine Hydrochloride (Potentiated or additive action). Products include:
Cardene Capsules ... 2095
Cardene I.V. ... 2709
Cardene SR Capsules ... 2097

Nifedipine (Potentiated or additive action). Products include:
Adalat Capsules (10 mg and 20 mg) ... 587
Adalat CC ... 589
Procardia Capsules ... 1971
Procardia XL Extended Release Tablets ... 1972

Nisoldipine (Potentiated or additive action).
No products indexed under this heading.

Nitroglycerin (Potentiated or additive action). Products include:
Deponit NTG Transdermal Delivery System ... 2397
Nitro-Bid IV ... 1523
Nitro-Bid Ointment ... 1524
Nitrodisc ... 2047
Nitro-Dur (nitroglycerin) Transdermal Infusion System ... 1326
Nitrolingual Spray ... 2027
Nitrostat Tablets ... 1925
Transderm-Nitro Transdermal Therapeutic System ... 859

Norepinephrine Bitartrate (Possible decreased response to pressor amines). Products include:
Levophed Bitartrate Injection ... 2315

Opium Alkaloids (Potentiation of orthostatic hypotension).
No products indexed under this heading.

Oxaprozin (Reduced diuretic, natriuretic, and antihypertensive effects of Moduretic). Products include:
Daypro Caplets ... 2426

Oxycodone Hydrochloride (Potentiation of orthostatic hypotension). Products include:
Percocet Tablets ... 938
Percodan Tablets ... 939
Percodan-Demi Tablets ... 940
Roxicodone Tablets, Oral Solution & Intensol (Oxycodone) ... 2244
Tylox Capsules ... 1584

Penbutolol Sulfate (Potentiated or additive action). Products include:
Levatol ... 2403

Pentobarbital Sodium (Potentiation of orthostatic hypotension). Products include:
Nembutal Sodium Capsules ... 436
Nembutal Sodium Solution ... 438
Nembutal Sodium Suppositories ... 440

Phenobarbital (Potentiation of orthostatic hypotension). Products include:
Arco-Lase Plus Tablets ... 512
Bellergal-S Tablets ... 2250
Donnatal ... 2060
Donnatal Extentabs ... 2061
Donnatal Tablets ... 2060
Phenobarbital Elixir and Tablets ... 1469

Quadrinal Tablets ... 1350

Phenoxybenzamine Hydrochloride (Potentiated or additive action). Products include:
Dibenzyline Capsules ... 2476

Phentolamine Mesylate (Potentiated or additive action). Products include:
Regitine ... 846

Phenylbutazone (Reduced diuretic, natriuretic, and antihypertensive effects of Moduretic).
No products indexed under this heading.

Pindolol (Potentiated or additive action). Products include:
Visken Tablets ... 2299

Piroxicam (Reduced diuretic, natriuretic, and antihypertensive effects of Moduretic). Products include:
Feldene Capsules ... 1965

Polythiazide (Potentiated or additive action). Products include:
Minizide Capsules ... 1938

Potassium Acid Phosphate (Potential for rapid increase in serum potassium levels). Products include:
K-Phos Original Formula 'Sodium Free' Tablets ... 639

Potassium Bicarbonate (Potential for rapid increase in serum potassium levels). Products include:
Alka-Seltzer Gold Effervescent Antacid ... 703

Potassium Chloride (Potential for rapid increase in serum potassium levels). Products include:
Chlor-3 Condiment ... 1004
K-Dur Microburst Release System (potassium chloride, USP) E.R. Tablets ... 1325
K-Lor Powder Packets ... 434
K-Norm Extended-Release Capsules ... 991
K-Tab Filmtab ... 434
Kolyum Liquid ... 992
Micro-K ... 2063
Micro-K LS Packets ... 2064
NuLYTELY ... 689
Cherry Flavor NuLYTELY ... 689
Rum-K Syrup ... 1005
Slow-K Extended-Release Tablets ... 851

Potassium Citrate (Potential for rapid increase in serum potassium levels). Products include:
Polycitra Syrup ... 578
Polycitra-K Crystals ... 579
Polycitra-K Oral Solution ... 579
Polycitra-LC ... 578

Potassium Gluconate (Potential for rapid increase in serum potassium levels). Products include:
Kolyum Liquid ... 992

Potassium Phosphate, Dibasic (Potential for rapid increase in serum potassium levels).
No products indexed under this heading.

Potassium Phosphate, Monobasic (Potential for rapid increase in serum potassium levels). Products include:
K-Phos Neutral Tablets ... 639
K-Phos Original Formula 'Sodium Free' Tablets ... 639

Prazosin Hydrochloride (Potentiated or additive action). Products include:
Minipress Capsules ... 1937
Minizide Capsules ... 1938

Prednisolone Acetate (Hypokalemia). Products include:
AK-CIDE ... ◉ 202
AK-CIDE Ointment ... ◉ 202
Blephamide Liquifilm Sterile Ophthalmic Suspension ... 476
Blephamide Ointment ... ◉ 237
Econopred & Econopred Plus Ophthalmic Suspensions ... ◉ 217
Poly-Pred Liquifilm ... ◉ 248

Pred Forte ... ◉ 250
Pred Mild ... ◉ 253
Pred-G Liquifilm Sterile Ophthalmic Suspension ... ◉ 251
Pred-G S.O.P. Sterile Ophthalmic Ointment ... ◉ 252
Vasocidin Ointment ... ◉ 268

Prednisolone Sodium Phosphate (Hypokalemia). Products include:
AK-Pred ... ◉ 204
Hydeltrasol Injection, Sterile ... 1665
Inflamase ... ◉ 265
Pediapred Oral Liquid ... 995
Vasocidin Ophthalmic Solution ... ◉ 270

Prednisolone Tebutate (Hypokalemia). Products include:
Hydeltra-T.B.A. Sterile Suspension ... 1667

Prednisone (Hypokalemia). Products include:
Deltasone Tablets ... 2595

Propoxyphene Hydrochloride (Potentiation of orthostatic hypotension). Products include:
Darvon ... 1435
Wygesic Tablets ... 2827

Propoxyphene Napsylate (Potentiation of orthostatic hypotension). Products include:
Darvon-N/Darvocet-N ... 1433

Propranolol Hydrochloride (Potentiated or additive action). Products include:
Inderal ... 2728
Inderal LA Long Acting Capsules ... 2730
Inderide Tablets ... 2732
Inderide LA Long Acting Capsules ... 2734

Quinapril Hydrochloride (Potentiated or additive action; increased risk of hyperkalemia). Products include:
Accupril Tablets ... 1893

Ramipril (Potentiated or additive action; increased risk of hyperkalemia). Products include:
Altace Capsules ... 1232

Rauwolfia Serpentina (Potentiated or additive action).
No products indexed under this heading.

Rescinnamine (Potentiated or additive action).
No products indexed under this heading.

Reserpine (Potentiated or additive action). Products include:
Diupres Tablets ... 1650
Hydropres Tablets ... 1675
Ser-Ap-Es Tablets ... 849

Secobarbital Sodium (Potentiation of orthostatic hypotension). Products include:
Seconal Sodium Pulvules ... 1474

Sodium Nitroprusside (Potentiated or additive action).
No products indexed under this heading.

Sotalol Hydrochloride (Potentiated or additive action). Products include:
Betapace Tablets ... 641

Spirapril Hydrochloride (Potentiated or additive action; increased risk of hyperkalemia).
No products indexed under this heading.

Spironolactone (Potential for rapid increase in serum potassium levels). Products include:
Aldactazide ... 2413
Aldactone ... 2414

Sufentanil Citrate (Potentiation of orthostatic hypotension). Products include:
Sufenta Injection ... 1309

Sulindac (Reduced diuretic, natriuretic, and antihypertensive effects of Moduretic). Products include:
Clinoril Tablets ... 1618

Terazosin Hydrochloride (Potentiated or additive action). Products include:
Hytrin Capsules ... 430

Thiamylal Sodium (Potentiation of orthostatic hypotension).
No products indexed under this heading.

Timolol Maleate (Potentiated or additive action). Products include:
Blocadren Tablets ... 1614
Timolide Tablets ... 1748
Timoptic in Ocudose ... 1753
Timoptic Sterile Ophthalmic Solution ... 1751
Timoptic-XE ... 1755

Tolazamide (Dosage adjustment of the antidiabetic drug may be required).
No products indexed under this heading.

Tolbutamide (Dosage adjustment of the antidiabetic drug may be required).
No products indexed under this heading.

Tolmetin Sodium (Reduced diuretic, natriuretic, and antihypertensive effects of Moduretic). Products include:
Tolectin (200, 400 and 600 mg) .. 1581

Torsemide (Potentiated or additive action; increased risk of hyperkalemia). Products include:
Demadex Tablets and Injection ... 686

Triamcinolone (Hypokalemia). Products include:
Aristocort Tablets ... 1022

Triamcinolone Acetonide (Hypokalemia). Products include:
Aristocort A 0.025% Cream ... 1027
Aristocort A 0.5% Cream ... 1031
Aristocort A 0.1% Cream ... 1029
Aristocort A 0.1% Ointment ... 1030
Azmacort Oral Inhaler ... 2011
Nasacort Nasal Inhaler ... 2024

Triamcinolone Diacetate (Hypokalemia). Products include:
Aristocort Suspension (Forte Parenteral) ... 1027
Aristocort Suspension (Intralesional) ... 1025

Triamcinolone Hexacetonide (Hypokalemia). Products include:
Aristospan Suspension (Intra-articular) ... 1033
Aristospan Suspension (Intralesional) ... 1032

Triamterene (Potential for rapid increase in serum potassium levels). Products include:
Dyazide ... 2479
Dyrenium Capsules ... 2481
Maxzide ... 1380

Trimethaphan Camsylate (Potentiated or additive action). Products include:
Arfonad Ampuls ... 2080

Tubocurarine Chloride (Increased responsiveness to tubocurarine).
No products indexed under this heading.

Verapamil Hydrochloride (Potentiated or additive action). Products include:
Calan SR Caplets ... 2422
Calan Tablets ... 2419
Isoptin Injectable ... 1344
Isoptin Oral Tablets ... 1346
Isoptin SR Tablets ... 1348
Verelan Capsules ... 1410
Verelan Capsules ... 2824

Food Interactions

Alcohol (Potentiation of orthostatic hypotension).

Diet, potassium-rich (Potential for rapid increases in serum potassium levels).

IMPORTANT NOTE: Always consult each drug listing in the patient's regimen for possible interactions.

Moisturel Cream Interactions Index 674

MOISTUREL CREAM
(Dimethicone, Petrolatum) 2688
None cited in PDR database.

MOISTUREL LOTION
(Dimethicone) 2688
None cited in PDR database.

8-MOP CAPSULES
(Methoxsalen) 1246
May interact with phenothiazines, tetracyclines, thiazides, sulfonamides, and certain other agents. Compounds in these categories include:

Anthralin (Concomitant therapy, either topically or systemically, with photosensitizing agents requires special care). Products include:
- Drithocreme 0.1%, 0.25%, 0.5%, 1.0% (HP) 905
- Dritho-Scalp 0.25%, 0.5% 906

Bendroflumethiazide (Concomitant therapy, either topically or systemically, with photosensitizing agents requires special care).
No products indexed under this heading.

Chlorothiazide (Concomitant therapy, either topically or systemically, with photosensitizing agents requires special care). Products include:
- Aldoclor Tablets 1598
- Diupres Tablets 1650
- Diuril Oral 1653

Chlorothiazide Sodium (Concomitant therapy, either topically or systemically, with photosensitizing agents requires special care). Products include:
- Diuril Sodium Intravenous 1652

Chlorpromazine (Concomitant therapy, either topically or systemically, with photosensitizing agents requires special care). Products include:
- Thorazine Suppositories 2523

Chlorpromazine Hydrochloride (Concomitant therapy, either topically or systemically, with photosensitizing agents requires special care). Products include:
- Thorazine 2523

Chlorpropamide (Concomitant therapy, either topically or systemically, with photosensitizing agents requires special care). Products include:
- Diabinese Tablets 1935

Coal Tar (Concomitant therapy, either topically or systemically, with photosensitizing agents requires special care). Products include:
- DHS 1932
- Fototar Cream 1253
- MG 217 .... ◙ 835
- P&S Plus Tar Gel .... ◙ 604
- Pentrax Anti-dandruff Shampoo 1055
- Tegrin Dandruff Shampoo .... ◙ 611
- Tegrin Skin Cream & Tegrin Medicated Soap .... ◙ 611
- X-Seb T Pearl Shampoo .... ◙ 606
- X-Seb T Plus Conditioning Shampoo .... ◙ 606

Demeclocycline Hydrochloride (Concomitant therapy, either topically or systemically, with photosensitizing agents requires special care). Products include:
- Declomycin Tablets 1371

Doxycycline Calcium (Concomitant therapy, either topically or systemically, with photosensitizing agents requires special care). Products include:
- Vibramycin Calcium Oral Suspension Syrup 1941

Doxycycline Hyclate (Concomitant therapy, either topically or systemically, with photosensitizing agents requires special care). Products include:
- Doryx Capsules 1913
- Vibramycin Hyclate Capsules 1941
- Vibramycin Hyclate Intravenous 2215
- Vibra-Tabs Film Coated Tablets 1941

Doxycycline Monohydrate (Concomitant therapy, either topically or systemically, with photosensitizing agents requires special care). Products include:
- Monodox Capsules 1805
- Vibramycin Monohydrate for Oral Suspension 1941

Fluphenazine Decanoate (Concomitant therapy, either topically or systemically, with photosensitizing agents requires special care). Products include:
- Prolixin Decanoate 509

Fluphenazine Enanthate (Concomitant therapy, either topically or systemically, with photosensitizing agents requires special care). Products include:
- Prolixin Enanthate 509

Fluphenazine Hydrochloride (Concomitant therapy, either topically or systemically, with photosensitizing agents requires special care). Products include:
- Prolixin 509

Glipizide (Concomitant therapy, either topically or systemically, with photosensitizing agents requires special care). Products include:
- Glucotrol Tablets 1967
- Glucotrol XL Extended Release Tablets 1968

Glyburide (Concomitant therapy, either topically or systemically, with photosensitizing agents requires special care). Products include:
- DiaBeta Tablets 1239
- Glynase PresTab Tablets 2609
- Micronase Tablets 2623

Griseofulvin (Concomitant therapy, either topically or systemically, with photosensitizing agents requires special care). Products include:
- Fulvicin P/G Tablets 2359
- Fulvicin P/G 165 & 330 Tablets 2359
- Grifulvin V (griseofulvin tablets) Microsize (griseofulvin oral suspension) Microsize 1888
- Gris-PEG Tablets, 125 mg & 250 mg 479

Hydrochlorothiazide (Concomitant therapy, either topically or systemically, with photosensitizing agents requires special care). Products include:
- Aldactazide 2413
- Aldoril Tablets 1604
- Apresazide Capsules 808
- Capozide 742
- Dyazide 2479
- Esidrix Tablets 821
- Esimil Tablets 822
- HydroDIURIL Tablets 1674
- Hydropres Tablets 1675
- Hyzaar Tablets 1677
- Inderide Tablets 2732
- Inderide LA Long Acting Capsules 2734
- Lopressor HCT Tablets 832
- Lotensin HCT 837
- Maxzide 1380
- Moduretic Tablets 1705
- Oretic Tablets 443
- Prinzide Tablets 1737
- Ser-Ap-Es Tablets 849
- Timolide Tablets 1748
- Vaseretic Tablets 1765
- Zestoretic 2850
- Ziac 1415

Hydroflumethiazide (Concomitant therapy, either topically or systemically, with photosensitizing agents requires special care). Products include:
- Diucardin Tablets 2718

Mesoridazine Besylate (Concomitant therapy, either topically or systemically, with photosensitizing agents requires special care). Products include:
- Serentil 684

Methacycline Hydrochloride (Concomitant therapy, either topically or systemically, with photosensitizing agents requires special care).
No products indexed under this heading.

Methotrimeprazine (Concomitant therapy, either topically or systemically, with photosensitizing agents requires special care). Products include:
- Levoprome 1274

Methyclothiazide (Concomitant therapy, either topically or systemically, with photosensitizing agents requires special care). Products include:
- Enduron Tablets 420

Methylene Blue (Concomitant therapy, either topically or systemically, with photosensitizing agents requires special care). Products include:
- Urised Tablets 1964

Minocycline Hydrochloride (Concomitant therapy, either topically or systemically, with photosensitizing agents requires special care). Products include:
- Dynacin Capsules 1590
- Minocin Intravenous 1382
- Minocin Oral Suspension 1385
- Minocin Pellet-Filled Capsules 1383

Nalidixic Acid (Concomitant therapy, either topically or systemically, with photosensitizing agents requires special care). Products include:
- NegGram 2323

Oxytetracycline Hydrochloride (Concomitant therapy, either topically or systemically, with photosensitizing agents requires special care). Products include:
- TERAK Ointment .... ⊙ 209
- Terra-Cortril Ophthalmic Suspension 2210
- Terramycin with Polymyxin B Sulfate Ophthalmic Ointment 2211
- Urobiotic-250 Capsules 2214

Perphenazine (Concomitant therapy, either topically or systemically, with photosensitizing agents requires special care). Products include:
- Etrafon 2355
- Triavil Tablets 1757
- Trilafon 2389

Polythiazide (Concomitant therapy, either topically or systemically, with photosensitizing agents requires special care). Products include:
- Minizide Capsules 1938

Prochlorperazine (Concomitant therapy, either topically or systemically, with photosensitizing agents requires special care). Products include:
- Compazine 2470

Promethazine Hydrochloride (Concomitant therapy, either topically or systemically, with photosensitizing agents requires special care). Products include:
- Mepergan Injection 2753
- Phenergan with Codeine 2777
- Phenergan with Dextromethorphan 2778
- Phenergan Injection 2773
- Phenergan Suppositories 2775
- Phenergan Syrup 2774
- Phenergan Tablets 2775
- Phenergan VC 2779
- Phenergan VC with Codeine 2781

Rose Bengal (Concomitant therapy, either topically or systemically, with photosensitizing agents requires special care).
No products indexed under this heading.

Sulfacytine (Concomitant therapy, either topically or systemically, with photosensitizing agents requires special care).

Sulfamethizole (Concomitant therapy, either topically or systemically, with photosensitizing agents requires special care). Products include:
- Urobiotic-250 Capsules 2214

Sulfamethoxazole (Concomitant therapy, either topically or systemically, with photosensitizing agents requires special care). Products include:
- Azo Gantanol Tablets 2080
- Bactrim DS Tablets 2084
- Bactrim I.V. Infusion 2082
- Bactrim 2084
- Gantanol Tablets 2119
- Septra 1174
- Septra I.V. Infusion 1169
- Septra I.V. Infusion ADD-Vantage Vials 1171
- Septra 1174

Sulfasalazine (Concomitant therapy, either topically or systemically, with photosensitizing agents requires special care). Products include:
- Azulfidine 1949

Sulfinpyrazone (Concomitant therapy, either topically or systemically, with photosensitizing agents requires special care). Products include:
- Anturane 807

Sulfisoxazole (Concomitant therapy, either topically or systemically, with photosensitizing agents requires special care). Products include:
- Azo Gantrisin Tablets 2081
- Gantrisin Tablets 2120

Sulfisoxazole Diolamine (Concomitant therapy, either topically or systemically, with photosensitizing agents requires special care).
No products indexed under this heading.

Tetracycline Hydrochloride (Concomitant therapy, either topically or systemically, with photosensitizing agents requires special care). Products include:
- Achromycin V Capsules 1367

Thioridazine Hydrochloride (Concomitant therapy, either topically or systemically, with photosensitizing agents requires special care). Products include:
- Mellaril 2269

Tolazamide (Concomitant therapy, either topically or systemically, with photosensitizing agents requires special care).
No products indexed under this heading.

Tolbutamide (Concomitant therapy, either topically or systemically, with photosensitizing agents requires special care).
No products indexed under this heading.

Trifluoperazine Hydrochloride (Concomitant therapy, either topically or systemically, with photosensitizing agents requires special care). Products include:
- Stelazine 2514

(◙ Described in PDR For Nonprescription Drugs) (⊙ Described in PDR For Ophthalmology)

675 **Interactions Index** **Monodox**

MONISTAT DUAL-PAK
(Miconazole Nitrate) 1850
None cited in PDR database.

MONISTAT 3 VAGINAL SUPPOSITORIES
(Miconazole Nitrate) 1850
None cited in PDR database.

MONISTAT-DERM (MICONAZOLE NITRATE 2%) CREAM
(Miconazole Nitrate) 1889
None cited in PDR database.

MONOCID INJECTION
(Cefonicid Sodium) 2497
May interact with aminoglycosides and certain other agents. Compounds in these categories include:

Amikacin Sulfate (Concomitant administration may result in nephrotoxicity). Products include:
Amikacin Sulfate Injection, USP 960
Amikin Injectable 501

Gentamicin Sulfate (Concomitant administration may result in nephrotoxicity). Products include:
Garamycin Injectable 2360
Genoptic Sterile Ophthalmic Solution ⊙ 243
Genoptic Sterile Ophthalmic Ointment ⊙ 243
Gentacidin Ointment ⊙ 264
Gentacidin Solution ⊙ 264
Gentak ⊙ 208
Pred-G Liquifilm Sterile Ophthalmic Suspension ⊙ 251
Pred-G S.O.P. Sterile Ophthalmic Ointment ⊙ 252

Kanamycin Sulfate (Concomitant administration may result in nephrotoxicity).
No products indexed under this heading.

Probenecid (Produces higher peak serum levels). Products include:
Benemid Tablets 1611
ColBENEMID Tablets 1622

Streptomycin Sulfate (Concomitant administration may result in nephrotoxicity). Products include:
Streptomycin Sulfate Injection 2208

Tobramycin Sulfate (Concomitant administration may result in nephrotoxicity). Products include:
Nebcin Vials, Hyporets & ADD-Vantage 1464
Tobramycin Sulfate Injection 968

MONOCLATE-P, FACTOR VIII:C, PASTEURIZED, MONOCLONAL ANTIBODY PURIFIED ANTIHEMOPHILIC FACTOR (HUMAN)
(Antihemophilic Factor (Human)) 521
None cited in PDR database.

MONODOX CAPSULES
(Doxycycline Monohydrate) 1805
May interact with barbiturates, oral contraceptives, penicillins, antacids containing aluminium, calcium and magnesium, oral anticoagulants, and certain other agents. Compounds in these categories include:

Aluminum Carbonate Gel (Absorption of tetracyclines is impaired). Products include:
Basaljel 2703

Aluminum Hydroxide (Absorption of tetracyclines is impaired). Products include:
ALternaGEL Liquid 1316
Maximum Strength Ascriptin ⊞ 630
Cama Arthritis Pain Reliever ⊞ 785
Gaviscon Extra Strength Relief Formula Antacid Tablets ⊞ 819
Gaviscon Extra Strength Relief Formula Liquid Antacid ⊞ 819
Gaviscon Liquid Antacid ⊞ 820
Gelusil Liquid & Tablets ⊞ 855
Maalox Heartburn Relief Suspension ⊞ 642
Maalox Heartburn Relief Tablets ⊞ 641
Maalox Magnesia and Alumina Oral Suspension ⊞ 642
Maalox Plus Tablets ⊞ 643
Extra Strength Maalox Antacid Plus Antigas Liquid and Tablets ⊞ 638
Tempo Soft Antacid ⊞ 835

Aluminum Hydroxide Gel (Absorption of tetracyclines is impaired). Products include:
ALternaGEL Liquid ⊞ 659
Aludrox Oral Suspension 2695
Amphojel Suspension 2695
Amphojel Suspension without Flavor 2695
Amphojel Tablets 2695
Arthritis Pain Ascriptin ⊞ 631
Regular Strength Ascriptin Tablets ⊞ 629
Gaviscon Antacid Tablets ⊞ 819
Gaviscon-2 Antacid Tablets ⊞ 820
Mylanta Liquid 1317
Mylanta Tablets ⊞ 660
Mylanta Double Strength Liquid 1317
Mylanta Double Strength Tablets ⊞ 660
Nephrox Suspension ⊞ 655

Amoxicillin Trihydrate (Interference with penicillins' bactericidal action). Products include:
Amoxil 2464
Augmentin 2468

Ampicillin (Interference with penicillins' bactericidal action). Products include:
Omnipen Capsules 2764
Omnipen for Oral Suspension 2765

Ampicillin Sodium (Interference with penicillins' bactericidal action). Products include:
Unasyn 2212

Aprobarbital (Decreases the half-life of doxycycline).
No products indexed under this heading.

Azlocillin Sodium (Interference with penicillins' bactericidal action).
No products indexed under this heading.

Bacampicillin Hydrochloride (Interference with penicillins' bactericidal action). Products include:
Spectrobid Tablets 2206

Butabarbital (Decreases the half-life of doxycycline).
No products indexed under this heading.

Butalbital (Decreases the half-life of doxycycline). Products include:
Esgic-plus Tablets 1013
Fioricet Tablets 2258
Fioricet with Codeine Capsules 2260
Fiorinal Capsules 2261
Fiorinal with Codeine Capsules 2262
Fiorinal Tablets 2261
Phrenilin 785
Sedapap Tablets 50 mg/650 mg 1543

Carbamazepine (Decrease the half-life of doxycycline). Products include:
Atretol Tablets 573
Tegretol Chewable Tablets 852
Tegretol Suspension 852
Tegretol Tablets 852

Carbenicillin Disodium (Interference with penicillins' bactericidal action).
No products indexed under this heading.

Carbenicillin Indanyl Sodium (Interference with penicillins' bactericidal action). Products include:
Geocillin Tablets 2199

Desogestrel (Concurrent use may render oral contraceptives less effective). Products include:
Desogen Tablets 1817
Ortho-Cept 1851

Dicloxacillin Sodium (Interference with penicillins' bactericidal action).
No products indexed under this heading.

Dicumarol (Depressed plasma prothrombin activity).
No products indexed under this heading.

Dihydroxyaluminum Sodium Carbonate (Absorption of tetracyclines is impaired).
No products indexed under this heading.

Ethinyl Estradiol (Concurrent use may render oral contraceptives less effective). Products include:
Brevicon 2088
Demulen 2428
Desogen Tablets 1817
Levlen/Tri-Levlen 651
Lo/Ovral Tablets 2746
Lo/Ovral-28 Tablets 2751
Modicon 1872
Nordette-21 Tablets 2755
Nordette-28 Tablets 2758
Norinyl 2088
Ortho-Cept 1851
Ortho-Cyclen/Ortho-Tri-Cyclen 1858
Ortho-Novum 1872
Ortho-Cyclen/Ortho Tri-Cyclen 1858
Ovcon 760
Ovral Tablets 2770
Ovral-28 Tablets 2770
Levlen/Tri-Levlen 651
Tri-Norinyl 2164
Triphasil-21 Tablets 2814
Triphasil-28 Tablets 2819

Ethynodiol Diacetate (Concurrent use may render oral contraceptives less effective). Products include:
Demulen 2428

Levonorgestrel (Concurrent use may render oral contraceptives less effective). Products include:
Levlen/Tri-Levlen 651
Nordette-21 Tablets 2755
Nordette-28 Tablets 2758
Norplant System 2759
Levlen/Tri-Levlen 651
Triphasil-21 Tablets 2814
Triphasil-28 Tablets 2819

Magaldrate (Absorption of tetracyclines is impaired).
No products indexed under this heading.

Magnesium Hydroxide (Absorption of tetracyclines is impaired). Products include:
Aludrox Oral Suspension 2695
Arthritis Pain Ascriptin ⊞ 631
Maximum Strength Ascriptin ⊞ 630
Regular Strength Ascriptin Tablets ⊞ 629
Di-Gel Antacid/Anti-Gas ⊞ 801
Gelusil Liquid & Tablets ⊞ 855
Maalox Magnesia and Alumina Oral Suspension ⊞ 642
Maalox Plus Tablets ⊞ 643
Extra Strength Maalox Antacid Plus Antigas Liquid and Tablets ⊞ 638
Mylanta Calcium Carbonate and Magnesium Hydroxide Tablets 1318
Mylanta Liquid 1317
Mylanta Tablets ⊞ 660
Mylanta Double Strength Liquid 1317
Mylanta Double Strength Tablets ⊞ 660
Phillips' Milk of Magnesia Liquid ⊞ 729
Rolaids Tablets ⊞ 843
Tempo Soft Antacid ⊞ 835

Magnesium Oxide (Absorption of tetracyclines is impaired). Products include:
Beelith Tablets 639
Bufferin Analgesic Tablets and Caplets ⊞ 613
Caltrate PLUS ⊞ 665
Cama Arthritis Pain Reliever ⊞ 785
Mag-Ox 400 668
Uro-Mag 668

Mephobarbital (Decreases the half-life of doxycycline). Products include:
Mebaral Tablets 2322

Mestranol (Concurrent use may render oral contraceptives less effective). Products include:
Norinyl 2088
Ortho-Novum 1872

Methoxyflurane (Potential for fatal renal toxicity).
No products indexed under this heading.

Mezlocillin Sodium (Interference with penicillins' bactericidal action). Products include:
Mezlin 601
Mezlin Pharmacy Bulk Package 604

Nafcillin Sodium (Interference with penicillins' bactericidal action).
No products indexed under this heading.

Norethindrone (Concurrent use may render oral contraceptives less effective). Products include:
Brevicon 2088
Micronor Tablets 1872
Modicon 1872
Norinyl 2088
Nor-Q D Tablets 2135
Ortho-Novum 1872
Ovcon 760
Tri-Norinyl 2164

Norethynodrel (Concurrent use may render oral contraceptives less effective).
No products indexed under this heading.

Norgestimate (Concurrent use may render oral contraceptives less effective). Products include:
Ortho-Cyclen/Ortho-Tri-Cyclen 1858
Ortho-Cyclen/Ortho Tri-Cyclen 1858

Norgestrel (Concurrent use may render oral contraceptives less effective). Products include:
Lo/Ovral Tablets 2746
Lo/Ovral-28 Tablets 2751
Ovral Tablets 2770
Ovral-28 Tablets 2770
Ovrette Tablets 2771

Penicillin G Benzathine (Interference with penicillins' bactericidal action). Products include:
Bicillin C-R Injection 2704
Bicillin C-R 900/300 Injection 2706
Bicillin L-A Injection 2707

Penicillin G Potassium (Interference with penicillins' bactericidal action). Products include:
Pfizerpen for Injection 2203

Penicillin G Procaine (Interference with penicillins' bactericidal action). Products include:
Bicillin C-R Injection 2704
Bicillin C-R 900/300 Injection 2706

Penicillin G Sodium (Interference with penicillins' bactericidal action).
No products indexed under this heading.

Penicillin V Potassium (Interference with penicillins' bactericidal action). Products include:
Pen•Vee K 2772

Pentobarbital Sodium (Decreases the half-life of doxycycline). Products include:
Nembutal Sodium Capsules 436
Nembutal Sodium Solution 438
Nembutal Sodium Suppositories 440

Phenobarbital (Decreases the half-life of doxycycline). Products include:
Arco-Lase Plus Tablets 512
Bellergal-S Tablets 2250
Donnatal 2060
Donnatal Extentabs 2061
Donnatal Tablets 2060
Phenobarbital Elixir and Tablets 1469
Quadrinal Tablets 1350

IMPORTANT NOTE: Always consult each drug listing in the patient's regimen for possible interactions.

Monodox Interactions Index 676

Phenytoin (Decreases the half-life of doxycycline). Products include:
- Dilantin Infatabs 1908
- Dilantin-125 Suspension 1911

Phenytoin Sodium (Decreases the half-life of doxycycline). Products include:
- Dilantin Kapseals 1906
- Dilantin Parenteral 1910

Secobarbital Sodium (Decreases the half-life of doxycycline). Products include:
- Seconal Sodium Pulvules 1474

Thiamylal Sodium (Decreases the half-life of doxycycline).
- No products indexed under this heading.

Ticarcillin Disodium (Interference with penicillins' bactericidal action). Products include:
- Ticar for Injection 2526
- Timentin for Injection 2528

Warfarin Sodium (Depressed plasma prothrombin activity). Products include:
- Coumadin 926

MONO-GESIC TABLETS

(Salsalate) 792

May interact with thyroid preparations, salicylates, antigout agents, anticoagulants, oral hypoglycemic agents, corticosteroids, and penicillins. Compounds in these categories include:

Acarbose (Hypoglycemic effect enhanced).
- No products indexed under this heading.

Allopurinol (Uricosuric action of gout drugs antagonized). Products include:
- Zyloprim Tablets 1226

Amoxicillin Trihydrate (Competition for protein-binding sites). Products include:
- Amoxil 2464
- Augmentin 2468

Ampicillin Sodium (Competition for protein-binding sites). Products include:
- Unasyn 2212

Aspirin (Potential toxicity). Products include:
- Alka-Seltzer Effervescent Antacid and Pain Reliever ▣ 701
- Alka-Seltzer Extra Strength Effervescent Antacid and Pain Reliever ▣ 703
- Alka-Seltzer Lemon Lime Effervescent Antacid and Pain Reliever ▣ 703
- Alka-Seltzer Plus Cold Medicine ▣ 705
- Alka-Seltzer Plus Cold & Cough Medicine ▣ 708
- Alka-Seltzer Plus Night-Time Cold Medicine ▣ 707
- Alka Seltzer Plus Sinus Medicine ▣ 707
- Arthritis Foundation Safety Coated Aspirin Tablets ▣ 675
- Arthritis Pain Ascriptin ▣ 631
- Maximum Strength Ascriptin ▣ 630
- Regular Strength Ascriptin Tablets ▣ 629
- Arthritis Strength BC Powder ▣ 609
- BC Cold Powder Multi-Symptom Formula (Cold-Sinus-Allergy) ▣ 609
- BC Cold Powder Non-Drowsy Formula (Cold-Sinus) ▣ 609
- BC Powder ▣ 609
- Bayer Children's Chewable Aspirin ▣ 711
- Genuine Bayer Aspirin Tablets & Caplets ▣ 713
- Extra Strength Bayer Arthritis Pain Regimen Formula ▣ 711
- Extra Strength Bayer Aspirin Caplets & Tablets ▣ 712
- Extended-Release Bayer 8-Hour Aspirin ▣ 712
- Extra Strength Bayer Plus Aspirin Caplets ▣ 713
- Extra Strength Bayer PM Aspirin ▣ 713
- Bayer Enteric Aspirin ▣ 709
- Bufferin Analgesic Tablets and Caplets ▣ 613
- Arthritis Strength Bufferin Analgesic Caplets ▣ 614
- Extra Strength Bufferin Analgesic Tablets ▣ 615
- Cama Arthritis Pain Reliever ▣ 785
- Darvon Compound-65 Pulvules 1435
- Easprin 1914
- Ecotrin 2455
- Ecotrin Enteric Coated Aspirin Maximum Strength Tablets and Caplets ▣ 816
- Ecotrin Enteric Coated Aspirin Regular Strength Tablets 2455
- Empirin Aspirin Tablets ▣ 854
- Empirin with Codeine Tablets 1093
- Excedrin Extra-Strength Analgesic Tablets & Caplets 732
- Fiorinal Capsules 2261
- Fiorinal with Codeine Capsules 2262
- Fiorinal Tablets 2261
- Halfprin 1362
- Healthprin Aspirin 2455
- Norgesic 1496
- Percodan Tablets 939
- Percodan-Demi Tablets 940
- Robaxisal Tablets 2071
- Soma Compound w/Codeine Tablets 2676
- Soma Compound Tablets 2675
- St. Joseph Adult Chewable Aspirin (81 mg.) ▣ 808
- Talwin Compound 2335
- Ursinus Inlay-Tabs ▣ 794
- Vanquish Analgesic Caplets ▣ 731

Azlocillin Sodium (Competition for protein-binding sites).
- No products indexed under this heading.

Bacampicillin Hydrochloride (Competition for protein-binding sites). Products include:
- Spectrobid Tablets 2206

Betamethasone Acetate (Competition for protein-binding sites). Products include:
- Celestone Soluspan Suspension 2347

Betamethasone Sodium Phosphate (Competition for protein-binding sites). Products include:
- Celestone Soluspan Suspension 2347

Carbenicillin Disodium (Competition for protein-binding sites).
- No products indexed under this heading.

Carbenicillin Indanyl Sodium (Competition for protein-binding sites). Products include:
- Geocillin Tablets 2199

Chlorpropamide (Hypoglycemic effect enhanced). Products include:
- Diabinese Tablets 1935

Choline Magnesium Trisalicylate (Potential toxicity). Products include:
- Trilisate 2000

Cortisone Acetate (Competition for protein-binding sites). Products include:
- Cortone Acetate Sterile Suspension 1623
- Cortone Acetate Tablets 1624

Dalteparin Sodium (Competition for protein binding predisposes to systemic bleeding). Products include:
- Fragmin 1954

Dexamethasone (Competition for protein-binding sites). Products include:
- AK-Trol Ointment & Suspension ⊙ 205
- Decadron Elixir 1633
- Decadron Tablets 1635
- Decaspray Topical Aerosol 1648
- Dexacidin Ointment ⊙ 263
- Maxitrol Ophthalmic Ointment and Suspension ⊙ 224
- TobraDex Ophthalmic Suspension and Ointment 473

Dexamethasone Acetate (Competition for protein-binding sites). Products include:
- Dalalone D.P. Injectable 1011
- Decadron-LA Sterile Suspension 1646

Dexamethasone Sodium Phosphate (Competition for protein-binding sites). Products include:
- Decadron Phosphate Injection 1637
- Decadron Phosphate Respihaler 1642
- Decadron Phosphate Sterile Ophthalmic Ointment 1641
- Decadron Phosphate Sterile Ophthalmic Solution 1642
- Decadron Phosphate Topical Cream 1644
- Decadron Phosphate Turbinaire 1645
- Decadron Phosphate with Xylocaine Injection, Sterile 1639
- Dexacort Phosphate in Respihaler 458
- Dexacort Phosphate in Turbinaire 459
- NeoDecadron Sterile Ophthalmic Ointment 1712
- NeoDecadron Sterile Ophthalmic Solution 1713
- NeoDecadron Topical Cream 1714

Dicloxacillin Sodium (Competition for protein-binding sites).
- No products indexed under this heading.

Dicumarol (Competition for protein binding predisposes to systemic bleeding).
- No products indexed under this heading.

Diflunisal (Potential toxicity). Products include:
- Dolobid Tablets 1654

Enoxaparin (Competition for protein binding predisposes to systemic bleeding). Products include:
- Lovenox Injection 2020

Fludrocortisone Acetate (Competition for protein-binding sites). Products include:
- Florinef Acetate Tablets 505

Glipizide (Hypoglycemic effect enhanced). Products include:
- Glucotrol Tablets 1967
- Glucotrol XL Extended Release Tablets 1968

Glyburide (Hypoglycemic effect enhanced). Products include:
- DiaBeta Tablets 1239
- Glynase PresTab Tablets 2609
- Micronase Tablets 2623

Heparin Calcium (Competition for protein binding predisposes to systemic bleeding).
- No products indexed under this heading.

Heparin Sodium (Competition for protein binding predisposes to systemic bleeding). Products include:
- Heparin Lock Flush Solution 2725
- Heparin Sodium Injection 2726
- Heparin Sodium Injection, USP, Sterile Solution 2615
- Heparin Sodium Vials 1441

Hydrocortisone (Competition for protein-binding sites). Products include:
- Anusol-HC Cream 2.5% 1896
- Aquanil HC Lotion 1931
- Bactine Hydrocortisone Anti-Itch Cream ▣ 709
- Caldecort Anti-Itch Hydrocortisone Spray ▣ 631
- Cortaid ▣ 836
- CORTENEMA 2535
- Cortisporin Ointment 1085
- Cortisporin Ophthalmic Ointment Sterile 1085
- Cortisporin Ophthalmic Suspension Sterile 1086
- Cortisporin Otic Solution Sterile 1087
- Cortisporin Otic Suspension Sterile 1088
- Cortizone-5 ▣ 831
- Cortizone-10 ▣ 831
- Hydrocortone Tablets 1672
- Hytone 907
- Massengill Medicated Soft Cloth Towelettes 2458
- PediOtic Suspension Sterile 1153
- Preparation H Hydrocortisone 1% Cream ▣ 872
- ProctoCream-HC 2.5% 2408
- VōSoL HC Otic Solution 2678

Hydrocortisone Acetate (Competition for protein-binding sites). Products include:
- Analpram-HC Rectal Cream 1% and 2.5% 977
- Anusol HC-1 Anti-Itch Hydrocortisone Ointment ▣ 847
- Anusol-HC Suppositories 1897
- Caldecort ▣ 631
- Carmol HC 924
- Coly-Mycin S Otic w/Neomycin & Hydrocortisone 1906
- Cortaid ▣ 836
- Cortifoam 2396
- Cortisporin Cream 1084
- Epifoam 2399
- Hydrocortone Acetate Sterile Suspension 1669
- Mantadil Cream 1135
- Nupercainal Hydrocortisone 1% Cream ▣ 645
- Ophthocort ⊙ 311
- Pramosone Cream, Lotion & Ointment 978
- ProctoCream-HC 2408
- ProctoFoam-HC 2409
- Terra-Cortril Ophthalmic Suspension 2210

Hydrocortisone Sodium Phosphate (Competition for protein-binding sites). Products include:
- Hydrocortone Phosphate Injection, Sterile 1670

Hydrocortisone Sodium Succinate (Competition for protein-binding sites). Products include:
- Solu-Cortef Sterile Powder 2641

Levothyroxine Sodium (Depressed plasma T4 value). Products include:
- Levothroid Tablets 1016
- Levoxyl Tablets 903
- Synthroid 1359

Liothyronine Sodium (Depressed plasma T4 value). Products include:
- Cytomel Tablets 2473
- Triostat Injection 2530

Magnesium Salicylate (Potential toxicity). Products include:
- Backache Caplets ▣ 613
- Bayer Select Backache Pain Relief Formula ▣ 715
- Doan's Extra-Strength Analgesic ▣ 633
- Extra Strength Doan's P.M. ▣ 633
- Doan's Regular Strength Analgesic ▣ 634
- Mobigesic Tablets ▣ 602

Metformin Hydrochloride (Hypoglycemic effect enhanced). Products include:
- Glucophage 752

Methotrexate Sodium (Competition for protein-binding sites). Products include:
- Methotrexate Sodium Tablets, Injection, for Injection and LPF Injection 1275

Methylprednisolone Acetate (Competition for protein-binding sites). Products include:
- Depo-Medrol Single-Dose Vial 2600
- Depo-Medrol Sterile Aqueous Suspension 2597

Methylprednisolone Sodium Succinate (Competition for protein-binding sites). Products include:
- Solu-Medrol Sterile Powder 2643

Mezlocillin Sodium (Competition for protein-binding sites). Products include:
- Mezlin 601
- Mezlin Pharmacy Bulk Package 604

Nafcillin Sodium (Competition for protein-binding sites).
- No products indexed under this heading.

(▣ Described in PDR For Nonprescription Drugs) (⊙ Described in PDR For Ophthalmology)

677 **Interactions Index** **Monopril**

Naproxen (Competition for protein-binding sites). Products include:
- Anaprox/Naprosyn 2117

Naproxen Sodium (Competition for protein-binding sites). Products include:
- Aleve 1975
- Anaprox/Naprosyn 2117

Penicillin G Benzathine (Competition for protein-binding sites). Products include:
- Bicillin C-R Injection 2704
- Bicillin C-R 900/300 Injection 2706
- Bicillin L-A Injection 2707

Penicillin G Potassium (Competition for protein-binding sites). Products include:
- Pfizerpen for Injection 2203

Penicillin G Procaine (Competition for protein-binding sites). Products include:
- Bicillin C-R Injection 2704
- Bicillin C-R 900/300 Injection 2706

Penicillin G Sodium (Competition for protein-binding sites).
- No products indexed under this heading.

Penicillin V Potassium (Competition for protein-binding sites). Products include:
- Pen•Vee K 2772

Phenytoin (Competition for protein-binding sites). Products include:
- Dilantin Infatabs 1908
- Dilantin-125 Suspension 1911

Phenytoin Sodium (Competition for protein-binding sites). Products include:
- Dilantin Kapseals 1906
- Dilantin Parenteral 1910

Prednisolone Acetate (Competition for protein-binding sites). Products include:
- AK-CIDE .... ◉ 202
- AK-CIDE Ointment .... ◉ 202
- Blephamide Liquifilm Sterile Ophthalmic Suspension 476
- Blephamide Ointment .... ◉ 237
- Econopred & Econopred Plus Ophthalmic Suspensions .... ◉ 217
- Poly-Pred Liquifilm .... ◉ 248
- Pred Forte .... ◉ 250
- Pred Mild .... ◉ 253
- Pred-G Liquifilm Sterile Ophthalmic Suspension .... ◉ 251
- Pred-G S.O.P. Sterile Ophthalmic Ointment .... ◉ 252
- Vasocidin Ointment .... ◉ 268

Prednisolone Sodium Phosphate (Competition for protein-binding sites). Products include:
- AK-Pred .... ◉ 204
- Hydeltrasol Injection, Sterile 1665
- Inflamase .... ◉ 265
- Pediapred Oral Liquid 995
- Vasocidin Ophthalmic Solution .... ◉ 270

Prednisolone Tebutate (Competition for protein-binding sites). Products include:
- Hydeltra-T.B.A. Sterile Suspension 1667

Prednisone (Competition for protein-binding sites). Products include:
- Deltasone Tablets 2595

Probenecid (Uricosuric action of gout drugs antagonized). Products include:
- Benemid Tablets 1611
- ColBENEMID Tablets 1622

Sulfinpyrazone (Uricosuric action of gout drugs antagonized). Products include:
- Anturane 807

Thyroxine (Depressed plasma T4 value; competition for protein-binding sites).
- No products indexed under this heading.

Thyroxine Sodium (Depressed plasma T4 value).
- No products indexed under this heading.

Ticarcillin Disodium (Competition for protein-binding sites). Products include:
- Ticar for Injection 2526
- Timentin for Injection 2528

Tolazamide (Hypoglycemic effect enhanced).
- No products indexed under this heading.

Tolbutamide (Hypoglycemic effect enhanced).
- No products indexed under this heading.

Triamcinolone (Competition for protein-binding sites). Products include:
- Aristocort Tablets 1022

Triamcinolone Acetonide (Competition for protein-binding sites). Products include:
- Aristocort A 0.025% Cream 1027
- Aristocort A 0.5% Cream 1031
- Aristocort A 0.1% Cream 1029
- Aristocort A 0.1% Ointment 1030
- Azmacort Oral Inhaler 2011
- Nasacort Nasal Inhaler 2024

Triamcinolone Diacetate (Competition for protein-binding sites). Products include:
- Aristocort Suspension (Forte Parenteral) 1027
- Aristocort Suspension (Intralesional) 1025

Triamcinolone Hexacetonide (Competition for protein-binding sites). Products include:
- Aristospan Suspension (Intra-articular) 1033
- Aristospan Suspension (Intralesional) 1032

l-Triiodothyronine (Competition for protein-binding sites).

Warfarin Sodium (Competition for protein binding predisposes to systemic bleeding). Products include:
- Coumadin 926

Food Interactions

Food that lowers urinary pH (Decreases urinary excretion and increases plasma levels).

Food that raises urinary pH (Increases renal clearance and urinary excretion of salicylic acid).

MONOKET
(Isosorbide Mononitrate) 2406
May interact with vasodilators, calcium channel blockers, and certain other agents. Compounds in these categories include:

Amlodipine Besylate (Combination therapy produces marked symptomatic orthostatic hypotension). Products include:
- Lotrel Capsules 840
- Norvasc Tablets 1940

Bepridil Hydrochloride (Combination therapy produces marked symptomatic orthostatic hypotension). Products include:
- Vascor (200, 300 and 400 mg) Tablets 1587

Diazoxide (Additive vasodilating effects). Products include:
- Hyperstat I.V. Injection 2363
- Proglycem 580

Diltiazem Hydrochloride (Combination therapy produces marked symptomatic orthostatic hypotension). Products include:
- Cardizem CD Capsules 1506
- Cardizem SR Capsules 1510
- Cardizem Injectable 1508
- Cardizem Tablets 1512
- Dilacor XR Extended-release Capsules 2018

Felodipine (Combination therapy produces marked symptomatic orthostatic hypotension). Products include:
- Plendil Extended-Release Tablets 527

Hydralazine Hydrochloride (Additive vasodilating effects). Products include:
- Apresazide Capsules 808
- Apresoline Hydrochloride Tablets 809
- Ser-Ap-Es Tablets 849

Isradipine (Combination therapy produces marked symptomatic orthostatic hypotension). Products include:
- DynaCirc Capsules 2256

Minoxidil (Additive vasodilating effects). Products include:
- Loniten Tablets 2618
- Rogaine Topical Solution 2637

Nicardipine Hydrochloride (Combination therapy produces marked symptomatic orthostatic hypotension). Products include:
- Cardene Capsules 2095
- Cardene I.V. 2709
- Cardene SR Capsules 2097

Nifedipine (Combination therapy produces marked symptomatic orthostatic hypotension). Products include:
- Adalat Capsules (10 mg and 20 mg) 587
- Adalat CC 589
- Procardia Capsules 1971
- Procardia XL Extended Release Tablets 1972

Nimodipine (Combination therapy produces marked symptomatic orthostatic hypotension). Products include:
- Nimotop Capsules 610

Nisoldipine (Combination therapy produces marked symptomatic orthostatic hypotension).
- No products indexed under this heading.

Verapamil Hydrochloride (Combination therapy produces marked symptomatic orthostatic hypotension). Products include:
- Calan SR Caplets 2422
- Calan Tablets 2419
- Isoptin Injectable 1344
- Isoptin Oral Tablets 1346
- Isoptin SR Tablets 1348
- Verelan Capsules 1410
- Verelan Capsules 2824

Food Interactions

Alcohol (Additive vasodilating effects).

MONONINE, COAGULATION FACTOR IX (HUMAN)
(Factor IX (Human)) 523
None cited in PDR database.

MONOPRIL TABLETS
(Fosinopril Sodium) 757
May interact with diuretics, potassium sparing diuretics, potassium preparations, lithium preparations, and certain other agents. Compounds in these categories include:

Aluminum Hydroxide (Antacids may impair absorption of fosinopril). Products include:
- ALternaGEL Liquid 1316
- Maximum Strength Ascriptin .... ▣ 630
- Cama Arthritis Pain Reliever .... ▣ 785
- Gaviscon Extra Strength Relief Formula Antacid Tablets .... ▣ 819
- Gaviscon Extra Strength Relief Formula Liquid Antacid .... ▣ 819
- Gaviscon Liquid Antacid .... ▣ 820
- Gelusil Liquid & Tablets .... ▣ 855
- Maalox Heartburn Relief Suspension .... ▣ 642
- Maalox Heartburn Relief Tablets .... ▣ 641
- Maalox Magnesia and Alumina Oral Suspension .... ▣ 642
- Maalox Plus Tablets .... ▣ 643
- Extra Strength Maalox Antacid Plus Antigas Liquid and Tablets ▣ 638
- Tempo Soft Antacid .... ▣ 835

Aluminum Hydroxide Gel (Antacids may impair absorption of fosinopril). Products include:
- ALternaGEL Liquid .... ▣ 659
- Aludrox Oral Suspension 2695
- Amphojel Suspension 2695
- Amphojel Suspension without Flavor 2695
- Amphojel Tablets 2695
- Arthritis Pain Ascriptin .... ▣ 631
- Regular Strength Ascriptin Tablets .... ▣ 629
- Gaviscon Antacid Tablets .... ▣ 819
- Gaviscon-2 Antacid Tablets .... ▣ 820
- Mylanta Liquid 1317
- Mylanta Tablets .... ▣ 660
- Mylanta Double Strength Liquid 1317
- Mylanta Double Strength Tablets .... ▣ 660
- Nephrox Suspension .... ▣ 655

Amiloride Hydrochloride (Potential for hyperkalemia; potential for excessive reduction in blood pressure after initiation of Monopril therapy). Products include:
- Midamor Tablets 1703
- Moduretic Tablets 1705

Bendroflumethiazide (Potential for excessive reduction in blood pressure after initiation of Monopril therapy).
- No products indexed under this heading.

Bumetanide (Potential for excessive reduction in blood pressure after initiation of Monopril therapy). Products include:
- Bumex 2093

Chlorothiazide (Potential for excessive reduction in blood pressure after initiation of Monopril therapy). Products include:
- Aldoclor Tablets 1598
- Diupres Tablets 1650
- Diuril Oral 1653

Chlorothiazide Sodium (Potential for excessive reduction in blood pressure after initiation of Monopril therapy). Products include:
- Diuril Sodium Intravenous 1652

Chlorthalidone (Potential for excessive reduction in blood pressure after initiation of Monopril therapy). Products include:
- Combipres Tablets 677
- Tenoretic Tablets 2845
- Thalitone 1245

Ethacrynic Acid (Potential for excessive reduction in blood pressure after initiation of Monopril therapy). Products include:
- Edecrin Tablets 1657

Furosemide (Potential for excessive reduction in blood pressure after initiation of Monopril therapy). Products include:
- Lasix Injection, Oral Solution and Tablets 1240

Hydrochlorothiazide (Potential for excessive reduction in blood pressure after initiation of Monopril therapy). Products include:
- Aldactazide 2413
- Aldoril Tablets 1604
- Apresazide Capsules 808
- Capozide 742
- Dyazide 2479
- Esidrix Tablets 821
- Esimil Tablets 822
- HydroDIURIL Tablets 1674
- Hydropres Tablets 1675
- Hyzaar Tablets 1677
- Inderide Tablets 2732
- Inderide LA Long Acting Capsules 2734
- Lopressor HCT Tablets 832
- Lotensin HCT 837
- Maxzide 1380

IMPORTANT NOTE: Always consult each drug listing in the patient's regimen for possible interactions.

Monopril | Interactions Index | 678

Moduretic Tablets ... 1705
Oretic Tablets ... 443
Prinzide Tablets ... 1737
Ser-Ap-Es Tablets ... 849
Timolide Tablets ... 1748
Vaseretic Tablets ... 1765
Zestoretic ... 2850
Ziac ... 1415

Hydroflumethiazide (Potential for excessive reduction in blood pressure after initiation of Monopril therapy). Products include:
Diucardin Tablets ... 2718

Indapamide (Potential for excessive reduction in blood pressure after initiation of Monopril therapy). Products include:
Lozol Tablets ... 2022

Lithium Carbonate (Potential for increased lithium levels and symptoms of lithium toxicity). Products include:
Eskalith ... 2485
Lithium Carbonate Capsules & Tablets ... 2230
Lithonate/Lithotabs/Lithobid ... 2543

Lithium Citrate (Potential for increased lithium levels and symptoms of lithium toxicity).
No products indexed under this heading.

Magaldrate (Antacids may impair absorption of fosinopril).
No products indexed under this heading.

Magnesium Hydroxide (Antacids may impair absorption of fosinopril). Products include:
Aludrox Oral Suspension ... 2695
Arthritis Pain Ascriptin ... ▣ 631
Maximum Strength Ascriptin ... ▣ 630
Regular Strength Ascriptin Tablets ... ▣ 629
Di-Gel Antacid/Anti-Gas ... ▣ 801
Gelusil Liquid & Tablets ... ▣ 855
Maalox Magnesia and Alumina Oral Suspension ... ▣ 642
Maalox Plus Tablets ... ▣ 643
Extra Strength Maalox Antacid Plus Antigas Liquid and Tablets ▣ 638
Mylanta Calcium Carbonate and Magnesium Hydroxide Tablets ... 1318
Mylanta Liquid ... 1317
Mylanta Tablets ... ▣ 660
Mylanta Double Strength Liquid ... 1317
Mylanta Double Strength Tablets .. ▣ 660
Phillips' Milk of Magnesia Liquid ... ▣ 729
Rolaids Tablets ... ▣ 843
Tempo Soft Antacid ... ▣ 835

Magnesium Oxide (Antacids may impair absorption of fosinopril). Products include:
Beelith Tablets ... 639
Bufferin Analgesic Tablets and Caplets ... ▣ 613
Caltrate PLUS ... ▣ 665
Cama Arthritis Pain Reliever ... ▣ 785
Mag-Ox 400 ... 668
Uro-Mag ... 668

Methyclothiazide (Potential for excessive reduction in blood pressure after initiation of Monopril therapy). Products include:
Enduron Tablets ... 420

Metolazone (Potential for excessive reduction in blood pressure after initiation of Monopril therapy). Products include:
Mykrox Tablets ... 993
Zaroxolyn Tablets ... 1000

Polythiazide (Potential for excessive reduction in blood pressure after initiation of Monopril therapy). Products include:
Minizide Capsules ... 1938

Potassium Acid Phosphate (Potential for hyperkalemia). Products include:
K-Phos Original Formula 'Sodium Free' Tablets ... 639

Potassium Bicarbonate (Potential for hyperkalemia). Products include:
Alka-Seltzer Gold Effervescent Antacid ... ▣ 703

Potassium Chloride (Potential for hyperkalemia). Products include:
Chlor-3 Condiment ... 1004
K-Dur Microburst Release System (potassium chloride, USP) E.R. Tablets ... 1325
K-Lor Powder Packets ... 434
K-Norm Extended-Release Capsules ... 991
K-Tab Filmtab ... 434
Kolyum Liquid ... 992
Micro-K ... 2063
Micro-K LS Packets ... 2064
NuLYTELY ... 689
Cherry Flavor NuLYTELY ... 689
Rum-K Syrup ... 1005
Slow-K Extended-Release Tablets ... 851

Potassium Citrate (Potential for hyperkalemia). Products include:
Polycitra Syrup ... 578
Polycitra-K Crystals ... 579
Polycitra-K Oral Solution ... 579
Polycitra-LC ... 578

Potassium Gluconate (Potential for hyperkalemia). Products include:
Kolyum Liquid ... 992

Potassium Phosphate, Dibasic (Potential for hyperkalemia).
No products indexed under this heading.

Potassium Phosphate, Monobasic (Potential for hyperkalemia). Products include:
K-Phos Neutral Tablets ... 639
K-Phos Original Formula 'Sodium Free' Tablets ... 639

Simethicone (Antacids may impair absorption of fosinopril). Products include:
Di-Gel Antacid/Anti-Gas ... ▣ 801
Gas-X ... ▣ 786
Gelusil Liquid & Tablets ... ▣ 855
Maalox Anti-Gas Tablets, Regular Strength ... ▣ 640
Maalox Anti-Gas Tablets, Extra Strength ... ▣ 640
Maalox Plus Tablets ... ▣ 643
Extra Strength Maalox Antacid Plus Antigas Liquid and Tablets ▣ 638
Mylanta Gas Relief Tablets-80 mg .. 1318
Maximum Strength Mylanta Gas Relief Tablets-125 mg ... 1318
Mylanta Liquid ... 1317
Mylanta Tablets ... ▣ 660
Mylanta Double Strength Liquid ... 1317
Mylanta Double Strength Tablets .. ▣ 660
Mylicon Infants' Drops ... 1317
Baby Orajel Tooth & Gum Cleanser ... ▣ 652
Phazyme Drops ... ▣ 767
Phazyme ... ▣ 767
Phazyme-125 Chewable Tablets .. ▣ 767
Phazyme-125 Softgels Maximum Strength ... ▣ 767
Tempo Soft Antacid ... ▣ 835
Titralac Plus ... ▣ 672
Tums Anti-gas/Antacid Formula Tablets, Assorted Fruit ... ▣ 827

Spironolactone (Potential for hyperkalemia; potential for excessive reduction in blood pressure after initiation of Monopril therapy). Products include:
Aldactazide ... 2413
Aldactone ... 2414

Torsemide (Potential for excessive reduction in blood pressure after initiation of Monopril therapy). Products include:
Demadex Tablets and Injection ... 686

Triamterene (Potential for hyperkalemia; potential for excessive reduction in blood pressure after initiation of Monopril therapy). Products include:
Dyazide ... 2479
Dyrenium Capsules ... 2481
Maxzide ... 1380

Food Interactions

Food, unspecified (Rate of absorption may be slowed by the presence of food in the GI tract; the extent of absorption is not affected).

MOTOFEN TABLETS

(Atropine Sulfate, Difenoxin Hydrochloride) ... 784

May interact with monoamine oxidase inhibitors, barbiturates, tranquilizers, narcotic analgesics, and certain other agents. Compounds in these categories include:

Alfentanil Hydrochloride (Effects potentiated). Products include:
Alfenta Injection ... 1286

Alprazolam (Effects potentiated). Products include:
Xanax Tablets ... 2649

Aprobarbital (Effects potentiated).
No products indexed under this heading.

Buprenorphine (Effects potentiated). Products include:
Buprenex Injectable ... 2006

Buspirone Hydrochloride (Effects potentiated). Products include:
BuSpar ... 737

Butabarbital (Effects potentiated).
No products indexed under this heading.

Butalbital (Effects potentiated). Products include:
Esgic-plus Tablets ... 1013
Fioricet Tablets ... 2258
Fioricet with Codeine Capsules ... 2260
Fiorinal Capsules ... 2261
Fiorinal with Codeine Capsules ... 2262
Fiorinal Tablets ... 2261
Phrenilin ... 785
Sedapap Tablets 50 mg/650 mg .. 1543

Chlordiazepoxide (Effects potentiated). Products include:
Libritabs Tablets ... 2177
Limbitrol ... 2180

Chlordiazepoxide Hydrochloride (Effects potentiated). Products include:
Librax Capsules ... 2176
Librium Capsules ... 2178
Librium Injectable ... 2179

Chlorpromazine (Effects potentiated). Products include:
Thorazine Suppositories ... 2523

Chlorprothixene (Effects potentiated).
No products indexed under this heading.

Chlorprothixene Hydrochloride (Effects potentiated).
No products indexed under this heading.

Clorazepate Dipotassium (Effects potentiated). Products include:
Tranxene ... 451

Codeine Phosphate (Effects potentiated). Products include:
Actifed with Codeine Cough Syrup.. 1067
Brontex ... 1981
Deconsal C Expectorant Syrup ... 456
Deconsal Pediatric Syrup ... 457
Dimetane-DC Cough Syrup ... 2059
Empirin with Codeine Tablets ... 1093
Fioricet with Codeine Capsules ... 2260
Fiorinal with Codeine Capsules ... 2262
Isoclor Expectorant ... 990
Novahistine DH ... 2462
Novahistine Expectorant ... 2463
Nucofed ... 2051
Phenergan with Codeine ... 2777
Phenergan VC with Codeine ... 2781
Robitussin A-C Syrup ... 2073
Robitussin-DAC Syrup ... 2074
Ryna ... ▣ 841
Soma Compound w/Codeine Tablets ... 2676
Tussi-Organidin NR Liquid and S NR Liquid ... 2677
Tylenol with Codeine ... 1583

Dezocine (Effects potentiated). Products include:
Dalgan Injection ... 538

Diazepam (Effects potentiated). Products include:
Dizac ... 1809
Valium Injectable ... 2182
Valium Tablets ... 2183
Valrelease Capsules ... 2169

Droperidol (Effects potentiated). Products include:
Inapsine Injection ... 1296

Fentanyl (Effects potentiated). Products include:
Duragesic Transdermal System ... 1288

Fentanyl Citrate (Effects potentiated). Products include:
Sublimaze Injection ... 1307

Fluphenazine Decanoate (Effects potentiated). Products include:
Prolixin Decanoate ... 509

Fluphenazine Enanthate (Effects potentiated). Products include:
Prolixin Enanthate ... 509

Fluphenazine Hydrochloride (Effects potentiated). Products include:
Prolixin ... 509

Furazolidone (Concurrent use may precipitate hypertensive crisis). Products include:
Furoxone ... 2046

Haloperidol (Effects potentiated). Products include:
Haldol Injection, Tablets and Concentrate ... 1575

Haloperidol Decanoate (Effects potentiated). Products include:
Haldol Decanoate ... 1577

Hydrocodone Bitartrate (Effects potentiated). Products include:
Anexsia 5/500 Elixir ... 1781
Anexia Tablets ... 1782
Codiclear DH Syrup ... 791
Deconamine CX Cough and Cold Liquid and Tablets ... 1319
Duratuss HD Elixir ... 2565
Hycodan Tablets and Syrup ... 930
Hycomine Compound Tablets ... 932
Hycomine ... 931
Hycotuss Expectorant Syrup ... 933
Hydrocet Capsules ... 782
Lorcet 10/650 ... 1018
Lortab ... 2566
Tussend ... 1783
Tussend Expectorant ... 1785
Vicodin Tablets ... 1356
Vicodin ES Tablets ... 1357
Vicodin Tuss Expectorant ... 1358
Zydone Capsules ... 949

Hydrocodone Polistirex (Effects potentiated). Products include:
Tussionex Pennkinetic Extended-Release Suspension ... 998

Hydroxyzine Hydrochloride (Effects potentiated). Products include:
Atarax Tablets & Syrup ... 2185
Marax Tablets & DF Syrup ... 2200
Vistaril Intramuscular Solution ... 2216

Isocarboxazid (Concurrent use may precipitate hypertensive crisis).
No products indexed under this heading.

Levorphanol Tartrate (Effects potentiated). Products include:
Levo-Dromoran ... 2129

Lorazepam (Effects potentiated). Products include:
Ativan Injection ... 2698
Ativan Tablets ... 2700

Loxapine Hydrochloride (Effects potentiated). Products include:
Loxitane ... 1378

Loxapine Succinate (Effects potentiated). Products include:
Loxitane Capsules ... 1378

Meperidine Hydrochloride (Effects potentiated). Products include:
Demerol ... 2308

(▣ Described in PDR For Nonprescription Drugs) (◉ Described in PDR For Ophthalmology)

Mepergan Injection 2753

Mephobarbital (Effects potentiated). Products include:

Mebaral Tablets 2322

Meprobamate (Effects potentiated). Products include:

Miltown Tablets 2672
PMB 200 and PMB 400 2783

Mesoridazine Besylate (Effects potentiated). Products include:

Serentil 684

Methadone Hydrochloride (Effects potentiated). Products include:

Methadone Hydrochloride Oral Concentrate 2233
Methadone Hydrochloride Oral Solution & Tablets 2235

Molindone Hydrochloride (Effects potentiated). Products include:

Moban Tablets and Concentrate 1048

Morphine Sulfate (Effects potentiated). Products include:

Astramorph/PF Injection, USP (Preservative-Free) 535
Duramorph 962
Infumorph 200 and Infumorph 500 Sterile Solutions 965
MS Contin Tablets 1994
MSIR 1997
Oramorph SR (Morphine Sulfate Sustained Release Tablets) 2236
RMS Suppositories 2657
Roxanol 2243

Opium Alkaloids (Effects potentiated).

No products indexed under this heading.

Oxazepam (Effects potentiated). Products include:

Serax Capsules 2810
Serax Tablets 2810

Oxycodone Hydrochloride (Effects potentiated). Products include:

Percocet Tablets 938
Percodan Tablets 939
Percodan-Demi Tablets 940
Roxicodone Tablets, Oral Solution & Intensol (Oxycodone) 2244
Tylox Capsules 1584

Pentobarbital Sodium (Effects potentiated). Products include:

Nembutal Sodium Capsules 436
Nembutal Sodium Solution 438
Nembutal Sodium Suppositories 440

Perphenazine (Effects potentiated). Products include:

Etrafon 2355
Triavil Tablets 1757
Trilafon 2389

Phenelzine Sulfate (Concurrent use may precipitate hypertensive crisis). Products include:

Nardil 1920

Phenobarbital (Effects potentiated). Products include:

Arco-Lase Plus Tablets 512
Bellergal-S Tablets 2250
Donnatal 2060
Donnatal Extentabs 2061
Donnatal Tablets 2060
Phenobarbital Elixir and Tablets 1469
Quadrinal Tablets 1350

Prazepam (Effects potentiated).

No products indexed under this heading.

Prochlorperazine (Effects potentiated). Products include:

Compazine 2470

Promethazine Hydrochloride (Effects potentiated). Products include:

Mepergan Injection 2753
Phenergan with Codeine 2777
Phenergan with Dextromethorphan 2778
Phenergan Injection 2773
Phenergan Suppositories 2775
Phenergan Syrup 2774
Phenergan Tablets 2775
Phenergan VC 2779
Phenergan VC with Codeine 2781

Propoxyphene Hydrochloride (Effects potentiated). Products include:

Darvon 1435
Wygesic Tablets 2827

Propoxyphene Napsylate (Effects potentiated). Products include:

Darvon-N/Darvocet-N 1433

Secobarbital Sodium (Effects potentiated). Products include:

Seconal Sodium Pulvules 1474

Selegiline Hydrochloride (Concurrent use may precipitate hypertensive crisis). Products include:

Eldepryl Tablets 2550

Sufentanil Citrate (Effects potentiated). Products include:

Sufenta Injection 1309

Thiamylal Sodium (Effects potentiated).

No products indexed under this heading.

Thioridazine Hydrochloride (Effects potentiated). Products include:

Mellaril 2269

Thiothixene (Effects potentiated). Products include:

Navane Capsules and Concentrate 2201
Navane Intramuscular 2202

Tranylcypromine Sulfate (Concurrent use may precipitate hypertensive crisis). Products include:

Parnate Tablets 2503

Trifluoperazine Hydrochloride (Effects potentiated). Products include:

Stelazine 2514

Food Interactions

Alcohol (Effects potentiated).

CHILDREN'S MOTRIN IBUPROFEN ORAL SUSPENSION

(Ibuprofen) 1546

May interact with oral anticoagulants, thiazides, lithium preparations, and certain other agents. Compounds in these categories include:

Aspirin (Yields a net decrease in anti-inflammatory activity with lowered blood levels of the non-aspirin drug in animal studies). Products include:

Alka-Seltzer Effervescent Antacid and Pain Reliever .... ®℗ 701
Alka-Seltzer Extra Strength Effervescent Antacid and Pain Reliever .... ®℗ 703
Alka-Seltzer Lemon Lime Effervescent Antacid and Pain Reliever .... ®℗ 703
Alka-Seltzer Plus Cold Medicine .... ®℗ 705
Alka-Seltzer Plus Cold & Cough Medicine .... ®℗ 708
Alka-Seltzer Plus Night-Time Cold Medicine .... ®℗ 707
Alka Seltzer Plus Sinus Medicine .. ®℗ 707
Arthritis Foundation Safety Coated Aspirin Tablets .... ®℗ 675
Arthritis Pain Ascriptin .... ®℗ 631
Maximum Strength Ascriptin .... ®℗ 630
Regular Strength Ascriptin Tablets .... ®℗ 629
Arthritis Strength BC Powder .... ®℗ 609
BC Cold Powder Multi-Symptom Formula (Cold-Sinus-Allergy) ...... ®℗ 609
BC Cold Powder Non-Drowsy Formula (Cold-Sinus) .... ®℗ 609
BC Powder .... ®℗ 609
Bayer Children's Chewable Aspirin .... ®℗ 711
Genuine Bayer Aspirin Tablets & Caplets .... ®℗ 713
Extra Strength Bayer Arthritis Pain Regimen Formula .... ®℗ 711
Extra Strength Bayer Aspirin Caplets & Tablets .... ®℗ 712
Extended-Release Bayer 8-Hour Aspirin .... ®℗ 712

Extra Strength Bayer Plus Aspirin Caplets .... ®℗ 713
Extra Strength Bayer PM Aspirin .. ®℗ 713
Bayer Enteric Aspirin .... ®℗ 709
Bufferin Analgesic Tablets and Caplets .... ®℗ 613
Arthritis Strength Bufferin Analgesic Caplets .... ®℗ 614
Extra Strength Bufferin Analgesic Tablets .... ®℗ 615
Cama Arthritis Pain Reliever .... ®℗ 785
Darvon Compound-65 Pulvules 1435
Easprin 1914
Ecotrin 2455
Ecotrin Enteric Coated Aspirin Maximum Strength Tablets and Caplets .... ®℗ 816
Ecotrin Enteric Coated Aspirin Regular Strength Tablets 2455
Empirin Aspirin Tablets .... ®℗ 854
Empirin with Codeine Tablets 1093
Excedrin Extra-Strength Analgesic Tablets & Caplets 732
Fiorinal Capsules 2261
Fiorinal with Codeine Capsules 2262
Fiorinal Tablets 2261
Halfprin 1362
Healthprin Aspirin 2455
Norgesic 1496
Percodan Tablets 939
Percodan-Demi Tablets 940
Robaxisal Tablets 2071
Soma Compound w/Codeine Tablets 2676
Soma Compound Tablets 2675
St. Joseph Adult Chewable Aspirin (81 mg.) .... ®℗ 808
Talwin Compound 2335
Ursinus Inlay-Tabs .... ®℗ 794
Vanquish Analgesic Caplets .... ®℗ 731

Bendroflumethiazide (Reduced natriuretic effect).

No products indexed under this heading.

Chlorothiazide (Reduced natriuretic effect). Products include:

Aldoclor Tablets 1598
Diupres Tablets 1650
Diuril Oral 1653

Chlorothiazide Sodium (Reduced natriuretic effect). Products include:

Diuril Sodium Intravenous 1652

Dicumarol (Potential for excessive bleeding).

No products indexed under this heading.

Furosemide (Reduced natriuretic effect). Products include:

Lasix Injection, Oral Solution and Tablets 1240

Hydrochlorothiazide (Reduced natriuretic effect). Products include:

Aldactazide 2413
Aldoril Tablets 1604
Apresazide Capsules 808
Capozide 742
Dyazide 2479
Esidrix Tablets 821
Esimil Tablets 822
HydroDIURIL Tablets 1674
Hydropres Tablets 1675
Hyzaar Tablets 1677
Inderide Tablets 2732
Inderide LA Long Acting Capsules .. 2734
Lopressor HCT Tablets 832
Lotensin HCT 837
Maxzide 1380
Moduretic Tablets 1705
Oretic Tablets 443
Prinzide Tablets 1737
Ser-Ap-Es Tablets 849
Timolide Tablets 1748
Vaseretic Tablets 1765
Zestoretic 2850
Ziac 1415

Hydroflumethiazide (Reduced natriuretic effect). Products include:

Diucardin Tablets 2718

Lithium Carbonate (Reduced renal lithium clearance and elevation of plasma lithium levels). Products include:

Eskalith 2485
Lithium Carbonate Capsules & Tablets 2230

Lithonate/Lithotabs/Lithobid 2543

Lithium Citrate (Reduced renal lithium clearance and elevation of plasma lithium levels).

No products indexed under this heading.

Methotrexate Sodium (Enhanced toxicity of methotrexate). Products include:

Methotrexate Sodium Tablets, Injection, for Injection and LPF Injection 1275

Methyclothiazide (Reduced natriuretic effect). Products include:

Enduron Tablets 420

Polythiazide (Reduced natriuretic effect). Products include:

Minizide Capsules 1938

Warfarin Sodium (Potential for excessive bleeding). Products include:

Coumadin 926

Food Interactions

Food, unspecified (The peak levels are somewhat lower (up to 30%) and the time to reach peak levels is slightly prolonged (up to 30 min.) although the extent of absorption is unchanged).

MOTRIN TABLETS

(Ibuprofen) 2625

May interact with oral anticoagulants, thiazides, and certain other agents. Compounds in these categories include:

Aspirin (May yield a net decrease in anti-inflammatory activity with lowered blood levels of the non-aspirin drug based on animal studies). Products include:

Alka-Seltzer Effervescent Antacid and Pain Reliever .... ®℗ 701
Alka-Seltzer Extra Strength Effervescent Antacid and Pain Reliever .... ®℗ 703
Alka-Seltzer Lemon Lime Effervescent Antacid and Pain Reliever .... ®℗ 703
Alka-Seltzer Plus Cold Medicine .... ®℗ 705
Alka-Seltzer Plus Cold & Cough Medicine .... ®℗ 708
Alka-Seltzer Plus Night-Time Cold Medicine .... ®℗ 707
Alka Seltzer Plus Sinus Medicine .. ®℗ 707
Arthritis Foundation Safety Coated Aspirin Tablets .... ®℗ 675
Arthritis Pain Ascriptin .... ®℗ 631
Maximum Strength Ascriptin .... ®℗ 630
Regular Strength Ascriptin Tablets .... ®℗ 629
Arthritis Strength BC Powder .... ®℗ 609
BC Cold Powder Multi-Symptom Formula (Cold-Sinus-Allergy) ...... ®℗ 609
BC Cold Powder Non-Drowsy Formula (Cold-Sinus) .... ®℗ 609
BC Powder .... ®℗ 609
Bayer Children's Chewable Aspirin .... ®℗ 711
Genuine Bayer Aspirin Tablets & Caplets .... ®℗ 713
Extra Strength Bayer Arthritis Pain Regimen Formula .... ®℗ 711
Extra Strength Bayer Aspirin Caplets & Tablets .... ®℗ 712
Extended-Release Bayer 8-Hour Aspirin .... ®℗ 712
Extra Strength Bayer Plus Aspirin Caplets .... ®℗ 713
Extra Strength Bayer PM Aspirin .. ®℗ 713
Bayer Enteric Aspirin .... ®℗ 709
Bufferin Analgesic Tablets and Caplets .... ®℗ 613
Arthritis Strength Bufferin Analgesic Caplets .... ®℗ 614
Extra Strength Bufferin Analgesic Tablets .... ®℗ 615
Cama Arthritis Pain Reliever .... ®℗ 785
Darvon Compound-65 Pulvules 1435
Easprin 1914
Ecotrin 2455
Ecotrin Enteric Coated Aspirin Maximum Strength Tablets and Caplets .... ®℗ 816

IMPORTANT NOTE: Always consult each drug listing in the patient's regimen for possible interactions.

Motrin **Interactions Index** **680**

- Ecotrin Enteric Coated Aspirin Regular Strength Tablets 2455
- Empirin Aspirin Tablets ▣ 854
- Empirin with Codeine Tablets 1093
- Excedrin Extra-Strength Analgesic Tablets & Caplets 732
- Fiorinal Capsules 2261
- Fiorinal with Codeine Capsules 2262
- Fiorinal Tablets 2261
- Halfprin 1362
- Healthprin Aspirin 2455
- Norgesic 1496
- Percodan Tablets 939
- Percodan-Demi Tablets 940
- Robaxisal Tablets 2071
- Soma Compound w/Codeine Tablets 2676
- Soma Compound Tablets 2675
- St. Joseph Adult Chewable Aspirin (81 mg.) ▣ 808
- Talwin Compound 2335
- Ursinus Inlay-Tabs ▣ 794
- Vanquish Analgesic Caplets ▣ 731

Bendroflumethiazide (Reduced natriuretic effects).
- No products indexed under this heading.

Chlorothiazide (Reduced natriuretic effects). Products include:
- Aldoclor Tablets 1598
- Diupres Tablets 1650
- Diuril Oral 1653

Chlorothiazide Sodium (Reduced natriuretic effects). Products include:
- Diuril Sodium Intravenous 1652

Dicumarol (Concurrent administration may cause bleeding).
- No products indexed under this heading.

Furosemide (Reduced natriuretic effects). Products include:
- Lasix Injection, Oral Solution and Tablets 1240

Hydrochlorothiazide (Reduced natriuretic effects). Products include:
- Aldactazide 2413
- Aldoril Tablets 1604
- Apresazide Capsules 808
- Capozide 742
- Dyazide 2479
- Esidrix Tablets 821
- Esimil Tablets 822
- HydroDIURIL Tablets 1674
- Hydropres Tablets 1675
- Hyzaar Tablets 1677
- Inderide Tablets 2732
- Inderide LA Long Acting Capsules 2734
- Lopressor HCT Tablets 832
- Lotensin HCT 837
- Maxzide 1380
- Moduretic Tablets 1705
- Oretic Tablets 443
- Prinzide Tablets 1737
- Ser-Ap-Es Tablets 849
- Timolide Tablets 1748
- Vaseretic Tablets 1765
- Zestoretic 2850
- Ziac 1415

Hydroflumethiazide (Reduced natriuretic effects). Products include:
- Diucardin Tablets 2718

Lithium Carbonate (Possible elevation of lithium serum levels and reduction in renal lithium clearance). Products include:
- Eskalith 2485
- Lithium Carbonate Capsules & Tablets 2230
- Lithonate/Lithotabs/Lithobid 2543

Lithium Citrate (Possible elevation of lithium serum levels and reduction in renal lithium clearance).
- No products indexed under this heading.

Methotrexate Sodium (Enhanced methotrexate toxicity). Products include:
- Methotrexate Sodium Tablets, Injection, for Injection and LPF Injection 1275

Methyclothiazide (Reduced natriuretic effects). Products include:
- Enduron Tablets 420

Polythiazide (Reduced natriuretic effects). Products include:
- Minizide Capsules 1938

Warfarin Sodium (Concurrent administration may cause bleeding). Products include:
- Coumadin 926

Food Interactions

Food, unspecified (A reduction in the rate of absorption but no appreciable decrease in the extent of absorption).

MOTRIN IB CAPLETS, TABLETS, AND GELTABS

(Ibuprofen) ▣ 838

May interact with aspirin and acetaminophen containing products. Compounds in this category include:

Acetaminophen (Concurrent use is not recommended except under a doctor's direction). Products include:
- Actifed Plus Caplets ▣ 845
- Actifed Plus Tablets ▣ 845
- Actifed Sinus Daytime/Nighttime Tablets and Caplets ▣ 846
- Alka-Seltzer Plus Cold Medicine Liqui-Gels ▣ 706
- Alka-Seltzer Plus Cold & Cough Medicine Liqui-Gels ▣ 705
- Alka-Seltzer Plus Night-Time Cold Medicine Liqui-Gels ▣ 706
- Allerest Headache Strength Tablets ▣ 627
- Allerest No Drowsiness Tablets ▣ 627
- Allerest Sinus Pain Formula ▣ 627
- Anexsia 5/500 Elixir 1781
- Anexia Tablets 1782
- Arthritis Foundation Aspirin Free Caplets ▣ 673
- Arthritis Foundation NightTime Caplets ▣ 674
- Bayer Select Headache Pain Relief Formula ▣ 716
- Bayer Select Menstrual Multi-Symptom Formula ▣ 716
- Bayer Select Night Time Pain Relief Formula ▣ 716
- Bayer Select Sinus Pain Relief Formula ▣ 717
- Benadryl Allergy Sinus Headache Formula Caplets ▣ 849
- Comtrex Multi-Symptom Cold Reliever Tablets/Caplets/Liqui-Gels/Liquid ▣ 615
- Allergy-Sinus Comtrex Multi-Symptom Allergy-Sinus Formula Tablets ▣ 617
- Comtrex Non-Drowsy ▣ 618
- Contac Day Allergy/Sinus Caplets ▣ 812
- Contac Day & Night ▣ 812
- Contac Night Allergy/Sinus Caplets ▣ 812
- Contac Severe Cold and Flu Formula Caplets ▣ 814
- Contac Severe Cold & Flu Non-Drowsy ▣ 815
- Coricidin 'D' Decongestant Tablets ▣ 800
- Coricidin Tablets ▣ 800
- DHCplus Capsules 1993
- Darvon-N/Darvocet-N 1433
- Drixoral Cold and Flu Extended-Release Tablets ▣ 803
- Drixoral Cough + Sore Throat Liquid Caps ▣ 802
- Drixoral Allergy/Sinus Extended Release Tablets ▣ 804
- Esgic-plus Tablets 1013
- Aspirin Free Excedrin Analgesic Caplets and Geltabs 732
- Excedrin Extra-Strength Analgesic Tablets & Caplets 732
- Excedrin P.M. Analgesic/Sleeping Aid Tablets, Caplets, Liquigels 733
- Fioricet Tablets 2258
- Fioricet with Codeine Capsules 2260
- Hycomine Compound Tablets 932
- Hydrocet Capsules 782
- Legatrin PM ▣ 651
- Lorcet 10/650 1018
- Lortab 2566
- Lurline PMS Tablets 982
- Maximum Strength Multi-Symptom Formula Midol ▣ 722
- PMS Multi-Symptom Formula Midol ▣ 723
- Teen Multi-Symptom Formula Midol ▣ 722
- Midrin Capsules 783
- Migralam Capsules 2038
- Panadol Tablets and Caplets ▣ 824
- Children's Panadol Chewable Tablets, Liquid, Infant's Drops ▣ 824
- Percocet Tablets 938
- Percogesic Analgesic Tablets ▣ 754
- Phrenilin 785
- Pyrroxate Caplets ▣ 772
- Sedapap Tablets 50 mg/650 mg 1543
- Sinarest Tablets ▣ 648
- Sinarest Extra Strength Tablets ▣ 648
- Sinarest No Drowsiness Tablets ▣ 648
- Sine-Aid Maximum Strength Sinus Medication Gelcaps, Caplets and Tablets 1554
- Sine-Off No Drowsiness Formula Caplets ▣ 824
- Sine-Off Sinus Medicine ▣ 825
- Singlet Tablets ▣ 825
- Sinulin Tablets 787
- Sinutab Sinus Allergy Medication, Maximum Strength Tablets and Caplets ▣ 860
- Sinutab Sinus Medication, Maximum Strength Without Drowsiness Formula, Tablets & Caplets ▣ 860
- Sinutab Sinus Medication, Regular Strength Without Drowsiness Formula ▣ 859
- Sudafed Cold and Cough Liquidcaps ▣ 862
- Sudafed Severe Cold Formula Caplets ▣ 863
- Sudafed Severe Cold Formula Tablets ▣ 864
- Sudafed Sinus Caplets ▣ 864
- Sudafed Sinus Tablets ▣ 864
- Talacen 2333
- TheraFlu ▣ 787
- TheraFlu Maximum Strength Nighttime Flu, Cold & Cough Medicine ▣ 788
- TheraFlu Maximum Strength Non-Drowsy Formula Flu, Cold & Cough Medicine ▣ 788
- Thera Flu Maximum Strength, Non-Drowsy Formula Flu, Cold and Cough Caplets ▣ 789
- Triaminic Sore Throat Formula ▣ 791
- Triaminicin Tablets ▣ 793
- Children's TYLENOL acetaminophen Chewable Tablets, Elixir, Suspension Liquid 1555
- Children's TYLENOL Cold Multi-Symptom Liquid Formula and Chewable Tablets 1561
- Children's TYLENOL Cold Plus Cough Multi Symptom Tablets and Liquid ▣ 681
- Infants' TYLENOL acetaminophen Drops and Suspension Drops 1555
- Infants' TYLENOL Cold Decongestant & Fever-Reducer Drops 1556
- TYLENOL Extended Relief Caplets 1558
- TYLENOL, Extra Strength, Acetaminophen Adult Liquid Pain Reliever 1560
- TYLENOL, Extra Strength, acetaminophen Gelcaps, Geltabs, Caplets, Tablets 1559
- TYLENOL, Extra Strength, Headache Plus Pain Reliever with Antacid Caplets 1559
- TYLENOL, Junior Strength, acetaminophen Coated Caplets, Grape and Fruit Chewable Tablets 1557
- TYLENOL Maximum Strength Allergy Sinus Medication Gelcaps and Caplets 1563
- TYLENOL Maximum Strength Allergy Sinus NightTime Medication Caplets 1555
- TYLENOL Flu Maximum Strength Gelcaps 1565
- TYLENOL Flu NightTime, Maximum Strength, Gelcaps 1566
- TYLENOL Maximum Strength Flu NightTime Hot Medication Packets 1562
- TYLENOL, Maximum Strength, Sinus Medication Geltabs, Gelcaps, Caplets and Tablets 1566
- TYLENOL Cold Multi-Symptom Formula Medication Tablets and Caplets 1561
- TYLENOL Cold Medication No Drowsiness Formula Gelcaps and Caplets 1562
- TYLENOL Cold Multi-Symptom Hot Medication Liquid Packets 1557
- TYLENOL Cough Multi-Symptom Medication 1564
- TYLENOL Cough Multi-Symptom Medication with Decongestant 1565
- TYLENOL, Regular Strength, acetaminophen Caplets and Tablets 1558
- TYLENOL PM, Extra Strength Pain Reliever/Sleep Aid Caplets, Geltabs, Gelcaps 1560
- TYLENOL Severe Allergy Medication Caplets 1564
- Tylenol with Codeine 1583
- Tylox Capsules 1584
- Unisom With Pain Relief-Nighttime Sleep Aid and Pain Reliever 1934
- Vanquish Analgesic Caplets ▣ 731
- Vicks 44 LiquiCaps Cough, Cold & Flu Relief ▣ 755
- Vicks 44M Cough, Cold & Flu Relief ▣ 756
- Vicks DayQuil ▣ 761
- Vicks Nyquil Hot Therapy ▣ 762
- Vicks NyQuil LiquiCaps Multi-Symptom Cold/Flu Relief ▣ 763
- Vicks NyQuil Multi-Symptom Cold/Flu Relief - (Original & Cherry Flavor) ▣ 763
- Vicodin Tablets 1356
- Vicodin ES Tablets 1357
- Wygesic Tablets 2827
- Zydone Capsules 949

Aspirin (Concurrent use is not recommended except under a doctor's direction). Products include:
- Alka-Seltzer Effervescent Antacid and Pain Reliever ▣ 701
- Alka-Seltzer Extra Strength Effervescent Antacid and Pain Reliever ▣ 703
- Alka-Seltzer Lemon Lime Effervescent Antacid and Pain Reliever ▣ 703
- Alka-Seltzer Plus Cold Medicine ▣ 705
- Alka-Seltzer Plus Cold & Cough Medicine ▣ 708
- Alka-Seltzer Plus Night-Time Cold Medicine ▣ 707
- Alka Seltzer Plus Sinus Medicine ▣ 707
- Arthritis Foundation Safety Coated Aspirin Tablets ▣ 675
- Arthritis Pain Ascriptin ▣ 631
- Maximum Strength Ascriptin ▣ 630
- Regular Strength Ascriptin Tablets ▣ 629
- Arthritis Strength BC Powder ▣ 609
- BC Cold Powder Multi-Symptom Formula (Cold-Sinus-Allergy) ▣ 609
- BC Cold Powder Non-Drowsy Formula (Cold-Sinus) ▣ 609
- BC Powder ▣ 609
- Bayer Children's Chewable Aspirin ▣ 711
- Genuine Bayer Aspirin Tablets & Caplets ▣ 713
- Extra Strength Bayer Arthritis Pain Regimen Formula ▣ 711
- Extra Strength Bayer Aspirin Caplets & Tablets ▣ 712
- Extended-Release Bayer 8-Hour Aspirin ▣ 712
- Extra Strength Bayer Plus Aspirin Caplets ▣ 713
- Extra Strength Bayer PM Aspirin ▣ 713
- Bayer Enteric Aspirin ▣ 709
- Bufferin Analgesic Tablets and Caplets ▣ 613
- Arthritis Strength Bufferin Analgesic Caplets ▣ 614
- Extra Strength Bufferin Analgesic Tablets ▣ 615
- Cama Arthritis Pain Reliever ▣ 785
- Darvon Compound-65 Pulvules 1435
- Easprin 1914
- Ecotrin 2455
- Ecotrin Enteric Coated Aspirin Maximum Strength Tablets and Caplets ▣ 816
- Ecotrin Enteric Coated Aspirin Regular Strength Tablets 2455
- Empirin Aspirin Tablets ▣ 854
- Empirin with Codeine Tablets 1093
- Excedrin Extra-Strength Analgesic Tablets & Caplets 732

(▣ Described in PDR For Nonprescription Drugs) (◉ Described in PDR For Ophthalmology)

Fiorinal Capsules 2261
Fiorinal with Codeine Capsules 2262
Fiorinal Tablets 2261
Halfprin 1362
Healthprin Aspirin 2455
Norgesic.. 1496
Percodan Tablets 939
Percodan-Demi Tablets 940
Robaxisal Tablets.. 2071
Soma Compound w/Codeine Tablets 2676
Soma Compound Tablets 2675
St. Joseph Adult Chewable Aspirin (81 mg.) .... ⊕ 808
Talwin Compound 2335
Ursinus Inlay-Tabs..................................... ⊕ 794
Vanquish Analgesic Caplets .... ⊕ 731

MOTRIN IB SINUS

(Ibuprofen, Pseudoephedrine Hydrochloride)... ⊕ 838

May interact with antidepressant drugs and antihypertensives. Compounds in these categories include:

Acebutolol Hydrochloride (Concurrent use is recommended under doctor's directions). Products include:

Sectral Capsules 2807

Amitriptyline Hydrochloride (Concurrent use is recommended under doctor's directions). Products include:

Elavil 2838
Endep Tablets 2174
Etrafon 2355
Limbitrol 2180
Triavil Tablets 1757

Amlodipine Besylate (Concurrent use is recommended under doctor's directions). Products include:

Lotrel Capsules 840
Norvasc Tablets 1940

Amoxapine (Concurrent use is recommended under doctor's directions). Products include:

Asendin Tablets 1369

Atenolol (Concurrent use is recommended under doctor's directions). Products include:

Tenoretic Tablets 2845
Tenormin Tablets and I.V. Injection 2847

Benazepril Hydrochloride (Concurrent use is recommended under doctor's directions). Products include:

Lotensin Tablets....................................... 834
Lotensin HCT... 837
Lotrel Capsules 840

Bendroflumethiazide (Concurrent use is recommended under doctor's directions).

No products indexed under this heading.

Betaxolol Hydrochloride (Concurrent use is recommended under doctor's directions). Products include:

Betoptic Ophthalmic Solution............ 469
Betoptic S Ophthalmic Suspension 471
Kerlone Tablets.. 2436

Bisoprolol Fumarate (Concurrent use is recommended under doctor's directions). Products include:

Zebeta Tablets 1413
Ziac 1415

Bupropion Hydrochloride (Concurrent use is recommended under doctor's directions). Products include:

Wellbutrin Tablets 1204

Captopril (Concurrent use is recommended under doctor's directions). Products include:

Capoten 739
Capozide 742

Carteolol Hydrochloride (Concurrent use is recommended under doctor's directions). Products include:

Cartrol Tablets 410
Ocupress Ophthalmic Solution, 1% Sterile.. ⊙ 309

Chlorothiazide (Concurrent use is recommended under doctor's directions). Products include:

Aldoclor Tablets 1598
Diupres Tablets 1650
Diuril Oral 1653

Chlorothiazide Sodium (Concurrent use is recommended under doctor's directions). Products include:

Diuril Sodium Intravenous 1652

Chlorthalidone (Concurrent use is recommended under doctor's directions). Products include:

Combipres Tablets 677
Tenoretic Tablets...................................... 2845
Thalitone 1245

Clonidine (Concurrent use is recommended under doctor's directions). Products include:

Catapres-TTS... 675

Clonidine Hydrochloride (Concurrent use is recommended under doctor's directions). Products include:

Catapres Tablets 674
Combipres Tablets 677

Deserpidine (Concurrent use is recommended under doctor's directions).

No products indexed under this heading.

Desipramine Hydrochloride (Concurrent use is recommended under doctor's directions). Products include:

Norpramin Tablets 1526

Diazoxide (Concurrent use is recommended under doctor's directions). Products include:

Hyperstat I.V. Injection 2363
Proglycem 580

Diltiazem Hydrochloride (Concurrent use is recommended under doctor's directions). Products include:

Cardizem CD Capsules 1506
Cardizem SR Capsules 1510
Cardizem Injectable 1508
Cardizem Tablets..................................... 1512
Dilacor XR Extended-release Capsules 2018

Doxazosin Mesylate (Concurrent use is recommended under doctor's directions). Products include:

Cardura Tablets 2186

Doxepin Hydrochloride (Concurrent use is recommended under doctor's directions). Products include:

Sinequan 2205
Zonalon Cream 1055

Enalapril Maleate (Concurrent use is recommended under doctor's directions). Products include:

Vaseretic Tablets 1765
Vasotec Tablets 1771

Enalaprilat (Concurrent use is recommended under doctor's directions). Products include:

Vasotec I.V.. 1768

Esmolol Hydrochloride (Concurrent use is recommended under doctor's directions). Products include:

Brevibloc Injection................................... 1808

Felodipine (Concurrent use is recommended under doctor's directions). Products include:

Plendil Extended-Release Tablets..... 527

Fluoxetine Hydrochloride (Concurrent use is recommended under doctor's directions). Products include:

Prozac Pulvules & Liquid, Oral Solution 919

Fosinopril Sodium (Concurrent use is recommended under doctor's directions). Products include:

Monopril Tablets 757

Furosemide (Concurrent use is recommended under doctor's directions). Products include:

Lasix Injection, Oral Solution and Tablets 1240

Guanabenz Acetate (Concurrent use is recommended under doctor's directions).

No products indexed under this heading.

Guanethidine Monosulfate (Concurrent use is recommended under doctor's directions). Products include:

Esimil Tablets 822
Ismelin Tablets 827

Hydralazine Hydrochloride (Concurrent use is recommended under doctor's directions). Products include:

Apresazide Capsules 808
Apresoline Hydrochloride Tablets .. 809
Ser-Ap-Es Tablets 849

Hydrochlorothiazide (Concurrent use is recommended under doctor's directions). Products include:

Aldactazide.. 2413
Aldoril Tablets.. 1604
Apresazide Capsules 808
Capozide 742
Dyazide 2479
Esidrix Tablets 821
Esimil Tablets 822
HydroDIURIL Tablets 1674
Hydropres Tablets.................................... 1675
Hyzaar Tablets 1677
Inderide Tablets 2732
Inderide LA Long Acting Capsules .. 2734
Lopressor HCT Tablets 832
Lotensin HCT... 837
Maxzide 1380
Moduretic Tablets 1705
Oretic Tablets 443
Prinzide Tablets 1737
Ser-Ap-Es Tablets 849
Timolide Tablets....................................... 1748
Vaseretic Tablets 1765
Zestoretic 2850
Ziac 1415

Hydroflumethiazide (Concurrent use is recommended under doctor's directions). Products include:

Diucardin Tablets..................................... 2718

Imipramine Hydrochloride (Concurrent use is recommended under doctor's directions). Products include:

Tofranil Ampuls 854
Tofranil Tablets 856

Imipramine Pamoate (Concurrent use is recommended under doctor's directions). Products include:

Tofranil-PM Capsules............................. 857

Indapamide (Concurrent use is recommended under doctor's directions). Products include:

Lozol Tablets 2022

Isocarboxazid (Concurrent use is recommended under doctor's directions).

No products indexed under this heading.

Isradipine (Concurrent use is recommended under doctor's directions). Products include:

DynaCirc Capsules 2256

Labetalol Hydrochloride (Concurrent use is recommended under doctor's directions). Products include:

Normodyne Injection 2377
Normodyne Tablets 2379
Trandate 1185

Levobunolol Hydrochloride (Concurrent use is recommended under doctor's directions). Products include:

Betagan .... ⊙ 233

Lisinopril (Concurrent use is recommended under doctor's directions). Products include:

Prinivil Tablets 1733
Prinzide Tablets 1737
Zestoretic 2850
Zestril Tablets 2854

Losartan Potassium (Concurrent use is recommended under doctor's directions). Products include:

Cozaar Tablets 1628
Hyzaar Tablets 1677

Maprotiline Hydrochloride (Concurrent use is recommended under doctor's directions). Products include:

Ludiomil Tablets...................................... 843

Mecamylamine Hydrochloride (Concurrent use is recommended under doctor's directions). Products include:

Inversine Tablets 1686

Methyclothiazide (Concurrent use is recommended under doctor's directions). Products include:

Enduron Tablets....................................... 420

Methyldopa (Concurrent use is recommended under doctor's directions). Products include:

Aldoclor Tablets 1598
Aldomet Oral 1600
Aldoril Tablets.. 1604

Methyldopate Hydrochloride (Concurrent use is recommended under doctor's directions). Products include:

Aldomet Ester HCl Injection 1602

Metipranolol Hydrochloride (Concurrent use is recommended under doctor's directions). Products include:

OptiPranolol (Metipranolol 0.3%) Sterile Ophthalmic Solution.......... ⊙ 258

Metolazone (Concurrent use is recommended under doctor's directions). Products include:

Mykrox Tablets.. 993
Zaroxolyn Tablets 1000

Metoprolol Succinate (Concurrent use is recommended under doctor's directions). Products include:

Toprol-XL Tablets 565

Metoprolol Tartrate (Concurrent use is recommended under doctor's directions). Products include:

Lopressor Ampuls 830
Lopressor HCT Tablets 832
Lopressor Tablets 830

Metyrosine (Concurrent use is recommended under doctor's directions). Products include:

Demser Capsules 1649

Minoxidil (Concurrent use is recommended under doctor's directions). Products include:

Loniten Tablets 2618
Rogaine Topical Solution 2637

Moexipril Hydrochloride (Concurrent use is recommended under doctor's directions). Products include:

Univasc Tablets 2410

Nadolol (Concurrent use is recommended under doctor's directions).

No products indexed under this heading.

IMPORTANT NOTE: Always consult each drug listing in the patient's regimen for possible interactions.

Nefazodone Hydrochloride (Concurrent use is recommended under doctor's directions). Products include:
- Serzone Tablets ... 771

Nicardipine Hydrochloride (Concurrent use is recommended under doctor's directions). Products include:
- Cardene Capsules ... 2095
- Cardene I.V. ... 2709
- Cardene SR Capsules ... 2097

Nifedipine (Concurrent use is recommended under doctor's directions). Products include:
- Adalat Capsules (10 mg and 20 mg) ... 587
- Adalat CC ... 589
- Procardia Capsules ... 1971
- Procardia XL Extended Release Tablets ... 1972

Nisoldipine (Concurrent use is recommended under doctor's directions).
- No products indexed under this heading.

Nitroglycerin (Concurrent use is recommended under doctor's directions). Products include:
- Deponit NTG Transdermal Delivery System ... 2397
- Nitro-Bid IV ... 1523
- Nitro-Bid Ointment ... 1524
- Nitrodisc ... 2047
- Nitro-Dur (nitroglycerin) Transdermal Infusion System ... 1326
- Nitrolingual Spray ... 2027
- Nitrostat Tablets ... 1925
- Transderm-Nitro Transdermal Therapeutic System ... 859

Nortriptyline Hydrochloride (Concurrent use is recommended under doctor's directions). Products include:
- Pamelor ... 2280

Paroxetine Hydrochloride (Concurrent use is recommended under doctor's directions). Products include:
- Paxil Tablets ... 2505

Penbutolol Sulfate (Concurrent use is recommended under doctor's directions). Products include:
- Levatol ... 2403

Phenelzine Sulfate (Concurrent use is recommended under doctor's directions). Products include:
- Nardil ... 1920

Phenoxybenzamine Hydrochloride (Concurrent use is recommended under doctor's directions). Products include:
- Dibenzyline Capsules ... 2476

Phentolamine Mesylate (Concurrent use is recommended under doctor's directions). Products include:
- Regitine ... 846

Pindolol (Concurrent use is recommended under doctor's directions). Products include:
- Visken Tablets ... 2299

Polythiazide (Concurrent use is recommended under doctor's directions). Products include:
- Minizide Capsules ... 1938

Prazosin Hydrochloride (Concurrent use is recommended under doctor's directions). Products include:
- Minipress Capsules ... 1937
- Minizide Capsules ... 1938

Propranolol Hydrochloride (Concurrent use is recommended under doctor's directions). Products include:
- Inderal ... 2728
- Inderal LA Long Acting Capsules ... 2730
- Inderide Tablets ... 2732
- Inderide LA Long Acting Capsules ... 2734

Protriptyline Hydrochloride (Concurrent use is recommended under doctor's directions). Products include:
- Vivactil Tablets ... 1774

Quinapril Hydrochloride (Concurrent use is recommended under doctor's directions). Products include:
- Accupril Tablets ... 1893

Ramipril (Concurrent use is recommended under doctor's directions). Products include:
- Altace Capsules ... 1232

Rauwolfia Serpentina (Concurrent use is recommended under doctor's directions).
- No products indexed under this heading.

Rescinnamine (Concurrent use is recommended under doctor's directions).
- No products indexed under this heading.

Reserpine (Concurrent use is recommended under doctor's directions). Products include:
- Diupres Tablets ... 1650
- Hydropres Tablets ... 1675
- Ser-Ap-Es Tablets ... 849

Sertraline Hydrochloride (Concurrent use is recommended under doctor's directions). Products include:
- Zoloft Tablets ... 2217

Sodium Nitroprusside (Concurrent use is recommended under doctor's directions).
- No products indexed under this heading.

Sotalol Hydrochloride (Concurrent use is recommended under doctor's directions). Products include:
- Betapace Tablets ... 641

Spirapril Hydrochloride (Concurrent use is recommended under doctor's directions).
- No products indexed under this heading.

Terazosin Hydrochloride (Concurrent use is recommended under doctor's directions). Products include:
- Hytrin Capsules ... 430

Timolol Maleate (Concurrent use is recommended under doctor's directions). Products include:
- Blocadren Tablets ... 1614
- Timolide Tablets ... 1748
- Timoptic in Ocudose ... 1753
- Timoptic Sterile Ophthalmic Solution ... 1751
- Timoptic-XE ... 1755

Torsemide (Concurrent use is recommended under doctor's directions). Products include:
- Demadex Tablets and Injection ... 686

Tranylcypromine Sulfate (Concurrent use is recommended under doctor's directions). Products include:
- Parnate Tablets ... 2503

Trazodone Hydrochloride (Concurrent use is recommended under doctor's directions). Products include:
- Desyrel and Desyrel Dividose ... 503

Trimethaphan Camsylate (Concurrent use is recommended under doctor's directions). Products include:
- Arfonad Ampuls ... 2080

Trimipramine Maleate (Concurrent use is recommended under doctor's directions). Products include:
- Surmontil Capsules ... 2811

Venlafaxine Hydrochloride (Concurrent use is recommended under doctor's directions). Products include:
- Effexor ... 2719

Verapamil Hydrochloride (Concurrent use is recommended under doctor's directions). Products include:
- Calan SR Caplets ... 2422
- Calan Tablets ... 2419
- Isoptin Injectable ... 1344
- Isoptin Oral Tablets ... 1346
- Isoptin SR Tablets ... 1348
- Verelan Capsules ... 1410
- Verelan Capsules ... 2824

MOTRIN IBUPROFEN SUSPENSION, ORAL DROPS, CHEWABLE TABLETS, CAPLETS

(Ibuprofen) ... 1546

May interact with oral anticoagulants, ACE inhibitors, thiazides, lithium preparations, and certain other agents. Compounds in these categories include:

Aspirin (Yields a net decrease in anti-inflammatory activity with lowered blood levels of non-aspirin drug in animal studies). Products include:
- Alka-Seltzer Effervescent Antacid and Pain Reliever ... ■ 701
- Alka-Seltzer Extra Strength Effervescent Antacid and Pain Reliever ... ■ 703
- Alka-Seltzer Lemon Lime Effervescent Antacid and Pain Reliever ... ■ 703
- Alka-Seltzer Plus Cold Medicine ... ■ 705
- Alka-Seltzer Plus Cold & Cough Medicine ... ■ 708
- Alka-Seltzer Plus Night-Time Cold Medicine ... ■ 707
- Alka Seltzer Plus Sinus Medicine ... ■ 707
- Arthritis Foundation Safety Coated Aspirin Tablets ... ■ 675
- Arthritis Pain Ascriptin ... ■ 631
- Maximum Strength Ascriptin ... ■ 630
- Regular Strength Ascriptin Tablets ... ■ 629
- Arthritis Strength BC Powder ... ■ 609
- BC Cold Powder Multi-Symptom Formula (Cold-Sinus-Allergy) ... ■ 609
- BC Cold Powder Non-Drowsy Formula (Cold-Sinus) ... ■ 609
- BC Powder ... ■ 609
- Bayer Children's Chewable Aspirin ... ■ 711
- Genuine Bayer Aspirin Tablets & Caplets ... ■ 713
- Extra Strength Bayer Arthritis Pain Regimen Formula ... ■ 711
- Extra Strength Bayer Aspirin Caplets & Tablets ... ■ 712
- Extended-Release Bayer 8-Hour Aspirin ... ■ 712
- Extra Strength Bayer Plus Aspirin Caplets ... ■ 713
- Extra Strength Bayer PM Aspirin ... ■ 713
- Bayer Enteric Aspirin ... ■ 709
- Bufferin Analgesic Tablets and Caplets ... ■ 613
- Arthritis Strength Bufferin Analgesic Caplets ... ■ 614
- Extra Strength Bufferin Analgesic Tablets ... ■ 615
- Cama Arthritis Pain Reliever ... ■ 785
- Darvon Compound-65 Pulvules ... 1435
- Easprin ... 1914
- Ecotrin ... 2455
- Ecotrin Enteric Coated Aspirin Maximum Strength Tablets and Caplets ... ■ 816
- Ecotrin Enteric Coated Aspirin Regular Strength Tablets ... 2455
- Empirin Aspirin Tablets ... ■ 854
- Empirin with Codeine Tablets ... 1093
- Excedrin Extra-Strength Analgesic Tablets & Caplets ... 732
- Fiorinal Capsules ... 2261
- Fiorinal with Codeine Capsules ... 2262
- Fiorinal Tablets ... 2261
- Halfprin ... 1362
- Healthprin Aspirin ... 2455
- Norgesic ... 1496
- Percodan Tablets ... 939
- Percodan-Demi Tablets ... 940
- Robaxisal Tablets ... 2071
- Soma Compound w/Codeine Tablets ... 2676
- Soma Compound Tablets ... 2675
- St. Joseph Adult Chewable Aspirin (81 mg.) ... ■ 808
- Talwin Compound ... 2335
- Ursinus Inlay-Tabs ... ■ 794
- Vanquish Analgesic Caplets ... ■ 731

Benazepril Hydrochloride (Ibuprofen may diminish the antihypertensive effect). Products include:
- Lotensin Tablets ... 834
- Lotensin HCT ... 837
- Lotrel Capsules ... 840

Bendroflumethiazide (Ibuprofen can reduce the natriuretic effect of thiazide diuretics in some patients).
- No products indexed under this heading.

Captopril (Ibuprofen may diminish the antihypertensive effect). Products include:
- Capoten ... 739
- Capozide ... 742

Chlorothiazide (Ibuprofen can reduce the natriuretic effect of thiazide diuretics in some patients). Products include:
- Aldoclor Tablets ... 1598
- Diupres Tablets ... 1650
- Diuril Oral ... 1653

Chlorothiazide Sodium (Ibuprofen can reduce the natriuretic effect of thiazide diuretics in some patients). Products include:
- Diuril Sodium Intravenous ... 1652

Dicumarol (Concurrent use may result in bleeding).
- No products indexed under this heading.

Enalapril Maleate (Ibuprofen may diminish the antihypertensive effect). Products include:
- Vaseretic Tablets ... 1765
- Vasotec Tablets ... 1771

Enalaprilat (Ibuprofen may diminish the antihypertensive effect). Products include:
- Vasotec I.V. ... 1768

Fosinopril Sodium (Ibuprofen may diminish the antihypertensive effect). Products include:
- Monopril Tablets ... 757

Furosemide (Ibuprofen can reduce the natriurectic effect furosemide). Products include:
- Lasix Injection, Oral Solution and Tablets ... 1240

Hydrochlorothiazide (Ibuprofen can reduce the natriuretic effect of thiazide diuretics in some patients). Products include:
- Aldactazide ... 2413
- Aldoril Tablets ... 1604
- Apresazide Capsules ... 808
- Capozide ... 742
- Dyazide ... 2479
- Esidrix Tablets ... 821
- Esimil Tablets ... 822
- HydroDIURIL Tablets ... 1674
- Hydropres Tablets ... 1675
- Hyzaar Tablets ... 1677
- Inderide Tablets ... 2732
- Inderide LA Long Acting Capsules ... 2734
- Lopressor HCT Tablets ... 832
- Lotensin HCT ... 837
- Maxzide ... 1380
- Moduretic Tablets ... 1705
- Oretic Tablets ... 443
- Prinzide Tablets ... 1737
- Ser-Ap-Es Tablets ... 849
- Timolide Tablets ... 1748
- Vaseretic Tablets ... 1765
- Zestoretic ... 2850
- Ziac ... 1415

Hydroflumethiazide (Ibuprofen can reduce the natriuretic effect of thiazide diuretics in some patients). Products include:
- Diucardin Tablets ... 2718

(■ Described in PDR For Nonprescription Drugs) (⊙ Described in PDR For Ophthalmology)

Lisinopril (Ibuprofen may diminish the antihypertensive effect). Products include:
- Prinivil Tablets ... 1733
- Prinzide Tablets ... 1737
- Zestoretic ... 2850
- Zestril Tablets ... 2854

Lithium Carbonate (Ibuprofen can produce an elevation of plasma lithium levels and a reduction in renal lithium clearance). Products include:
- Eskalith ... 2485
- Lithium Carbonate Capsules & Tablets ... 2230
- Lithonate/Lithotabs/Lithobid ... 2543

Lithium Citrate (Ibuprofen can produce an elevation of plasma lithium levels and a reduction in renal lithium clearance).
- No products indexed under this heading.

Methotrexate Sodium (Potential for enhanced methotrexate toxicity possibly resulting from competitively inhibiting methotrexate accumulation). Products include:
- Methotrexate Sodium Tablets, Injection, for Injection and LPF Injection ... 1275

Methyclothiazide (Ibuprofen can reduce the natriuretic effect of thiazide diuretics in some patients). Products include:
- Enduron Tablets ... 420

Moexipril Hydrochloride (Ibuprofen may diminish the antihypertensive effect). Products include:
- Univasc Tablets ... 2410

Polythiazide (Ibuprofen can reduce the natriuretic effect of thiazide diuretics in some patients). Products include:
- Minizide Capsules ... 1938

Quinapril Hydrochloride (Ibuprofen may diminish the antihypertensive effect). Products include:
- Accupril Tablets ... 1893

Ramipril (Ibuprofen may diminish the antihypertensive effect). Products include:
- Altace Capsules ... 1232

Spirapril Hydrochloride (Ibuprofen may diminish the antihypertensive effect).
- No products indexed under this heading.

Warfarin Sodium (Concurrent use may result in bleeding). Products include:
- Coumadin ... 926

Food Interactions

Food, unspecified (Food affects the rate but not the extent of absorption; T_{max} is delayed by approximately 30 to 60 minutes and peak levels are reduced by approximately 30 to 50%).

MSTA MUMPS SKIN TEST ANTIGEN
(Mumps Skin Test Antigen) ... 890
None cited in PDR database.

MUMPSVAX
(Mumps Virus Vaccine, Live) ... 1708
May interact with immunosuppressive agents. Compounds in this category include:

Azathioprine (Concurrent administration is containdicated). Products include:
- Imuran ... 1110

Cyclosporine (Concurrent administration is containdicated). Products include:
- Neoral ... 2276
- Sandimmune ... 2286

Immune Globulin (Human) (Concurrent administration is containdicated).
- No products indexed under this heading.

Immune Globulin Intravenous (Human) (Concurrent administration is containdicated).

Muromonab-CD3 (Concurrent administration is containdicated). Products include:
- Orthoclone OKT3 Sterile Solution ... 1837

Mycophenolate Mofetil (Concurrent administration is containdicated). Products include:
- CellCept Capsules ... 2099

Tacrolimus (Concurrent administration is containdicated). Products include:
- Prograf ... 1042

MURINE EAR DROPS
(Carbamide Peroxide) ... ▣ 780
None cited in PDR database.

MURINE EAR WAX REMOVAL SYSTEM
(Carbamide Peroxide) ... ▣ 780
None cited in PDR database.

MURINE TEARS LUBRICANT EYE DROPS
(Polyvinyl Alcohol, Povidone) ... ⊙ 316
None cited in PDR database.

MURINE TEARS PLUS LUBRICANT REDNESS RELIEVER EYE DROPS
(Polyvinyl Alcohol, Povidone, Tetrahydrozoline Hydrochloride) ... ⊙ 316
None cited in PDR database.

MURO 128 OPHTHALMIC OINTMENT
(Sodium Chloride) ... ⊙ 258
None cited in PDR database.

MURO 128 SOLUTION 2% AND 5%
(Sodium Chloride) ... ⊙ 258
None cited in PDR database.

MUSTARGEN
(Mechlorethamine Hydrochloride) ... 1709
May interact with antineoplastics. Compounds in this category include:

Altretamine (Hematopoiesis may be further compromised in patients who have been previously treated with chemotherapeutic agents). Products include:
- Hexalen Capsules ... 2571

Asparaginase (Hematopoiesis may be further compromised in patients who have been previously treated with chemotherapeutic agents). Products include:
- Elspar ... 1659

Bleomycin Sulfate (Hematopoiesis may be further compromised in patients who have been previously treated with chemotherapeutic agents). Products include:
- Blenoxane ... 692

Busulfan (Hematopoiesis may be further compromised in patients who have been previously treated with chemotherapeutic agents). Products include:
- Myleran Tablets ... 1143

Carboplatin (Hematopoiesis may be further compromised in patients who have been previously treated with chemotherapeutic agents). Products include:
- Paraplatin for Injection ... 705

Carmustine (BCNU) (Hematopoiesis may be further compromised in patients who have been previously treated with chemotherapeutic agents). Products include:
- BiCNU ... 691

Chlorambucil (Hematopoiesis may be further compromised in patients who have been previously treated with chemotherapeutic agents). Products include:
- Leukeran Tablets ... 1133

Cisplatin (Hematopoiesis may be further compromised in patients who have been previously treated with chemotherapeutic agents). Products include:
- Platinol ... 708
- Platinol-AQ Injection ... 710

Cyclophosphamide (Hematopoiesis may be further compromised in patients who have been previously treated with chemotherapeutic agents). Products include:
- Cytoxan ... 694
- NEOSAR Lyophilized/Neosar ... 1959

Dacarbazine (Hematopoiesis may be further compromised in patients who have been previously treated with chemotherapeutic agents). Products include:
- DTIC-Dome ... 600

Daunorubicin Hydrochloride (Hematopoiesis may be further compromised in patients who have been previously treated with chemotherapeutic agents). Products include:
- Cerubidine ... 795

Doxorubicin Hydrochloride (Hematopoiesis may be further compromised in patients who have been previously treated with chemotherapeutic agents). Products include:
- Adriamycin PFS ... 1947
- Adriamycin RDF ... 1947
- Doxorubicin Astra ... 540
- Rubex ... 712

Estramustine Phosphate Sodium (Hematopoiesis may be further compromised in patients who have been previously treated with chemotherapeutic agents). Products include:
- Emcyt Capsules ... 1953

Etoposide (Hematopoiesis may be further compromised in patients who have been previously treated with chemotherapeutic agents). Products include:
- VePesid Capsules and Injection ... 718

Floxuridine (Hematopoiesis may be further compromised in patients who have been previously treated with chemotherapeutic agents). Products include:
- Sterile FUDR ... 2118

Fluorouracil (Hematopoiesis may be further compromised in patients who have been previously treated with chemotherapeutic agents). Products include:
- Efudex ... 2113
- Fluoroplex Topical Solution & Cream 1% ... 479
- Fluorouracil Injection ... 2116

Flutamide (Hematopoiesis may be further compromised in patients who have been previously treated with chemotherapeutic agents). Products include:
- Eulexin Capsules ... 2358

Hydroxyurea (Hematopoiesis may be further compromised in patients who have been previously treated with chemotherapeutic agents). Products include:
- Hydrea Capsules ... 696

Idarubicin Hydrochloride (Hematopoiesis may be further compromised in patients who have been previously treated with chemotherapeutic agents). Products include:
- Idamycin ... 1955

Ifosfamide (Hematopoiesis may be further compromised in patients who have been previously treated with chemotherapeutic agents). Products include:
- IFEX ... 697

Interferon alfa-2A, Recombinant (Hematopoiesis may be further compromised in patients who have been previously treated with chemotherapeutic agents). Products include:
- Roferon-A Injection ... 2145

Interferon alfa-2B, Recombinant (Hematopoiesis may be further compromised in patients who have been previously treated with chemotherapeutic agents). Products include:
- Intron A ... 2364

Levamisole Hydrochloride (Hematopoiesis may be further compromised in patients who have been previously treated with chemotherapeutic agents). Products include:
- Ergamisol Tablets ... 1292

Lomustine (CCNU) (Hematopoiesis may be further compromised in patients who have been previously treated with chemotherapeutic agents). Products include:
- CeeNU ... 693

Megestrol Acetate (Hematopoiesis may be further compromised in patients who have been previously treated with chemotherapeutic agents). Products include:
- Megace Oral Suspension ... 699
- Megace Tablets ... 701

Melphalan (Hematopoiesis may be further compromised in patients who have been previously treated with chemotherapeutic agents). Products include:
- Alkeran Tablets ... 1071

Mercaptopurine (Hematopoiesis may be further compromised in patients who have been previously treated with chemotherapeutic agents). Products include:
- Purinethol Tablets ... 1156

Methotrexate Sodium (Hematopoiesis may be further compromised in patients who have been previously treated with chemotherapeutic agents). Products include:
- Methotrexate Sodium Tablets, Injection, for Injection and LPF Injection ... 1275

Mitomycin (Mitomycin-C) (Hematopoiesis may be further compromised in patients who have been previously treated with chemotherapeutic agents). Products include:
- Mutamycin ... 703

Mitotane (Hematopoiesis may be further compromised in patients who have been previously treated with chemotherapeutic agents). Products include:
- Lysodren ... 698

Mitoxantrone Hydrochloride (Hematopoiesis may be further compromised in patients who have been previously treated with chemotherapeutic agents). Products include:
- Novantrone ... 1279

IMPORTANT NOTE: Always consult each drug listing in the patient's regimen for possible interactions.

Mustargen

Paclitaxel (Hematopoiesis may be further compromised in patients who have been previously treated with chemotherapeutic agents). Products include:

Taxol 714

Procarbazine Hydrochloride (Hematopoiesis may be further compromised in patients who have been previously treated with chemotherapeutic agents). Products include:

Matulane Capsules 2131

Streptozocin (Hematopoiesis may be further compromised in patients who have been previously treated with chemotherapeutic agents). Products include:

Zanosar Sterile Powder 2653

Tamoxifen Citrate (Hematopoiesis may be further compromised in patients who have been previously treated with chemotherapeutic agents). Products include:

Nolvadex Tablets 2841

Teniposide (Hematopoiesis may be further compromised in patients who have been previously treated with chemotherapeutic agents). Products include:

Vumon 727

Thioguanine (Hematopoiesis may be further compromised in patients who have been previously treated with chemotherapeutic agents). Products include:

Thioguanine Tablets, Tabloid Brand 1181

Thiotepa (Hematopoiesis may be further compromised in patients who have been previously treated with chemotherapeutic agents). Products include:

Thioplex (Thiotepa For Injection) 1281

Vincristine Sulfate (Hematopoiesis may be further compromised in patients who have been previously treated with chemotherapeutic agents). Products include:

Oncovin Solution Vials & Hyporets 1466

Vinorelbine Tartrate (Hematopoiesis may be further compromised in patients who have been previously treated with chemotherapeutic agents). Products include:

Navelbine Injection 1145

MUTAMYCIN

(Mitomycin (Mitomycin-C))................... 703 May interact with antineoplastics, cytotoxic drugs, nitrogen-mustard-type alkylating agents, and certain other agents. Compounds in these categories include:

Altretamine (Adult respiratory distress syndrome). Products include:

Hexalen Capsules 2571

Asparaginase (Adult respiratory distress syndrome). Products include:

Elspar 1659

Bleomycin Sulfate (Hemolytic uremic syndrome; adult respiratory distress syndrome). Products include:

Blenoxane 692

Busulfan (Adult respiratory distress syndrome). Products include:

Myleran Tablets 1143

Carboplatin (Adult respiratory distress syndrome). Products include:

Paraplatin for Injection 705

Carmustine (BCNU) (Adult respiratory distress syndrome). Products include:

BiCNU 691

Chlorambucil (Adult respiratory distress syndrome). Products include:

Leukeran Tablets 1133

Cisplatin (Adult respiratory distress syndrome). Products include:

Platinol 708

Platinol-AQ Injection 710

Cyclophosphamide (Adult respiratory distress syndrome). Products include:

Cytoxan 694

NEOSAR Lyophilized/Neosar 1959

Dacarbazine (Hemolytic uremic syndrome; adult respiratory distress syndrome). Products include:

DTIC-Dome 600

Daunorubicin Hydrochloride (Hemolytic uremic syndrome; adult respiratory distress syndrome). Products include:

Cerubidine 795

Doxorubicin Hydrochloride (Hemolytic uremic syndrome; adult respiratory distress syndrome). Products include:

Adriamycin PFS 1947

Adriamycin RDF 1947

Doxorubicin Astra 540

Rubex 712

Estramustine Phosphate Sodium (Adult respiratory distress syndrome). Products include:

Emcyt Capsules 1953

Etoposide (Adult respiratory distress syndrome). Products include:

VePesid Capsules and Injection....... 718

Floxuridine (Adult respiratory distress syndrome). Products include:

Sterile FUDR 2118

Fluorouracil (Hemolytic uremic syndrome; adult respiratory distress syndrome). Products include:

Efudex 2113

Fluoroplex Topical Solution & Cream 1% 479

Fluorouracil Injection 2116

Flutamide (Adult respiratory distress syndrome). Products include:

Eulexin Capsules 2358

Hydroxyurea (Hemolytic uremic syndrome; adult respiratory distress syndrome). Products include:

Hydrea Capsules 696

Idarubicin Hydrochloride (Adult respiratory distress syndrome). Products include:

Idamycin 1955

Ifosfamide (Adult respiratory distress syndrome). Products include:

IFEX 697

Interferon alfa-2A, Recombinant (Adult respiratory distress syndrome). Products include:

Roferon-A Injection 2145

Interferon alfa-2B, Recombinant (Adult respiratory distress syndrome). Products include:

Intron A 2364

Levamisole Hydrochloride (Adult respiratory distress syndrome). Products include:

Ergamisol Tablets 1292

Lomustine (CCNU) (Adult respiratory distress syndrome). Products include:

CeeNU 693

Mechlorethamine Hydrochloride (Adult respiratory distress syndrome). Products include:

Mustargen... 1709

Megestrol Acetate (Adult respiratory distress syndrome). Products include:

Megace Oral Suspension 699

Megace Tablets 701

Melphalan (Adult respiratory distress syndrome). Products include:

Alkeran Tablets................................... 1071

Mercaptopurine (Adult respiratory distress syndrome). Products include:

Purinethol Tablets 1156

Methotrexate Sodium (Hemolytic uremic syndrome; adult respiratory distress syndrome). Products include:

Methotrexate Sodium Tablets, Injection, for Injection and LPF Injection 1275

Mitotane (Hemolytic uremic syndrome; adult respiratory distress syndrome). Products include:

Lysodren 698

Mitoxantrone Hydrochloride (Hemolytic uremic syndrome; adult respiratory distress syndrome). Products include:

Novantrone.. 1279

Paclitaxel (Adult respiratory distress syndrome). Products include:

Taxol 714

Procarbazine Hydrochloride (Hemolytic uremic syndrome; adult respiratory distress syndrome). Products include:

Matulane Capsules 2131

Streptozocin (Adult respiratory distress syndrome). Products include:

Zanosar Sterile Powder 2653

Tamoxifen Citrate (Hemolytic uremic syndrome; adult respiratory distress syndrome). Products include:

Nolvadex Tablets 2841

Teniposide (Adult respiratory distress syndrome). Products include:

Vumon 727

Thioguanine (Adult respiratory distress syndrome). Products include:

Thioguanine Tablets, Tabloid Brand 1181

Thiotepa (Adult respiratory distress syndrome). Products include:

Thioplex (Thiotepa For Injection) 1281

Vinblastine Sulfate (Acute shortness of breath; severe bronchospasm). Products include:

Velban Vials 1484

Vincristine Sulfate (Hemolytic uremic syndrome; adult respiratory distress syndrome). Products include:

Oncovin Solution Vials & Hyporets 1466

Vinorelbine Tartrate (Adult respiratory distress syndrome). Products include:

Navelbine Injection 1145

MYADEC TABLETS

(Vitamins with Minerals) ....ᴿᴰ 857 None cited in PDR database.

MYAMBUTOL TABLETS

(Ethambutol Hydrochloride)................1386 None cited in PDR database.

MYCELEX OTC CREAM ANTIFUNGAL

(Clotrimazole) ....ᴿᴰ 724 None cited in PDR database.

MYCELEX OTC SOLUTION ANTIFUNGAL

(Clotrimazole) ....ᴿᴰ 724 None cited in PDR database.

MYCELEX TROCHES

(Clotrimazole)...................................... 608 None cited in PDR database.

MYCELEX-7 VAGINAL CREAM ANTIFUNGAL

(Clotrimazole) ....ᴿᴰ 724 None cited in PDR database.

MYCELEX-7 VAGINAL INSERTS ANTIFUNGAL

(Clotrimazole) ....ᴿᴰ 725 None cited in PDR database.

MYCELEX-7 COMBINATION-PACK VAGINAL INSERTS & EXTERNAL VULVAR CREAM

(Clotrimazole) ....ᴿᴰ 725 None cited in PDR database.

MYCELEX-G 500 MG VAGINAL TABLETS

(Clotrimazole)...................................... 609 None cited in PDR database.

MYCITRACIN PLUS PAIN RELIEVER

(Bacitracin, Neomycin Sulfate, Lidocaine, Polymyxin B Sulfate) ......ᴿᴰ 839 None cited in PDR database.

MAXIMUM STRENGTH MYCITRACIN TRIPLE ANTIBIOTIC FIRST AID OINTMENT

(Bacitracin, Neomycin Sulfate, Polymyxin B Sulfate) ....ᴿᴰ 839 None cited in PDR database.

MYCOBUTIN CAPSULES

(Rifabutin) ....1957 May interact with narcotic analgesics, oral anticoagulants, corticosteroids, oral contraceptives, oral hypoglycemic agents, cardiac glycosides, barbiturates, beta blockers, progestins, xanthine bronchodilators, anticonvulsants, macrolide antibiotics, and certain other agents. Compounds in these categories include:

Acarbose (Potential for reduced activity of oral hypoglycemic agents through liver enzyme-inducing properties).

No products indexed under this heading.

Acebutolol Hydrochloride (Potential for decreased effects of concurrently administered beta-adrenergic blockers). Products include:

Sectral Capsules 2807

Alfentanil Hydrochloride (Potential for reduced activity of narcotics through liver enzyme-inducing properties). Products include:

Alfenta Injection 1286

Aminophylline (Potential for decreased effects of concurrently administered theophylline).

No products indexed under this heading.

Analgesics, unspecified (Potential for reduced activity of analgesics through liver enzyme-inducing properties).

Aprobarbital (Potential for decreased effects of concurrently administered barbiturates).

No products indexed under this heading.

Atenolol (Potential for decreased effects of concurrently administered beta-adrenergic blockers). Products include:

Tenoretic Tablets.................................. 2845

Tenormin Tablets and I.V. Injection 2847

(ᴿᴰ Described in PDR For Nonprescription Drugs) (◉ Described in PDR For Ophthalmology)

685 **Interactions Index** **Mycobutin**

Azithromycin (Concomitant administration with higher doses of rifabutin results in higher incidence of uveitis). Products include:

Zithromax 1944

Betamethasone Acetate (Potential for reduced activity of corticosteroids through liver enzyme-inducing properties). Products include:

Celestone Soluspan Suspension 2347

Betamethasone Sodium Phosphate (Potential for reduced activity of corticosteroids through liver enzyme-inducing properties). Products include:

Celestone Soluspan Suspension 2347

Betaxolol Hydrochloride (Potential for decreased effects of concurrently administered beta-adrenergic blockers). Products include:

Betoptic Ophthalmic Solution 469
Betoptic S Ophthalmic Suspension 471
Kerlone Tablets 2436

Bisoprolol Fumarate (Potential for decreased effects of concurrently administered beta-adrenergic blockers). Products include:

Zebeta Tablets 1413
Ziac 1415

Buprenorphine (Potential for reduced activity of narcotics through liver enzyme-inducing properties). Products include:

Buprenex Injectable 2006

Butabarbital (Potential for decreased effects of concurrently administered barbiturates).

No products indexed under this heading.

Butalbital (Potential for decreased effects of concurrently administered barbiturates). Products include:

Esgic-plus Tablets 1013
Fioricet Tablets 2258
Fioricet with Codeine Capsules 2260
Fiorinal Capsules 2261
Fiorinal with Codeine Capsules 2262
Fiorinal Tablets 2261
Phrenilin 785
Sedapap Tablets 50 mg/650 mg 1543

Carbamazepine (Potential for decreased effects of concurrently administered anticonvulsants). Products include:

Atretol Tablets 573
Tegretol Chewable Tablets 852
Tegretol Suspension 852
Tegretol Tablets 852

Carteolol Hydrochloride (Potential for decreased effects of concurrently administered beta-adrenergic blockers). Products include:

Cartrol Tablets 410
Ocupress Ophthalmic Solution, 1% Sterile .... ⊙ 309

Chloramphenicol (Potential for decreased effects of concurrently administered chloramphenicol). Products include:

Chloromycetin Ophthalmic Ointment, 1% .... ⊙ 310
Chloromycetin Ophthalmic Solution .... ⊙ 310
Chloroptic S.O.P. .... ⊙ 239
Chloroptic Sterile Ophthalmic Solution .... ⊙ 239
Elase-Chloromycetin Ointment 1040
Ophthocort .... ⊙ 311

Chloramphenicol Palmitate (Potential for decreased effects of concurrently administered chloramphenicol).

No products indexed under this heading.

Chloramphenicol Sodium Succinate (Potential for decreased effects of concurrently administered chloramphenicol). Products include:

Chloromycetin Sodium Succinate 1900

Chlorpropamide (Potential for reduced activity of oral hypoglycemic agents through liver enzyme-inducing properties). Products include:

Diabinese Tablets 1935

Clarithromycin (Concomitant administration with higher doses of rifabutin results in higher incidence of uveitis). Products include:

Biaxin 405

Clofibrate (Potential for decreased effects of concurrently administered clofibrate). Products include:

Atromid-S Capsules 2701

Codeine Phosphate (Potential for reduced activity of narcotics through liver enzyme-inducing properties). Products include:

Actifed with Codeine Cough Syrup 1067
Brontex 1981
Deconsal C Expectorant Syrup 456
Deconsal Pediatric Syrup 457
Dimetane-DC Cough Syrup 2059
Empirin with Codeine Tablets 1093
Fioricet with Codeine Capsules 2260
Fiorinal with Codeine Capsules 2262
Isoclor Expectorant 990
Novahistine DH 2462
Novahistine Expectorant 2463
Nucofed 2051
Phenergan with Codeine 2777
Phenergan VC with Codeine 2781
Robitussin A-C Syrup 2073
Robitussin-DAC Syrup 2074
Ryna .... ●○ 841
Soma Compound w/Codeine Tablets 2676
Tussi-Organidin NR Liquid and S NR Liquid 2677
Tylenol with Codeine 1583

Cortisone Acetate (Potential for reduced activity of corticosteroids through liver enzyme-inducing properties). Products include:

Cortone Acetate Sterile Suspension 1623
Cortone Acetate Tablets 1624

Cyclosporine (Potential for reduced activity of cyclosporine through liver enzyme-inducing properties). Products include:

Neoral 2276
Sandimmune 2286

Dapsone (Potential for reduced activity of dapsone through liver enzyme-inducing properties). Products include:

Dapsone Tablets USP 1284

Deslanoside (Potential for reduced activity of cardiac glycoside agents through liver enzyme-inducing properties).

No products indexed under this heading.

Desogestrel (Potential for reduced activity of oral contraceptives through liver enzyme-inducing properties). Products include:

Desogen Tablets 1817
Ortho-Cept 1851

Dexamethasone (Potential for reduced activity of corticosteroids through liver enzyme-inducing properties). Products include:

AK-Trol Ointment & Suspension .... ⊙ 205
Decadron Elixir 1633
Decadron Tablets 1635
Decaspray Topical Aerosol 1648
Dexacidin Ointment .... ⊙ 263
Maxitrol Ophthalmic Ointment and Suspension .... ⊙ 224
TobraDex Ophthalmic Suspension and Ointment 473

Dexamethasone Acetate (Potential for reduced activity of corticosteroids through liver enzyme-inducing properties). Products include:

Dalalone D.P. Injectable 1011
Decadron-LA Sterile Suspension 1646

Dexamethasone Sodium Phosphate (Potential for reduced activity of corticosteroids through liver enzyme-inducing properties). Products include:

Decadron Phosphate Injection 1637
Decadron Phosphate Respihaler 1642
Decadron Phosphate Sterile Ophthalmic Ointment 1641
Decadron Phosphate Sterile Ophthalmic Solution 1642
Decadron Phosphate Topical Cream 1644
Decadron Phosphate Turbinaire 1645
Decadron Phosphate with Xylocaine Injection, Sterile 1639
Dexacort Phosphate in Respihaler 458
Dexacort Phosphate in Turbinaire 459
NeoDecadron Sterile Ophthalmic Ointment 1712
NeoDecadron Sterile Ophthalmic Solution 1713
NeoDecadron Topical Cream 1714

Dezocine (Potential for reduced activity of narcotics through liver enzyme-inducing properties). Products include:

Dalgan Injection 538

Diazepam (Potential for decreased effects of concurrently administered diazepam). Products include:

Dizac 1809
Valium Injectable 2182
Valium Tablets 2183
Valrelease Capsules 2169

Dicumarol (Potential for reduced activity of anticoagulants through liver enzyme-inducing properties).

No products indexed under this heading.

Digitoxin (Potential for reduced activity of cardiac glycoside agents through liver enzyme-inducing properties). Products include:

Crystodigin Tablets 1433

Digoxin (Potential for reduced activity of cardiac glycoside agents through liver enzyme-inducing properties). Products include:

Lanoxicaps 1117
Lanoxin Elixir Pediatric 1120
Lanoxin Injection 1123
Lanoxin Injection Pediatric 1126
Lanoxin Tablets 1128

Disopyramide Phosphate (Potential for decreased effects of concurrently administered mexiletine). Products include:

Norpace 2444

Divalproex Sodium (Potential for decreased effects of concurrently administered anticonvulsants). Products include:

Depakote Tablets 415

Dyphylline (Potential for decreased effects of concurrently administered theophylline). Products include:

Lufyllin & Lufyllin-400 Tablets 2670
Lufyllin-GG Elixir & Tablets 2671

Erythromycin (Concomitant administration with higher doses of rifabutin results in higher incidence of uveitis). Products include:

A/T/S 2% Acne Topical Gel and Solution 1234
Benzamycin Topical Gel 905
E-Mycin Tablets 1341
Emgel 2% Topical Gel 1093
ERYC 1915
Erycette (erythromycin 2%) Topical Solution 1888
Ery-Tab Tablets 422
Erythromycin Base Filmtab 426
Erythromycin Delayed-Release Capsules, USP 427
Ilotycin Ophthalmic Ointment 912
PCE Dispertab Tablets 444
T-Stat 2.0% Topical Solution and Pads 2688

Theramycin Z Topical Solution 2% 1592

Erythromycin Estolate (Concomitant administration with higher doses of rifabutin results in higher incidence of uveitis). Products include:

Ilosone 911

Erythromycin Ethylsuccinate (Concomitant administration with higher doses of rifabutin results in higher incidence of uveitis). Products include:

E.E.S. 424
EryPed 421

Erythromycin Gluceptate (Concomitant administration with higher doses of rifabutin results in higher incidence of uveitis). Products include:

Ilotycin Gluceptate, IV, Vials 913

Erythromycin Stearate (Concomitant administration with higher doses of rifabutin results in higher incidence of uveitis). Products include:

Erythrocin Stearate Filmtab 425

Esmolol Hydrochloride (Potential for decreased effects of concurrently administered beta-adrenergic blockers). Products include:

Brevibloc Injection 1808

Ethinyl Estradiol (Potential for reduced activity of oral contraceptives through liver enzyme-inducing properties). Products include:

Brevicon 2088
Demulen 2428
Desogen Tablets 1817
Levlen/Tri-Levlen 651
Lo/Ovral Tablets 2746
Lo/Ovral-28 Tablets 2751
Modicon 1872
Nordette-21 Tablets 2755
Nordette-28 Tablets 2758
Norinyl 2088
Ortho-Cept 1851
Ortho-Cyclen/Ortho-Tri-Cyclen 1858
Ortho-Novum 1872
Ortho-Cyclen/Ortho Tri-Cyclen 1858
Ovcon 760
Ovral Tablets 2770
Ovral-28 Tablets 2770
Levlen/Tri-Levlen 651
Tri-Norinyl 2164
Triphasil-21 Tablets 2814
Triphasil-28 Tablets 2819

Ethosuximide (Potential for decreased effects of concurrently administered anticonvulsants). Products include:

Zarontin Capsules 1928
Zarontin Syrup 1929

Ethotoin (Potential for decreased effects of concurrently administered anticonvulsants). Products include:

Peganone Tablets 446

Ethynodiol Diacetate (Potential for reduced activity of oral contraceptives through liver enzyme-inducing properties). Products include:

Demulen 2428

Felbamate (Potential for decreased effects of concurrently administered anticonvulsants). Products include:

Felbatol 2666

Fentanyl (Potential for reduced activity of narcotics through liver enzyme-inducing properties). Products include:

Duragesic Transdermal System 1288

Fentanyl Citrate (Potential for reduced activity of narcotics through liver enzyme-inducing properties). Products include:

Sublimaze Injection 1307

IMPORTANT NOTE: Always consult each drug listing in the patient's regimen for possible interactions.

Mycobutin Interactions Index 686

Fluconazole (Concomitant administration with higher doses of rifabutin results in higher incidence of uveitis). Products include:
Diflucan Injection, Tablets, and Oral Suspension ... 2194

Fludrocortisone Acetate (Potential for reduced activity of corticosteroids through liver enzyme-inducing properties). Products include:
Florinef Acetate Tablets ... 505

Glipizide (Potential for reduced activity of oral hypoglycemic agents through liver enzyme-inducing properties). Products include:
Glucotrol Tablets ... 1967
Glucotrol XL Extended Release Tablets ... 1968

Glyburide (Potential for reduced activity of oral hypoglycemic agents through liver enzyme-inducing properties). Products include:
DiaBeta Tablets ... 1239
Glynase PresTab Tablets ... 2609
Micronase Tablets ... 2623

Hydrocodone Bitartrate (Potential for reduced activity of narcotics through liver enzyme-inducing properties). Products include:
Anexsia 5/500 Elixir ... 1781
Anexia Tablets ... 1782
Codiclear DH Syrup ... 791
Deconamine CX Cough and Cold Liquid and Tablets ... 1319
Duratuss HD Elixir ... 2565
Hycodan Tablets and Syrup ... 930
Hycomine Compound Tablets ... 932
Hycomine ... 931
Hycotuss Expectorant Syrup ... 933
Hydrocet Capsules ... 782
Lorcet 10/650 ... 1018
Lortab ... 2566
Tussend ... 1783
Tussend Expectorant ... 1785
Vicodin Tablets ... 1356
Vicodin ES Tablets ... 1357
Vicodin Tuss Expectorant ... 1358
Zydone Capsules ... 949

Hydrocodone Polistirex (Potential for reduced activity of narcotics through liver enzyme-inducing properties). Products include:
Tussionex Pennkinetic Extended-Release Suspension ... 998

Hydrocortisone (Potential for reduced activity of corticosteroids through liver enzyme-inducing properties). Products include:
Anusol-HC Cream 2.5% ... 1896
Aquanil HC Lotion ... 1931
Bactine Hydrocortisone Anti-Itch Cream ... ▣ 709
Caldecort Anti-Itch Hydrocortisone Spray ... ▣ 631
Cortaid ... ▣ 836
CORTENEMA ... 2535
Cortisporin Ointment ... 1085
Cortisporin Ophthalmic Ointment Sterile ... 1085
Cortisporin Ophthalmic Suspension Sterile ... 1086
Cortisporin Otic Solution Sterile ... 1087
Cortisporin Otic Suspension Sterile ... 1088
Cortizone-5 ... ▣ 831
Cortizone-10 ... ▣ 831
Hydrocortone Tablets ... 1672
Hytone ... 907
Massengill Medicated Soft Cloth Towelettes ... 2458
PediOtic Suspension Sterile ... 1153
Preparation H Hydrocortisone 1% Cream ... ▣ 872
ProctoCream-HC 2.5% ... 2408
VōSoL HC Otic Solution ... 2678

Hydrocortisone Acetate (Potential for reduced activity of corticosteroids through liver enzyme-inducing properties). Products include:
Analpram-HC Rectal Cream 1% and 2.5% ... 977
Anusol HC-1 Anti-Itch Hydrocortisone Ointment ... ▣ 847
Anusol-HC Suppositories ... 1897
Caldecort ... ▣ 631
Carmol HC ... 924
Coly-Mycin S Otic w/Neomycin & Hydrocortisone ... 1906
Cortaid ... ▣ 836
Cortifoam ... 2396
Cortisporin Cream ... 1084
Epifoam ... 2399
Hydrocortone Acetate Sterile Suspension ... 1669
Mantadil Cream ... 1135
Nupercainal Hydrocortisone 1% Cream ... ▣ 645
Ophthocort ... ◉ 311
Pramosone Cream, Lotion & Ointment ... 978
ProctoCream-HC ... 2408
ProctoFoam-HC ... 2409
Terra-Cortril Ophthalmic Suspension ... 2210

Hydrocortisone Sodium Phosphate (Potential for reduced activity of corticosteroids through liver enzyme-inducing properties). Products include:
Hydrocortone Phosphate Injection, Sterile ... 1670

Hydrocortisone Sodium Succinate (Potential for reduced activity of corticosteroids through liver enzyme-inducing properties). Products include:
Solu-Cortef Sterile Powder ... 2641

Ketoconazole (Potential for decreased effects of concurrently administered ketoconazole). Products include:
Nizoral 2% Cream ... 1297
Nizoral 2% Shampoo ... 1298
Nizoral Tablets ... 1298

Labetalol Hydrochloride (Potential for decreased effects of concurrently administered beta-adrenergic blockers). Products include:
Normodyne Injection ... 2377
Normodyne Tablets ... 2379
Trandate ... 1185

Lamotrigine (Potential for decreased effects of concurrently administered anticonvulsants). Products include:
Lamictal Tablets ... 1112

Levobunolol Hydrochloride (Potential for decreased effects of concurrently administered beta-adrenergic blockers). Products include:
Betagan ... ◉ 233

Levonorgestrel (Potential for reduced activity of oral contraceptives through liver enzyme-inducing properties). Products include:
Levlen/Tri-Levlen ... 651
Nordette-21 Tablets ... 2755
Nordette-28 Tablets ... 2758
Norplant System ... 2759
Levlen/Tri-Levlen ... 651
Triphasil-21 Tablets ... 2814
Triphasil-28 Tablets ... 2819

Levorphanol Tartrate (Potential for reduced activity of narcotics through liver enzyme-inducing properties). Products include:
Levo-Dromoran ... 2129

Medroxyprogesterone Acetate (Potential for decreased effects of concurrently administered progestins). Products include:
Amen Tablets ... 780
Cycrin Tablets ... 975
Depo-Provera Contraceptive Injection ... 2602
Depo-Provera Sterile Aqueous Suspension ... 2606
Premphase ... 2797
Prempro ... 2801
Provera Tablets ... 2636

Megestrol Acetate (Potential for decreased effects of concurrently administered progestins). Products include:
Megace Oral Suspension ... 699
Megace Tablets ... 701

Meperidine Hydrochloride (Potential for reduced activity of narcotics through liver enzyme-inducing properties). Products include:
Demerol ... 2308
Mepergan Injection ... 2753

Mephenytoin (Potential for decreased effects of concurrently administered anticonvulsants). Products include:
Mesantoin Tablets ... 2272

Mephobarbital (Potential for decreased effects of concurrently administered barbiturates). Products include:
Mebaral Tablets ... 2322

Mestranol (Potential for reduced activity of oral contraceptives through liver enzyme-inducing properties). Products include:
Norinyl ... 2088
Ortho-Novum ... 1872

Metformin Hydrochloride (Potential for reduced activity of oral hypoglycemic agents through liver enzyme-inducing properties). Products include:
Glucophage ... 752

Methadone Hydrochloride (Potential for reduced activity of methadone—and narcotics—through liver enzyme-inducing properties). Products include:
Methadone Hydrochloride Oral Concentrate ... 2233
Methadone Hydrochloride Oral Solution & Tablets ... 2235

Methsuximide (Potential for decreased effects of concurrently administered anticonvulsants). Products include:
Celontin Kapseals ... 1899

Methylprednisolone Acetate (Potential for reduced activity of corticosteroids through liver enzyme-inducing properties). Products include:
Depo-Medrol Single-Dose Vial ... 2600
Depo-Medrol Sterile Aqueous Suspension ... 2597

Methylprednisolone Sodium Succinate (Potential for reduced activity of corticosteroids through liver enzyme-inducing properties). Products include:
Solu-Medrol Sterile Powder ... 2643

Metipranolol Hydrochloride (Potential for decreased effects of concurrently administered beta-adrenergic blockers). Products include:
OptiPranolol (Metipranolol 0.3%) Sterile Ophthalmic Solution ... ◉ 258

Metoprolol Succinate (Potential for decreased effects of concurrently administered beta-adrenergic blockers). Products include:
Toprol-XL Tablets ... 565

Metoprolol Tartrate (Potential for decreased effects of concurrently administered beta-adrenergic blockers). Products include:
Lopressor Ampuls ... 830
Lopressor HCT Tablets ... 832
Lopressor Tablets ... 830

Morphine Sulfate (Potential for reduced activity of narcotics through liver enzyme-inducing properties). Products include:
Astramorph/PF Injection, USP (Preservative-Free) ... 535
Duramorph ... 962
Infumorph 200 and Infumorph 500 Sterile Solutions ... 965
MS Contin Tablets ... 1994
MSIR ... 1997
Oramorph SR (Morphine Sulfate Sustained Release Tablets) ... 2236
RMS Suppositories ... 2657
Roxanol ... 2243

Nadolol (Potential for decreased effects of concurrently administered beta-adrenergic blockers).
No products indexed under this heading.

Norethindrone (Potential for reduced activity of oral contraceptives through liver enzyme-inducing properties). Products include:
Brevicon ... 2088
Micronor Tablets ... 1872
Modicon ... 1872
Norinyl ... 2088
Nor-Q D Tablets ... 2135
Ortho-Novum ... 1872
Ovcon ... 760
Tri-Norinyl ... 2164

Norethynodrel (Potential for reduced activity of oral contraceptives through liver enzyme-inducing properties).
No products indexed under this heading.

Norgestimate (Potential for reduced activity of oral contraceptives through liver enzyme-inducing properties). Products include:
Ortho-Cyclen/Ortho-Tri-Cyclen ... 1858
Ortho-Cyclen/Ortho Tri-Cyclen ... 1858

Norgestrel (Potential for reduced activity of oral contraceptives through liver enzyme-inducing properties). Products include:
Lo/Ovral Tablets ... 2746
Lo/Ovral-28 Tablets ... 2751
Ovral Tablets ... 2770
Ovral-28 Tablets ... 2770
Ovrette Tablets ... 2771

Opium Alkaloids (Potential for reduced activity of narcotics through liver enzyme-inducing properties).
No products indexed under this heading.

Oxycodone Hydrochloride (Potential for reduced activity of narcotics through liver enzyme-inducing properties). Products include:
Percocet Tablets ... 938
Percodan Tablets ... 939
Percodan-Demi Tablets ... 940
Roxicodone Tablets, Oral Solution & Intensol (Oxycodone) ... 2244
Tylox Capsules ... 1584

Paramethadione (Potential for decreased effects of concurrently administered anticonvulsants).
No products indexed under this heading.

Penbutolol Sulfate (Potential for decreased effects of concurrently administered beta-adrenergic blockers). Products include:
Levatol ... 2403

Pentobarbital Sodium (Potential for decreased effects of concurrently administered barbiturates). Products include:
Nembutal Sodium Capsules ... 436
Nembutal Sodium Solution ... 438
Nembutal Sodium Suppositories ... 440

Phenacemide (Potential for decreased effects of concurrently administered anticonvulsants). Products include:
Phenurone Tablets ... 447

Phenobarbital (Potential for decreased effects of concurrently administered anticonvulsants and barbiturates). Products include:
Arco-Lase Plus Tablets ... 512
Bellergal-S Tablets ... 2250
Donnatal ... 2060
Donnatal Extentabs ... 2061
Donnatal Tablets ... 2060
Phenobarbital Elixir and Tablets ... 1469
Quadrinal Tablets ... 1350

Phensuximide (Potential for decreased effects of concurrently administered anticonvulsants). Products include:
Milontin Kapseals ... 1920

(▣ Described in PDR For Nonprescription Drugs) (◉ Described in PDR For Ophthalmology)

687 **Interactions Index** **Mykrox**

Phenytoin (Potential for decreased effects of concurrently administered anticonvulsants). Products include:
Dilantin Infatabs 1908
Dilantin-125 Suspension 1911

Phenytoin Sodium (Potential for decreased effects of concurrently administered anticonvulsants). Products include:
Dilantin Kapseals 1906
Dilantin Parenteral 1910

Pindolol (Potential for decreased effects of concurrently administered beta-adrenergic blockers). Products include:
Visken Tablets 2299

Prednisolone Acetate (Potential for reduced activity of corticosteroids through liver enzyme-inducing properties). Products include:
AK-CIDE .... ◉ 202
AK-CIDE Ointment .... ◉ 202
Blephamide Liquifilm Sterile Ophthalmic Suspension 476
Blephamide Ointment .... ◉ 237
Econopred & Econopred Plus Ophthalmic Suspensions .... ◉ 217
Poly-Pred Liquifilm .... ◉ 248
Pred Forte .... ◉ 250
Pred Mild .... ◉ 253
Pred-G Liquifilm Sterile Ophthalmic Suspension .... ◉ 251
Pred-G S.O.P. Sterile Ophthalmic Ointment .... ◉ 252
Vasocidin Ointment .... ◉ 268

Prednisolone Sodium Phosphate (Potential for reduced activity of corticosteroids through liver enzyme-inducing properties). Products include:
AK-Pred .... ◉ 204
Hydeltrasol Injection, Sterile 1665
Inflamase .... ◉ 265
Pediapred Oral Liquid 995
Vasocidin Ophthalmic Solution .... ◉ 270

Prednisolone Tebutate (Potential for reduced activity of corticosteroids through liver enzyme-inducing properties). Products include:
Hydeltra-T.B.A. Sterile Suspension 1667

Prednisone (Potential for reduced activity of corticosteroids through liver enzyme-inducing properties). Products include:
Deltasone Tablets 2595

Primidone (Potential for decreased effects of concurrently administered anticonvulsants). Products include:
Mysoline 2754

Propoxyphene Hydrochloride (Potential for reduced activity of narcotics through liver enzyme-inducing properties). Products include:
Darvon 1435
Wygesic Tablets 2827

Propoxyphene Napsylate (Potential for reduced activity of narcotics through liver enzyme-inducing properties). Products include:
Darvon-N/Darvocet-N 1433

Propranolol Hydrochloride (Potential for decreased effects of concurrently administered beta-adrenergic blockers). Products include:
Inderal 2728
Inderal LA Long Acting Capsules 2730
Inderide Tablets 2732
Inderide LA Long Acting Capsules .. 2734

Quinidine Gluconate (Potential for reduced activity of quinidine through liver enzyme-inducing properties). Products include:
Quinaglute Dura-Tabs Tablets 649

Quinidine Polygalacturonate (Potential for reduced activity of quinidine through liver enzyme-inducing properties).
No products indexed under this heading.

Quinidine Sulfate (Potential for reduced activity of quinidine through liver enzyme-inducing properties). Products include:
Quinidex Extentabs 2067

Secobarbital Sodium (Potential for decreased effects of concurrently administered barbiturates). Products include:
Seconal Sodium Pulvules 1474

Sotalol Hydrochloride (Potential for decreased effects of concurrently administered beta-adrenergic blockers). Products include:
Betapace Tablets 641

Sufentanil Citrate (Potential for reduced activity of narcotics through liver enzyme-inducing properties). Products include:
Sufenta Injection 1309

Theophylline (Potential for decreased effects of concurrently administered theophylline). Products include:
Marax Tablets & DF Syrup 2200
Quibron 2053

Theophylline Anhydrous (Potential for decreased effects of concurrently administered theophylline). Products include:
Aerolate 1004
Primatene Dual Action Formula .... ▣ 872
Primatene Tablets .... ▣ 873
Respbid Tablets 682
Slo-bid Gyrocaps 2033
Theo-24 Extended Release Capsules 2568
Theo-Dur Extended-Release Tablets 1327
Theo-X Extended-Release Tablets .. 788
Uni-Dur Extended-Release Tablets .. 1331
Uniphyl 400 mg Tablets 2001

Theophylline Calcium Salicylate (Potential for decreased effects of concurrently administered theophylline). Products include:
Quadrinal Tablets 1350

Theophylline Sodium Glycinate (Potential for decreased effects of concurrently administered theophylline).
No products indexed under this heading.

Thiamylal Sodium (Potential for decreased effects of concurrently administered barbiturates).
No products indexed under this heading.

Timolol Hemihydrate (Potential for decreased effects of concurrently administered beta-adrenergic blockers). Products include:
Betimol 0.25%, 0.5% .... ◉ 261

Timolol Maleate (Potential for decreased effects of concurrently administered beta-adrenergic blockers). Products include:
Blocadren Tablets 1614
Timolide Tablets 1748
Timoptic in Ocudose 1753
Timoptic Sterile Ophthalmic Solution 1751
Timoptic-XE 1755

Tolazamide (Potential for reduced activity of oral hypoglycemic agents through liver enzyme-inducing properties).
No products indexed under this heading.

Tolbutamide (Potential for reduced activity of oral hypoglycemic agents through liver enzyme-inducing properties).
No products indexed under this heading.

Triamcinolone (Potential for reduced activity of corticosteroids through liver enzyme-inducing properties). Products include:
Aristocort Tablets 1022

Triamcinolone Acetonide (Potential for reduced activity of corticosteroids through liver enzyme-inducing properties). Products include:
Aristocort A 0.025% Cream 1027
Aristocort A 0.5% Cream 1031
Aristocort A 0.1% Cream 1029
Aristocort A 0.1% Ointment 1030
Azmacort Oral Inhaler 2011
Nasacort Nasal Inhaler 2024

Triamcinolone Diacetate (Potential for reduced activity of corticosteroids through liver enzyme-inducing properties). Products include:
Aristocort Suspension (Forte Parenteral) 1027
Aristocort Suspension (Intralesional) 1025

Triamcinolone Hexacetonide (Potential for reduced activity of corticosteroids through liver enzyme-inducing properties). Products include:
Aristospan Suspension (Intra-articular) 1033
Aristospan Suspension (Intralesional) 1032

Trimethadione (Potential for decreased effects of concurrently administered anticonvulsants).
No products indexed under this heading.

Troleandomycin (Concomitant administration with higher doses of rifabutin results in higher incidence of uveitis). Products include:
Tao Capsules 2209

Valproic Acid (Potential for decreased effects of concurrently administered anticonvulsants). Products include:
Depakene 413

Verapamil Hydrochloride (Potential for decreased effects of concurrently administered verapamil). Products include:
Calan SR Caplets 2422
Calan Tablets 2419
Isoptin Injectable 1344
Isoptin Oral Tablets 1346
Isoptin SR Tablets 1348
Verelan Capsules 1410
Verelan Capsules 2824

Warfarin Sodium (Potential for reduced activity of anticoagulants through liver enzyme-inducing properties). Products include:
Coumadin 926

Zidovudine (Reduced steady-state plasma levels of zidovudine after repeated Mycobutin dosing). Products include:
Retrovir Capsules 1158
Retrovir I.V. Infusion 1163
Retrovir Syrup 1158

MYCOSTATIN CREAM, TOPICAL POWDER, AND OINTMENT
(Nystatin) 2688
None cited in PDR database.

MYCOSTATIN PASTILLES
(Nystatin) 704
None cited in PDR database.

MYKROX TABLETS
(Metolazone) 993
May interact with lithium preparations, antihypertensives, insulin, barbiturates, narcotic analgesics, loop diuretics, cardiac glycosides, corticosteroids, salicylates, non-steroidal anti-inflammatory agents, oral hypoglycemic agents, and certain other agents. Compounds in these categories include:

Acarbose (Blood glucose concentrations may be raised by metolazone in diabetics).
No products indexed under this heading.

Acebutolol Hydrochloride (Orthostatic hypotension may occur with concurrent therapy). Products include:
Sectral Capsules 2807

ACTH (Potential for increased hypokalemia).
No products indexed under this heading.

Alfentanil Hydrochloride (Potentiates orthostatic hypotensive effects). Products include:
Alfenta Injection 1286

Amlodipine Besylate (Orthostatic hypotension may occur with concurrent therapy). Products include:
Lotrel Capsules 840
Norvasc Tablets 1940

Aprobarbital (Potentiates orthostatic hypotensive effects).
No products indexed under this heading.

Aspirin (Antihypertensive effects of Mykrox may be decreased). Products include:
Alka-Seltzer Effervescent Antacid and Pain Reliever .... ▣ 701
Alka-Seltzer Extra Strength Effervescent Antacid and Pain Reliever .... ▣ 703
Alka-Seltzer Lemon Lime Effervescent Antacid and Pain Reliever .... ▣ 703
Alka-Seltzer Plus Cold Medicine .... ▣ 705
Alka-Seltzer Plus Cold & Cough Medicine .... ▣ 708
Alka-Seltzer Plus Night-Time Cold Medicine .... ▣ 707
Alka Seltzer Plus Sinus Medicine .. ▣ 707
Arthritis Foundation Safety Coated Aspirin Tablets .... ▣ 675
Arthritis Pain Ascriptin .... ▣ 631
Maximum Strength Ascriptin .... ▣ 630
Regular Strength Ascriptin Tablets .... ▣ 629
Arthritis Strength BC Powder .... ▣ 609
BC Cold Powder Multi-Symptom Formula (Cold-Sinus-Allergy) .... ▣ 609
BC Cold Powder Non-Drowsy Formula (Cold-Sinus) .... ▣ 609
BC Powder .... ▣ 609
Bayer Children's Chewable Aspirin .... ▣ 711
Genuine Bayer Aspirin Tablets & Caplets .... ▣ 713
Extra Strength Bayer Arthritis Pain Regimen Formula .... ▣ 711
Extra Strength Bayer Aspirin Caplets & Tablets .... ▣ 712
Extended-Release Bayer 8-Hour Aspirin .... ▣ 712
Extra Strength Bayer Plus Aspirin Caplets .... ▣ 713
Extra Strength Bayer PM Aspirin .. ▣ 713
Bayer Enteric Aspirin .... ▣ 709
Bufferin Analgesic Tablets and Caplets .... ▣ 613
Arthritis Strength Bufferin Analgesic Caplets .... ▣ 614
Extra Strength Bufferin Analgesic Tablets .... ▣ 615
Cama Arthritis Pain Reliever .... ▣ 785
Darvon Compound-65 Pulvules 1435
Easprin 1914
Ecotrin 2455
Ecotrin Enteric Coated Aspirin Maximum Strength Tablets and Caplets .... ▣ 816
Ecotrin Enteric Coated Aspirin Regular Strength Tablets 2455
Empirin Aspirin Tablets .... ▣ 854
Empirin with Codeine Tablets 1093
Excedrin Extra-Strength Analgesic Tablets & Caplets 732
Fiorinal Capsules 2261
Fiorinal with Codeine Capsules 2262
Fiorinal Tablets 2261
Halfprin 1362
Healthprin Aspirin 2455
Norgesic 1496
Percodan Tablets 939
Percodan-Demi Tablets 940
Robaxisal Tablets 2071

IMPORTANT NOTE: Always consult each drug listing in the patient's regimen for possible interactions.

Soma Compound w/Codeine Tablets 2676
Soma Compound Tablets 2675
St. Joseph Adult Chewable Aspirin (81 mg.) .... ▣ 808
Talwin Compound 2335
Ursinus Inlay-Tabs .... ▣ 794
Vanquish Analgesic Caplets .... ▣ 731

Atenolol (Orthostatic hypotension may occur with concurrent therapy). Products include:
Tenoretic Tablets 2845
Tenormin Tablets and I.V. Injection 2847

Benazepril Hydrochloride (Orthostatic hypotension may occur with concurrent therapy). Products include:
Lotensin Tablets 834
Lotensin HCT 837
Lotrel Capsules 840

Bendroflumethiazide (Orthostatic hypotension may occur with concurrent therapy).
No products indexed under this heading.

Betamethasone Acetate (Potential for increased hypokalemia). Products include:
Celestone Soluspan Suspension 2347

Betamethasone Sodium Phosphate (Potential for increased hypokalemia). Products include:
Celestone Soluspan Suspension 2347

Betaxolol Hydrochloride (Orthostatic hypotension may occur with concurrent therapy). Products include:
Betoptic Ophthalmic Solution 469
Betoptic S Ophthalmic Suspension 471
Kerlone Tablets 2436

Bisoprolol Fumarate (Orthostatic hypotension may occur with concurrent therapy). Products include:
Zebeta Tablets 1413
Ziac 1415

Bumetanide (Large or prolonged losses of fluids and electrolytes may result). Products include:
Bumex 2093

Buprenorphine (Potentiates orthostatic hypotensive effects). Products include:
Buprenex Injectable 2006

Butabarbital (Potentiates orthostatic hypotensive effects).
No products indexed under this heading.

Butalbital (Potentiates orthostatic hypotensive effects). Products include:
Esgic-plus Tablets 1013
Fioricet Tablets 2258
Fioricet with Codeine Capsules 2260
Fiorinal Capsules 2261
Fiorinal with Codeine Capsules 2262
Fiorinal Tablets 2261
Phrenilin 785
Sedapap Tablets 50 mg/650 mg .. 1543

Captopril (Orthostatic hypotension may occur with concurrent therapy). Products include:
Capoten 739
Capozide 742

Carteolol Hydrochloride (Orthostatic hypotension may occur with concurrent therapy). Products include:
Cartrol Tablets 410
Ocupress Ophthalmic Solution, 1% Sterile .... ⊙ 309

Chlorothiazide (Orthostatic hypotension may occur with concurrent therapy). Products include:
Aldoclor Tablets 1598
Diupres Tablets 1650
Diuril Oral 1653

Chlorothiazide Sodium (Orthostatic hypotension may occur with concurrent therapy). Products include:
Diuril Sodium Intravenous 1652

Chlorpropamide (Blood glucose concentrations may be raised by metolazone in diabetics). Products include:
Diabinese Tablets 1935

Chlorthalidone (Orthostatic hypotension may occur with concurrent therapy). Products include:
Combipres Tablets 677
Tenoretic Tablets 2845
Thalitone 1245

Choline Magnesium Trisalicylate (Antihypertensive effects of Mykrox may be decreased). Products include:
Trilisate 2000

Clonidine (Orthostatic hypotension may occur with concurrent therapy). Products include:
Catapres-TTS 675

Clonidine Hydrochloride (Orthostatic hypotension may occur with concurrent therapy). Products include:
Catapres Tablets 674
Combipres Tablets 677

Codeine Phosphate (Potentiates orthostatic hypotensive effects). Products include:
Actifed with Codeine Cough Syrup.. 1067
Brontex 1981
Deconsal C Expectorant Syrup 456
Deconsal Pediatric Syrup 457
Dimetane-DC Cough Syrup 2059
Empirin with Codeine Tablets 1093
Fioricet with Codeine Capsules 2260
Fiorinal with Codeine Capsules 2262
Isoclor Expectorant 990
Novahistine DH 2462
Novahistine Expectorant 2463
Nucofed 2051
Phenergan with Codeine 2777
Phenergan VC with Codeine 2781
Robitussin A-C Syrup 2073
Robitussin-DAC Syrup 2074
Ryna .... ▣ 841
Soma Compound w/Codeine Tablets 2676
Tussi-Organidin NR Liquid and S NR Liquid 2677
Tylenol with Codeine 1583

Cortisone Acetate (Potential for increased hypokalemia). Products include:
Cortone Acetate Sterile Suspension 1623
Cortone Acetate Tablets 1624

Deserpidine (Orthostatic hypotension may occur with concurrent therapy).
No products indexed under this heading.

Deslanoside (Hypokalemia increases sensitivity of the myocardium to digitalis toxicity).
No products indexed under this heading.

Dexamethasone (Potential for increased hypokalemia). Products include:
AK-Trol Ointment & Suspension .... ⊙ 205
Decadron Elixir 1633
Decadron Tablets 1635
Decaspray Topical Aerosol 1648
Dexacidin Ointment .... ⊙ 263
Maxitrol Ophthalmic Ointment and Suspension .... ⊙ 224
TobraDex Ophthalmic Suspension and Ointment 473

Dexamethasone Acetate (Potential for increased hypokalemia). Products include:
Dalalone D.P. Injectable 1011
Decadron-LA Sterile Suspension 1646

Dexamethasone Sodium Phosphate (Potential for increased hypokalemia). Products include:
Decadron Phosphate Injection 1637
Decadron Phosphate Respihaler 1642
Decadron Phosphate Sterile Ophthalmic Ointment 1641
Decadron Phosphate Sterile Ophthalmic Solution 1642
Decadron Phosphate Topical Cream 1644
Decadron Phosphate Turbinaire 1645
Decadron Phosphate with Xylocaine Injection, Sterile 1639
Dexacort Phosphate in Respihaler .. 458
Dexacort Phosphate in Turbinaire .. 459
NeoDecadron Sterile Ophthalmic Ointment 1712
NeoDecadron Sterile Ophthalmic Solution 1713
NeoDecadron Topical Cream 1714

Dezocine (Potentiates orthostatic hypotensive effects). Products include:
Dalgan Injection 538

Diazoxide (Orthostatic hypotension may occur with concurrent therapy). Products include:
Hyperstat I.V. Injection 2363
Proglycem 580

Diclofenac Potassium (Antihypertensive effects of Mykrox may be decreased). Products include:
Cataflam 816

Diclofenac Sodium (Antihypertensive effects of Mykrox may be decreased). Products include:
Voltaren Ophthalmic Sterile Ophthalmic Solution .... ⊙ 272
Voltaren Tablets 861

Dicumarol (May affect the hypoprothrombinemic response to anticoagulants; dosage adjustments may be necessary).
No products indexed under this heading.

Diflunisal (Antihypertensive effects of Mykrox may be decreased). Products include:
Dolobid Tablets 1654

Digitoxin (Hypokalemia increases sensitivity of the myocardium to digitalis toxicity). Products include:
Crystodigin Tablets 1433

Digoxin (Hypokalemia increases sensitivity of the myocardium to digitalis toxicity). Products include:
Lanoxicaps 1117
Lanoxin Elixir Pediatric 1120
Lanoxin Injection 1123
Lanoxin Injection Pediatric 1126
Lanoxin Tablets 1128

Diltiazem Hydrochloride (Orthostatic hypotension may occur with concurrent therapy). Products include:
Cardizem CD Capsules 1506
Cardizem SR Capsules 1510
Cardizem Injectable 1508
Cardizem Tablets 1512
Dilacor XR Extended-release Capsules 2018

Doxazosin Mesylate (Orthostatic hypotension may occur with concurrent therapy). Products include:
Cardura Tablets 2186

Enalapril Maleate (Orthostatic hypotension may occur with concurrent therapy). Products include:
Vaseretic Tablets 1765
Vasotec Tablets 1771

Enalaprilat (Orthostatic hypotension may occur with concurrent therapy). Products include:
Vasotec I.V. 1768

Esmolol Hydrochloride (Orthostatic hypotension may occur with concurrent therapy). Products include:
Brevibloc Injection 1808

Ethacrynic Acid (Large or prolonged losses of fluids and electrolytes may result). Products include:
Edecrin Tablets 1657

Etodolac (Antihypertensive effects of Mykrox may be decreased). Products include:
Lodine Capsules and Tablets 2743

Felodipine (Orthostatic hypotension may occur with concurrent therapy). Products include:
Plendil Extended-Release Tablets 527

Fenoprofen Calcium (Antihypertensive effects of Mykrox may be decreased). Products include:
Nalfon 200 Pulvules & Nalfon Tablets 917

Fentanyl (Potentiates orthostatic hypotensive effects). Products include:
Duragesic Transdermal System 1288

Fentanyl Citrate (Potentiates orthostatic hypotensive effects). Products include:
Sublimaze Injection 1307

Fludrocortisone Acetate (Potential for increased hypokalemia). Products include:
Florinef Acetate Tablets 505

Flurbiprofen (Antihypertensive effects of Mykrox may be decreased). Products include:
Ansaid Tablets 2579

Fosinopril Sodium (Orthostatic hypotension may occur with concurrent therapy). Products include:
Monopril Tablets 757

Furosemide (Large or prolonged losses of fluids and electrolytes may result; orthostatic hypotension may occur with concurrent therapy). Products include:
Lasix Injection, Oral Solution and Tablets 1240

Glipizide (Blood glucose concentrations may be raised by metolazone in diabetics). Products include:
Glucotrol Tablets 1967
Glucotrol XL Extended Release Tablets 1968

Glyburide (Blood glucose concentrations may be raised by metolazone in diabetics). Products include:
DiaBeta Tablets 1239
Glynase PresTab Tablets 2609
Micronase Tablets 2623

Guanabenz Acetate (Orthostatic hypotension may occur with concurrent therapy).
No products indexed under this heading.

Guanethidine Monosulfate (Orthostatic hypotension may occur with concurrent therapy). Products include:
Esimil Tablets 822
Ismelin Tablets 827

Hydralazine Hydrochloride (Orthostatic hypotension may occur with concurrent therapy). Products include:
Apresazide Capsules 808
Apresoline Hydrochloride Tablets .. 809
Ser-Ap-Es Tablets 849

Hydrochlorothiazide (Orthostatic hypotension may occur with concurrent therapy). Products include:
Aldactazide 2413
Aldoril Tablets 1604
Apresazide Capsules 808
Capozide 742
Dyazide 2479
Esidrix Tablets 821
Esimil Tablets 822
HydroDIURIL Tablets 1674
Hydropres Tablets 1675
Hyzaar Tablets 1677
Inderide Tablets 2732
Inderide LA Long Acting Capsules .. 2734
Lopressor HCT Tablets 832

(▣ Described in PDR For Nonprescription Drugs) (⊙ Described in PDR For Ophthalmology)

Lotensin HCT.. 837
Maxzide.. 1380
Moduretic Tablets.. 1705
Oretic Tablets... 443
Prinzide Tablets... 1737
Ser-Ap-Es Tablets.. 849
Timolide Tablets... 1748
Vaseretic Tablets.. 1765
Zestoretic... 2850
Ziac.. 1415

Hydrocodone Bitartrate (Potentiates orthostatic hypotensive effects). Products include:

Anexsia 5/500 Elixir.................................... 1781
Anexia Tablets... 1782
Codiclear DH Syrup.................................... 791
Deconamine CX Cough and Cold Liquid and Tablets.. 1319
Duratuss HD Elixir....................................... 2565
Hycodan Tablets and Syrup........................ 930
Hycomine Compound Tablets..................... 932
Hycomine.. 931
Hycotuss Expectorant Syrup...................... 933
Hydrocet Capsules...................................... 782
Lorcet 10/650... 1018
Lortab.. 2566
Tussend... 1783
Tussend Expectorant.................................. 1785
Vicodin Tablets.. 1356
Vicodin ES Tablets...................................... 1357
Vicodin Tuss Expectorant........................... 1358
Zydone Capsules... 949

Hydrocodone Polistirex (Potentiates orthostatic hypotensive effects). Products include:

Tussionex Pennkinetic Extended-Release Suspension..................................... 998

Hydrocortisone (Potential for increased hypokalemia). Products include:

Anusol-HC Cream 2.5%.............................. 1896
Aquanil HC Lotion....................................... 1931
Bactine Hydrocortisone Anti-Itch Cream... ᴾᴰ 709
Caldecort Anti-Itch Hydrocortisone Spray.. ᴾᴰ 631
Cortaid... ᴾᴰ 836
CORTENEMA.. 2535
Cortisporin Ointment.................................. 1085
Cortisporin Ophthalmic Ointment Sterile... 1085
Cortisporin Ophthalmic Suspension Sterile.. 1086
Cortisporin Otic Solution Sterile................. 1087
Cortisporin Otic Suspension Sterile............ 1088
Cortizone-5.. ᴾᴰ 831
Cortizone-10.. ᴾᴰ 831
Hydrocortone Tablets.................................. 1672
Hytone... 907
Massengill Medicated Soft Cloth Towelettes.. 2458
PediOtic Suspension Sterile........................ 1153
Preparation H Hydrocortisone 1% Cream.. ᴾᴰ 872
ProctoCream-HC 2.5%................................. 2408
VōSoL HC Otic Solution............................... 2678

Hydrocortisone Acetate (Potential for increased hypokalemia). Products include:

Analpram-HC Rectal Cream 1% and 2.5%.. 977
Anusol HC-1 Anti-Itch Hydrocortisone Ointment... ᴾᴰ 847
Anusol-HC Suppositories............................ 1897
Caldecort.. ᴾᴰ 631
Carmol HC.. 924
Coly-Mycin S Otic w/Neomycin & Hydrocortisone... 1906
Cortaid... ᴾᴰ 836
Cortifoam... 2396
Cortisporin Cream....................................... 1084
Epifoam... 2399
Hydrocortone Acetate Sterile Suspension.. 1669
Mantadil Cream... 1135
Nupercainal Hydrocortisone 1% Cream... ᴾᴰ 645
Ophthocort... ⓒ 311
Pramosone Cream, Lotion & Ointment... 978
ProctoCream-HC.. 2408
ProctoFoam-HC... 2409
Terra-Cortril Ophthalmic Suspension... 2210

Hydrocortisone Sodium Phosphate (Potential for increased hypokalemia). Products include:

Hydrocortone Phosphate Injection, Sterile... 1670

Hydrocortisone Sodium Succinate (Potential for increased hypokalemia). Products include:

Solu-Cortef Sterile Powder......................... 2641

Hydroflumethiazide (Orthostatic hypotension may occur with concurrent therapy). Products include:

Diucardin Tablets... 2718

Ibuprofen (Antihypertensive effects of Mykrox may be decreased). Products include:

Advil Cold and Sinus Caplets and Tablets (formerly CoAdvil)........................ ᴾᴰ 870
Advil Ibuprofen Tablets and Caplets... ᴾᴰ 870
Children's Advil Suspension........................ 2692
Arthritis Foundation Ibuprofen Tablets... ᴾᴰ 674
Bayer Select Ibuprofen Pain Relief Formula.. ᴾᴰ 715
Cramp End Tablets....................................... ᴾᴰ 735
Dimetapp Sinus Caplets.............................. ᴾᴰ 775
Haltran Tablets... ᴾᴰ 771
IBU Tablets... 1342
Ibuprohm... ᴾᴰ 735
Children's Motrin Ibuprofen Oral Suspension.. 1546
Motrin Tablets.. 2625
Motrin IB Caplets, Tablets, and Geltabs.. ᴾᴰ 838
Motrin IB Sinus.. ᴾᴰ 838
Motrin Ibuprofen Suspension, Oral Drops, Chewable Tablets, Caplets... 1546
Nuprin Ibuprofen/Analgesic Tablets & Caplets... ᴾᴰ 622
Sine-Aid IB Caplets...................................... 1554
Vicks DayQuil SINUS Pressure & PAIN Relief with IBUPROFEN........ ᴾᴰ 762

Indapamide (Orthostatic hypotension may occur with concurrent therapy). Products include:

Lozol Tablets.. 2022

Indomethacin (Antihypertensive effects of Mykrox may be decreased). Products include:

Indocin... 1680

Indomethacin Sodium Trihydrate (Antihypertensive effects of Mykrox may be decreased). Products include:

Indocin I.V... 1684

Insulin, Human (Blood glucose concentrations may be raised by metolazone in diabetics).

No products indexed under this heading.

Insulin, Human Isophane Suspension (Blood glucose concentrations may be raised by metolazone in diabetics). Products include:

Novolin N Human Insulin 10 ml Vials... 1795

Insulin, Human NPH (Blood glucose concentrations may be raised by metolazone in diabetics). Products include:

Humulin N, 100 Units.................................. 1448
Novolin N PenFill Cartridges Durable Insulin Delivery System........................ 1798
Novolin N Prefilled Syringe Disposable Insulin Delivery System........................ 1798

Insulin, Human Regular (Blood glucose concentrations may be raised by metolazone in diabetics). Products include:

Humulin R, 100 Units.................................. 1449
Novolin R Human Insulin 10 ml Vials... 1795
Novolin R PenFill Cartridges Durable Insulin Delivery System........................ 1798
Novolin R Prefilled Syringe Disposable Insulin Delivery System........................ 1798
Velosulin BR Human Insulin 10 ml Vials... 1795

Insulin, Human, Zinc Suspension (Blood glucose concentrations may be raised by metolazone in diabetics). Products include:

Humulin L, 100 Units.................................. 1446
Humulin U, 100 Units.................................. 1450
Novolin L Human Insulin 10 ml Vials... 1795

Insulin, NPH (Blood glucose concentrations may be raised by metolazone in diabetics). Products include:

NPH, 100 Units... 1450
Pork NPH, 100 Units................................... 1452
Purified Pork NPH Isophane Insulin... 1801

Insulin, Regular (Blood glucose concentrations may be raised by metolazone in diabetics). Products include:

Regular, 100 Units....................................... 1450
Pork Regular, 100 Units.............................. 1452
Pork Regular (Concentrated), 500 Units... 1453
Purified Pork Regular Insulin...................... 1801

Insulin, Zinc Crystals (Blood glucose concentrations may be raised by metolazone in diabetics). Products include:

NPH, 100 Units... 1450

Insulin, Zinc Suspension (Blood glucose concentrations may be raised by metolazone in diabetics). Products include:

Iletin I.. 1450
Lente, 100 Units.. 1450
Iletin II... 1452
Pork Lente, 100 Units.................................. 1452
Purified Pork Lente Insulin......................... 1801

Isradipine (Orthostatic hypotension may occur with concurrent therapy). Products include:

DynaCirc Capsules....................................... 2256

Ketoprofen (Antihypertensive effects of Mykrox may be decreased). Products include:

Orudis Capsules... 2766
Oruvail Capsules.. 2766

Ketorolac Tromethamine (Antihypertensive effects of Mykrox may be decreased). Products include:

Acular... 474
Acular... ⓒ 277
Toradol... 2159

Labetalol Hydrochloride (Orthostatic hypotension may occur with concurrent therapy). Products include:

Normodyne Injection................................... 2377
Normodyne Tablets...................................... 2379
Trandate... 1185

Levorphanol Tartrate (Potentiates orthostatic hypotensive effects). Products include:

Levo-Dromoran.. 2129

Lisinopril (Orthostatic hypotension may occur with concurrent therapy). Products include:

Prinivil Tablets... 1733
Prinzide Tablets... 1737
Zestoretic... 2850
Zestril Tablets.. 2854

Lithium Carbonate (Reduced renal clearance of lithium; high risk of lithium toxicity). Products include:

Eskalith.. 2485
Lithium Carbonate Capsules & Tablets... 2230
Lithonate/Lithotabs/Lithobid...................... 2543

Lithium Citrate (Reduced renal clearance of lithium; high risk of lithium toxicity).

No products indexed under this heading.

Losartan Potassium (Orthostatic hypotension may occur with concurrent therapy). Products include:

Cozaar Tablets... 1628
Hyzaar Tablets... 1677

Magnesium Salicylate (Antihypertensive effects of Mykrox may be decreased). Products include:

Backache Caplets... ᴾᴰ 613
Bayer Select Backache Pain Relief Formula.. ᴾᴰ 715
Doan's Extra-Strength Analgesic.... ᴾᴰ 633
Extra Strength Doan's P.M.......................... ᴾᴰ 633
Doan's Regular Strength Analgesic... ᴾᴰ 634
Mobigesic Tablets.. ᴾᴰ 602

Mecamylamine Hydrochloride (Orthostatic hypotension may occur with concurrent therapy). Products include:

Inversine Tablets.. 1686

Meclofenamate Sodium (Antihypertensive effects of Mykrox may be decreased).

No products indexed under this heading.

Mefenamic Acid (Antihypertensive effects of Mykrox may be decreased). Products include:

Ponstel... 1925

Meperidine Hydrochloride (Potentiates orthostatic hypotensive effects). Products include:

Demerol.. 2308
Mepergan Injection...................................... 2753

Mephobarbital (Potentiates orthostatic hypotensive effects). Products include:

Mebaral Tablets... 2322

Metformin Hydrochloride (Blood glucose concentrations may be raised by metolazone in diabetics). Products include:

Glucophage.. 752

Methadone Hydrochloride (Potentiates orthostatic hypotensive effects). Products include:

Methadone Hydrochloride Oral Concentrate.. 2233
Methadone Hydrochloride Oral Solution & Tablets....................................... 2235

Methenamine (Efficacy of methenamine may be decreased). Products include:

Urised Tablets.. 1964

Methenamine Hippurate (Efficacy of methenamine may be decreased).

No products indexed under this heading.

Methenamine Mandelate (Efficacy of methenamine may be decreased). Products include:

Uroqid-Acid No. 2 Tablets.......................... 640

Methylclothiazide (Orthostatic hypotension may occur with concurrent therapy). Products include:

Enduron Tablets... 420

Methyldopa (Orthostatic hypotension may occur with concurrent therapy). Products include:

Aldoclor Tablets... 1598
Aldomet Oral.. 1600
Aldoril Tablets.. 1604

Methyldopate Hydrochloride (Orthostatic hypotension may occur with concurrent therapy). Products include:

Aldomet Ester HCl Injection....................... 1602

Methylprednisolone Acetate (Potential for increased hypokalemia). Products include:

Depo-Medrol Single-Dose Vial.................... 2600
Depo-Medrol Sterile Aqueous Suspension.. 2597

Methylprednisolone Sodium Succinate (Potential for increased hypokalemia). Products include:

Solu-Medrol Sterile Powder........................ 2643

Metoprolol Succinate (Orthostatic hypotension may occur with concurrent therapy). Products include:

Toprol-XL Tablets.. 565

IMPORTANT NOTE: Always consult each drug listing in the patient's regimen for possible interactions.

Mykrox Interactions Index 690

Metoprolol Tartrate (Orthostatic hypotension may occur with concurrent therapy). Products include:
Lopressor Ampuls ... 830
Lopressor HCT Tablets ... 832
Lopressor Tablets ... 830

Metyrosine (Orthostatic hypotension may occur with concurrent therapy). Products include:
Demser Capsules ... 1649

Minoxidil (Orthostatic hypotension may occur with concurrent therapy). Products include:
Loniten Tablets ... 2618
Rogaine Topical Solution ... 2637

Moexipril Hydrochloride (Orthostatic hypotension may occur with concurrent therapy). Products include:
Univasc Tablets ... 2410

Morphine Sulfate (Potentiates orthostatic hypotensive effects). Products include:
Astramorph/PF Injection, USP (Preservative-Free) ... 535
Duramorph ... 962
Infumorph 200 and Infumorph 500 Sterile Solutions ... 965
MS Contin Tablets ... 1994
MSIR ... 1997
Oramorph SR (Morphine Sulfate Sustained Release Tablets) ... 2236
RMS Suppositories ... 2657
Roxanol ... 2243

Nabumetone (Antihypertensive effects of Mykrox may be decreased). Products include:
Relafen Tablets ... 2510

Nadolol (Orthostatic hypotension may occur with concurrent therapy).
No products indexed under this heading.

Naproxen (Antihypertensive effects of Mykrox may be decreased). Products include:
Anaprox/Naprosyn ... 2117

Naproxen Sodium (Antihypertensive effects of Mykrox may be decreased). Products include:
Aleve ... 1975
Anaprox/Naprosyn ... 2117

Nicardipine Hydrochloride (Orthostatic hypotension may occur with concurrent therapy). Products include:
Cardene Capsules ... 2095
Cardene I.V. ... 2709
Cardene SR Capsules ... 2097

Nifedipine (Orthostatic hypotension may occur with concurrent therapy). Products include:
Adalat Capsules (10 mg and 20 mg) ... 587
Adalat CC ... 589
Procardia Capsules ... 1971
Procardia XL Extended Release Tablets ... 1972

Nisoldipine (Orthostatic hypotension may occur with concurrent therapy).
No products indexed under this heading.

Nitroglycerin (Orthostatic hypotension may occur with concurrent therapy). Products include:
Deponit NTG Transdermal Delivery System ... 2397
Nitro-Bid IV ... 1523
Nitro-Bid Ointment ... 1524
Nitrodisc ... 2047
Nitro-Dur (nitroglycerin) Transdermal Infusion System ... 1326
Nitrolingual Spray ... 2027
Nitrostat Tablets ... 1925
Transderm-Nitro Transdermal Therapeutic System ... 859

Norepinephrine Bitartrate (Arterial responsiveness to norepinephrine may be decreased). Products include:
Levophed Bitartrate Injection ... 2315

Opium Alkaloids (Potentiates orthostatic hypotensive effects).
No products indexed under this heading.

Oxaprozin (Antihypertensive effects of Mykrox may be decreased). Products include:
Daypro Caplets ... 2426

Oxycodone Hydrochloride (Potentiates orthostatic hypotensive effects). Products include:
Percocet Tablets ... 938
Percodan Tablets ... 939
Percodan-Demi Tablets ... 940
Roxicodone Tablets, Oral Solution & Intensol (Oxycodone) ... 2244
Tylox Capsules ... 1584

Penbutolol Sulfate (Orthostatic hypotension may occur with concurrent therapy). Products include:
Levatol ... 2403

Pentobarbital Sodium (Potentiates orthostatic hypotensive effects). Products include:
Nembutal Sodium Capsules ... 436
Nembutal Sodium Solution ... 438
Nembutal Sodium Suppositories ... 440

Phenobarbital (Potentiates orthostatic hypotensive effects). Products include:
Arco-Lase Plus Tablets ... 512
Bellergal-S Tablets ... 2250
Donnatal ... 2060
Donnatal Extentabs ... 2061
Donnatal Tablets ... 2060
Phenobarbital Elixir and Tablets ... 1469
Quadrinal Tablets ... 1350

Phenoxybenzamine Hydrochloride (Orthostatic hypotension may occur with concurrent therapy). Products include:
Dibenzyline Capsules ... 2476

Phentolamine Mesylate (Orthostatic hypotension may occur with concurrent therapy). Products include:
Regitine ... 846

Phenylbutazone (Antihypertensive effects of Mykrox may be decreased).
No products indexed under this heading.

Pindolol (Orthostatic hypotension may occur with concurrent therapy). Products include:
Visken Tablets ... 2299

Piroxicam (Antihypertensive effects of Mykrox may be decreased). Products include:
Feldene Capsules ... 1965

Polythiazide (Orthostatic hypotension may occur with concurrent therapy). Products include:
Minizide Capsules ... 1938

Prazosin Hydrochloride (Orthostatic hypotension may occur with concurrent therapy). Products include:
Minipress Capsules ... 1937
Minizide Capsules ... 1938

Prednisolone Acetate (Potential for increased hypokalemia). Products include:
AK-CIDE ... ⊙ 202
AK-CIDE Ointment ... ⊙ 202
Blephamide Liquifilm Sterile Ophthalmic Suspension ... 476
Blephamide Ointment ... ⊙ 237
Econopred & Econopred Plus Ophthalmic Suspensions ... ⊙ 217
Poly-Pred Liquifilm ... ⊙ 248
Pred Forte ... ⊙ 250
Pred Mild ... ⊙ 253
Pred-G Liquifilm Sterile Ophthalmic Suspension ... ⊙ 251
Pred-G S.O.P. Sterile Ophthalmic Ointment ... ⊙ 252
Vasocidin Ointment ... ⊙ 268

Prednisolone Sodium Phosphate (Potential for increased hypokalemia). Products include:
AK-Pred ... ⊙ 204
Hydeltrasol Injection, Sterile ... 1665
Inflamase ... ⊙ 265
Pediapred Oral Liquid ... 995
Vasocidin Ophthalmic Solution ... ⊙ 270

Prednisolone Tebutate (Potential for increased hypokalemia). Products include:
Hydeltra-T.B.A. Sterile Suspension 1667

Prednisone (Potential for increased hypokalemia). Products include:
Deltasone Tablets ... 2595

Propoxyphene Hydrochloride (Potentiates orthostatic hypotensive effects). Products include:
Darvon ... 1435
Wygesic Tablets ... 2827

Propoxyphene Napsylate (Potentiates orthostatic hypotensive effects). Products include:
Darvon-N/Darvocet-N ... 1433

Propranolol Hydrochloride (Orthostatic hypotension may occur with concurrent therapy). Products include:
Inderal ... 2728
Inderal LA Long Acting Capsules ... 2730
Inderide Tablets ... 2732
Inderide LA Long Acting Capsules ... 2734

Quinapril Hydrochloride (Orthostatic hypotension may occur with concurrent therapy). Products include:
Accupril Tablets ... 1893

Ramipril (Orthostatic hypotension may occur with concurrent therapy). Products include:
Altace Capsules ... 1232

Rauwolfia Serpentina (Orthostatic hypotension may occur with concurrent therapy).
No products indexed under this heading.

Rescinnamine (Orthostatic hypotension may occur with concurrent therapy).
No products indexed under this heading.

Reserpine (Orthostatic hypotension may occur with concurrent therapy). Products include:
Diupres Tablets ... 1650
Hydropres Tablets ... 1675
Ser-Ap-Es Tablets ... 849

Salsalate (Antihypertensive effects of Mykrox may be decreased). Products include:
Mono-Gesic Tablets ... 792
Salflex Tablets ... 786

Secobarbital Sodium (Potentiates orthostatic hypotensive effects). Products include:
Seconal Sodium Pulvules ... 1474

Sodium Nitroprusside (Orthostatic hypotension may occur with concurrent therapy).
No products indexed under this heading.

Sotalol Hydrochloride (Orthostatic hypotension may occur with concurrent therapy). Products include:
Betapace Tablets ... 641

Spirapril Hydrochloride (Orthostatic hypotension may occur with concurrent therapy).
No products indexed under this heading.

Sufentanil Citrate (Potentiates orthostatic hypotensive effects). Products include:
Sufenta Injection ... 1309

Sulindac (Antihypertensive effects of Mykrox may be decreased). Products include:
Clinoril Tablets ... 1618

Terazosin Hydrochloride (Orthostatic hypotension may occur with concurrent therapy). Products include:
Hytrin Capsules ... 430

Thiamylal Sodium (Potentiates orthostatic hypotensive effects).
No products indexed under this heading.

Timolol Maleate (Orthostatic hypotension may occur with concurrent therapy). Products include:
Blocadren Tablets ... 1614
Timolide Tablets ... 1748
Timoptic in Ocudose ... 1753
Timoptic Sterile Ophthalmic Solution ... 1751
Timoptic-XE ... 1755

Tolazamide (Blood glucose concentrations may be raised by metolazone in diabetics).
No products indexed under this heading.

Tolbutamide (Blood glucose concentrations may be raised by metolazone in diabetics).
No products indexed under this heading.

Tolmetin Sodium (Antihypertensive effects of Mykrox may be decreased). Products include:
Tolectin (200, 400 and 600 mg) .. 1581

Torsemide (Orthostatic hypotension may occur with concurrent therapy). Products include:
Demadex Tablets and Injection ... 686

Triamcinolone (Potential for increased hypokalemia). Products include:
Aristocort Tablets ... 1022

Triamcinolone Acetonide (Potential for increased hypokalemia). Products include:
Aristocort A 0.025% Cream ... 1027
Aristocort A 0.5% Cream ... 1031
Aristocort A 0.1% Cream ... 1029
Aristocort A 0.1% Ointment ... 1030
Azmacort Oral Inhaler ... 2011
Nasacort Nasal Inhaler ... 2024

Triamcinolone Diacetate (Potential for increased hypokalemia). Products include:
Aristocort Suspension (Forte Parenteral) ... 1027
Aristocort Suspension (Intralesional) ... 1025

Triamcinolone Hexacetonide (Potential for increased hypokalemia). Products include:
Aristospan Suspension (Intra-articular) ... 1033
Aristospan Suspension (Intralesional) ... 1032

Trimethaphan Camsylate (Orthostatic hypotension may occur with concurrent therapy). Products include:
Arfonad Ampuls ... 2080

Tubocurarine Chloride (Neuromuscular blocking effects of curariform drugs may be enhanced).
No products indexed under this heading.

Verapamil Hydrochloride (Orthostatic hypotension may occur with concurrent therapy). Products include:
Calan SR Caplets ... 2422
Calan Tablets ... 2419
Isoptin Injectable ... 1344
Isoptin Oral Tablets ... 1346
Isoptin SR Tablets ... 1348
Verelan Capsules ... 1410
Verelan Capsules ... 2824

(▭ Described in PDR For Nonprescription Drugs) (⊙ Described in PDR For Ophthalmology)

Warfarin Sodium (May affect the hypoprothrombinemic response to anticoagulants; dosage adjustments may be necessary). Products include:
- Coumadin ... 926

Food Interactions

Alcohol (Potentiates orthostatic hypotensive effects).

MYLANTA CALCIUM CARBONATE AND MAGNESIUM HYDROXIDE TABLETS
(Calcium Carbonate, Magnesium Hydroxide) ... 1318
May interact with:

Prescription Drugs, unspecified (Resultant effects of concurrent use not specified).

MYLANTA GAS RELIEF TABLETS-80 MG
(Simethicone) ... 1318
None cited in PDR database.

MAXIMUM STRENGTH MYLANTA GAS RELIEF TABLETS-125 MG
(Simethicone) ... 1318
None cited in PDR database.

MYLANTA GELCAPS ANTACID
(Calcium Carbonate, Magnesium Carbonate) ... 662
May interact with:

Prescription Drugs, unspecified (Antacids may interact with certain unspecified prescription drugs).

MYLANTA LIQUID
(Aluminum Hydroxide, Magnesium Hydroxide, Simethicone) ... 1317
May interact with tetracyclines. Compounds in this category include:

Demeclocycline Hydrochloride (Effect not specified). Products include:
- Declomycin Tablets ... 1371

Doxycycline Calcium (Effect not specified). Products include:
- Vibramycin Calcium Oral Suspension Syrup ... 1941

Doxycycline Hyclate (Effect not specified). Products include:
- Doryx Capsules ... 1913
- Vibramycin Hyclate Capsules ... 1941
- Vibramycin Hyclate Intravenous ... 2215
- Vibra-Tabs Film Coated Tablets ... 1941

Doxycycline Monohydrate (Effect not specified). Products include:
- Monodox Capsules ... 1805
- Vibramycin Monohydrate for Oral Suspension ... 1941

Methacycline Hydrochloride (Effect not specified).
- No products indexed under this heading.

Minocycline Hydrochloride (Effect not specified). Products include:
- Dynacin Capsules ... 1590
- Minocin Intravenous ... 1382
- Minocin Oral Suspension ... 1385
- Minocin Pellet-Filled Capsules ... 1383

Oxytetracycline (Effect not specified). Products include:
- Terramycin Intramuscular Solution 2210

Oxytetracycline Hydrochloride (Effect not specified). Products include:
- TERAK Ointment ... ◉ 209
- Terra-Cortril Ophthalmic Suspension ... 2210
- Terramycin with Polymyxin B Sulfate Ophthalmic Ointment ... 2211
- Urobiotic-250 Capsules ... 2214

Tetracycline Hydrochloride (Effect not specified). Products include:
- Achromycin V Capsules ... 1367

MYLANTA NATURAL FIBER SUPPLEMENT
(Psyllium Preparations) ... 662
None cited in PDR database.

MYLANTA SOOTHING LOZENGES
(Calcium Carbonate) ... 1319
May interact with:

Prescription Drugs, unspecified (Concurrent use not recommended; consult your doctor).

MYLANTA TABLETS
(Aluminum Hydroxide, Magnesium Hydroxide, Simethicone) ... 660
See **Mylanta Liquid**

MYLANTA DOUBLE STRENGTH LIQUID
(Aluminum Hydroxide, Magnesium Hydroxide, Simethicone) ... 1317
See **Mylanta Liquid**

MYLANTA DOUBLE STRENGTH TABLETS
(Aluminum Hydroxide, Magnesium Hydroxide, Simethicone) ... 660
See **Mylanta Liquid**

MYLERAN TABLETS
(Busulfan) ... 1143
May interact with antineoplastics and certain other agents. Compounds in these categories include:

Altretamine (Potential for rare life-threatening hepatic veno-occlusive disease). Products include:
- Hexalen Capsules ... 2571

Asparaginase (Potential for rare life-threatening hepatic veno-occlusive disease). Products include:
- Elspar ... 1659

Bleomycin Sulfate (Potential for rare life-threatening hepatic veno-occlusive disease). Products include:
- Blenoxane ... 692

Bone Marrow Depressants, unspecified (Additive myelosuppression).

Carboplatin (Potential for rare life-threatening hepatic veno-occlusive disease). Products include:
- Paraplatin for Injection ... 705

Carmustine (BCNU) (Potential for rare life-threatening hepatic veno-occlusive disease). Products include:
- BiCNU ... 691

Chlorambucil (Potential for rare life-threatening hepatic veno-occlusive disease). Products include:
- Leukeran Tablets ... 1133

Cisplatin (Potential for rare life-threatening hepatic veno-occlusive disease). Products include:
- Platinol ... 708
- Platinol-AQ Injection ... 710

Cyclophosphamide (Potential for rare life-threatening hepatic veno-occlusive disease; potential for cardiac temponade). Products include:
- Cytoxan ... 694
- NEOSAR Lyophilized/Neosar ... 1959

Dacarbazine (Potential for rare life-threatening hepatic veno-occlusive disease). Products include:
- DTIC-Dome ... 600

Daunorubicin Hydrochloride (Potential for rare life-threatening hepatic veno-occlusive disease). Products include:
- Cerubidine ... 795

Doxorubicin Hydrochloride (Potential for rare life-threatening hepatic veno-occlusive disease). Products include:
- Adriamycin PFS ... 1947
- Adriamycin RDF ... 1947
- Doxorubicin Astra ... 540
- Rubex ... 712

Estramustine Phosphate Sodium (Potential for rare life-threatening hepatic veno-occlusive disease). Products include:
- Emcyt Capsules ... 1953

Etoposide (Potential for rare life-threatening hepatic veno-occlusive disease). Products include:
- VePesid Capsules and Injection ... 718

Floxuridine (Potential for rare life-threatening hepatic veno-occlusive disease). Products include:
- Sterile FUDR ... 2118

Fluorouracil (Potential for rare life-threatening hepatic veno-occlusive disease). Products include:
- Efudex ... 2113
- Fluoroplex Topical Solution & Cream 1% ... 479
- Fluorouracil Injection ... 2116

Flutamide (Potential for rare life-threatening hepatic veno-occlusive disease). Products include:
- Eulexin Capsules ... 2358

Hydroxyurea (Potential for rare life-threatening hepatic veno-occlusive disease). Products include:
- Hydrea Capsules ... 696

Idarubicin Hydrochloride (Potential for rare life-threatening hepatic veno-occlusive disease). Products include:
- Idamycin ... 1955

Ifosfamide (Potential for rare life-threatening hepatic veno-occlusive disease). Products include:
- IFEX ... 697

Interferon alfa-2A, Recombinant (Potential for rare life-threatening hepatic veno-occlusive disease). Products include:
- Roferon-A Injection ... 2145

Interferon alfa-2B, Recombinant (Potential for rare life-threatening hepatic veno-occlusive disease). Products include:
- Intron A ... 2364

Levamisole Hydrochloride (Potential for rare life-threatening hepatic veno-occlusive disease). Products include:
- Ergamisol Tablets ... 1292

Lomustine (CCNU) (Potential for rare life-threatening hepatic veno-occlusive disease). Products include:
- CeeNU ... 693

Mechlorethamine Hydrochloride (Potential for rare life-threatening hepatic veno-occlusive disease). Products include:
- Mustargen ... 1709

Megestrol Acetate (Potential for rare life-threatening hepatic veno-occlusive disease). Products include:
- Megace Oral Suspension ... 699
- Megace Tablets ... 701

Melphalan (Potential for rare life-threatening hepatic veno-occlusive disease). Products include:
- Alkeran Tablets ... 1071

Mercaptopurine (Potential for rare life-threatening hepatic veno-occlusive disease). Products include:
- Purinethol Tablets ... 1156

Methotrexate Sodium (Potential for rare life-threatening hepatic veno-occlusive disease). Products include:
- Methotrexate Sodium Tablets, Injection, for Injection and LPF Injection ... 1275

Mitomycin (Mitomycin-C) (Potential for rare life-threatening hepatic veno-occlusive disease). Products include:
- Mutamycin ... 703

Mitotane (Potential for rare life-threatening hepatic veno-occlusive disease). Products include:
- Lysodren ... 698

Mitoxantrone Hydrochloride (Potential for rare life-threatening hepatic veno-occlusive disease). Products include:
- Novantrone ... 1279

Paclitaxel (Potential for rare life-threatening hepatic veno-occlusive disease). Products include:
- Taxol ... 714

Procarbazine Hydrochloride (Potential for rare life-threatening hepatic veno-occlusive disease). Products include:
- Matulane Capsules ... 2131

Streptozocin (Potential for rare life-threatening hepatic veno-occlusive disease). Products include:
- Zanosar Sterile Powder ... 2653

Tamoxifen Citrate (Potential for rare life-threatening hepatic veno-occlusive disease). Products include:
- Nolvadex Tablets ... 2841

Teniposide (Potential for rare life-threatening hepatic veno-occlusive disease). Products include:
- Vumon ... 727

Thioguanine (Potential for esophageal varices associated with abnormal liver function tests; potential for rare life-threatening hepatic veno-occlusive disease). Products include:
- Thioguanine Tablets, Tabloid Brand ... 1181

Thiotepa (Potential for rare life-threatening hepatic veno-occlusive disease). Products include:
- Thioplex (Thiotepa For Injection) ... 1281

Vincristine Sulfate (Potential for rare life-threatening hepatic veno-occlusive disease). Products include:
- Oncovin Solution Vials & Hyporets 1466

Vinorelbine Tartrate (Potential for rare life-threatening hepatic veno-occlusive disease). Products include:
- Navelbine Injection ... 1145

MYLICON INFANTS' DROPS
(Simethicone) ... 1317
None cited in PDR database.

MYOCHRYSINE INJECTION
(Gold Sodium Thiomalate) ... 1711
May interact with cytotoxic drugs and certain other agents. Compounds in these categories include:

Bleomycin Sulfate (Safety of coadministration has NOT been established). Products include:
- Blenoxane ... 692

Daunorubicin Hydrochloride (Safety of coadministration has NOT been established). Products include:
- Cerubidine ... 795

Doxorubicin Hydrochloride (Safety of coadministration has NOT been established). Products include:
- Adriamycin PFS ... 1947
- Adriamycin RDF ... 1947
- Doxorubicin Astra ... 540
- Rubex ... 712

IMPORTANT NOTE: Always consult each drug listing in the patient's regimen for possible interactions.

Fluorouracil (Safety of coadministration has NOT been established). Products include:
- Efudex 2113
- Fluoroplex Topical Solution & Cream 1% 479
- Fluorouracil Injection 2116

Hydroxyurea (Safety of coadministration has NOT been established). Products include:
- Hydrea Capsules 696

Methotrexate Sodium (Safety of coadministration has NOT been established). Products include:
- Methotrexate Sodium Tablets, Injection, for Injection and LPF Injection 1275

Mitotane (Safety of coadministration has NOT been established). Products include:
- Lysodren 698

Mitoxantrone Hydrochloride (Safety of coadministration has NOT been established). Products include:
- Novantrone 1279

Penicillamine (Do not use concomitantly). Products include:
- Cuprimine Capsules 1630
- Depen Titratable Tablets 2662

Procarbazine Hydrochloride (Safety of coadministration has NOT been established). Products include:
- Matulane Capsules 2131

Tamoxifen Citrate (Safety of coadministration has NOT been established). Products include:
- Nolvadex Tablets 2841

Vincristine Sulfate (Safety of coadministration has NOT been established). Products include:
- Oncovin Solution Vials & Hyporets 1466

MYOFLEX EXTERNAL ANALGESIC CREME
(Trolamine Salicylate) ■ 643
None cited in PDR database.

MYSOLINE SUSPENSION
(Primidone) 2754
None cited in PDR database.

MYSOLINE TABLETS
(Primidone) 2754
None cited in PDR database.

NTZ LONG ACTING NASAL SPRAY & DROPS 0.05%
(Oxymetazoline Hydrochloride) ■ 727
None cited in PDR database.

NAFTIN CREAM 1%
(Naftifine Hydrochloride) 480
None cited in PDR database.

NAFTIN GEL 1%
(Naftifine Hydrochloride) 481
None cited in PDR database.

NALFON 200 PULVULES & NALFON TABLETS
(Fenoprofen Calcium) 917
May interact with sulfonamides, oral hypoglycemic agents, oral anticoagulants, loop diuretics, hydantoin anticonvulsants, salicylates, and certain other agents. Compounds in these categories include:

Acarbose (Sulfonylurea toxicity).
No products indexed under this heading.

Aspirin (Decreases half-life of fenoprofen). Products include:
- Alka-Seltzer Effervescent Antacid and Pain Reliever ■ 701
- Alka-Seltzer Extra Strength Effervescent Antacid and Pain Reliever ■ 703
- Alka-Seltzer Lemon Lime Effervescent Antacid and Pain Reliever ■ 703
- Alka-Seltzer Plus Cold Medicine ■ 705
- Alka-Seltzer Plus Cold & Cough Medicine ■ 708
- Alka-Seltzer Plus Night-Time Cold Medicine ■ 707
- Alka Seltzer Plus Sinus Medicine ■ 707
- Arthritis Foundation Safety Coated Aspirin Tablets ■ 675
- Arthritis Pain Ascriptin ■ 631
- Maximum Strength Ascriptin ■ 630
- Regular Strength Ascriptin Tablets ■ 629
- Arthritis Strength BC Powder ■ 609
- BC Cold Powder Multi-Symptom Formula (Cold-Sinus-Allergy) ■ 609
- BC Cold Powder Non-Drowsy Formula (Cold-Sinus) ■ 609
- BC Powder ■ 609
- Bayer Children's Chewable Aspirin ■ 711
- Genuine Bayer Aspirin Tablets & Caplets ■ 713
- Extra Strength Bayer Arthritis Pain Regimen Formula ■ 711
- Extra Strength Bayer Aspirin Caplets & Tablets ■ 712
- Extended-Release Bayer 8-Hour Aspirin ■ 712
- Extra Strength Bayer Plus Aspirin Caplets ■ 713
- Extra Strength Bayer PM Aspirin ■ 713
- Bayer Enteric Aspirin ■ 709
- Bufferin Analgesic Tablets and Caplets ■ 613
- Arthritis Strength Bufferin Analgesic Caplets ■ 614
- Extra Strength Bufferin Analgesic Tablets ■ 615
- Cama Arthritis Pain Reliever ■ 785
- Darvon Compound-65 Pulvules 1435
- Easprin 1914
- Ecotrin 2455
- Ecotrin Enteric Coated Aspirin Maximum Strength Tablets and Caplets ■ 816
- Ecotrin Enteric Coated Aspirin Regular Strength Tablets 2455
- Empirin Aspirin Tablets ■ 854
- Empirin with Codeine Tablets 1093
- Excedrin Extra-Strength Analgesic Tablets & Caplets 732
- Fiorinal Capsules 2261
- Fiorinal with Codeine Capsules 2262
- Fiorinal Tablets 2261
- Halfprin 1362
- Healthprin Aspirin 2455
- Norgesic 1496
- Percodan Tablets 939
- Percodan-Demi Tablets 940
- Robaxisal Tablets 2071
- Soma Compound w/Codeine Tablets 2676
- Soma Compound Tablets 2675
- St. Joseph Adult Chewable Aspirin (81 mg.) ■ 808
- Talwin Compound 2335
- Ursinus Inlay-Tabs ■ 794
- Vanquish Analgesic Caplets ■ 731

Bumetanide (Patients treated with Nalfon may be resistant to the effects of loop diuretics). Products include:
- Bumex 2093

Chlorpropamide (Sulfonylurea toxicity). Products include:
- Diabinese Tablets 1935

Choline Magnesium Trisalicylate (Decreases half-life of fenoprofen). Products include:
- Trilisate 2000

Dicumarol (Prolonged prothrombin time).
No products indexed under this heading.

Diflunisal (Decreases half-life of fenoprofen). Products include:
- Dolobid Tablets 1654

Ethacrynic Acid (Patients treated with Nalfon may be resistant to the effects of loop diuretics). Products include:
- Edecrin Tablets 1657

Ethotoin (Potential for increased activity and toxicity of ethotoin). Products include:
- Peganone Tablets 446

Furosemide (Patients treated with Nalfon may be resistant to the effects of loop diuretics). Products include:
- Lasix Injection, Oral Solution and Tablets 1240

Glipizide (Sulfonylurea toxicity). Products include:
- Glucotrol Tablets 1967
- Glucotrol XL Extended Release Tablets 1968

Glyburide (Sulfonylurea toxicity). Products include:
- DiaBeta Tablets 1239
- Glynase PresTab Tablets 2609
- Micronase Tablets 2623

Magnesium Salicylate (Decreases half-life of fenoprofen). Products include:
- Backache Caplets ■ 613
- Bayer Select Backache Pain Relief Formula ■ 715
- Doan's Extra-Strength Analgesic ■ 633
- Extra Strength Doan's P.M. ■ 633
- Doan's Regular Strength Analgesic ■ 634
- Mobigesic Tablets ■ 602

Mephenytoin (Potential for increased activity and toxicity of mephenytoin). Products include:
- Mesantoin Tablets 2272

Metformin Hydrochloride (Sulfonylurea toxicity). Products include:
- Glucophage 752

Phenobarbital (Decreases plasma half-life of fenoprofen). Products include:
- Arco-Lase Plus Tablets 512
- Bellergal-S Tablets 2250
- Donnatal 2060
- Donnatal Extentabs 2061
- Donnatal Tablets 2060
- Phenobarbital Elixir and Tablets 1469
- Quadrinal Tablets 1350

Phenytoin (Potential for increased activity and toxicity of phenytoin). Products include:
- Dilantin Infatabs 1908
- Dilantin-125 Suspension 1911

Phenytoin Sodium (Potential for increased activity and toxicity of phenytoin). Products include:
- Dilantin Kapseals 1906
- Dilantin Parenteral 1910

Salsalate (Decreases half-life of fenoprofen). Products include:
- Mono-Gesic Tablets 792
- Salflex Tablets 786

Sulfamethizole (Sulfonamide toxicity). Products include:
- Urobiotic-250 Capsules 2214

Sulfamethoxazole (Sulfonamide toxicity). Products include:
- Azo Gantanol Tablets 2080
- Bactrim DS Tablets 2084
- Bactrim I.V. Infusion 2082
- Bactrim 2084
- Gantanol Tablets 2119
- Septra 1174
- Septra I.V. Infusion 1169
- Septra I.V. Infusion ADD-Vantage Vials 1171
- Septra 1174

Sulfasalazine (Sulfonamide toxicity). Products include:
- Azulfidine 1949

Sulfinpyrazone (Sulfonamide toxicity). Products include:
- Anturane 807

Sulfisoxazole (Sulfonamide toxicity). Products include:
- Azo Gantrisin Tablets 2081
- Gantrisin Tablets 2120

Sulfisoxazole Diolamine (Sulfonamide toxicity).
No products indexed under this heading.

Tolazamide (Sulfonylurea toxicity).
No products indexed under this heading.

Tolbutamide (Sulfonylurea toxicity).
No products indexed under this heading.

Torsemide (Patients treated with Nalfon may be resistant to the effects of loop diuretics). Products include:
- Demadex Tablets and Injection 686

Warfarin Sodium (Prolonged prothrombin time). Products include:
- Coumadin 926

Food Interactions

Dairy products (Peak blood levels are delayed and diminished).

Meal, unspecified (Peak blood levels are delayed and diminished).

NAPHCON-A OPHTHALMIC SOLUTION
(Naphazoline Hydrochloride, Pheniramine Maleate) 473
None cited in PDR database.

NAPROSYN SUSPENSION
(Naproxen) 2117
See **EC-Naprosyn Delayed-Release Tablets**

NAPROSYN TABLETS
(Naproxen) 2117
See **EC-Naprosyn Delayed-Release Tablets**

NARCAN INJECTION
(Naloxone Hydrochloride) 934
May interact with:

Cardiotoxic drugs, unspecified (Narcan should be used with caution in patients who have received potentially cardiotoxic drugs).

NARDIL
(Phenelzine Sulfate) 1920
May interact with monoamine oxidase inhibitors, antihypertensives, sympathomimetics, dibenzazepines, tricyclic antidepressants, phenylpropanolamine containing anorectics, alpha adrenergic stimulants, antidepressant drugs, anorexiants, beta blockers, thiazides, narcotic analgesics, barbiturates, catecholamine depleting drugs, and certain other agents. Compounds in these categories include:

Acebutolol Hydrochloride (Exaggerated hypotensive effects). Products include:
- Sectral Capsules 2807

Albuterol (Hypertensive crises; potentiation of sympathomimetic substances). Products include:
- Proventil Inhalation Aerosol 2382
- Ventolin Inhalation Aerosol and Refill 1197

Albuterol Sulfate (Hypertensive crises; potentiation of sympathomimetic substances). Products include:
- Airet Solution for Inhalation 452
- Proventil Inhalation Solution 0.083% 2384
- Proventil Repetabs Tablets 2386
- Proventil Solution for Inhalation 0.5% 2383
- Proventil Syrup 2385
- Proventil Tablets 2386
- Ventolin Inhalation Solution 1198
- Ventolin Nebules Inhalation Solution 1199
- Ventolin Rotacaps for Inhalation 1200
- Ventolin Syrup 1202
- Ventolin Tablets 1203
- Volmax Extended-Release Tablets 1788

(■ Described in PDR For Nonprescription Drugs) (⊙ Described in PDR For Ophthalmology)

Interactions Index

Alfentanil Hydrochloride (Meperidine contraindication is extended to other narcotics). Products include:

Alfenta Injection 1286

Amitriptyline Hydrochloride (Concurrent or in rapid succession administration is contraindicated). Products include:

Elavil 2838
Endep Tablets 2174
Etrafon 2355
Limbitrol 2180
Triavil Tablets 1757

Amlodipine Besylate (Exaggerated hypotensive effects). Products include:

Lotrel Capsules 840
Norvasc Tablets 1940

Amoxapine (Concurrent or in rapid succession administration is contraindicated). Products include:

Asendin Tablets 1369

Amphetamine Resins (Concurrent administration is not recommended; hypertensive crises). Products include:

Biphetamine Capsules 983

Amphetamine Sulfate (Hypertensive crises; concurrent administration is not recommended).

No products indexed under this heading.

Aprobarbital (Potential for increased hypnosis).

No products indexed under this heading.

Atenolol (Exaggerated hypotensive effects). Products include:

Tenoretic Tablets 2845
Tenormin Tablets and I.V. Injection 2847

Benazepril Hydrochloride (Exaggerated hypotensive effects). Products include:

Lotensin Tablets 834
Lotensin HCT 837
Lotrel Capsules 840

Bendroflumethiazide (Exaggerated hypotensive effects).

No products indexed under this heading.

Benzphetamine Hydrochloride (Concurrent administration is not recommended). Products include:

Didrex Tablets 2607

Betaxolol Hydrochloride (Exaggerated hypotensive effects). Products include:

Betoptic Ophthalmic Solution............ 469
Betoptic S Ophthalmic Suspension 471
Kerlone Tablets 2436

Bisoprolol Fumarate (Exaggerated hypotensive effects). Products include:

Zebeta Tablets 1413
Ziac 1415

Buprenorphine (Meperidine contraindication is extended to other narcotics). Products include:

Buprenex Injectable 2006

Bupropion Hydrochloride (Concurrent administration is contraindicated; at least 14 days should elapse between discontinuation of an MAOI inhibitor and initiation of treatment with bupropion hydrochloride). Products include:

Wellbutrin Tablets 1204

Buspirone Hydrochloride (Elevated blood pressure; concurrent therapy is contraindicated). Products include:

BuSpar 737

Butabarbital (Potential for increased hypnosis).

No products indexed under this heading.

Butalbital (Potential for increased hypnosis). Products include:

Esgic-plus Tablets 1013
Fioricet Tablets 2258
Fioricet with Codeine Capsules 2260
Fiorinal Capsules 2261
Fiorinal with Codeine Capsules 2262
Fiorinal Tablets 2261
Phenrilin 785
Sedapap Tablets 50 mg/650 mg .. 1543

Caffeine-containing medications (Concurrent use with excessive caffeine intake should be avoided).

Captopril (Exaggerated hypotensive effects). Products include:

Capoten 739
Capozide 742

Carbamazepine (Concurrent or in rapid succession administration is contraindicated). Products include:

Atretol Tablets 573
Tegretol Chewable Tablets 852
Tegretol Suspension 852
Tegretol Tablets 852

Carteolol Hydrochloride (Exaggerated hypotensive effects). Products include:

Cartrol Tablets 410
Ocupress Ophthalmic Solution, 1 % Sterile... © 309

Chlorothiazide (Exaggerated hypotensive effects). Products include:

Aldoclor Tablets 1598
Diupres Tablets 1650
Diuril Oral 1653

Chlorothiazide Sodium (Exaggerated hypotensive effects). Products include:

Diuril Sodium Intravenous 1652

Chlorthalidone (Exaggerated hypotensive effects). Products include:

Combipres Tablets 677
Tenoretic Tablets 2845
Thalitone 1245

Clomipramine Hydrochloride (Concurrent or in rapid succession administration is contraindicated). Products include:

Anafranil Capsules 803

Clonidine (Exaggerated hypotensive effects). Products include:

Catapres-TTS 675

Clonidine Hydrochloride (Exaggerated hypotensive effects). Products include:

Catapres Tablets 674
Combipres Tablets 677

Clozapine (Concurrent or in rapid succession administration is contraindicated). Products include:

Clozaril Tablets 2252

Cocaine Hydrochloride (Hypertensive crises). Products include:

Cocaine Hydrochloride Topical Solution 537

Codeine Phosphate (Meperidine contraindication is extended to other narcotics). Products include:

Actifed with Codeine Cough Syrup.. 1067
Brontex 1981
Deconsal C Expectorant Syrup 456
Deconsal Pediatric Syrup 457
Dimetane-DC Cough Syrup 2059
Empirin with Codeine Tablets............ 1093
Fioricet with Codeine Capsules 2260
Fiorinal with Codeine Capsules 2262
Isoclor Expectorant 990
Novahistine DH 2462
Novahistine Expectorant 2463
Nucofed 2051
Phenergan with Codeine 2777
Phenergan VC with Codeine 2781
Robitussin A-C Syrup 2073
Robitussin-DAC Syrup 2074
Ryna .... ⊞ 841
Soma Compound w/Codeine Tablets 2676
Tussi-Organidin NR Liquid and S NR Liquid 2677
Tylenol with Codeine 1583

Cyclobenzaprine Hydrochloride (Possibility of unspecified adverse drug interaction; concurrent or in rapid succession administration should be avoided). Products include:

Flexeril Tablets 1661

Deserpidine (Exaggerated hypotensive effects; exercise caution).

No products indexed under this heading.

Desipramine Hydrochloride (Concurrent or in rapid succession administration is contraindicated). Products include:

Norpramin Tablets 1526

Dextroamphetamine (Hypertensive crises; concurrent administration is not recommended). Products include:

Biphetamine Capsules 983

Dextroamphetamine Sulfate (Hypertensive crises; concurrent administration is not recommended). Products include:

Dexedrine 2474
DextroStat Dextroamphetamine Tablets 2036

Dextromethorphan Hydrobromide (Concurrent administration is not recommended; may cause drowsiness and bizarre behavior). Products include:

Alka-Seltzer Plus Cold & Cough Medicine .... ⊞ 708
Alka-Seltzer Plus Cold & Cough Medicine Liqui-Gels .... ⊞ 705
Alka-Seltzer Plus Night-Time Cold Medicine .... ⊞ 707
Alka-Seltzer Plus Night-Time Cold Medicine Liqui-Gels .... ⊞ 706
Benylin Adult Formula Cough Suppressant .... ⊞ 852
Benylin Expectorant .... ⊞ 852
Benylin Multisymptom .... ⊞ 852
Benylin Pediatric Cough Suppressant .... ⊞ 853
Bromfed-DM Cough Syrup 1786
Buckley's Mixture .... ⊞ 624
Cerose DM .... ⊞ 878
Cheracol-D Cough Formula .... ⊞ 769
Cheracol Plus Head Cold/Cough Formula .... ⊞ 769
Children's Vicks NyQuil Cold/ Cough Relief .... ⊞ 758
Comtrex Multi-Symptom Cold Reliever Tablets/Caplets/Liqui-Gels/Liquid .... ⊞ 615
Comtrex Non-Drowsy .... ⊞ 618
Contac Day & Night Cold/Flu Caplets .... ⊞ 812
Contac Severe Cold and Flu Formula Caplets .... ⊞ 814
Contac Severe Cold & Flu Non-Drowsy .... ⊞ 815
Cough-X Lozenges .... ⊞ 602
Diabe-Tuss DM Syrup 1891
Dimetane-DX Cough Syrup 2059
Dimetapp DM Elixir .... ⊞ 774
Dorcol Children's Cough Syrup ....⊞ 785
Drixoral Cough Liquid Caps .... ⊞ 801
Drixoral Cough + Congestion Liquid Caps .... ⊞ 802
Drixoral Cough + Sore Throat Liquid Caps .... ⊞ 802
Humibid 462
Novahistine DMX .... ⊞ 822
PediaCare Cough-Cold Chewable Tablets 1553
PediaCare Cough-Cold Liquid 1553
PediCare Infant's Drops Decongestant Plus Cough 1553
PediaCare NightRest Cough-Cold Liquid 1553
Pediatric Vicks 44d Dry Hacking Cough & Head Congestion .... ⊞ 763
Pediatric Vicks 44e Chest Cough & Chest Congestion .... ⊞ 764
Pediatric Vicks 44m Cough & Cold Relief .... ⊞ 764
Phenergan with Dextromethorphan 2778
Robitussin Cold & Cough Liqui-Gels .... ⊞ 776
Robitussin Maximum Strength Cough Suppressant .... ⊞ 778

Robitussin Maximum Strength Cough & Cold .... ⊞ 778
Robitussin Pediatric Cough & Cold Formula .... ⊞ 779
Robitussin Pediatric Cough Suppressant .... ⊞ 779
Robitussin-CF .... ⊞ 777
Robitussin-DM .... ⊞ 777
Rondec-DM Oral Drops 954
Rondec-DM Syrup 954
Safe Tussin 30 1363
Sucrets 4-Hour Cough Suppressant .... ⊞ 826
Sudafed Cold and Cough Liquidcaps .... ⊞ 862
Sudafed Cough Syrup .... ⊞ 862
Sudafed Severe Cold Formula Caplets .... ⊞ 863
Sudafed Severe Cold Formula Tablets .... ⊞ 864
Syn-Rx DM Tablets 466
TheraFlu Flu, Cold and Cough Medicine .... ⊞ 787
TheraFlu Maximum Strength Nighttime Flu, Cold & Cough Medicine .... ⊞ 788
TheraFlu Maximum Strength Non-Drowsy Formula Flu, Cold & Cough Medicine .... ⊞ 788
Thera Flu Maximum Strength, Non-Drowsy Formula Flu, Cold and Cough Caplets .... ⊞ 789
Triaminic AM Cough and Decongestant Formula .... ⊞ 789
Triaminic Nite Light .... ⊞ 791
Triaminic Sore Throat Formula ...... ⊞ 791
Triaminic-DM Syrup .... ⊞ 792
Triaminicol Multi-Symptom Cold Tablets .... ⊞ 793
Triaminicol Multi-Symptom Relief ⊞ 794
Tussi-Organidin DM NR Liquid and DM-S NR Liquid 2677
Children's TYLENOL Cold Plus Cough Multi Symptom Tablets and Liquid .... ⊞ 681
TYLENOL Flu Maximum Strength Gelcaps 1565
TYLENOL Cold Multi-Symptom Formula Medication Tablets and Caplets 1561
TYLENOL Cold Medication No Drowsiness Formula Gelcaps and Caplets 1562
TYLENOL Cold Multi-Symptom Hot Medication Liquid Packets 1557
TYLENOL Cough Multi-Symptom Medication 1564
TYLENOL Cough Multi-Symptom Medication with Decongestant 1565
Vicks 44 Dry Hacking Cough .... ⊞ 755
Vicks 44 LiquiCaps Cough, Cold & Flu Relief .... ⊞ 755
Vicks 44 LiquiCaps Non-Drowsy Cough & Cold Relief .... ⊞ 756
Vicks 44D Dry Hacking Cough & Head Congestion .... ⊞ 755
Vicks 44E Chest Cough & Chest Congestion .... ⊞ 756
Vicks 44M Cough, Cold & Flu Relief .... ⊞ 756
Vicks DayQuil .... ⊞ 761
Vicks Nyquil Hot Therapy .... ⊞ 762
Vicks NyQuil LiquiCaps Multi-Symptom Cold/Flu Relief .... ⊞ 763
Vicks NyQuil Multi-Symptom Cold/Flu Relief - (Original & Cherry Flavor) .... ⊞ 763

Dextromethorphan Polistirex (Concurrent administration is not recommended; may cause drowsiness and bizarre behavior). Products include:

Delsym Extended-Release Suspension .... ⊞ 654

Dezocine (Meperidine contraindication is extended to other narcotics). Products include:

Dalgan Injection 538

Diazoxide (Exaggerated hypotensive effects). Products include:

Hyperstat I.V. Injection 2363
Proglycem 580

Diethylpropion Hydrochloride (Concurrent administration is not recommended).

No products indexed under this heading.

IMPORTANT NOTE: Always consult each drug listing in the patient's regimen for possible interactions.

Nardil
Interactions Index
694

Diltiazem Hydrochloride (Exaggerated hypotensive effects). Products include:
- Cardizem CD Capsules ... 1506
- Cardizem SR Capsules ... 1510
- Cardizem Injectable ... 1508
- Cardizem Tablets ... 1512
- Dilacor XR Extended-release Capsules ... 2018

Dobutamine Hydrochloride (Hypertensive crises; potentiation of sympathomimetic substances). Products include:
- Dobutrex Solution Vials ... 1439

Dopamine Hydrochloride (Hypertensive crises; potentiation of sympathomimetic substances).
- No products indexed under this heading.

Doxazosin Mesylate (Exaggerated hypotensive effects). Products include:
- Cardura Tablets ... 2186

Doxepin Hydrochloride (Concurrent or in rapid succession administration is contraindicated). Products include:
- Sinequan ... 2205
- Zonalon Cream ... 1055

Enalapril Maleate (Exaggerated hypotensive effects). Products include:
- Vaseretic Tablets ... 1765
- Vasotec Tablets ... 1771

Enalaprilat (Exaggerated hypotensive effects). Products include:
- Vasotec I.V. ... 1768

Ephedrine Hydrochloride (Hypertensive crises; potentiation of sympathomimetic substances). Products include:
- Primatene Dual Action Formula ... ▣ 872
- Primatene Tablets ... ▣ 873
- Quadrinal Tablets ... 1350

Ephedrine Sulfate (Hypertensive crises; potentiation of sympathomimetic substances). Products include:
- Bronkaid Caplets ... ▣ 717
- Marax Tablets & DF Syrup ... 2200

Ephedrine Tannate (Hypertensive crises; potentiation of sympathomimetic substances). Products include:
- Rynatuss ... 2673

Epinephrine (Hypertensive crises; potentiation of sympathomimetic substances). Products include:
- Bronkaid Mist ... ▣ 717
- EPIFRIN ... ⊚ 239
- EpiPen ... 790
- Marcaine Hydrochloride with Epinephrine 1:200,000 ... 2316
- Primatene Mist ... ▣ 873
- Sensorcaine with Epinephrine Injection ... 559
- Sus-Phrine Injection ... 1019
- Xylocaine with Epinephrine Injections ... 567

Epinephrine Bitartrate (Hypertensive crises; potentiation of sympathomimetic substances). Products include:
- Bronkaid Mist Suspension ... ▣ 718
- Sensorcaine-MPF with Epinephrine Injection ... 559

Epinephrine Hydrochloride (Hypertensive crises; potentiation of sympathomimetic substances). Products include:
- Ana-Kit Anaphylaxis Emergency Treatment Kit ... 617

Esmolol Hydrochloride (Exaggerated hypotensive effects). Products include:
- Brevibloc Injection ... 1808

Felodipine (Exaggerated hypotensive effects). Products include:
- Plendil Extended-Release Tablets ... 527

Fenfluramine Hydrochloride (Concurrent administration is not recommended). Products include:
- Pondimin Tablets ... 2066

Fentanyl (Meperidine contraindication is extended to other narcotics). Products include:
- Duragesic Transdermal System ... 1288

Fentanyl Citrate (Meperidine contraindication is extended to other narcotics). Products include:
- Sublimaze Injection ... 1307

Fluoxetine Hydrochloride (Concurrent or in rapid succession administration is contraindicated; serious reactions including hyperthermia, rigidity, myoclonic movements and death have been reported). Products include:
- Prozac Pulvules & Liquid, Oral Solution ... 919

Fosinopril Sodium (Exaggerated hypotensive effects). Products include:
- Monopril Tablets ... 757

Furazolidone (Hypertensive crises; at least 10 days should elapse between discontinuation of Nardil and institution of another MAOI). Products include:
- Furoxone ... 2046

Furosemide (Exaggerated hypotensive effects). Products include:
- Lasix Injection, Oral Solution and Tablets ... 1240

Guanabenz Acetate (Exaggerated hypotensive effects).
- No products indexed under this heading.

Guanethidine Monosulfate (Exaggerated hypotensive effects; contraindication). Products include:
- Esimil Tablets ... 822
- Ismelin Tablets ... 827

Hexobarbital (Potential for increased hypnosis).

Hydralazine Hydrochloride (Exaggerated hypotensive effects). Products include:
- Apresazide Capsules ... 808
- Apresoline Hydrochloride Tablets ... 809
- Ser-Ap-Es Tablets ... 849

Hydrochlorothiazide (Exaggerated hypotensive effects). Products include:
- Aldactazide ... 2413
- Aldoril Tablets ... 1604
- Apresazide Capsules ... 808
- Capozide ... 742
- Dyazide ... 2479
- Esidrix Tablets ... 821
- Esimil Tablets ... 822
- HydroDIURIL Tablets ... 1674
- Hydropres Tablets ... 1675
- Hyzaar Tablets ... 1677
- Inderide Tablets ... 2732
- Inderide LA Long Acting Capsules ... 2734
- Lopressor HCT Tablets ... 832
- Lotensin HCT ... 837
- Maxzide ... 1380
- Moduretic Tablets ... 1705
- Oretic Tablets ... 443
- Prinzide Tablets ... 1737
- Ser-Ap-Es Tablets ... 849
- Timolide Tablets ... 1748
- Vaseretic Tablets ... 1765
- Zestoretic ... 2850
- Ziac ... 1415

Hydrocodone Bitartrate (Meperidine contraindication is extended to other narcotics). Products include:
- Anexsia 5/500 Elixir ... 1781
- Anexia Tablets ... 1782
- Codiclear DH Syrup ... 791
- Deconamine CX Cough and Cold Liquid and Tablets ... 1319
- Duratuss HD Elixir ... 2565
- Hycodan Tablets and Syrup ... 930
- Hycomine Compound Tablets ... 932
- Hycomine ... 931
- Hycotuss Expectorant Syrup ... 933
- Hydrocet Capsules ... 782
- Lorcet 10/650 ... 1018
- Lortab ... 2566
- Tussend ... 1783
- Tussend Expectorant ... 1785
- Vicodin Tablets ... 1356
- Vicodin ES Tablets ... 1357
- Vicodin Tuss Expectorant ... 1358
- Zydone Capsules ... 949

Hydrocodone Polistirex (Meperidine contraindication is extended to other narcotics). Products include:
- Tussionex Pennkinetic Extended-Release Suspension ... 998

Hydroflumethiazide (Exaggerated hypotensive effects). Products include:
- Diucardin Tablets ... 2718

Imipramine Hydrochloride (Concurrent or in rapid succession administration is contraindicated). Products include:
- Tofranil Ampuls ... 854
- Tofranil Tablets ... 856

Imipramine Pamoate (Concurrent or in rapid succession administration is contraindicated). Products include:
- Tofranil-PM Capsules ... 857

Indapamide (Exaggerated hypotensive effects). Products include:
- Lozol Tablets ... 2022

Isocarboxazid (Hypertensive crises; at least 10 days should elapse between discontinuation of Nardil and institution of another MAOI).
- No products indexed under this heading.

Isoproterenol Hydrochloride (Hypertensive crises; potentiation of sympathomimetic substances). Products include:
- Isuprel Hydrochloride Injection 1:5000 ... 2311
- Isuprel Hydrochloride Solution 1:200 & 1:100 ... 2313
- Isuprel Mistometer ... 2312

Isoproterenol Sulfate (Hypertensive crises; potentiation of sympathomimetic substances). Products include:
- Norisodrine with Calcium Iodide Syrup ... 442

Isradipine (Exaggerated hypotensive effects). Products include:
- DynaCirc Capsules ... 2256

Labetalol Hydrochloride (Exaggerated hypotensive effects). Products include:
- Normodyne Injection ... 2377
- Normodyne Tablets ... 2379
- Trandate ... 1185

Levobunolol Hydrochloride (Exaggerated hypotensive effects). Products include:
- Betagan ... ⊚ 233

Levodopa (Concurrent use should be avoided). Products include:
- Atamet ... 572
- Larodopa Tablets ... 2129
- Sinemet Tablets ... 943
- Sinemet CR Tablets ... 944

Levorphanol Tartrate (Meperidine contraindication is extended to other narcotics). Products include:
- Levo-Dromoran ... 2129

Lisinopril (Exaggerated hypotensive effects). Products include:
- Prinivil Tablets ... 1733
- Prinzide Tablets ... 1737
- Zestoretic ... 2850
- Zestril Tablets ... 2854

Losartan Potassium (Exaggerated hypotensive effects). Products include:
- Cozaar Tablets ... 1628
- Hyzaar Tablets ... 1677

Maprotiline Hydrochloride (Concurrent or in rapid succession administration is contraindicated). Products include:
- Ludiomil Tablets ... 843

Mazindol (Concurrent administration is not recommended). Products include:
- Sanorex Tablets ... 2294

Mecamylamine Hydrochloride (Exaggerated hypotensive effects). Products include:
- Inversine Tablets ... 1686

Meperidine Hydrochloride (Concurrent therapy is contraindicated; circulatory collapse, seizures, coma and death have been reported). Products include:
- Demerol ... 2308
- Mepergan Injection ... 2753

Mephobarbital (Potential for increased hypnosis). Products include:
- Mebaral Tablets ... 2322

Metaproterenol Sulfate (Hypertensive crises; potentiation of sympathomimetic substances). Products include:
- Alupent ... 669
- Metaproterenol Sulfate Inhalation Solution, USP, Arm-a-Med ... 552

Metaraminol Bitartrate (Hypertensive crises; potentiation of sympathomimetic substances). Products include:
- Aramine Injection ... 1609

Methadone Hydrochloride (Meperidine contraindication is extended to other narcotics). Products include:
- Methadone Hydrochloride Oral Concentrate ... 2233
- Methadone Hydrochloride Oral Solution & Tablets ... 2235

Methamphetamine Hydrochloride (Concurrent administration is not recommended). Products include:
- Desoxyn Gradumet Tablets ... 419

Methoxamine Hydrochloride (Hypertensive crises; potentiation of sympathomimetic substances). Products include:
- Vasoxyl Injection ... 1196

Methyclothiazide (Exaggerated hypotensive effects). Products include:
- Enduron Tablets ... 420

Methyldopa (Hypertensive crises; exaggerated hypotensive effects). Products include:
- Aldoclor Tablets ... 1598
- Aldomet Oral ... 1600
- Aldoril Tablets ... 1604

Methyldopate Hydrochloride (Hypertensive crises; exaggerated hypotensive effects). Products include:
- Aldomet Ester HCl Injection ... 1602

Methylphenidate Hydrochloride (Hypertensive crises). Products include:
- Ritalin ... 848

Metipranolol Hydrochloride (Exaggerated hypotensive effects). Products include:
- OptiPranolol (Metipranolol 0.3%) Sterile Ophthalmic Solution ... ⊚ 258

Metolazone (Exaggerated hypotensive effects). Products include:
- Mykrox Tablets ... 993
- Zaroxolyn Tablets ... 1000

Metoprolol Succinate (Exaggerated hypotensive effects). Products include:
- Toprol-XL Tablets ... 565

Metoprolol Tartrate (Exaggerated hypotensive effects). Products include:
- Lopressor Ampuls ... 830
- Lopressor HCT Tablets ... 832

(▣ Described in PDR For Nonprescription Drugs)
(⊚ Described in PDR For Ophthalmology)

695 **Interactions Index** **Nardil**

Lopressor Tablets ... 830

Metyrosine (Exaggerated hypotensive effects). Products include:

Demser Capsules ... 1649

Minoxidil (Exaggerated hypotensive effects). Products include:

Loniten Tablets ... 2618
Rogaine Topical Solution ... 2637

Moexipril Hydrochloride (Exaggerated hypotensive effects). Products include:

Univasc Tablets ... 2410

Morphine Sulfate (Meperidine contraindication is extended to other narcotics). Products include:

Astramorph/PF Injection, USP (Preservative-Free) ... 535
Duramorph ... 962
Infumorph 200 and Infumorph 500 Sterile Solutions ... 965
MS Contin Tablets ... 1994
MSIR ... 1997
Oramorph SR (Morphine Sulfate Sustained Release Tablets) ... 2236
RMS Suppositories ... 2657
Roxanol ... 2243

Nadolol (Exaggerated hypotensive effects).

No products indexed under this heading.

Naphazoline Hydrochloride (Contraindicated). Products include:

Albalon Solution with Liquifilm ... ⊙ 231
Clear Eyes ACR Astringent/Lubricant Eye Redness Reliever Eye Drops ... ⊙ 316
Clear Eyes Lubricant Eye Redness Reliever ... ⊙ 316
4-Way Fast Acting Nasal Spray (regular & mentholated) ... ▣ 621
Naphcon-A Ophthalmic Solution ... 473
Privine ... ▣ 647
Vasocon-A ... ⊙ 271

Nefazodone Hydrochloride (Concurrent or in rapid succession administration is contraindicated). Products include:

Serzone Tablets ... 771

Nicardipine Hydrochloride (Exaggerated hypotensive effects). Products include:

Cardene Capsules ... 2095
Cardene I.V. ... 2709
Cardene SR Capsules ... 2097

Nifedipine (Exaggerated hypotensive effects). Products include:

Adalat Capsules (10 mg and 20 mg) ... 587
Adalat CC ... 589
Procardia Capsules ... 1971
Procardia XL Extended Release Tablets ... 1972

Nisoldipine (Exaggerated hypotensive effects).

No products indexed under this heading.

Nitroglycerin (Exaggerated hypotensive effects). Products include:

Deponit NTG Transdermal Delivery System ... 2397
Nitro-Bid IV ... 1523
Nitro-Bid Ointment ... 1524
Nitrodisc ... 2047
Nitro-Dur (nitroglycerin) Transdermal Infusion System ... 1326
Nitrolingual Spray ... 2027
Nitrostat Tablets ... 1925
Transderm-Nitro Transdermal Therapeutic System ... 859

Norepinephrine Bitartrate (Hypertensive crises; potentiation of sympathomimetic substances). Products include:

Levophed Bitartrate Injection ... 2315

Nortriptyline Hydrochloride (Hypertensive crises; concurrent or in rapid succession administration is contraindicated). Products include:

Pamelor ... 2280

Opium Alkaloids (Meperidine contraindication is extended to other narcotics).

No products indexed under this heading.

Oxycodone Hydrochloride (Meperidine contraindication is extended to other narcotics). Products include:

Percocet Tablets ... 938
Percodan Tablets ... 939
Percodan-Demi Tablets ... 940
Roxicodone Tablets, Oral Solution & Intensol (Oxycodone) ... 2244
Tylox Capsules ... 1584

Oxymetazoline Hydrochloride (Contraindicated). Products include:

Afrin ... ▣ 797
Cheracol Nasal Spray Pump ... ▣ 768
Duration 12 Hour Nasal Spray ... ▣ 805
4-Way Long Lasting Nasal Spray ... ▣ 621
NTZ Long Acting Nasal Spray & Drops 0.05% ... ▣ 727
Neo-Synephrine Maximum Strength 12 Hour Nasal Spray ... ▣ 726
Neo-Synephrine 12 Hour ... ▣ 726
Nōstrilla Long Acting Nasal Decongestant ... ▣ 644
Vicks Sinex 12-Hour Nasal Decongestant Spray and Ultra Fine Mist ... ▣ 765
Visine L.R. Eye Drops ... ▣ 746
Visine L.R. Eye Drops ... ⊙ 313

Paroxetine Hydrochloride (Concurrent or in rapid succession administration is contraindicated). Products include:

Paxil Tablets ... 2505

Penbutolol Sulfate (Exaggerated hypotensive effects). Products include:

Levatol ... 2403

Pentobarbital Sodium (Potential for increased hypnosis). Products include:

Nembutal Sodium Capsules ... 436
Nembutal Sodium Solution ... 438
Nembutal Sodium Suppositories ... 440

Phendimetrazine Tartrate (Concurrent administration is not recommended). Products include:

Bontril Slow-Release Capsules ... 781
Prelu-2 Timed Release Capsules ... 681

Phenmetrazine Hydrochloride (Concurrent administration is not recommended).

No products indexed under this heading.

Phenobarbital (Potential for increased hypnosis). Products include:

Arco-Lase Plus Tablets ... 512
Bellergal-S Tablets ... 2250
Donnatal ... 2060
Donnatal Extentabs ... 2061
Donnatal Tablets ... 2060
Phenobarbital Elixir and Tablets ... 1469
Quadrinal Tablets ... 1350

Phenoxybenzamine Hydrochloride (Exaggerated hypotensive effects). Products include:

Dibenzyline Capsules ... 2476

Phentolamine Mesylate (Exaggerated hypotensive effects). Products include:

Regitine ... 846

d-Phenylalanine (Concurrent use should be avoided).

L-Phenylalanine (Concurrent use should be avoided).

Phenylephrine Bitartrate (Hypertensive crises; potentiation of sympathomimetic substances).

No products indexed under this heading.

Phenylephrine Hydrochloride (Hypertensive crises; potentiation of sympathomimetic substances). Products include:

Atrohist Plus Tablets ... 454
Cerose DM ... ▣ 878
Comhist ... 2038
D.A. Chewable Tablets ... 951
Deconsal Pediatric Capsules ... 454
Dura-Vent/DA Tablets ... 953
Entex Capsules ... 1986
Entex Liquid ... 1986
Extendryl ... 1005
4-Way Fast Acting Nasal Spray (regular & mentholated) ... ▣ 621
Hemorid For Women ... ▣ 834
Hycomine Compound Tablets ... 932
Neo-Synephrine Hydrochloride 1% Carpuject ... 2324
Neo-Synephrine Hydrochloride 1% Injection ... 2324
Neo-Synephrine Hydrochloride (Ophthalmic) ... 2325
Neo-Synephrine ... ▣ 726
Nōstril ... ▣ 644
Novahistine Elixir ... ▣ 823
Phenergan VC ... 2779
Phenergan VC with Codeine ... 2781
Preparation H ... ▣ 871
Tympagesic Ear Drops ... 2342
Vasosulf ... ⊙ 271
Vicks Sinex Nasal Spray and Ultra Fine Mist ... ▣ 765

Phenylephrine Tannate (Hypertensive crises; potentiation of sympathomimetic substances). Products include:

Atrohist Pediatric Suspension ... 454
Ricobid-D Pediatric Suspension ... 2038
Ricobid Tablets and Pediatric Suspension ... 2038
Rynatan ... 2673
Rynatuss ... 2673

Phenylpropanolamine Containing Anorectics (Concurrent administration is not recommended).

Phenylpropanolamine Hydrochloride (Hypertensive crises; potentiation of sympathomimetic substances). Products include:

Acutrim ... ▣ 628
Allerest Children's Chewable Tablets ... ▣ 627
Allerest 12 Hour Caplets ... ▣ 627
Atrohist Plus Tablets ... 454
BC Cold Powder Multi-Symptom Formula (Cold-Sinus-Allergy) ... ▣ 609
BC Cold Powder Non-Drowsy Formula (Cold-Sinus) ... ▣ 609
Cheracol Plus Head Cold/Cough Formula ... ▣ 769
Comtrex Multi-Symptom Non-Drowsy Liqui-gels ... ▣ 618
Contac Continuous Action Nasal Decongestant/Antihistamine 12 Hour Capsules ... ▣ 813
Contac Maximum Strength Continuous Action Decongestant/Antihistamine 12 Hour Caplets ... ▣ 813
Contac Severe Cold and Flu Formula Caplets ... ▣ 814
Coricidin 'D' Decongestant Tablets ... ▣ 800
Dexatrim ... ▣ 832
Dexatrim Plus Vitamins Caplets ... ▣ 832
Dimetane-DC Cough Syrup ... 2059
Dimetapp Elixir ... ▣ 773
Dimetapp Extentabs ... ▣ 774
Dimetapp Tablets/Liqui-Gels ... ▣ 775
Dimetapp Cold & Allergy Chewable Tablets ... ▣ 773
Dimetapp DM Elixir ... ▣ 774
Dura-Vent Tablets ... 952
Entex Capsules ... 1986
Entex LA Tablets ... 1987
Entex Liquid ... 1986
Exgest LA Tablets ... 782
Hycomine ... 931
Isoclor Timesule Capsules ... ▣ 637
Nolamine Timed-Release Tablets ... 785
Ornade Spansule Capsules ... 2502
Propagest Tablets ... 786
Pyrroxate Caplets ... ▣ 772
Robitussin-CF ... ▣ 777
Sinulin Tablets ... 787
Tavist-D 12 Hour Relief Tablets ... ▣ 787
Teldrin 12 Hour Antihistamine/Nasal Decongestant Allergy Relief Capsules ... ▣ 826
Triaminic Allergy Tablets ... ▣ 789
Triaminic Cold Tablets ... ▣ 790
Triaminic Expectorant ... ▣ 790
Triaminic Syrup ... ▣ 792
Triaminic-12 Tablets ... ▣ 792
Triaminic-DM Syrup ... ▣ 792
Triaminicin Tablets ... ▣ 793
Triaminicol Multi-Symptom Cold Tablets ... ▣ 793
Triaminicol Multi-Symptom Relief ▣ 794
Vicks DayQuil Allergy Relief 12-Hour Extended Release Tablets ... ▣ 760
Vicks DayQuil Allergy Relief 4-Hour Tablets ... ▣ 760
Vicks DayQuil SINUS Pressure & CONGESTION Relief ... ▣ 761

Pindolol (Exaggerated hypotensive effects). Products include:

Visken Tablets ... 2299

Pirbuterol Acetate (Hypertensive crises; potentiation of sympathomimetic substances). Products include:

Maxair Autohaler ... 1492
Maxair Inhaler ... 1494

Polythiazide (Exaggerated hypotensive effects). Products include:

Minizide Capsules ... 1938

Prazosin Hydrochloride (Exaggerated hypotensive effects). Products include:

Minipress Capsules ... 1937
Minizide Capsules ... 1938

Propoxyphene Hydrochloride (Meperidine contraindication is extended to other narcotics). Products include:

Darvon ... 1435
Wygesic Tablets ... 2827

Propoxyphene Napsylate (Meperidine contraindication is extended to other narcotics). Products include:

Darvon-N/Darvocet-N ... 1433

Propranolol Hydrochloride (Exaggerated hypotensive effects). Products include:

Inderal ... 2728
Inderal LA Long Acting Capsules ... 2730
Inderide Tablets ... 2732
Inderide LA Long Acting Capsules ... 2734

Protriptyline Hydrochloride (Concurrent or in rapid succession administration is contraindicated). Products include:

Vivactil Tablets ... 1774

Pseudoephedrine Hydrochloride (Hypertensive crises; potentiation of sympathomimetic substances). Products include:

Actifed Allergy Daytime/Nighttime Caplets ... ▣ 844
Actifed Plus Caplets ... ▣ 845
Actifed Plus Tablets ... ▣ 845
Actifed with Codeine Cough Syrup ... 1067
Actifed Sinus Daytime/Nighttime Tablets and Caplets ... ▣ 846
Actifed Syrup ... ▣ 846
Actifed Tablets ... ▣ 844
Advil Cold and Sinus Caplets and Tablets (formerly CoAdvil) ... ▣ 870
Alka-Seltzer Plus Cold Medicine Liqui-Gels ... ▣ 706
Alka-Seltzer Plus Cold & Cough Medicine Liqui-Gels ... ▣ 705
Alka-Seltzer Plus Night-Time Cold Medicine Liqui-Gels ... ▣ 706
Allerest Headache Strength Tablets ... ▣ 627
Allerest Maximum Strength Tablets ... ▣ 627
Allerest No Drowsiness Tablets ... ▣ 627
Allerest Sinus Pain Formula ... ▣ 627
Anatuss LA Tablets ... 1542
Atrohist Pediatric Capsules ... 453
Bayer Select Sinus Pain Relief Formula ... ▣ 717
Benadryl Allergy Decongestant Liquid Medication ... ▣ 848
Benadryl Allergy Decongestant Tablets ... ▣ 848
Benadryl Allergy Sinus Headache Formula Caplets ... ▣ 849
Benylin Multisymptom ... ▣ 852
Bromfed Capsules (Extended-Release) ... 1785
Bromfed Syrup ... ▣ 733
Bromfed Tablets ... 1785
Bromfed-DM Cough Syrup ... 1786
Bromfed-PD Capsules (Extended-Release) ... 1785
Children's Vicks DayQuil Allergy Relief ... ▣ 757

IMPORTANT NOTE: Always consult each drug listing in the patient's regimen for possible interactions.

Nardil **Interactions Index** 696

Children's Vicks NyQuil Cold/Cough Relief ◘ 758
Comtrex Multi-Symptom Cold Reliever Tablets/Caplets/Liqui-Gels/Liquid ◘ 615
Allergy-Sinus Comtrex Multi-Symptom Allergy-Sinus Formula Tablets ◘ 617
Comtrex Multi-Symptom Non-Drowsy Caplets ◘ 618
Congess 1004
Contac Day Allergy/Sinus Caplets ◘ 812
Contac Day & Night ◘ 812
Contac Night Allergy/Sinus Caplets ◘ 812
Contac Severe Cold & Flu Non-Drowsy ◘ 815
Deconamine Chewable Tablets 1320
Deconamine CX Cough and Cold Liquid and Tablets 1319
Deconamine 1320
Deconsal C Expectorant Syrup 456
Deconsal Pediatric Syrup 457
Deconsal II Tablets 454
Dimetane-DX Cough Syrup 2059
Dimetapp Sinus Caplets ◘ 775
Dorcol Children's Cough Syrup ◘ 785
Drixoral Cough + Congestion Liquid Caps ◘ 802
Dura-Tap/PD Capsules 2867
Duratuss Tablets 2565
Duratuss HD Elixir 2565
Efidac/24 ◘ 635
Entex PSE Tablets 1987
Fedahist Gyrocaps 2401
Fedahist Timecaps 2401
Guaifed 1787
Guaifed Syrup ◘ 734
Guaimax-D Tablets 792
Guaitab Tablets ◘ 734
Isoclor Expectorant 990
Kronofed-A 977
Motrin IB Sinus ◘ 838
Novahistine DH 2462
Novahistine DMX ◘ 822
Novahistine Expectorant 2463
Nucofed 2051
PediaCare Cold Allergy Chewable Tablets ◘ 677
PediaCare Cough-Cold Chewable Tablets 1553
PediaCare 1553
PediaCare Infants' Decongestant Drops ◘ 677
PediCare Infant's Drops Decongestant Plus Cough 1553
PediaCare NightRest Cough-Cold Liquid 1553
Pediatric Vicks 44d Dry Hacking Cough & Head Congestion ◘ 763
Pediatric Vicks 44m Cough & Cold Relief ◘ 764
Robitussin Cold & Cough Liqui-Gels ◘ 776
Robitussin Maximum Strength Cough & Cold ◘ 778
Robitussin Pediatric Cough & Cold Formula ◘ 779
Robitussin Severe Congestion Liqui-Gels ◘ 776
Robitussin-DAC Syrup 2074
Robitussin-PE ◘ 778
Rondec Oral Drops 953
Rondec Syrup 953
Rondec Tablet 953
Rondec-DM Oral Drops 954
Rondec-DM Syrup 954
Rondec-TR Tablet 953
Ryna ◘ 841
Seldane-D Extended-Release Tablets 1538
Semprex-D Capsules 463
Semprex-D Capsules 1167
Sinarest Tablets ◘ 648
Sinarest Extra Strength Tablets ◘ 648
Sinarest No Drowsiness Tablets ◘ 648
Sine-Aid IB Caplets 1554
Sine-Aid Maximum Strength Sinus Medication Gelcaps, Caplets and Tablets 1554
Sine-Off No Drowsiness Formula Caplets ◘ 824
Sine-Off Sinus Medicine ◘ 825
Singlet Tablets ◘ 825
Sinutab Non-Drying Liquid Caps ◘ 859
Sinutab Sinus Allergy Medication, Maximum Strength Tablets and Caplets ◘ 860
Sinutab Sinus Medication, Maximum Strength Without Drowsiness Formula, Tablets & Caplets ◘ 860
Sinutab Sinus Medication, Regular Strength Without Drowsiness Formula ◘ 859
Sudafed Children's Liquid ◘ 861
Sudafed Cold and Cough Liquidcaps ◘ 862
Sudafed Cough Syrup ◘ 862
Sudafed Plus Liquid ◘ 862
Sudafed Plus Tablets ◘ 863
Sudafed Severe Cold Formula Caplets ◘ 863
Sudafed Severe Cold Formula Tablets ◘ 864
Sudafed Sinus Caplets ◘ 864
Sudafed Sinus Tablets ◘ 864
Sudafed Tablets, 30 mg ◘ 861
Sudafed Tablets, 60 mg ◘ 861
Sudafed 12 Hour Caplets ◘ 861
Syn-Rx Tablets 465
Syn-Rx DM Tablets 466
TheraFlu ◘ 787
TheraFlu Maximum Strength Nighttime Flu, Cold & Cough Medicine ◘ 788
TheraFlu Maximum Strength Non-Drowsy Formula Flu, Cold & Cough Medicine ◘ 788
Thera Flu Maximum Strength, Non-Drowsy Formula Flu, Cold and Cough Caplets ◘ 789
Triaminic AM Cough and Decongestant Formula ◘ 789
Triaminic AM Decongestant Formula ◘ 790
Triaminic Nite Light ◘ 791
Triaminic Sore Throat Formula ◘ 791
Tussend 1783
Tussend Expectorant 1785
Children's TYLENOL Cold Multi-Symptom Liquid Formula and Chewable Tablets 1561
Children's TYLENOL Cold Plus Cough Multi Symptom Tablets and Liquid ◘ 681
Infants' TYLENOL Cold Decongestant & Fever-Reducer Drops 1556
TYLENOL Maximum Strength Allergy Sinus Medication Gelcaps and Caplets 1563
TYLENOL Maximum Strength Allergy Sinus NightTime Medication Caplets 1555
TYLENOL Flu Maximum Strength Gelcaps 1565
TYLENOL Flu NightTime, Maximum Strength, Gelcaps 1566
TYLENOL Maximum Strength Flu NightTime Hot Medication Packets 1562
TYLENOL, Maximum Strength, Sinus Medication Geltabs, Gelcaps, Caplets and Tablets 1566
TYLENOL Cold Multi-Symptom Formula Medication Tablets and Caplets 1561
TYLENOL Cold Medication No Drowsiness Formula Gelcaps and Caplets 1562
TYLENOL Cold Multi-Symptom Hot Medication Liquid Packets 1557
TYLENOL Cough Multi-Symptom Medication with Decongestant 1565
Ursinus Inlay-Tabs ◘ 794
Vicks 44 LiquiCaps Cough, Cold & Flu Relief ◘ 755
Vicks 44 LiquiCaps Non-Drowsy Cough & Cold Relief ◘ 756
Vicks 44D Dry Hacking Cough & Head Congestion ◘ 755
Vicks 44M Cough, Cold & Flu Relief ◘ 756
Vicks DayQuil ◘ 761
Vicks DayQuil SINUS Pressure & PAIN Relief with IBUPROFEN ◘ 762
Vicks Nyquil Hot Therapy ◘ 762
Vicks NyQuil LiquiCaps Multi-Symptom Cold/Flu Relief ◘ 763
Vicks NyQuil Multi-Symptom Cold/Flu Relief - (Original & Cherry Flavor) ◘ 763

Pseudoephedrine Sulfate (Hypertensive crises; potentiation of sympathomimetic substances). Products include:
Cheracol Sinus ◘ 768
Chlor-Trimeton Allergy Decongestant Tablets ◘ 799
Claritin-D 2350
Drixoral Cold and Allergy Sustained-Action Tablets ◘ 802
Drixoral Cold and Flu Extended-Release Tablets ◘ 803
Drixoral Non-Drowsy Formula Extended-Release Tablets ◘ 803
Drixoral Allergy/Sinus Extended Release Tablets ◘ 804
Trinalin Repetabs Tablets 1330

Quinapril Hydrochloride (Exaggerated hypotensive effects). Products include:
Accupril Tablets 1893

Ramipril (Exaggerated hypotensive effects). Products include:
Altace Capsules 1232

Rauwolfia Serpentina (Exaggerated hypotensive effects; exercise caution).
No products indexed under this heading.

Rescinnamine (Exaggerated hypotensive effects; exercise caution).
No products indexed under this heading.

Reserpine (Exaggerated hypotensive effects; exercise caution). Products include:
Diupres Tablets 1650
Hydropres Tablets 1675
Ser-Ap-Es Tablets 849

Salmeterol Xinafoate (Hypertensive crises; potentiation of sympathomimetic substances). Products include:
Serevent Inhalation Aerosol 1176

Secobarbital Sodium (Potential for increased hypnosis). Products include:
Seconal Sodium Pulvules 1474

Selegiline Hydrochloride (Hypertensive crises; at least 10 days should elapse between discontinuation of Nardil and institution of another MAOI). Products include:
Eldepryl Tablets 2550

Sertraline Hydrochloride (Concurrent or in rapid succession administration is contraindicated). Products include:
Zoloft Tablets 2217

Sodium Nitroprusside (Exaggerated hypotensive effects).
No products indexed under this heading.

Sotalol Hydrochloride (Exaggerated hypotensive effects). Products include:
Betapace Tablets 641

Spirapril Hydrochloride (Exaggerated hypotensive effects).
No products indexed under this heading.

Sufentanil Citrate (Meperidine contraindication is extended to other narcotics). Products include:
Sufenta Injection 1309

Terazosin Hydrochloride (Exaggerated hypotensive effects). Products include:
Hytrin Capsules 430

Terbutaline Sulfate (Hypertensive crises; potentiation of sympathomimetic substances). Products include:
Brethaire Inhaler 813
Brethine Ampuls 815
Brethine Tablets 814
Bricanyl Subcutaneous Injection 1502
Bricanyl Tablets 1503

Tetrahydrozoline Hydrochloride (Contraindicated). Products include:
Collyrium Fresh ◉ 325
Murine Plus Lubricant Redness Reliever Eye Drops ◘ 781
Murine Tears Plus Lubricant Redness Reliever Eye Drops ◉ 316
Visine Maximum Strength Allergy Relief ◉ 313
Visine Moisturizing Eye Drops ◉ 313
Visine Original Eye Drops ◉ 314

Thiamylal Sodium (Potential for increased hypnosis).
No products indexed under this heading.

Timolol Hemihydrate (Exaggerated hypotensive effects). Products include:
Betimol 0.25%, 0.5% ◉ 261

Timolol Maleate (Exaggerated hypotensive effects). Products include:
Blocadren Tablets 1614
Timolide Tablets 1748
Timoptic in Ocudose 1753
Timoptic Sterile Ophthalmic Solution 1751
Timoptic-XE 1755

Torsemide (Exaggerated hypotensive effects). Products include:
Demadex Tablets and Injection 686

Tranylcypromine Sulfate (Hypertensive crises; at least 10 days should elapse between discontinuation of Nardil and institution of another MAOI). Products include:
Parnate Tablets 2503

Trimethaphan Camsylate (Exaggerated hypotensive effects). Products include:
Arfonad Ampuls 2080

Trimipramine Maleate (Concurrent or in rapid succession administration is contraindicated). Products include:
Surmontil Capsules 2811

L-Tryptophan (Concurrent use should be avoided).
No products indexed under this heading.

Tyramine (Concurrent use should be avoided).

L-Tyrosine (Concurrent use should be avoided). Products include:
Catemine Enteric Tablets (Tyrosine) 2565

Venlafaxine Hydrochloride (Concurrent or in rapid succession administration is contraindicated). Products include:
Effexor 2719

Verapamil Hydrochloride (Exaggerated hypotensive effects). Products include:
Calan SR Caplets 2422
Calan Tablets 2419
Isoptin Injectable 1344
Isoptin Oral Tablets 1346
Isoptin SR Tablets 1348
Verelan Capsules 1410
Verelan Capsules 2824

Food Interactions

Alcohol (Hypertensive crises).

Beans, broad (Concurrent and/or sequential intake must be avoided).

Beans, Fava (Concurrent and/or sequential intake must be avoided).

Beer, alcohol-free (Concurrent and/or sequential intake must be avoided).

Beer, reduced-alcohol (Concurrent and/or sequential intake must be avoided).

Beer, unspecified (Concurrent and/or sequential intake must be avoided).

Beverages, caffeine-containing (Excessive caffeine intake should be avoided).

Bologna, Lebanon (Concurrent and/or sequential intake must be avoided).

Cheese, aged (Concurrent and/or sequential intake must be avoided).

Cheese, unspecified (Concurrent and/or sequential intake must be avoided).

Chocolate (Concurrent and/or sequential intake must be avoided).

(◘ Described in PDR For Nonprescription Drugs) (◉ Described in PDR For Ophthalmology)

Fish, smoked (Concurrent and/or sequential intake must be avoided).

Food with high concentration of dopamine (Concurrent and/or sequential intake must be avoided).

Food with high concentration of tyramine (Concurrent and/or sequential intake must be avoided).

Herring, pickled (Concurrent and/or sequential intake must be avoided).

Liver (Concurrent and/or sequential intake must be avoided).

Meat extracts (Concurrent and/or sequential intake must be avoided).

Meat, unspecified (Concurrent and/or sequential intake must be avoided).

Pepperoni (Concurrent and/or sequential intake must be avoided).

Salami, hard (Concurrent and/or sequential intake must be avoided).

Salami, Genoa (Concurrent and/or sequential intake must be avoided).

Sauerkraut (Concurrent and/or sequential intake must be avoided).

Sausage, dry (Concurrent and/or sequential intake must be avoided).

Wine products (Concurrent and/or sequential intake must be avoided).

Wine, unspecified (Concurrent and/or sequential intake must be avoided).

Yeast extract (Concurrent and/or sequential intake must be avoided).

Yeast, brewer's (Concurrent and/or sequential intake must be avoided).

Yogurt (Concurrent and/or sequential intake must be avoided).

NASACORT NASAL INHALER

(Triamcinolone Acetonide) 2024

May interact with certain other agents. Compounds in this category include:

Prednisone (Potential for increased likelihood of HPA suppression). Products include:

Deltasone Tablets 2595

NASAL MOIST

(Sodium Chloride) .... ᴷᴰ 609

None cited in PDR database.

NāSAL MOISTURIZER AF NASAL DROPS

(Sodium Chloride) .... ᴷᴰ 726

None cited in PDR database.

NāSAL MOISTURIZER AF NASAL SPRAY

(Sodium Chloride) .... ᴷᴰ 726

None cited in PDR database.

NASALCROM NASAL SOLUTION

(Cromolyn Sodium) 994

None cited in PDR database.

NASALIDE NASAL SOLUTION 0.025%

(Flunisolide) 2110

None cited in PDR database.

NASAREL NASAL SOLUTION

(Flunisolide) 2133

None cited in PDR database.

NATACYN ANTIFUNGAL OPHTHALMIC SUSPENSION

(Natamycin) .... © 225

None cited in PDR database.

NATURE MADE ANTIOXIDANT FORMULA

(Vitamin A, Vitamin C, Vitamin E).... ᴷᴰ 748

None cited in PDR database.

NATURE MADE ESSENTIAL BALANCE MULTIVITAMIN

(Vitamins with Minerals) .... ᴷᴰ 748

None cited in PDR database.

NAVANE CAPSULES AND CONCENTRATE

(Thiothixene) 2201

May interact with phenothiazines, barbiturates, central nervous system depressants, belladona products, and certain other agents. Compounds in these categories include:

Alfentanil Hydrochloride (Dosage adjustments required). Products include:

Alfenta Injection 1286

Alprazolam (Dosage adjustments required). Products include:

Xanax Tablets 2649

Aprobarbital (Potentiated).

No products indexed under this heading.

Atropine Sulfate (Weak anticholinergic effect of Navane necessitates cautious use of atropine related drugs). Products include:

Arco-Lase Plus Tablets 512

Atrohist Plus Tablets 454

Atropine Sulfate Sterile Ophthalmic Solution .... © 233

Donnatal 2060

Donnatal Extentabs.............................. 2061

Donnatal Tablets 2060

Lomotil 2439

Motofen Tablets 784

Urised Tablets....................................... 1964

Belladonna Alkaloids (Weak anticholinergic effect of Navane necessitates cautious use of atropine related drugs). Products include:

Bellergal-S Tablets 2250

Hyland's Bed Wetting Tablets .... ᴷᴰ 828

Hyland's EnurAid Tablets.................. ᴷᴰ 829

Hyland's Teething Tablets .... ᴷᴰ 830

Buprenorphine (Dosage adjustments required). Products include:

Buprenex Injectable 2006

Buspirone Hydrochloride (Dosage adjustments required). Products include:

BuSpar 737

Butabarbital (Potentiated).

No products indexed under this heading.

Butalbital (Potentiated). Products include:

Esgic-plus Tablets 1013

Fioricet Tablets 2258

Fioricet with Codeine Capsules 2260

Fiorinal Capsules 2261

Fiorinal with Codeine Capsules 2262

Fiorinal Tablets 2261

Phrenilin 785

Sedapap Tablets 50 mg/650 mg .. 1543

Chlordiazepoxide (Dosage adjustments required). Products include:

Libritabs Tablets 2177

Limbitrol 2180

Chlordiazepoxide Hydrochloride (Dosage adjustments required). Products include:

Librax Capsules 2176

Librium Capsules................................. 2178

Librium Injectable 2179

Chlorpromazine (Likelihood of tardive dyskinesia). Products include:

Thorazine Suppositories 2523

Chlorprothixene (Dosage adjustments required).

No products indexed under this heading.

Chlorprothixene Hydrochloride (Dosage adjustments required).

No products indexed under this heading.

Clorazepate Dipotassium (Dosage adjustments required). Products include:

Tranxene 451

Clozapine (Dosage adjustments required). Products include:

Clozaril Tablets.................................... 2252

Codeine Phosphate (Dosage adjustments required). Products include:

Actifed with Codeine Cough Syrup.. 1067

Brontex 1981

Deconsal C Expectorant Syrup 456

Deconsal Pediatric Syrup.................... 457

Dimetane-DC Cough Syrup 2059

Empirin with Codeine Tablets............ 1093

Fioricet with Codeine Capsules 2260

Fiorinal with Codeine Capsules 2262

Isoclor Expectorant.............................. 990

Novahistine DH................................... 2462

Novahistine Expectorant..................... 2463

Nucofed 2051

Phenergan with Codeine 2777

Phenergan VC with Codeine 2781

Robitussin A-C Syrup 2073

Robitussin-DAC Syrup 2074

Ryna .... ᴷᴰ 841

Soma Compound w/Codeine Tablets 2676

Tussi-Organidin NR Liquid and S NR Liquid 2677

Tylenol with Codeine 1583

Desflurane (Dosage adjustments required). Products include:

Suprane 1813

Dezocine (Dosage adjustments required). Products include:

Dalgan Injection 538

Diazepam (Dosage adjustments required). Products include:

Dizac 1809

Valium Injectable 2182

Valium Tablets 2183

Valrelease Capsules 2169

Droperidol (Dosage adjustments required). Products include:

Inapsine Injection................................ 1296

Enflurane (Dosage adjustments required).

No products indexed under this heading.

Epinephrine Hydrochloride (Paradoxical hypotension may occur). Products include:

Ana-Kit Anaphylaxis Emergency Treatment Kit 617

Estazolam (Dosage adjustments required). Products include:

ProSom Tablets 449

Ethchlorvynol (Dosage adjustments required). Products include:

Placidyl Capsules................................. 448

Ethinamate (Dosage adjustments required).

No products indexed under this heading.

Fentanyl (Dosage adjustments required). Products include:

Duragesic Transdermal System........ 1288

Fentanyl Citrate (Dosage adjustments required). Products include:

Sublimaze Injection.............................. 1307

Fluphenazine Decanoate (Likelihood of tardive dyskinesia). Products include:

Prolixin Decanoate 509

Fluphenazine Enanthate (Likelihood of tardive dyskinesia). Products include:

Prolixin Enanthate 509

Fluphenazine Hydrochloride (Likelihood of tardive dyskinesia). Products include:

Prolixin 509

Flurazepam Hydrochloride (Dosage adjustments required). Products include:

Dalmane Capsules................................ 2173

Glutethimide (Dosage adjustments required).

No products indexed under this heading.

Haloperidol (Dosage adjustments required). Products include:

Haldol Injection, Tablets and Concentrate 1575

Haloperidol Decanoate (Dosage adjustments required). Products include:

Haldol Decanoate................................. 1577

Hydrocodone Bitartrate (Dosage adjustments required). Products include:

Anexsia 5/500 Elixir 1781

Anexia Tablets...................................... 1782

Codiclear DH Syrup 791

Deconamine CX Cough and Cold Liquid and Tablets............................... 1319

Duratuss HD Elixir............................... 2565

Hycodan Tablets and Syrup 930

Hycomine Compound Tablets 932

Hycomine 931

Hycotuss Expectorant Syrup 933

Hydrocet Capsules 782

Lorcet 10/650...................................... 1018

Lortab.. 2566

Tussend 1783

Tussend Expectorant 1785

Vicodin Tablets..................................... 1356

Vicodin ES Tablets 1357

Vicodin Tuss Expectorant 1358

Zydone Capsules 949

Hydrocodone Polistirex (Dosage adjustments required). Products include:

Tussionex Pennkinetic Extended-Release Suspension 998

Hydroxyzine Hydrochloride (Dosage adjustments required). Products include:

Atarax Tablets & Syrup....................... 2185

Marax Tablets & DF Syrup.................. 2200

Vistaril Intramuscular Solution.......... 2216

Hyoscyamine (Weak anticholinergic effect of Navane necessitates cautious use of atropine related drugs). Products include:

Cystospaz Tablets................................. 1963

Urised Tablets....................................... 1964

Hyoscyamine Sulfate (Weak anticholinergic effect of Navane necessitates cautious use of atropine related drugs). Products include:

Arco-Lase Plus Tablets 512

Atrohist Plus Tablets 454

Cystospaz-M Capsules 1963

Donnatal 2060

Donnatal Extentabs.............................. 2061

Donnatal Tablets 2060

Kutrase Capsules.................................. 2402

Levsin/Levsinex/Levbid 2405

Isoflurane (Dosage adjustments required).

No products indexed under this heading.

Ketamine Hydrochloride (Dosage adjustments required).

No products indexed under this heading.

Levomethadyl Acetate Hydrochloride (Dosage adjustments required). Products include:

Orlamm 2239

Levorphanol Tartrate (Dosage adjustments required). Products include:

Levo-Dromoran..................................... 2129

Lorazepam (Dosage adjustments required). Products include:

Ativan Injection.................................... 2698

Ativan Tablets 2700

Loxapine Hydrochloride (Dosage adjustments required). Products include:

Loxitane 1378

IMPORTANT NOTE: Always consult each drug listing in the patient's regimen for possible interactions.

Navane Oral — Interactions Index — 698

Loxapine Succinate (Dosage adjustments required). Products include:
- Loxitane Capsules ... 1378

Meperidine Hydrochloride (Dosage adjustments required). Products include:
- Demerol ... 2308
- Mepergan Injection ... 2753

Mephobarbital (Potentiating action of barbiturates). Products include:
- Mebaral Tablets ... 2322

Meprobamate (Dosage adjustments required). Products include:
- Miltown Tablets ... 2672
- PMB 200 and PMB 400 ... 2783

Mesoridazine Besylate (Likelihood of tardive dyskinesia). Products include:
- Serentil ... 684

Methadone Hydrochloride (Dosage adjustments required). Products include:
- Methadone Hydrochloride Oral Concentrate ... 2233
- Methadone Hydrochloride Oral Solution & Tablets ... 2235

Methohexital Sodium (Dosage adjustments required). Products include:
- Brevital Sodium Vials ... 1429

Methotrimeprazine (Dosage adjustments required). Products include:
- Levoprome ... 1274

Methoxyflurane (Dosage adjustments required).
- No products indexed under this heading.

Midazolam Hydrochloride (Dosage adjustments required). Products include:
- Versed Injection ... 2170

Molindone Hydrochloride (Dosage adjustments required). Products include:
- Moban Tablets and Concentrate ... 1048

Morphine Sulfate (Dosage adjustments required). Products include:
- Astramorph/PF Injection, USP (Preservative-Free) ... 535
- Duramorph ... 962
- Infumorph 200 and Infumorph 500 Sterile Solutions ... 965
- MS Contin Tablets ... 1994
- MSIR ... 1997
- Oramorph SR (Morphine Sulfate Sustained Release Tablets) ... 2236
- RMS Suppositories ... 2657
- Roxanol ... 2243

Opium Alkaloids (Dosage adjustments required).
- No products indexed under this heading.

Oxazepam (Dosage adjustments required). Products include:
- Serax Capsules ... 2810
- Serax Tablets ... 2810

Oxycodone Hydrochloride (Dosage adjustments required). Products include:
- Percocet Tablets ... 938
- Percodan Tablets ... 939
- Percodan-Demi Tablets ... 940
- Roxicodone Tablets, Oral Solution & Intensol (Oxycodone) ... 2244
- Tylox Capsules ... 1584

Pentobarbital Sodium (Potentiated). Products include:
- Nembutal Sodium Capsules ... 436
- Nembutal Sodium Solution ... 438
- Nembutal Sodium Suppositories ... 440

Perphenazine (Likelihood of tardive dyskinesia). Products include:
- Etrafon ... 2355
- Triavil Tablets ... 1757
- Trilafon ... 2389

Phenobarbital (Potentiated). Products include:
- Arco-Lase Plus Tablets ... 512
- Bellergal-S Tablets ... 2250
- Donnatal ... 2060
- Donnatal Extentabs ... 2061
- Donnatal Tablets ... 2060
- Phenobarbital Elixir and Tablets ... 1469
- Quadrinal Tablets ... 1350

Prazepam (Dosage adjustments required).
- No products indexed under this heading.

Prochlorperazine (Likelihood of tardive dyskinesia). Products include:
- Compazine ... 2470

Promethazine Hydrochloride (Likelihood of tardive dyskinesia). Products include:
- Mepergan Injection ... 2753
- Phenergan with Codeine ... 2777
- Phenergan with Dextromethorphan 2778
- Phenergan Injection ... 2773
- Phenergan Suppositories ... 2775
- Phenergan Syrup ... 2774
- Phenergan Tablets ... 2775
- Phenergan VC ... 2779
- Phenergan VC with Codeine ... 2781

Propofol (Dosage adjustments required). Products include:
- Diprivan Injection ... 2833

Propoxyphene Hydrochloride (Dosage adjustments required). Products include:
- Darvon ... 1435
- Wygesic Tablets ... 2827

Propoxyphene Napsylate (Dosage adjustments required). Products include:
- Darvon-N/Darvocet-N ... 1433

Quazepam (Dosage adjustments required). Products include:
- Doral Tablets ... 2664

Risperidone (Dosage adjustments required). Products include:
- Risperdal ... 1301

Scopolamine (Weak anticholinergic effect of Navane necessitates cautious use of atropine related drugs). Products include:
- Transderm Scōp Transdermal Therapeutic System ... 869

Scopolamine Hydrobromide (Weak anticholinergic effect of Navane necessitates cautious use of atropine related drugs). Products include:
- Atrohist Plus Tablets ... 454
- Donnatal ... 2060
- Donnatal Extentabs ... 2061
- Donnatal Tablets ... 2060

Secobarbital Sodium (Potentiated). Products include:
- Seconal Sodium Pulvules ... 1474

Sufentanil Citrate (Dosage adjustments required). Products include:
- Sufenta Injection ... 1309

Temazepam (Dosage adjustments required). Products include:
- Restoril Capsules ... 2284

Thiamylal Sodium (Potentiated).
- No products indexed under this heading.

Thioridazine Hydrochloride (Likelihood of tardive dyskinesia). Products include:
- Mellaril ... 2269

Triazolam (Dosage adjustments required). Products include:
- Halcion Tablets ... 2611

Trifluoperazine Hydrochloride (Likelihood of tardive dyskinesia). Products include:
- Stelazine ... 2514

Zolpidem Tartrate (Dosage adjustments required). Products include:
- Ambien Tablets ... 2416

NAVANE INTRAMUSCULAR
(Thiothixene) ... 2202
May interact with phenothiazines, barbiturates, central nervous system depressants, belladona products, and certain other agents. Compounds in these categories include:

Alfentanil Hydrochloride (Dosage adjustments required). Products include:
- Alfenta Injection ... 1286

Alprazolam (Dosage adjustments required). Products include:
- Xanax Tablets ... 2649

Aprobarbital (Potentiated).
- No products indexed under this heading.

Atropine Sulfate (Use with caution). Products include:
- Arco-Lase Plus Tablets ... 512
- Atrohist Plus Tablets ... 454
- Atropine Sulfate Sterile Ophthalmic Solution ... ⊙ 233
- Donnatal ... 2060
- Donnatal Extentabs ... 2061
- Donnatal Tablets ... 2060
- Lomotil ... 2439
- Motofen Tablets ... 784
- Urised Tablets ... 1964

Belladonna Alkaloids (Use with caution). Products include:
- Bellergal-S Tablets ... 2250
- Hyland's Bed Wetting Tablets ... ▣ 828
- Hyland's EnurAid Tablets ... ▣ 829
- Hyland's Teething Tablets ... ▣ 830

Buprenorphine (Dosage adjustments required). Products include:
- Buprenex Injectable ... 2006

Buspirone Hydrochloride (Dosage adjustments required). Products include:
- BuSpar ... 737

Butabarbital (Potentiated).
- No products indexed under this heading.

Butalbital (Potentiated). Products include:
- Esgic-plus Tablets ... 1013
- Fioricet Tablets ... 2258
- Fioricet with Codeine Capsules ... 2260
- Fiorinal Capsules ... 2261
- Fiorinal with Codeine Capsules ... 2262
- Fiorinal Tablets ... 2261
- Phrenilin ... 785
- Sedapap Tablets 50 mg/650 mg .. 1543

Chlordiazepoxide (Dosage adjustments required). Products include:
- Libritabs Tablets ... 2177
- Limbitrol ... 2180

Chlordiazepoxide Hydrochloride (Dosage adjustments required). Products include:
- Librax Capsules ... 2176
- Librium Capsules ... 2178
- Librium Injectable ... 2179

Chlorpromazine (Likelihood of tardive dyskinesia). Products include:
- Thorazine Suppositories ... 2523

Chlorprothixene (Dosage adjustments required).
- No products indexed under this heading.

Chlorprothixene Hydrochloride (Dosage adjustments required).
- No products indexed under this heading.

Clorazepate Dipotassium (Dosage adjustments required). Products include:
- Tranxene ... 451

Clozapine (Dosage adjustments required). Products include:
- Clozaril Tablets ... 2252

Codeine Phosphate (Dosage adjustments required). Products include:
- Actifed with Codeine Cough Syrup.. 1067
- Brontex ... 1981
- Deconsal C Expectorant Syrup ... 456
- Deconsal Pediatric Syrup ... 457
- Dimetane-DC Cough Syrup ... 2059
- Empirin with Codeine Tablets ... 1093
- Fioricet with Codeine Capsules ... 2260
- Fiorinal with Codeine Capsules ... 2262
- Isoclor Expectorant ... 990
- Novahistine DH ... 2462
- Novahistine Expectorant ... 2463
- Nucofed ... 2051
- Phenergan with Codeine ... 2777
- Phenergan VC with Codeine ... 2781
- Robitussin A-C Syrup ... 2073
- Robitussin-DAC Syrup ... 2074
- Ryna ... ▣ 841
- Soma Compound w/Codeine Tablets ... 2676
- Tussi-Organidin NR Liquid and S NR Liquid ... 2677
- Tylenol with Codeine ... 1583

Desflurane (Dosage adjustments required). Products include:
- Suprane ... 1813

Dezocine (Dosage adjustments required). Products include:
- Dalgan Injection ... 538

Diazepam (Dosage adjustments required). Products include:
- Dizac ... 1809
- Valium Injectable ... 2182
- Valium Tablets ... 2183
- Valrelease Capsules ... 2169

Droperidol (Dosage adjustments required). Products include:
- Inapsine Injection ... 1296

Enflurane (Dosage adjustments required).
- No products indexed under this heading.

Epinephrine Hydrochloride (Paradoxical hypotension may occur). Products include:
- Ana-Kit Anaphylaxis Emergency Treatment Kit ... 617

Estazolam (Dosage adjustments required). Products include:
- ProSom Tablets ... 449

Ethchlorvynol (Dosage adjustments required). Products include:
- Placidyl Capsules ... 448

Ethinamate (Dosage adjustments required).
- No products indexed under this heading.

Fentanyl (Dosage adjustments required). Products include:
- Duragesic Transdermal System ... 1288

Fentanyl Citrate (Dosage adjustments required). Products include:
- Sublimaze Injection ... 1307

Fluphenazine Decanoate (Likelihood of tardive dyskinesia). Products include:
- Prolixin Decanoate ... 509

Fluphenazine Enanthate (Likelihood of tardive dyskinesia). Products include:
- Prolixin Enanthate ... 509

Fluphenazine Hydrochloride (Likelihood of tardive dyskinesia). Products include:
- Prolixin ... 509

Flurazepam Hydrochloride (Dosage adjustments required). Products include:
- Dalmane Capsules ... 2173

Glutethimide (Dosage adjustments required).
- No products indexed under this heading.

Haloperidol (Dosage adjustments required). Products include:
- Haldol Injection, Tablets and Concentrate ... 1575

Haloperidol Decanoate (Dosage adjustments required). Products include:
- Haldol Decanoate ... 1577

(▣ Described in PDR For Nonprescription Drugs) (⊙ Described in PDR For Ophthalmology)

699 Interactions Index Nebcin Injection

Hydrocodone Bitartrate (Dosage adjustments required). Products include:
Anexsia 5/500 Elixir 1781
Anexia Tablets 1782
Codiclear DH Syrup 791
Deconamine CX Cough and Cold Liquid and Tablets 1319
Duratuss HD Elixir 2565
Hycodan Tablets and Syrup 930
Hycomine Compound Tablets 932
Hycomine 931
Hycotuss Expectorant Syrup 933
Hydrocet Capsules 782
Lorcet 10/650 1018
Lortab 2566
Tussend 1783
Tussend Expectorant 1785
Vicodin Tablets 1356
Vicodin ES Tablets 1357
Vicodin Tuss Expectorant 1358
Zydone Capsules 949

Hydrocodone Polistirex (Dosage adjustments required). Products include:
Tussionex Pennkinetic Extended-Release Suspension 998

Hydroxyzine Hydrochloride (Dosage adjustments required). Products include:
Atarax Tablets & Syrup 2185
Marax Tablets & DF Syrup 2200
Vistaril Intramuscular Solution 2216

Hyoscyamine (Use with caution). Products include:
Cystospaz Tablets 1963
Urised Tablets 1964

Hyoscyamine Sulfate (Use with caution). Products include:
Arco-Lase Plus Tablets 512
Atrohist Plus Tablets 454
Cystospaz-M Capsules 1963
Donnatal 2060
Donnatal Extentabs 2061
Donnatal Tablets 2060
Kutrase Capsules 2402
Levsin/Levsinex/Levbid 2405

Isoflurane (Dosage adjustments required).
No products indexed under this heading.

Ketamine Hydrochloride (Dosage adjustments required).
No products indexed under this heading.

Levomethadyl Acetate Hydrochloride (Dosage adjustments required). Products include:
Orlamm 2239

Levorphanol Tartrate (Dosage adjustments required). Products include:
Levo-Dromoran 2129

Lorazepam (Dosage adjustments required). Products include:
Ativan Injection 2698
Ativan Tablets 2700

Loxapine Hydrochloride (Dosage adjustments required). Products include:
Loxitane 1378

Loxapine Succinate (Dosage adjustments required). Products include:
Loxitane Capsules 1378

Meperidine Hydrochloride (Dosage adjustments required). Products include:
Demerol 2308
Mepergan Injection 2753

Mephobarbital (Potentiating action of barbiturates). Products include:
Mebaral Tablets 2322

Meprobamate (Dosage adjustments required). Products include:
Miltown Tablets 2672
PMB 200 and PMB 400 2783

Mesoridazine Besylate (Likelihood of tardive dyskinesia). Products include:
Serentil 684

Methadone Hydrochloride (Dosage adjustments required). Products include:
Methadone Hydrochloride Oral Concentrate 2233
Methadone Hydrochloride Oral Solution & Tablets 2235

Methohexital Sodium (Dosage adjustments required). Products include:
Brevital Sodium Vials 1429

Methotrimeprazine (Dosage adjustments required). Products include:
Levoprome 1274

Methoxyflurane (Dosage adjustments required).
No products indexed under this heading.

Midazolam Hydrochloride (Dosage adjustments required). Products include:
Versed Injection 2170

Molindone Hydrochloride (Dosage adjustments required). Products include:
Moban Tablets and Concentrate 1048

Morphine Sulfate (Dosage adjustments required). Products include:
Astramorph/PF Injection, USP (Preservative-Free) 535
Duramorph 962
Infumorph 200 and Infumorph 500 Sterile Solutions 965
MS Contin Tablets 1994
MSIR 1997
Oramorph SR (Morphine Sulfate Sustained Release Tablets) 2236
RMS Suppositories 2657
Roxanol 2243

Opium Alkaloids (Dosage adjustments required).
No products indexed under this heading.

Oxazepam (Dosage adjustments required). Products include:
Serax Capsules 2810
Serax Tablets 2810

Oxycodone Hydrochloride (Dosage adjustments required). Products include:
Percocet Tablets 938
Percodan Tablets 939
Percodan-Demi Tablets 940
Roxicodone Tablets, Oral Solution & Intensol (Oxycodone) 2244
Tylox Capsules 1584

Pentobarbital Sodium (Potentiated). Products include:
Nembutal Sodium Capsules 436
Nembutal Sodium Solution 438
Nembutal Sodium Suppositories 440

Perphenazine (Likelihood of tardive dyskinesia). Products include:
Etrafon 2355
Triavil Tablets 1757
Trilafon 2389

Phenobarbital (Potentiated). Products include:
Arco-Lase Plus Tablets 512
Bellergal-S Tablets 2250
Donnatal 2060
Donnatal Extentabs 2061
Donnatal Tablets 2060
Phenobarbital Elixir and Tablets 1469
Quadrinal Tablets 1350

Prazepam (Dosage adjustments required).
No products indexed under this heading.

Prochlorperazine (Likelihood of tardive dyskinesia). Products include:
Compazine 2470

Promethazine Hydrochloride (Likelihood of tardive dyskinesia). Products include:
Mepergan Injection 2753
Phenergan with Codeine 2777
Phenergan with Dextromethorphan 2778
Phenergan Injection 2773
Phenergan Suppositories 2775
Phenergan Syrup 2774
Phenergan Tablets 2775
Phenergan VC 2779
Phenergan VC with Codeine 2781

Propofol (Dosage adjustments required). Products include:
Diprivan Injection 2833

Propoxyphene Hydrochloride (Dosage adjustments required). Products include:
Darvon 1435
Wygesic Tablets 2827

Propoxyphene Napsylate (Dosage adjustments required). Products include:
Darvon-N/Darvocet-N 1433

Quazepam (Dosage adjustments required). Products include:
Doral Tablets 2664

Risperidone (Dosage adjustments required). Products include:
Risperdal 1301

Scopolamine (Use with caution). Products include:
Transderm Scōp Transdermal Therapeutic System 869

Scopolamine Hydrobromide (Use with caution). Products include:
Atrohist Plus Tablets 454
Donnatal 2060
Donnatal Extentabs 2061
Donnatal Tablets 2060

Secobarbital Sodium (Potentiated). Products include:
Seconal Sodium Pulvules 1474

Sufentanil Citrate (Dosage adjustments required). Products include:
Sufenta Injection 1309

Temazepam (Dosage adjustments required). Products include:
Restoril Capsules 2284

Thiamylal Sodium (Potentiated).
No products indexed under this heading.

Thioridazine Hydrochloride (Likelihood of tardive dyskinesia). Products include:
Mellaril 2269

Triazolam (Dosage adjustments required). Products include:
Halcion Tablets 2611

Trifluoperazine Hydrochloride (Likelihood of tardive dyskinesia). Products include:
Stelazine 2514

Zolpidem Tartrate (Dosage adjustments required). Products include:
Ambien Tablets 2416

NAVELBINE INJECTION
(Vinorelbine Tartrate) 1145
May interact with:

Cisplatin (Potential for higher incidence of granulocytopenia with vinorelbine used in combination with cisplatin). Products include:
Platinol 708
Platinol-AQ Injection 710

Mitomycin (Mitomycin-C) (Acute pulmonary reactions have been reported with vinorelbine and other vinca alkaloids used in conjunction with mitomycin). Products include:
Mutamycin 703

NEBCIN VIALS, HYPORETS & ADD-VANTAGE
(Tobramycin Sulfate) 1464
May interact with aminoglycosides, cephalosporins, and certain other agents. Compounds in these categories include:

Amikacin Sulfate (Avoid concurrent and sequential use). Products include:
Amikacin Sulfate Injection, USP 960
Amikin Injectable 501

Cefaclor (Increased incidence of nephrotoxicity). Products include:
Ceclor Pulvules & Suspension 1431

Cefadroxil Monohydrate (Increased incidence of nephrotoxicity). Products include:
Duricef 748

Cefamandole Nafate (Increased incidence of nephrotoxicity). Products include:
Mandol Vials, Faspak & ADD-Vantage 1461

Cefazolin Sodium (Increased incidence of nephrotoxicity). Products include:
Ancef Injection 2465
Kefzol Vials, Faspak & ADD-Vantage 1456

Cefixime (Increased incidence of nephrotoxicity). Products include:
Suprax 1399

Cefmetazole Sodium (Increased incidence of nephrotoxicity). Products include:
Zefazone 2654

Cefonicid Sodium (Increased incidence of nephrotoxicity). Products include:
Monocid Injection 2497

Cefoperazone Sodium (Increased incidence of nephrotoxicity). Products include:
Cefobid Intravenous/Intramuscular 2189
Cefobid Pharmacy Bulk Package - Not for Direct Infusion 2192

Ceforanide (Increased incidence of nephrotoxicity).
No products indexed under this heading.

Cefotaxime Sodium (Increased incidence of nephrotoxicity). Products include:
Claforan Sterile and Injection 1235

Cefotetan (Increased incidence of nephrotoxicity). Products include:
Cefotan 2829

Cefoxitin Sodium (Increased incidence of nephrotoxicity). Products include:
Mefoxin 1691
Mefoxin Premixed Intravenous Solution 1694

Cefpodoxime Proxetil (Increased incidence of nephrotoxicity). Products include:
Vantin for Oral Suspension and Vantin Tablets 2646

Cefprozil (Increased incidence of nephrotoxicity). Products include:
Cefzil Tablets and Oral Suspension 746

Ceftazidime (Increased incidence of nephrotoxicity). Products include:
Ceptaz 1081
Fortaz 1100
Tazicef for Injection 2519
Tazidime Vials, Faspak & ADD-Vantage 1478

Ceftizoxime Sodium (Increased incidence of nephrotoxicity). Products include:
Cefizox for Intramuscular or Intravenous Use 1034

IMPORTANT NOTE: Always consult each drug listing in the patient's regimen for possible interactions.

Nebcin Injection — Interactions Index — 700

Ceftriaxone Sodium (Increased incidence of nephrotoxicity). Products include:
- Rocephin Injectable Vials, ADD-Vantage, Galaxy Container ... 2142

Cefuroxime Axetil (Increased incidence of nephrotoxicity). Products include:
- Ceftin ... 1078

Cefuroxime Sodium (Increased incidence of nephrotoxicity). Products include:
- Kefurox Vials, Faspak & ADD-Vantage ... 1454
- Zinacef ... 1211

Cephalexin (Increased incidence of nephrotoxicity). Products include:
- Keflex Pulvules & Oral Suspension 914

Cephaloridine (Avoid concurrent and sequential use).

Cephalothin Sodium (Increased incidence of nephrotoxicity).

Cephapirin Sodium (Increased incidence of nephrotoxicity).
- No products indexed under this heading.

Cephradine (Increased incidence of nephrotoxicity).
- No products indexed under this heading.

Cisplatin (Avoid concurrent and sequential use). Products include:
- Platinol ... 708
- Platinol-AQ Injection ... 710

Colistin Sulfate (Avoid concurrent and sequential use). Products include:
- Coly-Mycin S Otic w/Neomycin & Hydrocortisone ... 1906

Decamethonium (Concurrent therapy in anesthetized patients may result in prolonged or secondary apnea).

Ethacrynic Acid (Do not use concurrently; ototoxicity). Products include:
- Edecrin Tablets ... 1657

Furosemide (Do not use concurrently; ototoxicity). Products include:
- Lasix Injection, Oral Solution and Tablets ... 1240

Gentamicin Sulfate (Avoid concurrent and sequential use). Products include:
- Garamycin Injectable ... 2360
- Genoptic Sterile Ophthalmic Solution ... ◉ 243
- Genoptic Sterile Ophthalmic Ointment ... ◉ 243
- Gentacidin Ointment ... ◉ 264
- Gentacidin Solution ... ◉ 264
- Gentak ... ◉ 208
- Pred-G Liquifilm Sterile Ophthalmic Suspension ... ◉ 251
- Pred-G S.O.P. Sterile Ophthalmic Ointment ... ◉ 252

Kanamycin Sulfate (Avoid concurrent and sequential use).
- No products indexed under this heading.

Loracarbef (Increased incidence of nephrotoxicity). Products include:
- Lorabid Suspension and Pulvules ... 1459

Neomycin Sulfate (Avoid concurrent and sequential use). Products include:
- AK-Spore ... ◉ 204
- AK-Trol Ointment & Suspension ... ◉ 205
- Bactine First Aid Antibiotic Plus Anesthetic Ointment ... ▣ 708
- Campho-Phenique Maximum Strength First Aid Antibiotic Plus Pain Reliever Ointment ... ▣ 719
- Coly-Mycin S Otic w/Neomycin & Hydrocortisone ... 1906
- Cortisporin Cream ... 1084
- Cortisporin Ointment ... 1085
- Cortisporin Ophthalmic Ointment Sterile ... 1085
- Cortisporin Ophthalmic Suspension Sterile ... 1086
- Cortisporin Otic Solution Sterile ... 1087
- Cortisporin Otic Suspension Sterile 1088
- Dexacidin Ointment ... ◉ 263
- Maxitrol Ophthalmic Ointment and Suspension ... ◉ 224
- Mycitracin ... ▣ 839
- NeoDecadron Sterile Ophthalmic Ointment ... 1712
- NeoDecadron Sterile Ophthalmic Solution ... 1713
- NeoDecadron Topical Cream ... 1714
- Neosporin G.U. Irrigant Sterile ... 1148
- Neosporin Ointment ... ▣ 857
- Neosporin Plus Maximum Strength Cream ... ▣ 858
- Neosporin Plus Maximum Strength Ointment ... ▣ 858
- Neosporin Ophthalmic Ointment Sterile ... 1148
- Neosporin Ophthalmic Solution Sterile ... 1149
- PediOtic Suspension Sterile ... 1153
- Poly-Pred Liquifilm ... ◉ 248

Paromomycin Sulfate (Avoid concurrent and sequential use).
- No products indexed under this heading.

Polymyxin B Sulfate (Avoid concurrent and sequential use). Products include:
- AK-Spore ... ◉ 204
- AK-Trol Ointment & Suspension ... ◉ 205
- Bactine First Aid Antibiotic Plus Anesthetic Ointment ... ▣ 708
- Betadine Brand First Aid Antibiotics & Moisturizer Ointment ... 1991
- Campho-Phenique Maximum Strength First Aid Antibiotic Plus Pain Reliever Ointment ... ▣ 719
- Cortisporin Cream ... 1084
- Cortisporin Ointment ... 1085
- Cortisporin Ophthalmic Ointment Sterile ... 1085
- Cortisporin Ophthalmic Suspension Sterile ... 1086
- Cortisporin Otic Solution Sterile ... 1087
- Cortisporin Otic Suspension Sterile 1088
- Dexacidin Ointment ... ◉ 263
- Maxitrol Ophthalmic Ointment and Suspension ... ◉ 224
- Mycitracin ... ▣ 839
- Neosporin G.U. Irrigant Sterile ... 1148
- Neosporin Ointment ... ▣ 857
- Neosporin Plus Maximum Strength Cream ... ▣ 858
- Neosporin Plus Maximum Strength Ointment ... ▣ 858
- Neosporin Ophthalmic Ointment Sterile ... 1148
- Neosporin Ophthalmic Solution Sterile ... 1149
- Ophthocort ... ◉ 311
- PediOtic Suspension Sterile ... 1153
- Polymyxin B Sulfate, Aerosporin Brand Sterile Powder ... 1154
- Poly-Pred Liquifilm ... ◉ 248
- Polysporin Ointment ... ▣ 858
- Polysporin Ophthalmic Ointment Sterile ... 1154
- Polysporin Powder ... ▣ 859
- Polytrim Ophthalmic Solution Sterile ... 482
- TERAK Ointment ... ◉ 209
- Terramycin with Polymyxin B Sulfate Ophthalmic Ointment ... 2211

Streptomycin Sulfate (Avoid concurrent and sequential use). Products include:
- Streptomycin Sulfate Injection ... 2208

Succinylcholine Chloride (Concurrent therapy in anesthetized patients may result in prolonged or secondary apnea). Products include:
- Anectine ... 1073

Tubocurarine Chloride (Concurrent therapy in anesthetized patients may result in prolonged or secondary apnea).
- No products indexed under this heading.

Vancomycin Hydrochloride (Avoid concurrent and sequential use). Products include:
- Vancocin HCl, Oral Solution & Pulvules ... 1483
- Vancocin HCl, Vials & ADD-Vantage ... 1481

Viomycin (Avoid concurrent and sequential use).

NEBUPENT FOR INHALATION SOLUTION

(Pentamidine Isethionate) ... 1040

None cited in PDR database.

NEGGRAM CAPLETS

(Nalidixic Acid) ... 2323

May interact with oral anticoagulants and certain other agents. Compounds in these categories include:

Dicumarol (Enhanced effects of oral anticoagulants).
- No products indexed under this heading.

Nitrofurantoin (Interference with therapeutic action of nalidixic acid). Products include:
- Macrodantin Capsules ... 1989

Nitrofurantoin Macrocrystals (Interference with therapeutic action of nalidixic acid).

Warfarin Sodium (Enhanced effect of oral anticoagulants). Products include:
- Coumadin ... 926

NEGGRAM SUSPENSION

(Nalidixic Acid) ... 2323

See **NegGram Caplets**

NEMBUTAL SODIUM CAPSULES

(Pentobarbital Sodium) ... 436

May interact with central nervous system depressants, oral anticoagulants, corticosteroids, monoamine oxidase inhibitors, estrogens, and certain other agents. Compounds in these categories include:

Alfentanil Hydrochloride (Additive CNS depressant effects). Products include:
- Alfenta Injection ... 1286

Alprazolam (Additive CNS depressant effects). Products include:
- Xanax Tablets ... 2649

Aprobarbital (Additive CNS depressant effects).
- No products indexed under this heading.

Betamethasone Acetate (Barbiturates enhance metabolism). Products include:
- Celestone Soluspan Suspension ... 2347

Betamethasone Sodium Phosphate (Barbiturates enhance metabolism). Products include:
- Celestone Soluspan Suspension ... 2347

Buprenorphine (Additive CNS depressant effects). Products include:
- Buprenex Injectable ... 2006

Buspirone Hydrochloride (Additive CNS depressant effects). Products include:
- BuSpar ... 737

Butabarbital (Additive CNS depressant effects).
- No products indexed under this heading.

Butalbital (Additive CNS depressant effects). Products include:
- Esgic-plus Tablets ... 1013
- Fioricet Tablets ... 2258
- Fioricet with Codeine Capsules ... 2260
- Fiorinal Capsules ... 2261
- Fiorinal with Codeine Capsules ... 2262
- Fiorinal Tablets ... 2261
- Phrenilin ... 785
- Sedapap Tablets 50 mg/650 mg .. 1543

Chlordiazepoxide (Additive CNS depressant effects). Products include:
- Libritabs Tablets ... 2177
- Limbitrol ... 2180

Chlordiazepoxide Hydrochloride (Additive CNS depressant effects). Products include:
- Librax Capsules ... 2176
- Librium Capsules ... 2178
- Librium Injectable ... 2179

Chlorotrianisene (Decreased effects of estrogens).
- No products indexed under this heading.

Chlorpromazine (Additive CNS depressant effects). Products include:
- Thorazine Suppositories ... 2523

Chlorprothixene (Additive CNS depressant effects).
- No products indexed under this heading.

Chlorprothixene Hydrochloride (Additive CNS depressant effects).
- No products indexed under this heading.

Chlorprothixene Lactate (Additive CNS depressant effects).
- No products indexed under this heading.

Clorazepate Dipotassium (Additive CNS depressant effects). Products include:
- Tranxene ... 451

Clozapine (Additive CNS depressant effects). Products include:
- Clozaril Tablets ... 2252

Codeine Phosphate (Additive CNS depressant effects). Products include:
- Actifed with Codeine Cough Syrup.. 1067
- Brontex ... 1981
- Deconsal C Expectorant Syrup ... 456
- Deconsal Pediatric Syrup ... 457
- Dimetane-DC Cough Syrup ... 2059
- Empirin with Codeine Tablets ... 1093
- Fioricet with Codeine Capsules ... 2260
- Fiorinal with Codeine Capsules ... 2262
- Isoclor Expectorant ... 990
- Novahistine DH ... 2462
- Novahistine Expectorant ... 2463
- Nucofed ... 2051
- Phenergan with Codeine ... 2777
- Phenergan VC with Codeine ... 2781
- Robitussin A-C Syrup ... 2073
- Robitussin-DAC Syrup ... 2074
- Ryna ... ▣ 841
- Soma Compound w/Codeine Tablets ... 2676
- Tussi-Organidin NR Liquid and S NR Liquid ... 2677
- Tylenol with Codeine ... 1583

Cortisone Acetate (Barbiturates enhance metabolism). Products include:
- Cortone Acetate Sterile Suspension ... 1623
- Cortone Acetate Tablets ... 1624

Desflurane (Additive CNS depressant effects). Products include:
- Suprane ... 1813

Dexamethasone (Barbiturates enchance metabolism). Products include:
- AK-Trol Ointment & Suspension ... ◉ 205
- Decadron Elixir ... 1633
- Decadron Tablets ... 1635
- Decaspray Topical Aerosol ... 1648
- Dexacidin Ointment ... ◉ 263
- Maxitrol Ophthalmic Ointment and Suspension ... ◉ 224
- TobraDex Ophthalmic Suspension and Ointment ... 473

Dexamethasone Acetate (Barbiturates enhance metabolism). Products include:
- Dalalone D.P. Injectable ... 1011
- Decadron-LA Sterile Suspension ... 1646

(▣ Described in PDR For Nonprescription Drugs) (◉ Described in PDR For Ophthalmology)

701 **Interactions Index** **Nembutal Sodium Capsules**

Dexamethasone Sodium Phosphate (Barbiturates enhance metabolism). Products include:
- Decadron Phosphate Injection ... 1637
- Decadron Phosphate Respihaler ... 1642
- Decadron Phosphate Sterile Ophthalmic Ointment ... 1641
- Decadron Phosphate Sterile Ophthalmic Solution ... 1642
- Decadron Phosphate Topical Cream ... 1644
- Decadron Phosphate Turbinaire ... 1645
- Decadron Phosphate with Xylocaine Injection, Sterile ... 1639
- Dexacort Phosphate in Respihaler .. 458
- Dexacort Phosphate in Turbinaire .. 459
- NeoDecadron Sterile Ophthalmic Ointment ... 1712
- NeoDecadron Sterile Ophthalmic Solution ... 1713
- NeoDecadron Topical Cream ... 1714

Dezocine (Additive CNS depressant effects). Products include:
- Dalgan Injection ... 538

Diazepam (Additive CNS depressant effects). Products include:
- Dizac ... 1809
- Valium Injectable ... 2182
- Valium Tablets ... 2183
- Valrelease Capsules ... 2169

Dicumarol (Increased metabolism, decreased anticoagulant response).
- No products indexed under this heading.

Dienestrol (Decreased effects of estrogens). Products include:
- Ortho Dienestrol Cream ... 1866

Diethylstilbestrol (Decreased effects of estrogens). Products include:
- Diethylstilbestrol Tablets ... 1437

Doxycycline Calcium (Barbiturates shortens half-life of doxycycline). Products include:
- Vibramycin Calcium Oral Suspension Syrup ... 1941

Doxycycline Hyclate (Barbiturates shorten half-life of doxycycline). Products include:
- Doryx Capsules ... 1913
- Vibramycin Hyclate Capsules ... 1941
- Vibramycin Hyclate Intravenous ... 2215
- Vibra-Tabs Film Coated Tablets ... 1941

Doxycycline Monohydrate (Barbiturates shorten half-life of doxycycline). Products include:
- Monodox Capsules ... 1805
- Vibramycin Monohydrate for Oral Suspension ... 1941

Droperidol (Additive CNS depressant effects). Products include:
- Inapsine Injection ... 1296

Enflurane (Additive CNS depressant effects).
- No products indexed under this heading.

Estazolam (Additive CNS depressant effects). Products include:
- ProSom Tablets ... 449

Estradiol (Decreased effects of estrogens). Products include:
- Climara Transdermal System ... 645
- Estrace Cream and Tablets ... 749
- Estraderm Transdermal System ... 824

Estrogens, Conjugated (Decreased effects of estrogens). Products include:
- PMB 200 and PMB 400 ... 2783
- Premarin Intravenous ... 2787
- Premarin with Methyltestosterone .. 2794
- Premarin Tablets ... 2789
- Premarin Vaginal Cream ... 2791
- Premphase ... 2797
- Prempro ... 2801

Estrogens, Esterified (Decreased effects of estrogens). Products include:
- ESTRATAB Tablets (0.3, 0.625, 1.25, 2.5 mg) ... 2536
- Estratest ... 2539
- Menest Tablets ... 2494

Estropipate (Decreased effects of estrogens). Products include:
- Ogen Tablets ... 2627
- Ogen Vaginal Cream ... 2630
- Ortho-Est ... 1869

Ethchlorvynol (Additive CNS depressant effects). Products include:
- Placidyl Capsules ... 448

Ethinamate (Additive CNS depressant effects).
- No products indexed under this heading.

Ethinyl Estradiol (Decreased effects on estrogens). Products include:
- Brevicon ... 2088
- Demulen ... 2428
- Desogen Tablets ... 1817
- Levlen/Tri-Levlen ... 651
- Lo/Ovral Tablets ... 2746
- Lo/Ovral-28 Tablets ... 2751
- Modicon ... 1872
- Nordette-21 Tablets ... 2755
- Nordette-28 Tablets ... 2758
- Norinyl ... 2088
- Ortho-Cept ... 1851
- Ortho-Cyclen/Ortho-Tri-Cyclen ... 1858
- Ortho-Novum ... 1872
- Ortho-Cyclen/Ortho Tri-Cyclen ... 1858
- Ovcon ... 760
- Ovral Tablets ... 2770
- Ovral-28 Tablets ... 2770
- Levlen/Tri-Levlen ... 651
- Tri-Norinyl ... 2164
- Triphasil-21 Tablets ... 2814
- Triphasil-28 Tablets ... 2819

Fentanyl (Additive CNS depressant effects). Products include:
- Duragesic Transdermal System ... 1288

Fentanyl Citrate (Additive CNS depressant effects). Products include:
- Sublimaze Injection ... 1307

Fludrocortisone Acetate (Barbiturates enhance metabolism). Products include:
- Florinef Acetate Tablets ... 505

Fluphenazine Decanoate (Additive CNS depressant effects). Products include:
- Prolixin Decanoate ... 509

Fluphenazine Enanthate (Additive CNS depressant effects). Products include:
- Prolixin Enanthate ... 509

Fluphenazine Hydrochloride (Additive CNS depressant effects). Products include:
- Prolixin ... 509

Flurazepam Hydrochloride (Additive CNS depressant effects). Products include:
- Dalmane Capsules ... 2173

Furazolidone (Prolongs effects of barbiturates). Products include:
- Furoxone ... 2046

Glutethimide (Additive CNS depressant effects).
- No products indexed under this heading.

Griseofulvin (Phenobarbital interferes with absorption). Products include:
- Fulvicin P/G Tablets ... 2359
- Fulvicin P/G 165 & 330 Tablets ... 2359
- Grifulvin V (griseofulvin tablets) Microsize (griseofulvin oral suspension) Microsize ... 1888
- Gris-PEG Tablets, 125 mg & 250 mg ... 479

Haloperidol (Additive CNS depressant effects). Products include:
- Haldol Injection, Tablets and Concentrate ... 1575

Haloperidol Decanoate (Additive CNS depressant effects). Products include:
- Haldol Decanoate ... 1577

Hydrocodone Bitartrate (Additive CNS depressant effects). Products include:
- Anexsia 5/500 Elixir ... 1781
- Anexia Tablets ... 1782
- Codiclear DH Syrup ... 791
- Deconamine CX Cough and Cold Liquid and Tablets ... 1319
- Duratuss HD Elixir ... 2565
- Hycodan Tablets and Syrup ... 930
- Hycomine Compound Tablets ... 932
- Hycomine ... 931
- Hycotuss Expectorant Syrup ... 933
- Hydrocet Capsules ... 782
- Lorcet 10/650 ... 1018
- Lortab ... 2566
- Tussend ... 1783
- Tussend Expectorant ... 1785
- Vicodin Tablets ... 1356
- Vicodin ES Tablets ... 1357
- Vicodin Tuss Expectorant ... 1358
- Zydone Capsules ... 949

Hydrocodone Polistirex (Additive CNS depressant effects). Products include:
- Tussionex Pennkinetic Extended-Release Suspension ... 998

Hydrocortisone (Barbiturates enhance metabolism). Products include:
- Anusol-HC Cream 2.5% ... 1896
- Aquanil HC Lotion ... 1931
- Bactine Hydrocortisone Anti-Itch Cream ... 709
- Caldecort Anti-Itch Hydrocortisone Spray ... 631
- Cortaid ... 836
- CORTENEMA ... 2535
- Cortisporin Ointment ... 1085
- Cortisporin Ophthalmic Ointment Sterile ... 1085
- Cortisporin Ophthalmic Suspension Sterile ... 1086
- Cortisporin Otic Solution Sterile ... 1087
- Cortisporin Otic Suspension Sterile ... 1088
- Cortizone-5 ... 831
- Cortizone-10 ... 831
- Hydrocortone Tablets ... 1672
- Hytone ... 907
- Massengill Medicated Soft Cloth Towelettes ... 2458
- PediOtic Suspension Sterile ... 1153
- Preparation H Hydrocortisone 1% Cream ... 872
- ProctoCream-HC 2.5% ... 2408
- VōSoL HC Otic Solution ... 2678

Hydrocortisone Acetate (Barbiturates enhance metabolism). Products include:
- Analpram-HC Rectal Cream 1% and 2.5% ... 977
- Anusol HC-1 Anti-Itch Hydrocortisone Ointment ... 847
- Anusol-HC Suppositories ... 1897
- Caldecort ... 631
- Carmol HC ... 924
- Coly-Mycin S Otic w/Neomycin & Hydrocortisone ... 1906
- Cortaid ... 836
- Cortifoam ... 2396
- Cortisporin Cream ... 1084
- Epifoam ... 2399
- Hydrocortone Acetate Sterile Suspension ... 1669
- Mantadil Cream ... 1135
- Nupercainal Hydrocortisone 1% Cream ... 645
- Ophthocort ... ⊙ 311
- Pramosone Cream, Lotion & Ointment ... 978
- ProctoCream-HC ... 2408
- ProctoFoam-HC ... 2409
- Terra-Cortril Ophthalmic Suspension ... 2210

Hydrocortisone Sodium Phosphate (Barbiturates enhance metabolism). Products include:
- Hydrocortone Phosphate Injection, Sterile ... 1670

Hydrocortisone Sodium Succinate (Barbiturates enhance metabolism). Products include:
- Solu-Cortef Sterile Powder ... 2641

Hydroxyzine Hydrochloride (Additive CNS depressant effects). Products include:
- Atarax Tablets & Syrup ... 2185
- Marax Tablets & DF Syrup ... 2200
- Vistaril Intramuscular Solution ... 2216

Isocarboxazid (Prolongs effects of barbiturates).
- No products indexed under this heading.

Isoflurane (Additive CNS depressant effects).
- No products indexed under this heading.

Ketamine Hydrochloride (Additive CNS depressant effects).
- No products indexed under this heading.

Levomethadyl Acetate Hydrochloride (Additive CNS depressant effects). Products include:
- Orlamm ... 2239

Levorphanol Tartrate (Additive CNS depressant effects). Products include:
- Levo-Dromoran ... 2129

Lorazepam (Additive CNS depressant effects). Products include:
- Ativan Injection ... 2698
- Ativan Tablets ... 2700

Loxapine Hydrochloride (Additive CNS depressant effects). Products include:
- Loxitane ... 1378

Loxapine Succinate (Additive CNS depressant effects). Products include:
- Loxitane Capsules ... 1378

Meperidine Hydrochloride (Additive CNS depressant effects). Products include:
- Demerol ... 2308
- Mepergan Injection ... 2753

Mephobarbital (Additive CNS depressant effects). Products include:
- Mebaral Tablets ... 2322

Meprobamate (Additive CNS depressant effects). Products include:
- Miltown Tablets ... 2672
- PMB 200 and PMB 400 ... 2783

Mesoridazine Besylate (Additive CNS depressant effects). Products include:
- Serentil ... 684

Methadone Hydrochloride (Additive CNS depressant effects). Products include:
- Methadone Hydrochloride Oral Concentrate ... 2233
- Methadone Hydrochloride Oral Solution & Tablets ... 2235

Methohexital Sodium (Additive CNS depressant effects). Products include:
- Brevital Sodium Vials ... 1429

Methotrimeprazine (Additive CNS depressant effects). Products include:
- Levoprome ... 1274

Methoxyflurane (Additive CNS depressant effects).
- No products indexed under this heading.

Methylprednisolone Acetate (Barbiturates enhance metabolism). Products include:
- Depo-Medrol Single-Dose Vial ... 2600
- Depo-Medrol Sterile Aqueous Suspension ... 2597

Methylprednisolone Sodium Succinate (Barbiturates enhance metabolism). Products include:
- Solu-Medrol Sterile Powder ... 2643

Midazolam Hydrochloride (Additive CNS depressant effects). Products include:
- Versed Injection ... 2170

Molindone Hydrochloride (Additive CNS depressant effects). Products include:
- Moban Tablets and Concentrate ... 1048

IMPORTANT NOTE: Always consult each drug listing in the patient's regimen for possible interactions.

Morphine Sulfate (Additive CNS depressant effects). Products include:
- Astramorph/PF Injection, USP (Preservative-Free) 535
- Duramorph 962
- Infumorph 200 and Infumorph 500 Sterile Solutions 965
- MS Contin Tablets 1994
- MSIR 1997
- Oramorph SR (Morphine Sulfate Sustained Release Tablets) 2236
- RMS Suppositories 2657
- Roxanol 2243

Opium Alkaloids (Additive CNS depressant effects).
- No products indexed under this heading.

Oxazepam (Additive CNS depressant effects). Products include:
- Serax Capsules 2810
- Serax Tablets 2810

Oxycodone Hydrochloride (Additive CNS depressant effects). Products include:
- Percocet Tablets 938
- Percodan Tablets 939
- Percodan-Demi Tablets 940
- Roxicodone Tablets, Oral Solution & Intensol (Oxycodone) 2244
- Tylox Capsules 1584

Perphenazine (Additive CNS depressant effects). Products include:
- Etrafon 2355
- Triavil Tablets 1757
- Trilafon 2389

Phenelzine Sulfate (Prolongs effects of barbiturates). Products include:
- Nardil 1920

Phenobarbital (Additive CNS depressant effects). Products include:
- Arco-Lase Plus Tablets 512
- Bellergal-S Tablets 2250
- Donnatal 2060
- Donnatal Extentabs 2061
- Donnatal Tablets 2060
- Phenobarbital Elixir and Tablets 1469
- Quadrinal Tablets 1350

Phenytoin (Variable effect on metabolism of phenytoin). Products include:
- Dilantin Infatabs 1908
- Dilantin-125 Suspension 1911

Phenytoin Sodium (Variable effect on metabolism of phenytoin). Products include:
- Dilantin Kapseals 1906
- Dilantin Parenteral 1910

Polyestradiol Phosphate (Decreased effects of estrogens).
- No products indexed under this heading.

Prazepam (Additive CNS depressant effects).
- No products indexed under this heading.

Prednisolone Acetate (Barbiturates enhance metabolism). Products include:
- AK-CIDE .... ⊙ 202
- AK-CIDE Ointment .... ⊙ 202
- Blephamide Liquifilm Sterile Ophthalmic Suspension 476
- Blephamide Ointment .... ⊙ 237
- Econopred & Econopred Plus Ophthalmic Suspensions .... ⊙ 217
- Poly-Pred Liquifilm .... ⊙ 248
- Pred Forte .... ⊙ 250
- Pred Mild .... ⊙ 253
- Pred-G Liquifilm Sterile Ophthalmic Suspension .... ⊙ 251
- Pred-G S.O.P. Sterile Ophthalmic Ointment .... ⊙ 252
- Vasocidin Ointment .... ⊙ 268

Prednisolone Sodium Phosphate (Barbiturates enhance metabolism). Products include:
- AK-Pred .... ⊙ 204
- Hydeltrasol Injection, Sterile 1665
- Inflamase .... ⊙ 265
- Pediapred Oral Liquid 995
- Vasocidin Ophthalmic Solution .... ⊙ 270

Prednisolone Tebutate (Barbiturates enhance metabolism). Products include:
- Hydeltra-T.B.A. Sterile Suspension 1667

Prednisone (Barbiturates enhance metabolism). Products include:
- Deltasone Tablets 2595

Prochlorperazine (Additive CNS depressant effects). Products include:
- Compazine 2470

Promethazine Hydrochloride (Additive CNS depressant effects). Products include:
- Mepergan Injection 2753
- Phenergan with Codeine 2777
- Phenergan with Dextromethorphan 2778
- Phenergan Injection 2773
- Phenergan Suppositories 2775
- Phenergan Syrup 2774
- Phenergan Tablets 2775
- Phenergan VC 2779
- Phenergan VC with Codeine 2781

Propofol (Additive CNS depressant effects). Products include:
- Diprivan Injection 2833

Propoxyphene Hydrochloride (Additive CNS depressant effects). Products include:
- Darvon 1435
- Wygesic Tablets 2827

Propoxyphene Napsylate (Additive CNS depressant effects). Products include:
- Darvon-N/Darvocet-N 1433

Quazepam (Additive CNS depressant effects). Products include:
- Doral Tablets 2664

Quinestrol (Decreased effects of estrogens).
- No products indexed under this heading.

Risperidone (Additive CNS depressant effects). Products include:
- Risperdal 1301

Secobarbital Sodium (Additive CNS depressant effects). Products include:
- Seconal Sodium Pulvules 1474

Selegiline Hydrochloride (Prolongs effects of barbiturates). Products include:
- Eldepryl Tablets 2550

Sufentanil Citrate (Additive CNS depressant effects). Products include:
- Sufenta Injection 1309

Temazepam (Additive CNS depressant effects). Products include:
- Restoril Capsules 2284

Thiamylal Sodium (Additive CNS depressant effects).
- No products indexed under this heading.

Thioridazine Hydrochloride (Additive CNS depressant effects). Products include:
- Mellaril 2269

Thiothixene (Additive CNS depressant effects). Products include:
- Navane Capsules and Concentrate 2201
- Navane Intramuscular 2202

Tranylcypromine Sulfate (Prolongs effects of barbiturates). Products include:
- Parnate Tablets 2503

Triamcinolone (Barbiturates enhance metabolism). Products include:
- Aristocort Tablets 1022

Triamcinolone Acetonide (Barbiturates enhance metabolism). Products include:
- Aristocort A 0.025% Cream 1027
- Aristocort A 0.5% Cream 1031
- Aristocort A 0.1% Cream 1029
- Aristocort A 0.1% Ointment 1030
- Azmacort Oral Inhaler 2011
- Nasacort Nasal Inhaler 2024

Triamcinolone Diacetate (Barbiturates enhance metabolism). Products include:
- Aristocort Suspension (Forte Parenteral) 1027
- Aristocort Suspension (Intralesional) 1025

Triamcinolone Hexacetonide (Barbiturates enhance metabolism). Products include:
- Aristospan Suspension (Intra-articular) 1033
- Aristospan Suspension (Intralesional) 1032

Triazolam (Additive CNS depressant effects). Products include:
- Halcion Tablets 2611

Trifluoperazine Hydrochloride (Additive CNS depressant effects). Products include:
- Stelazine 2514

Valproic Acid (Decreases barbiturate metabolism). Products include:
- Depakene 413

Warfarin Sodium (Increased metabolism, decreased anticoagulant response). Products include:
- Coumadin 926

Zolpidem Tartrate (Additive CNS depressant effects). Products include:
- Ambien Tablets 2416

NEMBUTAL SODIUM SOLUTION

(Pentobarbital Sodium) 438

May interact with central nervous system depressants, oral anticoagulants, corticosteroids, monoamine oxidase inhibitors, estrogens, and certain other agents. Compounds in these categories include:

Alfentanil Hydrochloride (Additive CNS depressant effects). Products include:
- Alfenta Injection 1286

Alprazolam (Additive CNS depressant effects). Products include:
- Xanax Tablets 2649

Aprobarbital (Additive CNS depressant effects).
- No products indexed under this heading.

Betamethasone Acetate (Barbiturates enhance metabolism). Products include:
- Celestone Soluspan Suspension 2347

Betamethasone Sodium Phosphate (Barbiturates enhance metabolism). Products include:
- Celestone Soluspan Suspension 2347

Buprenorphine (Additive CNS depressant effects). Products include:
- Buprenex Injectable 2006

Buspirone Hydrochloride (Additive CNS depressant effects). Products include:
- BuSpar 737

Butabarbital (Additive CNS depressant effects).
- No products indexed under this heading.

Butalbital (Additive CNS depressant effects). Products include:
- Esgic-plus Tablets 1013
- Fioricet Tablets 2258
- Fioricet with Codeine Capsules 2260
- Fiorinal Capsules 2261
- Fiorinal with Codeine Capsules 2262
- Fiorinal Tablets 2261
- Phrenilin 785
- Sedapap Tablets 50 mg/650 mg 1543

Chlordiazepoxide (Additive CNS depressant effects). Products include:
- Libritabs Tablets 2177
- Limbitrol 2180

Chlordiazepoxide Hydrochloride (Additive CNS depressant effects). Products include:
- Librax Capsules 2176
- Librium Capsules 2178
- Librium Injectable 2179

Chlorotrianisene (Decreased effects of estrogens).
- No products indexed under this heading.

Chlorpromazine (Additive CNS depressant effects). Products include:
- Thorazine Suppositories 2523

Chlorprothixene (Additive CNS depressant effects).
- No products indexed under this heading.

Chlorprothixene Hydrochloride (Additive CNS depressant effects).
- No products indexed under this heading.

Chlorprothixene Lactate (Additive CNS depressant effects).
- No products indexed under this heading.

Clorazepate Dipotassium (Additive CNS depressant effects). Products include:
- Tranxene 451

Clozapine (Additive CNS depressant effects). Products include:
- Clozaril Tablets 2252

Codeine Phosphate (Additive CNS depressant effects). Products include:
- Actifed with Codeine Cough Syrup 1067
- Brontex 1981
- Deconsal C Expectorant Syrup 456
- Deconsal Pediatric Syrup 457
- Dimetane-DC Cough Syrup 2059
- Empirin with Codeine Tablets 1093
- Fioricet with Codeine Capsules 2260
- Fiorinal with Codeine Capsules 2262
- Isoclor Expectorant 990
- Novahistine DH 2462
- Novahistine Expectorant 2463
- Nucofed 2051
- Phenergan with Codeine 2777
- Phenergan VC with Codeine 2781
- Robitussin A-C Syrup 2073
- Robitussin-DAC Syrup 2074
- Ryna .... ▣ 841
- Soma Compound w/Codeine Tablets 2676
- Tussi-Organidin NR Liquid and S NR Liquid 2677
- Tylenol with Codeine 1583

Cortisone Acetate (Barbiturates enhance metabolism). Products include:
- Cortone Acetate Sterile Suspension 1623
- Cortone Acetate Tablets 1624

Desflurane (Additive CNS depressant effects). Products include:
- Suprane 1813

Dexamethasone (Barbiturates enchance metabolism). Products include:
- AK-Trol Ointment & Suspension .... ⊙ 205
- Decadron Elixir 1633
- Decadron Tablets 1635
- Decaspray Topical Aerosol 1648
- Dexacidin Ointment .... ⊙ 263
- Maxitrol Ophthalmic Ointment and Suspension .... ⊙ 224
- TobraDex Ophthalmic Suspension and Ointment 473

Dexamethasone Acetate (Barbiturates enhance metabolism). Products include:
- Dalalone D.P. Injectable 1011
- Decadron-LA Sterile Suspension 1646

Dexamethasone Sodium Phosphate (Barbiturates enhance metabolism). Products include:
- Decadron Phosphate Injection 1637
- Decadron Phosphate Respihaler 1642
- Decadron Phosphate Sterile Ophthalmic Ointment 1641

(▣ Described in PDR For Nonprescription Drugs) (⊙ Described in PDR For Ophthalmology)

Interactions Index — Nembutal Sodium Solution

Decadron Phosphate Sterile Ophthalmic Solution 1642
Decadron Phosphate Topical Cream 1644
Decadron Phosphate Turbinaire ... 1645
Decadron Phosphate with Xylocaine Injection, Sterile 1639
Dexacort Phosphate in Respihaler .. 458
Dexacort Phosphate in Turbinaire .. 459
NeoDecadron Sterile Ophthalmic Ointment 1712
NeoDecadron Sterile Ophthalmic Solution 1713
NeoDecadron Topical Cream 1714

Dezocine (Additive CNS depressant effects). Products include:

Dalgan Injection 538

Diazepam (Additive CNS depressant effects). Products include:

Dizac 1809
Valium Injectable 2182
Valium Tablets 2183
Valrelease Capsules 2169

Dicumarol (Increased metabolism, decreased anticoagulant response).

No products indexed under this heading.

Dienestrol (Decreased effects of estrogens). Products include:

Ortho Dienestrol Cream 1866

Diethylstilbestrol (Decreased effects of estrogens). Products include:

Diethylstilbestrol Tablets 1437

Doxepin Hydrochloride (Phenobarbital shortens half-life). Products include:

Sinequan 2205
Zonalon Cream 1055

Doxycycline Calcium (Barbiturates shorten half-life of doxycycline). Products include:

Vibramycin Calcium Oral Suspension Syrup 1941

Doxycycline Hyclate (Barbiturates shorten half-life of doxycycline). Products include:

Doryx Capsules................................... 1913
Vibramycin Hyclate Capsules 1941
Vibramycin Hyclate Intravenous ... 2215
Vibra-Tabs Film Coated Tablets 1941

Doxycycline Monohydrate (Barbiturates shorten half-life of doxycycline). Products include:

Monodox Capsules 1805
Vibramycin Monohydrate for Oral Suspension 1941

Droperidol (Additive CNS depressant effects). Products include:

Inapsine Injection............................... 1296

Enflurane (Additive CNS depressant effects).

No products indexed under this heading.

Estazolam (Additive CNS depressant effects). Products include:

ProSom Tablets 449

Estradiol (Decreased effects of estrogens). Products include:

Climara Transdermal System 645
Estrace Cream and Tablets 749
Estraderm Transdermal System 824

Estrogens, Conjugated (Decreased effects of estrogens). Products include:

PMB 200 and PMB 400 2783
Premarin Intravenous 2787
Premarin with Methyltestosterone.. 2794
Premarin Tablets 2789
Premarin Vaginal Cream................... 2791
Premphase 2797
Prempro... 2801

Estrogens, Esterified (Decreased effects of estrogens). Products include:

ESTRATAB Tablets (0.3, 0.625, 1.25, 2.5 mg) 2536
Estratest 2539
Menest Tablets 2494

Estropipate (Decreased effects of estrogens). Products include:

Ogen Tablets 2627
Ogen Vaginal Cream.......................... 2630
Ortho-Est.. 1869

Ethchlorvynol (Additive CNS depressant effects). Products include:

Placidyl Capsules................................ 448

Ethinamate (Additive CNS depressant effects).

No products indexed under this heading.

Ethinyl Estradiol (Decreased effects of estrogens). Products include:

Brevicon... 2088
Demulen 2428
Desogen Tablets.................................. 1817
Levlen/Tri-Levlen 651
Lo/Ovral Tablets 2746
Lo/Ovral-28 Tablets........................... 2751
Modicon 1872
Nordette-21 Tablets............................ 2755
Nordette-28 Tablets............................ 2758
Norinyl 2088
Ortho-Cept 1851
Ortho-Cyclen/Ortho-Tri-Cyclen 1858
Ortho-Novum.. 1872
Ortho-Cyclen/Ortho Tri-Cyclen 1858
Ovcon 760
Ovral Tablets 2770
Ovral-28 Tablets 2770
Levlen/Tri-Levlen 651
Tri-Norinyl... 2164
Triphasil-21 Tablets 2814
Triphasil-28 Tablets............................ 2819

Fentanyl (Additive CNS depressant effects). Products include:

Duragesic Transdermal System........ 1288

Fentanyl Citrate (Additive CNS depressant effects). Products include:

Sublimaze Injection............................. 1307

Fludrocortisone Acetate (Barbiturates enhance metabolism). Products include:

Florinef Acetate Tablets 505

Fluphenazine Decanoate (Additive CNS depressant effects). Products include:

Prolixin Decanoate 509

Fluphenazine Enanthate (Additive CNS depressant effects). Products include:

Prolixin Enanthate 509

Fluphenazine Hydrochloride (Additive CNS depressant effects). Products include:

Prolixin 509

Flurazepam Hydrochloride (Additive CNS depressant effects). Products include:

Dalmane Capsules............................... 2173

Furazolidone (Prolongs effects of barbiturates). Products include:

Furoxone 2046

Glutethimide (Additive CNS depressant effects).

No products indexed under this heading.

Griseofulvin (Phenobarbital interferes with absorption). Products include:

Fulvicin P/G Tablets........................... 2359
Fulvicin P/G 165 & 330 Tablets 2359
Grifulvin V (griseofulvin tablets) Microsize (griseofulvin oral suspension) Microsize 1888
Gris-PEG Tablets, 125 mg & 250 mg 479

Haloperidol (Additive CNS depressant effects). Products include:

Haldol Injection, Tablets and Concentrate 1575

Haloperidol Decanoate (Additive CNS depressant effects). Products include:

Haldol Decanoate................................. 1577

Hydrocodone Bitartrate (Additive CNS depressant effects). Products include:

Anexsia 5/500 Elixir 1781
Anexia Tablets...................................... 1782
Codiclear DH Syrup 791
Deconamine CX Cough and Cold Liquid and Tablets............................... 1319
Duratuss HD Elixir.............................. 2565
Hycodan Tablets and Syrup 930
Hycomine Compound Tablets 932
Hycomine 931
Hycotuss Expectorant Syrup 933
Hydrocet Capsules 782
Lorcet 10/650...................................... 1018
Lortab 2566
Tussend 1783
Tussend Expectorant 1785
Vicodin Tablets..................................... 1356
Vicodin ES Tablets 1357
Vicodin Tuss Expectorant 1358
Zydone Capsules 949

Hydrocodone Polistirex (Additive CNS depressant effects). Products include:

Tussionex Pennkinetic Extended-Release Suspension 998

Hydrocortisone (Barbiturates enhance metabolism). Products include:

Anusol-HC Cream 2.5% 1896
Aquanil HC Lotion 1931
Bactine Hydrocortisone Anti-Itch Cream .... ⊕ 709
Caldecort Anti-Itch Hydrocortisone Spray .... ⊕ 631
Cortaid .... ⊕ 836
CORTENEMA... 2535
Cortisporin Ointment 1085
Cortisporin Ophthalmic Ointment Sterile 1085
Cortisporin Ophthalmic Suspension Sterile 1086
Cortisporin Otic Solution Sterile 1087
Cortisporin Otic Suspension Sterile 1088
Cortizone-5 .... ⊕ 831
Cortizone-10 .... ⊕ 831
Hydrocortone Tablets 1672
Hytone 907
Massengill Medicated Soft Cloth Towelettes.. 2458
PediOtic Suspension Sterile 1153
Preparation H Hydrocortisone 1% Cream .... ⊕ 872
ProctoCream-HC 2.5% 2408
VoSoL HC Otic Solution..................... 2678

Hydrocortisone Acetate (Barbiturates enhance metabolism). Products include:

Analpram-HC Rectal Cream 1% and 2.5% 977
Anusol HC-1 Anti-Itch Hydrocortisone Ointment....................................... ⊕ 847
Anusol-HC Suppositories 1897
Caldecort.. ⊕ 631
Carmol HC 924
Coly-Mycin S Otic w/Neomycin & Hydrocortisone 1906
Cortaid .... ⊕ 836
Cortifoam 2396
Cortisporin Cream............................... 1084
Epifoam 2399
Hydrocortone Acetate Sterile Suspension... 1669
Mantadil Cream 1135
Nupercainal Hydrocortisone 1% Cream .... ⊕ 645
Ophthocort .... ⓒ 311
Pramosone Cream, Lotion & Ointment 978
ProctoCream-HC 2408
ProctoFoam-HC 2409
Terra-Cortril Ophthalmic Suspension 2210

Hydrocortisone Sodium Phosphate (Barbiturates enhance metabolism). Products include:

Hydrocortone Phosphate Injection, Sterile 1670

Hydrocortisone Sodium Succinate (Barbiturates enhance metabolism). Products include:

Solu-Cortef Sterile Powder................ 2641

Hydroxyzine Hydrochloride (Additive CNS depressant effects). Products include:

Atarax Tablets & Syrup...................... 2185

Marax Tablets & DF Syrup................. 2200
Vistaril Intramuscular Solution......... 2216

Isocarboxazid (Prolongs effects of barbiturates).

No products indexed under this heading.

Isoflurane (Additive CNS depressant effects).

No products indexed under this heading.

Ketamine Hydrochloride (Additive CNS depressant effects).

No products indexed under this heading.

Levomethadyl Acetate Hydrochloride (Additive CNS depressant effects). Products include:

Orlaam 2239

Levorphanol Tartrate (Additive CNS depressant effects). Products include:

Levo-Dromoran 2129

Lorazepam (Additive CNS depressant effects). Products include:

Ativan Injection.................................... 2698
Ativan Tablets 2700

Loxapine Hydrochloride (Additive CNS depressant effects). Products include:

Loxitane 1378

Loxapine Succinate (Additive CNS depressant effects). Products include:

Loxitane Capsules 1378

Meperidine Hydrochloride (Additive CNS depressant effects). Products include:

Demerol 2308
Mepergan Injection 2753

Mephobarbital (Additive CNS depressant effects). Products include:

Mebaral Tablets 2322

Meprobamate (Additive CNS depressant effects). Products include:

Miltown Tablets 2672
PMB 200 and PMB 400 2783

Mesoridazine Besylate (Additive CNS depressant effects). Products include:

Serentil... 684

Methadone Hydrochloride (Additive CNS depressant effects). Products include:

Methadone Hydrochloride Oral Concentrate 2233
Methadone Hydrochloride Oral Solution & Tablets............................... 2235

Methohexital Sodium (Additive CNS depressant effects). Products include:

Brevital Sodium Vials 1429

Methotrimeprazine (Additive CNS depressant effects). Products include:

Levoprome 1274

Methoxyflurane (Additive CNS depressant effects).

No products indexed under this heading.

Methylprednisolone Acetate (Barbiturates enhance metabolism). Products include:

Depo-Medrol Single-Dose Vial 2600
Depo-Medrol Sterile Aqueous Suspension... 2597

Methylprednisolone Sodium Succinate (Barbiturates enhance metabolism). Products include:

Solu-Medrol Sterile Powder 2643

Midazolam Hydrochloride (Additive CNS depressant effects). Products include:

Versed Injection 2170

Molindone Hydrochloride (Additive CNS depressant effects). Products include:

Moban Tablets and Concentrate 1048

IMPORTANT NOTE: Always consult each drug listing in the patient's regimen for possible interactions.

Morphine Sulfate (Additive CNS depressant effects). Products include:
- Astramorph/PF Injection, USP (Preservative-Free) 535
- Duramorph 962
- Infumorph 200 and Infumorph 500 Sterile Solutions 965
- MS Contin Tablets 1994
- MSIR 1997
- Oramorph SR (Morphine Sulfate Sustained Release Tablets) 2236
- RMS Suppositories 2657
- Roxanol 2243

Opium Alkaloids (Additive CNS depressant effects).
- No products indexed under this heading.

Oxazepam (Additive CNS depressant effects). Products include:
- Serax Capsules 2810
- Serax Tablets 2810

Oxycodone Hydrochloride (Additive CNS depressant effects). Products include:
- Percocet Tablets 938
- Percodan Tablets 939
- Percodan-Demi Tablets 940
- Roxicodone Tablets, Oral Solution & Intensol (Oxycodone) 2244
- Tylox Capsules 1584

Perphenazine (Additive CNS depressant effects). Products include:
- Etrafon 2355
- Triavil Tablets 1757
- Trilafon 2389

Phenelzine Sulfate (Prolongs effects of barbiturates). Products include:
- Nardil 1920

Phenobarbital (Additive CNS depressant effects). Products include:
- Arco-Lase Plus Tablets 512
- Bellergal-S Tablets 2250
- Donnatal 2060
- Donnatal Extentabs 2061
- Donnatal Tablets 2060
- Phenobarbital Elixir and Tablets 1469
- Quadrinal Tablets 1350

Phenytoin (Variable effect on metabolism of phenytoin). Products include:
- Dilantin Infatabs 1908
- Dilantin-125 Suspension 1911

Phenytoin Sodium (Variable effect on metabolism of phenytoin). Products include:
- Dilantin Kapseals 1906
- Dilantin Parenteral 1910

Polyestradiol Phosphate (Decreased effects of estrogens).
- No products indexed under this heading.

Prazepam (Additive CNS depressant effects).
- No products indexed under this heading.

Prednisolone Acetate (Barbiturates enhance metabolism). Products include:
- AK-CIDE .... ⊙ 202
- AK-CIDE Ointment .... ⊙ 202
- Blephamide Liquifilm Sterile Ophthalmic Suspension 476
- Blephamide Ointment .... ⊙ 237
- Econopred & Econopred Plus Ophthalmic Suspensions .... ⊙ 217
- Poly-Pred Liquifilm .... ⊙ 248
- Pred Forte .... ⊙ 250
- Pred Mild .... ⊙ 253
- Pred-G Liquifilm Sterile Ophthalmic Suspension .... ⊙ 251
- Pred-G S.O.P. Sterile Ophthalmic Ointment .... ⊙ 252
- Vasocidin Ointment .... ⊙ 268

Prednisolone Sodium Phosphate (Barbiturates enhance metabolism). Products include:
- AK-Pred .... ⊙ 204
- Hydeltrasol Injection, Sterile 1665
- Inflamase .... ⊙ 265
- Pediapred Oral Liquid 995
- Vasocidin Ophthalmic Solution .... ⊙ 270

Prednisolone Tebutate (Barbiturates enhance metabolism). Products include:
- Hydeltra-T.B.A. Sterile Suspension 1667

Prednisone (Barbiturates enhance metabolism). Products include:
- Deltasone Tablets 2595

Prochlorperazine (Additive CNS depressant effects). Products include:
- Compazine 2470

Promethazine Hydrochloride (Additive CNS depressant effects). Products include:
- Mepergan Injection 2753
- Phenergan with Codeine 2777
- Phenergan with Dextromethorphan 2778
- Phenergan Injection 2773
- Phenergan Suppositories 2775
- Phenergan Syrup 2774
- Phenergan Tablets 2775
- Phenergan VC 2779
- Phenergan VC with Codeine 2781

Propofol (Additive CNS depressant effects). Products include:
- Diprivan Injection 2833

Propoxyphene Hydrochloride (Additive CNS depressant effects). Products include:
- Darvon 1435
- Wygesic Tablets 2827

Propoxyphene Napsylate (Additive CNS depressant effects). Products include:
- Darvon-N/Darvocet-N 1433

Quazepam (Additive CNS depressant effects). Products include:
- Doral Tablets 2664

Quinestrol (Decreased effects of estrogens).
- No products indexed under this heading.

Risperidone (Additive CNS depressant effects). Products include:
- Risperdal 1301

Secobarbital Sodium (Additive CNS depressant effects). Products include:
- Seconal Sodium Pulvules 1474

Selegiline Hydrochloride (Prolongs effects of barbiturates). Products include:
- Eldepryl Tablets 2550

Sufentanil Citrate (Additive CNS depressant effects). Products include:
- Sufenta Injection 1309

Temazepam (Additive CNS depressant effects). Products include:
- Restoril Capsules 2284

Thiamylal Sodium (Additive CNS depressant effects).
- No products indexed under this heading.

Thioridazine Hydrochloride (Additive CNS depressant effects). Products include:
- Mellaril 2269

Thiothixene (Additive CNS depressant effects). Products include:
- Navane Capsules and Concentrate 2201
- Navane Intramuscular 2202

Tranylcypromine Sulfate (Prolongs effects of barbiturates). Products include:
- Parnate Tablets 2503

Triamcinolone (Barbiturates enhance metabolism). Products include:
- Aristocort Tablets 1022

Triamcinolone Acetonide (Barbiturates enhance metabolism). Products include:
- Aristocort A 0.025% Cream 1027
- Aristocort A 0.5% Cream 1031
- Aristocort A 0.1% Cream 1029
- Aristocort A 0.1% Ointment 1030
- Azmacort Oral Inhaler 2011
- Nasacort Nasal Inhaler 2024

Triamcinolone Diacetate (Barbiturates enhance metabolism). Products include:
- Aristocort Suspension (Forte Parenteral) 1027
- Aristocort Suspension (Intralesional) 1025

Triamcinolone Hexacetonide (Barbiturates enhance metabolism). Products include:
- Aristospan Suspension (Intra-articular) 1033
- Aristospan Suspension (Intralesional) 1032

Triazolam (Additive CNS depressant effects). Products include:
- Halcion Tablets 2611

Trifluoperazine Hydrochloride (Additive CNS depressant effects). Products include:
- Stelazine 2514

Valproic Acid (Decreases barbiturate metabolism). Products include:
- Depakene 413

Warfarin Sodium (Decreased anticoagulant response). Products include:
- Coumadin 926

Zolpidem Tartrate (Additive CNS depressant effects). Products include:
- Ambien Tablets 2416

NEMBUTAL SODIUM SUPPOSITORIES

(Pentobarbital Sodium) 440

May interact with central nervous system depressants, oral anticoagulants, corticosteroids, monoamine oxidase inhibitors, estrogens, and certain other agents. Compounds in these categories include:

Alfentanil Hydrochloride (Additive CNS depressant effects). Products include:
- Alfenta Injection 1286

Alprazolam (Additive CNS depressant effects). Products include:
- Xanax Tablets 2649

Aprobarbital (Additive CNS depressant effects).
- No products indexed under this heading.

Betamethasone Acetate (Barbiturates enhance metabolism). Products include:
- Celestone Soluspan Suspension 2347

Betamethasone Sodium Phosphate (Barbiturates enhance metabolism). Products include:
- Celestone Soluspan Suspension 2347

Buprenorphine (Additive CNS depressant effects). Products include:
- Buprenex Injectable 2006

Buspirone Hydrochloride (Additive CNS depressant effects). Products include:
- BuSpar 737

Butabarbital (Additive CNS depressant effects).
- No products indexed under this heading.

Butalbital (Additive CNS depressant effects). Products include:
- Esgic-plus Tablets 1013
- Fioricet Tablets 2258
- Fioricet with Codeine Capsules 2260
- Fiorinal Capsules 2261
- Fiorinal with Codeine Capsules 2262
- Fiorinal Tablets 2261
- Phrenilin 785
- Sedapap Tablets 50 mg/650 mg 1543

Chlordiazepoxide (Additive CNS depressant effects). Products include:
- Libritabs Tablets 2177
- Limbitrol 2180

Chlordiazepoxide Hydrochloride (Additive CNS depressant effects). Products include:
- Librax Capsules 2176
- Librium Capsules 2178
- Librium Injectable 2179

Chlorotrianisene (Decreased effects of estrogens).
- No products indexed under this heading.

Chlorpromazine (Additive CNS depressant effects). Products include:
- Thorazine Suppositories 2523

Chlorprothixene (Additive CNS depressant effects).
- No products indexed under this heading.

Chlorprothixene Hydrochloride (Additive CNS depressant effects).
- No products indexed under this heading.

Chlorprothixene Lactate (Additive CNS depressant effects).
- No products indexed under this heading.

Clorazepate Dipotassium (Additive CNS depressant effects). Products include:
- Tranxene 451

Clozapine (Additive CNS depressant effects). Products include:
- Clozaril Tablets 2252

Codeine Phosphate (Additive CNS depressant effects). Products include:
- Actifed with Codeine Cough Syrup 1067
- Brontex 1981
- Deconsal C Expectorant Syrup 456
- Deconsal Pediatric Syrup 457
- Dimetane-DC Cough Syrup 2059
- Empirin with Codeine Tablets 1093
- Fioricet with Codeine Capsules 2260
- Fiorinal with Codeine Capsules 2262
- Isoclor Expectorant 990
- Novahistine DH 2462
- Novahistine Expectorant 2463
- Nucofed 2051
- Phenergan with Codeine 2777
- Phenergan VC with Codeine 2781
- Robitussin A-C Syrup 2073
- Robitussin-DAC Syrup 2074
- Ryna .... ▣ 841
- Soma Compound w/Codeine Tablets 2676
- Tussi-Organidin NR Liquid and S NR Liquid 2677
- Tylenol with Codeine 1583

Cortisone Acetate (Barbiturates enhance metabolism). Products include:
- Cortone Acetate Sterile Suspension 1623
- Cortone Acetate Tablets 1624

Desflurane (Additive CNS depressant effects). Products include:
- Suprane 1813

Dexamethasone (Barbiturates enhance metabolism). Products include:
- AK-Trol Ointment & Suspension .... ⊙ 205
- Decadron Elixir 1633
- Decadron Tablets 1635
- Decaspray Topical Aerosol 1648
- Dexacidin Ointment .... ⊙ 263
- Maxitrol Ophthalmic Ointment and Suspension .... ⊙ 224
- TobraDex Ophthalmic Suspension and Ointment 473

Dexamethasone Acetate (Barbiturates enhance metabolism). Products include:
- Dalalone D.P. Injectable 1011
- Decadron-LA Sterile Suspension 1646

Dexamethasone Sodium Phosphate (Barbiturates enhance metabolism). Products include:
- Decadron Phosphate Injection 1637
- Decadron Phosphate Respihaler 1642
- Decadron Phosphate Sterile Ophthalmic Ointment 1641

(▣ Described in PDR For Nonprescription Drugs) (⊙ Described in PDR For Ophthalmology)

Interactions Index

Nembutal Sodium Suppositories

Decadron Phosphate Sterile Ophthalmic Solution 1642
Decadron Phosphate Topical Cream 1644
Decadron Phosphate Turbinaire 1645
Decadron Phosphate with Xylocaine Injection, Sterile 1639
Dexacort Phosphate in Respihaler .. 458
Dexacort Phosphate in Turbinaire .. 459
NeoDecadron Sterile Ophthalmic Ointment 1712
NeoDecadron Sterile Ophthalmic Solution 1713
NeoDecadron Topical Cream 1714

Dezocine (Additive CNS depressant effects). Products include:

Dalgan Injection 538

Diazepam (Additive CNS depressant effects). Products include:

Dizac 1809
Valium Injectable 2182
Valium Tablets 2183
Valrelease Capsules 2169

Dicumarol (Decreased anticoagulant response).

No products indexed under this heading.

Dienestrol (Decreased effects of estrogens). Products include:

Ortho Dienestrol Cream 1866

Diethylstilbestrol (Decreased effects of estrogens). Products include:

Diethylstilbestrol Tablets 1437

Doxepin Hydrochloride (Phenobarbital shortens half-life). Products include:

Sinequan 2205
Zonalon Cream 1055

Doxycycline Hyclate (Barbiturates shorten half-life of doxycycline). Products include:

Doryx Capsules 1913
Vibramycin Hyclate Capsules 1941
Vibramycin Hyclate Intravenous 2215
Vibra-Tabs Film Coated Tablets 1941

Doxycycline Monohydrate (Barbiturates shorten half-life of doxycycline). Products include:

Monodox Capsules 1805
Vibramycin Monohydrate for Oral Suspension 1941

Droperidol (Additive CNS depressant effects). Products include:

Inapsine Injection 1296

Enflurane (Additive CNS depressant effects).

No products indexed under this heading.

Estazolam (Additive CNS depressant effects). Products include:

ProSom Tablets 449

Estradiol (Decreased effects of estrogens). Products include:

Climara Transdermal System 645
Estrace Cream and Tablets 749
Estraderm Transdermal System 824

Estrogens, Conjugated (Decreased effects of estrogens). Products include:

PMB 200 and PMB 400 2783
Premarin Intravenous 2787
Premarin with Methyltestosterone .. 2794
Premarin Tablets 2789
Premarin Vaginal Cream 2791
Premphase 2797
Prempro 2801

Estrogens, Esterified (Decreased effects of estrogens). Products include:

ESTRATAB Tablets (0.3, 0.625, 1.25, 2.5 mg) 2536
Estratest 2539
Menest Tablets 2494

Estropipate (Decreased effects of estrogens). Products include:

Ogen Tablets 2627
Ogen Vaginal Cream 2630
Ortho-Est 1869

Ethchlorvynol (Additive CNS depressant effects). Products include:

Placidyl Capsules 448

Ethinamate (Additive CNS depressant effects).

No products indexed under this heading.

Ethinyl Estradiol (Decreased effects of estrogens). Products include:

Brevicon 2088
Demulen 2428
Desogen Tablets 1817
Levlen/Tri-Levlen 651
Lo/Ovral Tablets 2746
Lo/Ovral-28 Tablets 2751
Modicon 1872
Nordette-21 Tablets 2755
Nordette-28 Tablets 2758
Norinyl 2088
Ortho-Cept 1851
Ortho-Cyclen/Ortho-Tri-Cyclen 1858
Ortho-Novum 1872
Ortho-Cyclen/Ortho Tri-Cyclen 1858
Ovcon 760
Ovral Tablets 2770
Ovral-28 Tablets 2770
Levlen/Tri-Levlen 651
Tri-Norinyl 2164
Triphasil-21 Tablets 2814
Triphasil-28 Tablets 2819

Fentanyl (Additive CNS depressant effects). Products include:

Duragesic Transdermal System 1288

Fentanyl Citrate (Additive CNS depressant effects). Products include:

Sublimaze Injection 1307

Fludrocortisone Acetate (Barbiturates enhance metabolism). Products include:

Florinef Acetate Tablets 505

Fluphenazine Decanoate (Additive CNS depressant effects). Products include:

Prolixin Decanoate 509

Fluphenazine Enanthate (Additive CNS depressant effects). Products include:

Prolixin Enanthate 509

Fluphenazine Hydrochloride (Additive CNS depressant effects). Products include:

Prolixin 509

Flurazepam Hydrochloride (Additive CNS depressant effects). Products include:

Dalmane Capsules 2173

Furazolidone (Prolongs effects of barbiturates). Products include:

Furoxone 2046

Glutethimide (Additive CNS depressant effects).

No products indexed under this heading.

Haloperidol (Additive CNS depressant effects). Products include:

Haldol Injection, Tablets and Concentrate 1575

Haloperidol Decanoate (Additive CNS depressant effects). Products include:

Haldol Decanoate 1577

Hydrocodone Bitartrate (Additive CNS depressant effects). Products include:

Anexsia 5/500 Elixir 1781
Anexia Tablets 1782
Codiclear DH Syrup 791
Deconamine CX Cough and Cold Liquid and Tablets 1319
Duratuss HD Elixir 2565
Hycodan Tablets and Syrup 930
Hycomine Compound Tablets 932
Hycomine 931
Hycotuss Expectorant Syrup 933
Hydrocet Capsules 782
Lorcet 10/650 1018
Lortab 2566
Tussend 1783

Tussend Expectorant 1785
Vicodin Tablets 1356
Vicodin ES Tablets 1357
Vicodin Tuss Expectorant 1358
Zydone Capsules 949

Hydrocodone Polistirex (Additive CNS depressant effects). Products include:

Tussionex Pennkinetic Extended-Release Suspension 998

Hydrocortisone (Barbiturates enhance metabolism). Products include:

Anusol-HC Cream 2.5% 1896
Aquanil HC Lotion 1931
Bactine Hydrocortisone Anti-Itch Cream .... ᴿᴰ 709
Caldecort Anti-Itch Hydrocortisone Spray .... ᴿᴰ 631
Cortaid .... ᴿᴰ 836
CORTENEMA 2535
Cortisporin Ointment 1085
Cortisporin Ophthalmic Ointment Sterile 1085
Cortisporin Ophthalmic Suspension Sterile 1086
Cortisporin Otic Solution Sterile 1087
Cortisporin Otic Suspension Sterile 1088
Cortizone-5 .... ᴿᴰ 831
Cortizone-10 .... ᴿᴰ 831
Hydrocortone Tablets 1672
Hytone 907
Massengill Medicated Soft Cloth Towelettes 2458
PediOtic Suspension Sterile 1153
Preparation H Hydrocortisone 1% Cream .... ᴿᴰ 872
ProctoCream-HC 2.5% 2408
VōSoL HC Otic Solution 2678

Hydrocortisone Acetate (Barbiturates enhance metabolism). Products include:

Analpram-HC Rectal Cream 1% and 2.5% 977
Anusol HC-1 Anti-Itch Hydrocortisone Ointment .... ᴿᴰ 847
Anusol-HC Suppositories 1897
Caldecort .... ᴿᴰ 631
Carmol HC 924
Coly-Mycin S Otic w/Neomycin & Hydrocortisone 1906
Cortaid .... ᴿᴰ 836
Cortifoam 2396
Cortisporin Cream 1084
Epifoam 2399
Hydrocortone Acetate Sterile Suspension 1669
Mantadil Cream 1135
Nupercainal Hydrocortisone 1% Cream .... ᴿᴰ 645
Ophthocort .... ⊙ 311
Pramosone Cream, Lotion & Ointment 978
ProctoCream-HC 2408
ProctoFoam-HC 2409
Terra-Cortril Ophthalmic Suspension 2210

Hydrocortisone Sodium Phosphate (Barbiturates enhance metabolism). Products include:

Hydrocortone Phosphate Injection, Sterile 1670

Hydrocortisone Sodium Succinate (Barbiturates enhance metabolism). Products include:

Solu-Cortef Sterile Powder 2641

Hydroxyzine Hydrochloride (Additive CNS depressant effects). Products include:

Atarax Tablets & Syrup 2185
Marax Tablets & DF Syrup 2200
Vistaril Intramuscular Solution 2216

Isocarboxazid (Prolongs effects of barbiturates).

No products indexed under this heading.

Isoflurane (Additive CNS depressant effects).

No products indexed under this heading.

Ketamine Hydrochloride (Additive CNS depressant effects).

No products indexed under this heading.

Levomethadyl Acetate Hydrochloride (Additive CNS depressant effects). Products include:

Orlaam 2239

Levorphanol Tartrate (Additive CNS depressant effects). Products include:

Levo-Dromoran 2129

Lorazepam (Additive CNS depressant effects). Products include:

Ativan Injection 2698
Ativan Tablets 2700

Loxapine Hydrochloride (Additive CNS depressant effects). Products include:

Loxitane 1378

Loxapine Succinate (Additive CNS depressant effects). Products include:

Loxitane Capsules 1378

Meperidine Hydrochloride (Additive CNS depressant effects). Products include:

Demerol 2308
Mepergan Injection 2753

Mephobarbital (Additive CNS depressant effects). Products include:

Mebaral Tablets 2322

Meprobamate (Additive CNS depressant effects). Products include:

Miltown Tablets 2672
PMB 200 and PMB 400 2783

Mesoridazine Besylate (Additive CNS depressant effects). Products include:

Serentil 684

Methadone Hydrochloride (Additive CNS depressant effects). Products include:

Methadone Hydrochloride Oral Concentrate 2233
Methadone Hydrochloride Oral Solution & Tablets 2235

Methohexital Sodium (Additive CNS depressant effects). Products include:

Brevital Sodium Vials 1429

Methotrimeprazine (Additive CNS depressant effects). Products include:

Levoprome 1274

Methoxyflurane (Additive CNS depressant effects).

No products indexed under this heading.

Methylprednisolone Acetate (Barbiturates enhance metabolism). Products include:

Depo-Medrol Single-Dose Vial 2600
Depo-Medrol Sterile Aqueous Suspension 2597

Methylprednisolone Sodium Succinate (Barbiturates enhance metabolism). Products include:

Solu-Medrol Sterile Powder 2643

Midazolam Hydrochloride (Additive CNS depressant effects). Products include:

Versed Injection 2170

Molindone Hydrochloride (Additive CNS depressant effects). Products include:

Moban Tablets and Concentrate 1048

Morphine Sulfate (Additive CNS depressant effects). Products include:

Astramorph/PF Injection, USP (Preservative-Free) 535
Duramorph 962
Infumorph 200 and Infumorph 500 Sterile Solutions 965
MS Contin Tablets 1994
MSIR 1997
Oramorph SR (Morphine Sulfate Sustained Release Tablets) 2236
RMS Suppositories 2657
Roxanol 2243

IMPORTANT NOTE: Always consult each drug listing in the patient's regimen for possible interactions.

Nembutal Sodium Suppositories Interactions Index

Opium Alkaloids (Additive CNS depressant effects).

No products indexed under this heading.

Oxazepam (Additive CNS depressant effects). Products include:

Serax Capsules 2810
Serax Tablets 2810

Oxycodone Hydrochloride (Additive CNS depressant effects). Products include:

Percocet Tablets 938
Percodan Tablets 939
Percodan-Demi Tablets 940
Roxicodone Tablets, Oral Solution & Intensol (Oxycodone) 2244
Tylox Capsules 1584

Perphenazine (Additive CNS depressant effects). Products include:

Etrafon 2355
Triavil Tablets 1757
Trilafon 2389

Phenelzine Sulfate (Prolongs effects of barbiturates). Products include:

Nardil 1920

Phenobarbital (Additive CNS depressant effects). Products include:

Arco-Lase Plus Tablets 512
Bellergal-S Tablets 2250
Donnatal 2060
Donnatal Extentabs 2061
Donnatal Tablets 2060
Phenobarbital Elixir and Tablets 1469
Quadrinal Tablets 1350

Phenytoin (Variable effect on metabolism of phenytoin). Products include:

Dilantin Infatabs 1908
Dilantin-125 Suspension 1911

Phenytoin Sodium (Variable effect on metabolism of phenytoin). Products include:

Dilantin Kapseals 1906
Dilantin Parenteral 1910

Polyestradiol Phosphate (Decreased effects of estrogens).

No products indexed under this heading.

Prazepam (Additive CNS depressant effects).

No products indexed under this heading.

Prednisolone Acetate (Barbiturates enhance metabolism). Products include:

AK-CIDE .... ◉ 202
AK-CIDE Ointment .... ◉ 202
Blephamide Liquifilm Sterile Ophthalmic Suspension 476
Blephamide Ointment .... ◉ 237
Econopred & Econopred Plus Ophthalmic Suspensions .... ◉ 217
Poly-Pred Liquifilm .... ◉ 248
Pred Forte .... ◉ 250
Pred Mild .... ◉ 253
Pred-G Liquifilm Sterile Ophthalmic Suspension .... ◉ 251
Pred-G S.O.P. Sterile Ophthalmic Ointment .... ◉ 252
Vasocidin Ointment .... ◉ 268

Prednisolone Sodium Phosphate (Barbiturates enhance metabolism). Products include:

AK-Pred .... ◉ 204
Hydeltrasol Injection, Sterile 1665
Inflamase .... ◉ 265
Pediapred Oral Liquid 995
Vasocidin Ophthalmic Solution ...... ◉ 270

Prednisolone Tebutate (Barbiturates enhance metabolism). Products include:

Hydeltra-T.B.A. Sterile Suspension 1667

Prednisone (Barbiturates enhance metabolism). Products include:

Deltasone Tablets 2595

Prochlorperazine (Additive CNS depressant effects). Products include:

Compazine 2470

Promethazine Hydrochloride (Additive CNS depressant effects). Products include:

Mepergan Injection 2753
Phenergan with Codeine 2777
Phenergan with Dextromethorphan 2778
Phenergan Injection 2773
Phenergan Suppositories 2775
Phenergan Syrup 2774
Phenergan Tablets 2775
Phenergan VC 2779
Phenergan VC with Codeine 2781

Propofol (Additive CNS depressant effects). Products include:

Diprivan Injection 2833

Propoxyphene Hydrochloride (Additive CNS depressant effects). Products include:

Darvon 1435
Wygesic Tablets 2827

Propoxyphene Napsylate (Additive CNS depressant effects). Products include:

Darvon-N/Darvocet-N 1433

Quazepam (Additive CNS depressant effects). Products include:

Doral Tablets 2664

Quinestrol (Decreased effects of estrogens).

No products indexed under this heading.

Risperidone (Additive CNS depressant effects). Products include:

Risperdal 1301

Secobarbital Sodium (Additive CNS depressant effects). Products include:

Seconal Sodium Pulvules 1474

Selegiline Hydrochloride (Prolongs effects of barbiturates). Products include:

Eldepryl Tablets 2550

Sufentanil Citrate (Additive CNS depressant effects). Products include:

Sufenta Injection 1309

Temazepam (Additive CNS depressant effects). Products include:

Restoril Capsules 2284

Thiamylal Sodium (Additive CNS depressant effects).

No products indexed under this heading.

Thioridazine Hydrochloride (Additive CNS depressant effects). Products include:

Mellaril 2269

Thiothixene (Additive CNS depressant effects). Products include:

Navane Capsules and Concentrate 2201
Navane Intramuscular 2202

Tranylcypromine Sulfate (Prolongs effects of barbiturates). Products include:

Parnate Tablets 2503

Triamcinolone (Barbiturates enhance metabolism). Products include:

Aristocort Tablets 1022

Triamcinolone Acetonide (Barbiturates enhance metabolism). Products include:

Aristocort A 0.025% Cream 1027
Aristocort A 0.5% Cream 1031
Aristocort A 0.1% Cream 1029
Aristocort A 0.1% Ointment 1030
Azmacort Oral Inhaler 2011
Nasacort Nasal Inhaler 2024

Triamcinolone Diacetate (Barbiturates enhance metabolism). Products include:

Aristocort Suspension (Forte Parenteral) 1027
Aristocort Suspension (Intralesional) 1025

Triamcinolone Hexacetonide (Barbiturates enhance metabolism). Products include:

Aristospan Suspension (Intra-articular) 1033
Aristospan Suspension (Intralesional) 1032

Triazolam (Additive CNS depressant effects). Products include:

Halcion Tablets 2611

Trifluoperazine Hydrochloride (Additive CNS depressant effects). Products include:

Stelazine 2514

Valproic Acid (Decreases barbiturates metabolism). Products include:

Depakene 413

Warfarin Sodium (Increased metabolism, decreased anticoagulant response). Products include:

Coumadin 926

Zolpidem Tartrate (Additive CNS depressant effects). Products include:

Ambien Tablets 2416

NEODECADRON STERILE OPHTHALMIC OINTMENT

(Neomycin Sulfate, Dexamethasone Sodium Phosphate) 1712
None cited in PDR database.

NEODECADRON STERILE OPHTHALMIC SOLUTION

(Neomycin Sulfate, Dexamethasone Sodium Phosphate) 1713
None cited in PDR database.

NEODECADRON TOPICAL CREAM

(Neomycin Sulfate, Dexamethasone Sodium Phosphate) 1714
None cited in PDR database.

NEORAL SOFT GELATIN CAPSULES FOR MICROEMULSION

(Cyclosporine) 2276
May interact with potassium sparing diuretics and certain other agents. Compounds in these categories include:

Allopurinol (Increases cyclosporine concentrations). Products include:

Zyloprim Tablets 1226

Amiloride Hydrochloride (Cyclosporine may cause hyperkalemia; concurrent use should be avoided). Products include:

Midamor Tablets 1703
Moduretic Tablets 1705

Amphotericin B (May potentiate renal dysfunction). Products include:

Fungizone Intravenous 506

Azathioprine (May potentiate renal dysfunction). Products include:

Imuran 1110

Bromocriptine Mesylate (Increases cyclosporine concentrations). Products include:

Parlodel 2281

Carbamazepine (Decreases cyclosporine concentrations). Products include:

Atretol Tablets 573
Tegretol Chewable Tablets 852
Tegretol Suspension 852
Tegretol Tablets 852

Cimetidine (May potentiate renal dysfunction). Products include:

Tagamet Tablets 2516

Cimetidine Hydrochloride (May potentiate renal dysfunction). Products include:

Tagamet 2516

Clarithromycin (Increases cyclosporine concentrations). Products include:

Biaxin 405

Danazol (Increases cyclosporine concentrations). Products include:

Danocrine Capsules 2307

Diclofenac Potassium (May potentiate renal dysfunction). Products include:

Cataflam 816

Diclofenac Sodium (May potentiate renal dysfunction). Products include:

Voltaren Ophthalmic Sterile Ophthalmic Solution .... ◉ 272
Voltaren Tablets 861

Digoxin (Reduced clearance of digoxin; decrease in the apparent volume of distribution of digoxin; severe digoxin toxicity can occur). Products include:

Lanoxicaps 1117
Lanoxin Elixir Pediatric 1120
Lanoxin Injection 1123
Lanoxin Injection Pediatric 1126
Lanoxin Tablets 1128

Diltiazem Hydrochloride (Increases cyclosporine concentrations). Products include:

Cardizem CD Capsules 1506
Cardizem SR Capsules 1510
Cardizem Injectable 1508
Cardizem Tablets 1512
Dilacor XR Extended-release Capsules 2018

Erythromycin (Increases cyclosporine concentrations). Products include:

A/T/S 2% Acne Topical Gel and Solution 1234
Benzamycin Topical Gel 905
E-Mycin Tablets 1341
Emgel 2% Topical Gel 1093
ERYC 1915
Erycette (erythromycin 2%) Topical Solution 1888
Ery-Tab Tablets 422
Erythromycin Base Filmtab 426
Erythromycin Delayed-Release Capsules, USP 427
Ilotycin Ophthalmic Ointment 912
PCE Dispertab Tablets 444
T-Stat 2.0% Topical Solution and Pads 2688
Theramycin Z Topical Solution 2% 1592

Erythromycin Estolate (Increases cyclosporine concentrations). Products include:

Ilosone 911

Erythromycin Ethylsuccinate (Increases cyclosporine concentrations). Products include:

E.E.S. 424
EryPed 421

Erythromycin Gluceptate (Increases cyclosporine concentrations). Products include:

Ilotycin Gluceptate, IV, Vials 913

Erythromycin Lactobionate (Increases cyclosporine concentrations).

No products indexed under this heading.

Erythromycin Stearate (Increases cyclosporine concentrations). Products include:

Erythrocin Stearate Filmtab 425

Fluconazole (Increases cyclosporine concentrations). Products include:

Diflucan Injection, Tablets, and Oral Suspension 2194

Gentamicin Sulfate (May potentiate renal dysfunction). Products include:

Garamycin Injectable 2360
Genoptic Sterile Ophthalmic Solution .... ◉ 243
Genoptic Sterile Ophthalmic Ointment .... ◉ 243
Gentacidin Ointment .... ◉ 264

(**◼** Described in PDR For Nonprescription Drugs) (◉ Described in PDR For Ophthalmology)

Gentacidin Solution ◉ 264
Gentak ◉ 208
Pred-G Liquifilm Sterile Ophthalmic Suspension ◉ 251
Pred-G S.O.P. Sterile Ophthalmic Ointment ◉ 252

Itraconazole (Increases cyclosporine concentrations). Products include:
Sporanox Capsules 1305

Ketoconazole (May potentiate renal dysfunction; increases cyclosporine concentrations). Products include:
Nizoral 2% Cream 1297
Nizoral 2% Shampoo 1298
Nizoral Tablets 1298

Lovastatin (Reduced clearance of lovastatin; potential for mycositis). Products include:
Mevacor Tablets 1699

Melphalan (May potentiate renal dysfunction). Products include:
Alkeran Tablets 1071

Methylprednisolone (Increases cyclosporine concentrations; potential for convulsion with high doses of methylprednisolone). Products include:
Medrol 2621

Methylprednisolone Acetate (Increases cyclosporine concentrations; potential for convulsion with high doses of methylprednisolone). Products include:
Depo-Medrol Single-Dose Vial 2600
Depo-Medrol Sterile Aqueous Suspension 2597

Methylprednisolone Sodium Succinate (Increases cyclosporine concentrations; potential for convulsion with high doses of methylprednisolone). Products include:
Solu-Medrol Sterile Powder 2643

Metoclopramide Hydrochloride (Increases cyclosporine concentrations). Products include:
Reglan 2068

Nafcillin Sodium (Decreases cyclosporine concentrations).
No products indexed under this heading.

Nephrotoxic Drugs (Potential for increased nephrotoxicity; careful monitoring of renal function is required).

Nicardipine Hydrochloride (Increases cyclosporine concentrations). Products include:
Cardene Capsules 2095
Cardene I.V. 2709
Cardene SR Capsules 2097

Nifedipine (Potential for frequent gingival hyperplasia). Products include:
Adalat Capsules (10 mg and 20 mg) 587
Adalat CC 589
Procardia Capsules 1971
Procardia XL Extended Release Tablets 1972

Octreotide Acetate (Decreases cyclosporine concentrations). Products include:
Sandostatin Injection 2292

Phenobarbital (Decreases cyclosporine concentrations). Products include:
Arco-Lase Plus Tablets 512
Bellergal-S Tablets 2250
Donnatal 2060
Donnatal Extentabs 2061
Donnatal Tablets 2060
Phenobarbital Elixir and Tablets 1469
Quadrinal Tablets 1350

Phenytoin (Decreases cyclosporine concentrations). Products include:
Dilantin Infatabs 1908
Dilantin-125 Suspension 1911

Phenytoin Sodium (Decreases cyclosporine concentrations). Products include:
Dilantin Kapseals 1906
Dilantin Parenteral 1910

Prednisolone (Reduced clearance of prednisolone). Products include:
Prelone Syrup 1787

Prednisolone Acetate (Reduced clearance of prednisolone). Products include:
AK-CIDE ◉ 202
AK-CIDE Ointment ◉ 202
Blephamide Liquifilm Sterile Ophthalmic Suspension 476
Blephamide Ointment ◉ 237
Econopred & Econopred Plus Ophthalmic Suspensions ◉ 217
Poly-Pred Liquifilm ◉ 248
Pred Forte ◉ 250
Pred Mild ◉ 253
Pred-G Liquifilm Sterile Ophthalmic Suspension ◉ 251
Pred-G S.O.P. Sterile Ophthalmic Ointment ◉ 252
Vasocidin Ointment ◉ 268

Prednisolone Sodium Phosphate (Reduced clearance of prednisolone). Products include:
AK-Pred ◉ 204
Hydeltrasol Injection, Sterile 1665
Inflamase ◉ 265
Pediapred Oral Liquid 995
Vasocidin Ophthalmic Solution ◉ 270

Ranitidine Hydrochloride (May potentiate renal dysfunction). Products include:
Zantac 1209
Zantac Injection 1207
Zantac Syrup 1209

Rifabutin (Caution should be exercised if used concurrently). Products include:
Mycobutin Capsules 1957

Rifampin (Decreases cyclosporine concentrations). Products include:
Rifadin 1528
Rifamate Capsules 1530
Rifater 1532
Rimactane Capsules 847

Spironolactone (Cyclosporine may cause hyperkalemia; concurrent use should be avoided). Products include:
Aldactazide 2413
Aldactone 2414

Sulfamethoxazole (May potentiate renal dysfunction). Products include:
Azo Gantanol Tablets 2080
Bactrim DS Tablets 2084
Bactrim I.V. Infusion 2082
Bactrim 2084
Gantanol Tablets 2119
Septra 1174
Septra I.V. Infusion 1169
Septra I.V. Infusion ADD-Vantage Vials 1171
Septra 1174

Tacrolimus (May potentiate renal dysfunction). Products include:
Prograf 1042

Ticlopidine Hydrochloride (Decreases cyclosporine concentrations). Products include:
Ticlid Tablets 2156

Tobramycin (May potentiate renal dysfunction). Products include:
AKTOB ◉ 206
TobraDex Ophthalmic Suspension and Ointment 473
Tobrex Ophthalmic Ointment and Solution ◉ 229

Tobramycin Sulfate (May potentiate renal dysfunction). Products include:
Nebcin Vials, Hyporets & ADD-Vantage 1464
Tobramycin Sulfate Injection 968

Triamterene (Cyclosporine may cause hyperkalemia; concurrent use should be avoided). Products include:
Dyazide 2479
Dyrenium Capsules 2481
Maxzide 1380

Trimethoprim (May potentiate renal dysfunction). Products include:
Bactrim DS Tablets 2084
Bactrim I.V. Infusion 2082
Bactrim 2084
Proloprim Tablets 1155
Septra 1174
Septra I.V. Infusion 1169
Septra I.V. Infusion ADD-Vantage Vials 1171
Septra 1174
Trimpex Tablets 2163

Vaccines (Live) (Vaccination may be less effective).

Vancomycin Hydrochloride (May potentiate renal dysfunction). Products include:
Vancocin HCl, Oral Solution & Pulvules 1483
Vancocin HCl, Vials & ADD-Vantage 1481

Verapamil Hydrochloride (Increases cyclosporine concentrations). Products include:
Calan SR Caplets 2422
Calan Tablets 2419
Isoptin Injectable 1344
Isoptin Oral Tablets 1346
Isoptin SR Tablets 1348
Verelan Capsules 1410
Verelan Capsules 2824

Food Interactions

Diet, high-lipid (A high fat meal consumed within one-half hour before Neoral administration decreased the AUC by 13% and C_{max} by 33%).

Food, unspecified (Administration of food with Neoral decreases the AUC and C_{max}).

Grapefruit (Affects the metabolism of cyclosporine and should be avoided).

Grapefruit Juice (Affects the metabolism of cyclosporine and should be avoided).

NEORAL ORAL SOLUTION FOR MICROEMULSION

(Cyclosporine) 2276
See **Neoral Soft Gelatin Capsules for Microemulsion**

NEOSAR LYOPHILIZED/NEOSAR

(Cyclophosphamide) 1959
May interact with cytotoxic drugs, general anesthetics, and certain other agents. Compounds in these categories include:

Bleomycin Sulfate (Possibility of combined drug action resulting in desirable or undesirable effects). Products include:
Blenoxane 692

Daunorubicin Hydrochloride (Possibility of combined drug action resulting in desirable or undesirable effects). Products include:
Cerubidine 795

Doxorubicin Hydrochloride (Doxorubicin-induced cardiotoxicity potentiated). Products include:
Adriamycin PFS 1947
Adriamycin RDF 1947
Doxorubicin Astra 540
Rubex 712

Enflurane (Effect not specified; anesthesiologist should be alerted).
No products indexed under this heading.

Fluorouracil (Possibility of combined drug action resulting in desirable or undesirable effects). Products include:
Efudex 2113
Fluoroplex Topical Solution & Cream 1% 479
Fluorouracil Injection 2116

Hydroxyurea (Possibility of combined drug action resulting in desirable or undesirable effects). Products include:
Hydrea Capsules 696

Isoflurane (Effect not specified; anesthesiologist should be alerted).
No products indexed under this heading.

Ketamine Hydrochloride (Effect not specified; anesthesiologist should be alerted).
No products indexed under this heading.

Methohexital Sodium (Effect not specified; anesthesiologist should be alerted). Products include:
Brevital Sodium Vials 1429

Methotrexate Sodium (Possibility of combined drug action resulting in desirable or undesirable effects). Products include:
Methotrexate Sodium Tablets, Injection, for Injection and LPF Injection 1275

Methoxyflurane (Effect not specified; anesthesiologist should be alerted).
No products indexed under this heading.

Mitotane (Possibility of combined drug action resulting in desirable or undesirable effects). Products include:
Lysodren 698

Mitoxantrone Hydrochloride (Possibility of combined drug action resulting in desirable or undesirable effects). Products include:
Novantrone 1279

Phenobarbital (Co-administration with chronic high doses of phenobarbital increases the rate of metabolism and the leukopenic activity of cyclophosphamide). Products include:
Arco-Lase Plus Tablets 512
Bellergal-S Tablets 2250
Donnatal 2060
Donnatal Extentabs 2061
Donnatal Tablets 2060
Phenobarbital Elixir and Tablets 1469
Quadrinal Tablets 1350

Procarbazine Hydrochloride (Possibility of combined drug action resulting in desirable or undesirable effects). Products include:
Matulane Capsules 2131

Propofol (Effect not specified; anesthesiologist should be alerted). Products include:
Diprivan Injection 2833

Succinylcholine Chloride (Marked and perisistent inhibition of cholinesterase activity; potentiates the effect of succinylcholine chloride). Products include:
Anectine 1073

Tamoxifen Citrate (Possibility of combined drug action resulting in desirable or undesirable effects). Products include:
Nolvadex Tablets 2841

Vincristine Sulfate (Possibility of combined drug action resulting in desirable or undesirable effects). Products include:
Oncovin Solution Vials & Hyporets 1466

IMPORTANT NOTE: Always consult each drug listing in the patient's regimen for possible interactions.

Neosar — Interactions Index

NEOSPORIN G.U. IRRIGANT STERILE (Neomycin Sulfate, Polymyxin B Sulfate) ....1148 None cited in PDR database.

NEOSPORIN OINTMENT (Bacitracin Zinc, Neomycin Sulfate, Polymyxin B Sulfate) .... ✦◎ 857 None cited in PDR database.

NEOSPORIN PLUS MAXIMUM STRENGTH CREAM (Polymyxin B Sulfate, Neomycin Sulfate, Lidocaine) .... ✦◎ 858 None cited in PDR database.

NEOSPORIN PLUS MAXIMUM STRENGTH OINTMENT (Polymyxin B Sulfate, Bacitracin Zinc, Neomycin Sulfate, Lidocaine) ✦◎ 858 None cited in PDR database.

NEOSPORIN OPHTHALMIC OINTMENT STERILE (Polymyxin B Sulfate, Bacitracin Zinc, Neomycin Sulfate) ....1148 None cited in PDR database.

NEOSPORIN OPHTHALMIC SOLUTION STERILE (Polymyxin B Sulfate, Neomycin Sulfate, Gramicidin) ....1149 None cited in PDR database.

NEOSTRATA AHA GEL FOR AGE SPOTS & SKIN LIGHTENING (Hydroquinone) ....1793 None cited in PDR database.

NEO-SYNEPHRINE MAXIMUM STRENGTH 12 HOUR NASAL SPRAY (Oxymetazoline Hydrochloride) ...... ✦◎ 726 None cited in PDR database.

NEO-SYNEPHRINE MAXIMUM STRENGTH 12 HOUR EXTRA MOISTURIZING NASAL SPRAY (Oxymetazoline Hydrochloride) ...... ✦◎ 726 None cited in PDR database.

NEO-SYNEPHRINE MAXIMUM STRENGTH 12 HOUR NASAL SPRAY PUMP (Oxymetazoline Hydrochloride) ...... ✦◎ 726 None cited in PDR database.

NEO-SYNEPHRINE HYDROCHLORIDE 1% CARPUJECT (Phenylephrine Hydrochloride) ....2324 May interact with monoamine oxidase inhibitors, tricyclic antidepressants, oxytocic drugs, and certain other agents. Compounds in these categories include:

Amitriptyline Hydrochloride (Pressor response potentiated). Products include:

Elavil .... 2838 Endep Tablets .... 2174 Etrafon .... 2355 Limbitrol .... 2180 Triavil Tablets 1757

Amoxapine (Pressor response potentiated). Products include:

Asendin Tablets 1369

Clomipramine Hydrochloride (Pressor response potentiated). Products include:

Anafranil Capsules 803

Desipramine Hydrochloride (Pressor response potentiated). Products include:

Norpramin Tablets 1526

Doxepin Hydrochloride (Pressor response potentiated). Products include:

Sinequan .... 2205 Zonalon Cream 1055

Ergonovine Maleate (Potentiates pressor effect).

No products indexed under this heading.

Furazolidone (Potentiates effect of sympathomimetic pressor amines). Products include:

Furoxone 2046

Halothane (May cause serious cardiac arrhythmias). Products include:

Fluothane 2724

Imipramine Hydrochloride (Pressor response potentiated). Products include:

Tofranil Ampuls .... 854 Tofranil Tablets 856

Imipramine Pamoate (Pressor response potentiated). Products include:

Tofranil-PM Capsules 857

Isocarboxazid (Potentiates effect of sympathomimetic pressor amines).

No products indexed under this heading.

Methylergonovine Maleate (Potentiates pressor effect). Products include:

Methergine 2272

Nortriptyline Hydrochloride (Pressor response potentiated). Products include:

Pamelor 2280

Oxytocin (Potentiates pressor effect). Products include:

Oxytocin Injection .... 2771 Syntocinon Injection 2296

Phenelzine Sulfate (Potentiates effect of sympathomimetic pressor amines). Products include:

Nardil 1920

Protriptyline Hydrochloride (Pressor response potentiated). Products include:

Vivactil Tablets 1774

Selegiline Hydrochloride (Potentiates effect of sympathomimetic pressor amines). Products include:

Eldepryl Tablets 2550

Tranylcypromine Sulfate (Potentiates effect of sympathomimetic pressor amines). Products include:

Parnate Tablets 2503

Trimipramine Maleate (Pressor response potentiated). Products include:

Surmontil Capsules 2811

NEO-SYNEPHRINE HYDROCHLORIDE 1% INJECTION (Phenylephrine Hydrochloride) ....2324 See Neo-Synephrine Hydrochloride 1% Carpuject

NEO-SYNEPHRINE HYDROCHLORIDE (OPHTHALMIC) (Phenylephrine Hydrochloride) ....2325 May interact with beta blockers, monoamine oxidase inhibitors, tricyclic antidepressants, inhalant anesthetics, and certain other agents. Compounds in these categories include:

Acebutolol Hydrochloride (Acute hypertension; ruptured congenital cerebral aneurysm may occur). Products include:

Sectral Capsules 2807

Amitriptyline Hydrochloride (Pressor response potentiated). Products include:

Elavil .... 2838 Endep Tablets .... 2174 Etrafon .... 2355 Limbitrol .... 2180 Triavil Tablets 1757

Amoxapine (Pressor response potentiated). Products include:

Asendin Tablets 1369

Atenolol (Acute hypertension; ruptured congenital cerebral aneurysm may occur). Products include:

Tenoretic Tablets .... 2845 Tenormin Tablets and I.V. Injection 2847

Betaxolol Hydrochloride (Acute hypertension; ruptured congenital cerebral aneurysm may occur). Products include:

Betoptic Ophthalmic Solution............ 469 Betoptic S Ophthalmic Suspension 471 Kerlone Tablets 2436

Bisoprolol Fumarate (Acute hypertension; ruptured congenital cerebral aneurysm may occur). Products include:

Zebeta Tablets .... 1413 Ziac 1415

Carteolol Hydrochloride (Acute hypertension; ruptured congenital cerebral aneurysm may occur). Products include:

Cartrol Tablets .... 410 Ocupress Ophthalmic Solution, 1% Sterile .... ◎ 309

Clomipramine Hydrochloride (Pressor response potentiated). Products include:

Anafranil Capsules 803

Desflurane (Neo-Synephrine may potentiate the cardiovascular depressant effects of potent inhalation anesthetic agents). Products include:

Suprane 1813

Desipramine Hydrochloride (Pressor response potentiated). Products include:

Norpramin Tablets 1526

Doxepin Hydrochloride (Pressor response potentiated). Products include:

Sinequan .... 2205 Zonalon Cream 1055

Enflurane (Neo-Synephrine may potentiate the cardiovascular depressant effects of potent inhalation anesthetic agents).

No products indexed under this heading.

Esmolol Hydrochloride (Acute hypertension; ruptured congenital cerebral aneurysm may occur). Products include:

Brevibloc Injection 1808

Furazolidone (Exaggerated adrenergic effects may occur). Products include:

Furoxone 2046

Guanethidine Monosulfate (Pressor response potentiated). Products include:

Ismelin Tablets .... 822 Ismelin Tablets 827

Halothane (Neo-Synephrine may potentiate the cardiovascular depressant effects of potent inhalation anesthetic agents). Products include:

Fluothane 2724

Imipramine Hydrochloride (Pressor response potentiated). Products include:

Tofranil Ampuls .... 854 Tofranil Tablets 856

Imipramine Pamoate (Pressor response potentiated). Products include:

Tofranil-PM Capsules 857

Isocarboxazid (Exaggerated adrenergic effects may occur).

No products indexed under this heading.

Isoflurane (Neo-Synephrine may potentiate the cardiovascular depressant effects of potent inhalation anesthetic agents).

No products indexed under this heading.

Labetalol Hydrochloride (Acute hypertension; ruptured congenital cerebral aneurysm may occur). Products include:

Normodyne Injection .... 2377 Normodyne Tablets .... 2379 Trandate 1185

Levobunolol Hydrochloride (Acute hypertension; ruptured congenital cerebral aneurysm may occur). Products include:

Betagan .... ◎ 233

Maprotiline Hydrochloride (Pressor response potentiated). Products include:

Ludiomil Tablets 843

Methoxyflurane (Neo-Synephrine may potentiate the cardiovascular depressant effects of potent inhalation anesthetic agents).

No products indexed under this heading.

Methyldopa (Pressor response potentiated). Products include:

Aldoclor Tablets .... 1598 Aldomet Oral .... 1600 Aldoril Tablets 1604

Methyldopate Hydrochloride (Pressor response potentiated). Products include:

Aldomet Ester HCl Injection 1602

Metipranolol Hydrochloride (Acute hypertension; ruptured congenital cerebral aneurysm may occur). Products include:

OptiPranolol (Metipranolol 0.3%) Sterile Ophthalmic Solution.......... ◎ 258

Metoprolol Succinate (Acute hypertension; ruptured congenital cerebral aneurysm may occur). Products include:

Toprol-XL Tablets 565

Metoprolol Tartrate (Acute hypertension; ruptured congenital cerebral aneurysm may occur). Products include:

Lopressor Ampuls .... 830 Lopressor HCT Tablets .... 832 Lopressor Tablets 830

Nadolol (Acute hypertension; ruptured congenital cerebral aneurysm may occur).

No products indexed under this heading.

Nortriptyline Hydrochloride (Pressor response potentiated). Products include:

Pamelor 2280

Penbutolol Sulfate (Acute hypertension; ruptured congenital cerebral aneurysm may occur). Products include:

Levatol 2403

Phenelzine Sulfate (Exaggerated adrenergic effects may occur). Products include:

Nardil 1920

(✦◎ Described in PDR For Nonprescription Drugs)   (◎ Described in PDR For Ophthalmology)

Interactions Index

Pindolol (Acute hypertension; ruptured congenital cerebral aneurysm may occur). Products include:

Visken Tablets....................................... 2299

Propranolol Hydrochloride (Acute hypertension; ruptured congenital cerebral aneurysm may occur). Products include:

Inderal 2728
Inderal LA Long Acting Capsules 2730
Inderide Tablets 2732
Inderide LA Long Acting Capsules .. 2734

Protriptyline Hydrochloride (Pressor response potentiated). Products include:

Vivactil Tablets 1774

Selegiline Hydrochloride (Exaggerated adrenergic effects may occur). Products include:

Eldepryl Tablets 2550

Sotalol Hydrochloride (Acute hypertension; ruptured congenital cerebral aneurysm may occur). Products include:

Betapace Tablets 641

Timolol Hemihydrate (Acute hypertension; ruptured congenital cerebral aneurysm may occur). Products include:

Betimol 0.25%, 0.5% .... ◎ 261

Timolol Maleate (Acute hypertension; ruptured congenital cerebral aneurysm may occur). Products include:

Blocadren Tablets 1614
Timolide Tablets...................................... 1748
Timoptic in Ocudose 1753
Timoptic Sterile Ophthalmic Solution... 1751
Timoptic-XE 1755

Tranylcypromine Sulfate (Exaggerated adrenergic effects may occur). Products include:

Parnate Tablets 2503

Trimipramine Maleate (Pressor response potentiated). Products include:

Surmontil Capsules................................ 2811

NEO-SYNEPHRINE NASAL DROPS, PEDIATRIC, MILD, REGULAR & EXTRA STRENGTH

(Phenylephrine Hydrochloride) .... ⊞ 726
None cited in PDR database.

NEO-SYNEPHRINE NASAL SPRAYS, PEDIATRIC, MILD, REGULAR & EXTRA STRENGTH

(Phenylephrine Hydrochloride) .... ⊞ 726
None cited in PDR database.

NEPHRAMINE

(Amino Acid Preparations) 2005
None cited in PDR database.

NEPHRO-CALCI TABLETS

(Calcium Carbonate) 2004
None cited in PDR database.

NEPHROCAPS

(Vitamins, Multiple) 1005
None cited in PDR database.

NEPHRO-FER TABLETS

(Ferrous Fumarate) 2004
None cited in PDR database.

NEPHRO-FER RX TABLETS

(Ferrous Fumarate, Folic Acid) 2005
None cited in PDR database.

NEPHRO-VITE + FE TABLETS

(Vitamins, Multiple, Ferrous Fumarate) 2006
None cited in PDR database.

NEPHRO-VITE RX TABLETS

(Vitamins with Minerals) 2006
None cited in PDR database.

NEPHROX SUSPENSION

(Aluminum Hydroxide Gel, Mineral Oil)... ⊞ 655
None cited in PDR database.

NEPRO SPECIALIZED LIQUID NUTRITION

(Nutritional Supplement) 2222
None cited in PDR database.

NEPTAZANE TABLETS

(Methazolamide) 1388
May interact with corticosteroids and certain other agents. Compounds in these categories include:

Aspirin (Concomitant use of high-dose aspirin and carbonic anhydrase inhibitors may produce anorexia, tachypnea, lethargy, coma, and death). Products include:

Alka-Seltzer Effervescent Antacid and Pain Reliever................................ ⊞ 701
Alka-Seltzer Extra Strength Effervescent Antacid and Pain Reliever .... ⊞ 703
Alka-Seltzer Lemon Lime Effervescent Antacid and Pain Reliever .... ⊞ 703
Alka-Seltzer Plus Cold Medicine .... ⊞ 705
Alka-Seltzer Plus Cold & Cough Medicine .... ⊞ 708
Alka-Seltzer Plus Night-Time Cold Medicine .... ⊞ 707
Alka Seltzer Plus Sinus Medicine .. ⊞ 707
Arthritis Foundation Safety Coated Aspirin Tablets .... ⊞ 675
Arthritis Pain Ascriptin .... ⊞ 631
Maximum Strength Ascriptin .... ⊞ 630
Regular Strength Ascriptin Tablets .... ⊞ 629
Arthritis Strength BC Powder......... ⊞ 609
BC Cold Powder Multi-Symptom Formula (Cold-Sinus-Allergy) ... ⊞ 609
BC Cold Powder Non-Drowsy Formula (Cold-Sinus)...................... ⊞ 609
BC Powder .... ⊞ 609
Bayer Children's Chewable Aspirin.. ⊞ 711
Genuine Bayer Aspirin Tablets & Caplets .... ⊞ 713
Extra Strength Bayer Arthritis Pain Regimen Formula .... ⊞ 711
Extra Strength Bayer Aspirin Caplets & Tablets .... ⊞ 712
Extended-Release Bayer 8-Hour Aspirin .... ⊞ 712
Extra Strength Bayer Plus Aspirin Caplets .... ⊞ 713
Extra Strength Bayer PM Aspirin .. ⊞ 713
Bayer Enteric Aspirin .... ⊞ 709
Bufferin Analgesic Tablets and Caplets .... ⊞ 613
Arthritis Strength Bufferin Analgesic Caplets .... ⊞ 614
Extra Strength Bufferin Analgesic Tablets .... ⊞ 615
Cama Arthritis Pain Reliever.......... ⊞ 785
Darvon Compound-65 Pulvules 1435
Easprin 1914
Ecotrin 2455
Ecotrin Enteric Coated Aspirin Maximum Strength Tablets and Caplets .... ⊞ 816
Ecotrin Enteric Coated Aspirin Regular Strength Tablets 2455
Empirin Aspirin Tablets .... ⊞ 854
Empirin with Codeine Tablets.......... 1093
Excedrin Extra-Strength Analgesic Tablets & Caplets 732
Fiorinal Capsules 2261
Fiorinal with Codeine Capsules 2262
Fiorinal Tablets 2261
Halfprin 1362
Healthprin Aspirin 2455
Norgesic.. 1496
Percodan Tablets.................................... 939
Percodan-Demi Tablets........................ 940
Robaxisal Tablets................................... 2071
Soma Compound w/Codeine Tablets 2676
Soma Compound Tablets 2675

St. Joseph Adult Chewable Aspirin (81 mg.) .... ⊞ 808
Talwin Compound 2335
Ursinus Inlay-Tabs................................ ⊞ 794
Vanquish Analgesic Caplets .... ⊞ 731

Betamethasone Acetate (Potential for developing hypokalemia). Products include:

Celestone Soluspan Suspension 2347

Betamethasone Sodium Phosphate (Potential for developing hypokalemia). Products include:

Celestone Soluspan Suspension 2347

Cortisone Acetate (Potential for developing hypokalemia). Products include:

Cortone Acetate Sterile Suspension 1623
Cortone Acetate Tablets..................... 1624

Dexamethasone (Potential for developing hypokalemia). Products include:

AK-Trol Ointment & Suspension ... ◎ 205
Decadron Elixir 1633
Decadron Tablets................................... 1635
Decaspray Topical Aerosol 1648
Dexacidin Ointment .... ◎ 263
Maxitrol Ophthalmic Ointment and Suspension .... ◎ 224
TobraDex Ophthalmic Suspension and Ointment...................................... 473

Dexamethasone Acetate (Potential for developing hypokalemia). Products include:

Dalalone D.P. Injectable 1011
Decadron-LA Sterile Suspension..... 1646

Dexamethasone Sodium Phosphate (Potential for developing hypokalemia). Products include:

Decadron Phosphate Injection 1637
Decadron Phosphate Respihaler..... 1642
Decadron Phosphate Sterile Ophthalmic Ointment 1641
Decadron Phosphate Sterile Ophthalmic Solution 1642
Decadron Phosphate Topical Cream.. 1644
Decadron Phosphate Turbinaire 1645
Decadron Phosphate with Xylocaine Injection, Sterile 1639
Dexacort Phosphate in Respihaler .. 458
Dexacort Phosphate in Turbinaire .. 459
NeoDecadron Sterile Ophthalmic Ointment... 1712
NeoDecadron Sterile Ophthalmic Solution 1713
NeoDecadron Topical Cream 1714

Fludrocortisone Acetate (Potential for developing hypokalemia). Products include:

Florinef Acetate Tablets 505

Hydrocortisone (Potential for developing hypokalemia). Products include:

Anusol-HC Cream 2.5% 1896
Aquanil HC Lotion 1931
Bactine Hydrocortisone Anti-Itch Cream... ⊞ 709
Caldecort Anti-Itch Hydrocortisone Spray .... ⊞ 631
Cortaid .... ⊞ 836
CORTENEMA.. 2535
Cortisporin Ointment 1085
Cortisporin Ophthalmic Ointment Sterile 1085
Cortisporin Ophthalmic Suspension Sterile 1086
Cortisporin Otic Solution Sterile 1087
Cortisporin Otic Suspension Sterile 1088
Cortizone-5 .... ⊞ 831
Cortizone-10 .... ⊞ 831
Hydrocortone Tablets 1672
Hytone 907
Massengill Medicated Soft Cloth Towelettes.. 2458
PediOtic Suspension Sterile 1153
Preparation H Hydrocortisone 1% Cream .... ⊞ 872
ProctoCream-HC 2.5% 2408
VōSoL HC Otic Solution....................... 2678

Hydrocortisone Acetate (Potential for developing hypokalemia). Products include:

Analpram-HC Rectal Cream 1% and 2.5% 977

Anusol HC-1 Anti-Itch Hydrocortisone Ointment...................................... ⊞ 847
Anusol-HC Suppositories 1897
Caldecort... ⊞ 631
Carmol HC 924
Coly-Mycin S Otic w/Neomycin & Hydrocortisone 1906
Cortaid .... ⊞ 836
Cortifoam 2396
Cortisporin Cream................................. 1084
Epifoam 2399
Hydrocortone Acetate Sterile Suspension... 1669
Mantadil Cream 1135
Nupercainal Hydrocortisone 1% Cream... ⊞ 645
Ophthocort .... ◎ 311
Pramosone Cream, Lotion & Ointment 978
ProctoCream-HC 2408
ProctoFoam-HC 2409
Terra-Cortril Ophthalmic Suspension 2210

Hydrocortisone Sodium Phosphate (Potential for developing hypokalemia). Products include:

Hydrocortone Phosphate Injection, Sterile 1670

Hydrocortisone Sodium Succinate (Potential for developing hypokalemia). Products include:

Solu-Cortef Sterile Powder................. 2641

Methylprednisolone Acetate (Potential for developing hypokalemia). Products include:

Depo-Medrol Single-Dose Vial 2600
Depo-Medrol Sterile Aqueous Suspension... 2597

Methylprednisolone Sodium Succinate (Potential for developing hypokalemia). Products include:

Solu-Medrol Sterile Powder 2643

Prednisolone Acetate (Potential for developing hypokalemia). Products include:

AK-CIDE .... ◎ 202
AK-CIDE Ointment................................ ◎ 202
Blephamide Liquifilm Sterile Ophthalmic Suspension................................ 476
Blephamide Ointment .... ◎ 237
Econopred & Econopred Plus Ophthalmic Suspensions .... ◎ 217
Poly-Pred Liquifilm .... ◎ 248
Pred Forte... ◎ 250
Pred Mild... ◎ 253
Pred-G Liquifilm Sterile Ophthalmic Suspension .... ◎ 251
Pred-G S.O.P. Sterile Ophthalmic Ointment... ◎ 252
Vasocidin Ointment .... ◎ 268

Prednisolone Sodium Phosphate (Potential for developing hypokalemia). Products include:

AK-Pred .... ◎ 204
Hydeltrasol Injection, Sterile............. 1665
Inflamase... ◎ 265
Pediapred Oral Liquid 995
Vasocidin Ophthalmic Solution .... ◎ 270

Prednisolone Tebutate (Potential for developing hypokalemia). Products include:

Hydeltra-T.B.A. Sterile Suspension 1667

Prednisone (Potential for developing hypokalemia). Products include:

Deltasone Tablets 2595

Triamcinolone (Potential for developing hypokalemia). Products include:

Aristocort Tablets 1022

Triamcinolone Acetonide (Potential for developing hypokalemia). Products include:

Aristocort A 0.025% Cream 1027
Aristocort A 0.5% Cream 1031
Aristocort A 0.1% Cream 1029
Aristocort A 0.1% Ointment 1030
Azmacort Oral Inhaler 2011
Nasacort Nasal Inhaler 2024

Triamcinolone Diacetate (Potential for developing hypokalemia). Products include:

Aristocort Suspension (Forte Parenteral).. 1027

IMPORTANT NOTE: Always consult each drug listing in the patient's regimen for possible interactions.

Neptazane Interactions Index 710

Aristocort Suspension (Intralesional) ... 1025

Triamcinolone Hexacetonide (Potential for developing hypokalemia). Products include:

Aristospan Suspension (Intra-articular) ... 1033
Aristospan Suspension (Intralesional) ... 1032

NESACAINE INJECTIONS
(Chloroprocaine Hydrochloride) ... 554
May interact with monoamine oxidase inhibitors, phenothiazines, sulfonamides, tricyclic antidepressants, vasopressors, and certain other agents. Compounds in these categories include:

Amitriptyline Hydrochloride (Severe, prolonged hypotension or hypertension). Products include:

Elavil ... 2838
Endep Tablets ... 2174
Etrafon ... 2355
Limbitrol ... 2180
Triavil Tablets ... 1757

Amoxapine (Severe, prolonged hypotension or hypertension). Products include:

Asendin Tablets ... 1369

Chlorpromazine (Severe, prolonged hypotension or hypertension). Products include:

Thorazine Suppositories ... 2523

Clomipramine Hydrochloride (Severe, prolonged hypotension or hypertension). Products include:

Anafranil Capsules ... 803

Desipramine Hydrochloride (Severe, prolonged hypotension or hypertension). Products include:

Norpramin Tablets ... 1526

Dopamine Hydrochloride (Severe, persistent hypertension or cerebrovascular accidents).

No products indexed under this heading.

Doxepin Hydrochloride (Severe, prolonged hypotension or hypertension). Products include:

Sinequan ... 2205
Zonalon Cream ... 1055

Epinephrine Bitartrate (Severe, persistent hypertension or cerebrovascular accidents). Products include:

Bronkaid Mist Suspension ... ▣ 718
Sensorcaine-MPF with Epinephrine Injection ... 559

Epinephrine Hydrochloride (Severe, persistent hypertension or cerebrovascular accidents). Products include:

Ana-Kit Anaphylaxis Emergency Treatment Kit ... 617

Ergonovine Maleate (Severe, persistent hypertension or cerebrovascular accidents).

No products indexed under this heading.

Fluphenazine Decanoate (Severe, prolonged hypotension or hypertension). Products include:

Prolixin Decanoate ... 509

Fluphenazine Enanthate (Severe, prolonged hypotension or hypertension). Products include:

Prolixin Enanthate ... 509

Fluphenazine Hydrochloride (Severe, prolonged hypotension or hypertension). Products include:

Prolixin ... 509

Furazolidone (Severe, prolonged hypotension or hypertension). Products include:

Furoxone ... 2046

Imipramine Hydrochloride (Severe, prolonged hypotension or hypertension). Products include:

Tofranil Ampuls ... 854
Tofranil Tablets ... 856

Imipramine Pamoate (Severe, prolonged hypotension or hypertension). Products include:

Tofranil-PM Capsules ... 857

Isocarboxazid (Severe, prolonged hypotension or hypertension).

No products indexed under this heading.

Maprotiline Hydrochloride (Severe, prolonged hypotension or hypertension). Products include:

Ludiomil Tablets ... 843

Mesoridazine Besylate (Severe, prolonged hypotension or hypertension). Products include:

Serentil ... 684

Metaraminol Bitartrate (Severe, persistent hypertension or cerebrovascular accidents). Products include:

Aramine Injection ... 1609

Methotrimeprazine (Severe, prolonged hypotension or hypertension). Products include:

Levoprome ... 1274

Methoxamine Hydrochloride (Severe, persistent hypertension or cerebrovascular accidents). Products include:

Vasoxyl Injection ... 1196

Methyclothiazide (Action of sulfonamides inhibited). Products include:

Enduron Tablets ... 420

Methylergonovine Maleate (Severe persistent hypertension or cerebrovascular accidents). Products include:

Methergine ... 2272

Norepinephrine Bitartrate (Severe, persistent hypertension or cerebrovascular accidents). Products include:

Levophed Bitartrate Injection ... 2315

Nortriptyline Hydrochloride (Severe, prolonged hypotension or hypertension). Products include:

Pamelor ... 2280

Perphenazine (Severe, prolonged hypotension or hypertension). Products include:

Etrafon ... 2355
Triavil Tablets ... 1757
Trilafon ... 2389

Phenelzine Sulfate (Severe, prolonged hypotension or hypertension). Products include:

Nardil ... 1920

Phenylephrine Hydrochloride (Severe, persistent hypertension or cerebrovascular accidents). Products include:

Atrohist Plus Tablets ... 454
Cerose DM ... ▣ 878
Comhist ... 2038
D.A. Chewable Tablets ... 951
Deconsal Pediatric Capsules ... 454
Dura-Vent/DA Tablets ... 953
Entex Capsules ... 1986
Entex Liquid ... 1986
Extendryl ... 1005
4-Way Fast Acting Nasal Spray (regular & mentholated) ... ▣ 621
Hemorid For Women ... ▣ 834
Hycomine Compound Tablets ... 932
Neo-Synephrine Hydrochloride 1% Carpuject ... 2324
Neo-Synephrine Hydrochloride 1% Injection ... 2324
Neo-Synephrine Hydrochloride (Ophthalmic) ... 2325
Neo-Synephrine ... ▣ 726
Nōstril ... ▣ 644
Novahistine Elixir ... ▣ 823
Phenergan VC ... 2779
Phenergan VC with Codeine ... 2781
Preparation H ... ▣ 871
Tympagesic Ear Drops ... 2342
Vasosulf ... ⊙ 271
Vicks Sinex Nasal Spray and Ultra Fine Mist ... ▣ 765

Prochlorperazine (Severe, prolonged hypotension or hypertension). Products include:

Compazine ... 2470

Promethazine Hydrochloride (Severe, prolonged hypotension or hypertension). Products include:

Mepergan Injection ... 2753
Phenergan with Codeine ... 2777
Phenergan with Dextromethorphan 2778
Phenergan Injection ... 2773
Phenergan Suppositories ... 2775
Phenergan Syrup ... 2774
Phenergan Tablets ... 2775
Phenergan VC ... 2779
Phenergan VC with Codeine ... 2781

Protriptyline Hydrochloride (Severe, prolonged hypotension or hypertension). Products include:

Vivactil Tablets ... 1774

Selegiline Hydrochloride (Severe, prolonged hypotension or hypertension). Products include:

Eldepryl Tablets ... 2550

Sulfamethizole (Action of sulfonamides inhibited). Products include:

Urobiotic-250 Capsules ... 2214

Sulfamethoxazole (Action of sulfonamides inhibited). Products include:

Azo Gantanol Tablets ... 2080
Bactrim DS Tablets ... 2084
Bactrim I.V. Infusion ... 2082
Bactrim ... 2084
Gantanol Tablets ... 2119
Septra ... 1174
Septra I.V. Infusion ... 1169
Septra I.V. Infusion ADD-Vantage Vials ... 1171
Septra ... 1174

Sulfasalazine (Action of sulfonamides inhibited). Products include:

Azulfidine ... 1949

Sulfinpyrazone (Action of sulfonamides inhibited). Products include:

Anturane ... 807

Sulfisoxazole (Action of sulfonamides inhibited). Products include:

Azo Gantrisin Tablets ... 2081
Gantrisin Tablets ... 2120

Sulfisoxazole Diolamine (Action of sulfonamides inhibited).

No products indexed under this heading.

Thioridazine Hydrochloride (Severe, prolonged hypotension or hypertension). Products include:

Mellaril ... 2269

Tranylcypromine Sulfate (Severe, prolonged hypotension or hypertension). Products include:

Parnate Tablets ... 2503

Trifluoperazine Hydrochloride (Severe, prolonged hypotension or hypertension). Products include:

Stelazine ... 2514

Trimipramine Maleate (Severe, prolonged hypotension or hypertension). Products include:

Surmontil Capsules ... 2811

NESACAINE-MPF INJECTION
(Chloroprocaine Hydrochloride) ... 554
See **Nesacaine Injections**

NESTABS FA TABLETS
(Vitamins with Minerals) ... 982
None cited in PDR database.

NETROMYCIN INJECTION 100 MG/ML
(Netilmicin Sulfate) ... 2373
May interact with nondepolarizing neuromuscular blocking agents, diuretics, cephalosporins, penicillins, and certain other agents. Compounds in these categories include:

Acyclovir (Neurotoxicity and/or nephrotoxicity). Products include:

Zovirax Capsules ... 1219
Zovirax Ointment 5% ... 1223
Zovirax ... 1219

Acyclovir Sodium (Neurotoxicity and/or nephrotoxicity). Products include:

Zovirax Sterile Powder ... 1223

Amikacin Sulfate (Neurotoxicity and/or nephrotoxicity). Products include:

Amikacin Sulfate Injection, USP ... 960
Amikin Injectable ... 501

Amiloride Hydrochloride (Ototoxicity). Products include:

Midamor Tablets ... 1703
Moduretic Tablets ... 1705

Amoxicillin Trihydrate (Mutual inactivation). Products include:

Amoxil ... 2464
Augmentin ... 2468

Amphotericin B (Neurotoxicity and/or nephrotoxicity). Products include:

Fungizone Intravenous ... 506

Ampicillin Sodium (Mutual inactivation). Products include:

Unasyn ... 2212

Atracurium Besylate (Potential for increased neuromuscular blockade and respiratory paralysis). Products include:

Tracrium Injection ... 1183

Azlocillin Sodium (Mutual inactivation).

No products indexed under this heading.

Bacampicillin Hydrochloride (Mutual inactivation). Products include:

Spectrobid Tablets ... 2206

Bacitracin (Neurotoxicity and/or nephrotoxicity). Products include:

Mycitracin ... ▣ 839

Bacitracin Zinc (Neurotoxicity and/or nephrotoxicity). Products include:

AK-Spore Ointment ... ⊙ 204
Bactine First Aid Antibiotic Plus Anesthetic Ointment ... ▣ 708
Betadine Brand First Aid Antibiotics & Moisturizer Ointment ... 1991
Campho-Phenique Maximum Strength First Aid Antibiotic Plus Pain Reliever Ointment ... ▣ 719
Cortisporin Ointment ... 1085
Cortisporin Ophthalmic Ointment Sterile ... 1085
Neosporin Ointment ... ▣ 857
Neosporin Plus Maximum Strength Ointment ... ▣ 858
Neosporin Ophthalmic Ointment Sterile ... 1148
Polysporin Ointment ... ▣ 858
Polysporin Ophthalmic Ointment Sterile ... 1154
Polysporin Powder ... ▣ 859

Bendroflumethiazide (Ototoxicity).

No products indexed under this heading.

Bumetanide (Ototoxicity). Products include:

Bumex ... 2093

Carbenicillin Disodium (Mutual inactivation).

No products indexed under this heading.

Carbenicillin Indanyl Sodium (Mutual inactivation). Products include:

Geocillin Tablets ... 2199

Cefaclor (Nephrotoxicity). Products include:

Ceclor Pulvules & Suspension ... 1431

(▣ Described in PDR For Nonprescription Drugs) (⊙ Described in PDR For Ophthalmology)

711 Interactions Index Netromycin

Cefadroxil Monohydrate (Nephrotoxicity). Products include:
Duricef 748
Cefamandole Nafate (Nephrotoxicity). Products include:
Mandol Vials, Faspak & ADD-Vantage 1461
Cefazolin Sodium (Nephrotoxicity). Products include:
Ancef Injection 2465
Kefzol Vials, Faspak & ADD-Vantage 1456
Cefixime (Nephrotoxicity). Products include:
Suprax 1399
Cefmetazole Sodium (Nephrotoxicity). Products include:
Zefazone 2654
Cefonicid Sodium (Nephrotoxicity). Products include:
Monocid Injection 2497
Cefoperazone Sodium (Nephrotoxicity). Products include:
Cefobid Intravenous/Intramuscular 2189
Cefobid Pharmacy Bulk Package - Not for Direct Infusion 2192
Ceforanide (Nephrotoxicity).
No products indexed under this heading.
Cefotaxime Sodium (Nephrotoxicity). Products include:
Claforan Sterile and Injection 1235
Cefotetan (Nephrotoxicity). Products include:
Cefotan 2829
Cefoxitin Sodium (Nephrotoxicity). Products include:
Mefoxin 1691
Mefoxin Premixed Intravenous Solution 1694
Cefpodoxime Proxetil (Nephrotoxicity). Products include:
Vantin for Oral Suspension and Vantin Tablets 2646
Cefprozil (Nephrotoxicity). Products include:
Cefzil Tablets and Oral Suspension 746
Ceftazidime (Nephrotoxicity). Products include:
Ceptaz 1081
Fortaz 1100
Tazicef for Injection 2519
Tazidime Vials, Faspak & ADD-Vantage 1478
Ceftizoxime Sodium (Nephrotoxicity). Products include:
Cefizox for Intramuscular or Intravenous Use 1034
Ceftriaxone Sodium (Nephrotoxicity). Products include:
Rocephin Injectable Vials, ADD-Vantage, Galaxy Container 2142
Cefuroxime Axetil (Nephrotoxicity). Products include:
Ceftin 1078
Cefuroxime Sodium (Nephrotoxicity). Products include:
Kefurox Vials, Faspak & ADD-Vantage 1454
Zinacef 1211
Cephalexin (Nephrotoxicity). Products include:
Keflex Pulvules & Oral Suspension 914
Cephalothin Sodium (Nephrotoxicity).
Cephapirin Sodium (Nephrotoxicity).
No products indexed under this heading.
Cephradine (Nephrotoxicity).
No products indexed under this heading.
Chlorothiazide (Ototoxicity). Products include:
Aldoclor Tablets 1598
Diupres Tablets 1650
Diuril Oral 1653
Chlorothiazide Sodium (Ototoxicity). Products include:
Diuril Sodium Intravenous 1652
Chlorthalidone (Ototoxicity). Products include:
Combipres Tablets 677
Tenoretic Tablets 2845
Thalitone 1245
Cisplatin (Neurotoxicity and/or nephrotoxicity). Products include:
Platinol 708
Platinol-AQ Injection 710
Colistin Sulfate (Neurotoxicity and/or nephrotoxicity). Products include:
Coly-Mycin S Otic w/Neomycin & Hydrocortisone 1906
Decamethonium (Potential for increased neuromuscular blockade and respiratory paralysis).
Dicloxacillin Sodium (Mutual inactivation).
No products indexed under this heading.
Ethacrynic Acid (Ototoxicity). Products include:
Edecrin Tablets 1657
Furosemide (Ototoxicity). Products include:
Lasix Injection, Oral Solution and Tablets 1240
Gentamicin (Neurotoxicity and/or nephrotoxicity).
No products indexed under this heading.
Gentamicin Sulfate (Neurotoxicity and/or nephrotoxicity). Products include:
Garamycin Injectable 2360
Genoptic Sterile Ophthalmic Solution ⊙ 243
Genoptic Sterile Ophthalmic Ointment ⊙ 243
Gentacidin Ointment ⊙ 264
Gentacidin Solution ⊙ 264
Gentak ⊙ 208
Pred-G Liquifilm Sterile Ophthalmic Suspension ⊙ 251
Pred-G S.O.P. Sterile Ophthalmic Ointment ⊙ 252
Hydrochlorothiazide (Ototoxicity). Products include:
Aldactazide 2413
Aldoril Tablets 1604
Apresazide Capsules 808
Capozide 742
Dyazide 2479
Esidrix Tablets 821
Esimil Tablets 822
HydroDIURIL Tablets 1674
Hydropres Tablets 1675
Hyzaar Tablets 1677
Inderide Tablets 2732
Inderide LA Long Acting Capsules 2734
Lopressor HCT Tablets 832
Lotensin HCT 837
Maxzide 1380
Moduretic Tablets 1705
Oretic Tablets 443
Prinzide Tablets 1737
Ser-Ap-Es Tablets 849
Timolide Tablets 1748
Vaseretic Tablets 1765
Zestoretic 2850
Ziac 1415
Hydroflumethiazide (Ototoxicity). Products include:
Diucardin Tablets 2718
Indapamide (Ototoxicity). Products include:
Lozol Tablets 2022
Kanamycin Sulfate (Neurotoxicity and/or nephrotoxicity).
No products indexed under this heading.
Loracarbef (Nephrotoxicity). Products include:
Lorabid Suspension and Pulvules 1459
Methyclothiazide (Ototoxicity). Products include:
Enduron Tablets 420
Metocurine Iodide (Potential for increased neuromuscular blockade and respiratory paralysis). Products include:
Metubine Iodide Vials 916
Metolazone (Ototoxicity). Products include:
Mykrox Tablets 993
Zaroxolyn Tablets 1000
Mezlocillin Sodium (Mutual inactivation). Products include:
Mezlin 601
Mezlin Pharmacy Bulk Package 604
Mivacurium Chloride (Potential for increased neuromuscular blockade and respiratory paralysis). Products include:
Mivacron 1138
Nafcillin Sodium (Mutual inactivation).
No products indexed under this heading.
Neomycin Sulfate (Neurotoxicity and/or nephrotoxicity). Products include:
AK-Spore ⊙ 204
AK-Trol Ointment & Suspension ⊙ 205
Bactine First Aid Antibiotic Plus Anesthetic Ointment ▣ 708
Campho-Phenique Maximum Strength First Aid Antibiotic Plus Pain Reliever Ointment ▣ 719
Coly-Mycin S Otic w/Neomycin & Hydrocortisone 1906
Cortisporin Cream 1084
Cortisporin Ointment 1085
Cortisporin Ophthalmic Ointment Sterile 1085
Cortisporin Ophthalmic Suspension Sterile 1086
Cortisporin Otic Solution Sterile 1087
Cortisporin Otic Suspension Sterile 1088
Dexacidin Ointment ⊙ 263
Maxitrol Ophthalmic Ointment and Suspension ⊙ 224
Mycitracin ▣ 839
NeoDecadron Sterile Ophthalmic Ointment 1712
NeoDecadron Sterile Ophthalmic Solution 1713
NeoDecadron Topical Cream 1714
Neosporin G.U. Irrigant Sterile 1148
Neosporin Ointment ▣ 857
Neosporin Plus Maximum Strength Cream ▣ 858
Neosporin Plus Maximum Strength Ointment ▣ 858
Neosporin Ophthalmic Ointment Sterile 1148
Neosporin Ophthalmic Solution Sterile 1149
PediOtic Suspension Sterile 1153
Poly-Pred Liquifilm ⊙ 248
Pancuronium Bromide Injection (Potential for increased neuromuscular blockade and respiratory paralysis).
No products indexed under this heading.
Paromomycin Sulfate (Neurotoxicity and/or nephrotoxicity).
No products indexed under this heading.
Penicillin G Benzathine (Mutual inactivation). Products include:
Bicillin C-R Injection 2704
Bicillin C-R 900/300 Injection 2706
Bicillin L-A Injection 2707
Penicillin G Potassium (Mutual inactivation). Products include:
Pfizerpen for Injection 2203
Penicillin G Procaine (Mutual inactivation). Products include:
Bicillin C-R Injection 2704
Bicillin C-R 900/300 Injection 2706
Penicillin G Sodium (Mutual inactivation).
No products indexed under this heading.
Penicillin V Potassium (Mutual inactivation). Products include:
Pen•Vee K 2772
Polymyxin B Sulfate (Neurotoxicity and/or nephrotoxicity). Products include:
AK-Spore ⊙ 204
AK-Trol Ointment & Suspension ⊙ 205
Bactine First Aid Antibiotic Plus Anesthetic Ointment ▣ 708
Betadine Brand First Aid Antibiotics & Moisturizer Ointment 1991
Campho-Phenique Maximum Strength First Aid Antibiotic Plus Pain Reliever Ointment ▣ 719
Cortisporin Cream 1084
Cortisporin Ointment 1085
Cortisporin Ophthalmic Ointment Sterile 1085
Cortisporin Ophthalmic Suspension Sterile 1086
Cortisporin Otic Solution Sterile 1087
Cortisporin Otic Suspension Sterile 1088
Dexacidin Ointment ⊙ 263
Maxitrol Ophthalmic Ointment and Suspension ⊙ 224
Mycitracin ▣ 839
Neosporin G.U. Irrigant Sterile 1148
Neosporin Ointment ▣ 857
Neosporin Plus Maximum Strength Cream ▣ 858
Neosporin Plus Maximum Strength Ointment ▣ 858
Neosporin Ophthalmic Ointment Sterile 1148
Neosporin Ophthalmic Solution Sterile 1149
Ophthocort ⊙ 311
PediOtic Suspension Sterile 1153
Polymyxin B Sulfate, Aerosporin Brand Sterile Powder 1154
Poly-Pred Liquifilm ⊙ 248
Polysporin Ointment ▣ 858
Polysporin Ophthalmic Ointment Sterile 1154
Polysporin Powder ▣ 859
Polytrim Ophthalmic Solution Sterile 482
TERAK Ointment ⊙ 209
Terramycin with Polymyxin B Sulfate Ophthalmic Ointment 2211
Polythiazide (Ototoxicity). Products include:
Minizide Capsules 1938
Rocuronium Bromide (Potential for increased neuromuscular blockade and respiratory paralysis). Products include:
Zemuron 1830
Spironolactone (Ototoxicity). Products include:
Aldactazide 2413
Aldactone 2414
Streptomycin Sulfate (Neurotoxicity and/or nephrotoxicity). Products include:
Streptomycin Sulfate Injection 2208
Succinylcholine Chloride (Potential for increased neuromuscular blockade and respiratory paralysis). Products include:
Anectine 1073
Ticarcillin Disodium (Mutual inactivation). Products include:
Ticar for Injection 2526
Timentin for Injection 2528
Tobramycin (Toxicity). Products include:
AKTOB ⊙ 206
TobraDex Ophthalmic Suspension and Ointment 473
Tobrex Ophthalmic Ointment and Solution ⊙ 229
Tobramycin Sulfate (Toxicity). Products include:
Nebcin Vials, Hyporets & ADD-Vantage 1464
Tobramycin Sulfate Injection 968
Torsemide (Ototoxicity). Products include:
Demadex Tablets and Injection 686
Triamterene (Ototoxicity). Products include:
Dyazide 2479
Dyrenium Capsules 2481
Maxzide 1380

IMPORTANT NOTE: Always consult each drug listing in the patient's regimen for possible interactions.

Vancomycin Hydrochloride (Toxicity). Products include:
- Vancocin HCl, Oral Solution & Pulvules 1483
- Vancocin HCl, Vials & ADD-Vantage 1481

Vecuronium Bromide (Potential for increased neuromuscular blockade and respiratory paralysis). Products include:
- Norcuron 1826

NEUPOGEN FOR INJECTION
(Filgrastim) 495

May interact with drugs which potentiate the release of neutrophils. Compounds in this category include:

Lithium Carbonate (Concurrent use should be undertaken with caution since lithium potentiates the release of neutrophils). Products include:
- Eskalith 2485
- Lithium Carbonate Capsules & Tablets 2230
- Lithonate/Lithotabs/Lithobid 2543

Lithium Citrate (Concurrent use should be undertaken with caution since lithium potentiates the release of neutrophils).
- No products indexed under this heading.

NEURONTIN CAPSULES
(Gabapentin) 1922

May interact with:

Aluminum Hydroxide (Coadministration reduces bioavailability of gabapentin by 20%; gabapentin should be taken at least 2 hours following antacid containing aluminum hydroxide and magnesium hydroxide). Products include:
- ALternaGEL Liquid 1316
- Maximum Strength Ascriptin .... ▣ 630
- Cama Arthritis Pain Reliever .... ▣ 785
- Gaviscon Extra Strength Relief Formula Antacid Tablets .... ▣ 819
- Gaviscon Extra Strength Relief Formula Liquid Antacid .... ▣ 819
- Gaviscon Liquid Antacid .... ▣ 820
- Gelusil Liquid & Tablets .... ▣ 855
- Maalox Heartburn Relief Suspension .... ▣ 642
- Maalox Heartburn Relief Tablets .... ▣ 641
- Maalox Magnesia and Alumina Oral Suspension .... ▣ 642
- Maalox Plus Tablets .... ▣ 643
- Extra Strength Maalox Antacid Plus Antigas Liquid and Tablets ▣ 638
- Tempo Soft Antacid .... ▣ 835

Cimetidine (Alters renal clearance of gabapentin and creatinine; this small decrease in excretion of gabapentin is not expected to be of clinical importance). Products include:
- Tagamet Tablets 2516

Cimetidine Hydrochloride (Alters renal clearance of gabapentin and creatinine; this small decrease in excretion of gabapentin is not expected to be of clinical importance). Products include:
- Tagamet 2516

Magnesium Hydroxide (Coadministration reduces bioavailability of gabapentin by 20%; gabapentin should be taken at least 2 hours following antacid containing aluminum hydroxide and magnesium hydroxide). Products include:
- Aludrox Oral Suspension 2695
- Arthritis Pain Ascriptin .... ▣ 631
- Maximum Strength Ascriptin .... ▣ 630
- Regular Strength Ascriptin Tablets .... ▣ 629
- Di-Gel Antacid/Anti-Gas .... ▣ 801
- Gelusil Liquid & Tablets .... ▣ 855
- Maalox Magnesia and Alumina Oral Suspension .... ▣ 642
- Maalox Plus Tablets .... ▣ 643
- Extra Strength Maalox Antacid Plus Antigas Liquid and Tablets ▣ 638
- Mylanta Calcium Carbonate and Magnesium Hydroxide Tablets........ 1318
- Mylanta Liquid 1317
- Mylanta Tablets .... ▣ 660
- Mylanta Double Strength Liquid 1317
- Mylanta Double Strength Tablets .. ▣ 660
- Phillips' Milk of Magnesia Liquid.... ▣ 729
- Rolaids Tablets .... ▣ 843
- Tempo Soft Antacid .... ▣ 835

Norethindrone (The Cmax of norethindrone was 13% higher when it was coadministered with gabapentin; this interaction is not expected to be of clinical importance). Products include:
- Brevicon 2088
- Micronor Tablets 1872
- Modicon 1872
- Norinyl 2088
- Nor-Q D Tablets 2135
- Ortho-Novum 1872
- Ovcon 760
- Tri-Norinyl 2164

Norethindrone Acetate (The Cmax of norethindrone was 13% higher when it was coadministered with gabapentin; this interaction is not expected to be of clinical importance). Products include:
- Aygestin Tablets 974

NEUTREXIN
(Trimetrexate Glucuronate) 2572

May interact with:

Acetaminophen (*In vitro* animal study indicates that acetaminophen alters the relative concentration of trimetrexate metabolites). Products include:
- Actifed Plus Caplets .... ▣ 845
- Actifed Plus Tablets .... ▣ 845
- Actifed Sinus Daytime/Nighttime Tablets and Caplets .... ▣ 846
- Alka-Seltzer Plus Cold Medicine Liqui-Gels .... ▣ 706
- Alka-Seltzer Plus Cold & Cough Medicine Liqui-Gels .... ▣ 705
- Alka-Seltzer Plus Night-Time Cold Medicine Liqui-Gels .... ▣ 706
- Allerest Headache Strength Tablets .... ▣ 627
- Allerest No Drowsiness Tablets .... ▣ 627
- Allerest Sinus Pain Formula .... ▣ 627
- Anexsia 5/500 Elixir 1781
- Anexia Tablets 1782
- Arthritis Foundation Aspirin Free Caplets .... ▣ 673
- Arthritis Foundation NightTime Caplets .... ▣ 674
- Bayer Select Headache Pain Relief Formula .... ▣ 716
- Bayer Select Menstrual Multi-Symptom Formula .... ▣ 716
- Bayer Select Night Time Pain Relief Formula .... ▣ 716
- Bayer Select Sinus Pain Relief Formula .... ▣ 717
- Benadryl Allergy Sinus Headache Formula Caplets .... ▣ 849
- Comtrex Multi-Symptom Cold Reliever Tablets/Caplets/Liqui-Gels/Liquid .... ▣ 615
- Allergy-Sinus Comtrex Multi-Symptom Allergy-Sinus Formula Tablets .... ▣ 617
- Comtrex Non-Drowsy .... ▣ 618
- Contac Day Allergy/Sinus Caplets ▣ 812
- Contac Day & Night .... ▣ 812
- Contac Night Allergy/Sinus Caplets .... ▣ 812
- Contac Severe Cold and Flu Formula Caplets .... ▣ 814
- Contac Severe Cold & Flu Non-Drowsy .... ▣ 815
- Coricidin 'D' Decongestant Tablets .... ▣ 800
- Coricidin Tablets .... ▣ 800
- DHCplus Capsules 1993
- Darvon-N/Darvocet-N 1433
- Drixoral Cold and Flu Extended-Release Tablets .... ▣ 803
- Drixoral Cough + Sore Throat Liquid Caps .... ▣ 802
- Drixoral Allergy/Sinus Extended Release Tablets .... ▣ 804
- Esgic-plus Tablets 1013
- Aspirin Free Excedrin Analgesic Caplets and Geltabs 732
- Excedrin Extra-Strength Analgesic Tablets & Caplets 732
- Excedrin P.M. Analgesic/Sleeping Aid Tablets, Caplets, Liquigels 733
- Fioricet Tablets 2258
- Fioricet with Codeine Capsules 2260
- Hycomine Compound Tablets 932
- Hydrocet Capsules 782
- Legatrin PM .... ▣ 651
- Lorcet 10/650 1018
- Lortab 2566
- Lurline PMS Tablets 982
- Maximum Strength Multi-Symptom Formula Midol .... ▣ 722
- PMS Multi-Symptom Formula Midol .... ▣ 723
- Teen Multi-Symptom Formula Midol .... ▣ 722
- Midrin Capsules 783
- Migralam Capsules 2038
- Panodol Tablets and Caplets .... ▣ 824
- Children's Panadol Chewable Tablets, Liquid, Infant's Drops.... ▣ 824
- Percocet Tablets 938
- Percogesic Analgesic Tablets .... ▣ 754
- Phrenilin 785
- Pyrroxate Caplets .... ▣ 772
- Sedapap Tablets 50 mg/650 mg .. 1543
- Sinarest Tablets .... ▣ 648
- Sinarest Extra Strength Tablets .... ▣ 648
- Sinarest No Drowsiness Tablets .... ▣ 648
- Sine-Aid Maximum Strength Sinus Medication Gelcaps, Caplets and Tablets 1554
- Sine-Off No Drowsiness Formula Caplets .... ▣ 824
- Sine-Off Sinus Medicine .... ▣ 825
- Singlet Tablets .... ▣ 825
- Sinulin Tablets 787
- Sinutab Sinus Allergy Medication, Maximum Strength Tablets and Caplets .... ▣ 860
- Sinutab Sinus Medication, Maximum Strength Without Drowsiness Formula, Tablets & Caplets .... ▣ 860
- Sinutab Sinus Medication, Regular Strength Without Drowsiness Formula .... ▣ 859
- Sudafed Cold and Cough Liquidcaps .... ▣ 862
- Sudafed Severe Cold Formula Caplets .... ▣ 863
- Sudafed Severe Cold Formula Tablets .... ▣ 864
- Sudafed Sinus Caplets .... ▣ 864
- Sudafed Sinus Tablets .... ▣ 864
- Talacen 2333
- TheraFlu .... ▣ 787
- TheraFlu Maximum Strength Nighttime Flu, Cold & Cough Medicine .... ▣ 788
- TheraFlu Maximum Strength Non-Drowsy Formula Flu, Cold & Cough Medicine .... ▣ 788
- Thera Flu Maximum Strength, Non-Drowsy Formula Flu, Cold and Cough Caplets .... ▣ 789
- Triaminic Sore Throat Formula .... ▣ 791
- Triaminicin Tablets .... ▣ 793
- Children's TYLENOL acetaminophen Chewable Tablets, Elixir, Suspension Liquid 1555
- Children's TYLENOL Cold Multi-Symptom Liquid Formula and Chewable Tablets 1561
- Children's TYLENOL Cold Plus Cough Multi Symptom Tablets and Liquid .... ▣ 681
- Infants' TYLENOL acetaminophen Drops and Suspension Drops 1555
- Infants' TYLENOL Cold Decongestant & Fever-Reducer Drops 1556
- TYLENOL Extended Relief Caplets.. 1558
- TYLENOL, Extra Strength, Acetaminophen Adult Liquid Pain Reliever 1560
- TYLENOL, Extra Strength, acetaminophen Gelcaps, Geltabs, Caplets, Tablets 1559
- TYLENOL, Extra Strength, Headache Plus Pain Reliever with Antacid Caplets 1559
- TYLENOL, Junior Strength, acetaminophen Coated Caplets, Grape and Fruit Chewable Tablets 1557
- TYLENOL Maximum Strength Allergy Sinus Medication Gelcaps and Caplets 1563
- TYLENOL Maximum Strength Allergy Sinus NightTime Medication Caplets 1555
- TYLENOL Flu Maximum Strength Gelcaps 1565
- TYLENOL Flu NightTime, Maximum Strength, Gelcaps 1566
- TYLENOL Maximum Strength Flu NightTime Hot Medication Packets 1562
- TYLENOL, Maximum Strength, Sinus Medication Geltabs, Gelcaps, Caplets and Tablets 1566
- TYLENOL Cold Multi-Symptom Formula Medication Tablets and Caplets 1561
- TYLENOL Cold Medication No Drowsiness Formula Gelcaps and Caplets 1562
- TYLENOL Cold Multi-Symptom Hot Medication Liquid Packets 1557
- TYLENOL Cough Multi-Symptom Medication 1564
- TYLENOL Cough Multi-Symptom Medication with Decongestant 1565
- TYLENOL, Regular Strength, acetaminophen Caplets and Tablets .. 1558
- TYLENOL PM, Extra Strength Pain Reliever/Sleep Aid Caplets, Geltabs, Gelcaps 1560
- TYLENOL Severe Allergy Medication Caplets 1564
- Tylenol with Codeine 1583
- Tylox Capsules 1584
- Unisom With Pain Relief-Nighttime Sleep Aid and Pain Reliever........ 1934
- Vanquish Analgesic Caplets .... ▣ 731
- Vicks 44 LiquiCaps Cough, Cold & Flu Relief .... ▣ 755
- Vicks 44M Cough, Cold & Flu Relief .... ▣ 756
- Vicks DayQuil .... ▣ 761
- Vicks Nyquil Hot Therapy .... ▣ 762
- Vicks NyQuil LiquiCaps Multi-Symptom Cold/Flu Relief .... ▣ 763
- Vicks NyQuil Multi-Symptom Cold/Flu Relief - (Original & Cherry Flavor) .... ▣ 763
- Vicodin Tablets 1356
- Vicodin ES Tablets 1357
- Wygesic Tablets 2827
- Zydone Capsules 949

Cimetidine (*In vitro* animal study indicates significant reduction in trimetrexate metabolism). Products include:
- Tagamet Tablets 2516

Cimetidine Hydrochloride (*In vitro* animal study indicates significant reduction in trimetrexate metabolism). Products include:
- Tagamet 2516

Clotrimazole (Based on *in vitro* animal model, nitrogen substituted imidazole drugs were potent, non-competitive inhibitors of trimetrexate metabolism). Products include:
- Prescription Strength Desenex Cream .... ▣ 633
- Gyne-Lotrimin .... ▣ 805
- Gyne-Lotrimin Pack .... ▣ 806
- Lotrimin 2371
- Lotrimin AF Antifungal Cream, Lotion and Solution .... ▣ 806
- Lotrisone Cream 2372
- Mycelex OTC Cream Antifungal .... ▣ 724
- Mycelex OTC Solution Antifungal .. ▣ 724
- Mycelex Troches 608
- Mycelex-7 Vaginal Cream Antifungal .... ▣ 724
- Mycelex-7 Vaginal Antifungal Cream with 7 Disposable Applicators .... ▣ 724
- Mycelex-7 Vaginal Inserts Antifungal .... ▣ 725
- Mycelex-7 Combination-Pack Vaginal Inserts & External Vulvar Cream .... ▣ 725
- Mycelex-G 500 mg Vaginal Tablets 609

(▣ Described in PDR For Nonprescription Drugs) (⊙ Described in PDR For Ophthalmology)

713 Interactions Index Nicobid

Erythromycin (May alter trimetrexate plasma concentrations). Products include:
A/T/S 2% Acne Topical Gel and Solution ... 1234
Benzamycin Topical Gel ... 905
E-Mycin Tablets ... 1341
Emgel 2% Topical Gel ... 1093
ERYC ... 1915
Erycette (erythromycin 2%) Topical Solution ... 1888
Ery-Tab Tablets ... 422
Erythromycin Base Filmtab ... 426
Erythromycin Delayed-Release Capsules, USP ... 427
Ilotycin Ophthalmic Ointment ... 912
PCE Dispertab Tablets ... 444
T-Stat 2.0% Topical Solution and Pads ... 2688
Theramycin Z Topical Solution 2% 1592

Erythromycin Estolate (May alter trimetrexate plasma concentrations). Products include:
Ilosone ... 911

Erythromycin Ethylsuccinate (May alter trimetrexate plasma concentrations). Products include:
E.E.S. ... 424
EryPed ... 421

Erythromycin Gluceptate (May alter trimetrexate plasma concentrations). Products include:
Ilotycin Gluceptate, IV, Vials ... 913

Erythromycin Stearate (May alter trimetrexate plasma concentrations). Products include:
Erythrocin Stearate Filmtab ... 425

Fluconazole (May alter trimetrexate plasma concentrations). Products include:
Diflucan Injection, Tablets, and Oral Suspension ... 2194

Ketoconazole (May alter trimetrexate plasma concentrations; based on *in vitro* animal model, nitrogen substituted imidazole drugs were potent, non-competitive inhibitors of trimetrexate metabolism). Products include:
Nizoral 2% Cream ... 1297
Nizoral 2% Shampoo ... 1298
Nizoral Tablets ... 1298

Miconazole (Based on *in vitro* animal model, nitrogen substituted imidazole drugs were potent, non-competitive inhibitors of trimetrexate metabolism).
No products indexed under this heading.

Rifabutin (May alter trimetrexate plasma concentrations). Products include:
Mycobutin Capsules ... 1957

Rifampin (May alter trimetrexate plasma concentrations). Products include:
Rifadin ... 1528
Rifamate Capsules ... 1530
Rifater ... 1532
Rimactane Capsules ... 847

N'ICE MEDICATED SUGARLESS SORE THROAT AND COUGH LOZENGES
(Menthol) ... 822
None cited in PDR database.

NICOBID
(Niacin) ... 2026
May interact with antihypertensives and lipid-lowering drugs. Compounds in these categories include:

Acebutolol Hydrochloride (Effect not specified; concomitant use requires a physician's consultation). Products include:
Sectral Capsules ... 2807

Amlodipine Besylate (Effect not specified; concomitant use requires a physician's consultation). Products include:
Lotrel Capsules ... 840
Norvasc Tablets ... 1940

Atenolol (Effect not specified; concomitant use requires a physician's consultation). Products include:
Tenoretic Tablets ... 2845
Tenormin Tablets and I.V. Injection 2847

Benazepril Hydrochloride (Effect not specified; concomitant use requires a physician's consultation). Products include:
Lotensin Tablets ... 834
Lotensin HCT ... 837
Lotrel Capsules ... 840

Bendroflumethiazide (Effect not specified; concomitant use requires a physician's consultation).
No products indexed under this heading.

Betaxolol Hydrochloride (Effect not specified; concomitant use requires a physician's consultation). Products include:
Betoptic Ophthalmic Solution ... 469
Betoptic S Ophthalmic Suspension 471
Kerlone Tablets ... 2436

Bisoprolol Fumarate (Effect not specified; concomitant use requires a physician's consultation). Products include:
Zebeta Tablets ... 1413
Ziac ... 1415

Captopril (Effect not specified; concomitant use requires a physician's consultation). Products include:
Capoten ... 739
Capozide ... 742

Carteolol Hydrochloride (Effect not specified; concomitant use requires a physician's consultation). Products include:
Cartrol Tablets ... 410
Ocupress Ophthalmic Solution, 1% Sterile ... ◉ 309

Chlorothiazide (Effect not specified; concomitant use requires a physician's consultation). Products include:
Aldoclor Tablets ... 1598
Diupres Tablets ... 1650
Diuril Oral ... 1653

Chlorothiazide Sodium (Effect not specified; concomitant use requires a physician's consultation). Products include:
Diuril Sodium Intravenous ... 1652

Chlorthalidone (Effect not specified; concomitant use requires a physician's consultation). Products include:
Combipres Tablets ... 677
Tenoretic Tablets ... 2845
Thalitone ... 1245

Cholestyramine (Effect not specified; concomitant use requires a physician's consultation). Products include:
Questran Light ... 769
Questran Powder ... 770

Clofibrate (Effect not specified; concomitant use requires a physician's consultation). Products include:
Atromid-S Capsules ... 2701

Clonidine (Effect not specified; concomitant use requires a physician's consultation). Products include:
Catapres-TTS ... 675

Clonidine Hydrochloride (Effect not specified; concomitant use requires a physician's consultation). Products include:
Catapres Tablets ... 674
Combipres Tablets ... 677

Colestipol Hydrochloride (Effect not specified; concomitant use requires a physician's consultation). Products include:
Colestid Tablets ... 2591

Deserpidine (Effect not specified; concomitant use requires a physician's consultation).
No products indexed under this heading.

Diazoxide (Effect not specified; concomitant use requires a physician's consultation). Products include:
Hyperstat I.V. Injection ... 2363
Proglycem ... 580

Diltiazem Hydrochloride (Effect not specified; concomitant use requires a physician's consultation). Products include:
Cardizem CD Capsules ... 1506
Cardizem SR Capsules ... 1510
Cardizem Injectable ... 1508
Cardizem Tablets ... 1512
Dilacor XR Extended-release Capsules ... 2018

Doxazosin Mesylate (Effect not specified; concomitant use requires a physician's consultation). Products include:
Cardura Tablets ... 2186

Enalapril Maleate (Effect not specified; concomitant use requires a physician's consultation). Products include:
Vaseretic Tablets ... 1765
Vasotec Tablets ... 1771

Enalaprilat (Effect not specified; concomitant use requires a physician's consultation). Products include:
Vasotec I.V. ... 1768

Esmolol Hydrochloride (Effect not specified; concomitant use requires a physician's consultation). Products include:
Brevibloc Injection ... 1808

Felodipine (Effect not specified; concomitant use requires a physician's consultation). Products include:
Plendil Extended-Release Tablets ... 527

Fluvastatin Sodium (Effect not specified; concomitant use requires a physician's consultation). Products include:
Lescol Capsules ... 2267

Fosinopril Sodium (Effect not specified; concomitant use requires a physician's consultation). Products include:
Monopril Tablets ... 757

Furosemide (Effect not specified; concomitant use requires a physician's consultation). Products include:
Lasix Injection, Oral Solution and Tablets ... 1240

Gemfibrozil (Effect not specified; concomitant use requires a physician's consultation). Products include:
Lopid Tablets ... 1917

Guanabenz Acetate (Effect not specified; concomitant use requires a physician's consultation).
No products indexed under this heading.

Guanethidine Monosulfate (Effect not specified; concomitant use requires a physician's consultation). Products include:
Esimil Tablets ... 822
Ismelin Tablets ... 827

Hydralazine Hydrochloride (Effect not specified; concomitant use requires a physician's consultation). Products include:
Apresazide Capsules ... 808
Apresoline Hydrochloride Tablets .. 809
Ser-Ap-Es Tablets ... 849

Hydrochlorothiazide (Effect not specified; concomitant use requires a physician's consultation). Products include:
Aldactazide ... 2413
Aldoril Tablets ... 1604
Apresazide Capsules ... 808
Capozide ... 742
Dyazide ... 2479
Esidrix Tablets ... 821
Esimil Tablets ... 822
HydroDIURIL Tablets ... 1674
Hydropres Tablets ... 1675
Hyzaar Tablets ... 1677
Inderide Tablets ... 2732
Inderide LA Long Acting Capsules .. 2734
Lopressor HCT Tablets ... 832
Lotensin HCT ... 837
Maxzide ... 1380
Moduretic Tablets ... 1705
Oretic Tablets ... 443
Prinzide Tablets ... 1737
Ser-Ap-Es Tablets ... 849
Timolide Tablets ... 1748
Vaseretic Tablets ... 1765
Zestoretic ... 2850
Ziac ... 1415

Hydroflumethiazide (Effect not specified; concomitant use requires a physician's consultation). Products include:
Diucardin Tablets ... 2718

Indapamide (Effect not specified; concomitant use requires a physician's consultation). Products include:
Lozol Tablets ... 2022

Isradipine (Effect not specified; concomitant use requires a physician's consultation). Products include:
DynaCirc Capsules ... 2256

Labetalol Hydrochloride (Effect not specified; concomitant use requires a physician's consultation). Products include:
Normodyne Injection ... 2377
Normodyne Tablets ... 2379
Trandate ... 1185

Lisinopril (Effect not specified; concomitant use requires a physician's consultation). Products include:
Prinivil Tablets ... 1733
Prinzide Tablets ... 1737
Zestoretic ... 2850
Zestril Tablets ... 2854

Losartan Potassium (Effect not specified; concomitant use requires a physician's consultation). Products include:
Cozaar Tablets ... 1628
Hyzaar Tablets ... 1677

Lovastatin (Effect not specified; concomitant use requires a physician's consultation). Products include:
Mevacor Tablets ... 1699

Mecamylamine Hydrochloride (Effect not specified; concomitant use requires a physician's consultation). Products include:
Inversine Tablets ... 1686

Methyclothiazide (Effect not specified; concomitant use requires a physician's consultation). Products include:
Enduron Tablets ... 420

Methyldopa (Effect not specified; concomitant use requires a physician's consultation). Products include:
Aldoclor Tablets ... 1598
Aldomet Oral ... 1600

IMPORTANT NOTE: Always consult each drug listing in the patient's regimen for possible interactions.

Nicobid | Interactions Index | 714

Aldoril Tablets ... 1604

Methyldopate Hydrochloride (Effect not specified; concomitant use requires a physician's consultation). Products include:

Aldomet Ester HCl Injection ... 1602

Metolazone (Effect not specified; concomitant use requires a physician's consultation). Products include:

Mykrox Tablets ... 993
Zaroxolyn Tablets ... 1000

Metoprolol Succinate (Effect not specified; concomitant use requires a physician's consultation). Products include:

Toprol-XL Tablets ... 565

Metoprolol Tartrate (Effect not specified; concomitant use requires a physician's consultation). Products include:

Lopressor Ampuls ... 830
Lopressor HCT Tablets ... 832
Lopressor Tablets ... 830

Metyrosine (Effect not specified; concomitant use requires a physician's consultation). Products include:

Demser Capsules ... 1649

Minoxidil (Effect not specified; concomitant use requires a physician's consultation). Products include:

Loniten Tablets ... 2618
Rogaine Topical Solution ... 2637

Moexipril Hydrochloride (Effect not specified; concomitant use requires a physician's consultation). Products include:

Univasc Tablets ... 2410

Nadolol (Effect not specified; concomitant use requires a physician's consultation).

No products indexed under this heading.

Nicardipine Hydrochloride (Effect not specified; concomitant use requires a physician's consultation). Products include:

Cardene Capsules ... 2095
Cardene I.V. ... 2709
Cardene SR Capsules ... 2097

Nifedipine (Effect not specified; concomitant use requires a physician's consultation). Products include:

Adalat Capsules (10 mg and 20 mg) ... 587
Adalat CC ... 589
Procardia Capsules ... 1971
Procardia XL Extended Release Tablets ... 1972

Nisoldipine (Effect not specified; concomitant use requires a physician's consultation).

No products indexed under this heading.

Nitroglycerin (Effect not specified; concomitant use requires a physician's consultation). Products include:

Deponit NTG Transdermal Delivery System ... 2397
Nitro-Bid IV ... 1523
Nitro-Bid Ointment ... 1524
Nitrodisc ... 2047
Nitro-Dur (nitroglycerin) Transdermal Infusion System ... 1326
Nitrolingual Spray ... 2027
Nitrostat Tablets ... 1925
Transderm-Nitro Transdermal Therapeutic System ... 859

Penbutolol Sulfate (Effect not specified; concomitant use requires a physician's consultation). Products include:

Levatol ... 2403

Phenoxybenzamine Hydrochloride (Effect not specified; concomitant use requires a physician's consultation). Products include:

Dibenzyline Capsules ... 2476

Phentolamine Mesylate (Effect not specified; concomitant use requires a physician's consultation). Products include:

Regitine ... 846

Pindolol (Effect not specified; concomitant use requires a physician's consultation). Products include:

Visken Tablets ... 2299

Polythiazide (Effect not specified; concomitant use requires a physician's consultation). Products include:

Minizide Capsules ... 1938

Pravastatin Sodium (Effect not specified; concomitant use requires a physician's consultation). Products include:

Pravachol ... 765

Prazosin Hydrochloride (Effect not specified; concomitant use requires a physician's consultation). Products include:

Minipress Capsules ... 1937
Minizide Capsules ... 1938

Probucol (Effect not specified; concomitant use requires a physician's consultation). Products include:

Lorelco Tablets ... 1517

Propranolol Hydrochloride (Effect not specified; concomitant use requires a physician's consultation). Products include:

Inderal ... 2728
Inderal LA Long Acting Capsules ... 2730
Inderide Tablets ... 2732
Inderide LA Long Acting Capsules ... 2734

Quinapril Hydrochloride (Effect not specified; concomitant use requires a physician's consultation). Products include:

Accupril Tablets ... 1893

Ramipril (Effect not specified; concomitant use requires a physician's consultation). Products include:

Altace Capsules ... 1232

Rauwolfia Serpentina (Effect not specified; concomitant use requires a physician's consultation).

No products indexed under this heading.

Rescinnamine (Effect not specified; concomitant use requires a physician's consultation).

No products indexed under this heading.

Reserpine (Effect not specified; concomitant use requires a physician's consultation). Products include:

Diupres Tablets ... 1650
Hydropres Tablets ... 1675
Ser-Ap-Es Tablets ... 849

Simvastatin (Effect not specified; concomitant use requires a physician's consultation). Products include:

Zocor Tablets ... 1775

Sodium Nitroprusside (Effect not specified; concomitant use requires a physician's consultation).

No products indexed under this heading.

Sotalol Hydrochloride (Effect not specified; concomitant use requires a physician's consultation). Products include:

Betapace Tablets ... 641

Spirapril Hydrochloride (Effect not specified; concomitant use requires a physician's consultation).

No products indexed under this heading.

Terazosin Hydrochloride (Effect not specified; concomitant use requires a physician's consultation). Products include:

Hytrin Capsules ... 430

Timolol Maleate (Effect not specified; concomitant use requires a physician's consultation). Products include:

Blocadren Tablets ... 1614
Timolide Tablets ... 1748
Timoptic in Ocudose ... 1753
Timoptic Sterile Ophthalmic Solution ... 1751
Timoptic-XE ... 1755

Torsemide (Effect not specified; concomitant use requires a physician's consultation). Products include:

Demadex Tablets and Injection ... 686

Trimethaphan Camsylate (Effect not specified; concomitant use requires a physician's consultation). Products include:

Arfonad Ampuls ... 2080

Verapamil Hydrochloride (Effect not specified; concomitant use requires a physician's consultation). Products include:

Calan SR Caplets ... 2422
Calan Tablets ... 2419
Isoptin Injectable ... 1344
Isoptin Oral Tablets ... 1346
Isoptin SR Tablets ... 1348
Verelan Capsules ... 1410
Verelan Capsules ... 2824

NICODERM (NICOTINE TRANSDERMAL SYSTEM)
(Nicotine) ... 1518

May interact with xanthine bronchodilators, insulin, sympathomimetics, and certain other agents. Compounds in these categories include:

Acetaminophen (Deinduction of hepatic enzymes on smoking cessation; may require a decrease in dose at cessation of smoking). Products include:

Actifed Plus Caplets ... ◙ 845
Actifed Plus Tablets ... ◙ 845
Actifed Sinus Daytime/Nighttime Tablets and Caplets ... ◙ 846
Alka-Seltzer Plus Cold Medicine Liqui-Gels ... ◙ 706
Alka-Seltzer Plus Cold & Cough Medicine Liqui-Gels ... ◙ 705
Alka-Seltzer Plus Night-Time Cold Medicine Liqui-Gels ... ◙ 706
Allerest Headache Strength Tablets ... ◙ 627
Allerest No Drowsiness Tablets ... ◙ 627
Allerest Sinus Pain Formula ... ◙ 627
Anexsia 5/500 Elixir ... 1781
Anexia Tablets ... 1782
Arthritis Foundation Aspirin Free Caplets ... ◙ 673
Arthritis Foundation NightTime Caplets ... ◙ 674
Bayer Select Headache Pain Relief Formula ... ◙ 716
Bayer Select Menstrual Multi-Symptom Formula ... ◙ 716
Bayer Select Night Time Pain Relief Formula ... ◙ 716
Bayer Select Sinus Pain Relief Formula ... ◙ 717
Benadryl Allergy Sinus Headache Formula Caplets ... ◙ 849
Comtrex Multi-Symptom Cold Reliever Tablets/Caplets/Liqui-Gels/Liquid ... ◙ 615
Allergy-Sinus Comtrex Multi-Symptom Allergy-Sinus Formula Tablets ... ◙ 617
Comtrex Non-Drowsy ... ◙ 618
Contac Day Allergy/Sinus Caplets ◙ 812
Contac Day & Night ... ◙ 812
Contac Night Allergy/Sinus Caplets ... ◙ 812
Contac Severe Cold and Flu Formula Caplets ... ◙ 814
Contac Severe Cold & Flu Non-Drowsy ... ◙ 815
Coricidin 'D' Decongestant Tablets ... ◙ 800
Coricidin Tablets ... ◙ 800
DHCplus Capsules ... 1993
Darvon-N/Darvocet-N ... 1433
Drixoral Cold and Flu Extended-Release Tablets ... ◙ 803
Drixoral Cough + Sore Throat Liquid Caps ... ◙ 802
Drixoral Allergy/Sinus Extended Release Tablets ... ◙ 804
Esgic-plus Tablets ... 1013
Aspirin Free Excedrin Analgesic Caplets and Geltabs ... 732
Excedrin Extra-Strength Analgesic Tablets & Caplets ... 732
Excedrin P.M. Analgesic/Sleeping Aid Tablets, Caplets, Liquigels ... 733
Fioricet Tablets ... 2258
Fioricet with Codeine Capsules ... 2260
Hycomine Compound Tablets ... 932
Hydrocet Capsules ... 782
Legatrin PM ... ◙ 651
Lorcet 10/650 ... 1018
Lortab ... 2566
Lurline PMS Tablets ... 982
Maximum Strength Multi-Symptom Formula Midol ... ◙ 722
PMS Multi-Symptom Formula Midol ... ◙ 723
Teen Multi-Symptom Formula Midol ... ◙ 722
Midrin Capsules ... 783
Migralam Capsules ... 2038
Panodol Tablets and Caplets ... ◙ 824
Children's Panadol Chewable Tablets, Liquid, Infant's Drops ... ◙ 824
Percocet Tablets ... 938
Percogesic Analgesic Tablets ... ◙ 754
Phrenilin ... 785
Pyrroxate Caplets ... ◙ 772
Sedapap Tablets 50 mg/650 mg .. 1543
Sinarest Tablets ... ◙ 648
Sinarest Extra Strength Tablets ... ◙ 648
Sinarest No Drowsiness Tablets ... ◙ 648
Sine-Aid Maximum Strength Sinus Medication Gelcaps, Caplets and Tablets ... 1554
Sine-Off No Drowsiness Formula Caplets ... ◙ 824
Sine-Off Sinus Medicine ... ◙ 825
Singlet Tablets ... ◙ 825
Sinulin Tablets ... 787
Sinutab Sinus Allergy Medication, Maximum Strength Tablets and Caplets ... ◙ 860
Sinutab Sinus Medication, Maximum Strength Without Drowsiness Formula, Tablets & Caplets ... ◙ 860
Sinutab Sinus Medication, Regular Strength Without Drowsiness Formula ... ◙ 859
Sudafed Cold and Cough Liquidcaps ... ◙ 862
Sudafed Severe Cold Formula Caplets ... ◙ 863
Sudafed Severe Cold Formula Tablets ... ◙ 864
Sudafed Sinus Caplets ... ◙ 864
Sudafed Sinus Tablets ... ◙ 864
Talacen ... 2333
TheraFlu ... ◙ 787
TheraFlu Maximum Strength Nighttime Flu, Cold & Cough Medicine ... ◙ 788
TheraFlu Maximum Strength Non-Drowsy Formula Flu, Cold & Cough Medicine ... ◙ 788
Thera Flu Maximum Strength, Non-Drowsy Formula Flu, Cold and Cough Caplets ... ◙ 789
Triaminic Sore Throat Formula ... ◙ 791
Triaminicin Tablets ... ◙ 793
Children's TYLENOL acetaminophen Chewable Tablets, Elixir, Suspension Liquid ... 1555
Children's TYLENOL Cold Multi-Symptom Liquid Formula and Chewable Tablets ... 1561
Children's TYLENOL Cold Plus Cough Multi Symptom Tablets and Liquid ... ◙ 681
Infants' TYLENOL acetaminophen Drops and Suspension Drops ... 1555

(◙ Described in PDR For Nonprescription Drugs) (⊙ Described in PDR For Ophthalmology)

Interactions Index — Nicoderm

Infants' TYLENOL Cold Decongestant & Fever-Reducer Drops 1556
TYLENOL Extended Relief Caplets.. 1558
TYLENOL, Extra Strength, Acetaminophen Adult Liquid Pain Reliever 1560
TYLENOL, Extra Strength, acetaminophen Gelcaps, Geltabs, Caplets, Tablets 1559
TYLENOL, Extra Strength, Headache Plus Pain Reliever with Antacid Caplets 1559
TYLENOL, Junior Strength, acetaminophen Coated Caplets, Grape and Fruit Chewable Tablets 1557
TYLENOL Maximum Strength Allergy Sinus Medication Gelcaps and Caplets 1563
TYLENOL Maximum Strength Allergy Sinus NightTime Medication Caplets 1555
TYLENOL Flu Maximum Strength Gelcaps 1565
TYLENOL Flu NightTime, Maximum Strength, Gelcaps 1566
TYLENOL Maximum Strength Flu NightTime Hot Medication Packets 1562
TYLENOL, Maximum Strength, Sinus Medication Geltabs, Gelcaps, Caplets and Tablets 1566
TYLENOL Cold Multi-Symptom Formula Medication Tablets and Caplets 1561
TYLENOL Cold Medication No Drowsiness Formula Gelcaps and Caplets 1562
TYLENOL Cold Multi-Symptom Hot Medication Liquid Packets.............. 1557
TYLENOL Cough Multi-Symptom Medication 1564
TYLENOL Cough Multi-Symptom Medication with Decongestant...... 1565
TYLENOL, Regular Strength, acetaminophen Caplets and Tablets .. 1558
TYLENOL PM, Extra Strength Pain Reliever/Sleep Aid Caplets, Geltabs, Gelcaps....................................... 1560
TYLENOL Severe Allergy Medication Caplets 1564
Tylenol with Codeine 1583
Tylox Capsules 1584
Unisom With Pain Relief-Nighttime Sleep Aid and Pain Reliever............ 1934
Vanquish Analgesic Caplets ....㊀ 731
Vicks 44 LiquiCaps Cough, Cold & Flu Relief.. ㊀ 755
Vicks 44M Cough, Cold & Flu Relief... ㊀ 756
Vicks DayQuil .... ㊀ 761
Vicks Nyquil Hot Therapy.................. ㊀ 762
Vicks NyQuil LiquiCaps Multi-Symptom Cold/Flu Relief .... ㊀ 763
Vicks NyQuil Multi-Symptom Cold/Flu Relief - (Original & Cherry Flavor)......................................㊀ 763
Vicodin Tablets 1356
Vicodin ES Tablets 1357
Wygesic Tablets 2827
Zydone Capsules 949

Albuterol (Decrease in circulating catecholamines with smoking cessation; may require an increase in dose at cessation of smoking). Products include:

Proventil Inhalation Aerosol 2382
Ventolin Inhalation Aerosol and Refill 1197

Albuterol Sulfate (Decrease in circulating catecholamines with smoking cessation; may require an increase in dose at cessation of smoking). Products include:

Airet Solution for Inhalation 452
Proventil Inhalation Solution 0.083% 2384
Proventil Repetabs Tablets 2386
Proventil Solution for Inhalation 0.5% 2383
Proventil Syrup...................................... 2385
Proventil Tablets 2386
Ventolin Inhalation Solution................ 1198
Ventolin Nebules Inhalation Solution... 1199
Ventolin Rotacaps for Inhalation 1200
Ventolin Syrup.. 1202
Ventolin Tablets 1203
Volmax Extended-Release Tablets .. 1788

Aminophylline (Deinduction of hepatic enzymes on smoking cessation; may require a decrease in dose at cessation of smoking).

No products indexed under this heading.

Caffeine-containing medications (Deinduction of hepatic enzymes on smoking cessation; may require a decrease in dose at cessation of smoking).

Dobutamine Hydrochloride (Decrease in circulating catecholamines with smoking cessation; may require an increase in dose at cessation of smoking). Products include:

Dobutrex Solution Vials........................ 1439

Dopamine Hydrochloride (Decrease in circulating catecholamines with smoking cessation; may require an increase in dose at cessation of smoking).

No products indexed under this heading.

Dyphylline (Deinduction of hepatic enzymes on smoking cessation; may require a decrease in dose at cessation of smoking). Products include:

Lufyllin & Lufyllin-400 Tablets 2670
Lufyllin-GG Elixir & Tablets 2671

Ephedrine Hydrochloride (Decrease in circulating catecholamines with smoking cessation; may require an increase in dose at cessation of smoking). Products include:

Primatene Dual Action Formula...... ㊀ 872
Primatene Tablets .... ㊀ 873
Quadrinal Tablets 1350

Ephedrine Sulfate (Decrease in circulating catecholamines with smoking cessation; may require an increase in dose at cessation of smoking). Products include:

Bronkaid Caplets ....㊀ 717
Marax Tablets & DF Syrup.................. 2200

Ephedrine Tannate (Decrease in circulating catecholamines with smoking cessation; may require an increase in dose at cessation of smoking). Products include:

Rynatuss 2673

Epinephrine (Decrease in circulating catecholamines with smoking cessation; may require an increase in dose at cessation of smoking). Products include:

Bronkaid Mist ....㊀ 717
EPIFRIN .... © 239
EpiPen 790
Marcaine Hydrochloride with Epinephrine 1:200,000 2316
Primatene Mist ....㊀ 873
Sensorcaine with Epinephrine Injection... 559
Sus-Phrine Injection 1019
Xylocaine with Epinephrine Injections... 567

Epinephrine Bitartrate (Decrease in circulating catecholamines with smoking cessation; may require an increase in dose at cessation of smoking). Products include:

Bronkaid Mist Suspension ....㊀ 718
Sensorcaine-MPF with Epinephrine Injection 559

Epinephrine Hydrochloride (Decrease in circulating catecholamines with smoking cessation; may require an increase in dose at cessation of smoking). Products include:

Ana-Kit Anaphylaxis Emergency Treatment Kit 617

Imipramine Hydrochloride (Deinduction of hepatic enzymes on smoking cessation; may require a decrease in dose at cessation of smoking). Products include:

Tofranil Ampuls 854
Tofranil Tablets 856

Imipramine Pamoate (Deinduction of hepatic enzymes on smoking cessation; may require a decrease in dose at cessation of smoking). Products include:

Tofranil-PM Capsules.......................... 857

Insulin, Human (Increase of subcutaneous insulin absorption with smoking cessation; may require a decrease in dose at cessation of smoking).

No products indexed under this heading.

Insulin, Human Isophane Suspension (Increase of subcutaneous insulin absorption with smoking cessation; may require a decrease in dose at cessation of smoking). Products include:

Novolin N Human Insulin 10 ml Vials... 1795

Insulin, Human NPH (Increase of subcutaneous insulin absorption with smoking cessation; may require a decrease in dose at cessation of smoking). Products include:

Humulin N, 100 Units 1448
Novolin N PenFill Cartridges Durable Insulin Delivery System 1798
Novolin N Prefilled Syringe Disposable Insulin Delivery System 1798

Insulin, Human Regular (Increase of subcutaneous insulin absorption with smoking cessation; may require a decrease in dose at cessation of smoking). Products include:

Humulin R, 100 Units 1449
Novolin R Human Insulin 10 ml Vials... 1795
Novolin R PenFill Cartridges Durable Insulin Delivery System 1798
Novolin R Prefilled Syringe Disposable Insulin Delivery System............ 1798
Velosulin BR Human Insulin 10 ml Vials... 1795

Insulin, Human, Zinc Suspension (Increase of subcutaneous insulin absorption with smoking cessation; may require a decrease in dose at cessation of smoking). Products include:

Humulin L, 100 Units 1446
Humulin U, 100 Units 1450
Novolin L Human Insulin 10 ml Vials... 1795

Insulin, NPH (Increase of subcutaneous insulin absorption with smoking cessation; may require a decrease in dose at cessation of smoking). Products include:

NPH, 100 Units 1450
Pork NPH, 100 Units.......................... 1452
Purified Pork NPH Isophane Insulin 1801

Insulin, Regular (Increase of subcutaneous insulin absorption with smoking cessation; may require a decrease in dose at cessation of smoking). Products include:

Regular, 100 Units 1450
Pork Regular, 100 Units 1452
Pork Regular (Concentrated), 500 Units 1453
Purified Pork Regular Insulin 1801

Insulin, Zinc Crystals (Increase of subcutaneous insulin absorption with smoking cessation; may require a decrease in dose at cessation of smoking). Products include:

NPH, 100 Units 1450

Insulin, Zinc Suspension (Increase of subcutaneous insulin absorption with smoking cessation; may require a decrease in dose at cessation of smoking). Products include:

Iletin I 1450
Lente, 100 Units 1450
Iletin II 1452
Pork Lente, 100 Units.......................... 1452

Purified Pork Lente Insulin 1801

Isoproterenol Hydrochloride (Decrease in circulating catecholamines with smoking cessation; may require an increase in dose at cessation of smoking). Products include:

Isuprel Hydrochloride Injection 1:5000 2311
Isuprel Hydrochloride Solution 1:200 & 1:100 2313
Isuprel Mistometer 2312

Isoproterenol Sulfate (Decrease in circulating catecholamines with smoking cessation; may require an increase in dose at cessation of smoking). Products include:

Norisodrine with Calcium Iodide Syrup... 442

Labetalol Hydrochloride (Decrease in circulating catecholamines with smoking cessation; may require a decrease in dose at cessation of smoking). Products include:

Normodyne Injection 2377
Normodyne Tablets 2379
Trandate 1185

Metaproterenol Sulfate (Decrease in circulating catecholamines with smoking cessation; may require an increase in dose at cessation of smoking). Products include:

Alupent.. 669
Metaproterenol Sulfate Inhalation Solution, USP, Arm-a-Med 552

Metaraminol Bitartrate (Decrease in circulating catecholamines with smoking cessation; may require an increase in dose at cessation of smoking). Products include:

Aramine Injection.................................. 1609

Methoxamine Hydrochloride (Decrease in circulating catecholamines with smoking cessation; may require an increase in dose at cessation of smoking). Products include:

Vasoxyl Injection 1196

Norepinephrine Bitartrate (Decrease in circulating catecholamines with smoking cessation; may require an increase in dose at cessation of smoking). Products include:

Levophed Bitartrate Injection 2315

Oxazepam (Deinduction of hepatic enzymes on smoking cessation; may require a decrease in dose at cessation of smoking). Products include:

Serax Capsules 2810
Serax Tablets.. 2810

Pentazocine Hydrochloride (Deinduction of hepatic enzymes on smoking cessation; may require a decrease in dose at cessation of smoking). Products include:

Talacen.. 2333
Talwin Compound 2335
Talwin Nx.. 2336

Pentazocine Lactate (Deinduction of hepatic enzymes on smoking cessation; may require a decrease in dose at cessation of smoking). Products include:

Talwin Injection...................................... 2334

Phenylephrine Bitartrate (Decrease in circulating catecholamines with smoking cessation; may require an increase in dose at cessation of smoking).

No products indexed under this heading.

Phenylephrine Hydrochloride (Decrease in circulating catecholamines with smoking cessation; may require an increase in dose at cessation of smoking). Products include:

Atrohist Plus Tablets 454
Cerose DM ....㊀ 878
Comhist 2038
D.A. Chewable Tablets.......................... 951
Deconsal Pediatric Capsules.............. 454
Dura-Vent/DA Tablets.......................... 953

IMPORTANT NOTE: Always consult each drug listing in the patient's regimen for possible interactions.

Nicoderm | Interactions Index | 716

Entex Capsules 1986
Entex Liquid 1986
Extendryl 1005
4-Way Fast Acting Nasal Spray (regular & mentholated) ▣ 621
Hemorid For Women ▣ 834
Hycomine Compound Tablets 932
Neo-Synephrine Hydrochloride 1% Carpuject 2324
Neo-Synephrine Hydrochloride 1% Injection 2324
Neo-Synephrine Hydrochloride (Ophthalmic) 2325
Neo-Synephrine ▣ 726
Nōstril ▣ 644
Novahistine Elixir ▣ 823
Phenergan VC 2779
Phenergan VC with Codeine 2781
Preparation H ▣ 871
Tympagesic Ear Drops 2342
Vasosulf ⊙ 271
Vicks Sinex Nasal Spray and Ultra Fine Mist ▣ 765

Phenylephrine Tannate (Decrease in circulating catecholamines with smoking cessation; may require an increase in dose at cessation of smoking). Products include:

Atrohist Pediatric Suspension 454
Ricobid-D Pediatric Suspension 2038
Ricobid Tablets and Pediatric Suspension 2038
Rynatan 2673
Rynatuss 2673

Phenylpropanolamine Hydrochloride (Decrease in circulating catecholamines with smoking cessation; may require an increase in dose at cessation of smoking). Products include:

Acutrim ▣ 628
Allerest Children's Chewable Tablets ▣ 627
Allerest 12 Hour Caplets ▣ 627
Atrohist Plus Tablets 454
BC Cold Powder Multi-Symptom Formula (Cold-Sinus-Allergy) ▣ 609
BC Cold Powder Non-Drowsy Formula (Cold-Sinus) ▣ 609
Cheracol Plus Head Cold/Cough Formula ▣ 769
Comtrex Multi-Symptom Non-Drowsy Liqui-gels ▣ 618
Contac Continuous Action Nasal Decongestant/Antihistamine 12 Hour Capsules ▣ 813
Contac Maximum Strength Continuous Action Decongestant/Antihistamine 12 Hour Caplets ▣ 813
Contac Severe Cold and Flu Formula Caplets ▣ 814
Coricidin 'D' Decongestant Tablets ▣ 800
Dexatrim ▣ 832
Dexatrim Plus Vitamins Caplets ▣ 832
Dimetane-DC Cough Syrup 2059
Dimetapp Elixir ▣ 773
Dimetapp Extentabs ▣ 774
Dimetapp Tablets/Liqui-Gels ▣ 775
Dimetapp Cold & Allergy Chewable Tablets ▣ 773
Dimetapp DM Elixir ▣ 774
Dura-Vent Tablets 952
Entex Capsules 1986
Entex LA Tablets 1987
Entex Liquid 1986
Exgest LA Tablets 782
Hycomine 931
Isoclor Timesule Capsules ▣ 637
Nolamine Timed-Release Tablets 785
Ornade Spansule Capsules 2502
Propagest Tablets 786
Pyrroxate Caplets ▣ 772
Robitussin-CF ▣ 777
Sinulin Tablets 787
Tavist-D 12 Hour Relief Tablets ▣ 787
Teldrin 12 Hour Antihistamine/Nasal Decongestant Allergy Relief Capsules ▣ 826
Triaminic Allergy Tablets ▣ 789
Triaminic Cold Tablets ▣ 790
Triaminic Expectorant ▣ 790
Triaminic Syrup ▣ 792
Triaminic-12 Tablets ▣ 792
Triaminic-DM Syrup ▣ 792
Triaminicin Tablets ▣ 793
Triaminicol Multi-Symptom Cold Tablets ▣ 793
Triaminicol Multi-Symptom Relief ▣ 794
Vicks DayQuil Allergy Relief 12-Hour Extended Release Tablets ▣ 760
Vicks DayQuil Allergy Relief 4-Hour Tablets ▣ 760
Vicks DayQuil SINUS Pressure & CONGESTION Relief ▣ 761

Pirbuterol Acetate (Decrease in circulating catecholamines with smoking cessation; may require an increase in dose at cessation of smoking). Products include:

Maxair Autohaler 1492
Maxair Inhaler 1494

Prazosin Hydrochloride (Decrease in circulating catecholamines with smoking cessation; may require a decrease in dose at cessation of smoking). Products include:

Minipress Capsules 1937
Minizide Capsules 1938

Propranolol Hydrochloride (Deinduction of hepatic enzymes on smoking cessation; may require a decrease in dose at cessation of smoking). Products include:

Inderal 2728
Inderal LA Long Acting Capsules 2730
Inderide Tablets 2732
Inderide LA Long Acting Capsules 2734

Pseudoephedrine Hydrochloride (Decrease in circulating catecholamines with smoking cessation; may require an increase in dose at cessation of smoking). Products include:

Actifed Allergy Daytime/Nighttime Caplets ▣ 844
Actifed Plus Caplets ▣ 845
Actifed Plus Tablets ▣ 845
Actifed with Codeine Cough Syrup 1067
Actifed Sinus Daytime/Nighttime Tablets and Caplets ▣ 846
Actifed Syrup ▣ 846
Actifed Tablets ▣ 844
Advil Cold and Sinus Caplets and Tablets (formerly CoAdvil) ▣ 870
Alka-Seltzer Plus Cold Medicine Liqui-Gels ▣ 706
Alka-Seltzer Plus Cold & Cough Medicine Liqui-Gels ▣ 705
Alka-Seltzer Plus Night-Time Cold Medicine Liqui-Gels ▣ 706
Allerest Headache Strength Tablets ▣ 627
Allerest Maximum Strength Tablets ▣ 627
Allerest No Drowsiness Tablets ▣ 627
Allerest Sinus Pain Formula ▣ 627
Anatuss LA Tablets 1542
Atrohist Pediatric Capsules 453
Bayer Select Sinus Pain Relief Formula ▣ 717
Benadryl Allergy Decongestant Liquid Medication ▣ 848
Benadryl Allergy Decongestant Tablets ▣ 848
Benadryl Allergy Sinus Headache Formula Caplets ▣ 849
Benylin Multisymptom ▣ 852
Bromfed Capsules (Extended-Release) 1785
Bromfed Syrup ▣ 733
Bromfed Tablets 1785
Bromfed-DM Cough Syrup 1786
Bromfed-PD Capsules (Extended-Release) 1785
Children's Vicks DayQuil Allergy Relief ▣ 757
Children's Vicks NyQuil Cold/Cough Relief ▣ 758
Comtrex Multi-Symptom Cold Reliever Tablets/Caplets/Liqui-Gels/Liquid ▣ 615
Allergy-Sinus Comtrex Multi-Symptom Allergy-Sinus Formula Tablets ▣ 617
Comtrex Multi-Symptom Non-Drowsy Caplets ▣ 618
Congess 1004
Contac Day Allergy/Sinus Caplets ▣ 812
Contac Day & Night ▣ 812
Contac Night Allergy/Sinus Caplets ▣ 812
Contac Severe Cold & Flu Non-Drowsy ▣ 815
Deconamine Chewable Tablets 1320
Deconamine CX Cough and Cold Liquid and Tablets 1319
Deconamine 1320
Deconsal C Expectorant Syrup 456
Deconsal Pediatric Syrup 457
Deconsal II Tablets 454
Dimetane-DX Cough Syrup 2059
Dimetapp Sinus Caplets ▣ 775
Dorcol Children's Cough Syrup ▣ 785
Drixoral Cough + Congestion Liquid Caps ▣ 802
Dura-Tap/PD Capsules 2867
Duratuss Tablets 2565
Duratuss HD Elixir 2565
Efidac/24 ▣ 635
Entex PSE Tablets 1987
Fedahist Gyrocaps 2401
Fedahist Timecaps 2401
Guaifed 1787
Guaifed Syrup ▣ 734
Guaimax-D Tablets 792
Guaitab Tablets ▣ 734
Isoclor Expectorant 990
Kronofed-A 977
Motrin IB Sinus ▣ 838
Novahistine DH 2462
Novahistine DMX ▣ 822
Novahistine Expectorant 2463
Nucofed 2051
PediaCare Cold Allergy Chewable Tablets ▣ 677
PediaCare Cough-Cold Chewable Tablets 1553
PediaCare 1553
PediaCare Infants' Decongestant Drops ▣ 677
PediCare Infant's Drops Decongestant Plus Cough 1553
PediaCare NightRest Cough-Cold Liquid 1553
Pediatric Vicks 44d Dry Hacking Cough & Head Congestion ▣ 763
Pediatric Vicks 44m Cough & Cold Relief ▣ 764
Robitussin Cold & Cough Liqui-Gels ▣ 776
Robitussin Maximum Strength Cough & Cold ▣ 778
Robitussin Pediatric Cough & Cold Formula ▣ 779
Robitussin Severe Congestion Liqui-Gels ▣ 776
Robitussin-DAC Syrup 2074
Robitussin-PE ▣ 778
Rondec Oral Drops 953
Rondec Syrup 953
Rondec Tablet 953
Rondec-DM Oral Drops 954
Rondec-DM Syrup 954
Rondec-TR Tablet 953
Ryna ▣ 841
Seldane-D Extended-Release Tablets 1538
Semprex-D Capsules 463
Semprex-D Capsules 1167
Sinarest Tablets ▣ 648
Sinarest Extra Strength Tablets ▣ 648
Sinarest No Drowsiness Tablets ▣ 648
Sine-Aid IB Caplets 1554
Sine-Aid Maximum Strength Sinus Medication Gelcaps, Caplets and Tablets 1554
Sine-Off No Drowsiness Formula Caplets ▣ 824
Sine-Off Sinus Medicine ▣ 825
Singlet Tablets ▣ 825
Sinutab Non-Drying Liquid Caps ▣ 859
Sinutab Sinus Allergy Medication, Maximum Strength Tablets and Caplets ▣ 860
Sinutab Sinus Medication, Maximum Strength Without Drowsiness Formula, Tablets & Caplets ▣ 860
Sinutab Sinus Medication, Regular Strength Without Drowsiness Formula ▣ 859
Sudafed Children's Liquid ▣ 861
Sudafed Cold and Cough Liquidcaps ▣ 862
Sudafed Cough Syrup ▣ 862
Sudafed Plus Liquid ▣ 862
Sudafed Plus Tablets ▣ 863
Sudafed Severe Cold Formula Caplets ▣ 863
Sudafed Severe Cold Formula Tablets ▣ 864
Sudafed Sinus Caplets ▣ 864
Sudafed Sinus Tablets ▣ 864
Sudafed Tablets, 30 mg ▣ 861
Sudafed Tablets, 60 mg ▣ 861
Sudafed 12 Hour Caplets ▣ 861
Syn-Rx Tablets 465
Syn-Rx DM Tablets 466
TheraFlu ▣ 787
TheraFlu Maximum Strength Nighttime Flu, Cold & Cough Medicine ▣ 788
TheraFlu Maximum Strength Non-Drowsy Formula Flu, Cold & Cough Medicine ▣ 788
Thera Flu Maximum Strength, Non-Drowsy Formula Flu, Cold and Cough Caplets ▣ 789
Triaminic AM Cough and Decongestant Formula ▣ 789
Triaminic AM Decongestant Formula ▣ 790
Triaminic Nite Light ▣ 791
Triaminic Sore Throat Formula ▣ 791
Tussend 1783
Tussend Expectorant 1785
Children's TYLENOL Cold Multi-Symptom Liquid Formula and Chewable Tablets 1561
Children's TYLENOL Cold Plus Cough Multi Symptom Tablets and Liquid ▣ 681
Infants' TYLENOL Cold Decongestant & Fever-Reducer Drops 1556
TYLENOL Maximum Strength Allergy Sinus Medication Gelcaps and Caplets 1563
TYLENOL Maximum Strength Allergy Sinus NightTime Medication Caplets 1555
TYLENOL Flu Maximum Strength Gelcaps 1565
TYLENOL Flu NightTime, Maximum Strength, Gelcaps 1566
TYLENOL Maximum Strength Flu NightTime Hot Medication Packets 1562
TYLENOL, Maximum Strength, Sinus Medication Geltabs, Gelcaps, Caplets and Tablets 1566
TYLENOL Cold Multi-Symptom Formula Medication Tablets and Caplets 1561
TYLENOL Cold Medication No Drowsiness Formula Gelcaps and Caplets 1562
TYLENOL Cold Multi-Symptom Hot Medication Liquid Packets 1557
TYLENOL Cough Multi-Symptom Medication with Decongestant 1565
Ursinus Inlay-Tabs ▣ 794
Vicks 44 LiquiCaps Cough, Cold & Flu Relief ▣ 755
Vicks 44 LiquiCaps Non-Drowsy Cough & Cold Relief ▣ 756
Vicks 44D Dry Hacking Cough & Head Congestion ▣ 755
Vicks 44M Cough, Cold & Flu Relief ▣ 756
Vicks DayQuil ▣ 761
Vicks DayQuil SINUS Pressure & PAIN Relief with IBUPROFEN ▣ 762
Vicks Nyquil Hot Therapy ▣ 762
Vicks NyQuil LiquiCaps Multi-Symptom Cold/Flu Relief ▣ 763
Vicks NyQuil Multi-Symptom Cold/Flu Relief - (Original & Cherry Flavor) ▣ 763

Pseudoephedrine Sulfate (Decrease in circulating catecholamines with smoking cessation; may require an increase in dose at cessation of smoking). Products include:

Cheracol Sinus ▣ 768
Chlor-Trimeton Allergy Decongestant Tablets ▣ 799
Claritin-D 2350
Drixoral Cold and Allergy Sustained-Action Tablets ▣ 802
Drixoral Cold and Flu Extended-Release Tablets ▣ 803
Drixoral Non-Drowsy Formula Extended-Release Tablets ▣ 803
Drixoral Allergy/Sinus Extended Release Tablets ▣ 804
Trinalin Repetabs Tablets 1330

Salmeterol Xinafoate (Decrease in circulating catecholamines with smoking cessation; may require an increase in dose at cessation of smoking). Products include:

Serevent Inhalation Aerosol 1176

(▣ Described in PDR For Nonprescription Drugs) (⊙ Described in PDR For Ophthalmology)

Interactions Index

Terbutaline Sulfate (Decrease in circulating catecholamines with smoking cessation; may require an increase in dose at cessation of smoking). Products include:

Brethaire Inhaler 813
Brethine Ampuls 815
Brethine Tablets 814
Bricanyl Subcutaneous Injection 1502
Bricanyl Tablets 1503

Theophylline (Deinduction of hepatic enzymes on smoking cessation; may require a decrease in dose at cessation of smoking). Products include:

Marax Tablets & DF Syrup 2200
Quibron 2053

Theophylline Anhydrous (Deinduction of hepatic enzymes on smoking cessation; may require a decrease in dose at cessation of smoking). Products include:

Aerolate 1004
Primatene Dual Action Formula ...... ⊕ 872
Primatene Tablets .... ⊕ 873
Respbid Tablets 682
Slo-bid Gyrocaps 2033
Theo-24 Extended Release Capsules 2568
Theo-Dur Extended-Release Tablets 1327
Theo-X Extended-Release Tablets .. 788
Uni-Dur Extended-Release Tablets .. 1331
Uniphyl 400 mg Tablets 2001

Theophylline Calcium Salicylate (Deinduction of hepatic enzymes on smoking cessation; may require a decrease in dose at cessation of smoking). Products include:

Quadrinal Tablets 1350

Theophylline Sodium Glycinate (Deinduction of hepatic enzymes on smoking cessation; may require a decrease in dose at cessation of smoking).

No products indexed under this heading.

NICOLAR TABLETS

(Niacin) 2026

May interact with insulin, oral hypoglycemic agents, nitrates and nitrites, calcium channel blockers, hmg-coa reductase inhibitors, and certain other agents. Compounds in these categories include:

Acarbose (Potential for dose-related rise in glucose intolerance; adjustment of diet and/or diabetic drug therapy may be necessary).

No products indexed under this heading.

Acebutolol Hydrochloride (Caution should be exercised when used concurrently with adrenergic blocking agents in patients with unstable angina or in the acute phase of myocardial infarction). Products include:

Sectral Capsules 2807

Amlodipine Besylate (Caution should be exercised when used concurrently in patients with unstable angina or in the acute phase of myocardial infarction). Products include:

Lotrel Capsules 840
Norvasc Tablets 1940

Amyl Nitrite (Caution should be exercised when used concurrently in patients with unstable angina or in the acute phase of myocardial infarction).

No products indexed under this heading.

Aspirin (Decreases metabolic clearance of nicotinic acid). Products include:

Alka-Seltzer Effervescent Antacid and Pain Reliever .... ⊕ 701
Alka-Seltzer Extra Strength Effervescent Antacid and Pain Reliever .... ⊕ 703
Alka-Seltzer Lemon Lime Effervescent Antacid and Pain Reliever .... ⊕ 703
Alka-Seltzer Plus Cold Medicine .... ⊕ 705
Alka-Seltzer Plus Cold & Cough Medicine .... ⊕ 708
Alka-Seltzer Plus Night-Time Cold Medicine .... ⊕ 707
Alka Seltzer Plus Sinus Medicine .. ⊕ 707
Arthritis Foundation Safety Coated Aspirin Tablets .... ⊕ 675
Arthritis Pain Ascriptin .... ⊕ 631
Maximum Strength Ascriptin .... ⊕ 630
Regular Strength Ascriptin Tablets .... ⊕ 629
Arthritis Strength BC Powder .... ⊕ 609
BC Cold Powder Multi-Symptom Formula (Cold-Sinus-Allergy) ...... ⊕ 609
BC Cold Powder Non-Drowsy Formula (Cold-Sinus) .... ⊕ 609
BC Powder .... ⊕ 609
Bayer Children's Chewable Aspirin .... ⊕ 711
Genuine Bayer Aspirin Tablets & Caplets .... ⊕ 713
Extra Strength Bayer Arthritis Pain Regimen Formula .... ⊕ 711
Extra Strength Bayer Aspirin Caplets & Tablets .... ⊕ 712
Extended-Release Bayer 8-Hour Aspirin .... ⊕ 712
Extra Strength Bayer Plus Aspirin Caplets .... ⊕ 713
Extra Strength Bayer PM Aspirin .. ⊕ 713
Bayer Enteric Aspirin .... ⊕ 709
Bufferin Analgesic Tablets and Caplets .... ⊕ 613
Arthritis Strength Bufferin Analgesic Caplets .... ⊕ 614
Extra Strength Bufferin Analgesic Tablets .... ⊕ 615
Cama Arthritis Pain Reliever .... ⊕ 785
Darvon Compound-65 Pulvules 1435
Easprin 1914
Ecotrin 2455
Ecotrin Enteric Coated Aspirin Maximum Strength Tablets and Caplets .... ⊕ 816
Ecotrin Enteric Coated Aspirin Regular Strength Tablets 2455
Empirin Aspirin Tablets .... ⊕ 854
Empirin with Codeine Tablets 1093
Excedrin Extra-Strength Analgesic Tablets & Caplets 732
Fiorinal Capsules 2261
Fiorinal with Codeine Capsules 2262
Fiorinal Tablets 2261
Halfprin 1362
Healthprin Aspirin 2455
Norgesic 1496
Percodan Tablets 939
Percodan-Demi Tablets 940
Robaxisal Tablets 2071
Soma Compound w/Codeine Tablets 2676
Soma Compound Tablets 2675
St. Joseph Adult Chewable Aspirin (81 mg.) .... ⊕ 808
Talwin Compound 2335
Ursinus Inlay-Tabs .... ⊕ 794
Vanquish Analgesic Caplets .... ⊕ 731

Atenolol (Caution should be exercised when used concurrently with adrenergic blocking agents in patients with unstable angina or in the acute phase of myocardial infarction). Products include:

Tenoretic Tablets 2845
Tenormin Tablets and I.V. Injection 2847

Bepridil Hydrochloride (Caution should be exercised when used concurrently in patients with unstable angina or in the acute phase of myocardial infarction). Products include:

Vascor (200, 300 and 400 mg) Tablets 1587

Betaxolol Hydrochloride (Caution should be exercised when used concurrently with adrenergic blocking agents in patients with unstable angina or in the acute phase of myocardial infarction). Products include:

Betoptic Ophthalmic Solution 469

Betoptic S Ophthalmic Suspension 471
Kerlone Tablets 2436

Bisoprolol Fumarate (Caution should be exercised when used concurrently with adrenergic blocking agents in patients with unstable angina or in the acute phase of myocardial infarction). Products include:

Zebeta Tablets 1413
Ziac 1415

Carteolol Hydrochloride (Caution should be exercised when used concurrently with adrenergic blocking agents in patients with unstable angina or in the acute phase of myocardial infarction). Products include:

Cartrol Tablets 410
Ocupress Ophthalmic Solution, 1% Sterile .... ⊙ 309

Chlorpropamide (Potential for dose-related rise in glucose intolerance; adjustment of diet and/or diabetic drug therapy may be necessary). Products include:

Diabinese Tablets 1935

Diltiazem Hydrochloride (Caution should be exercised when used concurrently in patients with unstable angina or in the acute phase of myocardial infarction). Products include:

Cardizem CD Capsules 1506
Cardizem SR Capsules 1510
Cardizem Injectable 1508
Cardizem Tablets 1512
Dilacor XR Extended-release Capsules 2018

Erythrityl Tetranitrate (Caution should be exercised when used concurrently in patients with unstable angina or in the acute phase of myocardial infarction).

No products indexed under this heading.

Esmolol Hydrochloride (Caution should be exercised when used concurrently with adrenergic blocking agents in patients with unstable angina or in the acute phase of myocardial infarction). Products include:

Brevibloc Injection 1808

Felodipine (Caution should be exercised when used concurrently in patients with unstable angina or in the acute phase of myocardial infarction). Products include:

Plendil Extended-Release Tablets 527

Fluvastatin Sodium (Concomitant administration with lipid-altering doses of nicotinic acid and HMG-CoA reductase inhibitors have been associated with rare cases of rhabdomyolysis). Products include:

Lescol Capsules 2267

Glipizide (Potential for dose-related rise in glucose intolerance; adjustment of diet and/or diabetic drug therapy may be necessary). Products include:

Glucotrol Tablets 1967
Glucotrol XL Extended Release Tablets 1968

Glyburide (Potential for dose-related rise in glucose intolerance; adjustment of diet and/or diabetic drug therapy may be necessary). Products include:

DiaBeta Tablets 1239
Glynase PresTab Tablets 2609
Micronase Tablets 2623

Insulin, Human (Potential for dose-related rise in glucose intolerance; adjustment of diet and/or diabetic drug therapy may be necessary).

No products indexed under this heading.

Insulin, Human Isophane Suspension (Potential for dose-related rise in glucose intolerance; adjustment of diet and/or diabetic drug therapy may be necessary). Products include:

Novolin N Human Insulin 10 ml Vials 1795

Insulin, Human NPH (Potential for dose-related rise in glucose intolerance; adjustment of diet and/or diabetic drug therapy may be necessary). Products include:

Humulin N, 100 Units 1448
Novolin N PenFill Cartridges Durable Insulin Delivery System 1798
Novolin N Prefilled Syringe Disposable Insulin Delivery System 1798

Insulin, Human Regular (Potential for dose-related rise in glucose intolerance; adjustment of diet and/or diabetic drug therapy may be necessary). Products include:

Humulin R, 100 Units 1449
Novolin R Human Insulin 10 ml Vials 1795
Novolin R PenFill Cartridges Durable Insulin Delivery System 1798
Novolin R Prefilled Syringe Disposable Insulin Delivery System 1798
Velosulin BR Human Insulin 10 ml Vials 1795

Insulin, Human, Zinc Suspension (Potential for dose-related rise in glucose intolerance; adjustment of diet and/or diabetic drug therapy may be necessary). Products include:

Humulin L, 100 Units 1446
Humulin U, 100 Units 1450
Novolin L Human Insulin 10 ml Vials 1795

Insulin, NPH (Potential for dose-related rise in glucose intolerance; adjustment of diet and/or diabetic drug therapy may be necessary). Products include:

NPH, 100 Units 1450
Pork NPH, 100 Units 1452
Purified Pork NPH Isophane Insulin 1801

Insulin, Regular (Potential for dose-related rise in glucose intolerance; adjustment of diet and/or diabetic drug therapy may be necessary). Products include:

Regular, 100 Units 1450
Pork Regular, 100 Units 1452
Pork Regular (Concentrated), 500 Units 1453
Purified Pork Regular Insulin 1801

Insulin, Zinc Crystals (Potential for dose-related rise in glucose intolerance; adjustment of diet and/or diabetic drug therapy may be necessary). Products include:

NPH, 100 Units 1450

Insulin, Zinc Suspension (Potential for dose-related rise in glucose intolerance; adjustment of diet and/or diabetic drug therapy may be necessary). Products include:

Iletin I 1450
Lente, 100 Units 1450
Iletin II 1452
Pork Lente, 100 Units 1452
Purified Pork Lente Insulin 1801

Isosorbide Dinitrate (Caution should be exercised when used concurrently in patients with unstable angina or in the acute phase of myocardial infarction). Products include:

Dilatrate-SR 2398
Isordil Sublingual Tablets 2739
Isordil Tembids 2741
Isordil Titradose Tablets 2742
Sorbitrate 2843

IMPORTANT NOTE: Always consult each drug listing in the patient's regimen for possible interactions.

Isosorbide Mononitrate (Caution should be exercised when used concurrently in patients with unstable angina or in the acute phase of myocardial infarction). Products include:

- Imdur 1323
- Ismo Tablets 2738
- Monoket 2406

Isradipine (Caution should be exercised when used concurrently in patients with unstable angina or in the acute phase of myocardial infarction). Products include:

- DynaCirc Capsules 2256

Labetalol Hydrochloride (Caution should be exercised when used concurrently with adrenergic blocking agents in patients with unstable angina or in the acute phase of myocardial infarction). Products include:

- Normodyne Injection 2377
- Normodyne Tablets 2379
- Trandate 1185

Lovastatin (Concomitant administration with lipid-altering doses of nicotinic acid and HMG-CoA reductase inhibitors have been associated with rare cases of rhabdomyolysis). Products include:

- Mevacor Tablets 1699

Mecamylamine Hydrochloride (Nicotinic acid may potentiate the effects of ganglionic blocking agents). Products include:

- Inversine Tablets 1686

Metformin Hydrochloride (Potential for dose-related rise in glucose intolerance; adjustment of diet and/or diabetic drug therapy may be necessary). Products include:

- Glucophage 752

Metoprolol Succinate (Caution should be exercised when used concurrently with adrenergic blocking agents in patients with unstable angina or in the acute phase of myocardial infarction). Products include:

- Toprol-XL Tablets 565

Metoprolol Tartrate (Caution should be exercised when used concurrently with adrenergic blocking agents in patients with unstable angina or in the acute phase of myocardial infarction). Products include:

- Lopressor Ampuls 830
- Lopressor HCT Tablets 832
- Lopressor Tablets 830

Nadolol (Caution should be exercised when used concurrently with adrenergic blocking agents in patients with unstable angina or in the acute phase of myocardial infarction).

No products indexed under this heading.

Nicardipine Hydrochloride (Caution should be exercised when used concurrently in patients with unstable angina or in the acute phase of myocardial infarction). Products include:

- Cardene Capsules 2095
- Cardene I.V. 2709
- Cardene SR Capsules 2097

Nifedipine (Caution should be exercised when used concurrently in patients with unstable angina or in the acute phase of myocardial infarction). Products include:

- Adalat Capsules (10 mg and 20 mg) 587
- Adalat CC 589
- Procardia Capsules 1971
- Procardia XL Extended Release Tablets 1972

Nimodipine (Caution should be exercised when used concurrently in patients with unstable angina or in the acute phase of myocardial infarction). Products include:

- Nimotop Capsules 610

Nisoldipine (Caution should be exercised when used concurrently in patients with unstable angina or in the acute phase of myocardial infarction).

No products indexed under this heading.

Nitroglycerin (Caution should be exercised when used concurrently in patients with unstable angina or in the acute phase of myocardial infarction). Products include:

- Deponit NTG Transdermal Delivery System 2397
- Nitro-Bid IV 1523
- Nitro-Bid Ointment 1524
- Nitrodisc 2047
- Nitro-Dur (nitroglycerin) Transdermal Infusion System 1326
- Nitrolingual Spray 2027
- Nitrostat Tablets 1925
- Transderm-Nitro Transdermal Therapeutic System 859

Penbutolol Sulfate (Caution should be exercised when used concurrently with adrenergic blocking agents in patients with unstable angina or in the acute phase of myocardial infarction). Products include:

- Levatol 2403

Pentaerythritol Tetranitrate (Caution should be exercised when used concurrently in patients with unstable angina or in the acute phase of myocardial infarction).

No products indexed under this heading.

Pindolol (Caution should be exercised when used concurrently with adrenergic blocking agents in patients with unstable angina or in the acute phase of myocardial infarction). Products include:

- Visken Tablets 2299

Pravastatin Sodium (Concomitant administration with lipid-altering doses of nicotinic acid and HMG-CoA reductase inhibitors have been associated with rare cases of rhabdomyolysis). Products include:

- Pravachol 765

Propranolol Hydrochloride (Caution should be exercised when used concurrently with adrenergic blocking agents in patients with unstable angina or in the acute phase of myocardial infarction). Products include:

- Inderal 2728
- Inderal LA Long Acting Capsules 2730
- Inderide Tablets 2732
- Inderide LA Long Acting Capsules 2734

Simvastatin (Concomitant administration with lipid-altering doses of nicotinic acid and HMG-CoA reductase inhibitors have been associated with rare cases of rhabdomyolysis). Products include:

- Zocor Tablets 1775

Sotalol Hydrochloride (Caution should be exercised when used concurrently with adrenergic blocking agents in patients with unstable angina or in the acute phase of myocardial infarction). Products include:

- Betapace Tablets 641

Timolol Maleate (Caution should be exercised when used concurrently with adrenergic blocking agents in patients with unstable angina or in the acute phase of myocardial infarction). Products include:

- Blocadren Tablets 1614
- Timolide Tablets 1748
- Timoptic in Ocudose 1753
- Timoptic Sterile Ophthalmic Solution 1751
- Timoptic-XE 1755

Tolazamide (Potential for dose-related rise in glucose intolerance; adjustment of diet and/or diabetic drug therapy may be necessary).

No products indexed under this heading.

Tolbutamide (Potential for dose-related rise in glucose intolerance; adjustment of diet and/or diabetic drug therapy may be necessary).

No products indexed under this heading.

Trimethaphan Camsylate (Nicotinic acid may potentiate the effects of ganglionic blocking agents). Products include:

- Arfonad Ampuls 2080

Verapamil Hydrochloride (Caution should be exercised when used concurrently in patients with unstable angina or in the acute phase of myocardial infarction). Products include:

- Calan SR Caplets 2422
- Calan Tablets 2419
- Isoptin Injectable 1344
- Isoptin Oral Tablets 1346
- Isoptin SR Tablets 1348
- Verelan Capsules 1410
- Verelan Capsules 2824

Food Interactions

Alcohol (May increase the side effects of flushing and pruritus).

Drinks, hot, unspecified (May increase the side effects of flushing and pruritus).

NICORETTE

(Nicotine Polacrilex) 2458

May interact with xanthine bronchodilators, insulin, sympathomimetics, and certain other agents. Compounds in these categories include:

Acetaminophen (Deinduction of hepatic enzymes on smoking cessation; may require a decrease in dose at cessation of smoking). Products include:

- Actifed Plus Caplets .... ▣ 845
- Actifed Plus Tablets .... ▣ 845
- Actifed Sinus Daytime/Nighttime Tablets and Caplets .... ▣ 846
- Alka-Seltzer Plus Cold Medicine Liqui-Gels .... ▣ 706
- Alka-Seltzer Plus Cold & Cough Medicine Liqui-Gels .... ▣ 705
- Alka-Seltzer Plus Night-Time Cold Medicine Liqui-Gels .... ▣ 706
- Allerest Headache Strength Tablets .... ▣ 627
- Allerest No Drowsiness Tablets .... ▣ 627
- Allerest Sinus Pain Formula .... ▣ 627
- Anexsia 5/500 Elixir 1781
- Anexia Tablets 1782
- Arthritis Foundation Aspirin Free Caplets .... ▣ 673
- Arthritis Foundation NightTime Caplets .... ▣ 674
- Bayer Select Headache Pain Relief Formula .... ▣ 716
- Bayer Select Menstrual Multi-Symptom Formula .... ▣ 716
- Bayer Select Night Time Pain Relief Formula .... ▣ 716
- Bayer Select Sinus Pain Relief Formula .... ▣ 717
- Benadryl Allergy Sinus Headache Formula Caplets .... ▣ 849
- Comtrex Multi-Symptom Cold Reliever Tablets/Caplets/Liqui-Gels/Liquid .... ▣ 615
- Allergy-Sinus Comtrex Multi-Symptom Allergy-Sinus Formula Tablets .... ▣ 617
- Comtrex Non-Drowsy .... ▣ 618
- Contac Day Allergy/Sinus Caplets ▣ 812
- Contac Day & Night .... ▣ 812
- Contac Night Allergy/Sinus Caplets .... ▣ 812
- Contac Severe Cold and Flu Formula Caplets .... ▣ 814
- Contac Severe Cold & Flu Non-Drowsy .... ▣ 815
- Coricidin 'D' Decongestant Tablets .... ▣ 800
- Coricidin Tablets .... ▣ 800
- DHCplus Capsules 1993
- Darvon-N/Darvocet-N 1433
- Drixoral Cold and Flu Extended-Release Tablets .... ▣ 803
- Drixoral Cough + Sore Throat Liquid Caps .... ▣ 802
- Drixoral Allergy/Sinus Extended Release Tablets .... ▣ 804
- Esgic-plus Tablets 1013
- Aspirin Free Excedrin Analgesic Caplets and Geltabs 732
- Excedrin Extra-Strength Analgesic Tablets & Caplets 732
- Excedrin P.M. Analgesic/Sleeping Aid Tablets, Caplets, Liquigels 733
- Fioricet Tablets 2258
- Fioricet with Codeine Capsules 2260
- Hycomine Compound Tablets 932
- Hydrocet Capsules 782
- Legatrin PM .... ▣ 651
- Lorcet 10/650 1018
- Lortab 2566
- Lurline PMS Tablets 982
- Maximum Strength Multi-Symptom Formula Midol .... ▣ 722
- PMS Multi-Symptom Formula Midol .... ▣ 723
- Teen Multi-Symptom Formula Midol .... ▣ 722
- Midrin Capsules 783
- Migralam Capsules 2038
- Panodol Tablets and Caplets .... ▣ 824
- Children's Panadol Chewable Tablets, Liquid, Infant's Drops .... ▣ 824
- Percocet Tablets 938
- Percogesic Analgesic Tablets .... ▣ 754
- Phrenilin 785
- Pyrroxate Caplets .... ▣ 772
- Sedapap Tablets 50 mg/650 mg 1543
- Sinarest Tablets .... ▣ 648
- Sinarest Extra Strength Tablets .... ▣ 648
- Sinarest No Drowsiness Tablets .... ▣ 648
- Sine-Aid Maximum Strength Sinus Medication Gelcaps, Caplets and Tablets 1554
- Sine-Off No Drowsiness Formula Caplets .... ▣ 824
- Sine-Off Sinus Medicine .... ▣ 825
- Singlet Tablets .... ▣ 825
- Sinulin Tablets 787
- Sinutab Sinus Allergy Medication, Maximum Strength Tablets and Caplets .... ▣ 860
- Sinutab Sinus Medication, Maximum Strength Without Drowsiness Formula, Tablets & Caplets .... ▣ 860
- Sinutab Sinus Medication, Regular Strength Without Drowsiness Formula .... ▣ 859
- Sudafed Cold and Cough Liquidcaps .... ▣ 862
- Sudafed Severe Cold Formula Caplets .... ▣ 863
- Sudafed Severe Cold Formula Tablets .... ▣ 864
- Sudafed Sinus Caplets .... ▣ 864
- Sudafed Sinus Tablets .... ▣ 864
- Talacen 2333
- TheraFlu .... ▣ 787
- TheraFlu Maximum Strength Nighttime Flu, Cold & Cough Medicine .... ▣ 788
- TheraFlu Maximum Strength Non-Drowsy Formula Flu, Cold & Cough Medicine .... ▣ 788
- Thera Flu Maximum Strength, Non-Drowsy Formula Flu, Cold and Cough Caplets .... ▣ 789
- Triaminic Sore Throat Formula .... ▣ 791
- Triaminicin Tablets .... ▣ 793
- Children's TYLENOL acetaminophen Chewable Tablets, Elixir, Suspension Liquid 1555
- Children's TYLENOL Cold Multi-Symptom Liquid Formula and Chewable Tablets 1561
- Children's TYLENOL Cold Plus Cough Multi Symptom Tablets and Liquid .... ▣ 681
- Infants' TYLENOL acetaminophen Drops and Suspension Drops 1555
- Infants' TYLENOL Cold Decongestant & Fever-Reducer Drops 1556

(▣ Described in PDR For Nonprescription Drugs) (◉ Described in PDR For Ophthalmology)

719 **Interactions Index** **Nicorette**

TYLENOL Extended Relief Caplets.. 1558
TYLENOL, Extra Strength, Acetaminophen Adult Liquid Pain Reliever 1560
TYLENOL, Extra Strength, acetaminophen Gelcaps, Geltabs, Caplets, Tablets 1559
TYLENOL, Extra Strength, Headache Plus Pain Reliever with Antacid Caplets 1559
TYLENOL, Junior Strength, acetaminophen Coated Caplets, Grape and Fruit Chewable Tablets 1557
TYLENOL Maximum Strength Allergy Sinus Medication Gelcaps and Caplets 1563
TYLENOL Maximum Strength Allergy Sinus NightTime Medication Caplets 1555
TYLENOL Flu Maximum Strength Gelcaps 1565
TYLENOL Flu NightTime, Maximum Strength, Gelcaps 1566
TYLENOL Maximum Strength Flu NightTime Hot Medication Packets 1562
TYLENOL, Maximum Strength, Sinus Medication Geltabs, Gelcaps, Caplets and Tablets 1566
TYLENOL Cold Multi-Symptom Formula Medication Tablets and Caplets 1561
TYLENOL Cold Medication No Drowsiness Formula Gelcaps and Caplets 1562
TYLENOL Cold Multi-Symptom Hot Medication Liquid Packets 1557
TYLENOL Cough Multi-Symptom Medication 1564
TYLENOL Cough Multi-Symptom Medication with Decongestant 1565
TYLENOL, Regular Strength, acetaminophen Caplets and Tablets .. 1558
TYLENOL PM, Extra Strength Pain Reliever/Sleep Aid Caplets, Geltabs, Gelcaps 1560
TYLENOL Severe Allergy Medication Caplets 1564
Tylenol with Codeine 1583
Tylox Capsules 1584
Unisom With Pain Relief-Nighttime Sleep Aid and Pain Reliever 1934
Vanquish Analgesic Caplets 731
Vicks 44 LiquiCaps Cough, Cold & Flu Relief 755
Vicks 44M Cough, Cold & Flu Relief 756
Vicks DayQuil 761
Vicks Nyquil Hot Therapy 762
Vicks NyQuil LiquiCaps Multi-Symptom Cold/Flu Relief 763
Vicks NyQuil Multi-Symptom Cold/Flu Relief - (Original & Cherry Flavor) 763
Vicodin Tablets 1356
Vicodin ES Tablets 1357
Wygesic Tablets 2827
Zydone Capsules 949

Albuterol (Decrease in circulating catecholamines with smoking cessation; may require an increase in dose at cessation of smoking). Products include:
Proventil Inhalation Aerosol 2382
Ventolin Inhalation Aerosol and Refill 1197

Albuterol Sulfate (Decrease in circulating catecholamines with smoking cessation; may require an increase in dose at cessation of smoking). Products include:
Airet Solution for Inhalation 452
Proventil Inhalation Solution 0.083% 2384
Proventil Repetabs Tablets 2386
Proventil Solution for Inhalation 0.5% 2383
Proventil Syrup 2385
Proventil Tablets 2386
Ventolin Inhalation Solution 1198
Ventolin Nebules Inhalation Solution 1199
Ventolin Rotacaps for Inhalation 1200
Ventolin Syrup 1202
Ventolin Tablets 1203
Volmax Extended-Release Tablets .. 1788

Aminophylline (Deinduction of hepatic enzymes on smoking cessation; may require a decrease in dose at cessation of smoking).
No products indexed under this heading.

Caffeine-containing medications (Deinduction of hepatic enzymes on smoking cessation; may require a decrease in dose at cessation of smoking).

Dobutamine Hydrochloride (Decrease in circulating catecholamines with smoking cessation; may require an increase in dose at cessation of smoking). Products include:
Dobutrex Solution Vials 1439

Dopamine Hydrochloride (Decrease in circulating catecholamines with smoking cessation; may require an increase in dose at cessation of smoking).
No products indexed under this heading.

Dyphylline (Deinduction of hepatic enzymes on smoking cessation; may require a decrease in dose at cessation of smoking). Products include:
Lufyllin & Lufyllin-400 Tablets 2670
Lufyllin-GG Elixir & Tablets 2671

Ephedrine Hydrochloride (Decrease in circulating catecholamines with smoking cessation; may require an increase in dose at cessation of smoking). Products include:
Primatene Dual Action Formula 872
Primatene Tablets 873
Quadrinal Tablets 1350

Ephedrine Sulfate (Decrease in circulating catecholamines with smoking cessation; may require an increase in dose at cessation of smoking). Products include:
Bronkaid Caplets 717
Marax Tablets & DF Syrup 2200

Ephedrine Tannate (Decrease in circulating catecholamines with smoking cessation; may require an increase in dose at cessation of smoking). Products include:
Rynatuss 2673

Epinephrine (Decrease in circulating catecholamines with smoking cessation; may require an increase in dose at cessation of smoking). Products include:
Bronkaid Mist 717
EPIFRIN ◉ 239
EpiPen 790
Marcaine Hydrochloride with Epinephrine 1:200,000 2316
Primatene Mist 873
Sensorcaine with Epinephrine Injection 559
Sus-Phrine Injection 1019
Xylocaine with Epinephrine Injections 567

Epinephrine Bitartrate (Decrease in circulating catecholamines with smoking cessation; may require an increase in dose at cessation of smoking). Products include:
Bronkaid Mist Suspension 718
Sensorcaine-MPF with Epinephrine Injection 559

Epinephrine Hydrochloride (Decrease in circulating catecholamines with smoking cessation; may require an increase in dose at cessation of smoking). Products include:
Ana-Kit Anaphylaxis Emergency Treatment Kit 617

Imipramine Hydrochloride (Deinduction of hepatic enzymes on smoking cessation; may require a decrease in dose at cessation of smoking). Products include:
Tofranil Ampuls 854
Tofranil Tablets 856

Imipramine Pamoate (Deinduction of hepatic enzymes on smoking cessation; may require a decrease in dose at cessation of smoking). Products include:
Tofranil-PM Capsules 857

Insulin, Human (Increase of subcutaneous insulin absorption with smoking cessation; may require a decrease in dose at cessation of smoking).
No products indexed under this heading.

Insulin, Human Isophane Suspension (Increase of subcutaneous insulin absorption with smoking cessation; may require a decrease in dose at cessation of smoking). Products include:
Novolin N Human Insulin 10 ml Vials 1795

Insulin, Human NPH (Increase of subcutaneous insulin absorption with smoking cessation; may require a decrease in dose at cessation of smoking). Products include:
Humulin N, 100 Units 1448
Novolin N PenFill Cartridges Durable Insulin Delivery System 1798
Novolin N Prefilled Syringe Disposable Insulin Delivery System 1798

Insulin, Human Regular (Increase of subcutaneous insulin absorption with smoking cessation; may require a decrease in dose at cessation of smoking). Products include:
Humulin R, 100 Units 1449
Novolin R Human Insulin 10 ml Vials 1795
Novolin R PenFill Cartridges Durable Insulin Delivery System 1798
Novolin R Prefilled Syringe Disposable Insulin Delivery System 1798
Velosulin BR Human Insulin 10 ml Vials 1795

Insulin, Human, Zinc Suspension (Increase of subcutaneous insulin absorption with smoking cessation; may require a decrease in dose at cessation of smoking). Products include:
Humulin L, 100 Units 1446
Humulin U, 100 Units 1450
Novolin L Human Insulin 10 ml Vials 1795

Insulin, NPH (Increase of subcutaneous insulin absorption with smoking cessation; may require a decrease in dose at cessation of smoking). Products include:
NPH, 100 Units 1450
Pork NPH, 100 Units 1452
Purified Pork NPH Isophane Insulin 1801

Insulin, Regular (Increase of subcutaneous insulin absorption with smoking cessation; may require a decrease in dose at cessation of smoking). Products include:
Regular, 100 Units 1450
Pork Regular, 100 Units 1452
Pork Regular (Concentrated), 500 Units 1453
Purified Pork Regular Insulin 1801

Insulin, Zinc Crystals (Increase of subcutaneous insulin absorption with smoking cessation; may require a decrease in dose at cessation of smoking). Products include:
NPH, 100 Units 1450

Insulin, Zinc Suspension (Increase of subcutaneous insulin absorption with smoking cessation; may require a decrease in dose at cessation of smoking). Products include:
Iletin I 1450
Lente, 100 Units 1450
Iletin II 1452
Pork Lente, 100 Units 1452
Purified Pork Lente Insulin 1801

Isoproterenol Hydrochloride (Decrease in circulating catecholamines with smoking cessation; may require an increase in dose at cessation of smoking). Products include:
Isuprel Hydrochloride Injection 1:5000 2311
Isuprel Hydrochloride Solution 1:200 & 1:100 2313
Isuprel Mistometer 2312

Isoproterenol Sulfate (Decrease in circulating catecholamines with smoking cessation; may require an increase in dose at cessation of smoking). Products include:
Norisodrine with Calcium Iodide Syrup 442

Labetalol Hydrochloride (Decrease in circulating catecholamines with smoking cessation; may require a decrease in dose at cessation of smoking). Products include:
Normodyne Injection 2377
Normodyne Tablets 2379
Trandate 1185

Metaproterenol Sulfate (Decrease in circulating catecholamines with smoking cessation; may require an increase in dose at cessation of smoking). Products include:
Alupent 669
Metaproterenol Sulfate Inhalation Solution, USP, Arm-a-Med 552

Metaraminol Bitartrate (Decrease in circulating catecholamines with smoking cessation; may require an increase in dose at cessation of smoking). Products include:
Aramine Injection 1609

Methoxamine Hydrochloride (Decrease in circulating catecholamines with smoking cessation; may require an increase in dose at cessation of smoking). Products include:
Vasoxyl Injection 1196

Norepinephrine Bitartrate (Decrease in circulating catecholamines with smoking cessation; may require an increase in dose at cessation of smoking). Products include:
Levophed Bitartrate Injection 2315

Oxazepam (Deinduction of hepatic enzymes on smoking cessation; may require a decrease in dose at cessation of smoking). Products include:
Serax Capsules 2810
Serax Tablets 2810

Pentazocine Hydrochloride (Deinduction of hepatic enzymes on smoking cessation; may require a decrease in dose at cessation of smoking). Products include:
Talacen 2333
Talwin Compound 2335
Talwin Nx 2336

Pentazocine Lactate (Deinduction of hepatic enzymes on smoking cessation; may require a decrease in dose at cessation of smoking). Products include:
Talwin Injection 2334

Phenylephrine Bitartrate (Decrease in circulating catecholamines with smoking cessation; may require an increase in dose at cessation of smoking).
No products indexed under this heading.

Phenylephrine Hydrochloride (Decrease in circulating catecholamines with smoking cessation; may require an increase in dose at cessation of smoking). Products include:
Atrohist Plus Tablets 454
Cerose DM 878
Comhist 2038
D.A. Chewable Tablets 951
Deconsal Pediatric Capsules 454
Dura-Vent/DA Tablets 953

IMPORTANT NOTE: Always consult each drug listing in the patient's regimen for possible interactions.

Nicorette **Interactions Index** **720**

Entex Capsules ... 1986
Entex Liquid ... 1986
Extendryl ... 1005
4-Way Fast Acting Nasal Spray (regular & mentholated) ... ▣ 621
Hemorid For Women ... ▣ 834
Hycomine Compound Tablets ... 932
Neo-Synephrine Hydrochloride 1% Carpuject ... 2324
Neo-Synephrine Hydrochloride 1% Injection ... 2324
Neo-Synephrine Hydrochloride (Ophthalmic) ... 2325
Neo-Synephrine ... ▣ 726
Nōstril ... ▣ 644
Novahistine Elixir ... ▣ 823
Phenergan VC ... 2779
Phenergan VC with Codeine ... 2781
Preparation H ... ▣ 871
Tympagesic Ear Drops ... 2342
Vasosulf ... ◉ 271
Vicks Sinex Nasal Spray and Ultra Fine Mist ... ▣ 765

Phenylephrine Tannate (Decrease in circulating catecholamines with smoking cessation; may require an increase in dose at cessation of smoking). Products include:
Atrohist Pediatric Suspension ... 454
Ricobid-D Pediatric Suspension ... 2038
Ricobid Tablets and Pediatric Suspension ... 2038
Rynatan ... 2673
Rynatuss ... 2673

Phenylpropanolamine Hydrochloride (Decrease in circulating catecholamines with smoking cessation; may require an increase in dose at cessation of smoking). Products include:
Acutrim ... ▣ 628
Allerest Children's Chewable Tablets ... ▣ 627
Allerest 12 Hour Caplets ... ▣ 627
Atrohist Plus Tablets ... 454
BC Cold Powder Multi-Symptom Formula (Cold-Sinus-Allergy) ... ▣ 609
BC Cold Powder Non-Drowsy Formula (Cold-Sinus) ... ▣ 609
Cheracol Plus Head Cold/Cough Formula ... ▣ 769
Comtrex Multi-Symptom Non-Drowsy Liqui-gels ... ▣ 618
Contac Continuous Action Nasal Decongestant/Antihistamine 12 Hour Capsules ... ▣ 813
Contac Maximum Strength Continuous Action Decongestant/Antihistamine 12 Hour Caplets ... ▣ 813
Contac Severe Cold and Flu Formula Caplets ... ▣ 814
Coricidin 'D' Decongestant Tablets ... ▣ 800
Dexatrim ... ▣ 832
Dexatrim Plus Vitamins Caplets ... ▣ 832
Dimetane-DC Cough Syrup ... 2059
Dimetapp Elixir ... ▣ 773
Dimetapp Extentabs ... ▣ 774
Dimetapp Tablets/Liqui-Gels ... ▣ 775
Dimetapp Cold & Allergy Chewable Tablets ... ▣ 773
Dimetapp DM Elixir ... ▣ 774
Dura-Vent Tablets ... 952
Entex Capsules ... 1986
Entex LA Tablets ... 1987
Entex Liquid ... 1986
Exgest LA Tablets ... 782
Hycomine ... 931
Isoclor Timesule Capsules ... ▣ 637
Nolamine Timed-Release Tablets ... 785
Ornade Spansule Capsules ... 2502
Propagest Tablets ... 786
Pyrroxate Caplets ... ▣ 772
Robitussin-CF ... ▣ 777
Sinulin Tablets ... 787
Tavist-D 12 Hour Relief Tablets ... ▣ 787
Teldrin 12 Hour Antihistamine/Nasal Decongestant Allergy Relief Capsules ... ▣ 826
Triaminic Allergy Tablets ... ▣ 789
Triaminic Cold Tablets ... ▣ 790
Triaminic Expectorant ... ▣ 790
Triaminic Syrup ... ▣ 792
Triaminic-12 Tablets ... ▣ 792
Triaminic-DM Syrup ... ▣ 792
Triaminicin Tablets ... ▣ 793
Triaminicol Multi-Symptom Cold Tablets ... ▣ 793
Triaminicol Multi-Symptom Relief ... ▣ 794
Vicks DayQuil Allergy Relief 12-Hour Extended Release Tablets ... ▣ 760
Vicks DayQuil Allergy Relief 4-Hour Tablets ... ▣ 760
Vicks DayQuil SINUS Pressure & CONGESTION Relief ... ▣ 761

Pirbuterol Acetate (Decrease in circulating catecholamines with smoking cessation; may require an increase in dose at cessation of smoking). Products include:
Maxair Autohaler ... 1492
Maxair Inhaler ... 1494

Prazosin Hydrochloride (Decrease in circulating catecholamines with smoking cessation; may require a decrease in dose at cessation of smoking). Products include:
Minipress Capsules ... 1937
Minizide Capsules ... 1938

Propranolol Hydrochloride (Deinduction of hepatic enzymes on smoking cessation; may require a decrease in dose at cessation of smoking). Products include:
Inderal ... 2728
Inderal LA Long Acting Capsules ... 2730
Inderide Tablets ... 2732
Inderide LA Long Acting Capsules ... 2734

Pseudoephedrine Hydrochloride (Decrease in circulating catecholamines with smoking cessation; may require an increase in dose at cessation of smoking). Products include:
Actifed Allergy Daytime/Nighttime Caplets ... ▣ 844
Actifed Plus Caplets ... ▣ 845
Actifed Plus Tablets ... ▣ 845
Actifed with Codeine Cough Syrup ... 1067
Actifed Sinus Daytime/Nighttime Tablets and Caplets ... ▣ 846
Actifed Syrup ... ▣ 846
Actifed Tablets ... ▣ 844
Advil Cold and Sinus Caplets and Tablets (formerly CoAdvil) ... ▣ 870
Alka-Seltzer Plus Cold Medicine Liqui-Gels ... ▣ 706
Alka-Seltzer Plus Cold & Cough Medicine Liqui-Gels ... ▣ 705
Alka-Seltzer Plus Night-Time Cold Medicine Liqui-Gels ... ▣ 706
Allerest Headache Strength Tablets ... ▣ 627
Allerest Maximum Strength Tablets ... ▣ 627
Allerest No Drowsiness Tablets ... ▣ 627
Allerest Sinus Pain Formula ... ▣ 627
Anatuss LA Tablets ... 1542
Atrohist Pediatric Capsules ... 453
Bayer Select Sinus Pain Relief Formula ... ▣ 717
Benadryl Allergy Decongestant Liquid Medication ... ▣ 848
Benadryl Allergy Decongestant Tablets ... ▣ 848
Benadryl Allergy Sinus Headache Formula Caplets ... ▣ 849
Benylin Multisymptom ... ▣ 852
Bromfed Capsules (Extended-Release) ... 1785
Bromfed Syrup ... ▣ 733
Bromfed Tablets ... 1785
Bromfed-DM Cough Syrup ... 1786
Bromfed-PD Capsules (Extended-Release) ... 1785
Children's Vicks DayQuil Allergy Relief ... ▣ 757
Children's Vicks NyQuil Cold/Cough Relief ... ▣ 758
Comtrex Multi-Symptom Cold Reliever Tablets/Caplets/Liqui-Gels/Liquid ... ▣ 615
Allergy-Sinus Comtrex Multi-Symptom Allergy-Sinus Formula Tablets ... ▣ 617
Comtrex Multi-Symptom Non-Drowsy Caplets ... ▣ 618
Congess ... 1004
Contac Day Allergy/Sinus Caplets ▣ 812
Contac Day & Night ... ▣ 812
Contac Night Allergy/Sinus Caplets ... ▣ 812
Contac Severe Cold & Flu Non-Drowsy ... ▣ 815
Deconamine Chewable Tablets ... 1320
Deconamine CX Cough and Cold Liquid and Tablets ... 1319
Deconamine ... 1320
Deconsal C Expectorant Syrup ... 456
Deconsal Pediatric Syrup ... 457
Deconsal II Tablets ... 454
Dimetane-DX Cough Syrup ... 2059
Dimetapp Sinus Caplets ... ▣ 775
Dorcol Children's Cough Syrup ... ▣ 785
Drixoral Cough + Congestion Liquid Caps ... ▣ 802
Dura-Tap/PD Capsules ... 2867
Duratuss Tablets ... 2565
Duratuss HD Elixir ... 2565
Efidac/24 ... ▣ 635
Entex PSE Tablets ... 1987
Fedahist Gyrocaps ... 2401
Fedahist Timecaps ... 2401
Guaifed ... 1787
Guaifed Syrup ... ▣ 734
Guaimax-D Tablets ... 792
Guaitab Tablets ... ▣ 734
Isoclor Expectorant ... 990
Kronofed-A ... 977
Motrin IB Sinus ... ▣ 838
Novahistine DH ... 2462
Novahistine DMX ... ▣ 822
Novahistine Expectorant ... 2463
Nucofed ... 2051
PediaCare Cold Allergy Chewable Tablets ... ▣ 677
PediaCare Cough-Cold Chewable Tablets ... 1553
PediaCare ... 1553
PediaCare Infants' Decongestant Drops ... ▣ 677
PediCare Infant's Drops Decongestant Plus Cough ... 1553
PediaCare NightRest Cough-Cold Liquid ... 1553
Pediatric Vicks 44d Dry Hacking Cough & Head Congestion ... ▣ 763
Pediatric Vicks 44m Cough & Cold Relief ... ▣ 764
Robitussin Cold & Cough Liqui-Gels ... ▣ 776
Robitussin Maximum Strength Cough & Cold ... ▣ 778
Robitussin Pediatric Cough & Cold Formula ... ▣ 779
Robitussin Severe Congestion Liqui-Gels ... ▣ 776
Robitussin-DAC Syrup ... 2074
Robitussin-PE ... ▣ 778
Rondec Oral Drops ... 953
Rondec Syrup ... 953
Rondec Tablet ... 953
Rondec-DM Oral Drops ... 954
Rondec-DM Syrup ... 954
Rondec-TR Tablet ... 953
Ryna ... ▣ 841
Seldane-D Extended-Release Tablets ... 1538
Semprex-D Capsules ... 463
Semprex-D Capsules ... 1167
Sinarest Tablets ... ▣ 648
Sinarest Extra Strength Tablets ... ▣ 648
Sinarest No Drowsiness Tablets ... ▣ 648
Sine-Aid IB Caplets ... 1554
Sine-Aid Maximum Strength Sinus Medication Gelcaps, Caplets and Tablets ... 1554
Sine-Off No Drowsiness Formula Caplets ... ▣ 824
Sine-Off Sinus Medicine ... ▣ 825
Singlet Tablets ... ▣ 825
Sinutab Non-Drying Liquid Caps ... ▣ 859
Sinutab Sinus Allergy Medication, Maximum Strength Tablets and Caplets ... ▣ 860
Sinutab Sinus Medication, Maximum Strength Without Drowsiness Formula, Tablets & Caplets ... ▣ 860
Sinutab Sinus Medication, Regular Strength Without Drowsiness Formula ... ▣ 859
Sudafed Children's Liquid ... ▣ 861
Sudafed Cold and Cough Liquidcaps ... ▣ 862
Sudafed Cough Syrup ... ▣ 862
Sudafed Plus Liquid ... ▣ 862
Sudafed Plus Tablets ... ▣ 863
Sudafed Severe Cold Formula Caplets ... ▣ 863
Sudafed Severe Cold Formula Tablets ... ▣ 864
Sudafed Sinus Caplets ... ▣ 864
Sudafed Sinus Tablets ... ▣ 864
Sudafed Tablets, 30 mg ... ▣ 861
Sudafed Tablets, 60 mg ... ▣ 861
Sudafed 12 Hour Caplets ... ▣ 861
Syn-Rx Tablets ... 465
Syn-Rx DM Tablets ... 466
TheraFlu ... ▣ 787
TheraFlu Maximum Strength Nighttime Flu, Cold & Cough Medicine ... ▣ 788
TheraFlu Maximum Strength Non-Drowsy Formula Flu, Cold & Cough Medicine ... ▣ 788
Thera Flu Maximum Strength, Non-Drowsy Formula Flu, Cold and Cough Caplets ... ▣ 789
Triaminic AM Cough and Decongestant Formula ... ▣ 789
Triaminic AM Decongestant Formula ... ▣ 790
Triaminic Nite Light ... ▣ 791
Triaminic Sore Throat Formula ... ▣ 791
Tussend ... 1783
Tussend Expectorant ... 1785
Children's TYLENOL Cold Multi-Symptom Liquid Formula and Chewable Tablets ... 1561
Children's TYLENOL Cold Plus Cough Multi Symptom Tablets and Liquid ... ▣ 681
Infants' TYLENOL Cold Decongestant & Fever-Reducer Drops ... 1556
TYLENOL Maximum Strength Allergy Sinus Medication Gelcaps and Caplets ... 1563
TYLENOL Maximum Strength Allergy Sinus NightTime Medication Caplets ... 1555
TYLENOL Flu Maximum Strength Gelcaps ... 1565
TYLENOL Flu NightTime, Maximum Strength, Gelcaps ... 1566
TYLENOL Maximum Strength Flu NightTime Hot Medication Packets ... 1562
TYLENOL, Maximum Strength, Sinus Medication Geltabs, Gelcaps, Caplets and Tablets ... 1566
TYLENOL Cold Multi-Symptom Formula Medication Tablets and Caplets ... 1561
TYLENOL Cold Medication No Drowsiness Formula Gelcaps and Caplets ... 1562
TYLENOL Cold Multi-Symptom Hot Medication Liquid Packets ... 1557
TYLENOL Cough Multi-Symptom Medication with Decongestant ... 1565
Ursinus Inlay-Tabs ... ▣ 794
Vicks 44 LiquiCaps Cough, Cold & Flu Relief ... ▣ 755
Vicks 44 LiquiCaps Non-Drowsy Cough & Cold Relief ... ▣ 756
Vicks 44D Dry Hacking Cough & Head Congestion ... ▣ 755
Vicks 44M Cough, Cold & Flu Relief ... ▣ 756
Vicks DayQuil ... ▣ 761
Vicks DayQuil SINUS Pressure & PAIN Relief with IBUPROFEN ... ▣ 762
Vicks Nyquil Hot Therapy ... ▣ 762
Vicks NyQuil LiquiCaps Multi-Symptom Cold/Flu Relief ... ▣ 763
Vicks NyQuil Multi-Symptom Cold/Flu Relief - (Original & Cherry Flavor) ... ▣ 763

Pseudoephedrine Sulfate (Decrease in circulating catecholamines with smoking cessation; may require an increase in dose at cessation of smoking). Products include:
Cheracol Sinus ... ▣ 768
Chlor-Trimeton Allergy Decongestant Tablets ... ▣ 799
Claritin-D ... 2350
Drixoral Cold and Allergy Sustained-Action Tablets ... ▣ 802
Drixoral Cold and Flu Extended-Release Tablets ... ▣ 803
Drixoral Non-Drowsy Formula Extended-Release Tablets ... ▣ 803
Drixoral Allergy/Sinus Extended Release Tablets ... ▣ 804
Trinalin Repetabs Tablets ... 1330

Salmeterol Xinafoate (Decrease in circulating catecholamines with smoking cessation; may require an increase in dose at cessation of smoking). Products include:
Serevent Inhalation Aerosol ... 1176

(▣ Described in PDR For Nonprescription Drugs) (◉ Described in PDR For Ophthalmology)

Interactions Index — Nicotrol

Terbutaline Sulfate (Decrease in circulating catecholamines with smoking cessation; may require an increase in dose at cessation of smoking). Products include:

Brethaire Inhaler 813
Brethine Ampuls 815
Brethine Tablets 814
Bricanyl Subcutaneous Injection 1502
Bricanyl Tablets 1503

Theophylline (Deinduction of hepatic enzymes on smoking cessation; may require a decrease in dose at cessation of smoking). Products include:

Marax Tablets & DF Syrup................. 2200
Quibron 2053

Theophylline Anhydrous (Deinduction of hepatic enzymes on smoking cessation; may require a decrease in dose at cessation of smoking). Products include:

Aerolate 1004
Primatene Dual Action Formula .... ⚫ 872
Primatene Tablets .... ⚫ 873
Respbid Tablets 682
Slo-bid Gyrocaps 2033
Theo-24 Extended Release Capsules 2568
Theo-Dur Extended-Release Tablets 1327
Theo-X Extended-Release Tablets .. 788
Uni-Dur Extended-Release Tablets.. 1331
Uniphyl 400 mg Tablets...................... 2001

Theophylline Calcium Salicylate (Deinduction of hepatic enzymes on smoking cessation; may require a decrease in dose at cessation of smoking). Products include:

Quadrinal Tablets 1350

Theophylline Sodium Glycinate (Deinduction of hepatic enzymes on smoking cessation; may require a decrease in dose at cessation of smoking).

No products indexed under this heading.

Food Interactions

Beverages, acidic (Interferes with buccal absorption of nicotine from Nicorette).

Beverages, caffeine-containing (Interferes with buccal absorption of nicotine from Nicorette).

Fruit juices, unspecified (Interferes with buccal absorption of nictoine from Nicorette).

Wine, unspecified (Interferes with buccal absorption of nicotine from Nicorette).

NICORETTE DS

(Nicotine Polacrilex) 2458
See Nicorette

NICOTINEX ELIXIR

(Niacin) .... ⚫ 655
None cited in PDR database.

NICOTROL NICOTINE TRANSDERMAL SYSTEM

(Nicotine) 1550
May interact with xanthine bronchodilators, insulin, sympathomimetics, and certain other agents. Compounds in these categories include:

Acetaminophen (Deinduction of hepatic enzymes on smoking cessation; may require a decrease in dose at cessation of smoking). Products include:

Actifed Plus Caplets .... ⚫ 845
Actifed Plus Tablets .... ⚫ 845
Actifed Sinus Daytime/Nighttime Tablets and Caplets .... ⚫ 846
Alka-Seltzer Plus Cold Medicine Liqui-Gels .... ⚫ 706
Alka-Seltzer Plus Cold & Cough Medicine Liqui-Gels........................... ⚫ 705
Alka-Seltzer Plus Night-Time Cold Medicine Liqui-Gels........................... ⚫ 706
Allerest Headache Strength Tablets .... ⚫ 627
Allerest No Drowsiness Tablets ...... ⚫ 627
Allerest Sinus Pain Formula .... ⚫ 627
Anexsia 5/500 Elixir 1781
Anexia Tablets.. 1782
Arthritis Foundation Aspirin Free Caplets .... ⚫ 673
Arthritis Foundation NightTime Caplets .... ⚫ 674
Bayer Select Headache Pain Relief Formula .... ⚫ 716
Bayer Select Menstrual Multi-Symptom Formula.............................. ⚫ 716
Bayer Select Night Time Pain Relief Formula.................................... ⚫ 716
Bayer Select Sinus Pain Relief Formula .... ⚫ 717
Benadryl Allergy Sinus Headache Formula Caplets................................. ⚫ 849
Comtrex Multi-Symptom Cold Reliever Tablets/Caplets/Liqui-Gels/Liquid.. ⚫ 615
Allergy-Sinus Comtrex Multi-Symptom Allergy-Sinus Formula Tablets .... ⚫ 617
Comtrex Non-Drowsy........................... ⚫ 618
Contac Day Allergy/Sinus Caplets ⚫ 812
Contac Day & Night .... ⚫ 812
Contac Night Allergy/Sinus Caplets .... ⚫ 812
Contac Severe Cold and Flu Formula Caplets .... ⚫ 814
Contac Severe Cold & Flu Non-Drowsy .... ⚫ 815
Coricidin 'D' Decongestant Tablets .... ⚫ 800
Coricidin Tablets .... ⚫ 800
DHCplus Capsules.................................. 1993
Darvon-N/Darvocet-N 1433
Drixoral Cold and Flu Extended-Release Tablets................................... ⚫ 803
Drixoral Cough + Sore Throat Liquid Caps .... ⚫ 802
Drixoral Allergy/Sinus Extended Release Tablets................................... ⚫ 804
Esgic-plus Tablets 1013
Aspirin Free Excedrin Analgesic Caplets and Geltabs 732
Excedrin Extra-Strength Analgesic Tablets & Caplets 732
Excedrin P.M. Analgesic/Sleeping Aid Tablets, Caplets, Liquigels....... 733
Fioricet Tablets 2258
Fioricet with Codeine Capsules 2260
Hycomine Compound Tablets 932
Hydrocet Capsules 782
Legatrin PM .... ⚫ 651
Lorcet 10/650.. 1018
Lortab 2566
Lurline PMS Tablets 982
Maximum Strength Multi-Symptom Formula Midol .... ⚫ 722
PMS Multi-Symptom Formula Midol .... ⚫ 723
Teen Multi-Symptom Formula Midol .... ⚫ 722
Midrin Capsules 783
Migralam Capsules 2038
Panodol Tablets and Caplets .... ⚫ 824
Children's Panadol Chewable Tablets, Liquid, Infant's Drops .... ⚫ 824
Percocet Tablets 938
Percogesic Analgesic Tablets .... ⚫ 754
Phrenilin 785
Pyrroxate Caplets .... ⚫ 772
Sedapap Tablets 50 mg/650 mg .. 1543
Sinarest Tablets .... ⚫ 648
Sinarest Extra Strength Tablets...... ⚫ 648
Sinarest No Drowsiness Tablets .... ⚫ 648
Sine-Aid Maximum Strength Sinus Medication Gelcaps, Caplets and Tablets 1554
Sine-Off No Drowsiness Formula Caplets .... ⚫ 824
Sine-Off Sinus Medicine .... ⚫ 825
Singlet Tablets .... ⚫ 825
Sinulin Tablets 787
Sinutab Sinus Allergy Medication, Maximum Strength Tablets and Caplets .... ⚫ 860
Sinutab Sinus Medication, Maximum Strength Without Drowsiness Formula, Tablets & Caplets .... ⚫ 860
Sinutab Sinus Medication, Regular Strength Without Drowsiness Formula .... ⚫ 859
Sudafed Cold and Cough Liquidcaps .... ⚫ 862
Sudafed Severe Cold Formula Caplets .... ⚫ 863
Sudafed Severe Cold Formula Tablets .... ⚫ 864
Sudafed Sinus Caplets......................... ⚫ 864
Sudafed Sinus Tablets......................... ⚫ 864
Talacen.. 2333
TheraFlu.. ⚫ 787
TheraFlu Maximum Strength Nighttime Flu, Cold & Cough Medicine .... ⚫ 788
TheraFlu Maximum Strength Non-Drowsy Formula Flu, Cold & Cough Medicine .... ⚫ 788
Thera Flu Maximum Strength, Non-Drowsy Formula Flu, Cold and Cough Caplets .... ⚫ 789
Triaminic Sore Throat Formula ...... ⚫ 791
Triaminicin Tablets .... ⚫ 793
Children's TYLENOL acetaminophen Chewable Tablets, Elixir, Suspension Liquid 1555
Children's TYLENOL Cold Multi-Symptom Liquid Formula and Chewable Tablets................................. 1561
Children's TYLENOL Cold Plus Cough Multi Symptom Tablets and Liquid .... ⚫ 681
Infants' TYLENOL acetaminophen Drops and Suspension Drops........ 1555
Infants' TYLENOL Cold Decongestant & Fever-Reducer Drops 1556
TYLENOL Extended Relief Caplets.. 1558
TYLENOL, Extra Strength, Acetaminophen Adult Liquid Pain Reliever 1560
TYLENOL, Extra Strength, acetaminophen Gelcaps, Geltabs, Caplets, Tablets 1559
TYLENOL, Extra Strength, Headache Plus Pain Reliever with Antacid Caplets 1559
TYLENOL, Junior Strength, acetaminophen Coated Caplets, Grape and Fruit Chewable Tablets 1557
TYLENOL Maximum Strength Allergy Sinus Medication Gelcaps and Caplets 1563
TYLENOL Maximum Strength Allergy Sinus NightTime Medication Caplets 1555
TYLENOL Flu Maximum Strength Gelcaps 1565
TYLENOL Flu NightTime, Maximum Strength, Gelcaps 1566
TYLENOL Maximum Strength Flu NightTime Hot Medication Packets 1562
TYLENOL, Maximum Strength, Sinus Medication Geltabs, Gelcaps, Caplets and Tablets 1566
TYLENOL Cold Multi-Symptom Formula Medication Tablets and Caplets 1561
TYLENOL Cold Medication No Drowsiness Formula Gelcaps and Caplets 1562
TYLENOL Cold Multi-Symptom Hot Medication Liquid Packets.............. 1557
TYLENOL Cough Multi-Symptom Medication 1564
TYLENOL Cough Multi-Symptom Medication with Decongestant...... 1565
TYLENOL, Regular Strength, acetaminophen Caplets and Tablets .. 1558
TYLENOL PM, Extra Strength Pain Reliever/Sleep Aid Caplets, Geltabs, Gelcaps...................................... 1560
TYLENOL Severe Allergy Medication Caplets 1564
Tylenol with Codeine 1583
Tylox Capsules 1584
Unisom With Pain Relief-Nighttime Sleep Aid and Pain Reliever.............. 1934
Vanquish Analgesic Caplets .... ⚫ 731
Vicks 44 LiquiCaps Cough, Cold & Flu Relief .... ⚫ 755
Vicks 44M Cough, Cold & Flu Relief .... ⚫ 756
Vicks DayQuil .... ⚫ 761
Vicks Nyquil Hot Therapy................... ⚫ 762
Vicks NyQuil LiquiCaps Multi-Symptom Cold/Flu Relief.............. ⚫ 763
Vicks NyQuil Multi-Symptom Cold/Flu Relief - (Original & Cherry Flavor) .... ⚫ 763
Vicodin Tablets 1356
Vicodin ES Tablets 1357
Wygesic Tablets 2827
Zydone Capsules 949

Albuterol (Decrease in circulating catecholamines with smoking cessation; may require an increase in dose at cessation of smoking). Products include:

Proventil Inhalation Aerosol 2382
Ventolin Inhalation Aerosol and Refill 1197

Albuterol Sulfate (Decrease in circulating catecholamines with smoking cessation; may require an increase in dose at cessation of smoking). Products include:

Airet Solution for Inhalation 452
Proventil Inhalation Solution 0.083% 2384
Proventil Repetabs Tablets 2386
Proventil Solution for Inhalation 0.5% 2383
Proventil Syrup 2385
Proventil Tablets 2386
Ventolin Inhalation Solution................. 1198
Ventolin Nebules Inhalation Solution 1199
Ventolin Rotacaps for Inhalation 1200
Ventolin Syrup.. 1202
Ventolin Tablets 1203
Volmax Extended-Release Tablets .. 1788

Aminophylline (Deinduction of hepatic enzymes on smoking cessation; may require a decrease in dose at cessation of smoking).

No products indexed under this heading.

Caffeine-containing medications (Deinduction of hepatic enzymes on smoking cessation; may require a decrease in dose at cessation of smoking).

Dobutamine Hydrochloride (Decrease in circulating catecholamines with smoking cessation; may require an increase in dose at cessation of smoking). Products include:

Dobutrex Solution Vials......................... 1439

Dopamine Hydrochloride (Decrease in circulating catecholamines with smoking cessation; may require an increase in dose at cessation of smoking).

No products indexed under this heading.

Dyphylline (Deinduction of hepatic enzymes on smoking cessation; may require a decrease in dose at cessation of smoking). Products include:

Lufyllin & Lufyllin-400 Tablets 2670
Lufyllin-GG Elixir & Tablets 2671

Ephedrine Hydrochloride (Decrease in circulating catecholamines with smoking cessation; may require an increase in dose at cessation of smoking). Products include:

Primatene Dual Action Formula...... ⚫ 872
Primatene Tablets .... ⚫ 873
Quadrinal Tablets 1350

Ephedrine Sulfate (Decrease in circulating catecholamines with smoking cessation; may require an increase in dose at cessation of smoking). Products include:

Bronkaid Caplets .... ⚫ 717
Marax Tablets & DF Syrup.................. 2200

Ephedrine Tannate (Decrease in circulating catecholamines with smoking cessation; may require an increase in dose at cessation of smoking). Products include:

Rynatuss 2673

Epinephrine (Decrease in circulating catecholamines with smoking cessation; may require an increase in dose at cessation of smoking). Products include:

Bronkaid Mist .... ⚫ 717
EPIFRIN .... ◉ 239
EpiPen 790
Marcaine Hydrochloride with Epinephrine 1:200,000 2316
Primatene Mist .... ⚫ 873

IMPORTANT NOTE: Always consult each drug listing in the patient's regimen for possible interactions.

Nicotrol **Interactions Index** 722

Sensorcaine with Epinephrine Injection 559
Sus-Phrine Injection 1019
Xylocaine with Epinephrine Injections 567

Epinephrine Bitartrate (Decrease in circulating catecholamines with smoking cessation; may require an increase in dose at cessation of smoking). Products include:
Bronkaid Mist Suspension ▣ 718
Sensorcaine-MPF with Epinephrine Injection 559

Epinephrine Hydrochloride (Decrease in circulating catecholamines with smoking cessation; may require an increase in dose at cessation of smoking). Products include:
Ana-Kit Anaphylaxis Emergency Treatment Kit 617

Imipramine Hydrochloride (Deinduction of hepatic enzymes on smoking cessation; may require a decrease in dose at cessation of smoking). Products include:
Tofranil Ampuls 854
Tofranil Tablets 856

Imipramine Pamoate (Deinduction of hepatic enzymes on smoking cessation; may require a decrease in dose at cessation of smoking). Products include:
Tofranil-PM Capsules 857

Insulin, Human (Increase of subcutaneous insulin absorption with smoking cessation; may require a decrease in dose at cessation of smoking).
No products indexed under this heading.

Insulin, Human Isophane Suspension (Increase of subcutaneous insulin absorption with smoking cessation; may require a decrease in dose at cessation of smoking). Products include:
Novolin N Human Insulin 10 ml Vials 1795

Insulin, Human NPH (Increase of subcutaneous insulin absorption with smoking cessation; may require a decrease in dose at cessation of smoking). Products include:
Humulin N, 100 Units 1448
Novolin N PenFill Cartridges Durable Insulin Delivery System 1798
Novolin N Prefilled Syringe Disposable Insulin Delivery System 1798

Insulin, Human Regular (Increase of subcutaneous insulin absorption with smoking cessation; may require a decrease in dose at cessation of smoking). Products include:
Humulin R, 100 Units 1449
Novolin R Human Insulin 10 ml Vials 1795
Novolin R PenFill Cartridges Durable Insulin Delivery System 1798
Novolin R Prefilled Syringe Disposable Insulin Delivery System 1798
Velosulin BR Human Insulin 10 ml Vials 1795

Insulin, Human, Zinc Suspension (Increase of subcutaneous insulin absorption with smoking cessation; may require a decrease in dose at cessation of smoking). Products include:
Humulin L, 100 Units 1446
Humulin U, 100 Units 1450
Novolin L Human Insulin 10 ml Vials 1795

Insulin, NPH (Increase of subcutaneous insulin absorption with smoking cessation; may require a decrease in dose at cessation of smoking). Products include:
NPH, 100 Units 1450
Pork NPH, 100 Units 1452
Purified Pork NPH Isophane Insulin 1801

Insulin, Regular (Increase of subcutaneous insulin absorption with smoking cessation; may require a decrease in dose at cessation of smoking). Products include:
Regular, 100 Units 1450
Pork Regular, 100 Units 1452
Pork Regular (Concentrated), 500 Units 1453
Purified Pork Regular Insulin 1801

Insulin, Zinc Crystals (Increase of subcutaneous insulin absorption with smoking cessation; may require a decrease in dose at cessation of smoking). Products include:
NPH, 100 Units 1450

Insulin, Zinc Suspension (Increase of subcutaneous insulin absorption with smoking cessation; may require a decrease in dose at cessation of smoking). Products include:
Iletin I 1450
Lente, 100 Units 1450
Iletin II 1452
Pork Lente, 100 Units 1452
Purified Pork Lente Insulin 1801

Isoproterenol Hydrochloride (Decrease in circulating catecholamines with smoking cessation; may require an increase in dose at cessation of smoking). Products include:
Isuprel Hydrochloride Injection 1:5000 2311
Isuprel Hydrochloride Solution 1:200 & 1:100 2313
Isuprel Mistometer 2312

Isoproterenol Sulfate (Decrease in circulating catecholamines with smoking cessation; may require an increase in dose at cessation of smoking). Products include:
Norisodrine with Calcium Iodide Syrup 442

Labetalol Hydrochloride (Decrease in circulating catecholamines with smoking cessation; may require a decrease in dose at cessation of smoking). Products include:
Normodyne Injection 2377
Normodyne Tablets 2379
Trandate 1185

Metaproterenol Sulfate (Decrease in circulating catecholamines with smoking cessation; may require an increase in dose at cessation of smoking). Products include:
Alupent 669
Metaproterenol Sulfate Inhalation Solution, USP, Arm-a-Med 552

Metaraminol Bitartrate (Decrease in circulating catecholamines with smoking cessation; may require an increase in dose at cessation of smoking). Products include:
Aramine Injection 1609

Methoxamine Hydrochloride (Decrease in circulating catecholamines with smoking cessation; may require an increase in dose at cessation of smoking). Products include:
Vasoxyl Injection 1196

Norepinephrine Bitartrate (Decrease in circulating catecholamines with smoking cessation; may require an increase in dose at cessation of smoking). Products include:
Levophed Bitartrate Injection 2315

Oxazepam (Deinduction of hepatic enzymes on smoking cessation; may require a decrease in dose at cessation of smoking). Products include:
Serax Capsules 2810
Serax Tablets 2810

Pentazocine Hydrochloride (Deinduction of hepatic enzymes on smoking cessation; may require a decrease in dose at cessation of smoking). Products include:
Talacen 2333
Talwin Compound 2335
Talwin Nx 2336

Pentazocine Lactate (Deinduction of hepatic enzymes on smoking cessation; may require a decrease in dose at cessation of smoking). Products include:
Talwin Injection 2334

Phenylephrine Bitartrate (Decrease in circulating catecholamines with smoking cessation; may require an increase in dose at cessation of smoking).
No products indexed under this heading.

Phenylephrine Hydrochloride (Decrease in circulating catecholamines with smoking cessation; may require an increase in dose at cessation of smoking). Products include:
Atrohist Plus Tablets 454
Cerose DM ▣ 878
Comhist 2038
D.A. Chewable Tablets 951
Deconsal Pediatric Capsules 454
Dura-Vent/DA Tablets 953
Entex Capsules 1986
Entex Liquid 1986
Extendryl 1005
4-Way Fast Acting Nasal Spray (regular & mentholated) ▣ 621
Hemorid For Women ▣ 834
Hycomine Compound Tablets 932
Neo-Synephrine Hydrochloride 1% Carpuject 2324
Neo-Synephrine Hydrochloride 1% Injection 2324
Neo-Synephrine Hydrochloride (Ophthalmic) 2325
Neo-Synephrine ▣ 726
Nōstril ▣ 644
Novahistine Elixir ▣ 823
Phenergan VC 2779
Phenergan VC with Codeine 2781
Preparation H ▣ 871
Tympagesic Ear Drops 2342
Vasosulf ⊙ 271
Vicks Sinex Nasal Spray and Ultra Fine Mist ▣ 765

Phenylephrine Tannate (Decrease in circulating catecholamines with smoking cessation; may require an increase in dose at cessation of smoking). Products include:
Atrohist Pediatric Suspension 454
Ricobid-D Pediatric Suspension 2038
Ricobid Tablets and Pediatric Suspension 2038
Rynatan 2673
Rynatuss 2673

Phenylpropanolamine Hydrochloride (Decrease in circulating catecholamines with smoking cessation; may require an increase in dose at cessation of smoking). Products include:
Acutrim ▣ 628
Allerest Children's Chewable Tablets ▣ 627
Allerest 12 Hour Caplets ▣ 627
Atrohist Plus Tablets 454
BC Cold Powder Multi-Symptom Formula (Cold-Sinus-Allergy) ▣ 609
BC Cold Powder Non-Drowsy Formula (Cold-Sinus) ▣ 609
Cheracol Plus Head Cold/Cough Formula ▣ 769
Comtrex Multi-Symptom Non-Drowsy Liqui-gels ▣ 618
Contac Continuous Action Nasal Decongestant/Antihistamine 12 Hour Capsules ▣ 813
Contac Maximum Strength Continuous Action Decongestant/Antihistamine 12 Hour Caplets ▣ 813
Contac Severe Cold and Flu Formula Caplets ▣ 814
Coricidin 'D' Decongestant Tablets ▣ 800
Dexatrim ▣ 832
Dexatrim Plus Vitamins Caplets ▣ 832
Dimetane-DC Cough Syrup 2059
Dimetapp Elixir ▣ 773
Dimetapp Extentabs ▣ 774
Dimetapp Tablets/Liqui-Gels ▣ 775
Dimetapp Cold & Allergy Chewable Tablets ▣ 773
Dimetapp DM Elixir ▣ 774
Dura-Vent Tablets 952
Entex Capsules 1986
Entex LA Tablets 1987
Entex Liquid 1986
Exgest LA Tablets 782
Hycomine 931
Isoclor Timesule Capsules ▣ 637
Nolamine Timed-Release Tablets 785
Ornade Spansule Capsules 2502
Propagest Tablets 786
Pyrroxate Caplets ▣ 772
Robitussin-CF ▣ 777
Sinulin Tablets 787
Tavist-D 12 Hour Relief Tablets ▣ 787
Teldrin 12 Hour Antihistamine/Nasal Decongestant Allergy Relief Capsules ▣ 826
Triaminic Allergy Tablets ▣ 789
Triaminic Cold Tablets ▣ 790
Triaminic Expectorant ▣ 790
Triaminic Syrup ▣ 792
Triaminic-12 Tablets ▣ 792
Triaminic-DM Syrup ▣ 792
Triaminicin Tablets ▣ 793
Triaminicol Multi-Symptom Cold Tablets ▣ 793
Triaminicol Multi-Symptom Relief ▣ 794
Vicks DayQuil Allergy Relief 12-Hour Extended Release Tablets ▣ 760
Vicks DayQuil Allergy Relief 4-Hour Tablets ▣ 760
Vicks DayQuil SINUS Pressure & CONGESTION Relief ▣ 761

Pirbuterol Acetate (Decrease in circulating catecholamines with smoking cessation; may require an increase in dose at cessation of smoking). Products include:
Maxair Autohaler 1492
Maxair Inhaler 1494

Prazosin Hydrochloride (Decrease in circulating catecholamines with smoking cessation; may require a decrease in dose at cessation of smoking). Products include:
Minipress Capsules 1937
Minizide Capsules 1938

Propranolol Hydrochloride (Deinduction of hepatic enzymes on smoking cessation; may require a decrease in dose at cessation of smoking). Products include:
Inderal 2728
Inderal LA Long Acting Capsules 2730
Inderide Tablets 2732
Inderide LA Long Acting Capsules 2734

Pseudoephedrine Hydrochloride (Decrease in circulating catecholamines with smoking cessation; may require an increase in dose at cessation of smoking). Products include:
Actifed Allergy Daytime/Nighttime Caplets ▣ 844
Actifed Plus Caplets ▣ 845
Actifed Plus Tablets ▣ 845
Actifed with Codeine Cough Syrup 1067
Actifed Sinus Daytime/Nighttime Tablets and Caplets ▣ 846
Actifed Syrup ▣ 846
Actifed Tablets ▣ 844
Advil Cold and Sinus Caplets and Tablets (formerly CoAdvil) ▣ 870
Alka-Seltzer Plus Cold Medicine Liqui-Gels ▣ 706
Alka-Seltzer Plus Cold & Cough Medicine Liqui-Gels ▣ 705
Alka-Seltzer Plus Night-Time Cold Medicine Liqui-Gels ▣ 706
Allerest Headache Strength Tablets ▣ 627
Allerest Maximum Strength Tablets ▣ 627
Allerest No Drowsiness Tablets ▣ 627
Allerest Sinus Pain Formula ▣ 627
Anatuss LA Tablets 1542
Atrohist Pediatric Capsules 453
Bayer Select Sinus Pain Relief Formula ▣ 717

(▣ Described in PDR For Nonprescription Drugs) (⊙ Described in PDR For Ophthalmology)

Interactions Index

Benadryl Allergy Decongestant Liquid Medication ....⊕ 848
Benadryl Allergy Decongestant Tablets ....⊕ 848
Benadryl Allergy Sinus Headache Formula Caplets ....⊕ 849
Benylin Multisymptom ....⊕ 852
Bromfed Capsules (Extended-Release) 1785
Bromfed Syrup ....⊕ 733
Bromfed Tablets 1785
Bromfed-DM Cough Syrup................ 1786
Bromfed-PD Capsules (Extended-Release) 1785
Children's Vicks DayQuil Allergy Relief ....⊕ 757
Children's Vicks NyQuil Cold/Cough Relief.......................................⊕ 758
Comtrex Multi-Symptom Cold Reliever Tablets/Caplets/Liqui-Gels/Liquid ....⊕ 615
Allergy-Sinus Comtrex Multi-Symptom Allergy-Sinus Formula Tablets ....⊕ 617
Comtrex Multi-Symptom Non-Drowsy Caplets.................................⊕ 618
Congess 1004
Contac Day Allergy/Sinus Caplets ⊕ 812
Contac Day & Night ....⊕ 812
Contac Night Allergy/Sinus Caplets ....⊕ 812
Contac Severe Cold & Flu Non-Drowsy ....⊕ 815
Deconamine Chewable Tablets 1320
Deconamine CX Cough and Cold Liquid and Tablets.............................. 1319
Deconamine 1320
Deconsal C Expectorant Syrup 456
Deconsal Pediatric Syrup 457
Deconsal II Tablets 454
Dimetane-DX Cough Syrup 2059
Dimetapp Sinus Caplets ....⊕ 775
Dorcol Children's Cough Syrup ......⊕ 785
Drixoral Cough + Congestion Liquid Caps ....⊕ 802
Dura-Tap/PD Capsules 2867
Duratuss Tablets 2565
Duratuss HD Elixir............................. 2565
Efidac/24 ....⊕ 635
Entex PSE Tablets 1987
Fedahist Gyrocaps.............................. 2401
Fedahist Timecaps 2401
Guaifed.. 1787
Guaifed Syrup ....⊕ 734
Guaimax-D Tablets 792
Guaitab Tablets ....⊕ 734
Isoclor Expectorant............................ 990
Kronofed-A 977
Motrin IB Sinus..................................⊕ 838
Novahistine DH.................................. 2462
Novahistine DMX ....⊕ 822
Novahistine Expectorant.................... 2463
Nucofed 2051
PediaCare Cold Allergy Chewable Tablets ....⊕ 677
PediaCare Cough-Cold Chewable Tablets 1553
PediaCare 1553
PediaCare Infants' Decongestant Drops ....⊕ 677
PediCare Infant's Drops Decongestant Plus Cough 1553
PediaCare NightRest Cough-Cold Liquid 1553
Pediatric Vicks 44d Dry Hacking Cough & Head Congestion..............⊕ 763
Pediatric Vicks 44m Cough & Cold Relief ....⊕ 764
Robitussin Cold & Cough Liqui-Gels ....⊕ 776
Robitussin Maximum Strength Cough & Cold ....⊕ 778
Robitussin Pediatric Cough & Cold Formula ....⊕ 779
Robitussin Severe Congestion Liqui-Gels ....⊕ 776
Robitussin-DAC Syrup 2074
Robitussin-PE ....⊕ 778
Rondec Oral Drops 953
Rondec Syrup 953
Rondec Tablet 953
Rondec-DM Oral Drops...................... 954
Rondec-DM Syrup 954
Rondec-TR Tablet 953
Ryna ....⊕ 841
Seldane-D Extended-Release Tablets 1538
Semprex-D Capsules 463
Semprex-D Capsules 1167
Sinarest Tablets ....⊕ 648

Sinarest Extra Strength Tablets......⊕ 648
Sinarest No Drowsiness Tablets ....⊕ 648
Sine-Aid IB Caplets 1554
Sine-Aid Maximum Strength Sinus Medication Gelcaps, Caplets and Tablets 1554
Sine-Off No Drowsiness Formula Caplets ....⊕ 824
Sine-Off Sinus Medicine ....⊕ 825
Singlet Tablets ....⊕ 825
Sinutab Non-Drying Liquid Caps ....⊕ 859
Sinutab Sinus Allergy Medication, Maximum Strength Tablets and Caplets ....⊕ 860
Sinutab Sinus Medication, Maximum Strength Without Drowsiness Formula, Tablets & Caplets ....⊕ 860
Sinutab Sinus Medication, Regular Strength Without Drowsiness Formula ....⊕ 859
Sudafed Children's Liquid ....⊕ 861
Sudafed Cold and Cough Liquidcaps ....⊕ 862
Sudafed Cough Syrup ....⊕ 862
Sudafed Plus Liquid ....⊕ 862
Sudafed Plus Tablets ....⊕ 863
Sudafed Severe Cold Formula Caplets ....⊕ 863
Sudafed Severe Cold Formula Tablets ....⊕ 864
Sudafed Sinus Caplets........................⊕ 864
Sudafed Sinus Tablets........................⊕ 864
Sudafed Tablets, 30 mg......................⊕ 861
Sudafed Tablets, 60 mg.....................⊕ 861
Sudafed 12 Hour Caplets ....⊕ 861
Syn-Rx Tablets 465
Syn-Rx DM Tablets 466
TheraFlu..⊕ 787
TheraFlu Maximum Strength Nighttime Flu, Cold & Cough Medicine ....⊕ 788
TheraFlu Maximum Strength Non-Drowsy Formula Flu, Cold & Cough Medicine ....⊕ 788
Thera Flu Maximum Strength, Non-Drowsy Formula Flu, Cold and Cough Caplets ....⊕ 789
Triaminic AM Cough and Decongestant Formula ....⊕ 789
Triaminic AM Decongestant Formula ....⊕ 790
Triaminic Nite Light ....⊕ 791
Triaminic Sore Throat Formula ......⊕ 791
Tussend 1783
Tussend Expectorant 1785
Children's TYLENOL Cold Multi-Symptom Liquid Formula and Chewable Tablets................................. 1561
Children's TYLENOL Cold Plus Cough Multi Symptom Tablets and Liquid ....⊕ 681
Infants' TYLENOL Cold Decongestant & Fever-Reducer Drops 1556
TYLENOL Maximum Strength Allergy Sinus Medication Gelcaps and Caplets 1563
TYLENOL Maximum Strength Allergy Sinus NightTime Medication Caplets 1555
TYLENOL Flu Maximum Strength Gelcaps 1565
TYLENOL Flu NightTime, Maximum Strength, Gelcaps 1566
TYLENOL Maximum Strength Flu NightTime Hot Medication Packets 1562
TYLENOL, Maximum Strength, Sinus Medication Geltabs, Gelcaps, Caplets and Tablets 1566
TYLENOL Cold Multi-Symptom Formula Medication Tablets and Caplets 1561
TYLENOL Cold Medication No Drowsiness Formula Gelcaps and Caplets 1562
TYLENOL Cold Multi-Symptom Hot Medication Liquid Packets............ 1557
TYLENOL Cough Multi-Symptom Medication with Decongestant 1565
Ursinus Inlay-Tabs.............................⊕ 794
Vicks 44 LiquiCaps Cough, Cold & Flu Relief ....⊕ 755
Vicks 44 LiquiCaps Non-Drowsy Cough & Cold Relief ....⊕ 756
Vicks 44D Dry Hacking Cough & Head Congestion ....⊕ 755
Vicks 44M Cough, Cold & Flu Relief ....⊕ 756
Vicks DayQuil ....⊕ 761

Vicks DayQuil SINUS Pressure & PAIN Relief with IBUPROFEN ......⊕ 762
Vicks Nyquil Hot Therapy..................⊕ 762
Vicks NyQuil LiquiCaps Multi-Symptom Cold/Flu Relief ....⊕ 763
Vicks NyQuil Multi-Symptom Cold/Flu Relief - (Original & Cherry Flavor) ....⊕ 763

Pseudoephedrine Sulfate (Decrease in circulating catecholamines with smoking cessation; may require an increase in dose at cessation of smoking). Products include:

Cheracol Sinus ....⊕ 768
Chlor-Trimeton Allergy Decongestant Tablets ....⊕ 799
Claritin-D 2350
Drixoral Cold and Allergy Sustained-Action Tablets ....⊕ 802
Drixoral Cold and Flu Extended-Release Tablets..................................⊕ 803
Drixoral Non-Drowsy Formula Extended-Release Tablets ....⊕ 803
Drixoral Allergy/Sinus Extended Release Tablets..................................⊕ 804
Trinalin Repetabs Tablets 1330

Salmeterol Xinafoate (Decrease in circulating catecholamines with smoking cessation; may require an increase in dose at cessation of smoking). Products include:

Serevent Inhalation Aerosol.............. 1176

Terbutaline Sulfate (Decrease in circulating catecholamines with smoking cessation; may require an increase in dose at cessation of smoking). Products include:

Brethaire Inhaler 813
Brethine Ampuls 815
Brethine Tablets.................................. 814
Bricanyl Subcutaneous Injection 1502
Bricanyl Tablets 1503

Theophylline (Deinduction of hepatic enzymes on smoking cessation; may require a decrease in dose at cessation of smoking). Products include:

Marax Tablets & DF Syrup................. 2200
Quibron 2053

Theophylline Anhydrous (Deinduction of hepatic enzymes on smoking cessation; may require a decrease in dose at cessation of smoking). Products include:

Aerolate 1004
Primatene Dual Action Formula......⊕ 872
Primatene Tablets ....⊕ 873
Respbid Tablets 682
Slo-bid Gyrocaps 2033
Theo-24 Extended Release Capsules 2568
Theo-Dur Extended-Release Tablets 1327
Theo-X Extended-Release Tablets .. 788
Uni-Dur Extended-Release Tablets.. 1331
Uniphyl 400 mg Tablets...................... 2001

Theophylline Calcium Salicylate (Deinduction of hepatic enzymes on smoking cessation; may require a decrease in dose at cessation of smoking). Products include:

Quadrinal Tablets 1350

Theophylline Sodium Glycinate (Deinduction of hepatic enzymes on smoking cessation; may require a decrease in dose at cessation of smoking).

No products indexed under this heading.

NIFEREX-150 CAPSULES

(Polysaccharide-Iron Complex) 793
None cited in PDR database.

NIFEREX ELIXIR

(Polysaccharide-Iron Complex) 793
None cited in PDR database.

NIFEREX-150 FORTE CAPSULES

(Polysaccharide-Iron Complex, Folic Acid, Cyanocobalamin) 794

None cited in PDR database.

NIFEREX FORTE ELIXIR

(Polysaccharide-Iron Complex) 794
None cited in PDR database.

NIFEREX TABLETS

(Polysaccharide-Iron Complex) 793
None cited in PDR database.

NIFEREX W/VITAMIN C TABLETS

(Polysaccharide-Iron Complex, Vitamin C) 793
None cited in PDR database.

NIFEREX-PN TABLETS

(Vitamins with Iron) 794
None cited in PDR database.

NIMOTOP CAPSULES

(Nimodipine)... 610
May interact with antihypertensives, calcium channel blockers, and certain other agents. Compounds in these categories include:

Acebutolol Hydrochloride (Concomitant administration results in intensified effect). Products include:

Sectral Capsules 2807

Amlodipine Besylate (Possibility of enhanced cardiovascular action). Products include:

Lotrel Capsules.................................... 840
Norvasc Tablets 1940

Atenolol (Concomitant administration results in intensified effect). Products include:

Tenoretic Tablets................................. 2845
Tenormin Tablets and I.V. Injection 2847

Benazepril Hydrochloride (Concomitant administration results in intensified effect). Products include:

Lotensin Tablets................................... 834
Lotensin HCT....................................... 837
Lotrel Capsules.................................... 840

Bendroflumethiazide (Concomitant administration results in intensified effect).

No products indexed under this heading.

Bepridil Hydrochloride (Possibility of enhanced cardiovascular action). Products include:

Vascor (200, 300 and 400 mg) Tablets 1587

Betaxolol Hydrochloride (Concomitant administration results in intensified effect). Products include:

Betoptic Ophthalmic Solution............ 469
Betoptic S Ophthalmic Suspension 471
Kerlone Tablets.................................... 2436

Bisoprolol Fumarate (Concomitant administration results in intensified effect). Products include:

Zebeta Tablets 1413
Ziac 1415

Captopril (Concomitant administration results in intensified effect). Products include:

Capoten 739
Capozide 742

Carteolol Hydrochloride (Concomitant administration results in intensified effect). Products include:

Cartrol Tablets 410
Ocupress Ophthalmic Solution, 1% Sterile.. ⊙ 309

Chlorothiazide (Concomitant administration results in intensified effect). Products include:

Aldoclor Tablets 1598
Diupres Tablets 1650
Diuril Oral 1653

Chlorothiazide Sodium (Concomitant administration results in intensified effect). Products include:

Diuril Sodium Intravenous 1652

IMPORTANT NOTE: Always consult each drug listing in the patient's regimen for possible interactions.

Nimotop Interactions Index 724

Chlorthalidone (Concomitant administration results in intensified effect). Products include:
Combipres Tablets ... 677
Tenoretic Tablets ... 2845
Thalitone ... 1245
Cimetidine (May increase peak nimodipine plasma concentrations and AUC). Products include:
Tagamet Tablets ... 2516
Cimetidine Hydrochloride (May increase peak nimodipine plasma concentrations and AUC). Products include:
Tagamet ... 2516
Clonidine (Concomitant administration results in intensified effect). Products include:
Catapres-TTS ... 675
Clonidine Hydrochloride (Concomitant administration results in intensified effect). Products include:
Catapres Tablets ... 674
Combipres Tablets ... 677
Deserpidine (Concomitant administration results in intensified effect).
No products indexed under this heading.
Diazoxide (Concomitant administration results in intensified effect). Products include:
Hyperstat I.V. Injection ... 2363
Proglycem ... 580
Diltiazem Hydrochloride (Possibility of enhanced cardiovascular action). Products include:
Cardizem CD Capsules ... 1506
Cardizem SR Capsules ... 1510
Cardizem Injectable ... 1508
Cardizem Tablets ... 1512
Dilacor XR Extended-release Capsules ... 2018
Doxazosin Mesylate (Concomitant administration results in intensified effect). Products include:
Cardura Tablets ... 2186
Enalapril Maleate (Concomitant administration results in intensified effect). Products include:
Vaseretic Tablets ... 1765
Vasotec Tablets ... 1771
Enalaprilat (Concomitant administration results in intensified effect). Products include:
Vasotec I.V. ... 1768
Esmolol Hydrochloride (Concomitant administration results in intensified effect). Products include:
Brevibloc Injection ... 1808
Felodipine (Possibility of enhanced cardiovascular action). Products include:
Plendil Extended-Release Tablets ... 527
Fosinopril Sodium (Concomitant administration results in intensified effect). Products include:
Monopril Tablets ... 757
Furosemide (Concomitant administration results in intensified effect). Products include:
Lasix Injection, Oral Solution and Tablets ... 1240
Guanabenz Acetate (Concomitant administration results in intensified effect).
No products indexed under this heading.
Guanethidine Monosulfate (Concomitant administration results in intensified effect). Products include:
Esimil Tablets ... 822
Ismelin Tablets ... 827
Hydralazine Hydrochloride (Concomitant administration results in intensified effect). Products include:
Apresazide Capsules ... 808
Apresoline Hydrochloride Tablets ... 809
Ser-Ap-Es Tablets ... 849
Hydrochlorothiazide (Concomitant administration results in intensified effect). Products include:
Aldactazide ... 2413
Aldoril Tablets ... 1604
Apresazide Capsules ... 808
Capozide ... 742
Dyazide ... 2479
Esidrix Tablets ... 821
Esimil Tablets ... 822
HydroDIURIL Tablets ... 1674
Hydropres Tablets ... 1675
Hyzaar Tablets ... 1677
Inderide Tablets ... 2732
Inderide LA Long Acting Capsules ... 2734
Lopressor HCT Tablets ... 832
Lotensin HCT ... 837
Maxzide ... 1380
Moduretic Tablets ... 1705
Oretic Tablets ... 443
Prinzide Tablets ... 1737
Ser-Ap-Es Tablets ... 849
Timolide Tablets ... 1748
Vaseretic Tablets ... 1765
Zestoretic ... 2850
Ziac ... 1415
Hydroflumethiazide (Concomitant administration results in intensified effect). Products include:
Diucardin Tablets ... 2718
Indapamide (Concomitant administration results in intensified effect). Products include:
Lozol Tablets ... 2022
Isradipine (Possibility of enhanced cardiovascular action). Products include:
DynaCirc Capsules ... 2256
Labetalol Hydrochloride (Concomitant administration results in intensified effect). Products include:
Normodyne Injection ... 2377
Normodyne Tablets ... 2379
Trandate ... 1185
Lisinopril (Concomitant administration results in intensified effect). Products include:
Prinivil Tablets ... 1733
Prinzide Tablets ... 1737
Zestoretic ... 2850
Zestril Tablets ... 2854
Losartan Potassium (Possibility of enhanced cardiovascular action). Products include:
Cozaar Tablets ... 1628
Hyzaar Tablets ... 1677
Mecamylamine Hydrochloride (Concomitant administration results in intensified effect). Products include:
Inversine Tablets ... 1686
Methyclothiazide (Concomitant administration results in intensified effect). Products include:
Enduron Tablets ... 420
Methyldopa (Concomitant administration results in intensified effect). Products include:
Aldoclor Tablets ... 1598
Aldomet Oral ... 1600
Aldoril Tablets ... 1604
Methyldopate Hydrochloride (Concomitant administration results in intensified effect). Products include:
Aldomet Ester HCl Injection ... 1602
Metolazone (Concomitant administration results in intensified effect). Products include:
Mykrox Tablets ... 993
Zaroxolyn Tablets ... 1000
Metoprolol Succinate (Concomitant administration results in intensified effect). Products include:
Toprol-XL Tablets ... 565
Metoprolol Tartrate (Concomitant administration results in intensified effect). Products include:
Lopressor Ampuls ... 830
Lopressor HCT Tablets ... 832
Lopressor Tablets ... 830
Metyrosine (Concomitant administration results in intensified effect). Products include:
Demser Capsules ... 1649
Minoxidil (Concomitant administration results in intensified effect). Products include:
Loniten Tablets ... 2618
Rogaine Topical Solution ... 2637
Moexipril Hydrochloride (Possibility of enhanced cardiovascular action). Products include:
Univasc Tablets ... 2410
Nadolol (Concomitant administration results in intensified effect).
No products indexed under this heading.
Nicardipine Hydrochloride (Possibility of enhanced cardiovascular action). Products include:
Cardene Capsules ... 2095
Cardene I.V. ... 2709
Cardene SR Capsules ... 2097
Nifedipine (Possibility of enhanced cardiovascular action). Products include:
Adalat Capsules (10 mg and 20 mg) ... 587
Adalat CC ... 589
Procardia Capsules ... 1971
Procardia XL Extended Release Tablets ... 1972
Nisoldipine (Possibility of enhanced cardiovascular action).
No products indexed under this heading.
Nitroglycerin (Concomitant administration results in intensified effect). Products include:
Deponit NTG Transdermal Delivery System ... 2397
Nitro-Bid IV ... 1523
Nitro-Bid Ointment ... 1524
Nitrodisc ... 2047
Nitro-Dur (nitroglycerin) Transdermal Infusion System ... 1326
Nitrolingual Spray ... 2027
Nitrostat Tablets ... 1925
Transderm-Nitro Transdermal Therapeutic System ... 859
Penbutolol Sulfate (Concomitant administration results in intensified effect). Products include:
Levatol ... 2403
Phenoxybenzamine Hydrochloride (Concomitant administration results in intensified effect). Products include:
Dibenzyline Capsules ... 2476
Phentolamine Mesylate (Concomitant administration results in intensified effect). Products include:
Regitine ... 846
Phenytoin (Potential for phenytoin toxicity). Products include:
Dilantin Infatabs ... 1908
Dilantin-125 Suspension ... 1911
Phenytoin Sodium (Potential for phenytoin toxicity). Products include:
Dilantin Kapseals ... 1906
Dilantin Parenteral ... 1910
Pindolol (Concomitant administration results in intensified effect). Products include:
Visken Tablets ... 2299
Polythiazide (Concomitant administration results in intensified effect). Products include:
Minizide Capsules ... 1938
Prazosin Hydrochloride (Concomitant administration results in intensified effect). Products include:
Minipress Capsules ... 1937
Minizide Capsules ... 1938
Propranolol Hydrochloride (Concomitant administration results in intensified effect). Products include:
Inderal ... 2728
Inderal LA Long Acting Capsules ... 2730
Inderide Tablets ... 2732
Inderide LA Long Acting Capsules ... 2734
Quinapril Hydrochloride (Concomitant administration results in intensified effect). Products include:
Accupril Tablets ... 1893
Ramipril (Concomitant administration results in intensified effect). Products include:
Altace Capsules ... 1232
Rauwolfia Serpentina (Concomitant administration results in intensified effect).
No products indexed under this heading.
Rescinnamine (Concomitant administration results in intensified effect).
No products indexed under this heading.
Reserpine (Concomitant administration results in intensified effect). Products include:
Diupres Tablets ... 1650
Hydropres Tablets ... 1675
Ser-Ap-Es Tablets ... 849
Sodium Nitroprusside (Concomitant administration results in intensified effect).
No products indexed under this heading.
Sotalol Hydrochloride (Concomitant administration results in intensified effect). Products include:
Betapace Tablets ... 641
Spirapril Hydrochloride (Concomitant administration results in intensified effect).
No products indexed under this heading.
Terazosin Hydrochloride (Concomitant administration results in intensified effect). Products include:
Hytrin Capsules ... 430
Timolol Maleate (Concomitant administration results in intensified effect). Products include:
Blocadren Tablets ... 1614
Timolide Tablets ... 1748
Timoptic in Ocudose ... 1753
Timoptic Sterile Ophthalmic Solution ... 1751
Timoptic-XE ... 1755
Torsemide (Concomitant administration results in intensified effect). Products include:
Demadex Tablets and Injection ... 686
Trimethaphan Camsylate (Concomitant administration results in intensified effect). Products include:
Arfonad Ampuls ... 2080
Verapamil Hydrochloride (Possibility of enhanced cardiovascular action). Products include:
Calan SR Caplets ... 2422
Calan Tablets ... 2419
Isoptin Injectable ... 1344
Isoptin Oral Tablets ... 1346
Isoptin SR Tablets ... 1348
Verelan Capsules ... 1410
Verelan Capsules ... 2824

Food Interactions

Meal, unspecified (Administration of nimodipine capsules following a standard breakfast resulted in 68% lower peak plasma concentration and 38% lower bioavailability).

NITRO-BID IV
(Nitroglycerin) ... 1523
May interact with vasodilators and certain other agents. Compounds in these categories include:

Diazoxide (Additive vasodilating effects). Products include:
Hyperstat I.V. Injection ... 2363
Proglycem ... 580

725 **Interactions Index** **Nitrostat Tablets**

Heparin Calcium (Intravenous nitroglycerin may interfere with the anticoagulant effect of heparin).
No products indexed under this heading.

Heparin Sodium (Intravenous nitroglycerin may interfere with the anticoagulant effect of heparin). Products include:
Heparin Lock Flush Solution 2725
Heparin Sodium Injection 2726
Heparin Sodium Injection, USP, Sterile Solution 2615
Heparin Sodium Vials 1441

Hydralazine Hydrochloride (Additive vasodilating effects). Products include:
Apresazide Capsules 808
Apresoline Hydrochloride Tablets .. 809
Ser-Ap-Es Tablets 849

Minoxidil (Additive vasodilating effects). Products include:
Loniten Tablets 2618
Rogaine Topical Solution 2637

NITRO-BID OINTMENT
(Nitroglycerin) 1524
May interact with calcium channel blockers, vasodilators, and certain other agents. Compounds in these categories include:

Amlodipine Besylate (May produce marked symptomatic orthostatic hypotension). Products include:
Lotrel Capsules 840
Norvasc Tablets 1940

Bepridil Hydrochloride (May produce marked symptomatic orthostatic hypotension). Products include:
Vascor (200, 300 and 400 mg) Tablets 1587

Diazoxide (Additive vasodilating effects). Products include:
Hyperstat I.V. Injection 2363
Proglycem 580

Diltiazem Hydrochloride (May produce marked symptomatic orthostatic hypotension). Products include:
Cardizem CD Capsules 1506
Cardizem SR Capsules 1510
Cardizem Injectable 1508
Cardizem Tablets 1512
Dilacor XR Extended-release Capsules 2018

Felodipine (May produce marked symptomatic orthostatic hypotension). Products include:
Plendil Extended-Release Tablets 527

Hydralazine Hydrochloride (Additive vasodilating effects). Products include:
Apresazide Capsules 808
Apresoline Hydrochloride Tablets .. 809
Ser-Ap-Es Tablets 849

Isradipine (May produce marked symptomatic orthostatic hypotension). Products include:
DynaCirc Capsules 2256

Minoxidil (Additive vasodilating effects). Products include:
Loniten Tablets 2618
Rogaine Topical Solution 2637

Nicardipine Hydrochloride (May produce marked symptomatic orthostatic hypotension). Products include:
Cardene Capsules 2095
Cardene I.V. 2709
Cardene SR Capsules 2097

Nifedipine (May produce marked symptomatic orthostatic hypotension). Products include:
Adalat Capsules (10 mg and 20 mg) 587
Adalat CC 589
Procardia Capsules 1971
Procardia XL Extended Release Tablets 1972

Nimodipine (May produce marked symptomatic orthostatic hypotension). Products include:
Nimotop Capsules 610

Nisoldipine (May produce marked symptomatic orthostatic hypotension).
No products indexed under this heading.

Verapamil Hydrochloride (May produce marked symptomatic orthostatic hypotension). Products include:
Calan SR Caplets 2422
Calan Tablets 2419
Isoptin Injectable 1344
Isoptin Oral Tablets 1346
Isoptin SR Tablets 1348
Verelan Capsules 1410
Verelan Capsules 2824

Food Interactions

Alcohol (Exhibits additive vasodilating effects).

NITRODISC
(Nitroglycerin) 2047
May interact with vasodilators and certain other agents. Compounds in these categories include:

Diazoxide (Vasodilating effects may be additive). Products include:
Hyperstat I.V. Injection 2363
Proglycem 580

Hydralazine Hydrochloride (Vasodilating effects may be additive). Products include:
Apresazide Capsules 808
Apresoline Hydrochloride Tablets .. 809
Ser-Ap-Es Tablets 849

Minoxidil (Vasodilating effects may be additive). Products include:
Loniten Tablets 2618
Rogaine Topical Solution 2637

Food Interactions

Alcohol (Exhibits additive effects).

NITRO-DUR (NITROGLYCERIN) TRANSDERMAL INFUSION SYSTEM
(Nitroglycerin) 1326
May interact with vasodilators. Compounds in this category include:

Diazoxide (Vasodilating effects of nitroglycerin may be additive with those of other vasodilators). Products include:
Hyperstat I.V. Injection 2363
Proglycem 580

Hydralazine Hydrochloride (Vasodilating effects of nitroglycerin may be additive with those of other vasodilators). Products include:
Apresazide Capsules 808
Apresoline Hydrochloride Tablets .. 809
Ser-Ap-Es Tablets 849

Minoxidil (Vasodilating effects of nitroglycerin may be additive with those of other vasodilators). Products include:
Loniten Tablets 2618
Rogaine Topical Solution 2637

Food Interactions

Alcohol (Enhances sensitivity to the hypotensive effects).

NITROLINGUAL SPRAY
(Nitroglycerin) 2027
May interact with calcium channel blockers and certain other agents. Compounds in these categories include:

Amlodipine Besylate (Marked symptomatic orthostatic hypotension). Products include:
Lotrel Capsules 840
Norvasc Tablets 1940

Bepridil Hydrochloride (Marked symptomatic orthostatic hypotension). Products include:
Vascor (200, 300 and 400 mg) Tablets 1587

Diltiazem Hydrochloride (Marked symptomatic orthostatic hypotension). Products include:
Cardizem CD Capsules 1506
Cardizem SR Capsules 1510
Cardizem Injectable 1508
Cardizem Tablets 1512
Dilacor XR Extended-release Capsules 2018

Drugs Depending On Vascular Smooth Muscle (Decreased or increased effect).

Felodipine (Marked symptomatic orthostatic hypotension). Products include:
Plendil Extended-Release Tablets 527

Isradipine (Marked symptomatic orthostatic hypotension). Products include:
DynaCirc Capsules 2256

Nicardipine Hydrochloride (Marked symptomatic orthostatic hypotension). Products include:
Cardene Capsules 2095
Cardene I.V. 2709
Cardene SR Capsules 2097

Nifedipine (Marked symptomatic orthostatic hypotension). Products include:
Adalat Capsules (10 mg and 20 mg) 587
Adalat CC 589
Procardia Capsules 1971
Procardia XL Extended Release Tablets 1972

Nimodipine (Marked symptomatic orthostatic hypotension). Products include:
Nimotop Capsules 610

Nisoldipine (Marked symptomatic orthostatic hypotension).
No products indexed under this heading.

Verapamil Hydrochloride (Marked symptomatic orthostatic hypotension). Products include:
Calan SR Caplets 2422
Calan Tablets 2419
Isoptin Injectable 1344
Isoptin Oral Tablets 1346
Isoptin SR Tablets 1348
Verelan Capsules 1410
Verelan Capsules 2824

Food Interactions

Alcohol (Enhanced sensitivity to hypotensive effects).

NITROSTAT TABLETS
(Nitroglycerin) 1925
May interact with antihypertensives, beta blockers, phenothiazines, and certain other agents. Compounds in these categories include:

Acebutolol Hydrochloride (Additive hypotensive effects). Products include:
Sectral Capsules 2807

Amlodipine Besylate (Additive hypotensive effects). Products include:
Lotrel Capsules 840
Norvasc Tablets 1940

Atenolol (Additive hypotensive effects). Products include:
Tenoretic Tablets 2845
Tenormin Tablets and I.V. Injection 2847

Benazepril Hydrochloride (Additive hypotensive effects). Products include:
Lotensin Tablets 834
Lotensin HCT 837
Lotrel Capsules 840

Bendroflumethiazide (Additive hypotensive effects).
No products indexed under this heading.

Betaxolol Hydrochloride (Additive hypotensive effects). Products include:
Betoptic Ophthalmic Solution 469
Betoptic S Ophthalmic Suspension 471
Kerlone Tablets 2436

Bisoprolol Fumarate (Additive hypotensive effects). Products include:
Zebeta Tablets 1413
Ziac 1415

Captopril (Additive hypotensive effects). Products include:
Capoten 739
Capozide 742

Carteolol Hydrochloride (Additive hypotensive effects). Products include:
Cartrol Tablets 410
Ocupress Ophthalmic Solution, 1% Sterile .... ◉ 309

Chlorothiazide (Additive hypotensive effects). Products include:
Aldoclor Tablets 1598
Diupres Tablets 1650
Diuril Oral 1653

Chlorothiazide Sodium (Additive hypotensive effects). Products include:
Diuril Sodium Intravenous 1652

Chlorpromazine (Additive hypotensive effects). Products include:
Thorazine Suppositories 2523

Chlorthalidone (Additive hypotensive effects). Products include:
Combipres Tablets 677
Tenoretic Tablets 2845
Thalitone 1245

Clonidine (Additive hypotensive effects). Products include:
Catapres-TTS 675

Clonidine Hydrochloride (Additive hypotensive effects). Products include:
Catapres Tablets 674
Combipres Tablets 677

Deserpidine (Additive hypotensive effects).
No products indexed under this heading.

Diazoxide (Additive hypotensive effects). Products include:
Hyperstat I.V. Injection 2363
Proglycem 580

Diltiazem Hydrochloride (Additive hypotensive effects). Products include:
Cardizem CD Capsules 1506
Cardizem SR Capsules 1510
Cardizem Injectable 1508
Cardizem Tablets 1512
Dilacor XR Extended-release Capsules 2018

Doxazosin Mesylate (Additive hypotensive effects). Products include:
Cardura Tablets 2186

Enalapril Maleate (Additive hypotensive effects). Products include:
Vaseretic Tablets 1765
Vasotec Tablets 1771

Enalaprilat (Additive hypotensive effects). Products include:
Vasotec I.V. 1768

Erythrityl Tetranitrate (Additive hypotensive effects).
No products indexed under this heading.

IMPORTANT NOTE: Always consult each drug listing in the patient's regimen for possible interactions.

Esmolol Hydrochloride (Additive hypotensive effects). Products include:
- Brevibloc Injection 1808

Felodipine (Additive hypotensive effects). Products include:
- Plendil Extended-Release Tablets 527

Fluphenazine Decanoate (Additive hypotensive effects). Products include:
- Prolixin Decanoate 509

Fluphenazine Enanthate (Additive hypotensive effects). Products include:
- Prolixin Enanthate 509

Fluphenazine Hydrochloride (Additive hypotensive effects). Products include:
- Prolixin 509

Fosinopril Sodium (Additive hypotensive effects). Products include:
- Monopril Tablets 757

Furosemide (Additive hypotensive effects). Products include:
- Lasix Injection, Oral Solution and Tablets 1240

Guanabenz Acetate (Additive hypotensive effects).
- No products indexed under this heading.

Guanethidine Monosulfate (Additive hypotensive effects). Products include:
- Esimil Tablets 822
- Ismelin Tablets 827

Hydralazine Hydrochloride (Additive hypotensive effects). Products include:
- Apresazide Capsules 808
- Apresoline Hydrochloride Tablets 809
- Ser-Ap-Es Tablets 849

Hydrochlorothiazide (Additive hypotensive effects). Products include:
- Aldactazide 2413
- Aldoril Tablets 1604
- Apresazide Capsules 808
- Capozide 742
- Dyazide 2479
- Esidrix Tablets 821
- Esimil Tablets 822
- HydroDIURIL Tablets 1674
- Hydropres Tablets 1675
- Hyzaar Tablets 1677
- Inderide Tablets 2732
- Inderide LA Long Acting Capsules 2734
- Lopressor HCT Tablets 832
- Lotensin HCT 837
- Maxzide 1380
- Moduretic Tablets 1705
- Oretic Tablets 443
- Prinzide Tablets 1737
- Ser-Ap-Es Tablets 849
- Timolide Tablets 1748
- Vaseretic Tablets 1765
- Zestoretic 2850
- Ziac 1415

Hydroflumethiazide (Additive hypotensive effects). Products include:
- Diucardin Tablets 2718

Indapamide (Additive hypotensive effects). Products include:
- Lozol Tablets 2022

Isosorbide Dinitrate (Additive hypotensive effects). Products include:
- Dilatrate-SR 2398
- Isordil Sublingual Tablets 2739
- Isordil Tembids 2741
- Isordil Titradose Tablets 2742
- Sorbitrate 2843

Isradipine (Additive hypotensive effects). Products include:
- DynaCirc Capsules 2256

Labetalol Hydrochloride (Additive hypotensive effects). Products include:
- Normodyne Injection 2377
- Normodyne Tablets 2379
- Trandate 1185

Levobunolol Hydrochloride (Additive hypotensive effects). Products include:
- Betagan .... ◉ 233

Lisinopril (Additive hypotensive effects). Products include:
- Prinivil Tablets 1733
- Prinzide Tablets 1737
- Zestoretic 2850
- Zestril Tablets 2854

Losartan Potassium (Additive hypotensive effects). Products include:
- Cozaar Tablets 1628
- Hyzaar Tablets 1677

Mecamylamine Hydrochloride (Additive hypotensive effects). Products include:
- Inversine Tablets 1686

Mesoridazine Besylate (Additive hypotensive effects). Products include:
- Serentil 684

Methotrimeprazine (Additive hypotensive effects). Products include:
- Levoprome 1274

Methyclothiazide (Additive hypotensive effects). Products include:
- Enduron Tablets 420

Methyldopa (Additive hypotensive effects). Products include:
- Aldoclor Tablets 1598
- Aldomet Oral 1600
- Aldoril Tablets 1604

Methyldopate Hydrochloride (Additive hypotensive effects). Products include:
- Aldomet Ester HCl Injection 1602

Metipranolol Hydrochloride (Additive hypotensive effects). Products include:
- OptiPranolol (Metipranolol 0.3%) Sterile Ophthalmic Solution .... ◉ 258

Metolazone (Additive hypotensive effects). Products include:
- Mykrox Tablets 993
- Zaroxolyn Tablets 1000

Metoprolol Succinate (Additive hypotensive effects). Products include:
- Toprol-XL Tablets 565

Metoprolol Tartrate (Additive hypotensive effects). Products include:
- Lopressor Ampuls 830
- Lopressor HCT Tablets 832
- Lopressor Tablets 830

Metyrosine (Additive hypotensive effects). Products include:
- Demser Capsules 1649

Minoxidil (Additive hypotensive effects). Products include:
- Loniten Tablets 2618
- Rogaine Topical Solution 2637

Moexipril Hydrochloride (Additive hypotensive effects). Products include:
- Univasc Tablets 2410

Nadolol (Additive hypotensive effects).
- No products indexed under this heading.

Nicardipine Hydrochloride (Additive hypotensive effects). Products include:
- Cardene Capsules 2095
- Cardene I.V. 2709
- Cardene SR Capsules 2097

Nifedipine (Additive hypotensive effects). Products include:
- Adalat Capsules (10 mg and 20 mg) 587
- Adalat CC 589
- Procardia Capsules 1971
- Procardia XL Extended Release Tablets 1972

Nisoldipine (Additive hypotensive effects).
- No products indexed under this heading.

Penbutolol Sulfate (Additive hypotensive effects). Products include:
- Levatol 2403

Pentaerythritol Tetranitrate (Additive hypotensive effects).
- No products indexed under this heading.

Perphenazine (Additive hypotensive effects). Products include:
- Etrafon 2355
- Triavil Tablets 1757
- Trilafon 2389

Phenoxybenzamine Hydrochloride (Additive hypotensive effects). Products include:
- Dibenzyline Capsules 2476

Phentolamine Mesylate (Additive hypotensive effects). Products include:
- Regitine 846

Pindolol (Additive hypotensive effects). Products include:
- Visken Tablets 2299

Polythiazide (Additive hypotensive effects). Products include:
- Minizide Capsules 1938

Prazosin Hydrochloride (Additive hypotensive effects). Products include:
- Minipress Capsules 1937
- Minizide Capsules 1938

Prochlorperazine (Additive hypotensive effects). Products include:
- Compazine 2470

Promethazine Hydrochloride (Additive hypotensive effects). Products include:
- Mepergan Injection 2753
- Phenergan with Codeine 2777
- Phenergan with Dextromethorphan 2778
- Phenergan Injection 2773
- Phenergan Suppositories 2775
- Phenergan Syrup 2774
- Phenergan Tablets 2775
- Phenergan VC 2779
- Phenergan VC with Codeine 2781

Propranolol Hydrochloride (Additive hypotensive effects). Products include:
- Inderal 2728
- Inderal LA Long Acting Capsules 2730
- Inderide Tablets 2732
- Inderide LA Long Acting Capsules 2734

Quinapril Hydrochloride (Additive hypotensive effects). Products include:
- Accupril Tablets 1893

Ramipril (Additive hypotensive effects). Products include:
- Altace Capsules 1232

Rauwolfia Serpentina (Additive hypotensive effects).
- No products indexed under this heading.

Rescinnamine (Additive hypotensive effects).
- No products indexed under this heading.

Reserpine (Additive hypotensive effects). Products include:
- Diupres Tablets 1650
- Hydropres Tablets 1675
- Ser-Ap-Es Tablets 849

Sodium Nitroprusside (Additive hypotensive effects).
- No products indexed under this heading.

Sotalol Hydrochloride (Additive hypotensive effects). Products include:
- Betapace Tablets 641

Spirapril Hydrochloride (Additive hypotensive effects).
- No products indexed under this heading.

Terazosin Hydrochloride (Additive hypotensive effects). Products include:
- Hytrin Capsules 430

Thioridazine Hydrochloride (Additive hypotensive effects). Products include:
- Mellaril 2269

Timolol Hemihydrate (Additive hypotensive effects). Products include:
- Betimol 0.25%, 0.5% .... ◉ 261

Timolol Maleate (Additive hypotensive effects). Products include:
- Blocadren Tablets 1614
- Timolide Tablets 1748
- Timoptic in Ocudose 1753
- Timoptic Sterile Ophthalmic Solution 1751
- Timoptic-XE 1755

Torsemide (Additive hypotensive effects). Products include:
- Demadex Tablets and Injection 686

Trifluoperazine Hydrochloride (Additive hypotensive effects). Products include:
- Stelazine 2514

Trimethaphan Camsylate (Additive hypotensive effects). Products include:
- Arfonad Ampuls 2080

Verapamil Hydrochloride (Additive hypotensive effects). Products include:
- Calan SR Caplets 2422
- Calan Tablets 2419
- Isoptin Injectable 1344
- Isoptin Oral Tablets 1346
- Isoptin SR Tablets 1348
- Verelan Capsules 1410
- Verelan Capsules 2824

Food Interactions

Alcohol (Hypotension).

NIX CREME RINSE

(Permethrin) .... ▣ 858

None cited in PDR database.

NIZORAL 2% CREAM

(Ketoconazole) 1297

None cited in PDR database.

NIZORAL 2% SHAMPOO

(Ketoconazole) 1298

None cited in PDR database.

NIZORAL TABLETS

(Ketoconazole) 1298

May interact with oral anticoagulants, oral hypoglycemic agents, anticholinergics, histamine h2-receptor antagonists, antacids, and certain other agents. Compounds in these categories include:

Acarbose (Possibility of severe hypoglycemia cannot be ruled out).
- No products indexed under this heading.

Aluminum Carbonate Gel (Nizoral requires acidity for dissolution, antacids should be given at least two hours after Nizoral administration). Products include:
- Basaljel 2703

Aluminum Hydroxide (Nizoral requires acidity for dissolution, antacids should be given at least two hours after Nizoral administration). Products include:
- ALternaGEL Liquid 1316
- Maximum Strength Ascriptin .... ▣ 630
- Cama Arthritis Pain Reliever .... ▣ 785
- Gaviscon Extra Strength Relief Formula Antacid Tablets .... ▣ 819

(▣ Described in PDR For Nonprescription Drugs) (◉ Described in PDR For Ophthalmology)

Gaviscon Extra Strength Relief Formula Liquid Antacid .... ✦D 819
Gaviscon Liquid Antacid .... ✦D 820
Gelusil Liquid & Tablets .... ✦D 855
Maalox Heartburn Relief Suspension .... ✦D 642
Maalox Heartburn Relief Tablets.... ✦D 641
Maalox Magnesia and Alumina Oral Suspension .... ✦D 642
Maalox Plus Tablets .... ✦D 643
Extra Strength Maalox Antacid Plus Antigas Liquid and Tablets ✦D 638
Tempo Soft Antacid .... ✦D 835

Aluminum Hydroxide Gel (Nizoral requires acidity for dissolution, antacids should be given at least two hours after Nizoral administration). Products include:

ALternaGEL Liquid .... ✦D 659
Aludrox Oral Suspension 2695
Amphojel Suspension 2695
Amphojel Suspension without Flavor 2695
Amphojel Tablets................................... 2695
Arthritis Pain Ascriptin .... ✦D 631
Regular Strength Ascriptin Tablets .... ✦D 629
Gaviscon Antacid Tablets................... ✦D 819
Gaviscon-2 Antacid Tablets .... ✦D 820
Mylanta Liquid 1317
Mylanta Tablets .... ✦D 660
Mylanta Double Strength Liquid 1317
Mylanta Double Strength Tablets .. ✦D 660
Nephrox Suspension .... ✦D 655

Astemizole (Coadministration is contraindicated; elevated plasma levels of astemizole resulting in prolonged QT intervals). Products include:

Hismanal Tablets 1293

Atropine Sulfate (Nizoral requires acidity for dissolution, these drugs should be given at least two hours after Nizoral administration). Products include:

Arco-Lase Plus Tablets 512
Atrohist Plus Tablets 454
Atropine Sulfate Sterile Ophthalmic Solution .... ◊ 233
Donnatal 2060
Donnatal Extentabs.............................. 2061
Donnatal Tablets 2060
Lomotil 2439
Motofen Tablets 784
Urised Tablets... 1964

Belladonna Alkaloids (Nizoral requires acidity for dissolution, these drugs should be given at least two hours after Nizoral administration). Products include:

Bellergal-S Tablets 2250
Hyland's Bed Wetting Tablets .... ✦D 828
Hyland's EnurAid Tablets................... ✦D 829
Hyland's Teething Tablets .... ✦D 830

Benztropine Mesylate (Nizoral requires acidity for dissolution, these drugs should be given at least two hours after Nizoral administration). Products include:

Cogentin 1621

Biperiden Hydrochloride (Nizoral requires acidity for dissolution, these drugs should be given at least two hours after Nizoral administration). Products include:

Akineton 1333

Chlorpropamide (Possibility of severe hypoglycemia cannot be ruled out). Products include:

Diabinese Tablets 1935

Cimetidine (Nizoral requires acidity for dissolution, these drugs should be given at least two hours after Nizoral administration). Products include:

Tagamet Tablets 2516

Cimetidine Hydrochloride (Nizoral requires acidity for dissolution, these drugs should be given at least two hours after Nizoral administration). Products include:

Tagamet... 2516

Cisapride (Marked elevation in cisapride plasma concentrations and prolonged QT interval, and has rarely been associated with ventricular arrhythmias and torsades de pointes; concurrent use is contraindicated). Products include:

Propulsid 1300

Clidinium Bromide (Nizoral requires acidity for dissolution, these drugs should be given at least two hours after Nizoral administration). Products include:

Librax Capsules 2176
Quarzan Capsules 2181

Cyclosporine (Co-administration may alter the metabolism of cyclosporine resulting in increased plasma concentration of cyclosporine). Products include:

Neoral 2276
Sandimmune 2286

Dicumarol (Anticoagulant effect enhanced).

No products indexed under this heading.

Dicyclomine Hydrochloride (Nizoral requires acidity for dissolution, these drugs should be given at least two hours after Nizoral administration). Products include:

Bentyl 1501

Digoxin (Rare cases of elevated plasma concentrations of digoxin; monitor digoxin concentration). Products include:

Lanoxicaps 1117
Lanoxin Elixir Pediatric 1120
Lanoxin Injection 1123
Lanoxin Injection Pediatric................ 1126
Lanoxin Tablets 1128

Famotidine (Nizoral requires acidity for dissolution, these drugs should be given at least two hours after Nizoral administration). Products include:

Pepcid AC 1319
Pepcid Injection 1722
Pepcid... 1720

Glipizide (Possibility of severe hypoglycemia cannot be ruled out). Products include:

Glucotrol Tablets 1967
Glucotrol XL Extended Release Tablets 1968

Glyburide (Possibility of severe hypoglycemia cannot be ruled out). Products include:

DiaBeta Tablets 1239
Glynase PresTab Tablets 2609
Micronase Tablets 2623

Glycopyrrolate (Nizoral requires acidity for dissolution, these drugs should be given at least two hours after Nizoral administration). Products include:

Robinul Forte Tablets........................... 2072
Robinul Injectable 2072
Robinul Tablets....................................... 2072

Hyoscyamine (Nizoral requires acidity for dissolution, these drugs should be given at least two hours after Nizoral administration). Products include:

Cystospaz Tablets 1963
Urised Tablets... 1964

Hyoscyamine Sulfate (Nizoral requires acidity for dissolution, these drugs should be given at least two hours after Nizoral administration). Products include:

Arco-Lase Plus Tablets 512
Atrohist Plus Tablets 454
Cystospaz-M Capsules 1963
Donnatal 2060
Donnatal Extentabs.............................. 2061
Donnatal Tablets 2060
Kutrase Capsules................................... 2402
Levsin/Levsinex/Levbid 2405

Ipratropium Bromide (Nizoral requires acidity for dissolution, these drugs should be given at least two hours after Nizoral administration). Products include:

Atrovent Inhalation Aerosol.............. 671
Atrovent Inhalation Solution 673

Isoniazid (Affects ketoconazole concentrations adversely). Products include:

Nydrazid Injection 508
Rifamate Capsules 1530
Rifater... 1532

Loratadine (AUC and C_{max} of loratadine averaged 302% and 251% respectively following coadministration; no cardiac changes were noted). Products include:

Claritin 2349
Claritin-D 2350

Magaldrate (Nizoral requires acidity for dissolution, antacids should be given at least two hours after Nizoral administration).

No products indexed under this heading.

Magnesium Hydroxide (Nizoral requires acidity for dissolution, antacids should be given at least two hours after Nizoral administration). Products include:

Aludrox Oral Suspension 2695
Arthritis Pain Ascriptin .... ✦D 631
Maximum Strength Ascriptin .... ✦D 630
Regular Strength Ascriptin Tablets .... ✦D 629
Di-Gel Antacid/Anti-Gas .... ✦D 801
Gelusil Liquid & Tablets .... ✦D 855
Maalox Magnesia and Alumina Oral Suspension .... ✦D 642
Maalox Plus Tablets .... ✦D 643
Extra Strength Maalox Antacid Plus Antigas Liquid and Tablets ✦D 638
Mylanta Calcium Carbonate and Magnesium Hydroxide Tablets...... 1318
Mylanta Liquid 1317
Mylanta Tablets .... ✦D 660
Mylanta Double Strength Liquid 1317
Mylanta Double Strength Tablets .. ✦D 660
Phillips' Milk of Magnesia Liquid.... ✦D 729
Rolaids Tablets....................................... ✦D 843
Tempo Soft Antacid .... ✦D 835

Magnesium Oxide (Nizoral requires acidity for dissolution, antacids should be given at least two hours after Nizoral administration). Products include:

Beelith Tablets 639
Bufferin Analgesic Tablets and Caplets.. ✦D 613
Caltrate PLUS .... ✦D 665
Cama Arthritis Pain Reliever............ ✦D 785
Mag-Ox 400 668
Uro-Mag... 668

Mepenzolate Bromide (Nizoral requires acidity for dissolution, these drugs should be given at least two hours after Nizoral administration).

No products indexed under this heading.

Metformin Hydrochloride (Possibility of severe hypoglycemia cannot be ruled out). Products include:

Glucophage 752

Methylprednisolone (Co-administration may alter the metabolism of methylprednisolone resulting in increased plasma concentration; dosage of methylprednisolone may have to be adjusted). Products include:

Medrol 2621

Methylprednisolone Acetate (Co-administration may alter the metabolism of methylprednisolone resulting in increased plasma concentration; dosage of methylprednisolone may have to be adjusted). Products include:

Depo-Medrol Single-Dose Vial 2600
Depo-Medrol Sterile Aqueous Suspension.. 2597

Methylprednisolone Sodium Succinate (Co-administration may alter the metabolism of methylprednisolone resulting in increased plasma concentration; dosage of methylprednisolone may have to be adjusted). Products include:

Solu-Medrol Sterile Powder 2643

Midazolam Hydrochloride (Co-administration with oral midazolam has resulted in elevated plasma concentration of midazolam resulting in prolonged hypnotic and sedative effects; concurrent oral use should be avoided). Products include:

Versed Injection 2170

Nizatidine (Nizoral requires acidity for dissolution, these drugs should be given at least two hours after Nizoral administration). Products include:

Axid Pulvules 1427

Oxybutynin Chloride (Nizoral requires acidity for dissolution, these drugs should be given at least two hours after Nizoral administration). Products include:

Ditropan... 1516

Phenytoin (May alter metabolism of one or both drugs). Products include:

Dilantin Infatabs 1908
Dilantin-125 Suspension 1911

Phenytoin Sodium (May alter metabolism of one or both drugs). Products include:

Dilantin Kapseals 1906
Dilantin Parenteral 1910

Procyclidine Hydrochloride (Nizoral requires acidity for dissolution, these drugs should be given at least two hours after Nizoral administration). Products include:

Kemadrin Tablets 1112

Propantheline Bromide (Nizoral requires acidity for dissolution, these drugs should be given at least two hours after Nizoral administration). Products include:

Pro-Banthine Tablets 2052

Ranitidine Hydrochloride (Nizoral requires acidity for dissolution, these drugs should be given at least two hours after Nizoral administration). Products include:

Zantac... 1209
Zantac Injection 1207
Zantac Syrup 1209

Rifampin (Reduces blood levels of ketoconazole). Products include:

Rifadin 1528
Rifamate Capsules 1530
Rifater... 1532
Rimactane Capsules.............................. 847

Scopolamine (Nizoral requires acidity for dissolution, these drugs should be given at least two hours after Nizoral administration). Products include:

Transderm Scōp Transdermal Therapeutic System 869

Scopolamine Hydrobromide (Nizoral requires acidity for dissolution, these drugs should be given at least two hours after Nizoral administration). Products include:

Atrohist Plus Tablets 454
Donnatal 2060
Donnatal Extentabs.............................. 2061
Donnatal Tablets 2060

Sodium Bicarbonate (Nizoral requires acidity for dissolution, antacids should be given at least two hours after Nizoral administration). Products include:

Alka-Seltzer Effervescent Antacid and Pain Reliever .... ✦D 701

IMPORTANT NOTE: Always consult each drug listing in the patient's regimen for possible interactions.

Nizoral Interactions Index 728

Alka-Seltzer Extra Strength Effervescent Antacid and Pain Reliever ... ◙ 703
Alka-Seltzer Gold Effervescent Antacid ... ◙ 703
Alka-Seltzer Lemon Lime Effervescent Antacid and Pain Reliever ... ◙ 703
Arm & Hammer Pure Baking Soda ... ◙ 627
Ceo-Two Rectal Suppositories ... 666
Citrocarbonate Antacid ... ◙ 770
Massengill Disposable Douches ... ◙ 820
Massengill Liquid Concentrate ... ◙ 820
NuLYTELY ... 689
Cherry Flavor NuLYTELY ... 689

Tacrolimus (Co-administration may alter the metabolism of tacrolimus resulting in increased plasma concentration; dosage of tacrolimus may have to be adjusted). Products include:
Prograf ... 1042

Terfenadine (Produces QT interval prolongation/ventricular dysrhythmias; potential for cardiac arrest, torsades de pointes and fatalities; concurrent use is contraindicated). Products include:
Seldane Tablets ... 1536
Seldane-D Extended-Release Tablets ... 1538

Tolazamide (Possibility of severe hypoglycemia cannot be ruled out).
No products indexed under this heading.

Tolbutamide (Possibility of severe hypoglycemia cannot be ruled out).
No products indexed under this heading.

Triazolam (Co-administration has resulted in elevated plasma concentration of triazolam resulting in prolonged hypnotic and sedative effects; concurrent use with oral triazolam is contraindicated). Products include:
Halcion Tablets ... 2611

Tridihexethyl Chloride (Nizoral requires acidity for dissolution, these drugs should be given at least two hours after Nizoral administration).
No products indexed under this heading.

Trihexyphenidyl Hydrochloride (Nizoral requires acidity for dissolution, these drugs should be given at least two hours after Nizoral administration). Products include:
Artane ... 1368

Warfarin Sodium (Anticoagulant effect enhanced). Products include:
Coumadin ... 926

Food Interactions

Alcohol (Potential for disulfiram-like reaction to alcohol resulting in flushing, rash, peripheral edema, nausea and headache).

NO DOZ MAXIMUM STRENGTH CAPLETS

(Caffeine) ... ◙ 622
May interact with:

Caffeine-containing medications (May cause sleeplessness, irritability, nervousness and rapid heart beat).

Food Interactions

Beverages, caffeine-containing (May cause sleeplessness, irritability, nervousness and rapid heart beat).

Food, caffeine containing (May cause sleeplessness, irritability, nervousness and rapid heart beat).

NOLAHIST TABLETS

(Phenindamine Tartrate) ... 785
May interact with tranquilizers, hypnotics and sedatives, and certain other agents. Compounds in these categories include:

Alprazolam (May increase drowsiness effect). Products include:
Xanax Tablets ... 2649

Buspirone Hydrochloride (May increase drowsiness effect). Products include:
BuSpar ... 737

Chlordiazepoxide (May increase drowsiness effect). Products include:
Libritabs Tablets ... 2177
Limbitrol ... 2180

Chlordiazepoxide Hydrochloride (May increase drowsiness effect). Products include:
Librax Capsules ... 2176
Librium Capsules ... 2178
Librium Injectable ... 2179

Chlorpromazine (May increase drowsiness effect). Products include:
Thorazine Suppositories ... 2523

Chlorpromazine Hydrochloride (May increase drowsiness effect). Products include:
Thorazine ... 2523

Chlorprothixene (May increase drowsiness effect).
No products indexed under this heading.

Chlorprothixene Hydrochloride (May increase drowsiness effect).
No products indexed under this heading.

Clorazepate Dipotassium (May increase drowsiness effect). Products include:
Tranxene ... 451

Diazepam (May increase drowsiness effect). Products include:
Dizac ... 1809
Valium Injectable ... 2182
Valium Tablets ... 2183
Valrelease Capsules ... 2169

Droperidol (May increase drowsiness effect). Products include:
Inapsine Injection ... 1296

Estazolam (May increase drowsiness effect). Products include:
ProSom Tablets ... 449

Ethchlorvynol (May increase drowsiness effect). Products include:
Placidyl Capsules ... 448

Ethinamate (May increase drowsiness effect).
No products indexed under this heading.

Fluphenazine Decanoate (May increase drowsiness effect). Products include:
Prolixin Decanoate ... 509

Fluphenazine Enanthate (May increase drowsiness effect). Products include:
Prolixin Enanthate ... 509

Fluphenazine Hydrochloride (May increase drowsiness effect). Products include:
Prolixin ... 509

Flurazepam Hydrochloride (May increase drowsiness effect). Products include:
Dalmane Capsules ... 2173

Glutethimide (May increase drowsiness effect).
No products indexed under this heading.

Haloperidol (May increase drowsiness effect). Products include:
Haldol Injection, Tablets and Concentrate ... 1575

Haloperidol Decanoate (May increase drowsiness effect). Products include:
Haldol Decanoate ... 1577

Hydroxyzine Hydrochloride (May increase drowsiness effect). Products include:
Atarax Tablets & Syrup ... 2185
Marax Tablets & DF Syrup ... 2200
Vistaril Intramuscular Solution ... 2216

Lorazepam (May increase drowsiness effect). Products include:
Ativan Injection ... 2698
Ativan Tablets ... 2700

Loxapine Hydrochloride (May increase drowsiness effect). Products include:
Loxitane ... 1378

Loxapine Succinate (May increase drowsiness effect). Products include:
Loxitane Capsules ... 1378

Meprobamate (May increase drowsiness effect). Products include:
Miltown Tablets ... 2672
PMB 200 and PMB 400 ... 2783

Mesoridazine Besylate (May increase drowsiness effect). Products include:
Serentil ... 684

Midazolam Hydrochloride (May increase drowsiness effect). Products include:
Versed Injection ... 2170

Molindone Hydrochloride (May increase drowsiness effect). Products include:
Moban Tablets and Concentrate ... 1048

Oxazepam (May increase drowsiness effect). Products include:
Serax Capsules ... 2810
Serax Tablets ... 2810

Perphenazine (May increase drowsiness effect). Products include:
Etrafon ... 2355
Triavil Tablets ... 1757
Trilafon ... 2389

Prazepam (May increase drowsiness effect).
No products indexed under this heading.

Prochlorperazine (May increase drowsiness effect). Products include:
Compazine ... 2470

Promethazine Hydrochloride (May increase drowsiness effect). Products include:
Mepergan Injection ... 2753
Phenergan with Codeine ... 2777
Phenergan with Dextromethorphan ... 2778
Phenergan Injection ... 2773
Phenergan Suppositories ... 2775
Phenergan Syrup ... 2774
Phenergan Tablets ... 2775
Phenergan VC ... 2779
Phenergan VC with Codeine ... 2781

Propofol (May increase drowsiness effect). Products include:
Diprivan Injection ... 2833

Quazepam (May increase drowsiness effect). Products include:
Doral Tablets ... 2664

Secobarbital Sodium (May increase drowsiness effect). Products include:
Seconal Sodium Pulvules ... 1474

Temazepam (May increase drowsiness effect). Products include:
Restoril Capsules ... 2284

Thioridazine Hydrochloride (May increase drowsiness effect). Products include:
Mellaril ... 2269

Thiothixene (May increase drowsiness effect). Products include:
Navane Capsules and Concentrate ... 2201
Navane Intramuscular ... 2202

Triazolam (May increase drowsiness effect). Products include:
Halcion Tablets ... 2611

Trifluoperazine Hydrochloride (May increase drowsiness effect). Products include:
Stelazine ... 2514

Zolpidem Tartrate (May increase drowsiness effect). Products include:
Ambien Tablets ... 2416

Food Interactions

Alcohol (Increased drowsiness).

NOLAMINE TIMED-RELEASE TABLETS

(Phenindamine Tartrate, Phenylpropanolamine Hydrochloride, Chlorpheniramine Maleate) ... 785
May interact with monoamine oxidase inhibitors. Compounds in this category include:

Furazolidone (Concurrent therapy contraindicated). Products include:
Furoxone ... 2046

Isocarboxazid (Concurrent therapy contraindicated).
No products indexed under this heading.

Phenelzine Sulfate (Concurrent therapy contraindicated). Products include:
Nardil ... 1920

Selegiline Hydrochloride (Concurrent therapy contraindicated). Products include:
Eldepryl Tablets ... 2550

Tranylcypromine Sulfate (Concurrent therapy contraindicated). Products include:
Parnate Tablets ... 2503

NOLVADEX TABLETS

(Tamoxifen Citrate) ... 2841
May interact with oral anticoagulants, cytotoxic drugs, and certain other agents. Compounds in these categories include:

Bleomycin Sulfate (Increased incidence of thromboembolic events when cytotoxic agents are combined with Nolvadex). Products include:
Blenoxane ... 692

Bromocriptine Mesylate (Concomitant therapy has been shown to elevate serum tamoxifen and N-desmethyl-tamoxifen). Products include:
Parlodel ... 2281

Daunorubicin Hydrochloride (Increased incidence of thromboembolic events when cytotoxic agents are combined with Nolvadex). Products include:
Cerubidine ... 795

Dicumarol (Increased anticoagulant effect; monitor patient's prothrombin time).
No products indexed under this heading.

Doxorubicin Hydrochloride (Increased incidence of thromboembolic events when cytotoxic agents are combined with Nolvadex). Products include:
Adriamycin PFS ... 1947
Adriamycin RDF ... 1947
Doxorubicin Astra ... 540
Rubex ... 712

Fluorouracil (Increased incidence of thromboembolic events when cytotoxic agents are combined with Nolvadex). Products include:
Efudex ... 2113
Fluoroplex Topical Solution & Cream 1% ... 479
Fluorouracil Injection ... 2116

(◙ Described in PDR For Nonprescription Drugs) (⊚ Described in PDR For Ophthalmology)

729 **Interactions Index** **Nordette-21**

Hydroxyurea (Increased incidence of thromboembolic events when cytotoxic agents are combined with Nolvadex). Products include:
Hydrea Capsules 696

Methotrexate Sodium (Increased incidence of thromboembolic events when cytotoxic agents are combined with Nolvadex). Products include:
Methotrexate Sodium Tablets, Injection, for Injection and LPF Injection 1275

Mitotane (Increased incidence of thromboembolic events when cytotoxic agents are combined with Nolvadex). Products include:
Lysodren 698

Mitoxantrone Hydrochloride (Increased incidence of thromboembolic events when cytotoxic agents are combined with Nolvadex). Products include:
Novantrone 1279

Phenobarbital (Concomitant therapy in one patient resulted in lower steady state serum level of tamoxifen). Products include:
Arco-Lase Plus Tablets 512
Bellergal-S Tablets 2250
Donnatal 2060
Donnatal Extentabs 2061
Donnatal Tablets 2060
Phenobarbital Elixir and Tablets 1469
Quadrinal Tablets 1350

Procarbazine Hydrochloride (Increased incidence of thromboembolic events when cytotoxic agents are combined with Nolvadex). Products include:
Matulane Capsules 2131

Vincristine Sulfate (Increased incidence of thromboembolic events when cytotoxic agents are combined with Nolvadex). Products include:
Oncovin Solution Vials & Hyporets 1466

Warfarin Sodium (Increased anticoagulant effect; monitor patient's prothrombin time). Products include:
Coumadin 926

NORCURON
(Vecuronium Bromide) 1826
May interact with nondepolarizing neuromuscular blocking agents, inhalant anesthetics, aminoglycosides, tetracyclines, and certain other agents. Compounds in these categories include:

Amikacin Sulfate (Possible prolongation of neuromuscular blockade). Products include:
Amikacin Sulfate Injection, USP 960
Amikin Injectable 501

Atracurium Besylate (Additive effect). Products include:
Tracrium Injection 1183

Bacitracin (Possible prolongation of neuromuscular blockade). Products include:
Mycitracin .... ▣ 839

Colistimethate Sodium (Possible prolongation of neuromuscular blockade). Products include:
Coly-Mycin M Parenteral 1905

Colistin Sulfate (Possible prolongation of neuromuscular blockade). Products include:
Coly-Mycin S Otic w/Neomycin & Hydrocortisone 1906

Demeclocycline Hydrochloride (Possible prolongation of neuromuscular blockade). Products include:
Declomycin Tablets 1371

Desflurane (Pronounced enhancement of neuromuscular blockade). Products include:
Suprane 1813

Doxycycline Calcium (Possible prolongation of neuromuscular blockade). Products include:
Vibramycin Calcium Oral Suspension Syrup 1941

Doxycycline Hyclate (Possible prolongation of neuromuscular blockade). Products include:
Doryx Capsules 1913
Vibramycin Hyclate Capsules 1941
Vibramycin Hyclate Intravenous 2215
Vibra-Tabs Film Coated Tablets 1941

Doxycycline Monohydrate (Possible prolongation of neuromuscular blockade). Products include:
Monodox Capsules 1805
Vibramycin Monohydrate for Oral Suspension 1941

Enflurane (Pronounced enhancement of neuromuscular blockade).
No products indexed under this heading.

Gentamicin Sulfate (Possible prolongation of neuromuscular blockade). Products include:
Garamycin Injectable 2360
Genoptic Sterile Ophthalmic Solution .... ⊙ 243
Genoptic Sterile Ophthalmic Ointment .... ⊙ 243
Gentacidin Ointment .... ⊙ 264
Gentacidin Solution .... ⊙ 264
Gentak .... ⊙ 208
Pred-G Liquifilm Sterile Ophthalmic Suspension .... ⊙ 251
Pred-G S.O.P. Sterile Ophthalmic Ointment .... ⊙ 252

Halothane (Pronounced enhancement of neuromuscular blockade). Products include:
Fluothane 2724

Isoflurane (Pronounced enhancement of neuromuscular blockade).
No products indexed under this heading.

Kanamycin Sulfate (Possible prolongation of neuromuscular blockade).
No products indexed under this heading.

Magnesium Sulfate Injection (May enhance the neuromuscular blockade).

Methacycline Hydrochloride (Possible prolongation of neuromuscular blockade).
No products indexed under this heading.

Methoxyflurane (Pronounced enhancement of neuromuscular blockade).
No products indexed under this heading.

Metocurine Iodide (Additive effect). Products include:
Metubine Iodide Vials 916

Minocycline Hydrochloride (Possible prolongation of neuromuscular blockade). Products include:
Dynacin Capsules 1590
Minocin Intravenous 1382
Minocin Oral Suspension 1385
Minocin Pellet-Filled Capsules 1383

Mivacurium Chloride (Additive effect). Products include:
Mivacron 1138

Neomycin, oral (Possible prolongation of neuromuscular blockade).

Oxytetracycline (Possible prolongation of neuromuscular blockade). Products include:
Terramycin Intramuscular Solution 2210

Oxytetracycline Hydrochloride (Possible prolongation of neuromuscular blockade). Products include:
TERAK Ointment .... ⊙ 209
Terra-Cortril Ophthalmic Suspension 2210
Terramycin with Polymyxin B Sulfate Ophthalmic Ointment 2211
Urobiotic-250 Capsules 2214

Pancuronium Bromide Injection (Additive effect).
No products indexed under this heading.

Polymyxin B Sulfate (Possible prolongation of neuromuscular blockade). Products include:
AK-Spore .... ⊙ 204
AK-Trol Ointment & Suspension .... ⊙ 205
Bactine First Aid Antibiotic Plus Anesthetic Ointment .... ▣ 708
Betadine Brand First Aid Antibiotics & Moisturizer Ointment 1991
Campho-Phenique Maximum Strength First Aid Antibiotic Plus Pain Reliever Ointment .... ▣ 719
Cortisporin Cream 1084
Cortisporin Ointment 1085
Cortisporin Ophthalmic Ointment Sterile 1085
Cortisporin Ophthalmic Suspension Sterile 1086
Cortisporin Otic Solution Sterile 1087
Cortisporin Otic Suspension Sterile 1088
Dexacidin Ointment .... ⊙ 263
Maxitrol Ophthalmic Ointment and Suspension .... ⊙ 224
Mycitracin .... ▣ 839
Neosporin G.U. Irrigant Sterile 1148
Neosporin Ointment .... ▣ 857
Neosporin Plus Maximum Strength Cream .... ▣ 858
Neosporin Plus Maximum Strength Ointment .... ▣ 858
Neosporin Ophthalmic Ointment Sterile 1148
Neosporin Ophthalmic Solution Sterile 1149
Ophthocort .... ⊙ 311
PediOtic Suspension Sterile 1153
Polymyxin B Sulfate, Aerosporin Brand Sterile Powder 1154
Poly-Pred Liquifilm .... ⊙ 248
Polysporin Ointment .... ▣ 858
Polysporin Ophthalmic Ointment Sterile 1154
Polysporin Powder .... ▣ 859
Polytrim Ophthalmic Solution Sterile 482
TERAK Ointment .... ⊙ 209
Terramycin with Polymyxin B Sulfate Ophthalmic Ointment 2211

Quinidine Gluconate (Possible recurrent paralysis). Products include:
Quinaglute Dura-Tabs Tablets 649

Quinidine Polygalacturonate (Possible recurrent paralysis).
No products indexed under this heading.

Quinidine Sulfate (Possible recurrent paralysis). Products include:
Quinidex Extentabs 2067

Rocuronium Bromide (Additive effect). Products include:
Zemuron 1830

Streptomycin Sulfate (Possible prolongation of neuromuscular blockade). Products include:
Streptomycin Sulfate Injection 2208

Succinylcholine Chloride (Prior administration may enhance neuromuscular blocking effect and duration of action of Norcuron). Products include:
Anectine 1073

Tetracycline Hydrochloride (Possible prolongation of neuromuscular blockade). Products include:
Achromycin V Capsules 1367

Tobramycin (Possible prolongation of neuromuscular blockade). Products include:
AKTOB .... ⊙ 206
TobraDex Ophthalmic Suspension and Ointment 473
Tobrex Ophthalmic Ointment and Solution .... ⊙ 229

Tobramycin Sulfate (Possible prolongation of neuromuscular blockade). Products include:
Nebcin Vials, Hyporets & ADD-Vantage 1464
Tobramycin Sulfate Injection 968

NORDETTE-21 TABLETS
(Levonorgestrel, Ethinyl Estradiol) 2755
May interact with barbiturates and certain other agents. Compounds in these categories include:

Ampicillin Sodium (Reduced efficacy; increased incidence of breakthrough bleeding). Products include:
Unasyn 2212

Aprobarbital (Reduced efficacy; increased incidence of breakthrough bleeding).
No products indexed under this heading.

Butabarbital (Reduced efficacy; increased incidence of breakthrough bleeding).
No products indexed under this heading.

Butalbital (Reduced efficacy; increased incidence of breakthrough bleeding). Products include:
Esgic-plus Tablets 1013
Fioricet Tablets 2258
Fioricet with Codeine Capsules 2260
Fiorinal Capsules 2261
Fiorinal with Codeine Capsules 2262
Fiorinal Tablets 2261
Phrenilin 785
Sedapap Tablets 50 mg/650 mg .. 1543

Mephobarbital (Reduced efficacy; increased incidence of breakthrough bleeding). Products include:
Mebaral Tablets 2322

Oxytetracycline (Reduced efficacy; increased incidence of breakthrough bleeding). Products include:
Terramycin Intramuscular Solution 2210

Oxytetracycline Hydrochloride (Reduced efficacy; increased incidence of breakthrough bleeding). Products include:
TERAK Ointment .... ⊙ 209
Terra-Cortril Ophthalmic Suspension 2210
Terramycin with Polymyxin B Sulfate Ophthalmic Ointment 2211
Urobiotic-250 Capsules 2214

Pentobarbital Sodium (Reduced efficacy; increased incidence of breakthrough bleeding). Products include:
Nembutal Sodium Capsules 436
Nembutal Sodium Solution 438
Nembutal Sodium Suppositories 440

Phenobarbital (Reduced efficacy; increased incidence of breakthrough bleeding). Products include:
Arco-Lase Plus Tablets 512
Bellergal-S Tablets 2250
Donnatal 2060
Donnatal Extentabs 2061
Donnatal Tablets 2060
Phenobarbital Elixir and Tablets 1469
Quadrinal Tablets 1350

Phenylbutazone (Reduced efficacy; increased incidence of breakthrough bleeding).
No products indexed under this heading.

Phenytoin Sodium (Reduced efficacy; increased incidence of breakthrough bleeding). Products include:
Dilantin Kapseals 1906
Dilantin Parenteral 1910

Rifampin (Reduced efficacy; increased incidence of breakthrough bleeding). Products include:
Rifadin 1528
Rifamate Capsules 1530
Rifater 1532
Rimactane Capsules 847

Secobarbital Sodium (Reduced efficacy; increased incidence of breakthrough bleeding). Products include:
Seconal Sodium Pulvules 1474

IMPORTANT NOTE: Always consult each drug listing in the patient's regimen for possible interactions.

Nordette-21 Interactions Index 730

Tetracycline Hydrochloride (Reduced efficacy; increased incidence of breakthrough bleeding). Products include:
Achromycin V Capsules ... 1367
Thiamylal Sodium (Reduced efficacy; increased incidence of breakthrough bleeding).
No products indexed under this heading.

NORDETTE-28 TABLETS
(Levonorgestrel, Ethinyl Estradiol) ... 2758
See **Nordette-21 Tablets**

NORFLEX INJECTION
(Orphenadrine Citrate) ... 1496
See **Norflex Extended-Release Tablets**

NORFLEX EXTENDED-RELEASE TABLETS
(Orphenadrine Citrate) ... 1496
May interact with:

Propoxyphene Hydrochloride (Concomitant use results in confusion, anxiety and tremors). Products include:
Darvon ... 1435
Wygesic Tablets ... 2827
Propoxyphene Napsylate (Concomitant use results in confusion, anxiety and tremors). Products include:
Darvon-N/Darvocet-N ... 1433

NORGESIC FORTE TABLETS
(Orphenadrine Citrate, Aspirin) ... 1496
See **Norgesic Tablets**

NORGESIC TABLETS
(Orphenadrine Citrate, Aspirin) ... 1496
May interact with:

Propoxyphene Hydrochloride (Potential for confusion, anxiety and tremors). Products include:
Darvon ... 1435
Wygesic Tablets ... 2827
Propoxyphene Napsylate (Potential for confusion, anxiety and tremors). Products include:
Darvon-N/Darvocet-N ... 1433

NORINYL 1+35 21-DAY TABLETS
(Ethinyl Estradiol, Norethindrone) ... 2088
See **Brevicon 21-Day Tablets**

NORINYL 1+35 28-DAY TABLETS
(Norethindrone, Ethinyl Estradiol) ... 2088
See **Brevicon 21-Day Tablets**

NORINYL 1+50 21-DAY TABLETS
(Norethindrone, Mestranol) ... 2088
See **Brevicon 21-Day Tablets**

NORINYL 1+50 28-DAY TABLETS
(Norethindrone, Mestranol) ... 2088
See **Brevicon 21-Day Tablets**

NORISODRINE WITH CALCIUM IODIDE SYRUP
(Calcium Iodide, Isoproterenol Sulfate) ... 442
May interact with monoamine oxidase inhibitors, sympathomimetics, and certain other agents. Compounds in these categories include:

Albuterol (Co-administration with other adrenergic agent produces additive effects). Products include:
Proventil Inhalation Aerosol ... 2382
Ventolin Inhalation Aerosol and Refill ... 1197
Albuterol Sulfate (Co-administration with other adrenergic agent produces additive effects). Products include:
Airet Solution for Inhalation ... 452
Proventil Inhalation Solution 0.083% ... 2384
Proventil Repetabs Tablets ... 2386
Proventil Solution for Inhalation 0.5% ... 2383
Proventil Syrup ... 2385
Proventil Tablets ... 2386
Ventolin Inhalation Solution ... 1198
Ventolin Nebules Inhalation Solution ... 1199
Ventolin Rotacaps for Inhalation ... 1200
Ventolin Syrup ... 1202
Ventolin Tablets ... 1203
Volmax Extended-Release Tablets .. 1788
Dobutamine Hydrochloride (Co-administration with other adrenergic agent produces additive effects). Products include:
Dobutrex Solution Vials ... 1439
Dopamine Hydrochloride (Co-administration with other adrenergic agent produces additive effects).
No products indexed under this heading.
Ephedrine Hydrochloride (Co-administration with other adrenergic agent produces additive effects). Products include:
Primatene Dual Action Formula ... ▣ 872
Primatene Tablets ... ▣ 873
Quadrinal Tablets ... 1350
Ephedrine Sulfate (Co-administration with other adrenergic agent produces additive effects). Products include:
Bronkaid Caplets ... ▣ 717
Marax Tablets & DF Syrup ... 2200
Ephedrine Tannate (Co-administration with other adrenergic agent produces additive effects). Products include:
Rynatuss ... 2673
Epinephrine (Co-administration with other adrenergic agent produces additive effects). Products include:
Bronkaid Mist ... ▣ 717
EPIFRIN ... ⊙ 239
EpiPen ... 790
Marcaine Hydrochloride with Epinephrine 1:200,000 ... 2316
Primatene Mist ... ▣ 873
Sensorcaine with Epinephrine Injection ... 559
Sus-Phrine Injection ... 1019
Xylocaine with Epinephrine Injections ... 567
Epinephrine Bitartrate (Co-administration with other adrenergic agent produces additive effects). Products include:
Bronkaid Mist Suspension ... ▣ 718
Sensorcaine-MPF with Epinephrine Injection ... 559
Epinephrine Hydrochloride (Co-administration with other adrenergic agent produces additive effects). Products include:
Ana-Kit Anaphylaxis Emergency Treatment Kit ... 617
Furazolidone (Co-administration may induce hypertensive crisis). Products include:
Furoxone ... 2046
Isocarboxazid (Co-administration may induce hypertensive crisis).
No products indexed under this heading.
Isoproterenol Hydrochloride (Co-administration with other adrenergic agent produces additive effects). Products include:
Isuprel Hydrochloride Injection 1:5000 ... 2311
Isuprel Hydrochloride Solution 1:200 & 1:100 ... 2313
Isuprel Mistometer ... 2312
Lithium Carbonate (Concurrant use may enhance the hypothyroid and goitrogenic effects of either drug). Products include:
Eskalith ... 2485
Lithium Carbonate Capsules & Tablets ... 2230
Lithonate/Lithotabs/Lithobid ... 2543
Metaproterenol Sulfate (Co-administration with other adrenergic agent produces additive effects). Products include:
Alupent ... 669
Metaproterenol Sulfate Inhalation Solution, USP, Arm-a-Med ... 552
Metaraminol Bitartrate (Co-administration with other adrenergic agent produces additive effects). Products include:
Aramine Injection ... 1609
Methoxamine Hydrochloride (Co-administration with other adrenergic agent produces additive effects). Products include:
Vasoxyl Injection ... 1196
Norepinephrine Bitartrate (Co-administration with other adrenergic agent produces additive effects). Products include:
Levophed Bitartrate Injection ... 2315
Phenelzine Sulfate (Co-administration may induce hypertensive crisis). Products include:
Nardil ... 1920
Phenylephrine Bitartrate (Co-administration with other adrenergic agent produces additive effects).
No products indexed under this heading.
Phenylephrine Hydrochloride (Co-administration with other adrenergic agent produces additive effects). Products include:
Atrohist Plus Tablets ... 454
Cerose DM ... ▣ 878
Comhist ... 2038
D.A. Chewable Tablets ... 951
Deconsal Pediatric Capsules ... 454
Dura-Vent/DA Tablets ... 953
Entex Capsules ... 1986
Entex Liquid ... 1986
Extendryl ... 1005
4-Way Fast Acting Nasal Spray (regular & mentholated) ... ▣ 621
Hemorid For Women ... ▣ 834
Hycomine Compound Tablets ... 932
Neo-Synephrine Hydrochloride 1% Carpuject ... 2324
Neo-Synephrine Hydrochloride 1% Injection ... 2324
Neo-Synephrine Hydrochloride (Ophthalmic) ... 2325
Neo-Synephrine ... ▣ 726
Nōstril ... ▣ 644
Novahistine Elixir ... ▣ 823
Phenergan VC ... 2779
Phenergan VC with Codeine ... 2781
Preparation H ... ▣ 871
Tympagesic Ear Drops ... 2342
Vasosulf ... ⊙ 271
Vicks Sinex Nasal Spray and Ultra Fine Mist ... ▣ 765
Phenylephrine Tannate (Co-administration with other adrenergic agent produces additive effects). Products include:
Atrohist Pediatric Suspension ... 454
Ricobid-D Pediatric Suspension ... 2038
Ricobid Tablets and Pediatric Suspension ... 2038
Rynatan ... 2673
Rynatuss ... 2673
Phenylpropanolamine Hydrochloride (Co-administration with other adrenergic agent produces additive effects). Products include:
Acutrim ... ▣ 628
Allerest Children's Chewable Tablets ... ▣ 627
Allerest 12 Hour Caplets ... ▣ 627
Atrohist Plus Tablets ... 454
BC Cold Powder Multi-Symptom Formula (Cold-Sinus-Allergy) ... ▣ 609
BC Cold Powder Non-Drowsy Formula (Cold-Sinus) ... ▣ 609
Cheracol Plus Head Cold/Cough Formula ... ▣ 769
Comtrex Multi-Symptom Non-Drowsy Liqui-gels ... ▣ 618
Contac Continuous Action Nasal Decongestant/Antihistamine 12 Hour Capsules ... ▣ 813
Contac Maximum Strength Continuous Action Decongestant/Antihistamine 12 Hour Caplets ... ▣ 813
Contac Severe Cold and Flu Formula Caplets ... ▣ 814
Coricidin 'D' Decongestant Tablets ... ▣ 800
Dexatrim ... ▣ 832
Dexatrim Plus Vitamins Caplets ... ▣ 832
Dimetane-DC Cough Syrup ... 2059
Dimetapp Elixir ... ▣ 773
Dimetapp Extentabs ... ▣ 774
Dimetapp Tablets/Liqui-Gels ... ▣ 775
Dimetapp Cold & Allergy Chewable Tablets ... ▣ 773
Dimetapp DM Elixir ... ▣ 774
Dura-Vent Tablets ... 952
Entex Capsules ... 1986
Entex LA Tablets ... 1987
Entex Liquid ... 1986
Exgest LA Tablets ... 782
Hycomine ... 931
Isoclor Timesule Capsules ... ▣ 637
Nolamine Timed-Release Tablets ... 785
Ornade Spansule Capsules ... 2502
Propagest Tablets ... 786
Pyrroxate Caplets ... ▣ 772
Robitussin-CF ... ▣ 777
Sinulin Tablets ... 787
Tavist-D 12 Hour Relief Tablets ... ▣ 787
Teldrin 12 Hour Antihistamine/Nasal Decongestant Allergy Relief Capsules ... ▣ 826
Triaminic Allergy Tablets ... ▣ 789
Triaminic Cold Tablets ... ▣ 790
Triaminic Expectorant ... ▣ 790
Triaminic Syrup ... ▣ 792
Triaminic-12 Tablets ... ▣ 792
Triaminic-DM Syrup ... ▣ 792
Triaminicin Tablets ... ▣ 793
Triaminicol Multi-Symptom Cold Tablets ... ▣ 793
Triaminicol Multi-Symptom Relief ... ▣ 794
Vicks DayQuil Allergy Relief 12-Hour Extended Release Tablets ... ▣ 760
Vicks DayQuil Allergy Relief 4-Hour Tablets ... ▣ 760
Vicks DayQuil SINUS Pressure & CONGESTION Relief ... ▣ 761
Pirbuterol Acetate (Co-administration with other adrenergic agent produces additive effects). Products include:
Maxair Autohaler ... 1492
Maxair Inhaler ... 1494
Propranolol Hydrochloride (Antagonizes isoproterenol). Products include:
Inderal ... 2728
Inderal LA Long Acting Capsules ... 2730
Inderide Tablets ... 2732
Inderide LA Long Acting Capsules .. 2734
Pseudoephedrine Hydrochloride (Co-administration with other adrenergic agent produces additive effects). Products include:
Actifed Allergy Daytime/Nighttime Caplets ... ▣ 844
Actifed Plus Caplets ... ▣ 845
Actifed Plus Tablets ... ▣ 845
Actifed with Codeine Cough Syrup .. 1067
Actifed Sinus Daytime/Nighttime Tablets and Caplets ... ▣ 846
Actifed Syrup ... ▣ 846
Actifed Tablets ... ▣ 844
Advil Cold and Sinus Caplets and Tablets (formerly CoAdvil) ... ▣ 870
Alka-Seltzer Plus Cold Medicine Liqui-Gels ... ▣ 706
Alka-Seltzer Plus Cold & Cough Medicine Liqui-Gels ... ▣ 705
Alka-Seltzer Plus Night-Time Cold Medicine Liqui-Gels ... ▣ 706
Allerest Headache Strength Tablets ... ▣ 627
Allerest Maximum Strength Tablets ... ▣ 627

(▣ Described in PDR For Nonprescription Drugs) (⊙ Described in PDR For Ophthalmology)

Interactions Index

Normodyne Injection

Allerest No Drowsiness Tablets ...... ®D 627
Allerest Sinus Pain Formula .... ®D 627
Anatuss LA Tablets 1542
Atrohist Pediatric Capsules 453
Bayer Select Sinus Pain Relief Formula .... ®D 717
Benadryl Allergy Decongestant Liquid Medication .... ®D 848
Benadryl Allergy Decongestant Tablets .... ®D 848
Benadryl Allergy Sinus Headache Formula Caplets .... ®D 849
Benylin Multisymptom .... ®D 852
Bromfed Capsules (Extended-Release) 1785
Bromfed Syrup .... ®D 733
Bromfed Tablets 1785
Bromfed-DM Cough Syrup 1786
Bromfed-PD Capsules (Extended-Release) 1785
Children's Vicks DayQuil Allergy Relief .... ®D 757
Children's Vicks NyQuil Cold/ Cough Relief .... ®D 758
Comtrex Multi-Symptom Cold Reliever Tablets/Caplets/Liqui-Gels/Liquid .... ®D 615
Allergy-Sinus Comtrex Multi-Symptom Allergy-Sinus Formula Tablets .... ®D 617
Comtrex Multi-Symptom Non-Drowsy Caplets .... ®D 618
Congess 1004
Contac Day Allergy/Sinus Caplets ®D 812
Contac Day & Night .... ®D 812
Contac Night Allergy/Sinus Caplets .... ®D 812
Contac Severe Cold & Flu Non-Drowsy .... ®D 815
Deconamine Chewable Tablets 1320
Deconamine CX Cough and Cold Liquid and Tablets 1319
Deconamine 1320
Deconsal C Expectorant Syrup 456
Deconsal Pediatric Syrup 457
Deconsal II Tablets 454
Dimetane-DX Cough Syrup 2059
Dimetapp Sinus Caplets .... ®D 775
Dorcol Children's Cough Syrup ...... ®D 785
Drixoral Cough + Congestion Liquid Caps .... ®D 802
Dura-Tap/PD Capsules 2867
Duratuss Tablets 2565
Duratuss HD Elixir 2565
Efidac/24 .... ®D 635
Entex PSE Tablets 1987
Fedahist Gyrocaps 2401
Fedahist Timecaps 2401
Guaifed 1787
Guaifed Syrup .... ®D 734
Guaimax-D Tablets 792
Guaitab Tablets .... ®D 734
Isoclor Expectorant 990
Kronofed-A 977
Motrin IB Sinus .... ®D 838
Novahistine DH 2462
Novahistine DMX .... ®D 822
Novahistine Expectorant 2463
Nucofed 2051
PediaCare Cold Allergy Chewable Tablets .... ®D 677
PediaCare Cough-Cold Chewable Tablets 1553
PediaCare 1553
PediaCare Infants' Decongestant Drops .... ®D 677
PediCare Infant's Drops Decongestant Plus Cough 1553
PediaCare NightRest Cough-Cold Liquid 1553
Pediatric Vicks 44d Dry Hacking Cough & Head Congestion .... ®D 763
Pediatric Vicks 44m Cough & Cold Relief .... ®D 764
Robitussin Cold & Cough Liqui-Gels .... ®D 776
Robitussin Maximum Strength Cough & Cold .... ®D 778
Robitussin Pediatric Cough & Cold Formula .... ®D 779
Robitussin Severe Congestion Liqui-Gels .... ®D 776
Robitussin-DAC Syrup 2074
Robitussin-PE .... ®D 778
Rondec Oral Drops 953
Rondec Syrup 953
Rondec Tablet 953
Rondec-DM Oral Drops 954
Rondec-DM Syrup 954
Rondec-TR Tablet 953
Ryna .... ®D 841
Seldane-D Extended-Release Tablets 1538
Semprex-D Capsules 463
Semprex-D Capsules 1167
Sinarest Tablets .... ®D 648
Sinarest Extra Strength Tablets ...... ®D 648
Sinarest No Drowsiness Tablets .... ®D 648
Sine-Aid IB Caplets 1554
Sine-Aid Maximum Strength Sinus Medication Gelcaps, Caplets and Tablets 1554
Sine-Off No Drowsiness Formula Caplets .... ®D 824
Sine-Off Sinus Medicine .... ®D 825
Singlet Tablets .... ®D 825
Sinutab Non-Drying Liquid Caps .... ®D 859
Sinutab Sinus Allergy Medication, Maximum Strength Tablets and Caplets .... ®D 860
Sinutab Sinus Medication, Maximum Strength Without Drowsiness Formula, Tablets & Caplets .... ®D 860
Sinutab Sinus Medication, Regular Strength Without Drowsiness Formula .... ®D 859
Sudafed Children's Liquid .... ®D 861
Sudafed Cold and Cough Liquidcaps .... ®D 862
Sudafed Cough Syrup .... ®D 862
Sudafed Plus Liquid .... ®D 862
Sudafed Plus Tablets .... ®D 863
Sudafed Severe Cold Formula Caplets .... ®D 863
Sudafed Severe Cold Formula Tablets .... ®D 864
Sudafed Sinus Caplets .... ®D 864
Sudafed Sinus Tablets .... ®D 864
Sudafed Tablets, 30 mg .... ®D 861
Sudafed Tablets, 60 mg .... ®D 861
Sudafed 12 Hour Caplets .... ®D 861
Syn-Rx Tablets 465
Syn-Rx DM Tablets 466
TheraFlu .... ®D 787
TheraFlu Maximum Strength Nighttime Flu, Cold & Cough Medicine .... ®D 788
TheraFlu Maximum Strength Non-Drowsy Formula Flu, Cold & Cough Medicine .... ®D 788
Thera Flu Maximum Strength, Non-Drowsy Formula Flu, Cold and Cough Caplets .... ®D 789
Triaminic AM Cough and Decongestant Formula .... ®D 789
Triaminic AM Decongestant Formula .... ®D 790
Triaminic Nite Light .... ®D 791
Triaminic Sore Throat Formula ...... ®D 791
Tussend 1783
Tussend Expectorant 1785
Children's TYLENOL Cold Multi-Symptom Liquid Formula and Chewable Tablets 1561
Children's TYLENOL Cold Plus Cough Multi Symptom Tablets and Liquid .... ®D 681
Infants' TYLENOL Cold Decongestant & Fever-Reducer Drops 1556
TYLENOL Maximum Strength Allergy Sinus Medication Gelcaps and Caplets 1563
TYLENOL Maximum Strength Allergy Sinus NightTime Medication Caplets 1555
TYLENOL Flu Maximum Strength Gelcaps 1565
TYLENOL Flu NightTime, Maximum Strength, Gelcaps 1566
TYLENOL Maximum Strength Flu NightTime Hot Medication Packets 1562
TYLENOL, Maximum Strength, Sinus Medication Geltabs, Gelcaps, Caplets and Tablets 1566
TYLENOL Cold Multi-Symptom Formula Medication Tablets and Caplets 1561
TYLENOL Cold Medication No Drowsiness Formula Gelcaps and Caplets 1562
TYLENOL Cold Multi-Symptom Hot Medication Liquid Packets 1557
TYLENOL Cough Multi-Symptom Medication with Decongestant 1565
Ursinus Inlay-Tabs .... ®D 794
Vicks 44 LiquiCaps Cough, Cold & Flu Relief .... ®D 755
Vicks 44 LiquiCaps Non-Drowsy Cough & Cold Relief .... ®D 756
Vicks 44D Dry Hacking Cough & Head Congestion .... ®D 755
Vicks 44M Cough, Cold & Flu Relief .... ®D 756
Vicks DayQuil .... ®D 761
Vicks DayQuil SINUS Pressure & PAIN Relief with IBUPROFEN .... ®D 762
Vicks Nyquil Hot Therapy .... ®D 762
Vicks NyQuil LiquiCaps Multi-Symptom Cold/Flu Relief .... ®D 763
Vicks NyQuil Multi-Symptom Cold/Flu Relief - (Original & Cherry Flavor) .... ®D 763

Pseudoephedrine Sulfate (Co-administration with other adrenergic agent produces additive effects). Products include:

Cheracol Sinus .... ®D 768
Chlor-Trimeton Allergy Decongestant Tablets .... ®D 799
Claritin-D 2350
Drixoral Cold and Allergy Sustained-Action Tablets .... ®D 802
Drixoral Cold and Flu Extended-Release Tablets .... ®D 803
Drixoral Non-Drowsy Formula Extended-Release Tablets .... ®D 803
Drixoral Allergy/Sinus Extended Release Tablets .... ®D 804
Trinalin Repetabs Tablets 1330

Salmeterol Xinafoate (Co-administration with other adrenergic agent produces additive effects). Products include:

Serevent Inhalation Aerosol 1176

Selegiline Hydrochloride (Co-administration may induce hypertensive crisis). Products include:

Eldepryl Tablets 2550

Terbutaline Sulfate (Co-administration with other adrenergic agent produces additive effects). Products include:

Brethaire Inhaler 813
Brethine Ampuls 815
Brethine Tablets 814
Bricanyl Subcutaneous Injection 1502
Bricanyl Tablets 1503

Tranylcypromine Sulfate (Co-administration may induce hypertensive crisis). Products include:

Parnate Tablets 2503

NORMODYNE INJECTION

(Labetalol Hydrochloride) 2377

May interact with oral hypoglycemic agents, insulin, tricyclic antidepressants, sympathomimetic bronchodilators, diphenylalkylamine-type calcium antagonists, and certain other agents. Compounds in these categories include:

Acarbose (Altered dosage requirements).

No products indexed under this heading.

Albuterol (Beta-blocker can blunt the bronchodilator effect of beta-receptor agonists in patients with bronchospasm; greater than normal anti-asthmatic dose of beta-agonist may be required). Products include:

Proventil Inhalation Aerosol 2382
Ventolin Inhalation Aerosol and Refill 1197

Albuterol Sulfate (Beta-blocker can blunt the bronchodilator effect of beta-receptor agonists in patients with bronchospasm; greater than normal anti-asthmatic dose of beta-agonist may be required). Products include:

Airet Solution for Inhalation 452
Proventil Inhalation Solution 0.083% 2384
Proventil Repetabs Tablets 2386
Proventil Solution for Inhalation 0.5% 2383
Proventil Syrup 2385
Proventil Tablets 2386
Ventolin Inhalation Solution 1198
Ventolin Nebules Inhalation Solution 1199

Ventolin Rotacaps for Inhalation 1200
Ventolin Syrup 1202
Ventolin Tablets 1203
Volmax Extended-Release Tablets .. 1788

Amitriptyline Hydrochloride (Potential for tremor). Products include:

Elavil 2838
Endep Tablets 2174
Etrafon 2355
Limbitrol 2180
Triavil Tablets 1757

Amoxapine (Potential for tremor). Products include:

Asendin Tablets 1369

Bitolterol Mesylate (Beta-blocker can blunt the bronchodilator effect of beta-receptor agonists in patients with bronchospasm; greater than normal anti-asthmatic dose of beta-agonist may be required). Products include:

Tornalate Solution for Inhalation, 0.2% 956
Tornalate Metered Dose Inhaler 957

Chlorpropamide (Altered dosage requirements). Products include:

Diabinese Tablets 1935

Cimetidine (Increases bioavailability of labetalol). Products include:

Tagamet Tablets 2516

Cimetidine Hydrochloride (Increases bioavailability of labetalol). Products include:

Tagamet 2516

Clomipramine Hydrochloride (Potential for tremor). Products include:

Anafranil Capsules 803

Desipramine Hydrochloride (Potential for tremor). Products include:

Norpramin Tablets 1526

Doxepin Hydrochloride (Potential for tremor). Products include:

Sinequan 2205
Zonalon Cream 1055

Ephedrine Hydrochloride (Beta-blocker can blunt the bronchodilator effect of beta-receptor agonists in patients with bronchospasm; greater than normal anti-asthmatic dose of beta-agonist may be required). Products include:

Primatene Dual Action Formula ...... ®D 872
Primatene Tablets .... ®D 873
Quadrinal Tablets 1350

Ephedrine Sulfate (Beta-blocker can blunt the bronchodilator effect of beta-receptor agonists in patients with bronchospasm; greater than normal anti-asthmatic dose of beta-agonist may be required). Products include:

Bronkaid Caplets .... ®D 717
Marax Tablets & DF Syrup 2200

Ephedrine Tannate (Beta-blocker can blunt the bronchodilator effect of beta-receptor agonists in patients with bronchospasm; greater than normal anti-asthmatic dose of beta-agonist may be required). Products include:

Rynatuss 2673

Epinephrine (Beta-blocker can blunt the bronchodilator effect of beta-receptor agonists in patients with bronchospasm; greater than normal anti-asthmatic dose of beta-agonist may be required). Products include:

Bronkaid Mist .... ®D 717
EPIFRIN .... Ⓒ 239
EpiPen 790
Marcaine Hydrochloride with Epinephrine 1:200,000 2316
Primatene Mist .... ®D 873
Sensorcaine with Epinephrine Injection 559
Sus-Phrine Injection 1019

IMPORTANT NOTE: Always consult each drug listing in the patient's regimen for possible interactions.

Normodyne Injection — Interactions Index — 732

Xylocaine with Epinephrine Injections ... 567

Epinephrine Hydrochloride (Beta-blocker can blunt the bronchodilator effect of beta-receptor agonists in patients with bronchospasm; greater than normal anti-asthmatic dose of beta-agonist may be required). Products include:
- Ana-Kit Anaphylaxis Emergency Treatment Kit ... 617

Ethylnorepinephrine Hydrochloride (Beta-blocker can blunt the bronchodilator effect of beta-receptor agonists in patients with bronchospasm; greater than normal anti-asthmatic dose of beta-agonist may be required).
- No products indexed under this heading.

Glipizide (Altered dosage requirements). Products include:
- Glucotrol Tablets ... 1967
- Glucotrol XL Extended Release Tablets ... 1968

Glyburide (Altered dosage requirements). Products include:
- DiaBeta Tablets ... 1239
- Glynase PresTab Tablets ... 2609
- Micronase Tablets ... 2623

Halothane (Synergism has been reported between labetalol I.V. and halothane anesthesia; potential increased hypotensive effect, reduction in cardiac output and increase in central venous pressure). Products include:
- Fluothane ... 2724

Imipramine Hydrochloride (Potential for tremor). Products include:
- Tofranil Ampuls ... 854
- Tofranil Tablets ... 856

Imipramine Pamoate (Potential for tremor). Products include:
- Tofranil-PM Capsules ... 857

Insulin, Human (Altered dosage requirements).
- No products indexed under this heading.

Insulin, Human Isophane Suspension (Altered dosage requirements). Products include:
- Novolin N Human Insulin 10 ml Vials ... 1795

Insulin, Human NPH (Altered dosage requirements). Products include:
- Humulin N, 100 Units ... 1448
- Novolin N PenFill Cartridges Durable Insulin Delivery System ... 1798
- Novolin N Prefilled Syringe Disposable Insulin Delivery System ... 1798

Insulin, Human Regular (Altered dosage requirements). Products include:
- Humulin R, 100 Units ... 1449
- Novolin R Human Insulin 10 ml Vials ... 1795
- Novolin R PenFill Cartridges Durable Insulin Delivery System ... 1798
- Novolin R Prefilled Syringe Disposable Insulin Delivery System ... 1798
- Velosulin BR Human Insulin 10 ml Vials ... 1795

Insulin, Human, Zinc Suspension (Altered dosage requirements). Products include:
- Humulin L, 100 Units ... 1446
- Humulin U, 100 Units ... 1450
- Novolin L Human Insulin 10 ml Vials ... 1795

Insulin, NPH (Altered dosage requirements). Products include:
- NPH, 100 Units ... 1450
- Pork NPH, 100 Units ... 1452
- Purified Pork NPH Isophane Insulin ... 1801

Insulin, Regular (Altered dosage requirements). Products include:
- Regular, 100 Units ... 1450
- Pork Regular, 100 Units ... 1452
- Pork Regular (Concentrated), 500 Units ... 1453
- Purified Pork Regular Insulin ... 1801

Insulin, Zinc Crystals (Altered dosage requirements). Products include:
- NPH, 100 Units ... 1450

Insulin, Zinc Suspension (Altered dosage requirements). Products include:
- Iletin I ... 1450
- Lente, 100 Units ... 1450
- Iletin II ... 1452
- Pork Lente, 100 Units ... 1452
- Purified Pork Lente Insulin ... 1801

Isoetharine (Beta-blocker can blunt the bronchodilator effect of beta-receptor agonists in patients with bronchospasm; greater than normal anti-asthmatic dose of beta-agonist may be required). Products include:
- Bronkometer Aerosol ... 2302
- Bronkosol Solution ... 2302
- Isoetharine Inhalation Solution, USP, Arm-a-Med ... 551

Isoproterenol Hydrochloride (Beta-blocker can blunt the bronchodilator effect of beta-receptor agonists in patients with bronchospasm; greater than normal anti-asthmatic dose of beta-agonist may be required). Products include:
- Isuprel Hydrochloride Injection 1:5000 ... 2311
- Isuprel Hydrochloride Solution 1:200 & 1:100 ... 2313
- Isuprel Mistometer ... 2312

Isoproterenol Sulfate (Beta-blocker can blunt the bronchodilator effect of beta-receptor agonists in patients with bronchospasm; greater than normal anti-asthmatic dose of beta-agonist may be required). Products include:
- Norisodrine with Calcium Iodide Syrup ... 442

Maprotiline Hydrochloride (Potential for tremor). Products include:
- Ludiomil Tablets ... 843

Metaproterenol Sulfate (Beta-blocker can blunt the bronchodilator effect of beta-receptor agonists in patients with bronchospasm; greater than normal anti-asthmatic dose of beta-agonist may be required). Products include:
- Alupent ... 669
- Metaproterenol Sulfate Inhalation Solution, USP, Arm-a-Med ... 552

Metformin Hydrochloride (Altered dosage requirements). Products include:
- Glucophage ... 752

Nitroglycerin (Reflex tachycardia produced by nitroglycerin blunted). Products include:
- Deponit NTG Transdermal Delivery System ... 2397
- Nitro-Bid IV ... 1523
- Nitro-Bid Ointment ... 1524
- Nitrodisc ... 2047
- Nitro-Dur (nitroglycerin) Transdermal Infusion System ... 1326
- Nitrolingual Spray ... 2027
- Nitrostat Tablets ... 1925
- Transderm-Nitro Transdermal Therapeutic System ... 859

Nortriptyline Hydrochloride (Potential for tremor). Products include:
- Pamelor ... 2280

Pirbuterol Acetate (Beta-blocker can blunt the bronchodilator effect of beta-receptor agonists in patients with bronchospasm; greater than normal anti-asthmatic dose of beta-agonist may be required). Products include:
- Maxair Autohaler ... 1492
- Maxair Inhaler ... 1494

Protriptyline Hydrochloride (Potential for tremor). Products include:
- Vivactil Tablets ... 1774

Salmeterol Xinafoate (Beta-blocker can blunt the bronchodilator effect of beta-receptor agonists in patients with bronchospasm; greater than normal anti-asthmatic dose of beta-agonist may be required). Products include:
- Serevent Inhalation Aerosol ... 1176

Terbutaline Sulfate (Beta-blocker can blunt the bronchodilator effect of beta-receptor agonists in patients with bronchospasm; greater than normal anti-asthmatic dose of beta-agonist may be required). Products include:
- Brethaire Inhaler ... 813
- Brethine Ampuls ... 815
- Brethine Tablets ... 814
- Bricanyl Subcutaneous Injection ... 1502
- Bricanyl Tablets ... 1503

Tolazamide (Altered dosage requirements).
- No products indexed under this heading.

Tolbutamide (Altered dosage requirements).
- No products indexed under this heading.

Trimipramine Maleate (Potential for tremor). Products include:
- Surmontil Capsules ... 2811

Verapamil Hydrochloride (Care should be taken if coadministered; effects of concomitant use not specified). Products include:
- Calan SR Caplets ... 2422
- Calan Tablets ... 2419
- Isoptin Injectable ... 1344
- Isoptin Oral Tablets ... 1346
- Isoptin SR Tablets ... 1348
- Verelan Capsules ... 1410
- Verelan Capsules ... 2824

NORMODYNE TABLETS

(Labetalol Hydrochloride) ... 2379

May interact with oral hypoglycemic agents, tricyclic antidepressants, sympathomimetic bronchodilators, diphenylalkylamine-type calcium antagonists, insulin, and certain other agents. Compounds in these categories include:

Acarbose (Altered dosage requirements).
- No products indexed under this heading.

Albuterol (Beta-blocker can blunt the bronchodilator effect of beta-receptor agonists in patients with bronchospasm; greater than normal anti-asthmatic dose of beta-agonist may be required). Products include:
- Proventil Inhalation Aerosol ... 2382
- Ventolin Inhalation Aerosol and Refill ... 1197

Albuterol Sulfate (Beta-blocker can blunt the bronchodilator effect of beta-receptor agonists in patients with bronchospasm; greater than normal anti-asthmatic dose of beta-agonist may be required). Products include:
- Airet Solution for Inhalation ... 452
- Proventil Inhalation Solution 0.083% ... 2384
- Proventil Repetabs Tablets ... 2386
- Proventil Solution for Inhalation 0.5% ... 2383
- Proventil Syrup ... 2385
- Proventil Tablets ... 2386
- Ventolin Inhalation Solution ... 1198
- Ventolin Nebules Inhalation Solution ... 1199
- Ventolin Rotacaps for Inhalation ... 1200
- Ventolin Syrup ... 1202
- Ventolin Tablets ... 1203
- Volmax Extended-Release Tablets ... 1788

Amitriptyline Hydrochloride (Potential for tremor). Products include:
- Elavil ... 2838
- Endep Tablets ... 2174
- Etrafon ... 2355
- Limbitrol ... 2180
- Triavil Tablets ... 1757

Amoxapine (Potential for tremor). Products include:
- Asendin Tablets ... 1369

Bitolterol Mesylate (Beta-blocker can blunt the bronchodilator effect of beta-receptor agonists in patients with bronchospasm; greater than normal anti-asthmatic dose of beta-agonist may be required). Products include:
- Tornalate Solution for Inhalation, 0.2% ... 956
- Tornalate Metered Dose Inhaler ... 957

Chlorpropamide (Altered dosage requirements). Products include:
- Diabinese Tablets ... 1935

Cimetidine (Increases bioavailability of labetalol). Products include:
- Tagamet Tablets ... 2516

Cimetidine Hydrochloride (Increases bioavailability of labetalol). Products include:
- Tagamet ... 2516

Clomipramine Hydrochloride (Potential for tremor). Products include:
- Anafranil Capsules ... 803

Desipramine Hydrochloride (Potential for tremor). Products include:
- Norpramin Tablets ... 1526

Doxepin Hydrochloride (Potential for tremor). Products include:
- Sinequan ... 2205
- Zonalon Cream ... 1055

Ephedrine Hydrochloride (Beta-blocker can blunt the bronchodilator effect of beta-receptor agonists in patients with bronchospasm; greater than normal anti-asthmatic dose of beta-agonist may be required). Products include:
- Primatene Dual Action Formula ... ▣ 872
- Primatene Tablets ... ▣ 873
- Quadrinal Tablets ... 1350

Ephedrine Sulfate (Beta-blocker can blunt the bronchodilator effect of beta-receptor agonists in patients with bronchospasm; greater than normal anti-asthmatic dose of beta-agonist may be required). Products include:
- Bronkaid Caplets ... ▣ 717
- Marax Tablets & DF Syrup ... 2200

Ephedrine Tannate (Beta-blocker can blunt the bronchodilator effect of beta-receptor agonists in patients with bronchospasm; greater than normal anti-asthmatic dose of beta-agonist may be required). Products include:
- Rynatuss ... 2673

Epinephrine (Potential for unresponsiveness to the usual dose of epinephrine to treat allergic reaction). Products include:
- Bronkaid Mist ... ▣ 717
- EPIFRIN ... ⊙ 239
- EpiPen ... 790
- Marcaine Hydrochloride with Epinephrine 1:200,000 ... 2316
- Primatene Mist ... ▣ 873
- Sensorcaine with Epinephrine Injection ... 559
- Sus-Phrine Injection ... 1019
- Xylocaine with Epinephrine Injections ... 567

(▣ Described in PDR For Nonprescription Drugs) (⊙ Described in PDR For Ophthalmology)

Interactions Index

Epinephrine Hydrochloride (Potential for unresponsiveness to the usual dose of epinephrine to treat allergic reaction). Products include:

Ana-Kit Anaphylaxis Emergency Treatment Kit 617

Ethylnorepinephrine Hydrochloride (Beta-blocker can blunt the bronchodilator effect of beta-receptor agonists in patients with bronchospasm; greater than normal anti-asthmatic dose of beta-agonist may be required).

No products indexed under this heading.

Glipizide (Altered dosage requirements). Products include:

Glucotrol Tablets 1967
Glucotrol XL Extended Release Tablets 1968

Glyburide (Altered dosage requirements). Products include:

DiaBeta Tablets 1239
Glynase PresTab Tablets 2609
Micronase Tablets 2623

Halothane (Synergism has been reported between labetalol I.V. and halothane anesthesia; potential increased hypotensive effect, reduction in cardiac output and increase in central venous pressure). Products include:

Fluothane 2724

Imipramine Hydrochloride (Potential for tremor). Products include:

Tofranil Ampuls 854
Tofranil Tablets 856

Imipramine Pamoate (Potential for tremor). Products include:

Tofranil-PM Capsules 857

Insulin, Human (Altered dosage requirements).

No products indexed under this heading.

Insulin, Human Isophane Suspension (Altered dosage requirements). Products include:

Novolin N Human Insulin 10 ml Vials 1795

Insulin, Human NPH (Altered dosage requirements). Products include:

Humulin N, 100 Units 1448
Novolin N PenFill Cartridges Durable Insulin Delivery System 1798
Novolin N Prefilled Syringe Disposable Insulin Delivery System 1798

Insulin, Human Regular (Altered dosage requirements). Products include:

Humulin R, 100 Units 1449
Novolin R Human Insulin 10 ml Vials 1795
Novolin R PenFill Cartridges Durable Insulin Delivery System 1798
Novolin R Prefilled Syringe Disposable Insulin Delivery System 1798
Velosulin BR Human Insulin 10 ml Vials 1795

Insulin, Human, Zinc Suspension (Altered dosage requirements). Products include:

Humulin L, 100 Units 1446
Humulin U, 100 Units 1450
Novolin L Human Insulin 10 ml Vials 1795

Insulin, NPH (Altered dosage requirements). Products include:

NPH, 100 Units 1450
Pork NPH, 100 Units 1452
Purified Pork NPH Isophane Insulin 1801

Insulin, Regular (Altered dosage requirements). Products include:

Regular, 100 Units 1450
Pork Regular, 100 Units 1452
Pork Regular (Concentrated), 500 Units 1453

Purified Pork Regular Insulin 1801

Insulin, Zinc Crystals (Altered dosage requirements). Products include:

NPH, 100 Units 1450

Insulin, Zinc Suspension (Altered dosage requirements). Products include:

Iletin I 1450
Lente, 100 Units 1450
Iletin II 1452
Pork Lente, 100 Units 1452
Purified Pork Lente Insulin 1801

Isoetharine (Beta-blocker can blunt the bronchodilator effect of beta-receptor agonists in patients with bronchospasm; greater than normal anti-asthmatic dose of beta-agonist may be required). Products include:

Bronkometer Aerosol 2302
Bronkosol Solution 2302
Isoetharine Inhalation Solution, USP, Arm-a-Med 551

Isoproterenol Hydrochloride (Beta-blocker can blunt the bronchodilator effect of beta-receptor agonists in patients with bronchospasm; greater than normal anti-asthmatic dose of beta-agonist may be required). Products include:

Isuprel Hydrochloride Injection 1:5000 2311
Isuprel Hydrochloride Solution 1:200 & 1:100 2313
Isuprel Mistometer 2312

Isoproterenol Sulfate (Beta-blocker can blunt the bronchodilator effect of beta-receptor agonists in patients with bronchospasm; greater than normal anti-asthmatic dose of beta-agonist may be required). Products include:

Norisodrine with Calcium Iodide Syrup 442

Maprotiline Hydrochloride (Potential for tremor). Products include:

Ludiomil Tablets 843

Metaproterenol Sulfate (Beta-blocker can blunt the bronchodilator effect of beta-receptor agonists in patients with bronchospasm; greater than normal anti-asthmatic dose of beta-agonist may be required). Products include:

Alupent 669
Metaproterenol Sulfate Inhalation Solution, USP, Arm-a-Med 552

Metformin Hydrochloride (Altered dosage requirements). Products include:

Glucophage 752

Nitroglycerin (Reflex tachycardia produced by nitroglycerin blunted). Products include:

Deponit NTG Transdermal Delivery System 2397
Nitro-Bid IV 1523
Nitro-Bid Ointment 1524
Nitrodisc 2047
Nitro-Dur (nitroglycerin) Transdermal Infusion System 1326
Nitrolingual Spray 2027
Nitrostat Tablets 1925
Transderm-Nitro Transdermal Therapeutic System 859

Nortriptyline Hydrochloride (Potential for tremor). Products include:

Pamelor 2280

Pirbuterol Acetate (Beta-blocker can blunt the bronchodilator effect of beta-receptor agonists in patients with bronchospasm; greater than normal anti-asthmatic dose of beta-agonist may be required). Products include:

Maxair Autohaler 1492
Maxair Inhaler 1494

Protriptyline Hydrochloride (Potential for tremor). Products include:

Vivactil Tablets 1774

Salmeterol Xinafoate (Beta-blocker can blunt the bronchodilator effect of beta-receptor agonists in patients with bronchospasm; greater than normal anti-asthmatic dose of beta-agonist may be required). Products include:

Serevent Inhalation Aerosol 1176

Terbutaline Sulfate (Beta-blocker can blunt the bronchodilator effect of beta-receptor agonists in patients with bronchospasm; greater than normal anti-asthmatic dose of beta-agonist may be required). Products include:

Brethaire Inhaler 813
Brethine Ampuls 815
Brethine Tablets 814
Bricanyl Subcutaneous Injection 1502
Bricanyl Tablets 1503

Tolazamide (Altered dosage requirements).

No products indexed under this heading.

Tolbutamide (Altered dosage requirements).

No products indexed under this heading.

Trimipramine Maleate (Potential for tremor). Products include:

Surmontil Capsules 2811

Verapamil Hydrochloride (Care should be taken if coadministered; effects of concomitant use not specified). Products include:

Calan SR Caplets 2422
Calan Tablets 2419
Isoptin Injectable 1344
Isoptin Oral Tablets 1346
Isoptin SR Tablets 1348
Verelan Capsules 1410
Verelan Capsules 2824

NOROXIN TABLETS

(Norfloxacin) 1715

May interact with antacids, xanthine bronchodilators, oral anticoagulants, and certain other agents. Compounds in these categories include:

Aluminum Carbonate Gel (Concomitant administration not recommended). Products include:

Basaljel 2703

Aluminum Hydroxide (Concomitant administration not recommended). Products include:

ALternaGEL Liquid 1316
Maximum Strength Ascriptin .... ⊕ 630
Cama Arthritis Pain Reliever .... ⊕ 785
Gaviscon Extra Strength Relief Formula Antacid Tablets .... ⊕ 819
Gaviscon Extra Strength Relief Formula Liquid Antacid .... ⊕ 819
Gaviscon Liquid Antacid .... ⊕ 820
Gelusil Liquid & Tablets .... ⊕ 855
Maalox Heartburn Relief Suspension .... ⊕ 642
Maalox Heartburn Relief Tablets .... ⊕ 641
Maalox Magnesia and Alumina Oral Suspension .... ⊕ 642
Maalox Plus Tablets .... ⊕ 643
Extra Strength Maalox Antacid Plus Antigas Liquid and Tablets ⊕ 638
Tempo Soft Antacid .... ⊕ 835

Aluminum Hydroxide Gel (Concomitant administration not recommended). Products include:

ALternaGEL Liquid .... ⊕ 659
Aludrox Oral Suspension 2695
Amphojel Suspension 2695
Amphojel Suspension without Flavor 2695
Amphojel Tablets 2695
Arthritis Pain Ascriptin .... ⊕ 631
Regular Strength Ascriptin Tablets .... ⊕ 629
Gaviscon Antacid Tablets .... ⊕ 819

Gaviscon-2 Antacid Tablets .... ⊕ 820
Mylanta Liquid 1317
Mylanta Tablets .... ⊕ 660
Mylanta Double Strength Liquid 1317
Mylanta Double Strength Tablets .. ⊕ 660
Nephrox Suspension .... ⊕ 655

Aminophylline (Elevated theophylline plasma levels).

No products indexed under this heading.

Caffeine (May interfere with the metabolism of caffeine). Products include:

Arthritis Strength BC Powder .... ⊕ 609
BC Powder .... ⊕ 609
Bayer Select Headache Pain Relief Formula .... ⊕ 716
Cafergot 2251
DHCplus Capsules 1993
Darvon Compound-65 Pulvules 1435
Esgic-plus Tablets 1013
Aspirin Free Excedrin Analgesic Caplets and Geltabs 732
Excedrin Extra-Strength Analgesic Tablets & Caplets 732
Fioricet Tablets 2258
Fioricet with Codeine Capsules 2260
Fiorinal Capsules 2261
Fiorinal with Codeine Capsules 2262
Fiorinal Tablets 2261
Maximum Strength Multi-Symptom Formula Midol .... ⊕ 722
Migralam Capsules 2038
No Doz Maximum Strength Caplets .... ⊕ 622
Norgesic 1496
Vanquish Analgesic Caplets .... ⊕ 731
Wigraine Tablets & Suppositories .. 1829

Cyclosporine (Elevated serum levels of cyclosporine). Products include:

Neoral 2276
Sandimmune 2286

Dicumarol (Potential for enhanced effects of oral anticoagulant).

No products indexed under this heading.

Dihydroxyaluminum Sodium Carbonate (Concomitant administration not recommended).

No products indexed under this heading.

Dyphylline (Elevated theophylline plasma levels). Products include:

Lufyllin & Lufyllin-400 Tablets 2670
Lufyllin-GG Elixir & Tablets 2671

Magaldrate (Concomitant administration not recommended).

No products indexed under this heading.

Magnesium Hydroxide (Concomitant administration not recommended). Products include:

Aludrox Oral Suspension 2695
Arthritis Pain Ascriptin .... ⊕ 631
Maximum Strength Ascriptin .... ⊕ 630
Regular Strength Ascriptin Tablets .... ⊕ 629
Di-Gel Antacid/Anti-Gas .... ⊕ 801
Gelusil Liquid & Tablets .... ⊕ 855
Maalox Magnesia and Alumina Oral Suspension .... ⊕ 642
Maalox Plus Tablets .... ⊕ 643
Extra Strength Maalox Antacid Plus Antigas Liquid and Tablets ⊕ 638
Mylanta Calcium Carbonate and Magnesium Hydroxide Tablets 1318
Mylanta Liquid 1317
Mylanta Tablets .... ⊕ 660
Mylanta Double Strength Liquid 1317
Mylanta Double Strength Tablets .. ⊕ 660
Phillips' Milk of Magnesia Liquid .... ⊕ 729
Rolaids Tablets .... ⊕ 843
Tempo Soft Antacid .... ⊕ 835

Magnesium Oxide (Concomitant administration not recommended). Products include:

Beelith Tablets 639
Bufferin Analgesic Tablets and Caplets .... ⊕ 613
Caltrate PLUS .... ⊕ 665
Cama Arthritis Pain Reliever .... ⊕ 785
Mag-Ox 400 668
Uro-Mag 668

IMPORTANT NOTE: Always consult each drug listing in the patient's regimen for possible interactions.

Nitrofurantoin (Concomitant use not recommended; antagonizes antibacterial effect of norfloxacin in urinary tract). Products include:

Macrodantin Capsules 1989

Probenecid (Diminished urinary excretion of norfloxacin). Products include:

Benemid Tablets 1611
ColBENEMID Tablets 1622

Sucralfate (May interfere with absorption resulting in lower levels of norfloxacin). Products include:

Carafate Suspension 1505
Carafate Tablets 1504

Theophylline (Elevated theophylline plasma levels). Products include:

Marax Tablets & DF Syrup 2200
Quibron 2053

Theophylline Anhydrous (Elevated theophylline plasma levels). Products include:

Aerolate 1004
Primatene Dual Action Formula .... ◘ 872
Primatene Tablets .... ◘ 873
Respbid Tablets 682
Slo-bid Gyrocaps 2033
Theo-24 Extended Release Capsules 2568
Theo-Dur Extended-Release Tablets 1327
Theo-X Extended-Release Tablets .. 788
Uni-Dur Extended-Release Tablets .. 1331
Uniphyl 400 mg Tablets 2001

Theophylline Calcium Salicylate (Elevated theophylline plasma levels). Products include:

Quadrinal Tablets 1350

Theophylline Sodium Glycinate (Elevated theophylline plasma levels).

No products indexed under this heading.

Vitamins with Iron (May result in lower serum and urine levels of norfloxacin). Products include:

Bugs Bunny/Flintstones .... ◘ 718
Iberet Tablets 433
Iberet-500 Liquid 433
Iberet-Folic-500 Filmtab 429
Iberet-Liquid 433
Materna Tablets 1379
Nephro-Vite + Fe Tablets 2006
Niferex-PN Tablets 794
Stresstabs + Iron .... ◘ 671
Sunkist Children's Chewable Multivitamins - Plus Iron .... ◘ 649
Trinsicon Capsules 2570

Warfarin Sodium (Potential for enhanced effects of oral anticoagulant). Products include:

Coumadin 926

Zinc Sulfate (May result in lower serum and urine levels of norfloxacin). Products include:

Clear Eyes ACR Astringent/Lubricant Eye Redness Reliever Eye Drops .... ⊙ 316
Visine Maximum Strength Allergy Relief .... ⊙ 313

Food Interactions

Food, unspecified (The presence of food may decrease the absorption).

NOROXIN TABLETS

(Norfloxacin) 2048

May interact with antacids, xanthine bronchodilators, oral anticoagulants, and certain other agents. Compounds in these categories include:

Aluminum Carbonate Gel (Concomitant administration not recommended). Products include:

Basaljel 2703

Aluminum Hydroxide (Concomitant administration not recommended). Products include:

ALternaGEL Liquid 1316
Maximum Strength Ascriptin .... ◘ 630
Cama Arthritis Pain Reliever .... ◘ 785
Gaviscon Extra Strength Relief Formula Antacid Tablets .... ◘ 819
Gaviscon Extra Strength Relief Formula Liquid Antacid .... ◘ 819
Gaviscon Liquid Antacid .... ◘ 820
Gelusil Liquid & Tablets .... ◘ 855
Maalox Heartburn Relief Suspension .... ◘ 642
Maalox Heartburn Relief Tablets .... ◘ 641
Maalox Magnesia and Alumina Oral Suspension .... ◘ 642
Maalox Plus Tablets .... ◘ 643
Extra Strength Maalox Antacid Plus Antigas Liquid and Tablets ◘ 638
Tempo Soft Antacid .... ◘ 835

Aluminum Hydroxide Gel (Concomitant administration not recommended). Products include:

ALternaGEL Liquid .... ◘ 659
Aludrox Oral Suspension 2695
Amphojel Suspension 2695
Amphojel Suspension without Flavor 2695
Amphojel Tablets 2695
Arthritis Pain Ascriptin .... ◘ 631
Regular Strength Ascriptin Tablets .... ◘ 629
Gaviscon Antacid Tablets .... ◘ 819
Gaviscon-2 Antacid Tablets .... ◘ 820
Mylanta Liquid 1317
Mylanta Tablets .... ◘ 660
Mylanta Double Strength Liquid 1317
Mylanta Double Strength Tablets .. ◘ 660
Nephrox Suspension .... ◘ 655

Aminophylline (Elevated theophylline plasma levels).

No products indexed under this heading.

Caffeine (May interfere with the metabolism of caffeine). Products include:

Arthritis Strength BC Powder .... ◘ 609
BC Powder .... ◘ 609
Bayer Select Headache Pain Relief Formula .... ◘ 716
Cafergot 2251
DHCplus Capsules 1993
Darvon Compound-65 Pulvules 1435
Esgic-plus Tablets 1013
Aspirin Free Excedrin Analgesic Caplets and Geltabs 732
Excedrin Extra-Strength Analgesic Tablets & Caplets 732
Fioricet Tablets 2258
Fioricet with Codeine Capsules 2260
Fiorinal Capsules 2261
Fiorinal with Codeine Capsules 2262
Fiorinal Tablets 2261
Maximum Strength Multi-Symptom Formula Midol .... ◘ 722
Migralam Capsules 2038
No Doz Maximum Strength Caplets .... ◘ 622
Norgesic 1496
Vanquish Analgesic Caplets .... ◘ 731
Wigraine Tablets & Suppositories .. 1829

Cyclosporine (Elevated serum levels of cyclosporine). Products include:

Neoral 2276
Sandimmune 2286

Dicumarol (Potential for enhanced effects of oral anticoagulant).

No products indexed under this heading.

Dihydroxyaluminum Sodium Carbonate (Concomitant administration not recommended).

No products indexed under this heading.

Dyphylline (Elevated theophylline plasma levels). Products include:

Lufyllin & Lufyllin-400 Tablets 2670
Lufyllin-GG Elixir & Tablets 2671

Magaldrate (Concomitant administration not recommended).

No products indexed under this heading.

Magnesium Hydroxide (Concomitant administration not recommended). Products include:

Aludrox Oral Suspension 2695
Arthritis Pain Ascriptin .... ◘ 631
Maximum Strength Ascriptin .... ◘ 630
Regular Strength Ascriptin Tablets .... ◘ 629
Di-Gel Antacid/Anti-Gas .... ◘ 801
Gelusil Liquid & Tablets .... ◘ 855
Maalox Magnesia and Alumina Oral Suspension .... ◘ 642
Maalox Plus Tablets .... ◘ 643
Extra Strength Maalox Antacid Plus Antigas Liquid and Tablets ◘ 638
Mylanta Calcium Carbonate and Magnesium Hydroxide Tablets 1318
Mylanta Liquid 1317
Mylanta Tablets .... ◘ 660
Mylanta Double Strength Liquid 1317
Mylanta Double Strength Tablets .. ◘ 660
Phillips' Milk of Magnesia Liquid .... ◘ 729
Rolaids Tablets .... ◘ 843
Tempo Soft Antacid .... ◘ 835

Magnesium Oxide (Concomitant administration not recommended). Products include:

Beelith Tablets 639
Bufferin Analgesic Tablets and Caplets .... ◘ 613
Caltrate PLUS .... ◘ 665
Cama Arthritis Pain Reliever .... ◘ 785
Mag-Ox 400 668
Uro-Mag 668

Nitrofurantoin (Concomitant use not recommended; antagonizes antibacterial effect of norfloxacin in urinary tract). Products include:

Macrodantin Capsules 1989

Probenecid (Diminished urinary excretion of norfloxacin). Products include:

Benemid Tablets 1611
ColBENEMID Tablets 1622

Sucralfate (May interfere with absorption resulting in lower levels of norfloxacin). Products include:

Carafate Suspension 1505
Carafate Tablets 1504

Theophylline (Elevated theophylline plasma levels). Products include:

Marax Tablets & DF Syrup 2200
Quibron 2053

Theophylline Anhydrous (Elevated theophylline plasma levels). Products include:

Aerolate 1004
Primatene Dual Action Formula ...... ◘ 872
Primatene Tablets .... ◘ 873
Respbid Tablets 682
Slo-bid Gyrocaps 2033
Theo-24 Extended Release Capsules 2568
Theo-Dur Extended-Release Tablets 1327
Theo-X Extended-Release Tablets .. 788
Uni-Dur Extended-Release Tablets .. 1331
Uniphyl 400 mg Tablets 2001

Theophylline Calcium Salicylate (Elevated theophylline plasma levels). Products include:

Quadrinal Tablets 1350

Theophylline Sodium Glycinate (Elevated theophylline plasma levels).

No products indexed under this heading.

Vitamins with Iron (May result in lower serum and urine levels of norfloxacin). Products include:

Bugs Bunny/Flintstones .... ◘ 718
Iberet Tablets 433
Iberet-500 Liquid 433
Iberet-Folic-500 Filmtab 429
Iberet-Liquid 433
Materna Tablets 1379
Nephro-Vite + Fe Tablets 2006
Niferex-PN Tablets 794
Stresstabs + Iron .... ◘ 671
Sunkist Children's Chewable Multivitamins - Plus Iron .... ◘ 649
Trinsicon Capsules 2570

Warfarin Sodium (Potential for enhanced effects of oral anticoagulant). Products include:

Coumadin 926

Zinc Sulfate (May result in lower serum and urine levels of norfloxacin). Products include:

Clear Eyes ACR Astringent/Lubricant Eye Redness Reliever Eye Drops .... ⊙ 316
Visine Maximum Strength Allergy Relief .... ⊙ 313

Food Interactions

Food, unspecified (The presence of food may decrease the absorption).

NORPACE CAPSULES

(Disopyramide Phosphate) 2444

May interact with antiarrhythmics, hepatic microsomal enzyme inducers, and certain other agents. Compounds in these categories include:

Acebutolol Hydrochloride (Excessive widening of QRS complex and prolongation of Q-T interval). Products include:

Sectral Capsules 2807

Adenosine (Excessive widening of QRS complex and prolongation of Q-T interval). Products include:

Adenocard Injection 1021
Adenoscan 1024

Amiodarone Hydrochloride (Excessive widening of QRS complex and prolongation of Q-T interval). Products include:

Cordarone Intravenous 2715
Cordarone Tablets 2712

Bretylium Tosylate (Excessive widening of QRS complex and prolongation of Q-T interval).

No products indexed under this heading.

Carbamazepine (Concurrent administration with hepatic enzyme inducers may lower plasma levels of disopyramide). Products include:

Atretol Tablets 573
Tegretol Chewable Tablets 852
Tegretol Suspension 852
Tegretol Tablets 852

Chlorpropamide (Concurrent administration with hepatic enzyme inducers may lower plasma levels of disopyramide). Products include:

Diabinese Tablets 1935

Glipizide (Concurrent administration with hepatic enzyme inducers may lower plasma levels of disopyramide). Products include:

Glucotrol Tablets 1967
Glucotrol XL Extended Release Tablets 1968

Glyburide (Concurrent administration with hepatic enzyme inducers may lower plasma levels of disopyramide). Products include:

DiaBeta Tablets 1239
Glynase PresTab Tablets 2609
Micronase Tablets 2623

Lidocaine Hydrochloride (Excessive widening of QRS complex and prolongation of Q-T interval). Products include:

Bactine Antiseptic/Anesthetic First Aid Liquid .... ◘ 708
Campho-Phenique Maximum Strength First Aid Antibiotic Plus Pain Reliever Ointment .... ◘ 719
Decadron Phosphate with Xylocaine Injection, Sterile 1639
Xylocaine Injections 567

Mexiletine Hydrochloride (Excessive widening of QRS complex and prolongation of Q-T interval). Products include:

Mexitil Capsules 678

Moricizine Hydrochloride (Excessive widening of QRS complex and prolongation of Q-T interval). Products include:

Ethmozine Tablets 2041

Phenobarbital (Concurrent administration with hepatic enzyme inducers may lower plasma levels of disopyramide). Products include:

Arco-Lase Plus Tablets 512
Bellergal-S Tablets 2250
Donnatal 2060

(◘ Described in PDR For Nonprescription Drugs) (⊙ Described in PDR For Ophthalmology)

Donnatal Extentabs 2061
Donnatal Tablets 2060
Phenobarbital Elixir and Tablets 1469
Quadrinal Tablets 1350

Phenylbutazone (Concurrent administration with hepatic enzyme inducers may lower plasma levels of disopyramide).
No products indexed under this heading.

Phenytoin (Concurrent administration with hepatic enzyme inducers may lower plasma levels of disopyramide). Products include:
Dilantin Infatabs 1908
Dilantin-125 Suspension 1911

Phenytoin Sodium (Concurrent administration with hepatic enzyme inducers may lower plasma levels of disopyramide). Products include:
Dilantin Kapseals 1906
Dilantin Parenteral 1910

Procainamide Hydrochloride (Excessive widening of QRS complex and prolongation of Q-T interval). Products include:
Procan SR Tablets 1926

Propafenone Hydrochloride (Excessive widening of QRS complex and prolongation of Q-T interval). Products include:
Rythmol Tablets–150mg, 225mg, 300mg 1352

Propranolol Hydrochloride (Excessive widening of QRS complex and prolongation of Q-T interval). Products include:
Inderal 2728
Inderal LA Long Acting Capsules 2730
Inderide Tablets 2732
Inderide LA Long Acting Capsules 2734

Quinidine Gluconate (Excessive widening of QRS complex and prolongation of Q-T interval). Products include:
Quinaglute Dura-Tabs Tablets 649

Quinidine Polygalacturonate (Excessive widening of QRS complex and prolongation of Q-T interval).
No products indexed under this heading.

Quinidine Sulfate (Excessive widening of QRS complex and prolongation of Q-T interval). Products include:
Quinidex Extentabs 2067

Rifampin (Concurrent administration with hepatic enzyme inducers may lower plasma levels of disopyramide). Products include:
Rifadin 1528
Rifamate Capsules 1530
Rifater 1532
Rimactane Capsules 847

Sotalol Hydrochloride (Excessive widening of QRS complex and prolongation of Q-T interval). Products include:
Betapace Tablets 641

Tocainide Hydrochloride (Excessive widening of QRS complex and prolongation of Q-T interval). Products include:
Tonocard Tablets 531

Tolazamide (Concurrent administration with hepatic enzyme inducers may lower plasma levels of disopyramide).
No products indexed under this heading.

Tolbutamide (Concurrent administration with hepatic enzyme inducers may lower plasma levels of disopyramide).
No products indexed under this heading.

Verapamil Hydrochloride (Excessive widening of QRS complex and prolongation of Q-T interval; disopyramide should not be administered within 48 hours before or 24 hours after verapamil administration). Products include:
Calan SR Caplets 2422
Calan Tablets 2419
Isoptin Injectable 1344
Isoptin Oral Tablets 1346
Isoptin SR Tablets 1348
Verelan Capsules 1410
Verelan Capsules 2824

NORPACE CR CAPSULES
(Disopyramide Phosphate) 2444
See **Norpace Capsules**

NORPLANT SYSTEM
(Levonorgestrel) 2759
May interact with:

Carbamazepine (Reduces efficacy (pregnancy)). Products include:
Atretol Tablets 573
Tegretol Chewable Tablets 852
Tegretol Suspension 852
Tegretol Tablets 852

Phenytoin (Reduces efficacy (pregnancy)). Products include:
Dilantin Infatabs 1908
Dilantin-125 Suspension 1911

Phenytoin Sodium (Reduces efficacy (pregnancy)). Products include:
Dilantin Kapseals 1906
Dilantin Parenteral 1910

NORPRAMIN TABLETS
(Desipramine Hydrochloride) 1526
May interact with thyroid preparations, anticholinergics, sympathomimetics, benzodiazepines, phenothiazines, tranquilizers, monoamine oxidase inhibitors, tricyclic antidepressants, antidepressant drugs, barbiturates, and certain other agents. Compounds in these categories include:

Albuterol (Close supervision and careful dosage adjustment required). Products include:
Proventil Inhalation Aerosol 2382
Ventolin Inhalation Aerosol and Refill 1197

Albuterol Sulfate (Close supervision and careful dosage adjustment required). Products include:
Airet Solution for Inhalation 452
Proventil Inhalation Solution 0.083% 2384
Proventil Repetabs Tablets 2386
Proventil Solution for Inhalation 0.5% 2383
Proventil Syrup 2385
Proventil Tablets 2386
Ventolin Inhalation Solution 1198
Ventolin Nebules Inhalation Solution 1199
Ventolin Rotacaps for Inhalation 1200
Ventolin Syrup 1202
Ventolin Tablets 1203
Volmax Extended-Release Tablets 1788

Alprazolam (Sedative effects of both drugs are additive). Products include:
Xanax Tablets 2649

Amitriptyline Hydrochloride (An individual who is stable on a given dose of tricyclic may become abruptly toxic when given with drugs that inhibit cytochrome P4502D6 and drugs that are substrates for P4502D6; careful adjustment of dosage is required). Products include:
Elavil 2838
Endep Tablets 2174
Etrafon 2355
Limbitrol 2180
Triavil Tablets 1757

Amoxapine (An individual who is stable on a given dose of tricyclic may become abruptly toxic when given with drugs that inhibit cytochrome P4502D6 and drugs that are substrates for P4502D6; careful adjustment of dosage is required). Products include:
Asendin Tablets 1369

Aprobarbital (Induces liver enzyme activity thereby reduces tricyclic antidepressant plasma levels).
No products indexed under this heading.

Atropine Sulfate (Close supervision and careful dosage adjustment required). Products include:
Arco-Lase Plus Tablets 512
Atrohist Plus Tablets 454
Atropine Sulfate Sterile Ophthalmic Solution .... ◉ 233
Donnatal 2060
Donnatal Extentabs 2061
Donnatal Tablets 2060
Lomotil 2439
Motofen Tablets 784
Urised Tablets 1964

Belladonna Alkaloids (Close supervision and careful dosage adjustment required). Products include:
Bellergal-S Tablets 2250
Hyland's Bed Wetting Tablets .... ▣ 828
Hyland's EnurAid Tablets .... ▣ 829
Hyland's Teething Tablets .... ▣ 830

Benztropine Mesylate (Close supervision and careful dosage adjustment required). Products include:
Cogentin 1621

Biperiden Hydrochloride (Close supervision and careful dosage adjustment required). Products include:
Akineton 1333

Bupropion Hydrochloride (An individual who is stable on a given dose of tricyclic may become abruptly toxic when given with drugs that inhibit cytochrome P4502D6 and drugs that are substrates for P4502D6; careful adjustment of dosage is required). Products include:
Wellbutrin Tablets 1204

Buspirone Hydrochloride (Additive sedative and anticholinergic effects). Products include:
BuSpar 737

Butabarbital (Induces liver enzyme activity thereby reduces tricyclic antidepressant plasma levels).
No products indexed under this heading.

Butalbital (Induces liver enzyme activity thereby reduces tricyclic antidepressant plasma levels). Products include:
Esgic-plus Tablets 1013
Fioricet Tablets 2258
Fioricet with Codeine Capsules 2260
Fiorinal Capsules 2261
Fiorinal with Codeine Capsules 2262
Fiorinal Tablets 2261
Phrenilin 785
Sedapap Tablets 50 mg/650 mg 1543

Carbamazepine (An individual who is stable on a given dose of tricyclic may become abruptly toxic when given with drugs that inhibit cytochrome P4502D6 and drugs that are substrates for P4502D6; careful adjustment of dosage is required). Products include:
Atretol Tablets 573
Tegretol Chewable Tablets 852
Tegretol Suspension 852
Tegretol Tablets 852

Chlordiazepoxide (Sedative effects of both drugs are additive). Products include:
Libritabs Tablets 2177
Limbitrol 2180

Chlordiazepoxide Hydrochloride (Sedative effects of both drugs are additive). Products include:
Librax Capsules 2176
Librium Capsules 2178
Librium Injectable 2179

Chlorpromazine (Additive sedative and anticholinergic effects; increases plasma levels; an individual who is stable on a given dose of tricyclic may become abruptly toxic when given with drugs that inhibit cytochrome P4502D6 and drugs that are substrates for P4502D6; careful adjustment of dosage is required). Products include:
Thorazine Suppositories 2523

Chlorpromazine Hydrochloride (Additive sedative and anticholinergic effects; increases plasma levels; an individual who is stable on a given dose of tricyclic may become abruptly toxic when given with drugs that inhibit cytochrome P4502D6 and drugs that are substrates for P4502D6; careful adjustment of dosage is required). Products include:
Thorazine 2523

Chlorprothixene (Additive sedative and anticholinergic effects).
No products indexed under this heading.

Chlorprothixene Hydrochloride (Additive sedative and anticholinergic effects).
No products indexed under this heading.

Cimetidine (Significant increases in tricyclic antidepressant plasma levels; decreases plasma levels of tricyclic antidepressant upon discontinuation of cimetidine which may result in loss of therapeutic efficacy of the tricyclic antidepressant). Products include:
Tagamet Tablets 2516

Cimetidine Hydrochloride (Significant increases in tricyclic antidepressant plasma levels; decreases plasma levels of tricyclic antidepressant upon discontinuation of cimetidine which may result in loss of therapeutic efficacy of the tricyclic antidepressant). Products include:
Tagamet 2516

Clidinium Bromide (Close supervision and careful dosage adjustment required). Products include:
Librax Capsules 2176
Quarzan Capsules 2181

Clorazepate Dipotassium (Sedative effects of both drugs are additive). Products include:
Tranxene 451

Diazepam (Sedative effects of both drugs are additive). Products include:
Dizac 1809
Valium Injectable 2182
Valium Tablets 2183
Valrelease Capsules 2169

Dicyclomine Hydrochloride (Close supervision and careful dosage adjustment required). Products include:
Bentyl 1501

Dobutamine Hydrochloride (Close supervision and careful dosage adjustment required). Products include:
Dobutrex Solution Vials 1439

IMPORTANT NOTE: Always consult each drug listing in the patient's regimen for possible interactions.

Norpramin Interactions Index 736

Dopamine Hydrochloride (Close supervision and careful dosage adjustment required).
No products indexed under this heading.

Doxepin Hydrochloride (An individual who is stable on a given dose of tricyclic may become abruptly toxic when given with drugs that inhibit cytochrome P4502D6 and drugs that are substrates for P4502D6; careful adjustment of dosage is required). Products include:
Sinequan ... 2205
Zonalon Cream ... 1055

Droperidol (Additive sedative and anticholinergic effects). Products include:
Inapsine Injection ... 1296

Ephedrine Hydrochloride (Close supervision and careful dosage adjustment required). Products include:
Primatene Dual Action Formula ◘ 872
Primatene Tablets ◘ 873
Quadrinal Tablets ... 1350

Ephedrine Sulfate (Close supervision and careful dosage adjustments required). Products include:
Bronkaid Caplets ◘ 717
Marax Tablets & DF Syrup ... 2200

Ephedrine Tannate (Close supervision and careful dosage adjustment required). Products include:
Rynatuss ... 2673

Epinephrine (Close supervision and careful dosage adjustment required). Products include:
Bronkaid Mist ◘ 717
EPIFRIN ⊙ 239
EpiPen ... 790
Marcaine Hydrochloride with Epinephrine 1:200,000 ... 2316
Primatene Mist ◘ 873
Sensorcaine with Epinephrine Injection ... 559
Sus-Phrine Injection ... 1019
Xylocaine with Epinephrine Injections ... 567

Epinephrine Bitartrate (Close supervision and careful dosage adjustment required). Products include:
Bronkaid Mist Suspension ◘ 718
Sensorcaine-MPF with Epinephrine Injection ... 559

Epinephrine Hydrochloride (Close supervision and careful dosage adjustment required). Products include:
Ana-Kit Anaphylaxis Emergency Treatment Kit ... 617

Estazolam (Sedative effects of both drugs are additive). Products include:
ProSom Tablets ... 449

Flecainide Acetate (An individual who is stable on a given dose of tricyclic may become abruptly toxic when given with drugs that inhibit cytochrome P4502D6 and drugs that are substrates for P4502D6; careful adjustment of dosage is required). Products include:
Tambocor Tablets ... 1497

Fluoxetine Hydrochloride (An individual who is stable on a given dose of tricyclic may become abruptly toxic when given with drugs that inhibit cytochrome P4502D6 and drugs that are substrates for P4502D6; careful adjustment of dosage is required). Products include:
Prozac Pulvules & Liquid, Oral Solution ... 919

Fluphenazine Decanoate (Additive sedative and anticholinergic effects; increases plasma levels; an individual who is stable on a given dose of tricyclic may become abruptly toxic when given with drugs that inhibit cytochrome P4502D6 and drugs that are substrates for P4502D6; careful adjustment of dosage is required). Products include:
Prolixin Decanoate ... 509

Fluphenazine Enanthate (Additive sedative and anticholinergic effects; increases plasma levels; an individual who is stable on a given dose of tricyclic may become abruptly toxic when given with drugs that inhibit cytochrome P4502D6 and drugs that are substrates for P4502D6; careful adjustment of dosage is required). Products include:
Prolixin Enanthate ... 509

Fluphenazine Hydrochloride (Additive sedative and anticholinergic effects; increases plasma levels; an individual who is stable on a given dose of tricyclic may become abruptly toxic when given with drugs that inhibit cytochrome P4502D6 and drugs that are substrates for P4502D6; careful adjustment of dosage is required). Products include:
Prolixin ... 509

Flurazepam Hydrochloride (Sedative effects of both drugs are additive). Products include:
Dalmane Capsules ... 2173

Furazolidone (Contraindication; hyperpyretic crises; severe convulsions; death). Products include:
Furoxone ... 2046

Glycopyrrolate (Close supervision and careful dosage adjustment required). Products include:
Robinul Forte Tablets ... 2072
Robinul Injectable ... 2072
Robinul Tablets ... 2072

Guanethidine Monosulfate (Antihypertensive effect blocked). Products include:
Esimil Tablets ... 822
Ismelin Tablets ... 827

Halazepam (Sedative effects of both drugs are additive).
No products indexed under this heading.

Haloperidol (Additive sedative and anticholinergic effects). Products include:
Haldol Injection, Tablets and Concentrate ... 1575

Haloperidol Decanoate (Additive sedative and anticholinergic effects). Products include:
Haldol Decanoate ... 1577

Hydroxyzine Hydrochloride (Additive sedative and anticholinergic effects). Products include:
Atarax Tablets & Syrup ... 2185
Marax Tablets & DF Syrup ... 2200
Vistaril Intramuscular Solution ... 2216

Hyoscyamine (Close supervision and careful dosage adjustment required). Products include:
Cystospaz Tablets ... 1963
Urised Tablets ... 1964

Hyoscyamine Sulfate (Close supervision and careful dosage adjustment required). Products include:
Arco-Lase Plus Tablets ... 512
Atrohist Plus Tablets ... 454
Cystospaz-M Capsules ... 1963
Donnatal ... 2060
Donnatal Extentabs ... 2061
Donnatal Tablets ... 2060
Kutrase Capsules ... 2402
Levsin/Levsinex/Levbid ... 2405

Imipramine Hydrochloride (An individual who is stable on a given dose of tricyclic may become abruptly toxic when given with drugs that inhibit cytochrome P4502D6 and drugs that are substrates for P4502D6; careful adjustment of dosage is required). Products include:
Tofranil Ampuls ... 854
Tofranil Tablets ... 856

Imipramine Pamoate (An individual who is stable on a given dose of tricyclic may become abruptly toxic when given with drugs that inhibit cytochrome P4502D6 and drugs that are substrates for P4502D6; careful adjustment of dosage is required). Products include:
Tofranil-PM Capsules ... 857

Ipratropium Bromide (Close supervision and careful dosage adjustment required). Products include:
Atrovent Inhalation Aerosol ... 671
Atrovent Inhalation Solution ... 673

Isocarboxazid (An individual who is stable on a given dose of tricyclic may become abruptly toxic when given with drugs that inhibit cytochrome P4502D6 and drugs that are substrates for P4502D6; careful adjustment of dosage is required).
No products indexed under this heading.

Isoproterenol Hydrochloride (Close supervision and careful dosage adjustment required). Products include:
Isuprel Hydrochloride Injection 1:5000 ... 2311
Isuprel Hydrochloride Solution 1:200 & 1:100 ... 2313
Isuprel Mistometer ... 2312

Isoproterenol Sulfate (Close supervision and careful dosage adjustment required). Products include:
Norisodrine with Calcium Iodide Syrup ... 442

Lorazepam (Sedative effects of both drugs are additive). Products include:
Ativan Injection ... 2698
Ativan Tablets ... 2700

Loxapine Hydrochloride (Additive sedative and anticholinergic effects). Products include:
Loxitane ... 1378

Loxapine Succinate (Additive sedative and anticholinergic effects). Products include:
Loxitane Capsules ... 1378

Maprotiline Hydrochloride (An individual who is stable on a given dose of tricyclic may become abruptly toxic when given with drugs that inhibit cytochrome P4502D6 and drugs that are substrates for P4502D6; careful adjustment of dosage is required). Products include:
Ludiomil Tablets ... 843

Mepenzolate Bromide (Close supervision and careful dosage adjustment required).
No products indexed under this heading.

Mephobarbital (Induces liver enzyme activity thereby reduces tricyclic antidepressant plasma levels). Products include:
Mebaral Tablets ... 2322

Meprobamate (Additive sedative and anticholinergic effects). Products include:
Miltown Tablets ... 2672
PMB 200 and PMB 400 ... 2783

Mesoridazine Besylate (Additive sedative and anticholinergic effects; increases plasma levels; an individual who is stable on a given dose of tricyclic may become abruptly toxic when given with drugs that inhibit cytochrome P4502D6 and drugs that are substrates for P4502D6; careful adjustment of dosage is required). Products include:
Serentil ... 684

Metaproterenol Sulfate (Close supervision and careful dosage adjustment required). Products include:
Alupent ... 669
Metaproterenol Sulfate Inhalation Solution, USP, Arm-a-Med ... 552

Metaraminol Bitartrate (Close supervision and careful dosage adjustment required). Products include:
Aramine Injection ... 1609

Methotrimeprazine (Additive sedative and anticholinergic effects; increases plasma levels; an individual who is stable on a given dose of tricyclic may become abruptly toxic when given with drugs that inhibit cytochrome P4502D6 and drugs that are substrates forP4502D6; careful adjustment of dosage is required). Products include:
Levoprome ... 1274

Methoxamine Hydrochloride (Close supervision and careful dosage adjustment required). Products include:
Vasoxyl Injection ... 1196

Midazolam Hydrochloride (Sedative effects of both drugs are additive). Products include:
Versed Injection ... 2170

Molindone Hydrochloride (Additive sedative and anticholinergic effects). Products include:
Moban Tablets and Concentrate ... 1048

Nefazodone Hydrochloride (An individual who is stable on a given dose of tricyclic may become abruptly toxic when given with drugs that inhibit cytochrome P4502D6 and drugs that are substrates for P4502D6; careful adjustment of dosage is required). Products include:
Serzone Tablets ... 771

Norepinephrine Bitartrate (Close supervision and careful dosage adjustment required). Products include:
Levophed Bitartrate Injection ... 2315

Nortriptyline Hydrochloride (An individual who is stable on a given dose of tricyclic may become abruptly toxic when given with drugs that inhibit cytochrome P4502D6 and drugs that are substrates for P4502D6; careful adjustment of dosage is required). Products include:
Pamelor ... 2280

Oxazepam (Sedative effects of both drugs are additive). Products include:
Serax Capsules ... 2810
Serax Tablets ... 2810

Oxybutynin Chloride (Close supervision and careful dosage adjustment required). Products include:
Ditropan ... 1516

(◘ Described in PDR For Nonprescription Drugs) (⊙ Described in PDR For Ophthalmology)

Interactions Index

Norpramin

Paroxetine Hydrochloride (An individual who is stable on a given dose of tricyclic may become abruptly toxic when given with drugs that inhibit cytochrome P4502D6 and drugs that are substrates for P4502D6; careful adjustment of dosage is required). Products include:

Paxil Tablets 2505

Pentobarbital Sodium (Induces liver enzyme activity thereby reduces tricyclic antidepressant plasma levels). Products include:

Nembutal Sodium Capsules 436
Nembutal Sodium Solution 438
Nembutal Sodium Suppositories....... 440

Perphenazine (Additive sedative and anticholinergic effects; increases plasma levels; an individual who is stable on a given dose of tricyclic may become abruptly toxic when given with drugs that inhibit cytochrome P4502D6 and drugs that are substrates for P4502D6; careful adjustment of dosage is required). Products include:

Etrafon 2355
Triavil Tablets 1757
Trilafon.. 2389

Phenelzine Sulfate (An individual who is stable on a given dose of tricyclic may become abruptly toxic when given with drugs that inhibit cytochrome P4502D6 and drugs that are substrates for P4502D6; careful adjustment of dosage is required). Products include:

Nardil 1920

Phenobarbital (Induces liver enzyme activity thereby reduces tricyclic antidepressant plasma levels). Products include:

Arco-Lase Plus Tablets 512
Bellergal-S Tablets 2250
Donnatal 2060
Donnatal Extentabs............................. 2061
Donnatal Tablets 2060
Phenobarbital Elixir and Tablets 1469
Quadrinal Tablets 1350

Phenylephrine Hydrochloride (Close supervision and careful dosage adjustment required). Products include:

Atrohist Plus Tablets 454
Cerose DM ....⊞ 878
Comhist 2038
D.A. Chewable Tablets....................... 951
Deconsal Pediatric Capsules.............. 454
Dura-Vent/DA Tablets 953
Entex Capsules.................................... 1986
Entex Liquid 1986
Extendryl 1005
4-Way Fast Acting Nasal Spray (regular & mentholated) ....⊞ 621
Hemorid For Women ....⊞ 834
Hycomine Compound Tablets 932
Neo-Synephrine Hydrochloride 1% Carpuject... 2324
Neo-Synephrine Hydrochloride 1% Injection 2324
Neo-Synephrine Hydrochloride (Ophthalmic) 2325
Neo-Synephrine ....⊞ 726
Nōstril ....⊞ 644
Novahistine Elixir ....⊞ 823
Phenergan VC 2779
Phenergan VC with Codeine 2781
Preparation H ....⊞ 871
Tympagesic Ear Drops 2342
Vasosulf .... ⓒ 271
Vicks Sinex Nasal Spray and Ultra Fine Mist ....⊞ 765

Phenylephrine Tannate (Close supervision and careful dosage adjustment required). Products include:

Atrohist Pediatric Suspension 454
Ricobid-D Pediatric Suspension....... 2038
Ricobid Tablets and Pediatric Suspension... 2038
Rynatan 2673
Rynatuss 2673

Phenylpropanolamine Hydrochloride (Close supervision and careful dosage adjustment required). Products include:

Acutrim ....⊞ 628
Allerest Children's Chewable Tablets ....⊞ 627
Allerest 12 Hour Caplets ....⊞ 627
Atrohist Plus Tablets 454
BC Cold Powder Multi-Symptom Formula (Cold-Sinus-Allergy) ......⊞ 609
BC Cold Powder Non-Drowsy Formula (Cold-Sinus) ....⊞ 609
Cheracol Plus Head Cold/Cough Formula ....⊞ 769
Comtrex Multi-Symptom Non-Drowsy Liqui-gels...............................⊞ 618
Contac Continuous Action Nasal Decongestant/Antihistamine 12 Hour Capsules.....................................⊞ 813
Contac Maximum Strength Continuous Action Decongestant/ Antihistamine 12 Hour Caplets..⊞ 813
Contac Severe Cold and Flu Formula Caplets ....⊞ 814
Coricidin 'D' Decongestant Tablets ....⊞ 800
Dexatrim ....⊞ 832
Dexatrim Plus Vitamins Caplets ....⊞ 832
Dimetane-DC Cough Syrup 2059
Dimetapp Elixir ....⊞ 773
Dimetapp Extentabs ....⊞ 774
Dimetapp Tablets/Liqui-Gels ....⊞ 775
Dimetapp Cold & Allergy Chewable Tablets ....⊞ 773
Dimetapp DM Elixir ....⊞ 774
Dura-Vent Tablets 952
Entex Capsules.................................... 1986
Entex LA Tablets 1987
Entex Liquid 1986
Exgest LA Tablets 782
Hycomine 931
Isoclor Timesule Capsules ....⊞ 637
Nolamine Timed-Release Tablets 785
Ornade Spansule Capsules 2502
Propagest Tablets 786
Pyrroxate Caplets ....⊞ 772
Robitussin-CF ....⊞ 777
Sinulin Tablets 787
Tavist-D 12 Hour Relief Tablets ....⊞ 787
Teldrin 12 Hour Antihistamine/ Nasal Decongestant Allergy Relief Capsules ....⊞ 826
Triaminic Allergy Tablets ....⊞ 789
Triaminic Cold Tablets ....⊞ 790
Triaminic Expectorant ....⊞ 790
Triaminic Syrup ....⊞ 792
Triaminic-12 Tablets ....⊞ 792
Triaminic-DM Syrup ....⊞ 792
Triaminicin Tablets.............................⊞ 793
Triaminicol Multi-Symptom Cold Tablets ....⊞ 793
Triaminicol Multi-Symptom Relief ⊞ 794
Vicks DayQuil Allergy Relief 12-Hour Extended Release Tablets..⊞ 760
Vicks DayQuil Allergy Relief 4-Hour Tablets ....⊞ 760
Vicks DayQuil SINUS Pressure & CONGESTION Relief.........................⊞ 761

Pirbuterol Acetate (Close supervision and careful dosage adjustment required). Products include:

Maxair Autohaler 1492
Maxair Inhaler 1494

Prazepam (Sedative effects of both drugs are additive).

No products indexed under this heading.

Prochlorperazine (Additive sedative and anticholinergic effects; increases plasma levels; an individual who is stable on a given dose of tricyclic may become abruptly toxic when given with drugs that inhibit cytochrome P4502D6 and drugs that are substrates for P4502D6; careful adjustment of dosage is required). Products include:

Compazine 2470

Procyclidine Hydrochloride (Close supervision and careful dosage adjustment required). Products include:

Kemadrin Tablets 1112

Promethazine Hydrochloride (Additive sedative and anticholinergic effects; increases plasma levels; an individual who is stable on a given dose of tricyclic may become abruptly toxic when given with drugs that inhibit cytochrome P4502D6 and drugs that are substrates for P4502D6; careful adjustment of dosage is required). Products include:

Mepergan Injection 2753
Phenergan with Codeine..................... 2777
Phenergan with Dextromethorphan 2778
Phenergan Injection 2773
Phenergan Suppositories 2775
Phenergan Syrup 2774
Phenergan Tablets 2775
Phenergan VC 2779
Phenergan VC with Codeine 2781

Propafenone Hydrochloride (An individual who is stable on a given dose of tricyclic may become abruptly toxic when given with drugs that inhibit cytochrome P4502D6 and drugs that are substrates for P4502D6; careful adjustment of dosage is required). Products include:

Rythmol Tablets–150mg, 225mg, 300mg.. 1352

Propantheline Bromide (Close supervision and careful dosage adjustment required). Products include:

Pro-Banthine Tablets........................... 2052

Protriptyline Hydrochloride (An individual who is stable on a given dose of tricyclic may become abruptly toxic when given with drugs that inhibit cytochrome P4502D6 and drugs that are substrates for P4502D6; careful adjustment of dosage is required). Products include:

Vivactil Tablets 1774

Pseudoephedrine Hydrochloride (Close supervision and careful dosage adjustment required). Products include:

Actifed Allergy Daytime/Nighttime Caplets...⊞ 844
Actifed Plus Caplets ....⊞ 845
Actifed Plus Tablets ....⊞ 845
Actifed with Codeine Cough Syrup.. 1067
Actifed Sinus Daytime/Nighttime Tablets and Caplets ....⊞ 846
Actifed Syrup.......................................⊞ 846
Actifed Tablets ....⊞ 844
Advil Cold and Sinus Caplets and Tablets (formerly CoAdvil) ....⊞ 870
Alka-Seltzer Plus Cold Medicine Liqui-Gels ....⊞ 706
Alka-Seltzer Plus Cold & Cough Medicine Liqui-Gels..........................⊞ 705
Alka-Seltzer Plus Night-Time Cold Medicine Liqui-Gels..........................⊞ 706
Allerest Headache Strength Tablets ....⊞ 627
Allerest Maximum Strength Tablets ....⊞ 627
Allerest No Drowsiness Tablets ......⊞ 627
Allerest Sinus Pain Formula ....⊞ 627
Anatuss LA Tablets.............................. 1542
Atrohist Pediatric Capsules................ 453
Bayer Select Sinus Pain Relief Formula ....⊞ 717
Benadryl Allergy Decongestant Liquid Medication ....⊞ 848
Benadryl Allergy Decongestant Tablets ....⊞ 848
Benadryl Allergy Sinus Headache Formula Caplets ....⊞ 849
Benylin Multisymptom ....⊞ 852
Bromfed Capsules (Extended-Release) 1785
Bromfed Syrup ....⊞ 733
Bromfed Tablets 1785
Bromfed-DM Cough Syrup................. 1786
Bromfed-PD Capsules (Extended-Release).. 1785
Children's Vicks DayQuil Allergy Relief ....⊞ 757
Children's Vicks NyQuil Cold/ Cough Relief.......................................⊞ 758

Comtrex Multi-Symptom Cold Reliever Tablets/Caplets/Liqui-Gels/Liquid...⊞ 615
Allergy-Sinus Comtrex Multi-Symptom Allergy-Sinus Formula Tablets ....⊞ 617
Comtrex Multi-Symptom Non-Drowsy Caplets...................................⊞ 618
Congess 1004
Contac Day Allergy/Sinus Caplets ⊞ 812
Contac Day & Night ....⊞ 812
Contac Night Allergy/Sinus Caplets ....⊞ 812
Contac Severe Cold & Flu Non-Drowsy ....⊞ 815
Deconamine Chewable Tablets 1320
Deconamine CX Cough and Cold Liquid and Tablets.............................. 1319
Deconamine 1320
Deconsal C Expectorant Syrup 456
Deconsal Pediatric Syrup 457
Deconsal II Tablets 454
Dimetane-DX Cough Syrup 2059
Dimetapp Sinus Caplets ....⊞ 775
Dorcol Children's Cough Syrup ......⊞ 785
Drixoral Cough + Congestion Liquid Caps ....⊞ 802
Dura-Tap/PD Capsules 2867
Duratuss Tablets 2565
Duratuss HD Elixir............................... 2565
Efidac/24 ....⊞ 635
Entex PSE Tablets 1987
Fedahist Gyrocaps............................... 2401
Fedahist Timecaps 2401
Guaifed.. 1787
Guaifed Syrup ....⊞ 734
Guaimax-D Tablets 792
Guaitab Tablets ....⊞ 734
Isoclor Expectorant.............................. 990
Kronofed-A 977
Motrin IB Sinus ....⊞ 838
Novahistine DH.................................... 2462
Novahistine DMX ....⊞ 822
Novahistine Expectorant..................... 2463
Nucofed 2051
PediaCare Cold Allergy Chewable Tablets ....⊞ 677
PediaCare Cough-Cold Chewable Tablets 1553
PediaCare 1553
PediaCare Infants' Decongestant Drops ....⊞ 677
PediaCare Infant's Drops Decongestant Plus Cough 1553
PediaCare NightRest Cough-Cold Liquid 1553
Pediatric Vicks 44d Dry Hacking Cough & Head Congestion...............⊞ 763
Pediatric Vicks 44m Cough & Cold Relief ....⊞ 764
Robitussin Cold & Cough Liqui-Gels ....⊞ 776
Robitussin Maximum Strength Cough & Cold ....⊞ 778
Robitussin Pediatric Cough & Cold Formula ....⊞ 779
Robitussin Severe Congestion Liqui-Gels ....⊞ 776
Robitussin-DAC Syrup 2074
Robitussin-PE ....⊞ 778
Rondec Oral Drops 953
Rondec Syrup 953
Rondec Tablet....................................... 953
Rondec-DM Oral Drops 954
Rondec-DM Syrup 954
Rondec-TR Tablet 953
Ryna ....⊞ 841
Seldane-D Extended-Release Tablets 1538
Semprex-D Capsules 463
Semprex-D Capsules 1167
Sinarest Tablets ....⊞ 648
Sinarest Extra Strength Tablets.......⊞ 648
Sinarest No Drowsiness Tablets ....⊞ 648
Sine-Aid IB Caplets 1554
Sine-Aid Maximum Strength Sinus Medication Gelcaps, Caplets and Tablets 1554
Sine-Off No Drowsiness Formula Caplets ....⊞ 824
Sine-Off Sinus Medicine ....⊞ 825
Singlet Tablets ....⊞ 825
Sinutab Non-Drying Liquid Caps....⊞ 859
Sinutab Sinus Allergy Medication, Maximum Strength Tablets and Caplets ....⊞ 860
Sinutab Sinus Medication, Maximum Strength Without Drowsiness Formula, Tablets & Caplets ....⊞ 860

IMPORTANT NOTE: Always consult each drug listing in the patient's regimen for possible interactions.

- Sinutab Sinus Medication, Regular Strength Without Drowsiness Formula ◘ 859
- Sudafed Children's Liquid ◘ 861
- Sudafed Cold and Cough Liquid-caps ◘ 862
- Sudafed Cough Syrup ◘ 862
- Sudafed Plus Liquid ◘ 862
- Sudafed Plus Tablets ◘ 863
- Sudafed Severe Cold Formula Caplets ◘ 863
- Sudafed Severe Cold Formula Tablets ◘ 864
- Sudafed Sinus Caplets ◘ 864
- Sudafed Sinus Tablets ◘ 864
- Sudafed Tablets, 30 mg ◘ 861
- Sudafed Tablets, 60 mg ◘ 861
- Sudafed 12 Hour Caplets ◘ 861
- Syn-Rx Tablets 465
- Syn-Rx DM Tablets 466
- TheraFlu ◘ 787
- TheraFlu Maximum Strength Nighttime Flu, Cold & Cough Medicine ◘ 788
- TheraFlu Maximum Strength Non-Drowsy Formula Flu, Cold & Cough Medicine ◘ 788
- Thera Flu Maximum Strength, Non-Drowsy Formula Flu, Cold and Cough Caplets ◘ 789
- Triaminic AM Cough and Decongestant Formula ◘ 789
- Triaminic AM Decongestant Formula ◘ 790
- Triaminic Nite Light ◘ 791
- Triaminic Sore Throat Formula ◘ 791
- Tussend 1783
- Tussend Expectorant 1785
- Children's TYLENOL Cold Multi-Symptom Liquid Formula and Chewable Tablets 1561
- Children's TYLENOL Cold Plus Cough Multi Symptom Tablets and Liquid ◘ 681
- Infants' TYLENOL Cold Decongestant & Fever-Reducer Drops 1556
- TYLENOL Maximum Strength Allergy Sinus Medication Gelcaps and Caplets 1563
- TYLENOL Maximum Strength Allergy Sinus NightTime Medication Caplets 1555
- TYLENOL Flu Maximum Strength Gelcaps 1565
- TYLENOL Flu NightTime, Maximum Strength, Gelcaps 1566
- TYLENOL Maximum Strength Flu NightTime Hot Medication Packets 1562
- TYLENOL, Maximum Strength, Sinus Medication Geltabs, Gelcaps, Caplets and Tablets 1566
- TYLENOL Cold Multi-Symptom Formula Medication Tablets and Caplets 1561
- TYLENOL Cold Medication No Drowsiness Formula Gelcaps and Caplets 1562
- TYLENOL Cold Multi-Symptom Hot Medication Liquid Packets 1557
- TYLENOL Cough Multi-Symptom Medication with Decongestant 1565
- Ursinus Inlay-Tabs ◘ 794
- Vicks 44 LiquiCaps Cough, Cold & Flu Relief ◘ 755
- Vicks 44 LiquiCaps Non-Drowsy Cough & Cold Relief ◘ 756
- Vicks 44D Dry Hacking Cough & Head Congestion ◘ 755
- Vicks 44M Cough, Cold & Flu Relief ◘ 756
- Vicks DayQuil ◘ 761
- Vicks DayQuil SINUS Pressure & PAIN Relief with IBUPROFEN ◘ 762
- Vicks Nyquil Hot Therapy ◘ 762
- Vicks NyQuil LiquiCaps Multi-Symptom Cold/Flu Relief ◘ 763
- Vicks NyQuil Multi-Symptom Cold/Flu Relief - (Original & Cherry Flavor) ◘ 763

Pseudoephedrine Sulfate (Close supervision and careful dosage adjustment required). Products include:

- Cheracol Sinus ◘ 768
- Chlor-Trimeton Allergy Decongestant Tablets ◘ 799
- Claritin-D 2350
- Drixoral Cold and Allergy Sustained-Action Tablets ◘ 802
- Drixoral Cold and Flu Extended-Release Tablets ◘ 803
- Drixoral Non-Drowsy Formula Extended-Release Tablets ◘ 803
- Drixoral Allergy/Sinus Extended Release Tablets ◘ 804
- Trinalin Repetabs Tablets 1330

Quazepam (Sedative effects of both drugs are additive). Products include:

- Doral Tablets 2664

Quinidine Gluconate (An individual who is stable on a given dose of tricyclic may become abruptly toxic when given with drugs that inhibit cytochrome P4502D6 and drugs that are substrates for P4502D6; careful adjustment of dosage is required). Products include:

- Quinaglute Dura-Tabs Tablets 649

Quinidine Polygalacturonate (An individual who is stable on a given dose of tricyclic may become abruptly toxic when given with drugs that inhibit cytochrome P4502D6 and drugs that are substrates for P4502D6; careful adjustment of dosage is required).

No products indexed under this heading.

Quinidine Sulfate (An individual who is stable on a given dose of tricyclic may become abruptly toxic when given with drugs that inhibit cytochrome P4502D6 and drugs that are substrates for P4502D6; careful adjustment of dosage is required). Products include:

- Quinidex Extentabs 2067

Salmeterol Xinafoate (Close supervision and careful dosage adjustment required). Products include:

- Serevent Inhalation Aerosol 1176

Scopolamine (Close supervision and careful dosage adjustment required). Products include:

- Transderm Scōp Transdermal Therapeutic System 869

Scopolamine Hydrobromide (Close supervision and careful dosage adjustment required). Products include:

- Atrohist Plus Tablets 454
- Donnatal 2060
- Donnatal Extentabs 2061
- Donnatal Tablets 2060

Secobarbital Sodium (Induces liver enzyme activity thereby reduces tricyclic antidepressant plasma levels). Products include:

- Seconal Sodium Pulvules 1474

Selegiline Hydrochloride (Contraindication; hyperpyretic crises; severe convulsions; death). Products include:

- Eldepryl Tablets 2550

Sertraline Hydrochloride (An individual who is stable on a given dose of tricyclic may become abruptly toxic when given with drugs that inhibit cytochrome P4502D6 and drugs that are substrates for P4502D6; careful adjustment of dosage is required). Products include:

- Zoloft Tablets 2217

Temazepam (Sedative effects of both drugs are additive). Products include:

- Restoril Capsules 2284

Terbutaline Sulfate (Close supervision and careful dosage adjustment required). Products include:

- Brethaire Inhaler 813
- Brethine Ampuls 815
- Brethine Tablets 814
- Bricanyl Subcutaneous Injection 1502
- Bricanyl Tablets 1503

Thiamylal Sodium (Induces liver enzyme activity thereby reduces tricyclic antidepressant plasma levels).

No products indexed under this heading.

Thioridazine Hydrochloride (Additive sedative and anticholinergic effects; increases plasma levels; an individual who is stable on a given dose of tricyclic may become abruptly toxic when given with drugs that inhibit cytochrome P4502D6 and drugs that are substrates for P4502D6; careful adjustment of dosage is required). Products include:

- Mellaril 2269

Thiothixene (Additive sedative and anticholinergic effects). Products include:

- Navane Capsules and Concentrate 2201
- Navane Intramuscular 2202

Thyroid (Cardiovascular toxicity, including arrhythmias).

No products indexed under this heading.

Tranylcypromine Sulfate (An individual who is stable on a given dose of tricyclic may become abruptly toxic when given with drugs that inhibit cytochrome P4502D6 and drugs that are substrates for P4502D6; careful adjustment of dosage is required). Products include:

- Parnate Tablets 2503

Trazodone Hydrochloride (An individual who is stable on a given dose of tricyclic may become abruptly toxic when given with drugs that inhibit cytochrome P4502D6 and drugs that are substrates for P4502D6; careful adjustment of dosage is required). Products include:

- Desyrel and Desyrel Dividose 503

Triazolam (Sedative effects of both drugs are additive). Products include:

- Halcion Tablets 2611

Tridihexethyl Chloride (Close supervision and careful dosage adjustment required).

No products indexed under this heading.

Trifluoperazine Hydrochloride (Additive sedative and anticholinergic effects; increases plasma levels; an individual who is stable on a given dose of tricyclic may become abruptly toxic when given with drugs that inhibit cytochrome P4502D6 and drugs that are substrates for P4502D6; careful adjustment of dosage is required). Products include:

- Stelazine 2514

Trihexyphenidyl Hydrochloride (Close supervision and careful dosage adjustments required). Products include:

- Artane 1368

Trimipramine Maleate (An individual who is stable on a given dose of tricyclic may become abruptly toxic when given with drugs that inhibit cytochrome P4502D6 and drugs that are substrates for P4502D6; careful adjustment of dosage is required). Products include:

- Surmontil Capsules 2811

Venlafaxine Hydrochloride (An individual who is stable on a given dose of tricyclic may become abruptly toxic when given with drugs that inhibit cytochrome P4502D6 and drugs that are substrates for P4502D6; careful adjustment of dosage is required). Products include:

- Effexor 2719

Food Interactions

Alcohol (Exaggerated response to alcohol; increased danger of suicide or overdose; induces liver enzyme activity thereby reduces tricyclic antidepressant plasma levels).

NOR-Q D TABLETS

(Norethindrone) 2135

See **Brevicon 21-Day Tablets**

NORVASC TABLETS

(Amlodipine Besylate) 1940

None cited in PDR database.

NŌSTRIL 1/4% MILD NASAL DECONGESTANT

(Phenylephrine Hydrochloride) ◘ 644

None cited in PDR database.

NŌSTRIL 1/2% REGULAR NASAL DECONGESTANT

(Phenylephrine Hydrochloride) ◘ 644

None cited in PDR database.

NŌSTRILLA LONG ACTING NASAL DECONGESTANT

(Oxymetazoline Hydrochloride) ◘ 644

None cited in PDR database.

NOVACET LOTION

(Sulfur, Sulfacetamide Sodium) 1054

None cited in PDR database.

NOVAHISTINE DH

(Codeine Phosphate, Pseudoephedrine Hydrochloride, Chlorpheniramine Maleate) 2462

May interact with tricyclic antidepressants, monoamine oxidase inhibitors, central nervous system depressants, beta blockers, veratrum alkaloids, and certain other agents. Compounds in these categories include:

Acebutolol Hydrochloride (Potentiates effects of pseudoephedrine). Products include:

- Sectral Capsules 2807

Alfentanil Hydrochloride (Potentiated effects). Products include:

- Alfenta Injection 1286

Alprazolam (Potentiated effects). Products include:

- Xanax Tablets 2649

Amitriptyline Hydrochloride (Potentiated effects). Products include:

- Elavil 2838
- Endep Tablets 2174
- Etrafon 2355
- Limbitrol 2180
- Triavil Tablets 1757

Amoxapine (Potentiated effects). Products include:

- Asendin Tablets 1369

Aprobarbital (Potentiated effects).

No products indexed under this heading.

Atenolol (Potentiates effects of pseudoephedrine). Products include:

- Tenoretic Tablets 2845
- Tenormin Tablets and I.V. Injection 2847

Betaxolol Hydrochloride (Potentiates effects of pseudoephedrine). Products include:

- Betoptic Ophthalmic Solution 469
- Betoptic S Ophthalmic Suspension 471

(◘ Described in PDR For Nonprescription Drugs) (◉ Described in PDR For Ophthalmology)

Kerlone Tablets ... 2436

Bisoprolol Fumarate (Potentiates effects of pseudoephedrine). Products include:

Zebeta Tablets ... 1413
Ziac ... 1415

Buprenorphine (Potentiated effects). Products include:

Buprenex Injectable ... 2006

Buspirone Hydrochloride (Potentiated effects). Products include:

BuSpar ... 737

Butabarbital (Potentiated effects).

No products indexed under this heading.

Butalbital (Potentiated effects). Products include:

Esgic-plus Tablets ... 1013
Fioricet Tablets ... 2258
Fioricet with Codeine Capsules ... 2260
Fiorinal Capsules ... 2261
Fiorinal with Codeine Capsules ... 2262
Fiorinal Tablets ... 2261
Phrenilin ... 785
Sedapap Tablets 50 mg/650 mg .. 1543

Carteolol Hydrochloride (Potentiates effects of pseudoephedrine). Products include:

Cartrol Tablets ... 410
Ocupress Ophthalmic Solution, 1% Sterile ... ⊙ 309

Chlordiazepoxide (Potentiated effects). Products include:

Libritabs Tablets ... 2177
Limbitrol ... 2180

Chlordiazepoxide Hydrochloride (Potentiated effects). Products include:

Librax Capsules ... 2176
Librium Capsules ... 2178
Librium Injectable ... 2179

Chlorpromazine (Potentiated effects). Products include:

Thorazine Suppositories ... 2523

Chlorpromazine Hydrochloride (Potentiated effects). Products include:

Thorazine ... 2523

Chlorprothixene (Potentiated effects).

No products indexed under this heading.

Chlorprothixene Hydrochloride (Potentiated effects).

No products indexed under this heading.

Clomipramine Hydrochloride (Potentiated effects). Products include:

Anafranil Capsules ... 803

Clorazepate Dipotassium (Potentiated effects). Products include:

Tranxene ... 451

Clozapine (Potentiated effects). Products include:

Clozaril Tablets ... 2252

Cryptenamine Preparations (Reduced antihypertensive effects).

Desflurane (Potentiated effects). Products include:

Suprane ... 1813

Desipramine Hydrochloride (Potentiated effects). Products include:

Norpramin Tablets ... 1526

Dezocine (Potentiated effects). Products include:

Dalgan Injection ... 538

Diazepam (Potentiated effects). Products include:

Dizac ... 1809
Valium Injectable ... 2182
Valium Tablets ... 2183
Valrelease Capsules ... 2169

Doxepin Hydrochloride (Potentiated effects). Products include:

Sinequan ... 2205
Zonalon Cream ... 1055

Droperidol (Potentiated effects). Products include:

Inapsine Injection ... 1296

Enflurane (Potentiated effects).

No products indexed under this heading.

Esmolol Hydrochloride (Potentiates effects of pseudoephedrine). Products include:

Brevibloc Injection ... 1808

Estazolam (Potentiated effects). Products include:

ProSom Tablets ... 449

Ethchlorvynol (Potentiated effects). Products include:

Placidyl Capsules ... 448

Ethinamate (Potentiated effects).

No products indexed under this heading.

Fentanyl (Potentiated effects). Products include:

Duragesic Transdermal System ... 1288

Fentanyl Citrate (Potentiated effects). Products include:

Sublimaze Injection ... 1307

Fluphenazine Decanoate (Potentiated effects). Products include:

Prolixin Decanoate ... 509

Fluphenazine Enanthate (Potentiated effects). Products include:

Prolixin Enanthate ... 509

Fluphenazine Hydrochloride (Potentiated effects). Products include:

Prolixin ... 509

Flurazepam Hydrochloride (Potentiated effects). Products include:

Dalmane Capsules ... 2173

Furazolidone (Potentiated effects of MAO inhibitors; potentiated effects of pseudoephedrine). Products include:

Furoxone ... 2046

Glutethimide (Potentiated effects).

No products indexed under this heading.

Haloperidol (Potentiated effects). Products include:

Haldol Injection, Tablets and Concentrate ... 1575

Haloperidol Decanoate (Potentiated effects). Products include:

Haldol Decanoate ... 1577

Hydrocodone Bitartrate (Potentiated effects). Products include:

Anexsia 5/500 Elixir ... 1781
Anexia Tablets ... 1782
Codiclear DH Syrup ... 791
Deconamine CX Cough and Cold Liquid and Tablets ... 1319
Duratuss HD Elixir ... 2565
Hycodan Tablets and Syrup ... 930
Hycomine Compound Tablets ... 932
Hycomine ... 931
Hycotuss Expectorant Syrup ... 933
Hydrocet Capsules ... 782
Lorcet 10/650 ... 1018
Lortab ... 2566
Tussend ... 1783
Tussend Expectorant ... 1785
Vicodin Tablets ... 1356
Vicodin ES Tablets ... 1357
Vicodin Tuss Expectorant ... 1358
Zydone Capsules ... 949

Hydrocodone Polistirex (Potentiated effects). Products include:

Tussionex Pennkinetic Extended-Release Suspension ... 998

Hydroxyzine Hydrochloride (Potentiated effects). Products include:

Atarax Tablets & Syrup ... 2185
Marax Tablets & DF Syrup ... 2200
Vistaril Intramuscular Solution ... 2216

Imipramine Hydrochloride (Potentiated effects). Products include:

Tofranil Ampuls ... 854
Tofranil Tablets ... 856

Imipramine Pamoate (Potentiated effects). Products include:

Tofranil-PM Capsules ... 857

Isocarboxazid (Potentiated effects of MAO inhibitors; potentiated effects of pseudoephedrine).

No products indexed under this heading.

Isoflurane (Potentiated effects).

No products indexed under this heading.

Ketamine Hydrochloride (Potentiated effects).

No products indexed under this heading.

Labetalol Hydrochloride (Potentiates effects of pseudoephedrine). Products include:

Normodyne Injection ... 2377
Normodyne Tablets ... 2379
Trandate ... 1185

Levobunolol Hydrochloride (Potentiates effects of pseudoephedrine). Products include:

Betagan ... ⊙ 233

Levomethadyl Acetate Hydrochloride (Potentiated effects). Products include:

Orlamm ... 2239

Levorphanol Tartrate (Potentiated effects). Products include:

Levo-Dromoran ... 2129

Lorazepam (Potentiated effects). Products include:

Ativan Injection ... 2698
Ativan Tablets ... 2700

Loxapine Hydrochloride (Potentiated effects). Products include:

Loxitane ... 1378

Loxapine Succinate (Potentiated effects). Products include:

Loxitane Capsules ... 1378

Maprotiline Hydrochloride (Potentiated effects). Products include:

Ludiomil Tablets ... 843

Mecamylamine Hydrochloride (Reduced antihypertensive effects). Products include:

Inversine Tablets ... 1686

Meperidine Hydrochloride (Potentiated effects). Products include:

Demerol ... 2308
Mepergan Injection ... 2753

Mephobarbital (Potentiated effects). Products include:

Mebaral Tablets ... 2322

Meprobamate (Potentiated effects). Products include:

Miltown Tablets ... 2672
PMB 200 and PMB 400 ... 2783

Mesoridazine (Potentiated effects).

Methadone Hydrochloride (Potentiated effects). Products include:

Methadone Hydrochloride Oral Concentrate ... 2233
Methadone Hydrochloride Oral Solution & Tablets ... 2235

Methohexital Sodium (Potentiated effects). Products include:

Brevital Sodium Vials ... 1429

Methotrimeprazine (Potentiated effects). Products include:

Levoprome ... 1274

Methoxyflurane (Potentiated effects).

No products indexed under this heading.

Methyldopa (Reduced antihypertensive effects). Products include:

Aldoclor Tablets ... 1598
Aldomet Oral ... 1600
Aldoril Tablets ... 1604

Metipranolol Hydrochloride (Potentiates effects of pseudoephedrine). Products include:

OptiPranolol (Metipranolol 0.3%) Sterile Ophthalmic Solution ... ⊙ 258

Metoprolol Succinate (Potentiates effects of pseudoephedrine). Products include:

Toprol-XL Tablets ... 565

Metoprolol Tartrate (Potentiates effects of pseudoephedrine). Products include:

Lopressor Ampuls ... 830
Lopressor HCT Tablets ... 832
Lopressor Tablets ... 830

Midazolam Hydrochloride (Potentiated effects). Products include:

Versed Injection ... 2170

Molindone Hydrochloride (Potentiated effects). Products include:

Moban Tablets and Concentrate ... 1048

Morphine Sulfate (Potentiated effects). Products include:

Astramorph/PF Injection, USP (Preservative-Free) ... 535
Duramorph ... 962
Infumorph 200 and Infumorph 500 Sterile Solutions ... 965
MS Contin Tablets ... 1994
MSIR ... 1997
Oramorph SR (Morphine Sulfate Sustained Release Tablets) ... 2236
RMS Suppositories ... 2657
Roxanol ... 2243

Nadolol (Potentiates effects of pseudoephedrine).

No products indexed under this heading.

Nortriptyline Hydrochloride (Potentiated effects). Products include:

Pamelor ... 2280

Opium Alkaloids (Potentiated effects).

No products indexed under this heading.

Oxazepam (Potentiated effects). Products include:

Serax Capsules ... 2810
Serax Tablets ... 2810

Oxycodone Hydrochloride (Potentiated effects). Products include:

Percocet Tablets ... 938
Percodan Tablets ... 939
Percodan-Demi Tablets ... 940
Roxicodone Tablets, Oral Solution & Intensol (Oxycodone) ... 2244
Tylox Capsules ... 1584

Penbutolol Sulfate (Potentiates effects of pseudoephedrine). Products include:

Levatol ... 2403

Pentobarbital Sodium (Potentiated effects). Products include:

Nembutal Sodium Capsules ... 436
Nembutal Sodium Solution ... 438
Nembutal Sodium Suppositories ... 440

Perphenazine (Potentiated effects). Products include:

Etrafon ... 2355
Triavil Tablets ... 1757
Trilafon ... 2389

Phenelzine Sulfate (Potentiated effects of MAO inhibitors; potentiated effects of pseudoephedrine). Products include:

Nardil ... 1920

Phenobarbital (Potentiated effects). Products include:

Arco-Lase Plus Tablets ... 512
Bellergal-S Tablets ... 2250
Donnatal ... 2060
Donnatal Extentabs ... 2061
Donnatal Tablets ... 2060
Phenobarbital Elixir and Tablets ... 1469
Quadrinal Tablets ... 1350

Pindolol (Potentiates effects of pseudoephedrine). Products include:

Visken Tablets ... 2299

Prazepam (Potentiated effects).

No products indexed under this heading.

Prochlorperazine (Potentiated effects). Products include:

Compazine ... 2470

IMPORTANT NOTE: Always consult each drug listing in the patient's regimen for possible interactions.

Promethazine Hydrochloride (Potentiated effects). Products include:
- Mepergan Injection ... 2753
- Phenergan with Codeine ... 2777
- Phenergan with Dextromethorphan 2778
- Phenergan Injection ... 2773
- Phenergan Suppositories ... 2775
- Phenergan Syrup ... 2774
- Phenergan Tablets ... 2775
- Phenergan VC ... 2779
- Phenergan VC with Codeine ... 2781

Propofol (Potentiated effects). Products include:
- Diprivan Injection ... 2833

Propoxyphene Hydrochloride (Potentiated effects). Products include:
- Darvon ... 1435
- Wygesic Tablets ... 2827

Propoxyphene Napsylate (Potentiated effects). Products include:
- Darvon-N/Darvocet-N ... 1433

Propranolol Hydrochloride (Potentiates effects of pseudoephedrine). Products include:
- Inderal ... 2728
- Inderal LA Long Acting Capsules ... 2730
- Inderide Tablets ... 2732
- Inderide LA Long Acting Capsules .. 2734

Protriptyline Hydrochloride (Potentiated effects). Products include:
- Vivactil Tablets ... 1774

Quazepam (Potentiated effects). Products include:
- Doral Tablets ... 2664

Reserpine (Reduced antihypertensive effects). Products include:
- Diupres Tablets ... 1650
- Hydropres Tablets ... 1675
- Ser-Ap-Es Tablets ... 849

Risperidone (Potentiated effects). Products include:
- Risperdal ... 1301

Secobarbital Sodium (Potentiated effects). Products include:
- Seconal Sodium Pulvules ... 1474

Selegiline Hydrochloride (Potentiated effects of MAO inhibitors; potentiated effects of pseudoephedrine). Products include:
- Eldepryl Tablets ... 2550

Sotalol Hydrochloride (Potentiates effects of pseudoephedrine). Products include:
- Betapace Tablets ... 641

Sufentanil Citrate (Potentiated effects). Products include:
- Sufenta Injection ... 1309

Temazepam (Potentiated effects). Products include:
- Restoril Capsules ... 2284

Thiamylal Sodium (Potentiated effects).
- No products indexed under this heading.

Thioridazine Hydrochloride (Potentiated effects). Products include:
- Mellaril ... 2269

Thiothixene (Potentiated effects). Products include:
- Navane Capsules and Concentrate 2201
- Navane Intramuscular ... 2202

Timolol Hemihydrate (Potentiates effects of pseudoephedrine). Products include:
- Betimol 0.25%, 0.5% ... ◉ 261

Timolol Maleate (Potentiates effects of pseudoephedrine). Products include:
- Blocadren Tablets ... 1614
- Timolide Tablets ... 1748
- Timoptic in Ocudose ... 1753
- Timoptic Sterile Ophthalmic Solution ... 1751
- Timoptic-XE ... 1755

Tranylcypromine Sulfate (Potentiated effects of MAO inhibitors; potentiated effects of pseudoephedrine). Products include:
- Parnate Tablets ... 2503

Triazolam (Potentiated effects). Products include:
- Halcion Tablets ... 2611

Trifluoperazine Hydrochloride (Potentiated effects). Products include:
- Stelazine ... 2514

Trimipramine Maleate (Potentiated effects). Products include:
- Surmontil Capsules ... 2811

Zolpidem Tartrate (Potentiated effects). Products include:
- Ambien Tablets ... 2416

Food Interactions

Alcohol (Potentiated effects).

NOVAHISTINE DMX

(Dextromethorphan Hydrobromide, Guaifenesin, Pseudoephedrine Hydrochloride) ... ▣ 822

May interact with monoamine oxidase inhibitors. Compounds in this category include:

Furazolidone (Concurrent and/or sequential use is contraindicated). Products include:
- Furoxone ... 2046

Isocarboxazid (Concurrent and/or sequential use is contraindicated).
- No products indexed under this heading.

Phenelzine Sulfate (Concurrent and/or sequential use is contraindicated). Products include:
- Nardil ... 1920

Selegiline Hydrochloride (Concurrent and/or sequential use is contraindicated). Products include:
- Eldepryl Tablets ... 2550

Tranylcypromine Sulfate (Concurrent and/or sequential use is contraindicated). Products include:
- Parnate Tablets ... 2503

NOVAHISTINE ELIXIR

(Chlorpheniramine Maleate, Phenylephrine Hydrochloride) ... ▣ 823

May interact with monoamine oxidase inhibitors, hypnotics and sedatives, tranquilizers, and certain other agents. Compounds in these categories include:

Alprazolam (May increase the drowsiness effect; avoid concurrent use). Products include:
- Xanax Tablets ... 2649

Buspirone Hydrochloride (May increase the drowsiness effect; avoid concurrent use). Products include:
- BuSpar ... 737

Chlordiazepoxide (May increase the drowsiness effect; avoid concurrent use). Products include:
- Libritabs Tablets ... 2177
- Limbitrol ... 2180

Chlordiazepoxide Hydrochloride (May increase the drowsiness effect; avoid concurrent use). Products include:
- Librax Capsules ... 2176
- Librium Capsules ... 2178
- Librium Injectable ... 2179

Chlorpromazine (May increase the drowsiness effect; avoid concurrent use). Products include:
- Thorazine Suppositories ... 2523

Chlorpromazine Hydrochloride (May increase the drowsiness effect; avoid concurrent use). Products include:
- Thorazine ... 2523

Chlorprothixene (May increase the drowsiness effect; avoid concurrent use).
- No products indexed under this heading.

Chlorprothixene Hydrochloride (May increase the drowsiness effect; avoid concurrent use).
- No products indexed under this heading.

Clorazepate Dipotassium (May increase the drowsiness effect; avoid concurrent use). Products include:
- Tranxene ... 451

Diazepam (May increase the drowsiness effect; avoid concurrent use). Products include:
- Dizac ... 1809
- Valium Injectable ... 2182
- Valium Tablets ... 2183
- Valrelease Capsules ... 2169

Droperidol (May increase the drowsiness effect; avoid concurrent use). Products include:
- Inapsine Injection ... 1296

Estazolam (May increase the drowsiness effect; avoid concurrent use). Products include:
- ProSom Tablets ... 449

Ethchlorvynol (May increase the drowsiness effect; avoid concurrent use). Products include:
- Placidyl Capsules ... 448

Ethinamate (May increase the drowsiness effect; avoid concurrent use).
- No products indexed under this heading.

Fluphenazine Decanoate (May increase the drowsiness effect; avoid concurrent use). Products include:
- Prolixin Decanoate ... 509

Fluphenazine Enanthate (May increase the drowsiness effect; avoid concurrent use). Products include:
- Prolixin Enanthate ... 509

Fluphenazine Hydrochloride (May increase the drowsiness effect; avoid concurrent use). Products include:
- Prolixin ... 509

Flurazepam Hydrochloride (May increase the drowsiness effect; avoid concurrent use). Products include:
- Dalmane Capsules ... 2173

Furazolidone (Concurrent and/or sequential use is contraindicated). Products include:
- Furoxone ... 2046

Glutethimide (May increase the drowsiness effect; avoid concurrent use).
- No products indexed under this heading.

Haloperidol (May increase the drowsiness effect; avoid concurrent use). Products include:
- Haldol Injection, Tablets and Concentrate ... 1575

Haloperidol Decanoate (May increase the drowsiness effect; avoid concurrent use). Products include:
- Haldol Decanoate ... 1577

Hydroxyzine Hydrochloride (May increase the drowsiness effect; avoid concurrent use). Products include:
- Atarax Tablets & Syrup ... 2185
- Marax Tablets & DF Syrup ... 2200
- Vistaril Intramuscular Solution ... 2216

Isocarboxazid (Concurrent and/or sequential use is contraindicated).
- No products indexed under this heading.

Lorazepam (May increase the drowsiness effect; avoid concurrent use). Products include:
- Ativan Injection ... 2698
- Ativan Tablets ... 2700

Loxapine Hydrochloride (May increase the drowsiness effect; avoid concurrent use). Products include:
- Loxitane ... 1378

Loxapine Succinate (May increase the drowsiness effect; avoid concurrent use). Products include:
- Loxitane Capsules ... 1378

Meprobamate (May increase the drowsiness effect; avoid concurrent use). Products include:
- Miltown Tablets ... 2672
- PMB 200 and PMB 400 ... 2783

Mesoridazine Besylate (May increase the drowsiness effect; avoid concurrent use). Products include:
- Serentil ... 684

Midazolam Hydrochloride (May increase the drowsiness effect; avoid concurrent use). Products include:
- Versed Injection ... 2170

Molindone Hydrochloride (May increase the drowsiness effect; avoid concurrent use). Products include:
- Moban Tablets and Concentrate ... 1048

Oxazepam (May increase the drowsiness effect; avoid concurrent use). Products include:
- Serax Capsules ... 2810
- Serax Tablets ... 2810

Perphenazine (May increase the drowsiness effect; avoid concurrent use). Products include:
- Etrafon ... 2355
- Triavil Tablets ... 1757
- Trilafon ... 2389

Phenelzine Sulfate (Concurrent and/or sequential use is contraindicated). Products include:
- Nardil ... 1920

Prazepam (May increase the drowsiness effect; avoid concurrent use).
- No products indexed under this heading.

Prochlorperazine (May increase the drowsiness effect; avoid concurrent use). Products include:
- Compazine ... 2470

Promethazine Hydrochloride (May increase the drowsiness effect; avoid concurrent use). Products include:
- Mepergan Injection ... 2753
- Phenergan with Codeine ... 2777
- Phenergan with Dextromethorphan 2778
- Phenergan Injection ... 2773
- Phenergan Suppositories ... 2775
- Phenergan Syrup ... 2774
- Phenergan Tablets ... 2775
- Phenergan VC ... 2779
- Phenergan VC with Codeine ... 2781

Propofol (May increase the drowsiness effect; avoid concurrent use). Products include:
- Diprivan Injection ... 2833

Quazepam (May increase the drowsiness effect; avoid concurrent use). Products include:
- Doral Tablets ... 2664

Secobarbital Sodium (May increase the drowsiness effect; avoid concurrent use). Products include:
- Seconal Sodium Pulvules ... 1474

Selegiline Hydrochloride (Concurrent and/or sequential use is contraindicated). Products include:
- Eldepryl Tablets ... 2550

Temazepam (May increase the drowsiness effect; avoid concurrent use). Products include:
- Restoril Capsules ... 2284

Thioridazine Hydrochloride (May increase the drowsiness effect; avoid concurrent use). Products include:
- Mellaril ... 2269

(▣ Described in PDR For Nonprescription Drugs) (◉ Described in PDR For Ophthalmology)

Thiothixene (May increase the drowsiness effect; avoid concurrent use). Products include:

Navane Capsules and Concentrate ... 2201
Navane Intramuscular ... 2202

Tranylcypromine Sulfate (Concurrent and/or sequential use is contraindicated). Products include:

Parnate Tablets ... 2503

Triazolam (May increase the drowsiness effect; avoid concurrent use). Products include:

Halcion Tablets ... 2611

Trifluoperazine Hydrochloride (May increase the drowsiness effect; avoid concurrent use). Products include:

Stelazine ... 2514

Zolpidem Tartrate (May increase the drowsiness effect; avoid concurrent use). Products include:

Ambien Tablets ... 2416

Food Interactions

Alcohol (May increase the drowsiness effect; avoid concurrent use).

NOVAHISTINE EXPECTORANT

(Codeine Phosphate, Pseudoephedrine Hydrochloride, Guaifenesin) ... 2463

May interact with tricyclic antidepressants, monoamine oxidase inhibitors, central nervous system depressants, beta blockers, veratrum alkaloids, hypnotics and sedatives, tranquilizers, narcotic analgesics, general anesthetics, and certain other agents. Compounds in these categories include:

Acebutolol Hydrochloride (Potentiates the sympathomimetic effects of pseudoephedrine). Products include:

Sectral Capsules ... 2807

Alfentanil Hydrochloride (Codeine may potentiate CNS depressant effects). Products include:

Alfenta Injection ... 1286

Alprazolam (Codeine may potentiate CNS depressant effects). Products include:

Xanax Tablets ... 2649

Amitriptyline Hydrochloride (Codeine may potentiate CNS depressant effects). Products include:

Elavil ... 2838
Endep Tablets ... 2174
Etrafon ... 2355
Limbitrol ... 2180
Triavil Tablets ... 1757

Amoxapine (Codeine may potentiate CNS depressant effects). Products include:

Asendin Tablets ... 1369

Aprobarbital (Codeine may potentiate CNS depressant effects).

No products indexed under this heading.

Atenolol (Potentiates the sympathomimetic effects of pseudoephedrine). Products include:

Tenoretic Tablets ... 2845
Tenormin Tablets and I.V. Injection 2847

Betaxolol Hydrochloride (Potentiates the sympathomimetic effects of pseudoephedrine). Products include:

Betoptic Ophthalmic Solution ... 469
Betoptic S Ophthalmic Suspension 471
Kerlone Tablets ... 2436

Bisoprolol Fumarate (Potentiates the sympathomimetic effects of pseudoephedrine). Products include:

Zebeta Tablets ... 1413
Ziac ... 1415

Buprenorphine (Codeine may potentiate CNS depressant effects). Products include:

Buprenex Injectable ... 2006

Buspirone Hydrochloride (Codeine may potentiate CNS depressant effects). Products include:

BuSpar ... 737

Butabarbital (Codeine may potentiate CNS depressant effects).

No products indexed under this heading.

Butalbital (Codeine may potentiate CNS depressant effects). Products include:

Esgic-plus Tablets ... 1013
Fioricet Tablets ... 2258
Fioricet with Codeine Capsules ... 2260
Fiorinal Capsules ... 2261
Fiorinal with Codeine Capsules ... 2262
Fiorinal Tablets ... 2261
Phrenilin ... 785
Sedapap Tablets 50 mg/650 mg .. 1543

Carteolol Hydrochloride (Potentiates the sympathomimetic effects of pseudoephedrine). Products include:

Cartrol Tablets ... 410
Ocupress Ophthalmic Solution, 1% Sterile ... ◉ 309

Chlordiazepoxide (Codeine may potentiate CNS depressant effects). Products include:

Libritabs Tablets ... 2177
Limbitrol ... 2180

Chlordiazepoxide Hydrochloride (Codeine may potentiate CNS depressant effects). Products include:

Librax Capsules ... 2176
Librium Capsules ... 2178
Librium Injectable ... 2179

Chlorpromazine (Codeine may potentiate CNS depressant effects). Products include:

Thorazine Suppositories ... 2523

Chlorpromazine Hydrochloride (Codeine may potentiate CNS depressant effects). Products include:

Thorazine ... 2523

Chlorprothixene (Codeine may potentiate CNS depressant effects).

No products indexed under this heading.

Chlorprothixene Hydrochloride (Codeine may potentiate CNS depressant effects).

No products indexed under this heading.

Clomipramine Hydrochloride (Codeine may potentiate CNS depressant effects). Products include:

Anafranil Capsules ... 803

Clorazepate Dipotassium (Codeine may potentiate CNS depressant effects). Products include:

Tranxene ... 451

Clozapine (Codeine may potentiate CNS depressant effects). Products include:

Clozaril Tablets ... 2252

Cryptenamine Preparations (Sympathomimetic may reduce the antihypertensive effects of veratrum alkaloids).

Desflurane (Codeine may potentiate CNS depressant effects). Products include:

Suprane ... 1813

Desipramine Hydrochloride (Codeine may potentiate CNS depressant effects). Products include:

Norpramin Tablets ... 1526

Dezocine (Codeine may potentiate CNS depressant effects). Products include:

Dalgan Injection ... 538

Diazepam (Codeine may potentiate CNS depressant effects). Products include:

Dizac ... 1809
Valium Injectable ... 2182
Valium Tablets ... 2183
Valrelease Capsules ... 2169

Doxepin Hydrochloride (Codeine may potentiate CNS depressant effects). Products include:

Sinequan ... 2205
Zonalon Cream ... 1055

Droperidol (Codeine may potentiate CNS depressant effects). Products include:

Inapsine Injection ... 1296

Enflurane (Codeine may potentiate CNS depressant effects).

No products indexed under this heading.

Esmolol Hydrochloride (Potentiates the sympathomimetic effects of pseudoephedrine). Products include:

Brevibloc Injection ... 1808

Estazolam (Codeine may potentiate CNS depressant effects). Products include:

ProSom Tablets ... 449

Ethchlorvynol (Codeine may potentiate CNS depressant effects). Products include:

Placidyl Capsules ... 448

Ethinamate (Codeine may potentiate CNS depressant effects).

No products indexed under this heading.

Fentanyl (Codeine may potentiate CNS depressant effects). Products include:

Duragesic Transdermal System ... 1288

Fentanyl Citrate (Codeine may potentiate CNS depressant effects). Products include:

Sublimaze Injection ... 1307

Fluphenazine Decanoate (Codeine may potentiate CNS depressant effects). Products include:

Prolixin Decanoate ... 509

Fluphenazine Enanthate (Codeine may potentiate CNS depressant effects). Products include:

Prolixin Enanthate ... 509

Fluphenazine Hydrochloride (Codeine may potentiate CNS depressant effects). Products include:

Prolixin ... 509

Flurazepam Hydrochloride (Codeine may potentiate CNS depressant effects). Products include:

Dalmane Capsules ... 2173

Furazolidone (Potentiates the sympathomimetic effects of pseudoephedrine; codeine may potentiate CNS depressant effects; concurrent and/or sequential use is contraindicated). Products include:

Furoxone ... 2046

Glutethimide (Codeine may potentiate CNS depressant effects).

No products indexed under this heading.

Haloperidol (Codeine may potentiate CNS depressant effects). Products include:

Haldol Injection, Tablets and Concentrate ... 1575

Haloperidol Decanoate (Codeine may potentiate CNS depressant effects). Products include:

Haldol Decanoate ... 1577

Hydrocodone Bitartrate (Codeine may potentiate CNS depressant effects). Products include:

Anexsia 5/500 Elixir ... 1781
Anexia Tablets ... 1782
Codiclear DH Syrup ... 791
Deconamine CX Cough and Cold Liquid and Tablets ... 1319
Duratuss HD Elixir ... 2565
Hycodan Tablets and Syrup ... 930
Hycomine Compound Tablets ... 932
Hycomine ... 931
Hycotuss Expectorant Syrup ... 933
Hydrocet Capsules ... 782
Lorcet 10/650 ... 1018
Lortab ... 2566
Tussend ... 1783
Tussend Expectorant ... 1785
Vicodin Tablets ... 1356
Vicodin ES Tablets ... 1357
Vicodin Tuss Expectorant ... 1358
Zydone Capsules ... 949

Hydrocodone Polistirex (Codeine may potentiate CNS depressant effects). Products include:

Tussionex Pennkinetic Extended-Release Suspension ... 998

Hydroxyzine Hydrochloride (Codeine may potentiate CNS depressant effects). Products include:

Atarax Tablets & Syrup ... 2185
Marax Tablets & DF Syrup ... 2200
Vistaril Intramuscular Solution ... 2216

Imipramine Hydrochloride (Codeine may potentiate CNS depressant effects). Products include:

Tofranil Ampuls ... 854
Tofranil Tablets ... 856

Imipramine Pamoate (Codeine may potentiate CNS depressant effects). Products include:

Tofranil-PM Capsules ... 857

Isocarboxazid (Potentiates the sympathomimetic effects of pseudoephedrine; codeine may potentiate CNS depressant effects; concurrent and/or sequential use is contraindicated).

No products indexed under this heading.

Isoflurane (Codeine may potentiate CNS depressant effects).

No products indexed under this heading.

Ketamine Hydrochloride (Codeine may potentiate CNS depressant effects).

No products indexed under this heading.

Labetalol Hydrochloride (Potentiates the sympathomimetic effects of pseudoephedrine). Products include:

Normodyne Injection ... 2377
Normodyne Tablets ... 2379
Trandate ... 1185

Levobunolol Hydrochloride (Potentiates the sympathomimetic effects of pseudoephedrine). Products include:

Betagan ... ◉ 233

Levomethadyl Acetate Hydrochloride (Codeine may potentiate CNS depressant effects). Products include:

Orlamm ... 2239

Levorphanol Tartrate (Codeine may potentiate CNS depressant effects). Products include:

Levo-Dromoran ... 2129

Lorazepam (Codeine may potentiate CNS depressant effects). Products include:

Ativan Injection ... 2698
Ativan Tablets ... 2700

Loxapine Hydrochloride (Codeine may potentiate CNS depressant effects). Products include:

Loxitane ... 1378

Loxapine Succinate (Codeine may potentiate CNS depressant effects). Products include:

Loxitane Capsules ... 1378

Maprotiline Hydrochloride (Codeine may potentiate CNS depressant effects). Products include:

Ludiomil Tablets ... 843

IMPORTANT NOTE: Always consult each drug listing in the patient's regimen for possible interactions.

Novahistine Expectorant Interactions Index 742

Mecamylamine Hydrochloride (Sympathomimetic may reduce the antihypertensive effects). Products include:
Inversine Tablets ... 1686

Meperidine Hydrochloride (Codeine may potentiate CNS depressant effects). Products include:
Demerol ... 2308
Mepergan Injection ... 2753

Mephobarbital (Codeine may potentiate CNS depressant effects). Products include:
Mebaral Tablets ... 2322

Meprobamate (Codeine may potentiate CNS depressant effects). Products include:
Miltown Tablets ... 2672
PMB 200 and PMB 400 ... 2783

Mesoridazine Besylate (Codeine may potentiate CNS depressant effects). Products include:
Serentil ... 684

Methadone Hydrochloride (Codeine may potentiate CNS depressant effects). Products include:
Methadone Hydrochloride Oral Concentrate ... 2233
Methadone Hydrochloride Oral Solution & Tablets ... 2235

Methohexital Sodium (Codeine may potentiate CNS depressant effects). Products include:
Brevital Sodium Vials ... 1429

Methotrimeprazine (Codeine may potentiate CNS depressant effects). Products include:
Levoprome ... 1274

Methoxyflurane (Codeine may potentiate CNS depressant effects).
No products indexed under this heading.

Methyldopa (Sympathomimetic may reduce the antihypertensive effects). Products include:
Aldoclor Tablets ... 1598
Aldomet Oral ... 1600
Aldoril Tablets ... 1604

Methyldopate Hydrochloride (Sympathomimetic may reduce the antihypertensive effects). Products include:
Aldomet Ester HCl Injection ... 1602

Metipranolol Hydrochloride (Potentiates the sympathomimetic effects of pseudoephedrine). Products include:
OptiPranolol (Metipranolol 0.3%) Sterile Ophthalmic Solution ... ⊙ 258

Metoprolol Succinate (Potentiates the sympathomimetic effects of pseudoephedrine). Products include:
Toprol-XL Tablets ... 565

Metoprolol Tartrate (Potentiates the sympathomimetic effects of pseudoephedrine). Products include:
Lopressor Ampuls ... 830
Lopressor HCT Tablets ... 832
Lopressor Tablets ... 830

Midazolam Hydrochloride (Codeine may potentiate CNS depressant effects). Products include:
Versed Injection ... 2170

Molindone Hydrochloride (Codeine may potentiate CNS depressant effects). Products include:
Moban Tablets and Concentrate ... 1048

Morphine Sulfate (Codeine may potentiate CNS depressant effects). Products include:
Astramorph/PF Injection, USP (Preservative-Free) ... 535
Duramorph ... 962
Infumorph 200 and Infumorph 500 Sterile Solutions ... 965
MS Contin Tablets ... 1994
MSIR ... 1997
Oramorph SR (Morphine Sulfate Sustained Release Tablets) ... 2236
RMS Suppositories ... 2657
Roxanol ... 2243

Nadolol (Potentiates the sympathomimetic effects of pseudoephedrine).
No products indexed under this heading.

Nortriptyline Hydrochloride (Codeine may potentiate CNS depressant effects). Products include:
Pamelor ... 2280

Opium Alkaloids (Codeine may potentiate CNS depressant effects).
No products indexed under this heading.

Oxazepam (Codeine may potentiate CNS depressant effects). Products include:
Serax Capsules ... 2810
Serax Tablets ... 2810

Oxycodone Hydrochloride (Codeine may potentiate CNS depressant effects). Products include:
Percocet Tablets ... 938
Percodan Tablets ... 939
Percodan-Demi Tablets ... 940
Roxicodone Tablets, Oral Solution & Intensol (Oxycodone) ... 2244
Tylox Capsules ... 1584

Penbutolol Sulfate (Potentiates the sympathomimetic effects of pseudoephedrine). Products include:
Levatol ... 2403

Pentobarbital Sodium (Codeine may potentiate CNS depressant effects). Products include:
Nembutal Sodium Capsules ... 436
Nembutal Sodium Solution ... 438
Nembutal Sodium Suppositories ... 440

Perphenazine (Codeine may potentiate CNS depressant effects). Products include:
Etrafon ... 2355
Triavil Tablets ... 1757
Trilafon ... 2389

Phenelzine Sulfate (Potentiates the sympathomimetic effects of pseudoephedrine; codeine may potentiate CNS depressant effects; concurrent and/or sequential use is contraindicated). Products include:
Nardil ... 1920

Phenobarbital (Codeine may potentiate CNS depressant effects). Products include:
Arco-Lase Plus Tablets ... 512
Bellergal-S Tablets ... 2250
Donnatal ... 2060
Donnatal Extentabs ... 2061
Donnatal Tablets ... 2060
Phenobarbital Elixir and Tablets ... 1469
Quadrinal Tablets ... 1350

Pindolol (Potentiates the sympathomimetic effects of pseudoephedrine). Products include:
Visken Tablets ... 2299

Prazepam (Codeine may potentiate CNS depressant effects).
No products indexed under this heading.

Prochlorperazine (Codeine may potentiate CNS depressant effects). Products include:
Compazine ... 2470

Promethazine Hydrochloride (Codeine may potentiate CNS depressant effects). Products include:
Mepergan Injection ... 2753
Phenergan with Codeine ... 2777
Phenergan with Dextromethorphan ... 2778
Phenergan Injection ... 2773
Phenergan Suppositories ... 2775
Phenergan Syrup ... 2774
Phenergan Tablets ... 2775
Phenergan VC ... 2779
Phenergan VC with Codeine ... 2781

Propofol (Codeine may potentiate CNS depressant effects). Products include:
Diprivan Injection ... 2833

Propoxyphene Hydrochloride (Codeine may potentiate CNS depressant effects). Products include:
Darvon ... 1435
Wygesic Tablets ... 2827

Propoxyphene Napsylate (Codeine may potentiate CNS depressant effects). Products include:
Darvon-N/Darvocet-N ... 1433

Propranolol Hydrochloride (Potentiates the sympathomimetic effects of pseudoephedrine). Products include:
Inderal ... 2728
Inderal LA Long Acting Capsules ... 2730
Inderide Tablets ... 2732
Inderide LA Long Acting Capsules ... 2734

Protriptyline Hydrochloride (Codeine may potentiate CNS depressant effects). Products include:
Vivactil Tablets ... 1774

Quazepam (Codeine may potentiate CNS depressant effects). Products include:
Doral Tablets ... 2664

Reserpine (Sympathomimetic may reduce the antihypertensive effects). Products include:
Diupres Tablets ... 1650
Hydropres Tablets ... 1675
Ser-Ap-Es Tablets ... 849

Risperidone (Codeine may potentiate CNS depressant effects). Products include:
Risperdal ... 1301

Secobarbital Sodium (Codeine may potentiate CNS depressant effects). Products include:
Seconal Sodium Pulvules ... 1474

Selegiline Hydrochloride (Potentiates the sympathomimetic effects of pseudoephedrine; codeine may potentiate CNS depressant effects; concurrent and/or sequential use is contraindicated). Products include:
Eldepryl Tablets ... 2550

Sotalol Hydrochloride (Potentiates the sympathomimetic effects of pseudoephedrine). Products include:
Betapace Tablets ... 641

Sufentanil Citrate (Codeine may potentiate CNS depressant effects). Products include:
Sufenta Injection ... 1309

Temazepam (Codeine may potentiate CNS depressant effects). Products include:
Restoril Capsules ... 2284

Thiamylal Sodium (Codeine may potentiate CNS depressant effects).
No products indexed under this heading.

Thioridazine Hydrochloride (Codeine may potentiate CNS depressant effects). Products include:
Mellaril ... 2269

Thiothixene (Codeine may potentiate CNS depressant effects). Products include:
Navane Capsules and Concentrate ... 2201
Navane Intramuscular ... 2202

Tranylcypromine Sulfate (Potentiates the sympathomimetic effects of pseudoephedrine; codeine may potentiate CNS depressant effects; concurrent and/or sequential use is contraindicated). Products include:
Parnate Tablets ... 2503

Triazolam (Codeine may potentiate CNS depressant effects). Products include:
Halcion Tablets ... 2611

Trifluoperazine Hydrochloride (Codeine may potentiate CNS depressant effects). Products include:
Stelazine ... 2514

Trimipramine Maleate (Codeine may potentiate CNS depressant effects). Products include:
Surmontil Capsules ... 2811

Zolpidem Tartrate (Codeine may potentiate CNS depressant effects). Products include:
Ambien Tablets ... 2416

Food Interactions

Alcohol (Codeine may potentiate CNS depressant effects).

NOVANTRONE
(Mitoxantrone Hydrochloride) ... 1279
May interact with:

Daunorubicin Hydrochloride (Possible danger of cardiac effects). Products include:
Cerubidine ... 795

Doxorubicin Hydrochloride (Possible danger of cardiac effects). Products include:
Adriamycin PFS ... 1947
Adriamycin RDF ... 1947
Doxorubicin Astra ... 540
Rubex ... 712

NOVOCAIN HYDROCHLORIDE FOR SPINAL ANESTHESIA
(Procaine Hydrochloride) ... 2326
May interact with sulfonamides. Compounds in this category include:

Sulfamethizole (Action of sulfonamides inhibited). Products include:
Urobiotic-250 Capsules ... 2214

Sulfamethoxazole (Action of sulfonamides inhibited). Products include:
Azo Gantanol Tablets ... 2080
Bactrim DS Tablets ... 2084
Bactrim I.V. Infusion ... 2082
Bactrim ... 2084
Gantanol Tablets ... 2119
Septra ... 1174
Septra I.V. Infusion ... 1169
Septra I.V. Infusion ADD-Vantage Vials ... 1171
Septra ... 1174

Sulfasalazine (Action of sulfonamides inhibited). Products include:
Azulfidine ... 1949

Sulfinpyrazone (Action of sulfonamides inhibited). Products include:
Anturane ... 807

Sulfisoxazole (Action of sulfonamides inhibited). Products include:
Azo Gantrisin Tablets ... 2081
Gantrisin Tablets ... 2120

Sulfisoxazole Diolamine (Action of sulfonamides inhibited).
No products indexed under this heading.

NOVOLIN L HUMAN INSULIN 10 ML VIALS
(Insulin, Human, Zinc Suspension) ... 1795
None cited in PDR database.

NOVOLIN N HUMAN INSULIN 10 ML VIALS
(Insulin, Human Isophane Suspension) ... 1795
None cited in PDR database.

NOVOLIN N PENFILL CARTRIDGES DURABLE INSULIN DELIVERY SYSTEM
(Insulin, Human NPH) ... 1798
None cited in PDR database.

NOVOLIN N PREFILLED SYRINGE DISPOSABLE INSULIN DELIVERY SYSTEM
(Insulin, Human NPH) ... 1798
None cited in PDR database.

(▣ Described in PDR For Nonprescription Drugs) (⊙ Described in PDR For Ophthalmology)

Interactions Index — Nubain Injection

NOVOLIN 70/30 HUMAN INSULIN 10 ML VIALS
(Insulin, Human Regular and Human NPH Mixture) 1794
None cited in PDR database.

NOVOLIN 70/30 PENFILL CARTRIDGES DURABLE INSULIN DELIVERY SYSTEM
(Insulin, Human Regular and Human NPH Mixture) 1797
None cited in PDR database.

NOVOLIN 70/30 PREFILLED DISPOSABLE INSULIN DELIVERY SYSTEM
(Insulin, Human Regular and Human NPH Mixture) 1798
None cited in PDR database.

NOVOLIN R HUMAN INSULIN 10 ML VIALS
(Insulin, Human Regular) 1795
None cited in PDR database.

NOVOLIN R PENFILL CARTRIDGES DURABLE INSULIN DELIVERY SYSTEM
(Insulin, Human Regular) 1798
None cited in PDR database.

NOVOLIN R PREFILLED SYRINGE DISPOSABLE INSULIN DELIVERY SYSTEM
(Insulin, Human Regular) 1798
None cited in PDR database.

NUBAIN INJECTION
(Nalbuphine Hydrochloride) 935
May interact with narcotic analgesics, anesthetics, phenothiazines, tranquilizers, hypnotics and sedatives, central nervous system depressants, general anesthetics, and certain other agents. Compounds in these categories include:

Alfentanil Hydrochloride (Additive CNS depression). Products include:

Alfenta Injection 1286

Alprazolam (Additive CNS depression). Products include:

Xanax Tablets 2649

Aprobarbital (Additive CNS depression).

No products indexed under this heading.

Buprenorphine (Additive CNS depression). Products include:

Buprenex Injectable 2006

Buspirone Hydrochloride (Additive CNS depression). Products include:

BuSpar 737

Butabarbital (Additive CNS depression).

No products indexed under this heading.

Butalbital (Additive CNS depression). Products include:

Esgic-plus Tablets 1013
Fioricet Tablets 2258
Fioricet with Codeine Capsules 2260
Fiorinal Capsules 2261
Fiorinal with Codeine Capsules 2262
Fiorinal Tablets 2261
Phrenilin 785
Sedapap Tablets 50 mg/650 mg .. 1543

Chlordiazepoxide (Additive CNS depression). Products include:

Libritabs Tablets 2177
Limbitrol 2180

Chlordiazepoxide Hydrochloride (Additive CNS depression). Products include:

Librax Capsules 2176
Librium Capsules 2178
Librium Injectable 2179

Chlorpromazine (Additive CNS depression). Products include:

Thorazine Suppositories 2523

Chlorpromazine Hydrochloride (Additive CNS depression). Products include:

Thorazine 2523

Chlorprothixene (Additive CNS depression).

No products indexed under this heading.

Chlorprothixene Hydrochloride (Additive CNS depression).

No products indexed under this heading.

Clorazepate Dipotassium (Additive CNS depression). Products include:

Tranxene 451

Clozapine (Additive CNS depression). Products include:

Clozaril Tablets 2252

Codeine Phosphate (Additive CNS depression). Products include:

Actifed with Codeine Cough Syrup.. 1067
Brontex 1981
Deconsal C Expectorant Syrup 456
Deconsal Pediatric Syrup 457
Dimetane-DC Cough Syrup 2059
Empirin with Codeine Tablets............ 1093
Fioricet with Codeine Capsules 2260
Fiorinal with Codeine Capsules 2262
Isoclor Expectorant 990
Novahistine DH 2462
Novahistine Expectorant 2463
Nucofed 2051
Phenergan with Codeine 2777
Phenergan VC with Codeine 2781
Robitussin A-C Syrup 2073
Robitussin-DAC Syrup 2074
Ryna .... ᴿᴰ 841
Soma Compound w/Codeine Tablets 2676
Tussi-Organidin NR Liquid and S NR Liquid 2677
Tylenol with Codeine 1583

Desflurane (Additive CNS depression). Products include:

Suprane 1813

Dezocine (Additive CNS depression). Products include:

Dalgan Injection 538

Diazepam (Additive CNS depression). Products include:

Dizac 1809
Valium Injectable 2182
Valium Tablets 2183
Valrelease Capsules 2169

Droperidol (Additive CNS depression). Products include:

Inapsine Injection 1296

Enflurane (Additive CNS depression).

No products indexed under this heading.

Estazolam (Additive CNS depression). Products include:

ProSom Tablets 449

Ethchlorvynol (Additive CNS depression). Products include:

Placidyl Capsules 448

Ethinamate (Additive CNS depression).

No products indexed under this heading.

Fentanyl (Additive CNS depression). Products include:

Duragesic Transdermal System......... 1288

Fentanyl Citrate (Additive CNS depression). Products include:

Sublimaze Injection 1307

Fluphenazine Decanoate (Additive CNS depression). Products include:

Prolixin Decanoate 509

Fluphenazine Enanthate (Additive CNS depression). Products include:

Prolixin Enanthate 509

Fluphenazine Hydrochloride (Additive CNS depression). Products include:

Prolixin 509

Flurazepam Hydrochloride (Additive CNS depression). Products include:

Dalmane Capsules 2173

Glutethimide (Additive CNS depression).

No products indexed under this heading.

Haloperidol (Additive CNS depression). Products include:

Haldol Injection, Tablets and Concentrate 1575

Haloperidol Decanoate (Additive CNS depression). Products include:

Haldol Decanoate 1577

Halothane (Additive CNS depression). Products include:

Fluothane 2724

Hydrocodone Bitartrate (Additive CNS depression). Products include:

Anexsia 5/500 Elixir 1781
Anexia Tablets 1782
Codiclear DH Syrup 791
Deconamine CX Cough and Cold Liquid and Tablets 1319
Duratuss HD Elixir 2565
Hycodan Tablets and Syrup 930
Hycomine Compound Tablets 932
Hycomine 931
Hycotuss Expectorant Syrup 933
Hydrocet Capsules 782
Lorcet 10/650 1018
Lortab 2566
Tussend 1783
Tussend Expectorant 1785
Vicodin Tablets 1356
Vicodin ES Tablets 1357
Vicodin Tuss Expectorant 1358
Zydone Capsules 949

Hydrocodone Polistirex (Additive CNS depression). Products include:

Tussionex Pennkinetic Extended-Release Suspension 998

Hydroxyzine Hydrochloride (Additive CNS depression). Products include:

Atarax Tablets & Syrup 2185
Marax Tablets & DF Syrup 2200
Vistaril Intramuscular Solution 2216

Isoflurane (Additive CNS depression).

No products indexed under this heading.

Ketamine Hydrochloride (Additive CNS depression).

No products indexed under this heading.

Levomethadyl Acetate Hydrochloride (Additive CNS depression). Products include:

Orlamm 2239

Levorphanol Tartrate (Additive CNS depression). Products include:

Levo-Dromoran 2129

Lorazepam (Additive CNS depression). Products include:

Ativan Injection 2698
Ativan Tablets 2700

Loxapine Hydrochloride (Additive CNS depression). Products include:

Loxitane 1378

Loxapine Succinate (Additive CNS depression). Products include:

Loxitane Capsules 1378

Meperidine Hydrochloride (Additive CNS depression). Products include:

Demerol 2308
Mepergan Injection 2753

Mephobarbital (Additive CNS depression). Products include:

Mebaral Tablets 2322

Meprobamate (Additive CNS depression). Products include:

Miltown Tablets 2672
PMB 200 and PMB 400 2783

Mesoridazine Besylate (Additive CNS depression). Products include:

Serentil 684

Methadone Hydrochloride (Additive CNS depression). Products include:

Methadone Hydrochloride Oral Concentrate 2233
Methadone Hydrochloride Oral Solution & Tablets 2235

Methohexital Sodium (Additive CNS depression). Products include:

Brevital Sodium Vials 1429

Methotrimeprazine (Additive CNS depression). Products include:

Levoprome 1274

Methoxyflurane (Additive CNS depression).

No products indexed under this heading.

Midazolam Hydrochloride (Additive CNS depression). Products include:

Versed Injection 2170

Molindone Hydrochloride (Additive CNS depression). Products include:

Moban Tablets and Concentrate 1048

Morphine Sulfate (Additive CNS depression). Products include:

Astramorph/PF Injection, USP (Preservative-Free) 535
Duramorph 962
Infumorph 200 and Infumorph 500 Sterile Solutions 965
MS Contin Tablets 1994
MSIR 1997
Oramorph SR (Morphine Sulfate Sustained Release Tablets) 2236
RMS Suppositories 2657
Roxanol 2243

Opium Alkaloids (Additive CNS depression).

No products indexed under this heading.

Oxazepam (Additive CNS depression). Products include:

Serax Capsules 2810
Serax Tablets 2810

Oxycodone Hydrochloride (Additive CNS depression). Products include:

Percocet Tablets 938
Percodan Tablets 939
Percodan-Demi Tablets 940
Roxicodone Tablets, Oral Solution & Intensol (Oxycodone) 2244
Tylox Capsules 1584

Pentobarbital Sodium (Additive CNS depression). Products include:

Nembutal Sodium Capsules 436
Nembutal Sodium Solution 438
Nembutal Sodium Suppositories 440

Perphenazine (Additive CNS depression). Products include:

Etrafon 2355
Triavil Tablets 1757
Trilafon 2389

Phenobarbital (Additive CNS depression). Products include:

Arco-Lase Plus Tablets 512
Bellergal-S Tablets 2250
Donnatal 2060
Donnatal Extentabs 2061
Donnatal Tablets 2060

IMPORTANT NOTE: Always consult each drug listing in the patient's regimen for possible interactions.

Nubain Injection — Interactions Index — 744

Phenobarbital Elixir and Tablets 1469
Quadrinal Tablets 1350

Prazepam (Additive CNS depression).
No products indexed under this heading.

Prochlorperazine (Additive CNS depression). Products include:
Compazine 2470

Promethazine Hydrochloride (Additive CNS depression). Products include:
Mepergan Injection 2753
Phenergan with Codeine 2777
Phenergan with Dextromethorphan 2778
Phenergan Injection 2773
Phenergan Suppositories 2775
Phenergan Syrup 2774
Phenergan Tablets 2775
Phenergan VC 2779
Phenergan VC with Codeine 2781

Propofol (Additive CNS depression). Products include:
Diprivan Injection 2833

Propoxyphene Hydrochloride (Additive CNS depression). Products include:
Darvon 1435
Wygesic Tablets 2827

Propoxyphene Napsylate (Additive CNS depression). Products include:
Darvon-N/Darvocet-N 1433

Quazepam (Additive CNS depression). Products include:
Doral Tablets 2664

Risperidone (Additive CNS depression). Products include:
Risperdal 1301

Secobarbital Sodium (Additive CNS depression). Products include:
Seconal Sodium Pulvules 1474

Sufentanil Citrate (Additive CNS depression). Products include:
Sufenta Injection 1309

Temazepam (Additive CNS depression). Products include:
Restoril Capsules 2284

Thiamylal Sodium (Additive CNS depression).
No products indexed under this heading.

Thioridazine Hydrochloride (Additive CNS depression). Products include:
Mellaril 2269

Thiothixene (Additive CNS depression). Products include:
Navane Capsules and Concentrate 2201
Navane Intramuscular 2202

Triazolam (Additive CNS depression). Products include:
Halcion Tablets 2611

Trifluoperazine Hydrochloride (Additive CNS depression). Products include:
Stelazine 2514

Zolpidem Tartrate (Additive CNS depression). Products include:
Ambien Tablets 2416

Food Interactions

Alcohol (Additive CNS depression).

NUCOFED EXPECTORANT

(Codeine Phosphate, Pseudoephedrine Hydrochloride, Guaifenesin) 2051
See **Nucofed Syrup and Capsules**

NUCOFED PEDIATRIC EXPECTORANT

(Codeine Phosphate, Pseudoephedrine Hydrochloride, Guaifenesin) 2051
See **Nucofed Syrup and Capsules**

NUCOFED SYRUP AND CAPSULES

(Codeine Phosphate, Pseudoephedrine Hydrochloride) 2051
May interact with beta blockers, veratrum alkaloids, sympathomimetics, tricyclic antidepressants, central nervous system depressants, general anesthetics, anticholinergics, monoamine oxidase inhibitors, cardiac glycosides, and certain other agents. Compounds in these categories include:

Acebutolol Hydrochloride (Increased pressor effect of pseudoephedrine). Products include:
Sectral Capsules 2807

Albuterol (Increased effect of either agent; increased potential for side effects). Products include:
Proventil Inhalation Aerosol 2382
Ventolin Inhalation Aerosol and Refill 1197

Albuterol Sulfate (Increased effect of either agent; increased potential for side effects). Products include:
Airet Solution for Inhalation 452
Proventil Inhalation Solution 0.083% 2384
Proventil Repetabs Tablets 2386
Proventil Solution for Inhalation 0.5% 2383
Proventil Syrup 2385
Proventil Tablets 2386
Ventolin Inhalation Solution 1198
Ventolin Nebules Inhalation Solution 1199
Ventolin Rotacaps for Inhalation 1200
Ventolin Syrup 1202
Ventolin Tablets 1203
Volmax Extended-Release Tablets .. 1788

Alfentanil Hydrochloride (May increase the depressant effects of codeine). Products include:
Alfenta Injection 1286

Alprazolam (May increase the depressant effects of codeine). Products include:
Xanax Tablets 2649

Amitriptyline Hydrochloride (May antagonize effects of pseudoephedrine; increased effects of antidepressants or the codeine). Products include:
Elavil 2838
Endep Tablets 2174
Etrafon 2355
Limbitrol 2180
Triavil Tablets 1757

Amoxapine (May antagonize effects of pseudoephedrine; increased effects of antidepressants or the codeine). Products include:
Asendin Tablets 1369

Aprobarbital (May increase the depressant effects of codeine).
No products indexed under this heading.

Atenolol (Increased pressor effect of pseudoephedrine). Products include:
Tenoretic Tablets 2845
Tenormin Tablets and I.V. Injection 2847

Atropine Sulfate (Concurrent use may result in paralytic ileus). Products include:
Arco-Lase Plus Tablets 512
Atrohist Plus Tablets 454
Atropine Sulfate Sterile Ophthalmic Solution ...... ◉ 233
Donnatal 2060
Donnatal Extentabs 2061
Donnatal Tablets 2060
Lomotil 2439
Motofen Tablets 784
Urised Tablets 1964

Belladonna Alkaloids (Concurrent use may result in paralytic ileus). Products include:
Bellergal-S Tablets 2250
Hyland's Bed Wetting Tablets ...... ◘ 828
Hyland's EnurAid Tablets ...... ◘ 829
Hyland's Teething Tablets ...... ◘ 830

Benztropine Mesylate (Concurrent use may result in paralytic ileus). Products include:
Cogentin 1621

Betaxolol Hydrochloride (Increased pressor effect of pseudoephedrine). Products include:
Betoptic Ophthalmic Solution 469
Betoptic S Ophthalmic Suspension 471
Kerlone Tablets 2436

Biperiden Hydrochloride (Concurrent use may result in paralytic ileus). Products include:
Akineton 1333

Bisoprolol Fumarate (Increased pressor effect of pseudoephedrine). Products include:
Zebeta Tablets 1413
Ziac 1415

Buprenorphine (May increase the depressant effects of codeine). Products include:
Buprenex Injectable 2006

Buspirone Hydrochloride (May increase the depressant effects of codeine). Products include:
BuSpar 737

Butabarbital (May increase the depressant effects of codeine).
No products indexed under this heading.

Butalbital (May increase the depressant effects of codeine). Products include:
Esgic-plus Tablets 1013
Fioricet Tablets 2258
Fioricet with Codeine Capsules 2260
Fiorinal Capsules 2261
Fiorinal with Codeine Capsules 2262
Fiorinal Tablets 2261
Phrenilin 785
Sedapap Tablets 50 mg/650 mg .. 1543

Carteolol Hydrochloride (Increased pressor effect of pseudoephedrine). Products include:
Cartrol Tablets 410
Ocupress Ophthalmic Solution, 1% Sterile ...... ◉ 309

Chlordiazepoxide (May increase the depressant effects of codeine). Products include:
Libritabs Tablets 2177
Limbitrol 2180

Chlordiazepoxide Hydrochloride (May increase the depressant effects of codeine). Products include:
Librax Capsules 2176
Librium Capsules 2178
Librium Injectable 2179

Chlorpromazine (May increase the depressant effects of codeine). Products include:
Thorazine Suppositories 2523

Chlorpromazine Hydrochloride (May increase the depressant effects of codeine). Products include:
Thorazine 2523

Chlorprothixene (May increase the depressant effects of codeine).
No products indexed under this heading.

Chlorprothixene Hydrochloride (May increase the depressant effects of codeine).
No products indexed under this heading.

Clidinium Bromide (Concurrent use may result in paralytic ileus). Products include:
Librax Capsules 2176
Quarzan Capsules 2181

Clomipramine Hydrochloride (May antagonize effects of pseudoephedrine; increased effects of antidepressants or the codeine). Products include:
Anafranil Capsules 803

Clorazepate Dipotassium (May increase the depressant effects of codeine). Products include:
Tranxene 451

Clozapine (May increase the depressant effects of codeine). Products include:
Clozaril Tablets 2252

Cryptenamine Preparations (Decreased hypotensive effects).

Desflurane (May increase the depressant effects of codeine). Products include:
Suprane 1813

Desipramine Hydrochloride (May antagonize effects of pseudoephedrine; increased effects of antidepressants or the codeine). Products include:
Norpramin Tablets 1526

Deslanoside (Possibility of cardiac arrhythmias).
No products indexed under this heading.

Dezocine (May increase the depressant effects of codeine). Products include:
Dalgan Injection 538

Diazepam (May increase the depressant effects of codeine). Products include:
Dizac 1809
Valium Injectable 2182
Valium Tablets 2183
Valrelease Capsules 2169

Dicyclomine Hydrochloride (Concurrent use may result in paralytic ileus). Products include:
Bentyl 1501

Digitoxin (Possibility of cardiac arrhythmias). Products include:
Crystodigin Tablets 1433

Digoxin (Possibility of cardiac arrhythmias). Products include:
Lanoxicaps 1117
Lanoxin Elixir Pediatric 1120
Lanoxin Injection 1123
Lanoxin Injection Pediatric 1126
Lanoxin Tablets 1128

Dobutamine Hydrochloride (Increased effect of either agent; increased potential for side effects). Products include:
Dobutrex Solution Vials 1439

Dopamine Hydrochloride (Increased effect of either agent; increased potential for side effects).
No products indexed under this heading.

Doxepin Hydrochloride (May antagonize effects of pseudoephedrine; increased effects of antidepressants or the codeine). Products include:
Sinequan 2205
Zonalon Cream 1055

Droperidol (May increase the depressant effects of codeine). Products include:
Inapsine Injection 1296

Enflurane (May increase the depressant effects of codeine).
No products indexed under this heading.

Ephedrine Hydrochloride (Increased effect of either agent; increased potential for side effects). Products include:
Primatene Dual Action Formula ...... ◘ 872
Primatene Tablets ...... ◘ 873
Quadrinal Tablets 1350

Ephedrine Sulfate (Increased effect of either agent; increased potential for side effects). Products include:
Bronkaid Caplets ...... ◘ 717
Marax Tablets & DF Syrup 2200

(◘ Described in PDR For Nonprescription Drugs) (◉ Described in PDR For Ophthalmology)

Ephedrine Tannate (Increased effect of either agent; increased potential for side effects). Products include:
- Rynatuss 2673

Epinephrine (Increased effect of either agent; increased potential for side effects). Products include:
- Bronkaid Mist .... ⊡ 717
- EPIFRIN .... ⊙ 239
- EpiPen 790
- Marcaine Hydrochloride with Epinephrine 1:200,000 2316
- Primatene Mist .... ⊡ 873
- Sensorcaine with Epinephrine Injection 559
- Sus-Phrine Injection 1019
- Xylocaine with Epinephrine Injections 567

Epinephrine Bitartrate (Increased effect of either agent; increased potential for side effects). Products include:
- Bronkaid Mist Suspension .... ⊡ 718
- Sensorcaine-MPF with Epinephrine Injection 559

Epinephrine Hydrochloride (Increased effect of either agent; increased potential for side effects). Products include:
- Ana-Kit Anaphylaxis Emergency Treatment Kit 617

Esmolol Hydrochloride (Increased pressor effect of pseudoephedrine). Products include:
- Brevibloc Injection 1808

Estazolam (May increase the depressant effects of codeine). Products include:
- ProSom Tablets 449

Ethchlorvynol (May increase the depressant effects of codeine). Products include:
- Placidyl Capsules 448

Ethinamate (May increase the depressant effects of codeine).
- No products indexed under this heading.

Fentanyl (May increase the depressant effects of codeine). Products include:
- Duragesic Transdermal System 1288

Fentanyl Citrate (May increase the depressant effects of codeine). Products include:
- Sublimaze Injection 1307

Fluphenazine Decanoate (May increase the depressant effects of codeine). Products include:
- Prolixin Decanoate 509

Fluphenazine Enanthate (May increase the depressant effects of codeine). Products include:
- Prolixin Enanthate 509

Fluphenazine Hydrochloride (May increase the depressant effects of codeine). Products include:
- Prolixin 509

Flurazepam Hydrochloride (May increase the depressant effects of codeine). Products include:
- Dalmane Capsules 2173

Furazolidone (Concurrent and/or sequential use in contraindication; potential for hypertensive crisis). Products include:
- Furoxone 2046

Glutethimide (May increase the depressant effects of codeine).
- No products indexed under this heading.

Glycopyrrolate (Concurrent use may result in paralytic ileus). Products include:
- Robinul Forte Tablets 2072
- Robinul Injectable 2072
- Robinul Tablets 2072

Haloperidol (May increase the depressant effects of codeine). Products include:
- Haldol Injection, Tablets and Concentrate 1575

Haloperidol Decanoate (May increase the depressant effects of codeine). Products include:
- Haldol Decanoate 1577

Hydrocodone Bitartrate (May increase the depressant effects of codeine). Products include:
- Anexsia 5/500 Elixir 1781
- Anexia Tablets 1782
- Codiclear DH Syrup 791
- Deconamine CX Cough and Cold Liquid and Tablets 1319
- Duratuss HD Elixir 2565
- Hycodan Tablets and Syrup 930
- Hycomine Compound Tablets 932
- Hycomine 931
- Hycotuss Expectorant Syrup 933
- Hydrocet Capsules 782
- Lorcet 10/650 1018
- Lortab 2566
- Tussend 1783
- Tussend Expectorant 1785
- Vicodin Tablets 1356
- Vicodin ES Tablets 1357
- Vicodin Tuss Expectorant 1358
- Zydone Capsules 949

Hydrocodone Polistirex (May increase the depressant effects of codeine). Products include:
- Tussionex Pennkinetic Extended-Release Suspension 998

Hydroxyzine Hydrochloride (May increase the depressant effects of codeine). Products include:
- Atarax Tablets & Syrup 2185
- Marax Tablets & DF Syrup 2200
- Vistaril Intramuscular Solution 2216

Hyoscyamine (Concurrent use may result in paralytic ileus). Products include:
- Cystospaz Tablets 1963
- Urised Tablets 1964

Hyoscyamine Sulfate (Concurrent use may result in paralytic ileus). Products include:
- Arco-Lase Plus Tablets 512
- Atrohist Plus Tablets 454
- Cystospaz-M Capsules 1963
- Donnatal 2060
- Donnatal Extentabs 2061
- Donnatal Tablets 2060
- Kutrase Capsules 2402
- Levsin/Levsinex/Levbid 2405

Imipramine Hydrochloride (May antagonize effects of pseudoephedrine; increased effects of antidepressants or the codeine). Products include:
- Tofranil Ampuls 854
- Tofranil Tablets 856

Imipramine Pamoate (May antagonize effects of pseudoephedrine; increased effects of antidepressants or the codeine). Products include:
- Tofranil-PM Capsules 857

Ipratropium Bromide (Concurrent use may result in paralytic ileus). Products include:
- Atrovent Inhalation Aerosol 671
- Atrovent Inhalation Solution 673

Isocarboxazid (Concurrent and/or sequential use in contraindication; potential for hypertensive crisis).
- No products indexed under this heading.

Isoflurane (May increase the depressant effects of codeine).
- No products indexed under this heading.

Isoproterenol Hydrochloride (Increased effect of either agent; increased potential for side effects). Products include:
- Isuprel Hydrochloride Injection 1:5000 2311
- Isuprel Hydrochloride Solution 1:200 & 1:100 2313
- Isuprel Mistometer 2312

Isoproterenol Sulfate (Increased effect of either agent; increased potential for side effects). Products include:
- Norisodrine with Calcium Iodide Syrup 442

Ketamine Hydrochloride (May increase the depressant effects of codeine).
- No products indexed under this heading.

Labetalol Hydrochloride (Increased pressor effect of pseudoephedrine). Products include:
- Normodyne Injection 2377
- Normodyne Tablets 2379
- Trandate 1185

Levobunolol Hydrochloride (Increased pressor effect of pseudoephedrine). Products include:
- Betagan .... ⊙ 233

Levomethadyl Acetate Hydrochloride (May increase the depressant effects of codeine). Products include:
- Orlamm 2239

Levorphanol Tartrate (May increase the depressant effects of codeine). Products include:
- Levo-Dromoran 2129

Lorazepam (May increase the depressant effects of codeine). Products include:
- Ativan Injection 2698
- Ativan Tablets 2700

Loxapine Hydrochloride (May increase the depressant effects of codeine). Products include:
- Loxitane 1378

Loxapine Succinate (May increase the depressant effects of codeine). Products include:
- Loxitane Capsules 1378

Maprotiline Hydrochloride (May antagonize effects of pseudoephedrine; increased effects of antidepressants or the codeine). Products include:
- Ludiomil Tablets 843

Mepenzolate Bromide (Concurrent use may result in paralytic ileus).
- No products indexed under this heading.

Meperidine Hydrochloride (May increase the depressant effects of codeine). Products include:
- Demerol 2308
- Mepergan Injection 2753

Mephobarbital (May increase the depressant effects of codeine). Products include:
- Mebaral Tablets 2322

Meprobamate (May increase the depressant effects of codeine). Products include:
- Miltown Tablets 2672
- PMB 200 and PMB 400 2783

Mesoridazine Besylate (May increase the depressant effects of codeine). Products include:
- Serentil 684

Metaproterenol Sulfate (Increased effect of either agent; increased potential for side effects). Products include:
- Alupent 669
- Metaproterenol Sulfate Inhalation Solution, USP, Arm-a-Med 552

Metaraminol Bitartrate (Increased effect of either agent; increased potential for side effects). Products include:
- Aramine Injection 1609

Methadone Hydrochloride (May increase the depressant effects of codeine). Products include:
- Methadone Hydrochloride Oral Concentrate 2233
- Methadone Hydrochloride Oral Solution & Tablets 2235

Methohexital Sodium (May increase the depressant effects of codeine). Products include:
- Brevital Sodium Vials 1429

Methotrimeprazine (May increase the depressant effects of codeine). Products include:
- Levoprome 1274

Methoxamine Hydrochloride (Increased effect of either agent; increased potential for side effects). Products include:
- Vasoxyl Injection 1196

Methoxyflurane (May increase the depressant effects of codeine).
- No products indexed under this heading.

Metipranolol Hydrochloride (Increased pressor effect of pseudoephedrine). Products include:
- OptiPranolol (Metipranolol 0.3%) Sterile Ophthalmic Solution .... ⊙ 258

Metoprolol Succinate (Increased pressor effect of pseudoephedrine). Products include:
- Toprol-XL Tablets 565

Metoprolol Tartrate (Increased pressor effect of pseudoephedrine). Products include:
- Lopressor Ampuls 830
- Lopressor HCT Tablets 832
- Lopressor Tablets 830

Midazolam Hydrochloride (May increase the depressant effects of codeine). Products include:
- Versed Injection 2170

Molindone Hydrochloride (May increase the depressant effects of codeine). Products include:
- Moban Tablets and Concentrate 1048

Morphine Sulfate (May increase the depressant effects of codeine). Products include:
- Astramorph/PF Injection, USP (Preservative-Free) 535
- Duramorph 962
- Infumorph 200 and Infumorph 500 Sterile Solutions 965
- MS Contin Tablets 1994
- MSIR 1997
- Oramorph SR (Morphine Sulfate Sustained Release Tablets) 2236
- RMS Suppositories 2657
- Roxanol 2243

Nadolol (Increased pressor effect of pseudoephedrine).
- No products indexed under this heading.

Norepinephrine Bitartrate (Increased effect of either agent; increased potential for side effects). Products include:
- Levophed Bitartrate Injection 2315

Nortriptyline Hydrochloride (May antagonize effects of pseudoephedrine; increased effects of antidepressants or the codeine). Products include:
- Pamelor 2280

Opium Alkaloids (May increase the depressant effects of codeine).
- No products indexed under this heading.

Oxazepam (May increase the depressant effects of codeine). Products include:
- Serax Capsules 2810
- Serax Tablets 2810

Oxybutynin Chloride (Concurrent use may result in paralytic ileus). Products include:
- Ditropan 1516

IMPORTANT NOTE: Always consult each drug listing in the patient's regimen for possible interactions.

Oxycodone Hydrochloride (May increase the depressant effects of codeine). Products include:
- Percocet Tablets ... 938
- Percodan Tablets ... 939
- Percodan-Demi Tablets ... 940
- Roxicodone Tablets, Oral Solution & Intensol (Oxycodone) ... 2244
- Tylox Capsules ... 1584

Penbutolol Sulfate (Increased pressor effect of pseudoephedrine). Products include:
- Levatol ... 2403

Pentobarbital Sodium (May increase the depressant effects of codeine). Products include:
- Nembutal Sodium Capsules ... 436
- Nembutal Sodium Solution ... 438
- Nembutal Sodium Suppositories ... 440

Perphenazine (May increase the depressant effects of codeine). Products include:
- Etrafon ... 2355
- Triavil Tablets ... 1757
- Trilafon ... 2389

Phenelzine Sulfate (Concurrent and/or sequential use in contraindication; potential for hypertensive crisis). Products include:
- Nardil ... 1920

Phenobarbital (May increase the depressant effects of codeine). Products include:
- Arco-Lase Plus Tablets ... 512
- Bellergal-S Tablets ... 2250
- Donnatal ... 2060
- Donnatal Extentabs ... 2061
- Donnatal Tablets ... 2060
- Phenobarbital Elixir and Tablets ... 1469
- Quadrinal Tablets ... 1350

Phenylephrine Bitartrate (Increased effect of either agent; increased potential for side effects).
- No products indexed under this heading.

Phenylephrine Hydrochloride (Increased effect of either agent; increased potential for side effects). Products include:
- Atrohist Plus Tablets ... 454
- Cerose DM ... ◘ 878
- Comhist ... 2038
- D.A. Chewable Tablets ... 951
- Deconsal Pediatric Capsules ... 454
- Dura-Vent/DA Tablets ... 953
- Entex Capsules ... 1986
- Entex Liquid ... 1986
- Extendryl ... 1005
- 4-Way Fast Acting Nasal Spray (regular & mentholated) ... ◘ 621
- Hemorid For Women ... ◘ 834
- Hycomine Compound Tablets ... 932
- Neo-Synephrine Hydrochloride 1% Carpuject ... 2324
- Neo-Synephrine Hydrochloride 1% Injection ... 2324
- Neo-Synephrine Hydrochloride (Ophthalmic) ... 2325
- Neo-Synephrine ... ◘ 726
- Nōstril ... ◘ 644
- Novahistine Elixir ... ◘ 823
- Phenergan VC ... 2779
- Phenergan VC with Codeine ... 2781
- Preparation H ... ◘ 871
- Tympagesic Ear Drops ... 2342
- Vasosulf ... ⊙ 271
- Vicks Sinex Nasal Spray and Ultra Fine Mist ... ◘ 765

Phenylephrine Tannate (Increased effect of either agent; increased potential for side effects). Products include:
- Atrohist Pediatric Suspension ... 454
- Ricobid-D Pediatric Suspension ... 2038
- Ricobid Tablets and Pediatric Suspension ... 2038
- Rynatan ... 2673
- Rynatuss ... 2673

Phenylpropanolamine Hydrochloride (Increased effect of either agent; increased potential for side effects). Products include:
- Acutrim ... ◘ 628
- Allerest Children's Chewable Tablets ... ◘ 627
- Allerest 12 Hour Caplets ... ◘ 627
- Atrohist Plus Tablets ... 454
- BC Cold Powder Multi-Symptom Formula (Cold-Sinus-Allergy) ... ◘ 609
- BC Cold Powder Non-Drowsy Formula (Cold-Sinus) ... ◘ 609
- Cheracol Plus Head Cold/Cough Formula ... ◘ 769
- Comtrex Multi-Symptom Non-Drowsy Liqui-gels ... ◘ 618
- Contac Continuous Action Nasal Decongestant/Antihistamine 12 Hour Capsules ... ◘ 813
- Contac Maximum Strength Continuous Action Decongestant/Antihistamine 12 Hour Caplets ... ◘ 813
- Contac Severe Cold and Flu Formula Caplets ... ◘ 814
- Coricidin 'D' Decongestant Tablets ... ◘ 800
- Dexatrim ... ◘ 832
- Dexatrim Plus Vitamins Caplets ... ◘ 832
- Dimetane-DC Cough Syrup ... 2059
- Dimetapp Elixir ... ◘ 773
- Dimetapp Extentabs ... ◘ 774
- Dimetapp Tablets/Liqui-Gels ... ◘ 775
- Dimetapp Cold & Allergy Chewable Tablets ... ◘ 773
- Dimetapp DM Elixir ... ◘ 774
- Dura-Vent Tablets ... 952
- Entex Capsules ... 1986
- Entex LA Tablets ... 1987
- Entex Liquid ... 1986
- Exgest LA Tablets ... 782
- Hycomine ... 931
- Isoclor Timesule Capsules ... ◘ 637
- Nolamine Timed-Release Tablets ... 785
- Ornade Spansule Capsules ... 2502
- Propagest Tablets ... 786
- Pyrroxate Caplets ... ◘ 772
- Robitussin-CF ... ◘ 777
- Sinulin Tablets ... 787
- Tavist-D 12 Hour Relief Tablets ... ◘ 787
- Teldrin 12 Hour Antihistamine/Nasal Decongestant Allergy Relief Capsules ... ◘ 826
- Triaminic Allergy Tablets ... ◘ 789
- Triaminic Cold Tablets ... ◘ 790
- Triaminic Expectorant ... ◘ 790
- Triaminic Syrup ... ◘ 792
- Triaminic-12 Tablets ... ◘ 792
- Triaminic-DM Syrup ... ◘ 792
- Triaminicin Tablets ... ◘ 793
- Triaminicol Multi-Symptom Cold Tablets ... ◘ 793
- Triaminicol Multi-Symptom Relief ◘ 794
- Vicks DayQuil Allergy Relief 12-Hour Extended Release Tablets ... ◘ 760
- Vicks DayQuil Allergy Relief 4-Hour Tablets ... ◘ 760
- Vicks DayQuil SINUS Pressure & CONGESTION Relief ... ◘ 761

Pindolol (Increased pressor effect of pseudoephedrine). Products include:
- Visken Tablets ... 2299

Pirbuterol Acetate (Increased effect of either agent; increased potential for side effects). Products include:
- Maxair Autohaler ... 1492
- Maxair Inhaler ... 1494

Prazepam (May increase the depressant effects of codeine).
- No products indexed under this heading.

Prochlorperazine (May increase the depressant effects of codeine). Products include:
- Compazine ... 2470

Procyclidine Hydrochloride (Concurrent use may result in paralytic ileus). Products include:
- Kemadrin Tablets ... 1112

Promethazine Hydrochloride (May increase the depressant effects of codeine). Products include:
- Mepergan Injection ... 2753
- Phenergan with Codeine ... 2777
- Phenergan with Dextromethorphan 2778
- Phenergan Injection ... 2773
- Phenergan Suppositories ... 2775
- Phenergan Syrup ... 2774
- Phenergan Tablets ... 2775
- Phenergan VC ... 2779
- Phenergan VC with Codeine ... 2781

Propantheline Bromide (Concurrent use may result in paralytic ileus). Products include:
- Pro-Banthīne Tablets ... 2052

Propofol (May increase the depressant effects of codeine). Products include:
- Diprivan Injection ... 2833

Propoxyphene Hydrochloride (May increase the depressant effects of codeine). Products include:
- Darvon ... 1435
- Wygesic Tablets ... 2827

Propoxyphene Napsylate (May increase the depressant effects of codeine). Products include:
- Darvon-N/Darvocet-N ... 1433

Propranolol Hydrochloride (Increased pressor effect of pseudoephedrine). Products include:
- Inderal ... 2728
- Inderal LA Long Acting Capsules ... 2730
- Inderide Tablets ... 2732
- Inderide LA Long Acting Capsules .. 2734

Protriptyline Hydrochloride (May antagonize effects of pseudoephedrine; increased effects of antidepressants or the codeine). Products include:
- Vivactil Tablets ... 1774

Pseudoephedrine Sulfate (Increased effect of either agent; increased potential for side effects). Products include:
- Cheracol Sinus ... ◘ 768
- Chlor-Trimeton Allergy Decongestant Tablets ... ◘ 799
- Claritin-D ... 2350
- Drixoral Cold and Allergy Sustained-Action Tablets ... ◘ 802
- Drixoral Cold and Flu Extended-Release Tablets ... ◘ 803
- Drixoral Non-Drowsy Formula Extended-Release Tablets ... ◘ 803
- Drixoral Allergy/Sinus Extended Release Tablets ... ◘ 804
- Trinalin Repetabs Tablets ... 1330

Quazepam (May increase the depressant effects of codeine). Products include:
- Doral Tablets ... 2664

Risperidone (May increase the depressant effects of codeine). Products include:
- Risperdal ... 1301

Salmeterol Xinafoate (Increased effect of either agent; increased potential for side effects). Products include:
- Serevent Inhalation Aerosol ... 1176

Scopolamine (Concurrent use may result in paralytic ileus). Products include:
- Transderm Scōp Transdermal Therapeutic System ... 869

Scopolamine Hydrobromide (Concurrent use may result in paralytic ileus). Products include:
- Atrohist Plus Tablets ... 454
- Donnatal ... 2060
- Donnatal Extentabs ... 2061
- Donnatal Tablets ... 2060

Secobarbital Sodium (May increase the depressant effects of codeine). Products include:
- Seconal Sodium Pulvules ... 1474

Selegiline Hydrochloride (Concurrent and/or sequential use in contraindication; potential for hypertensive crisis). Products include:
- Eldepryl Tablets ... 2550

Sotalol Hydrochloride (Increased pressor effect of pseudoephedrine). Products include:
- Betapace Tablets ... 641

Sufentanil Citrate (May increase the depressant effects of codeine). Products include:
- Sufenta Injection ... 1309

Temazepam (May increase the depressant effects of codeine). Products include:
- Restoril Capsules ... 2284

Terbutaline Sulfate (Increased effect of either agent; increased potential for side effects). Products include:
- Brethaire Inhaler ... 813
- Brethine Ampuls ... 815
- Brethine Tablets ... 814
- Bricanyl Subcutaneous Injection ... 1502
- Bricanyl Tablets ... 1503

Thiamylal Sodium (May increase the depressant effects of codeine).
- No products indexed under this heading.

Thioridazine Hydrochloride (May increase the depressant effects of codeine). Products include:
- Mellaril ... 2269

Thiothixene (May increase the depressant effects of codeine). Products include:
- Navane Capsules and Concentrate 2201
- Navane Intramuscular ... 2202

Timolol Maleate (Increased pressor effect of pseudoephedrine). Products include:
- Blocadren Tablets ... 1614
- Timolide Tablets ... 1748
- Timoptic in Ocudose ... 1753
- Timoptic Sterile Ophthalmic Solution ... 1751
- Timoptic-XE ... 1755

Tranylcypromine Sulfate (Concurrent and/or sequential use in contraindication; potential for hypertensive crisis). Products include:
- Parnate Tablets ... 2503

Triazolam (May increase the depressant effects of codeine). Products include:
- Halcion Tablets ... 2611

Tridihexethyl Chloride (Concurrent use may result in paralytic ileus).
- No products indexed under this heading.

Trifluoperazine Hydrochloride (May increase the depressant effects of codeine). Products include:
- Stelazine ... 2514

Trihexyphenidyl Hydrochloride (Concurrent use may result in paralytic ileus). Products include:
- Artane ... 1368

Trimipramine Maleate (May antagonize effects of pseudoephedrine; increased effects of antidepressants or the codeine). Products include:
- Surmontil Capsules ... 2811

Zolpidem Tartrate (May increase the depressant effects of codeine). Products include:
- Ambien Tablets ... 2416

Food Interactions

Alcohol (May increase the depressant effects of codeine).

NU-IRON 150 CAPSULES

(Polysaccharide-Iron Complex) ... 1543
None cited in PDR database.

NU-IRON ELIXIR

(Polysaccharide-Iron Complex) ... 1543
None cited in PDR database.

NULYTELY

(Polyethylene Glycol) ... 689
May interact with:

Oral Medications, unspecified (Oral medications may not be absorbed if given within one hour).

(◘ Described in PDR For Nonprescription Drugs) (⊙ Described in PDR For Ophthalmology)

747 Interactions Index Numorphan Injection

Food Interactions

Food, unspecified (Solid food should not be given for at least two hours before the solution is given).

CHERRY FLAVOR NULYTELY
(Polyethylene Glycol, Sodium Bicarbonate, Sodium Chloride, Potassium Chloride) ... 689
May interact with:

Oral Medications, unspecified (Oral medication administered within one hour of the start of administration of Nulytely may be flushed from gastrointestinal tract and not absorbed).

NUMORPHAN INJECTION
(Oxymorphone Hydrochloride) ... 936
May interact with narcotic analgesics, anesthetics, phenothiazines, tranquilizers, hypnotics and sedatives, central nervous system depressants, and certain other agents. Compounds in these categories include:

Alfentanil Hydrochloride (Additive CNS depression). Products include:
Alfenta Injection ... 1286

Alprazolam (Additive CNS depression). Products include:
Xanax Tablets ... 2649

Aprobarbital (Additive CNS depression).
No products indexed under this heading.

Buprenorphine (Additive CNS depression). Products include:
Buprenex Injectable ... 2006

Buspirone Hydrochloride (Additive CNS depression). Products include:
BuSpar ... 737

Butabarbital (Additive CNS depression).
No products indexed under this heading.

Butalbital (Additive CNS depression). Products include:
Esgic-plus Tablets ... 1013
Fioricet Tablets ... 2258
Fioricet with Codeine Capsules ... 2260
Fiorinal Capsules ... 2261
Fiorinal with Codeine Capsules ... 2262
Fiorinal Tablets ... 2261
Phrenilin ... 785
Sedapap Tablets 50 mg/650 mg .. 1543

Chlordiazepoxide (Additive CNS depression). Products include:
Libritabs Tablets ... 2177
Limbitrol ... 2180

Chlordiazepoxide Hydrochloride (Additive CNS depression). Products include:
Librax Capsules ... 2176
Librium Capsules ... 2178
Librium Injectable ... 2179

Chlorpromazine (Additive CNS depression). Products include:
Thorazine Suppositories ... 2523

Chlorprothixene (Additive CNS depression).
No products indexed under this heading.

Chlorprothixene Hydrochloride (Additive CNS depression).
No products indexed under this heading.

Clorazepate Dipotassium (Additive CNS depression). Products include:
Tranxene ... 451

Clozapine (Additive CNS depression). Products include:
Clozaril Tablets ... 2252

Codeine Phosphate (Additive CNS depression). Products include:
Actifed with Codeine Cough Syrup.. 1067
Brontex ... 1981
Deconsal C Expectorant Syrup ... 456
Deconsal Pediatric Syrup ... 457
Dimetane-DC Cough Syrup ... 2059
Empirin with Codeine Tablets ... 1093
Fioricet with Codeine Capsules ... 2260
Fiorinal with Codeine Capsules ... 2262
Isoclor Expectorant ... 990
Novahistine DH ... 2462
Novahistine Expectorant ... 2463
Nucofed ... 2051
Phenergan with Codeine ... 2777
Phenergan VC with Codeine ... 2781
Robitussin A-C Syrup ... 2073
Robitussin-DAC Syrup ... 2074
Ryna ... 841
Soma Compound w/Codeine Tablets ... 2676
Tussi-Organidin NR Liquid and S NR Liquid ... 2677
Tylenol with Codeine ... 1583

Desflurane (Additive CNS depression). Products include:
Suprane ... 1813

Dezocine (Additive CNS depression). Products include:
Dalgan Injection ... 538

Diazepam (Additive CNS depression). Products include:
Dizac ... 1809
Valium Injectable ... 2182
Valium Tablets ... 2183
Valrelease Capsules ... 2169

Droperidol (Additive CNS depression). Products include:
Inapsine Injection ... 1296

Enflurane (Additive CNS depression).
No products indexed under this heading.

Estazolam (Additive CNS depression). Products include:
ProSom Tablets ... 449

Ethchlorvynol (Additive CNS depression). Products include:
Placidyl Capsules ... 448

Ethinamate (Additive CNS depression).
No products indexed under this heading.

Fentanyl (Additive CNS depression). Products include:
Duragesic Transdermal System ... 1288

Fentanyl Citrate (Additive CNS depression). Products include:
Sublimaze Injection ... 1307

Fluphenazine Decanoate (Additive CNS depression). Products include:
Prolixin Decanoate ... 509

Fluphenazine Enanthate (Additive CNS depression). Products include:
Prolixin Enanthate ... 509

Fluphenazine Hydrochloride (Additive CNS depression). Products include:
Prolixin ... 509

Flurazepam Hydrochloride (Additive CNS depression). Products include:
Dalmane Capsules ... 2173

Glutethimide (Additive CNS depression).
No products indexed under this heading.

Haloperidol (Additive CNS depression). Products include:
Haldol Injection, Tablets and Concentrate ... 1575

Haloperidol Decanoate (Additive CNS depression). Products include:
Haldol Decanoate ... 1577

Halothane (Additive CNS depression). Products include:
Fluothane ... 2724

Hydrocodone Bitartrate (Additive CNS depression). Products include:
Anexsia 5/500 Elixir ... 1781
Anexia Tablets ... 1782
Codiclear DH Syrup ... 791
Deconamine CX Cough and Cold Liquid and Tablets ... 1319
Duratuss HD Elixir ... 2565
Hycodan Tablets and Syrup ... 930
Hycomine Compound Tablets ... 932
Hycomine ... 931
Hycotuss Expectorant Syrup ... 933
Hydrocet Capsules ... 782
Lorcet 10/650 ... 1018
Lortab ... 2566
Tussend ... 1783
Tussend Expectorant ... 1785
Vicodin Tablets ... 1356
Vicodin ES Tablets ... 1357
Vicodin Tuss Expectorant ... 1358
Zydone Capsules ... 949

Hydrocodone Polistirex (Additive CNS depression). Products include:
Tussionex Pennkinetic Extended-Release Suspension ... 998

Hydroxyzine Hydrochloride (Additive CNS depression). Products include:
Atarax Tablets & Syrup ... 2185
Marax Tablets & DF Syrup ... 2200
Vistaril Intramuscular Solution ... 2216

Isoflurane (Additive CNS depression).
No products indexed under this heading.

Ketamine Hydrochloride (Additive CNS depression).
No products indexed under this heading.

Levomethadyl Acetate Hydrochloride (Additive CNS depression). Products include:
Orlamm ... 2239

Levorphanol Tartrate (Additive CNS depression). Products include:
Levo-Dromoran ... 2129

Lorazepam (Additive CNS depression). Products include:
Ativan Injection ... 2698
Ativan Tablets ... 2700

Loxapine Hydrochloride (Additive CNS depression). Products include:
Loxitane ... 1378

Loxapine Succinate (Additive CNS depression). Products include:
Loxitane Capsules ... 1378

Meperidine Hydrochloride (Additive CNS depression). Products include:
Demerol ... 2308
Mepergan Injection ... 2753

Mephobarbital (Additive CNS depression). Products include:
Mebaral Tablets ... 2322

Meprobamate (Additive CNS depression). Products include:
Miltown Tablets ... 2672
PMB 200 and PMB 400 ... 2783

Mesoridazine Besylate (Additive CNS depression). Products include:
Serentil ... 684

Methadone Hydrochloride (Additive CNS depression). Products include:
Methadone Hydrochloride Oral Concentrate ... 2233
Methadone Hydrochloride Oral Solution & Tablets ... 2235

Methohexital Sodium (Additive CNS depression). Products include:
Brevital Sodium Vials ... 1429

Methotrimeprazine (Additive CNS depression). Products include:
Levoprome ... 1274

Methoxyflurane (Additive CNS depression).
No products indexed under this heading.

Midazolam Hydrochloride (Additive CNS depression). Products include:
Versed Injection ... 2170

Molindone Hydrochloride (Additive CNS depression). Products include:
Moban Tablets and Concentrate ... 1048

Morphine Sulfate (Additive CNS depression). Products include:
Astramorph/PF Injection, USP (Preservative-Free) ... 535
Duramorph ... 962
Infumorph 200 and Infumorph 500 Sterile Solutions ... 965
MS Contin Tablets ... 1994
MSIR ... 1997
Oramorph SR (Morphine Sulfate Sustained Release Tablets) ... 2236
RMS Suppositories ... 2657
Roxanol ... 2243

Opium Alkaloids (Additive CNS depression).
No products indexed under this heading.

Oxazepam (Additive CNS depression). Products include:
Serax Capsules ... 2810
Serax Tablets ... 2810

Oxycodone Hydrochloride (Additive CNS depression). Products include:
Percocet Tablets ... 938
Percodan Tablets ... 939
Percodan-Demi Tablets ... 940
Roxicodone Tablets, Oral Solution & Intensol (Oxycodone) ... 2244
Tylox Capsules ... 1584

Pentobarbital Sodium (Additive CNS depression). Products include:
Nembutal Sodium Capsules ... 436
Nembutal Sodium Solution ... 438
Nembutal Sodium Suppositories ... 440

Perphenazine (Additive CNS depression). Products include:
Etrafon ... 2355
Triavil Tablets ... 1757
Trilafon ... 2389

Phenobarbital (Additive CNS depression). Products include:
Arco-Lase Plus Tablets ... 512
Bellergal-S Tablets ... 2250
Donnatal ... 2060
Donnatal Extentabs ... 2061
Donnatal Tablets ... 2060
Phenobarbital Elixir and Tablets ... 1469
Quadrinal Tablets ... 1350

Prazepam (Additive CNS depression).
No products indexed under this heading.

Prochlorperazine (Additive CNS depression). Products include:
Compazine ... 2470

Promethazine Hydrochloride (Additive CNS depression). Products include:
Mepergan Injection ... 2753
Phenergan with Codeine ... 2777
Phenergan with Dextromethorphan 2778
Phenergan Injection ... 2773
Phenergan Suppositories ... 2775
Phenergan Syrup ... 2774
Phenergan Tablets ... 2775
Phenergan VC ... 2779
Phenergan VC with Codeine ... 2781

Propofol (Additive CNS depression). Products include:
Diprivan Injection ... 2833

Propoxyphene Hydrochloride (Additive CNS depression). Products include:
Darvon ... 1435
Wygesic Tablets ... 2827

Propoxyphene Napsylate (Additive CNS depression). Products include:
Darvon-N/Darvocet-N ... 1433

IMPORTANT NOTE: Always consult each drug listing in the patient's regimen for possible interactions.

Quazepam (Additive CNS depression). Products include:
Doral Tablets 2664

Risperidone (Additive CNS depression). Products include:
Risperdal 1301

Secobarbital Sodium (Additive CNS depression). Products include:
Seconal Sodium Pulvules 1474

Sufentanil Citrate (Additive CNS depression). Products include:
Sufenta Injection 1309

Temazepam (Additive CNS depression). Products include:
Restoril Capsules 2284

Thiamylal Sodium (Additive CNS depression).
No products indexed under this heading.

Thioridazine Hydrochloride (Additive CNS depression). Products include:
Mellaril 2269

Thiothixene (Additive CNS depression). Products include:
Navane Capsules and Concentrate 2201
Navane Intramuscular 2202

Triazolam (Additive CNS depression). Products include:
Halcion Tablets 2611

Trifluoperazine Hydrochloride (Additive CNS depression). Products include:
Stelazine 2514

Zolpidem Tartrate (Additive CNS depression). Products include:
Ambien Tablets 2416

Food Interactions

Alcohol (Additive CNS depression).

NUMORPHAN SUPPOSITORIES

(Oxymorphone Hydrochloride) 937

May interact with narcotic analgesics, tranquilizers, hypnotics and sedatives, general anesthetics, phenothiazines, central nervous system depressants, and certain other agents. Compounds in these categories include:

Alfentanil Hydrochloride (Additive CNS depression). Products include:
Alfenta Injection 1286

Alprazolam (Additive CNS depression). Products include:
Xanax Tablets 2649

Aprobarbital (Additive CNS depression).
No products indexed under this heading.

Buprenorphine (Additive CNS depression). Products include:
Buprenex Injectable 2006

Buspirone Hydrochloride (Additive CNS depression). Products include:
BuSpar 737

Butabarbital (Additive CNS depression).
No products indexed under this heading.

Butalbital (Additive CNS depression). Products include:
Esgic-plus Tablets 1013
Fioricet Tablets 2258
Fioricet with Codeine Capsules 2260
Fiorinal Capsules 2261
Fiorinal with Codeine Capsules 2262
Fiorinal Tablets 2261
Phrenilin 785
Sedapap Tablets 50 mg/650 mg 1543

Chlordiazepoxide (Additive CNS depression). Products include:
Libritabs Tablets 2177
Limbitrol 2180

Chlordiazepoxide Hydrochloride (Additive CNS depression). Products include:
Librax Capsules 2176
Librium Capsules 2178
Librium Injectable 2179

Chlorpromazine (Additive CNS depression). Products include:
Thorazine Suppositories 2523

Chlorprothixene (Additive CNS depression).
No products indexed under this heading.

Chlorprothixene Hydrochloride (Additive CNS depression).
No products indexed under this heading.

Clorazepate Dipotassium (Additive CNS depression). Products include:
Tranxene 451

Clozapine (Additive CNS depression). Products include:
Clozaril Tablets 2252

Codeine Phosphate (Additive CNS depression). Products include:
Actifed with Codeine Cough Syrup 1067
Brontex 1981
Deconsal C Expectorant Syrup 456
Deconsal Pediatric Syrup 457
Dimetane-DC Cough Syrup 2059
Empirin with Codeine Tablets 1093
Fioricet with Codeine Capsules 2260
Fiorinal with Codeine Capsules 2262
Isoclor Expectorant 990
Novahistine DH 2462
Novahistine Expectorant 2463
Nucofed 2051
Phenergan with Codeine 2777
Phenergan VC with Codeine 2781
Robitussin A-C Syrup 2073
Robitussin-DAC Syrup 2074
Ryna ▣ 841
Soma Compound w/Codeine Tablets 2676
Tussi-Organidin NR Liquid and S NR Liquid 2677
Tylenol with Codeine 1583

Desflurane (Additive CNS depression). Products include:
Suprane 1813

Dezocine (Additive CNS depression). Products include:
Dalgan Injection 538

Diazepam (Additive CNS depression). Products include:
Dizac 1809
Valium Injectable 2182
Valium Tablets 2183
Valrelease Capsules 2169

Droperidol (Additive CNS depression). Products include:
Inapsine Injection 1296

Enflurane (Additive CNS depression).
No products indexed under this heading.

Estazolam (Additive CNS depression). Products include:
ProSom Tablets 449

Ethchlorvynol (Additive CNS depression). Products include:
Placidyl Capsules 448

Ethinamate (Additive CNS depression).
No products indexed under this heading.

Fentanyl (Additive CNS depression). Products include:
Duragesic Transdermal System 1288

Fentanyl Citrate (Additive CNS depression). Products include:
Sublimaze Injection 1307

Fluphenazine Decanoate (Additive CNS depression). Products include:
Prolixin Decanoate 509

Fluphenazine Enanthate (Additive CNS depression). Products include:
Prolixin Enanthate 509

Fluphenazine Hydrochloride (Additive CNS depression). Products include:
Prolixin 509

Flurazepam Hydrochloride (Additive CNS depression). Products include:
Dalmane Capsules 2173

Glutethimide (Additive CNS depression).
No products indexed under this heading.

Haloperidol (Additive CNS depression). Products include:
Haldol Injection, Tablets and Concentrate 1575

Haloperidol Decanoate (Additive CNS depression). Products include:
Haldol Decanoate 1577

Hydrocodone Bitartrate (Additive CNS depression). Products include:
Anexsia 5/500 Elixir 1781
Anexia Tablets 1782
Codiclear DH Syrup 791
Deconamine CX Cough and Cold Liquid and Tablets 1319
Duratuss HD Elixir 2565
Hycodan Tablets and Syrup 930
Hycomine Compound Tablets 932
Hycomine 931
Hycotuss Expectorant Syrup 933
Hydrocet Capsules 782
Lorcet 10/650 1018
Lortab 2566
Tussend 1783
Tussend Expectorant 1785
Vicodin Tablets 1356
Vicodin ES Tablets 1357
Vicodin Tuss Expectorant 1358
Zydone Capsules 949

Hydrocodone Polistirex (Additive CNS depression). Products include:
Tussionex Pennkinetic Extended-Release Suspension 998

Hydroxyzine Hydrochloride (Additive CNS depression). Products include:
Atarax Tablets & Syrup 2185
Marax Tablets & DF Syrup 2200
Vistaril Intramuscular Solution 2216

Isoflurane (Additive CNS depression).
No products indexed under this heading.

Ketamine Hydrochloride (Additive CNS depression).
No products indexed under this heading.

Levomethadyl Acetate Hydrochloride (Additive CNS depression). Products include:
Orlamm 2239

Levorphanol Tartrate (Additive CNS depression). Products include:
Levo-Dromoran 2129

Lorazepam (Additive CNS depression). Products include:
Ativan Injection 2698
Ativan Tablets 2700

Loxapine Hydrochloride (Additive CNS depression). Products include:
Loxitane 1378

Loxapine Succinate (Additive CNS depression). Products include:
Loxitane Capsules 1378

Meperidine Hydrochloride (Additive CNS depression). Products include:
Demerol 2308
Mepergan Injection 2753

Mephobarbital (Additive CNS depression). Products include:
Mebaral Tablets 2322

Meprobamate (Additive CNS depression). Products include:
Miltown Tablets 2672
PMB 200 and PMB 400 2783

Mesoridazine Besylate (Additive CNS depression). Products include:
Serentil 684

Methadone Hydrochloride (Additive CNS depression). Products include:
Methadone Hydrochloride Oral Concentrate 2233
Methadone Hydrochloride Oral Solution & Tablets 2235

Methohexital Sodium (Additive CNS depression). Products include:
Brevital Sodium Vials 1429

Methotrimeprazine (Additive CNS depression). Products include:
Levoprome 1274

Methoxyflurane (Additive CNS depression).
No products indexed under this heading.

Midazolam Hydrochloride (Additive CNS depression). Products include:
Versed Injection 2170

Molindone Hydrochloride (Additive CNS depression). Products include:
Moban Tablets and Concentrate 1048

Morphine Sulfate (Additive CNS depression). Products include:
Astramorph/PF Injection, USP (Preservative-Free) 535
Duramorph 962
Infumorph 200 and Infumorph 500 Sterile Solutions 965
MS Contin Tablets 1994
MSIR 1997
Oramorph SR (Morphine Sulfate Sustained Release Tablets) 2236
RMS Suppositories 2657
Roxanol 2243

Opium Alkaloids (Additive CNS depression).
No products indexed under this heading.

Oxazepam (Additive CNS depression). Products include:
Serax Capsules 2810
Serax Tablets 2810

Oxycodone Hydrochloride (Additive CNS depression). Products include:
Percocet Tablets 938
Percodan Tablets 939
Percodan-Demi Tablets 940
Roxicodone Tablets, Oral Solution & Intensol (Oxycodone) 2244
Tylox Capsules 1584

Pentobarbital Sodium (Additive CNS depression). Products include:
Nembutal Sodium Capsules 436
Nembutal Sodium Solution 438
Nembutal Sodium Suppositories 440

Perphenazine (Additive CNS depression). Products include:
Etrafon 2355
Triavil Tablets 1757
Trilafon 2389

Phenobarbital (Additive CNS depression). Products include:
Arco-Lase Plus Tablets 512
Bellergal-S Tablets 2250
Donnatal 2060
Donnatal Extentabs 2061
Donnatal Tablets 2060
Phenobarbital Elixir and Tablets 1469
Quadrinal Tablets 1350

Prazepam (Additive CNS depression).
No products indexed under this heading.

Prochlorperazine (Additive CNS depression). Products include:
Compazine 2470

(▣ Described in PDR For Nonprescription Drugs) (◉ Described in PDR For Ophthalmology)

Promethazine Hydrochloride (Additive CNS depression). Products include:

Mepergan Injection 2753
Phenergan with Codeine 2777
Phenergan with Dextromethorphan 2778
Phenergan Injection 2773
Phenergan Suppositories 2775
Phenergan Syrup 2774
Phenergan Tablets 2775
Phenergan VC 2779
Phenergan VC with Codeine 2781

Propofol (Additive CNS depression). Products include:

Diprivan Injection 2833

Propoxyphene Hydrochloride (Additive CNS depression). Products include:

Darvon 1435
Wygesic Tablets 2827

Propoxyphene Napsylate (Additive CNS depression). Products include:

Darvon-N/Darvocet-N 1433

Quazepam (Additive CNS depression). Products include:

Doral Tablets 2664

Risperidone (Additive CNS depression). Products include:

Risperdal 1301

Secobarbital Sodium (Additive CNS depression). Products include:

Seconal Sodium Pulvules 1474

Sufentanil Citrate (Additive CNS depression). Products include:

Sufenta Injection 1309

Temazepam (Additive CNS depression). Products include:

Restoril Capsules 2284

Thiamylal Sodium (Additive CNS depression).

No products indexed under this heading.

Thioridazine Hydrochloride (Additive CNS depression). Products include:

Mellaril 2269

Thiothixene (Additive CNS depression). Products include:

Navane Capsules and Concentrate 2201
Navane Intramuscular 2202

Triazolam (Additive CNS depression). Products include:

Halcion Tablets 2611

Trifluoperazine Hydrochloride (Additive CNS depression). Products include:

Stelazine 2514

Zolpidem Tartrate (Additive CNS depression). Products include:

Ambien Tablets 2416

Food Interactions

Alcohol (Additive CNS depression).

NUPERCAINAL HEMORRHOIDAL AND ANESTHETIC OINTMENT

(Dibucaine) .... ◆D 644
None cited in PDR database.

NUPERCAINAL HYDROCORTISONE 1% CREAM

(Hydrocortisone Acetate) .... ◆D 645
None cited in PDR database.

NUPERCAINAL PAIN RELIEF CREAM

(Dibucaine) .... ◆D 645
None cited in PDR database.

NUPERCAINAL SUPPOSITORIES

(Cocoa Butter, Zinc Oxide) .... ◆D 645
None cited in PDR database.

NUPRIN IBUPROFEN/ANALGESIC TABLETS & CAPLETS

(Ibuprofen) .... ◆D 622

May interact with aspirin and acetaminophen containing products. Compounds in this category include:

Acetaminophen (Concomitant administration recommended only under a doctor's direction). Products include:

Actifed Plus Caplets .... ◆D 845
Actifed Plus Tablets .... ◆D 845
Actifed Sinus Daytime/Nighttime Tablets and Caplets .... ◆D 846
Alka-Seltzer Plus Cold Medicine Liqui-Gels .... ◆D 706
Alka-Seltzer Plus Cold & Cough Medicine Liqui-Gels .... ◆D 705
Alka-Seltzer Plus Night-Time Cold Medicine Liqui-Gels .... ◆D 706
Allerest Headache Strength Tablets .... ◆D 627
Allerest No Drowsiness Tablets ...... ◆D 627
Allerest Sinus Pain Formula .... ◆D 627
Anexsia 5/500 Elixir 1781
Anexia Tablets 1782
Arthritis Foundation Aspirin Free Caplets .... ◆D 673
Arthritis Foundation NightTime Caplets .... ◆D 674
Bayer Select Headache Pain Relief Formula .... ◆D 716
Bayer Select Menstrual Multi-Symptom Formula .... ◆D 716
Bayer Select Night Time Pain Relief Formula .... ◆D 716
Bayer Select Sinus Pain Relief Formula .... ◆D 717
Benadryl Allergy Sinus Headache Formula Caplets .... ◆D 849
Comtrex Multi-Symptom Cold Reliever Tablets/Caplets/Liqui-Gels/Liquid .... ◆D 615
Allergy-Sinus Comtrex Multi-Symptom Allergy-Sinus Formula Tablets .... ◆D 617
Comtrex Non-Drowsy .... ◆D 618
Contac Day Allergy/Sinus Caplets ◆D 812
Contac Day & Night .... ◆D 812
Contac Night Allergy/Sinus Caplets .... ◆D 812
Contac Severe Cold and Flu Formula Caplets .... ◆D 814
Contac Severe Cold & Flu Non-Drowsy .... ◆D 815
Coricidin 'D' Decongestant Tablets .... ◆D 800
Coricidin Tablets .... ◆D 800
DHCplus Capsules 1993
Darvon-N/Darvocet-N 1433
Drixoral Cold and Flu Extended-Release Tablets .... ◆D 803
Drixoral Cough + Sore Throat Liquid Caps .... ◆D 802
Drixoral Allergy/Sinus Extended Release Tablets .... ◆D 804
Esgic-plus Tablets 1013
Aspirin Free Excedrin Analgesic Caplets and Geltabs 732
Excedrin Extra-Strength Analgesic Tablets & Caplets 732
Excedrin P.M. Analgesic/Sleeping Aid Tablets, Caplets, Liquigels 733
Fioricet Tablets 2258
Fioricet with Codeine Capsules 2260
Hycomine Compound Tablets 932
Hydrocet Capsules 782
Legatrin PM .... ◆D 651
Lorcet 10/650 1018
Lortab 2566
Lurline PMS Tablets 982
Maximum Strength Multi-Symptom Formula Midol .... ◆D 722
PMS Multi-Symptom Formula Midol .... ◆D 723
Teen Multi-Symptom Formula Midol .... ◆D 722
Midrin Capsules 783
Migralam Capsules 2038
Panodol Tablets and Caplets .... ◆D 824
Children's Panadol Chewable Tablets, Liquid, Infant's Drops .... ◆D 824
Percocet Tablets 938
Percogesic Analgesic Tablets .... ◆D 754
Phrenilin 785
Pyrroxate Caplets .... ◆D 772
Sedapap Tablets 50 mg/650 mg .. 1543
Sinarest Tablets .... ◆D 648
Sinarest Extra Strength Tablets ...... ◆D 648
Sinarest No Drowsiness Tablets .... ◆D 648
Sine-Aid Maximum Strength Sinus Medication Gelcaps, Caplets and Tablets 1554
Sine-Off No Drowsiness Formula Caplets .... ◆D 824
Sine-Off Sinus Medicine .... ◆D 825
Singlet Tablets .... ◆D 825
Sinulin Tablets 787
Sinutab Sinus Allergy Medication, Maximum Strength Tablets and Caplets .... ◆D 860
Sinutab Sinus Medication, Maximum Strength Without Drowsiness Formula, Tablets & Caplets .... ◆D 860
Sinutab Sinus Medication, Regular Strength Without Drowsiness Formula .... ◆D 859
Sudafed Cold and Cough Liquidcaps .... ◆D 862
Sudafed Severe Cold Formula Caplets .... ◆D 863
Sudafed Severe Cold Formula Tablets .... ◆D 864
Sudafed Sinus Caplets .... ◆D 864
Sudafed Sinus Tablets .... ◆D 864
Talacen 2333
TheraFlu .... ◆D 787
TheraFlu Maximum Strength Nighttime Flu, Cold & Cough Medicine .... ◆D 788
TheraFlu Maximum Strength Non-Drowsy Formula Flu, Cold & Cough Medicine .... ◆D 788
Thera Flu Maximum Strength, Non-Drowsy Formula Flu, Cold and Cough Caplets .... ◆D 789
Triaminic Sore Throat Formula ...... ◆D 791
Triaminicin Tablets .... ◆D 793
Children's TYLENOL acetaminophen Chewable Tablets, Elixir, Suspension Liquid 1555
Children's TYLENOL Cold Multi-Symptom Liquid Formula and Chewable Tablets 1561
Children's TYLENOL Cold Plus Cough Multi Symptom Tablets and Liquid .... ◆D 681
Infants' TYLENOL acetaminophen Drops and Suspension Drops 1555
Infants' TYLENOL Cold Decongestant & Fever-Reducer Drops 1556
TYLENOL Extended Relief Caplets.. 1558
TYLENOL, Extra Strength, Acetaminophen Adult Liquid Pain Reliever 1560
TYLENOL, Extra Strength, acetaminophen Gelcaps, Geltabs, Caplets, Tablets 1559
TYLENOL, Extra Strength, Headache Plus Pain Reliever with Antacid Caplets 1559
TYLENOL, Junior Strength, acetaminophen Coated Caplets, Grape and Fruit Chewable Tablets 1557
TYLENOL Maximum Strength Allergy Sinus Medication Gelcaps and Caplets 1563
TYLENOL Maximum Strength Allergy Sinus NightTime Medication Caplets 1555
TYLENOL Flu Maximum Strength Gelcaps 1565
TYLENOL Flu NightTime, Maximum Strength, Gelcaps 1566
TYLENOL Maximum Strength Flu NightTime Hot Medication Packets 1562
TYLENOL, Maximum Strength, Sinus Medication Geltabs, Gelcaps, Caplets and Tablets 1566
TYLENOL Cold Multi-Symptom Formula Medication Tablets and Caplets 1561
TYLENOL Cold Medication No Drowsiness Formula Gelcaps and Caplets 1562
TYLENOL Cold Multi-Symptom Hot Medication Liquid Packets 1557
TYLENOL Cough Multi-Symptom Medication 1564
TYLENOL Cough Multi-Symptom Medication with Decongestant 1565
TYLENOL, Regular Strength, acetaminophen Caplets and Tablets .. 1558
TYLENOL PM, Extra Strength Pain Reliever/Sleep Aid Caplets, Geltabs, Gelcaps 1560
TYLENOL Severe Allergy Medication Caplets 1564
Tylenol with Codeine 1583
Tylox Capsules 1584
Unisom With Pain Relief-Nighttime Sleep Aid and Pain Reliever 1934
Vanquish Analgesic Caplets .... ◆D 731
Vicks 44 LiquiCaps Cough, Cold & Flu Relief .... ◆D 755
Vicks 44M Cough, Cold & Flu Relief .... ◆D 756
Vicks DayQuil .... ◆D 761
Vicks Nyquil Hot Therapy .... ◆D 762
Vicks NyQuil LiquiCaps Multi-Symptom Cold/Flu Relief .... ◆D 763
Vicks NyQuil Multi-Symptom Cold/Flu Relief - (Original & Cherry Flavor) .... ◆D 763
Vicodin Tablets 1356
Vicodin ES Tablets 1357
Wygesic Tablets 2827
Zydone Capsules 949

Aspirin (Concomitant administration recommended only under a doctor's direction). Products include:

Alka-Seltzer Effervescent Antacid and Pain Reliever .... ◆D 701
Alka-Seltzer Extra Strength Effervescent Antacid and Pain Reliever .... ◆D 703
Alka-Seltzer Lemon Lime Effervescent Antacid and Pain Reliever .... ◆D 703
Alka-Seltzer Plus Cold Medicine .... ◆D 705
Alka-Seltzer Plus Cold & Cough Medicine .... ◆D 708
Alka-Seltzer Plus Night-Time Cold Medicine .... ◆D 707
Alka Seltzer Plus Sinus Medicine .. ◆D 707
Arthritis Foundation Safety Coated Aspirin Tablets .... ◆D 675
Arthritis Pain Ascriptin .... ◆D 631
Maximum Strength Ascriptin .... ◆D 630
Regular Strength Ascriptin Tablets .... ◆D 629
Arthritis Strength BC Powder .... ◆D 609
BC Cold Powder Multi-Symptom Formula (Cold-Sinus-Allergy) ...... ◆D 609
BC Cold Powder Non-Drowsy Formula (Cold-Sinus) .... ◆D 609
BC Powder .... ◆D 609
Bayer Children's Chewable Aspirin .... ◆D 711
Genuine Bayer Aspirin Tablets & Caplets .... ◆D 713
Extra Strength Bayer Arthritis Pain Regimen Formula .... ◆D 711
Extra Strength Bayer Aspirin Caplets & Tablets .... ◆D 712
Extended-Release Bayer 8-Hour Aspirin .... ◆D 712
Extra Strength Bayer Plus Aspirin Caplets .... ◆D 713
Extra Strength Bayer PM Aspirin .. ◆D 713
Bayer Enteric Aspirin .... ◆D 709
Bufferin Analgesic Tablets and Caplets .... ◆D 613
Arthritis Strength Bufferin Analgesic Caplets .... ◆D 614
Extra Strength Bufferin Analgesic Tablets .... ◆D 615
Cama Arthritis Pain Reliever .... ◆D 785
Darvon Compound-65 Pulvules 1435
Easprin 1914
Ecotrin 2455
Ecotrin Enteric Coated Aspirin Maximum Strength Tablets and Caplets .... ◆D 816
Ecotrin Enteric Coated Aspirin Regular Strength Tablets 2455
Empirin Aspirin Tablets .... ◆D 854
Empirin with Codeine Tablets 1093
Excedrin Extra-Strength Analgesic Tablets & Caplets 732
Fiorinal Capsules 2261
Fiorinal with Codeine Capsules 2262
Fiorinal Tablets 2261
Halfprin 1362
Healthprin Aspirin 2455
Norgesic 1496
Percodan Tablets 939
Percodan-Demi Tablets 940
Robaxisal Tablets 2071
Soma Compound w/Codeine Tablets 2676
Soma Compound Tablets 2675
St. Joseph Adult Chewable Aspirin (81 mg.) .... ◆D 808
Talwin Compound 2335
Ursinus Inlay-Tabs .... ◆D 794
Vanquish Analgesic Caplets .... ◆D 731

IMPORTANT NOTE: Always consult each drug listing in the patient's regimen for possible interactions.

NUROMAX INJECTION
(Doxacurium Chloride) 1149
May interact with inhalant anesthetics, aminoglycosides, tetracyclines, lithium preparations, local anesthetics, and certain other agents. Compounds in these categories include:

Amikacin Sulfate (Enhances the neuromuscular blocking action). Products include:
- Amikacin Sulfate Injection, USP 960
- Amikin Injectable 501

Bacitracin (Enhances the neuromuscular blocking action). Products include:
- Mycitracin ...... ▣ 839

Bupivacaine Hydrochloride (Enhances the neuromuscular blocking action). Products include:
- Marcaine Hydrochloride with Epinephrine 1:200,000 2316
- Marcaine Hydrochloride Injection...... 2316
- Marcaine Spinal 2319
- Sensorcaine 559

Carbamazepine (The time of onset of neuromuscular block is lengthened and the duration of block is shortened). Products include:
- Atretol Tablets 573
- Tegretol Chewable Tablets 852
- Tegretol Suspension...... 852
- Tegretol Tablets 852

Chloroprocaine Hydrochloride (Enhances the neuromuscular blocking action). Products include:
- Nescaine/Nescaine MPF...... 554

Clindamycin Hydrochloride (Enhances the neuromuscular blocking action).
- No products indexed under this heading.

Clindamycin Palmitate Hydrochloride (Enhances the neuromuscular blocking action).
- No products indexed under this heading.

Clindamycin Phosphate (Enhances the neuromuscular blocking action). Products include:
- Cleocin Phosphate Injection 2586
- Cleocin T Topical 2590
- Cleocin Vaginal Cream...... 2589

Colistimethate Sodium (Enhances the neuromuscular blocking action). Products include:
- Coly-Mycin M Parenteral...... 1905

Colistin Sulfate (Enhances the neuromuscular blocking action). Products include:
- Coly-Mycin S Otic w/Neomycin & Hydrocortisone 1906

Demeclocycline Hydrochloride (Enhances the neuromuscular blocking action). Products include:
- Declomycin Tablets...... 1371

Desflurane (Decreases the ED_{50} by 30% to 45%; prolongs the clinically effective duration of action by up to 25%). Products include:
- Suprane 1813

Doxycycline Calcium (Enhances the neuromuscular blocking action). Products include:
- Vibramycin Calcium Oral Suspension Syrup...... 1941

Doxycycline Hyclate (Enhances the neuromuscular blocking action). Products include:
- Doryx Capsules...... 1913
- Vibramycin Hyclate Capsules...... 1941
- Vibramycin Hyclate Intravenous 2215
- Vibra-Tabs Film Coated Tablets 1941

Doxycycline Monohydrate (Enhances the neuromuscular blocking action). Products include:
- Monodox Capsules 1805
- Vibramycin Monohydrate for Oral Suspension 1941

Enflurane (Decreases the ED_{50} by 30% to 45%; prolongs the clinically effective duration of action by up to 25%).
- No products indexed under this heading.

Etidocaine Hydrochloride (Enhances the neuromuscular blocking action). Products include:
- Duranest Injections 542

Gentamicin Sulfate (Enhances the neuromuscular blocking action). Products include:
- Garamycin Injectable 2360
- Genoptic Sterile Ophthalmic Solution...... ⊙ 243
- Genoptic Sterile Ophthalmic Ointment ...... ⊙ 243
- Gentacidin Ointment ...... ⊙ 264
- Gentacidin Solution...... ⊙ 264
- Gentak ...... ⊙ 208
- Pred-G Liquifilm Sterile Ophthalmic Suspension ...... ⊙ 251
- Pred-G S.O.P. Sterile Ophthalmic Ointment ...... ⊙ 252

Halothane (Decreases the ED_{50} by 30% to 45%; prolongs the clinically effective duration of action by up to 25%). Products include:
- Fluothane 2724

Isoflurane (Decreases the ED_{50} by 30% to 45%; prolongs the clinically effective duration of action by up to 25%).
- No products indexed under this heading.

Kanamycin Sulfate (Enhances the neuromuscular blocking action).
- No products indexed under this heading.

Lidocaine Hydrochloride (Enhances the neuromuscular blocking action). Products include:
- Bactine Antiseptic/Anesthetic First Aid Liquid ...... ▣ 708
- Campho-Phenique Maximum Strength First Aid Antibiotic Plus Pain Reliever Ointment ...... ▣ 719
- Decadron Phosphate with Xylocaine Injection, Sterile 1639
- Xylocaine Injections 567

Lincomycin Hydrochloride Monohydrate (Enhances the neuromuscular blocking action).
- No products indexed under this heading.

Lithium Carbonate (Enhances the neuromuscular blocking action). Products include:
- Eskalith 2485
- Lithium Carbonate Capsules & Tablets 2230
- Lithonate/Lithotabs/Lithobid 2543

Lithium Citrate (Enhances the neuromuscular blocking action).
- No products indexed under this heading.

Magnesium Salts (Enhances the neuromuscular blocking action).

Mepivacaine Hydrochloride Injection (Enhances the neuromuscular blocking action). Products include:
- Carbocaine Hydrochloride Injection 2303

Methacycline Hydrochloride (Enhances the neuromuscular blocking action).
- No products indexed under this heading.

Methoxyflurane (Decreases the ED_{50} by 30% to 45%; prolongs the clinically effective duration of action by up to 25%).
- No products indexed under this heading.

Minocycline Hydrochloride (Enhances the neuromuscular blocking action). Products include:
- Dynacin Capsules 1590
- Minocin Intravenous 1382
- Minocin Oral Suspension 1385
- Minocin Pellet-Filled Capsules 1383

Oxytetracycline Hydrochloride (Enhances the neuromuscular blocking action). Products include:
- TERAK Ointment ...... ⊙ 209
- Terra-Cortril Ophthalmic Suspension 2210
- Terramycin with Polymyxin B Sulfate Ophthalmic Ointment 2211
- Urobiotic-250 Capsules 2214

Phenytoin (The time of onset of neuromuscular block is lengthened and the duration of block is shortened). Products include:
- Dilantin Infatabs 1908
- Dilantin-125 Suspension 1911

Phenytoin Sodium (The time of onset of neuromuscular block is lengthened and the duration of block is shortened). Products include:
- Dilantin Kapseals 1906
- Dilantin Parenteral 1910

Polymyxin Preparations (Enhances the neuromuscular blocking action).

Procainamide Hydrochloride (Enhances the neuromuscular blocking action). Products include:
- Procan SR Tablets...... 1926

Procaine Hydrochloride (Enhances the neuromuscular blocking action). Products include:
- Novocain Hydrochloride for Spinal Anesthesia 2326

Quinidine Gluconate (Enhances the neuromuscular blocking action). Products include:
- Quinaglute Dura-Tabs Tablets 649

Quinidine Polygalacturonate (Enhances the neuromuscular blocking action).
- No products indexed under this heading.

Quinidine Sulfate (Enhances the neuromuscular blocking action). Products include:
- Quinidex Extentabs 2067

Streptomycin Sulfate (Enhances the neuromuscular blocking action). Products include:
- Streptomycin Sulfate Injection...... 2208

Tetracaine Hydrochloride (Enhances the neuromuscular blocking action). Products include:
- Cetacaine Topical Anesthetic 794
- Pontocaine Hydrochloride for Spinal Anesthesia...... 2330

Tetracycline Hydrochloride (Enhances the neuromuscular blocking action). Products include:
- Achromycin V Capsules 1367

Tobramycin (Enhances the neuromuscular blocking action). Products include:
- AKTOB ...... ⊙ 206
- TobraDex Ophthalmic Suspension and Ointment...... 473
- Tobrex Ophthalmic Ointment and Solution ...... ⊙ 229

Tobramycin Sulfate (Enhances the neuromuscular blocking action). Products include:
- Nebcin Vials, Hyporets & ADD-Vantage 1464
- Tobramycin Sulfate Injection 968

NURSOY, SOY PROTEIN FORMULA FOR INFANTS, CONCENTRATED LIQUID, READY-TO-FEED, AND POWDER
(Protein Preparations)....................2763
None cited in PDR database.

NUTR-E-SOL
(Vitamin E) 468
None cited in PDR database.

NUTROPIN
(Somatropin) 1061
May interact with glucocorticoids. Compounds in this category include:

Betamethasone Acetate (Concomitant glucocorticoid therapy may inhibit the growth promoting effect, especially in patients with chronic renal failure). Products include:
- Celestone Soluspan Suspension 2347

Betamethasone Sodium Phosphate (Concomitant glucocorticoid therapy may inhibit the growth promoting effect, especially in patients with chronic renal failure). Products include:
- Celestone Soluspan Suspension 2347

Cortisone Acetate (Concomitant glucocorticoid therapy may inhibit the growth promoting effect, especially in patients with chronic renal failure). Products include:
- Cortone Acetate Sterile Suspension 1623
- Cortone Acetate Tablets...... 1624

Dexamethasone (Concomitant glucocorticoid therapy may inhibit the growth promoting effect, especially in patients with chronic renal failure). Products include:
- AK-Trol Ointment & Suspension ...... ⊙ 205
- Decadron Elixir 1633
- Decadron Tablets...... 1635
- Decaspray Topical Aerosol 1648
- Dexacidin Ointment ...... ⊙ 263
- Maxitrol Ophthalmic Ointment and Suspension ...... ⊙ 224
- TobraDex Ophthalmic Suspension and Ointment...... 473

Dexamethasone Acetate (Concomitant glucocorticoid therapy may inhibit the growth promoting effect, especially in patients with chronic renal failure). Products include:
- Dalalone D.P. Injectable 1011
- Decadron-LA Sterile Suspension...... 1646

Dexamethasone Sodium Phosphate (Concomitant glucocorticoid therapy may inhibit the growth promoting effect, especially in patients with chronic renal failure). Products include:
- Decadron Phosphate Injection 1637
- Decadron Phosphate Respihaler 1642
- Decadron Phosphate Sterile Ophthalmic Ointment 1641
- Decadron Phosphate Sterile Ophthalmic Solution 1642
- Decadron Phosphate Topical Cream 1644
- Decadron Phosphate Turbinaire 1645
- Decadron Phosphate with Xylocaine Injection, Sterile 1639
- Dexacort Phosphate in Respihaler .. 458
- Dexacort Phosphate in Turbinaire .. 459
- NeoDecadron Sterile Ophthalmic Ointment 1712
- NeoDecadron Sterile Ophthalmic Solution 1713
- NeoDecadron Topical Cream 1714

Fludrocortisone Acetate (Concomitant glucocorticoid therapy may inhibit the growth promoting effect, especially in patients with chronic renal failure). Products include:
- Florinef Acetate Tablets 505

Hydrocortisone (Concomitant glucocorticoid therapy may inhibit the growth promoting effect, especially in patients with chronic renal failure). Products include:
- Anusol-HC Cream 2.5% 1896
- Aquanil HC Lotion 1931
- Bactine Hydrocortisone Anti-Itch Cream ...... ▣ 709
- Caldecort Anti-Itch Hydrocortisone Spray ...... ▣ 631
- Cortaid ...... ▣ 836
- CORTENEMA...... 2535
- Cortisporin Ointment 1085
- Cortisporin Ophthalmic Ointment Sterile 1085

(▣ Described in PDR For Nonprescription Drugs) (⊙ Described in PDR For Ophthalmology)

Cortisporin Ophthalmic Suspension Sterile ... 1086
Cortisporin Otic Solution Sterile ... 1087
Cortisporin Otic Suspension Sterile ... 1088
Cortizone-5 ... ▣ 831
Cortizone-10 ... ▣ 831
Hydrocortone Tablets ... 1672
Hytone ... 907
Massengill Medicated Soft Cloth Towelettes ... 2458
PediOtic Suspension Sterile ... 1153
Preparation H Hydrocortisone 1% Cream ... ▣ 872
ProctoCream-HC 2.5% ... 2408
VōSoL HC Otic Solution ... 2678

Hydrocortisone Acetate (Concomitant glucocorticoid therapy may inhibit the growth promoting effect, especially in patients with chronic renal failure). Products include:
Analpram-HC Rectal Cream 1% and 2.5% ... 977
Anusol HC-1 Anti-Itch Hydrocortisone Ointment ... ▣ 847
Anusol-HC Suppositories ... 1897
Caldecort ... ▣ 631
Carmol HC ... 924
Coly-Mycin S Otic w/Neomycin & Hydrocortisone ... 1906
Cortaid ... ▣ 836
Cortifoam ... 2396
Cortisporin Cream ... 1084
Epifoam ... 2399
Hydrocortone Acetate Sterile Suspension ... 1669
Mantadil Cream ... 1135
Nupercainal Hydrocortisone 1% Cream ... ▣ 645
Ophthocort ... ⊙ 311
Pramosone Cream, Lotion & Ointment ... 978
ProctoCream-HC ... 2408
ProctoFoam-HC ... 2409
Terra-Cortril Ophthalmic Suspension ... 2210

Hydrocortisone Sodium Phosphate (Concomitant glucocorticoid therapy may inhibit the growth promoting effect, especially in patients with chronic renal failure). Products include:
Hydrocortone Phosphate Injection, Sterile ... 1670

Hydrocortisone Sodium Succinate (Concomitant glucocorticoid therapy may inhibit the growth promoting effect, especially in patients with chronic renal failure). Products include:
Solu-Cortef Sterile Powder ... 2641

Methylprednisolone Acetate (Concomitant glucocorticoid therapy may inhibit the growth promoting effect, especially in patients with chronic renal failure). Products include:
Depo-Medrol Single-Dose Vial ... 2600
Depo-Medrol Sterile Aqueous Suspension ... 2597

Methylprednisolone Sodium Succinate (Concomitant glucocorticoid therapy may inhibit the growth promoting effect, especially in patients with chronic renal failure). Products include:
Solu-Medrol Sterile Powder ... 2643

Prednisolone Acetate (Concomitant glucocorticoid therapy may inhibit the growth promoting effect, especially in patients with chronic renal failure). Products include:
AK-CIDE ... ⊙ 202
AK-CIDE Ointment ... ⊙ 202
Blephamide Liquifilm Sterile Ophthalmic Suspension ... 476
Blephamide Ointment ... ⊙ 237
Econopred & Econopred Plus Ophthalmic Suspensions ... ⊙ 217
Poly-Pred Liquifilm ... ⊙ 248
Pred Forte ... ⊙ 250
Pred Mild ... ⊙ 253
Pred-G Liquifilm Sterile Ophthalmic Suspension ... ⊙ 251
Pred-G S.O.P. Sterile Ophthalmic Ointment ... ⊙ 252
Vasocidin Ointment ... ⊙ 268

Prednisolone Sodium Phosphate (Concomitant glucocorticoid therapy may inhibit the growth promoting effect, especially in patients with chronic renal failure). Products include:
AK-Pred ... ⊙ 204
Hydeltrasol Injection, Sterile ... 1665
Inflamase ... ⊙ 265
Pediapred Oral Liquid ... 995
Vasocidin Ophthalmic Solution ... ⊙ 270

Prednisolone Tebutate (Concomitant glucocorticoid therapy may inhibit the growth promoting effect, especially in patients with chronic renal failure). Products include:
Hydeltra-T.B.A. Sterile Suspension 1667

Prednisone (Concomitant glucocorticoid therapy may inhibit the growth promoting effect, especially in patients with chronic renal failure). Products include:
Deltasone Tablets ... 2595

Triamcinolone (Concomitant glucocorticoid therapy may inhibit the growth promoting effect, especially in patients with chronic renal failure). Products include:
Aristocort Tablets ... 1022

Triamcinolone Acetonide (Concomitant glucocorticoid therapy may inhibit the growth promoting effect, especially in patients with chronic renal failure). Products include:
Aristocort A 0.025% Cream ... 1027
Aristocort A 0.5% Cream ... 1031
Aristocort A 0.1% Cream ... 1029
Aristocort A 0.1% Ointment ... 1030
Azmacort Oral Inhaler ... 2011
Nasacort Nasal Inhaler ... 2024

Triamcinolone Diacetate (Concomitant glucocorticoid therapy may inhibit the growth promoting effect, especially in patients with chronic renal failure). Products include:
Aristocort Suspension (Forte Parenteral) ... 1027
Aristocort Suspension (Intralesional) ... 1025

Triamcinolone Hexacetonide (Concomitant glucocorticoid therapy may inhibit the growth promoting effect, especially in patients with chronic renal failure). Products include:
Aristospan Suspension (Intra-articular) ... 1033
Aristospan Suspension (Intralesional) ... 1032

NYDRAZID INJECTION

(Isoniazid) ... 508
May interact with:

Phenytoin (Co-administration may decrease the excretion of phenytoin resulting in enhanced effects and phenytoin intoxication; appropriate dosage adjustment of the anticonvulsant should be made). Products include:
Dilantin Infatabs ... 1908
Dilantin-125 Suspension ... 1911

Phenytoin Sodium (Co-administration may decrease the excretion of phenytoin resulting in enhanced effects and phenytoin intoxication; appropriate dosage adjustment of the anticonvulsant should be made). Products include:
Dilantin Kapseals ... 1906
Dilantin Parenteral ... 1910

Food Interactions

Alcohol (Daily ingestion of alcohol may be associated with a higher incidence of isoniazid hepatitis).

MAXIMUM STRENGTH NYTOL CAPLETS

(Doxylamine Succinate) ... ▣ 610

Food Interactions

Alcohol (When consuming alcohol, use Nytol with caution).

NYTOL QUICKCAPS CAPLETS

(Diphenhydramine Hydrochloride) .. ▣ 610
May interact with central nervous system depressants, monoamine oxidase inhibitors, and certain other agents. Compounds in these categories include:

Alfentanil Hydrochloride (Heightens depressant effect). Products include:
Alfenta Injection ... 1286

Alprazolam (Heightens depressant effect). Products include:
Xanax Tablets ... 2649

Aprobarbital (Heightens depressant effect).
No products indexed under this heading.

Buprenorphine (Heightens depressant effect). Products include:
Buprenex Injectable ... 2006

Buspirone Hydrochloride (Heightens depressant effect). Products include:
BuSpar ... 737

Butabarbital (Heightens depressant effect).
No products indexed under this heading.

Butalbital (Heightens depressant effect). Products include:
Esgic-plus Tablets ... 1013
Fioricet Tablets ... 2258
Fioricet with Codeine Capsules ... 2260
Fiorinal Capsules ... 2261
Fiorinal with Codeine Capsules ... 2262
Fiorinal Tablets ... 2261
Phrenilin ... 785
Sedapap Tablets 50 mg/650 mg .. 1543

Chlordiazepoxide (Heightens depressant effect). Products include:
Libritabs Tablets ... 2177
Limbitrol ... 2180

Chlordiazepoxide Hydrochloride (Heightens depressant effect). Products include:
Librax Capsules ... 2176
Librium Capsules ... 2178
Librium Injectable ... 2179

Chlorpromazine (Heightens depressant effect). Products include:
Thorazine Suppositories ... 2523

Chlorpromazine Hydrochloride (Heightens depressant effect). Products include:
Thorazine ... 2523

Chlorprothixene (Heightens depressant effect).
No products indexed under this heading.

Chlorprothixene Hydrochloride (Heightens depressant effect).
No products indexed under this heading.

Clorazepate Dipotassium (Heightens depressant effect). Products include:
Tranxene ... 451

Clozapine (Heightens depressant effect). Products include:
Clozaril Tablets ... 2252

Codeine Phosphate (Heightens depressant effect). Products include:
Actifed with Codeine Cough Syrup.. 1067
Brontex ... 1981
Deconsal C Expectorant Syrup ... 456
Deconsal Pediatric Syrup ... 457
Dimetane-DC Cough Syrup ... 2059
Empirin with Codeine Tablets ... 1093
Fioricet with Codeine Capsules ... 2260
Fiorinal with Codeine Capsules ... 2262
Isoclor Expectorant ... 990
Novahistine DH ... 2462
Novahistine Expectorant ... 2463
Nucofed ... 2051
Phenergan with Codeine ... 2777
Phenergan VC with Codeine ... 2781
Robitussin A-C Syrup ... 2073
Robitussin-DAC Syrup ... 2074
Ryna ... ▣ 841
Soma Compound w/Codeine Tablets ... 2676
Tussi-Organidin NR Liquid and S NR Liquid ... 2677
Tylenol with Codeine ... 1583

Desflurane (Heightens depressant effect). Products include:
Suprane ... 1813

Dezocine (Heightens depressant effect). Products include:
Dalgan Injection ... 538

Diazepam (Heightens depressant effect). Products include:
Dizac ... 1809
Valium Injectable ... 2182
Valium Tablets ... 2183
Valrelease Capsules ... 2169

Droperidol (Heightens depressant effect). Products include:
Inapsine Injection ... 1296

Enflurane (Heightens depressant effect).
No products indexed under this heading.

Estazolam (Heightens depressant effect). Products include:
ProSom Tablets ... 449

Ethchlorvynol (Heightens depressant effect). Products include:
Placidyl Capsules ... 448

Ethinamate (Heightens depressant effect).
No products indexed under this heading.

Fentanyl (Heightens depressant effect). Products include:
Duragesic Transdermal System ... 1288

Fentanyl Citrate (Heightens depressant effect). Products include:
Sublimaze Injection ... 1307

Fluphenazine Decanoate (Heightens depressant effect). Products include:
Prolixin Decanoate ... 509

Fluphenazine Enanthate (Heightens depressant effect). Products include:
Prolixin Enanthate ... 509

Fluphenazine Hydrochloride (Heightens depressant effect). Products include:
Prolixin ... 509

Flurazepam Hydrochloride (Heightens depressant effect). Products include:
Dalmane Capsules ... 2173

Furazolidone (Prolongs and intensifies anticholinergic effects). Products include:
Furoxone ... 2046

Glutethimide (Heightens depressant effect).
No products indexed under this heading.

Haloperidol (Heightens depressant effect). Products include:
Haldol Injection, Tablets and Concentrate ... 1575

Haloperidol Decanoate (Heightens depressant effect). Products include:
Haldol Decanoate ... 1577

Hydrocodone Bitartrate (Heightens depressant effect). Products include:
Anexsia 5/500 Elixir ... 1781
Anexia Tablets ... 1782
Codiclear DH Syrup ... 791
Deconamine CX Cough and Cold Liquid and Tablets ... 1319
Duratuss HD Elixir ... 2565

IMPORTANT NOTE: Always consult each drug listing in the patient's regimen for possible interactions.

Nytol QuickCaps | Interactions Index | 752

Hycodan Tablets and Syrup 930
Hycomine Compound Tablets 932
Hycomine 931
Hycotuss Expectorant Syrup 933
Hydrocet Capsules 782
Lorcet 10/650.................................. 1018
Lortab.. 2566
Tussend 1783
Tussend Expectorant 1785
Vicodin Tablets 1356
Vicodin ES Tablets 1357
Vicodin Tuss Expectorant 1358
Zydone Capsules 949

Hydrocodone Polistirex (Heightens depressant effect). Products include:

Tussionex Pennkinetic Extended-Release Suspension 998

Hydroxyzine Hydrochloride (Heightens depressant effect). Products include:

Atarax Tablets & Syrup................... 2185
Marax Tablets & DF Syrup.............. 2200
Vistaril Intramuscular Solution....... 2216

Isocarboxazid (Prolongs and intensifies anticholinergic effects).

No products indexed under this heading.

Isoflurane (Heightens depressant effect).

No products indexed under this heading.

Ketamine Hydrochloride (Heightens depressant effect).

No products indexed under this heading.

Levomethadyl Acetate Hydrochloride (Heightens depressant effect). Products include:

Orlamm 2239

Levorphanol Tartrate (Heightens depressant effect). Products include:

Levo-Dromoran 2129

Lorazepam (Heightens depressant effect). Products include:

Ativan Injection 2698
Ativan Tablets 2700

Loxapine Hydrochloride (Heightens depressant effect). Products include:

Loxitane 1378

Loxapine Succinate (Heightens depressant effect). Products include:

Loxitane Capsules 1378

Meperidine Hydrochloride (Heightens depressant effect). Products include:

Demerol 2308
Mepergan Injection 2753

Mephobarbital (Heightens depressant effect). Products include:

Mebaral Tablets 2322

Meprobamate (Heightens depressant effect). Products include:

Miltown Tablets 2672
PMB 200 and PMB 400 2783

Mesoridazine (Heightens depressant effect).

Methadone Hydrochloride (Heightens depressant effect). Products include:

Methadone Hydrochloride Oral Concentrate 2233
Methadone Hydrochloride Oral Solution & Tablets 2235

Methohexital Sodium (Heightens depressant effect). Products include:

Brevital Sodium Vials 1429

Methotrimeprazine (Heightens depressant effect). Products include:

Levoprome 1274

Methoxyflurane (Heightens depressant effect).

No products indexed under this heading.

Midazolam Hydrochloride (Heightens depressant effect). Products include:

Versed Injection 2170

Molindone Hydrochloride (Heightens depressant effect). Products include:

Moban Tablets and Concentrate 1048

Morphine Sulfate (Heightens depressant effect). Products include:

Astramorph/PF Injection, USP (Preservative-Free) 535
Duramorph 962
Infumorph 200 and Infumorph 500 Sterile Solutions........................ 965
MS Contin Tablets............................ 1994
MSIR 1997
Oramorph SR (Morphine Sulfate Sustained Release Tablets) 2236
RMS Suppositories 2657
Roxanol 2243

Opium Alkaloids (Heightens depressant effect).

No products indexed under this heading.

Oxazepam (Heightens depressant effect). Products include:

Serax Capsules 2810
Serax Tablets.................................... 2810

Oxycodone Hydrochloride (Heightens depressant effect). Products include:

Percocet Tablets 938
Percodan Tablets.............................. 939
Percodan-Demi Tablets.................... 940
Roxicodone Tablets, Oral Solution & Intensol (Oxycodone) 2244
Tylox Capsules 1584

Pentobarbital Sodium (Heightens depressant effect). Products include:

Nembutal Sodium Capsules 436
Nembutal Sodium Solution 438
Nembutal Sodium Suppositories..... 440

Perphenazine (Heightens depressant effect). Products include:

Etrafon 2355
Triavil Tablets 1757
Trilafon... 2389

Phenelzine Sulfate (Prolongs and intensifies anticholinergic effects). Products include:

Nardil 1920

Phenobarbital (Heightens depressant effect). Products include:

Arco-Lase Plus Tablets 512
Bellergal-S Tablets 2250
Donnatal 2060
Donnatal Extentabs.......................... 2061
Donnatal Tablets 2060
Phenobarbital Elixir and Tablets 1469
Quadrinal Tablets 1350

Prazepam (Heightens depressant effect).

No products indexed under this heading.

Prochlorperazine (Heightens depressant effect). Products include:

Compazine 2470

Promethazine Hydrochloride (Heightens depressant effect). Products include:

Mepergan Injection 2753
Phenergan with Codeine.................. 2777
Phenergan with Dextromethorphan 2778
Phenergan Injection 2773
Phenergan Suppositories 2775
Phenergan Syrup 2774
Phenergan Tablets 2775
Phenergan VC 2779
Phenergan VC with Codeine 2781

Propofol (Heightens depressant effect). Products include:

Diprivan Injection............................. 2833

Propoxyphene Hydrochloride (Heightens depressant effect). Products include:

Darvon 1435
Wygesic Tablets 2827

Propoxyphene Napsylate (Heightens depressant effect). Products include:

Darvon-N/Darvocet-N 1433

Quazepam (Heightens depressant effect). Products include:

Doral Tablets 2664

Risperidone (Heightens depressant effect). Products include:

Risperdal 1301

Secobarbital Sodium (Heightens depressant effect). Products include:

Seconal Sodium Pulvules 1474

Selegiline Hydrochloride (Prolongs and intensifies anticholinergic effects). Products include:

Eldepryl Tablets 2550

Sufentanil Citrate (Heightens depressant effect). Products include:

Sufenta Injection 1309

Temazepam (Heightens depressant effect). Products include:

Restoril Capsules 2284

Thiamylal Sodium (Heightens depressant effect).

No products indexed under this heading.

Thioridazine Hydrochloride (Heightens depressant effect). Products include:

Mellaril 2269

Thiothixene (Heightens depressant effect). Products include:

Navane Capsules and Concentrate 2201
Navane Intramuscular 2202

Tranylcypromine Sulfate (Prolongs and intensifies anticholinergic effects). Products include:

Parnate Tablets 2503

Triazolam (Heightens depressant effect). Products include:

Halcion Tablets................................. 2611

Trifluoperazine Hydrochloride (Heightens depressant effect). Products include:

Stelazine 2514

Zolpidem Tartrate (Heightens depressant effect). Products include:

Ambien Tablets................................. 2416

Food Interactions

Alcohol (Heightens depressant effect).

OCCLUSAL-HP

(Salicylic Acid) 1054
None cited in PDR database.

OCUCOAT

(Hydroxypropyl Methylcellulose) .... ◉ 321
None cited in PDR database.

OCUCOAT AND OCUCOAT PF EYE DROPS

(Dextran 70, Hydroxypropyl Methylcellulose)............................ ◉ 322
None cited in PDR database.

OCEAN NASAL MIST

(Sodium Chloride)............................ ▣ 655
None cited in PDR database.

OCUFEN

(Flurbiprofen Sodium) .... ◉ 245
May interact with:

Acetylcholine Chloride (Ineffective when used in patients treated with Ocufen). Products include:

Miochol-E with Iocare Steri-Tags and Miochol-E System Pak .... ◉ 273

Carbachol (Ineffective when used in patients treated with Ocufen). Products include:

Isopto Carbachol Ophthalmic Solution .... ◉ 223
MIOSTAT Intraocular Solution .... ◉ 224

OCUFLOX

(Ofloxacin) 481
None cited in PDR database.

OCUPRESS OPHTHALMIC SOLUTION, 1% STERILE

(Carteolol Hydrochloride) .... ◉ 309
May interact with beta blockers and catecholamine depleting drugs. Compounds in these categories include:

Acebutolol Hydrochloride (Potential for additive effects). Products include:

Sectral Capsules 2807

Atenolol (Potential for additive effects). Products include:

Tenoretic Tablets.............................. 2845
Tenormin Tablets and I.V. Injection 2847

Betaxolol Hydrochloride (Potential for additive effects). Products include:

Betoptic Ophthalmic Solution........... 469
Betoptic S Ophthalmic Suspension 471
Kerlone Tablets................................. 2436

Bisoprolol Fumarate (Potential for additive effects). Products include:

Zebeta Tablets 1413
Ziac 1415

Deserpidine (Possible additive effects and the production of hypotension and/or marked bradycardia).

No products indexed under this heading.

Esmolol Hydrochloride (Potential for additive effects). Products include:

Brevibloc Injection........................... 1808

Guanethidine Monosulfate (Possible additive effects and the production of hypotension and/or marked bradycardia). Products include:

Esimil Tablets 822
Ismelin Tablets 827

Labetalol Hydrochloride (Potential for additive effects). Products include:

Normodyne Injection 2377
Normodyne Tablets 2379
Trandate 1185

Levobunolol Hydrochloride (Potential for additive effects). Products include:

Betagan .... ◉ 233

Metipranolol Hydrochloride (Potential for additive effects). Products include:

OptiPranolol (Metipranolol 0.3%) Sterile Ophthalmic Solution......... ◉ 258

Metoprolol Succinate (Potential for additive effects). Products include:

Toprol-XL Tablets 565

Metoprolol Tartrate (Potential for additive effects). Products include:

Lopressor Ampuls............................. 830
Lopressor HCT Tablets..................... 832
Lopressor Tablets 830

Nadolol (Potential for additive effects).

No products indexed under this heading.

Penbutolol Sulfate (Potential for additive effects). Products include:

Levatol 2403

Pindolol (Potential for additive effects). Products include:

Visken Tablets.................................. 2299

Propranolol Hydrochloride (Potential for additive effects). Products include:

Inderal 2728
Inderal LA Long Acting Capsules 2730
Inderide Tablets 2732
Inderide LA Long Acting Capsules .. 2734

Rauwolfia Serpentina (Possible additive effects and the production of hypotension and/or marked bradycardia).

No products indexed under this heading.

(▣ Described in PDR For Nonprescription Drugs) (◉ Described in PDR For Ophthalmology)

Rescinnamine (Possible additive effects and the production of hypotension and/or marked bradycardia).
No products indexed under this heading.

Reserpine (Possible additive effects and the production of hypotension and/or marked bradycardia). Products include:
Diupres Tablets 1650
Hydropres Tablets 1675
Ser-Ap-Es Tablets 849

Sotalol Hydrochloride (Potential for additive effects). Products include:
Betapace Tablets 641

Timolol Hemihydrate (Potential for additive effects). Products include:
Betimol 0.25%, 0.5% .... ◉ 261

Timolol Maleate (Potential for additive effects). Products include:
Blocadren Tablets 1614
Timolide Tablets 1748
Timoptic in Ocudose 1753
Timoptic Sterile Ophthalmic Solution 1751
Timoptic-XE 1755

OCUSERT PILO-20 AND PILO-40 OCULAR THERAPEUTIC SYSTEMS
(Pilocarpine) .... ◉ 254
May interact with:

Epinephrine (Increased rate of absorption from the eye). Products include:
Bronkaid Mist .... ◘ 717
EPIFRIN .... ◉ 239
EpiPen 790
Marcaine Hydrochloride with Epinephrine 1:200,000 2316
Primatene Mist .... ◘ 873
Sensorcaine with Epinephrine Injection 559
Sus-Phrine Injection 1019
Xylocaine with Epinephrine Injections 567

Epinephrine Bitartrate (Increased rate of absorption from the eye). Products include:
Bronkaid Mist Suspension .... ◘ 718
Sensorcaine-MPF with Epinephrine Injection 559

OCUVITE VITAMIN AND MINERAL SUPPLEMENT
(Vitamins with Minerals) .... ◉ 322
None cited in PDR database.

OCUVITE EXTRA VITAMIN AND MINERAL SUPPLEMENT
(Vitamins with Minerals) .... ◉ 323
None cited in PDR database.

OGEN TABLETS
(Estropipate) 2627
May interact with progestins. Compounds in this category include:

Desogestrel (Possible adverse effects on lipoprotein metabolism; impairment of glucose tolerance and possible enhancement of mitotic activity in breast epithelial tissues). Products include:
Desogen Tablets 1817
Ortho-Cept 1851

Medroxyprogesterone Acetate (Possible adverse effects on lipoprotein metabolism; impairment of glucose tolerance and possible enhancement of mitotic activity in breast epithelial tissues). Products include:
Amen Tablets 780
Cycrin Tablets 975
Depo-Provera Contraceptive Injection 2602
Depo-Provera Sterile Aqueous Suspension 2606
Premphase 2797
Prempro 2801
Provera Tablets 2636

Megestrol Acetate (Possible adverse effects on lipoprotein metabolism; impairment of glucose tolerance and possible enhancement of mitotic activity in breast epithelial tissues). Products include:
Megace Oral Suspension 699
Megace Tablets 701

Norgestimate (Possible adverse effects on lipoprotein metabolism; impairment of glucose tolerance and possible enhancement of mitotic activity in breast epithelial tissues). Products include:
Ortho-Cyclen/Ortho-Tri-Cyclen 1858
Ortho-Cyclen/Ortho Tri-Cyclen 1858

OGEN VAGINAL CREAM
(Estropipate) 2630
May interact with progestins. Compounds in this category include:

Desogestrel (Potential for adverse effects on carbohydrate and lipid metabolism). Products include:
Desogen Tablets 1817
Ortho-Cept 1851

Medroxyprogesterone Acetate (Potential for adverse effects on carbohydrate and lipid metabolism). Products include:
Amen Tablets 780
Cycrin Tablets 975
Depo-Provera Contraceptive Injection 2602
Depo-Provera Sterile Aqueous Suspension 2606
Premphase 2797
Prempro 2801
Provera Tablets 2636

Megestrol Acetate (Potential for adverse effects on carbohydrate and lipid metabolism). Products include:
Megace Oral Suspension 699
Megace Tablets 701

Norgestimate (Potential for adverse effects on carbohydrate and lipid metabolism). Products include:
Ortho-Cyclen/Ortho-Tri-Cyclen 1858
Ortho-Cyclen/Ortho Tri-Cyclen 1858

OIL OF OLAY DAILY UV PROTECTANT SPF 15 BEAUTY FLUID-ORIGINAL AND FRAGRANCE FREE (OLAY CO. INC.)
(Octyl Methoxycinnamate, Phenylbenzimidazole-5-Sulfonic Acid) .... ◘ 751
None cited in PDR database.

OMNIHIB
(Haemophilus B Conjugate Vaccine) .. 2499
None cited in PDR database.

OMNIPEN CAPSULES
(Ampicillin) 2764
See **Omnipen for Oral Suspension**

OMNIPEN FOR ORAL SUSPENSION
(Ampicillin) 2765
May interact with bacteriostatic antibiotics and oral contraceptives. Compounds in these categories include:

Allopurinol (Increased possibility of skin rash, particularly in hyperuricemic patients, may occur). Products include:
Zyloprim Tablets 1226

Chloramphenicol (Bacteriostatic antibiotics may interfere with the bactericidal effect of penicillin; clinical significance of this interaction is not well-documented). Products include:
Chloromycetin Ophthalmic Ointment, 1% .... ◉ 310
Chloromycetin Ophthalmic Solution .... ◉ 310
Chloroptic S.O.P. .... ◉ 239
Chloroptic Sterile Ophthalmic Solution .... ◉ 239
Elase-Chloromycetin Ointment 1040
Ophthocort .... ◉ 311

Chloramphenicol Palmitate (Bacteriostatic antibiotics may interfere with the bactericidal effect of penicillin; clinical significance of this interaction is not well-documented).
No products indexed under this heading.

Chloramphenicol Sodium Succinate (Bacteriostatic antibiotics may interfere with the bactericidal effect of penicillin; clinical significance of this interaction is not well-documented). Products include:
Chloromycetin Sodium Succinate 1900

Demeclocycline Hydrochloride (Bacteriostatic antibiotics may interfere with the bactericidal effect of penicillin; clinical significance of this interaction is not well-documented). Products include:
Declomycin Tablets 1371

Desogestrel (Oral contraceptives may be less effective and potential for increased breakthrough bleeding). Products include:
Desogen Tablets 1817
Ortho-Cept 1851

Doxycycline Calcium (Bacteriostatic antibiotics may interfere with the bactericidal effect of penicillin; clinical significance of this interaction is not well-documented). Products include:
Vibramycin Calcium Oral Suspension Syrup 1941

Doxycycline Hyclate (Bacteriostatic antibiotics may interfere with the bactericidal effect of penicillin; clinical significance of this interaction is not well-documented). Products include:
Doryx Capsules 1913
Vibramycin Hyclate Capsules 1941
Vibramycin Hyclate Intravenous 2215
Vibra-Tabs Film Coated Tablets 1941

Doxycycline Monohydrate (Bacteriostatic antibiotics may interfere with the bactericidal effect of penicillin; clinical significance of this interaction is not well-documented). Products include:
Monodox Capsules 1805
Vibramycin Monohydrate for Oral Suspension 1941

Erythromycin (Bacteriostatic antibiotics may interfere with the bactericidal effect of penicillin; clinical significance of this interaction is not well-documented). Products include:
A/T/S 2% Acne Topical Gel and Solution 1234
Benzamycin Topical Gel 905
E-Mycin Tablets 1341
Emgel 2% Topical Gel 1093
ERYC 1915
Erycette (erythromycin 2%) Topical Solution 1888
Ery-Tab Tablets 422
Erythromycin Base Filmtab 426
Erythromycin Delayed-Release Capsules, USP 427
Ilotycin Ophthalmic Ointment 912
PCE Dispertab Tablets 444
T-Stat 2.0% Topical Solution and Pads 2688
Theramycin Z Topical Solution 2% 1592

Erythromycin Estolate (Bacteriostatic antibiotics may interfere with the bactericidal effect of penicillin; clinical significance of this interaction is not well-documented). Products include:
Ilosone 911

Erythromycin Ethylsuccinate (Bacteriostatic antibiotics may interfere with the bactericidal effect of penicillin; clinical significance of this interaction is not well-documented). Products include:
E.E.S. 424
EryPed 421

Erythromycin Gluceptate (Bacteriostatic antibiotics may interfere with the bactericidal effect of penicillin; clinical significance of this interaction is not well-documented). Products include:
Ilotycin Gluceptate, IV, Vials 913

Erythromycin Stearate (Bacteriostatic antibiotics may interfere with the bactericidal effect of penicillin; clinical significance of this interaction is not well-documented). Products include:
Erythrocin Stearate Filmtab 425

Ethinyl Estradiol (Oral contraceptives may be less effective and potential for increased breakthrough bleeding). Products include:
Brevicon 2088
Demulen 2428
Desogen Tablets 1817
Levlen/Tri-Levlen 651
Lo/Ovral Tablets 2746
Lo/Ovral-28 Tablets 2751
Modicon 1872
Nordette-21 Tablets 2755
Nordette-28 Tablets 2758
Norinyl 2088
Ortho-Cept 1851
Ortho-Cyclen/Ortho-Tri-Cyclen 1858
Ortho-Novum 1872
Ortho-Cyclen/Ortho Tri-Cyclen 1858
Ovcon 760
Ovral Tablets 2770
Ovral-28 Tablets 2770
Levlen/Tri-Levlen 651
Tri-Norinyl 2164
Triphasil-21 Tablets 2814
Triphasil-28 Tablets 2819

Ethynodiol Diacetate (Oral contraceptives may be less effective and potential for increased breakthrough bleeding). Products include:
Demulen 2428

Levonorgestrel (Oral contraceptives may be less effective and potential for increased breakthrough bleeding). Products include:
Levlen/Tri-Levlen 651
Nordette-21 Tablets 2755
Nordette-28 Tablets 2758
Norplant System 2759
Levlen/Tri-Levlen 651
Triphasil-21 Tablets 2814
Triphasil-28 Tablets 2819

Mestranol (Oral contraceptives may be less effective and potential for increased breakthrough bleeding). Products include:
Norinyl 2088
Ortho-Novum 1872

Methacycline Hydrochloride (Bacteriostatic antibiotics may interfere with the bactericidal effect of penicillin; clinical significance of this interaction is not well-documented).
No products indexed under this heading.

Minocycline Hydrochloride (Bacteriostatic antibiotics may interfere with the bactericidal effect of penicillin; clinical significance of this interaction is not well-documented). Products include:
Dynacin Capsules 1590
Minocin Intravenous 1382
Minocin Oral Suspension 1385

IMPORTANT NOTE: Always consult each drug listing in the patient's regimen for possible interactions.

Omnipen **Interactions Index** 754

Minocin Pellet-Filled Capsules 1383

Norethindrone (Oral contraceptives may be less effective and potential for increased breakthrough bleeding). Products include:

Brevicon........................ 2088
Micronor Tablets 1872
Modicon........................ 1872
Norinyl 2088
Nor-Q D Tablets 2135
Ortho-Novum........................ 1872
Ovcon 760
Tri-Norinyl........................ 2164

Norethynodrel (Oral contraceptives may be less effective and potential for increased breakthrough bleeding).

No products indexed under this heading.

Norgestimate (Oral contraceptives may be less effective and potential for increased breakthrough bleeding). Products include:

Ortho-Cyclen/Ortho-Tri-Cyclen 1858
Ortho-Cyclen/Ortho Tri-Cyclen 1858

Norgestrel (Oral contraceptives may be less effective and potential for increased breakthrough bleeding). Products include:

Lo/Ovral Tablets 2746
Lo/Ovral-28 Tablets........................ 2751
Ovral Tablets 2770
Ovral-28 Tablets 2770
Ovrette Tablets........................ 2771

Oxytetracycline Hydrochloride (Bacteriostatic antibiotics may interfere with the bactericidal effect of penicillin; clinical significance of this interaction is not well-documented). Products include:

TERAK Ointment .... ⊙ 209
Terra-Cortril Ophthalmic Suspension 2210
Terramycin with Polymyxin B Sulfate Ophthalmic Ointment 2211
Urobiotic-250 Capsules 2214

Probenecid (Decreases renal tubular secretion of ampicillin resulting in increased blood levels and/or ampicillin toxicity). Products include:

Benemid Tablets 1611
ColBENEMID Tablets 1622

Sulfamethizole (Bacteriostatic antibiotics may interfere with the bactericidal effect of penicillin; clinical significance of this interaction is not well-documented). Products include:

Urobiotic-250 Capsules 2214

Sulfamethoxazole (Bacteriostatic antibiotics may interfere with the bactericidal effect of penicillin; clinical significance of this interaction is not well-documented). Products include:

Azo Gantanol Tablets........................ 2080
Bactrim DS Tablets........................ 2084
Bactrim I.V. Infusion 2082
Bactrim 2084
Gantanol Tablets 2119
Septra........................ 1174
Septra I.V. Infusion 1169
Septra I.V. Infusion ADD-Vantage Vials........................ 1171
Septra........................ 1174

Sulfinpyrazone (Bacteriostatic antibiotics may interfere with the bactericidal effect of penicillin; clinical significance of this interaction is not well-documented). Products include:

Anturane 807

Sulfisoxazole (Bacteriostatic antibiotics may interfere with the bactericidal effect of penicillin; clinical significance of this interaction is not well-documented). Products include:

Azo Gantrisin Tablets........................ 2081
Gantrisin Tablets 2120

Tetracycline Hydrochloride (Bacteriostatic antibiotics may interfere with the bactericidal effect of penicillin; clinical significance of this interaction is not well-documented). Products include:

Achromycin V Capsules 1367

ONCASPAR
(Pegaspargase) 2028
May interact with anticoagulants, non-steroidal anti-inflammatory agents, antineoplastics, highly protein bound drugs (selected), and certain other agents. Compounds in these categories include:

Altretamine (Potential for unspecified unfavorable interactions). Products include:

Hexalen Capsules 2571

Amiodarone Hydrochloride (Depletion of serum proteins by pegaspargase may increase the toxicity of other drugs which are protein bound). Products include:

Cordarone Intravenous 2715
Cordarone Tablets........................ 2712

Amitriptyline Hydrochloride (Depletion of serum proteins by pegaspargase may increase the toxicity of other drugs which are protein bound). Products include:

Elavil 2838
Endep Tablets 2174
Etrafon 2355
Limbitrol 2180
Triavil Tablets 1757

Asparaginase (Potential for unspecified unfavorable interactions). Products include:

Elspar 1659

Aspirin (Increased risk of bleeding and/or thrombosis). Products include:

Alka-Seltzer Effervescent Antacid and Pain Reliever .... ▣ 701
Alka-Seltzer Extra Strength Effervescent Antacid and Pain Reliever .... ▣ 703
Alka-Seltzer Lemon Lime Effervescent Antacid and Pain Reliever .... ▣ 703
Alka-Seltzer Plus Cold Medicine .... ▣ 705
Alka-Seltzer Plus Cold & Cough Medicine .... ▣ 708
Alka-Seltzer Plus Night-Time Cold Medicine .... ▣ 707
Alka Seltzer Plus Sinus Medicine .. ▣ 707
Arthritis Foundation Safety Coated Aspirin Tablets .... ▣ 675
Arthritis Pain Ascriptin .... ▣ 631
Maximum Strength Ascriptin .... ▣ 630
Regular Strength Ascriptin Tablets .... ▣ 629
Arthritis Strength BC Powder......... ▣ 609
BC Cold Powder Multi-Symptom Formula (Cold-Sinus-Allergy) .... ▣ 609
BC Cold Powder Non-Drowsy Formula (Cold-Sinus)............ ▣ 609
BC Powder .... ▣ 609
Bayer Children's Chewable Aspirin .... ▣ 711
Genuine Bayer Aspirin Tablets & Caplets .... ▣ 713
Extra Strength Bayer Arthritis Pain Regimen Formula .... ▣ 711
Extra Strength Bayer Aspirin Caplets & Tablets .... ▣ 712
Extended-Release Bayer 8-Hour Aspirin .... ▣ 712
Extra Strength Bayer Plus Aspirin Caplets........................ ▣ 713
Extra Strength Bayer PM Aspirin .. ▣ 713
Bayer Enteric Aspirin .... ▣ 709
Bufferin Analgesic Tablets and Caplets .... ▣ 613
Arthritis Strength Bufferin Analgesic Caplets .... ▣ 614
Extra Strength Bufferin Analgesic Tablets .... ▣ 615
Cama Arthritis Pain Reliever............ ▣ 785
Darvon Compound-65 Pulvules 1435
Easprin........................ 1914
Ecotrin 2455
Ecotrin Enteric Coated Aspirin Maximum Strength Tablets and Caplets .... ▣ 816
Ecotrin Enteric Coated Aspirin Regular Strength Tablets 2455
Empirin Aspirin Tablets .... ▣ 854
Empirin with Codeine Tablets............ 1093
Excedrin Extra-Strength Analgesic Tablets & Caplets 732
Fiorinal Capsules 2261
Fiorinal with Codeine Capsules 2262
Fiorinal Tablets........................ 2261
Halfprin 1362
Healthprin Aspirin........................ 2455
Norgesic........................ 1496
Percodan Tablets........................ 939
Percodan-Demi Tablets........................ 940
Robaxisal Tablets........................ 2071
Soma Compound w/Codeine Tablets 2676
Soma Compound Tablets........................ 2675
St. Joseph Adult Chewable Aspirin (81 mg.) .... ▣ 808
Talwin Compound 2335
Ursinus Inlay-Tabs........................ ▣ 794
Vanquish Analgesic Caplets .... ▣ 731

Atovaquone (Depletion of serum proteins by pegaspargase may increase the toxicity of other drugs which are protein bound). Products include:

Mepron Suspension 1135

Bleomycin Sulfate (Potential for unspecified unfavorable interactions). Products include:

Blenoxane 692

Busulfan (Potential for unspecified unfavorable interactions). Products include:

Myleran Tablets 1143

Carboplatin (Potential for unspecified unfavorable interactions). Products include:

Paraplatin for Injection 705

Carmustine (BCNU) (Potential for unspecified unfavorable interactions). Products include:

BiCNU........................ 691

Cefonicid Sodium (Depletion of serum proteins by pegaspargase may increase the toxicity of other drugs which are protein bound). Products include:

Monocid Injection 2497

Chlorambucil (Potential for unspecified unfavorable interactions). Products include:

Leukeran Tablets 1133

Chlordiazepoxide (Depletion of serum proteins by pegaspargase may increase the toxicity of other drugs which are protein bound). Products include:

Libritabs Tablets 2177
Limbitrol 2180

Chlordiazepoxide Hydrochloride (Depletion of serum proteins by pegaspargase may increase the toxicity of other drugs which are protein bound). Products include:

Librax Capsules 2176
Librium Capsules........................ 2178
Librium Injectable 2179

Chlorpromazine (Depletion of serum proteins by pegaspargase may increase the toxicity of other drugs which are protein bound). Products include:

Thorazine Suppositories........................ 2523

Chlorpromazine Hydrochloride (Depletion of serum proteins by pegaspargase may increase the toxicity of other drugs which are protein bound). Products include:

Thorazine 2523

Cisplatin (Potential for unspecified unfavorable interactions). Products include:

Platinol 708
Platinol-AQ Injection........................ 710

Clomipramine Hydrochloride (Depletion of serum proteins by pegaspargase may increase the toxicity of other drugs which are protein bound). Products include:

Anafranil Capsules 803

Clozapine (Depletion of serum proteins by pegaspargase may increase the toxicity of other drugs which are protein bound). Products include:

Clozaril Tablets........................ 2252

Cyclophosphamide (Potential for unspecified unfavorable interactions). Products include:

Cytoxan 694
NEOSAR Lyophilized/Neosar 1959

Cyclosporine (Depletion of serum proteins by pegaspargase may increase the toxicity of other drugs which are protein bound). Products include:

Neoral 2276
Sandimmune 2286

Dacarbazine (Potential for unspecified unfavorable interactions). Products include:

DTIC-Dome........................ 600

Dalteparin Sodium (Increased risk of bleeding and/or thrombosis). Products include:

Fragmin 1954

Daunorubicin Hydrochloride (Potential for unspecified unfavorable interactions). Products include:

Cerubidine 795

Diazepam (Depletion of serum proteins by pegaspargase may increase the toxicity of other drugs which are protein bound). Products include:

Dizac 1809
Valium Injectable........................ 2182
Valium Tablets 2183
Valrelease Capsules 2169

Diclofenac Potassium (Depletion of serum proteins by pegaspargase may increase the toxicity of other drugs which are protein bound; increased risk of bleeding and/or thrombosis). Products include:

Cataflam 816

Diclofenac Sodium (Depletion of serum proteins by pegaspargase may increase the toxicity of other drugs which are protein bound; increased risk of bleeding and/or thrombosis). Products include:

Voltaren Ophthalmic Sterile Ophthalmic Solution .... ⊙ 272
Voltaren Tablets........................ 861

Dicumarol (Increased risk of bleeding and/or thrombosis).

No products indexed under this heading.

Dipyridamole (Increased risk of bleeding and/or thrombosis). Products include:

Persantine Tablets 681

Doxorubicin Hydrochloride (Potential for unspecified unfavorable interactions). Products include:

Adriamycin PFS 1947
Adriamycin RDF 1947
Doxorubicin Astra 540
Rubex 712

Enoxaparin (Increased risk of bleeding and/or thrombosis). Products include:

Lovenox Injection........................ 2020

Estramustine Phosphate Sodium (Potential for unspecified unfavorable interactions). Products include:

Emcyt Capsules 1953

(▣ Described in PDR For Nonprescription Drugs) (⊙ Described in PDR For Ophthalmology)

755 Interactions Index Oncaspar

Etodolac (Increased risk of bleeding and/or thrombosis). Products include:
Lodine Capsules and Tablets ... 2743

Etoposide (Potential for unspecified unfavorable interactions). Products include:
VePesid Capsules and Injection ... 718

Fenoprofen Calcium (Depletion of serum proteins by pegaspargase may increase the toxicity of other drugs which are protein bound; increased risk of bleeding and/or thrombosis). Products include:
Nalfon 200 Pulvules & Nalfon Tablets ... 917

Floxuridine (Potential for unspecified unfavorable interactions). Products include:
Sterile FUDR ... 2118

Fluorouracil (Potential for unspecified unfavorable interactions). Products include:
Efudex ... 2113
Fluoroplex Topical Solution & Cream 1% ... 479
Fluorouracil Injection ... 2116

Flurazepam Hydrochloride (Depletion of serum proteins by pegaspargase may increase the toxicity of other drugs which are protein bound). Products include:
Dalmane Capsules ... 2173

Flurbiprofen (Depletion of serum proteins by pegaspargase may increase the toxicity of other drugs which are protein bound; increased risk of bleeding and/or thrombosis). Products include:
Ansaid Tablets ... 2579

Flutamide (Potential for unspecified unfavorable interactions). Products include:
Eulexin Capsules ... 2358

Glipizide (Depletion of serum proteins by pegaspargase may increase the toxicity of other drugs which are protein bound). Products include:
Glucotrol Tablets ... 1967
Glucotrol XL Extended Release Tablets ... 1968

Heparin Calcium (Increased risk of bleeding and/or thrombosis).
No products indexed under this heading.

Heparin Sodium (Increased risk of bleeding and/or thrombosis). Products include:
Heparin Lock Flush Solution ... 2725
Heparin Sodium Injection ... 2726
Heparin Sodium Injection, USP, Sterile Solution ... 2615
Heparin Sodium Vials ... 1441

Hydroxyurea (Potential for unspecified unfavorable interactions). Products include:
Hydrea Capsules ... 696

Ibuprofen (Depletion of serum proteins by pegaspargase may increase the toxicity of other drugs which are protein bound; increased risk of bleeding and/or thrombosis). Products include:
Advil Cold and Sinus Caplets and Tablets (formerly CoAdvil) ... ◘ 870
Advil Ibuprofen Tablets and Caplets ... ◘ 870
Children's Advil Suspension ... 2692
Arthritis Foundation Ibuprofen Tablets ... ◘ 674
Bayer Select Ibuprofen Pain Relief Formula ... ◘ 715
Cramp End Tablets ... ◘ 735
Dimetapp Sinus Caplets ... ◘ 775
Haltran Tablets ... ◘ 771
IBU Tablets ... 1342
Ibuprohm ... ◘ 735
Children's Motrin Ibuprofen Oral Suspension ... 1546
Motrin Tablets ... 2625
Motrin IB Caplets, Tablets, and Geltabs ... ◘ 838
Motrin IB Sinus ... ◘ 838
Motrin Ibuprofen Suspension, Oral Drops, Chewable Tablets, Caplets ... 1546
Nuprin Ibuprofen/Analgesic Tablets & Caplets ... ◘ 622
Sine-Aid IB Caplets ... 1554
Vicks DayQuil SINUS Pressure & PAIN Relief with IBUPROFEN ... ◘ 762

Idarubicin Hydrochloride (Potential for unspecified unfavorable interactions). Products include:
Idamycin ... 1955

Ifosfamide (Potential for unspecified unfavorable interactions). Products include:
IFEX ... 697

Imipramine Hydrochloride (Depletion of serum proteins by pegaspargase may increase the toxicity of other drugs which are protein bound). Products include:
Tofranil Ampuls ... 854
Tofranil Tablets ... 856

Imipramine Pamoate (Depletion of serum proteins by pegaspargase may increase the toxicity of other drugs which are protein bound). Products include:
Tofranil-PM Capsules ... 857

Indomethacin (Depletion of serum proteins by pegaspargase may increase the toxicity of other drugs which are protein bound; increased risk of bleeding and/or thrombosis). Products include:
Indocin ... 1680

Indomethacin Sodium Trihydrate (Depletion of serum proteins by pegaspargase may increase the toxicity of other drugs which are protein bound; increased risk of bleeding and/or thrombosis). Products include:
Indocin I.V. ... 1684

Interferon alfa-2A, Recombinant (Potential for unspecified unfavorable interactions). Products include:
Roferon-A Injection ... 2145

Interferon alfa-2B, Recombinant (Potential for unspecified unfavorable interactions). Products include:
Intron A ... 2364

Ketoprofen (Depletion of serum proteins by pegaspargase may increase the toxicity of other drugs which are protein bound; increased risk of bleeding and/or thrombosis). Products include:
Orudis Capsules ... 2766
Oruvail Capsules ... 2766

Ketorolac Tromethamine (Depletion of serum proteins by pegaspargase may increase the toxicity of other drugs which are protein bound; increased risk of bleeding and/or thrombosis). Products include:
Acular ... 474
Acular ... ⊙ 277
Toradol ... 2159

Levamisole Hydrochloride (Potential for unspecified unfavorable interactions). Products include:
Ergamisol Tablets ... 1292

Lomustine (CCNU) (Potential for unspecified unfavorable interactions). Products include:
CeeNU ... 693

Mechlorethamine Hydrochloride (Potential for unspecified unfavorable interactions). Products include:
Mustargen ... 1709

Meclofenamate Sodium (Depletion of serum proteins by pegaspargase may increase the toxicity of other drugs which are protein bound; increased risk of bleeding and/or thrombosis).
No products indexed under this heading.

Mefenamic Acid (Depletion of serum proteins by pegaspargase may increase the toxicity of other drugs which are protein bound; increased risk of bleeding and/or thrombosis). Products include:
Ponstel ... 1925

Megestrol Acetate (Potential for unspecified unfavorable interactions). Products include:
Megace Oral Suspension ... 699
Megace Tablets ... 701

Melphalan (Potential for unspecified unfavorable interactions). Products include:
Alkeran Tablets ... 1071

Mercaptopurine (Potential for unspecified unfavorable interactions). Products include:
Purinethol Tablets ... 1156

Methotrexate Sodium (Pegaspargase inhibits protein synthesis and cell replication and thus interferes with the action of methotrexate which requires cell replication for its lethal effect; potential for unspecified unfavorable interactions). Products include:
Methotrexate Sodium Tablets, Injection, for Injection and LPF Injection ... 1275

Midazolam Hydrochloride (Depletion of serum proteins by pegaspargase may increase the toxicity of other drugs which are protein bound). Products include:
Versed Injection ... 2170

Mitomycin (Mitomycin-C) (Potential for unspecified unfavorable interactions). Products include:
Mutamycin ... 703

Mitotane (Potential for unspecified unfavorable interactions). Products include:
Lysodren ... 698

Mitoxantrone Hydrochloride (Potential for unspecified unfavorable interactions). Products include:
Novantrone ... 1279

Nabumetone (Increased risk of bleeding and/or thrombosis). Products include:
Relafen Tablets ... 2510

Naproxen (Depletion of serum proteins by pegaspargase may increase the toxicity of other drugs which are protein bound; increased risk of bleeding and/or thrombosis). Products include:
Anaprox/Naprosyn ... 2117

Naproxen Sodium (Depletion of serum proteins by pegaspargase may increase the toxicity of other drugs which are protein bound; increased risk of bleeding and/or thrombosis). Products include:
Aleve ... 1975
Anaprox/Naprosyn ... 2117

Nortriptyline Hydrochloride (Depletion of serum proteins by pegaspargase may increase the toxicity of other drugs which are protein bound). Products include:
Pamelor ... 2280

Oxaprozin (Depletion of serum proteins by pegaspargase may increase the toxicity of other drugs which are protein bound; increased risk of bleeding and/or thrombosis). Products include:
Daypro Caplets ... 2426

Oxazepam (Depletion of serum proteins by pegaspargase may increase the toxicity of other drugs which are protein bound). Products include:
Serax Capsules ... 2810
Serax Tablets ... 2810

Paclitaxel (Potential for unspecified unfavorable interactions). Products include:
Taxol ... 714

Phenylbutazone (Depletion of serum proteins by pegaspargase may increase the toxicity of other drugs which are protein bound; increased risk of bleeding and/or thrombosis).
No products indexed under this heading.

Piroxicam (Depletion of serum proteins by pegaspargase may increase the toxicity of other drugs which are protein bound; increased risk of bleeding and/or thrombosis). Products include:
Feldene Capsules ... 1965

Procarbazine Hydrochloride (Potential for unspecified unfavorable interactions). Products include:
Matulane Capsules ... 2131

Propranolol Hydrochloride (Depletion of serum proteins by pegaspargase may increase the toxicity of other drugs which are protein bound). Products include:
Inderal ... 2728
Inderal LA Long Acting Capsules ... 2730
Inderide Tablets ... 2732
Inderide LA Long Acting Capsules ... 2734

Streptozocin (Potential for unspecified unfavorable interactions). Products include:
Zanosar Sterile Powder ... 2653

Sulindac (Depletion of serum proteins by pegaspargase may increase the toxicity of other drugs which are protein bound; increased risk of bleeding and/or thrombosis). Products include:
Clinoril Tablets ... 1618

Tamoxifen Citrate (Potential for unspecified unfavorable interactions). Products include:
Nolvadex Tablets ... 2841

Temazepam (Depletion of serum proteins by pegaspargase may increase the toxicity of other drugs which are protein bound). Products include:
Restoril Capsules ... 2284

Teniposide (Potential for unspecified unfavorable interactions). Products include:
Vumon ... 727

Thioguanine (Potential for unspecified unfavorable interactions). Products include:
Thioguanine Tablets, Tabloid Brand ... 1181

Thiotepa (Potential for unspecified unfavorable interactions). Products include:
Thioplex (Thiotepa For Injection) ... 1281

Tolbutamide (Depletion of serum proteins by pegaspargase may increase the toxicity of other drugs which are protein bound).
No products indexed under this heading.

IMPORTANT NOTE: Always consult each drug listing in the patient's regimen for possible interactions.

Oncaspar | Interactions Index | 756

Tolmetin Sodium (Depletion of serum proteins by pegaspargase may increase the toxicity of other drugs which are protein bound; increased risk of bleeding and/or thrombosis). Products include:
- Tolectin (200, 400 and 600 mg) .. 1581

Trimipramine Maleate (Depletion of serum proteins by pegaspargase may increase the toxicity of other drugs which are protein bound). Products include:
- Surmontil Capsules ... 2811

Vincristine Sulfate (Potential for unspecified unfavorable interactions). Products include:
- Oncovin Solution Vials & Hyporets 1466

Vinorelbine Tartrate (Potential for unspecified unfavorable interactions). Products include:
- Navelbine Injection ... 1145

Warfarin Sodium (Depletion of serum proteins by pegaspargase may increase the toxicity of other drugs which are protein bound; increased risk of bleeding and/or thrombosis). Products include:
- Coumadin ... 926

ONCOVIN SOLUTION VIALS & HYPORETS
(Vincristine Sulfate) ... 1466
May interact with:

Mitomycin (Mitomycin-C) (Acute shortness of breath; severe bronchospasm). Products include:
- Mutamycin ... 703

Neurotoxic Drugs (Potential for increased neurotoxicity).

Phenytoin (Increased seizure activity due to reduced phenytoin blood levels). Products include:
- Dilantin Infatabs ... 1908
- Dilantin-125 Suspension ... 1911

Phenytoin Sodium (Increased seizure activity due to reduced phenytoin blood levels). Products include:
- Dilantin Kapseals ... 1906
- Dilantin Parenteral ... 1910

ONE-A-DAY ESSENTIAL VITAMINS WITH BETA CAROTENE
(Vitamins with Minerals) ... ⊡ 727
None cited in PDR database.

ONE-A-DAY EXTRAS ANTIOXIDANT
(Vitamin A, Vitamin C, Vitamin E, Zinc Oxide) ... ⊡ 728
None cited in PDR database.

ONE-A-DAY EXTRAS GARLIC
(Garlic Extract) ... ⊡ 728
None cited in PDR database.

ONE-A-DAY EXTRAS VITAMIN C
(Vitamin C) ... ⊡ 728
None cited in PDR database.

ONE-A-DAY EXTRAS VITAMIN E
(Vitamin E) ... ⊡ 728
None cited in PDR database.

ONE-A-DAY MAXIMUM
(Vitamins with Minerals) ... ⊡ 728
None cited in PDR database.

ONE-A-DAY MEN'S
(Vitamins, Multiple) ... ⊡ 729
None cited in PDR database.

ONE-A-DAY WOMEN'S
(Vitamins with Minerals) ... ⊡ 729
None cited in PDR database.

ONE-A-DAY 55 PLUS
(Vitamins with Minerals) ... ⊡ 727
None cited in PDR database.

OPHTHALGAN
(Glycerin) ... ⊙ 326
None cited in PDR database.

OPHTHETIC
(Proparacaine Hydrochloride) ... ⊙ 247
None cited in PDR database.

OPHTHOCORT
(Chloramphenicol, Polymyxin B Sulfate, Hydrocortisone Acetate) .... ⊙ 311
None cited in PDR database.

OPTIPRANOLOL (METIPRANOLOL 0.3%) STERILE OPHTHALMIC SOLUTION
(Metipranolol Hydrochloride) ... ⊙ 258
May interact with beta blockers, catecholamine depleting drugs, adrenergic augmenting psychotropics, calcium channel blockers, cardiac glycosides, and certain other agents. Compounds in these categories include:

Acebutolol Hydrochloride (Potential for additive effects). Products include:
- Sectral Capsules ... 2807

Amlodipine Besylate (Possible precipitation of left ventricular failure and hypotension). Products include:
- Lotrel Capsules ... 840
- Norvasc Tablets ... 1940

Atenolol (Potential for additive effects). Products include:
- Tenoretic Tablets ... 2845
- Tenormin Tablets and I.V. Injection 2847

Bepridil Hydrochloride (Possible precipitation of left ventricular failure and hypotension). Products include:
- Vascor (200, 300 and 400 mg) Tablets ... 1587

Betaxolol Hydrochloride (Potential for additive effects). Products include:
- Betoptic Ophthalmic Solution ... 469
- Betoptic S Ophthalmic Suspension 471
- Kerlone Tablets ... 2436

Bisoprolol Fumarate (Potential for additive effects). Products include:
- Zebeta Tablets ... 1413
- Ziac ... 1415

Carteolol Hydrochloride (Potential for additive effects). Products include:
- Cartrol Tablets ... 410
- Ocupress Ophthalmic Solution, 1% Sterile ... ⊙ 309

Deserpidine (Possible additive effects and the production of hypotension and/or bradycardia).
- No products indexed under this heading.

Deslanoside (The concomitant use of beta-adrenergic receptor blocking agents with digitalis and calcium channel antagonists may have additive effects, prolonging arterioventricular conduction time).
- No products indexed under this heading.

Digitoxin (The concomitant use of beta-adrenergic receptor blocking agents with digitalis and calcium channel antagonists may have additive effects, prolonging arterioventricular conduction time). Products include:
- Crystodigin Tablets ... 1433

Digoxin (The concomitant use of beta-adrenergic receptor blocking agents with digitalis and calcium channel antagonists may have additive effects, prolonging arterioventricular conduction time). Products include:
- Lanoxicaps ... 1117
- Lanoxin Elixir Pediatric ... 1120
- Lanoxin Injection ... 1123
- Lanoxin Injection Pediatric ... 1126
- Lanoxin Tablets ... 1128

Diltiazem Hydrochloride (Possible precipitation of left ventricular failure and hypotension). Products include:
- Cardizem CD Capsules ... 1506
- Cardizem SR Capsules ... 1510
- Cardizem Injectable ... 1508
- Cardizem Tablets ... 1512
- Dilacor XR Extended-release Capsules ... 2018

Esmolol Hydrochloride (Potential for additive effects). Products include:
- Brevibloc Injection ... 1808

Felodipine (Possible precipitation of left ventricular failure and hypotension). Products include:
- Plendil Extended-Release Tablets 527

Guanethidine Monosulfate (Possible additive effects and the production of hypotension and/or bradycardia). Products include:
- Esimil Tablets ... 822
- Ismelin Tablets ... 827

Isocarboxazid (Caution should be used in patients using concomitant adrenergic psychotropic drugs).
- No products indexed under this heading.

Isradipine (Possible precipitation of left ventricular failure and hypotension). Products include:
- DynaCirc Capsules ... 2256

Labetalol Hydrochloride (Potential for additive effects). Products include:
- Normodyne Injection ... 2377
- Normodyne Tablets ... 2379
- Trandate ... 1185

Levobunolol Hydrochloride (Potential for additve effects). Products include:
- Betagan ... ⊙ 233

Metoprolol Succinate (Potential for additive effects). Products include:
- Toprol-XL Tablets ... 565

Metoprolol Tartrate (Potential for additive effects). Products include:
- Lopressor Ampuls ... 830
- Lopressor HCT Tablets ... 832
- Lopressor Tablets ... 830

Nadolol (Potential for additive effects).
- No products indexed under this heading.

Naphazoline Hydrochloride (Caution should be used in patients using concomitant adrenergic psychotropic drugs). Products include:
- Albalon Solution with Liquifilm ... ⊙ 231
- Clear Eyes ACR Astringent/Lubricant Eye Redness Reliever Eye Drops ... ⊙ 316
- Clear Eyes Lubricant Eye Redness Reliever ... ⊙ 316
- 4-Way Fast Acting Nasal Spray (regular & mentholated) ... ⊡ 621
- Naphcon-A Ophthalmic Solution ... 473
- Privine ... ⊡ 647
- Vasocon-A ... ⊙ 271

Nicardipine Hydrochloride (Possible precipitation of left ventricular failure and hypotension). Products include:
- Cardene Capsules ... 2095
- Cardene I.V. ... 2709
- Cardene SR Capsules ... 2097

Nifedipine (Possible precipitation of left ventricular failure and hypotension). Products include:
- Adalat Capsules (10 mg and 20 mg) ... 587
- Adalat CC ... 589
- Procardia Capsules ... 1971
- Procardia XL Extended Release Tablets ... 1972

Nimodipine (Possible precipitation of left ventricular failure and hypotension). Products include:
- Nimotop Capsules ... 610

Nisoldipine (Possible precipitation of left ventricular failure and hypotension).
- No products indexed under this heading.

Oxymetazoline Hydrochloride (Caution should be used in patients using concomitant adrenergic psychotropic drugs). Products include:
- Afrin ... ⊡ 797
- Cheracol Nasal Spray Pump ... ⊡ 768
- Duration 12 Hour Nasal Spray ... ⊡ 805
- 4-Way Long Lasting Nasal Spray ... ⊡ 621
- NTZ Long Acting Nasal Spray & Drops 0.05% ... ⊡ 727
- Neo-Synephrine Maximum Strength 12 Hour Nasal Spray .. ⊡ 726
- Neo-Synephrine 12 Hour ... ⊡ 726
- Nōstrilla Long Acting Nasal Decongestant ... ⊡ 644
- Vicks Sinex 12-Hour Nasal Decongestant Spray and Ultra Fine Mist ... ⊡ 765
- Visine L.R. Eye Drops ... ⊡ 746
- Visine L.R. Eye Drops ... ⊙ 313

Pargyline Hydrochloride (Caution should be used in patients using concomitant adrenergic psychotropic drugs).
- No products indexed under this heading.

Penbutolol Sulfate (Potential for additive effects). Products include:
- Levatol ... 2403

Phenelzine Sulfate (Caution should be used in patients using concomitant adrenergic psychotropic drugs). Products include:
- Nardil ... 1920

Phenylephrine Hydrochloride (Caution should be used in patients using concomitant adrenergic psychotropic drugs). Products include:
- Atrohist Plus Tablets ... 454
- Cerose DM ... ⊡ 878
- Comhist ... 2038
- D.A. Chewable Tablets ... 951
- Deconsal Pediatric Capsules ... 454
- Dura-Vent/DA Tablets ... 953
- Entex Capsules ... 1986
- Entex Liquid ... 1986
- Extendryl ... 1005
- 4-Way Fast Acting Nasal Spray (regular & mentholated) ... ⊡ 621
- Hemorid For Women ... ⊡ 834
- Hycomine Compound Tablets ... 932
- Neo-Synephrine Hydrochloride 1% Carpuject ... 2324
- Neo-Synephrine Hydrochloride 1% Injection ... 2324
- Neo-Synephrine Hydrochloride (Ophthalmic) ... 2325
- Neo-Synephrine ... ⊡ 726
- Nōstril ... ⊡ 644
- Novahistine Elixir ... ⊡ 823
- Phenergan VC ... 2779
- Phenergan VC with Codeine ... 2781
- Preparation H ... ⊡ 871
- Tympagesic Ear Drops ... 2342
- Vasosulf ... ⊙ 271
- Vicks Sinex Nasal Spray and Ultra Fine Mist ... ⊡ 765

(⊡ Described in PDR For Nonprescription Drugs) (⊙ Described in PDR For Ophthalmology)

757 **Interactions Index** **Baby Orajel**

Phenylpropanolamine Hydrochloride (Caution should be used in patients using concomitant adrenergic psychotropic drugs). Products include:
- Acutrim ... 628
- Allerest Children's Chewable Tablets ... 627
- Allerest 12 Hour Caplets ... 627
- Atrohist Plus Tablets ... 454
- BC Cold Powder Multi-Symptom Formula (Cold-Sinus-Allergy) ... 609
- BC Cold Powder Non-Drowsy Formula (Cold-Sinus) ... 609
- Cheracol Plus Head Cold/Cough Formula ... 769
- Comtrex Multi-Symptom Non-Drowsy Liqui-gels ... 618
- Contac Continuous Action Nasal Decongestant/Antihistamine 12 Hour Capsules ... 813
- Contac Maximum Strength Continuous Action Decongestant/Antihistamine 12 Hour Caplets ... 813
- Contac Severe Cold and Flu Formula Caplets ... 814
- Coricidin 'D' Decongestant Tablets ... 800
- Dexatrim ... 832
- Dexatrim Plus Vitamins Caplets ... 832
- Dimetane-DC Cough Syrup ... 2059
- Dimetapp Elixir ... 773
- Dimetapp Extentabs ... 774
- Dimetapp Tablets/Liqui-Gels ... 775
- Dimetapp Cold & Allergy Chewable Tablets ... 773
- Dimetapp DM Elixir ... 774
- Dura-Vent Tablets ... 952
- Entex Capsules ... 1986
- Entex LA Tablets ... 1987
- Entex Liquid ... 1986
- Exgest LA Tablets ... 782
- Hycomine ... 931
- Isoclor Timesule Capsules ... 637
- Nolamine Timed-Release Tablets ... 785
- Ornade Spansule Capsules ... 2502
- Propagest Tablets ... 786
- Pyrroxate Caplets ... 772
- Robitussin-CF ... 777
- Sinulin Tablets ... 787
- Tavist-D 12 Hour Relief Tablets ... 787
- Teldrin 12 Hour Antihistamine/Nasal Decongestant Allergy Relief Capsules ... 826
- Triaminic Allergy Tablets ... 789
- Triaminic Cold Tablets ... 790
- Triaminic Expectorant ... 790
- Triaminic Syrup ... 792
- Triaminic-12 Tablets ... 792
- Triaminic-DM Syrup ... 792
- Triaminicin Tablets ... 793
- Triaminicol Multi-Symptom Cold Tablets ... 793
- Triaminicol Multi-Symptom Relief ... 794
- Vicks DayQuil Allergy Relief 12-Hour Extended Release Tablets ... 760
- Vicks DayQuil Allergy Relief 4-Hour Tablets ... 760
- Vicks DayQuil SINUS Pressure & CONGESTION Relief ... 761

Pindolol (Potential for additive effects). Products include:
- Visken Tablets ... 2299

Propranolol Hydrochloride (Potential for additive effects). Products include:
- Inderal ... 2728
- Inderal LA Long Acting Capsules ... 2730
- Inderide Tablets ... 2732
- Inderide LA Long Acting Capsules ... 2734

Pseudoephedrine Hydrochloride (Caution should be used in patients using concomitant adrenergic psychotropic drugs). Products include:
- Actifed Allergy Daytime/Nighttime Caplets ... 844
- Actifed Plus Caplets ... 845
- Actifed Plus Tablets ... 845
- Actifed with Codeine Cough Syrup ... 1067
- Actifed Sinus Daytime/Nighttime Tablets and Caplets ... 846
- Actifed Syrup ... 846
- Actifed Tablets ... 844
- Advil Cold and Sinus Caplets and Tablets (formerly CoAdvil) ... 870
- Alka-Seltzer Plus Cold Medicine Liqui-Gels ... 706
- Alka-Seltzer Plus Cold & Cough Medicine Liqui-Gels ... 705
- Alka-Seltzer Plus Night-Time Cold Medicine Liqui-Gels ... 706
- Allerest Headache Strength Tablets ... 627
- Allerest Maximum Strength Tablets ... 627
- Allerest No Drowsiness Tablets ... 627
- Allerest Sinus Pain Formula ... 627
- Anatuss LA Tablets ... 1542
- Atrohist Pediatric Capsules ... 453
- Bayer Select Sinus Pain Relief Formula ... 717
- Benadryl Allergy Decongestant Liquid Medication ... 848
- Benadryl Allergy Decongestant Tablets ... 848
- Benadryl Allergy Sinus Headache Formula Caplets ... 849
- Benylin Multisymptom ... 852
- Bromfed Capsules (Extended-Release) ... 1785
- Bromfed Syrup ... 733
- Bromfed Tablets ... 1785
- Bromfed-DM Cough Syrup ... 1786
- Bromfed-PD Capsules (Extended-Release) ... 1785
- Children's Vicks DayQuil Allergy Relief ... 757
- Children's Vicks NyQuil Cold/Cough Relief ... 758
- Comtrex Multi-Symptom Cold Reliever Tablets/Caplets/Liqui-Gels/Liquid ... 615
- Allergy-Sinus Comtrex Multi-Symptom Allergy-Sinus Formula Tablets ... 617
- Comtrex Multi-Symptom Non-Drowsy Caplets ... 618
- Congess ... 1004
- Contac Day Allergy/Sinus Caplets ... 812
- Contac Day & Night ... 812
- Contac Night Allergy/Sinus Caplets ... 812
- Contac Severe Cold & Flu Non-Drowsy ... 815
- Deconamine Chewable Tablets ... 1320
- Deconamine CX Cough and Cold Liquid and Tablets ... 1319
- Deconamine ... 1320
- Deconsal C Expectorant Syrup ... 456
- Deconsal Pediatric Syrup ... 457
- Deconsal II Tablets ... 454
- Dimetane-DX Cough Syrup ... 2059
- Dimetapp Sinus Caplets ... 775
- Dorcol Children's Cough Syrup ... 785
- Drixoral Cough + Congestion Liquid Caps ... 802
- Dura-Tap/PD Capsules ... 2867
- Duratuss Tablets ... 2565
- Duratuss HD Elixir ... 2565
- Efidac/24 ... 635
- Entex PSE Tablets ... 1987
- Fedahist Gyrocaps ... 2401
- Fedahist Timecaps ... 2401
- Guaifed ... 1787
- Guaifed Syrup ... 734
- Guaimax-D Tablets ... 792
- Guaitab Tablets ... 734
- Isoclor Expectorant ... 990
- Kronofed-A ... 977
- Motrin IB Sinus ... 838
- Novahistine DH ... 2462
- Novahistine DMX ... 822
- Novahistine Expectorant ... 2463
- Nucofed ... 2051
- PediaCare Cold Allergy Chewable Tablets ... 677
- PediaCare Cough-Cold Chewable Tablets ... 1553
- PediaCare ... 1553
- PediaCare Infants' Decongestant Drops ... 677
- PediCare Infant's Drops Decongestant Plus Cough ... 1553
- PediaCare NightRest Cough-Cold Liquid ... 1553
- Pediatric Vicks 44d Dry Hacking Cough & Head Congestion ... 763
- Pediatric Vicks 44m Cough & Cold Relief ... 764
- Robitussin Cold & Cough Liqui-Gels ... 776
- Robitussin Maximum Strength Cough & Cold ... 778
- Robitussin Pediatric Cough & Cold Formula ... 779
- Robitussin Severe Congestion Liqui-Gels ... 776
- Robitussin-DAC Syrup ... 2074
- Robitussin-PE ... 778
- Rondec Oral Drops ... 953
- Rondec Syrup ... 953
- Rondec Tablet ... 953
- Rondec-DM Oral Drops ... 954
- Rondec-DM Syrup ... 954
- Rondec-TR Tablet ... 953
- Ryna ... 841
- Seldane-D Extended-Release Tablets ... 1538
- Semprex-D Capsules ... 463
- Semprex-D Capsules ... 1167
- Sinarest Tablets ... 648
- Sinarest Extra Strength Tablets ... 648
- Sinarest No Drowsiness Tablets ... 648
- Sine-Aid IB Caplets ... 1554
- Sine-Aid Maximum Strength Sinus Medication Gelcaps, Caplets and Tablets ... 1554
- Sine-Off No Drowsiness Formula Caplets ... 824
- Sine-Off Sinus Medicine ... 825
- Singlet Tablets ... 825
- Sinutab Non-Drying Liquid Caps ... 859
- Sinutab Sinus Allergy Medication, Maximum Strength Tablets and Caplets ... 860
- Sinutab Sinus Medication, Maximum Strength Without Drowsiness Formula, Tablets & Caplets ... 860
- Sinutab Sinus Medication, Regular Strength Without Drowsiness Formula ... 859
- Sudafed Children's Liquid ... 861
- Sudafed Cold and Cough Liquidcaps ... 862
- Sudafed Cough Syrup ... 862
- Sudafed Plus Liquid ... 862
- Sudafed Plus Tablets ... 863
- Sudafed Severe Cold Formula Caplets ... 863
- Sudafed Severe Cold Formula Tablets ... 864
- Sudafed Sinus Caplets ... 864
- Sudafed Sinus Tablets ... 864
- Sudafed Tablets, 30 mg ... 861
- Sudafed Tablets, 60 mg ... 861
- Sudafed 12 Hour Caplets ... 861
- Syn-Rx Tablets ... 465
- Syn-Rx DM Tablets ... 466
- TheraFlu ... 787
- TheraFlu Maximum Strength Nighttime Flu, Cold & Cough Medicine ... 788
- TheraFlu Maximum Strength Non-Drowsy Formula Flu, Cold & Cough Medicine ... 788
- Thera Flu Maximum Strength, Non-Drowsy Formula Flu, Cold and Cough Caplets ... 789
- Triaminic AM Cough and Decongestant Formula ... 789
- Triaminic AM Decongestant Formula ... 790
- Triaminic Nite Light ... 791
- Triaminic Sore Throat Formula ... 791
- Tussend ... 1783
- Tussend Expectorant ... 1785
- Children's TYLENOL Cold Multi-Symptom Liquid Formula and Chewable Tablets ... 1561
- Children's TYLENOL Cold Plus Cough Multi Symptom Tablets and Liquid ... 681
- Infants' TYLENOL Cold Decongestant & Fever-Reducer Drops ... 1556
- TYLENOL Maximum Strength Allergy Sinus Medication Gelcaps and Caplets ... 1563
- TYLENOL Maximum Strength Allergy Sinus NightTime Medication Caplets ... 1555
- TYLENOL Flu Maximum Strength Gelcaps ... 1565
- TYLENOL Flu NightTime, Maximum Strength, Gelcaps ... 1566
- TYLENOL Maximum Strength Flu NightTime Hot Medication Packets ... 1562
- TYLENOL, Maximum Strength, Sinus Medication Geltabs, Gelcaps, Caplets and Tablets ... 1566
- TYLENOL Cold Multi-Symptom Formula Medication Tablets and Caplets ... 1561
- TYLENOL Cold Medication No Drowsiness Formula Gelcaps and Caplets ... 1562
- TYLENOL Cold Multi-Symptom Hot Medication Liquid Packets ... 1557
- TYLENOL Cough Multi-Symptom Medication with Decongestant ... 1565
- Ursinus Inlay-Tabs ... 794
- Vicks 44 LiquiCaps Cough, Cold & Flu Relief ... 755
- Vicks 44 LiquiCaps Non-Drowsy Cough & Cold Relief ... 756
- Vicks 44D Dry Hacking Cough & Head Congestion ... 755
- Vicks 44M Cough, Cold & Flu Relief ... 756
- Vicks DayQuil ... 761
- Vicks DayQuil SINUS Pressure & PAIN Relief with IBUPROFEN ... 762
- Vicks Nyquil Hot Therapy ... 762
- Vicks NyQuil LiquiCaps Multi-Symptom Cold/Flu Relief ... 763
- Vicks NyQuil Multi-Symptom Cold/Flu Relief - (Original & Cherry Flavor) ... 763

Rauwolfia Serpentina (Possible additive effects and the production of hypotension and/or bradycardia).
- No products indexed under this heading.

Rescinnamine (Possible additive effects and the production of hypotension and/or bradycardia).
- No products indexed under this heading.

Reserpine (Possible additive effects and the production of hypotension and/or bradycardia). Products include:
- Diupres Tablets ... 1650
- Hydropres Tablets ... 1675
- Ser-Ap-Es Tablets ... 849

Sotalol Hydrochloride (Potential for additive effects). Products include:
- Betapace Tablets ... 641

Tetrahydrozoline Hydrochloride (Caution should be used in patients using concomitant adrenergic psychotropic drugs). Products include:
- Collyrium Fresh ... 325
- Murine Plus Lubricant Redness Reliever Eye Drops ... 781
- Murine Tears Plus Lubricant Redness Reliever Eye Drops ... 316
- Visine Maximum Strength Allergy Relief ... 313
- Visine Moisturizing Eye Drops ... 313
- Visine Original Eye Drops ... 314

Timolol Hemihydrate (Potential for additive effects). Products include:
- Betimol 0.25%, 0.5% ... 261

Timolol Maleate (Potential for additive effects). Products include:
- Blocadren Tablets ... 1614
- Timolide Tablets ... 1748
- Timoptic in Ocudose ... 1753
- Timoptic Sterile Ophthalmic Solution ... 1751
- Timoptic-XE ... 1755

Tranylcypromine Sulfate (Caution should be used in patients using concomitant adrenergic psychotropic drugs). Products include:
- Parnate Tablets ... 2503

Verapamil Hydrochloride (Possible precipitation of left ventricular failure and hypotension). Products include:
- Calan SR Caplets ... 2422
- Calan Tablets ... 2419
- Isoptin Injectable ... 1344
- Isoptin Oral Tablets ... 1346
- Isoptin SR Tablets ... 1348
- Verelan Capsules ... 1410
- Verelan Capsules ... 2824

BABY ORAJEL TEETHING PAIN MEDICINE
(Benzocaine) ... 652
None cited in PDR database.

BABY ORAJEL TOOTH & GUM CLEANSER
(Simethicone) ... 652
None cited in PDR database.

IMPORTANT NOTE: Always consult each drug listing in the patient's regimen for possible interactions.

Orajel | Interactions Index | 758

ORAJEL MAXIMUM STRENGTH TOOTHACHE MEDICATION
(Benzocaine) ▣ 652
None cited in PDR database.

ORAJEL MOUTH-AID FOR CANKER AND COLD SORES
(Benzocaine, Benzalkonium Chloride, Zinc Chloride) ▣ 652
None cited in PDR database.

ORAJEL PERIOSEPTIC OXYGENATING LIQUID
(Carbamide Peroxide) ▣ 653
None cited in PDR database.

ORAMORPH SR (MORPHINE SULFATE SUSTAINED RELEASE TABLETS)
(Morphine Sulfate) 2236
May interact with central nervous system depressants, hypnotics and sedatives, antihistamines, psychotropics, and certain other agents. Compounds in these categories include:

Acrivastine (CNS depressant effects are potentiated). Products include:
Semprex-D Capsules 463
Semprex-D Capsules 1167

Alfentanil Hydrochloride (CNS depressant effects are potentiated). Products include:
Alfenta Injection 1286

Alprazolam (CNS depressant effects are potentiated). Products include:
Xanax Tablets 2649

Amitriptyline Hydrochloride (CNS depressant effects are potentiated). Products include:
Elavil 2838
Endep Tablets 2174
Etrafon 2355
Limbitrol 2180
Triavil Tablets 1757

Amoxapine (CNS depressant effects are potentiated). Products include:
Asendin Tablets 1369

Aprobarbital (CNS depressant effects are potentiated).
No products indexed under this heading.

Astemizole (CNS depressant effects are potentiated). Products include:
Hismanal Tablets 1293

Azatadine Maleate (CNS depressant effects are potentiated). Products include:
Trinalin Repetabs Tablets 1330

Bromodiphenhydramine Hydrochloride (CNS depressant effects are potentiated).
No products indexed under this heading.

Brompheniramine Maleate (CNS depressant effects are potentiated). Products include:
Alka Seltzer Plus Sinus Medicine ▣ 707
Bromfed Capsules (Extended-Release) 1785
Bromfed Syrup ▣ 733
Bromfed Tablets 1785
Bromfed-DM Cough Syrup 1786
Bromfed-PD Capsules (Extended-Release) 1785
Dimetane-DC Cough Syrup 2059
Dimetane-DX Cough Syrup 2059
Dimetapp Elixir ▣ 773
Dimetapp Extentabs ▣ 774
Dimetapp Tablets/Liqui-Gels ▣ 775
Dimetapp Cold & Allergy Chewable Tablets ▣ 773
Dimetapp DM Elixir ▣ 774
Vicks DayQuil Allergy Relief 12-Hour Extended Release Tablets ▣ 760
Vicks DayQuil Allergy Relief 4-Hour Tablets ▣ 760

Buprenorphine (CNS depressant effects are potentiated; may alter analgesic effect or may precipitate withdrawal symptoms). Products include:
Buprenex Injectable 2006

Buspirone Hydrochloride (CNS depressant effects are potentiated). Products include:
BuSpar 737

Butabarbital (CNS depressant effects are potentiated).
No products indexed under this heading.

Butalbital (CNS depressant effects are potentiated). Products include:
Esgic-plus Tablets 1013
Fioricet Tablets 2258
Fioricet with Codeine Capsules 2260
Fiorinal Capsules 2261
Fiorinal with Codeine Capsules 2262
Fiorinal Tablets 2261
Phrenilin 785
Sedapap Tablets 50 mg/650 mg 1543

Butorphanol Tartrate (May alter analgesic effect or may precipitate withdrawal symptoms). Products include:
Stadol 775

Chlordiazepoxide (CNS depressant effects are potentiated). Products include:
Libritabs Tablets 2177
Limbitrol 2180

Chlordiazepoxide Hydrochloride (CNS depressant effects are potentiated). Products include:
Librax Capsules 2176
Librium Capsules 2178
Librium Injectable 2179

Chlorpheniramine Maleate (CNS depressant effects are potentiated). Products include:
Alka-Seltzer Plus Cold Medicine ▣ 705
Alka-Seltzer Plus Cold Medicine Liqui-Gels ▣ 706
Alka-Seltzer Plus Cold & Cough Medicine ▣ 708
Alka-Seltzer Plus Cold & Cough Medicine Liqui-Gels ▣ 705
Allerest Children's Chewable Tablets ▣ 627
Allerest Headache Strength Tablets ▣ 627
Allerest Maximum Strength Tablets ▣ 627
Allerest Sinus Pain Formula ▣ 627
Allerest 12 Hour Caplets ▣ 627
Ana-Kit Anaphylaxis Emergency Treatment Kit 617
Atrohist Pediatric Capsules 453
Atrohist Plus Tablets 454
BC Cold Powder Multi-Symptom Formula (Cold-Sinus-Allergy) ▣ 609
Cerose DM ▣ 878
Cheracol Plus Head Cold/Cough Formula ▣ 769
Children's Vicks DayQuil Allergy Relief ▣ 757
Children's Vicks NyQuil Cold/Cough Relief ▣ 758
Chlor-Trimeton Allergy Decongestant Tablets ▣ 799
Chlor-Trimeton Allergy Tablets ▣ 798
Comhist 2038
Comtrex Multi-Symptom Cold Reliever Tablets/Caplets/Liqui-Gels/Liquid ▣ 615
Allergy-Sinus Comtrex Multi-Symptom Allergy-Sinus Formula Tablets ▣ 617
Contac Continuous Action Nasal Decongestant/Antihistamine 12 Hour Capsules ▣ 813
Contac Maximum Strength Continuous Action Decongestant/Antihistamine 12 Hour Caplets ▣ 813
Contac Severe Cold and Flu Formula Caplets ▣ 814
Coricidin 'D' Decongestant Tablets ▣ 800
Coricidin Tablets ▣ 800
D.A. Chewable Tablets 951
Deconamine 1320
Dura-Tap/PD Capsules 2867
Dura-Vent/DA Tablets 953
Extendryl 1005
Fedahist Gyrocaps 2401
Fedahist Timecaps 2401
Hycomine Compound Tablets 932
Isoclor Timesule Capsules ▣ 637
Kronofed-A 977
Nolamine Timed-Release Tablets 785
Novahistine DH 2462
Novahistine Elixir ▣ 823
Ornade Spansule Capsules 2502
PediaCare Cold Allergy Chewable Tablets ▣ 677
PediaCare Cough-Cold Chewable Tablets 1553
PediaCare Cough-Cold Liquid 1553
PediaCare NightRest Cough-Cold Liquid 1553
Pediatric Vicks 44m Cough & Cold Relief ▣ 764
Pyrroxate Caplets ▣ 772
Ryna ▣ 841
Sinarest Tablets ▣ 648
Sinarest Extra Strength Tablets ▣ 648
Sine-Off Sinus Medicine ▣ 825
Singlet Tablets ▣ 825
Sinulin Tablets 787
Sinutab Sinus Allergy Medication, Maximum Strength Tablets and Caplets ▣ 860
Sudafed Plus Liquid ▣ 862
Sudafed Plus Tablets ▣ 863
Teldrin 12 Hour Antihistamine/Nasal Decongestant Allergy Relief Capsules ▣ 826
TheraFlu ▣ 787
TheraFlu Maximum Strength Nighttime Flu, Cold & Cough Medicine ▣ 788
Triaminic Allergy Tablets ▣ 789
Triaminic Cold Tablets ▣ 790
Triaminic Nite Light ▣ 791
Triaminic Syrup ▣ 792
Triaminic-12 Tablets ▣ 792
Triaminicin Tablets ▣ 793
Triaminicol Multi-Symptom Cold Tablets ▣ 793
Triaminicol Multi-Symptom Relief ▣ 794
Tussend 1783
Children's TYLENOL Cold Multi-Symptom Liquid Formula and Chewable Tablets 1561
Children's TYLENOL Cold Plus Cough Multi Symptom Tablets and Liquid ▣ 681
TYLENOL Maximum Strength Allergy Sinus Medication Gelcaps and Caplets 1563
TYLENOL Cold Multi-Symptom Formula Medication Tablets and Caplets 1561
TYLENOL Cold Multi-Symptom Hot Medication Liquid Packets 1557
Vicks 44 LiquiCaps Cough, Cold & Flu Relief ▣ 755
Vicks 44M Cough, Cold & Flu Relief ▣ 756

Chlorpheniramine Polistirex (CNS depressant effects are potentiated). Products include:
Tussionex Pennkinetic Extended-Release Suspension 998

Chlorpheniramine Tannate (CNS depressant effects are potentiated). Products include:
Atrohist Pediatric Suspension 454
Ricobid Tablets and Pediatric Suspension 2038
Rynatan 2673
Rynatuss 2673

Chlorpromazine (CNS depressant effects are potentiated). Products include:
Thorazine Suppositories 2523

Chlorprothixene (CNS depressant effects are potentiated).
No products indexed under this heading.

Chlorprothixene Hydrochloride (CNS depressant effects are potentiated).
No products indexed under this heading.

Clemastine Fumarate (CNS depressant effects are potentiated). Products include:
Tavist Syrup 2297
Tavist Tablets 2298
Tavist-1 12 Hour Relief Tablets ▣ 787
Tavist-D 12 Hour Relief Tablets ▣ 787

Clorazepate Dipotassium (CNS depressant effects are potentiated). Products include:
Tranxene 451

Clozapine (CNS depressant effects are potentiated). Products include:
Clozaril Tablets 2252

Codeine Phosphate (CNS depressant effects are potentiated). Products include:
Actifed with Codeine Cough Syrup 1067
Brontex 1981
Deconsal C Expectorant Syrup 456
Deconsal Pediatric Syrup 457
Dimetane-DC Cough Syrup 2059
Empirin with Codeine Tablets 1093
Fioricet with Codeine Capsules 2260
Fiorinal with Codeine Capsules 2262
Isoclor Expectorant 990
Novahistine DH 2462
Novahistine Expectorant 2463
Nucofed 2051
Phenergan with Codeine 2777
Phenergan VC with Codeine 2781
Robitussin A-C Syrup 2073
Robitussin-DAC Syrup 2074
Ryna ▣ 841
Soma Compound w/Codeine Tablets 2676
Tussi-Organidin NR Liquid and S NR Liquid 2677
Tylenol with Codeine 1583

Cyproheptadine Hydrochloride (CNS depressant effects are potentiated). Products include:
Periactin 1724

Desflurane (CNS depressant effects are potentiated). Products include:
Suprane 1813

Desipramine Hydrochloride (CNS depressant effects are potentiated). Products include:
Norpramin Tablets 1526

Dexchlorpheniramine Maleate (CNS depressant effects are potentiated).
No products indexed under this heading.

Dezocine (CNS depressant effects are potentiated). Products include:
Dalgan Injection 538

Diazepam (CNS depressant effects are potentiated). Products include:
Dizac 1809
Valium Injectable 2182
Valium Tablets 2183
Valrelease Capsules 2169

Diphenhydramine Citrate (CNS depressant effects are potentiated). Products include:
Excedrin P.M. Analgesic/Sleeping Aid Tablets, Caplets, Liquigels 733

Diphenhydramine Hydrochloride (CNS depressant effects are potentiated). Products include:
Actifed Allergy Daytime/Nighttime Caplets ▣ 844
Actifed Sinus Daytime/Nighttime Tablets and Caplets ▣ 846
Arthritis Foundation NightTime Caplets ▣ 674
Extra Strength Bayer PM Aspirin ▣ 713
Bayer Select Night Time Pain Relief Formula ▣ 716
Benadryl Allergy Decongestant Liquid Medication ▣ 848
Benadryl Allergy Decongestant Tablets ▣ 848
Benadryl Allergy Liquid Medication ▣ 849
Benadryl Allergy ▣ 848
Benadryl Allergy Sinus Headache Formula Caplets ▣ 849
Benadryl Capsules 1898
Benadryl Dye-Free Allergy Liquigel Softgels ▣ 850

(▣ Described in PDR For Nonprescription Drugs) (⊙ Described in PDR For Ophthalmology)

Interactions Index

Oramorph SR

Benadryl Dye-Free Allergy Liquid Medication .... ✦D 850

Benadryl Itch Relief Cream, Children's Formula and Maximum Strength 2% .... ✦D 851

Benadryl Itch Relief Spray, Children's Formula and Maximum Strength 2% .... ✦D 851

Benadryl Itch Relief Stick Maximum Strength 2% .... ✦D 850

Benadryl Itch Stopping Gel, Children's Formula and Maximum Strength 2% .... ✦D 851

Benadryl Kapseals 1898

Benadryl Injection 1898

Contac Day & Night Cold/Flu Night Caplets .... ✦D 812

Contac Night Allergy/Sinus Caplets .... ✦D 812

Extra Strength Doan's P.M. .... ✦D 633

Legatrin PM .... ✦D 651

Miles Nervine Nighttime Sleep-Aid ✦D 723

Nytol QuickCaps Caplets .... ✦D 610

Sleepinal Night-time Sleep Aid Capsules and Softgels .... ✦D 834

TYLENOL Maximum Strength Allergy Sinus NightTime Medication Caplets 1555

TYLENOL Flu NightTime, Maximum Strength, Gelcaps 1566

TYLENOL Maximum Strength Flu NightTime Hot Medication Packets 1562

TYLENOL PM, Extra Strength Pain Reliever/Sleep Aid Caplets, Geltabs, Gelcaps 1560

TYLENOL Severe Allergy Medication Caplets 1564

Maximum Strength Unisom Sleepgels 1934

Unisom With Pain Relief-Nighttime Sleep Aid and Pain Reliever............ 1934

Doxepin Hydrochloride (CNS depressant effects are potentiated). Products include:

Sinequan 2205

Zonalon Cream 1055

Droperidol (CNS depressant effects are potentiated). Products include:

Inapsine Injection 1296

Enflurane (CNS depressant effects are potentiated).

No products indexed under this heading.

Estazolam (CNS depressant effects are potentiated). Products include:

ProSom Tablets 449

Ethchlorvynol (CNS depressant effects are potentiated). Products include:

Placidyl Capsules 448

Ethinamate (CNS depressant effects are potentiated).

No products indexed under this heading.

Fentanyl (CNS depressant effects are potentiated). Products include:

Duragesic Transdermal System......... 1288

Fentanyl Citrate (CNS depressant effects are potentiated). Products include:

Sublimaze Injection 1307

Fluphenazine Decanoate (CNS depressant effects are potentiated). Products include:

Prolixin Decanoate 509

Fluphenazine Enanthate (CNS depressant effects are potentiated). Products include:

Prolixin Enanthate 509

Fluphenazine Hydrochloride (CNS depressant effects are potentiated). Products include:

Prolixin 509

Flurazepam Hydrochloride (CNS depressant effects are potentiated). Products include:

Dalmane Capsules 2173

Glutethimide (CNS depressant effects are potentiated).

No products indexed under this heading.

Haloperidol (CNS depressant effects are potentiated). Products include:

Haldol Injection, Tablets and Concentrate 1575

Haloperidol Decanoate (CNS depressant effects are potentiated). Products include:

Haldol Decanoate 1577

Hydrocodone Bitartrate (CNS depressant effects are potentiated). Products include:

Anexsia 5/500 Elixir 1781

Anexia Tablets 1782

Codiclear DH Syrup 791

Deconamine CX Cough and Cold Liquid and Tablets 1319

Duratuss HD Elixir 2565

Hycodan Tablets and Syrup 930

Hycomine Compound Tablets 932

Hycomine 931

Hycotuss Expectorant Syrup 933

Hydrocet Capsules 782

Lorcet 10/650 1018

Lortab 2566

Tussend 1783

Tussend Expectorant 1785

Vicodin Tablets 1356

Vicodin ES Tablets 1357

Vicodin Tuss Expectorant 1358

Zydone Capsules 949

Hydrocodone Polistirex (CNS depressant effects are potentiated). Products include:

Tussionex Pennkinetic Extended-Release Suspension 998

Hydroxyzine Hydrochloride (CNS depressant effects are potentiated). Products include:

Atarax Tablets & Syrup 2185

Marax Tablets & DF Syrup 2200

Vistaril Intramuscular Solution 2216

Imipramine Hydrochloride (CNS depressant effects are potentiated). Products include:

Tofranil Ampuls 854

Tofranil Tablets 856

Imipramine Pamoate (CNS depressant effects are potentiated). Products include:

Tofranil-PM Capsules 857

Isocarboxazid (CNS depressant effects are potentiated).

No products indexed under this heading.

Isoflurane (CNS depressant effects are potentiated).

No products indexed under this heading.

Ketamine Hydrochloride (CNS depressant effects are potentiated).

No products indexed under this heading.

Levomethadyl Acetate Hydrochloride (CNS depressant effects are potentiated). Products include:

Orlaam 2239

Levorphanol Tartrate (CNS depressant effects are potentiated). Products include:

Levo-Dromoran 2129

Lithium Carbonate (CNS depressant effects are potentiated). Products include:

Eskalith 2485

Lithium Carbonate Capsules & Tablets 2230

Lithonate/Lithotabs/Lithobid 2543

Lithium Citrate (CNS depressant effects are potentiated).

No products indexed under this heading.

Loratadine (CNS depressant effects are potentiated). Products include:

Claritin 2349

Claritin-D 2350

Lorazepam (CNS depressant effects are potentiated). Products include:

Ativan Injection 2698

Ativan Tablets 2700

Loxapine Hydrochloride (CNS depressant effects are potentiated). Products include:

Loxitane 1378

Loxapine Succinate (CNS depressant effects are potentiated). Products include:

Loxitane Capsules 1378

Maprotiline Hydrochloride (CNS depressant effects are potentiated). Products include:

Ludiomil Tablets 843

Meperidine Hydrochloride (CNS depressant effects are potentiated). Products include:

Demerol 2308

Mepergan Injection 2753

Mephobarbital (CNS depressant effects are potentiated). Products include:

Mebaral Tablets 2322

Meprobamate (CNS depressant effects are potentiated). Products include:

Miltown Tablets 2672

PMB 200 and PMB 400 2783

Mesoridazine Besylate (CNS depressant effects are potentiated). Products include:

Serentil 684

Methadone Hydrochloride (CNS depressant effects are potentiated). Products include:

Methadone Hydrochloride Oral Concentrate 2233

Methadone Hydrochloride Oral Solution & Tablets 2235

Methdilazine Hydrochloride (CNS depressant effects are potentiated).

No products indexed under this heading.

Methohexital Sodium (CNS depressant effects are potentiated). Products include:

Brevital Sodium Vials 1429

Methotrimeprazine (CNS depressant effects are potentiated). Products include:

Levoprome 1274

Methoxyflurane (CNS depressant effects are potentiated).

No products indexed under this heading.

Midazolam Hydrochloride (CNS depressant effects are potentiated). Products include:

Versed Injection 2170

Molindone Hydrochloride (CNS depressant effects are potentiated). Products include:

Moban Tablets and Concentrate 1048

Nalbuphine Hydrochloride (May alter analgesic effect or may precipitate withdrawal symptoms). Products include:

Nubain Injection 935

Nortriptyline Hydrochloride (CNS depressant effects are potentiated). Products include:

Pamelor 2280

Opium Alkaloids (CNS depressant effects are potentiated).

No products indexed under this heading.

Oxazepam (CNS depressant effects are potentiated). Products include:

Serax Capsules 2810

Serax Tablets 2810

Oxycodone Hydrochloride (CNS depressant effects are potentiated). Products include:

Percocet Tablets 938

Percodan Tablets 939

Percodan-Demi Tablets 940

Roxicodone Tablets, Oral Solution & Intensol (Oxycodone) 2244

Tylox Capsules 1584

Pentazocine Hydrochloride (May alter analgesic effect or may precipitate withdrawal symptoms). Products include:

Talacen 2333

Talwin Compound 2335

Talwin Nx 2336

Pentazocine Lactate (May alter analgesic effect or may precipitate withdrawal symptoms). Products include:

Talwin Injection 2334

Pentobarbital Sodium (CNS depressant effects are potentiated). Products include:

Nembutal Sodium Capsules 436

Nembutal Sodium Solution 438

Nembutal Sodium Suppositories 440

Perphenazine (CNS depressant effects are potentiated). Products include:

Etrafon 2355

Triavil Tablets 1757

Trilafon 2389

Phenelzine Sulfate (CNS depressant effects are potentiated). Products include:

Nardil 1920

Phenobarbital (CNS depressant effects are potentiated). Products include:

Arco-Lase Plus Tablets 512

Bellergal-S Tablets 2250

Donnatal 2060

Donnatal Extentabs 2061

Donnatal Tablets 2060

Phenobarbital Elixir and Tablets 1469

Quadrinal Tablets 1350

Prazepam (CNS depressant effects are potentiated).

No products indexed under this heading.

Prochlorperazine (CNS depressant effects are potentiated). Products include:

Compazine 2470

Promethazine Hydrochloride (CNS depressant effects are potentiated). Products include:

Mepergan Injection 2753

Phenergan with Codeine 2777

Phenergan with Dextromethorphan 2778

Phenergan Injection 2773

Phenergan Suppositories 2775

Phenergan Syrup 2774

Phenergan Tablets 2775

Phenergan VC 2779

Phenergan VC with Codeine 2781

Propofol (CNS depressant effects are potentiated). Products include:

Diprivan Injection 2833

Propoxyphene Hydrochloride (CNS depressant effects are potentiated). Products include:

Darvon 1435

Wygesic Tablets 2827

Propoxyphene Napsylate (CNS depressant effects are potentiated). Products include:

Darvon-N/Darvocet-N 1433

Protriptyline Hydrochloride (CNS depressant effects are potentiated). Products include:

Vivactil Tablets 1774

Pyrilamine Maleate (CNS depressant effects are potentiated). Products include:

4-Way Fast Acting Nasal Spray (regular & mentholated) .... ✦D 621

Maximum Strength Multi-Symptom Formula Midol .... ✦D 722

IMPORTANT NOTE: Always consult each drug listing in the patient's regimen for possible interactions.

Oramorph SR — Interactions Index — 760

PMS Multi-Symptom Formula Midol ▣ 723

Pyrilamine Tannate (CNS depressant effects are potentiated). Products include:
Atrohist Pediatric Suspension 454
Rynatan 2673

Quazepam (CNS depressant effects are potentiated). Products include:
Doral Tablets 2664

Risperidone (CNS depressant effects are potentiated). Products include:
Risperdal 1301

Secobarbital Sodium (CNS depressant effects are potentiated). Products include:
Seconal Sodium Pulvules 1474

Sufentanil Citrate (CNS depressant effects are potentiated). Products include:
Sufenta Injection 1309

Temazepam (CNS depressant effects are potentiated). Products include:
Restoril Capsules 2284

Terfenadine (CNS depressant effects are potentiated). Products include:
Seldane Tablets 1536
Seldane-D Extended-Release Tablets 1538

Thiamylal Sodium (CNS depressant effects are potentiated).
No products indexed under this heading.

Thioridazine Hydrochloride (CNS depressant effects are potentiated). Products include:
Mellaril 2269

Thiothixene (CNS depressant effects are potentiated). Products include:
Navane Capsules and Concentrate 2201
Navane Intramuscular 2202

Tranylcypromine Sulfate (CNS depressant effects are potentiated). Products include:
Parnate Tablets 2503

Triazolam (CNS depressant effects are potentiated). Products include:
Halcion Tablets 2611

Trifluoperazine Hydrochloride (CNS depressant effects are potentiated). Products include:
Stelazine 2514

Trimeprazine Tartrate (CNS depressant effects are potentiated). Products include:
Temaril Tablets, Syrup and Spansule Extended-Release Capsules 483

Trimipramine Maleate (CNS depressant effects are potentiated). Products include:
Surmontil Capsules 2811

Tripelennamine Hydrochloride (CNS depressant effects are potentiated). Products include:
PBZ Tablets 845
PBZ-SR Tablets 844

Triprolidine Hydrochloride (CNS depressant effects are potentiated). Products include:
Actifed Plus Caplets ▣ 845
Actifed Plus Tablets ▣ 845
Actifed with Codeine Cough Syrup 1067
Actifed Syrup ▣ 846
Actifed Tablets ▣ 844

Zolpidem Tartrate (CNS depressant effects are potentiated). Products include:
Ambien Tablets 2416

Food Interactions

Alcohol (CNS depressant effects are potentiated).

ORAP TABLETS
(Pimozide) 1050
May interact with phenothiazines, tricyclic antidepressants, antiarrhythmics, hypnotics and sedatives, narcotic analgesics, tranquilizers, central nervous system depressants, and certain other agents. Compounds in these categories include:

Acebutolol Hydrochloride (Additive effect on QT prolongation). Products include:
Sectral Capsules 2807

Adenosine (Additive effect on QT prolongation). Products include:
Adenocard Injection 1021
Adenoscan 1024

Alfentanil Hydrochloride (CNS depression potentiated). Products include:
Alfenta Injection 1286

Alprazolam (CNS depression potentiated). Products include:
Xanax Tablets 2649

Amiodarone Hydrochloride (Additive effect on QT prolongation). Products include:
Cordarone Intravenous 2715
Cordarone Tablets 2712

Amitriptyline Hydrochloride (Additive effect on QT prolongation; CNS depression potentiated). Products include:
Elavil 2838
Endep Tablets 2174
Etrafon 2355
Limbitrol 2180
Triavil Tablets 1757

Amoxapine (Additive effect on QT prolongation; CNS depression potentiated). Products include:
Asendin Tablets 1369

Aprobarbital (CNS depression potentiated).
No products indexed under this heading.

Bretylium Tosylate (Additive effect on QT prolongation).
No products indexed under this heading.

Buprenorphine (CNS depression potentiated). Products include:
Buprenex Injectable 2006

Buspirone Hydrochloride (CNS depression potentiated). Products include:
BuSpar 737

Butabarbital (CNS depression potentiated).
No products indexed under this heading.

Butalbital (CNS depression potentiated). Products include:
Esgic-plus Tablets 1013
Fioricet Tablets 2258
Fioricet with Codeine Capsules 2260
Fiorinal Capsules 2261
Fiorinal with Codeine Capsules 2262
Fiorinal Tablets 2261
Phrenilin 785
Sedapap Tablets 50 mg/650 mg 1543

Chlordiazepoxide (CNS depression potentiated). Products include:
Libritabs Tablets 2177
Limbitrol 2180

Chlordiazepoxide Hydrochloride (CNS depression potentiated). Products include:
Librax Capsules 2176
Librium Capsules 2178
Librium Injectable 2179

Chlorpromazine (Additive effect on QT prolongation; CNS depression potentiated). Products include:
Thorazine Suppositories 2523

Chlorpromazine Hydrochloride (Additive effect on QT prolongation; CNS depression potentiated). Products include:
Thorazine 2523

Chlorprothixene (CNS depression potentiated).
No products indexed under this heading.

Chlorprothixene Hydrochloride (CNS depression potentiated).
No products indexed under this heading.

Clomipramine Hydrochloride (Additive effect on QT prolongation; CNS depression potentiated). Products include:
Anafranil Capsules 803

Clorazepate Dipotassium (CNS depression potentiated). Products include:
Tranxene 451

Clozapine (CNS depression potentiated). Products include:
Clozaril Tablets 2252

Codeine Phosphate (CNS depression potentiated). Products include:
Actifed with Codeine Cough Syrup 1067
Brontex 1981
Deconsal C Expectorant Syrup 456
Deconsal Pediatric Syrup 457
Dimetane-DC Cough Syrup 2059
Empirin with Codeine Tablets 1093
Fioricet with Codeine Capsules 2260
Fiorinal with Codeine Capsules 2262
Isoclor Expectorant 990
Novahistine DH 2462
Novahistine Expectorant 2463
Nucofed 2051
Phenergan with Codeine 2777
Phenergan VC with Codeine 2781
Robitussin A-C Syrup 2073
Robitussin-DAC Syrup 2074
Ryna ▣ 841
Soma Compound w/Codeine Tablets 2676
Tussi-Organidin NR Liquid and S NR Liquid 2677
Tylenol with Codeine 1583

Desflurane (CNS depression potentiated). Products include:
Suprane 1813

Desipramine Hydrochloride (Additive effect on QT prolongation; CNS depression potentiated). Products include:
Norpramin Tablets 1526

Dezocine (CNS depression potentiated). Products include:
Dalgan Injection 538

Diazepam (CNS depression potentiated). Products include:
Dizac 1809
Valium Injectable 2182
Valium Tablets 2183
Valrelease Capsules 2169

Disopyramide Phosphate (Additive effect on QT prolongation). Products include:
Norpace 2444

Doxepin Hydrochloride (Additive effect on QT prolongation; CNS depression potentiated). Products include:
Sinequan 2205
Zonalon Cream 1055

Droperidol (CNS depression potentiated). Products include:
Inapsine Injection 1296

Enflurane (CNS depression potentiated).
No products indexed under this heading.

Estazolam (CNS depression potentiated). Products include:
ProSom Tablets 449

Ethchlorvynol (CNS depression potentiated). Products include:
Placidyl Capsules 448

Ethinamate (CNS depression potentiated).
No products indexed under this heading.

Fentanyl (CNS depression potentiated). Products include:
Duragesic Transdermal System 1288

Fentanyl Citrate (CNS depression potentiated). Products include:
Sublimaze Injection 1307

Flecainide Acetate (Additive effect on QT prolongation). Products include:
Tambocor Tablets 1497

Fluphenazine Decanoate (Additive effect on QT prolongation; CNS depression potentiated). Products include:
Prolixin Decanoate 509

Fluphenazine Enanthate (Additive effect on QT prolongation; CNS depression potentiated). Products include:
Prolixin Enanthate 509

Fluphenazine Hydrochloride (Additive effect on QT prolongation; CNS depression potentiated). Products include:
Prolixin 509

Flurazepam Hydrochloride (CNS depression potentiated). Products include:
Dalmane Capsules 2173

Glutethimide (CNS depression potentiated).
No products indexed under this heading.

Haloperidol (CNS depression potentiated). Products include:
Haldol Injection, Tablets and Concentrate 1575

Haloperidol Decanoate (CNS depression potentiated). Products include:
Haldol Decanoate 1577

Hydrocodone Bitartrate (CNS depression potentiated). Products include:
Anexsia 5/500 Elixir 1781
Anexia Tablets 1782
Codiclear DH Syrup 791
Deconamine CX Cough and Cold Liquid and Tablets 1319
Duratuss HD Elixir 2565
Hycodan Tablets and Syrup 930
Hycomine Compound Tablets 932
Hycomine 931
Hycotuss Expectorant Syrup 933
Hydrocet Capsules 782
Lorcet 10/650 1018
Lortab 2566
Tussend 1783
Tussend Expectorant 1785
Vicodin Tablets 1356
Vicodin ES Tablets 1357
Vicodin Tuss Expectorant 1358
Zydone Capsules 949

Hydrocodone Polistirex (CNS depression potentiated). Products include:
Tussionex Pennkinetic Extended-Release Suspension 998

Hydroxyzine Hydrochloride (CNS depression potentiated). Products include:
Atarax Tablets & Syrup 2185
Marax Tablets & DF Syrup 2200
Vistaril Intramuscular Solution 2216

Imipramine Hydrochloride (Additive effect on QT prolongation; CNS depression potentiated). Products include:
Tofranil Ampuls 854
Tofranil Tablets 856

Imipramine Pamoate (Additive effect on QT prolongation; CNS depression potentiated). Products include:
Tofranil-PM Capsules 857

(▣ Described in PDR For Nonprescription Drugs) (◉ Described in PDR For Ophthalmology)

Interactions Index

Isoflurane (CNS depression potentiated).

No products indexed under this heading.

Ketamine Hydrochloride (CNS depression potentiated).

No products indexed under this heading.

Levomethadyl Acetate Hydrochloride (CNS depression potentiated). Products include:

Orlamm 2239

Levorphanol Tartrate (CNS depression potentiated). Products include:

Levo-Dromoran 2129

Lidocaine Hydrochloride (Additive effect on QT prolongation). Products include:

Bactine Antiseptic/Anesthetic First Aid Liquid .... ◆ 708
Campho-Phenique Maximum Strength First Aid Antibiotic Plus Pain Reliever Ointment ...... ◆ 719
Decadron Phosphate with Xylocaine Injection, Sterile 1639
Xylocaine Injections 567

Lorazepam (CNS depression potentiated). Products include:

Ativan Injection 2698
Ativan Tablets 2700

Loxapine Hydrochloride (CNS depression potentiated). Products include:

Loxitane 1378

Loxapine Succinate (CNS depression potentiated). Products include:

Loxitane Capsules 1378

Maprotiline Hydrochloride (Additive effect on QT prolongation; CNS depression potentiated). Products include:

Ludiomil Tablets 843

Meperidine Hydrochloride (CNS depression potentiated). Products include:

Demerol 2308
Mepergan Injection 2753

Mephobarbital (CNS depression potentiated). Products include:

Mebaral Tablets 2322

Meprobamate (CNS depression potentiated). Products include:

Miltown Tablets 2672
PMB 200 and PMB 400 2783

Mesoridazine Besylate (Additive effect on QT prolongation; CNS depression potentiated). Products include:

Serentil 684

Methadone Hydrochloride (CNS depression potentiated). Products include:

Methadone Hydrochloride Oral Concentrate 2233
Methadone Hydrochloride Oral Solution & Tablets 2235

Methohexital Sodium (CNS depression potentiated). Products include:

Brevital Sodium Vials 1429

Methotrimeprazine (Additive effect on QT prolongation; CNS depression potentiated). Products include:

Levoprome 1274

Methoxyflurane (CNS depression potentiated).

No products indexed under this heading.

Mexiletine Hydrochloride (Additive effect on QT prolongation). Products include:

Mexitil Capsules 678

Midazolam Hydrochloride (CNS depression potentiated). Products include:

Versed Injection 2170

Molindone Hydrochloride (CNS depression potentiated). Products include:

Moban Tablets and Concentrate 1048

Moricizine Hydrochloride (Additive effect on QT prolongation). Products include:

Ethmozine Tablets 2041

Morphine Sulfate (CNS depression potentiated). Products include:

Astramorph/PF Injection, USP (Preservative-Free) 535
Duramorph 962
Infumorph 200 and Infumorph 500 Sterile Solutions 965
MS Contin Tablets 1994
MSIR 1997
Oramorph SR (Morphine Sulfate Sustained Release Tablets) 2236
RMS Suppositories 2657
Roxanol 2243

Nortriptyline Hydrochloride (Additive effect on QT prolongation; CNS depression potentiated). Products include:

Pamelor 2280

Opium Alkaloids (CNS depression potentiated).

No products indexed under this heading.

Oxazepam (CNS depression potentiated). Products include:

Serax Capsules 2810
Serax Tablets 2810

Oxycodone Hydrochloride (CNS depression potentiated). Products include:

Percocet Tablets 938
Percodan Tablets 939
Percodan-Demi Tablets 940
Roxicodone Tablets, Oral Solution & Intensol (Oxycodone) 2244
Tylox Capsules 1584

Pentobarbital Sodium (CNS depression potentiated). Products include:

Nembutal Sodium Capsules 436
Nembutal Sodium Solution 438
Nembutal Sodium Suppositories 440

Perphenazine (Additive effect on QT prolongation; CNS depression potentiated). Products include:

Etrafon 2355
Triavil Tablets 1757
Trilafon 2389

Phenobarbital (CNS depression potentiated). Products include:

Arco-Lase Plus Tablets 512
Bellergal-S Tablets 2250
Donnatal 2060
Donnatal Extentabs 2061
Donnatal Tablets 2060
Phenobarbital Elixir and Tablets 1469
Quadrinal Tablets 1350

Prazepam (CNS depression potentiated).

No products indexed under this heading.

Procainamide Hydrochloride (Additive effect on QT prolongation). Products include:

Procan SR Tablets 1926

Prochlorperazine (Additive effect on QT prolongation; CNS depression potentiated). Products include:

Compazine 2470

Promethazine Hydrochloride (Additive effect on QT prolongation; CNS depression potentiated). Products include:

Mepergan Injection 2753
Phenergan with Codeine 2777
Phenergan with Dextromethorphan 2778
Phenergan Injection 2773
Phenergan Suppositories 2775
Phenergan Syrup 2774
Phenergan Tablets 2775
Phenergan VC 2779
Phenergan VC with Codeine 2781

Propafenone Hydrochloride (Additive effect on QT prolongation). Products include:

Rythmol Tablets–150mg, 225mg, 300mg 1352

Propofol (CNS depression potentiated). Products include:

Diprivan Injection 2833

Propoxyphene Hydrochloride (CNS depression potentiated). Products include:

Darvon 1435
Wygesic Tablets 2827

Propoxyphene Napsylate (CNS depression potentiated). Products include:

Darvon-N/Darvocet-N 1433

Propranolol Hydrochloride (Additive effect on QT prolongation). Products include:

Inderal 2728
Inderal LA Long Acting Capsules 2730
Inderide Tablets 2732
Inderide LA Long Acting Capsules .. 2734

Protriptyline Hydrochloride (Additive effect on QT prolongation; CNS depression potentiated). Products include:

Vivactil Tablets 1774

Quazepam (CNS depression potentiated). Products include:

Doral Tablets 2664

Quinidine Gluconate (Additive effect on QT prolongation). Products include:

Quinaglute Dura-Tabs Tablets 649

Quinidine Polygalacturonate (Additive effect on QT prolongation).

No products indexed under this heading.

Quinidine Sulfate (Additive effect on QT prolongation). Products include:

Quinidex Extentabs 2067

Risperidone (CNS depression potentiated). Products include:

Risperdal 1301

Secobarbital Sodium (CNS depression potentiated). Products include:

Seconal Sodium Pulvules 1474

Sotalol Hydrochloride (Additive effect on QT prolongation). Products include:

Betapace Tablets 641

Sufentanil Citrate (CNS depression potentiated). Products include:

Sufenta Injection 1309

Temazepam (CNS depression potentiated). Products include:

Restoril Capsules 2284

Thiamylal Sodium (CNS depression potentiated).

No products indexed under this heading.

Thioridazine Hydrochloride (Additive effect on QT prolongation; CNS depression potentiated). Products include:

Mellaril 2269

Thiothixene (CNS depression potentiated). Products include:

Navane Capsules and Concentrate 2201
Navane Intramuscular 2202

Tocainide Hydrochloride (Additive effect on QT prolongation). Products include:

Tonocard Tablets 531

Triazolam (CNS depression potentiated). Products include:

Halcion Tablets 2611

Trifluoperazine Hydrochloride (Additive effect on QT prolongation; CNS depression potentiated). Products include:

Stelazine 2514

Trimipramine Maleate (Additive effect on QT prolongation; CNS depression potentiated). Products include:

Surmontil Capsules 2811

Verapamil Hydrochloride (Additive effect on QT prolongation). Products include:

Calan SR Caplets 2422
Calan Tablets 2419
Isoptin Injectable 1344
Isoptin Oral Tablets 1346
Isoptin SR Tablets 1348
Verelan Capsules 1410
Verelan Capsules 2824

Zolpidem Tartrate (CNS depression potentiated). Products include:

Ambien Tablets 2416

Food Interactions

Alcohol (CNS depression potentiated).

ORCHID FRESH II PERINEAL/OSTOMY CLEANSER

(Benzethonium Chloride) .... ◆ 625

None cited in PDR database.

ORETIC TABLETS

(Hydrochlorothiazide) 443

May interact with antihypertensives, ganglionic blocking agents, peripheral adrenergic blockers, corticosteroids, cardiac glycosides, insulin, barbiturates, narcotic analgesics, and certain other agents. Compounds in these categories include:

Acebutolol Hydrochloride (Additive or potentiative effects). Products include:

Sectral Capsules 2807

ACTH (Hypokalemia).

No products indexed under this heading.

Alfentanil Hydrochloride (May aggravate orthostatic hypotension). Products include:

Alfenta Injection 1286

Amlodipine Besylate (Additive or potentiative effects). Products include:

Lotrel Capsules 840
Norvasc Tablets 1940

Aprobarbital (May aggravate orthostatic hypotension).

No products indexed under this heading.

Atenolol (Additive or potentiative effects). Products include:

Tenoretic Tablets 2845
Tenormin Tablets and I.V. Injection 2847

Benazepril Hydrochloride (Additive or potentiative effects). Products include:

Lotensin Tablets 834
Lotensin HCT 837
Lotrel Capsules 840

Bendroflumethiazide (Additive or potentiative effects).

No products indexed under this heading.

Betamethasone Acetate (Hypokalemia). Products include:

Celestone Soluspan Suspension 2347

Betamethasone Sodium Phosphate (Hypokalemia). Products include:

Celestone Soluspan Suspension 2347

Betaxolol Hydrochloride (Additive or potentiative effects). Products include:

Betoptic Ophthalmic Solution 469
Betoptic S Ophthalmic Suspension 471
Kerlone Tablets 2436

Bisoprolol Fumarate (Additive or potentiative effects). Products include:

Zebeta Tablets 1413
Ziac 1415

IMPORTANT NOTE: Always consult each drug listing in the patient's regimen for possible interactions.

Oretic | Interactions Index | 762

Buprenorphine (May aggravate orthostatic hypotension). Products include:
- Buprenex Injectable ... 2006

Butabarbital (May aggravate orthostatic hypotension).
- No products indexed under this heading.

Butalbital (May aggravate orthostatic hypotension). Products include:
- Esgic-plus Tablets ... 1013
- Fioricet Tablets ... 2258
- Fioricet with Codeine Capsules ... 2260
- Fiorinal Capsules ... 2261
- Fiorinal with Codeine Capsules ... 2262
- Fiorinal Tablets ... 2261
- Phrenilin ... 785
- Sedapap Tablets 50 mg/650 mg ... 1543

Captopril (Additive or potentiative effects). Products include:
- Capoten ... 739
- Capozide ... 742

Carteolol Hydrochloride (Additive or potentiative effects). Products include:
- Cartrol Tablets ... 410
- Ocupress Ophthalmic Solution, 1% Sterile ... ⊙ 309

Chlorothiazide (Additive or potentiative effects). Products include:
- Aldoclor Tablets ... 1598
- Diupres Tablets ... 1650
- Diuril Oral ... 1653

Chlorothiazide Sodium (Additive or potentiative effects). Products include:
- Diuril Sodium Intravenous ... 1652

Chlorthalidone (Additive or potentiative effects). Products include:
- Combipres Tablets ... 677
- Tenoretic Tablets ... 2845
- Thalitone ... 1245

Clonidine (Additive or potentiative effects). Products include:
- Catapres-TTS ... 675

Clonidine Hydrochloride (Additive or potentiative effects). Products include:
- Catapres Tablets ... 674
- Combipres Tablets ... 677

Codeine Phosphate (May aggravate orthostatic hypotension). Products include:
- Actifed with Codeine Cough Syrup ... 1067
- Brontex ... 1981
- Deconsal C Expectorant Syrup ... 456
- Deconsal Pediatric Syrup ... 457
- Dimetane-DC Cough Syrup ... 2059
- Empirin with Codeine Tablets ... 1093
- Fioricet with Codeine Capsules ... 2260
- Fiorinal with Codeine Capsules ... 2262
- Isoclor Expectorant ... 990
- Novahistine DH ... 2462
- Novahistine Expectorant ... 2463
- Nucofed ... 2051
- Phenergan with Codeine ... 2777
- Phenergan VC with Codeine ... 2781
- Robitussin A-C Syrup ... 2073
- Robitussin-DAC Syrup ... 2074
- Ryna ... ▣ 841
- Soma Compound w/Codeine Tablets ... 2676
- Tussi-Organidin NR Liquid and S NR Liquid ... 2677
- Tylenol with Codeine ... 1583

Cortisone Acetate (Hypokalemia). Products include:
- Cortone Acetate Sterile Suspension ... 1623
- Cortone Acetate Tablets ... 1624

Deserpidine (Potentiation occurs).
- No products indexed under this heading.

Deslanoside (Increased sensitization to effects).
- No products indexed under this heading.

Dexamethasone (Hypokalemia). Products include:
- AK-Trol Ointment & Suspension ... ⊙ 205
- Decadron Elixir ... 1633
- Decadron Tablets ... 1635
- Decaspray Topical Aerosol ... 1648
- Dexacidin Ointment ... ⊙ 263
- Maxitrol Ophthalmic Ointment and Suspension ... ⊙ 224
- TobraDex Ophthalmic Suspension and Ointment ... 473

Dexamethasone Acetate (Hypokalemia). Products include:
- Dalalone D.P. Injectable ... 1011
- Decadron-LA Sterile Suspension ... 1646

Dexamethasone Sodium Phosphate (Hypokalemia). Products include:
- Decadron Phosphate Injection ... 1637
- Decadron Phosphate Respihaler ... 1642
- Decadron Phosphate Sterile Ophthalmic Ointment ... 1641
- Decadron Phosphate Sterile Ophthalmic Solution ... 1642
- Decadron Phosphate Topical Cream ... 1644
- Decadron Phosphate Turbinaire ... 1645
- Decadron Phosphate with Xylocaine Injection, Sterile ... 1639
- Dexacort Phosphate in Respihaler ... 458
- Dexacort Phosphate in Turbinaire ... 459
- NeoDecadron Sterile Ophthalmic Ointment ... 1712
- NeoDecadron Sterile Ophthalmic Solution ... 1713
- NeoDecadron Topical Cream ... 1714

Dezocine (May aggravate orthostatic hypotension). Products include:
- Dalgan Injection ... 538

Diazoxide (Additive or potentiative effects). Products include:
- Hyperstat I.V. Injection ... 2363
- Proglycem ... 580

Digitoxin (Increased sensitization to effects). Products include:
- Crystodigin Tablets ... 1433

Digoxin (Increased sensitization to effects). Products include:
- Lanoxicaps ... 1117
- Lanoxin Elixir Pediatric ... 1120
- Lanoxin Injection ... 1123
- Lanoxin Injection Pediatric ... 1126
- Lanoxin Tablets ... 1128

Diltiazem Hydrochloride (Additive or potentiative effects). Products include:
- Cardizem CD Capsules ... 1506
- Cardizem SR Capsules ... 1510
- Cardizem Injectable ... 1508
- Cardizem Tablets ... 1512
- Dilacor XR Extended-release Capsules ... 2018

Doxazosin Mesylate (Additive or potentiative effects). Products include:
- Cardura Tablets ... 2186

Enalapril Maleate (Additive or potentiative effects). Products include:
- Vaseretic Tablets ... 1765
- Vasotec Tablets ... 1771

Enalaprilat (Additive of potentiative effects). Products include:
- Vasotec I.V. ... 1768

Esmolol Hydrochloride (Additive or potentiative effects). Products include:
- Brevibloc Injection ... 1808

Felodipine (Additive or potentiative effects). Products include:
- Plendil Extended-Release Tablets ... 527

Fentanyl (May aggravate orthostatic hypotension). Products include:
- Duragesic Transdermal System ... 1288

Fentanyl Citrate (May aggravate orthostatic hypotension). Products include:
- Sublimaze Injection ... 1307

Fludrocortisone Acetate (Hypokalemia). Products include:
- Florinef Acetate Tablets ... 505

Fosinopril Sodium (Additive or potentiative effects). Products include:
- Monopril Tablets ... 757

Furosemide (Additive or potentiative effects). Products include:
- Lasix Injection, Oral Solution and Tablets ... 1240

Guanabenz Acetate (Additive or potentiative effects).
- No products indexed under this heading.

Guanethidine Monosulfate (Potentiation occurs). Products include:
- Esimil Tablets ... 822
- Ismelin Tablets ... 827

Hydralazine Hydrochloride (Additive or potentiative effects). Products include:
- Apresazide Capsules ... 808
- Apresoline Hydrochloride Tablets ... 809
- Ser-Ap-Es Tablets ... 849

Hydrocodone Bitartrate (May aggravate orthostatic hypotension). Products include:
- Anexsia 5/500 Elixir ... 1781
- Anexia Tablets ... 1782
- Codiclear DH Syrup ... 791
- Deconamine CX Cough and Cold Liquid and Tablets ... 1319
- Duratuss HD Elixir ... 2565
- Hycodan Tablets and Syrup ... 930
- Hycomine Compound Tablets ... 932
- Hycomine ... 931
- Hycotuss Expectorant Syrup ... 933
- Hydrocet Capsules ... 782
- Lorcet 10/650 ... 1018
- Lortab ... 2566
- Tussend ... 1783
- Tussend Expectorant ... 1785
- Vicodin Tablets ... 1356
- Vicodin ES Tablets ... 1357
- Vicodin Tuss Expectorant ... 1358
- Zydone Capsules ... 949

Hydrocodone Polistirex (May aggravate orthostatic hypotension). Products include:
- Tussionex Pennkinetic Extended-Release Suspension ... 998

Hydrocortisone (Hypokalemia). Products include:
- Anusol-HC Cream 2.5% ... 1896
- Aquanil HC Lotion ... 1931
- Bactine Hydrocortisone Anti-Itch Cream ... ▣ 709
- Caldecort Anti-Itch Hydrocortisone Spray ... ▣ 631
- Cortaid ... ▣ 836
- CORTENEMA ... 2535
- Cortisporin Ointment ... 1085
- Cortisporin Ophthalmic Ointment Sterile ... 1085
- Cortisporin Ophthalmic Suspension Sterile ... 1086
- Cortisporin Otic Solution Sterile ... 1087
- Cortisporin Otic Suspension Sterile ... 1088
- Cortizone-5 ... ▣ 831
- Cortizone-10 ... ▣ 831
- Hydrocortone Tablets ... 1672
- Hytone ... 907
- Massengill Medicated Soft Cloth Towelettes ... 2458
- PediOtic Suspension Sterile ... 1153
- Preparation H Hydrocortisone 1% Cream ... ▣ 872
- ProctoCream-HC 2.5% ... 2408
- VōSoL HC Otic Solution ... 2678

Hydrocortisone Acetate (Hypokalemia). Products include:
- Analpram-HC Rectal Cream 1% and 2.5% ... 977
- Anusol HC-1 Anti-Itch Hydrocortisone Ointment ... ▣ 847
- Anusol-HC Suppositories ... 1897
- Caldecort ... ▣ 631
- Carmol HC ... 924
- Coly-Mycin S Otic w/Neomycin & Hydrocortisone ... 1906
- Cortaid ... ▣ 836
- Cortifoam ... 2396
- Cortisporin Cream ... 1084
- Epifoam ... 2399
- Hydrocortone Acetate Sterile Suspension ... 1669
- Mantadil Cream ... 1135
- Nupercainal Hydrocortisone 1% Cream ... ▣ 645
- Ophthocort ... ⊙ 311
- Pramosone Cream, Lotion & Ointment ... 978
- ProctoCream-HC ... 2408
- ProctoFoam-HC ... 2409
- Terra-Cortril Ophthalmic Suspension ... 2210

Hydrocortisone Sodium Phosphate (Hypokalemia). Products include:
- Hydrocortone Phosphate Injection, Sterile ... 1670

Hydrocortisone Sodium Succinate (Hypokalemia). Products include:
- Solu-Cortef Sterile Powder ... 2641

Hydroflumethiazide (Additive or potentiative effects). Products include:
- Diucardin Tablets ... 2718

Indapamide (Additive or potentiative effects). Products include:
- Lozol Tablets ... 2022

Insulin, Human (Increased or decreased insulin requirements).
- No products indexed under this heading.

Insulin, Human Isophane Suspension (Increased or decreased insulin requirements). Products include:
- Novolin N Human Insulin 10 ml Vials ... 1795

Insulin, Human NPH (Increased or decreased insulin requirements). Products include:
- Humulin N, 100 Units ... 1448
- Novolin N PenFill Cartridges Durable Insulin Delivery System ... 1798
- Novolin N Prefilled Syringe Disposable Insulin Delivery System ... 1798

Insulin, Human Regular (Increased or decreased insulin requirements). Products include:
- Humulin R, 100 Units ... 1449
- Novolin R Human Insulin 10 ml Vials ... 1795
- Novolin R PenFill Cartridges Durable Insulin Delivery System ... 1798
- Novolin R Prefilled Syringe Disposable Insulin Delivery System ... 1798
- Velosulin BR Human Insulin 10 ml Vials ... 1795

Insulin, Human, Zinc Suspension (Increased or decreased insulin requirements). Products include:
- Humulin L, 100 Units ... 1446
- Humulin U, 100 Units ... 1450
- Novolin L Human Insulin 10 ml Vials ... 1795

Insulin, NPH (Increased or decreased insulin requirements). Products include:
- NPH, 100 Units ... 1450
- Pork NPH, 100 Units ... 1452
- Purified Pork NPH Isophane Insulin ... 1801

Insulin, Regular (Increased or decreased insulin requirements). Products include:
- Regular, 100 Units ... 1450
- Pork Regular, 100 Units ... 1452
- Pork Regular (Concentrated), 500 Units ... 1453
- Purified Pork Regular Insulin ... 1801

Insulin, Zinc Crystals (Increased or decreased insulin requirements). Products include:
- NPH, 100 Units ... 1450

Insulin, Zinc Suspension (Increased or decreased insulin requirements). Products include:
- Iletin I ... 1450
- Lente, 100 Units ... 1450
- Iletin II ... 1452
- Pork Lente, 100 Units ... 1452
- Purified Pork Lente Insulin ... 1801

Isradipine (Additive or potentiative effects). Products include:
- DynaCirc Capsules ... 2256

(▣ Described in PDR For Nonprescription Drugs) (⊙ Described in PDR For Ophthalmology)

Labetalol Hydrochloride (Additive or potentiative effects). Products include:
- Normodyne Injection ... 2377
- Normodyne Tablets ... 2379
- Trandate ... 1185

Levorphanol Tartrate (May aggravate orthostatic hypotension). Products include:
- Levo-Dromoran ... 2129

Lisinopril (Additive or potentiative effects). Products include:
- Prinivil Tablets ... 1733
- Prinzide Tablets ... 1737
- Zestoretic ... 2850
- Zestril Tablets ... 2854

Losartan Potassium (Additive or potentiative effects). Products include:
- Cozaar Tablets ... 1628
- Hyzaar Tablets ... 1677

Mecamylamine Hydrochloride (Potentiation occurs). Products include:
- Inversine Tablets ... 1686

Meperidine Hydrochloride (May aggravate orthostatic hypotension). Products include:
- Demerol ... 2308
- Mepergan Injection ... 2753

Mephobarbital (May aggravate orthostatic hypotension). Products include:
- Mebaral Tablets ... 2322

Methadone Hydrochloride (May aggravate orthostatic hypotension). Products include:
- Methadone Hydrochloride Oral Concentrate ... 2233
- Methadone Hydrochloride Oral Solution & Tablets ... 2235

Methyclothiazide (Additive or potentiative effects). Products include:
- Enduron Tablets ... 420

Methyldopa (Additive or potentiative effects). Products include:
- Aldoclor Tablets ... 1598
- Aldomet Oral ... 1600
- Aldoril Tablets ... 1604

Methyldopate Hydrochloride (Additive or potentiated effects). Products include:
- Aldomet Ester HCl Injection ... 1602

Methylprednisolone Acetate (Hypokalemia). Products include:
- Depo-Medrol Single-Dose Vial ... 2600
- Depo-Medrol Sterile Aqueous Suspension ... 2597

Methylprednisolone Sodium Succinate (Hypokalemia). Products include:
- Solu-Medrol Sterile Powder ... 2643

Metolazone (Additive or potentiative effects). Products include:
- Mykrox Tablets ... 993
- Zaroxolyn Tablets ... 1000

Metoprolol Succinate (Additive or potentiative effects). Products include:
- Toprol-XL Tablets ... 565

Metoprolol Tartrate (Additive or potentiative effects). Products include:
- Lopressor Ampuls ... 830
- Lopressor HCT Tablets ... 832
- Lopressor Tablets ... 830

Metyrosine (Additive or potentiative effects). Products include:
- Demser Capsules ... 1649

Minoxidil (Additive or potentiative effects). Products include:
- Loniten Tablets ... 2618
- Rogaine Topical Solution ... 2637

Moexipril Hydrochloride (Additive or potentiative effects). Products include:
- Univasc Tablets ... 2410

Morphine Sulfate (May aggravate orthostatic hypotension). Products include:
- Astramorph/PF Injection, USP (Preservative-Free) ... 535
- Duramorph ... 962
- Infumorph 200 and Infumorph 500 Sterile Solutions ... 965
- MS Contin Tablets ... 1994
- MSIR ... 1997
- Oramorph SR (Morphine Sulfate Sustained Release Tablets) ... 2236
- RMS Suppositories ... 2657
- Roxanol ... 2243

Nadolol (Additive or potentiative effects).
- No products indexed under this heading.

Nicardipine Hydrochloride (Additive or potentiative effects). Products include:
- Cardene Capsules ... 2095
- Cardene I.V. ... 2709
- Cardene SR Capsules ... 2097

Nifedipine (Additive or potentiative effects). Products include:
- Adalat Capsules (10 mg and 20 mg) ... 587
- Adalat CC ... 589
- Procardia Capsules ... 1971
- Procardia XL Extended Release Tablets ... 1972

Nisoldipine (Additive or potentiative effects).
- No products indexed under this heading.

Nitroglycerin (Additive or potentiative effects). Products include:
- Deponit NTG Transdermal Delivery System ... 2397
- Nitro-Bid IV ... 1523
- Nitro-Bid Ointment ... 1524
- Nitrodisc ... 2047
- Nitro-Dur (nitroglycerin) Transdermal Infusion System ... 1326
- Nitrolingual Spray ... 2027
- Nitrostat Tablets ... 1925
- Transderm-Nitro Transdermal Therapeutic System ... 859

Norepinephrine Bitartrate (Decreased arterial responsiveness). Products include:
- Levophed Bitartrate Injection ... 2315

Opium Alkaloids (May aggravate orthostatic hypotension).
- No products indexed under this heading.

Oxycodone Hydrochloride (May aggravate orthostatic hypotension). Products include:
- Percocet Tablets ... 938
- Percodan Tablets ... 939
- Percodan-Demi Tablets ... 940
- Roxicodone Tablets, Oral Solution & Intensol (Oxycodone) ... 2244
- Tylox Capsules ... 1584

Pancuronium Bromide Injection (Decreased serum levels).
- No products indexed under this heading.

Penbutolol Sulfate (Additive or potentiative effects). Products include:
- Levatol ... 2403

Pentobarbital Sodium (May aggravate orthostatic hypotension). Products include:
- Nembutal Sodium Capsules ... 436
- Nembutal Sodium Solution ... 438
- Nembutal Sodium Suppositories ... 440

Phenobarbital (May aggravate orthostatic hypotension). Products include:
- Arco-Lase Plus Tablets ... 512
- Bellergal-S Tablets ... 2250
- Donnatal ... 2060
- Donnatal Extentabs ... 2061
- Donnatal Tablets ... 2060
- Phenobarbital Elixir and Tablets ... 1469
- Quadrinal Tablets ... 1350

Phenoxybenzamine Hydrochloride (Additive or potentiative effects). Products include:
- Dibenzyline Capsules ... 2476

Phentolamine Mesylate (Additive or potentiative effects). Products include:
- Regitine ... 846

Pindolol (Additive or potentiative effects). Products include:
- Visken Tablets ... 2299

Polythiazide (Additive or potentiative effects). Products include:
- Minizide Capsules ... 1938

Prazosin Hydrochloride (Potentiation occurs). Products include:
- Minipress Capsules ... 1937
- Minizide Capsules ... 1938

Prednisolone Acetate (Hypokalemia). Products include:
- AK-CIDE ... ⊙ 202
- AK-CIDE Ointment ... ⊙ 202
- Blephamide Liquifilm Sterile Ophthalmic Suspension ... 476
- Blephamide Ointment ... ⊙ 237
- Econopred & Econopred Plus Ophthalmic Suspensions ... ⊙ 217
- Poly-Pred Liquifilm ... ⊙ 248
- Pred Forte ... ⊙ 250
- Pred Mild ... ⊙ 253
- Pred-G Liquifilm Sterile Ophthalmic Suspension ... ⊙ 251
- Pred-G S.O.P. Sterile Ophthalmic Ointment ... ⊙ 252
- Vasocidin Ointment ... ⊙ 268

Prednisolone Sodium Phosphate (Hypokalemia). Products include:
- AK-Pred ... ⊙ 204
- Hydeltrasol Injection, Sterile ... 1665
- Inflamase ... ⊙ 265
- Pediapred Oral Liquid ... 995
- Vasocidin Ophthalmic Solution ... ⊙ 270

Prednisolone Tebutate (Hypokalemia). Products include:
- Hydeltra-T.B.A. Sterile Suspension 1667

Prednisone (Hypokalemia). Products include:
- Deltasone Tablets ... 2595

Propoxyphene Hydrochloride (May aggravate orthostatic hypotension). Products include:
- Darvon ... 1435
- Wygesic Tablets ... 2827

Propoxyphene Napsylate (May aggravate orthostatic hypotension). Products include:
- Darvon-N/Darvocet-N ... 1433

Propranolol Hydrochloride (Additive or potentiative effects). Products include:
- Inderal ... 2728
- Inderal LA Long Acting Capsules ... 2730
- Inderide Tablets ... 2732
- Inderide LA Long Acting Capsules .. 2734

Quinapril Hydrochloride (Additive or potentiative effects). Products include:
- Accupril Tablets ... 1893

Ramipril (Additive or potentiative effects). Products include:
- Altace Capsules ... 1232

Rauwolfia Serpentina (Potentiation occurs).
- No products indexed under this heading.

Rescinnamine (Potentiation occurs).
- No products indexed under this heading.

Reserpine (Potentiation occurs). Products include:
- Diupres Tablets ... 1650
- Hydropres Tablets ... 1675
- Ser-Ap-Es Tablets ... 849

Secobarbital Sodium (May aggravate orthostatic hypotension). Products include:
- Seconal Sodium Pulvules ... 1474

Sodium Nitroprusside (Additive or potentiative effects).
- No products indexed under this heading.

Sotalol Hydrochloride (Additive or potentiative effects). Products include:
- Betapace Tablets ... 641

Spirapril Hydrochloride (Additive or potentiative effects).
- No products indexed under this heading.

Sufentanil Citrate (May aggravate orthostatic hypotension). Products include:
- Sufenta Injection ... 1309

Terazosin Hydrochloride (Additive or potentiative effects). Products include:
- Hytrin Capsules ... 430

Thiamylal Sodium (May aggravate orthostatic hypotension).
- No products indexed under this heading.

Timolol Maleate (Additive or potentiative effects). Products include:
- Blocadren Tablets ... 1614
- Timolide Tablets ... 1748
- Timoptic in Ocudose ... 1753
- Timoptic Sterile Ophthalmic Solution ... 1751
- Timoptic-XE ... 1755

Torsemide (Additive or potentiative effects). Products include:
- Demadex Tablets and Injection ... 686

Triamcinolone (Hypokalemia). Products include:
- Aristocort Tablets ... 1022

Triamcinolone Acetonide (Hypokalemia). Products include:
- Aristocort A 0.025% Cream ... 1027
- Aristocort A 0.5% Cream ... 1031
- Aristocort A 0.1% Cream ... 1029
- Aristocort A 0.1% Ointment ... 1030
- Azmacort Oral Inhaler ... 2011
- Nasacort Nasal Inhaler ... 2024

Triamcinolone Diacetate (Hypokalemia). Products include:
- Aristocort Suspension (Forte Parenteral) ... 1027
- Aristocort Suspension (Intralesional) ... 1025

Triamcinolone Hexacetonide (Hypokalemia). Products include:
- Aristospan Suspension (Intra-articular) ... 1033
- Aristospan Suspension (Intralesional) ... 1032

Trimethaphan Camsylate (Potentiation occurs). Products include:
- Arfonad Ampuls ... 2080

Tubocurarine Chloride (Increased responsiveness).
- No products indexed under this heading.

Verapamil Hydrochloride (Additive or potentiative effects). Products include:
- Calan SR Caplets ... 2422
- Calan Tablets ... 2419
- Isoptin Injectable ... 1344
- Isoptin Oral Tablets ... 1346
- Isoptin SR Tablets ... 1348
- Verelan Capsules ... 1410
- Verelan Capsules ... 2824

Food Interactions

Alcohol (May aggravate orthostatic hypotension).

ORETON METHYL
(Methyltestosterone) ... 1255
May interact with oral anticoagulants, insulin, and certain other

IMPORTANT NOTE: Always consult each drug listing in the patient's regimen for possible interactions.

Oreton | Interactions Index | 764

agents. Compounds in these categories include:

Dicumarol (Decreased anticoagulant requirements).
No products indexed under this heading.

Insulin, Human (Androgens may decrease blood glucose and insulin requirements in diabetics).
No products indexed under this heading.

Insulin, Human Isophane Suspension (Androgens may decrease blood glucose and insulin requirements in diabetics). Products include:
Novolin N Human Insulin 10 ml Vials 1795

Insulin, Human NPH (Androgens may decrease blood glucose and insulin requirements in diabetics). Products include:
Humulin N, 100 Units 1448
Novolin N PenFill Cartridges Durable Insulin Delivery System 1798
Novolin N Prefilled Syringe Disposable Insulin Delivery System 1798

Insulin, Human Regular (Androgens may decrease blood glucose and insulin requirements in diabetics). Products include:
Humulin R, 100 Units 1449
Novolin R Human Insulin 10 ml Vials 1795
Novolin R PenFill Cartridges Durable Insulin Delivery System 1798
Novolin R Prefilled Syringe Disposable Insulin Delivery System 1798
Velosulin BR Human Insulin 10 ml Vials 1795

Insulin, Human, Zinc Suspension (Androgens may decrease blood glucose and insulin requirements in diabetics). Products include:
Humulin L, 100 Units 1446
Humulin U, 100 Units 1450
Novolin L Human Insulin 10 ml Vials 1795

Insulin, NPH (Androgens may decrease blood glucose and insulin requirements in diabetics). Products include:
NPH, 100 Units 1450
Pork NPH, 100 Units 1452
Purified Pork NPH Isophane Insulin 1801

Insulin, Regular (Androgens may decrease blood glucose and insulin requirements in diabetics). Products include:
Regular, 100 Units 1450
Pork Regular, 100 Units 1452
Pork Regular (Concentrated), 500 Units 1453
Purified Pork Regular Insulin 1801

Insulin, Zinc Crystals (Androgens may decrease blood glucose and insulin requirements in diabetics). Products include:
NPH, 100 Units 1450

Insulin, Zinc Suspension (Androgens may decrease blood glucose and insulin requirements in diabetics). Products include:
Iletin I 1450
Lente, 100 Units 1450
Iletin II 1452
Pork Lente, 100 Units 1452
Purified Pork Lente Insulin 1801

Oxyphenbutazone (Co-administration may result in elevated serum levels of oxyphenbutazone).

Warfarin Sodium (Decreased anticoagulant requirements). Products include:
Coumadin 926

ORGANIDIN NR TABLETS AND LIQUID
(Guaifenesin) 2672
None cited in PDR database.

ORIMUNE
(Poliovirus Vaccine, Live, Oral, Trivalent, Types 1,2,3 (Sabin)) 1388
May interact with antineoplastics and corticosteroids. Compounds in these categories include:

Altretamine (Contraindicated). Products include:
Hexalen Capsules 2571

Asparaginase (Contraindicated). Products include:
Elspar 1659

Betamethasone Acetate (Contraindicated). Products include:
Celestone Soluspan Suspension 2347

Betamethasone Sodium Phosphate (Contraindicated). Products include:
Celestone Soluspan Suspension 2347

Bleomycin Sulfate (Contraindicated). Products include:
Blenoxane 692

Busulfan (Contraindicated). Products include:
Myleran Tablets 1143

Carboplatin (Contraindicated). Products include:
Paraplatin for Injection 705

Carmustine (BCNU) (Contraindicated). Products include:
BiCNU 691

Chlorambucil (Contraindicated). Products include:
Leukeran Tablets 1133

Cisplatin (Contraindicated). Products include:
Platinol 708
Platinol-AQ Injection 710

Cortisone Acetate (Contraindicated). Products include:
Cortone Acetate Sterile Suspension 1623
Cortone Acetate Tablets 1624

Cyclophosphamide (Contraindicated). Products include:
Cytoxan 694
NEOSAR Lyophilized/Neosar 1959

Dacarbazine (Contraindicated). Products include:
DTIC-Dome 600

Daunorubicin Hydrochloride (Contraindicated). Products include:
Cerubidine 795

Dexamethasone (Contraindicated). Products include:
AK-Trol Ointment & Suspension .... ⊙ 205
Decadron Elixir 1633
Decadron Tablets 1635
Decaspray Topical Aerosol 1648
Dexacidin Ointment .... ⊙ 263
Maxitrol Ophthalmic Ointment and Suspension .... ⊙ 224
TobraDex Ophthalmic Suspension and Ointment 473

Dexamethasone Acetate (Contraindicated). Products include:
Dalalone D.P. Injectable 1011
Decadron-LA Sterile Suspension 1646

Dexamethasone Sodium Phosphate (Contraindicated). Products include:
Decadron Phosphate Injection 1637
Decadron Phosphate Respihaler 1642
Decadron Phosphate Sterile Ophthalmic Ointment 1641
Decadron Phosphate Sterile Ophthalmic Solution 1642
Decadron Phosphate Topical Cream 1644
Decadron Phosphate Turbinaire 1645
Decadron Phosphate with Xylocaine Injection, Sterile 1639
Dexacort Phosphate in Respihaler .. 458
Dexacort Phosphate in Turbinaire .. 459

NeoDecadron Sterile Ophthalmic Ointment 1712
NeoDecadron Sterile Ophthalmic Solution 1713
NeoDecadron Topical Cream 1714

Doxorubicin Hydrochloride (Contraindicated). Products include:
Adriamycin PFS 1947
Adriamycin RDF 1947
Doxorubicin Astra 540
Rubex 712

Estramustine Phosphate Sodium (Contraindicated). Products include:
Emcyt Capsules 1953

Etoposide (Contraindicated). Products include:
VePesid Capsules and Injection 718

Floxuridine (Contraindicated). Products include:
Sterile FUDR 2118

Fludrocortisone Acetate (Contraindicated). Products include:
Florinef Acetate Tablets 505

Fluorouracil (Contraindicated). Products include:
Efudex 2113
Fluoroplex Topical Solution & Cream 1% 479
Fluorouracil Injection 2116

Flutamide (Contraindicated). Products include:
Eulexin Capsules 2358

Hydrocortisone (Contraindicated). Products include:
Anusol-HC Cream 2.5% 1896
Aquanil HC Lotion 1931
Bactine Hydrocortisone Anti-Itch Cream .... ▣ 709
Caldecort Anti-Itch Hydrocortisone Spray .... ▣ 631
Cortaid .... ▣ 836
CORTENEMA 2535
Cortisporin Ointment 1085
Cortisporin Ophthalmic Ointment Sterile 1085
Cortisporin Ophthalmic Suspension Sterile 1086
Cortisporin Otic Solution Sterile 1087
Cortisporin Otic Suspension Sterile 1088
Cortizone-5 .... ▣ 831
Cortizone-10 .... ▣ 831
Hydrocortone Tablets 1672
Hytone 907
Massengill Medicated Soft Cloth Towelettes 2458
PediOtic Suspension Sterile 1153
Preparation H Hydrocortisone 1% Cream .... ▣ 872
ProctoCream-HC 2.5% 2408
VōSoL HC Otic Solution 2678

Hydrocortisone Acetate (Contraindicated). Products include:
Analpram-HC Rectal Cream 1% and 2.5% 977
Anusol HC-1 Anti-Itch Hydrocortisone Ointment .... ▣ 847
Anusol-HC Suppositories 1897
Caldecort .... ▣ 631
Carmol HC 924
Coly-Mycin S Otic w/Neomycin & Hydrocortisone 1906
Cortaid .... ▣ 836
Cortifoam 2396
Cortisporin Cream 1084
Epifoam 2399
Hydrocortone Acetate Sterile Suspension 1669
Mantadil Cream 1135
Nupercainal Hydrocortisone 1% Cream .... ▣ 645
Ophthocort .... ⊙ 311
Pramosone Cream, Lotion & Ointment 978
ProctoCream-HC 2408
ProctoFoam-HC 2409
Terra-Cortril Ophthalmic Suspension 2210

Hydrocortisone Sodium Phosphate (Contraindicated). Products include:
Hydrocortone Phosphate Injection, Sterile 1670

Hydrocortisone Sodium Succinate (Contraindicated). Products include:
Solu-Cortef Sterile Powder 2641

Hydroxyurea (Contraindicated). Products include:
Hydrea Capsules 696

Idarubicin Hydrochloride (Contraindicated). Products include:
Idamycin 1955

Ifosfamide (Contraindicated). Products include:
IFEX 697

Interferon alfa-2A, Recombinant (Contraindicated). Products include:
Roferon-A Injection 2145

Interferon alfa-2B, Recombinant (Contraindicated). Products include:
Intron A 2364

Levamisole Hydrochloride (Contraindicated). Products include:
Ergamisol Tablets 1292

Lomustine (CCNU) (Contraindicated). Products include:
CeeNU 693

Mechlorethamine Hydrochloride (Contraindicated). Products include:
Mustargen 1709

Megestrol Acetate (Contraindicated). Products include:
Megace Oral Suspension 699
Megace Tablets 701

Melphalan (Contraindicated). Products include:
Alkeran Tablets 1071

Mercaptopurine (Contraindicated). Products include:
Purinethol Tablets 1156

Methotrexate Sodium (Contraindicated). Products include:
Methotrexate Sodium Tablets, Injection, for Injection and LPF Injection 1275

Methylprednisolone Acetate (Contraindicated). Products include:
Depo-Medrol Single-Dose Vial 2600
Depo-Medrol Sterile Aqueous Suspension 2597

Methylprednisolone Sodium Succinate (Contraindicated). Products include:
Solu-Medrol Sterile Powder 2643

Mitomycin (Mitomycin-C) (Contraindicated). Products include:
Mutamycin 703

Mitotane (Contraindicated). Products include:
Lysodren 698

Mitoxantrone Hydrochloride (Contraindicated). Products include:
Novantrone 1279

Paclitaxel (Contraindicated). Products include:
Taxol 714

Prednisolone Acetate (Contraindicated). Products include:
AK-CIDE .... ⊙ 202
AK-CIDE Ointment .... ⊙ 202
Blephamide Liquifilm Sterile Ophthalmic Suspension 476
Blephamide Ointment .... ⊙ 237
Econopred & Econopred Plus Ophthalmic Suspensions .... ⊙ 217
Poly-Pred Liquifilm .... ⊙ 248
Pred Forte .... ⊙ 250
Pred Mild .... ⊙ 253
Pred-G Liquifilm Sterile Ophthalmic Suspension .... ⊙ 251
Pred-G S.O.P. Sterile Ophthalmic Ointment .... ⊙ 252
Vasocidin Ointment .... ⊙ 268

Prednisolone Sodium Phosphate (Contraindicated). Products include:
AK-Pred .... ⊙ 204
Hydeltrasol Injection, Sterile 1665

(▣ Described in PDR For Nonprescription Drugs) (⊙ Described in PDR For Ophthalmology)

Interactions Index

Orlamm

Inflamase .... © 265
Pediapred Oral Liquid 995
Vasocidin Ophthalmic Solution ...... © 270

Prednisolone Tebutate (Contraindicated). Products include:

Hydeltra-T.B.A. Sterile Suspension 1667

Prednisone (Contraindicated). Products include:

Deltasone Tablets 2595

Procarbazine Hydrochloride (Contraindicated). Products include:

Matulane Capsules 2131

Streptozocin (Contraindicated). Products include:

Zanosar Sterile Powder 2653

Tamoxifen Citrate (Contraindicated). Products include:

Nolvadex Tablets 2841

Teniposide (Contraindicated). Products include:

Vumon 727

Thioguanine (Contraindicated). Products include:

Thioguanine Tablets, Tabloid Brand 1181

Thiotepa (Contraindicated). Products include:

Thioplex (Thiotepa For Injection) 1281

Triamcinolone (Contraindicated). Products include:

Aristocort Tablets 1022

Triamcinolone Acetonide (Contraindicated). Products include:

Aristocort A 0.025% Cream 1027
Aristocort A 0.5% Cream 1031
Aristocort A 0.1% Cream 1029
Aristocort A 0.1% Ointment 1030
Azmacort Oral Inhaler 2011
Nasacort Nasal Inhaler 2024

Triamcinolone Diacetate (Contraindicated). Products include:

Aristocort Suspension (Forte Parenteral) 1027
Aristocort Suspension (Intralesional) 1025

Triamcinolone Hexacetonide (Contraindicated). Products include:

Aristospan Suspension (Intra-articular) 1033
Aristospan Suspension (Intralesional) 1032

Vincristine Sulfate (Contraindicated). Products include:

Oncovin Solution Vials & Hyporets 1466

Vinorelbine Tartrate (Contraindicated). Products include:

Navelbine Injection 1145

ORLAMM

(Levomethadyl Acetate Hydrochloride) 2239

May interact with mixed agonist/antagonist opioid analgesics, hypnotics and sedatives, narcotic analgesics, antihistamines, benzodiazepines, tranquilizers, phenothiazines, antidepressant drugs, central nervous system depressants, and certain other agents. Compounds in these categories include:

Acrivastine (Potential for serious side effects, including respiratory depression, hypotension, profound sedation and coma, if used concurrently). Products include:

Semprex-D Capsules 463
Semprex-D Capsules 1167

Alfentanil Hydrochloride (Potential for serious side effects, including respiratory depression, hypotension, profound sedation and coma, if used concurrently). Products include:

Alfenta Injection 1286

Alprazolam (Potential for serious side effects, including respiratory depression, hypotension, profound sedation and coma, if used concurrently). Products include:

Xanax Tablets 2649

Amitriptyline Hydrochloride (Potential for serious side effects, including respiratory depression, hypotension, profound sedation and coma, if used concurrently). Products include:

Elavil 2838
Endep Tablets 2174
Etrafon 2355
Limbitrol 2180
Triavil Tablets 1757

Amoxapine (Potential for serious side effects, including respiratory depression, hypotension, profound sedation and coma, if used concurrently). Products include:

Asendin Tablets 1369

Aprobarbital (Potential for serious side effects, including respiratory depression, hypotension, profound sedation and coma, if used concurrently).

No products indexed under this heading.

Astemizole (Potential for serious side effects, including respiratory depression, hypotension, profound sedation and coma, if used concurrently). Products include:

Hismanal Tablets 1293

Azatadine Maleate (Potential for serious side effects, including respiratory depression, hypotension, profound sedation and coma, if used concurrently). Products include:

Trinalin Repetabs Tablets 1330

Bromodiphenhydramine Hydrochloride (Potential for serious side effects, including respiratory depression, hypotension, profound sedation and coma, if used concurrently).

No products indexed under this heading.

Brompheniramine Maleate (Potential for serious side effects, including respiratory depression, hypotension, profound sedation and coma, if used concurrently). Products include:

Alka Seltzer Plus Sinus Medicine ..⊞ 707
Bromfed Capsules (Extended-Release) 1785
Bromfed Syrup .... ⊞ 733
Bromfed Tablets 1785
Bromfed-DM Cough Syrup.................. 1786
Bromfed-PD Capsules (Extended-Release) 1785
Dimetane-DC Cough Syrup 2059
Dimetane-DX Cough Syrup 2059
Dimetapp Elixir .... ⊞ 773
Dimetapp Extentabs .... ⊞ 774
Dimetapp Tablets/Liqui-Gels .... ⊞ 775
Dimetapp Cold & Allergy Chewable Tablets .... ⊞ 773
Dimetapp DM Elixir .... ⊞ 774
Vicks DayQuil Allergy Relief 12-Hour Extended Release Tablets.. ⊞ 760
Vicks DayQuil Allergy Relief 4-Hour Tablets .... ⊞ 760

Buprenorphine (Potential for serious side effects, including respiratory depression, hypotension, profound sedation and coma, if used concurrently; patients maintained on levomethadyl acetate hydrochloride may experience withdrawal symptoms when administered mixed agonists/antagonists). Products include:

Buprenex Injectable 2006

Bupropion Hydrochloride (Potential for serious side effects, including respiratory depression, hypotension, profound sedation and coma, if used concurrently). Products include:

Wellbutrin Tablets 1204

Buspirone Hydrochloride (Potential for serious side effects, including respiratory depression, hypotension, profound sedation and coma, if used concurrently). Products include:

BuSpar 737

Butabarbital (Potential for serious side effects, including respiratory depression, hypotension, profound sedation and coma, if used concurrently).

No products indexed under this heading.

Butalbital (Potential for serious side effects, including respiratory depression, hypotension, profound sedation and coma, if used concurrently). Products include:

Esgic-plus Tablets 1013
Fioricet Tablets 2258
Fioricet with Codeine Capsules 2260
Fiorinal Capsules 2261
Fiorinal with Codeine Capsules 2262
Fiorinal Tablets 2261
Phrenilin 785
Sedapap Tablets 50 mg/650 mg .. 1543

Butorphanol Tartrate (Patients maintained on levomethadyl acetate hydrochloride may experience withdrawal symptoms when administered mixed agonists/antagonists). Products include:

Stadol 775

Carbamazepine (May increase levomethadyl acetate hydrochloride's peak activity and/or shorten its duration of action). Products include:

Atretol Tablets 573
Tegretol Chewable Tablets 852
Tegretol Suspension 852
Tegretol Tablets 852

Chlordiazepoxide (Potential for serious side effects, including respiratory depression, hypotension, profound sedation and coma, if used concurrently). Products include:

Libritabs Tablets 2177
Limbitrol 2180

Chlordiazepoxide Hydrochloride (Potential for serious side effects, including respiratory depression, hypotension, profound sedation and coma, if used concurrently). Products include:

Librax Capsules 2176
Librium Capsules 2178
Librium Injectable 2179

Chlorpheniramine Maleate (Potential for serious side effects, including respiratory depression, hypotension, profound sedation and coma, if used concurrently). Products include:

Alka-Seltzer Plus Cold Medicine .... ⊞ 705
Alka-Seltzer Plus Cold Medicine Liqui-Gels .... ⊞ 706
Alka-Seltzer Plus Cold & Cough Medicine .... ⊞ 708
Alka-Seltzer Plus Cold & Cough Medicine Liqui-Gels .... ⊞ 705
Allerest Children's Chewable Tablets .... ⊞ 627
Allerest Headache Strength Tablets .... ⊞ 627
Allerest Maximum Strength Tablets .... ⊞ 627
Allerest Sinus Pain Formula .... ⊞ 627
Allerest 12 Hour Caplets .... ⊞ 627
Ana-Kit Anaphylaxis Emergency Treatment Kit 617
Atrohist Pediatric Capsules 453
Atrohist Plus Tablets 454
BC Cold Powder Multi-Symptom Formula (Cold-Sinus-Allergy) ...... ⊞ 609
Cerose DM .... ⊞ 878
Cheracol Plus Head Cold/Cough Formula .... ⊞ 769
Children's Vicks DayQuil Allergy Relief .... ⊞ 757
Children's Vicks NyQuil Cold/Cough Relief .... ⊞ 758
Chlor-Trimeton Allergy Decongestant Tablets .... ⊞ 799
Chlor-Trimeton Allergy Tablets ...... ⊞ 798
Comhist 2038
Comtrex Multi-Symptom Cold Reliever Tablets/Caplets/Liqui-Gels/Liquid .... ⊞ 615
Allergy-Sinus Comtrex Multi-Symptom Allergy-Sinus Formula Tablets .... ⊞ 617
Contac Continuous Action Nasal Decongestant/Antihistamine 12 Hour Capsules .... ⊞ 813
Contac Maximum Strength Continuous Action Decongestant/Antihistamine 12 Hour Caplets.. ⊞ 813
Contac Severe Cold and Flu Formula Caplets .... ⊞ 814
Coricidin 'D' Decongestant Tablets .... ⊞ 800
Coricidin Tablets .... ⊞ 800
D.A. Chewable Tablets 951
Deconamine 1320
Dura-Tap/PD Capsules 2867
Dura-Vent/DA Tablets 953
Extendryl 1005
Fedahist Gyrocaps 2401
Fedahist Timecaps 2401
Hycomine Compound Tablets 932
Isoclor Timesule Capsules .... ⊞ 637
Kronofed-A 977
Nolamine Timed-Release Tablets 785
Novahistine DH 2462
Novahistine Elixir .... ⊞ 823
Ornade Spansule Capsules 2502
PediaCare Cold Allergy Chewable Tablets .... ⊞ 677
PediaCare Cough-Cold Chewable Tablets 1553
PediaCare Cough-Cold Liquid 1553
PediaCare NightRest Cough-Cold Liquid 1553
Pediatric Vicks 44m Cough & Cold Relief .... ⊞ 764
Pyrroxate Caplets .... ⊞ 772
Ryna .... ⊞ 841
Sinarest Tablets .... ⊞ 648
Sinarest Extra Strength Tablets ...... ⊞ 648
Sine-Off Sinus Medicine .... ⊞ 825
Singlet Tablets .... ⊞ 825
Sinulin Tablets 787
Sinutab Sinus Allergy Medication, Maximum Strength Tablets and Caplets .... ⊞ 860
Sudafed Plus Liquid .... ⊞ 862
Sudafed Plus Tablets .... ⊞ 863
Teldrin 12 Hour Antihistamine/Nasal Decongestant Allergy Relief Capsules .... ⊞ 826
TheraFlu .... ⊞ 787
TheraFlu Maximum Strength Nighttime Flu, Cold & Cough Medicine .... ⊞ 788
Triaminic Allergy Tablets .... ⊞ 789
Triaminic Cold Tablets .... ⊞ 790
Triaminic Nite Light .... ⊞ 791
Triaminic Syrup .... ⊞ 792
Triaminic-12 Tablets .... ⊞ 792
Triaminicin Tablets .... ⊞ 793
Triaminicol Multi-Symptom Cold Tablets .... ⊞ 793
Triaminicol Multi-Symptom Relief ⊞ 794
Tussend 1783
Children's TYLENOL Cold Multi-Symptom Liquid Formula and Chewable Tablets 1561
Children's TYLENOL Cold Plus Cough Multi Symptom Tablets and Liquid .... ⊞ 681
TYLENOL Maximum Strength Allergy Sinus Medication Gelcaps and Caplets 1563
TYLENOL Cold Multi-Symptom Formula Medication Tablets and Caplets 1561
TYLENOL Cold Multi-Symptom Hot Medication Liquid Packets 1557
Vicks 44 LiquiCaps Cough, Cold & Flu Relief .... ⊞ 755
Vicks 44M Cough, Cold & Flu Relief .... ⊞ 756

Chlorpheniramine Polistirex (Potential for serious side effects, including respiratory depression, hypotension, profound sedation and coma, if used concurrently). Products include:

Tussionex Pennkinetic Extended-Release Suspension 998

IMPORTANT NOTE: Always consult each drug listing in the patient's regimen for possible interactions.

Chlorpheniramine Tannate (Potential for serious side effects, including respiratory depression, hypotension, profound sedation and coma, if used concurrently). Products include:
- Atrohist Pediatric Suspension ... 454
- Ricobid Tablets and Pediatric Suspension ... 2038
- Rynatan ... 2673
- Rynatuss ... 2673

Chlorpromazine (Potential for serious side effects, including respiratory depression, hypotension, profound sedation and coma, if used concurrently). Products include:
- Thorazine Suppositories ... 2523

Chlorpromazine Hydrochloride (Potential for serious side effects, including respiratory depression, hypotension, profound sedation and coma, if used concurrently). Products include:
- Thorazine ... 2523

Chlorprothixene (Potential for serious side effects, including respiratory depression, hypotension, profound sedation and coma, if used concurrently).
- No products indexed under this heading.

Chlorprothixene Hydrochloride (Potential for serious side effects, including respiratory depression, hypotension, profound sedation and coma, if used concurrently).
- No products indexed under this heading.

Cimetidine (May slow the onset, lower the activity and/or increase the duration of action of levomethadyl acetate hydrochloride). Products include:
- Tagamet Tablets ... 2516

Cimetidine Hydrochloride (May slow the onset, lower the activity and/or increase the duration of action of levomethadyl acetate hydrochloride). Products include:
- Tagamet ... 2516

Clemastine Fumarate (Potential for serious side effects, including respiratory depression, hypotension, profound sedation and coma, if used concurrently). Products include:
- Tavist Syrup ... 2297
- Tavist Tablets ... 2298
- Tavist-1 12 Hour Relief Tablets ... ▣ 787
- Tavist-D 12 Hour Relief Tablets ... ▣ 787

Clorazepate Dipotassium (Potential for serious side effects, including respiratory depression, hypotension, profound sedation and coma, if used concurrently). Products include:
- Tranxene ... 451

Clozapine (Potential for serious side effects, including respiratory depression, hypotension, profound sedation and coma, if used concurrently). Products include:
- Clozaril Tablets ... 2252

Codeine Phosphate (Potential for serious side effects, including respiratory depression, hypotension, profound sedation and coma, if used concurrently). Products include:
- Actifed with Codeine Cough Syrup.. 1067
- Brontex ... 1981
- Deconsal C Expectorant Syrup ... 456
- Deconsal Pediatric Syrup ... 457
- Dimetane-DC Cough Syrup ... 2059
- Empirin with Codeine Tablets ... 1093
- Fioricet with Codeine Capsules ... 2260
- Fiorinal with Codeine Capsules ... 2262
- Isoclor Expectorant ... 990
- Novahistine DH ... 2462
- Novahistine Expectorant ... 2463
- Nucofed ... 2051
- Phenergan with Codeine ... 2777
- Phenergan VC with Codeine ... 2781
- Robitussin A-C Syrup ... 2073
- Robitussin-DAC Syrup ... 2074
- Ryna ... ▣ 841
- Soma Compound w/Codeine Tablets ... 2676
- Tussi-Organidin NR Liquid and S NR Liquid ... 2677
- Tylenol with Codeine ... 1583

Cyproheptadine Hydrochloride (Potential for serious side effects, including respiratory depression, hypotension, profound sedation and coma, if used concurrently). Products include:
- Periactin ... 1724

Desflurane (Potential for serious side effects, including respiratory depression, hypotension, profound sedation and coma, if used concurrently). Products include:
- Suprane ... 1813

Desipramine Hydrochloride (Potential for serious side effects, including respiratory depression, hypotension, profound sedation and coma, if used concurrently). Products include:
- Norpramin Tablets ... 1526

Dexchlorpheniramine Maleate (Potential for serious side effects, including respiratory depression, hypotension, profound sedation and coma, if used concurrently).
- No products indexed under this heading.

Dezocine (Potential for serious side effects, including respiratory depression, hypotension, profound sedation and coma, if used concurrently). Products include:
- Dalgan Injection ... 538

Diazepam (Potential for serious side effects, including respiratory depression, hypotension, profound sedation and coma, if used concurrently). Products include:
- Dizac ... 1809
- Valium Injectable ... 2182
- Valium Tablets ... 2183
- Valrelease Capsules ... 2169

Diphenhydramine Citrate (Potential for serious side effects, including respiratory depression, hypotension, profound sedation and coma, if used concurrently). Products include:
- Excedrin P.M. Analgesic/Sleeping Aid Tablets, Caplets, Liquigels ... 733

Diphenhydramine Hydrochloride (Potential for serious side effects, including respiratory depression, hypotension, profound sedation and coma, if used concurrently). Products include:
- Actifed Allergy Daytime/Nighttime Caplets ... ▣ 844
- Actifed Sinus Daytime/Nighttime Tablets and Caplets ... ▣ 846
- Arthritis Foundation NightTime Caplets ... ▣ 674
- Extra Strength Bayer PM Aspirin .. ▣ 713
- Bayer Select Night Time Pain Relief Formula ... ▣ 716
- Benadryl Allergy Decongestant Liquid Medication ... ▣ 848
- Benadryl Allergy Decongestant Tablets ... ▣ 848
- Benadryl Allergy Liquid Medication ... ▣ 849
- Benadryl Allergy ... ▣ 848
- Benadryl Allergy Sinus Headache Formula Caplets ... ▣ 849
- Benadryl Capsules ... 1898
- Benadryl Dye-Free Allergy Liquigel Softgels ... ▣ 850
- Benadryl Dye-Free Allergy Liquid Medication ... ▣ 850
- Benadryl Itch Relief Cream, Children's Formula and Maximum Strength 2% ... ▣ 851
- Benadryl Itch Relief Spray, Children's Formula and Maximum Strength 2% ... ▣ 851
- Benadryl Itch Relief Stick Maximum Strength 2% ... ▣ 850
- Benadryl Itch Stopping Gel, Children's Formula and Maximum Strength 2% ... ▣ 851
- Benadryl Kapseals ... 1898
- Benadryl Injection ... 1898
- Contac Day & Night Cold/Flu Night Caplets ... ▣ 812
- Contac Night Allergy/Sinus Caplets ... ▣ 812
- Extra Strength Doan's P.M. ... ▣ 633
- Legatrin PM ... ▣ 651
- Miles Nervine Nighttime Sleep-Aid ▣ 723
- Nytol QuickCaps Caplets ... ▣ 610
- Sleepinal Night-time Sleep Aid Capsules and Softgels ... ▣ 834
- TYLENOL Maximum Strength Allergy Sinus NightTime Medication Caplets ... 1555
- TYLENOL Flu NightTime, Maximum Strength, Gelcaps ... 1566
- TYLENOL Maximum Strength Flu NightTime Hot Medication Packets ... 1562
- TYLENOL PM, Extra Strength Pain Reliever/Sleep Aid Caplets, Geltabs, Gelcaps ... 1560
- TYLENOL Severe Allergy Medication Caplets ... 1564
- Maximum Strength Unisom Sleepgels ... 1934
- Unisom With Pain Relief-Nighttime Sleep Aid and Pain Reliever ... 1934

Diphenylpyraline Hydrochloride (Potential for serious side effects, including respiratory depression, hypotension, profound sedation and coma, if used concurrently).
- No products indexed under this heading.

Doxepin Hydrochloride (Potential for serious side effects, including respiratory depression, hypotension, profound sedation and coma, if used concurrently). Products include:
- Sinequan ... 2205
- Zonalon Cream ... 1055

Droperidol (Potential for serious side effects, including respiratory depression, hypotension, profound sedation and coma, if used concurrently). Products include:
- Inapsine Injection ... 1296

Enflurane (Potential for serious side effects, including respiratory depression, hypotension, profound sedation and coma, if used concurrently).
- No products indexed under this heading.

Erythromycin (May slow the onset, lower the activity and/or increase the duration of action of levomethadyl acetate hydrochloride). Products include:
- A/T/S 2% Acne Topical Gel and Solution ... 1234
- Benzamycin Topical Gel ... 905
- E-Mycin Tablets ... 1341
- Emgel 2% Topical Gel ... 1093
- ERYC ... 1915
- Erycette (erythromycin 2%) Topical Solution ... 1888
- Ery-Tab Tablets ... 422
- Erythromycin Base Filmtab ... 426
- Erythromycin Delayed-Release Capsules, USP ... 427
- Ilotycin Ophthalmic Ointment ... 912
- PCE Dispertab Tablets ... 444
- T-Stat 2.0% Topical Solution and Pads ... 2688
- Theramycin Z Topical Solution 2% 1592

Erythromycin Estolate (May slow the onset, lower the activity and/or increase the duration of action of levomethadyl acetate hydrochloride). Products include:
- Ilosone ... 911

Erythromycin Ethylsuccinate (May slow the onset, lower the activity and/or increase the duration of action of levomethadyl acetate hydrochloride). Products include:
- E.E.S. ... 424
- EryPed ... 421

Erythromycin Gluceptate (May slow the onset, lower the activity and/or increase the duration of action of levomethadyl acetate hydrochloride). Products include:
- Ilotycin Gluceptate, IV, Vials ... 913

Erythromycin Lactobionate (May slow the onset, lower the activity and/or increase the duration of action of levomethadyl acetate hydrochloride).
- No products indexed under this heading.

Erythromycin Stearate (May slow the onset, lower the activity and/or increase the duration of action of levomethadyl acetate hydrochloride). Products include:
- Erythrocin Stearate Filmtab ... 425

Estazolam (Potential for serious side effects, including respiratory depression, hypotension, profound sedation and coma, if used concurrently). Products include:
- ProSom Tablets ... 449

Ethchlorvynol (Potential for serious side effects, including respiratory depression, hypotension, profound sedation and coma, if used concurrently). Products include:
- Placidyl Capsules ... 448

Ethinamate (Potential for serious side effects, including respiratory depression, hypotension, profound sedation and coma, if used concurrently).
- No products indexed under this heading.

Fentanyl (Potential for serious side effects, including respiratory depression, hypotension, profound sedation and coma, if used concurrently). Products include:
- Duragesic Transdermal System ... 1288

Fentanyl Citrate (Potential for serious side effects, including respiratory depression, hypotension, profound sedation and coma, if used concurrently). Products include:
- Sublimaze Injection ... 1307

Fluoxetine Hydrochloride (Potential for serious side effects, including respiratory depression, hypotension, profound sedation and coma, if used concurrently). Products include:
- Prozac Pulvules & Liquid, Oral Solution ... 919

Fluphenazine Decanoate (Potential for serious side effects, including respiratory depression, hypotension, profound sedation and coma, if used concurrently). Products include:
- Prolixin Decanoate ... 509

Fluphenazine Enanthate (Potential for serious side effects, including respiratory depression, hypotension, profound sedation and coma, if used concurrently). Products include:
- Prolixin Enanthate ... 509

Fluphenazine Hydrochloride (Potential for serious side effects, including respiratory depression, hypotension, profound sedation and coma, if used concurrently). Products include:
- Prolixin ... 509

(▣ Described in PDR For Nonprescription Drugs) (◉ Described in PDR For Ophthalmology)

767 Interactions Index Orlamm

Flurazepam Hydrochloride (Potential for serious side effects, including respiratory depression, hypotension, profound sedation and coma, if used concurrently). Products include:
Dalmane Capsules ... 2173

Glutethimide (Potential for serious side effects, including respiratory depression, hypotension, profound sedation and coma, if used concurrently).
No products indexed under this heading.

Halazepam (Potential for serious side effects, including respiratory depression, hypotension, profound sedation and coma, if used concurrently).
No products indexed under this heading.

Haloperidol (Potential for serious side effects, including respiratory depression, hypotension, profound sedation and coma, if used concurrently). Products include:
Haldol Injection, Tablets and Concentrate ... 1575

Haloperidol Decanoate (Potential for serious side effects, including respiratory depression, hypotension, profound sedation and coma, if used concurrently). Products include:
Haldol Decanoate ... 1577

Hydrocodone Bitartrate (Potential for serious side effects, including respiratory depression, hypotension, profound sedation and coma, if used concurrently). Products include:
Anexsia 5/500 Elixir ... 1781
Anexia Tablets ... 1782
Codiclear DH Syrup ... 791
Deconamine CX Cough and Cold Liquid and Tablets ... 1319
Duratuss HD Elixir ... 2565
Hycodan Tablets and Syrup ... 930
Hycomine Compound Tablets ... 932
Hycomine ... 931
Hycotuss Expectorant Syrup ... 933
Hydrocet Capsules ... 782
Lorcet 10/650 ... 1018
Lortab ... 2566
Tussend ... 1783
Tussend Expectorant ... 1785
Vicodin Tablets ... 1356
Vicodin ES Tablets ... 1357
Vicodin Tuss Expectorant ... 1358
Zydone Capsules ... 949

Hydrocodone Polistirex (Potential for serious side effects, including respiratory depression, hypotension, profound sedation and coma, if used concurrently). Products include:
Tussionex Pennkinetic Extended-Release Suspension ... 998

Hydroxyzine Hydrochloride (Potential for serious side effects, including respiratory depression, hypotension, profound sedation and coma, if used concurrently). Products include:
Atarax Tablets & Syrup ... 2185
Marax Tablets & DF Syrup ... 2200
Vistaril Intramuscular Solution ... 2216

Imipramine Hydrochloride (Potential for serious side effects, including respiratory depression, hypotension, profound sedation and coma, if used concurrently). Products include:
Tofranil Ampuls ... 854
Tofranil Tablets ... 856

Imipramine Pamoate (Potential for serious side effects, including respiratory depression, hypotension, profound sedation and coma, if used concurrently). Products include:
Tofranil-PM Capsules ... 857

Isocarboxazid (Potential for serious side effects, including respiratory depression, hypotension, profound sedation and coma, if used concurrently).
No products indexed under this heading.

Isoflurane (Potential for serious side effects, including respiratory depression, hypotension, profound sedation and coma, if used concurrently).
No products indexed under this heading.

Ketamine Hydrochloride (Potential for serious side effects, including respiratory depression, hypotension, profound sedation and coma, if used concurrently).
No products indexed under this heading.

Ketoconazole (May slow the onset, lower the activity and/or increase the duration of action of levomethadyl acetate hydrochloride). Products include:
Nizoral 2% Cream ... 1297
Nizoral 2% Shampoo ... 1298
Nizoral Tablets ... 1298

Levorphanol Tartrate (Potential for serious side effects, including respiratory depression, hypotension, profound sedation and coma, if used concurrently). Products include:
Levo-Dromoran ... 2129

Loratadine (Potential for serious side effects, including respiratory depression, hypotension, profound sedation and coma, if used concurrently). Products include:
Claritin ... 2349
Claritin-D ... 2350

Lorazepam (Potential for serious side effects, including respiratory depression, hypotension, profound sedation and coma, if used concurrently). Products include:
Ativan Injection ... 2698
Ativan Tablets ... 2700

Loxapine Hydrochloride (Potential for serious side effects, including respiratory depression, hypotension, profound sedation and coma, if used concurrently). Products include:
Loxitane ... 1378

Loxapine Succinate (Potential for serious side effects, including respiratory depression, hypotension, profound sedation and coma, if used concurrently). Products include:
Loxitane Capsules ... 1378

Maprotiline Hydrochloride (Potential for serious side effects, including respiratory depression, hypotension, profound sedation and coma, if used concurrently). Products include:
Ludiomil Tablets ... 843

Meperidine Hydrochloride (Agonists, such as meperidine, should not be used concurrently because they would be ineffective unless given at high doses; potential for serious side effects, including respiratory depression, hypotension, profound sedation and coma, if used concurrently). Products include:
Demerol ... 2308
Mepergan Injection ... 2753

Mephobarbital (Potential for serious side effects, including respiratory depression, hypotension, profound sedation and coma, if used concurrently). Products include:
Mebaral Tablets ... 2322

Meprobamate (Potential for serious side effects, including respiratory depression, hypotension, profound sedation and coma, if used concurrently). Products include:
Miltown Tablets ... 2672
PMB 200 and PMB 400 ... 2783

Mesoridazine Besylate (Potential for serious side effects, including respiratory depression, hypotension, profound sedation and coma, if used concurrently). Products include:
Serentil ... 684

Methadone Hydrochloride (Potential for serious side effects, including respiratory depression, hypotension, profound sedation and coma, if used concurrently). Products include:
Methadone Hydrochloride Oral Concentrate ... 2233
Methadone Hydrochloride Oral Solution & Tablets ... 2235

Methdilazine Hydrochloride (Potential for serious side effects, including respiratory depression, hypotension, profound sedation and coma, if used concurrently).
No products indexed under this heading.

Methohexital Sodium (Potential for serious side effects, including respiratory depression, hypotension, profound sedation and coma, if used concurrently). Products include:
Brevital Sodium Vials ... 1429

Methotrimeprazine (Potential for serious side effects, including respiratory depression, hypotension, profound sedation and coma, if used concurrently). Products include:
Levoprome ... 1274

Methoxyflurane (Potential for serious side effects, including respiratory depression, hypotension, profound sedation and coma, if used concurrently).
No products indexed under this heading.

Midazolam Hydrochloride (Potential for serious side effects, including respiratory depression, hypotension, profound sedation and coma, if used concurrently). Products include:
Versed Injection ... 2170

Molindone Hydrochloride (Potential for serious side effects, including respiratory depression, hypotension, profound sedation and coma, if used concurrently). Products include:
Moban Tablets and Concentrate ... 1048

Morphine Sulfate (Potential for serious side effects, including respiratory depression, hypotension, profound sedation and coma, if used concurrently). Products include:
Astramorph/PF Injection, USP (Preservative-Free) ... 535
Duramorph ... 962
Infumorph 200 and Infumorph 500 Sterile Solutions ... 965
MS Contin Tablets ... 1994
MSIR ... 1997
Oramorph SR (Morphine Sulfate Sustained Release Tablets) ... 2236
RMS Suppositories ... 2657
Roxanol ... 2243

Nalbuphine Hydrochloride (Patients maintained on levomethadyl acetate hydrochloride may experience withdrawal symptoms when administered mixed agonists/antagonists). Products include:
Nubain Injection ... 935

Naloxone Hydrochloride (Patients maintained on levomethadyl acetate hydrochloride may experience withdrawal symptoms when administered naloxone). Products include:
Narcan Injection ... 934
Talwin Nx ... 2336

Naltrexone Hydrochloride (Patients maintained on levomethadyl acetate hydrochloride may experience withdrawal symptoms when administered naltrexone). Products include:
ReVia Tablets ... 940

Nefazodone Hydrochloride (Potential for serious side effects, including respiratory depression, hypotension, profound sedation and coma, if used concurrently). Products include:
Serzone Tablets ... 771

Nortriptyline Hydrochloride (Potential for serious side effects, including respiratory depression, hypotension, profound sedation and coma, if used concurrently). Products include:
Pamelor ... 2280

Opium Alkaloids (Potential for serious side effects, including respiratory depression, hypotension, profound sedation and coma, if used concurrently).
No products indexed under this heading.

Oxazepam (Potential for serious side effects, including respiratory depression, hypotension, profound sedation and coma, if used concurrently). Products include:
Serax Capsules ... 2810
Serax Tablets ... 2810

Oxycodone Hydrochloride (Potential for serious side effects, including respiratory depression, hypotension, profound sedation and coma, if used concurrently). Products include:
Percocet Tablets ... 938
Percodan Tablets ... 939
Percodan-Demi Tablets ... 940
Roxicodone Tablets, Oral Solution & Intensol (Oxycodone) ... 2244
Tylox Capsules ... 1584

Paroxetine Hydrochloride (Potential for serious side effects, including respiratory depression, hypotension, profound sedation and coma, if used concurrently). Products include:
Paxil Tablets ... 2505

Pentazocine Hydrochloride (Patients maintained on levomethadyl acetate hydrochloride may experience withdrawal symptoms when administered mixed agonists/antagonists). Products include:
Talacen ... 2333
Talwin Compound ... 2335
Talwin Nx ... 2336

Pentazocine Lactate (Patients maintained on levomethadyl acetate hydrochloride may experience withdrawal symptoms when administered mixed agonists/antagonists). Products include:
Talwin Injection ... 2334

Pentobarbital Sodium (Potential for serious side effects, including respiratory depression, hypotension, profound sedation and coma, if used concurrently). Products include:
Nembutal Sodium Capsules ... 436
Nembutal Sodium Solution ... 438
Nembutal Sodium Suppositories ... 440

IMPORTANT NOTE: Always consult each drug listing in the patient's regimen for possible interactions.

Orlamm **Interactions Index** 768

Perphenazine (Potential for serious side effects, including respiratory depression, hypotension, profound sedation and coma, if used concurrently). Products include:

Etrafon 2355
Triavil Tablets 1757
Trilafon 2389

Phenelzine Sulfate (Potential for serious side effects, including respiratory depression, hypotension, profound sedation and coma, if used concurrently). Products include:

Nardil 1920

Phenobarbital (May increase levomethadyl acetate hydrochloride's peak activity and/or shorten its duration of action). Products include:

Arco-Lase Plus Tablets 512
Bellergal-S Tablets 2250
Donnatal 2060
Donnatal Extentabs 2061
Donnatal Tablets 2060
Phenobarbital Elixir and Tablets 1469
Quadrinal Tablets 1350

Phenytoin (May increase levomethadyl acetate hydrochloride's peak activity and/or shorten its duration of action). Products include:

Dilantin Infatabs 1908
Dilantin-125 Suspension 1911

Phenytoin Sodium (May increase levomethadyl acetate hydrochloride's peak activity and/or shorten its duration of action). Products include:

Dilantin Kapseals 1906
Dilantin Parenteral 1910

Prazepam (Potential for serious side effects, including respiratory depression, hypotension, profound sedation and coma, if used concurrently).

No products indexed under this heading.

Prochlorperazine (Potential for serious side effects, including respiratory depression, hypotension, profound sedation and coma, if used concurrently). Products include:

Compazine 2470

Promethazine Hydrochloride (Potential for serious side effects, including respiratory depression, hypotension, profound sedation and coma, if used concurrently). Products include:

Mepergan Injection 2753
Phenergan with Codeine 2777
Phenergan with Dextromethorphan 2778
Phenergan Injection 2773
Phenergan Suppositories 2775
Phenergan Syrup 2774
Phenergan Tablets 2775
Phenergan VC 2779
Phenergan VC with Codeine 2781

Propofol (Potential for serious side effects, including respiratory depression, hypotension, profound sedation and coma, if used concurrently). Products include:

Diprivan Injection 2833

Propoxyphene Hydrochloride (Agonists, such as propoxyphene, should not be used concurrently because they would be ineffective unless given at high doses; potential for serious side effects, including respiratory depression, hypotension, profound sedation and coma, if used concurrently). Products include:

Darvon 1435
Wygesic Tablets 2827

Propoxyphene Napsylate (Agonists, such as propoxyphene, should not be used concurrently because they would be ineffective unless given at high doses; potential for serious side effects, including respiratory depression, hypotension, profound sedation and coma, if used concurrently). Products include:

Darvon-N/Darvocet-N 1433

Protriptyline Hydrochloride (Potential for serious side effects, including respiratory depression, hypotension, profound sedation and coma, if used concurrently). Products include:

Vivactil Tablets 1774

Pyrilamine Maleate (Potential for serious side effects, including respiratory depression, hypotension, profound sedation and coma, if used concurrently). Products include:

4-Way Fast Acting Nasal Spray (regular & mentholated) .... ▣ 621
Maximum Strength Multi-Symptom Formula Midol .... ▣ 722
PMS Multi-Symptom Formula Midol .... ▣ 723

Pyrilamine Tannate (Potential for serious side effects, including respiratory depression, hypotension, profound sedation and coma, if used concurrently). Products include:

Atrohist Pediatric Suspension 454
Rynatan 2673

Quazepam (Potential for serious side effects, including respiratory depression, hypotension, profound sedation and coma, if used concurrently). Products include:

Doral Tablets 2664

Rifampin (May increase levomethadyl acetate hydrochloride's peak activity and/or shorten its duration of action). Products include:

Rifadin 1528
Rifamate Capsules 1530
Rifater 1532
Rimactane Capsules 847

Risperidone (Potential for serious side effects, including respiratory depression, hypotension, profound sedation and coma, if used concurrently). Products include:

Risperdal 1301

Secobarbital Sodium (Potential for serious side effects, including respiratory depression, hypotension, profound sedation and coma, if used concurrently). Products include:

Seconal Sodium Pulvules 1474

Sertraline Hydrochloride (Potential for serious side effects, including respiratory depression, hypotension, profound sedation and coma, if used concurrently). Products include:

Zoloft Tablets 2217

Sufentanil Citrate (Potential for serious side effects, including respiratory depression, hypotension, profound sedation and coma, if used concurrently). Products include:

Sufenta Injection 1309

Temazepam (Potential for serious side effects, including respiratory depression, hypotension, profound sedation and coma, if used concurrently). Products include:

Restoril Capsules 2284

Terfenadine (Potential for serious side effects, including respiratory depression, hypotension, profound sedation and coma, if used concurrently). Products include:

Seldane Tablets 1536
Seldane-D Extended-Release Tablets 1538

Thiamylal Sodium (Potential for serious side effects, including respiratory depression, hypotension, profound sedation and coma, if used concurrently).

No products indexed under this heading.

Thioridazine Hydrochloride (Potential for serious side effects, including respiratory depression, hypotension, profound sedation and coma, if used concurrently). Products include:

Mellaril 2269

Thiothixene (Potential for serious side effects, including respiratory depression, hypotension, profound sedation and coma, if used concurrently). Products include:

Navane Capsules and Concentrate 2201
Navane Intramuscular 2202

Tranylcypromine Sulfate (Potential for serious side effects, including respiratory depression, hypotension, profound sedation and coma, if used concurrently). Products include:

Parnate Tablets 2503

Trazodone Hydrochloride (Potential for serious side effects, including respiratory depression, hypotension, profound sedation and coma, if used concurrently). Products include:

Desyrel and Desyrel Dividose 503

Triazolam (Potential for serious side effects, including respiratory depression, hypotension, profound sedation and coma, if used concurrently). Products include:

Halcion Tablets 2611

Trifluoperazine Hydrochloride (Potential for serious side effects, including respiratory depression, hypotension, profound sedation and coma, if used concurrently). Products include:

Stelazine 2514

Trimeprazine Tartrate (Potential for serious side effects, including respiratory depression, hypotension, profound sedation and coma, if used concurrently). Products include:

Temaril Tablets, Syrup and Spansule Extended-Release Capsules 483

Trimipramine Maleate (Potential for serious side effects, including respiratory depression, hypotension, profound sedation and coma, if used concurrently). Products include:

Surmontil Capsules 2811

Tripelennamine Hydrochloride (Potential for serious side effects, including respiratory depression, hypotension, profound sedation and coma, if used concurrently). Products include:

PBZ Tablets 845
PBZ-SR Tablets 844

Triprolidine Hydrochloride (Potential for serious side effects, including respiratory depression, hypotension, profound sedation and coma, if used concurrently). Products include:

Actifed Plus Caplets .... ▣ 845
Actifed Plus Tablets .... ▣ 845
Actifed with Codeine Cough Syrup.. 1067
Actifed Syrup .... ▣ 846
Actifed Tablets .... ▣ 844

Venlafaxine Hydrochloride (Potential for serious side effects, including respiratory depression, hypotension, profound sedation and coma, if used concurrently). Products include:

Effexor 2719

Zolpidem Tartrate (Potential for serious side effects, including respiratory depression, hypotension, profound sedation and coma, if used concurrently). Products include:

Ambien Tablets 2416

Food Interactions

Alcohol (Potential for serious side effects, including respiratory depression, hypotension, profound sedation and coma, if used concurrently).

ORNADE SPANSULE CAPSULES

(Phenylpropanolamine Hydrochloride, Chlorpheniramine Maleate) 2502

May interact with central nervous system depressants, monoamine oxidase inhibitors, oral anticoagulants, ganglionic blocking agents, beta blockers, alpha adrenergic blockers, anticholinergics, corticosteroids, phenothiazines, and certain other agents. Compounds in these categories include:

Acebutolol Hydrochloride (Hypotensive action antagonized). Products include:

Sectral Capsules 2807

Alfentanil Hydrochloride (Potentiated). Products include:

Alfenta Injection 1286

Alprazolam (Potentiated). Products include:

Xanax Tablets 2649

Amphetamine Resins (Additive effects). Products include:

Biphetamine Capsules 983

Aprobarbital (Potentiated).

No products indexed under this heading.

Atenolol (Hypotensive action antagonized). Products include:

Tenoretic Tablets 2845
Tenormin Tablets and I.V. Injection 2847

Atropine Sulfate (Potentiation of CNS depressant and atropine-like effects). Products include:

Arco-Lase Plus Tablets 512
Atrohist Plus Tablets 454
Atropine Sulfate Sterile Ophthalmic Solution .... ⊙ 233
Donnatal 2060
Donnatal Extentabs 2061
Donnatal Tablets 2060
Lomotil 2439
Motofen Tablets 784
Urised Tablets 1964

Belladonna Alkaloids (Potentiation of CNS depressant and atropine-like effects). Products include:

Bellergal-S Tablets 2250
Hyland's Bed Wetting Tablets .... ▣ 828
Hyland's EnurAid Tablets .... ▣ 829
Hyland's Teething Tablets .... ▣ 830

Benztropine Mesylate (Potentiation of CNS depressant and atropine-like effects). Products include:

Cogentin 1621

Betamethasone Acetate (Decreased effects of corticosteroids). Products include:

Celestone Soluspan Suspension 2347

Betamethasone Sodium Phosphate (Decreased effects of corticosteroids). Products include:

Celestone Soluspan Suspension 2347

Betaxolol Hydrochloride (Hypotensive action antagonized). Products include:

Betoptic Ophthalmic Solution 469
Betoptic S Ophthalmic Suspension 471
Kerlone Tablets 2436

Biperiden Hydrochloride (Potentiation of CNS depressant and atropine-like effects). Products include:

Akineton 1333

(▣ Described in PDR For Nonprescription Drugs) (⊙ Described in PDR For Ophthalmology)

Interactions Index

Ornade Spansule

Bisoprolol Fumarate (Hypotensive action antagonized). Products include:

Zebeta Tablets 1413
Ziac 1415

Buprenorphine (Potentiated). Products include:

Buprenex Injectable 2006

Buspirone Hydrochloride (Potentiated). Products include:

BuSpar 737

Butabarbital (Potentiated).

No products indexed under this heading.

Butalbital (Potentiated). Products include:

Esgic-plus Tablets 1013
Fioricet Tablets 2258
Fioricet with Codeine Capsules 2260
Fiorinal Capsules 2261
Fiorinal with Codeine Capsules 2262
Fiorinal Tablets 2261
Phrenilin 785
Sedapap Tablets 50 mg/650 mg .. 1543

Carteolol Hydrochloride (Hypotensive action antagonized). Products include:

Cartrol Tablets 410
Ocupress Ophthalmic Solution, 1% Sterile .... ◎ 309

Chlordiazepoxide (Potentiated). Products include:

Libritabs Tablets 2177
Limbitrol 2180

Chlordiazepoxide Hydrochloride (Potentiated). Products include:

Librax Capsules 2176
Librium Capsules 2178
Librium Injectable 2179

Chlorpromazine (Additive CNS depressant effect; urinary retention; glaucoma;). Products include:

Thorazine Suppositories 2523

Chlorprothixene (Potentiated).

No products indexed under this heading.

Chlorprothixene Hydrochloride (Potentiated).

No products indexed under this heading.

Clidinium Bromide (Potentiation of CNS depressant and atropine-like effects). Products include:

Librax Capsules 2176
Quarzan Capsules 2181

Clorazepate Dipotassium (Potentiated). Products include:

Tranxene 451

Clozapine (Potentiated). Products include:

Clozaril Tablets 2252

Codeine Phosphate (Potentiated). Products include:

Actifed with Codeine Cough Syrup.. 1067
Brontex 1981
Deconsal C Expectorant Syrup 456
Deconsal Pediatric Syrup 457
Dimetane-DC Cough Syrup 2059
Empirin with Codeine Tablets 1093
Fioricet with Codeine Capsules 2260
Fiorinal with Codeine Capsules 2262
Isoclor Expectorant 990
Novahistine DH 2462
Novahistine Expectorant 2463
Nucofed 2051
Phenergan with Codeine 2777
Phenergan VC with Codeine 2781
Robitussin A-C Syrup 2073
Robitussin-DAC Syrup 2074
Ryna .... ◙ 841
Soma Compound w/Codeine Tablets 2676
Tussi-Organidin NR Liquid and S NR Liquid 2677
Tylenol with Codeine 1583

Cortisone Acetate (Decreased effects of corticosteroids). Products include:

Cortone Acetate Sterile Suspension 1623
Cortone Acetate Tablets 1624

Desflurane (Potentiated). Products include:

Suprane 1813

Dexamethasone (Decreased effects). Products include:

AK-Trol Ointment & Suspension .... ◎ 205
Decadron Elixir 1633
Decadron Tablets 1635
Decaspray Topical Aerosol 1648
Dexacidin Ointment .... ◎ 263
Maxitrol Ophthalmic Ointment and Suspension .... ◎ 224
TobraDex Ophthalmic Suspension and Ointment 473

Dexamethasone Acetate (Decreased effects of corticosteroids). Products include:

Dalalone D.P. Injectable 1011
Decadron-LA Sterile Suspension 1646

Dexamethasone Sodium Phosphate (Decreased effects of corticosteroids). Products include:

Decadron Phosphate Injection 1637
Decadron Phosphate Respihaler 1642
Decadron Phosphate Sterile Ophthalmic Ointment 1641
Decadron Phosphate Sterile Ophthalmic Solution 1642
Decadron Phosphate Topical Cream 1644
Decadron Phosphate Turbinaire 1645
Decadron Phosphate with Xylocaine Injection, Sterile 1639
Dexacort Phosphate in Respihaler .. 458
Dexacort Phosphate in Turbinaire .. 459
NeoDecadron Sterile Ophthalmic Ointment 1712
NeoDecadron Sterile Ophthalmic Solution 1713
NeoDecadron Topical Cream 1714

Dextroamphetamine Sulfate (Additive effects). Products include:

Dexedrine 2474
DextroStat Dextroamphetamine Tablets 2036

Dezocine (Potentiated). Products include:

Dalgan Injection 538

Diazepam (Potentiated). Products include:

Dizac 1809
Valium Injectable 2182
Valium Tablets 2183
Valrelease Capsules 2169

Dicumarol (Action of oral anticoagulants may be inhibited).

No products indexed under this heading.

Dicyclomine Hydrochloride (Potentiation of CNS depressant and atropine-like effects). Products include:

Bentyl 1501

Doxazosin Mesylate (Hypotensive action antagonized). Products include:

Cardura Tablets 2186

Droperidol (Potentiated). Products include:

Inapsine Injection 1296

Enflurane (Potentiated).

No products indexed under this heading.

Esmolol Hydrochloride (Hypotensive action antagonized). Products include:

Brevibloc Injection 1808

Estazolam (Potentiated). Products include:

ProSom Tablets 449

Ethchlorvynol (Potentiated). Products include:

Placidyl Capsules 448

Ethinamate (Potentiated).

No products indexed under this heading.

Fentanyl (Potentiated). Products include:

Duragesic Transdermal System 1288

Fentanyl Citrate (Potentiated). Products include:

Sublimaze Injection 1307

Fludrocortisone Acetate (Decreased effects of corticosteroids). Products include:

Florinef Acetate Tablets 505

Fluphenazine Decanoate (Additive CNS depressant effect; urinary retention; glaucoma). Products include:

Prolixin Decanoate 509

Fluphenazine Enanthate (Additive CNS depressant effect; urinary retention; glaucoma). Products include:

Prolixin Enanthate 509

Fluphenazine Hydrochloride (Additive CNS depressant effect; urinary retention; glaucoma). Products include:

Prolixin 509

Flurazepam Hydrochloride (Potentiated). Products include:

Dalmane Capsules 2173

Furazolidone (Contraindicated; prolongs and intensifies the anticholinergic effects and potentiates the pressor effects). Products include:

Furoxone 2046

Glutethimide (Potentiated).

No products indexed under this heading.

Glycopyrrolate (Potentiation of CNS depressant and atropine-like effects). Products include:

Robinul Forte Tablets 2072
Robinul Injectable 2072
Robinul Tablets 2072

Guanethidine Monosulfate (Hypotensive action antagonized). Products include:

Esimil Tablets 822
Ismelin Tablets 827

Haloperidol (Potentiated). Products include:

Haldol Injection, Tablets and Concentrate 1575

Haloperidol Decanoate (Potentiated). Products include:

Haldol Decanoate 1577

Hydrocodone Bitartrate (Potentiated). Products include:

Anexsia 5/500 Elixir 1781
Anexia Tablets 1782
Codiclear DH Syrup 791
Deconamine CX Cough and Cold Liquid and Tablets 1319
Duratuss HD Elixir 2565
Hycodan Tablets and Syrup 930
Hycomine Compound Tablets 932
Hycomine 931
Hycotuss Expectorant Syrup 933
Hydrocet Capsules 782
Lorcet 10/650 1018
Lortab 2566
Tussend 1783
Tussend Expectorant 1785
Vicodin Tablets 1356
Vicodin ES Tablets 1357
Vicodin Tuss Expectorant 1358
Zydone Capsules 949

Hydrocodone Polistirex (Potentiated). Products include:

Tussionex Pennkinetic Extended-Release Suspension 998

Hydrocortisone (Decreased effects of corticosteroids). Products include:

Anusol-HC Cream 2.5% 1896
Aquanil HC Lotion 1931
Bactine Hydrocortisone Anti-Itch Cream .... ◙ 709
Caldecort Anti-Itch Hydrocortisone Spray .... ◙ 631
Cortaid .... ◙ 836
CORTENEMA 2535
Cortisporin Ointment 1085
Cortisporin Ophthalmic Ointment Sterile 1085

Cortisporin Ophthalmic Suspension Sterile 1086
Cortisporin Otic Solution Sterile 1087
Cortisporin Otic Suspension Sterile 1088
Cortizone-5 .... ◙ 831
Cortizone-10 .... ◙ 831
Hydrocortone Tablets 1672
Hytone 907
Massengill Medicated Soft Cloth Towelettes 2458
PediOtic Suspension Sterile 1153
Preparation H Hydrocortisone 1% Cream .... ◙ 872
ProctoCream-HC 2.5% 2408
VōSoL HC Otic Solution 2678

Hydrocortisone Acetate (Decreased effects of corticosteroids). Products include:

Analpram-HC Rectal Cream 1% and 2.5% 977
Anusol HC-1 Anti-Itch Hydrocortisone Ointment .... ◙ 847
Anusol-HC Suppositories 1897
Caldecort .... ◙ 631
Ca;mol HC 924
Coly-Mycin S Otic w/Neomycin & Hydrocortisone 1906
Cortaid .... ◙ 836
Cortifoam 2396
Cortisporin Cream 1084
Epifoam 2399
Hydrocortone Acetate Sterile Suspension 1669
Mantadil Cream 1135
Nupercainal Hydrocortisone 1% Cream .... ◙ 645
Ophthocort .... ◎ 311
Pramosone Cream, Lotion & Ointment 978
ProctoCream-HC 2408
ProctoFoam-HC 2409
Terra-Cortril Ophthalmic Suspension 2210

Hydrocortisone Sodium Phosphate (Decreased effects of corticosteroids). Products include:

Hydrocortone Phosphate Injection, Sterile 1670

Hydrocortisone Sodium Succinate (Decreased effects of corticosteroids). Products include:

Solu-Cortef Sterile Powder 2641

Hydroxyzine Hydrochloride (Potentiated). Products include:

Atarax Tablets & Syrup 2185
Marax Tablets & DF Syrup 2200
Vistaril Intramuscular Solution 2216

Hyoscyamine (Potentiation of CNS depressant and atropine-like effects). Products include:

Cystospaz Tablets 1963
Urised Tablets 1964

Hyoscyamine Sulfate (Potentiation of CNS depressant and atropine-like effects). Products include:

Arco-Lase Plus Tablets 512
Atrohist Plus Tablets 454
Cystospaz-M Capsules 1963
Donnatal 2060
Donnatal Extentabs 2061
Donnatal Tablets 2060
Kutrase Capsules 2402
Levsin/Levsinex/Levbid 2405

Imipramine Hydrochloride (Potentiation of CNS depressant and atropine-like effects). Products include:

Tofranil Ampuls 854
Tofranil Tablets 856

Imipramine Pamoate (Potentiation of CNS depressant and atropine-like effects). Products include:

Tofranil-PM Capsules 857

Ipratropium Bromide (Potentiation of CNS depressant and atropine-like effects). Products include:

Atrovent Inhalation Aerosol 671
Atrovent Inhalation Solution 673

Isocarboxazid (Contraindicated; prolongs and intensifies the anticholinergic effects and potentiates the pressor effects).

No products indexed under this heading.

IMPORTANT NOTE: Always consult each drug listing in the patient's regimen for possible interactions.

Ornade Spansule Interactions Index 770

Isoflurane (Potentiated).
No products indexed under this heading.

Ketamine Hydrochloride (Potentiated).
No products indexed under this heading.

Labetalol Hydrochloride (Hypotensive action antagonized). Products include:
Normodyne Injection ... 2377
Normodyne Tablets ... 2379
Trandate ... 1185

Levobunolol Hydrochloride (Hypotensive action antagonized). Products include:
Betagan ... ⊙ 233

Levomethadyl Acetate Hydrochloride (Potentiated). Products include:
Orlamm ... 2239

Levorphanol Tartrate (Potentiated). Products include:
Levo-Dromoran ... 2129

Lorazepam (Potentiated). Products include:
Ativan Injection ... 2698
Ativan Tablets ... 2700

Loxapine Hydrochloride (Potentiated). Products include:
Loxitane ... 1378

Loxapine Succinate (Potentiated). Products include:
Loxitane Capsules ... 1378

Mecamylamine Hydrochloride (Potentiates reactions of sympathomimetics). Products include:
Inversine Tablets ... 1686

Mepenzolate Bromide (Potentiation of CNS depressant and atropine-like effects).
No products indexed under this heading.

Meperidine Hydrochloride (Potentiated). Products include:
Demerol ... 2308
Mepergan Injection ... 2753

Mephobarbital (Potentiated). Products include:
Mebaral Tablets ... 2322

Meprobamate (Potentiated). Products include:
Miltown Tablets ... 2672
PMB 200 and PMB 400 ... 2783

Mesoridazine Besylate (Additive CNS depressant effect; urinary retention; glaucoma). Products include:
Serentil ... 684

Methadone Hydrochloride (Potentiated). Products include:
Methadone Hydrochloride Oral Concentrate ... 2233
Methadone Hydrochloride Oral Solution & Tablets ... 2235

Methamphetamine Hydrochloride (Additive effects). Products include:
Desoxyn Gradumet Tablets ... 419

Methohexital Sodium (Potentiated). Products include:
Brevital Sodium Vials ... 1429

Methotrimeprazine (Potentiated). Products include:
Levoprome ... 1274

Methoxyflurane (Potentiated).
No products indexed under this heading.

Methylprednisolone (Decreased effects of corticosteroids). Products include:
Medrol ... 2621

Methylprednisolone Acetate (Decreased effects of corticosteroids). Products include:
Depo-Medrol Single-Dose Vial ... 2600
Depo-Medrol Sterile Aqueous Suspension ... 2597

Methylprednisolone Sodium Succinate (Decreased effects of corticosteroids). Products include:
Solu-Medrol Sterile Powder ... 2643

Metipranolol Hydrochloride (Hypotensive action antagonized). Products include:
OptiPranolol (Metipranolol 0.3%) Sterile Ophthalmic Solution ... ⊙ 258

Metoprolol Succinate (Hypotensive action antagonized). Products include:
Toprol-XL Tablets ... 565

Metoprolol Tartrate (Hypotensive action antagonized). Products include:
Lopressor Ampuls ... 830
Lopressor HCT Tablets ... 832
Lopressor Tablets ... 830

Midazolam Hydrochloride (Potentiated). Products include:
Versed Injection ... 2170

Molindone Hydrochloride (Potentiated). Products include:
Moban Tablets and Concentrate ... 1048

Morphine Sulfate (Potentiated). Products include:
Astramorph/PF Injection, USP (Preservative-Free) ... 535
Duramorph ... 962
Infumorph 200 and Infumorph 500 Sterile Solutions ... 965
MS Contin Tablets ... 1994
MSIR ... 1997
Oramorph SR (Morphine Sulfate Sustained Release Tablets) ... 2236
RMS Suppositories ... 2657
Roxanol ... 2243

Nadolol (Hypotensive action antagonized).
No products indexed under this heading.

Norepinephrine Bitartrate (Cardiovascular effects potentiated). Products include:
Levophed Bitartrate Injection ... 2315

Opium Alkaloids (Potentiated).
No products indexed under this heading.

Oxazepam (Potentiated). Products include:
Serax Capsules ... 2810
Serax Tablets ... 2810

Oxybutynin Chloride (Potentiation of CNS depressant and atropine-like effects). Products include:
Ditropan ... 1516

Oxycodone Hydrochloride (Potentiated). Products include:
Percocet Tablets ... 938
Percodan Tablets ... 939
Percodan-Demi Tablets ... 940
Roxicodone Tablets, Oral Solution & Intensol (Oxycodone) ... 2244
Tylox Capsules ... 1584

Penbutolol Sulfate (Hypotensive action antagonized). Products include:
Levatol ... 2403

Pentobarbital Sodium (Potentiated). Products include:
Nembutal Sodium Capsules ... 436
Nembutal Sodium Solution ... 438
Nembutal Sodium Suppositories ... 440

Perphenazine (Additive CNS depressant effect; urinary retention; glaucoma). Products include:
Etrafon ... 2355
Triavil Tablets ... 1757
Trilafon ... 2389

Phenelzine Sulfate (Contraindicated; prolongs and intensifies the anticholinergic effects and potentiates the pressor effects). Products include:
Nardil ... 1920

Phenobarbital (Potentiated). Products include:
Arco-Lase Plus Tablets ... 512
Bellergal-S Tablets ... 2250
Donnatal ... 2060
Donnatal Extentabs ... 2061
Donnatal Tablets ... 2060
Phenobarbital Elixir and Tablets ... 1469
Quadrinal Tablets ... 1350

Pindolol (Hypotensive action antagonized). Products include:
Visken Tablets ... 2299

Prazepam (Potentiated).
No products indexed under this heading.

Prazosin Hydrochloride (Hypotensive action antagonized). Products include:
Minipress Capsules ... 1937
Minizide Capsules ... 1938

Prednisolone Acetate (Decreased effects of corticosteroids). Products include:
AK-CIDE ... ⊙ 202
AK-CIDE Ointment ... ⊙ 202
Blephamide Liquifilm Sterile Ophthalmic Suspension ... 476
Blephamide Ointment ... ⊙ 237
Econopred & Econopred Plus Ophthalmic Suspensions ... ⊙ 217
Poly-Pred Liquifilm ... ⊙ 248
Pred Forte ... ⊙ 250
Pred Mild ... ⊙ 253
Pred-G Liquifilm Sterile Ophthalmic Suspension ... ⊙ 251
Pred-G S.O.P. Sterile Ophthalmic Ointment ... ⊙ 252
Vasocidin Ointment ... ⊙ 268

Prednisolone Sodium Phosphate (Decreased effects of corticosteroids). Products include:
AK-Pred ... ⊙ 204
Hydeltrasol Injection, Sterile ... 1665
Inflamase ... ⊙ 265
Pediapred Oral Liquid ... 995
Vasocidin Ophthalmic Solution ... ⊙ 270

Prednisolone Tebutate (Decreased effects of corticosteroids). Products include:
Hydeltra-T.B.A. Sterile Suspension 1667

Prednisone (Decreased effects of corticosteroids). Products include:
Deltasone Tablets ... 2595

Prochlorperazine (Additive CNS depressant effect; urinary retention; glaucoma;). Products include:
Compazine ... 2470

Procyclidine Hydrochloride (Potentiation of CNS depressant and atropine-like effects). Products include:
Kemadrin Tablets ... 1112

Promethazine Hydrochloride (Additive CNS depressant effect; urinary retention; glaucoma). Products include:
Mepergan Injection ... 2753
Phenergan with Codeine ... 2777
Phenergan with Dextromethorphan 2778
Phenergan Injection ... 2773
Phenergan Suppositories ... 2775
Phenergan Syrup ... 2774
Phenergan Tablets ... 2775
Phenergan VC ... 2779
Phenergan VC with Codeine ... 2781

Propantheline Bromide (Potentiation of CNS depressant and atropine-like effects). Products include:
Pro-Banthine Tablets ... 2052

Propofol (Potentiated). Products include:
Diprivan Injection ... 2833

Propoxyphene Hydrochloride (Potentiated). Products include:
Darvon ... 1435
Wygesic Tablets ... 2827

Propoxyphene Napsylate (Potentiated). Products include:
Darvon-N/Darvocet-N ... 1433

Propranolol Hydrochloride (Hypotensive action antagonized). Products include:
Inderal ... 2728
Inderal LA Long Acting Capsules ... 2730
Inderide Tablets ... 2732
Inderide LA Long Acting Capsules ... 2734

Quazepam (Potentiated). Products include:
Doral Tablets ... 2664

Risperidone (Potentiated). Products include:
Risperdal ... 1301

Scopolamine (Potentiation of CNS depressant and atropine-like effects). Products include:
Transderm Scōp Transdermal Therapeutic System ... 869

Scopolamine Hydrobromide (Potentiation of CNS depressant and atropine-like effects). Products include:
Atrohist Plus Tablets ... 454
Donnatal ... 2060
Donnatal Extentabs ... 2061
Donnatal Tablets ... 2060

Secobarbital Sodium (Potentiated). Products include:
Seconal Sodium Pulvules ... 1474

Selegiline Hydrochloride (Contraindicated; prolongs and intensifies the anticholinergic effects and potentiates the pressor effects). Products include:
Eldepryl Tablets ... 2550

Sotalol Hydrochloride (Hypotensive action antagonized). Products include:
Betapace Tablets ... 641

Sufentanil Citrate (Potentiated). Products include:
Sufenta Injection ... 1309

Temazepam (Potentiated). Products include:
Restoril Capsules ... 2284

Terazosin Hydrochloride (Hypotensive action antagonized). Products include:
Hytrin Capsules ... 430

Thiamylal Sodium (Potentiated).
No products indexed under this heading.

Thioridazine Hydrochloride (Additive CNS depressant effect; urinary retention; glaucoma). Products include:
Mellaril ... 2269

Thiothixene (Additive effects). Products include:
Navane Capsules and Concentrate 2201
Navane Intramuscular ... 2202

Timolol Hemihydrate (Hypotensive action antagonized). Products include:
Betimol 0.25%, 0.5% ... ⊙ 261

Timolol Maleate (Hypotensive action antagonized). Products include:
Blocadren Tablets ... 1614
Timolide Tablets ... 1748
Timoptic in Ocudose ... 1753
Timoptic Sterile Ophthalmic Solution ... 1751
Timoptic-XE ... 1755

Tranylcypromine Sulfate (Contraindicated; prolongs and intensifies the anticholinergic effects and potentiates the pressor effects). Products include:
Parnate Tablets ... 2503

Triamcinolone (Decreased effects of corticosteroids). Products include:
Aristocort Tablets ... 1022

Triamcinolone Acetonide (Decreased effects of corticosteroids). Products include:
Aristocort A 0.025% Cream ... 1027
Aristocort A 0.5% Cream ... 1031
Aristocort A 0.1% Cream ... 1029
Aristocort A 0.1% Ointment ... 1030
Azmacort Oral Inhaler ... 2011
Nasacort Nasal Inhaler ... 2024

(Described in PDR For Nonprescription Drugs) (⊙ Described in PDR For Ophthalmology)

Triamcinolone Diacetate (Decreased effects of corticosteroids). Products include:

Aristocort Suspension (Forte Parenteral) 1027
Aristocort Suspension (Intralesional) 1025

Triamcinolone Hexacetonide (Decreased effects of corticosteroids). Products include:

Aristospan Suspension (Intra-articular) 1033
Aristospan Suspension (Intralesional) 1032

Triazolam (Potentiated). Products include:

Halcion Tablets 2611

Tridihexethyl Chloride (Potentiation of CNS depressant and atropine-like effects).

No products indexed under this heading.

Trifluoperazine Hydrochloride (Additive CNS depressant effect; urinary retention; glaucoma). Products include:

Stelazine 2514

Trihexyphenidyl Hydrochloride (Potentiation of CNS depressant and atropine-like effects). Products include:

Artane 1368

Trimethaphan Camsylate (Reactions potentiated). Products include:

Arfonad Ampuls 2080

Warfarin Sodium (Action of oral anticoagulants may be inhibited; should not be taken together). Products include:

Coumadin 926

Zolpidem Tartrate (Potentiated). Products include:

Ambien Tablets 2416

Food Interactions

Alcohol (Potentiated).

ORTHO-CEPT 21 TABLETS

(Desogestrel, Ethinyl Estradiol) 1851

May interact with barbiturates and tetracyclines. Compounds in these categories include:

Ampicillin (Potential for reduced efficacy and increased incidence of breakthrough bleeding and menstrual irregularities). Products include:

Omnipen Capsules 2764
Omnipen for Oral Suspension 2765

Ampicillin Sodium (Potential for reduced efficacy and increased incidence of breakthrough bleeding and menstrual irregularities). Products include:

Unasyn 2212

Aprobarbital (Potential for reduced efficacy and increased incidence of breakthrough bleeding and menstrual irregularities).

No products indexed under this heading.

Butabarbital (Potential for reduced efficacy and increased incidence of breakthrough bleeding and menstrual irregularities).

No products indexed under this heading.

Butalbital (Potential for reduced efficacy and increased incidence of breakthrough bleeding and menstrual irregularities). Products include:

Esgic-plus Tablets 1013
Fioricet Tablets 2258
Fioricet with Codeine Capsules 2260
Fiorinal Capsules 2261
Fiorinal with Codeine Capsules 2262
Fiorinal Tablets 2261
Phrenilin 785

Sedapap Tablets 50 mg/650 mg .. 1543

Demeclocycline Hydrochloride (Potential for reduced efficacy and increased incidence of breakthrough bleeding and menstrual irregularities). Products include:

Declomycin Tablets 1371

Doxycycline Calcium (Potential for reduced efficacy and increased incidence of breakthrough bleeding and menstrual irregularities). Products include:

Vibramycin Calcium Oral Suspension Syrup 1941

Doxycycline Hyclate (Potential for reduced efficacy and increased incidence of breakthrough bleeding and menstrual irregularities). Products include:

Doryx Capsules 1913
Vibramycin Hyclate Capsules 1941
Vibramycin Hyclate Intravenous 2215
Vibra-Tabs Film Coated Tablets 1941

Doxycycline Monohydrate (Potential for reduced efficacy and increased incidence of breakthrough bleeding and menstrual irregularities). Products include:

Monodox Capsules 1805
Vibramycin Monohydrate for Oral Suspension 1941

Griseofulvin (Potential for reduced efficacy and increased incidence of breakthrough bleeding and menstrual irregularities). Products include:

Fulvicin P/G Tablets 2359
Fulvicin P/G 165 & 330 Tablets 2359
Grifulvin V (griseofulvin tablets)
Microsize (griseofulvin oral suspension) Microsize 1888
Gris-PEG Tablets, 125 mg & 250 mg 479

Mephobarbital (Potential for reduced efficacy and increased incidence of breakthrough bleeding and menstrual irregularities). Products include:

Mebaral Tablets 2322

Methacycline Hydrochloride (Potential for reduced efficacy and increased incidence of breakthrough bleeding and menstrual irregularities).

No products indexed under this heading.

Minocycline Hydrochloride (Potential for reduced efficacy and increased incidence of breakthrough bleeding and menstrual irregularities). Products include:

Dynacin Capsules 1590
Minocin Intravenous 1382
Minocin Oral Suspension 1385
Minocin Pellet-Filled Capsules 1383

Oxytetracycline Hydrochloride (Potential for reduced efficacy and increased incidence of breakthrough bleeding and menstrual irregularities). Products include:

TERAK Ointment .... ⊙ 209
Terra-Cortril Ophthalmic Suspension 2210
Terramycin with Polymyxin B Sulfate Ophthalmic Ointment 2211
Urobiotic-250 Capsules 2214

Pentobarbital Sodium (Potential for reduced efficacy and increased incidence of breakthrough bleeding and menstrual irregularities). Products include:

Nembutal Sodium Capsules 436
Nembutal Sodium Solution 438
Nembutal Sodium Suppositories 440

Phenobarbital (Potential for reduced efficacy and increased incidence of breakthrough bleeding and menstrual irregularities). Products include:

Arco-Lase Plus Tablets 512

Bellergal-S Tablets 2250
Donnatal 2060
Donnatal Extentabs 2061
Donnatal Tablets 2060
Phenobarbital Elixir and Tablets 1469
Quadrinal Tablets 1350

Phenylbutazone (Potential for reduced efficacy and increased incidence of breakthrough bleeding and menstrual irregularities).

No products indexed under this heading.

Phenytoin Sodium (Potential for reduced efficacy and increased incidence of breakthrough bleeding and menstrual irregularities). Products include:

Dilantin Kapseals 1906
Dilantin Parenteral 1910

Rifampin (Potential for reduced efficacy and increased incidence of breakthrough bleeding and menstrual irregularities). Products include:

Rifadin 1528
Rifamate Capsules 1530
Rifater 1532
Rimactane Capsules 847

Secobarbital Sodium (Potential for reduced efficacy and increased incidence of breakthrough bleeding and menstrual irregularities). Products include:

Seconal Sodium Pulvules 1474

Tetracycline Hydrochloride (Potential for reduced efficacy and increased incidence of breakthrough bleeding and menstrual irregularities). Products include:

Achromycin V Capsules 1367

Thiamylal Sodium (Potential for reduced efficacy and increased incidence of breakthrough bleeding and menstrual irregularities).

No products indexed under this heading.

ORTHO-CEPT 28 TABLETS

(Desogestrel, Ethinyl Estradiol) 1851
See Ortho-Cept 21 Tablets

ORTHO-CYCLEN 21 TABLETS

(Norgestimate, Ethinyl Estradiol) 1858

May interact with barbiturates and tetracyclines. Compounds in these categories include:

Ampicillin (Potential for reduced efficacy and increased incidence of breakthrough bleeding and menstrual irregularities). Products include:

Omnipen Capsules 2764
Omnipen for Oral Suspension 2765

Ampicillin Sodium (Potential for reduced efficacy and increased incidence of breakthrough bleeding and menstrual irregularities). Products include:

Unasyn 2212

Aprobarbital (Potential for reduced efficacy and increased incidence of breakthrough bleeding and menstrual irregularities).

No products indexed under this heading.

Butabarbital (Potential for reduced efficacy and increased incidence of breakthrough bleeding and menstrual irregularities).

No products indexed under this heading.

Butalbital (Potential for reduced efficacy and increased incidence of breakthrough bleeding and menstrual irregularities). Products include:

Esgic-plus Tablets 1013

Fioricet Tablets 2258
Fioricet with Codeine Capsules 2260
Fiorinal Capsules 2261
Fiorinal with Codeine Capsules 2262
Fiorinal Tablets 2261
Phrenilin 785
Sedapap Tablets 50 mg/650 mg .. 1543

Carbamazepine (Potential for reduced efficacy and increased incidence of breakthrough bleeding and menstrual irregularities). Products include:

Atretol Tablets 573
Tegretol Chewable Tablets 852
Tegretol Suspension 852
Tegretol Tablets 852

Demeclocycline Hydrochloride (Potential for reduced efficacy and increased incidence of breakthrough bleeding and menstrual irregularities). Products include:

Declomycin Tablets 1371

Doxycycline Calcium (Potential for reduced efficacy and increased incidence of breakthrough bleeding and menstrual irregularities). Products include:

Vibramycin Calcium Oral Suspension Syrup 1941

Doxycycline Hyclate (Potential for reduced efficacy and increased incidence of breakthrough bleeding and menstrual irregularities). Products include:

Doryx Capsules 1913
Vibramycin Hyclate Capsules 1941
Vibramycin Hyclate Intravenous 2215
Vibra-Tabs Film Coated Tablets 1941

Doxycycline Monohydrate (Potential for reduced efficacy and increased incidence of breakthrough bleeding and menstrual irregularities). Products include:

Monodox Capsules 1805
Vibramycin Monohydrate for Oral Suspension 1941

Griseofulvin (Potential for reduced efficacy and increased incidence of breakthrough bleeding and menstrual irregularities). Products include:

Fulvicin P/G Tablets 2359
Fulvicin P/G 165 & 330 Tablets 2359
Grifulvin V (griseofulvin tablets)
Microsize (griseofulvin oral suspension) Microsize 1888
Gris-PEG Tablets, 125 mg & 250 mg 479

Mephobarbital (Potential for reduced efficacy and increased incidence of breakthrough bleeding and menstrual irregularities). Products include:

Mebaral Tablets 2322

Methacycline Hydrochloride (Potential for reduced efficacy and increased incidence of breakthrough bleeding and menstrual irregularities).

No products indexed under this heading.

Minocycline Hydrochloride (Potential for reduced efficacy and increased incidence of breakthrough bleeding and menstrual irregularities). Products include:

Dynacin Capsules 1590
Minocin Intravenous 1382
Minocin Oral Suspension 1385
Minocin Pellet-Filled Capsules 1383

Oxytetracycline Hydrochloride (Potential for reduced efficacy and increased incidence of breakthrough bleeding and menstrual irregularities). Products include:

TERAK Ointment .... ⊙ 209
Terra-Cortril Ophthalmic Suspension 2210
Terramycin with Polymyxin B Sulfate Ophthalmic Ointment 2211
Urobiotic-250 Capsules 2214

IMPORTANT NOTE: Always consult each drug listing in the patient's regimen for possible interactions.

Ortho-Cyclen/Ortho-Tri-Cyclen — Interactions Index — 772

Pentobarbital Sodium (Potential for reduced efficacy and increased incidence of breakthrough bleeding and menstrual irregularities). Products include:
- Nembutal Sodium Capsules ... 436
- Nembutal Sodium Solution ... 438
- Nembutal Sodium Suppositories ... 440

Phenobarbital (Potential for reduced efficacy and increased incidence of breakthrough bleeding and menstrual irregularities). Products include:
- Arco-Lase Plus Tablets ... 512
- Bellergal-S Tablets ... 2250
- Donnatal ... 2060
- Donnatal Extentabs ... 2061
- Donnatal Tablets ... 2060
- Phenobarbital Elixir and Tablets ... 1469
- Quadrinal Tablets ... 1350

Phenylbutazone (Potential for reduced efficacy and increased incidence of breakthrough bleeding and menstrual irregularities).
- No products indexed under this heading.

Phenytoin Sodium (Potential for reduced efficacy and increased incidence of breakthrough bleeding and menstrual irregularities). Products include:
- Dilantin Kapseals ... 1906
- Dilantin Parenteral ... 1910

Rifampin (Potential for reduced efficacy and increased incidence of breakthrough bleeding and menstrual irregularities). Products include:
- Rifadin ... 1528
- Rifamate Capsules ... 1530
- Rifater ... 1532
- Rimactane Capsules ... 847

Secobarbital Sodium (Potential for reduced efficacy and increased incidence of breakthrough bleeding and menstrual irregularities). Products include:
- Seconal Sodium Pulvules ... 1474

Tetracycline Hydrochloride (Potential for reduced efficacy and increased incidence of breakthrough bleeding and menstrual irregularities). Products include:
- Achromycin V Capsules ... 1367

Thiamylal Sodium (Potential for reduced efficacy and increased incidence of breakthrough bleeding and menstrual irregularities).
- No products indexed under this heading.

ORTHO-CYCLEN 28 TABLETS
(Norgestimate, Ethinyl Estradiol) ... 1858
See **Ortho-Cyclen 21 Tablets**

ORTHO DIAPHRAGM KITS—ALL-FLEX ARCING SPRING; ORTHO COIL SPRING; ORTHO-WHITE FLAT SPRING
(Diaphragm) ... 1865
None cited in PDR database.

ORTHO DIAPHRAGM KIT-COIL SPRING
(Diaphragm) ... 1865
None cited in PDR database.

ORTHO DIENESTROL CREAM
(Dienestrol) ... 1866
None cited in PDR database.

ORTHO-EST .625 TABLETS
(Estropipate) ... 1869
May interact with progestins. Compounds in this category include:

Desogestrel (Potential risk of adverse effects on carbohydrate and lipid metabolism; the choice of progestin and dosage may be important in minimizing these adverse effects). Products include:
- Desogen Tablets ... 1817
- Ortho-Cept ... 1851

Medroxyprogesterone Acetate (Potential risk of adverse effects on carbohydrate and lipid metabolism; the choice of progestin and dosage may be important in minimizing these adverse effects). Products include:
- Amen Tablets ... 780
- Cycrin Tablets ... 975
- Depo-Provera Contraceptive Injection ... 2602
- Depo-Provera Sterile Aqueous Suspension ... 2606
- Premphase ... 2797
- Prempro ... 2801
- Provera Tablets ... 2636

Megestrol Acetate (Potential risk of adverse effects on carbohydrate and lipid metabolism; the choice of progestin and dosage may be important in minimizing these adverse effects). Products include:
- Megace Oral Suspension ... 699
- Megace Tablets ... 701

Norgestimate (Potential risk of adverse effects on carbohydrate and lipid metabolism; the choice of progestin and dosage may be important in minimizing these adverse effects). Products include:
- Ortho-Cyclen/Ortho-Tri-Cyclen ... 1858
- Ortho-Cyclen/Ortho Tri-Cyclen ... 1858

ORTHO-EST 1.25 TABLETS
(Estropipate) ... 1869
See **Ortho-Est .625 Tablets**

ORTHO-GYNOL CONTRACEPTIVE JELLY
(Nonoxynol-9) ... ⊡ 740
None cited in PDR database.

ORTHO-NOVUM 1/35□21 TABLETS
(Norethindrone, Ethinyl Estradiol) ... 1872
See **Ortho-Novum 7/7/7 □21 Tablets**

ORTHO-NOVUM 1/35□28 TABLETS
(Norethindrone, Ethinyl Estradiol) ... 1872
See **Ortho-Novum 7/7/7 □21 Tablets**

ORTHO-NOVUM 1/50□21 TABLETS
(Norethindrone, Mestranol) ... 1872
See **Ortho-Novum 7/7/7 □21 Tablets**

ORTHO-NOVUM 1/50□28 TABLETS
(Norethindrone, Mestranol) ... 1872
See **Ortho-Novum 7/7/7 □21 Tablets**

ORTHO-NOVUM 7/7/7 □21 TABLETS
(Norethindrone, Ethinyl Estradiol) ... 1872
May interact with tetracyclines, barbiturates, and certain other agents. Compounds in these categories include:

Ampicillin (Potential for reduced efficacy and increased incidence of breakthrough bleeding and menstrual irregularities). Products include:
- Omnipen Capsules ... 2764
- Omnipen for Oral Suspension ... 2765

Ampicillin Sodium (Potential for reduced efficacy and increased incidence of breakthrough bleeding and menstrual irregularities). Products include:
- Unasyn ... 2212

Aprobarbital (Potential for reduced efficacy and increased incidence of breakthrough bleeding and menstrual irregularities).
- No products indexed under this heading.

Butabarbital (Potential for reduced efficacy and increased incidence of breakthrough bleeding and menstrual irregularities).
- No products indexed under this heading.

Butalbital (Potential for reduced efficacy and increased incidence of breakthrough bleeding and menstrual irregularities). Products include:
- Esgic-plus Tablets ... 1013
- Fioricet Tablets ... 2258
- Fioricet with Codeine Capsules ... 2260
- Fiorinal Capsules ... 2261
- Fiorinal with Codeine Capsules ... 2262
- Fiorinal Tablets ... 2261
- Phrenilin ... 785
- Sedapap Tablets 50 mg/650 mg .. 1543

Carbamazepine (Potential for reduced efficacy and increased incidence of breakthrough bleeding and menstrual irregularities). Products include:
- Atretol Tablets ... 573
- Tegretol Chewable Tablets ... 852
- Tegretol Suspension ... 852
- Tegretol Tablets ... 852

Demeclocycline Hydrochloride (Potential for reduced efficacy and increased incidence of breakthrough bleeding and menstrual irregularities). Products include:
- Declomycin Tablets ... 1371

Doxycycline Calcium (Potential for reduced efficacy and increased incidence of breakthrough bleeding and menstrual irregularities). Products include:
- Vibramycin Calcium Oral Suspension Syrup ... 1941

Doxycycline Hyclate (Potential for reduced efficacy and increased incidence of breakthrough bleeding and menstrual irregularities). Products include:
- Doryx Capsules ... 1913
- Vibramycin Hyclate Capsules ... 1941
- Vibramycin Hyclate Intravenous ... 2215
- Vibra-Tabs Film Coated Tablets ... 1941

Doxycycline Monohydrate (Potential for reduced efficacy and increased incidence of breakthrough bleeding and menstrual irregularities). Products include:
- Monodox Capsules ... 1805
- Vibramycin Monohydrate for Oral Suspension ... 1941

Griseofulvin (Potential for reduced efficacy and increased incidence of breakthrough bleeding and menstrual irregularities). Products include:
- Fulvicin P/G Tablets ... 2359
- Fulvicin P/G 165 & 330 Tablets ... 2359
- Grifulvin V (griseofulvin tablets) Microsize (griseofulvin oral suspension) Microsize ... 1888
- Gris-PEG Tablets, 125 mg & 250 mg ... 479

Mephobarbital (Potential for reduced efficacy and increased incidence of breakthrough bleeding and menstrual irregularities). Products include:
- Mebaral Tablets ... 2322

Methacycline Hydrochloride (Potential for reduced efficacy and increased incidence of breakthrough bleeding and menstrual irregularities).
- No products indexed under this heading.

Minocycline Hydrochloride (Potential for reduced efficacy and increased incidence of breakthrough bleeding and menstrual irregularities). Products include:
- Dynacin Capsules ... 1590
- Minocin Intravenous ... 1382
- Minocin Oral Suspension ... 1385
- Minocin Pellet-Filled Capsules ... 1383

Oxytetracycline Hydrochloride (Potential for reduced efficacy and increased incidence of breakthrough bleeding and menstrual irregularities). Products include:
- TERAK Ointment ... ⊙ 209
- Terra-Cortril Ophthalmic Suspension ... 2210
- Terramycin with Polymyxin B Sulfate Ophthalmic Ointment ... 2211
- Urobiotic-250 Capsules ... 2214

Pentobarbital Sodium (Potential for reduced efficacy and increased incidence of breakthrough bleeding and menstrual irregularities). Products include:
- Nembutal Sodium Capsules ... 436
- Nembutal Sodium Solution ... 438
- Nembutal Sodium Suppositories ... 440

Phenobarbital (Potential for reduced efficacy and increased incidence of breakthrough bleeding and menstrual irregularities). Products include:
- Arco-Lase Plus Tablets ... 512
- Bellergal-S Tablets ... 2250
- Donnatal ... 2060
- Donnatal Extentabs ... 2061
- Donnatal Tablets ... 2060
- Phenobarbital Elixir and Tablets ... 1469
- Quadrinal Tablets ... 1350

Phenylbutazone (Potential for reduced efficacy and increased incidence of breakthrough bleeding and menstrual irregularities).
- No products indexed under this heading.

Phenytoin (Potential for reduced efficacy and increased incidence of breakthrough bleeding and menstrual irregularities). Products include:
- Dilantin Infatabs ... 1908
- Dilantin-125 Suspension ... 1911

Phenytoin Sodium (Potential for reduced efficacy and increased incidence of breakthrough bleeding and menstrual irregularities). Products include:
- Dilantin Kapseals ... 1906
- Dilantin Parenteral ... 1910

Rifampin (Concomitant use results in reduced efficacy and increased incidence of breakthrough bleeding and menstrual irregularities). Products include:
- Rifadin ... 1528
- Rifamate Capsules ... 1530
- Rifater ... 1532
- Rimactane Capsules ... 847

Secobarbital Sodium (Potential for reduced efficacy and increased incidence of breakthrough bleeding and menstrual irregularities). Products include:
- Seconal Sodium Pulvules ... 1474

Tetracycline Hydrochloride (Potential for reduced efficacy and increased incidence of breakthrough bleeding and menstrual irregularities). Products include:
- Achromycin V Capsules ... 1367

Thiamylal Sodium (Potential for reduced efficacy and increased incidence of breakthrough bleeding and menstrual irregularities).
No products indexed under this heading.

ORTHO-NOVUM 7/7/7 □28 TABLETS
(Norethindrone, Ethinyl Estradiol)......1872
See **Ortho-Novum 7/7/7 □21 Tablets**

ORTHO-NOVUM 10/11□21 TABLETS
(Norethindrone, Ethinyl Estradiol)......1872
See **Ortho-Novum 7/7/7 □21 Tablets**

ORTHO-NOVUM 10/11□28 TABLETS
(Norethindrone, Ethinyl Estradiol)......1872
See **Ortho-Novum 7/7/7 □21 Tablets**

ORTHO TRI-CYCLEN 21 TABLETS
(Norgestimate, Ethinyl Estradiol)........1858
See **Ortho-Cyclen 21 Tablets**

ORTHO TRI-CYCLEN 28 TABLETS
(Norgestimate, Ethinyl Estradiol)........1858
See **Ortho-Cyclen 21 Tablets**

ORTHO-WHITE DIAPHRAGM KIT-FLAT SPRING (SEE ALSO ORTHO DIAPHRAGM KITS)
(Diaphragm)..1865
None cited in PDR database.

ORTHOCLONE OKT3 STERILE SOLUTION
(Muromonab-CD3) 1837
May interact with corticosteroids and certain other agents. Compounds in these categories include:

Azathioprine (Infection or malignancies have been reported with azathioprine alone and in conjunction with muromonab-CD3). Products include:
Imuran 1110

Betamethasone Acetate (Psychosis and infection have been reported in patients treated with corticosteroids alone and in conjunction with muromonab-CD3). Products include:
Celestone Soluspan Suspension 2347

Betamethasone Sodium Phosphate (Psychosis and infection have been reported in patients treated with corticosteroids alone and in conjunction with muromonab-CD3). Products include:
Celestone Soluspan Suspension 2347

Cortisone Acetate (Psychosis and infection have been reported in patients treated with corticosteroids alone and in conjunction with muromonab-CD3). Products include:
Cortone Acetate Sterile Suspension 1623
Cortone Acetate Tablets.................. 1624

Cyclosporine (Seizures, encephalopathy, infections, malignancies, and thrombotic events have been reported in patients receiving cyclosporine alone and in conjunction with muromonab-CD3). Products include:
Neoral 2276
Sandimmune 2286

Dexamethasone (Psychosis and infection have been reported in patients treated with corticosteroids alone and in conjunction with muromonab-CD3). Products include:
AK-Trol Ointment & Suspension .... ⊙ 205
Decadron Elixir 1633
Decadron Tablets................................ 1635
Decaspray Topical Aerosol 1648
Dexacidin Ointment .... ⊙ 263
Maxitrol Ophthalmic Ointment and Suspension .... ⊙ 224
TobraDex Ophthalmic Suspension and Ointment.................................... 473

Dexamethasone Acetate (Psychosis and infection have been reported in patients treated with corticosteroids alone and in conjunction with muromonab-CD3). Products include:
Dalalone D.P. Injectable 1011
Decadron-LA Sterile Suspension...... 1646

Dexamethasone Sodium Phosphate (Psychosis and infection have been reported in patients treated with corticosteroids alone and in conjunction with muromonab-CD3). Products include:
Decadron Phosphate Injection 1637
Decadron Phosphate Respihaler 1642
Decadron Phosphate Sterile Ophthalmic Ointment 1641
Decadron Phosphate Sterile Ophthalmic Solution 1642
Decadron Phosphate Topical Cream 1644
Decadron Phosphate Turbinaire 1645
Decadron Phosphate with Xylocaine Injection, Sterile 1639
Dexacort Phosphate in Respihaler .. 458
Dexacort Phosphate in Turbinaire .. 459
NeoDecadron Sterile Ophthalmic Ointment 1712
NeoDecadron Sterile Ophthalmic Solution 1713
NeoDecadron Topical Cream 1714

Fludrocortisone Acetate (Psychosis and infection have been reported in patients treated with corticosteroids alone and in conjunction with muromonab-CD-3). Products include:
Florinef Acetate Tablets 505

Hydrocortisone (Psychosis and infection have been reported in patients treated with corticosteroids alone and in conjunction with muromonab-CD3). Products include:
Anusol-HC Cream 2.5% 1896
Aquanil HC Lotion 1931
Bactine Hydrocortisone Anti-Itch Cream .... ▣ 709
Caldecort Anti-Itch Hydrocortisone Spray .... ▣ 631
Cortaid .... ▣ 836
CORTENEMA...................................... 2535
Cortisporin Ointment 1085
Cortisporin Ophthalmic Ointment Sterile 1085
Cortisporin Ophthalmic Suspension Sterile 1086
Cortisporin Otic Solution Sterile 1087
Cortisporin Otic Suspension Sterile 1088
Cortizone-5 .... ▣ 831
Cortizone-10 .... ▣ 831
Hydrocortone Tablets 1672
Hytone 907
Massengill Medicated Soft Cloth Towelettes.. 2458
PediOtic Suspension Sterile 1153
Preparation H Hydrocortisone 1% Cream .... ▣ 872
ProctoCream-HC 2.5% 2408
VōSoL HC Otic Solution.................... 2678

Hydrocortisone Acetate (Psychosis and infection have been reported in patients treated with corticosteroids alone and in conjunction with muromonab-CD3). Products include:
Analpram-HC Rectal Cream 1% and 2.5% 977
Anusol HC-1 Anti-Itch Hydrocortisone Ointment .... ▣ 847
Anusol-HC Suppositories 1897
Caldecort.. ▣ 631
Carmol HC 924
Coly-Mycin S Otic w/Neomycin & Hydrocortisone 1906
Cortaid .... ▣ 836
Cortifoam 2396
Cortisporin Cream.............................. 1084
Epifoam 2399
Hydrocortone Acetate Sterile Suspension.. 1669
Mantadil Cream 1135
Nupercainal Hydrocortisone 1% Cream .... ▣ 645
Ophthocort .... ⊙ 311
Pramosone Cream, Lotion & Ointment 978
ProctoCream-HC 2408
ProctoFoam-HC 2409
Terra-Cortril Ophthalmic Suspension 2210

Hydrocortisone Sodium Phosphate (Psychosis and infection have been reported in patients treated with corticosteroids alone and in conjunction with muromonab-CD3). Products include:
Hydrocortone Phosphate Injection, Sterile 1670

Hydrocortisone Sodium Succinate (Psychosis and infection have been reported in patients treated with corticosteroids alone and in conjunction with muromonab-CD3). Products include:
Solu-Cortef Sterile Powder................ 2641

Indomethacin (Encephalopathy and other CNS effects have been reported in patients treated with indomethacin alone and in conjunction with muromonab-CD3). Products include:
Indocin 1680

Indomethacin Sodium Trihydrate (Encephalopathy and other CNS effects have been reported in patients treated with indomethacin alone and in conjunction with muromonab-CD3). Products include:
Indocin I.V. 1684

Methylprednisolone Acetate (Psychosis and infection have been reported in patients treated with corticosteroids alone and in conjunction with muromonab-CD3). Products include:
Depo-Medrol Single-Dose Vial 2600
Depo-Medrol Sterile Aqueous Suspension.. 2597

Methylprednisolone Sodium Succinate (Psychosis and infection have been reported in patients treated with corticosteroids alone and in conjunction with muromonab-CD3). Products include:
Solu-Medrol Sterile Powder................ 2643

Prednisolone Acetate (Psychosis and infection have been reported in patients treated with corticosteroids alone and in conjunction with muromonab-CD3). Products include:
AK-CIDE .... ⊙ 202
AK-CIDE Ointment.......................... ⊙ 202
Blephamide Liquifilm Sterile Ophthalmic Suspension 476
Blephamide Ointment .... ⊙ 237
Econopred & Econopred Plus Ophthalmic Suspensions .... ⊙ 217
Poly-Pred Liquifilm .... ⊙ 248
Pred Forte.. ⊙ 250
Pred Mild.. ⊙ 253
Pred-G Liquifilm Sterile Ophthalmic Suspension .... ⊙ 251
Pred-G S.O.P. Sterile Ophthalmic Ointment .... ⊙ 252
Vasocidin Ointment .... ⊙ 268

Prednisolone Sodium Phosphate (Psychosis and infection have been reported in patients treated with corticosteroids alone and in conjunction with muromonab-CD3). Products include:
AK-Pred .... ⊙ 204
Hydeltrasol Injection, Sterile 1665
Inflamase.. ⊙ 265
Pediapred Oral Liquid 995
Vasocidin Ophthalmic Solution ...... ⊙ 270

Prednisolone Tebutate (Psychosis and infection have been reported in patients treated with corticosteroids alone and in conjunction with muromonab-CD3). Products include:
Hydeltra-T.B.A. Sterile Suspension 1667

Prednisone (Psychosis and infection have been reported in patients treated with corticosteroids alone and in conjunction with muromonab-CD3). Products include:
Deltasone Tablets 2595

Triamcinolone (Psychosis and infection have been reported in patients treated with corticosteroids alone and in conjunction with muromonab-CD3). Products include:
Aristocort Tablets 1022

Triamcinolone Acetonide (Psychosis and infection have been reported in patients treated with corticosteroids alone and in conjunction with muromonab-CD3). Products include:
Aristocort A 0.025% Cream 1027
Aristocort A 0.5% Cream 1031
Aristocort A 0.1% Cream 1029
Aristocort A 0.1% Ointment 1030
Azmacort Oral Inhaler 2011
Nasacort Nasal Inhaler 2024

Triamcinolone Diacetate (Psychosis and infection have been reported in patients treated with corticosteroids alone and in conjunction with muromonab-CD3). Products include:
Aristocort Suspension (Forte Parenteral).. 1027
Aristocort Suspension (Intralesional).. 1025

Triamcinolone Hexacetonide (Psychosis and infection have been reported in patients treated with corticosteroids alone and in conjunction with muromonab-CD3). Products include:
Aristospan Suspension (Intra-articular) 1033
Aristospan Suspension (Intralesional).. 1032

ORUDIS CAPSULES
(Ketoprofen) 2766
May interact with lithium preparations, diuretics, and certain other agents. Compounds in these categories include:

Amiloride Hydrochloride (Reduced urinary potassium and chloride excretion). Products include:
Midamor Tablets 1703
Moduretic Tablets 1705

Aspirin (Decreased protein-binding and increased plasma clearance of ketoprofen). Products include:
Alka-Seltzer Effervescent Antacid and Pain Reliever .... ▣ 701
Alka-Seltzer Extra Strength Effervescent Antacid and Pain Reliever .... ▣ 703
Alka-Seltzer Lemon Lime Effervescent Antacid and Pain Reliever .... ▣ 703
Alka-Seltzer Plus Cold Medicine .... ▣ 705
Alka-Seltzer Plus Cold & Cough Medicine .... ▣ 708
Alka-Seltzer Plus Night-Time Cold Medicine .... ▣ 707
Alka Seltzer Plus Sinus Medicine .. ▣ 707
Arthritis Foundation Safety Coated Aspirin Tablets .... ▣ 675
Arthritis Pain Ascriptin .... ▣ 631
Maximum Strength Ascriptin .... ▣ 630
Regular Strength Ascriptin Tablets .... ▣ 629
Arthritis Strength BC Powder.......... ▣ 609
BC Cold Powder Multi-Symptom Formula (Cold-Sinus-Allergy) .... ▣ 609

IMPORTANT NOTE: Always consult each drug listing in the patient's regimen for possible interactions.

Orudis/Oruvail **Interactions Index** 774

BC Cold Powder Non-Drowsy Formula (Cold-Sinus) ▣ 609
BC Powder ▣ 609
Bayer Children's Chewable Aspirin ▣ 711
Genuine Bayer Aspirin Tablets & Caplets ▣ 713
Extra Strength Bayer Arthritis Pain Regimen Formula ▣ 711
Extra Strength Bayer Aspirin Caplets & Tablets ▣ 712
Extended-Release Bayer 8-Hour Aspirin ▣ 712
Extra Strength Bayer Plus Aspirin Caplets ▣ 713
Extra Strength Bayer PM Aspirin .. ▣ 713
Bayer Enteric Aspirin ▣ 709
Bufferin Analgesic Tablets and Caplets ▣ 613
Arthritis Strength Bufferin Analgesic Caplets ▣ 614
Extra Strength Bufferin Analgesic Tablets ▣ 615
Cama Arthritis Pain Reliever ▣ 785
Darvon Compound-65 Pulvules 1435
Easprin 1914
Ecotrin 2455
Ecotrin Enteric Coated Aspirin Maximum Strength Tablets and Caplets ▣ 816
Ecotrin Enteric Coated Aspirin Regular Strength Tablets 2455
Empirin Aspirin Tablets ▣ 854
Empirin with Codeine Tablets 1093
Excedrin Extra-Strength Analgesic Tablets & Caplets 732
Fiorinal Capsules 2261
Fiorinal with Codeine Capsules 2262
Fiorinal Tablets 2261
Halfprin 1362
Healthprin Aspirin 2455
Norgesic 1496
Percodan Tablets 939
Percodan-Demi Tablets 940
Robaxisal Tablets 2071
Soma Compound w/Codeine Tablets 2676
Soma Compound Tablets 2675
St. Joseph Adult Chewable Aspirin (81 mg.) ▣ 808
Talwin Compound 2335
Ursinus Inlay-Tabs ▣ 794
Vanquish Analgesic Caplets ▣ 731

Bendroflumethiazide (Reduced urinary potassium and chloride excretion).
No products indexed under this heading.

Bumetanide (Reduced urinary potassium and chloride excretion). Products include:
Bumex 2093

Chlorothiazide (Reduced urinary potassium and chloride excretion). Products include:
Aldoclor Tablets 1598
Diupres Tablets 1650
Diuril Oral 1653

Chlorothiazide Sodium (Reduced urinary potassium and chloride excretion). Products include:
Diuril Sodium Intravenous 1652

Chlorthalidone (Reduced urinary potassium and chloride excretion). Products include:
Combipres Tablets 677
Tenoretic Tablets 2845
Thalitone 1245

Ethacrynic Acid (Reduced urinary potassium and chloride excretion). Products include:
Edecrin Tablets 1657

Furosemide (Reduced urinary potassium and chloride excretion). Products include:
Lasix Injection, Oral Solution and Tablets 1240

Hydrochlorothiazide (Reduced urinary potassium and chloride excretion). Products include:
Aldactazide 2413
Aldoril Tablets 1604
Apresazide Capsules 808
Capozide 742
Dyazide 2479
Esidrix Tablets 821
Esimil Tablets 822
HydroDIURIL Tablets 1674
Hydropres Tablets 1675
Hyzaar Tablets 1677
Inderide Tablets 2732
Inderide LA Long Acting Capsules .. 2734
Lopressor HCT Tablets 832
Lotensin HCT 837
Maxzide 1380
Moduretic Tablets 1705
Oretic Tablets 443
Prinzide Tablets 1737
Ser-Ap-Es Tablets 849
Timolide Tablets 1748
Vaseretic Tablets 1765
Zestoretic 2850
Ziac 1415

Hydroflumethiazide (Reduced urinary potassium and chloride excretion). Products include:
Diucardin Tablets 2718

Indapamide (Reduced urinary potassium and chloride excretion). Products include:
Lozol Tablets 2022

Lithium Carbonate (Increased steady-state plasma lithium levels). Products include:
Eskalith 2485
Lithium Carbonate Capsules & Tablets 2230
Lithonate/Lithotabs/Lithobid 2543

Lithium Citrate (Increased steady-state plasma lithium levels).
No products indexed under this heading.

Methotrexate Sodium (Increased toxicity; avoid coadministration). Products include:
Methotrexate Sodium Tablets, Injection, for Injection and LPF Injection 1275

Methyclothiazide (Reduced urinary potassium and chloride excretion). Products include:
Enduron Tablets 420

Metolazone (Reduced urinary potassium and chloride excretion). Products include:
Mykrox Tablets 993
Zaroxolyn Tablets 1000

Polythiazide (Reduced urinary potassium and chloride excretion). Products include:
Minizide Capsules 1938

Probenecid (Decreased protein-binding and increased plasma clearance of ketoprofen). Products include:
Benemid Tablets 1611
ColBENEMID Tablets 1622

Spironolactone (Reduced urinary potassium and chloride excretion). Products include:
Aldactazide 2413
Aldactone 2414

Torsemide (Reduced urinary potassium and chloride excretion). Products include:
Demadex Tablets and Injection 686

Triamterene (Reduced urinary potassium and chloride excretion). Products include:
Dyazide 2479
Dyrenium Capsules 2481
Maxzide 1380

Warfarin Sodium (Concurrent therapy requires close monitoring of patients on both drugs). Products include:
Coumadin 926

Food Interactions

Food, unspecified (Slows rate of absorption resulting in delayed and reduced peak concentrations).

ORUVAIL CAPSULES
(Ketoprofen) 2766
See **Orudis Capsules**

OSCILLOCOCCINUM
(Homeopathic Medications) ▣ 612
None cited in PDR database.

OSM_GLYN ORAL OSMOTIC AGENT
(Glycerin) ⊙ 226
None cited in PDR database.

OSMOLITE ISOTONIC LIQUID NUTRITION
(Nutritional Supplement) 2222
None cited in PDR database.

OSMOLITE HN HIGH NITROGEN ISOTONIC LIQUID NUTRITION
(Nutritional Supplement) 2222
None cited in PDR database.

OTIC DOMEBORO SOLUTION
(Acetic Acid) 611
None cited in PDR database.

OTRIVIN NASAL DROPS
(Xylometazoline Hydrochloride) ▣ 645
None cited in PDR database.

OTRIVIN PEDIATRIC NASAL DROPS
(Xylometazoline Hydrochloride) ▣ 645
None cited in PDR database.

OVCON 35
(Norethindrone, Ethinyl Estradiol) 760
May interact with barbiturates, tetracyclines, and certain other agents. Compounds in these categories include:

Ampicillin (Possibility for reduced efficacy and increased breakthrough bleeding and menstrual irregularities with concomitant use). Products include:
Omnipen Capsules 2764
Omnipen for Oral Suspension 2765

Ampicillin Sodium (Possibility for reduced efficacy and increased breakthrough bleeding and menstrual irregularities with concomitant use). Products include:
Unasyn 2212

Aprobarbital (Potential for reduced efficacy and increased breakthrough bleeding and menstrual irregularities with concomitant use).
No products indexed under this heading.

Butabarbital (Potential for reduced efficacy and increased breakthrough bleeding and menstrual irregularities with concomitant use).
No products indexed under this heading.

Butalbital (Potential for reduced efficacy and increased breakthrough bleeding and menstrual irregularities with concomitant use). Products include:
Esgic-plus Tablets 1013
Fioricet Tablets 2258
Fioricet with Codeine Capsules 2260
Fiorinal Capsules 2261
Fiorinal with Codeine Capsules 2262
Fiorinal Tablets 2261
Phrenilin 785
Sedapap Tablets 50 mg/650 mg .. 1543

Demeclocycline Hydrochloride (Possibility for reduced efficacy and increased breakthrough bleeding and menstrual irregularities with concomitant use of tetracyclines). Products include:
Declomycin Tablets 1371

Doxycycline Calcium (Possibility for reduced efficacy and increased breakthrough bleeding and menstrual irregularities with concomitant use of tetracyclines). Products include:
Vibramycin Calcium Oral Suspension Syrup 1941

Doxycycline Hyclate (Possibility for reduced efficacy and increased breakthrough bleeding and menstrual irregularities with concomitant use of tetracyclines). Products include:
Doryx Capsules 1913
Vibramycin Hyclate Capsules 1941
Vibramycin Hyclate Intravenous 2215
Vibra-Tabs Film Coated Tablets 1941

Doxycycline Monohydrate (Possibility for reduced efficacy and increased breakthrough bleeding and menstrual irregularities with concomitant use of tetracyclines). Products include:
Monodox Capsules 1805
Vibramycin Monohydrate for Oral Suspension 1941

Griseofulvin (Possibility for reduced efficacy and increased breakthrough bleeding and menstrual irregularities with concomitant use). Products include:
Fulvicin P/G Tablets 2359
Fulvicin P/G 165 & 330 Tablets 2359
Grifulvin V (griseofulvin tablets) Microsize (griseofulvin oral suspension) Microsize 1888
Gris-PEG Tablets, 125 mg & 250 mg 479

Mephobarbital (Potential for reduced efficacy and increased breakthrough bleeding and menstrual irregularities with concomitant use). Products include:
Mebaral Tablets 2322

Methacycline Hydrochloride (Possibility for reduced efficacy and increased breakthrough bleeding and menstrual irregularities with concomitant use of tetracyclines).
No products indexed under this heading.

Minocycline Hydrochloride (Possibility for reduced efficacy and increased breakthrough bleeding and menstrual irregularities with concomitant use of tetracyclines). Products include:
Dynacin Capsules 1590
Minocin Intravenous 1382
Minocin Oral Suspension 1385
Minocin Pellet-Filled Capsules 1383

Oxytetracycline Hydrochloride (Possibility for reduced efficacy and increased breakthrough bleeding and menstrual irregularities with concomitant use of tetracyclines). Products include:
TERAK Ointment ⊙ 209
Terra-Cortril Ophthalmic Suspension 2210
Terramycin with Polymyxin B Sulfate Ophthalmic Ointment 2211
Urobiotic-250 Capsules 2214

Pentobarbital Sodium (Potential for reduced efficacy and increased breakthrough bleeding and menstrual irregularities with concomitant use). Products include:
Nembutal Sodium Capsules 436
Nembutal Sodium Solution 438
Nembutal Sodium Suppositories 440

Phenobarbital (Potential for reduced efficacy and increased breakthrough bleeding and menstrual irregularities with concomitant use). Products include:
Arco-Lase Plus Tablets 512
Bellergal-S Tablets 2250
Donnatal 2060
Donnatal Extentabs 2061

(▣ Described in PDR For Nonprescription Drugs) (⊙ Described in PDR For Ophthalmology)

775 **Interactions Index** **Oxsoralen Lotion**

Donnatal Tablets ... 2060
Phenobarbital Elixir and Tablets ... 1469
Quadrinal Tablets ... 1350

Phenylbutazone (Potential for reduced efficacy and increased breakthrough bleeding and menstrual irregularities with concomitant use).
No products indexed under this heading.

Phenytoin (Potential for reduced efficacy and increased breakthrough bleeding and menstrual irregularities with concomitant use). Products include:
Dilantin Infatabs ... 1908
Dilantin-125 Suspension ... 1911

Phenytoin Sodium (Potential for reduced efficacy and increased breakthrough bleeding and menstrual irregularities with concomitant use). Products include:
Dilantin Kapseals ... 1906
Dilantin Parenteral ... 1910

Rifampin (Potential for reduced efficacy and increased breakthrough bleeding and menstrual irregularities with concomitant use). Products include:
Rifadin ... 1528
Rifamate Capsules ... 1530
Rifater ... 1532
Rimactane Capsules ... 847

Secobarbital Sodium (Potential for reduced efficacy and increased breakthrough bleeding and menstrual irregularities with concomitant use). Products include:
Seconal Sodium Pulvules ... 1474

Tetracycline Hydrochloride (Possibility for reduced efficacy and increased breakthrough bleeding and menstrual irregularities with concomitant use of tetracyclines). Products include:
Achromycin V Capsules ... 1367

Thiamylal Sodium (Potential for reduced efficacy and increased breakthrough bleeding and menstrual irregularities with concomitant use).
No products indexed under this heading.

OVCON 50
(Norethindrone, Ethinyl Estradiol) ... 760
See **Ovcon 35**

OVRAL TABLETS
(Norgestrel, Ethinyl Estradiol) ... 2770
See **Lo/Ovral Tablets**

OVRAL-28 TABLETS
(Norgestrel, Ethinyl Estradiol) ... 2770
See **Lo/Ovral Tablets**

OVRETTE TABLETS
(Norgestrel) ... 2771
See **Lo/Ovral Tablets**

OXANDRIN
(Oxandrolone) ... 2862
May interact with oral anticoagulants, oral hypoglycemic agents, corticosteroids, and certain other agents. Compounds in these categories include:

Acarbose (Oxandrolone may inhibit the metabolism of oral hypoglycemic agents).
No products indexed under this heading.

ACTH (Increased risk of edema).
No products indexed under this heading.

Betamethasone Acetate (Increased risk of edema). Products include:
Celestone Soluspan Suspension ... 2347

Betamethasone Sodium Phosphate (Increased risk of edema). Products include:
Celestone Soluspan Suspension ... 2347

Chlorpropamide (Oxandrolone may inhibit the metabolism of oral hypoglycemic agents). Products include:
Diabinese Tablets ... 1935

Cortisone Acetate (Increased risk of edema). Products include:
Cortone Acetate Sterile Suspension ... 1623
Cortone Acetate Tablets ... 1624

Dexamethasone (Increased risk of edema). Products include:
AK-Trol Ointment & Suspension ... ⊙ 205
Decadron Elixir ... 1633
Decadron Tablets ... 1635
Decaspray Topical Aerosol ... 1648
Dexacidin Ointment ... ⊙ 263
Maxitrol Ophthalmic Ointment and Suspension ... ⊙ 224
TobraDex Ophthalmic Suspension and Ointment ... 473

Dexamethasone Acetate (Increased risk of edema). Products include:
Dalalone D.P. Injectable ... 1011
Decadron-LA Sterile Suspension ... 1646

Dexamethasone Sodium Phosphate (Increased risk of edema). Products include:
Decadron Phosphate Injection ... 1637
Decadron Phosphate Respihaler ... 1642
Decadron Phosphate Sterile Ophthalmic Ointment ... 1641
Decadron Phosphate Sterile Ophthalmic Solution ... 1642
Decadron Phosphate Topical Cream ... 1644
Decadron Phosphate Turbinaire ... 1645
Decadron Phosphate with Xylocaine Injection, Sterile ... 1639
Dexacort Phosphate in Respihaler .. 458
Dexacort Phosphate in Turbinaire .. 459
NeoDecadron Sterile Ophthalmic Ointment ... 1712
NeoDecadron Sterile Ophthalmic Solution ... 1713
NeoDecadron Topical Cream ... 1714

Dicumarol (Anabolic steroids may increase the sensitivity to oral anticoagulants; dosage of the anticoagulants may have to be decreased in order to maintain desired prothrombin time).
No products indexed under this heading.

Fludrocortisone Acetate (Increased risk of edema). Products include:
Florinef Acetate Tablets ... 505

Glipizide (Oxandrolone may inhibit the metabolism of oral hypoglycemic agents). Products include:
Glucotrol Tablets ... 1967
Glucotrol XL Extended Release Tablets ... 1968

Glyburide (Oxandrolone may inhibit the metabolism of oral hypoglycemic agents). Products include:
DiaBeta Tablets ... 1239
Glynase PresTab Tablets ... 2609
Micronase Tablets ... 2623

Hydrocortisone (Increased risk of edema). Products include:
Anusol-HC Cream 2.5% ... 1896
Aquanil HC Lotion ... 1931
Bactine Hydrocortisone Anti-Itch Cream ... ◘ 709
Caldecort Anti-Itch Hydrocortisone Spray ... ◘ 631
Cortaid ... ◘ 836
CORTENEMA ... 2535
Cortisporin Ointment ... 1085
Cortisporin Ophthalmic Ointment Sterile ... 1085
Cortisporin Ophthalmic Suspension Sterile ... 1086
Cortisporin Otic Solution Sterile ... 1087
Cortisporin Otic Suspension Sterile 1088
Cortizone-5 ... ◘ 831
Cortizone-10 ... ◘ 831
Hydrocortone Tablets ... 1672
Hytone ... 907
Massengill Medicated Soft Cloth Towelettes ... 2458
PediOtic Suspension Sterile ... 1153
Preparation H Hydrocortisone 1% Cream ... ◘ 872
ProctoCream-HC 2.5% ... 2408
VōSoL HC Otic Solution ... 2678

Hydrocortisone Acetate (Increased risk of edema). Products include:
Analpram-HC Rectal Cream 1% and 2.5% ... 977
Anusol HC-1 Anti-Itch Hydrocortisone Ointment ... ◘ 847
Anusol-HC Suppositories ... 1897
Caldecort ... ◘ 631
Carmol HC ... 924
Coly-Mycin S Otic w/Neomycin & Hydrocortisone ... 1906
Cortaid ... ◘ 836
Cortifoam ... 2396
Cortisporin Cream ... 1084
Epifoam ... 2399
Hydrocortone Acetate Sterile Suspension ... 1669
Mantadil Cream ... 1135
Nupercainal Hydrocortisone 1% Cream ... ◘ 645
Ophthocort ... ⊙ 311
Pramosone Cream, Lotion & Ointment ... 978
ProctoCream-HC ... 2408
ProctoFoam-HC ... 2409
Terra-Cortril Ophthalmic Suspension ... 2210

Hydrocortisone Sodium Phosphate (Increased risk of edema). Products include:
Hydrocortone Phosphate Injection, Sterile ... 1670

Hydrocortisone Sodium Succinate (Increased risk of edema). Products include:
Solu-Cortef Sterile Powder ... 2641

Metformin Hydrochloride (Oxandrolone may inhibit the metabolism of oral hypoglycemic agents). Products include:
Glucophage ... 752

Methylprednisolone Acetate (Increased risk of edema). Products include:
Depo-Medrol Single-Dose Vial ... 2600
Depo-Medrol Sterile Aqueous Suspension ... 2597

Methylprednisolone Sodium Succinate (Increased risk of edema). Products include:
Solu-Medrol Sterile Powder ... 2643

Prednisolone Acetate (Increased risk of edema). Products include:
AK-CIDE ... ⊙ 202
AK-CIDE Ointment ... ⊙ 202
Blephamide Liquifilm Sterile Ophthalmic Suspension ... 476
Blephamide Ointment ... ⊙ 237
Econopred & Econopred Plus Ophthalmic Suspensions ... ⊙ 217
Poly-Pred Liquifilm ... ⊙ 248
Pred Forte ... ⊙ 250
Pred Mild ... ⊙ 253
Pred-G Liquifilm Sterile Ophthalmic Suspension ... ⊙ 251
Pred-G S.O.P. Sterile Ophthalmic Ointment ... ⊙ 252
Vasocidin Ointment ... ⊙ 268

Prednisolone Sodium Phosphate (Increased risk of edema). Products include:
AK-Pred ... ⊙ 204
Hydeltrasol Injection, Sterile ... 1665
Inflamase ... ⊙ 265
Pediapred Oral Liquid ... 995
Vasocidin Ophthalmic Solution ... ⊙ 270

Prednisolone Tebutate (Increased risk of edema). Products include:
Hydeltra-T.B.A. Sterile Suspension 1667

Prednisone (Increased risk of edema). Products include:
Deltasone Tablets ... 2595

Tolazamide (Oxandrolone may inhibit the metabolism of oral hypoglycemic agents).
No products indexed under this heading.

Tolbutamide (Oxandrolone may inhibit the metabolism of oral hypoglycemic agents).
No products indexed under this heading.

Triamcinolone (Increased risk of edema). Products include:
Aristocort Tablets ... 1022

Triamcinolone Acetonide (Increased risk of edema). Products include:
Aristocort A 0.025% Cream ... 1027
Aristocort A 0.5% Cream ... 1031
Aristocort A 0.1% Cream ... 1029
Aristocort A 0.1% Ointment ... 1030
Azmacort Oral Inhaler ... 2011
Nasacort Nasal Inhaler ... 2024

Triamcinolone Diacetate (Increased risk of edema). Products include:
Aristocort Suspension (Forte Parenteral) ... 1027
Aristocort Suspension (Intralesional) ... 1025

Triamcinolone Hexacetonide (Increased risk of edema). Products include:
Aristospan Suspension (Intra-articular) ... 1033
Aristospan Suspension (Intralesional) ... 1032

Warfarin Sodium (Anabolic steroids may increase the sensitivity to oral anticoagulants; dosage of the anticoagulants may have to be decreased in order to maintain desired prothrombin time). Products include:
Coumadin ... 926

OXISTAT CREAM
(Oxiconazole Nitrate) ... 1152
None cited in PDR database.

OXISTAT LOTION
(Oxiconazole Nitrate) ... 1152
None cited in PDR database.

OXSORALEN LOTION 1%
(Methoxsalen) ... 1256
May interact with phenothiazines, sulfonamides, tetracyclines, thiazides, and certain other agents. Compounds in these categories include:

Anthralin (Possible photosensitivity effects). Products include:
Drithocreme 0.1%, 0.25%, 0.5%, 1.0% (HP) ... 905
Dritho-Scalp 0.25%, 0.5% ... 906

Bendroflumethiazide (Possible photosensitivity effects).
No products indexed under this heading.

Chlorothiazide (Possible photosensitivity effects). Products include:
Aldoclor Tablets ... 1598
Diupres Tablets ... 1650
Diuril Oral ... 1653

Chlorothiazide Sodium (Possible photosensitivity effects). Products include:
Diuril Sodium Intravenous ... 1652

Chlorpromazine (Possible photosensitivity effects). Products include:
Thorazine Suppositories ... 2523

Coal Tar (Possible photosensitivity effects). Products include:
DHS ... 1932
Fototar Cream ... 1253
MG 217 ... ◘ 835
P&S Plus Tar Gel ... ◘ 604
Pentrax Anti-dandruff Shampoo ... 1055
Tegrin Dandruff Shampoo ... ◘ 611
Tegrin Skin Cream & Tegrin Medicated Soap ... ◘ 611

IMPORTANT NOTE: Always consult each drug listing in the patient's regimen for possible interactions.

X-Seb T Pearl Shampoo ⊡ 606
X-Seb T Plus Conditioning Shampoo ⊡ 606

Demeclocycline Hydrochloride (Possible photosensitivity effects). Products include:
Declomycin Tablets 1371

Doxycycline Calcium (Possible photosensitivity effects). Products include:
Vibramycin Calcium Oral Suspension Syrup 1941

Doxycycline Hyclate (Possible photosensitivity effects). Products include:
Doryx Capsules 1913
Vibramycin Hyclate Capsules 1941
Vibramycin Hyclate Intravenous 2215
Vibra-Tabs Film Coated Tablets 1941

Doxycycline Monohydrate (Possible photosensitivity effects). Products include:
Monodox Capsules 1805
Vibramycin Monohydrate for Oral Suspension 1941

Fluphenazine Decanoate (Possible photosensitivity effects). Products include:
Prolixin Decanoate 509

Fluphenazine Enanthate (Possible photosensitivity effects). Products include:
Prolixin Enanthate 509

Fluphenazine Hydrochloride (Possible photosensitivity effects). Products include:
Prolixin 509

Griseofulvin (Possible photosensitivity effects). Products include:
Fulvicin P/G Tablets 2359
Fulvicin P/G 165 & 330 Tablets 2359
Grifulvin V (griseofulvin tablets) Microsize (griseofulvin oral suspension) Microsize 1888
Gris-PEG Tablets, 125 mg & 250 mg 479

Hydrochlorothiazide (Possible photosensitivity effects). Products include:
Aldactazide 2413
Aldoril Tablets 1604
Apresazide Capsules 808
Capozide 742
Dyazide 2479
Esidrix Tablets 821
Esimil Tablets 822
HydroDIURIL Tablets 1674
Hydropres Tablets 1675
Hyzaar Tablets 1677
Inderide Tablets 2732
Inderide LA Long Acting Capsules 2734
Lopressor HCT Tablets 832
Lotensin HCT 837
Maxzide 1380
Moduretic Tablets 1705
Oretic Tablets 443
Prinzide Tablets 1737
Ser-Ap-Es Tablets 849
Timolide Tablets 1748
Vaseretic Tablets 1765
Zestoretic 2850
Ziac 1415

Hydroflumethiazide (Possible photosensitivity effects). Products include:
Diucardin Tablets 2718

Mesoridazine Besylate (Possible photosensitivity effects). Products include:
Serentil 684

Methacycline Hydrochloride (Possible photosensitivity effects).
No products indexed under this heading.

Methotrimeprazine (Possible photosensitivity effects). Products include:
Levoprome 1274

Methyclothiazide (Possible photosensitivity effects). Products include:
Enduron Tablets 420

Methylene Blue (Possible photosensitivity effects). Products include:
Urised Tablets 1964

Minocycline Hydrochloride (Possible photosensitivity effects). Products include:
Dynacin Capsules 1590
Minocin Intravenous 1382
Minocin Oral Suspension 1385
Minocin Pellet-Filled Capsules 1383

Nalidixic Acid (Possible photosensitivity effects). Products include:
NegGram 2323

Oxytetracycline (Possible photosensitivity effects). Products include:
Terramycin Intramuscular Solution 2210

Oxytetracycline Hydrochloride (Possible photosensitivity effects). Products include:
TERAK Ointment ⊙ 209
Terra-Cortril Ophthalmic Suspension 2210
Terramycin with Polymyxin B Sulfate Ophthalmic Ointment 2211
Urobiotic-250 Capsules 2214

Perphenazine (Possible photosensitivity effects). Products include:
Etrafon 2355
Triavil Tablets 1757
Trilafon 2389

Polythiazide (Possible photosensitivity effects). Products include:
Minizide Capsules 1938

Prochlorperazine (Possible photosensitivity effects). Products include:
Compazine 2470

Promethazine Hydrochloride (Possible photosensitivity effects). Products include:
Mepergan Injection 2753
Phenergan with Codeine 2777
Phenergan with Dextromethorphan 2778
Phenergan Injection 2773
Phenergan Suppositories 2775
Phenergan Syrup 2774
Phenergan Tablets 2775
Phenergan VC 2779
Phenergan VC with Codeine 2781

Sulfamethizole (Possible photosensitivity effects). Products include:
Urobiotic-250 Capsules 2214

Sulfamethoxazole (Possible photosensitivity effects). Products include:
Azo Gantanol Tablets 2080
Bactrim DS Tablets 2084
Bactrim I.V. Infusion 2082
Bactrim 2084
Gantanol Tablets 2119
Septra 1174
Septra I.V. Infusion 1169
Septra I.V. Infusion ADD-Vantage Vials 1171
Septra 1174

Sulfasalazine (Possible photosensitivity effects). Products include:
Azulfidine 1949

Sulfinpyrazone (Possible photosensitivity effects). Products include:
Anturane 807

Sulfisoxazole (Possible photosensitivity effects). Products include:
Azo Gantrisin Tablets 2081
Gantrisin Tablets 2120

Sulfisoxazole Diolamine (Possible photosensitivity effects).
No products indexed under this heading.

Tetracycline Hydrochloride (Possible photosensitivity effects). Products include:
Achromycin V Capsules 1367

Thioridazine Hydrochloride (Possible photosensitivity effects). Products include:
Mellaril 2269

Trifluoperazine Hydrochloride (Possible photosensitivity effects). Products include:
Stelazine 2514

OXSORALEN-ULTRA CAPSULES

(Methoxsalen) 1257

May interact with phenothiazines, sulfonamides, tetracyclines, thiazides, and certain other agents. Compounds in these categories include:

Anthralin (Possible photosensitivity effects). Products include:
Drithocreme 0.1%, 0.25%, 0.5%, 1.0% (HP) 905
Dritho-Scalp 0.25%, 0.5% 906

Bendroflumethiazide (Possible photosensitivity effects).
No products indexed under this heading.

Chlorothiazide (Possible photosensitivity effects). Products include:
Aldoclor Tablets 1598
Diupres Tablets 1650
Diuril Oral 1653

Chlorothiazide Sodium (Possible photosensitivity effects). Products include:
Diuril Sodium Intravenous 1652

Chlorpromazine (Possible photosensitivity effects). Products include:
Thorazine Suppositories 2523

Coal Tar (Possible photosensitivity effects). Products include:
DHS 1932
Fototar Cream 1253
MG 217 ⊡ 835
P&S Plus Tar Gel ⊡ 604
Pentrax Anti-dandruff Shampoo 1055
Tegrin Dandruff Shampoo ⊡ 611
Tegrin Skin Cream & Tegrin Medicated Soap ⊡ 611
X-Seb T Pearl Shampoo ⊡ 606
X-Seb T Plus Conditioning Shampoo ⊡ 606

Demeclocycline Hydrochloride (Possible photosensitivity effects). Products include:
Declomycin Tablets 1371

Doxycycline Calcium (Possible photosensitivity effects). Products include:
Vibramycin Calcium Oral Suspension Syrup 1941

Doxycycline Hyclate (Possible photosensitivity effects). Products include:
Doryx Capsules 1913
Vibramycin Hyclate Capsules 1941
Vibramycin Hyclate Intravenous 2215
Vibra-Tabs Film Coated Tablets 1941

Doxycycline Monohydrate (Possible photosensitivity effects). Products include:
Monodox Capsules 1805
Vibramycin Monohydrate for Oral Suspension 1941

Fluphenazine Decanoate (Possible photosensitivity effects). Products include:
Prolixin Decanoate 509

Fluphenazine Enanthate (Possible photosensitivity effects). Products include:
Prolixin Enanthate 509

Fluphenazine Hydrochloride (Possible photosensitivity effects). Products include:
Prolixin 509

Griseofulvin (Possible photosensitivity effects). Products include:
Fulvicin P/G Tablets 2359
Fulvicin P/G 165 & 330 Tablets 2359
Grifulvin V (griseofulvin tablets) Microsize (griseofulvin oral suspension) Microsize 1888
Gris-PEG Tablets, 125 mg & 250 mg 479

Hydrochlorothiazide (Possible photosensitivity effects). Products include:
Aldactazide 2413
Aldoril Tablets 1604
Apresazide Capsules 808
Capozide 742
Dyazide 2479
Esidrix Tablets 821
Esimil Tablets 822
HydroDIURIL Tablets 1674
Hydropres Tablets 1675
Hyzaar Tablets 1677
Inderide Tablets 2732
Inderide LA Long Acting Capsules 2734
Lopressor HCT Tablets 832
Lotensin HCT 837
Maxzide 1380
Moduretic Tablets 1705
Oretic Tablets 443
Prinzide Tablets 1737
Ser-Ap-Es Tablets 849
Timolide Tablets 1748
Vaseretic Tablets 1765
Zestoretic 2850
Ziac 1415

Hydroflumethiazide (Possible photosensitivity effects). Products include:
Diucardin Tablets 2718

Mesoridazine Besylate (Possible photosensitivity effects). Products include:
Serentil 684

Methacycline Hydrochloride (Possible photosensitivity effects).
No products indexed under this heading.

Methotrimeprazine (Possible photosensitivity effects). Products include:
Levoprome 1274

Methyclothiazide (Possible photosensitivity effects). Products include:
Enduron Tablets 420

Methylene Blue (Possible photosensitivity effects). Products include:
Urised Tablets 1964

Minocycline Hydrochloride (Possible photosensitivity effects). Products include:
Dynacin Capsules 1590
Minocin Intravenous 1382
Minocin Oral Suspension 1385
Minocin Pellet-Filled Capsules 1383

Nalidixic Acid (Possible photosensitivity effects). Products include:
NegGram 2323

Oxytetracycline (Possible photosensitivity effects). Products include:
Terramycin Intramuscular Solution 2210

Oxytetracycline Hydrochloride (Possible photosensitivity effects). Products include:
TERAK Ointment ⊙ 209
Terra-Cortril Ophthalmic Suspension 2210
Terramycin with Polymyxin B Sulfate Ophthalmic Ointment 2211
Urobiotic-250 Capsules 2214

Perphenazine (Possible photosensitivity effects). Products include:
Etrafon 2355
Triavil Tablets 1757
Trilafon 2389

Polythiazide (Possible photosensitivity effects). Products include:
Minizide Capsules 1938

Prochlorperazine (Possible photosensitivity effects). Products include:
Compazine 2470

Promethazine Hydrochloride (Possible photosensitivity effects). Products include:
Mepergan Injection 2753
Phenergan with Codeine 2777
Phenergan with Dextromethorphan 2778
Phenergan Injection 2773
Phenergan Suppositories 2775
Phenergan Syrup 2774
Phenergan Tablets 2775
Phenergan VC 2779
Phenergan VC with Codeine 2781

(⊡ Described in PDR For Nonprescription Drugs) (⊙ Described in PDR For Ophthalmology)

Sulfamethizole (Possible photosensitivity effects). Products include:
Urobiotic-250 Capsules ... 2214

Sulfamethoxazole (Possible photosensitivity effects). Products include:
Azo Gantanol Tablets ... 2080
Bactrim DS Tablets ... 2084
Bactrim I.V. Infusion ... 2082
Bactrim ... 2084
Gantanol Tablets ... 2119
Septra ... 1174
Septra I.V. Infusion ... 1169
Septra I.V. Infusion ADD-Vantage Vials ... 1171
Septra ... 1174

Sulfasalazine (Possible photosensitivity effects). Products include:
Azulfidine ... 1949

Sulfinpyrazone (Possible photosensitivity effects). Products include:
Anturane ... 807

Sulfisoxazole (Possible photosensitivity effects). Products include:
Azo Gantrisin Tablets ... 2081
Gantrisin Tablets ... 2120

Sulfisoxazole Diolamine (Possible photosensitivity effects).
No products indexed under this heading.

Tetracycline Hydrochloride (Possible photosensitivity effects). Products include:
Achromycin V Capsules ... 1367

Thioridazine Hydrochloride (Possible photosensitivity effects). Products include:
Mellaril ... 2269

Trifluoperazine Hydrochloride (Possible photosensitivity effects). Products include:
Stelazine ... 2514

OXYTOCIN INJECTION

(Oxytocin) ... 2771
May interact with vasopressors and certain other agents. Compounds in these categories include:

Cyclopropane (Hypotension; maternal sinus bradycardia with abnormal atrioventricular rhythms).

Dopamine Hydrochloride (Severe hypertension).
No products indexed under this heading.

Epinephrine Hydrochloride (Severe hypertension). Products include:
Ana-Kit Anaphylaxis Emergency Treatment Kit ... 617

Metaraminol Bitartrate (Severe hypertension). Products include:
Aramine Injection ... 1609

Methoxamine Hydrochloride (Severe hypertension). Products include:
Vasoxyl Injection ... 1196

Norepinephrine Bitartrate (Severe hypertension). Products include:
Levophed Bitartrate Injection ... 2315

PBZ TABLETS

(Tripelennamine Hydrochloride) ... 845
May interact with central nervous system depressants and certain other agents. Compounds in these categories include:

Alfentanil Hydrochloride (CNS effects may be additive). Products include:
Alfenta Injection ... 1286

Alprazolam (CNS effects may be additive). Products include:
Xanax Tablets ... 2649

Aprobarbital (CNS effects may be additive).
No products indexed under this heading.

Buprenorphine (CNS effects may be additive). Products include:
Buprenex Injectable ... 2006

Buspirone Hydrochloride (CNS effects may be additive). Products include:
BuSpar ... 737

Butabarbital (CNS effects may be additive).
No products indexed under this heading.

Butalbital (CNS effects may be additive). Products include:
Esgic-plus Tablets ... 1013
Fioricet Tablets ... 2258
Fioricet with Codeine Capsules ... 2260
Fiorinal Capsules ... 2261
Fiorinal with Codeine Capsules ... 2262
Fiorinal Tablets ... 2261
Phrenilin ... 785
Sedapap Tablets 50 mg/650 mg ... 1543

Chlordiazepoxide (CNS effects may be additive). Products include:
Libritabs Tablets ... 2177
Limbitrol ... 2180

Chlordiazepoxide Hydrochloride (CNS effects may be additive). Products include:
Librax Capsules ... 2176
Librium Capsules ... 2178
Librium Injectable ... 2179

Chlorpromazine (CNS effects may be additive). Products include:
Thorazine Suppositories ... 2523

Chlorprothixene (CNS effects may be additive).
No products indexed under this heading.

Chlorprothixene Hydrochloride (CNS effects may be additive).
No products indexed under this heading.

Chlorprothixene Lactate (CNS effects may be additive).
No products indexed under this heading.

Clorazepate Dipotassium (CNS effects may be additive). Products include:
Tranxene ... 451

Clozapine (CNS effects may be additive). Products include:
Clozaril Tablets ... 2252

Codeine Phosphate (CNS effects may be additive). Products include:
Actifed with Codeine Cough Syrup ... 1067
Brontex ... 1981
Deconsal C Expectorant Syrup ... 456
Deconsal Pediatric Syrup ... 457
Dimetane-DC Cough Syrup ... 2059
Empirin with Codeine Tablets ... 1093
Fioricet with Codeine Capsules ... 2260
Fiorinal with Codeine Capsules ... 2262
Isoclor Expectorant ... 990
Novahistine DH ... 2462
Novahistine Expectorant ... 2463
Nucofed ... 2051
Phenergan with Codeine ... 2777
Phenergan VC with Codeine ... 2781
Robitussin A-C Syrup ... 2073
Robitussin-DAC Syrup ... 2074
Ryna ... 841
Soma Compound w/Codeine Tablets ... 2676
Tussi-Organidin NR Liquid and S NR Liquid ... 2677
Tylenol with Codeine ... 1583

Desflurane (CNS effects may be additive). Products include:
Suprane ... 1813

Dezocine (CNS effects may be additive). Products include:
Dalgan Injection ... 538

Diazepam (CNS effects may be additive). Products include:
Dizac ... 1809
Valium Injectable ... 2182
Valium Tablets ... 2183
Valrelease Capsules ... 2169

Droperidol (CNS effects may be additive). Products include:
Inapsine Injection ... 1296

Enflurane (CNS effects may be additive).
No products indexed under this heading.

Estazolam (CNS effects may be additive). Products include:
ProSom Tablets ... 449

Ethchlorvynol (CNS effects may be additive). Products include:
Placidyl Capsules ... 448

Ethinamate (CNS effects may be additive).
No products indexed under this heading.

Fentanyl (CNS effects may be additive). Products include:
Duragesic Transdermal System ... 1288

Fentanyl Citrate (CNS effects may be additive). Products include:
Sublimaze Injection ... 1307

Fluphenazine Decanoate (CNS effects may be additive). Products include:
Prolixin Decanoate ... 509

Fluphenazine Enanthate (CNS effects may be additive). Products include:
Prolixin Enanthate ... 509

Fluphenazine Hydrochloride (CNS effects may be additive). Products include:
Prolixin ... 509

Flurazepam Hydrochloride (CNS effects may be additive). Products include:
Dalmane Capsules ... 2173

Glutethimide (CNS effects may be additive).
No products indexed under this heading.

Haloperidol (CNS effects may be additive). Products include:
Haldol Injection, Tablets and Concentrate ... 1575

Haloperidol Decanoate (CNS effects may be additive). Products include:
Haldol Decanoate ... 1577

Hydrocodone Bitartrate (CNS effects may be additive). Products include:
Anexsia 5/500 Elixir ... 1781
Anexia Tablets ... 1782
Codiclear DH Syrup ... 791
Deconamine CX Cough and Cold Liquid and Tablets ... 1319
Duratuss HD Elixir ... 2565
Hycodan Tablets and Syrup ... 930
Hycomine Compound Tablets ... 932
Hycomine ... 931
Hycotuss Expectorant Syrup ... 933
Hydrocet Capsules ... 782
Lorcet 10/650 ... 1018
Lortab ... 2566
Tussend ... 1783
Tussend Expectorant ... 1785
Vicodin Tablets ... 1356
Vicodin ES Tablets ... 1357
Vicodin Tuss Expectorant ... 1358
Zydone Capsules ... 949

Hydrocodone Polistirex (CNS effects may be additive). Products include:
Tussionex Pennkinetic Extended-Release Suspension ... 998

Hydroxyzine Hydrochloride (CNS effects may be additive). Products include:
Atarax Tablets & Syrup ... 2185
Marax Tablets & DF Syrup ... 2200
Vistaril Intramuscular Solution ... 2216

Isoflurane (CNS effects may be additive).
No products indexed under this heading.

Ketamine Hydrochloride (CNS effects may be additive).
No products indexed under this heading.

Levomethadyl Acetate Hydrochloride (CNS effects may be additive). Products include:
Orlamm ... 2239

Levorphanol Tartrate (CNS effects may be additive). Products include:
Levo-Dromoran ... 2129

Lorazepam (CNS effects may be additive). Products include:
Ativan Injection ... 2698
Ativan Tablets ... 2700

Loxapine Hydrochloride (CNS effects may be additive). Products include:
Loxitane ... 1378

Loxapine Succinate (CNS effects may be additive). Products include:
Loxitane Capsules ... 1378

Meperidine Hydrochloride (CNS effects may be additive). Products include:
Demerol ... 2308
Mepergan Injection ... 2753

Mephobarbital (CNS effects may be additive). Products include:
Mebaral Tablets ... 2322

Meprobamate (CNS effects may be additive). Products include:
Miltown Tablets ... 2672
PMB 200 and PMB 400 ... 2783

Mesoridazine Besylate (CNS effects may be additive). Products include:
Serentil ... 684

Methadone Hydrochloride (CNS effects may be additive). Products include:
Methadone Hydrochloride Oral Concentrate ... 2233
Methadone Hydrochloride Oral Solution & Tablets ... 2235

Methohexital Sodium (CNS effects may be additive). Products include:
Brevital Sodium Vials ... 1429

Methotrimeprazine (CNS effects may be additive). Products include:
Levoprome ... 1274

Methoxyflurane (CNS effects may be additive).
No products indexed under this heading.

Midazolam Hydrochloride (CNS effects may be additive). Products include:
Versed Injection ... 2170

Molindone Hydrochloride (CNS effects may be additive). Products include:
Moban Tablets and Concentrate ... 1048

Morphine Sulfate (CNS effects may be additive). Products include:
Astramorph/PF Injection, USP (Preservative-Free) ... 535
Duramorph ... 962
Infumorph 200 and Infumorph 500 Sterile Solutions ... 965
MS Contin Tablets ... 1994
MSIR ... 1997
Oramorph SR (Morphine Sulfate Sustained Release Tablets) ... 2236
RMS Suppositories ... 2657
Roxanol ... 2243

Opium Alkaloids (CNS effects may be additive).
No products indexed under this heading.

Oxazepam (CNS effects may be additive). Products include:
Serax Capsules ... 2810
Serax Tablets ... 2810

IMPORTANT NOTE: Always consult each drug listing in the patient's regimen for possible interactions.

Oxycodone Hydrochloride (CNS effects may be additive). Products include:

- Percocet Tablets ... 938
- Percodan Tablets ... 939
- Percodan-Demi Tablets ... 940
- Roxicodone Tablets, Oral Solution & Intensol (Oxycodone) ... 2244
- Tylox Capsules ... 1584

Pentobarbital Sodium (CNS effects may be additive). Products include:

- Nembutal Sodium Capsules ... 436
- Nembutal Sodium Solution ... 438
- Nembutal Sodium Suppositories ... 440

Perphenazine (CNS effects may be additive). Products include:

- Etrafon ... 2355
- Triavil Tablets ... 1757
- Trilafon ... 2389

Phenobarbital (CNS effects may be additive). Products include:

- Arco-Lase Plus Tablets ... 512
- Bellergal-S Tablets ... 2250
- Donnatal ... 2060
- Donnatal Extentabs ... 2061
- Donnatal Tablets ... 2060
- Phenobarbital Elixir and Tablets ... 1469
- Quadrinal Tablets ... 1350

Prazepam (CNS effects may be additive).

No products indexed under this heading.

Prochlorperazine (CNS effects may be additive). Products include:

- Compazine ... 2470

Promethazine Hydrochloride (CNS effects may be additive). Products include:

- Mepergan Injection ... 2753
- Phenergan with Codeine ... 2777
- Phenergan with Dextromethorphan 2778
- Phenergan Injection ... 2773
- Phenergan Suppositories ... 2775
- Phenergan Syrup ... 2774
- Phenergan Tablets ... 2775
- Phenergan VC ... 2779
- Phenergan VC with Codeine ... 2781

Propofol (CNS effects may be additive). Products include:

- Diprivan Injection ... 2833

Propoxyphene Hydrochloride (CNS effects may be additive). Products include:

- Darvon ... 1435
- Wygesic Tablets ... 2827

Propoxyphene Napsylate (CNS effects may be additive). Products include:

- Darvon-N/Darvocet-N ... 1433

Quazepam (CNS effects may be additive). Products include:

- Doral Tablets ... 2664

Risperidone (CNS effects may be additive). Products include:

- Risperdal ... 1301

Secobarbital Sodium (CNS effects may be additive). Products include:

- Seconal Sodium Pulvules ... 1474

Sufentanil Citrate (CNS effects may be additive). Products include:

- Sufenta Injection ... 1309

Temazepam (CNS effects may be additive). Products include:

- Restoril Capsules ... 2284

Thiamylal Sodium (CNS effects may be additive).

No products indexed under this heading.

Thioridazine Hydrochloride (CNS effects may be additive). Products include:

- Mellaril ... 2269

Thiothixene (CNS effects may be additive). Products include:

- Navane Capsules and Concentrate 2201
- Navane Intramuscular ... 2202

Triazolam (CNS effects may be additive). Products include:

- Halcion Tablets ... 2611

Trifluoperazine Hydrochloride (CNS effects may be additive). Products include:

- Stelazine ... 2514

Zolpidem Tartrate (CNS effects may be additive). Products include:

- Ambien Tablets ... 2416

Food Interactions

Alcohol (CNS effects may be additive).

PBZ-SR TABLETS

(Tripelennamine Hydrochloride) ... **844**

May interact with central nervous system depressants, monoamine oxidase inhibitors, and certain other agents. Compounds in these categories include:

Alfentanil Hydrochloride (CNS effects may be additive). Products include:

- Alfenta Injection ... 1286

Alprazolam (CNS effects may be additive). Products include:

- Xanax Tablets ... 2649

Aprobarbital (CNS effects may be additive).

No products indexed under this heading.

Buprenorphine (CNS effects may be additive). Products include:

- Buprenex Injectable ... 2006

Buspirone Hydrochloride (CNS effects may be additive). Products include:

- BuSpar ... 737

Butabarbital (CNS effects may be additive).

No products indexed under this heading.

Butalbital (CNS effects may be additive). Products include:

- Esgic-plus Tablets ... 1013
- Fioricet Tablets ... 2258
- Fioricet with Codeine Capsules ... 2260
- Fiorinal Capsules ... 2261
- Fiorinal with Codeine Capsules ... 2262
- Fiorinal Tablets ... 2261
- Phrenilin ... 785
- Sedapap Tablets 50 mg/650 mg .. 1543

Chlordiazepoxide (CNS effects may be additive). Products include:

- Libritabs Tablets ... 2177
- Limbitrol ... 2180

Chlordiazepoxide Hydrochloride (CNS effects may be additive). Products include:

- Librax Capsules ... 2176
- Librium Capsules ... 2178
- Librium Injectable ... 2179

Chlorpromazine (CNS effects may be additive). Products include:

- Thorazine Suppositories ... 2523

Chlorprothixene (CNS effects may be additive).

No products indexed under this heading.

Chlorprothixene Hydrochloride (CNS effects may be additive).

No products indexed under this heading.

Chlorprothixene Lactate (CNS effects may be additive).

No products indexed under this heading.

Clorazepate Dipotassium (CNS effects may be additive). Products include:

- Tranxene ... 451

Clozapine (CNS effects may be additive). Products include:

- Clozaril Tablets ... 2252

Codeine Phosphate (CNS effects may be additive). Products include:

- Actifed with Codeine Cough Syrup.. 1067
- Brontex ... 1981
- Deconsal C Expectorant Syrup ... 456
- Deconsal Pediatric Syrup ... 457
- Dimetane-DC Cough Syrup ... 2059
- Empirin with Codeine Tablets ... 1093
- Fioricet with Codeine Capsules ... 2260
- Fiorinal with Codeine Capsules ... 2262
- Isoclor Expectorant ... 990
- Novahistine DH ... 2462
- Novahistine Expectorant ... 2463
- Nucofed ... 2051
- Phenergan with Codeine ... 2777
- Phenergan VC with Codeine ... 2781
- Robitussin A-C Syrup ... 2073
- Robitussin-DAC Syrup ... 2074
- Ryna ... ◘ 841
- Soma Compound w/Codeine Tablets ... 2676
- Tussi-Organidin NR Liquid and S NR Liquid ... 2677
- Tylenol with Codeine ... 1583

Desflurane (CNS effects may be additive). Products include:

- Suprane ... 1813

Dezocine (CNS effects may be additive). Products include:

- Dalgan Injection ... 538

Diazepam (CNS effects may be additive). Products include:

- Dizac ... 1809
- Valium Injectable ... 2182
- Valium Tablets ... 2183
- Valrelease Capsules ... 2169

Droperidol (CNS effects may be additive). Products include:

- Inapsine Injection ... 1296

Enflurane (CNS effects may be additive).

No products indexed under this heading.

Estazolam (CNS effects may be additive). Products include:

- ProSom Tablets ... 449

Ethchlorvynol (CNS effects may be additive). Products include:

- Placidyl Capsules ... 448

Ethinamate (CNS effects may be additive).

No products indexed under this heading.

Fentanyl (CNS effects may be additive). Products include:

- Duragesic Transdermal System ... 1288

Fentanyl Citrate (CNS effects may be additive). Products include:

- Sublimaze Injection ... 1307

Fluphenazine Decanoate (CNS effects may be additive). Products include:

- Prolixin Decanoate ... 509

Fluphenazine Enanthate (CNS effects may be additive). Products include:

- Prolixin Enanthate ... 509

Fluphenazine Hydrochloride (CNS effects may be additive). Products include:

- Prolixin ... 509

Flurazepam Hydrochloride (CNS effects may be additive). Products include:

- Dalmane Capsules ... 2173

Furazolidone (Concurrent use contraindicated). Products include:

- Furoxone ... 2046

Glutethimide (CNS effects may be additive).

No products indexed under this heading.

Haloperidol (CNS effects may be additive). Products include:

- Haldol Injection, Tablets and Concentrate ... 1575

Haloperidol Decanoate (CNS effects may be additive). Products include:

- Haldol Decanoate ... 1577

Hydrocodone Bitartrate (CNS effects may be additive). Products include:

- Anexsia 5/500 Elixir ... 1781
- Anexia Tablets ... 1782
- Codiclear DH Syrup ... 791
- Deconamine CX Cough and Cold Liquid and Tablets ... 1319
- Duratuss HD Elixir ... 2565
- Hycodan Tablets and Syrup ... 930
- Hycomine Compound Tablets ... 932
- Hycomine ... 931
- Hycotuss Expectorant Syrup ... 933
- Hydrocet Capsules ... 782
- Lorcet 10/650 ... 1018
- Lortab ... 2566
- Tussend ... 1783
- Tussend Expectorant ... 1785
- Vicodin Tablets ... 1356
- Vicodin ES Tablets ... 1357
- Vicodin Tuss Expectorant ... 1358
- Zydone Capsules ... 949

Hydrocodone Polistirex (CNS effects may be additive). Products include:

- Tussionex Pennkinetic Extended-Release Suspension ... 998

Hydroxyzine Hydrochloride (CNS effects may be additive). Products include:

- Atarax Tablets & Syrup ... 2185
- Marax Tablets & DF Syrup ... 2200
- Vistaril Intramuscular Solution ... 2216

Isocarboxazid (Concurrent use contraindicated).

No products indexed under this heading.

Isoflurane (CNS effects may be additive).

No products indexed under this heading.

Ketamine Hydrochloride (CNS effects may be additive).

No products indexed under this heading.

Levomethadyl Acetate Hydrochloride (CNS effects may be additive). Products include:

- Orlamm ... 2239

Levorphanol Tartrate (CNS effects may be additive). Products include:

- Levo-Dromoran ... 2129

Lorazepam (CNS effects may be additive). Products include:

- Ativan Injection ... 2698
- Ativan Tablets ... 2700

Loxapine Hydrochloride (CNS effects may be additive). Products include:

- Loxitane ... 1378

Loxapine Succinate (CNS effects may be additive). Products include:

- Loxitane Capsules ... 1378

Meperidine Hydrochloride (CNS effects may be additive). Products include:

- Demerol ... 2308
- Mepergan Injection ... 2753

Mephobarbital (CNS effects may be additive). Products include:

- Mebaral Tablets ... 2322

Meprobamate (CNS effects may be additive). Products include:

- Miltown Tablets ... 2672
- PMB 200 and PMB 400 ... 2783

Mesoridazine Besylate (CNS effects may be additive). Products include:

- Serentil ... 684

Methadone Hydrochloride (CNS effects may be additive). Products include:

- Methadone Hydrochloride Oral Concentrate ... 2233
- Methadone Hydrochloride Oral Solution & Tablets ... 2235

Methohexital Sodium (CNS effects may be additive). Products include:

- Brevital Sodium Vials ... 1429

Methotrimeprazine (CNS effects may be additive). Products include:

- Levoprome ... 1274

(◘ Described in PDR For Nonprescription Drugs) (◉ Described in PDR For Ophthalmology)

Interactions Index

Methoxyflurane (CNS effects may be additive).

No products indexed under this heading.

Midazolam Hydrochloride (CNS effects may be additive). Products include:

Versed Injection 2170

Molindone Hydrochloride (CNS effects may be additive). Products include:

Moban Tablets and Concentrate 1048

Morphine Sulfate (CNS effects may be additive). Products include:

Astramorph/PF Injection, USP (Preservative-Free) 535
Duramorph 962
Infumorph 200 and Infumorph 500 Sterile Solutions 965
MS Contin Tablets 1994
MSIR 1997
Oramorph SR (Morphine Sulfate Sustained Release Tablets) 2236
RMS Suppositories 2657
Roxanol 2243

Opium Alkaloids (CNS effects may be additive).

No products indexed under this heading.

Oxazepam (CNS effects may be additive). Products include:

Serax Capsules 2810
Serax Tablets 2810

Oxycodone Hydrochloride (CNS effects may be additive). Products include:

Percocet Tablets 938
Percodan Tablets 939
Percodan-Demi Tablets 940
Roxicodone Tablets, Oral Solution & Intensol (Oxycodone) 2244
Tylox Capsules 1584

Pentobarbital Sodium (CNS effects may be additive). Products include:

Nembutal Sodium Capsules 436
Nembutal Sodium Solution 438
Nembutal Sodium Suppositories 440

Perphenazine (CNS effects may be additive). Products include:

Etrafon 2355
Triavil Tablets 1757
Trilafon 2389

Phenelzine Sulfate (Concurrent use contraindicated). Products include:

Nardil 1920

Phenobarbital (CNS effects may be additive). Products include:

Arco-Lase Plus Tablets 512
Bellergal-S Tablets 2250
Donnatal 2060
Donnatal Extentabs 2061
Donnatal Tablets 2060
Phenobarbital Elixir and Tablets 1469
Quadrinal Tablets 1350

Prazepam (CNS effects may be additive).

No products indexed under this heading.

Prochlorperazine (CNS effects may be additive). Products include:

Compazine 2470

Promethazine Hydrochloride (CNS effects may be additive). Products include:

Mepergan Injection 2753
Phenergan with Codeine 2777
Phenergan with Dextromethorphan 2778
Phenergan Injection 2773
Phenergan Suppositories 2775
Phenergan Syrup 2774
Phenergan Tablets 2775
Phenergan VC 2779
Phenergan VC with Codeine 2781

Propofol (CNS effects may be additive). Products include:

Diprivan Injection 2833

Propoxyphene Hydrochloride (CNS effects may be additive). Products include:

Darvon 1435
Wygesic Tablets 2827

Propoxyphene Napsylate (CNS effects may be additive). Products include:

Darvon-N/Darvocet-N 1433

Quazepam (CNS effects may be additive). Products include:

Doral Tablets 2664

Risperidone (CNS effects may be additive). Products include:

Risperdal 1301

Secobarbital Sodium (CNS effects may be additive). Products include:

Seconal Sodium Pulvules 1474

Selegiline Hydrochloride (Concurrent use contraindicated). Products include:

Eldepryl Tablets 2550

Sufentanil Citrate (CNS effects may be additive). Products include:

Sufenta Injection 1309

Temazepam (CNS effects may be additive). Products include:

Restoril Capsules 2284

Thiamylal Sodium (CNS effects may be additive).

No products indexed under this heading.

Thioridazine Hydrochloride (CNS effects may be additive). Products include:

Mellaril 2269

Thiothixene (CNS effects may be additive). Products include:

Navane Capsules and Concentrate 2201
Navane Intramuscular 2202

Tranylcypromine Sulfate (Concurrent use contraindicated). Products include:

Parnate Tablets 2503

Triazolam (CNS effects may be additive). Products include:

Halcion Tablets 2611

Trifluoperazine Hydrochloride (CNS effects may be additive). Products include:

Stelazine 2514

Zolpidem Tartrate (CNS effects may be additive). Products include:

Ambien Tablets 2416

Food Interactions

Alcohol (CNS effects may be additive).

PCE DISPERTAB TABLETS (Erythromycin) 444

May interact with oral anticoagulants, xanthine bronchodilators, and certain other agents. Compounds in these categories include:

Alfentanil Hydrochloride (Elevations in serum erythromycin and alfentanil concentration). Products include:

Alfenta Injection 1286

Aminophylline (Concomitant administration with high doses of theophylline may be associated with increased theophylline levels and potential toxicity).

No products indexed under this heading.

Bromocriptine Mesylate (Elevations in serum erythromycin and bromocriptine concentration). Products include:

Parlodel 2281

Carbamazepine (Elevations in serum erythromycin and carbamazepine concentration). Products include:

Atretol Tablets 573

Tegretol Chewable Tablets 852
Tegretol Suspension 852
Tegretol Tablets 852

Cyclosporine (Elevations in serum erythromycin and cyclosporine concentration). Products include:

Neoral 2276
Sandimmune 2286

Dicumarol (Increased anticoagulant effects).

No products indexed under this heading.

Digoxin (Elevated digoxin serum levels). Products include:

Lanoxicaps 1117
Lanoxin Elixir Pediatric 1120
Lanoxin Injection 1123
Lanoxin Injection Pediatric 1126
Lanoxin Tablets 1128

Dihydroergotamine Mesylate (Potential for acute ergot toxicity characterized by severe peripheral vasospasm and dysesthesia). Products include:

D.H.E. 45 Injection 2255

Disopyramide Phosphate (Elevations in serum erythromycin and disopyramide concentration). Products include:

Norpace 2444

Dyphylline (Concomitant administration with high doses of theophylline may be associated with increased theophylline levels and potential toxicity). Products include:

Lufyllin & Lufyllin-400 Tablets 2670
Lufyllin-GG Elixir & Tablets 2671

Ergotamine Tartrate (Potential for acute ergot toxicity characterized by severe peripheral vasospasm and dysesthesia). Products include:

Bellergal-S Tablets 2250
Cafergot 2251
Ergomar 1486
Wigraine Tablets & Suppositories .. 1829

Hexobarbital (Elevations in serum erythromycin and hexobarbital concentration).

Lovastatin (Potential for rhabdomyolysis in seriously ill patients; elevations in serum erythromycin and lovastatin concentration). Products include:

Mevacor Tablets 1699

Midazolam Hydrochloride (Decreased clearance of midazolam and increase in the pharmacologic effect of midazolam). Products include:

Versed Injection 2170

Phenytoin (Elevations in serum erythromycin and phenytoin concentration). Products include:

Dilantin Infatabs 1908
Dilantin-125 Suspension 1911

Phenytoin Sodium (Elevations in serum erythromycin and phenytoin concentration). Products include:

Dilantin Kapseals 1906
Dilantin Parenteral 1910

Terfenadine (Concomitant use alters the metabolism of terfenadine; rare cases of serious cardiovascular adverse events, including deaths, cardiac arrest, torsades de pointes, and other ventricular arrhythmias; concurrent use is contraindicated). Products include:

Seldane Tablets 1536
Seldane-D Extended-Release Tablets 1538

Theophylline (Concomitant administration with high doses of theophylline may be associated with increased theophylline levels and potential toxicity). Products include:

Marax Tablets & DF Syrup 2200
Quibron 2053

Theophylline Anhydrous (Concomitant administration with high doses of theophylline may be associated with increased theophylline levels and potential toxicity). Products include:

Aerolate 1004
Primatene Dual Action Formula ...... ⊕ 872
Primatene Tablets .... ⊕ 873
Respbid Tablets 682
Slo-bid Gyrocaps 2033
Theo-24 Extended Release Capsules 2568
Theo-Dur Extended-Release Tablets 1327
Theo-X Extended-Release Tablets .. 788
Uni-Dur Extended-Release Tablets .. 1331
Uniphyl 400 mg Tablets 2001

Theophylline Calcium Salicylate (Concomitant administration with high doses of theophylline may be associated with increased theophylline levels and potential toxicity). Products include:

Quadrinal Tablets 1350

Theophylline Sodium Glycinate (Concomitant administration with high doses of theophylline may be associated with increased theophylline levels and potential toxicity).

No products indexed under this heading.

Triazolam (Decreased clearance of triazolam and increase in the pharmacologic effect of triazolam). Products include:

Halcion Tablets 2611

Warfarin Sodium (Increased anticoagulant effects; effect more pronounced in elderly). Products include:

Coumadin 926

Food Interactions

Meal, unspecified (Optimal blood levels are obtained when PCE is given in the fasting state).

PHISOHEX (Hexachlorophene) 2327

None cited in PDR database.

PMB 200 AND PMB 400 (Estrogens, Conjugated, Meprobamate) 2783

May interact with central nervous system depressants, psychotropics, narcotic analgesics, progestins, and certain other agents. Compounds in these categories include:

Alfentanil Hydrochloride (Additive effects). Products include:

Alfenta Injection 1286

Alprazolam (Additive effects). Products include:

Xanax Tablets 2649

Amitriptyline Hydrochloride (Additive effects). Products include:

Elavil 2838
Endep Tablets 2174
Etrafon 2355
Limbitrol 2180
Triavil Tablets 1757

Amoxapine (Additive effects). Products include:

Asendin Tablets 1369

Aprobarbital (Additive effects).

No products indexed under this heading.

Buprenorphine (Additive effects). Products include:

Buprenex Injectable 2006

Buspirone Hydrochloride (Additive effects). Products include:

BuSpar 737

Butabarbital (Additive effects).

No products indexed under this heading.

IMPORTANT NOTE: Always consult each drug listing in the patient's regimen for possible interactions.

PMB

Interactions Index

Butalbital (Additive effects). Products include:

Esgic-plus Tablets 1013
Fioricet Tablets 2258
Fioricet with Codeine Capsules 2260
Fiorinal Capsules 2261
Fiorinal with Codeine Capsules 2262
Fiorinal Tablets 2261
Phrenilin 785
Sedapap Tablets 50 mg/650 mg .. 1543

Chlordiazepoxide (Additive effects). Products include:

Libritabs Tablets 2177
Limbitrol 2180

Chlordiazepoxide Hydrochloride (Additive effects). Products include:

Librax Capsules 2176
Librium Capsules 2178
Librium Injectable 2179

Chlorpromazine (Additive effects). Products include:

Thorazine Suppositories 2523

Chlorprothixene (Additive effects).

No products indexed under this heading.

Chlorprothixene Hydrochloride (Additive effects).

No products indexed under this heading.

Clonidine (Additive effects). Products include:

Catapres-TTS 675

Clonidine Hydrochloride (Additive effects). Products include:

Catapres Tablets 674
Combipres Tablets 677

Clorazepate Dipotassium (Additive effects). Products include:

Tranxene 451

Clozapine (Additive effects). Products include:

Clozaril Tablets 2252

Codeine Phosphate (Additive effects). Products include:

Actifed with Codeine Cough Syrup.. 1067
Brontex 1981
Deconsal C Expectorant Syrup 456
Deconsal Pediatric Syrup 457
Dimetane-DC Cough Syrup 2059
Empirin with Codeine Tablets........... 1093
Fioricet with Codeine Capsules 2260
Fiorinal with Codeine Capsules 2262
Isoclor Expectorant 990
Novahistine DH 2462
Novahistine Expectorant 2463
Nucofed 2051
Phenergan with Codeine 2777
Phenergan VC with Codeine 2781
Robitussin A-C Syrup 2073
Robitussin-DAC Syrup 2074
Ryna .... ◆◻ 841
Soma Compound w/Codeine Tablets 2676
Tussi-Organidin NR Liquid and S NR Liquid 2677
Tylenol with Codeine 1583

Desflurane (Additive effects). Products include:

Suprane 1813

Desipramine Hydrochloride (Additive effects). Products include:

Norpramin Tablets 1526

Desogestrel (Adverse effects on carbohydrate and lipid metabolism). Products include:

Desogen Tablets 1817
Ortho-Cept 1851

Dezocine (Additive effects). Products include:

Dalgan Injection 538

Diazepam (Additive effects). Products include:

Dizac 1809
Valium Injectable 2182
Valium Tablets 2183
Valrelease Capsules 2169

Doxepin Hydrochloride (Additive effects). Products include:

Sinequan 2205
Zonalon Cream 1055

Droperidol (Additive effects). Products include:

Inapsine Injection 1296

Enflurane (Additive effects).

No products indexed under this heading.

Estazolam (Additive effects). Products include:

ProSom Tablets 449

Ethchlorvynol (Additive effects). Products include:

Placidyl Capsules 448

Ethinamate (Additive effects).

No products indexed under this heading.

Fentanyl (Additive effects). Products include:

Duragesic Transdermal System........ 1288

Fentanyl Citrate (Additive effects). Products include:

Sublimaze Injection 1307

Fluphenazine Decanoate (Additive effects). Products include:

Prolixin Decanoate 509

Fluphenazine Enanthate (Additive effects). Products include:

Prolixin Enanthate 509

Fluphenazine Hydrochloride (Additive effects). Products include:

Prolixin 509

Flurazepam Hydrochloride (Additive effects). Products include:

Dalmane Capsules 2173

Glutethimide (Additive effects).

No products indexed under this heading.

Haloperidol (Additive effects). Products include:

Haldol Injection, Tablets and Concentrate 1575

Haloperidol Decanoate (Additive effects). Products include:

Haldol Decanoate 1577

Hydrocodone Bitartrate (Additive effects). Products include:

Anexsia 5/500 Elixir 1781
Anexia Tablets 1782
Codiclear DH Syrup 791
Deconamine CX Cough and Cold Liquid and Tablets 1319
Duratuss HD Elixir 2565
Hycodan Tablets and Syrup 930
Hycomine Compound Tablets 932
Hycomine 931
Hycotuss Expectorant Syrup 933
Hydrocet Capsules 782
Lorcet 10/650 1018
Lortab 2566
Tussend 1783
Tussend Expectorant 1785
Vicodin Tablets 1356
Vicodin ES Tablets 1357
Vicodin Tuss Expectorant 1358
Zydone Capsules 949

Hydrocodone Polistirex (Additive effects). Products include:

Tussionex Pennkinetic Extended-Release Suspension 998

Hydroxyzine Hydrochloride (Additive effects). Products include:

Atarax Tablets & Syrup 2185
Marax Tablets & DF Syrup 2200
Vistaril Intramuscular Solution 2216

Imipramine Hydrochloride (Additive effects). Products include:

Tofranil Ampuls 854
Tofranil Tablets 856

Imipramine Pamoate (Additive effects). Products include:

Tofranil-PM Capsules 857

Isocarboxazid (Additive effects).

No products indexed under this heading.

Isoflurane (Additive effects).

No products indexed under this heading.

Ketamine Hydrochloride (Additive effects).

No products indexed under this heading.

Levomethadyl Acetate Hydrochloride (Additive effects). Products include:

Orlaam 2239

Levorphanol Tartrate (Additive effects). Products include:

Levo-Dromoran 2129

Lithium Carbonate (Additive effects). Products include:

Eskalith 2485
Lithium Carbonate Capsules & Tablets 2230
Lithonate/Lithotabs/Lithobid 2543

Lithium Citrate (Additive effects).

No products indexed under this heading.

Lorazepam (Additive effects). Products include:

Ativan Injection 2698
Ativan Tablets 2700

Loxapine Hydrochloride (Additive effects). Products include:

Loxitane 1378

Loxapine Succinate (Additive effects). Products include:

Loxitane Capsules 1378

Maprotiline Hydrochloride (Additive effects). Products include:

Ludiomil Tablets 843

Medroxyprogesterone Acetate (Adverse effects on carbohydrate and lipid metabolism). Products include:

Amen Tablets 780
Cycrin Tablets 975
Depo-Provera Contraceptive Injection 2602
Depo-Provera Sterile Aqueous Suspension 2606
Premphase 2797
Prempro 2801
Provera Tablets 2636

Megestrol Acetate (Adverse effects on carbohydrate and lipid metabolism). Products include:

Megace Oral Suspension 699
Megace Tablets 701

Meperidine Hydrochloride (Additive effects). Products include:

Demerol 2308
Mepergan Injection 2753

Mephobarbital (Additive effects). Products include:

Mebaral Tablets 2322

Mesoridazine Besylate (Additive effects). Products include:

Serentil 684

Methadone Hydrochloride (Additive effects). Products include:

Methadone Hydrochloride Oral Concentrate 2233
Methadone Hydrochloride Oral Solution & Tablets 2235

Methohexital Sodium (Additive effects). Products include:

Brevital Sodium Vials 1429

Methotrimeprazine (Additive effects). Products include:

Levoprome 1274

Methoxyflurane (Additive effects).

No products indexed under this heading.

Midazolam Hydrochloride (Additive effects). Products include:

Versed Injection 2170

Molindone Hydrochloride (Additive effects). Products include:

Moban Tablets and Concentrate 1048

Morphine Sulfate (Additive effects). Products include:

Astramorph/PF Injection, USP (Preservative-Free) 535
Duramorph 962
Infumorph 200 and Infumorph 500 Sterile Solutions 965
MS Contin Tablets 1994
MSIR 1997
Oramorph SR (Morphine Sulfate Sustained Release Tablets) 2236

RMS Suppositories 2657
Roxanol 2243

Norgestimate (Adverse effects on carbohydrate and lipid metabolism). Products include:

Ortho-Cyclen/Ortho-Tri-Cyclen 1858
Ortho-Cyclen/Ortho Tri-Cyclen 1858

Nortriptyline Hydrochloride (Additive effects). Products include:

Pamelor 2280

Opium Alkaloids (Additive effects).

No products indexed under this heading.

Oxazepam (Additive effects). Products include:

Serax Capsules 2810
Serax Tablets 2810

Oxycodone Hydrochloride (Additive effects). Products include:

Percocet Tablets 938
Percodan Tablets 939
Percodan-Demi Tablets 940
Roxicodone Tablets, Oral Solution & Intensol (Oxycodone) 2244
Tylox Capsules 1584

Pentobarbital Sodium (Additive effects). Products include:

Nembutal Sodium Capsules 436
Nembutal Sodium Solution 438
Nembutal Sodium Suppositories 440

Perphenazine (Additive effects). Products include:

Etrafon 2355
Triavil Tablets 1757
Trilafon 2389

Phenelzine Sulfate (Additive effects). Products include:

Nardil 1920

Phenobarbital (Additive effects). Products include:

Arco-Lase Plus Tablets 512
Bellergal-S Tablets 2250
Donnatal 2060
Donnatal Extentabs 2061
Donnatal Tablets 2060
Phenobarbital Elixir and Tablets 1469
Quadrinal Tablets 1350

Prazepam (Additive effects).

No products indexed under this heading.

Prochlorperazine (Additive effects). Products include:

Compazine 2470

Promethazine Hydrochloride (Additive effects). Products include:

Mepergan Injection 2753
Phenergan with Codeine 2777
Phenergan with Dextromethorphan 2778
Phenergan Injection 2773
Phenergan Suppositories 2775
Phenergan Syrup 2774
Phenergan Tablets 2775
Phenergan VC 2779
Phenergan VC with Codeine 2781

Propofol (Additive effects). Products include:

Diprivan Injection 2833

Propoxyphene Hydrochloride (Additive effects). Products include:

Darvon 1435
Wygesic Tablets 2827

Propoxyphene Napsylate (Additive effects). Products include:

Darvon-N/Darvocet-N 1433

Protriptyline Hydrochloride (Additive effects). Products include:

Vivactil Tablets 1774

Quazepam (Additive effects). Products include:

Doral Tablets 2664

Risperidone (Additive effects). Products include:

Risperdal 1301

Secobarbital Sodium (Additive effects). Products include:

Seconal Sodium Pulvules 1474

Sufentanil Citrate (Additive effects). Products include:

Sufenta Injection 1309

(◆◻ Described in PDR For Nonprescription Drugs) (◉ Described in PDR For Ophthalmology)

Temazepam (Additive effects). Products include:
Restoril Capsules 2284

Thiamylal Sodium (Additive effects).
No products indexed under this heading.

Thioridazine Hydrochloride (Additive effects). Products include:
Mellaril 2269

Thiothixene (Additive effects). Products include:
Navane Capsules and Concentrate 2201
Navane Intramuscular 2202

Tranylcypromine Sulfate (Additive effects). Products include:
Parnate Tablets 2503

Triazolam (Additive effects). Products include:
Halcion Tablets 2611

Trifluoperazine Hydrochloride (Additive effects). Products include:
Stelazine 2514

Trimipramine Maleate (Additive effects). Products include:
Surmontil Capsules 2811

Zolpidem Tartrate (Additive effects). Products include:
Ambien Tablets 2416

Food Interactions

Alcohol (Additive effects).

PPD TINE TEST

(Tuberculin, Purified Protein Derivative, Multiple Puncture Device) 2874
May interact with corticosteroids and immunosuppressive agents. Compounds in these categories include:

Azathioprine (Reactivity to the test may be suppressed). Products include:
Imuran 1110

Betamethasone Acetate (Reactivity to the test may be suppressed). Products include:
Celestone Soluspan Suspension 2347

Betamethasone Sodium Phosphate (Reactivity to the test may be suppressed). Products include:
Celestone Soluspan Suspension 2347

Cortisone Acetate (Reactivity to the test may be suppressed). Products include:
Cortone Acetate Sterile Suspension 1623
Cortone Acetate Tablets 1624

Cyclosporine (Reactivity to the test may be suppressed). Products include:
Neoral 2276
Sandimmune 2286

Desoximetasone (Reactivity to the test may be suppressed). Products include:
Topicort 1243

Dexamethasone Acetate (Reactivity to the test may be suppressed). Products include:
Dalalone D.P. Injectable 1011
Decadron-LA Sterile Suspension 1646

Dexamethasone Sodium Phosphate (Reactivity to the test may be suppressed). Products include:
Decadron Phosphate Injection 1637
Decadron Phosphate Respihaler 1642
Decadron Phosphate Sterile Ophthalmic Ointment 1641
Decadron Phosphate Sterile Ophthalmic Solution 1642
Decadron Phosphate Topical Cream 1644
Decadron Phosphate Turbinaire 1645
Decadron Phosphate with Xylocaine Injection, Sterile 1639
Dexacort Phosphate in Respihaler .. 458
Dexacort Phosphate in Turbinaire .. 459
NeoDecadron Sterile Ophthalmic Ointment 1712
NeoDecadron Sterile Ophthalmic Solution 1713
NeoDecadron Topical Cream 1714

Fludrocortisone Acetate (Reactivity to the test may be suppressed). Products include:
Florinef Acetate Tablets 505

Hydrocortisone (Reactivity to the test may be suppressed). Products include:
Anusol-HC Cream 2.5% 1896
Aquanil HC Lotion 1931
Bactine Hydrocortisone Anti-Itch Cream .... ■ 709
Caldecort Anti-Itch Hydrocortisone Spray .... ■ 631
Cortaid .... ■ 836
CORTENEMA 2535
Cortisporin Ointment 1085
Cortisporin Ophthalmic Ointment Sterile 1085
Cortisporin Ophthalmic Suspension Sterile 1086
Cortisporin Otic Solution Sterile 1087
Cortisporin Otic Suspension Sterile 1088
Cortizone-5 .... ■ 831
Cortizone-10 .... ■ 831
Hydrocortone Tablets 1672
Hytone 907
Massengill Medicated Soft Cloth Towelettes 2458
PediOtic Suspension Sterile 1153
Preparation H Hydrocortisone 1% Cream .... ■ 872
ProctoCream-HC 2.5% 2408
VōSoL HC Otic Solution 2678

Hydrocortisone Acetate (Reactivity to the test may be suppressed). Products include:
Analpram-HC Rectal Cream 1% and 2.5% 977
Anusol HC-1 Anti-Itch Hydrocortisone Ointment .... ■ 847
Anusol-HC Suppositories 1897
Caldecort .... ■ 631
Carmol HC 924
Coly-Mycin S Otic w/Neomycin & Hydrocortisone 1906
Cortaid .... ■ 836
Cortifoam 2396
Cortisporin Cream 1084
Epifoam 2399
Hydrocortone Acetate Sterile Suspension 1669
Mantadil Cream 1135
Nupercainal Hydrocortisone 1% Cream .... ■ 645
Ophthocort .... ⊙ 311
Pramosone Cream, Lotion & Ointment 978
ProctoCream-HC 2408
ProctoFoam-HC 2409
Terra-Cortril Ophthalmic Suspension 2210

Hydrocortisone Sodium Phosphate (Reactivity to the test may be suppressed). Products include:
Hydrocortone Phosphate Injection, Sterile 1670

Hydrocortisone Sodium Succinate (Reactivity to the test may be suppressed). Products include:
Solu-Cortef Sterile Powder 2641

Immune Globulin (Human) (Reactivity to the test may be suppressed).
No products indexed under this heading.

Immune Globulin Intravenous (Human) (Reactivity to the test may be suppressed).

Methylprednisolone Acetate (Reactivity to the test may be suppressed). Products include:
Depo-Medrol Single-Dose Vial 2600
Depo-Medrol Sterile Aqueous Suspension 2597

Methylprednisolone Sodium Succinate (Reactivity to the test may be suppressed). Products include:
Solu-Medrol Sterile Powder 2643

Muromonab-CD3 (Reactivity to the test may be suppressed). Products include:
Orthoclone OKT3 Sterile Solution .. 1837

Mycophenolate Mofetil (Reactivity to the test may be suppressed). Products include:
CellCept Capsules 2099

Prednisolone Acetate (Reactivity to the test may be suppressed). Products include:
AK-CIDE .... ⊙ 202
AK-CIDE Ointment .... ⊙ 202
Blephamide Liquifilm Sterile Ophthalmic Suspension 476
Blephamide Ointment .... ⊙ 237
Econopred & Econopred Plus Ophthalmic Suspensions .... ⊙ 217
Poly-Pred Liquifilm .... ⊙ 248
Pred Forte .... ⊙ 250
Pred Mild .... ⊙ 253
Pred-G Liquifilm Sterile Ophthalmic Suspension .... ⊙ 251
Pred-G S.O.P. Sterile Ophthalmic Ointment .... ⊙ 252
Vasocidin Ointment .... ⊙ 268

Prednisolone Sodium Phosphate (Reactivity to the test may be suppressed). Products include:
AK-Pred .... ⊙ 204
Hydeltrasol Injection, Sterile 1665
Inflamase .... ⊙ 265
Pediapred Oral Liquid 995
Vasocidin Ophthalmic Solution .... ⊙ 270

Prednisolone Tebutate (Reactivity to the test may be suppressed). Products include:
Hydeltra-T.B.A. Sterile Suspension 1667

Prednisone (Reactivity to the test may be suppressed). Products include:
Deltasone Tablets 2595

Tacrolimus (Reactivity to the test may be suppressed). Products include:
Prograf 1042

Triamcinolone (Reactivity to the test may be suppressed). Products include:
Aristocort Tablets 1022

Triamcinolone Acetonide (Reactivity to the test may be suppressed). Products include:
Aristocort A 0.025% Cream 1027
Aristocort A 0.5% Cream 1031
Aristocort A 0.1% Cream 1029
Aristocort A 0.1% Ointment 1030
Azmacort Oral Inhaler 2011
Nasacort Nasal Inhaler 2024

Triamcinolone Diacetate (Reactivity to the test may be suppressed). Products include:
Aristocort Suspension (Forte Parenteral) 1027
Aristocort Suspension (Intralesional) 1025

Triamcinolone Hexacetonide (Reactivity to the test may be suppressed). Products include:
Aristospan Suspension (Intra-articular) 1033
Aristospan Suspension (Intralesional) 1032

P&S LIQUID

(Mineral Oil) .... ■ 604
None cited in PDR database.

P&S PLUS TAR GEL

(Coal Tar) .... ■ 604
None cited in PDR database.

P&S SHAMPOO

(Salicylic Acid) .... ■ 605
None cited in PDR database.

PAMELOR CAPSULES

(Nortriptyline Hydrochloride) 2280
May interact with anticholinergics, sympathomimetics, monoamine oxidase inhibitors, thyroid preparations, drugs that inhibit cytochrome p450iid6, antidepressant drugs, phenothiazines, selective serotonin reuptake inhibitors, and certain other agents. Compounds in these categories include:

Albuterol (Effects of concurrent use not specified; careful adjustment of dosage and close supervision are required). Products include:
Proventil Inhalation Aerosol 2382
Ventolin Inhalation Aerosol and Refill 1197

Albuterol Sulfate (Effects of concurrent use not specified; careful adjustment of dosage and close supervision are required). Products include:
Airet Solution for Inhalation 452
Proventil Inhalation Solution 0.083% 2384
Proventil Repetabs Tablets 2386
Proventil Solution for Inhalation 0.5% 2383
Proventil Syrup 2385
Proventil Tablets 2386
Ventolin Inhalation Solution 1198
Ventolin Nebules Inhalation Solution 1199
Ventolin Rotacaps for Inhalation 1200
Ventolin Syrup 1202
Ventolin Tablets 1203
Volmax Extended-Release Tablets .. 1788

Amitriptyline Hydrochloride (Concurrent use with drugs that are substrate for cytochrome $P_{450}IID_6$ may make normal metabolizer resemble poor metabolizer leading to higher than expected plasma concentrations of TCA with resultant toxicity). Products include:
Elavil 2838
Endep Tablets 2174
Etrafon 2355
Limbitrol 2180
Triavil Tablets 1757

Amoxapine (Concurrent use with drugs that are substrate for cytochrome $P_{450}IID_6$ may make normal metabolizer resemble poor metabolizer leading to higher than expected plasma concentrations of TCA with resultant toxicity). Products include:
Asendin Tablets 1369

Atropine Sulfate (Effects of concurrent use not specified; careful adjustment of dosage and close supervision are required). Products include:
Arco-Lase Plus Tablets 512
Atrohist Plus Tablets 454
Atropine Sulfate Sterile Ophthalmic Solution .... ⊙ 233
Donnatal 2060
Donnatal Extentabs 2061
Donnatal Tablets 2060
Lomotil 2439
Motofen Tablets 784
Urised Tablets 1964

Belladonna Alkaloids (Effects of concurrent use not specified; careful adjustment of dosage and close supervision are required). Products include:
Bellergal-S Tablets 2250
Hyland's Bed Wetting Tablets .... ■ 828
Hyland's EnurAid Tablets .... ■ 829
Hyland's Teething Tablets .... ■ 830

Benztropine Mesylate (Effects of concurrent use not specified; careful adjustment of dosage and close supervision are required). Products include:
Cogentin 1621

Biperiden Hydrochloride (Effects of concurrent use not specified; careful adjustment of dosage and close supervision are required). Products include:
Akineton 1333

IMPORTANT NOTE: Always consult each drug listing in the patient's regimen for possible interactions.

Pamelor | Interactions Index | 782

Bupropion Hydrochloride (Concurrent use with drugs that are substrate for cytochrome $P_{450}IID_6$ may make normal metabolizer resemble poor metabolizer leading to higher than expected plasma concentrations of TCA with resultant toxicity). Products include:
- Wellbutrin Tablets 1204

Chlorpromazine (Concurrent use with drugs that are substrate for cytochrome $P_{450}IID_6$ may make normal metabolizer resemble poor metabolizer leading to higher than expected plasma concentrations of TCA with resultant toxicity). Products include:
- Thorazine Suppositories 2523

Chlorpromazine Hydrochloride (Concurrent use with drugs that are substrate for cytochrome $P_{450}IID_6$ may make normal metabolizer resemble poor metabolizer leading to higher than expected plasma concentrations of TCA with resultant toxicity). Products include:
- Thorazine 2523

Chlorpropamide (Potential for significant hypoglycemia in type II diabetics). Products include:
- Diabinese Tablets 1935

Cimetidine (Concurrent administration can produce clinically significant increases in the plasma concentrations of the tricyclic antidepressant). Products include:
- Tagamet Tablets 2516

Cimetidine Hydrochloride (Concurrent administration can produce clinically significant increases in the plasma concentrations of the tricyclic antidepressant). Products include:
- Tagamet 2516

Clidinium Bromide (Effects of concurrent use not specified; careful adjustment of dosage and close supervision are required). Products include:
- Librax Capsules 2176
- Quarzan Capsules 2181

Clonidine (Protryptyline may block the antihypertensive effect). Products include:
- Catapres-TTS 675

Clonidine Hydrochloride (Protryptyline may block the antihypertensive effect). Products include:
- Catapres Tablets 674
- Combipres Tablets 677

Desipramine Hydrochloride (Concurrent use with drugs that are substrate for cytochrome $P_{450}IID_6$ may make normal metabolizer resemble poor metabolizer leading to higher than expected plasma concentrations of TCA with resultant toxicity). Products include:
- Norpramin Tablets 1526

Dicyclomine Hydrochloride (Effects of concurrent use not specified; careful adjustment of dosage and close supervision are required). Products include:
- Bentyl 1501

Dobutamine Hydrochloride (Effects of concurrent use not specified; careful adjustment of dosage and close supervision are required). Products include:
- Dobutrex Solution Vials 1439

Dopamine Hydrochloride (Effects of concurrent use not specified; careful adjustment of dosage and close supervision are required).
- No products indexed under this heading.

Doxepin Hydrochloride (Concurrent use with drugs that are substrate for cytochrome $P_{450}IID_6$ may make normal metabolizer resemble poor metabolizer leading to higher than expected plasma concentrations of TCA with resultant toxicity). Products include:
- Sinequan 2205
- Zonalon Cream 1055

Ephedrine Hydrochloride (Effects of concurrent use not specified; careful adjustment of dosage and close supervision are required). Products include:
- Primatene Dual Action Formula ..... ◼ 872
- Primatene Tablets ..... ◼ 873
- Quadrinal Tablets 1350

Ephedrine Sulfate (Effects of concurrent use not specified; careful adjustment of dosage and close supervision are required). Products include:
- Bronkaid Caplets ..... ◼ 717
- Marax Tablets & DF Syrup 2200

Ephedrine Tannate (Effects of concurrent use not specified; careful adjustment of dosage and close supervision are required). Products include:
- Rynatuss 2673

Epinephrine (Effects of concurrent use not specified; careful adjustment of dosage and close supervision are required). Products include:
- Bronkaid Mist ..... ◼ 717
- EPIFRIN ..... ⊙ 239
- EpiPen 790
- Marcaine Hydrochloride with Epinephrine 1:200,000 2316
- Primatene Mist ..... ◼ 873
- Sensorcaine with Epinephrine Injection 559
- Sus-Phrine Injection 1019
- Xylocaine with Epinephrine Injections 567

Epinephrine Bitartrate (Effects of concurrent use not specified; careful adjustment of dosage and close supervision are required). Products include:
- Bronkaid Mist Suspension ..... ◼ 718
- Sensorcaine-MPF with Epinephrine Injection 559

Epinephrine Hydrochloride (Effects of concurrent use not specified; careful adjustment of dosage and close supervision are required). Products include:
- Ana-Kit Anaphylaxis Emergency Treatment Kit 617

Flecainide Acetate (Concurrent use with drugs that are substrate for cytochrome $P_{450}IID_6$ may make normal metabolizer resemble poor metabolizer leading to higher than expected plasma concentrations of TCA with resultant toxicity). Products include:
- Tambocor Tablets 1497

Fluoxetine Hydrochloride (Concurrent use with drugs that are substrate for cytochrome $P_{450}IID_6$ may make normal matabolizer resemble poor metabolizer leading to higher than expected plasma concentrations of TCA with resultant toxicity; due to variation in the extent of inhibition of $P_{450}IID_6$ and long half-life of fluoxetine and active metabolite sufficient time must elapse, at least 5 weeks, before switching to TCA). Products include:
- Prozac Pulvules & Liquid, Oral Solution 919

Fluphenazine Decanoate (Concurrent use with drugs that are substrate for cytochrome $P_{450}IID_6$ may make normal metabolizer resemble poor metabolizer leading to higher than expected plasma concentrations of TCA with resultant toxicity). Products include:
- Prolixin Decanoate 509

Fluphenazine Enanthate (Concurrent use with drugs that are substrate for cytochrome $P_{450}IID_6$ may make normal metabolizer resemble poor metabolizer leading to higher than expected plasma concentrations of TCA with resultant toxicity). Products include:
- Prolixin Enanthate 509

Fluphenazine Hydrochloride (Concurrent use with drugs that are substrate for cytochrome $P_{450}IID_6$ may make normal metabolizer resemble poor metabolizer leading to higher than expected plasma concentrations of TCA with resultant toxicity). Products include:
- Prolixin 509

Fluvoxamine Maleate (Concurrent use with drugs that are substrate for cytochrome $P_{450}IID_6$ may make normal metabolizer resemble poor metabolizer leading to higher than expected plasma concentrations of TCA with resultant toxicity). Products include:
- Luvox Tablets 2544

Furazolidone (Potential for hyperpyretic crises, severe convulsions, and fatalities; concurrent and/or sequential use is contraindicated). Products include:
- Furoxone 2046

Glycopyrrolate (Effects of concurrent use not specified; careful adjustment of dosage and close supervision are required). Products include:
- Robinul Forte Tablets 2072
- Robinul Injectable 2072
- Robinul Tablets 2072

Guanadrel Sulfate (Protryptyline may block the antihypertensive effect). Products include:
- Hylorel Tablets 985

Guanethidine Monosulfate (Protryptyline may block the antihypertensive effect of guanethidine or similarly acting compounds). Products include:
- Esimil Tablets 822
- Ismelin Tablets 827

Hyoscyamine (Effects of concurrent use not specified; careful adjustment of dosage and close supervision are required). Products include:
- Cystospaz Tablets 1963
- Urised Tablets 1964

Hyoscyamine Sulfate (Effects of concurrent use not specified; careful adjustment of dosage and close supervision are required). Products include:
- Arco-Lase Plus Tablets 512
- Atrohist Plus Tablets 454
- Cystospaz-M Capsules 1963
- Donnatal 2060
- Donnatal Extentabs 2061
- Donnatal Tablets 2060
- Kutrase Capsules 2402
- Levsin/Levsinex/Levbid 2405

Imipramine Hydrochloride (Concurrent use with drugs that are substrate for cytochrome $P_{450}IID_6$ may make normal metabolizer resemble poor metabolizer leading to higher than expected plasma concentrations of TCA with resultant toxicity). Products include:
- Tofranil Ampuls 854
- Tofranil Tablets 856

Imipramine Pamoate (Concurrent use with drugs that are substrate for cytochrome $P_{450}IID_6$ may make normal metabolizer resemble poor metabolizer leading to higher than expected plasma concentrations of TCA with resultant toxicity). Products include:
- Tofranil-PM Capsules 857

Ipratropium Bromide (Effects of concurrent use not specified; careful adjustment of dosage and close supervision are required). Products include:
- Atrovent Inhalation Aerosol 671
- Atrovent Inhalation Solution 673

Isocarboxazid (Potential for hyperpyretic crises, severe convulsions, and fatalities; concurrent and/or sequential use is contraindicated).
- No products indexed under this heading.

Isoproterenol Hydrochloride (Effects of concurrent use not specified; careful adjustment of dosage and close supervision are required). Products include:
- Isuprel Hydrochloride Injection 1:5000 2311
- Isuprel Hydrochloride Solution 1:200 & 1:100 2313
- Isuprel Mistometer 2312

Isoproterenol Sulfate (Effects of concurrent use not specified; careful adjustment of dosage and close supervision are required). Products include:
- Norisodrine with Calcium Iodide Syrup 442

Levothyroxine Sodium (Co-administration may produce cardiac arrhythmias). Products include:
- Levothroid Tablets 1016
- Levoxyl Tablets 903
- Synthroid 1359

Liothyronine Sodium (Co-administration may produce cardiac arrhythmias). Products include:
- Cytomel Tablets 2473
- Triostat Injection 2530

Liotrix (Co-administration may produce cardiac arrhythmias).
- No products indexed under this heading.

Maprotiline Hydrochloride (Concurrent use with drugs that are substrate for cytochrome $P_{450}IID_6$ may make normal metabolizer resemble poor metabolizer leading to higher than expected plasma concentrations of TCA with resultant toxicity). Products include:
- Ludiomil Tablets 843

Mepenzolate Bromide (Effects of concurrent use not specified; careful adjustment of dosage and close supervision are required).
- No products indexed under this heading.

Mesoridazine Besylate (Concurrent use with drugs that are substrate for cytochrome $P_{450}IID_6$ may make normal metabolizer resemble poor metabolizer leading to higher than expected plasma concentrations of TCA with resultant toxicity). Products include:
- Serentil 684

(◼ Described in PDR For Nonprescription Drugs) (⊙ Described in PDR For Ophthalmology)

Interactions Index

Metaproterenol Sulfate (Effects of concurrent use not specified; careful adjustment of dosage and close supervision are required). Products include:

Alupent 669
Metaproterenol Sulfate Inhalation Solution, USP, Arm-a-Med 552

Metaraminol Bitartrate (Effects of concurrent use not specified; careful adjustment of dosage and close supervision are required). Products include:

Aramine Injection 1609

Methotrimeprazine (Concurrent use with drugs that are substrate for cytochrome $P_{450}IID_6$ may make normal metabolizer resemble poor metabolizer leading to higher than expected plasma concentrations of TCA with resultant toxicity). Products include:

Levoprome 1274

Methoxamine Hydrochloride (Effects of concurrent use not specified; careful adjustment of dosage and close supervision are required). Products include:

Vasoxyl Injection 1196

Nefazodone Hydrochloride (Concurrent use with drugs that are substrate for cytochrome $P_{450}IID_6$ may make normal metabolizer resemble poor metabolizer leading to higher than expected plasma concentrations of TCA with resultant toxicity). Products include:

Serzone Tablets 771

Norepinephrine Bitartrate (Effects of concurrent use not specified; careful adjustment of dosage and close supervision are required). Products include:

Levophed Bitartrate Injection 2315

Oxybutynin Chloride (Effects of concurrent use not specified; careful adjustment of dosage and close supervision are required). Products include:

Ditropan 1516

Paroxetine Hydrochloride (Concurrent use with drugs that are substrate for cytochrome $P_{450}IID_6$ may make normal metabolizer resemble poor metabolizer leading to higher than expected plasma concentrations of TCA with resultant toxicity; due to variation in the extent of inhibition of $P_{450}IID_6$ caution is indicated; if co-administered sufficient time should elapse before switching to TCA). Products include:

Paxil Tablets 2505

Perphenazine (Concurrent use with drugs that are substrate for cytochrome $P_{450}IID_6$ may make normal metabolizer resemble poor metabolizer leading to higher than expected plasma concentrations of TCA with resultant toxicity). Products include:

Etrafon 2355
Triavil Tablets 1757
Trilafon 2389

Phenelzine Sulfate (Potential for hyperpyretic crises, severe convulsions, and fatalities; concurrent and/or sequential use is contraindicated). Products include:

Nardil 1920

Phenylephrine Bitartrate (Effects of concurrent use not specified; careful adjustment of dosage and close supervision are required).

No products indexed under this heading.

Phenylephrine Hydrochloride (Effects of concurrent use not specified; careful adjustment of dosage and close supervision are required). Products include:

Atrohist Plus Tablets 454
Cerose DM .... ®D 878
Comhist 2038
D.A. Chewable Tablets 951
Deconsal Pediatric Capsules 454
Dura-Vent/DA Tablets 953
Entex Capsules 1986
Entex Liquid 1986
Extendryl 1005
4-Way Fast Acting Nasal Spray (regular & mentholated) .... ®D 621
Hemorid For Women .... ®D 834
Hycomine Compound Tablets 932
Neo-Synephrine Hydrochloride 1% Carpuject 2324
Neo-Synephrine Hydrochloride 1% Injection 2324
Neo-Synephrine Hydrochloride (Ophthalmic) 2325
Neo-Synephrine .... ®D 726
Nöstril .... ®D 644
Novahistine Elixir .... ®D 823
Phenergan VC 2779
Phenergan VC with Codeine 2781
Preparation H .... ®D 871
Tympagesic Ear Drops 2342
Vasosulf .... © 271
Vicks Sinex Nasal Spray and Ultra Fine Mist .... ®D 765

Phenylephrine Tannate (Effects of concurrent use not specified; careful adjustment of dosage and close supervision are required). Products include:

Atrohist Pediatric Suspension 454
Ricobid-D Pediatric Suspension 2038
Ricobid Tablets and Pediatric Suspension 2038
Rynatan 2673
Rynatuss 2673

Phenylpropanolamine Hydrochloride (Effects of concurrent use not specified; careful adjustment of dosage and close supervision are required). Products include:

Acutrim .... ®D 628
Allerest Children's Chewable Tablets .... ®D 627
Allerest 12 Hour Caplets .... ®D 627
Atrohist Plus Tablets 454
BC Cold Powder Multi-Symptom Formula (Cold-Sinus-Allergy) ...... ®D 609
BC Cold Powder Non-Drowsy Formula (Cold-Sinus) .... ®D 609
Cheracol Plus Head Cold/Cough Formula .... ®D 769
Comtrex Multi-Symptom Non-Drowsy Liqui-gels .... ®D 618
Contac Continuous Action Nasal Decongestant/Antihistamine 12 Hour Capsules .... ®D 813
Contac Maximum Strength Continuous Action Decongestant/ Antihistamine 12 Hour Caplets.. ®D 813
Contac Severe Cold and Flu Formula Caplets .... ®D 814
Coricidin 'D' Decongestant Tablets .... ®D 800
Dexatrim .... ®D 832
Dexatrim Plus Vitamins Caplets .... ®D 832
Dimetane-DC Cough Syrup 2059
Dimetapp Elixir .... ®D 773
Dimetapp Extentabs .... ®D 774
Dimetapp Tablets/Liqui-Gels .... ®D 775
Dimetapp Cold & Allergy Chewable Tablets .... ®D 773
Dimetapp DM Elixir .... ®D 774
Dura-Vent Tablets 952
Entex Capsules 1986
Entex LA Tablets 1987
Entex Liquid 1986
Exgest LA Tablets 782
Hycomine 931
Isoclor Timesule Capsules .... ®D 637
Nolamine Timed-Release Tablets 785
Ornade Spansule Capsules 2502
Propagest Tablets 786
Pyrroxate Caplets .... ®D 772
Robitussin-CF .... ®D 777
Sinulin Tablets 787
Tavist-D 12 Hour Relief Tablets .... ®D 787
Teldrin 12 Hour Antihistamine/ Nasal Decongestant Allergy Relief Capsules .... ®D 826

Triaminic Allergy Tablets .... ®D 789
Triaminic Cold Tablets .... ®D 790
Triaminic Expectorant .... ®D 790
Triaminic Syrup .... ®D 792
Triaminic-12 Tablets .... ®D 792
Triaminic-DM Syrup .... ®D 792
Triaminicin Tablets .... ®D 793
Triaminicol Multi-Symptom Cold Tablets .... ®D 793
Triaminicol Multi-Symptom Relief ®D 794
Vicks DayQuil Allergy Relief 12-Hour Extended Release Tablets.. ®D 760
Vicks DayQuil Allergy Relief 4-Hour Tablets .... ®D 760
Vicks DayQuil SINUS Pressure & CONGESTION Relief .... ®D 761

Pirbuterol Acetate (Effects of concurrent use not specified; careful adjustment of dosage and close supervision are required). Products include:

Maxair Autohaler 1492
Maxair Inhaler 1494

Prochlorperazine (Concurrent use with drugs that are substrate for cytochrome $P_{450}IID_6$ may make normal metabolizer resemble poor metabolizer leading to higher than expected plasma concentrations of TCA with resultant toxicity). Products include:

Compazine 2470

Procyclidine Hydrochloride (Effects of concurrent use not specified; careful adjustment of dosage and close supervision are required). Products include:

Kemadrin Tablets 1112

Promethazine Hydrochloride (Concurrent use with drugs that are substrate for cytochrome $P_{450}IID_6$ may make normal metabolizer resemble poor metabolizer leading to higher than expected plasma concentrations of TCA with resultant toxicity). Products include:

Mepergan Injection 2753
Phenergan with Codeine 2777
Phenergan with Dextromethorphan 2778
Phenergan Injection 2773
Phenergan Suppositories 2775
Phenergan Syrup 2774
Phenergan Tablets 2775
Phenergan VC 2779
Phenergan VC with Codeine 2781

Propafenone Hydrochloride (Concurrent use with drugs that are substrate for cytochrome $P_{450}IID_6$ may make normal metabolizer resemble poor metabolizer leading to higher than expected plasma concentrations of TCA with resultant toxicity). Products include:

Rythmol Tablets–150mg, 225mg, 300mg 1352

Propantheline Bromide (Effects of concurrent use not specified; careful adjustment of dosage and close supervision are required). Products include:

Pro-Banthine Tablets 2052

Protriptyline Hydrochloride (Concurrent use with drugs that are substrate for cytochrome $P_{450}IID_6$ may make normal metabolizer resemble poor metabolizer leading to higher than expected plasma concentrations of TCA with resultant toxicity). Products include:

Vivactil Tablets 1774

Pseudoephedrine Hydrochloride (Effects of concurrent use not specified; careful adjustment of dosage and close supervision are required). Products include:

Actifed Allergy Daytime/Nighttime Caplets .... ®D 844
Actifed Plus Caplets .... ®D 845
Actifed Plus Tablets .... ®D 845
Actifed with Codeine Cough Syrup.. 1067
Actifed Sinus Daytime/Nighttime Tablets and Caplets .... ®D 846

Pamelor

Actifed Syrup .... ®D 846
Actifed Tablets .... ®D 844
Advil Cold and Sinus Caplets and Tablets (formerly CoAdvil) .... ®D 870
Alka-Seltzer Plus Cold Medicine Liqui-Gels .... ®D 706
Alka-Seltzer Plus Cold & Cough Medicine Liqui-Gels .... ®D 705
Alka-Seltzer Plus Night-Time Cold Medicine Liqui-Gels .... ®D 706
Allerest Headache Strength Tablets .... ®D 627
Allerest Maximum Strength Tablets .... ®D 627
Allerest No Drowsiness Tablets ...... ®D 627
Allerest Sinus Pain Formula .... ®D 627
Anatuss LA Tablets 1542
Atrohist Pediatric Capsules 453
Bayer Select Sinus Pain Relief Formula .... ®D 717
Benadryl Allergy Decongestant Liquid Medication .... ®D 848
Benadryl Allergy Decongestant Tablets .... ®D 848
Benadryl Allergy Sinus Headache Formula Caplets .... ®D 849
Benylin Multisymptom .... ®D 852
Bromfed Capsules (Extended-Release) 1785
Bromfed Syrup .... ®D 733
Bromfed Tablets 1785
Bromfed-DM Cough Syrup 1786
Bromfed-PD Capsules (Extended-Release) 1785
Children's Vicks DayQuil Allergy Relief .... ®D 757
Children's Vicks NyQuil Cold/ Cough Relief .... ®D 758
Comtrex Multi-Symptom Cold Reliever Tablets/Caplets/Liqui-Gels/Liquid .... ®D 615
Allergy-Sinus Comtrex Multi-Symptom Allergy-Sinus Formula Tablets .... ®D 617
Comtrex Multi-Symptom Non-Drowsy Caplets .... ®D 618
Congess 1004
Contac Day Allergy/Sinus Caplets ®D 812
Contac Day & Night .... ®D 812
Contac Night Allergy/Sinus Caplets .... ®D 812
Contac Severe Cold & Flu Non-Drowsy .... ®D 815
Deconamine Chewable Tablets 1320
Deconamine CX Cough and Cold Liquid and Tablets 1319
Deconamine 1320
Deconsal C Expectorant Syrup 456
Deconsal Pediatric Syrup 457
Deconsal II Tablets 454
Dimetane-DX Cough Syrup 2059
Dimetapp Sinus Caplets .... ®D 775
Dorcol Children's Cough Syrup ...... ®D 785
Drixoral Cough + Congestion Liquid Caps .... ®D 802
Dura-Tap/PD Capsules 2867
Duratuss Tablets 2565
Duratuss HD Elixir 2565
Efidac/24 .... ®D 635
Entex PSE Tablets 1987
Fedahist Gyrocaps 2401
Fedahist Timecaps 2401
Guaifed 1787
Guaifed Syrup .... ®D 734
Guaimax-D Tablets 792
Guaitab Tablets .... ®D 734
Isoclor Expectorant 990
Kronofed-A 977
Motrin IB Sinus .... ®D 838
Novahistine DH 2462
Novahistine DMX .... ®D 822
Novahistine Expectorant 2463
Nucofed 2051
PediaCare Cold Allergy Chewable Tablets .... ®D 677
PediaCare Cough-Cold Chewable Tablets 1553
PediaCare 1553
PediaCare Infants' Decongestant Drops .... ®D 677
PediCare Infant's Drops Decongestant Plus Cough 1553
PediaCare NightRest Cough-Cold Liquid 1553
Pediatric Vicks 44d Dry Hacking Cough & Head Congestion .... ®D 763
Pediatric Vicks 44m Cough & Cold Relief .... ®D 764
Robitussin Cold & Cough Liqui-Gels .... ®D 776

IMPORTANT NOTE: Always consult each drug listing in the patient's regimen for possible interactions.

Pamelor **Interactions Index** **784**

Robitussin Maximum Strength Cough & Cold ▣ 778
Robitussin Pediatric Cough & Cold Formula ▣ 779
Robitussin Severe Congestion Liqui-Gels ▣ 776
Robitussin-DAC Syrup 2074
Robitussin-PE ▣ 778
Rondec Oral Drops 953
Rondec Syrup 953
Rondec Tablet 953
Rondec-DM Oral Drops 954
Rondec-DM Syrup 954
Rondec-TR Tablet 953
Ryna ▣ 841
Seldane-D Extended-Release Tablets 1538
Semprex-D Capsules 463
Semprex-D Capsules 1167
Sinarest Tablets ▣ 648
Sinarest Extra Strength Tablets ▣ 648
Sinarest No Drowsiness Tablets ▣ 648
Sine-Aid IB Caplets 1554
Sine-Aid Maximum Strength Sinus Medication Gelcaps, Caplets and Tablets 1554
Sine-Off No Drowsiness Formula Caplets ▣ 824
Sine-Off Sinus Medicine ▣ 825
Singlet Tablets ▣ 825
Sinutab Non-Drying Liquid Caps ▣ 859
Sinutab Sinus Allergy Medication, Maximum Strength Tablets and Caplets ▣ 860
Sinutab Sinus Medication, Maximum Strength Without Drowsiness Formula, Tablets & Caplets ▣ 860
Sinutab Sinus Medication, Regular Strength Without Drowsiness Formula ▣ 859
Sudafed Children's Liquid ▣ 861
Sudafed Cold and Cough Liquidcaps ▣ 862
Sudafed Cough Syrup ▣ 862
Sudafed Plus Liquid ▣ 862
Sudafed Plus Tablets ▣ 863
Sudafed Severe Cold Formula Caplets ▣ 863
Sudafed Severe Cold Formula Tablets ▣ 864
Sudafed Sinus Caplets ▣ 864
Sudafed Sinus Tablets ▣ 864
Sudafed Tablets, 30 mg ▣ 861
Sudafed Tablets, 60 mg ▣ 861
Sudafed 12 Hour Caplets ▣ 861
Syn-Rx Tablets 465
Syn-Rx DM Tablets 466
TheraFlu ▣ 787
TheraFlu Maximum Strength Nighttime Flu, Cold & Cough Medicine ▣ 788
TheraFlu Maximum Strength Non-Drowsy Formula Flu, Cold & Cough Medicine ▣ 788
Thera Flu Maximum Strength, Non-Drowsy Formula Flu, Cold and Cough Caplets ▣ 789
Triaminic AM Cough and Decongestant Formula ▣ 789
Triaminic AM Decongestant Formula ▣ 790
Triaminic Nite Light ▣ 791
Triaminic Sore Throat Formula ▣ 791
Tussend 1783
Tussend Expectorant 1785
Children's TYLENOL Cold Multi-Symptom Liquid Formula and Chewable Tablets 1561
Children's TYLENOL Cold Plus Cough Multi Symptom Tablets and Liquid ▣ 681
Infants' TYLENOL Cold Decongestant & Fever-Reducer Drops 1556
TYLENOL Maximum Strength Allergy Sinus Medication Gelcaps and Caplets 1563
TYLENOL Maximum Strength Allergy Sinus NightTime Medication Caplets 1555
TYLENOL Flu Maximum Strength Gelcaps 1565
TYLENOL Flu NightTime, Maximum Strength, Gelcaps 1566
TYLENOL Maximum Strength Flu NightTime Hot Medication Packets 1562
TYLENOL, Maximum Strength, Sinus Medication Geltabs, Gelcaps, Caplets and Tablets 1566
TYLENOL Cold Multi-Symptom Formula Medication Tablets and Caplets 1561
TYLENOL Cold Medication No Drowsiness Formula Gelcaps and Caplets 1562
TYLENOL Cold Multi-Symptom Hot Medication Liquid Packets 1557
TYLENOL Cough Multi-Symptom Medication with Decongestant 1565
Ursinus Inlay-Tabs ▣ 794
Vicks 44 LiquiCaps Cough, Cold & Flu Relief ▣ 755
Vicks 44 LiquiCaps Non-Drowsy Cough & Cold Relief ▣ 756
Vicks 44D Dry Hacking Cough & Head Congestion ▣ 755
Vicks 44M Cough, Cold & Flu Relief ▣ 756
Vicks DayQuil ▣ 761
Vicks DayQuil SINUS Pressure & PAIN Relief with IBUPROFEN ▣ 762
Vicks Nyquil Hot Therapy ▣ 762
Vicks NyQuil LiquiCaps Multi-Symptom Cold/Flu Relief ▣ 763
Vicks NyQuil Multi-Symptom Cold/Flu Relief - (Original & Cherry Flavor) ▣ 763

Pseudoephedrine Sulfate (Effects of concurrent use not specified; careful adjustment of dosage and close supervision are required). Products include:
Cheracol Sinus ▣ 768
Chlor-Trimeton Allergy Decongestant Tablets ▣ 799
Claritin-D 2350
Drixoral Cold and Allergy Sustained-Action Tablets ▣ 802
Drixoral Cold and Flu Extended-Release Tablets ▣ 803
Drixoral Non-Drowsy Formula Extended-Release Tablets ▣ 803
Drixoral Allergy/Sinus Extended Release Tablets ▣ 804
Trinalin Repetabs Tablets 1330

Quinidine Gluconate (Co-administration may result in longer plasma half-life, higher AUC and lower clearance of nortriptyline). Products include:
Quinaglute Dura-Tabs Tablets 649

Quinidine Polygalacturonate (Co-administration may result in longer plasma half-life, higher AUC and lower clearance of nortriptyline).
No products indexed under this heading.

Quinidine Sulfate (Co-administration may result in longer plasma half-life, higher AUC and lower clearance of nortriptyline). Products include:
Quinidex Extentabs 2067

Reserpine (Co-administration may produce a "stimulating" effect in some depressed patients). Products include:
Diupres Tablets 1650
Hydropres Tablets 1675
Ser-Ap-Es Tablets 849

Salmeterol Xinafoate (Effects of concurrent use not specified; careful adjustment of dosage and close supervision are required). Products include:
Serevent Inhalation Aerosol 1176

Scopolamine (Effects of concurrent use not specified; careful adjustment of dosage and close supervision are required). Products include:
Transderm Scōp Transdermal Therapeutic System 869

Scopolamine Hydrobromide (Effects of concurrent use not specified; careful adjustment of dosage and close supervision are required). Products include:
Atrohist Plus Tablets 454
Donnatal 2060
Donnatal Extentabs 2061
Donnatal Tablets 2060

Selegiline Hydrochloride (Potential for hyperpyretic crises, severe convulsions, and fatalities; concurrent and/or sequential use is contraindicated). Products include:
Eldepryl Tablets 2550

Sertraline Hydrochloride (Concurrent use with drugs that are substrate for cytochrome $P_{450}IID_6$ may make normal metabolizer resemble poor metabolizer leading to higher than expected plasma concentrations of TCA with resultant toxicity; due to variation in the extent of inhibition of $P_{450}IID_6$ caution is indicated; if co-administered sufficient time should elapse before switching to TCA). Products include:
Zoloft Tablets 2217

Terbutaline Sulfate (Effects of concurrent use not specified; careful adjustment of dosage and close supervision are required). Products include:
Brethaire Inhaler 813
Brethine Ampuls 815
Brethine Tablets 814
Bricanyl Subcutaneous Injection 1502
Bricanyl Tablets 1503

Thioridazine Hydrochloride (Concurrent use with drugs that are substrate for cytochrome $P_{450}IID_6$ may make normal metabolizer resemble poor metabolizer leading to higher than expected plasma concentrations of TCA with resultant toxicity). Products include:
Mellaril 2269

Thyroglobulin (Co-administration may produce cardiac arrhythmias).
No products indexed under this heading.

Thyroid (Co-administration may produce cardiac arrhythmias).
No products indexed under this heading.

Thyroxine (Co-administration may produce cardiac arrhythmias).
No products indexed under this heading.

Thyroxine Sodium (Co-administration may produce cardiac arrhythmias).
No products indexed under this heading.

Tranylcypromine Sulfate (Potential for hyperpyretic crises, severe convulsions, and fatalities; concurrent and/or sequential use is contraindicated). Products include:
Parnate Tablets 2503

Trazodone Hydrochloride (Concurrent use with drugs that are substrate for cytochrome $P_{450}IID_6$ may make normal metabolizer resemble poor metabolizer leading to higher than expected plasma concentrations of TCA with resultant toxicity). Products include:
Desyrel and Desyrel Dividose 503

Tridihexethyl Chloride (Effects of concurrent use not specified; careful adjustment of dosage and close supervision are required).
No products indexed under this heading.

Trifluoperazine Hydrochloride (Concurrent use with drugs that are substrate for cytochrome $P_{450}IID_6$ may make normal metabolizer resemble poor metabolizer leading to higher than expected plasma concentrations of TCA with resultant toxicity). Products include:
Stelazine 2514

Trihexyphenidyl Hydrochloride (Effects of concurrent use not specified; careful adjustment of dosage and close supervision are required). Products include:
Artane 1368

Trimipramine Maleate (Concurrent use with drugs that are substrate for cytochrome $P_{450}IID_6$ may make normal metabolizer resemble poor metabolizer leading to higher than expected plasma concentrations of TCA with resultant toxicity). Products include:
Surmontil Capsules 2811

Venlafaxine Hydrochloride (Concurrent use with drugs that are substrate for cytochrome $P_{450}IID_6$ may make normal metabolizer resemble poor metabolizer leading to higher than expected plasma concentrations of TCA with resultant toxicity; due to variation in the extent of inhibition of $P_{450}IID_6$ caution is indicated; if co-administered sufficient time should elapse before switching to TCA). Products include:
Effexor 2719

Food Interactions

Alcohol (Excessive consumption of alcohol with nortriptyline may have a potentiating effect and exaggerated response to alcohol).

PAMELOR SOLUTION
(Nortriptyline Hydrochloride) 2280
See **Pamelor Capsules**

PANODOL TABLETS AND CAPLETS
(Acetaminophen) ▣ 824
None cited in PDR database.

CHILDREN'S PANADOL CHEWABLE TABLETS, LIQUID, INFANT'S DROPS
(Acetaminophen) ▣ 824
None cited in PDR database.

PANAFIL OINTMENT
(Papain, Chlorophyllin Copper Complex, Urea) 2246
May interact with:

Heavy metal salts, unspecified (Papain may be inactivated by the salts of heavy metals).

Hydrogen Peroxide (May inactivate papain). Products include:
Oxysept Disinfection System ⊙ 340
Oxysept 1 Disinfecting Solution ⊙ 339
UltraCare System ⊙ 342

PANAFIL-WHITE OINTMENT
(Papain, Urea) 2247
May interact with:

Heavy metal salts, unspecified (Papain may be inactivated by the salts of heavy metals).

Hydrogen Peroxide (May inactivate papain). Products include:
Oxysept Disinfection System ⊙ 340
Oxysept 1 Disinfecting Solution ⊙ 339
UltraCare System ⊙ 342

PANCREASE CAPSULES
(Pancrelipase) 1579
None cited in PDR database.

PANCREASE MT CAPSULES
(Pancrelipase) 1579
None cited in PDR database.

(▣ Described in PDR For Nonprescription Drugs) (⊙ Described in PDR For Ophthalmology)

785 **Interactions Index** **Paraflex**

PANHEMATIN
(Hemin For Injection) 443

May interact with oral anticoagulants, estrogens, and barbiturates. Compounds in these categories include:

Aprobarbital (Increases delta-aminolevalinic acid synthetase).
- No products indexed under this heading.

Butabarbital (Increases delta-aminolevalinic acid synthetase).
- No products indexed under this heading.

Butalbital (Increases delta-aminolevalinic acid synthetase). Products include:
- Esgic-plus Tablets 1013
- Fioricet Tablets 2258
- Fioricet with Codeine Capsules 2260
- Fiorinal Capsules 2261
- Fiorinal with Codeine Capsules 2262
- Fiorinal Tablets 2261
- Phrenilin 785
- Sedapap Tablets 50 mg/650 mg .. 1543

Chlorotrianisene (Increases delta-aminolevalinic acid synthetase).
- No products indexed under this heading.

Dicumarol (Hypocoagulable state).
- No products indexed under this heading.

Dienestrol (Increases delta-aminolevalinic acid synthetase). Products include:
- Ortho Dienestrol Cream 1866

Diethylstilbestrol (Increases delta-aminolevalinic acid synthetase). Products include:
- Diethylstilbestrol Tablets 1437

Estradiol (Increases delta-aminolevalinic acid synthetase). Products include:
- Climara Transdermal System 645
- Estrace Cream and Tablets 749
- Estraderm Transdermal System 824

Estrogens, Conjugated (Increases delta-aminolevalinic acid synthetase). Products include:
- PMB 200 and PMB 400 2783
- Premarin Intravenous 2787
- Premarin with Methyltestosterone .. 2794
- Premarin Tablets 2789
- Premarin Vaginal Cream 2791
- Premphase 2797
- Prempro 2801

Estrogens, Esterified (Increases delta-aminolevalinic acid synthetase). Products include:
- ESTRATAB Tablets (0.3, 0.625, 1.25, 2.5 mg) 2536
- Estratest 2539
- Menest Tablets 2494

Estropipate (Increases delta-aminolevalinic acid synthetase). Products include:
- Ogen Tablets 2627
- Ogen Vaginal Cream 2630
- Ortho-Est 1869

Ethinyl Estradiol (Increases delta-aminolevalinic acid synthetase). Products include:
- Brevicon 2088
- Demulen 2428
- Desogen Tablets 1817
- Levlen/Tri-Levlen 651
- Lo/Ovral Tablets 2746
- Lo/Ovral-28 Tablets 2751
- Modicon 1872
- Nordette-21 Tablets 2755
- Nordette-28 Tablets 2758
- Norinyl 2088
- Ortho-Cept 1851
- Ortho-Cyclen/Ortho-Tri-Cyclen 1858
- Ortho-Novum 1872
- Ortho-Cyclen/Ortho Tri-Cyclen 1858
- Ovcon 760
- Ovral Tablets 2770
- Ovral-28 Tablets 2770
- Levlen/Tri-Levlen 651
- Tri-Norinyl 2164
- Triphasil-21 Tablets 2814
- Triphasil-28 Tablets 2819

Mephobarbital (Increases delta-aminolevalinic acid synthetase). Products include:
- Mebaral Tablets 2322

Pentobarbital Sodium (Increases delta-aminolevalinic acid synthetase). Products include:
- Nembutal Sodium Capsules 436
- Nembutal Sodium Solution 438
- Nembutal Sodium Suppositories 440

Phenobarbital (Increases delta-aminolevalinic acid synthetase). Products include:
- Arco-Lase Plus Tablets 512
- Bellergal-S Tablets 2250
- Donnatal 2060
- Donnatal Extentabs 2061
- Donnatal Tablets 2060
- Phenobarbital Elixir and Tablets 1469
- Quadrinal Tablets 1350

Polyestradiol Phosphate (Increases delta-aminolevalinic acid synthetase).
- No products indexed under this heading.

Quinestrol (Increases delta-aminolevalinic acid synthetase).
- No products indexed under this heading.

Secobarbital Sodium (Increases delta-aminolevalinic acid synthetase). Products include:
- Seconal Sodium Pulvules 1474

Thiamylal Sodium (Increases delta-aminolevalinic acid synthetase).
- No products indexed under this heading.

Warfarin Sodium (Hypocoagulable state). Products include:
- Coumadin 926

PAPAVERINE HYDROCHLORIDE VIALS AND AMPOULES
(Papaverine Hydrochloride) 1468

None cited in PDR database.

PARAFLEX CAPLETS
(Chlorzoxazone) 1580

May interact with central nervous system depressants and certain other agents. Compounds in these categories include:

Alfentanil Hydrochloride (May produce additive effect). Products include:
- Alfenta Injection 1286

Alprazolam (May produce additive effect). Products include:
- Xanax Tablets 2649

Aprobarbital (May produce additive effect).
- No products indexed under this heading.

Buprenorphine (May produce additive effect). Products include:
- Buprenex Injectable 2006

Buspirone Hydrochloride (May produce additive effect). Products include:
- BuSpar 737

Butabarbital (May produce additive effect).
- No products indexed under this heading.

Butalbital (May produce additive effect). Products include:
- Esgic-plus Tablets 1013
- Fioricet Tablets 2258
- Fioricet with Codeine Capsules 2260
- Fiorinal Capsules 2261
- Fiorinal with Codeine Capsules 2262
- Fiorinal Tablets 2261
- Phrenilin 785
- Sedapap Tablets 50 mg/650 mg .. 1543

Chlordiazepoxide (May produce additive effect). Products include:
- Libritabs Tablets 2177
- Limbitrol 2180

Chlordiazepoxide Hydrochloride (May produce additive effect). Products include:
- Librax Capsules 2176
- Librium Capsules 2178
- Librium Injectable 2179

Chlorpromazine (May produce additive effect). Products include:
- Thorazine Suppositories 2523

Chlorpromazine Hydrochloride (May produce additive effect). Products include:
- Thorazine 2523

Chlorprothixene (May produce additive effect).
- No products indexed under this heading.

Chlorprothixene Hydrochloride (May produce additive effect).
- No products indexed under this heading.

Clorazepate Dipotassium (May produce additive effect). Products include:
- Tranxene 451

Clozapine (May produce additive effect). Products include:
- Clozaril Tablets 2252

Codeine Phosphate (May produce additive effect). Products include:
- Actifed with Codeine Cough Syrup.. 1067
- Brontex 1981
- Deconsal C Expectorant Syrup 456
- Deconsal Pediatric Syrup 457
- Dimetane-DC Cough Syrup 2059
- Empirin with Codeine Tablets 1093
- Fioricet with Codeine Capsules 2260
- Fiorinal with Codeine Capsules 2262
- Isoclor Expectorant 990
- Novahistine DH 2462
- Novahistine Expectorant 2463
- Nucofed 2051
- Phenergan with Codeine 2777
- Phenergan VC with Codeine 2781
- Robitussin A-C Syrup 2073
- Robitussin-DAC Syrup 2074
- Ryna 841
- Soma Compound w/Codeine Tablets 2676
- Tussi-Organidin NR Liquid and S NR Liquid 2677
- Tylenol with Codeine 1583

Desflurane (May produce additive effect). Products include:
- Suprane 1813

Dezocine (May produce additive effect). Products include:
- Dalgan Injection 538

Diazepam (May produce additive effect). Products include:
- Dizac 1809
- Valium Injectable 2182
- Valium Tablets 2183
- Valrelease Capsules 2169

Droperidol (May produce additive effect). Products include:
- Inapsine Injection 1296

Enflurane (May produce additive effect).
- No products indexed under this heading.

Estazolam (May produce additive effect). Products include:
- ProSom Tablets 449

Ethchlorvynol (May produce additive effect). Products include:
- Placidyl Capsules 448

Ethinamate (May produce additive effect).
- No products indexed under this heading.

Fentanyl (May produce additive effect). Products include:
- Duragesic Transdermal System 1288

Fentanyl Citrate (May produce additive effect). Products include:
- Sublimaze Injection 1307

Fluphenazine Decanoate (May produce additive effect). Products include:
- Prolixin Decanoate 509

Fluphenazine Enanthate (May produce additive effect). Products include:
- Prolixin Enanthate 509

Fluphenazine Hydrochloride (May produce additive effect). Products include:
- Prolixin 509

Flurazepam Hydrochloride (May produce additive effect). Products include:
- Dalmane Capsules 2173

Glutethimide (May produce additive effect).
- No products indexed under this heading.

Haloperidol (May produce additive effect). Products include:
- Haldol Injection, Tablets and Concentrate 1575

Haloperidol Decanoate (May produce additive effect). Products include:
- Haldol Decanoate 1577

Hydrocodone Bitartrate (May produce additive effect). Products include:
- Anexsia 5/500 Elixir 1781
- Anexia Tablets 1782
- Codiclear DH Syrup 791
- Deconamine CX Cough and Cold Liquid and Tablets 1319
- Duratuss HD Elixir 2565
- Hycodan Tablets and Syrup 930
- Hycomine Compound Tablets 932
- Hycomine 931
- Hycotuss Expectorant Syrup 933
- Hydrocet Capsules 782
- Lorcet 10/650 1018
- Lortab 2566
- Tussend 1783
- Tussend Expectorant 1785
- Vicodin Tablets 1356
- Vicodin ES Tablets 1357
- Vicodin Tuss Expectorant 1358
- Zydone Capsules 949

Hydrocodone Polistirex (May produce additive effect). Products include:
- Tussionex Pennkinetic Extended-Release Suspension 998

Hydroxyzine Hydrochloride (May produce additive effect). Products include:
- Atarax Tablets & Syrup 2185
- Marax Tablets & DF Syrup 2200
- Vistaril Intramuscular Solution 2216

Isoflurane (May produce additive effect).
- No products indexed under this heading.

Ketamine Hydrochloride (May produce additive effect).
- No products indexed under this heading.

Levomethadyl Acetate Hydrochloride (May produce additive effect). Products include:
- Orlamm 2239

Levorphanol Tartrate (May produce additive effect). Products include:
- Levo-Dromoran 2129

Lorazepam (May produce additive effect). Products include:
- Ativan Injection 2698
- Ativan Tablets 2700

Loxapine Hydrochloride (May produce additive effect). Products include:
- Loxitane 1378

Loxapine Succinate (May produce additive effect). Products include:
- Loxitane Capsules 1378

IMPORTANT NOTE: Always consult each drug listing in the patient's regimen for possible interactions.

Paraflex   Interactions Index   786

Meperidine Hydrochloride (May produce additive effect). Products include:
- Demerol ... 2308
- Mepergan Injection ... 2753

Mephobarbital (May produce additive effect). Products include:
- Mebaral Tablets ... 2322

Meprobamate (May produce additive effect). Products include:
- Miltown Tablets ... 2672
- PMB 200 and PMB 400 ... 2783

Mesoridazine Besylate (May produce additive effect). Products include:
- Serentil ... 684

Methadone Hydrochloride (May produce additive effect). Products include:
- Methadone Hydrochloride Oral Concentrate ... 2233
- Methadone Hydrochloride Oral Solution & Tablets ... 2235

Methohexital Sodium (May produce additive effect). Products include:
- Brevital Sodium Vials ... 1429

Methotrimeprazine (May produce additive effect). Products include:
- Levoprome ... 1274

Methoxyflurane (May produce additive effect).
- No products indexed under this heading.

Midazolam Hydrochloride (May produce additive effect). Products include:
- Versed Injection ... 2170

Molindone Hydrochloride (May produce additive effect). Products include:
- Moban Tablets and Concentrate ... 1048

Morphine Sulfate (May produce additive effect). Products include:
- Astramorph/PF Injection, USP (Preservative-Free) ... 535
- Duramorph ... 962
- Infumorph 200 and Infumorph 500 Sterile Solutions ... 965
- MS Contin Tablets ... 1994
- MSIR ... 1997
- Oramorph SR (Morphine Sulfate Sustained Release Tablets) ... 2236
- RMS Suppositories ... 2657
- Roxanol ... 2243

Opium Alkaloids (May produce additive effect).
- No products indexed under this heading.

Oxazepam (May produce additive effect). Products include:
- Serax Capsules ... 2810
- Serax Tablets ... 2810

Oxycodone Hydrochloride (May produce additive effect). Products include:
- Percocet Tablets ... 938
- Percodan Tablets ... 939
- Percodan-Demi Tablets ... 940
- Roxicodone Tablets, Oral Solution & Intensol (Oxycodone) ... 2244
- Tylox Capsules ... 1584

Pentobarbital Sodium (May produce additive effect). Products include:
- Nembutal Sodium Capsules ... 436
- Nembutal Sodium Solution ... 438
- Nembutal Sodium Suppositories ... 440

Perphenazine (May produce additive effect). Products include:
- Etrafon ... 2355
- Triavil Tablets ... 1757
- Trilafon ... 2389

Phenobarbital (May produce additive effect). Products include:
- Arco-Lase Plus Tablets ... 512
- Bellergal-S Tablets ... 2250
- Donnatal ... 2060
- Donnatal Extentabs ... 2061
- Donnatal Tablets ... 2060
- Phenobarbital Elixir and Tablets ... 1469
- Quadrinal Tablets ... 1350

Prazepam (May produce additive effect).
- No products indexed under this heading.

Prochlorperazine (May produce additive effect). Products include:
- Compazine ... 2470

Promethazine Hydrochloride (May produce additive effect). Products include:
- Mepergan Injection ... 2753
- Phenergan with Codeine ... 2777
- Phenergan with Dextromethorphan ... 2778
- Phenergan Injection ... 2773
- Phenergan Suppositories ... 2775
- Phenergan Syrup ... 2774
- Phenergan Tablets ... 2775
- Phenergan VC ... 2779
- Phenergan VC with Codeine ... 2781

Propofol (May produce additive effect). Products include:
- Diprivan Injection ... 2833

Propoxyphene Hydrochloride (May produce additive effect). Products include:
- Darvon ... 1435
- Wygesic Tablets ... 2827

Propoxyphene Napsylate (May produce additive effect). Products include:
- Darvon-N/Darvocet-N ... 1433

Quazepam (May produce additive effect). Products include:
- Doral Tablets ... 2664

Risperidone (May produce additive effect). Products include:
- Risperdal ... 1301

Secobarbital Sodium (May produce additive effect). Products include:
- Seconal Sodium Pulvules ... 1474

Sufentanil Citrate (May produce additive effect). Products include:
- Sufenta Injection ... 1309

Temazepam (May produce additive effect). Products include:
- Restoril Capsules ... 2284

Thiamylal Sodium (May produce additive effect).
- No products indexed under this heading.

Thioridazine Hydrochloride (May produce additive effect). Products include:
- Mellaril ... 2269

Thiothixene (May produce additive effect). Products include:
- Navane Capsules and Concentrate ... 2201
- Navane Intramuscular ... 2202

Triazolam (May produce additive effect). Products include:
- Halcion Tablets ... 2611

Trifluoperazine Hydrochloride (May produce additive effect). Products include:
- Stelazine ... 2514

Zolpidem Tartrate (May produce additive effect). Products include:
- Ambien Tablets ... 2416

Food Interactions

Alcohol (May produce additive effect).

PARAFON FORTE DSC CAPLETS
(Chlorzoxazone) ... 1581
May interact with central nervous system depressants and certain other agents. Compounds in these categories include:

Alfentanil Hydrochloride (May produce additive effect). Products include:
- Alfenta Injection ... 1286

Alprazolam (May produce additive effect). Products include:
- Xanax Tablets ... 2649

Aprobarbital (May produce additive effect).
- No products indexed under this heading.

Buprenorphine (May produce additive effect). Products include:
- Buprenex Injectable ... 2006

Buspirone Hydrochloride (May produce additive effect). Products include:
- BuSpar ... 737

Butabarbital (May produce additive effect).
- No products indexed under this heading.

Butalbital (May produce additive effect). Products include:
- Esgic-plus Tablets ... 1013
- Fioricet Tablets ... 2258
- Fioricet with Codeine Capsules ... 2260
- Fiorinal Capsules ... 2261
- Fiorinal with Codeine Capsules ... 2262
- Fiorinal Tablets ... 2261
- Phrenilin ... 785
- Sedapap Tablets 50 mg/650 mg ... 1543

Chlordiazepoxide (May produce additive effect). Products include:
- Libritabs Tablets ... 2177
- Limbitrol ... 2180

Chlordiazepoxide Hydrochloride (May produce additive effect). Products include:
- Librax Capsules ... 2176
- Librium Capsules ... 2178
- Librium Injectable ... 2179

Chlorpromazine (May produce additive effect). Products include:
- Thorazine Suppositories ... 2523

Chlorpromazine Hydrochloride (May produce additive effect). Products include:
- Thorazine ... 2523

Chlorprothixene (May produce additive effect).
- No products indexed under this heading.

Chlorprothixene Hydrochloride (May produce additive effect).
- No products indexed under this heading.

Clorazepate Dipotassium (May produce additive effect). Products include:
- Tranxene ... 451

Clozapine (May produce additive effect). Products include:
- Clozaril Tablets ... 2252

Codeine Phosphate (May produce additive effect). Products include:
- Actifed with Codeine Cough Syrup .. 1067
- Brontex ... 1981
- Deconsal C Expectorant Syrup ... 456
- Deconsal Pediatric Syrup ... 457
- Dimetane-DC Cough Syrup ... 2059
- Empirin with Codeine Tablets ... 1093
- Fioricet with Codeine Capsules ... 2260
- Fiorinal with Codeine Capsules ... 2262
- Isoclor Expectorant ... 990
- Novahistine DH ... 2462
- Novahistine Expectorant ... 2463
- Nucofed ... 2051
- Phenergan with Codeine ... 2777
- Phenergan VC with Codeine ... 2781
- Robitussin A-C Syrup ... 2073
- Robitussin-DAC Syrup ... 2074
- Ryna ... ▣ 841
- Soma Compound w/Codeine Tablets ... 2676
- Tussi-Organidin NR Liquid and S NR Liquid ... 2677
- Tylenol with Codeine ... 1583

Desflurane (May produce additive effect). Products include:
- Suprane ... 1813

Dezocine (May produce additive effect). Products include:
- Dalgan Injection ... 538

Diazepam (May produce additive effect). Products include:
- Dizac ... 1809
- Valium Injectable ... 2182
- Valium Tablets ... 2183
- Valrelease Capsules ... 2169

Droperidol (May produce additive effect). Products include:
- Inapsine Injection ... 1296

Enflurane (May produce additive effect).
- No products indexed under this heading.

Estazolam (May produce additive effect). Products include:
- ProSom Tablets ... 449

Ethchlorvynol (May produce additive effect). Products include:
- Placidyl Capsules ... 448

Ethinamate (May produce additive effect).
- No products indexed under this heading.

Fentanyl (May produce additive effect). Products include:
- Duragesic Transdermal System ... 1288

Fentanyl Citrate (May produce additive effect). Products include:
- Sublimaze Injection ... 1307

Fluphenazine Decanoate (May produce additive effect). Products include:
- Prolixin Decanoate ... 509

Fluphenazine Enanthate (May produce additive effect). Products include:
- Prolixin Enanthate ... 509

Fluphenazine Hydrochloride (May produce additive effect). Products include:
- Prolixin ... 509

Flurazepam Hydrochloride (May produce additive effect). Products include:
- Dalmane Capsules ... 2173

Glutethimide (May produce additive effect).
- No products indexed under this heading.

Haloperidol (May produce additive effect). Products include:
- Haldol Injection, Tablets and Concentrate ... 1575

Haloperidol Decanoate (May produce additive effect). Products include:
- Haldol Decanoate ... 1577

Hydrocodone Bitartrate (May produce additive effect). Products include:
- Anexsia 5/500 Elixir ... 1781
- Anexia Tablets ... 1782
- Codiclear DH Syrup ... 791
- Deconamine CX Cough and Cold Liquid and Tablets ... 1319
- Duratuss HD Elixir ... 2565
- Hycodan Tablets and Syrup ... 930
- Hycomine Compound Tablets ... 932
- Hycomine ... 931
- Hycotuss Expectorant Syrup ... 933
- Hydrocet Capsules ... 782
- Lorcet 10/650 ... 1018
- Lortab ... 2566
- Tussend ... 1783
- Tussend Expectorant ... 1785
- Vicodin Tablets ... 1356
- Vicodin ES Tablets ... 1357
- Vicodin Tuss Expectorant ... 1358
- Zydone Capsules ... 949

Hydrocodone Polistirex (May produce additive effect). Products include:
- Tussionex Pennkinetic Extended-Release Suspension ... 998

Hydroxyzine Hydrochloride (May produce additive effect). Products include:
- Atarax Tablets & Syrup ... 2185
- Marax Tablets & DF Syrup ... 2200
- Vistaril Intramuscular Solution ... 2216

(▣ Described in PDR For Nonprescription Drugs)   (⊙ Described in PDR For Ophthalmology)

787 Interactions Index Parlodel

Isoflurane (May produce additive effect).
No products indexed under this heading.

Ketamine Hydrochloride (May produce additive effect).
No products indexed under this heading.

Levomethadyl Acetate Hydrochloride (May produce additive effect). Products include:
Orlamm 2239

Levorphanol Tartrate (May produce additive effect). Products include:
Levo-Dromoran 2129

Lorazepam (May produce additive effect). Products include:
Ativan Injection 2698
Ativan Tablets 2700

Loxapine Hydrochloride (May produce additive effect). Products include:
Loxitane 1378

Loxapine Succinate (May produce additive effect). Products include:
Loxitane Capsules 1378

Meperidine Hydrochloride (May produce additive effect). Products include:
Demerol 2308
Mepergan Injection 2753

Mephobarbital (May produce additive effect). Products include:
Mebaral Tablets 2322

Meprobamate (May produce additive effect). Products include:
Miltown Tablets 2672
PMB 200 and PMB 400 2783

Mesoridazine Besylate (May produce additive effect). Products include:
Serentil 684

Methadone Hydrochloride (May produce additive effect). Products include:
Methadone Hydrochloride Oral Concentrate 2233
Methadone Hydrochloride Oral Solution & Tablets 2235

Methohexital Sodium (May produce additive effect). Products include:
Brevital Sodium Vials 1429

Methotrimeprazine (May produce additive effect). Products include:
Levoprome 1274

Methoxyflurane (May produce additive effect).
No products indexed under this heading.

Midazolam Hydrochloride (May produce additive effect). Products include:
Versed Injection 2170

Molindone Hydrochloride (May produce additive effect). Products include:
Moban Tablets and Concentrate 1048

Morphine Sulfate (May produce additive effect). Products include:
Astramorph/PF Injection, USP (Preservative-Free) 535
Duramorph 962
Infumorph 200 and Infumorph 500 Sterile Solutions 965
MS Contin Tablets 1994
MSIR 1997
Oramorph SR (Morphine Sulfate Sustained Release Tablets) 2236
RMS Suppositories 2657
Roxanol 2243

Opium Alkaloids (May produce additive effect).
No products indexed under this heading.

Oxazepam (May produce additive effect). Products include:
Serax Capsules 2810
Serax Tablets 2810

Oxycodone Hydrochloride (May produce additive effect). Products include:
Percocet Tablets 938
Percodan Tablets 939
Percodan-Demi Tablets 940
Roxicodone Tablets, Oral Solution & Intensol (Oxycodone) 2244
Tylox Capsules 1584

Pentobarbital Sodium (May produce additive effect). Products include:
Nembutal Sodium Capsules 436
Nembutal Sodium Solution 438
Nembutal Sodium Suppositories 440

Perphenazine (May produce additive effect). Products include:
Etrafon 2355
Triavil Tablets 1757
Trilafon 2389

Phenobarbital (May produce additive effect). Products include:
Arco-Lase Plus Tablets 512
Bellergal-S Tablets 2250
Donnatal 2060
Donnatal Extentabs 2061
Donnatal Tablets 2060
Phenobarbital Elixir and Tablets 1469
Quadrinal Tablets 1350

Prazepam (May produce additive effect).
No products indexed under this heading.

Prochlorperazine (May produce additive effect). Products include:
Compazine 2470

Promethazine Hydrochloride (May produce additive effect). Products include:
Mepergan Injection 2753
Phenergan with Codeine 2777
Phenergan with Dextromethorphan 2778
Phenergan Injection 2773
Phenergan Suppositories 2775
Phenergan Syrup 2774
Phenergan Tablets 2775
Phenergan VC 2779
Phenergan VC with Codeine 2781

Propofol (May produce additive effect). Products include:
Diprivan Injection 2833

Propoxyphene Hydrochloride (May produce additive effect). Products include:
Darvon 1435
Wygesic Tablets 2827

Propoxyphene Napsylate (May produce additive effect). Products include:
Darvon-N/Darvocet-N 1433

Quazepam (May produce additive effect). Products include:
Doral Tablets 2664

Risperidone (May produce additive effect). Products include:
Risperdal 1301

Secobarbital Sodium (May produce additive effect). Products include:
Seconal Sodium Pulvules 1474

Sufentanil Citrate (May produce additive effect). Products include:
Sufenta Injection 1309

Temazepam (May produce additive effect). Products include:
Restoril Capsules 2284

Thiamylal Sodium (May produce additive effect).
No products indexed under this heading.

Thioridazine Hydrochloride (May produce additive effect). Products include:
Mellaril 2269

Thiothixene (May produce additive effect). Products include:
Navane Capsules and Concentrate 2201
Navane Intramuscular 2202

Triazolam (May produce additive effect). Products include:
Halcion Tablets 2611

Trifluoperazine Hydrochloride (May produce additive effect). Products include:
Stelazine 2514

Zolpidem Tartrate (May produce additive effect). Products include:
Ambien Tablets 2416

Food Interactions

Alcohol (May produce additive effect).

PARAGARD T380A INTRAUTERINE COPPER CONTRACEPTIVE
(Intrauterine device) 1880
None cited in PDR database.

PARAPLATIN FOR INJECTION
(Carboplatin) 705
May interact with aminoglycosides and certain other agents. Compounds in these categories include:

Amikacin Sulfate (Concomitant treatment has resulted in increased renal and/or audiologic toxicity). Products include:
Amikacin Sulfate Injection, USP 960
Amikin Injectable 501

Gentamicin Sulfate (Concomitant treatment has resulted in increased renal and/or audiologic toxicity). Products include:
Garamycin Injectable 2360
Genoptic Sterile Ophthalmic Solution .... ⊙ 243
Genoptic Sterile Ophthalmic Ointment .... ⊙ 243
Gentacidin Ointment .... ⊙ 264
Gentacidin Solution .... ⊙ 264
Gentak .... ⊙ 208
Pred-G Liquifilm Sterile Ophthalmic Suspension .... ⊙ 251
Pred-G S.O.P. Sterile Ophthalmic Ointment .... ⊙ 252

Kanamycin Sulfate (Concomitant treatment has resulted in increased renal and/or audiologic toxicity).
No products indexed under this heading.

Nephrotoxic Drugs (Renal effects may be potentiated).

Streptomycin Sulfate (Concomitant treatment has resulted in increased renal and/or audiologic toxicity). Products include:
Streptomycin Sulfate Injection 2208

Tobramycin (Concomitant treatment has resulted in increased renal and/or audiologic toxicity). Products include:
AKTOB .... ⊙ 206
TobraDex Ophthalmic Suspension and Ointment 473
Tobrex Ophthalmic Ointment and Solution .... ⊙ 229

Tobramycin Sulfate (Concomitant treatment has resulted in increased renal and/or audiologic toxicity). Products include:
Nebcin Vials, Hyporets & ADD-Vantage 1464
Tobramycin Sulfate Injection 968

PAREMYD
(Hydroxyamphetamine Hydrobromide, Tropicamide) .... ⊙ 247
None cited in PDR database.

PARLODEL CAPSULES
(Bromocriptine Mesylate) 2281
May interact with dopamine antagonists, butyrophenones, ergot-containing drugs, and certain other agents. Compounds in these categories include:

Chlorpromazine (Decrease in efficacy of Parlodel). Products include:
Thorazine Suppositories 2523

Chlorpromazine Hydrochloride (Decrease in efficacy of Parlodel). Products include:
Thorazine 2523

Clozapine (Decrease in efficacy of Parlodel). Products include:
Clozaril Tablets 2252

Dihydroergotamine Mesylate (Concomitant use is not recommended). Products include:
D.H.E. 45 Injection 2255

Ergoloid Mesylates (Concomitant use is not recommended). Products include:
Hydergine 2265

Ergotamine Tartrate (Concomitant use is not recommended). Products include:
Bellergal-S Tablets 2250
Cafergot 2251
Ergomar 1486
Wigraine Tablets & Suppositories 1829

Fluphenazine Decanoate (Decrease in efficacy of Parlodel). Products include:
Prolixin Decanoate 509

Fluphenazine Enanthate (Decrease in efficacy of Parlodel). Products include:
Prolixin Enanthate 509

Fluphenazine Hydrochloride (Decrease in efficacy of Parlodel). Products include:
Prolixin 509

Haloperidol (Decrease in efficacy of Parlodel). Products include:
Haldol Injection, Tablets and Concentrate 1575

Haloperidol Decanoate (Decrease in efficacy of Parlodel). Products include:
Haldol Decanoate 1577

Mesoridazine Besylate (Decrease in efficacy of Parlodel). Products include:
Serentil 684

Methotrimeprazine (Decrease in efficacy of Parlodel). Products include:
Levoprome 1274

Methylergonovine Maleate (Concomitant use is not recommended). Products include:
Methergine 2272

Methysergide Maleate (Concomitant use is not recommended). Products include:
Sansert Tablets 2295

Metoclopramide Hydrochloride (Decrease in efficacy of Parlodel). Products include:
Reglan 2068

Perphenazine (Decrease in efficacy of Parlodel). Products include:
Etrafon 2355
Triavil Tablets 1757
Trilafon 2389

Pimozide (Decrease in efficacy of Parlodel). Products include:
Orap Tablets 1050

Prochlorperazine (Decrease in efficacy of Parlodel). Products include:
Compazine 2470

Promethazine Hydrochloride (Decrease in efficacy of Parlodel). Products include:
Mepergan Injection 2753
Phenergan with Codeine 2777

IMPORTANT NOTE: Always consult each drug listing in the patient's regimen for possible interactions.

Parlodel — Interactions Index — 788

Phenergan with Dextromethorphan 2778
Phenergan Injection 2773
Phenergan Suppositories 2775
Phenergan Syrup 2774
Phenergan Tablets 2775
Phenergan VC 2779
Phenergan VC with Codeine 2781

Thioridazine Hydrochloride (Decrease in efficacy of Parlodel). Products include:
Mellaril 2269

Trifluoperazine Hydrochloride (Decrease in efficacy of Parlodel). Products include:
Stelazine 2514

PARLODEL SNAPTABS
(Bromocriptine Mesylate) 2281
See **Parlodel Capsules**

PARNATE TABLETS
(Tranylcypromine Sulfate) 2503

May interact with monoamine oxidase inhibitors, dibenzazepines, tricyclic antidepressants, sympathomimetics, antihypertensives, phenothiazines, insulin, oral hypoglycemic agents, narcotic analgesics, antihistamines, general anesthetics, anticholinergic-type anitparkinsonism drugs, central nervous system depressants, diuretics, hypnotics and sedatives, alpha adrenergic stimulants, phenylpropanolamine containing anorectics, anorexiants, and certain other agents. Compounds in these categories include:

Acarbose (Hypoglycemic episodes).
No products indexed under this heading.

Acebutolol Hydrochloride (Contraindicated; potentiated). Products include:
Sectral Capsules 2807

Acrivastine (Contraindicated). Products include:
Semprex-D Capsules 463
Semprex-D Capsules 1167

Albuterol (Contraindicated; hypertension, headache and related symptoms precipitated). Products include:
Proventil Inhalation Aerosol 2382
Ventolin Inhalation Aerosol and Refill 1197

Albuterol Sulfate (Contraindicated; hypertension, headache and related symptoms precipitated). Products include:
Airet Solution for Inhalation 452
Proventil Inhalation Solution 0.083% 2384
Proventil Repetabs Tablets 2386
Proventil Solution for Inhalation 0.5% 2383
Proventil Syrup 2385
Proventil Tablets 2386
Ventolin Inhalation Solution 1198
Ventolin Nebules Inhalation Solution 1199
Ventolin Rotacaps for Inhalation 1200
Ventolin Syrup 1202
Ventolin Tablets 1203
Volmax Extended-Release Tablets 1788

Alfentanil Hydrochloride (Contraindicated; potentiated). Products include:
Alfenta Injection 1286

Alprazolam (Contraindicated; potentiated). Products include:
Xanax Tablets 2649

Amitriptyline Hydrochloride (Contraindicated; hypertensive crises; severe convulsive seizures). Products include:
Elavil 2838
Endep Tablets 2174
Etrafon 2355
Limbitrol 2180
Triavil Tablets 1757

Amlodipine Besylate (Contraindicated; potentiated). Products include:
Lotrel Capsules 840
Norvasc Tablets 1940

Amoxapine (Contraindicated; hypertensive crises; severe convulsive seizures). Products include:
Asendin Tablets 1369

Amphetamine Resins (Combined use contraindicated). Products include:
Biphetamine Capsules 983

Aprobarbital (Contraindicated; potentiated).
No products indexed under this heading.

Astemizole (Contraindicated). Products include:
Hismanal Tablets 1293

Atenolol (Contraindicated; potentiated). Products include:
Tenoretic Tablets 2845
Tenormin Tablets and I.V. Injection 2847

Azatadine Maleate (Contraindicated). Products include:
Trinalin Repetabs Tablets 1330

Benazepril Hydrochloride (Contraindicated; potentiated). Products include:
Lotensin Tablets 834
Lotensin HCT 837
Lotrel Capsules 840

Bendroflumethiazide (Contraindicated; potentiated).
No products indexed under this heading.

Benzphetamine Hydrochloride (Combined use contraindicated). Products include:
Didrex Tablets 2607

Benztropine Mesylate (Combined use contraindicated; severe reactions reported). Products include:
Cogentin 1621

Betaxolol Hydrochloride (Contraindicated; potentiated). Products include:
Betoptic Ophthalmic Solution 469
Betoptic S Ophthalmic Suspension 471
Kerlone Tablets 2436

Biperiden Hydrochloride (Combined use contraindicated; severe reactions reported). Products include:
Akineton 1333

Bisoprolol Fumarate (Contraindicated; potentiated). Products include:
Zebeta Tablets 1413
Ziac 1415

Brompheniramine Maleate (Contraindicated). Products include:
Alka Seltzer Plus Sinus Medicine ◙ 707
Bromfed Capsules (Extended-Release) 1785
Bromfed Syrup ◙ 733
Bromfed Tablets 1785
Bromfed-DM Cough Syrup 1786
Bromfed-PD Capsules (Extended-Release) 1785
Dimetane-DC Cough Syrup 2059
Dimetane-DX Cough Syrup 2059
Dimetapp Elixir ◙ 773
Dimetapp Extentabs ◙ 774
Dimetapp Tablets/Liqui-Gels ◙ 775
Dimetapp Cold & Allergy Chewable Tablets ◙ 773
Dimetapp DM Elixir ◙ 774
Vicks DayQuil Allergy Relief 12-Hour Extended Release Tablets ◙ 760
Vicks DayQuil Allergy Relief 4-Hour Tablets ◙ 760

Buprenorphine (Contraindicated; potentiated). Products include:
Buprenex Injectable 2006

Bupropion Hydrochloride (Concurrent use is contraindicated; at least 14 days should elapse between discontinuation of a MAOI and initiation of treatment with bupropion). Products include:
Wellbutrin Tablets 1204

Buspirone Hydrochloride (Combined use contraindicated; several cases of elevated blood pressure have been reported). Products include:
BuSpar 737

Butabarbital (Contraindicated; potentiated).
No products indexed under this heading.

Butalbital (Contraindicated; potentiated). Products include:
Esgic-plus Tablets 1013
Fioricet Tablets 2258
Fioricet with Codeine Capsules 2260
Fiorinal Capsules 2261
Fiorinal with Codeine Capsules 2262
Fiorinal Tablets 2261
Phrenilin 785
Sedapap Tablets 50 mg/650 mg 1543

Caffeine (Excessive use contraindicated). Products include:
Arthritis Strength BC Powder ◙ 609
BC Powder ◙ 609
Bayer Select Headache Pain Relief Formula ◙ 716
Cafergot 2251
DHCplus Capsules 1993
Darvon Compound-65 Pulvules 1435
Esgic-plus Tablets 1013
Aspirin Free Excedrin Analgesic Caplets and Geltabs 732
Excedrin Extra-Strength Analgesic Tablets & Caplets 732
Fioricet Tablets 2258
Fioricet with Codeine Capsules 2260
Fiorinal Capsules 2261
Fiorinal with Codeine Capsules 2262
Fiorinal Tablets 2261
Maximum Strength Multi-Symptom Formula Midol ◙ 722
Migralam Capsules 2038
No Doz Maximum Strength Caplets ◙ 622
Norgesic 1496
Vanquish Analgesic Caplets ◙ 731
Wigraine Tablets & Suppositories 1829

Captopril (Contraindicated; potentiated). Products include:
Capoten 739
Capozide 742

Carbamazepine (Contraindicated; hypertensive crises; severe convulsive seizures). Products include:
Atretol Tablets 573
Tegretol Chewable Tablets 852
Tegretol Suspension 852
Tegretol Tablets 852

Carteolol Hydrochloride (Contraindicated; potentiated). Products include:
Cartrol Tablets 410
Ocupress Ophthalmic Solution, 1% Sterile ◉ 309

Chlordiazepoxide (Contraindicated; potentiated). Products include:
Libritabs Tablets 2177
Limbitrol 2180

Chlordiazepoxide Hydrochloride (Contraindicated; potentiated). Products include:
Librax Capsules 2176
Librium Capsules 2178
Librium Injectable 2179

Chlorothiazide (Contraindicated; potentiated). Products include:
Aldoclor Tablets 1598
Diupres Tablets 1650
Diuril Oral 1653

Chlorothiazide Sodium (Contraindicated; potentiated). Products include:
Diuril Sodium Intravenous 1652

Chlorpheniramine Maleate (Contraindicated). Products include:
Alka-Seltzer Plus Cold Medicine ◙ 705
Alka-Seltzer Plus Cold Medicine Liqui-Gels ◙ 706
Alka-Seltzer Plus Cold & Cough Medicine ◙ 708
Alka-Seltzer Plus Cold & Cough Medicine Liqui-Gels ◙ 705
Allerest Children's Chewable Tablets ◙ 627
Allerest Headache Strength Tablets ◙ 627
Allerest Maximum Strength Tablets ◙ 627
Allerest Sinus Pain Formula ◙ 627
Allerest 12 Hour Caplets ◙ 627
Ana-Kit Anaphylaxis Emergency Treatment Kit 617
Atrohist Pediatric Capsules 453
Atrohist Plus Tablets 454
BC Cold Powder Multi-Symptom Formula (Cold-Sinus-Allergy) ◙ 609
Cerose DM ◙ 878
Cheracol Plus Head Cold/Cough Formula ◙ 769
Children's Vicks DayQuil Allergy Relief ◙ 757
Children's Vicks NyQuil Cold/Cough Relief ◙ 758
Chlor-Trimeton Allergy Decongestant Tablets ◙ 799
Chlor-Trimeton Allergy Tablets ◙ 798
Comhist 2038
Comtrex Multi-Symptom Cold Reliever Tablets/Caplets/Liqui-Gels/Liquid ◙ 615
Allergy-Sinus Comtrex Multi-Symptom Allergy-Sinus Formula Tablets ◙ 617
Contac Continuous Action Nasal Decongestant/Antihistamine 12 Hour Capsules ◙ 813
Contac Maximum Strength Continuous Action Decongestant/Antihistamine 12 Hour Caplets ◙ 813
Contac Severe Cold and Flu Formula Caplets ◙ 814
Coricidin 'D' Decongestant Tablets ◙ 800
Coricidin Tablets ◙ 800
D.A. Chewable Tablets 951
Deconamine 1320
Dura-Tap/PD Capsules 2867
Dura-Vent/DA Tablets 953
Extendryl 1005
Fedahist Gyrocaps 2401
Fedahist Timecaps 2401
Hycomine Compound Tablets 932
Isoclor Timesule Capsules ◙ 637
Kronofed-A 977
Nolamine Timed-Release Tablets 785
Novahistine DH 2462
Novahistine Elixir ◙ 823
Ornade Spansule Capsules 2502
PediaCare Cold Allergy Chewable Tablets ◙ 677
PediaCare Cough-Cold Chewable Tablets 1553
PediaCare Cough-Cold Liquid 1553
PediaCare NightRest Cough-Cold Liquid 1553
Pediatric Vicks 44m Cough & Cold Relief ◙ 764
Pyrroxate Caplets ◙ 772
Ryna ◙ 841
Sinarest Tablets ◙ 648
Sinarest Extra Strength Tablets ◙ 648
Sine-Off Sinus Medicine ◙ 825
Singlet Tablets ◙ 825
Sinulin Tablets 787
Sinutab Sinus Allergy Medication, Maximum Strength Tablets and Caplets ◙ 860
Sudafed Plus Liquid ◙ 862
Sudafed Plus Tablets ◙ 863
Teldrin 12 Hour Antihistamine/Nasal Decongestant Allergy Relief Capsules ◙ 826
TheraFlu ◙ 787
TheraFlu Maximum Strength Nighttime Flu, Cold & Cough Medicine ◙ 788
Triaminic Allergy Tablets ◙ 789
Triaminic Cold Tablets ◙ 790
Triaminic Nite Light ◙ 791
Triaminic Syrup ◙ 792
Triaminic-12 Tablets ◙ 792
Triaminicin Tablets ◙ 793
Triaminicol Multi-Symptom Cold Tablets ◙ 793

(◙ Described in PDR For Nonprescription Drugs) (◉ Described in PDR For Ophthalmology)

Triaminicol Multi-Symptom Relief ◾️ 794
Tussend 1783
Children's TYLENOL Cold Multi-Symptom Liquid Formula and Chewable Tablets 1561
Children's TYLENOL Cold Plus Cough Multi Symptom Tablets and Liquid .... ◾️ 681
TYLENOL Maximum Strength Allergy Sinus Medication Gelcaps and Caplets 1563
TYLENOL Cold Multi-Symptom Formula Medication Tablets and Caplets 1561
TYLENOL Cold Multi-Symptom Hot Medication Liquid Packets 1557
Vicks 44 LiquiCaps Cough, Cold & Flu Relief .... ◾️ 755
Vicks 44M Cough, Cold & Flu Relief .... ◾️ 756

Chlorpheniramine Polistirex (Contraindicated). Products include:

Tussionex Pennkinetic Extended-Release Suspension 998

Chlorpheniramine Tannate (Contraindicated). Products include:

Atrohist Pediatric Suspension 454
Ricobid Tablets and Pediatric Suspension 2038
Rynatan 2673
Rynatuss 2673

Chlorpromazine (Additive hypotensive effects). Products include:

Thorazine Suppositories 2523

Chlorpropamide (Hypoglycemic episodes). Products include:

Diabinese Tablets 1935

Chlorprothixene (Contraindicated; potentiated).

No products indexed under this heading.

Chlorprothixene Hydrochloride (Contraindicated; potentiated).

No products indexed under this heading.

Chlorthalidone (Contraindicated; potentiated). Products include:

Combipres Tablets 677
Tenoretic Tablets 2845
Thalitone 1245

Clemastine Fumarate (Contraindicated). Products include:

Tavist Syrup 2297
Tavist Tablets 2298
Tavist-1 12 Hour Relief Tablets .... ◾️ 787
Tavist-D 12 Hour Relief Tablets .... ◾️ 787

Clomipramine Hydrochloride (Contraindicated). Products include:

Anafranil Capsules 803

Clonidine (Contraindicated; potentiated). Products include:

Catapres-TTS 675

Clonidine Hydrochloride (Contraindicated; potentiated). Products include:

Catapres Tablets 674
Combipres Tablets 677

Clorazepate Dipotassium (Contraindicated; potentiated). Products include:

Tranxene 451

Clozapine (Contraindicated). Products include:

Clozaril Tablets 2252

Codeine Phosphate (Contraindicated; potentiated). Products include:

Actifed with Codeine Cough Syrup.. 1067
Brontex 1981
Deconsal C Expectorant Syrup 456
Deconsal Pediatric Syrup 457
Dimetane-DC Cough Syrup 2059
Empirin with Codeine Tablets 1093
Fioricet with Codeine Capsules 2260
Fiorinal with Codeine Capsules 2262
Isoclor Expectorant 990
Novahistine DH 2462
Novahistine Expectorant 2463
Nucofed 2051
Phenergan with Codeine 2777
Phenergan VC with Codeine 2781
Robitussin A-C Syrup 2073
Robitussin-DAC Syrup 2074

Ryna .... ◾️ 841
Soma Compound w/Codeine Tablets 2676
Tussi-Organidin NR Liquid and S NR Liquid 2677
Tylenol with Codeine 1583

Cyclobenzaprine Hydrochloride (Contraindicated; hypertensive crises; severe convulsive seizures). Products include:

Flexeril Tablets 1661

Cyproheptadine Hydrochloride (Contraindicated). Products include:

Periactin 1724

Deserpidine (Contraindicated; potentiated).

No products indexed under this heading.

Desflurane (Contraindicated; potentiated). Products include:

Suprane 1813

Desipramine Hydrochloride (Contraindicated; hypertensive crises; severe convulsive seizures). Products include:

Norpramin Tablets 1526

Dexchlorpheniramine Maleate (Contraindicated).

No products indexed under this heading.

Dextroamphetamine Sulfate (Combined use contraindicated). Products include:

Dexedrine 2474
DextroStat Dextroamphetamine Tablets 2036

Dextromethorphan Hydrobromide (May cause brief episodes of psychosis or bizarre behavior; concurrent use is contraindicated). Products include:

Alka-Seltzer Plus Cold & Cough Medicine .... ◾️ 708
Alka-Seltzer Plus Cold & Cough Medicine Liqui-Gels .... ◾️ 705
Alka-Seltzer Plus Night-Time Cold Medicine .... ◾️ 707
Alka-Seltzer Plus Night-Time Cold Medicine Liqui-Gels .... ◾️ 706
Benylin Adult Formula Cough Suppressant .... ◾️ 852
Benylin Expectorant .... ◾️ 852
Benylin Multisymptom .... ◾️ 852
Benylin Pediatric Cough Suppressant .... ◾️ 853
Bromfed-DM Cough Syrup 1786
Buckley's Mixture .... ◾️ 624
Cerose DM .... ◾️ 878
Cheracol-D Cough Formula .... ◾️ 769
Cheracol Plus Head Cold/Cough Formula .... ◾️ 769
Children's Vicks NyQuil Cold/Cough Relief .... ◾️ 758
Comtrex Multi-Symptom Cold Reliever Tablets/Caplets/Liqui-Gels/Liquid .... ◾️ 615
Comtrex Non-Drowsy .... ◾️ 618
Contac Day & Night Cold/Flu Caplets .... ◾️ 812
Contac Severe Cold and Flu Formula Caplets .... ◾️ 814
Contac Severe Cold & Flu Non-Drowsy .... ◾️ 815
Cough-X Lozenges .... ◾️ 602
Diabe-Tuss DM Syrup 1891
Dimetane-DX Cough Syrup 2059
Dimetapp DM Elixir .... ◾️ 774
Dorcol Children's Cough Syrup ...... ◾️ 785
Drixoral Cough Liquid Caps .... ◾️ 801
Drixoral Cough + Congestion Liquid Caps .... ◾️ 802
Drixoral Cough + Sore Throat Liquid Caps .... ◾️ 802
Humibid 462
Novahistine DMX .... ◾️ 822
PediaCare Cough-Cold Chewable Tablets 1553
PediaCare Cough-Cold Liquid 1553
PediCare Infant's Drops Decongestant Plus Cough 1553
PediaCare NightRest Cough-Cold Liquid 1553
Pediatric Vicks 44d Dry Hacking Cough & Head Congestion .... ◾️ 763
Pediatric Vicks 44e Chest Cough & Chest Congestion .... ◾️ 764

Pediatric Vicks 44m Cough & Cold Relief .... ◾️ 764
Phenergan with Dextromethorphan 2778
Robitussin Cold & Cough Liqui-Gels .... ◾️ 776
Robitussin Maximum Strength Cough Suppressant .... ◾️ 778
Robitussin Maximum Strength Cough & Cold .... ◾️ 778
Robitussin Pediatric Cough & Cold Formula .... ◾️ 779
Robitussin Pediatric Cough Suppressant .... ◾️ 779
Robitussin-CF .... ◾️ 777
Robitussin-DM .... ◾️ 777
Rondec-DM Oral Drops 954
Rondec-DM Syrup 954
Safe Tussin 30 1363
Sucrets 4-Hour Cough Suppressant .... ◾️ 826
Sudafed Cold and Cough Liquidcaps .... ◾️ 862
Sudafed Cough Syrup .... ◾️ 862
Sudafed Severe Cold Formula Caplets .... ◾️ 863
Sudafed Severe Cold Formula Tablets .... ◾️ 864
Syn-Rx DM Tablets 466
TheraFlu Flu, Cold and Cough Medicine .... ◾️ 787
TheraFlu Maximum Strength Nighttime Flu, Cold & Cough Medicine .... ◾️ 788
TheraFlu Maximum Strength Non-Drowsy Formula Flu, Cold & Cough Medicine .... ◾️ 788
Thera Flu Maximum Strength, Non-Drowsy Formula Flu, Cold and Cough Caplets .... ◾️ 789
Triaminic AM Cough and Decongestant Formula .... ◾️ 789
Triaminic Nite Light .... ◾️ 791
Triaminic Sore Throat Formula ...... ◾️ 791
Triaminic-DM Syrup .... ◾️ 792
Triaminicol Multi-Symptom Cold Tablets .... ◾️ 793
Triaminicol Multi-Symptom Relief ◾️ 794
Tussi-Organidin DM NR Liquid and DM-S NR Liquid 2677
Children's TYLENOL Cold Plus Cough Multi Symptom Tablets and Liquid .... ◾️ 681
TYLENOL Flu Maximum Strength Gelcaps 1565
TYLENOL Cold Multi-Symptom Formula Medication Tablets and Caplets 1561
TYLENOL Cold Medication No Drowsiness Formula Gelcaps and Caplets 1562
TYLENOL Cold Multi-Symptom Hot Medication Liquid Packets 1557
TYLENOL Cough Multi-Symptom Medication 1564
TYLENOL Cough Multi-Symptom Medication with Decongestant 1565
Vicks 44 Dry Hacking Cough .... ◾️ 755
Vicks 44 LiquiCaps Cough, Cold & Flu Relief .... ◾️ 755
Vicks 44 LiquiCaps Non-Drowsy Cough & Cold Relief .... ◾️ 756
Vicks 44D Dry Hacking Cough & Head Congestion .... ◾️ 755
Vicks 44E Chest Cough & Chest Congestion .... ◾️ 756
Vicks 44M Cough, Cold & Flu Relief .... ◾️ 756
Vicks DayQuil .... ◾️ 761
Vicks Nyquil Hot Therapy .... ◾️ 762
Vicks NyQuil LiquiCaps Multi-Symptom Cold/Flu Relief .... ◾️ 763
Vicks NyQuil Multi-Symptom Cold/Flu Relief - (Original & Cherry Flavor) .... ◾️ 763

Dextromethorphan Polistirex (May cause brief episodes of psychosis or bizarre behavior; concurrent use is contraindicated). Products include:

Delsym Extended-Release Suspension .... ◾️ 654

Dezocine (Contraindicated; potentiated). Products include:

Dalgan Injection 538

Diazepam (Contraindicated; potentiated). Products include:

Dizac 1809
Valium Injectable 2182
Valium Tablets 2183

Valrelease Capsules 2169

Diazoxide (Contraindicated; potentiated). Products include:

Hyperstat I.V. Injection 2363
Proglycem 580

Diethylpropion Hydrochloride (Combined use contraindicated).

No products indexed under this heading.

Diltiazem Hydrochloride (Contraindicated; potentiated). Products include:

Cardizem CD Capsules 1506
Cardizem SR Capsules 1510
Cardizem Injectable 1508
Cardizem Tablets 1512
Dilacor XR Extended-release Capsules 2018

Diphenhydramine Citrate (Contraindicated). Products include:

Excedrin P.M. Analgesic/Sleeping Aid Tablets, Caplets, Liquigels 733

Diphenhydramine Hydrochloride (Contraindicated; combined use contraindicated; severe reactions reported). Products include:

Actifed Allergy Daytime/Nighttime Caplets .... ◾️ 844
Actifed Sinus Daytime/Nighttime Tablets and Caplets .... ◾️ 846
Arthritis Foundation NightTime Caplets .... ◾️ 674
Extra Strength Bayer PM Aspirin .. ◾️ 713
Bayer Select Night Time Pain Relief Formula .... ◾️ 716
Benadryl Allergy Decongestant Liquid Medication .... ◾️ 848
Benadryl Allergy Decongestant Tablets .... ◾️ 848
Benadryl Allergy Liquid Medication .... ◾️ 849
Benadryl Allergy .... ◾️ 848
Benadryl Allergy Sinus Headache Formula Caplets .... ◾️ 849
Benadryl Capsules 1898
Benadryl Dye-Free Allergy Liquigel Softgels .... ◾️ 850
Benadryl Dye-Free Allergy Liquid Medication .... ◾️ 850
Benadryl Itch Relief Cream, Children's Formula and Maximum Strength 2% .... ◾️ 851
Benadryl Itch Relief Spray, Children's Formula and Maximum Strength 2% .... ◾️ 851
Benadryl Itch Relief Stick Maximum Strength 2% .... ◾️ 850
Benadryl Itch Stopping Gel, Children's Formula and Maximum Strength 2% .... ◾️ 851
Benadryl Kapseals 1898
Benadryl Injection 1898
Contac Day & Night Cold/Flu Night Caplets .... ◾️ 812
Contac Night Allergy/Sinus Caplets .... ◾️ 812
Extra Strength Doan's P.M. .... ◾️ 633
Legatrin PM .... ◾️ 651
Miles Nervine Nighttime Sleep-Aid ◾️ 723
Nytol QuickCaps Caplets .... ◾️ 610
Sleepinal Night-time Sleep Aid Capsules and Softgels .... ◾️ 834
TYLENOL Maximum Strength Allergy Sinus NightTime Medication Caplets 1555
TYLENOL Flu NightTime, Maximum Strength, Gelcaps 1566
TYLENOL Maximum Strength Flu NightTime Hot Medication Packets 1562
TYLENOL PM, Extra Strength Pain Reliever/Sleep Aid Caplets, Geltabs, Gelcaps 1560
TYLENOL Severe Allergy Medication Caplets 1564
Maximum Strength Unisom Sleepgels 1934
Unisom With Pain Relief-Nighttime Sleep Aid and Pain Reliever 1934

Diphenylpyraline Hydrochloride (Contraindicated).

No products indexed under this heading.

Disulfiram (Administer with caution). Products include:

Antabuse Tablets 2695

IMPORTANT NOTE: Always consult each drug listing in the patient's regimen for possible interactions.

Parnate | Interactions Index | 790

Dobutamine Hydrochloride (Contraindicated; hypertension, headache and related symptoms precipitated). Products include:
Dobutrex Solution Vials ... 1439
Dopamine Hydrochloride (Contraindicated; hypertension, headache and related symptoms precipitated).
No products indexed under this heading.
Doxazosin Mesylate (Contraindicated; potentiated). Products include:
Cardura Tablets ... 2186
Doxepin Hydrochloride (Contraindicated; hypertensive crises; severe convulsive seizures). Products include:
Sinequan ... 2205
Zonalon Cream ... 1055
Droperidol (Contraindicated; potentiated). Products include:
Inapsine Injection ... 1296
Enalapril Maleate (Contraindicated; potentiated). Products include:
Vaseretic Tablets ... 1765
Vasotec Tablets ... 1771
Enalaprilat (Contraindicated; potentiated). Products include:
Vasotec I.V. ... 1768
Enflurane (Contraindicated; potentiated).
No products indexed under this heading.
Ephedrine Hydrochloride (Contraindicated; hypertension, headache and related symptoms precipitated). Products include:
Primatene Dual Action Formula ... ▣ 872
Primatene Tablets ... ▣ 873
Quadrinal Tablets ... 1350
Ephedrine Sulfate (Contraindicated; hypertension, headache and related symptoms precipitated). Products include:
Bronkaid Caplets ... ▣ 717
Marax Tablets & DF Syrup ... 2200
Ephedrine Tannate (Contraindicated; hypertension, headache and related symptoms precipitated). Products include:
Rynatuss ... 2673
Epinephrine (Contraindicated; hypertension, headache and related symptoms precipitated). Products include:
Bronkaid Mist ... ▣ 717
EPIFRIN ... ⊙ 239
EpiPen ... 790
Marcaine Hydrochloride with Epinephrine 1:200,000 ... 2316
Primatene Mist ... ▣ 873
Sensorcaine with Epinephrine Injection ... 559
Sus-Phrine Injection ... 1019
Xylocaine with Epinephrine Injections ... 567
Epinephrine Bitartrate (Contraindicated; hypertension, headache and related symptoms precipitated). Products include:
Bronkaid Mist Suspension ... ▣ 718
Sensorcaine-MPF with Epinephrine Injection ... 559
Epinephrine Hydrochloride (Contraindicated; hypertension, headache and related symptoms precipitated). Products include:
Ana-Kit Anaphylaxis Emergency Treatment Kit ... 617
Esmolol Hydrochloride (Contraindicated; potentiated). Products include:
Brevibloc Injection ... 1808
Estazolam (Contraindicated; potentiated). Products include:
ProSom Tablets ... 449
Ethchlorvynol (Contraindicated; potentiated). Products include:
Placidyl Capsules ... 448
Ethinamate (Contraindicated; potentiated).
No products indexed under this heading.
Felodipine (Contraindicated; potentiated). Products include:
Plendil Extended-Release Tablets ... 527
Fenfluramine Hydrochloride (Combined use contraindicated). Products include:
Pondimin Tablets ... 2066
Fentanyl (Contraindicated; potentiated). Products include:
Duragesic Transdermal System ... 1288
Fentanyl Citrate (Contraindicated; potentiated). Products include:
Sublimaze Injection ... 1307
Fluoxetine Hydrochloride (Potential for fatal reactions including hyperthermia, rigidity, myoclonus, and autonomic instability; concurrent use is contraindicated; at least 5 weeks should be allowed after stopping SSRI before starting Parnate). Products include:
Prozac Pulvules & Liquid, Oral Solution ... 919
Fluphenazine Decanoate (Additive hypotensive effects; contraindicated; potentiated). Products include:
Prolixin Decanoate ... 509
Fluphenazine Enanthate (Additive hypotensive effects; contraindicated; potentiated). Products include:
Prolixin Enanthate ... 509
Fluphenazine Hydrochloride (Additive hypotensive effects; contraindicated; potentiated). Products include:
Prolixin ... 509
Flurazepam Hydrochloride (Contraindicated; potentiated). Products include:
Dalmane Capsules ... 2173
Fosinopril Sodium (Contraindicated; potentiated). Products include:
Monopril Tablets ... 757
Furazolidone (Contraindicated; hypertensive crises; severe convulsive seizures). Products include:
Furoxone ... 2046
Furosemide (Contraindicated; potentiated). Products include:
Lasix Injection, Oral Solution and Tablets ... 1240
Glipizide (Hypoglycemic episodes). Products include:
Glucotrol Tablets ... 1967
Glucotrol XL Extended Release Tablets ... 1968
Glutethimide (Contraindicated; potentiated).
No products indexed under this heading.
Glyburide (Hypoglycemic episodes). Products include:
DiaBeta Tablets ... 1239
Glynase PresTab Tablets ... 2609
Micronase Tablets ... 2623
Guanabenz Acetate (Contraindicated; potentiated).
No products indexed under this heading.
Guanethidine Monosulfate (Contraindicated; potentiated). Products include:
Esimil Tablets ... 822
Ismelin Tablets ... 827
Haloperidol (Contraindicated; potentiated). Products include:
Haldol Injection, Tablets and Concentrate ... 1575
Haloperidol Decanoate (Contraindicated; potentiated). Products include:
Haldol Decanoate ... 1577
Hydralazine Hydrochloride (Contraindicated; potentiated). Products include:
Apresazide Capsules ... 808
Apresoline Hydrochloride Tablets ... 809
Ser-Ap-Es Tablets ... 849
Hydrochlorothiazide (Contraindicated; potentiated). Products include:
Aldactazide ... 2413
Aldoril Tablets ... 1604
Apresazide Capsules ... 808
Capozide ... 742
Dyazide ... 2479
Esidrix Tablets ... 821
Esimil Tablets ... 822
HydroDIURIL Tablets ... 1674
Hydropres Tablets ... 1675
Hyzaar Tablets ... 1677
Inderide Tablets ... 2732
Inderide LA Long Acting Capsules ... 2734
Lopressor HCT Tablets ... 832
Lotensin HCT ... 837
Maxzide ... 1380
Moduretic Tablets ... 1705
Oretic Tablets ... 443
Prinzide Tablets ... 1737
Ser-Ap-Es Tablets ... 849
Timolide Tablets ... 1748
Vaseretic Tablets ... 1765
Zestoretic ... 2850
Ziac ... 1415
Hydrocodone Bitartrate (Contraindicated; potentiated). Products include:
Anexsia 5/500 Elixir ... 1781
Anexia Tablets ... 1782
Codiclear DH Syrup ... 791
Deconamine CX Cough and Cold Liquid and Tablets ... 1319
Duratuss HD Elixir ... 2565
Hycodan Tablets and Syrup ... 930
Hycomine Compound Tablets ... 932
Hycomine ... 931
Hycotuss Expectorant Syrup ... 933
Hydrocet Capsules ... 782
Lorcet 10/650 ... 1018
Lortab ... 2566
Tussend ... 1783
Tussend Expectorant ... 1785
Vicodin Tablets ... 1356
Vicodin ES Tablets ... 1357
Vicodin Tuss Expectorant ... 1358
Zydone Capsules ... 949
Hydrocodone Polistirex (Contraindicated; potentiated). Products include:
Tussionex Pennkinetic Extended-Release Suspension ... 998
Hydroflumethiazide (Contraindicated; potentiated). Products include:
Diucardin Tablets ... 2718
Hydroxyzine Hydrochloride (Contraindicated; potentiated). Products include:
Atarax Tablets & Syrup ... 2185
Marax Tablets & DF Syrup ... 2200
Vistaril Intramuscular Solution ... 2216
Imipramine Hydrochloride (Contraindicated; hypertensive crises; severe convulsive seizures). Products include:
Tofranil Ampuls ... 854
Tofranil Tablets ... 856
Imipramine Pamoate (Contraindicated; hypertensive crises; severe convulsive seizures). Products include:
Tofranil-PM Capsules ... 857
Indapamide (Contraindicated; potentiated). Products include:
Lozol Tablets ... 2022
Insulin, Human (Hypoglycemic episodes).
No products indexed under this heading.
Insulin, Human Isophane Suspension (Hypoglycemic episodes). Products include:
Novolin N Human Insulin 10 ml Vials ... 1795
Insulin, Human NPH (Hypoglycemic episodes). Products include:
Humulin N, 100 Units ... 1448
Novolin N PenFill Cartridges Durable Insulin Delivery System ... 1798
Novolin N Prefilled Syringe Disposable Insulin Delivery System ... 1798
Insulin, Human Regular (Hypoglycemic episodes). Products include:
Humulin R, 100 Units ... 1449
Novolin R Human Insulin 10 ml Vials ... 1795
Novolin R PenFill Cartridges Durable Insulin Delivery System ... 1798
Novolin R Prefilled Syringe Disposable Insulin Delivery System ... 1798
Velosulin BR Human Insulin 10 ml Vials ... 1795
Insulin, Human, Zinc Suspension (Hypoglycemic episodes). Products include:
Humulin L, 100 Units ... 1446
Humulin U, 100 Units ... 1450
Novolin L Human Insulin 10 ml Vials ... 1795
Insulin, NPH (Hypoglycemic episodes). Products include:
NPH, 100 Units ... 1450
Pork NPH, 100 Units ... 1452
Purified Pork NPH Isophane Insulin ... 1801
Insulin, Regular (Hypoglycemic episodes). Products include:
Regular, 100 Units ... 1450
Pork Regular, 100 Units ... 1452
Pork Regular (Concentrated), 500 Units ... 1453
Purified Pork Regular Insulin ... 1801
Insulin, Zinc Crystals (Hypoglycemic episodes). Products include:
NPH, 100 Units ... 1450
Insulin, Zinc Suspension (Hypoglycemic episodes). Products include:
Iletin I ... 1450
Lente, 100 Units ... 1450
Iletin II ... 1452
Pork Lente, 100 Units ... 1452
Purified Pork Lente Insulin ... 1801
Isocarboxazid (Contraindicated; hypertensive crises; severe convulsive seizures).
No products indexed under this heading.
Isoflurane (Contraindicated; potentiated).
No products indexed under this heading.
Isoproterenol Hydrochloride (Contraindicated; hypertension, headache and related symptoms precipitated). Products include:
Isuprel Hydrochloride Injection 1:5000 ... 2311
Isuprel Hydrochloride Solution 1:200 & 1:100 ... 2313
Isuprel Mistometer ... 2312
Isoproterenol Sulfate (Contraindicated; hypertension, headache and related symptoms precipitated). Products include:
Norisodrine with Calcium Iodide Syrup ... 442
Isradipine (Contraindicated; potentiated). Products include:
DynaCirc Capsules ... 2256
Ketamine Hydrochloride (Contraindicated; potentiated).
No products indexed under this heading.
Labetalol Hydrochloride (Contraindicated; potentiated). Products include:
Normodyne Injection ... 2377
Normodyne Tablets ... 2379
Trandate ... 1185

791 **Interactions Index** **Parnate**

Levodopa (Contraindicated; hypertension, headache and related symptoms precipitated). Products include:
Atamet ... 572
Larodopa Tablets ... 2129
Sinemet Tablets ... 943
Sinemet CR Tablets ... 944
Levomethadyl Acetate Hydrochloride (Contraindicated; potentiated). Products include:
Orlamm ... 2239
Levorphanol Tartrate (Contraindicated; potentiated). Products include:
Levo-Dromoran ... 2129
Lisinopril (Contraindicated; potentiated). Products include:
Prinivil Tablets ... 1733
Prinzide Tablets ... 1737
Zestoretic ... 2850
Zestril Tablets ... 2854
Loratadine (Contraindicated). Products include:
Claritin ... 2349
Claritin-D ... 2350
Lorazepam (Contraindicated; potentiated). Products include:
Ativan Injection ... 2698
Ativan Tablets ... 2700
Losartan Potassium (Contraindicated; potentiated). Products include:
Cozaar Tablets ... 1628
Hyzaar Tablets ... 1677
Loxapine Hydrochloride (Contraindicated; potentiated). Products include:
Loxitane ... 1378
Loxapine Succinate (Contraindicated; potentiated). Products include:
Loxitane Capsules ... 1378
Maprotiline Hydrochloride (Contraindicated; hypertensive crises; severe convulsive seizures). Products include:
Ludiomil Tablets ... 843
Mazindol (Combined use contraindicated). Products include:
Sanorex Tablets ... 2294
Mecamylamine Hydrochloride (Contraindicated; potentiated). Products include:
Inversine Tablets ... 1686
Meperidine Hydrochloride (Contraindicated; potentiated; serious reactions precipitated). Products include:
Demerol ... 2308
Mepergan Injection ... 2753
Mephobarbital (Contraindicated; potentiated). Products include:
Mebaral Tablets ... 2322
Meprobamate (Contraindicated; potentiated). Products include:
Miltown Tablets ... 2672
PMB 200 and PMB 400 ... 2783
Mesoridazine Besylate (Additive hypotensive effects). Products include:
Serentil ... 684
Metaproterenol Sulfate (Contraindicated; hypertension, headache and related symptoms precipitated). Products include:
Alupent ... 669
Metaproterenol Sulfate Inhalation Solution, USP, Arm-a-Med ... 552
Metaraminol Bitartrate (Contraindicated; hypertension, headache and related symptoms precipitated). Products include:
Aramine Injection ... 1609
Metformin Hydrochloride (Hypoglycemic episodes). Products include:
Glucophage ... 752
Methadone Hydrochloride (Contraindicated; potentiated). Products include:
Methadone Hydrochloride Oral Concentrate ... 2233
Methadone Hydrochloride Oral Solution & Tablets ... 2235
Methamphetamine Hydrochloride (Combined use contraindicated). Products include:
Desoxyn Gradumet Tablets ... 419
Methdilazine Hydrochloride (Contraindicated).
No products indexed under this heading.
Methohexital Sodium (Contraindicated; potentiated). Products include:
Brevital Sodium Vials ... 1429
Methotrimeprazine (Contraindicated; potentiated). Products include:
Levoprome ... 1274
Methoxamine Hydrochloride (Contraindicated; hypertension, headache and related symptoms precipitated). Products include:
Vasoxyl Injection ... 1196
Methoxyflurane (Contraindicated; potentiated).
No products indexed under this heading.
Methyclothiazide (Contraindicated; potentiated; hypertensive crises; severe convulsive seizures). Products include:
Enduron Tablets ... 420
Methyldopa (Contraindicated; potentiated; hypertension headache and related symptoms precipitated). Products include:
Aldoclor Tablets ... 1598
Aldomet Oral ... 1600
Aldoril Tablets ... 1604
Methyldopate Hydrochloride (Contraindicated; potentiated; hypertension headache and related symptoms precipitated). Products include:
Aldomet Ester HCl Injection ... 1602
Metolazone (Contraindicated; potentiated). Products include:
Mykrox Tablets ... 993
Zaroxolyn Tablets ... 1000
Metoprolol Succinate (Contraindicated; potentiated). Products include:
Toprol-XL Tablets ... 565
Metoprolol Tartrate (Contraindicated; potentiated). Products include:
Lopressor Ampuls ... 830
Lopressor HCT Tablets ... 832
Lopressor Tablets ... 830
Metyrosine (Contraindicated; potentiated). Products include:
Demser Capsules ... 1649
Midazolam Hydrochloride (Contraindicated; potentiated). Products include:
Versed Injection ... 2170
Minoxidil (Contraindicated; potentiated). Products include:
Loniten Tablets ... 2618
Rogaine Topical Solution ... 2637
Moexipril Hydrochloride (Contraindicated; potentiated). Products include:
Univasc Tablets ... 2410
Molindone Hydrochloride (Contraindicated; potentiated). Products include:
Moban Tablets and Concentrate ... 1048
Morphine Sulfate (Contraindicated; potentiated). Products include:
Astramorph/PF Injection, USP (Preservative-Free) ... 535
Duramorph ... 962
Infumorph 200 and Infumorph 500 Sterile Solutions ... 965
MS Contin Tablets ... 1994
MSIR ... 1997
Oramorph SR (Morphine Sulfate Sustained Release Tablets) ... 2236
RMS Suppositories ... 2657
Roxanol ... 2243
Nadolol (Contraindicated; potentiated).
No products indexed under this heading.
Naphazoline Hydrochloride (Combined use contraindicated). Products include:
Albalon Solution with Liquifilm ... ◉ 231
Clear Eyes ACR Astringent/Lubricant Eye Redness Reliever Eye Drops ... ◉ 316
Clear Eyes Lubricant Eye Redness Reliever ... ◉ 316
4-Way Fast Acting Nasal Spray (regular & mentholated) ... ▣ 621
Naphcon-A Ophthalmic Solution ... 473
Privine ... ▣ 647
Vasocon-A ... ◉ 271
Nicardipine Hydrochloride (Contraindicated; potentiated). Products include:
Cardene Capsules ... 2095
Cardene I.V. ... 2709
Cardene SR Capsules ... 2097
Nifedipine (Contraindicated; potentiated). Products include:
Adalat Capsules (10 mg and 20 mg) ... 587
Adalat CC ... 589
Procardia Capsules ... 1971
Procardia XL Extended Release Tablets ... 1972
Nisoldipine (Contraindicated; potentiated).
No products indexed under this heading.
Nitroglycerin (Contraindicated; potentiated). Products include:
Deponit NTG Transdermal Delivery System ... 2397
Nitro-Bid IV ... 1523
Nitro-Bid Ointment ... 1524
Nitrodisc ... 2047
Nitro-Dur (nitroglycerin) Transdermal Infusion System ... 1326
Nitrolingual Spray ... 2027
Nitrostat Tablets ... 1925
Transderm-Nitro Transdermal Therapeutic System ... 859
Norepinephrine Bitartrate (Contraindicated; hypertension, headache and related symptoms precipitated). Products include:
Levophed Bitartrate Injection ... 2315
Nortriptyline Hydrochloride (Contraindicated; hypertensive crises; severe convulsive seizures). Products include:
Pamelor ... 2280
Opium Alkaloids (Contraindicated; potentiated).
No products indexed under this heading.
Oxazepam (Contraindicated; potentiated). Products include:
Serax Capsules ... 2810
Serax Tablets ... 2810
Oxycodone Hydrochloride (Contraindicated; potentiated). Products include:
Percocet Tablets ... 938
Percodan Tablets ... 939
Percodan-Demi Tablets ... 940
Roxicodone Tablets, Oral Solution & Intensol (Oxycodone) ... 2244
Tylox Capsules ... 1584
Oxymetazoline Hydrochloride (Combined use contraindicated). Products include:
Afrin ... ▣ 797
Cheracol Nasal Spray Pump ... ▣ 768
Duration 12 Hour Nasal Spray ... ▣ 805
4-Way Long Lasting Nasal Spray ... ▣ 621
NTZ Long Acting Nasal Spray & Drops 0.05% ... ▣ 727
Neo-Synephrine Maximum Strength 12 Hour Nasal Spray ... ▣ 726
Neo-Synephrine 12 Hour ... ▣ 726
Nōstrilla Long Acting Nasal Decongestant ... ▣ 644
Vicks Sinex 12-Hour Nasal Decongestant Spray and Ultra Fine Mist ... ▣ 765
Visine L.R. Eye Drops ... ▣ 746
Visine L.R. Eye Drops ... ◉ 313
Paroxetine Hydrochloride (Potential for fatal reactions including hyperthermia, rigidity, myoclonus, and autonomic instability; concurrent use is contraindicated; at least 2 weeks should be allowed after stopping SSRI before starting Parnate). Products include:
Paxil Tablets ... 2505
Penbutolol Sulfate (Contraindicated; potentiated). Products include:
Levatol ... 2403
Pentobarbital Sodium (Contraindicated; potentiated). Products include:
Nembutal Sodium Capsules ... 436
Nembutal Sodium Solution ... 438
Nembutal Sodium Suppositories ... 440
Perphenazine (Contraindicated; additive hypertensive effects; potentiated; hypertensive crises; severe convulsive seizures). Products include:
Etrafon ... 2355
Triavil Tablets ... 1757
Trilafon ... 2389
Phendimetrazine Tartrate (Combined use contraindicated). Products include:
Bontril Slow-Release Capsules ... 781
Prelu-2 Timed Release Capsules ... 681
Phenelzine Sulfate (Contraindicated; hypertensive crises; severe convulsive seizures). Products include:
Nardil ... 1920
Phenmetrazine Hydrochloride (Combined use contraindicated).
No products indexed under this heading.
Phenobarbital (Contraindicated; potentiated). Products include:
Arco-Lase Plus Tablets ... 512
Bellergal-S Tablets ... 2250
Donnatal ... 2060
Donnatal Extentabs ... 2061
Donnatal Tablets ... 2060
Phenobarbital Elixir and Tablets ... 1469
Quadrinal Tablets ... 1350
Phenoxybenzamine Hydrochloride (Contraindicated; potentiated). Products include:
Dibenzyline Capsules ... 2476
Phentolamine Mesylate (Contraindicated; potentiated). Products include:
Regitine ... 846
Phenylephrine Bitartrate (Contraindicated; hypertension, headache and related symptoms precipitated).
No products indexed under this heading.
Phenylephrine Hydrochloride (Contraindicated; hypertension, headache and related symptoms precipitated; combined use contraindicated). Products include:
Atrohist Plus Tablets ... 454
Cerose DM ... ▣ 878
Comhist ... 2038
D.A. Chewable Tablets ... 951
Deconsal Pediatric Capsules ... 454
Dura-Vent/DA Tablets ... 953
Entex Capsules ... 1986
Entex Liquid ... 1986
Extendryl ... 1005
4-Way Fast Acting Nasal Spray (regular & mentholated) ... ▣ 621
Hemorid For Women ... ▣ 834
Hycomine Compound Tablets ... 932

IMPORTANT NOTE: Always consult each drug listing in the patient's regimen for possible interactions.

Parnate **Interactions Index** 792

Neo-Synephrine Hydrochloride 1% Carpuject ... 2324
Neo-Synephrine Hydrochloride 1% Injection ... 2324
Neo-Synephrine Hydrochloride (Ophthalmic) ... 2325
Neo-Synephrine ... ▣ 726
Nōstril ... ▣ 644
Novahistine Elixir ... ▣ 823
Phenergan VC ... 2779
Phenergan VC with Codeine ... 2781
Preparation H ... ▣ 871
Tympagesic Ear Drops ... 2342
Vasosulf ... ⊙ 271
Vicks Sinex Nasal Spray and Ultra Fine Mist ... ▣ 765

Phenylephrine Tannate (Contraindicated; hypertension, headache and related symptoms precipitated). Products include:
Atrohist Pediatric Suspension ... 454
Ricobid-D Pediatric Suspension ... 2038
Ricobid Tablets and Pediatric Suspension ... 2038
Rynatan ... 2673
Rynatuss ... 2673

Phenylpropanolamine Containing Anorectics (Combined use contraindicated).

Phenylpropanolamine Hydrochloride (Contraindicated; hypertension, headache and related symptoms precipitated). Products include:
Acutrim ... ▣ 628
Allerest Children's Chewable Tablets ... ▣ 627
Allerest 12 Hour Caplets ... ▣ 627
Atrohist Plus Tablets ... 454
BC Cold Powder Multi-Symptom Formula (Cold-Sinus-Allergy) ... ▣ 609
BC Cold Powder Non-Drowsy Formula (Cold-Sinus) ... ▣ 609
Cheracol Plus Head Cold/Cough Formula ... ▣ 769
Comtrex Multi-Symptom Non-Drowsy Liqui-gels ... ▣ 618
Contac Continuous Action Nasal Decongestant/Antihistamine 12 Hour Capsules ... ▣ 813
Contac Maximum Strength Continuous Action Decongestant/Antihistamine 12 Hour Caplets ... ▣ 813
Contac Severe Cold and Flu Formula Caplets ... ▣ 814
Coricidin 'D' Decongestant Tablets ... ▣ 800
Dexatrim ... ▣ 832
Dexatrim Plus Vitamins Caplets ... ▣ 832
Dimetane-DC Cough Syrup ... 2059
Dimetapp Elixir ... ▣ 773
Dimetapp Extentabs ... ▣ 774
Dimetapp Tablets/Liqui-Gels ... ▣ 775
Dimetapp Cold & Allergy Chewable Tablets ... ▣ 773
Dimetapp DM Elixir ... ▣ 774
Dura-Vent Tablets ... 952
Entex Capsules ... 1986
Entex LA Tablets ... 1987
Entex Liquid ... 1986
Exgest LA Tablets ... 782
Hycomine ... 931
Isoclor Timesule Capsules ... ▣ 637
Nolamine Timed-Release Tablets ... 785
Ornade Spansule Capsules ... 2502
Propagest Tablets ... 786
Pyrroxate Caplets ... ▣ 772
Robitussin-CF ... ▣ 777
Sinulin Tablets ... 787
Tavist-D 12 Hour Relief Tablets ... ▣ 787
Teldrin 12 Hour Antihistamine/Nasal Decongestant Allergy Relief Capsules ... ▣ 826
Triaminic Allergy Tablets ... ▣ 789
Triaminic Cold Tablets ... ▣ 790
Triaminic Expectorant ... ▣ 790
Triaminic Syrup ... ▣ 792
Triaminic-12 Tablets ... ▣ 792
Triaminic-DM Syrup ... ▣ 792
Triaminicin Tablets ... ▣ 793
Triaminicol Multi-Symptom Cold Tablets ... ▣ 793
Triaminicol Multi-Symptom Relief ▣ 794
Vicks DayQuil Allergy Relief 12-Hour Extended Release Tablets ... ▣ 760
Vicks DayQuil Allergy Relief 4-Hour Tablets ... ▣ 760
Vicks DayQuil SINUS Pressure & CONGESTION Relief ... ▣ 761

Pindolol (Contraindicated; potentiated). Products include:
Visken Tablets ... 2299

Pirbuterol Acetate (Contraindicated; hypertension, headache and related symptoms precipitated). Products include:
Maxair Autohaler ... 1492
Maxair Inhaler ... 1494

Polythiazide (Contraindicated; potentiated). Products include:
Minizide Capsules ... 1938

Prazepam (Contraindicated; potentiated).
No products indexed under this heading.

Prazosin Hydrochloride (Contraindicated; potentiated). Products include:
Minipress Capsules ... 1937
Minizide Capsules ... 1938

Prochlorperazine (Additive hypotensive effects). Products include:
Compazine ... 2470

Procyclidine Hydrochloride (Combined use contraindicated; severe reactions reported). Products include:
Kemadrin Tablets ... 1112

Promethazine Hydrochloride (Contraindicated; potentiated; additive hypotensive effects). Products include:
Mepergan Injection ... 2753
Phenergan with Codeine ... 2777
Phenergan with Dextromethorphan 2778
Phenergan Injection ... 2773
Phenergan Suppositories ... 2775
Phenergan Syrup ... 2774
Phenergan Tablets ... 2775
Phenergan VC ... 2779
Phenergan VC with Codeine ... 2781

Propofol (Contraindicated; potentiated). Products include:
Diprivan Injection ... 2833

Propoxyphene Hydrochloride (Contraindicated; potentiated). Products include:
Darvon ... 1435
Wygesic Tablets ... 2827

Propoxyphene Napsylate (Contraindicated; potentiated). Products include:
Darvon-N/Darvocet-N ... 1433

Propranolol Hydrochloride (Contraindicated; potentiated). Products include:
Inderal ... 2728
Inderal LA Long Acting Capsules ... 2730
Inderide Tablets ... 2732
Inderide LA Long Acting Capsules .. 2734

Protriptyline Hydrochloride (Contraindicated; hypertensive crises; severe convulsive seizures). Products include:
Vivactil Tablets ... 1774

Pseudoephedrine Hydrochloride (Contraindicated; hypertension, headache and related symptoms precipitated; combined use contraindicated). Products include:
Actifed Allergy Daytime/Nighttime Caplets ... ▣ 844
Actifed Plus Caplets ... ▣ 845
Actifed Plus Tablets ... ▣ 845
Actifed with Codeine Cough Syrup .. 1067
Actifed Sinus Daytime/Nighttime Tablets and Caplets ... ▣ 846
Actifed Syrup ... ▣ 846
Actifed Tablets ... ▣ 844
Advil Cold and Sinus Caplets and Tablets (formerly CoAdvil) ... ▣ 870
Alka-Seltzer Plus Cold Medicine Liqui-Gels ... ▣ 706
Alka-Seltzer Plus Cold & Cough Medicine Liqui-Gels ... ▣ 705
Alka-Seltzer Plus Night-Time Cold Medicine Liqui-Gels ... ▣ 706
Allerest Headache Strength Tablets ... ▣ 627
Allerest Maximum Strength Tablets ... ▣ 627
Allerest No Drowsiness Tablets ... ▣ 627
Allerest Sinus Pain Formula ... ▣ 627
Anatuss LA Tablets ... 1542
Atrohist Pediatric Capsules ... 453
Bayer Select Sinus Pain Relief Formula ... ▣ 717
Benadryl Allergy Decongestant Liquid Medication ... ▣ 848
Benadryl Allergy Decongestant Tablets ... ▣ 848
Benadryl Allergy Sinus Headache Formula Caplets ... ▣ 849
Benylin Multisymptom ... ▣ 852
Bromfed Capsules (Extended-Release) ... 1785
Bromfed Syrup ... ▣ 733
Bromfed Tablets ... 1785
Bromfed-DM Cough Syrup ... 1786
Bromfed-PD Capsules (Extended-Release) ... 1785
Children's Vicks DayQuil Allergy Relief ... ▣ 757
Children's Vicks NyQuil Cold/Cough Relief ... ▣ 758
Comtrex Multi-Symptom Cold Reliever Tablets/Caplets/Liqui-Gels/Liquid ... ▣ 615
Allergy-Sinus Comtrex Multi-Symptom Allergy-Sinus Formula Tablets ... ▣ 617
Comtrex Multi-Symptom Non-Drowsy Caplets ... ▣ 618
Congess ... 1004
Contac Day Allergy/Sinus Caplets ▣ 812
Contac Day & Night ... ▣ 812
Contac Night Allergy/Sinus Caplets ... ▣ 812
Contac Severe Cold & Flu Non-Drowsy ... ▣ 815
Deconamine Chewable Tablets ... 1320
Deconamine CX Cough and Cold Liquid and Tablets ... 1319
Deconamine ... 1320
Deconsal C Expectorant Syrup ... 456
Deconsal Pediatric Syrup ... 457
Deconsal II Tablets ... 454
Dimetane-DX Cough Syrup ... 2059
Dimetapp Sinus Caplets ... ▣ 775
Dorcol Children's Cough Syrup ... ▣ 785
Drixoral Cough + Congestion Liquid Caps ... ▣ 802
Dura-Tap/PD Capsules ... 2867
Duratuss Tablets ... 2565
Duratuss HD Elixir ... 2565
Efidac/24 ... ▣ 635
Entex PSE Tablets ... 1987
Fedahist Gyrocaps ... 2401
Fedahist Timecaps ... 2401
Guaifed ... 1787
Guaifed Syrup ... ▣ 734
Guaimax-D Tablets ... 792
Guaitab Tablets ... ▣ 734
Isoclor Expectorant ... 990
Kronofed-A ... 977
Motrin IB Sinus ... ▣ 838
Novahistine DH ... 2462
Novahistine DMX ... ▣ 822
Novahistine Expectorant ... 2463
Nucofed ... 2051
PediaCare Cold Allergy Chewable Tablets ... ▣ 677
PediaCare Cough-Cold Chewable Tablets ... 1553
PediaCare ... 1553
PediaCare Infants' Decongestant Drops ... ▣ 677
PediCare Infant's Drops Decongestant Plus Cough ... 1553
PediaCare NightRest Cough-Cold Liquid ... 1553
Pediatric Vicks 44d Dry Hacking Cough & Head Congestion ... ▣ 763
Pediatric Vicks 44m Cough & Cold Relief ... ▣ 764
Robitussin Cold & Cough Liqui-Gels ... ▣ 776
Robitussin Maximum Strength Cough & Cold ... ▣ 778
Robitussin Pediatric Cough & Cold Formula ... ▣ 779
Robitussin Severe Congestion Liqui-Gels ... ▣ 776
Robitussin-DAC Syrup ... 2074
Robitussin-PE ... ▣ 778
Rondec Oral Drops ... 953
Rondec Syrup ... 953
Rondec Tablet ... 953
Rondec-DM Oral Drops ... 954
Rondec-DM Syrup ... 954
Rondec-TR Tablet ... 953
Ryna ... ▣ 841
Seldane-D Extended-Release Tablets ... 1538
Semprex-D Capsules ... 463
Semprex-D Capsules ... 1167
Sinarest Tablets ... ▣ 648
Sinarest Extra Strength Tablets ... ▣ 648
Sinarest No Drowsiness Tablets ... ▣ 648
Sine-Aid IB Caplets ... 1554
Sine-Aid Maximum Strength Sinus Medication Gelcaps, Caplets and Tablets ... 1554
Sine-Off No Drowsiness Formula Caplets ... ▣ 824
Sine-Off Sinus Medicine ... ▣ 825
Singlet Tablets ... ▣ 825
Sinutab Non-Drying Liquid Caps ... ▣ 859
Sinutab Sinus Allergy Medication, Maximum Strength Tablets and Caplets ... ▣ 860
Sinutab Sinus Medication, Maximum Strength Without Drowsiness Formula, Tablets & Caplets ... ▣ 860
Sinutab Sinus Medication, Regular Strength Without Drowsiness Formula ... ▣ 859
Sudafed Children's Liquid ... ▣ 861
Sudafed Cold and Cough Liquid-caps ... ▣ 862
Sudafed Cough Syrup ... ▣ 862
Sudafed Plus Liquid ... ▣ 862
Sudafed Plus Tablets ... ▣ 863
Sudafed Severe Cold Formula Caplets ... ▣ 863
Sudafed Severe Cold Formula Tablets ... ▣ 864
Sudafed Sinus Caplets ... ▣ 864
Sudafed Sinus Tablets ... ▣ 864
Sudafed Tablets, 30 mg ... ▣ 861
Sudafed Tablets, 60 mg ... ▣ 861
Sudafed 12 Hour Caplets ... ▣ 861
Syn-Rx Tablets ... 465
Syn-Rx DM Tablets ... 466
TheraFlu ... ▣ 787
TheraFlu Maximum Strength Nighttime Flu, Cold & Cough Medicine ... ▣ 788
TheraFlu Maximum Strength Non-Drowsy Formula Flu, Cold & Cough Medicine ... ▣ 788
Thera Flu Maximum Strength, Non-Drowsy Formula Flu, Cold and Cough Caplets ... ▣ 789
Triaminic AM Cough and Decongestant Formula ... ▣ 789
Triaminic AM Decongestant Formula ... ▣ 790
Triaminic Nite Light ... ▣ 791
Triaminic Sore Throat Formula ... ▣ 791
Tussend ... 1783
Tussend Expectorant ... 1785
Children's TYLENOL Cold Multi-Symptom Liquid Formula and Chewable Tablets ... 1561
Children's TYLENOL Cold Plus Cough Multi Symptom Tablets and Liquid ... ▣ 681
Infants' TYLENOL Cold Decongestant & Fever-Reducer Drops ... 1556
TYLENOL Maximum Strength Allergy Sinus Medication Gelcaps and Caplets ... 1563
TYLENOL Maximum Strength Allergy Sinus NightTime Medication Caplets ... 1555
TYLENOL Flu Maximum Strength Gelcaps ... 1565
TYLENOL Flu NightTime, Maximum Strength, Gelcaps ... 1566
TYLENOL Maximum Strength Flu NightTime Hot Medication Packets ... 1562
TYLENOL, Maximum Strength, Sinus Medication Geltabs, Gelcaps, Caplets and Tablets ... 1566
TYLENOL Cold Multi-Symptom Formula Medication Tablets and Caplets ... 1561
TYLENOL Cold Medication No Drowsiness Formula Gelcaps and Caplets ... 1562
TYLENOL Cold Multi-Symptom Hot Medication Liquid Packets ... 1557
TYLENOL Cough Multi-Symptom Medication with Decongestant ... 1565
Ursinus Inlay-Tabs ... ▣ 794
Vicks 44 LiquiCaps Cough, Cold & Flu Relief ... ▣ 755
Vicks 44 LiquiCaps Non-Drowsy Cough & Cold Relief ... ▣ 756

(▣ Described in PDR For Nonprescription Drugs) (⊙ Described in PDR For Ophthalmology)

Vicks 44D Dry Hacking Cough & Head Congestion .... ⊕ 755
Vicks 44M Cough, Cold & Flu Relief .... ⊕ 756
Vicks DayQuil .... ⊕ 761
Vicks DayQuil SINUS Pressure & PAIN Relief with IBUPROFEN ..... ⊕ 762
Vicks Nyquil Hot Therapy.................... ⊕ 762
Vicks NyQuil LiquiCaps Multi-Symptom Cold/Flu Relief .... ⊕ 763
Vicks NyQuil Multi-Symptom Cold/Flu Relief - (Original & Cherry Flavor) .... ⊕ 763

Pseudoephedrine Sulfate (Contraindicated; hypertension, headache and related symptoms precipitated). Products include:

Cheracol Sinus .... ⊕ 768
Chlor-Trimeton Allergy Decongestant Tablets .... ⊕ 799
Claritin-D 2350
Drixoral Cold and Allergy Sustained-Action Tablets .... ⊕ 802
Drixoral Cold and Flu Extended-Release Tablets.................................... ⊕ 803
Drixoral Non-Drowsy Formula Extended-Release Tablets .... ⊕ 803
Drixoral Allergy/Sinus Extended Release Tablets.................................... ⊕ 804
Trinalin Repetabs Tablets 1330

Pyrilamine Maleate (Contraindicated). Products include:

4-Way Fast Acting Nasal Spray (regular & mentholated) .... ⊕ 621
Maximum Strength Multi-Symptom Formula Midol .... ⊕ 722
PMS Multi-Symptom Formula Midol .... ⊕ 723

Pyrilamine Tannate (Contraindicated). Products include:

Atrohist Pediatric Suspension 454
Rynatan 2673

Quazepam (Contraindicated; potentiated). Products include:

Doral Tablets 2664

Quinapril Hydrochloride (Contraindicated; potentiated). Products include:

Accupril Tablets 1893

Ramipril (Contraindicated; potentiated). Products include:

Altace Capsules 1232

Rauwolfia Serpentina (Contraindicated; potentiated).

No products indexed under this heading.

Rescinnamine (Contraindicated; potentiated).

No products indexed under this heading.

Reserpine (Contraindicated; potentiated). Products include:

Diupres Tablets 1650
Hydropres Tablets.................................. 1675
Ser-Ap-Es Tablets 849

Risperidone (Contraindicated; potentiated). Products include:

Risperdal 1301

Salmeterol Xinafoate (Contraindicated; hypertension, headache and related symptoms precipitated). Products include:

Serevent Inhalation Aerosol................ 1176

Secobarbital Sodium (Contraindicated; potentiated). Products include:

Seconal Sodium Pulvules 1474

Selegiline Hydrochloride (Contraindicated; hypertensive crises; severe convulsive seizures). Products include:

Eldepryl Tablets 2550

Sertraline Hydrochloride (Potential for fatal reactions including hyperthermia, rigidity, myoclonus, and autonomic instability; concurrent use is contraindicated; at least 2 weeks should be allowed after stopping SSRI before starting Parnate). Products include:

Zoloft Tablets 2217

Sodium Nitroprusside (Contraindicated; potentiated).

No products indexed under this heading.

Sotalol Hydrochloride (Contraindicated; potentiated). Products include:

Betapace Tablets 641

Spirapril Hydrochloride (Contraindicated; potentiated).

No products indexed under this heading.

Sufentanil Citrate (Contraindicated; potentiated). Products include:

Sufenta Injection 1309

Temazepam (Contraindicated; potentiated). Products include:

Restoril Capsules 2284

Terazosin Hydrochloride (Contraindicated; potentiated). Products include:

Hytrin Capsules 430

Terbutaline Sulfate (Contraindicated; hypertension, headache and related symptoms precipitated). Products include:

Brethaire Inhaler 813
Brethine Ampuls 815
Brethine Tablets...................................... 814
Bricanyl Subcutaneous Injection 1502
Bricanyl Tablets 1503

Terfenadine (Contraindicated). Products include:

Seldane Tablets 1536
Seldane-D Extended-Release Tablets 1538

Tetrahydrozoline Hydrochloride (Combined use contraindicated). Products include:

Collyrium Fresh .... ◉ 325
Murine Plus Lubricant Redness Reliever Eye Drops .... ⊕ 781
Murine Tears Plus Lubricant Redness Reliever Eye Drops .... ◉ 316
Visine Maximum Strength Allergy Relief .... ◉ 313
Visine Moisturizing Eye Drops .... ◉ 313
Visine Original Eye Drops.................. ◉ 314

Thiamylal Sodium (Contraindicated; potentiated).

No products indexed under this heading.

Thioridazine Hydrochloride (Additive hypotensive effects). Products include:

Mellaril 2269

Thiothixene (Contraindicated; potentiated). Products include:

Navane Capsules and Concentrate 2201
Navane Intramuscular 2202

Timolol Maleate (Contraindicated; potentiated). Products include:

Blocadren Tablets 1614
Timolide Tablets...................................... 1748
Timoptic in Ocudose 1753
Timoptic Sterile Ophthalmic Solution... 1751
Timoptic-XE 1755

Tolazamide (Hypoglycemic episodes).

No products indexed under this heading.

Tolbutamide (Hypoglycemic episodes).

No products indexed under this heading.

Torsemide (Contraindicated; potentiated). Products include:

Demadex Tablets and Injection 686

Triazolam (Contraindicated; potentiated). Products include:

Halcion Tablets.. 2611

Trifluoperazine Hydrochloride (Additive hypotensive effects). Products include:

Stelazine 2514

Trihexyphenidyl Hydrochloride (Combined use contraindicated; severe reactions reported). Products include:

Artane.. 1368

Trimeprazine Tartrate (Contraindicated). Products include:

Temaril Tablets, Syrup and Spansule Extended-Release Capsules.. 483

Trimethaphan Camsylate (Contraindicated; potentiated). Products include:

Arfonad Ampuls 2080

Trimipramine Maleate (Contraindicated; hypertensive crises; severe convulsive seizures). Products include:

Surmontil Capsules 2811

Tripelennamine Hydrochloride (Contraindicated). Products include:

PBZ Tablets 845
PBZ-SR Tablets.. 844

Triprolidine Hydrochloride (Contraindicated). Products include:

Actifed Plus Caplets .... ⊕ 845
Actifed Plus Tablets .... ⊕ 845
Actifed with Codeine Cough Syrup.. 1067
Actifed Syrup... ⊕ 846
Actifed Tablets .... ⊕ 844

L-Tryptophan (Contraindicated; hypertension, headache and related symptoms precipitated).

No products indexed under this heading.

Venlafaxine Hydrochloride (Potential for fatal reactions including hyperthermia, rigidity, myoclonus, and autonomic instability; concurrent use is contraindicated; at least 2 weeks should be allowed after stopping SSRI before starting Parnate). Products include:

Effexor 2719

Verapamil Hydrochloride (Contraindicated; potentiated). Products include:

Calan SR Caplets 2422
Calan Tablets.. 2419
Isoptin Injectable 1344
Isoptin Oral Tablets 1346
Isoptin SR Tablets 1348
Verelan Capsules 1410
Verelan Capsules 2824

Zolpidem Tartrate (Contraindicated; potentiated). Products include:

Ambien Tablets.. 2416

Food Interactions

Alcohol (Contraindicated; potentiated).

Anchovies (Potential for hypertensive crisis).

Avocados (Potential for hypertensive crisis).

Bananas (Potential for hypertensive crisis).

Beans, broad (Potential for hypertensive crisis).

Beans, Fava (Potential for hypertensive crisis).

Beer, alcohol-free (Potential for hypertensive crisis).

Beer, unspecified (Potential for hypertensive crisis).

Caviar (Potential for hypertensive crisis).

Cheese, aged (Potential for hypertensive crisis).

Cheese, strong, unpasteurized (Potential for hypertensive crisis).

Cheese, unspecified (Potential for hypertensive crisis).

Chocolate (Potential for hypertensive crisis).

Cream, sour (Potential for hypertensive crisis).

Figs, canned (Potential for hypertensive crisis).

Food with high concentration of tyramine (Potential for hypertensive crisis).

Herring, pickled (Potential for hypertensive crisis).

Liquers (Potential for hypertensive crisis).

Liver (Potential for hypertensive crisis).

Meat extracts (Potential for hypertensive crisis).

Meat prepared with tenderizers (Potential for hypertensive crisis).

Raisins (Potential for hypertensive crisis).

Sauerkraut (Potential for hypertensive crisis).

Sherry (Potential for hypertensive crisis).

Soy sauce (Potential for hypertensive crisis).

Wine, Chianti (Potential for hypertensive crisis).

Yeast extract (Potential for hypertensive crisis).

Yogurt (Potential for hypertensive crisis).

PASER GRANULES

(Aminosalicylic Acid) 1285

May interact with:

Digoxin (Potential for reduced digoxin levels). Products include:

Lanoxicaps 1117
Lanoxin Elixir Pediatric 1120
Lanoxin Injection 1123
Lanoxin Injection Pediatric.................. 1126
Lanoxin Tablets 1128

Isoniazid (Concurrent use with a rapidly available form of aminosalicylic acid has been reported to produce a 20% reduction in the acetylation of INH; the lower serum levels produced by delayed release preparation will result in a reduced effect on the acetylation of INH). Products include:

Nydrazid Injection 508
Rifamate Capsules 1530
Rifater.. 1532

Rifampin (May block the absorption of rifampin; PASER granules do not contain excipient that blocks the absorption). Products include:

Rifadin 1528
Rifamate Capsules 1530
Rifater.. 1532
Rimactane Capsules 847

Vitamin B_{12} (Reduced absorption of vitamin B_{12} with clinically significant erythrocyte abnormalities developing after depletion). Products include:

Ener-B Vitamin B_{12} Nasal Gel Dietary Supplement 1792
Mega-B 512
Niferex Forte Elixir 794
Stuart Prenatal Tablets .... ⊕ 881
The Stuart Formula Tablets.............. ⊕ 663
Trinsicon Capsules 2570

PAXIL TABLETS

(Paroxetine Hydrochloride) 2505

May interact with monoamine oxidase inhibitors, oral anticoagulants, antidepressant drugs, phenothiazines, type 1 antiarrhythmic drugs, highly protein bound drugs (selected), lithium preparations, and certain other agents. Compounds in these categories include:

Amiodarone Hydrochloride (Potential for increase in adverse effects of either drug). Products include:

Cordarone Intravenous 2715
Cordarone Tablets.................................. 2712

IMPORTANT NOTE: Always consult each drug listing in the patient's regimen for possible interactions.

Paxil Interactions Index 794

Amitriptyline Hydrochloride (Potential for increase in adverse effects of either drug; Paroxetine may significantly inhibit the activity of cytochrome isoenzyme $P_{450}IID_6$; coadministration should be approached with caution). Products include:

Elavil ... 2838
Endep Tablets ... 2174
Etrafon ... 2355
Limbitrol ... 2180
Triavil Tablets ... 1757

Amoxapine (Paroxetine may significantly inhibit the activity of cytochrome isoenzyme P_{450} IID_6; coadministration should be approached with caution). Products include:

Asendin Tablets ... 1369

Atovaquone (Potential for increase in adverse effects of either drug). Products include:

Mepron Suspension ... 1135

Bupropion Hydrochloride (Paroxetine may significantly inhibit the activity of cytochrome isoenzyme $P_{450}IID_6$; co-administration should be approached with caution). Products include:

Wellbutrin Tablets ... 1204

Cefonicid Sodium (Potential for increase in adverse effects of either drug). Products include:

Monocid Injection ... 2497

Chlordiazepoxide (Potential for increase in adverse effects of either drug). Products include:

Libritabs Tablets ... 2177
Limbitrol ... 2180

Chlordiazepoxide Hydrochloride (Potential for increase in adverse effects of either drug). Products include:

Librax Capsules ... 2176
Librium Capsules ... 2178
Librium Injectable ... 2179

Chlorpromazine (Potential for increase in adverse effects of either drug; Paroxetine may significantly inhibit the activity of cytochrome isoenzyme $P_{450}IID_6$; coadministration should be approached with caution). Products include:

Thorazine Suppositories ... 2523

Chlorpromazine Hydrochloride (Potential for increase in adverse effects of either drug; Paroxetine may significantly inhibit the activity of cytochrome isoenzyme $P_{450}IID_6$; coadministration should be approached with caution). Products include:

Thorazine ... 2523

Cimetidine (Potential for increased steady-state plasma concentration of paroxetine). Products include:

Tagamet Tablets ... 2516

Cimetidine Hydrochloride (Potential for increased steady-state plasma concentration of paroxetine). Products include:

Tagamet ... 2516

Clomipramine Hydrochloride (Potential for increase in adverse effects of either drug). Products include:

Anafranil Capsules ... 803

Clozapine (Potential for increase in adverse effects of either drug). Products include:

Clozaril Tablets ... 2252

Cyclosporine (Potential for increase in adverse effects of either drug). Products include:

Neoral ... 2276
Sandimmune ... 2286

Desipramine Hydrochloride (Paroxetine may significantly inhibit the activity of cytochrome isoenzyme $P_{450}IID_6$; coadministration should be approached with caution). Products include:

Norpramin Tablets ... 1526

Diazepam (Potential for increase in adverse effects of either drug). Products include:

Dizac ... 1809
Valium Injectable ... 2182
Valium Tablets ... 2183
Valrelease Capsules ... 2169

Diclofenac Potassium (Potential for increase in adverse effects of either drug). Products include:

Cataflam ... 816

Diclofenac Sodium (Potential for increase in adverse effects of either drug). Products include:

Voltaren Ophthalmic Sterile Ophthalmic Solution ... ⊙ 272
Voltaren Tablets ... 861

Dicumarol (Potential for increased bleeding diathesis in the face of unaltered prothrombin time).

No products indexed under this heading.

Digoxin (Potential for decrease in mean digoxin AUC). Products include:

Lanoxicaps ... 1117
Lanoxin Elixir Pediatric ... 1120
Lanoxin Injection ... 1123
Lanoxin Injection Pediatric ... 1126
Lanoxin Tablets ... 1128

Dipyridamole (Potential for increase in adverse effects of either drug). Products include:

Persantine Tablets ... 681

Disopyramide Phosphate (Paroxetine may significantly inhibit the activity of cytochrome isoenzyme $P_{450}IID_6$; coadministration should be approached with caution). Products include:

Norpace ... 2444

Doxepin Hydrochloride (Paroxetine may significantly inhibit the activity of cytochrome isoenzyme $P_{450}IID_6$; coadministration should be approached with caution). Products include:

Sinequan ... 2205
Zonalon Cream ... 1055

Fenoprofen Calcium (Potential for increase in adverse effects of either drug). Products include:

Nalfon 200 Pulvules & Nalfon Tablets ... 917

Fluoxetine Hydrochloride (Paroxetine may significantly inhibit the activity of cytochrome isoenzyme P_{450} IID_6; coadministration should be approached with caution). Products include:

Prozac Pulvules & Liquid, Oral Solution ... 919

Fluphenazine Decanoate (Paroxetine may significantly inhibit the activity of cytochrome isoenzyme $P_{450}IID_6$; coadministration should be approached with caution). Products include:

Prolixin Decanoate ... 509

Fluphenazine Enanthate (Paroxetine may significantly inhibit the activity of cytochrome isoenzyme $P_{450}IID_6$; coadministration should be approached with caution). Products include:

Prolixin Enanthate ... 509

Fluphenazine Hydrochloride (Paroxetine may significantly inhibit the activity of cytochrome isoenzyme $P_{450}IID_6$; coadministration should be approached with caution). Products include:

Prolixin ... 509

Flurazepam Hydrochloride (Potential for increase in adverse effects of either drug). Products include:

Dalmane Capsules ... 2173

Flurbiprofen (Potential for increase in adverse effects of either drug). Products include:

Ansaid Tablets ... 2579

Furazolidone (Potential for serious and fatal reactions including hyperthermia, rigidity, myoclonus and other serious reactions; concurrent and/or sequential use is contraindicated). Products include:

Furoxone ... 2046

Glipizide (Potential for increase in adverse effects of either drug). Products include:

Glucotrol Tablets ... 1967
Glucotrol XL Extended Release Tablets ... 1968

Ibuprofen (Potential for increase in adverse effects of either drug). Products include:

Advil Cold and Sinus Caplets and Tablets (formerly CoAdvil) ... ▣ 870
Advil Ibuprofen Tablets and Caplets ... ▣ 870
Children's Advil Suspension ... 2692
Arthritis Foundation Ibuprofen Tablets ... ▣ 674
Bayer Select Ibuprofen Pain Relief Formula ... ▣ 715
Cramp End Tablets ... ▣ 735
Dimetapp Sinus Caplets ... ▣ 775
Haltran Tablets ... ▣ 771
IBU Tablets ... 1342
Ibuprohm ... ▣ 735
Children's Motrin Ibuprofen Oral Suspension ... 1546
Motrin Tablets ... 2625
Motrin IB Caplets, Tablets, and Geltabs ... ▣ 838
Motrin IB Sinus ... ▣ 838
Motrin Ibuprofen Suspension, Oral Drops, Chewable Tablets, Caplets ... 1546
Nuprin Ibuprofen/Analgesic Tablets & Caplets ... ▣ 622
Sine-Aid IB Caplets ... 1554
Vicks DayQuil SINUS Pressure & PAIN Relief with IBUPROFEN ... ▣ 762

Imipramine Hydrochloride (Potential for increase in adverse effects of either drug; Paroxetine may significantly inhibit the activity of cytochrome isoenzyme $P_{450}IID_6$; coadministration should be approached with caution). Products include:

Tofranil Ampuls ... 854
Tofranil Tablets ... 856

Imipramine Pamoate (Potential for increase in adverse effects of either drug; Paroxetine may significantly inhibit the activity of cytochrome isoenzyme $P_{450}IID_6$; coadministration should be approached with caution). Products include:

Tofranil-PM Capsules ... 857

Indomethacin (Potential for increase in adverse effects of either drug). Products include:

Indocin ... 1680

Indomethacin Sodium Trihydrate (Potential for increase in adverse effects of either drug). Products include:

Indocin I.V. ... 1684

Isocarboxazid (Potential for serious and fatal reactions including hyperthermia, rigidity, myoclonus and other serious reactions; concurrent and/or sequential use is contraindicated).

No products indexed under this heading.

Ketoprofen (Potential for increase in adverse effects of either drug). Products include:

Orudis Capsules ... 2766
Oruvail Capsules ... 2766

Ketorolac Tromethamine (Potential for increase in adverse effects of either drug). Products include:

Acular ... 474
Acular ... ⊙ 277
Toradol ... 2159

Lithium Carbonate (Concurrent administration should be undertaken with caution). Products include:

Eskalith ... 2485
Lithium Carbonate Capsules & Tablets ... 2230
Lithonate/Lithotabs/Lithobid ... 2543

Lithium Citrate (Concurrent administration should be undertaken with caution).

No products indexed under this heading.

Maprotiline Hydrochloride (Paroxetine may significantly inhibit the activity of cytochrome isoenzyme $P_{450}IID_6$; coadministration should be approached with caution). Products include:

Ludiomil Tablets ... 843

Meclofenamate Sodium (Potential for increase in adverse effects of either drug).

No products indexed under this heading.

Mefenamic Acid (Potential for increase in adverse effects of either drug). Products include:

Ponstel ... 1925

Mesoridazine Besylate (Paroxetine may significantly inhibit the activity of cytochrome isoenzyme $P_{450}IID_6$; coadministration should be approached with caution). Products include:

Serentil ... 684

Methotrimeprazine (Potential for increase in adverse effects of either drug; Paroxetine may significantly inhibit the activity of cytochrome isoenzyme $P_{450}IID_6$; coadministration should be approached with caution). Products include:

Levoprome ... 1274

Midazolam Hydrochloride (Potential for increase in adverse effects of either drug). Products include:

Versed Injection ... 2170

Moricizine Hydrochloride (Paroxetine may significantly inhibit the activity of cytochrome isoenzyme $P_{450}IID_6$; coadministration should be approached with caution). Products include:

Ethmozine Tablets ... 2041

Naproxen (Potential for increase in adverse effects of either drug). Products include:

Anaprox/Naprosyn ... 2117

Naproxen Sodium (Potential for increase in adverse effects of either drug). Products include:

Aleve ... 1975
Anaprox/Naprosyn ... 2117

(▣ Described in PDR For Nonprescription Drugs) (⊙ Described in PDR For Ophthalmology)

Nefazodone Hydrochloride (Potential for increase in adverse effects of either drug; Paroxetine may significantly inhibit the activity of cytochrome isoenzyme $P_{450}IID_6$; coadministration should be approached with caution). Products include:

Serzone Tablets 771

Nortriptyline Hydrochloride (Potential for increase in adverse effects of either drug; Paroxetine may significantly inhibit the activity of cytochrome isoenzyme $P_{450}IID_6$; coadministration should be approached with caution). Products include:

Pamelor 2280

Oxaprozin (Potential for increase in adverse effects of either drug). Products include:

Daypro Caplets 2426

Oxazepam (Potential for increase in adverse effects of either drug). Products include:

Serax Capsules 2810
Serax Tablets.. 2810

Perphenazine (Paroxetine may significantly inhibit the activity of cytochrome isoenzyme $P_{450}IID_6$; coadministration should be approached with caution). Products include:

Etrafon 2355
Triavil Tablets 1757
Trilafon.. 2389

Phenelzine Sulfate (Potential for serious and fatal reactions including hyperthermia, rigidity, myoclonus and other serious reactions; concurrent and/or sequential use is contraindicated). Products include:

Nardil 1920

Phenobarbital (Potential for reduction paroxetine AUC and half-life). Products include:

Arco-Lase Plus Tablets 512
Bellergal-S Tablets 2250
Donnatal 2060
Donnatal Extentabs.............................. 2061
Donnatal Tablets 2060
Phenobarbital Elixir and Tablets 1469
Quadrinal Tablets 1350

Phenylbutazone (Potential for increase in adverse effects of either drug).

No products indexed under this heading.

Phenytoin (Potential for reduction paroxetine AUC and half-life). Products include:

Dilantin Infatabs 1908
Dilantin-125 Suspension 1911

Phenytoin Sodium (Potential for reduction paroxetine AUC and half-life). Products include:

Dilantin Kapseals 1906
Dilantin Parenteral 1910

Pimozide (Concomitant use has been associated with extrapyramidal symptoms including dystonia, akathesia, bradykinesia, cogwheel rigidity, hypertonia, and oculogyric crisis). Products include:

Orap Tablets 1050

Piroxicam (Potential for increase in adverse effects of either drug). Products include:

Feldene Capsules................................. 1965

Procainamide Hydrochloride (Paroxetine may significantly inhibit the activity of cytochrome isoenzyme $P_{450}IID_6$; coadministration should be approached with caution). Products include:

Procan SR Tablets................................ 1926

Prochlorperazine (Paroxetine may significantly inhibit the activity of cytochrome isoenzyme $P_{450}IID_6$; coadministration should be approached with caution). Products include:

Compazine 2470

Procyclidine Hydrochloride (Increased steady-state AUC, C_{max} and C_{min} values of procyclidine with concurrent use). Products include:

Kemadrin Tablets 1112

Promethazine Hydrochloride (Paroxetine may significantly inhibit the activity of cytochrome isoenzyme $P_{450}IID_6$; coadministration should be approached with caution). Products include:

Mepergan Injection 2753
Phenergan with Codeine..................... 2777
Phenergan with Dextromethorphan 2778
Phenergan Injection 2773
Phenergan Suppositories 2775
Phenergan Syrup 2774
Phenergan Tablets 2775
Phenergan VC 2779
Phenergan VC with Codeine 2781

Propafenone Hydrochloride (Paroxetine may significantly inhibit the activity of cytochrome isoenzyme $P_{450}IID_6$; coadministration should be approached with caution). Products include:

Rythmol Tablets–150mg, 225mg, 300mg.. 1352

Propranolol Hydrochloride (Potential for increase in adverse effects of either drug). Products include:

Inderal 2728
Inderal LA Long Acting Capsules 2730
Inderide Tablets 2732
Inderide LA Long Acting Capsules .. 2734

Protriptyline Hydrochloride (Paroxetine may significantly inhibit the activity of cytochrome isoenzyme $P_{450}IID_6$; coadministration should be approached with caution). Products include:

Vivactil Tablets 1774

Quinidine Gluconate (Paroxetine may significantly inhibit the activity of cytochrome isoenzyme $P_{450}IID_6$; coadministration should be approached with caution). Products include:

Quinaglute Dura-Tabs Tablets 649

Quinidine Polygalacturonate (Paroxetine may significantly inhibit the activity of cytochrome isoenzyme $P_{450}IID_6$; coadministration should be approached with caution).

No products indexed under this heading.

Quinidine Sulfate (Paroxetine may significantly inhibit the activity of cytochrome isoenzyme $P_{450}IID_6$; coadministration should be approached with caution). Products include:

Quinidex Extentabs.............................. 2067

Selegiline Hydrochloride (Potential for serious and fatal reactions including hyperthermia, rigidity, myoclonus and other serious reactions; concurrent and/or sequential use is contraindicated). Products include:

Eldepryl Tablets 2550

Sertraline Hydrochloride (Paroxetine may significantly inhibit the activity of cytochrome isoenzyme $P_{450}IID_6$; coadministration should be approached with caution). Products include:

Zoloft Tablets 2217

Sulindac (Potential for increase in adverse effects of either drug). Products include:

Clinoril Tablets 1618

Temazepam (Potential for increase in adverse effects of either drug). Products include:

Restoril Capsules................................. 2284

Thioridazine Hydrochloride (Paroxetine may significantly inhibit the activity of cytochrome isoenzyme $P_{450}IID_6$; coadministration should be approached with caution). Products include:

Mellaril 2269

Tolbutamide (Potential for increase in adverse effects of either drug).

No products indexed under this heading.

Tolmetin Sodium (Potential for increase in adverse effects of either drug). Products include:

Tolectin (200, 400 and 600 mg) .. 1581

Tranylcypromine Sulfate (Potential for serious and fatal reactions including hyperthermia, rigidity, myoclonus and other serious reactions; concurrent and/or sequential use is contraindicated). Products include:

Parnate Tablets 2503

Trazodone Hydrochloride (Paroxetine may significantly inhibit the activity of cytochrome isoenzyme $P_{450}IID_6$; coadministration should be approached with caution). Products include:

Desyrel and Desyrel Dividose 503

Trifluoperazine Hydrochloride (Paroxetine may significantly inhibit the activity of cytochrome isoenzyme $P_{450}IID_6$; coadministration should be approached with caution). Products include:

Stelazine 2514

Trimipramine Maleate (Potential for increase in adverse effects of either drug; Paroxetine may significantly inhibit the activity of cytochrome isoenzyme $P_{450}IID_6$; coadministration should be approached with caution). Products include:

Surmontil Capsules.............................. 2811

L-Tryptophan (Potential for headache, nausea, sweating and dizziness; concomitant use is not recommended).

No products indexed under this heading.

Venlafaxine Hydrochloride (Potential for increase in adverse effects of either drug; Paroxetine may significantly inhibit the activity of cytochrome isoenzyme $P_{450}IID_6$; coadministration should be approached with caution). Products include:

Effexor 2719

Warfarin Sodium (Potential for increase in adverse effects of either drug; potential for increased bleeding diathesis in the face of unaltered prothrombin time). Products include:

Coumadin 926

Food Interactions

Alcohol (Concurrent use should be avoided).

PEDIACARE COLD ALLERGY CHEWABLE TABLETS

(Pseudoephedrine Hydrochloride, Chlorpheniramine Maleate) .... ◈ 677

May interact with hypnotics and sedatives, tranquilizers, monoamine oxidase inhibitors, and certain other agents. Compounds in these categories include:

Alprazolam (May increase the drowsiness effect). Products include:

Xanax Tablets 2649

Buspirone Hydrochloride (May increase the drowsiness effect). Products include:

BuSpar 737

Chlordiazepoxide (May increase the drowsiness effect). Products include:

Libritabs Tablets 2177
Limbitrol 2180

Chlordiazepoxide Hydrochloride (May increase the drowsiness effect). Products include:

Librax Capsules 2176
Librium Capsules 2178
Librium Injectable 2179

Chlorpromazine (May increase the drowsiness effect). Products include:

Thorazine Suppositories 2523

Chlorpromazine Hydrochloride (May increase the drowsiness effect). Products include:

Thorazine 2523

Chlorprothixene (May increase the drowsiness effect).

No products indexed under this heading.

Chlorprothixene Hydrochloride (May increase the drowsiness effect).

No products indexed under this heading.

Clorazepate Dipotassium (May increase the drowsiness effect). Products include:

Tranxene 451

Diazepam (May increase the drowsiness effect). Products include:

Dizac 1809
Valium Injectable 2182
Valium Tablets 2183
Valrelease Capsules 2169

Droperidol (May increase the drowsiness effect). Products include:

Inapsine Injection................................. 1296

Estazolam (May increase the drowsiness effect). Products include:

ProSom Tablets 449

Ethchlorvynol (May increase the drowsiness effect). Products include:

Placidyl Capsules................................. 448

Ethinamate (May increase the drowsiness effect).

No products indexed under this heading.

Fluphenazine Decanoate (May increase the drowsiness effect). Products include:

Prolixin Decanoate 509

Fluphenazine Enanthate (May increase the drowsiness effect). Products include:

Prolixin Enanthate 509

Fluphenazine Hydrochloride (May increase the drowsiness effect). Products include:

Prolixin 509

Flurazepam Hydrochloride (May increase the drowsiness effect). Products include:

Dalmane Capsules................................ 2173

Furazolidone (Concurrent and/or sequential use is not recommended). Products include:

Furoxone 2046

Glutethimide (May increase the drowsiness effect).

No products indexed under this heading.

Haloperidol (May increase the drowsiness effect). Products include:

Haldol Injection, Tablets and Concentrate 1575

Haloperidol Decanoate (May increase the drowsiness effect). Products include:

Haldol Decanoate................................. 1577

IMPORTANT NOTE: Always consult each drug listing in the patient's regimen for possible interactions.

PediaCare | Interactions Index | 796

Hydroxyzine Hydrochloride (May increase the drowsiness effect). Products include:
- Atarax Tablets & Syrup 2185
- Marax Tablets & DF Syrup 2200
- Vistaril Intramuscular Solution 2216

Isocarboxazid (Concurrent and/or sequential use is not recommended).
- No products indexed under this heading.

Lorazepam (May increase the drowsiness effect). Products include:
- Ativan Injection 2698
- Ativan Tablets 2700

Loxapine Hydrochloride (May increase the drowsiness effect). Products include:
- Loxitane 1378

Loxapine Succinate (May increase the drowsiness effect). Products include:
- Loxitane Capsules 1378

Meprobamate (May increase the drowsiness effect). Products include:
- Miltown Tablets 2672
- PMB 200 and PMB 400 2783

Mesoridazine Besylate (May increase the drowsiness effect). Products include:
- Serentil 684

Midazolam Hydrochloride (May increase the drowsiness effect). Products include:
- Versed Injection 2170

Molindone Hydrochloride (May increase the drowsiness effect). Products include:
- Moban Tablets and Concentrate 1048

Oxazepam (May increase the drowsiness effect). Products include:
- Serax Capsules 2810
- Serax Tablets 2810

Perphenazine (May increase the drowsiness effect). Products include:
- Etrafon 2355
- Triavil Tablets 1757
- Trilafon 2389

Phenelzine Sulfate (Concurrent and/or sequential use is not recommended). Products include:
- Nardil 1920

Prazepam (May increase the drowsiness effect).
- No products indexed under this heading.

Prochlorperazine (May increase the drowsiness effect). Products include:
- Compazine 2470

Promethazine Hydrochloride (May increase the drowsiness effect). Products include:
- Mepergan Injection 2753
- Phenergan with Codeine 2777
- Phenergan with Dextromethorphan 2778
- Phenergan Injection 2773
- Phenergan Suppositories 2775
- Phenergan Syrup 2774
- Phenergan Tablets 2775
- Phenergan VC 2779
- Phenergan VC with Codeine 2781

Propofol (May increase the drowsiness effect). Products include:
- Diprivan Injection 2833

Quazepam (May increase the drowsiness effect). Products include:
- Doral Tablets 2664

Secobarbital Sodium (May increase the drowsiness effect). Products include:
- Seconal Sodium Pulvules 1474

Selegiline Hydrochloride (Concurrent and/or sequential use is not recommended). Products include:
- Eldepryl Tablets 2550

Temazepam (May increase the drowsiness effect). Products include:
- Restoril Capsules 2284

Thioridazine Hydrochloride (May increase the drowsiness effect). Products include:
- Mellaril 2269

Thiothixene (May increase the drowsiness effect). Products include:
- Navane Capsules and Concentrate 2201
- Navane Intramuscular 2202

Tranylcypromine Sulfate (Concurrent and/or sequential use is not recommended). Products include:
- Parnate Tablets 2503

Triazolam (May increase the drowsiness effect). Products include:
- Halcion Tablets 2611

Trifluoperazine Hydrochloride (May increase the drowsiness effect). Products include:
- Stelazine 2514

Zolpidem Tartrate (May increase the drowsiness effect). Products include:
- Ambien Tablets 2416

PEDIACARE COUGH-COLD CHEWABLE TABLETS

(Chlorpheniramine Maleate, Pseudoephedrine Hydrochloride, Dextromethorphan Hydrobromide) 1553

See **PediaCare NightRest Cough-Cold Liquid**

PEDIACARE COUGH-COLD LIQUID

(Pseudoephedrine Hydrochloride, Chlorpheniramine Maleate, Dextromethorphan Hydrobromide) 1553

See **PediaCare NightRest Cough-Cold Liquid**

PEDIACARE INFANTS DROPS DECONGESTANT

(Pseudoephedrine Hydrochloride) 1553

See **PediaCare NightRest Cough-Cold Liquid**

PEDI-CARE INFANT'S DROPS DECONGESTANT PLUS COUGH

(Dextromethorphan Hydrobromide, Pseudoephedrine Hydrochloride) 1553

See **PediaCare NightRest Cough-Cold Liquid**

PEDIACARE NIGHTREST COUGH-COLD LIQUID

(Chlorpheniramine Maleate, Dextromethorphan Hydrobromide, Pseudoephedrine Hydrochloride) 1553

May interact with monoamine oxidase inhibitors, hypnotics and sedatives, and tranquilizers. Compounds in these categories include:

Alprazolam (Increases the drowsiness effect). Products include:
- Xanax Tablets 2649

Buspirone Hydrochloride (Increases the drowsiness effect). Products include:
- BuSpar 737

Chlordiazepoxide (Increases the drowsiness effect). Products include:
- Libritabs Tablets 2177
- Limbitrol 2180

Chlordiazepoxide Hydrochloride (Increases the drowsiness effect). Products include:
- Librax Capsules 2176
- Librium Capsules 2178
- Librium Injectable 2179

Chlorpromazine (Increases the drowsiness effect). Products include:
- Thorazine Suppositories 2523

Chlorpromazine Hydrochloride (Increases the drowsiness effect). Products include:
- Thorazine 2523

Chlorprothixene (Increases the drowsiness effect).
- No products indexed under this heading.

Chlorprothixene Hydrochloride (Increases the drowsiness effect).
- No products indexed under this heading.

Clorazepate Dipotassium (Increases the drowsiness effect). Products include:
- Tranxene 451

Diazepam (Increases the drowsiness effect). Products include:
- Dizac 1809
- Valium Injectable 2182
- Valium Tablets 2183
- Valrelease Capsules 2169

Droperidol (Increases the drowsiness effect). Products include:
- Inapsine Injection 1296

Estazolam (Increases the drowsiness effect). Products include:
- ProSom Tablets 449

Ethchlorvynol (Increases the drowsiness effect). Products include:
- Placidyl Capsules 448

Ethinamate (Increases the drowsiness effect).
- No products indexed under this heading.

Fluphenazine Decanoate (Increases the drowsiness effect). Products include:
- Prolixin Decanoate 509

Fluphenazine Enanthate (Increases the drowsiness effect). Products include:
- Prolixin Enanthate 509

Fluphenazine Hydrochloride (Increases the drowsiness effect). Products include:
- Prolixin 509

Flurazepam Hydrochloride (Increases the drowsiness effect). Products include:
- Dalmane Capsules 2173

Furazolidone (Concurrent and/or sequential use is not recommended). Products include:
- Furoxone 2046

Glutethimide (Increases the drowsiness effect).
- No products indexed under this heading.

Haloperidol (Increases the drowsiness effect). Products include:
- Haldol Injection, Tablets and Concentrate 1575

Haloperidol Decanoate (Increases the drowsiness effect). Products include:
- Haldol Decanoate 1577

Hydroxyzine Hydrochloride (Increases the drowsiness effect). Products include:
- Atarax Tablets & Syrup 2185
- Marax Tablets & DF Syrup 2200
- Vistaril Intramuscular Solution 2216

Isocarboxazid (Concurrent and/or sequential use is not recommended).
- No products indexed under this heading.

Lorazepam (Increases the drowsiness effect). Products include:
- Ativan Injection 2698
- Ativan Tablets 2700

Loxapine Hydrochloride (Increases the drowsiness effect). Products include:
- Loxitane 1378

Loxapine Succinate (Increases the drowsiness effect). Products include:
- Loxitane Capsules 1378

Meprobamate (Increases the drowsiness effect). Products include:
- Miltown Tablets 2672
- PMB 200 and PMB 400 2783

Mesoridazine Besylate (Increases the drowsiness effect). Products include:
- Serentil 684

Midazolam Hydrochloride (Increases the drowsiness effect). Products include:
- Versed Injection 2170

Molindone Hydrochloride (Increases the drowsiness effect). Products include:
- Moban Tablets and Concentrate 1048

Oxazepam (Increases the drowsiness effect). Products include:
- Serax Capsules 2810
- Serax Tablets 2810

Perphenazine (Increases the drowsiness effect). Products include:
- Etrafon 2355
- Triavil Tablets 1757
- Trilafon 2389

Phenelzine Sulfate (Concurrent and/or sequential use is not recommended). Products include:
- Nardil 1920

Prazepam (Increases the drowsiness effect).
- No products indexed under this heading.

Prochlorperazine (Increases the drowsiness effect). Products include:
- Compazine 2470

Promethazine Hydrochloride (Increases the drowsiness effect). Products include:
- Mepergan Injection 2753
- Phenergan with Codeine 2777
- Phenergan with Dextromethorphan 2778
- Phenergan Injection 2773
- Phenergan Suppositories 2775
- Phenergan Syrup 2774
- Phenergan Tablets 2775
- Phenergan VC 2779
- Phenergan VC with Codeine 2781

Propofol (Increases the drowsiness effect). Products include:
- Diprivan Injection 2833

Quazepam (Increases the drowsiness effect). Products include:
- Doral Tablets 2664

Secobarbital Sodium (Increases the drowsiness effect). Products include:
- Seconal Sodium Pulvules 1474

Selegiline Hydrochloride (Concurrent and/or sequential use is not recommended). Products include:
- Eldepryl Tablets 2550

Temazepam (Increases the drowsiness effect). Products include:
- Restoril Capsules 2284

Thioridazine Hydrochloride (Increases the drowsiness effect). Products include:
- Mellaril 2269

Thiothixene (Increases the drowsiness effect). Products include:
- Navane Capsules and Concentrate 2201
- Navane Intramuscular 2202

Tranylcypromine Sulfate (Concurrent and/or sequential use is not recommended). Products include:
- Parnate Tablets 2503

Triazolam (Increases the drowsiness effect). Products include:
- Halcion Tablets 2611

Trifluoperazine Hydrochloride (Increases the drowsiness effect). Products include:
- Stelazine 2514

Zolpidem Tartrate (Increases the drowsiness effect). Products include:
- Ambien Tablets 2416

PEDIALYTE ORAL ELECTROLYTE MAINTENANCE SOLUTION

(Electrolyte Supplement) 2222
None cited in PDR database.

PEDIAPRED ORAL LIQUID

(Prednisolone Sodium Phosphate) **995**
May interact with barbiturates, oral hypoglycemic agents, insulin, and certain other agents. Compounds in these categories include:

Acarbose (Increased requirement of hypoglycemic agents in diabetes).
No products indexed under this heading.

Aprobarbital (Induces hepatic microsomal drug metabolizing enzyme activity which may result in enhanced metabolism of prednisolone; dosage of prednisolone may need to be increased).
No products indexed under this heading.

Aspirin (Aspirin should be used cautiously in conjunction with corticosteroids in hypoprothrombinemia). Products include:

Alka-Seltzer Effervescent Antacid and Pain Reliever .... ✦◻ 701
Alka-Seltzer Extra Strength Effervescent Antacid and Pain Reliever .... ✦◻ 703
Alka-Seltzer Lemon Lime Effervescent Antacid and Pain Reliever .... ✦◻ 703
Alka-Seltzer Plus Cold Medicine .... ✦◻ 705
Alka-Seltzer Plus Cold & Cough Medicine .... ✦◻ 708
Alka-Seltzer Plus Night-Time Cold Medicine .... ✦◻ 707
Alka Seltzer Plus Sinus Medicine .. ✦◻ 707
Arthritis Foundation Safety Coated Aspirin Tablets .... ✦◻ 675
Arthritis Pain Ascriptin .... ✦◻ 631
Maximum Strength Ascriptin .... ✦◻ 630
Regular Strength Ascriptin Tablets .... ✦◻ 629
Arthritis Strength BC Powder......... ✦◻ 609
BC Cold Powder Multi-Symptom Formula (Cold-Sinus-Allergy) ...... ✦◻ 609
BC Cold Powder Non-Drowsy Formula (Cold-Sinus) .... ✦◻ 609
BC Powder .... ✦◻ 609
Bayer Children's Chewable Aspirin .... ✦◻ 711
Genuine Bayer Aspirin Tablets & Caplets .... ✦◻ 713
Extra Strength Bayer Arthritis Pain Regimen Formula .... ✦◻ 711
Extra Strength Bayer Aspirin Caplets & Tablets .... ✦◻ 712
Extended-Release Bayer 8-Hour Aspirin .... ✦◻ 712
Extra Strength Bayer Plus Aspirin Caplets .... ✦◻ 713
Extra Strength Bayer PM Aspirin .. ✦◻ 713
Bayer Enteric Aspirin .... ✦◻ 709
Bufferin Analgesic Tablets and Caplets .... ✦◻ 613
Arthritis Strength Bufferin Analgesic Caplets .... ✦◻ 614
Extra Strength Bufferin Analgesic Tablets .... ✦◻ 615
Cama Arthritis Pain Reliever........... ✦◻ 785
Darvon Compound-65 Pulvules 1435
Easprin 1914
Ecotrin 2455
Ecotrin Enteric Coated Aspirin Maximum Strength Tablets and Caplets .... ✦◻ 816
Ecotrin Enteric Coated Aspirin Regular Strength Tablets 2455
Empirin Aspirin Tablets .... ✦◻ 854
Empirin with Codeine Tablets........... 1093
Excedrin Extra-Strength Analgesic Tablets & Caplets 732
Fiorinal Capsules 2261
Fiorinal with Codeine Capsules 2262
Fiorinal Tablets 2261
Halfprin 1362
Healthprin Aspirin 2455
Norgesic.. 1496
Percodan Tablets.................................... 939
Percodan-Demi Tablets........................ 940
Robaxisal Tablets.................................... 2071

Soma Compound w/Codeine Tablets 2676
Soma Compound Tablets.................... 2675
St. Joseph Adult Chewable Aspirin (81 mg.) .... ✦◻ 808
Talwin Compound 2335
Ursinus Inlay-Tabs................................ ✦◻ 794
Vanquish Analgesic Caplets .... ◎ 731

Butabarbital (Induces hepatic microsomal drug metabolizing enzyme activity which may result in enhanced metabolism of prednisolone; dosage of prednisolone may need to be increased).
No products indexed under this heading.

Butalbital (Induces hepatic microsomal drug metabolizing enzyme activity which may result in enhanced metabolism of prednisolone; dosage of prednisolone may need to be increased). Products include:

Esgic-plus Tablets 1013
Fioricet Tablets 2258
Fioricet with Codeine Capsules 2260
Fiorinal Capsules 2261
Fiorinal with Codeine Capsules 2262
Fiorinal Tablets 2261
Phrenilin 785
Sedapap Tablets 50 mg/650 mg .. 1543

Chlorpropamide (Increased requirement of hypoglycemic agents in diabetes). Products include:

Diabinese Tablets 1935

Glipizide (Increased requirement of hypoglycemic agents in diabetes). Products include:

Glucotrol Tablets 1967
Glucotrol XL Extended Release Tablets 1968

Glyburide (Increased requirement of hypoglycemic agents in diabetes). Products include:

DiaBeta Tablets 1239
Glynase PresTab Tablets 2609
Micronase Tablets 2623

Insulin, Human (Increased requirement of insulin in diabetes).
No products indexed under this heading.

Insulin, Human Isophane Suspension (Increased requirement of insulin in diabetes). Products include:

Novolin N Human Insulin 10 ml Vials.. 1795

Insulin, Human NPH (Increased requirement of insulin in diabetes). Products include:

Humulin N, 100 Units 1448
Novolin N PenFill Cartridges Durable Insulin Delivery System 1798
Novolin N Prefilled Syringe Disposable Insulin Delivery System 1798

Insulin, Human Regular (Increased requirement of insulin in diabetes). Products include:

Humulin R, 100 Units 1449
Novolin R Human Insulin 10 ml Vials.. 1795
Novolin R PenFill Cartridges Durable Insulin Delivery System 1798
Novolin R Prefilled Syringe Disposable Insulin Delivery System 1798
Velosulin BR Human Insulin 10 ml Vials.. 1795

Insulin, Human, Zinc Suspension (Increased requirement of insulin in diabetes). Products include:

Humulin L, 100 Units 1446
Humulin U, 100 Units 1450
Novolin L Human Insulin 10 ml Vials.. 1795

Insulin, NPH (Increased requirement of insulin in diabetes). Products include:

NPH, 100 Units 1450
Pork NPH, 100 Units.......................... 1452
Purified Pork NPH Isophane Insulin 1801

Insulin, Regular (Increased requirement of insulin in diabetes). Products include:

Regular, 100 Units 1450
Pork Regular, 100 Units 1452
Pork Regular (Concentrated), 500 Units 1453
Purified Pork Regular Insulin 1801

Insulin, Zinc Crystals (Increased requirement of insulin in diabetes). Products include:

NPH, 100 Units 1450

Insulin, Zinc Suspension (Increased requirement of insulin in diabetes). Products include:

Iletin I 1450
Lente, 100 Units 1450
Iletin II.. 1452
Pork Lente, 100 Units.......................... 1452
Purified Pork Lente Insulin 1801

Mephobarbital (Induces hepatic microsomal drug metabolizing enzyme activity which may result in enhanced metabolism of prednisolone; dosage of prednisolone may need to be increased). Products include:

Mebaral Tablets 2322

Metformin Hydrochloride (Increased requirement of hypoglycemic agents in diabetes). Products include:

Glucophage 752

Pentobarbital Sodium (Induces hepatic microsomal drug metabolizing enzyme activity which may result in enhanced metabolism of prednisolone; dosage of prednisolone may need to be increased). Products include:

Nembutal Sodium Capsules 436
Nembutal Sodium Solution 438
Nembutal Sodium Suppositories...... 440

Phenobarbital (Induces hepatic microsomal drug metabolizing enzyme activity which may result in enhanced metabolism of prednisolone; dosage of prednisolone may need to be increased). Products include:

Arco-Lase Plus Tablets 512
Bellergal-S Tablets 2250
Donnatal 2060
Donnatal Extentabs.............................. 2061
Donnatal Tablets 2060
Phenobarbital Elixir and Tablets...... 1469
Quadrinal Tablets 1350

Secobarbital Sodium (Induces hepatic microsomal drug metabolizing enzyme activity which may result in enhanced metabolism of prednisolone; dosage of prednisolone may need to be increased). Products include:

Seconal Sodium Pulvules 1474

Thiamylal Sodium (Induces hepatic microsomal drug metabolizing enzyme activity which may result in enhanced metabolism of prednisolone; dosage of prednisolone may need to be increased).
No products indexed under this heading.

Tolazamide (Increased requirement of hypoglycemic agents in diabetes).
No products indexed under this heading.

Tolbutamide (Increased requirement of hypoglycemic agents in diabetes).
No products indexed under this heading.

PEDIASURE COMPLETE LIQUID NUTRITION

(Nutritional Supplement) 2222
None cited in PDR database.

PEDIASURE WITH FIBER COMPLETE LIQUID NUTRITION

(Nutritional Supplement) 2223
None cited in PDR database.

PEDIATRIC VICKS 44D DRY HACKING COUGH & HEAD CONGESTION

(Dextromethorphan Hydrobromide, Pseudoephedrine Hydrochloride) .... ✦◻ 763
May interact with monoamine oxidase inhibitors. Compounds in this category include:

Furazolidone (Concurrent and/or sequential use is not recommended). Products include:

Furoxone 2046

Isocarboxazid (Concurrent and/or sequential use is not recommended).
No products indexed under this heading.

Phenelzine Sulfate (Concurrent and/or sequential use is not recommended). Products include:

Nardil 1920

Selegiline Hydrochloride (Concurrent and/or sequential use is not recommended). Products include:

Eldepryl Tablets 2550

Tranylcypromine Sulfate (Concurrent and/or sequential use is not recommended). Products include:

Parnate Tablets 2503

PEDIATRIC VICKS 44E CHEST COUGH & CHEST CONGESTION

(Dextromethorphan Hydrobromide, Guaifenesin).. ✦◻ 764
May interact with monoamine oxidase inhibitors. Compounds in this category include:

Furazolidone (Concurrent and/or sequential use is not recommended). Products include:

Furoxone 2046

Isocarboxazid (Concurrent and/or sequential use is not recommended).
No products indexed under this heading.

Phenelzine Sulfate (Concurrent and/or sequential use is not recommended). Products include:

Nardil 1920

Selegiline Hydrochloride (Concurrent and/or sequential use is not recommended). Products include:

Eldepryl Tablets 2550

Tranylcypromine Sulfate (Concurrent and/or sequential use is not recommended). Products include:

Parnate Tablets 2503

PEDIATRIC VICKS 44M COUGH & COLD RELIEF

(Chlorpheniramine Maleate, Dextromethorphan Hydrobromide, Pseudoephedrine Hydrochloride) .... ✦◻ 764
May interact with hypnotics and sedatives, tranquilizers, monoamine oxidase inhibitors, and certain other agents. Compounds in these categories include:

Alprazolam (May increase drowsiness effect). Products include:

Xanax Tablets 2649

Buspirone Hydrochloride (May increase drowsiness effect). Products include:

BuSpar 737

Chlordiazepoxide (May increase drowsiness effect). Products include:

Libritabs Tablets 2177
Limbitrol 2180

IMPORTANT NOTE: Always consult each drug listing in the patient's regimen for possible interactions.

Pediatric Vicks 44m C & C — Interactions Index — 798

Chlordiazepoxide Hydrochloride (May increase drowsiness effect). Products include:
- Librax Capsules ... 2176
- Librium Capsules ... 2178
- Librium Injectable ... 2179

Chlorpromazine (May increase drowsiness effect). Products include:
- Thorazine Suppositories ... 2523

Chlorpromazine Hydrochloride (May increase drowsiness effect). Products include:
- Thorazine ... 2523

Chlorprothixene (May increase drowsiness effect).
- No products indexed under this heading.

Chlorprothixene Hydrochloride (May increase drowsiness effect).
- No products indexed under this heading.

Clorazepate Dipotassium (May increase drowsiness effect). Products include:
- Tranxene ... 451

Diazepam (May increase drowsiness effect). Products include:
- Dizac ... 1809
- Valium Injectable ... 2182
- Valium Tablets ... 2183
- Valrelease Capsules ... 2169

Droperidol (May increase drowsiness effect). Products include:
- Inapsine Injection ... 1296

Estazolam (May increase drowsiness effect). Products include:
- ProSom Tablets ... 449

Ethchlorvynol (May increase drowsiness effect). Products include:
- Placidyl Capsules ... 448

Ethinamate (May increase drowsiness effect).
- No products indexed under this heading.

Fluphenazine Decanoate (May increase drowsiness effect). Products include:
- Prolixin Decanoate ... 509

Fluphenazine Enanthate (May increase drowsiness effect). Products include:
- Prolixin Enanthate ... 509

Fluphenazine Hydrochloride (May increase drowsiness effect). Products include:
- Prolixin ... 509

Flurazepam Hydrochloride (May increase drowsiness effect). Products include:
- Dalmane Capsules ... 2173

Furazolidone (Concurrent and/or sequential use is not recommended). Products include:
- Furoxone ... 2046

Glutethimide (May increase drowsiness effect).
- No products indexed under this heading.

Haloperidol (May increase drowsiness effect). Products include:
- Haldol Injection, Tablets and Concentrate ... 1575

Haloperidol Decanoate (May increase drowsiness effect). Products include:
- Haldol Decanoate ... 1577

Hydroxyzine Hydrochloride (May increase drowsiness effect). Products include:
- Atarax Tablets & Syrup ... 2185
- Marax Tablets & DF Syrup ... 2200
- Vistaril Intramuscular Solution ... 2216

Isocarboxazid (Concurrent and/or sequential use is not recommended).
- No products indexed under this heading.

Lorazepam (May increase drowsiness effect). Products include:
- Ativan Injection ... 2698
- Ativan Tablets ... 2700

Loxapine Hydrochloride (May increase drowsiness effect). Products include:
- Loxitane ... 1378

Loxapine Succinate (May increase drowsiness effect). Products include:
- Loxitane Capsules ... 1378

Meprobamate (May increase drowsiness effect). Products include:
- Miltown Tablets ... 2672
- PMB 200 and PMB 400 ... 2783

Mesoridazine Besylate (May increase drowsiness effect). Products include:
- Serentil ... 684

Midazolam Hydrochloride (May increase drowsiness effect). Products include:
- Versed Injection ... 2170

Molindone Hydrochloride (May increase drowsiness effect). Products include:
- Moban Tablets and Concentrate ... 1048

Oxazepam (May increase drowsiness effect). Products include:
- Serax Capsules ... 2810
- Serax Tablets ... 2810

Perphenazine (May increase drowsiness effect). Products include:
- Etrafon ... 2355
- Triavil Tablets ... 1757
- Trilafon ... 2389

Phenelzine Sulfate (Concurrent and/or sequential use is not recommended). Products include:
- Nardil ... 1920

Prazepam (May increase drowsiness effect).
- No products indexed under this heading.

Prochlorperazine (May increase drowsiness effect). Products include:
- Compazine ... 2470

Promethazine Hydrochloride (May increase drowsiness effect). Products include:
- Mepergan Injection ... 2753
- Phenergan with Codeine ... 2777
- Phenergan with Dextromethorphan ... 2778
- Phenergan Injection ... 2773
- Phenergan Suppositories ... 2775
- Phenergan Syrup ... 2774
- Phenergan Tablets ... 2775
- Phenergan VC ... 2779
- Phenergan VC with Codeine ... 2781

Propofol (May increase drowsiness effect). Products include:
- Diprivan Injection ... 2833

Quazepam (May increase drowsiness effect). Products include:
- Doral Tablets ... 2664

Secobarbital Sodium (May increase drowsiness effect). Products include:
- Seconal Sodium Pulvules ... 1474

Selegiline Hydrochloride (Concurrent and/or sequential use is not recommended). Products include:
- Eldepryl Tablets ... 2550

Temazepam (May increase drowsiness effect). Products include:
- Restoril Capsules ... 2284

Thioridazine Hydrochloride (May increase drowsiness effect). Products include:
- Mellaril ... 2269

Thiothixene (May increase drowsiness effect). Products include:
- Navane Capsules and Concentrate ... 2201
- Navane Intramuscular ... 2202

Tranylcypromine Sulfate (Concurrent and/or sequential use is not recommended). Products include:
- Parnate Tablets ... 2503

Triazolam (May increase drowsiness effect). Products include:
- Halcion Tablets ... 2611

Trifluoperazine Hydrochloride (May increase drowsiness effect). Products include:
- Stelazine ... 2514

Zolpidem Tartrate (May increase drowsiness effect). Products include:
- Ambien Tablets ... 2416

Food Interactions

Alcohol (May increase drowsiness effect).

PEDIOTIC SUSPENSION STERILE

(Polymyxin B Sulfate, Neomycin Sulfate, Hydrocortisone) ... 1153
None cited in PDR database.

PEDVAXHIB

(Haemophilus B Conjugate Vaccine) .. 1718
May interact with immunosuppressive agents. Compounds in this category include:

Azathioprine (Expected immune response may not be observed). Products include:
- Imuran ... 1110

Cyclosporine (Expected immune response may not be observed). Products include:
- Neoral ... 2276
- Sandimmune ... 2286

Immune Globulin (Human) (Expected immune response may not be observed).
- No products indexed under this heading.

Immune Globulin Intravenous (Human) (Expected immune response may not be observed).

Muromonab-CD3 (Expected immune response may not be observed). Products include:
- Orthoclone OKT3 Sterile Solution .. 1837

Mycophenolate Mofetil (Expected immune response may not be observed). Products include:
- CellCept Capsules ... 2099

Tacrolimus (Expected immune response may not be observed). Products include:
- Prograf ... 1042

PEGANONE TABLETS

(Ethotoin) ... 446
May interact with oral anticoagulants and certain other agents. Compounds in these categories include:

Dicumarol (Possible interactions, not yet documented).
- No products indexed under this heading.

Folic Acid (Interferes with folic acid metabolism). Products include:
- Cefol Filmtab ... 412
- Fero-Folic-500 Filmtab ... 429
- Iberet-Folic-500 Filmtab ... 429
- Materna Tablets ... 1379
- Mega-B ... 512
- Megadose ... 512
- Nephro-Fer Rx Tablets ... 2005
- Nephro-Vite + Fe Tablets ... 2006
- Nephro-Vite Rx Tablets ... 2006
- Niferex-150 Forte Capsules ... 794
- Niferex Forte Elixir ... 794
- Sigtab Tablets ... ◘ 772
- Slow Fe with Folic Acid ... 869
- Stuart Prenatal Tablets ... ◘ 881
- The Stuart Formula Tablets ... ◘ 663
- Trinsicon Capsules ... 2570
- Zymacap Capsules ... ◘ 772

Phenacemide (Paranoid symptoms). Products include:
- Phenurone Tablets ... 447

Warfarin Sodium (Possible interactions, not yet documented). Products include:
- Coumadin ... 926

PEN•KERA CREME

(Glycerin, Polyamide Sugar Condensate, Urea) ... ◘ 603
None cited in PDR database.

PEN•VEE K FOR ORAL SOLUTION

(Penicillin V Potassium) ... 2772
None cited in PDR database.

PEN•VEE K TABLETS

(Penicillin V Potassium) ... 2772
None cited in PDR database.

PENETREX TABLETS

(Enoxacin) ... 2031
May interact with xanthine bronchodilators, antacids containing aluminium, calcium and magnesium, iron containing oral preparations, and certain other agents. Compounds in these categories include:

Aluminum Carbonate Gel (Reduces the oral absorption of enoxacin). Products include:
- Basaljel ... 2703

Aluminum Hydroxide (Reduces the oral absorption of enoxacin). Products include:
- ALternaGEL Liquid ... 1316
- Maximum Strength Ascriptin ... ◘ 630
- Cama Arthritis Pain Reliever ... ◘ 785
- Gaviscon Extra Strength Relief Formula Antacid Tablets ... ◘ 819
- Gaviscon Extra Strength Relief Formula Liquid Antacid ... ◘ 819
- Gaviscon Liquid Antacid ... ◘ 820
- Gelusil Liquid & Tablets ... ◘ 855
- Maalox Heartburn Relief Suspension ... ◘ 642
- Maalox Heartburn Relief Tablets ... ◘ 641
- Maalox Magnesia and Alumina Oral Suspension ... ◘ 642
- Maalox Plus Tablets ... ◘ 643
- Extra Strength Maalox Antacid Plus Antigas Liquid and Tablets ◘ 638
- Tempo Soft Antacid ... ◘ 835

Aluminum Hydroxide Gel (Reduces the oral absorption of enoxacin). Products include:
- ALternaGEL Liquid ... ◘ 659
- Aludrox Oral Suspension ... 2695
- Amphojel Suspension ... 2695
- Amphojel Suspension without Flavor ... 2695
- Amphojel Tablets ... 2695
- Arthritis Pain Ascriptin ... ◘ 631
- Regular Strength Ascriptin Tablets ... ◘ 629
- Gaviscon Antacid Tablets ... ◘ 819
- Gaviscon-2 Antacid Tablets ... ◘ 820
- Mylanta Liquid ... 1317
- Mylanta Tablets ... ◘ 660
- Mylanta Double Strength Liquid ... 1317
- Mylanta Double Strength Tablets .. ◘ 660
- Nephrox Suspension ... ◘ 655

Aluminum Hydroxide Gel, Dried (Reduces the oral absorption of enoxacin).

Aminophylline (Decreased theophylline clearance and increase in theophylline serum levels).
- No products indexed under this heading.

Bismuth Subsalicylate (Decreases bioavailability of enoxacin by 25%). Products include:
- Maximum Strength Pepto-Bismol Liquid ... ◘ 753
- Pepto-Bismol Original Liquid, Original and Cherry Tablets and Easy-To-Swallow Caplets ... 1976
- Pepto-Bismol Maximum Strength Liquid ... 1976

(◘ Described in PDR For Nonprescription Drugs) (⊙ Described in PDR For Ophthalmology)

Caffeine (Decreased caffeine clearance and increased caffeine serum levels). Products include:

Arthritis Strength BC Powder......... ⊕D 609
BC Powder .... ⊕D 609
Bayer Select Headache Pain Relief Formula .... ⊕D 716
Cafergot 2251
DHCplus Capsules............................... 1993
Darvon Compound-65 Pulvules 1435
Esgic-plus Tablets 1013
Aspirin Free Excedrin Analgesic Caplets and Geltabs 732
Excedrin Extra-Strength Analgesic Tablets & Caplets 732
Fioricet Tablets 2258
Fioricet with Codeine Capsules 2260
Fiorinal Capsules 2261
Fiorinal with Codeine Capsules 2262
Fiorinal Tablets 2261
Maximum Strength Multi-Symptom Formula Midol .... ⊕D 722
Migralam Capsules 2038
No Doz Maximum Strength Caplets .... ⊕D 622
Norgesic... 1496
Vanquish Analgesic Caplets .... ⊕D 731
Wigraine Tablets & Suppositories .. 1829

Cyclosporine (Potential for elevated serum levels of cyclosporin). Products include:

Neoral 2276
Sandimmune 2286

Digoxin (Enoxacin may raise serum digoxin levels). Products include:

Lanoxicaps 1117
Lanoxin Elixir Pediatric 1120
Lanoxin Injection 1123
Lanoxin Injection Pediatric............... 1126
Lanoxin Tablets 1128

Dihydroxyaluminum Sodium Carbonate (Reduces the oral absorption of enoxacin).

No products indexed under this heading.

Dyphylline (Decreased theophylline clearance and increase in theophylline serum levels). Products include:

Lufyllin & Lufyllin-400 Tablets 2670
Lufyllin-GG Elixir & Tablets 2671

Fenbufen (Potential for seizures).

Ferrous Fumarate (Reduces the oral absorption of enoxacin). Products include:

Chromagen Capsules 2339
Ferro-Sequels .... ⊕D 669
Nephro-Fer Tablets 2004
Nephro-Fer Rx Tablets........................ 2005
Nephro-Vite + Fe Tablets 2006
Sigtab-M Tablets .... ⊕D 772
Stresstabs + Iron .... ⊕D 671
The Stuart Formula Tablets............... ⊕D 663
Theragran-M Tablets with Beta Carotene .... ⊕D 623
Trinsicon Capsules 2570
Vitron-C Tablets .... ⊕D 650

Ferrous Gluconate (Reduces the oral absorption of enoxacin). Products include:

Fergon Iron Supplement Tablets.... ⊕D 721
Megadose 512

Ferrous Sulfate (Reduces the oral absorption of enoxacin). Products include:

Feosol Capsules 2456
Feosol Elixir 2456
Feosol Tablets 2457
Fero-Folic-500 Filmtab 429
Fero-Grad-500 Filmtab...................... 429
Fero-Gradumet Filmtab..................... 429
Iberet Tablets 433
Iberet-500 Liquid 433
Iberet-Folic-500 Filmtab.................... 429
Iberet-Liquid.. 433
Irospan 982
Slow Fe Tablets................................... 869
Slow Fe with Folic Acid 869

Magaldrate (Reduces the oral absorption of enoxacin).

No products indexed under this heading.

Magnesium Hydroxide (Reduces the oral absorption of enoxacin). Products include:

Aludrox Oral Suspension 2695
Arthritis Pain Ascriptin .... ⊕D 631
Maximum Strength Ascriptin .... ⊕D 630
Regular Strength Ascriptin Tablets .... ⊕D 629
Di-Gel Antacid/Anti-Gas .... ⊕D 801
Gelusil Liquid & Tablets .... ⊕D 855
Maalox Magnesia and Alumina Oral Suspension .... ⊕D 642
Maalox Plus Tablets .... ⊕D 643
Extra Strength Maalox Antacid Plus Antigas Liquid and Tablets ⊕D 638
Mylanta Calcium Carbonate and Magnesium Hydroxide Tablets...... 1318
Mylanta Liquid 1317
Mylanta Tablets .... ⊕D 660
Mylanta Double Strength Liquid 1317
Mylanta Double Strength Tablets .. ⊕D 660
Phillips' Milk of Magnesia Liquid.... ⊕D 729
Rolaids Tablets .... ⊕D 843
Tempo Soft Antacid .... ⊕D 835

Magnesium Oxide (Reduces the oral absorption of enoxacin). Products include:

Beelith Tablets 639
Bufferin Analgesic Tablets and Caplets .... ⊕D 613
Caltrate PLUS .... ⊕D 665
Cama Arthritis Pain Reliever............ ⊕D 785
Mag-Ox 400 668
Uro-Mag.. 668

Polysaccharide-Iron Complex (Reduces the oral absorption of enoxacin). Products include:

Niferex-150 Capsules 793
Niferex Elixir 793
Niferex-150 Forte Capsules 794
Niferex Forte Elixir 794
Niferex 793
Niferex-PN Tablets 794
Nu-Iron 150 Capsules......................... 1543
Nu-Iron Elixir 1543
Sunkist Children's Chewable Multivitamins - Plus Iron........................... ⊕D 649

Sucralfate (Reduces the oral absorption of enoxacin). Products include:

Carafate Suspension 1505
Carafate Tablets.................................. 1504

Theophylline (Decreased theophylline clearance and increase in theophylline serum levels). Products include:

Marax Tablets & DF Syrup................. 2200
Quibron 2053

Theophylline Anhydrous (Decreased theophylline clearance and increase in theophylline serum levels). Products include:

Aerolate 1004
Primatene Dual Action Formula...... ⊕D 872
Primatene Tablets .... ⊕D 873
Respbid Tablets 682
Slo-bid Gyrocaps 2033
Theo-24 Extended Release Capsules 2568
Theo-Dur Extended-Release Tablets 1327
Theo-X Extended-Release Tablets .. 788
Uni-Dur Extended-Release Tablets.. 1331
Uniphyl 400 mg Tablets..................... 2001

Theophylline Calcium Salicylate (Decreased theophylline clearance and increase in theophylline serum levels). Products include:

Quadrinal Tablets 1350

Theophylline Sodium Glycinate (Decreased theophylline clearance and increase in theophylline serum levels).

No products indexed under this heading.

Warfarin Sodium (Potential for decreased clearance of R-warfarin isomer). Products include:

Coumadin 926

Zinc Sulfate (Reduces the oral absorption of enoxacin). Products include:

Clear Eyes ACR Astringent/Lubricant Eye Redness Reliever Eye Drops .... ◎ 316
Visine Maximum Strength Allergy Relief .... ◎ 313

PENTAM 300 INJECTION

(Pentamidine Isethionate)....................1041
None cited in PDR database.

PENTASA

(Mesalamine) 1527
None cited in PDR database.

PENTASPAN INJECTION

(Pentastarch) 937
None cited in PDR database.

PENTRAX ANTI-DANDRUFF SHAMPOO

(Coal Tar) 1055
None cited in PDR database.

PEPCID AC

(Famotidine) 1319
None cited in PDR database.

PEPCID INJECTION

(Famotidine) 1722
None cited in PDR database.

PEPCID INJECTION PREMIXED

(Famotidine) 1722
None cited in PDR database.

PEPCID ORAL SUSPENSION

(Famotidine) 1720
May interact with antacids and certain other agents. Compounds in these categories include:

Aluminum Carbonate Gel (Bioavailability may be slightly decreased by antacids). Products include:

Basaljel.. 2703

Aluminum Hydroxide (Bioavailability may be slightly decreased by antacids). Products include:

ALternaGEL Liquid 1316
Maximum Strength Ascriptin .... ⊕D 630
Cama Arthritis Pain Reliever............ ⊕D 785
Gaviscon Extra Strength Relief Formula Antacid Tablets................. ⊕D 819
Gaviscon Extra Strength Relief Formula Liquid Antacid.................. ⊕D 819
Gaviscon Liquid Antacid .... ⊕D 820
Gelusil Liquid & Tablets .... ⊕D 855
Maalox Heartburn Relief Suspension .... ⊕D 642
Maalox Heartburn Relief Tablets.... ⊕D 641
Maalox Magnesia and Alumina Oral Suspension .... ⊕D 642
Maalox Plus Tablets .... ⊕D 643
Extra Strength Maalox Antacid Plus Antigas Liquid and Tablets ⊕D 638
Tempo Soft Antacid .... ⊕D 835

Aluminum Hydroxide Gel (Bioavailability may be slightly decreased by antacids). Products include:

ALternaGEL Liquid .... ⊕D 659
Aludrox Oral Suspension 2695
Amphojel Suspension 2695
Amphojel Suspension without Flavor 2695
Amphojel Tablets................................. 2695
Arthritis Pain Ascriptin .... ⊕D 631
Regular Strength Ascriptin Tablets .... ⊕D 629
Gaviscon Antacid Tablets................... ⊕D 819
Gaviscon-2 Antacid Tablets .... ⊕D 820
Mylanta Liquid 1317
Mylanta Tablets .... ⊕D 660
Mylanta Double Strength Liquid 1317
Mylanta Double Strength Tablets .. ⊕D 660
Nephrox Suspension .... ⊕D 655

Dihydroxyaluminum Sodium Carbonate (Bioavailability may be slightly decreased by antacids).

No products indexed under this heading.

Magaldrate (Bioavailability may be slightly decreased by antacids).

No products indexed under this heading.

Magnesium Hydroxide (Bioavailability may be slightly decreased by antacids). Products include:

Aludrox Oral Suspension 2695
Arthritis Pain Ascriptin .... ⊕D 631
Maximum Strength Ascriptin .... ⊕D 630
Regular Strength Ascriptin Tablets .... ⊕D 629
Di-Gel Antacid/Anti-Gas .... ⊕D 801
Gelusil Liquid & Tablets .... ⊕D 855
Maalox Magnesia and Alumina Oral Suspension .... ⊕D 642
Maalox Plus Tablets........................... ⊕D 643
Extra Strength Maalox Antacid Plus Antigas Liquid and Tablets ⊕D 638
Mylanta Calcium Carbonate and Magnesium Hydroxide Tablets...... 1318
Mylanta Liquid 1317
Mylanta Tablets .... ⊕D 660
Mylanta Double Strength Liquid 1317
Mylanta Double Strength Tablets .. ⊕D 660
Phillips' Milk of Magnesia Liquid.... ⊕D 729
Rolaids Tablets .... ⊕D 843
Tempo Soft Antacid .... ⊕D 835

Magnesium Oxide (Bioavailability may be slightly decreased by antacids). Products include:

Beelith Tablets 639
Bufferin Analgesic Tablets and Caplets .... ⊕D 613
Caltrate PLUS .... ⊕D 665
Cama Arthritis Pain Reliever............ ⊕D 785
Mag-Ox 400 668
Uro-Mag.. 668

Sodium Bicarbonate (Bioavailability may be slightly decreased by antacids). Products include:

Alka-Seltzer Effervescent Antacid and Pain Reliever............................. ⊕D 701
Alka-Seltzer Extra Strength Effervescent Antacid and Pain Reliever .... ⊕D 703
Alka-Seltzer Gold Effervescent Antacid.. ⊕D 703
Alka-Seltzer Lemon Lime Effervescent Antacid and Pain Reliever .... ⊕D 703
Arm & Hammer Pure Baking Soda .... ⊕D 627
Ceo-Two Rectal Suppositories 666
Citrocarbonate Antacid...................... ⊕D 770
Massengill Disposable Douches...... ⊕D 820
Massengill Liquid Concentrate........ ⊕D 820
NuLYTELY... 689
Cherry Flavor NuLYTELY 689

Food Interactions

Food, unspecified (Bioavailability may be slightly increased by antacids).

PEPCID TABLETS

(Famotidine) 1720
See Pepcid Oral Suspension

PEPTAVLON

(Pentagastrin).......................................2878
None cited in PDR database.

PEPTO-BISMOL ORIGINAL LIQUID, ORIGINAL AND CHERRY TABLETS AND EASY-TO-SWALLOW CAPLETS

(Bismuth Subsalicylate) 1976
May interact with oral anticoagulants, oral hypoglycemic agents, and antigout agents. Compounds in these categories include:

Acarbose (Use cautiously).

No products indexed under this heading.

Allopurinol (Use cautiously). Products include:

Zyloprim Tablets 1226

IMPORTANT NOTE: Always consult each drug listing in the patient's regimen for possible interactions.

Chlorpropamide (Use cautiously). Products include:
- Diabinese Tablets 1935

Dicumarol (Use cautiously).
- No products indexed under this heading.

Glipizide (Use cautiously). Products include:
- Glucotrol Tablets 1967
- Glucotrol XL Extended Release Tablets 1968

Glyburide (Use cautiously). Products include:
- DiaBeta Tablets 1239
- Glynase PresTab Tablets 2609
- Micronase Tablets 2623

Metformin Hydrochloride (Use cautiously). Products include:
- Glucophage 752

Probenecid (Use cautiously). Products include:
- Benemid Tablets 1611
- ColBENEMID Tablets 1622

Sulfinpyrazone (Use cautiously). Products include:
- Anturane 807

Tolazamide (Use cautiously).
- No products indexed under this heading.

Tolbutamide (Use cautiously).
- No products indexed under this heading.

Warfarin Sodium (Use cautiously). Products include:
- Coumadin 926

PEPTO-BISMOL MAXIMUM STRENGTH LIQUID

(Bismuth Subsalicylate) **1976**
May interact with oral anticoagulants, antigout agents, and oral hypoglycemic agents. Compounds in these categories include:

Acarbose (Use cautiously).
- No products indexed under this heading.

Allopurinol (Use cautiously). Products include:
- Zyloprim Tablets 1226

Chlorpropamide (Use cautiously). Products include:
- Diabinese Tablets 1935

Dicumarol (Use cautiously).
- No products indexed under this heading.

Glipizide (Use cautiously). Products include:
- Glucotrol Tablets 1967
- Glucotrol XL Extended Release Tablets 1968

Glyburide (Use cautiously). Products include:
- DiaBeta Tablets 1239
- Glynase PresTab Tablets 2609
- Micronase Tablets 2623

Metformin Hydrochloride (Use cautiously). Products include:
- Glucophage 752

Probenecid (Use cautiously). Products include:
- Benemid Tablets 1611
- ColBENEMID Tablets 1622

Sulfinpyrazone (Use cautiously). Products include:
- Anturane 807

Tolazamide (Use cautiously).
- No products indexed under this heading.

Tolbutamide (Use cautiously).
- No products indexed under this heading.

Warfarin Sodium (Use cautiously). Products include:
- Coumadin 926

PEPTO DIARRHEA CONTROL

(Loperamide Hydrochloride) **1976**
May interact with:

Antibiotics, unspecified (Effect not specified).

PERATIVE SPECIALIZED LIQUID NUTRITION

(Nutritional Beverage) **2223**
None cited in PDR database.

PERCOCET TABLETS

(Oxycodone Hydrochloride, Acetaminophen) **938**
May interact with narcotic analgesics, general anesthetics, phenothiazines, tranquilizers, hypnotics and sedatives, central nervous system depressants, monoamine oxidase inhibitors, tricyclic antidepressants, anticholinergics, and certain other agents. Compounds in these categories include:

Alfentanil Hydrochloride (Additive CNS depression; dose of one or both agents should be reduced). Products include:
- Alfenta Injection 1286

Alprazolam (Additive CNS depression; dose of one or both agents should be reduced). Products include:
- Xanax Tablets 2649

Amitriptyline Hydrochloride (Increased effect of antidepressant or oxycodone). Products include:
- Elavil 2838
- Endep Tablets 2174
- Etrafon 2355
- Limbitrol 2180
- Triavil Tablets 1757

Amoxapine (Increased effect of antidepressant or oxycodone). Products include:
- Asendin Tablets 1369

Aprobarbital (Additive CNS depression; dose of one or both agents should be reduced).
- No products indexed under this heading.

Atropine Sulfate (May produce paralytic ileus). Products include:
- Arco-Lase Plus Tablets 512
- Atrohist Plus Tablets 454
- Atropine Sulfate Sterile Ophthalmic Solution ..... ⊙ 233
- Donnatal 2060
- Donnatal Extentabs 2061
- Donnatal Tablets 2060
- Lomotil 2439
- Motofen Tablets 784
- Urised Tablets 1964

Belladonna Alkaloids (May produce paralytic ileus). Products include:
- Bellergal-S Tablets 2250
- Hyland's Bed Wetting Tablets ..... ▣ 828
- Hyland's EnurAid Tablets ..... ▣ 829
- Hyland's Teething Tablets ..... ▣ 830

Benztropine Mesylate (May produce paralytic ileus). Products include:
- Cogentin 1621

Biperiden Hydrochloride (May produce paralytic ileus). Products include:
- Akineton 1333

Buprenorphine (Additive CNS depression; dose of one or both agents should be reduced). Products include:
- Buprenex Injectable 2006

Buspirone Hydrochloride (Additive CNS depression; dose of one or both agents should be reduced). Products include:
- BuSpar 737

Butabarbital (Additive CNS depression; dose of one or both agents should be reduced).
- No products indexed under this heading.

Butalbital (Additive CNS depression; dose of one or both agents should be reduced). Products include:
- Esgic-plus Tablets 1013
- Fioricet Tablets 2258
- Fioricet with Codeine Capsules 2260
- Fiorinal Capsules 2261
- Fiorinal with Codeine Capsules 2262
- Fiorinal Tablets 2261
- Phrenilin 785
- Sedapap Tablets 50 mg/650 mg 1543

Chlordiazepoxide (Additive CNS depression; dose of one or both agents should be reduced). Products include:
- Libritabs Tablets 2177
- Limbitrol 2180

Chlordiazepoxide Hydrochloride (Additive CNS depression; dose of one or both agents should be reduced). Products include:
- Librax Capsules 2176
- Librium Capsules 2178
- Librium Injectable 2179

Chlorpromazine (Additive CNS depression; dose of one or both agents should be reduced). Products include:
- Thorazine Suppositories 2523

Chlorpromazine Hydrochloride (Additive CNS depression; dose of one or both agents should be reduced). Products include:
- Thorazine 2523

Chlorprothixene (Additive CNS depression; dose of one or both agents should be reduced).
- No products indexed under this heading.

Chlorprothixene Hydrochloride (Additive CNS depression; dose of one or both agents should be reduced).
- No products indexed under this heading.

Clidinium Bromide (May produce paralytic ileus). Products include:
- Librax Capsules 2176
- Quarzan Capsules 2181

Clomipramine Hydrochloride (Increased effect of antidepressant or oxycodone). Products include:
- Anafranil Capsules 803

Clorazepate Dipotassium (Additive CNS depression; dose of one or both agents should be reduced). Products include:
- Tranxene 451

Clozapine (Additive CNS depression; dose of one or both agents should be reduced). Products include:
- Clozaril Tablets 2252

Codeine Phosphate (Additive CNS depression; dose of one or both agents should be reduced). Products include:
- Actifed with Codeine Cough Syrup 1067
- Brontex 1981
- Deconsal C Expectorant Syrup 456
- Deconsal Pediatric Syrup 457
- Dimetane-DC Cough Syrup 2059
- Empirin with Codeine Tablets 1093
- Fioricet with Codeine Capsules 2260
- Fiorinal with Codeine Capsules 2262
- Isoclor Expectorant 990
- Novahistine DH 2462
- Novahistine Expectorant 2463
- Nucofed 2051
- Phenergan with Codeine 2777
- Phenergan VC with Codeine 2781
- Robitussin A-C Syrup 2073
- Robitussin-DAC Syrup 2074
- Ryna ..... ▣ 841
- Soma Compound w/Codeine Tablets 2676
- Tussi-Organidin NR Liquid and S NR Liquid 2677
- Tylenol with Codeine 1583

Desflurane (Additive CNS depression; dose of one or both agents should be reduced). Products include:
- Suprane 1813

Desipramine Hydrochloride (Increased effect of antidepressant or oxycodone). Products include:
- Norpramin Tablets 1526

Dezocine (Additive CNS depression; dose of one or both agents should be reduced). Products include:
- Dalgan Injection 538

Diazepam (Additive CNS depression; dose of one or both agents should be reduced). Products include:
- Dizac 1809
- Valium Injectable 2182
- Valium Tablets 2183
- Valrelease Capsules 2169

Dicyclomine Hydrochloride (May produce paralytic ileus). Products include:
- Bentyl 1501

Doxepin Hydrochloride (Increased effect of antidepressant or oxycodone). Products include:
- Sinequan 2205
- Zonalon Cream 1055

Droperidol (Additive CNS depression; dose of one or both agents should be reduced). Products include:
- Inapsine Injection 1296

Enflurane (Additive CNS depression; dose of one or both agents should be reduced).
- No products indexed under this heading.

Estazolam (Additive CNS depression; dose of one or both agents should be reduced). Products include:
- ProSom Tablets 449

Ethchlorvynol (Additive CNS depression; dose of one or both agents should be reduced). Products include:
- Placidyl Capsules 448

Ethinamate (Additive CNS depression; dose of one or both agents should be reduced).
- No products indexed under this heading.

Ethopropazine Hydrochloride (May produce paralytic ileus).

Fentanyl (Additive CNS depression; dose of one or both agents should be reduced). Products include:
- Duragesic Transdermal System 1288

Fentanyl Citrate (Additive CNS depression; dose of one or both agents should be reduced). Products include:
- Sublimaze Injection 1307

Fluphenazine Decanoate (Additive CNS depression; dose of one or both agents should be reduced). Products include:
- Prolixin Decanoate 509

Fluphenazine Enanthate (Additive CNS depression; dose of one or both agents should be reduced). Products include:
- Prolixin Enanthate 509

Fluphenazine Hydrochloride (Additive CNS depression; dose of one or both agents should be reduced). Products include:
- Prolixin 509

Flurazepam Hydrochloride (Additive CNS depression; dose of one or both agents should be reduced). Products include:

Dalmane Capsules 2173

Furazolidone (Increased effect of either oxycodone or MAO inhibitor). Products include:

Furoxone 2046

Glutethimide (Additive CNS depression; dose of one or both agents should be reduced).

No products indexed under this heading.

Glycopyrrolate (May produce paralytic ileus). Products include:

Robinul Forte Tablets.............................. 2072
Robinul Injectable 2072
Robinul Tablets....................................... 2072

Haloperidol (Additive CNS depression; dose of one or both agents should be reduced). Products include:

Haldol Injection, Tablets and Concentrate 1575

Haloperidol Decanoate (Additive CNS depression; dose of one or both agents should be reduced). Products include:

Haldol Decanoate................................... 1577

Hydrocodone Bitartrate (Additive CNS depression; dose of one or both agents should be reduced). Products include:

Anexsia 5/500 Elixir 1781
Anexia Tablets.. 1782
Codiclear DH Syrup 791
Deconamine CX Cough and Cold Liquid and Tablets................................... 1319
Duratuss HD Elixir 2565
Hycodan Tablets and Syrup 930
Hycomine Compound Tablets 932
Hycomine 931
Hycotuss Expectorant Syrup 933
Hydrocet Capsules 782
Lorcet 10/650... 1018
Lortab 2566
Tussend 1783
Tussend Expectorant 1785
Vicodin Tablets 1356
Vicodin ES Tablets 1357
Vicodin Tuss Expectorant 1358
Zydone Capsules 949

Hydrocodone Polistirex (Additive CNS depression; dose of one or both agents should be reduced). Products include:

Tussionex Pennkinetic Extended-Release Suspension 998

Hydroxyzine Hydrochloride (Additive CNS depression; dose of one or both agents should be reduced). Products include:

Atarax Tablets & Syrup........................... 2185
Marax Tablets & DF Syrup...................... 2200
Vistaril Intramuscular Solution........ 2216

Hyoscyamine (May produce paralytic ileus). Products include:

Cystospaz Tablets 1963
Urised Tablets... 1964

Hyoscyamine Sulfate (May produce paralytic ileus). Products include:

Arco-Lase Plus Tablets 512
Atrohist Plus Tablets 454
Cystospaz-M Capsules 1963
Donnatal 2060
Donnatal Extentabs................................. 2061
Donnatal Tablets 2060
Kutrase Capsules.................................... 2402
Levsin/Levsinex/Levbid 2405

Imipramine Hydrochloride (Increased effect of antidepressant or oxycodone). Products include:

Tofranil Ampuls 854
Tofranil Tablets 856

Imipramine Pamoate (Increased effect of antidepressant or oxycodone). Products include:

Tofranil-PM Capsules............................. 857

Ipratropium Bromide (May produce paralytic ileus). Products include:

Atrovent Inhalation Aerosol.................... 671
Atrovent Inhalation Solution 673

Isocarboxazid (Increased effect of either oxycodone or MAO inhibitor).

No products indexed under this heading.

Isoflurane (Additive CNS depression; dose of one or both agents should be reduced).

No products indexed under this heading.

Ketamine Hydrochloride (Additive CNS depression; dose of one or both agents should be reduced).

No products indexed under this heading.

Levomethadyl Acetate Hydrochloride (Additive CNS depression; dose of one or both agents should be reduced). Products include:

Orlaam 2239

Levorphanol Tartrate (Additive CNS depression; dose of one or both agents should be reduced). Products include:

Levo-Dromoran 2129

Lorazepam (Additive CNS depression; dose of one or both agents should be reduced). Products include:

Ativan Injection 2698
Ativan Tablets 2700

Loxapine Hydrochloride (Additive CNS depression; dose of one or both agents should be reduced). Products include:

Loxitane 1378

Loxapine Succinate (Additive CNS depression; dose of one or both agents should be reduced). Products include:

Loxitane Capsules 1378

Maprotiline Hydrochloride (Increased effect of antidepressant or oxycodone). Products include:

Ludiomil Tablets...................................... 843

Mepenzolate Bromide (May produce paralytic ileus).

No products indexed under this heading.

Meperidine Hydrochloride (Additive CNS depression; dose of one or both agents should be reduced). Products include:

Demerol 2308
Mepergan Injection 2753

Mephobarbital (Additive CNS depression; dose of one or both agents should be reduced). Products include:

Mebaral Tablets 2322

Meprobamate (Additive CNS depression; dose of one or both agents should be reduced). Products include:

Miltown Tablets 2672
PMB 200 and PMB 400 2783

Mesoridazine Besylate (Additive CNS depression; dose of one or both agents should be reduced). Products include:

Serentil 684

Methadone Hydrochloride (Additive CNS depression; dose of one or both agents should be reduced). Products include:

Methadone Hydrochloride Oral Concentrate 2233
Methadone Hydrochloride Oral Solution & Tablets.................................... 2235

Methohexital Sodium (Additive CNS depression; dose of one or both agents should be reduced). Products include:

Brevital Sodium Vials.............................. 1429

Methotrimeprazine (Additive CNS depression; dose of one or both agents should be reduced). Products include:

Levoprome 1274

Methoxyflurane (Additive CNS depression; dose of one or both agents should be reduced).

No products indexed under this heading.

Midazolam Hydrochloride (Additive CNS depression; dose of one or both agents should be reduced). Products include:

Versed Injection 2170

Molindone Hydrochloride (Additive CNS depression; dose of one or both agents should be reduced). Products include:

Moban Tablets and Concentrate...... 1048

Morphine Sulfate (Additive CNS depression; dose of one or both agents should be reduced). Products include:

Astramorph/PF Injection, USP (Preservative-Free) 535
Duramorph 962
Infumorph 200 and Infumorph 500 Sterile Solutions............................. 965
MS Contin Tablets................................... 1994
MSIR 1997
Oramorph SR (Morphine Sulfate Sustained Release Tablets) 2236
RMS Suppositories 2657
Roxanol 2243

Nortriptyline Hydrochloride (Increased effect of antidepressant or oxycodone). Products include:

Pamelor 2280

Opium Alkaloids (Additive CNS depression; dose of one or both agents should be reduced).

No products indexed under this heading.

Oxazepam (Additive CNS depression; dose of one or both agents should be reduced; increased effect of antidepressant). Products include:

Serax Capsules 2810
Serax Tablets... 2810

Oxybutynin Chloride (May produce paralytic ileus). Products include:

Ditropan... 1516

Oxyphenonium Bromide (May produce paralytic ileus).

Pentobarbital Sodium (Additive CNS depression; dose of one or both agents should be reduced). Products include:

Nembutal Sodium Capsules 436
Nembutal Sodium Solution 438
Nembutal Sodium Suppositories...... 440

Perphenazine (Additive CNS depression; dose of one or both agents should be reduced). Products include:

Etrafon 2355
Triavil Tablets 1757
Trilafon... 2389

Phenelzine Sulfate (Increased effect of either oxycodone or MAO inhibitor). Products include:

Nardil 1920

Phenobarbital (Additive CNS depression; dose of one or both agents should be reduced). Products include:

Arco-Lase Plus Tablets 512
Bellergal-S Tablets 2250
Donnatal 2060
Donnatal Extentabs................................. 2061
Donnatal Tablets 2060
Phenobarbital Elixir and Tablets...... 1469
Quadrinal Tablets 1350

Prazepam (Additive CNS depression; dose of one or both agents should be reduced).

No products indexed under this heading.

Prochlorperazine (Additive CNS depression; dose of one or both agents should be reduced). Products include:

Compazine 2470

Procyclidine Hydrochloride (May produce paralytic ileus). Products include:

Kemadrin Tablets 1112

Promethazine Hydrochloride (Additive CNS depression; dose of one or both agents should be reduced). Products include:

Mepergan Injection 2753
Phenergan with Codeine 2777
Phenergan with Dextromethorphan 2778
Phenergan Injection 2773
Phenergan Suppositories 2775
Phenergan Syrup.................................... 2774
Phenergan Tablets 2775
Phenergan VC 2779
Phenergan VC with Codeine 2781

Propantheline Bromide (May produce paralytic ileus). Products include:

Pro-Banthine Tablets............................... 2052

Propofol (Additive CNS depression; dose of one or both agents should be reduced). Products include:

Diprivan Injection.................................... 2833

Propoxyphene Hydrochloride (Additive CNS depression; dose of one or both agents should be reduced). Products include:

Darvon 1435
Wygesic Tablets 2827

Propoxyphene Napsylate (Additive CNS depression; dose of one or both agents should be reduced). Products include:

Darvon-N/Darvocet-N 1433

Protriptyline Hydrochloride (Increased effect of antidepressant or oxycodone). Products include:

Vivactil Tablets 1774

Quazepam (Additive CNS depression; dose of one or both agents should be reduced). Products include:

Doral Tablets 2664

Risperidone (Additive CNS depression; dose of one or both agents should be reduced). Products include:

Risperdal 1301

Scopolamine (May produce paralytic ileus). Products include:

Transderm Scōp Transdermal Therapeutic System 869

Scopolamine Hydrobromide (May produce paralytic ileus). Products include:

Atrohist Plus Tablets 454
Donnatal 2060
Donnatal Extentabs................................. 2061
Donnatal Tablets 2060

Secobarbital Sodium (Additive CNS depression; dose of one or both agents should be reduced). Products include:

Seconal Sodium Pulvules 1474

Selegiline Hydrochloride (Increased effect of either oxycodone or MAO inhibitor). Products include:

Eldepryl Tablets 2550

Sufentanil Citrate (Additive CNS depression; dose of one or both agents should be reduced). Products include:

Sufenta Injection 1309

Temazepam (Additive CNS depression; dose of one or both agents should be reduced). Products include:

Restoril Capsules.................................... 2284

IMPORTANT NOTE: Always consult each drug listing in the patient's regimen for possible interactions.

Thiamylal Sodium (Additive CNS depression; dose of one or both agents should be reduced).
No products indexed under this heading.

Thioridazine Hydrochloride (Additive CNS depression; dose of one or both agents should be reduced). Products include:
Mellaril 2269

Thiothixene (Additive CNS depression; dose of one or both agents should be reduced). Products include:
Navane Capsules and Concentrate 2201
Navane Intramuscular 2202

Tranylcypromine Sulfate (Increased effect of either oxycodone or MAO inhibitor). Products include:
Parnate Tablets 2503

Triazolam (Additive CNS depression; dose of one or both agents should be reduced). Products include:
Halcion Tablets 2611

Tridihexethyl Chloride (May produce paralytic ileus).
No products indexed under this heading.

Trifluoperazine Hydrochloride (Additive CNS depression; dose of one or both agents should be reduced). Products include:
Stelazine 2514

Trihexyphenidyl Hydrochloride (May produce paralytic ileus). Products include:
Artane 1368

Trimipramine Maleate (Increased effect of antidepressant or oxycodone). Products include:
Surmontil Capsules 2811

Zolpidem Tartrate (Additive CNS depression; dose of one or both agents should be reduced). Products include:
Ambien Tablets 2416

Food Interactions

Alcohol (Additive CNS depression).

PERCODAN TABLETS

(Oxycodone Hydrochloride, Oxycodone Terephthalate, Aspirin) 939

May interact with narcotic analgesics, general anesthetics, phenothiazines, tranquilizers, hypnotics and sedatives, anticoagulants, central nervous system depressants, and certain other agents. Compounds in these categories include:

Alfentanil Hydrochloride (Additive CNS depression). Products include:
Alfenta Injection 1286

Alprazolam (Additive CNS depression). Products include:
Xanax Tablets 2649

Aprobarbital (Additive CNS depression).
No products indexed under this heading.

Buprenorphine (Additive CNS depression). Products include:
Buprenex Injectable 2006

Buspirone Hydrochloride (Additive CNS depression). Products include:
BuSpar 737

Butabarbital (Additive CNS depression).
No products indexed under this heading.

Butalbital (Additive CNS depression). Products include:
Esgic-plus Tablets 1013
Fioricet Tablets 2258
Fioricet with Codeine Capsules 2260
Fiorinal Capsules 2261
Fiorinal with Codeine Capsules 2262
Fiorinal Tablets 2261
Phrenilin 785
Sedapap Tablets 50 mg/650 mg 1543

Chlordiazepoxide (Additive CNS depression). Products include:
Libritabs Tablets 2177
Limbitrol 2180

Chlordiazepoxide Hydrochloride (Additive CNS depression). Products include:
Librax Capsules 2176
Librium Capsules 2178
Librium Injectable 2179

Chlorpromazine (Additive CNS depression). Products include:
Thorazine Suppositories 2523

Chlorpromazine Hydrochloride (Additive CNS depression). Products include:
Thorazine 2523

Chlorprothixene (Additive CNS depression).
No products indexed under this heading.

Chlorprothixene Hydrochloride (Additive CNS depression).
No products indexed under this heading.

Clorazepate Dipotassium (Additive CNS depression). Products include:
Tranxene 451

Clozapine (Additive CNS depression). Products include:
Clozaril Tablets 2252

Codeine Phosphate (Additive CNS depression). Products include:
Actifed with Codeine Cough Syrup 1067
Brontex 1981
Deconsal C Expectorant Syrup 456
Deconsal Pediatric Syrup 457
Dimetane-DC Cough Syrup 2059
Empirin with Codeine Tablets 1093
Fioricet with Codeine Capsules 2260
Fiorinal with Codeine Capsules 2262
Isoclor Expectorant 990
Novahistine DH 2462
Novahistine Expectorant 2463
Nucofed 2051
Phenergan with Codeine 2777
Phenergan VC with Codeine 2781
Robitussin A-C Syrup 2073
Robitussin-DAC Syrup 2074
Ryna ■ 841
Soma Compound w/Codeine Tablets 2676
Tussi-Organidin NR Liquid and S NR Liquid 2677
Tylenol with Codeine 1583

Dalteparin Sodium (Enhanced effect of anticoagulant). Products include:
Fragmin 1954

Desflurane (Additive CNS depression). Products include:
Suprane 1813

Dezocine (Additive CNS depression). Products include:
Dalgan Injection 538

Diazepam (Additive CNS depression). Products include:
Dizac 1809
Valium Injectable 2182
Valium Tablets 2183
Valrelease Capsules 2169

Dicumarol (Enhanced effect of anticoagulant).
No products indexed under this heading.

Droperidol (Additive CNS depression). Products include:
Inapsine Injection 1296

Enflurane (Additive CNS depression).
No products indexed under this heading.

Enoxaparin (Enhanced effect of anticoagulant). Products include:
Lovenox Injection 2020

Estazolam (Additive CNS depression). Products include:
ProSom Tablets 449

Ethchlorvynol (Additive CNS depression). Products include:
Placidyl Capsules 448

Ethinamate (Additive CNS depression).
No products indexed under this heading.

Fentanyl (Additive CNS depression). Products include:
Duragesic Transdermal System 1288

Fentanyl Citrate (Additive CNS depression). Products include:
Sublimaze Injection 1307

Fluphenazine Decanoate (Additive CNS depression). Products include:
Prolixin Decanoate 509

Fluphenazine Enanthate (Additive CNS depression). Products include:
Prolixin Enanthate 509

Fluphenazine Hydrochloride (Additive CNS depression). Products include:
Prolixin 509

Flurazepam Hydrochloride (Additive CNS depression). Products include:
Dalmane Capsules 2173

Glutethimide (Additive CNS depression).
No products indexed under this heading.

Haloperidol (Additive CNS depression). Products include:
Haldol Injection, Tablets and Concentrate 1575

Haloperidol Decanoate (Additive CNS depression). Products include:
Haldol Decanoate 1577

Heparin Calcium (Enhanced effect of anticoagulant).
No products indexed under this heading.

Heparin Sodium (Enhanced effect of anticoagulant). Products include:
Heparin Lock Flush Solution 2725
Heparin Sodium Injection 2726
Heparin Sodium Injection, USP, Sterile Solution 2615
Heparin Sodium Vials 1441

Hydrocodone Bitartrate (Additive CNS depression). Products include:
Anexsia 5/500 Elixir 1781
Anexia Tablets 1782
Codiclear DH Syrup 791
Deconamine CX Cough and Cold Liquid and Tablets 1319
Duratuss HD Elixir 2565
Hycodan Tablets and Syrup 930
Hycomine Compound Tablets 932
Hycomine 931
Hycotuss Expectorant Syrup 933
Hydrocet Capsules 782
Lorcet 10/650 1018
Lortab 2566
Tussend 1783
Tussend Expectorant 1785
Vicodin Tablets 1356
Vicodin ES Tablets 1357
Vicodin Tuss Expectorant 1358
Zydone Capsules 949

Hydrocodone Polistirex (Additive CNS depression). Products include:
Tussionex Pennkinetic Extended-Release Suspension 998

Hydroxyzine Hydrochloride (Additive CNS depression). Products include:
Atarax Tablets & Syrup 2185
Marax Tablets & DF Syrup 2200
Vistaril Intramuscular Solution 2216

Isoflurane (Additive CNS depression).
No products indexed under this heading.

Ketamine Hydrochloride (Additive CNS depression).
No products indexed under this heading.

Levomethadyl Acetate Hydrochloride (Additive CNS depression). Products include:
Orlamm 2239

Levorphanol Tartrate (Additive CNS depression). Products include:
Levo-Dromoran 2129

Lorazepam (Additive CNS depression). Products include:
Ativan Injection 2698
Ativan Tablets 2700

Loxapine Hydrochloride (Additive CNS depression). Products include:
Loxitane 1378

Loxapine Succinate (Additive CNS depression). Products include:
Loxitane Capsules 1378

Meperidine Hydrochloride (Additive CNS depression). Products include:
Demerol 2308
Mepergan Injection 2753

Mephobarbital (Additive CNS depression). Products include:
Mebaral Tablets 2322

Meprobamate (Additive CNS depression). Products include:
Miltown Tablets 2672
PMB 200 and PMB 400 2783

Mesoridazine (Additive CNS depression).

Mesoridazine Besylate (Additive CNS depression). Products include:
Serentil 684

Methadone Hydrochloride (Additive CNS depression). Products include:
Methadone Hydrochloride Oral Concentrate 2233
Methadone Hydrochloride Oral Solution & Tablets 2235

Methohexital Sodium (Additive CNS depression). Products include:
Brevital Sodium Vials 1429

Methotrimeprazine (Additive CNS depression). Products include:
Levoprome 1274

Methoxyflurane (Additive CNS depression).
No products indexed under this heading.

Midazolam Hydrochloride (Additive CNS depression). Products include:
Versed Injection 2170

Molindone Hydrochloride (Additive CNS depression). Products include:
Moban Tablets and Concentrate 1048

Morphine Sulfate (Additive CNS depression). Products include:
Astramorph/PF Injection, USP (Preservative-Free) 535
Duramorph 962
Infumorph 200 and Infumorph 500 Sterile Solutions 965
MS Contin Tablets 1994
MSIR 1997
Oramorph SR (Morphine Sulfate Sustained Release Tablets) 2236
RMS Suppositories 2657
Roxanol 2243

Opium Alkaloids (Additive CNS depression).
No products indexed under this heading.

Oxazepam (Additive CNS depression). Products include:
Serax Capsules 2810
Serax Tablets 2810

803 Interactions Index Percodan-Demi

Pentobarbital Sodium (Additive CNS depression). Products include:
Nembutal Sodium Capsules 436
Nembutal Sodium Solution 438
Nembutal Sodium Suppositories 440

Perphenazine (Additive CNS depression). Products include:
Etrafon 2355
Triavil Tablets 1757
Trilafon 2389

Phenobarbital (Additive CNS depression). Products include:
Arco-Lase Plus Tablets 512
Bellergal-S Tablets 2250
Donnatal 2060
Donnatal Extentabs 2061
Donnatal Tablets 2060
Phenobarbital Elixir and Tablets 1469
Quadrinal Tablets 1350

Prazepam (Additive CNS depression).
No products indexed under this heading.

Probenecid (Aspirin may inhibit the uricosuric effects). Products include:
Benemid Tablets 1611
ColBENEMID Tablets 1622

Prochlorperazine (Additive CNS depression). Products include:
Compazine 2470

Promethazine Hydrochloride (Additive CNS depression). Products include:
Mepergan Injection 2753
Phenergan with Codeine 2777
Phenergan with Dextromethorphan 2778
Phenergan Injection 2773
Phenergan Suppositories 2775
Phenergan Syrup 2774
Phenergan Tablets 2775
Phenergan VC 2779
Phenergan VC with Codeine 2781

Propofol (Additive CNS depression). Products include:
Diprivan Injection 2833

Propoxyphene Hydrochloride (Additive CNS depression). Products include:
Darvon 1435
Wygesic Tablets 2827

Propoxyphene Napsylate (Additive CNS depression). Products include:
Darvon-N/Darvocet-N 1433

Quazepam (Additive CNS depression). Products include:
Doral Tablets 2664

Risperidone (Additive CNS depression). Products include:
Risperdal 1301

Secobarbital Sodium (Additive CNS depression). Products include:
Seconal Sodium Pulvules 1474

Sufentanil Citrate (Additive CNS depression). Products include:
Sufenta Injection 1309

Sulfinpyrazone (Aspirin may inhibit the uricosuric effects). Products include:
Anturane 807

Temazepam (Additive CNS depression). Products include:
Restoril Capsules 2284

Thiamylal Sodium (Additive CNS depression).
No products indexed under this heading.

Thioridazine Hydrochloride (Additive CNS depression). Products include:
Mellaril 2269

Thiothixene (Additive CNS depression). Products include:
Navane Capsules and Concentrate 2201
Navane Intramuscular 2202

Triazolam (Additive CNS depression). Products include:
Halcion Tablets 2611

Trifluoperazine Hydrochloride (Additive CNS depression). Products include:
Stelazine 2514

Warfarin Sodium (Enhanced effect of anticoagulant). Products include:
Coumadin 926

Zolpidem Tartrate (Additive CNS depression). Products include:
Ambien Tablets 2416

Food Interactions

Alcohol (Additive CNS depression).

PERCODAN-DEMI TABLETS
(Oxycodone Hydrochloride, Oxycodone Terephthalate, Aspirin) 940
May interact with central nervous system depressants, anticoagulants, antigout agents, general anesthetics, hypnotics and sedatives, tranquilizers, phenothiazines, and certain other agents. Compounds in these categories include:

Alfentanil Hydrochloride (CNS depressant effects of Percodan-Demi may be additive). Products include:
Alfenta Injection 1286

Allopurinol (Aspirin inhibits the uricosuric effect of uricosuric agents). Products include:
Zyloprim Tablets 1226

Alprazolam (CNS depressant effects of Percodan-Demi may be additive). Products include:
Xanax Tablets 2649

Aprobarbital (CNS depressant effects of Percodan-Demi may be additive).
No products indexed under this heading.

Buprenorphine (CNS depressant effects of Percodan-Demi may be additive). Products include:
Buprenex Injectable 2006

Buspirone Hydrochloride (CNS depressant effects of Percodan-Demi may be additive). Products include:
BuSpar 737

Butabarbital (CNS depressant effects of Percodan-Demi may be additive).
No products indexed under this heading.

Butalbital (CNS depressant effects of Percodan-Demi may be additive). Products include:
Esgic-plus Tablets 1013
Fioricet Tablets 2258
Fioricet with Codeine Capsules 2260
Fiorinal Capsules 2261
Fiorinal with Codeine Capsules 2262
Fiorinal Tablets 2261
Phrenilin 785
Sedapap Tablets 50 mg/650 mg .. 1543

Chlordiazepoxide (CNS depressant effects of Percodan-Demi may be additive). Products include:
Libritabs Tablets 2177
Limbitrol 2180

Chlordiazepoxide Hydrochloride (CNS depressant effects of Percodan-Demi may be additive). Products include:
Librax Capsules 2176
Librium Capsules 2178
Librium Injectable 2179

Chlorpromazine (CNS depressant effects of Percodan-Demi may be additive). Products include:
Thorazine Suppositories 2523

Chlorpromazine Hydrochloride (CNS depressant effects of Percodan-Demi may be additive). Products include:
Thorazine 2523

Chlorprothixene (CNS depressant effects of Percodan-Demi may be additive).
No products indexed under this heading.

Chlorprothixene Hydrochloride (CNS depressant effects of Percodan-Demi may be additive).
No products indexed under this heading.

Clorazepate Dipotassium (CNS depressant effects of Percodan-Demi may be additive). Products include:
Tranxene 451

Clozapine (CNS depressant effects of Percodan-Demi may be additive). Products include:
Clozaril Tablets 2252

Codeine Phosphate (CNS depressant effects of Percodan-Demi may be additive). Products include:
Actifed with Codeine Cough Syrup.. 1067
Brontex 1981
Deconsal C Expectorant Syrup 456
Deconsal Pediatric Syrup 457
Dimetane-DC Cough Syrup 2059
Empirin with Codeine Tablets 1093
Fioricet with Codeine Capsules 2260
Fiorinal with Codeine Capsules 2262
Isoclor Expectorant 990
Novahistine DH 2462
Novahistine Expectorant 2463
Nucofed 2051
Phenergan with Codeine 2777
Phenergan VC with Codeine 2781
Robitussin A-C Syrup 2073
Robitussin-DAC Syrup 2074
Ryna 841
Soma Compound w/Codeine Tablets 2676
Tussi-Organidin NR Liquid and S NR Liquid 2677
Tylenol with Codeine 1583

Dalteparin Sodium (Enhanced effect of anticoagulants). Products include:
Fragmin 1954

Desflurane (CNS depressant effects of Percodan-Demi may be additive). Products include:
Suprane 1813

Dezocine (CNS depressant effects of Percodan-Demi may be additive). Products include:
Dalgan Injection 538

Diazepam (CNS depressant effects of Percodan-Demi may be additive). Products include:
Dizac 1809
Valium Injectable 2182
Valium Tablets 2183
Valrelease Capsules 2169

Dicumarol (Enhanced effect of anticoagulants).
No products indexed under this heading.

Droperidol (CNS depressant effects of Percodan-Demi may be additive). Products include:
Inapsine Injection 1296

Enflurane (CNS depressant effects of Percodan-Demi may be additive).
No products indexed under this heading.

Enoxaparin (Enhanced effect of anticoagulants). Products include:
Lovenox Injection 2020

Estazolam (CNS depressant effects of Percodan-Demi may be additive). Products include:
ProSom Tablets 449

Ethchlorvynol (CNS depressant effects of Percodan-Demi may be additive). Products include:
Placidyl Capsules 448

Ethinamate (CNS depressant effects of Percodan-Demi may be additive).
No products indexed under this heading.

Fentanyl (CNS depressant effects of Percodan-Demi may be additive). Products include:
Duragesic Transdermal System 1288

Fentanyl Citrate (CNS depressant effects of Percodan-Demi may be additive). Products include:
Sublimaze Injection 1307

Fluphenazine Decanoate (CNS depressant effects of Percodan-Demi may be additive). Products include:
Prolixin Decanoate 509

Fluphenazine Enanthate (CNS depressant effects of Percodan-Demi may be additive). Products include:
Prolixin Enanthate 509

Fluphenazine Hydrochloride (CNS depressant effects of Percodan-Demi may be additive). Products include:
Prolixin 509

Flurazepam Hydrochloride (CNS depressant effects of Percodan-Demi may be additive). Products include:
Dalmane Capsules 2173

Glutethimide (CNS depressant effects of Percodan-Demi may be additive).
No products indexed under this heading.

Haloperidol (CNS depressant effects of Percodan-Demi may be additive). Products include:
Haldol Injection, Tablets and Concentrate 1575

Haloperidol Decanoate (CNS depressant effects of Percodan-Demi may be additive). Products include:
Haldol Decanoate 1577

Heparin Calcium (Enhanced effect of anticoagulants).
No products indexed under this heading.

Heparin Sodium (Enhanced effect of anticoagulants). Products include:
Heparin Lock Flush Solution 2725
Heparin Sodium Injection 2726
Heparin Sodium Injection, USP, Sterile Solution 2615
Heparin Sodium Vials 1441

Hydrocodone Bitartrate (CNS depressant effects of Percodan-Demi may be additive). Products include:
Anexsia 5/500 Elixir 1781
Anexia Tablets 1782
Codiclear DH Syrup 791
Deconamine CX Cough and Cold Liquid and Tablets 1319
Duratuss HD Elixir 2565
Hycodan Tablets and Syrup 930
Hycomine Compound Tablets 932
Hycomine 931
Hycotuss Expectorant Syrup 933
Hydrocet Capsules 782
Lorcet 10/650 1018
Lortab 2566
Tussend 1783
Tussend Expectorant 1785
Vicodin Tablets 1356
Vicodin ES Tablets 1357
Vicodin Tuss Expectorant 1358
Zydone Capsules 949

Hydrocodone Polistirex (CNS depressant effects of Percodan-Demi may be additive). Products include:
Tussionex Pennkinetic Extended-Release Suspension 998

Hydroxyzine Hydrochloride (CNS depressant effects of Percodan-Demi may be additive). Products include:
Atarax Tablets & Syrup 2185
Marax Tablets & DF Syrup 2200
Vistaril Intramuscular Solution 2216

Isoflurane (CNS depressant effects of Percodan-Demi may be additive).
No products indexed under this heading.

IMPORTANT NOTE: Always consult each drug listing in the patient's regimen for possible interactions.

Ketamine Hydrochloride (CNS depressant effects of Percodan-Demi may be additive).
No products indexed under this heading.

Levomethadyl Acetate Hydrochloride (CNS depressant effects of Percodan-Demi may be additive). Products include:
Orlamm ... 2239

Levorphanol Tartrate (CNS depressant effects of Percodan-Demi may be additive). Products include:
Levo-Dromoran ... 2129

Lorazepam (CNS depressant effects of Percodan-Demi may be additive). Products include:
Ativan Injection ... 2698
Ativan Tablets ... 2700

Loxapine Hydrochloride (CNS depressant effects of Percodan-Demi may be additive). Products include:
Loxitane ... 1378

Loxapine Succinate (CNS depressant effects of Percodan-Demi may be additive). Products include:
Loxitane Capsules ... 1378

Meperidine Hydrochloride (CNS depressant effects of Percodan-Demi may be additive). Products include:
Demerol ... 2308
Mepergan Injection ... 2753

Mephobarbital (CNS depressant effects of Percodan-Demi may be additive). Products include:
Mebaral Tablets ... 2322

Meprobamate (CNS depressant effects of Percodan-Demi may be additive). Products include:
Miltown Tablets ... 2672
PMB 200 and PMB 400 ... 2783

Mesoridazine (CNS depressant effects of Percodan-Demi may be additive).

Methadone Hydrochloride (CNS depressant effects of Percodan-Demi may be additive). Products include:
Methadone Hydrochloride Oral Concentrate ... 2233
Methadone Hydrochloride Oral Solution & Tablets ... 2235

Methohexital Sodium (CNS depressant effects of Percodan-Demi may be additive). Products include:
Brevital Sodium Vials ... 1429

Methotrimeprazine (CNS depressant effects of Percodan-Demi may be additive). Products include:
Levoprome ... 1274

Methoxyflurane (CNS depressant effects of Percodan-Demi may be additive).
No products indexed under this heading.

Midazolam Hydrochloride (CNS depressant effects of Percodan-Demi may be additive). Products include:
Versed Injection ... 2170

Molindone Hydrochloride (CNS depressant effects of Percodan-Demi may be additive). Products include:
Moban Tablets and Concentrate ... 1048

Morphine Sulfate (CNS depressant effects of Percodan-Demi may be additive). Products include:
Astramorph/PF Injection, USP (Preservative-Free) ... 535
Duramorph ... 962
Infumorph 200 and Infumorph 500 Sterile Solutions ... 965
MS Contin Tablets ... 1994
MSIR ... 1997
Oramorph SR (Morphine Sulfate Sustained Release Tablets) ... 2236
RMS Suppositories ... 2657
Roxanol ... 2243

Opium Alkaloids (CNS depressant effects of Percodan-Demi may be additive).
No products indexed under this heading.

Oxazepam (CNS depressant effects of Percodan-Demi may be additive). Products include:
Serax Capsules ... 2810
Serax Tablets ... 2810

Pentobarbital Sodium (CNS depressant effects of Percodan-Demi may be additive). Products include:
Nembutal Sodium Capsules ... 436
Nembutal Sodium Solution ... 438
Nembutal Sodium Suppositories ... 440

Perphenazine (CNS depressant effects of Percodan-Demi may be additive). Products include:
Etrafon ... 2355
Triavil Tablets ... 1757
Trilafon ... 2389

Phenobarbital (CNS depressant effects of Percodan-Demi may be additive). Products include:
Arco-Lase Plus Tablets ... 512
Bellergal-S Tablets ... 2250
Donnatal ... 2060
Donnatal Extentabs ... 2061
Donnatal Tablets ... 2060
Phenobarbital Elixir and Tablets ... 1469
Quadrinal Tablets ... 1350

Prazepam (CNS depressant effects of Percodan-Demi may be additive).
No products indexed under this heading.

Probenecid (Aspirin inhibits the uricosuric effect of uricosuric agents). Products include:
Benemid Tablets ... 1611
ColBENEMID Tablets ... 1622

Prochlorperazine (CNS depressant effects of Percodan-Demi may be additive). Products include:
Compazine ... 2470

Promethazine Hydrochloride (CNS depressant effects of Percodan-Demi may be additive). Products include:
Mepergan Injection ... 2753
Phenergan with Codeine ... 2777
Phenergan with Dextromethorphan 2778
Phenergan Injection ... 2773
Phenergan Suppositories ... 2775
Phenergan Syrup ... 2774
Phenergan Tablets ... 2775
Phenergan VC ... 2779
Phenergan VC with Codeine ... 2781

Propofol (CNS depressant effects of Percodan-Demi may be additive). Products include:
Diprivan Injection ... 2833

Propoxyphene Hydrochloride (CNS depressant effects of Percodan-Demi may be additive). Products include:
Darvon ... 1435
Wygesic Tablets ... 2827

Propoxyphene Napsylate (CNS depressant effects of Percodan-Demi may be additive). Products include:
Darvon-N/Darvocet-N ... 1433

Quazepam (CNS depressant effects of Percodan-Demi may be additive). Products include:
Doral Tablets ... 2664

Risperidone (CNS depressant effects of Percodan-Demi may be additive). Products include:
Risperdal ... 1301

Secobarbital Sodium (CNS depressant effects of Percodan-Demi may be additive). Products include:
Seconal Sodium Pulvules ... 1474

Sufentanil Citrate (CNS depressant effects of Percodan-Demi may be additive). Products include:
Sufenta Injection ... 1309

Sulfinpyrazone (Aspirin inhibits the uricosuric effect of uricosuric agents). Products include:
Anturane ... 807

Temazepam (CNS depressant effects of Percodan-Demi may be additive). Products include:
Restoril Capsules ... 2284

Thiamylal Sodium (CNS depressant effects of Percodan-Demi may be additive).
No products indexed under this heading.

Thioridazine Hydrochloride (CNS depressant effects of Percodan-Demi may be additive). Products include:
Mellaril ... 2269

Thiothixene (CNS depressant effects of Percodan-Demi may be additive). Products include:
Navane Capsules and Concentrate 2201
Navane Intramuscular ... 2202

Triazolam (CNS depressant effects of Percodan-Demi may be additive). Products include:
Halcion Tablets ... 2611

Trifluoperazine Hydrochloride (CNS depressant effects of Percodan-Demi may be additive). Products include:
Stelazine ... 2514

Warfarin Sodium (Enhanced effect of anticoagulants). Products include:
Coumadin ... 926

Zolpidem Tartrate (CNS depressant effects of Percodan-Demi may be additive). Products include:
Ambien Tablets ... 2416

Food Interactions

Alcohol (CNS depressant effects of Percodan-Demi may be additive).

PERCOGESIC ANALGESIC TABLETS

(Acetaminophen, Phenyltoloxamine Citrate) ... ▣ 754
May interact with tranquilizers, hypnotics and sedatives, and certain other agents. Compounds in these categories include:

Alprazolam (May increase the drowsiness effect). Products include:
Xanax Tablets ... 2649

Buspirone Hydrochloride (May increase the drowsiness effect). Products include:
BuSpar ... 737

Chlordiazepoxide (May increase the drowsiness effect). Products include:
Libritabs Tablets ... 2177
Limbitrol ... 2180

Chlordiazepoxide Hydrochloride (May increase the drowsiness effect). Products include:
Librax Capsules ... 2176
Librium Capsules ... 2178
Librium Injectable ... 2179

Chlorpromazine (May increase the drowsiness effect). Products include:
Thorazine Suppositories ... 2523

Chlorprothixene (May increase the drowsiness effect).
No products indexed under this heading.

Chlorprothixene Hydrochloride (May increase the drowsiness effect).
No products indexed under this heading.

Clorazepate Dipotassium (May increase the drowsiness effect). Products include:
Tranxene ... 451

Diazepam (May increase the drowsiness effect). Products include:
Dizac ... 1809
Valium Injectable ... 2182
Valium Tablets ... 2183
Valrelease Capsules ... 2169

Droperidol (May increase the drowsiness effect). Products include:
Inapsine Injection ... 1296

Estazolam (May increase the drowsiness effect). Products include:
ProSom Tablets ... 449

Ethchlorvynol (May increase the drowsiness effect). Products include:
Placidyl Capsules ... 448

Ethinamate (May increase the drowsiness effect).
No products indexed under this heading.

Fluphenazine Decanoate (May increase the drowsiness effect). Products include:
Prolixin Decanoate ... 509

Fluphenazine Enanthate (May increase the drowsiness effect). Products include:
Prolixin Enanthate ... 509

Fluphenazine Hydrochloride (May increase the drowsiness effect). Products include:
Prolixin ... 509

Flurazepam Hydrochloride (May increase the drowsiness effect). Products include:
Dalmane Capsules ... 2173

Glutethimide (May increase the drowsiness effect).
No products indexed under this heading.

Haloperidol (May increase the drowsiness effect). Products include:
Haldol Injection, Tablets and Concentrate ... 1575

Haloperidol Decanoate (May increase the drowsiness effect). Products include:
Haldol Decanoate ... 1577

Hydroxyzine Hydrochloride (May increase the drowsiness effect). Products include:
Atarax Tablets & Syrup ... 2185
Marax Tablets & DF Syrup ... 2200
Vistaril Intramuscular Solution ... 2216

Lorazepam (May increase the drowsiness effect). Products include:
Ativan Injection ... 2698
Ativan Tablets ... 2700

Loxapine Hydrochloride (May increase the drowsiness effect). Products include:
Loxitane ... 1378

Loxapine Succinate (May increase the drowsiness effect). Products include:
Loxitane Capsules ... 1378

Meprobamate (May increase the drowsiness effect). Products include:
Miltown Tablets ... 2672
PMB 200 and PMB 400 ... 2783

Mesoridazine Besylate (May increase the drowsiness effect). Products include:
Serentil ... 684

Midazolam Hydrochloride (May increase the drowsiness effect). Products include:
Versed Injection ... 2170

Molindone Hydrochloride (May increase the drowsiness effect). Products include:
Moban Tablets and Concentrate ... 1048

Oxazepam (May increase the drowsiness effect). Products include:
Serax Capsules ... 2810
Serax Tablets ... 2810

Perphenazine (May increase the drowsiness effect). Products include:
Etrafon ... 2355

Triavil Tablets 1757
Trilafon 2389

Prazepam (May increase the drowsiness effect).
No products indexed under this heading.

Prochlorperazine (May increase the drowsiness effect). Products include:
Compazine 2470

Promethazine Hydrochloride (May increase the drowsiness effect). Products include:
Mepergan Injection 2753
Phenergan with Codeine 2777
Phenergan with Dextromethorphan 2778
Phenergan Injection 2773
Phenergan Suppositories 2775
Phenergan Syrup 2774
Phenergan Tablets 2775
Phenergan VC 2779
Phenergan VC with Codeine 2781

Propofol (May increase the drowsiness effect). Products include:
Diprivan Injection 2833

Quazepam (May increase the drowsiness effect). Products include:
Doral Tablets 2664

Secobarbital Sodium (May increase the drowsiness effect). Products include:
Seconal Sodium Pulvules 1474

Temazepam (May increase the drowsiness effect). Products include:
Restoril Capsules 2284

Thioridazine Hydrochloride (May increase the drowsiness effect). Products include:
Mellaril 2269

Thiothixene (May increase the drowsiness effect). Products include:
Navane Capsules and Concentrate 2201
Navane Intramuscular 2202

Triazolam (May increase the drowsiness effect). Products include:
Halcion Tablets 2611

Trifluoperazine Hydrochloride (May increase the drowsiness effect). Products include:
Stelazine 2514

Zolpidem Tartrate (May increase the drowsiness effect). Products include:
Ambien Tablets 2416

Food Interactions

Alcohol (May increase the drowsiness effect).

PERDIEM FIBER BULK-FORMING LAXATIVE

(Psyllium Preparations) 869
None cited in PDR database.

PERDIEM BULK-FORMING LAXATIVE

(Psyllium Preparations, Senna Concentrates) 869
None cited in PDR database.

PERGONAL (MENOTROPINS FOR INJECTION, USP)

(Menotropins) 2448
None cited in PDR database.

PERIACTIN SYRUP

(Cyproheptadine Hydrochloride) 1724
May interact with central nervous system depressants and monoamine oxidase inhibitors. Compounds in these categories include:

Alfentanil Hydrochloride (Additive effects). Products include:
Alfenta Injection 1286

Alprazolam (Additive effects). Products include:
Xanax Tablets 2649

Aprobarbital (Additive effects).
No products indexed under this heading.

Buprenorphine (Additive effects). Products include:
Buprenex Injectable 2006

Buspirone Hydrochloride (Additive effects). Products include:
BuSpar 737

Butabarbital (Additive effects).
No products indexed under this heading.

Butalbital (Additive effects). Products include:
Esgic-plus Tablets 1013
Fioricet Tablets 2258
Fioricet with Codeine Capsules 2260
Fiorinal Capsules 2261
Fiorinal with Codeine Capsules 2262
Fiorinal Tablets 2261
Phrenilin 785
Sedapap Tablets 50 mg/650 mg .. 1543

Chlordiazepoxide (Additive effects). Products include:
Libritabs Tablets 2177
Limbitrol 2180

Chlordiazepoxide Hydrochloride (Additive effects). Products include:
Librax Capsules 2176
Librium Capsules 2178
Librium Injectable 2179

Chlorpromazine (Additive effects). Products include:
Thorazine Suppositories 2523

Chlorprothixene (Additive effects).
No products indexed under this heading.

Chlorprothixene Hydrochloride (Additive effects).
No products indexed under this heading.

Chlorprothixene Lactate (Additive effects).
No products indexed under this heading.

Clorazepate Dipotassium (Additive effects). Products include:
Tranxene 451

Clozapine (Additive effects). Products include:
Clozaril Tablets 2252

Codeine Phosphate (Additive effects). Products include:
Actifed with Codeine Cough Syrup.. 1067
Brontex 1981
Deconsal C Expectorant Syrup 456
Deconsal Pediatric Syrup 457
Dimetane-DC Cough Syrup 2059
Empirin with Codeine Tablets 1093
Fioricet with Codeine Capsules 2260
Fiorinal with Codeine Capsules 2262
Isoclor Expectorant 990
Novahistine DH 2462
Novahistine Expectorant 2463
Nucofed 2051
Phenergan with Codeine 2777
Phenergan VC with Codeine 2781
Robitussin A-C Syrup 2073
Robitussin-DAC Syrup 2074
Ryna 841
Soma Compound w/Codeine Tablets 2676
Tussi-Organidin NR Liquid and S NR Liquid 2677
Tylenol with Codeine 1583

Desflurane (Additive effects). Products include:
Suprane 1813

Dezocine (Additive effects). Products include:
Dalgan Injection 538

Diazepam (Additive effects). Products include:
Dizac 1809
Valium Injectable 2182
Valium Tablets 2183
Valrelease Capsules 2169

Droperidol (Additive effects). Products include:
Inapsine Injection 1296

Enflurane (Additive effects).
No products indexed under this heading.

Estazolam (Additive effects). Products include:
ProSom Tablets 449

Ethchlorvynol (Additive effects). Products include:
Placidyl Capsules 448

Ethinamate (Additive effects).
No products indexed under this heading.

Fentanyl (Additive effects). Products include:
Duragesic Transdermal System 1288

Fentanyl Citrate (Additive effects). Products include:
Sublimaze Injection 1307

Fluphenazine Decanoate (Additive effects). Products include:
Prolixin Decanoate 509

Fluphenazine Enanthate (Additive effects). Products include:
Prolixin Enanthate 509

Fluphenazine Hydrochloride (Additive effects). Products include:
Prolixin 509

Flurazepam Hydrochloride (Additive effects). Products include:
Dalmane Capsules 2173

Furazolidone (Contraindication; anticholinergic effects of antihistamines prolonged and intensified). Products include:
Furoxone 2046

Glutethimide (Additive effects).
No products indexed under this heading.

Haloperidol (Additive effects). Products include:
Haldol Injection, Tablets and Concentrate 1575

Haloperidol Decanoate (Additive effects). Products include:
Haldol Decanoate 1577

Hydrocodone Bitartrate (Additive effects). Products include:
Anexsia 5/500 Elixir 1781
Anexia Tablets 1782
Codiclear DH Syrup 791
Deconamine CX Cough and Cold Liquid and Tablets 1319
Duratuss HD Elixir 2565
Hycodan Tablets and Syrup 930
Hycomine Compound Tablets 932
Hycomine 931
Hycotuss Expectorant Syrup 933
Hydrocet Capsules 782
Lorcet 10/650 1018
Lortab 2566
Tussend 1783
Tussend Expectorant 1785
Vicodin Tablets 1356
Vicodin ES Tablets 1357
Vicodin Tuss Expectorant 1358
Zydone Capsules 949

Hydrocodone Polistirex (Additive effects). Products include:
Tussionex Pennkinetic Extended-Release Suspension 998

Hydroxyzine Hydrochloride (Additive effects). Products include:
Atarax Tablets & Syrup 2185
Marax Tablets & DF Syrup 2200
Vistaril Intramuscular Solution 2216

Isocarboxazid (Contraindication; anticholinergic effects of antihistamines prolonged and intensified).
No products indexed under this heading.

Isoflurane (Additive effects).
No products indexed under this heading.

Ketamine Hydrochloride (Additive effects).
No products indexed under this heading.

Levomethadyl Acetate Hydrochloride (Additive effects). Products include:
Orlamm 2239

Levorphanol Tartrate (Additive effects). Products include:
Levo-Dromoran 2129

Lorazepam (Additive effects). Products include:
Ativan Injection 2698
Ativan Tablets 2700

Loxapine Hydrochloride (Additive effects). Products include:
Loxitane 1378

Loxapine Succinate (Additive effects). Products include:
Loxitane Capsules 1378

Meperidine Hydrochloride (Additive effects). Products include:
Demerol 2308
Mepergan Injection 2753

Mephobarbital (Additive effects). Products include:
Mebaral Tablets 2322

Meprobamate (Additive effects). Products include:
Miltown Tablets 2672
PMB 200 and PMB 400 2783

Mesoridazine Besylate (Additive effects). Products include:
Serentil 684

Methadone Hydrochloride (Additive effects). Products include:
Methadone Hydrochloride Oral Concentrate 2233
Methadone Hydrochloride Oral Solution & Tablets 2235

Methohexital Sodium (Additive effects). Products include:
Brevital Sodium Vials 1429

Methotrimeprazine (Additive effects). Products include:
Levoprome 1274

Methoxyflurane (Additive effects).
No products indexed under this heading.

Midazolam Hydrochloride (Additive effects). Products include:
Versed Injection 2170

Molindone Hydrochloride (Additive effects). Products include:
Moban Tablets and Concentrate 1048

Morphine Sulfate (Additive effects). Products include:
Astramorph/PF Injection, USP (Preservative-Free) 535
Duramorph 962
Infumorph 200 and Infumorph 500 Sterile Solutions 965
MS Contin Tablets 1994
MSIR 1997
Oramorph SR (Morphine Sulfate Sustained Release Tablets) 2236
RMS Suppositories 2657
Roxanol 2243

Opium Alkaloids (Additive effects).
No products indexed under this heading.

Oxazepam (Additive effects). Products include:
Serax Capsules 2810
Serax Tablets 2810

Oxycodone Hydrochloride (Additive effects). Products include:
Percocet Tablets 938
Percodan Tablets 939
Percodan-Demi Tablets 940
Roxicodone Tablets, Oral Solution & Intensol (Oxycodone) 2244
Tylox Capsules 1584

Pentobarbital Sodium (Additive effects). Products include:
Nembutal Sodium Capsules 436
Nembutal Sodium Solution 438
Nembutal Sodium Suppositories 440

Perphenazine (Additive effects). Products include:
Etrafon 2355

IMPORTANT NOTE: Always consult each drug listing in the patient's regimen for possible interactions.

Periactin | Interactions Index | 806

Triavil Tablets ... 1757
Trilafon ... 2389

Phenelzine Sulfate (Contraindication; anticholinergic effects of antihistamines prolonged and intensified). Products include:
Nardil ... 1920

Phenobarbital (Additive effects). Products include:
Arco-Lase Plus Tablets ... 512
Bellergal-S Tablets ... 2250
Donnatal ... 2060
Donnatal Extentabs ... 2061
Donnatal Tablets ... 2060
Phenobarbital Elixir and Tablets ... 1469
Quadrinal Tablets ... 1350

Prazepam (Additive effects).
No products indexed under this heading.

Prochlorperazine (Additive effects). Products include:
Compazine ... 2470

Promethazine Hydrochloride (Additive effects). Products include:
Mepergan Injection ... 2753
Phenergan with Codeine ... 2777
Phenergan with Dextromethorphan 2778
Phenergan Injection ... 2773
Phenergan Suppositories ... 2775
Phenergan Syrup ... 2774
Phenergan Tablets ... 2775
Phenergan VC ... 2779
Phenergan VC with Codeine ... 2781

Propofol (Additive effects). Products include:
Diprivan Injection ... 2833

Propoxyphene Hydrochloride (Additive effects). Products include:
Darvon ... 1435
Wygesic Tablets ... 2827

Propoxyphene Napsylate (Additive effects). Products include:
Darvon-N/Darvocet-N ... 1433

Quazepam (Additive effects). Products include:
Doral Tablets ... 2664

Risperidone (Additive effects). Products include:
Risperdal ... 1301

Secobarbital Sodium (Additive effects). Products include:
Seconal Sodium Pulvules ... 1474

Selegiline Hydrochloride (Contraindication; anticholinergic effects of antihistamines prolonged and intensified). Products include:
Eldepryl Tablets ... 2550

Sufentanil Citrate (Additive effects). Products include:
Sufenta Injection ... 1309

Temazepam (Additive effects). Products include:
Restoril Capsules ... 2284

Thiamylal Sodium (Additive effects).
No products indexed under this heading.

Thioridazine Hydrochloride (Additive effects). Products include:
Mellaril ... 2269

Thiothixene (Additive effects). Products include:
Navane Capsules and Concentrate 2201
Navane Intramuscular ... 2202

Tranylcypromine Sulfate (Contraindication; anticholinergic effects of antihistamines prolonged and intensified). Products include:
Parnate Tablets ... 2503

Triazolam (Additive effects). Products include:
Halcion Tablets ... 2611

Trifluoperazine Hydrochloride (Additive effects). Products include:
Stelazine ... 2514

Zolpidem Tartrate (Additive effects). Products include:
Ambien Tablets ... 2416

Food Interactions

Alcohol (Additive effects).

PERIACTIN TABLETS
(Cyproheptadine Hydrochloride) ... 1724
See **Periactin Syrup**

PERI-COLACE
(Casanthranol, Docusate Sodium) ... 2052
None cited in PDR database.

PERIDEX
(Chlorhexidine Gluconate) ... 1978
None cited in PDR database.

PERMAX TABLETS
(Pergolide Mesylate) ... 575
May interact with dopamine antagonists, highly protein bound drugs (selected), and certain other agents. Compounds in these categories include:

Amiodarone Hydrochloride (Caution should be exercised if coadministered). Products include:
Cordarone Intravenous ... 2715
Cordarone Tablets ... 2712

Amitriptyline Hydrochloride (Caution should be exercised if coadministered). Products include:
Elavil ... 2838
Endep Tablets ... 2174
Etrafon ... 2355
Limbitrol ... 2180
Triavil Tablets ... 1757

Atovaquone (Caution should be exercised if coadministered). Products include:
Mepron Suspension ... 1135

Cefonicid Sodium (Caution should be exercised if coadministered). Products include:
Monocid Injection ... 2497

Chlordiazepoxide (Caution should be exercised if coadministered). Products include:
Libritabs Tablets ... 2177
Limbitrol ... 2180

Chlordiazepoxide Hydrochloride (Caution should be exercised if coadministered). Products include:
Librax Capsules ... 2176
Librium Capsules ... 2178
Librium Injectable ... 2179

Chlorpromazine (May diminish the effectiveness of Permax; caution should be exercised if coadministered). Products include:
Thorazine Suppositories ... 2523

Clomipramine Hydrochloride (Caution should be exercised if coadministered). Products include:
Anafranil Capsules ... 803

Clozapine (May diminish the effectiveness of Permax). Products include:
Clozaril Tablets ... 2252

Cyclosporine (Caution should be exercised if coadministered). Products include:
Neoral ... 2276
Sandimmune ... 2286

Diazepam (Caution should be exercised if coadministered). Products include:
Dizac ... 1809
Valium Injectable ... 2182
Valium Tablets ... 2183
Valrelease Capsules ... 2169

Diclofenac Potassium (Caution should be exercised if coadministered). Products include:
Cataflam ... 816

Diclofenac Sodium (Caution should be exercised if coadministered). Products include:
Voltaren Ophthalmic Sterile Ophthalmic Solution ... ⊙ 272
Voltaren Tablets ... 861

Dipyridamole (Caution should be exercised if coadministered). Products include:
Persantine Tablets ... 681

Fenoprofen Calcium (Caution should be exercised if coadministered). Products include:
Nalfon 200 Pulvules & Nalfon Tablets ... 917

Fluphenazine Decanoate (May diminish the effectiveness of Permax). Products include:
Prolixin Decanoate ... 509

Fluphenazine Enanthate (May diminish the effectiveness of Permax). Products include:
Prolixin Enanthate ... 509

Fluphenazine Hydrochloride (May diminish the effectiveness of Permax). Products include:
Prolixin ... 509

Flurazepam Hydrochloride (Caution should be exercised if coadministered). Products include:
Dalmane Capsules ... 2173

Flurbiprofen (Caution should be exercised if coadministered). Products include:
Ansaid Tablets ... 2579

Glipizide (Caution should be exercised if coadministered). Products include:
Glucotrol Tablets ... 1967
Glucotrol XL Extended Release Tablets ... 1968

Haloperidol (May diminish the effectiveness of Permax). Products include:
Haldol Injection, Tablets and Concentrate ... 1575

Haloperidol Decanoate (May diminish the effectiveness of Permax). Products include:
Haldol Decanoate ... 1577

Ibuprofen (Caution should be exercised if coadministered). Products include:
Advil Cold and Sinus Caplets and Tablets (formerly CoAdvil) ... ⊡ 870
Advil Ibuprofen Tablets and Caplets ... ⊡ 870
Children's Advil Suspension ... 2692
Arthritis Foundation Ibuprofen Tablets ... ⊡ 674
Bayer Select Ibuprofen Pain Relief Formula ... ⊡ 715
Cramp End Tablets ... ⊡ 735
Dimetapp Sinus Caplets ... ⊡ 775
Haltran Tablets ... ⊡ 771
IBU Tablets ... 1342
Ibuprohm ... ⊡ 735
Children's Motrin Ibuprofen Oral Suspension ... 1546
Motrin Tablets ... 2625
Motrin IB Caplets, Tablets, and Geltabs ... ⊡ 838
Motrin IB Sinus ... ⊡ 838
Motrin Ibuprofen Suspension, Oral Drops, Chewable Tablets, Caplets ... 1546
Nuprin Ibuprofen/Analgesic Tablets & Caplets ... ⊡ 622
Sine-Aid IB Caplets ... 1554
Vicks DayQuil SINUS Pressure & PAIN Relief with IBUPROFEN ... ⊡ 762

Imipramine Hydrochloride (Caution should be exercised if coadministered). Products include:
Tofranil Ampuls ... 854
Tofranil Tablets ... 856

Imipramine Pamoate (Caution should be exercised if coadministered). Products include:
Tofranil-PM Capsules ... 857

Indomethacin (Caution should be exercised if coadministered). Products include:
Indocin ... 1680

Indomethacin Sodium Trihydrate (Caution should be exercised if coadministered). Products include:
Indocin I.V. ... 1684

Ketoprofen (Caution should be exercised if coadministered). Products include:
Orudis Capsules ... 2766
Oruvail Capsules ... 2766

Ketorolac Tromethamine (Caution should be exercised if coadministered). Products include:
Acular ... 474
Acular ... ⊙ 277
Toradol ... 2159

Levodopa (Concomitant use may cause and/or exacerbate preexisting states of confusion and hallucination). Products include:
Atamet ... 572
Larodopa Tablets ... 2129
Sinemet Tablets ... 943
Sinemet CR Tablets ... 944

Meclofenamate Sodium (Caution should be exercised if coadministered).
No products indexed under this heading.

Mefenamic Acid (Caution should be exercised if coadministered). Products include:
Ponstel ... 1925

Mesoridazine Besylate (May diminish the effectiveness of Permax). Products include:
Serentil ... 684

Metoclopramide Hydrochloride (May diminish the effectiveness of Permax). Products include:
Reglan ... 2068

Midazolam Hydrochloride (Caution should be exercised if coadministered). Products include:
Versed Injection ... 2170

Naproxen (Caution should be exercised if coadministered). Products include:
Anaprox/Naprosyn ... 2117

Naproxen Sodium (Caution should be exercised if coadministered). Products include:
Aleve ... 1975
Anaprox/Naprosyn ... 2117

Nortriptyline Hydrochloride (Caution should be exercised if coadministered). Products include:
Pamelor ... 2280

Oxaprozin (Caution should be exercised if coadministered). Products include:
Daypro Caplets ... 2426

Oxazepam (Caution should be exercised if coadministered). Products include:
Serax Capsules ... 2810
Serax Tablets ... 2810

Perphenazine (May diminish the effectiveness of Permax). Products include:
Etrafon ... 2355
Triavil Tablets ... 1757
Trilafon ... 2389

Phenylbutazone (Caution should be exercised if coadministered).
No products indexed under this heading.

Pimozide (May diminish the effectiveness of Permax). Products include:
Orap Tablets ... 1050

Piroxicam (Caution should be exercised if coadministered). Products include:
Feldene Capsules ... 1965

Prochlorperazine (May diminish the effectiveness of Permax). Products include:
Compazine ... 2470

(⊡ Described in PDR For Nonprescription Drugs) (⊙ Described in PDR For Ophthalmology)

807 Interactions Index Phenergan with Codeine

Promethazine Hydrochloride (May diminish the effectiveness of Permax). Products include:
Mepergan Injection ... 2753
Phenergan with Codeine ... 2777
Phenergan with Dextromethorphan 2778
Phenergan Injection ... 2773
Phenergan Suppositories ... 2775
Phenergan Syrup ... 2774
Phenergan Tablets ... 2775
Phenergan VC ... 2779
Phenergan VC with Codeine ... 2781

Propranolol Hydrochloride (Caution should be exercised if coadministered). Products include:
Inderal ... 2728
Inderal LA Long Acting Capsules ... 2730
Inderide Tablets ... 2732
Inderide LA Long Acting Capsules .. 2734

Sulindac (Caution should be exercised if coadministered). Products include:
Clinoril Tablets ... 1618

Temazepam (Caution should be exercised if coadministered). Products include:
Restoril Capsules ... 2284

Thioridazine Hydrochloride (May diminish the effectiveness of Permax). Products include:
Mellaril ... 2269

Thiothixene (May diminish the effectiveness of Permax). Products include:
Navane Capsules and Concentrate 2201
Navane Intramuscular ... 2202

Tolbutamide (Caution should be exercised if coadministered).
No products indexed under this heading.

Tolmetin Sodium (Caution should be exercised if coadministered). Products include:
Tolectin (200, 400 and 600 mg) .. 1581

Trifluoperazine Hydrochloride (May diminish the effectiveness of Permax). Products include:
Stelazine ... 2514

Trimipramine Maleate (Caution should be exercised if coadministered). Products include:
Surmontil Capsules ... 2811

Warfarin Sodium (Caution should be exercised if coadministered). Products include:
Coumadin ... 926

PERSANTINE TABLETS
(Dipyridamole) ... 681
None cited in PDR database.

PFIZERPEN FOR INJECTION
(Penicillin G Potassium) ... 2203
May interact with tetracyclines and certain other agents. Compounds in these categories include:

Demeclocycline Hydrochloride (May diminish bactericidal effects of penicillins). Products include:
Declomycin Tablets ... 1371

Doxycycline Calcium (May diminish bactericidal effects of penicillins). Products include:
Vibramycin Calcium Oral Suspension Syrup ... 1941

Doxycycline Hyclate (May diminish bactericidal effects of penicillins). Products include:
Doryx Capsules ... 1913
Vibramycin Hyclate Capsules ... 1941
Vibramycin Hyclate Intravenous ... 2215
Vibra-Tabs Film Coated Tablets ... 1941

Doxycycline Monohydrate (May diminish bactericidal effects of penicillins). Products include:
Monodox Capsules ... 1805
Vibramycin Monohydrate for Oral Suspension ... 1941

Erythromycin (May diminish bactericidal effects of penicillin). Products include:
A/T/S 2% Acne Topical Gel and Solution ... 1234
Benzamycin Topical Gel ... 905
E-Mycin Tablets ... 1341
Emgel 2% Topical Gel ... 1093
ERYC ... 1915
Erycette (erythromycin 2%) Topical Solution ... 1888
Ery-Tab Tablets ... 422
Erythromycin Base Filmtab ... 426
Erythromycin Delayed-Release Capsules, USP ... 427
Ilotycin Ophthalmic Ointment ... 912
PCE Dispertab Tablets ... 444
T-Stat 2.0% Topical Solution and Pads ... 2688
Theramycin Z Topical Solution 2% 1592

Erythromycin Estolate (May diminish bactericidal effects of penicillin). Products include:
Ilosone ... 911

Erythromycin Ethylsuccinate (May diminish bactericidal effects of penicillin). Products include:
E.E.S. ... 424
EryPed ... 421

Erythromycin Gluceptate (May diminish bactericidal effects of penicillin). Products include:
Ilotycin Gluceptate, IV, Vials ... 913

Erythromycin Stearate (May diminish bactericidal effects of penicillin). Products include:
Erythrocin Stearate Filmtab ... 425

Methacycline Hydrochloride (May diminish bactericidal effects of penicillins).
No products indexed under this heading.

Minocycline Hydrochloride (May diminish bactericidal effects of penicillins). Products include:
Dynacin Capsules ... 1590
Minocin Intravenous ... 1382
Minocin Oral Suspension ... 1385
Minocin Pellet-Filled Capsules ... 1383

Oxytetracycline Hydrochloride (May diminish bactericidal effects of penicillins). Products include:
TERAK Ointment ... ⊙ 209
Terra-Cortril Ophthalmic Suspension ... 2210
Terramycin with Polymyxin B Sulfate Ophthalmic Ointment ... 2211
Urobiotic-250 Capsules ... 2214

Probenecid (Penicillin blood levels may be prolonged). Products include:
Benemid Tablets ... 1611
ColBENEMID Tablets ... 1622

Tetracycline Hydrochloride (May diminish bactericidal effects of penicillins). Products include:
Achromycin V Capsules ... 1367

PHAZYME DROPS
(Simethicone) ... ▣ 767
None cited in PDR database.

PHAZYME TABLETS
(Simethicone) ... ▣ 767
None cited in PDR database.

PHAZYME-95 TABLETS
(Simethicone) ... ▣ 767
None cited in PDR database.

PHAZYME-125 CHEWABLE TABLETS
(Simethicone) ... ▣ 767
None cited in PDR database.

PHAZYME-125 SOFTGELS MAXIMUM STRENGTH
(Simethicone) ... ▣ 767
None cited in PDR database.

PHENERGAN WITH CODEINE
(Codeine Phosphate, Promethazine Hydrochloride) ... 2777
May interact with narcotic analgesics, hypnotics and sedatives, tricyclic antidepressants, tranquilizers, monoamine oxidase inhibitors, and certain other agents. Compounds in these categories include:

Alfentanil Hydrochloride (Additive sedative effects). Products include:
Alfenta Injection ... 1286

Alprazolam (Additive sedative effects). Products include:
Xanax Tablets ... 2649

Amitriptyline Hydrochloride (Additive sedative effects). Products include:
Elavil ... 2838
Endep Tablets ... 2174
Etrafon ... 2355
Limbitrol ... 2180
Triavil Tablets ... 1757

Amoxapine (Additive sedative effects). Products include:
Asendin Tablets ... 1369

Buprenorphine (Additive sedative effects). Products include:
Buprenex Injectable ... 2006

Buspirone Hydrochloride (Additive sedative effects). Products include:
BuSpar ... 737

Chlordiazepoxide (Additive sedative effects). Products include:
Libritabs Tablets ... 2177
Limbitrol ... 2180

Chlordiazepoxide Hydrochloride (Additive sedative effects). Products include:
Librax Capsules ... 2176
Librium Capsules ... 2178
Librium Injectable ... 2179

Chlorpromazine (Additive sedative effects). Products include:
Thorazine Suppositories ... 2523

Chlorprothixene (Additive sedative effects).
No products indexed under this heading.

Chlorprothixene Hydrochloride (Additive sedative effects).
No products indexed under this heading.

Clomipramine Hydrochloride (Additive sedative effects). Products include:
Anafranil Capsules ... 803

Clorazepate Dipotassium (Additive sedative effects). Products include:
Tranxene ... 451

Desipramine Hydrochloride (Additive sedative effects). Products include:
Norpramin Tablets ... 1526

Dezocine (Additive sedative effects). Products include:
Dalgan Injection ... 538

Diazepam (Additive sedative effects). Products include:
Dizac ... 1809
Valium Injectable ... 2182
Valium Tablets ... 2183
Valrelease Capsules ... 2169

Doxepin Hydrochloride (Additive sedative effects). Products include:
Sinequan ... 2205
Zonalon Cream ... 1055

Droperidol (Additive sedative effects). Products include:
Inapsine Injection ... 1296

Estazolam (Additive sedative effects). Products include:
ProSom Tablets ... 449

Ethchlorvynol (Additive sedative effects). Products include:
Placidyl Capsules ... 448

Ethinamate (Additive sedative effects).
No products indexed under this heading.

Fentanyl (Additive sedative effects). Products include:
Duragesic Transdermal System ... 1288

Fentanyl Citrate (Additive sedative effects). Products include:
Sublimaze Injection ... 1307

Fluphenazine Decanoate (Additive sedative effects). Products include:
Prolixin Decanoate ... 509

Fluphenazine Enanthate (Additive sedative effects). Products include:
Prolixin Enanthate ... 509

Fluphenazine Hydrochloride (Additive sedative effects). Products include:
Prolixin ... 509

Flurazepam Hydrochloride (Additive sedative effects). Products include:
Dalmane Capsules ... 2173

Furazolidone (Excessive narcotic effects). Products include:
Furoxone ... 2046

Glutethimide (Additive sedative effects).
No products indexed under this heading.

Haloperidol (Additive sedative effects). Products include:
Haldol Injection, Tablets and Concentrate ... 1575

Haloperidol Decanoate (Additive sedative effects). Products include:
Haldol Decanoate ... 1577

Hydrocodone Bitartrate (Additive sedative effects). Products include:
Anexsia 5/500 Elixir ... 1781
Anexia Tablets ... 1782
Codiclear DH Syrup ... 791
Deconamine CX Cough and Cold Liquid and Tablets ... 1319
Duratuss HD Elixir ... 2565
Hycodan Tablets and Syrup ... 930
Hycomine Compound Tablets ... 932
Hycomine ... 931
Hycotuss Expectorant Syrup ... 933
Hydrocet Capsules ... 782
Lorcet 10/650 ... 1018
Lortab ... 2566
Tussend ... 1783
Tussend Expectorant ... 1785
Vicodin Tablets ... 1356
Vicodin ES Tablets ... 1357
Vicodin Tuss Expectorant ... 1358
Zydone Capsules ... 949

Hydrocodone Polistirex (Additive sedative effects). Products include:
Tussionex Pennkinetic Extended-Release Suspension ... 998

Hydroxyzine Hydrochloride (Additive sedative effects). Products include:
Atarax Tablets & Syrup ... 2185
Marax Tablets & DF Syrup ... 2200
Vistaril Intramuscular Solution ... 2216

Imipramine Hydrochloride (Additive sedative effects). Products include:
Tofranil Ampuls ... 854
Tofranil Tablets ... 856

Imipramine Pamoate (Additive sedative effects). Products include:
Tofranil-PM Capsules ... 857

Isocarboxazid (Excessive narcotic effects).
No products indexed under this heading.

IMPORTANT NOTE: Always consult each drug listing in the patient's regimen for possible interactions.

Levorphanol Tartrate (Additive sedative effects). Products include:
Levo-Dromoran 2129

Lorazepam (Additive sedative effects). Products include:
Ativan Injection 2698
Ativan Tablets 2700

Loxapine Hydrochloride (Additive sedative effects). Products include:
Loxitane 1378

Maprotiline Hydrochloride (Additive sedative effects). Products include:
Ludiomil Tablets 843

Meperidine Hydrochloride (Additive sedative effects). Products include:
Demerol 2308
Mepergan Injection 2753

Meprobamate (Additive sedative effects). Products include:
Miltown Tablets 2672
PMB 200 and PMB 400 2783

Mesoridazine Besylate (Additive sedative effects). Products include:
Serentil 684

Methadone Hydrochloride (Additive sedative effects). Products include:
Methadone Hydrochloride Oral Concentrate 2233
Methadone Hydrochloride Oral Solution & Tablets 2235

Midazolam Hydrochloride (Additive sedative effects). Products include:
Versed Injection 2170

Molindone Hydrochloride (Additive sedative effects). Products include:
Moban Tablets and Concentrate 1048

Morphine Sulfate (Additive sedative effects). Products include:
Astramorph/PF Injection, USP (Preservative-Free) 535
Duramorph 962
Infumorph 200 and Infumorph 500 Sterile Solutions 965
MS Contin Tablets 1994
MSIR 1997
Oramorph SR (Morphine Sulfate Sustained Release Tablets) 2236
RMS Suppositories 2657
Roxanol 2243

Nortriptyline Hydrochloride (Additive sedative effects). Products include:
Pamelor 2280

Opium Alkaloids (Additive sedative effects).
No products indexed under this heading.

Oxazepam (Additive sedative effects). Products include:
Serax Capsules 2810
Serax Tablets 2810

Oxycodone Hydrochloride (Additive sedative effects). Products include:
Percocet Tablets 938
Percodan Tablets 939
Percodan-Demi Tablets 940
Roxicodone Tablets, Oral Solution & Intensol (Oxycodone) 2244
Tylox Capsules 1584

Perphenazine (Additive sedative effects). Products include:
Etrafon 2355
Triavil Tablets 1757
Trilafon 2389

Phenelzine Sulfate (Excessive narcotic effects). Products include:
Nardil 1920

Prazepam (Additive sedative effects).
No products indexed under this heading.

Prochlorperazine (Additive sedative effects). Products include:
Compazine 2470

Propofol (Additive sedative effects). Products include:
Diprivan Injection 2833

Propoxyphene Hydrochloride (Additive sedative effects). Products include:
Darvon 1435
Wygesic Tablets 2827

Propoxyphene Napsylate (Additive sedative effects). Products include:
Darvon-N/Darvocet-N 1433

Protriptyline Hydrochloride (Additive sedative effects). Products include:
Vivactil Tablets 1774

Quazepam (Additive sedative effects). Products include:
Doral Tablets 2664

Secobarbital Sodium (Additive sedative effects). Products include:
Seconal Sodium Pulvules 1474

Selegiline Hydrochloride (Excessive narcotic effects). Products include:
Eldepryl Tablets 2550

Sufentanil Citrate (Additive sedative effects). Products include:
Sufenta Injection 1309

Temazepam (Additive sedative effects). Products include:
Restoril Capsules 2284

Thioridazine Hydrochloride (Additive sedative effects). Products include:
Mellaril 2269

Thiothixene (Additive sedative effects). Products include:
Navane Capsules and Concentrate 2201
Navane Intramuscular 2202

Tranylcypromine Sulfate (Excessive narcotic effects). Products include:
Parnate Tablets 2503

Triazolam (Additive sedative effects). Products include:
Halcion Tablets 2611

Trifluoperazine Hydrochloride (Additive sedative effects). Products include:
Stelazine 2514

Trimipramine Maleate (Additive sedative effects). Products include:
Surmontil Capsules 2811

Zolpidem Tartrate (Additive sedative effects). Products include:
Ambien Tablets 2416

Food Interactions

Alcohol (Additive sedative effects).

PHENERGAN WITH DEXTROMETHORPHAN

(Promethazine Hydrochloride, Dextromethorphan Hydrobromide) 2778
May interact with narcotic analgesics, hypnotics and sedatives, tricyclic antidepressants, tranquilizers, and certain other agents. Compounds in these categories include:

Alfentanil Hydrochloride (Additive sedative effects). Products include:
Alfenta Injection 1286

Alprazolam (Additive sedative effects). Products include:
Xanax Tablets 2649

Amitriptyline Hydrochloride (Additive sedative effects). Products include:
Elavil 2838
Endep Tablets 2174
Etrafon 2355
Limbitrol 2180
Triavil Tablets 1757

Amoxapine (Additive sedative effects). Products include:
Asendin Tablets 1369

Buprenorphine (Additive sedative effects). Products include:
Buprenex Injectable 2006

Buspirone Hydrochloride (Additive sedative effects). Products include:
BuSpar 737

Chlordiazepoxide (Additive sedative effects). Products include:
Libritabs Tablets 2177
Limbitrol 2180

Chlordiazepoxide Hydrochloride (Additive sedative effects). Products include:
Librax Capsules 2176
Librium Capsules 2178
Librium Injectable 2179

Chlorpromazine (Additive sedative effects). Products include:
Thorazine Suppositories 2523

Clomipramine Hydrochloride (Additive sedative effects). Products include:
Anafranil Capsules 803

Clorazepate Dipotassium (Additive sedative effects). Products include:
Tranxene 451

Codeine Phosphate (Additive sedative effects). Products include:
Actifed with Codeine Cough Syrup 1067
Brontex 1981
Deconsal C Expectorant Syrup 456
Deconsal Pediatric Syrup 457
Dimetane-DC Cough Syrup 2059
Empirin with Codeine Tablets 1093
Fioricet with Codeine Capsules 2260
Fiorinal with Codeine Capsules 2262
Isoclor Expectorant 990
Novahistine DH 2462
Novahistine Expectorant 2463
Nucofed 2051
Phenergan with Codeine 2777
Phenergan VC with Codeine 2781
Robitussin A-C Syrup 2073
Robitussin-DAC Syrup 2074
Ryna ▣ 841
Soma Compound w/Codeine Tablets 2676
Tussi-Organidin NR Liquid and S NR Liquid 2677
Tylenol with Codeine 1583

Desipramine Hydrochloride (Additive sedative effects). Products include:
Norpramin Tablets 1526

Dezocine (Additive sedative effects). Products include:
Dalgan Injection 538

Diazepam (Additive sedative effects). Products include:
Dizac 1809
Valium Injectable 2182
Valium Tablets 2183
Valrelease Capsules 2169

Doxepin Hydrochloride (Additive sedative effects). Products include:
Sinequan 2205
Zonalon Cream 1055

Droperidol (Additive sedative effects). Products include:
Inapsine Injection 1296

Estazolam (Additive sedative effects). Products include:
ProSom Tablets 449

Ethchlorvynol (Additive sedative effects). Products include:
Placidyl Capsules 448

Ethinamate (Additive sedative effects).
No products indexed under this heading.

Fentanyl (Additive sedative effects). Products include:
Duragesic Transdermal System 1288

Fentanyl Citrate (Additive sedative effects). Products include:
Sublimaze Injection 1307

Fluphenazine Decanoate (Additive sedative effects). Products include:
Prolixin Decanoate 509

Fluphenazine Enanthate (Additive sedative effects). Products include:
Prolixin Enanthate 509

Fluphenazine Hydrochloride (Additive sedative effects). Products include:
Prolixin 509

Flurazepam Hydrochloride (Additive sedative effects). Products include:
Dalmane Capsules 2173

Glutethimide (Additive sedative effects).
No products indexed under this heading.

Haloperidol (Additive sedative effects). Products include:
Haldol Injection, Tablets and Concentrate 1575

Haloperidol Decanoate (Additive sedative effects). Products include:
Haldol Decanoate 1577

Hydrocodone Bitartrate (Additive sedative effects). Products include:
Anexsia 5/500 Elixir 1781
Anexia Tablets 1782
Codiclear DH Syrup 791
Deconamine CX Cough and Cold Liquid and Tablets 1319
Duratuss HD Elixir 2565
Hycodan Tablets and Syrup 930
Hycomine Compound Tablets 932
Hycomine 931
Hycotuss Expectorant Syrup 933
Hydrocet Capsules 782
Lorcet 10/650 1018
Lortab 2566
Tussend 1783
Tussend Expectorant 1785
Vicodin Tablets 1356
Vicodin ES Tablets 1357
Vicodin Tuss Expectorant 1358
Zydone Capsules 949

Hydrocodone Polistirex (Additive sedative effects). Products include:
Tussionex Pennkinetic Extended-Release Suspension 998

Hydroxyzine Hydrochloride (Additive sedative effects). Products include:
Atarax Tablets & Syrup 2185
Marax Tablets & DF Syrup 2200
Vistaril Intramuscular Solution 2216

Imipramine Hydrochloride (Additive sedative effects). Products include:
Tofranil Ampuls 854
Tofranil Tablets 856

Imipramine Pamoate (Additive sedative effects). Products include:
Tofranil-PM Capsules 857

Levorphanol Tartrate (Additive sedative effects). Products include:
Levo-Dromoran 2129

Lorazepam (Additive sedative effects). Products include:
Ativan Injection 2698
Ativan Tablets 2700

Loxapine Hydrochloride (Additive sedative effects). Products include:
Loxitane 1378

Maprotiline Hydrochloride (Additive sedative effects). Products include:
Ludiomil Tablets 843

Meperidine Hydrochloride (Additive sedative effects). Products include:
Demerol 2308

809 **Interactions Index** **Phenergan Injection**

Mepergan Injection 2753

Meprobamate (Additive sedative effects). Products include:

Miltown Tablets 2672
PMB 200 and PMB 400 2783

Mesoridazine Besylate (Additive sedative effects). Products include:

Serentil 684

Methadone Hydrochloride (Additive sedative effects). Products include:

Methadone Hydrochloride Oral Concentrate 2233
Methadone Hydrochloride Oral Solution & Tablets 2235

Midazolam Hydrochloride (Additive sedative effects). Products include:

Versed Injection 2170

Molindone Hydrochloride (Additive sedative effects). Products include:

Moban Tablets and Concentrate 1048

Morphine Sulfate (Additive sedative effects). Products include:

Astramorph/PF Injection, USP (Preservative-Free) 535
Duramorph 962
Infumorph 200 and Infumorph 500 Sterile Solutions 965
MS Contin Tablets 1994
MSIR 1997
Oramorph SR (Morphine Sulfate Sustained Release Tablets) 2236
RMS Suppositories 2657
Roxanol 2243

Nortriptyline Hydrochloride (Additive sedative effects). Products include:

Pamelor 2280

Opium Alkaloids (Additive sedative effects).

No products indexed under this heading.

Oxazepam (Additive sedative effects). Products include:

Serax Capsules 2810
Serax Tablets 2810

Oxycodone Hydrochloride (Additive sedative effects). Products include:

Percocet Tablets 938
Percodan Tablets 939
Percodan-Demi Tablets 940
Roxicodone Tablets, Oral Solution & Intensol (Oxycodone) 2244
Tylox Capsules 1584

Perphenazine (Additive sedative effects). Products include:

Etrafon 2355
Triavil Tablets 1757
Trilafon 2389

Prazepam (Additive sedative effects).

No products indexed under this heading.

Prochlorperazine (Additive sedative effects). Products include:

Compazine 2470

Propofol (Additive sedative effects). Products include:

Diprivan Injection 2833

Propoxyphene Hydrochloride (Additive sedative effects). Products include:

Darvon 1435
Wygesic Tablets 2827

Propoxyphene Napsylate (Additive sedative effects). Products include:

Darvon-N/Darvocet-N 1433

Protriptyline Hydrochloride (Additive sedative effects). Products include:

Vivactil Tablets 1774

Quazepam (Additive sedative effects). Products include:

Doral Tablets 2664

Secobarbital Sodium (Additive sedative effects). Products include:

Seconal Sodium Pulvules 1474

Sufentanil Citrate (Additive sedative effects). Products include:

Sufenta Injection 1309

Temazepam (Additive sedative effects). Products include:

Restoril Capsules 2284

Thioridazine Hydrochloride (Additive sedative effects). Products include:

Mellaril 2269

Thiothixene (Additive sedative effects). Products include:

Navane Capsules and Concentrate 2201
Navane Intramuscular 2202

Triazolam (Additive sedative effects). Products include:

Halcion Tablets 2611

Trifluoperazine Hydrochloride (Additive sedative effects). Products include:

Stelazine 2514

Trimipramine Maleate (Additive sedative effects). Products include:

Surmontil Capsules 2811

Zolpidem Tartrate (Additive sedative effects). Products include:

Ambien Tablets 2416

Food Interactions

Alcohol (Additive sedative effects).

PHENERGAN INJECTION

(Promethazine Hydrochloride) 2773

May interact with narcotic analgesics, barbiturates, hypnotics and sedatives, general anesthetics, tranquilizers, central nervous system depressants, monoamine oxidase inhibitors, and certain other agents. Compounds in these categories include:

Alfentanil Hydrochloride (Additive sedative effects). Products include:

Alfenta Injection 1286

Alprazolam (Additive sedative effects). Products include:

Xanax Tablets 2649

Aprobarbital (Additive sedative effects).

No products indexed under this heading.

Buprenorphine (Additive sedative effects). Products include:

Buprenex Injectable 2006

Buspirone Hydrochloride (Additive sedative effects). Products include:

BuSpar 737

Butabarbital (Additive sedative effects).

No products indexed under this heading.

Butalbital (Additive sedative effects). Products include:

Esgic-plus Tablets 1013
Fioricet Tablets 2258
Fioricet with Codeine Capsules 2260
Fiorinal Capsules 2261
Fiorinal with Codeine Capsules 2262
Fiorinal Tablets 2261
Phrenilin 785
Sedapap Tablets 50 mg/650 mg 1543

Chlordiazepoxide (Additive sedative effects). Products include:

Libritabs Tablets 2177
Limbitrol 2180

Chlordiazepoxide Hydrochloride (Additive sedative effects). Products include:

Librax Capsules 2176
Librium Capsules 2178
Librium Injectable 2179

Chlorpromazine (Additive sedative effects). Products include:

Thorazine Suppositories 2523

Chlorprothixene (Additive sedative effects).

No products indexed under this heading.

Chlorprothixene Hydrochloride (Additive sedative effects).

No products indexed under this heading.

Clorazepate Dipotassium (Additive sedative effects). Products include:

Tranxene 451

Clozapine (Additive sedative effects). Products include:

Clozaril Tablets 2252

Codeine Phosphate (Additive sedative effects). Products include:

Actifed with Codeine Cough Syrup 1067
Brontex 1981
Deconsal C Expectorant Syrup 456
Deconsal Pediatric Syrup 457
Dimetane-DC Cough Syrup 2059
Empirin with Codeine Tablets 1093
Fioricet with Codeine Capsules 2260
Fiorinal with Codeine Capsules 2262
Isoclor Expectorant 990
Novahistine DH 2462
Novahistine Expectorant 2463
Nucofed 2051
Phenergan with Codeine 2777
Phenergan VC with Codeine 2781
Robitussin A-C Syrup 2073
Robitussin-DAC Syrup 2074
Ryna 841
Soma Compound w/Codeine Tablets 2676
Tussi-Organidin NR Liquid and S NR Liquid 2677
Tylenol with Codeine 1583

Desflurane (Additive sedative effects). Products include:

Suprane 1813

Dezocine (Additive sedative effects). Products include:

Dalgan Injection 538

Diazepam (Additive sedative effects). Products include:

Dizac 1809
Valium Injectable 2182
Valium Tablets 2183
Valrelease Capsules 2169

Droperidol (Additive sedative effects). Products include:

Inapsine Injection 1296

Enflurane (Additive sedative effects).

No products indexed under this heading.

Epinephrine Hydrochloride (Potential for reversal of the vasopressor effect). Products include:

Ana-Kit Anaphylaxis Emergency Treatment Kit 617

Estazolam (Additive sedative effects). Products include:

ProSom Tablets 449

Ethchlorvynol (Additive sedative effects). Products include:

Placidyl Capsules 448

Ethinamate (Additive sedative effects).

No products indexed under this heading.

Fentanyl (Additive sedative effects). Products include:

Duragesic Transdermal System 1288

Fentanyl Citrate (Additive sedative effects). Products include:

Sublimaze Injection 1307

Fluphenazine Decanoate (Additive sedative effects). Products include:

Prolixin Decanoate 509

Fluphenazine Enanthate (Additive sedative effects). Products include:

Prolixin Enanthate 509

Fluphenazine Hydrochloride (Additive sedative effects). Products include:

Prolixin 509

Flurazepam Hydrochloride (Additive sedative effects). Products include:

Dalmane Capsules 2173

Furazolidone (Possibility of increased incidence of extrapyramidal effects). Products include:

Furoxone 2046

Glutethimide (Additive sedative effects).

No products indexed under this heading.

Haloperidol (Additive sedative effects). Products include:

Haldol Injection, Tablets and Concentrate 1575

Haloperidol Decanoate (Additive sedative effects). Products include:

Haldol Decanoate 1577

Hydrocodone Bitartrate (Additive sedative effects). Products include:

Anexsia 5/500 Elixir 1781
Anexia Tablets 1782
Codiclear DH Syrup 791
Deconamine CX Cough and Cold Liquid and Tablets 1319
Duratuss HD Elixir 2565
Hycodan Tablets and Syrup 930
Hycomine Compound Tablets 932
Hycomine 931
Hycotuss Expectorant Syrup 933
Hydrocet Capsules 782
Lorcet 10/650 1018
Lortab 2566
Tussend 1783
Tussend Expectorant 1785
Vicodin Tablets 1356
Vicodin ES Tablets 1357
Vicodin Tuss Expectorant 1358
Zydone Capsules 949

Hydrocodone Polistirex (Additive sedative effects). Products include:

Tussionex Pennkinetic Extended-Release Suspension 998

Hydroxyzine Hydrochloride (Additive sedative effects). Products include:

Atarax Tablets & Syrup 2185
Marax Tablets & DF Syrup 2200
Vistaril Intramuscular Solution 2216

Isocarboxazid (Possibility of increased incidence of extrapyramidal effects).

No products indexed under this heading.

Isoflurane (Additive sedative effects).

No products indexed under this heading.

Ketamine Hydrochloride (Additive sedative effects).

No products indexed under this heading.

Levomethadyl Acetate Hydrochloride (Additive sedative effects). Products include:

Orlamm 2239

Levorphanol Tartrate (Additive sedative effects). Products include:

Levo-Dromoran 2129

Lorazepam (Additive sedative effects). Products include:

Ativan Injection 2698
Ativan Tablets 2700

Loxapine Hydrochloride (Additive sedative effects). Products include:

Loxitane 1378

Loxapine Succinate (Additive sedative effects). Products include:

Loxitane Capsules 1378

IMPORTANT NOTE: Always consult each drug listing in the patient's regimen for possible interactions.

Meperidine Hydrochloride (Additive sedative effects). Products include:
- Demerol ... 2308
- Mepergan Injection ... 2753

Mephobarbital (Additive sedative effects). Products include:
- Mebaral Tablets ... 2322

Meprobamate (Additive sedative effects). Products include:
- Miltown Tablets ... 2672
- PMB 200 and PMB 400 ... 2783

Mesoridazine Besylate (Additive sedative effects). Products include:
- Serentil ... 684

Methadone Hydrochloride (Additive sedative effects). Products include:
- Methadone Hydrochloride Oral Concentrate ... 2233
- Methadone Hydrochloride Oral Solution & Tablets ... 2235

Methohexital Sodium (Additive sedative effects). Products include:
- Brevital Sodium Vials ... 1429

Methotrimeprazine (Additive sedative effects). Products include:
- Levoprome ... 1274

Methoxyflurane (Additive sedative effects).
- No products indexed under this heading.

Midazolam Hydrochloride (Additive sedative effects). Products include:
- Versed Injection ... 2170

Molindone Hydrochloride (Additive sedative effects). Products include:
- Moban Tablets and Concentrate ... 1048

Morphine Sulfate (Additive sedative effects). Products include:
- Astramorph/PF Injection, USP (Preservative-Free) ... 535
- Duramorph ... 962
- Infumorph 200 and Infumorph 500 Sterile Solutions ... 965
- MS Contin Tablets ... 1994
- MSIR ... 1997
- Oramorph SR (Morphine Sulfate Sustained Release Tablets) ... 2236
- RMS Suppositories ... 2657
- Roxanol ... 2243

Opium Alkaloids (Additive sedative effects).
- No products indexed under this heading.

Oxazepam (Additive sedative effects). Products include:
- Serax Capsules ... 2810
- Serax Tablets ... 2810

Oxycodone Hydrochloride (Additive sedative effects). Products include:
- Percocet Tablets ... 938
- Percodan Tablets ... 939
- Percodan-Demi Tablets ... 940
- Roxicodone Tablets, Oral Solution & Intensol (Oxycodone) ... 2244
- Tylox Capsules ... 1584

Pentobarbital Sodium (Additive sedative effects). Products include:
- Nembutal Sodium Capsules ... 436
- Nembutal Sodium Solution ... 438
- Nembutal Sodium Suppositories ... 440

Perphenazine (Additive sedative effects). Products include:
- Etrafon ... 2355
- Triavil Tablets ... 1757
- Trilafon ... 2389

Phenelzine Sulfate (Possibility of increased incidence of extrapyramidal effects). Products include:
- Nardil ... 1920

Phenobarbital (Additive sedative effects). Products include:
- Arco-Lase Plus Tablets ... 512
- Bellergal-S Tablets ... 2250
- Donnatal ... 2060
- Donnatal Extentabs ... 2061
- Donnatal Tablets ... 2060
- Phenobarbital Elixir and Tablets ... 1469
- Quadrinal Tablets ... 1350

Prazepam (Additive sedative effects).
- No products indexed under this heading.

Prochlorperazine (Additive sedative effects). Products include:
- Compazine ... 2470

Propofol (Additive sedative effects). Products include:
- Diprivan Injection ... 2833

Propoxyphene Hydrochloride (Additive sedative effects). Products include:
- Darvon ... 1435
- Wygesic Tablets ... 2827

Propoxyphene Napsylate (Additive sedative effects). Products include:
- Darvon-N/Darvocet-N ... 1433

Quazepam (Additive sedative effects). Products include:
- Doral Tablets ... 2664

Risperidone (Additive sedative effects). Products include:
- Risperdal ... 1301

Secobarbital Sodium (Additive sedative effects). Products include:
- Seconal Sodium Pulvules ... 1474

Selegiline Hydrochloride (Possibility of increased incidence of extrapyramidal effects). Products include:
- Eldepryl Tablets ... 2550

Sufentanil Citrate (Additive sedative effects). Products include:
- Sufenta Injection ... 1309

Temazepam (Additive sedative effects). Products include:
- Restoril Capsules ... 2284

Thiamylal Sodium (Additive sedative effects).
- No products indexed under this heading.

Thioridazine Hydrochloride (Additive sedative effects). Products include:
- Mellaril ... 2269

Thiothixene (Additive sedative effects). Products include:
- Navane Capsules and Concentrate ... 2201
- Navane Intramuscular ... 2202

Tranylcypromine Sulfate (Possibility of increased incidence of extrapyramidal effects). Products include:
- Parnate Tablets ... 2503

Triazolam (Additive sedative effects). Products include:
- Halcion Tablets ... 2611

Trifluoperazine Hydrochloride (Additive sedative effects). Products include:
- Stelazine ... 2514

Zolpidem Tartrate (Additive sedative effects). Products include:
- Ambien Tablets ... 2416

Food Interactions

Alcohol (Additive sedative effects).

PHENERGAN SUPPOSITORIES

(Promethazine Hydrochloride) ... 2775

May interact with narcotic analgesics, hypnotics and sedatives, tricyclic antidepressants, tranquilizers, central nervous system depressants, barbiturates, and certain other agents. Compounds in these categories include:

Alfentanil Hydrochloride (Additive sedative effects). Products include:
- Alfenta Injection ... 1286

Alprazolam (Additive sedative effects). Products include:
- Xanax Tablets ... 2649

Amitriptyline Hydrochloride (Additive sedative effects). Products include:
- Elavil ... 2838
- Endep Tablets ... 2174
- Etrafon ... 2355
- Limbitrol ... 2180
- Triavil Tablets ... 1757

Amoxapine (Additive sedative effects). Products include:
- Asendin Tablets ... 1369

Aprobarbital (Additive sedative effects; reduce the dose of barbiturate by one-half).
- No products indexed under this heading.

Buprenorphine (Additive sedative effects). Products include:
- Buprenex Injectable ... 2006

Buspirone Hydrochloride (Additive sedative effects). Products include:
- BuSpar ... 737

Butabarbital (Additive sedative effects; reduce the dose of barbiturate by one-half).
- No products indexed under this heading.

Butalbital (Additive sedative effects; reduce the dose of barbiturate by one-half). Products include:
- Esgic-plus Tablets ... 1013
- Fioricet Tablets ... 2258
- Fioricet with Codeine Capsules ... 2260
- Fiorinal Capsules ... 2261
- Fiorinal with Codeine Capsules ... 2262
- Fiorinal Tablets ... 2261
- Phrenilin ... 785
- Sedapap Tablets 50 mg/650 mg ... 1543

Chlordiazepoxide (Additive sedative effects). Products include:
- Libritabs Tablets ... 2177
- Limbitrol ... 2180

Chlordiazepoxide Hydrochloride (Additive sedative effects). Products include:
- Librax Capsules ... 2176
- Librium Capsules ... 2178
- Librium Injectable ... 2179

Chlorpromazine (Additive sedative effects). Products include:
- Thorazine Suppositories ... 2523

Chlorprothixene (Additive sedative effects).
- No products indexed under this heading.

Chlorprothixene Hydrochloride (Additive sedative effects).
- No products indexed under this heading.

Clomipramine Hydrochloride (Additive sedative effects). Products include:
- Anafranil Capsules ... 803

Clorazepate Dipotassium (Additive sedative effects). Products include:
- Tranxene ... 451

Clozapine (Additive sedative effects). Products include:
- Clozaril Tablets ... 2252

Codeine Phosphate (Additive sedative effects). Products include:
- Actifed with Codeine Cough Syrup ... 1067
- Brontex ... 1981
- Deconsal C Expectorant Syrup ... 456
- Deconsal Pediatric Syrup ... 457
- Dimetane-DC Cough Syrup ... 2059
- Empirin with Codeine Tablets ... 1093
- Fioricet with Codeine Capsules ... 2260
- Fiorinal with Codeine Capsules ... 2262
- Isoclor Expectorant ... 990
- Novahistine DH ... 2462
- Novahistine Expectorant ... 2463
- Nucofed ... 2051
- Phenergan with Codeine ... 2777
- Phenergan VC with Codeine ... 2781
- Robitussin A-C Syrup ... 2073
- Robitussin-DAC Syrup ... 2074
- Ryna ... ▣ 841
- Soma Compound w/Codeine Tablets ... 2676
- Tussi-Organidin NR Liquid and S NR Liquid ... 2677
- Tylenol with Codeine ... 1583

Desflurane (Additive sedative effects). Products include:
- Suprane ... 1813

Desipramine Hydrochloride (Additive sedative effects). Products include:
- Norpramin Tablets ... 1526

Dezocine (Additive sedative effects). Products include:
- Dalgan Injection ... 538

Diazepam (Additive sedative effects). Products include:
- Dizac ... 1809
- Valium Injectable ... 2182
- Valium Tablets ... 2183
- Valrelease Capsules ... 2169

Doxepin Hydrochloride (Additive sedative effects). Products include:
- Sinequan ... 2205
- Zonalon Cream ... 1055

Droperidol (Additive sedative effects). Products include:
- Inapsine Injection ... 1296

Enflurane (Additive sedative effects).
- No products indexed under this heading.

Epinephrine (Potential for reversal of the vasopressor effect). Products include:
- Bronkaid Mist ... ▣ 717
- EPIFRIN ... ⊙ 239
- EpiPen ... 790
- Marcaine Hydrochloride with Epinephrine 1:200,000 ... 2316
- Primatene Mist ... ▣ 873
- Sensorcaine with Epinephrine Injection ... 559
- Sus-Phrine Injection ... 1019
- Xylocaine with Epinephrine Injections ... 567

Estazolam (Additive sedative effects). Products include:
- ProSom Tablets ... 449

Ethchlorvynol (Additive sedative effects). Products include:
- Placidyl Capsules ... 448

Ethinamate (Additive sedative effects).
- No products indexed under this heading.

Fentanyl (Additive sedative effects). Products include:
- Duragesic Transdermal System ... 1288

Fentanyl Citrate (Additive sedative effects). Products include:
- Sublimaze Injection ... 1307

Fluphenazine Decanoate (Additive sedative effects). Products include:
- Prolixin Decanoate ... 509

Fluphenazine Enanthate (Additive sedative effects). Products include:
- Prolixin Enanthate ... 509

Fluphenazine Hydrochloride (Additive sedative effects). Products include:
- Prolixin ... 509

Flurazepam Hydrochloride (Additive sedative effects). Products include:
- Dalmane Capsules ... 2173

Glutethimide (Additive sedative effects).
- No products indexed under this heading.

Haloperidol (Additive sedative effects). Products include:
- Haldol Injection, Tablets and Concentrate ... 1575

Haloperidol Decanoate (Additive sedative effects). Products include:
- Haldol Decanoate ... 1577

(▣ Described in PDR For Nonprescription Drugs) (⊙ Described in PDR For Ophthalmology)

Hydrocodone Bitartrate (Additive sedative effects). Products include:
Anexsia 5/500 Elixir ... 1781
Anexia Tablets ... 1782
Codiclear DH Syrup ... 791
Deconamine CX Cough and Cold Liquid and Tablets ... 1319
Duratuss HD Elixir ... 2565
Hycodan Tablets and Syrup ... 930
Hycomine Compound Tablets ... 932
Hycomine ... 931
Hycotuss Expectorant Syrup ... 933
Hydrocet Capsules ... 782
Lorcet 10/650 ... 1018
Lortab ... 2566
Tussend ... 1783
Tussend Expectorant ... 1785
Vicodin Tablets ... 1356
Vicodin ES Tablets ... 1357
Vicodin Tuss Expectorant ... 1358
Zydone Capsules ... 949

Hydrocodone Polistirex (Additive sedative effects). Products include:
Tussionex Pennkinetic Extended-Release Suspension ... 998

Hydroxyzine Hydrochloride (Additive sedative effects). Products include:
Atarax Tablets & Syrup ... 2185
Marax Tablets & DF Syrup ... 2200
Vistaril Intramuscular Solution ... 2216

Imipramine Hydrochloride (Additive sedative effects). Products include:
Tofranil Ampuls ... 854
Tofranil Tablets ... 856

Imipramine Pamoate (Additive sedative effects). Products include:
Tofranil-PM Capsules ... 857

Isoflurane (Additive sedative effects).
No products indexed under this heading.

Ketamine Hydrochloride (Additive sedative effects).
No products indexed under this heading.

Levomethadyl Acetate Hydrochloride (Additive sedative effects). Products include:
Orlamm ... 2239

Levorphanol Tartrate (Additive sedative effects). Products include:
Levo-Dromoran ... 2129

Lorazepam (Additive sedative effects). Products include:
Ativan Injection ... 2698
Ativan Tablets ... 2700

Loxapine Hydrochloride (Additive sedative effects). Products include:
Loxitane ... 1378

Loxapine Succinate (Additive sedative effects). Products include:
Loxitane Capsules ... 1378

Maprotiline Hydrochloride (Additive sedative effects). Products include:
Ludiomil Tablets ... 843

Meperidine Hydrochloride (Additive sedative effects; reduce meperidine dose by one-fourth to one-half). Products include:
Demerol ... 2308
Mepergan Injection ... 2753

Mephobarbital (Additive sedative effects; reduce the dose of barbiturate by one-half). Products include:
Mebaral Tablets ... 2322

Meprobamate (Additive sedative effects). Products include:
Miltown Tablets ... 2672
PMB 200 and PMB 400 ... 2783

Mesoridazine Besylate (Additive sedative effects). Products include:
Serentil ... 684

Methadone Hydrochloride (Additive sedative effects). Products include:
Methadone Hydrochloride Oral Concentrate ... 2233
Methadone Hydrochloride Oral Solution & Tablets ... 2235

Methohexital Sodium (Additive sedative effects). Products include:
Brevital Sodium Vials ... 1429

Methotrimeprazine (Additive sedative effects). Products include:
Levoprome ... 1274

Methoxyflurane (Additive sedative effects).
No products indexed under this heading.

Midazolam Hydrochloride (Additive sedative effects). Products include:
Versed Injection ... 2170

Molindone Hydrochloride (Additive sedative effects). Products include:
Moban Tablets and Concentrate ... 1048

Morphine Sulfate (Additive sedative effects; reduce the dose of morphine by one-fourth to one-half). Products include:
Astramorph/PF Injection, USP (Preservative-Free) ... 535
Duramorph ... 962
Infumorph 200 and Infumorph 500 Sterile Solutions ... 965
MS Contin Tablets ... 1994
MSIR ... 1997
Oramorph SR (Morphine Sulfate Sustained Release Tablets) ... 2236
RMS Suppositories ... 2657
Roxanol ... 2243

Nortriptyline Hydrochloride (Additive sedative effects). Products include:
Pamelor ... 2280

Opium Alkaloids (Additive sedative effects).
No products indexed under this heading.

Oxazepam (Additive sedative effects). Products include:
Serax Capsules ... 2810
Serax Tablets ... 2810

Oxycodone Hydrochloride (Additive sedative effects). Products include:
Percocet Tablets ... 938
Percodan Tablets ... 939
Percodan-Demi Tablets ... 940
Roxicodone Tablets, Oral Solution & Intensol (Oxycodone) ... 2244
Tylox Capsules ... 1584

Pentobarbital Sodium (Additive sedative effects; reduce the dose of barbiturate by one-half). Products include:
Nembutal Sodium Capsules ... 436
Nembutal Sodium Solution ... 438
Nembutal Sodium Suppositories ... 440

Perphenazine (Additive sedative effects). Products include:
Etrafon ... 2355
Triavil Tablets ... 1757
Trilafon ... 2389

Phenobarbital (Additive sedative effects; reduce the dose of barbiturate by one-half). Products include:
Arco-Lase Plus Tablets ... 512
Bellergal-S Tablets ... 2250
Donnatal ... 2060
Donnatal Extentabs ... 2061
Donnatal Tablets ... 2060
Phenobarbital Elixir and Tablets ... 1469
Quadrinal Tablets ... 1350

Prazepam (Additive sedative effects).
No products indexed under this heading.

Prochlorperazine (Additive sedative effects). Products include:
Compazine ... 2470

Propofol (Additive sedative effects). Products include:
Diprivan Injection ... 2833

Propoxyphene Hydrochloride (Additive sedative effects). Products include:
Darvon ... 1435
Wygesic Tablets ... 2827

Propoxyphene Napsylate (Additive sedative effects). Products include:
Darvon-N/Darvocet-N ... 1433

Protriptyline Hydrochloride (Additive sedative effects). Products include:
Vivactil Tablets ... 1774

Quazepam (Additive sedative effects). Products include:
Doral Tablets ... 2664

Risperidone (Additive sedative effects). Products include:
Risperdal ... 1301

Secobarbital Sodium (Additive sedative effects; reduce the dose of barbiturate by one-half). Products include:
Seconal Sodium Pulvules ... 1474

Sufentanil Citrate (Additive sedative effects). Products include:
Sufenta Injection ... 1309

Temazepam (Additive sedative effects). Products include:
Restoril Capsules ... 2284

Thiamylal Sodium (Additive sedative effects; reduce the dose of barbiturate by one-half).
No products indexed under this heading.

Thioridazine Hydrochloride (Additive sedative effects). Products include:
Mellaril ... 2269

Thiothixene (Additive sedative effects). Products include:
Navane Capsules and Concentrate 2201
Navane Intramuscular ... 2202

Triazolam (Additive sedative effects). Products include:
Halcion Tablets ... 2611

Trifluoperazine Hydrochloride (Additive sedative effects). Products include:
Stelazine ... 2514

Trimipramine Maleate (Additive sedative effects). Products include:
Surmontil Capsules ... 2811

Zolpidem Tartrate (Additive sedative effects). Products include:
Ambien Tablets ... 2416

Food Interactions

Alcohol (Additive sedative effects).

PHENERGAN SYRUP FORTIS

(Promethazine Hydrochloride) ... 2774

May interact with narcotic analgesics, hypnotics and sedatives, tricyclic antidepressants, tranquilizers, and certain other agents. Compounds in these categories include:

Alfentanil Hydrochloride (Additive sedative effects). Products include:
Alfenta Injection ... 1286

Alprazolam (Additive sedative effects). Products include:
Xanax Tablets ... 2649

Amitriptyline Hydrochloride (Additive sedative effects). Products include:
Elavil ... 2838
Endep Tablets ... 2174
Etrafon ... 2355
Limbitrol ... 2180
Triavil Tablets ... 1757

Amoxapine (Additive sedative effects). Products include:
Asendin Tablets ... 1369

Buprenorphine (Additive sedative effects). Products include:
Buprenex Injectable ... 2006

Buspirone Hydrochloride (Additive sedative effects). Products include:
BuSpar ... 737

Chlordiazepoxide (Additive sedative effects). Products include:
Libritabs Tablets ... 2177
Limbitrol ... 2180

Chlordiazepoxide Hydrochloride (Additive sedative effects). Products include:
Librax Capsules ... 2176
Librium Capsules ... 2178
Librium Injectable ... 2179

Chlorpromazine (Additive sedative effects). Products include:
Thorazine Suppositories ... 2523

Chlorprothixene (Additive sedative effects).
No products indexed under this heading.

Chlorprothixene Hydrochloride (Additive sedative effects).
No products indexed under this heading.

Clomipramine Hydrochloride (Additive sedative effects). Products include:
Anafranil Capsules ... 803

Clorazepate Dipotassium (Additive sedative effects). Products include:
Tranxene ... 451

Codeine Phosphate (Additive sedative effects). Products include:
Actifed with Codeine Cough Syrup .. 1067
Brontex ... 1981
Deconsal C Expectorant Syrup ... 456
Deconsal Pediatric Syrup ... 457
Dimetane-DC Cough Syrup ... 2059
Empirin with Codeine Tablets ... 1093
Fioricet with Codeine Capsules ... 2260
Fiorinal with Codeine Capsules ... 2262
Isoclor Expectorant ... 990
Novahistine DH ... 2462
Novahistine Expectorant ... 2463
Nucofed ... 2051
Phenergan with Codeine ... 2777
Phenergan VC with Codeine ... 2781
Robitussin A-C Syrup ... 2073
Robitussin-DAC Syrup ... 2074
Ryna ... 841
Soma Compound w/Codeine Tablets ... 2676
Tussi-Organidin NR Liquid and S NR Liquid ... 2677
Tylenol with Codeine ... 1583

Desipramine Hydrochloride (Additive sedative effects). Products include:
Norpramin Tablets ... 1526

Dezocine (Additive sedative effects). Products include:
Dalgan Injection ... 538

Diazepam (Additive sedative effects). Products include:
Dizac ... 1809
Valium Injectable ... 2182
Valium Tablets ... 2183
Valrelease Capsules ... 2169

Doxepin Hydrochloride (Additive sedative effects). Products include:
Sinequan ... 2205
Zonalon Cream ... 1055

Droperidol (Additive sedative effects). Products include:
Inapsine Injection ... 1296

Estazolam (Additive sedative effects). Products include:
ProSom Tablets ... 449

Ethchlorvynol (Additive sedative effects). Products include:
Placidyl Capsules ... 448

IMPORTANT NOTE: Always consult each drug listing in the patient's regimen for possible interactions.

Phenergan Syrup

Interactions Index

Ethinamate (Additive sedative effects).

No products indexed under this heading.

Fentanyl (Additive sedative effects). Products include:

Duragesic Transdermal System....... 1288

Fentanyl Citrate (Additive sedative effects). Products include:

Sublimaze Injection................................ 1307

Fluphenazine Decanoate (Additive sedative effects). Products include:

Prolixin Decanoate 509

Fluphenazine Enanthate (Additive sedative effects). Products include:

Prolixin Enanthate 509

Fluphenazine Hydrochloride (Additive sedative effects). Products include:

Prolixin 509

Flurazepam Hydrochloride (Additive sedative effects). Products include:

Dalmane Capsules.................................. 2173

Glutethimide (Additive sedative effects).

No products indexed under this heading.

Haloperidol (Additive sedative effects). Products include:

Haldol Injection, Tablets and Concentrate 1575

Haloperidol Decanoate (Additive sedative effects). Products include:

Haldol Decanoate................................... 1577

Hydrocodone Bitartrate (Additive sedative effects). Products include:

Anexsia 5/500 Elixir	1781
Anexia Tablets	1782
Codiclear DH Syrup	791
Deconamine CX Cough and Cold Liquid and Tablets	1319
Duratuss HD Elixir	2565
Hycodan Tablets and Syrup	930
Hycomine Compound Tablets	932
Hycomine	931
Hycotuss Expectorant Syrup	933
Hydrocet Capsules	782
Lorcet 10/650	1018
Lortab	2566
Tussend	1783
Tussend Expectorant	1785
Vicodin Tablets	1356
Vicodin ES Tablets	1357
Vicodin Tuss Expectorant	1358
Zydone Capsules	949

Hydrocodone Polistirex (Additive sedative effects). Products include:

Tussionex Pennkinetic Extended-Release Suspension 998

Hydroxyzine Hydrochloride (Additive sedative effects). Products include:

Atarax Tablets & Syrup	2185
Marax Tablets & DF Syrup	2200
Vistaril Intramuscular Solution	2216

Imipramine Hydrochloride (Additive sedative effects). Products include:

Tofranil Ampuls	854
Tofranil Tablets	856

Imipramine Pamoate (Additive sedative effects). Products include:

Tofranil-PM Capsules............................ 857

Levorphanol Tartrate (Additive sedative effects). Products include:

Levo-Dromoran.. 2129

Lorazepam (Additive sedative effects). Products include:

Ativan Injection	2698
Ativan Tablets	2700

Loxapine Hydrochloride (Additive sedative effects). Products include:

Loxitane 1378

Loxapine Succinate (Additive sedative effects). Products include:

Loxitane Capsules 1378

Maprotiline Hydrochloride (Additive sedative effects). Products include:

Ludiomil Tablets..................................... 843

Meperidine Hydrochloride (Additive sedative effects). Products include:

Demerol	2308
Mepergan Injection	2753

Meprobamate (Additive sedative effects). Products include:

Miltown Tablets	2672
PMB 200 and PMB 400	2783

Mesoridazine Besylate (Additive sedative effects). Products include:

Serentil 684

Methadone Hydrochloride (Additive sedative effects). Products include:

Methadone Hydrochloride Oral Concentrate	2233
Methadone Hydrochloride Oral Solution & Tablets	2235

Midazolam Hydrochloride (Additive sedative effects). Products include:

Versed Injection 2170

Molindone Hydrochloride (Additive sedative effects). Products include:

Moban Tablets and Concentrate...... 1048

Morphine Sulfate (Additive sedative effects). Products include:

Astramorph/PF Injection, USP (Preservative-Free)	535
Duramorph	962
Infumorph 200 and Infumorph 500 Sterile Solutions	965
MS Contin Tablets	1994
MSIR	1997
Oramorph SR (Morphine Sulfate Sustained Release Tablets)	2236
RMS Suppositories	2657
Roxanol	2243

Nortriptyline Hydrochloride (Additive sedative effects). Products include:

Pamelor 2280

Opium Alkaloids (Additive sedative effects).

No products indexed under this heading.

Oxazepam (Additive sedative effects). Products include:

Serax Capsules	2810
Serax Tablets	2810

Oxycodone Hydrochloride (Additive sedative effects). Products include:

Percocet Tablets	938
Percodan Tablets	939
Percodan-Demi Tablets	940
Roxicodone Tablets, Oral Solution & Intensol (Oxycodone)	2244
Tylox Capsules	1584

Perphenazine (Additive sedative effects). Products include:

Etrafon	2355
Triavil Tablets	1757
Trilafon	2389

Prazepam (Additive sedative effects).

No products indexed under this heading.

Prochlorperazine (Additive sedative effects). Products include:

Compazine 2470

Propofol (Additive sedative effects). Products include:

Diprivan Injection................................... 2833

Propoxyphene Hydrochloride (Additive sedative effects). Products include:

Darvon	1435
Wygesic Tablets	2827

Propoxyphene Napsylate (Additive sedative effects). Products include:

Darvon-N/Darvocet-N 1433

Protriptyline Hydrochloride (Additive sedative effects). Products include:

Vivactil Tablets 1774

Quazepam (Additive sedative effects). Products include:

Doral Tablets... 2664

Secobarbital Sodium (Additive sedative effects). Products include:

Seconal Sodium Pulvules 1474

Sufentanil Citrate (Additive sedative effects). Products include:

Sufenta Injection 1309

Temazepam (Additive sedative effects). Products include:

Restoril Capsules.................................... 2284

Thioridazine Hydrochloride (Additive sedative effects). Products include:

Mellaril 2269

Thiothixene (Additive sedative effects). Products include:

Navane Capsules and Concentrate	2201
Navane Intramuscular	2202

Triazolam (Additive sedative effects). Products include:

Halcion Tablets....................................... 2611

Trifluoperazine Hydrochloride (Additive sedative effects). Products include:

Stelazine 2514

Trimipramine Maleate (Additive sedative effects). Products include:

Surmontil Capsules................................ 2811

Zolpidem Tartrate (Additive sedative effects). Products include:

Ambien Tablets....................................... 2416

Food Interactions

Alcohol (Additive sedative effects).

PHENERGAN SYRUP PLAIN

(Promethazine Hydrochloride)............2774
See Phenergan Syrup Fortis

PHENERGAN TABLETS

(Promethazine Hydrochloride)............2775
See Phenergan Suppositories

PHENERGAN VC

(Promethazine Hydrochloride, Phenylephrine Hydrochloride) 2779
May interact with narcotic analgesics, hypnotics and sedatives, tricyclic antidepressants, tranquilizers, monoamine oxidase inhibitors, sympathomimetics, sympathomimetic bronchodilators, beta blockers, alpha adrenergic blockers, and certain other agents. Compounds in these categories include:

Acebutolol Hydrochloride (Cardiostimulating effects blocked). Products include:

Sectral Capsules 2807

Albuterol (Tachycardia or arrhythmias may occur). Products include:

Proventil Inhalation Aerosol	2382
Ventolin Inhalation Aerosol and Refill	1197

Albuterol Sulfate (Tachycardia or arrhythmias may occur). Products include:

Airet Solution for Inhalation	452
Proventil Inhalation Solution 0.083%	2384
Proventil Repetabs Tablets	2386
Proventil Solution for Inhalation 0.5%	2383
Proventil Syrup	2385
Proventil Tablets	2386
Ventolin Inhalation Solution	1198
Ventolin Nebules Inhalation Solution	1199
Ventolin Rotacaps for Inhalation	1200

Ventolin Syrup	1202
Ventolin Tablets	1203
Volmax Extended-Release Tablets	1788

Alfentanil Hydrochloride (Additive sedative effects). Products include:

Alfenta Injection 1286

Alprazolam (Additive sedative effects). Products include:

Xanax Tablets 2649

Amitriptyline Hydrochloride (Additive sedative effects; increased pressor response). Products include:

Elavil	2838
Endep Tablets	2174
Etrafon	2355
Limbitrol	2180
Triavil Tablets	1757

Amoxapine (Additive sedative effects; increased pressor response). Products include:

Asendin Tablets 1369

Amphetamine Aspartate (Synergistic adrenergic response).

No products indexed under this heading.

Amphetamine Resins (Synergistic adrenergic response). Products include:

Biphetamine Capsules........................... 983

Amphetamine Sulfate (Synergistic adrenergic response).

No products indexed under this heading.

Atenolol (Cardiostimulating effects blocked). Products include:

Tenoretic Tablets	2845
Tenormin Tablets and I.V. Injection	2847

Atropine Sulfate (Enhanced pressor response; reflex bradycardia blocked). Products include:

Arco-Lase Plus Tablets	512
Atrohist Plus Tablets	454
Atropine Sulfate Sterile Ophthalmic Solution	◉ 233
Donnatal	2060
Donnatal Extentabs	2061
Donnatal Tablets	2060
Lomotil	2439
Motofen Tablets	784
Urised Tablets	1964

Betaxolol Hydrochloride (Cardiostimulating effects blocked). Products include:

Betoptic Ophthalmic Solution	469
Betoptic S Ophthalmic Suspension	471
Kerlone Tablets	2436

Bisoprolol Fumarate (Cardiostimulating effects blocked). Products include:

Zebeta Tablets	1413
Ziac	1415

Bitolterol Mesylate (Tachycardia or arrhythmias may occur). Products include:

Tornalate Solution for Inhalation, 0.2%	956
Tornalate Metered Dose Inhaler	957

Buprenorphine (Additive sedative effects). Products include:

Buprenex Injectable 2006

Buspirone Hydrochloride (Additive sedative effects). Products include:

BuSpar 737

Carteolol Hydrochloride (Cardiostimulating effects blocked). Products include:

Cartrol Tablets	410
Ocupress Ophthalmic Solution, 1% Sterile	◉ 309

Chlordiazepoxide (Additive sedative effects). Products include:

Libritabs Tablets	2177
Limbitrol	2180

Chlordiazepoxide Hydrochloride (Additive sedative effects). Products include:

Librax Capsules	2176
Librium Capsules	2178

(⊞ Described in PDR For Nonprescription Drugs)

(◉ Described in PDR For Ophthalmology)

813 Interactions Index Phenergan VC

Librium Injectable 2179

Chlorpromazine (Additive sedative effects). Products include:
Thorazine Suppositories 2523

Chlorprothixene (Additive sedative effects).
No products indexed under this heading.

Chlorprothixene Hydrochloride (Additive sedative effects).
No products indexed under this heading.

Clomipramine Hydrochloride (Additive sedative effects; increased pressor response). Products include:
Anafranil Capsules 803

Clorazepate Dipotassium (Additive sedative effects). Products include:
Tranxene 451

Codeine Phosphate (Additive sedative effects). Products include:
Actifed with Codeine Cough Syrup.. 1067
Brontex 1981
Deconsal C Expectorant Syrup 456
Deconsal Pediatric Syrup 457
Dimetane-DC Cough Syrup 2059
Empirin with Codeine Tablets 1093
Fioricet with Codeine Capsules 2260
Fiorinal with Codeine Capsules 2262
Isoclor Expectorant 990
Novahistine DH 2462
Novahistine Expectorant 2463
Nucofed 2051
Phenergan with Codeine 2777
Phenergan VC with Codeine 2781
Robitussin A-C Syrup 2073
Robitussin-DAC Syrup 2074
Ryna .... ▣ 841
Soma Compound w/Codeine Tablets 2676
Tussi-Organidin NR Liquid and S NR Liquid 2677
Tylenol with Codeine 1583

Desipramine Hydrochloride (Additive sedative effects; increased pressor response). Products include:
Norpramin Tablets 1526

Dezocine (Additive sedative effects). Products include:
Dalgan Injection 538

Diazepam (Additive sedative effects). Products include:
Dizac 1809
Valium Injectable 2182
Valium Tablets 2183
Valrelease Capsules 2169

Dobutamine Hydrochloride (Tachycardia or arrhythmias may occur). Products include:
Dobutrex Solution Vials 1439

Dopamine Hydrochloride (Tachycardia or arrhythmias may occur).
No products indexed under this heading.

Doxazosin Mesylate (Decreased pressor response). Products include:
Cardura Tablets 2186

Doxepin Hydrochloride (Additive sedative effects; increased pressor response). Products include:
Sinequan 2205
Zonalon Cream 1055

Droperidol (Additive sedative effects). Products include:
Inapsine Injection 1296

Ephedrine Hydrochloride (Tachycardia or arrhythmias may occur). Products include:
Primatene Dual Action Formula .... ▣ 872
Primatene Tablets .... ▣ 873
Quadrinal Tablets 1350

Ephedrine Sulfate (Tachycardia or arrhythmias may occur). Products include:
Bronkaid Caplets .... ▣ 717
Marax Tablets & DF Syrup 2200

Ephedrine Tannate (Tachycardia or arrhythmias may occur). Products include:
Rynatuss 2673

Epinephrine (Tachycardia or arrhythmias may occur). Products include:
Bronkaid Mist .... ▣ 717
EPIFRIN .... ⊙ 239
EpiPen 790
Marcaine Hydrochloride with Epinephrine 1:200,000 2316
Primatene Mist .... ▣ 873
Sensorcaine with Epinephrine Injection 559
Sus-Phrine Injection 1019
Xylocaine with Epinephrine Injections 567

Epinephrine Bitartrate (Tachycardia or arrhythmias may occur). Products include:
Bronkaid Mist Suspension .... ▣ 718
Sensorcaine-MPF with Epinephrine Injection 559

Epinephrine Hydrochloride (Tachycardia or arrhythmias may occur). Products include:
Ana-Kit Anaphylaxis Emergency Treatment Kit 617

Ergotamine Tartrate (Excessive rise in blood pressure). Products include:
Bellergal-S Tablets 2250
Cafergot 2251
Ergomar 1486
Wigraine Tablets & Suppositories .. 1829

Esmolol Hydrochloride (Cardiostimulating effects blocked). Products include:
Brevibloc Injection 1808

Estazolam (Additive sedative effects). Products include:
ProSom Tablets 449

Ethchlorvynol (Additive sedative effects). Products include:
Placidyl Capsules 448

Ethinamate (Additive sedative effects).
No products indexed under this heading.

Ethylnorepinephrine Hydrochloride (Tachycardia or arrhythmias may occur).
No products indexed under this heading.

Fentanyl (Additive sedative effects). Products include:
Duragesic Transdermal System 1288

Fentanyl Citrate (Additive sedative effects). Products include:
Sublimaze Injection 1307

Fluphenazine Decanoate (Additive sedative effects). Products include:
Prolixin Decanoate 509

Fluphenazine Enanthate (Additive sedative effects). Products include:
Prolixin Enanthate 509

Fluphenazine Hydrochloride (Additive sedative effects). Products include:
Prolixin 509

Flurazepam Hydrochloride (Additive sedative effects). Products include:
Dalmane Capsules 2173

Furazolidone (Acute hypertensive crisis; concurrent use is contraindicated). Products include:
Furoxone 2046

Glutethimide (Additive sedative effects).
No products indexed under this heading.

Haloperidol (Additive sedative effects). Products include:
Haldol Injection, Tablets and Concentrate 1575

Haloperidol Decanoate (Additive sedative effects). Products include:
Haldol Decanoate 1577

Hydrocodone Bitartrate (Additive sedative effects). Products include:
Anexsia 5/500 Elixir 1781
Anexia Tablets 1782
Codiclear DH Syrup 791
Deconamine CX Cough and Cold Liquid and Tablets 1319
Duratuss HD Elixir 2565
Hycodan Tablets and Syrup 930
Hycomine Compound Tablets 932
Hycomine 931
Hycotuss Expectorant Syrup 933
Hydrocet Capsules 782
Lorcet 10/650 1018
Lortab 2566
Tussend 1783
Tussend Expectorant 1785
Vicodin Tablets 1356
Vicodin ES Tablets 1357
Vicodin Tuss Expectorant 1358
Zydone Capsules 949

Hydrocodone Polistirex (Additive sedative effects). Products include:
Tussionex Pennkinetic Extended-Release Suspension 998

Hydroxyzine Hydrochloride (Additive sedative effects). Products include:
Atarax Tablets & Syrup 2185
Marax Tablets & DF Syrup 2200
Vistaril Intramuscular Solution 2216

Imipramine Hydrochloride (Additive sedative effects; increased pressor response). Products include:
Tofranil Ampuls 854
Tofranil Tablets 856

Imipramine Pamoate (Additive sedative effects; increased pressor response). Products include:
Tofranil-PM Capsules 857

Isocarboxazid (Acute hypertensive crisis; concurrent use is contraindicated).
No products indexed under this heading.

Isoetharine (Tachycardia or arrhythmias may occur). Products include:
Bronkometer Aerosol 2302
Bronkosol Solution 2302
Isoetharine Inhalation Solution, USP, Arm-a-Med 551

Isoproterenol Hydrochloride (Tachycardia or arrhythmias may occur). Products include:
Isuprel Hydrochloride Injection 1:5000 2311
Isuprel Hydrochloride Solution 1:200 & 1:100 2313
Isuprel Mistometer 2312

Isoproterenol Sulfate (Tachycardia or arrhythmias may occur). Products include:
Norisodrine with Calcium Iodide Syrup 442

Labetalol Hydrochloride (Cardiostimulating effects blocked). Products include:
Normodyne Injection 2377
Normodyne Tablets 2379
Trandate 1185

Levobunolol Hydrochloride (Cardiostimulating effects blocked). Products include:
Betagan .... ⊙ 233

Levorphanol Tartrate (Additive sedative effects). Products include:
Levo-Dromoran 2129

Lorazepam (Additive sedative effects). Products include:
Ativan Injection 2698
Ativan Tablets 2700

Loxapine Hydrochloride (Additive sedative effects). Products include:
Loxitane 1378

Maprotiline Hydrochloride (Additive sedative effects; increased pressor response). Products include:
Ludiomil Tablets 843

Meperidine Hydrochloride (Additive sedative effects). Products include:
Demerol 2308
Mepergan Injection 2753

Meprobamate (Additive sedative effects). Products include:
Miltown Tablets 2672
PMB 200 and PMB 400 2783

Mesoridazine Besylate (Additive sedative effects). Products include:
Serentil 684

Metaproterenol Sulfate (Tachycardia or arrhythmias may occur). Products include:
Alupent 669
Metaproterenol Sulfate Inhalation Solution, USP, Arm-a-Med 552

Metaraminol Bitartrate (Tachycardia or arrhythmias may occur). Products include:
Aramine Injection 1609

Methadone Hydrochloride (Additive sedative effects). Products include:
Methadone Hydrochloride Oral Concentrate 2233
Methadone Hydrochloride Oral Solution & Tablets 2235

Methoxamine Hydrochloride (Tachycardia or arrhythmias may occur). Products include:
Vasoxyl Injection 1196

Metipranolol Hydrochloride (Cardiostimulating effects blocked). Products include:
OptiPranolol (Metipranolol 0.3%) Sterile Ophthalmic Solution .... ⊙ 258

Metoprolol Succinate (Cardiostimulating effects blocked). Products include:
Toprol-XL Tablets 565

Metoprolol Tartrate (Cardiostimulating effects blocked). Products include:
Lopressor Ampuls 830
Lopressor HCT Tablets 832
Lopressor Tablets 830

Midazolam Hydrochloride (Additive sedative effects). Products include:
Versed Injection 2170

Molindone Hydrochloride (Additive sedative effects). Products include:
Moban Tablets and Concentrate 1048

Morphine Sulfate (Additive sedative effects). Products include:
Astramorph/PF Injection, USP (Preservative-Free) 535
Duramorph 962
Infumorph 200 and Infumorph 500 Sterile Solutions 965
MS Contin Tablets 1994
MSIR 1997
Oramorph SR (Morphine Sulfate Sustained Release Tablets) 2236
RMS Suppositories 2657
Roxanol 2243

Nadolol (Cardiostimulating effects blocked).
No products indexed under this heading.

Norepinephrine Bitartrate (Tachycardia or arrhythmias may occur). Products include:
Levophed Bitartrate Injection 2315

Nortriptyline Hydrochloride (Additive sedative effects; increased pressor response). Products include:
Pamelor 2280

Opium Alkaloids (Additive sedative effects).
No products indexed under this heading.

IMPORTANT NOTE: Always consult each drug listing in the patient's regimen for possible interactions.

Phenergan VC
Interactions Index
814

Oxazepam (Additive sedative effects). Products include:
Serax Capsules 2810
Serax Tablets 2810
Oxycodone Hydrochloride (Additive sedative effects). Products include:
Percocet Tablets 938
Percodan Tablets 939
Percodan-Demi Tablets 940
Roxicodone Tablets, Oral Solution & Intensol (Oxycodone) 2244
Tylox Capsules 1584
Penbutolol Sulfate (Cardiostimulating effects blocked). Products include:
Levatol 2403
Perphenazine (Additive sedative effects). Products include:
Etrafon 2355
Triavil Tablets 1757
Trilafon 2389
Phenelzine Sulfate (Acute hypertensive crisis; concurrent use is contraindicated). Products include:
Nardil 1920
Phentolamine Mesylate (Decreased pressor response). Products include:
Regitine 846
Phenylephrine Bitartrate (Tachycardia or arrhythmias may occur).
No products indexed under this heading.
Phenylephrine Tannate (Tachycardia or arrhythmias may occur). Products include:
Atrohist Pediatric Suspension 454
Ricobid-D Pediatric Suspension 2038
Ricobid Tablets and Pediatric Suspension 2038
Rynatan 2673
Rynatuss 2673
Phenylpropanolamine Hydrochloride (Tachycardia or arrhythmias may occur). Products include:
Acutrim ◘ 628
Allerest Children's Chewable Tablets ◘ 627
Allerest 12 Hour Caplets ◘ 627
Atrohist Plus Tablets 454
BC Cold Powder Multi-Symptom Formula (Cold-Sinus-Allergy) ◘ 609
BC Cold Powder Non-Drowsy Formula (Cold-Sinus) ◘ 609
Cheracol Plus Head Cold/Cough Formula ◘ 769
Comtrex Multi-Symptom Non-Drowsy Liqui-gels ◘ 618
Contac Continuous Action Nasal Decongestant/Antihistamine 12 Hour Capsules ◘ 813
Contac Maximum Strength Continuous Action Decongestant/Antihistamine 12 Hour Caplets ◘ 813
Contac Severe Cold and Flu Formula Caplets ◘ 814
Coricidin 'D' Decongestant Tablets ◘ 800
Dexatrim ◘ 832
Dexatrim Plus Vitamins Caplets ◘ 832
Dimetane-DC Cough Syrup 2059
Dimetapp Elixir ◘ 773
Dimetapp Extentabs ◘ 774
Dimetapp Tablets/Liqui-Gels ◘ 775
Dimetapp Cold & Allergy Chewable Tablets ◘ 773
Dimetapp DM Elixir ◘ 774
Dura-Vent Tablets 952
Entex Capsules 1986
Entex LA Tablets 1987
Entex Liquid 1986
Exgest LA Tablets 782
Hycomine 931
Isoclor Timesule Capsules ◘ 637
Nolamine Timed-Release Tablets 785
Ornade Spansule Capsules 2502
Propagest Tablets 786
Pyrroxate Caplets ◘ 772
Robitussin-CF ◘ 777
Sinulin Tablets 787
Tavist-D 12 Hour Relief Tablets ◘ 787
Teldrin 12 Hour Antihistamine/Nasal Decongestant Allergy Relief Capsules ◘ 826
Triaminic Allergy Tablets ◘ 789
Triaminic Cold Tablets ◘ 790
Triaminic Expectorant ◘ 790
Triaminic Syrup ◘ 792
Triaminic-12 Tablets ◘ 792
Triaminic-DM Syrup ◘ 792
Triaminicin Tablets ◘ 793
Triaminicol Multi-Symptom Cold Tablets ◘ 793
Triaminicol Multi-Symptom Relief ◘ 794
Vicks DayQuil Allergy Relief 12-Hour Extended Release Tablets ◘ 760
Vicks DayQuil Allergy Relief 4-Hour Tablets ◘ 760
Vicks DayQuil SINUS Pressure & CONGESTION Relief ◘ 761
Pindolol (Cardiostimulating effects blocked). Products include:
Visken Tablets 2299
Pirbuterol Acetate (Tachycardia or arrhythmias may occur). Products include:
Maxair Autohaler 1492
Maxair Inhaler 1494
Prazepam (Additive sedative effects).
No products indexed under this heading.
Prazosin Hydrochloride (Decreased pressor response). Products include:
Minipress Capsules 1937
Minizide Capsules 1938
Prochlorperazine (Additive sedative effects). Products include:
Compazine 2470
Propofol (Additive sedative effects). Products include:
Diprivan Injection 2833
Propoxyphene Hydrochloride (Additive sedative effects). Products include:
Darvon 1435
Wygesic Tablets 2827
Propoxyphene Napsylate (Additive sedative effects). Products include:
Darvon-N/Darvocet-N 1433
Propranolol Hydrochloride (Cardiostimulating effects blocked). Products include:
Inderal 2728
Inderal LA Long Acting Capsules 2730
Inderide Tablets 2732
Inderide LA Long Acting Capsules 2734
Protriptyline Hydrochloride (Additive sedative effects; increased pressor response). Products include:
Vivactil Tablets 1774
Pseudoephedrine Hydrochloride (Tachycardia or arrhythmias may occur). Products include:
Actifed Allergy Daytime/Nighttime Caplets ◘ 844
Actifed Plus Caplets ◘ 845
Actifed Plus Tablets ◘ 845
Actifed with Codeine Cough Syrup 1067
Actifed Sinus Daytime/Nighttime Tablets and Caplets ◘ 846
Actifed Syrup ◘ 846
Actifed Tablets ◘ 844
Advil Cold and Sinus Caplets and Tablets (formerly CoAdvil) ◘ 870
Alka-Seltzer Plus Cold Medicine Liqui-Gels ◘ 706
Alka-Seltzer Plus Cold & Cough Medicine Liqui-Gels ◘ 705
Alka-Seltzer Plus Night-Time Cold Medicine Liqui-Gels ◘ 706
Allerest Headache Strength Tablets ◘ 627
Allerest Maximum Strength Tablets ◘ 627
Allerest No Drowsiness Tablets ◘ 627
Allerest Sinus Pain Formula ◘ 627
Anatuss LA Tablets 1542
Atrohist Pediatric Capsules 453
Bayer Select Sinus Pain Relief Formula ◘ 717
Benadryl Allergy Decongestant Liquid Medication ◘ 848
Benadryl Allergy Decongestant Tablets ◘ 848
Benadryl Allergy Sinus Headache Formula Caplets ◘ 849
Benylin Multisymptom ◘ 852
Bromfed Capsules (Extended-Release) 1785
Bromfed Syrup ◘ 733
Bromfed Tablets 1785
Bromfed-DM Cough Syrup 1786
Bromfed-PD Capsules (Extended-Release) 1785
Children's Vicks DayQuil Allergy Relief ◘ 757
Children's Vicks NyQuil Cold/Cough Relief ◘ 758
Comtrex Multi-Symptom Cold Reliever Tablets/Caplets/Liqui-Gels/Liquid ◘ 615
Allergy-Sinus Comtrex Multi-Symptom Allergy-Sinus Formula Tablets ◘ 617
Comtrex Multi-Symptom Non-Drowsy Caplets ◘ 618
Congess 1004
Contac Day Allergy/Sinus Caplets ◘ 812
Contac Day & Night ◘ 812
Contac Night Allergy/Sinus Caplets ◘ 812
Contac Severe Cold & Flu Non-Drowsy ◘ 815
Deconamine Chewable Tablets 1320
Deconamine CX Cough and Cold Liquid and Tablets 1319
Deconamine 1320
Deconsal C Expectorant Syrup 456
Deconsal Pediatric Syrup 457
Deconsal II Tablets 454
Dimetane-DX Cough Syrup 2059
Dimetapp Sinus Caplets ◘ 775
Dorcol Children's Cough Syrup ◘ 785
Drixoral Cough + Congestion Liquid Caps ◘ 802
Dura-Tap/PD Capsules 2867
Duratuss Tablets 2565
Duratuss HD Elixir 2565
Efidac/24 ◘ 635
Entex PSE Tablets 1987
Fedahist Gyrocaps 2401
Fedahist Timecaps 2401
Guaifed 1787
Guaifed Syrup ◘ 734
Guaimax-D Tablets 792
Guaitab Tablets ◘ 734
Isoclor Expectorant 990
Kronofed-A 977
Motrin IB Sinus ◘ 838
Novahistine DH 2462
Novahistine DMX ◘ 822
Novahistine Expectorant 2463
Nucofed 2051
PediaCare Cold Allergy Chewable Tablets ◘ 677
PediaCare Cough-Cold Chewable Tablets 1553
PediaCare 1553
PediaCare Infants' Decongestant Drops ◘ 677
PediCare Infant's Drops Decongestant Plus Cough 1553
PediaCare NightRest Cough-Cold Liquid 1553
Pediatric Vicks 44d Dry Hacking Cough & Head Congestion ◘ 763
Pediatric Vicks 44m Cough & Cold Relief ◘ 764
Robitussin Cold & Cough Liqui-Gels ◘ 776
Robitussin Maximum Strength Cough & Cold ◘ 778
Robitussin Pediatric Cough & Cold Formula ◘ 779
Robitussin Severe Congestion Liqui-Gels ◘ 776
Robitussin-DAC Syrup 2074
Robitussin-PE ◘ 778
Rondec Oral Drops 953
Rondec Syrup 953
Rondec Tablet 953
Rondec-DM Oral Drops 954
Rondec-DM Syrup 954
Rondec-TR Tablet 953
Ryna ◘ 841
Seldane-D Extended-Release Tablets 1538
Semprex-D Capsules 463
Semprex-D Capsules 1167
Sinarest Tablets ◘ 648
Sinarest Extra Strength Tablets ◘ 648
Sinarest No Drowsiness Tablets ◘ 648
Sine-Aid IB Caplets 1554
Sine-Aid Maximum Strength Sinus Medication Gelcaps, Caplets and Tablets 1554
Sine-Off No Drowsiness Formula Caplets ◘ 824
Sine-Off Sinus Medicine ◘ 825
Singlet Tablets ◘ 825
Sinutab Non-Drying Liquid Caps ◘ 859
Sinutab Sinus Allergy Medication, Maximum Strength Tablets and Caplets ◘ 860
Sinutab Sinus Medication, Maximum Strength Without Drowsiness Formula, Tablets & Caplets ◘ 860
Sinutab Sinus Medication, Regular Strength Without Drowsiness Formula ◘ 859
Sudafed Children's Liquid ◘ 861
Sudafed Cold and Cough Liquidcaps ◘ 862
Sudafed Cough Syrup ◘ 862
Sudafed Plus Liquid ◘ 862
Sudafed Plus Tablets ◘ 863
Sudafed Severe Cold Formula Caplets ◘ 863
Sudafed Severe Cold Formula Tablets ◘ 864
Sudafed Sinus Caplets ◘ 864
Sudafed Sinus Tablets ◘ 864
Sudafed Tablets, 30 mg ◘ 861
Sudafed Tablets, 60 mg ◘ 861
Sudafed 12 Hour Caplets ◘ 861
Syn-Rx Tablets 465
Syn-Rx DM Tablets 466
TheraFlu ◘ 787
TheraFlu Maximum Strength Nighttime Flu, Cold & Cough Medicine ◘ 788
TheraFlu Maximum Strength Non-Drowsy Formula Flu, Cold & Cough Medicine ◘ 788
Thera Flu Maximum Strength, Non-Drowsy Formula Flu, Cold and Cough Caplets ◘ 789
Triaminic AM Cough and Decongestant Formula ◘ 789
Triaminic AM Decongestant Formula ◘ 790
Triaminic Nite Light ◘ 791
Triaminic Sore Throat Formula ◘ 791
Tussend 1783
Tussend Expectorant 1785
Children's TYLENOL Cold Multi-Symptom Liquid Formula and Chewable Tablets 1561
Children's TYLENOL Cold Plus Cough Multi Symptom Tablets and Liquid ◘ 681
Infants' TYLENOL Cold Decongestant & Fever-Reducer Drops 1556
TYLENOL Maximum Strength Allergy Sinus Medication Gelcaps and Caplets 1563
TYLENOL Maximum Strength Allergy Sinus NightTime Medication Caplets 1555
TYLENOL Flu Maximum Strength Gelcaps 1565
TYLENOL Flu NightTime, Maximum Strength, Gelcaps 1566
TYLENOL Maximum Strength Flu NightTime Hot Medication Packets 1562
TYLENOL, Maximum Strength, Sinus Medication Geltabs, Gelcaps, Caplets and Tablets 1566
TYLENOL Cold Multi-Symptom Formula Medication Tablets and Caplets 1561
TYLENOL Cold Medication No Drowsiness Formula Gelcaps and Caplets 1562
TYLENOL Cold Multi-Symptom Hot Medication Liquid Packets 1557
TYLENOL Cough Multi-Symptom Medication with Decongestant 1565
Ursinus Inlay-Tabs ◘ 794
Vicks 44 LiquiCaps Cough, Cold & Flu Relief ◘ 755
Vicks 44 LiquiCaps Non-Drowsy Cough & Cold Relief ◘ 756
Vicks 44D Dry Hacking Cough & Head Congestion ◘ 755
Vicks 44M Cough, Cold & Flu Relief ◘ 756
Vicks DayQuil ◘ 761
Vicks DayQuil SINUS Pressure & PAIN Relief with IBUPROFEN ◘ 762
Vicks Nyquil Hot Therapy ◘ 762
Vicks NyQuil LiquiCaps Multi-Symptom Cold/Flu Relief ◘ 763

(◘ Described in PDR For Nonprescription Drugs)
(◉ Described in PDR For Ophthalmology)

815 **Interactions Index** **Phenergan VC with Codeine**

Vicks NyQuil Multi-Symptom Cold/Flu Relief - (Original & Cherry Flavor) ▣ 763

Pseudoephedrine Sulfate (Tachycardia or arrhythmias may occur). Products include:
- Cheracol Sinus ▣ 768
- Chlor-Trimeton Allergy Decongestant Tablets ▣ 799
- Claritin-D 2350
- Drixoral Cold and Allergy Sustained-Action Tablets ▣ 802
- Drixoral Cold and Flu Extended-Release Tablets ▣ 803
- Drixoral Non-Drowsy Formula Extended-Release Tablets ▣ 803
- Drixoral Allergy/Sinus Extended Release Tablets ▣ 804
- Trinalin Repetabs Tablets 1330

Quazepam (Additive sedative effects). Products include:
- Doral Tablets 2664

Salmeterol Xinafoate (Tachycardia or arrhythmias may occur). Products include:
- Serevent Inhalation Aerosol 1176

Secobarbital Sodium (Additive sedative effects). Products include:
- Seconal Sodium Pulvules 1474

Selegiline Hydrochloride (Acute hypertensive crisis; concurrent use is contraindicated). Products include:
- Eldepryl Tablets 2550

Sotalol Hydrochloride (Cardiostimulating effects blocked). Products include:
- Betapace Tablets 641

Sufentanil Citrate (Additive sedative effects). Products include:
- Sufenta Injection 1309

Temazepam (Additive sedative effects). Products include:
- Restoril Capsules 2284

Terazosin Hydrochloride (Decreased pressor response). Products include:
- Hytrin Capsules 430

Terbutaline Sulfate (Tachycardia or arrhythmias may occur). Products include:
- Brethaire Inhaler 813
- Brethine Ampuls 815
- Brethine Tablets 814
- Bricanyl Subcutaneous Injection 1502
- Bricanyl Tablets 1503

Thioridazine Hydrochloride (Additive sedative effects). Products include:
- Mellaril 2269

Thiothixene (Additive sedative effects). Products include:
- Navane Capsules and Concentrate 2201
- Navane Intramuscular 2202

Timolol Hemihydrate (Cardiostimulating effects blocked). Products include:
- Betimol 0.25%, 0.5% ⊙ 261

Timolol Maleate (Cardiostimulating effects blocked). Products include:
- Blocadren Tablets 1614
- Timolide Tablets 1748
- Timoptic in Ocudose 1753
- Timoptic Sterile Ophthalmic Solution 1751
- Timoptic-XE 1755

Tranylcypromine Sulfate (Acute hypertensive crisis; concurrent use is contraindicated). Products include:
- Parnate Tablets 2503

Triazolam (Additive sedative effects). Products include:
- Halcion Tablets 2611

Trifluoperazine Hydrochloride (Additive sedative effects). Products include:
- Stelazine 2514

Trimipramine Maleate (Additive sedative effects; increased pressor response). Products include:
- Surmontil Capsules 2811

Zolpidem Tartrate (Additive sedative effects). Products include:
- Ambien Tablets 2416

Food Interactions

Alcohol (Additive sedative effects).

PHENERGAN VC WITH CODEINE

(Codeine Phosphate, Promethazine Hydrochloride, Phenylephrine Hydrochloride) 2781

May interact with narcotic analgesics, hypnotics and sedatives, tricyclic antidepressants, tranquilizers, monoamine oxidase inhibitors, sympathomimetics, sympathomimetic bronchodilators, beta blockers, alpha adrenergic blockers, and certain other agents. Compounds in these categories include:

Acebutolol Hydrochloride (Cardiostimulating effects blocked). Products include:
- Sectral Capsules 2807

Albuterol (Tachycardia or arrhythmias may occur). Products include:
- Proventil Inhalation Aerosol 2382
- Ventolin Inhalation Aerosol and Refill 1197

Albuterol Sulfate (Tachycardia or arrhythmias may occur). Products include:
- Airet Solution for Inhalation 452
- Proventil Inhalation Solution 0.083% 2384
- Proventil Repetabs Tablets 2386
- Proventil Solution for Inhalation 0.5% 2383
- Proventil Syrup 2385
- Proventil Tablets 2386
- Ventolin Inhalation Solution 1198
- Ventolin Nebules Inhalation Solution 1199
- Ventolin Rotacaps for Inhalation 1200
- Ventolin Syrup 1202
- Ventolin Tablets 1203
- Volmax Extended-Release Tablets 1788

Alfentanil Hydrochloride (Additive sedative effects). Products include:
- Alfenta Injection 1286

Alprazolam (Additive sedative effects). Products include:
- Xanax Tablets 2649

Amitriptyline Hydrochloride (Additive sedative effects; increased pressor response). Products include:
- Elavil 2838
- Endep Tablets 2174
- Etrafon 2355
- Limbitrol 2180
- Triavil Tablets 1757

Amoxapine (Additive sedative effects; increased pressor response). Products include:
- Asendin Tablets 1369

Atenolol (Cardiostimulating effects blocked). Products include:
- Tenoretic Tablets 2845
- Tenormin Tablets and I.V. Injection 2847

Atropine Sulfate (Enhanced pressor response; reflex bradycardia blocked). Products include:
- Arco-Lase Plus Tablets 512
- Atrohist Plus Tablets 454
- Atropine Sulfate Sterile Ophthalmic Solution ⊙ 233
- Donnatal 2060
- Donnatal Extentabs 2061
- Donnatal Tablets 2060
- Lomotil 2439
- Motofen Tablets 784
- Urised Tablets 1964

Betaxolol Hydrochloride (Cardiostimulating effects blocked). Products include:
- Betoptic Ophthalmic Solution 469
- Betoptic S Ophthalmic Suspension 471
- Kerlone Tablets 2436

Bisoprolol Fumarate (Cardiostimulating effects blocked). Products include:
- Zebeta Tablets 1413
- Ziac 1415

Bitolterol Mesylate (Tachycardia or arrhythmias may occur). Products include:
- Tornalate Solution for Inhalation, 0.2% 956
- Tornalate Metered Dose Inhaler 957

Buprenorphine (Additive sedative effects). Products include:
- Buprenex Injectable 2006

Buspirone Hydrochloride (Additive sedative effects). Products include:
- BuSpar 737

Carteolol Hydrochloride (Cardiostimulating effects blocked). Products include:
- Cartrol Tablets 410
- Ocupress Ophthalmic Solution, 1% Sterile ⊙ 309

Chlordiazepoxide (Additive sedative effects). Products include:
- Libritabs Tablets 2177
- Limbitrol 2180

Chlordiazepoxide Hydrochloride (Additive sedative effects). Products include:
- Librax Capsules 2176
- Librium Capsules 2178
- Librium Injectable 2179

Chlorpromazine (Additive sedative effects). Products include:
- Thorazine Suppositories 2523

Chlorprothixene (Additive sedative effects).
- No products indexed under this heading.

Chlorprothixene Hydrochloride (Additive sedative effects).
- No products indexed under this heading.

Clomipramine Hydrochloride (Additive sedative effects; increased pressor response). Products include:
- Anafranil Capsules 803

Clorazepate Dipotassium (Additive sedative effects). Products include:
- Tranxene 451

Desipramine Hydrochloride (Additive sedative effects; increased pressor response). Products include:
- Norpramin Tablets 1526

Dezocine (Additive sedative effects). Products include:
- Dalgan Injection 538

Diazepam (Additive sedative effects). Products include:
- Dizac 1809
- Valium Injectable 2182
- Valium Tablets 2183
- Valrelease Capsules 2169

Dobutamine Hydrochloride (Tachycardia or arrhythmias may occur). Products include:
- Dobutrex Solution Vials 1439

Dopamine Hydrochloride (Tachycardia or arrhythmias may occur).
- No products indexed under this heading.

Doxazosin Mesylate (Pressor response decreased). Products include:
- Cardura Tablets 2186

Doxepin Hydrochloride (Additive sedative effects; increased pressor response). Products include:
- Sinequan 2205
- Zonalon Cream 1055

Droperidol (Additive sedative effects). Products include:
- Inapsine Injection 1296

Ephedrine Hydrochloride (Tachycardia or arrhythmias may occur). Products include:
- Primatene Dual Action Formula ▣ 872
- Primatene Tablets ▣ 873
- Quadrinal Tablets 1350

Ephedrine Sulfate (Tachycardia or arrhythmias may occur). Products include:
- Bronkaid Caplets ▣ 717
- Marax Tablets & DF Syrup 2200

Ephedrine Tannate (Tachycardia or arrhythmias may occur). Products include:
- Rynatuss 2673

Epinephrine (Tachycardia or arrhythmias may occur). Products include:
- Bronkaid Mist ▣ 717
- EPIFRIN ⊙ 239
- EpiPen 790
- Marcaine Hydrochloride with Epinephrine 1:200,000 2316
- Primatene Mist ▣ 873
- Sensorcaine with Epinephrine Injection 559
- Sus-Phrine Injection 1019
- Xylocaine with Epinephrine Injections 567

Epinephrine Bitartrate (Tachycardia or arrhythmias may occur). Products include:
- Bronkaid Mist Suspension ▣ 718
- Sensorcaine-MPF with Epinephrine Injection 559

Epinephrine Hydrochloride (Tachycardia or arrhythmias may occur). Products include:
- Ana-Kit Anaphylaxis Emergency Treatment Kit 617

Ergotamine Tartrate (Excessive rise in blood pressure). Products include:
- Bellergal-S Tablets 2250
- Cafergot 2251
- Ergomar 1486
- Wigraine Tablets & Suppositories 1829

Esmolol Hydrochloride (Cardiostimulating effects blocked). Products include:
- Brevibloc Injection 1808

Estazolam (Additive sedative effects). Products include:
- ProSom Tablets 449

Ethchlorvynol (Additive sedative effects). Products include:
- Placidyl Capsules 448

Ethinamate (Additive sedative effects).
- No products indexed under this heading.

Ethylnorepinephrine Hydrochloride (Tachycardia or arrhythmias may occur).
- No products indexed under this heading.

Fentanyl (Additive sedative effects). Products include:
- Duragesic Transdermal System 1288

Fentanyl Citrate (Additive sedative effects). Products include:
- Sublimaze Injection 1307

Fluphenazine Decanoate (Additive sedative effects). Products include:
- Prolixin Decanoate 509

Fluphenazine Enanthate (Additive sedative effects). Products include:
- Prolixin Enanthate 509

Fluphenazine Hydrochloride (Additive sedative effects). Products include:
- Prolixin 509

Flurazepam Hydrochloride (Additive sedative effects). Products include:
- Dalmane Capsules 2173

IMPORTANT NOTE: Always consult each drug listing in the patient's regimen for possible interactions.

Phenergan VC with Codeine

Interactions Index

Furazolidone (Acute hypertensive crisis; concurrent use is contraindicated). Products include:

Furoxone 2046

Glutethimide (Additive sedative effects).

No products indexed under this heading.

Haloperidol (Additive sedative effects). Products include:

Haldol Injection, Tablets and Concentrate 1575

Haloperidol Decanoate (Additive sedative effects). Products include:

Haldol Decanoate.................................. 1577

Hydrocodone Bitartrate (Additive sedative effects). Products include:

Anexsia 5/500 Elixir 1781
Anexia Tablets....................................... 1782
Codiclear DH Syrup 791
Deconamine CX Cough and Cold Liquid and Tablets............................... 1319
Duratuss HD Elixir 2565
Hycodan Tablets and Syrup 930
Hycomine Compound Tablets 932
Hycomine 931
Hycotuss Expectorant Syrup 933
Hydrocet Capsules 782
Lorcet 10/650....................................... 1018
Lortab 2566
Tussend 1783
Tussend Expectorant 1785
Vicodin Tablets...................................... 1356
Vicodin ES Tablets 1357
Vicodin Tuss Expectorant 1358
Zydone Capsules 949

Hydrocodone Polistirex (Additive sedative effects). Products include:

Tussionex Pennkinetic Extended-Release Suspension 998

Hydroxyzine Hydrochloride (Additive sedative effects). Products include:

Atarax Tablets & Syrup........................ 2185
Marax Tablets & DF Syrup................... 2200
Vistaril Intramuscular Solution.......... 2216

Imipramine Hydrochloride (Additive sedative effects; increased pressor response). Products include:

Tofranil Ampuls 854
Tofranil Tablets 856

Imipramine Pamoate (Additive sedative effects; increased pressor response). Products include:

Tofranil-PM Capsules........................... 857

Isocarboxazid (Acute hypertensive crisis; concurrent use is contraindicated).

No products indexed under this heading.

Isoetharine (Tachycardia or arrhythmias may occur). Products include:

Bronkometer Aerosol 2302
Bronkosol Solution 2302
Isoetharine Inhalation Solution, USP, Arm-a-Med................................... 551

Isoproterenol Hydrochloride (Tachycardia or arrhythmias may occur). Products include:

Isuprel Hydrochloride Injection 1:5000 2311
Isuprel Hydrochloride Solution 1:200 & 1:100 2313
Isuprel Mistometer 2312

Isoproterenol Sulfate (Tachycardia or arrhythmias may occur). Products include:

Norisodrine with Calcium Iodide Syrup.. 442

Labetalol Hydrochloride (Cardiostimulating effects blocked). Products include:

Normodyne Injection 2377
Normodyne Tablets 2379
Trandate 1185

Levobunolol Hydrochloride (Cardiostimulating effects blocked). Products include:

Betagan .... ◉ 233

Levorphanol Tartrate (Additive sedative effects). Products include:

Levo-Dromoran 2129

Lorazepam (Additive sedative effects). Products include:

Ativan Injection..................................... 2698
Ativan Tablets 2700

Loxapine Hydrochloride (Additive sedative effects). Products include:

Loxitane 1378

Maprotiline Hydrochloride (Additive sedative effects; increased pressor response). Products include:

Ludiomil Tablets................................... 843

Meperidine Hydrochloride (Additive sedative effects). Products include:

Demerol 2308
Mepergan Injection 2753

Meprobamate (Additive sedative effects). Products include:

Miltown Tablets 2672
PMB 200 and PMB 400 2783

Mesoridazine Besylate (Additive sedative effects). Products include:

Serentil... 684

Metaproterenol Sulfate (Tachycardia or arrhythmias may occur). Products include:

Alupent... 669
Metaproterenol Sulfate Inhalation Solution, USP, Arm-a-Med 552

Metaraminol Bitartrate (Tachycardia or arrhythmias may occur). Products include:

Aramine Injection.................................. 1609

Methadone Hydrochloride (Additive sedative effects). Products include:

Methadone Hydrochloride Oral Concentrate 2233
Methadone Hydrochloride Oral Solution & Tablets................................ 2235

Methoxamine Hydrochloride (Tachycardia or arrhythmias may occur). Products include:

Vasoxyl Injection 1196

Metipranolol Hydrochloride (Cardiostimulating effects blocked). Products include:

OptiPranolol (Metipranolol 0.3%) Sterile Ophthalmic Solution........... ◉ 258

Metoprolol Succinate (Cardiostimulating effects blocked). Products include:

Toprol-XL Tablets 565

Metoprolol Tartrate (Cardiostimulating effects blocked). Products include:

Lopressor Ampuls 830
Lopressor HCT Tablets 832
Lopressor Tablets 830

Midazolam Hydrochloride (Additive sedative effects). Products include:

Versed Injection 2170

Molindone Hydrochloride (Additive sedative effects). Products include:

Moban Tablets and Concentrate.......... 1048

Morphine Sulfate (Additive sedative effects). Products include:

Astramorph/PF Injection, USP (Preservative-Free) 535
Duramorph 962
Infumorph 200 and Infumorph 500 Sterile Solutions.............................. 965
MS Contin Tablets 1994
MSIR 1997
Oramorph SR (Morphine Sulfate Sustained Release Tablets) 2236
RMS Suppositories 2657
Roxanol 2243

Nadolol (Cardiostimulating effects blocked).

No products indexed under this heading.

Norepinephrine Bitartrate (Tachycardia or arrhythmias may occur). Products include:

Levophed Bitartrate Injection 2315

Nortriptyline Hydrochloride (Additive sedative effects; increased pressor response). Products include:

Pamelor 2280

Opium Alkaloids (Additive sedative effects).

No products indexed under this heading.

Oxazepam (Additive sedative effects). Products include:

Serax Capsules 2810
Serax Tablets... 2810

Oxycodone Hydrochloride (Additive sedative effects). Products include:

Percocet Tablets 938
Percodan Tablets................................... 939
Percodan-Demi Tablets......................... 940
Roxicodone Tablets, Oral Solution & Intensol (Oxycodone) 2244
Tylox Capsules 1584

Penbutolol Sulfate (Cardiostimulating effects blocked). Products include:

Levatol 2403

Perphenazine (Additive sedative effects). Products include:

Etrafon 2355
Triavil Tablets 1757
Trilafon... 2389

Phenelzine Sulfate (Acute hypertensive crisis; concurrent use is contraindicated). Products include:

Nardil 1920

Phentolamine Mesylate (Decreased pressor response). Products include:

Regitine 846

Phenylephrine Bitartrate (Tachycardia or arrhythmias may occur).

No products indexed under this heading.

Phenylephrine Tannate (Tachycardia or arrhythmias may occur). Products include:

Atrohist Pediatric Suspension 454
Ricobid-D Pediatric Suspension......... 2038
Ricobid Tablets and Pediatric Suspension.. 2038
Rynatan 2673
Rynatuss 2673

Phenylpropanolamine Hydrochloride (Tachycardia or arrhythmias may occur). Products include:

Acutrim .... ᴹᴰ 628
Allerest Children's Chewable Tablets .... ᴹᴰ 627
Allerest 12 Hour Caplets .... ᴹᴰ 627
Atrohist Plus Tablets 454
BC Cold Powder Multi-Symptom Formula (Cold-Sinus-Allergy) ...... ᴹᴰ 609
BC Cold Powder Non-Drowsy Formula (Cold-Sinus) .... ᴹᴰ 609
Cheracol Plus Head Cold/Cough Formula .... ᴹᴰ 769
Comtrex Multi-Symptom Non-Drowsy Liqui-gels............................... ᴹᴰ 618
Contac Continuous Action Nasal Decongestant/Antihistamine 12 Hour Capsules..................................... ᴹᴰ 813
Contac Maximum Strength Continuous Action Decongestant/Antihistamine 12 Hour Caplets.. ᴹᴰ 813
Contac Severe Cold and Flu Formula Caplets .... ᴹᴰ 814
Coricidin 'D' Decongestant Tablets .... ᴹᴰ 800
Dexatrim .... ᴹᴰ 832
Dexatrim Plus Vitamins Caplets .... ᴹᴰ 832
Dimetane-DC Cough Syrup 2059
Dimetapp Elixir .... ᴹᴰ 773
Dimetapp Extentabs .... ᴹᴰ 774
Dimetapp Tablets/Liqui-Gels .... ᴹᴰ 775
Dimetapp Cold & Allergy Chewable Tablets .... ᴹᴰ 773
Dimetapp DM Elixir .... ᴹᴰ 774
Dura-Vent Tablets 952
Entex Capsules 1986
Entex LA Tablets 1987
Entex Liquid 1986

Exgest LA Tablets 782
Hycomine 931
Isoclor Timesule Capsules .... ᴹᴰ 637
Nolamine Timed-Release Tablets 785
Ornade Spansule Capsules 2502
Propagest Tablets 786
Pyrroxate Caplets .... ᴹᴰ 772
Robitussin-CF .... ᴹᴰ 777
Sinulin Tablets 787
Tavist-D 12 Hour Relief Tablets .... ᴹᴰ 787
Teldrin 12 Hour Antihistamine/Nasal Decongestant Allergy Relief Capsules .... ᴹᴰ 826
Triaminic Allergy Tablets .... ᴹᴰ 789
Triaminic Cold Tablets .... ᴹᴰ 790
Triaminic Expectorant .... ᴹᴰ 790
Triaminic Syrup .... ᴹᴰ 792
Triaminic-12 Tablets .... ᴹᴰ 792
Triaminic-DM Syrup .... ᴹᴰ 792
Triaminicin Tablets .... ᴹᴰ 793
Triaminicol Multi-Symptom Cold Tablets .... ᴹᴰ 793
Triaminicol Multi-Symptom Relief ᴹᴰ 794
Vicks DayQuil Allergy Relief 12-Hour Extended Release Tablets.. ᴹᴰ 760
Vicks DayQuil Allergy Relief 4-Hour Tablets .... ᴹᴰ 760
Vicks DayQuil SINUS Pressure & CONGESTION Relief........................ ᴹᴰ 761

Pindolol (Cardiostimulating effects blocked). Products include:

Visken Tablets.. 2299

Pirbuterol Acetate (Tachycardia or arrhythmias may occur). Products include:

Maxair Autohaler 1492
Maxair Inhaler 1494

Prazepam (Additive sedative effects).

No products indexed under this heading.

Prazosin Hydrochloride (Pressor response decreased). Products include:

Minipress Capsules................................ 1937
Minizide Capsules 1938

Prochlorperazine (Additive sedative effects). Products include:

Compazine 2470

Propofol (Additive sedative effects). Products include:

Diprivan Injection................................. 2833

Propoxyphene Hydrochloride (Additive sedative effects). Products include:

Darvon 1435
Wygesic Tablets 2827

Propoxyphene Napsylate (Additive sedative effects). Products include:

Darvon-N/Darvocet-N 1433

Propranolol Hydrochloride (Cardiostimulating effects blocked). Products include:

Inderal 2728
Inderal LA Long Acting Capsules 2730
Inderide Tablets 2732
Inderide LA Long Acting Capsules .. 2734

Protriptyline Hydrochloride (Additive sedative effects; increased pressor response). Products include:

Vivactil Tablets 1774

Pseudoephedrine Hydrochloride (Tachycardia or arrhythmias may occur). Products include:

Actifed Allergy Daytime/Nighttime Caplets.. ᴹᴰ 844
Actifed Plus Caplets .... ᴹᴰ 845
Actifed Plus Tablets .... ᴹᴰ 845
Actifed with Codeine Cough Syrup.. 1067
Actifed Sinus Daytime/Nighttime Tablets and Caplets .... ᴹᴰ 846
Actifed Syrup... ᴹᴰ 846
Actifed Tablets .... ᴹᴰ 844
Advil Cold and Sinus Caplets and Tablets (formerly CoAdvil) .... ᴹᴰ 870
Alka-Seltzer Plus Cold Medicine Liqui-Gels .... ᴹᴰ 706
Alka-Seltzer Plus Cold & Cough Medicine Liqui-Gels.......................... ᴹᴰ 705
Alka-Seltzer Plus Night-Time Cold Medicine Liqui-Gels.......................... ᴹᴰ 706
Allerest Headache Strength Tablets .... ᴹᴰ 627

(ᴹᴰ Described in PDR For Nonprescription Drugs) (◉ Described in PDR For Ophthalmology)

Interactions Index

Allerest Maximum Strength Tablets .... ✦D 627
Allerest No Drowsiness Tablets ...... ✦D 627
Allerest Sinus Pain Formula .... ✦D 627
Anatuss LA Tablets 1542
Atrohist Pediatric Capsules 453
Bayer Select Sinus Pain Relief Formula .... ✦D 717
Benadryl Allergy Decongestant Liquid Medication .... ✦D 848
Benadryl Allergy Decongestant Tablets .... ✦D 848
Benadryl Allergy Sinus Headache Formula Caplets .... ✦D 849
Benylin Multisymptom .... ✦D 852
Bromfed Capsules (Extended-Release) 1785
Bromfed Syrup .... ✦D 733
Bromfed Tablets 1785
Bromfed-DM Cough Syrup 1786
Bromfed-PD Capsules (Extended-Release) 1785
Children's Vicks DayQuil Allergy Relief .... ✦D 757
Children's Vicks NyQuil Cold/ Cough Relief .... ✦D 758
Comtrex Multi-Symptom Cold Reliever Tablets/Caplets/Liqui-Gels/Liquid .... ✦D 615
Allergy-Sinus Comtrex Multi-Symptom Allergy-Sinus Formula Tablets .... ✦D 617
Comtrex Multi-Symptom Non-Drowsy Caplets .... ✦D 618
Congess 1004
Contac Day Allergy/Sinus Caplets ✦D 812
Contac Day & Night .... ✦D 812
Contac Night Allergy/Sinus Caplets .... ✦D 812
Contac Severe Cold & Flu Non-Drowsy .... ✦D 815
Deconamine Chewable Tablets 1320
Deconamine CX Cough and Cold Liquid and Tablets 1319
Deconamine 1320
Deconsal C Expectorant Syrup 456
Deconsal Pediatric Syrup 457
Deconsal II Tablets 454
Dimetane-DX Cough Syrup 2059
Dimetapp Sinus Caplets .... ✦D 775
Dorcol Children's Cough Syrup ..... ✦D 785
Drixoral Cough + Congestion Liquid Caps .... ✦D 802
Dura-Tap/PD Capsules 2867
Duratuss Tablets 2565
Duratuss HD Elixir 2565
Efidac/24 .... ✦D 635
Entex PSE Tablets 1987
Fedahist Gyrocaps 2401
Fedahist Timecaps 2401
Guaifed 1787
Guaifed Syrup .... ✦D 734
Guaimax-D Tablets 792
Guaitab Tablets .... ✦D 734
Isoclor Expectorant 990
Kronofed-A 977
Motrin IB Sinus .... ✦D 838
Novahistine DH 2462
Novahistine DMX .... ✦D 822
Novahistine Expectorant 2463
Nucofed 2051
PediaCare Cold Allergy Chewable Tablets .... ✦D 677
PediaCare Cough-Cold Chewable Tablets 1553
PediaCare 1553
PediaCare Infants' Decongestant Drops .... ✦D 677
PediCare Infant's Drops Decongestant Plus Cough 1553
PediaCare NightRest Cough-Cold Liquid 1553
Pediatric Vicks 44d Dry Hacking Cough & Head Congestion .... ✦D 763
Pediatric Vicks 44m Cough & Cold Relief .... ✦D 764
Robitussin Cold & Cough Liqui-Gels .... ✦D 776
Robitussin Maximum Strength Cough & Cold .... ✦D 778
Robitussin Pediatric Cough & Cold Formula .... ✦D 779
Robitussin Severe Congestion Liqui-Gels .... ✦D 776
Robitussin-DAC Syrup 2074
Robitussin-PE .... ✦D 778
Rondec Oral Drops 953
Rondec Syrup 953
Rondec Tablet 953
Rondec-DM Oral Drops 954
Rondec-DM Syrup 954

Rondec-TR Tablet 953
Ryna .... ✦D 841
Seldane-D Extended-Release Tablets 1538
Semprex-D Capsules 463
Semprex-D Capsules 1167
Sinarest Tablets .... ✦D 648
Sinarest Extra Strength Tablets .... ✦D 648
Sinarest No Drowsiness Tablets .... ✦D 648
Sine-Aid IB Caplets 1554
Sine-Aid Maximum Strength Sinus Medication Gelcaps, Caplets and Tablets 1554
Sine-Off No Drowsiness Formula Caplets .... ✦D 824
Sine-Off Sinus Medicine .... ✦D 825
Singlet Tablets .... ✦D 825
Sinutab Non-Drying Liquid Caps .... ✦D 859
Sinutab Sinus Allergy Medication, Maximum Strength Tablets and Caplets .... ✦D 860
Sinutab Sinus Medication, Maximum Strength Without Drowsiness Formula, Tablets & Caplets .... ✦D 860
Sinutab Sinus Medication, Regular Strength Without Drowsiness Formula .... ✦D 859
Sudafed Children's Liquid .... ✦D 861
Sudafed Cold and Cough Liquidcaps .... ✦D 862
Sudafed Cough Syrup .... ✦D 862
Sudafed Plus Liquid .... ✦D 862
Sudafed Plus Tablets .... ✦D 863
Sudafed Severe Cold Formula Caplets .... ✦D 863
Sudafed Severe Cold Formula Tablets .... ✦D 864
Sudafed Sinus Caplets .... ✦D 864
Sudafed Sinus Tablets .... ✦D 864
Sudafed Tablets, 30 mg .... ✦D 861
Sudafed Tablets, 60 mg .... ✦D 861
Sudafed 12 Hour Caplets .... ✦D 861
Syn-Rx Tablets 465
Syn-Rx DM Tablets 466
TheraFlu .... ✦D 787
TheraFlu Maximum Strength Nighttime Flu, Cold & Cough Medicine .... ✦D 788
TheraFlu Maximum Strength Non-Drowsy Formula Flu, Cold & Cough Medicine .... ✦D 788
Thera Flu Maximum Strength, Non-Drowsy Formula Flu, Cold and Cough Caplets .... ✦D 789
Triaminic AM Cough and Decongestant Formula .... ✦D 789
Triaminic AM Decongestant Formula .... ✦D 790
Triaminic Nite Light .... ✦D 791
Triaminic Sore Throat Formula ..... ✦D 791
Tussend 1783
Tussend Expectorant 1785
Children's TYLENOL Cold Multi-Symptom Liquid Formula and Chewable Tablets 1561
Children's TYLENOL Cold Plus Cough Multi Symptom Tablets and Liquid .... ✦D 681
Infants' TYLENOL Cold Decongestant & Fever-Reducer Drops 1556
TYLENOL Maximum Strength Allergy Sinus Medication Gelcaps and Caplets 1563
TYLENOL Maximum Strength Allergy Sinus NightTime Medication Caplets 1555
TYLENOL Flu Maximum Strength Gelcaps 1565
TYLENOL Flu NightTime, Maximum Strength, Gelcaps 1566
TYLENOL Maximum Strength Flu NightTime Hot Medication Packets 1562
TYLENOL, Maximum Strength, Sinus Medication Geltabs, Gelcaps, Caplets and Tablets 1566
TYLENOL Cold Multi-Symptom Formula Medication Tablets and Caplets 1561
TYLENOL Cold Medication No Drowsiness Formula Gelcaps and Caplets 1562
TYLENOL Cold Multi-Symptom Hot Medication Liquid Packets 1557
TYLENOL Cough Multi-Symptom Medication with Decongestant 1565
Ursinus Inlay-Tabs .... ✦D 794
Vicks 44 LiquiCaps Cough, Cold & Flu Relief .... ✦D 755

Vicks 44 LiquiCaps Non-Drowsy Cough & Cold Relief .... ✦D 756
Vicks 44D Dry Hacking Cough & Head Congestion .... ✦D 755
Vicks 44M Cough, Cold & Flu Relief .... ✦D 756
Vicks DayQuil .... ✦D 761
Vicks DayQuil SINUS Pressure & PAIN Relief with IBUPROFEN ..... ✦D 762
Vicks Nyquil Hot Therapy .... ✦D 762
Vicks NyQuil LiquiCaps Multi-Symptom Cold/Flu Relief .... ✦D 763
Vicks NyQuil Multi-Symptom Cold/Flu Relief - (Original & Cherry Flavor) .... ✦D 763

Pseudoephedrine Sulfate (Tachycardia or arrhythmias may occur). Products include:

Cheracol Sinus .... ✦D 768
Chlor-Trimeton Allergy Decongestant Tablets .... ✦D 799
Claritin-D 2350
Drixoral Cold and Allergy Sustained-Action Tablets .... ✦D 802
Drixoral Cold and Flu Extended-Release Tablets .... ✦D 803
Drixoral Non-Drowsy Formula Extended-Release Tablets .... ✦D 803
Drixoral Allergy/Sinus Extended Release Tablets .... ✦D 804
Trinalin Repetabs Tablets 1330

Quazepam (Additive sedative effects). Products include:

Doral Tablets 2664

Salmeterol Xinafoate (Tachycardia or arrhythmias may occur). Products include:

Serevent Inhalation Aerosol 1176

Secobarbital Sodium (Additive sedative effects). Products include:

Seconal Sodium Pulvules 1474

Selegiline Hydrochloride (Acute hypertensive crisis; concurrent use is contraindicated). Products include:

Eldepryl Tablets 2550

Sotalol Hydrochloride (Cardio-stimulating effects blocked). Products include:

Betapace Tablets 641

Sufentanil Citrate (Additive sedative effects). Products include:

Sufenta Injection 1309

Temazepam (Additive sedative effects). Products include:

Restoril Capsules 2284

Terazosin Hydrochloride (Pressor response decreased). Products include:

Hytrin Capsules 430

Terbutaline Sulfate (Tachycardia or arrhythmias may occur). Products include:

Brethaire Inhaler 813
Brethine Ampuls 815
Brethine Tablets 814
Bricanyl Subcutaneous Injection ... 1502
Bricanyl Tablets 1503

Thioridazine Hydrochloride (Additive sedative effects). Products include:

Mellaril 2269

Thiothixene (Additive sedative effects). Products include:

Navane Capsules and Concentrate 2201
Navane Intramuscular 2202

Timolol Hemihydrate (Cardio-stimulating effects blocked). Products include:

Betimol 0.25%, 0.5% .... © 261

Timolol Maleate (Cardiostimulating effects blocked). Products include:

Blocadren Tablets 1614
Timolide Tablets 1748
Timoptic in Ocudose 1753
Timoptic Sterile Ophthalmic Solution 1751
Timoptic-XE 1755

Tranylcypromine Sulfate (Acute hypertensive crisis; concurrent use is contraindicated). Products include:

Parnate Tablets 2503

Phenobarbital

Triazolam (Additive sedative effects). Products include:

Halcion Tablets 2611

Trifluoperazine Hydrochloride (Additive sedative effects). Products include:

Stelazine 2514

Trimipramine Maleate (Additive sedative effects; increased pressor response). Products include:

Surmontil Capsules 2811

Zolpidem Tartrate (Additive sedative effects). Products include:

Ambien Tablets 2416

Food Interactions

Alcohol (Additive sedative effects).

PHENOBARBITAL ELIXIR AND TABLETS

(Phenobarbital) 1469

May interact with oral anticoagulants, corticosteroids, central nervous system depressants, antihistamines, tranquilizers, monoamine oxidase inhibitors, oral contraceptives, hypnotics and sedatives, and certain other agents. Compounds in these categories include:

Acrivastine (Additive depressant effects). Products include:

Semprex-D Capsules 463
Semprex-D Capsules 1167

Alfentanil Hydrochloride (Additive depressant effects). Products include:

Alfenta Injection 1286

Alprazolam (Additive depressant effects). Products include:

Xanax Tablets 2649

Aprobarbital (Additive depressant effects).

No products indexed under this heading.

Astemizole (Additive depressant effects). Products include:

Hismanal Tablets 1293

Azatadine Maleate (Additive depressant effects). Products include:

Trinalin Repetabs Tablets 1330

Betamethasone Acetate (Enhanced metabolism of exogenous corticosteroids). Products include:

Celestone Soluspan Suspension 2347

Betamethasone Sodium Phosphate (Enhanced metabolism of exogenous corticosteroids). Products include:

Celestone Soluspan Suspension 2347

Bromodiphenhydramine Hydrochloride (Additive depressant effects).

No products indexed under this heading.

Brompheniramine Maleate (Additive depressant effects). Products include:

Alka Seltzer Plus Sinus Medicine .. ✦D 707
Bromfed Capsules (Extended-Release) 1785
Bromfed Syrup .... ✦D 733
Bromfed Tablets 1785
Bromfed-DM Cough Syrup 1786
Bromfed-PD Capsules (Extended-Release) 1785
Dimetane-DC Cough Syrup 2059
Dimetane-DX Cough Syrup 2059
Dimetapp Elixir .... ✦D 773
Dimetapp Extentabs .... ✦D 774
Dimetapp Tablets/Liqui-Gels .... ✦D 775
Dimetapp Cold & Allergy Chewable Tablets .... ✦D 773
Dimetapp DM Elixir .... ✦D 774
Vicks DayQuil Allergy Relief 12-Hour Extended Release Tablets .. ✦D 760
Vicks DayQuil Allergy Relief 4-Hour Tablets .... ✦D 760

IMPORTANT NOTE: Always consult each drug listing in the patient's regimen for possible interactions.

Phenobarbital Interactions Index 818

Buprenorphine (Additive depressant effects). Products include:

Buprenex Injectable ... 2006

Buspirone Hydrochloride (Additive depressant effects). Products include:

BuSpar ... 737

Butabarbital (Additive depressant effects).

No products indexed under this heading.

Butalbital (Additive depressant effects). Products include:

Esgic-plus Tablets ... 1013
Fioricet Tablets ... 2258
Fioricet with Codeine Capsules ... 2260
Fiorinal Capsules ... 2261
Fiorinal with Codeine Capsules ... 2262
Fiorinal Tablets ... 2261
Phrenilin ... 785
Sedapap Tablets 50 mg/650 mg .. 1543

Chlordiazepoxide (Additive depressant effects). Products include:

Libritabs Tablets ... 2177
Limbitrol ... 2180

Chlordiazepoxide Hydrochloride (Additive depressant effects). Products include:

Librax Capsules ... 2176
Librium Capsules ... 2178
Librium Injectable ... 2179

Chlorpheniramine Maleate (Additive depressant effects). Products include:

Alka-Seltzer Plus Cold Medicine ... ▣ 705
Alka-Seltzer Plus Cold Medicine Liqui-Gels ... ▣ 706
Alka-Seltzer Plus Cold & Cough Medicine ... ▣ 708
Alka-Seltzer Plus Cold & Cough Medicine Liqui-Gels ... ▣ 705
Allerest Children's Chewable Tablets ... ▣ 627
Allerest Headache Strength Tablets ... ▣ 627
Allerest Maximum Strength Tablets ... ▣ 627
Allerest Sinus Pain Formula ... ▣ 627
Allerest 12 Hour Caplets ... ▣ 627
Ana-Kit Anaphylaxis Emergency Treatment Kit ... 617
Atrohist Pediatric Capsules ... 453
Atrohist Plus Tablets ... 454
BC Cold Powder Multi-Symptom Formula (Cold-Sinus-Allergy) ... ▣ 609
Cerose DM ... ▣ 878
Cheracol Plus Head Cold/Cough Formula ... ▣ 769
Children's Vicks DayQuil Allergy Relief ... ▣ 757
Children's Vicks NyQuil Cold/Cough Relief ... ▣ 758
Chlor-Trimeton Allergy Decongestant Tablets ... ▣ 799
Chlor-Trimeton Allergy Tablets ... ▣ 798
Comhist ... 2038
Comtrex Multi-Symptom Cold Reliever Tablets/Caplets/Liqui-Gels/Liquid ... ▣ 615
Allergy-Sinus Comtrex Multi-Symptom Allergy-Sinus Formula Tablets ... ▣ 617
Contac Continuous Action Nasal Decongestant/Antihistamine 12 Hour Capsules ... ▣ 813
Contac Maximum Strength Continuous Action Decongestant/Antihistamine 12 Hour Caplets .. ▣ 813
Contac Severe Cold and Flu Formula Caplets ... ▣ 814
Coricidin 'D' Decongestant Tablets ... ▣ 800
Coricidin Tablets ... ▣ 800
D.A. Chewable Tablets ... 951
Deconamine ... 1320
Dura-Tap/PD Capsules ... 2867
Dura-Vent/DA Tablets ... 953
Extendryl ... 1005
Fedahist Gyrocaps ... 2401
Fedahist Timecaps ... 2401
Hycomine Compound Tablets ... 932
Isoclor Timesule Capsules ... ▣ 637
Kronofed-A ... 977
Nolamine Timed-Release Tablets ... 785
Novahistine DH ... 2462
Novahistine Elixir ... ▣ 823
Ornade Spansule Capsules ... 2502
PediaCare Cold Allergy Chewable Tablets ... ▣ 677
PediaCare Cough-Cold Chewable Tablets ... 1553
PediaCare Cough-Cold Liquid ... 1553
PediaCare NightRest Cough-Cold Liquid ... 1553
Pediatric Vicks 44m Cough & Cold Relief ... ▣ 764
Pyrroxate Caplets ... ▣ 772
Ryna ... ▣ 841
Sinarest Tablets ... ▣ 648
Sinarest Extra Strength Tablets ... ▣ 648
Sine-Off Sinus Medicine ... ▣ 825
Singlet Tablets ... ▣ 825
Sinulin Tablets ... 787
Sinutab Sinus Allergy Medication, Maximum Strength Tablets and Caplets ... ▣ 860
Sudafed Plus Liquid ... ▣ 862
Sudafed Plus Tablets ... ▣ 863
Teldrin 12 Hour Antihistamine/Nasal Decongestant Allergy Relief Capsules ... ▣ 826
TheraFlu ... ▣ 787
TheraFlu Maximum Strength Nighttime Flu, Cold & Cough Medicine ... ▣ 788
Triaminic Allergy Tablets ... ▣ 789
Triaminic Cold Tablets ... ▣ 790
Triaminic Nite Light ... ▣ 791
Triaminic Syrup ... ▣ 792
Triaminic-12 Tablets ... ▣ 792
Triaminicin Tablets ... ▣ 793
Triaminicol Multi-Symptom Cold Tablets ... ▣ 793
Triaminicol Multi-Symptom Relief ▣ 794
Tussend ... 1783
Children's TYLENOL Cold Multi-Symptom Liquid Formula and Chewable Tablets ... 1561
Children's TYLENOL Cold Plus Cough Multi Symptom Tablets and Liquid ... ▣ 681
TYLENOL Maximum Strength Allergy Sinus Medication Gelcaps and Caplets ... 1563
TYLENOL Cold Multi-Symptom Formula Medication Tablets and Caplets ... 1561
TYLENOL Cold Multi-Symptom Hot Medication Liquid Packets ... 1557
Vicks 44 LiquiCaps Cough, Cold & Flu Relief ... ▣ 755
Vicks 44M Cough, Cold & Flu Relief ... ▣ 756

Chlorpheniramine Polistirex (Additive depressant effects). Products include:

Tussionex Pennkinetic Extended-Release Suspension ... 998

Chlorpheniramine Tannate (Additive depressant effects). Products include:

Atrohist Pediatric Suspension ... 454
Ricobid Tablets and Pediatric Suspension ... 2038
Rynatan ... 2673
Rynatuss ... 2673

Chlorpromazine (Additive depressant effects). Products include:

Thorazine Suppositories ... 2523

Chlorprothixene (Additive depressant effects).

No products indexed under this heading.

Chlorprothixene Hydrochloride (Additive depressant effects).

No products indexed under this heading.

Clemastine Fumarate (Additive depressant effects). Products include:

Tavist Syrup ... 2297
Tavist Tablets ... 2298
Tavist-1 12 Hour Relief Tablets ... ▣ 787
Tavist-D 12 Hour Relief Tablets ... ▣ 787

Clorazepate Dipotassium (Additive depressant effects). Products include:

Tranxene ... 451

Clozapine (Additive depressant effects). Products include:

Clozaril Tablets ... 2252

Codeine Phosphate (Additive depressant effects). Products include:

Actifed with Codeine Cough Syrup.. 1067
Brontex ... 1981
Deconsal C Expectorant Syrup ... 456
Deconsal Pediatric Syrup ... 457
Dimetane-DC Cough Syrup ... 2059
Empirin with Codeine Tablets ... 1093
Fioricet with Codeine Capsules ... 2260
Fiorinal with Codeine Capsules ... 2262
Isoclor Expectorant ... 990
Novahistine DH ... 2462
Novahistine Expectorant ... 2463
Nucofed ... 2051
Phenergan with Codeine ... 2777
Phenergan VC with Codeine ... 2781
Robitussin A-C Syrup ... 2073
Robitussin-DAC Syrup ... 2074
Ryna ... ▣ 841
Soma Compound w/Codeine Tablets ... 2676
Tussi-Organidin NR Liquid and S NR Liquid ... 2677
Tylenol with Codeine ... 1583

Cortisone Acetate (Enhanced metabolism of exogenous corticosteroids). Products include:

Cortone Acetate Sterile Suspension ... 1623
Cortone Acetate Tablets ... 1624

Cyproheptadine Hydrochloride (Additive depressant effects). Products include:

Periactin ... 1724

Desflurane (Additive depressant effects). Products include:

Suprane ... 1813

Desogestrel (Decreased estrogen effect). Products include:

Desogen Tablets ... 1817
Ortho-Cept ... 1851

Dexamethasone (Enhanced metabolism of exogenous corticosteroids). Products include:

AK-Trol Ointment & Suspension ... ⊙ 205
Decadron Elixir ... 1633
Decadron Tablets ... 1635
Decaspray Topical Aerosol ... 1648
Dexacidin Ointment ... ⊙ 263
Maxitrol Ophthalmic Ointment and Suspension ... ⊙ 224
TobraDex Ophthalmic Suspension and Ointment ... 473

Dexamethasone Acetate (Enhanced metabolism of exogenous corticosteroids). Products include:

Dalalone D.P. Injectable ... 1011
Decadron-LA Sterile Suspension ... 1646

Dexamethasone Sodium Phosphate (Enhanced metabolism of exogenous corticosteroids). Products include:

Decadron Phosphate Injection ... 1637
Decadron Phosphate Respihaler ... 1642
Decadron Phosphate Sterile Ophthalmic Ointment ... 1641
Decadron Phosphate Sterile Ophthalmic Solution ... 1642
Decadron Phosphate Topical Cream ... 1644
Decadron Phosphate Turbinaire ... 1645
Decadron Phosphate with Xylocaine Injection, Sterile ... 1639
Dexacort Phosphate in Respihaler .. 458
Dexacort Phosphate in Turbinaire .. 459
NeoDecadron Sterile Ophthalmic Ointment ... 1712
NeoDecadron Sterile Ophthalmic Solution ... 1713
NeoDecadron Topical Cream ... 1714

Dexchlorpheniramine Maleate (Additive depressant effects).

No products indexed under this heading.

Dezocine (Additive depressant effects). Products include:

Dalgan Injection ... 538

Diazepam (Additive depressant effects). Products include:

Dizac ... 1809
Valium Injectable ... 2182
Valium Tablets ... 2183
Valrelease Capsules ... 2169

Dicumarol (Lowered plasma levels and decreased anticoagulant activity).

No products indexed under this heading.

Diphenhydramine Citrate (Additive depressant effects). Products include:

Excedrin P.M. Analgesic/Sleeping Aid Tablets, Caplets, Liquigels ... 733

Diphenhydramine Hydrochloride (Additive depressant effects). Products include:

Actifed Allergy Daytime/Nighttime Caplets ... ▣ 844
Actifed Sinus Daytime/Nighttime Tablets and Caplets ... ▣ 846
Arthritis Foundation NightTime Caplets ... ▣ 674
Extra Strength Bayer PM Aspirin .. ▣ 713
Bayer Select Night Time Pain Relief Formula ... ▣ 716
Benadryl Allergy Decongestant Liquid Medication ... ▣ 848
Benadryl Allergy Decongestant Tablets ... ▣ 848
Benadryl Allergy Liquid Medication ... ▣ 849
Benadryl Allergy ... ▣ 848
Benadryl Allergy Sinus Headache Formula Caplets ... ▣ 849
Benadryl Capsules ... 1898
Benadryl Dye-Free Allergy Liqui-gel Softgels ... ▣ 850
Benadryl Dye-Free Allergy Liquid Medication ... ▣ 850
Benadryl Itch Relief Cream, Children's Formula and Maximum Strength 2% ... ▣ 851
Benadryl Itch Relief Spray, Children's Formula and Maximum Strength 2% ... ▣ 851
Benadryl Itch Relief Stick Maximum Strength 2% ... ▣ 850
Benadryl Itch Stopping Gel, Children's Formula and Maximum Strength 2% ... ▣ 851
Benadryl Kapseals ... 1898
Benadryl Injection ... 1898
Contac Day & Night Cold/Flu Night Caplets ... ▣ 812
Contac Night Allergy/Sinus Caplets ... ▣ 812
Extra Strength Doan's P.M. ... ▣ 633
Legatrin PM ... ▣ 651
Miles Nervine Nighttime Sleep-Aid ▣ 723
Nytol QuickCaps Caplets ... ▣ 610
Sleepinal Night-time Sleep Aid Capsules and Softgels ... ▣ 834
TYLENOL Maximum Strength Allergy Sinus NightTime Medication Caplets ... 1555
TYLENOL Flu NightTime, Maximum Strength, Gelcaps ... 1566
TYLENOL Maximum Strength Flu NightTime Hot Medication Packets ... 1562
TYLENOL PM, Extra Strength Pain Reliever/Sleep Aid Caplets, Geltabs, Gelcaps ... 1560
TYLENOL Severe Allergy Medication Caplets ... 1564
Maximum Strength Unisom Sleepgels ... 1934
Unisom With Pain Relief-Nighttime Sleep Aid and Pain Reliever ... 1934

Divalproex Sodium (Increases the phenobarbital serum levels). Products include:

Depakote Tablets ... 415

Doxycycline Calcium (Shortened half-life of doxycycline). Products include:

Vibramycin Calcium Oral Suspension Syrup ... 1941

Doxycycline Hyclate (Shortened half-life of doxycycline). Products include:

Doryx Capsules ... 1913
Vibramycin Hyclate Capsules ... 1941
Vibramycin Hyclate Intravenous ... 2215
Vibra-Tabs Film Coated Tablets ... 1941

Doxycycline Monohydrate (Shortened half-life of doxycycline). Products include:

Monodox Capsules ... 1805

(▣ Described in PDR For Nonprescription Drugs) (⊙ Described in PDR For Ophthalmology)

Interactions Index — Phenobarbital

Vibramycin Monohydrate for Oral Suspension 1941

Droperidol (Additive depressant effects). Products include:

Inapsine Injection 1296

Enflurane (Additive depressant effects).

No products indexed under this heading.

Estazolam (Additive depressant effects). Products include:

ProSom Tablets 449

Ethchlorvynol (Additive depressant effects). Products include:

Placidyl Capsules 448

Ethinamate (Additive depressant effects).

No products indexed under this heading.

Ethinyl Estradiol (Decreased estrogen effect). Products include:

Brevicon 2088
Demulen 2428
Desogen Tablets 1817
Levlen/Tri-Levlen 651
Lo/Ovral Tablets 2746
Lo/Ovral-28 Tablets 2751
Modicon 1872
Nordette-21 Tablets 2755
Nordette-28 Tablets 2758
Norinyl 2088
Ortho-Cept 1851
Ortho-Cyclen/Ortho-Tri-Cyclen 1858
Ortho-Novum 1872
Ortho-Cyclen/Ortho Tri-Cyclen 1858
Ovcon 760
Ovral Tablets 2770
Ovral-28 Tablets 2770
Levlen/Tri-Levlen 651
Tri-Norinyl 2164
Triphasil-21 Tablets 2814
Triphasil-28 Tablets 2819

Ethynodiol Diacetate (Decreased estrogen effect). Products include:

Demulen 2428

Fentanyl (Additive depressant effects). Products include:

Duragesic Transdermal System 1288

Fentanyl Citrate (Additive depressant effects). Products include:

Sublimaze Injection 1307

Fludrocortisone Acetate (Enhanced metabolism of exogenous corticosteroids). Products include:

Florinef Acetate Tablets 505

Fluphenazine Decanoate (Additive depressant effects). Products include:

Prolixin Decanoate 509

Fluphenazine Enanthate (Additive depressant effects). Products include:

Prolixin Enanthate 509

Fluphenazine Hydrochloride (Additive depressant effects). Products include:

Prolixin 509

Flurazepam Hydrochloride (Additive depressant effects). Products include:

Dalmane Capsules 2173

Furazolidone (Prolongs the effects of barbiturates). Products include:

Furoxone 2046

Glutethimide (Additive depressant effects).

No products indexed under this heading.

Griseofulvin (Interference with griseofulvin absorption; decreased blood levels). Products include:

Fulvicin P/G Tablets 2359
Fulvicin P/G 165 & 330 Tablets 2359
Grifulvin V (griseofulvin tablets) Microsize (griseofulvin oral suspension) Microsize 1888
Gris-PEG Tablets, 125 mg & 250 mg 479

Haloperidol (Additive depressant effects). Products include:

Haldol Injection, Tablets and Concentrate 1575

Haloperidol Decanoate (Additive depressant effects). Products include:

Haldol Decanoate 1577

Hydrocodone Bitartrate (Additive depressant effects). Products include:

Anexsia 5/500 Elixir 1781
Anexia Tablets 1782
Codiclear DH Syrup 791
Deconamine CX Cough and Cold Liquid and Tablets 1319
Duratuss HD Elixir 2565
Hycodan Tablets and Syrup 930
Hycomine Compound Tablets 932
Hycomine 931
Hycotuss Expectorant Syrup 933
Hydrocet Capsules 782
Lorcet 10/650 1018
Lortab 2566
Tussend 1783
Tussend Expectorant 1785
Vicodin Tablets 1356
Vicodin ES Tablets 1357
Vicodin Tuss Expectorant 1358
Zydone Capsules 949

Hydrocodone Polistirex (Additive depressant effects). Products include:

Tussionex Pennkinetic Extended-Release Suspension 998

Hydrocortisone (Enhanced metabolism of exogenous corticosteroids). Products include:

Anusol-HC Cream 2.5% 1896
Aquanil HC Lotion 1931
Bactine Hydrocortisone Anti-Itch Cream .... ®D 709
Caldecort Anti-Itch Hydrocortisone Spray .... ®D 631
Cortaid .... ®D 836
CORTENEMA 2535
Cortisporin Ointment 1085
Cortisporin Ophthalmic Ointment Sterile 1085
Cortisporin Ophthalmic Suspension Sterile 1086
Cortisporin Otic Solution Sterile 1087
Cortisporin Otic Suspension Sterile 1088
Cortizone-5 .... ®D 831
Cortizone-10 .... ®D 831
Hydrocortone Tablets 1672
Hytone 907
Massengill Medicated Soft Cloth Towelettes 2458
PediOtic Suspension Sterile 1153
Preparation H Hydrocortisone 1% Cream .... ®D 872
ProctoCream-HC 2.5% 2408
VöSoL HC Otic Solution 2678

Hydrocortisone Acetate (Enhanced metabolism of exogenous corticosteroids). Products include:

Analpram-HC Rectal Cream 1% and 2.5% 977
Anusol HC-1 Anti-Itch Hydrocortisone Ointment .... ®D 847
Anusol-HC Suppositories 1897
Caldecort .... ®D 631
Carmol HC 924
Coly-Mycin S Otic w/Neomycin & Hydrocortisone 1906
Cortaid .... ®D 836
Cortifoam 2396
Cortisporin Cream 1084
Epifoam 2399
Hydrocortone Acetate Sterile Suspension 1669
Mantadil Cream 1135
Nupercainal Hydrocortisone 1% Cream .... ®D 645
Ophthocort .... ⊙ 311
Pramosone Cream, Lotion & Ointment 978
ProctoCream-HC 2408
ProctoFoam-HC 2409
Terra-Cortril Ophthalmic Suspension 2210

Hydrocortisone Sodium Phosphate (Enhanced metabolism of exogenous corticosteroids). Products include:

Hydrocortone Phosphate Injection, Sterile 1670

Hydrocortisone Sodium Succinate (Enhanced metabolism of exogenous corticosteroids). Products include:

Solu-Cortef Sterile Powder 2641

Hydroxyzine Hydrochloride (Additive depressant effects). Products include:

Atarax Tablets & Syrup 2185
Marax Tablets & DF Syrup 2200
Vistaril Intramuscular Solution 2216

Isocarboxazid (Prolongs the effects of barbiturates).

No products indexed under this heading.

Isoflurane (Additive depressant effects).

No products indexed under this heading.

Ketamine Hydrochloride (Additive depressant effects).

No products indexed under this heading.

Levomethadyl Acetate Hydrochloride (Additive depressant effects). Products include:

Orlaam 2239

Levonorgestrel (Decreased estrogen effect). Products include:

Levlen/Tri-Levlen 651
Nordette-21 Tablets 2755
Nordette-28 Tablets 2758
Norplant System 2759
Levlen/Tri-Levlen 651
Triphasil-21 Tablets 2814
Triphasil-28 Tablets 2819

Levorphanol Tartrate (Additive depressant effects). Products include:

Levo-Dromoran 2129

Loratadine (Additive depressant effects). Products include:

Claritin 2349
Claritin-D 2350

Lorazepam (Additive depressant effects). Products include:

Ativan Injection 2698
Ativan Tablets 2700

Loxapine Hydrochloride (Additive depressant effects). Products include:

Loxitane 1378

Loxapine Succinate (Additive depressant effects). Products include:

Loxitane Capsules 1378

Meperidine Hydrochloride (Additive depressant effects). Products include:

Demerol 2308
Mepergan Injection 2753

Mephobarbital (Additive depressant effects). Products include:

Mebaral Tablets 2322

Meprobamate (Additive depressant effects). Products include:

Miltown Tablets 2672
PMB 200 and PMB 400 2783

Mesoridazine Besylate (Additive depressant effects). Products include:

Serentil 684

Mestranol (Decreased estrogen effect). Products include:

Norinyl 2088
Ortho-Novum 1872

Methadone Hydrochloride (Additive depressant effects). Products include:

Methadone Hydrochloride Oral Concentrate 2233
Methadone Hydrochloride Oral Solution & Tablets 2235

Methdilazine Hydrochloride (Additive depressant effects).

No products indexed under this heading.

Methohexital Sodium (Additive depressant effects). Products include:

Brevital Sodium Vials 1429

Methotrimeprazine (Additive depressant effects). Products include:

Levoprome 1274

Methoxyflurane (Additive depressant effects).

No products indexed under this heading.

Methylprednisolone Acetate (Enhanced metabolism of exogenous corticosteroids). Products include:

Depo-Medrol Single-Dose Vial 2600
Depo-Medrol Sterile Aqueous Suspension 2597

Methylprednisolone Sodium Succinate (Enhanced metabolism of exogenous corticosteroids). Products include:

Solu-Medrol Sterile Powder 2643

Midazolam Hydrochloride (Additive depressant effects). Products include:

Versed Injection 2170

Molindone Hydrochloride (Additive depressant effects). Products include:

Moban Tablets and Concentrate 1048

Morphine Sulfate (Additive depressant effects). Products include:

Astramorph/PF Injection, USP (Preservative-Free) 535
Duramorph 962
Infumorph 200 and Infumorph 500 Sterile Solutions 965
MS Contin Tablets 1994
MSIR 1997
Oramorph SR (Morphine Sulfate Sustained Release Tablets) 2236
RMS Suppositories 2657
Roxanol 2243

Norethindrone (Decreased estrogen effect). Products include:

Brevicon 2088
Micronor Tablets 1872
Modicon 1872
Norinyl 2088
Nor-Q D Tablets 2135
Ortho-Novum 1872
Ovcon 760
Tri-Norinyl 2164

Norethynodrel (Decreased estrogen effect).

No products indexed under this heading.

Norgestimate (Decreased estrogen effect). Products include:

Ortho-Cyclen/Ortho-Tri-Cyclen 1858
Ortho-Cyclen/Ortho Tri-Cyclen 1858

Norgestrel (Decreased estrogen effect). Products include:

Lo/Ovral Tablets 2746
Lo/Ovral-28 Tablets 2751
Ovral Tablets 2770
Ovral-28 Tablets 2770
Ovrette Tablets 2771

Opium Alkaloids (Additive depressant effects).

No products indexed under this heading.

Oxazepam (Additive depressant effects). Products include:

Serax Capsules 2810
Serax Tablets 2810

Oxycodone Hydrochloride (Additive depressant effects). Products include:

Percocet Tablets 938
Percodan Tablets 939
Percodan-Demi Tablets 940
Roxicodone Tablets, Oral Solution & Intensol (Oxycodone) 2244
Tylox Capsules 1584

IMPORTANT NOTE: Always consult each drug listing in the patient's regimen for possible interactions.

Pentobarbital Sodium (Additive depressant effects). Products include:
- Nembutal Sodium Capsules 436
- Nembutal Sodium Solution 438
- Nembutal Sodium Suppositories 440

Perphenazine (Additive depressant effects). Products include:
- Etrafon 2355
- Triavil Tablets 1757
- Trilafon 2389

Phenelzine Sulfate (Prolongs the effects of barbiturates). Products include:
- Nardil 1920

Phenytoin (Variable effect on the metabolism of phenytoin). Products include:
- Dilantin Infatabs 1908
- Dilantin-125 Suspension 1911

Phenytoin Sodium (Variable effect on the metabolism of phenytoin). Products include:
- Dilantin Kapseals 1906
- Dilantin Parenteral 1910

Prazepam (Additive depressant effects).
- No products indexed under this heading.

Prednisolone Acetate (Enhanced metabolism of exogenous corticosteroids). Products include:
- AK-CIDE ◉ 202
- AK-CIDE Ointment ◉ 202
- Blephamide Liquifilm Sterile Ophthalmic Suspension 476
- Blephamide Ointment ◉ 237
- Econopred & Econopred Plus Ophthalmic Suspensions ◉ 217
- Poly-Pred Liquifilm ◉ 248
- Pred Forte ◉ 250
- Pred Mild ◉ 253
- Pred-G Liquifilm Sterile Ophthalmic Suspension ◉ 251
- Pred-G S.O.P. Sterile Ophthalmic Ointment ◉ 252
- Vasocidin Ointment ◉ 268

Prednisolone Sodium Phosphate (Enhanced metabolism of exogenous corticosteroids). Products include:
- AK-Pred ◉ 204
- Hydeltrasol Injection, Sterile 1665
- Inflamase ◉ 265
- Pediapred Oral Liquid 995
- Vasocidin Ophthalmic Solution ◉ 270

Prednisolone Tebutate (Enhanced metabolism of exogenous corticosteroids). Products include:
- Hydeltra-T.B.A. Sterile Suspension 1667

Prednisone (Enhanced metabolism of exogenous corticosteroids). Products include:
- Deltasone Tablets 2595

Prochlorperazine (Additive depressant effects). Products include:
- Compazine 2470

Promethazine Hydrochloride (Additive depressant effects). Products include:
- Mepergan Injection 2753
- Phenergan with Codeine 2777
- Phenergan with Dextromethorphan 2778
- Phenergan Injection 2773
- Phenergan Suppositories 2775
- Phenergan Syrup 2774
- Phenergan Tablets 2775
- Phenergan VC 2779
- Phenergan VC with Codeine 2781

Propofol (Additive depressant effects). Products include:
- Diprivan Injection 2833

Propoxyphene Hydrochloride (Additive depressant effects). Products include:
- Darvon 1435
- Wygesic Tablets 2827

Propoxyphene Napsylate (Additive depressant effects). Products include:
- Darvon-N/Darvocet-N 1433

Pyrilamine Maleate (Additive depressant effects). Products include:
- 4-Way Fast Acting Nasal Spray (regular & mentholated) ▣ 621
- Maximum Strength Multi-Symptom Formula Midol ▣ 722
- PMS Multi-Symptom Formula Midol ▣ 723

Pyrilamine Tannate (Additive depressant effects). Products include:
- Atrohist Pediatric Suspension 454
- Rynatan 2673

Quazepam (Additive depressant effects). Products include:
- Doral Tablets 2664

Risperidone (Additive depressant effects). Products include:
- Risperdal 1301

Secobarbital Sodium (Additive depressant effects). Products include:
- Seconal Sodium Pulvules 1474

Selegiline Hydrochloride (Prolongs the effects of barbiturates). Products include:
- Eldepryl Tablets 2550

Sodium Valproate (Increases the phenobarbital serum levels).

Sufentanil Citrate (Additive depressant effects). Products include:
- Sufenta Injection 1309

Temazepam (Additive depressant effects). Products include:
- Restoril Capsules 2284

Terfenadine (Additive depressant effects). Products include:
- Seldane Tablets 1536
- Seldane-D Extended-Release Tablets 1538

Thiamylal Sodium (Additive depressant effects).
- No products indexed under this heading.

Thioridazine Hydrochloride (Additive depressant effects). Products include:
- Mellaril 2269

Thiothixene (Additive depressant effects). Products include:
- Navane Capsules and Concentrate 2201
- Navane Intramuscular 2202

Tranylcypromine Sulfate (Prolongs the effects of barbiturates). Products include:
- Parnate Tablets 2503

Triamcinolone (Enhanced metabolism of exogenous corticosteroids). Products include:
- Aristocort Tablets 1022

Triamcinolone Acetonide (Enhanced metabolism of exogenous corticosteroids). Products include:
- Aristocort A 0.025% Cream 1027
- Aristocort A 0.5% Cream 1031
- Aristocort A 0.1% Cream 1029
- Aristocort A 0.1% Ointment 1030
- Azmacort Oral Inhaler 2011
- Nasacort Nasal Inhaler 2024

Triamcinolone Diacetate (Enhanced metabolism of exogenous corticosteroids). Products include:
- Aristocort Suspension (Forte Parenteral) 1027
- Aristocort Suspension (Intralesional) 1025

Triamcinolone Hexacetonide (Enhanced metabolism of exogenous corticosteroids). Products include:
- Aristospan Suspension (Intra-articular) 1033
- Aristospan Suspension (Intralesional) 1032

Triazolam (Additive depressant effects). Products include:
- Halcion Tablets 2611

Trifluoperazine Hydrochloride (Additive depressant effects). Products include:
- Stelazine 2514

Trimeprazine Tartrate (Additive depressant effects). Products include:
- Temaril Tablets, Syrup and Spansule Extended-Release Capsules 483

Tripelennamine Hydrochloride (Additive depressant effects). Products include:
- PBZ Tablets 845
- PBZ-SR Tablets 844

Triprolidine Hydrochloride (Additive depressant effects). Products include:
- Actifed Plus Caplets ▣ 845
- Actifed Plus Tablets ▣ 845
- Actifed with Codeine Cough Syrup 1067
- Actifed Syrup ▣ 846
- Actifed Tablets ▣ 844

Valproic Acid (Increases the phenobarbital serum levels). Products include:
- Depakene 413

Warfarin Sodium (Lowered plasma levels and decreased anticoagulant activity). Products include:
- Coumadin 926

Zolpidem Tartrate (Additive depressant effects). Products include:
- Ambien Tablets 2416

Food Interactions

Alcohol (Additive depressant effects).

PHENURONE TABLETS
(Phenacemide) 447

May interact with anticonvulsants and certain other agents. Compounds in these categories include:

Carbamazepine (Concurrent use requires extreme caution). Products include:
- Atretol Tablets 573
- Tegretol Chewable Tablets 852
- Tegretol Suspension 852
- Tegretol Tablets 852

Divalproex Sodium (Concurrent use requires extreme caution). Products include:
- Depakote Tablets 415

Ethosuximide (Concurrent use requires extreme caution). Products include:
- Zarontin Capsules 1928
- Zarontin Syrup 1929

Ethotoin (May result in paranoid symptoms). Products include:
- Peganone Tablets 446

Felbamate (Concurrent use requires extreme caution). Products include:
- Felbatol 2666

Lamotrigine (Concurrent use requires extreme caution). Products include:
- Lamictal Tablets 1112

Mephenytoin (Concurrent use requires extreme caution). Products include:
- Mesantoin Tablets 2272

Methsuximide (Concurrent use requires extreme caution). Products include:
- Celontin Kapseals 1899

Paramethadione (Concurrent use requires extreme caution).
- No products indexed under this heading.

Phenobarbital (Concurrent use requires extreme caution). Products include:
- Arco-Lase Plus Tablets 512
- Bellergal-S Tablets 2250
- Donnatal 2060
- Donnatal Extentabs 2061
- Donnatal Tablets 2060
- Phenobarbital Elixir and Tablets 1469
- Quadrinal Tablets 1350

Phensuximide (Concurrent use requires extreme caution). Products include:
- Milontin Kapseals 1920

Phenytoin (Concurrent use requires extreme caution). Products include:
- Dilantin Infatabs 1908
- Dilantin-125 Suspension 1911

Phenytoin Sodium (Concurrent use requires extreme caution). Products include:
- Dilantin Kapseals 1906
- Dilantin Parenteral 1910

Primidone (Concurrent use requires extreme caution). Products include:
- Mysoline 2754

Trimethadione (Concurrent use requires extreme caution).
- No products indexed under this heading.

Valproic Acid (Concurrent use requires extreme caution). Products include:
- Depakene 413

PHILLIPS' GELCAPS
(Docusate Sodium, Phenolphthalein) ▣ 729

May interact with:

Mineral Oil (Concurrent oral use is not recommended). Products include:
- Anusol Ointment ▣ 847
- Aquaphor Healing Ointment 640
- Aquaphor Healing Ointment, Original Formula 640
- Eucerin Original Moisturizing Creme (Unscented) 641
- Eucerin Original Moisturizing Lotion 641
- Eucerin Plus Dry Skin Care Moisturizing Lotion 641
- Eucerin Plus Moisturizing Creme 641
- Fleet Mineral Oil Enema 1002
- Hemorid For Women Creme ▣ 834
- Keri Lotion - Original Formula ▣ 622
- Kondremul ▣ 637
- Lubriderm Bath and Shower Oil ▣ 856
- Nephrox Suspension ▣ 655
- Preparation H Hemorrhoidal Ointment ▣ 871
- Refresh PM Lubricant Eye Ointment ◉ 254
- Replens Vaginal Moisturizer ▣ 859
- Tears Renewed Ointment ◉ 209

PHILLIPS' MILK OF MAGNESIA LIQUID
(Magnesium Hydroxide) ▣ 729

May interact with:

Prescription Drugs, unspecified (Effect not specified).

PHOSCHOL CONCENTRATE
(Phosphatidylcholine) 488

None cited in PDR database.

PHOSCHOL 900 SOFTGELS
(Phosphatidylcholine) 488

None cited in PDR database.

PHOSLO TABLETS
(Calcium Acetate) 690

May interact with cardiac glycosides, tetracyclines, and certain other agents. Compounds in these categories include:

Antacids, unspecified (Concurrent use should be avoided).

Demeclocycline Hydrochloride (Bioavailability of oral tetracyclines may be decreased). Products include:

Declomycin Tablets................................. 1371

Deslanoside (Hypercalcemia may precipitate cardiac arrhythmia).

No products indexed under this heading.

Digitoxin (Hypercalcemia may precipitate cardiac arrhythmia). Products include:

Crystodigin Tablets................................. 1433

Digoxin (Hypercalcemia may precipitate cardiac arrhythmia). Products include:

Lanoxicaps 1117
Lanoxin Elixir Pediatric 1120
Lanoxin Injection 1123
Lanoxin Injection Pediatric.................... 1126
Lanoxin Tablets 1128

Doxycycline Calcium (Bioavailability of oral tetracyclines may be decreased). Products include:

Vibramycin Calcium Oral Suspension Syrup... 1941

Doxycycline Hyclate (Bioavailability of oral tetracyclines may be decreased). Products include:

Doryx Capsules.. 1913
Vibramycin Hyclate Capsules 1941
Vibramycin Hyclate Intravenous 2215
Vibra-Tabs Film Coated Tablets 1941

Doxycycline Monohydrate (Bioavailability of oral tetracyclines may be decreased). Products include:

Monodox Capsules 1805
Vibramycin Monohydrate for Oral Suspension 1941

Methacycline Hydrochloride (Bioavailability of oral tetracyclines may be decreased).

No products indexed under this heading.

Minocycline Hydrochloride (Bioavailability of oral tetracyclines may be decreased). Products include:

Dynacin Capsules 1590
Minocin Intravenous............................... 1382
Minocin Oral Suspension 1385
Minocin Pellet-Filled Capsules 1383

Oxytetracycline Hydrochloride (Bioavailability of oral tetracyclines may be decreased). Products include:

TERAK Ointment .... ⊙ 209
Terra-Cortril Ophthalmic Suspension 2210
Terramycin with Polymyxin B Sulfate Ophthalmic Ointment 2211
Urobiotic-250 Capsules 2214

Tetracycline Hydrochloride (Bioavailability of oral tetracyclines may be decreased). Products include:

Achromycin V Capsules 1367

PHOSPHOLINE IODIDE

(Echothiophate Iodide)........................ ⊙ 326

May interact with:

Succinylcholine Chloride (Possible additive effects). Products include:

Anectine... 1073

PHRENILIN FORTE CAPSULES

(Butalbital, Acetaminophen)................ 785

May interact with monoamine oxidase inhibitors, central nervous system depressants, narcotic analgesics, general anesthetics, tranquilizers, hypnotics and sedatives, and certain other agents. Compounds in these categories include:

Alfentanil Hydrochloride (Potential for increased CNS depression). Products include:

Alfenta Injection 1286

Alprazolam (Potential for increased CNS depression). Products include:

Xanax Tablets 2649

Aprobarbital (Potential for increased CNS depression).

No products indexed under this heading.

Buprenorphine (Potential for increased CNS depression). Products include:

Buprenex Injectable 2006

Buspirone Hydrochloride (Potential for increased CNS depression). Products include:

BuSpar 737

Butabarbital (Potential for increased CNS depression).

No products indexed under this heading.

Chlordiazepoxide (Potential for increased CNS depression). Products include:

Libritabs Tablets 2177
Limbitrol 2180

Chlordiazepoxide Hydrochloride (Potential for increased CNS depression). Products include:

Librax Capsules 2176
Librium Capsules.................................... 2178
Librium Injectable 2179

Chlorpromazine (Potential for increased CNS depression). Products include:

Thorazine Suppositories....................... 2523

Chlorpromazine Hydrochloride (Potential for levels of both drugs). Products include:

Thorazine 2523

Chlorprothixene (Potential for increased CNS depression).

No products indexed under this heading.

Chlorprothixene Hydrochloride (Potential for increased CNS depression).

No products indexed under this heading.

Clorazepate Dipotassium (Potential for increased CNS depression). Products include:

Tranxene 451

Clozapine (Potential for increased CNS depression). Products include:

Clozaril Tablets.. 2252

Codeine Phosphate (Potential for increased CNS depression). Products include:

Actifed with Codeine Cough Syrup.. 1067
Brontex 1981
Deconsal C Expectorant Syrup 456
Deconsal Pediatric Syrup 457
Dimetane-DC Cough Syrup 2059
Empirin with Codeine Tablets............ 1093
Fioricet with Codeine Capsules 2260
Fiorinal with Codeine Capsules 2262
Isoclor Expectorant................................ 990
Novahistine DH....................................... 2462
Novahistine Expectorant...................... 2463
Nucofed 2051
Phenergan with Codeine....................... 2777
Phenergan VC with Codeine 2781
Robitussin A-C Syrup............................ 2073
Robitussin-DAC Syrup........................... 2074
Ryna .... ⊞ 841
Soma Compound w/Codeine Tablets 2676
Tussi-Organidin NR Liquid and S NR Liquid 2677
Tylenol with Codeine 1583

Desflurane (Potential for increased CNS depression). Products include:

Suprane 1813

Dezocine (Potential for increased CNS depression). Products include:

Dalgan Injection 538

Diazepam (Potential for increased CNS depression). Products include:

Dizac 1809
Valium Injectable 2182
Valium Tablets 2183

Valrelease Capsules 2169

Droperidol (Potential for increased CNS depression). Products include:

Inapsine Injection................................... 1296

Enflurane (Potential for increased CNS depression).

No products indexed under this heading.

Estazolam (Potential for increased CNS depression). Products include:

ProSom Tablets 449

Ethchlorvynol (Potential for increased CNS depression). Products include:

Placidyl Capsules.................................... 448

Ethinamate (Potential for increased CNS depression).

No products indexed under this heading.

Fentanyl (Potential for increased CNS depression). Products include:

Duragesic Transdermal System........ 1288

Fentanyl Citrate (Potential for increased CNS depression). Products include:

Sublimaze Injection................................ 1307

Fluphenazine Decanoate (Potential for increased CNS depression). Products include:

Prolixin Decanoate 509

Fluphenazine Enanthate (Potential for increased CNS depression). Products include:

Prolixin Enanthate 509

Fluphenazine Hydrochloride (Potential for increased CNS depression). Products include:

Prolixin 509

Flurazepam Hydrochloride (Potential for increased CNS depression). Products include:

Dalmane Capsules.................................. 2173

Furazolidone (Enhances the CNS effects of butalbital). Products include:

Furoxone 2046

Glutethimide (Potential for increased CNS depression).

No products indexed under this heading.

Haloperidol (Potential for increased CNS depression). Products include:

Haldol Injection, Tablets and Concentrate 1575

Haloperidol Decanoate (Potential for increased CNS depression). Products include:

Haldol Decanoate.................................... 1577

Hydrocodone Bitartrate (Potential for increased CNS depression). Products include:

Anexsia 5/500 Elixir 1781
Anexia Tablets... 1782
Codiclear DH Syrup 791
Deconamine CX Cough and Cold Liquid and Tablets................................. 1319
Duratuss HD Elixir.................................. 2565
Hycodan Tablets and Syrup 930
Hycomine Compound Tablets 932
Hycomine 931
Hycotuss Expectorant Syrup 933
Hydrocet Capsules 782
Lorcet 10/650... 1018
Lortab 2566
Tussend 1783
Tussend Expectorant 1785
Vicodin Tablets.. 1356
Vicodin ES Tablets 1357
Vicodin Tuss Expectorant 1358
Zydone Capsules 949

Hydrocodone Polistirex (Potential for increased CNS depression). Products include:

Tussionex Pennkinetic Extended-Release Suspension 998

Hydroxyzine Hydrochloride (Potential for increased CNS depression). Products include:

Atarax Tablets & Syrup........................ 2185

Marax Tablets & DF Syrup................... 2200
Vistaril Intramuscular Solution.......... 2216

Isocarboxazid (Enhances the CNS effects of butalbital).

No products indexed under this heading.

Isoflurane (Potential for increased CNS depression).

No products indexed under this heading.

Ketamine Hydrochloride (Potential for increased CNS depression).

No products indexed under this heading.

Levomethadyl Acetate Hydrochloride (Potential for increased CNS depression). Products include:

Orlamm 2239

Levorphanol Tartrate (Potential for increased CNS depression). Products include:

Levo-Dromoran.. 2129

Lorazepam (Potential for increased CNS depression). Products include:

Ativan Injection.. 2698
Ativan Tablets 2700

Loxapine Hydrochloride (Potential for increased CNS depression). Products include:

Loxitane 1378

Loxapine Succinate (Potential for increased CNS depression). Products include:

Loxitane Capsules 1378

Meperidine Hydrochloride (Potential for increased CNS depression). Products include:

Demerol 2308
Mepergan Injection 2753

Mephobarbital (Potential for increased CNS depression). Products include:

Mebaral Tablets 2322

Meprobamate (Potential for increased CNS depression). Products include:

Miltown Tablets 2672
PMB 200 and PMB 400 2783

Mesoridazine (Potential for increased CNS depression).

Mesoridazine Besylate (Potential for increased CNS depression). Products include:

Serentil... 684

Methadone Hydrochloride (Potential for increased CNS depression). Products include:

Methadone Hydrochloride Oral Concentrate 2233
Methadone Hydrochloride Oral Solution & Tablets................................ 2235

Methohexital Sodium (Potential for increased CNS depression). Products include:

Brevital Sodium Vials............................ 1429

Methotrimeprazine (Potential for increased CNS depression). Products include:

Levoprome 1274

Methoxyflurane (Potential for increased CNS depression).

No products indexed under this heading.

Midazolam Hydrochloride (Potential for increased CNS depression). Products include:

Versed Injection 2170

Molindone Hydrochloride (Potential for increased CNS depression). Products include:

Moban Tablets and Concentrate...... 1048

Morphine Sulfate (Potential for increased CNS depression). Products include:

Astramorph/PF Injection, USP (Preservative-Free) 535
Duramorph 962

IMPORTANT NOTE: Always consult each drug listing in the patient's regimen for possible interactions.

Phrenilin **Interactions Index** 822

Infumorph 200 and Infumorph 500 Sterile Solutions ... 965
MS Contin Tablets ... 1994
MSIR ... 1997
Oramorph SR (Morphine Sulfate Sustained Release Tablets) ... 2236
RMS Suppositories ... 2657
Roxanol ... 2243

Opium Alkaloids (Potential for increased CNS depression).
No products indexed under this heading.

Oxazepam (Potential for increased CNS depression). Products include:
Serax Capsules ... 2810
Serax Tablets ... 2810

Oxycodone Hydrochloride (Potential for increased CNS depression). Products include:
Percocet Tablets ... 938
Percodan Tablets ... 939
Percodan-Demi Tablets ... 940
Roxicodone Tablets, Oral Solution & Intensol (Oxycodone) ... 2244
Tylox Capsules ... 1584

Pentobarbital Sodium (Potential for increased CNS depression). Products include:
Nembutal Sodium Capsules ... 436
Nembutal Sodium Solution ... 438
Nembutal Sodium Suppositories ... 440

Perphenazine (Potential for increased CNS depression). Products include:
Etrafon ... 2355
Triavil Tablets ... 1757
Trilafon ... 2389

Phenelzine Sulfate (Enhances the CNS effects of butalbital). Products include:
Nardil ... 1920

Phenobarbital (Potential for increased CNS depression). Products include:
Arco-Lase Plus Tablets ... 512
Bellergal-S Tablets ... 2250
Donnatal ... 2060
Donnatal Extentabs ... 2061
Donnatal Tablets ... 2060
Phenobarbital Elixir and Tablets ... 1469
Quadrinal Tablets ... 1350

Prazepam (Potential for increased CNS depression).
No products indexed under this heading.

Prochlorperazine (Potential for increased CNS depression). Products include:
Compazine ... 2470

Promethazine Hydrochloride (Potential for increased CNS depression). Products include:
Mepergan Injection ... 2753
Phenergan with Codeine ... 2777
Phenergan with Dextromethorphan ... 2778
Phenergan Injection ... 2773
Phenergan Suppositories ... 2775
Phenergan Syrup ... 2774
Phenergan Tablets ... 2775
Phenergan VC ... 2779
Phenergan VC with Codeine ... 2781

Propofol (Potential for increased CNS depression). Products include:
Diprivan Injection ... 2833

Propoxyphene Hydrochloride (Potential for increased CNS depression). Products include:
Darvon ... 1435
Wygesic Tablets ... 2827

Propoxyphene Napsylate (Potential for increased CNS depression). Products include:
Darvon-N/Darvocet-N ... 1433

Quazepam (Potential for increased CNS depression). Products include:
Doral Tablets ... 2664

Risperidone (Potential for increased CNS depression). Products include:
Risperdal ... 1301

Secobarbital Sodium (Potential for increased CNS depression). Products include:
Seconal Sodium Pulvules ... 1474

Selegiline Hydrochloride (Enhances the CNS effects of butalbital). Products include:
Eldepryl Tablets ... 2550

Sufentanil Citrate (Potential for increased CNS depression). Products include:
Sufenta Injection ... 1309

Temazepam (Potential for increased CNS depression). Products include:
Restoril Capsules ... 2284

Thiamylal Sodium (Potential for increased CNS depression).
No products indexed under this heading.

Thioridazine Hydrochloride (Potential for increased CNS depression). Products include:
Mellaril ... 2269

Thiothixene (Potential for increased CNS depression). Products include:
Navane Capsules and Concentrate ... 2201
Navane Intramuscular ... 2202

Tranylcypromine Sulfate (Enhances the CNS effects of butalbital). Products include:
Parnate Tablets ... 2503

Triazolam (Potential for increased CNS depression). Products include:
Halcion Tablets ... 2611

Trifluoperazine Hydrochloride (Potential for increased CNS depression). Products include:
Stelazine ... 2514

Zolpidem Tartrate (Potential for increased CNS depression). Products include:
Ambien Tablets ... 2416

Food Interactions

Alcohol (Potential for increased CNS depression).

PHRENILIN TABLETS
(Butalbital, Acetaminophen) ... 785
See **Phrenilin Forte Capsules**

PILAGAN LIQUIFILM STERILE OPHTHALMIC SOLUTION
(Pilocarpine Nitrate) ... ◉ 248
None cited in PDR database.

PILAGEN LIQUIFILM STERILE OPHTHALMIC SOLUTION WITH C CAP COMPLIANCE CAP
(Pilocarpine Nitrate) ... ◉ 248
None cited in PDR database.

PILOCAR
(Pilocarpine Hydrochloride) ... ◉ 268
None cited in PDR database.

PILOCAR TWIN PACK
(Pilocarpine Hydrochloride) ... ◉ 268
None cited in PDR database.

PILOPINE HS OPHTHALMIC GEL
(Pilocarpine Hydrochloride) ... ◉ 226
None cited in PDR database.

PIMA SYRUP
(Potassium Iodide) ... 1005
None cited in PDR database.

PIN-X PINWORM TREATMENT
(Pyrantel Pamoate) ... ▣ 654
None cited in PDR database.

PIPRACIL
(Piperacillin Sodium) ... 1390
May interact with aminoglycosides, nondepolarizing neuromuscular blocking agents, and certain other agents. Compounds in these categories include:

Amikacin Sulfate (Substantial inactivation of aminoglycosides *in vitro*). Products include:
Amikacin Sulfate Injection, USP ... 960
Amikin Injectable ... 501

Atracurium Besylate (Co-administration with vecuronium has been implicated in the prolongation of the neuromuscular blockage; due to similar mechanism of action, same interaction can be expected with other non-depolarizing muscle relaxants). Products include:
Tracrium Injection ... 1183

Gentamicin Sulfate (Substantial inactivation of aminoglycosides *in vitro*). Products include:
Garamycin Injectable ... 2360
Genoptic Sterile Ophthalmic Solution ... ◉ 243
Genoptic Sterile Ophthalmic Ointment ... ◉ 243
Gentacidin Ointment ... ◉ 264
Gentacidin Solution ... ◉ 264
Gentak ... ◉ 208
Pred-G Liquifilm Sterile Ophthalmic Suspension ... ◉ 251
Pred-G S.O.P. Sterile Ophthalmic Ointment ... ◉ 252

Kanamycin Sulfate (Substantial inactivation of aminoglycosides *in vitro*).
No products indexed under this heading.

Metocurine Iodide (Co-administration with vecuronium has been implicated in the prolongation of the neuromuscular blockage; due to similar mechanism of action, same interaction can be expected with other non-depolarizing muscle relaxants). Products include:
Metubine Iodide Vials ... 916

Mivacurium Chloride (Co-administration with vecuronium has been implicated in the prolongation of the neuromuscular blockage; due to similar mechanism of action, same interaction can be expected with other non-depolarizing muscle relaxants). Products include:
Mivacron ... 1138

Pancuronium Bromide Injection (Co-administration with vecuronium has been implicated in the prolongation of the neuromuscular blockage; due to similar mechanism of action, same interaction can be expected with other non-depolarizing muscle relaxants).
No products indexed under this heading.

Probenecid (Increases peak serum level and area under the curve). Products include:
Benemid Tablets ... 1611
ColBENEMID Tablets ... 1622

Rocuronium Bromide (Co-administration with vecuronium has been implicated in the prolongation of the neuromuscular blockage; due to similar mechanism of action, same interaction can be expected with other non-depolarizing muscle relaxants). Products include:
Zemuron ... 1830

Streptomycin Sulfate (Substantial inactivation of aminoglycosides *in vitro*). Products include:
Streptomycin Sulfate Injection ... 2208

Tobramycin Sulfate (Substantial inactivation of aminoglycosides *in vitro*). Products include:
Nebcin Vials, Hyporets & ADD-Vantage ... 1464
Tobramycin Sulfate Injection ... 968

Vecuronium Bromide (Co-administration with vecuronium has been implicated in the prolongation of the neuromuscular blockage; due to similar mechanism of action, same interaction can be expected with other non-depolarizing muscle relaxants). Products include:
Norcuron ... 1826

PLACIDYL CAPSULES
(Ethchlorvynol) ... 448
May interact with central nervous system depressants, monoamine oxidase inhibitors, oral anticoagulants, and tricyclic antidepressants. Compounds in these categories include:

Alfentanil Hydrochloride (Exaggerated depressant effects). Products include:
Alfenta Injection ... 1286

Alprazolam (Exaggerated depressant effects). Products include:
Xanax Tablets ... 2649

Amitriptyline Hydrochloride (Transient delirium). Products include:
Elavil ... 2838
Endep Tablets ... 2174
Etrafon ... 2355
Limbitrol ... 2180
Triavil Tablets ... 1757

Amoxapine (Transient delirium). Products include:
Asendin Tablets ... 1369

Aprobarbital (Exaggerated depressant effects).
No products indexed under this heading.

Buprenorphine (Exaggerated depressant effects). Products include:
Buprenex Injectable ... 2006

Buspirone Hydrochloride (Exaggerated depressant effects). Products include:
BuSpar ... 737

Butabarbital (Exaggerated depressant effects).
No products indexed under this heading.

Butalbital (Exaggerated depressant effects). Products include:
Esgic-plus Tablets ... 1013
Fioricet Tablets ... 2258
Fioricet with Codeine Capsules ... 2260
Fiorinal Capsules ... 2261
Fiorinal with Codeine Capsules ... 2262
Fiorinal Tablets ... 2261
Phrenilin ... 785
Sedapap Tablets 50 mg/650 mg ... 1543

Chlordiazepoxide (Exaggerated depressant effects). Products include:
Libritabs Tablets ... 2177
Limbitrol ... 2180

Chlordiazepoxide Hydrochloride (Exaggerated depressant effects). Products include:
Librax Capsules ... 2176
Librium Capsules ... 2178
Librium Injectable ... 2179

Chlorpromazine (Exaggerated depressant effects). Products include:
Thorazine Suppositories ... 2523

Chlorprothixene (Exaggerated depressant effects).
No products indexed under this heading.

(▣ Described in PDR For Nonprescription Drugs) (◉ Described in PDR For Ophthalmology)

Interactions Index — Placidyl

Chlorprothixene Hydrochloride (Exxaggerated depressant effects).

No products indexed under this heading.

Clomipramine Hydrochloride (Transient delirium). Products include:

Anafranil Capsules 803

Clorazepate Dipotassium (Exaggerated depressant effects). Products include:

Tranxene 451

Clozapine (Exaggerated depressant effects). Products include:

Clozaril Tablets 2252

Codeine Phosphate (Exaggerated depressant effects). Products include:

Actifed with Codeine Cough Syrup.. 1067
Brontex 1981
Deconsal C Expectorant Syrup 456
Deconsal Pediatric Syrup 457
Dimetane-DC Cough Syrup 2059
Empirin with Codeine Tablets............ 1093
Fioricet with Codeine Capsules 2260
Fiorinal with Codeine Capsules 2262
Isoclor Expectorant 990
Novahistine DH 2462
Novahistine Expectorant...................... 2463
Nucofed 2051
Phenergan with Codeine 2777
Phenergan VC with Codeine 2781
Robitussin A-C Syrup 2073
Robitussin-DAC Syrup 2074
Ryna .... ◆◻ 841
Soma Compound w/Codeine Tablets 2676
Tussi-Organidin NR Liquid and S NR Liquid 2677
Tylenol with Codeine 1583

Desflurane (Exaggerated depressant effects). Products include:

Suprane 1813

Desipramine Hydrochloride (Transient delirium). Products include:

Norpramin Tablets 1526

Dezocine (Exaggerated depressant effects). Products include:

Dalgan Injection 538

Diazepam (Exaggerated depressant effects). Products include:

Dizac 1809
Valium Injectable 2182
Valium Tablets 2183
Valrelease Capsules 2169

Dicumarol (Decreased prothrombin time response).

No products indexed under this heading.

Doxepin Hydrochloride (Transient delirium). Products include:

Sinequan 2205
Zonalon Cream 1055

Droperidol (Exaggerated depressant effects). Products include:

Inapsine Injection 1296

Enflurane (Exaggerated depressant effects).

No products indexed under this heading.

Estazolam (Exaggerated depressant effects). Products include:

ProSom Tablets 449

Ethinamate (Exaggerated depressant effects).

No products indexed under this heading.

Fentanyl (Exaggerated depressant effects). Products include:

Duragesic Transdermal System........ 1288

Fentanyl Citrate (Exaggerated depressant effects). Products include:

Sublimaze Injection 1307

Fluphenazine Decanoate (Exaggerated depressant effects). Products include:

Prolixin Decanoate 509

Fluphenazine Enanthate (Exaggerated depressant effects). Products include:

Prolixin Enanthate 509

Fluphenazine Hydrochloride (Exaggerated depressant effects). Products include:

Prolixin 509

Flurazepam Hydrochloride (Exaggerated depressant effects). Products include:

Dalmane Capsules 2173

Furazolidone (Exaggerated depressant effects). Products include:

Furoxone 2046

Glutethimide (Exaggerated depressant effects).

No products indexed under this heading.

Haloperidol (Exaggerated depressant effects). Products include:

Haldol Injection, Tablets and Concentrate 1575

Haloperidol Decanoate (Exaggerated depressant effects). Products include:

Haldol Decanoate 1577

Hydrocodone Bitartrate (Exaggerated depressant effects). Products include:

Anexsia 5/500 Elixir 1781
Anexia Tablets 1782
Codiclear DH Syrup 791
Deconamine CX Cough and Cold Liquid and Tablets 1319
Duratuss HD Elixir 2565
Hycodan Tablets and Syrup 930
Hycomine Compound Tablets 932
Hycomine 931
Hycotuss Expectorant Syrup 933
Hydrocet Capsules 782
Lorcet 10/650 1018
Lortab 2566
Tussend 1783
Tussend Expectorant 1785
Vicodin Tablets 1356
Vicodin ES Tablets 1357
Vicodin Tuss Expectorant 1358
Zydone Capsules 949

Hydrocodone Polistirex (Exaggerated depressant effects). Products include:

Tussionex Pennkinetic Extended-Release Suspension 998

Hydroxyzine Hydrochloride (Exaggerated depressant effects). Products include:

Atarax Tablets & Syrup 2185
Marax Tablets & DF Syrup 2200
Vistaril Intramuscular Solution 2216

Imipramine Hydrochloride (Transient delirium). Products include:

Tofranil Ampuls 854
Tofranil Tablets 856

Imipramine Pamoate (Transient delirium). Products include:

Tofranil-PM Capsules 857

Isocarboxazid (Exaggerated depressant effects).

No products indexed under this heading.

Isoflurane (Exaggerated depressant effects).

No products indexed under this heading.

Ketamine Hydrochloride (Exaggerated depressant effects).

No products indexed under this heading.

Levomethadyl Acetate Hydrochloride (Exaggerated depressant effects). Products include:

Orlaam 2239

Levorphanol Tartrate (Exaggerated depressant effects). Products include:

Levo-Dromoran 2129

Lorazepam (Exaggerated depressant effects). Products include:

Ativan Injection 2698
Ativan Tablets 2700

Loxapine Hydrochloride (Exaggerated depressant effects). Products include:

Loxitane 1378

Loxapine Succinate (Exaggerated depressant effects). Products include:

Loxitane Capsules 1378

Maprotiline Hydrochloride (Transient delirium). Products include:

Ludiomil Tablets 843

Meperidine Hydrochloride (Exaggerated depressant effects). Products include:

Demerol 2308
Mepergan Injection 2753

Mephobarbital (Exaggerated depressant effects). Products include:

Mebaral Tablets 2322

Meprobamate (Exaggerated depressant effects). Products include:

Miltown Tablets 2672
PMB 200 and PMB 400 2783

Mesoridazine Besylate (Exaggerated depressant effects). Products include:

Serentil 684

Methadone Hydrochloride (Exaggerated depressant effects). Products include:

Methadone Hydrochloride Oral Concentrate 2233
Methadone Hydrochloride Oral Solution & Tablets 2235

Methohexital Sodium (Exaggerated depressant effects). Products include:

Brevital Sodium Vials 1429

Methotrimeprazine (Exaggerated depressant effects). Products include:

Levoprome 1274

Methoxyflurane (Exaggerated depressant effects).

No products indexed under this heading.

Midazolam Hydrochloride (Exaggerated depressant effects). Products include:

Versed Injection 2170

Molindone Hydrochloride (Exaggerated depressant effects). Products include:

Moban Tablets and Concentrate 1048

Morphine Sulfate (Exaggerated depressant effects). Products include:

Astramorph/PF Injection, USP (Preservative-Free) 535
Duramorph 962
Infumorph 200 and Infumorph 500 Sterile Solutions 965
MS Contin Tablets 1994
MSIR 1997
Oramorph SR (Morphine Sulfate Sustained Release Tablets) 2236
RMS Suppositories 2657
Roxanol 2243

Nortriptyline Hydrochloride (Transient delirium). Products include:

Pamelor 2280

Opium Alkaloids (Exaggerated depressant effects).

No products indexed under this heading.

Oxazepam (Exaggerated depressant effects). Products include:

Serax Capsules 2810
Serax Tablets 2810

Oxycodone Hydrochloride (Exaggerated depressant effects). Products include:

Percocet Tablets 938

Percodan Tablets 939
Percodan-Demi Tablets 940
Roxicodone Tablets, Oral Solution & Intensol (Oxycodone) 2244
Tylox Capsules 1584

Pentobarbital Sodium (Exaggerated depressant effects). Products include:

Nembutal Sodium Capsules 436
Nembutal Sodium Solution 438
Nembutal Sodium Suppositories 440

Perphenazine (Exaggerated depressant effects). Products include:

Etrafon 2355
Triavil Tablets 1757
Trilafon 2389

Phenelzine Sulfate (Exaggerated depressant effects). Products include:

Nardil 1920

Phenobarbital (Exaggerated depressant effects). Products include:

Arco-Lase Plus Tablets 512
Bellergal-S Tablets 2250
Donnatal 2060
Donnatal Extentabs 2061
Donnatal Tablets 2060
Phenobarbital Elixir and Tablets 1469
Quadrinal Tablets 1350

Prazepam (Exaggerated depressant effects).

No products indexed under this heading.

Prochlorperazine (Exaggerated depressant effects). Products include:

Compazine 2470

Promethazine Hydrochloride (Exaggerated depressant effects). Products include:

Mepergan Injection 2753
Phenergan with Codeine 2777
Phenergan with Dextromethorphan 2778
Phenergan Injection 2773
Phenergan Suppositories 2775
Phenergan Syrup 2774
Phenergan Tablets 2775
Phenergan VC 2779
Phenergan VC with Codeine 2781

Propofol (Exaggerated depressant effects). Products include:

Diprivan Injection 2833

Propoxyphene Hydrochloride (Exaggerated depressant effects). Products include:

Darvon 1435
Wygesic Tablets 2827

Propoxyphene Napsylate (Exaggerated depressant effects). Products include:

Darvon-N/Darvocet-N 1433

Protriptyline Hydrochloride (Transient delirium). Products include:

Vivactil Tablets 1774

Quazepam (Exaggerated depressant effects). Products include:

Doral Tablets 2664

Risperidone (Exaggerated depressant effects). Products include:

Risperdal 1301

Secobarbital Sodium (Exaggerated depressant effects). Products include:

Seconal Sodium Pulvules 1474

Selegiline Hydrochloride (Exaggerated depressant effects). Products include:

Eldepryl Tablets 2550

Sufentanil Citrate (Exaggerated depressant effects). Products include:

Sufenta Injection 1309

Temazepam (Exaggerated depressant effects). Products include:

Restoril Capsules 2284

Thiamylal Sodium (Exaggerated depressant effects).

No products indexed under this heading.

IMPORTANT NOTE: Always consult each drug listing in the patient's regimen for possible interactions.

Placidyl — Interactions Index — 824

Thioridazine Hydrochloride (Exaggerated depressant effects). Products include:
- Mellaril ... 2269

Thiothixene (Exaggerated depressant effects). Products include:
- Navane Capsules and Concentrate 2201
- Navane Intramuscular ... 2202

Tranylcypromine Sulfate (Exaggerated depressant effects). Products include:
- Parnate Tablets ... 2503

Triazolam (Exaggerated depressant effects). Products include:
- Halcion Tablets ... 2611

Trifluoperazine Hydrochloride (Exaggerated depressant effects). Products include:
- Stelazine ... 2514

Trimipramine Maleate (Transient delirium). Products include:
- Surmontil Capsules ... 2811

Warfarin Sodium (Decreased prothrombin time response). Products include:
- Coumadin ... 926

Zolpidem Tartrate (Exaggerated depressant effects). Products include:
- Ambien Tablets ... 2416

PLAQUENIL SULFATE TABLETS

(Hydroxychloroquine Sulfate) ... 2328

May interact with:

Hepatotoxic Drugs, unspecified (Use with caution).

PLASMA-PLEX, PLASMA PROTEIN FRACTION (HUMAN) 5%

(Plasma Protein Fraction (Human)) .. 524

None cited in PDR database.

PLATINOL

(Cisplatin) ... 708

May interact with aminoglycosides, anticonvulsants, and certain other agents. Compounds in these categories include:

Amikacin Sulfate (Potentiation of cumulative nephrotoxicity). Products include:
- Amikacin Sulfate Injection, USP ... 960
- Amikin Injectable ... 501

Carbamazepine (Plasma levels of anticonvulsant agents may become subtherapeutic). Products include:
- Atretol Tablets ... 573
- Tegretol Chewable Tablets ... 852
- Tegretol Suspension ... 852
- Tegretol Tablets ... 852

Divalproex Sodium (Plasma levels of anticonvulsant agents may become subtherapeutic). Products include:
- Depakote Tablets ... 415

Ethosuximide (Plasma levels of anticonvulsant agents may become subtherapeutic). Products include:
- Zarontin Capsules ... 1928
- Zarontin Syrup ... 1929

Ethotoin (Plasma levels of anticonvulsant agents may become subtherapeutic). Products include:
- Peganone Tablets ... 446

Felbamate (Plasma levels of anticonvulsant agents may become subtherapeutic). Products include:
- Felbatol ... 2666

Gentamicin Sulfate (Potentiation of cumulative nephrotoxicity). Products include:
- Garamycin Injectable ... 2360
- Genoptic Sterile Ophthalmic Solution ... ⊙ 243
- Genoptic Sterile Ophthalmic Ointment ... ⊙ 243
- Gentacidin Ointment ... ⊙ 264
- Gentacidin Solution ... ⊙ 264
- Gentak ... ⊙ 208
- Pred-G Liquifilm Sterile Ophthalmic Suspension ... ⊙ 251
- Pred-G S.O.P. Sterile Ophthalmic Ointment ... ⊙ 252

Kanamycin Sulfate (Potentiation of cumulative nephrotoxicity).
- No products indexed under this heading.

Lamotrigine (Plasma levels of anticonvulsant agents may become subtherapeutic). Products include:
- Lamictal Tablets ... 1112

Mephenytoin (Plasma levels of anticonvulsant agents may become subtherapeutic). Products include:
- Mesantoin Tablets ... 2272

Methsuximide (Plasma levels of anticonvulsant agents may become subtherapeutic). Products include:
- Celontin Kapseals ... 1899

Paramethadione (Plasma levels of anticonvulsant agents may become subtherapeutic).
- No products indexed under this heading.

Phenacemide (Plasma levels of anticonvulsant agents may become subtherapeutic). Products include:
- Phenurone Tablets ... 447

Phenobarbital (Plasma levels of anticonvulsant agents may become subtherapeutic). Products include:
- Arco-Lase Plus Tablets ... 512
- Bellergal-S Tablets ... 2250
- Donnatal ... 2060
- Donnatal Extentabs ... 2061
- Donnatal Tablets ... 2060
- Phenobarbital Elixir and Tablets ... 1469
- Quadrinal Tablets ... 1350

Phensuximide (Plasma levels of anticonvulsant agents may become subtherapeutic). Products include:
- Milontin Kapseals ... 1920

Phenytoin (Plasma levels of anticonvulsant agents may become subtherapeutic). Products include:
- Dilantin Infatabs ... 1908
- Dilantin-125 Suspension ... 1911

Phenytoin Sodium (Plasma levels of anticonvulsant agents may become subtherapeutic). Products include:
- Dilantin Kapseals ... 1906
- Dilantin Parenteral ... 1910

Primidone (Plasma levels of anticonvulsant agents may become subtherapeutic). Products include:
- Mysoline ... 2754

Pyridoxine Hydrochloride (Response duration may be adversely affected when pyridoxine is used in combination with altretamine and Platinol).
- No products indexed under this heading.

Streptomycin Sulfate (Potentiation of cumulative nephrotoxicity). Products include:
- Streptomycin Sulfate Injection ... 2208

Tobramycin (Potentiation of cumulative nephrotoxicity). Products include:
- AKTOB ... ⊙ 206
- TobraDex Ophthalmic Suspension and Ointment ... 473
- Tobrex Ophthalmic Ointment and Solution ... ⊙ 229

Tobramycin Sulfate (Potentiation of cumulative nephrotoxicity). Products include:
- Nebcin Vials, Hyporets & ADD-Vantage ... 1464
- Tobramycin Sulfate Injection ... 968

Trimethadione (Plasma levels of anticonvulsant agents may become subtherapeutic).
- No products indexed under this heading.

Valproic Acid (Plasma levels of anticonvulsant agents may become subtherapeutic). Products include:
- Depakene ... 413

PLATINOL-AQ INJECTION

(Cisplatin) ... 710

May interact with aminoglycosides, anticonvulsants, and certain other agents. Compounds in these categories include:

Amikacin Sulfate (Concomitant administration potentiates nephrotoxicity). Products include:
- Amikacin Sulfate Injection, USP ... 960
- Amikin Injectable ... 501

Carbamazepine (Plasma levels of anticonvulsant agents may become subtherapeutic). Products include:
- Atretol Tablets ... 573
- Tegretol Chewable Tablets ... 852
- Tegretol Suspension ... 852
- Tegretol Tablets ... 852

Divalproex Sodium (Plasma levels of anticonvulsant agents may become subtherapeutic). Products include:
- Depakote Tablets ... 415

Ethosuximide (Plasma levels of anticonvulsant agents may become subtherapeutic). Products include:
- Zarontin Capsules ... 1928
- Zarontin Syrup ... 1929

Ethotoin (Plasma levels of anticonvulsant agents may become subtherapeutic). Products include:
- Peganone Tablets ... 446

Felbamate (Plasma levels of anticonvulsant agents may become subtherapeutic). Products include:
- Felbatol ... 2666

Gentamicin Sulfate (Concomitant administration potentiates nephrotoxicity). Products include:
- Garamycin Injectable ... 2360
- Genoptic Sterile Ophthalmic Solution ... ⊙ 243
- Genoptic Sterile Ophthalmic Ointment ... ⊙ 243
- Gentacidin Ointment ... ⊙ 264
- Gentacidin Solution ... ⊙ 264
- Gentak ... ⊙ 208
- Pred-G Liquifilm Sterile Ophthalmic Suspension ... ⊙ 251
- Pred-G S.O.P. Sterile Ophthalmic Ointment ... ⊙ 252

Kanamycin Sulfate (Concomitant administration potentiates nephrotoxicity).
- No products indexed under this heading.

Lamotrigine (Plasma levels of anticonvulsant agents may become subtherapeutic). Products include:
- Lamictal Tablets ... 1112

Mephenytoin (Plasma levels of anticonvulsant agents may become subtherapeutic). Products include:
- Mesantoin Tablets ... 2272

Methsuximide (Plasma levels of anticonvulsant agents may become subtherapeutic). Products include:
- Celontin Kapseals ... 1899

Paramethadione (Plasma levels of anticonvulsant agents may become subtherapeutic).
- No products indexed under this heading.

Phenacemide (Plasma levels of anticonvulsant agents may become subtherapeutic). Products include:
- Phenurone Tablets ... 447

Phenobarbital (Plasma levels of anticonvulsant agents may become subtherapeutic). Products include:
- Arco-Lase Plus Tablets ... 512
- Bellergal-S Tablets ... 2250
- Donnatal ... 2060
- Donnatal Extentabs ... 2061
- Donnatal Tablets ... 2060
- Phenobarbital Elixir and Tablets ... 1469
- Quadrinal Tablets ... 1350

Phensuximide (Plasma levels of anticonvulsant agents may become subtherapeutic). Products include:
- Milontin Kapseals ... 1920

Phenytoin (Plasma levels of anticonvulsant agents may become subtherapeutic). Products include:
- Dilantin Infatabs ... 1908
- Dilantin-125 Suspension ... 1911

Phenytoin Sodium (Plasma levels of anticonvulsant agents may become subtherapeutic). Products include:
- Dilantin Kapseals ... 1906
- Dilantin Parenteral ... 1910

Primidone (Plasma levels of anticonvulsant agents may become subtherapeutic). Products include:
- Mysoline ... 2754

Pyridoxine Hydrochloride (Response duration may be adversely affected when pyridoxine is used in combination with altretamine and Platinol).
- No products indexed under this heading.

Streptomycin Sulfate (Concomitant administration potentiates nephrotoxicity). Products include:
- Streptomycin Sulfate Injection ... 2208

Tobramycin (Concomitant administration potentiates nephrotoxicity). Products include:
- AKTOB ... ⊙ 206
- TobraDex Ophthalmic Suspension and Ointment ... 473
- Tobrex Ophthalmic Ointment and Solution ... ⊙ 229

Tobramycin Sulfate (Concomitant administration potentiates nephrotoxicity). Products include:
- Nebcin Vials, Hyporets & ADD-Vantage ... 1464
- Tobramycin Sulfate Injection ... 968

Trimethadione (Plasma levels of anticonvulsant agents may become subtherapeutic).
- No products indexed under this heading.

Valproic Acid (Plasma levels of anticonvulsant agents may become subtherapeutic). Products include:
- Depakene ... 413

PLENDIL EXTENDED-RELEASE TABLETS

(Felodipine) ... 527

May interact with anticonvulsants, beta blockers, and certain other agents. Compounds in these categories include:

Acebutolol Hydrochloride (Caution should be exercised when using Plendil in patients with heart failure or compromised ventricular function, particularly in combination with beta blocker). Products include:
- Sectral Capsules ... 2807

Atenolol (Caution should be exercised when using Plendil in patients with heart failure or compromised ventricular function, particularly in combination with beta blocker). Products include:
- Tenoretic Tablets ... 2845
- Tenormin Tablets and I.V. Injection 2847

(▭ Described in PDR For Nonprescription Drugs) (⊙ Described in PDR For Ophthalmology)

Betaxolol Hydrochloride (Caution should be exercised when using Plendil in patients with heart failure or compromised ventricular function, particularly in combination with beta blocker). Products include:

Betoptic Ophthalmic Solution........... 469
Betoptic S Ophthalmic Suspension 471
Kerlone Tablets....................................... 2436

Bisoprolol Fumarate (Caution should be exercised when using Plendil in patients with heart failure or compromised ventricular function, particularly in combination with beta blocker). Products include:

Zebeta Tablets 1413
Ziac 1415

Carbamazepine (Potential for low maximum plasma concentrations of felodipine in epileptic patients on long-term anticonvulsant therapy). Products include:

Atretol Tablets 573
Tegretol Chewable Tablets 852
Tegretol Suspension............................. 852
Tegretol Tablets 852

Carteolol Hydrochloride (Caution should be exercised when using Plendil in patients with heart failure or compromised ventricular function, particularly in combination with beta blocker). Products include:

Cartrol Tablets 410
Ocupress Ophthalmic Solution, 1% Sterile.. ⊕ 309

Cimetidine (Increases AUC and C_{max} by approximately 50%; low doses of Plendil should be used). Products include:

Tagamet Tablets 2516

Cimetidine Hydrochloride (Increases AUC and C_{max} by approximately 50%; low doses of Plendil should be used). Products include:

Tagamet.. 2516

Digoxin (Co-administration does not significantly alter the pharmacokinetics of digoxin in patients with heart failure). Products include:

Lanoxicaps 1117
Lanoxin Elixir Pediatric 1120
Lanoxin Injection 1123
Lanoxin Injection Pediatric................ 1126
Lanoxin Tablets 1128

Divalproex Sodium (Potential for low maximum plasma concentrations of felodipine in epileptic patients on long-term anticonvulsant therapy). Products include:

Depakote Tablets................................... 415

Esmolol Hydrochloride (Caution should be exercised when using Plendil in 31% with 38% respectively compromised ventricular function, particularly in combination with beta blocker). Products include:

Brevibloc Injection................................. 1808

Ethosuximide (Potential for low maximum plasma concentrations of felodipine in epileptic patients on long-term anticonvulsant therapy). Products include:

Zarontin Capsules 1928
Zarontin Syrup 1929

Ethotoin (Potential for low maximum plasma concentrations of felodipine in epileptic patients on long-term anticonvulsant therapy). Products include:

Peganone Tablets 446

Felbamate (Potential for low maximum plasma concentrations of felodipine in epileptic patients on long-term anticonvulsant therapy). Products include:

Felbatol 2666

Labetalol Hydrochloride (Caution should be exercised when using Plendil in patients with heart failure or compromised ventricular function, particularly in combination with beta blocker). Products include:

Normodyne Injection 2377
Normodyne Tablets 2379
Trandate 1185

Lamotrigine (Potential for low maximum plasma concentrations of felodipine in epileptic patients on long-term anticonvulsant therapy). Products include:

Lamictal Tablets..................................... 1112

Levobunolol Hydrochloride (Caution should be exercised when using Plendil in patients with heart failure or compromised ventricular function, particularly in combination with beta blocker). Products include:

Betagan .... ⊕ 233

Mephenytoin (Potential for low maximum plasma concentrations of felodipine in epileptic patients on long-term anticonvulsant therapy). Products include:

Mesantoin Tablets 2272

Methsuximide (Potential for low maximum plasma concentrations of felodipine in epileptic patients on long-term anticonvulsant therapy). Products include:

Celontin Kapseals 1899

Metipranolol Hydrochloride (Caution should be exercised when using Plendil in patients with heart failure or compromised ventricular function, particularly in combination with beta blocker). Products include:

OptiPranolol (Metipranolol 0.3%)
Sterile Ophthalmic Solution...... ⊕ 258

Metoprolol Succinate (Increased AUC and C_{max} of metoprolol approximately 31% and 38% respectively). Products include:

Toprol-XL Tablets 565

Metoprolol Tartrate (Increased AUC and C_{max} of metoprolol approximately 31% and 38% respectively). Products include:

Lopressor Ampuls 830
Lopressor HCT Tablets 832
Lopressor Tablets 830

Nadolol (Caution should be exercised when using Plendil in patients with heart failure or compromised ventricular function, particularly in combination with beta blocker).

No products indexed under this heading.

Paramethadione (Potential for low maximum plasma concentrations of felodipine in epileptic patients on long-term anticonvulsant therapy).

No products indexed under this heading.

Penbutolol Sulfate (Caution should be exercised when using Plendil in patients with heart failure or compromised ventricular function, particularly in combination with beta blocker). Products include:

Levatol 2403

Phenacemide (Potential for low maximum plasma concentrations of felodipine in epileptic patients on long-term anticonvulsant therapy). Products include:

Phenurone Tablets 447

Phenobarbital (Potential for low maximum plasma concentrations of felodipine in epileptic patients on long-term anticonvulsant therapy). Products include:

Arco-Lase Plus Tablets 512
Bellergal-S Tablets 2250
Donnatal 2060
Donnatal Extentabs.............................. 2061

Donnatal Tablets 2060
Phenobarbital Elixir and Tablets 1469
Quadrinal Tablets 1350

Phensuximide (Potential for low maximum plasma concentrations of felodipine in epileptic patients on long-term anticonvulsant therapy). Products include:

Milontin Kapseals.................................. 1920

Phenytoin (Potential for low maximum plasma concentrations of felodipine in epileptic patients on long-term anticonvulsant therapy). Products include:

Dilantin Infatabs.................................... 1908
Dilantin-125 Suspension 1911

Phenytoin Sodium (Potential for low maximum plasma concentrations of felodipine in epileptic patients on long-term anticonvulsant therapy). Products include:

Dilantin Kapseals.................................. 1906
Dilantin Parenteral 1910

Pindolol (Caution should be exercised when using Plendil in patients with heart failure or compromised ventricular function, particularly in combination with beta blocker). Products include:

Visken Tablets.. 2299

Primidone (Potential for low maximum plasma concentrations of felodipine in epileptic patients on long-term anticonvulsant therapy). Products include:

Mysoline... 2754

Propranolol Hydrochloride (Caution should be exercised when using Plendil in patients with heart failure or compromised ventricular function, particularly in combination with beta blocker). Products include:

Inderal 2728
Inderal LA Long Acting Capsules 2730
Inderide Tablets 2732
Inderide LA Long Acting Capsules .. 2734

Sotalol Hydrochloride (Caution should be exercised when using Plendil in patients with heart failure or compromised ventricular function, particularly in combination with beta blocker). Products include:

Betapace Tablets 641

Timolol Hemihydrate (Caution should be exercised when using Plendil in patients with heart failure or compromised ventricular function, particularly in combination with beta blocker). Products include:

Betimol 0.25%, 0.5% .... ⊕ 261

Timolol Maleate (Caution should be exercised when using Plendil in patients with heart failure or compromised ventricular function, particularly in combination with beta blocker). Products include:

Blocadren Tablets 1614
Timolide Tablets.................................... 1748
Timoptic in Ocudose 1753
Timoptic Sterile Ophthalmic Solution.. 1751
Timoptic-XE 1755

Trimethadione (Potential for low maximum plasma concentrations of felodipine in epileptic patients on long-term anticonvulsant therapy).

No products indexed under this heading.

Valproic Acid (Potential for low maximum plasma concentrations of felodipine in epileptic patients on long-term anticonvulsant therapy). Products include:

Depakene 413

Food Interactions

Grapefruit juice, doubly concentrated (Increases bioavailability more than two-fold).

PNEUMOVAX 23

(Pneumococcal Vaccine, Polyvalent)..1725
May interact with immunosuppressive agents. Compounds in this category include:

Azathioprine (Expected serum antibody response may not be obtained). Products include:

Imuran 1110

Cyclosporine (Expected serum antibody response may not be obtained). Products include:

Neoral.. 2276
Sandimmune 2286

Immune Globulin (Human) (Expected serum antibody response may not be obtained).

No products indexed under this heading.

Immune Globulin Intravenous (Human) (Expected serum antibody response may not be obtained).

Muromonab-CD3 (Expected serum antibody response may not be obtained). Products include:

Orthoclone OKT3 Sterile Solution .. 1837

Mycophenolate Mofetil (Expected serum antibody response may not be obtained). Products include:

CellCept Capsules 2099

Tacrolimus (Expected serum antibody response may not be obtained). Products include:

Prograf 1042

PNU-IMUNE 23

(Pneumococcal Vaccine, Polyvalent)..1393
May interact with immunosuppressive agents and antineoplastics. Compounds in these categories include:

Altretamine (Possible impaired serum antibody response to vaccine). Products include:

Hexalen Capsules 2571

Asparaginase (Possible impaired serum antibody response to vaccine). Products include:

Elspar 1659

Azathioprine (Reduction of antibody levels). Products include:

Imuran 1110

Bleomycin Sulfate (Possible impaired serum antibody response to vaccine). Products include:

Blenoxane 692

Busulfan (Possible impaired serum antibody response to vaccine). Products include:

Myleran Tablets 1143

Carboplatin (Possible impaired serum antibody response to vaccine). Products include:

Paraplatin for Injection 705

Carmustine (BCNU) (Possible impaired serum antibody response to vaccine). Products include:

BiCNU 691

Chlorambucil (Possible impaired serum antibody response to vaccine). Products include:

Leukeran Tablets 1133

Cisplatin (Possible impaired serum antibody response to vaccine). Products include:

Platinol 708
Platinol-AQ Injection............................ 710

Cyclophosphamide (Possible impaired serum antibody response to vaccine). Products include:

Cytoxan 694
NEOSAR Lyophilized/Neosar 1959

Cyclosporine (Reduction of antibody levels). Products include:

Neoral.. 2276

IMPORTANT NOTE: Always consult each drug listing in the patient's regimen for possible interactions.

Sandimmune 2286

Dacarbazine (Possible impaired serum antibody response to vaccine). Products include:

DTIC-Dome 600

Daunorubicin Hydrochloride (Possible impaired serum antibody response to vaccine). Products include:

Cerubidine 795

Doxorubicin Hydrochloride (Possible impaired serum antibody response to vaccine). Products include:

Adriamycin PFS 1947
Adriamycin RDF 1947
Doxorubicin Astra 540
Rubex 712

Estramustine Phosphate Sodium (Possible impaired serum antibody response to vaccine). Products include:

Emcyt Capsules 1953

Etoposide (Possible impaired serum antibody response to vaccine). Products include:

VePesid Capsules and Injection 718

Floxuridine (Possible impaired serum antibody response to vaccine). Products include:

Sterile FUDR 2118

Fluorouracil (Possible impaired serum antibody response to vaccine). Products include:

Efudex 2113
Fluoroplex Topical Solution & Cream 1% 479
Fluorouracil Injection 2116

Flutamide (Possible impaired serum antibody response to vaccine). Products include:

Eulexin Capsules 2358

Hydroxyurea (Possible impaired serum antibody response to vaccine). Products include:

Hydrea Capsules 696

Idarubicin Hydrochloride (Possible impaired serum antibody response to vaccine). Products include:

Idamycin 1955

Ifosfamide (Possible impaired serum antibody response to vaccine). Products include:

IFEX 697

Immune Globulin (Human) (Reduction of antibody levels).

No products indexed under this heading.

Immune Globulin Intravenous (Human) (Reduction of antibody levels).

Interferon alfa-2A, Recombinant (Possible impaired serum antibody response to vaccine). Products include:

Roferon-A Injection 2145

Interferon alfa-2B, Recombinant (Possible impaired serum antibody response to vaccine). Products include:

Intron A 2364

Levamisole Hydrochloride (Possible impaired serum antibody response to vaccine). Products include:

Ergamisol Tablets 1292

Lomustine (CCNU) (Possible impaired serum antibody response to vaccine). Products include:

CeeNU 693

Mechlorethamine Hydrochloride (Possible impaired serum antibody response to vaccine). Products include:

Mustargen 1709

Megestrol Acetate (Possible impaired serum antibody response to vaccine). Products include:

Megace Oral Suspension 699
Megace Tablets 701

Melphalan (Possible impaired serum antibody response to vaccine). Products include:

Alkeran Tablets 1071

Mercaptopurine (Possible impaired serum antibody response to vaccine). Products include:

Purinethol Tablets 1156

Methotrexate Sodium (Possible impaired serum antibody response to vaccine). Products include:

Methotrexate Sodium Tablets, Injection, for Injection and LPF Injection 1275

Mitomycin (Mitomycin-C) (Possible impaired serum antibody response to vaccine). Products include:

Mutamycin 703

Mitotane (Possible impaired serum antibody response to vaccine). Products include:

Lysodren 698

Mitoxantrone Hydrochloride (Possible impaired serum antibody response to vaccine). Products include:

Novantrone 1279

Muromonab-CD3 (Reduction of antibody levels). Products include:

Orthoclone OKT3 Sterile Solution .. 1837

Mycophenolate Mofetil (Reduction of antibody levels). Products include:

CellCept Capsules 2099

Paclitaxel (Possible impaired serum antibody response to vaccine). Products include:

Taxol 714

Procarbazine Hydrochloride (Possible impaired serum antibody response to vaccine). Products include:

Matulane Capsules 2131

Streptozocin (Possible impaired serum antibody response to vaccine). Products include:

Zanosar Sterile Powder 2653

Tacrolimus (Reduction of antibody levels). Products include:

Prograf 1042

Tamoxifen Citrate (Possible impaired serum antibody response to vaccine). Products include:

Nolvadex Tablets 2841

Teniposide (Possible impaired serum antibody response to vaccine). Products include:

Vumon 727

Thioguanine (Possible impaired serum antibody response to vaccine). Products include:

Thioguanine Tablets, Tabloid Brand 1181

Thiotepa (Possible impaired serum antibody response to vaccine). Products include:

Thioplex (Thiotepa For Injection) 1281

Vincristine Sulfate (Possible impaired serum antibody response to vaccine). Products include:

Oncovin Solution Vials & Hyporets 1466

Vinorelbine Tartrate (Possible impaired serum antibody response to vaccine). Products include:

Navelbine Injection 1145

PODOCON-25

(Podophyllin) 1891
None cited in PDR database.

POLIOVAX

(Poliovirus Vaccine Inactivated, Trivalent Types 1,2,3) 891
None cited in PDR database.

POLYCITRA SYRUP

(Potassium Citrate, Sodium Citrate, Citric Acid) 578
May interact with potassium preparations, potassium sparing diuretics, cardiac glycosides, ACE inhibitors, and certain other agents. Compounds in these categories include:

Aluminum Carbonate Gel (Patients with low urinary output or reduced glomerular filtration rates should avoid concomitant use of aluminum-based antacids). Products include:

Basaljel 2703

Aluminum Hydroxide (Patients with low urinary output or reduced glomerular filtration rates should avoid concomitant use of aluminum-based antacids). Products include:

ALternaGEL Liquid 1316
Maximum Strength Ascriptin .... ▣ 630
Cama Arthritis Pain Reliever .... ▣ 785
Gaviscon Extra Strength Relief Formula Antacid Tablets .... ▣ 819
Gaviscon Extra Strength Relief Formula Liquid Antacid .... ▣ 819
Gaviscon Liquid Antacid .... ▣ 820
Gelusil Liquid & Tablets .... ▣ 855
Maalox Heartburn Relief Suspension .... ▣ 642
Maalox Heartburn Relief Tablets .... ▣ 641
Maalox Magnesia and Alumina Oral Suspension .... ▣ 642
Maalox Plus Tablets .... ▣ 643
Extra Strength Maalox Antacid Plus Antigas Liquid and Tablets ▣ 638
Tempo Soft Antacid .... ▣ 835

Aluminum Hydroxide Gel (Patients with low urinary output or reduced glomerular filtration rates should avoid concomitant use of aluminum-based antacids). Products include:

ALternaGEL Liquid .... ▣ 659
Aludrox Oral Suspension 2695
Amphojel Suspension 2695
Amphojel Suspension without Flavor 2695
Amphojel Tablets 2695
Arthritis Pain Ascriptin .... ▣ 631
Regular Strength Ascriptin Tablets .... ▣ 629
Gaviscon Antacid Tablets .... ▣ 819
Gaviscon-2 Antacid Tablets .... ▣ 820
Mylanta Liquid 1317
Mylanta Tablets .... ▣ 660
Mylanta Double Strength Liquid 1317
Mylanta Double Strength Tablets .. ▣ 660
Nephrox Suspension .... ▣ 655

Amiloride Hydrochloride (Potential toxicity). Products include:

Midamor Tablets 1703
Moduretic Tablets 1705

Benazepril Hydrochloride (Potential toxicity). Products include:

Lotensin Tablets 834
Lotensin HCT 837
Lotrel Capsules 840

Captopril (Potential toxicity). Products include:

Capoten 739
Capozide 742

Deslanoside (Potential toxicity).

No products indexed under this heading.

Digitoxin (Potential toxicity). Products include:

Crystodigin Tablets 1433

Digoxin (Potential toxicity). Products include:

Lanoxicaps 1117
Lanoxin Elixir Pediatric 1120
Lanoxin Injection 1123
Lanoxin Injection Pediatric 1126
Lanoxin Tablets 1128

Enalapril Maleate (Potential toxicity). Products include:

Vaseretic Tablets 1765
Vasotec Tablets 1771

Enalaprilat (Potential toxicity). Products include:

Vasotec I.V. 1768

Fosinopril Sodium (Potential toxicity). Products include:

Monopril Tablets 757

Lisinopril (Potential toxicity). Products include:

Prinivil Tablets 1733
Prinzide Tablets 1737
Zestoretic 2850
Zestril Tablets 2854

Moexipril Hydrochloride (Potential toxicity). Products include:

Univasc Tablets 2410

Potassium Acid Phosphate (Potential toxicity). Products include:

K-Phos Original Formula 'Sodium Free' Tablets 639

Potassium Bicarbonate (Potential toxicity). Products include:

Alka-Seltzer Gold Effervescent Antacid .... ▣ 703

Potassium Chloride (Potential toxicity). Products include:

Chlor-3 Condiment 1004
K-Dur Microburst Release System (potassium chloride, USP) E.R. Tablets 1325
K-Lor Powder Packets 434
K-Norm Extended-Release Capsules 991
K-Tab Filmtab 434
Kolyum Liquid 992
Micro-K 2063
Micro-K LS Packets 2064
NuLYTELY 689
Cherry Flavor NuLYTELY 689
Rum-K Syrup 1005
Slow-K Extended-Release Tablets 851

Potassium Gluconate (Potential toxicity). Products include:

Kolyum Liquid 992

Potassium Phosphate, Dibasic (Potential toxicity).

No products indexed under this heading.

Potassium Phosphate, Monobasic (Potential toxicity). Products include:

K-Phos Neutral Tablets 639
K-Phos Original Formula 'Sodium Free' Tablets 639

Quinapril Hydrochloride (Potential toxicity). Products include:

Accupril Tablets 1893

Ramipril (Potential toxicity). Products include:

Altace Capsules 1232

Spirapril Hydrochloride (Potential toxicity).

No products indexed under this heading.

Spironolactone (Potential toxicity). Products include:

Aldactazide 2413
Aldactone 2414

Triamterene (Potential toxicity). Products include:

Dyazide 2479
Dyrenium Capsules 2481
Maxzide 1380

POLYCITRA-K CRYSTALS

(Potassium Citrate, Citric Acid) 579
May interact with potassium preparations, potassium sparing diuretics, ACE inhibitors, and cardiac glycosides. Compounds in these categories include:

Amiloride Hydrochloride (Potential toxicity). Products include:

Midamor Tablets 1703
Moduretic Tablets 1705

Benazepril Hydrochloride (Potential toxicity). Products include:

Lotensin Tablets 834
Lotensin HCT 837
Lotrel Capsules 840

827 Interactions Index Polysporin Ophthalmic Ointment

Captopril (Potential toxicity). Products include:
- Capoten ... 739
- Capozide ... 742

Deslanoside (Potential toxicity).
- No products indexed under this heading.

Digitoxin (Potential toxicity). Products include:
- Crystodigin Tablets ... 1433

Digoxin (Potential toxicity). Products include:
- Lanoxicaps ... 1117
- Lanoxin Elixir Pediatric ... 1120
- Lanoxin Injection ... 1123
- Lanoxin Injection Pediatric ... 1126
- Lanoxin Tablets ... 1128

Enalapril Maleate (Potential toxicity). Products include:
- Vaseretic Tablets ... 1765
- Vasotec Tablets ... 1771

Enalaprilat (Potential toxicity). Products include:
- Vasotec I.V. ... 1768

Fosinopril Sodium (Potential toxicity). Products include:
- Monopril Tablets ... 757

Lisinopril (Potential toxicity). Products include:
- Prinivil Tablets ... 1733
- Prinzide Tablets ... 1737
- Zestoretic ... 2850
- Zestril Tablets ... 2854

Moexipril Hydrochloride (Potential toxicity). Products include:
- Univasc Tablets ... 2410

Potassium Acid Phosphate (Potential toxicity). Products include:
- K-Phos Original Formula 'Sodium Free' Tablets ... 639

Potassium Bicarbonate (Potential toxicity). Products include:
- Alka-Seltzer Gold Effervescent Antacid ... ▣ 703

Potassium Chloride (Potential toxicity). Products include:
- Chlor-3 Condiment ... 1004
- K-Dur Microburst Release System (potassium chloride, USP) E.R. Tablets ... 1325
- K-Lor Powder Packets ... 434
- K-Norm Extended-Release Capsules ... 991
- K-Tab Filmtab ... 434
- Kolyum Liquid ... 992
- Micro-K ... 2063
- Micro-K LS Packets ... 2064
- NuLYTELY ... 689
- Cherry Flavor NuLYTELY ... 689
- Rum-K Syrup ... 1005
- Slow-K Extended-Release Tablets ... 851

Potassium Gluconate (Potential toxicity). Products include:
- Kolyum Liquid ... 992

Potassium Phosphate, Dibasic (Potential toxicity).
- No products indexed under this heading.

Potassium Phosphate, Monobasic (Potential toxicity). Products include:
- K-Phos Neutral Tablets ... 639
- K-Phos Original Formula 'Sodium Free' Tablets ... 639

Quinapril Hydrochloride (Potential toxicity). Products include:
- Accupril Tablets ... 1893

Ramipril (Potential toxicity). Products include:
- Altace Capsules ... 1232

Spirapril Hydrochloride (Potential toxicity).
- No products indexed under this heading.

Spironolactone (Potential toxicity). Products include:
- Aldactazide ... 2413
- Aldactone ... 2414

Triamterene (Potential toxicity). Products include:
- Dyazide ... 2479
- Dyrenium Capsules ... 2481
- Maxzide ... 1380

POLYCITRA-K ORAL SOLUTION

(Potassium Citrate, Citric Acid) ... 579

May interact with ACE inhibitors, potassium sparing diuretics, potassium preparations, and cardiac glycosides. Compounds in these categories include:

Amiloride Hydrochloride (Increased risk of hyperkalemia). Products include:
- Midamor Tablets ... 1703
- Moduretic Tablets ... 1705

Benazepril Hydrochloride (Increased risk of hyperkalemia). Products include:
- Lotensin Tablets ... 834
- Lotensin HCT ... 837
- Lotrel Capsules ... 840

Captopril (Increased risk of hyperkalemia). Products include:
- Capoten ... 739
- Capozide ... 742

Deslanoside (Increased risk of hyperkalemia).
- No products indexed under this heading.

Digitoxin (Increased risk of hyperkalemia). Products include:
- Crystodigin Tablets ... 1433

Digoxin (Increased risk of hyperkalemia). Products include:
- Lanoxicaps ... 1117
- Lanoxin Elixir Pediatric ... 1120
- Lanoxin Injection ... 1123
- Lanoxin Injection Pediatric ... 1126
- Lanoxin Tablets ... 1128

Enalapril Maleate (Increased risk of hyperkalemia). Products include:
- Vaseretic Tablets ... 1765
- Vasotec Tablets ... 1771

Enalaprilat (Increased risk of hyperkalemia). Products include:
- Vasotec I.V. ... 1768

Fosinopril Sodium (Increased risk of hyperkalemia). Products include:
- Monopril Tablets ... 757

Lisinopril (Increased risk of hyperkalemia). Products include:
- Prinivil Tablets ... 1733
- Prinzide Tablets ... 1737
- Zestoretic ... 2850
- Zestril Tablets ... 2854

Moexipril Hydrochloride (Increased risk of hyperkalemia). Products include:
- Univasc Tablets ... 2410

Potassium Acid Phosphate (Increased risk of hyperkalemia). Products include:
- K-Phos Original Formula 'Sodium Free' Tablets ... 639

Potassium Bicarbonate (Increased risk of hyperkalemia). Products include:
- Alka-Seltzer Gold Effervescent Antacid ... ▣ 703

Potassium Chloride (Increased risk of hyperkalemia). Products include:
- Chlor-3 Condiment ... 1004
- K-Dur Microburst Release System (potassium chloride, USP) E.R. Tablets ... 1325
- K-Lor Powder Packets ... 434
- K-Norm Extended-Release Capsules ... 991
- K-Tab Filmtab ... 434
- Kolyum Liquid ... 992
- Micro-K ... 2063
- Micro-K LS Packets ... 2064
- NuLYTELY ... 689
- Cherry Flavor NuLYTELY ... 689
- Rum-K Syrup ... 1005
- Slow-K Extended-Release Tablets ... 851

Potassium Gluconate (Increased risk of hyperkalemia). Products include:
- Kolyum Liquid ... 992

Potassium Phosphate, Dibasic (Increased risk of hyperkalemia).
- No products indexed under this heading.

Potassium Phosphate, Monobasic (Increased risk of hyperkalemia). Products include:
- K-Phos Neutral Tablets ... 639
- K-Phos Original Formula 'Sodium Free' Tablets ... 639

Quinapril Hydrochloride (Increased risk of hyperkalemia). Products include:
- Accupril Tablets ... 1893

Ramipril (Increased risk of hyperkalemia). Products include:
- Altace Capsules ... 1232

Spirapril Hydrochloride (Increased risk of hyperkalemia).
- No products indexed under this heading.

Spironolactone (Increased risk of hyperkalemia). Products include:
- Aldactazide ... 2413
- Aldactone ... 2414

Triamterene (Increased risk of hyperkalemia). Products include:
- Dyazide ... 2479
- Dyrenium Capsules ... 2481
- Maxzide ... 1380

POLYCITRA-LC

(Potassium Citrate, Citric Acid, Sodium Citrate) ... 578

See **Polycitra Syrup**

POLYCOSE GLUCOSE POLYMERS

(Glucose Polymers) ... 2223

None cited in PDR database.

POLYMYXIN B SULFATE, AEROSPORIN BRAND STERILE POWDER

(Polymyxin B Sulfate) ... 1154

May interact with aminoglycosides and certain other agents. Compounds in these categories include:

Amikacin Sulfate (Nephrotoxic/neurotoxic effects enhanced). Products include:
- Amikacin Sulfate Injection, USP ... 960
- Amikin Injectable ... 501

Cephaloridine (Nephrotoxic/neurotoxic effects enhanced).

Colistin Sulfate (Nephrotoxic/neurotoxic effects enhanced). Products include:
- Coly-Mycin S Otic w/Neomycin & Hydrocortisone ... 1906

Decamethonium (Precipitation of respiratory depression).

Ether (Precipitation of respiratory depression).

Gallamine (Precipitation of respiratory depression).

Gentamicin Sulfate (Nephrotoxic/neurotoxic effects enhanced). Products include:
- Garamycin Injectable ... 2360
- Genoptic Sterile Ophthalmic Solution ... ⊙ 243
- Genoptic Sterile Ophthalmic Ointment ... ⊙ 243
- Gentacidin Ointment ... ⊙ 264
- Gentacidin Solution ... ⊙ 264
- Gentak ... ⊙ 208
- Pred-G Liquifilm Sterile Ophthalmic Suspension ... ⊙ 251
- Pred-G S.O.P. Sterile Ophthalmic Ointment ... ⊙ 252

Kanamycin Sulfate (Nephrotoxic/neurotoxic effects enhanced).
- No products indexed under this heading.

Neomycin Sulfate (Nephrotoxic/neurotoxic effects enhanced). Products include:
- AK-Spore ... ⊙ 204
- AK-Trol Ointment & Suspension ... ⊙ 205
- Bactine First Aid Antibiotic Plus Anesthetic Ointment ... ▣ 708
- Campho-Phenique Maximum Strength First Aid Antibiotic Plus Pain Reliever Ointment ... ▣ 719
- Coly-Mycin S Otic w/Neomycin & Hydrocortisone ... 1906
- Cortisporin Cream ... 1084
- Cortisporin Ointment ... 1085
- Cortisporin Ophthalmic Ointment Sterile ... 1085
- Cortisporin Ophthalmic Suspension Sterile ... 1086
- Cortisporin Otic Solution Sterile ... 1087
- Cortisporin Otic Suspension Sterile ... 1088
- Dexacidin Ointment ... ⊙ 263
- Maxitrol Ophthalmic Ointment and Suspension ... ⊙ 224
- Mycitracin ... ▣ 839
- NeoDecadron Sterile Ophthalmic Ointment ... 1712
- NeoDecadron Sterile Ophthalmic Solution ... 1713
- NeoDecadron Topical Cream ... 1714
- Neosporin G.U. Irrigant Sterile ... 1148
- Neosporin Ointment ... ▣ 857
- Neosporin Plus Maximum Strength Cream ... ▣ 858
- Neosporin Plus Maximum Strength Ointment ... ▣ 858
- Neosporin Ophthalmic Ointment Sterile ... 1148
- Neosporin Ophthalmic Solution Sterile ... 1149
- PediOtic Suspension Sterile ... 1153
- Poly-Pred Liquifilm ... ⊙ 248

Paromomycin Sulfate (Nephrotoxic/neurotoxic effects enhanced).
- No products indexed under this heading.

Sodium Citrate, Injection (Precipitation of respiratory depression).

Streptomycin Sulfate (Nephrotoxic/neurotoxic effects enhanced). Products include:
- Streptomycin Sulfate Injection ... 2208

Succinylcholine Chloride (Precipitation of respiratory depression). Products include:
- Anectine ... 1073

Tobramycin (Nephrotoxic/neurotoxic effects enhanced). Products include:
- AKTOB ... ⊙ 206
- TobraDex Ophthalmic Suspension and Ointment ... 473
- Tobrex Ophthalmic Ointment and Solution ... ⊙ 229

Tobramycin Sulfate (Nephrotoxic/neurotoxic effects enhanced). Products include:
- Nebcin Vials, Hyporets & ADD-Vantage ... 1464
- Tobramycin Sulfate Injection ... 968

Tubocurarine Chloride (Precipitation of respiratory depression).
- No products indexed under this heading.

Viomycin (Nephrotoxic/neurotoxic effects enhanced).

POLY-PRED LIQUIFILM

(Neomycin Sulfate, Polymyxin B Sulfate, Prednisolone Acetate) ... ⊙ 248

None cited in PDR database.

POLYSPORIN OINTMENT

(Bacitracin Zinc, Polymyxin B Sulfate) ... ▣ 858

None cited in PDR database.

IMPORTANT NOTE: Always consult each drug listing in the patient's regimen for possible interactions.

POLYSPORIN OPHTHALMIC OINTMENT STERILE
(Polymyxin B Sulfate, Bacitracin Zinc) 1154
None cited in PDR database.

POLYSPORIN POWDER
(Bacitracin Zinc, Polymyxin B Sulfate) ▣ 859
None cited in PDR database.

POLYTRIM OPHTHALMIC SOLUTION STERILE
(Polymyxin B Sulfate, Trimethoprim Sulfate) 482
None cited in PDR database.

PONARIS NASAL MUCOSAL EMOLLIENT
(Oil Based Products, Iodine Preparations) ▣ 658
None cited in PDR database.

PONDIMIN TABLETS
(Fenfluramine Hydrochloride) 2066
May interact with central nervous system depressants, monoamine oxidase inhibitors, and certain other agents. Compounds in these categories include:

Alfentanil Hydrochloride (Possible additive effects of CNS depressants). Products include:
- Alfenta Injection 1286

Alprazolam (Possible additive effects of CNS depressants). Products include:
- Xanax Tablets 2649

Aprobarbital (Possible additive effects of CNS depressants).
- No products indexed under this heading.

Buprenorphine (Possible additive effects of CNS depressants). Products include:
- Buprenex Injectable 2006

Buspirone Hydrochloride (Possible additive effects of CNS depressants). Products include:
- BuSpar 737

Butabarbital (Possible additive effects of CNS depressants).
- No products indexed under this heading.

Butalbital (Possible additive effects of CNS depressants). Products include:
- Esgic-plus Tablets 1013
- Fioricet Tablets 2258
- Fioricet with Codeine Capsules 2260
- Fiorinal Capsules 2261
- Fiorinal with Codeine Capsules 2262
- Fiorinal Tablets 2261
- Phrenilin 785
- Sedapap Tablets 50 mg/650 mg 1543

Chlordiazepoxide (Possible additive effects of CNS depressants). Products include:
- Libritabs Tablets 2177
- Limbitrol 2180

Chlordiazepoxide Hydrochloride (Possible additive effects of CNS depressants). Products include:
- Librax Capsules 2176
- Librium Capsules 2178
- Librium Injectable 2179

Chlorpromazine (Possible additive effects of CNS depressants). Products include:
- Thorazine Suppositories 2523

Chlorprothixene (Possible additive effects of CNS depressants).
- No products indexed under this heading.

Chlorprothixene Hydrochloride (Possible additive effects of CNS depressants).
- No products indexed under this heading.

Clorazepate Dipotassium (Possible additive effects of CNS depressants). Products include:
- Tranxene 451

Clozapine (Possible additive effects of CNS depressants). Products include:
- Clozaril Tablets 2252

Codeine Phosphate (Possible additive effects of CNS depressants). Products include:
- Actifed with Codeine Cough Syrup 1067
- Brontex 1981
- Deconsal C Expectorant Syrup 456
- Deconsal Pediatric Syrup 457
- Dimetane-DC Cough Syrup 2059
- Empirin with Codeine Tablets 1093
- Fioricet with Codeine Capsules 2260
- Fiorinal with Codeine Capsules 2262
- Isoclor Expectorant 990
- Novahistine DH 2462
- Novahistine Expectorant 2463
- Nucofed 2051
- Phenergan with Codeine 2777
- Phenergan VC with Codeine 2781
- Robitussin A-C Syrup 2073
- Robitussin-DAC Syrup 2074
- Ryna ▣ 841
- Soma Compound w/Codeine Tablets 2676
- Tussi-Organidin NR Liquid and S NR Liquid 2677
- Tylenol with Codeine 1583

Deserpidine (Increased effect of hypertensives).
- No products indexed under this heading.

Desflurane (Possible additive effects of CNS depressants). Products include:
- Suprane 1813

Dezocine (Possible additive effects of CNS depressants). Products include:
- Dalgan Injection 538

Diazepam (Possible additive effects of CNS depressants). Products include:
- Dizac 1809
- Valium Injectable 2182
- Valium Tablets 2183
- Valrelease Capsules 2169

Droperidol (Possible additive effects of CNS depressants). Products include:
- Inapsine Injection 1296

Enflurane (Possible additive effects of CNS depressants).
- No products indexed under this heading.

Estazolam (Possible additive effects of CNS depressants). Products include:
- ProSom Tablets 449

Ethchlorvynol (Possible additive effects of CNS depressants). Products include:
- Placidyl Capsules 448

Ethinamate (Possible additive effects of CNS depressants).
- No products indexed under this heading.

Fentanyl (Possible additive effects of CNS depressants). Products include:
- Duragesic Transdermal System 1288

Fentanyl Citrate (Possible additive effects of CNS depressants). Products include:
- Sublimaze Injection 1307

Fluphenazine Decanoate (Possible additive effects of CNS depressants). Products include:
- Prolixin Decanoate 509

Fluphenazine Enanthate (Possible additive effects of CNS depressants). Products include:
- Prolixin Enanthate 509

Fluphenazine Hydrochloride (Possible additive effects of CNS depressants). Products include:
- Prolixin 509

Flurazepam Hydrochloride (Possible additive effects of CNS depressants). Products include:
- Dalmane Capsules 2173

Furazolidone (Hypertensive crisis may result). Products include:
- Furoxone 2046

Glutethimide (Possible additive effects of CNS depressants).
- No products indexed under this heading.

Guanadrel Sulfate (Increased effect of hypertensives). Products include:
- Hylorel Tablets 985

Guanethidine Monosulfate (Potential for slight increase in antihypertensive effect). Products include:
- Esimil Tablets 822
- Ismelin Tablets 827

Haloperidol (Possible additive effects of CNS depressants). Products include:
- Haldol Injection, Tablets and Concentrate 1575

Haloperidol Decanoate (Possible additive effects of CNS depressants). Products include:
- Haldol Decanoate 1577

Hydrocodone Bitartrate (Possible additive effects of CNS depressants). Products include:
- Anexsia 5/500 Elixir 1781
- Anexia Tablets 1782
- Codiclear DH Syrup 791
- Deconamine CX Cough and Cold Liquid and Tablets 1319
- Duratuss HD Elixir 2565
- Hycodan Tablets and Syrup 930
- Hycomine Compound Tablets 932
- Hycomine 931
- Hycotuss Expectorant Syrup 933
- Hydrocet Capsules 782
- Lorcet 10/650 1018
- Lortab 2566
- Tussend 1783
- Tussend Expectorant 1785
- Vicodin Tablets 1356
- Vicodin ES Tablets 1357
- Vicodin Tuss Expectorant 1358
- Zydone Capsules 949

Hydrocodone Polistirex (Possible additive effects of CNS depressants). Products include:
- Tussionex Pennkinetic Extended-Release Suspension 998

Hydroxyzine Hydrochloride (Possible additive effects of CNS depressants). Products include:
- Atarax Tablets & Syrup 2185
- Marax Tablets & DF Syrup 2200
- Vistaril Intramuscular Solution 2216

Isocarboxazid (Hypertensive crisis may result; concurrent or sequential use within 14 days is contraindicated).
- No products indexed under this heading.

Isoflurane (Possible additive effects of CNS depressants).
- No products indexed under this heading.

Ketamine Hydrochloride (Possible additive effects of CNS depressants).
- No products indexed under this heading.

Levomethadyl Acetate Hydrochloride (Possible additive effects of CNS depressants). Products include:
- Orlamm 2239

Levorphanol Tartrate (Possible additive effects of CNS depressants). Products include:
- Levo-Dromoran 2129

Lorazepam (Possible additive effects of CNS depressants). Products include:
- Ativan Injection 2698
- Ativan Tablets 2700

Loxapine Hydrochloride (Possible additive effects of CNS depressants). Products include:
- Loxitane 1378

Loxapine Succinate (Possible additive effects of CNS depressants). Products include:
- Loxitane Capsules 1378

Meperidine Hydrochloride (Possible additive effects of CNS depressants). Products include:
- Demerol 2308
- Mepergan Injection 2753

Mephobarbital (Possible additive effects of CNS depressants). Products include:
- Mebaral Tablets 2322

Meprobamate (Possible additive effects of CNS depressants). Products include:
- Miltown Tablets 2672
- PMB 200 and PMB 400 2783

Mesoridazine Besylate (Possible additive effects of CNS depressants). Products include:
- Serentil 684

Methadone Hydrochloride (Possible additive effects of CNS depressants). Products include:
- Methadone Hydrochloride Oral Concentrate 2233
- Methadone Hydrochloride Oral Solution & Tablets 2235

Methohexital Sodium (Possible additive effects of CNS depressants). Products include:
- Brevital Sodium Vials 1429

Methotrimeprazine (Possible additive effects of CNS depressants). Products include:
- Levoprome 1274

Methoxyflurane (Possible additive effects of CNS depressants).
- No products indexed under this heading.

Methyldopa (Potential for slight increase in antihypertensive effect). Products include:
- Aldoclor Tablets 1598
- Aldomet Oral 1600
- Aldoril Tablets 1604

Methyldopate Hydrochloride (Potential for slight increase in antihypertensive effect). Products include:
- Aldomet Ester HCl Injection 1602

Midazolam Hydrochloride (Possible additive effects of CNS depressants). Products include:
- Versed Injection 2170

Molindone Hydrochloride (Possible additive effects of CNS depressants). Products include:
- Moban Tablets and Concentrate 1048

Morphine Sulfate (Possible additive effects of CNS depressants). Products include:
- Astramorph/PF Injection, USP (Preservative-Free) 535
- Duramorph 962
- Infumorph 200 and Infumorph 500 Sterile Solutions 965
- MS Contin Tablets 1994
- MSIR 1997
- Oramorph SR (Morphine Sulfate Sustained Release Tablets) 2236
- RMS Suppositories 2657
- Roxanol 2243

Opium Alkaloids (Possible additive effects of CNS depressants).
- No products indexed under this heading.

(▣ Described in PDR For Nonprescription Drugs) (◉ Described in PDR For Ophthalmology)

829 **Interactions Index** **Pravachol**

Oxazepam (Possible additive effects of CNS depressants). Products include:
- Serax Capsules 2810
- Serax Tablets 2810

Oxycodone Hydrochloride (Possible additive effects of CNS depressants). Products include:
- Percocet Tablets 938
- Percodan Tablets 939
- Percodan-Demi Tablets 940
- Roxicodone Tablets, Oral Solution & Intensol (Oxycodone) 2244
- Tylox Capsules 1584

Pentobarbital Sodium (Possible additive effects of CNS depressants). Products include:
- Nembutal Sodium Capsules 436
- Nembutal Sodium Solution 438
- Nembutal Sodium Suppositories 440

Perphenazine (Possible additive effects of CNS depressants). Products include:
- Etrafon 2355
- Triavil Tablets 1757
- Trilafon 2389

Phenelzine Sulfate (Hypertensive crisis may result; concurrent or sequential use within 14 days is contraindicated). Products include:
- Nardil 1920

Phenobarbital (Possible additive effects of CNS depressants). Products include:
- Arco-Lase Plus Tablets 512
- Bellergal-S Tablets 2250
- Donnatal 2060
- Donnatal Extentabs 2061
- Donnatal Tablets 2060
- Phenobarbital Elixir and Tablets 1469
- Quadrinal Tablets 1350

Prazepam (Possible additive effects of CNS depressants).
- No products indexed under this heading.

Prochlorperazine (Possible additive effects of CNS depressants). Products include:
- Compazine 2470

Promethazine Hydrochloride (Possible additive effects of CNS depressants). Products include:
- Mepergan Injection 2753
- Phenergan with Codeine 2777
- Phenergan with Dextromethorphan 2778
- Phenergan Injection 2773
- Phenergan Suppositories 2775
- Phenergan Syrup 2774
- Phenergan Tablets 2775
- Phenergan VC 2779
- Phenergan VC with Codeine 2781

Propofol (Possible additive effects of CNS depressants). Products include:
- Diprivan Injection 2833

Propoxyphene Hydrochloride (Possible additive effects of CNS depressants). Products include:
- Darvon 1435
- Wygesic Tablets 2827

Propoxyphene Napsylate (Possible additive effects of CNS depressants). Products include:
- Darvon-N/Darvocet-N 1433

Quazepam (Possible additive effects of CNS depressants). Products include:
- Doral Tablets 2664

Rauwolfia Serpentina (Potential for slight increase in antihypertensive effect).
- No products indexed under this heading.

Rescinnamine (Potential for slight increase in antihypertensive effect).
- No products indexed under this heading.

Reserpine (Potential for slight increase in antihypertensive effect). Products include:
- Diupres Tablets 1650
- Hydropres Tablets 1675
- Ser-Ap-Es Tablets 849

Risperidone (Possible additive effects of CNS depressants). Products include:
- Risperdal 1301

Secobarbital Sodium (Possible additive effects of CNS depressants). Products include:
- Seconal Sodium Pulvules 1474

Selegiline Hydrochloride (Hypertensive crisis may result; concurrent or sequential use within 14 days is contraindicated). Products include:
- Eldepryl Tablets 2550

Sufentanil Citrate (Possible additive effects of CNS depressants). Products include:
- Sufenta Injection 1309

Temazepam (Possible additive effects of CNS depressants). Products include:
- Restoril Capsules 2284

Thiamylal Sodium (Possible additive effects of CNS depressants).
- No products indexed under this heading.

Thioridazine Hydrochloride (Possible additive effects of CNS depressants). Products include:
- Mellaril 2269

Thiothixene (Possible additive effects of CNS depressants). Products include:
- Navane Capsules and Concentrate 2201
- Navane Intramuscular 2202

Tranylcypromine Sulfate (Hypertensive crisis may result; concurrent or sequential use within 14 days is contraindicated). Products include:
- Parnate Tablets 2503

Triazolam (Possible additive effects of CNS depressants). Products include:
- Halcion Tablets 2611

Trifluoperazine Hydrochloride (Possible additive effects of CNS depressants). Products include:
- Stelazine 2514

Zolpidem Tartrate (Possible additive effects of CNS depressants). Products include:
- Ambien Tablets 2416

PONSTEL
(Mefenamic Acid) 1925
May interact with oral anticoagulants. Compounds in this category include:

Dicumarol (Prolonged prothrombin time).
- No products indexed under this heading.

Warfarin Sodium (Prolonged prothrombin time). Products include:
- Coumadin 926

PONTOCAINE HYDROCHLORIDE FOR SPINAL ANESTHESIA
(Tetracaine Hydrochloride) 2330
May interact with sulfonamides. Compounds in this category include:

Sulfamethizole (Inhibited sulfonamide action). Products include:
- Urobiotic-250 Capsules 2214

Sulfamethoxazole (Inhibited sulfonamide action). Products include:
- Azo Gantanol Tablets 2080
- Bactrim DS Tablets 2084
- Bactrim I.V. Infusion 2082
- Bactrim 2084
- Gantanol Tablets 2119
- Septra 1174
- Septra I.V. Infusion 1169
- Septra I.V. Infusion ADD-Vantage Vials 1171
- Septra 1174

Sulfasalazine (Inhibited sulfonamide action). Products include:
- Azulfidine 1949

Sulfinpyrazone (Inhibited sulfonamide action). Products include:
- Anturane 807

Sulfisoxazole (Inhibited sulfonamide action). Products include:
- Azo Gantrisin Tablets 2081
- Gantrisin Tablets 2120

Sulfisoxazole Diolamine (Inhibited sulfonamide action).
- No products indexed under this heading.

POTABA
(Aminobenzoate Potassium) 1229
May interact with sulfonamides. Compounds in this category include:

Bendroflumethiazide (Concurrent administration contraindicated).
- No products indexed under this heading.

Chlorothiazide (Concurrent administration contraindicated). Products include:
- Aldoclor Tablets 1598
- Diupres Tablets 1650
- Diuril Oral 1653

Chlorothiazide Sodium (Concurrent administration contraindicated). Products include:
- Diuril Sodium Intravenous 1652

Chlorpropamide (Concurrent administration contraindicated). Products include:
- Diabinese Tablets 1935

Glipizide (Concurrent administration contraindicated). Products include:
- Glucotrol Tablets 1967
- Glucotrol XL Extended Release Tablets 1968

Glyburide (Concurrent administration contraindicated). Products include:
- DiaBeta Tablets 1239
- Glynase PresTab Tablets 2609
- Micronase Tablets 2623

Hydrochlorothiazide (Concurrent administration contraindicated). Products include:
- Aldactazide 2413
- Aldoril Tablets 1604
- Apresazide Capsules 808
- Capozide 742
- Dyazide 2479
- Esidrix Tablets 821
- Esimil Tablets 822
- HydroDIURIL Tablets 1674
- Hydropres Tablets 1675
- Hyzaar Tablets 1677
- Inderide Tablets 2732
- Inderide LA Long Acting Capsules .. 2734
- Lopressor HCT Tablets 832
- Lotensin HCT 837
- Maxzide 1380
- Moduretic Tablets 1705
- Oretic Tablets 443
- Prinzide Tablets 1737
- Ser-Ap-Es Tablets 849
- Timolide Tablets 1748
- Vaseretic Tablets 1765
- Zestoretic 2850
- Ziac 1415

Hydroflumethiazide (Concurrent administration contraindicated). Products include:
- Diucardin Tablets 2718

Methyclothiazide (Concurrent administration contraindicated). Products include:
- Enduron Tablets 420

Polythiazide (Concurrent administration contraindicated). Products include:
- Minizide Capsules 1938

Sulfamethizole (Concurrent administration contraindicated). Products include:
- Urobiotic-250 Capsules 2214

Sulfamethoxazole (Concurrent administration contraindicated). Products include:
- Azo Gantanol Tablets 2080
- Bactrim DS Tablets 2084
- Bactrim I.V. Infusion 2082
- Bactrim 2084
- Gantanol Tablets 2119
- Septra 1174
- Septra I.V. Infusion 1169
- Septra I.V. Infusion ADD-Vantage Vials 1171
- Septra 1174

Sulfasalazine (Concurrent administration contraindicated). Products include:
- Azulfidine 1949

Sulfinpyrazone (Concurrent administration contraindicated). Products include:
- Anturane 807

Sulfisoxazole (Concurrent administration contraindicated). Products include:
- Azo Gantrisin Tablets 2081
- Gantrisin Tablets 2120

Sulfisoxazole Diolamine (Concurrent administration contraindicated).
- No products indexed under this heading.

Tolazamide (Concurrent administration contraindicated).
- No products indexed under this heading.

Tolbutamide (Concurrent administration contraindicated).
- No products indexed under this heading.

PRAMEGEL
(Pramoxine Hydrochloride) 1055
None cited in PDR database.

PRAMOSONE CREAM, LOTION & OINTMENT
(Hydrocortisone Acetate, Pramoxine Hydrochloride) 978
None cited in PDR database.

PRAVACHOL
(Pravastatin Sodium) 765
May interact with immunosuppressive agents, fibrates, oral anticoagulants, and certain other agents. Compounds in these categories include:

Azathioprine (Potential for increased risk of myopathy resulted with immunosuppressive drug cyclosporine). Products include:
- Imuran 1110

Cholestyramine (Decreases mean AUC by 40 to 50%; may be administered 1 hour before or 4 hours after cholestyramine administration). Products include:
- Questran Light 769
- Questran Powder 770

Cimetidine (A significant difference was observed between the AUC's for pravastatin when given with cimetidine compared to when given with antacids). Products include:
- Tagamet Tablets 2516

IMPORTANT NOTE: Always consult each drug listing in the patient's regimen for possible interactions.

Cimetidine Hydrochloride (A significant difference was observed between the AUC's for pravastatin when given with cimetidine compared to when given with antacids). Products include:
- Tagamet ... 2516

Clofibrate (Potential for increased risk of myopathy; combined use should be avoided). Products include:
- Atromid-S Capsules ... 2701

Colestipol Hydrochloride (Decreases mean AUC by 40 to 50%; may be administered 1 hour before colestipol administration). Products include:
- Colestid Tablets ... 2591

Cyclosporine (Potential for increased risk of myopathy; no meaniful elevations in cyclosporine levels; potential for increased pravastatin levels in cardiac transplant patients). Products include:
- Neoral ... 2276
- Sandimmune ... 2286

Dicumarol (Potential for bleeding and prolongation of PT).
- No products indexed under this heading.

Erythromycin (Potential for increased risk of myopathy). Products include:
- A/T/S 2% Acne Topical Gel and Solution ... 1234
- Benzamycin Topical Gel ... 905
- E-Mycin Tablets ... 1341
- Emgel 2% Topical Gel ... 1093
- ERYC ... 1915
- Erycette (erythromycin 2%) Topical Solution ... 1888
- Ery-Tab Tablets ... 422
- Erythromycin Base Filmtab ... 426
- Erythromycin Delayed-Release Capsules, USP ... 427
- Ilotycin Ophthalmic Ointment ... 912
- PCE Dispertab Tablets ... 444
- T-Stat 2.0% Topical Solution and Pads ... 2688
- Theramycin Z Topical Solution 2% ... 1592

Erythromycin Estolate (Potential for increased risk of myopathy). Products include:
- Ilosone ... 911

Erythromycin Ethylsuccinate (Potential for increased risk of myopathy). Products include:
- E.E.S. ... 424
- EryPed ... 421

Erythromycin Gluceptate (Potential for increased risk of myopathy). Products include:
- Ilotycin Gluceptate, IV, Vials ... 913

Erythromycin Stearate (Potential for increased risk of myopathy). Products include:
- Erythrocin Stearate Filmtab ... 425

Gemfibrozil (Potential for increased risk of myopathy; combined use should be avoided). Products include:
- Lopid Tablets ... 1917

Muromonab-CD3 (Potential for increased risk of myopathy resulted with immunosuppressive drug cyclosporin). Products include:
- Orthoclone OKT3 Sterile Solution .. 1837

Mycophenolate Mofetil (Potential for increased risk of myopathy resulted with immunosuppressive drug cyclosporine). Products include:
- CellCept Capsules ... 2099

Nicotinic Acid (Potential for increased risk of myopathy with lipid lowering doses of nicotinic acid).
- No products indexed under this heading.

Tacrolimus (Potential for increased risk of myopathy resulted with immunosuppressive drug cyclosporine). Products include:
- Prograf ... 1042

Warfarin Sodium (Potential for bleeding and prolongation of PT). Products include:
- Coumadin ... 926

PRECARE PRENATAL MULTI-VITAMIN/MINERAL
(Vitamins with Minerals) ... 2568
None cited in PDR database.

PRED FORTE
(Prednisolone Acetate) ... ⊙ 250
None cited in PDR database.

PRED MILD
(Prednisolone Acetate) ... ⊙ 253
None cited in PDR database.

PRED-G LIQUIFILM STERILE OPHTHALMIC SUSPENSION
(Gentamicin Sulfate, Prednisolone Acetate) ... ⊙ 251
None cited in PDR database.

PRED-G S.O.P. STERILE OPHTHALMIC OINTMENT
(Gentamicin Sulfate, Prednisolone Acetate) ... ⊙ 252
None cited in PDR database.

PREGNYL
(Chorionic Gonadotropin) ... 1828
None cited in PDR database.

PRELONE SYRUP
(Prednisolone) ... 1787
May interact with:

Aspirin (Aspirin should be used cautiously in conjunction with corticosteroids in hypoprothrombinemia). Products include:
- Alka-Seltzer Effervescent Antacid and Pain Reliever ... ▣ 701
- Alka-Seltzer Extra Strength Effervescent Antacid and Pain Reliever ... ▣ 703
- Alka-Seltzer Lemon Lime Effervescent Antacid and Pain Reliever ... ▣ 703
- Alka-Seltzer Plus Cold Medicine ... ▣ 705
- Alka-Seltzer Plus Cold & Cough Medicine ... ▣ 708
- Alka-Seltzer Plus Night-Time Cold Medicine ... ▣ 707
- Alka Seltzer Plus Sinus Medicine ... ▣ 707
- Arthritis Foundation Safety Coated Aspirin Tablets ... ▣ 675
- Arthritis Pain Ascriptin ... ▣ 631
- Maximum Strength Ascriptin ... ▣ 630
- Regular Strength Ascriptin Tablets ... ▣ 629
- Arthritis Strength BC Powder ... ▣ 609
- BC Cold Powder Multi-Symptom Formula (Cold-Sinus-Allergy) ... ▣ 609
- BC Cold Powder Non-Drowsy Formula (Cold-Sinus) ... ▣ 609
- BC Powder ... ▣ 609
- Bayer Children's Chewable Aspirin ... ▣ 711
- Genuine Bayer Aspirin Tablets & Caplets ... ▣ 713
- Extra Strength Bayer Arthritis Pain Regimen Formula ... ▣ 711
- Extra Strength Bayer Aspirin Caplets & Tablets ... ▣ 712
- Extended-Release Bayer 8-Hour Aspirin ... ▣ 712
- Extra Strength Bayer Plus Aspirin Caplets ... ▣ 713
- Extra Strength Bayer PM Aspirin .. ▣ 713
- Bayer Enteric Aspirin ... ▣ 709
- Bufferin Analgesic Tablets and Caplets ... ▣ 613
- Arthritis Strength Bufferin Analgesic Caplets ... ▣ 614
- Extra Strength Bufferin Analgesic Tablets ... ▣ 615
- Cama Arthritis Pain Reliever ... ▣ 785
- Darvon Compound-65 Pulvules ... 1435
- Easprin ... 1914
- Ecotrin ... 2455
- Ecotrin Enteric Coated Aspirin Maximum Strength Tablets and Caplets ... ▣ 816
- Ecotrin Enteric Coated Aspirin Regular Strength Tablets ... 2455
- Empirin Aspirin Tablets ... ▣ 854
- Empirin with Codeine Tablets ... 1093
- Excedrin Extra-Strength Analgesic Tablets & Caplets ... 732
- Fiorinal Capsules ... 2261
- Fiorinal with Codeine Capsules ... 2262
- Fiorinal Tablets ... 2261
- Halfprin ... 1362
- Healthprin Aspirin ... 2455
- Norgesic ... 1496
- Percodan Tablets ... 939
- Percodan-Demi Tablets ... 940
- Robaxisal Tablets ... 2071
- Soma Compound w/Codeine Tablets ... 2676
- Soma Compound Tablets ... 2675
- St. Joseph Adult Chewable Aspirin (81 mg.) ... ▣ 808
- Talwin Compound ... 2335
- Ursinus Inlay-Tabs ... ▣ 794
- Vanquish Analgesic Caplets ... ▣ 731

PRELU-2 TIMED RELEASE CAPSULES
(Phendimetrazine Tartrate) ... 681
May interact with monoamine oxidase inhibitors, insulin, and certain other agents. Compounds in these categories include:

Furazolidone (Contraindicated; hypertensive crises may result). Products include:
- Furoxone ... 2046

Guanethidine Monosulfate (Decreased hypotensive effect). Products include:
- Esimil Tablets ... 822
- Ismelin Tablets ... 827

Insulin, Human (Altered insulin requirements).
- No products indexed under this heading.

Insulin, Human Isophane Suspension (Altered insulin requirements). Products include:
- Novolin N Human Insulin 10 ml Vials ... 1795

Insulin, Human NPH (Altered insulin requirements). Products include:
- Humulin N, 100 Units ... 1448
- Novolin N PenFill Cartridges Durable Insulin Delivery System ... 1798
- Novolin N Prefilled Syringe Disposable Insulin Delivery System ... 1798

Insulin, Human Regular (Altered insulin requirements). Products include:
- Humulin R, 100 Units ... 1449
- Novolin R Human Insulin 10 ml Vials ... 1795
- Novolin R PenFill Cartridges Durable Insulin Delivery System ... 1798
- Novolin R Prefilled Syringe Disposable Insulin Delivery System ... 1798
- Velosulin BR Human Insulin 10 ml Vials ... 1795

Insulin, Human, Zinc Suspension (Altered insulin requirements). Products include:
- Humulin L, 100 Units ... 1446
- Humulin U, 100 Units ... 1450
- Novolin L Human Insulin 10 ml Vials ... 1795

Insulin, NPH (Altered insulin requirements). Products include:
- NPH, 100 Units ... 1450
- Pork NPH, 100 Units ... 1452
- Purified Pork NPH Isophane Insulin ... 1801

Insulin, Regular (Altered insulin requirements). Products include:
- Regular, 100 Units ... 1450
- Pork Regular, 100 Units ... 1452
- Pork Regular (Concentrated), 500 Units ... 1453
- Purified Pork Regular Insulin ... 1801

Insulin, Zinc Crystals (Altered insulin requirements). Products include:
- NPH, 100 Units ... 1450

Insulin, Zinc Suspension (Altered insulin requirements). Products include:
- Iletin I ... 1450
- Lente, 100 Units ... 1450
- Iletin II ... 1452
- Pork Lente, 100 Units ... 1452
- Purified Pork Lente Insulin ... 1801

Isocarboxazid (Contraindicated; hypertensive crises may result).
- No products indexed under this heading.

Phenelzine Sulfate (Contraindicated; hypertensive crises may result). Products include:
- Nardil ... 1920

Selegiline Hydrochloride (Contraindicated); hypertensive crises may result). Products include:
- Eldepryl Tablets ... 2550

Tranylcypromine Sulfate (Contraindicated; hypertensive crises may result). Products include:
- Parnate Tablets ... 2503

PREMARIN INTRAVENOUS
(Estrogens, Conjugated) ... 2787
None cited in PDR database.

PREMARIN WITH METHYLTESTOSTERONE
(Estrogens, Conjugated, Methyltestosterone) ... 2794
May interact with oral anticoagulants, insulin, progestins, and certain other agents. Compounds in these categories include:

Desogestrel (Adverse effects on carbohydrate and lipid metabolism). Products include:
- Desogen Tablets ... 1817
- Ortho-Cept ... 1851

Dicumarol (Decreased anticoagulant requirements).
- No products indexed under this heading.

Insulin, Human (Decreased blood glucose and insulin requirements).
- No products indexed under this heading.

Insulin, Human Isophane Suspension (Decreased blood glucose and insulin requirements). Products include:
- Novolin N Human Insulin 10 ml Vials ... 1795

Insulin, Human NPH (Decreased blood glucose and insulin requirements). Products include:
- Humulin N, 100 Units ... 1448
- Novolin N PenFill Cartridges Durable Insulin Delivery System ... 1798
- Novolin N Prefilled Syringe Disposable Insulin Delivery System ... 1798

Insulin, Human Regular (Decreased blood glucose and insulin requirements). Products include:
- Humulin R, 100 Units ... 1449
- Novolin R Human Insulin 10 ml Vials ... 1795
- Novolin R PenFill Cartridges Durable Insulin Delivery System ... 1798
- Novolin R Prefilled Syringe Disposable Insulin Delivery System ... 1798
- Velosulin BR Human Insulin 10 ml Vials ... 1795

Insulin, Human, Zinc Suspension (Decreased blood glucose and insulin requirements). Products include:
- Humulin L, 100 Units ... 1446
- Humulin U, 100 Units ... 1450

(▣ Described in PDR For Nonprescription Drugs) (⊙ Described in PDR For Ophthalmology)

Novolin L Human Insulin 10 ml Vials 1795

Insulin, NPH (Decreased blood glucose and insulin requirements). Products include:

NPH, 100 Units 1450
Pork NPH, 100 Units 1452
Purified Pork NPH Isophane Insulin 1801

Insulin, Regular (Decreased blood glucose and insulin requirements). Products include:

Regular, 100 Units 1450
Pork Regular, 100 Units 1452
Pork Regular (Concentrated), 500 Units 1453
Purified Pork Regular Insulin 1801

Insulin, Zinc Crystals (Decreased blood glucose and insulin requirements). Products include:

NPH, 100 Units 1450

Insulin, Zinc Suspension (Decreased blood glucose and insulin requirements). Products include:

Iletin I 1450
Lente, 100 Units 1450
Iletin II 1452
Pork Lente, 100 Units 1452
Purified Pork Lente Insulin 1801

Medroxyprogesterone Acetate (Adverse effects on carbohydrate and lipid metabolism). Products include:

Amen Tablets 780
Cycrin Tablets 975
Depo-Provera Contraceptive Injection 2602
Depo-Provera Sterile Aqueous Suspension 2606
Premphase 2797
Prempro 2801
Provera Tablets 2636

Megestrol Acetate (Adverse effects on carbohydrate and lipid metabolism). Products include:

Megace Oral Suspension 699
Megace Tablets 701

Norgestimate (Adverse effects on carbohydrate and lipid metabolism). Products include:

Ortho-Cyclen/Ortho-Tri-Cyclen 1858
Ortho-Cyclen/Ortho Tri-Cyclen 1858

Oxyphenbutazone (Elevated serum levels of oxyphenbutazone).

Warfarin Sodium (Decreased anticoagulant requirements). Products include:

Coumadin 926

PREMARIN TABLETS

(Estrogens, Conjugated) **2789**
May interact with progestins. Compounds in this category include:

Desogestrel (Potential adverse effects on carbohydrate and lipid metabolism). Products include:

Desogen Tablets 1817
Ortho-Cept 1851

Medroxyprogesterone Acetate (Potential adverse effects on carbohydrate and lipid metabolism). Products include:

Amen Tablets 780
Cycrin Tablets 975
Depo-Provera Contraceptive Injection 2602
Depo-Provera Sterile Aqueous Suspension 2606
Premphase 2797
Prempro 2801
Provera Tablets 2636

Megestrol Acetate (Potential adverse effects on carbohydrate and lipid metabolism). Products include:

Megace Oral Suspension 699
Megace Tablets 701

Norgestimate (Potential adverse effects on carbohydrate and lipid metabolism). Products include:

Ortho-Cyclen/Ortho-Tri-Cyclen 1858
Ortho-Cyclen/Ortho Tri-Cyclen 1858

PREMARIN VAGINAL CREAM

(Estrogens, Conjugated) **2791**
May interact with progestins. Compounds in this category include:

Desogestrel (Potential adverse effects on carbohydrate and lipid metabolism). Products include:

Desogen Tablets 1817
Ortho-Cept 1851

Medroxyprogesterone Acetate (Potential adverse effects on carbohydrate and lipid metabolism). Products include:

Amen Tablets 780
Cycrin Tablets 975
Depo-Provera Contraceptive Injection 2602
Depo-Provera Sterile Aqueous Suspension 2606
Premphase 2797
Prempro 2801
Provera Tablets 2636

Megestrol Acetate (Potential adverse effects on carbohydrate and lipid metabolism). Products include:

Megace Oral Suspension 699
Megace Tablets 701

Norgestimate (Potential adverse effects on carbohydrate and lipid metabolism). Products include:

Ortho-Cyclen/Ortho-Tri-Cyclen 1858
Ortho-Cyclen/Ortho Tri-Cyclen 1858

PREMPHASE

(Estrogens, Conjugated, Medroxyprogesterone Acetate) **2797**
May interact with:

Aminoglutethimide (Aminoglutethimide administered concomitantly with medroxyprogesterone acetate (MPA) may significantly depress the bioavailability of MPA). Products include:

Cytadren Tablets 819

Food Interactions

Food, unspecified (Administration with food approximately doubles MPA C_{max} and increases MPA AUC by approximately 30%).

PREMPRO

(Estrogens, Conjugated, Medroxyprogesterone Acetate) **2801**
May interact with:

Aminoglutethimide (Aminoglutethimide administered concomitantly with medroxyprogesterone acetate (MPA) may significantly depress the bioavailability of MPA). Products include:

Cytadren Tablets 819

Food Interactions

Food, unspecified (Administration with food approximately doubles MPA C_{max} and increases MPA AUC by approximately 30%).

SYNTHROID INJECTION

(Levothyroxine Sodium) **1359**
See **Synthroid Tablets**

PREPARATION H HEMORRHOIDAL CREAM

(Glycerin, Petrolatum, Phenylephrine Hydrochloride, Shark Liver Oil) **871**
None cited in PDR database.

PREPARATION H HEMORRHOIDAL OINTMENT

(Mineral Oil, Petrolatum, Phenylephrine Hydrochloride, Shark Liver Oil) **871**
None cited in PDR database.

PREPARATION H HEMORRHOIDAL SUPPOSITORIES

(Yeast Cell Derivative, Live) **871**
None cited in PDR database.

PREPARATION H HYDROCORTISONE 1% CREAM

(Hydrocortisone) **872**
None cited in PDR database.

PREPIDIL GEL

(Dinoprostone) **2633**
May interact with oxytocic drugs. Compounds in this category include:

Ergonovine Maleate (Prepidil may augment the activity of other oxytocic drugs; co-administration is not recommended).

No products indexed under this heading.

Methylergonovine Maleate (Prepidil may augment the activity of other oxytocic drugs; co-administration is not recommended). Products include:

Methergine 2272

Oxytocin (Injection) (Prepidil may augment the activity of other oxytocic drugs; co-administration is not recommended).

PREVACID DELAYED-RELEASE CAPSULES

(Lansoprazole) **2562**
May interact with absorption of drugs where gastric ph is an important determinant in their bioavailability, xanthine bronchodilators, and certain other agents. Compounds in these categories include:

Aminophylline (Co-administration has resulted in a minor increase (10%) in the clearance of theophylline; this interaction is unlikely to be of clinical concern, nonetheless monitor blood levels).

No products indexed under this heading.

Bacampicillin Hydrochloride (Lansoprazole causes a profound and long lasting inhibition of gastric acid secretion; therefore, it is theoretically possible that it may interfere with the oral absorption of drugs where gastric pH is an important determinant of bioavailability). Products include:

Spectrobid Tablets 2206

Digoxin (Lansoprazole causes a profound and long lasting inhibition of gastric acid secretion; therefore, it is theoretically possible that it may interfere with the oral absorption of drugs where gastric pH is an important determinant of bioavailability, such as digoxin). Products include:

Lanoxicaps 1117
Lanoxin Elixir Pediatric 1120
Lanoxin Injection 1123
Lanoxin Injection Pediatric 1126
Lanoxin Tablets 1128

Dyphylline (Co-administration has resulted in a minor increase (10%) in the clearance of theophylline; this interaction is unlikely to be of clinical concern, nonetheless monitor blood levels). Products include:

Lufyllin & Lufyllin-400 Tablets 2670
Lufyllin-GG Elixir & Tablets 2671

Ferrous Fumarate (Lansoprazole causes a profound and long lasting inhibition of gastric acid secretion; therefore, it is theoretically possible that it may interfere with the oral absorption of drugs where gastric pH is an important determinant of bioavailability). Products include:

Chromagen Capsules 2339
Ferro-Sequels 669
Nephro-Fer Tablets 2004
Nephro-Fer Rx Tablets 2005
Nephro-Vite + Fe Tablets 2006
Sigtab-M Tablets 772
Stresstabs + Iron 671
The Stuart Formula Tablets 663
Theragran-M Tablets with Beta Carotene 623
Trinsicon Capsules 2570
Vitron-C Tablets 650

Ferrous Gluconate (Lansoprazole causes a profound and long lasting inhibition of gastric acid secretion; therefore, it is theoretically possible that it may interfere with the oral absorption of drugs where gastric pH is an important determinant of bioavailability). Products include:

Fergon Iron Supplement Tablets 721
Megadose 512

Ferrous Sulfate (Lansoprazole causes a profound and long lasting inhibition of gastric acid secretion; therefore, it is theoretically possible that it may interfere with the oral absorption of drugs where gastric pH is an important determinant of bioavailability). Products include:

Feosol Capsules 2456
Feosol Elixir 2456
Feosol Tablets 2457
Fero-Folic-500 Filmtab 429
Fero-Grad-500 Filmtab 429
Fero-Gradumet Filmtab 429
Iberet Tablets 433
Iberet-500 Liquid 433
Iberet-Folic-500 Filmtab 429
Iberet-Liquid 433
Irospan 982
Slow Fe Tablets 869
Slow Fe with Folic Acid 869

Ketoconazole (Lansoprazole causes a profound and long lasting inhibition of gastric acid secretion; therefore, it is theoretically possible that it may interfere with the oral absorption of drugs where gastric pH is an important determinant of bioavailability). Products include:

Nizoral 2% Cream 1297
Nizoral 2% Shampoo 1298
Nizoral Tablets 1298

Sucralfate (Co-administration delays absorption and reduces bioavailability of lansoprazole by about 30%, therefore lansoprazole should be taken at least 30 minutes prior to sucralfate). Products include:

Carafate Suspension 1505
Carafate Tablets 1504

Theophylline (Co-administration has resulted in a minor increase (10%) in the clearance of theophylline; this interaction is unlikely to be of clinical concern, nonetheless monitor blood levels). Products include:

Marax Tablets & DF Syrup 2200
Quibron 2053

Theophylline Anhydrous (Co-administration has resulted in a minor increase (10%) in the clearance of theophylline; this interaction is unlikely to be of clinical concern, nonetheless monitor blood levels). Products include:

Aerolate 1004
Primatene Dual Action Formula 872
Primatene Tablets 873
Respbid Tablets 682
Slo-bid Gyrocaps 2033
Theo-24 Extended Release Capsules 2568

IMPORTANT NOTE: Always consult each drug listing in the patient's regimen for possible interactions.

Theo-Dur Extended-Release Tablets ... 1327
Theo-X Extended-Release Tablets ... 788
Uni-Dur Extended-Release Tablets ... 1331
Uniphyl 400 mg Tablets ... 2001

Theophylline Calcium Salicylate (Co-administration has resulted in a minor increase (10%) in the clearance of theophylline; this interaction is unlikely to be of clinical concern, nonetheless monitor blood levels). Products include:

Quadrinal Tablets ... 1350

Theophylline Sodium Glycinate (Co-administration has resulted in a minor increase (10%) in the clearance of theophylline; this interaction is unlikely to be of clinical concern, nonetheless monitor blood levels).

No products indexed under this heading.

Food Interactions

Food, unspecified (Cmax and AUC are diminished by about 50% if the drug is given 30 minutes after food as opposed to the fasting condition).

PRILOSEC DELAYED-RELEASE CAPSULES

(Omeprazole) ... 529

May interact with absorption of drugs where gastric ph is an important determinant in their bioavailability, benzodiazepines, and certain other agents. Compounds in these categories include:

Alprazolam (Potential for metabolism interaction via cytochrome P-450 system). Products include:

Xanax Tablets ... 2649

Bacampicillin Hydrochloride (Omeprazole may interfere with the gastric absorption). Products include:

Spectrobid Tablets ... 2206

Chlordiazepoxide (Potential for metabolism interaction via cytochrome P-450 system). Products include:

Libritabs Tablets ... 2177
Limbitrol ... 2180

Chlordiazepoxide Hydrochloride (Potential for metabolism interaction via cytochrome P-450 system). Products include:

Librax Capsules ... 2176
Librium Capsules ... 2178
Librium Injectable ... 2179

Clorazepate Dipotassium (Potential for metabolism interaction via cytochrome P-450 system). Products include:

Tranxene ... 451

Cyclosporine (Potential of metabolism interaction via the cytochrome P-450 system). Products include:

Neoral ... 2276
Sandimmune ... 2286

Diazepam (Potential for metabolism interaction via cytochrome P-450 system; prolonged elimination of diazepam). Products include:

Dizac ... 1809
Valium Injectable ... 2182
Valium Tablets ... 2183
Valrelease Capsules ... 2169

Disulfiram (Potential of metabolism interaction via the cytochrome P-450 system). Products include:

Antabuse Tablets ... 2695

Drugs which undergo biotransformation by cytochrome P-450 mixed function oxidase (Potential of metabolism interaction via the cytochrome P-450 system).

Estazolam (Potential for metabolism interaction via cytochrome P-450 system). Products include:

ProSom Tablets ... 449

Ferrous Fumarate (Omeprazole may interfere with the gastric absorption). Products include:

Chromagen Capsules ... 2339
Ferro-Sequels ... ■ 669
Nephro-Fer Tablets ... 2004
Nephro-Fer Rx Tablets ... 2005
Nephro-Vite + Fe Tablets ... 2006
Sigtab-M Tablets ... ■ 772
Stresstabs + Iron ... ■ 671
The Stuart Formula Tablets ... ■ 663
Theragran-M Tablets with Beta Carotene ... ■ 623
Trinsicon Capsules ... 2570
Vitron-C Tablets ... ■ 650

Ferrous Gluconate (Omeprazole may interfere with the gastric absorption). Products include:

Fergon Iron Supplement Tablets ... ■ 721
Megadose ... 512

Ferrous Sulfate (Omeprazole may interfere with the gastric absorption). Products include:

Feosol Capsules ... 2456
Feosol Elixir ... 2456
Feosol Tablets ... 2457
Fero-Folic-500 Filmtab ... 429
Fero-Grad-500 Filmtab ... 429
Fero-Gradumet Filmtab ... 429
Iberet Tablets ... 433
Iberet-500 Liquid ... 433
Iberet-Folic-500 Filmtab ... 429
Iberet-Liquid ... 433
Irospan ... 982
Slow Fe Tablets ... 869
Slow Fe with Folic Acid ... 869

Flurazepam Hydrochloride (Potential for metabolism interaction via cytochrome P-450 system). Products include:

Dalmane Capsules ... 2173

Halazepam (Potential for metabolism interaction via cytochrome P-450 system).

No products indexed under this heading.

Ketoconazole (Omeprazole may interfere with the gastric absorption). Products include:

Nizoral 2% Cream ... 1297
Nizoral 2% Shampoo ... 1298
Nizoral Tablets ... 1298

Lorazepam (Potential for metabolism interaction via cytochrome P-450 system). Products include:

Ativan Injection ... 2698
Ativan Tablets ... 2700

Midazolam Hydrochloride (Potential for metabolism interaction via cytochrome P-450 system). Products include:

Versed Injection ... 2170

Oxazepam (Potential for metabolism interaction via cytochrome P-450 system). Products include:

Serax Capsules ... 2810
Serax Tablets ... 2810

Phenytoin (Prolonged elimination of phenytoin). Products include:

Dilantin Infatabs ... 1908
Dilantin-125 Suspension ... 1911

Phenytoin Sodium (Prolonged elimination of phenytoin). Products include:

Dilantin Kapseals ... 1906
Dilantin Parenteral ... 1910

Prazepam (Potential for metabolism interaction via cytochrome P-450 system).

No products indexed under this heading.

Quazepam (Potential for metabolism interaction via cytochrome P-450 system). Products include:

Doral Tablets ... 2664

Temazepam (Potential for metabolism interaction via cytochrome P-450 system). Products include:

Restoril Capsules ... 2284

Triazolam (Potential for metabolism interaction via cytochrome P-450 system). Products include:

Halcion Tablets ... 2611

Warfarin Sodium (Prolonged elimination of warfarin). Products include:

Coumadin ... 926

PRIMACOR INJECTION

(Milrinone Lactate) ... 2331

May interact with:

Furosemide (Immediate chemical interaction which is evidenced by the formation of a precipitate when furosemide is injected into IV line of an infusion of Primacor). Products include:

Lasix Injection, Oral Solution and Tablets ... 1240

PRIMATENE DUAL ACTION FORMULA

(Ephedrine Hydrochloride, Guaifenesin, Theophylline Anhydrous) ... ■ 872

May interact with monoamine oxidase inhibitors. Compounds in this category include:

Furazolidone (Concurrent and/or sequential use is not recommended). Products include:

Furoxone ... 2046

Isocarboxazid (Concurrent and/or sequential use is not recommended).

No products indexed under this heading.

Phenelzine Sulfate (Concurrent and/or sequential use is not recommended). Products include:

Nardil ... 1920

Selegiline Hydrochloride (Concurrent and/or sequential use is not recommended). Products include:

Eldepryl Tablets ... 2550

Tranylcypromine Sulfate (Concurrent and/or sequential use is not recommended). Products include:

Parnate Tablets ... 2503

PRIMATENE MIST

(Epinephrine) ... ■ 873

May interact with monoamine oxidase inhibitors. Compounds in this category include:

Furazolidone (Concurrent and/or sequential use is not recommended). Products include:

Furoxone ... 2046

Isocarboxazid (Concurrent and/or sequential use is not recommended).

No products indexed under this heading.

Phenelzine Sulfate (Concurrent and/or sequential use is not recommended). Products include:

Nardil ... 1920

Selegiline Hydrochloride (Concurrent and/or sequential use is not recommended). Products include:

Eldepryl Tablets ... 2550

Tranylcypromine Sulfate (Concurrent and/or sequential use is not recommended). Products include:

Parnate Tablets ... 2503

PRIMATENE TABLETS

(Theophylline Anhydrous, Ephedrine Hydrochloride) ... ■ 873

May interact with monoamine oxidase inhibitors. Compounds in this category include:

Furazolidone (Concurrent and/or sequential use is not recommended). Products include:

Furoxone ... 2046

Isocarboxazid (Concurrent and/or sequential use is not recommended).

No products indexed under this heading.

Phenelzine Sulfate (Concurrent and/or sequential use is not recommended). Products include:

Nardil ... 1920

Selegiline Hydrochloride (Concurrent and/or sequential use is not recommended). Products include:

Eldepryl Tablets ... 2550

Tranylcypromine Sulfate (Concurrent and/or sequential use is not recommended). Products include:

Parnate Tablets ... 2503

PRIMAXIN I.M.

(Imipenem-Cilastatin Sodium) ... 1727

May interact with:

Probenecid (Concomitant administration results in only minimal increase in plasma levels of imipenem). Products include:

Benemid Tablets ... 1611
ColBENEMID Tablets ... 1622

PRIMAXIN I.V.

(Imipenem-Cilastatin Sodium) ... 1729

May interact with:

Ganciclovir Sodium (Concomitant administration may result in generalized seizures). Products include:

Cytovene-IV ... 2103

Probenecid (Concomitant administration results in only minimal increase in plasma levels of imipenem; concomitant administration not recommended). Products include:

Benemid Tablets ... 1611
ColBENEMID Tablets ... 1622

PRINIVIL TABLETS

(Lisinopril) ... 1733

May interact with diuretics, potassium sparing diuretics, potassium preparations, thiazides, lithium preparations, and certain other agents. Compounds in these categories include:

Amiloride Hydrochloride (Potential for significant hyperkalemia; possibility of excessive reduction in blood pressure). Products include:

Midamor Tablets ... 1703
Moduretic Tablets ... 1705

Bendroflumethiazide (Thiazide-induced potassium loss attenuated; possibility of excessive reduction in blood pressure).

No products indexed under this heading.

Bumetanide (Possibility of excessive reduction in blood pressure). Products include:

Bumex ... 2093

Chlorothiazide (Thiazide-induced potassium loss attenuated; possibility of excessive reduction in blood pressure). Products include:

Aldoclor Tablets ... 1598
Diupres Tablets ... 1650
Diuril Oral ... 1653

Chlorothiazide Sodium (Thiazide-induced potassium loss attenuated; possibility of excessive reduction in blood pressure). Products include:

Diuril Sodium Intravenous ... 1652

Chlorthalidone (Possibility of excessive reduction in blood pressure). Products include:

Combipres Tablets ... 677
Tenoretic Tablets ... 2845
Thalitone ... 1245

Ethacrynic Acid (Possibility of excessive reduction in blood pressure). Products include:

Edecrin Tablets ... 1657

Furosemide (Possibility of excessive reduction in blood pressure). Products include:

Lasix Injection, Oral Solution and Tablets ... 1240

Hydrochlorothiazide (Thiazide-induced potassium loss attenuated; possibility of excessive reduction in blood pressure). Products include:

Aldactazide ... 2413
Aldoril Tablets ... 1604
Apresazide Capsules ... 808
Capozide ... 742
Dyazide ... 2479
Esidrix Tablets ... 821
Esimil Tablets ... 822
HydroDIURIL Tablets ... 1674
Hydropres Tablets ... 1675
Hyzaar Tablets ... 1677
Inderide Tablets ... 2732
Inderide LA Long Acting Capsules .. 2734
Lopressor HCT Tablets ... 832
Lotensin HCT ... 837
Maxzide ... 1380
Moduretic Tablets ... 1705
Oretic Tablets ... 443
Prinzide Tablets ... 1737
Ser-Ap-Es Tablets ... 849
Timolide Tablets ... 1748
Vaseretic Tablets ... 1765
Zestoretic ... 2850
Ziac ... 1415

Hydroflumethiazide (Thiazide-induced potassium loss attenuated; possibility of excessive reduction in blood pressure). Products include:

Diucardin Tablets ... 2718

Indapamide (Possibility of excessive reduction in blood pressure). Products include:

Lozol Tablets ... 2022

Indomethacin (Reduces antihypertensive effect). Products include:

Indocin ... 1680

Indomethacin Sodium Trihydrate (Reduces antihypertensive effect). Products include:

Indocin I.V. ... 1684

Lithium Carbonate (Potential for reversible lithium toxicity; frequent monitoring of lithium levels is recommended). Products include:

Eskalith ... 2485
Lithium Carbonate Capsules & Tablets ... 2230
Lithonate/Lithotabs/Lithobid ... 2543

Lithium Citrate (Potential for reversible lithium toxicity; frequent monitoring of lithium levels is recommended).

No products indexed under this heading.

Methyclothiazide (Thiazide-induced potassium loss attenuated; possibility of excessive reduction in blood pressure). Products include:

Enduron Tablets ... 420

Metolazone (Possibility of excessive reduction in blood pressure). Products include:

Mykrox Tablets ... 993
Zaroxolyn Tablets ... 1000

Polythiazide (Thiazide-induced potassium loss attenuated; possibility of excessive reduction in blood pressure). Products include:

Minizide Capsules ... 1938

Potassium Acid Phosphate (Potential for significant hyperkalemia). Products include:

K-Phos Original Formula 'Sodium Free' Tablets ... 639

Potassium Bicarbonate (Potential for significant hyperkalemia). Products include:

Alka-Seltzer Gold Effervescent Antacid ... ▣ 703

Potassium Chloride (Potential for significant hyperkalemia). Products include:

Chlor-3 Condiment ... 1004
K-Dur Microburst Release System (potassium chloride, USP) E.R. Tablets ... 1325
K-Lor Powder Packets ... 434
K-Norm Extended-Release Capsules ... 991
K-Tab Filmtab ... 434
Kolyum Liquid ... 992
Micro-K ... 2063
Micro-K LS Packets ... 2064
NuLYTELY ... 689
Cherry Flavor NuLYTELY ... 689
Rum-K Syrup ... 1005
Slow-K Extended-Release Tablets ... 851

Potassium Citrate (Potential for significant hyperkalemia). Products include:

Polycitra Syrup ... 578
Polycitra-K Crystals ... 579
Polycitra-K Oral Solution ... 579
Polycitra-LC ... 578

Potassium Gluconate (Potential for significant hyperkalemia). Products include:

Kolyum Liquid ... 992

Potassium Phosphate, Dibasic (Potential for significant hyperkalemia).

No products indexed under this heading.

Potassium Phosphate, Monobasic (Potential for significant hyperkalemia). Products include:

K-Phos Neutral Tablets ... 639
K-Phos Original Formula 'Sodium Free' Tablets ... 639

Spironolactone (Potential for significant hyperkalemia; possibility of excessive reduction in blood pressure). Products include:

Aldactazide ... 2413
Aldactone ... 2414

Torsemide (Possibility of excessive reduction in blood pressure). Products include:

Demadex Tablets and Injection ... 686

Triamterene (Potential for significant hyperkalemia; possibility of excessive reduction in blood pressure). Products include:

Dyazide ... 2479
Dyrenium Capsules ... 2481
Maxzide ... 1380

PRINZIDE TABLETS

(Lisinopril, Hydrochlorothiazide) ... 1737

May interact with barbiturates, narcotic analgesics, potassium sparing diuretics, potassium preparations, antihypertensives, corticosteroids, lithium preparations, non-steroidal anti-inflammatory agents, diuretics, insulin, oral hypoglycemic agents, nondepolarizing neuromuscular blocking agents, bile acid sequestering agents, and certain other agents. Compounds in these categories include:

Acarbose (Dosage adjustment of the antidiabetic drug may be required).

No products indexed under this heading.

Acebutolol Hydrochloride (Additive effect or potentiation). Products include:

Sectral Capsules ... 2807

ACTH (Intensified electrolyte depletion, particularly hypokalemia).

No products indexed under this heading.

Alfentanil Hydrochloride (Potentiates orthostatic hypotension). Products include:

Alfenta Injection ... 1286

Amiloride Hydrochloride (Concomitant therapy may lead to hyperkalemia). Products include:

Midamor Tablets ... 1703
Moduretic Tablets ... 1705

Amlodipine Besylate (Additive effect or potentiation). Products include:

Lotrel Capsules ... 840
Norvasc Tablets ... 1940

Aprobarbital (Potentiates orthostatic hypotension).

No products indexed under this heading.

Atenolol (Additive effect or potentiation). Products include:

Tenoretic Tablets ... 2845
Tenormin Tablets and I.V. Injection 2847

Atracurium Besylate (Possible increased responsiveness to the muscle relaxant). Products include:

Tracrium Injection ... 1183

Benazepril Hydrochloride (Additive effect or potentiation). Products include:

Lotensin Tablets ... 834
Lotensin HCT ... 837
Lotrel Capsules ... 840

Bendroflumethiazide (Additive effect or potentiation).

No products indexed under this heading.

Betamethasone Acetate (Intensified electrolyte depletion, particularly hypokalemia). Products include:

Celestone Soluspan Suspension ... 2347

Betamethasone Sodium Phosphate (Intensified electrolyte depletion, particularly hypokalemia). Products include:

Celestone Soluspan Suspension ... 2347

Betaxolol Hydrochloride (Additive effect or potentiation). Products include:

Betoptic Ophthalmic Solution ... 469
Betoptic S Ophthalmic Suspension ... 471
Kerlone Tablets ... 2436

Bisoprolol Fumarate (Additive effect or potentiation). Products include:

Zebeta Tablets ... 1413
Ziac ... 1415

Buprenorphine (Potentiates orthostatic hypotension). Products include:

Buprenex Injectable ... 2006

Butabarbital (Potentiates orthostatic hypotension).

No products indexed under this heading.

Butalbital (Potentiates orthostatic hypotension). Products include:

Esgic-plus Tablets ... 1013
Fioricet Tablets ... 2258
Fioricet with Codeine Capsules ... 2260
Fiorinal Capsules ... 2261
Fiorinal with Codeine Capsules ... 2262
Fiorinal Tablets ... 2261
Phrenilin ... 785
Sedapap Tablets 50 mg/650 mg .. 1543

Captopril (Additive effect or potentiation). Products include:

Capoten ... 739
Capozide ... 742

Carteolol Hydrochloride (Additive effect or potentiation). Products include:

Cartrol Tablets ... 410
Ocupress Ophthalmic Solution, 1% Sterile ... ⊚ 309

Chlorothiazide (Additive effect or potentiation). Products include:

Aldoclor Tablets ... 1598
Diupres Tablets ... 1650
Diuril Oral ... 1653

Chlorothiazide Sodium (Additive effect or potentiation). Products include:

Diuril Sodium Intravenous ... 1652

Chlorpropamide (Dosage adjustment of the antidiabetic drug may be required). Products include:

Diabinese Tablets ... 1935

Chlorthalidone (Additive effect or potentiation). Products include:

Combipres Tablets ... 677
Tenoretic Tablets ... 2845
Thalitone ... 1245

Cholestyramine (Binds the hydrochlorothiazide and reduces its absorption by 85% from the gastrointestinal tract). Products include:

Questran Light ... 769
Questran Powder ... 770

Clonidine (Additive effect or potentiation). Products include:

Catapres-TTS ... 675

Clonidine Hydrochloride (Additive effect or potentiation). Products include:

Catapres Tablets ... 674
Combipres Tablets ... 677

Codeine Phosphate (Potentiates orthostatic hypotension). Products include:

Actifed with Codeine Cough Syrup.. 1067
Brontex ... 1981
Deconsal C Expectorant Syrup ... 456
Deconsal Pediatric Syrup ... 457
Dimetane-DC Cough Syrup ... 2059
Empirin with Codeine Tablets ... 1093
Fioricet with Codeine Capsules ... 2260
Fiorinal with Codeine Capsules ... 2262
Isoclor Expectorant ... 990
Novahistine DH ... 2462
Novahistine Expectorant ... 2463
Nucofed ... 2051
Phenergan with Codeine ... 2777
Phenergan VC with Codeine ... 2781
Robitussin A-C Syrup ... 2073
Robitussin-DAC Syrup ... 2074
Ryna ... ▣ 841
Soma Compound w/Codeine Tablets ... 2676
Tussi-Organidin NR Liquid and S NR Liquid ... 2677
Tylenol with Codeine ... 1583

Colestipol Hydrochloride (Binds the hydrochlorothiazide and reduces its absorption by 43% from the gastrointestinal tract). Products include:

Colestid Tablets ... 2591

Cortisone Acetate (Intensified electrolyte depletion, particularly hypokalemia). Products include:

Cortone Acetate Sterile Suspension ... 1623
Cortone Acetate Tablets ... 1624

Deserpidine (Additive effect or potentiation).

No products indexed under this heading.

Dexamethasone (Intensified electrolyte depletion, particularly hypokalemia). Products include:

AK-Trol Ointment & Suspension ... ⊚ 205
Decadron Elixir ... 1633
Decadron Tablets ... 1635
Decaspray Topical Aerosol ... 1648
Dexacidin Ointment ... ⊚ 263
Maxitrol Ophthalmic Ointment and Suspension ... ⊚ 224
TobraDex Ophthalmic Suspension and Ointment ... 473

Dexamethasone Acetate (Intensified electrolyte depletion, particularly hypokalemia). Products include:

Dalalone D.P. Injectable ... 1011
Decadron-LA Sterile Suspension ... 1646

IMPORTANT NOTE: Always consult each drug listing in the patient's regimen for possible interactions.

Dexamethasone Sodium Phosphate (Intensified electrolyte depletion, particularly hypokalemia). Products include:

- Decadron Phosphate Injection 1637
- Decadron Phosphate Respihaler 1642
- Decadron Phosphate Sterile Ophthalmic Ointment 1641
- Decadron Phosphate Sterile Ophthalmic Solution 1642
- Decadron Phosphate Topical Cream 1644
- Decadron Phosphate Turbinaire 1645
- Decadron Phosphate with Xylocaine Injection, Sterile 1639
- Dexacort Phosphate in Respihaler .. 458
- Dexacort Phosphate in Turbinaire .. 459
- NeoDecadron Sterile Ophthalmic Ointment 1712
- NeoDecadron Sterile Ophthalmic Solution 1713
- NeoDecadron Topical Cream 1714

Dezocine (Potentiates orthostatic hypotension). Products include:

- Dalgan Injection 538

Diazoxide (Additive effect or potentiation). Products include:

- Hyperstat I.V. Injection 2363
- Proglycem 580

Diclofenac Potassium (Reduces the diuretic, naturetic, and antihypertensive effects of thiazides). Products include:

- Cataflam 816

Diclofenac Sodium (Reduces the diuretic, naturetic, and antihypertensive effects of thiazides). Products include:

- Voltaren Ophthalmic Sterile Ophthalmic Solution .... ◉ 272
- Voltaren Tablets 861

Diltiazem Hydrochloride (Additive effect or potentiation). Products include:

- Cardizem CD Capsules 1506
- Cardizem SR Capsules 1510
- Cardizem Injectable 1508
- Cardizem Tablets 1512
- Dilacor XR Extended-release Capsules 2018

Doxazosin Mesylate (Additive effect or potentiation). Products include:

- Cardura Tablets 2186

Enalapril Maleate (Additive effect or potentiation). Products include:

- Vaseretic Tablets 1765
- Vasotec Tablets 1771

Enalaprilat (Additive effect or potentiation). Products include:

- Vasotec I.V. 1768

Esmolol Hydrochloride (Additive effect or potentiation). Products include:

- Brevibloc Injection 1808

Etodolac (Reduces the diuretic, naturetic, and antihypertensive effects of thiazides). Products include:

- Lodine Capsules and Tablets 2743

Felodipine (Additive effect or potentiation). Products include:

- Plendil Extended-Release Tablets 527

Fenoprofen Calcium (Reduces the diuretic, naturetic, and antihypertensive effects of thiazides). Products include:

- Nalfon 200 Pulvules & Nalfon Tablets 917

Fentanyl (Potentiates orthostatic hypotension). Products include:

- Duragesic Transdermal System 1288

Fentanyl Citrate (Potentiates orthostatic hypotension). Products include:

- Sublimaze Injection 1307

Fludrocortisone Acetate (Intensified electrolyte depletion, particularly hypokalemia). Products include:

- Florinef Acetate Tablets 505

Flurbiprofen (Reduces the diuretic, naturetic, and antihypertensive effects of thiazides). Products include:

- Ansaid Tablets 2579

Fosinopril Sodium (Additive effect or potentiation). Products include:

- Monopril Tablets 757

Furosemide (Additive effect or potentiation). Products include:

- Lasix Injection, Oral Solution and Tablets 1240

Glipizide (Dosage adjustment of the antidiabetic drug may be required). Products include:

- Glucotrol Tablets 1967
- Glucotrol XL Extended Release Tablets 1968

Glyburide (Dosage adjustment of the antidiabetic drug may be required). Products include:

- DiaBeta Tablets 1239
- Glynase PresTab Tablets 2609
- Micronase Tablets 2623

Guanabenz Acetate (Additive effect or potentiation).

- No products indexed under this heading.

Guanethidine Monosulfate (Additive effect or potentiation). Products include:

- Esimil Tablets 822
- Ismelin Tablets 827

Hydralazine Hydrochloride (Additive effect or potentiation). Products include:

- Apresazide Capsules 808
- Apresoline Hydrochloride Tablets .. 809
- Ser-Ap-Es Tablets 849

Hydrocodone Bitartrate (Potentiates orthostatic hypotension). Products include:

- Anexsia 5/500 Elixir 1781
- Anexia Tablets 1782
- Codiclear DH Syrup 791
- Deconamine CX Cough and Cold Liquid and Tablets 1319
- Duratuss HD Elixir 2565
- Hycodan Tablets and Syrup 930
- Hycomine Compound Tablets 932
- Hycomine 931
- Hycotuss Expectorant Syrup 933
- Hydrocet Capsules 782
- Lorcet 10/650 1018
- Lortab 2566
- Tussend 1783
- Tussend Expectorant 1785
- Vicodin Tablets 1356
- Vicodin ES Tablets 1357
- Vicodin Tuss Expectorant 1358
- Zydone Capsules 949

Hydrocodone Polistirex (Potentiates orthostatic hypotension). Products include:

- Tussionex Pennkinetic Extended-Release Suspension 998

Hydrocortisone (Intensified electrolyte depletion, particularly hypokalemia). Products include:

- Anusol-HC Cream 2.5% 1896
- Aquanil HC Lotion 1931
- Bactine Hydrocortisone Anti-Itch Cream .... ▣ 709
- Caldecort Anti-Itch Hydrocortisone Spray .... ▣ 631
- Cortaid .... ▣ 836
- CORTENEMA 2535
- Cortisporin Ointment 1085
- Cortisporin Ophthalmic Ointment Sterile 1085
- Cortisporin Ophthalmic Suspension Sterile 1086
- Cortisporin Otic Solution Sterile 1087
- Cortisporin Otic Suspension Sterile 1088
- Cortizone-5 .... ▣ 831
- Cortizone-10 .... ▣ 831
- Hydrocortone Tablets 1672
- Hytone 907
- Massengill Medicated Soft Cloth Towelettes 2458
- PediOtic Suspension Sterile 1153
- Preparation H Hydrocortisone 1% Cream .... ▣ 872
- ProctoCream-HC 2.5% 2408
- VōSoL HC Otic Solution 2678

Hydrocortisone Acetate (Intensified electrolyte depletion, particularly hypokalemia). Products include:

- Analpram-HC Rectal Cream 1% and 2.5% 977
- Anusol HC-1 Anti-Itch Hydrocortisone Ointment .... ▣ 847
- Anusol-HC Suppositories 1897
- Caldecort .... ▣ 631
- Carmol HC 924
- Coly-Mycin S Otic w/Neomycin & Hydrocortisone 1906
- Cortaid .... ▣ 836
- Cortifoam 2396
- Cortisporin Cream 1084
- Epifoam 2399
- Hydrocortone Acetate Sterile Suspension 1669
- Mantadil Cream 1135
- Nupercainal Hydrocortisone 1% Cream .... ▣ 645
- Ophthocort .... ◉ 311
- Pramosone Cream, Lotion & Ointment 978
- ProctoCream-HC 2408
- ProctoFoam-HC 2409
- Terra-Cortril Ophthalmic Suspension 2210

Hydrocortisone Sodium Phosphate (Intensified electrolyte depletion, particularly hypokalemia). Products include:

- Hydrocortone Phosphate Injection, Sterile 1670

Hydrocortisone Sodium Succinate (Intensified electrolyte depletion, particularly hypokalemia). Products include:

- Solu-Cortef Sterile Powder 2641

Hydroflumethiazide (Additive effect or potentiation). Products include:

- Diucardin Tablets 2718

Ibuprofen (Reduces the diuretic, naturetic, and antihypertensive effects of thiazides). Products include:

- Advil Cold and Sinus Caplets and Tablets (formerly CoAdvil) .... ▣ 870
- Advil Ibuprofen Tablets and Caplets .... ▣ 870
- Children's Advil Suspension 2692
- Arthritis Foundation Ibuprofen Tablets .... ▣ 674
- Bayer Select Ibuprofen Pain Relief Formula .... ▣ 715
- Cramp End Tablets .... ▣ 735
- Dimetapp Sinus Caplets .... ▣ 775
- Haltran Tablets .... ▣ 771
- IBU Tablets 1342
- Ibuprohm .... ▣ 735
- Children's Motrin Ibuprofen Oral Suspension 1546
- Motrin Tablets 2625
- Motrin IB Caplets, Tablets, and Geltabs .... ▣ 838
- Motrin IB Sinus .... ▣ 838
- Motrin Ibuprofen Suspension, Oral Drops, Chewable Tablets, Caplets 1546
- Nuprin Ibuprofen/Analgesic Tablets & Caplets .... ▣ 622
- Sine-Aid IB Caplets 1554
- Vicks DayQuil SINUS Pressure & PAIN Relief with IBUPROFEN ...... ▣ 762

Indapamide (Additive effect or potentiation). Products include:

- Lozol Tablets 2022

Indomethacin (Reduces lisinopril effects; reduces the diuretic, naturetic and antihypertensive effects of thiazides). Products include:

- Indocin 1680

Indomethacin Sodium Trihydrate (Reduces the diuretic, naturetic, and antihypertensive effects of thiazides; reduces lisinopril effects). Products include:

- Indocin I.V. 1684

Insulin, Human (Dosage adjustment of the antidiabetic drug may be required).

- No products indexed under this heading.

Insulin, Human Isophane Suspension (Dosage adjustment of the antidiabetic drug may be required). Products include:

- Novolin N Human Insulin 10 ml Vials 1795

Insulin, Human NPH (Dosage adjustment of the antidiabetic drug may be required). Products include:

- Humulin N, 100 Units 1448
- Novolin N PenFill Cartridges Durable Insulin Delivery System 1798
- Novolin N Prefilled Syringe Disposable Insulin Delivery System 1798

Insulin, Human Regular (Dosage adjustment of the antidiabetic drug may be required). Products include:

- Humulin R, 100 Units 1449
- Novolin R Human Insulin 10 ml Vials 1795
- Novolin R PenFill Cartridges Durable Insulin Delivery System 1798
- Novolin R Prefilled Syringe Disposable Insulin Delivery System 1798
- Velosulin BR Human Insulin 10 ml Vials 1795

Insulin, Human, Zinc Suspension (Dosage adjustment of the antidiabetic drug may be required). Products include:

- Humulin L, 100 Units 1446
- Humulin U, 100 Units 1450
- Novolin L Human Insulin 10 ml Vials 1795

Insulin, NPH (Dosage adjustment of the antidiabetic drug may be required). Products include:

- NPH, 100 Units 1450
- Pork NPH, 100 Units 1452
- Purified Pork NPH Isophane Insulin 1801

Insulin, Regular (Dosage adjustment of the antidiabetic drug may be required). Products include:

- Regular, 100 Units 1450
- Pork Regular, 100 Units 1452
- Pork Regular (Concentrated), 500 Units 1453
- Purified Pork Regular Insulin 1801

Insulin, Zinc Crystals (Dosage adjustment of the antidiabetic drug may be required). Products include:

- NPH, 100 Units 1450

Insulin, Zinc Suspension (Dosage adjustment of the antidiabetic drug may be required). Products include:

- Iletin I 1450
- Lente, 100 Units 1450
- Iletin II 1452
- Pork Lente, 100 Units 1452
- Purified Pork Lente Insulin 1801

Isradipine (Additive effect or potentiation). Products include:

- DynaCirc Capsules 2256

Ketoprofen (Reduces the diuretic, naturetic, and antihypertensive effects of thiazides). Products include:

- Orudis Capsules 2766
- Oruvail Capsules 2766

Ketorolac Tromethamine (Reduces the diuretic, naturetic, and antihypertensive effects of thiazides). Products include:

- Acular 474
- Acular .... ◉ 277
- Toradol 2159

Labetalol Hydrochloride (Additive effect or potentiation). Products include:

- Normodyne Injection 2377
- Normodyne Tablets 2379
- Trandate 1185

(▣ Described in PDR For Nonprescription Drugs) (◉ Described in PDR For Ophthalmology)

Levorphanol Tartrate (Potentiates orthostatic hypotension). Products include:

Levo-Dromoran 2129

Lithium Carbonate (Potential for lithium toxicity; monitor lithium levels frequently). Products include:

Eskalith 2485
Lithium Carbonate Capsules & Tablets 2230
Lithonate/Lithotabs/Lithobid 2543

Lithium Citrate (Potential for lithium toxicity; monitor lithium levels frequently).

No products indexed under this heading.

Losartan Potassium (Additive effect or potentiation). Products include:

Cozaar Tablets 1628
Hyzaar Tablets 1677

Mecamylamine Hydrochloride (Additive effect or potentiation). Products include:

Inversine Tablets 1686

Meclofenamate Sodium (Reduces the diuretic, naturetic, and antihypertensive effects of thiazides).

No products indexed under this heading.

Mefenamic Acid (Reduces the diuretic, naturetic, and antihypertensive effects of thiazides). Products include:

Ponstel 1925

Meperidine Hydrochloride (Potentiates orthostatic hypotension). Products include:

Demerol 2308
Mepergan Injection 2753

Mephobarbital (Potentiates orthostatic hypotension). Products include:

Mebaral Tablets 2322

Metformin Hydrochloride (Dosage adjustment of the antidiabetic drug may be required). Products include:

Glucophage 752

Methadone Hydrochloride (Potentiates orthostatic hypotension). Products include:

Methadone Hydrochloride Oral Concentrate 2233
Methadone Hydrochloride Oral Solution & Tablets 2235

Methyclothiazide (Additive effect or potentiation). Products include:

Enduron Tablets 420

Methyldopa (Additive effect or potentiation). Products include:

Aldoclor Tablets 1598
Aldomet Oral 1600
Aldoril Tablets 1604

Methyldopate Hydrochloride (Additive effect or potentiation). Products include:

Aldomet Ester HCl Injection 1602

Methylprednisolone Acetate (Intensified electrolyte depletion, particularly hypokalemia). Products include:

Depo-Medrol Single-Dose Vial 2600
Depo-Medrol Sterile Aqueous Suspension 2597

Methylprednisolone Sodium Succinate (Intensified electrolyte depletion, particularly hypokalemia). Products include:

Solu-Medrol Sterile Powder 2643

Metocurine Iodide (Possible increased responsiveness to the muscle relaxant). Products include:

Metubine Iodide Vials 916

Metolazone (Additive effect or potentiation). Products include:

Mykrox Tablets 993

Zaroxolyn Tablets 1000

Metoprolol Succinate (Additive effect or potentiation). Products include:

Toprol-XL Tablets 565

Metoprolol Tartrate (Additive effect or potentiation). Products include:

Lopressor Ampuls 830
Lopressor HCT Tablets 832
Lopressor Tablets 830

Metyrosine (Additive effect or potentiation). Products include:

Demser Capsules 1649

Minoxidil (Additive effect or potentiation). Products include:

Loniten Tablets 2618
Rogaine Topical Solution 2637

Mivacurium Chloride (Possible increased responsiveness to the muscle relaxant). Products include:

Mivacron 1138

Moexipril Hydrochloride (Additive effect or potentiation). Products include:

Univasc Tablets 2410

Morphine Sulfate (Potentiates orthostatic hypotension). Products include:

Astramorph/PF Injection, USP (Preservative-Free) 535
Duramorph 962
Infumorph 200 and Infumorph 500 Sterile Solutions 965
MS Contin Tablets 1994
MSIR 1997
Oramorph SR (Morphine Sulfate Sustained Release Tablets) 2236
RMS Suppositories 2657
Roxanol 2243

Nabumetone (Reduces the diuretic, naturetic, and antihypertensive effects of thiazides). Products include:

Relafen Tablets 2510

Nadolol (Additive effect or potentiation).

No products indexed under this heading.

Naproxen (Reduces the diuretic, naturetic, and antihypertensive effects of thiazides). Products include:

Anaprox/Naprosyn 2117

Naproxen Sodium (Reduces the diuretic, naturetic, and antihypertensive effects of thiazides). Products include:

Aleve 1975
Anaprox/Naprosyn 2117

Nicardipine Hydrochloride (Additive effect or potentiation). Products include:

Cardene Capsules 2095
Cardene I.V. 2709
Cardene SR Capsules 2097

Nifedipine (Additive effect or potentiation). Products include:

Adalat Capsules (10 mg and 20 mg) 587
Adalat CC 589
Procardia Capsules 1971
Procardia XL Extended Release Tablets 1972

Nisoldipine (Additive effect or potentiation).

No products indexed under this heading.

Nitroglycerin (Additive effect or potentiation). Products include:

Deponit NTG Transdermal Delivery System 2397
Nitro-Bid IV 1523
Nitro-Bid Ointment 1524
Nitrodisc 2047
Nitro-Dur (nitroglycerin) Transdermal Infusion System 1326
Nitrolingual Spray 2027
Nitrostat Tablets 1925
Transderm-Nitro Transdermal Therapeutic System 859

Norepinephrine Bitartrate (Possible decreased response to pressor amines). Products include:

Levophed Bitartrate Injection 2315

Opium Alkaloids (Potentiates orthostatic hypotension).

No products indexed under this heading.

Oxaprozin (Reduces the diuretic, naturetic, and antihypertensive effects of thiazides). Products include:

Daypro Caplets 2426

Oxycodone Hydrochloride (Potentiates orthostatic hypotension). Products include:

Percocet Tablets 938
Percodan Tablets 939
Percodan-Demi Tablets 940
Roxicodone Tablets, Oral Solution & Intensol (Oxycodone) 2244
Tylox Capsules 1584

Pancuronium Bromide Injection (Possible increased responsiveness to the muscle relaxant).

No products indexed under this heading.

Penbutolol Sulfate (Additive effect or potentiation). Products include:

Levatol 2403

Pentobarbital Sodium (Potentiates orthostatic hypotension). Products include:

Nembutal Sodium Capsules 436
Nembutal Sodium Solution 438
Nembutal Sodium Suppositories 440

Phenobarbital (Potentiates orthostatic hypotension). Products include:

Arco-Lase Plus Tablets 512
Bellergal-S Tablets 2250
Donnatal 2060
Donnatal Extentabs 2061
Donnatal Tablets 2060
Phenobarbital Elixir and Tablets 1469
Quadrinal Tablets 1350

Phenoxybenzamine Hydrochloride (Additive effect or potentiation). Products include:

Dibenzyline Capsules 2476

Phentolamine Mesylate (Additive effect or potentiation). Products include:

Regitine 846

Phenylbutazone (Reduces the diuretic, naturetic, and antihypertensive effects of thiazides).

No products indexed under this heading.

Pindolol (Additive effect or potentiation). Products include:

Visken Tablets 2299

Piroxicam (Reduces the diuretic, naturetic, and antihypertensive effects of thiazides). Products include:

Feldene Capsules 1965

Polythiazide (Additive effect or potentiation). Products include:

Minizide Capsules 1938

Potassium Acid Phosphate (Concomitant therapy may lead to hyperkalemia). Products include:

K-Phos Original Formula 'Sodium Free' Tablets 639

Potassium Bicarbonate (Concomitant therapy may lead to hyperkalemia). Products include:

Alka-Seltzer Gold Effervescent Antacid .... ◻◻ 703

Potassium Chloride (Concomitant therapy may lead to hyperkalemia). Products include:

Chlor-3 Condiment 1004
K-Dur Microburst Release System (potassium chloride, USP) E.R. Tablets 1325
K-Lor Powder Packets 434
K-Norm Extended-Release Capsules 991

K-Tab Filmtab 434
Kolyum Liquid 992
Micro-K 2063
Micro-K LS Packets 2064
NuLYTELY 689
Cherry Flavor NuLYTELY 689
Rum-K Syrup 1005
Slow-K Extended-Release Tablets 851

Potassium Citrate (Concomitant therapy may lead to hyperkalemia). Products include:

Polycitra Syrup 578
Polycitra-K Crystals 579
Polycitra-K Oral Solution 579
Polycitra-LC 578

Potassium Gluconate (Concomitant therapy may lead to hyperkalemia). Products include:

Kolyum Liquid 992

Potassium Phosphate, Dibasic (Concomitant therapy may lead to hyperkalemia).

No products indexed under this heading.

Potassium Phosphate, Monobasic (Concomitant therapy may lead to hyperkalemia). Products include:

K-Phos Neutral Tablets 639
K-Phos Original Formula 'Sodium Free' Tablets 639

Prazosin Hydrochloride (Additive effect or potentiation). Products include:

Minipress Capsules 1937
Minizide Capsules 1938

Prednisolone Acetate (Intensified electrolyte depletion, particularly hypokalemia). Products include:

AK-CIDE .... ◎ 202
AK-CIDE Ointment .... ◎ 202
Blephamide Liquifilm Sterile Ophthalmic Suspension 476
Blephamide Ointment .... ◎ 237
Econopred & Econopred Plus Ophthalmic Suspensions .... ◎ 217
Poly-Pred Liquifilm .... ◎ 248
Pred Forte .... ◎ 250
Pred Mild .... ◎ 253
Pred-G Liquifilm Sterile Ophthalmic Suspension .... ◎ 251
Pred-G S.O.P. Sterile Ophthalmic Ointment .... ◎ 252
Vasocidin Ointment .... ◎ 268

Prednisolone Sodium Phosphate (Intensified electrolyte depletion, particularly hypokalemia). Products include:

AK-Pred .... ◎ 204
Hydeltrasol Injection, Sterile 1665
Inflamase .... ◎ 265
Pediapred Oral Liquid 995
Vasocidin Ophthalmic Solution .... ◎ 270

Prednisolone Tebutate (Intensified electrolyte depletion, particularly hypokalemia). Products include:

Hydeltra-T.B.A. Sterile Suspension 1667

Prednisone (Intensified electrolyte depletion, particularly hypokalemia). Products include:

Deltasone Tablets 2595

Propoxyphene Hydrochloride (Potentiates orthostatic hypotension). Products include:

Darvon 1435
Wygesic Tablets 2827

Propoxyphene Napsylate (Potentiates orthostatic hypotension). Products include:

Darvon-N/Darvocet-N 1433

Propranolol Hydrochloride (Additive effect or potentiation). Products include:

Inderal 2728
Inderal LA Long Acting Capsules 2730
Inderide Tablets 2732
Inderide LA Long Acting Capsules .. 2734

Quinapril Hydrochloride (Additive effect or potentiation). Products include:

Accupril Tablets 1893

IMPORTANT NOTE: Always consult each drug listing in the patient's regimen for possible interactions.

Ramipril (Additive effect or potentiation). Products include:
- Altace Capsules ... 1232

Rauwolfia Serpentina (Additive effect or potentiation).
- No products indexed under this heading.

Rescinnamine (Additive effect or potentiation).
- No products indexed under this heading.

Reserpine (Additive effect or potentiation). Products include:
- Diupres Tablets ... 1650
- Hydropres Tablets ... 1675
- Ser-Ap-Es Tablets ... 849

Rocuronium Bromide (Possible increased responsiveness to the muscle relaxant). Products include:
- Zemuron ... 1830

Secobarbital Sodium (Potentiates orthostatic hypotension). Products include:
- Seconal Sodium Pulvules ... 1474

Sodium Nitroprusside (Additive effect or potentiation).
- No products indexed under this heading.

Sotalol Hydrochloride (Additive effect or potentiation). Products include:
- Betapace Tablets ... 641

Spirapril Hydrochloride (Additive effect or potentiation).
- No products indexed under this heading.

Spironolactone (Concomitant therapy may lead to hyperkalemia). Products include:
- Aldactazide ... 2413
- Aldactone ... 2414

Sufentanil Citrate (Potentiates orthostatic hypotension). Products include:
- Sufenta Injection ... 1309

Sulindac (Reduces the diuretic, naturetic, and antihypertensive effects of thiazides). Products include:
- Clinoril Tablets ... 1618

Terazosin Hydrochloride (Additive effect or potentiation). Products include:
- Hytrin Capsules ... 430

Thiamylal Sodium (Potentiates orthostatic hypotension).
- No products indexed under this heading.

Timolol Maleate (Additive effect or potentiation). Products include:
- Blocadren Tablets ... 1614
- Timolide Tablets ... 1748
- Timoptic in Ocudose ... 1753
- Timoptic Sterile Ophthalmic Solution ... 1751
- Timoptic-XE ... 1755

Tolazamide (Dosage adjustment of the antidiabetic drug may be required).
- No products indexed under this heading.

Tolbutamide (Dosage adjustment of the antidiabetic drug may be required).
- No products indexed under this heading.

Tolmetin Sodium (Reduces the diuretic, naturetic, and antihypertensive effects of thiazides). Products include:
- Tolectin (200, 400 and 600 mg) .. 1581

Torsemide (Additive effect or potentiation). Products include:
- Demadex Tablets and Injection ... 686

Triamcinolone (Intensified electrolyte depletion, particularly hypokalemia). Products include:
- Aristocort Tablets ... 1022

Triamcinolone Acetonide (Intensified electrolyte depletion, particularly hypokalemia). Products include:
- Aristocort A 0.025% Cream ... 1027
- Aristocort A 0.5% Cream ... 1031
- Aristocort A 0.1% Cream ... 1029
- Aristocort A 0.1% Ointment ... 1030
- Azmacort Oral Inhaler ... 2011
- Nasacort Nasal Inhaler ... 2024

Triamcinolone Diacetate (Intensified electrolyte depletion, particularly hypokalemia). Products include:
- Aristocort Suspension (Forte Parenteral) ... 1027
- Aristocort Suspension (Intralesional) ... 1025

Triamcinolone Hexacetonide (Intensified electrolyte depletion, particularly hypokalemia). Products include:
- Aristospan Suspension (Intra-articular) ... 1033
- Aristospan Suspension (Intralesional) ... 1032

Triamterene (Concomitant therapy may lead to hyperkalemia). Products include:
- Dyazide ... 2479
- Dyrenium Capsules ... 2481
- Maxzide ... 1380

Trimethaphan Camsylate (Additive effect or potentiation). Products include:
- Arfonad Ampuls ... 2080

Vecuronium Bromide (Possible increased responsiveness to the muscle relaxant). Products include:
- Norcuron ... 1826

Verapamil Hydrochloride (Additive effect or potentiation). Products include:
- Calan SR Caplets ... 2422
- Calan Tablets ... 2419
- Isoptin Injectable ... 1344
- Isoptin Oral Tablets ... 1346
- Isoptin SR Tablets ... 1348
- Verelan Capsules ... 1410
- Verelan Capsules ... 2824

Food Interactions

Alcohol (Potentiates orthostatic hypotension).

PRISCOLINE HYDROCHLORIDE AMPULS

(Tolazoline Hydrochloride) ... 845
None cited in PDR database.

PRIVINE NASAL SOLUTION AND DROPS

(Naphazoline Hydrochloride) ... ◘ 647
None cited in PDR database.

PRIVINE NASAL SPRAY

(Naphazoline Hydrochloride) ... ◘ 647
None cited in PDR database.

PRO-BANTHINE TABLETS

(Propantheline Bromide) ... 2052
May interact with antiarrhythmics, antihistamines, phenothiazines, tricyclic antidepressants, corticosteroids, anticholinergics, belladona products, narcotic analgesics, and certain other agents. Compounds in these categories include:

Acebutolol Hydrochloride (Excessive cholinergic blockade). Products include:
- Sectral Capsules ... 2807

Acrivastine (Excessive cholinergic blockade). Products include:
- Semprex-D Capsules ... 463
- Semprex-D Capsules ... 1167

Adenosine (Excessive cholinergic blockade). Products include:
- Adenocard Injection ... 1021
- Adenoscan ... 1024

Alfentanil Hydrochloride (Excessive cholinergic blockade). Products include:
- Alfenta Injection ... 1286

Amiodarone Hydrochloride (Excessive cholinergic blockade). Products include:
- Cordarone Intravenous ... 2715
- Cordarone Tablets ... 2712

Amitriptyline Hydrochloride (Excessive cholinergic blockade). Products include:
- Elavil ... 2838
- Endep Tablets ... 2174
- Etrafon ... 2355
- Limbitrol ... 2180
- Triavil Tablets ... 1757

Amoxapine (Excessive cholinergic blockade). Products include:
- Asendin Tablets ... 1369

Astemizole (Excessive cholinergic blockade). Products include:
- Hismanal Tablets ... 1293

Atropine Sulfate (Excessive cholinergic blockade; increased intraocular pressure). Products include:
- Arco-Lase Plus Tablets ... 512
- Atrohist Plus Tablets ... 454
- Atropine Sulfate Sterile Ophthalmic Solution ... ⊙ 233
- Donnatal ... 2060
- Donnatal Extentabs ... 2061
- Donnatal Tablets ... 2060
- Lomotil ... 2439
- Motofen Tablets ... 784
- Urised Tablets ... 1964

Azatadine Maleate (Excessive cholinergic blockade). Products include:
- Trinalin Repetabs Tablets ... 1330

Belladonna Alkaloids (Excessive cholinergic blockade; increased intraocular pressure). Products include:
- Bellergal-S Tablets ... 2250
- Hyland's Bed Wetting Tablets ... ◘ 828
- Hyland's EnurAid Tablets ... ◘ 829
- Hyland's Teething Tablets ... ◘ 830

Benztropine Mesylate (Excessive cholinergic blockade; increased intraocular pressure). Products include:
- Cogentin ... 1621

Betamethasone Acetate (Increased intraocular pressure). Products include:
- Celestone Soluspan Suspension ... 2347

Betamethasone Sodium Phosphate (Increased intraocular pressure). Products include:
- Celestone Soluspan Suspension ... 2347

Biperiden Hydrochloride (Excessive cholinergic blockade; increased intraocular pressure). Products include:
- Akineton ... 1333

Bretylium Tosylate (Excessive cholinergic blockade).
- No products indexed under this heading.

Bromodiphenhydramine Hydrochloride (Excessive cholinergic blockade).
- No products indexed under this heading.

Brompheniramine Maleate (Excessive cholinergic blockade). Products include:
- Alka Seltzer Plus Sinus Medicine .. ◘ 707
- Bromfed Capsules (Extended-Release) ... 1785
- Bromfed Syrup ... ◘ 733
- Bromfed Tablets ... 1785
- Bromfed-DM Cough Syrup ... 1786
- Bromfed-PD Capsules (Extended-Release) ... 1785
- Dimetane-DC Cough Syrup ... 2059
- Dimetane-DX Cough Syrup ... 2059
- Dimetapp Elixir ... ◘ 773
- Dimetapp Extentabs ... ◘ 774
- Dimetapp Tablets/Liqui-Gels ... ◘ 775
- Dimetapp Cold & Allergy Chewable Tablets ... ◘ 773
- Dimetapp DM Elixir ... ◘ 774
- Vicks DayQuil Allergy Relief 12-Hour Extended Release Tablets .. ◘ 760
- Vicks DayQuil Allergy Relief 4-Hour Tablets ... ◘ 760

Buprenorphine (Excessive cholinergic blockade). Products include:
- Buprenex Injectable ... 2006

Chlorpheniramine Maleate (Excessive cholinergic blockade). Products include:
- Alka-Seltzer Plus Cold Medicine ... ◘ 705
- Alka-Seltzer Plus Cold Medicine Liqui-Gels ... ◘ 706
- Alka-Seltzer Plus Cold & Cough Medicine ... ◘ 708
- Alka-Seltzer Plus Cold & Cough Medicine Liqui-Gels ... ◘ 705
- Allerest Children's Chewable Tablets ... ◘ 627
- Allerest Headache Strength Tablets ... ◘ 627
- Allerest Maximum Strength Tablets ... ◘ 627
- Allerest Sinus Pain Formula ... ◘ 627
- Allerest 12 Hour Caplets ... ◘ 627
- Ana-Kit Anaphylaxis Emergency Treatment Kit ... 617
- Atrohist Pediatric Capsules ... 453
- Atrohist Plus Tablets ... 454
- BC Cold Powder Multi-Symptom Formula (Cold-Sinus-Allergy) ... ◘ 609
- Cerose DM ... ◘ 878
- Cheracol Plus Head Cold/Cough Formula ... ◘ 769
- Children's Vicks DayQuil Allergy Relief ... ◘ 757
- Children's Vicks NyQuil Cold/Cough Relief ... ◘ 758
- Chlor-Trimeton Allergy Decongestant Tablets ... ◘ 799
- Chlor-Trimeton Allergy Tablets ... ◘ 798
- Comhist ... 2038
- Comtrex Multi-Symptom Cold Reliever Tablets/Caplets/Liqui-Gels/Liquid ... ◘ 615
- Allergy-Sinus Comtrex Multi-Symptom Allergy-Sinus Formula Tablets ... ◘ 617
- Contac Continuous Action Nasal Decongestant/Antihistamine 12 Hour Capsules ... ◘ 813
- Contac Maximum Strength Continuous Action Decongestant/Antihistamine 12 Hour Caplets .. ◘ 813
- Contac Severe Cold and Flu Formula Caplets ... ◘ 814
- Coricidin 'D' Decongestant Tablets ... ◘ 800
- Coricidin Tablets ... ◘ 800
- D.A. Chewable Tablets ... 951
- Deconamine ... 1320
- Dura-Tap/PD Capsules ... 2867
- Dura-Vent/DA Tablets ... 953
- Extendryl ... 1005
- Fedahist Gyrocaps ... 2401
- Fedahist Timecaps ... 2401
- Hycomine Compound Tablets ... 932
- Isoclor Timesule Capsules ... ◘ 637
- Kronofed-A ... 977
- Nolamine Timed-Release Tablets ... 785
- Novahistine DH ... 2462
- Novahistine Elixir ... ◘ 823
- Ornade Spansule Capsules ... 2502
- PediaCare Cold Allergy Chewable Tablets ... ◘ 677
- PediaCare Cough-Cold Chewable Tablets ... 1553
- PediaCare Cough-Cold Liquid ... 1553
- PediaCare NightRest Cough-Cold Liquid ... 1553
- Pediatric Vicks 44m Cough & Cold Relief ... ◘ 764
- Pyrroxate Caplets ... ◘ 772
- Ryna ... ◘ 841
- Sinarest Tablets ... ◘ 648
- Sinarest Extra Strength Tablets ... ◘ 648
- Sine-Off Sinus Medicine ... ◘ 825
- Singlet Tablets ... ◘ 825
- Sinulin Tablets ... 787
- Sinutab Sinus Allergy Medication, Maximum Strength Tablets and Caplets ... ◘ 860
- Sudafed Plus Liquid ... ◘ 862
- Sudafed Plus Tablets ... ◘ 863
- Teldrin 12 Hour Antihistamine/Nasal Decongestant Allergy Relief Capsules ... ◘ 826

(◘ Described in PDR For Nonprescription Drugs) (⊙ Described in PDR For Ophthalmology)

Interactions Index

TheraFlu .... ⊕ 787
TheraFlu Maximum Strength Nighttime Flu, Cold & Cough Medicine .... ⊕ 788
Triaminic Allergy Tablets .... ⊕ 789
Triaminic Cold Tablets .... ⊕ 790
Triaminic Nite Light .... ⊕ 791
Triaminic Syrup .... ⊕ 792
Triaminic-12 Tablets .... ⊕ 792
Triaminicin Tablets .... ⊕ 793
Triaminicol Multi-Symptom Cold Tablets .... ⊕ 793
Triaminicol Multi-Symptom Relief ⊕ 794
Tussend 1783
Children's TYLENOL Cold Multi-Symptom Liquid Formula and Chewable Tablets................................ 1561
Children's TYLENOL Cold Plus Cough Multi Symptom Tablets and Liquid .... ⊕ 681
TYLENOL Maximum Strength Allergy Sinus Medication Gelcaps and Caplets 1563
TYLENOL Cold Multi-Symptom Formula Medication Tablets and Caplets 1561
TYLENOL Cold Multi-Symptom Hot Medication Liquid Packets 1557
Vicks 44 LiquiCaps Cough, Cold & Flu Relief .... ⊕ 755
Vicks 44M Cough, Cold & Flu Relief .... ⊕ 756

Chlorpheniramine Polistirex (Excessive cholinergic blockade). Products include:

Tussionex Pennkinetic Extended-Release Suspension 998

Chlorpheniramine Tannate (Excessive cholinergic blockade). Products include:

Atrohist Pediatric Suspension 454
Ricobid Tablets and Pediatric Suspension.. 2038
Rynatan 2673
Rynatuss 2673

Chlorpromazine (Excessive cholinergic blockade; potentiated sedative effect). Products include:

Thorazine Suppositories 2523

Chlorpromazine Hydrochloride (Excessive cholinergic blockade; potentiated sedative effect). Products include:

Thorazine 2523

Clemastine Fumarate (Excessive cholinergic blockade). Products include:

Tavist Syrup 2297
Tavist Tablets 2298
Tavist-1 12 Hour Relief Tablets .... ⊕ 787
Tavist-D 12 Hour Relief Tablets .... ⊕ 787

Clidinium Bromide (Excessive cholinergic blockade; increased intraocular pressure). Products include:

Librax Capsules 2176
Quarzan Capsules 2181

Clomipramine Hydrochloride (Excessive cholinergic blockade). Products include:

Anafranil Capsules 803

Codeine Phosphate (Excessive cholinergic blockade). Products include:

Actifed with Codeine Cough Syrup.. 1067
Brontex 1981
Deconsal C Expectorant Syrup 456
Deconsal Pediatric Syrup 457
Dimetane-DC Cough Syrup 2059
Empirin with Codeine Tablets........... 1093
Fioricet with Codeine Capsules 2260
Fiorinal with Codeine Capsules 2262
Isoclor Expectorant............................. 990
Novahistine DH................................... 2462
Novahistine Expectorant.................... 2463
Nucofed 2051
Phenergan with Codeine 2777
Phenergan VC with Codeine 2781
Robitussin A-C Syrup.......................... 2073
Robitussin-DAC Syrup 2074
Ryna .... ⊕ 841
Soma Compound w/Codeine Tablets 2676
Tussi-Organidin NR Liquid and S NR Liquid 2677

Tylenol with Codeine 1583

Cortisone Acetate (Increased intraocular pressure). Products include:

Cortone Acetate Sterile Suspension 1623
Cortone Acetate Tablets 1624

Cyproheptadine Hydrochloride (Excessive cholinergic blockade). Products include:

Periactin 1724

Desipramine Hydrochloride (Excessive cholinergic blockade). Products include:

Norpramin Tablets 1526

Dexamethasone (Increased intraocular pressure). Products include:

AK-Trol Ointment & Suspension .... ⊙ 205
Decadron Elixir 1633
Decadron Tablets................................. 1635
Decaspray Topical Aerosol 1648
Dexacidin Ointment .... ⊙ 263
Maxitrol Ophthalmic Ointment and Suspension .... ⊙ 224
TobraDex Ophthalmic Suspension and Ointment.. 473

Dexamethasone Acetate (Increased intraocular pressure). Products include:

Dalalone D.P. Injectable 1011
Decadron-LA Sterile Suspension 1646

Dexamethasone Sodium Phosphate (Increased intraocular pressure). Products include:

Decadron Phosphate Injection 1637
Decadron Phosphate Respihaler 1642
Decadron Phosphate Sterile Ophthalmic Ointment................................. 1641
Decadron Phosphate Sterile Ophthalmic Solution 1642
Decadron Phosphate Topical Cream 1644
Decadron Phosphate Turbinaire 1645
Decadron Phosphate with Xylocaine Injection, Sterile 1639
Dexacort Phosphate in Respihaler .. 458
Dexacort Phosphate in Turbinaire .. 459
NeoDecadron Sterile Ophthalmic Ointment 1712
NeoDecadron Sterile Ophthalmic Solution 1713
NeoDecadron Topical Cream 1714

Dexchlorpheniramine Maleate (Excessive cholinergic blockade).

No products indexed under this heading.

Dezocine (Excessive cholinergic blockade). Products include:

Dalgan Injection 538

Dicyclomine Hydrochloride (Excessive cholinergic blockade; increased intraocular pressure). Products include:

Bentyl 1501

Digoxin (Increased serum digoxin levels in patients who are taking slow-dissolving tablets of digoxin). Products include:

Lanoxicaps 1117
Lanoxin Elixir Pediatric 1120
Lanoxin Injection 1123
Lanoxin Injection Pediatric................. 1126
Lanoxin Tablets 1128

Diphenhydramine Citrate (Excessive cholinergic blockade). Products include:

Excedrin P.M. Analgesic/Sleeping Aid Tablets, Caplets, Liquigels 733

Diphenhydramine Hydrochloride (Excessive cholinergic blockade). Products include:

Actifed Allergy Daytime/Nighttime Caplets .... ⊕ 844
Actifed Sinus Daytime/Nighttime Tablets and Caplets .... ⊕ 846
Arthritis Foundation NightTime Caplets .... ⊕ 674
Extra Strength Bayer PM Aspirin .. ⊕ 713
Bayer Select Night Time Pain Relief Formula .... ⊕ 716
Benadryl Allergy Decongestant Liquid Medication .... ⊕ 848
Benadryl Allergy Decongestant Tablets .... ⊕ 848
Benadryl Allergy Liquid Medication.. ⊕ 849
Benadryl Allergy .... ⊕ 848
Benadryl Allergy Sinus Headache Formula Caplets .... ⊕ 849
Benadryl Capsules............................... 1898
Benadryl Dye-Free Allergy Liquigel Softgels... ⊕ 850
Benadryl Dye-Free Allergy Liquid Medication .... ⊕ 850
Benadryl Itch Relief Cream, Children's Formula and Maximum Strength 2% .... ⊕ 851
Benadryl Itch Relief Spray, Children's Formula and Maximum Strength 2% .... ⊕ 851
Benadryl Itch Relief Stick Maximum Strength 2% .... ⊕ 850
Benadryl Itch Stopping Gel, Children's Formula and Maximum Strength 2% .... ⊕ 851
Benadryl Kapseals 1898
Benadryl Injection 1898
Contac Day & Night Cold/Flu Night Caplets... ⊕ 812
Contac Night Allergy/Sinus Caplets .... ⊕ 812
Extra Strength Doan's P.M.................. ⊕ 633
Legatrin PM .... ⊕ 651
Miles Nervine Nighttime Sleep-Aid ⊕ 723
Nytol QuickCaps Caplets .... ⊕ 610
Sleepinal Night-time Sleep Aid Capsules and Softgels .... ⊕ 834
TYLENOL Maximum Strength Allergy Sinus NightTime Medication Caplets 1555
TYLENOL Flu NightTime, Maximum Strength, Gelcaps 1566
TYLENOL Maximum Strength Flu NightTime Hot Medication Packets 1562
TYLENOL PM, Extra Strength Pain Reliever/Sleep Aid Caplets, Geltabs, Gelcaps 1560
TYLENOL Severe Allergy Medication Caplets 1564
Maximum Strength Unisom Sleepgels 1934
Unisom With Pain Relief-Nighttime Sleep Aid and Pain Reliever............ 1934

Diphenylpyraline Hydrochloride (Excessive cholinergic blockade).

No products indexed under this heading.

Disopyramide Phosphate (Excessive cholinergic blockade). Products include:

Norpace 2444

Doxepin Hydrochloride (Excessive cholinergic blockade). Products include:

Sinequan 2205
Zonalon Cream 1055

Drugs, Oral, unspecified (Delayed absorption of other medications given concomitantly).

Fentanyl (Excessive cholinergic blockade). Products include:

Duragesic Transdermal System......... 1288

Fentanyl Citrate (Excessive cholinergic blockade). Products include:

Sublimaze Injection.............................. 1307

Flecainide Acetate (Excessive cholinergic blockade). Products include:

Tambocor Tablets 1497

Fludrocortisone Acetate (Increased intraocular pressure). Products include:

Florinef Acetate Tablets 505

Fluphenazine Decanoate (Excessive cholinergic blockade; potentiated sedative effect). Products include:

Prolixin Decanoate 509

Fluphenazine Enanthate (Excessive cholinergic blockade; potentiated sedative effect). Products include:

Prolixin Enanthate 509

Fluphenazine Hydrochloride (Excessive cholinergic blockade; potentiated sedative effect). Products include:

Prolixin 509

Glycopyrrolate (Excessive cholinergic blockade; increased intraocular pressure). Products include:

Robinul Forte Tablets........................... 2072
Robinul Injectable 2072
Robinul Tablets..................................... 2072

Hydrocodone Bitartrate (Excessive cholinergic blockade). Products include:

Anexsia 5/500 Elixir 1781
Anexia Tablets....................................... 1782
Codiclear DH Syrup 791
Deconamine CX Cough and Cold Liquid and Tablets............................... 1319
Duratuss HD Elixir............................... 2565
Hycodan Tablets and Syrup 930
Hycomine Compound Tablets 932
Hycomine 931
Hycotuss Expectorant Syrup 933
Hydrocet Capsules 782
Lorcet 10/650....................................... 1018
Lortab 2566
Tussend 1783
Tussend Expectorant 1785
Vicodin Tablets 1356
Vicodin ES Tablets 1357
Vicodin Tuss Expectorant 1358
Zydone Capsules 949

Hydrocodone Polistirex (Excessive cholinergic blockade). Products include:

Tussionex Pennkinetic Extended-Release Suspension 998

Hydrocortisone (Increased intraocular pressure). Products include:

Anusol-HC Cream 2.5% 1896
Aquanil HC Lotion 1931
Bactine Hydrocortisone Anti-Itch Cream.. ⊕ 709
Caldecort Anti-Itch Hydrocortisone Spray .... ⊕ 631
Cortaid .... ⊕ 836
CORTENEMA.. 2535
Cortisporin Ointment 1085
Cortisporin Ophthalmic Ointment Sterile 1085
Cortisporin Ophthalmic Suspension Sterile 1086
Cortisporin Otic Solution Sterile 1087
Cortisporin Otic Suspension Sterile 1088
Cortizone-5 .... ⊕ 831
Cortizone-10 .... ⊕ 831
Hydrocortone Tablets 1672
Hytone 907
Massengill Medicated Soft Cloth Towelettes... 2458
PediOtic Suspension Sterile 1153
Preparation H Hydrocortisone 1% Cream .... ⊕ 872
ProctoCream-HC 2.5% 2408
VōSoL HC Otic Solution...................... 2678

Hydrocortisone Acetate (Increased intraocular pressure). Products include:

Analpram-HC Rectal Cream 1% and 2.5% 977
Anusol HC-1 Anti-Itch Hydrocortisone Ointment................................... ⊕ 847
Anusol-HC Suppositories 1897
Caldecort.. ⊕ 631
Carmol HC 924
Coly-Mycin S Otic w/Neomycin & Hydrocortisone 1906
Cortaid .... ⊕ 836
Cortifoam 2396
Cortisporin Cream................................ 1084
Epifoam 2399
Hydrocortone Acetate Sterile Suspension.. 1669
Mantadil Cream 1135
Nupercainal Hydrocortisone 1% Cream.. ⊕ 645
Ophthocort .... ⊙ 311
Pramosone Cream, Lotion & Ointment 978
ProctoCream-HC 2408
ProctoFoam-HC 2409
Terra-Cortril Ophthalmic Suspension 2210

IMPORTANT NOTE: Always consult each drug listing in the patient's regimen for possible interactions.

Pro-Banthine **Interactions Index** 838

Hydrocortisone Sodium Phosphate (Increased intraocular pressure). Products include:
Hydrocortone Phosphate Injection, Sterile ... 1670

Hydrocortisone Sodium Succinate (Increased intraocular pressure). Products include:
Solu-Cortef Sterile Powder ... 2641

Hyoscyamine (Excessive cholinergic blockade; increased intraocular pressure). Products include:
Cystospaz Tablets ... 1963
Urised Tablets ... 1964

Hyoscyamine Sulfate (Excessive cholinergic blockade; increased intraocular pressure). Products include:
Arco-Lase Plus Tablets ... 512
Atrohist Plus Tablets ... 454
Cystospaz-M Capsules ... 1963
Donnatal ... 2060
Donnatal Extentabs ... 2061
Donnatal Tablets ... 2060
Kutrase Capsules ... 2402
Levsin/Levsinex/Levbid ... 2405

Imipramine Hydrochloride (Excessive cholinergic blockade). Products include:
Tofranil Ampuls ... 854
Tofranil Tablets ... 856

Imipramine Pamoate (Excessive cholinergic blockade). Products include:
Tofranil-PM Capsules ... 857

Ipratropium Bromide (Excessive cholinergic blockade; increased intraocular pressure). Products include:
Atrovent Inhalation Aerosol ... 671
Atrovent Inhalation Solution ... 673

Levorphanol Tartrate (Excessive cholinergic blockade). Products include:
Levo-Dromoran ... 2129

Lidocaine Hydrochloride (Excessive cholinergic blockade). Products include:
Bactine Antiseptic/Anesthetic First Aid Liquid ... ▣ 708
Campho-Phenique Maximum Strength First Aid Antibiotic Plus Pain Reliever Ointment ... ▣ 719
Decadron Phosphate with Xylocaine Injection, Sterile ... 1639
Xylocaine Injections ... 567

Loratadine (Excessive cholinergic blockade). Products include:
Claritin ... 2349
Claritin-D ... 2350

Maprotiline Hydrochloride (Excessive cholinergic blockade). Products include:
Ludiomil Tablets ... 843

Mepenzolate Bromide (Excessive cholinergic blockade; increased intraocular pressure).
No products indexed under this heading.

Meperidine Hydrochloride (Excessive cholinergic blockade). Products include:
Demerol ... 2308
Mepergan Injection ... 2753

Mesoridazine Besylate (Excessive cholinergic blockade; potentiated sedative effect). Products include:
Serentil ... 684

Methadone Hydrochloride (Excessive cholinergic blockade). Products include:
Methadone Hydrochloride Oral Concentrate ... 2233
Methadone Hydrochloride Oral Solution & Tablets ... 2235

Methdilazine Hydrochloride (Excessive cholinergic blockade).
No products indexed under this heading.

Methotrimeprazine (Excessive cholinergic blockade; potentiated sedative effect). Products include:
Levoprome ... 1274

Methylprednisolone Acetate (Increased intraocular pressure). Products include:
Depo-Medrol Single-Dose Vial ... 2600
Depo-Medrol Sterile Aqueous Suspension ... 2597

Methylprednisolone Sodium Succinate (Increased intraocular pressure). Products include:
Solu-Medrol Sterile Powder ... 2643

Mexiletine Hydrochloride (Excessive cholinergic blockade). Products include:
Mexitil Capsules ... 678

Moricizine Hydrochloride (Excessive cholinergic blockade). Products include:
Ethmozine Tablets ... 2041

Morphine Sulfate (Excessive cholinergic blockade). Products include:
Astramorph/PF Injection, USP (Preservative-Free) ... 535
Duramorph ... 962
Infumorph 200 and Infumorph 500 Sterile Solutions ... 965
MS Contin Tablets ... 1994
MSIR ... 1997
Oramorph SR (Morphine Sulfate Sustained Release Tablets) ... 2236
RMS Suppositories ... 2657
Roxanol ... 2243

Nortriptyline Hydrochloride (Excessive cholinergic blockade). Products include:
Pamelor ... 2280

Opium Alkaloids (Excessive cholinergic blockade).
No products indexed under this heading.

Oxybutynin Chloride (Excessive cholinergic blockade; increased intraocular pressure). Products include:
Ditropan ... 1516

Oxycodone Hydrochloride (Excessive cholinergic blockade). Products include:
Percocet Tablets ... 938
Percodan Tablets ... 939
Percodan-Demi Tablets ... 940
Roxicodone Tablets, Oral Solution & Intensol (Oxycodone) ... 2244
Tylox Capsules ... 1584

Perphenazine (Excessive cholinergic blockade; potentiated sedative effect). Products include:
Etrafon ... 2355
Triavil Tablets ... 1757
Trilafon ... 2389

Prednisolone Acetate (Increased intraocular pressure). Products include:
AK-CIDE ... ◉ 202
AK-CIDE Ointment ... ◉ 202
Blephamide Liquifilm Sterile Ophthalmic Suspension ... 476
Blephamide Ointment ... ◉ 237
Econopred & Econopred Plus Ophthalmic Suspensions ... ◉ 217
Poly-Pred Liquifilm ... ◉ 248
Pred Forte ... ◉ 250
Pred Mild ... ◉ 253
Pred-G Liquifilm Sterile Ophthalmic Suspension ... ◉ 251
Pred-G S.O.P. Sterile Ophthalmic Ointment ... ◉ 252
Vasocidin Ointment ... ◉ 268

Prednisolone Sodium Phosphate (Increased intraocular pressure). Products include:
AK-Pred ... ◉ 204
Hydeltrasol Injection, Sterile ... 1665
Inflamase ... ◉ 265
Pediapred Oral Liquid ... 995
Vasocidin Ophthalmic Solution ... ◉ 270

Prednisolone Tebutate (Increased intraocular pressure). Products include:
Hydeltra-T.B.A. Sterile Suspension ... 1667

Prednisone (Increased intraocular pressure). Products include:
Deltasone Tablets ... 2595

Procainamide Hydrochloride (Excessive cholinergic blockade). Products include:
Procan SR Tablets ... 1926

Prochlorperazine (Excessive cholinergic blockade; potentiated sedative effect). Products include:
Compazine ... 2470

Procyclidine Hydrochloride (Excessive cholinergic blockade; increased intraocular pressure). Products include:
Kemadrin Tablets ... 1112

Promethazine Hydrochloride (Excessive cholinergic blockade; potentiated sedative effect). Products include:
Mepergan Injection ... 2753
Phenergan with Codeine ... 2777
Phenergan with Dextromethorphan ... 2778
Phenergan Injection ... 2773
Phenergan Suppositories ... 2775
Phenergan Syrup ... 2774
Phenergan Tablets ... 2775
Phenergan VC ... 2779
Phenergan VC with Codeine ... 2781

Propafenone Hydrochloride (Excessive cholinergic blockade). Products include:
Rythmol Tablets–150mg, 225mg, 300mg ... 1352

Propoxyphene Hydrochloride (Excessive cholinergic blockade). Products include:
Darvon ... 1435
Wygesic Tablets ... 2827

Propoxyphene Napsylate (Excessive cholinergic blockade). Products include:
Darvon-N/Darvocet-N ... 1433

Propranolol Hydrochloride (Excessive cholinergic blockade). Products include:
Inderal ... 2728
Inderal LA Long Acting Capsules ... 2730
Inderide Tablets ... 2732
Inderide LA Long Acting Capsules ... 2734

Protriptyline Hydrochloride (Excessive cholinergic blockade). Products include:
Vivactil Tablets ... 1774

Pyrilamine Maleate (Excessive cholinergic blockade). Products include:
4-Way Fast Acting Nasal Spray (regular & mentholated) ... ▣ 621
Maximum Strength Multi-Symptom Formula Midol ... ▣ 722
PMS Multi-Symptom Formula Midol ... ▣ 723

Pyrilamine Tannate (Excessive cholinergic blockade). Products include:
Atrohist Pediatric Suspension ... 454
Rynatan ... 2673

Quinidine Gluconate (Excessive cholinergic blockade). Products include:
Quinaglute Dura-Tabs Tablets ... 649

Quinidine Polygalacturonate (Excessive cholinergic blockade).
No products indexed under this heading.

Quinidine Sulfate (Excessive cholinergic blockade). Products include:
Quinidex Extentabs ... 2067

Scopolamine (Excessive cholinergic blockade; increased intraocular pressure). Products include:
Transderm Scōp Transdermal Therapeutic System ... 869

Scopolamine Hydrobromide (Excessive cholinergic blockade; increased intraocular pressure). Products include:
Atrohist Plus Tablets ... 454
Donnatal ... 2060
Donnatal Extentabs ... 2061
Donnatal Tablets ... 2060

Sotalol Hydrochloride (Excessive cholinergic blockade). Products include:
Betapace Tablets ... 641

Sufentanil Citrate (Excessive cholinergic blockade). Products include:
Sufenta Injection ... 1309

Terfenadine (Excessive cholinergic blockade). Products include:
Seldane Tablets ... 1536
Seldane-D Extended-Release Tablets ... 1538

Thioridazine Hydrochloride (Excessive cholinergic blockade; potentiated sedative effect). Products include:
Mellaril ... 2269

Tocainide Hydrochloride (Excessive cholinergic blockade). Products include:
Tonocard Tablets ... 531

Triamcinolone (Increased intraocular pressure). Products include:
Aristocort Tablets ... 1022

Triamcinolone Acetonide (Increased intraocular pressure). Products include:
Aristocort A 0.025% Cream ... 1027
Aristocort A 0.5% Cream ... 1031
Aristocort A 0.1% Cream ... 1029
Aristocort A 0.1% Ointment ... 1030
Azmacort Oral Inhaler ... 2011
Nasacort Nasal Inhaler ... 2024

Triamcinolone Diacetate (Increased intraocular pressure). Products include:
Aristocort Suspension (Forte Parenteral) ... 1027
Aristocort Suspension (Intralesional) ... 1025

Triamcinolone Hexacetonide (Increased intraocular pressure). Products include:
Aristospan Suspension (Intra-articular) ... 1033
Aristospan Suspension (Intralesional) ... 1032

Tridihexethyl Chloride (Excessive cholinergic blockade; increased intraocular pressure).
No products indexed under this heading.

Trifluoperazine Hydrochloride (Excessive cholinergic blockade; potentiated sedative effect). Products include:
Stelazine ... 2514

Trihexyphenidyl Hydrochloride (Excessive cholinergic blockade; increased intraocular pressure). Products include:
Artane ... 1368

Trimeprazine Tartrate (Excessive cholinergic blockade). Products include:
Temaril Tablets, Syrup and Spansule Extended-Release Capsules ... 483

Trimipramine Maleate (Excessive cholinergic blockade). Products include:
Surmontil Capsules ... 2811

Tripelennamine Hydrochloride (Excessive cholinergic blockade). Products include:
PBZ Tablets ... 845
PBZ-SR Tablets ... 844

Triprolidine Hydrochloride (Excessive cholinergic blockade). Products include:
Actifed Plus Caplets ... ▣ 845
Actifed Plus Tablets ... ▣ 845

(▣ Described in PDR For Nonprescription Drugs) (◉ Described in PDR For Ophthalmology)

839 **Interactions Index** **Procardia**

Actifed with Codeine Cough Syrup.. 1067
Actifed Syrup ⊡ 846
Actifed Tablets ⊡ 844

Verapamil Hydrochloride (Excessive cholinergic blockade). Products include:
Calan SR Caplets 2422
Calan Tablets 2419
Isoptin Injectable 1344
Isoptin Oral Tablets 1346
Isoptin SR Tablets 1348
Verelan Capsules 1410
Verelan Capsules 2824

PROCAN SR TABLETS

(Procainamide Hydrochloride) 1926

May interact with antiarrhythmics, anticholinergics, type 1 antiarrhythmic drugs, cardiac glycosides, and certain other agents. Compounds in these categories include:

Acebutolol Hydrochloride (Additive cardiac effects). Products include:
Sectral Capsules 2807

Adenosine (Additive cardiac effects). Products include:
Adenocard Injection 1021
Adenoscan 1024

Amiodarone Hydrochloride (Additive cardiac effects). Products include:
Cordarone Intravenous 2715
Cordarone Tablets 2712

Atracurium Besylate (Potentiation of effects of skeletal muscle relaxants). Products include:
Tracrium Injection 1183

Atropine Sulfate (Enhanced anticholinergic effects). Products include:
Arco-Lase Plus Tablets 512
Atrohist Plus Tablets 454
Atropine Sulfate Sterile Ophthalmic Solution ◉ 233
Donnatal 2060
Donnatal Extentabs 2061
Donnatal Tablets 2060
Lomotil 2439
Motofen Tablets 784
Urised Tablets 1964

Belladonna Alkaloids (Enhanced anticholinergic effects). Products include:
Bellergal-S Tablets 2250
Hyland's Bed Wetting Tablets ⊡ 828
Hyland's EnurAid Tablets ⊡ 829
Hyland's Teething Tablets ⊡ 830

Benztropine Mesylate (Enhanced anticholinergic effects). Products include:
Cogentin 1621

Biperiden Hydrochloride (Enhanced anticholinergic effects). Products include:
Akineton 1333

Bretylium Tosylate (Additive cardiac effects; additive toxic effects).
No products indexed under this heading.

Clidinium Bromide (Enhanced anticholinergic effects). Products include:
Librax Capsules 2176
Quarzan Capsules 2181

Deslanoside (Additional depression of conduction and ventricular asystole or fibrillation may result in certain patients).
No products indexed under this heading.

Dicyclomine Hydrochloride (Enhanced anticholinergic effects). Products include:
Bentyl 1501

Digitoxin (Additional depression of conduction and ventricular asystole or fibrillation may result in certain patients). Products include:
Crystodigin Tablets 1433

Digoxin (Additional depression of conduction and ventricular asystole or fibrillation may result in certain patients). Products include:
Lanoxicaps 1117
Lanoxin Elixir Pediatric 1120
Lanoxin Injection 1123
Lanoxin Injection Pediatric 1126
Lanoxin Tablets 1128

Disopyramide Phosphate (Enhanced prolongation of conduction or depression of contractility and hypotension). Products include:
Norpace 2444

Edrophonium Chloride (Antagonized effect). Products include:
Tensilon Injectable 1261

Glycopyrrolate (Enhanced anticholinergic effects). Products include:
Robinul Forte Tablets 2072
Robinul Injectable 2072
Robinul Tablets 2072

Hyoscyamine (Enhanced anticholinergic effects). Products include:
Cystospaz Tablets 1963
Urised Tablets 1964

Hyoscyamine Sulfate (Enhanced anticholinergic effects). Products include:
Arco-Lase Plus Tablets 512
Atrohist Plus Tablets 454
Cystospaz-M Capsules 1963
Donnatal 2060
Donnatal Extentabs 2061
Donnatal Tablets 2060
Kutrase Capsules 2402
Levsin/Levsinex/Levbid 2405

Ipratropium Bromide (Enhanced anticholinergic effects). Products include:
Atrovent Inhalation Aerosol 671
Atrovent Inhalation Solution 673

Lidocaine Hydrochloride (Additive cardiac effects). Products include:
Bactine Antiseptic/Anesthetic First Aid Liquid ⊡ 708
Campho-Phenique Maximum Strength First Aid Antibiotic Plus Pain Reliever Ointment ⊡ 719
Decadron Phosphate with Xylocaine Injection, Sterile 1639
Xylocaine Injections 567

Mepenzolate Bromide (Enhanced anticholinergic effects).
No products indexed under this heading.

Metocurine Iodide (Potentiation of effects of skeletal muscle relaxants). Products include:
Metubine Iodide Vials 916

Mexiletine Hydrochloride (Potential for agranulocytosis and additive cardiac effects). Products include:
Mexitil Capsules 678

Moricizine Hydrochloride (Additive cardiac effects). Products include:
Ethmozine Tablets 2041

Oxybutynin Chloride (Enhanced anticholinergic effects). Products include:
Ditropan 1516

Pancuronium Bromide Injection (Potentiation of effects of skeletal muscle relaxants).
No products indexed under this heading.

Procyclidine Hydrochloride (Enhanced anticholinergic effects). Products include:
Kemadrin Tablets 1112

Propafenone Hydrochloride (Additive cardiac effects). Products include:
Rythmol Tablets–150mg, 225mg, 300mg 1352

Propantheline Bromide (Enhanced anticholinergic effects). Products include:
Pro-Banthīne Tablets 2052

Propranolol Hydrochloride (Additive cardiac effects). Products include:
Inderal 2728
Inderal LA Long Acting Capsules 2730
Inderide Tablets 2732
Inderide LA Long Acting Capsules .. 2734

Quinidine Gluconate (Enhanced prolongation of conduction or depression of contractility and hypotension). Products include:
Quinaglute Dura-Tabs Tablets 649

Quinidine Polygalacturonate (Enhanced prolongation of conduction or depression of contractility and hypotension).
No products indexed under this heading.

Quinidine Sulfate (Enhanced prolongation of conduction or depression of contractility and hypotension). Products include:
Quinidex Extentabs 2067

Scopolamine (Enhanced anticholinergic effects). Products include:
Transderm Scōp Transdermal Therapeutic System 869

Scopolamine Hydrobromide (Enhanced anticholinergic effects). Products include:
Atrohist Plus Tablets 454
Donnatal 2060
Donnatal Extentabs 2061
Donnatal Tablets 2060

Sotalol Hydrochloride (Additive cardiac effects). Products include:
Betapace Tablets 641

Succinylcholine Chloride (Procainamide reduces acetycholine release). Products include:
Anectine 1073

Tocainide Hydrochloride (Additive cardiac effects). Products include:
Tonocard Tablets 531

Trichlormethiazide (Potentiation of hypotensive effects of thiazide diuretics).
No products indexed under this heading.

Tridihexethyl Chloride (Enhanced anticholinergic effects).
No products indexed under this heading.

Trihexyphenidyl Hydrochloride (Enhanced anticholinergic effects). Products include:
Artane 1368

Trimethaphan Camsylate (Potentiation of hypotensive effects of antihypertensives). Products include:
Arfonad Ampuls 2080

Vecuronium Bromide (Potentiation of effects of skeletal muscle relaxants). Products include:
Norcuron 1826

Verapamil Hydrochloride (Additive cardiac effects). Products include:
Calan SR Caplets 2422
Calan Tablets 2419
Isoptin Injectable 1344
Isoptin Oral Tablets 1346
Isoptin SR Tablets 1348
Verelan Capsules 1410
Verelan Capsules 2824

PROCARDIA CAPSULES

(Nifedipine) 1971

May interact with beta blockers, oral anticoagulants, cardiac glycosides, and certain other agents. Compounds in these categories include:

Acebutolol Hydrochloride (Increased likelihood of congestive heart failure, severe hypotension or exacerbation of angina). Products include:
Sectral Capsules 2807

Atenolol (Increased likelihood of congestive heart failure, severe hypotension or exacerbation of angina). Products include:
Tenoretic Tablets 2845
Tenormin Tablets and I.V. Injection 2847

Betaxolol Hydrochloride (Increased likelihood of congestive heart failure, severe hypotension or exacerbation of angina). Products include:
Betoptic Ophthalmic Solution 469
Betoptic S Ophthalmic Suspension 471
Kerlone Tablets 2436

Bisoprolol Fumarate (Increased likelihood of congestive heart failure, severe hypotension or exacerbation of angina). Products include:
Zebeta Tablets 1413
Ziac 1415

Carteolol Hydrochloride (Increased likelihood of congestive heart failure, severe hypotension or exacerbation of angina). Products include:
Cartrol Tablets 410
Ocupress Ophthalmic Solution, 1% Sterile ◉ 309

Cimetidine (Increases peak nifedipine plasma levels). Products include:
Tagamet Tablets 2516

Cimetidine Hydrochloride (Increases peak nifedipine plasma levels). Products include:
Tagamet 2516

Deslanoside (Potential for increased digoxin levels).
No products indexed under this heading.

Dicumarol (Increased prothrombin time).
No products indexed under this heading.

Digitoxin (Potential for increased digoxin levels). Products include:
Crystodigin Tablets 1433

Digoxin (Potential for increased digoxin levels). Products include:
Lanoxicaps 1117
Lanoxin Elixir Pediatric 1120
Lanoxin Injection 1123
Lanoxin Injection Pediatric 1126
Lanoxin Tablets 1128

Esmolol Hydrochloride (Increased likelihood of congestive heart failure, severe hypotension or exacerbation of angina). Products include:
Brevibloc Injection 1808

Labetalol Hydrochloride (Increased likelihood of congestive heart failure, severe hypotension or exacerbation of angina). Products include:
Normodyne Injection 2377
Normodyne Tablets 2379
Trandate 1185

Levobunolol Hydrochloride (Increased likelihood of congestive heart failure, severe hypotension or exacerbation of angina). Products include:
Betagan ◉ 233

IMPORTANT NOTE: Always consult each drug listing in the patient's regimen for possible interactions.

Metipranolol Hydrochloride (Increased likelihood of congestive heart failure, severe hypotension or exacerbation of angina). Products include:
OptiPranolol (Metipranolol 0.3%) Sterile Ophthalmic Solution .... ◉ 258
Metoprolol Succinate (Increased likelihood of congestive heart failure, severe hypotension or exacerbation of angina). Products include:
Toprol-XL Tablets 565
Metoprolol Tartrate (Increased likelihood of congestive heart failure, severe hypotension or exacerbation of angina). Products include:
Lopressor Ampuls 830
Lopressor HCT Tablets 832
Lopressor Tablets 830
Nadolol (Increased likelihood of congestive heart failure, severe hypotension or exacerbation of angina).
No products indexed under this heading.
Penbutolol Sulfate (Increased likelihood of congestive heart failure, severe hypotension or exacerbation of angina). Products include:
Levatol 2403
Pindolol (Increased likelihood of congestive heart failure, severe hypotension or exacerbation of angina). Products include:
Visken Tablets 2299
Propranolol Hydrochloride (Increased likelihood of congestive heart failure, severe hypotension or exacerbation of angina). Products include:
Inderal 2728
Inderal LA Long Acting Capsules 2730
Inderide Tablets 2732
Inderide LA Long Acting Capsules 2734
Ranitidine Hydrochloride (Co-administration produces smaller non-significant increases in nifedipine level). Products include:
Zantac 1209
Zantac Injection 1207
Zantac Syrup 1209
Sotalol Hydrochloride (Increased likelihood of congestive heart failure, severe hypotension or exacerbation of angina). Products include:
Betapace Tablets 641
Timolol Hemihydrate (Increased likelihood of congestive heart failure, severe hypotension or exacerbation of angina). Products include:
Betimol 0.25%, 0.5% .... ◉ 261
Timolol Maleate (Increased likelihood of congestive heart failure, severe hypotension or exacerbation of angina). Products include:
Blocadren Tablets 1614
Timolide Tablets 1748
Timoptic in Ocudose 1753
Timoptic Sterile Ophthalmic Solution 1751
Timoptic-XE 1755
Warfarin Sodium (Increased prothrombin time). Products include:
Coumadin 926

PROCARDIA XL EXTENDED RELEASE TABLETS

(Nifedipine) 1972

May interact with beta blockers, oral anticoagulants, diuretics, cardiac glycosides, and certain other agents. Compounds in these categories include:

Acebutolol Hydrochloride (Potential for congestive heart failure, severe hypotension, or exacerbation of angina). Products include:
Sectral Capsules 2807
Amiloride Hydrochloride (Serum potassium slightly decreased). Products include:
Midamor Tablets 1703
Moduretic Tablets 1705
Atenolol (Potential for congestive heart failure, severe hypotension, or exacerbation of angina). Products include:
Tenoretic Tablets 2845
Tenormin Tablets and I.V. Injection 2847
Bendroflumethiazide (Serum potassium slightly decreased).
No products indexed under this heading.
Betaxolol Hydrochloride (Potential for congestive heart failure, severe hypotension, or exacerbation of angina). Products include:
Betoptic Ophthalmic Solution 469
Betoptic S Ophthalmic Suspension 471
Kerlone Tablets 2436
Bisoprolol Fumarate (Potential for congestive heart failure, severe hypotension, or exacerbation of angina). Products include:
Zebeta Tablets 1413
Ziac 1415
Bumetanide (Serum potassium slightly decreased). Products include:
Bumex 2093
Carteolol Hydrochloride (Potential for congestive heart failure, severe hypotension, or exacerbation of angina). Products include:
Cartrol Tablets 410
Ocupress Ophthalmic Solution, 1% Sterile .... ◉ 309
Chlorothiazide (Serum potassium slightly decreased). Products include:
Aldoclor Tablets 1598
Diupres Tablets 1650
Diuril Oral 1653
Chlorothiazide Sodium (Serum potassium slightly decreased). Products include:
Diuril Sodium Intravenous 1652
Chlorthalidone (Serum potassium slightly decreased). Products include:
Combipres Tablets 677
Tenoretic Tablets 2845
Thalitone 1245
Cimetidine (Significant increase peak nifedipine plasma levels and AUC). Products include:
Tagamet Tablets 2516
Cimetidine Hydrochloride (Significant increase in peak nifedipine plasma levels and AUC). Products include:
Tagamet 2516
Deslanoside (Potential for elevated digoxin levels).
No products indexed under this heading.
Dicumarol (Rare reports of increased prothrombin time).
No products indexed under this heading.
Digitoxin (Potential for elevated digoxin levels). Products include:
Crystodigin Tablets 1433
Digoxin (Potential for elevated digoxin levels). Products include:
Lanoxicaps 1117
Lanoxin Elixir Pediatric 1120
Lanoxin Injection 1123
Lanoxin Injection Pediatric 1126
Lanoxin Tablets 1128
Esmolol Hydrochloride (Potential for congestive heart failure, severe hypotension, or exacerbation of angina). Products include:
Brevibloc Injection 1808
Ethacrynic Acid (Serum potassium slightly decreased). Products include:
Edecrin Tablets 1657
Fentanyl Citrate (Severe hypotension and/or increased fluid volume requirements have been reported in patients receiving nifedipine together with a beta blocker undergoing high dose fentanyl anesthesia). Products include:
Sublimaze Injection 1307
Furosemide (Serum potassium slightly decreased). Products include:
Lasix Injection, Oral Solution and Tablets 1240
Hydrochlorothiazide (Serum potassium slightly decreased). Products include:
Aldactazide 2413
Aldoril Tablets 1604
Apresazide Capsules 808
Capozide 742
Dyazide 2479
Esidrix Tablets 821
Esimil Tablets 822
HydroDIURIL Tablets 1674
Hydropres Tablets 1675
Hyzaar Tablets 1677
Inderide Tablets 2732
Inderide LA Long Acting Capsules 2734
Lopressor HCT Tablets 832
Lotensin HCT 837
Maxzide 1380
Moduretic Tablets 1705
Oretic Tablets 443
Prinzide Tablets 1737
Ser-Ap-Es Tablets 849
Timolide Tablets 1748
Vaseretic Tablets 1765
Zestoretic 2850
Ziac 1415
Hydroflumethiazide (Serum potassium slightly decreased). Products include:
Diucardin Tablets 2718
Indapamide (Serum potassium slightly decreased). Products include:
Lozol Tablets 2022
Labetalol Hydrochloride (Potential for congestive heart failure, severe hypotension, or exacerbation of angina). Products include:
Normodyne Injection 2377
Normodyne Tablets 2379
Trandate 1185
Levobunolol Hydrochloride (Potential for congestive heart failure, severe hypotension, or exacerbation of angina). Products include:
Betagan .... ◉ 233
Methyclothiazide (Serum potassium slightly decreased). Products include:
Enduron Tablets 420
Metipranolol Hydrochloride (Potential for congestive heart failure, severe hypotension, or exacerbation of angina). Products include:
OptiPranolol (Metipranolol 0.3%) Sterile Ophthalmic Solution .... ◉ 258
Metolazone (Serum potassium slightly decreased). Products include:
Mykrox Tablets 993
Zaroxolyn Tablets 1000
Metoprolol Succinate (Potential for congestive heart failure, severe hypotension, or exacerbation of angina). Products include:
Toprol-XL Tablets 565
Metoprolol Tartrate (Potential for congestive heart failure, severe hypotension, or exacerbation of angina). Products include:
Lopressor Ampuls 830
Lopressor HCT Tablets 832
Lopressor Tablets 830
Nadolol (Potential for congestive heart failure, severe hypotension, or exacerbation of angina).
No products indexed under this heading.
Penbutolol Sulfate (Potential for congestive heart failure, severe hypotension, or exacerbation of angina). Products include:
Levatol 2403
Pindolol (Potential for congestive heart failure, severe hypotension, or exacerbation of angina). Products include:
Visken Tablets 2299
Polythiazide (Serum potassium slightly decreased). Products include:
Minizide Capsules 1938
Propranolol Hydrochloride (Potential for congestive heart failure, severe hypotension, or exacerbation of angina). Products include:
Inderal 2728
Inderal LA Long Acting Capsules 2730
Inderide Tablets 2732
Inderide LA Long Acting Capsules 2734
Ranitidine Hydrochloride (Co-administration produces smaller non-significant increases in nifedipine level). Products include:
Zantac 1209
Zantac Injection 1207
Zantac Syrup 1209
Sotalol Hydrochloride (Potential for congestive heart failure, severe hypotension, or exacerbation of angina). Products include:
Betapace Tablets 641
Spironolactone (Serum potassium slightly decreased). Products include:
Aldactazide 2413
Aldactone 2414
Timolol Hemihydrate (Potential for congestive heart failure, severe hypotension, or exacerbation of angina). Products include:
Betimol 0.25%, 0.5% .... ◉ 261
Timolol Maleate (Potential for congestive heart failure, severe hypotension, or exacerbation of angina). Products include:
Blocadren Tablets 1614
Timolide Tablets 1748
Timoptic in Ocudose 1753
Timoptic Sterile Ophthalmic Solution 1751
Timoptic-XE 1755
Torsemide (Serum potassium slightly decreased). Products include:
Demadex Tablets and Injection 686
Triamterene (Serum potassium slightly decreased). Products include:
Dyazide 2479
Dyrenium Capsules 2481
Maxzide 1380
Warfarin Sodium (Rare reports of increased prothrombin time). Products include:
Coumadin 926

Food Interactions

Food, unspecified (Presence of food slightly alters the early rate of drug absorption).

PRO-CLUDE TRANSPARENT WOUND DRESSING

(Dressings, sterile) 2867

None cited in PDR database.

PROCRIT FOR INJECTION

(Epoetin Alfa) 1841

None cited in PDR database.

PROCTOCREAM-HC
(Hydrocortisone Acetate, Pramoxine Hydrochloride) 2408
None cited in PDR database.

PROCTOCREAM-HC 2.5%
(Hydrocortisone) 2408
None cited in PDR database.

PROCTOFOAM-HC
(Hydrocortisone Acetate, Pramoxine Hydrochloride) 2409
None cited in PDR database.

PRODIUM
(Phenazopyridine Hydrochloride) 690
None cited in PDR database.

PROFASI (CHORIONIC GONADOTROPIN FOR INJECTION, USP)
(Chorionic Gonadotropin) 2450
None cited in PDR database.

PROFENAL 1% STERILE OPHTHALMIC SOLUTION
(Suprofen) .... ⊙ 227
May interact with oral anticoagulants and certain other agents. Compounds in these categories include:

Dicumarol (Use with caution).
No products indexed under this heading.

Warfarin Sodium (Use with caution). Products include:
Coumadin 926

PROGLYCEM CAPSULES
(Diazoxide) 580
May interact with oral anticoagulants, thiazides, diuretics, and certain other agents. Compounds in these categories include:

Amiloride Hydrochloride (Concomitant administration may potentiate the hyperglycemic and hyperuricemic effects of diazoxide). Products include:
Midamor Tablets 1703
Moduretic Tablets 1705

Bendroflumethiazide (Concomitant administration may potentiate the hyperglycemic and hyperuricemic effects of diazoxide).
No products indexed under this heading.

Bumetanide (Concomitant administration may potentiate the hyperglycemic and hyperuricemic effects of diazoxide). Products include:
Bumex 2093

Chlorothiazide (Concomitant administration may potentiate the hyperglycemic and hyperuricemic effects of diazoxide). Products include:
Aldoclor Tablets 1598
Diupres Tablets 1650
Diuril Oral 1653

Chlorothiazide Sodium (Concomitant administration may potentiate the hyperglycemic and hyperuricemic effects of diazoxide). Products include:
Diuril Sodium Intravenous 1652

Chlorthalidone (Concomitant administration may potentiate the hyperglycemic and hyperuricemic effects of diazoxide). Products include:
Combipres Tablets 677
Tenoretic Tablets 2845
Thalitone 1245

Dicumarol (Increased blood levels of coumarin derivatives).
No products indexed under this heading.

Ethacrynic Acid (Concomitant administration may potentiate the hyperglycemic and hyperuricemic effects of diazoxide). Products include:
Edecrin Tablets 1657

Furosemide (Concomitant administration may potentiate the hyperglycemic and hyperuricemic effects of diazoxide). Products include:
Lasix Injection, Oral Solution and Tablets 1240

Hydrochlorothiazide (Concomitant administration may potentiate the hyperglycemic and hyperuricemic effects of diazoxide). Products include:
Aldactazide 2413
Aldoril Tablets 1604
Apresazide Capsules 808
Capozide 742
Dyazide 2479
Esidrix Tablets 821
Esimil Tablets 822
HydroDIURIL Tablets 1674
Hydropres Tablets 1675
Hyzaar Tablets 1677
Inderide Tablets 2732
Inderide LA Long Acting Capsules .. 2734
Lopressor HCT Tablets 832
Lotensin HCT 837
Maxzide 1380
Moduretic Tablets 1705
Oretic Tablets 443
Prinzide Tablets 1737
Ser-Ap-Es Tablets 849
Timolide Tablets 1748
Vaseretic Tablets 1765
Zestoretic 2850
Ziac 1415

Hydroflumethiazide (Concomitant administration may potentiate the hyperglycemic and hyperuricemic effects of diazoxide). Products include:
Diucardin Tablets 2718

Indapamide (Concomitant administration may potentiate the hyperglycemic and hyperuricemic effects of diazoxide). Products include:
Lozol Tablets 2022

Methyclothiazide (Concomitant administration may potentiate the hyperglycemic and hyperuricemic effects of diazoxide). Products include:
Enduron Tablets 420

Metolazone (Concomitant administration may potentiate the hyperglycemic and hyperuricemic effects of diazoxide). Products include:
Mykrox Tablets 993
Zaroxolyn Tablets 1000

Phenytoin (Concomitant administration with oral diazoxide may result in a loss of seizure control). Products include:
Dilantin Infatabs 1908
Dilantin-125 Suspension 1911

Phenytoin Sodium (Concomitant administration with oral diazoxide may result in a loss of seizure control). Products include:
Dilantin Kapseals 1906
Dilantin Parenteral 1910

Polythiazide (Concomitant administration may potentiate the hyperglycemic and hyperuricemic effects of diazoxide). Products include:
Minizide Capsules 1938

Spironolactone (Concomitant administration may potentiate the hyperglycemic and hyperuricemic effects of diazoxide). Products include:
Aldactazide 2413
Aldactone 2414

Torsemide (Concomitant administration may potentiate the hyperglycemic and hyperuricemic effects of diazoxide). Products include:
Demadex Tablets and Injection 686

Triamterene (Concomitant administration may potentiate the hyperglycemic and hyperuricemic effects of diazoxide). Products include:
Dyazide 2479
Dyrenium Capsules 2481
Maxzide 1380

Warfarin Sodium (Increased blood levels of coumarin derivatives). Products include:
Coumadin 926

PROGLYCEM SUSPENSION
(Diazoxide) 580
See **Proglycem Capsules**

PROGRAF
(Tacrolimus) 1042
May interact with immunosuppressive agents, potassium sparing diuretics, aminoglycosides, and certain other agents. Compounds in these categories include:

Amikacin Sulfate (Potential for additive or synergistic impairment of renal function). Products include:
Amikacin Sulfate Injection, USP 960
Amikin Injectable 501

Amiloride Hydrochloride (Mild to severe hyperkalemia has been reported with tacrolimus; concurrent use with potassium sparing diuretics should be avoided). Products include:
Midamor Tablets 1703
Moduretic Tablets 1705

Amphotericin B (Potential for additive or synergistic impairment of renal function). Products include:
Fungizone Intravenous 506

Azathioprine (Concurrent use should be avoided). Products include:
Imuran 1110

Bromocriptine Mesylate (May increase tacrolimus blood levels). Products include:
Parlodel 2281

Carbamazepine (May decrease tacrolimus blood levels). Products include:
Atretol Tablets 573
Tegretol Chewable Tablets 852
Tegretol Suspension 852
Tegretol Tablets 852

Cimetidine (May increase tacrolimus blood levels). Products include:
Tagamet Tablets 2516

Cimetidine Hydrochloride (May increase tacrolimus blood levels). Products include:
Tagamet 2516

Cisplatin (Potential for additive or synergistic impairment of renal function). Products include:
Platinol 708
Platinol-AQ Injection 710

Clarithromycin (May increase tacrolimus blood levels). Products include:
Biaxin 405

Clotrimazole (May increase tacrolimus blood levels). Products include:
Prescription Strength Desenex Cream .... ⊡ 633
Gyne-Lotrimin .... ⊡ 805
Gyne-Lotrimin Pack .... ⊡ 806
Lotrimin 2371
Lotrimin AF Antifungal Cream, Lotion and Solution .... ⊡ 806
Lotrisone Cream 2372
Mycelex OTC Cream Antifungal .... ⊡ 724
Mycelex OTC Solution Antifungal .. ⊡ 724
Mycelex Troches 608
Mycelex-7 Vaginal Cream Antifungal .... ⊡ 724
Mycelex-7 Vaginal Antifungal Cream with 7 Disposable Applicators .... ⊡ 724
Mycelex-7 Vaginal Inserts Antifungal .... ⊡ 725
Mycelex-7 Combination-Pack Vaginal Inserts & External Vulvar Cream .... ⊡ 725
Mycelex-G 500 mg Vaginal Tablets 609

Cyclosporine (Increases tacrolimus blood levels resulting in additive/synergistic nephrotoxicity; Prograf should not be used simultaneously with cyclosporine; Prograf or cyclosporine should be discontinued at least 24 hours or more prior to initiating the other). Products include:
Neoral 2276
Sandimmune 2286

Danazol (May increase tacrolimus blood levels). Products include:
Danocrine Capsules 2307

Diltiazem Hydrochloride (May increase tacrolimus blood levels). Products include:
Cardizem CD Capsules 1506
Cardizem SR Capsules 1510
Cardizem Injectable 1508
Cardizem Tablets 1512
Dilacor XR Extended-release Capsules 2018

Erythromycin (May increase tacrolimus blood levels). Products include:
A/T/S 2% Acne Topical Gel and Solution 1234
Benzamycin Topical Gel 905
E-Mycin Tablets 1341
Emgel 2% Topical Gel 1093
ERYC 1915
Erycette (erythromycin 2%) Topical Solution 1888
Ery-Tab Tablets 422
Erythromycin Base Filmtab 426
Erythromycin Delayed-Release Capsules, USP 427
Ilotycin Ophthalmic Ointment 912
PCE Dispertab Tablets 444
T-Stat 2.0% Topical Solution and Pads 2688
Theramycin Z Topical Solution 2% 1592

Erythromycin Estolate (May increase tacrolimus blood levels). Products include:
Ilosone 911

Erythromycin Ethylsuccinate (May increase tacrolimus blood levels). Products include:
E.E.S. 424
EryPed 421

Erythromycin Gluceptate (May increase tacrolimus blood levels). Products include:
Ilotycin Gluceptate, IV, Vials 913

Erythromycin Stearate (May increase tacrolimus blood levels). Products include:
Erythrocin Stearate Filmtab 425

Fluconazole (May increase tacrolimus blood levels). Products include:
Diflucan Injection, Tablets, and Oral Suspension 2194

Gentamicin Sulfate (Potential for additive or synergistic impairment of renal function). Products include:
Garamycin Injectable 2360
Genoptic Sterile Ophthalmic Solution .... ⊙ 243
Genoptic Sterile Ophthalmic Ointment .... ⊙ 243
Gentacidin Ointment .... ⊙ 264
Gentacidin Solution .... ⊙ 264
Gentak .... ⊙ 208
Pred-G Liquifilm Sterile Ophthalmic Suspension .... ⊙ 251
Pred-G S.O.P. Sterile Ophthalmic Ointment .... ⊙ 252

IMPORTANT NOTE: Always consult each drug listing in the patient's regimen for possible interactions.

Itraconazole (May increase tacrolimus blood levels). Products include:

Sporanox Capsules 1305

Kanamycin Sulfate (Potential for additive or synergistic impairment of renal function).

No products indexed under this heading.

Ketoconazole (May increase tacrolimus blood levels). Products include:

Nizoral 2% Cream 1297
Nizoral 2% Shampoo 1298
Nizoral Tablets 1298

Measles Virus Vaccine Live (During treatment with tacrolimus, vaccination may be less effective). Products include:

Attenuvax 1610

Measles & Rubella Virus Vaccine Live (During treatment with tacrolimus, vaccination may be less effective). Products include:

M-R-VAX II 1689

Measles, Mumps & Rubella Virus Vaccine Live (During treatment with tacrolimus, vaccination may be less effective). Products include:

M-M-R II 1687

Methylprednisolone (May increase tacrolimus blood levels). Products include:

Medrol 2621

Methylprednisolone Acetate (May increase tacrolimus blood levels). Products include:

Depo-Medrol Single-Dose Vial 2600
Depo-Medrol Sterile Aqueous Suspension 2597

Methylprednisolone Sodium Succinate (May increase tacrolimus blood levels). Products include:

Solu-Medrol Sterile Powder 2643

Metoclopramide Hydrochloride (May increase tacrolimus blood levels). Products include:

Reglan 2068

Muromonab-CD3 (Concurrent use should be avoided). Products include:

Orthoclone OKT3 Sterile Solution .. 1837

Mycophenolate Mofetil (Concurrent use should be avoided). Products include:

CellCept Capsules 2099

Nicardipine Hydrochloride (May increase tacrolimus blood levels). Products include:

Cardene Capsules 2095
Cardene I.V. 2709
Cardene SR Capsules 2097

Phenobarbital (May decrease tacrolimus blood levels). Products include:

Arco-Lase Plus Tablets 512
Bellergal-S Tablets 2250
Donnatal 2060
Donnatal Extentabs 2061
Donnatal Tablets 2060
Phenobarbital Elixir and Tablets 1469
Quadrinal Tablets 1350

Phenytoin (May decrease tacrolimus blood levels). Products include:

Dilantin Infatabs 1908
Dilantin-125 Suspension 1911

Phenytoin Sodium (May decrease tacrolimus blood levels). Products include:

Dilantin Kapseals 1906
Dilantin Parenteral 1910

Poliovirus Vaccine Inactivated, Trivalent Types 1,2,3 (During treatment with tacrolimus, vaccination may be less effective). Products include:

IPOL Poliovirus Vaccine Inactivated 885
Poliovax 891

Poliovirus Vaccine, Live, Oral, Trivalent, Types 1,2,3 (Sabin) (During treatment with tacrolimus, vaccination may be less effective). Products include:

Orimune 1388

Rifabutin (May decrease tacrolimus blood levels). Products include:

Mycobutin Capsules 1957

Rifampin (May decrease tacrolimus blood levels). Products include:

Rifadin 1528
Rifamate Capsules 1530
Rifater 1532
Rimactane Capsules 847

Spironolactone (Mild to severe hyperkalemia has been reported with tacrolimus; concurrent use with potassium sparing diuretics should be avoided). Products include:

Aldactazide 2413
Aldactone 2414

Streptomycin Sulfate (Potential for additive or synergistic impairment of renal function). Products include:

Streptomycin Sulfate Injection 2208

Tobramycin (Potential for additive or synergistic impairment of renal function). Products include:

AKTOB .... ◉ 206
TobraDex Ophthalmic Suspension and Ointment 473
Tobrex Ophthalmic Ointment and Solution .... ◉ 229

Tobramycin Sulfate (Potential for additive or synergistic impairment of renal function). Products include:

Nebcin Vials, Hyporets & ADD-Vantage 1464
Tobramycin Sulfate Injection 968

Triamterene (Mild to severe hyperkalemia has been reported with tacrolimus; concurrent use with potassium sparing diuretics should be avoided). Products include:

Dyazide 2479
Dyrenium Capsules 2481
Maxzide 1380

Troleandomycin (Increases tacrolimus blood levels). Products include:

Tao Capsules 2209

Typhoid Vaccine Live Oral TY21a (During treatment with tacrolimus, vaccination may be less effective). Products include:

Vivotif Berna 665

Vaccines (Live) (During treatment with tacrolimus, vaccination may be less effective).

Verapamil Hydrochloride (May increase tacrolimus blood levels). Products include:

Calan SR Caplets 2422
Calan Tablets 2419
Isoptin Injectable 1344
Isoptin Oral Tablets 1346
Isoptin SR Tablets 1348
Verelan Capsules 1410
Verelan Capsules 2824

Yellow Fever Vaccine (During treatment with tacrolimus, vaccination may be less effective).

No products indexed under this heading.

Food Interactions

Meal, unspecified (The presence of food reduces the absorption of tacrolimus (decrease in AUC and C_{max}, and increase in T_{max}).

PRO-HEPATONE CAPSULES

(Vitamins with Minerals, Amino Acid Preparations) 1542
None cited in PDR database.

PROLASTIN ALPHA$_1$-PROTEINASE INHIBITOR (HUMAN)

(Alpha$_1$-Proteinase Inhibitor (Human)) 635
None cited in PDR database.

PROLEUKIN FOR INJECTION

(Aldesleukin) 797

May interact with beta blockers, antihypertensives, narcotic analgesics, hypnotics and sedatives, tranquilizers, aminoglycosides, radiographic iodinated contrast media, cytotoxic drugs, glucocorticoids, and certain other agents. Compounds in these categories include:

Acebutolol Hydrochloride (May potentiate the hypotension seen with aldesleukin). Products include:

Sectral Capsules 2807

Alfentanil Hydrochloride (Potential for unspecified effect on central nervous function). Products include:

Alfenta Injection 1286

Alprazolam (Potential for unspecified effect on central nervous function). Products include:

Xanax Tablets 2649

Amikacin Sulfate (Potential for increased nephrotoxicity). Products include:

Amikacin Sulfate Injection, USP 960
Amikin Injectable 501

Amlodipine Besylate (May potentiate the hypotension seen with aldesleukin). Products include:

Lotrel Capsules 840
Norvasc Tablets 1940

Asparaginase (Potential for increased hepatic toxicity). Products include:

Elspar 1659

Atenolol (May potentiate the hypotension seen with aldesleukin). Products include:

Tenoretic Tablets 2845
Tenormin Tablets and I.V. Injection 2847

Benazepril Hydrochloride (May potentiate the hypotension seen with aldesleukin). Products include:

Lotensin Tablets 834
Lotensin HCT 837
Lotrel Capsules 840

Bendroflumethiazide (May potentiate the hypotension seen with aldesleukin).

No products indexed under this heading.

Betamethasone Acetate (May reduce the antitumor effectiveness of aldesleukin). Products include:

Celestone Soluspan Suspension 2347

Betamethasone Sodium Phosphate (May reduce the antitumor effectiveness of aldesleukin). Products include:

Celestone Soluspan Suspension 2347

Betaxolol Hydrochloride (May potentiate the hypotension seen with aldesleukin). Products include:

Betoptic Ophthalmic Solution 469
Betoptic S Ophthalmic Suspension 471
Kerlone Tablets 2436

Bisoprolol Fumarate (May potentiate the hypotension seen with aldesleukin). Products include:

Zebeta Tablets 1413
Ziac 1415

Bleomycin Sulfate (Potential for increased myelotoxicity). Products include:

Blenoxane 692

Buprenorphine (Potential for unspecified effect on central nervous function). Products include:

Buprenex Injectable 2006

Buspirone Hydrochloride (Potential for unspecified effect on central nervous function). Products include:

BuSpar 737

Captopril (May potentiate the hypotension seen with aldesleukin). Products include:

Capoten 739
Capozide 742

Carteolol Hydrochloride (May potentiate the hypotension seen with aldesleukin). Products include:

Cartrol Tablets 410
Ocupress Ophthalmic Solution, 1% Sterile .... ◉ 309

Chlordiazepoxide (Potential for unspecified effect on central nervous function). Products include:

Libritabs Tablets 2177
Limbitrol 2180

Chlordiazepoxide Hydrochloride (Potential for unspecified effect on central nervous function). Products include:

Librax Capsules 2176
Librium Capsules 2178
Librium Injectable 2179

Chlorothiazide (May potentiate the hypotension seen with aldesleukin). Products include:

Aldoclor Tablets 1598
Diupres Tablets 1650
Diuril Oral 1653

Chlorothiazide Sodium (May potentiate the hypotension seen with aldesleukin). Products include:

Diuril Sodium Intravenous 1652

Chlorpromazine (Potential for unspecified effect on central nervous function). Products include:

Thorazine Suppositories 2523

Chlorprothixene (Potential for unspecified effect on central nervous function).

No products indexed under this heading.

Chlorprothixene Hydrochloride (Potential for unspecified effect on central nervous function).

No products indexed under this heading.

Chlorthalidone (May potentiate the hypotension seen with aldesleukin). Products include:

Combipres Tablets 677
Tenoretic Tablets 2845
Thalitone 1245

Clonidine (May potentiate the hypotension seen with aldesleukin). Products include:

Catapres-TTS 675

Clonidine Hydrochloride (May potentiate the hypotension seen with aldesleukin). Products include:

Catapres Tablets 674
Combipres Tablets 677

Clorazepate Dipotassium (Potential for unspecified effect on central nervous function). Products include:

Tranxene 451

Codeine Phosphate (Potential for unspecified effect on central nervous function). Products include:

Actifed with Codeine Cough Syrup.. 1067
Brontex 1981
Deconsal C Expectorant Syrup 456
Deconsal Pediatric Syrup 457
Dimetane-DC Cough Syrup 2059

843 **Interactions Index** **Proleukin**

Empirin with Codeine Tablets ... 1093
Fioricet with Codeine Capsules ... 2260
Fiorinal with Codeine Capsules ... 2262
Isoclor Expectorant ... 990
Novahistine DH ... 2462
Novahistine Expectorant ... 2463
Nucofed ... 2051
Phenergan with Codeine ... 2777
Phenergan VC with Codeine ... 2781
Robitussin A-C Syrup ... 2073
Robitussin-DAC Syrup ... 2074
Ryna ... ▣ 841
Soma Compound w/Codeine Tablets ... 2676
Tussi-Organidin NR Liquid and S NR Liquid ... 2677
Tylenol with Codeine ... 1583

Cortisone Acetate (May reduce the antitumor effectiveness of aldesleukin). Products include:
Cortone Acetate Sterile Suspension ... 1623
Cortone Acetate Tablets ... 1624

Daunorubicin Hydrochloride (Potential for increased myelotoxicity). Products include:
Cerubidine ... 795

Deserpidine (May potentiate the hypotension seen with aldesleukin).
No products indexed under this heading.

Dexamethasone (May reduce the antitumor effectiveness of aldesleukin). Products include:
AK-Trol Ointment & Suspension ... ◉ 205
Decadron Elixir ... 1633
Decadron Tablets ... 1635
Decaspray Topical Aerosol ... 1648
Dexacidin Ointment ... ◉ 263
Maxitrol Ophthalmic Ointment and Suspension ... ◉ 224
TobraDex Ophthalmic Suspension and Ointment ... 473

Dexamethasone Acetate (May reduce the antitumor effectiveness of aldesleukin). Products include:
Dalalone D.P. Injectable ... 1011
Decadron-LA Sterile Suspension ... 1646

Dexamethasone Sodium Phosphate (May reduce the antitumor effectiveness of aldesleukin). Products include:
Decadron Phosphate Injection ... 1637
Decadron Phosphate Respihaler ... 1642
Decadron Phosphate Sterile Ophthalmic Ointment ... 1641
Decadron Phosphate Sterile Ophthalmic Solution ... 1642
Decadron Phosphate Topical Cream ... 1644
Decadron Phosphate Turbinaire ... 1645
Decadron Phosphate with Xylocaine Injection, Sterile ... 1639
Dexacort Phosphate in Respihaler ... 458
Dexacort Phosphate in Turbinaire ... 459
NeoDecadron Sterile Ophthalmic Ointment ... 1712
NeoDecadron Sterile Ophthalmic Solution ... 1713
NeoDecadron Topical Cream ... 1714

Dezocine (Potential for unspecified effect on central nervous function). Products include:
Dalgan Injection ... 538

Diatrizoate Meglumine (Potential for delayed adverse reactions to iodinated contrast media including fever, chills, nausea, vomiting, pruritus, rash, diarrhea, hypotension, edema, and oliguria).

Diatrizoate Sodium (Potential for delayed adverse reactions to iodinated contrast media including fever, chills, nausea, vomiting, pruritus, rash, diarrhea, hypotension, edema, and oliguria).

Diazepam (Potential for unspecified effect on central nervous function). Products include:
Dizac ... 1809
Valium Injectable ... 2182
Valium Tablets ... 2183
Valrelease Capsules ... 2169

Diazoxide (May potentiate the hypotension seen with aldesleukin). Products include:
Hyperstat I.V. Injection ... 2363
Proglycem ... 580

Diltiazem Hydrochloride (May potentiate the hypotension seen with aldesleukin). Products include:
Cardizem CD Capsules ... 1506
Cardizem SR Capsules ... 1510
Cardizem Injectable ... 1508
Cardizem Tablets ... 1512
Dilacor XR Extended-release Capsules ... 2018

Doxazosin Mesylate (May potentiate the hypotension seen with aldesleukin). Products include:
Cardura Tablets ... 2186

Doxorubicin Hydrochloride (Potential for increased cardiotoxicity and myelotoxicity). Products include:
Adriamycin PFS ... 1947
Adriamycin RDF ... 1947
Doxorubicin Astra ... 540
Rubex ... 712

Droperidol (Potential for unspecified effect on central nervous function). Products include:
Inapsine Injection ... 1296

Enalapril Maleate (May potentiate the hypotension seen with aldesleukin). Products include:
Vaseretic Tablets ... 1765
Vasotec Tablets ... 1771

Enalaprilat (May potentiate the hypotension seen with aldesleukin). Products include:
Vasotec I.V. ... 1768

Esmolol Hydrochloride (May potentiate the hypotension seen with aldesleukin). Products include:
Brevibloc Injection ... 1808

Estazolam (Potential for unspecified effect on central nervous function). Products include:
ProSom Tablets ... 449

Ethchlorvynol (Potential for unspecified effect on central nervous function). Products include:
Placidyl Capsules ... 448

Ethinamate (Potential for unspecified effect on central nervous function).
No products indexed under this heading.

Ethiodized Oil (Potential for delayed adverse reactions to iodinated contrast media including fever, chills, nausea, vomiting, pruritus, rash, diarrhea, hypotension, edema, and oliguria).
No products indexed under this heading.

Felodipine (May potentiate the hypotension seen with aldesleukin). Products include:
Plendil Extended-Release Tablets ... 527

Fentanyl (Potential for unspecified effect on central nervous function). Products include:
Duragesic Transdermal System ... 1288

Fentanyl Citrate (Potential for unspecified effect on central nervous function). Products include:
Sublimaze Injection ... 1307

Fludrocortisone Acetate (May reduce the antitumor effectiveness of aldesleukin). Products include:
Florinef Acetate Tablets ... 505

Fluorouracil (Potential for increased myelotoxicity). Products include:
Efudex ... 2113
Fluoroplex Topical Solution & Cream 1% ... 479
Fluorouracil Injection ... 2116

Fluphenazine Decanoate (Potential for unspecified effect on central nervous function). Products include:
Prolixin Decanoate ... 509

Fluphenazine Enanthate (Potential for unspecified effect on central nervous function). Products include:
Prolixin Enanthate ... 509

Fluphenazine Hydrochloride (Potential for unspecified effect on central nervous function). Products include:
Prolixin ... 509

Flurazepam Hydrochloride (Potential for unspecified effect on central nervous function). Products include:
Dalmane Capsules ... 2173

Fosinopril Sodium (May potentiate the hypotension seen with aldesleukin). Products include:
Monopril Tablets ... 757

Furosemide (May potentiate the hypotension seen with aldesleukin). Products include:
Lasix Injection, Oral Solution and Tablets ... 1240

Gadopentetate Dimeglumine (Potential for delayed adverse reactions to iodinated contrast media including fever, chills, nausea, vomiting, pruritus, rash, diarrhea, hypotension, edema, and oliguria).
No products indexed under this heading.

Gentamicin Sulfate (Potential for increased nephrotoxicity). Products include:
Garamycin Injectable ... 2360
Genoptic Sterile Ophthalmic Solution ... ◉ 243
Genoptic Sterile Ophthalmic Ointment ... ◉ 243
Gentacidin Ointment ... ◉ 264
Gentacidin Solution ... ◉ 264
Gentak ... ◉ 208
Pred-G Liquifilm Sterile Ophthalmic Suspension ... ◉ 251
Pred-G S.O.P. Sterile Ophthalmic Ointment ... ◉ 252

Glutethimide (Potential for unspecified effect on central nervous function).
No products indexed under this heading.

Guanabenz Acetate (May potentiate the hypotension seen with aldesleukin).
No products indexed under this heading.

Guanethidine Monosulfate (May potentiate the hypotension seen with aldesleukin). Products include:
Esimil Tablets ... 822
Ismelin Tablets ... 827

Haloperidol (Potential for unspecified effect on central nervous function). Products include:
Haldol Injection, Tablets and Concentrate ... 1575

Haloperidol Decanoate (Potential for unspecified effect on central nervous function). Products include:
Haldol Decanoate ... 1577

Hepatotoxic Drugs, unspecified (Potential for increased hepatic toxicity).

Hydralazine Hydrochloride (May potentiate the hypotension seen with aldesleukin). Products include:
Apresazide Capsules ... 808
Apresoline Hydrochloride Tablets ... 809
Ser-Ap-Es Tablets ... 849

Hydrochlorothiazide (May potentiate the hypotension seen with aldesleukin). Products include:
Aldactazide ... 2413
Aldoril Tablets ... 1604
Apresazide Capsules ... 808
Capozide ... 742
Dyazide ... 2479
Esidrix Tablets ... 821
Esimil Tablets ... 822
HydroDIURIL Tablets ... 1674
Hydropres Tablets ... 1675
Hyzaar Tablets ... 1677
Inderide Tablets ... 2732
Inderide LA Long Acting Capsules ... 2734
Lopressor HCT Tablets ... 832
Lotensin HCT ... 837
Maxzide ... 1380
Moduretic Tablets ... 1705
Oretic Tablets ... 443
Prinzide Tablets ... 1737
Ser-Ap-Es Tablets ... 849
Timolide Tablets ... 1748
Vaseretic Tablets ... 1765
Zestoretic ... 2850
Ziac ... 1415

Hydrocodone Bitartrate (Potential for unspecified effect on central nervous function). Products include:
Anexsia 5/500 Elixir ... 1781
Anexia Tablets ... 1782
Codiclear DH Syrup ... 791
Deconamine CX Cough and Cold Liquid and Tablets ... 1319
Duratuss HD Elixir ... 2565
Hycodan Tablets and Syrup ... 930
Hycomine Compound Tablets ... 932
Hycomine ... 931
Hycotuss Expectorant Syrup ... 933
Hydrocet Capsules ... 782
Lorcet 10/650 ... 1018
Lortab ... 2566
Tussend ... 1783
Tussend Expectorant ... 1785
Vicodin Tablets ... 1356
Vicodin ES Tablets ... 1357
Vicodin Tuss Expectorant ... 1358
Zydone Capsules ... 949

Hydrocodone Polistirex (Potential for unspecified effect on central nervous function). Products include:
Tussionex Pennkinetic Extended-Release Suspension ... 998

Hydrocortisone (May reduce the antitumor effectiveness of aldesleukin). Products include:
Anusol-HC Cream 2.5% ... 1896
Aquanil HC Lotion ... 1931
Bactine Hydrocortisone Anti-Itch Cream ... ▣ 709
Caldecort Anti-Itch Hydrocortisone Spray ... ▣ 631
Cortaid ... ▣ 836
CORTENEMA ... 2535
Cortisporin Ointment ... 1085
Cortisporin Ophthalmic Ointment Sterile ... 1085
Cortisporin Ophthalmic Suspension Sterile ... 1086
Cortisporin Otic Solution Sterile ... 1087
Cortisporin Otic Suspension Sterile ... 1088
Cortizone-5 ... ▣ 831
Cortizone-10 ... ▣ 831
Hydrocortone Tablets ... 1672
Hytone ... 907
Massengill Medicated Soft Cloth Towelettes ... 2458
PediOtic Suspension Sterile ... 1153
Preparation H Hydrocortisone 1% Cream ... ▣ 872
ProctoCream-HC 2.5% ... 2408
VōSoL HC Otic Solution ... 2678

Hydrocortisone Acetate (May reduce the antitumor effectiveness of aldesleukin). Products include:
Analpram-HC Rectal Cream 1% and 2.5% ... 977
Anusol HC-1 Anti-Itch Hydrocortisone Ointment ... ▣ 847
Anusol-HC Suppositories ... 1897
Caldecort ... ▣ 631
Carmol HC ... 924
Coly-Mycin S Otic w/Neomycin & Hydrocortisone ... 1906
Cortaid ... ▣ 836
Cortifoam ... 2396
Cortisporin Cream ... 1084
Epifoam ... 2399
Hydrocortone Acetate Sterile Suspension ... 1669
Mantadil Cream ... 1135
Nupercainal Hydrocortisone 1% Cream ... ▣ 645

IMPORTANT NOTE: Always consult each drug listing in the patient's regimen for possible interactions.

Proleukin Interactions Index 844

Ophthocort ⊙ 311
Pramosone Cream, Lotion & Ointment 978
ProctoCream-HC 2408
ProctoFoam-HC 2409
Terra-Cortril Ophthalmic Suspension 2210

Hydrocortisone Sodium Phosphate (May reduce the antitumor effectiveness of aldesleukin). Products include:
Hydrocortone Phosphate Injection, Sterile 1670

Hydrocortisone Sodium Succinate (May reduce the antitumor effectiveness of aldesleukin). Products include:
Solu-Cortef Sterile Powder 2641

Hydroflumethiazide (May potentiate the hypotension seen with aldesleukin). Products include:
Diucardin Tablets 2718

Hydroxyurea (Potential for increased myelotoxicity). Products include:
Hydrea Capsules 696

Hydroxyzine Hydrochloride (Potential for unspecified effect on central nervous function). Products include:
Atarax Tablets & Syrup 2185
Marax Tablets & DF Syrup 2200
Vistaril Intramuscular Solution 2216

Indapamide (May potentiate the hypotension seen with aldesleukin). Products include:
Lozol Tablets 2022

Indomethacin (Potential for increased nephrotoxicity). Products include:
Indocin 1680

Iodamide Meglumine (Potential for delayed adverse reactions to iodinated contrast media including fever, chills, nausea, vomiting, pruritus, rash, diarrhea, hypotension, edema, and oliguria).
No products indexed under this heading.

Iohexol (Potential for delayed adverse reactions to iodinated contrast media including fever, chills, nausea, vomiting, pruritus, rash, diarrhea, hypotension, edema, and oliguria).
No products indexed under this heading.

Iopamidol (Potential for delayed adverse reactions to iodinated contrast media including fever, chills, nausea, vomiting, pruritus, rash, diarrhea, hypotension, edema, and oliguria).
No products indexed under this heading.

Iothalamate Meglumine (Potential for delayed adverse reactions to iodinated contrast media including fever, chills, nausea, vomiting, pruritus, rash, diarrhea, hypotension, edema, and oliguria).
No products indexed under this heading.

Iopanoic Acid (Potential for delayed adverse reactions to iodinated contrast media including fever, chills, nausea, vomiting, pruritus, rash, diarrhea, hypotension, edema, and oliguria).

Ioxaglate Meglumine (Potential for delayed adverse reactions to iodinated contrast media including fever, chills, nausea, vomiting, pruritus, rash, diarrhea, hypotension, edema, and oliguria).
No products indexed under this heading.

Ioxaglate Sodium (Potential for delayed adverse reactions to iodinated contrast media including fever, chills, nausea, vomiting, pruritus, rash, diarrhea, hypotension, edema, and oliguria).
No products indexed under this heading.

Isradipine (May potentiate the hypotension seen with aldesleukin). Products include:
DynaCirc Capsules 2256

Kanamycin Sulfate (Potential for increased nephrotoxicity).
No products indexed under this heading.

Labetalol Hydrochloride (May potentiate the hypotension seen with aldesleukin). Products include:
Normodyne Injection 2377
Normodyne Tablets 2379
Trandate 1185

Levobunolol Hydrochloride (May potentiate the hypotension seen with aldesleukin). Products include:
Betagan ⊙ 233

Levorphanol Tartrate (Potential for unspecified effect on central nervous function). Products include:
Levo-Dromoran 2129

Lisinopril (May potentiate the hypotension seen with aldesleukin). Products include:
Prinivil Tablets 1733
Prinzide Tablets 1737
Zestoretic 2850
Zestril Tablets 2854

Lorazepam (Potential for unspecified effect on central nervous function). Products include:
Ativan Injection 2698
Ativan Tablets 2700

Losartan Potassium (May potentiate the hypotension seen with aldesleukin). Products include:
Cozaar Tablets 1628
Hyzaar Tablets 1677

Loxapine Hydrochloride (Potential for unspecified effect on central nervous function). Products include:
Loxitane 1378

Loxapine Succinate (Potential for unspecified effect on central nervous function). Products include:
Loxitane Capsules 1378

Mecamylamine Hydrochloride (May potentiate the hypotension seen with aldesleukin). Products include:
Inversine Tablets 1686

Meperidine Hydrochloride (Potential for unspecified effect on central nervous function). Products include:
Demerol 2308
Mepergan Injection 2753

Meprobamate (Potential for unspecified effect on central nervous function). Products include:
Miltown Tablets 2672
PMB 200 and PMB 400 2783

Mesoridazine Besylate (Potential for unspecified effect on central nervous function). Products include:
Serentil 684

Methadone Hydrochloride (Potential for unspecified effect on central nervous function). Products include:
Methadone Hydrochloride Oral Concentrate 2233
Methadone Hydrochloride Oral Solution & Tablets 2235

Methotrexate Sodium (Potential for increased hepatic toxicity and myelotoxicity). Products include:
Methotrexate Sodium Tablets, Injection, for Injection and LPF Injection 1275

Methyclothiazide (May potentiate the hypotension seen with aldesleukin). Products include:
Enduron Tablets 420

Methyldopa (May potentiate the hypotension seen with aldesleukin). Products include:
Aldoclor Tablets 1598
Aldomet Oral 1600
Aldoril Tablets 1604

Methyldopate Hydrochloride (May potentiate the hypotension seen with aldesleukin). Products include:
Aldomet Ester HCl Injection 1602

Methylprednisolone Acetate (May reduce the antitumor effectiveness of aldesleukin). Products include:
Depo-Medrol Single-Dose Vial 2600
Depo-Medrol Sterile Aqueous Suspension 2597

Methylprednisolone Sodium Succinate (May reduce the antitumor effectiveness of aldesleukin). Products include:
Solu-Medrol Sterile Powder 2643

Metipranolol Hydrochloride (May potentiate the hypotension seen with aldesleukin). Products include:
OptiPranolol (Metipranolol 0.3%) Sterile Ophthalmic Solution ⊙ 258

Metolazone (May potentiate the hypotension seen with aldesleukin). Products include:
Mykrox Tablets 993
Zaroxolyn Tablets 1000

Metoprolol Succinate (May potentiate the hypotension seen with aldesleukin). Products include:
Toprol-XL Tablets 565

Metoprolol Tartrate (May potentiate the hypotension seen with aldesleukin). Products include:
Lopressor Ampuls 830
Lopressor HCT Tablets 832
Lopressor Tablets 830

Metyrosine (May potentiate the hypotension seen with aldesleukin). Products include:
Demser Capsules 1649

Midazolam Hydrochloride (Potential for unspecified effect on central nervous function). Products include:
Versed Injection 2170

Minoxidil (May potentiate the hypotension seen with aldesleukin). Products include:
Loniten Tablets 2618
Rogaine Topical Solution 2637

Mitotane (Potential for increased myelotoxicity). Products include:
Lysodren 698

Mitoxantrone Hydrochloride (Potential for increased myelotoxicity). Products include:
Novantrone 1279

Moexipril Hydrochloride (May potentiate the hypotension seen with aldesleukin). Products include:
Univasc Tablets 2410

Molindone Hydrochloride (Potential for unspecified effect on central nervous function). Products include:
Moban Tablets and Concentrate 1048

Morphine Sulfate (Potential for unspecified effect on central nervous function). Products include:
Astramorph/PF Injection, USP (Preservative-Free) 535
Duramorph 962
Infumorph 200 and Infumorph 500 Sterile Solutions 965
MS Contin Tablets 1994
MSIR 1997
Oramorph SR (Morphine Sulfate Sustained Release Tablets) 2236
RMS Suppositories 2657
Roxanol 2243

Nadolol (May potentiate the hypotension seen with aldesleukin).
No products indexed under this heading.

Nephrotoxic Drugs (Potential for increased nephrotoxicity).

Nicardipine Hydrochloride (May potentiate the hypotension seen with aldesleukin). Products include:
Cardene Capsules 2095
Cardene I.V. 2709
Cardene SR Capsules 2097

Nifedipine (May potentiate the hypotension seen with aldesleukin). Products include:
Adalat Capsules (10 mg and 20 mg) 587
Adalat CC 589
Procardia Capsules 1971
Procardia XL Extended Release Tablets 1972

Nisoldipine (May potentiate the hypotension seen with aldesleukin).
No products indexed under this heading.

Nitroglycerin (May potentiate the hypotension seen with aldesleukin). Products include:
Deponit NTG Transdermal Delivery System 2397
Nitro-Bid IV 1523
Nitro-Bid Ointment 1524
Nitrodisc 2047
Nitro-Dur (nitroglycerin) Transdermal Infusion System 1326
Nitrolingual Spray 2027
Nitrostat Tablets 1925
Transderm-Nitro Transdermal Therapeutic System 859

Opium Alkaloids (Potential for unspecified effect on central nervous function).
No products indexed under this heading.

Oxazepam (Potential for unspecified effect on central nervous function). Products include:
Serax Capsules 2810
Serax Tablets 2810

Oxycodone Hydrochloride (Potential for unspecified effect on central nervous function). Products include:
Percocet Tablets 938
Percodan Tablets 939
Percodan-Demi Tablets 940
Roxicodone Tablets, Oral Solution & Intensol (Oxycodone) 2244
Tylox Capsules 1584

Penbutolol Sulfate (May potentiate the hypotension seen with aldesleukin). Products include:
Levatol 2403

Perphenazine (Potential for unspecified effect on central nervous function). Products include:
Etrafon 2355
Triavil Tablets 1757
Trilafon 2389

Phenoxybenzamine Hydrochloride (May potentiate the hypotension seen with aldesleukin). Products include:
Dibenzyline Capsules 2476

Phentolamine Mesylate (May potentiate the hypotension seen with aldesleukin). Products include:
Regitine 846

(▭ Described in PDR For Nonprescription Drugs) (⊙ Described in PDR For Ophthalmology)

845 **Interactions Index** **Prolixin**

Pindolol (May potentiate the hypotension seen with aldesleukin). Products include:
Visken Tablets ... 2299
Polythiazide (May potentiate the hypotension seen with aldesleukin). Products include:
Minizide Capsules ... 1938
Prazepam (Potential for unspecified effect on central nervous function).
No products indexed under this heading.
Prazosin Hydrochloride (May potentiate the hypotension seen with aldesleukin). Products include:
Minipress Capsules ... 1937
Minizide Capsules ... 1938
Prednisolone Acetate (May reduce the antitumor effectiveness of aldesleukin). Products include:
AK-CIDE ... ⊙ 202
AK-CIDE Ointment ... ⊙ 202
Blephamide Liquifilm Sterile Ophthalmic Suspension ... 476
Blephamide Ointment ... ⊙ 237
Econopred & Econopred Plus Ophthalmic Suspensions ... ⊙ 217
Poly-Pred Liquifilm ... ⊙ 248
Pred Forte ... ⊙ 250
Pred Mild ... ⊙ 253
Pred-G Liquifilm Sterile Ophthalmic Suspension ... ⊙ 251
Pred-G S.O.P. Sterile Ophthalmic Ointment ... ⊙ 252
Vasocidin Ointment ... ⊙ 268
Prednisolone Sodium Phosphate (May reduce the antitumor effectiveness of aldesleukin). Products include:
AK-Pred ... ⊙ 204
Hydeltrasol Injection, Sterile ... 1665
Inflamase ... ⊙ 265
Pediapred Oral Liquid ... 995
Vasocidin Ophthalmic Solution ... ⊙ 270
Prednisolone Tebutate (May reduce the antitumor effectiveness of aldesleukin). Products include:
Hydeltra-T.B.A. Sterile Suspension 1667
Prednisone (May reduce the antitumor effectiveness of aldesleukin). Products include:
Deltasone Tablets ... 2595
Procarbazine Hydrochloride (Potential for increased myelotoxicity). Products include:
Matulane Capsules ... 2131
Prochlorperazine (Potential for unspecified effect on central nervous function). Products include:
Compazine ... 2470
Promethazine Hydrochloride (Potential for unspecified effect on central nervous function). Products include:
Mepergan Injection ... 2753
Phenergan with Codeine ... 2777
Phenergan with Dextromethorphan 2778
Phenergan Injection ... 2773
Phenergan Suppositories ... 2775
Phenergan Syrup ... 2774
Phenergan Tablets ... 2775
Phenergan VC ... 2779
Phenergan VC with Codeine ... 2781
Propofol (Potential for unspecified effect on central nervous function). Products include:
Diprivan Injection ... 2833
Propoxyphene Hydrochloride (Potential for unspecified effect on central nervous function). Products include:
Darvon ... 1435
Wygesic Tablets ... 2827
Propoxyphene Napsylate (Potential for unspecified effect on central nervous function). Products include:
Darvon-N/Darvocet-N ... 1433
Propranolol Hydrochloride (May potentiate the hypotension seen with aldesleukin). Products include:
Inderal ... 2728
Inderal LA Long Acting Capsules ... 2730
Inderide Tablets ... 2732
Inderide LA Long Acting Capsules .. 2734
Quazepam (Potential for unspecified effect on central nervous function). Products include:
Doral Tablets ... 2664
Quinapril Hydrochloride (May potentiate the hypotension seen with aldesleukin). Products include:
Accupril Tablets ... 1893
Ramipril (May potentiate the hypotension seen with aldesleukin). Products include:
Altace Capsules ... 1232
Rauwolfia Serpentina (May potentiate the hypotension seen with aldesleukin).
No products indexed under this heading.
Rescinnamine (May potentiate the hypotension seen with aldesleukin).
No products indexed under this heading.
Reserpine (May potentiate the hypotension seen with aldesleukin). Products include:
Diupres Tablets ... 1650
Hydropres Tablets ... 1675
Ser-Ap-Es Tablets ... 849
Secobarbital Sodium (Potential for unspecified effect on central nervous function). Products include:
Seconal Sodium Pulvules ... 1474
Sodium Nitroprusside (May potentiate the hypotension seen with aldesleukin).
No products indexed under this heading.
Sotalol Hydrochloride (May potentiate the hypotension seen with aldesleukin). Products include:
Betapace Tablets ... 641
Spirapril Hydrochloride (May potentiate the hypotension seen with aldesleukin).
No products indexed under this heading.
Streptomycin Sulfate (Potential for increased nephrotoxicity). Products include:
Streptomycin Sulfate Injection ... 2208
Sufentanil Citrate (Potential for unspecified effect on central nervous function). Products include:
Sufenta Injection ... 1309
Tamoxifen Citrate (Potential for increased myelotoxicity). Products include:
Nolvadex Tablets ... 2841
Temazepam (Potential for unspecified effect on central nervous function). Products include:
Restoril Capsules ... 2284
Terazosin Hydrochloride (May potentiate the hypotension seen with aldesleukin). Products include:
Hytrin Capsules ... 430
Thioridazine Hydrochloride (Potential for unspecified effect on central nervous function). Products include:
Mellaril ... 2269
Thiothixene (Potential for unspecified effect on central nervous function). Products include:
Navane Capsules and Concentrate 2201
Navane Intramuscular ... 2202
Timolol Hemihydrate (May potentiate the hypotension seen with aldesleukin). Products include:
Betimol 0.25%, 0.5% ... ⊙ 261
Timolol Maleate (May potentiate the hypotension seen with aldesleukin). Products include:
Blocadren Tablets ... 1614
Timolide Tablets ... 1748
Timoptic in Ocudose ... 1753
Timoptic Sterile Ophthalmic Solution ... 1751
Timoptic-XE ... 1755
Tobramycin (Potential for increased nephrotoxicity). Products include:
AKTOB ... ⊙ 206
TobraDex Ophthalmic Suspension and Ointment ... 473
Tobrex Ophthalmic Ointment and Solution ... ⊙ 229
Tobramycin Sulfate (Potential for increased nephrotoxicity). Products include:
Nebcin Vials, Hyporets & ADD-Vantage ... 1464
Tobramycin Sulfate Injection ... 968
Torsemide (May potentiate the hypotension seen with aldesleukin). Products include:
Demadex Tablets and Injection ... 686
Triamcinolone (May reduce the antitumor effectiveness of aldesleukin). Products include:
Aristocort Tablets ... 1022
Triamcinolone Acetonide (May reduce the antitumor effectiveness of aldesleukin). Products include:
Aristocort A 0.025% Cream ... 1027
Aristocort A 0.5% Cream ... 1031
Aristocort A 0.1% Cream ... 1029
Aristocort A 0.1% Ointment ... 1030
Azmacort Oral Inhaler ... 2011
Nasacort Nasal Inhaler ... 2024
Triamcinolone Diacetate (May reduce the antitumor effectiveness of aldesleukin). Products include:
Aristocort Suspension (Forte Parenteral) ... 1027
Aristocort Suspension (Intralesional) ... 1025
Triamcinolone Hexacetonide (May reduce the antitumor effectiveness of aldesleukin). Products include:
Aristospan Suspension (Intra-articular) ... 1033
Aristospan Suspension (Intralesional) ... 1032
Triazolam (Potential for unspecified effect on central nervous function). Products include:
Halcion Tablets ... 2611
Trifluoperazine Hydrochloride (Potential for unspecified effect on central nervous function). Products include:
Stelazine ... 2514
Trimethaphan Camsylate (May potentiate the hypotension seen with aldesleukin). Products include:
Arfonad Ampuls ... 2080
Tyropanoate Sodium (Potential for delayed adverse reactions to iodinated contrast media including fever, chills, nausea, vomiting, pruritus, rash, diarrhea, hypotension, edema, and oliguria).
No products indexed under this heading.
Verapamil Hydrochloride (May potentiate the hypotension seen with aldesleukin). Products include:
Calan SR Caplets ... 2422
Calan Tablets ... 2419
Isoptin Injectable ... 1344
Isoptin Oral Tablets ... 1346
Isoptin SR Tablets ... 1348
Verelan Capsules ... 1410
Verelan Capsules ... 2824
Vincristine Sulfate (Potential for increased myelotoxicity). Products include:
Oncovin Solution Vials & Hyporets 1466
Zolpidem Tartrate (Potential for unspecified effect on central nervous function). Products include:
Ambien Tablets ... 2416

PROLIXIN DECANOATE
(Fluphenazine Decanoate) ... 509
May interact with central nervous system depressants, narcotic analgesics, antihistamines, barbiturates, and certain other agents. Compounds in these categories include:
Acrivastine (Potentiation of CNS depressant effect may occur). Products include:
Semprex-D Capsules ... 463
Semprex-D Capsules ... 1167
Alfentanil Hydrochloride (Potentiation of CNS depressant effect may occur). Products include:
Alfenta Injection ... 1286
Alprazolam (Potentiation of CNS depressant effect may occur). Products include:
Xanax Tablets ... 2649
Aprobarbital (Potentiation of CNS depressant effect may occur).
No products indexed under this heading.
Astemizole (Potentiation of CNS depressant effect may occur). Products include:
Hismanal Tablets ... 1293
Atropine Sulfate (Additive anticholinergic effects). Products include:
Arco-Lase Plus Tablets ... 512
Atrohist Plus Tablets ... 454
Atropine Sulfate Sterile Ophthalmic Solution ... ⊙ 233
Donnatal ... 2060
Donnatal Extentabs ... 2061
Donnatal Tablets ... 2060
Lomotil ... 2439
Motofen Tablets ... 784
Urised Tablets ... 1964
Azatadine Maleate (Potentiation of CNS depressant effect may occur). Products include:
Trinalin Repetabs Tablets ... 1330
Bromodiphenhydramine Hydrochloride (Potentiation of CNS depressant effect may occur).
No products indexed under this heading.
Brompheniramine Maleate (Potentiation of CNS depressant effect may occur). Products include:
Alka Seltzer Plus Sinus Medicine .. ▣ 707
Bromfed Capsules (Extended-Release) ... 1785
Bromfed Syrup ... ▣ 733
Bromfed Tablets ... 1785
Bromfed-DM Cough Syrup ... 1786
Bromfed-PD Capsules (Extended-Release) ... 1785
Dimetane-DC Cough Syrup ... 2059
Dimetane-DX Cough Syrup ... 2059
Dimetapp Elixir ... ▣ 773
Dimetapp Extentabs ... ▣ 774
Dimetapp Tablets/Liqui-Gels ... ▣ 775
Dimetapp Cold & Allergy Chewable Tablets ... ▣ 773
Dimetapp DM Elixir ... ▣ 774
Vicks DayQuil Allergy Relief 12-Hour Extended Release Tablets.. ▣ 760
Vicks DayQuil Allergy Relief 4-Hour Tablets ... ▣ 760
Buprenorphine (Potentiation of CNS depressant effect may occur). Products include:
Buprenex Injectable ... 2006
Buspirone Hydrochloride (Potentiation of CNS depressant effect may occur). Products include:
BuSpar ... 737
Butabarbital (Potentiation of CNS depressant effect may occur).
No products indexed under this heading.

IMPORTANT NOTE: Always consult each drug listing in the patient's regimen for possible interactions.

Prolixin

Butalbital (Potentiation of CNS depressant effect may occur). Products include:

Esgic-plus Tablets 1013
Fioricet Tablets 2258
Fioricet with Codeine Capsules 2260
Fiorinal Capsules 2261
Fiorinal with Codeine Capsules 2262
Fiorinal Tablets 2261
Phrenilin 785
Sedapap Tablets 50 mg/650 mg .. 1543

Chlordiazepoxide (Potentiation of CNS depressant effect may occur). Products include:

Libritabs Tablets 2177
Limbitrol 2180

Chlordiazepoxide Hydrochloride (Potentiation of CNS depressant effect may occur). Products include:

Librax Capsules 2176
Librium Capsules 2178
Librium Injectable 2179

Chlorpheniramine Maleate (Potentiation of CNS depressant effect may occur). Products include:

Alka-Seltzer Plus Cold Medicine ....⊕D 705
Alka-Seltzer Plus Cold Medicine Liqui-Gels .... ⊕D 706
Alka-Seltzer Plus Cold & Cough Medicine .... ⊕D 708
Alka-Seltzer Plus Cold & Cough Medicine Liqui-Gels.......................... ⊕D 705
Allerest Children's Chewable Tablets .... ⊕D 627
Allerest Headache Strength Tablets .... ⊕D 627
Allerest Maximum Strength Tablets .... ⊕D 627
Allerest Sinus Pain Formula .... ⊕D 627
Allerest 12 Hour Caplets .... ⊕D 627
Ana-Kit Anaphylaxis Emergency Treatment Kit 617
Atrohist Pediatric Capsules 453
Atrohist Plus Tablets 454
BC Cold Powder Multi-Symptom Formula (Cold-Sinus-Allergy) ...... ⊕D 609
Cerose DM .... ⊕D 878
Cheracol Plus Head Cold/Cough Formula .... ⊕D 769
Children's Vicks DayQuil Allergy Relief .... ⊕D 757
Children's Vicks NyQuil Cold/ Cough Relief .... ⊕D 758
Chlor-Trimeton Allergy Decongestant Tablets .... ⊕D 799
Chlor-Trimeton Allergy Tablets ...... ⊕D 798
Comhist 2038
Comtrex Multi-Symptom Cold Reliever Tablets/Caplets/Liqui-Gels/Liquid .... ⊕D 615
Allergy-Sinus Comtrex Multi-Symptom Allergy-Sinus Formula Tablets .... ⊕D 617
Contac Continuous Action Nasal Decongestant/Antihistamine 12 Hour Capsules .... ⊕D 813
Contac Maximum Strength Continuous Action Decongestant/ Antihistamine 12 Hour Caplets.. ⊕D 813
Contac Severe Cold and Flu Formula Caplets .... ⊕D 814
Coricidin 'D' Decongestant Tablets .... ⊕D 800
Coricidin Tablets .... ⊕D 800
D.A. Chewable Tablets......................... 951
Deconamine 1320
Dura-Tap/PD Capsules 2867
Dura-Vent/DA Tablets 953
Extendryl 1005
Fedahist Gyrocaps 2401
Fedahist Timecaps 2401
Hycomine Compound Tablets 932
Isoclor Timesule Capsules .... ⊕D 637
Kronofed-A 977
Nolamine Timed-Release Tablets 785
Novahistine DH 2462
Novahistine Elixir .... ⊕D 823
Ornade Spansule Capsules 2502
PediaCare Cold Allergy Chewable Tablets .... ⊕D 677
PediaCare Cough-Cold Chewable Tablets 1553
PediaCare Cough-Cold Liquid............ 1553
PediaCare NightRest Cough-Cold Liquid 1553
Pediatric Vicks 44m Cough & Cold Relief .... ⊕D 764
Pyrroxate Caplets .... ⊕D 772
Ryna .... ⊕D 841
Sinarest Tablets .... ⊕D 648
Sinarest Extra Strength Tablets...... ⊕D 648
Sine-Off Sinus Medicine .... ⊕D 825
Singlet Tablets .... ⊕D 825
Sinulin Tablets 787
Sinutab Sinus Allergy Medication, Maximum Strength Tablets and Caplets .... ⊕D 860
Sudafed Plus Liquid .... ⊕D 862
Sudafed Plus Tablets .... ⊕D 863
Teldrin 12 Hour Antihistamine/ Nasal Decongestant Allergy Relief Capsules .... ⊕D 826
TheraFlu .... ⊕D 787
TheraFlu Maximum Strength Nighttime Flu, Cold & Cough Medicine .... ⊕D 788
Triaminic Allergy Tablets .... ⊕D 789
Triaminic Cold Tablets .... ⊕D 790
Triaminic Nite Light .... ⊕D 791
Triaminic Syrup .... ⊕D 792
Triaminic-12 Tablets .... ⊕D 792
Triaminicin Tablets .... ⊕D 793
Triaminicol Multi-Symptom Cold Tablets .... ⊕D 793
Triaminicol Multi-Symptom Relief ⊕D 794
Tussend 1783
Children's TYLENOL Cold Multi-Symptom Liquid Formula and Chewable Tablets............................. 1561
Children's TYLENOL Cold Plus Cough Multi Symptom Tablets and Liquid .... ⊕D 681
TYLENOL Maximum Strength Allergy Sinus Medication Gelcaps and Caplets 1563
TYLENOL Cold Multi-Symptom Formula Medication Tablets and Caplets 1561
TYLENOL Cold Multi-Symptom Hot Medication Liquid Packets............. 1557
Vicks 44 LiquiCaps Cough, Cold & Flu Relief .... ⊕D 755
Vicks 44M Cough, Cold & Flu Relief .... ⊕D 756

Chlorpheniramine Polistirex (Potentiation of CNS depressant effect may occur). Products include:

Tussionex Pennkinetic Extended-Release Suspension 998

Chlorpheniramine Tannate (Potentiation of CNS depressant effect may occur). Products include:

Atrohist Pediatric Suspension 454
Ricobid Tablets and Pediatric Suspension 2038
Rynatan 2673
Rynatuss 2673

Chlorpromazine (Potentiation of CNS depressant effect may occur). Products include:

Thorazine Suppositories 2523

Chlorprothixene (Potentiation of CNS depressant effect may occur).

No products indexed under this heading.

Chlorprothixene Hydrochloride (Potentiation of CNS depressant effect may occur).

No products indexed under this heading.

Clemastine Fumarate (Potentiation of CNS depressant effect may occur). Products include:

Tavist Syrup 2297
Tavist Tablets 2298
Tavist-1 12 Hour Relief Tablets .... ⊕D 787
Tavist-D 12 Hour Relief Tablets .... ⊕D 787

Clorazepate Dipotassium (Potentiation of CNS depressant effect may occur). Products include:

Tranxene 451

Clozapine (Potentiation of CNS depressant effect may occur). Products include:

Clozaril Tablets 2252

Codeine Phosphate (Potentiation of CNS depressant effect may occur). Products include:

Actifed with Codeine Cough Syrup.. 1067
Brontex 1981
Deconsal C Expectorant Syrup 456
Deconsal Pediatric Syrup 457
Dimetane-DC Cough Syrup 2059
Empirin with Codeine Tablets........... 1093
Fioricet with Codeine Capsules 2260
Fiorinal with Codeine Capsules 2262
Isoclor Expectorant 990
Novahistine DH 2462
Novahistine Expectorant 2463
Nucofed 2051
Phenergan with Codeine 2777
Phenergan VC with Codeine 2781
Robitussin A-C Syrup 2073
Robitussin-DAC Syrup 2074
Ryna .... ⊕D 841
Soma Compound w/Codeine Tablets 2676
Tussi-Organidin NR Liquid and S NR Liquid 2677
Tylenol with Codeine 1583

Cyproheptadine Hydrochloride (Potentiation of CNS depressant effect may occur). Products include:

Periactin 1724

Desflurane (Potentiation of CNS depressant effect may occur). Products include:

Suprane 1813

Dexchlorpheniramine Maleate (Potentiation of CNS depressant effect may occur).

No products indexed under this heading.

Dezocine (Potentiation of CNS depressant effect may occur). Products include:

Dalgan Injection 538

Diazepam (Potentiation of CNS depressant effect may occur). Products include:

Dizac 1809
Valium Injectable 2182
Valium Tablets 2183
Valrelease Capsules 2169

Diphenhydramine Citrate (Potentiation of CNS depressant effect may occur). Products include:

Excedrin P.M. Analgesic/Sleeping Aid Tablets, Caplets, Liquigels 733

Diphenhydramine Hydrochloride (Potentiation of CNS depressant effect may occur). Products include:

Actifed Allergy Daytime/Nighttime Caplets .... ⊕D 844
Actifed Sinus Daytime/Nighttime Tablets and Caplets .... ⊕D 846
Arthritis Foundation NightTime Caplets .... ⊕D 674
Extra Strength Bayer PM Aspirin .. ⊕D 713
Bayer Select Night Time Pain Relief Formula .... ⊕D 716
Benadryl Allergy Decongestant Liquid Medication .... ⊕D 848
Benadryl Allergy Decongestant Tablets .... ⊕D 848
Benadryl Allergy Liquid Medication .... ⊕D 849
Benadryl Allergy .... ⊕D 848
Benadryl Allergy Sinus Headache Formula Caplets .... ⊕D 849
Benadryl Capsules 1898
Benadryl Dye-Free Allergy Liquigel Softgels .... ⊕D 850
Benadryl Dye-Free Allergy Liquid Medication .... ⊕D 850
Benadryl Itch Relief Cream, Children's Formula and Maximum Strength 2% .... ⊕D 851
Benadryl Itch Relief Spray, Children's Formula and Maximum Strength 2% .... ⊕D 851
Benadryl Itch Relief Stick Maximum Strength 2% .... ⊕D 850
Benadryl Itch Stopping Gel, Children's Formula and Maximum Strength 2% .... ⊕D 851
Benadryl Kapseals 1898
Benadryl Injection 1898
Contac Day & Night Cold/Flu Night Caplets .... ⊕D 812
Contac Night Allergy/Sinus Caplets .... ⊕D 812
Extra Strength Doan's P.M. .... ⊕D 633
Legatrin PM .... ⊕D 651
Miles Nervine Nighttime Sleep-Aid ⊕D 723
Nytol QuickCaps Caplets .... ⊕D 610
Sleepinal Night-time Sleep Aid Capsules and Softgels .... ⊕D 834

TYLENOL Maximum Strength Allergy Sinus NightTime Medication Caplets 1555
TYLENOL Flu NightTime, Maximum Strength, Gelcaps 1566
TYLENOL Maximum Strength Flu NightTime Hot Medication Packets 1562
TYLENOL PM, Extra Strength Pain Reliever/Sleep Aid Caplets, Geltabs, Gelcaps 1560
TYLENOL Severe Allergy Medication Caplets 1564
Maximum Strength Unisom Sleepgels 1934
Unisom With Pain Relief-Nighttime Sleep Aid and Pain Reliever........... 1934

Diphenylpyraline Hydrochloride (Potentiation of CNS depressant effect may occur).

No products indexed under this heading.

Droperidol (Potentiation of CNS depressant effect may occur). Products include:

Inapsine Injection 1296

Enflurane (Potentiation of CNS depressant effect may occur).

No products indexed under this heading.

Estazolam (Potentiation of CNS depressant effect may occur). Products include:

ProSom Tablets 449

Ethchlorvynol (Potentiation of CNS depressant effect may occur). Products include:

Placidyl Capsules 448

Ethinamate (Potentiation of CNS depressant effect may occur).

No products indexed under this heading.

Fentanyl (Potentiation of CNS depressant effect may occur). Products include:

Duragesic Transdermal System........ 1288

Fentanyl Citrate (Potentiation of CNS depressant effect may occur). Products include:

Sublimaze Injection 1307

Fluphenazine Enanthate (Potentiation of CNS depressant effect may occur). Products include:

Prolixin Enanthate 509

Fluphenazine Hydrochloride (Potentiation of CNS depressant effect may occur). Products include:

Prolixin 509

Flurazepam Hydrochloride (Potentiation of CNS depressant effect may occur). Products include:

Dalmane Capsules 2173

Glutethimide (Potentiation of CNS depressant effect may occur).

No products indexed under this heading.

Haloperidol (Potentiation of CNS depressant effect may occur). Products include:

Haldol Injection, Tablets and Concentrate 1575

Haloperidol Decanoate (Potentiation of CNS depressant effect may occur). Products include:

Haldol Decanoate 1577

Hydrocodone Bitartrate (Potentiation of CNS depressant effect may occur). Products include:

Anexsia 5/500 Elixir 1781
Anexia Tablets 1782
Codiclear DH Syrup 791
Deconamine CX Cough and Cold Liquid and Tablets 1319
Duratuss HD Elixir 2565
Hycodan Tablets and Syrup 930
Hycomine Compound Tablets 932
Hycomine 931
Hycotuss Expectorant Syrup 933
Hydrocet Capsules 782
Lorcet 10/650 1018
Lortab 2566

(⊕D Described in PDR For Nonprescription Drugs) (◉ Described in PDR For Ophthalmology)

Tussend 1783
Tussend Expectorant 1785
Vicodin Tablets 1356
Vicodin ES Tablets 1357
Vicodin Tuss Expectorant 1358
Zydone Capsules 949

Hydrocodone Polistirex (Potentiation of CNS depressant effect may occur). Products include:

Tussionex Pennkinetic Extended-Release Suspension 998

Hydroxyzine Hydrochloride (Potentiation of CNS depressant effect may occur). Products include:

Atarax Tablets & Syrup 2185
Marax Tablets & DF Syrup 2200
Vistaril Intramuscular Solution 2216

Isoflurane (Potentiation of CNS depressant effect may occur).

No products indexed under this heading.

Ketamine Hydrochloride (Potentiation of CNS depressant effect may occur).

No products indexed under this heading.

Levomethadyl Acetate Hydrochloride (Potentiation of CNS depressant effect may occur). Products include:

Orlamm 2239

Levorphanol Tartrate (Potentiation of CNS depressant effect may occur). Products include:

Levo-Dromoran 2129

Loratadine (Potentiation of CNS depressant effect may occur). Products include:

Claritin 2349
Claritin-D 2350

Lorazepam (Potentiation of CNS depressant effect may occur). Products include:

Ativan Injection 2698
Ativan Tablets 2700

Loxapine Hydrochloride (Potentiation of CNS depressant effect may occur). Products include:

Loxitane 1378

Loxapine Succinate (Potentiation of CNS depressant effect may occur). Products include:

Loxitane Capsules 1378

Meperidine Hydrochloride (Potentiation of CNS depressant effect may occur). Products include:

Demerol 2308
Mepergan Injection 2753

Mephobarbital (Potentiation of CNS depressant effect may occur). Products include:

Mebaral Tablets 2322

Meprobamate (Potentiation of CNS depressant effect may occur). Products include:

Miltown Tablets 2672
PMB 200 and PMB 400 2783

Mesoridazine Besylate (Potentiation of CNS depressant effect may occur). Products include:

Serentil 684

Methadone Hydrochloride (Potentiation of CNS depressant effect may occur). Products include:

Methadone Hydrochloride Oral Concentrate 2233
Methadone Hydrochloride Oral Solution & Tablets 2235

Methdilazine Hydrochloride (Potentiation of CNS depressant effect may occur).

No products indexed under this heading.

Methohexital Sodium (Potentiation of CNS depressant effect may occur). Products include:

Brevital Sodium Vials 1429

Methotrimeprazine (Potentiation of CNS depressant effect may occur). Products include:

Levoprome 1274

Methoxyflurane (Potentiation of CNS depressant effect may occur).

No products indexed under this heading.

Midazolam Hydrochloride (Potentiation of CNS depressant effect may occur). Products include:

Versed Injection 2170

Molindone Hydrochloride (Potentiation of CNS depressant effect may occur). Products include:

Moban Tablets and Concentrate 1048

Morphine Sulfate (Potentiation of CNS depressant effect may occur). Products include:

Astramorph/PF Injection, USP (Preservative-Free) 535
Duramorph 962
Infumorph 200 and Infumorph 500 Sterile Solutions 965
MS Contin Tablets 1994
MSIR 1997
Oramorph SR (Morphine Sulfate Sustained Release Tablets) 2236
RMS Suppositories 2657
Roxanol 2243

Opium Alkaloids (Potentiation of CNS depressant effect may occur).

No products indexed under this heading.

Oxazepam (Potentiation of CNS depressant effect may occur). Products include:

Serax Capsules 2810
Serax Tablets 2810

Oxycodone Hydrochloride (Potentiation of CNS depressant effect may occur). Products include:

Percocet Tablets 938
Percodan Tablets 939
Percodan-Demi Tablets 940
Roxicodone Tablets, Oral Solution & Intensol (Oxycodone) 2244
Tylox Capsules 1584

Pentobarbital Sodium (Potentiation of CNS depressant effect may occur). Products include:

Nembutal Sodium Capsules 436
Nembutal Sodium Solution 438
Nembutal Sodium Suppositories 440

Perphenazine (Potentiation of CNS depressant effect may occur). Products include:

Etrafon 2355
Triavil Tablets 1757
Trilafon 2389

Phenobarbital (Potentiation of CNS depressant effect may occur). Products include:

Arco-Lase Plus Tablets 512
Bellergal-S Tablets 2250
Donnatal 2060
Donnatal Extentabs 2061
Donnatal Tablets 2060
Phenobarbital Elixir and Tablets 1469
Quadrinal Tablets 1350

Prazepam (Potentiation of CNS depressant effect may occur).

No products indexed under this heading.

Prochlorperazine (Potentiation of CNS depressant effect may occur). Products include:

Compazine 2470

Promethazine Hydrochloride (Potentiation of CNS depressant effect may occur). Products include:

Mepergan Injection 2753
Phenergan with Codeine 2777
Phenergan with Dextromethorphan 2778
Phenergan Injection 2773
Phenergan Suppositories 2775
Phenergan Syrup 2774
Phenergan Tablets 2775
Phenergan VC 2779

Phenergan VC with Codeine 2781

Propofol (Potentiation of CNS depressant effect may occur). Products include:

Diprivan Injection 2833

Propoxyphene Hydrochloride (Potentiation of CNS depressant effect may occur). Products include:

Darvon 1435
Wygesic Tablets 2827

Propoxyphene Napsylate (Potentiation of CNS depressant effect may occur). Products include:

Darvon-N/Darvocet-N 1433

Pyrilamine Maleate (Potentiation of CNS depressant effect may occur). Products include:

4-Way Fast Acting Nasal Spray (regular & mentholated) .... ⊕ 621
Maximum Strength Multi-Symptom Formula Midol .... ⊕ 722
PMS Multi-Symptom Formula Midol .... ⊕ 723

Pyrilamine Tannate (Potentiation of CNS depressant effect may occur). Products include:

Atrohist Pediatric Suspension 454
Rynatan 2673

Quazepam (Potentiation of CNS depressant effect may occur). Products include:

Doral Tablets 2664

Risperidone (Potentiation of CNS depressant effect may occur). Products include:

Risperdal 1301

Secobarbital Sodium (Potentiation of CNS depressant effect may occur). Products include:

Seconal Sodium Pulvules 1474

Sufentanil Citrate (Potentiation of CNS depressant effect may occur). Products include:

Sufenta Injection 1309

Temazepam (Potentiation of CNS depressant effect may occur). Products include:

Restoril Capsules 2284

Terfenadine (Potentiation of CNS depressant effect may occur). Products include:

Seldane Tablets 1536
Seldane-D Extended-Release Tablets 1538

Thiamylal Sodium (Potentiation of CNS depressant effect may occur).

No products indexed under this heading.

Thioridazine Hydrochloride (Potentiation of CNS depressant effect may occur). Products include:

Mellaril 2269

Thiothixene (Potentiation of CNS depressant effect may occur). Products include:

Navane Capsules and Concentrate 2201
Navane Intramuscular 2202

Triazolam (Potentiation of CNS depressant effect may occur). Products include:

Halcion Tablets 2611

Trifluoperazine Hydrochloride (Potentiation of CNS depressant effect may occur). Products include:

Stelazine 2514

Trimeprazine Tartrate (Potentiation of CNS depressant effect may occur). Products include:

Temaril Tablets, Syrup and Spansule Extended-Release Capsules .. 483

Tripelennamine Hydrochloride (Potentiation of CNS depressant effect may occur). Products include:

PBZ Tablets 845
PBZ-SR Tablets 844

Triprolidine Hydrochloride (Potentiation of CNS depressant effect may occur). Products include:

Actifed Plus Caplets .... ⊕ 845
Actifed Plus Tablets .... ⊕ 845
Actifed with Codeine Cough Syrup.. 1067
Actifed Syrup .... ⊕ 846
Actifed Tablets .... ⊕ 844

Zolpidem Tartrate (Potentiation of CNS depressant effect may occur). Products include:

Ambien Tablets 2416

Food Interactions

Alcohol (Potentiation of the effect of alcohol may occur).

PROLIXIN ELIXIR

(Fluphenazine Hydrochloride) 509
See Prolixin Decanoate

PROLIXIN ENANTHATE

(Fluphenazine Enanthate) 509
See Prolixin Decanoate

PROLIXIN INJECTION

(Fluphenazine Hydrochloride) 509
See Prolixin Decanoate

PROLIXIN ORAL CONCENTRATE

(Fluphenazine Hydrochloride) 509
See Prolixin Decanoate

PROLOPRIM TABLETS

(Trimethoprim) 1155
May interact with:

Phenytoin (Increased phenytoin half-life and decreased phenytoin metabolic clearance rate; possible excessive phenytoin effect). Products include:

Dilantin Infatabs 1908
Dilantin-125 Suspension 1911

Phenytoin Sodium (Increased phenytoin half-life and decreased phenytoin metabolic clearance rate; possible excessive phenytoin effect). Products include:

Dilantin Kapseals 1906
Dilantin Parenteral 1910

PROMISE SENSITIVE TOOTHPASTE

(Potassium Nitrate, Sodium Monofluorophosphate) .... ⊕ 610
None cited in PDR database.

PROMOTE HIGH PROTEIN LIQUID NUTRITION

(Nutritional Supplement) 2223
None cited in PDR database.

PROMOTE WITH FIBER, HIGH-PROTEIN LIQUID NUTRITION

(Nutritional Beverage) 2224
None cited in PDR database.

PRONTO LICE KILLING SHAMPOO & CONDITIONER IN ONE KIT

(Pyrethrins, Piperonyl Butoxide) .... ⊕ 653
None cited in PDR database.

PROPAGEST TABLETS

(Phenylpropanolamine Hydrochloride) 786
May interact with antihypertensives and antidepressant drugs. Compounds in these categories include:

Acebutolol Hydrochloride (Concurrent administration is not recommended). Products include:

Sectral Capsules 2807

IMPORTANT NOTE: Always consult each drug listing in the patient's regimen for possible interactions.

Propagest | Interactions Index | 848

Amitriptyline Hydrochloride (Concurrent administration is not recommended). Products include:
Elavil ... 2838
Endep Tablets ... 2174
Etrafon ... 2355
Limbitrol ... 2180
Triavil Tablets ... 1757

Amlodipine Besylate (Concurrent administration is not recommended). Products include:
Lotrel Capsules ... 840
Norvasc Tablets ... 1940

Amoxapine (Concurrent administration is not recommended). Products include:
Asendin Tablets ... 1369

Atenolol (Concurrent administration is not recommended). Products include:
Tenoretic Tablets ... 2845
Tenormin Tablets and I.V. Injection 2847

Benazepril Hydrochloride (Concurrent administration is not recommended). Products include:
Lotensin Tablets ... 834
Lotensin HCT ... 837
Lotrel Capsules ... 840

Bendroflumethiazide (Concurrent administration is not recommended).
No products indexed under this heading.

Betaxolol Hydrochloride (Concurrent administration is not recommended). Products include:
Betoptic Ophthalmic Solution ... 469
Betoptic S Ophthalmic Suspension 471
Kerlone Tablets ... 2436

Bisoprolol Fumarate (Concurrent administration is not recommended). Products include:
Zebeta Tablets ... 1413
Ziac ... 1415

Bupropion Hydrochloride (Concurrent administration is not recommended). Products include:
Wellbutrin Tablets ... 1204

Captopril (Concurrent administration is not recommended). Products include:
Capoten ... 739
Capozide ... 742

Carteolol Hydrochloride (Concurrent administration is not recommended). Products include:
Cartrol Tablets ... 410
Ocupress Ophthalmic Solution, 1% Sterile ... ◎ 309

Chlorothiazide (Concurrent administration is not recommended). Products include:
Aldoclor Tablets ... 1598
Diupres Tablets ... 1650
Diuril Oral ... 1653

Chlorothiazide Sodium (Concurrent administration is not recommended). Products include:
Diuril Sodium Intravenous ... 1652

Chlorthalidone (Concurrent administration is not recommended). Products include:
Combipres Tablets ... 677
Tenoretic Tablets ... 2845
Thalitone ... 1245

Clonidine (Concurrent administration is not recommended). Products include:
Catapres-TTS ... 675

Clonidine Hydrochloride (Concurrent administration is not recommended). Products include:
Catapres Tablets ... 674
Combipres Tablets ... 677

Deserpidine (Concurrent administration is not recommended).
No products indexed under this heading.

Desipramine Hydrochloride (Concurrent administration is not recommended). Products include:
Norpramin Tablets ... 1526

Diazoxide (Concurrent administration is not recommended). Products include:
Hyperstat I.V. Injection ... 2363
Proglycem ... 580

Diltiazem Hydrochloride (Concurrent administration is not recommended). Products include:
Cardizem CD Capsules ... 1506
Cardizem SR Capsules ... 1510
Cardizem Injectable ... 1508
Cardizem Tablets ... 1512
Dilacor XR Extended-release Capsules ... 2018

Doxazosin Mesylate (Concurrent administration is not recommended). Products include:
Cardura Tablets ... 2186

Doxepin Hydrochloride (Concurrent administration is not recommended). Products include:
Sinequan ... 2205
Zonalon Cream ... 1055

Enalapril Maleate (Concurrent administration is not recommended). Products include:
Vaseretic Tablets ... 1765
Vasotec Tablets ... 1771

Enalaprilat (Concurrent administration is not recommended). Products include:
Vasotec I.V. ... 1768

Esmolol Hydrochloride (Concurrent administration is not recommended). Products include:
Brevibloc Injection ... 1808

Felodipine (Concurrent administration is not recommended). Products include:
Plendil Extended-Release Tablets ... 527

Fluoxetine Hydrochloride (Concurrent administration is not recommended). Products include:
Prozac Pulvules & Liquid, Oral Solution ... 919

Fosinopril Sodium (Concurrent administration is not recommended). Products include:
Monopril Tablets ... 757

Furosemide (Concurrent administration is not recommended). Products include:
Lasix Injection, Oral Solution and Tablets ... 1240

Guanabenz Acetate (Concurrent administration is not recommended).
No products indexed under this heading.

Guanethidine Monosulfate (Concurrent administration is not recommended). Products include:
Esimil Tablets ... 822
Ismelin Tablets ... 827

Hydralazine Hydrochloride (Concurrent administration is not recommended). Products include:
Apresazide Capsules ... 808
Apresoline Hydrochloride Tablets .. 809
Ser-Ap-Es Tablets ... 849

Hydrochlorothiazide (Concurrent administration is not recommended). Products include:
Aldactazide ... 2413
Aldoril Tablets ... 1604
Apresazide Capsules ... 808
Capozide ... 742
Dyazide ... 2479
Esidrix Tablets ... 821
Esimil Tablets ... 822
HydroDIURIL Tablets ... 1674
Hydropres Tablets ... 1675
Hyzaar Tablets ... 1677
Inderide Tablets ... 2732
Inderide LA Long Acting Capsules .. 2734
Lopressor HCT Tablets ... 832
Lotensin HCT ... 837
Maxzide ... 1380
Moduretic Tablets ... 1705
Oretic Tablets ... 443
Prinzide Tablets ... 1737
Ser-Ap-Es Tablets ... 849
Timolide Tablets ... 1748
Vaseretic Tablets ... 1765
Zestoretic ... 2850
Ziac ... 1415

Hydroflumethiazide (Concurrent administration is not recommended). Products include:
Diucardin Tablets ... 2718

Imipramine Hydrochloride (Concurrent administration is not recommended). Products include:
Tofranil Ampuls ... 854
Tofranil Tablets ... 856

Imipramine Pamoate (Concurrent administration is not recommended). Products include:
Tofranil-PM Capsules ... 857

Indapamide (Concurrent administration is not recommended). Products include:
Lozol Tablets ... 2022

Isocarboxazid (Concurrent administration is not recommended).
No products indexed under this heading.

Isradipine (Concurrent administration is not recommended). Products include:
DynaCirc Capsules ... 2256

Labetalol Hydrochloride (Concurrent administration is not recommended). Products include:
Normodyne Injection ... 2377
Normodyne Tablets ... 2379
Trandate ... 1185

Lisinopril (Concurrent administration is not recommended). Products include:
Prinivil Tablets ... 1733
Prinzide Tablets ... 1737
Zestoretic ... 2850
Zestril Tablets ... 2854

Losartan Potassium (Concurrent administration is not recommended). Products include:
Cozaar Tablets ... 1628
Hyzaar Tablets ... 1677

Maprotiline Hydrochloride (Concurrent administration is not recommended). Products include:
Ludiomil Tablets ... 843

Mecamylamine Hydrochloride (Concurrent administration is not recommended). Products include:
Inversine Tablets ... 1686

Methyclothiazide (Concurrent administration is not recommended). Products include:
Enduron Tablets ... 420

Methyldopa (Concurrent administration is not recommended). Products include:
Aldoclor Tablets ... 1598
Aldomet Oral ... 1600
Aldoril Tablets ... 1604

Methyldopate Hydrochloride (Concurrent administration is not recommended). Products include:
Aldomet Ester HCl Injection ... 1602

Metolazone (Concurrent administration is not recommended). Products include:
Mykrox Tablets ... 993
Zaroxolyn Tablets ... 1000

Metoprolol Succinate (Concurrent administration is not recommended). Products include:
Toprol-XL Tablets ... 565

Metoprolol Tartrate (Concurrent administration is not recommended). Products include:
Lopressor Ampuls ... 830
Lopressor HCT Tablets ... 832
Lopressor Tablets ... 830

Metyrosine (Concurrent administration is not recommended). Products include:
Demser Capsules ... 1649

Minoxidil (Concurrent administration is not recommended). Products include:
Loniten Tablets ... 2618
Rogaine Topical Solution ... 2637

Moexipril Hydrochloride (Concurrent administration is not recommended). Products include:
Univasc Tablets ... 2410

Nadolol (Concurrent administration is not recommended).
No products indexed under this heading.

Nefazodone Hydrochloride (Concurrent administration is not recommended). Products include:
Serzone Tablets ... 771

Nicardipine Hydrochloride (Concurrent administration is not recommended). Products include:
Cardene Capsules ... 2095
Cardene I.V. ... 2709
Cardene SR Capsules ... 2097

Nifedipine (Concurrent administration is not recommended). Products include:
Adalat Capsules (10 mg and 20 mg) ... 587
Adalat CC ... 589
Procardia Capsules ... 1971
Procardia XL Extended Release Tablets ... 1972

Nisoldipine (Concurrent administration is not recommended).
No products indexed under this heading.

Nitroglycerin (Concurrent administration is not recommended). Products include:
Deponit NTG Transdermal Delivery System ... 2397
Nitro-Bid IV ... 1523
Nitro-Bid Ointment ... 1524
Nitrodisc ... 2047
Nitro-Dur (nitroglycerin) Transdermal Infusion System ... 1326
Nitrolingual Spray ... 2027
Nitrostat Tablets ... 1925
Transderm-Nitro Transdermal Therapeutic System ... 859

Nortriptyline Hydrochloride (Concurrent administration is not recommended). Products include:
Pamelor ... 2280

Paroxetine Hydrochloride (Concurrent administration is not recommended). Products include:
Paxil Tablets ... 2505

Penbutolol Sulfate (Concurrent administration is not recommended). Products include:
Levatol ... 2403

Phenelzine Sulfate (Concurrent administration is not recommended). Products include:
Nardil ... 1920

Phenoxybenzamine Hydrochloride (Concurrent administration is not recommended). Products include:
Dibenzyline Capsules ... 2476

Phentolamine Mesylate (Concurrent administration is not recommended). Products include:
Regitine ... 846

Pindolol (Concurrent administration is not recommended). Products include:
Visken Tablets ... 2299

Polythiazide (Concurrent administration is not recommended). Products include:
Minizide Capsules ... 1938

(▣ Described in PDR For Nonprescription Drugs) (◎ Described in PDR For Ophthalmology)

Prazosin Hydrochloride (Concurrent administration is not recommended). Products include:

Minipress Capsules 1937
Minizide Capsules 1938

Propranolol Hydrochloride (Concurrent administration is not recommended). Products include:

Inderal 2728
Inderal LA Long Acting Capsules 2730
Inderide Tablets 2732
Inderide LA Long Acting Capsules .. 2734

Protriptyline Hydrochloride (Concurrent administration is not recommended). Products include:

Vivactil Tablets 1774

Quinapril Hydrochloride (Concurrent administration is not recommended). Products include:

Accupril Tablets 1893

Ramipril (Concurrent administration is not recommended). Products include:

Altace Capsules 1232

Rauwolfia Serpentina (Concurrent administration is not recommended).

No products indexed under this heading.

Rescinnamine (Concurrent administration is not recommended).

No products indexed under this heading.

Reserpine (Concurrent administration is not recommended). Products include:

Diupres Tablets 1650
Hydropres Tablets..................................... 1675
Ser-Ap-Es Tablets 849

Sertraline Hydrochloride (Concurrent administration is not recommended). Products include:

Zoloft Tablets 2217

Sodium Nitroprusside (Concurrent administration is not recommended).

No products indexed under this heading.

Sotalol Hydrochloride (Concurrent administration is not recommended). Products include:

Betapace Tablets 641

Spirapril Hydrochloride (Concurrent administration is not recommended).

No products indexed under this heading.

Terazosin Hydrochloride (Concurrent administration is not recommended). Products include:

Hytrin Capsules 430

Timolol Maleate (Concurrent administration is not recommended). Products include:

Blocadren Tablets 1614
Timolide Tablets.. 1748
Timoptic in Ocudose 1753
Timoptic Sterile Ophthalmic Solution... 1751
Timoptic-XE 1755

Torsemide (Concurrent administration is not recommended). Products include:

Demadex Tablets and Injection 686

Tranylcypromine Sulfate (Concurrent administration is not recommended). Products include:

Parnate Tablets 2503

Trazodone Hydrochloride (Concurrent administration is not recommended). Products include:

Desyrel and Desyrel Dividose 503

Trimethaphan Camsylate (Concurrent administration is not recommended). Products include:

Arfonad Ampuls 2080

Trimipramine Maleate (Concurrent administration is not recommended). Products include:

Surmontil Capsules................................... 2811

Venlafaxine Hydrochloride (Concurrent administration is not recommended). Products include:

Effexor 2719

Verapamil Hydrochloride (Concurrent administration is not recommended). Products include:

Calan SR Caplets 2422
Calan Tablets.. 2419
Isoptin Injectable 1344
Isoptin Oral Tablets 1346
Isoptin SR Tablets 1348
Verelan Capsules 1410
Verelan Capsules 2824

PROPHYLLIN CCC TOPICAL EMOLLIENT OINTMENT

(Petrolatum, White) 2247
None cited in PDR database.

PROPINE WITH C CAP COMPLIANCE CAP

(Dipivefrin Hydrochloride) .... ⊙ 253
None cited in PDR database.

PROPULSID

(Cisapride) 1300

May interact with narcotic analgesics, benzodiazepines, and certain other agents. Compounds in these categories include:

Alprazolam (Sedative effects of benzodiazepines may be accelerated). Products include:

Xanax Tablets 2649

Atropine Sulfate (Concurrent use of anticholinergic compounds would be expected to compromise the beneficial effects of cisapride). Products include:

Arco-Lase Plus Tablets 512
Atrohist Plus Tablets 454
Atropine Sulfate Sterile Ophthalmic Solution .... ⊙ 233
Donnatal 2060
Donnatal Extentabs................................... 2061
Donnatal Tablets 2060
Lomotil 2439
Motofen Tablets 784
Urised Tablets... 1964

Belladonna Alkaloids (Concurrent use of anticholinergic compounds would be expected to compromise the beneficial effects of cisapride). Products include:

Bellergal-S Tablets 2250
Hyland's Bed Wetting Tablets .... ⊕ 828
Hyland's EnurAid Tablets................... ⊕ 829
Hyland's Teething Tablets .... ⊕ 830

Benztropine Mesylate (Concurrent use of anticholinergic compounds would be expected to compromise the beneficial effects of cisapride). Products include:

Cogentin 1621

Biperiden Hydrochloride (Concurrent use of anticholinergic compounds would be expected to compromise the beneficial effects of cisapride). Products include:

Akineton 1333

Chlordiazepoxide (Sedative effects of benzodiazepines may be accelerated). Products include:

Libritabs Tablets 2177
Limbitrol 2180

Chlordiazepoxide Hydrochloride (Sedative effects of benzodiazepines may be accelerated). Products include:

Librax Capsules 2176
Librium Capsules 2178
Librium Injectable 2179

Cimetidine (Coadministration leads to an increased peak plasma concentration and AUC of cisapride; GI absorption of cimetidine is accelerated when coadministered). Products include:

Tagamet Tablets 2516

Cimetidine Hydrochloride (Coadministration leads to an increased peak plasma concentration and AUC of cisapride; GI absorption of cimetidine is accelerated when coadministered). Products include:

Tagamet.. 2516

Clidinium Bromide (Concurrent use of anticholinergic compounds would be expected to compromise the beneficial effects of cisapride). Products include:

Librax Capsules 2176
Quarzan Capsules 2181

Clorazepate Dipotassium (Sedative effects of benzodiazepines may be accelerated). Products include:

Tranxene 451

Diazepam (Sedative effects of benzodiazepines may be accelerated). Products include:

Dizac 1809
Valium Injectable 2182
Valium Tablets 2183
Valrelease Capsules 2169

Dicumarol (Potential for increased coagulation times).

No products indexed under this heading.

Dicyclomine Hydrochloride (Concurrent use of anticholinergic compounds would be expected to compromise the beneficial effects of cisapride). Products include:

Bentyl 1501

Erythromycin (Due to weak *In Vitro* inhibition of cytochrome P_{450} 3A4, the clinical effect on cisapride metabolism is unknown). Products include:

A/T/S 2% Acne Topical Gel and Solution 1234
Benzamycin Topical Gel 905
E-Mycin Tablets 1341
Emgel 2% Topical Gel........................... 1093
ERYC.. 1915
Erycette (erythromycin 2%) Topical Solution... 1888
Ery-Tab Tablets 422
Erythromycin Base Filmtab 426
Erythromycin Delayed-Release Capsules, USP.................................... 427
Ilotycin Ophthalmic Ointment............. 912
PCE Dispertab Tablets 444
T-Stat 2.0% Topical Solution and Pads 2688
Theramycin Z Topical Solution 2% 1592

Erythromycin Estolate (Due to weak *In Vitro* inhibition of cytochrome P_{450} 3A4, the clinical effect on cisapride metabolism is unknown). Products include:

Ilosone 911

Erythromycin Ethylsuccinate (Due to weak *In Vitro* inhibition of cytochrome P_{450} 3A4, the clinical effect on cisapride metabolism is unknown). Products include:

E.E.S... 424
EryPed 421

Erythromycin Gluceptate (Due to weak *In Vitro* inhibition of cytochrome P_{450} 3A4, the clinical effect on cisapride metabolism is unknown). Products include:

Ilotycin Gluceptate, IV, Vials 913

Erythromycin Stearate (Due to weak *In Vitro* inhibition of cytochrome P_{450} 3A4, the clinical effect on cisapride metabolism is unknown). Products include:

Erythrocin Stearate Filmtab 425

Estazolam (Sedative effects of benzodiazepines may be accelerated). Products include:

ProSom Tablets 449

Fluconazole (Due to weak *In Vitro* inhibition of cytochrome P_{450} 3A4, the clinical effect on cisapride metabolism is unknown). Products include:

Diflucan Injection, Tablets, and Oral Suspension................................... 2194

Flurazepam Hydrochloride (Sedative effects of benzodiazepines may be accelerated). Products include:

Dalmane Capsules..................................... 2173

Glycopyrrolate (Concurrent use of anticholinergic compounds would be expected to compromise the beneficial effects of cisapride). Products include:

Robinul Forte Tablets............................... 2072
Robinul Injectable 2072
Robinul Tablets.. 2072

Halazepam (Sedative effects of benzodiazepines may be accelerated).

No products indexed under this heading.

Hyoscyamine (Concurrent use of anticholinergic compounds would be expected to compromise the beneficial effects of cisapride). Products include:

Cystospaz Tablets 1963
Urised Tablets... 1964

Hyoscyamine Sulfate (Concurrent use of anticholinergic compounds would be expected to compromise the beneficial effects of cisapride). Products include:

Arco-Lase Plus Tablets 512
Atrohist Plus Tablets 454
Cystospaz-M Capsules 1963
Donnatal 2060
Donnatal Extentabs................................... 2061
Donnatal Tablets 2060
Kutrase Capsules....................................... 2402
Levsin/Levsinex/Levbid 2405

Ipratropium Bromide (Concurrent use of anticholinergic compounds would be expected to compromise the beneficial effects of cisapride). Products include:

Atrovent Inhalation Aerosol.................. 671
Atrovent Inhalation Solution 673

Itraconazole (Due to *In Vitro* inhibition of cytochrome P_{450} 3A4, itraconazole is expected to markedly raise cisapride plasma levels; concurrent use is contraindicated). Products include:

Sporanox Capsules 1305

Ketoconazole (Oral ketoconazole potently inhibits the metabolism of cisapride resulting in a mean eightfold increase in AUC and prolonged QT intervals with rarely ventricular arrhythmias and torsade de pointes; concurrent use is contraindicated). Products include:

Nizoral 2% Cream 1297
Nizoral 2% Shampoo............................... 1298
Nizoral Tablets 1298

Lorazepam (Sedative effects of benzodiazepines may be accelerated). Products include:

Ativan Injection... 2698
Ativan Tablets 2700

Mepenzolate Bromide (Concurrent use of anticholinergic compounds would be expected to compromise the beneficial effects of cisapride).

No products indexed under this heading.

IMPORTANT NOTE: Always consult each drug listing in the patient's regimen for possible interactions.

Propulsid — **Interactions Index** — **850**

Miconazole (Due to *In Vitro* inhibition of cytochrome P_{450} 3A4, miconazole is expected to markedly raise cisapride plasma levels; concurrent use is contraindicated).
No products indexed under this heading.

Midazolam Hydrochloride (Sedative effects of benzodiazepines may be accelerated). Products include:
Versed Injection ... 2170

Oxazepam (Sedative effects of benzodiazepines may be accelerated). Products include:
Serax Capsules ... 2810
Serax Tablets ... 2810

Oxybutynin Chloride (Concurrent use of anticholinergic compounds would be expected to compromise the beneficial effects of cisapride). Products include:
Ditropan ... 1516

Prazepam (Sedative effects of benzodiazepines may be accelerated).
No products indexed under this heading.

Procyclidine Hydrochloride (Concurrent use of anticholinergic compounds would be expected to compromise the beneficial effects of cisapride). Products include:
Kemadrin Tablets ... 1112

Propantheline Bromide (Concurrent use of anticholinergic compounds would be expected to compromise the beneficial effects of cisapride). Products include:
Pro-Banthīne Tablets ... 2052

Quazepam (Sedative effects of benzodiazepines may be accelerated). Products include:
Doral Tablets ... 2664

Ranitidine Hydrochloride (GI absorption of ranitidine is accelerated when coadministered). Products include:
Zantac ... 1209
Zantac Injection ... 1207
Zantac Syrup ... 1209

Scopolamine (Concurrent use of anticholinergic compounds would be expected to compromise the beneficial effects of cisapride). Products include:
Transderm Scōp Transdermal Therapeutic System ... 869

Scopolamine Hydrobromide (Concurrent use of anticholinergic compounds would be expected to compromise the beneficial effects of cisapride). Products include:
Atrohist Plus Tablets ... 454
Donnatal ... 2060
Donnatal Extentabs ... 2061
Donnatal Tablets ... 2060

Temazepam (Sedative effects of benzodiazepines may be accelerated). Products include:
Restoril Capsules ... 2284

Triazolam (Sedative effects of benzodiazepines may be accelerated). Products include:
Halcion Tablets ... 2611

Tridihexethyl Chloride (Concurrent use of anticholinergic compounds would be expected to compromise the beneficial effects of cisapride).
No products indexed under this heading.

Trihexyphenidyl Hydrochloride (Concurrent use of anticholinergic compounds would be expected to compromise the beneficial effects of cisapride). Products include:
Artane ... 1368

Troleandomycin (Due to *In Vitro* inhibition of cytochrome P_{450} 3A4, troleandomycin is expected to markedly raise cisapride plasma levels; concurrent use is contraindicated). Products include:
Tao Capsules ... 2209

Warfarin Sodium (Potential for increased coagulation times). Products include:
Coumadin ... 926

Food Interactions

Alcohol (Sedative effects of alcohol may be accelerated).

PROSCAR TABLETS
(Finasteride) ... 1741
May interact with xanthine bronchodilators. Compounds in this category include:

Aminophylline (Increased theophylline clearance by 7% and decreased its half-life by 10%).
No products indexed under this heading.

Dyphylline (Increased theophylline clearance by 7% and decreased its half-life by 10%). Products include:
Lufyllin & Lufyllin-400 Tablets ... 2670
Lufyllin-GG Elixir & Tablets ... 2671

Theophylline (Increased theophylline clearance by 7% and decreased its half-life by 10%). Products include:
Marax Tablets & DF Syrup ... 2200
Quibron ... 2053

Theophylline Anhydrous (Increased theophylline clearance by 7% and decreased its half-life by 10%). Products include:
Aerolate ... 1004
Primatene Dual Action Formula ... ▣ 872
Primatene Tablets ... ▣ 873
Respbid Tablets ... 682
Slo-bid Gyrocaps ... 2033
Theo-24 Extended Release Capsules ... 2568
Theo-Dur Extended-Release Tablets ... 1327
Theo-X Extended-Release Tablets ... 788
Uni-Dur Extended-Release Tablets ... 1331
Uniphyl 400 mg Tablets ... 2001

Theophylline Calcium Salicylate (Increased theophylline clearance by 7% and decreased its half-life by 10%). Products include:
Quadrinal Tablets ... 1350

Theophylline Sodium Glycinate (Increased theophylline clearance by 7% and decreased its half-life by 10%).
No products indexed under this heading.

PROSOM TABLETS
(Estazolam) ... 449
May interact with central nervous system depressants, anticonvulsants, antihistamines, barbiturates, monoamine oxidase inhibitors, narcotic analgesics, phenothiazines, and certain other agents. Compounds in these categories include:

Acrivastine (Potentiates the action of benzodiazepines). Products include:
Semprex-D Capsules ... 463
Semprex-D Capsules ... 1167

Alfentanil Hydrochloride (Potentiates the action of benzodiazepines). Products include:
Alfenta Injection ... 1286

Alprazolam (Potentiates the action of benzodiazepines). Products include:
Xanax Tablets ... 2649

Aprobarbital (Potentiates the action of benzodiazepines).
No products indexed under this heading.

Astemizole (Potentiates the action of benzodiazepines). Products include:
Hismanal Tablets ... 1293

Azatadine Maleate (Potentiates the action of benzodiazepines). Products include:
Trinalin Repetabs Tablets ... 1330

Bromodiphenhydramine Hydrochloride (Potentiates the action of benzodiazepines).
No products indexed under this heading.

Brompheniramine Maleate (Potentiates the action of benzodiazepines). Products include:
Alka Seltzer Plus Sinus Medicine ... ▣ 707
Bromfed Capsules (Extended-Release) ... 1785
Bromfed Syrup ... ▣ 733
Bromfed Tablets ... 1785
Bromfed-DM Cough Syrup ... 1786
Bromfed-PD Capsules (Extended-Release) ... 1785
Dimetane-DC Cough Syrup ... 2059
Dimetane-DX Cough Syrup ... 2059
Dimetapp Elixir ... ▣ 773
Dimetapp Extentabs ... ▣ 774
Dimetapp Tablets/Liqui-Gels ... ▣ 775
Dimetapp Cold & Allergy Chewable Tablets ... ▣ 773
Dimetapp DM Elixir ... ▣ 774
Vicks DayQuil Allergy Relief 12-Hour Extended Release Tablets ... ▣ 760
Vicks DayQuil Allergy Relief 4-Hour Tablets ... ▣ 760

Buprenorphine (Potentiates the action of benzodiazepines). Products include:
Buprenex Injectable ... 2006

Buspirone Hydrochloride (Potentiates the action of benzodiazepines). Products include:
BuSpar ... 737

Butabarbital (Potentiates the action of benzodiazepines).
No products indexed under this heading.

Butalbital (Potentiates the action of benzodiazepines). Products include:
Esgic-plus Tablets ... 1013
Fioricet Tablets ... 2258
Fioricet with Codeine Capsules ... 2260
Fiorinal Capsules ... 2261
Fiorinal with Codeine Capsules ... 2262
Fiorinal Tablets ... 2261
Phrenilin ... 785
Sedapap Tablets 50 mg/650 mg ... 1543

Carbamazepine (Potentiates the action of benzodiazepines). Products include:
Atretol Tablets ... 573
Tegretol Chewable Tablets ... 852
Tegretol Suspension ... 852
Tegretol Tablets ... 852

Chlordiazepoxide (Potentiates the action of benzodiazepines). Products include:
Libritabs Tablets ... 2177
Limbitrol ... 2180

Chlordiazepoxide Hydrochloride (Potentiates the action of benzodiazepines). Products include:
Librax Capsules ... 2176
Librium Capsules ... 2178
Librium Injectable ... 2179

Chlorpheniramine Maleate (Potentiates the action of benzodiazepines). Products include:
Alka-Seltzer Plus Cold Medicine ... ▣ 705
Alka-Seltzer Plus Cold Medicine Liqui-Gels ... ▣ 706
Alka-Seltzer Plus Cold & Cough Medicine ... ▣ 708
Alka-Seltzer Plus Cold & Cough Medicine Liqui-Gels ... ▣ 705
Allerest Children's Chewable Tablets ... ▣ 627
Allerest Headache Strength Tablets ... ▣ 627
Allerest Maximum Strength Tablets ... ▣ 627
Allerest Sinus Pain Formula ... ▣ 627
Allerest 12 Hour Caplets ... ▣ 627
Ana-Kit Anaphylaxis Emergency Treatment Kit ... 617
Atrohist Pediatric Capsules ... 453
Atrohist Plus Tablets ... 454
BC Cold Powder Multi-Symptom Formula (Cold-Sinus-Allergy) ... ▣ 609
Cerose DM ... ▣ 878
Cheracol Plus Head Cold/Cough Formula ... ▣ 769
Children's Vicks DayQuil Allergy Relief ... ▣ 757
Children's Vicks NyQuil Cold/Cough Relief ... ▣ 758
Chlor-Trimeton Allergy Decongestant Tablets ... ▣ 799
Chlor-Trimeton Allergy Tablets ... ▣ 798
Comhist ... 2038
Comtrex Multi-Symptom Cold Reliever Tablets/Caplets/Liqui-Gels/Liquid ... ▣ 615
Allergy-Sinus Comtrex Multi-Symptom Allergy-Sinus Formula Tablets ... ▣ 617
Contac Continuous Action Nasal Decongestant/Antihistamine 12 Hour Capsules ... ▣ 813
Contac Maximum Strength Continuous Action Decongestant/Antihistamine 12 Hour Caplets ... ▣ 813
Contac Severe Cold and Flu Formula Caplets ... ▣ 814
Coricidin 'D' Decongestant Tablets ... ▣ 800
Coricidin Tablets ... ▣ 800
D.A. Chewable Tablets ... 951
Deconamine ... 1320
Dura-Tap/PD Capsules ... 2867
Dura-Vent/DA Tablets ... 953
Extendryl ... 1005
Fedahist Gyrocaps ... 2401
Fedahist Timecaps ... 2401
Hycomine Compound Tablets ... 932
Isoclor Timesule Capsules ... ▣ 637
Kronofed-A ... 977
Nolamine Timed-Release Tablets ... 785
Novahistine DH ... 2462
Novahistine Elixir ... ▣ 823
Ornade Spansule Capsules ... 2502
PediaCare Cold Allergy Chewable Tablets ... ▣ 677
PediaCare Cough-Cold Chewable Tablets ... 1553
PediaCare Cough-Cold Liquid ... 1553
PediaCare NightRest Cough-Cold Liquid ... 1553
Pediatric Vicks 44m Cough & Cold Relief ... ▣ 764
Pyrroxate Caplets ... ▣ 772
Ryna ... ▣ 841
Sinarest Tablets ... ▣ 648
Sinarest Extra Strength Tablets ... ▣ 648
Sine-Off Sinus Medicine ... ▣ 825
Singlet Tablets ... ▣ 825
Sinulin Tablets ... 787
Sinutab Sinus Allergy Medication, Maximum Strength Tablets and Caplets ... ▣ 860
Sudafed Plus Liquid ... ▣ 862
Sudafed Plus Tablets ... ▣ 863
Teldrin 12 Hour Antihistamine/Nasal Decongestant Allergy Relief Capsules ... ▣ 826
TheraFlu ... ▣ 787
TheraFlu Maximum Strength Nighttime Flu, Cold & Cough Medicine ... ▣ 788
Triaminic Allergy Tablets ... ▣ 789
Triaminic Cold Tablets ... ▣ 790
Triaminic Nite Light ... ▣ 791
Triaminic Syrup ... ▣ 792
Triaminic-12 Tablets ... ▣ 792
Triaminicin Tablets ... ▣ 793
Triaminicol Multi-Symptom Cold Tablets ... ▣ 793
Triaminicol Multi-Symptom Relief ... ▣ 794
Tussend ... 1783
Children's TYLENOL Cold Multi-Symptom Liquid Formula and Chewable Tablets ... 1561
Children's TYLENOL Cold Plus Cough Multi Symptom Tablets and Liquid ... ▣ 681
TYLENOL Maximum Strength Allergy Sinus Medication Gelcaps and Caplets ... 1563

(▣ Described in PDR For Nonprescription Drugs) (⊙ Described in PDR For Ophthalmology)

TYLENOL Cold Multi-Symptom Formula Medication Tablets and Caplets 1561
TYLENOL Cold Multi-Symptom Hot Medication Liquid Packets 1557
Vicks 44 LiquiCaps Cough, Cold & Flu Relief .... ◆D 755
Vicks 44M Cough, Cold & Flu Relief .... ◆D 756

Chlorpheniramine Polistirex (Potentiates the action of benzodiazepines). Products include:

Tussionex Pennkinetic Extended-Release Suspension 998

Chlorpheniramine Tannate (Potentiates the action of benzodiazepines). Products include:

Atrohist Pediatric Suspension 454
Ricobid Tablets and Pediatric Suspension 2038
Rynatan 2673
Rynatuss 2673

Chlorpromazine (Potentiates the action of benzodiazepines). Products include:

Thorazine Suppositories 2523

Chlorpromazine Hydrochloride (Potentiates the action of benzodiazepines). Products include:

Thorazine 2523

Chlorprothixene (Potentiates the action of benzodiazepines).

No products indexed under this heading.

Chlorprothixene Hydrochloride (Potentiates the action of benzodiazepines).

No products indexed under this heading.

Clemastine Fumarate (Potentiates the action of benzodiazepines). Products include:

Tavist Syrup 2297
Tavist Tablets 2298
Tavist-1 12 Hour Relief Tablets ....◆D 787
Tavist-D 12 Hour Relief Tablets ...◆D 787

Clorazepate Dipotassium (Potentiates the action of benzodiazepines). Products include:

Tranxene 451

Clozapine (Potentiates the action of benzodiazepines). Products include:

Clozaril Tablets 2252

Codeine Phosphate (Potentiates the action of benzodiazepines). Products include:

Actifed with Codeine Cough Syrup.. 1067
Brontex 1981
Deconsal C Expectorant Syrup 456
Deconsal Pediatric Syrup 457
Dimetane-DC Cough Syrup 2059
Empirin with Codeine Tablets 1093
Fioricet with Codeine Capsules 2260
Fiorinal with Codeine Capsules 2262
Isoclor Expectorant 990
Novahistine DH 2462
Novahistine Expectorant 2463
Nucofed 2051
Phenergan with Codeine 2777
Phenergan VC with Codeine 2781
Robitussin A-C Syrup 2073
Robitussin-DAC Syrup 2074
Ryna .... ◆D 841
Soma Compound w/Codeine Tablets 2676
Tussi-Organidin NR Liquid and S NR Liquid 2677
Tylenol with Codeine 1583

Cyproheptadine Hydrochloride (Potentiates the action of benzodiazepines). Products include:

Periactin 1724

Desflurane (Potentiates the action of benzodiazepines). Products include:

Suprane 1813

Dexchlorpheniramine Maleate (Potentiates the action of benzodiazepines).

No products indexed under this heading.

Dezocine (Potentiates the action of benzodiazepines). Products include:

Dalgan Injection 538

Diazepam (Potentiates the action of benzodiazepines). Products include:

Dizac 1809
Valium Injectable 2182
Valium Tablets 2183
Valrelease Capsules 2169

Diphenhydramine Citrate (Potentiates the action of benzodiazepines). Products include:

Excedrin P.M. Analgesic/Sleeping Aid Tablets, Caplets, Liquigels 733

Diphenhydramine Hydrochloride (Potentiates the action of benzodiazepines). Products include:

Actifed Allergy Daytime/Nighttime Caplets .... ◆D 844
Actifed Sinus Daytime/Nighttime Tablets and Caplets .... ◆D 846
Arthritis Foundation NightTime Caplets .... ◆D 674
Extra Strength Bayer PM Aspirin ..◆D 713
Bayer Select Night Time Pain Relief Formula .... ◆D 716
Benadryl Allergy Decongestant Liquid Medication .... ◆D 848
Benadryl Allergy Decongestant Tablets .... ◆D 848
Benadryl Allergy Liquid Medication .... ◆D 849
Benadryl Allergy .... ◆D 848
Benadryl Allergy Sinus Headache Formula Caplets .... ◆D 849
Benadryl Capsules 1898
Benadryl Dye-Free Allergy Liquigel Softgels .... ◆D 850
Benadryl Dye-Free Allergy Liquid Medication .... ◆D 850
Benadryl Itch Relief Cream, Children's Formula and Maximum Strength 2% .... ◆D 851
Benadryl Itch Relief Spray, Children's Formula and Maximum Strength 2% .... ◆D 851
Benadryl Itch Relief Stick Maximum Strength 2% .... ◆D 850
Benadryl Itch Stopping Gel, Children's Formula and Maximum Strength 2% .... ◆D 851
Benadryl Kapseals 1898
Benadryl Injection 1898
Contac Day & Night Cold/Flu Night Caplets .... ◆D 812
Contac Night Allergy/Sinus Caplets .... ◆D 812
Extra Strength Doan's P.M. .... ◆D 633
Legatrin PM .... ◆D 651
Miles Nervine Nighttime Sleep-Aid ◆D 723
Nytol QuickCaps Caplets .... ◆D 610
Sleepinal Night-time Sleep Aid Capsules and Softgels .... ◆D 834
TYLENOL Maximum Strength Allergy Sinus NightTime Medication Caplets 1555
TYLENOL Flu NightTime, Maximum Strength, Gelcaps 1566
TYLENOL Maximum Strength Flu NightTime Hot Medication Packets 1562
TYLENOL PM, Extra Strength Pain Reliever/Sleep Aid Caplets, Geltabs, Gelcaps 1560
TYLENOL Severe Allergy Medication Caplets 1564
Maximum Strength Unisom Sleepgels 1934
Unisom With Pain Relief-Nighttime Sleep Aid and Pain Reliever 1934

Diphenylpyraline Hydrochloride (Potentiates the action of benzodiazepines).

No products indexed under this heading.

Divalproex Sodium (Potentiates the action of benzodiazepines). Products include:

Depakote Tablets 415

Droperidol (Potentiates the action of benzodiazepines). Products include:

Inapsine Injection 1296

Enflurane (Potentiates the action of benzodiazepines).

No products indexed under this heading.

Ethchlorvynol (Potentiates the action of benzodiazepines). Products include:

Placidyl Capsules 448

Ethinamate (Potentiates the action of benzodiazepines).

No products indexed under this heading.

Ethosuximide (Potentiates the action of benzodiazepines). Products include:

Zarontin Capsules 1928
Zarontin Syrup 1929

Ethotoin (Potentiates the action of benzodiazepines). Products include:

Peganone Tablets 446

Felbamate (Potentiates the action of benzodiazepines). Products include:

Felbatol 2666

Fentanyl (Potentiates the action of benzodiazepines). Products include:

Duragesic Transdermal System 1288

Fentanyl Citrate (Potentiates the action of benzodiazepines). Products include:

Sublimaze Injection 1307

Fluphenazine Decanoate (Potentiates the action of benzodiazepines). Products include:

Prolixin Decanoate 509

Fluphenazine Enanthate (Potentiates the action of benzodiazepines). Products include:

Prolixin Enanthate 509

Fluphenazine Hydrochloride (Potentiates the action of benzodiazepines). Products include:

Prolixin 509

Flurazepam Hydrochloride (Potentiates the action of benzodiazepines). Products include:

Dalmane Capsules 2173

Furazolidone (Potentiates the action of benzodiazepines). Products include:

Furoxone 2046

Glutethimide (Potentiates the action of benzodiazepines).

No products indexed under this heading.

Haloperidol (Potentiates the action of benzodiazepines). Products include:

Haldol Injection, Tablets and Concentrate 1575

Haloperidol Decanoate (Potentiates the action of benzodiazepines). Products include:

Haldol Decanoate 1577

Hydrocodone Bitartrate (Potentiates the action of benzodiazepines). Products include:

Anexsia 5/500 Elixir 1781
Anexia Tablets 1782
Codiclear DH Syrup 791
Deconamine CX Cough and Cold Liquid and Tablets 1319
Duratuss HD Elixir 2565
Hycodan Tablets and Syrup 930
Hycomine Compound Tablets 932
Hycomine 931
Hycotuss Expectorant Syrup 933
Hydrocet Capsules 782
Lorcet 10/650 1018
Lortab 2566
Tussend 1783
Tussend Expectorant 1785
Vicodin Tablets 1356
Vicodin ES Tablets 1357

Vicodin Tuss Expectorant 1358
Zydone Capsules 949

Hydrocodone Polistirex (Potentiates the action of benzodiazepines). Products include:

Tussionex Pennkinetic Extended-Release Suspension 998

Hydroxyzine Hydrochloride (Potentiates the action of benzodiazepines). Products include:

Atarax Tablets & Syrup 2185
Marax Tablets & DF Syrup 2200
Vistaril Intramuscular Solution 2216

Isocarboxazid (Potentiates the action of benzodiazepines).

No products indexed under this heading.

Isoflurane (Potentiates the action of benzodiazepines).

No products indexed under this heading.

Ketamine Hydrochloride (Potentiates the action of benzodiazepines).

No products indexed under this heading.

Lamotrigine (Potentiates the action of benzodiazepines). Products include:

Lamictal Tablets 1112

Levomethadyl Acetate Hydrochloride (Potentiates the action of benzodiazepines). Products include:

Orlamm 2239

Levorphanol Tartrate (Potentiates the action of benzodiazepines). Products include:

Levo-Dromoran 2129

Loratadine (Potentiates the action of benzodiazepines). Products include:

Claritin 2349
Claritin-D 2350

Lorazepam (Potentiates the action of benzodiazepines). Products include:

Ativan Injection 2698
Ativan Tablets 2700

Loxapine Hydrochloride (Potentiates the action of benzodiazepines). Products include:

Loxitane 1378

Loxapine Succinate (Potentiates the action of benzodiazepines). Products include:

Loxitane Capsules 1378

Meperidine Hydrochloride (Potentiates the action of benzodiazepines). Products include:

Demerol 2308
Mepergan Injection 2753

Mephenytoin (Potentiates the action of benzodiazepines). Products include:

Mesantoin Tablets 2272

Mephobarbital (Potentiates the action of benzodiazepines). Products include:

Mebaral Tablets 2322

Meprobamate (Potentiates the action of benzodiazepines). Products include:

Miltown Tablets 2672
PMB 200 and PMB 400 2783

Mesoridazine (Potentiates the action of benzodiazepines).

Mesoridazine Besylate (Potentiates the action of benzodiazepines). Products include:

Serentil 684

Methadone Hydrochloride (Potentiates the action of benzodiazepines). Products include:

Methadone Hydrochloride Oral Concentrate 2233
Methadone Hydrochloride Oral Solution & Tablets 2235

IMPORTANT NOTE: Always consult each drug listing in the patient's regimen for possible interactions.

Methdilazine Hydrochloride (Potentiates the action of benzodiazepines).
No products indexed under this heading.

Methohexital Sodium (Potentiates the action of benzodiazepines). Products include:
Brevital Sodium Vials ... 1429

Methotrimeprazine (Potentiates the action of benzodiazepines). Products include:
Levoprome ... 1274

Methoxyflurane (Potentiates the action of benzodiazepines).
No products indexed under this heading.

Methsuximide (Potentiates the action of benzodiazepines). Products include:
Celontin Kapseals ... 1899

Midazolam Hydrochloride (Potentiates the action of benzodiazepines). Products include:
Versed Injection ... 2170

Molindone Hydrochloride (Potentiates the action of benzodiazepines). Products include:
Moban Tablets and Concentrate ... 1048

Morphine Sulfate (Potentiates the action of benzodiazepines). Products include:
Astramorph/PF Injection, USP (Preservative-Free) ... 535
Duramorph ... 962
Infumorph 200 and Infumorph 500 Sterile Solutions ... 965
MS Contin Tablets ... 1994
MSIR ... 1997
Oramorph SR (Morphine Sulfate Sustained Release Tablets) ... 2236
RMS Suppositories ... 2657
Roxanol ... 2243

Opium Alkaloids (Potentiates the action of benzodiazepines).
No products indexed under this heading.

Oxazepam (Potentiates the action of benzodiazepines). Products include:
Serax Capsules ... 2810
Serax Tablets ... 2810

Oxycodone Hydrochloride (Potentiates the action of benzodiazepines). Products include:
Percocet Tablets ... 938
Percodan Tablets ... 939
Percodan-Demi Tablets ... 940
Roxicodone Tablets, Oral Solution & Intensol (Oxycodone) ... 2244
Tylox Capsules ... 1584

Paramethadione (Potentiates the action of benzodiazepines).
No products indexed under this heading.

Pentobarbital Sodium (Potentiates the action of benzodiazepines). Products include:
Nembutal Sodium Capsules ... 436
Nembutal Sodium Solution ... 438
Nembutal Sodium Suppositories ... 440

Perphenazine (Potentiates the action of benzodiazepines). Products include:
Etrafon ... 2355
Triavil Tablets ... 1757
Trilafon ... 2389

Phenacemide (Potentiates the action of benzodiazepines). Products include:
Phenurone Tablets ... 447

Phenelzine Sulfate (Potentiates the action of benzodiazepines). Products include:
Nardil ... 1920

Phenobarbital (Potentiates the action of benzodiazepines). Products include:
Arco-Lase Plus Tablets ... 512
Bellergal-S Tablets ... 2250
Donnatal ... 2060
Donnatal Extentabs ... 2061
Donnatal Tablets ... 2060
Phenobarbital Elixir and Tablets ... 1469
Quadrinal Tablets ... 1350

Phensuximide (Potentiates the action of benzodiazepines). Products include:
Milontin Kapseals ... 1920

Phenytoin (Potentiates the action of benzodiazepines). Products include:
Dilantin Infatabs ... 1908
Dilantin-125 Suspension ... 1911

Phenytoin Sodium (Potentiates the action of benzodiazepines). Products include:
Dilantin Kapseals ... 1906
Dilantin Parenteral ... 1910

Prazepam (Potentiates the action of benzodiazepines).
No products indexed under this heading.

Primidone (Potentiates the action of benzodiazepines). Products include:
Mysoline ... 2754

Prochlorperazine (Potentiates the action of benzodiazepines). Products include:
Compazine ... 2470

Promethazine Hydrochloride (Potentiates the action of benzodiazepines). Products include:
Mepergan Injection ... 2753
Phenergan with Codeine ... 2777
Phenergan with Dextromethorphan ... 2778
Phenergan Injection ... 2773
Phenergan Suppositories ... 2775
Phenergan Syrup ... 2774
Phenergan Tablets ... 2775
Phenergan VC ... 2779
Phenergan VC with Codeine ... 2781

Propofol (Potentiates the action of benzodiazepines). Products include:
Diprivan Injection ... 2833

Propoxyphene Hydrochloride (Potentiates the action of benzodiazepines). Products include:
Darvon ... 1435
Wygesic Tablets ... 2827

Propoxyphene Napsylate (Potentiates the action of benzodiazepines). Products include:
Darvon-N/Darvocet-N ... 1433

Pyrilamine Maleate (Potentiates the action of benzodiazepines). Products include:
4-Way Fast Acting Nasal Spray (regular & mentholated) ... ▣ 621
Maximum Strength Multi-Symptom Formula Midol ... ▣ 722
PMS Multi-Symptom Formula Midol ... ▣ 723

Pyrilamine Tannate (Potentiates the action of benzodiazepines). Products include:
Atrohist Pediatric Suspension ... 454
Rynatan ... 2673

Quazepam (Potentiates the action of benzodiazepines). Products include:
Doral Tablets ... 2664

Risperidone (Potentiates the action of benzodiazepines). Products include:
Risperdal ... 1301

Secobarbital Sodium (Potentiates the action of benzodiazepines). Products include:
Seconal Sodium Pulvules ... 1474

Selegiline Hydrochloride (Potentiates the action of benzodiazepines). Products include:
Eldepryl Tablets ... 2550

Sufentanil Citrate (Potentiates the action of benzodiazepines). Products include:
Sufenta Injection ... 1309

Temazepam (Potentiates the action of benzodiazepines). Products include:
Restoril Capsules ... 2284

Terfenadine (Potentiates the action of benzodiazepines). Products include:
Seldane Tablets ... 1536
Seldane-D Extended-Release Tablets ... 1538

Thiamylal Sodium (Potentiates the action of benzodiazepines).
No products indexed under this heading.

Thioridazine Hydrochloride (Potentiates the action of benzodiazepines). Products include:
Mellaril ... 2269

Thiothixene (Potentiates the action of benzodiazepines). Products include:
Navane Capsules and Concentrate ... 2201
Navane Intramuscular ... 2202

Tranylcypromine Sulfate (Potentiates the action of benzodiazepines). Products include:
Parnate Tablets ... 2503

Triazolam (Potentiates the action of benzodiazepines). Products include:
Halcion Tablets ... 2611

Trifluoperazine Hydrochloride (Potentiates the action of benzodiazepines). Products include:
Stelazine ... 2514

Trimeprazine Tartrate (Potentiates the action of benzodiazepines). Products include:
Temaril Tablets, Syrup and Spansule Extended-Release Capsules ... 483

Trimethadione (Potentiates the action of benzodiazepines).
No products indexed under this heading.

Tripelennamine Hydrochloride (Potentiates the action of benzodiazepines). Products include:
PBZ Tablets ... 845
PBZ-SR Tablets ... 844

Triprolidine Hydrochloride (Potentiates the action of benzodiazepines). Products include:
Actifed Plus Caplets ... ▣ 845
Actifed Plus Tablets ... ▣ 845
Actifed with Codeine Cough Syrup ... 1067
Actifed Syrup ... ▣ 846
Actifed Tablets ... ▣ 844

Valproic Acid (Potentiates the action of benzodiazepines). Products include:
Depakene ... 413

Zolpidem Tartrate (Potentiates the action of benzodiazepines). Products include:
Ambien Tablets ... 2416

Food Interactions

Alcohol (Potentiates the action of benzodiazepines).

PROS-TECH PLUS

(Nutritional Supplement) ... 668
None cited in PDR database.

PROSTEP (NICOTINE TRANSDERMAL SYSTEM)

(Nicotine) ... 1394
May interact with xanthine bronchodilators, insulin, and certain other agents. Compounds in these categories include:

Acetaminophen (Deinduction of hepatic enzymes on smoking cessation; may require a decrease in dose at cessation of smoking). Products include:
Actifed Plus Caplets ... ▣ 845
Actifed Plus Tablets ... ▣ 845
Actifed Sinus Daytime/Nighttime Tablets and Caplets ... ▣ 846
Alka-Seltzer Plus Cold Medicine Liqui-Gels ... ▣ 706
Alka-Seltzer Plus Cold & Cough Medicine Liqui-Gels ... ▣ 705
Alka-Seltzer Plus Night-Time Cold Medicine Liqui-Gels ... ▣ 706
Allerest Headache Strength Tablets ... ▣ 627
Allerest No Drowsiness Tablets ... ▣ 627
Allerest Sinus Pain Formula ... ▣ 627
Anexsia 5/500 Elixir ... 1781
Anexia Tablets ... 1782
Arthritis Foundation Aspirin Free Caplets ... ▣ 673
Arthritis Foundation NightTime Caplets ... ▣ 674
Bayer Select Headache Pain Relief Formula ... ▣ 716
Bayer Select Menstrual Multi-Symptom Formula ... ▣ 716
Bayer Select Night Time Pain Relief Formula ... ▣ 716
Bayer Select Sinus Pain Relief Formula ... ▣ 717
Benadryl Allergy Sinus Headache Formula Caplets ... ▣ 849
Comtrex Multi-Symptom Cold Reliever Tablets/Caplets/Liqui-Gels/Liquid ... ▣ 615
Allergy-Sinus Comtrex Multi-Symptom Allergy-Sinus Formula Tablets ... ▣ 617
Comtrex Non-Drowsy ... ▣ 618
Contac Day Allergy/Sinus Caplets ▣ 812
Contac Day & Night ... ▣ 812
Contac Night Allergy/Sinus Caplets ... ▣ 812
Contac Severe Cold and Flu Formula Caplets ... ▣ 814
Contac Severe Cold & Flu Non-Drowsy ... ▣ 815
Coricidin 'D' Decongestant Tablets ... ▣ 800
Coricidin Tablets ... ▣ 800
DHCplus Capsules ... 1993
Darvon-N/Darvocet-N ... 1433
Drixoral Cold and Flu Extended-Release Tablets ... ▣ 803
Drixoral Cough + Sore Throat Liquid Caps ... ▣ 802
Drixoral Allergy/Sinus Extended Release Tablets ... ▣ 804
Esgic-plus Tablets ... 1013
Aspirin Free Excedrin Analgesic Caplets and Geltabs ... 732
Excedrin Extra-Strength Analgesic Tablets & Caplets ... 732
Excedrin P.M. Analgesic/Sleeping Aid Tablets, Caplets, Liquigels ... 733
Fioricet Tablets ... 2258
Fioricet with Codeine Capsules ... 2260
Hycomine Compound Tablets ... 932
Hydrocet Capsules ... 782
Legatrin PM ... ▣ 651
Lorcet 10/650 ... 1018
Lortab ... 2566
Lurline PMS Tablets ... 982
Maximum Strength Multi-Symptom Formula Midol ... ▣ 722
PMS Multi-Symptom Formula Midol ... ▣ 723
Teen Multi-Symptom Formula Midol ... ▣ 722
Midrin Capsules ... 783
Migralam Capsules ... 2038
Panodol Tablets and Caplets ... ▣ 824
Children's Panadol Chewable Tablets, Liquid, Infant's Drops ... ▣ 824
Percocet Tablets ... 938
Percogesic Analgesic Tablets ... ▣ 754
Phrenilin ... 785
Pyrroxate Caplets ... ▣ 772
Sedapap Tablets 50 mg/650 mg ... 1543
Sinarest Tablets ... ▣ 648
Sinarest Extra Strength Tablets ... ▣ 648
Sinarest No Drowsiness Tablets ... ▣ 648
Sine-Aid Maximum Strength Sinus Medication Gelcaps, Caplets and Tablets ... 1554
Sine-Off No Drowsiness Formula Caplets ... ▣ 824
Sine-Off Sinus Medicine ... ▣ 825
Singlet Tablets ... ▣ 825
Sinulin Tablets ... 787
Sinutab Sinus Allergy Medication, Maximum Strength Tablets and Caplets ... ▣ 860
Sinutab Sinus Medication, Maximum Strength Without Drowsi-

(▣ Described in PDR For Nonprescription Drugs) (◉ Described in PDR For Ophthalmology)

Interactions Index

ness Formula, Tablets & Caplets .... ®© 860
Sinutab Sinus Medication, Regular Strength Without Drowsiness Formula .... ®© 859
Sudafed Cold and Cough Liquidcaps .... ®© 862
Sudafed Severe Cold Formula Caplets .... ®© 863
Sudafed Severe Cold Formula Tablets .... ®© 864
Sudafed Sinus Caplets........................ ®© 864
Sudafed Sinus Tablets........................ ®© 864
Talacen 2333
TheraFlu....................................... ®© 787
TheraFlu Maximum Strength Nighttime Flu, Cold & Cough Medicine .... ®© 788
TheraFlu Maximum Strength Non-Drowsy Formula Flu, Cold & Cough Medicine .... ®© 788
Thera Flu Maximum Strength, Non-Drowsy Formula Flu, Cold and Cough Caplets .... ®© 789
Triaminic Sore Throat Formula ...... ®© 791
Triaminicin Tablets .... ®© 793
Children's TYLENOL acetaminophen Chewable Tablets, Elixir, Suspension Liquid 1555
Children's TYLENOL Cold Multi-Symptom Liquid Formula and Chewable Tablets................................ 1561
Children's TYLENOL Cold Plus Cough Multi Symptom Tablets and Liquid.. ®© 681
Infants' TYLENOL acetaminophen Drops and Suspension Drops........ 1555
Infants' TYLENOL Cold Decongestant & Fever-Reducer Drops 1556
TYLENOL Extended Relief Caplets.. 1558
TYLENOL, Extra Strength, Acetaminophen Adult Liquid Pain Reliever 1560
TYLENOL, Extra Strength, acetaminophen Gelcaps, Geltabs, Caplets, Tablets 1559
TYLENOL, Extra Strength, Headache Plus Pain Reliever with Antacid Caplets 1559
TYLENOL, Junior Strength, acetaminophen Coated Caplets, Grape and Fruit Chewable Tablets 1557
TYLENOL Maximum Strength Allergy Sinus Medication Gelcaps and Caplets 1563
TYLENOL Maximum Strength Allergy Sinus NightTime Medication Caplets 1555
TYLENOL Flu Maximum Strength Gelcaps 1565
TYLENOL Flu NightTime, Maximum Strength, Gelcaps 1566
TYLENOL Maximum Strength Flu NightTime Hot Medication Packets 1562
TYLENOL, Maximum Strength, Sinus Medication Geltabs, Gelcaps, Caplets and Tablets 1566
TYLENOL Cold Multi-Symptom Formula Medication Tablets and Caplets 1561
TYLENOL Cold Medication No Drowsiness Formula Gelcaps and Caplets 1562
TYLENOL Cold Multi-Symptom Hot Medication Liquid Packets............. 1557
TYLENOL Cough Multi-Symptom Medication 1564
TYLENOL Cough Multi-Symptom Medication with Decongestant...... 1565
TYLENOL, Regular Strength, acetaminophen Caplets and Tablets .. 1558
TYLENOL PM, Extra Strength Pain Reliever/Sleep Aid Caplets, Geltabs, Gelcaps....................................... 1560
TYLENOL Severe Allergy Medication Caplets 1564
Tylenol with Codeine 1583
Tylox Capsules 1584
Unisom With Pain Relief-Nighttime Sleep Aid and Pain Reliever............ 1934
Vanquish Analgesic Caplets .... ®© 731
Vicks 44 LiquiCaps Cough, Cold & Flu Relief....................................... ®© 755
Vicks 44M Cough, Cold & Flu Relief....................................... ®© 756
Vicks DayQuil .... ®© 761
Vicks Nyquil Hot Therapy.................. ®© 762
Vicks NyQuil LiquiCaps Multi-Symptom Cold/Flu Relief .... ®© 763

Vicks NyQuil Multi-Symptom Cold/Flu Relief - (Original & Cherry Flavor)....................................... ®© 763
Vicodin Tablets 1356
Vicodin ES Tablets 1357
Wygesic Tablets 2827
Zydone Capsules 949

Aminophylline (Deinduction of hepatic enzymes on smoking cessation; may require a decrease in dose at cessation of smoking).

No products indexed under this heading.

Caffeine (Deinduction of hepatic enzymes on smoking cessation; may require a decrease in dose at cessation of smoking). Products include:

Arthritis Strength BC Powder.......... ®© 609
BC Powder .... ®© 609
Bayer Select Headache Pain Relief Formula .... ®© 716
Cafergot....................................... 2251
DHCplus Capsules....................................... 1993
Darvon Compound-65 Pulvules 1435
Esgic-plus Tablets 1013
Aspirin Free Excedrin Analgesic Caplets and Geltabs 732
Excedrin Extra-Strength Analgesic Tablets & Caplets 732
Fioricet Tablets....................................... 2258
Fioricet with Codeine Capsules 2260
Fiorinal Capsules 2261
Fiorinal with Codeine Capsules 2262
Fiorinal Tablets....................................... 2261
Maximum Strength Multi-Symptom Formula Midol .... ®© 722
Migralam Capsules 2038
No Doz Maximum Strength Caplets .... ®© 622
Norgesic....................................... 1496
Vanquish Analgesic Caplets .... ®© 731
Wigraine Tablets & Suppositories .. 1829

Caffeine Anhydrous (Deinduction of hepatic enzymes on smoking cessation; may require a decrease in dose at cessation of smoking).

No products indexed under this heading.

Caffeine Citrate (Deinduction of hepatic enzymes on smoking cessation; may require a decrease in dose at cessation of smoking).

No products indexed under this heading.

Caffeine Sodium Benzoate (Deinduction of hepatic enzymes on smoking cessation; may require a decrease in dose at cessation of smoking).

No products indexed under this heading.

Dyphylline (Deinduction of hepatic enzymes on smoking cessation; may require a decrease in dose at cessation of smoking). Products include:

Lufyllin & Lufyllin-400 Tablets 2670
Lufyllin-GG Elixir & Tablets 2671

Imipramine Hydrochloride (Deinduction of hepatic enzymes on smoking cessation; may require a decrease in dose at cessation of smoking). Products include:

Tofranil Ampuls 854
Tofranil Tablets 856

Imipramine Pamoate (Deinduction of hepatic enzymes on smoking cessation; may require a decrease in dose at cessation of smoking). Products include:

Tofranil-PM Capsules............................ 857

Insulin, Human (Increased subcutaneous insulin absorption with smoking cessation).

No products indexed under this heading.

Insulin, Human Isophane Suspension (Increased subcutaneous insulin absorption with smoking cessation). Products include:

Novolin N Human Insulin 10 ml Vials....................................... 1795

Insulin, Human NPH (Increased subcutaneous insulin absorption with smoking cessation). Products include:

Humulin N, 100 Units.......................... 1448
Novolin N PenFill Cartridges Durable Insulin Delivery System 1798
Novolin N Prefilled Syringe Disposable Insulin Delivery System 1798

Insulin, Human Regular (Increased subcutaneous insulin absorption with smoking cessation). Products include:

Humulin R, 100 Units 1449
Novolin R Human Insulin 10 ml Vials....................................... 1795
Novolin R PenFill Cartridges Durable Insulin Delivery System 1798
Novolin R Prefilled Syringe Disposable Insulin Delivery System 1798
Velosulin BR Human Insulin 10 ml Vials....................................... 1795

Insulin, Human, Zinc Suspension (Increased subcutaneous insulin absorption with smoking cessation). Products include:

Humulin L, 100 Units 1446
Humulin U, 100 Units 1450
Novolin L Human Insulin 10 ml Vials....................................... 1795

Insulin, NPH (Increased subcutaneous insulin absorption with smoking cessation). Products include:

NPH, 100 Units 1450
Pork NPH, 100 Units............................ 1452
Purified Pork NPH Isophane Insulin 1801

Insulin, Regular (Increased subcutaneous insulin absorption with smoking cessation). Products include:

Regular, 100 Units 1450
Pork Regular, 100 Units 1452
Pork Regular (Concentrated), 500 Units 1453
Purified Pork Regular Insulin 1801

Insulin, Zinc Crystals (Increased subcutaneous insulin absorption with smoking cessation). Products include:

NPH, 100 Units 1450

Insulin, Zinc Suspension (Increased subcutaneous insulin absorption with smoking cessation). Products include:

Iletin I 1450
Lente, 100 Units 1450
Iletin II....................................... 1452
Pork Lente, 100 Units.......................... 1452
Purified Pork Lente Insulin 1801

Isoproterenol Hydrochloride (Decrease in circulating catecholamines with smoking cessation). Products include:

Isuprel Hydrochloride Injection 1:5000 2311
Isuprel Hydrochloride Solution 1:200 & 1:100 2313
Isuprel Mistometer 2312

Labetalol Hydrochloride (Decrease in circulating catecholamines with smoking cessation). Products include:

Normodyne Injection 2377
Normodyne Tablets 2379
Trandate 1185

Oxazepam (Deinduction of hepatic enzymes on smoking cessation; may require a decrease in dose at cessation of smoking). Products include:

Serax Capsules 2810
Serax Tablets....................................... 2810

Pentazocine Hydrochloride (Deinduction of hepatic enzymes on smoking cessation; may require a decrease in dose at cessation of smoking). Products include:

Talacen....................................... 2333
Talwin Compound 2335
Talwin Nx....................................... 2336

Pentazocine Lactate (Deinduction of hepatic enzymes on smoking cessation; may require a decrease in dose at cessation of smoking). Products include:

Talwin Injection....................................... 2334

Phenylephrine Hydrochloride (Decrease in circulating catecholamines with smoking cessation). Products include:

Atrohist Plus Tablets 454
Cerose DM .... ®© 878
Comhist 2038
D.A. Chewable Tablets.......................... 951
Deconsal Pediatric Capsules.............. 454
Dura-Vent/DA Tablets 953
Entex Capsules 1986
Entex Liquid 1986
Extendryl 1005
4-Way Fast Acting Nasal Spray (regular & mentholated) .... ®© 621
Hemorid For Women .... ®© 834
Hycomine Compound Tablets 932
Neo-Synephrine Hydrochloride 1% Carpuject....................................... 2324
Neo-Synephrine Hydrochloride 1% Injection 2324
Neo-Synephrine Hydrochloride (Ophthalmic) 2325
Neo-Synephrine .... ®© 726
Nöstril....................................... ®© 644
Novahistine Elixir .... ®© 823
Phenergan VC 2779
Phenergan VC with Codeine 2781
Preparation H .... ®© 871
Tympagesic Ear Drops 2342
Vasosulf .... © 271
Vicks Sinex Nasal Spray and Ultra Fine Mist .... ®© 765

Prazosin Hydrochloride (Decrease in circulating catecholamines with smoking cessation). Products include:

Minipress Capsules................................ 1937
Minizide Capsules 1938

Propranolol Hydrochloride (Deinduction of hepatic enzymes on smoking cessation; may require a decrease in dose at cessation of smoking). Products include:

Inderal 2728
Inderal LA Long Acting Capsules 2730
Inderide Tablets 2732
Inderide LA Long Acting Capsules .. 2734

Theophylline (Deinduction of hepatic enzymes on smoking cessation; may require a decrease in dose at cessation of smoking). Products include:

Marax Tablets & DF Syrup.................. 2200
Quibron 2053

Theophylline Anhydrous (Deinduction of hepatic enzymes on smoking cessation; may require a decrease in dose at cessation of smoking). Products include:

Aerolate 1004
Primatene Dual Action Formula...... ®© 872
Primatene Tablets .... ®© 873
Respbid Tablets 682
Slo-bid Gyrocaps 2033
Theo-24 Extended Release Capsules 2568
Theo-Dur Extended-Release Tablets 1327
Theo-X Extended-Release Tablets .. 788
Uni-Dur Extended-Release Tablets.. 1331
Uniphyl 400 mg Tablets........................ 2001

Theophylline Calcium Salicylate (Deinduction of hepatic enzymes on smoking cessation; may require a decrease in dose at cessation of smoking). Products include:

Quadrinal Tablets 1350

Theophylline Sodium Glycinate (Deinduction of hepatic enzymes on smoking cessation; may require a decrease in dose at cessation of smoking).

No products indexed under this heading.

IMPORTANT NOTE: Always consult each drug listing in the patient's regimen for possible interactions.

PROSTIGMIN INJECTABLE
(Neostigmine Methylsulfate) 1260
May interact with antiarrhythmics, general anesthetics, and certain other agents. Compounds in these categories include:

Acebutolol Hydrochloride (Interferes with neuromuscular transmission). Products include:
Sectral Capsules 2807

Adenosine (Interferes with neuromuscular transmission). Products include:
Adenocard Injection 1021
Adenoscan 1024

Amiodarone Hydrochloride (Interferes with neuromuscular transmission). Products include:
Cordarone Intravenous 2715
Cordarone Tablets 2712

Bretylium Tosylate (Interferes with neuromuscular transmission).
No products indexed under this heading.

Decamethonium (Phase I block of depolarizing muscle relaxants may be prolonged).

Disopyramide Phosphate (Interferes with neuromuscular transmission). Products include:
Norpace 2444

Enflurane (Caution should be exercised if used concurrently in myasthenia gravis).
No products indexed under this heading.

Isoflurane (Caution should be exercised if used concurrently in myasthenia gravis).
No products indexed under this heading.

Kanamycin Sulfate (May accentuate neuromuscular block).
No products indexed under this heading.

Ketamine Hydrochloride (Caution should be exercised if used concurrently in myasthenia gravis).
No products indexed under this heading.

Lidocaine Hydrochloride (Interferes with neuromuscular transmission). Products include:
Bactine Antiseptic/Anesthetic First Aid Liquid .... ◙ 708
Campho-Phenique Maximum Strength First Aid Antibiotic Plus Pain Reliever Ointment .... ◙ 719
Decadron Phosphate with Xylocaine Injection, Sterile 1639
Xylocaine Injections 567

Local Anesthetics (Prostigmin dosage increase may be required).

Methohexital Sodium (Caution should be exercised if used concurrently in myasthenia gravis). Products include:
Brevital Sodium Vials 1429

Methoxyflurane (Caution should be exercised if used concurrently in myasthenia gravis).
No products indexed under this heading.

Mexiletine Hydrochloride (Interferes with neuromuscular transmission). Products include:
Mexitil Capsules 678

Moricizine Hydrochloride (Interferes with neuromuscular transmission). Products include:
Ethmozine Tablets 2041

Neomycin Sulfate (May accentuate neuromuscular block). Products include:
AK-Spore .... ⊙ 204
AK-Trol Ointment & Suspension .... ⊙ 205
Bactine First Aid Antibiotic Plus Anesthetic Ointment .... ◙ 708
Campho-Phenique Maximum Strength First Aid Antibiotic Plus Pain Reliever Ointment .... ◙ 719
Coly-Mycin S Otic w/Neomycin & Hydrocortisone 1906
Cortisporin Cream 1084
Cortisporin Ointment 1085
Cortisporin Ophthalmic Ointment Sterile 1085
Cortisporin Ophthalmic Suspension Sterile 1086
Cortisporin Otic Solution Sterile 1087
Cortisporin Otic Suspension Sterile 1088
Dexacidin Ointment .... ⊙ 263
Maxitrol Ophthalmic Ointment and Suspension .... ⊙ 224
Mycitracin .... ◙ 839
NeoDecadron Sterile Ophthalmic Ointment 1712
NeoDecadron Sterile Ophthalmic Solution 1713
NeoDecadron Topical Cream 1714
Neosporin G.U. Irrigant Sterile 1148
Neosporin Ointment .... ◙ 857
Neosporin Plus Maximum Strength Cream .... ◙ 858
Neosporin Plus Maximum Strength Ointment .... ◙ 858
Neosporin Ophthalmic Ointment Sterile 1148
Neosporin Ophthalmic Solution Sterile 1149
PediOtic Suspension Sterile 1153
Poly-Pred Liquifilm .... ⊙ 248

Procainamide Hydrochloride (Interferes with neuromuscular transmission). Products include:
Procan SR Tablets 1926

Propafenone Hydrochloride (Interferes with neuromuscular transmission). Products include:
Rythmol Tablets–150mg, 225mg, 300mg 1352

Propofol (Caution should be exercised if used concurrently in myasthenia gravis). Products include:
Diprivan Injection 2833

Propranolol Hydrochloride (Interferes with neuromuscular transmission). Products include:
Inderal 2728
Inderal LA Long Acting Capsules 2730
Inderide Tablets 2732
Inderide LA Long Acting Capsules 2734

Quinidine Gluconate (Interferes with neuromuscular transmission). Products include:
Quinaglute Dura-Tabs Tablets 649

Quinidine Polygalacturonate (Interferes with neuromuscular transmission).
No products indexed under this heading.

Quinidine Sulfate (Interferes with neuromuscular transmission). Products include:
Quinidex Extentabs 2067

Sotalol Hydrochloride (Interferes with neuromuscular transmission). Products include:
Betapace Tablets 641

Streptomycin Sulfate (May accentuate neuromuscular block). Products include:
Streptomycin Sulfate Injection 2208

Succinylcholine Chloride (Phase I block of depolarizing muscle relaxants may be prolonged). Products include:
Anectine 1073

Tocainide Hydrochloride (Interferes with neuromuscular transmission). Products include:
Tonocard Tablets 531

Verapamil Hydrochloride (Interferes with neuromuscular transmission). Products include:
Calan SR Caplets 2422
Calan Tablets 2419
Isoptin Injectable 1344
Isoptin Oral Tablets 1346
Isoptin SR Tablets 1348
Verelan Capsules 1410
Verelan Capsules 2824

PROSTIGMIN TABLETS
(Neostigmine Bromide) 1261
May interact with anticholinergics, antiarrhythmics, and certain other agents. Compounds in these categories include:

Acebutolol Hydrochloride (Interferes with neuromuscular transmission). Products include:
Sectral Capsules 2807

Adenosine (Interferes with neuromuscular transmission). Products include:
Adenocard Injection 1021
Adenoscan 1024

Amiodarone Hydrochloride (Interferes with neuromuscular transmission). Products include:
Cordarone Intravenous 2715
Cordarone Tablets 2712

Atropine Sulfate (Decreased intestinal motility). Products include:
Arco-Lase Plus Tablets 512
Atrohist Plus Tablets 454
Atropine Sulfate Sterile Ophthalmic Solution .... ⊙ 233
Donnatal 2060
Donnatal Extentabs 2061
Donnatal Tablets 2060
Lomotil 2439
Motofen Tablets 784
Urised Tablets 1964

Belladonna Alkaloids (Decreased intestinal motility). Products include:
Bellergal-S Tablets 2250
Hyland's Bed Wetting Tablets .... ◙ 828
Hyland's EnurAid Tablets .... ◙ 829
Hyland's Teething Tablets .... ◙ 830

Benztropine Mesylate (Decreased intestinal motility). Products include:
Cogentin 1621

Biperiden Hydrochloride (Decreased intestinal motility). Products include:
Akineton 1333

Bretylium Tosylate (Interferes with neuromuscular transmission).
No products indexed under this heading.

Clidinium Bromide (Decreased intestinal motility). Products include:
Librax Capsules 2176
Quarzan Capsules 2181

Dicyclomine Hydrochloride (Decreased intestinal motility). Products include:
Bentyl 1501

Disopyramide Phosphate (Interferes with neuromuscular transmission). Products include:
Norpace 2444

Ethopropazine Hydrochloride (Decreased intestinal motility).

Glycopyrrolate (Decreased intestinal motility). Products include:
Robinul Forte Tablets 2072
Robinul Injectable 2072
Robinul Tablets 2072

Hyoscyamine (Decreased intestinal motility). Products include:
Cystospaz Tablets 1963
Urised Tablets 1964

Hyoscyamine Sulfate (Decreased intestinal motility). Products include:
Arco-Lase Plus Tablets 512
Atrohist Plus Tablets 454
Cystospaz-M Capsules 1963
Donnatal 2060
Donnatal Extentabs 2061
Donnatal Tablets 2060
Kutrase Capsules 2402
Levsin/Levsinex/Levbid 2405

Ipratropium Bromide (Decreased intestinal motility). Products include:
Atrovent Inhalation Aerosol 671
Atrovent Inhalation Solution 673

Kanamycin Sulfate (May accentuate neuromuscular block).
No products indexed under this heading.

Lidocaine Hydrochloride (Interferes with neuromuscular transmission). Products include:
Bactine Antiseptic/Anesthetic First Aid Liquid .... ◙ 708
Campho-Phenique Maximum Strength First Aid Antibiotic Plus Pain Reliever Ointment .... ◙ 719
Decadron Phosphate with Xylocaine Injection, Sterile 1639
Xylocaine Injections 567

Local Anesthetics (Prostigmin dosage increase may be required).

Mepenzolate Bromide (Decreased intestinal motility).
No products indexed under this heading.

Mexiletine Hydrochloride (Interferes with neuromuscular transmission). Products include:
Mexitil Capsules 678

Moricizine Hydrochloride (Interferes with neuromuscular transmission). Products include:
Ethmozine Tablets 2041

Oxybutynin Chloride (Decreased intestinal motility). Products include:
Ditropan 1516

Oxyphenonium Bromide (Decreased intestinal motility).

Procainamide Hydrochloride (Interferes with neuromuscular transmission). Products include:
Procan SR Tablets 1926

Procyclidine Hydrochloride (Decreased intestinal motility). Products include:
Kemadrin Tablets 1112

Propafenone Hydrochloride (Interferes with neuromuscular transmission). Products include:
Rythmol Tablets–150mg, 225mg, 300mg 1352

Propantheline Bromide (Decreased intestinal motility). Products include:
Pro-Banthīne Tablets 2052

Propranolol Hydrochloride (Interferes with neuromuscular transmission). Products include:
Inderal 2728
Inderal LA Long Acting Capsules 2730
Inderide Tablets 2732
Inderide LA Long Acting Capsules 2734

Quinidine Gluconate (Interferes with neuromuscular transmission). Products include:
Quinaglute Dura-Tabs Tablets 649

Quinidine Polygalacturonate (Interferes with neuromuscular transmission).
No products indexed under this heading.

Quinidine Sulfate (Interferes with neuromuscular transmission). Products include:
Quinidex Extentabs 2067

Scopolamine (Decreased intestinal motility). Products include:
Transderm Scōp Transdermal Therapeutic System 869

Scopolamine Hydrobromide (Decreased intestinal motility). Products include:
Atrohist Plus Tablets 454
Donnatal 2060
Donnatal Extentabs 2061
Donnatal Tablets 2060

Sotalol Hydrochloride (Interferes with neuromuscular transmission). Products include:
Betapace Tablets 641

(◙ Described in PDR For Nonprescription Drugs) (⊙ Described in PDR For Ophthalmology)

Streptomycin Sulfate (May accentuate neuromuscular block). Products include:

Streptomycin Sulfate Injection.......... 2208

Tocainide Hydrochloride (Interferes with neuromuscular transmission). Products include:

Tonocard Tablets.. 531

Tridihexethyl Chloride (Decreased intestinal motility).

No products indexed under this heading.

Trihexyphenidyl Hydrochloride (Decreased intestinal motility). Products include:

Artane... 1368

Verapamil Hydrochloride (Interferes with neuromuscular transmission). Products include:

Calan SR Caplets.. 2422
Calan Tablets.. 2419
Isoptin Injectable....................................... 1344
Isoptin Oral Tablets................................... 1346
Isoptin SR Tablets...................................... 1348
Verelan Capsules.. 1410
Verelan Capsules.. 2824

PROSTIN E2 SUPPOSITORY

(Dinoprostone)..2634

May interact with oxytocic drugs. Compounds in this category include:

Ergonovine Maleate (Prostin E2 may augment the activity of other oxytocic drugs; coadministration is not recommended).

No products indexed under this heading.

Methylergonovine Maleate (Prostin E2 may augment the activity of other oxytocic drugs; coadministration is not recommended). Products include:

Methergine... 2272

Oxytocin (Injection) (Prostin E2 may augment the activity of other oxytocic drugs; coadministration is not recommended).

PROSTIN VR PEDIATRIC STERILE SOLUTION

(Alprostadil)..2635

None cited in PDR database.

PROTAMINE SULFATE AMPOULES & VIALS

(Protamine Sulfate)..................................1471

May interact with:

Antibiotics, unspecified (Incompatible with unspecified cephalosporins and penicillins in vitro).

PROTEGRA ANTIOXIDANT VITAMIN & MINERAL SUPPLEMENT

(Vitamin C, Vitamin E, Beta Carotene)..ⓂⒹ 670

None cited in PDR database.

PROTOPAM CHLORIDE FOR INJECTION

(Pralidoxime Chloride)...........................2806

May interact with barbiturates, xanthine bronchodilators, phenothiazines, and certain other agents. Compounds in these categories include:

Aminophylline (Concurrent use should be avoided in patients with organophosphate poisoning).

No products indexed under this heading.

Aprobarbital (Barbiturates are potentiated by the anticholinesterases, they should be used cautiously in the treatment of convulsions).

No products indexed under this heading.

Atropine Nitrate, Methyl (Signs of atropinization may occur earlier than expected).

No products indexed under this heading.

Atropine Sulfate (Signs of atropinization may occur earlier than expected). Products include:

Arco-Lase Plus Tablets............................ 512
Atrohist Plus Tablets................................ 454
Atropine Sulfate Sterile Ophthalmic Solution.. © 233
Donnatal... 2060
Donnatal Extentabs.................................. 2061
Donnatal Tablets....................................... 2060
Lomotil.. 2439
Motofen Tablets... 784
Urised Tablets.. 1964

Butabarbital (Barbiturates are potentiated by the anticholinesterases, they should be used cautiously in the treatment of convulsions).

No products indexed under this heading.

Butalbital (Barbiturates are potentiated by the anticholinesterases, they should be used cautiously in the treatment of convulsions). Products include:

Esgic-plus Tablets..................................... 1013
Fioricet Tablets.. 2258
Fioricet with Codeine Capsules.......... 2260
Fiorinal Capsules...................................... 2261
Fiorinal with Codeine Capsules.......... 2262
Fiorinal Tablets.. 2261
Phrenilin... 785
Sedapap Tablets 50 mg/650 mg.. 1543

Chlorpromazine (Concurrent use should be avoided in patients with organophosphate poisoning). Products include:

Thorazine Suppositories......................... 2523

Dyphylline (Concurrent use should be avoided in patients with organophosphate poisoning). Products include:

Lufyllin & Lufyllin-400 Tablets.......... 2670
Lufyllin-GG Elixir & Tablets................ 2671

Fluphenazine Decanoate (Concurrent use should be avoided in patients with organophosphate poisoning). Products include:

Prolixin Decanoate.................................... 509

Fluphenazine Enanthate (Concurrent use should be avoided in patients with organophosphate poisoning). Products include:

Prolixin Enanthate.................................... 509

Fluphenazine Hydrochloride (Concurrent use should be avoided in patients with organophosphate poisoning). Products include:

Prolixin.. 509

Mephobarbital (Barbiturates are potentiated by the anticholinesterases, they should be used cautiously in the treatment of convulsions). Products include:

Mebaral Tablets... 2322

Mesoridazine Besylate (Concurrent use should be avoided in patients with organophosphate poisoning). Products include:

Serentil... 684

Methotrimeprazine (Concurrent use should be avoided in patients with organophosphate poisoning). Products include:

Levoprome.. 1274

Morphine Sulfate (Concurrent use should be avoided in patients with organophosphate poisoning). Products include:

Astramorph/PF Injection, USP (Preservative-Free)............................... 535
Duramorph.. 962
Infumorph 200 and Infumorph 500 Sterile Solutions............................ 965
MS Contin Tablets..................................... 1994
MSIR.. 1997
Oramorph SR (Morphine Sulfate Sustained Release Tablets).............. 2236
RMS Suppositories................................... 2657
Roxanol.. 2243

Pentobarbital Sodium (Barbiturates are potentiated by the anticholinesterases, they should be used cautiously in the treatment of convulsions). Products include:

Nembutal Sodium Capsules................ 436
Nembutal Sodium Solution.................. 438
Nembutal Sodium Suppositories...... 440

Perphenazine (Concurrent use should be avoided in patients with organophosphate poisoning). Products include:

Etrafon... 2355
Triavil Tablets... 1757
Trilafon.. 2389

Phenobarbital (Barbiturates are potentiated by the anticholinesterases, they should be used cautiously in the treatment of convulsions). Products include:

Arco-Lase Plus Tablets............................ 512
Bellergal-S Tablets.................................... 2250
Donnatal.. 2060
Donnatal Extentabs.................................. 2061
Donnatal Tablets....................................... 2060
Phenobarbital Elixir and Tablets...... 1469
Quadrinal Tablets..................................... 1350

Prochlorperazine (Concurrent use should be avoided in patients with organophosphate poisoning). Products include:

Compazine.. 2470

Promethazine Hydrochloride (Concurrent use should be avoided in patients with organophosphate poisoning). Products include:

Mepergan Injection................................... 2753
Phenergan with Codeine......................... 2777
Phenergan with Dextromethorphan 2778
Phenergan Injection................................. 2773
Phenergan Suppositories........................ 2775
Phenergan Syrup....................................... 2774
Phenergan Tablets..................................... 2775
Phenergan VC... 2779
Phenergan VC with Codeine.................. 2781

Reserpine (Concurrent use should be avoided in patients with organophosphate poisoning). Products include:

Diupres Tablets.. 1650
Hydropres Tablets..................................... 1675
Ser-Ap-Es Tablets...................................... 849

Secobarbital Sodium (Barbiturates are potentiated by the anticholinesterases, they should be used cautiously in the treatment of convulsions). Products include:

Seconal Sodium Pulvules....................... 1474

Succinylcholine Chloride (Concurrent use should be avoided in patients with organophosphate poisoning). Products include:

Anectine... 1073

Theophylline (Concurrent use should be avoided in patients with organophosphate poisoning). Products include:

Marax Tablets & DF Syrup..................... 2200
Quibron.. 2053

Theophylline Anhydrous (Concurrent use should be avoided in patients with organophosphate poisoning). Products include:

Aerolate.. 1004
Primatene Dual Action Formula......ⓂⒹ 872
Primatene Tablets.....................................ⓂⒹ 873
Respbid Tablets.. 682
Slo-bid Gyrocaps....................................... 2033
Theo-24 Extended Release Capsules.. 2568
Theo-Dur Extended-Release Tablets.. 1327
Theo-X Extended-Release Tablets.. 788
Uni-Dur Extended-Release Tablets.. 1331
Uniphyl 400 mg Tablets.......................... 2001

Theophylline Calcium Salicylate (Concurrent use should be avoided in patients with organophosphate poisoning). Products include:

Quadrinal Tablets...................................... 1350

Theophylline Sodium Glycinate (Concurrent use should be avoided in patients with organophosphate poisoning).

No products indexed under this heading.

Thiamylal Sodium (Barbiturates are potentiated by the anticholinesterases, they should be used cautiously in the treatment of convulsions).

No products indexed under this heading.

Thioridazine Hydrochloride (Concurrent use should be avoided in patients with organophosphate poisoning). Products include:

Mellaril... 2269

Trifluoperazine Hydrochloride (Concurrent use should be avoided in patients with organophosphate poisoning). Products include:

Stelazine.. 2514

PROTOSTAT TABLETS

(Metronidazole).......................................1883

May interact with oral anticoagulants, lithium preparations, and certain other agents. Compounds in these categories include:

Cimetidine (Prolongs the half-life and decreases plasma clearance of metronidazole). Products include:

Tagamet Tablets... 2516

Cimetidine Hydrochloride (Prolongs the half-life and decreases plasma clearance of metronidazole). Products include:

Tagamet.. 2516

Dicumarol (Potentiation of anticoagulant effect).

No products indexed under this heading.

Disulfiram (Potential for psychotic reactions in alcoholic patients who are using metronidazole and disulfiram concurrently). Products include:

Antabuse Tablets....................................... 2695

Lithium Carbonate (Elevated serum lithium levels and potential for Lithium toxicity). Products include:

Eskalith.. 2485
Lithium Carbonate Capsules & Tablets.. 2230
Lithonate/Lithotabs/Lithobid............. 2543

Lithium Citrate (Elevated serum lithium levels and potential for Lithium toxicity).

No products indexed under this heading.

Phenobarbital (May accelerate the elimination of metronidazole reduced plasma levels). Products include:

Arco-Lase Plus Tablets............................ 512
Bellergal-S Tablets.................................... 2250
Donnatal.. 2060
Donnatal Extentabs.................................. 2061
Donnatal Tablets....................................... 2060
Phenobarbital Elixir and Tablets...... 1469
Quadrinal Tablets..................................... 1350

Phenytoin (May accelerate the elimination of metronidazole reduced plasma levels). Products include:

Dilantin Infatabs....................................... 1908

IMPORTANT NOTE: Always consult each drug listing in the patient's regimen for possible interactions.

Protostat | Interactions Index | 856

Dilantin-125 Suspension ... 1911

Phenytoin Sodium (May accelerate the elimination of metronidazole reduced plasma levels). Products include:

Dilantin Kapseals ... 1906
Dilantin Parenteral ... 1910

Warfarin Sodium (Potentiation of anticoagulant effect). Products include:

Coumadin ... 926

Food Interactions

Alcohol (Abdominal cramps, nausea, vomiting, headache, and flushing may occur; alcohol should not be consumed during and for at least one day after therapy).

PROTROPIN

(Somatrem) ... 1063

May interact with glucocorticoids. Compounds in this category include:

Betamethasone Acetate (May inhibit growth-promoting effect of Protropin growth hormone). Products include:

Celestone Soluspan Suspension ... 2347

Betamethasone Sodium Phosphate (May inhibit growth-promoting effect of Protropin growth hormone). Products include:

Celestone Soluspan Suspension ... 2347

Cortisone Acetate (May inhibit growth-promoting effect of Protropin growth hormone). Products include:

Cortone Acetate Sterile Suspension ... 1623
Cortone Acetate Tablets ... 1624

Dexamethasone (May inhibit growth-promoting effect of Protropin growth hormone). Products include:

AK-Trol Ointment & Suspension ... ◉ 205
Decadron Elixir ... 1633
Decadron Tablets ... 1635
Decaspray Topical Aerosol ... 1648
Dexacidin Ointment ... ◉ 263
Maxitrol Ophthalmic Ointment and Suspension ... ◉ 224
TobraDex Ophthalmic Suspension and Ointment ... 473

Dexamethasone Acetate (May inhibit growth-promoting effect of Protropin growth hormone). Products include:

Dalalone D.P. Injectable ... 1011
Decadron-LA Sterile Suspension ... 1646

Dexamethasone Sodium Phosphate (May inhibit growth-promoting effect of Protropin growth hormone). Products include:

Decadron Phosphate Injection ... 1637
Decadron Phosphate Respihaler ... 1642
Decadron Phosphate Sterile Ophthalmic Ointment ... 1641
Decadron Phosphate Sterile Ophthalmic Solution ... 1642
Decadron Phosphate Topical Cream ... 1644
Decadron Phosphate Turbinaire ... 1645
Decadron Phosphate with Xylocaine Injection, Sterile ... 1639
Dexacort Phosphate in Respihaler ... 458
Dexacort Phosphate in Turbinaire ... 459
NeoDecadron Sterile Ophthalmic Ointment ... 1712
NeoDecadron Sterile Ophthalmic Solution ... 1713
NeoDecadron Topical Cream ... 1714

Fludrocortisone Acetate (May inhibit growth-promoting effect of Protropin growth hormone). Products include:

Florinef Acetate Tablets ... 505

Hydrocortisone (May inhibit growth-promoting effect of Protropin growth hormone). Products include:

Anusol-HC Cream 2.5% ... 1896
Aquanil HC Lotion ... 1931
Bactine Hydrocortisone Anti-Itch Cream ... ▣ 709
Caldecort Anti-Itch Hydrocortisone Spray ... ▣ 631
Cortaid ... ▣ 836
CORTENEMA ... 2535
Cortisporin Ointment ... 1085
Cortisporin Ophthalmic Ointment Sterile ... 1085
Cortisporin Ophthalmic Suspension Sterile ... 1086
Cortisporin Otic Solution Sterile ... 1087
Cortisporin Otic Suspension Sterile 1088
Cortizone-5 ... ▣ 831
Cortizone-10 ... ▣ 831
Hydrocortone Tablets ... 1672
Hytone ... 907
Massengill Medicated Soft Cloth Towelettes ... 2458
PediOtic Suspension Sterile ... 1153
Preparation H Hydrocortisone 1% Cream ... ▣ 872
ProctoCream-HC 2.5% ... 2408
VōSoL HC Otic Solution ... 2678

Hydrocortisone Acetate (May inhibit growth-promoting effect of Protropin growth hormone). Products include:

Analpram-HC Rectal Cream 1% and 2.5% ... 977
Anusol HC-1 Anti-Itch Hydrocortisone Ointment ... ▣ 847
Anusol-HC Suppositories ... 1897
Caldecort ... ▣ 631
Carmol HC ... 924
Coly-Mycin S Otic w/Neomycin & Hydrocortisone ... 1906
Cortaid ... ▣ 836
Cortifoam ... 2396
Cortisporin Cream ... 1084
Epifoam ... 2399
Hydrocortone Acetate Sterile Suspension ... 1669
Mantadil Cream ... 1135
Nupercainal Hydrocortisone 1% Cream ... ▣ 645
Ophthocort ... ◉ 311
Pramosone Cream, Lotion & Ointment ... 978
ProctoCream-HC ... 2408
ProctoFoam-HC ... 2409
Terra-Cortril Ophthalmic Suspension ... 2210

Hydrocortisone Sodium Phosphate (May inhibit growth-promoting effect of Protropin growth hormone). Products include:

Hydrocortone Phosphate Injection, Sterile ... 1670

Hydrocortisone Sodium Succinate (May inhibit growth-promoting effect of Protropin growth hormone). Products include:

Solu-Cortef Sterile Powder ... 2641

Methylprednisolone Acetate (May inhibit growth-promoting effect of Protropin growth hormone). Products include:

Depo-Medrol Single-Dose Vial ... 2600
Depo-Medrol Sterile Aqueous Suspension ... 2597

Methylprednisolone Sodium Succinate (May inhibit growth-promoting effect of Protropin growth hormone). Products include:

Solu-Medrol Sterile Powder ... 2643

Prednisolone Acetate (May inhibit growth-promoting effect of Protropin growth hormone). Products include:

AK-CIDE ... ◉ 202
AK-CIDE Ointment ... ◉ 202
Blephamide Liquifilm Sterile Ophthalmic Suspension ... 476
Blephamide Ointment ... ◉ 237
Econopred & Econopred Plus Ophthalmic Suspensions ... ◉ 217
Poly-Pred Liquifilm ... ◉ 248
Pred Forte ... ◉ 250
Pred Mild ... ◉ 253
Pred-G Liquifilm Sterile Ophthalmic Suspension ... ◉ 251
Pred-G S.O.P. Sterile Ophthalmic Ointment ... ◉ 252
Vasocidin Ointment ... ◉ 268

Prednisolone Sodium Phosphate (May inhibit growth-promoting effect of Protropin growth hormone). Products include:

AK-Pred ... ◉ 204
Hydeltrasol Injection, Sterile ... 1665
Inflamase ... ◉ 265
Pediapred Oral Liquid ... 995
Vasocidin Ophthalmic Solution ... ◉ 270

Prednisolone Tebutate (May inhibit growth-promoting effect of Protropin growth hormone). Products include:

Hydeltra-T.B.A. Sterile Suspension 1667

Prednisone (May inhibit growth-promoting effect of Protropin growth hormone). Products include:

Deltasone Tablets ... 2595

Triamcinolone (May inhibit growth-promoting effect of Protropin growth hormone). Products include:

Aristocort Tablets ... 1022

Triamcinolone Acetonide (May inhibit growth-promoting effect of Protropin growth hormone). Products include:

Aristocort A 0.025% Cream ... 1027
Aristocort A 0.5% Cream ... 1031
Aristocort A 0.1% Cream ... 1029
Aristocort A 0.1% Ointment ... 1030
Azmacort Oral Inhaler ... 2011
Nasacort Nasal Inhaler ... 2024

Triamcinolone Diacetate (May inhibit growth-promoting effect of Protropin growth hormone). Products include:

Aristocort Suspension (Forte Parenteral) ... 1027
Aristocort Suspension (Intralesional) ... 1025

Triamcinolone Hexacetonide (May inhibit growth-promoting effect of Protropin growth hormone). Products include:

Aristospan Suspension (Intra-articular) ... 1033
Aristospan Suspension (Intralesional) ... 1032

PROVENTIL INHALATION AEROSOL

(Albuterol) ... 2382

May interact with sympathomimetic aerosol bronchodilators, monoamine oxidase inhibitors, tricyclic antidepressants, drugs which lower serum potassium (selected), and beta blockers. Compounds in these categories include:

Acebutolol Hydrochloride (Inhibited effects of both drugs). Products include:

Sectral Capsules ... 2807

Amitriptyline Hydrochloride (Potentiates albuterol's effects on the vascular system). Products include:

Elavil ... 2838
Endep Tablets ... 2174
Etrafon ... 2355
Limbitrol ... 2180
Triavil Tablets ... 1757

Amoxapine (Potentiates albuterol's effects on the vascular system). Products include:

Asendin Tablets ... 1369

Atenolol (Inhibited effects of both drugs). Products include:

Tenoretic Tablets ... 2845
Tenormin Tablets and I.V. Injection 2847

Bendroflumethiazide (Potential for additive hypokalemic effect with concurrent use).

No products indexed under this heading.

Betamethasone Acetate (Potential for additive hypokalemic effect with concurrent use). Products include:

Celestone Soluspan Suspension ... 2347

Betamethasone Sodium Phosphate (Potential for additive hypokalemic effect with concurrent use). Products include:

Celestone Soluspan Suspension ... 2347

Betaxolol Hydrochloride (Inhibited effects of both drugs). Products include:

Betoptic Ophthalmic Solution ... 469
Betoptic S Ophthalmic Suspension ... 471
Kerlone Tablets ... 2436

Bisoprolol Fumarate (Inhibited effects of both drugs). Products include:

Zebeta Tablets ... 1413
Ziac ... 1415

Bitolterol Mesylate (Potentiates cardiovascular effects). Products include:

Tornalate Solution for Inhalation, 0.2% ... 956
Tornalate Metered Dose Inhaler ... 957

Carteolol Hydrochloride (Inhibited effects of both drugs). Products include:

Cartrol Tablets ... 410
Ocupress Ophthalmic Solution, 1% Sterile ... ◉ 309

Chlorothiazide (Potential for additive hypokalemic effect with concurrent use). Products include:

Aldoclor Tablets ... 1598
Diupres Tablets ... 1650
Diuril Oral ... 1653

Chlorothiazide Sodium (Potential for additive hypokalemic effect with concurrent use). Products include:

Diuril Sodium Intravenous ... 1652

Clomipramine Hydrochloride (Potentiates albuterol's effects on the vascular system). Products include:

Anafranil Capsules ... 803

Cortisone Acetate (Potential for additive hypokalemic effect with concurrent use). Products include:

Cortone Acetate Sterile Suspension ... 1623
Cortone Acetate Tablets ... 1624

Desipramine Hydrochloride (Potentiates albuterol's effects on the vascular system). Products include:

Norpramin Tablets ... 1526

Dexamethasone (Potential for additive hypokalemic effect with concurrent use). Products include:

AK-Trol Ointment & Suspension ... ◉ 205
Decadron Elixir ... 1633
Decadron Tablets ... 1635
Decaspray Topical Aerosol ... 1648
Dexacidin Ointment ... ◉ 263
Maxitrol Ophthalmic Ointment and Suspension ... ◉ 224
TobraDex Ophthalmic Suspension and Ointment ... 473

Dexamethasone Acetate (Potential for additive hypokalemic effect with concurrent use). Products include:

Dalalone D.P. Injectable ... 1011
Decadron-LA Sterile Suspension ... 1646

Dexamethasone Sodium Phosphate (Potential for additive hypokalemic effect with concurrent use). Products include:

Decadron Phosphate Injection ... 1637
Decadron Phosphate Respihaler ... 1642
Decadron Phosphate Sterile Ophthalmic Ointment ... 1641
Decadron Phosphate Sterile Ophthalmic Solution ... 1642
Decadron Phosphate Topical Cream ... 1644
Decadron Phosphate Turbinaire ... 1645
Decadron Phosphate with Xylocaine Injection, Sterile ... 1639
Dexacort Phosphate in Respihaler ... 458
Dexacort Phosphate in Turbinaire ... 459
NeoDecadron Sterile Ophthalmic Ointment ... 1712

NeoDecadron Sterile Ophthalmic Solution ... 1713
NeoDecadron Topical Cream ... 1714

Doxepin Hydrochloride (Potentiates albuterol's effects on the vascular system). Products include:
Sinequan ... 2205
Zonalon Cream ... 1055

Furazolidone (Potentiates albuterol's effects on the vascular system). Products include:
Furoxone ... 2046

Hydrochlorothiazide (Potential for additive hypokalemic effect with concurrent use). Products include:
Aldactazide ... 2413
Aldoril Tablets ... 1604
Apresazide Capsules ... 808
Capozide ... 742
Dyazide ... 2479
Esidrix Tablets ... 821
Esimil Tablets ... 822
HydroDIURIL Tablets ... 1674
Hydropres Tablets ... 1675
Hyzaar Tablets ... 1677
Inderide Tablets ... 2732
Inderide LA Long Acting Capsules .. 2734
Lopressor HCT Tablets ... 832
Lotensin HCT ... 837
Maxzide ... 1380
Moduretic Tablets ... 1705
Oretic Tablets ... 443
Prinzide Tablets ... 1737
Ser-Ap-Es Tablets ... 849
Timolide Tablets ... 1748
Vaseretic Tablets ... 1765
Zestoretic ... 2850
Ziac ... 1415

Hydrocortisone (Potential for additive hypokalemic effect with concurrent use). Products include:
Anusol-HC Cream 2.5% ... 1896
Aquanil HC Lotion ... 1931
Bactine Hydrocortisone Anti-Itch Cream ... ▣ 709
Caldecort Anti-Itch Hydrocortisone Spray ... ▣ 631
Cortaid ... ▣ 836
CORTENEMA ... 2535
Cortisporin Ointment ... 1085
Cortisporin Ophthalmic Ointment Sterile ... 1085
Cortisporin Ophthalmic Suspension Sterile ... 1086
Cortisporin Otic Solution Sterile ... 1087
Cortisporin Otic Suspension Sterile 1088
Cortizone-5 ... ▣ 831
Cortizone-10 ... ▣ 831
Hydrocortone Tablets ... 1672
Hytone ... 907
Massengill Medicated Soft Cloth Towelettes ... 2458
PediOtic Suspension Sterile ... 1153
Preparation H Hydrocortisone 1% Cream ... ▣ 872
ProctoCream-HC 2.5% ... 2408
VōSoL HC Otic Solution ... 2678

Hydrocortisone Acetate (Potential for additive hypokalemic effect with concurrent use). Products include:
Analpram-HC Rectal Cream 1% and 2.5% ... 977
Anusol HC-1 Anti-Itch Hydrocortisone Ointment ... ▣ 847
Anusol-HC Suppositories ... 1897
Caldecort ... ▣ 631
Carmol HC ... 924
Coly-Mycin S Otic w/Neomycin & Hydrocortisone ... 1906
Cortaid ... ▣ 836
Cortifoam ... 2396
Cortisporin Cream ... 1084
Epifoam ... 2399
Hydrocortone Acetate Sterile Suspension ... 1669
Mantadil Cream ... 1135
Nupercainal Hydrocortisone 1% Cream ... ▣ 645
Ophthocort ... ◉ 311
Pramosone Cream, Lotion & Ointment ... 978
ProctoCream-HC ... 2408
ProctoFoam-HC ... 2409
Terra-Cortril Ophthalmic Suspension ... 2210

Hydrocortisone Sodium Phosphate (Potential for additive hypokalemic effect with concurrent use). Products include:
Hydrocortone Phosphate Injection, Sterile ... 1670

Hydrocortisone Sodium Succinate (Potential for additive hypokalemic effect with concurrent use). Products include:
Solu-Cortef Sterile Powder ... 2641

Hydroflumethiazide (Potential for additive hypokalemic effect with concurrent use). Products include:
Diucardin Tablets ... 2718

Imipramine Hydrochloride (Potentiates albuterol's effects on the vascular system). Products include:
Tofranil Ampuls ... 854
Tofranil Tablets ... 856

Imipramine Pamoate (Potentiates albuterol's effects on the vascular system). Products include:
Tofranil-PM Capsules ... 857

Isocarboxazid (Potentiates albuterol's effects on the vascular system).
No products indexed under this heading.

Isoetharine (Potentiates cardiovascular effects). Products include:
Bronkometer Aerosol ... 2302
Bronkosol Solution ... 2302
Isoetharine Inhalation Solution, USP, Arm-a-Med ... 551

Isoproterenol Hydrochloride (Potentiates cardiovascular effects). Products include:
Isuprel Hydrochloride Injection 1:5000 ... 2311
Isuprel Hydrochloride Solution 1:200 & 1:100 ... 2313
Isuprel Mistometer ... 2312

Labetalol Hydrochloride (Inhibited effects of both drugs). Products include:
Normodyne Injection ... 2377
Normodyne Tablets ... 2379
Trandate ... 1185

Levobunolol Hydrochloride (Inhibited effects of both drugs). Products include:
Betagan ... ◉ 233

Maprotiline Hydrochloride (Potentiates albuterol's effects on the vascular system). Products include:
Ludiomil Tablets ... 843

Metaproterenol Sulfate (Potentiates cardiovascular effects). Products include:
Alupent ... 669
Metaproterenol Sulfate Inhalation Solution, USP, Arm-a-Med ... 552

Methyclothiazide (Potential for additive hypokalemic effect with concurrent use). Products include:
Enduron Tablets ... 420

Methylprednisolone Acetate (Potential for additive hypokalemic effect with concurrent use). Products include:
Depo-Medrol Single-Dose Vial ... 2600
Depo-Medrol Sterile Aqueous Suspension ... 2597

Methylprednisolone Sodium Succinate (Potential for additive hypokalemic effect with concurrent use). Products include:
Solu-Medrol Sterile Powder ... 2643

Metipranolol Hydrochloride (Inhibited effects of both drugs). Products include:
OptiPranolol (Metipranolol 0.3%) Sterile Ophthalmic Solution ... ◉ 258

Metoprolol Succinate (Inhibited effects of both drugs). Products include:
Toprol-XL Tablets ... 565

Metoprolol Tartrate (Inhibited effects of both drugs). Products include:
Lopressor Ampuls ... 830
Lopressor HCT Tablets ... 832
Lopressor Tablets ... 830

Nadolol (Inhibited effects of both drugs).
No products indexed under this heading.

Nortriptyline Hydrochloride (Potentiates albuterol's effects on the vascular system). Products include:
Pamelor ... 2280

Penbutolol Sulfate (Inhibited effects of both drugs). Products include:
Levatol ... 2403

Phenelzine Sulfate (Potentiates albuterol's effects on the vascular system). Products include:
Nardil ... 1920

Pindolol (Inhibited effects of both drugs). Products include:
Visken Tablets ... 2299

Pirbuterol Acetate (Potentiates cardiovascular effects). Products include:
Maxair Autohaler ... 1492
Maxair Inhaler ... 1494

Polythiazide (Potential for additive hypokalemic effect with concurrent use). Products include:
Minizide Capsules ... 1938

Prednisolone Acetate (Potential for additive hypokalemic effect with concurrent use). Products include:
AK-CIDE ... ◉ 202
AK-CIDE Ointment ... ◉ 202
Blephamide Liquifilm Sterile Ophthalmic Suspension ... 476
Blephamide Ointment ... ◉ 237
Econopred & Econopred Plus Ophthalmic Suspensions ... ◉ 217
Poly-Pred Liquifilm ... ◉ 248
Pred Forte ... ◉ 250
Pred Mild ... ◉ 253
Pred-G Liquifilm Sterile Ophthalmic Suspension ... ◉ 251
Pred-G S.O.P. Sterile Ophthalmic Ointment ... ◉ 252
Vasocidin Ointment ... ◉ 268

Prednisolone Sodium Phosphate (Potential for additive hypokalemic effect with concurrent use). Products include:
AK-Pred ... ◉ 204
Hydeltrasol Injection, Sterile ... 1665
Inflamase ... ◉ 265
Pediapred Oral Liquid ... 995
Vasocidin Ophthalmic Solution ... ◉ 270

Prednisolone Tebutate (Potential for additive hypokalemic effect with concurrent use). Products include:
Hydeltra-T.B.A. Sterile Suspension 1667

Prednisone (Potential for additive hypokalemic effect with concurrent use). Products include:
Deltasone Tablets ... 2595

Propranolol Hydrochloride (Inhibited effects of both drugs). Products include:
Inderal ... 2728
Inderal LA Long Acting Capsules ... 2730
Inderide Tablets ... 2732
Inderide LA Long Acting Capsules .. 2734

Protriptyline Hydrochloride (Potentiates albuterol's effects on the vascular system). Products include:
Vivactil Tablets ... 1774

Salmeterol Xinafoate (Potentiates cardiovascular effects). Products include:
Serevent Inhalation Aerosol ... 1176

Selegiline Hydrochloride (Potentiates albuterol's effects on the vascular system). Products include:
Eldepryl Tablets ... 2550

Sotalol Hydrochloride (Inhibited effects of both drugs). Products include:
Betapace Tablets ... 641

Terbutaline Sulfate (Potentiates cardiovascular effects). Products include:
Brethaire Inhaler ... 813
Brethine Ampuls ... 815
Brethine Tablets ... 814
Bricanyl Subcutaneous Injection ... 1502
Bricanyl Tablets ... 1503

Timolol Hemihydrate (Inhibited effects of both drugs). Products include:
Betimol 0.25%, 0.5% ... ◉ 261

Timolol Maleate (Inhibited effects of both drugs). Products include:
Blocadren Tablets ... 1614
Timolide Tablets ... 1748
Timoptic in Ocudose ... 1753
Timoptic Sterile Ophthalmic Solution ... 1751
Timoptic-XE ... 1755

Tranylcypromine Sulfate (Potentiates albuterol's effects on the vascular system). Products include:
Parnate Tablets ... 2503

Triamcinolone (Potential for additive hypokalemic effect with concurrent use). Products include:
Aristocort Tablets ... 1022

Triamcinolone Acetonide (Potential for additive hypokalemic effect with concurrent use). Products include:
Aristocort A 0.025% Cream ... 1027
Aristocort A 0.5% Cream ... 1031
Aristocort A 0.1% Cream ... 1029
Aristocort A 0.1% Ointment ... 1030
Azmacort Oral Inhaler ... 2011
Nasacort Nasal Inhaler ... 2024

Triamcinolone Diacetate (Potential for additive hypokalemic effect with concurrent use). Products include:
Aristocort Suspension (Forte Parenteral) ... 1027
Aristocort Suspension (Intralesional) ... 1025

Triamcinolone Hexacetonide (Potential for additive hypokalemic effect with concurrent use). Products include:
Aristospan Suspension (Intra-articular) ... 1033
Aristospan Suspension (Intralesional) ... 1032

Trimipramine Maleate (Potentiates albuterol's effects on the vascular system). Products include:
Surmontil Capsules ... 2811

PROVENTIL INHALATION SOLUTION 0.083%

(Albuterol Sulfate) ... 2384
May interact with sympathomimetic aerosol bronchodilators, monoamine oxidase inhibitors, tricyclic antidepressants, drugs which lower serum potassium (selected), and beta blockers. Compounds in these categories include:

Acebutolol Hydrochloride (Effects of both drugs inhibited). Products include:
Sectral Capsules ... 2807

Albuterol (Effect not specified; concurrent use should be avoided). Products include:
Proventil Inhalation Aerosol ... 2382
Ventolin Inhalation Aerosol and Refill ... 1197

IMPORTANT NOTE: Always consult each drug listing in the patient's regimen for possible interactions.

Proventil Solution 0.083% | Interactions Index | 858

Amitriptyline Hydrochloride (Action of albuterol on the vascular system may be potentiated). Products include:
- Elavil ... 2838
- Endep Tablets ... 2174
- Etrafon ... 2355
- Limbitrol ... 2180
- Triavil Tablets ... 1757

Amoxapine (Action of albuterol on the vascular system may be potentiated). Products include:
- Asendin Tablets ... 1369

Atenolol (Effects of both drugs inhibited). Products include:
- Tenoretic Tablets ... 2845
- Tenormin Tablets and I.V. Injection 2847

Bendroflumethiazide (Potential for additive hypokalemic effect with concurrent use).
- No products indexed under this heading.

Betamethasone Acetate (Potential for additive hypokalemic effect with concurrent use). Products include:
- Celestone Soluspan Suspension ... 2347

Betamethasone Sodium Phosphate (Potential for additive hypokalemic effect with concurrent use). Products include:
- Celestone Soluspan Suspension ... 2347

Betaxolol Hydrochloride (Effects of both drugs inhibited). Products include:
- Betoptic Ophthalmic Solution ... 469
- Betoptic S Ophthalmic Suspension 471
- Kerlone Tablets ... 2436

Bisoprolol Fumarate (Effects of both drugs inhibited). Products include:
- Zebeta Tablets ... 1413
- Ziac ... 1415

Bitolterol Mesylate (Effect not specified; concurrent use should be avoided). Products include:
- Tornalate Solution for Inhalation, 0.2% ... 956
- Tornalate Metered Dose Inhaler ... 957

Carteolol Hydrochloride (Effects of both drugs inhibited). Products include:
- Cartrol Tablets ... 410
- Ocupress Ophthalmic Solution, 1% Sterile ... ◉ 309

Chlorothiazide (Potential for additive hypokalemic effect with concurrent use). Products include:
- Aldoclor Tablets ... 1598
- Diupres Tablets ... 1650
- Diuril Oral ... 1653

Chlorothiazide Sodium (Potential for additive hypokalemic effect with concurrent use). Products include:
- Diuril Sodium Intravenous ... 1652

Clomipramine Hydrochloride (Action of albuterol on the vascular system may be potentiated). Products include:
- Anafranil Capsules ... 803

Cortisone Acetate (Potential for additive hypokalemic effect with concurrent use). Products include:
- Cortone Acetate Sterile Suspension ... 1623
- Cortone Acetate Tablets ... 1624

Desipramine Hydrochloride (Action of albuterol on the vascular system may be potentiated). Products include:
- Norpramin Tablets ... 1526

Dexamethasone (Potential for additive hypokalemic effect with concurrent use). Products include:
- AK-Trol Ointment & Suspension ... ◉ 205
- Decadron Elixir ... 1633
- Decadron Tablets ... 1635
- Decaspray Topical Aerosol ... 1648
- Dexacidin Ointment ... ◉ 263
- Maxitrol Ophthalmic Ointment and Suspension ... ◉ 224
- TobraDex Ophthalmic Suspension and Ointment ... 473

Dexamethasone Acetate (Potential for additive hypokalemic effect with concurrent use). Products include:
- Dalalone D.P. Injectable ... 1011
- Decadron-LA Sterile Suspension ... 1646

Dexamethasone Sodium Phosphate (Potential for additive hypokalemic effect with concurrent use). Products include:
- Decadron Phosphate Injection ... 1637
- Decadron Phosphate Respihaler ... 1642
- Decadron Phosphate Sterile Ophthalmic Ointment ... 1641
- Decadron Phosphate Sterile Ophthalmic Solution ... 1642
- Decadron Phosphate Topical Cream ... 1644
- Decadron Phosphate Turbinaire ... 1645
- Decadron Phosphate with Xylocaine Injection, Sterile ... 1639
- Dexacort Phosphate in Respihaler .. 458
- Dexacort Phosphate in Turbinaire .. 459
- NeoDecadron Sterile Ophthalmic Ointment ... 1712
- NeoDecadron Sterile Ophthalmic Solution ... 1713
- NeoDecadron Topical Cream ... 1714

Doxepin Hydrochloride (Action of albuterol on the vascular system may be potentiated). Products include:
- Sinequan ... 2205
- Zonalon Cream ... 1055

Esmolol Hydrochloride (Effects of both drugs inhibited). Products include:
- Brevibloc Injection ... 1808

Furazolidone (Action of albuterol on the vascular system may be potentiated). Products include:
- Furoxone ... 2046

Hydrochlorothiazide (Potential for additive hypokalemic effect with concurrent use). Products include:
- Aldactazide ... 2413
- Aldoril Tablets ... 1604
- Apresazide Capsules ... 808
- Capozide ... 742
- Dyazide ... 2479
- Esidrix Tablets ... 821
- Esimil Tablets ... 822
- HydroDIURIL Tablets ... 1674
- Hydropres Tablets ... 1675
- Hyzaar Tablets ... 1677
- Inderide Tablets ... 2732
- Inderide LA Long Acting Capsules .. 2734
- Lopressor HCT Tablets ... 832
- Lotensin HCT ... 837
- Maxzide ... 1380
- Moduretic Tablets ... 1705
- Oretic Tablets ... 443
- Prinzide Tablets ... 1737
- Ser-Ap-Es Tablets ... 849
- Timolide Tablets ... 1748
- Vaseretic Tablets ... 1765
- Zestoretic ... 2850
- Ziac ... 1415

Hydrocortisone (Potential for additive hypokalemic effect with concurrent use). Products include:
- Anusol-HC Cream 2.5% ... 1896
- Aquanil HC Lotion ... 1931
- Bactine Hydrocortisone Anti-Itch Cream ... ▣ 709
- Caldecort Anti-Itch Hydrocortisone Spray ... ▣ 631
- Cortaid ... ▣ 836
- CORTENEMA ... 2535
- Cortisporin Ointment ... 1085
- Cortisporin Ophthalmic Ointment Sterile ... 1085
- Cortisporin Ophthalmic Suspension Sterile ... 1086
- Cortisporin Otic Solution Sterile ... 1087
- Cortisporin Otic Suspension Sterile 1088
- Cortizone-5 ... ▣ 831
- Cortizone-10 ... ▣ 831
- Hydrocortone Tablets ... 1672
- Hytone ... 907
- Massengill Medicated Soft Cloth Towelettes ... 2458
- PediOtic Suspension Sterile ... 1153
- Preparation H Hydrocortisone 1% Cream ... ▣ 872
- ProctoCream-HC 2.5% ... 2408
- VōSoL HC Otic Solution ... 2678

Hydrocortisone Acetate (Potential for additive hypokalemic effect with concurrent use). Products include:
- Analpram-HC Rectal Cream 1% and 2.5% ... 977
- Anusol HC-1 Anti-Itch Hydrocortisone Ointment ... ▣ 847
- Anusol-HC Suppositories ... 1897
- Caldecort ... ▣ 631
- Carmol HC ... 924
- Coly-Mycin S Otic w/Neomycin & Hydrocortisone ... 1906
- Cortaid ... ▣ 836
- Cortifoam ... 2396
- Cortisporin Cream ... 1084
- Epifoam ... 2399
- Hydrocortone Acetate Sterile Suspension ... 1669
- Mantadil Cream ... 1135
- Nupercainal Hydrocortisone 1% Cream ... ▣ 645
- Ophthocort ... ◉ 311
- Pramosone Cream, Lotion & Ointment ... 978
- ProctoCream-HC ... 2408
- ProctoFoam-HC ... 2409
- Terra-Cortril Ophthalmic Suspension ... 2210

Hydrocortisone Sodium Phosphate (Potential for additive hypokalemic effect with concurrent use). Products include:
- Hydrocortone Phosphate Injection, Sterile ... 1670

Hydrocortisone Sodium Succinate (Potential for additive hypokalemic effect with concurrent use). Products include:
- Solu-Cortef Sterile Powder ... 2641

Hydroflumethiazide (Potential for additive hypokalemic effect with concurrent use). Products include:
- Diucardin Tablets ... 2718

Imipramine Hydrochloride (Action of albuterol on the vascular system may be potentiated). Products include:
- Tofranil Ampuls ... 854
- Tofranil Tablets ... 856

Imipramine Pamoate (Action of albuterol on the vascular system may be potentiated). Products include:
- Tofranil-PM Capsules ... 857

Isocarboxazid (Action of albuterol on the vascular system may be potentiated).
- No products indexed under this heading.

Isoetharine (Effect not specified; concurrent use should be avoided). Products include:
- Bronkometer Aerosol ... 2302
- Bronkosol Solution ... 2302
- Isoetharine Inhalation Solution, USP, Arm-a-Med ... 551

Isoproterenol Hydrochloride (Effect not specified; concurrent use should be avoided). Products include:
- Isuprel Hydrochloride Injection 1:5000 ... 2311
- Isuprel Hydrochloride Solution 1:200 & 1:100 ... 2313
- Isuprel Mistometer ... 2312

Labetalol Hydrochloride (Effects of both drugs inhibited). Products include:
- Normodyne Injection ... 2377
- Normodyne Tablets ... 2379
- Trandate ... 1185

Levobunolol Hydrochloride (Effects of both drugs inhibited). Products include:
- Betagan ... ◉ 233

Maprotiline Hydrochloride (Action of albuterol on the vascular system may be potentiated). Products include:
- Ludiomil Tablets ... 843

Metaproterenol Sulfate (Effect not specified; concurrent use should be avoided). Products include:
- Alupent ... 669
- Metaproterenol Sulfate Inhalation Solution, USP, Arm-a-Med ... 552

Methyclothiazide (Potential for additive hypokalemic effect with concurrent use). Products include:
- Enduron Tablets ... 420

Methylprednisolone Acetate (Potential for additive hypokalemic effect with concurrent use). Products include:
- Depo-Medrol Single-Dose Vial ... 2600
- Depo-Medrol Sterile Aqueous Suspension ... 2597

Methylprednisolone Sodium Succinate (Potential for additive hypokalemic effect with concurrent use). Products include:
- Solu-Medrol Sterile Powder ... 2643

Metipranolol Hydrochloride (Effects of both drugs inhibited). Products include:
- OptiPranolol (Metipranolol 0.3%) Sterile Ophthalmic Solution ... ◉ 258

Metoprolol Succinate (Effects of both drugs inhibited). Products include:
- Toprol-XL Tablets ... 565

Metoprolol Tartrate (Effects of both drugs inhibited). Products include:
- Lopressor Ampuls ... 830
- Lopressor HCT Tablets ... 832
- Lopressor Tablets ... 830

Nadolol (Effects of both drugs inhibited).
- No products indexed under this heading.

Nortriptyline Hydrochloride (Action of albuterol on the vascular system may be potentiated). Products include:
- Pamelor ... 2280

Penbutolol Sulfate (Effects of both drugs inhibited). Products include:
- Levatol ... 2403

Phenelzine Sulfate (Action of albuterol on the vascular system may be potentiated). Products include:
- Nardil ... 1920

Pindolol (Effects of both drugs inhibited). Products include:
- Visken Tablets ... 2299

Pirbuterol Acetate (Effect not specified; concurrent use should be avoided). Products include:
- Maxair Autohaler ... 1492
- Maxair Inhaler ... 1494

Polythiazide (Potential for additive hypokalemic effect with concurrent use). Products include:
- Minizide Capsules ... 1938

Prednisolone Acetate (Potential for additive hypokalemic effect with concurrent use). Products include:
- AK-CIDE ... ◉ 202
- AK-CIDE Ointment ... ◉ 202
- Blephamide Liquifilm Sterile Ophthalmic Suspension ... 476
- Blephamide Ointment ... ◉ 237
- Econopred & Econopred Plus Ophthalmic Suspensions ... ◉ 217
- Poly-Pred Liquifilm ... ◉ 248
- Pred Forte ... ◉ 250
- Pred Mild ... ◉ 253
- Pred-G Liquifilm Sterile Ophthalmic Suspension ... ◉ 251
- Pred-G S.O.P. Sterile Ophthalmic Ointment ... ◉ 252
- Vasocidin Ointment ... ◉ 268

(▣ Described in PDR For Nonprescription Drugs) (◉ Described in PDR For Ophthalmology)

859 **Interactions Index** **Proventil**

Prednisolone Sodium Phosphate (Potential for additive hypokalemic effect with concurrent use). Products include:
AK-Pred ◉ 204
Hydeltrasol Injection, Sterile 1665
Inflamase ◉ 265
Pediapred Oral Liquid 995
Vasocidin Ophthalmic Solution ◉ 270

Prednisolone Tebutate (Potential for additive hypokalemic effect with concurrent use). Products include:
Hydeltra-T.B.A. Sterile Suspension 1667

Prednisone (Potential for additive hypokalemic effect with concurrent use). Products include:
Deltasone Tablets 2595

Propranolol Hydrochloride (Effects of both drugs inhibited). Products include:
Inderal 2728
Inderal LA Long Acting Capsules 2730
Inderide Tablets 2732
Inderide LA Long Acting Capsules 2734

Protriptyline Hydrochloride (Action of albuterol on the vascular system may be potentiated). Products include:
Vivactil Tablets 1774

Salmeterol Xinafoate (Effect not specified; concurrent use should be avoided). Products include:
Serevent Inhalation Aerosol 1176

Selegiline Hydrochloride (Action of albuterol on the vascular system may be potentiated). Products include:
Eldepryl Tablets 2550

Sotalol Hydrochloride (Effects of both drugs inhibited). Products include:
Betapace Tablets 641

Terbutaline Sulfate (Effect not specified; concurrent use should be avoided). Products include:
Brethaire Inhaler 813
Brethine Ampuls 815
Brethine Tablets 814
Bricanyl Subcutaneous Injection 1502
Bricanyl Tablets 1503

Timolol Hemihydrate (Effects of both drugs inhibited). Products include:
Betimol 0.25%, 0.5% ◉ 261

Timolol Maleate (Effects of both drugs inhibited). Products include:
Blocadren Tablets 1614
Timolide Tablets 1748
Timoptic in Ocudose 1753
Timoptic Sterile Ophthalmic Solution 1751
Timoptic-XE 1755

Tranylcypromine Sulfate (Action of albuterol on the vascular system may be potentiated). Products include:
Parnate Tablets 2503

Triamcinolone (Potential for additive hypokalemic effect with concurrent use). Products include:
Aristocort Tablets 1022

Triamcinolone Acetonide (Potential for additive hypokalemic effect with concurrent use). Products include:
Aristocort A 0.025% Cream 1027
Aristocort A 0.5% Cream 1031
Aristocort A 0.1% Cream 1029
Aristocort A 0.1% Ointment 1030
Azmacort Oral Inhaler 2011
Nasacort Nasal Inhaler 2024

Triamcinolone Diacetate (Potential for additive hypokalemic effect with concurrent use). Products include:
Aristocort Suspension (Forte Parenteral) 1027
Aristocort Suspension (Intralesional) 1025

Triamcinolone Hexacetonide (Potential for additive hypokalemic effect with concurrent use). Products include:
Aristospan Suspension (Intra-articular) 1033
Aristospan Suspension (Intralesional) 1032

Trimipramine Maleate (Action of albuterol on the vascular system may be potentiated). Products include:
Surmontil Capsules 2811

PROVENTIL REPETABS TABLETS

(Albuterol Sulfate) 2386

May interact with sympathomimetic bronchodilators, monoamine oxidase inhibitors, tricyclic antidepressants, beta blockers, drugs which lower serum potassium (selected), and certain other agents. Compounds in these categories include:

Acebutolol Hydrochloride (Effect of both drugs inhibited). Products include:
Sectral Capsules 2807

Amitriptyline Hydrochloride (Potentiation of albuterol's action on vascular system). Products include:
Elavil 2838
Endep Tablets 2174
Etrafon 2355
Limbitrol 2180
Triavil Tablets 1757

Amoxapine (Potentiation of albuterol's action on vascular system). Products include:
Asendin Tablets 1369

Atenolol (Effect of both drugs inhibited). Products include:
Tenoretic Tablets 2845
Tenormin Tablets and I.V. Injection 2847

Bendroflumethiazide (Potential for additive hypokalemic effect with concurrent use).
No products indexed under this heading.

Betamethasone Acetate (Potential for additive hypokalemic effect with concurrent use). Products include:
Celestone Soluspan Suspension 2347

Betamethasone Sodium Phosphate (Potential for additive hypokalemic effect with concurrent use). Products include:
Celestone Soluspan Suspension 2347

Betaxolol Hydrochloride (Effect of both drugs inhibited). Products include:
Betoptic Ophthalmic Solution 469
Betoptic S Ophthalmic Suspension 471
Kerlone Tablets 2436

Bisoprolol Fumarate (Effect of both drugs inhibited). Products include:
Zebeta Tablets 1413
Ziac 1415

Bitolterol Mesylate (Deleterious cardiovascular effects). Products include:
Tornalate Solution for Inhalation, 0.2% 956
Tornalate Metered Dose Inhaler 957

Carteolol Hydrochloride (Effect of both drugs inhibited). Products include:
Cartrol Tablets 410
Ocupress Ophthalmic Solution, 1% Sterile ◉ 309

Chlorothiazide (Potential for additive hypokalemic effect with concurrent use). Products include:
Aldoclor Tablets 1598
Diupres Tablets 1650
Diuril Oral 1653

Chlorothiazide Sodium (Potential for additive hypokalemic effect with concurrent use). Products include:
Diuril Sodium Intravenous 1652

Clomipramine Hydrochloride (Potentiation of albuterol's action on vascular system). Products include:
Anafranil Capsules 803

Cortisone Acetate (Potential for additive hypokalemic effect with concurrent use). Products include:
Cortone Acetate Sterile Suspension 1623
Cortone Acetate Tablets 1624

Desipramine Hydrochloride (Potentiation of albuterol's action on vascular system). Products include:
Norpramin Tablets 1526

Dexamethasone (Potential for additive hypokalemic effect with concurrent use). Products include:
AK-Trol Ointment & Suspension ◉ 205
Decadron Elixir 1633
Decadron Tablets 1635
Decaspray Topical Aerosol 1648
Dexacidin Ointment ◉ 263
Maxitrol Ophthalmic Ointment and Suspension ◉ 224
TobraDex Ophthalmic Suspension and Ointment 473

Dexamethasone Acetate (Potential for additive hypokalemic effect with concurrent use). Products include:
Dalalone D.P. Injectable 1011
Decadron-LA Sterile Suspension 1646

Dexamethasone Sodium Phosphate (Potential for additive hypokalemic effect with concurrent use). Products include:
Decadron Phosphate Injection 1637
Decadron Phosphate Respihaler 1642
Decadron Phosphate Sterile Ophthalmic Ointment 1641
Decadron Phosphate Sterile Ophthalmic Solution 1642
Decadron Phosphate Topical Cream 1644
Decadron Phosphate Turbinaire 1645
Decadron Phosphate with Xylocaine Injection, Sterile 1639
Dexacort Phosphate in Respihaler 458
Dexacort Phosphate in Turbinaire 459
NeoDecadron Sterile Ophthalmic Ointment 1712
NeoDecadron Sterile Ophthalmic Solution 1713
NeoDecadron Topical Cream 1714

Digoxin (Decreased serum digoxin levels (16%-22%); the clinical significance of these findings for patients with COPD who are concurrently taking these drugs on a chronic basis is unclear). Products include:
Lanoxicaps 1117
Lanoxin Elixir Pediatric 1120
Lanoxin Injection 1123
Lanoxin Injection Pediatric 1126
Lanoxin Tablets 1128

Doxepin Hydrochloride (Potentiation of albuterol's action on vascular system). Products include:
Sinequan 2205
Zonalon Cream 1055

Ephedrine Hydrochloride (Deleterious cardiovascular effects). Products include:
Primatene Dual Action Formula ⊡ 872
Primatene Tablets ⊡ 873
Quadrinal Tablets 1350

Ephedrine Sulfate (Deleterious cardiovascular effects). Products include:
Bronkaid Caplets ⊡ 717
Marax Tablets & DF Syrup 2200

Ephedrine Tannate (Deleterious cardiovascular effects). Products include:
Rynatuss 2673

Epinephrine (Deleterious cardiovascular effects). Products include:
Bronkaid Mist ⊡ 717
EPIFRIN ◉ 239
EpiPen 790
Marcaine Hydrochloride with Epinephrine 1:200,000 2316
Primatene Mist ⊡ 873
Sensorcaine with Epinephrine Injection 559
Sus-Phrine Injection 1019
Xylocaine with Epinephrine Injections 567

Epinephrine Bitartrate (Deleterious cardiovascular effects). Products include:
Bronkaid Mist Suspension ⊡ 718
Sensorcaine-MPF with Epinephrine Injection 559

Epinephrine Hydrochloride (Deleterious cardiovascular effects). Products include:
Ana-Kit Anaphylaxis Emergency Treatment Kit 617

Esmolol Hydrochloride (Effect of both drugs inhibited). Products include:
Brevibloc Injection 1808

Ethylnorepinephrine Hydrochloride (Deleterious cardiovascular effects).
No products indexed under this heading.

Furazolidone (Potentiation of albuterol's action on vascular system). Products include:
Furoxone 2046

Hydrochlorothiazide (Potential for additive hypokalemic effect with concurrent use). Products include:
Aldactazide 2413
Aldoril Tablets 1604
Apresazide Capsules 808
Capozide 742
Dyazide 2479
Esidrix Tablets 821
Esimil Tablets 822
HydroDIURIL Tablets 1674
Hydropres Tablets 1675
Hyzaar Tablets 1677
Inderide Tablets 2732
Inderide LA Long Acting Capsules 2734
Lopressor HCT Tablets 832
Lotensin HCT 837
Maxzide 1380
Moduretic Tablets 1705
Oretic Tablets 443
Prinzide Tablets 1737
Ser-Ap-Es Tablets 849
Timolide Tablets 1748
Vaseretic Tablets 1765
Zestoretic 2850
Ziac 1415

Hydrocortisone (Potential for additive hypokalemic effect with concurrent use). Products include:
Anusol-HC Cream 2.5% 1896
Aquanil HC Lotion 1931
Bactine Hydrocortisone Anti-Itch Cream ⊡ 709
Caldecort Anti-Itch Hydrocortisone Spray ⊡ 631
Cortaid ⊡ 836
CORTENEMA 2535
Cortisporin Ointment 1085
Cortisporin Ophthalmic Ointment Sterile 1085
Cortisporin Ophthalmic Suspension Sterile 1086
Cortisporin Otic Solution Sterile 1087
Cortisporin Otic Suspension Sterile 1088
Cortizone-5 ⊡ 831
Cortizone-10 ⊡ 831
Hydrocortone Tablets 1672
Hytone 907
Massengill Medicated Soft Cloth Towelettes 2458
PediOtic Suspension Sterile 1153
Preparation H Hydrocortisone 1% Cream ⊡ 872
ProctoCream-HC 2.5% 2408
VōSoL HC Otic Solution 2678

IMPORTANT NOTE: Always consult each drug listing in the patient's regimen for possible interactions.

Hydrocortisone Acetate (Potential for additive hypokalemic effect with concurrent use). Products include:
- Analpram-HC Rectal Cream 1% and 2.5% ... 977
- Anusol HC-1 Anti-Itch Hydrocortisone Ointment ... ▣ 847
- Anusol-HC Suppositories ... 1897
- Caldecort ... ▣ 631
- Carmol HC ... 924
- Coly-Mycin S Otic w/Neomycin & Hydrocortisone ... 1906
- Cortaid ... ▣ 836
- Cortifoam ... 2396
- Cortisporin Cream ... 1084
- Epifoam ... 2399
- Hydrocortone Acetate Sterile Suspension ... 1669
- Mantadil Cream ... 1135
- Nupercainal Hydrocortisone 1% Cream ... ▣ 645
- Ophthocort ... ⊙ 311
- Pramosone Cream, Lotion & Ointment ... 978
- ProctoCream-HC ... 2408
- ProctoFoam-HC ... 2409
- Terra-Cortril Ophthalmic Suspension ... 2210

Hydrocortisone Sodium Phosphate (Potential for additive hypokalemic effect with concurrent use). Products include:
- Hydrocortone Phosphate Injection, Sterile ... 1670

Hydrocortisone Sodium Succinate (Potential for additive hypokalemic effect with concurrent use). Products include:
- Solu-Cortef Sterile Powder ... 2641

Hydroflumethiazide (Potential for additive hypokalemic effect with concurrent use). Products include:
- Diucardin Tablets ... 2718

Imipramine Hydrochloride (Potentiation of albuterol's action on vascular system). Products include:
- Tofranil Ampuls ... 854
- Tofranil Tablets ... 856

Imipramine Pamoate (Potentiation of albuterol's action on vascular system). Products include:
- Tofranil-PM Capsules ... 857

Isocarboxazid (Potentiation of albuterol's action on vascular system).
- No products indexed under this heading.

Isoetharine (Deleterious cardiovascular effects). Products include:
- Bronkometer Aerosol ... 2302
- Bronkosol Solution ... 2302
- Isoetharine Inhalation Solution, USP, Arm-a-Med ... 551

Isoproterenol Hydrochloride (Deleterious cardiovascular effects). Products include:
- Isuprel Hydrochloride Injection 1:5000 ... 2311
- Isuprel Hydrochloride Solution 1:200 & 1:100 ... 2313
- Isuprel Mistometer ... 2312

Isoproterenol Sulfate (Deleterious cardiovascular effects). Products include:
- Norisodrine with Calcium Iodide Syrup ... 442

Labetalol Hydrochloride (Effect of both drugs inhibited). Products include:
- Normodyne Injection ... 2377
- Normodyne Tablets ... 2379
- Trandate ... 1185

Levobunolol Hydrochloride (Effect of both drugs inhibited). Products include:
- Betagan ... ⊙ 233

Maprotiline Hydrochloride (Potentiation of albuterol's action on vascular system). Products include:
- Ludiomil Tablets ... 843

Metaproterenol Sulfate (Deleterious cardiovascular effects). Products include:
- Alupent ... 669
- Metaproterenol Sulfate Inhalation Solution, USP, Arm-a-Med ... 552

Methyclothiazide (Potential for additive hypokalemic effect with concurrent use). Products include:
- Enduron Tablets ... 420

Methylprednisolone Acetate (Potential for additive hypokalemic effect with concurrent use). Products include:
- Depo-Medrol Single-Dose Vial ... 2600
- Depo-Medrol Sterile Aqueous Suspension ... 2597

Methylprednisolone Sodium Succinate (Potential for additive hypokalemic effect with concurrent use). Products include:
- Solu-Medrol Sterile Powder ... 2643

Metipranolol Hydrochloride (Effect of both drugs inhibited). Products include:
- OptiPranolol (Metipranolol 0.3%) Sterile Ophthalmic Solution ... ⊙ 258

Metoprolol Succinate (Effect of both drugs inhibited). Products include:
- Toprol-XL Tablets ... 565

Metoprolol Tartrate (Effect of both drugs inhibited). Products include:
- Lopressor Ampuls ... 830
- Lopressor HCT Tablets ... 832
- Lopressor Tablets ... 830

Nadolol (Effect of both drugs inhibited).
- No products indexed under this heading.

Nortriptyline Hydrochloride (Potentiation of albuterol's action on vascular system). Products include:
- Pamelor ... 2280

Penbutolol Sulfate (Effect of both drugs inhibited). Products include:
- Levatol ... 2403

Phenelzine Sulfate (Potentiation of albuterol's action on vascular system). Products include:
- Nardil ... 1920

Pindolol (Effect of both drugs inhibited). Products include:
- Visken Tablets ... 2299

Pirbuterol Acetate (Deleterious cardiovascular effects). Products include:
- Maxair Autohaler ... 1492
- Maxair Inhaler ... 1494

Polythiazide (Potential for additive hypokalemic effect with concurrent use). Products include:
- Minizide Capsules ... 1938

Prednisolone Acetate (Potential for additive hypokalemic effect with concurrent use). Products include:
- AK-CIDE ... ⊙ 202
- AK-CIDE Ointment ... ⊙ 202
- Blephamide Liquifilm Sterile Ophthalmic Suspension ... 476
- Blephamide Ointment ... ⊙ 237
- Econopred & Econopred Plus Ophthalmic Suspensions ... ⊙ 217
- Poly-Pred Liquifilm ... ⊙ 248
- Pred Forte ... ⊙ 250
- Pred Mild ... ⊙ 253
- Pred-G Liquifilm Sterile Ophthalmic Suspension ... ⊙ 251
- Pred-G S.O.P. Sterile Ophthalmic Ointment ... ⊙ 252
- Vasocidin Ointment ... ⊙ 268

Prednisolone Sodium Phosphate (Potential for additive hypokalemic effect with concurrent use). Products include:
- AK-Pred ... ⊙ 204
- Hydeltrasol Injection, Sterile ... 1665
- Inflamase ... ⊙ 265
- Pediapred Oral Liquid ... 995
- Vasocidin Ophthalmic Solution ... ⊙ 270

Prednisolone Tebutate (Potential for additive hypokalemic effect with concurrent use). Products include:
- Hydeltra-T.B.A. Sterile Suspension 1667

Prednisone (Potential for additive hypokalemic effect with concurrent use). Products include:
- Deltasone Tablets ... 2595

Propranolol Hydrochloride (Effect of both drugs inhibited). Products include:
- Inderal ... 2728
- Inderal LA Long Acting Capsules ... 2730
- Inderide Tablets ... 2732
- Inderide LA Long Acting Capsules ... 2734

Protriptyline Hydrochloride (Potentiation of albuterol's action on vascular system). Products include:
- Vivactil Tablets ... 1774

Salmeterol Xinafoate (Deleterious cardiovascular effects). Products include:
- Serevent Inhalation Aerosol ... 1176

Selegiline Hydrochloride (Potentiation of albuterol's action on vascular system). Products include:
- Eldepryl Tablets ... 2550

Sotalol Hydrochloride (Effect of both drugs inhibited). Products include:
- Betapace Tablets ... 641

Terbutaline Sulfate (Deleterious cardiovascular effects). Products include:
- Brethaire Inhaler ... 813
- Brethine Ampuls ... 815
- Brethine Tablets ... 814
- Bricanyl Subcutaneous Injection ... 1502
- Bricanyl Tablets ... 1503

Timolol Hemihydrate (Effect of both drugs inhibited). Products include:
- Betimol 0.25%, 0.5% ... ⊙ 261

Timolol Maleate (Effect of both drugs inhibited). Products include:
- Blocadren Tablets ... 1614
- Timolide Tablets ... 1748
- Timoptic in Ocudose ... 1753
- Timoptic Sterile Ophthalmic Solution ... 1751
- Timoptic-XE ... 1755

Tranylcypromine Sulfate (Potentiation of albuterol's action on vascular system). Products include:
- Parnate Tablets ... 2503

Triamcinolone (Potential for additive hypokalemic effect with concurrent use). Products include:
- Aristocort Tablets ... 1022

Triamcinolone Acetonide (Potential for additive hypokalemic effect with concurrent use). Products include:
- Aristocort A 0.025% Cream ... 1027
- Aristocort A 0.5% Cream ... 1031
- Aristocort A 0.1% Cream ... 1029
- Aristocort A 0.1% Ointment ... 1030
- Azmacort Oral Inhaler ... 2011
- Nasacort Nasal Inhaler ... 2024

Triamcinolone Diacetate (Potential for additive hypokalemic effect with concurrent use). Products include:
- Aristocort Suspension (Forte Parenteral) ... 1027
- Aristocort Suspension (Intralesional) ... 1025

Triamcinolone Hexacetonide (Potential for additive hypokalemic effect with concurrent use). Products include:
- Aristospan Suspension (Intra-articular) ... 1033
- Aristospan Suspension (Intralesional) ... 1032

Trimipramine Maleate (Potentiation of albuterol's action on vascular system). Products include:
- Surmontil Capsules ... 2811

PROVENTIL SOLUTION FOR INHALATION 0.5%
(Albuterol Sulfate) ... 2383

May interact with sympathomimetic aerosol bronchodilators, monoamine oxidase inhibitors, tricyclic antidepressants, beta blockers, and drugs which lower serum potassium (selected). Compounds in these categories include:

Acebutolol Hydrochloride (Effects of both drugs inhibited). Products include:
- Sectral Capsules ... 2807

Albuterol (Effect not specified; concurrent use should be avoided). Products include:
- Proventil Inhalation Aerosol ... 2382
- Ventolin Inhalation Aerosol and Refill ... 1197

Amitriptyline Hydrochloride (Potentiation of albuterol's action on vascular system). Products include:
- Elavil ... 2838
- Endep Tablets ... 2174
- Etrafon ... 2355
- Limbitrol ... 2180
- Triavil Tablets ... 1757

Amoxapine (Potentiation of albuterol's action on vascular system). Products include:
- Asendin Tablets ... 1369

Atenolol (Effects of both drugs inhibited). Products include:
- Tenoretic Tablets ... 2845
- Tenormin Tablets and I.V. Injection 2847

Bendroflumethiazide (Potential for additive hypokalemic effect with concurrent use).
- No products indexed under this heading.

Betamethasone Acetate (Potential for additive hypokalemic effect with concurrent use). Products include:
- Celestone Soluspan Suspension ... 2347

Betamethasone Sodium Phosphate (Potential for additive hypokalemic effect with concurrent use). Products include:
- Celestone Soluspan Suspension ... 2347

Betaxolol Hydrochloride (Effects of both drugs inhibited). Products include:
- Betoptic Ophthalmic Solution ... 469
- Betoptic S Ophthalmic Suspension 471
- Kerlone Tablets ... 2436

Bisoprolol Fumarate (Effects of both drugs inhibited). Products include:
- Zebeta Tablets ... 1413
- Ziac ... 1415

Bitolterol Mesylate (Effect not specified; concurrent use should be avoided). Products include:
- Tornalate Solution for Inhalation, 0.2% ... 956
- Tornalate Metered Dose Inhaler ... 957

Carteolol Hydrochloride (Effects of both drugs inhibited). Products include:
- Cartrol Tablets ... 410
- Ocupress Ophthalmic Solution, 1% Sterile ... ⊙ 309

Chlorothiazide (Potential for additive hypokalemic effect with concurrent use). Products include:
- Aldoclor Tablets ... 1598
- Diupres Tablets ... 1650
- Diuril Oral ... 1653

(▣ Described in PDR For Nonprescription Drugs) (⊙ Described in PDR For Ophthalmology)

861 **Interactions Index** **Proventil Solution 0.5%**

Chlorothiazide Sodium (Potential for additive hypokalemic effect with concurrent use). Products include:
- Diuril Sodium Intravenous ... 1652

Clomipramine Hydrochloride (Potentiation of albuterol's action on vascular system). Products include:
- Anafranil Capsules ... 803

Cortisone Acetate (Potential for additive hypokalemic effect with concurrent use). Products include:
- Cortone Acetate Sterile Suspension ... 1623
- Cortone Acetate Tablets ... 1624

Desipramine Hydrochloride (Potentiation of albuterol's action on vascular system). Products include:
- Norpramin Tablets ... 1526

Dexamethasone (Potential for additive hypokalemic effect with concurrent use). Products include:
- AK-Trol Ointment & Suspension ... ⊙ 205
- Decadron Elixir ... 1633
- Decadron Tablets ... 1635
- Decaspray Topical Aerosol ... 1648
- Dexacidin Ointment ... ⊙ 263
- Maxitrol Ophthalmic Ointment and Suspension ... ⊙ 224
- TobraDex Ophthalmic Suspension and Ointment ... 473

Dexamethasone Acetate (Potential for additive hypokalemic effect with concurrent use). Products include:
- Dalalone D.P. Injectable ... 1011
- Decadron-LA Sterile Suspension ... 1646

Dexamethasone Sodium Phosphate (Potential for additive hypokalemic effect with concurrent use). Products include:
- Decadron Phosphate Injection ... 1637
- Decadron Phosphate Respihaler ... 1642
- Decadron Phosphate Sterile Ophthalmic Ointment ... 1641
- Decadron Phosphate Sterile Ophthalmic Solution ... 1642
- Decadron Phosphate Topical Cream ... 1644
- Decadron Phosphate Turbinaire ... 1645
- Decadron Phosphate with Xylocaine Injection, Sterile ... 1639
- Dexacort Phosphate in Respihaler ... 458
- Dexacort Phosphate in Turbinaire ... 459
- NeoDecadron Sterile Ophthalmic Ointment ... 1712
- NeoDecadron Sterile Ophthalmic Solution ... 1713
- NeoDecadron Topical Cream ... 1714

Doxepin Hydrochloride (Potentiation of albuterol's action on vascular system). Products include:
- Sinequan ... 2205
- Zonalon Cream ... 1055

Epinephrine (Should not be used concomitantly). Products include:
- Bronkaid Mist ... ▣ 717
- EPIFRIN ... ⊙ 239
- EpiPen ... 790
- Marcaine Hydrochloride with Epinephrine 1:200,000 ... 2316
- Primatene Mist ... ▣ 873
- Sensorcaine with Epinephrine Injection ... 559
- Sus-Phrine Injection ... 1019
- Xylocaine with Epinephrine Injections ... 567

Epinephrine Hydrochloride (Should not be used concomitantly). Products include:
- Ana-Kit Anaphylaxis Emergency Treatment Kit ... 617

Esmolol Hydrochloride (Effects of both drugs inhibited). Products include:
- Brevibloc Injection ... 1808

Ethylnorepinephrine Hydrochloride (Should not be used concomitantly).
- No products indexed under this heading.

Furazolidone (Potentiation of albuterol's action on vascular system). Products include:
- Furoxone ... 2046

Hydrochlorothiazide (Potential for additive hypokalemic effect with concurrent use). Products include:
- Aldactazide ... 2413
- Aldoril Tablets ... 1604
- Apresazide Capsules ... 808
- Capozide ... 742
- Dyazide ... 2479
- Esidrix Tablets ... 821
- Esimil Tablets ... 822
- HydroDIURIL Tablets ... 1674
- Hydropres Tablets ... 1675
- Hyzaar Tablets ... 1677
- Inderide Tablets ... 2732
- Inderide LA Long Acting Capsules ... 2734
- Lopressor HCT Tablets ... 832
- Lotensin HCT ... 837
- Maxzide ... 1380
- Moduretic Tablets ... 1705
- Oretic Tablets ... 443
- Prinzide Tablets ... 1737
- Ser-Ap-Es Tablets ... 849
- Timolide Tablets ... 1748
- Vaseretic Tablets ... 1765
- Zestoretic ... 2850
- Ziac ... 1415

Hydrocortisone (Potential for additive hypokalemic effect with concurrent use). Products include:
- Anusol-HC Cream 2.5% ... 1896
- Aquanil HC Lotion ... 1931
- Bactine Hydrocortisone Anti-Itch Cream ... ▣ 709
- Caldecort Anti-Itch Hydrocortisone Spray ... ▣ 631
- Cortaid ... ▣ 836
- CORTENEMA ... 2535
- Cortisporin Ointment ... 1085
- Cortisporin Ophthalmic Ointment Sterile ... 1085
- Cortisporin Ophthalmic Suspension Sterile ... 1086
- Cortisporin Otic Solution Sterile ... 1087
- Cortisporin Otic Suspension Sterile ... 1088
- Cortizone-5 ... ▣ 831
- Cortizone-10 ... ▣ 831
- Hydrocortone Tablets ... 1672
- Hytone ... 907
- Massengill Medicated Soft Cloth Towelettes ... 2458
- PediOtic Suspension Sterile ... 1153
- Preparation H Hydrocortisone 1% Cream ... ▣ 872
- ProctoCream-HC 2.5% ... 2408
- VōSoL HC Otic Solution ... 2678

Hydrocortisone Acetate (Potential for additive hypokalemic effect with concurrent use). Products include:
- Analpram-HC Rectal Cream 1% and 2.5% ... 977
- Anusol HC-1 Anti-Itch Hydrocortisone Ointment ... ▣ 847
- Anusol-HC Suppositories ... 1897
- Caldecort ... ▣ 631
- Carmol HC ... 924
- Coly-Mycin S Otic w/Neomycin & Hydrocortisone ... 1906
- Cortaid ... ▣ 836
- Cortifoam ... 2396
- Cortisporin Cream ... 1084
- Epifoam ... 2399
- Hydrocortone Acetate Sterile Suspension ... 1669
- Mantadil Cream ... 1135
- Nupercainal Hydrocortisone 1% Cream ... ▣ 645
- Ophthocort ... ⊙ 311
- Pramosone Cream, Lotion & Ointment ... 978
- ProctoCream-HC ... 2408
- ProctoFoam-HC ... 2409
- Terra-Cortril Ophthalmic Suspension ... 2210

Hydrocortisone Sodium Phosphate (Potential for additive hypokalemic effect with concurrent use). Products include:
- Hydrocortone Phosphate Injection, Sterile ... 1670

Hydrocortisone Sodium Succinate (Potential for additive hypokalemic effect with concurrent use). Products include:
- Solu-Cortef Sterile Powder ... 2641

Hydroflumethiazide (Potential for additive hypokalemic effect with concurrent use). Products include:
- Diucardin Tablets ... 2718

Imipramine Hydrochloride (Potentiation of albuterol's action on vascular system). Products include:
- Tofranil Ampuls ... 854
- Tofranil Tablets ... 856

Imipramine Pamoate (Potentiation of albuterol's action on vascular system). Products include:
- Tofranil-PM Capsules ... 857

Isocarboxazid (Potentiation of albuterol's action on vascular system).
- No products indexed under this heading.

Isoetharine (Effect not specified; concurrent use should be avoided). Products include:
- Bronkometer Aerosol ... 2302
- Bronkosol Solution ... 2302
- Isoetharine Inhalation Solution, USP, Arm-a-Med ... 551

Isoproterenol Hydrochloride (Effect not specified; concurrent use should be avoided). Products include:
- Isuprel Hydrochloride Injection 1:5000 ... 2311
- Isuprel Hydrochloride Solution 1:200 & 1:100 ... 2313
- Isuprel Mistometer ... 2312

Labetalol Hydrochloride (Effects of both drugs inhibited). Products include:
- Normodyne Injection ... 2377
- Normodyne Tablets ... 2379
- Trandate ... 1185

Levobunolol Hydrochloride (Effects of both drugs inhibited). Products include:
- Betagan ... ⊙ 233

Maprotiline Hydrochloride (Potentiation of albuterol's action on vascular system). Products include:
- Ludiomil Tablets ... 843

Metaproterenol Sulfate (Effect not specified; concurrent use should be avoided). Products include:
- Alupent ... 669
- Metaproterenol Sulfate Inhalation Solution, USP, Arm-a-Med ... 552

Methyclothiazide (Potential for additive hypokalemic effect with concurrent use). Products include:
- Enduron Tablets ... 420

Methylprednisolone Acetate (Potential for additive hypokalemic effect with concurrent use). Products include:
- Depo-Medrol Single-Dose Vial ... 2600
- Depo-Medrol Sterile Aqueous Suspension ... 2597

Methylprednisolone Sodium Succinate (Potential for additive hypokalemic effect with concurrent use). Products include:
- Solu-Medrol Sterile Powder ... 2643

Metipranolol Hydrochloride (Effects of both drugs inhibited). Products include:
- OptiPranolol (Metipranolol 0.3%) Sterile Ophthalmic Solution ... ⊙ 258

Metoprolol Succinate (Effects of both drugs inhibited). Products include:
- Toprol-XL Tablets ... 565

Metoprolol Tartrate (Effects of both drugs inhibited). Products include:
- Lopressor Ampuls ... 830
- Lopressor HCT Tablets ... 832
- Lopressor Tablets ... 830

Nadolol (Effects of both drugs inhibited).
- No products indexed under this heading.

Nortriptyline Hydrochloride (Potentiation of albuterol's action on vascular system). Products include:
- Pamelor ... 2280

Penbutolol Sulfate (Effects of both drugs inhibited). Products include:
- Levatol ... 2403

Phenelzine Sulfate (Potentiation of albuterol's action on vascular system). Products include:
- Nardil ... 1920

Pindolol (Effects of both drugs inhibited). Products include:
- Visken Tablets ... 2299

Pirbuterol Acetate (Effect not specified; concurrent use should be avoided). Products include:
- Maxair Autohaler ... 1492
- Maxair Inhaler ... 1494

Polythiazide (Potential for additive hypokalemic effect with concurrent use). Products include:
- Minizide Capsules ... 1938

Prednisolone Acetate (Potential for additive hypokalemic effect with concurrent use). Products include:
- AK-CIDE ... ⊙ 202
- AK-CIDE Ointment ... ⊙ 202
- Blephamide Liquifilm Sterile Ophthalmic Suspension ... 476
- Blephamide Ointment ... ⊙ 237
- Econopred & Econopred Plus Ophthalmic Suspensions ... ⊙ 217
- Poly-Pred Liquifilm ... ⊙ 248
- Pred Forte ... ⊙ 250
- Pred Mild ... ⊙ 253
- Pred-G Liquifilm Sterile Ophthalmic Suspension ... ⊙ 251
- Pred-G S.O.P. Sterile Ophthalmic Ointment ... ⊙ 252
- Vasocidin Ointment ... ⊙ 268

Prednisolone Sodium Phosphate (Potential for additive hypokalemic effect with concurrent use). Products include:
- AK-Pred ... ⊙ 204
- Hydeltrasol Injection, Sterile ... 1665
- Inflamase ... ⊙ 265
- Pediapred Oral Liquid ... 995
- Vasocidin Ophthalmic Solution ... ⊙ 270

Prednisolone Tebutate (Potential for additive hypokalemic effect with concurrent use). Products include:
- Hydeltra-T.B.A. Sterile Suspension 1667

Prednisone (Potential for additive hypokalemic effect with concurrent use). Products include:
- Deltasone Tablets ... 2595

Propranolol Hydrochloride (Effects of both drugs inhibited). Products include:
- Inderal ... 2728
- Inderal LA Long Acting Capsules ... 2730
- Inderide Tablets ... 2732
- Inderide LA Long Acting Capsules ... 2734

Protriptyline Hydrochloride (Potentiation of albuterol's action on vascular system). Products include:
- Vivactil Tablets ... 1774

Salmeterol Xinafoate (Effect not specified; concurrent use should be avoided). Products include:
- Serevent Inhalation Aerosol ... 1176

Selegiline Hydrochloride (Potentiation of albuterol's action on vascular system). Products include:
- Eldepryl Tablets ... 2550

Sotalol Hydrochloride (Effects of both drugs inhibited). Products include:
- Betapace Tablets ... 641

IMPORTANT NOTE: Always consult each drug listing in the patient's regimen for possible interactions.

Terbutaline Sulfate (Effect not specified; concurrent use should be avoided). Products include:
- Brethaire Inhaler ... 813
- Brethine Ampuls ... 815
- Brethine Tablets ... 814
- Bricanyl Subcutaneous Injection ... 1502
- Bricanyl Tablets ... 1503

Timolol Hemihydrate (Effects of both drugs inhibited). Products include:
- Betimol 0.25%, 0.5% ... ◉ 261

Timolol Maleate (Effects of both drugs inhibited). Products include:
- Blocadren Tablets ... 1614
- Timolide Tablets ... 1748
- Timoptic in Ocudose ... 1753
- Timoptic Sterile Ophthalmic Solution ... 1751
- Timoptic-XE ... 1755

Tranylcypromine Sulfate (Potentiation of albuterol's action on vascular system). Products include:
- Parnate Tablets ... 2503

Triamcinolone (Potential for additive hypokalemic effect with concurrent use). Products include:
- Aristocort Tablets ... 1022

Triamcinolone Acetonide (Potential for additive hypokalemic effect with concurrent use). Products include:
- Aristocort A 0.025% Cream ... 1027
- Aristocort A 0.5% Cream ... 1031
- Aristocort A 0.1% Cream ... 1029
- Aristocort A 0.1% Ointment ... 1030
- Azmacort Oral Inhaler ... 2011
- Nasacort Nasal Inhaler ... 2024

Triamcinolone Diacetate (Potential for additive hypokalemic effect with concurrent use). Products include:
- Aristocort Suspension (Forte Parenteral) ... 1027
- Aristocort Suspension (Intralesional) ... 1025

Triamcinolone Hexacetonide (Potential for additive hypokalemic effect with concurrent use). Products include:
- Aristospan Suspension (Intra-articular) ... 1033
- Aristospan Suspension (Intralesional) ... 1032

Trimipramine Maleate (Potentiation of albuterol's action on vascular system). Products include:
- Surmontil Capsules ... 2811

PROVENTIL SYRUP

(Albuterol Sulfate) ... 2385

May interact with monoamine oxidase inhibitors, tricyclic antidepressants, beta blockers, sympathomimetics, drugs which lower serum potassium (selected), and certain other agents. Compounds in these categories include:

Acebutolol Hydrochloride (Effects of both drugs inhibited). Products include:
- Sectral Capsules ... 2807

Albuterol (Concomitant use with other oral sympathomimetic agents is not recommended since such use may lead to deleterious cardiovascular effects). Products include:
- Proventil Inhalation Aerosol ... 2382
- Ventolin Inhalation Aerosol and Refill ... 1197

Amitriptyline Hydrochloride (Potentiation of albuterol's action on vascular system). Products include:
- Elavil ... 2838
- Endep Tablets ... 2174
- Etrafon ... 2355
- Limbitrol ... 2180
- Triavil Tablets ... 1757

Amoxapine (Potentiation of albuterol's action on vascular system). Products include:
- Asendin Tablets ... 1369

Atenolol (Effects of both drugs inhibited). Products include:
- Tenoretic Tablets ... 2845
- Tenormin Tablets and I.V. Injection 2847

Bendroflumethiazide (Potential for additive hypokalemic effect with concurrent use).
- No products indexed under this heading.

Betamethasone Acetate (Potential for additive hypokalemic effect with concurrent use). Products include:
- Celestone Soluspan Suspension ... 2347

Betamethasone Sodium Phosphate (Potential for additive hypokalemic effect with concurrent use). Products include:
- Celestone Soluspan Suspension ... 2347

Betaxolol Hydrochloride (Effects of both drugs inhibited). Products include:
- Betoptic Ophthalmic Solution ... 469
- Betoptic S Ophthalmic Suspension 471
- Kerlone Tablets ... 2436

Bisoprolol Fumarate (Effects of both drugs inhibited). Products include:
- Zebeta Tablets ... 1413
- Ziac ... 1415

Carteolol Hydrochloride (Effects of both drugs inhibited). Products include:
- Cartrol Tablets ... 410
- Ocupress Ophthalmic Solution, 1% Sterile ... ◉ 309

Chlorothiazide (Potential for additive hypokalemic effect with concurrent use). Products include:
- Aldoclor Tablets ... 1598
- Diupres Tablets ... 1650
- Diuril Oral ... 1653

Chlorothiazide Sodium (Potential for additive hypokalemic effect with concurrent use). Products include:
- Diuril Sodium Intravenous ... 1652

Clomipramine Hydrochloride (Potentiation of albuterol's action on vascular system). Products include:
- Anafranil Capsules ... 803

Cortisone Acetate (Potential for additive hypokalemic effect with concurrent use). Products include:
- Cortone Acetate Sterile Suspension ... 1623
- Cortone Acetate Tablets ... 1624

Desipramine Hydrochloride (Potentiation of albuterol's action on vascular system). Products include:
- Norpramin Tablets ... 1526

Dexamethasone (Potential for additive hypokalemic effect with concurrent use). Products include:
- AK-Trol Ointment & Suspension ... ◉ 205
- Decadron Elixir ... 1633
- Decadron Tablets ... 1635
- Decaspray Topical Aerosol ... 1648
- Dexacidin Ointment ... ◉ 263
- Maxitrol Ophthalmic Ointment and Suspension ... ◉ 224
- TobraDex Ophthalmic Suspension and Ointment ... 473

Dexamethasone Acetate (Potential for additive hypokalemic effect with concurrent use). Products include:
- Dalalone D.P. Injectable ... 1011
- Decadron-LA Sterile Suspension ... 1646

Dexamethasone Sodium Phosphate (Potential for additive hypokalemic effect with concurrent use). Products include:
- Decadron Phosphate Injection ... 1637
- Decadron Phosphate Respihaler ... 1642
- Decadron Phosphate Sterile Ophthalmic Ointment ... 1641
- Decadron Phosphate Sterile Ophthalmic Solution ... 1642
- Decadron Phosphate Topical Cream ... 1644
- Decadron Phosphate Turbinaire ... 1645
- Decadron Phosphate with Xylocaine Injection, Sterile ... 1639
- Dexacort Phosphate in Respihaler .. 458
- Dexacort Phosphate in Turbinaire .. 459
- NeoDecadron Sterile Ophthalmic Ointment ... 1712
- NeoDecadron Sterile Ophthalmic Solution ... 1713
- NeoDecadron Topical Cream ... 1714

Digoxin (Decreased serum digoxin levels (16%-22%); the clinical significance of these findings for patients with COPD who are concurrently taking these drugs on a chronic basis is unclear). Products include:
- Lanoxicaps ... 1117
- Lanoxin Elixir Pediatric ... 1120
- Lanoxin Injection ... 1123
- Lanoxin Injection Pediatric ... 1126
- Lanoxin Tablets ... 1128

Dobutamine Hydrochloride (Concomitant use with other oral sympathomimetic agents is not recommended since such use may lead to deleterious cardiovascular effects). Products include:
- Dobutrex Solution Vials ... 1439

Dopamine Hydrochloride (Concomitant use with other oral sympathomimetic agents is not recommended since such use may lead to deleterious cardiovascular effects).
- No products indexed under this heading.

Doxepin Hydrochloride (Potentiation of albuterol's action on vascular system). Products include:
- Sinequan ... 2205
- Zonalon Cream ... 1055

Ephedrine Hydrochloride (Concomitant use with other oral sympathomimetic agents is not recommended since such use may lead to deleterious cardiovascular effects). Products include:
- Primatene Dual Action Formula ... ▣ 872
- Primatene Tablets ... ▣ 873
- Quadrinal Tablets ... 1350

Ephedrine Sulfate (Concomitant use with other oral sympathomimetic agents is not recommended since such use may lead to deleterious cardiovascular effects). Products include:
- Bronkaid Caplets ... ▣ 717
- Marax Tablets & DF Syrup ... 2200

Ephedrine Tannate (Concomitant use with other oral sympathomimetic agents is not recommended since such use may lead to deleterious cardiovascular effects). Products include:
- Rynatuss ... 2673

Esmolol Hydrochloride (Effects of both drugs inhibited). Products include:
- Brevibloc Injection ... 1808

Furazolidone (Potentiation of albuterol's action on vascular system). Products include:
- Furoxone ... 2046

Hydrochlorothiazide (Potential for additive hypokalemic effect with concurrent use). Products include:
- Aldactazide ... 2413
- Aldoril Tablets ... 1604
- Apresazide Capsules ... 808
- Capozide ... 742
- Dyazide ... 2479
- Esidrix Tablets ... 821
- Esimil Tablets ... 822
- HydroDIURIL Tablets ... 1674
- Hydropres Tablets ... 1675
- Hyzaar Tablets ... 1677
- Inderide Tablets ... 2732
- Inderide LA Long Acting Capsules .. 2734
- Lopressor HCT Tablets ... 832
- Lotensin HCT ... 837
- Maxzide ... 1380
- Moduretic Tablets ... 1705
- Oretic Tablets ... 443
- Prinzide Tablets ... 1737
- Ser-Ap-Es Tablets ... 849
- Timolide Tablets ... 1748
- Vaseretic Tablets ... 1765
- Zestoretic ... 2850
- Ziac ... 1415

Hydrocortisone (Potential for additive hypokalemic effect with concurrent use). Products include:
- Anusol-HC Cream 2.5% ... 1896
- Aquanil HC Lotion ... 1931
- Bactine Hydrocortisone Anti-Itch Cream ... ▣ 709
- Caldecort Anti-Itch Hydrocortisone Spray ... ▣ 631
- Cortaid ... ▣ 836
- CORTENEMA ... 2535
- Cortisporin Ointment ... 1085
- Cortisporin Ophthalmic Ointment Sterile ... 1085
- Cortisporin Ophthalmic Suspension Sterile ... 1086
- Cortisporin Otic Solution Sterile ... 1087
- Cortisporin Otic Suspension Sterile 1088
- Cortizone-5 ... ▣ 831
- Cortizone-10 ... ▣ 831
- Hydrocortone Tablets ... 1672
- Hytone ... 907
- Massengill Medicated Soft Cloth Towelettes ... 2458
- PediOtic Suspension Sterile ... 1153
- Preparation H Hydrocortisone 1% Cream ... ▣ 872
- ProctoCream-HC 2.5% ... 2408
- VōSoL HC Otic Solution ... 2678

Hydrocortisone Acetate (Potential for additive hypokalemic effect with concurrent use). Products include:
- Analpram-HC Rectal Cream 1% and 2.5% ... 977
- Anusol HC-1 Anti-Itch Hydrocortisone Ointment ... ▣ 847
- Anusol-HC Suppositories ... 1897
- Caldecort ... ▣ 631
- Carmol HC ... 924
- Coly-Mycin S Otic w/Neomycin & Hydrocortisone ... 1906
- Cortaid ... ▣ 836
- Cortifoam ... 2396
- Cortisporin Cream ... 1084
- Epifoam ... 2399
- Hydrocortone Acetate Sterile Suspension ... 1669
- Mantadil Cream ... 1135
- Nupercainal Hydrocortisone 1% Cream ... ▣ 645
- Ophthocort ... ◉ 311
- Pramosone Cream, Lotion & Ointment ... 978
- ProctoCream-HC ... 2408
- ProctoFoam-HC ... 2409
- Terra-Cortril Ophthalmic Suspension ... 2210

Hydrocortisone Sodium Phosphate (Potential for additive hypokalemic effect with concurrent use). Products include:
- Hydrocortone Phosphate Injection, Sterile ... 1670

Hydrocortisone Sodium Succinate (Potential for additive hypokalemic effect with concurrent use). Products include:
- Solu-Cortef Sterile Powder ... 2641

Hydroflumethiazide (Potential for additive hypokalemic effect with concurrent use). Products include:
- Diucardin Tablets ... 2718

Imipramine Hydrochloride (Potentiation of albuterol's action on vascular system). Products include:
- Tofranil Ampuls ... 854
- Tofranil Tablets ... 856

Imipramine Pamoate (Potentiation of albuterol's action on vascular system). Products include:
- Tofranil-PM Capsules ... 857

(▣ Described in PDR For Nonprescription Drugs) (◉ Described in PDR For Ophthalmology)

Interactions Index — Proventil Syrup

Isocarboxazid (Potentiation of albuterol's action on vascular system).

No products indexed under this heading.

Isoproterenol Sulfate (Concomitant use with other oral sympathomimetic agents is not recommended since such use may lead to deleterious cardiovascular effects). Products include:

Norisodrine with Calcium Iodide Syrup 442

Labetalol Hydrochloride (Effects of both drugs inhibited). Products include:

Normodyne Injection 2377
Normodyne Tablets 2379
Trandate 1185

Levobunolol Hydrochloride (Effects of both drugs inhibited). Products include:

Betagan .... ⊙ 233

Maprotiline Hydrochloride (Potentiation of albuterol's action on vascular system). Products include:

Ludiomil Tablets................................ 843

Metaproterenol Sulfate (Concomitant use with other oral sympathomimetic agents is not recommended since such use may lead to deleterious cardiovascular effects). Products include:

Alupent... 669
Metaproterenol Sulfate Inhalation Solution, USP, Arm-a-Med 552

Methyclothiazide (Potential for additive hypokalemic effect with concurrent use). Products include:

Enduron Tablets................................ 420

Methylprednisolone Acetate (Potential for additive hypokalemic effect with concurrent use). Products include:

Depo-Medrol Single-Dose Vial 2600
Depo-Medrol Sterile Aqueous Suspension 2597

Methylprednisolone Sodium Succinate (Potential for additive hypokalemic effect with concurrent use). Products include:

Solu-Medrol Sterile Powder.............. 2643

Metipranolol Hydrochloride (Effects of both drugs inhibited). Products include:

OptiPranolol (Metipranolol 0.3%) Sterile Ophthalmic Solution.......... ⊙ 258

Metoprolol Succinate (Effects of both drugs inhibited). Products include:

Toprol-XL Tablets 565

Metoprolol Tartrate (Effects of both drugs inhibited). Products include:

Lopressor Ampuls 830
Lopressor HCT Tablets 832
Lopressor Tablets 830

Nadolol (Effects of both drugs inhibited).

No products indexed under this heading.

Nortriptyline Hydrochloride (Potentiation of albuterol's action on vascular system). Products include:

Pamelor 2280

Penbutolol Sulfate (Effects of both drugs inhibited). Products include:

Levatol 2403

Phenelzine Sulfate (Potentiation of albuterol's action on vascular system). Products include:

Nardil 1920

Phenylephrine Bitartrate (Concomitant use with other oral sympathomimetic agents is not recommended since such use may lead to deleterious cardiovascular effects).

No products indexed under this heading.

Phenylephrine Hydrochloride (Concomitant use with other oral sympathomimetic agents is not recommended since such use may lead to deleterious cardiovascular effects). Products include:

Atrohist Plus Tablets 454
Cerose DM .... ᴹᴰ 878
Comhist 2038
D.A. Chewable Tablets...................... 951
Deconsal Pediatric Capsules............. 454
Dura-Vent/DA Tablets....................... 953
Entex Capsules 1986
Entex Liquid 1986
Extendryl 1005
4-Way Fast Acting Nasal Spray (regular & mentholated).................. ᴹᴰ 621
Hemorid For Women .... ᴹᴰ 834
Hycomine Compound Tablets 932
Neo-Synephrine Hydrochloride 1% Carpuject.. 2324
Neo-Synephrine Hydrochloride 1% Injection 2324
Neo-Synephrine Hydrochloride (Ophthalmic) 2325
Neo-Synephrine .... ᴹᴰ 726
Nōstril .... ᴹᴰ 644
Novahistine Elixir .... ᴹᴰ 823
Phenergan VC 2779
Phenergan VC with Codeine 2781
Preparation H .... ᴹᴰ 871
Tympagesic Ear Drops 2342
Vasosulf .... ⊙ 271
Vicks Sinex Nasal Spray and Ultra Fine Mist .... ᴹᴰ 765

Phenylephrine Tannate (Concomitant use with other oral sympathomimetic agents is not recommended since such use may lead to deleterious cardiovascular effects). Products include:

Atrohist Pediatric Suspension 454
Ricobid-D Pediatric Suspension....... 2038
Ricobid Tablets and Pediatric Suspension 2038
Rynatan 2673
Rynatuss 2673

Phenylpropanolamine Hydrochloride (Concomitant use with other oral sympathomimetic agents is not recommended since such use may lead to deleterious cardiovascular effects). Products include:

Acutrim .... ᴹᴰ 628
Allerest Children's Chewable Tablets .... ᴹᴰ 627
Allerest 12 Hour Caplets .... ᴹᴰ 627
Atrohist Plus Tablets 454
BC Cold Powder Multi-Symptom Formula (Cold-Sinus-Allergy) .... ᴹᴰ 609
BC Cold Powder Non-Drowsy Formula (Cold-Sinus)........................ ᴹᴰ 609
Cheracol Plus Head Cold/Cough Formula .... ᴹᴰ 769
Comtrex Multi-Symptom Non-Drowsy Liqui-gels............................ ᴹᴰ 618
Contac Continuous Action Nasal Decongestant/Antihistamine 12 Hour Capsules................................... ᴹᴰ 813
Contac Maximum Strength Continuous Action Decongestant/ Antihistamine 12 Hour Caplets.. ᴹᴰ 813
Contac Severe Cold and Flu Formula Caplets .... ᴹᴰ 814
Coricidin 'D' Decongestant Tablets .... ᴹᴰ 800
Dexatrim .... ᴹᴰ 832
Dexatrim Plus Vitamins Caplets ... ᴹᴰ 832
Dimetane-DC Cough Syrup 2059
Dimetapp Elixir .... ᴹᴰ 773
Dimetapp Extentabs.......................... ᴹᴰ 774
Dimetapp Tablets/Liqui-Gels .... ᴹᴰ 775
Dimetapp Cold & Allergy Chewable Tablets .... ᴹᴰ 773
Dimetapp DM Elixir........................... ᴹᴰ 774
Dura-Vent Tablets 952
Entex Capsules 1986
Entex LA Tablets 1987
Entex Liquid 1986
Exgest LA Tablets 782

Hycomine 931
Isoclor Timesule Capsules .... ᴹᴰ 637
Nolamine Timed-Release Tablets 785
Ornade Spansule Capsules 2502
Propagest Tablets 786
Pyrroxate Caplets .... ᴹᴰ 772
Robitussin-CF .... ᴹᴰ 777
Sinulin Tablets 787
Tavist-D 12 Hour Relief Tablets ... ᴹᴰ 787
Teldrin 12 Hour Antihistamine/ Nasal Decongestant Allergy Relief Capsules................................... ᴹᴰ 826
Triaminic Allergy Tablets .... ᴹᴰ 789
Triaminic Cold Tablets .... ᴹᴰ 790
Triaminic Expectorant .... ᴹᴰ 790
Triaminic Syrup .... ᴹᴰ 792
Triaminic-12 Tablets .... ᴹᴰ 792
Triaminic-DM Syrup .... ᴹᴰ 792
Triaminicin Tablets .... ᴹᴰ 793
Triaminicol Multi-Symptom Cold Tablets .... ᴹᴰ 793
Triaminicol Multi-Symptom Relief ᴹᴰ 794
Vicks DayQuil Allergy Relief 12-Hour Extended Release Tablets.. ᴹᴰ 760
Vicks DayQuil Allergy Relief 4-Hour Tablets .... ᴹᴰ 760
Vicks DayQuil SINUS Pressure & CONGESTION Relief.......................... ᴹᴰ 761

Pindolol (Effects of both drugs inhibited). Products include:

Visken Tablets................................... 2299

Polythiazide (Potential for additive hypokalemic effect with concurrent use). Products include:

Minizide Capsules 1938

Prednisolone Acetate (Potential for additive hypokalemic effect with concurrent use). Products include:

AK-CIDE... ⊙ 202
AK-CIDE Ointment............................ ⊙ 202
Blephamide Liquifilm Sterile Ophthalmic Suspension........................... 476
Blephamide Ointment .... ⊙ 237
Econopred & Econopred Plus Ophthalmic Suspensions .... ⊙ 217
Poly-Pred Liquifilm .... ⊙ 248
Pred Forte.. ⊙ 250
Pred Mild.. ⊙ 253
Pred-G Liquifilm Sterile Ophthalmic Suspension .... ⊙ 251
Pred-G S.O.P. Sterile Ophthalmic Ointment .... ⊙ 252
Vasocidin Ointment .... ⊙ 268

Prednisolone Sodium Phosphate (Potential for additive hypokalemic effect with concurrent use). Products include:

AK-Pred .... ⊙ 204
Hydeltrasol Injection, Sterile............ 1665
Inflammase.. ⊙ 265
Pediapred Oral Liquid 995
Vasocidin Ophthalmic Solution .... ⊙ 270

Prednisolone Tebutate (Potential for additive hypokalemic effect with concurrent use). Products include:

Hydeltra-T.B.A. Sterile Suspension 1667

Prednisone (Potential for additive hypokalemic effect with concurrent use). Products include:

Deltasone Tablets 2595

Propranolol Hydrochloride (Effects of both drugs inhibited). Products include:

Inderal 2728
Inderal LA Long Acting Capsules 2730
Inderide Tablets 2732
Inderide LA Long Acting Capsules.. 2734

Protriptyline Hydrochloride (Potentiation of albuterol's action on vascular system). Products include:

Vivactil Tablets 1774

Pseudoephedrine Hydrochloride (Concomitant use with other oral sympathomimetic agents is not recommended since such use may lead to deleterious cardiovascular effects). Products include:

Actifed Allergy Daytime/Nighttime Caplets.. ᴹᴰ 844
Actifed Plus Caplets .... ᴹᴰ 845
Actifed Plus Tablets .... ᴹᴰ 845
Actifed with Codeine Cough Syrup.. 1067
Actifed Sinus Daytime/Nighttime Tablets and Caplets .... ᴹᴰ 846

Actifed Syrup..................................... ᴹᴰ 846
Actifed Tablets .... ᴹᴰ 844
Advil Cold and Sinus Caplets and Tablets (formerly CoAdvil) .... ᴹᴰ 870
Alka-Seltzer Plus Cold Medicine Liqui-Gels .... ᴹᴰ 706
Alka-Seltzer Plus Cold & Cough Medicine Liqui-Gels......................... ᴹᴰ 705
Alka-Seltzer Plus Night-Time Cold Medicine Liqui-Gels......................... ᴹᴰ 706
Allerest Headache Strength Tablets .... ᴹᴰ 627
Allerest Maximum Strength Tablets .... ᴹᴰ 627
Allerest No Drowsiness Tablets.... ᴹᴰ 627
Allerest Sinus Pain Formula .... ᴹᴰ 627
Anatuss LA Tablets............................ 1542
Atrohist Pediatric Capsules.............. 453
Bayer Select Sinus Pain Relief Formula .... ᴹᴰ 717
Benadryl Allergy Decongestant Liquid Medication .... ᴹᴰ 848
Benadryl Allergy Decongestant Tablets .... ᴹᴰ 848
Benadryl Allergy Sinus Headache Formula Caplets............................... ᴹᴰ 849
Benylin Multisymptom...................... ᴹᴰ 852
Bromfed Capsules (Extended-Release) 1785
Bromfed Syrup.................................. ᴹᴰ 733
Bromfed Tablets 1785
Bromfed-DM Cough Syrup............... 1786
Bromfed-PD Capsules (Extended-Release)... 1785
Children's Vicks DayQuil Allergy Relief .... ᴹᴰ 757
Children's Vicks NyQuil Cold/ Cough Relief..................................... ᴹᴰ 758
Comtrex Multi-Symptom Cold Reliever Tablets/Caplets/Liqui-Gels/Liquid.. ᴹᴰ 615
Allergy-Sinus Comtrex Multi-Symptom Allergy-Sinus Formula Tablets .... ᴹᴰ 617
Comtrex Multi-Symptom Non-Drowsy Caplets................................. ᴹᴰ 618
Congess 1004
Contac Day Allergy/Sinus Caplets ᴹᴰ 812
Contac Day & Night .... ᴹᴰ 812
Contac Night Allergy/Sinus Caplets .... ᴹᴰ 812
Contac Severe Cold & Flu Non-Drowsy .... ᴹᴰ 815
Deconamine Chewable Tablets 1320
Deconamine CX Cough and Cold Liquid and Tablets............................. 1319
Deconamine 1320
Deconsal C Expectorant Syrup 456
Deconsal Pediatric Syrup 457
Deconsal II Tablets 454
Dimetane-DX Cough Syrup 2059
Dimetapp Sinus Caplets .... ᴹᴰ 775
Dorcol Children's Cough Syrup ...ᴹᴰ 785
Drixoral Cough + Congestion Liquid Caps .... ᴹᴰ 802
Dura-Tap/PD Capsules 2867
Duratuss Tablets 2565
Duratuss HD Elixir 2565
Efidac/24 .... ᴹᴰ 635
Entex PSE Tablets 1987
Fedahist Gyrocaps............................. 2401
Fedahist Timecaps 2401
Guaifed... 1787
Guaifed Syrup .... ᴹᴰ 734
Guaimax-D Tablets 792
Guaitab Tablets .... ᴹᴰ 734
Isoclor Expectorant........................... 990
Kronofed-A... 977
Motrin IB Sinus .... ᴹᴰ 838
Novahistine DH.................................. 2462
Novahistine DMX .... ᴹᴰ 822
Novahistine Expectorant................... 2463
Nucofed 2051
PediaCare Cold Allergy Chewable Tablets .... ᴹᴰ 677
PediaCare Cough-Cold Chewable Tablets 1553
PediaCare 1553
PediaCare Infants' Decongestant Drops .... ᴹᴰ 677
PediCare Infant's Drops Decongestant Plus Cough 1553
PediaCare NightRest Cough-Cold Liquid 1553
Pediatric Vicks 44d Dry Hacking Cough & Head Congestion.............. ᴹᴰ 763
Pediatric Vicks 44m Cough & Cold Relief .... ᴹᴰ 764
Robitussin Cold & Cough Liqui-Gels .... ᴹᴰ 776

IMPORTANT NOTE: Always consult each drug listing in the patient's regimen for possible interactions.

Proventil Syrup **Interactions Index** **864**

Robitussin Maximum Strength Cough & Cold ▣ 778
Robitussin Pediatric Cough & Cold Formula ▣ 779
Robitussin Severe Congestion Liqui-Gels ▣ 776
Robitussin-DAC Syrup 2074
Robitussin-PE ▣ 778
Rondec Oral Drops 953
Rondec Syrup 953
Rondec Tablet 953
Rondec-DM Oral Drops 954
Rondec-DM Syrup 954
Rondec-TR Tablet 953
Ryna ▣ 841
Seldane-D Extended-Release Tablets 1538
Semprex-D Capsules 463
Semprex-D Capsules 1167
Sinarest Tablets ▣ 648
Sinarest Extra Strength Tablets ▣ 648
Sinarest No Drowsiness Tablets ▣ 648
Sine-Aid IB Caplets 1554
Sine-Aid Maximum Strength Sinus Medication Gelcaps, Caplets and Tablets 1554
Sine-Off No Drowsiness Formula Caplets ▣ 824
Sine-Off Sinus Medicine ▣ 825
Singlet Tablets ▣ 825
Sinutab Non-Drying Liquid Caps ▣ 859
Sinutab Sinus Allergy Medication, Maximum Strength Tablets and Caplets ▣ 860
Sinutab Sinus Medication, Maximum Strength Without Drowsiness Formula, Tablets & Caplets ▣ 860
Sinutab Sinus Medication, Regular Strength Without Drowsiness Formula ▣ 859
Sudafed Children's Liquid ▣ 861
Sudafed Cold and Cough Liquidcaps ▣ 862
Sudafed Cough Syrup ▣ 862
Sudafed Plus Liquid ▣ 862
Sudafed Plus Tablets ▣ 863
Sudafed Severe Cold Formula Caplets ▣ 863
Sudafed Severe Cold Formula Tablets ▣ 864
Sudafed Sinus Caplets ▣ 864
Sudafed Sinus Tablets ▣ 864
Sudafed Tablets, 30 mg ▣ 861
Sudafed Tablets, 60 mg ▣ 861
Sudafed 12 Hour Caplets ▣ 861
Syn-Rx Tablets 465
Syn-Rx DM Tablets 466
TheraFlu ▣ 787
TheraFlu Maximum Strength Nighttime Flu, Cold & Cough Medicine ▣ 788
TheraFlu Maximum Strength Non-Drowsy Formula Flu, Cold & Cough Medicine ▣ 788
Thera Flu Maximum Strength, Non-Drowsy Formula Flu, Cold and Cough Caplets ▣ 789
Triaminic AM Cough and Decongestant Formula ▣ 789
Triaminic AM Decongestant Formula ▣ 790
Triaminic Nite Light ▣ 791
Triaminic Sore Throat Formula ▣ 791
Tussend 1783
Tussend Expectorant 1785
Children's TYLENOL Cold Multi-Symptom Liquid Formula and Chewable Tablets 1561
Children's TYLENOL Cold Plus Cough Multi Symptom Tablets and Liquid ▣ 681
Infants' TYLENOL Cold Decongestant & Fever-Reducer Drops 1556
TYLENOL Maximum Strength Allergy Sinus Medication Gelcaps and Caplets 1563
TYLENOL Maximum Strength Allergy Sinus NightTime Medication Caplets 1555
TYLENOL Flu Maximum Strength Gelcaps 1565
TYLENOL Flu NightTime, Maximum Strength, Gelcaps 1566
TYLENOL Maximum Strength Flu NightTime Hot Medication Packets 1562
TYLENOL, Maximum Strength, Sinus Medication Geltabs, Gelcaps, Caplets and Tablets 1566
TYLENOL Cold Multi-Symptom Formula Medication Tablets and Caplets 1561
TYLENOL Cold Medication No Drowsiness Formula Gelcaps and Caplets 1562
TYLENOL Cold Multi-Symptom Hot Medication Liquid Packets 1557
TYLENOL Cough Multi-Symptom Medication with Decongestant 1565
Ursinus Inlay-Tabs ▣ 794
Vicks 44 LiquiCaps Cough, Cold & Flu Relief ▣ 755
Vicks 44 LiquiCaps Non-Drowsy Cough & Cold Relief ▣ 756
Vicks 44D Dry Hacking Cough & Head Congestion ▣ 755
Vicks 44M Cough, Cold & Flu Relief ▣ 756
Vicks DayQuil ▣ 761
Vicks DayQuil SINUS Pressure & PAIN Relief with IBUPROFEN ▣ 762
Vicks Nyquil Hot Therapy ▣ 762
Vicks NyQuil LiquiCaps Multi-Symptom Cold/Flu Relief ▣ 763
Vicks NyQuil Multi-Symptom Cold/Flu Relief - (Original & Cherry Flavor) ▣ 763

Pseudoephedrine Sulfate (Concomitant use with other oral sympathomimetic agents is not recommended since such use may lead to deleterious cardiovascular effects). Products include:
Cheracol Sinus ▣ 768
Chlor-Trimeton Allergy Decongestant Tablets ▣ 799
Claritin-D 2350
Drixoral Cold and Allergy Sustained-Action Tablets ▣ 802
Drixoral Cold and Flu Extended-Release Tablets ▣ 803
Drixoral Non-Drowsy Formula Extended-Release Tablets ▣ 803
Drixoral Allergy/Sinus Extended Release Tablets ▣ 804
Trinalin Repetabs Tablets 1330

Salmeterol Xinafoate (Concomitant use with other oral sympathomimetic agents is not recommended since such use may lead to deleterious cardiovascular effects). Products include:
Serevent Inhalation Aerosol 1176

Selegiline Hydrochloride (Potentiation of albuterol's action on vascular system). Products include:
Eldepryl Tablets 2550

Sotalol Hydrochloride (Effects of both drugs inhibited). Products include:
Betapace Tablets 641

Terbutaline Sulfate (Concomitant use with other oral sympathomimetic agents is not recommended since such use may lead to deleterious cardiovascular effects). Products include:
Brethaire Inhaler 813
Brethine Ampuls 815
Brethine Tablets 814
Bricanyl Subcutaneous Injection 1502
Bricanyl Tablets 1503

Timolol Hemihydrate (Effects of both drugs inhibited). Products include:
Betimol 0.25%, 0.5% ⊙ 261

Timolol Maleate (Effects of both drugs inhibited). Products include:
Blocadren Tablets 1614
Timolide Tablets 1748
Timoptic in Ocudose 1753
Timoptic Sterile Ophthalmic Solution 1751
Timoptic-XE 1755

Tranylcypromine Sulfate (Potentiation of albuterol's action on vascular system). Products include:
Parnate Tablets 2503

Triamcinolone (Potential for additive hypokalemic effect with concurrent use). Products include:
Aristocort Tablets 1022

Triamcinolone Acetonide (Potential for additive hypokalemic effect with concurrent use). Products include:
Aristocort A 0.025% Cream 1027
Aristocort A 0.5% Cream 1031
Aristocort A 0.1% Cream 1029
Aristocort A 0.1% Ointment 1030
Azmacort Oral Inhaler 2011
Nasacort Nasal Inhaler 2024

Triamcinolone Diacetate (Potential for additive hypokalemic effect with concurrent use). Products include:
Aristocort Suspension (Forte Parenteral) 1027
Aristocort Suspension (Intralesional) 1025

Triamcinolone Hexacetonide (Potential for additive hypokalemic effect with concurrent use). Products include:
Aristospan Suspension (Intra-articular) 1033
Aristospan Suspension (Intralesional) 1032

Trimipramine Maleate (Potentiation of albuterol's action on vascular system). Products include:
Surmontil Capsules 2811

PROVENTIL TABLETS
(Albuterol Sulfate) 2386
See **Proventil Repetabs Tablets**

PROVERA TABLETS
(Medroxyprogesterone Acetate) 2636
May interact with estrogens and certain other agents. Compounds in these categories include:

Aminoglutethimide (Significantly depresses the bioavailability of Provera). Products include:
Cytadren Tablets 819

Chlorotrianisene (Potential for adverse effects on carbohydrate and lipid metabolism).
No products indexed under this heading.

Dienestrol (Potential for adverse effects on carbohydrate and lipid metabolism). Products include:
Ortho Dienestrol Cream 1866

Diethylstilbestrol (Potential for adverse effects on carbohydrate and lipid metabolism). Products include:
Diethylstilbestrol Tablets 1437

Estradiol (Potential for adverse effects on carbohydrate and lipid metabolism). Products include:
Climara Transdermal System 645
Estrace Cream and Tablets 749
Estraderm Transdermal System 824

Estrogens, Conjugated (Potential for adverse effects on carbohydrate and lipid metabolism). Products include:
PMB 200 and PMB 400 2783
Premarin Intravenous 2787
Premarin with Methyltestosterone 2794
Premarin Tablets 2789
Premarin Vaginal Cream 2791
Premphase 2797
Prempro 2801

Estrogens, Esterified (Potential for adverse effects on carbohydrate and lipid metabolism). Products include:
ESTRATAB Tablets (0.3, 0.625, 1.25, 2.5 mg) 2536
Estratest 2539
Menest Tablets 2494

Estropipate (Potential for adverse effects on carbohydrate and lipid metabolism). Products include:
Ogen Tablets 2627
Ogen Vaginal Cream 2630
Ortho-Est 1869

Ethinyl Estradiol (Potential for adverse effects on carbohydrate and lipid metabolism). Products include:
Brevicon 2088
Demulen 2428
Desogen Tablets 1817
Levlen/Tri-Levlen 651
Lo/Ovral Tablets 2746
Lo/Ovral-28 Tablets 2751
Modicon 1872
Nordette-21 Tablets 2755
Nordette-28 Tablets 2758
Norinyl 2088
Ortho-Cept 1851
Ortho-Cyclen/Ortho-Tri-Cyclen 1858
Ortho-Novum 1872
Ortho-Cyclen/Ortho Tri-Cyclen 1858
Ovcon 760
Ovral Tablets 2770
Ovral-28 Tablets 2770
Levlen/Tri-Levlen 651
Tri-Norinyl 2164
Triphasil-21 Tablets 2814
Triphasil-28 Tablets 2819

Polyestradiol Phosphate (Potential for adverse effects on carbohydrate and lipid metabolism).
No products indexed under this heading.

Quinestrol (Potential for adverse effects on carbohydrate and lipid metabolism).
No products indexed under this heading.

PROVOCHOLINE FOR INHALATION
(Methacholine Chloride) 2140
May interact with beta blockers. Compounds in this category include:

Acebutolol Hydrochloride (Response to methacholine can be exaggerated or prolonged). Products include:
Sectral Capsules 2807

Atenolol (Response to methacholine can be exaggerated or prolonged). Products include:
Tenoretic Tablets 2845
Tenormin Tablets and I.V. Injection 2847

Betaxolol Hydrochloride (Response to methacholine can be exaggerated or prolonged). Products include:
Betoptic Ophthalmic Solution 469
Betoptic S Ophthalmic Suspension 471
Kerlone Tablets 2436

Bisoprolol Fumarate (Response to methacholine can be exaggerated or prolonged). Products include:
Zebeta Tablets 1413
Ziac 1415

Carteolol Hydrochloride (Response to methacholine can be exaggerated or prolonged). Products include:
Cartrol Tablets 410
Ocupress Ophthalmic Solution, 1% Sterile ⊙ 309

Esmolol Hydrochloride (Response to methacholine can be exaggerated or prolonged). Products include:
Brevibloc Injection 1808

Labetalol Hydrochloride (Response to methacholine can be exaggerated or prolonged). Products include:
Normodyne Injection 2377
Normodyne Tablets 2379
Trandate 1185

Levobunolol Hydrochloride (Response to methacholine can be exaggerated or prolonged). Products include:
Betagan ⊙ 233

(▣ Described in PDR For Nonprescription Drugs) (⊙ Described in PDR For Ophthalmology)

Metipranolol Hydrochloride (Response to methacholine can be exaggerated or prolonged). Products include:

OptiPranolol (Metipranolol 0.3%) Sterile Ophthalmic Solution ⊙ 258

Metoprolol Succinate (Response to methacholine can be exaggerated or prolonged). Products include:

Toprol-XL Tablets 565

Metoprolol Tartrate (Response to methacholine can be exaggerated or prolonged). Products include:

Lopressor Ampuls 830
Lopressor HCT Tablets 832
Lopressor Tablets 830

Nadolol (Response to methacholine can be exaggerated or prolonged).

No products indexed under this heading.

Penbutolol Sulfate (Response to methacholine can be exaggerated or prolonged). Products include:

Levatol 2403

Pindolol (Response to methacholine can be exaggerated or prolonged). Products include:

Visken Tablets 2299

Propranolol Hydrochloride (Response to methacholine can be exaggerated or prolonged). Products include:

Inderal 2728
Inderal LA Long Acting Capsules 2730
Inderide Tablets 2732
Inderide LA Long Acting Capsules 2734

Sotalol Hydrochloride (Response to methacholine can be exaggerated or prolonged). Products include:

Betapace Tablets 641

Timolol Hemihydrate (Response to methacholine can be exaggerated or prolonged). Products include:

Betimol 0.25%, 0.5% ⊙ 261

Timolol Maleate (Response to methacholine can be exaggerated or prolonged). Products include:

Blocadren Tablets 1614
Timolide Tablets 1748
Timoptic in Ocudose 1753
Timoptic Sterile Ophthalmic Solution 1751
Timoptic-XE 1755

PROZAC PULVULES & LIQUID, ORAL SOLUTION

(Fluoxetine Hydrochloride) 919

May interact with monoamine oxidase inhibitors, oral anticoagulants, antidepressant drugs, insulin, oral hypoglycemic agents, drugs that are predominantly metabolized by the p450iid6 system, and certain other agents. Compounds in these categories include:

Acarbose (Prozac may alter glycemic control; oral hypoglycemic dosage may need to be adjusted).

No products indexed under this heading.

Amitriptyline Hydrochloride (Inhibition of the activity of isoenzyme p450iid6 making normal metabolizers resemble "poor metabolizers"; therapy with drugs that are predominantly metabolized by the p450iid6 system and have relatively narrow therapeutic index should be initiated at low end of the dose range if a patient is receiving Prozac concurrently or has taken it in the previous 5 weeks). Products include:

Elavil 2838
Endep Tablets 2174
Etrafon 2355
Limbitrol 2180
Triavil Tablets 1757

Amoxapine (Inhibition of the activity of isoenzyme p450iid6 making normal metabolizers resemble "poor metabolizers"; therapy with drugs that are predominantly metabolized by the p450iid6 system and have relatively narrow therapeutic index should be initiated at low end of the dose range if a patient is receiving Prozac concurrently or has taken it in the previous 5 weeks). Products include:

Asendin Tablets 1369

Bupropion Hydrochloride (Inhibition of the activity of isoenzyme p450iid6 making normal metabolizers resemble "poor metabolizers"; therapy with drugs that are predominantly metabolized by the p450iid6 system and have relatively narrow therapeutic index should be initiated at low end of the dose range if a patient is receiving Prozac concurrently or has taken it in the previous 5 weeks; concomitant administration may result in greater increase in previously stable plasma levels of other antidepressants). Products include:

Wellbutrin Tablets 1204

Carbamazepine (Inhibition of the activity of isoenzyme p450iid6 making normal metabolizers resemble "poor metabolizers"; therapy with drugs that are predominantly metabolized by the p450iid6 system and have relatively narrow therapeutic index should be initiated at low end of the dose range if a patient is receiving Prozac concurrently or has taken it in the previous 5 weeks). Products include:

Atretol Tablets 573
Tegretol Chewable Tablets 852
Tegretol Suspension 852
Tegretol Tablets 852

Chlorpropamide (Prozac may alter glycemic control; oral hypoglycemic dosage may need to be adjusted). Products include:

Diabinese Tablets 1935

Clomipramine Hydrochloride (Inhibition of the activity of isoenzyme p450iid6 making normal metabolizers resemble "poor metabolizers"; therapy with drugs that are predominantly metabolized by the p450iid6 system and have relatively narrow therapeutic index should be initiated at low end of the dose range if a patient is receiving Prozac concurrently or has taken it in the previous 5 weeks). Products include:

Anafranil Capsules 803

Desipramine Hydrochloride (Inhibition of the activity of isoenzyme p450iid6 making normal metabolizers resemble "poor metabolizers"; therapy with drugs that are predominantly metabolized by the p450iid6 system and have relatively narrow therapeutic index should be initiated at low end of the dose range if a patient is receiving Prozac concurrently or has taken it in the previous 5 weeks). Products include:

Norpramin Tablets 1526

Diazepam (Half-life of concurrently administered diazepam may be prolonged). Products include:

Dizac 1809
Valium Injectable 2182
Valium Tablets 2183
Valrelease Capsules 2169

Dicumarol (Potential for adverse effects of either drug).

No products indexed under this heading.

Digitoxin (Potential for adverse effects of either drug). Products include:

Crystodigin Tablets 1433

Doxepin Hydrochloride (Inhibition of the activity of isoenzyme p450iid6 making normal metabolizers resemble "poor metabolizers"; therapy with drugs that are predominantly metabolized by the p450iid6 system and have relatively narrow therapeutic index should be initiated at low end of the dose range if a patient is receiving Prozac concurrently or has taken it in the previous 5 weeks). Products include:

Sinequan 2205
Zonalon Cream 1055

Encainide Hydrochloride (Inhibition of the activity of isoenzyme p450iid6 making normal metabolizers resemble "poor metabolizers"; therapy with drugs that are predominantly metabolized by the p450iid6 system and have relatively narrow therapeutic index should be initiated at low end of the dose range if a patient is receiving Prozac concurrently or has taken it in the previous 5 weeks).

No products indexed under this heading.

Flecainide Acetate (Inhibition of the activity of isoenzyme p450iid6 making normal metabolizers resemble "poor metabolizers"; therapy with drugs that are predominantly metabolized by the p450iid6 system and have relatively narrow therapeutic index should be initiated at low end of the dose range if a patient is receiving Prozac concurrently or has taken it in the previous 5 weeks). Products include:

Tambocor Tablets 1497

Furazolidone (Co-administration may result in serious, sometimes fatal, reactions including hyperthermia, rigidity, myoclonus, autonomic instability and coma; concurrent and/or sequential use is contraindicated and at least 5 weeks or longer should be allowed after stopping Prozac before starting MAO inhibitor). Products include:

Furoxone 2046

Glipizide (Prozac may alter glycemic control; oral hypoglycemic dosage may need to be adjusted). Products include:

Glucotrol Tablets 1967
Glucotrol XL Extended Release Tablets 1968

Glyburide (Prozac may alter glycemic control; oral hypoglycemic dosage may need to be adjusted). Products include:

DiaBeta Tablets 1239
Glynase PresTab Tablets 2609
Micronase Tablets 2623

Imipramine Hydrochloride (Inhibition of the activity of isoenzyme p450iid6 making normal metabolizers resemble "poor metabolizers"; therapy with drugs that are predominantly metabolized by the p450iid6 system and have relatively narrow therapeutic index should be initiated at low end of the dose range if a patient is receiving Prozac concurrently or has taken it in the previous 5 weeks). Products include:

Tofranil Ampuls 854
Tofranil Tablets 856

Imipramine Pamoate (Inhibition of the activity of isoenzyme p450iid6 making normal metabolizers resemble "poor metabolizers"; therapy with drugs that are predominantly metabolized by the p450iid6 system and have relatively narrow therapeutic index should be initiated at low end of the dose range if a patient is receiving Prozac concurrently or has taken it in the previous 5 weeks). Products include:

Tofranil-PM Capsules 857

Insulin, Human (Prozac may alter glycemic control; insulin dosage may need to be adjusted).

No products indexed under this heading.

Insulin, Human Isophane Suspension (Prozac may alter glycemic control; insulin dosage may need to be adjusted). Products include:

Novolin N Human Insulin 10 ml Vials 1795

Insulin, Human NPH (Prozac may alter glycemic control; insulin dosage may need to be adjusted). Products include:

Humulin N, 100 Units 1448
Novolin N PenFill Cartridges Durable Insulin Delivery System 1798
Novolin N Prefilled Syringe Disposable Insulin Delivery System 1798

Insulin, Human Regular (Prozac may alter glycemic control; insulin dosage may need to be adjusted). Products include:

Humulin R, 100 Units 1449
Novolin R Human Insulin 10 ml Vials 1795
Novolin R PenFill Cartridges Durable Insulin Delivery System 1798
Novolin R Prefilled Syringe Disposable Insulin Delivery System 1798
Velosulin BR Human Insulin 10 ml Vials 1795

Insulin, Human, Zinc Suspension (Prozac may alter glycemic control; insulin dosage may need to be adjusted). Products include:

Humulin L, 100 Units 1446
Humulin U, 100 Units 1450
Novolin L Human Insulin 10 ml Vials 1795

Insulin, NPH (Prozac may alter glycemic control; insulin dosage may need to be adjusted). Products include:

NPH, 100 Units 1450
Pork NPH, 100 Units 1452
Purified Pork NPH Isophane Insulin 1801

Insulin, Regular (Prozac may alter glycemic control; insulin dosage may need to be adjusted). Products include:

Regular, 100 Units 1450
Pork Regular, 100 Units 1452
Pork Regular (Concentrated), 500 Units 1453
Purified Pork Regular Insulin 1801

Insulin, Zinc Crystals (Prozac may alter glycemic control; insulin dosage may need to be adjusted). Products include:

NPH, 100 Units 1450

Insulin, Zinc Suspension (Prozac may alter glycemic control; insulin dosage may need to be adjusted). Products include:

Iletin I 1450
Lente, 100 Units 1450
Iletin II 1452
Pork Lente, 100 Units 1452
Purified Pork Lente Insulin 1801

IMPORTANT NOTE: Always consult each drug listing in the patient's regimen for possible interactions.

Prozac

Interactions Index

Isocarboxazid (Co-administration may result in serious, sometimes fatal, reactions including hyperthermia, rigidity, myoclonus, autonomic instability and coma; concurrent and/or sequential use is contraindicated and at least 5 weeks or longer should be allowed after stopping Prozac before starting MAO inhibitor).

No products indexed under this heading.

Lithium Carbonate (Increased and decreased lithium levels; potential for lithium toxicity). Products include:

Eskalith 2485
Lithium Carbonate Capsules & Tablets 2230
Lithonate/Lithotabs/Lithobid 2543

Lithium Citrate (Increased and decreased lithium levels; potential for lithium toxicity).

No products indexed under this heading.

Maprotiline Hydrochloride (Inhibition of the activity of isoenzyme p450iid6 making normal metabolizers resemble "poor metabolizers"; therapy with drugs that are predominantly metabolized by the p450iid6 system and have relatively narrow therapeutic index should be initiated at low end of the dose range if a patient is receiving Prozac concurrently or has taken it in the previous 5 weeks; concomitant administration may result in greater increase in previously stable plasma levels of other antidepressants). Products include:

Ludiomil Tablets................................... 843

Metformin Hydrochloride (Prozac may alter glycemic control; oral hypoglycemic dosage may need to be adjusted). Products include:

Glucophage 752

Nefazodone Hydrochloride (Inhibition of the activity of isoenzyme p450iid6 making normal metabolizers resemble "poor metabolizers"; therapy with drugs that are predominantly metabolized by the p450iid6 system and have relatively narrow therapeutic index should be initiated at low end of the dose range if a patient is receiving Prozac concurrently or has taken it in the previous 5 weeks). Products include:

Serzone Tablets 771

Nortriptyline Hydrochloride (Inhibition of the activity of isoenzyme p450iid6 making normal metabolizers resemble "poor metabolizers"; therapy with drugs that are predominantly metabolized by the p450iid6 system and have relatively narrow therapeutic index should be initiated at low end of the dose range if a patient is receiving Prozac concurrently or has taken it in the previous 5 weeks). Products include:

Pamelor 2280

Paroxetine Hydrochloride (Inhibition of the activity of isoenzyme p450iid6 making normal metabolizers resemble "poor metabolizers"; therapy with drugs that are predominantly metabolized by the p450iid6 system and have relatively narrow therapeutic index should be initiated at low end of the dose range if a patient is receiving Prozac concurrently or has taken it in the previous 5 weeks; concomitant administration may result in greater increase in previously stable plasma levels of other antidepressants). Products include:

Paxil Tablets 2505

Phenelzine Sulfate (Co-administration may result in serious, sometimes fatal, reactions including hyperthermia, rigidity, myoclonus, autonomic instability and coma; concurrent and/or sequential use is contraindicated and at least 5 weeks or longer should be allowed after stopping Prozac before starting MAO inhibitor). Products include:

Nardil 1920

Phenytoin (Patients on stable doses of phenytoin have developed elevated plasma phenytoin concentrations and clinical phenytoin toxicity following initiation of fluoxetine treatment). Products include:

Dilantin Infatabs.................................. 1908
Dilantin-125 Suspension 1911

Phenytoin Sodium (Patients on stable doses of phenytoin have developed elevated plasma phenytoin concentrations and clinical phenytoin toxicity following initiation of fluoxetine treatment). Products include:

Dilantin Kapseals 1906
Dilantin Parenteral 1910

Protriptyline Hydrochloride (Inhibition of the activity of isoenzyme p450iid6 making normal metabolizers resemble "poor metabolizers"; therapy with drugs that are predominantly metabolized by the p450iid6 system and have relatively narrow therapeutic index should be initiated at low end of the dose range if a patient is receiving Prozac concurrently or has taken it in the previous 5 weeks). Products include:

Vivactil Tablets 1774

Selegiline Hydrochloride (Co-administration may result in serious, sometimes fatal, reactions including hyperthermia, rigidity, myoclonus, autonomic instability and coma; concurrent and/or sequential use is contraindicated and at least 5 weeks or longer should be allowed after stopping Prozac before starting MAO inhibitor). Products include:

Eldepryl Tablets 2550

Sertraline Hydrochloride (Inhibition of the activity of isoenzyme $P_{450}IID_6$ making normal metabolizers resemble "poor metabolizers"; therapy with drugs that are predominantly metabolized by the $P_{450}IID_6$ system and have relatively narrow therapeutic index should be initiated at low end of the dose range if a patient is receiving Prozac or has taken it in the previous 5 weeks). Products include:

Zoloft Tablets 2217

Tolazamide (Prozac may alter glycemic control; oral hypoglycemic dosage may need to be adjusted).

No products indexed under this heading.

Tolbutamide (Prozac may alter glycemic control; oral hypoglycemic dosage may need to be adjusted).

No products indexed under this heading.

Tranylcypromine Sulfate (Co-administration may result in serious, sometimes fatal, reactions including hyperthermia, rigidity, myoclonus, autonomic instability and coma; concurrent and/or sequential use is contraindicated and at least 5 weeks or longer should be allowed after stopping Prozac before starting MAO inhibitor). Products include:

Parnate Tablets 2503

Trazodone Hydrochloride (Inhibition of the activity of isoenzyme p450iid6 making normal metabolizers resemble "poor metabolizers"; therapy with drugs that are predominantly metabolized by the p450iid6 system and have relatively narrow therapeutic index should be initiated at low end of the dose range if a patient is receiving Prozac concurrently or has taken it in the previous 5 weeks; concomitant administration may result in greater increase in previously stable plasma levels of other antidepressants). Products include:

Desyrel and Desyrel Dividose 503

Trimipramine Maleate (Inhibition of the activity of isoenzyme p450iid6 making normal metabolizers resemble "poor metabolizers"; therapy with drugs that are predominantly metabolized by the p450iid6 system and have relatively narrow therapeutic index should be initiated at low end of the dose range if a patient is receiving Prozac concurrently or has taken it in the previous 5 weeks). Products include:

Surmontil Capsules.............................. 2811

L-Tryptophan (Potential for agitation, restlessness and gastrointestinal distress).

No products indexed under this heading.

Venlafaxine Hydrochloride (Inhibition of the activity of isoenzyme p450iid6 making normal metabolizers resemble "poor metabolizers"; therapy with drugs that are predominantly metabolized by the p450iid6 system and have relatively narrow therapeutic index should be initiated at low end of the dose range if a patient is receiving Prozac concurrently or has taken it in the previous 5 weeks). Products include:

Effexor 2719

Vinblastine Sulfate (Inhibition of the activity of isoenzyme p450iid6 making normal metabolizers resemble "poor metabolizers"; therapy with drugs that are predominantly metabolized by the p450iid6 system and have relatively narrow therapeutic index should be initiated at low end of the dose range if a patient is receiving Prozac concurrently or has taken it in the previous 5 weeks). Products include:

Velban Vials 1484

Warfarin Sodium (Potential for adverse effects of either drug). Products include:

Coumadin 926

Food Interactions

Food, unspecified (May delay absorption of fluoxetine inconsequentially).

PSORCON CREAM 0.05%

(Diflorasone Diacetate) 909
None cited in PDR database.

PSORCON OINTMENT 0.05%

(Diflorasone Diacetate) 908
None cited in PDR database.

PULMOCARE SPECIALIZED NUTRITION FOR PULMONARY PATIENTS

(Nutritional Supplement) 2224
None cited in PDR database.

PULMOZYME INHALATION

(Dornase Alfa) 1064
None cited in PDR database.

PURGE CONCENTRATE

(Castor Oil) .... �◻ 655
None cited in PDR database.

PURI-CLENS, WOUND DEODORIZER AND CLEANSER SPRAY GEL

(Benzethonium Chloride) 2554
None cited in PDR database.

PURIFIED PORK LENTE INSULIN

(Insulin, Zinc Suspension)....................1801
None cited in PDR database.

PURINETHOL TABLETS

(Mercaptopurine)..................................1156
May interact with:

Allopurinol (Concomitant use at the regular dose results in delayed catabolism of mercaptopurine; substantial dosage reductions may be required to avoid the development of life-threatening bone marrow depression). Products include:

Zyloprim Tablets 1226

Doxorubicin Hydrochloride (Potential for increased hepatotoxicity). Products include:

Adriamycin PFS 1947
Adriamycin RDF 1947
Doxorubicin Astra 540
Rubex 712

Hepatotoxic Drugs, unspecified (Hepatotoxicity).

Sulfamethoxazole (Enhanced bone marrow suppression has been noted in some of the patients also receiving trimethoprim-sulfamethoxazole). Products include:

Azo Gantanol Tablets........................... 2080
Bactrim DS Tablets............................... 2084
Bactrim I.V. Infusion........................... 2082
Bactrim 2084
Gantanol Tablets 2119
Septra... 1174
Septra I.V. Infusion 1169
Septra I.V. Infusion ADD-Vantage Vials.. 1171
Septra... 1174

Thioguanine (Complete cross-resistance). Products include:

Thioguanine Tablets, Tabloid Brand 1181

Trimethoprim (Enhanced bone marrow suppression has been noted in some of the patients also receiving trimethoprim-sulfamethoxazole). Products include:

Bactrim DS Tablets............................... 2084
Bactrim I.V. Infusion........................... 2082
Bactrim 2084
Proloprim Tablets 1155
Septra... 1174
Septra I.V. Infusion 1169
Septra I.V. Infusion ADD-Vantage Vials.. 1171
Septra... 1174
Trimpex Tablets 2163

(◻ Described in PDR For Nonprescription Drugs) (◉ Described in PDR For Ophthalmology)

867 Interactions Index Quadrinal

PYRAZINAMIDE TABLETS
(Pyrazinamide) 1398
None cited in PDR database.

PYRIDIUM
(Phenazopyridine Hydrochloride) 1928
None cited in PDR database.

PYRROXATE CAPLETS
(Acetaminophen, Chlorpheniramine Maleate, Phenylpropanolamine Hydrochloride) .... ▣ 772
May interact with monoamine oxidase inhibitors and certain other agents. Compounds in these categories include:

Furazolidone (Product labeling recommends physician's supervision for concurrent administration of these drugs). Products include:
- Furoxone 2046

Isocarboxazid (Product labeling recommends physician's supervision for concurrent administration of these drugs).
- No products indexed under this heading.

Phenelzine Sulfate (Product labeling recommends physician's supervision for concurrent administration of these drugs). Products include:
- Nardil 1920

Selegiline Hydrochloride (Product labeling recommends physician's supervision for concurrent administration of these drugs). Products include:
- Eldepryl Tablets 2550

Tranylcypromine Sulfate (Product labeling recommends physician's supervision for concurrent administration of these drugs). Products include:
- Parnate Tablets 2503

Food Interactions

Alcohol (Concurrent use not recommended).

QUADRINAL TABLETS
(Ephedrine Hydrochloride, Phenobarbital, Potassium Iodide, Theophylline Calcium Salicylate) 1350
May interact with cardiac glycosides, general anesthetics, monoamine oxidase inhibitors, sympathomimetics, tricyclic antidepressants, central nervous system depressants, oral anticoagulants, corticosteroids, and certain other agents. Compounds in these categories include:

Albuterol (Increased effects). Products include:
- Proventil Inhalation Aerosol 2382
- Ventolin Inhalation Aerosol and Refill 1197

Albuterol Sulfate (Increased effects). Products include:
- Airet Solution for Inhalation 452
- Proventil Inhalation Solution 0.083% 2384
- Proventil Repetabs Tablets 2386
- Proventil Solution for Inhalation 0.5% 2383
- Proventil Syrup 2385
- Proventil Tablets 2386
- Ventolin Inhalation Solution 1198
- Ventolin Nebules Inhalation Solution 1199
- Ventolin Rotacaps for Inhalation 1200
- Ventolin Syrup 1202
- Ventolin Tablets 1203
- Volmax Extended-Release Tablets .. 1788

Alfentanil Hydrochloride (Increased effects). Products include:
- Alfenta Injection 1286

Alprazolam (Increased effects). Products include:
- Xanax Tablets 2649

Amitriptyline Hydrochloride (Decreased effects; possible antagonized pressor effect of ephedrine). Products include:
- Elavil 2838
- Endep Tablets 2174
- Etrafon 2355
- Limbitrol 2180
- Triavil Tablets 1757

Amoxapine (Decreased effects; possible antagonized pressor effect of ephedrine). Products include:
- Asendin Tablets 1369

Aprobarbital (Increased effects).
- No products indexed under this heading.

Betamethasone Acetate (Decreased effects). Products include:
- Celestone Soluspan Suspension 2347

Betamethasone Sodium Phosphate (Decreased effects). Products include:
- Celestone Soluspan Suspension 2347

Buprenorphine (Increased effects). Products include:
- Buprenex Injectable 2006

Buspirone Hydrochloride (Increased effects). Products include:
- BuSpar 737

Butabarbital (Increased effects).
- No products indexed under this heading.

Butalbital (Increased effects). Products include:
- Esgic-plus Tablets 1013
- Fioricet Tablets 2258
- Fioricet with Codeine Capsules 2260
- Fiorinal Capsules 2261
- Fiorinal with Codeine Capsules 2262
- Fiorinal Tablets 2261
- Phrenilin 785
- Sedapap Tablets 50 mg/650 mg .. 1543

Chlordiazepoxide (Fatty acid mobilization; increased effects). Products include:
- Libritabs Tablets 2177
- Limbitrol 2180

Chlordiazepoxide Hydrochloride (Fatty acid mobilization; increased effects). Products include:
- Librax Capsules 2176
- Librium Capsules 2178
- Librium Injectable 2179

Chlorpromazine (Increased effects). Products include:
- Thorazine Suppositories 2523

Chlorprothixene (Increased effects).
- No products indexed under this heading.

Chlorprothixene Hydrochloride (Increased effects).
- No products indexed under this heading.

Cimetidine (Increased theophylline blood levels). Products include:
- Tagamet Tablets 2516

Cimetidine Hydrochloride (Increased theophylline blood levels). Products include:
- Tagamet 2516

Clindamycin Hydrochloride (Increased theophylline plasma levels).
- No products indexed under this heading.

Clindamycin Palmitate Hydrochloride (Increased theophylline plasma levels).
- No products indexed under this heading.

Clindamycin Phosphate (Increased theophylline plasma levels). Products include:
- Cleocin Phosphate Injection 2586
- Cleocin T Topical 2590
- Cleocin Vaginal Cream 2589

Clomipramine Hydrochloride (Decreased effects; possible antagonized pressor effect of ephedrine). Products include:
- Anafranil Capsules 803

Clorazepate Dipotassium (Increased effects). Products include:
- Tranxene 451

Clozapine (Increased effects). Products include:
- Clozaril Tablets 2252

Codeine Phosphate (Increased effects). Products include:
- Actifed with Codeine Cough Syrup.. 1067
- Brontex 1981
- Deconsal C Expectorant Syrup 456
- Deconsal Pediatric Syrup 457
- Dimetane-DC Cough Syrup 2059
- Empirin with Codeine Tablets 1093
- Fioricet with Codeine Capsules 2260
- Fiorinal with Codeine Capsules 2262
- Isoclor Expectorant 990
- Novahistine DH 2462
- Novahistine Expectorant 2463
- Nucofed 2051
- Phenergan with Codeine 2777
- Phenergan VC with Codeine 2781
- Robitussin A-C Syrup 2073
- Robitussin-DAC Syrup 2074
- Ryna .... ▣ 841
- Soma Compound w/Codeine Tablets 2676
- Tussi-Organidin NR Liquid and S NR Liquid 2677
- Tylenol with Codeine 1583

Cortisone Acetate (Decreased effects). Products include:
- Cortone Acetate Sterile Suspension 1623
- Cortone Acetate Tablets 1624

Desflurane (Increased effects). Products include:
- Suprane 1813

Desipramine Hydrochloride (Decreased effects; possible antagonized pressor effect of ephedrine). Products include:
- Norpramin Tablets 1526

Deslanoside (Decreased effects; possible cardiac arrhythmias).
- No products indexed under this heading.

Dexamethasone (Decreased effects). Products include:
- AK-Trol Ointment & Suspension .... ◉ 205
- Decadron Elixir 1633
- Decadron Tablets 1635
- Decaspray Topical Aerosol 1648
- Dexacidin Ointment .... ◉ 263
- Maxitrol Ophthalmic Ointment and Suspension .... ◉ 224
- TobraDex Ophthalmic Suspension and Ointment 473

Dexamethasone Acetate (Decreased effects). Products include:
- Dalalone D.P. Injectable 1011
- Decadron-LA Sterile Suspension 1646

Dexamethasone Sodium Phosphate (Decreased effects). Products include:
- Decadron Phosphate Injection 1637
- Decadron Phosphate Respihaler 1642
- Decadron Phosphate Sterile Ophthalmic Ointment 1641
- Decadron Phosphate Sterile Ophthalmic Solution 1642
- Decadron Phosphate Topical Cream 1644
- Decadron Phosphate Turbinaire 1645
- Decadron Phosphate with Xylocaine Injection, Sterile 1639
- Dexacort Phosphate in Respihaler .. 458
- Dexacort Phosphate in Turbinaire .. 459
- NeoDecadron Sterile Ophthalmic Ointment 1712
- NeoDecadron Sterile Ophthalmic Solution 1713
- NeoDecadron Topical Cream 1714

Dezocine (Increased effects). Products include:
- Dalgan Injection 538

Diazepam (Increased effects). Products include:
- Dizac 1809
- Valium Injectable 2182
- Valium Tablets 2183
- Valrelease Capsules 2169

Dicumarol (Decreased anticoagulant effects).
- No products indexed under this heading.

Digitoxin (Decreased effects; possible cardiac arrhythmias). Products include:
- Crystodigin Tablets 1433

Digoxin (Decreased effects; possible cardiac arrhythmias). Products include:
- Lanoxicaps 1117
- Lanoxin Elixir Pediatric 1120
- Lanoxin Injection 1123
- Lanoxin Injection Pediatric 1126
- Lanoxin Tablets 1128

Dobutamine Hydrochloride (Increased effects). Products include:
- Dobutrex Solution Vials 1439

Dopamine Hydrochloride (Increased effects).
- No products indexed under this heading.

Doxepin Hydrochloride (Decreased effects; possible antagonized pressor effect of ephedrine). Products include:
- Sinequan 2205
- Zonalon Cream 1055

Doxycycline Calcium (Decreased effects). Products include:
- Vibramycin Calcium Oral Suspension Syrup 1941

Doxycycline Hyclate (Decreased effects). Products include:
- Doryx Capsules 1913
- Vibramycin Hyclate Capsules 1941
- Vibramycin Hyclate Intravenous 2215
- Vibra-Tabs Film Coated Tablets 1941

Doxycycline Monohydrate (Decreased effects). Products include:
- Monodox Capsules 1805
- Vibramycin Monohydrate for Oral Suspension 1941

Droperidol (Increased effects). Products include:
- Inapsine Injection 1296

Enflurane (Increased effects of medication; cardiac arrhythmias).
- No products indexed under this heading.

Epinephrine (Increased effects). Products include:
- Bronkaid Mist .... ▣ 717
- EPIFRIN .... ◉ 239
- EpiPen 790
- Marcaine Hydrochloride with Epinephrine 1:200,000 2316
- Primatene Mist .... ▣ 873
- Sensorcaine with Epinephrine Injection 559
- Sus-Phrine Injection 1019
- Xylocaine with Epinephrine Injections 567

Epinephrine Bitartrate (Increased effects). Products include:
- Bronkaid Mist Suspension .... ▣ 718
- Sensorcaine-MPF with Epinephrine Injection 559

Epinephrine Hydrochloride (Increased effects). Products include:
- Ana-Kit Anaphylaxis Emergency Treatment Kit 617

Ergonovine Maleate (Hypertension).
- No products indexed under this heading.

Erythromycin (Increased theophylline plasma levels). Products include:
- A/T/S 2% Acne Topical Gel and Solution 1234
- Benzamycin Topical Gel 905
- E-Mycin Tablets 1341
- Emgel 2% Topical Gel 1093
- ERYC 1915
- Erycette (erythromycin 2%) Topical Solution 1888

IMPORTANT NOTE: Always consult each drug listing in the patient's regimen for possible interactions.

Quadrinal Interactions Index 868

Ery-Tab Tablets 422
Erythromycin Base Filmtab 426
Erythromycin Delayed-Release Capsules, USP 427
Ilotycin Ophthalmic Ointment 912
PCE Dispertab Tablets 444
T-Stat 2.0% Topical Solution and Pads 2688
Theramycin Z Topical Solution 2% 1592

Erythromycin Estolate (Increased theophylline plasma levels). Products include:
Ilosone 911

Erythromycin Ethylsuccinate (Increased theophylline plasma levels). Products include:
E.E.S. 424
EryPed 421

Erythromycin Gluceptate (Increased theophylline plasma levels). Products include:
Ilotycin Gluceptate, IV, Vials 913

Erythromycin Lactobionate (Increased theophylline plasma levels).
No products indexed under this heading.

Erythromycin Stearate (Increased theophylline plasma levels). Products include:
Erythrocin Stearate Filmtab 425

Estazolam (Increased effects). Products include:
ProSom Tablets 449

Ethchlorvynol (Increased effects). Products include:
Placidyl Capsules 448

Ethinamate (Increased effects).
No products indexed under this heading.

Fentanyl (Increased effects). Products include:
Duragesic Transdermal System 1288

Fentanyl Citrate (Increased effects). Products include:
Sublimaze Injection 1307

Fludrocortisone Acetate (Decreased effects). Products include:
Florinef Acetate Tablets 505

Fluphenazine Decanoate (Increased effects). Products include:
Prolixin Decanoate 509

Fluphenazine Enanthate (Increased effects). Products include:
Prolixin Enanthate 509

Fluphenazine Hydrochloride (Increased effects). Products include:
Prolixin 509

Flurazepam Hydrochloride (Increased effects). Products include:
Dalmane Capsules 2173

Furazolidone (Potentiated pressor effect of ephedrine). Products include:
Furoxone 2046

Furosemide (Increased diuresis). Products include:
Lasix Injection, Oral Solution and Tablets 1240

Glutethimide (Increased effects).
No products indexed under this heading.

Griseofulvin (Decreased effects). Products include:
Fulvicin P/G Tablets 2359
Fulvicin P/G 165 & 330 Tablets 2359
Grifulvin V (griseofulvin tablets) Microsize (griseofulvin oral suspension) Microsize 1888
Gris-PEG Tablets, 125 mg & 250 mg 479

Guanethidine Monosulfate (Decreased hypotensive effect). Products include:
Esimil Tablets 822
Ismelin Tablets 827

Haloperidol (Increased effects). Products include:
Haldol Injection, Tablets and Concentrate 1575

Haloperidol Decanoate (Increased effects). Products include:
Haldol Decanoate 1577

Hexamethonium (Decreased hexamethonium-induced chronotropic effect).

Hydrocodone Bitartrate (Increased effects). Products include:
Anexsia 5/500 Elixir 1781
Anexia Tablets 1782
Codiclear DH Syrup 791
Deconamine CX Cough and Cold Liquid and Tablets 1319
Duratuss HD Elixir 2565
Hycodan Tablets and Syrup 930
Hycomine Compound Tablets 932
Hycomine 931
Hycotuss Expectorant Syrup 933
Hydrocet Capsules 782
Lorcet 10/650 1018
Lortab 2566
Tussend 1783
Tussend Expectorant 1785
Vicodin Tablets 1356
Vicodin ES Tablets 1357
Vicodin Tuss Expectorant 1358
Zydone Capsules 949

Hydrocodone Polistirex (Increased effects). Products include:
Tussionex Pennkinetic Extended-Release Suspension 998

Hydrocortisone (Decreased effects). Products include:
Anusol-HC Cream 2.5% 1896
Aquanil HC Lotion 1931
Bactine Hydrocortisone Anti-Itch Cream .... [NP] 709
Caldecort Anti-Itch Hydrocortisone Spray .... [NP] 631
Cortaid .... [NP] 836
CORTENEMA 2535
Cortisporin Ointment 1085
Cortisporin Ophthalmic Ointment Sterile 1085
Cortisporin Ophthalmic Suspension Sterile 1086
Cortisporin Otic Solution Sterile 1087
Cortisporin Otic Suspension Sterile 1088
Cortizone-5 .... [NP] 831
Cortizone-10 .... [NP] 831
Hydrocortone Tablets 1672
Hytone 907
Massengill Medicated Soft Cloth Towelettes 2458
PediOtic Suspension Sterile 1153
Preparation H Hydrocortisone 1% Cream .... [NP] 872
ProctoCream-HC 2.5% 2408
VōSoL HC Otic Solution 2678

Hydrocortisone Acetate (Decreased effects). Products include:
Analpram-HC Rectal Cream 1% and 2.5% 977
Anusol HC-1 Anti-Itch Hydrocortisone Ointment .... [NP] 847
Anusol-HC Suppositories 1897
Caldecort .... [NP] 631
Carmol HC 924
Coly-Mycin S Otic w/Neomycin & Hydrocortisone 1906
Cortaid .... [NP] 836
Cortifoam 2396
Cortisporin Cream 1084
Epifoam 2399
Hydrocortone Acetate Sterile Suspension 1669
Mantadil Cream 1135
Nupercainal Hydrocortisone 1% Cream .... [NP] 645
Ophthocort .... ⊙ 311
Pramosone Cream, Lotion & Ointment 978
ProctoCream-HC 2408
ProctoFoam-HC 2409
Terra-Cortril Ophthalmic Suspension 2210

Hydrocortisone Sodium Phosphate (Decreased effects). Products include:
Hydrocortone Phosphate Injection, Sterile 1670

Hydrocortisone Sodium Succinate (Decreased effects). Products include:
Solu-Cortef Sterile Powder 2641

Hydroxyzine Hydrochloride (Increased effects). Products include:
Atarax Tablets & Syrup 2185
Marax Tablets & DF Syrup 2200
Vistaril Intramuscular Solution 2216

Imipramine Hydrochloride (Decreased effects; possible antagonized pressor effect of ephedrine). Products include:
Tofranil Ampuls 854
Tofranil Tablets 856

Imipramine Pamoate (Decreased effects; possible antagonized pressor effect of ephedrine). Products include:
Tofranil-PM Capsules 857

Isocarboxazid (Potentiated pressor effect of ephedrine).
No products indexed under this heading.

Isoflurane (Increased effects of medication; cardiac arrhythmias).
No products indexed under this heading.

Isoproterenol Hydrochloride (Increased effects). Products include:
Isuprel Hydrochloride Injection 1:5000 2311
Isuprel Hydrochloride Solution 1:200 & 1:100 2313
Isuprel Mistometer 2312

Isoproterenol Sulfate (Increased effects). Products include:
Norisodrine with Calcium Iodide Syrup 442

Ketamine Hydrochloride (Increased effects of medication; cardiac arrhythmias).
No products indexed under this heading.

Levomethadyl Acetate Hydrochloride (Increased effects). Products include:
Orlamm 2239

Levorphanol Tartrate (Increased effects). Products include:
Levo-Dromoran 2129

Lincomycin Hydrochloride Monohydrate (Increased theophylline plasma levels).
No products indexed under this heading.

Lithium Carbonate (Increased excretion of lithium carbonate). Products include:
Eskalith 2485
Lithium Carbonate Capsules & Tablets 2230
Lithonate/Lithotabs/Lithobid 2543

Lorazepam (Increased effects). Products include:
Ativan Injection 2698
Ativan Tablets 2700

Loxapine Hydrochloride (Increased effects). Products include:
Loxitane 1378

Loxapine Succinate (Increased effects). Products include:
Loxitane Capsules 1378

Maprotiline Hydrochloride (Decreased effects; possible antagonized pressor effect of ephedrine). Products include:
Ludiomil Tablets 843

Meperidine Hydrochloride (Increased effects). Products include:
Demerol 2308
Mepergan Injection 2753

Mephobarbital (Increased effects). Products include:
Mebaral Tablets 2322

Meprobamate (Increased effects). Products include:
Miltown Tablets 2672
PMB 200 and PMB 400 2783

Mesoridazine Besylate (Increased effects). Products include:
Serentil 684

Metaproterenol Sulfate (Increased effects). Products include:
Alupent 669
Metaproterenol Sulfate Inhalation Solution, USP, Arm-a-Med 552

Metaraminol Bitartrate (Increased effects). Products include:
Aramine Injection 1609

Methadone Hydrochloride (Increased effects). Products include:
Methadone Hydrochloride Oral Concentrate 2233
Methadone Hydrochloride Oral Solution & Tablets 2235

Methohexital Sodium (Increased effects of medication; cardiac arrhythmias). Products include:
Brevital Sodium Vials 1429

Methotrimeprazine (Increased effects). Products include:
Levoprome 1274

Methoxamine Hydrochloride (Increased effects). Products include:
Vasoxyl Injection 1196

Methoxyflurane (Increased effects of medication; cardiac arrhythmias).
No products indexed under this heading.

Methylergonovine Maleate (Hypertension). Products include:
Methergine 2272

Methylprednisolone Acetate (Decreased effects). Products include:
Depo-Medrol Single-Dose Vial 2600
Depo-Medrol Sterile Aqueous Suspension 2597

Methylprednisolone Sodium Succinate (Decreased effects). Products include:
Solu-Medrol Sterile Powder 2643

Midazolam Hydrochloride (Increased effects). Products include:
Versed Injection 2170

Molindone Hydrochloride (Increased effects). Products include:
Moban Tablets and Concentrate 1048

Morphine Sulfate (Increased effects). Products include:
Astramorph/PF Injection, USP (Preservative-Free) 535
Duramorph 962
Infumorph 200 and Infumorph 500 Sterile Solutions 965
MS Contin Tablets 1994
MSIR 1997
Oramorph SR (Morphine Sulfate Sustained Release Tablets) 2236
RMS Suppositories 2657
Roxanol 2243

Norepinephrine Bitartrate (Increased effects). Products include:
Levophed Bitartrate Injection 2315

Nortriptyline Hydrochloride (Decreased effects; possible antagonized pressor effect of ephedrine). Products include:
Pamelor 2280

Opium Alkaloids (Increased effects).
No products indexed under this heading.

Oxazepam (Increased effects). Products include:
Serax Capsules 2810
Serax Tablets 2810

Oxycodone Hydrochloride (Increased effects). Products include:
Percocet Tablets 938
Percodan Tablets 939
Percodan-Demi Tablets 940

([NP] Described in PDR For Nonprescription Drugs) (⊙ Described in PDR For Ophthalmology)

Roxicodone Tablets, Oral Solution & Intensol (Oxycodone) 2244
Tylox Capsules 1584

Oxytocin (Hypertension). Products include:

Oxytocin Injection 2771
Syntocinon Injection 2296

Oxytocin (Nasal Spray) (Hypertension).

Pentobarbital Sodium (Increased effects). Products include:

Nembutal Sodium Capsules 436
Nembutal Sodium Solution 438
Nembutal Sodium Suppositories...... 440

Perphenazine (Increased effects). Products include:

Etrafon 2355
Triavil Tablets 1757
Trilafon.. 2389

Phenelzine Sulfate (Potentiated pressor effect of ephedrine). Products include:

Nardil 1920

Phenylephrine Bitartrate (Increased effects).

No products indexed under this heading.

Phenylephrine Hydrochloride (Increased effects). Products include:

Atrohist Plus Tablets 454
Cerose DM .... ⊕ 878
Comhist 2038
D.A. Chewable Tablets........................... 951
Deconsal Pediatric Capsules............... 454
Dura-Vent/DA Tablets 953
Entex Capsules 1986
Entex Liquid 1986
Extendryl 1005
4-Way Fast Acting Nasal Spray (regular & mentholated) .... ⊕ 621
Hemorid For Women .... ⊕ 834
Hycomine Compound Tablets 932
Neo-Synephrine Hydrochloride 1% Carpuject... 2324
Neo-Synephrine Hydrochloride 1% Injection 2324
Neo-Synephrine Hydrochloride (Ophthalmic) 2325
Neo-Synephrine .... ⊕ 726
Nostril .... ⊕ 644
Novahistine Elixir .... ⊕ 823
Phenergan VC 2779
Phenergan VC with Codeine 2781
Preparation H .... ⊕ 871
Tympagesic Ear Drops 2342
Vasosulf .... © 271
Vicks Sinex Nasal Spray and Ultra Fine Mist .... ⊕ 765

Phenylephrine Tannate (Increased effects). Products include:

Atrohist Pediatric Suspension 454
Ricobid-D Pediatric Suspension........ 2038
Ricobid Tablets and Pediatric Suspension.. 2038
Rynatan 2673
Rynatuss 2673

Phenylpropanolamine Hydrochloride (Increased effects). Products include:

Acutrim .... ⊕ 628
Allerest Children's Chewable Tablets .... ⊕ 627
Allerest 12 Hour Caplets .... ⊕ 627
Atrohist Plus Tablets 454
BC Cold Powder Multi-Symptom Formula (Cold-Sinus-Allergy) ...... ⊕ 609
BC Cold Powder Non-Drowsy Formula (Cold-Sinus) .... ⊕ 609
Cheracol Plus Head Cold/Cough Formula .... ⊕ 769
Comtrex Multi-Symptom Non-Drowsy Liqui-gels................................. ⊕ 618
Contac Continuous Action Nasal Decongestant/Antihistamine 12 Hour Capsules.. ⊕ 813
Contac Maximum Strength Continuous Action Decongestant/ Antihistamine 12 Hour Caplets.. ⊕ 813
Contac Severe Cold and Flu Formula Caplets .... ⊕ 814
Coricidin 'D' Decongestant Tablets .... ⊕ 800
Dexatrim .... ⊕ 832
Dexatrim Plus Vitamins Caplets .... ⊕ 832
Dimetane-DC Cough Syrup 2059
Dimetapp Elixir .... ⊕ 773
Dimetapp Extentabs .... ⊕ 774
Dimetapp Tablets/Liqui-Gels .... ⊕ 775
Dimetapp Cold & Allergy Chewable Tablets .... ⊕ 773
Dimetapp DM Elixir................................ ⊕ 774
Dura-Vent Tablets 952
Entex Capsules 1986
Entex LA Tablets 1987
Entex Liquid 1986
Exgest LA Tablets 782
Hycomine 931
Isoclor Timesule Capsules .... ⊕ 637
Nolamine Timed-Release Tablets 785
Ornade Spansule Capsules 2502
Propagest Tablets 786
Pyrroxate Caplets .... ⊕ 772
Robitussin-CF .... ⊕ 777
Sinulin Tablets 787
Tavist-D 12 Hour Relief Tablets.... ⊕ 787
Teldrin 12 Hour Antihistamine/ Nasal Decongestant Allergy Relief Capsules .... ⊕ 826
Triaminic Allergy Tablets .... ⊕ 789
Triaminic Cold Tablets .... ⊕ 790
Triaminic Expectorant .... ⊕ 790
Triaminic Syrup .... ⊕ 792
Triaminic-12 Tablets .... ⊕ 792
Triaminic-DM Syrup .... ⊕ 792
Triaminicin Tablets .... ⊕ 793
Triaminicol Multi-Symptom Cold Tablets .... ⊕ 793
Triaminicol Multi-Symptom Relief ⊕ 794
Vicks DayQuil Allergy Relief 12-Hour Extended Release Tablets.. ⊕ 760
Vicks DayQuil Allergy Relief 4-Hour Tablets .... ⊕ 760
Vicks DayQuil SINUS Pressure & CONGESTION Relief........................... ⊕ 761

Phenytoin (Decreased effects; decreased phenytoin levels). Products include:

Dilantin Infatabs....................................... 1908
Dilantin-125 Suspension 1911

Phenytoin Sodium (Decreased effects; decreased phenytoin levels). Products include:

Dilantin Kapseals 1906
Dilantin Parenteral 1910

Pirbuterol Acetate (Increased effects). Products include:

Maxair Autohaler 1492
Maxair Inhaler 1494

Prazepam (Increased effects).

No products indexed under this heading.

Prednisolone Acetate (Decreased effects). Products include:

AK-CIDE .... © 202
AK-CIDE Ointment................................. © 202
Blephamide Liquifilm Sterile Ophthalmic Suspension.............................. 476
Blephamide Ointment .... © 237
Econopred & Econopred Plus Ophthalmic Suspensions .... © 217
Poly-Pred Liquifilm .... © 248
Pred Forte... © 250
Pred Mild... © 253
Pred-G Liquifilm Sterile Ophthalmic Suspension .... © 251
Pred-G S.O.P. Sterile Ophthalmic Ointment .... © 252
Vasocidin Ointment .... © 268

Prednisolone Sodium Phosphate (Decreased effects). Products include:

AK-Pred .... © 204
Hydeltrasol Injection, Sterile.............. 1665
Inflamase... © 265
Pediapred Oral Liquid 995
Vasocidin Ophthalmic Solution ...... © 270

Prednisolone Tebutate (Decreased effects). Products include:

Hydeltra-T.B.A. Sterile Suspension 1667

Prednisone (Decreased effects). Products include:

Deltasone Tablets 2595

Prochlorperazine (Increased effects). Products include:

Compazine 2470

Promethazine Hydrochloride (Increased effects). Products include:

Mepergan Injection 2753
Phenergan with Codeine...................... 2777
Phenergan with Dextromethorphan 2778
Phenergan Injection 2773
Phenergan Suppositories 2775
Phenergan Syrup 2774
Phenergan Tablets 2775
Phenergan VC 2779
Phenergan VC with Codeine 2781

Propofol (Increased effects). Products include:

Diprivan Injection.................................... 2833

Propoxyphene Hydrochloride (Increased effects). Products include:

Darvon 1435
Wygesic Tablets 2827

Propoxyphene Napsylate (Increased effects). Products include:

Darvon-N/Darvocet-N 1433

Propranolol Hydrochloride (Antagonism of propranolol effect). Products include:

Inderal 2728
Inderal LA Long Acting Capsules 2730
Inderide Tablets 2732
Inderide LA Long Acting Capsules .. 2734

Protriptyline Hydrochloride (Decreased effects; possible antagonized pressor effect of ephedrine). Products include:

Vivactil Tablets 1774

Pseudoephedrine Hydrochloride (Increased effects). Products include:

Actifed Allergy Daytime/Nighttime Caplets .... ⊕ 844
Actifed Plus Caplets .... ⊕ 845
Actifed Plus Tablets .... ⊕ 845
Actifed with Codeine Cough Syrup.. 1067
Actifed Sinus Daytime/Nighttime Tablets and Caplets .... ⊕ 846
Actifed Syrup... ⊕ 846
Actifed Tablets .... ⊕ 844
Advil Cold and Sinus Caplets and Tablets (formerly CoAdvil) .... ⊕ 870
Alka-Seltzer Plus Cold Medicine Liqui-Gels .... ⊕ 706
Alka-Seltzer Plus Cold & Cough Medicine Liqui-Gels.............................. ⊕ 705
Alka-Seltzer Plus Night-Time Cold Medicine Liqui-Gels.............................. ⊕ 706
Allerest Headache Strength Tablets .... ⊕ 627
Allerest Maximum Strength Tablets .... ⊕ 627
Allerest No Drowsiness Tablets....... ⊕ 627
Allerest Sinus Pain Formula .... ⊕ 627
Anatuss LA Tablets.................................. 1542
Atrohist Pediatric Capsules................ 453
Bayer Select Sinus Pain Relief Formula .... ⊕ 717
Benadryl Allergy Decongestant Liquid Medication .... ⊕ 848
Benadryl Allergy Decongestant Tablets .... ⊕ 848
Benadryl Allergy Sinus Headache Formula Caplets .... ⊕ 849
Benylin Multisymptom.......................... ⊕ 852
Bromfed Capsules (Extended-Release) 1785
Bromfed Syrup .... ⊕ 733
Bromfed Tablets 1785
Bromfed-DM Cough Syrup.................. 1786
Bromfed-PD Capsules (Extended-Release) 1785
Children's Vicks DayQuil Allergy Relief .... ⊕ 757
Children's Vicks NyQuil Cold/ Cough Relief... ⊕ 758
Comtrex Multi-Symptom Cold Reliever Tablets/Caplets/Liqui-Gels/Liquid.. ⊕ 615
Allergy-Sinus Comtrex Multi-Symptom Allergy-Sinus Formula Tablets .... ⊕ 617
Comtrex Multi-Symptom Non-Drowsy Caplets.. ⊕ 618
Congess 1004
Contac Day Allergy/Sinus Caplets ⊕ 812
Contac Day & Night .... ⊕ 812
Contac Night Allergy/Sinus Caplets .... ⊕ 812
Contac Severe Cold & Flu Non-Drowsy .... ⊕ 815
Deconamine Chewable Tablets 1320
Deconamine CX Cough and Cold Liquid and Tablets................................... 1319
Deconamine 1320
Deconsal C Expectorant Syrup 456
Deconsal Pediatric Syrup 457
Deconsal II Tablets 454
Dimetane-DX Cough Syrup 2059
Dimetapp Sinus Caplets .... ⊕ 775
Dorcol Children's Cough Syrup ...... ⊕ 785
Drixoral Cough + Congestion Liquid Caps .... ⊕ 802
Dura-Tap/PD Capsules 2867
Duratuss Tablets 2565
Duratuss HD Elixir................................... 2565
Efidac/24 .... ⊕ 635
Entex PSE Tablets 1987
Fedahist Gyrocaps................................... 2401
Fedahist Timecaps 2401
Guaifed.. 1787
Guaifed Syrup.. ⊕ 734
Guaimax-D Tablets 792
Guaitab Tablets .... ⊕ 734
Isoclor Expectorant 990
Kronofed-A 977
Motrin IB Sinus .... ⊕ 838
Novahistine DH 2462
Novahistine DMX .... ⊕ 822
Novahistine Expectorant...................... 2463
Nucofed 2051
PediaCare Cold Allergy Chewable Tablets .... ⊕ 677
PediaCare Cough-Cold Chewable Tablets 1553
PediaCare 1553
PediaCare Infants' Decongestant Drops .... ⊕ 677
PediCare Infant's Drops Decongestant Plus Cough 1553
PediaCare NightRest Cough-Cold Liquid 1553
Pediatric Vicks 44d Dry Hacking Cough & Head Congestion.............. ⊕ 763
Pediatric Vicks 44m Cough & Cold Relief .... ⊕ 764
Robitussin Cold & Cough Liqui-Gels .... ⊕ 776
Robitussin Maximum Strength Cough & Cold .... ⊕ 778
Robitussin Pediatric Cough & Cold Formula .... ⊕ 779
Robitussin Severe Congestion Liqui-Gels .... ⊕ 776
Robitussin-DAC Syrup 2074
Robitussin-PE .... ⊕ 778
Rondec Oral Drops 953
Rondec Syrup 953
Rondec Tablet.. 953
Rondec-DM Oral Drops......................... 954
Rondec-DM Syrup 954
Rondec-TR Tablet 953
Ryna .... ⊕ 841
Seldane-D Extended-Release Tablets 1538
Semprex-D Capsules 463
Semprex-D Capsules 1167
Sinarest Tablets .... ⊕ 648
Sinarest Extra Strength Tablets....... ⊕ 648
Sinarest No Drowsiness Tablets .... ⊕ 648
Sine-Aid IB Caplets 1554
Sine-Aid Maximum Strength Sinus Medication Gelcaps, Caplets and Tablets 1554
Sine-Off No Drowsiness Formula Caplets .... ⊕ 824
Sine-Off Sinus Medicine .... ⊕ 825
Singlet Tablets .... ⊕ 825
Sinutab Non-Drying Liquid Caps .... ⊕ 859
Sinutab Sinus Allergy Medication, Maximum Strength Tablets and Caplets .... ⊕ 860
Sinutab Sinus Medication, Maximum Strength Without Drowsiness Formula, Tablets & Caplets .... ⊕ 860
Sinutab Sinus Medication, Regular Strength Without Drowsiness Formula .... ⊕ 859
Sudafed Children's Liquid .... ⊕ 861
Sudafed Cold and Cough Liquidcaps .... ⊕ 862
Sudafed Cough Syrup .... ⊕ 862
Sudafed Plus Liquid .... ⊕ 862
Sudafed Plus Tablets .... ⊕ 863
Sudafed Severe Cold Formula Caplets .... ⊕ 863
Sudafed Severe Cold Formula Tablets .... ⊕ 864
Sudafed Sinus Caplets........................... ⊕ 864
Sudafed Sinus Tablets............................ ⊕ 864
Sudafed Tablets, 30 mg......................... ⊕ 861
Sudafed Tablets, 60 mg......................... ⊕ 861
Sudafed 12 Hour Caplets .... ⊕ 861
Syn-Rx Tablets 465
Syn-Rx DM Tablets 466
TheraFlu.. ⊕ 787

IMPORTANT NOTE: Always consult each drug listing in the patient's regimen for possible interactions.

TheraFlu Maximum Strength Nighttime Flu, Cold & Cough Medicine ▣ 788
TheraFlu Maximum Strength Non-Drowsy Formula Flu, Cold & Cough Medicine ▣ 788
Thera Flu Maximum Strength, Non-Drowsy Formula Flu, Cold and Cough Caplets ▣ 789
Triaminic AM Cough and Decongestant Formula ▣ 789
Triaminic AM Decongestant Formula ▣ 790
Triaminic Nite Light ▣ 791
Triaminic Sore Throat Formula ▣ 791
Tussend 1783
Tussend Expectorant 1785
Children's TYLENOL Cold Multi-Symptom Liquid Formula and Chewable Tablets 1561
Children's TYLENOL Cold Plus Cough Multi Symptom Tablets and Liquid ▣ 681
Infants' TYLENOL Cold Decongestant & Fever-Reducer Drops 1556
TYLENOL Maximum Strength Allergy Sinus Medication Gelcaps and Caplets 1563
TYLENOL Maximum Strength Allergy Sinus NightTime Medication Caplets 1555
TYLENOL Flu Maximum Strength Gelcaps 1565
TYLENOL Flu NightTime, Maximum Strength, Gelcaps 1566
TYLENOL Maximum Strength Flu NightTime Hot Medication Packets 1562
TYLENOL, Maximum Strength, Sinus Medication Geltabs, Gelcaps, Caplets and Tablets 1566
TYLENOL Cold Multi-Symptom Formula Medication Tablets and Caplets 1561
TYLENOL Cold Medication No Drowsiness Formula Gelcaps and Caplets 1562
TYLENOL Cold Multi-Symptom Hot Medication Liquid Packets 1557
TYLENOL Cough Multi-Symptom Medication with Decongestant 1565
Ursinus Inlay-Tabs ▣ 794
Vicks 44 LiquiCaps Cough, Cold & Flu Relief ▣ 755
Vicks 44 LiquiCaps Non-Drowsy Cough & Cold Relief ▣ 756
Vicks 44D Dry Hacking Cough & Head Congestion ▣ 755
Vicks 44M Cough, Cold & Flu Relief ▣ 756
Vicks DayQuil ▣ 761
Vicks DayQuil SINUS Pressure & PAIN Relief with IBUPROFEN ▣ 762
Vicks Nyquil Hot Therapy ▣ 762
Vicks NyQuil LiquiCaps Multi-Symptom Cold/Flu Relief ▣ 763
Vicks NyQuil Multi-Symptom Cold/Flu Relief - (Original & Cherry Flavor) ▣ 763

Pseudoephedrine Sulfate (Increased effects). Products include:
Cheracol Sinus ▣ 768
Chlor-Trimeton Allergy Decongestant Tablets ▣ 799
Claritin-D 2350
Drixoral Cold and Allergy Sustained-Action Tablets ▣ 802
Drixoral Cold and Flu Extended-Release Tablets ▣ 803
Drixoral Non-Drowsy Formula Extended-Release Tablets ▣ 803
Drixoral Allergy/Sinus Extended Release Tablets ▣ 804
Trinalin Repetabs Tablets 1330

Quazepam (Increased effects). Products include:
Doral Tablets 2664

Reserpine (Tachycardia; decreased pressor effect of ephedrine). Products include:
Diupres Tablets 1650
Hydropres Tablets 1675
Ser-Ap-Es Tablets 849

Risperidone (Increased effects). Products include:
Risperdal 1301

Salmeterol Xinafoate (Increased effects). Products include:
Serevent Inhalation Aerosol 1176

Secobarbital Sodium (Increased effects). Products include:
Seconal Sodium Pulvules 1474

Selegiline Hydrochloride (Potentiated pressor effect of ephedrine). Products include:
Eldepryl Tablets 2550

Sufentanil Citrate (Increased effects). Products include:
Sufenta Injection 1309

Temazepam (Increased effects). Products include:
Restoril Capsules 2284

Terbutaline Sulfate (Increased effects). Products include:
Brethaire Inhaler 813
Brethine Ampuls 815
Brethine Tablets 814
Bricanyl Subcutaneous Injection 1502
Bricanyl Tablets 1503

Thiamylal Sodium (Increased effects).
No products indexed under this heading.

Thioridazine Hydrochloride (Increased effects). Products include:
Mellaril 2269

Thiothixene (Increased effects). Products include:
Navane Capsules and Concentrate 2201
Navane Intramuscular 2202

Tranylcypromine Sulfate (Potentiated pressor effect of ephedrine). Products include:
Parnate Tablets 2503

Triamcinolone (Decreased effects). Products include:
Aristocort Tablets 1022

Triamcinolone Acetonide (Decreased effects). Products include:
Aristocort A 0.025% Cream 1027
Aristocort A 0.5% Cream 1031
Aristocort A 0.1% Cream 1029
Aristocort A 0.1% Ointment 1030
Azmacort Oral Inhaler 2011
Nasacort Nasal Inhaler 2024

Triamcinolone Diacetate (Decreased effects). Products include:
Aristocort Suspension (Forte Parenteral) 1027
Aristocort Suspension (Intralesional) 1025

Triamcinolone Hexacetonide (Decreased effects). Products include:
Aristospan Suspension (Intra-articular) 1033
Aristospan Suspension (Intralesional) 1032

Triazolam (Increased effects). Products include:
Halcion Tablets 2611

Trifluoperazine Hydrochloride (Increased effects). Products include:
Stelazine 2514

Trimipramine Maleate (Decreased effects; possible antagonized pressor effect of ephedrine). Products include:
Surmontil Capsules 2811

Troleandomycin (Increased theophylline plasma levels). Products include:
Tao Capsules 2209

Warfarin Sodium (Decreased anticoagulant effects). Products include:
Coumadin 926

Zolpidem Tartrate (Increased effects). Products include:
Ambien Tablets 2416

Food Interactions

Alcohol (Increased effects).

QUARZAN CAPSULES

(Clidinium Bromide) 2181
None cited in PDR database.

QUESTRAN LIGHT

(Cholestyramine) 769
May interact with tetracyclines, thyroid preparations, cardiac glycosides, hmg-coa reductase inhibitors, and certain other agents. Compounds in these categories include:

Chlorothiazide (Delayed or reduced absorption of concomitantly administered oral chlorothiazide (acidic)). Products include:
Aldoclor Tablets 1598
Diupres Tablets 1650
Diuril Oral 1653

Demeclocycline Hydrochloride (Delayed or reduced absorption of concomitantly administered oral tetracycline). Products include:
Declomycin Tablets 1371

Deslanoside (Delayed or reduced absorption of concomitantly administered oral digitalis).
No products indexed under this heading.

Digitoxin (Delayed or reduced absorption of concomitantly administered oral digitalis). Products include:
Crystodigin Tablets 1433

Digoxin (Delayed or reduced absorption of concomitantly administered oral digitalis). Products include:
Lanoxicaps 1117
Lanoxin Elixir Pediatric 1120
Lanoxin Injection 1123
Lanoxin Injection Pediatric 1126
Lanoxin Tablets 1128

Doxycycline Calcium (Delayed or reduced absorption of concomitantly administered oral tetracycline). Products include:
Vibramycin Calcium Oral Suspension Syrup 1941

Doxycycline Hyclate (Delayed or reduced absorption of concomitantly administered oral tetracycline). Products include:
Doryx Capsules 1913
Vibramycin Hyclate Capsules 1941
Vibramycin Hyclate Intravenous 2215
Vibra-Tabs Film Coated Tablets 1941

Doxycycline Monohydrate (Delayed or reduced absorption of concomitantly administered oral tetracycline). Products include:
Monodox Capsules 1805
Vibramycin Monohydrate for Oral Suspension 1941

Fluvastatin Sodium (Enhances lipid-lowering effects). Products include:
Lescol Capsules 2267

Levothyroxine Sodium (Delayed or reduced absorption of concomitantly administered oral thyroid preparations). Products include:
Levothroid Tablets 1016
Levoxyl Tablets 903
Synthroid 1359

Liothyronine Sodium (Delayed or reduced absorption of concomitantly administered oral thyroid preparations). Products include:
Cytomel Tablets 2473
Triostat Injection 2530

Liotrix (Delayed or reduced absorption of concomitantly administered oral thyroid preparations).
No products indexed under this heading.

Lovastatin (Enhances lipid-lowering effects). Products include:
Mevacor Tablets 1699

Methacycline Hydrochloride (Delayed or reduced absorption of concomitantly administered oral tetracycline).
No products indexed under this heading.

Minocycline Hydrochloride (Delayed or reduced absorption of concomitantly administered oral tetracycline). Products include:
Dynacin Capsules 1590
Minocin Intravenous 1382
Minocin Oral Suspension 1385
Minocin Pellet-Filled Capsules 1383

Nicotinic Acid (Combined therapy produces additive effects on LDL-cholesterol lowering).
No products indexed under this heading.

Oxytetracycline Hydrochloride (Delayed or reduced absorption of concomitantly administered oral tetracycline). Products include:
TERAK Ointment ◉ 209
Terra-Cortril Ophthalmic Suspension 2210
Terramycin with Polymyxin B Sulfate Ophthalmic Ointment 2211
Urobiotic-250 Capsules 2214

Penicillin G Potassium (Delayed or reduced absorption of concomitantly administered oral penicillin G). Products include:
Pfizerpen for Injection 2203

Phenobarbital (Delayed or reduced absorption of concomitantly administered oral phenobarbital). Products include:
Arco-Lase Plus Tablets 512
Bellergal-S Tablets 2250
Donnatal 2060
Donnatal Extentabs 2061
Donnatal Tablets 2060
Phenobarbital Elixir and Tablets 1469
Quadrinal Tablets 1350

Phenylbutazone (Delayed or reduced absorption of concomitantly administered oral phenylbutazone).
No products indexed under this heading.

Potassium Phosphate, Monobasic (Possible interference with the absorption of oral phosphate supplements). Products include:
K-Phos Neutral Tablets 639
K-Phos Original Formula 'Sodium Free' Tablets 639

Pravastatin Sodium (Enhances lipid-lowering effects). Products include:
Pravachol 765

Propranolol Hydrochloride (Delayed or reduced absorption of concomitantly administered oral propranolol (basic)). Products include:
Inderal 2728
Inderal LA Long Acting Capsules 2730
Inderide Tablets 2732
Inderide LA Long Acting Capsules 2734

Simvastatin (Enhances lipid-lowering effects). Products include:
Zocor Tablets 1775

Tetracycline Hydrochloride (Delayed or reduced absorption of concomitantly administered oral tetracycline). Products include:
Achromycin V Capsules 1367

Thyroglobulin (Delayed or reduced absorption of concomitantly administered oral thyroid preparations).
No products indexed under this heading.

Thyroid (Delayed or reduced absorption of concomitantly administered oral thyroid preparations).
No products indexed under this heading.

(▣ Described in PDR For Nonprescription Drugs) (◉ Described in PDR For Ophthalmology)

Interactions Index

Thyroxine (Delayed or reduced absorption of concomitantly administered oral thyroid preparations).

No products indexed under this heading.

Thyroxine Sodium (Delayed or reduced absorption of concomitantly administered oral thyroid preparations).

No products indexed under this heading.

Vitamin A (Cholestyramine may interfere with oral absorption and digestion of fat soluble vitamin A). Products include:

Aquasol A Vitamin A Capsules, USP 534
Aquasol A Parenteral 534
Materna Tablets 1379
Megadose 512
Nature Made Antioxidant Formula **◆D** 748
One-A-Day Extras Antioxidant .... **◆D** 728
Theragran Antioxidant .... **◆D** 623
Zymacap Capsules .... **◆D** 772

Vitamin D (Cholestyramine may interfere with oral absorption and digestion of fat soluble vitamin D). Products include:

Caltrate PLUS .... **◆D** 665
Caltrate 600 + D .... **◆D** 665
Citracal Caplets+ D 1780
Dical-D Tablets & Wafers 420
Drisdol .... **◆D** 794
Materna Tablets 1379
Megadose 512
Zymacap Capsules .... **◆D** 772

Vitamin K (Cholestyramine may interfere with oral absorption and digestion of fat soluble vitamin K).

No products indexed under this heading.

Vitamin K_1 (Cholestyramine may interfere with oral absorption and digestion of fat soluble vitamin K). Products include:

AquaMEPHYTON Injection 1608
Konakion Injection 2127
Mephyton Tablets 1696

Warfarin Sodium (Delayed or reduced absorption of concomitantly administered oral warfarin). Products include:

Coumadin 926

QUESTRAN POWDER

(Cholestyramine) 770

May interact with thyroid preparations, cardiac glycosides, tetracyclines, hmg-coa reductase inhibitors, and certain other agents. Compounds in these categories include:

Chlorothiazide (Delayed or reduced absorption of concomitantly administered oral chlorothiazide (acidic)). Products include:

Aldoclor Tablets 1598
Diupres Tablets 1650
Diuril Oral 1653

Demeclocycline Hydrochloride (Delayed or reduced absorption of concomitantly administered oral tetracycline). Products include:

Declomycin Tablets 1371

Deslanoside (Delayed or reduced absorption of concomitantly administered oral digitalis).

No products indexed under this heading.

Digitoxin (Delayed or reduced absorption of concomitantly administered oral digitalis). Products include:

Crystodigin Tablets 1433

Digoxin (Delayed or reduced absorption of concomitantly administered oral digitalis). Products include:

Lanoxicaps 1117
Lanoxin Elixir Pediatric 1120
Lanoxin Injection 1123

Lanoxin Injection Pediatric 1126
Lanoxin Tablets 1128

Doxycycline Calcium (Delayed or reduced absorption of concomitantly administered oral tetracycline). Products include:

Vibramycin Calcium Oral Suspension Syrup 1941

Doxycycline Hyclate (Delayed or reduced absorption of concomitantly administered oral tetracycline). Products include:

Doryx Capsules 1913
Vibramycin Hyclate Capsules 1941
Vibramycin Hyclate Intravenous 2215
Vibra-Tabs Film Coated Tablets 1941

Doxycycline Monohydrate (Delayed or reduced absorption of concomitantly administered oral tetracycline). Products include:

Monodox Capsules 1805
Vibramycin Monohydrate for Oral Suspension 1941

Fluvastatin Sodium (Enhances lipid-lowering effects). Products include:

Lescol Capsules 2267

Levothyroxine Sodium (Delayed or reduced absorption of concomitantly administered oral thyroid preparations). Products include:

Levothroid Tablets 1016
Levoxyl Tablets 903
Synthroid 1359

Liothyronine Sodium (Delayed or reduced absorption of concomitantly administered oral thyroid preparations). Products include:

Cytomel Tablets 2473
Triostat Injection 2530

Liotrix (Delayed or reduced absorption of concomitantly administered oral thyroid preparations).

No products indexed under this heading.

Lovastatin (Enhances lipid-lowering effects). Products include:

Mevacor Tablets 1699

Methacycline Hydrochloride (Delayed or reduced absorption of concomitantly administered oral tetracycline).

No products indexed under this heading.

Minocycline Hydrochloride (Delayed or reduced absorption of concomitantly administered oral tetracycline). Products include:

Dynacin Capsules 1590
Minocin Intravenous 1382
Minocin Oral Suspension 1385
Minocin Pellet-Filled Capsules 1383

Nicotinic Acid (Combined therapy produces additive effects on LDL-cholesterol lowering).

No products indexed under this heading.

Oxytetracycline Hydrochloride (Delayed or reduced absorption of concomitantly administered oral tetracycline). Products include:

TERAK Ointment .... © 209
Terra-Cortril Ophthalmic Suspension 2210
Terramycin with Polymyxin B Sulfate Ophthalmic Ointment 2211
Urobiotic-250 Capsules 2214

Penicillin G Potassium (Delayed or reduced absorption of concomitantly administered oral penicillin G). Products include:

Pfizerpen for Injection 2203

Phenobarbital (Delayed or reduced absorption of concomitantly administered oral phenobarbital). Products include:

Arco-Lase Plus Tablets 512
Bellergal-S Tablets 2250
Donnatal 2060
Donnatal Extentabs 2061

Donnatal Tablets 2060
Phenobarbital Elixir and Tablets 1469
Quadrinal Tablets 1350

Phenylbutazone (Delayed or reduced absorption of concomitantly administered oral phenylbutazone).

No products indexed under this heading.

Potassium Phosphate, Monobasic (Possible interference with the absorption of oral phosphate supplements). Products include:

K-Phos Neutral Tablets 639
K-Phos Original Formula 'Sodium Free' Tablets 639

Pravastatin Sodium (Enhances lipid-lowering effects). Products include:

Pravachol 765

Propranolol Hydrochloride (Delayed or reduced absorption of concomitantly administered oral propranolol (basic)). Products include:

Inderal 2728
Inderal LA Long Acting Capsules 2730
Inderide Tablets 2732
Inderide LA Long Acting Capsules .. 2734

Simvastatin (Enhances lipid-lowering effects). Products include:

Zocor Tablets 1775

Tetracycline Hydrochloride (Delayed or reduced absorption of concomitantly administered oral tetracycline). Products include:

Achromycin V Capsules 1367

Thyroglobulin (Delayed or reduced absorption of concomitantly administered oral thyroid preparations).

No products indexed under this heading.

Thyroid (Delayed or reduced absorption of concomitantly administered oral thyroid preparations).

No products indexed under this heading.

Vitamin A (Cholestyramine may interfere with oral absorption and digestion of fat soluble vitamin A). Products include:

Aquasol A Vitamin A Capsules, USP 534
Aquasol A Parenteral 534
Materna Tablets 1379
Megadose 512
Nature Made Antioxidant Formula **◆D** 748
One-A-Day Extras Antioxidant .... **◆D** 728
Theragran Antioxidant .... **◆D** 623
Zymacap Capsules .... **◆D** 772

Vitamin D (Cholestyramine may interfere with oral absorption and digestion of fat soluble vitamin D). Products include:

Caltrate PLUS .... **◆D** 665
Caltrate 600 + D .... **◆D** 665
Citracal Caplets+ D 1780
Dical-D Tablets & Wafers 420
Drisdol .... **◆D** 794
Materna Tablets 1379
Megadose 512
Zymacap Capsules .... **◆D** 772

Vitamin K (Cholestyramine may interfere with oral absorption and digestion of fat soluble vitamin K).

No products indexed under this heading.

Vitamin K_1 (Cholestyramine may interfere with oral absorption and digestion of fat soluble vitamin K). Products include:

AquaMEPHYTON Injection 1608
Konakion Injection 2127
Mephyton Tablets 1696

Warfarin Sodium (Delayed or reduced absorption of concomitantly administered oral warfarin). Products include:

Coumadin 926

QUIBRON CAPSULES

(Theophylline, Guaifenesin) 2053
See Quibron-T/SR Tablets

QUIBRON-300 CAPSULES

(Theophylline, Guaifenesin) 2053
See Quibron-T/SR Tablets

QUIBRON-T TABLETS

(Theophylline) 2053
See Quibron-T/SR Tablets

QUIBRON-T/SR TABLETS

(Theophylline) 2053

May interact with oral contraceptives, sympathomimetic bronchodilators, and certain other agents. Compounds in these categories include:

Albuterol (Toxic synergism may occur). Products include:

Proventil Inhalation Aerosol 2382
Ventolin Inhalation Aerosol and Refill 1197

Albuterol Sulfate (Toxic synergism may occur). Products include:

Airet Solution for Inhalation 452
Proventil Inhalation Solution 0.083% 2384
Proventil Repetabs Tablets 2386
Proventil Solution for Inhalation 0.5% 2383
Proventil Syrup 2385
Proventil Tablets 2386
Ventolin Inhalation Solution 1198
Ventolin Nebules Inhalation Solution 1199
Ventolin Rotacaps for Inhalation 1200
Ventolin Syrup 1202
Ventolin Tablets 1203
Volmax Extended-Release Tablets .. 1788

Allopurinol (High doses of allopurinol increase serum theophylline levels). Products include:

Zyloprim Tablets 1226

Bitolterol Mesylate (Toxic synergism may occur). Products include:

Tornalate Solution for Inhalation, 0.2% 956
Tornalate Metered Dose Inhaler 957

Cimetidine (Increases serum theophylline levels). Products include:

Tagamet Tablets 2516

Cimetidine Hydrochloride (Increases serum theophylline levels). Products include:

Tagamet 2516

Ciprofloxacin (Increases serum theophylline levels). Products include:

Cipro I.V. 595
Cipro I.V. Pharmacy Bulk Package .. 597

Ciprofloxacin Hydrochloride (Increases serum theophylline levels). Products include:

Ciloxan Ophthalmic Solution 472
Cipro Tablets 592

Desogestrel (Increases serum theophylline levels). Products include:

Desogen Tablets 1817
Ortho-Cept 1851

Ephedrine Hydrochloride (Toxic synergism may occur). Products include:

Primatene Dual Action Formula ...... **◆D** 872
Primatene Tablets .... **◆D** 873
Quadrinal Tablets 1350

Ephedrine Sulfate (Toxic synergism may occur). Products include:

Bronkaid Caplets .... **◆D** 717
Marax Tablets & DF Syrup 2200

Ephedrine Tannate (Toxic synergism may occur). Products include:

Rynatuss 2673

Epinephrine (Toxic synergism may occur). Products include:

Bronkaid Mist .... **◆D** 717
EPIFRIN .... © 239
EpiPen 790
Marcaine Hydrochloride with Epinephrine 1:200,000 2316

IMPORTANT NOTE: Always consult each drug listing in the patient's regimen for possible interactions.

Quibron **Interactions Index** 872

- Primatene Mist ▣ 873
- Sensorcaine with Epinephrine Injection 559
- Sus-Phrine Injection 1019
- Xylocaine with Epinephrine Injections 567

Epinephrine Hydrochloride (Toxic synergism may occur). Products include:
- Ana-Kit Anaphylaxis Emergency Treatment Kit 617

Erythromycin (Increases serum theophylline levels). Products include:
- A/T/S 2% Acne Topical Gel and Solution 1234
- Benzamycin Topical Gel 905
- E-Mycin Tablets 1341
- Emgel 2% Topical Gel 1093
- ERYC 1915
- Erycette (erythromycin 2%) Topical Solution 1888
- Ery-Tab Tablets 422
- Erythromycin Base Filmtab 426
- Erythromycin Delayed-Release Capsules, USP 427
- Ilotycin Ophthalmic Ointment 912
- PCE Dispertab Tablets 444
- T-Stat 2.0% Topical Solution and Pads 2688
- Theramycin Z Topical Solution 2% 1592

Erythromycin Estolate (Increases serum theophylline levels). Products include:
- Ilosone 911

Erythromycin Ethylsuccinate (Increases serum theophylline levels). Products include:
- E.E.S. 424
- EryPed 421

Erythromycin Gluceptate (Increases serum theophylline levels). Products include:
- Ilotycin Gluceptate, IV, Vials 913

Erythromycin Stearate (Increases serum theophylline levels). Products include:
- Erythrocin Stearate Filmtab 425

Ethinyl Estradiol (Increases serum theophylline levels). Products include:
- Brevicon 2088
- Demulen 2428
- Desogen Tablets 1817
- Levlen/Tri-Levlen 651
- Lo/Ovral Tablets 2746
- Lo/Ovral-28 Tablets 2751
- Modicon 1872
- Nordette-21 Tablets 2755
- Nordette-28 Tablets 2758
- Norinyl 2088
- Ortho-Cept 1851
- Ortho-Cyclen/Ortho Tri Cyclen 1858
- Ortho-Novum 1872
- Ortho-Cyclen/Ortho Tri-Cyclen 1858
- Ovcon 760
- Ovral Tablets 2770
- Ovral-28 Tablets 2770
- Levlen/Tri-Levlen 651
- Tri-Norinyl 2164
- Triphasil-21 Tablets 2814
- Triphasil-28 Tablets 2819

Ethylnorepinephrine Hydrochloride (Toxic synergism may occur).
- No products indexed under this heading.

Ethynodiol Diacetate (Increases serum theophylline levels). Products include:
- Demulen 2428

Isoetharine (Toxic synergism may occur). Products include:
- Bronkometer Aerosol 2302
- Bronkosol Solution 2302
- Isoetharine Inhalation Solution, USP, Arm-a-Med 551

Isoproterenol Hydrochloride (Toxic synergism may occur). Products include:
- Isuprel Hydrochloride Injection 1:5000 2311
- Isuprel Hydrochloride Solution 1:200 & 1:100 2313
- Isuprel Mistometer 2312

Isoproterenol Sulfate (Toxic synergism may occur). Products include:
- Norisodrine with Calcium Iodide Syrup 442

Levonorgestrel (Increases serum theophylline levels). Products include:
- Levlen/Tri-Levlen 651
- Nordette-21 Tablets 2755
- Nordette-28 Tablets 2758
- Norplant System 2759
- Levlen/Tri-Levlen 651
- Triphasil-21 Tablets 2814
- Triphasil-28 Tablets 2819

Lithium Carbonate (Increased renal excretion of lithium). Products include:
- Eskalith 2485
- Lithium Carbonate Capsules & Tablets 2230
- Lithonate/Lithotabs/Lithobid 2543

Mestranol (Increases serum theophylline levels). Products include:
- Norinyl 2088
- Ortho-Novum 1872

Metaproterenol Sulfate (Toxic synergism may occur). Products include:
- Alupent 669
- Metaproterenol Sulfate Inhalation Solution, USP, Arm-a-Med 552

Norethindrone (Increases serum theophylline levels). Products include:
- Brevicon 2088
- Micronor Tablets 1872
- Modicon 1872
- Norinyl 2088
- Nor-Q D Tablets 2135
- Ortho-Novum 1872
- Ovcon 760
- Tri-Norinyl 2164

Norethynodrel (Increases serum theophylline levels).
- No products indexed under this heading.

Norgestimate (Increases serum theophylline levels). Products include:
- Ortho-Cyclen/Ortho-Tri-Cyclen 1858
- Ortho-Cyclen/Ortho Tri-Cyclen 1858

Norgestrel (Increases serum theophylline levels). Products include:
- Lo/Ovral Tablets 2746
- Lo/Ovral-28 Tablets 2751
- Ovral Tablets 2770
- Ovral-28 Tablets 2770
- Ovrette Tablets 2771

Phenytoin (Decreased theophylline and phenytoin serum levels). Products include:
- Dilantin Infatabs 1908
- Dilantin-125 Suspension 1911

Phenytoin Sodium (Decreased theophylline and phenytoin serum levels). Products include:
- Dilantin Kapseals 1906
- Dilantin Parenteral 1910

Pirbuterol Acetate (Toxic synergism may occur). Products include:
- Maxair Autohaler 1492
- Maxair Inhaler 1494

Propranolol Hydrochloride (Increases serum theophylline levels). Products include:
- Inderal 2728
- Inderal LA Long Acting Capsules 2730
- Inderide Tablets 2732
- Inderide LA Long Acting Capsules 2734

Rifampin (Decreased serum theophylline levels). Products include:
- Rifadin 1528
- Rifamate Capsules 1530
- Rifater 1532
- Rimactane Capsules 847

Salmeterol Xinafoate (Toxic synergism may occur). Products include:
- Serevent Inhalation Aerosol 1176

Terbutaline Sulfate (Toxic synergism may occur). Products include:
- Brethaire Inhaler 813
- Brethine Ampuls 815
- Brethine Tablets 814
- Bricanyl Subcutaneous Injection 1502
- Bricanyl Tablets 1503

Troleandomycin (Increases serum theophylline levels). Products include:
- Tao Capsules 2209

Food Interactions

Food, unspecified (Food ingestion may influence the absorption characteristics of some or all theophylline controlled-release products).

QUINAGLUTE DURA-TABS TABLETS

(Quinidine Gluconate) 649

May interact with carbonic anhydrase inhibitors, thiazides, phenothiazines, tricyclic antidepressants, neuromuscular blocking agents, anticholinergics, negative inotropic agents, vasodilators, cholinergic agents, vasopressors, and certain other agents. Compounds in these categories include:

Acebutolol Hydrochloride (Quinidine's negative inotropic actions may be additive to those of other similar agents). Products include:
- Sectral Capsules 2807

Acetazolamide (Reduces renal elimination of quinidine by alkalinizing the urine). Products include:
- Diamox Sequels (Sustained Release) 1373
- Diamox Sequels (Sustained Release) ⊙ 319
- Diamox Tablets 1372
- Diamox Tablets ⊙ 317

Amiodarone Hydrochloride (Co-administration may increase quinidine levels). Products include:
- Cordarone Intravenous 2715
- Cordarone Tablets 2712

Amitriptyline Hydrochloride (Therapeutic serum levels of quinidine inhibit the action of cytochrome P450IID6 and most polycyclic antidepressants are metabolized by this enzyme; caution should be exercised). Products include:
- Elavil 2838
- Endep Tablets 2174
- Etrafon 2355
- Limbitrol 2180
- Triavil Tablets 1757

Amoxapine (Therapeutic serum levels of quinidine inhibit the action of cytochrome P450IID6 and most polycyclic antidepressants are metabolized by this enzyme; caution should be exercised). Products include:
- Asendin Tablets 1369

Atenolol (Quinidine's negative inotropic actions may be additive to those of other similar agents). Products include:
- Tenoretic Tablets 2845
- Tenormin Tablets and I.V. Injection 2847

Atracurium Besylate (Quinidine potentiates the action of neuromuscular blocking agents). Products include:
- Tracrium Injection 1183

Atropine Sulfate (Quinidine's anticholinergic actions may be additive to those of other anticholinergic drugs). Products include:
- Arco-Lase Plus Tablets 512
- Atrohist Plus Tablets 454
- Atropine Sulfate Sterile Ophthalmic Solution ⊙ 233
- Donnatal 2060
- Donnatal Extentabs 2061
- Donnatal Tablets 2060
- Lomotil 2439
- Motofen Tablets 784
- Urised Tablets 1964

Belladonna Alkaloids (Quinidine's anticholinergic actions may be additive to those of other anticholinergic drugs). Products include:
- Bellergal-S Tablets 2250
- Hyland's Bed Wetting Tablets ▣ 828
- Hyland's EnurAid Tablets ▣ 829
- Hyland's Teething Tablets ▣ 830

Bendroflumethiazide (Reduces renal elimination of quinidine by alkalinizing the urine).
- No products indexed under this heading.

Benztropine Mesylate (Quinidine's anticholinergic actions may be additive to those of other anticholinergic drugs). Products include:
- Cogentin 1621

Betaxolol Hydrochloride (Quinidine's negative inotropic actions may be additive to those of other similar agents). Products include:
- Betoptic Ophthalmic Solution 469
- Betoptic S Ophthalmic Suspension 471
- Kerlone Tablets 2436

Biperiden Hydrochloride (Quinidine's anticholinergic actions may be additive to those of other anticholinergic drugs). Products include:
- Akineton 1333

Carteolol Hydrochloride (Quinidine's negative inotropic actions may be additive to those of other similar agents). Products include:
- Cartrol Tablets 410
- Ocupress Ophthalmic Solution, 1% Sterile ⊙ 309

Chlorothiazide (Reduces renal elimination of quinidine by alkalinizing the urine). Products include:
- Aldoclor Tablets 1598
- Diupres Tablets 1650
- Diuril Oral 1653

Chlorothiazide Sodium (Reduces renal elimination of quinidine by alkalinizing the urine). Products include:
- Diuril Sodium Intravenous 1652

Chlorpromazine (Therapeutic serum levels of quinidine inhibit the action of cytochrome P450IID6 and certain unspecified phenothiazines are metabolized by this enzyme; caution should be exercised). Products include:
- Thorazine Suppositories 2523

Chlorpromazine Hydrochloride (Therapeutic serum levels of quinidine inhibit the action of cytochrome P450IID6 and certain unspecified phenothiazines are metabolized by this enzyme; caution should be exercised). Products include:
- Thorazine 2523

Cimetidine (Co-administration may increase quinidine levels). Products include:
- Tagamet Tablets 2516

Cimetidine Hydrochloride (Co-administration may increase quinidine levels). Products include:
- Tagamet 2516

Clidinium Bromide (Quinidine's anticholinergic actions may be additive to those of other anticholinergic drugs). Products include:
- Librax Capsules 2176
- Quarzan Capsules 2181

(▣ Described in PDR For Nonprescription Drugs) (⊙ Described in PDR For Ophthalmology)

873 **Interactions Index** **Quinaglute**

Clomipramine Hydrochloride (Therapeutic serum levels of quinidine inhibit the action of cytochrome P450IID6 and most polycyclic antidepressants are metabolized by this enzyme; caution should be exercised). Products include:
Anafranil Capsules ... 803

Decamethonium (Quinidine potentiates the action of neuromuscular blocking agent).

Desipramine Hydrochloride (Therapeutic serum levels of quinidine inhibit the action of cytochrome P450IID6 and most polycyclic antidepressants are metabolized by this enzyme; caution should be exercised). Products include:
Norpramin Tablets ... 1526

Diazoxide (Quinidine's vasodilating actions may be additive to those of other vasodilators). Products include:
Hyperstat I.V. Injection ... 2363
Proglycem ... 580

Dichlorphenamide (Reduces renal elimination of quinidine by alkalinizing the urine). Products include:
Daranide Tablets ... 1633

Dicyclomine Hydrochloride (Quinidine's anticholinergic actions may be additive to those of other anticholinergic drugs). Products include:
Bentyl ... 1501

Digoxin (Quinidine slows the elimination of digoxin and simultaneously reduces digoxin's apparent volume of distribution resulting in elevated serum digoxin levels). Products include:
Lanoxicaps ... 1117
Lanoxin Elixir Pediatric ... 1120
Lanoxin Injection ... 1123
Lanoxin Injection Pediatric ... 1126
Lanoxin Tablets ... 1128

Dopamine Hydrochloride (Quinidine's vasodilating actions may be antagonistic to those of vasopressors).
No products indexed under this heading.

Dorzolamide Hydrochloride (Reduces renal elimination of quinidine by alkalinizing the urine). Products include:
Trusopt Sterile Ophthalmic Solution ... 1760

Doxacurium Chloride (Quinidine potentiates the action of neuromuscular blocking agents). Products include:
Nuromax Injection ... 1149

Doxepin Hydrochloride (Therapeutic serum levels of quinidine inhibit the action of cytochrome P450IID6 and most polycyclic antidepressants are metabolized by this enzyme; caution should be exercised). Products include:
Sinequan ... 2205
Zonalon Cream ... 1055

Edrophonium Chloride (Quinidine's anticholinergic actions may be antagonistic to those of cholinergic agents). Products include:
Tensilon Injectable ... 1261

Epinephrine Bitartrate (Quinidine's vasodilating actions may be antagonistic to those of vasopressors). Products include:
Bronkaid Mist Suspension ... ⊞ 718
Sensorcaine-MPF with Epinephrine Injection ... 559

Epinephrine Hydrochloride (Quinidine's vasodilating actions may be antagonistic to those of vasopressors). Products include:
Ana-Kit Anaphylaxis Emergency Treatment Kit ... 617

Esmolol Hydrochloride (Quinidine's negative inotropic actions may be additive to those of other similar agents). Products include:
Brevibloc Injection ... 1808

Felodipine (Potential for variable slowing of the metabolism of felodipine). Products include:
Plendil Extended-Release Tablets ... 527

Fluphenazine Decanoate (Therapeutic serum levels of quinidine inhibit the action of cytochrome P450IID6 and certain unspecified phenothiazines are metabolized by this enzyme; caution should be exercised). Products include:
Prolixin Decanoate ... 509

Fluphenazine Enanthate (Therapeutic serum levels of quinidine inhibit the action of cytochrome P450IID6 and certain unspecified phenothiazines are metabolized by this enzyme; caution should be exercised). Products include:
Prolixin Enanthate ... 509

Fluphenazine Hydrochloride (Therapeutic serum levels of quinidine inhibit the action of cytochrome P450IID6 and certain unspecified phenothiazines are metabolized by this enzyme; caution should be exercised). Products include:
Prolixin ... 509

Glycopyrrolate (Quinidine's anticholinergic actions may be additive to those of other anticholinergic drugs). Products include:
Robinul Forte Tablets ... 2072
Robinul Injectable ... 2072
Robinul Tablets ... 2072

Haloperidol (Serum levels of haloperidol are increased when quinidine is co-administered). Products include:
Haldol Injection, Tablets and Concentrate ... 1575

Haloperidol Decanoate (Serum levels of haloperidol are increased when quinidine is co-administered). Products include:
Haldol Decanoate ... 1577

Hydralazine Hydrochloride (Quinidine's vasodilating actions may be additive to those of other vasodilators). Products include:
Apresazide Capsules ... 808
Apresoline Hydrochloride Tablets ... 809
Ser-Ap-Es Tablets ... 849

Hydrochlorothiazide (Reduces renal elimination of quinidine by alkalinizing the urine). Products include:
Aldactazide ... 2413
Aldoril Tablets ... 1604
Apresazide Capsules ... 808
Capozide ... 742
Dyazide ... 2479
Esidrix Tablets ... 821
Esimil Tablets ... 822
HydroDIURIL Tablets ... 1674
Hydropres Tablets ... 1675
Hyzaar Tablets ... 1677
Inderide Tablets ... 2732
Inderide LA Long Acting Capsules ... 2734
Lopressor HCT Tablets ... 832
Lotensin HCT ... 837
Maxzide ... 1380
Moduretic Tablets ... 1705
Oretic Tablets ... 443
Prinzide Tablets ... 1737
Ser-Ap-Es Tablets ... 849
Timolide Tablets ... 1748
Vaseretic Tablets ... 1765
Zestoretic ... 2850
Ziac ... 1415

Hydroflumethiazide (Reduces renal elimination of quinidine by alkalinizing the urine). Products include:
Diucardin Tablets ... 2718

Hyoscyamine (Quinidine's anticholinergic actions may be additive to those of other anticholinergic drugs). Products include:
Cystospaz Tablets ... 1963
Urised Tablets ... 1964

Hyoscyamine Sulfate (Quinidine's anticholinergic actions may be additive to those of other anticholinergic drugs). Products include:
Arco-Lase Plus Tablets ... 512
Atrohist Plus Tablets ... 454
Cystospaz-M Capsules ... 1963
Donnatal ... 2060
Donnatal Extentabs ... 2061
Donnatal Tablets ... 2060
Kutrase Capsules ... 2402
Levsin/Levsinex/Levbid ... 2405

Imipramine Hydrochloride (Therapeutic serum levels of quinidine inhibit the action of cytochrome P450IID6 and most polycyclic antidepressants are metabolized by this enzyme; caution should be exercised). Products include:
Tofranil Ampuls ... 854
Tofranil Tablets ... 856

Imipramine Pamoate (Therapeutic serum levels of quinidine inhibit the action of cytochrome P450IID6 and most polycyclic antidepressants are metabolized by this enzyme; caution should be exercised). Products include:
Tofranil-PM Capsules ... 857

Ipratropium Bromide (Quinidine's anticholinergic actions may be additive to those of other anticholinergic drugs). Products include:
Atrovent Inhalation Aerosol ... 671
Atrovent Inhalation Solution ... 673

Ketoconazole (Co-administration may increase quinidine levels). Products include:
Nizoral 2% Cream ... 1297
Nizoral 2% Shampoo ... 1298
Nizoral Tablets ... 1298

Labetalol Hydrochloride (Quinidine's negative inotropic actions may be additive to those of other similar agents). Products include:
Normodyne Injection ... 2377
Normodyne Tablets ... 2379
Trandate ... 1185

Maprotiline Hydrochloride (Therapeutic serum levels of quinidine inhibit the action of cytochrome P450IID6 and most polycyclic antidepressants are metabolized by this enzyme; caution should be exercised). Products include:
Ludiomil Tablets ... 843

Mepenzolate Bromide (Quinidine's anticholinergic actions may be additive to those of other anticholinergic drugs).
No products indexed under this heading.

Mesoridazine Besylate (Therapeutic serum levels of quinidine inhibit the action of cytochrome P450IID6 and certain unspecified phenothiazines are metabolized by this enzyme; caution should be exercised). Products include:
Serentil ... 684

Metaraminol Bitartrate (Quinidine's vasodilating actions may be antagonistic to those of vasopressors). Products include:
Aramine Injection ... 1609

Methazolamide (Reduces renal elimination of quinidine by alkalinizing the urine). Products include:
Glauctabs ... ⊙ 208
MZM ... ⊙ 267
Neptazane Tablets ... 1388
Neptazane Tablets ... ⊙ 320

Methotrimeprazine (Therapeutic serum levels of quinidine inhibit the action of cytochrome P450IID6 and certain unspecified phenothiazines are metabolized by this enzyme; caution should be exercised). Products include:
Levoprome ... 1274

Methoxamine Hydrochloride (Quinidine's vasodilating actions may be antagonistic to those of vasopressors). Products include:
Vasoxyl Injection ... 1196

Methyclothiazide (Reduces renal elimination of quinidine by alkalinizing the urine). Products include:
Enduron Tablets ... 420

Metocurine Iodide (Quinidine potentiates the action of neuromuscular blocking agents). Products include:
Metubine Iodide Vials ... 916

Metoprolol Tartrate (Quinidine's negative inotropic actions may be additive to those of other similar agents). Products include:
Lopressor Ampuls ... 830
Lopressor HCT Tablets ... 832
Lopressor Tablets ... 830

Mexiletine Hydrochloride (Therapeutic serum levels of quinidine inhibit the action of cytochrome P450IID6 and mexiletine is metabolized by this enzyme; caution should be exercised). Products include:
Mexitil Capsules ... 678

Minoxidil (Quinidine's vasodilating actions may be additive to those of other vasodilators). Products include:
Loniten Tablets ... 2618
Rogaine Topical Solution ... 2637

Mivacurium Chloride (Quinidine potentiates the action of neuromuscular blocking agents). Products include:
Mivacron ... 1138

Nadolol (Quinidine's negative inotropic actions may be additive to those of other similar agents).
No products indexed under this heading.

Neostigmine Bromide (Quinidine's anticholinergic actions may be antagonistic to those of cholinergic agents). Products include:
Prostigmin Tablets ... 1261

Neostigmine Methylsulfate (Quinidine's anticholinergic actions may be antagonistic to those of cholinergic agents). Products include:
Prostigmin Injectable ... 1260

Nicardipine Hydrochloride (Potential for variable slowing of the metabolism of nicardipine). Products include:
Cardene Capsules ... 2095
Cardene I.V. ... 2709
Cardene SR Capsules ... 2097

Nifedipine (Very rarely co-administration may decrease quinidine levels; quinidine causes variable slowing of the metabolism of nifedipine). Products include:
Adalat Capsules (10 mg and 20 mg) ... 587
Adalat CC ... 589
Procardia Capsules ... 1971
Procardia XL Extended Release Tablets ... 1972

IMPORTANT NOTE: Always consult each drug listing in the patient's regimen for possible interactions.

Nimodipine (Potential for variable slowing of the metabolism of nimodipine). Products include:
- Nimotop Capsules ... 610

Norepinephrine Bitartrate (Quinidine's vasodilating actions may be antagonistic to those of vasopressors). Products include:
- Levophed Bitartrate Injection ... 2315

Nortriptyline Hydrochloride (Therapeutic serum levels of quinidine inhibit the action of cytochrome P450IID6 and most polycyclic antidepressants are metabolized by this enzyme; caution should be exercised). Products include:
- Pamelor ... 2280

Oxybutynin Chloride (Quinidine's anticholinergic actions may be additive to those of other anticholinergic drugs). Products include:
- Ditropan ... 1516

Pancuronium Bromide Injection (Quinidine potentiates the action of neuromuscular blocking agents).
- No products indexed under this heading.

Penbutolol Sulfate (Quinidine's negative inotropic actions may be additive to those of other similar agents). Products include:
- Levatol ... 2403

Perphenazine (Therapeutic serum levels of quinidine inhibit the action of cytochrome P450IID6 and certain unspecified phenothiazines are metabolized by this enzyme; caution should be exercised). Products include:
- Etrafon ... 2355
- Triavil Tablets ... 1757
- Trilafon ... 2389

Phenobarbital (Hepatic elimination of quinidine may be accelerated by co-administration). Products include:
- Arco-Lase Plus Tablets ... 512
- Bellergal-S Tablets ... 2250
- Donnatal ... 2060
- Donnatal Extentabs ... 2061
- Donnatal Tablets ... 2060
- Phenobarbital Elixir and Tablets ... 1469
- Quadrinal Tablets ... 1350

Phenylephrine Hydrochloride (Quinidine's vasodilating actions may be antagonistic to those of vasopressors). Products include:
- Atrohist Plus Tablets ... 454
- Cerose DM ... ◙ 878
- Comhist ... 2038
- D.A. Chewable Tablets ... 951
- Deconsal Pediatric Capsules ... 454
- Dura-Vent/DA Tablets ... 953
- Entex Capsules ... 1986
- Entex Liquid ... 1986
- Extendryl ... 1005
- 4-Way Fast Acting Nasal Spray (regular & mentholated) ... ◙ 621
- Hemorid For Women ... ◙ 834
- Hycomine Compound Tablets ... 932
- Neo-Synephrine Hydrochloride 1% Carpuject ... 2324
- Neo-Synephrine Hydrochloride 1% Injection ... 2324
- Neo-Synephrine Hydrochloride (Ophthalmic) ... 2325
- Neo-Synephrine ... ◙ 726
- Nōstril ... ◙ 644
- Novahistine Elixir ... ◙ 823
- Phenergan VC ... 2779
- Phenergan VC with Codeine ... 2781
- Preparation H ... ◙ 871
- Tympagesic Ear Drops ... 2342
- Vasosulf ... ⊙ 271
- Vicks Sinex Nasal Spray and Ultra Fine Mist ... ◙ 765

Phenytoin (Hepatic elimination of quinidine may be accelerated by co-administration). Products include:
- Dilantin Infatabs ... 1908
- Dilantin-125 Suspension ... 1911

Phenytoin Sodium (Hepatic elimination of quinidine may be accelerated by co-administration). Products include:
- Dilantin Kapseals ... 1906
- Dilantin Parenteral ... 1910

Pindolol (Quinidine's negative inotropic actions may be additive to those of other similar agents). Products include:
- Visken Tablets ... 2299

Polythiazide (Reduces renal elimination of quinidine by alkalinizing the urine). Products include:
- Minizide Capsules ... 1938

Procainamide Hydrochloride (Co-administration causes an increase in serum levels of procainamide). Products include:
- Procan SR Tablets ... 1926

Prochlorperazine (Therapeutic serum levels of quinidine inhibit the action of cytochrome P450IID6 and certain unspecified phenothiazines are metabolized by this enzyme; caution should be exercised). Products include:
- Compazine ... 2470

Procyclidine Hydrochloride (Quinidine's anticholinergic actions may be additive to those of other anticholinergic drugs). Products include:
- Kemadrin Tablets ... 1112

Promethazine Hydrochloride (Therapeutic serum levels of quinidine inhibit the action of cytochrome P450IID6 and certain unspecified phenothiazines are metabolized by this enzyme; caution should be exercised). Products include:
- Mepergan Injection ... 2753
- Phenergan with Codeine ... 2777
- Phenergan with Dextromethorphan ... 2778
- Phenergan Injection ... 2773
- Phenergan Suppositories ... 2775
- Phenergan Syrup ... 2774
- Phenergan Tablets ... 2775
- Phenergan VC ... 2779
- Phenergan VC with Codeine ... 2781

Propantheline Bromide (Quinidine's anticholinergic actions may be additive to those of other anticholinergic drugs). Products include:
- Pro-Banthīne Tablets ... 2052

Propranolol Hydrochloride (Co-administration may cause increase in the peak serum levels of quinidine; decrease in quinidine's volume of distribution, and decrease in total quinidine clearance). Products include:
- Inderal ... 2728
- Inderal LA Long Acting Capsules ... 2730
- Inderide Tablets ... 2732
- Inderide LA Long Acting Capsules ... 2734

Protriptyline Hydrochloride (Therapeutic serum levels of quinidine inhibit the action of cytochrome P450IID6 and most polycyclic antidepressants are metabolized by this enzyme; caution should be exercised). Products include:
- Vivactil Tablets ... 1774

Pyridostigmine Bromide (Quinidine's anticholinergic actions may be antagonistic to those of cholinergic agents). Products include:
- Mestinon Injectable ... 1253
- Mestinon ... 1254

Rifampin (Hepatic elimination of quinidine may be accelerated by co-administration). Products include:
- Rifadin ... 1528
- Rifamate Capsules ... 1530
- Rifater ... 1532
- Rimactane Capsules ... 847

Rocuronium Bromide (Quinidine potentiates the action of neuromuscular blocking agents). Products include:
- Zemuron ... 1830

Scopolamine (Quinidine's anticholinergic actions may be additive to those of other anticholinergic drugs). Products include:
- Transderm Scōp Transdermal Therapeutic System ... 869

Scopolamine Hydrobromide (Quinidine's anticholinergic actions may be additive to those of other anticholinergic drugs). Products include:
- Atrohist Plus Tablets ... 454
- Donnatal ... 2060
- Donnatal Extentabs ... 2061
- Donnatal Tablets ... 2060

Sodium Bicarbonate (Systemic sodium bicarbonate reduces renal elimination of quinidine by alkalinizing the urine). Products include:
- Alka-Seltzer Effervescent Antacid and Pain Reliever ... ◙ 701
- Alka-Seltzer Extra Strength Effervescent Antacid and Pain Reliever ... ◙ 703
- Alka-Seltzer Gold Effervescent Antacid ... ◙ 703
- Alka-Seltzer Lemon Lime Effervescent Antacid and Pain Reliever ... ◙ 703
- Arm & Hammer Pure Baking Soda ... ◙ 627
- Ceo-Two Rectal Suppositories ... 666
- Citrocarbonate Antacid ... ◙ 770
- Massengill Disposable Douches ... ◙ 820
- Massengill Liquid Concentrate ... ◙ 820
- NuLYTELY ... 689
- Cherry Flavor NuLYTELY ... 689

Succinylcholine Chloride (Quinidine potentiates the action of neuromuscular blocking agents). Products include:
- Anectine ... 1073

Thioridazine Hydrochloride (Therapeutic serum levels of quinidine inhibit the action of cytochrome P450IID6 and certain unspecified phenothiazines are metabolized by this enzyme; caution should be exercised). Products include:
- Mellaril ... 2269

Timolol Maleate (Quinidine's negative inotropic actions may be additive to those of other similar agents). Products include:
- Blocadren Tablets ... 1614
- Timolide Tablets ... 1748
- Timoptic in Ocudose ... 1753
- Timoptic Sterile Ophthalmic Solution ... 1751
- Timoptic-XE ... 1755

Trazodone Hydrochloride (Therapeutic serum levels of quinidine inhibit the action of cytochrome P450IID6 and most polycyclic antidepressants are metabolized by this enzyme; caution should be exercised). Products include:
- Desyrel and Desyrel Dividose ... 503

Tridihexethyl Chloride (Quinidine's anticholinergic actions may be additive to those of other anticholinergic drugs).
- No products indexed under this heading.

Trifluoperazine Hydrochloride (Therapeutic serum levels of quinidine inhibit the action of cytochrome P450IID6 and certain unspecified phenothiazines are metabolized by this enzyme; caution should be exercised). Products include:
- Stelazine ... 2514

Trihexyphenidyl Hydrochloride (Quinidine's anticholinergic actions may be additive to those of other anticholinergic drugs). Products include:
- Artane ... 1368

Trimipramine Maleate (Therapeutic serum levels of quinidine inhibit the action of cytochrome P450IID6 and most polycyclic antidepressants are metabolized by this enzyme; caution should be exercised). Products include:
- Surmontil Capsules ... 2811

Tubocurarine Chloride (Potentiation of neuromuscular blockade).
- No products indexed under this heading.

Vecuronium Bromide (Quinidine potentiates the action of neuromuscular blocking agents). Products include:
- Norcuron ... 1826

Verapamil Hydrochloride (Hepatic clearance of quinidine is significantly reduced with co-administration resulting in corresponding increase in serum levels and half-life). Products include:
- Calan SR Caplets ... 2422
- Calan Tablets ... 2419
- Isoptin Injectable ... 1344
- Isoptin Oral Tablets ... 1346
- Isoptin SR Tablets ... 1348
- Verelan Capsules ... 1410
- Verelan Capsules ... 2824

Warfarin Sodium (Quinidine may potentiate anticoagulant action of warfarin). Products include:
- Coumadin ... 926

Food Interactions

Food, unspecified (Increases absorption of quinidine in both rate (27%) and extent (17%)).

QUINIDEX EXTENTABS

(Quinidine Sulfate) ... 2067

May interact with anticholinergics, carbonic anhydrase inhibitors, thiazides, oral anticoagulants, nondepolarizing neuromuscular blocking agents, cholinergic agents, phenothiazines, and certain other agents. Compounds in these categories include:

Acetazolamide (Alkalinization of urine resulting in decreased excretion of quinidine). Products include:
- Diamox Sequels (Sustained Release) ... 1373
- Diamox Sequels (Sustained Release) ... ⊙ 319
- Diamox Tablets ... 1372
- Diamox Tablets ... ⊙ 317

Amiodarone Hydrochloride (Increased serum concentration of quinidine). Products include:
- Cordarone Intravenous ... 2715
- Cordarone Tablets ... 2712

Atracurium Besylate (Potentiation of neuromuscular blockade). Products include:
- Tracrium Injection ... 1183

Atropine Sulfate (Additive vagolytic effect). Products include:
- Arco-Lase Plus Tablets ... 512
- Atrohist Plus Tablets ... 454
- Atropine Sulfate Sterile Ophthalmic Solution ... ⊙ 233
- Donnatal ... 2060
- Donnatal Extentabs ... 2061
- Donnatal Tablets ... 2060
- Lomotil ... 2439
- Motofen Tablets ... 784
- Urised Tablets ... 1964

Belladonna Alkaloids (Additive vagolytic effect). Products include:
- Bellergal-S Tablets ... 2250
- Hyland's Bed Wetting Tablets ... ◙ 828
- Hyland's EnurAid Tablets ... ◙ 829

(◙ Described in PDR For Nonprescription Drugs) (⊙ Described in PDR For Ophthalmology)

875 **Interactions Index** **Quinidex**

Hyland's Teething Tablets ■ 830

Bendroflumethiazide (Alkalinization of urine resulting in decreased excretion of quinidine).
No products indexed under this heading.

Benztropine Mesylate (Additive vagolytic effect). Products include:
Cogentin 1621

Biperiden Hydrochloride (Additive vagolytic effect). Products include:
Akineton 1333

Chlorothiazide (Alkalinization of urine resulting in decreased excretion of quinidine). Products include:
Aldoclor Tablets 1598
Diupres Tablets 1650
Diuril Oral 1653

Chlorothiazide Sodium (Alkalinization of urine resulting in decreased excretion of quinidine). Products include:
Diuril Sodium Intravenous 1652

Chlorpromazine (Additive cardiac depressive effects). Products include:
Thorazine Suppositories 2523

Cimetidine (Prolonged quinidine half-life; increase in serum quinidine level). Products include:
Tagamet Tablets 2516

Cimetidine Hydrochloride (Prolonged quinidine half-life; increase in serum quinidine level). Products include:
Tagamet 2516

Clidinium Bromide (Additive vagolytic effect). Products include:
Librax Capsules 2176
Quarzan Capsules 2181

Decamethonium (Potentiation of neuromuscular blockade).

Dichlorphenamide (Alkalinization of urine resulting in decreased excretion of quinidine). Products include:
Daranide Tablets 1633

Dicumarol (Reduction of clotting factor concentrations).
No products indexed under this heading.

Dicyclomine Hydrochloride (Additive vagolytic effect). Products include:
Bentyl 1501

Digitoxin (Increased serum concentration of digitoxin). Products include:
Crystodigin Tablets 1433

Digoxin (Increased serum concentration of digoxin). Products include:
Lanoxicaps 1117
Lanoxin Elixir Pediatric 1120
Lanoxin Injection 1123
Lanoxin Injection Pediatric 1126
Lanoxin Tablets 1128

Dorzolamide Hydrochloride (Alkalinization of urine resulting in decreased excretion of quinidine). Products include:
Trusopt Sterile Ophthalmic Solution 1760

Edrophonium Chloride (Antagonism of cholinergic effects). Products include:
Tensilon Injectable 1261

Ethopropazine Hydrochloride (Additive vagolytic effect).

Fluphenazine Decanoate (Additive cardiac depressive effects). Products include:
Prolixin Decanoate 509

Fluphenazine Enanthate (Additive cardiac depressive effects). Products include:
Prolixin Enanthate 509

Fluphenazine Hydrochloride (Additive cardiac depressive effects). Products include:
Prolixin 509

Glycopyrrolate (Additive vagolytic effect). Products include:
Robinul Forte Tablets 2072
Robinul Injectable 2072
Robinul Tablets 2072

Guanidine Hydrochloride (Antagonism of cholinergic effects).
No products indexed under this heading.

Hydrochlorothiazide (Alkalinization of urine resulting in decreased excretion of quinidine). Products include:
Aldactazide 2413
Aldoril Tablets 1604
Apresazide Capsules 808
Capozide 742
Dyazide 2479
Esidrix Tablets 821
Esimil Tablets 822
HydroDIURIL Tablets 1674
Hydropres Tablets 1675
Hyzaar Tablets 1677
Inderide Tablets 2732
Inderide LA Long Acting Capsules 2734
Lopressor HCT Tablets 832
Lotensin HCT 837
Maxzide 1380
Moduretic Tablets 1705
Oretic Tablets 443
Prinzide Tablets 1737
Ser-Ap-Es Tablets 849
Timolide Tablets 1748
Vaseretic Tablets 1765
Zestoretic 2850
Ziac 1415

Hydroflumethiazide (Alkalinization of urine resulting in decreased excretion of quinidine). Products include:
Diucardin Tablets 2718

Hyoscyamine (Additive vagolytic effect). Products include:
Cystospaz Tablets 1963
Urised Tablets 1964

Hyoscyamine Sulfate (Additive vagolytic effect). Products include:
Arco-Lase Plus Tablets 512
Atrohist Plus Tablets 454
Cystospaz-M Capsules 1963
Donnatal 2060
Donnatal Extentabs 2061
Donnatal Tablets 2060
Kutrase Capsules 2402
Levsin/Levsinex/Levbid 2405

Ipratropium Bromide (Additive vagolytic effect). Products include:
Atrovent Inhalation Aerosol 671
Atrovent Inhalation Solution 673

Mepenzolate Bromide (Additive vagolytic effect).
No products indexed under this heading.

Mesoridazine Besylate (Additive cardiac depressive effects). Products include:
Serentil 684

Methazolamide (Alkalinization of urine resulting in decreased excretion of quinidine). Products include:
Glauctabs ◉ 208
MZM ◉ 267
Neptazane Tablets 1388
Neptazane Tablets ◉ 320

Methotrimeprazine (Additive cardiac depressive effects). Products include:
Levoprome 1274

Methyclothiazide (Alkalinization of urine resulting in decreased excretion of quinidine). Products include:
Enduron Tablets 420

Metocurine Iodide (Potentiation of neuromuscular blockade). Products include:
Metubine Iodide Vials 916

Mivacurium Chloride (Potentiation of neuromuscular blockade). Products include:
Mivacron 1138

Neostigmine Bromide (Antagonism of cholinergic effects). Products include:
Prostigmin Tablets 1261

Neostigmine Methylsulfate (Antagonism of cholinergic effects). Products include:
Prostigmin Injectable 1260

Nifedipine (Decreased serum concentrations of quinidine). Products include:
Adalat Capsules (10 mg and 20 mg) 587
Adalat CC 589
Procardia Capsules 1971
Procardia XL Extended Release Tablets 1972

Oxybutynin Chloride (Additive vagolytic effect). Products include:
Ditropan 1516

Oxyphenonium Bromide (Additive vagolytic effect).

Pancuronium Bromide Injection (Potentiation of neuromuscular blockade).
No products indexed under this heading.

Perphenazine (Additive cardiac depressive effects). Products include:
Etrafon 2355
Triavil Tablets 1757
Trilafon 2389

Phenobarbital (Decreased plasma half-life of quinidine). Products include:
Arco-Lase Plus Tablets 512
Bellergal-S Tablets 2250
Donnatal 2060
Donnatal Extentabs 2061
Donnatal Tablets 2060
Phenobarbital Elixir and Tablets 1469
Quadrinal Tablets 1350

Phenytoin (Decreased plasma half-life of quinidine). Products include:
Dilantin Infatabs 1908
Dilantin-125 Suspension 1911

Phenytoin Sodium (Decreased plasma half-life of quinidine). Products include:
Dilantin Kapseals 1906
Dilantin Parenteral 1910

Polythiazide (Alkalinization of urine resulting in decreased excretion of quinidine). Products include:
Minizide Capsules 1938

Prochlorperazine (Additive cardiac depressive effects). Products include:
Compazine 2470

Procyclidine Hydrochloride (Additive vagolytic effect). Products include:
Kemadrin Tablets 1112

Promethazine Hydrochloride (Additive cardiac depressive effects). Products include:
Mepergan Injection 2753
Phenergan with Codeine 2777
Phenergan with Dextromethorphan 2778
Phenergan Injection 2773
Phenergan Suppositories 2775
Phenergan Syrup 2774
Phenergan Tablets 2775
Phenergan VC 2779
Phenergan VC with Codeine 2781

Propantheline Bromide (Additive vagolytic effect). Products include:
Pro-Banthine Tablets 2052

Pyridostigmine Bromide (Antagonism of cholinergic effects). Products include:
Mestinon Injectable 1253
Mestinon 1254

Ranitidine Hydrochloride (Premature ventricular contractions and/or bigeminy). Products include:
Zantac 1209
Zantac Injection 1207
Zantac Syrup 1209

Reserpine (Additive cardiac depressive effects). Products include:
Diupres Tablets 1650
Hydropres Tablets 1675
Ser-Ap-Es Tablets 849

Rifampin (Decreased plasma half-life of quinidine). Products include:
Rifadin 1528
Rifamate Capsules 1530
Rifater 1532
Rimactane Capsules 847

Rocuronium Bromide (Potentiation of neuromuscular blockade). Products include:
Zemuron 1830

Scopolamine (Additive vagolytic effect). Products include:
Transderm Scōp Transdermal Therapeutic System 869

Scopolamine Hydrobromide (Additive vagolytic effect). Products include:
Atrohist Plus Tablets 454
Donnatal 2060
Donnatal Extentabs 2061
Donnatal Tablets 2060

Sodium Bicarbonate (Alkalinization of urine resulting in decreased excretion of quinidine). Products include:
Alka-Seltzer Effervescent Antacid and Pain Reliever ■ 701
Alka-Seltzer Extra Strength Effervescent Antacid and Pain Reliever ■ 703
Alka-Seltzer Gold Effervescent Antacid ■ 703
Alka-Seltzer Lemon Lime Effervescent Antacid and Pain Reliever ■ 703
Arm & Hammer Pure Baking Soda ■ 627
Ceo-Two Rectal Suppositories 666
Citrocarbonate Antacid ■ 770
Massengill Disposable Douches ■ 820
Massengill Liquid Concentrate ■ 820
NuLYTELY 689
Cherry Flavor NuLYTELY 689

Succinylcholine Chloride (Potentiation of neuromuscular blockade). Products include:
Anectine 1073

Tridihexethyl Chloride (Additive vagolytic effect).
No products indexed under this heading.

Trifluoperazine Hydrochloride (Additive cardiac depressive effects). Products include:
Stelazine 2514

Trihexyphenidyl Hydrochloride (Additive vagolytic effect). Products include:
Artane 1368

Vecuronium Bromide (Potentiation of neuromuscular blockade). Products include:
Norcuron 1826

Verapamil Hydrochloride (Increased quinidine half-life and increase in serum quinidine level; potential hypotensive reactions). Products include:
Calan SR Caplets 2422
Calan Tablets 2419
Isoptin Injectable 1344
Isoptin Oral Tablets 1346
Isoptin SR Tablets 1348
Verelan Capsules 1410
Verelan Capsules 2824

Warfarin Sodium (Reduction of clotting factor concentrations). Products include:
Coumadin 926

IMPORTANT NOTE: Always consult each drug listing in the patient's regimen for possible interactions.

PURIFIED PORK NPH ISOPHANE INSULIN
(Insulin, NPH) 1801
None cited in PDR database.

PURIFIED PORK REGULAR INSULIN
(Insulin, Regular) 1801
None cited in PDR database.

RMS SUPPOSITORIES
(Morphine Sulfate)...................................2657
May interact with narcotic analgesics, general anesthetics, antihistamines, phenothiazines, barbiturates, tranquilizers, hypnotics and sedatives, tricyclic antidepressants, central nervous system depressants, and certain other agents. Compounds in these categories include:

Acrivastine (Additive CNS depressant effect). Products include:
- Semprex-D Capsules 463
- Semprex-D Capsules 1167

Alfentanil Hydrochloride (Additive CNS depressant effect). Products include:
- Alfenta Injection 1286

Alprazolam (Additive CNS depressant effect). Products include:
- Xanax Tablets 2649

Amitriptyline Hydrochloride (Additive CNS depressant effect). Products include:
- Elavil 2838
- Endep Tablets 2174
- Etrafon 2355
- Limbitrol 2180
- Triavil Tablets 1757

Amoxapine (Additive CNS depressant effect). Products include:
- Asendin Tablets 1369

Aprobarbital (Additive CNS depressant effect).
- No products indexed under this heading.

Astemizole (Additive CNS depressant effect). Products include:
- Hismanal Tablets 1293

Azatadine Maleate (Additive CNS depressant effect). Products include:
- Trinalin Repetabs Tablets 1330

Bromodiphenhydramine Hydrochloride (Additive CNS depressant effect).
- No products indexed under this heading.

Brompheniramine Maleate (Additive CNS depressant effect). Products include:
- Alka Seltzer Plus Sinus Medicine .. ▣ 707
- Bromfed Capsules (Extended-Release) 1785
- Bromfed Syrup .... ▣ 733
- Bromfed Tablets 1785
- Bromfed-DM Cough Syrup 1786
- Bromfed-PD Capsules (Extended-Release) 1785
- Dimetane-DC Cough Syrup 2059
- Dimetane-DX Cough Syrup 2059
- Dimetapp Elixir .... ▣ 773
- Dimetapp Extentabs .... ▣ 774
- Dimetapp Tablets/Liqui-Gels .... ▣ 775
- Dimetapp Cold & Allergy Chewable Tablets .... ▣ 773
- Dimetapp DM Elixir .... ▣ 774
- Vicks DayQuil Allergy Relief 12-Hour Extended Release Tablets.. ▣ 760
- Vicks DayQuil Allergy Relief 4-Hour Tablets .... ▣ 760

Buprenorphine (Additive CNS depressant effect). Products include:
- Buprenex Injectable 2006

Buspirone Hydrochloride (Additive CNS depressant effect). Products include:
- BuSpar 737

Butabarbital (Additive CNS depressant effect).
- No products indexed under this heading.

Butalbital (Additive CNS depressant effect). Products include:
- Esgic-plus Tablets 1013
- Fioricet Tablets 2258
- Fioricet with Codeine Capsules 2260
- Fiorinal Capsules 2261
- Fiorinal with Codeine Capsules 2262
- Fiorinal Tablets 2261
- Phrenilin 785
- Sedapap Tablets 50 mg/650 mg .. 1543

Chlordiazepoxide (Additive CNS depressant effect). Products include:
- Libritabs Tablets 2177
- Limbitrol 2180

Chlordiazepoxide Hydrochloride (Additive CNS depressant effect). Products include:
- Librax Capsules 2176
- Librium Capsules 2178
- Librium Injectable 2179

Chlorpheniramine Maleate (Additive CNS depressant effect). Products include:
- Alka-Seltzer Plus Cold Medicine .... ▣ 705
- Alka-Seltzer Plus Cold Medicine Liqui-Gels .... ▣ 706
- Alka-Seltzer Plus Cold & Cough Medicine .... ▣ 708
- Alka-Seltzer Plus Cold & Cough Medicine Liqui-Gels .... ▣ 705
- Allerest Children's Chewable Tablets .... ▣ 627
- Allerest Headache Strength Tablets .... ▣ 627
- Allerest Maximum Strength Tablets .... ▣ 627
- Allerest Sinus Pain Formula .... ▣ 627
- Allerest 12 Hour Caplets .... ▣ 627
- Ana-Kit Anaphylaxis Emergency Treatment Kit 617
- Atrohist Pediatric Capsules 453
- Atrohist Plus Tablets 454
- BC Cold Powder Multi-Symptom Formula (Cold-Sinus-Allergy) .... ▣ 609
- Cerose DM .... ▣ 878
- Cheracol Plus Head Cold/Cough Formula .... ▣ 769
- Children's Vicks DayQuil Allergy Relief .... ▣ 757
- Children's Vicks NyQuil Cold/Cough Relief .... ▣ 758
- Chlor-Trimeton Allergy Decongestant Tablets .... ▣ 799
- Chlor-Trimeton Allergy Tablets .... ▣ 798
- Comhist 2038
- Comtrex Multi-Symptom Cold Reliever Tablets/Caplets/Liqui-Gels/Liquid .... ▣ 615
- Allergy-Sinus Comtrex Multi-Symptom Allergy-Sinus Formula Tablets .... ▣ 617
- Contac Continuous Action Nasal Decongestant/Antihistamine 12 Hour Capsules .... ▣ 813
- Contac Maximum Strength Continuous Action Decongestant/Antihistamine 12 Hour Caplets.. ▣ 813
- Contac Severe Cold and Flu Formula Caplets .... ▣ 814
- Coricidin 'D' Decongestant Tablets .... ▣ 800
- Coricidin Tablets .... ▣ 800
- D.A. Chewable Tablets 951
- Deconamine 1320
- Dura-Tap/PD Capsules 2867
- Dura-Vent/DA Tablets 953
- Extendryl 1005
- Fedahist Gyrocaps 2401
- Fedahist Timecaps 2401
- Hycomine Compound Tablets 932
- Isoclor Timesule Capsules .... ▣ 637
- Kronofed-A 977
- Nolamine Timed-Release Tablets 785
- Novahistine DH 2462
- Novahistine Elixir .... ▣ 823
- Ornade Spansule Capsules 2502
- PediaCare Cold Allergy Chewable Tablets .... ▣ 677
- PediaCare Cough-Cold Chewable Tablets 1553
- PediaCare Cough-Cold Liquid 1553
- PediaCare NightRest Cough-Cold Liquid 1553
- Pediatric Vicks 44m Cough & Cold Relief .... ▣ 764
- Pyrroxate Caplets .... ▣ 772
- Ryna .... ▣ 841
- Sinarest Tablets .... ▣ 648
- Sinarest Extra Strength Tablets .... ▣ 648
- Sine-Off Sinus Medicine .... ▣ 825
- Singlet Tablets .... ▣ 825
- Sinulin Tablets 787
- Sinutab Sinus Allergy Medication, Maximum Strength Tablets and Caplets .... ▣ 860
- Sudafed Plus Liquid .... ▣ 862
- Sudafed Plus Tablets .... ▣ 863
- Teldrin 12 Hour Antihistamine/Nasal Decongestant Allergy Relief Capsules .... ▣ 826
- TheraFlu .... ▣ 787
- TheraFlu Maximum Strength Nighttime Flu, Cold & Cough Medicine .... ▣ 788
- Triaminic Allergy Tablets .... ▣ 789
- Triaminic Cold Tablets .... ▣ 790
- Triaminic Nite Light .... ▣ 791
- Triaminic Syrup .... ▣ 792
- Triaminic-12 Tablets .... ▣ 792
- Triaminicin Tablets .... ▣ 793
- Triaminicol Multi-Symptom Cold Tablets .... ▣ 793
- Triaminicol Multi-Symptom Relief ▣ 794
- Tussend 1783
- Children's TYLENOL Cold Multi-Symptom Liquid Formula and Chewable Tablets 1561
- Children's TYLENOL Cold Plus Cough Multi Symptom Tablets and Liquid .... ▣ 681
- TYLENOL Maximum Strength Allergy Sinus Medication Gelcaps and Caplets 1563
- TYLENOL Cold Multi-Symptom Formula Medication Tablets and Caplets 1561
- TYLENOL Cold Multi-Symptom Hot Medication Liquid Packets 1557
- Vicks 44 LiquiCaps Cough, Cold & Flu Relief .... ▣ 755
- Vicks 44M Cough, Cold & Flu Relief .... ▣ 756

Chlorpheniramine Polistirex (Additive CNS depressant effect). Products include:
- Tussionex Pennkinetic Extended-Release Suspension 998

Chlorpheniramine Tannate (Additive CNS depressant effect). Products include:
- Atrohist Pediatric Suspension 454
- Ricobid Tablets and Pediatric Suspension 2038
- Rynatan 2673
- Rynatuss 2673

Chlorpromazine (Additive CNS depressant effect). Products include:
- Thorazine Suppositories 2523

Chlorpromazine Hydrochloride (Additive CNS depressant effect). Products include:
- Thorazine 2523

Chlorprothixene (Additive CNS depressant effect).
- No products indexed under this heading.

Chlorprothixene Hydrochloride (Additive CNS depressant effect).
- No products indexed under this heading.

Clemastine Fumarate (Additive CNS depressant effect). Products include:
- Tavist Syrup 2297
- Tavist Tablets 2298
- Tavist-1 12 Hour Relief Tablets .... ▣ 787
- Tavist-D 12 Hour Relief Tablets .... ▣ 787

Clomipramine Hydrochloride (Additive CNS depressant effect). Products include:
- Anafranil Capsules 803

Clorazepate Dipotassium (Additive CNS depressant effect). Products include:
- Tranxene 451

Clozapine (Additive CNS depressant effect). Products include:
- Clozaril Tablets 2252

Codeine Phosphate (Additive CNS depressant effect). Products include:
- Actifed with Codeine Cough Syrup.. 1067
- Brontex 1981
- Deconsal C Expectorant Syrup 456
- Deconsal Pediatric Syrup 457
- Dimetane-DC Cough Syrup 2059
- Empirin with Codeine Tablets 1093
- Fioricet with Codeine Capsules 2260
- Fiorinal with Codeine Capsules 2262
- Isoclor Expectorant 990
- Novahistine DH 2462
- Novahistine Expectorant 2463
- Nucofed 2051
- Phenergan with Codeine 2777
- Phenergan VC with Codeine 2781
- Robitussin A-C Syrup 2073
- Robitussin-DAC Syrup 2074
- Ryna .... ▣ 841
- Soma Compound w/Codeine Tablets 2676
- Tussi-Organidin NR Liquid and S NR Liquid 2677
- Tylenol with Codeine 1583

Cyproheptadine Hydrochloride (Additive CNS depressant effect). Products include:
- Periactin 1724

Desflurane (Additive CNS depressant effect). Products include:
- Suprane 1813

Desipramine Hydrochloride (Additive CNS depressant effect). Products include:
- Norpramin Tablets 1526

Dexchlorpheniramine Maleate (Additive CNS depressant effect).
- No products indexed under this heading.

Dezocine (Additive CNS depressant effect). Products include:
- Dalgan Injection 538

Diazepam (Additive CNS depressant effect). Products include:
- Dizac 1809
- Valium Injectable 2182
- Valium Tablets 2183
- Valrelease Capsules 2169

Diphenhydramine Citrate (Additive CNS depressant effect). Products include:
- Excedrin P.M. Analgesic/Sleeping Aid Tablets, Caplets, Liquigels 733

Diphenhydramine Hydrochloride (Additive CNS depressant effect). Products include:
- Actifed Allergy Daytime/Nighttime Caplets .... ▣ 844
- Actifed Sinus Daytime/Nighttime Tablets and Caplets .... ▣ 846
- Arthritis Foundation NightTime Caplets .... ▣ 674
- Extra Strength Bayer PM Aspirin .. ▣ 713
- Bayer Select Night Time Pain Relief Formula .... ▣ 716
- Benadryl Allergy Decongestant Liquid Medication .... ▣ 848
- Benadryl Allergy Decongestant Tablets .... ▣ 848
- Benadryl Allergy Liquid Medication .... ▣ 849
- Benadryl Allergy .... ▣ 848
- Benadryl Allergy Sinus Headache Formula Caplets .... ▣ 849
- Benadryl Capsules 1898
- Benadryl Dye-Free Allergy Liqui-gel Softgels .... ▣ 850
- Benadryl Dye-Free Allergy Liquid Medication .... ▣ 850
- Benadryl Itch Relief Cream, Children's Formula and Maximum Strength 2% .... ▣ 851
- Benadryl Itch Relief Spray, Children's Formula and Maximum Strength 2% .... ▣ 851
- Benadryl Itch Relief Stick Maximum Strength 2% .... ▣ 850
- Benadryl Itch Stopping Gel, Children's Formula and Maximum Strength 2% .... ▣ 851
- Benadryl Kapseals 1898
- Benadryl Injection 1898
- Contac Day & Night Cold/Flu Night Caplets .... ▣ 812
- Contac Night Allergy/Sinus Caplets .... ▣ 812
- Extra Strength Doan's P.M. .... ▣ 633
- Legatrin PM .... ▣ 651
- Miles Nervine Nighttime Sleep-Aid ▣ 723
- Nytol QuickCaps Caplets .... ▣ 610
- Sleepinal Night-time Sleep Aid Capsules and Softgels .... ▣ 834

(▣ Described in PDR For Nonprescription Drugs) (⊙ Described in PDR For Ophthalmology)

TYLENOL Maximum Strength Allergy Sinus NightTime Medication Caplets 1555
TYLENOL Flu NightTime, Maximum Strength, Gelcaps 1566
TYLENOL Maximum Strength Flu NightTime Hot Medication Packets 1562
TYLENOL PM, Extra Strength Pain Reliever/Sleep Aid Caplets, Geltabs, Gelcaps 1560
TYLENOL Severe Allergy Medication Caplets 1564
Maximum Strength Unisom Sleepgels 1934
Unisom With Pain Relief-Nighttime Sleep Aid and Pain Reliever............ 1934

Diphenylpyraline Hydrochloride (Additive CNS depressant effect).

No products indexed under this heading.

Doxepin Hydrochloride (Additive CNS depressant effect). Products include:

Sinequan 2205
Zonalon Cream 1055

Droperidol (Additive CNS depressant effect). Products include:

Inapsine Injection............................... 1296

Enflurane (Additive CNS depressant effect).

No products indexed under this heading.

Estazolam (Additive CNS depressant effect). Products include:

ProSom Tablets 449

Ethchlorvynol (Additive CNS depressant effect). Products include:

Placidyl Capsules................................ 448

Ethinamate (Additive CNS depressant effect).

No products indexed under this heading.

Fentanyl (Additive CNS depressant effect). Products include:

Duragesic Transdermal System........ 1288

Fentanyl Citrate (Additive CNS depressant effect). Products include:

Sublimaze Injection............................. 1307

Fluphenazine Decanoate (Additive CNS depressant effect). Products include:

Prolixin Decanoate 509

Fluphenazine Enanthate (Additive CNS depressant effect). Products include:

Prolixin Enanthate 509

Fluphenazine Hydrochloride (Additive CNS depressant effect). Products include:

Prolixin 509

Flurazepam Hydrochloride (Additive CNS depressant effect). Products include:

Dalmane Capsules.............................. 2173

Glutethimide (Additive CNS depressant effect).

No products indexed under this heading.

Haloperidol (Additive CNS depressant effect). Products include:

Haldol Injection, Tablets and Concentrate 1575

Haloperidol Decanoate (Additive CNS depressant effect). Products include:

Haldol Decanoate................................ 1577

Hydrocodone Bitartrate (Additive CNS depressant effect). Products include:

Anexsia 5/500 Elixir 1781
Anexia Tablets..................................... 1782
Codiclear DH Syrup 791
Deconamine CX Cough and Cold Liquid and Tablets................................ 1319
Duratuss HD Elixir.............................. 2565
Hycodan Tablets and Syrup 930
Hycomine Compound Tablets 932
Hycomine 931

Hycotuss Expectorant Syrup 933
Hydrocet Capsules 782
Lorcet 10/650...................................... 1018
Lortab 2566
Tussend 1783
Tussend Expectorant 1785
Vicodin Tablets 1356
Vicodin ES Tablets 1357
Vicodin Tuss Expectorant 1358
Zydone Capsules 949

Hydrocodone Polistirex (Additive CNS depressant effect). Products include:

Tussionex Pennkinetic Extended-Release Suspension 998

Hydroxyzine Hydrochloride (Additive CNS depressant effect). Products include:

Atarax Tablets & Syrup...................... 2185
Marax Tablets & DF Syrup................. 2200
Vistaril Intramuscular Solution......... 2216

Imipramine Hydrochloride (Additive CNS depressant effect). Products include:

Tofranil Ampuls 854
Tofranil Tablets 856

Imipramine Pamoate (Additive CNS depressant effect). Products include:

Tofranil-PM Capsules......................... 857

Isoflurane (Additive CNS depressant effect).

No products indexed under this heading.

Ketamine Hydrochloride (Additive CNS depressant effect).

No products indexed under this heading.

Levomethadyl Acetate Hydrochloride (Additive CNS depressant effect). Products include:

Orlaam 2239

Levorphanol Tartrate (Additive CNS depressant effect). Products include:

Levo-Dromoran................................... 2129

Loratadine (Additive CNS depressant effect). Products include:

Claritin 2349
Claritin-D 2350

Lorazepam (Additive CNS depressant effect). Products include:

Ativan Injection................................... 2698
Ativan Tablets 2700

Loxapine Hydrochloride (Additive CNS depressant effect). Products include:

Loxitane 1378

Loxapine Succinate (Additive CNS depressant effect). Products include:

Loxitane Capsules 1378

Maprotiline Hydrochloride (Additive CNS depressant effect). Products include:

Ludiomil Tablets.................................. 843

Meperidine Hydrochloride (Additive CNS depressant effect). Products include:

Demerol 2308
Mepergan Injection 2753

Mephobarbital (Additive CNS depressant effect). Products include:

Mebaral Tablets 2322

Meprobamate (Additive CNS depressant effect). Products include:

Miltown Tablets 2672
PMB 200 and PMB 400 2783

Mesoridazine Besylate (Additive CNS depressant effect). Products include:

Serentil 684

Methadone Hydrochloride (Additive CNS depressant effect). Products include:

Methadone Hydrochloride Oral Concentrate 2233
Methadone Hydrochloride Oral Solution & Tablets................................ 2235

Methdilazine Hydrochloride (Additive CNS depressant effect).

No products indexed under this heading.

Methohexital Sodium (Additive CNS depressant effect). Products include:

Brevital Sodium Vials......................... 1429

Methotrimeprazine (Additive CNS depressant effect). Products include:

Levoprome 1274

Methoxyflurane (Additive CNS depressant effect).

No products indexed under this heading.

Midazolam Hydrochloride (Additive CNS depressant effect). Products include:

Versed Injection 2170

Molindone Hydrochloride (Additive CNS depressant effect). Products include:

Moban Tablets and Concentrate...... 1048

Nortriptyline Hydrochloride (Additive CNS depressant effect). Products include:

Pamelor 2280

Opium Alkaloids (Additive CNS depressant effect).

No products indexed under this heading.

Oxazepam (Additive CNS depressant effect). Products include:

Serax Capsules 2810
Serax Tablets....................................... 2810

Oxycodone Hydrochloride (Additive CNS depressant effect). Products include:

Percocet Tablets 938
Percodan Tablets................................. 939
Percodan-Demi Tablets...................... 940
Roxicodone Tablets, Oral Solution & Intensol (Oxycodone) 2244
Tylox Capsules 1584

Pentobarbital Sodium (Additive CNS depressant effect). Products include:

Nembutal Sodium Capsules 436
Nembutal Sodium Solution 438
Nembutal Sodium Suppositories...... 440

Perphenazine (Additive CNS depressant effect). Products include:

Etrafon 2355
Triavil Tablets 1757
Trilafon... 2389

Phenobarbital (Additive CNS depressant effect). Products include:

Arco-Lase Plus Tablets 512
Bellergal-S Tablets 2250
Donnatal 2060
Donnatal Extentabs............................. 2061
Donnatal Tablets 2060
Phenobarbital Elixir and Tablets...... 1469
Quadrinal Tablets 1350

Prazepam (Additive CNS depressant effect).

No products indexed under this heading.

Prochlorperazine (Additive CNS depressant effect). Products include:

Compazine 2470

Promethazine Hydrochloride (Additive CNS depressant effect). Products include:

Mepergan Injection 2753
Phenergan with Codeine.................... 2777
Phenergan with Dextromethorphan 2778
Phenergan Injection 2773
Phenergan Suppositories 2775
Phenergan Syrup 2774
Phenergan Tablets 2775
Phenergan VC 2779
Phenergan VC with Codeine 2781

Propofol (Additive CNS depressant effect). Products include:

Diprivan Injection................................ 2833

Propoxyphene Hydrochloride (Additive CNS depressant effect). Products include:

Darvon 1435
Wygesic Tablets 2827

Propoxyphene Napsylate (Additive CNS depressant effect). Products include:

Darvon-N/Darvocet-N 1433

Protriptyline Hydrochloride (Additive CNS depressant effect). Products include:

Vivactil Tablets 1774

Pyrilamine Maleate (Additive CNS depressant effect). Products include:

4-Way Fast Acting Nasal Spray (regular & mentholated) .... ᴾᴰ 621
Maximum Strength Multi-Symptom Formula Midol .... ᴾᴰ 722
PMS Multi-Symptom Formula Midol .... ᴾᴰ 723

Pyrilamine Tannate (Additive CNS depressant effect). Products include:

Atrohist Pediatric Suspension 454
Rynatan 2673

Quazepam (Additive CNS depressant effect). Products include:

Doral Tablets 2664

Risperidone (Additive CNS depressant effect). Products include:

Risperdal 1301

Secobarbital Sodium (Additive CNS depressant effect). Products include:

Seconal Sodium Pulvules 1474

Sufentanil Citrate (Additive CNS depressant effect). Products include:

Sufenta Injection 1309

Temazepam (Additive CNS depressant effect). Products include:

Restoril Capsules................................ 2284

Terfenadine (Additive CNS depressant effect). Products include:

Seldane Tablets 1536
Seldane-D Extended-Release Tablets 1538

Thiamylal Sodium (Additive CNS depressant effect).

No products indexed under this heading.

Thioridazine Hydrochloride (Additive CNS depressant effect). Products include:

Mellaril 2269

Thiothixene (Additive CNS depressant effect). Products include:

Navane Capsules and Concentrate 2201
Navane Intramuscular 2202

Triazolam (Additive CNS depressant effect). Products include:

Halcion Tablets.................................... 2611

Trifluoperazine Hydrochloride (Additive CNS depressant effect). Products include:

Stelazine 2514

Trimeprazine Tartrate (Additive CNS depressant effect). Products include:

Temaril Tablets, Syrup and Spansule Extended-Release Capsules.. 483

Trimipramine Maleate (Additive CNS depressant effect). Products include:

Surmontil Capsules............................. 2811

Tripelennamine Hydrochloride (Additive CNS depressant effect). Products include:

PBZ Tablets 845
PBZ-SR Tablets................................... 844

Triprolidine Hydrochloride (Additive CNS depressant effect). Products include:

Actifed Plus Caplets .... ᴾᴰ 845
Actifed Plus Tablets .... ᴾᴰ 845
Actifed with Codeine Cough Syrup.. 1067
Actifed Syrup....................................... ᴾᴰ 846
Actifed Tablets .... ᴾᴰ 844

IMPORTANT NOTE: Always consult each drug listing in the patient's regimen for possible interactions.

RMS

Zolpidem Tartrate (Additive CNS depressant effect). Products include:

Ambien Tablets....................................... 2416

Food Interactions

Alcohol (Additive CNS depressant effect).

RABIES VACCINE ADSORBED

(Rabies Vaccine) 2508

May interact with immunosuppressive agents. Compounds in this category include:

Azathioprine (Interferes with development of active immunity and may reduce the effectiveness of rabies vaccine). Products include:

Imuran 1110

Cyclosporine (Interferes with development of active immunity and may reduce the effectiveness of rabies vaccine). Products include:

Neoral... 2276
Sandimmune 2286

Immune Globulin (Human) (Interferes with development of active immunity and may reduce the effectiveness of rabies vaccine).

No products indexed under this heading.

Immune Globulin Intravenous (Human) (Interferes with development of active immunity and may reduce the effectiveness of rabies vaccine).

Muromonab-CD3 (Interferes with development of active immunity and may reduce the effectiveness of rabies vaccine). Products include:

Orthoclone OKT3 Sterile Solution .. 1837

Mycophenolate Mofetil (Interferes with development of active immunity and may reduce the effectiveness of rabies vaccine). Products include:

CellCept Capsules 2099

Tacrolimus (Interferes with development of active immunity and may reduce the effectiveness of rabies vaccine). Products include:

Prograf... 1042

RABIES VACCINE, IMOVAX RABIES I.D.

(Rabies Vaccine) 883

May interact with:

Chloroquine Hydrochloride (Reduced antibody response). Products include:

Aralen Hydrochloride Injection 2301

Chloroquine Phosphate (Reduced antibody response). Products include:

Aralen Phosphate Tablets 2301

RADICAL PC

(Nutritional Supplement) 1807

None cited in PDR database.

RECOMBIVAX HB

(Hepatitis B Vaccine)............................1744

None cited in PDR database.

REFRESH PLUS CELLUFRESH FORMULA LUBRICANT EYE DROPS

(Carboxymethylcellulose Sodium) .. ◉ 254

None cited in PDR database.

REFRESH PM LUBRICANT EYE OINTMENT

(Petrolatum, White, Mineral Oil) ...... ◉ 254

None cited in PDR database.

REGITINE

(Phentolamine Mesylate) 846

May interact with:

Withhold all medications, except those deemed essential,

for at least 24 hours prior to Regitine blocking test for pheochromocytoma

REGLAN INJECTABLE

(Metoclopramide Hydrochloride)........2068

May interact with anticholinergics, narcotic analgesics, central nervous system depressants, hypnotics and sedatives, tranquilizers, cardiac glycosides, insulin, monoamine oxidase inhibitors, and certain other agents. Compounds in these categories include:

Acetaminophen (Increased rate and/or extent of absorption from the small bowel). Products include:

Actifed Plus Caplets............................ ᴹᴰ 845
Actifed Plus Tablets .... ᴹᴰ 845
Actifed Sinus Daytime/Nighttime Tablets and Caplets .... ᴹᴰ 846
Alka-Seltzer Plus Cold Medicine Liqui-Gels .... ᴹᴰ 706
Alka-Seltzer Plus Cold & Cough Medicine Liqui-Gels.......................... ᴹᴰ 705
Alka-Seltzer Plus Night-Time Cold Medicine Liqui-Gels.......................... ᴹᴰ 706
Allerest Headache Strength Tablets .... ᴹᴰ 627
Allerest No Drowsiness Tablets...... ᴹᴰ 627
Allerest Sinus Pain Formula .... ᴹᴰ 627
Anexsia 5/500 Elixir 1781
Anexia Tablets...................................... 1782
Arthritis Foundation Aspirin Free Caplets .... ᴹᴰ 673
Arthritis Foundation NightTime Caplets .... ᴹᴰ 674
Bayer Select Headache Pain Relief Formula .... ᴹᴰ 716
Bayer Select Menstrual Multi-Symptom Formula............................... ᴹᴰ 716
Bayer Select Night Time Pain Relief Formula.................................... ᴹᴰ 716
Bayer Select Sinus Pain Relief Formula .... ᴹᴰ 717
Benadryl Allergy Sinus Headache Formula Caplets............................. ᴹᴰ 849
Comtrex Multi-Symptom Cold Reliever Tablets/Caplets/Liqui-Gels/Liquid.. ᴹᴰ 615
Allergy-Sinus Comtrex Multi-Symptom Allergy-Sinus Formula Tablets .... ᴹᴰ 617
Comtrex Non-Drowsy .... ᴹᴰ 618
Contac Day Allergy/Sinus Caplets ᴹᴰ 812
Contac Day & Night .... ᴹᴰ 812
Contac Night Allergy/Sinus Caplets .... ᴹᴰ 812
Contac Severe Cold and Flu Formula Caplets .... ᴹᴰ 814
Contac Severe Cold & Flu Non-Drowsy .... ᴹᴰ 815
Coricidin 'D' Decongestant Tablets .... ᴹᴰ 800
Coricidin Tablets .... ᴹᴰ 800
DHCplus Capsules................................ 1993
Darvon-N/Darvocet-N 1433
Drixoral Cold and Flu Extended-Release Tablets.................................... ᴹᴰ 803
Drixoral Cough + Sore Throat Liquid Caps .... ᴹᴰ 802
Drixoral Allergy/Sinus Extended Release Tablets.................................... ᴹᴰ 804
Esgic-plus Tablets 1013
Aspirin Free Excedrin Analgesic Caplets and Geltabs 732
Excedrin Extra-Strength Analgesic Tablets & Caplets 732
Excedrin P.M. Analgesic/Sleeping Aid Tablets, Caplets, Liquigels...... 733
Fioricet Tablets...................................... 2258
Fioricet with Codeine Capsules 2260
Hycomine Compound Tablets 932
Hydrocet Capsules 782
Legatrin PM .... ᴹᴰ 651
Lorcet 10/650.. 1018
Lortab 2566
Lurline PMS Tablets 982
Maximum Strength Multi-Symptom Formula Midol .... ᴹᴰ 722
PMS Multi-Symptom Formula Midol .... ᴹᴰ 723
Teen Multi-Symptom Formula Midol .... ᴹᴰ 722
Midrin Capsules 783
Migralam Capsules 2038
Panodol Tablets and Caplets .... ᴹᴰ 824

Children's Panadol Chewable Tablets, Liquid, Infant's Drops.... ᴹᴰ 824
Percocet Tablets 938
Percogesic Analgesic Tablets .... ᴹᴰ 754
Phrenilin 785
Pyrroxate Caplets .... ᴹᴰ 772
Sedapap Tablets 50 mg/650 mg .. 1543
Sinarest Tablets .... ᴹᴰ 648
Sinarest Extra Strength Tablets...... ᴹᴰ 648
Sinarest No Drowsiness Tablets .... ᴹᴰ 648
Sine-Aid Maximum Strength Sinus Medication Gelcaps, Caplets and Tablets 1554
Sine-Off No Drowsiness Formula Caplets .... ᴹᴰ 824
Sine-Off Sinus Medicine .... ᴹᴰ 825
Singlet Tablets .... ᴹᴰ 825
Sinulin Tablets 787
Sinutab Sinus Allergy Medication, Maximum Strength Tablets and Caplets .... ᴹᴰ 860
Sinutab Sinus Medication, Maximum Strength Without Drowsiness Formula, Tablets & Caplets .... ᴹᴰ 860
Sinutab Sinus Medication, Regular Strength Without Drowsiness Formula .... ᴹᴰ 859
Sudafed Cold and Cough Liquidcaps .... ᴹᴰ 862
Sudafed Severe Cold Formula Caplets .... ᴹᴰ 863
Sudafed Severe Cold Formula Tablets .... ᴹᴰ 864
Sudafed Sinus Caplets....................... ᴹᴰ 864
Sudafed Sinus Tablets....................... ᴹᴰ 864
Talacen... 2333
TheraFlu... ᴹᴰ 787
TheraFlu Maximum Strength Nighttime Flu, Cold & Cough Medicine .... ᴹᴰ 788
TheraFlu Maximum Strength Non-Drowsy Formula Flu, Cold & Cough Medicine .... ᴹᴰ 788
Thera Flu Maximum Strength, Non-Drowsy Formula Flu, Cold and Cough Caplets .... ᴹᴰ 789
Triaminic Sore Throat Formula ...... ᴹᴰ 791
Triaminicin Tablets.............................. ᴹᴰ 793
Children's TYLENOL acetaminophen Chewable Tablets, Elixir, Suspension Liquid 1555
Children's TYLENOL Cold Multi-Symptom Liquid Formula and Chewable Tablets................................. 1561
Children's TYLENOL Cold ,Plus Cough Multi Symptom Tablets and Liquid .... ᴹᴰ 681
Infants' TYLENOL acetaminophen Drops and Suspension Drops........ 1555
Infants' TYLENOL Cold Decongestant & Fever-Reducer Drops.......... 1556
TYLENOL Extended Relief Caplets.. 1558
TYLENOL, Extra Strength, Acetaminophen Adult Liquid Pain Reliever 1560
TYLENOL, Extra Strength, acetaminophen Gelcaps, Geltabs, Caplets, Tablets....................................... 1559
TYLENOL, Extra Strength, Headache Plus Pain Reliever with Antacid Caplets 1559
TYLENOL, Junior Strength, acetaminophen Coated Caplets, Grape and Fruit Chewable Tablets 1557
TYLENOL Maximum Strength Allergy Sinus Medication Gelcaps and Caplets 1563
TYLENOL Maximum Strength Allergy Sinus NightTime Medication Caplets 1555
TYLENOL Flu Maximum Strength Gelcaps 1565
TYLENOL Flu NightTime, Maximum Strength, Gelcaps 1566
TYLENOL Maximum Strength Flu NightTime Hot Medication Packets 1562
TYLENOL, Maximum Strength, Sinus Medication Geltabs, Gelcaps, Caplets and Tablets 1566
TYLENOL Cold Multi-Symptom Formula Medication Tablets and Caplets 1561
TYLENOL Cold Medication No Drowsiness Formula Gelcaps and Caplets 1562
TYLENOL Cold Multi-Symptom Hot Medication Liquid Packets.............. 1557

TYLENOL Cough Multi-Symptom Medication 1564
TYLENOL Cough Multi-Symptom Medication with Decongestant...... 1565
TYLENOL, Regular Strength, acetaminophen Caplets and Tablets .. 1558
TYLENOL PM, Extra Strength Pain Reliever/Sleep Aid Caplets, Geltabs, Gelcaps....................................... 1560
TYLENOL Severe Allergy Medication Caplets 1564
Tylenol with Codeine 1583
Tylox Capsules 1584
Unisom With Pain Relief-Nighttime Sleep Aid and Pain Reliever............ 1934
Vanquish Analgesic Caplets .... ᴹᴰ 731
Vicks 44 LiquiCaps Cough, Cold & Flu Relief... ᴹᴰ 755
Vicks 44M Cough, Cold & Flu Relief .... ᴹᴰ 756
Vicks DayQuil .... ᴹᴰ 761
Vicks Nyquil Hot Therapy.................. ᴹᴰ 762
Vicks NyQuil LiquiCaps Multi-Symptom Cold/Flu Relief.............. ᴹᴰ 763
Vicks NyQuil Multi-Symptom Cold/Flu Relief - (Original & Cherry Flavor).................................... ᴹᴰ 763
Vicodin Tablets...................................... 1356
Vicodin ES Tablets 1357
Wygesic Tablets 2827
Zydone Capsules 949

Alfentanil Hydrochloride (Additive sedative effects; antagonizes gastrointestinal motility effects). Products include:

Alfenta Injection 1286

Alprazolam (Additive sedative effects). Products include:

Xanax Tablets 2649

Aprobarbital (Additive sedative effects).

No products indexed under this heading.

Atropine Sulfate (Antagonizes gastrointestinal motility effects). Products include:

Arco-Lase Plus Tablets 512
Atrohist Plus Tablets 454
Atropine Sulfate Sterile Ophthalmic Solution .... ◉ 233
Donnatal 2060
Donnatal Extentabs.............................. 2061
Donnatal Tablets 2060
Lomotil 2439
Motofen Tablets 784
Urised Tablets.. 1964

Belladonna Alkaloids (Antagonizes gastrointestinal motility effects). Products include:

Bellergal-S Tablets 2250
Hyland's Bed Wetting Tablets .... ᴹᴰ 828
Hyland's EnurAid Tablets.................. ᴹᴰ 829
Hyland's Teething Tablets................. ᴹᴰ 830

Benztropine Mesylate (Antagonizes gastrointestinal motility effects). Products include:

Cogentin 1621

Biperiden Hydrochloride (Antagonizes gastrointestinal motility effects). Products include:

Akineton 1333

Buprenorphine (Additive sedative effects; antagonizes gastrointestinal motility effects). Products include:

Buprenex Injectable 2006

Buspirone Hydrochloride (Additive sedative effects). Products include:

BuSpar 737

Butabarbital (Additive sedative effects).

No products indexed under this heading.

Butalbital (Additive sedative effects). Products include:

Esgic-plus Tablets 1013
Fioricet Tablets....................................... 2258
Fioricet with Codeine Capsules 2260
Fiorinal Capsules 2261
Fiorinal with Codeine Capsules 2262
Fiorinal Tablets...................................... 2261
Phrenilin 785
Sedapap Tablets 50 mg/650 mg .. 1543

(ᴹᴰ Described in PDR For Nonprescription Drugs) (◉ Described in PDR For Ophthalmology)

Chlordiazepoxide (Additive sedative effects). Products include:

Libritabs Tablets 2177
Limbitrol 2180

Chlordiazepoxide Hydrochloride (Additive sedative effects). Products include:

Librax Capsules 2176
Librium Capsules 2178
Librium Injectable 2179

Chlorpromazine (Additive sedative effects). Products include:

Thorazine Suppositories 2523

Chlorpromazine Hydrochloride (Additive sedative effects). Products include:

Thorazine 2523

Chlorprothixene (Additive sedative effects).

No products indexed under this heading.

Chlorprothixene Hydrochloride (Additive sedative effects).

No products indexed under this heading.

Clidinium Bromide (Antagonizes gastrointestinal motility effects). Products include:

Librax Capsules 2176
Quarzan Capsules 2181

Clorazepate Dipotassium (Additive sedative effects). Products include:

Tranxene 451

Clozapine (Additive sedative effects; antagonizes gastrointestinal motility effects). Products include:

Clozaril Tablets 2252

Codeine Phosphate (Additive sedative effects; antagonizes gastrointestinal motility effects). Products include:

Actifed with Codeine Cough Syrup.. 1067
Brontex 1981
Deconsal C Expectorant Syrup 456
Deconsal Pediatric Syrup 457
Dimetane-DC Cough Syrup 2059
Empirin with Codeine Tablets............ 1093
Fioricet with Codeine Capsules 2260
Fiorinal with Codeine Capsules 2262
Isoclor Expectorant 990
Novahistine DH..................................... 2462
Novahistine Expectorant...................... 2463
Nucofed 2051
Phenergan with Codeine...................... 2777
Phenergan VC with Codeine 2781
Robitussin A-C Syrup........................... 2073
Robitussin-DAC Syrup 2074
Ryna .... ◙ 841
Soma Compound w/Codeine Tablets 2676
Tussi-Organidin NR Liquid and S NR Liquid 2677
Tylenol with Codeine 1583

Cyclosporine (Increased rate and/or extent of absorption from the small bowel). Products include:

Neoral 2276
Sandimmune 2286

Desflurane (Additive sedative effects; antagonizes gastrointestinal motility effects). Products include:

Suprane 1813

Deslanoside (Diminished absorption from the stomach).

No products indexed under this heading.

Dezocine (Additive sedative effects; antagonizes gastrointestinal motility effects). Products include:

Dalgan Injection 538

Diazepam (Additive sedative effects). Products include:

Dizac 1809
Valium Injectable 2182
Valium Tablets 2183
Valrelease Capsules 2169

Dicyclomine Hydrochloride (Antagonizes gastrointestinal motility effects). Products include:

Bentyl 1501

Digitoxin (Diminished absorption from the stomach). Products include:

Crystodigin Tablets............................... 1433

Digoxin (Diminished absorption from the stomach). Products include:

Lanoxicaps 1117
Lanoxin Elixir Pediatric 1120
Lanoxin Injection 1123
Lanoxin Injection Pediatric.................. 1126
Lanoxin Tablets 1128

Droperidol (Additive sedative effects). Products include:

Inapsine Injection.................................. 1296

Enflurane (Additive sedative effects).

No products indexed under this heading.

Estazolam (Additive sedative effects; antagonizes gastrointestinal motility effects). Products include:

ProSom Tablets 449

Ethchlorvynol (Additive sedative effects). Products include:

Placidyl Capsules.................................. 448

Ethinamate (Additive sedative effects).

No products indexed under this heading.

Fentanyl (Additive sedative effects; antagonizes gastrointestinal motility effects). Products include:

Duragesic Transdermal System......... 1288

Fentanyl Citrate (Additive sedative effects; antagonizes gastrointestinal motility effects). Products include:

Sublimaze Injection............................... 1307

Fluphenazine Decanoate (Additive sedative effects). Products include:

Prolixin Decanoate 509

Fluphenazine Enanthate (Additive sedative effects). Products include:

Prolixin Enanthate 509

Fluphenazine Hydrochloride (Additive sedative effects). Products include:

Prolixin 509

Flurazepam Hydrochloride (Additive sedative effects). Products include:

Dalmane Capsules................................. 2173

Furazolidone (Metoclopramide releases catecholamines in patients with essential hypertension hence it should be used cautiously in patients receiving MAO inhibitors). Products include:

Furoxone 2046

Glutethimide (Additive sedative effects).

No products indexed under this heading.

Glycopyrrolate (Antagonizes gastrointestinal motility effects). Products include:

Robinul Forte Tablets............................ 2072
Robinul Injectable 2072
Robinul Tablets...................................... 2072

Haloperidol (Additive sedative effects). Products include:

Haldol Injection, Tablets and Concentrate 1575

Haloperidol Decanoate (Additive sedative effects). Products include:

Haldol Decanoate.................................. 1577

Hydrocodone Bitartrate (Additive sedative effects; antagonizes gastrointestinal motility effects). Products include:

Anexsia 5/500 Elixir 1781
Anexia Tablets....................................... 1782
Codiclear DH Syrup 791
Deconamine CX Cough and Cold Liquid and Tablets................................ 1319
Duratuss HD Elixir................................ 2565
Hycodan Tablets and Syrup 930
Hycomine Compound Tablets 932
Hycomine 931
Hycotuss Expectorant Syrup 933
Hydrocet Capsules 782
Lorcet 10/650.. 1018
Lortab 2566
Tussend 1783
Tussend Expectorant 1785
Vicodin Tablets...................................... 1356
Vicodin ES Tablets 1357
Vicodin Tuss Expectorant 1358
Zydone Capsules 949

Hydrocodone Polistirex (Additive sedative effects; antagonizes gastrointestinal motility effects). Products include:

Tussionex Pennkinetic Extended-Release Suspension 998

Hydroxyzine Hydrochloride (Additive sedative effects). Products include:

Atarax Tablets & Syrup........................ 2185
Marax Tablets & DF Syrup................... 2200
Vistaril Intramuscular Solution........... 2216

Hyoscyamine (Antagonizes gastrointestinal motility effects). Products include:

Cystospaz Tablets 1963
Urised Tablets.. 1964

Hyoscyamine Sulfate (Antagonizes gastrointestinal motility effects). Products include:

Arco-Lase Plus Tablets 512
Atrohist Plus Tablets 454
Cystospaz-M Capsules 1963
Donnatal 2060
Donnatal Extentabs............................... 2061
Donnatal Tablets 2060
Kutrase Capsules.................................. 2402
Levsin/Levsinex/Levbid 2405

Insulin, Human (Exogenous insulin may begin to act before food has left the stomach and lead to hypoglycemia in diabetic patients with gastroparesis; insulin dosage or timing of dosage may require adjustment).

No products indexed under this heading.

Insulin, Human Isophane Suspension (Exogenous insulin may begin to act before food has left the stomach and lead to hypoglycemia in diabetic patients with gastroparesis; insulin dosage or timing of dosage may require adjustment). Products include:

Novolin N Human Insulin 10 ml Vials.. 1795

Insulin, Human NPH (Exogenous insulin may begin to act before food has left the stomach and lead to hypoglycemia in diabetic patients with gastroparesis; insulin dosage or timing of dosage may require adjustment). Products include:

Humulin N, 100 Units 1448
Novolin N PenFill Cartridges Durable Insulin Delivery System 1798
Novolin N Prefilled Syringe Disposable Insulin Delivery System 1798

Insulin, Human Regular (Exogenous insulin may begin to act before food has left the stomach and lead to hypoglycemia in diabetic patients with gastroparesis; insulin dosage or timing of dosage may require adjustment). Products include:

Humulin R, 100 Units 1449
Novolin R Human Insulin 10 ml Vials.. 1795
Novolin R PenFill Cartridges Durable Insulin Delivery System 1798
Novolin R Prefilled Syringe Disposable Insulin Delivery System 1798
Velosulin BR Human Insulin 10 ml Vials.. 1795

Insulin, Human, Zinc Suspension (Exogenous insulin may begin to act before food has left the stomach and lead to hypoglycemia in diabetic patients with gastroparesis; insulin dosage or timing of dosage may require adjustment). Products include:

Humulin L, 100 Units 1446
Humulin U, 100 Units 1450
Novolin L Human Insulin 10 ml Vials.. 1795

Insulin, NPH (Exogenous insulin may begin to act before food has left the stomach and lead to hypoglycemia in diabetic patients with gastroparesis; insulin dosage or timing of dosage may require adjustment). Products include:

NPH, 100 Units 1450
Pork NPH, 100 Units............................ 1452
Purified Pork NPH Isophane Insulin 1801

Insulin, Regular (Exogenous insulin may begin to act before food has left the stomach and lead to hypoglycemia in diabetic patients with gastroparesis; insulin dosage or timing of dosage may require adjustment). Products include:

Regular, 100 Units 1450
Pork Regular, 100 Units 1452
Pork Regular (Concentrated), 500 Units 1453
Purified Pork Regular Insulin 1801

Insulin, Zinc Crystals (Exogenous insulin may begin to act before food has left the stomach and lead to hypoglycemia in diabetic patients with gastroparesis; insulin dosage or timing of dosage may require adjustment). Products include:

NPH, 100 Units 1450

Insulin, Zinc Suspension (Exogenous insulin may begin to act before food has left the stomach and lead to hypoglycemia in diabetic patients with gastroparesis; insulin dosage or timing of dosage may require adjustment). Products include:

Iletin I 1450
Lente, 100 Units 1450
Iletin II... 1452
Pork Lente, 100 Units........................... 1452
Purified Pork Lente Insulin 1801

Ipratropium Bromide (Antagonizes gastrointestinal motility effects). Products include:

Atrovent Inhalation Aerosol................ 671
Atrovent Inhalation Solution 673

Isocarboxazid (Metoclopramide releases catecholamines in patients with essential hypertension hence it should be used cautiously in patients receiving MAO inhibitors).

No products indexed under this heading.

Ketamine Hydrochloride (Additive sedative effects; antagonizes gastrointestinal motility effects).

No products indexed under this heading.

Levodopa (Increased rate and/or extent of absorption from the small bowel). Products include:

Atamet 572
Larodopa Tablets................................... 2129
Sinemet Tablets 943
Sinemet CR Tablets 944

Levomethadyl Acetate Hydrochloride (Additive sedative effects; antagonizes gastrointestinal motility effects). Products include:

Orlamm 2239

Levorphanol Tartrate (Additive sedative effects; antagonizes gastrointestinal motility effects). Products include:

Levo-Dromoran...................................... 2129

IMPORTANT NOTE: Always consult each drug listing in the patient's regimen for possible interactions.

Reglan Interactions Index 880

Lorazepam (Additive sedative effects). Products include:
- Ativan Injection 2698
- Ativan Tablets 2700

Loxapine Hydrochloride (Additive sedative effects). Products include:
- Loxitane 1378

Loxapine Succinate (Additive sedative effects; antagonizes gastrointestinal motility effects). Products include:
- Loxitane Capsules 1378

Mepenzolate Bromide (Antagonizes gastrointestinal motility effects).
- No products indexed under this heading.

Meperidine Hydrochloride (Additive sedative effects; antagonizes gastrointestinal motility effects). Products include:
- Demerol 2308
- Mepergan Injection 2753

Mephobarbital (Additive sedative effects). Products include:
- Mebaral Tablets 2322

Meprobamate (Additive sedative effects). Products include:
- Miltown Tablets 2672
- PMB 200 and PMB 400 2783

Mesoridazine Besylate (Additive sedative effects). Products include:
- Serentil 684

Methadone Hydrochloride (Additive sedative effects; antagonizes gastrointestinal motility effects). Products include:
- Methadone Hydrochloride Oral Concentrate 2233
- Methadone Hydrochloride Oral Solution & Tablets 2235

Methohexital Sodium (Additive sedative effects). Products include:
- Brevital Sodium Vials 1429

Methotrimeprazine (Additive sedative effects; antagonizes gastrointestinal motility effects). Products include:
- Levoprome 1274

Methoxyflurane (Additive sedative effects).
- No products indexed under this heading.

Midazolam Hydrochloride (Additive sedative effects). Products include:
- Versed Injection 2170

Molindone Hydrochloride (Additive sedative effects). Products include:
- Moban Tablets and Concentrate 1048

Morphine Sulfate (Additive sedative effects; antagonizes gastrointestinal motility effects). Products include:
- Astramorph/PF Injection, USP (Preservative-Free) 535
- Duramorph 962
- Infumorph 200 and Infumorph 500 Sterile Solutions 965
- MS Contin Tablets 1994
- MSIR 1997
- Oramorph SR (Morphine Sulfate Sustained Release Tablets) 2236
- RMS Suppositories 2657
- Roxanol 2243

Opium Alkaloids (Additive sedative effects; antagonizes gastrointestinal motility effects).
- No products indexed under this heading.

Oxazepam (Additive sedative effects). Products include:
- Serax Capsules 2810
- Serax Tablets 2810

Oxybutynin Chloride (Antagonizes gastrointestinal motility effects). Products include:
- Ditropan 1516

Oxycodone Hydrochloride (Additive sedative effects; antagonizes gastrointestinal motility effects). Products include:
- Percocet Tablets 938
- Percodan Tablets 939
- Percodan-Demi Tablets 940
- Roxicodone Tablets, Oral Solution & Intensol (Oxycodone) 2244
- Tylox Capsules 1584

Pentobarbital Sodium (Additive sedative effects). Products include:
- Nembutal Sodium Capsules 436
- Nembutal Sodium Solution 438
- Nembutal Sodium Suppositories 440

Perphenazine (Additive sedative effects). Products include:
- Etrafon 2355
- Triavil Tablets 1757
- Trilafon 2389

Phenelzine Sulfate (Metoclopramide releases catecholamines in patients with essential hypertension hence it should be used cautiously in patients receiving MAO inhibitors). Products include:
- Nardil 1920

Phenobarbital (Additive sedative effects). Products include:
- Arco-Lase Plus Tablets 512
- Bellergal-S Tablets 2250
- Donnatal 2060
- Donnatal Extentabs 2061
- Donnatal Tablets 2060
- Phenobarbital Elixir and Tablets 1469
- Quadrinal Tablets 1350

Prazepam (Additive sedative effects).
- No products indexed under this heading.

Prochlorperazine (Additive sedative effects). Products include:
- Compazine 2470

Procyclidine Hydrochloride (Antagonizes gastrointestinal motility effects). Products include:
- Kemadrin Tablets 1112

Promethazine Hydrochloride (Additive sedative effects). Products include:
- Mepergan Injection 2753
- Phenergan with Codeine 2777
- Phenergan with Dextromethorphan 2778
- Phenergan Injection 2773
- Phenergan Suppositories 2775
- Phenergan Syrup 2774
- Phenergan Tablets 2775
- Phenergan VC 2779
- Phenergan VC with Codeine 2781

Propantheline Bromide (Antagonizes gastrointestinal motility effects). Products include:
- Pro-Banthine Tablets 2052

Propofol (Additive sedative effects; antagonizes gastrointestinal motility effects). Products include:
- Diprivan Injection 2833

Propoxyphene Hydrochloride (Additive sedative effects; antagonizes gastrointestinal motility effects). Products include:
- Darvon 1435
- Wygesic Tablets 2827

Propoxyphene Napsylate (Additive sedative effects; antagonizes gastrointestinal motility effects). Products include:
- Darvon-N/Darvocet-N 1433

Quazepam (Additive sedative effects; antagonizes gastrointestinal motility effects). Products include:
- Doral Tablets 2664

Risperidone (Additive sedative effects; antagonizes gastrointestinal motility effects). Products include:
- Risperdal 1301

Scopolamine (Antagonizes gastrointestinal motility effects). Products include:
- Transderm Scōp Transdermal Therapeutic System 869

Scopolamine Hydrobromide (Antagonizes gastrointestinal motility effects). Products include:
- Atrohist Plus Tablets 454
- Donnatal 2060
- Donnatal Extentabs 2061
- Donnatal Tablets 2060

Secobarbital Sodium (Additive sedative effects; antagonizes gastrointestinal motility effects). Products include:
- Seconal Sodium Pulvules 1474

Selegiline Hydrochloride (Metoclopramide releases catecholamines in patients with essential hypertension hence it should be used cautiously in patients receiving MAO inhibitors). Products include:
- Eldepryl Tablets 2550

Sufentanil Citrate (Additive sedative effects; antagonizes gastrointestinal motility effects). Products include:
- Sufenta Injection 1309

Temazepam (Additive sedative effects). Products include:
- Restoril Capsules 2284

Tetracycline Hydrochloride (Increased rate and/or extent of absorption from the small bowel). Products include:
- Achromycin V Capsules 1367

Thiamylal Sodium (Additive sedative effects).
- No products indexed under this heading.

Thioridazine Hydrochloride (Additive sedative effects). Products include:
- Mellaril 2269

Thiothixene (Additive sedative effects). Products include:
- Navane Capsules and Concentrate 2201
- Navane Intramuscular 2202

Tranylcypromine Sulfate (Metoclopramide releases catecholamines in patients with essential hypertension hence it should be used cautiously in patients receiving MAO inhibitors). Products include:
- Parnate Tablets 2503

Triazolam (Additive sedative effects). Products include:
- Halcion Tablets 2611

Tridihexethyl Chloride (Antagonizes gastrointestinal motility effects).
- No products indexed under this heading.

Trifluoperazine Hydrochloride (Additive sedative effects). Products include:
- Stelazine 2514

Trihexyphenidyl Hydrochloride (Antagonizes gastrointestinal motility effects). Products include:
- Artane 1368

Zolpidem Tartrate (Additive sedative effects; antagonizes gastrointestinal motility effects). Products include:
- Ambien Tablets 2416

Food Interactions

Alcohol (Increased rate and/or extent of absorption from the small bowel; additive sedative effects).

REGLAN SYRUP
(Metoclopramide Hydrochloride) 2068
- See **Reglan Injectable**

REGLAN TABLETS
(Metoclopramide Hydrochloride) 2068
- See **Reglan Injectable**

REHYDRALYTE ORAL ELECTROLYTE REHYDRATION SOLUTION
(Electrolyte Supplement) 2224
None cited in PDR database.

RELAFEN TABLETS
(Nabumetone) 2510
May interact with highly protein bound drugs (selected). Compounds in this category include:

Amiodarone Hydrochloride (In vitro studies have shown that 6 MNA, an active metabolite of nabumetone, may displace other protein bound drugs from their binding site). Products include:
- Cordarone Intravenous 2715
- Cordarone Tablets 2712

Amitriptyline Hydrochloride (In vitro studies have shown that 6 MNA, an active metabolite of nabumetone, may displace other protein bound drugs from their binding site). Products include:
- Elavil 2838
- Endep Tablets 2174
- Etrafon 2355
- Limbitrol 2180
- Triavil Tablets 1757

Atovaquone (In vitro studies have shown that 6 MNA, an active metabolite of nabumetone, may displace other protein bound drugs from their binding site). Products include:
- Mepron Suspension 1135

Cefonicid Sodium (In vitro studies have shown that 6 MNA, an active metabolite of nabumetone, may displace other protein bound drugs from their binding site). Products include:
- Monocid Injection 2497

Chlordiazepoxide (In vitro studies have shown that 6 MNA, an active metabolite of nabumetone, may displace other protein bound drugs from their binding site). Products include:
- Libritabs Tablets 2177
- Limbitrol 2180

Chlordiazepoxide Hydrochloride (In vitro studies have shown that 6 MNA, an active metabolite of nabumetone, may displace other protein bound drugs from their binding site). Products include:
- Librax Capsules 2176
- Librium Capsules 2178
- Librium Injectable 2179

Chlorpromazine (In vitro studies have shown that 6 MNA, an active metabolite of nabumetone, may displace other protein bound drugs from their binding site). Products include:
- Thorazine Suppositories 2523

Chlorpromazine Hydrochloride (In vitro studies have shown that 6 MNA, an active metabolite of nabumetone, may displace other protein bound drugs from their binding site). Products include:
- Thorazine 2523

Clomipramine Hydrochloride (In vitro studies have shown that 6 MNA, an active metabolite of nabumetone, may displace other protein bound drugs from their binding site). Products include:
- Anafranil Capsules 803

Clozapine (In vitro studies have shown that 6 MNA, an active metabolite of nabumetone, may displace other protein bound drugs from their binding site). Products include:
- Clozaril Tablets 2252

Cyclosporine (In vitro studies have shown that 6 MNA, an active metabolite of nabumetone, may displace other protein bound drugs from their binding site). Products include:
- Neoral 2276
- Sandimmune 2286

Diazepam (In vitro studies have shown that 6 MNA, an active metabolite of nabumetone, may displace other protein bound drugs from their binding site). Products include:
- Dizac 1809
- Valium Injectable 2182
- Valium Tablets 2183
- Valrelease Capsules 2169

Diclofenac Potassium (In vitro studies have shown that 6 MNA, an active metabolite of nabumetone, may displace other protein bound drugs from their binding site). Products include:
- Cataflam 816

Diclofenac Sodium (In vitro studies have shown that 6 MNA, an active metabolite of nabumetone, may displace other protein bound drugs from their binding site). Products include:
- Voltaren Ophthalmic Sterile Ophthalmic Solution .... ⊙ 272
- Voltaren Tablets 861

Dipyridamole (In vitro studies have shown that 6 MNA, an active metabolite of nabumetone, may displace other protein bound drugs from their binding site). Products include:
- Persantine Tablets 681

Fenoprofen Calcium (In vitro studies have shown that 6 MNA, an active metabolite of nabumetone, may displace other protein bound drugs from their binding site). Products include:
- Nalfon 200 Pulvules & Nalfon Tablets 917

Flurazepam Hydrochloride (In vitro studies have shown that 6 MNA, an active metabolite of nabumetone, may displace other protein bound drugs from their binding site). Products include:
- Dalmane Capsules 2173

Flurbiprofen (In vitro studies have shown that 6 MNA, an active metabolite of nabumetone, may displace other protein bound drugs from their binding site). Products include:
- Ansaid Tablets 2579

Glipizide (In vitro studies have shown that 6 MNA, an active metabolite of nabumetone, may displace other protein bound drugs from their binding site). Products include:
- Glucotrol Tablets 1967
- Glucotrol XL Extended Release Tablets 1968

Ibuprofen (In vitro studies have shown that 6 MNA, an active metabolite of nabumetone, may displace other protein bound drugs from their binding site). Products include:
- Advil Cold and Sinus Caplets and Tablets (formerly CoAdvil) .... ⊡ 870
- Advil Ibuprofen Tablets and Caplets .... ⊡ 870
- Children's Advil Suspension 2692
- Arthritis Foundation Ibuprofen Tablets .... ⊡ 674
- Bayer Select Ibuprofen Pain Relief Formula .... ⊡ 715
- Cramp End Tablets .... ⊡ 735
- Dimetapp Sinus Caplets .... ⊡ 775
- Haltran Tablets .... ⊡ 771
- IBU Tablets 1342
- Ibuprohm .... ⊡ 735
- Children's Motrin Ibuprofen Oral Suspension 1546
- Motrin Tablets 2625
- Motrin IB Caplets, Tablets, and Geltabs .... ⊡ 838
- Motrin IB Sinus .... ⊡ 838
- Motrin Ibuprofen Suspension, Oral Drops, Chewable Tablets, Caplets 1546
- Nuprin Ibuprofen/Analgesic Tablets & Caplets .... ⊡ 622
- Sine-Aid IB Caplets 1554
- Vicks DayQuil SINUS Pressure & PAIN Relief with IBUPROFEN .... ⊡ 762

Imipramine Hydrochloride (In vitro studies have shown that 6 MNA, an active metabolite of nabumetone, may displace other protein bound drugs from their binding site). Products include:
- Tofranil Ampuls 854
- Tofranil Tablets 856

Imipramine Pamoate (In vitro studies have shown that 6 MNA, an active metabolite of nabumetone, may displace other protein bound drugs from their binding site). Products include:
- Tofranil-PM Capsules 857

Indomethacin (In vitro studies have shown that 6 MNA, an active metabolite of nabumetone, may displace other protein bound drugs from their binding site). Products include:
- Indocin 1680

Indomethacin Sodium Trihydrate (In vitro studies have shown that 6 MNA, an active metabolite of nabumetone, may displace other protein bound drugs from their binding site). Products include:
- Indocin I.V. 1684

Ketoprofen (In vitro studies have shown that 6 MNA, an active metabolite of nabumetone, may displace other protein bound drugs from their binding site). Products include:
- Orudis Capsules 2766
- Oruvail Capsules 2766

Ketorolac Tromethamine (In vitro studies have shown that 6 MNA, an active metabolite of nabumetone, may displace other protein bound drugs from their binding site). Products include:
- Acular 474
- Acular .... ⊙ 277
- Toradol 2159

Meclofenamate Sodium (In vitro studies have shown that 6 MNA, an active metabolite of nabumetone, may displace other protein bound drugs from their binding site).
- No products indexed under this heading.

Mefenamic Acid (In vitro studies have shown that 6 MNA, an active metabolite of nabumetone, may displace other protein bound drugs from their binding site). Products include:
- Ponstel 1925

Midazolam Hydrochloride (In vitro studies have shown that 6 MNA, an active metabolite of nabumetone, may displace other protein bound drugs from their binding site). Products include:
- Versed Injection 2170

Naproxen (In vitro studies have shown that 6 MNA, an active metabolite of nabumetone, may displace other protein bound drugs from their binding site). Products include:
- Anaprox/Naprosyn 2117

Naproxen Sodium (In vitro studies have shown that 6 MNA, an active metabolite of nabumetone, may displace other protein bound drugs from their binding site). Products include:
- Aleve 1975
- Anaprox/Naprosyn 2117

Nortriptyline Hydrochloride (In vitro studies have shown that 6 MNA, an active metabolite of nabumetone, may displace other protein bound drugs from their binding site). Products include:
- Pamelor 2280

Oxaprozin (In vitro studies have shown that 6 MNA, an active metabolite of nabumetone, may displace other protein bound drugs from their binding site). Products include:
- Daypro Caplets 2426

Oxazepam (In vitro studies have shown that 6 MNA, an active metabolite of nabumetone, may displace other protein bound drugs from their binding site). Products include:
- Serax Capsules 2810
- Serax Tablets 2810

Phenylbutazone (In vitro studies have shown that 6 MNA, an active metabolite of nabumetone, may displace other protein bound drugs from their binding site).
- No products indexed under this heading.

Piroxicam (In vitro studies have shown that 6 MNA, an active metabolite of nabumetone, may displace other protein bound drugs from their binding site). Products include:
- Feldene Capsules 1965

Propranolol Hydrochloride (In vitro studies have shown that 6 MNA, an active metabolite of nabumetone, may displace other protein bound drugs from their binding site). Products include:
- Inderal 2728
- Inderal LA Long Acting Capsules 2730
- Inderide Tablets 2732
- Inderide LA Long Acting Capsules .. 2734

Sulindac (In vitro studies have shown that 6 MNA, an active metabolite of nabumetone, may displace other protein bound drugs from their binding site). Products include:
- Clinoril Tablets 1618

Temazepam (In vitro studies have shown that 6 MNA, an active metabolite of nabumetone, may displace other protein bound drugs from their binding site). Products include:
- Restoril Capsules 2284

Tolbutamide (In vitro studies have shown that 6 MNA, an active metabolite of nabumetone, may displace other protein bound drugs from their binding site).
- No products indexed under this heading.

Tolmetin Sodium (In vitro studies have shown that 6 MNA, an active metabolite of nabumetone, may displace other protein bound drugs from their binding site). Products include:
- Tolectin (200, 400 and 600 mg) .. 1581

Trimipramine Maleate (In vitro studies have shown that 6 MNA, an active metabolite of nabumetone, may displace other protein bound drugs from their binding site). Products include:
- Surmontil Capsules 2811

Warfarin Sodium (Effects not specified; caution should be exercised; in vitro studies have shown that 6 MNA, an active metabolite of nabumetone, may displace other protein bound drugs from their binding site). Products include:
- Coumadin 926

Food Interactions

Dairy products (Potential for more rapid absorption, however, the total amount of GMNA in the plasma is unchanged).

Food, unspecified (Potential for more rapid absorption, however, the total amount of GMNA in the plasma is unchanged).

REOPRO VIALS

(Abciximab) 1471

May interact with non-steroidal anti-inflammatory agents, anticoagulants, thrombolytics, and platelet inhibitors. Compounds in these categories include:

Alteplase, Recombinant (Abciximab inhibits platelet aggregation; concurrent use may be associated with an increase in bleeding). Products include:
- Activase 1058

Anistreplase (Abciximab inhibits platelet aggregation; concurrent use may be associated with an increase in bleeding). Products include:
- Eminase 2039

Aspirin (Abciximab inhibits platelet aggregation; concurrent use may be associated with an increase in bleeding). Products include:
- Alka-Seltzer Effervescent Antacid and Pain Reliever .... ⊡ 701
- Alka-Seltzer Extra Strength Effervescent Antacid and Pain Reliever .... ⊡ 703
- Alka-Seltzer Lemon Lime Effervescent Antacid and Pain Reliever .... ⊡ 703
- Alka-Seltzer Plus Cold Medicine .... ⊡ 705
- Alka-Seltzer Plus Cold & Cough Medicine .... ⊡ 708
- Alka-Seltzer Plus Night-Time Cold Medicine .... ⊡ 707
- Alka Seltzer Plus Sinus Medicine .. ⊡ 707
- Arthritis Foundation Safety Coated Aspirin Tablets .... ⊡ 675
- Arthritis Pain Ascriptin .... ⊡ 631
- Maximum Strength Ascriptin .... ⊡ 630
- Regular Strength Ascriptin Tablets .... ⊡ 629
- Arthritis Strength BC Powder .... ⊡ 609
- BC Cold Powder Multi-Symptom Formula (Cold-Sinus-Allergy) .... ⊡ 609
- BC Cold Powder Non-Drowsy Formula (Cold-Sinus) .... ⊡ 609
- BC Powder .... ⊡ 609
- Bayer Children's Chewable Aspirin .... ⊡ 711
- Genuine Bayer Aspirin Tablets & Caplets .... ⊡ 713
- Extra Strength Bayer Arthritis Pain Regimen Formula .... ⊡ 711
- Extra Strength Bayer Aspirin Caplets & Tablets .... ⊡ 712
- Extended-Release Bayer 8-Hour Aspirin .... ⊡ 712
- Extra Strength Bayer Plus Aspirin Caplets .... ⊡ 713
- Extra Strength Bayer PM Aspirin .. ⊡ 713
- Bayer Enteric Aspirin .... ⊡ 709
- Bufferin Analgesic Tablets and Caplets .... ⊡ 613
- Arthritis Strength Bufferin Analgesic Caplets .... ⊡ 614
- Extra Strength Bufferin Analgesic Tablets .... ⊡ 615
- Cama Arthritis Pain Reliever .... ⊡ 785
- Darvon Compound-65 Pulvules 1435
- Easprin 1914
- Ecotrin 2455
- Ecotrin Enteric Coated Aspirin Maximum Strength Tablets and Caplets .... ⊡ 816

IMPORTANT NOTE: Always consult each drug listing in the patient's regimen for possible interactions.

ReoPro **Interactions Index** 882

Ecotrin Enteric Coated Aspirin Regular Strength Tablets ... 2455
Empirin Aspirin Tablets ... ◘ 854
Empirin with Codeine Tablets ... 1093
Excedrin Extra-Strength Analgesic Tablets & Caplets ... 732
Fiorinal Capsules ... 2261
Fiorinal with Codeine Capsules ... 2262
Fiorinal Tablets ... 2261
Halfprin ... 1362
Healthprin Aspirin ... 2455
Norgesic ... 1496
Percodan Tablets ... 939
Percodan-Demi Tablets ... 940
Robaxisal Tablets ... 2071
Soma Compound w/Codeine Tablets ... 2676
Soma Compound Tablets ... 2675
St. Joseph Adult Chewable Aspirin (81 mg.) ... ◘ 808
Talwin Compound ... 2335
Ursinus Inlay-Tabs ... ◘ 794
Vanquish Analgesic Caplets ... ◘ 731

Azlocillin Sodium (Abciximab inhibits platelet aggregation; concurrent use may be associated with an increase in bleeding).
No products indexed under this heading.

Carbenicillin Indanyl Sodium (Abciximab inhibits platelet aggregation; concurrent use may be associated with an increase in bleeding). Products include:
Geocillin Tablets ... 2199

Choline Magnesium Trisalicylate (Abciximab inhibits platelet aggregation; concurrent use may be associated with an increase in bleeding). Products include:
Trilisate ... 2000

Dalteparin Sodium (Abciximab inhibits platelet aggregation; concurrent use may be associated with an increase in bleeding). Products include:
Fragmin ... 1954

Diclofenac Potassium (Abciximab inhibits platelet aggregation; concurrent use may be associated with an increase in bleeding). Products include:
Cataflam ... 816

Diclofenac Sodium (Abciximab inhibits platelet aggregation; concurrent use may be associated with an increase in bleeding). Products include:
Voltaren Ophthalmic Sterile Ophthalmic Solution ... ⊙ 272
Voltaren Tablets ... 861

Dicumarol (Abciximab inhibits platelet aggregation; concurrent use may be associated with an increase in bleeding).
No products indexed under this heading.

Diflunisal (Abciximab inhibits platelet aggregation; concurrent use may be associated with an increase in bleeding). Products include:
Dolobid Tablets ... 1654

Dipyridamole (Abciximab inhibits platelet aggregation; concurrent use may be associated with an increase in bleeding). Products include:
Persantine Tablets ... 681

Enoxaparin (Abciximab inhibits platelet aggregation; concurrent use may be associated with an increase in bleeding). Products include:
Lovenox Injection ... 2020

Etodolac (Abciximab inhibits platelet aggregation; concurrent use may be associated with an increase in bleeding). Products include:
Lodine Capsules and Tablets ... 2743

Fenoprofen Calcium (Abciximab inhibits platelet aggregation; concurrent use may be associated with an increase in bleeding). Products include:
Nalfon 200 Pulvules & Nalfon Tablets ... 917

Flurbiprofen (Abciximab inhibits platelet aggregation; concurrent use may be associated with an increase in bleeding). Products include:
Ansaid Tablets ... 2579

Heparin Calcium (Abciximab inhibits platelet aggregation; concurrent use may be associated with an increase in bleeding).
No products indexed under this heading.

Heparin Sodium (Abciximab inhibits platelet aggregation; concurrent use may be associated with an increase in bleeding). Products include:
Heparin Lock Flush Solution ... 2725
Heparin Sodium Injection ... 2726
Heparin Sodium Injection, USP, Sterile Solution ... 2615
Heparin Sodium Vials ... 1441

Ibuprofen (Abciximab inhibits platelet aggregation; concurrent use may be associated with an increase in bleeding). Products include:
Advil Cold and Sinus Caplets and Tablets (formerly CoAdvil) ... ◘ 870
Advil Ibuprofen Tablets and Caplets ... ◘ 870
Children's Advil Suspension ... 2692
Arthritis Foundation Ibuprofen Tablets ... ◘ 674
Bayer Select Ibuprofen Pain Relief Formula ... ◘ 715
Cramp End Tablets ... ◘ 735
Dimetapp Sinus Caplets ... ◘ 775
Haltran Tablets ... ◘ 771
IBU Tablets ... 1342
Ibuprohm ... ◘ 735
Children's Motrin Ibuprofen Oral Suspension ... 1546
Motrin Tablets ... 2625
Motrin IB Caplets, Tablets, and Geltabs ... ◘ 838
Motrin IB Sinus ... ◘ 838
Motrin Ibuprofen Suspension, Oral Drops, Chewable Tablets, Caplets ... 1546
Nuprin Ibuprofen/Analgesic Tablets & Caplets ... ◘ 622
Sine-Aid IB Caplets ... 1554
Vicks DayQuil SINUS Pressure & PAIN Relief with IBUPROFEN ... ◘ 762

Indomethacin (Abciximab inhibits platelet aggregation; concurrent use may be associated with an increase in bleeding). Products include:
Indocin ... 1680

Indomethacin Sodium Trihydrate (Abciximab inhibits platelet aggregation; concurrent use may be associated with an increase in bleeding). Products include:
Indocin I.V. ... 1684

Ketoprofen (Abciximab inhibits platelet aggregation; concurrent use may be associated with an increase in bleeding). Products include:
Orudis Capsules ... 2766
Oruvail Capsules ... 2766

Ketorolac Tromethamine (Abciximab inhibits platelet aggregation; concurrent use may be associated with an increase in bleeding). Products include:
Acular ... 474
Acular ... ⊙ 277
Toradol ... 2159

Magnesium Salicylate (Abciximab inhibits platelet aggregation; concurrent use may be associated with an increase in bleeding). Products include:
Backache Caplets ... ◘ 613
Bayer Select Backache Pain Relief Formula ... ◘ 715
Doan's Extra-Strength Analgesic ... ◘ 633
Extra Strength Doan's P.M. ... ◘ 633
Doan's Regular Strength Analgesic ... ◘ 634
Mobigesic Tablets ... ◘ 602

Meclofenamate Sodium (Abciximab inhibits platelet aggregation; concurrent use may be associated with an increase in bleeding).
No products indexed under this heading.

Mefenamic Acid (Abciximab inhibits platelet aggregation; concurrent use may be associated with an increase in bleeding). Products include:
Ponstel ... 1925

Mezlocillin Sodium (Abciximab inhibits platelet aggregation; concurrent use may be associated with an increase in bleeding). Products include:
Mezlin ... 601
Mezlin Pharmacy Bulk Package ... 604

Nabumetone (Abciximab inhibits platelet aggregation; concurrent use may be associated with an increase in bleeding). Products include:
Relafen Tablets ... 2510

Nafcillin Sodium (Abciximab inhibits platelet aggregation; concurrent use may be associated with an increase in bleeding).
No products indexed under this heading.

Naproxen (Abciximab inhibits platelet aggregation; concurrent use may be associated with an increase in bleeding). Products include:
Anaprox/Naprosyn ... 2117

Naproxen Sodium (Abciximab inhibits platelet aggregation; concurrent use may be associated with an increase in bleeding). Products include:
Aleve ... 1975
Anaprox/Naprosyn ... 2117

Oxaprozin (Abciximab inhibits platelet aggregation; concurrent use may be associated with an increase in bleeding). Products include:
Daypro Caplets ... 2426

Penicillin G Benzathine (Abciximab inhibits platelet aggregation; concurrent use may be associated with an increase in bleeding). Products include:
Bicillin C-R Injection ... 2704
Bicillin C-R 900/300 Injection ... 2706
Bicillin L-A Injection ... 2707

Penicillin G Procaine (Abciximab inhibits platelet aggregation; concurrent use may be associated with an increase in bleeding). Products include:
Bicillin C-R Injection ... 2704
Bicillin C-R 900/300 Injection ... 2706

Phenylbutazone (Abciximab inhibits platelet aggregation; concurrent use may be associated with an increase in bleeding).
No products indexed under this heading.

Piroxicam (Abciximab inhibits platelet aggregation; concurrent use may be associated with an increase in bleeding). Products include:
Feldene Capsules ... 1965

Salsalate (Abciximab inhibits platelet aggregation; concurrent use may be associated with an increase in bleeding). Products include:
Mono-Gesic Tablets ... 792
Salflex Tablets ... 786

Streptokinase (Abciximab inhibits platelet aggregation; concurrent use may be associated with an increase in bleeding). Products include:
Streptase for Infusion ... 562

Sulindac (Abciximab inhibits platelet aggregation; concurrent use may be associated with an increase in bleeding). Products include:
Clinoril Tablets ... 1618

Ticarcillin Disodium (Abciximab inhibits platelet aggregation; concurrent use may be associated with an increase in bleeding). Products include:
Ticar for Injection ... 2526
Timentin for Injection ... 2528

Ticlopidine Hydrochloride (Abciximab inhibits platelet aggregation; concurrent use may be associated with an increase in bleeding). Products include:
Ticlid Tablets ... 2156

Tolmetin Sodium (Abciximab inhibits platelet aggregation; concurrent use may be associated with an increase in bleeding). Products include:
Tolectin (200, 400 and 600 mg) ... 1581

Urokinase (Abciximab inhibits platelet aggregation; concurrent use may be associated with an increase in bleeding). Products include:
Abbokinase ... 403
Abbokinase Open-Cath ... 405

Warfarin Sodium (Abciximab inhibits platelet aggregation; concurrent use may be associated with an increase in bleeding). Products include:
Coumadin ... 926

REPLENS VAGINAL MOISTURIZER
(Glycerin, Lubricant) ... ◘ 859
None cited in PDR database.

RESPBID TABLETS
(Theophylline Anhydrous) ... 682
May interact with sympathomimetic bronchodilators, oral contraceptives, macrolide antibiotics, and certain other agents. Compounds in these categories include:

Albuterol (Toxic synergism). Products include:
Proventil Inhalation Aerosol ... 2382
Ventolin Inhalation Aerosol and Refill ... 1197

Albuterol Sulfate (Toxic synergism). Products include:
Airet Solution for Inhalation ... 452
Proventil Inhalation Solution 0.083% ... 2384
Proventil Repetabs Tablets ... 2386
Proventil Solution for Inhalation 0.5% ... 2383
Proventil Syrup ... 2385
Proventil Tablets ... 2386
Ventolin Inhalation Solution ... 1198
Ventolin Nebules Inhalation Solution ... 1199
Ventolin Rotacaps for Inhalation ... 1200
Ventolin Syrup ... 1202
Ventolin Tablets ... 1203
Volmax Extended-Release Tablets ... 1788

Allopurinol (Increased serum theophylline levels with high-dose allopurinol). Products include:
Zyloprim Tablets ... 1226

Azithromycin (Increases theophylline blood levels). Products include:
Zithromax ... 1944

Bitolterol Mesylate (Toxic synergism). Products include:
Tornalate Solution for Inhalation, 0.2% ... 956
Tornalate Metered Dose Inhaler ... 957

(◘ Described in PDR For Nonprescription Drugs) (⊙ Described in PDR For Ophthalmology)

Interactions Index

Restoril

Cimetidine (Increased theophylline blood levels). Products include:

Tagamet Tablets 2516

Ciprofloxacin (Increased serum theophylline levels). Products include:

Cipro I.V. 595
Cipro I.V. Pharmacy Bulk Package.. 597

Ciprofloxacin Hydrochloride (Increased serum theophylline levels). Products include:

Ciloxan Ophthalmic Solution.............. 472
Cipro Tablets 592

Clarithromycin (Increases theophylline blood levels). Products include:

Biaxin 405

Desogestrel (Increased serum theophylline levels). Products include:

Desogen Tablets...................................... 1817
Ortho-Cept 1851

Ephedrine Hydrochloride (Toxic synergism). Products include:

Primatene Dual Action Formula...... ᴴᴰ 872
Primatene Tablets .... ᴴᴰ 873
Quadrinal Tablets 1350

Ephedrine Sulfate (Toxic synergism). Products include:

Bronkaid Caplets .... ᴴᴰ 717
Marax Tablets & DF Syrup.................. 2200

Ephedrine Tannate (Toxic synergism). Products include:

Rynatuss 2673

Epinephrine (Toxic synergism). Products include:

Bronkaid Mist .... ᴴᴰ 717
EPIFRIN .... ◎ 239
EpiPen 790
Marcaine Hydrochloride with Epinephrine 1:200,000 2316
Primatene Mist .... ᴴᴰ 873
Sensorcaine with Epinephrine Injection... 559
Sus-Phrine Injection 1019
Xylocaine with Epinephrine Injections... 567

Epinephrine Bitartrate (Toxic synergism). Products include:

Bronkaid Mist Suspension .... ᴴᴰ 718
Sensorcaine-MPF with Epinephrine Injection 559

Epinephrine Hydrochloride (Toxic synergism). Products include:

Ana-Kit Anaphylaxis Emergency Treatment Kit 617

Erythromycin (Increases theophylline blood levels). Products include:

A/T/S 2% Acne Topical Gel and Solution 1234
Benzamycin Topical Gel 905
E-Mycin Tablets...................................... 1341
Emgel 2% Topical Gel.......................... 1093
ERYC 1915
Erycette (erythromycin 2%) Topical Solution 1888
Ery-Tab Tablets 422
Erythromycin Base Filmtab 426
Erythromycin Delayed-Release Capsules, USP 427
Ilotycin Ophthalmic Ointment............ 912
PCE Dispertab Tablets 444
T-Stat 2.0% Topical Solution and Pads 2688
Theramycin Z Topical Solution 2% 1592

Erythromycin Estolate (Increases theophylline blood levels). Products include:

Ilosone 911

Erythromycin Ethylsuccinate (Increases theophylline blood levels). Products include:

E.E.S. 424
EryPed 421

Erythromycin Gluceptate (Increases theophylline blood levels). Products include:

Ilotycin Gluceptate, IV, Vials 913

Erythromycin Stearate (Increases theophylline blood levels). Products include:

Erythrocin Stearate Filmtab 425

Ethinyl Estradiol (Increased serum theophylline levels). Products include:

Brevicon.. 2088
Demulen 2428
Desogen Tablets....................................... 1817
Levlen/Tri-Levlen.................................... 651
Lo/Ovral Tablets 2746
Lo/Ovral-28 Tablets............................... 2751
Modicon 1872
Nordette-21 Tablets................................ 2755
Nordette-28 Tablets................................ 2758
Norinyl 2088
Ortho-Cept 1851
Ortho-Cyclen/Ortho-Tri-Cyclen 1858
Ortho-Novum... 1872
Ortho-Cyclen/Ortho Tri-Cyclen 1858
Ovcon 760
Ovral Tablets 2770
Ovral-28 Tablets 2770
Levlen/Tri-Levlen.................................... 651
Tri-Norinyl.. 2164
Triphasil-21 Tablets 2814
Triphasil-28 Tablets 2819

Ethylnorepinephrine Hydrochloride (Toxic synergism).

No products indexed under this heading.

Ethynodiol Diacetate (Increased serum theophylline levels). Products include:

Demulen 2428

Isoetharine (Toxic synergism). Products include:

Bronkometer Aerosol 2302
Bronkosol Solution 2302
Isoetharine Inhalation Solution, USP, Arm-a-Med....................................... 551

Isoproterenol Hydrochloride (Toxic synergism). Products include:

Isuprel Hydrochloride Injection 1:5000 2311
Isuprel Hydrochloride Solution 1:200 & 1:100 2313
Isuprel Mistometer 2312

Isoproterenol Sulfate (Toxic synergism). Products include:

Norisodrine with Calcium Iodide Syrup.. 442

Levonorgestrel (Increased serum theophylline levels). Products include:

Levlen/Tri-Levlen.................................... 651
Nordette-21 Tablets................................ 2755
Nordette-28 Tablets................................ 2758
Norplant System 2759
Levlen/Tri-Levlen.................................... 651
Triphasil-21 Tablets................................ 2814
Triphasil-28 Tablets................................ 2819

Lithium Carbonate (Increased excretion of lithium carbonate). Products include:

Eskalith 2485
Lithium Carbonate Capsules & Tablets 2230
Lithonate/Lithotabs/Lithobid 2543

Mestranol (Increased serum theophylline levels). Products include:

Norinyl 2088
Ortho-Novum... 1872

Metaproterenol Sulfate (Toxic synergism). Products include:

Alupent.. 669
Metaproterenol Sulfate Inhalation Solution, USP, Arm-a-Med 552

Norethindrone (Increased serum theophylline levels). Products include:

Brevicon... 2088
Micronor Tablets 1872
Modicon... 1872
Norinyl 2088
Nor-Q D Tablets 2135
Ortho-Novum... 1872
Ovcon 760
Tri-Norinyl.. 2164

Norethynodrel (Increased serum theophylline levels).

No products indexed under this heading.

Norgestimate (Increased serum theophylline levels). Products include:

Ortho-Cyclen/Ortho-Tri-Cyclen 1858
Ortho-Cyclen/Ortho Tri-Cyclen 1858

Norgestrel (Increased serum theophylline levels). Products include:

Lo/Ovral Tablets 2746
Lo/Ovral-28 Tablets............................... 2751
Ovral Tablets 2770
Ovral-28 Tablets 2770
Ovrette Tablets... 2771

Phenytoin (Decreased theophylline and phenytoin serum levels). Products include:

Dilantin Infatabs 1908
Dilantin-125 Suspension 1911

Phenytoin Sodium (Decreased theophylline and phenytoin serum levels). Products include:

Dilantin Kapseals 1906
Dilantin Parenteral 1910

Pirbuterol Acetate (Toxic synergism). Products include:

Maxair Autohaler 1492
Maxair Inhaler 1494

Propranolol Hydrochloride (Increases serum theophylline levels). Products include:

Inderal 2728
Inderal LA Long Acting Capsules 2730
Inderide Tablets 2732
Inderide LA Long Acting Capsules .. 2734

Rifampin (Decreases serum theophylline levels). Products include:

Rifadin 1528
Rifamate Capsules 1530
Rifater.. 1532
Rimactane Capsules................................ 847

Salmeterol Xinafoate (Toxic synergism). Products include:

Serevent Inhalation Aerosol................. 1176

Terbutaline Sulfate (Toxic synergism). Products include:

Brethaire Inhaler 813
Brethine Ampuls 815
Brethine Tablets....................................... 814
Bricanyl Subcutaneous Injection 1502
Bricanyl Tablets 1503

Troleandomycin (Increases theophylline blood levels). Products include:

Tao Capsules 2209

Food Interactions

Beverages, caffeine-containing (Avoid large quantities; increased side effects).

Chocolate (Eating large quantity of chocolate increases theophylline side effects).

Cola (Drinking large quantity of cola increases theophylline side effects).

Diet, high-lipid (Reduced plasma concentration levels; delay in time of peak plasma levels).

RESTORIL CAPSULES

(Temazepam) 2284

May interact with central nervous system depressants, hypnotics and sedatives, and certain other agents. Compounds in these categories include:

Alfentanil Hydrochloride (Additive effects). Products include:

Alfenta Injection 1286

Alprazolam (Additive effects). Products include:

Xanax Tablets 2649

Aprobarbital (Additive effects).

No products indexed under this heading.

Buprenorphine (Additive effects). Products include:

Buprenex Injectable 2006

Buspirone Hydrochloride (Additive effects). Products include:

BuSpar 737

Butabarbital (Additive effects).

No products indexed under this heading.

Butalbital (Additive effects). Products include:

Esgic-plus Tablets 1013
Fioricet Tablets... 2258
Fioricet with Codeine Capsules 2260
Fiorinal Capsules 2261
Fiorinal with Codeine Capsules 2262
Fiorinal Tablets 2261
Phrenilin 785
Sedapap Tablets 50 mg/650 mg .. 1543

Chlordiazepoxide (Additive effects). Products include:

Libritabs Tablets 2177
Limbitrol 2180

Chlordiazepoxide Hydrochloride (Additive effects). Products include:

Librax Capsules 2176
Librium Capsules..................................... 2178
Librium Injectable 2179

Chlorpromazine (Additive effects). Products include:

Thorazine Suppositories 2523

Chlorprothixene (Additive effects).

No products indexed under this heading.

Chlorprothixene Hydrochloride (Additive effects).

No products indexed under this heading.

Clorazepate Dipotassium (Additive effects). Products include:

Tranxene 451

Clozapine (Additive effects). Products include:

Clozaril Tablets... 2252

Codeine Phosphate (Additive effects). Products include:

Actifed with Codeine Cough Syrup.. 1067
Brontex 1981
Deconsal C Expectorant Syrup 456
Deconsal Pediatric Syrup 457
Dimetane-DC Cough Syrup 2059
Empirin with Codeine Tablets............ 1093
Fioricet with Codeine Capsules 2260
Fiorinal with Codeine Capsules 2262
Isoclor Expectorant................................. 990
Novahistine DH.. 2462
Novahistine Expectorant....................... 2463
Nucofed 2051
Phenergan with Codeine....................... 2777
Phenergan VC with Codeine 2781
Robitussin A-C Syrup............................. 2073
Robitussin-DAC Syrup........................... 2074
Ryna .... ᴴᴰ 841
Soma Compound w/Codeine Tablets 2676
Tussi-Organidin NR Liquid and S NR Liquid 2677
Tylenol with Codeine 1583

Desflurane (Additive effects). Products include:

Suprane 1813

Dezocine (Additive effects). Products include:

Dalgan Injection 538

Diazepam (Additive effects). Products include:

Dizac 1809
Valium Injectable 2182
Valium Tablets 2183
Valrelease Capsules 2169

Diphenhydramine Hydrochloride (Synergistic effect is possible). Products include:

Actifed Allergy Daytime/Nighttime Caplets.. ᴴᴰ 844
Actifed Sinus Daytime/Nighttime Tablets and Caplets .... ᴴᴰ 846
Arthritis Foundation NightTime Caplets .... ᴴᴰ 674
Extra Strength Bayer PM Aspirin .. ᴴᴰ 713
Bayer Select Night Time Pain Relief Formula..................................... ᴴᴰ 716
Benadryl Allergy Decongestant Liquid Medication .... ᴴᴰ 848
Benadryl Allergy Decongestant Tablets .... ᴴᴰ 848

IMPORTANT NOTE: Always consult each drug listing in the patient's regimen for possible interactions.

Restoril　Interactions Index　884

Benadryl Allergy Liquid Medication ▪ 849
Benadryl Allergy ▪ 848
Benadryl Allergy Sinus Headache Formula Caplets ▪ 849
Benadryl Capsules 1898
Benadryl Dye-Free Allergy Liqui-gel Softgels ▪ 850
Benadryl Dye-Free Allergy Liquid Medication ▪ 850
Benadryl Itch Relief Cream, Children's Formula and Maximum Strength 2% ▪ 851
Benadryl Itch Relief Spray, Children's Formula and Maximum Strength 2% ▪ 851
Benadryl Itch Relief Stick Maximum Strength 2% ▪ 850
Benadryl Itch Stopping Gel, Children's Formula and Maximum Strength 2% ▪ 851
Benadryl Kapseals 1898
Benadryl Injection 1898
Contac Day & Night Cold/Flu Night Caplets ▪ 812
Contac Night Allergy/Sinus Caplets ▪ 812
Extra Strength Doan's P.M. ▪ 633
Legatrin PM ▪ 651
Miles Nervine Nighttime Sleep-Aid ▪ 723
Nytol QuickCaps Caplets ▪ 610
Sleepinal Night-time Sleep Aid Capsules and Softgels ▪ 834
TYLENOL Maximum Strength Allergy Sinus NightTime Medication Caplets 1555
TYLENOL Flu NightTime, Maximum Strength, Gelcaps 1566
TYLENOL Maximum Strength Flu NightTime Hot Medication Packets 1562
TYLENOL PM, Extra Strength Pain Reliever/Sleep Aid Caplets, Geltabs, Gelcaps 1560
TYLENOL Severe Allergy Medication Caplets 1564
Maximum Strength Unisom Sleepgels 1934
Unisom With Pain Relief-Nighttime Sleep Aid and Pain Reliever 1934

Droperidol (Additive effects). Products include:
Inapsine Injection 1296

Enflurane (Additive effects).
No products indexed under this heading.

Estazolam (Additive effects). Products include:
ProSom Tablets 449

Ethchlorvynol (Additive effects). Products include:
Placidyl Capsules 448

Ethinamate (Additive effects).
No products indexed under this heading.

Fentanyl (Additive effects). Products include:
Duragesic Transdermal System 1288

Fentanyl Citrate (Additive effects). Products include:
Sublimaze Injection 1307

Fluphenazine Decanoate (Additive effects). Products include:
Prolixin Decanoate 509

Fluphenazine Enanthate (Additive effects). Products include:
Prolixin Enanthate 509

Fluphenazine Hydrochloride (Additive effects). Products include:
Prolixin 509

Flurazepam Hydrochloride (Additive effects). Products include:
Dalmane Capsules 2173

Glutethimide (Additive effects).
No products indexed under this heading.

Haloperidol (Additive effects). Products include:
Haldol Injection, Tablets and Concentrate 1575

Haloperidol Decanoate (Additive effects). Products include:
Haldol Decanoate 1577

Hydrocodone Bitartrate (Additive effects). Products include:
Anexsia 5/500 Elixir 1781
Anexia Tablets 1782
Codiclear DH Syrup 791
Deconamine CX Cough and Cold Liquid and Tablets 1319
Duratuss HD Elixir 2565
Hycodan Tablets and Syrup 930
Hycomine Compound Tablets 932
Hycomine 931
Hycotuss Expectorant Syrup 933
Hydrocet Capsules 782
Lorcet 10/650 1018
Lortab 2566
Tussend 1783
Tussend Expectorant 1785
Vicodin Tablets 1356
Vicodin ES Tablets 1357
Vicodin Tuss Expectorant 1358
Zydone Capsules 949

Hydrocodone Polistirex (Additive effects). Products include:
Tussionex Pennkinetic Extended-Release Suspension 998

Hydroxyzine Hydrochloride (Additive effects). Products include:
Atarax Tablets & Syrup 2185
Marax Tablets & DF Syrup 2200
Vistaril Intramuscular Solution 2216

Isoflurane (Additive effects).
No products indexed under this heading.

Ketamine Hydrochloride (Additive effects).
No products indexed under this heading.

Levomethadyl Acetate Hydrochloride (Additive effects). Products include:
Orlamm 2239

Levorphanol Tartrate (Additive effects). Products include:
Levo-Dromoran 2129

Lorazepam (Additive effects). Products include:
Ativan Injection 2698
Ativan Tablets 2700

Loxapine Hydrochloride (Additive effects). Products include:
Loxitane 1378

Loxapine Succinate (Additive effects). Products include:
Loxitane Capsules 1378

Meperidine Hydrochloride (Additive effects). Products include:
Demerol 2308
Mepergan Injection 2753

Mephobarbital (Additive effects). Products include:
Mebaral Tablets 2322

Meprobamate (Additive effects). Products include:
Miltown Tablets 2672
PMB 200 and PMB 400 2783

Mesoridazine Besylate (Additive effects). Products include:
Serentil 684

Methadone Hydrochloride (Additive effects). Products include:
Methadone Hydrochloride Oral Concentrate 2233
Methadone Hydrochloride Oral Solution & Tablets 2235

Methohexital Sodium (Additive effects). Products include:
Brevital Sodium Vials 1429

Methotrimeprazine (Additive effects). Products include:
Levoprome 1274

Methoxyflurane (Additive effects).
No products indexed under this heading.

Midazolam Hydrochloride (Additive effects). Products include:
Versed Injection 2170

Molindone Hydrochloride (Additive effects). Products include:
Moban Tablets and Concentrate 1048

Morphine Sulfate (Additive effects). Products include:
Astramorph/PF Injection, USP (Preservative-Free) 535
Duramorph 962
Infumorph 200 and Infumorph 500 Sterile Solutions 965
MS Contin Tablets 1994
MSIR 1997
Oramorph SR (Morphine Sulfate Sustained Release Tablets) 2236
RMS Suppositories 2657
Roxanol 2243

Opium Alkaloids (Additive effects).
No products indexed under this heading.

Oxazepam (Additive effects). Products include:
Serax Capsules 2810
Serax Tablets 2810

Oxycodone Hydrochloride (Additive effects). Products include:
Percocet Tablets 938
Percodan Tablets 939
Percodan-Demi Tablets 940
Roxicodone Tablets, Oral Solution & Intensol (Oxycodone) 2244
Tylox Capsules 1584

Pentobarbital Sodium (Additive effects). Products include:
Nembutal Sodium Capsules 436
Nembutal Sodium Solution 438
Nembutal Sodium Suppositories 440

Perphenazine (Additive effects). Products include:
Etrafon 2355
Triavil Tablets 1757
Trilafon 2389

Phenobarbital (Additive effects). Products include:
Arco-Lase Plus Tablets 512
Bellergal-S Tablets 2250
Donnatal 2060
Donnatal Extentabs 2061
Donnatal Tablets 2060
Phenobarbital Elixir and Tablets 1469
Quadrinal Tablets 1350

Prazepam (Additive effects).
No products indexed under this heading.

Prochlorperazine (Additive effects). Products include:
Compazine 2470

Promethazine Hydrochloride (Additive effects). Products include:
Mepergan Injection 2753
Phenergan with Codeine 2777
Phenergan with Dextromethorphan 2778
Phenergan Injection 2773
Phenergan Suppositories 2775
Phenergan Syrup 2774
Phenergan Tablets 2775
Phenergan VC 2779
Phenergan VC with Codeine 2781

Propofol (Additive effects). Products include:
Diprivan Injection 2833

Propoxyphene Hydrochloride (Additive effects). Products include:
Darvon 1435
Wygesic Tablets 2827

Propoxyphene Napsylate (Additive effects). Products include:
Darvon-N/Darvocet-N 1433

Quazepam (Additive effects). Products include:
Doral Tablets 2664

Risperidone (Additive effects). Products include:
Risperdal 1301

Secobarbital Sodium (Additive effects). Products include:
Seconal Sodium Pulvules 1474

Sufentanil Citrate (Additive effects). Products include:
Sufenta Injection 1309

Thiamylal Sodium (Additive effects).
No products indexed under this heading.

Thioridazine Hydrochloride (Additive effects). Products include:
Mellaril 2269

Thiothixene (Additive effects). Products include:
Navane Capsules and Concentrate 2201
Navane Intramuscular 2202

Triazolam (Additive effects). Products include:
Halcion Tablets 2611

Trifluoperazine Hydrochloride (Additive effects). Products include:
Stelazine 2514

Zolpidem Tartrate (Additive effects). Products include:
Ambien Tablets 2416

Food Interactions

Alcohol (Additive effects).

RETIN-A (TRETINOIN) CREAM/GEL/LIQUID
(Tretinoin) 1889
May interact with:

Concomitant Topical Acne Therapy (Effect not specified).

Resorcinol (Caution should be exercised). Products include:
BiCozene Creme ▪ 785

Salicylic Acid (Caution should be exercised). Products include:
DuoFilm Liquid Wart Remover ▪ 804
DuoFilm Patch Wart Remover ▪ 804
DuoPlant Gel Plantar Wart Remover ▪ 804
MG 217 Medicated Tar-Free Shampoo ▪ 835
Occlusal-HP 1054
P&S Shampoo ▪ 605
SalAc 1055
Stri-Dex Clear Gel ▪ 730
Stri-Dex ▪ 730
Wart-Off Wart Remover ▪ 747

Sulfur (Caution should be exercised). Products include:
MG 217 Medicated Tar-Free Shampoo ▪ 835
Novacet Lotion 1054
Sulfacet-R MVL Lotion 909

Topical Medications (Effect not specified).

RETROVIR CAPSULES
(Zidovudine) 1158
May interact with aspirin and acetaminophen containing products, cytotoxic drugs, experimental nucleoside analogues (selected) for aids and arc, and certain other agents. Compounds in these categories include:

Acetaminophen (May competitively inhibit glucuronidation; possible increased incidence of granulocytopenia). Products include:
Actifed Plus Caplets ▪ 845
Actifed Plus Tablets ▪ 845
Actifed Sinus Daytime/Nighttime Tablets and Caplets ▪ 846
Alka-Seltzer Plus Cold Medicine Liqui-Gels ▪ 706
Alka-Seltzer Plus Cold & Cough Medicine Liqui-Gels ▪ 705
Alka-Seltzer Plus Night-Time Cold Medicine Liqui-Gels ▪ 706
Allerest Headache Strength Tablets ▪ 627
Allerest No Drowsiness Tablets ▪ 627
Allerest Sinus Pain Formula ▪ 627
Anexsia 5/500 Elixir 1781
Anexia Tablets 1782
Arthritis Foundation Aspirin Free Caplets ▪ 673
Arthritis Foundation NightTime Caplets ▪ 674
Bayer Select Headache Pain Relief Formula ▪ 716
Bayer Select Menstrual Multi-Symptom Formula ▪ 716
Bayer Select Night Time Pain Relief Formula ▪ 716

(▪ Described in PDR For Nonprescription Drugs)　(⊙ Described in PDR For Ophthalmology)

Interactions Index

Retrovir

Bayer Select Sinus Pain Relief Formula .... ᴾᴰ 717
Benadryl Allergy Sinus Headache Formula Caplets .... ᴾᴰ 849
Comtrex Multi-Symptom Cold Reliever Tablets/Caplets/Liqui-Gels/Liquid .... ᴾᴰ 615
Allergy-Sinus Comtrex Multi-Symptom Allergy-Sinus Formula Tablets .... ᴾᴰ 617
Comtrex Non-Drowsy .... ᴾᴰ 618
Contac Day Allergy/Sinus Caplets ᴾᴰ 812
Contac Day & Night .... ᴾᴰ 812
Contac Night Allergy/Sinus Caplets .... ᴾᴰ 812
Contac Severe Cold and Flu Formula Caplets .... ᴾᴰ 814
Contac Severe Cold & Flu Non-Drowsy .... ᴾᴰ 815
Coricidin 'D' Decongestant Tablets .... ᴾᴰ 800
Coricidin Tablets .... ᴾᴰ 800
DHCplus Capsules 1993
Darvon-N/Darvocet-N 1433
Drixoral Cold and Flu Extended-Release Tablets .... ᴾᴰ 803
Drixoral Cough + Sore Throat Liquid Caps .... ᴾᴰ 802
Drixoral Allergy/Sinus Extended Release Tablets .... ᴾᴰ 804
Esgic-plus Tablets 1013
Aspirin Free Excedrin Analgesic Caplets and Geltabs 732
Excedrin Extra-Strength Analgesic Tablets & Caplets 732
Excedrin P.M. Analgesic/Sleeping Aid Tablets, Caplets, Liquigels 733
Fioricet Tablets 2258
Fioricet with Codeine Capsules 2260
Hycomine Compound Tablets 932
Hydrocet Capsules 782
Legatrin PM .... ᴾᴰ 651
Lorcet 10/650 1018
Lortab 2566
Lurline PMS Tablets 982
Maximum Strength Multi-Symptom Formula Midol .... ᴾᴰ 722
PMS Multi-Symptom Formula Midol .... ᴾᴰ 723
Teen Multi-Symptom Formula Midol .... ᴾᴰ 722
Midrin Capsules 783
Migralam Capsules 2038
Panodol Tablets and Caplets .... ᴾᴰ 824
Children's Panadol Chewable Tablets, Liquid, Infant's Drops .... ᴾᴰ 824
Percocet Tablets 938
Percogesic Analgesic Tablets .... ᴾᴰ 754
Phrenilin 785
Pyrroxate Caplets .... ᴾᴰ 772
Sedapap Tablets 50 mg/650 mg .. 1543
Sinarest Tablets .... ᴾᴰ 648
Sinarest Extra Strength Tablets ...... ᴾᴰ 648
Sinarest No Drowsiness Tablets .... ᴾᴰ 648
Sine-Aid Maximum Strength Sinus Medication Gelcaps, Caplets and Tablets 1554
Sine-Off No Drowsiness Formula Caplets .... ᴾᴰ 824
Sine-Off Sinus Medicine .... ᴾᴰ 825
Singlet Tablets .... ᴾᴰ 825
Sinulin Tablets 787
Sinutab Sinus Allergy Medication, Maximum Strength Tablets and Caplets .... ᴾᴰ 860
Sinutab Sinus Medication, Maximum Strength Without Drowsiness Formula, Tablets & Caplets .... ᴾᴰ 860
Sinutab Sinus Medication, Regular Strength Without Drowsiness Formula .... ᴾᴰ 859
Sudafed Cold and Cough Liquidcaps .... ᴾᴰ 862
Sudafed Severe Cold Formula Caplets .... ᴾᴰ 863
Sudafed Severe Cold Formula Tablets .... ᴾᴰ 864
Sudafed Sinus Caplets .... ᴾᴰ 864
Sudafed Sinus Tablets .... ᴾᴰ 864
Talacen 2333
TheraFlu .... ᴾᴰ 787
TheraFlu Maximum Strength Nighttime Flu, Cold & Cough Medicine .... ᴾᴰ 788
TheraFlu Maximum Strength Non-Drowsy Formula Flu, Cold & Cough Medicine .... ᴾᴰ 788
Thera Flu Maximum Strength, Non-Drowsy Formula Flu, Cold and Cough Caplets .... ᴾᴰ 789
Triaminic Sore Throat Formula ...... ᴾᴰ 791
Triaminicin Tablets .... ᴾᴰ 793
Children's TYLENOL acetaminophen Chewable Tablets, Elixir, Suspension Liquid 1555
Children's TYLENOL Cold Multi-Symptom Liquid Formula and Chewable Tablets 1561
Children's TYLENOL Cold Plus Cough Multi Symptom Tablets and Liquid .... ᴾᴰ 681
Infants' TYLENOL acetaminophen Drops and Suspension Drops 1555
Infants' TYLENOL Cold Decongestant & Fever-Reducer Drops 1556
TYLENOL Extended Relief Caplets.. 1558
TYLENOL, Extra Strength, Acetaminophen Adult Liquid Pain Reliever 1560
TYLENOL, Extra Strength, acetaminophen Gelcaps, Geltabs, Caplets, Tablets 1559
TYLENOL, Extra Strength, Headache Plus Pain Reliever with Antacid Caplets 1559
TYLENOL, Junior Strength, acetaminophen Coated Caplets, Grape and Fruit Chewable Tablets 1557
TYLENOL Maximum Strength Allergy Sinus Medication Gelcaps and Caplets 1563
TYLENOL Maximum Strength Allergy Sinus NightTime Medication Caplets 1555
TYLENOL Flu Maximum Strength Gelcaps 1565
TYLENOL Flu NightTime, Maximum Strength, Gelcaps 1566
TYLENOL Maximum Strength Flu NightTime Hot Medication Packets 1562
TYLENOL, Maximum Strength, Sinus Medication Geltabs, Gelcaps, Caplets and Tablets 1566
TYLENOL Cold Multi-Symptom Formula Medication Tablets and Caplets 1561
TYLENOL Cold Medication No Drowsiness Formula Gelcaps and Caplets 1562
TYLENOL Cold Multi-Symptom Hot Medication Liquid Packets 1557
TYLENOL Cough Multi-Symptom Medication 1564
TYLENOL Cough Multi-Symptom Medication with Decongestant 1565
TYLENOL, Regular Strength, acetaminophen Caplets and Tablets .. 1558
TYLENOL PM, Extra Strength Pain Reliever/Sleep Aid Caplets, Geltabs, Gelcaps 1560
TYLENOL Severe Allergy Medication Caplets 1564
Tylenol with Codeine 1583
Tylox Capsules 1584
Unisom With Pain Relief-Nighttime Sleep Aid and Pain Reliever 1934
Vanquish Analgesic Caplets .... ᴾᴰ 731
Vicks 44 LiquiCaps Cough, Cold & Flu Relief .... ᴾᴰ 755
Vicks 44M Cough, Cold & Flu Relief .... ᴾᴰ 756
Vicks DayQuil .... ᴾᴰ 761
Vicks Nyquil Hot Therapy .... ᴾᴰ 762
Vicks NyQuil LiquiCaps Multi-Symptom Cold/Flu Relief .... ᴾᴰ 763
Vicks NyQuil Multi-Symptom Cold/Flu Relief - (Original & Cherry Flavor) .... ᴾᴰ 763
Vicodin Tablets 1356
Vicodin ES Tablets 1357
Wygesic Tablets 2827
Zydone Capsules 949

Acyclovir (Concomitant use may result in neurotoxicity (profound lethargy)). Products include:

Zovirax Capsules 1219
Zovirax Ointment 5% 1223
Zovirax 1219

Acyclovir Sodium (Concomitant use may result in neurotoxicity (profound lethargy)). Products include:

Zovirax Sterile Powder 1223

Amphotericin B (Increased risk of nephrotoxicity). Products include:

Fungizone Intravenous 506

Aspirin (May competitively inhibit glucuronidation; possible increased incidence of granulocytopenia). Products include:

Alka-Seltzer Effervescent Antacid and Pain Reliever .... ᴾᴰ 701
Alka-Seltzer Extra Strength Effervescent Antacid and Pain Reliever .... ᴾᴰ 703
Alka-Seltzer Lemon Lime Effervescent Antacid and Pain Reliever .... ᴾᴰ 703
Alka-Seltzer Plus Cold Medicine .... ᴾᴰ 705
Alka-Seltzer Plus Cold & Cough Medicine .... ᴾᴰ 708
Alka-Seltzer Plus Night-Time Cold Medicine .... ᴾᴰ 707
Alka Seltzer Plus Sinus Medicine .. ᴾᴰ 707
Arthritis Foundation Safety Coated Aspirin Tablets .... ᴾᴰ 675
Arthritis Pain Ascriptin .... ᴾᴰ 631
Maximum Strength Ascriptin .... ᴾᴰ 630
Regular Strength Ascriptin Tablets .... ᴾᴰ 629
Arthritis Strength BC Powder .... ᴾᴰ 609
BC Cold Powder Multi-Symptom Formula (Cold-Sinus-Allergy) ...... ᴾᴰ 609
BC Cold Powder Non-Drowsy Formula (Cold-Sinus) .... ᴾᴰ 609
BC Powder .... ᴾᴰ 609
Bayer Children's Chewable Aspirin .... ᴾᴰ 711
Genuine Bayer Aspirin Tablets & Caplets .... ᴾᴰ 713
Extra Strength Bayer Arthritis Pain Regimen Formula .... ᴾᴰ 711
Extra Strength Bayer Aspirin Caplets & Tablets .... ᴾᴰ 712
Extended-Release Bayer 8-Hour Aspirin .... ᴾᴰ 712
Extra Strength Bayer Plus Aspirin Caplets .... ᴾᴰ 713
Extra Strength Bayer PM Aspirin .. ᴾᴰ 713
Bayer Enteric Aspirin .... ᴾᴰ 709
Bufferin Analgesic Tablets and Caplets .... ᴾᴰ 613
Arthritis Strength Bufferin Analgesic Caplets .... ᴾᴰ 614
Extra Strength Bufferin Analgesic Tablets .... ᴾᴰ 615
Cama Arthritis Pain Reliever .... ᴾᴰ 785
Darvon Compound-65 Pulvules 1435
Easprin 1914
Ecotrin 2455
Ecotrin Enteric Coated Aspirin Maximum Strength Tablets and Caplets .... ᴾᴰ 816
Ecotrin Enteric Coated Aspirin Regular Strength Tablets 2455
Empirin Aspirin Tablets .... ᴾᴰ 854
Empirin with Codeine Tablets 1093
Excedrin Extra-Strength Analgesic Tablets & Caplets 732
Fiorinal Capsules 2261
Fiorinal with Codeine Capsules 2262
Fiorinal Tablets 2261
Halfprin 1362
Healthprin Aspirin 2455
Norgesic 1496
Percodan Tablets 939
Percodan-Demi Tablets 940
Robaxisal Tablets 2071
Soma Compound w/Codeine Tablets 2676
Soma Compound Tablets 2675
St. Joseph Adult Chewable Aspirin (81 mg.) .... ᴾᴰ 808
Talwin Compound 2335
Ursinus Inlay-Tabs .... ᴾᴰ 794
Vanquish Analgesic Caplets .... ᴾᴰ 731

Atovaquone (Co-administration shows a 24% +/-12% decrease in zidovudine oral clearance, leading to a 35% +/-23% increase in plasma zidovudine AUC; this effect is minor and would not expect to produce clinically significant events). Products include:

Mepron Suspension 1135

Bleomycin Sulfate (Increased risk of hematological toxicity). Products include:

Blenoxane 692

Dapsone (Increased risk of hematological toxicity). Products include:

Dapsone Tablets USP 1284

Daunorubicin Hydrochloride (Increased risk of hematological toxicity). Products include:

Cerubidine 795

Divalproex Sodium (Valproic acid increases the oral bioavailability of zidovudine through the inhibition of first-pass hepatic metabolism; patients should be monitored closely for zidovudine-related adverse effects). Products include:

Depakote Tablets 415

Doxorubicin Hydrochloride (Increased risk of hematological toxicity). Products include:

Adriamycin PFS 1947
Adriamycin RDF 1947
Doxorubicin Astra 540
Rubex 712

Fluconazole (Co-administration may interfere with the oral clearance and metabolism of zidovudine). Products include:

Diflucan Injection, Tablets, and Oral Suspension 2194

Flucytosine (Increased risk of hematological toxicity). Products include:

Ancobon Capsules 2079

Fluorouracil (Increased risk of hematological toxicity). Products include:

Efudex 2113
Fluoroplex Topical Solution & Cream 1% 479
Fluorouracil Injection 2116

Ganciclovir Sodium (May increase the potential for hematological toxicity). Products include:

Cytovene-IV 2103

Hydroxyurea (Increased risk of hematological toxicity). Products include:

Hydrea Capsules 696

Indomethacin (Inhibits glucuronidation of Retrovir). Products include:

Indocin 1680

Indomethacin Sodium Trihydrate (Inhibits glucuronidation of Retrovir). Products include:

Indocin I.V. 1684

Interferon alfa-2A, Recombinant (Increased risk of hematological toxicity). Products include:

Roferon-A Injection 2145

Interferon alfa-2B, Recombinant (Increased risk of hematological toxicity). Products include:

Intron A 2364

Methadone Hydrochloride (Elevates plasma levels in some patients and while remaining unchanged in others). Products include:

Methadone Hydrochloride Oral Concentrate 2233
Methadone Hydrochloride Oral Solution & Tablets 2235

Methotrexate Sodium (Increased risk of hematological toxicity). Products include:

Methotrexate Sodium Tablets, Injection, for Injection and LPF Injection 1275

Mitotane (Increased risk of toxicity). Products include:

Lysodren 698

Mitoxantrone Hydrochloride (Increased risk of hematological toxicity). Products include:

Novantrone 1279

Nephrotoxic Drugs (Increased risk of toxicity).

Pentamidine Isethionate (Increased risk of toxicity). Products include:

NebuPent for Inhalation Solution 1040
Pentam 300 Injection 1041

IMPORTANT NOTE: Always consult each drug listing in the patient's regimen for possible interactions.

Phenytoin (Possible alteration in the phenytoin plasma levels; low levels in some patients; high level documented in one case). Products include:
- Dilantin Infatabs ... 1908
- Dilantin-125 Suspension ... 1911

Phenytoin Sodium (Possible alteration in the phenytoin plasma levels; low levels in some patients; high level documented in one case). Products include:
- Dilantin Kapseals ... 1906
- Dilantin Parenteral ... 1910

Probenecid (Inhibits glucuronidation of Retrovir; may reduce renal excretion of Retrovir; concomitant use may result in flu-like symptoms consisting of myalgia, malaise and/or fever and maculopapular rash). Products include:
- Benemid Tablets ... 1611
- ColBENEMID Tablets ... 1622

Procarbazine Hydrochloride (Increased risk of hematological toxicity). Products include:
- Matulane Capsules ... 2131

Ribavirin (Some experimental nucleoside analogues affecting DNA replication, such as ribavirin, antagonizes the *in vitro* antiviral activity of Retrovir against HIV and thus concomitant use of such drugs should be avoided). Products include:
- Virazole ... 1264

Rifampin (Coadministration decreases the area under the plasma concentration curve by an average of 48% +/- 34%). Products include:
- Rifadin ... 1528
- Rifamate Capsules ... 1530
- Rifater ... 1532
- Rimactane Capsules ... 847

Tamoxifen Citrate (Increased risk of hematological toxicity). Products include:
- Nolvadex Tablets ... 2841

Valproic Acid (Increases the oral bioavailability of zidovudine through the inhibition of first-pass hepatic metabolism). Products include:
- Depakene ... 413

Vinblastine Sulfate (Increased risk of hematological toxicity). Products include:
- Velban Vials ... 1484

Vincristine Sulfate (Increased risk of hematological toxicity). Products include:
- Oncovin Solution Vials & Hyporets 1466

Food Interactions

Food, unspecified (Administration of Retrovir Capsules with food decreased peak plasma concentrations by greater than 50%, however, bioavailability as determined by AUC may not be affected).

RETROVIR I.V. INFUSION

(Zidovudine) ... 1163

May interact with cytotoxic drugs, aspirin and acetaminophen containing products, experimental nucleoside analogues (selected) for aids and arc, and certain other agents. Compounds in these categories include:

Acetaminophen (May competitively inhibit glucuronidation; possible increased incidence of granulocytopenia). Products include:
- Actifed Plus Caplets ... ▣ 845
- Actifed Plus Tablets ... ▣ 845
- Actifed Sinus Daytime/Nighttime Tablets and Caplets ... ▣ 846
- Alka-Seltzer Plus Cold Medicine Liqui-Gels ... ▣ 706
- Alka-Seltzer Plus Cold & Cough Medicine Liqui-Gels ... ▣ 705
- Alka-Seltzer Plus Night-Time Cold Medicine Liqui-Gels ... ▣ 706
- Allerest Headache Strength Tablets ... ▣ 627
- Allerest No Drowsiness Tablets ... ▣ 627
- Allerest Sinus Pain Formula ... ▣ 627
- Anexsia 5/500 Elixir ... 1781
- Anexia Tablets ... 1782
- Arthritis Foundation Aspirin Free Caplets ... ▣ 673
- Arthritis Foundation NightTime Caplets ... ▣ 674
- Bayer Select Headache Pain Relief Formula ... ▣ 716
- Bayer Select Menstrual Multi-Symptom Formula ... ▣ 716
- Bayer Select Night Time Pain Relief Formula ... ▣ 716
- Bayer Select Sinus Pain Relief Formula ... ▣ 717
- Benadryl Allergy Sinus Headache Formula Caplets ... ▣ 849
- Comtrex Multi-Symptom Cold Reliever Tablets/Caplets/Liqui-Gels/Liquid ... ▣ 615
- Allergy-Sinus Comtrex Multi-Symptom Allergy-Sinus Formula Tablets ... ▣ 617
- Comtrex Non-Drowsy ... ▣ 618
- Contac Day Allergy/Sinus Caplets ▣ 812
- Contac Day & Night ... ▣ 812
- Contac Night Allergy/Sinus Caplets ... ▣ 812
- Contac Severe Cold and Flu Formula Caplets ... ▣ 814
- Contac Severe Cold & Flu Non-Drowsy ... ▣ 815
- Coricidin 'D' Decongestant Tablets ... ▣ 800
- Coricidin Tablets ... ▣ 800
- DHCplus Capsules ... 1993
- Darvon-N/Darvocet-N ... 1433
- Drixoral Cold and Flu Extended-Release Tablets ... ▣ 803
- Drixoral Cough + Sore Throat Liquid Caps ... ▣ 802
- Drixoral Allergy/Sinus Extended Release Tablets ... ▣ 804
- Esgic-plus Tablets ... 1013
- Aspirin Free Excedrin Analgesic Caplets and Geltabs ... 732
- Excedrin Extra-Strength Analgesic Tablets & Caplets ... 732
- Excedrin P.M. Analgesic/Sleeping Aid Tablets, Caplets, Liquigels ... 733
- Fioricet Tablets ... 2258
- Fioricet with Codeine Capsules ... 2260
- Hycomine Compound Tablets ... 932
- Hydrocet Capsules ... 782
- Legatrin PM ... ▣ 651
- Lorcet 10/650 ... 1018
- Lortab ... 2566
- Lurline PMS Tablets ... 982
- Maximum Strength Multi-Symptom Formula Midol ... ▣ 722
- PMS Multi-Symptom Formula Midol ... ▣ 723
- Teen Multi-Symptom Formula Midol ... ▣ 722
- Midrin Capsules ... 783
- Migralam Capsules ... 2038
- Panodol Tablets and Caplets ... ▣ 824
- Children's Panadol Chewable Tablets, Liquid, Infant's Drops ... ▣ 824
- Percocet Tablets ... 938
- Percogesic Analgesic Tablets ... ▣ 754
- Phrenilin ... 785
- Pyrroxate Caplets ... ▣ 772
- Sedapap Tablets 50 mg/650 mg ... 1543
- Sinarest Tablets ... ▣ 648
- Sinarest Extra Strength Tablets ... ▣ 648
- Sinarest No Drowsiness Tablets ... ▣ 648
- Sine-Aid Maximum Strength Sinus Medication Gelcaps, Caplets and Tablets ... 1554
- Sine-Off No Drowsiness Formula Caplets ... ▣ 824
- Sine-Off Sinus Medicine ... ▣ 825
- Singlet Tablets ... ▣ 825
- Sinulin Tablets ... 787
- Sinutab Sinus Allergy Medication, Maximum Strength Tablets and Caplets ... ▣ 860
- Sinutab Sinus Medication, Maximum Strength Without Drowsiness Formula, Tablets & Caplets ... ▣ 860
- Sinutab Sinus Medication, Regular Strength Without Drowsiness Formula ... ▣ 859
- Sudafed Cold and Cough Liquidcaps ... ▣ 862
- Sudafed Severe Cold Formula Caplets ... ▣ 863
- Sudafed Severe Cold Formula Tablets ... ▣ 864
- Sudafed Sinus Caplets ... ▣ 864
- Sudafed Sinus Tablets ... ▣ 864
- Talacen ... 2333
- TheraFlu ... ▣ 787
- TheraFlu Maximum Strength Nighttime Flu, Cold & Cough Medicine ... ▣ 788
- TheraFlu Maximum Strength Non-Drowsy Formula Flu, Cold & Cough Medicine ... ▣ 788
- Thera Flu Maximum Strength, Non-Drowsy Formula Flu, Cold and Cough Caplets ... ▣ 789
- Triaminic Sore Throat Formula ... ▣ 791
- Triaminicin Tablets ... ▣ 793
- Children's TYLENOL acetaminophen Chewable Tablets, Elixir, Suspension Liquid ... 1555
- Children's TYLENOL Cold Multi-Symptom Liquid Formula and Chewable Tablets ... 1561
- Children's TYLENOL Cold Plus Cough Multi Symptom Tablets and Liquid ... ▣ 681
- Infants' TYLENOL acetaminophen Drops and Suspension Drops ... 1555
- Infants' TYLENOL Cold Decongestant & Fever-Reducer Drops ... 1556
- TYLENOL Extended Relief Caplets .. 1558
- TYLENOL, Extra Strength, Acetaminophen Adult Liquid Pain Reliever ... 1560
- TYLENOL, Extra Strength, acetaminophen Gelcaps, Geltabs, Caplets, Tablets ... 1559
- TYLENOL, Extra Strength, Headache Plus Pain Reliever with Antacid Caplets ... 1559
- TYLENOL, Junior Strength, acetaminophen Coated Caplets, Grape and Fruit Chewable Tablets ... 1557
- TYLENOL Maximum Strength Allergy Sinus Medication Gelcaps and Caplets ... 1563
- TYLENOL Maximum Strength Allergy Sinus NightTime Medication Caplets ... 1555
- TYLENOL Flu Maximum Strength Gelcaps ... 1565
- TYLENOL Flu NightTime, Maximum Strength, Gelcaps ... 1566
- TYLENOL Maximum Strength Flu NightTime Hot Medication Packets ... 1562
- TYLENOL, Maximum Strength, Sinus Medication Geltabs, Gelcaps, Caplets and Tablets ... 1566
- TYLENOL Cold Multi-Symptom Formula Medication Tablets and Caplets ... 1561
- TYLENOL Cold Medication No Drowsiness Formula Gelcaps and Caplets ... 1562
- TYLENOL Cold Multi-Symptom Hot Medication Liquid Packets ... 1557
- TYLENOL Cough Multi-Symptom Medication ... 1564
- TYLENOL Cough Multi-Symptom Medication with Decongestant ... 1565
- TYLENOL, Regular Strength, acetaminophen Caplets and Tablets .. 1558
- TYLENOL PM, Extra Strength Pain Reliever/Sleep Aid Caplets, Geltabs, Gelcaps ... 1560
- TYLENOL Severe Allergy Medication Caplets ... 1564
- Tylenol with Codeine ... 1583
- Tylox Capsules ... 1584
- Unisom With Pain Relief-Nighttime Sleep Aid and Pain Reliever ... 1934
- Vanquish Analgesic Caplets ... ▣ 731
- Vicks 44 LiquiCaps Cough, Cold & Flu Relief ... ▣ 755
- Vicks 44M Cough, Cold & Flu Relief ... ▣ 756
- Vicks DayQuil ... ▣ 761
- Vicks Nyquil Hot Therapy ... ▣ 762
- Vicks NyQuil LiquiCaps Multi-Symptom Cold/Flu Relief ... ▣ 763
- Vicks NyQuil Multi-Symptom Cold/Flu Relief - (Original & Cherry Flavor) ... ▣ 763
- Vicodin Tablets ... 1356
- Vicodin ES Tablets ... 1357
- Wygesic Tablets ... 2827
- Zydone Capsules ... 949

Acyclovir (One published report of neurotoxicity (profound lethargy) associated with concomitant use; may increase the potential for hematological toxicity). Products include:
- Zovirax Capsules ... 1219
- Zovirax Ointment 5% ... 1223
- Zovirax ... 1219

Acyclovir Sodium (One published report of neurotoxicity (profound lethargy) associated with concomitant use; may increase the potential for hematological toxicity). Products include:
- Zovirax Sterile Powder ... 1223

Amphotericin B (Increased risk of nephrotoxicity). Products include:
- Fungizone Intravenous ... 506

Aspirin (May competitively inhibit glucuronidation; possible increased incidence of granulocytopenia). Products include:
- Alka-Seltzer Effervescent Antacid and Pain Reliever ... ▣ 701
- Alka-Seltzer Extra Strength Effervescent Antacid and Pain Reliever ... ▣ 703
- Alka-Seltzer Lemon Lime Effervescent Antacid and Pain Reliever ... ▣ 703
- Alka-Seltzer Plus Cold Medicine ... ▣ 705
- Alka-Seltzer Plus Cold & Cough Medicine ... ▣ 708
- Alka-Seltzer Plus Night-Time Cold Medicine ... ▣ 707
- Alka Seltzer Plus Sinus Medicine .. ▣ 707
- Arthritis Foundation Safety Coated Aspirin Tablets ... ▣ 675
- Arthritis Pain Ascriptin ... ▣ 631
- Maximum Strength Ascriptin ... ▣ 630
- Regular Strength Ascriptin Tablets ... ▣ 629
- Arthritis Strength BC Powder ... ▣ 609
- BC Cold Powder Multi-Symptom Formula (Cold-Sinus-Allergy) ... ▣ 609
- BC Cold Powder Non-Drowsy Formula (Cold-Sinus) ... ▣ 609
- BC Powder ... ▣ 609
- Bayer Children's Chewable Aspirin ... ▣ 711
- Genuine Bayer Aspirin Tablets & Caplets ... ▣ 713
- Extra Strength Bayer Arthritis Pain Regimen Formula ... ▣ 711
- Extra Strength Bayer Aspirin Caplets & Tablets ... ▣ 712
- Extended-Release Bayer 8-Hour Aspirin ... ▣ 712
- Extra Strength Bayer Plus Aspirin Caplets ... ▣ 713
- Extra Strength Bayer PM Aspirin .. ▣ 713
- Bayer Enteric Aspirin ... ▣ 709
- Bufferin Analgesic Tablets and Caplets ... ▣ 613
- Arthritis Strength Bufferin Analgesic Caplets ... ▣ 614
- Extra Strength Bufferin Analgesic Tablets ... ▣ 615
- Cama Arthritis Pain Reliever ... ▣ 785
- Darvon Compound-65 Pulvules ... 1435
- Easprin ... 1914
- Ecotrin ... 2455
- Ecotrin Enteric Coated Aspirin Maximum Strength Tablets and Caplets ... ▣ 816
- Ecotrin Enteric Coated Aspirin Regular Strength Tablets ... 2455
- Empirin Aspirin Tablets ... ▣ 854
- Empirin with Codeine Tablets ... 1093
- Excedrin Extra-Strength Analgesic Tablets & Caplets ... 732
- Fiorinal Capsules ... 2261
- Fiorinal with Codeine Capsules ... 2262
- Fiorinal Tablets ... 2261
- Halfprin ... 1362
- Healthprin Aspirin ... 2455
- Norgesic ... 1496
- Percodan Tablets ... 939
- Percodan-Demi Tablets ... 940
- Robaxisal Tablets ... 2071
- Soma Compound w/Codeine Tablets ... 2676
- Soma Compound Tablets ... 2675
- St. Joseph Adult Chewable Aspirin (81 mg.) ... ▣ 808
- Talwin Compound ... 2335

(▣ Described in PDR For Nonprescription Drugs) (⊙ Described in PDR For Ophthalmology)

887 **Interactions Index** **Rhinocort**

Ursinus Inlay-Tabs ▣ 794
Vanquish Analgesic Caplets ▣ 731

Atovaquone (Co-administration shows a 24% +/-12% decrease in zidovudine oral clearance, leading to a 35% +/-23% increase in plasma zidovudine AUC; this effect is minor and would not expect to produce clinically significant events). Products include:
Mepron Suspension 1135

Bleomycin Sulfate (Increased risk of hematological toxicity). Products include:
Blenoxane 692

Dapsone (Increased risk of hematological toxicity). Products include:
Dapsone Tablets USP 1284

Daunorubicin Hydrochloride (Increased risk of hematological toxicity). Products include:
Cerubidine 795

Divalproex Sodium (Increases the oral bioavailability of zidovudine through the inhibition of first-pass hepatic metabolism). Products include:
Depakote Tablets 415

Doxorubicin Hydrochloride (Increased risk of hematological toxicity). Products include:
Adriamycin PFS 1947
Adriamycin RDF 1947
Doxorubicin Astra 540
Rubex 712

Fluconazole (Co-administration may interfere with the oral clearance and metabolism of zidovudine). Products include:
Diflucan Injection, Tablets, and Oral Suspension 2194

Flucytosine (Increased risk of hematological toxicity). Products include:
Ancobon Capsules 2079

Fluorouracil (Increased risk of hematological toxicity). Products include:
Efudex 2113
Fluoroplex Topical Solution & Cream 1% 479
Fluorouracil Injection 2116

Ganciclovir Sodium (May increase the potential for hematological toxicity). Products include:
Cytovene-IV 2103

Hydroxyurea (Increased risk of hematological toxicity). Products include:
Hydrea Capsules 696

Indomethacin (May competitively inhibit glucuronidation). Products include:
Indocin 1680

Indomethacin Sodium Trihydrate (May competitively inhibit glucuronidation). Products include:
Indocin I.V. 1684

Interferon alfa-2A, Recombinant (Increased risk of hematological toxicity). Products include:
Roferon-A Injection 2145

Interferon alfa-2B, Recombinant (Increased risk of hematological toxicity). Products include:
Intron A 2364

Methotrexate Sodium (Increased risk of hematological toxicity). Products include:
Methotrexate Sodium Tablets, Injection, for Injection and LPF Injection 1275

Mitotane (Increased risk of toxicity). Products include:
Lysodren 698

Mitoxantrone Hydrochloride (Increased risk of toxicity). Products include:
Novantrone 1279

Nephrotoxic Drugs (Increased risk of toxicity).

Pentamidine Isethionate (Increased risk of toxicity). Products include:
NebuPent for Inhalation Solution 1040
Pentam 300 Injection 1041

Phenytoin (Low phenytoin levels reported in some patients; high level documented in one case). Products include:
Dilantin Infatabs 1908
Dilantin-125 Suspension 1911

Phenytoin Sodium (Low phenytoin levels reported in some patients; high level documented in one case). Products include:
Dilantin Kapseals 1906
Dilantin Parenteral 1910

Probenecid (May inhibit glucuronidation and/or reduce renal excretion of zidovudine). Products include:
Benemid Tablets 1611
ColBENEMID Tablets 1622

Procarbazine Hydrochloride (Increased risk of hematological toxicity). Products include:
Matulane Capsules 2131

Tamoxifen Citrate (Increased risk of hematological toxicity). Products include:
Nolvadex Tablets 2841

Valproic Acid (Increases the oral bioavailability of zidovudine through the inhibition of first-pass hepatic metabolism). Products include:
Depakene 413

Vinblastine Sulfate (Increased risk of hematological toxicity). Products include:
Velban Vials 1484

Vincristine Sulfate (Increased risk of hematological toxicity). Products include:
Oncovin Solution Vials & Hyporets 1466

RETROVIR SYRUP
(Zidovudine) 1158
See **Retrovir Capsules**

RēV-EYES OPHTHALMIC EYEDROPS 0.5%
(Dapiprazole Hydrochloride) ◉ 323
None cited in PDR database.

REVIA TABLETS
(Naltrexone Hydrochloride) 940
May interact with narcotic analgesics and certain other agents. Compounds in these categories include:

Alfentanil Hydrochloride (Concurrent use is contraindicated; severe withdrawal syndromes may be precipitated by the concurrent ingestion of opioids). Products include:
Alfenta Injection 1286

Buprenorphine (Concurrent use is contraindicated; severe withdrawal syndromes may be precipitated by the concurrent ingestion of opioids). Products include:
Buprenex Injectable 2006

Codeine Phosphate (Concurrent use is contraindicated; severe withdrawal syndromes may be precipitated by the concurrent ingestion of opioids). Products include:
Actifed with Codeine Cough Syrup 1067
Brontex 1981
Deconsal C Expectorant Syrup 456
Deconsal Pediatric Syrup 457
Dimetane-DC Cough Syrup 2059
Empirin with Codeine Tablets 1093
Fioricet with Codeine Capsules 2260
Fiorinal with Codeine Capsules 2262
Isoclor Expectorant 990
Novahistine DH 2462
Novahistine Expectorant 2463
Nucofed 2051
Phenergan with Codeine 2777
Phenergan VC with Codeine 2781
Robitussin A-C Syrup 2073
Robitussin-DAC Syrup 2074
Ryna ▣ 841
Soma Compound w/Codeine Tablets 2676
Tussi-Organidin NR Liquid and S NR Liquid 2677
Tylenol with Codeine 1583

Dezocine (Concurrent use is contraindicated; severe withdrawal syndromes may be precipitated by the concurrent ingestion of opioids). Products include:
Dalgan Injection 538

Difenoxin Hydrochloride (Patients may not benefit from opioid-containing antidiarrheal preparations). Products include:
Motofen Tablets 784

Diphenoxylate Hydrochloride (Patients may not benefit from opioid-containing antidiarrheal preparations). Products include:
Lomotil 2439

Fentanyl (Concurrent use is contraindicated; severe withdrawal syndromes may be precipitated by the concurrent ingestion of opioids). Products include:
Duragesic Transdermal System 1288

Fentanyl Citrate (Concurrent use is contraindicated; severe withdrawal syndromes may be precipitated by the concurrent ingestion of opioids). Products include:
Sublimaze Injection 1307

Hydrocodone Bitartrate (Concurrent use is contraindicated; severe withdrawal syndromes may be precipitated by the concurrent ingestion of opioids). Products include:
Anexsia 5/500 Elixir 1781
Anexia Tablets 1782
Codiclear DH Syrup 791
Deconamine CX Cough and Cold Liquid and Tablets 1319
Duratuss HD Elixir 2565
Hycodan Tablets and Syrup 930
Hycomine Compound Tablets 932
Hycomine 931
Hycotuss Expectorant Syrup 933
Hydrocet Capsules 782
Lorcet 10/650 1018
Lortab 2566
Tussend 1783
Tussend Expectorant 1785
Vicodin Tablets 1356
Vicodin ES Tablets 1357
Vicodin Tuss Expectorant 1358
Zydone Capsules 949

Hydrocodone Polistirex (Concurrent use is contraindicated; severe withdrawal syndromes may be precipitated by the concurrent ingestion of opioids). Products include:
Tussionex Pennkinetic Extended-Release Suspension 998

Levorphanol Tartrate (Concurrent use is contraindicated; severe withdrawal syndromes may be precipitated by the concurrent ingestion of opioids). Products include:
Levo-Dromoran 2129

Meperidine Hydrochloride (Concurrent use is contraindicated; severe withdrawal syndromes may be precipitated by the concurrent ingestion of opioids). Products include:
Demerol 2308
Mepergan Injection 2753

Methadone Hydrochloride (Concurrent use is contraindicated; severe withdrawal syndromes may be precipitated by the concurrent ingestion of opioids). Products include:
Methadone Hydrochloride Oral Concentrate 2233
Methadone Hydrochloride Oral Solution & Tablets 2235

Morphine Sulfate (Concurrent use is contraindicated; severe withdrawal syndromes may be precipitated by the concurrent ingestion of opioids). Products include:
Astramorph/PF Injection, USP (Preservative-Free) 535
Duramorph 962
Infumorph 200 and Infumorph 500 Sterile Solutions 965
MS Contin Tablets 1994
MSIR 1997
Oramorph SR (Morphine Sulfate Sustained Release Tablets) 2236
RMS Suppositories 2657
Roxanol 2243

Opium Alkaloids (Concurrent use is contraindicated; severe withdrawal syndromes may be precipitated by the concurrent ingestion of opioids).
No products indexed under this heading.

Oxycodone Hydrochloride (Concurrent use is contraindicated; severe withdrawal syndromes may be precipitated by the concurrent ingestion of opioids). Products include:
Percocet Tablets 938
Percodan Tablets 939
Percodan-Demi Tablets 940
Roxicodone Tablets, Oral Solution & Intensol (Oxycodone) 2244
Tylox Capsules 1584

Propoxyphene Hydrochloride (Concurrent use is contraindicated; severe withdrawal syndromes may be precipitated by the concurrent ingestion of opioids). Products include:
Darvon 1435
Wygesic Tablets 2827

Propoxyphene Napsylate (Concurrent use is contraindicated; severe withdrawal syndromes may be precipitated by the concurrent ingestion of opioids). Products include:
Darvon-N/Darvocet-N 1433

Sufentanil Citrate (Concurrent use is contraindicated; severe withdrawal syndromes may be precipitated by the concurrent ingestion of opioids). Products include:
Sufenta Injection 1309

Thioridazine Hydrochloride (Lethargy and somnolence have been reported following doses of ReVia and thioridazine). Products include:
Mellaril 2269

REVEX
(Nalmefene Hydrochloride) 1811
May interact with:

Flumazenil (Co-administration may produce seizures). Products include:
Romazicon 2147

RHEABAN MAXIMUM STRENGTH FAST ACTING CAPLETS
(Attapulgite, Activated) ▣ 743
None cited in PDR database.

RHINOCORT NASAL INHALER
(Budesonide) 556
None cited in PDR database.

IMPORTANT NOTE: Always consult each drug listing in the patient's regimen for possible interactions.

RHOGAM RH$_0$(D) IMMUNE GLOBULIN (HUMAN)
(Immune Globulin (Human)) 1847
None cited in PDR database.

RICOBID-D PEDIATRIC SUSPENSION
(Phenylephrine Tannate)....................2038
None cited in PDR database.

RICOBID TABLETS AND PEDIATRIC SUSPENSION
(Chlorpheniramine Tannate, Phenylephrine Tannate) 2038
None cited in PDR database.

RID LICE CONTROL SPRAY
(Permethrin)....................1933
None cited in PDR database.

RID LICE KILLING SHAMPOO
(Pyrethrum Extract, Piperonyl Butoxide)....................1933
None cited in PDR database.

RIDAURA CAPSULES
(Auranofin) 2513
May interact with:

Phenytoin (Increased phenytoin blood levels). Products include:
- Dilantin Infatabs 1908
- Dilantin-125 Suspension 1911

Phenytoin Sodium (Increased phenytoin blood levels). Products include:
- Dilantin Kapseals 1906
- Dilantin Parenteral 1910

RIFADIN CAPSULES
(Rifampin)....................1528
May interact with oral anticoagulants, corticosteroids, cardiac glycosides, oral contraceptives, oral hypoglycemic agents, narcotic analgesics, barbiturates, beta blockers, anticonvulsants, xanthine bronchodilators, progestins, and certain other agents. Compounds in these categories include:

Acarbose (Reduced activity of oral hypoglycemic agent).
- No products indexed under this heading.

Acebutolol Hydrochloride (Diminished effects of concurrently administered beta blocker). Products include:
- Sectral Capsules 2807

Alfentanil Hydrochloride (Reduced activity of narcotics). Products include:
- Alfenta Injection 1286

Aminophylline (Diminished effects of concurrently administered theophylline).
- No products indexed under this heading.

Aprobarbital (Diminished effects of concurrently administered barbiturate).
- No products indexed under this heading.

Atenolol (Diminished effects of concurrently administered beta blocker). Products include:
- Tenoretic Tablets 2845
- Tenormin Tablets and I.V. Injection 2847

Betamethasone Acetate (Reduced activity of corticosteroid). Products include:
- Celestone Soluspan Suspension 2347

Betamethasone Sodium Phosphate (Reduced activity of corticosteroid). Products include:
- Celestone Soluspan Suspension 2347

Betaxolol Hydrochloride (Diminished effects of concurrently administered beta blocker). Products include:
- Betoptic Ophthalmic Solution.......... 469
- Betoptic S Ophthalmic Suspension 471
- Kerlone Tablets.................... 2436

Bisoprolol Fumarate (Diminished effects of concurrently administered beta blocker). Products include:
- Zebeta Tablets 1413
- Ziac 1415

Buprenorphine (Reduced activity of narcotics). Products include:
- Buprenex Injectable 2006

Butabarbital (Diminished effects of concurrently administered barbiturate).
- No products indexed under this heading.

Butalbital (Diminished effects of concurrently administered barbiturate). Products include:
- Esgic-plus Tablets 1013
- Fioricet Tablets 2258
- Fioricet with Codeine Capsules 2260
- Fiorinal Capsules 2261
- Fiorinal with Codeine Capsules 2262
- Fiorinal Tablets 2261
- Phrenilin 785
- Sedapap Tablets 50 mg/650 mg .. 1543

Carbamazepine (Diminished effects of concurrently administered anticonvulsant). Products include:
- Atretol Tablets 573
- Tegretol Chewable Tablets 852
- Tegretol Suspension.................... 852
- Tegretol Tablets 852

Carteolol Hydrochloride (Diminished effects of concurrently administered beta blocker). Products include:
- Cartrol Tablets 410
- Ocupress Ophthalmic Solution, 1% Sterile.................... ⊙ 309

Chloramphenicol (Diminished effects of concurrently administered chloramphenicol). Products include:
- Chloromycetin Ophthalmic Ointment, 1% .... ⊙ 310
- Chloromycetin Ophthalmic Solution.................... ⊙ 310
- Chloroptic S.O.P. .... ⊙ 239
- Chloroptic Sterile Ophthalmic Solution .... ⊙ 239
- Elase-Chloromycetin Ointment 1040
- Ophthocort .... ⊙ 311

Chloramphenicol Palmitate (Diminished effects of concurrently administered chloramphenicol).
- No products indexed under this heading.

Chloramphenicol Sodium Succinate (Diminished effects of concurrently administered chloramphenicol). Products include:
- Chloromycetin Sodium Succinate.... 1900

Chlorpropamide (Reduced activity of oral hypoglycemic agent). Products include:
- Diabinese Tablets 1935

Clofibrate (Diminished effects of concurrently administered clofibrate). Products include:
- Atromid-S Capsules 2701

Codeine Phosphate (Reduced activity of narcotics). Products include:
- Actifed with Codeine Cough Syrup.. 1067
- Brontex 1981
- Deconsal C Expectorant Syrup 456
- Deconsal Pediatric Syrup.................... 457
- Dimetane-DC Cough Syrup 2059
- Empirin with Codeine Tablets........... 1093
- Fioricet with Codeine Capsules 2260
- Fiorinal with Codeine Capsules 2262
- Isoclor Expectorant.................... 990
- Novahistine DH.................... 2462
- Novahistine Expectorant.................... 2463
- Nucofed 2051
- Phenergan with Codeine.................... 2777
- Phenergan VC with Codeine 2781
- Robitussin A-C Syrup 2073
- Robitussin-DAC Syrup 2074
- Ryna .... ▣ 841
- Soma Compound w/Codeine Tablets 2676
- Tussi-Organidin NR Liquid and S NR Liquid 2677
- Tylenol with Codeine 1583

Cortisone Acetate (Reduced activity of corticosteroid). Products include:
- Cortone Acetate Sterile Suspension 1623
- Cortone Acetate Tablets 1624

Cyclosporine (Reduced activity of cyclosporin). Products include:
- Neoral 2276
- Sandimmune 2286

Dapsone (Reduced activity of dapsone). Products include:
- Dapsone Tablets USP 1284

Deslanoside (Reduced activity of cardiac glycoside).
- No products indexed under this heading.

Desogestrel (Reduced activity of oral contraceptives; patients using oral contraceptives should be advised to change to nonhormonal methods of birth control). Products include:
- Desogen Tablets.................... 1817
- Ortho-Cept 1851

Dexamethasone (Reduced activity of corticosteroid). Products include:
- AK-Trol Ointment & Suspension .... ⊙ 205
- Decadron Elixir 1633
- Decadron Tablets.................... 1635
- Decaspray Topical Aerosol 1648
- Dexacidin Ointment .... ⊙ 263
- Maxitrol Ophthalmic Ointment and Suspension .... ⊙ 224
- TobraDex Ophthalmic Suspension and Ointment.................... 473

Dexamethasone Acetate (Reduced activity of corticosteroid). Products include:
- Dalalone D.P. Injectable 1011
- Decadron-LA Sterile Suspension...... 1646

Dexamethasone Sodium Phosphate (Reduced activity of corticosteroid). Products include:
- Decadron Phosphate Injection 1637
- Decadron Phosphate Respihaler...... 1642
- Decadron Phosphate Sterile Ophthalmic Ointment.................... 1641
- Decadron Phosphate Sterile Ophthalmic Solution 1642
- Decadron Phosphate Topical Cream.................... 1644
- Decadron Phosphate Turbinaire 1645
- Decadron Phosphate with Xylocaine Injection, Sterile 1639
- Dexacort Phosphate in Respihaler .. 458
- Dexacort Phosphate in Turbinaire .. 459
- NeoDecadron Sterile Ophthalmic Ointment 1712
- NeoDecadron Sterile Ophthalmic Solution 1713
- NeoDecadron Topical Cream 1714

Dezocine (Reduced activity of narcotics). Products include:
- Dalgan Injection 538

Diazepam (Diminished effects of concurrently administered diazepam). Products include:
- Dizac 1809
- Valium Injectable 2182
- Valium Tablets 2183
- Valrelease Capsules 2169

Dicumarol (Reduced activity of anticoagulant).
- No products indexed under this heading.

Digitoxin (Reduced activity of cardiac glycoside). Products include:
- Crystodigin Tablets.................... 1433

Digoxin (Reduced activity of cardiac glycoside). Products include:
- Lanoxicaps 1117
- Lanoxin Elixir Pediatric 1120
- Lanoxin Injection 1123
- Lanoxin Injection Pediatric................. 1126
- Lanoxin Tablets 1128

Disopyramide Phosphate (Diminished effects of concurrently administered disopyramide). Products include:
- Norpace 2444

Divalproex Sodium (Diminished effects of concurrently administered anticonvulsant). Products include:
- Depakote Tablets.................... 415

Dyphylline (Diminished effects of concurrently administered theophylline). Products include:
- Lufyllin & Lufyllin-400 Tablets 2670
- Lufyllin-GG Elixir & Tablets 2671

Esmolol Hydrochloride (Diminished effects of concurrently administered beta blocker). Products include:
- Brevibloc Injection 1808

Ethinyl Estradiol (Reduced activity of oral contraceptives; patients using oral contraceptives should be advised to change to nonhormonal methods of birth control). Products include:
- Brevicon.................... 2088
- Demulen 2428
- Desogen Tablets.................... 1817
- Levlen/Tri-Levlen.................... 651
- Lo/Ovral Tablets 2746
- Lo/Ovral-28 Tablets.................... 2751
- Modicon.................... 1872
- Nordette-21 Tablets.................... 2755
- Nordette-28 Tablets.................... 2758
- Norinyl 2088
- Ortho-Cept 1851
- Ortho-Cyclen/Ortho-Tri-Cyclen 1858
- Ortho-Novum.................... 1872
- Ortho-Cyclen/Ortho Tri-Cyclen 1858
- Ovcon 760
- Ovral Tablets 2770
- Ovral-28 Tablets 2770
- Levlen/Tri-Levlen.................... 651
- Tri-Norinyl.................... 2164
- Triphasil-21 Tablets 2814
- Triphasil-28 Tablets.................... 2819

Ethosuximide (Diminished effects of concurrently administered anticonvulsant). Products include:
- Zarontin Capsules 1928
- Zarontin Syrup 1929

Ethotoin (Diminished effects of concurrently administered anticonvulsant). Products include:
- Peganone Tablets 446

Ethynodiol Diacetate (Reduced activity of oral contraceptives; patients using oral contraceptives should be advised to change to nonhormonal methods of birth control). Products include:
- Demulen 2428

Felbamate (Diminished effects of concurrently administered anticonvulsant). Products include:
- Felbatol 2666

Fentanyl (Reduced activity of narcotics). Products include:
- Duragesic Transdermal System......... 1288

Fentanyl Citrate (Reduced activity of narcotics). Products include:
- Sublimaze Injection.................... 1307

Fludrocortisone Acetate (Reduced activity of corticosteroid). Products include:
- Florinef Acetate Tablets 505

Glipizide (Reduced activity of oral hypoglycemic agent). Products include:
- Glucotrol Tablets 1967
- Glucotrol XL Extended Release Tablets 1968

Glyburide (Reduced activity of oral hypoglycemic agent). Products include:
- DiaBeta Tablets 1239
- Glynase PresTab Tablets 2609
- Micronase Tablets.................... 2623

(▣ Described in PDR For Nonprescription Drugs) (⊙ Described in PDR For Ophthalmology)

Halothane (Increased hepatotoxicity of both drugs). Products include:
Fluothane ... 2724

Hydrocodone Bitartrate (Reduced activity of narcotics). Products include:
Anexsia 5/500 Elixir ... 1781
Anexia Tablets ... 1782
Codiclear DH Syrup ... 791
Deconamine CX Cough and Cold Liquid and Tablets ... 1319
Duratuss HD Elixir ... 2565
Hycodan Tablets and Syrup ... 930
Hycomine Compound Tablets ... 932
Hycomine ... 931
Hycotuss Expectorant Syrup ... 933
Hydrocet Capsules ... 782
Lorcet 10/650 ... 1018
Lortab ... 2566
Tussend ... 1783
Tussend Expectorant ... 1785
Vicodin Tablets ... 1356
Vicodin ES Tablets ... 1357
Vicodin Tuss Expectorant ... 1358
Zydone Capsules ... 949

Hydrocodone Polistirex (Reduced activity of narcotics). Products include:
Tussionex Pennkinetic Extended-Release Suspension ... 998

Hydrocortisone (Reduced activity of corticosteroid). Products include:
Anusol-HC Cream 2.5% ... 1896
Aquanil HC Lotion ... 1931
Bactine Hydrocortisone Anti-Itch Cream ... ▣ 709
Caldecort Anti-Itch Hydrocortisone Spray ... ▣ 631
Cortaid ... ▣ 836
CORTENEMA ... 2535
Cortisporin Ointment ... 1085
Cortisporin Ophthalmic Ointment Sterile ... 1085
Cortisporin Ophthalmic Suspension Sterile ... 1086
Cortisporin Otic Solution Sterile ... 1087
Cortisporin Otic Suspension Sterile 1088
Cortizone-5 ... ▣ 831
Cortizone-10 ... ▣ 831
Hydrocortone Tablets ... 1672
Hytone ... 907
Massengill Medicated Soft Cloth Towelettes ... 2458
PediOtic Suspension Sterile ... 1153
Preparation H Hydrocortisone 1% Cream ... ▣ 872
ProctoCream-HC 2.5% ... 2408
VōSoL HC Otic Solution ... 2678

Hydrocortisone Acetate (Reduced activity of corticosteroid). Products include:
Analpram-HC Rectal Cream 1% and 2.5% ... 977
Anusol HC-1 Anti-Itch Hydrocortisone Ointment ... ▣ 847
Anusol-HC Suppositories ... 1897
Caldecort ... ▣ 631
Carmol HC ... 924
Coly-Mycin S Otic w/Neomycin & Hydrocortisone ... 1906
Cortaid ... ▣ 836
Cortifoam ... 2396
Cortisporin Cream ... 1084
Epifoam ... 2399
Hydrocortone Acetate Sterile Suspension ... 1669
Mantadil Cream ... 1135
Nupercainal Hydrocortisone 1% Cream ... ▣ 645
Ophthocort ... ◉ 311
Pramosone Cream, Lotion & Ointment ... 978
ProctoCream-HC ... 2408
ProctoFoam-HC ... 2409
Terra-Cortril Ophthalmic Suspension ... 2210

Hydrocortisone Sodium Phosphate (Reduced activity of corticosteroid). Products include:
Hydrocortone Phosphate Injection, Sterile ... 1670

Hydrocortisone Sodium Succinate (Reduced activity of corticosteroid). Products include:
Solu-Cortef Sterile Powder ... 2641

Ketoconazole (Diminished serum concentrations of both drugs). Products include:
Nizoral 2% Cream ... 1297
Nizoral 2% Shampoo ... 1298
Nizoral Tablets ... 1298

Labetalol Hydrochloride (Diminished effects of concurrently administered beta blocker). Products include:
Normodyne Injection ... 2377
Normodyne Tablets ... 2379
Trandate ... 1185

Lamotrigine (Diminished effects of concurrently administered anticonvulsant). Products include:
Lamictal Tablets ... 1112

Levobunolol Hydrochloride (Diminished effects of concurrently administered beta blocker). Products include:
Betagan ... ◉ 233

Levonorgestrel (Reduced activity of oral contraceptives; patients using oral contraceptives should be advised to change to nonhormonal methods of birth control). Products include:
Levlen/Tri-Levlen ... 651
Nordette-21 Tablets ... 2755
Nordette-28 Tablets ... 2758
Norplant System ... 2759
Levlen/Tri-Levlen ... 651
Triphasil-21 Tablets ... 2814
Triphasil-28 Tablets ... 2819

Levorphanol Tartrate (Reduced activity of narcotics). Products include:
Levo-Dromoran ... 2129

Medroxyprogesterone Acetate (Diminished effects of concurrently administered progestin). Products include:
Amen Tablets ... 780
Cycrin Tablets ... 975
Depo-Provera Contraceptive Injection ... 2602
Depo-Provera Sterile Aqueous Suspension ... 2606
Premphase ... 2797
Prempro ... 2801
Provera Tablets ... 2636

Megestrol Acetate (Diminished effects of concurrently administered progestin). Products include:
Megace Oral Suspension ... 699
Megace Tablets ... 701

Meperidine Hydrochloride (Reduced activity of narcotics). Products include:
Demerol ... 2308
Mepergan Injection ... 2753

Mephenytoin (Diminished effects of concurrently administered anticonvulsant). Products include:
Mesantoin Tablets ... 2272

Mephobarbital (Diminished effects of concurrently administered barbiturate). Products include:
Mebaral Tablets ... 2322

Mestranol (Reduced activity of oral contraceptives; patients using oral contraceptives should be advised to change to nonhormonal methods of birth control). Products include:
Norinyl ... 2088
Ortho-Novum ... 1872

Metformin Hydrochloride (Reduced activity of oral hypoglycemic agent). Products include:
Glucophage ... 752

Methadone Hydrochloride (Diminished effects of concurrently administered methadone). Products include:
Methadone Hydrochloride Oral Concentrate ... 2233
Methadone Hydrochloride Oral Solution & Tablets ... 2235

Methsuximide (Diminished effects of concurrently administered anticonvulsant). Products include:
Celontin Kapseals ... 1899

Methylprednisolone Acetate (Reduced activity of corticosteroid). Products include:
Depo-Medrol Single-Dose Vial ... 2600
Depo-Medrol Sterile Aqueous Suspension ... 2597

Methylprednisolone Sodium Succinate (Reduced activity of corticosteroid). Products include:
Solu-Medrol Sterile Powder ... 2643

Metipranolol Hydrochloride (Diminished effects of concurrently administered beta blocker). Products include:
OptiPranolol (Metipranolol 0.3%) Sterile Ophthalmic Solution ... ◉ 258

Metoprolol Succinate (Diminished effects of concurrently administered beta blocker). Products include:
Toprol-XL Tablets ... 565

Metoprolol Tartrate (Diminished effects of concurrently administered beta blocker). Products include:
Lopressor Ampuls ... 830
Lopressor HCT Tablets ... 832
Lopressor Tablets ... 830

Mexiletine Hydrochloride (Diminished effects of concurrently administered mexiletine). Products include:
Mexitil Capsules ... 678

Morphine Sulfate (Reduced activity of narcotics). Products include:
Astramorph/PF Injection, USP (Preservative-Free) ... 535
Duramorph ... 962
Infumorph 200 and Infumorph 500 Sterile Solutions ... 965
MS Contin Tablets ... 1994
MSIR ... 1997
Oramorph SR (Morphine Sulfate Sustained Release Tablets) ... 2236
RMS Suppositories ... 2657
Roxanol ... 2243

Nadolol (Diminished effects of concurrently administered beta blocker).
No products indexed under this heading.

Norethindrone (Reduced activity of oral contraceptives; patients using oral contraceptives should be advised to change to nonhormonal methods of birth control). Products include:
Brevicon ... 2088
Micronor Tablets ... 1872
Modicon ... 1872
Norinyl ... 2088
Nor-Q D Tablets ... 2135
Ortho-Novum ... 1872
Ovcon ... 760
Tri-Norinyl ... 2164

Norethynodrel (Reduced activity of oral contraceptives; patients using oral contraceptives should be advised to change to nonhormonal methods of birth control).
No products indexed under this heading.

Norgestimate (Reduced activity of oral contraceptives; patients using oral contraceptives should be advised to change to nonhormonal methods of birth control). Products include:
Ortho-Cyclen/Ortho-Tri-Cyclen ... 1858
Ortho-Cyclen/Ortho Tri-Cyclen ... 1858

Norgestrel (Reduced activity of oral contraceptives; patients using oral contraceptives should be advised to change to nonhormonal methods of birth control). Products include:
Lo/Ovral Tablets ... 2746
Lo/Ovral-28 Tablets ... 2751
Ovral Tablets ... 2770
Ovral-28 Tablets ... 2770
Ovrette Tablets ... 2771

Opium Alkaloids (Reduced activity of narcotics).
No products indexed under this heading.

Oxycodone Hydrochloride (Reduced activity of narcotics). Products include:
Percocet Tablets ... 938
Percodan Tablets ... 939
Percodan-Demi Tablets ... 940
Roxicodone Tablets, Oral Solution & Intensol (Oxycodone) ... 2244
Tylox Capsules ... 1584

Para-Aminosalicylic Acid (Decreases serum rifampin levels; the drugs should be taken at least 8 hours apart).

Paramethadione (Diminished effects of concurrently administered anticonvulsant).
No products indexed under this heading.

Penbutolol Sulfate (Diminished effects of concurrently administered beta blocker). Products include:
Levatol ... 2403

Pentobarbital Sodium (Diminished effects of concurrently administered barbiturate). Products include:
Nembutal Sodium Capsules ... 436
Nembutal Sodium Solution ... 438
Nembutal Sodium Suppositories ... 440

Phenacemide (Diminished effects of concurrently administered anticonvulsant). Products include:
Phenurone Tablets ... 447

Phenobarbital (Diminished effects of concurrently administered barbiturate). Products include:
Arco-Lase Plus Tablets ... 512
Bellergal-S Tablets ... 2250
Donnatal ... 2060
Donnatal Extentabs ... 2061
Donnatal Tablets ... 2060
Phenobarbital Elixir and Tablets ... 1469
Quadrinal Tablets ... 1350

Phensuximide (Diminished effects of concurrently administered anticonvulsant). Products include:
Milontin Kapseals ... 1920

Phenytoin (Diminished effects of concurrently administered anticonvulsant). Products include:
Dilantin Infatabs ... 1908
Dilantin-125 Suspension ... 1911

Phenytoin Sodium (Diminished effects of concurrently administered anticonvulsant). Products include:
Dilantin Kapseals ... 1906
Dilantin Parenteral ... 1910

Pindolol (Diminished effects of concurrently administered beta blocker). Products include:
Visken Tablets ... 2299

Prednisolone Acetate (Reduced activity of corticosteroid). Products include:
AK-CIDE ... ◉ 202
AK-CIDE Ointment ... ◉ 202
Blephamide Liquifilm Sterile Ophthalmic Suspension ... 476
Blephamide Ointment ... ◉ 237
Econopred & Econopred Plus Ophthalmic Suspensions ... ◉ 217
Poly-Pred Liquifilm ... ◉ 248
Pred Forte ... ◉ 250
Pred Mild ... ◉ 253
Pred-G Liquifilm Sterile Ophthalmic Suspension ... ◉ 251
Pred-G S.O.P. Sterile Ophthalmic Ointment ... ◉ 252
Vasocidin Ointment ... ◉ 268

Prednisolone Sodium Phosphate (Reduced activity of corticosteroid). Products include:
AK-Pred ... ◉ 204
Hydeltrasol Injection, Sterile ... 1665

IMPORTANT NOTE: Always consult each drug listing in the patient's regimen for possible interactions.

Rifadin

Inflamase ◉ 265
Pediapred Oral Liquid 995
Vasocidin Ophthalmic Solution ◉ 270

Prednisolone Tebutate (Reduced activity of corticosteroid). Products include:

Hydeltra-T.B.A. Sterile Suspension 1667

Prednisone (Reduced activity of corticosteroid). Products include:

Deltasone Tablets 2595

Primidone (Diminished effects of concurrently administered anticonvulsant). Products include:

Mysoline 2754

Probenecid (Increases rifampin blood levels). Products include:

Benemid Tablets 1611
ColBENEMID Tablets 1622

Propoxyphene Hydrochloride (Reduced activity of narcotics). Products include:

Darvon 1435
Wygesic Tablets 2827

Propoxyphene Napsylate (Reduced activity of narcotics). Products include:

Darvon-N/Darvocet-N 1433

Propranolol Hydrochloride (Diminished effects of concurrently administered beta blocker). Products include:

Inderal 2728
Inderal LA Long Acting Capsules 2730
Inderide Tablets 2732
Inderide LA Long Acting Capsules .. 2734

Quinidine Gluconate (Reduced activity of quinidine). Products include:

Quinaglute Dura-Tabs Tablets 649

Quinidine Polygalacturonate (Reduced activity of quinidine).

No products indexed under this heading.

Quinidine Sulfate (Reduced activity of quinidine). Products include:

Quinidex Extentabs 2067

Secobarbital Sodium (Diminished effects of concurrently administered barbiturate). Products include:

Seconal Sodium Pulvules 1474

Sotalol Hydrochloride (Diminished effects of concurrently administered beta blocker). Products include:

Betapace Tablets 641

Sufentanil Citrate (Reduced activity of narcotics). Products include:

Sufenta Injection 1309

Theophylline (Diminished effects of concurrently administered theophylline). Products include:

Marax Tablets & DF Syrup 2200
Quibron 2053

Theophylline Anhydrous (Diminished effects of concurrently administered theophylline). Products include:

Aerolate 1004
Primatene Dual Action Formula ᴷᴰ 872
Primatene Tablets ᴷᴰ 873
Respbid Tablets 682
Slo-bid Gyrocaps 2033
Theo-24 Extended Release Capsules 2568
Theo-Dur Extended-Release Tablets 1327
Theo-X Extended-Release Tablets .. 788
Uni-Dur Extended-Release Tablets.. 1331
Uniphyl 400 mg Tablets 2001

Theophylline Calcium Salicylate (Diminished effects of concurrently administered theophylline). Products include:

Quadrinal Tablets 1350

Theophylline Sodium Glycinate (Diminished effects of concurrently administered theophylline).

No products indexed under this heading.

Thiamylal Sodium (Diminished effects of concurrently administered barbiturate).

No products indexed under this heading.

Timolol Hemihydrate (Diminished effects of concurrently administered beta blocker). Products include:

Betimol 0.25%, 0.5% ◉ 261

Timolol Maleate (Diminished effects of concurrently administered beta blocker). Products include:

Blocadren Tablets 1614
Timolide Tablets 1748
Timoptic in Ocudose 1753
Timoptic Sterile Ophthalmic Solution 1751
Timoptic-XE 1755

Tolazamide (Reduced activity of oral hypoglycemic agent).

No products indexed under this heading.

Tolbutamide (Reduced activity of oral hypoglycemic agent).

No products indexed under this heading.

Triamcinolone (Reduced activity of corticosteroid). Products include:

Aristocort Tablets 1022

Triamcinolone Acetonide (Reduced activity of corticosteroid). Products include:

Aristocort A 0.025% Cream 1027
Aristocort A 0.5% Cream 1031
Aristocort A 0.1% Cream 1029
Aristocort A 0.1% Ointment 1030
Azmacort Oral Inhaler 2011
Nasacort Nasal Inhaler 2024

Triamcinolone Diacetate (Reduced activity of corticosteroid). Products include:

Aristocort Suspension (Forte Parenteral) 1027
Aristocort Suspension (Intralesional) 1025

Triamcinolone Hexacetonide (Reduced activity of corticosteroid). Products include:

Aristospan Suspension (Intra-articular) 1033
Aristospan Suspension (Intralesional) 1032

Trimethadione (Diminished effects of concurrently administered anticonvulsant).

No products indexed under this heading.

Valproic Acid (Diminished effects of concurrently administered anticonvulsant). Products include:

Depakene 413

Verapamil Hydrochloride (Diminished effects of concurrently administered verapamil). Products include:

Calan SR Caplets 2422
Calan Tablets 2419
Isoptin Injectable 1344
Isoptin Oral Tablets 1346
Isoptin SR Tablets 1348
Verelan Capsules 1410
Verelan Capsules 2824

Vitamin D (Effect not specified when used with rifampin-INH). Products include:

Caltrate PLUS ᴷᴰ 665
Caltrate 600 + D ᴷᴰ 665
Citracal Caplets + D 1780
Dical-D Tablets & Wafers 420
Drisdol ᴷᴰ 794
Materna Tablets 1379
Megadose 512
Zymacap Capsules ᴷᴰ 772

Warfarin Sodium (Reduced activity of anticoagulant). Products include:

Coumadin 926

RIFADIN I.V.

(Rifampin) 1528
See Rifadin Capsules

RIFAMATE CAPSULES

(Rifampin, Isoniazid) 1530

May interact with oral anticoagulants, oral contraceptives, oral hypoglycemic agents, cardiac glycosides, and certain other agents. Compounds in these categories include:

Acarbose (Pharmacologic activity decreased when rifampin is given with other antituberculosis drugs).

No products indexed under this heading.

Betamethasone (Pharmacologic activity decreased when rifampin is given in combination with other antituberculosis drugs).

No products indexed under this heading.

Betamethasone Acetate (Pharmacologic activity decreased when rifampin is given with other antituberculosis drugs). Products include:

Celestone Soluspan Suspension 2347

Betamethasone Sodium Phosphate (Pharmacologic activity decreased when rifampin is given with other antituberculosis drugs). Products include:

Celestone Soluspan Suspension 2347

Chlorpropamide (Pharmacologic activity decreased when rifampin is given with other antituberculosis drugs). Products include:

Diabinese Tablets 1935

Cortisone Acetate (Pharmacologic activity decreased when rifampin is given with other antituberculosis drugs). Products include:

Cortone Acetate Sterile Suspension 1623
Cortone Acetate Tablets 1624

Dapsone (Pharmacologic activity decreased when rifampin is given with other antituberculosis drugs). Products include:

Dapsone Tablets USP 1284

Deslanoside (Pharmacologic activity decreased when rifampin is given with other antituberculosis drugs).

No products indexed under this heading.

Desogestrel (Reliability of oral contraceptive affected). Products include:

Desogen Tablets 1817
Ortho-Cept 1851

Dexamethasone (Pharmacologic activity decreased when rifampin is given with other antituberculosis drugs). Products include:

AK-Trol Ointment & Suspension ◉ 205
Decadron Elixir 1633
Decadron Tablets 1635
Decaspray Topical Aerosol 1648
Dexacidin Ointment ◉ 263
Maxitrol Ophthalmic Ointment and Suspension ◉ 224
TobraDex Ophthalmic Suspension and Ointment 473

Dexamethasone Acetate (Pharmacologic activity decreased when rifampin is given with other antituberculosis drugs). Products include:

Dalalone D.P. Injectable 1011
Decadron-LA Sterile Suspension 1646

Dexamethasone Phosphate (Pharmacologic activity decreased when rifampin is given with other antituberculosis drugs).

No products indexed under this heading.

Dexamethasone Sodium Phosphate (Pharmacologic activity decreased when rifampin is given with other antituberculosis drugs). Products include:

Decadron Phosphate Injection 1637
Decadron Phosphate Respihaler 1642
Decadron Phosphate Sterile Ophthalmic Ointment 1641
Decadron Phosphate Sterile Ophthalmic Solution 1642
Decadron Phosphate Topical Cream 1644
Decadron Phosphate Turbinaire 1645
Decadron Phosphate with Xylocaine Injection, Sterile 1639
Dexacort Phosphate in Respihaler .. 458
Dexacort Phosphate in Turbinaire .. 459
NeoDecadron Sterile Ophthalmic Ointment 1712
NeoDecadron Sterile Ophthalmic Solution 1713
NeoDecadron Topical Cream 1714

Dicumarol (Decreased anticoagulant dosage requirements).

No products indexed under this heading.

Digitoxin (Pharmacologic activity decreased when rifampin is given with other antituberculosis drugs). Products include:

Crystodigin Tablets 1433

Digoxin (Pharmacologic activity decreased when rifampin is given with other antituberculosis drugs). Products include:

Lanoxicaps 1117
Lanoxin Elixir Pediatric 1120
Lanoxin Injection 1123
Lanoxin Injection Pediatric 1126
Lanoxin Tablets 1128

Disopyramide Phosphate (Pharmacologic activity decreased when rifampin is given with other antituberculosis drugs). Products include:

Norpace 2444

Ethambutol Hydrochloride (Potential for thrombocytopenia). Products include:

Myambutol Tablets 1386

Ethinyl Estradiol (Reliability of oral contraceptive affected). Products include:

Brevicon 2088
Demulen 2428
Desogen Tablets 1817
Levlen/Tri-Levlen 651
Lo/Ovral Tablets 2746
Lo/Ovral-28 Tablets 2751
Modicon 1872
Nordette-21 Tablets 2755
Nordette-28 Tablets 2758
Norinyl 2088
Ortho-Cept 1851
Ortho-Cyclen/Ortho-Tri-Cyclen 1858
Ortho-Novum 1872
Ortho-Cyclen/Ortho Tri-Cyclen 1858
Ovcon 760
Ovral Tablets 2770
Ovral-28 Tablets 2770
Levlen/Tri-Levlen 651
Tri-Norinyl 2164
Triphasil-21 Tablets 2814
Triphasil-28 Tablets 2819

Ethynodiol Diacetate (Reliability of oral contraceptive affected). Products include:

Demulen 2428

Glipizide (Pharmacologic activity decreased when rifampin is given with other antituberculosis drugs). Products include:

Glucotrol Tablets 1967
Glucotrol XL Extended Release Tablets 1968

Glyburide (Pharmacologic activity decreased when rifampin is given with other antituberculosis drugs). Products include:

DiaBeta Tablets 1239
Glynase PresTab Tablets 2609
Micronase Tablets 2623

(ᴷᴰ Described in PDR For Nonprescription Drugs) (◉ Described in PDR For Ophthalmology)

Hepatotoxic Drugs, unspecified (Fatalities associated with jaundice).

Hydrocortisone (Pharmacologic activity decreased when rifampin is given with other antituberculosis drugs). Products include:
- Anusol-HC Cream 2.5% 1896
- Aquanil HC Lotion 1931
- Bactine Hydrocortisone Anti-Itch Cream ..... ▣ 709
- Caldecort Anti-Itch Hydrocortisone Spray ..... ▣ 631
- Cortaid ..... ▣ 836
- CORTENEMA 2535
- Cortisporin Ointment 1085
- Cortisporin Ophthalmic Ointment Sterile 1085
- Cortisporin Ophthalmic Suspension Sterile 1086
- Cortisporin Otic Solution Sterile 1087
- Cortisporin Otic Suspension Sterile 1088
- Cortizone-5 ..... ▣ 831
- Cortizone-10 ..... ▣ 831
- Hydrocortone Tablets 1672
- Hytone 907
- Massengill Medicated Soft Cloth Towelettes 2458
- PediOtic Suspension Sterile 1153
- Preparation H Hydrocortisone 1% Cream ..... ▣ 872
- ProctoCream-HC 2.5% 2408
- VōSoL HC Otic Solution 2678

Hydrocortisone Acetate (Pharmacologic activity decreased when rifampin is given with other antituberculosis drugs). Products include:
- Analpram-HC Rectal Cream 1% and 2.5% 977
- Anusol HC-1 Anti-Itch Hydrocortisone Ointment ..... ▣ 847
- Anusol-HC Suppositories 1897
- Caldecort ..... ▣ 631
- Carmol HC 924
- Coly-Mycin S Otic w/Neomycin & Hydrocortisone 1906
- Cortaid ..... ▣ 836
- Cortifoam 2396
- Cortisporin Cream 1084
- Epifoam 2399
- Hydrocortone Acetate Sterile Suspension 1669
- Mantadil Cream 1135
- Nupercainal Hydrocortisone 1% Cream ..... ▣ 645
- Ophthocort ..... ◉ 311
- Pramosone Cream, Lotion & Ointment 978
- ProctoCream-HC 2408
- ProctoFoam-HC 2409
- Terra-Cortril Ophthalmic Suspension 2210

Hydrocortisone Sodium Phosphate (Pharmacologic activity decreased when rifampin is given with other antituberculosis drugs). Products include:
- Hydrocortone Phosphate Injection, Sterile 1670

Hydrocortisone Sodium Succinate (Pharmacologic activity decreased when rifampin is given with other antituberculosis drugs). Products include:
- Solu-Cortef Sterile Powder 2641

Levonorgestrel (Reliability of oral contraceptive affected). Products include:
- Levlen/Tri-Levlen 651
- Nordette-21 Tablets 2755
- Nordette-28 Tablets 2758
- Norplant System 2759
- Levlen/Tri-Levlen 651
- Triphasil-21 Tablets 2814
- Triphasil-28 Tablets 2819

Mestranol (Reliability of oral contraceptive affected). Products include:
- Norinyl 2088
- Ortho-Novum 1872

Metformin Hydrochloride (Pharmacologic activity decreased when rifampin is given with other antituberculosis drugs). Products include:
- Glucophage 752

Methadone Hydrochloride (Pharmacologic activity decreased when rifampin is given with other antituberculosis drugs). Products include:
- Methadone Hydrochloride Oral Concentrate 2233
- Methadone Hydrochloride Oral Solution & Tablets 2235

Methylprednisolone Acetate (Pharmacologic activity decreased when rifampin is given with other antituberculosis drugs). Products include:
- Depo-Medrol Single-Dose Vial 2600
- Depo-Medrol Sterile Aqueous Suspension 2597

Methylprednisolone Sodium Succinate (Pharmacologic activity decreased when rifampin is given with other antituberculosis drugs). Products include:
- Solu-Medrol Sterile Powder 2643

Norethindrone (Reliability of oral contraceptive affected). Products include:
- Brevicon 2088
- Micronor Tablets 1872
- Modicon 1872
- Norinyl 2088
- Nor-Q D Tablets 2135
- Ortho-Novum 1872
- Ovcon 760
- Tri-Norinyl 2164

Norethynodrel (Reliability of oral contraceptive affected).
- No products indexed under this heading.

Norgestimate (Reliability of oral contraceptive affected). Products include:
- Ortho-Cyclen/Ortho-Tri-Cyclen 1858
- Ortho-Cyclen/Ortho Tri-Cyclen 1858

Norgestrel (Reliability of oral contraceptive affected). Products include:
- Lo/Ovral Tablets 2746
- Lo/Ovral-28 Tablets 2751
- Ovral Tablets 2770
- Ovral-28 Tablets 2770
- Ovrette Tablets 2771

Phenytoin (Phenytoin intoxication). Products include:
- Dilantin Infatabs 1908
- Dilantin-125 Suspension 1911

Phenytoin Sodium (Phenytoin intoxication). Products include:
- Dilantin Kapseals 1906
- Dilantin Parenteral 1910

Prednisolone (Pharmacologic activity decreased when rifampin is given with other antituberculosis drugs). Products include:
- Prelone Syrup 1787

Prednisolone Acetate (Pharmacologic activity decreased when rifampin is given with other antituberculosis drugs). Products include:
- AK-CIDE ..... ◉ 202
- AK-CIDE Ointment ..... ◉ 202
- Blephamide Liquifilm Sterile Ophthalmic Suspension 476
- Blephamide Ointment ..... ◉ 237
- Econopred & Econopred Plus Ophthalmic Suspensions ..... ◉ 217
- Poly-Pred Liquifilm ..... ◉ 248
- Pred Forte ..... ◉ 250
- Pred Mild ..... ◉ 253
- Pred-G Liquifilm Sterile Ophthalmic Suspension ..... ◉ 251
- Pred-G S.O.P. Sterile Ophthalmic Ointment ..... ◉ 252
- Vasocidin Ointment ..... ◉ 268

Prednisolone Sodium Phosphate (Pharmacologic activity decreased when rifampin is given with other antituberculosis drugs). Products include:
- AK-Pred ..... ◉ 204
- Hydeltrasol Injection, Sterile 1665
- Inflamase ..... ◉ 265
- Pediapred Oral Liquid 995
- Vasocidin Ophthalmic Solution ..... ◉ 270

Prednisolone Tebutate (Pharmacologic activity decreased when rifampin is given with other antituberculosis drugs). Products include:
- Hydeltra-T.B.A. Sterile Suspension 1667

Prednisone (Pharmacologic activity decreased when rifampin is given with other antituberculosis drugs). Products include:
- Deltasone Tablets 2595

Quinidine Gluconate (Pharmacologic activity decreased when rifampin is given with other antituberculosis drugs). Products include:
- Quinaglute Dura-Tabs Tablets 649

Quinidine Polygalacturonate (Pharmacologic activity decreased when rifampin is given with other antituberculosis drugs).
- No products indexed under this heading.

Quinidine Sulfate (Pharmacologic activity decreased when rifampin is given with other antituberculosis drugs). Products include:
- Quinidex Extentabs 2067

Tolazamide (Pharmacologic activity decreased when rifampin is given with other antituberculosis drugs).
- No products indexed under this heading.

Tolbutamide (Pharmacologic activity decreased when rifampin is given with other antituberculosis drugs).
- No products indexed under this heading.

Triamcinolone (Pharmacologic activity decreased when rifampin is given with other antituberculosis drugs). Products include:
- Aristocort Tablets 1022

Triamcinolone Acetonide (Pharmacologic activity decreased when rifampin is given with other antituberculosis drugs). Products include:
- Aristocort A 0.025% Cream 1027
- Aristocort A 0.5% Cream 1031
- Aristocort A 0.1% Cream 1029
- Aristocort A 0.1% Ointment 1030
- Azmacort Oral Inhaler 2011
- Nasacort Nasal Inhaler 2024

Triamcinolone Diacetate (Pharmacologic activity decreased when rifampin is given with other antituberculosis drugs). Products include:
- Aristocort Suspension (Forte Parenteral) 1027
- Aristocort Suspension (Intralesional) 1025

Triamcinolone Hexacetonide (Pharmacologic activity decreased when rifampin is given with other antituberculosis drugs). Products include:
- Aristospan Suspension (Intra-articular) 1033
- Aristospan Suspension (Intralesional) 1032

Warfarin Sodium (Increased anticoagulant dosage requirements). Products include:
- Coumadin 926

Food Interactions

Alcohol (Increased incidence of Isoniazid hepatitis).

RIFATER

(Rifampin, Isoniazid, Pyrazinamide) ..1532

May interact with barbiturates, oral anticoagulants, beta blockers, narcotic analgesics, xanthine bronchodilators, oral hypoglycemic agents, oral contraceptives, cardiac glycosides, corticosteroids, progestins, antacids, and certain other agents. Compounds in these categories include:

Acarbose (Rifampin accelerates the metabolism of oral hypoglycemic agent; isoniazid may produce hyperglycemia and lead to loss of glucose control; dosage adjustment may be required when starting or stoppiing concomitantly administered rifampin).
- No products indexed under this heading.

Acebutolol Hydrochloride (Rifampin accelerates the metabolism of beta blocker; dosage adjustment may be required when starting or stopping concomitantly administered rifampin). Products include:
- Sectral Capsules 2807

Alfentanil Hydrochloride (Rifampin accelerates the metabolism of narcotic; dosage adjustment may be required when starting or stopping concomitantly administered rifampin). Products include:
- Alfenta Injection 1286

Aluminum Carbonate Gel (Reduces absorption of rifampin and isoniazid). Products include:
- Basaljel 2703

Aluminum Hydroxide (Reduces absorption of rifampin and isoniazid). Products include:
- ALternaGEL Liquid 1316
- Maximum Strength Ascriptin ..... ▣ 630
- Cama Arthritis Pain Reliever ..... ▣ 785
- Gaviscon Extra Strength Relief Formula Antacid Tablets ..... ▣ 819
- Gaviscon Extra Strength Relief Formula Liquid Antacid ..... ▣ 819
- Gaviscon Liquid Antacid ..... ▣ 820
- Gelusil Liquid & Tablets ..... ▣ 855
- Maalox Heartburn Relief Suspension ..... ▣ 642
- Maalox Heartburn Relief Tablets ..... ▣ 641
- Maalox Magnesia and Alumina Oral Suspension ..... ▣ 642
- Maalox Plus Tablets ..... ▣ 643
- Extra Strength Maalox Antacid Plus Antigas Liquid and Tablets ▣ 638
- Tempo Soft Antacid ..... ▣ 835

Aluminum Hydroxide Gel (Reduces absorption of rifampin and isoniazid). Products include:
- ALternaGEL Liquid ..... ▣ 659
- Aludrox Oral Suspension 2695
- Amphojel Suspension 2695
- Amphojel Suspension without Flavor 2695
- Amphojel Tablets 2695
- Arthritis Pain Ascriptin ..... ▣ 631
- Regular Strength Ascriptin Tablets ..... ▣ 629
- Gaviscon Antacid Tablets ..... ▣ 819
- Gaviscon-2 Antacid Tablets ..... ▣ 820
- Mylanta Liquid 1317
- Mylanta Tablets ..... ▣ 660
- Mylanta Double Strength Liquid 1317
- Mylanta Double Strength Tablets ..... ▣ 660
- Nephrox Suspension ..... ▣ 655

Aminosalicylic Acid (Increases the plasma concentration and elimination half-life of isoniazid). Products include:
- PASER Granules 1285

IMPORTANT NOTE: Always consult each drug listing in the patient's regimen for possible interactions.

Aminophylline (Rifampin accelerates the metabolism of theophylline and isoniazid inhibits the metabolism; dosage adjustment may be required when starting stopping concomitantly administered rifampin).
- No products indexed under this heading.

Aprobarbital (Rifampin accelerates the metabolism of barbiturates; dosage adjustment may be required when starting or stopping concomitantly administered rifampin).
- No products indexed under this heading.

Atenolol (Rifampin accelerates the metabolism of beta blocker; dosage adjustment may be required when starting or stopping concomitantly administered rifampin). Products include:
- Tenoretic Tablets 2845
- Tenormin Tablets and I.V. Injection 2847

Betamethasone Acetate (Rifampin accelerates the metabolism of corticosteroid; dosage adjustment may be required when starting or stopping concomitantly administered rifampin). Products include:
- Celestone Soluspan Suspension 2347

Betamethasone Sodium Phosphate (Rifampin accelerates the metabolism of corticosteroid; dosage adjustment may be required when starting or stopping concomitantly administered rifampin). Products include:
- Celestone Soluspan Suspension 2347

Betaxolol Hydrochloride (Rifampin accelerates the metabolism of beta blocker; dosage adjustment may be required when starting or stopping concomitantly administered rifampin). Products include:
- Betoptic Ophthalmic Solution........ 469
- Betoptic S Ophthalmic Suspension 471
- Kerlone Tablets........ 2436

Bisoprolol Fumarate (Rifampin accelerates the metabolism of beta blocker; dosage adjustment may be required when starting or stopping concomitantly administered rifampin). Products include:
- Zebeta Tablets 1413
- Ziac 1415

Buprenorphine (Rifampin accelerates the metabolism of narcotic; dosage adjustment may be required when starting or stopping concomitantly administered rifampin). Products include:
- Buprenex Injectable 2006

Butabarbital (Rifampin accelerates the metabolism of barbiturates; dosage adjustment may be required when starting or stopping concomitantly administered rifampin).
- No products indexed under this heading.

Butalbital (Rifampin accelerates the metabolism of barbiturates; dosage adjustment may be required when starting or stopping concomitantly administered rifampin). Products include:
- Esgic-plus Tablets 1013
- Fioricet Tablets........ 2258
- Fioricet with Codeine Capsules 2260
- Fiorinal Capsules 2261
- Fiorinal with Codeine Capsules 2262
- Fiorinal Tablets........ 2261
- Phrenilin 785
- Sedapap Tablets 50 mg/650 mg .. 1543

Carbamazepine (Isoniazid inhibits the metabolism of carbamazepine). Products include:
- Atretol Tablets 573
- Tegretol Chewable Tablets 852
- Tegretol Suspension........ 852
- Tegretol Tablets 852

Carteolol Hydrochloride (Rifampin accelerates the metabolism of beta blocker; dosage adjustment may be required when starting or stopping concomitantly administered rifampin). Products include:
- Cartrol Tablets 410
- Ocupress Ophthalmic Solution, 1% Sterile........ ⊙ 309

Chloramphenicol (Rifampin accelerates the metabolism of chloramphenicol; dosage adjustment may be required when starting or stopping concomitantly administered rifampin). Products include:
- Chloromycetin Ophthalmic Ointment, 1% .... ⊙ 310
- Chloromycetin Ophthalmic Solution........ ⊙ 310
- Chloroptic S.O.P. .... ⊙ 239
- Chloroptic Sterile Ophthalmic Solution .... ⊙ 239
- Elase-Chloromycetin Ointment 1040
- Ophthocort .... ⊙ 311

Chloramphenicol Palmitate (Rifampin accelerates the metabolism of chloramphenicol; dosage adjustment may be required when starting or stopping concomitantly administered rifampin).
- No products indexed under this heading.

Chloramphenicol Sodium Succinate (Rifampin accelerates the metabolism of chloramphenicol; dosage adjustment may be required when starting or stopping concomitantly administered rifampin). Products include:
- Chloromycetin Sodium Succinate.... 1900

Chlorpropamide (Rifampin accelerates the metabolism of oral hypoglycemic agent; isoniazid may produce hyperglycemia and lead to loss of glucose control; dosage adjustment may be required when starting or stoppiing concomitantly administered rifampin). Products include:
- Diabinese Tablets 1935

Ciprofloxacin (Rifampin accelerates the metabolism of ciprofloxacin; dosage adjustment may be required when starting or stopping concomitantly administered rifampin). Products include:
- Cipro I.V. 595
- Cipro I.V. Pharmacy Bulk Package.. 597

Ciprofloxacin Hydrochloride (Rifampin accelerates the metabolism of ciprofloxacin; dosage adjustment may be required when starting or stopping concomitantly administered rifampin). Products include:
- Ciloxan Ophthalmic Solution........ 472
- Cipro Tablets 592

Clofibrate (Rifampin accelerates the metabolism of clofibrate; dosage adjustment may be required when starting or stopping concomitantly administered rifampin). Products include:
- Atromid-S Capsules 2701

Codeine Phosphate (Rifampin accelerates the metabolism of narcotic; dosage adjustment may be required when starting or stopping concomitantly administered rifampin). Products include:
- Actifed with Codeine Cough Syrup.. 1067
- Brontex 1981
- Deconsal C Expectorant Syrup 456
- Deconsal Pediatric Syrup 457
- Dimetane-DC Cough Syrup 2059
- Empirin with Codeine Tablets........ 1093
- Fioricet with Codeine Capsules 2260
- Fiorinal with Codeine Capsules 2262
- Isoclor Expectorant........ 990
- Novahistine DH........ 2462
- Novahistine Expectorant........ 2463
- Nucofed 2051
- Phenergan with Codeine........ 2777
- Phenergan VC with Codeine 2781
- Robitussin A-C Syrup 2073
- Robitussin-DAC Syrup 2074
- Ryna .... ▣ 841
- Soma Compound w/Codeine Tablets 2676
- Tussi-Organidin NR Liquid and S NR Liquid 2677
- Tylenol with Codeine 1583

Cortisone Acetate (Rifampin accelerates the metabolism of corticosteroid; dosage adjustment may be required when starting or stopping concomitantly administered rifampin). Products include:
- Cortone Acetate Sterile Suspension 1623
- Cortone Acetate Tablets 1624

Cycloserine (Rifater exaggerates drowsiness and dizziness). Products include:
- Seromycin Pulvules........ 1476

Cyclosporine (Rifampin accelerates the metabolism of cyclosporine; dosage adjustment may be required when starting or stopping concomitantly administered rifampin). Products include:
- Neoral........ 2276
- Sandimmune 2286

Deslanoside (Rifampin accelerates the metabolism of cardiac glycosides; dosage adjustment may be required when starting or stopping concomitantly administered rifampin).
- No products indexed under this heading.

Desogestrel (Rifampin accelerates the metabolism of oral contraceptive or progestin; dosage adjustment may be required when starting or stopping concomitantly administered rifampin). Products include:
- Desogen Tablets........ 1817
- Ortho-Cept 1851

Dexamethasone (Rifampin accelerates the metabolism of corticosteroid; dosage adjustment may be required when starting or stopping concomitantly administered rifampin). Products include:
- AK-Trol Ointment & Suspension .... ⊙ 205
- Decadron Elixir 1633
- Decadron Tablets........ 1635
- Decaspray Topical Aerosol 1648
- Dexacidin Ointment .... ⊙ 263
- Maxitrol Ophthalmic Ointment and Suspension .... ⊙ 224
- TobraDex Ophthalmic Suspension and Ointment........ 473

Dexamethasone Acetate (Rifampin accelerates the metabolism of corticosteroid; dosage adjustment may be required when starting or stopping concomitantly administered rifampin). Products include:
- Dalalone D.P. Injectable 1011
- Decadron-LA Sterile Suspension...... 1646

Dexamethasone Sodium Phosphate (Rifampin accelerates the metabolism of corticosteroid; dosage adjustment may be required when starting or stopping concomitantly administered rifampin). Products include:
- Decadron Phosphate Injection 1637
- Decadron Phosphate Respihaler...... 1642
- Decadron Phosphate Sterile Ophthalmic Ointment........ 1641
- Decadron Phosphate Sterile Ophthalmic Solution 1642
- Decadron Phosphate Topical Cream........ 1644
- Decadron Phosphate Turbinaire 1645
- Decadron Phosphate with Xylocaine Injection, Sterile 1639
- Dexacort Phosphate in Respihaler .. 458
- Dexacort Phosphate in Turbinaire .. 459
- NeoDecadron Sterile Ophthalmic Ointment 1712
- NeoDecadron Sterile Ophthalmic Solution 1713
- NeoDecadron Topical Cream 1714

Dezocine (Rifampin accelerates the metabolism of narcotic; dosage adjustment may be required when starting or stopping concomitantly administered rifampin). Products include:
- Dalgan Injection 538

Diazepam (Rifampin accelerates the metabolism of diazepam and isoniazid inhibits the metabolism of diazepam; dosage adjustment may be required when starting or stopping concomitantly administered rifampin). Products include:
- Dizac........ 1809
- Valium Injectable 2182
- Valium Tablets 2183
- Valrelease Capsules 2169

Dicumarol (Rifampin accelerates the metabolism of anticoagulants and isoniazid inhibits the metabolism; increased requirements of coumarin type anticoagulant; dosage adjustment may be required when starting or stopping concomitantly administered rifampin).
- No products indexed under this heading.

Digitoxin (Rifampin accelerates the metabolism of cardiac glycosides; dosage adjustment may be required when starting or stopping concomitantly administered rifampin). Products include:
- Crystodigin Tablets........ 1433

Digoxin (Rifampin accelerates the metabolism of cardiac glycosides; dosage adjustment may be required when starting or stopping concomitantly administered rifampin). Products include:
- Lanoxicaps 1117
- Lanoxin Elixir Pediatric 1120
- Lanoxin Injection 1123
- Lanoxin Injection Pediatric........ 1126
- Lanoxin Tablets 1128

Dihydroxyaluminum Sodium Carbonate (Reduces absorption of rifampin and isoniazid).
- No products indexed under this heading.

Diltiazem Hydrochloride (Rifampin accelerates the metabolism of diltiazem; dosage adjustment may be required when starting or stopping concomitantly administered rifampin). Products include:
- Cardizem CD Capsules 1506
- Cardizem SR Capsules 1510
- Cardizem Injectable 1508
- Cardizem Tablets........ 1512
- Dilacor XR Extended-release Capsules 2018

Disopyramide Phosphate (Rifampin accelerates the metabolism of disopyramide; dosage adjustment may be required when starting or stopping concomitantly administered rifampin). Products include:
- Norpace 2444

Disulfiram (Rifater exaggerates acute behavioral and coordination changes). Products include:
- Antabuse Tablets........ 2695

Divalproex Sodium (Isoniazid inhibits the metabolism of valproic acid). Products include:
- Depakote Tablets........ 415

Dyphylline (Rifampin accelerates the metabolism of theophylline and isoniazid inhibits the metabolism; dosage adjustment may be required when starting stopping concomitantly administered rifampin). Products include:
- Lufyllin & Lufyllin-400 Tablets 2670
- Lufyllin-GG Elixir & Tablets 2671

(▣ Described in PDR For Nonprescription Drugs) (⊙ Described in PDR For Ophthalmology)

893 **Interactions Index** **Rifater**

Enalapril Maleate (Concurrent use results in decreased concentrations of enalaprilat, the active metabolite). Products include:

Vaseretic Tablets 1765
Vasotec Tablets 1771

Enflurane (Fast acetylation of isoniazid may produce high concentrations of hydrazine which facilitate defloration).

No products indexed under this heading.

Esmolol Hydrochloride (Rifampin accelerates the metabolism of beta blocker; dosage adjustment may be required when starting or stopping concomitantly administered rifampin). Products include:

Brevibloc Injection 1808

Ethinyl Estradiol (Rifampin accelerates the metabolism of oral contraceptive; dosage adjustment may be required when starting or stopping concomitantly administered rifampin). Products include:

Brevicon 2088
Demulen 2428
Desogen Tablets 1817
Levlen/Tri-Levlen 651
Lo/Ovral Tablets 2746
Lo/Ovral-28 Tablets 2751
Modicon 1872
Nordette-21 Tablets 2755
Nordette-28 Tablets 2758
Norinyl 2088
Ortho-Cept 1851
Ortho-Cyclen/Ortho-Tri-Cyclen 1858
Ortho-Novum 1872
Ortho-Cyclen/Ortho Tri-Cyclen 1858
Ovcon 760
Ovral Tablets 2770
Ovral-28 Tablets 2770
Levlen/Tri-Levlen 651
Tri-Norinyl 2164
Triphasil-21 Tablets 2814
Triphasil-28 Tablets 2819

Ethynodiol Diacetate (Rifampin accelerates the metabolism of oral contraceptive; dosage adjustment may be required when starting or stopping concomitantly administered rifampin). Products include:

Demulen 2428

Fentanyl (Rifampin accelerates the metabolism of narcotic; dosage adjustment may be required when starting or stopping concomitantly administered rifampin). Products include:

Duragesic Transdermal System 1288

Fentanyl Citrate (Rifampin accelerates the metabolism of narcotic; dosage adjustment may be required when starting or stopping concomitantly administered rifampin). Products include:

Sublimaze Injection 1307

Fluconazole (Rifampin accelerates the metabolism of fluconazole; dosage adjustment may be required when starting or stopping concomitantly administered rifampin). Products include:

Diflucan Injection, Tablets, and Oral Suspension 2194

Fludrocortisone Acetate (Rifampin accelerates the metabolism of corticosteroid; dosage adjustment may be required when starting or stopping concomitantly administered rifampin). Products include:

Florinef Acetate Tablets 505

Glipizide (Rifampin accelerates the metabolism of oral hypoglycemic agent; isoniazid may produce hyperglycemia and lead to loss of glucose control; dosage adjustment may be required when starting or stopping concomitantly administered rifampin). Products include:

Glucotrol Tablets 1967
Glucotrol XL Extended Release Tablets 1968

Glyburide (Rifampin accelerates the metabolism of oral hypoglycemic agent; isoniazid may produce hyperglycemia and lead to loss of glucose control; dosage adjustment may be required when starting or stopping concomitantly administered rifampin). Products include:

DiaBeta Tablets 1239
Glynase PresTab Tablets 2609
Micronase Tablets 2623

Haloperidol (Rifampin accelerates the metabolism of haloperidol and isoniazid inhibits the metabolism of haloperidol; dosage adjustment may be required when starting or stopping concomitantly administered rifampin). Products include:

Haldol Injection, Tablets and Concentrate 1575

Haloperidol Decanoate (Rifampin accelerates the metabolism of haloperidol and isoniazid inhibits the metabolism of haloperidol; dosage adjustment may be required when starting or stopping concomitantly administered rifampin). Products include:

Haldol Decanoate 1577

Halothane (Incresed potential for hepatotoxicity). Products include:

Fluothane 2724

Hydrocodone Bitartrate (Rifampin accelerates the metabolism of narcotic; dosage adjustment may be required when starting or stopping concomitantly administered rifampin). Products include:

Anexsia 5/500 Elixir 1781
Anexia Tablets 1782
Codiclear DH Syrup 791
Deconamine CX Cough and Cold Liquid and Tablets 1319
Duratuss HD Elixir 2565
Hycodan Tablets and Syrup 930
Hycomine Compound Tablets 932
Hycomine 931
Hycotuss Expectorant Syrup 933
Hydrocet Capsules 782
Lorcet 10/650 1018
Lortab 2566
Tussend 1783
Tussend Expectorant 1785
Vicodin Tablets 1356
Vicodin ES Tablets 1357
Vicodin Tuss Expectorant 1358
Zydone Capsules 949

Hydrocodone Polistirex (Rifampin accelerates the metabolism of narcotic; dosage adjustment may be required when starting or stopping concomitantly administered rifampin). Products include:

Tussionex Pennkinetic Extended-Release Suspension 998

Hydrocortisone (Rifampin accelerates the metabolism of corticosteroid; dosage adjustment may be required when starting or stopping concomitantly administered rifampin). Products include:

Anusol-HC Cream 2.5% 1896
Aquanil HC Lotion 1931
Bactine Hydrocortisone Anti-Itch Cream .... ⊞ 709
Caldecort Anti-Itch Hydrocortisone Spray .... ⊞ 631
Cortaid .... ⊞ 836
CORTENEMA 2535
Cortisporin Ointment 1085
Cortisporin Ophthalmic Ointment Sterile 1085
Cortisporin Ophthalmic Suspension Sterile 1086
Cortisporin Otic Solution Sterile 1087
Cortisporin Otic Suspension Sterile 1088
Cortizone-5 .... ⊞ 831
Cortizone-10 .... ⊞ 831
Hydrocortone Tablets 1672
Hytone 907
Massengill Medicated Soft Cloth Towelettes 2458
PediOtic Suspension Sterile 1153
Preparation H Hydrocortisone 1% Cream .... ⊞ 872
ProctoCream-HC 2.5% 2408
VōSoL HC Otic Solution 2678

Hydrocortisone Acetate (Rifampin accelerates the metabolism of corticosteroid; dosage adjustment may be required when starting or stopping concomitantly administered rifampin). Products include:

Analpram-HC Rectal Cream 1% and 2.5% 977
Anusol HC-1 Anti-Itch Hydrocortisone Ointment .... ⊞ 847
Anusol-HC Suppositories 1897
Caldecort .... ⊞ 631
Carmol HC 924
Coly-Mycin S Otic w/Neomycin & Hydrocortisone 1906
Cortaid .... ⊞ 836
Cortifoam 2396
Cortisporin Cream 1084
Epifoam 2399
Hydrocortone Acetate Sterile Suspension 1669
Mantadil Cream 1135
Nupercainal Hydrocortisone 1% Cream .... ⊞ 645
Ophthocort .... ◉ 311
Pramosone Cream, Lotion & Ointment 978
ProctoCream-HC 2408
ProctoFoam-HC 2409
Terra-Cortril Ophthalmic Suspension 2210

Hydrocortisone Sodium Phosphate (Rifampin accelerates the metabolism of corticosteroid; dosage adjustment may be required when starting or stopping concomitantly administered rifampin). Products include:

Hydrocortone Phosphate Injection, Sterile 1670

Hydrocortisone Sodium Succinate (Rifampin accelerates the metabolism of corticosteroid; dosage adjustment may be required when starting or stopping concomitantly administered rifampin). Products include:

Solu-Cortef Sterile Powder 2641

Itraconazole (Rifampin accelerates the metabolism of itraconazole; dosage adjustment may be required when starting or stopping concomitantly administered rifampin). Products include:

Sporanox Capsules 1305

Ketoconazole (Rifampin accelerates the metabolism of ketoconazole; dosage adjustment may be required when starting or stopping concomitantly administered rifampin). Products include:

Nizoral 2% Cream 1297
Nizoral 2% Shampoo 1298
Nizoral Tablets 1298

Labetalol Hydrochloride (Rifampin accelerates the metabolism of beta blocker; dosage adjustment may be required when starting or stopping concomitantly administered rifampin). Products include:

Normodyne Injection 2377
Normodyne Tablets 2379
Trandate 1185

Levobunolol Hydrochloride (Rifampin accelerates the metabolism of beta blocker; dosage adjustment may be required when starting or stopping concomitantly administered rifampin). Products include:

Betagan .... ◉ 233

Levodopa (Concurrent use may produce symptoms of excess catecholamine stimulation (agitation, flushing, palpitations) or lack of levodopa effect). Products include:

Atamet 572
Larodopa Tablets 2129
Sinemet Tablets 943
Sinemet CR Tablets 944

Levonorgestrel (Rifampin accelerates the metabolism of oral contraceptive; dosage adjustment may be required when starting or stopping concomitantly administered rifampin). Products include:

Levlen/Tri-Levlen 651
Nordette-21 Tablets 2755
Nordette-28 Tablets 2758
Norplant System 2759
Levlen/Tri-Levlen 651
Triphasil-21 Tablets 2814
Triphasil-28 Tablets 2819

Levorphanol Tartrate (Rifampin accelerates the metabolism of narcotic; dosage adjustment may be required when starting or stopping concomitantly administered rifampin). Products include:

Levo-Dromoran 2129

Magaldrate (Reduces absorption of rifampin and isoniazid).

No products indexed under this heading.

Magnesium Hydroxide (Reduces absorption of rifampin and isoniazid). Products include:

Aludrox Oral Suspension 2695
Arthritis Pain Ascriptin .... ⊞ 631
Maximum Strength Ascriptin .... ⊞ 630
Regular Strength Ascriptin Tablets .... ⊞ 629
Di-Gel Antacid/Anti-Gas .... ⊞ 801
Gelusil Liquid & Tablets .... ⊞ 855
Maalox Magnesia and Alumina Oral Suspension .... ⊞ 642
Maalox Plus Tablets .... ⊞ 643
Extra Strength Maalox Antacid Plus Antigas Liquid and Tablets ⊞ 638
Mylanta Calcium Carbonate and Magnesium Hydroxide Tablets 1318
Mylanta Liquid 1317
Mylanta Tablets .... ⊞ 660
Mylanta Double Strength Liquid 1317
Mylanta Double Strength Tablets .... ⊞ 660
Phillips' Milk of Magnesia Liquid .... ⊞ 729
Rolaids Tablets .... ⊞ 843
Tempo Soft Antacid .... ⊞ 835

Magnesium Oxide (Reduces absorption of rifampin and isoniazid). Products include:

Beelith Tablets 639
Bufferin Analgesic Tablets and Caplets .... ⊞ 613
Caltrate PLUS .... ⊞ 665
Cama Arthritis Pain Reliever .... ⊞ 785
Mag-Ox 400 668
Uro-Mag 668

Medroxyprogesterone Acetate (Rifampin accelerates the metabolism of progestin; dosage adjustment may be required when starting or stopping concomitantly administered rifampin). Products include:

Amen Tablets 780
Cycrin Tablets 975
Depo-Provera Contraceptive Injection 2602
Depo-Provera Sterile Aqueous Suspension 2606
Premphase 2797
Prempro 2801
Provera Tablets 2636

IMPORTANT NOTE: Always consult each drug listing in the patient's regimen for possible interactions.

Rifater

Interactions Index

Megestrol Acetate (Rifampin accelerates the metabolism of progestin; dosage adjustment may be required when starting or stopping concomitantly administered rifampin). Products include:

Megace Oral Suspension 699
Megace Tablets 701

Meperidine Hydrochloride (Rifampin accelerates the metabolism of narcotic; dosage adjustment may be required when starting or stopping concomitantly administered rifampin; Rifater exaggerates drowsiness). Products include:

Demerol 2308
Mepergan Injection 2753

Mephobarbital (Rifampin accelerates the metabolism of barbiturates; dosage adjustment may be required when starting or stopping concomitantly administered rifampin). Products include:

Mebaral Tablets 2322

Mestranol (Rifampin accelerates the metabolism of oral contraceptive; dosage adjustment may be required when starting or stopping concomitantly administered rifampin). Products include:

Norinyl 2088
Ortho-Novum 1872

Metformin Hydrochloride (Rifampin accelerates the metabolism of oral hypoglycemic agent; isoniazid may produce hyperglycemia and lead to loss of glucose control; dosage adjustment may be required when starting or stoppiing concomitantly administered rifampin). Products include:

Glucophage 752

Methadone Hydrochloride (Rifampin accelerates the metabolism of narcotic; dosage adjustment may be required when starting or stopping concomitantly administered rifampin). Products include:

Methadone Hydrochloride Oral Concentrate 2233
Methadone Hydrochloride Oral Solution & Tablets 2235

Methylprednisolone Acetate (Rifampin accelerates the metabolism of corticosteroid; dosage adjustment may be required when starting or stopping concomitantly administered rifampin). Products include:

Depo-Medrol Single-Dose Vial 2600
Depo-Medrol Sterile Aqueous Suspension 2597

Methylprednisolone Sodium Succinate (Rifampin accelerates the metabolism of corticosteroid; dosage adjustment may be required when starting or stopping concomitantly administered rifampin). Products include:

Solu-Medrol Sterile Powder 2643

Metipranolol Hydrochloride (Rifampin accelerates the metabolism of beta blocker; dosage adjustment may be required when starting or stopping concomitantly administered rifampin). Products include:

OptiPranolol (Metipranolol 0.3%) Sterile Ophthalmic Solution .... ◉ 258

Metoprolol Succinate (Rifampin accelerates the metabolism of beta blocker; dosage adjustment may be required when starting or stopping concomitantly administered rifampin). Products include:

Toprol-XL Tablets 565

Metoprolol Tartrate (Rifampin accelerates the metabolism of beta blocker; dosage adjustment may be required when starting or stopping concomitantly administered rifampin). Products include:

Lopressor Ampuls 830
Lopressor HCT Tablets 832
Lopressor Tablets 830

Mexiletine Hydrochloride (Rifampin accelerates the metabolism of mexiletine; dosage adjustment may be required when starting or stopping concomitantly administered rifampin). Products include:

Mexitil Capsules 678

Morphine Sulfate (Rifampin accelerates the metabolism of narcotic; dosage adjustment may be required when starting or stopping concomitantly administered rifampin). Products include:

Astramorph/PF Injection, USP (Preservative-Free) 535
Duramorph 962
Infumorph 200 and Infumorph 500 Sterile Solutions 965
MS Contin Tablets 1994
MSIR 1997
Oramorph SR (Morphine Sulfate Sustained-Release Tablets) 2236
RMS Suppositories 2657
Roxanol 2243

Nadolol (Rifampin accelerates the metabolism of beta blocker; dosage adjustment may be required when starting or stopping concomitantly administered rifampin).

No products indexed under this heading.

Nifedipine (Rifampin accelerates the metabolism of nifedipine; dosage adjustment may be required when starting or stopping concomitantly administered rifampin). Products include:

Adalat Capsules (10 mg and 20 mg) 587
Adalat CC 589
Procardia Capsules 1971
Procardia XL Extended Release Tablets 1972

Norethindrone (Rifampin accelerates the metabolism of oral contraceptive; dosage adjustment may be required when starting or stopping concomitantly administered rifampin). Products include:

Brevicon 2088
Micronor Tablets 1872
Modicon 1872
Norinyl 2088
Nor-Q D Tablets 2135
Ortho-Novum 1872
Ovcon 760
Tri-Norinyl 2164

Norethynodrel (Rifampin accelerates the metabolism of oral contraceptive; dosage adjustment may be required when starting or stopping concomitantly administered rifampin).

No products indexed under this heading.

Norgestimate (Rifampin accelerates the metabolism of oral contraceptive or progestin; dosage adjustment may be required when starting or stopping concomitantly administered rifampin). Products include:

Ortho-Cyclen/Ortho-Tri-Cyclen 1858
Ortho-Cyclen/Ortho Tri-Cyclen 1858

Norgestrel (Rifampin accelerates the metabolism of oral contraceptive; dosage adjustment may be required when starting or stopping concomitantly administered rifampin). Products include:

Lo/Ovral Tablets 2746

Lo/Ovral-28 Tablets 2751
Ovral Tablets 2770
Ovral-28 Tablets 2770
Ovrette Tablets 2771

Nortriptyline Hydrochloride (Rifampin accelerates the metabolism of nortriptyline; dosage adjustment may be required when starting or stopping concomitantly administered rifampin). Products include:

Pamelor 2280

Opium Alkaloids (Rifampin accelerates the metabolism of narcotic; dosage adjustment may be required when starting or stopping concomitantly administered rifampin).

No products indexed under this heading.

Oxycodone Hydrochloride (Rifampin accelerates the metabolism of narcotic; dosage adjustment may be required when starting or stopping concomitantly administered rifampin). Products include:

Percocet Tablets 938
Percodan Tablets 939
Percodan-Demi Tablets 940
Roxicodone Tablets, Oral Solution & Intensol (Oxycodone) 2244
Tylox Capsules 1584

Para-Aminosalicylic Acid (Increases the plasma concentration and elimination half-life of isoniazid).

Penbutolol Sulfate (Rifampin accelerates the metabolism of beta blocker; dosage adjustment may be required when starting or stopping concomitantly administered rifampin). Products include:

Levatol 2403

Pentobarbital Sodium (Rifampin accelerates the metabolism of barbiturates; dosage adjustment may be required when starting or stopping concomitantly administered rifampin). Products include:

Nembutal Sodium Capsules 436
Nembutal Sodium Solution 438
Nembutal Sodium Suppositories 440

Phenobarbital (Rifampin accelerates the metabolism of barbiturates; dosage adjustment may be required when starting or stopping concomitantly administered rifampin). Products include:

Arco-Lase Plus Tablets 512
Bellergal-S Tablets 2250
Donnatal 2060
Donnatal Extentabs 2061
Donnatal Tablets 2060
Phenobarbital Elixir and Tablets 1469
Quadrinal Tablets 1350

Phenytoin (Rifampin accelerates the matabolism and isoniazid inhibits the metabolism of phenytoin; dosage adjustment may be required when starting or stopping concomitantly administered rifampin). Products include:

Dilantin Infatabs 1908
Dilantin-125 Suspension 1911

Phenytoin Sodium (Rifampin accelerates the metabolism and isoniazid inhibits the metabolism of phenytoin; dosage adjustment may be required when starting or stopping concomitantly administered rifampin). Products include:

Dilantin Kapseals 1906
Dilantin Parenteral 1910

Pindolol (Rifampin accelerates the metabolism of beta blocker; dosage adjustment may be required when starting or stopping concomitantly administered rifampin). Products include:

Visken Tablets 2299

Prednisolone Acetate (Rifampin accelerates the metabolism of corticosteroid; dosage adjustment may be required when starting or stopping concomitantly administered rifampin; may increase the serum concentration of isoniazid by increasing acetylation rate and/or renal clearance). Products include:

AK-CIDE .... ◉ 202
AK-CIDE Ointment .... ◉ 202
Blephamide Liquifilm Sterile Ophthalmic Suspension 476
Blephamide Ointment .... ◉ 237
Econopred & Econopred Plus Ophthalmic Suspensions .... ◉ 217
Poly-Pred Liquifilm .... ◉ 248
Pred Forte .... ◉ 250
Pred Mild .... ◉ 253
Pred-G Liquifilm Sterile Ophthalmic Suspension .... ◉ 251
Pred-G S.O.P. Sterile Ophthalmic Ointment .... ◉ 252
Vasocidin Ointment .... ◉ 268

Prednisolone Sodium Phosphate (Rifampin accelerates the metabolism of corticosteroid; dosage adjustment may be required when starting or stopping concomitantly administered rifampin; may increase the serum concentration of isoniazid by increasing acetylation rate and/or renal clearance). Products include:

AK-Pred .... ◉ 204
Hydeltrasol Injection, Sterile 1665
Inflamase .... ◉ 265
Pediapred Oral Liquid 995
Vasocidin Ophthalmic Solution ...... ◉ 270

Prednisolone Tebutate (Rifampin accelerates the metabolism of corticosteroid; dosage adjustment may be required when starting or stopping concomitantly administered rifampin; may increase the serum concentration of isoniazid by increasing acetylation rate and/or renal clearance). Products include:

Hydeltra-T.B.A. Sterile Suspension 1667

Prednisone (Rifampin accelerates the metabolism of corticosteroid; dosage adjustment may be required when starting or stopping concomitantly administered rifampin). Products include:

Deltasone Tablets 2595

Primidone (Isoniazid inhibits the metabolism of primidone). Products include:

Mysoline 2754

Probenecid (Increases blood levels of rifampin). Products include:

Benemid Tablets 1611
ColBENEMID Tablets 1622

Propoxyphene Hydrochloride (Rifampin accelerates the metabolism of narcotic; dosage adjustment may be required when starting or stopping concomitantly administered rifampin). Products include:

Darvon 1435
Wygesic Tablets 2827

Propoxyphene Napsylate (Rifampin accelerates the metabolism of narcotic; dosage adjustment may be required when starting or stopping concomitantly administered rifampin). Products include:

Darvon-N/Darvocet-N 1433

Propranolol Hydrochloride (Rifampin accelerates the metabolism of beta blocker; dosage adjustment may be required when starting or stopping concomitantly administered rifampin). Products include:

Inderal 2728
Inderal LA Long Acting Capsules 2730
Inderide Tablets 2732
Inderide LA Long Acting Capsules .. 2734

(**◙** Described in PDR For Nonprescription Drugs) (◉ Described in PDR For Ophthalmology)

Quinidine Gluconate (Rifampin accelerates the metabolism of quinidine; dosage adjustment may be required when starting or stopping concomitantly administered rifampin). Products include:

Quinaglute Dura-Tabs Tablets 649

Quinidine Polygalacturonate (Rifampin accelerates the metabolism of quinidine; dosage adjustment may be required when starting or stopping concomitantly administered rifampin).

No products indexed under this heading.

Quinidine Sulfate (Rifampin accelerates the metabolism of tocainide; dosage adjustment may be required when starting or stopping concomitantly administered rifampin). Products include:

Quinidex Extentabs 2067

Secobarbital Sodium (Rifampin accelerates the metabolism of barbiturates; dosage adjustment may be required when starting or stopping concomitantly administered rifampin). Products include:

Seconal Sodium Pulvules 1474

Sodium Bicarbonate (Reduces absorption of rifampin and isoniazid). Products include:

Alka-Seltzer Effervescent Antacid and Pain Reliever .... ⊕ 701

Alka-Seltzer Extra Strength Effervescent Antacid and Pain Reliever .... ⊕ 703

Alka-Seltzer Gold Effervescent Antacid .... ⊕ 703

Alka-Seltzer Lemon Lime Effervescent Antacid and Pain Reliever .... ⊕ 703

Arm & Hammer Pure Baking Soda .... ⊕ 627

Ceo-Two Rectal Suppositories 666

Citrocarbonate Antacid .... ⊕ 770

Massengill Disposable Douches ...... ⊕ 820

Massengill Liquid Concentrate .... ⊕ 820

NuLYTELY 689

Cherry Flavor NuLYTELY 689

Sotalol Hydrochloride (Rifampin accelerates the metabolism of beta blocker; dosage adjustment may be required when starting or stopping concomitantly administered rifampin). Products include:

Betapace Tablets 641

Sufentanil Citrate (Rifampin accelerates the metabolism of narcotic; dosage adjustment may be required when starting or stopping concomitantly administered rifampin). Products include:

Sufenta Injection 1309

Sulfamethoxazole (Increases blood levels of rifampin). Products include:

Azo Gantanol Tablets 2080

Bactrim DS Tablets 2084

Bactrim I.V. Infusion 2082

Bactrim 2084

Gantanol Tablets 2119

Septra 1174

Septra I.V. Infusion 1169

Septra I.V. Infusion ADD-Vantage Vials 1171

Septra 1174

Sulfasalazine (Reduced plasma concentration of sulfapyridine by rifampin due to alteration in colonic bacteria responsible for reduction of sulfasalazine to sulfapyridine). Products include:

Azulfidine 1949

Theophylline (Rifampin accelerates the metabolism of theophylline and isoniazid inhibits the metabolism; dosage adjustment may be required when starting stopping concomitantly administered rifampin). Products include:

Marax Tablets & DF Syrup 2200

Quibron 2053

Theophylline Anhydrous (Rifampin accelerates the metabolism of theophylline and isoniazid inhibits the metabolism; dosage adjustment may be required when starting stopping concomitantly administered rifampin). Products include:

Aerolate 1004

Primatene Dual Action Formula ...... ⊕ 872

Primatene Tablets .... ⊕ 873

Respbid Tablets 682

Slo-bid Gyrocaps 2033

Theo-24 Extended Release Capsules 2568

Theo-Dur Extended-Release Tablets 1327

Theo-X Extended-Release Tablets .. 788

Uni-Dur Extended-Release Tablets .. 1331

Uniphyl 400 mg Tablets 2001

Theophylline Calcium Salicylate (Rifampin accelerates the metabolism of theophylline and isoniazid inhibits the metabolism; dosage adjustment may be required when starting stopping concomitantly administered rifampin). Products include:

Quadrinal Tablets 1350

Theophylline Sodium Glycinate (Rifampin accelerates the metabolism of theophylline and isoniazid inhibits the metabolism; dosage adjustment may be required when starting stopping concomitantly administered rifampin).

No products indexed under this heading.

Thiamylal Sodium (Rifampin accelerates the metabolism of barbiturates; dosage adjustment may be required when starting or stopping concomitantly administered rifampin).

No products indexed under this heading.

Timolol Hemihydrate (Rifampin accelerates the metabolism of beta blocker; dosage adjustment may be required when starting or stopping concomitantly administered rifampin). Products include:

Betimol 0.25%, 0.5% .... © 261

Timolol Maleate (Rifampin accelerates the metabolism of beta blocker; dosage adjustment may be required when starting or stopping concomitantly administered rifampin). Products include:

Blocadren Tablets 1614

Timolide Tablets 1748

Timoptic in Ocudose 1753

Timoptic Sterile Ophthalmic Solution 1751

Timoptic-XE 1755

Tocainide Hydrochloride (Rifampin accelerates the metabolism of tocainide; dosage adjustment may be required when starting or stopping concomitantly administered rifampin). Products include:

Tonocard Tablets 531

Tolazamide (Rifampin accelerates the metabolism of oral hypoglycemic agent; isoniazid may produce hyperglycemia and lead to loss of glucose control; dosage adjustment may be required when starting or stopping concomitantly administered rifampin).

No products indexed under this heading.

Tolbutamide (Rifampin accelerates the metabolism of oral hypoglycemic agent; isoniazid may produce hyperglycemia and lead to loss of glucose control; dosage adjustment may be required when starting or stopping/concomitantly administered rifampin).

No products indexed under this heading.

Triamcinolone (Rifampin accelerates the metabolism of corticosteroid; dosage adjustment may be required when starting or stopping concomitantly administered rifampin). Products include:

Aristocort Tablets 1022

Triamcinolone Acetonide (Rifampin accelerates the metabolism of corticosteroid; dosage adjustment may be required when starting or stopping concomitantly administered rifampin). Products include:

Aristocort A 0.025% Cream 1027

Aristocort A 0.5% Cream 1031

Aristocort A 0.1% Cream 1029

Aristocort A 0.1% Ointment 1030

Azmacort Oral Inhaler 2011

Nasacort Nasal Inhaler 2024

Triamcinolone Diacetate (Rifampin accelerates the metabolism of corticosteroid; dosage adjustment may be required when starting or stopping concomitantly administered rifampin). Products include:

Aristocort Suspension (Forte Parenteral) 1027

Aristocort Suspension (Intralesional) 1025

Triamcinolone Hexacetonide (Rifampin accelerates the metabolism of corticosteroid; dosage adjustment may be required when starting or stopping concomitantly administered rifampin). Products include:

Aristospan Suspension (Intra-articular) 1033

Aristospan Suspension (Intralesional) 1032

Trimethoprim (Increases blood levels of rifampin). Products include:

Bactrim DS Tablets 2084

Bactrim I.V. Infusion 2082

Bactrim 2084

Proloprim Tablets 1155

Septra 1174

Septra I.V. Infusion 1169

Septra I.V. Infusion ADD-Vantage Vials 1171

Septra 1174

Trimpex Tablets 2163

Valproic Acid (Isoniazid inhibits the metabolism of valproic acid). Products include:

Depakene 413

Verapamil Hydrochloride (Rifampin accelerates the metabolism of verapamil; dosage adjustment may be required when starting or stopping concomitantly administered rifampin). Products include:

Calan SR Caplets 2422

Calan Tablets 2419

Isoptin Injectable 1344

Isoptin Oral Tablets 1346

Isoptin SR Tablets 1348

Verelan Capsules 1410

Verelan Capsules 2824

Warfarin Sodium (Rifampin accelerates the metabolism of anticoagulants and isoniazid inhibits the metabolism; increased requirements of coumarin type anticoagulant; dosage adjustment may be required when starting or stopping concomitantly administered rifampin). Products include:

Coumadin 926

Food Interactions

Alcohol (Daily ingestion of alcohol may be associated with higher incidence of isoniazid hepatitis).

Cheese, unspecified (Isoniazid has some MAO inhibiting activity, an interaction with tyramine containing food may occur).

Fish, tropical (Isoniazid may inhibit diamine oxidase, causing exaggerated response (headache, sweating, palpitations, flushing, hypotension) to food containing histamine).

Food with high concentration of tyramine (Isoniazid has some MAO inhibiting activity, an interaction with tyramine containing food may occur).

Skipjack fish (Isoniazid may inhibit diamine oxidase, causing exaggerated response (headache, sweating, palpitations, flushing, hypotension) to food containing histamine).

Tuna fish (Isoniazid may inhibit diamine oxidase, causing exaggerated response (headache, sweating, palpitations, flushing, hypotension) to food containing histamine).

Wine, red (Isoniazid has some MAO inhibiting activity, an interaction with tyramine containing food may occur).

RIMACTANE CAPSULES

(Rifampin) 847

May interact with oral anticoagulants, oral contraceptives, oral hypoglycemic agents, corticosteroids, and cardiac glycosides. Compounds in these categories include:

Acarbose (Diminished effects).

No products indexed under this heading.

Betamethasone Acetate (Diminished effects). Products include:

Celestone Soluspan Suspension 2347

Betamethasone Sodium Phosphate (Diminished effects). Products include:

Celestone Soluspan Suspension 2347

Chlorpropamide (Diminished effects). Products include:

Diabinese Tablets 1935

Cortisone Acetate (Diminished effects). Products include:

Cortone Acetate Sterile Suspension 1623

Cortone Acetate Tablets 1624

Dapsone (Diminished effects). Products include:

Dapsone Tablets USP 1284

Deslanoside (Diminished effects).

No products indexed under this heading.

Desogestrel (Reliability of oral contraceptive affected). Products include:

Desogen Tablets 1817

Ortho-Cept 1851

Dexamethasone (Diminished effects). Products include:

AK-Trol Ointment & Suspension .... © 205

Decadron Elixir 1633

Decadron Tablets 1635

Decaspray Topical Aerosol 1648

Dexacidin Ointment .... © 263

Maxitrol Ophthalmic Ointment and Suspension .... © 224

TobraDex Ophthalmic Suspension and Ointment 473

Dexamethasone Acetate (Diminished effects). Products include:

Dalalone D.P. Injectable 1011

Decadron-LA Sterile Suspension 1646

Dexamethasone Sodium Phosphate (Diminished effects). Products include:

Decadron Phosphate Injection 1637

Decadron Phosphate Respihaler 1642

IMPORTANT NOTE: Always consult each drug listing in the patient's regimen for possible interactions.

Rimactane | Interactions Index | 896

Decadron Phosphate Sterile Ophthalmic Ointment ... 1641
Decadron Phosphate Sterile Ophthalmic Solution ... 1642
Decadron Phosphate Topical Cream ... 1644
Decadron Phosphate Turbinaire ... 1645
Decadron Phosphate with Xylocaine Injection, Sterile ... 1639
Dexacort Phosphate in Respihaler .. 458
Dexacort Phosphate in Turbinaire .. 459
NeoDecadron Sterile Ophthalmic Ointment ... 1712
NeoDecadron Sterile Ophthalmic Solution ... 1713
NeoDecadron Topical Cream ... 1714

Dicumarol (Increased requirements).
No products indexed under this heading.

Digitoxin (Diminished effects). Products include:
Crystodigin Tablets ... 1433

Digoxin (Diminished effects). Products include:
Lanoxicaps ... 1117
Lanoxin Elixir Pediatric ... 1120
Lanoxin Injection ... 1123
Lanoxin Injection Pediatric ... 1126
Lanoxin Tablets ... 1128

Ethambutol Hydrochloride (Potential for thrombocytopenia). Products include:
Myambutol Tablets ... 1386

Ethinyl Estradiol (Reliability of oral contraceptive affected). Products include:
Brevicon ... 2088
Demulen ... 2428
Desogen Tablets ... 1817
Levlen/Tri-Levlen ... 651
Lo/Ovral Tablets ... 2746
Lo/Ovral-28 Tablets ... 2751
Modicon ... 1872
Nordette-21 Tablets ... 2755
Nordette-28 Tablets ... 2758
Norinyl ... 2088
Ortho-Cept ... 1851
Ortho-Cyclen/Ortho-Tri-Cyclen ... 1858
Ortho-Novum ... 1872
Ortho-Cyclen/Ortho Tri-Cyclen ... 1858
Ovcon ... 760
Ovral Tablets ... 2770
Ovral-28 Tablets ... 2770
Levlen/Tri-Levlen ... 651
Tri-Norinyl ... 2164
Triphasil-21 Tablets ... 2814
Triphasil-28 Tablets ... 2819

Ethynodiol Diacetate (Reliability of oral contraceptive affected). Products include:
Demulen ... 2428

Fludrocortisone Acetate (Diminished effects). Products include:
Florinef Acetate Tablets ... 505

Glipizide (Diminished effects). Products include:
Glucotrol Tablets ... 1967
Glucotrol XL Extended Release Tablets ... 1968

Glyburide (Diminished effects). Products include:
DiaBeta Tablets ... 1239
Glynase PresTab Tablets ... 2609
Micronase Tablets ... 2623

Hepatotoxic Drugs, unspecified (Increased risk of liver toxicity).

Hydrocortisone (Diminished effects). Products include:
Anusol-HC Cream 2.5% ... 1896
Aquanil HC Lotion ... 1931
Bactine Hydrocortisone Anti-Itch Cream ... ▣ 709
Caldecort Anti-Itch Hydrocortisone Spray ... ▣ 631
Cortaid ... ▣ 836
CORTENEMA ... 2535
Cortisporin Ointment ... 1085
Cortisporin Ophthalmic Ointment Sterile ... 1085
Cortisporin Ophthalmic Suspension Sterile ... 1086
Cortisporin Otic Solution Sterile ... 1087
Cortisporin Otic Suspension Sterile 1088
Cortizone-5 ... ▣ 831
Cortizone-10 ... ▣ 831
Hydrocortone Tablets ... 1672
Hytone ... 907
Massengill Medicated Soft Cloth Towelettes ... 2458
PediOtic Suspension Sterile ... 1153
Preparation H Hydrocortisone 1% Cream ... ▣ 872
ProctoCream-HC 2.5% ... 2408
VōSoL HC Otic Solution ... 2678

Hydrocortisone Acetate (Diminished effects). Products include:
Analpram-HC Rectal Cream 1% and 2.5% ... 977
Anusol HC-1 Anti-Itch Hydrocortisone Ointment ... ▣ 847
Anusol-HC Suppositories ... 1897
Caldecort ... ▣ 631
Carmol HC ... 924
Coly-Mycin S Otic w/Neomycin & Hydrocortisone ... 1906
Cortaid ... ▣ 836
Cortifoam ... 2396
Cortisporin Cream ... 1084
Epifoam ... 2399
Hydrocortone Acetate Sterile Suspension ... 1669
Mantadil Cream ... 1135
Nupercainal Hydrocortisone 1% Cream ... ▣ 645
Ophthocort ... ◉ 311
Pramosone Cream, Lotion & Ointment ... 978
ProctoCream-HC ... 2408
ProctoFoam-HC ... 2409
Terra-Cortril Ophthalmic Suspension ... 2210

Hydrocortisone Sodium Phosphate (Diminished effects). Products include:
Hydrocortone Phosphate Injection, Sterile ... 1670

Hydrocortisone Sodium Succinate (Diminished effects). Products include:
Solu-Cortef Sterile Powder ... 2641

Levonorgestrel (Reliability of oral contraceptive affected). Products include:
Levlen/Tri-Levlen ... 651
Nordette-21 Tablets ... 2755
Nordette-28 Tablets ... 2758
Norplant System ... 2759
Levlen/Tri-Levlen ... 651
Triphasil-21 Tablets ... 2814
Triphasil-28 Tablets ... 2819

Mestranol (Reliability of oral contraceptive affected). Products include:
Norinyl ... 2088
Ortho-Novum ... 1872

Metformin Hydrochloride (Diminished effects). Products include:
Glucophage ... 752

Methadone Hydrochloride (Diminished effects). Products include:
Methadone Hydrochloride Oral Concentrate ... 2233
Methadone Hydrochloride Oral Solution & Tablets ... 2235

Methylprednisolone Acetate (Diminished effects). Products include:
Depo-Medrol Single-Dose Vial ... 2600
Depo-Medrol Sterile Aqueous Suspension ... 2597

Methylprednisolone Sodium Succinate (Diminished effects). Products include:
Solu-Medrol Sterile Powder ... 2643

Norethindrone (Reliability of oral contraceptive affected). Products include:
Brevicon ... 2088
Micronor Tablets ... 1872
Modicon ... 1872
Norinyl ... 2088
Nor-Q D Tablets ... 2135
Ortho-Novum ... 1872
Ovcon ... 760
Tri-Norinyl ... 2164

Norethynodrel (Reliability of oral contraceptive affected).
No products indexed under this heading.

Norgestimate (Reliability of oral contraceptive affected). Products include:
Ortho-Cyclen/Ortho-Tri-Cyclen ... 1858
Ortho-Cyclen/Ortho Tri-Cyclen ... 1858

Norgestrel (Reliability of oral contraceptive affected). Products include:
Lo/Ovral Tablets ... 2746
Lo/Ovral-28 Tablets ... 2751
Ovral Tablets ... 2770
Ovral-28 Tablets ... 2770
Ovrette Tablets ... 2771

Prednisolone Acetate (Diminished effects). Products include:
AK-CIDE ... ◉ 202
AK-CIDE Ointment ... ◉ 202
Blephamide Liquifilm Sterile Ophthalmic Suspension ... 476
Blephamide Ointment ... ◉ 237
Econopred & Econopred Plus Ophthalmic Suspensions ... ◉ 217
Poly-Pred Liquifilm ... ◉ 248
Pred Forte ... ◉ 250
Pred Mild ... ◉ 253
Pred-G Liquifilm Sterile Ophthalmic Suspension ... ◉ 251
Pred-G S.O.P. Sterile Ophthalmic Ointment ... ◉ 252
Vasocidin Ointment ... ◉ 268

Prednisolone Sodium Phosphate (Diminished effects). Products include:
AK-Pred ... ◉ 204
Hydeltrasol Injection, Sterile ... 1665
Inflamase ... ◉ 265
Pediapred Oral Liquid ... 995
Vasocidin Ophthalmic Solution ... ◉ 270

Prednisolone Tebutate (Diminished effects). Products include:
Hydeltra-T.B.A. Sterile Suspension 1667

Prednisone (Diminished effects). Products include:
Deltasone Tablets ... 2595

Tolazamide (Diminished effects).
No products indexed under this heading.

Tolbutamide (Diminished effects).
No products indexed under this heading.

Triamcinolone (Diminished effects). Products include:
Aristocort Tablets ... 1022

Triamcinolone Acetonide (Diminished effects). Products include:
Aristocort A 0.025% Cream ... 1027
Aristocort A 0.5% Cream ... 1031
Aristocort A 0.1% Cream ... 1029
Aristocort A 0.1% Ointment ... 1030
Azmacort Oral Inhaler ... 2011
Nasacort Nasal Inhaler ... 2024

Triamcinolone Diacetate (Diminished effects). Products include:
Aristocort Suspension (Forte Parenteral) ... 1027
Aristocort Suspension (Intralesional) ... 1025

Triamcinolone Hexacetonide (Diminished effects). Products include:
Aristospan Suspension (Intra-articular) ... 1033
Aristospan Suspension (Intralesional) ... 1032

Verapamil Hydrochloride (Reduced bioavailability and efficacy). Products include:
Calan SR Caplets ... 2422
Calan Tablets ... 2419
Isoptin Injectable ... 1344
Isoptin Oral Tablets ... 1346
Isoptin SR Tablets ... 1348
Verelan Capsules ... 1410
Verelan Capsules ... 2824

Warfarin Sodium (Increased requirements). Products include:
Coumadin ... 926

RISPERDAL
(Risperidone) ... 1301
May interact with antihypertensives, dopamine agonists, central nervous system depressants, drugs that inhibit cytochrome p450iid6 and other p450 isoenzymes, and certain other agents. Compounds in these categories include:

Acebutolol Hydrochloride (Because of its potential for inducing hypotension, risperidone may enhance the hypotensive effect of therapeutic agents with a potential for producing hypotension). Products include:
Sectral Capsules ... 2807

Alfentanil Hydrochloride (Effects not specified; caution should be used when used concurrently). Products include:
Alfenta Injection ... 1286

Alprazolam (Effects not specified; caution should be used when used concurrently). Products include:
Xanax Tablets ... 2649

Amitriptyline Hydrochloride (Inhibitors of cytochrome P450IID6 could interfere with the conversion of risperidone to 9-hydroxyrisperidone). Products include:
Elavil ... 2838
Endep Tablets ... 2174
Etrafon ... 2355
Limbitrol ... 2180
Triavil Tablets ... 1757

Amlodipine Besylate (Because of its potential for inducing hypotension, risperidone may enhance the hypotensive effect of therapeutic agents with a potential for producing hypotension). Products include:
Lotrel Capsules ... 840
Norvasc Tablets ... 1940

Aprobarbital (Effects not specified; caution should be used when used concurrently).
No products indexed under this heading.

Atenolol (Because of its potential for inducing hypotension, risperidone may enhance the hypotensive effect of therapeutic agents with a potential for producing hypotension). Products include:
Tenoretic Tablets ... 2845
Tenormin Tablets and I.V. Injection 2847

Benazepril Hydrochloride (Because of its potential for inducing hypotension, risperidone may enhance the hypotensive effect of therapeutic agents with a potential for producing hypotension). Products include:
Lotensin Tablets ... 834
Lotensin HCT ... 837
Lotrel Capsules ... 840

Bendroflumethiazide (Because of its potential for inducing hypotension, risperidone may enhance the hypotensive effect of therapeutic agents with a potential for producing hypotension).
No products indexed under this heading.

Betaxolol Hydrochloride (Because of its potential for inducing hypotension, risperidone may enhance the hypotensive effect of therapeutic agents with a potential for producing hypotension). Products include:
Betoptic Ophthalmic Solution ... 469
Betoptic S Ophthalmic Suspension 471
Kerlone Tablets ... 2436

(▣ Described in PDR For Nonprescription Drugs) (◉ Described in PDR For Ophthalmology)

897 Interactions Index Risperdal

Bisoprolol Fumarate (Because of its potential for inducing hypotension, risperidone may enhance the hypotensive effect of therapeutic agents with a potential for producing hypotension). Products include:

Zebeta Tablets ... 1413
Ziac ... 1415

Bromocriptine Mesylate (Risperidone may antagonize the effect of dopamine agonists). Products include:

Parlodel ... 2281

Buprenorphine (Effects not specified; caution should be used when used concurrently). Products include:

Buprenex Injectable ... 2006

Buspirone Hydrochloride (Effects not specified; caution should be used when used concurrently). Products include:

BuSpar ... 737

Butabarbital (Effects not specified; caution should be used when used concurrently).

No products indexed under this heading.

Butalbital (Effects not specified; caution should be used when used concurrently). Products include:

Esgic-plus Tablets ... 1013
Fioricet Tablets ... 2258
Fioricet with Codeine Capsules ... 2260
Fiorinal Capsules ... 2261
Fiorinal with Codeine Capsules ... 2262
Fiorinal Tablets ... 2261
Phrenilin ... 785
Sedapap Tablets 50 mg/650 mg .. 1543

Captopril (Because of its potential for inducing hypotension, risperidone may enhance the hypotensive effect of therapeutic agents with a potential for producing hypotension). Products include:

Capoten ... 739
Capozide ... 742

Carbamazepine (Chronic administration of carbamazepine may increase the clearance of risperidone). Products include:

Atretol Tablets ... 573
Tegretol Chewable Tablets ... 852
Tegretol Suspension ... 852
Tegretol Tablets ... 852

Carteolol Hydrochloride (Because of its potential for inducing hypotension, risperidone may enhance the hypotensive effect of therapeutic agents with a potential for producing hypotension). Products include:

Cartrol Tablets ... 410
Ocupress Ophthalmic Solution, 1% Sterile ... ◉ 309

Chlordiazepoxide (Effects not specified; caution should be used when used concurrently). Products include:

Libritabs Tablets ... 2177
Limbitrol ... 2180

Chlordiazepoxide Hydrochloride (Effects not specified; caution should be used when used concurrently). Products include:

Librax Capsules ... 2176
Librium Capsules ... 2178
Librium Injectable ... 2179

Chlorothiazide (Because of its potential for inducing hypotension, risperidone may enhance the hypotensive effect of therapeutic agents with a potential for producing hypotension). Products include:

Aldoclor Tablets ... 1598
Diupres Tablets ... 1650
Diuril Oral ... 1653

Chlorothiazide Sodium (Because of its potential for inducing hypotension, risperidone may enhance the hypotensive effect of therapeutic agents with a potential for producing hypotension). Products include:

Diuril Sodium Intravenous ... 1652

Chlorpromazine (Inhibitors of cytochrome P450IID6 could interfere with the conversion of risperidone to 9-hydroxyrisperidone; caution should be used when used concurrently). Products include:

Thorazine Suppositories ... 2523

Chlorpromazine Hydrochloride (Inhibitors of cytochrome P450IID6 could interfere with the conversion of risperidone to 9-hydroxyrisperidone; caution should be used when used concurrently). Products include:

Thorazine ... 2523

Chlorprothixene (Effects not specified; caution should be used when used concurrently).

No products indexed under this heading.

Chlorprothixene Hydrochloride (Effects not specified; caution should be used when used concurrently).

No products indexed under this heading.

Chlorthalidone (Because of its potential for inducing hypotension, risperidone may enhance the hypotensive effect of therapeutic agents with a potential for producing hypotension). Products include:

Combipres Tablets ... 677
Tenoretic Tablets ... 2845
Thalitone ... 1245

Clonidine (Because of its potential for inducing hypotension, risperidone may enhance the hypotensive effect of therapeutic agents with a potential for producing hypotension). Products include:

Catapres-TTS ... 675

Clonidine Hydrochloride (Because of its potential for inducing hypotension, risperidone may enhance the hypotensive effect of therapeutic agents with a potential for producing hypotension). Products include:

Catapres Tablets ... 674
Combipres Tablets ... 677

Clorazepate Dipotassium (Effects not specified; caution should be used when used concurrently). Products include:

Tranxene ... 451

Clozapine (Chronic administration of clozapine with risperidone may decrease the clearance of risperidone; caution should be used when used concurrently). Products include:

Clozaril Tablets ... 2252

CNS-Active Drugs, unspecified (Effects not specified; caution should be used when used concurrently).

Codeine Phosphate (Effects not specified; caution should be used when used concurrently). Products include:

Actifed with Codeine Cough Syrup.. 1067
Brontex ... 1981
Deconsal C Expectorant Syrup ... 456
Deconsal Pediatric Syrup ... 457
Dimetane-DC Cough Syrup ... 2059
Empirin with Codeine Tablets ... 1093
Fioricet with Codeine Capsules ... 2260
Fiorinal with Codeine Capsules ... 2262
Isoclor Expectorant ... 990
Novahistine DH ... 2462
Novahistine Expectorant ... 2463
Nucofed ... 2051
Phenergan with Codeine ... 2777
Phenergan VC with Codeine ... 2781
Robitussin A-C Syrup ... 2073
Robitussin-DAC Syrup ... 2074
Ryna ... 841
Soma Compound w/Codeine Tablets ... 2676
Tussi-Organidin NR Liquid and S NR Liquid ... 2677
Tylenol with Codeine ... 1583

Deserpidine (Because of its potential for inducing hypotension, risperidone may enhance the hypotensive effect of therapeutic agents with a potential for producing hypotension).

No products indexed under this heading.

Desflurane (Effects not specified; caution should be used when used concurrently). Products include:

Suprane ... 1813

Dezocine (Effects not specified; caution should be used when used concurrently). Products include:

Dalgan Injection ... 538

Diazepam (Effects not specified; caution should be used when used concurrently). Products include:

Dizac ... 1809
Valium Injectable ... 2182
Valium Tablets ... 2183
Valrelease Capsules ... 2169

Diazoxide (Because of its potential for inducing hypotension, risperidone may enhance the hypotensive effect of therapeutic agents with a potential for producing hypotension). Products include:

Hyperstat I.V. Injection ... 2363
Proglycem ... 580

Diltiazem Hydrochloride (Because of its potential for inducing hypotension, risperidone may enhance the hypotensive effect of therapeutic agents with a potential for producing hypotension). Products include:

Cardizem CD Capsules ... 1506
Cardizem SR Capsules ... 1510
Cardizem Injectable ... 1508
Cardizem Tablets ... 1512
Dilacor XR Extended-release Capsules ... 2018

Dopamine Hydrochloride (Risperidone may antagonize the effect of dopamine agonists).

No products indexed under this heading.

Doxazosin Mesylate (Because of its potential for inducing hypotension, risperidone may enhance the hypotensive effect of therapeutic agents with a potential for producing hypotension). Products include:

Cardura Tablets ... 2186

Droperidol (Effects not specified; caution should be used when used concurrently). Products include:

Inapsine Injection ... 1296

Enalapril Maleate (Because of its potential for inducing hypotension, risperidone may enhance the hypotensive effect of therapeutic agents with a potential for producing hypotension). Products include:

Vaseretic Tablets ... 1765
Vasotec Tablets ... 1771

Enalaprilat (Because of its potential for inducing hypotension, risperidone may enhance the hypotensive effect of therapeutic agents with a potential for producing hypotension). Products include:

Vasotec I.V. ... 1768

Enflurane (Effects not specified; caution should be used when used concurrently).

No products indexed under this heading.

Esmolol Hydrochloride (Because of its potential for inducing hypotension, risperidone may enhance the hypotensive effect of therapeutic agents with a potential for producing hypotension). Products include:

Brevibloc Injection ... 1808

Estazolam (Effects not specified; caution should be used when used concurrently). Products include:

ProSom Tablets ... 449

Ethchlorvynol (Effects not specified; caution should be used when used concurrently). Products include:

Placidyl Capsules ... 448

Ethinamate (Effects not specified; caution should be used when used concurrently).

No products indexed under this heading.

Felodipine (Because of its potential for inducing hypotension, risperidone may enhance the hypotensive effect of therapeutic agents with a potential for producing hypotension). Products include:

Plendil Extended-Release Tablets ... 527

Fentanyl (Effects not specified; caution should be used when used concurrently). Products include:

Duragesic Transdermal System ... 1288

Fentanyl Citrate (Effects not specified; caution should be used when used concurrently). Products include:

Sublimaze Injection ... 1307

Fluoxetine Hydrochloride (Inhibitors of cytochrome P450IID6 could interfere with the conversion of risperidone to 9-hydroxyrisperidone). Products include:

Prozac Pulvules & Liquid, Oral Solution ... 919

Fluphenazine Decanoate (Effects not specified; caution should be used when used concurrently). Products include:

Prolixin Decanoate ... 509

Fluphenazine Enanthate (Effects not specified; caution should be used when used concurrently). Products include:

Prolixin Enanthate ... 509

Fluphenazine Hydrochloride (Effects not specified; caution should be used when used concurrently). Products include:

Prolixin ... 509

Flurazepam Hydrochloride (Effects not specified; caution should be used when used concurrently). Products include:

Dalmane Capsules ... 2173

Fosinopril Sodium (Because of its potential for inducing hypotension, risperidone may enhance the hypotensive effect of therapeutic agents with a potential for producing hypotension). Products include:

Monopril Tablets ... 757

Furosemide (Because of its potential for inducing hypotension, risperidone may enhance the hypotensive effect of therapeutic agents with a potential for producing hypotension). Products include:

Lasix Injection, Oral Solution and Tablets ... 1240

Glutethimide (Effects not specified; caution should be used when used concurrently).

No products indexed under this heading.

IMPORTANT NOTE: Always consult each drug listing in the patient's regimen for possible interactions.

Guanabenz Acetate (Because of its potential for inducing hypotension, risperidone may enhance the hypotensive effect of therapeutic agents with a potential for producing hypotension).

No products indexed under this heading.

Guanethidine Monosulfate (Because of its potential for inducing hypotension, risperidone may enhance the hypotensive effect of therapeutic agents with a potential for producing hypotension). Products include:

Esimil Tablets 822
Ismelin Tablets 827

Haloperidol (Inhibitors of cytochrome P450IID6 could interfere with the conversion of risperidone to 9-hydroxyrisperidone; caution should be used when used concurrently). Products include:

Haldol Injection, Tablets and Concentrate 1575

Haloperidol Decanoate (Inhibitors of cytochrome P450IID6 could interfere with the conversion of risperidone to 9-hydroxyrisperidone; caution should be used when used concurrently). Products include:

Haldol Decanoate 1577

Hydralazine Hydrochloride (Because of its potential for inducing hypotension, risperidone may enhance the hypotensive effect of therapeutic agents with a potential for producing hypotension). Products include:

Apresazide Capsules 808
Apresoline Hydrochloride Tablets .. 809
Ser-Ap-Es Tablets 849

Hydrochlorothiazide (Because of its potential for inducing hypotension, risperidone may enhance the hypotensive effect of therapeutic agents with a potential for producing hypotension). Products include:

Aldactazide 2413
Aldoril Tablets 1604
Apresazide Capsules 808
Capozide 742
Dyazide 2479
Esidrix Tablets 821
Esimil Tablets 822
HydroDIURIL Tablets 1674
Hydropres Tablets 1675
Hyzaar Tablets 1677
Inderide Tablets 2732
Inderide LA Long Acting Capsules .. 2734
Lopressor HCT Tablets 832
Lotensin HCT 837
Maxzide 1380
Moduretic Tablets 1705
Oretic Tablets 443
Prinzide Tablets 1737
Ser-Ap-Es Tablets 849
Timolide Tablets 1748
Vaseretic Tablets 1765
Zestoretic 2850
Ziac 1415

Hydrocodone Bitartrate (Effects not specified; caution should be used when used concurrently). Products include:

Anexsia 5/500 Elixir 1781
Anexia Tablets 1782
Codiclear DH Syrup 791
Deconamine CX Cough and Cold Liquid and Tablets 1319
Duratuss HD Elixir 2565
Hycodan Tablets and Syrup 930
Hycomine Compound Tablets 932
Hycomine 931
Hycotuss Expectorant Syrup 933
Hydrocet Capsules 782
Lorcet 10/650 1018
Lortab 2566
Tussend 1783
Tussend Expectorant 1785
Vicodin Tablets 1356
Vicodin ES Tablets 1357
Vicodin Tuss Expectorant 1358
Zydone Capsules 949

Hydrocodone Polistirex (Effects not specified; caution should be used when used concurrently). Products include:

Tussionex Pennkinetic Extended-Release Suspension 998

Hydroflumethiazide (Because of its potential for inducing hypotension, risperidone may enhance the hypotensive effect of therapeutic agents with a potential for producing hypotension). Products include:

Diucardin Tablets 2718

Hydroxyzine Hydrochloride (Effects not specified; caution should be used when used concurrently). Products include:

Atarax Tablets & Syrup 2185
Marax Tablets & DF Syrup 2200
Vistaril Intramuscular Solution 2216

Imipramine Hydrochloride (Inhibitors of cytochrome P450IID6 could interfere with the conversion of risperidone to 9-hydroxyrisperidone). Products include:

Tofranil Ampuls 854
Tofranil Tablets 856

Indapamide (Because of its potential for inducing hypotension, risperidone may enhance the hypotensive effect of therapeutic agents with a potential for producing hypotension). Products include:

Lozol Tablets 2022

Isoflurane (Effects not specified; caution should be used when used concurrently).

No products indexed under this heading.

Isradipine (Because of its potential for inducing hypotension, risperidone may enhance the hypotensive effect of therapeutic agents with a potential for producing hypotension). Products include:

DynaCirc Capsules 2256

Ketamine Hydrochloride (Effects not specified; caution should be used when used concurrently).

No products indexed under this heading.

Labetalol Hydrochloride (Because of its potential for inducing hypotension, risperidone may enhance the hypotensive effect of therapeutic agents with a potential for producing hypotension). Products include:

Normodyne Injection 2377
Normodyne Tablets 2379
Trandate 1185

Levobunolol Hydrochloride (Because of its potential for inducing hypotension, risperidone may enhance the hypotensive effect of therapeutic agents with a potential for producing hypotension). Products include:

Betagan .... ◉ 233

Levodopa (Risperidone may antagonize the effect of levodopa). Products include:

Atamet 572
Larodopa Tablets 2129
Sinemet Tablets 943
Sinemet CR Tablets 944

Levorphanol Tartrate (Effects not specified; caution should be used when used concurrently). Products include:

Levo-Dromoran 2129

Lisinopril (Because of its potential for inducing hypotension, risperidone may enhance the hypotensive effect of therapeutic agents with a potential for producing hypotension). Products include:

Prinivil Tablets 1733
Prinzide Tablets 1737
Zestoretic 2850
Zestril Tablets 2854

Lorazepam (Effects not specified; caution should be used when used concurrently). Products include:

Ativan Injection 2698
Ativan Tablets 2700

Losartan Potassium (Because of its potential for inducing hypotension, risperidone may enhance the hypotensive effect of therapeutic agents with a potential for producing hypotension). Products include:

Cozaar Tablets 1628
Hyzaar Tablets 1677

Loxapine Hydrochloride (Effects not specified; caution should be used when used concurrently). Products include:

Loxitane 1378

Loxapine Succinate (Effects not specified; caution should be used when used concurrently). Products include:

Loxitane Capsules 1378

Mecamylamine Hydrochloride (Because of its potential for inducing hypotension, risperidone may enhance the hypotensive effect of therapeutic agents with a potential for producing hypotension). Products include:

Inversine Tablets 1686

Meperidine Hydrochloride (Effects not specified; caution should be used when used concurrently). Products include:

Demerol 2308
Mepergan Injection 2753

Mephobarbital (Effects not specified; caution should be used when used concurrently). Products include:

Mebaral Tablets 2322

Meprobamate (Effects not specified; caution should be used when used concurrently). Products include:

Miltown Tablets 2672
PMB 200 and PMB 400 2783

Mesoridazine Besylate (Effects not specified; caution should be used when used concurrently). Products include:

Serentil 684

Methadone Hydrochloride (Effects not specified; caution should be used when used concurrently). Products include:

Methadone Hydrochloride Oral Concentrate 2233
Methadone Hydrochloride Oral Solution & Tablets 2235

Methohexital Sodium (Effects not specified; caution should be used when used concurrently). Products include:

Brevital Sodium Vials 1429

Methotrimeprazine (Effects not specified; caution should be used when used concurrently). Products include:

Levoprome 1274

Methoxyflurane (Effects not specified; caution should be used when used concurrently).

No products indexed under this heading.

Methyclothiazide (Because of its potential for inducing hypotension, risperidone may enhance the hypotensive effect of therapeutic agents with a potential for producing hypotension). Products include:

Enduron Tablets 420

Methyldopa (Because of its potential for inducing hypotension, risperidone may enhance the hypotensive effect of therapeutic agents with a potential for producing hypotension). Products include:

Aldoclor Tablets 1598
Aldomet Oral 1600
Aldoril Tablets 1604

Methyldopate Hydrochloride (Because of its potential for inducing hypotension, risperidone may enhance the hypotensive effect of therapeutic agents with a potential for producing hypotension). Products include:

Aldomet Ester HCl Injection 1602

Metipranolol Hydrochloride (Because of its potential for inducing hypotension, risperidone may enhance the hypotensive effect of therapeutic agents with a potential for producing hypotension). Products include:

OptiPranolol (Metipranolol 0.3%) Sterile Ophthalmic Solution .... ◉ 258

Metolazone (Because of its potential for inducing hypotension, risperidone may enhance the hypotensive effect of therapeutic agents with a potential for producing hypotension). Products include:

Mykrox Tablets 993
Zaroxolyn Tablets 1000

Metoprolol Succinate (Because of its potential for inducing hypotension, risperidone may enhance the hypotensive effect of therapeutic agents with a potential for producing hypotension). Products include:

Toprol-XL Tablets 565

Metoprolol Tartrate (Because of its potential for inducing hypotension, risperidone may enhance the hypotensive effect of therapeutic agents with a potential for producing hypotension). Products include:

Lopressor Ampuls 830
Lopressor HCT Tablets 832
Lopressor Tablets 830

Metyrosine (Because of its potential for inducing hypotension, risperidone may enhance the hypotensive effect of therapeutic agents with a potential for producing hypotension). Products include:

Demser Capsules 1649

Midazolam Hydrochloride (Effects not specified; caution should be used when used concurrently). Products include:

Versed Injection 2170

Minoxidil (Because of its potential for inducing hypotension, risperidone may enhance the hypotensive effect of therapeutic agents with a potential for producing hypotension). Products include:

Loniten Tablets 2618
Rogaine Topical Solution 2637

Molindone Hydrochloride (Effects not specified; caution should be used when used concurrently). Products include:

Moban Tablets and Concentrate 1048

Morphine Sulfate (Effects not specified; caution should be used when used concurrently). Products include:

Astramorph/PF Injection, USP (Preservative-Free) 535
Duramorph 962
Infumorph 200 and Infumorph 500 Sterile Solutions 965
MS Contin Tablets 1994
MSIR 1997
Oramorph SR (Morphine Sulfate Sustained Release Tablets) 2236
RMS Suppositories 2657
Roxanol 2243

(▭ Described in PDR For Nonprescription Drugs) (◉ Described in PDR For Ophthalmology)

Nadolol (Because of its potential for inducing hypotension, risperidone may enhance the hypotensive effect of therapeutic agents with a potential for producing hypotension).

No products indexed under this heading.

Nicardipine Hydrochloride (Because of its potential for inducing hypotension, risperidone may enhance the hypotensive effect of therapeutic agents with a potential for producing hypotension). Products include:

Cardene Capsules 2095
Cardene I.V. 2709
Cardene SR Capsules 2097

Nifedipine (Because of its potential for inducing hypotension, risperidone may enhance the hypotensive effect of therapeutic agents with a potential for producing hypotension). Products include:

Adalat Capsules (10 mg and 20 mg) 587
Adalat CC 589
Procardia Capsules 1971
Procardia XL Extended Release Tablets 1972

Nisoldipine (Because of its potential for inducing hypotension, risperidone may enhance the hypotensive effect of therapeutic agents with a potential for producing hypotension).

No products indexed under this heading.

Nitroglycerin (Because of its potential for inducing hypotension, risperidone may enhance the hypotensive effect of therapeutic agents with a potential for producing hypotension). Products include:

Deponit NTG Transdermal Delivery System 2397
Nitro-Bid IV 1523
Nitro-Bid Ointment 1524
Nitrodisc 2047
Nitro-Dur (nitroglycerin) Transdermal Infusion System 1326
Nitrolingual Spray 2027
Nitrostat Tablets 1925
Transderm-Nitro Transdermal Therapeutic System 859

Opium Alkaloids (Effects not specified; caution should be used when used concurrently).

No products indexed under this heading.

Oxazepam (Effects not specified; caution should be used when used concurrently). Products include:

Serax Capsules 2810
Serax Tablets 2810

Oxycodone Hydrochloride (Effects not specified; caution should be used when used concurrently). Products include:

Percocet Tablets 938
Percodan Tablets 939
Percodan-Demi Tablets 940
Roxicodone Tablets, Oral Solution & Intensol (Oxycodone) 2244
Tylox Capsules 1584

Penbutolol Sulfate (Because of its potential for inducing hypotension, risperidone may enhance the hypotensive effect of therapeutic agents with a potential for producing hypotension). Products include:

Levatol 2403

Pentobarbital Sodium (Effects not specified; caution should be used when used concurrently). Products include:

Nembutal Sodium Capsules 436
Nembutal Sodium Solution 438
Nembutal Sodium Suppositories 440

Pergolide Mesylate (Risperidone may antagonize the effect of dopamine agonists). Products include:

Permax Tablets 575

Perphenazine (Effects not specified; caution should be used when used concurrently). Products include:

Etrafon 2355
Triavil Tablets 1757
Trilafon 2389

Phenobarbital (Effects not specified; caution should be used when used concurrently). Products include:

Arco-Lase Plus Tablets 512
Bellergal-S Tablets 2250
Donnatal 2060
Donnatal Extentabs 2061
Donnatal Tablets 2060
Phenobarbital Elixir and Tablets 1469
Quadrinal Tablets 1350

Phenoxybenzamine Hydrochloride (Because of its potential for inducing hypotension, risperidone may enhance the hypotensive effect of therapeutic agents with a potential for producing hypotension). Products include:

Dibenzyline Capsules 2476

Phentolamine Mesylate (Because of its potential for inducing hypotension, risperidone may enhance the hypotensive effect of therapeutic agents with a potential for producing hypotension). Products include:

Regitine 846

Pindolol (Because of its potential for inducing hypotension, risperidone may enhance the hypotensive effect of therapeutic agents with a potential for producing hypotension). Products include:

Visken Tablets 2299

Polythiazide (Because of its potential for inducing hypotension, risperidone may enhance the hypotensive effect of therapeutic agents with a potential for producing hypotension). Products include:

Minizide Capsules 1938

Prazepam (Effects not specified; caution should be used when used concurrently).

No products indexed under this heading.

Prazosin Hydrochloride (Because of its potential for inducing hypotension, risperidone may enhance the hypotensive effect of therapeutic agents with a potential for producing hypotension). Products include:

Minipress Capsules 1937
Minizide Capsules 1938

Prochlorperazine (Effects not specified; caution should be used when used concurrently). Products include:

Compazine 2470

Promethazine Hydrochloride (Effects not specified; caution should be used when used concurrently). Products include:

Mepergan Injection 2753
Phenergan with Codeine 2777
Phenergan with Dextromethorphan 2778
Phenergan Injection 2773
Phenergan Suppositories 2775
Phenergan Syrup 2774
Phenergan Tablets 2775
Phenergan VC 2779
Phenergan VC with Codeine 2781

Propofol (Effects not specified; caution should be used when used concurrently). Products include:

Diprivan Injection 2833

Propoxyphene Hydrochloride (Effects not specified; caution should be used when used concurrently). Products include:

Darvon 1435
Wygesic Tablets 2827

Propoxyphene Napsylate (Effects not specified; caution should be used when used concurrently). Products include:

Darvon-N/Darvocet-N 1433

Propranolol Hydrochloride (Because of its potential for inducing hypotension, risperidone may enhance the hypotensive effect of therapeutic agents with a potential for producing hypotension). Products include:

Inderal 2728
Inderal LA Long Acting Capsules 2730
Inderide Tablets 2732
Inderide LA Long Acting Capsules .. 2734

Quazepam (Effects not specified; caution should be used when used concurrently). Products include:

Doral Tablets 2664

Quinapril Hydrochloride (Because of its potential for inducing hypotension, risperidone may enhance the hypotensive effect of therapeutic agents with a potential for producing hypotension). Products include:

Accupril Tablets 1893

Quinidine Gluconate (Inhibitors of cytochrome P450IID6 could interfere with the conversion of risperidone to 9-hydroxyrisperidone). Products include:

Quinaglute Dura-Tabs Tablets 649

Quinidine Polygalacturonate (Inhibitors of cytochrome P450IID6 could interfere with the conversion of risperidone to 9-hydroxyrisperidone).

No products indexed under this heading.

Quinidine Sulfate (Inhibitors of cytochrome P450IID6 could interfere with the conversion of risperidone to 9-hydroxyrisperidone). Products include:

Quinidex Extentabs 2067

Ramipril (Because of its potential for inducing hypotension, risperidone may enhance the hypotensive effect of therapeutic agents with a potential for producing hypotension). Products include:

Altace Capsules 1232

Rauwolfia Serpentina (Because of its potential for inducing hypotension, risperidone may enhance the hypotensive effect of therapeutic agents with a potential for producing hypotension).

No products indexed under this heading.

Rescinnamine (Because of its potential for inducing hypotension, risperidone may enhance the hypotensive effect of therapeutic agents with a potential for producing hypotension).

No products indexed under this heading.

Reserpine (Because of its potential for inducing hypotension, risperidone may enhance the hypotensive effect of therapeutic agents with a potential for producing hypotension). Products include:

Diupres Tablets 1650
Hydropres Tablets 1675
Ser-Ap-Es Tablets 849

Secobarbital Sodium (Effects not specified; caution should be used when used concurrently). Products include:

Seconal Sodium Pulvules 1474

Sodium Nitroprusside (Because of its potential for inducing hypotension, risperidone may enhance the hypotensive effect of therapeutic agents with a potential for producing hypotension).

No products indexed under this heading.

Sotalol Hydrochloride (Because of its potential for inducing hypotension, risperidone may enhance the hypotensive effect of therapeutic agents with a potential for producing hypotension). Products include:

Betapace Tablets 641

Spirapril Hydrochloride (Because of its potential for inducing hypotension, risperidone may enhance the hypotensive effect of therapeutic agents with a potential for producing hypotension).

No products indexed under this heading.

Sufentanil Citrate (Effects not specified; caution should be used when used concurrently). Products include:

Sufenta Injection 1309

Temazepam (Effects not specified; caution should be used when used concurrently). Products include:

Restoril Capsules 2284

Terazosin Hydrochloride (Because of its potential for inducing hypotension, risperidone may enhance the hypotensive effect of therapeutic agents with a potential for producing hypotension). Products include:

Hytrin Capsules 430

Thiamylal Sodium (Effects not specified; caution should be used when used concurrently).

No products indexed under this heading.

Thioridazine Hydrochloride (Effects not specified; caution should be used when used concurrently). Products include:

Mellaril 2269

Thiothixene (Effects not specified; caution should be used when used concurrently). Products include:

Navane Capsules and Concentrate 2201
Navane Intramuscular 2202

Timolol Maleate (Because of its potential for inducing hypotension, risperidone may enhance the hypotensive effect of therapeutic agents with a potential for producing hypotension). Products include:

Blocadren Tablets 1614
Timolide Tablets 1748
Timoptic in Ocudose 1753
Timoptic Sterile Ophthalmic Solution 1751
Timoptic-XE 1755

Torsemide (Because of its potential for inducing hypotension, risperidone may enhance the hypotensive effect of therapeutic agents with a potential for producing hypotension). Products include:

Demadex Tablets and Injection 686

Triazolam (Effects not specified; caution should be used when used concurrently). Products include:

Halcion Tablets 2611

Trifluoperazine Hydrochloride (Effects not specified; caution should be used when used concurrently). Products include:

Stelazine 2514

IMPORTANT NOTE: Always consult each drug listing in the patient's regimen for possible interactions.

Trimethaphan Camsylate (Because of its potential for inducing hypotension, risperidone may enhance the hypotensive effect of therapeutic agents with a potential for producing hypotension). Products include:

Arfonad Ampuls 2080

Verapamil Hydrochloride (Because of its potential for inducing hypotension, risperidone may enhance the hypotensive effect of therapeutic agents with a potential for producing hypotension). Products include:

Calan SR Caplets 2422
Calan Tablets 2419
Isoptin Injectable 1344
Isoptin Oral Tablets 1346
Isoptin SR Tablets 1348
Verelan Capsules 1410
Verelan Capsules 2824

Zolpidem Tartrate (Effects not specified; caution should be used when used concurrently). Products include:

Ambien Tablets 2416

Food Interactions

Alcohol (Effects not specified; concurrent use should be avoided).

RITALIN HYDROCHLORIDE TABLETS

(Methylphenidate Hydrochloride) 848

May interact with oral anticoagulants, vasopressors, monoamine oxidase inhibitors, tricyclic antidepressants, and certain other agents. Compounds in these categories include:

Amitriptyline Hydrochloride (Metabolism inhibited; downward dosage adjustment of antidepressant may be required). Products include:

Elavil 2838
Endep Tablets 2174
Etrafon 2355
Limbitrol 2180
Triavil Tablets 1757

Amoxapine (Metabolism inhibited; downward dosage adjustment of antidepressant may be required). Products include:

Asendin Tablets 1369

Clomipramine Hydrochloride (Metabolism inhibited; downward dosage adjustment of antidepressant may be required). Products include:

Anafranil Capsules 803

Desipramine Hydrochloride (Metabolism inhibited; downward dosage adjustment of antidepressant may be required). Products include:

Norpramin Tablets 1526

Dicumarol (Metabolism inhibited).

No products indexed under this heading.

Dopamine Hydrochloride (Concomitant use requires caution).

No products indexed under this heading.

Doxepin Hydrochloride (Metabolism inhibited; downward dosage adjustment of antidepressant may be required). Products include:

Sinequan 2205
Zonalon Cream 1055

Epinephrine Hydrochloride (Concomitant use requires caution). Products include:

Ana-Kit Anaphylaxis Emergency Treatment Kit 617

Furazolidone (Concomitant use requires caution). Products include:

Furoxone 2046

Guanethidine Monosulfate (Decreased hypotensive effect). Products include:

Esimil Tablets 822
Ismelin Tablets 827

Imipramine Hydrochloride (Metabolism inhibited; downward dosage adjustment of antidepressant may be required). Products include:

Tofranil Ampuls 854
Tofranil Tablets 856

Imipramine Pamoate (Metabolism inhibited; downward dosage adjustment of antidepressant may be required). Products include:

Tofranil-PM Capsules 857

Isocarboxazid (Concomitant use requires caution).

No products indexed under this heading.

Maprotiline Hydrochloride (Metabolism inhibited; downward dosage adjustment of antidepressant may be required). Products include:

Ludiomil Tablets 843

Metaraminol Bitartrate (Concomitant use requires caution). Products include:

Aramine Injection 1609

Methoxamine Hydrochloride (Concomitant use requires caution). Products include:

Vasoxyl Injection 1196

Norepinephrine Bitartrate (Concomitant use requires caution). Products include:

Levophed Bitartrate Injection 2315

Nortriptyline Hydrochloride (Metabolism inhibited; downward dosage adjustment of antidepressant may be required). Products include:

Pamelor 2280

Phenelzine Sulfate (Concomitant use requires caution). Products include:

Nardil 1920

Phenylbutazone (Metabolism inhibited; downward dosage adjustment of phenylbutazone may be required).

No products indexed under this heading.

Phenylephrine Hydrochloride (Concomitant use requires caution). Products include:

Atrohist Plus Tablets 454
Cerose DM .... ▣ 878
Comhist 2038
D.A. Chewable Tablets 951
Deconsal Pediatric Capsules 454
Dura-Vent/DA Tablets 953
Entex Capsules 1986
Entex Liquid 1986
Extendryl 1005
4-Way Fast Acting Nasal Spray (regular & mentholated) .... ▣ 621
Hemorid For Women .... ▣ 834
Hycomine Compound Tablets 932
Neo-Synephrine Hydrochloride 1% Carpuject 2324
Neo-Synephrine Hydrochloride 1% Injection 2324
Neo-Synephrine Hydrochloride (Ophthalmic) 2325
Neo-Synephrine .... ▣ 726
Nōstril .... ▣ 644
Novahistine Elixir .... ▣ 823
Phenergan VC 2779
Phenergan VC with Codeine 2781
Preparation H .... ▣ 871
Tympagesic Ear Drops 2342
Vasosulf .... ◎ 271
Vicks Sinex Nasal Spray and Ultra Fine Mist .... ▣ 765

Phenytoin (Metabolism inhibited; downward dosage adjustment of anticonvulsant may be required). Products include:

Dilantin Infatabs 1908
Dilantin-125 Suspension 1911

Phenytoin Sodium (Metabolism inhibited; downward dosage adjustment of anticonvulsant may be required). Products include:

Dilantin Kapseals 1906
Dilantin Parenteral 1910

Primidone (Metabolism inhibited; downward dosage adjustment of anticonvulsant may be required). Products include:

Mysoline 2754

Protriptyline Hydrochloride (Metabolism inhibited; downward dosage adjustment of antidepressant may be required). Products include:

Vivactil Tablets 1774

Selegiline Hydrochloride (Concomitant use requires caution). Products include:

Eldepryl Tablets 2550

Tranylcypromine Sulfate (Concomitant use requires caution). Products include:

Parnate Tablets 2503

Trimipramine Maleate (Metabolism inhibited; downward dosage adjustment of antidepressant may be required). Products include:

Surmontil Capsules 2811

Warfarin Sodium (Metabolism inhibited). Products include:

Coumadin 926

RITALIN-SR TABLETS

(Methylphenidate Hydrochloride) 848

See **Ritalin Hydrochloride Tablets**

ROBAXIN INJECTABLE

(Methocarbamol) 2070

May interact with central nervous system depressants and certain other agents. Compounds in these categories include:

Alfentanil Hydrochloride (Increased CNS depressant effect). Products include:

Alfenta Injection 1286

Alprazolam (Increased CNS depressant effect). Products include:

Xanax Tablets 2649

Aprobarbital (Increased CNS depressant effect).

No products indexed under this heading.

Buprenorphine (Increased CNS depressant effect). Products include:

Buprenex Injectable 2006

Buspirone Hydrochloride (Increased CNS depressant effect). Products include:

BuSpar 737

Butabarbital (Increased CNS depressant effect).

No products indexed under this heading.

Butalbital (Increased CNS depressant effect). Products include:

Esgic-plus Tablets 1013
Fioricet Tablets 2258
Fioricet with Codeine Capsules 2260
Fiorinal Capsules 2261
Fiorinal with Codeine Capsules 2262
Fiorinal Tablets 2261
Phrenilin 785
Sedapap Tablets 50 mg/650 mg 1543

Chlordiazepoxide (Increased CNS depressant effect). Products include:

Libritabs Tablets 2177
Limbitrol 2180

Chlordiazepoxide Hydrochloride (Increased CNS depressant effect). Products include:

Librax Capsules 2176
Librium Capsules 2178
Librium Injectable 2179

Chlorpromazine (Increased CNS depressant effect). Products include:

Thorazine Suppositories 2523

Chlorprothixene (Increased CNS depressant effect).

No products indexed under this heading.

Chlorprothixene Hydrochloride (Increased CNS depressant effect).

No products indexed under this heading.

Chlorprothixene Lactate (Increased CNS depressant effect).

No products indexed under this heading.

Clorazepate Dipotassium (Increased CNS depressant effect). Products include:

Tranxene 451

Clozapine (Increased CNS depressant effect). Products include:

Clozaril Tablets 2252

Codeine Phosphate (Increased CNS depressant effect). Products include:

Actifed with Codeine Cough Syrup 1067
Brontex 1981
Deconsal C Expectorant Syrup 456
Deconsal Pediatric Syrup 457
Dimetane-DC Cough Syrup 2059
Empirin with Codeine Tablets 1093
Fioricet with Codeine Capsules 2260
Fiorinal with Codeine Capsules 2262
Isoclor Expectorant 990
Novahistine DH 2462
Novahistine Expectorant 2463
Nucofed 2051
Phenergan with Codeine 2777
Phenergan VC with Codeine 2781
Robitussin A-C Syrup 2073
Robitussin-DAC Syrup 2074
Ryna .... ▣ 841
Soma Compound w/Codeine Tablets 2676
Tussi-Organidin NR Liquid and S NR Liquid 2677
Tylenol with Codeine 1583

Desflurane (Increased CNS depressant effect). Products include:

Suprane 1813

Dezocine (Increased CNS depressant effect). Products include:

Dalgan Injection 538

Diazepam (Increased CNS depressant effect). Products include:

Dizac 1809
Valium Injectable 2182
Valium Tablets 2183
Valrelease Capsules 2169

Droperidol (Increased CNS depressant effect). Products include:

Inapsine Injection 1296

Enflurane (Increased CNS depressant effect).

No products indexed under this heading.

Estazolam (Increased CNS depressant effect). Products include:

ProSom Tablets 449

Ethchlorvynol (Increased CNS depressant effect). Products include:

Placidyl Capsules 448

Ethinamate (Increased CNS depressant effect).

No products indexed under this heading.

Fentanyl (Increased CNS depressant effect). Products include:

Duragesic Transdermal System 1288

Fentanyl Citrate (Increased CNS depressant effect). Products include:

Sublimaze Injection 1307

Fluphenazine Decanoate (Increased CNS depressant effect). Products include:

Prolixin Decanoate 509

Fluphenazine Enanthate (Increased CNS depressant effect). Products include:

Prolixin Enanthate 509

(▣ Described in PDR For Nonprescription Drugs) (◎ Described in PDR For Ophthalmology)

901 Interactions Index Robaxin Tablets

Fluphenazine Hydrochloride (Increased CNS depressant effect). Products include:
Prolixin ... 509

Flurazepam Hydrochloride (Increased CNS depressant effect). Products include:
Dalmane Capsules ... 2173

Glutethimide (Increased CNS depressant effect).
No products indexed under this heading.

Haloperidol (Increased CNS depressant effect). Products include:
Haldol Injection, Tablets and Concentrate ... 1575

Haloperidol Decanoate (Increased CNS depressant effect). Products include:
Haldol Decanoate ... 1577

Hydrocodone Bitartrate (Increased CNS depressant effect). Products include:
Anexsia 5/500 Elixir ... 1781
Anexia Tablets ... 1782
Codiclear DH Syrup ... 791
Deconamine CX Cough and Cold Liquid and Tablets ... 1319
Duratuss HD Elixir ... 2565
Hycodan Tablets and Syrup ... 930
Hycomine Compound Tablets ... 932
Hycomine ... 931
Hycotuss Expectorant Syrup ... 933
Hydrocet Capsules ... 782
Lorcet 10/650 ... 1018
Lortab ... 2566
Tussend ... 1783
Tussend Expectorant ... 1785
Vicodin Tablets ... 1356
Vicodin ES Tablets ... 1357
Vicodin Tuss Expectorant ... 1358
Zydone Capsules ... 949

Hydrocodone Polistirex (Increased CNS depressant effect). Products include:
Tussionex Pennkinetic Extended-Release Suspension ... 998

Hydroxyzine Hydrochloride (Increased CNS depressant effect). Products include:
Atarax Tablets & Syrup ... 2185
Marax Tablets & DF Syrup ... 2200
Vistaril Intramuscular Solution ... 2216

Isoflurane (Increased CNS depressant effect).
No products indexed under this heading.

Ketamine Hydrochloride (Increased CNS depressant effect).
No products indexed under this heading.

Levomethadyl Acetate Hydrochloride (Increased CNS depressant effect). Products include:
Orlamm ... 2239

Levorphanol Tartrate (Increased CNS depressant effect). Products include:
Levo-Dromoran ... 2129

Lorazepam (Increased CNS depressant effect). Products include:
Ativan Injection ... 2698
Ativan Tablets ... 2700

Loxapine Hydrochloride (Increased CNS depressant effect). Products include:
Loxitane ... 1378

Loxapine Succinate (Increased CNS depressant effect). Products include:
Loxitane Capsules ... 1378

Meperidine Hydrochloride (Increased CNS depressant effect). Products include:
Demerol ... 2308
Mepergan Injection ... 2753

Mephobarbital (Increased CNS depressant effect). Products include:
Mebaral Tablets ... 2322

Meprobamate (Increased CNS depressant effect). Products include:
Miltown Tablets ... 2672
PMB 200 and PMB 400 ... 2783

Mesoridazine Besylate (Increased CNS depressant effect). Products include:
Serentil ... 684

Methadone Hydrochloride (Increased CNS depressant effect). Products include:
Methadone Hydrochloride Oral Concentrate ... 2233
Methadone Hydrochloride Oral Solution & Tablets ... 2235

Methohexital Sodium (Increased CNS depressant effect). Products include:
Brevital Sodium Vials ... 1429

Methotrimeprazine (Increased CNS depressant effect). Products include:
Levoprome ... 1274

Methoxyflurane (Increased CNS depressant effect).
No products indexed under this heading.

Midazolam Hydrochloride (Increased CNS depressant effect). Products include:
Versed Injection ... 2170

Molindone Hydrochloride (Increased CNS depressant effect). Products include:
Moban Tablets and Concentrate ... 1048

Morphine Sulfate (Increased CNS depressant effect). Products include:
Astramorph/PF Injection, USP (Preservative-Free) ... 535
Duramorph ... 962
Infumorph 200 and Infumorph 500 Sterile Solutions ... 965
MS Contin Tablets ... 1994
MSIR ... 1997
Oramorph SR (Morphine Sulfate Sustained Release Tablets) ... 2236
RMS Suppositories ... 2657
Roxanol ... 2243

Opium Alkaloids (Increased CNS depressant effect).
No products indexed under this heading.

Oxazepam (Increased CNS depressant effect). Products include:
Serax Capsules ... 2810
Serax Tablets ... 2810

Oxycodone Hydrochloride (Increased CNS depressant effect). Products include:
Percocet Tablets ... 938
Percodan Tablets ... 939
Percodan-Demi Tablets ... 940
Roxicodone Tablets, Oral Solution & Intensol (Oxycodone) ... 2244
Tylox Capsules ... 1584

Pentobarbital Sodium (Increased additive effect). Products include:
Nembutal Sodium Capsules ... 436
Nembutal Sodium Solution ... 438
Nembutal Sodium Suppositories ... 440

Perphenazine (Increased CNS depressant effect). Products include:
Etrafon ... 2355
Triavil Tablets ... 1757
Trilafon ... 2389

Phenobarbital (Increased CNS depressant effect). Products include:
Arco-Lase Plus Tablets ... 512
Bellergal-S Tablets ... 2250
Donnatal ... 2060
Donnatal Extentabs ... 2061
Donnatal Tablets ... 2060
Phenobarbital Elixir and Tablets ... 1469
Quadrinal Tablets ... 1350

Prazepam (Increased CNS depressant effect).
No products indexed under this heading.

Prochlorperazine (Increased CNS depressant effect). Products include:
Compazine ... 2470

Promethazine Hydrochloride (Increased CNS depressant effect). Products include:
Mepergan Injection ... 2753
Phenergan with Codeine ... 2777
Phenergan with Dextromethorphan ... 2778
Phenergan Injection ... 2773
Phenergan Suppositories ... 2775
Phenergan Syrup ... 2774
Phenergan Tablets ... 2775
Phenergan VC ... 2779
Phenergan VC with Codeine ... 2781

Propofol (Increased CNS depressant effect). Products include:
Diprivan Injection ... 2833

Propoxyphene Hydrochloride (Increased CNS depressant effect). Products include:
Darvon ... 1435
Wygesic Tablets ... 2827

Propoxyphene Napsylate (Increased CNS depressant effect). Products include:
Darvon-N/Darvocet-N ... 1433

Quazepam (Increased CNS depressant effect). Products include:
Doral Tablets ... 2664

Risperidone (Increased CNS depressant effect). Products include:
Risperdal ... 1301

Secobarbital Sodium (Increased CNS depressant effect). Products include:
Seconal Sodium Pulvules ... 1474

Sufentanil Citrate (Increased CNS depressant effect). Products include:
Sufenta Injection ... 1309

Temazepam (Increased CNS depressant effect). Products include:
Restoril Capsules ... 2284

Thiamylal Sodium (Increased CNS depressant effect).
No products indexed under this heading.

Thioridazine Hydrochloride (Increased CNS depressant effect). Products include:
Mellaril ... 2269

Thiothixene (Increased CNS depressant effect). Products include:
Navane Capsules and Concentrate ... 2201
Navane Intramuscular ... 2202

Triazolam (Increased CNS depressant effect). Products include:
Halcion Tablets ... 2611

Trifluoperazine Hydrochloride (Increased CNS depressant effect). Products include:
Stelazine ... 2514

Zolpidem Tartrate (Increased CNS depressant effect). Products include:
Ambien Tablets ... 2416

Food Interactions

Alcohol (Increased depressant effect).

ROBAXIN TABLETS

(Methocarbamol) ... 2071
May interact with central nervous system depressants and certain other agents. Compounds in these categories include:

Alfentanil Hydrochloride (Increased CNS depressant effect). Products include:
Alfenta Injection ... 1286

Alprazolam (Increased CNS depressant effect). Products include:
Xanax Tablets ... 2649

Aprobarbital (Increased CNS depressant effect).
No products indexed under this heading.

Buprenorphine (Increased CNS depressant effect). Products include:
Buprenex Injectable ... 2006

Buspirone Hydrochloride (Increased CNS depressant effect). Products include:
BuSpar ... 737

Butabarbital (Increased CNS depressant effect).
No products indexed under this heading.

Butalbital (Increased CNS depressant effect). Products include:
Esgic-plus Tablets ... 1013
Fioricet Tablets ... 2258
Fioricet with Codeine Capsules ... 2260
Fiorinal Capsules ... 2261
Fiorinal with Codeine Capsules ... 2262
Fiorinal Tablets ... 2261
Phrenilin ... 785
Sedapap Tablets 50 mg/650 mg ... 1543

Chlordiazepoxide (Increased CNS depressant effect). Products include:
Libritabs Tablets ... 2177
Limbitrol ... 2180

Chlordiazepoxide Hydrochloride (Increased CNS depressant effect). Products include:
Librax Capsules ... 2176
Librium Capsules ... 2178
Librium Injectable ... 2179

Chlorpromazine (Increased CNS depressant effect). Products include:
Thorazine Suppositories ... 2523

Chlorprothixene (Increased CNS depressant effect).
No products indexed under this heading.

Chlorprothixene Hydrochloride (Increased CNS depressant effect).
No products indexed under this heading.

Chlorprothixene Lactate (Increased CNS depressant effect).
No products indexed under this heading.

Clorazepate Dipotassium (Increased CNS depressant effect). Products include:
Tranxene ... 451

Clozapine (Increased CNS depressant effect). Products include:
Clozaril Tablets ... 2252

Codeine Phosphate (Increased CNS depressant effect). Products include:
Actifed with Codeine Cough Syrup ... 1067
Brontex ... 1981
Deconsal C Expectorant Syrup ... 456
Deconsal Pediatric Syrup ... 457
Dimetane-DC Cough Syrup ... 2059
Empirin with Codeine Tablets ... 1093
Fioricet with Codeine Capsules ... 2260
Fiorinal with Codeine Capsules ... 2262
Isoclor Expectorant ... 990
Novahistine DH ... 2462
Novahistine Expectorant ... 2463
Nucofed ... 2051
Phenergan with Codeine ... 2777
Phenergan VC with Codeine ... 2781
Robitussin A-C Syrup ... 2073
Robitussin-DAC Syrup ... 2074
Ryna ... 841
Soma Compound w/Codeine Tablets ... 2676
Tussi-Organidin NR Liquid and S NR Liquid ... 2677
Tylenol with Codeine ... 1583

Desflurane (Increased CNS depressant effect). Products include:
Suprane ... 1813

Dezocine (Increased CNS depressant effect). Products include:
Dalgan Injection ... 538

Diazepam (Increased CNS depressant effect). Products include:
Dizac ... 1809
Valium Injectable ... 2182
Valium Tablets ... 2183
Valrelease Capsules ... 2169

Droperidol (Increased CNS depressant effect). Products include:
Inapsine Injection ... 1296

IMPORTANT NOTE: Always consult each drug listing in the patient's regimen for possible interactions.

Robaxin Tablets — Interactions Index — 902

Enflurane (Increased CNS depressant effect).
No products indexed under this heading.

Estazolam (Increased CNS depressant effect). Products include:
ProSom Tablets ... 449

Ethchlorvynol (Increased CNS depressant effect). Products include:
Placidyl Capsules ... 448

Ethinamate (Increased CNS depressant effect).
No products indexed under this heading.

Fentanyl (Increased CNS depressant effect). Products include:
Duragesic Transdermal System ... 1288

Fentanyl Citrate (Increased CNS depressant effect). Products include:
Sublimaze Injection ... 1307

Fluphenazine Decanoate (Increased CNS depressant effect). Products include:
Prolixin Decanoate ... 509

Fluphenazine Enanthate (Increased CNS depressant effect). Products include:
Prolixin Enanthate ... 509

Fluphenazine Hydrochloride (Increased CNS depressant effect). Products include:
Prolixin ... 509

Flurazepam Hydrochloride (Increased CNS depressant effect). Products include:
Dalmane Capsules ... 2173

Glutethimide (Increased CNS depressant effect).
No products indexed under this heading.

Haloperidol (Increased CNS depressant effect). Products include:
Haldol Injection, Tablets and Concentrate ... 1575

Haloperidol Decanoate (Increased CNS depressant effect). Products include:
Haldol Decanoate ... 1577

Hydrocodone Bitartrate (Increased CNS depressant effect). Products include:
Anexsia 5/500 Elixir ... 1781
Anexia Tablets ... 1782
Codiclear DH Syrup ... 791
Deconamine CX Cough and Cold Liquid and Tablets ... 1319
Duratuss HD Elixir ... 2565
Hycodan Tablets and Syrup ... 930
Hycomine Compound Tablets ... 932
Hycomine ... 931
Hycotuss Expectorant Syrup ... 933
Hydrocet Capsules ... 782
Lorcet 10/650 ... 1018
Lortab ... 2566
Tussend ... 1783
Tussend Expectorant ... 1785
Vicodin Tablets ... 1356
Vicodin ES Tablets ... 1357
Vicodin Tuss Expectorant ... 1358
Zydone Capsules ... 949

Hydrocodone Polistirex (Increased CNS depressant effect). Products include:
Tussionex Pennkinetic Extended-Release Suspension ... 998

Hydroxyzine Hydrochloride (Increased CNS depressant effect). Products include:
Atarax Tablets & Syrup ... 2185
Marax Tablets & DF Syrup ... 2200
Vistaril Intramuscular Solution ... 2216

Isoflurane (Increased CNS depressant effect).
No products indexed under this heading.

Ketamine Hydrochloride (Increased CNS depressant effect).
No products indexed under this heading.

Levomethadyl Acetate Hydrochloride (Increased CNS depressant effect). Products include:
Orlamm ... 2239

Levorphanol Tartrate (Increased CNS depressant effect). Products include:
Levo-Dromoran ... 2129

Lorazepam (Increased CNS depressant effect). Products include:
Ativan Injection ... 2698
Ativan Tablets ... 2700

Loxapine Hydrochloride (Increased CNS depressant effect). Products include:
Loxitane ... 1378

Loxapine Succinate (Increased CNS depressant effect). Products include:
Loxitane Capsules ... 1378

Meperidine Hydrochloride (Increased CNS depressant effect). Products include:
Demerol ... 2308
Mepergan Injection ... 2753

Mephobarbital (Increased CNS depressant effect). Products include:
Mebaral Tablets ... 2322

Meprobamate (Increased CNS depressant effect). Products include:
Miltown Tablets ... 2672
PMB 200 and PMB 400 ... 2783

Mesoridazine Besylate (Increased CNS depressant effect). Products include:
Serentil ... 684

Methadone Hydrochloride (Increased CNS depressant effect). Products include:
Methadone Hydrochloride Oral Concentrate ... 2233
Methadone Hydrochloride Oral Solution & Tablets ... 2235

Methohexital Sodium (Increased CNS depressant effect). Products include:
Brevital Sodium Vials ... 1429

Methotrimeprazine (Increased CNS depressant effect). Products include:
Levoprome ... 1274

Methoxyflurane (Increased CNS depressant effect).
No products indexed under this heading.

Midazolam Hydrochloride (Increased CNS depressant effect). Products include:
Versed Injection ... 2170

Molindone Hydrochloride (Increased CNS depressant effect). Products include:
Moban Tablets and Concentrate ... 1048

Morphine Sulfate (Increased CNS depressant effect). Products include:
Astramorph/PF Injection, USP (Preservative-Free) ... 535
Duramorph ... 962
Infumorph 200 and Infumorph 500 Sterile Solutions ... 965
MS Contin Tablets ... 1994
MSIR ... 1997
Oramorph SR (Morphine Sulfate Sustained Release Tablets) ... 2236
RMS Suppositories ... 2657
Roxanol ... 2243

Opium Alkaloids (Increased CNS depressant effect).
No products indexed under this heading.

Oxazepam (Increased CNS depressant effect). Products include:
Serax Capsules ... 2810
Serax Tablets ... 2810

Oxycodone Hydrochloride (Increased CNS depressant effect). Products include:
Percocet Tablets ... 938
Percodan Tablets ... 939
Percodan-Demi Tablets ... 940
Roxicodone Tablets, Oral Solution & Intensol (Oxycodone) ... 2244
Tylox Capsules ... 1584

Pentobarbital Sodium (Increased CNS depressant effect). Products include:
Nembutal Sodium Capsules ... 436
Nembutal Sodium Solution ... 438
Nembutal Sodium Suppositories ... 440

Perphenazine (Increased CNS depressant effect). Products include:
Etrafon ... 2355
Triavil Tablets ... 1757
Trilafon ... 2389

Phenobarbital (Increased CNS depressant effect). Products include:
Arco-Lase Plus Tablets ... 512
Bellergal-S Tablets ... 2250
Donnatal ... 2060
Donnatal Extentabs ... 2061
Donnatal Tablets ... 2060
Phenobarbital Elixir and Tablets ... 1469
Quadrinal Tablets ... 1350

Prazepam (Increased CNS depressant effect).
No products indexed under this heading.

Prochlorperazine (Increased CNS depressant effect). Products include:
Compazine ... 2470

Promethazine Hydrochloride (Increased CNS depressant effect). Products include:
Mepergan Injection ... 2753
Phenergan with Codeine ... 2777
Phenergan with Dextromethorphan ... 2778
Phenergan Injection ... 2773
Phenergan Suppositories ... 2775
Phenergan Syrup ... 2774
Phenergan Tablets ... 2775
Phenergan VC ... 2779
Phenergan VC with Codeine ... 2781

Propofol (Increased CNS depressant effect). Products include:
Diprivan Injection ... 2833

Propoxyphene Hydrochloride (Increased CNS depressant effect). Products include:
Darvon ... 1435
Wygesic Tablets ... 2827

Propoxyphene Napsylate (Increased CNS depressant effect). Products include:
Darvon-N/Darvocet-N ... 1433

Quazepam (Increased CNS depressant effect). Products include:
Doral Tablets ... 2664

Risperidone (Increased CNS depressant effect). Products include:
Risperdal ... 1301

Secobarbital Sodium (Increased CNS depressant effect). Products include:
Seconal Sodium Pulvules ... 1474

Sufentanil Citrate (Increased CNS depressant effect). Products include:
Sufenta Injection ... 1309

Temazepam (Increased CNS depressant effect). Products include:
Restoril Capsules ... 2284

Thiamylal Sodium (Increased CNS depressant effect).
No products indexed under this heading.

Thioridazine Hydrochloride (Increased CNS depressant effect). Products include:
Mellaril ... 2269

Thiothixene (Increased CNS depressant effect). Products include:
Navane Capsules and Concentrate ... 2201
Navane Intramuscular ... 2202

Triazolam (Increased CNS depressant effect). Products include:
Halcion Tablets ... 2611

Trifluoperazine Hydrochloride (Increased CNS depressant effect). Products include:
Stelazine ... 2514

Zolpidem Tartrate (Increased CNS depressant effect). Products include:
Ambien Tablets ... 2416

Food Interactions

Alcohol (Increased CNS depressant effect).

ROBAXIN-750 TABLETS
(Methocarbamol) ... 2071
See **Robaxin Tablets**

ROBAXISAL TABLETS
(Methocarbamol, Aspirin) ... 2071
May interact with central nervous system depressants, anticoagulants, and certain other agents. Compounds in these categories include:

Alfentanil Hydrochloride (Increased depressant effect). Products include:
Alfenta Injection ... 1286

Alprazolam (Increased depressant effect). Products include:
Xanax Tablets ... 2649

Aprobarbital (Increased depressant effect).
No products indexed under this heading.

Buprenorphine (Increased depressant effect). Products include:
Buprenex Injectable ... 2006

Buspirone Hydrochloride (Increased depressant effect). Products include:
BuSpar ... 737

Butabarbital (Increased depressant effect).
No products indexed under this heading.

Butalbital (Increased depressant effect). Products include:
Esgic-plus Tablets ... 1013
Fioricet Tablets ... 2258
Fioricet with Codeine Capsules ... 2260
Fiorinal Capsules ... 2261
Fiorinal with Codeine Capsules ... 2262
Fiorinal Tablets ... 2261
Phrenilin ... 785
Sedapap Tablets 50 mg/650 mg ... 1543

Chlordiazepoxide (Increased depressant effect). Products include:
Libritabs Tablets ... 2177
Limbitrol ... 2180

Chlordiazepoxide Hydrochloride (Increased depressant effect). Products include:
Librax Capsules ... 2176
Librium Capsules ... 2178
Librium Injectable ... 2179

Chlorpromazine (Increased depressant effect). Products include:
Thorazine Suppositories ... 2523

Chlorprothixene (Increased depressant effect).
No products indexed under this heading.

Chlorprothixene Hydrochloride (Increased depressant effect).
No products indexed under this heading.

Chlorprothixene Lactate (Increased depressant effect).
No products indexed under this heading.

Clorazepate Dipotassium (Increased depressant effect). Products include:
Tranxene ... 451

Clozapine (Increased depressant effect). Products include:
Clozaril Tablets ... 2252

Codeine Phosphate (Increased depressant effect). Products include:
Actifed with Codeine Cough Syrup ... 1067
Brontex ... 1981
Deconsal C Expectorant Syrup ... 456
Deconsal Pediatric Syrup ... 457

(▣ Described in PDR For Nonprescription Drugs) (◉ Described in PDR For Ophthalmology)

903 Interactions Index Robitussin A-C

Dimetane-DC Cough Syrup 2059
Empirin with Codeine Tablets 1093
Fioricet with Codeine Capsules 2260
Fiorinal with Codeine Capsules 2262
Isoclor Expectorant 990
Novahistine DH 2462
Novahistine Expectorant 2463
Nucofed 2051
Phenergan with Codeine 2777
Phenergan VC with Codeine 2781
Robitussin A-C Syrup 2073
Robitussin-DAC Syrup 2074
Ryna 841
Soma Compound w/Codeine Tablets 2676
Tussi-Organidin NR Liquid and S NR Liquid 2677
Tylenol with Codeine 1583

Dalteparin Sodium (Increased anticoagulant effect). Products include:
Fragmin 1954

Desflurane (Increased depressant effect). Products include:
Suprane 1813

Dezocine (Increased depressant effect). Products include:
Dalgan Injection 538

Diazepam (Increased depressant effect). Products include:
Dizac 1809
Valium Injectable 2182
Valium Tablets 2183
Valrelease Capsules 2169

Dicumarol (Increased anticoagulant effect).
No products indexed under this heading.

Droperidol (Increased depressant effect). Products include:
Inapsine Injection 1296

Enflurane (Increased depressant effect).
No products indexed under this heading.

Enoxaparin (Increased anticoagulant effect). Products include:
Lovenox Injection 2020

Estazolam (Increased depressant effect). Products include:
ProSom Tablets 449

Ethchlorvynol (Increased depressant effect). Products include:
Placidyl Capsules 448

Ethinamate (Increased depressant effect).
No products indexed under this heading.

Fentanyl (Increased depressant effect). Products include:
Duragesic Transdermal System 1288

Fentanyl Citrate (Increased depressant effect). Products include:
Sublimaze Injection 1307

Fluphenazine Decanoate (Increased depressant effect). Products include:
Prolixin Decanoate 509

Fluphenazine Enanthate (Increased depressant effect). Products include:
Prolixin Enanthate 509

Fluphenazine Hydrochloride (Increased depressant effect). Products include:
Prolixin 509

Flurazepam Hydrochloride (Increased depressant effect). Products include:
Dalmane Capsules 2173

Glutethimide (Increased depressant effect).
No products indexed under this heading.

Haloperidol (Increased depressant effect). Products include:
Haldol Injection, Tablets and Concentrate 1575

Haloperidol Decanoate (Increased depressant effect). Products include:
Haldol Decanoate 1577

Heparin Calcium (Increased anticoagulant effect).
No products indexed under this heading.

Heparin Sodium (Increased anticoagulant effect). Products include:
Heparin Lock Flush Solution 2725
Heparin Sodium Injection 2726
Heparin Sodium Injection, USP, Sterile Solution 2615
Heparin Sodium Vials 1441

Hydrocodone Bitartrate (Increased depressant effect). Products include:
Anexsia 5/500 Elixir 1781
Anexia Tablets 1782
Codiclear DH Syrup 791
Deconamine CX Cough and Cold Liquid and Tablets 1319
Duratuss HD Elixir 2565
Hycodan Tablets and Syrup 930
Hycomine Compound Tablets 932
Hycomine 931
Hycotuss Expectorant Syrup 933
Hydrocet Capsules 782
Lorcet 10/650 1018
Lortab 2566
Tussend 1783
Tussend Expectorant 1785
Vicodin Tablets 1356
Vicodin ES Tablets 1357
Vicodin Tuss Expectorant 1358
Zydone Capsules 949

Hydrocodone Polistirex (Increased depressant effect). Products include:
Tussionex Pennkinetic Extended-Release Suspension 998

Hydroxyzine Hydrochloride (Increased depressant effect). Products include:
Atarax Tablets & Syrup 2185
Marax Tablets & DF Syrup 2200
Vistaril Intramuscular Solution 2216

Isoflurane (Increased depressant effect).
No products indexed under this heading.

Ketamine Hydrochloride (Increased depressant effect).
No products indexed under this heading.

Levomethadyl Acetate Hydrochloride (Increased depressant effect). Products include:
Orlamm 2239

Levorphanol Tartrate (Increased depressant effect). Products include:
Levo-Dromoran 2129

Lorazepam (Increased depressant effect). Products include:
Ativan Injection 2698
Ativan Tablets 2700

Loxapine Hydrochloride (Increased depressant effect). Products include:
Loxitane 1378

Loxapine Succinate (Increased depressant effect). Products include:
Loxitane Capsules 1378

Meperidine Hydrochloride (Increased depressant effect). Products include:
Demerol 2308
Mepergan Injection 2753

Mephobarbital (Increased depressant effect). Products include:
Mebaral Tablets 2322

Meprobamate (Increased depressant effect). Products include:
Miltown Tablets 2672
PMB 200 and PMB 400 2783

Mesoridazine Besylate (Increased depressant effect). Products include:
Serentil 684

Methadone Hydrochloride (Increased depressant effect). Products include:
Methadone Hydrochloride Oral Concentrate 2233
Methadone Hydrochloride Oral Solution & Tablets 2235

Methohexital Sodium (Increased depressant effect). Products include:
Brevital Sodium Vials 1429

Methotrimeprazine (Increased depressant effect). Products include:
Levoprome 1274

Methoxyflurane (Increased depressant effect).
No products indexed under this heading.

Midazolam Hydrochloride (Increased depressant effect). Products include:
Versed Injection 2170

Molindone Hydrochloride (Increased depressant effect). Products include:
Moban Tablets and Concentrate 1048

Morphine Sulfate (Increased depressant effect). Products include:
Astramorph/PF Injection, USP (Preservative-Free) 535
Duramorph 962
Infumorph 200 and Infumorph 500 Sterile Solutions 965
MS Contin Tablets 1994
MSIR 1997
Oramorph SR (Morphine Sulfate Sustained Release Tablets) 2236
RMS Suppositories 2657
Roxanol 2243

Opium Alkaloids (Increased depressant effect).
No products indexed under this heading.

Oxazepam (Increased depressant effect). Products include:
Serax Capsules 2810
Serax Tablets 2810

Oxycodone Hydrochloride (Increased depressant effect). Products include:
Percocet Tablets 938
Percodan Tablets 939
Percodan-Demi Tablets 940
Roxicodone Tablets, Oral Solution & Intensol (Oxycodone) 2244
Tylox Capsules 1584

Pentobarbital Sodium (Increased depressant effect). Products include:
Nembutal Sodium Capsules 436
Nembutal Sodium Solution 438
Nembutal Sodium Suppositories 440

Perphenazine (Increased depressant effect). Products include:
Etrafon 2355
Triavil Tablets 1757
Trilafon 2389

Phenobarbital (Increased depressant effect). Products include:
Arco-Lase Plus Tablets 512
Bellergal-S Tablets 2250
Donnatal 2060
Donnatal Extentabs 2061
Donnatal Tablets 2060
Phenobarbital Elixir and Tablets 1469
Quadrinal Tablets 1350

Prazepam (Increased depressant effect).
No products indexed under this heading.

Prochlorperazine (Increased depressant effect). Products include:
Compazine 2470

Promethazine Hydrochloride (Increased depressant effect). Products include:
Mepergan Injection 2753
Phenergan with Codeine 2777
Phenergan with Dextromethorphan 2778
Phenergan Injection 2773
Phenergan Suppositories 2775
Phenergan Syrup 2774
Phenergan Tablets 2775
Phenergan VC 2779
Phenergan VC with Codeine 2781

Propofol (Increased depressant effect). Products include:
Diprivan Injection 2833

Propoxyphene Hydrochloride (Increased depressant effect). Products include:
Darvon 1435
Wygesic Tablets 2827

Propoxyphene Napsylate (Increased depressant effect). Products include:
Darvon-N/Darvocet-N 1433

Quazepam (Increased depressant effect). Products include:
Doral Tablets 2664

Risperidone (Increased depressant effect). Products include:
Risperdal 1301

Secobarbital Sodium (Increased depressant effect). Products include:
Seconal Sodium Pulvules 1474

Sufentanil Citrate (Increased depressant effect). Products include:
Sufenta Injection 1309

Temazepam (Increased depressant effect). Products include:
Restoril Capsules 2284

Thiamylal Sodium (Increased depressant effect).
No products indexed under this heading.

Thioridazine Hydrochloride (Increased depressant effect). Products include:
Mellaril 2269

Thiothixene (Increased depressant effect). Products include:
Navane Capsules and Concentrate 2201
Navane Intramuscular 2202

Triazolam (Increased depressant effect). Products include:
Halcion Tablets 2611

Trifluoperazine Hydrochloride (Increased depressant effect). Products include:
Stelazine 2514

Warfarin Sodium (Increased anticoagulant effect). Products include:
Coumadin 926

Zolpidem Tartrate (Increased depressant effect). Products include:
Ambien Tablets 2416

Food Interactions

Alcohol (Increased depressant effect).

ROBINUL FORTE TABLETS
(Glycopyrrolate) 2072
None cited in PDR database.

ROBINUL INJECTABLE
(Glycopyrrolate) 2072
May interact with:

Cyclopropane (Potential ventricular arrhythmias).

ROBINUL TABLETS
(Glycopyrrolate) 2072
None cited in PDR database.

ROBITUSSIN
(Guaifenesin) 777
None cited in PDR database.

ROBITUSSIN A-C SYRUP
(Codeine Phosphate, Guaifenesin) 2073
May interact with hypnotics and sedatives, tranquilizers, and monoamine oxidase inhibitors. Compounds in these categories include:

Alprazolam (Concurrent therapy may cause greater sedation). Products include:
Xanax Tablets 2649

IMPORTANT NOTE: Always consult each drug listing in the patient's regimen for possible interactions.

Buspirone Hydrochloride (Concurrent therapy may cause greater sedation). Products include:
- BuSpar ... 737

Chlordiazepoxide (Concurrent therapy may cause greater sedation). Products include:
- Libritabs Tablets ... 2177
- Limbitrol ... 2180

Chlordiazepoxide Hydrochloride (Concurrent therapy may cause greater sedation). Products include:
- Librax Capsules ... 2176
- Librium Capsules ... 2178
- Librium Injectable ... 2179

Chlorpromazine (Concurrent therapy may cause greater sedation). Products include:
- Thorazine Suppositories ... 2523

Chlorprothixene (Concurrent therapy may cause greater sedation).
- No products indexed under this heading.

Chlorprothixene Hydrochloride (Concurrent therapy may cause greater sedation).
- No products indexed under this heading.

Clorazepate Dipotassium (Concurrent therapy may cause greater sedation). Products include:
- Tranxene ... 451

Diazepam (Concurrent therapy may cause greater sedation). Products include:
- Dizac ... 1809
- Valium Injectable ... 2182
- Valium Tablets ... 2183
- Valrelease Capsules ... 2169

Droperidol (Concurrent therapy may cause greater sedation). Products include:
- Inapsine Injection ... 1296

Estazolam (Concurrent therapy may cause greater sedation). Products include:
- ProSom Tablets ... 449

Ethchlorvynol (Concurrent therapy may cause greater sedation). Products include:
- Placidyl Capsules ... 448

Ethinamate (Concurrent therapy may cause greater sedation).
- No products indexed under this heading.

Fluphenazine Decanoate (Concurrent therapy may cause greater sedation). Products include:
- Prolixin Decanoate ... 509

Fluphenazine Enanthate (Concurrent therapy may cause greater sedation). Products include:
- Prolixin Enanthate ... 509

Fluphenazine Hydrochloride (Concurrent therapy may cause greater sedation). Products include:
- Prolixin ... 509

Flurazepam Hydrochloride (Concurrent therapy may cause greater sedation). Products include:
- Dalmane Capsules ... 2173

Furazolidone (Concurrent therapy may cause greater sedation). Products include:
- Furoxone ... 2046

Glutethimide (Concurrent therapy may cause greater sedation).
- No products indexed under this heading.

Haloperidol (Concurrent therapy may cause greater sedation). Products include:
- Haldol Injection, Tablets and Concentrate ... 1575

Haloperidol Decanoate (Concurrent therapy may cause greater sedation). Products include:
- Haldol Decanoate ... 1577

Hydroxyzine Hydrochloride (Concurrent therapy may cause greater sedation). Products include:
- Atarax Tablets & Syrup ... 2185
- Marax Tablets & DF Syrup ... 2200
- Vistaril Intramuscular Solution ... 2216

Isocarboxazid (Concurrent therapy may cause greater sedation).
- No products indexed under this heading.

Lorazepam (Concurrent therapy may cause greater sedation). Products include:
- Ativan Injection ... 2698
- Ativan Tablets ... 2700

Loxapine Hydrochloride (Concurrent therapy may cause greater sedation). Products include:
- Loxitane ... 1378

Loxapine Succinate (Concurrent therapy may cause greater sedation). Products include:
- Loxitane Capsules ... 1378

Meprobamate (Concurrent therapy may cause greater sedation). Products include:
- Miltown Tablets ... 2672
- PMB 200 and PMB 400 ... 2783

Mesoridazine Besylate (Concurrent therapy may cause greater sedation). Products include:
- Serentil ... 684

Midazolam Hydrochloride (Concurrent therapy may cause greater sedation). Products include:
- Versed Injection ... 2170

Molindone Hydrochloride (Concurrent therapy may cause greater sedation). Products include:
- Moban Tablets and Concentrate ... 1048

Oxazepam (Concurrent therapy may cause greater sedation). Products include:
- Serax Capsules ... 2810
- Serax Tablets ... 2810

Perphenazine (Concurrent therapy may cause greater sedation). Products include:
- Etrafon ... 2355
- Triavil Tablets ... 1757
- Trilafon ... 2389

Phenelzine Sulfate (Concurrent therapy may cause greater sedation). Products include:
- Nardil ... 1920

Prazepam (Concurrent therapy may cause greater sedation).
- No products indexed under this heading.

Prochlorperazine (Concurrent therapy may cause greater sedation). Products include:
- Compazine ... 2470

Promethazine Hydrochloride (Concurrent therapy may cause greater sedation). Products include:
- Mepergan Injection ... 2753
- Phenergan with Codeine ... 2777
- Phenergan with Dextromethorphan ... 2778
- Phenergan Injection ... 2773
- Phenergan Suppositories ... 2775
- Phenergan Syrup ... 2774
- Phenergan Tablets ... 2775
- Phenergan VC ... 2779
- Phenergan VC with Codeine ... 2781

Propofol (Concurrent therapy may cause greater sedation). Products include:
- Diprivan Injection ... 2833

Quazepam (Concurrent therapy may cause greater sedation). Products include:
- Doral Tablets ... 2664

Secobarbital Sodium (Concurrent therapy may cause greater sedation). Products include:
- Seconal Sodium Pulvules ... 1474

Selegiline Hydrochloride (Concurrent therapy may cause greater sedation). Products include:
- Eldepryl Tablets ... 2550

Temazepam (Concurrent therapy may cause greater sedation). Products include:
- Restoril Capsules ... 2284

Thioridazine Hydrochloride (Concurrent therapy may cause greater sedation). Products include:
- Mellaril ... 2269

Thiothixene (Concurrent therapy may cause greater sedation). Products include:
- Navane Capsules and Concentrate 2201
- Navane Intramuscular ... 2202

Tranylcypromine Sulfate (Concurrent therapy may cause greater sedation). Products include:
- Parnate Tablets ... 2503

Triazolam (Concurrent therapy may cause greater sedation). Products include:
- Halcion Tablets ... 2611

Trifluoperazine Hydrochloride (Concurrent therapy may cause greater sedation). Products include:
- Stelazine ... 2514

Zolpidem Tartrate (Concurrent therapy may cause greater sedation). Products include:
- Ambien Tablets ... 2416

ROBITUSSIN COLD & COUGH LIQUI-GELS

(Guaifenesin, Dextromethorphan Hydrobromide, Pseudoephedrine Hydrochloride) ... ▣ 776

May interact with monoamine oxidase inhibitors. Compounds in this category include:

Furazolidone (Concurrent and/or sequential use is not recommended). Products include:
- Furoxone ... 2046

Isocarboxazid (Concurrent and/or sequential use is not recommended).
- No products indexed under this heading.

Phenelzine Sulfate (Concurrent and/or sequential use is not recommended). Products include:
- Nardil ... 1920

Selegiline Hydrochloride (Concurrent and/or sequential use is not recommended). Products include:
- Eldepryl Tablets ... 2550

Tranylcypromine Sulfate (Concurrent and/or sequential use is not recommended). Products include:
- Parnate Tablets ... 2503

ROBITUSSIN MAXIMUM STRENGTH COUGH & COLD

(Dextromethorphan Hydrobromide, Pseudoephedrine Hydrochloride) ... ▣ 778

May interact with monoamine oxidase inhibitors. Compounds in this category include:

Furazolidone (Concurrent and/or sequential use is not recommended). Products include:
- Furoxone ... 2046

Isocarboxazid (Concurrent and/or sequential use is not recommended).
- No products indexed under this heading.

Phenelzine Sulfate (Concurrent and/or sequential use is not recommended). Products include:
- Nardil ... 1920

Selegiline Hydrochloride (Concurrent and/or sequential use is not recommended). Products include:
- Eldepryl Tablets ... 2550

Tranylcypromine Sulfate (Concurrent and/or sequential use is not recommended). Products include:
- Parnate Tablets ... 2503

ROBITUSSIN MAXIMUM STRENGTH COUGH SUPPRESSANT

(Dextromethorphan Hydrobromide) ... ▣ 778

May interact with monoamine oxidase inhibitors. Compounds in this category include:

Furazolidone (Concurrent and/or sequential use is not recommended). Products include:
- Furoxone ... 2046

Isocarboxazid (Concurrent and/or sequential use is not recommended).
- No products indexed under this heading.

Phenelzine Sulfate (Concurrent and/or sequential use is not recommended). Products include:
- Nardil ... 1920

Selegiline Hydrochloride (Concurrent and/or sequential use is not recommended). Products include:
- Eldepryl Tablets ... 2550

Tranylcypromine Sulfate (Concurrent and/or sequential use is not recommended). Products include:
- Parnate Tablets ... 2503

ROBITUSSIN PEDIATRIC COUGH & COLD FORMULA

(Dextromethorphan Hydrobromide, Pseudoephedrine Hydrochloride) ... ▣ 779

May interact with monoamine oxidase inhibitors. Compounds in this category include:

Furazolidone (Concurrent and/or sequential use should be avoided). Products include:
- Furoxone ... 2046

Isocarboxazid (Concurrent and/or sequential use should be avoided).
- No products indexed under this heading.

Phenelzine Sulfate (Concurrent and/or sequential use should be avoided). Products include:
- Nardil ... 1920

Selegiline Hydrochloride (Concurrent and/or sequential use should be avoided). Products include:
- Eldepryl Tablets ... 2550

Tranylcypromine Sulfate (Concurrent and/or sequential use should be avoided). Products include:
- Parnate Tablets ... 2503

ROBITUSSIN PEDIATRIC COUGH SUPPRESSANT

(Dextromethorphan Hydrobromide) ... ▣ 779

May interact with monoamine oxidase inhibitors. Compounds in this category include:

Furazolidone (Concurrent and/or sequential use should be avoided). Products include:
- Furoxone ... 2046

Isocarboxazid (Concurrent and/or sequential use should be avoided).
- No products indexed under this heading.

(▣ Described in PDR For Nonprescription Drugs) (⊛ Described in PDR For Ophthalmology)

Phenelzine Sulfate (Concurrent and/or sequential use should be avoided). Products include:

Nardil 1920

Selegiline Hydrochloride (Concurrent and/or sequential use should be avoided). Products include:

Eldepryl Tablets 2550

Tranylcypromine Sulfate (Concurrent and/or sequential use should be avoided). Products include:

Parnate Tablets 2503

ROBITUSSIN SEVERE CONGESTION LIQUI-GELS

(Guaifenesin, Pseudoephedrine Hydrochloride)....................................... ⊕D 776

May interact with monoamine oxidase inhibitors. Compounds in this category include:

Furazolidone (Concurrent and/or sequential use is not recommended). Products include:

Furoxone 2046

Isocarboxazid (Concurrent and/or sequential use is not recommended).

No products indexed under this heading.

Phenelzine Sulfate (Concurrent and/or sequential use is not recommended). Products include:

Nardil 1920

Selegiline Hydrochloride (Concurrent and/or sequential use is not recommended). Products include:

Eldepryl Tablets 2550

Tranylcypromine Sulfate (Concurrent and/or sequential use is not recommended). Products include:

Parnate Tablets 2503

ROBITUSSIN-CF

(Dextromethorphan Hydrobromide, Guaifenesin, Phenylpropanolamine Hydrochloride)....................................... ⊕D 777

May interact with monoamine oxidase inhibitors. Compounds in this category include:

Furazolidone (Concurrent and/or sequential use is not recommended). Products include:

Furoxone 2046

Isocarboxazid (Concurrent and/or sequential use is not recommended).

No products indexed under this heading.

Phenelzine Sulfate (Concurrent and/or sequential use is not recommended). Products include:

Nardil 1920

Selegiline Hydrochloride (Concurrent and/or sequential use is not recommended). Products include:

Eldepryl Tablets 2550

Tranylcypromine Sulfate (Concurrent and/or sequential use is not recommended). Products include:

Parnate Tablets 2503

ROBITUSSIN-DAC SYRUP

(Codeine Phosphate, Guaifenesin, Pseudoephedrine Hydrochloride) 2074

May interact with monoamine oxidase inhibitors. Compounds in this category include:

Furazolidone (Concurrent use is not recommended). Products include:

Furoxone 2046

Isocarboxazid (Concurrent use is not recommended).

No products indexed under this heading.

Phenelzine Sulfate (Concurrent use is not recommended). Products include:

Nardil 1920

Selegiline Hydrochloride (Concurrent use is not recommended). Products include:

Eldepryl Tablets 2550

Tranylcypromine Sulfate (Concurrent and/or sequential use is not recommended). Products include:

Parnate Tablets 2503

ROBITUSSIN-DM

(Dextromethorphan Hydrobromide, Guaifenesin)... ⊕D 777

May interact with monoamine oxidase inhibitors. Compounds in this category include:

Furazolidone (Concurrent and/or sequential use is not recommended). Products include:

Furoxone 2046

Isocarboxazid (Concurrent and/or sequential use is not recommended).

No products indexed under this heading.

Phenelzine Sulfate (Concurrent and/or sequential use is not recommended). Products include:

Nardil 1920

Selegiline Hydrochloride (Concurrent and/or sequential use is not recommended). Products include:

Eldepryl Tablets 2550

Tranylcypromine Sulfate (Concurrent and/or sequential use is not recommended). Products include:

Parnate Tablets 2503

ROBITUSSIN-PE

(Guaifenesin, Pseudoephedrine Hydrochloride)....................................... ⊕D 778

May interact with monoamine oxidase inhibitors. Compounds in this category include:

Furazolidone (Concurrent and/or sequential use is not recommended). Products include:

Furoxone 2046

Isocarboxazid (Concurrent and/or sequential use is not recommended).

No products indexed under this heading.

Phenelzine Sulfate (Concurrent and/or sequential use is not recommended). Products include:

Nardil 1920

Selegiline Hydrochloride (Concurrent and/or sequential use is not recommended). Products include:

Eldepryl Tablets 2550

Tranylcypromine Sulfate (Concurrent and/or sequential use is not recommended). Products include:

Parnate Tablets 2503

ROCALTROL CAPSULES

(Calcitriol) 2141

May interact with cardiac glycosides, magnesium-containing antacids, and certain other agents. Compounds in these categories include:

Cholestyramine (Reduced intestinal absorption of Rocaltrol). Products include:

Questran Light 769
Questran Powder 770

Deslanoside (Increased risk of cardiac arrhythmias).

No products indexed under this heading.

Digitoxin (Increased risk of cardiac arrhythmias). Products include:

Crystodigin Tablets................................ 1433

Digoxin (Increased risk of cardiac arrhythmias). Products include:

Lanoxicaps 1117
Lanoxin Elixir Pediatric 1120
Lanoxin Injection 1123
Lanoxin Injection Pediatric.................... 1126
Lanoxin Tablets 1128

Magaldrate (Potential for hypermagnesemia in patients on chronic renal dialysis).

No products indexed under this heading.

Magnesium Carbonate (Potential for hypermagnesemia in patients on chronic renal dialysis). Products include:

Gaviscon Extra Strength Relief Formula Antacid Tablets................ ⊕D 819
Gaviscon Extra Strength Relief Formula Liquid Antacid.................. ⊕D 819
Gaviscon Liquid Antacid..................... ⊕D 820
Maalox Heartburn Relief Suspension .... ⊕D 642
Maalox Heartburn Relief Tablets.... ⊕D 641
Marblen .... ⊕D 655
Mylanta Gelcaps Antacid .... ⊕D 662

Magnesium Hydroxide (Potential for hypermagnesemia in patients on chronic renal dialysis). Products include:

Aludrox Oral Suspension 2695
Arthritis Pain Ascriptin .... ⊕D 631
Maximum Strength Ascriptin .... ⊕D 630
Regular Strength Ascriptin Tablets .... ⊕D 629
Di-Gel Antacid/Anti-Gas .... ⊕D 801
Gelusil Liquid & Tablets .... ⊕D 855
Maalox Magnesia and Alumina Oral Suspension .... ⊕D 642
Maalox Plus Tablets .... ⊕D 643
Extra Strength Maalox Antacid Plus Antigas Liquid and Tablets ⊕D 638
Mylanta Calcium Carbonate and Magnesium Hydroxide Tablets...... 1318
Mylanta Liquid 1317
Mylanta Tablets .... ⊕D 660
Mylanta Double Strength Liquid 1317
Mylanta Double Strength Tablets .. ⊕D 660
Phillips' Milk of Magnesia Liquid... ⊕D 729
Rolaids Tablets .... ⊕D 843
Tempo Soft Antacid .... ⊕D 835

Magnesium Trisilicate (Potential for hypermagnesemia in patients on chronic renal dialysis). Products include:

Gaviscon Antacid Tablets................... ⊕D 819
Gaviscon-2 Antacid Tablets .... ⊕D 820

Vitamin D (Possible additive effect and hypercalcemia). Products include:

Caltrate PLUS .... ⊕D 665
Caltrate 600 + D .... ⊕D 665
Citracal Caplets + D 1780
Dical-D Tablets & Wafers 420
Drisdol .... ⊕D 794
Materna Tablets 1379
Megadose 512
Zymacap Capsules .... ⊕D 772

ROCEPHIN INJECTABLE VIALS, ADD-VANTAGE, GALAXY CONTAINER

(Ceftriaxone Sodium) 2142

None cited in PDR database.

ROFERON-A INJECTION

(Interferon alfa-2A, Recombinant) 2145

May interact with:

Aminophylline (Reduced clearance of theophylline).

No products indexed under this heading.

Bone Marrow Depressants, unspecified (Caution should be exercised when administered concomitantly with myelosuppressive agents).

Dyphylline (Reduced clearance of theophylline). Products include:

Lufyllin & Lufyllin-400 Tablets 2670

Lufyllin-GG Elixir & Tablets 2671

Theophylline (Reduced clearance of theophylline). Products include:

Marax Tablets & DF Syrup.................. 2200
Quibron 2053

Theophylline Anhydrous (Reduced clearance of theophylline). Products include:

Aerolate 1004
Primatene Dual Action Formula...... ⊕D 872
Primatene Tablets .... ⊕D 873
Respbid Tablets 682
Slo-bid Gyrocaps 2033
Theo-24 Extended Release Capsules 2568
Theo-Dur Extended-Release Tablets 1327
Theo-X Extended-Release Tablets .. 788
Uni-Dur Extended-Release Tablets.. 1331
Uniphyl 400 mg Tablets....................... 2001

Theophylline Calcium Salicylate (Reduced clearance of theophylline). Products include:

Quadrinal Tablets 1350

Theophylline Sodium Glycinate (Reduced clearance of theophylline).

No products indexed under this heading.

Zidovudine (Concomitant therapy may result in synergistic toxicity). Products include:

Retrovir Capsules 1158
Retrovir I.V. Infusion........................... 1163
Retrovir Syrup...................................... 1158

ROGAINE TOPICAL SOLUTION

(Minoxidil) 2637

May interact with:

Guanethidine Monosulfate (Theoretical possibility of potentiation of orthostatic hypotension). Products include:

Esimil Tablets 822
Ismelin Tablets 827

ROLAIDS TABLETS

(Calcium Carbonate, Magnesium Hydroxide) .... ⊕D 843

May interact with:

Drugs, Oral, unspecified (Antacids may interact with certain unspecified prescription drugs).

ROLAIDS (CALCIUM RICH/SODIUM FREE) TABLETS

(Calcium Carbonate) .... ⊕D 843

May interact with:

Drugs, Oral, unspecified (Antacids may interact with certain unspecified prescription drugs).

ROMAZICON

(Flumazenil) 2147

May interact with antidepressant drugs, neuromuscular blocking agents, and certain other agents. Compounds in these categories include:

Amitriptyline Hydrochloride (Toxic effects of cyclic antidepressant may emerge with the reversal of the benzodiazepine effect). Products include:

Elavil 2838
Endep Tablets 2174
Etrafon 2355
Limbitrol 2180
Triavil Tablets 1757

Amoxapine (Toxic effects of cyclic antidepressant may emerge with the reversal of the benzodiazepine effect). Products include:

Asendin Tablets 1369

IMPORTANT NOTE: Always consult each drug listing in the patient's regimen for possible interactions.

Romazicon Interactions Index 906

Atracurium Besylate (Romazicon should not be used until the effects of neuromuscular blockade have been fully reversed). Products include:
Tracrium Injection 1183

Desipramine Hydrochloride (Toxic effects of cyclic antidepressant may emerge with the reversal of the benzodiazepine effect). Products include:
Norpramin Tablets 1526

Doxacurium Chloride (Romazicon should not be used until the effects of neuromuscular blockade have been fully reversed). Products include:
Nuromax Injection 1149

Doxepin Hydrochloride (Toxic effects of cyclic antidepressant may emerge with the reversal of the benzodiazepine effect). Products include:
Sinequan 2205
Zonalon Cream 1055

Imipramine Hydrochloride (Toxic effects of cyclic antidepressant may emerge with the reversal of the benzodiazepine effect). Products include:
Tofranil Ampuls 854
Tofranil Tablets 856

Imipramine Pamoate (Toxic effects of cyclic antidepressant may emerge with the reversal of the benzodiazepine effect). Products include:
Tofranil-PM Capsules 857

Maprotiline Hydrochloride (Toxic effects of cyclic antidepressant may emerge with the reversal of the benzodiazepine effect). Products include:
Ludiomil Tablets 843

Metocurine Iodide (Romazicon should not be used until the effects of neuromuscular blockade have been fully reversed). Products include:
Metubine Iodide Vials 916

Mivacurium Chloride (Romazicon should not be used until the effects of neuromuscular blockade have been fully reversed). Products include:
Mivacron 1138

Nefazodone Hydrochloride (Toxic effects of cyclic antidepressant may emerge with the reversal of the benzodiazepine effect). Products include:
Serzone Tablets 771

Nortriptyline Hydrochloride (Toxic effects of cyclic antidepressant may emerge with the reversal of the benzodiazepine effect). Products include:
Pamelor 2280

Pancuronium Bromide Injection (Romazicon should not be used until the effects of neuromuscular blockade have been fully reversed).
No products indexed under this heading.

Paroxetine Hydrochloride (Toxic effects of cyclic antidepressant may emerge with the reversal of the benzodiazepine effect). Products include:
Paxil Tablets 2505

Protriptyline Hydrochloride (Toxic effects of cyclic antidepressant may emerge with the reversal of the benzodiazepine effect). Products include:
Vivactil Tablets 1774

Rocuronium Bromide (Romazicon should not be used until the effects of neuromuscular blockade have been fully reversed). Products include:
Zemuron 1830

Sertraline Hydrochloride (Toxic effects of cyclic antidepressant may emerge with the reversal of the benzodiazepine effect). Products include:
Zoloft Tablets 2217

Succinylcholine Chloride (Romazicon should not be used until the effects of neuromuscular blockade have been fully reversed). Products include:
Anectine 1073

Trazodone Hydrochloride (Toxic effects of cyclic antidepressant may emerge with the reversal of the benzodiazepine effect). Products include:
Desyrel and Desyrel Dividose 503

Trimipramine Maleate (Toxic effects of cyclic antidepressant may emerge with the reversal of the benzodiazepine effect). Products include:
Surmontil Capsules 2811

Vecuronium Bromide (Romazicon should not be used until the effects of neuromuscular blockade have been fully reversed). Products include:
Norcuron 1826

Venlafaxine Hydrochloride (Toxic effects of cyclic antidepressant may emerge with the reversal of the benzodiazepine effect). Products include:
Effexor 2719

Food Interactions

Alcohol (Concurrent use should be avoided).

RONDEC ORAL DROPS

(Carbinoxamine Maleate, Pseudoephedrine Hydrochloride) 953
May interact with tricyclic antidepressants, central nervous system depressants, monoamine oxidase inhibitors, veratrum alkaloids, beta blockers, and certain other agents. Compounds in these categories include:

Acebutolol Hydrochloride (Effects of sympathomimetics increased). Products include:
Sectral Capsules 2807

Alfentanil Hydrochloride (Enhanced effects of CNS depressants). Products include:
Alfenta Injection 1286

Alprazolam (Enhanced effects of CNS depressants). Products include:
Xanax Tablets 2649

Amitriptyline Hydrochloride (Enhanced effects of tricyclic antidepressants). Products include:
Elavil 2838
Endep Tablets 2174
Etrafon 2355
Limbitrol 2180
Triavil Tablets 1757

Amoxapine (Enhanced effects of tricyclic antidepressants). Products include:
Asendin Tablets 1369

Aprobarbital (Enhanced effects of CNS depressants).
No products indexed under this heading.

Atenolol (Effects of sympathomimetics increased). Products include:
Tenoretic Tablets 2845
Tenormin Tablets and I.V. Injection 2847

Betaxolol Hydrochloride (Effects of sympathomimetics increased). Products include:
Betoptic Ophthalmic Solution 469
Betoptic S Ophthalmic Suspension 471
Kerlone Tablets 2436

Bisoprolol Fumarate (Effects of sympathomimetics increased). Products include:
Zebeta Tablets 1413
Ziac 1415

Buprenorphine (Enhanced effects of CNS depressants). Products include:
Buprenex Injectable 2006

Buspirone Hydrochloride (Enhanced effects of CNS depressants). Products include:
BuSpar 737

Butabarbital (Enhanced effects of CNS depressants).
No products indexed under this heading.

Butalbital (Enhanced effects of CNS depressants). Products include:
Esgic-plus Tablets 1013
Fioricet Tablets 2258
Fioricet with Codeine Capsules 2260
Fiorinal Capsules 2261
Fiorinal with Codeine Capsules 2262
Fiorinal Tablets 2261
Phrenilin 785
Sedapap Tablets 50 mg/650 mg .. 1543

Carteolol Hydrochloride (Effects of sympathomimetics increased). Products include:
Cartrol Tablets 410
Ocupress Ophthalmic Solution, 1% Sterile ..... ⊙ 309

Chlordiazepoxide (Enhanced effects of CNS depressants). Products include:
Libritabs Tablets 2177
Limbitrol 2180

Chlordiazepoxide Hydrochloride (Enhanced effects of CNS depressants). Products include:
Librax Capsules 2176
Librium Capsules 2178
Librium Injectable 2179

Chlorpromazine (Enhanced effects of CNS depressants). Products include:
Thorazine Suppositories 2523

Chlorprothixene (Enhanced effects of CNS depressants).
No products indexed under this heading.

Chlorprothixene Hydrochloride (Enhanced effects of CNS depressants).
No products indexed under this heading.

Clomipramine Hydrochloride (Enhanced effects of tricyclic antidepressants). Products include:
Anafranil Capsules 803

Clorazepate Dipotassium (Enhanced effects of CNS depressants). Products include:
Tranxene 451

Clozapine (Enhanced effects of CNS depressants). Products include:
Clozaril Tablets 2252

Codeine Phosphate (Enhanced effects of CNS depressants). Products include:
Actifed with Codeine Cough Syrup.. 1067
Brontex 1981
Deconsal C Expectorant Syrup 456
Deconsal Pediatric Syrup 457
Dimetane-DC Cough Syrup 2059
Empirin with Codeine Tablets 1093
Fioricet with Codeine Capsules 2260
Fiorinal with Codeine Capsules 2262
Isoclor Expectorant 990
Novahistine DH 2462
Novahistine Expectorant 2463
Nucofed 2051
Phenergan with Codeine 2777
Phenergan VC with Codeine 2781
Robitussin A-C Syrup 2073
Robitussin-DAC Syrup 2074
Ryna ..... ▣ 841
Soma Compound w/Codeine Tablets 2676
Tussi-Organidin NR Liquid and S NR Liquid 2677
Tylenol with Codeine 1583

Cryptenamine Preparations (Reduced antihypertensive effects).

Desflurane (Enhanced effects of CNS depressants). Products include:
Suprane 1813

Desipramine Hydrochloride (Enhanced effects of tricyclic antidepressants). Products include:
Norpramin Tablets 1526

Dezocine (Enhanced effects of CNS depressants). Products include:
Dalgan Injection 538

Diazepam (Enhanced effects of CNS depressants). Products include:
Dizac 1809
Valium Injectable 2182
Valium Tablets 2183
Valrelease Capsules 2169

Doxepin Hydrochloride (Enhanced effects of tricyclic antidepressants). Products include:
Sinequan 2205
Zonalon Cream 1055

Droperidol (Enhanced effects of CNS depressants). Products include:
Inapsine Injection 1296

Enflurane (Enhanced effects of CNS depressants).
No products indexed under this heading.

Esmolol Hydrochloride (Effects of sympathomimetics increased). Products include:
Brevibloc Injection 1808

Estazolam (Enhanced effects of CNS depressants). Products include:
ProSom Tablets 449

Ethchlorvynol (Enhanced effects of CNS depressants). Products include:
Placidyl Capsules 448

Ethinamate (Enhanced effects of CNS depressants).
No products indexed under this heading.

Fentanyl (Enhanced effects of CNS depressants). Products include:
Duragesic Transdermal System 1288

Fentanyl Citrate (Enhanced effects of CNS depressants). Products include:
Sublimaze Injection 1307

Fluphenazine Decanoate (Enhanced effects of CNS depressants). Products include:
Prolixin Decanoate 509

Fluphenazine Enanthate (Enhanced effects of CNS depressants). Products include:
Prolixin Enanthate 509

Fluphenazine Hydrochloride (Enhanced effects of CNS depressants). Products include:
Prolixin 509

Flurazepam Hydrochloride (Enhanced effects of CNS depressants). Products include:
Dalmane Capsules 2173

Furazolidone (Effects of sympathomimetics increased; anticholinergic effects of antihistamines prolonged and intensified; concurrent use is contraindicated). Products include:
Furoxone 2046

Glutethimide (Enhanced effects of CNS depressants).
No products indexed under this heading.

(▣ Described in PDR For Nonprescription Drugs) (⊙ Described in PDR For Ophthalmology)

Haloperidol (Enhanced effects of CNS depressants). Products include:
- Haldol Injection, Tablets and Concentrate ... 1575

Haloperidol Decanoate (Enhanced effects of CNS depressants). Products include:
- Haldol Decanoate ... 1577

Hydrocodone Bitartrate (Enhanced effects of CNS depressants). Products include:
- Anexsia 5/500 Elixir ... 1781
- Anexia Tablets ... 1782
- Codiclear DH Syrup ... 791
- Deconamine CX Cough and Cold Liquid and Tablets ... 1319
- Duratuss HD Elixir ... 2565
- Hycodan Tablets and Syrup ... 930
- Hycomine Compound Tablets ... 932
- Hycomine ... 931
- Hycotuss Expectorant Syrup ... 933
- Hydrocet Capsules ... 782
- Lorcet 10/650 ... 1018
- Lortab ... 2566
- Tussend ... 1783
- Tussend Expectorant ... 1785
- Vicodin Tablets ... 1356
- Vicodin ES Tablets ... 1357
- Vicodin Tuss Expectorant ... 1358
- Zydone Capsules ... 949

Hydrocodone Polistirex (Enhanced effects of CNS depressants). Products include:
- Tussionex Pennkinetic Extended-Release Suspension ... 998

Hydroxyzine Hydrochloride (Enhanced effects of CNS depressants). Products include:
- Atarax Tablets & Syrup ... 2185
- Marax Tablets & DF Syrup ... 2200
- Vistaril Intramuscular Solution ... 2216

Imipramine Hydrochloride (Enhanced effects of tricyclic antidepressants). Products include:
- Tofranil Ampuls ... 854
- Tofranil Tablets ... 856

Imipramine Pamoate (Enhanced effects of tricyclic antidepressants). Products include:
- Tofranil-PM Capsules ... 857

Isocarboxazid (Effects of sympathomimetics increased; anticholinergic effects of antihistamines prolonged and intensified; concurrent use is contraindicated).
- No products indexed under this heading.

Isoflurane (Enhanced effects of CNS depressants).
- No products indexed under this heading.

Ketamine Hydrochloride (Enhanced effects of CNS depressants).
- No products indexed under this heading.

Labetalol Hydrochloride (Effects of sympathomimetics increased). Products include:
- Normodyne Injection ... 2377
- Normodyne Tablets ... 2379
- Trandate ... 1185

Levobunolol Hydrochloride (Effects of sympathomimetics increased). Products include:
- Betagan ... ⊙ 233

Levorphanol Tartrate (Enhanced effects of CNS depressants). Products include:
- Levo-Dromoran ... 2129

Lorazepam (Enhanced effects of CNS depressants). Products include:
- Ativan Injection ... 2698
- Ativan Tablets ... 2700

Loxapine Hydrochloride (Enhanced effects of CNS depressants). Products include:
- Loxitane ... 1378

Loxapine Succinate (Enhanced effects of CNS depressants). Products include:
- Loxitane Capsules ... 1378

Maprotiline Hydrochloride (Enhanced effects of tricyclic antidepressants). Products include:
- Ludiomil Tablets ... 843

Mecamylamine Hydrochloride (Reduced antihypertensive effects). Products include:
- Inversine Tablets ... 1686

Meperidine Hydrochloride (Enhanced effects of CNS depressants). Products include:
- Demerol ... 2308
- Mepergan Injection ... 2753

Mephobarbital (Enhanced effects of CNS depressants). Products include:
- Mebaral Tablets ... 2322

Meprobamate (Enhanced effects of CNS depressants). Products include:
- Miltown Tablets ... 2672
- PMB 200 and PMB 400 ... 2783

Mesoridazine Besylate (Enhanced effects of CNS depressants). Products include:
- Serentil ... 684

Methadone Hydrochloride (Enhanced effects of CNS depressants). Products include:
- Methadone Hydrochloride Oral Concentrate ... 2233
- Methadone Hydrochloride Oral Solution & Tablets ... 2235

Methohexital Sodium (Enhanced effects of CNS depressants). Products include:
- Brevital Sodium Vials ... 1429

Methotrimeprazine (Enhanced effects of CNS depressants). Products include:
- Levoprome ... 1274

Methoxyflurane (Enhanced effects of CNS depressants).
- No products indexed under this heading.

Methyldopa (Reduced antihypertensive effects). Products include:
- Aldoclor Tablets ... 1598
- Aldomet Oral ... 1600
- Aldoril Tablets ... 1604

Metipranolol Hydrochloride (Effects of sympathomimetics increased). Products include:
- OptiPranolol (Metipranolol 0.3%) Sterile Ophthalmic Solution ... ⊙ 258

Metoprolol Succinate (Effects of sympathomimetics increased). Products include:
- Toprol-XL Tablets ... 565

Metoprolol Tartrate (Effects of sympathomimetics increased). Products include:
- Lopressor Ampuls ... 830
- Lopressor HCT Tablets ... 832
- Lopressor Tablets ... 830

Midazolam Hydrochloride (Enhanced effects of CNS depressants). Products include:
- Versed Injection ... 2170

Molindone Hydrochloride (Enhanced effects of CNS depressants). Products include:
- Moban Tablets and Concentrate ... 1048

Morphine Sulfate (Enhanced effects of CNS depressants). Products include:
- Astramorph/PF Injection, USP (Preservative-Free) ... 535
- Duramorph ... 962
- Infumorph 200 and Infumorph 500 Sterile Solutions ... 965
- MS Contin Tablets ... 1994
- MSIR ... 1997
- Oramorph SR (Morphine Sulfate Sustained Release Tablets) ... 2236
- RMS Suppositories ... 2657
- Roxanol ... 2243

Nadolol (Effects of sympathomimetics increased).
- No products indexed under this heading.

Nortriptyline Hydrochloride (Enhanced effects of tricyclic antidepressants). Products include:
- Pamelor ... 2280

Opium Alkaloids (Enhanced effects of CNS depressants).
- No products indexed under this heading.

Oxazepam (Enhanced effects of CNS depressants). Products include:
- Serax Capsules ... 2810
- Serax Tablets ... 2810

Oxycodone Hydrochloride (Enhanced effects of CNS depressants). Products include:
- Percocet Tablets ... 938
- Percodan Tablets ... 939
- Percodan-Demi Tablets ... 940
- Roxicodone Tablets, Oral Solution & Intensol (Oxycodone) ... 2244
- Tylox Capsules ... 1584

Penbutolol Sulfate (Effects of sympathomimetics increased). Products include:
- Levatol ... 2403

Pentobarbital Sodium (Enhanced effects of CNS depressants). Products include:
- Nembutal Sodium Capsules ... 436
- Nembutal Sodium Solution ... 438
- Nembutal Sodium Suppositories ... 440

Perphenazine (Enhanced effects of CNS depressants). Products include:
- Etrafon ... 2355
- Triavil Tablets ... 1757
- Trilafon ... 2389

Phenelzine Sulfate (Effects of sympathomimetics increased; anticholinergic effects of antihistamines prolonged and intensified; concurrent use is contraindicated). Products include:
- Nardil ... 1920

Phenobarbital (Enhanced effects of CNS depressants). Products include:
- Arco-Lase Plus Tablets ... 512
- Bellergal-S Tablets ... 2250
- Donnatal ... 2060
- Donnatal Extentabs ... 2061
- Donnatal Tablets ... 2060
- Phenobarbital Elixir and Tablets ... 1469
- Quadrinal Tablets ... 1350

Pindolol (Effects of sympathomimetics increased). Products include:
- Visken Tablets ... 2299

Prazepam (Enhanced effects of CNS depressants).
- No products indexed under this heading.

Prochlorperazine (Enhanced effects of CNS depressants). Products include:
- Compazine ... 2470

Promethazine Hydrochloride (Enhanced effects of CNS depressants). Products include:
- Mepergan Injection ... 2753
- Phenergan with Codeine ... 2777
- Phenergan with Dextromethorphan ... 2778
- Phenergan Injection ... 2773
- Phenergan Suppositories ... 2775
- Phenergan Syrup ... 2774
- Phenergan Tablets ... 2775
- Phenergan VC ... 2779
- Phenergan VC with Codeine ... 2781

Propofol (Enhanced effects of CNS depressants). Products include:
- Diprivan Injection ... 2833

Propoxyphene Hydrochloride (Enhanced effects of CNS depressants). Products include:
- Darvon ... 1435
- Wygesic Tablets ... 2827

Propoxyphene Napsylate (Enhanced effects of CNS depressants). Products include:
- Darvon-N/Darvocet-N ... 1433

Propranolol Hydrochloride (Effects of sympathomimetics increased). Products include:
- Inderal ... 2728
- Inderal LA Long Acting Capsules ... 2730
- Inderide Tablets ... 2732
- Inderide LA Long Acting Capsules ... 2734

Protriptyline Hydrochloride (Enhanced effects of tricyclic antidepressants). Products include:
- Vivactil Tablets ... 1774

Quazepam (Enhanced effects of CNS depressants). Products include:
- Doral Tablets ... 2664

Reserpine (Reduced antihypertensive effects). Products include:
- Diupres Tablets ... 1650
- Hydropres Tablets ... 1675
- Ser-Ap-Es Tablets ... 849

Risperidone (Enhanced effects of CNS depressants). Products include:
- Risperdal ... 1301

Secobarbital Sodium (Enhanced effects of CNS depressants). Products include:
- Seconal Sodium Pulvules ... 1474

Selegiline Hydrochloride (Effects of sympathomimetics increased; anticholinergic effects of antihistamines prolonged and intensified; concurrent use is contraindicated). Products include:
- Eldepryl Tablets ... 2550

Sotalol Hydrochloride (Effects of sympathomimetics increased). Products include:
- Betapace Tablets ... 641

Sufentanil Citrate (Enhanced effects of CNS depressants). Products include:
- Sufenta Injection ... 1309

Temazepam (Enhanced effects of CNS depressants). Products include:
- Restoril Capsules ... 2284

Thiamylal Sodium (Enhanced effects of CNS depressants).
- No products indexed under this heading.

Thioridazine Hydrochloride (Enhanced effects of CNS depressants). Products include:
- Mellaril ... 2269

Thiothixene (Enhanced effects of CNS depressants). Products include:
- Navane Capsules and Concentrate ... 2201
- Navane Intramuscular ... 2202

Timolol Maleate (Effects of sympathomimetics increased). Products include:
- Blocadren Tablets ... 1614
- Timolide Tablets ... 1748
- Timoptic in Ocudose ... 1753
- Timoptic Sterile Ophthalmic Solution ... 1751
- Timoptic-XE ... 1755

Tranylcypromine Sulfate (Effects of sympathomimetics increased; anticholinergic effects of antihistamines prolonged and intensified; concurrent use is contraindicated). Products include:
- Parnate Tablets ... 2503

Triazolam (Enhanced effects of CNS depressants). Products include:
- Halcion Tablets ... 2611

Trifluoperazine Hydrochloride (Enhanced effects of CNS depressants). Products include:
- Stelazine ... 2514

Trimipramine Maleate (Enhanced effects of tricyclic antidepressants). Products include:
- Surmontil Capsules ... 2811

IMPORTANT NOTE: Always consult each drug listing in the patient's regimen for possible interactions.

Rondec Interactions Index 908

Zolpidem Tartrate (Enhanced effects of CNS depressants). Products include:
Ambien Tablets ... 2416

Food Interactions

Alcohol (Enhanced effects of alcohol).

RONDEC SYRUP
(Carbinoxamine Maleate, Pseudoephedrine Hydrochloride) ... 953
See **Rondec Oral Drops**

RONDEC TABLET
(Carbinoxamine Maleate, Pseudoephedrine Hydrochloride) ... 953
See **Rondec Oral Drops**

RONDEC-DM ORAL DROPS
(Carbinoxamine Maleate, Pseudoephedrine Hydrochloride, Dextromethorphan Hydrobromide) ... 954
May interact with tricyclic antidepressants, central nervous system depressants, monoamine oxidase inhibitors, veratrum alkaloids, beta blockers, and certain other agents. Compounds in these categories include:

Acebutolol Hydrochloride (Effects of sympathomimetics increased). Products include:
Sectral Capsules ... 2807

Alfentanil Hydrochloride (Enhanced effects of CNS depressants). Products include:
Alfenta Injection ... 1286

Alprazolam (Enhanced effects of CNS depressants). Products include:
Xanax Tablets ... 2649

Amitriptyline Hydrochloride (Enhanced effects of tricyclic antidepressants). Products include:
Elavil ... 2838
Endep Tablets ... 2174
Etrafon ... 2355
Limbitrol ... 2180
Triavil Tablets ... 1757

Amoxapine (Enhanced effects of tricyclic antidepressants). Products include:
Asendin Tablets ... 1369

Aprobarbital (Enhanced effects of CNS depressants).
No products indexed under this heading.

Atenolol (Effects of sympathomimetics increased). Products include:
Tenoretic Tablets ... 2845
Tenormin Tablets and I.V. Injection ... 2847

Betaxolol Hydrochloride (Effects of sympathomimetics increased). Products include:
Betoptic Ophthalmic Solution ... 469
Betoptic S Ophthalmic Suspension ... 471
Kerlone Tablets ... 2436

Bisoprolol Fumarate (Effects of sympathomimetics increased). Products include:
Zebeta Tablets ... 1413
Ziac ... 1415

Buprenorphine (Enhanced effects of CNS depressants). Products include:
Buprenex Injectable ... 2006

Buspirone Hydrochloride (Enhanced effects of CNS depressants). Products include:
BuSpar ... 737

Butabarbital (Enhanced effects of CNS depressants).
No products indexed under this heading.

Butalbital (Enhanced effects of CNS depressants). Products include:
Esgic-plus Tablets ... 1013
Fioricet Tablets ... 2258
Fioricet with Codeine Capsules ... 2260
Fiorinal Capsules ... 2261
Fiorinal with Codeine Capsules ... 2262
Fiorinal Tablets ... 2261
Phrenilin ... 785
Sedapap Tablets 50 mg/650 mg ... 1543

Carteolol Hydrochloride (Effects of sympathomimetics increased). Products include:
Cartrol Tablets ... 410
Ocupress Ophthalmic Solution, 1% Sterile ... ◉ 309

Chlordiazepoxide (Enhanced effects of CNS depressants). Products include:
Libritabs Tablets ... 2177
Limbitrol ... 2180

Chlordiazepoxide Hydrochloride (Enhanced effects of CNS depressants). Products include:
Librax Capsules ... 2176
Librium Capsules ... 2178
Librium Injectable ... 2179

Chlorpromazine (Enhanced effects of CNS depressants). Products include:
Thorazine Suppositories ... 2523

Chlorpromazine Hydrochloride (Enhanced effects of CNS depressants). Products include:
Thorazine ... 2523

Chlorprothixene (Enhanced effects of CNS depressants).
No products indexed under this heading.

Chlorprothixene Hydrochloride (Enhanced effects of CNS depressants).
No products indexed under this heading.

Clomipramine Hydrochloride (Enhanced effects of tricyclic antidepressants). Products include:
Anafranil Capsules ... 803

Clorazepate Dipotassium (Enhanced effects of CNS depressants). Products include:
Tranxene ... 451

Clozapine (Enhanced effects of CNS depressants). Products include:
Clozaril Tablets ... 2252

Codeine Phosphate (Enhanced effects of CNS depressants). Products include:
Actifed with Codeine Cough Syrup ... 1067
Brontex ... 1981
Deconsal C Expectorant Syrup ... 456
Deconsal Pediatric Syrup ... 457
Dimetane-DC Cough Syrup ... 2059
Empirin with Codeine Tablets ... 1093
Fioricet with Codeine Capsules ... 2260
Fiorinal with Codeine Capsules ... 2262
Isoclor Expectorant ... 990
Novahistine DH ... 2462
Novahistine Expectorant ... 2463
Nucofed ... 2051
Phenergan with Codeine ... 2777
Phenergan VC with Codeine ... 2781
Robitussin A-C Syrup ... 2073
Robitussin-DAC Syrup ... 2074
Ryna ... ▣ 841
Soma Compound w/Codeine Tablets ... 2676
Tussi-Organidin NR Liquid and S NR Liquid ... 2677
Tylenol with Codeine ... 1583

Cryptenamine Preparations (Reduced antihypertensive effects).

Desflurane (Enhanced effects of CNS depressants). Products include:
Suprane ... 1813

Desipramine Hydrochloride (Enhanced effects of tricyclic antidepressants). Products include:
Norpramin Tablets ... 1526

Dezocine (Enhanced effects of CNS depressants). Products include:
Dalgan Injection ... 538

Diazepam (Enhanced effects of CNS depressants). Products include:
Dizac ... 1809
Valium Injectable ... 2182
Valium Tablets ... 2183
Valrelease Capsules ... 2169

Doxepin Hydrochloride (Enhanced effects of tricyclic antidepressants). Products include:
Sinequan ... 2205
Zonalon Cream ... 1055

Droperidol (Enhanced effects of CNS depressants). Products include:
Inapsine Injection ... 1296

Enflurane (Enhanced effects of CNS depressants).
No products indexed under this heading.

Esmolol Hydrochloride (Effects of sympathomimetics increased). Products include:
Brevibloc Injection ... 1808

Estazolam (Enhanced effects of CNS depressants). Products include:
ProSom Tablets ... 449

Ethchlorvynol (Enhanced effects of CNS depressants). Products include:
Placidyl Capsules ... 448

Ethinamate (Enhanced effects of CNS depressants).
No products indexed under this heading.

Fentanyl (Enhanced effects of CNS depressants). Products include:
Duragesic Transdermal System ... 1288

Fentanyl Citrate (Enhanced effects of CNS depressants). Products include:
Sublimaze Injection ... 1307

Fluphenazine Decanoate (Enhanced effects of CNS depressants). Products include:
Prolixin Decanoate ... 509

Fluphenazine Enanthate (Enhanced effects of CNS depressants). Products include:
Prolixin Enanthate ... 509

Fluphenazine Hydrochloride (Enhanced effects of CNS depressants). Products include:
Prolixin ... 509

Flurazepam Hydrochloride (Enhanced effects of CNS depressants). Products include:
Dalmane Capsules ... 2173

Furazolidone (Increased effects of sympathomimetics; anticholinergic effects of antihistamines prolonged and intensified; concurrent use is contraindicated). Products include:
Furoxone ... 2046

Glutethimide (Enhanced effects of CNS depressants).
No products indexed under this heading.

Haloperidol (Enhanced effects of CNS depressants). Products include:
Haldol Injection, Tablets and Concentrate ... 1575

Haloperidol Decanoate (Enhanced effects of CNS depressants). Products include:
Haldol Decanoate ... 1577

Hydrocodone Bitartrate (Enhanced effects of CNS depressants). Products include:
Anexsia 5/500 Elixir ... 1781
Anexia Tablets ... 1782
Codiclear DH Syrup ... 791
Deconamine CX Cough and Cold Liquid and Tablets ... 1319
Duratuss HD Elixir ... 2565
Hycodan Tablets and Syrup ... 930
Hycomine Compound Tablets ... 932
Hycomine ... 931
Hycotuss Expectorant Syrup ... 933
Hydrocet Capsules ... 782
Lorcet 10/650 ... 1018
Lortab ... 2566
Tussend ... 1783
Tussend Expectorant ... 1785
Vicodin Tablets ... 1356
Vicodin ES Tablets ... 1357
Vicodin Tuss Expectorant ... 1358
Zydone Capsules ... 949

Hydrocodone Polistirex (Enhanced effects of CNS depressants). Products include:
Tussionex Pennkinetic Extended-Release Suspension ... 998

Hydroxyzine Hydrochloride (Enhanced effects of CNS depressants). Products include:
Atarax Tablets & Syrup ... 2185
Marax Tablets & DF Syrup ... 2200
Vistaril Intramuscular Solution ... 2216

Imipramine Hydrochloride (Enhanced effects of tricyclic antidepressants). Products include:
Tofranil Ampuls ... 854
Tofranil Tablets ... 856

Imipramine Pamoate (Enhanced effects of tricyclic antidepressants). Products include:
Tofranil-PM Capsules ... 857

Isocarboxazid (Increased effects of sympathomimetics; anticholinergic effects of antihistamines prolonged and intensified; concurrent use is contraindicated).
No products indexed under this heading.

Isoflurane (Enhanced effects of CNS depressants).
No products indexed under this heading.

Ketamine Hydrochloride (Enhanced effects of CNS depressants).
No products indexed under this heading.

Labetalol Hydrochloride (Effects of sympathomimetics increased). Products include:
Normodyne Injection ... 2377
Normodyne Tablets ... 2379
Trandate ... 1185

Levobunolol Hydrochloride (Effects of sympathomimetics increased). Products include:
Betagan ... ◉ 233

Levorphanol Tartrate (Enhanced effects of CNS depressants). Products include:
Levo-Dromoran ... 2129

Lorazepam (Enhanced effects of CNS depressants). Products include:
Ativan Injection ... 2698
Ativan Tablets ... 2700

Loxapine Hydrochloride (Enhanced effects of CNS depressants). Products include:
Loxitane ... 1378

Loxapine Succinate (Enhanced effects of CNS depressants). Products include:
Loxitane Capsules ... 1378

Maprotiline Hydrochloride (Enhanced effects of tricyclic antidepressants). Products include:
Ludiomil Tablets ... 843

Mecamylamine Hydrochloride (Reduced antihypertensive effects). Products include:
Inversine Tablets ... 1686

Meperidine Hydrochloride (Enhanced effects of CNS depressants). Products include:
Demerol ... 2308
Mepergan Injection ... 2753

Mephobarbital (Enhanced effects of CNS depressants). Products include:
Mebaral Tablets ... 2322

Meprobamate (Enhanced effects of CNS depressants). Products include:
Miltown Tablets ... 2672
PMB 200 and PMB 400 ... 2783

Mesoridazine Besylate (Enhanced effects of CNS depressants). Products include:
Serentil ... 684

(▣ Described in PDR For Nonprescription Drugs) (◉ Described in PDR For Ophthalmology)

909 **Interactions Index** **Roxanol**

Methadone Hydrochloride (Enhanced effects of CNS depressants). Products include:
- Methadone Hydrochloride Oral Concentrate 2233
- Methadone Hydrochloride Oral Solution & Tablets 2235

Methohexital Sodium (Enhanced effects of CNS depressants). Products include:
- Brevital Sodium Vials 1429

Methotrimeprazine (Enhanced effects of CNS depressants). Products include:
- Levoprome 1274

Methoxyflurane (Enhanced effects of CNS depressants).
- No products indexed under this heading.

Methyldopa (Reduced antihypertensive effects). Products include:
- Aldoclor Tablets 1598
- Aldomet Oral 1600
- Aldoril Tablets 1604

Methyldopate Hydrochloride (Reduced antihypertensive effects). Products include:
- Aldomet Ester HCl Injection 1602

Metipranolol Hydrochloride (Effects of sympathomimetics increased). Products include:
- OptiPranolol (Metipranolol 0.3%) Sterile Ophthalmic Solution .... ◉ 258

Metoprolol Succinate (Effects of sympathomimetics increased). Products include:
- Toprol-XL Tablets 565

Metoprolol Tartrate (Effects of sympathomimetics increased). Products include:
- Lopressor Ampuls 830
- Lopressor HCT Tablets 832
- Lopressor Tablets 830

Midazolam Hydrochloride (Enhanced effects of CNS depressants). Products include:
- Versed Injection 2170

Molindone Hydrochloride (Enhanced effects of CNS depressants). Products include:
- Moban Tablets and Concentrate 1048

Morphine Sulfate (Enhanced effects of CNS depressants). Products include:
- Astramorph/PF Injection, USP (Preservative-Free) 535
- Duramorph 962
- Infumorph 200 and Infumorph 500 Sterile Solutions 965
- MS Contin Tablets 1994
- MSIR 1997
- Oramorph SR (Morphine Sulfate Sustained Release Tablets) 2236
- RMS Suppositories 2657
- Roxanol 2243

Nadolol (Effects of sympathomimetics increased).
- No products indexed under this heading.

Nortriptyline Hydrochloride (Enhanced effects of tricyclic antidepressants). Products include:
- Pamelor 2280

Opium Alkaloids (Enhanced effects of CNS depressants).
- No products indexed under this heading.

Oxazepam (Enhanced effects of CNS depressants). Products include:
- Serax Capsules 2810
- Serax Tablets 2810

Oxycodone Hydrochloride (Enhanced effects of CNS depressants). Products include:
- Percocet Tablets 938
- Percodan Tablets 939
- Percodan-Demi Tablets 940
- Roxicodone Tablets, Oral Solution & Intensol (Oxycodone) 2244
- Tylox Capsules 1584

Penbutolol Sulfate (Effects of sympathomimetics increased). Products include:
- Levatol 2403

Pentobarbital Sodium (Enhanced effects of CNS depressants). Products include:
- Nembutal Sodium Capsules 436
- Nembutal Sodium Solution 438
- Nembutal Sodium Suppositories 440

Perphenazine (Enhanced effects of CNS depressants). Products include:
- Etrafon 2355
- Triavil Tablets 1757
- Trilafon 2389

Phenelzine Sulfate (Increased effects of sympathomimetics; anticholinergic effects of antihistamines prolonged and intensified; concurrent use is contraindicated). Products include:
- Nardil 1920

Phenobarbital (Enhanced effects of CNS depressants). Products include:
- Arco-Lase Plus Tablets 512
- Bellergal-S Tablets 2250
- Donnatal 2060
- Donnatal Extentabs 2061
- Donnatal Tablets 2060
- Phenobarbital Elixir and Tablets 1469
- Quadrinal Tablets 1350

Pindolol (Effects of sympathomimetics increased). Products include:
- Visken Tablets 2299

Prazepam (Enhanced effects of CNS depressants).
- No products indexed under this heading.

Prochlorperazine (Enhanced effects of CNS depressants). Products include:
- Compazine 2470

Promethazine Hydrochloride (Enhanced effects of CNS depressants). Products include:
- Mepergan Injection 2753
- Phenergan with Codeine 2777
- Phenergan with Dextromethorphan 2778
- Phenergan Injection 2773
- Phenergan Suppositories 2775
- Phenergan Syrup 2774
- Phenergan Tablets 2775
- Phenergan VC 2779
- Phenergan VC with Codeine 2781

Propofol (Enhanced effects of CNS depressants). Products include:
- Diprivan Injection 2833

Propoxyphene Hydrochloride (Enhanced effects of CNS depressants). Products include:
- Darvon 1435
- Wygesic Tablets 2827

Propoxyphene Napsylate (Enhanced effects of CNS depressants). Products include:
- Darvon-N/Darvocet-N 1433

Propranolol Hydrochloride (Effects of sympathomimetics increased). Products include:
- Inderal 2728
- Inderal LA Long Acting Capsules 2730
- Inderide Tablets 2732
- Inderide LA Long Acting Capsules 2734

Protriptyline Hydrochloride (Enhanced effects of tricyclic antidepressants). Products include:
- Vivactil Tablets 1774

Quazepam (Enhanced effects of CNS depressants). Products include:
- Doral Tablets 2664

Reserpine (Reduced antihypertensive effects). Products include:
- Diupres Tablets 1650
- Hydropres Tablets 1675
- Ser-Ap-Es Tablets 849

Risperidone (Enhanced effects of CNS depressants). Products include:
- Risperdal 1301

Secobarbital Sodium (Enhanced effects of CNS depressants). Products include:
- Seconal Sodium Pulvules 1474

Selegiline Hydrochloride (Increased effects of sympathomimetics; anticholinergic effects of antihistamines prolonged and intensified; concurrent use is contraindicated). Products include:
- Eldepryl Tablets 2550

Sotalol Hydrochloride (Effects of sympathomimetics increased). Products include:
- Betapace Tablets 641

Sufentanil Citrate (Enhanced effects of CNS depressants). Products include:
- Sufenta Injection 1309

Temazepam (Enhanced effects of CNS depressants). Products include:
- Restoril Capsules 2284

Thiamylal Sodium (Enhanced effects of CNS depressants).
- No products indexed under this heading.

Thioridazine Hydrochloride (Enhanced effects of CNS depressants). Products include:
- Mellaril 2269

Thiothixene (Enhanced effects of CNS depressants). Products include:
- Navane Capsules and Concentrate 2201
- Navane Intramuscular 2202

Timolol Maleate (Effects of sympathomimetics increased). Products include:
- Blocadren Tablets 1614
- Timolide Tablets 1748
- Timoptic in Ocudose 1753
- Timoptic Sterile Ophthalmic Solution 1751
- Timoptic-XE 1755

Tranylcypromine Sulfate (Increased effects of sympathomimetics; anticholinergic effects of antihistamines prolonged and intensified; concurrent use is contraindicated). Products include:
- Parnate Tablets 2503

Triazolam (Enhanced effects of CNS depressants). Products include:
- Halcion Tablets 2611

Trifluoperazine Hydrochloride (Enhanced effects of CNS depressants). Products include:
- Stelazine 2514

Trimipramine Maleate (Enhanced effects of tricyclic antidepressants). Products include:
- Surmontil Capsules 2811

Zolpidem Tartrate (Enhanced effects of CNS depressants). Products include:
- Ambien Tablets 2416

Food Interactions

Alcohol (Enhanced effects of alcohol).

RONDEC-DM SYRUP
(Carbinoxamine Maleate, Pseudoephedrine Hydrochloride, Dextromethorphan Hydrobromide) 954
See **Rondec-DM Oral Drops**

RONDEC-TR TABLET
(Carbinoxamine Maleate, Pseudoephedrine Hydrochloride) 953
See **Rondec Oral Drops**

ROWASA RECTAL SUPPOSITORIES, 500 MG
(Mesalamine) 2548
See **ROWASA Rectal Suspension Enema 4.0 grams/unit (60 mL)**

ROWASA RECTAL SUSPENSION ENEMA 4.0 GRAMS/UNIT (60 ML)
(Mesalamine) 2548
May interact with:

Sulfasalazine (Patients on concurrent oral products which liberate mesalamine should be carefully monitored with urinalysis). Products include:
- Azulfidine 1949

ROXANOL (MORPHINE SULFATE CONCENTRATED ORAL SOLUTION)
(Morphine Sulfate) 2243
May interact with tricyclic antidepressants, central nervous system depressants, urinary alkalizing agents, monoamine oxidase inhibitors, antihistamines, beta blockers, anticoagulants, and certain other agents. Compounds in these categories include:

Acebutolol Hydrochloride (Depressant effects of morphine may be enhanced). Products include:
- Sectral Capsules 2807

Acrivastine (Depressant effects of morphine may be enhanced). Products include:
- Semprex-D Capsules 463
- Semprex-D Capsules 1167

Alfentanil Hydrochloride (Respiratory depression, hypotension, and profound sedation or coma may result; depressant effects of morphine may be enhanced). Products include:
- Alfenta Injection 1286

Alprazolam (Respiratory depression, hypotension, and profound sedation or coma may result; depressant effects of morphine may be enhanced). Products include:
- Xanax Tablets 2649

Amitriptyline Hydrochloride (Respiratory depression, hypotension, and profound sedation or coma may result). Products include:
- Elavil 2838
- Endep Tablets 2174
- Etrafon 2355
- Limbitrol 2180
- Triavil Tablets 1757

Amoxapine (Respiratory depression, hypotension, and profound sedation or coma may result). Products include:
- Asendin Tablets 1369

Aprobarbital (Respiratory depression, hypotension, and profound sedation or coma may result; depressant effects of morphine may be enhanced).
- No products indexed under this heading.

Astemizole (Depressant effects of morphine may be enhanced). Products include:
- Hismanal Tablets 1293

Atenolol (Depressant effects of morphine may be enhanced). Products include:
- Tenoretic Tablets 2845
- Tenormin Tablets and I.V. Injection 2847

Azatadine Maleate (Depressant effects of morphine may be enhanced). Products include:
- Trinalin Repetabs Tablets 1330

Betaxolol Hydrochloride (Depressant effects of morphine may be enhanced). Products include:
- Betoptic Ophthalmic Solution 469
- Betoptic S Ophthalmic Suspension 471
- Kerlone Tablets 2436

IMPORTANT NOTE: Always consult each drug listing in the patient's regimen for possible interactions.

Roxanol

Interactions Index

Bisoprolol Fumarate (Depressant effects of morphine may be enhanced). Products include:

Zebeta Tablets 1413
Ziac 1415

Bromodiphenhydramine Hydrochloride (Depressant effects of morphine may be enhanced).

No products indexed under this heading.

Brompheniramine Maleate (Depressant effects of morphine may be enhanced). Products include:

Alka Seltzer Plus Sinus Medicine ..ᵃᴰ 707
Bromfed Capsules (Extended-Release) 1785
Bromfed Syrup ....ᵃᴰ 733
Bromfed Tablets 1785
Bromfed-DM Cough Syrup................... 1786
Bromfed-PD Capsules (Extended-Release) 1785
Dimetane-DC Cough Syrup 2059
Dimetane-DX Cough Syrup 2059
Dimetapp Elixir ....ᵃᴰ 773
Dimetapp Extentabs ....ᵃᴰ 774
Dimetapp Tablets/Liqui-Gels ....ᵃᴰ 775
Dimetapp Cold & Allergy Chewable Tablets ....ᵃᴰ 773
Dimetapp DM Elixir ....ᵃᴰ 774
Vicks DayQuil Allergy Relief 12-Hour Extended Release Tablets..ᵃᴰ 760
Vicks DayQuil Allergy Relief 4-Hour Tablets ....ᵃᴰ 760

Buprenorphine (Respiratory depression, hypotension, and profound sedation or coma may result; depressant effects of morphine may be enhanced). Products include:

Buprenex Injectable 2006

Buspirone Hydrochloride (Respiratory depression, hypotension, and profound sedation or coma may result; depressant effects of morphine may be enhanced). Products include:

BuSpar 737

Butabarbital (Respiratory depression, hypotension, and profound sedation or coma may result; depressant effects of morphine may be enhanced).

No products indexed under this heading.

Butalbital (Respiratory depression, hypotension, and profound sedation or coma may result; depressant effects of morphine may be enhanced). Products include:

Esgic-plus Tablets 1013
Fioricet Tablets 2258
Fioricet with Codeine Capsules 2260
Fiorinal Capsules 2261
Fiorinal with Codeine Capsules 2262
Fiorinal Tablets 2261
Phrenilin 785
Sedapap Tablets 50 mg/650 mg .. 1543

Carteolol Hydrochloride (Depressant effects of morphine may be enhanced). Products include:

Cartrol Tablets 410
Ocupress Ophthalmic Solution, 1% Sterile.. ◎ 309

Chloral Hydrate (Depressant effects of morphine may be enhanced).

No products indexed under this heading.

Chlordiazepoxide (Respiratory depression, hypotension, and profound sedation or coma may result; depressant effects of morphine may be enhanced). Products include:

Libritabs Tablets 2177
Limbitrol 2180

Chlordiazepoxide Hydrochloride (Respiratory depression, hypotension, and profound sedation or coma may result; depressant effects of morphine may be enhanced). Products include:

Librax Capsules 2176
Librium Capsules 2178

Librium Injectable 2179

Chlorpheniramine Maleate (Depressant effects of morphine may be enhanced). Products include:

Alka-Seltzer Plus Cold Medicine ....ᵃᴰ 705
Alka-Seltzer Plus Cold Medicine Liqui-Gels ....ᵃᴰ 706
Alka-Seltzer Plus Cold & Cough Medicine ....ᵃᴰ 708
Alka-Seltzer Plus Cold & Cough Medicine Liqui-Gels ....ᵃᴰ 705
Allerest Children's Chewable Tablets ....ᵃᴰ 627
Allerest Headache Strength Tablets ....ᵃᴰ 627
Allerest Maximum Strength Tablets ....ᵃᴰ 627
Allerest Sinus Pain Formula ....ᵃᴰ 627
Allerest 12 Hour Caplets ....ᵃᴰ 627
Ana-Kit Anaphylaxis Emergency Treatment Kit 617
Atrohist Pediatric Capsules 453
Atrohist Plus Tablets 454
BC Cold Powder Multi-Symptom Formula (Cold-Sinus-Allergy) ......ᵃᴰ 609
Cerose DM ....ᵃᴰ 878
Cheracol Plus Head Cold/Cough Formula ....ᵃᴰ 769
Children's Vicks DayQuil Allergy Relief ....ᵃᴰ 757
Children's Vicks NyQuil Cold/Cough Relief ....ᵃᴰ 758
Chlor-Trimeton Allergy Decongestant Tablets ....ᵃᴰ 799
Chlor-Trimeton Allergy Tablets ......ᵃᴰ 798
Comhist 2038
Comtrex Multi-Symptom Cold Reliever Tablets/Caplets/Liqui-Gels/Liquid ....ᵃᴰ 615
Allergy-Sinus Comtrex Multi-Symptom Allergy-Sinus Formula Tablets ....ᵃᴰ 617
Contac Continuous Action Nasal Decongestant/Antihistamine 12 Hour Capsules ....ᵃᴰ 813
Contac Maximum Strength Continuous Action Decongestant/Antihistamine 12 Hour Caplets..ᵃᴰ 813
Contac Severe Cold and Flu Formula Caplets ....ᵃᴰ 814
Coricidin 'D' Decongestant Tablets ....ᵃᴰ 800
Coricidin Tablets ....ᵃᴰ 800
D.A. Chewable Tablets 951
Deconamine 1320
Dura-Tap/PD Capsules 2867
Dura-Vent/DA Tablets 953
Extendryl 1005
Fedahist Gyrocaps 2401
Fedahist Timecaps 2401
Hycomine Compound Tablets 932
Isoclor Timesule Capsules ....ᵃᴰ 637
Kronofed-A 977
Nolamine Timed-Release Tablets 785
Novahistine DH 2462
Novahistine Elixir ....ᵃᴰ 823
Ornade Spansule Capsules 2502
PediaCare Cold Allergy Chewable Tablets ....ᵃᴰ 677
PediaCare Cough-Cold Chewable Tablets 1553
PediaCare Cough-Cold Liquid 1553
PediaCare NightRest Cough-Cold Liquid 1553
Pediatric Vicks 44m Cough & Cold Relief ....ᵃᴰ 764
Pyrroxate Caplets ....ᵃᴰ 772
Ryna ....ᵃᴰ 841
Sinarest Tablets ....ᵃᴰ 648
Sinarest Extra Strength Tablets......ᵃᴰ 648
Sine-Off Sinus Medicine ....ᵃᴰ 825
Singlet Tablets ....ᵃᴰ 825
Sinulin Tablets 787
Sinutab Sinus Allergy Medication, Maximum Strength Tablets and Caplets ....ᵃᴰ 860
Sudafed Plus Liquid ....ᵃᴰ 862
Sudafed Plus Tablets ....ᵃᴰ 863
Teldrin 12 Hour Antihistamine/Nasal Decongestant Allergy Relief Capsules ....ᵃᴰ 826
TheraFlu ....ᵃᴰ 787
TheraFlu Maximum Strength Nighttime Flu, Cold & Cough Medicine ....ᵃᴰ 788
Triaminic Allergy Tablets ....ᵃᴰ 789
Triaminic Cold Tablets ....ᵃᴰ 790
Triaminic Nite Light ....ᵃᴰ 791
Triaminic Syrup ....ᵃᴰ 792
Triaminic-12 Tablets ....ᵃᴰ 792
Triaminicin Tablets ....ᵃᴰ 793

Triaminicol Multi-Symptom Cold Tablets ....ᵃᴰ 793
Triaminicol Multi-Symptom Relief ᵃᴰ 794
Tussend 1783
Children's TYLENOL Cold Multi-Symptom Liquid Formula and Chewable Tablets 1561
Children's TYLENOL Cold Plus Cough Multi Symptom Tablets and Liquid ....ᵃᴰ 681
TYLENOL Maximum Strength Allergy Sinus Medication Gelcaps and Caplets 1563
TYLENOL Cold Multi-Symptom Formula Medication Tablets and Caplets 1561
TYLENOL Cold Multi-Symptom Hot Medication Liquid Packets 1557
Vicks 44 LiquiCaps Cough, Cold & Flu Relief ....ᵃᴰ 755
Vicks 44M Cough, Cold & Flu Relief ....ᵃᴰ 756

Chlorpheniramine Polistirex (Depressant effects of morphine may be enhanced). Products include:

Tussionex Pennkinetic Extended-Release Suspension 998

Chlorpheniramine Tannate (Depressant effects of morphine may be enhanced). Products include:

Atrohist Pediatric Suspension 454
Ricobid Tablets and Pediatric Suspension 2038
Rynatan 2673
Rynatuss 2673

Chlorpromazine (Respiratory depression, hypotension, and profound sedation or coma may result; depressant effects of morphine may be enhanced; analgesic effect of morphine potentiated). Products include:

Thorazine Suppositories 2523

Chlorprothixene (Respiratory depression, hypotension, and profound sedation or coma may result; depressant effects of morphine may be enhanced).

No products indexed under this heading.

Chlorprothixene Hydrochloride (Respiratory depression, hypotension, and profound sedation or coma may result; depressant effects of morphine may be enhanced).

No products indexed under this heading.

Clemastine Fumarate (Depressant effects of morphine may be enhanced). Products include:

Tavist Syrup 2297
Tavist Tablets 2298
Tavist-1 12 Hour Relief Tablets ....ᵃᴰ 787
Tavist-D 12 Hour Relief Tablets ....ᵃᴰ 787

Clomipramine Hydrochloride (Respiratory depression, hypotension, and profound sedation or coma may result). Products include:

Anafranil Capsules 803

Clorazepate Dipotassium (Respiratory depression, hypotension, and profound sedation or coma may result; depressant effects of morphine may be enhanced). Products include:

Tranxene 451

Clozapine (Respiratory depression, hypotension, and profound sedation or coma may result; depressant effects of morphine may be enhanced). Products include:

Clozaril Tablets 2252

Codeine Phosphate (Respiratory depression, hypotension, and profound sedation or coma may result; depressant effects of morphine may be enhanced). Products include:

Actifed with Codeine Cough Syrup.. 1067
Brontex 1981
Deconsal C Expectorant Syrup 456
Deconsal Pediatric Syrup 457
Dimetane-DC Cough Syrup 2059
Empirin with Codeine Tablets 1093

Fioricet with Codeine Capsules 2260
Fiorinal with Codeine Capsules 2262
Isoclor Expectorant 990
Novahistine DH 2462
Novahistine Expectorant 2463
Nucofed 2051
Phenergan with Codeine 2777
Phenergan VC with Codeine 2781
Robitussin A-C Syrup 2073
Robitussin-DAC Syrup 2074
Ryna ....ᵃᴰ 841
Soma Compound w/Codeine Tablets 2676
Tussi-Organidin NR Liquid and S NR Liquid 2677
Tylenol with Codeine 1583

Cyproheptadine Hydrochloride (Depressant effects of morphine may be enhanced). Products include:

Periactin 1724

Dalteparin Sodium (Anticoagulant activity may be increased). Products include:

Fragmin 1954

Desflurane (Respiratory depression, hypotension, and profound sedation or coma may result; depressant effects of morphine may be enhanced). Products include:

Suprane 1813

Desipramine Hydrochloride (Respiratory depression, hypotension, and profound sedation or coma may result). Products include:

Norpramin Tablets 1526

Dexchlorpheniramine Maleate (Depressant effects of morphine may be enhanced).

No products indexed under this heading.

Dezocine (Respiratory depression, hypotension, and profound sedation or coma may result; depressant effects of morphine may be enhanced). Products include:

Dalgan Injection 538

Diazepam (Respiratory depression, hypotension, and profound sedation or coma may result; depressant effects of morphine may be enhanced). Products include:

Dizac 1809
Valium Injectable 2182
Valium Tablets 2183
Valrelease Capsules 2169

Dicumarol (Anticoagulant activity may be increased).

No products indexed under this heading.

Diphenhydramine Citrate (Depressant effects of morphine may be enhanced). Products include:

Excedrin P.M. Analgesic/Sleeping Aid Tablets, Caplets, Liquigels 733

Diphenhydramine Hydrochloride (Depressant effects of morphine may be enhanced). Products include:

Actifed Allergy Daytime/Nighttime Caplets ....ᵃᴰ 844
Actifed Sinus Daytime/Nighttime Tablets and Caplets ....ᵃᴰ 846
Arthritis Foundation NightTime Caplets ....ᵃᴰ 674
Extra Strength Bayer PM Aspirin ..ᵃᴰ 713
Bayer Select Night Time Pain Relief Formula ....ᵃᴰ 716
Benadryl Allergy Decongestant Liquid Medication ....ᵃᴰ 848
Benadryl Allergy Decongestant Tablets ....ᵃᴰ 848
Benadryl Allergy Liquid Medication ....ᵃᴰ 849
Benadryl Allergy ....ᵃᴰ 848
Benadryl Allergy Sinus Headache Formula Caplets ....ᵃᴰ 849
Benadryl Capsules 1898
Benadryl Dye-Free Allergy Liquigel Softgels ....ᵃᴰ 850
Benadryl Dye-Free Allergy Liquid Medication ....ᵃᴰ 850
Benadryl Itch Relief Cream, Children's Formula and Maximum Strength 2% ....ᵃᴰ 851

(ᵃᴰ Described in PDR For Nonprescription Drugs) (◎ Described in PDR For Ophthalmology)

Interactions Index Roxanol

Benadryl Itch Relief Spray, Children's Formula and Maximum Strength 2% .... ◆D 851

Benadryl Itch Relief Stick Maximum Strength 2% .... ◆D 850

Benadryl Itch Stopping Gel, Children's Formula and Maximum Strength 2% .... ◆D 851

Benadryl Kapseals 1898

Benadryl Injection 1898

Contac Day & Night Cold/Flu Night Caplets .... ◆D 812

Contac Night Allergy/Sinus Caplets .... ◆D 812

Extra Strength Doan's P.M. .... ◆D 633

Legatrin PM .... ◆D 651

Miles Nervine Nighttime Sleep-Aid ◆D 723

Nytol QuickCaps Caplets .... ◆D 610

Sleepinal Night-time Sleep Aid Capsules and Softgels .... ◆D 834

TYLENOL Maximum Strength Allergy Sinus NightTime Medication Caplets 1555

TYLENOL Flu NightTime, Maximum Strength, Gelcaps 1566

TYLENOL Maximum Strength Flu NightTime Hot Medication Packets 1562

TYLENOL PM, Extra Strength Pain Reliever/Sleep Aid Caplets, Geltabs, Gelcaps 1560

TYLENOL Severe Allergy Medication Caplets 1564

Maximum Strength Unisom Sleepgels 1934

Unisom With Pain Relief-Nighttime Sleep Aid and Pain Reliever............. 1934

Diphenylpyraline Hydrochloride (Depressant effects of morphine may be enhanced).

No products indexed under this heading.

Doxepin Hydrochloride (Respiratory depression, hypotension, and profound sedation or coma may result). Products include:

Sinequan 2205

Zonalon Cream 1055

Droperidol (Respiratory depression, hypotension, and profound sedation or coma may result; depressant effects of morphine may be enhanced). Products include:

Inapsine Injection................................... 1296

Enflurane (Respiratory depression, hypotension, and profound sedation or coma may result; depressant effects of morphine may be enhanced).

No products indexed under this heading.

Enoxaparin (Anticoagulant activity may be increased). Products include:

Lovenox Injection 2020

Esmolol Hydrochloride (Depressant effects of morphine may be enhanced). Products include:

Brevibloc Injection.................................. 1808

Estazolam (Respiratory depression, hypotension, and profound sedation or coma may result; depressant effects of morphine may be enhanced). Products include:

ProSom Tablets 449

Ethchlorvynol (Respiratory depression, hypotension, and profound sedation or coma may result; depressant effects of morphine may be enhanced). Products include:

Placidyl Capsules................................... 448

Ethinamate (Respiratory depression, hypotension, and profound sedation or coma may result; depressant effects of morphine may be enhanced).

No products indexed under this heading.

Fentanyl (Respiratory depression, hypotension, and profound sedation or coma may result; depressant effects of morphine may be enhanced). Products include:

Duragesic Transdermal System........ 1288

Fentanyl Citrate (Respiratory depression, hypotension, and profound sedation or coma may result; depressant effects of morphine may be enhanced). Products include:

Sublimaze Injection................................ 1307

Fluphenazine Decanoate (Respiratory depression, hypotension, and profound sedation or coma may result; depressant effects of morphine may be enhanced). Products include:

Prolixin Decanoate 509

Fluphenazine Enanthate (Respiratory depression, hypotension, and profound sedation or coma may result; depressant effects of morphine may be enhanced). Products include:

Prolixin Enanthate 509

Fluphenazine Hydrochloride (Respiratory depression, hypotension, and profound sedation or coma may result; depressant effects of morphine may be enhanced). Products include:

Prolixin 509

Flurazepam Hydrochloride (Respiratory depression, hypotension, and profound sedation or coma may result; depressant effects of morphine may be enhanced). Products include:

Dalmane Capsules.................................. 2173

Furazolidone (Depressant effects of morphine may be enhanced). Products include:

Furoxone 2046

Glutethimide (Respiratory depression, hypotension, and profound sedation or coma may result; depressant effects of morphine may be enhanced).

No products indexed under this heading.

Haloperidol (Respiratory depression, hypotension, and profound sedation or coma may result; depressant effects of morphine may be enhanced). Products include:

Haldol Injection, Tablets and Concentrate 1575

Haloperidol Decanoate (Respiratory depression, hypotension, and profound sedation or coma may result; depressant effects of morphine may be enhanced). Products include:

Haldol Decanoate.................................... 1577

Heparin Calcium (Anticoagulant activity may be increased).

No products indexed under this heading.

Heparin Sodium (Anticoagulant activity may be increased). Products include:

Heparin Lock Flush Solution 2725

Heparin Sodium Injection..................... 2726

Heparin Sodium Injection, USP, Sterile Solution 2615

Heparin Sodium Vials............................ 1441

Hydrocodone Bitartrate (Respiratory depression, hypotension, and profound sedation or coma may result; depressant effects of morphine may be enhanced). Products include:

Anexsia 5/500 Elixir 1781

Anexia Tablets.. 1782

Codiclear DH Syrup 791

Deconamine CX Cough and Cold Liquid and Tablets.................................. 1319

Duratuss HD Elixir................................... 2565

Hycodan Tablets and Syrup 930

Hycomine Compound Tablets 932

Hycomine 931

Hycotuss Expectorant Syrup 933

Hydrocet Capsules 782

Lorcet 10/650... 1018

Lortab 2566

Tussend 1783

Tussend Expectorant 1785

Vicodin Tablets... 1356

Vicodin ES Tablets 1357

Vicodin Tuss Expectorant 1358

Zydone Capsules 949

Hydrocodone Polistirex (Respiratory depression, hypotension, and profound sedation or coma may result; depressant effects of morphine may be enhanced). Products include:

Tussionex Pennkinetic Extended-Release Suspension 998

Hydroxyzine Hydrochloride (Respiratory depression, hypotension, and profound sedation or coma may result; depressant effects of morphine may be enhanced). Products include:

Atarax Tablets & Syrup......................... 2185

Marax Tablets & DF Syrup.................... 2200

Vistaril Intramuscular Solution........... 2216

Imipramine Hydrochloride (Respiratory depression, hypotension, and profound sedation or coma may result). Products include:

Tofranil Ampuls 854

Tofranil Tablets 856

Imipramine Pamoate (Respiratory depression, hypotension, and profound sedation or coma may result). Products include:

Tofranil-PM Capsules............................. 857

Isocarboxazid (Depressant effects of morphine may be enhanced).

No products indexed under this heading.

Isoflurane (Respiratory depression, hypotension, and profound sedation or coma may result; depressant effects of morphine may be enhanced).

No products indexed under this heading.

Ketamine Hydrochloride (Respiratory depression, hypotension, and profound sedation or coma may result; depressant effects of morphine may be enhanced).

No products indexed under this heading.

Labetalol Hydrochloride (Depressant effects of morphine may be enhanced). Products include:

Normodyne Injection 2377

Normodyne Tablets 2379

Trandate 1185

Levobunolol Hydrochloride (Depressant effects of morphine may be enhanced). Products include:

Betagan .... ◉ 233

Levomethadyl Acetate Hydrochloride (Respiratory depression, hypotension, and profound sedation or coma may result; depressant effects of morphine may be enhanced). Products include:

Orlamm 2239

Levorphanol Tartrate (Respiratory depression, hypotension, and profound sedation or coma may result; depressant effects of morphine may be enhanced). Products include:

Levo-Dromoran 2129

Loratadine (Depressant effects of morphine may be enhanced). Products include:

Claritin 2349

Claritin-D 2350

Lorazepam (Respiratory depression, hypotension, and profound sedation or coma may result; depressant effects of morphine may be enhanced). Products include:

Ativan Injection... 2698

Ativan Tablets 2700

Loxapine Hydrochloride (Respiratory depression, hypotension, and profound sedation or coma may result; depressant effects of morphine may be enhanced). Products include:

Loxitane 1378

Loxapine Succinate (Respiratory depression, hypotension, and profound sedation or coma may result; depressant effects of morphine may be enhanced). Products include:

Loxitane Capsules................................... 1378

Maprotiline Hydrochloride (Respiratory depression, hypotension, and profound sedation or coma may result). Products include:

Ludiomil Tablets....................................... 843

Meperidine Hydrochloride (Respiratory depression, hypotension, and profound sedation or coma may result; depressant effects of morphine may be enhanced). Products include:

Demerol 2308

Mepergan Injection 2753

Mephobarbital (Respiratory depression, hypotension, and profound sedation or coma may result; depressant effects of morphine may be enhanced). Products include:

Mebaral Tablets 2322

Meprobamate (Respiratory depression, hypotension, and profound sedation or coma may result; depressant effects of morphine may be enhanced). Products include:

Miltown Tablets 2672

PMB 200 and PMB 400 2783

Mesoridazine Besylate (Respiratory depression, hypotension, and profound sedation or coma may result; depressant effects of morphine may be enhanced). Products include:

Serentil 684

Methadone Hydrochloride (Respiratory depression, hypotension, and profound sedation or coma may result; depressant effects of morphine may be enhanced). Products include:

Methadone Hydrochloride Oral Concentrate 2233

Methadone Hydrochloride Oral Solution & Tablets................................. 2235

Methdilazine Hydrochloride (Depressant effects of morphine may be enhanced).

No products indexed under this heading.

Methocarbamol (Analgesic effect of morphine potentiated). Products include:

Robaxin Injectable................................... 2070

Robaxin Tablets 2071

Robaxisal Tablets..................................... 2071

Methohexital Sodium (Respiratory depression, hypotension, and profound sedation or coma may result; depressant effects of morphine may be enhanced). Products include:

Brevital Sodium Vials 1429

Methotrimeprazine (Respiratory depression, hypotension, and profound sedation or coma may result; depressant effects of morphine may be enhanced). Products include:

Levoprome 1274

Methoxyflurane (Respiratory depression, hypotension, and profound sedation or coma may result; depressant effects of morphine may be enhanced).

No products indexed under this heading.

IMPORTANT NOTE: Always consult each drug listing in the patient's regimen for possible interactions.

Roxanol | Interactions Index | 912

Metipranolol Hydrochloride (Depressant effects of morphine may be enhanced). Products include:
- OptiPranolol (Metipranolol 0.3%) Sterile Ophthalmic Solution .... ◉ 258

Metoprolol Succinate (Depressant effects of morphine may be enhanced). Products include:
- Toprol-XL Tablets 565

Metoprolol Tartrate (Depressant effects of morphine may be enhanced). Products include:
- Lopressor Ampuls 830
- Lopressor HCT Tablets 832
- Lopressor Tablets 830

Midazolam Hydrochloride (Respiratory depression, hypotension, and profound sedation or coma may result; depressant effects of morphine may be enhanced). Products include:
- Versed Injection 2170

Molindone Hydrochloride (Respiratory depression, hypotension, and profound sedation or coma may result; depressant effects of morphine may be enhanced). Products include:
- Moban Tablets and Concentrate 1048

Nadolol (Depressant effects of morphine may be enhanced).
- No products indexed under this heading.

Nortriptyline Hydrochloride (Respiratory depression, hypotension, and profound sedation or coma may result). Products include:
- Pamelor 2280

Opium Alkaloids (Respiratory depression hypotension, and profound sedation or coma may result; depressant effects of morphine may be enhanced).
- No products indexed under this heading.

Oxazepam (Respiratory depression, hypotension, and profound sedation or coma may result; depressant effects of morphine may be enhanced). Products include:
- Serax Capsules 2810
- Serax Tablets 2810

Oxycodone Hydrochloride (Respiratory depression, hypotension, and profound sedation or coma may result; depressant effects of morphine may be enhanced). Products include:
- Percocet Tablets 938
- Percodan Tablets 939
- Percodan-Demi Tablets 940
- Roxicodone Tablets, Oral Solution & Intensol (Oxycodone) 2244
- Tylox Capsules 1584

Penbutolol Sulfate (Depressant effects of morphine may be enhanced). Products include:
- Levatol 2403

Pentobarbital Sodium (Respiratory depression, hypotension, and profound sedation or coma may result; depressant effects of morphine sulfate may be enhanced). Products include:
- Nembutal Sodium Capsules 436
- Nembutal Sodium Solution 438
- Nembutal Sodium Suppositories 440

Perphenazine (Respiratory depression, hypotension, and profound sedation or coma may result; depressant effects of morphine may be enhanced). Products include:
- Etrafon 2355
- Triavil Tablets 1757
- Trilafon 2389

Phenelzine Sulfate (Depressant effects of morphine may be enhanced). Products include:
- Nardil 1920

Phenobarbital (Respiratory depression, hypotension, and profound sedation or coma may result; depressant effects of morphine may be enhanced). Products include:
- Arco-Lase Plus Tablets 512
- Bellergal-S Tablets 2250
- Donnatal 2060
- Donnatal Extentabs 2061
- Donnatal Tablets 2060
- Phenobarbital Elixir and Tablets 1469
- Quadrinal Tablets 1350

Pindolol (Depressant effects of morphine may be enhanced). Products include:
- Visken Tablets 2299

Potassium Acid Phosphate (Effects of morphine may be antagonized). Products include:
- K-Phos Original Formula 'Sodium Free' Tablets 639

Potassium Citrate (Effects of morphine may be potentiated). Products include:
- Polycitra Syrup 578
- Polycitra-K Crystals 579
- Polycitra-K Oral Solution 579
- Polycitra-LC 578

Prazepam (Respiratory depression, hypotension, and profound sedation or coma may result; depressant effects of morphine may be enhanced).
- No products indexed under this heading.

Procarbazine Hydrochloride (Depressant effects of morphine may be enhanced). Products include:
- Matulane Capsules 2131

Prochlorperazine (Respiratory depression, hypotension, and profound sedation or coma may result; depressant effects of morphine may be enhanced; analgesic effect of morphine potentiated). Products include:
- Compazine 2470

Promethazine Hydrochloride (Respiratory depression, hypotension, and profound sedation or coma may result; depressant effects of morphine may be enhanced). Products include:
- Mepergan Injection 2753
- Phenergan with Codeine 2777
- Phenergan with Dextromethorphan 2778
- Phenergan Injection 2773
- Phenergan Suppositories 2775
- Phenergan Syrup 2774
- Phenergan Tablets 2775
- Phenergan VC 2779
- Phenergan VC with Codeine 2781

Propofol (Respiratory depression, hypotension, and profound sedation or coma may result; depressant effects of morphine may be enhanced). Products include:
- Diprivan Injection 2833

Propoxyphene Hydrochloride (Respiratory depression, hypotension, and profound sedation or coma may result; depressant effects of morphine may be enhanced). Products include:
- Darvon 1435
- Wygesic Tablets 2827

Propoxyphene Napsylate (Respiratory depression, hypotension, and profound sedation or coma may result; depressant effects of morphine may be enhanced). Products include:
- Darvon-N/Darvocet-N 1433

Propranolol Hydrochloride (Depressant effects of morphine may be enhanced). Products include:
- Inderal 2728
- Inderal LA Long Acting Capsules 2730
- Inderide Tablets 2732
- Inderide LA Long Acting Capsules 2734

Protriptyline Hydrochloride (Respiratory depression, hypotension, and profound sedation or coma may result). Products include:
- Vivactil Tablets 1774

Pyrilamine Maleate (Depressant effects of morphine may be enhanced). Products include:
- 4-Way Fast Acting Nasal Spray (regular & mentholated) .... ▣ 621
- Maximum Strength Multi-Symptom Formula Midol .... ▣ 722
- PMS Multi-Symptom Formula Midol .... ▣ 723

Pyrilamine Tannate (Depressant effects of morphine may be enhanced). Products include:
- Atrohist Pediatric Suspension 454
- Rynatan 2673

Quazepam (Respiratory depression, hypotension, and profound sedation or coma may result; depressant effects of morphine may be enhanced). Products include:
- Doral Tablets 2664

Risperidone (Respiratory depression, hypotension, and profound sedation or coma may result; depressant effects of morphine may be enhanced). Products include:
- Risperdal 1301

Secobarbital Sodium (Respiratory depression, hypotension, and profound sedation or coma may result; depressant effects of morphine may be enhanced). Products include:
- Seconal Sodium Pulvules 1474

Selegiline Hydrochloride (Depressant effects of morphine may be enhanced). Products include:
- Eldepryl Tablets 2550

Sodium Acid Phosphate (Effects of morphine may be antagonized). Products include:
- Uroqid-Acid No. 2 Tablets 640

Sodium Citrate (Effects of morphine may be potentiated). Products include:
- Bicitra 578
- Citrocarbonate Antacid .... ▣ 770
- Polycitra 578
- Salix SST Lozenges Saliva Stimulant .... ▣ 797

Sotalol Hydrochloride (Depressant effects of morphine may be enhanced). Products include:
- Betapace Tablets 641

Sufentanil Citrate (Respiratory depression, hypotension, and profound sedation or coma may result; depressant effects of morphine may be enhanced). Products include:
- Sufenta Injection 1309

Temazepam (Respiratory depression, hypotension, and profound sedation or coma may result; depressant effects of morphine may be enhanced). Products include:
- Restoril Capsules 2284

Terfenadine (Depressant effects of morphine may be enhanced). Products include:
- Seldane Tablets 1536
- Seldane-D Extended-Release Tablets 1538

Thiamylal Sodium (Respiratory depression, hypotension, and profound sedation or coma may result; depressant effects of morphine may be enhanced).
- No products indexed under this heading.

Thioridazine Hydrochloride (Respiratory depression, hypotension, and profound sedation or coma may result; depressant effects of morphine may be enhanced). Products include:
- Mellaril 2269

Thiothixene (Respiratory depression, hypotension, and profoundsedation or coma may result; depressant effects of morphine may be enhanced). Products include:
- Navane Capsules and Concentrate 2201
- Navane Intramuscular 2202

Timolol Hemihydrate (Depressant effects of morphine may be enhanced). Products include:
- Betimol 0.25%, 0.5% .... ◉ 261

Timolol Maleate (Depressant effects of morphine may be enhanced). Products include:
- Blocadren Tablets 1614
- Timolide Tablets 1748
- Timoptic in Ocudose 1753
- Timoptic Sterile Ophthalmic Solution 1751
- Timoptic-XE 1755

Tranylcypromine Sulfate (Depressant effects of morphine may be enhanced). Products include:
- Parnate Tablets 2503

Triazolam (Respiratory depression, hypotension, and profound sedation or coma may result; depressant effects of morphine may be enhanced). Products include:
- Halcion Tablets 2611

Trifluoperazine Hydrochloride (Respiratory depression, hypotension, and profound sedation or coma may result; depressant effects of morphine may be enhanced). Products include:
- Stelazine 2514

Trimeprazine Tartrate (Depressant effects of morphine may be enhanced). Products include:
- Temaril Tablets, Syrup and Spansule Extended-Release Capsules 483

Trimipramine Maleate (Respiratory depression, hypotension, and profound sedation or coma may result). Products include:
- Surmontil Capsules 2811

Tripelennamine Hydrochloride (Depressant effects of morphine may be enhanced). Products include:
- PBZ Tablets 845
- PBZ-SR Tablets 844

Triprolidine Hydrochloride (Depressant effects of morphine may be enhanced). Products include:
- Actifed Plus Caplets .... ▣ 845
- Actifed Plus Tablets .... ▣ 845
- Actifed with Codeine Cough Syrup 1067
- Actifed Syrup .... ▣ 846
- Actifed Tablets .... ▣ 844

Warfarin Sodium (Anticoagulant activity may be increased). Products include:
- Coumadin 926

Zolpidem Tartrate (Respiratory depression, hypotension, and profound sedation or coma may result; depressant effects of morphine may be enhanced). Products include:
- Ambien Tablets 2416

Food Interactions

Alcohol (Respiratory depression, hypotension, and profound sedation or coma may result; depressant effects of morphine may be enhanced).

(▣ Described in PDR For Nonprescription Drugs) (◉ Described in PDR For Ophthalmology)

913 **Interactions Index** **Roxicodone**

ROXANOL 100 (MORPHINE SULFATE CONCENTRATED ORAL SOLUTION)
(Morphine Sulfate) 2243
See **Roxanol (Morphine Sulfate Concentrated Oral Solution)**

ROXICODONE TABLETS, ORAL SOLUTION & INTENSOL (OXYCODONE)
(Oxycodone Hydrochloride) 2244
May interact with central nervous system depressants and certain other agents. Compounds in these categories include:

Alfentanil Hydrochloride (Possible additive CNS depression). Products include:
Alfenta Injection 1286

Alprazolam (Possible additive CNS depression). Products include:
Xanax Tablets 2649

Aprobarbital (Possible additive CNS depression).
No products indexed under this heading.

Buprenorphine (Possible additive CNS depression). Products include:
Buprenex Injectable 2006

Buspirone Hydrochloride (Possible additive CNS depression). Products include:
BuSpar 737

Butabarbital (Possible additive CNS depression).
No products indexed under this heading.

Butalbital (Possible additive CNS depression). Products include:
Esgic-plus Tablets 1013
Fioricet Tablets 2258
Fioricet with Codeine Capsules 2260
Fiorinal Capsules 2261
Fiorinal with Codeine Capsules 2262
Fiorinal Tablets 2261
Phrenilin 785
Sedapap Tablets 50 mg/650 mg 1543

Chlordiazepoxide (Possible additive CNS depression). Products include:
Libritabs Tablets 2177
Limbitrol 2180

Chlordiazepoxide Hydrochloride (Possible additive CNS depression). Products include:
Librax Capsules 2176
Librium Capsules 2178
Librium Injectable 2179

Chlorpromazine (Possible additive CNS depression). Products include:
Thorazine Suppositories 2523

Chlorprothixene (Possible additive CNS depression).
No products indexed under this heading.

Chlorprothixene Hydrochloride (Possible additive CNS depression).
No products indexed under this heading.

Chlorprothixene Lactate (Possible additive CNS depression).
No products indexed under this heading.

Clorazepate Dipotassium (Possible additive CNS depression). Products include:
Tranxene 451

Clozapine (Possible additive CNS depression). Products include:
Clozaril Tablets 2252

Codeine Phosphate (Possible additive CNS depression). Products include:
Actifed with Codeine Cough Syrup 1067
Brontex 1981
Deconsal C Expectorant Syrup 456
Deconsal Pediatric Syrup 457
Dimetane-DC Cough Syrup 2059
Empirin with Codeine Tablets 1093
Fioricet with Codeine Capsules 2260
Fiorinal with Codeine Capsules 2262
Isoclor Expectorant 990
Novahistine DH 2462
Novahistine Expectorant 2463
Nucofed 2051
Phenergan with Codeine 2777
Phenergan VC with Codeine 2781
Robitussin A-C Syrup 2073
Robitussin-DAC Syrup 2074
Ryna 841
Soma Compound w/Codeine Tablets 2676
Tussi-Organidin NR Liquid and S NR Liquid 2677
Tylenol with Codeine 1583

Desflurane (Possible additive CNS depression). Products include:
Suprane 1813

Dezocine (Possible additive CNS depression). Products include:
Dalgan Injection 538

Diazepam (Possible additive CNS depression). Products include:
Dizac 1809
Valium Injectable 2182
Valium Tablets 2183
Valrelease Capsules 2169

Droperidol (Possible additive CNS depression). Products include:
Inapsine Injection 1296

Enflurane (Possible additive CNS depression).
No products indexed under this heading.

Estazolam (Possible additive CNS depression). Products include:
ProSom Tablets 449

Ethchlorvynol (Possible additive CNS depression). Products include:
Placidyl Capsules 448

Ethinamate (Possible additive CNS depression).
No products indexed under this heading.

Fentanyl (Possible additive CNS depression). Products include:
Duragesic Transdermal System 1288

Fentanyl Citrate (Possible additive CNS depression). Products include:
Sublimaze Injection 1307

Fluphenazine Decanoate (Possible additive CNS depression). Products include:
Prolixin Decanoate 509

Fluphenazine Enanthate (Possible additive CNS depression). Products include:
Prolixin Enanthate 509

Fluphenazine Hydrochloride (Possible additive CNS depression). Products include:
Prolixin 509

Flurazepam Hydrochloride (Possible additive CNS depression). Products include:
Dalmane Capsules 2173

Glutethimide (Possible additive CNS depression).
No products indexed under this heading.

Haloperidol (Possible additive CNS depression). Products include:
Haldol Injection, Tablets and Concentrate 1575

Haloperidol Decanoate (Possible additive CNS depression). Products include:
Haldol Decanoate 1577

Hydrocodone Bitartrate (Possible additive CNS depression). Products include:
Anexsia 5/500 Elixir 1781
Anexia Tablets 1782
Codiclear DH Syrup 791
Deconamine CX Cough and Cold Liquid and Tablets 1319
Duratuss HD Elixir 2565
Hycodan Tablets and Syrup 930
Hycomine Compound Tablets 932
Hycomine 931
Hycotuss Expectorant Syrup 933
Hydrocet Capsules 782
Lorcet 10/650 1018
Lortab 2566
Tussend 1783
Tussend Expectorant 1785
Vicodin Tablets 1356
Vicodin ES Tablets 1357
Vicodin Tuss Expectorant 1358
Zydone Capsules 949

Hydrocodone Polistirex (Possible additive CNS depression). Products include:
Tussionex Pennkinetic Extended-Release Suspension 998

Hydroxyzine Hydrochloride (Possible additive CNS depression). Products include:
Atarax Tablets & Syrup 2185
Marax Tablets & DF Syrup 2200
Vistaril Intramuscular Solution 2216

Isoflurane (Possible additive CNS depression).
No products indexed under this heading.

Ketamine Hydrochloride (Possible additive CNS depression).
No products indexed under this heading.

Levomethadyl Acetate Hydrochloride (Possible additive CNS depression). Products include:
Orlamm 2239

Levorphanol Tartrate (Possible additive CNS depression). Products include:
Levo-Dromoran 2129

Lorazepam (Possible additive CNS depression). Products include:
Ativan Injection 2698
Ativan Tablets 2700

Loxapine Hydrochloride (Possible additive CNS depression). Products include:
Loxitane 1378

Loxapine Succinate (Possible additive CNS depression). Products include:
Loxitane Capsules 1378

Meperidine Hydrochloride (Possible additive CNS depression). Products include:
Demerol 2308
Mepergan Injection 2753

Mephobarbital (Possible additive CNS depression). Products include:
Mebaral Tablets 2322

Meprobamate (Possible additive CNS depression). Products include:
Miltown Tablets 2672
PMB 200 and PMB 400 2783

Mesoridazine Besylate (Possible additive CNS depression). Products include:
Serentil 684

Methadone Hydrochloride (Possible additive CNS depression). Products include:
Methadone Hydrochloride Oral Concentrate 2233
Methadone Hydrochloride Oral Solution & Tablets 2235

Methohexital Sodium (Possible additive CNS depression). Products include:
Brevital Sodium Vials 1429

Methotrimeprazine (Possible additive CNS depression). Products include:
Levoprome 1274

Methoxyflurane (Possible additive CNS depression).
No products indexed under this heading.

Midazolam Hydrochloride (Possible additive CNS depression). Products include:
Versed Injection 2170

Molindone Hydrochloride (Possible additive CNS depression). Products include:
Moban Tablets and Concentrate 1048

Morphine Sulfate (Possible additive CNS depression). Products include:
Astramorph/PF Injection, USP (Preservative-Free) 535
Duramorph 962
Infumorph 200 and Infumorph 500 Sterile Solutions 965
MS Contin Tablets 1994
MSIR 1997
Oramorph SR (Morphine Sulfate Sustained Release Tablets) 2236
RMS Suppositories 2657
Roxanol 2243

Opium Alkaloids (Possible additive CNS depression).
No products indexed under this heading.

Oxazepam (Possible additive CNS depression). Products include:
Serax Capsules 2810
Serax Tablets 2810

Pentobarbital Sodium (Possible additive CNS depression). Products include:
Nembutal Sodium Capsules 436
Nembutal Sodium Solution 438
Nembutal Sodium Suppositories 440

Perphenazine (Possible additive CNS depression). Products include:
Etrafon 2355
Triavil Tablets 1757
Trilafon 2389

Phenobarbital (Possible additive CNS depression). Products include:
Arco-Lase Plus Tablets 512
Bellergal-S Tablets 2250
Donnatal 2060
Donnatal Extentabs 2061
Donnatal Tablets 2060
Phenobarbital Elixir and Tablets 1469
Quadrinal Tablets 1350

Prazepam (Possible additive CNS depression).
No products indexed under this heading.

Prochlorperazine (Possible additive CNS depression). Products include:
Compazine 2470

Promethazine Hydrochloride (Possible additive CNS depression). Products include:
Mepergan Injection 2753
Phenergan with Codeine 2777
Phenergan with Dextromethorphan 2778
Phenergan Injection 2773
Phenergan Suppositories 2775
Phenergan Syrup 2774
Phenergan Tablets 2775
Phenergan VC 2779
Phenergan VC with Codeine 2781

Propofol (Possible additive CNS depression). Products include:
Diprivan Injection 2833

Propoxyphene Hydrochloride (Possible additive CNS depression). Products include:
Darvon 1435
Wygesic Tablets 2827

Propoxyphene Napsylate (Possible additive CNS depression). Products include:
Darvon-N/Darvocet-N 1433

Quazepam (Possible additive CNS depression). Products include:
Doral Tablets 2664

Risperidone (Possible additive CNS depression). Products include:
Risperdal 1301

IMPORTANT NOTE: Always consult each drug listing in the patient's regimen for possible interactions.

Secobarbital Sodium (Possible additive CNS depression). Products include:
Seconal Sodium Pulvules 1474

Sufentanil Citrate (Possible additive CNS depression). Products include:
Sufenta Injection 1309

Temazepam (Possible additive CNS depression). Products include:
Restoril Capsules 2284

Thiamylal Sodium (Possible additive CNS depression).
No products indexed under this heading.

Thioridazine Hydrochloride (Possible additive CNS depression). Products include:
Mellaril 2269

Thiothixene (Possible additive CNS depression). Products include:
Navane Capsules and Concentrate 2201
Navane Intramuscular 2202

Triazolam (Possible additive CNS depression). Products include:
Halcion Tablets 2611

Trifluoperazine Hydrochloride (Possible additive CNS depression). Products include:
Stelazine 2514

Zolpidem Tartrate (Possible additive CNS depression). Products include:
Ambien Tablets 2416

Food Interactions

Alcohol (Possible additive CNS depression).

RUBEX

(Doxorubicin Hydrochloride) 712
May interact with antineoplastics and certain other agents. Compounds in these categories include:

Altretamine (Doxorubicin may potentiate the toxicity of other anticancer therapies). Products include:
Hexalen Capsules 2571

Asparaginase (Doxorubicin may potentiate the toxicity of other anticancer therapies). Products include:
Elspar 1659

Bleomycin Sulfate (Doxorubicin may potentiate the toxicity of other anticancer therapies). Products include:
Blenoxane 692

Busulfan (Doxorubicin may potentiate the toxicity of other anticancer therapies). Products include:
Myleran Tablets 1143

Carboplatin (Doxorubicin may potentiate the toxicity of other anticancer therapies). Products include:
Paraplatin for Injection 705

Carmustine (BCNU) (Doxorubicin may potentiate the toxicity of other anticancer therapies). Products include:
BiCNU 691

Chlorambucil (Doxorubicin may potentiate the toxicity of other anticancer therapies). Products include:
Leukeran Tablets 1133

Cisplatin (Doxorubicin may potentiate the toxicity of other anticancer therapies). Products include:
Platinol 708
Platinol-AQ Injection 710

Cyclophosphamide (Doxorubicin may potentiate the toxicity of other anticancer therapies; serious irreversible myocardial toxicity; exacerbation of cyclopyhosphamide-induced hemorrhagic cystitis). Products include:
Cytoxan 694
NEOSAR Lyophilized/Neosar 1959

Cytarabine (Combination therapy results in necrotizing colitis, typhilitis, bloody stools and severe infections). Products include:
Cytosar-U Sterile Powder 2592

Dacarbazine (Doxorubicin may potentiate the toxicity of other anticancer therapies). Products include:
DTIC-Dome 600

Daunorubicin Hydrochloride (Doxorubicin may potentiate the toxicity of other anticancer therapies). Products include:
Cerubidine 795

Estramustine Phosphate Sodium (Doxorubicin may potentiate the toxicity of other anticancer therapies). Products include:
Emcyt Capsules 1953

Etoposide (Doxorubicin may potentiate the toxicity of other anticancer therapies). Products include:
VePesid Capsules and Injection 718

Floxuridine (Doxorubicin may potentiate the toxicity of other anticancer therapies). Products include:
Sterile FUDR 2118

Fluorouracil (Doxorubicin may potentiate the toxicity of other anticancer therapies). Products include:
Efudex 2113
Fluoroplex Topical Solution & Cream 1% 479
Fluorouracil Injection 2116

Flutamide (Doxorubicin may potentiate the toxicity of other anticancer therapies). Products include:
Eulexin Capsules 2358

Hydroxyurea (Doxorubicin may potentiate the toxicity of other anticancer therapies). Products include:
Hydrea Capsules 696

Idarubicin Hydrochloride (Doxorubicin may potentiate the toxicity of other anticancer therapies). Products include:
Idamycin 1955

Ifosfamide (Doxorubicin may potentiate the toxicity of other anticancer therapies). Products include:
IFEX 697

Interferon alfa-2A, Recombinant (Doxorubicin may potentiate the toxicity of other anticancer therapies). Products include:
Roferon-A Injection 2145

Interferon alfa-2B, Recombinant (Doxorubicin may potentiate the toxicity of other anticancer therapies). Products include:
Intron A 2364

Levamisole Hydrochloride (Doxorubicin may potentiate the toxicity of other anticancer therapies). Products include:
Ergamisol Tablets 1292

Lomustine (CCNU) (Doxorubicin may potentiate the toxicity of other anticancer therapies). Products include:
CeeNU 693

Mechlorethamine Hydrochloride (Doxorubicin may potentiate the toxicity of other anticancer therapies). Products include:
Mustargen 1709

Megestrol Acetate (Doxorubicin may potentiate the toxicity of other anticancer therapies). Products include:
Megace Oral Suspension 699
Megace Tablets 701

Melphalan (Doxorubicin may potentiate the toxicity of other anticancer therapies). Products include:
Alkeran Tablets 1071

Mercaptopurine (Doxorubicin may potentiate the toxicity of other anticancer therapies; enhanced hepatotoxicity of 6-mercaptopurine). Products include:
Purinethol Tablets 1156

Methotrexate Sodium (Doxorubicin may potentiate the toxicity of other anticancer therapies). Products include:
Methotrexate Sodium Tablets, Injection, for Injection and LPF Injection 1275

Mitomycin (Mitomycin-C) (Doxorubicin may potentiate the toxicity of other anticancer therapies). Products include:
Mutamycin 703

Mitotane (Doxorubicin may potentiate the toxicity of other anticancer therapies). Products include:
Lysodren 698

Mitoxantrone Hydrochloride (Doxorubicin may potentiate the toxicity of other anticancer therapies). Products include:
Novantrone 1279

Paclitaxel (Doxorubicin may potentiate the toxicity of other anticancer therapies). Products include:
Taxol 714

Procarbazine Hydrochloride (Doxorubicin may potentiate the toxicity of other anticancer therapies). Products include:
Matulane Capsules 2131

Streptozocin (Doxorubicin may potentiate the toxicity of other anticancer therapies). Products include:
Zanosar Sterile Powder 2653

Tamoxifen Citrate (Doxorubicin may potentiate the toxicity of other anticancer therapies). Products include:
Nolvadex Tablets 2841

Teniposide (Doxorubicin may potentiate the toxicity of other anticancer therapies). Products include:
Vumon 727

Thioguanine (Doxorubicin may potentiate the toxicity of other anticancer therapies). Products include:
Thioguanine Tablets, Tabloid Brand 1181

Thiotepa (Doxorubicin may potentiate the toxicity of other anticancer therapies). Products include:
Thioplex (Thiotepa For Injection) 1281

Vincristine Sulfate (Doxorubicin may potentiate the toxicity of other anticancer therapies). Products include:
Oncovin Solution Vials & Hyporets 1466

Vinorelbine Tartrate (Doxorubicin may potentiate the toxicity of other anticancer therapies). Products include:
Navelbine Injection 1145

RUM-K SYRUP

(Potassium Chloride) 1005
None cited in PDR database.

RYNA LIQUID

(Chlorpheniramine Maleate, Pseudoephedrine Hydrochloride) .... ■ 841
May interact with:

Furazolidone (Concurrent and/or sequential use is not recommended). Products include:
Furoxone 2046

Isocarboxazid (Concurrent and/or sequential use is not recommended).
No products indexed under this heading.

Phenelzine Sulfate (Concurrent and/or sequential use is not recommended). Products include:
Nardil 1920

Selegiline Hydrochloride (Concurrent and/or sequential use is not recommended). Products include:
Eldepryl Tablets 2550

Tranylcypromine Sulfate (Concurrent and/or sequential use is not recommended). Products include:
Parnate Tablets 2503

RYNA-C LIQUID

(Chlorpheniramine Maleate, Codeine Phosphate, Pseudoephedrine Hydrochloride) .... ■ 841
May interact with monoamine oxidase inhibitors and certain other agents. Compounds in these categories include:

Furazolidone (Concurrent and/or sequential use is not recommended). Products include:
Furoxone 2046

Isocarboxazid (Concurrent and/or sequential use is not recommended).
No products indexed under this heading.

Phenelzine Sulfate (Concurrent and/or sequential use is not recommended). Products include:
Nardil 1920

Selegiline Hydrochloride (Concurrent and/or sequential use is not recommended). Products include:
Eldepryl Tablets 2550

Tranylcypromine Sulfate (Concurrent and/or sequential use is not recommended). Products include:
Parnate Tablets 2503

Food Interactions

Alcohol (May increase drowsiness effect).

RYNA-CX LIQUID

(Codeine Phosphate, Guaifenesin, Pseudoephedrine Hydrochloride) .... ■ 841
See **Ryna-C Liquid**

RYNATAN TABLETS

(Chlorpheniramine Tannate, Pyrilamine Tannate, Phenylephrine Tannate) 2673
See **Rynatan-S Pediatric Suspension**

RYNATAN-S PEDIATRIC SUSPENSION

(Phenylephrine Tannate, Chlorpheniramine Tannate, Pyrilamine Tannate) 2673
May interact with monoamine oxidase inhibitors, central nervous system depressants, hypnotics and sedatives, tranquilizers, and certain other agents. Compounds in these categories include:

Alfentanil Hydrochloride (Additive CNS effects). Products include:
Alfenta Injection 1286

Alprazolam (Additive CNS effects). Products include:
Xanax Tablets 2649

Aprobarbital (Additive CNS effects).
No products indexed under this heading.

Buprenorphine (Additive CNS effects). Products include:
Buprenex Injectable 2006

Buspirone Hydrochloride (Additive CNS effects). Products include:
BuSpar 737

915 **Interactions Index** **Rynatan**

Butabarbital (Additive CNS effects).
No products indexed under this heading.

Butalbital (Additive CNS effects). Products include:
- Esgic-plus Tablets ... 1013
- Fioricet Tablets ... 2258
- Fioricet with Codeine Capsules ... 2260
- Fiorinal Capsules ... 2261
- Fiorinal with Codeine Capsules ... 2262
- Fiorinal Tablets ... 2261
- Phrenilin ... 785
- Sedapap Tablets 50 mg/650 mg .. 1543

Chlordiazepoxide (Additive CNS effects). Products include:
- Libritabs Tablets ... 2177
- Limbitrol ... 2180

Chlordiazepoxide Hydrochloride (Additive CNS effects). Products include:
- Librax Capsules ... 2176
- Librium Capsules ... 2178
- Librium Injectable ... 2179

Chlorpromazine (Additive CNS effects). Products include:
- Thorazine Suppositories ... 2523

Chlorpromazine Hydrochloride (Additive CNS effects). Products include:
- Thorazine ... 2523

Chlorprothixene (Additive CNS effects).
No products indexed under this heading.

Chlorprothixene Hydrochloride (Additive CNS effects).
No products indexed under this heading.

Clorazepate Dipotassium (Additive CNS effects). Products include:
- Tranxene ... 451

Clozapine (Additive CNS effects). Products include:
- Clozaril Tablets ... 2252

Codeine Phosphate (Additive CNS effects). Products include:
- Actifed with Codeine Cough Syrup.. 1067
- Brontex ... 1981
- Deconsal C Expectorant Syrup ... 456
- Deconsal Pediatric Syrup ... 457
- Dimetane-DC Cough Syrup ... 2059
- Empirin with Codeine Tablets ... 1093
- Fioricet with Codeine Capsules ... 2260
- Fiorinal with Codeine Capsules ... 2262
- Isoclor Expectorant ... 990
- Novahistine DH ... 2462
- Novahistine Expectorant ... 2463
- Nucofed ... 2051
- Phenergan with Codeine ... 2777
- Phenergan VC with Codeine ... 2781
- Robitussin A-C Syrup ... 2073
- Robitussin-DAC Syrup ... 2074
- Ryna ... ◙ 841
- Soma Compound w/Codeine Tablets ... 2676
- Tussi-Organidin NR Liquid and S NR Liquid ... 2677
- Tylenol with Codeine ... 1583

Desflurane (Additive CNS effects). Products include:
- Suprane ... 1813

Dezocine (Additive CNS effects). Products include:
- Dalgan Injection ... 538

Diazepam (Additive CNS effects). Products include:
- Dizac ... 1809
- Valium Injectable ... 2182
- Valium Tablets ... 2183
- Valrelease Capsules ... 2169

Droperidol (Additive CNS effects). Products include:
- Inapsine Injection ... 1296

Enflurane (Additive CNS effects).
No products indexed under this heading.

Estazolam (Additive CNS effects). Products include:
- ProSom Tablets ... 449

Ethchlorvynol (Additive CNS effects). Products include:
- Placidyl Capsules ... 448

Ethinamate (Additive CNS effects).
No products indexed under this heading.

Fentanyl (Additive CNS effects). Products include:
- Duragesic Transdermal System ... 1288

Fentanyl Citrate (Additive CNS effects). Products include:
- Sublimaze Injection ... 1307

Fluphenazine Decanoate (Additive CNS effects). Products include:
- Prolixin Decanoate ... 509

Fluphenazine Enanthate (Additive CNS effects). Products include:
- Prolixin Enanthate ... 509

Fluphenazine Hydrochloride (Additive CNS effects). Products include:
- Prolixin ... 509

Flurazepam Hydrochloride (Additive CNS effects). Products include:
- Dalmane Capsules ... 2173

Furazolidone (Prolongs and intensifies anticholinergic effects of antihistamines and overall effects of sympathomimetics; use with caution or avoid concurrent use). Products include:
- Furoxone ... 2046

Glutethimide (Additive CNS effects).
No products indexed under this heading.

Haloperidol (Additive CNS effects). Products include:
- Haldol Injection, Tablets and Concentrate ... 1575

Haloperidol Decanoate (Additive CNS effects). Products include:
- Haldol Decanoate ... 1577

Hydrocodone Bitartrate (Additive CNS effects). Products include:
- Anexsia 5/500 Elixir ... 1781
- Anexia Tablets ... 1782
- Codiclear DH Syrup ... 791
- Deconamine CX Cough and Cold Liquid and Tablets ... 1319
- Duratuss HD Elixir ... 2565
- Hycodan Tablets and Syrup ... 930
- Hycomine Compound Tablets ... 932
- Hycomine ... 931
- Hycotuss Expectorant Syrup ... 933
- Hydrocet Capsules ... 782
- Lorcet 10/650 ... 1018
- Lortab ... 2566
- Tussend ... 1783
- Tussend Expectorant ... 1785
- Vicodin Tablets ... 1356
- Vicodin ES Tablets ... 1357
- Vicodin Tuss Expectorant ... 1358
- Zydone Capsules ... 949

Hydrocodone Polistirex (Additive CNS effects). Products include:
- Tussionex Pennkinetic Extended-Release Suspension ... 998

Hydroxyzine Hydrochloride (Additive CNS effects). Products include:
- Atarax Tablets & Syrup ... 2185
- Marax Tablets & DF Syrup ... 2200
- Vistaril Intramuscular Solution ... 2216

Isocarboxazid (Prolongs and intensifies anticholinergic effects of antihistamines and overall effects of sympathomimetics; use with caution or avoid concurrent use).
No products indexed under this heading.

Isoflurane (Additive CNS effects).
No products indexed under this heading.

Ketamine Hydrochloride (Additive CNS effects).
No products indexed under this heading.

Levomethadyl Acetate Hydrochloride (Additive CNS effects). Products include:
- Orlamm ... 2239

Levorphanol Tartrate (Additive CNS effects). Products include:
- Levo-Dromoran ... 2129

Lorazepam (Additive CNS effects). Products include:
- Ativan Injection ... 2698
- Ativan Tablets ... 2700

Loxapine Hydrochloride (Additive CNS effects). Products include:
- Loxitane ... 1378

Loxapine Succinate (Additive CNS effects). Products include:
- Loxitane Capsules ... 1378

Meperidine Hydrochloride (Additive CNS effects). Products include:
- Demerol ... 2308
- Mepergan Injection ... 2753

Mephobarbital (Additive CNS effects). Products include:
- Mebaral Tablets ... 2322

Meprobamate (Additive CNS effects). Products include:
- Miltown Tablets ... 2672
- PMB 200 and PMB 400 ... 2783

Mesoridazine Besylate (Additive CNS effects). Products include:
- Serentil ... 684

Methadone Hydrochloride (Additive CNS effects). Products include:
- Methadone Hydrochloride Oral Concentrate ... 2233
- Methadone Hydrochloride Oral Solution & Tablets ... 2235

Methohexital Sodium (Additive CNS effects). Products include:
- Brevital Sodium Vials ... 1429

Methotrimeprazine (Additive CNS effects). Products include:
- Levoprome ... 1274

Methoxyflurane (Additive CNS effects).
No products indexed under this heading.

Midazolam Hydrochloride (Additive CNS effects). Products include:
- Versed Injection ... 2170

Molindone Hydrochloride (Additive CNS effects). Products include:
- Moban Tablets and Concentrate ... 1048

Morphine Sulfate (Additive CNS effects). Products include:
- Astramorph/PF Injection, USP (Preservative-Free) ... 535
- Duramorph ... 962
- Infumorph 200 and Infumorph 500 Sterile Solutions ... 965
- MS Contin Tablets ... 1994
- MSIR ... 1997
- Oramorph SR (Morphine Sulfate Sustained Release Tablets) ... 2236
- RMS Suppositories ... 2657
- Roxanol ... 2243

Opium Alkaloids (Additive CNS effects).
No products indexed under this heading.

Oxazepam (Additive CNS effects). Products include:
- Serax Capsules ... 2810
- Serax Tablets ... 2810

Oxycodone Hydrochloride (Additive CNS effects). Products include:
- Percocet Tablets ... 938
- Percodan Tablets ... 939
- Percodan-Demi Tablets ... 940
- Roxicodone Tablets, Oral Solution & Intensol (Oxycodone) ... 2244
- Tylox Capsules ... 1584

Pentobarbital Sodium (Additive CNS effects). Products include:
- Nembutal Sodium Capsules ... 436
- Nembutal Sodium Solution ... 438
- Nembutal Sodium Suppositories ... 440

Perphenazine (Additive CNS effects). Products include:
- Etrafon ... 2355
- Triavil Tablets ... 1757
- Trilafon ... 2389

Phenelzine Sulfate (Prolongs and intensifies anticholinergic effects of antihistamines and overall effects of sympathomimetics; use with caution or avoid concurrent use). Products include:
- Nardil ... 1920

Phenobarbital (Additive CNS effects). Products include:
- Arco-Lase Plus Tablets ... 512
- Bellergal-S Tablets ... 2250
- Donnatal ... 2060
- Donnatal Extentabs ... 2061
- Donnatal Tablets ... 2060
- Phenobarbital Elixir and Tablets ... 1469
- Quadrinal Tablets ... 1350

Prazepam (Additive CNS effects).
No products indexed under this heading.

Prochlorperazine (Additive CNS effects). Products include:
- Compazine ... 2470

Promethazine Hydrochloride (Additive CNS effects). Products include:
- Mepergan Injection ... 2753
- Phenergan with Codeine ... 2777
- Phenergan with Dextromethorphan 2778
- Phenergan Injection ... 2773
- Phenergan Suppositories ... 2775
- Phenergan Syrup ... 2774
- Phenergan Tablets ... 2775
- Phenergan VC ... 2779
- Phenergan VC with Codeine ... 2781

Propofol (Additive CNS effects). Products include:
- Diprivan Injection ... 2833

Propoxyphene Hydrochloride (Additive CNS effects). Products include:
- Darvon ... 1435
- Wygesic Tablets ... 2827

Propoxyphene Napsylate (Additive CNS effects). Products include:
- Darvon-N/Darvocet-N ... 1433

Quazepam (Additive CNS effects). Products include:
- Doral Tablets ... 2664

Risperidone (Additive CNS effects). Products include:
- Risperdal ... 1301

Secobarbital Sodium (Additive CNS effects). Products include:
- Seconal Sodium Pulvules ... 1474

Selegiline Hydrochloride (Prolongs and intensifies anticholinergic effects of antihistamines and overall effects of sympathomimetics; use with caution or avoid concurrent use). Products include:
- Eldepryl Tablets ... 2550

Sufentanil Citrate (Additive CNS effects). Products include:
- Sufenta Injection ... 1309

Temazepam (Additive CNS effects). Products include:
- Restoril Capsules ... 2284

Thiamylal Sodium (Additive CNS effects).
No products indexed under this heading.

Thioridazine Hydrochloride (Additive CNS effects). Products include:
- Mellaril ... 2269

Thiothixene (Additive CNS effects). Products include:
- Navane Capsules and Concentrate 2201
- Navane Intramuscular ... 2202

IMPORTANT NOTE: Always consult each drug listing in the patient's regimen for possible interactions.

Rynatan **Interactions Index** 916

Tranylcypromine Sulfate (Prolongs and intensifies anticholinergic effects of antihistamines and overall effects of sympathomimetics; use with caution or avoid concurrent use). Products include:

Parnate Tablets 2503

Triazolam (Additive CNS effects). Products include:

Halcion Tablets 2611

Trifluoperazine Hydrochloride (Additive CNS effects). Products include:

Stelazine 2514

Zolpidem Tartrate (Additive CNS effects). Products include:

Ambien Tablets 2416

Food Interactions

Alcohol (Additive CNS effects).

RYNATUSS PEDIATRIC SUSPENSION

(Carbetapentane Tannate, Chlorpheniramine Tannate, Ephedrine Tannate, Phenylephrine Tannate) 2673

May interact with monoamine oxidase inhibitors and central nervous system depressants. Compounds in these categories include:

Alfentanil Hydrochloride (Additive CNS effects). Products include:

Alfenta Injection 1286

Alprazolam (Additive CNS effects). Products include:

Xanax Tablets 2649

Aprobarbital (Additive CNS effects).

No products indexed under this heading.

Buprenorphine (Additive CNS effects). Products include:

Buprenex Injectable 2006

Buspirone Hydrochloride (Additive CNS effects). Products include:

BuSpar 737

Butabarbital (Additive CNS effects).

No products indexed under this heading.

Butalbital (Additive CNS effects). Products include:

Esgic-plus Tablets 1013
Fioricet Tablets 2258
Fioricet with Codeine Capsules 2260
Fiorinal Capsules 2261
Fiorinal with Codeine Capsules 2262
Fiorinal Tablets 2261
Phrenilin 785
Sedapap Tablets 50 mg/650 mg 1543

Chlordiazepoxide (Additive CNS effects). Products include:

Libritabs Tablets 2177
Limbitrol 2180

Chlordiazepoxide Hydrochloride (Additive CNS effects). Products include:

Librax Capsules 2176
Librium Capsules 2178
Librium Injectable 2179

Chlorpromazine (Additive CNS effects). Products include:

Thorazine Suppositories 2523

Chlorprothixene (Additive CNS effects).

No products indexed under this heading.

Chlorprothixene Hydrochloride (Additive CNS effects).

No products indexed under this heading.

Clorazepate Dipotassium (Additive CNS effects). Products include:

Tranxene 451

Clozapine (Additive CNS effects). Products include:

Clozaril Tablets 2252

Codeine Phosphate (Additive CNS effects). Products include:

Actifed with Codeine Cough Syrup.. 1067
Brontex 1981
Deconsal C Expectorant Syrup 456
Deconsal Pediatric Syrup 457
Dimetane-DC Cough Syrup 2059
Empirin with Codeine Tablets 1093
Fioricet with Codeine Capsules 2260
Fiorinal with Codeine Capsules 2262
Isoclor Expectorant 990
Novahistine DH 2462
Novahistine Expectorant 2463
Nucofed 2051
Phenergan with Codeine 2777
Phenergan VC with Codeine 2781
Robitussin A-C Syrup 2073
Robitussin-DAC Syrup 2074
Ryna 841
Soma Compound w/Codeine Tablets 2676
Tussi-Organidin NR Liquid and S NR Liquid 2677
Tylenol with Codeine 1583

Desflurane (Additive CNS effects). Products include:

Suprane 1813

Dezocine (Additive CNS effects). Products include:

Dalgan Injection 538

Diazepam (Additive CNS effects). Products include:

Dizac 1809
Valium Injectable 2182
Valium Tablets 2183
Valrelease Capsules 2169

Droperidol (Additive CNS effects). Products include:

Inapsine Injection 1296

Enflurane (Additive CNS effects).

No products indexed under this heading.

Estazolam (Additive CNS effects). Products include:

ProSom Tablets 449

Ethchlorvynol (Additive CNS effects). Products include:

Placidyl Capsules 448

Ethinamate (Additive CNS effects).

No products indexed under this heading.

Fentanyl (Additive CNS effects). Products include:

Duragesic Transdermal System 1288

Fentanyl Citrate (Additive CNS effects). Products include:

Sublimaze Injection 1307

Fluphenazine Decanoate (Additive CNS effects). Products include:

Prolixin Decanoate 509

Fluphenazine Enanthate (Additive CNS effects). Products include:

Prolixin Enanthate 509

Fluphenazine Hydrochloride (Additive CNS effects). Products include:

Prolixin 509

Flurazepam Hydrochloride (Additive CNS effects). Products include:

Dalmane Capsules 2173

Furazolidone (MAOIs may prolong and intensify anticholinergic effects of antihistamines and overall effects of sympathomimetics). Products include:

Furoxone 2046

Glutethimide (Additive CNS effects).

No products indexed under this heading.

Haloperidol (Additive CNS effects). Products include:

Haldol Injection, Tablets and Concentrate 1575

Haloperidol Decanoate (Additive CNS effects). Products include:

Haldol Decanoate 1577

Hydrocodone Bitartrate (Additive CNS effects). Products include:

Anexsia 5/500 Elixir 1781
Anexia Tablets 1782
Codiclear DH Syrup 791
Deconamine CX Cough and Cold Liquid and Tablets 1319
Duratuss HD Elixir 2565
Hycodan Tablets and Syrup 930
Hycomine Compound Tablets 932
Hycomine 931
Hycotuss Expectorant Syrup 933
Hydrocet Capsules 782
Lorcet 10/650 1018
Lortab 2566
Tussend 1783
Tussend Expectorant 1785
Vicodin Tablets 1356
Vicodin ES Tablets 1357
Vicodin Tuss Expectorant 1358
Zydone Capsules 949

Hydrocodone Polistirex (Additive CNS effects). Products include:

Tussionex Pennkinetic Extended-Release Suspension 998

Hydroxyzine Hydrochloride (Additive CNS effects). Products include:

Atarax Tablets & Syrup 2185
Marax Tablets & DF Syrup 2200
Vistaril Intramuscular Solution 2216

Isocarboxazid (MAOIs may prolong and intensify anticholinergic effects of antihistamines and overall effects of sympathomimetics).

No products indexed under this heading.

Isoflurane (Additive CNS effects).

No products indexed under this heading.

Ketamine Hydrochloride (Additive CNS effects).

No products indexed under this heading.

Levomethadyl Acetate Hydrochloride (Additive CNS effects). Products include:

Orlamm 2239

Levorphanol Tartrate (Additive CNS effects). Products include:

Levo-Dromoran 2129

Lorazepam (Additive CNS effects). Products include:

Ativan Injection 2698
Ativan Tablets 2700

Loxapine Hydrochloride (Additive CNS effects). Products include:

Loxitane 1378

Loxapine Succinate (Additive CNS effects). Products include:

Loxitane Capsules 1378

Meperidine Hydrochloride (Additive CNS effects). Products include:

Demerol 2308
Mepergan Injection 2753

Mephobarbital (Additive CNS effects). Products include:

Mebaral Tablets 2322

Meprobamate (Additive CNS effects). Products include:

Miltown Tablets 2672
PMB 200 and PMB 400 2783

Mesoridazine Besylate (Additive CNS effects). Products include:

Serentil 684

Methadone Hydrochloride (Additive CNS effects). Products include:

Methadone Hydrochloride Oral Concentrate 2233
Methadone Hydrochloride Oral Solution & Tablets 2235

Methohexital Sodium (Additive CNS effects). Products include:

Brevital Sodium Vials 1429

Methotrimeprazine (Additive CNS effects). Products include:

Levoprome 1274

Methoxyflurane (Additive CNS effects).

No products indexed under this heading.

Midazolam Hydrochloride (Additive CNS effects). Products include:

Versed Injection 2170

Molindone Hydrochloride (Additive CNS effects). Products include:

Moban Tablets and Concentrate 1048

Morphine Sulfate (Additive CNS effects). Products include:

Astramorph/PF Injection, USP (Preservative-Free) 535
Duramorph 962
Infumorph 200 and Infumorph 500 Sterile Solutions 965
MS Contin Tablets 1994
MSIR 1997
Oramorph SR (Morphine Sulfate Sustained Release Tablets) 2236
RMS Suppositories 2657
Roxanol 2243

Opium Alkaloids (Additive CNS effects).

No products indexed under this heading.

Oxazepam (Additive CNS effects). Products include:

Serax Capsules 2810
Serax Tablets 2810

Oxycodone Hydrochloride (Additive CNS effects). Products include:

Percocet Tablets 938
Percodan Tablets 939
Percodan-Demi Tablets 940
Roxicodone Tablets, Oral Solution & Intensol (Oxycodone) 2244
Tylox Capsules 1584

Pentobarbital Sodium (Additive CNS effects). Products include:

Nembutal Sodium Capsules 436
Nembutal Sodium Solution 438
Nembutal Sodium Suppositories 440

Perphenazine (Additive CNS effects). Products include:

Etrafon 2355
Triavil Tablets 1757
Trilafon 2389

Phenelzine Sulfate (MAOIs may prolong and intensify anticholinergic effects of antihistamines and overall effects of sympathomimetics). Products include:

Nardil 1920

Phenobarbital (Additive CNS effects). Products include:

Arco-Lase Plus Tablets 512
Bellergal-S Tablets 2250
Donnatal 2060
Donnatal Extentabs 2061
Donnatal Tablets 2060
Phenobarbital Elixir and Tablets 1469
Quadrinal Tablets 1350

Prazepam (Additive CNS effects).

No products indexed under this heading.

Prochlorperazine (Additive CNS effects). Products include:

Compazine 2470

Promethazine Hydrochloride (Additive CNS effects). Products include:

Mepergan Injection 2753
Phenergan with Codeine 2777
Phenergan with Dextromethorphan 2778
Phenergan Injection 2773
Phenergan Suppositories 2775
Phenergan Syrup 2774
Phenergan Tablets 2775
Phenergan VC 2779
Phenergan VC with Codeine 2781

Propofol (Additive CNS effects). Products include:

Diprivan Injection 2833

Propoxyphene Hydrochloride (Additive CNS effects). Products include:

Darvon 1435
Wygesic Tablets 2827

(Described in PDR For Nonprescription Drugs) (Described in PDR For Ophthalmology)

Propoxyphene Napsylate (Additive CNS effects). Products include:

Darvon-N/Darvocet-N 1433

Quazepam (Additive CNS effects). Products include:

Doral Tablets 2664

Risperidone (Additive CNS effects). Products include:

Risperdal 1301

Secobarbital Sodium (Additive CNS effects). Products include:

Seconal Sodium Pulvules 1474

Selegiline Hydrochloride (MAOIs may prolong and intensify anticholinergic effects of antihistamines and overall effects of sympathomimetics). Products include:

Eldepryl Tablets 2550

Sufentanil Citrate (Additive CNS effects). Products include:

Sufenta Injection 1309

Temazepam (Additive CNS effects). Products include:

Restoril Capsules 2284

Thiamylal Sodium (Additive CNS effects).

No products indexed under this heading.

Thioridazine Hydrochloride (Additive CNS effects). Products include:

Mellaril 2269

Thiothixene (Additive CNS effects). Products include:

Navane Capsules and Concentrate 2201
Navane Intramuscular 2202

Tranylcypromine Sulfate (MAOIs may prolong and intensify anticholinergic effects of antihistamines and overall effects of sympathomimetics). Products include:

Parnate Tablets 2503

Triazolam (Additive CNS effects). Products include:

Halcion Tablets 2611

Trifluoperazine Hydrochloride (Additive CNS effects). Products include:

Stelazine 2514

Zolpidem Tartrate (Additive CNS effects). Products include:

Ambien Tablets... 2416

Food Interactions

Alcohol (Additive CNS effects).

RYNATUSS TABLETS

(Chlorpheniramine Tannate, Carbetapentane Tannate, Phenylephrine Tannate, Ephedrine Tannate) 2673

See Rynatuss Pediatric Suspension

RYTHMOL TABLETS–150MG, 225MG, 300MG

(Propafenone Hydrochloride)..............1352

May interact with beta blockers, cardiac glycosides, local anesthetics, and certain other agents. Compounds in these categories include:

Acebutolol Hydrochloride (Potential for increased plasma concentration and elimination half-life of beta blockers; dosage reduction of beta-antagonist may be necessary). Products include:

Sectral Capsules 2807

Atenolol (Potential for increased plasma concentration and elimination half-life of beta blockers; dosage reduction of beta-antagonist may be necessary). Products include:

Tenoretic Tablets..................................... 2845
Tenormin Tablets and I.V. Injection 2847

Betaxolol Hydrochloride (Potential for increased plasma concentration and elimination half-life of beta blockers; dosage reduction of beta-antagonist may be necessary). Products include:

Betoptic Ophthalmic Solution............ 469
Betoptic S Ophthalmic Suspension 471
Kerlone Tablets.. 2436

Bisoprolol Fumarate (Potential for increased plasma concentration and elimination half-life of beta blockers; dosage reduction of beta-antagonist may be necessary). Products include:

Zebeta Tablets 1413
Ziac 1415

Bupivacaine Hydrochloride (Concomitant use of local anesthetics may increase the risk of CNS side effects). Products include:

Marcaine Hydrochloride with Epinephrine 1:200,000 2316
Marcaine Hydrochloride Injection.... 2316
Marcaine Spinal 2319
Sensorcaine 559

Carteolol Hydrochloride (Potential for increased plasma concentration and elimination half-life of beta blockers; dosage reduction of beta-antagonist may be necessary). Products include:

Cartrol Tablets 410
Ocupress Ophthalmic Solution, 1% Sterile... ◉ 309

Chloroprocaine Hydrochloride (Concomitant use of local anesthetics may increase the risk of CNS side effects). Products include:

Nescaine/Nescaine MPF....................... 554

Cimetidine (Increases steady-state plasma concentrations with no detectable changes in electrocardiographic parameters). Products include:

Tagamet Tablets 2516

Cimetidine Hydrochloride (Increases steady-state plasma concentrations with no detectable changes in electrocardiographic parameters). Products include:

Tagamet.. 2516

Deslanoside (Potential for elevated digoxin levels; dosage reduction of digitalis may be necessary).

No products indexed under this heading.

Digitoxin (Potential for elevated digoxin levels; dosage reduction of digitalis may be necessary). Products include:

Crystodigin Tablets................................. 1433

Digoxin (Potential for elevated digoxin levels; dosage reduction of digitalis may be necessary). Products include:

Lanoxicaps 1117
Lanoxin Elixir Pediatric 1120
Lanoxin Injection 1123
Lanoxin Injection Pediatric.................. 1126
Lanoxin Tablets 1128

Esmolol Hydrochloride (Potential for increased plasma concentration and elimination half-life of beta blockers; dosage reduction of beta-antagonist may be necessary). Products include:

Brevibloc Injection.................................. 1808

Etidocaine Hydrochloride (Concomitant use of local anesthetics may increase the risk of CNS side effects). Products include:

Duranest Injections 542

Labetalol Hydrochloride (Potential for increased plasma concentration and elimination half-life of beta blockers; dosage reduction of beta-antagonist may be necessary). Products include:

Normodyne Injection 2377
Normodyne Tablets 2379
Trandate 1185

Levobunolol Hydrochloride (Potential for increased plasma concentration and elimination half-life of beta blockers; dosage reduction of beta-antagonist may be necessary). Products include:

Betagan .... ◉ 233

Lidocaine Hydrochloride (Concomitant use of local anesthetics may increase the risk of CNS side effects). Products include:

Bactine Antiseptic/Anesthetic First Aid Liquid .... ⊕⊡ 708
Campho-Phenique Maximum Strength First Aid Antibiotic Plus Pain Reliever Ointment .... ⊕⊡ 719
Decadron Phosphate with Xylocaine Injection, Sterile 1639
Xylocaine Injections 567

Mepivacaine Hydrochloride Injection (Concomitant use of local anesthetics may increase the risk of CNS side effects). Products include:

Carbocaine Hydrochloride Injection 2303

Metipranolol Hydrochloride (Potential for increased plasma concentration and elimination half-life of beta blockers; dosage reduction of beta-antagonist may be necessary). Products include:

OptiPranolol (Metipranolol 0.3%) Sterile Ophthalmic Solution.......... ◉ 258

Metoprolol Succinate (Potential for increased plasma concentration and elimination half-life of beta blockers; dosage reduction of beta-antagonist may be necessary). Products include:

Toprol-XL Tablets 565

Metoprolol Tartrate (Potential for increased plasma concentration and elimination half-life of beta blockers; dosage reduction of beta-antagonist may be necessary). Products include:

Lopressor Ampuls 830
Lopressor HCT Tablets 832
Lopressor Tablets 830

Nadolol (Potential for increased plasma concentration and elimination half-life of beta blockers; dosage reduction of beta-antagonist may be necessary).

No products indexed under this heading.

Penbutolol Sulfate (Potential for increased plasma concentration and elimination half-life of beta blockers; dosage reduction of beta-antagonist may be necessary). Products include:

Levatol 2403

Pindolol (Potential for increased plasma concentration and elimination half-life of beta blockers; dosage reduction of beta-antagonist may be necessary). Products include:

Visken Tablets... 2299

Procaine Hydrochloride (Concomitant use of local anesthetics may increase the risk of CNS side effects). Products include:

Novocain Hydrochloride for Spinal Anesthesia 2326

Propranolol Hydrochloride (Potential for increased plasma concentration and elimination half-life of beta blockers; dosage reduction of beta-antagonist may be necessary). Products include:

Inderal 2728
Inderal LA Long Acting Capsules 2730
Inderide Tablets 2732
Inderide LA Long Acting Capsules.. 2734

Quinidine Gluconate (Small doses of quinidine completely inhibit the hydroxylation metabolic pathway). Products include:

Quinaglute Dura-Tabs Tablets 649

Quinidine Polygalacturonate (Small doses of quinidine completely inhibit the hydroxylation metabolic pathway).

No products indexed under this heading.

Quinidine Sulfate (Small doses of quinidine completely inhibit the hydroxylation metabolic pathway). Products include:

Quinidex Extentabs 2067

Sotalol Hydrochloride (Potential for increased plasma concentration and elimination half-life of beta blockers; dosage reduction of beta-antagonist may be necessary). Products include:

Betapace Tablets 641

Tetracaine Hydrochloride (Concomitant use of local anesthetics may increase the risk of CNS side effects). Products include:

Cetacaine Topical Anesthetic 794
Pontocaine Hydrochloride for Spinal Anesthesia 2330

Timolol Hemihydrate (Potential for increased plasma concentration and elimination half-life of beta blockers; dosage reduction of beta-antagonist may be necessary). Products include:

Betimol 0.25%, 0.5% .... ◉ 261

Timolol Maleate (Potential for increased plasma concentration and elimination half-life of beta blockers; dosage reduction of beta-antagonist may be necessary). Products include:

Blocadren Tablets 1614
Timolide Tablets....................................... 1748
Timoptic in Ocudose 1753
Timoptic Sterile Ophthalmic Solution.. 1751
Timoptic-XE 1755

Warfarin Sodium (Increase in mean steady-state plasma levels of warfarin resulting in increased prothrombin time). Products include:

Coumadin 926

Food Interactions

Food, unspecified (Increased peak blood level and bioavailability in a single dose study).

SMA IRON FORTIFIED INFANT FORMULA, CONCENTRATED, READY-TO-FEED AND POWDER

(Nutritional Supplement) 2811
None cited in PDR database.

SMA LO-IRON INFANT FORMULA, CONCENTRATED, READY-TO-FEED AND POWDER

(Nutritional Supplement) 2811
None cited in PDR database.

SSD CREAM

(Silver Sulfadiazine)...............................1355

IMPORTANT NOTE: Always consult each drug listing in the patient's regimen for possible interactions.

May interact with:

Cimetidine (Higher incidence of leukopenia). Products include:

Tagamet Tablets 2516

Cimetidine Hydrochloride (Higher incidence of leukopenia). Products include:

Tagamet........ 2516

SSD AF CREAM
(Silver Sulfadiazine)........1355
See **SSD Cream**

SSKI SOLUTION
(Potassium Iodide)........2658
May interact with lithium preparations, antithyroid agents, ACE inhibitors, potassium preparations, and potassium sparing diuretics. Compounds in these categories include:

Amiloride Hydrochloride (Potential for hyperkalemia, cardiac arrhythmias or cardiac arrest). Products include:

Midamor Tablets 1703
Moduretic Tablets 1705

Benazepril Hydrochloride (Potential for hyperkalemia, cardiac arrhythmias or cardiac arrest). Products include:

Lotensin Tablets........ 834
Lotensin HCT........ 837
Lotrel Capsules........ 840

Captopril (Potential for hyperkalemia, cardiac arrhythmias or cardiac arrest). Products include:

Capoten 739
Capozide 742

Enalapril Maleate (Potential for hyperkalemia, cardiac arrhythmias or cardiac arrest). Products include:

Vaseretic Tablets........ 1765
Vasotec Tablets 1771

Enalaprilat (Potential for hyperkalemia, cardiac arrhythmias or cardiac arrest). Products include:

Vasotec I.V........ 1768

Fosinopril Sodium (Potential for hyperkalemia, cardiac arrhythmias or cardiac arrest). Products include:

Monopril Tablets 757

Lisinopril (Potential for hyperkalemia, cardiac arrhythmias or cardiac arrest). Products include:

Prinivil Tablets 1733
Prinzide Tablets 1737
Zestoretic 2850
Zestril Tablets 2854

Lithium Carbonate (Concurrent use may potentiate the hypothyroid and goitrogenic effect). Products include:

Eskalith 2485
Lithium Carbonate Capsules & Tablets........ 2230
Lithonate/Lithotabs/Lithobid 2543

Lithium Citrate (Concurrent use may potentiate the hypothyroid and goitrogenic effect).

No products indexed under this heading.

Methimazole (Concurrent use may potentiate the hypothyroid and goitrogenic effect). Products include:

Tapazole Tablets 1477

Moexipril Hydrochloride (Potential for hyperkalemia, cardiac arrhythmias or cardiac arrest). Products include:

Univasc Tablets 2410

Potassium Acid Phosphate (Potential for hyperkalemia, cardiac arrhythmias or cardiac arrest). Products include:

K-Phos Original Formula 'Sodium Free' Tablets 639

Potassium Bicarbonate (Potential for hyperkalemia, cardiac arrhythmias or cardiac arrest). Products include:

Alka-Seltzer Gold Effervescent Antacid........ ⊡ 703

Potassium Chloride (Potential for hyperkalemia, cardiac arrhythmias or cardiac arrest). Products include:

Chlor-3 Condiment 1004
K-Dur Microburst Release System (potassium chloride, USP) E.R. Tablets 1325
K-Lor Powder Packets 434
K-Norm Extended-Release Capsules 991
K-Tab Filmtab 434
Kolyum Liquid 992
Micro-K........ 2063
Micro-K LS Packets........ 2064
NuLYTELY........ 689
Cherry Flavor NuLYTELY 689
Rum-K Syrup 1005
Slow-K Extended-Release Tablets........ 851

Potassium Citrate (Potential for hyperkalemia, cardiac arrhythmias or cardiac arrest). Products include:

Polycitra Syrup 578
Polycitra-K Crystals 579
Polycitra-K Oral Solution 579
Polycitra-LC 578

Potassium Gluconate (Potential for hyperkalemia, cardiac arrhythmias or cardiac arrest). Products include:

Kolyum Liquid 992

Potassium Phosphate, Dibasic (Potential for hyperkalemia, cardiac arrhythmias or cardiac arrest).

No products indexed under this heading.

Potassium Phosphate, Monobasic (Potential for hyperkalemia, cardiac arrhythmias or cardiac arrest). Products include:

K-Phos Neutral Tablets 639
K-Phos Original Formula 'Sodium Free' Tablets 639

Quinapril Hydrochloride (Potential for hyperkalemia, cardiac arrhythmias or cardiac arrest). Products include:

Accupril Tablets 1893

Ramipril (Potential for hyperkalemia, cardiac arrhythmias or cardiac arrest). Products include:

Altace Capsules 1232

Spirapril Hydrochloride (Potential for hyperkalemia, cardiac arrhythmias or cardiac arrest).

No products indexed under this heading.

Spironolactone (Potential for hyperkalemia, cardiac arrhythmias or cardiac arrest). Products include:

Aldactazide........ 2413
Aldactone 2414

Triamterene (Potential for hyperkalemia, cardiac arrhythmias or cardiac arrest). Products include:

Dyazide 2479
Dyrenium Capsules........ 2481
Maxzide 1380

SAFE TUSSIN 30
(Dextromethorphan Hydrobromide, Guaifenesin) 1363
None cited in PDR database.

SAF-GEL
(Dressings, sterile)........2867
None cited in PDR database.

SALAC
(Salicylic Acid) 1055
None cited in PDR database.

SALAGEN TABLETS
(Pilocarpine Hydrochloride) 1489
May interact with beta blockers, parasympathomimetics, anticholinergics, and certain other agents. Compounds in these categories include:

Acebutolol Hydrochloride (Potential for conduction disturbances). Products include:

Sectral Capsules 2807

Atenolol (Potential for conduction disturbances). Products include:

Tenoretic Tablets........ 2845
Tenormin Tablets and I.V. Injection 2847

Atropine Sulfate (Pilocarpine might antagonize the anticholinergic effects of drugs used concomitantly). Products include:

Arco-Lase Plus Tablets 512
Atrohist Plus Tablets 454
Atropine Sulfate Sterile Ophthalmic Solution .... ⊙ 233
Donnatal 2060
Donnatal Extentabs........ 2061
Donnatal Tablets 2060
Lomotil........ 2439
Motofen Tablets 784
Urised Tablets........ 1964

Belladonna Alkaloids (Pilocarpine might antagonize the anticholinergic effects of drugs used concomitantly). Products include:

Bellergal-S Tablets 2250
Hyland's Bed Wetting Tablets .... ⊡ 828
Hyland's EnurAid Tablets........ ⊡ 829
Hyland's Teething Tablets .... ⊡ 830

Benztropine Mesylate (Pilocarpine might antagonize the anticholinergic effects of drugs used concomitantly). Products include:

Cogentin 1621

Betaxolol Hydrochloride (Potential for conduction disturbances). Products include:

Betoptic Ophthalmic Solution........ 469
Betoptic S Ophthalmic Suspension 471
Kerlone Tablets........ 2436

Biperiden Hydrochloride (Pilocarpine might antagonize the anticholinergic effects of drugs used concomitantly). Products include:

Akineton 1333

Bisoprolol Fumarate (Potential for conduction disturbances). Products include:

Zebeta Tablets 1413
Ziac 1415

Carteolol Hydrochloride (Potential for conduction disturbances). Products include:

Cartrol Tablets 410
Ocupress Ophthalmic Solution, 1% Sterile........ ⊙ 309

Clidinium Bromide (Pilocarpine might antagonize the anticholinergic effects of drugs used concomitantly). Products include:

Librax Capsules 2176
Quarzan Capsules 2181

Dicyclomine Hydrochloride (Pilocarpine might antagonize the anticholinergic effects of drugs used concomitantly). Products include:

Bentyl 1501

Edrophonium Chloride (Additive pharmacologic effect). Products include:

Tensilon Injectable 1261

Esmolol Hydrochloride (Potential for conduction disturbances). Products include:

Brevibloc Injection........ 1808

Glycopyrrolate (Pilocarpine might antagonize the anticholinergic effects of drugs used concomitantly). Products include:

Robinul Forte Tablets........ 2072
Robinul Injectable 2072
Robinul Tablets........ 2072

Hyoscyamine (Pilocarpine might antagonize the anticholinergic effects of drugs used concomitantly). Products include:

Cystospaz Tablets 1963
Urised Tablets 1964

Hyoscyamine Sulfate (Pilocarpine might antagonize the anticholinergic effects of drugs used concomitantly). Products include:

Arco-Lase Plus Tablets 512
Atrohist Plus Tablets 454
Cystospaz-M Capsules 1963
Donnatal 2060
Donnatal Extentabs........ 2061
Donnatal Tablets 2060
Kutrase Capsules........ 2402
Levsin/Levsinex/Levbid 2405

Ipratropium Bromide (Pilocarpine might antagonize the anticholinergic effects of drugs used concomitantly). Products include:

Atrovent Inhalation Aerosol........ 671
Atrovent Inhalation Solution 673

Labetalol Hydrochloride (Potential for conduction disturbances). Products include:

Normodyne Injection 2377
Normodyne Tablets 2379
Trandate 1185

Levobunolol Hydrochloride (Potential for conduction disturbances). Products include:

Betagan .... ⊙ 233

Mepenzolate Bromide (Pilocarpine might antagonize the anticholinergic effects of drugs used concomitantly).

No products indexed under this heading.

Metipranolol Hydrochloride (Potential for conduction disturbances). Products include:

OptiPranolol (Metipranolol 0.3%) Sterile Ophthalmic Solution........ ⊙ 258

Metoprolol Succinate (Potential for conduction disturbances). Products include:

Toprol-XL Tablets 565

Metoprolol Tartrate (Potential for conduction disturbances). Products include:

Lopressor Ampuls 830
Lopressor HCT Tablets 832
Lopressor Tablets 830

Nadolol (Potential for conduction disturbances).

No products indexed under this heading.

Neostigmine Bromide (Additive pharmacologic effect). Products include:

Prostigmin Tablets 1261

Neostigmine Methylsulfate (Additive pharmacologic effect). Products include:

Prostigmin Injectable 1260

Oxybutynin Chloride (Pilocarpine might antagonize the anticholinergic effects of drugs used concomitantly). Products include:

Ditropan........ 1516

Penbutolol Sulfate (Potential for conduction disturbances). Products include:

Levatol 2403

Pindolol (Potential for conduction disturbances). Products include:

Visken Tablets........ 2299

Procyclidine Hydrochloride (Pilocarpine might antagonize the anticholinergic effects of drugs used concomitantly). Products include:

Kemadrin Tablets 1112

Propantheline Bromide (Pilocarpine might antagonize the anticholinergic effects of drugs used concomitantly). Products include:

Pro-Banthine Tablets 2052

(⊡ Described in PDR For Nonprescription Drugs) (⊙ Described in PDR For Ophthalmology)

919 **Interactions Index** **Salflex**

Propranolol Hydrochloride (Potential for conduction disturbances). Products include:
- Inderal ... 2728
- Inderal LA Long Acting Capsules ... 2730
- Inderide Tablets ... 2732
- Inderide LA Long Acting Capsules .. 2734

Pyridostigmine Bromide (Additive pharmacologic effect). Products include:
- Mestinon Injectable ... 1253
- Mestinon ... 1254

Scopolamine (Pilocarpine might antagonize the anticholinergic effects of drugs used concomitantly). Products include:
- Transderm Scōp Transdermal Therapeutic System ... 869

Scopolamine Hydrobromide (Pilocarpine might antagonize the anticholinergic effects of drugs used concomitantly). Products include:
- Atrohist Plus Tablets ... 454
- Donnatal ... 2060
- Donnatal Extentabs ... 2061
- Donnatal Tablets ... 2060

Sotalol Hydrochloride (Potential for conduction disturbances). Products include:
- Betapace Tablets ... 641

Timolol Hemihydrate (Potential for conduction disturbances). Products include:
- Betimol 0.25%, 0.5% ... ⊙ 261

Timolol Maleate (Potential for conduction disturbances). Products include:
- Blocadren Tablets ... 1614
- Timolide Tablets ... 1748
- Timoptic in Ocudose ... 1753
- Timoptic Sterile Ophthalmic Solution ... 1751
- Timoptic-XE ... 1755

Tridihexethyl Chloride (Pilocarpine might antagonize the anticholinergic effects of drugs used concomitantly).
- No products indexed under this heading.

Trihexyphenidyl Hydrochloride (Pilocarpine might antagonize the anticholinergic effects of drugs used concomitantly). Products include:
- Artane ... 1368

Food Interactions

Diet, high-lipid (Decrease in the rate of absorption of pilocarpine when taken with high fat meal).

SALFLEX TABLETS

(Salsalate) ... 786

May interact with antigout agents, salicylates, urinary alkalizing agents, oral anticoagulants, oral hypoglycemic agents, penicillins, corticosteroids, and certain other agents. Compounds in these categories include:

Acarbose (Hypoglycemic effect may be enhanced).
- No products indexed under this heading.

Allopurinol (Uricosuric action antagonized). Products include:
- Zyloprim Tablets ... 1226

Amoxicillin Trihydrate (Competition for protein binding site). Products include:
- Amoxil ... 2464
- Augmentin ... 2468

Ampicillin Sodium (Competition for protein binding site). Products include:
- Unasyn ... 2212

Aspirin (Potential for additive effect and toxicity). Products include:
- Alka-Seltzer Effervescent Antacid and Pain Reliever ... ◙ 701
- Alka-Seltzer Extra Strength Effervescent Antacid and Pain Reliever ... ◙ 703
- Alka-Seltzer Lemon Lime Effervescent Antacid and Pain Reliever ... ◙ 703
- Alka-Seltzer Plus Cold Medicine ... ◙ 705
- Alka-Seltzer Plus Cold & Cough Medicine ... ◙ 708
- Alka-Seltzer Plus Night-Time Cold Medicine ... ◙ 707
- Alka Seltzer Plus Sinus Medicine .. ◙ 707
- Arthritis Foundation Safety Coated Aspirin Tablets ... ◙ 675
- Arthritis Pain Ascriptin ... ◙ 631
- Maximum Strength Ascriptin ... ◙ 630
- Regular Strength Ascriptin Tablets ... ◙ 629
- Arthritis Strength BC Powder ... ◙ 609
- BC Cold Powder Multi-Symptom Formula (Cold-Sinus-Allergy) ... ◙ 609
- BC Cold Powder Non-Drowsy Formula (Cold-Sinus) ... ◙ 609
- BC Powder ... ◙ 609
- Bayer Children's Chewable Aspirin ... ◙ 711
- Genuine Bayer Aspirin Tablets & Caplets ... ◙ 713
- Extra Strength Bayer Arthritis Pain Regimen Formula ... ◙ 711
- Extra Strength Bayer Aspirin Caplets & Tablets ... ◙ 712
- Extended-Release Bayer 8-Hour Aspirin ... ◙ 712
- Extra Strength Bayer Plus Aspirin Caplets ... ◙ 713
- Extra Strength Bayer PM Aspirin .. ◙ 713
- Bayer Enteric Aspirin ... ◙ 709
- Bufferin Analgesic Tablets and Caplets ... ◙ 613
- Arthritis Strength Bufferin Analgesic Caplets ... ◙ 614
- Extra Strength Bufferin Analgesic Tablets ... ◙ 615
- Cama Arthritis Pain Reliever ... ◙ 785
- Darvon Compound-65 Pulvules ... 1435
- Easprin ... 1914
- Ecotrin ... 2455
- Ecotrin Enteric Coated Aspirin Maximum Strength Tablets and Caplets ... ◙ 816
- Ecotrin Enteric Coated Aspirin Regular Strength Tablets ... 2455
- Empirin Aspirin Tablets ... ◙ 854
- Empirin with Codeine Tablets ... 1093
- Excedrin Extra-Strength Analgesic Tablets & Caplets ... 732
- Fiorinal Capsules ... 2261
- Fiorinal with Codeine Capsules ... 2262
- Fiorinal Tablets ... 2261
- Halfprin ... 1362
- Healthprin Aspirin ... 2455
- Norgesic ... 1496
- Percodan Tablets ... 939
- Percodan-Demi Tablets ... 940
- Robaxisal Tablets ... 2071
- Soma Compound w/Codeine Tablets ... 2676
- Soma Compound Tablets ... 2675
- St. Joseph Adult Chewable Aspirin (81 mg.) ... ◙ 808
- Talwin Compound ... 2335
- Ursinus Inlay-Tabs ... ◙ 794
- Vanquish Analgesic Caplets ... ◙ 731

Azlocillin Sodium (Competition for protein binding site).
- No products indexed under this heading.

Bacampicillin Hydrochloride (Competition for protein binding site). Products include:
- Spectrobid Tablets ... 2206

Betamethasone Acetate (Competition for protein binding sites). Products include:
- Celestone Soluspan Suspension ... 2347

Betamethasone Sodium Phosphate (Competition for protein binding sites). Products include:
- Celestone Soluspan Suspension ... 2347

Carbenicillin Disodium (Competition for protein binding site).
- No products indexed under this heading.

Carbenicillin Indanyl Sodium (Competition for protein binding site). Products include:
- Geocillin Tablets ... 2199

Chlorpropamide (Hypoglycemic effect may be enhanced). Products include:
- Diabinese Tablets ... 1935

Choline Magnesium Trisalicylate (Potential for additive effect and toxicity). Products include:
- Trilisate ... 2000

Cortisone Acetate (Competition for protein binding sites). Products include:
- Cortone Acetate Sterile Suspension ... 1623
- Cortone Acetate Tablets ... 1624

Dexamethasone (Competition for protein binding sites). Products include:
- AK-Trol Ointment & Suspension ... ⊙ 205
- Decadron Elixir ... 1633
- Decadron Tablets ... 1635
- Decaspray Topical Aerosol ... 1648
- Dexacidin Ointment ... ⊙ 263
- Maxitrol Ophthalmic Ointment and Suspension ... ⊙ 224
- TobraDex Ophthalmic Suspension and Ointment ... 473

Dexamethasone Acetate (Competition for protein binding sites). Products include:
- Dalalone D.P. Injectable ... 1011
- Decadron-LA Sterile Suspension ... 1646

Dexamethasone Sodium Phosphate (Competition for protein binding sites). Products include:
- Decadron Phosphate Injection ... 1637
- Decadron Phosphate Respihaler ... 1642
- Decadron Phosphate Sterile Ophthalmic Ointment ... 1641
- Decadron Phosphate Sterile Ophthalmic Solution ... 1642
- Decadron Phosphate Topical Cream ... 1644
- Decadron Phosphate Turbinaire ... 1645
- Decadron Phosphate with Xylocaine Injection, Sterile ... 1639
- Dexacort Phosphate in Respihaler .. 458
- Dexacort Phosphate in Turbinaire .. 459
- NeoDecadron Sterile Ophthalmic Ointment ... 1712
- NeoDecadron Sterile Ophthalmic Solution ... 1713
- NeoDecadron Topical Cream ... 1714

Dicloxacillin Sodium (Competition for protein binding site).
- No products indexed under this heading.

Dicumarol (Increased potential for systemic bleeding).
- No products indexed under this heading.

Diflunisal (Potential for additive effect and toxicity). Products include:
- Dolobid Tablets ... 1654

Fludrocortisone Acetate (Competition for protein binding sites). Products include:
- Florinef Acetate Tablets ... 505

Glipizide (Hypoglycemic effect may be enhanced). Products include:
- Glucotrol Tablets ... 1967
- Glucotrol XL Extended Release Tablets ... 1968

Glyburide (Hypoglycemic effect may be enhanced). Products include:
- DiaBeta Tablets ... 1239
- Glynase PresTab Tablets ... 2609
- Micronase Tablets ... 2623

Hydrocortisone (Competition for protein binding sites). Products include:
- Anusol-HC Cream 2.5% ... 1896
- Aquanil HC Lotion ... 1931
- Bactine Hydrocortisone Anti-Itch Cream ... ◙ 709
- Caldecort Anti-Itch Hydrocortisone Spray ... ◙ 631
- Cortaid ... ◙ 836
- CORTENEMA ... 2535
- Cortisporin Ointment ... 1085
- Cortisporin Ophthalmic Ointment Sterile ... 1085
- Cortisporin Ophthalmic Suspension Sterile ... 1086
- Cortisporin Otic Solution Sterile ... 1087
- Cortisporin Otic Suspension Sterile 1088
- Cortizone-5 ... ◙ 831
- Cortizone-10 ... ◙ 831
- Hydrocortone Tablets ... 1672
- Hytone ... 907
- Massengill Medicated Soft Cloth Towelettes ... 2458
- PediOtic Suspension Sterile ... 1153
- Preparation H Hydrocortisone 1% Cream ... ◙ 872
- ProctoCream-HC 2.5% ... 2408
- VōSoL HC Otic Solution ... 2678

Hydrocortisone Acetate (Competition for protein binding sites). Products include:
- Analpram-HC Rectal Cream 1% and 2.5% ... 977
- Anusol HC-1 Anti-Itch Hydrocortisone Ointment ... ◙ 847
- Anusol-HC Suppositories ... 1897
- Caldecort ... ◙ 631
- Carmol HC ... 924
- Coly-Mycin S Otic w/Neomycin & Hydrocortisone ... 1906
- Cortaid ... ◙ 836
- Cortifoam ... 2396
- Cortisporin Cream ... 1084
- Epifoam ... 2399
- Hydrocortone Acetate Sterile Suspension ... 1669
- Mantadil Cream ... 1135
- Nupercainal Hydrocortisone 1% Cream ... ◙ 645
- Ophthocort ... ⊙ 311
- Pramosone Cream, Lotion & Ointment ... 978
- ProctoCream-HC ... 2408
- ProctoFoam-HC ... 2409
- Terra-Cortril Ophthalmic Suspension ... 2210

Hydrocortisone Sodium Phosphate (Competition for protein binding sites). Products include:
- Hydrocortone Phosphate Injection, Sterile ... 1670

Hydrocortisone Sodium Succinate (Competition for protein binding sites). Products include:
- Solu-Cortef Sterile Powder ... 2641

Magnesium Salicylate (Potential for additive effect and toxicity). Products include:
- Backache Caplets ... ◙ 613
- Bayer Select Backache Pain Relief Formula ... ◙ 715
- Doan's Extra-Strength Analgesic ... ◙ 633
- Extra Strength Doan's P.M. ... ◙ 633
- Doan's Regular Strength Analgesic ... ◙ 634
- Mobigesic Tablets ... ◙ 602

Metformin Hydrochloride (Hypoglycemic effect may be enhanced). Products include:
- Glucophage ... 752

Methotrexate Sodium (Competition for protein binding site). Products include:
- Methotrexate Sodium Tablets, Injection, for Injection and LPF Injection ... 1275

Methylprednisolone Acetate (Competition for protein binding sites). Products include:
- Depo-Medrol Single-Dose Vial ... 2600
- Depo-Medrol Sterile Aqueous Suspension ... 2597

Methylprednisolone Sodium Succinate (Competition for protein binding sites). Products include:
- Solu-Medrol Sterile Powder ... 2643

Mezlocillin Sodium (Competition for protein binding site). Products include:
- Mezlin ... 601
- Mezlin Pharmacy Bulk Package ... 604

Nafcillin Sodium (Competition for protein binding site).
- No products indexed under this heading.

IMPORTANT NOTE: Always consult each drug listing in the patient's regimen for possible interactions.

Salflex **Interactions Index** 920

Naproxen (Competition for protein binding site). Products include:
- Anaprox/Naprosyn 2117

Naproxen Sodium (Competition for protein binding site). Products include:
- Aleve 1975
- Anaprox/Naprosyn 2117

Penicillin G Benzathine (Competition for protein binding site). Products include:
- Bicillin C-R Injection 2704
- Bicillin C-R 900/300 Injection 2706
- Bicillin L-A Injection 2707

Penicillin G Potassium (Competition for protein binding site). Products include:
- Pfizerpen for Injection 2203

Penicillin G Procaine (Competition for protein binding site). Products include:
- Bicillin C-R Injection 2704
- Bicillin C-R 900/300 Injection 2706

Penicillin G Sodium (Competition for protein binding site).
- No products indexed under this heading.

Penicillin V Potassium (Competition for protein binding site). Products include:
- Pen•Vee K 2772

Phenytoin (Competition for protein binding site). Products include:
- Dilantin Infatabs 1908
- Dilantin-125 Suspension 1911

Phenytoin Sodium (Competition for protein binding site). Products include:
- Dilantin Kapseals 1906
- Dilantin Parenteral 1910

Potassium Citrate (Lowers plasma levels of salicylic acid). Products include:
- Polycitra Syrup 578
- Polycitra-K Crystals 579
- Polycitra-K Oral Solution 579
- Polycitra-LC 578

Prednisolone Acetate (Competition for protein binding sites). Products include:
- AK-CIDE .... ⊙ 202
- AK-CIDE Ointment .... ⊙ 202
- Blephamide Liquifilm Sterile Ophthalmic Suspension 476
- Blephamide Ointment .... ⊙ 237
- Econopred & Econopred Plus Ophthalmic Suspensions .... ⊙ 217
- Poly-Pred Liquifilm .... ⊙ 248
- Pred Forte .... ⊙ 250
- Pred Mild .... ⊙ 253
- Pred-G Liquifilm Sterile Ophthalmic Suspension .... ⊙ 251
- Pred-G S.O.P. Sterile Ophthalmic Ointment .... ⊙ 252
- Vasocidin Ointment .... ⊙ 268

Prednisolone Sodium Phosphate (Competition for protein binding sites). Products include:
- AK-Pred .... ⊙ 204
- Hydeltrasol Injection, Sterile 1665
- Inflamase .... ⊙ 265
- Pediapred Oral Liquid 995
- Vasocidin Ophthalmic Solution .... ⊙ 270

Prednisolone Tebutate (Competition for protein binding sites). Products include:
- Hydeltra-T.B.A. Sterile Suspension 1667

Prednisone (Competition for protein binding sites). Products include:
- Deltasone Tablets 2595

Probenecid (Uricosuric action antagonized). Products include:
- Benemid Tablets 1611
- ColBENEMID Tablets 1622

Sodium Citrate (Lowers plasma levels of salicylic acid). Products include:
- Bicitra 578
- Citrocarbonate Antacid .... ⊞ 770
- Polycitra 578

- Salix SST Lozenges Saliva Stimulant .... ⊞ 797

Sulfinpyrazone (Uricosuric action antagonized). Products include:
- Anturane 807

Thyroxine Sodium (Competition for protein binding site).
- No products indexed under this heading.

Ticarcillin Disodium (Competition for protein binding site). Products include:
- Ticar for Injection 2526
- Timentin for Injection 2528

Tolazamide (Hypoglycemic effect may be enhanced).
- No products indexed under this heading.

Tolbutamide (Hypoglycemic effect may be enhanced).
- No products indexed under this heading.

Triamcinolone (Competition for protein binding sites). Products include:
- Aristocort Tablets 1022

Triamcinolone Acetonide (Competition for protein binding sites). Products include:
- Aristocort A 0.025% Cream 1027
- Aristocort A 0.5% Cream 1031
- Aristocort A 0.1% Cream 1029
- Aristocort A 0.1% Ointment 1030
- Azmacort Oral Inhaler 2011
- Nasacort Nasal Inhaler 2024

Triamcinolone Diacetate (Competition for protein binding sites). Products include:
- Aristocort Suspension (Forte Parenteral) 1027
- Aristocort Suspension (Intralesional) 1025

Triamcinolone Hexacetonide (Competition for protein binding sites). Products include:
- Aristospan Suspension (Intra-articular) 1033
- Aristospan Suspension (Intralesional) 1032

l-Triiodothyronine (Competition for protein binding site).

Warfarin Sodium (Increased potential for systemic bleeding; competition for protein binding site). Products include:
- Coumadin 926

Food Interactions

Food, unspecified (Slows the absorption).

SALINEX NASAL MIST AND DROPS
(Sodium Chloride) .... ⊞ 734
None cited in PDR database.

SALIVART SALIVA SUBSTITUTE
(Sodium Carboxymethylcellulose) .. ⊞ 656
None cited in PDR database.

SALIX SST LOZENGES SALIVA STIMULANT
(Sorbitol, Malic Acid, Sodium Citrate, Citric Acid, Dicalcium Phosphate) .... ⊞ 797
None cited in PDR database.

SANDIMMUNE I.V. AMPULS FOR INFUSION
(Cyclosporine) 2286
May interact with immunosuppressive agents, potassium sparing diuretics, and certain other agents. Compounds in these categories include:

Amiloride Hydrochloride (Cyclosporine may cause hyperkalemia, concurrent use should be avoided). Products include:
- Midamor Tablets 1703
- Moduretic Tablets 1705

Amphotericin B (Potential synergies of nephrotoxicity may occur). Products include:
- Fungizone Intravenous 506

Antibiotics, unspecified (Potential synergies of nephrotoxicity may occur).

Azapropazon (Potential nephrotoxic synergy).

Azathioprine (Increases susceptibility to infection). Products include:
- Imuran 1110

Bromocriptine Mesylate (Increases cyclosporine levels; dosage adjustments are essential). Products include:
- Parlodel 2281

Carbamazepine (Decreases cyclosporine plasma concentrations; dosage adjustments are essential). Products include:
- Atretol Tablets 573
- Tegretol Chewable Tablets 852
- Tegretol Suspension 852
- Tegretol Tablets 852

Cimetidine (Potential nephrotoxic synergy). Products include:
- Tagamet Tablets 2516

Cimetidine Hydrochloride (Potential nephrotoxic synergy). Products include:
- Tagamet 2516

Danazol (Increases cyclosporine plasma concentrations; dosage adjustments are essential). Products include:
- Danocrine Capsules 2307

Diclofenac Potassium (Potential nephrotoxic synergy). Products include:
- Cataflam 816

Diclofenac Sodium (Potential nephrotoxic synergy). Products include:
- Voltaren Ophthalmic Sterile Ophthalmic Solution .... ⊙ 272
- Voltaren Tablets 861

Digoxin (Reduced clearance of digoxin and potential for severe digitalis toxicity). Products include:
- Lanoxicaps 1117
- Lanoxin Elixir Pediatric 1120
- Lanoxin Injection 1123
- Lanoxin Injection Pediatric 1126
- Lanoxin Tablets 1128

Diltiazem Hydrochloride (Increases cyclosporine plasma concentrations; dosage adjustments are essential). Products include:
- Cardizem CD Capsules 1506
- Cardizem SR Capsules 1510
- Cardizem Injectable 1508
- Cardizem Tablets 1512
- Dilacor XR Extended-release Capsules 2018

Erythromycin (Increases cyclosporine plasma concentrations; dosage adjustments are essential). Products include:
- A/T/S 2% Acne Topical Gel and Solution 1234
- Benzamycin Topical Gel 905
- E-Mycin Tablets 1341
- Emgel 2% Topical Gel 1093
- ERYC 1915
- Erycette (erythromycin 2%) Topical Solution 1888
- Ery-Tab Tablets 422
- Erythromycin Base Filmtab 426
- Erythromycin Delayed-Release Capsules, USP 427
- Ilotycin Ophthalmic Ointment 912
- PCE Dispertab Tablets 444
- T-Stat 2.0% Topical Solution and Pads 2688
- Theramycin Z Topical Solution 2% 1592

Erythromycin Estolate (Increases cyclosporine plasma concentrations; dosage adjustments are essential). Products include:
- Ilosone 911

Erythromycin Ethylsuccinate (Increases cyclosporine plasma concentrations; dosage adjustments are essential). Products include:
- E.E.S. 424
- EryPed 421

Erythromycin Gluceptate (Increases cyclosporine plasma concentrations; dosage adjustments are essential). Products include:
- Ilotycin Gluceptate, IV, Vials 913

Erythromycin Lactobionate (Increases cyclosporine plasma concentrations; dosage adjustments are essential).
- No products indexed under this heading.

Erythromycin Stearate (Increases cyclosporine plasma concentrations; dosage adjustments are essential). Products include:
- Erythrocin Stearate Filmtab 425

Fluconazole (Increases cyclosporine levels; dosage adjustments are essential). Products include:
- Diflucan Injection, Tablets, and Oral Suspension 2194

Gentamicin Sulfate (Potential synergies of nephrotoxicity may occur). Products include:
- Garamycin Injectable 2360
- Genoptic Sterile Ophthalmic Solution .... ⊙ 243
- Genoptic Sterile Ophthalmic Ointment .... ⊙ 243
- Gentacidin Ointment .... ⊙ 264
- Gentacidin Solution .... ⊙ 264
- Gentak .... ⊙ 208
- Pred-G Liquifilm Sterile Ophthalmic Suspension .... ⊙ 251
- Pred-G S.O.P. Sterile Ophthalmic Ointment .... ⊙ 252

Immune Globulin (Human) (Increases susceptibility to infection).
- No products indexed under this heading.

Immune Globulin Intravenous (Human) (Increases susceptibility to infection).

Itraconazole (Increases cyclosporine levels; dosage adjustments are essential). Products include:
- Sporanox Capsules 1305

Ketoconazole (Potential nephrotoxic synergy; increases cyclosporine plasma concentrations; dosage adjustments are essential). Products include:
- Nizoral 2% Cream 1297
- Nizoral 2% Shampoo 1298
- Nizoral Tablets 1298

Lovastatin (Reduced clearance of lovastatin; concomitant administration associated with development of myositis). Products include:
- Mevacor Tablets 1699

Melphalan (Potential nephrotoxic synergy). Products include:
- Alkeran Tablets 1071

Methylprednisolone (Increases cyclosporine plasma concentrations; dosage adjustments are essential; convulsions have occurred with high dose methylprednisolone). Products include:
- Medrol 2621

Methylprednisolone Acetate (Increases cyclosporine plasma concentrations; dosage adjustments are essential; convulsions have occurred with high dose methylprednisolone). Products include:
- Depo-Medrol Single-Dose Vial 2600

(⊞ Described in PDR For Nonprescription Drugs) (⊙ Described in PDR For Ophthalmology)

921 **Interactions Index** **Sandostatin**

Depo-Medrol Sterile Aqueous Suspension 2597

Methylprednisolone Sodium Succinate (Increases cyclosporine plasma concentrations; dosage adjustments are essential; convulsions have occurred with high dose methylprednisolone). Products include:
Solu-Medrol Sterile Powder 2643

Metoclopramide Hydrochloride (Increases cyclosporine levels; dosage adjustments are essential). Products include:
Reglan 2068

Muromonab-CD3 (Increased susceptibility to infection and increased risk for development of lymphomas and malignancies). Products include:
Orthoclone OKT3 Sterile Solution .. 1837

Mycophenolate Mofetil (Increases susceptibility to infection). Products include:
CellCept Capsules 2099

Nephrotoxic Drugs (Potential synergics of nephrotoxicity).

Nicardipine Hydrochloride (Increases cyclosporine plasma concentrations; dosage adjustments are essential). Products include:
Cardene Capsules 2095
Cardene I.V. 2709
Cardene SR Capsules 2097

Nifedipine (Potential for frequent gingival hyperplasia). Products include:
Adalat Capsules (10 mg and 20 mg) 587
Adalat CC 589
Procardia Capsules 1971
Procardia XL Extended Release Tablets 1972

Phenobarbital (Decreases cyclosporine plasma levels; dosage adjustments are essential). Products include:
Arco-Lase Plus Tablets 512
Bellergal-S Tablets 2250
Donnatal 2060
Donnatal Extentabs 2061
Donnatal Tablets 2060
Phenobarbital Elixir and Tablets 1469
Quadrinal Tablets 1350

Phenytoin (Decreases cyclosporine plasma levels; dosage adjustments are essential). Products include:
Dilantin Infatabs 1908
Dilantin-125 Suspension 1911

Phenytoin Sodium (Decreases cyclosporine plasma levels; dosage adjustments are essential). Products include:
Dilantin Kapseals 1906
Dilantin Parenteral 1910

Prednisolone (Reduced clearance of prednisolone). Products include:
Prelone Syrup 1787

Prednisolone Acetate (Reduced clearance of prednisolone). Products include:
AK-CIDE .... ⊙ 202
AK-CIDE Ointment .... ⊙ 202
Blephamide Liquifilm Sterile Ophthalmic Suspension 476
Blephamide Ointment .... ⊙ 237
Econopred & Econopred Plus Ophthalmic Suspensions .... ⊙ 217
Poly-Pred Liquifilm .... ⊙ 248
Pred Forte .... ⊙ 250
Pred Mild .... ⊙ 253
Pred-G Liquifilm Sterile Ophthalmic Suspension .... ⊙ 251
Pred-G S.O.P. Sterile Ophthalmic Ointment .... ⊙ 252
Vasocidin Ointment .... ⊙ 268

Prednisolone Sodium Phosphate (Reduced clearance of prednisolone). Products include:
AK-Pred .... ⊙ 204
Hydeltrasol Injection, Sterile 1665
Inflamase .... ⊙ 265
Pediapred Oral Liquid 995
Vasocidin Ophthalmic Solution .... ⊙ 270

Prednisolone Tebutate (Reduced clearance of prednisolone). Products include:
Hydeltra-T.B.A. Sterile Suspension 1667

Ranitidine Hydrochloride (Potential nephrotoxic synergy). Products include:
Zantac 1209
Zantac Injection 1207
Zantac Syrup 1209

Rifampin (Decreases cyclosporine plasma levels; dosage adjustments are essential). Products include:
Rifadin 1528
Rifamate Capsules 1530
Rifater 1532
Rimactane Capsules 847

Spironolactone (Cyclosporine may cause hyperkalemia, concurrent use should be avoided). Products include:
Aldactazide 2413
Aldactone 2414

Sulfamethoxazole (Potential nephrotoxic synergy; decreases cyclosporine plasma levels; dosage adjustments are essential). Products include:
Azo Gantanol Tablets 2080
Bactrim DS Tablets 2084
Bactrim I.V. Infusion 2082
Bactrim 2084
Gantanol Tablets 2119
Septra 1174
Septra I.V. Infusion 1169
Septra I.V. Infusion ADD-Vantage Vials 1171
Septra 1174

Tacrolimus (Increases susceptibility to infection). Products include:
Prograf 1042

Tobramycin (Potential synergies of nephrotoxicity may occur). Products include:
AKTOB .... ⊙ 206
TobraDex Ophthalmic Suspension and Ointment 473
Tobrex Ophthalmic Ointment and Solution .... ⊙ 229

Tobramycin Sulfate (Potential synergies of nephrotoxicity may occur). Products include:
Nebcin Vials, Hyporets & ADD-Vantage 1464
Tobramycin Sulfate Injection 968

Triamterene (Cyclosporine may cause hyperkalemia, concurrent use should be avoided). Products include:
Dyazide 2479
Dyrenium Capsules 2481
Maxzide 1380

Trimethoprim (Potential nephrotoxic synergy; decreases cyclosporine plasma levels; dosage adjustments are essential). Products include:
Bactrim DS Tablets 2084
Bactrim I.V. Infusion 2082
Bactrim 2084
Proloprim Tablets 1155
Septra 1174
Septra I.V. Infusion 1169
Septra I.V. Infusion ADD-Vantage Vials 1171
Septra 1174
Trimpex Tablets 2163

Vancomycin Hydrochloride (Potential nephrotoxic synergy). Products include:
Vancocin HCl, Oral Solution & Pulvules 1483
Vancocin HCl, Vials & ADD-Vantage 1481

Verapamil Hydrochloride (Increases cyclosporine levels; dosage adjustments are essential). Products include:
Calan SR Caplets 2422
Calan Tablets 2419
Isoptin Injectable 1344
Isoptin Oral Tablets 1346
Isoptin SR Tablets 1348
Verelan Capsules 1410
Verelan Capsules 2824

SANDIMMUNE ORAL SOLUTION
(Cyclosporine) 2286
See **Sandimmune I.V. Ampuls for Infusion**

SANDIMMUNE SOFT GELATIN CAPSULES
(Cyclosporine) 2286
See **Sandimmune I.V. Ampuls for Infusion**

SANDOGLOBULIN I.V.
(Globulin, Immune (Human)) 2290
May interact with:

Measles, Mumps & Rubella Virus Vaccine Live (Antibodies in Immune Globulin may interfere with the response to live viral vaccines). Products include:
M-M-R II 1687

SANDOSTATIN INJECTION
(Octreotide Acetate) 2292
May interact with oral hypoglycemic agents, insulin, beta blockers, calcium channel blockers, and certain other agents. Compounds in these categories include:

Acarbose (Adjustment of the dosage of hypoglycemic agents may be required).
No products indexed under this heading.

Acebutolol Hydrochloride (Adjustment of the dosage of beta blockers may be required). Products include:
Sectral Capsules 2807

Amlodipine Besylate (Adjustment of the dosage of calcium channel blocker may be required). Products include:
Lotrel Capsules 840
Norvasc Tablets 1940

Atenolol (Adjustment of the dosage of beta blockers may be required). Products include:
Tenoretic Tablets 2845
Tenormin Tablets and I.V. Injection 2847

Bepridil Hydrochloride (Adjustment of the dosage of calcium channel blocker may be required). Products include:
Vascor (200, 300 and 400 mg) Tablets 1587

Betaxolol Hydrochloride (Adjustment of the dosage of beta blockers may be required). Products include:
Betoptic Ophthalmic Solution 469
Betoptic S Ophthalmic Suspension 471
Kerlone Tablets 2436

Bisoprolol Fumarate (Adjustment of the dosage of beta blockers may be required). Products include:
Zebeta Tablets 1413
Ziac 1415

Carteolol Hydrochloride (Adjustment of the dosage of beta blockers may be required). Products include:
Cartrol Tablets 410
Ocupress Ophthalmic Solution, 1% Sterile .... ⊙ 309

Chlorpropamide (Adjustment of the dosage of hypoglycemic agents may be required). Products include:
Diabinese Tablets 1935

Cyclosporine (Co-administration may decrease blood levels of cyclosporine and may result in transplant rejection). Products include:
Neoral 2276
Sandimmune 2286

Diazoxide (Adjustment of the dosage of diazoxide may be required). Products include:
Hyperstat I.V. Injection 2363
Proglycem 580

Diltiazem Hydrochloride (Adjustment of the dosage of calcium channel blocker may be required). Products include:
Cardizem CD Capsules 1506
Cardizem SR Capsules 1510
Cardizem Injectable 1508
Cardizem Tablets 1512
Dilacor XR Extended-release Capsules 2018

Esmolol Hydrochloride (Adjustment of the dosage of beta blockers may be required). Products include:
Brevibloc Injection 1808

Felodipine (Adjustment of the dosage of calcium channel blocker may be required). Products include:
Plendil Extended-Release Tablets 527

Glipizide (Adjustment of the dosage of hypoglycemic agents may be required). Products include:
Glucotrol Tablets 1967
Glucotrol XL Extended Release Tablets 1968

Glyburide (Adjustment of the dosage of hypoglycemic agents may be required). Products include:
DiaBeta Tablets 1239
Glynase PresTab Tablets 2609
Micronase Tablets 2623

Insulin, Human (Adjustment of the dosage of insulin may be required).
No products indexed under this heading.

Insulin, Human Isophane Suspension (Adjustment of the dosage of insulin may be required). Products include:
Novolin N Human Insulin 10 ml Vials 1795

Insulin, Human NPH (Adjustment of the dosage of insulin may be required). Products include:
Humulin N, 100 Units 1448
Novolin N PenFill Cartridges Durable Insulin Delivery System 1798
Novolin N Prefilled Syringe Disposable Insulin Delivery System 1798

Insulin, Human Regular (Adjustment of the dosage of insulin may be required). Products include:
Humulin R, 100 Units 1449
Novolin R Human Insulin 10 ml Vials 1795
Novolin R PenFill Cartridges Durable Insulin Delivery System 1798
Novolin R Prefilled Syringe Disposable Insulin Delivery System 1798
Velosulin BR Human Insulin 10 ml Vials 1795

Insulin, Human, Zinc Suspension (Adjustment of the dosage of insulin may be required). Products include:
Humulin L, 100 Units 1446
Humulin U, 100 Units 1450
Novolin L Human Insulin 10 ml Vials 1795

Insulin, NPH (Adjustment of the dosage of insulin may be required). Products include:
NPH, 100 Units 1450
Pork NPH, 100 Units 1452
Purified Pork NPH Isophane Insulin 1801

Insulin, Regular (Adjustment of the dosage of insulin may be required). Products include:
Regular, 100 Units 1450

IMPORTANT NOTE: Always consult each drug listing in the patient's regimen for possible interactions.

Sandostatin **Interactions Index** **922**

Pork Regular, 100 Units 1452
Pork Regular (Concentrated), 500 Units 1453
Purified Pork Regular Insulin 1801

Insulin, Zinc Crystals (Adjustment of the dosage of insulin may be required). Products include:
NPH, 100 Units 1450

Insulin, Zinc Suspension (Adjustment of the dosage of insulin may be required). Products include:
Iletin I 1450
Lente, 100 Units 1450
Iletin II 1452
Pork Lente, 100 Units 1452
Purified Pork Lente Insulin 1801

Isradipine (Adjustment of the dosage of calcium channel blocker may be required). Products include:
DynaCirc Capsules 2256

Labetalol Hydrochloride (Adjustment of the dosage of beta blockers may be required). Products include:
Normodyne Injection 2377
Normodyne Tablets 2379
Trandate 1185

Levobunolol Hydrochloride (Adjustment of the dosage of beta blockers may be required). Products include:
Betagan ..... ◉ 233

Metformin Hydrochloride (Adjustment of the dosage of hypoglycemic agents may be required). Products include:
Glucophage 752

Metipranolol Hydrochloride (Adjustment of the dosage of beta blockers may be required). Products include:
OptiPranolol (Metipranolol 0.3%) Sterile Ophthalmic Solution ..... ◉ 258

Metoprolol Succinate (Adjustment of the dosage of beta blockers may be required). Products include:
Toprol-XL Tablets 565

Metoprolol Tartrate (Adjustment of the dosage of beta blockers may be required). Products include:
Lopressor Ampuls 830
Lopressor HCT Tablets 832
Lopressor Tablets 830

Nadolol (Adjustment of the dosage of beta blockers may be required).
No products indexed under this heading.

Nicardipine Hydrochloride (Adjustment of the dosage of calcium channel blocker may be required). Products include:
Cardene Capsules 2095
Cardene I.V. 2709
Cardene SR Capsules 2097

Nifedipine (Adjustment of the dosage of calcium channel blocker may be required). Products include:
Adalat Capsules (10 mg and 20 mg) 587
Adalat CC 589
Procardia Capsules 1971
Procardia XL Extended Release Tablets 1972

Nimodipine (Adjustment of the dosage of calcium channel blocker may be required). Products include:
Nimotop Capsules 610

Nisoldipine (Adjustment of the dosage of calcium channel blocker may be required).
No products indexed under this heading.

Penbutolol Sulfate (Adjustment of the dosage of beta blockers may be required). Products include:
Levatol 2403

Pindolol (Adjustment of the dosage of beta blockers may be required). Products include:
Visken Tablets 2299

Propranolol Hydrochloride (Adjustment of the dosage of beta blockers may be required). Products include:
Inderal 2728
Inderal LA Long Acting Capsules 2730
Inderide Tablets 2732
Inderide LA Long Acting Capsules 2734

Sotalol Hydrochloride (Adjustment of the dosage of beta blockers may be required). Products include:
Betapace Tablets 641

Timolol Hemihydrate (Adjustment of the dosage of beta blockers may be required). Products include:
Betimol 0.25%, 0.5% ..... ◉ 261

Timolol Maleate (Adjustment of the dosage of beta blockers may be required). Products include:
Blocadren Tablets 1614
Timolide Tablets 1748
Timoptic in Ocudose 1753
Timoptic Sterile Ophthalmic Solution 1751
Timoptic-XE 1755

Tolazamide (Adjustment of the dosage of hypoglycemic agents may be required).
No products indexed under this heading.

Tolbutamide (Adjustment of the dosage of hypoglycemic agents may be required).
No products indexed under this heading.

Verapamil Hydrochloride (Adjustment of the dosage of calcium channel blocker may be required). Products include:
Calan SR Caplets 2422
Calan Tablets 2419
Isoptin Injectable 1344
Isoptin Oral Tablets 1346
Isoptin SR Tablets 1348
Verelan Capsules 1410
Verelan Capsules 2824

SANOREX TABLETS

(Mazindol) 2294

May interact with monoamine oxidase inhibitors, insulin, vasopressors, sympathomimetics, and certain other agents. Compounds in these categories include:

Albuterol (Mazindol may potentiate blood pressure increases in those patients taking sympathomimetics). Products include:
Proventil Inhalation Aerosol 2382
Ventolin Inhalation Aerosol and Refill 1197

Albuterol Sulfate (Mazindol may potentiate blood pressure increases in those patients taking sympathomimetics). Products include:
Airet Solution for Inhalation 452
Proventil Inhalation Solution 0.083% 2384
Proventil Repetabs Tablets 2386
Proventil Solution for Inhalation 0.5% 2383
Proventil Syrup 2385
Proventil Tablets 2386
Ventolin Inhalation Solution 1198
Ventolin Nebules Inhalation Solution 1199
Ventolin Rotacaps for Inhalation 1200
Ventolin Syrup 1202
Ventolin Tablets 1203
Volmax Extended-Release Tablets 1788

Dobutamine Hydrochloride (Mazindol may potentiate blood pressure increases in those patients taking sympathomimetics). Products include:
Dobutrex Solution Vials 1439

Dopamine Hydrochloride (Potentiated pressor effects; Mazindol may potentiate blood pressure increases in those patients taking sympathomimetics).
No products indexed under this heading.

Ephedrine Hydrochloride (Mazindol may potentiate blood pressure increases in those patients taking sympathomimetics). Products include:
Primatene Dual Action Formula ..... ▣ 872
Primatene Tablets ..... ▣ 873
Quadrinal Tablets 1350

Ephedrine Sulfate (Mazindol may potentiate blood pressure increases in those patients taking sympathomimetics). Products include:
Bronkaid Caplets ..... ▣ 717
Marax Tablets & DF Syrup 2200

Ephedrine Tannate (Mazindol may potentiate blood pressure increases in those patients taking sympathomimetics). Products include:
Rynatuss 2673

Epinephrine (Mazindol may potentiate blood pressure increases in those patients taking sympathomimetics). Products include:
Bronkaid Mist ..... ▣ 717
EPIFRIN ..... ◉ 239
EpiPen 790
Marcaine Hydrochloride with Epinephrine 1:200,000 2316
Primatene Mist ..... ▣ 873
Sensorcaine with Epinephrine Injection 559
Sus-Phrine Injection 1019
Xylocaine with Epinephrine Injections 567

Epinephrine Bitartrate (Mazindol may potentiate blood pressure increases in those patients taking sympathomimetics). Products include:
Bronkaid Mist Suspension ..... ▣ 718
Sensorcaine-MPF with Epinephrine Injection 559

Epinephrine Hydrochloride (Potentiated pressor effects; Mazindol may potentiate blood pressure increases in those patients taking sympathomimetics). Products include:
Ana-Kit Anaphylaxis Emergency Treatment Kit 617

Furazolidone (Concurrent use is contraindicated; potential for hypertensive crises). Products include:
Furoxone 2046

Guanethidine Monosulfate (Decreased hypotensive effect). Products include:
Esimil Tablets 822
Ismelin Tablets 827

Insulin, Human (Altered insulin requirements).
No products indexed under this heading.

Insulin, Human Isophane Suspension (Altered insulin requirements). Products include:
Novolin N Human Insulin 10 ml Vials 1795

Insulin, Human NPH (Altered insulin requirements). Products include:
Humulin N, 100 Units 1448
Novolin N PenFill Cartridges Durable Insulin Delivery System 1798
Novolin N Prefilled Syringe Disposable Insulin Delivery System 1798

Insulin, Human Regular (Altered insulin requirements). Products include:
Humulin R, 100 Units 1449
Novolin R Human Insulin 10 ml Vials 1795
Novolin R PenFill Cartridges Durable Insulin Delivery System 1798
Novolin R Prefilled Syringe Disposable Insulin Delivery System 1798
Velosulin BR Human Insulin 10 ml Vials 1795

Insulin, Human, Zinc Suspension (Altered insulin requirements). Products include:
Humulin L, 100 Units 1446
Humulin U, 100 Units 1450
Novolin L Human Insulin 10 ml Vials 1795

Insulin, NPH (Altered insulin requirements). Products include:
NPH, 100 Units 1450
Pork NPH, 100 Units 1452
Purified Pork NPH Isophane Insulin 1801

Insulin, Regular (Altered insulin requirements). Products include:
Regular, 100 Units 1450
Pork Regular, 100 Units 1452
Pork Regular (Concentrated), 500 Units 1453
Purified Pork Regular Insulin 1801

Insulin, Zinc Crystals (Altered insulin requirements). Products include:
NPH, 100 Units 1450

Insulin, Zinc Suspension (Altered insulin requirements). Products include:
Iletin I 1450
Lente, 100 Units 1450
Iletin II 1452
Pork Lente, 100 Units 1452
Purified Pork Lente Insulin 1801

Isocarboxazid (Concurrent use is contraindicated; potential for hypertensive crises).
No products indexed under this heading.

Isoproterenol Hydrochloride (Mazindol may potentiate blood pressure increases in those patients taking sympathomimetics). Products include:
Isuprel Hydrochloride Injection 1:5000 2311
Isuprel Hydrochloride Solution 1:200 & 1:100 2313
Isuprel Mistometer 2312

Isoproterenol Sulfate (Mazindol may potentiate blood pressure increases in those patients taking sympathomimetics). Products include:
Norisodrine with Calcium Iodide Syrup 442

Metaproterenol Sulfate (Mazindol may potentiate blood pressure increases in those patients taking sympathomimetics). Products include:
Alupent 669
Metaproterenol Sulfate Inhalation Solution, USP, Arm-a-Med 552

Metaraminol Bitartrate (Potentiated pressor effects; Mazindol may potentiate blood pressure increases in those patients taking sympathomimetics). Products include:
Aramine Injection 1609

Methoxamine Hydrochloride (Potentiated pressor effects; Mazindol may potentiate blood pressure increases in those patients taking sympathomimetics). Products include:
Vasoxyl Injection 1196

Norepinephrine Bitartrate (Potentiated pressor effects; Mazindol may potentiate blood pressure increases in those patients taking sympathomimetics). Products include:
Levophed Bitartrate Injection 2315

Phenelzine Sulfate (Concurrent use is contraindicated; potential for hypertensive crises). Products include:
Nardil 1920

(▣ Described in PDR For Nonprescription Drugs) (◉ Described in PDR For Ophthalmology)

Phenylephrine Bitartrate

(Mazindol may potentiate blood pressure increases in those patients taking sympathomimetics).

No products indexed under this heading.

Phenylephrine Hydrochloride

(Potentiated pressor effects; Mazindol may potentiate blood pressure increases in those patients taking sympathomimetics). Products include:

Atrohist Plus Tablets 454
Cerose DM .... ◉ 878
Comhist 2038
D.A. Chewable Tablets......................... 951
Deconsal Pediatric Capsules................ 454
Dura-Vent/DA Tablets 953
Entex Capsules 1986
Entex Liquid 1986
Extendryl 1005
4-Way Fast Acting Nasal Spray (regular & mentholated) .... ◉ 621
Hemorid For Women .... ◉ 834
Hycomine Compound Tablets 932
Neo-Synephrine Hydrochloride 1% Carpuject.. 2324
Neo-Synephrine Hydrochloride 1% Injection 2324
Neo-Synephrine Hydrochloride (Ophthalmic) 2325
Neo-Synephrine .... ◉ 726
Nöstril .... ◉ 644
Novahistine Elixir .... ◉ 823
Phenergan VC 2779
Phenergan VC with Codeine 2781
Preparation H .... ◉ 871
Tympagesic Ear Drops 2342
Vasosulf .... © 271
Vicks Sinex Nasal Spray and Ultra Fine Mist .... ◉ 765

Phenylephrine Tannate

(Mazindol may potentiate blood pressure increases in those patients taking sympathomimetics). Products include:

Atrohist Pediatric Suspension 454
Ricobid-D Pediatric Suspension........ 2038
Ricobid Tablets and Pediatric Suspension.. 2038
Rynatan 2673
Rynatuss 2673

Phenylpropanolamine Hydrochloride

(Mazindol may potentiate blood pressure increases in those patients taking sympathomimetics). Products include:

Acutrim .... ◉ 628
Allerest Children's Chewable Tablets .... ◉ 627
Allerest 12 Hour Caplets .... ◉ 627
Atrohist Plus Tablets 454
BC Cold Powder Multi-Symptom Formula (Cold-Sinus-Allergy) ...... ◉ 609
BC Cold Powder Non-Drowsy Formula (Cold-Sinus) .... ◉ 609
Cheracol Plus Head Cold/Cough Formula .... ◉ 769
Comtrex Multi-Symptom Non-Drowsy Liqui-gels............................... ◉ 618
Contac Continuous Action Nasal Decongestant/Antihistamine 12 Hour Capsules..................................... ◉ 813
Contac Maximum Strength Continuous Action Decongestant/Antihistamine 12 Hour Caplets.. ◉ 813
Contac Severe Cold and Flu Formula Caplets .... ◉ 814
Coricidin 'D' Decongestant Tablets .... ◉ 800
Dexatrim .... ◉ 832
Dexatrim Plus Vitamins Caplets .... ◉ 832
Dimetane-DC Cough Syrup 2059
Dimetapp Elixir .... ◉ 773
Dimetapp Extentabs .... ◉ 774
Dimetapp Tablets/Liqui-Gels .... ◉ 775
Dimetapp Cold & Allergy Chewable Tablets .... ◉ 773
Dimetapp DM Elixir .... ◉ 774
Dura-Vent Tablets 952
Entex Capsules 1986
Entex LA Tablets 1987
Entex Liquid 1986
Exgest LA Tablets 782
Hycomine 931
Isoclor Timesule Capsules .... ◉ 637
Nolamine Timed-Release Tablets 785

Ornade Spansule Capsules 2502
Propagest Tablets 786
Pyrroxate Caplets .... ◉ 772
Robitussin-CF .... ◉ 777
Sinulin Tablets 787
Tavist-D 12 Hour Relief Tablets .... ◉ 787
Teldrin 12 Hour Antihistamine/Nasal Decongestant Allergy Relief Capsules.................................... ◉ 826
Triaminic Allergy Tablets .... ◉ 789
Triaminic Cold Tablets .... ◉ 790
Triaminic Expectorant .... ◉ 790
Triaminic Syrup .... ◉ 792
Triaminic-12 Tablets .... ◉ 792
Triaminic-DM Syrup .... ◉ 792
Triaminicin Tablets .... ◉ 793
Triaminicol Multi-Symptom Cold Tablets .... ◉ 793
Triaminicol Multi-Symptom Relief ◉ 794
Vicks DayQuil Allergy Relief 12-Hour Extended Release Tablets.. ◉ 760
Vicks DayQuil Allergy Relief 4-Hour Tablets .... ◉ 760
Vicks DayQuil SINUS Pressure & CONGESTION Relief........................ ◉ 761

Pirbuterol Acetate

(Mazindol may potentiate blood pressure increases in those patients taking sympathomimetics). Products include:

Maxair Autohaler 1492
Maxair Inhaler 1494

Pseudoephedrine Hydrochloride

(Mazindol may potentiate blood pressure increases in those patients taking sympathomimetics). Products include:

Actifed Allergy Daytime/Nighttime Caplets.. ◉ 844
Actifed Plus Caplets .... ◉ 845
Actifed Plus Tablets .... ◉ 845
Actifed with Codeine Cough Syrup.. 1067
Actifed Sinus Daytime/Nighttime Tablets and Caplets .... ◉ 846
Actifed Syrup.. ◉ 846
Actifed Tablets .... ◉ 844
Advil Cold and Sinus Caplets and Tablets (formerly CoAdvil) .... ◉ 870
Alka-Seltzer Plus Cold Medicine Liqui-Gels .... ◉ 706
Alka-Seltzer Plus Cold & Cough Medicine Liqui-Gels.......................... ◉ 705
Alka-Seltzer Plus Night-Time Cold Medicine Liqui-Gels.......................... ◉ 706
Allerest Headache Strength Tablets .... ◉ 627
Allerest Maximum Strength Tablets .... ◉ 627
Allerest No Drowsiness Tablets...... ◉ 627
Allerest Sinus Pain Formula .... ◉ 627
Anatuss LA Tablets.............................. 1542
Atrohist Pediatric Capsules................ 453
Bayer Select Sinus Pain Relief Formula .... ◉ 717
Benadryl Allergy Decongestant Liquid Medication .... ◉ 848
Benadryl Allergy Decongestant Tablets .... ◉ 848
Benadryl Allergy Sinus Headache Formula Caplets .... ◉ 849
Benylin Multisymptom....................... ◉ 852
Bromfed Capsules (Extended-Release) 1785
Bromfed Syrup .... ◉ 733
Bromfed Tablets 1785
Bromfed-DM Cough Syrup................. 1786
Bromfed-PD Capsules (Extended-Release) 1785
Children's Vicks DayQuil Allergy Relief .... ◉ 757
Children's Vicks NyQuil Cold/Cough Relief.. ◉ 758
Comtrex Multi-Symptom Cold Reliever Tablets/Caplets/Liqui-Gels/Liquid .... ◉ 615
Allergy-Sinus Comtrex Multi-Symptom Allergy-Sinus Formula Tablets .... ◉ 617
Comtrex Multi-Symptom Non-Drowsy Caplets.................................... ◉ 618
Congress 1004
Contac Day Allergy/Sinus Caplets ◉ 812
Contac Day & Night .... ◉ 812
Contac Night Allergy/Sinus Caplets .... ◉ 812
Contac Severe Cold & Flu Non-Drowsy .... ◉ 815
Deconamine Chewable Tablets 1320
Deconamine CX Cough and Cold Liquid and Tablets............................... 1319

Deconamine 1320
Deconsal C Expectorant Syrup 456
Deconsal Pediatric Syrup 457
Deconsal II Tablets 454
Dimetane-DX Cough Syrup 2059
Dimetapp Sinus Caplets .... ◉ 775
Dorcol Children's Cough Syrup ...... ◉ 785
Drixoral Cough + Congestion Liquid Caps .... ◉ 802
Dura-Tap/PD Capsules 2867
Duratuss Tablets 2565
Duratuss HD Elixir............................... 2565
Efidac/24 .... ◉ 635
Entex PSE Tablets................................ 1987
Fedahist Gyrocaps............................... 2401
Fedahist Timecaps 2401
Guaifed.. 1787
Guaifed Syrup .... ◉ 734
Guaimax-D Tablets 792
Guaitab Tablets .... ◉ 734
Isoclor Expectorant............................. 990
Kronofed-A 977
Motrin IB Sinus.................................... ◉ 838
Novahistine DH.................................... 2462
Novahistine DMX .... ◉ 822
Novahistine Expectorant..................... 2463
Nucofed 2051
PediaCare Cold Allergy Chewable Tablets .... ◉ 677
PediaCare Cough-Cold Chewable Tablets 1553
PediaCare 1553
PediaCare Infants' Decongestant Drops .... ◉ 677
PediCare Infant's Drops Decongestant Plus Cough 1553
PediaCare NightRest Cough-Cold Liquid 1553
Pediatric Vicks 44d Dry Hacking Cough & Head Congestion.............. ◉ 763
Pediatric Vicks 44m Cough & Cold Relief .... ◉ 764
Robitussin Cold & Cough Liqui-Gels .... ◉ 776
Robitussin Maximum Strength Cough & Cold .... ◉ 778
Robitussin Pediatric Cough & Cold Formula .... ◉ 779
Robitussin Severe Congestion Liqui-Gels .... ◉ 776
Robitussin-DAC Syrup 2074
Robitussin-PE .... ◉ 778
Rondec Oral Drops 953
Rondec Syrup 953
Rondec Tablet....................................... 953
Rondec-DM Oral Drops 954
Rondec-DM Syrup 954
Rondec-TR Tablet 953
Ryna .... ◉ 841
Seldane-D Extended-Release Tablets 1538
Semprex-D Capsules 463
Semprex-D Capsules 1167
Sinarest Tablets .... ◉ 648
Sinarest Extra Strength Tablets...... ◉ 648
Sinarest No Drowsiness Tablets .... ◉ 648
Sine-Aid IB Caplets 1554
Sine-Aid Maximum Strength Sinus Medication Gelcaps, Caplets and Tablets 1554
Sine-Off No Drowsiness Formula Caplets .... ◉ 824
Sine-Off Sinus Medicine .... ◉ 825
Singlet Tablets .... ◉ 825
Sinutab Non-Drying Liquid Caps.... ◉ 859
Sinutab Sinus Allergy Medication, Maximum Strength Tablets and Caplets .... ◉ 860
Sinutab Sinus Medication, Maximum Strength Without Drowsiness Formula, Tablets & Caplets .... ◉ 860
Sinutab Sinus Medication, Regular Strength Without Drowsiness Formula .... ◉ 859
Sudafed Children's Liquid .... ◉ 861
Sudafed Cold and Cough Liquidcaps.. ◉ 862
Sudafed Cough Syrup .... ◉ 862
Sudafed Plus Liquid .... ◉ 862
Sudafed Plus Tablets .... ◉ 863
Sudafed Severe Cold Formula Caplets .... ◉ 863
Sudafed Severe Cold Formula Tablets .... ◉ 864
Sudafed Sinus Caplets........................ ◉ 864
Sudafed Sinus Tablets......................... ◉ 864
Sudafed Tablets, 30 mg....................... ◉ 861
Sudafed Tablets, 60 mg....................... ◉ 861
Sudafed 12 Hour Caplets .... ◉ 861
Syn-Rx Tablets 465

Syn-Rx DM Tablets 466
TheraFlu.. ◉ 787
TheraFlu Maximum Strength Nighttime Flu, Cold & Cough Medicine .... ◉ 788
TheraFlu Maximum Strength Non-Drowsy Formula Flu, Cold & Cough Medicine .... ◉ 788
Thera Flu Maximum Strength, Non-Drowsy Formula Flu, Cold and Cough Caplets .... ◉ 789
Triaminic AM Cough and Decongestant Formula .... ◉ 789
Triaminic AM Decongestant Formula .... ◉ 790
Triaminic Nite Light .... ◉ 791
Triaminic Sore Throat Formula ..... ◉ 791
Tussend 1783
Tussend Expectorant 1785
Children's TYLENOL Cold Multi-Symptom Liquid Formula and Chewable Tablets................................. 1561
Children's TYLENOL Cold Plus Cough Multi Symptom Tablets and Liquid .... ◉ 681
Infants' TYLENOL Cold Decongestant & Fever-Reducer Drops 1556
TYLENOL Maximum Strength Allergy Sinus Medication Gelcaps and Caplets 1563
TYLENOL Maximum Strength Allergy Sinus NightTime Medication Caplets 1555
TYLENOL Flu Maximum Strength Gelcaps 1565
TYLENOL Flu NightTime, Maximum Strength, Gelcaps 1566
TYLENOL Maximum Strength Flu NightTime Hot Medication Packets 1562
TYLENOL, Maximum Strength, Sinus Medication Geltabs, Gelcaps, Caplets and Tablets 1566
TYLENOL Cold Multi-Symptom Formula Medication Tablets and Caplets 1561
TYLENOL Cold Medication No Drowsiness Formula Gelcaps and Caplets 1562
TYLENOL Cold Multi-Symptom Hot Medication Liquid Packets.............. 1557
TYLENOL Cough Multi-Symptom Medication with Decongestant 1565
Ursinus Inlay-Tabs............................... ◉ 794
Vicks 44 LiquiCaps Cough, Cold & Flu Relief.. ◉ 755
Vicks 44 LiquiCaps Non-Drowsy Cough & Cold Relief .... ◉ 756
Vicks 44D Dry Hacking Cough & Head Congestion .... ◉ 755
Vicks 44M Cough, Cold & Flu Relief .... ◉ 756
Vicks DayQuil .... ◉ 761
Vicks DayQuil SINUS Pressure & PAIN Relief with IBUPROFEN ...... ◉ 762
Vicks Nyquil Hot Therapy.................... ◉ 762
Vicks NyQuil LiquiCaps Multi-Symptom Cold/Flu Relief .... ◉ 763
Vicks NyQuil Multi-Symptom Cold/Flu Relief - (Original & Cherry Flavor)..................................... ◉ 763

Pseudoephedrine Sulfate

(Mazindol may potentiate blood pressure increases in those patients taking sympathomimetics). Products include:

Cheracol Sinus .... ◉ 768
Chlor-Trimeton Allergy Decongestant Tablets .... ◉ 799
Claritin-D 2350
Drixoral Cold and Allergy Sustained-Action Tablets .... ◉ 802
Drixoral Cold and Flu Extended-Release Tablets.................................... ◉ 803
Drixoral Non-Drowsy Formula Extended-Release Tablets .... ◉ 803
Drixoral Allergy/Sinus Extended Release Tablets.................................... ◉ 804
Trinalin Repetabs Tablets 1330

Salmeterol Xinafoate

(Mazindol may potentiate blood pressure increases in those patients taking sympathomimetics). Products include:

Serevent Inhalation Aerosol................ 1176

Selegiline Hydrochloride

(Concurrent use is contraindicated; potential for hypertensive crises). Products include:

Eldepryl Tablets 2550

IMPORTANT NOTE: Always consult each drug listing in the patient's regimen for possible interactions.

Terbutaline Sulfate (Mazindol may potentiate blood pressure increases in those patients taking sympathomimetics). Products include:

- Brethaire Inhaler 813
- Brethine Ampuls 815
- Brethine Tablets 814
- Bricanyl Subcutaneous Injection 1502
- Bricanyl Tablets 1503

Tranylcypromine Sulfate (Concurrent use is contraindicated; potential for hypertensive crises). Products include:

- Parnate Tablets 2503

SANSERT TABLETS

(Methysergide Maleate) **2295**

May interact with narcotic analgesics. Compounds in this category include:

Alfentanil Hydrochloride (Methysergide may reverse the analgesic activity of narcotic analgesics). Products include:

- Alfenta Injection 1286

Buprenorphine (Methysergide may reverse the analgesic activity of narcotic analgesics). Products include:

- Buprenex Injectable 2006

Codeine Phosphate (Methysergide may reverse the analgesic activity of narcotic analgesics). Products include:

- Actifed with Codeine Cough Syrup .. 1067
- Brontex 1981
- Deconsal C Expectorant Syrup 456
- Deconsal Pediatric Syrup 457
- Dimetane-DC Cough Syrup 2059
- Empirin with Codeine Tablets 1093
- Fioricet with Codeine Capsules 2260
- Fiorinal with Codeine Capsules 2262
- Isoclor Expectorant 990
- Novahistine DH 2462
- Novahistine Expectorant 2463
- Nucofed 2051
- Phenergan with Codeine 2777
- Phenergan VC with Codeine 2781
- Robitussin A-C Syrup 2073
- Robitussin-DAC Syrup 2074
- Ryna .... ■ 841
- Soma Compound w/Codeine Tablets 2676
- Tussi-Organidin NR Liquid and S NR Liquid 2677
- Tylenol with Codeine 1583

Dezocine (Methysergide may reverse the analgesic activity of narcotic analgesics). Products include:

- Dalgan Injection 538

Fentanyl (Methysergide may reverse the analgesic activity of narcotic analgesics). Products include:

- Duragesic Transdermal System 1288

Fentanyl Citrate (Methysergide may reverse the analgesic activity of narcotic analgesics). Products include:

- Sublimaze Injection 1307

Hydrocodone Bitartrate (Methysergide may reverse the analgesic activity of narcotic analgesics). Products include:

- Anexsia 5/500 Elixir 1781
- Anexia Tablets 1782
- Codiclear DH Syrup 791
- Deconamine CX Cough and Cold Liquid and Tablets 1319
- Duratuss HD Elixir 2565
- Hycodan Tablets and Syrup 930
- Hycomine Compound Tablets 932
- Hycomine 931
- Hycotuss Expectorant Syrup 933
- Hydrocet Capsules 782
- Lorcet 10/650 1018
- Lortab 2566
- Tussend 1783
- Tussend Expectorant 1785
- Vicodin Tablets 1356
- Vicodin ES Tablets 1357
- Vicodin Tuss Expectorant 1358
- Zydone Capsules 949

Hydrocodone Polistirex (Methysergide may reverse the analgesic activity of narcotic analgesics). Products include:

- Tussionex Pennkinetic Extended-Release Suspension 998

Levorphanol Tartrate (Methysergide may reverse the analgesic activity of narcotic analgesics). Products include:

- Levo-Dromoran 2129

Meperidine Hydrochloride (Methysergide may reverse the analgesic activity of narcotic analgesics). Products include:

- Demerol 2308
- Mepergan Injection 2753

Methadone Hydrochloride (Methysergide may reverse the analgesic activity of narcotic analgesics). Products include:

- Methadone Hydrochloride Oral Concentrate 2233
- Methadone Hydrochloride Oral Solution & Tablets 2235

Morphine Sulfate (Methysergide may reverse the analgesic activity of narcotic analgesics). Products include:

- Astramorph/PF Injection, USP (Preservative-Free) 535
- Duramorph 962
- Infumorph 200 and Infumorph 500 Sterile Solutions 965
- MS Contin Tablets 1994
- MSIR 1997
- Oramorph SR (Morphine Sulfate Sustained Release Tablets) 2236
- RMS Suppositories 2657
- Roxanol 2243

Opium Alkaloids (Methysergide may reverse the analgesic activity of narcotic analgesics).

No products indexed under this heading.

Oxycodone Hydrochloride (Methysergide may reverse the analgesic activity of narcotic analgesics). Products include:

- Percocet Tablets 938
- Percodan Tablets 939
- Percodan-Demi Tablets 940
- Roxicodone Tablets, Oral Solution & Intensol (Oxycodone) 2244
- Tylox Capsules 1584

Propoxyphene Hydrochloride (Methysergide may reverse the analgesic activity of narcotic analgesics). Products include:

- Darvon 1435
- Wygesic Tablets 2827

Propoxyphene Napsylate (Methysergide may reverse the analgesic activity of narcotic analgesics). Products include:

- Darvon-N/Darvocet-N 1433

Sufentanil Citrate (Methysergide may reverse the analgesic activity of narcotic analgesics). Products include:

- Sufenta Injection 1309

SARAPIN

(Sarracenia purpurea, Pitcher Plant Distillate) **1231**

None cited in PDR database.

SATIN ANTIMICROBIAL SKIN CLEANSER FOR DIABETIC/CANCER PATIENT CARE

(Chloroxylenol) .... ■ **625**

None cited in PDR database.

SCLEROMATE

(Morrhuate Sodium) **1891**

None cited in PDR database.

SEA-CLENS, WOUND CLEANSER

(Sodium Chloride) **2554**

None cited in PDR database.

SECONAL SODIUM PULVULES

(Secobarbital Sodium) **1474**

May interact with central nervous system depressants, narcotic analgesics, tranquilizers, antihistamines, oral anticoagulants, corticosteroids, monoamine oxidase inhibitors, oral contraceptives, and certain other agents. Compounds in these categories include:

Acrivastine (Concomitant use may produce additive CNS-depressant effects). Products include:

- Semprex-D Capsules 463
- Semprex-D Capsules 1167

Alfentanil Hydrochloride (Concomitant use may produce additive CNS-depressant effects). Products include:

- Alfenta Injection 1286

Alprazolam (Concomitant use may produce additive CNS-depressant effects). Products include:

- Xanax Tablets 2649

Aprobarbital (Concomitant use may produce additive CNS-depressant effects).

No products indexed under this heading.

Astemizole (Concomitant use may produce additive CNS-depressant effects). Products include:

- Hismanal Tablets 1293

Azatadine Maleate (Concomitant use may produce additive CNS-depressant effects). Products include:

- Trinalin Repetabs Tablets 1330

Betamethasone Acetate (Enhanced metabolism of exogenous corticosteroids). Products include:

- Celestone Soluspan Suspension 2347

Betamethasone Sodium Phosphate (Enhanced metabolism of exogenous corticosteroids). Products include:

- Celestone Soluspan Suspension 2347

Bromodiphenhydramine Hydrochloride (Concomitant use may produce additive CNS-depressant effects).

No products indexed under this heading.

Brompheniramine Maleate (Concomitant use may produce additive CNS-depressant effects). Products include:

- Alka Seltzer Plus Sinus Medicine .. ■ 707
- Bromfed Capsules (Extended-Release) 1785
- Bromfed Syrup .... ■ 733
- Bromfed Tablets 1785
- Bromfed-DM Cough Syrup 1786
- Bromfed-PD Capsules (Extended-Release) 1785
- Dimetane-DC Cough Syrup 2059
- Dimetane-DX Cough Syrup 2059
- Dimetapp Elixir .... ■ 773
- Dimetapp Extentabs .... ■ 774
- Dimetapp Tablets/Liqui-Gels .... ■ 775
- Dimetapp Cold & Allergy Chewable Tablets .... ■ 773
- Dimetapp DM Elixir .... ■ 774
- Vicks DayQuil Allergy Relief 12-Hour Extended Release Tablets .. ■ 760
- Vicks DayQuil Allergy Relief 4-Hour Tablets .... ■ 760

Buprenorphine (Concomitant use may produce additive CNS-depressant effects). Products include:

- Buprenex Injectable 2006

Buspirone Hydrochloride (Concomitant use may produce additive CNS-depressant effects). Products include:

- BuSpar 737

Butabarbital (Concomitant use may produce additive CNS-depressant effects).

No products indexed under this heading.

Butalbital (Concomitant use may produce additive CNS-depressant effects). Products include:

- Esgic-plus Tablets 1013
- Fioricet Tablets 2258
- Fioricet with Codeine Capsules 2260
- Fiorinal Capsules 2261
- Fiorinal with Codeine Capsules 2262
- Fiorinal Tablets 2261
- Phrenilin 785
- Sedapap Tablets 50 mg/650 mg .. 1543

Chlordiazepoxide (Concomitant use may produce additive CNS-depressant effects). Products include:

- Libritabs Tablets 2177
- Limbitrol 2180

Chlordiazepoxide Hydrochloride (Concomitant use may produce additive CNS-depressant effects). Products include:

- Librax Capsules 2176
- Librium Capsules 2178
- Librium Injectable 2179

Chlorpheniramine Maleate (Concomitant use may produce additive CNS-depressant effects). Products include:

- Alka-Seltzer Plus Cold Medicine .... ■ 705
- Alka-Seltzer Plus Cold Medicine Liqui-Gels .... ■ 706
- Alka-Seltzer Plus Cold & Cough Medicine .... ■ 708
- Alka-Seltzer Plus Cold & Cough Medicine Liqui-Gels .... ■ 705
- Allerest Children's Chewable Tablets .... ■ 627
- Allerest Headache Strength Tablets .... ■ 627
- Allerest Maximum Strength Tablets .... ■ 627
- Allerest Sinus Pain Formula .... ■ 627
- Allerest 12 Hour Caplets .... ■ 627
- Ana-Kit Anaphylaxis Emergency Treatment Kit 617
- Atrohist Pediatric Capsules 453
- Atrohist Plus Tablets 454
- BC Cold Powder Multi-Symptom Formula (Cold-Sinus-Allergy) .... ■ 609
- Cerose DM .... ■ 878
- Cheracol Plus Head Cold/Cough Formula .... ■ 769
- Children's Vicks DayQuil Allergy Relief .... ■ 757
- Children's Vicks NyQuil Cold/Cough Relief .... ■ 758
- Chlor-Trimeton Allergy Decongestant Tablets .... ■ 799
- Chlor-Trimeton Allergy Tablets .... ■ 798
- Comhist 2038
- Comtrex Multi-Symptom Cold Reliever Tablets/Caplets/Liqui-Gels/Liquid .... ■ 615
- Allergy-Sinus Comtrex Multi-Symptom Allergy-Sinus Formula Tablets .... ■ 617
- Contac Continuous Action Nasal Decongestant/Antihistamine 12 Hour Capsules .... ■ 813
- Contac Maximum Strength Continuous Action Decongestant/Antihistamine 12 Hour Caplets .. ■ 813
- Contac Severe Cold and Flu Formula Caplets .... ■ 814
- Coricidin 'D' Decongestant Tablets .... ■ 800
- Coricidin Tablets .... ■ 800
- D.A. Chewable Tablets 951
- Deconamine 1320
- Dura-Tap/PD Capsules 2867
- Dura-Vent/DA Tablets 953
- Extendryl 1005
- Fedahist Gyrocaps 2401
- Fedahist Timecaps 2401
- Hycomine Compound Tablets 932
- Isoclor Timesule Capsules .... ■ 637
- Kronofed-A 977
- Nolamine Timed-Release Tablets 785
- Novahistine DH 2462
- Novahistine Elixir .... ■ 823
- Ornade Spansule Capsules 2502
- PediaCare Cold Allergy Chewable Tablets .... ■ 677

(■ Described in PDR For Nonprescription Drugs) (◉ Described in PDR For Ophthalmology)

Interactions Index

PediaCare Cough-Cold Chewable Tablets 1553
PediaCare Cough-Cold Liquid............ 1553
PediaCare NightRest Cough-Cold Liquid 1553
Pediatric Vicks 44m Cough & Cold Relief .... ⊕ 764
Pyrroxate Caplets .... ⊕ 772
Ryna .... ⊕ 841
Sinarest Tablets .... ⊕ 648
Sinarest Extra Strength Tablets...... ⊕ 648
Sine-Off Sinus Medicine .... ⊕ 825
Singlet Tablets .... ⊕ 825
Sinulin Tablets 787
Sinutab Sinus Allergy Medication, Maximum Strength Tablets and Caplets .... ⊕ 860
Sudafed Plus Liquid .... ⊕ 862
Sudafed Plus Tablets .... ⊕ 863
Teldrin 12 Hour Antihistamine/ Nasal Decongestant Allergy Relief Capsules .... ⊕ 826
TheraFlu... ⊕ 787
TheraFlu Maximum Strength Nighttime Flu, Cold & Cough Medicine .... ⊕ 788
Triaminic Allergy Tablets .... ⊕ 789
Triaminic Cold Tablets .... ⊕ 790
Triaminic Nite Light .... ⊕ 791
Triaminic Syrup .... ⊕ 792
Triaminic-12 Tablets .... ⊕ 792
Triaminicin Tablets................................ ⊕ 793
Triaminicol Multi-Symptom Cold Tablets .... ⊕ 793
Triaminicol Multi-Symptom Relief ⊕ 794
Tussend 1783
Children's TYLENOL Cold Multi-Symptom Liquid Formula and Chewable Tablets................................ 1561
Children's TYLENOL Cold Plus Cough Multi Symptom Tablets and Liquid .... ⊕ 681
TYLENOL Maximum Strength Allergy Sinus Medication Gelcaps and Caplets 1563
TYLENOL Cold Multi-Symptom Formula Medication Tablets and Caplets 1561
TYLENOL Cold Multi-Symptom Hot Medication Liquid Packets.............. 1557
Vicks 44 LiquiCaps Cough, Cold & Flu Relief... ⊕ 755
Vicks 44M Cough, Cold & Flu Relief .... ⊕ 756

Chlorpheniramine Polistirex (Concomitant use may produce additive CNS-depressant effects). Products include:

Tussionex Pennkinetic Extended-Release Suspension 998

Chlorpheniramine Tannate (Concomitant use may produce additive CNS-depressant effects). Products include:

Atrohist Pediatric Suspension 454
Ricobid Tablets and Pediatric Suspension.. 2038
Rynatan 2673
Rynatuss 2673

Chlorpromazine (Concomitant use may produce additive CNS-depressant effects). Products include:

Thorazine Suppositories 2523

Chlorprothixene (Concomitant use may produce additive CNS-depressant effects).

No products indexed under this heading.

Chlorprothixene Hydrochloride (Concomitant use may produce additive CNS-depressant effects).

No products indexed under this heading.

Clemastine Fumarate (Concomitant use may produce additive CNS-depressant effects). Products include:

Tavist Syrup... 2297
Tavist Tablets 2298
Tavist-1 12 Hour Relief Tablets .... ⊕ 787
Tavist-D 12 Hour Relief Tablets .... ⊕ 787

Clorazepate Dipotassium (Concomitant use may produce additive CNS-depressant effects). Products include:

Tranxene 451

Clozapine (Concomitant use may produce additive CNS-depressant effects). Products include:

Clozaril Tablets...................................... 2252

Codeine Phosphate (Concomitant use may produce additive CNS-depressant effects). Products include:

Actifed with Codeine Cough Syrup.. 1067
Brontex 1981
Deconsal C Expectorant Syrup 456
Deconsal Pediatric Syrup.................... 457
Dimetane-DC Cough Syrup 2059
Empirin with Codeine Tablets........... 1093
Fioricet with Codeine Capsules 2260
Fiorinal with Codeine Capsules 2262
Isoclor Expectorant............................... 990
Novahistine DH...................................... 2462
Novahistine Expectorant..................... 2463
Nucofed 2051
Phenergan with Codeine 2777
Phenergan VC with Codeine 2781
Robitussin A-C Syrup............................ 2073
Robitussin-DAC Syrup 2074
Ryna .... ⊕ 841
Soma Compound w/Codeine Tablets 2676
Tussi-Organidin NR Liquid and S NR Liquid 2677
Tylenol with Codeine 1583

Cortisone Acetate (Enhanced metabolism of exogenous corticosteroids). Products include:

Cortone Acetate Sterile Suspension 1623
Cortone Acetate Tablets...................... 1624

Cyproheptadine Hydrochloride (Concomitant use may produce additive CNS-depressant effects). Products include:

Periactin 1724

Desflurane (Concomitant use may produce additive CNS-depressant effects). Products include:

Suprane 1813

Desogestrel (Decreased effect of estradiol by increasing its metabolism). Products include:

Desogen Tablets.................................... 1817
Ortho-Cept 1851

Dexamethasone (Enhanced metabolism of exogenous corticosteroids). Products include:

AK-Trol Ointment & Suspension .... ⊙ 205
Decadron Elixir 1633
Decadron Tablets................................... 1635
Decaspray Topical Aerosol 1648
Dexacidin Ointment .... ⊙ 263
Maxitrol Ophthalmic Ointment and Suspension .... ⊙ 224
TobraDex Ophthalmic Suspension and Ointment... 473

Dexamethasone Acetate (Enhanced metabolism of exogenous corticosteroids). Products include:

Dalalone D.P. Injectable 1011
Decadron-LA Sterile Suspension...... 1646

Dexamethasone Sodium Phosphate (Enhanced metabolism of exogenous corticosteroids). Products include:

Decadron Phosphate Injection.......... 1637
Decadron Phosphate Respihaler 1642
Decadron Phosphate Sterile Ophthalmic Ointment 1641
Decadron Phosphate Sterile Ophthalmic Solution 1642
Decadron Phosphate Topical Cream.. 1644
Decadron Phosphate Turbinaire 1645
Decadron Phosphate with Xylocaine Injection, Sterile 1639
Dexacort Phosphate in Respihaler.. 458
Dexacort Phosphate in Turbinaire .. 459
NeoDecadron Sterile Ophthalmic Ointment 1712
NeoDecadron Sterile Ophthalmic Solution 1713
NeoDecadron Topical Cream 1714

Dexchlorpheniramine Maleate (Concomitant use may produce additive CNS-depressant effects).

No products indexed under this heading.

Dezocine (Concomitant use may produce additive CNS-depressant effects). Products include:

Dalgan Injection 538

Diazepam (Concomitant use may produce additive CNS-depressant effects). Products include:

Dizac 1809
Valium Injectable 2182
Valium Tablets 2183
Valrelease Capsules 2169

Dicumarol (Barbiturates can induce hepatic microsomal enzymes, resulting in increased or decreased anticoagulant response).

No products indexed under this heading.

Diphenhydramine Citrate (Concomitant use may produce additive CNS-depressant effects). Products include:

Excedrin P.M. Analgesic/Sleeping Aid Tablets, Caplets, Liquigels 733

Diphenhydramine Hydrochloride (Concomitant use may produce additive CNS-depressant effects). Products include:

Actifed Allergy Daytime/Nighttime Caplets.. ⊕ 844
Actifed Sinus Daytime/Nighttime Tablets and Caplets .... ⊕ 846
Arthritis Foundation NightTime Caplets .... ⊕ 674
Extra Strength Bayer PM Aspirin .. ⊕ 713
Bayer Select Night Time Pain Relief Formula.. ⊕ 716
Benadryl Allergy Decongestant Liquid Medication .... ⊕ 848
Benadryl Allergy Decongestant Tablets .... ⊕ 848
Benadryl Allergy Liquid Medication.. ⊕ 849
Benadryl Allergy................................... ⊕ 848
Benadryl Allergy Sinus Headache Formula Caplets................................. ⊕ 849
Benadryl Capsules................................ 1898
Benadryl Dye-Free Allergy Liquigel Softgels... ⊕ 850
Benadryl Dye-Free Allergy Liquid Medication .... ⊕ 850
Benadryl Itch Relief Cream, Children's Formula and Maximum Strength 2% .... ⊕ 851
Benadryl Itch Relief Spray, Children's Formula and Maximum Strength 2% .... ⊕ 851
Benadryl Itch Relief Stick Maximum Strength 2% .... ⊕ 850
Benadryl Itch Stopping Gel, Children's Formula and Maximum Strength 2% .... ⊕ 851
Benadryl Kapseals................................ 1898
Benadryl Injection 1898
Contac Day & Night Cold/Flu Night Caplets.. ⊕ 812
Contac Night Allergy/Sinus Caplets .... ⊕ 812
Extra Strength Doan's P.M. .... ⊕ 633
Legatrin PM .... ⊕ 651
Miles Nervine Nighttime Sleep-Aid ⊕ 723
Nytol QuickCaps Caplets .... ⊕ 610
Sleepinal Night-time Sleep Aid Capsules and Softgels........................ ⊕ 834
TYLENOL Maximum Strength Allergy Sinus NightTime Medication Caplets 1555
TYLENOL Flu NightTime, Maximum Strength, Gelcaps 1566
TYLENOL Maximum Strength Flu NightTime Hot Medication Packets 1562
TYLENOL PM, Extra Strength Pain Reliever/Sleep Aid Caplets, Geltabs, Gelcaps 1560
TYLENOL Severe Allergy Medication Caplets 1564
Maximum Strength Unisom Sleepgels 1934
Unisom With Pain Relief-Nighttime Sleep Aid and Pain Reliever........... 1934

Divalproex Sodium (Increases blood levels of secobarbital sodium). Products include:

Depakote Tablets................................... 415

Doxycycline Calcium (Half-life of doxycycline may be shortened). Products include:

Vibramycin Calcium Oral Suspension Syrup... 1941

Doxycycline Hyclate (Half-life of doxycycline may be shortened). Products include:

Doryx Capsules...................................... 1913
Vibramycin Hyclate Capsules............ 1941
Vibramycin Hyclate Intravenous 2215
Vibra-Tabs Film Coated Tablets 1941

Doxycycline Monohydrate (Half-life of doxycycline may be shortened). Products include:

Monodox Capsules 1805
Vibramycin Monohydrate for Oral Suspension 1941

Droperidol (Concomitant use may produce additive CNS-depressant effects). Products include:

Inapsine Injection.................................. 1296

Enflurane (Concomitant use may produce additive CNS-depressant effects).

No products indexed under this heading.

Estazolam (Concomitant use may produce additive CNS-depressant effects). Products include:

ProSom Tablets 449

Ethchlorvynol (Concomitant use may produce additive CNS-depressant effects). Products include:

Placidyl Capsules................................... 448

Ethinamate (Concomitant use may produce additive CNS-depressant effects).

No products indexed under this heading.

Ethinyl Estradiol (Decreased effect of estradiol by increasing its metabolism). Products include:

Brevicon.. 2088
Demulen 2428
Desogen Tablets..................................... 1817
Levlen/Tri-Levlen................................... 651
Lo/Ovral Tablets 2746
Lo/Ovral-28 Tablets............................... 2751
Modicon... 1872
Nordette-21 Tablets............................... 2755
Nordette-28 Tablets............................... 2758
Norinyl 2088
Ortho-Cept 1851
Ortho-Cyclen/Ortho-Tri-Cyclen 1858
Ortho-Novum... 1872
Ortho-Cyclen/Ortho Tri-Cyclen 1858
Ovcon 760
Ovral Tablets.. 2770
Ovral-28 Tablets 2770
Levlen/Tri-Levlen................................... 651
Tri-Norinyl.. 2164
Triphasil-21 Tablets............................... 2814
Triphasil-28 Tablets............................... 2819

Ethynodiol Diacetate (Decreased effect of estradiol by increasing its metabolism). Products include:

Demulen 2428

Fentanyl (Concomitant use may produce additive CNS-depressant effects). Products include:

Duragesic Transdermal System......... 1288

Fentanyl Citrate (Concomitant use may produce additive CNS-depressant effects). Products include:

Sublimaze Injection............................... 1307

Fludrocortisone Acetate (Enhanced metabolism of exogenous corticosteroids). Products include:

Florinet Acetate Tablets 505

Fluphenazine Decanoate (Concomitant use may produce additive CNS-depressant effects). Products include:

Prolixin Decanoate 509

Fluphenazine Enanthate (Concomitant use may produce additive CNS-depressant effects). Products include:

Prolixin Enanthate 509

IMPORTANT NOTE: Always consult each drug listing in the patient's regimen for possible interactions.

Seconal **Interactions Index** 926

Fluphenazine Hydrochloride (Concomitant use may produce additive CNS-depressant effects). Products include:
Prolixin 509

Flurazepam Hydrochloride (Concomitant use may produce additive CNS-depressant effects). Products include:
Dalmane Capsules 2173

Furazolidone (Prolongs the effects of barbiturates). Products include:
Furoxone 2046

Glutethimide (Concomitant use may produce additive CNS-depressant effects).
No products indexed under this heading.

Griseofulvin (Interference with absorption of orally administered griseofulvin, thus decreasing its blood level). Products include:
Fulvicin P/G Tablets 2359
Fulvicin P/G 165 & 330 Tablets 2359
Grifulvin V (griseofulvin tablets) Microsize (griseofulvin oral suspension) Microsize 1888
Gris-PEG Tablets, 125 mg & 250 mg 479

Haloperidol (Concomitant use may produce additive CNS-depressant effects). Products include:
Haldol Injection, Tablets and Concentrate 1575

Haloperidol Decanoate (Concomitant use may produce additive CNS-depressant effects). Products include:
Haldol Decanoate 1577

Hydrocodone Bitartrate (Concomitant use may produce additive CNS-depressant effects). Products include:
Anexsia 5/500 Elixir 1781
Anexia Tablets 1782
Codiclear DH Syrup 791
Deconamine CX Cough and Cold Liquid and Tablets 1319
Duratuss HD Elixir 2565
Hycodan Tablets and Syrup 930
Hycomine Compound Tablets 932
Hycomine 931
Hycotuss Expectorant Syrup 933
Hydrocet Capsules 782
Lorcet 10/650 1018
Lortab 2566
Tussend 1783
Tussend Expectorant 1785
Vicodin Tablets 1356
Vicodin ES Tablets 1357
Vicodin Tuss Expectorant 1358
Zydone Capsules 949

Hydrocodone Polistirex (Concomitant use may produce additive CNS-depressant effects). Products include:
Tussionex Pennkinetic Extended-Release Suspension 998

Hydrocortisone (Enhanced metabolism of exogenous corticosteroids). Products include:
Anusol-HC Cream 2.5% 1896
Aquanil HC Lotion 1931
Bactine Hydrocortisone Anti-Itch Cream .... ◘ 709
Caldecort Anti-Itch Hydrocortisone Spray .... ◘ 631
Cortaid .... ◘ 836
CORTENEMA 2535
Cortisporin Ointment 1085
Cortisporin Ophthalmic Ointment Sterile 1085
Cortisporin Ophthalmic Suspension Sterile 1086
Cortisporin Otic Solution Sterile 1087
Cortisporin Otic Suspension Sterile 1088
Cortizone-5 .... ◘ 831
Cortizone-10 .... ◘ 831
Hydrocortone Tablets 1672
Hytone 907
Massengill Medicated Soft Cloth Towelettes 2458
PediOtic Suspension Sterile 1153
Preparation H Hydrocortisone 1% Cream .... ◘ 872
ProctoCream-HC 2.5% 2408
VōSoL HC Otic Solution 2678

Hydrocortisone Acetate (Enhanced metabolism of exogenous corticosteroids). Products include:
Analpram-HC Rectal Cream 1% and 2.5% 977
Anusol HC-1 Anti-Itch Hydrocortisone Ointment .... ◘ 847
Anusol-HC Suppositories 1897
Caldecort .... ◘ 631
Carmol HC 924
Coly-Mycin S Otic w/Neomycin & Hydrocortisone 1906
Cortaid .... ◘ 836
Cortifoam 2396
Cortisporin Cream 1084
Epifoam 2399
Hydrocortone Acetate Sterile Suspension 1669
Mantadil Cream 1135
Nupercainal Hydrocortisone 1% Cream .... ◘ 645
Ophthocort .... ⊙ 311
Pramosone Cream, Lotion & Ointment 978
ProctoCream-HC 2408
ProctoFoam-HC 2409
Terra-Cortril Ophthalmic Suspension 2210

Hydrocortisone Sodium Phosphate (Enhanced metabolism of exogenous corticosteroids). Products include:
Hydrocortone Phosphate Injection, Sterile 1670

Hydrocortisone Sodium Succinate (Enhanced metabolism of exogenous corticosteroids). Products include:
Solu-Cortef Sterile Powder 2641

Hydroxyzine Hydrochloride (Concomitant use may produce additive CNS-depressant effects). Products include:
Atarax Tablets & Syrup 2185
Marax Tablets & DF Syrup 2200
Vistaril Intramuscular Solution 2216

Isocarboxazid (Prolongs the effects of barbiturates).
No products indexed under this heading.

Isoflurane (Concomitant use may produce additive CNS-depressant effects).
No products indexed under this heading.

Ketamine Hydrochloride (Concomitant use may produce additive CNS-depressant effects).
No products indexed under this heading.

Levomethadyl Acetate Hydrochloride (Concomitant use may produce additive CNS-depressant effects). Products include:
Orlamm 2239

Levonorgestrel (Decreased effect of estradiol by increasing its metabolism). Products include:
Levlen/Tri-Levlen 651
Nordette-21 Tablets 2755
Nordette-28 Tablets 2758
Norplant System 2759
Levlen/Tri-Levlen 651
Triphasil-21 Tablets 2814
Triphasil-28 Tablets 2819

Levorphanol Tartrate (Concomitant use may produce additive CNS-depressant effects). Products include:
Levo-Dromoran 2129

Loratadine (Concomitant use may produce additive CNS-depressant effects). Products include:
Claritin 2349
Claritin-D 2350

Lorazepam (Concomitant use may produce additive CNS-depressant effects). Products include:
Ativan Injection 2698
Ativan Tablets 2700

Loxapine Hydrochloride (Concomitant use may produce additive CNS-depressant effects). Products include:
Loxitane 1378

Loxapine Succinate (Concomitant use may produce additive CNS-depressant effects). Products include:
Loxitane Capsules 1378

Meperidine Hydrochloride (Concomitant use may produce additive CNS-depressant effects). Products include:
Demerol 2308
Mepergan Injection 2753

Mephobarbital (Concomitant use may produce additive CNS-depressant effects). Products include:
Mebaral Tablets 2322

Meprobamate (Concomitant use may produce additive CNS-depressant effects). Products include:
Miltown Tablets 2672
PMB 200 and PMB 400 2783

Mesoridazine Besylate (Concomitant use may produce additive CNS-depressant effects). Products include:
Serentil 684

Mestranol (Decreased effect of estradiol by increasing its metabolism). Products include:
Norinyl 2088
Ortho-Novum 1872

Methadone Hydrochloride (Concomitant use may produce additive CNS-depressant effects). Products include:
Methadone Hydrochloride Oral Concentrate 2233
Methadone Hydrochloride Oral Solution & Tablets 2235

Methdilazine Hydrochloride (Concomitant use may produce additive CNS-depressant effects).
No products indexed under this heading.

Methohexital Sodium (Concomitant use may produce additive CNS-depressant effects). Products include:
Brevital Sodium Vials 1429

Methotrimeprazine (Concomitant use may produce additive CNS-depressant effects). Products include:
Levoprome 1274

Methoxyflurane (Concomitant use may produce additive CNS-depressant effects).
No products indexed under this heading.

Methylprednisolone Acetate (Enhanced metabolism of exogenous corticosteroids). Products include:
Depo-Medrol Single-Dose Vial 2600
Depo-Medrol Sterile Aqueous Suspension 2597

Methylprednisolone Sodium Succinate (Enhanced metabolism of exogenous corticosteroids). Products include:
Solu-Medrol Sterile Powder 2643

Midazolam Hydrochloride (Concomitant use may produce additive CNS-depressant effects). Products include:
Versed Injection 2170

Molindone Hydrochloride (Concomitant use may produce additive CNS-depressant effects). Products include:
Moban Tablets and Concentrate 1048

Morphine Sulfate (Concomitant use may produce additive CNS-depressant effects). Products include:
Astramorph/PF Injection, USP (Preservative-Free) 535
Duramorph 962
Infumorph 200 and Infumorph 500 Sterile Solutions 965
MS Contin Tablets 1994
MSIR 1997
Oramorph SR (Morphine Sulfate Sustained Release Tablets) 2236
RMS Suppositories 2657
Roxanol 2243

Norethindrone (Decreased effect of estradiol by increasing its metabolism). Products include:
Brevicon 2088
Micronor Tablets 1872
Modicon 1872
Norinyl 2088
Nor-Q D Tablets 2135
Ortho-Novum 1872
Ovcon 760
Tri-Norinyl 2164

Norethynodrel (Decreased effect of estradiol by increasing its metabolism).
No products indexed under this heading.

Norgestimate (Decreased effect of estradiol by increasing its metabolism). Products include:
Ortho-Cyclen/Ortho-Tri-Cyclen 1858
Ortho-Cyclen/Ortho Tri-Cyclen 1858

Norgestrel (Decreased effect of estradiol by increasing its metabolism). Products include:
Lo/Ovral Tablets 2746
Lo/Ovral-28 Tablets 2751
Ovral Tablets 2770
Ovral-28 Tablets 2770
Ovrette Tablets 2771

Opium Alkaloids (Concomitant use may produce additive CNS-depressant effects).
No products indexed under this heading.

Oxazepam (Concomitant use may produce additive CNS-depressant effects). Products include:
Serax Capsules 2810
Serax Tablets 2810

Oxycodone Hydrochloride (Concomitant use may produce additive CNS-depressant effects). Products include:
Percocet Tablets 938
Percodan Tablets 939
Percodan-Demi Tablets 940
Roxicodone Tablets, Oral Solution & Intensol (Oxycodone) 2244
Tylox Capsules 1584

Pentobarbital Sodium (Concomitant use may produce additive CNS-depressant effects). Products include:
Nembutal Sodium Capsules 436
Nembutal Sodium Solution 438
Nembutal Sodium Suppositories 440

Perphenazine (Concomitant use may produce additive CNS-depressant effects). Products include:
Etrafon 2355
Triavil Tablets 1757
Trilafon 2389

Phenelzine Sulfate (Prolongs the effects of barbiturates). Products include:
Nardil 1920

Phenobarbital (Concomitant use may produce additive CNS-depressant effects). Products include:
Arco-Lase Plus Tablets 512
Bellergal-S Tablets 2250
Donnatal 2060
Donnatal Extentabs 2061
Donnatal Tablets 2060
Phenobarbital Elixir and Tablets 1469
Quadrinal Tablets 1350

(◘ Described in PDR For Nonprescription Drugs) (⊙ Described in PDR For Ophthalmology)

Phenytoin (Variable effect on the metabolism of phenytoin). Products include:
- Dilantin Infatabs ... 1908
- Dilantin-125 Suspension ... 1911

Phenytoin Sodium (Variable effect on the metabolism of phenytoin). Products include:
- Dilantin Kapseals ... 1906
- Dilantin Parenteral ... 1910

Prazepam (Concomitant use may produce additive CNS-depressant effects).
- No products indexed under this heading.

Prednisolone Acetate (Enhanced metabolism of exogenous corticosteroids). Products include:
- AK-CIDE ... ◉ 202
- AK-CIDE Ointment ... ◉ 202
- Blephamide Liquifilm Sterile Ophthalmic Suspension ... 476
- Blephamide Ointment ... ◉ 237
- Econopred & Econopred Plus Ophthalmic Suspensions ... ◉ 217
- Poly-Pred Liquifilm ... ◉ 248
- Pred Forte ... ◉ 250
- Pred Mild ... ◉ 253
- Pred-G Liquifilm Sterile Ophthalmic Suspension ... ◉ 251
- Pred-G S.O.P. Sterile Ophthalmic Ointment ... ◉ 252
- Vasocidin Ointment ... ◉ 268

Prednisolone Sodium Phosphate (Enhanced metabolism of exogenous corticosteroids). Products include:
- AK-Pred ... ◉ 204
- Hydeltrasol Injection, Sterile ... 1665
- Inflamase ... ◉ 265
- Pediapred Oral Liquid ... 995
- Vasocidin Ophthalmic Solution ... ◉ 270

Prednisolone Tebutate (Enhanced metabolism of exogenous corticosteroids). Products include:
- Hydeltra-T.B.A. Sterile Suspension 1667

Prednisone (Enhanced metabolism of exogenous corticosteroids). Products include:
- Deltasone Tablets ... 2595

Prochlorperazine (Concomitant use may produce additive CNS-depressant effects). Products include:
- Compazine ... 2470

Promethazine Hydrochloride (Concomitant use may produce additive CNS-depressant effects). Products include:
- Mepergan Injection ... 2753
- Phenergan with Codeine ... 2777
- Phenergan with Dextromethorphan 2778
- Phenergan Injection ... 2773
- Phenergan Suppositories ... 2775
- Phenergan Syrup ... 2774
- Phenergan Tablets ... 2775
- Phenergan VC ... 2779
- Phenergan VC with Codeine ... 2781

Propofol (Concomitant use may produce additive CNS-depressant effects). Products include:
- Diprivan Injection ... 2833

Propoxyphene Hydrochloride (Concomitant use may produce additive CNS-depressant effects). Products include:
- Darvon ... 1435
- Wygesic Tablets ... 2827

Propoxyphene Napsylate (Concomitant use may produce additive CNS-depressant effects). Products include:
- Darvon-N/Darvocet-N ... 1433

Pyrilamine Maleate (Concomitant use may produce additive CNS-depressant effects). Products include:
- 4-Way Fast Acting Nasal Spray (regular & mentholated) ... 🕮 621
- Maximum Strength Multi-Symptom Formula Midol ... 🕮 722
- PMS Multi-Symptom Formula Midol ... 🕮 723

Pyrilamine Tannate (Concomitant use may produce additive CNS-depressant effects). Products include:
- Atrohist Pediatric Suspension ... 454
- Rynatan ... 2673

Quazepam (Concomitant use may produce additive CNS-depressant effects). Products include:
- Doral Tablets ... 2664

Risperidone (Concomitant use may produce additive CNS-depressant effects). Products include:
- Risperdal ... 1301

Selegiline Hydrochloride (Prolongs the effects of barbiturates). Products include:
- Eldepryl Tablets ... 2550

Sufentanil Citrate (Concomitant use may produce additive CNS-depressant effects). Products include:
- Sufenta Injection ... 1309

Temazepam (Concomitant use may produce additive CNS-depressant effects). Products include:
- Restoril Capsules ... 2284

Terfenadine (Concomitant use may produce additive CNS-depressant effects). Products include:
- Seldane Tablets ... 1536
- Seldane-D Extended-Release Tablets ... 1538

Thiamylal Sodium (Concomitant use may produce additive CNS-depressant effects).
- No products indexed under this heading.

Thioridazine Hydrochloride (Concomitant use may produce additive CNS-depressant effects). Products include:
- Mellaril ... 2269

Thiothixene (Concomitant use may produce additive CNS-depressant effects). Products include:
- Navane Capsules and Concentrate 2201
- Navane Intramuscular ... 2202

Tranylcypromine Sulfate (Prolongs the effects of barbiturates). Products include:
- Parnate Tablets ... 2503

Triamcinolone (Enhanced metabolism of exogenous corticosteroids). Products include:
- Aristocort Tablets ... 1022

Triamcinolone Acetonide (Enhanced metabolism of exogenous corticosteroids). Products include:
- Aristocort A 0.025% Cream ... 1027
- Aristocort A 0.5% Cream ... 1031
- Aristocort A 0.1% Cream ... 1029
- Aristocort A 0.1% Ointment ... 1030
- Azmacort Oral Inhaler ... 2011
- Nasacort Nasal Inhaler ... 2024

Triamcinolone Diacetate (Enhanced metabolism of exogenous corticosteroids). Products include:
- Aristocort Suspension (Forte Parenteral) ... 1027
- Aristocort Suspension (Intralesional) ... 1025

Triamcinolone Hexacetonide (Enhanced metabolism of exogenous corticosteroids). Products include:
- Aristospan Suspension (Intra-articular) ... 1033
- Aristospan Suspension (Intralesional) ... 1032

Triazolam (Concomitant use may produce additive CNS-depressant effects). Products include:
- Halcion Tablets ... 2611

Trifluoperazine Hydrochloride (Concomitant use may produce additive CNS-depressant effects). Products include:
- Stelazine ... 2514

Trimeprazine Tartrate (Concomitant use may produce additive CNS-depressant effects). Products include:
- Temaril Tablets, Syrup and Spansule Extended-Release Capsules .. 483

Tripelennamine Hydrochloride (Concomitant use may produce additive CNS-depressant effects). Products include:
- PBZ Tablets ... 845
- PBZ-SR Tablets ... 844

Triprolidine Hydrochloride (Concomitant use may produce additive CNS-depressant effects). Products include:
- Actifed Plus Caplets ... 🕮 845
- Actifed Plus Tablets ... 🕮 845
- Actifed with Codeine Cough Syrup.. 1067
- Actifed Syrup ... 🕮 846
- Actifed Tablets ... 🕮 844

Valproic Acid (Increases blood levels of secobarbital sodium). Products include:
- Depakene ... 413

Warfarin Sodium (Barbiturates can induce hepatic microsomal enzymes, resulting in increased or decreased anticoagulant response). Products include:
- Coumadin ... 926

Zolpidem Tartrate (Concomitant use may produce additive CNS-depressant effects). Products include:
- Ambien Tablets ... 2416

Food Interactions

Alcohol (Concomitant use may produce additive CNS-depressant effects).

SECRETIN-FERRING

(Secretin) ... 2872

None cited in PDR database.

SECTRAL CAPSULES

(Acebutolol Hydrochloride) ... 2807

May interact with catecholamine depleting drugs, non-steroidal anti-inflammatory agents, alpha adrenergic stimulants, and insulin. Compounds in these categories include:

Deserpidine (Additive effect).
- No products indexed under this heading.

Diclofenac Potassium (Blunting of the antihypertensive effect). Products include:
- Cataflam ... 816

Diclofenac Sodium (Blunting of the antihypertensive effect). Products include:
- Voltaren Ophthalmic Sterile Ophthalmic Solution ... ◉ 272
- Voltaren Tablets ... 861

Etodolac (Blunting of the antihypertensive effect). Products include:
- Lodine Capsules and Tablets ... 2743

Fenoprofen Calcium (Blunting of the antihypertensive effect). Products include:
- Nalfon 200 Pulvules & Nalfon Tablets ... 917

Flurbiprofen (Blunting of the antihypertensive effect). Products include:
- Ansaid Tablets ... 2579

Guanethidine Monosulfate (Additive effect). Products include:
- Esimil Tablets ... 822
- Ismelin Tablets ... 827

Ibuprofen (Blunting of the antihypertensive effect). Products include:
- Advil Cold and Sinus Caplets and Tablets (formerly CoAdvil) ... 🕮 870
- Advil Ibuprofen Tablets and Caplets ... 🕮 870
- Children's Advil Suspension ... 2692
- Arthritis Foundation Ibuprofen Tablets ... 🕮 674
- Bayer Select Ibuprofen Pain Relief Formula ... 🕮 715
- Cramp End Tablets ... 🕮 735
- Dimetapp Sinus Caplets ... 🕮 775
- Haltran Tablets ... 🕮 771
- IBU Tablets ... 1342
- Ibuprohm ... 🕮 735
- Children's Motrin Ibuprofen Oral Suspension ... 1546
- Motrin Tablets ... 2625
- Motrin IB Caplets, Tablets, and Geltabs ... 🕮 838
- Motrin IB Sinus ... 🕮 838
- Motrin Ibuprofen Suspension, Oral Drops, Chewable Tablets, Caplets ... 1546
- Nuprin Ibuprofen/Analgesic Tablets & Caplets ... 🕮 622
- Sine-Aid IB Caplets ... 1554
- Vicks DayQuil SINUS Pressure & PAIN Relief with IBUPROFEN ... 🕮 762

Indomethacin (Blunting of the antihypertensive effect). Products include:
- Indocin ... 1680

Indomethacin Sodium Trihydrate (Blunting of the antihypertensive effect). Products include:
- Indocin I.V. ... 1684

Insulin, Human (Beta-blockers may potentiate insulin-induced hypoglycemia).
- No products indexed under this heading.

Insulin, Human Isophane Suspension (Beta-blockers may potentiate insulin-induced hypoglycemia). Products include:
- Novolin N Human Insulin 10 ml Vials ... 1795

Insulin, Human NPH (Beta-blockers may potentiate insulin-induced hypoglycemia). Products include:
- Humulin N, 100 Units ... 1448
- Novolin N PenFill Cartridges Durable Insulin Delivery System ... 1798
- Novolin N Prefilled Syringe Disposable Insulin Delivery System ... 1798

Insulin, Human Regular (Beta-blockers may potentiate insulin-induced hypoglycemia). Products include:
- Humulin R, 100 Units ... 1449
- Novolin R Human Insulin 10 ml Vials ... 1795
- Novolin R PenFill Cartridges Durable Insulin Delivery System ... 1798
- Novolin R Prefilled Syringe Disposable Insulin Delivery System ... 1798
- Velosulin BR Human Insulin 10 ml Vials ... 1795

Insulin, Human, Zinc Suspension (Beta-blockers may potentiate insulin-induced hypoglycemia). Products include:
- Humulin L, 100 Units ... 1446
- Humulin U, 100 Units ... 1450
- Novolin L Human Insulin 10 ml Vials ... 1795

Insulin, NPH (Beta-blockers may potentiate insulin-induced hypoglycemia). Products include:
- NPH, 100 Units ... 1450
- Pork NPH, 100 Units ... 1452
- Purified Pork NPH Isophane Insulin ... 1801

Insulin, Regular (Beta-blockers may potentiate insulin-induced hypoglycemia). Products include:
- Regular, 100 Units ... 1450
- Pork Regular, 100 Units ... 1452
- Pork Regular (Concentrated), 500 Units ... 1453
- Purified Pork Regular Insulin ... 1801

Insulin, Zinc Crystals (Beta-blockers may potentiate insulin-induced hypoglycemia). Products include:
- NPH, 100 Units ... 1450

IMPORTANT NOTE: Always consult each drug listing in the patient's regimen for possible interactions.

Sectral **Interactions Index** 928

Insulin, Zinc Suspension (Beta-blockers may potentiate insulin-induced hypoglycemia). Products include:
Iletin I 1450
Lente, 100 Units 1450
Iletin II 1452
Pork Lente, 100 Units 1452
Purified Pork Lente Insulin 1801

Ketoprofen (Blunting of the antihypertensive effect). Products include:
Orudis Capsules 2766
Oruvail Capsules 2766

Ketorolac Tromethamine (Blunting of the antihypertensive effect). Products include:
Acular 474
Acular ◉ 277
Toradol 2159

Meclofenamate Sodium (Blunting of the antihypertensive effect).
No products indexed under this heading.

Mefenamic Acid (Blunting of the antihypertensive effect). Products include:
Ponstel 1925

Nabumetone (Blunting of the antihypertensive effect). Products include:
Relafen Tablets 2510

Naphazoline Hydrochloride (Potential for exaggerated hypertensive response). Products include:
Albalon Solution with Liquifilm ◉ 231
Clear Eyes ACR Astringent/Lubricant Eye Redness Reliever Eye Drops ◉ 316
Clear Eyes Lubricant Eye Redness Reliever ◉ 316
4-Way Fast Acting Nasal Spray (regular & mentholated) ▣ 621
Naphcon-A Ophthalmic Solution 473
Privine ▣ 647
Vasocon-A ◉ 271

Naproxen (Blunting of the antihypertensive effect). Products include:
Anaprox/Naprosyn 2117

Naproxen Sodium (Blunting of the antihypertensive effect). Products include:
Aleve 1975
Anaprox/Naprosyn 2117

Oxaprozin (Blunting of the antihypertensive effect). Products include:
Daypro Caplets 2426

Oxymetazoline Hydrochloride (Potential for exaggerated hypertensive response). Products include:
Afrin ▣ 797
Cheracol Nasal Spray Pump ▣ 768
Duration 12 Hour Nasal Spray ▣ 805
4-Way Long Lasting Nasal Spray ▣ 621
NTZ Long Acting Nasal Spray & Drops 0.05% ▣ 727
Neo-Synephrine Maximum Strength 12 Hour Nasal Spray ▣ 726
Neo-Synephrine 12 Hour ▣ 726
Nōstrilla Long Acting Nasal Decongestant ▣ 644
Vicks Sinex 12-Hour Nasal Decongestant Spray and Ultra Fine Mist ▣ 765
Visine L.R. Eye Drops ▣ 746
Visine L.R. Eye Drops ◉ 313

Phenylbutazone (Blunting of the antihypertensive effect).
No products indexed under this heading.

Phenylephrine Hydrochloride (Potential for exaggerated hypertensive response). Products include:
Atrohist Plus Tablets 454
Cerose DM ▣ 878
Comhist 2038
D.A. Chewable Tablets 951
Deconsal Pediatric Capsules 454
Dura-Vent/DA Tablets 953
Entex Capsules 1986
Entex Liquid 1986
Extendryl 1005
4-Way Fast Acting Nasal Spray (regular & mentholated) ▣ 621
Hemorid For Women ▣ 834
Hycomine Compound Tablets 932
Neo-Synephrine Hydrochloride 1% Carpuject 2324
Neo-Synephrine Hydrochloride 1% Injection 2324
Neo-Synephrine Hydrochloride (Ophthalmic) 2325
Neo-Synephrine ▣ 726
Nōstril ▣ 644
Novahistine Elixir ▣ 823
Phenergan VC 2779
Phenergan VC with Codeine 2781
Preparation H ▣ 871
Tympagesic Ear Drops 2342
Vasosulf ◉ 271
Vicks Sinex Nasal Spray and Ultra Fine Mist ▣ 765

Phenylpropanolamine Hydrochloride (Potential for exaggerated hypertensive response). Products include:
Acutrim ▣ 628
Allerest Children's Chewable Tablets ▣ 627
Allerest 12 Hour Caplets ▣ 627
Atrohist Plus Tablets 454
BC Cold Powder Multi-Symptom Formula (Cold-Sinus-Allergy) ▣ 609
BC Cold Powder Non-Drowsy Formula (Cold-Sinus) ▣ 609
Cheracol Plus Head Cold/Cough Formula ▣ 769
Comtrex Multi-Symptom Non-Drowsy Liqui-gels ▣ 618
Contac Continuous Action Nasal Decongestant/Antihistamine 12 Hour Capsules ▣ 813
Contac Maximum Strength Continuous Action Decongestant/Antihistamine 12 Hour Caplets ▣ 813
Contac Severe Cold and Flu Formula Caplets ▣ 814
Coricidin 'D' Decongestant Tablets ▣ 800
Dexatrim ▣ 832
Dexatrim Plus Vitamins Caplets ▣ 832
Dimetane-DC Cough Syrup 2059
Dimetapp Elixir ▣ 773
Dimetapp Extentabs ▣ 774
Dimetapp Tablets/Liqui-Gels ▣ 775
Dimetapp Cold & Allergy Chewable Tablets ▣ 773
Dimetapp DM Elixir ▣ 774
Dura-Vent Tablets 952
Entex Capsules 1986
Entex LA Tablets 1987
Entex Liquid 1986
Exgest LA Tablets 782
Hycomine 931
Isoclor Timesule Capsules ▣ 637
Nolamine Timed-Release Tablets 785
Ornade Spansule Capsules 2502
Propagest Tablets 786
Pyrroxate Caplets ▣ 772
Robitussin-CF ▣ 777
Sinulin Tablets 787
Tavist-D 12 Hour Relief Tablets ▣ 787
Teldrin 12 Hour Antihistamine/Nasal Decongestant Allergy Relief Capsules ▣ 826
Triaminic Allergy Tablets ▣ 789
Triaminic Cold Tablets ▣ 790
Triaminic Expectorant ▣ 790
Triaminic Syrup ▣ 792
Triaminic-12 Tablets ▣ 792
Triaminic-DM Syrup ▣ 792
Triaminicin Tablets ▣ 793
Triaminicol Multi-Symptom Cold Tablets ▣ 793
Triaminicol Multi-Symptom Relief ▣ 794
Vicks DayQuil Allergy Relief 12-Hour Extended Release Tablets ▣ 760
Vicks DayQuil Allergy Relief 4-Hour Tablets ▣ 760
Vicks DayQuil SINUS Pressure & CONGESTION Relief ▣ 761

Piroxicam (Blunting of the antihypertensive effect). Products include:
Feldene Capsules 1965

Pseudoephedrine Hydrochloride (Potential for exaggerated hypertensive response). Products include:
Actifed Allergy Daytime/Nighttime Caplets ▣ 844
Actifed Plus Caplets ▣ 845
Actifed Plus Tablets ▣ 845
Actifed with Codeine Cough Syrup 1067
Actifed Sinus Daytime/Nighttime Tablets and Caplets ▣ 846
Actifed Syrup ▣ 846
Actifed Tablets ▣ 844
Advil Cold and Sinus Caplets and Tablets (formerly CoAdvil) ▣ 870
Alka-Seltzer Plus Cold Medicine Liqui-Gels ▣ 706
Alka-Seltzer Plus Cold & Cough Medicine Liqui-Gels ▣ 705
Alka-Seltzer Plus Night-Time Cold Medicine Liqui-Gels ▣ 706
Allerest Headache Strength Tablets ▣ 627
Allerest Maximum Strength Tablets ▣ 627
Allerest No Drowsiness Tablets ▣ 627
Allerest Sinus Pain Formula ▣ 627
Anatuss LA Tablets 1542
Atrohist Pediatric Capsules 453
Bayer Select Sinus Pain Relief Formula ▣ 717
Benadryl Allergy Decongestant Liquid Medication ▣ 848
Benadryl Allergy Decongestant Tablets ▣ 848
Benadryl Allergy Sinus Headache Formula Caplets ▣ 849
Benylin Multisymptom ▣ 852
Bromfed Capsules (Extended-Release) 1785
Bromfed Syrup ▣ 733
Bromfed Tablets 1785
Bromfed-DM Cough Syrup 1786
Bromfed-PD Capsules (Extended-Release) 1785
Children's Vicks DayQuil Allergy Relief ▣ 757
Children's Vicks NyQuil Cold/Cough Relief ▣ 758
Comtrex Multi-Symptom Cold Reliever Tablets/Caplets/Liqui-Gels/Liquid ▣ 615
Allergy-Sinus Comtrex Multi-Symptom Allergy-Sinus Formula Tablets ▣ 617
Comtrex Multi-Symptom Non-Drowsy Caplets ▣ 618
Congess 1004
Contac Day Allergy/Sinus Caplets ▣ 812
Contac Day & Night ▣ 812
Contac Night Allergy/Sinus Caplets ▣ 812
Contac Severe Cold & Flu Non-Drowsy ▣ 815
Deconamine Chewable Tablets 1320
Deconamine CX Cough and Cold Liquid and Tablets 1319
Deconamine 1320
Deconsal C Expectorant Syrup 456
Deconsal Pediatric Syrup 457
Deconsal II Tablets 454
Dimetane-DX Cough Syrup 2059
Dimetapp Sinus Caplets ▣ 775
Dorcol Children's Cough Syrup ▣ 785
Drixoral Cough + Congestion Liquid Caps ▣ 802
Dura-Tap/PD Capsules 2867
Duratuss Tablets 2565
Duratuss HD Elixir 2565
Efidac/24 ▣ 635
Entex PSE Tablets 1987
Fedahist Gyrocaps 2401
Fedahist Timecaps 2401
Guaifed 1787
Guaifed Syrup ▣ 734
Guaimax-D Tablets 792
Guaitab Tablets ▣ 734
Isoclor Expectorant 990
Kronofed-A 977
Motrin IB Sinus ▣ 838
Novahistine DH 2462
Novahistine DMX ▣ 822
Novahistine Expectorant 2463
Nucofed 2051
PediaCare Cold Allergy Chewable Tablets ▣ 677
PediaCare Cough-Cold Chewable Tablets 1553
PediaCare 1553
PediaCare Infants' Decongestant Drops ▣ 677
PediCare Infant's Drops Decongestant Plus Cough 1553
PediaCare NightRest Cough-Cold Liquid 1553
Pediatric Vicks 44d Dry Hacking Cough & Head Congestion ▣ 763
Pediatric Vicks 44m Cough & Cold Relief ▣ 764
Robitussin Cold & Cough Liqui-Gels ▣ 776
Robitussin Maximum Strength Cough & Cold ▣ 778
Robitussin Pediatric Cough & Cold Formula ▣ 779
Robitussin Severe Congestion Liqui-Gels ▣ 776
Robitussin-DAC Syrup 2074
Robitussin-PE ▣ 778
Rondec Oral Drops 953
Rondec Syrup 953
Rondec Tablet 953
Rondec-DM Oral Drops 954
Rondec-DM Syrup 954
Rondec-TR Tablet 953
Ryna ▣ 841
Seldane-D Extended-Release Tablets 1538
Semprex-D Capsules 463
Semprex-D Capsules 1167
Sinarest Tablets ▣ 648
Sinarest Extra Strength Tablets ▣ 648
Sinarest No Drowsiness Tablets ▣ 648
Sine-Aid IB Caplets 1554
Sine-Aid Maximum Strength Sinus Medication Gelcaps, Caplets and Tablets 1554
Sine-Off No Drowsiness Formula Caplets ▣ 824
Sine-Off Sinus Medicine ▣ 825
Singlet Tablets ▣ 825
Sinutab Non-Drying Liquid Caps ▣ 859
Sinutab Sinus Allergy Medication, Maximum Strength Tablets and Caplets ▣ 860
Sinutab Sinus Medication, Maximum Strength Without Drowsiness Formula, Tablets & Caplets ▣ 860
Sinutab Sinus Medication, Regular Strength Without Drowsiness Formula ▣ 859
Sudafed Children's Liquid ▣ 861
Sudafed Cold and Cough Liquidcaps ▣ 862
Sudafed Cough Syrup ▣ 862
Sudafed Plus Liquid ▣ 862
Sudafed Plus Tablets ▣ 863
Sudafed Severe Cold Formula Caplets ▣ 863
Sudafed Severe Cold Formula Tablets ▣ 864
Sudafed Sinus Caplets ▣ 864
Sudafed Sinus Tablets ▣ 864
Sudafed Tablets, 30 mg ▣ 861
Sudafed Tablets, 60 mg ▣ 861
Sudafed 12 Hour Caplets ▣ 861
Syn-Rx Tablets 465
Syn-Rx DM Tablets 466
TheraFlu ▣ 787
TheraFlu Maximum Strength Nighttime Flu, Cold & Cough Medicine ▣ 788
TheraFlu Maximum Strength Non-Drowsy Formula Flu, Cold & Cough Medicine ▣ 788
Thera Flu Maximum Strength, Non-Drowsy Formula Flu, Cold and Cough Caplets ▣ 789
Triaminic AM Cough and Decongestant Formula ▣ 789
Triaminic AM Decongestant Formula ▣ 790
Triaminic Nite Light ▣ 791
Triaminic Sore Throat Formula ▣ 791
Tussend 1783
Tussend Expectorant 1785
Children's TYLENOL Cold Multi-Symptom Liquid Formula and Chewable Tablets 1561
Children's TYLENOL Cold Plus Cough Multi Symptom Tablets and Liquid ▣ 681
Infants' TYLENOL Cold Decongestant & Fever-Reducer Drops 1556
TYLENOL Maximum Strength Allergy Sinus Medication Gelcaps and Caplets 1563
TYLENOL Maximum Strength Allergy Sinus NightTime Medication Caplets 1555
TYLENOL Flu Maximum Strength Gelcaps 1565
TYLENOL Flu NightTime, Maximum Strength, Gelcaps 1566
TYLENOL Maximum Strength Flu NightTime Hot Medication Packets 1562

(▣ Described in PDR For Nonprescription Drugs) (◉ Described in PDR For Ophthalmology)

TYLENOL, Maximum Strength, Sinus Medication Geltabs, Gelcaps, Caplets and Tablets 1566
TYLENOL Cold Multi-Symptom Formula Medication Tablets and Caplets 1561
TYLENOL Cold Medication No Drowsiness Formula Gelcaps and Caplets 1562
TYLENOL Cold Multi-Symptom Hot Medication Liquid Packets 1557
TYLENOL Cough Multi-Symptom Medication with Decongestant 1565
Ursinus Inlay-Tabs .... ◘ 794
Vicks 44 LiquiCaps Cough, Cold & Flu Relief .... ◘ 755
Vicks 44 LiquiCaps Non-Drowsy Cough & Cold Relief .... ◘ 756
Vicks 44D Dry Hacking Cough & Head Congestion .... ◘ 755
Vicks 44M Cough, Cold & Flu Relief .... ◘ 756
Vicks DayQuil .... ◘ 761
Vicks DayQuil SINUS Pressure & PAIN Relief with IBUPROFEN .... ◘ 762
Vicks Nyquil Hot Therapy .... ◘ 762
Vicks NyQuil LiquiCaps Multi-Symptom Cold/Flu Relief .... ◘ 763
Vicks NyQuil Multi-Symptom Cold/Flu Relief - (Original & Cherry Flavor) .... ◘ 763

Rauwolfia Serpentina (Additive effect).
No products indexed under this heading.

Rescinnamine (Additive effect).
No products indexed under this heading.

Reserpine (Additive effect). Products include:
Diupres Tablets 1650
Hydropres Tablets 1675
Ser-Ap-Es Tablets 849

Sulindac (Blunting of the antihypertensive effect). Products include:
Clinoril Tablets 1618

Tetrahydrozoline Hydrochloride (Potential for exaggerated hypertensive response). Products include:
Collyrium Fresh .... ⊙ 325
Murine Plus Lubricant Redness Reliever Eye Drops .... ◘ 781
Murine Tears Plus Lubricant Redness Reliever Eye Drops .... ⊙ 316
Visine Maximum Strength Allergy Relief .... ⊙ 313
Visine Moisturizing Eye Drops .... ⊙ 313
Visine Original Eye Drops .... ⊙ 314

Tolmetin Sodium (Blunting of the antihypertensive effect). Products include:
Tolectin (200, 400 and 600 mg) .. 1581

Food Interactions

Food, unspecified (Slightly decreases absorption and peak concentration).

SEDAPAP TABLETS 50 MG/650 MG

(Acetaminophen, Butalbital) **1543**
May interact with central nervous system depressants, narcotic analgesics, tranquilizers, psychotropics, tricyclic antidepressants, monoamine oxidase inhibitors, general anesthetics, and certain other agents. Compounds in these categories include:

Alfentanil Hydrochloride (Additive CNS depression). Products include:
Alfenta Injection 1286

Alprazolam (Additive CNS depression). Products include:
Xanax Tablets 2649

Amitriptyline Hydrochloride (Additive CNS depression). Products include:
Elavil 2838
Endep Tablets 2174
Etrafon 2355
Limbitrol 2180
Triavil Tablets 1757

Amoxapine (Additive CNS depression). Products include:
Asendin Tablets 1369

Aprobarbital (Additive CNS depression).
No products indexed under this heading.

Buprenorphine (Additive CNS depression). Products include:
Buprenex Injectable 2006

Buspirone Hydrochloride (Additive CNS depression). Products include:
BuSpar 737

Butabarbital (Additive CNS depression).
No products indexed under this heading.

Chlordiazepoxide (Additive CNS depression). Products include:
Libritabs Tablets 2177
Limbitrol 2180

Chlordiazepoxide Hydrochloride (Additive CNS depression). Products include:
Librax Capsules 2176
Librium Capsules 2178
Librium Injectable 2179

Chlorpromazine (Additive CNS depression). Products include:
Thorazine Suppositories 2523

Chlorpromazine Hydrochloride (Additive CNS depression). Products include:
Thorazine 2523

Chlorprothixene (Additive CNS depression).
No products indexed under this heading.

Chlorprothixene Hydrochloride (Additive CNS depression).
No products indexed under this heading.

Clomipramine Hydrochloride (Additive CNS depression). Products include:
Anafranil Capsules 803

Clorazepate Dipotassium (Additive CNS depression). Products include:
Tranxene 451

Clozapine (Additive CNS depression). Products include:
Clozaril Tablets 2252

Codeine Phosphate (Additive CNS depression). Products include:
Actifed with Codeine Cough Syrup.. 1067
Brontex 1981
Deconsal C Expectorant Syrup 456
Deconsal Pediatric Syrup 457
Dimetane-DC Cough Syrup 2059
Empirin with Codeine Tablets 1093
Fioricet with Codeine Capsules 2260
Fiorinal with Codeine Capsules 2262
Isoclor Expectorant 990
Novahistine DH 2462
Novahistine Expectorant 2463
Nucofed 2051
Phenergan with Codeine 2777
Phenergan VC with Codeine 2781
Robitussin A-C Syrup 2073
Robitussin-DAC Syrup 2074
Ryna .... ◘ 841
Soma Compound w/Codeine Tablets 2676
Tussi-Organidin NR Liquid and S NR Liquid 2677
Tylenol with Codeine 1583

Desflurane (Additive CNS depression). Products include:
Suprane 1813

Desipramine Hydrochloride (Additive CNS depression). Products include:
Norpramin Tablets 1526

Dezocine (Additive CNS depression). Products include:
Dalgan Injection 538

Diazepam (Additive CNS depression). Products include:
Dizac 1809
Valium Injectable 2182
Valium Tablets 2183
Valrelease Capsules 2169

Doxepin Hydrochloride (Additive CNS depression). Products include:
Sinequan 2205
Zonalon Cream 1055

Droperidol (Additive CNS depression). Products include:
Inapsine Injection 1296

Enflurane (Additive CNS depression).
No products indexed under this heading.

Estazolam (Additive CNS depression). Products include:
ProSom Tablets 449

Ethchlorvynol (Additive CNS depression). Products include:
Placidyl Capsules 448

Ethinamate (Additive CNS depression).
No products indexed under this heading.

Fentanyl (Additive CNS depression). Products include:
Duragesic Transdermal System 1288

Fentanyl Citrate (Additive CNS depression). Products include:
Sublimaze Injection 1307

Fluphenazine Decanoate (Additive CNS depression). Products include:
Prolixin Decanoate 509

Fluphenazine Enanthate (Additive CNS depression). Products include:
Prolixin Enanthate 509

Fluphenazine Hydrochloride (Additive CNS depression). Products include:
Prolixin 509

Flurazepam Hydrochloride (Additive CNS depression). Products include:
Dalmane Capsules 2173

Furazolidone (Additive CNS depression). Products include:
Furoxone 2046

Glutethimide (Additive CNS depression).
No products indexed under this heading.

Haloperidol (Additive CNS depression). Products include:
Haldol Injection, Tablets and Concentrate 1575

Haloperidol Decanoate (Additive CNS depression). Products include:
Haldol Decanoate 1577

Hydrocodone Bitartrate (Additive CNS depression). Products include:
Anexsia 5/500 Elixir 1781
Anexia Tablets 1782
Codiclear DH Syrup 791
Deconamine CX Cough and Cold Liquid and Tablets 1319
Duratuss HD Elixir 2565
Hycodan Tablets and Syrup 930
Hycomine Compound Tablets 932
Hycomine 931
Hycotuss Expectorant Syrup 933
Hydrocet Capsules 782
Lorcet 10/650 1018
Lortab 2566
Tussend 1783
Tussend Expectorant 1785
Vicodin Tablets 1356
Vicodin ES Tablets 1357
Vicodin Tuss Expectorant 1358
Zydone Capsules 949

Hydrocodone Polistirex (Additive CNS depression). Products include:
Tussionex Pennkinetic Extended-Release Suspension 998

Hydroxyzine Hydrochloride (Additive CNS depression). Products include:
Atarax Tablets & Syrup 2185
Marax Tablets & DF Syrup 2200
Vistaril Intramuscular Solution 2216

Imipramine Hydrochloride (Additive CNS depression). Products include:
Tofranil Ampuls 854
Tofranil Tablets 856

Imipramine Pamoate (Additive CNS depression). Products include:
Tofranil-PM Capsules 857

Isocarboxazid (Additive CNS depression).
No products indexed under this heading.

Isoflurane (Additive CNS depression).
No products indexed under this heading.

Ketamine Hydrochloride (Additive CNS depression).
No products indexed under this heading.

Levomethadyl Acetate Hydrochloride (Additive CNS depression). Products include:
Orlamm 2239

Levorphanol Tartrate (Additive CNS depression). Products include:
Levo-Dromoran 2129

Lithium Carbonate (Additive CNS depression). Products include:
Eskalith 2485
Lithium Carbonate Capsules & Tablets 2230
Lithonate/Lithotabs/Lithobid 2543

Lithium Citrate (Additive CNS depression).
No products indexed under this heading.

Lorazepam (Additive CNS depression). Products include:
Ativan Injection 2698
Ativan Tablets 2700

Loxapine Hydrochloride (Additive CNS depression). Products include:
Loxitane 1378

Loxapine Succinate (Additive CNS depression). Products include:
Loxitane Capsules 1378

Maprotiline Hydrochloride (Additive CNS depression). Products include:
Ludiomil Tablets 843

Meperidine Hydrochloride (Additive CNS depression). Products include:
Demerol 2308
Mepergan Injection 2753

Mephobarbital (Additive CNS depression). Products include:
Mebaral Tablets 2322

Meprobamate (Additive CNS depression). Products include:
Miltown Tablets 2672
PMB 200 and PMB 400 2783

Mesoridazine Besylate (Additive CNS depression). Products include:
Serentil 684

Methadone Hydrochloride (Additive CNS depression). Products include:
Methadone Hydrochloride Oral Concentrate 2233
Methadone Hydrochloride Oral Solution & Tablets 2235

Methohexital Sodium (Additive CNS depression). Products include:
Brevital Sodium Vials 1429

Methotrimeprazine (Additive CNS depression). Products include:
Levoprome 1274

IMPORTANT NOTE: Always consult each drug listing in the patient's regimen for possible interactions.

Sedapap Interactions Index 930

Methoxyflurane (Additive CNS depression).
No products indexed under this heading.

Midazolam Hydrochloride (Additive CNS depression). Products include:
Versed Injection 2170

Molindone Hydrochloride (Additive CNS depression). Products include:
Moban Tablets and Concentrate 1048

Morphine Sulfate (Additive CNS depression). Products include:
Astramorph/PF Injection, USP (Preservative-Free) 535
Duramorph 962
Infumorph 200 and Infumorph 500 Sterile Solutions 965
MS Contin Tablets 1994
MSIR 1997
Oramorph SR (Morphine Sulfate Sustained Release Tablets) 2236
RMS Suppositories 2657
Roxanol 2243

Nortriptyline Hydrochloride (Additive CNS depression). Products include:
Pamelor 2280

Opium Alkaloids (Additive CNS depression).
No products indexed under this heading.

Oxazepam (Additive CNS depression). Products include:
Serax Capsules 2810
Serax Tablets 2810

Oxycodone Hydrochloride (Additive CNS depression). Products include:
Percocet Tablets 938
Percodan Tablets 939
Percodan-Demi Tablets 940
Roxicodone Tablets, Oral Solution & Intensol (Oxycodone) 2244
Tylox Capsules 1584

Pentobarbital Sodium (Additive CNS depression). Products include:
Nembutal Sodium Capsules 436
Nembutal Sodium Solution 438
Nembutal Sodium Suppositories 440

Perphenazine (Additive CNS depression). Products include:
Etrafon 2355
Triavil Tablets 1757
Trilafon 2389

Phenelzine Sulfate (Additive CNS depression). Products include:
Nardil 1920

Phenobarbital (Additive CNS depression). Products include:
Arco-Lase Plus Tablets 512
Bellergal-S Tablets 2250
Donnatal 2060
Donnatal Extentabs 2061
Donnatal Tablets 2060
Phenobarbital Elixir and Tablets 1469
Quadrinal Tablets 1350

Prazepam (Additive CNS depression).
No products indexed under this heading.

Prochlorperazine (Additive CNS depression). Products include:
Compazine 2470

Promethazine Hydrochloride (Additive CNS depression). Products include:
Mepergan Injection 2753
Phenergan with Codeine 2777
Phenergan with Dextromethorphan 2778
Phenergan Injection 2773
Phenergan Suppositories 2775
Phenergan Syrup 2774
Phenergan Tablets 2775
Phenergan VC 2779
Phenergan VC with Codeine 2781

Propofol (Additive CNS depression). Products include:
Diprivan Injection 2833

Propoxyphene Hydrochloride (Additive CNS depression). Products include:
Darvon 1435
Wygesic Tablets 2827

Propoxyphene Napsylate (Additive CNS depression). Products include:
Darvon-N/Darvocet-N 1433

Protriptyline Hydrochloride (Additive CNS depression; decreased blood levels of the antidepressant). Products include:
Vivactil Tablets 1774

Quazepam (Additive CNS depression). Products include:
Doral Tablets 2664

Risperidone (Additive CNS depression). Products include:
Risperdal 1301

Secobarbital Sodium (Additive CNS depression). Products include:
Seconal Sodium Pulvules 1474

Selegiline Hydrochloride (Additive CNS depression). Products include:
Eldepryl Tablets 2550

Sufentanil Citrate (Additive CNS depression). Products include:
Sufenta Injection 1309

Temazepam (Additive CNS depression). Products include:
Restoril Capsules 2284

Thiamylal Sodium (Additive CNS depression).
No products indexed under this heading.

Thioridazine Hydrochloride (Additive CNS depression). Products include:
Mellaril 2269

Thiothixene (Additive CNS depression). Products include:
Navane Capsules and Concentrate 2201
Navane Intramuscular 2202

Tranylcypromine Sulfate (Additive CNS depression). Products include:
Parnate Tablets 2503

Triazolam (Additive CNS depression). Products include:
Halcion Tablets 2611

Trifluoperazine Hydrochloride (Additive CNS depression). Products include:
Stelazine 2514

Trimipramine Maleate (Additive CNS depression). Products include:
Surmontil Capsules 2811

Zolpidem Tartrate (Additive CNS depression). Products include:
Ambien Tablets 2416

Food Interactions

Alcohol (Additive CNS depression).

SELDANE TABLETS

(Terfenadine) **1536**

May interact with macrolide antibiotics and certain other agents. Compounds in these categories include:

Azithromycin (Co-administration is contraindicated; potential for QT interval prolongation with ventricular arrhythmia including Torsades de pointes). Products include:
Zithromax 1944

Clarithromycin (Co-administration is contraindicated; potential for QT interval prolongation with ventricular arrhythmia including Torsades de pointes). Products include:
Biaxin 405

Erythromycin (Co-administration is contraindicated; potential for QT interval prolongation with ventricular arrhythmia including Torsades de pointes). Products include:
A/T/S 2% Acne Topical Gel and Solution 1234
Benzamycin Topical Gel 905
E-Mycin Tablets 1341
Emgel 2% Topical Gel 1093
ERYC 1915
Erycette (erythromycin 2%) Topical Solution 1888
Ery-Tab Tablets 422
Erythromycin Base Filmtab 426
Erythromycin Delayed-Release Capsules, USP 427
Ilotycin Ophthalmic Ointment 912
PCE Dispertab Tablets 444
T-Stat 2.0% Topical Solution and Pads 2688
Theramycin Z Topical Solution 2% 1592

Erythromycin Estolate (Co-administration is contraindicated; potential for QT interval prolongation with ventricular arrhythmia including Torsades de pointes). Products include:
Ilosone 911

Erythromycin Ethylsuccinate (Co-administration is contraindicated; potential for QT interval prolongation with ventricular arrhythmia including Torsades de pointes). Products include:
E.E.S. 424
EryPed 421

Erythromycin Gluceptate (Co-administration is contraindicated; potential for QT interval prolongation with ventricular arrhythmia including Torsades de pointes). Products include:
Ilotycin Gluceptate, IV, Vials 913

Erythromycin Stearate (Co-administration is contraindicated; potential for QT interval prolongation with ventricular arrhythmia including Torsades de pointes). Products include:
Erythrocin Stearate Filmtab 425

Fluconazole (Co-administration is not recommended; due to chemical similarity of fluconazole to ketoconazole). Products include:
Diflucan Injection, Tablets, and Oral Suspension 2194

Itraconazole (Co-administration is contraindicated; potential for QT interval prolongation and rare serious cardiac events, e.g. death, cardiac arrest, and ventricular arrhythmia including Torsades de pointes). Products include:
Sporanox Capsules 1305

Ketoconazole (Co-administration is contraindicated; potential for QT interval prolongation and rare serious cardiac events, e.g. death, cardiac arrest, and ventricular arrhythmia including Torsade de pointes). Products include:
Nizoral 2% Cream 1297
Nizoral 2% Shampoo 1298
Nizoral Tablets 1298

Metronidazole (Co-administration is not recommended; due to chemical similarity of metronidazole to ketoconazole). Products include:
Flagyl 375 Capsules 2434
Flagyl I.V. RTU 2247
MetroGel 1047
MetroGel-Vaginal 902
Protostat Tablets 1883

Metronidazole Hydrochloride (Co-administration is not recommended; due to chemical similarity of metronidazole to ketaconazole). Products include:
Flagyl I.V. 2247

Miconazole (Co-administration is not recommended; due to chemical similarity of miconazole to ketoconazole).
No products indexed under this heading.

Troleandomycin (Co-administration is contraindicated; potential for QT interval prolongation with ventricular arrhythmia including Torsades de pointes). Products include:
Tao Capsules 2209

SELDANE-D EXTENDED-RELEASE TABLETS

(Pseudoephedrine Hydrochloride, Terfenadine) **1538**

May interact with monoamine oxidase inhibitors, macrolide antibiotics, beta blockers, sympathomimetics, and certain other agents. Compounds in these categories include:

Acebutolol Hydrochloride (Increases the effect of sympathomimetic amines). Products include:
Sectral Capsules 2807

Albuterol (Co-administration may produce combined harmful effects on cardiovascular system). Products include:
Proventil Inhalation Aerosol 2382
Ventolin Inhalation Aerosol and Refill 1197

Albuterol Sulfate (Co-administration may produce combined harmful effects on cardiovascular system). Products include:
Airet Solution for Inhalation 452
Proventil Inhalation Solution 0.083% 2384
Proventil Repetabs Tablets 2386
Proventil Solution for Inhalation 0.5% 2383
Proventil Syrup 2385
Proventil Tablets 2386
Ventolin Inhalation Solution 1198
Ventolin Nebules Inhalation Solution 1199
Ventolin Rotacaps for Inhalation 1200
Ventolin Syrup 1202
Ventolin Tablets 1203
Volmax Extended-Release Tablets .. 1788

Atenolol (Increases the effect of sympathomimetic amines). Products include:
Tenoretic Tablets 2845
Tenormin Tablets and I.V. Injection 2847

Azithromycin (Co-administration is contraindicated; potential for QT interval prolongation with ventricular arrhythmia including Torsades de pointes). Products include:
Zithromax 1944

Betaxolol Hydrochloride (Increases the effect of sympathomimetic amines). Products include:
Betoptic Ophthalmic Solution 469
Betoptic S Ophthalmic Suspension 471
Kerlone Tablets 2436

Bisoprolol Fumarate (Increases the effect of sympathomimetic amines). Products include:
Zebeta Tablets 1413
Ziac 1415

Carteolol Hydrochloride (Increases the effect of sympathomimetic amines). Products include:
Cartrol Tablets 410
Ocupress Ophthalmic Solution, 1% Sterile .... ⊙ 309

Clarithromycin (Co-administration is contraindicated; potential for QT interval prolongation with ventricular arrhythmia including Torsades de pointes). Products include:
Biaxin 405

(▭ Described in PDR For Nonprescription Drugs) (⊙ Described in PDR For Ophthalmology)

Deserpidine (Reduced antihypertensive effect).
No products indexed under this heading.

Dobutamine Hydrochloride (Co-administration may produce combined harmful effects on cardiovascular system). Products include:
Dobutrex Solution Vials 1439

Dopamine Hydrochloride (Co-administration may produce combined harmful effects on cardiovascular system).
No products indexed under this heading.

Ephedrine Hydrochloride (Co-administration may produce combined harmful effects on cardiovascular system). Products include:
Primatene Dual Action Formula .... ⊞ 872
Primatene Tablets .... ⊞ 873
Quadrinal Tablets 1350

Ephedrine Sulfate (Co-administration may produce combined harmful effects on cardiovascular system). Products include:
Bronkaid Caplets .... ⊞ 717
Marax Tablets & DF Syrup 2200

Ephedrine Tannate (Co-administration may produce combined harmful effects on cardiovascular system). Products include:
Rynatuss 2673

Epinephrine (Co-administration may produce combined harmful effects on cardiovascular system). Products include:
Bronkaid Mist .... ⊞ 717
EPIFRIN .... ⊙ 239
EpiPen 790
Marcaine Hydrochloride with Epinephrine 1:200,000 2316
Primatene Mist .... ⊞ 873
Sensorcaine with Epinephrine Injection 559
Sus-Phrine Injection 1019
Xylocaine with Epinephrine Injections 567

Epinephrine Bitartrate (Co-administration may produce combined harmful effects on cardiovascular system). Products include:
Bronkaid Mist Suspension .... ⊞ 718
Sensorcaine-MPF with Epinephrine Injection 559

Epinephrine Hydrochloride (Co-administration may produce combined harmful effects on cardiovascular system). Products include:
Ana-Kit Anaphylaxis Emergency Treatment Kit 617

Erythromycin (Co-administration is contraindicated; potential for QT interval prolongation with ventricular arrhythmia including Torsades de pointes). Products include:
A/T/S 2% Acne Topical Gel and Solution 1234
Benzamycin Topical Gel 905
E-Mycin Tablets 1341
Emgel 2% Topical Gel 1093
ERYC 1915
Erycette (erythromycin 2%) Topical Solution 1888
Ery-Tab Tablets 422
Erythromycin Base Filmtab 426
Erythromycin Delayed-Release Capsules, USP 427
Ilotycin Ophthalmic Ointment 912
PCE Dispertab Tablets 444
T-Stat 2.0% Topical Solution and Pads 2688
Theramycin Z Topical Solution 2% 1592

Erythromycin Estolate (Co-administration is contraindicated; potential for QT interval prolongation with ventricular arrhythmia including Torsades de pointes). Products include:
Ilosone 911

Erythromycin Ethylsuccinate (Co-administration is contraindicated; potential for QT interval prolongation with ventricular arrhythmia including Torsades de pointes). Products include:
E.E.S. 424
EryPed 421

Erythromycin Gluceptate (Co-administration is contraindicated; potential for QT interval prolongation with ventricular arrhythmia including Torsades de pointes). Products include:
Ilotycin Gluceptate, IV, Vials 913

Erythromycin Stearate (Co-administration is contraindicated; potential for QT interval prolongation with ventricular arrhythmia including Torsades de pointes). Products include:
Erythrocin Stearate Filmtab 425

Esmolol Hydrochloride (Increases the effect of sympathomimetic amines). Products include:
Brevibloc Injection 1808

Fluconazole (Co-administration is not recommended; due to chemical similarity of fluconazole to ketoconazole). Products include:
Diflucan Injection, Tablets, and Oral Suspension 2194

Furazolidone (Increases the effect of sympathomimetic amines; prolongs and intensifies effects of antihistamines; concurrent use is contraindicated). Products include:
Furoxone 2046

Isocarboxazid (Increases the effect of sympathomimetic amines; prolongs and intensifies effects of antihistamines; concurrent use is contraindicated).
No products indexed under this heading.

Isoproterenol Hydrochloride (Co-administration may produce combined harmful effects on cardiovascular system). Products include:
Isuprel Hydrochloride Injection 1:5000 2311
Isuprel Hydrochloride Solution 1:200 & 1:100 2313
Isuprel Mistometer 2312

Isoproterenol Sulfate (Co-administration may produce combined harmful effects on cardiovascular system). Products include:
Norisodrine with Calcium Iodide Syrup 442

Itraconazole (Co-administration is contraindicated; potential for QT interval prolongation and rare serious cardiac events, e.g. death, cardiac arrest, and ventricular arrhythmia including Torsades de pointes.). Products include:
Sporanox Capsules 1305

Ketoconazole (Co-administration is contraindicated; potential for QT interval prolongation and rare serious cardiac events, e.g. death, cardiac arrest, and ventricular arrhythmia including Torsades de pointes.). Products include:
Nizoral 2% Cream 1297
Nizoral 2% Shampoo 1298
Nizoral Tablets 1298

Labetalol Hydrochloride (Increases the effect of sympathomimetic amines). Products include:
Normodyne Injection 2377
Normodyne Tablets 2379
Trandate 1185

Levobunolol Hydrochloride (Increases the effect of sympathomimetic amines). Products include:
Betagan .... ⊙ 233

Mecamylamine Hydrochloride (Reduced antihypertensive effect). Products include:
Inversine Tablets 1686

Metaproterenol Sulfate (Co-administration may produce combined harmful effects on cardiovascular system). Products include:
Alupent 669
Metaproterenol Sulfate Inhalation Solution, USP, Arm-a-Med 552

Metaraminol Bitartrate (Co-administration may produce combined harmful effects on cardiovascular system). Products include:
Aramine Injection 1609

Methoxamine Hydrochloride (Co-administration may produce combined harmful effects on cardiovascular system). Products include:
Vasoxyl Injection 1196

Methyldopa (Reduced antihypertensive effect). Products include:
Aldoclor Tablets 1598
Aldomet Oral 1600
Aldoril Tablets 1604

Methyldopate Hydrochloride (Reduced antihypertensive effect). Products include:
Aldomet Ester HCl Injection 1602

Metipranolol Hydrochloride (Increases the effect of sympathomimetic amines). Products include:
OptiPranolol (Metipranolol 0.3%) Sterile Ophthalmic Solution .... ⊙ 258

Metoprolol Succinate (Increases the effect of sympathomimetic amines). Products include:
Toprol-XL Tablets 565

Metoprolol Tartrate (Increases the effect of sympathomimetic amines). Products include:
Lopressor Ampuls 830
Lopressor HCT Tablets 832
Lopressor Tablets 830

Metronidazole (Co-administration is not recommended; due to chemical similarity of metronidazole to ketoconazole). Products include:
Flagyl 375 Capsules 2434
Flagyl I.V. RTU 2247
MetroGel 1047
MetroGel-Vaginal 902
Protostat Tablets 1883

Metronidazole Hydrochloride (Co-administration is not recommended; due to chemical similarity of metronidazole to ketaconazole). Products include:
Flagyl I.V. 2247

Miconazole (Co-administration is not recommended; due to chemical similarity of miconazole to ketoconazole).
No products indexed under this heading.

Nadolol (Increases the effect of sympathomimetic amines).
No products indexed under this heading.

Norepinephrine Bitartrate (Co-administration may produce combined harmful effects on cardiovascular system). Products include:
Levophed Bitartrate Injection 2315

Penbutolol Sulfate (Increases the effect of sympathomimetic amines). Products include:
Levatol 2403

Phenelzine Sulfate (Increases the effect of sympathomimetic amines; prolongs and intensifies effects of antihistamines; concurrent use is contraindicated). Products include:
Nardil 1920

Phenylephrine Bitartrate (Co-administration may produce combined harmful effects on cardiovascular system).
No products indexed under this heading.

Phenylephrine Hydrochloride (Co-administration may produce combined harmful effects on cardiovascular system). Products include:
Atrohist Plus Tablets 454
Cerose DM .... ⊞ 878
Comhist 2038
D.A. Chewable Tablets 951
Deconsal Pediatric Capsules 454
Dura-Vent/DA Tablets 953
Entex Capsules 1986
Entex Liquid 1986
Extendryl 1005
4-Way Fast Acting Nasal Spray (regular & mentholated) .... ⊞ 621
Hemorid For Women .... ⊞ 834
Hycomine Compound Tablets 932
Neo-Synephrine Hydrochloride 1% Carpuject 2324
Neo-Synephrine Hydrochloride 1% Injection 2324
Neo-Synephrine Hydrochloride (Ophthalmic) 2325
Neo-Synephrine .... ⊞ 726
Nōstril .... ⊞ 644
Novahistine Elixir .... ⊞ 823
Phenergan VC 2779
Phenergan VC with Codeine 2781
Preparation H .... ⊞ 871
Tympagesic Ear Drops 2342
Vasosulf .... ⊙ 271
Vicks Sinex Nasal Spray and Ultra Fine Mist .... ⊞ 765

Phenylephrine Tannate (Co-administration may produce combined harmful effects on cardiovascular system). Products include:
Atrohist Pediatric Suspension 454
Ricobid-D Pediatric Suspension 2038
Ricobid Tablets and Pediatric Suspension 2038
Rynatan 2673
Rynatuss 2673

Phenylpropanolamine Hydrochloride (Co-administration may produce combined harmful effects on cardiovascular system). Products include:
Acutrim .... ⊞ 628
Allerest Children's Chewable Tablets .... ⊞ 627
Allerest 12 Hour Caplets .... ⊞ 627
Atrohist Plus Tablets 454
BC Cold Powder Multi-Symptom Formula (Cold-Sinus-Allergy) .... ⊞ 609
BC Cold Powder Non-Drowsy Formula (Cold-Sinus) .... ⊞ 609
Cheracol Plus Head Cold/Cough Formula .... ⊞ 769
Comtrex Multi-Symptom Non-Drowsy Liqui-gels .... ⊞ 618
Contac Continuous Action Nasal Decongestant/Antihistamine 12 Hour Capsules .... ⊞ 813
Contac Maximum Strength Continuous Action Decongestant/Antihistamine 12 Hour Caplets .... ⊞ 813
Contac Severe Cold and Flu Formula Caplets .... ⊞ 814
Coricidin 'D' Decongestant Tablets .... ⊞ 800
Dexatrim .... ⊞ 832
Dexatrim Plus Vitamins Caplets .... ⊞ 832
Dimetane-DC Cough Syrup 2059
Dimetapp Elixir .... ⊞ 773
Dimetapp Extentabs .... ⊞ 774
Dimetapp Tablets/Liqui-Gels .... ⊞ 775
Dimetapp Cold & Allergy Chewable Tablets .... ⊞ 773
Dimetapp DM Elixir .... ⊞ 774
Dura-Vent Tablets 952
Entex Capsules 1986
Entex LA Tablets 1987
Entex Liquid 1986
Exgest LA Tablets 782
Hycomine 931
Isoclor Timesule Capsules .... ⊞ 637
Nolamine Timed-Release Tablets 785
Ornade Spansule Capsules 2502
Propagest Tablets 786
Pyrroxate Caplets .... ⊞ 772
Robitussin-CF .... ⊞ 777

IMPORTANT NOTE: Always consult each drug listing in the patient's regimen for possible interactions.

Seldane-D **Interactions Index** 932

Sinulin Tablets 787
Tavist-D 12 Hour Relief Tablets .... ▣ 787
Teldrin 12 Hour Antihistamine/Nasal Decongestant Allergy Relief Capsules .... ▣ 826
Triaminic Allergy Tablets .... ▣ 789
Triaminic Cold Tablets .... ▣ 790
Triaminic Expectorant .... ▣ 790
Triaminic Syrup .... ▣ 792
Triaminic-12 Tablets .... ▣ 792
Triaminic-DM Syrup .... ▣ 792
Triaminicin Tablets .... ▣ 793
Triaminicol Multi-Symptom Cold Tablets .... ▣ 793
Triaminicol Multi-Symptom Relief ▣ 794
Vicks DayQuil Allergy Relief 12-Hour Extended Release Tablets.. ▣ 760
Vicks DayQuil Allergy Relief 4-Hour Tablets .... ▣ 760
Vicks DayQuil SINUS Pressure & CONGESTION Relief........ ▣ 761

Pindolol (Increases the effect of sympathomimetic amines). Products include:
Visken Tablets........ 2299

Pirbuterol Acetate (Co-administration may produce combined harmful effects on cardiovascular system). Products include:
Maxair Autohaler 1492
Maxair Inhaler 1494

Propranolol Hydrochloride (Increases the effect of sympathomimetic amines). Products include:
Inderal 2728
Inderal LA Long Acting Capsules 2730
Inderide Tablets 2732
Inderide LA Long Acting Capsules .. 2734

Pseudoephedrine Sulfate (Co-administration may produce combined harmful effects on cardiovascular system). Products include:
Cheracol Sinus .... ▣ 768
Chlor-Trimeton Allergy Decongestant Tablets .... ▣ 799
Claritin-D 2350
Drixoral Cold and Allergy Sustained-Action Tablets .... ▣ 802
Drixoral Cold and Flu Extended-Release Tablets........ ▣ 803
Drixoral Non-Drowsy Formula Extended-Release Tablets .... ▣ 803
Drixoral Allergy/Sinus Extended Release Tablets........ ▣ 804
Trinalin Repetabs Tablets 1330

Rauwolfia Serpentina (Reduced antihypertensive effect).
No products indexed under this heading.

Rescinnamine (Reduced antihypertensive effect).
No products indexed under this heading.

Reserpine (Reduced antihypertensive effect). Products include:
Diupres Tablets 1650
Hydropres Tablets........ 1675
Ser-Ap-Es Tablets 849

Salmeterol Xinafoate (Co-administration may produce combined harmful effects on cardiovascular system). Products include:
Serevent Inhalation Aerosol........ 1176

Selegiline Hydrochloride (Increases the effect of sympathomimetic amines; prolongs and intensifies effects of antihistamines; concurrent use is contraindicated). Products include:
Eldepryl Tablets 2550

Sotalol Hydrochloride (Increases the effect of sympathomimetic amines). Products include:
Betapace Tablets 641

Terbutaline Sulfate (Co-administration may produce combined harmful effects on cardiovascular system). Products include:
Brethaire Inhaler 813
Brethine Ampuls 815
Brethine Tablets........ 814
Bricanyl Subcutaneous Injection...... 1502
Bricanyl Tablets 1503

Timolol Hemihydrate (Increases the effect of sympathomimetic amines). Products include:
Betimol 0.25%, 0.5% .... ⊙ 261

Timolol Maleate (Increases the effect of sympathomimetic amines). Products include:
Blocadren Tablets 1614
Timolide Tablets........ 1748
Timoptic in Ocudose 1753
Timoptic Sterile Ophthalmic Solution........ 1751
Timoptic-XE 1755

Tranylcypromine Sulfate (Increases the effect of sympathomimetic amines; prolongs and intensifies effects of antihistamines; concurrent use is contraindicated). Products include:
Parnate Tablets 2503

Troleandomycin (Co-administration is contraindicated; potential for QT interval prolongation with ventricular arrhythmia including Torsades de pointes). Products include:
Tao Capsules........ 2209

SELSUN BLUE DANDRUFF SHAMPOO
(Selenium Sulfide)........ ▣ 783
None cited in PDR database.

SELSUN BLUE DANDRUFF SHAMPOO MEDICATED TREATMENT FORMULA
(Selenium Sulfide)........ ▣ 783
None cited in PDR database.

SELSUN BLUE EXTRA CONDITIONING FORMULA DANDRUFF SHAMPOO
(Selenium Sulfide)........ ▣ 783
None cited in PDR database.

SELSUN GOLD FOR WOMEN DANDRUFF SHAMPOO
(Selenium Sulfide)........ ▣ 783
None cited in PDR database.

SELSUN RX 2.5% SELENIUM SULFIDE LOTION, USP
(Selenium Sulfide) 2225
None cited in PDR database.

SEMICID VAGINAL CONTRACEPTIVE INSERTS
(Nonoxynol-9)........ ▣ 874
None cited in PDR database.

SEMPREX-D CAPSULES
(Acrivastine, Pseudoephedrine Hydrochloride) 463
May interact with monoamine oxidase inhibitors, sympathomimetics, central nervous system depressants, catecholamine depleting drugs, veratrum alkaloids, and certain other agents. Compounds in these categories include:

Albuterol (Beta-adrenergic agonists (other sympathomimetics) increase the effects of pseudoephedrine and combined effects on cardiovascular system may be harmful). Products include:
Proventil Inhalation Aerosol 2382
Ventolin Inhalation Aerosol and Refill 1197

Albuterol Sulfate (Beta-adrenergic agonists (other sympathomimetics) increase the effects of pseudoephedrine and combined effects on cardiovascular system may be harmful). Products include:
Airet Solution for Inhalation 452
Proventil Inhalation Solution 0.083%........ 2384
Proventil Repetabs Tablets 2386
Proventil Solution for Inhalation 0.5%........ 2383
Proventil Syrup 2385
Proventil Tablets 2386
Ventolin Inhalation Solution........ 1198
Ventolin Nebules Inhalation Solution........ 1199
Ventolin Rotacaps for Inhalation...... 1200
Ventolin Syrup........ 1202
Ventolin Tablets 1203
Volmax Extended-Release Tablets .. 1788

Alfentanil Hydrochloride (Co-administration may result in additional reduction in alertness and impairment of CNS performance and should be avoided). Products include:
Alfenta Injection 1286

Alprazolam (Co-administration may result in additional reduction in alertness and impairment of CNS performance and should be avoided). Products include:
Xanax Tablets 2649

Aprobarbital (Co-administration may result in additional reduction in alertness and impairment of CNS performance and should be avoided).
No products indexed under this heading.

Buprenorphine (Co-administration may result in additional reduction in alertness and impairment of CNS performance and should be avoided). Products include:
Buprenex Injectable 2006

Buspirone Hydrochloride (Co-administration may result in additional reduction in alertness and impairment of CNS performance and should be avoided). Products include:
BuSpar 737

Butabarbital (Co-administration may result in additional reduction in alertness and impairment of CNS performance and should be avoided).
No products indexed under this heading.

Butalbital (Co-administration may result in additional reduction in alertness and impairment of CNS performance and should be avoided). Products include:
Esgic-plus Tablets 1013
Fioricet Tablets........ 2258
Fioricet with Codeine Capsules 2260
Fiorinal Capsules 2261
Fiorinal with Codeine Capsules 2262
Fiorinal Tablets........ 2261
Phrenilin 785
Sedapap Tablets 50 mg/650 mg .. 1543

Chlordiazepoxide (Co-administration may result in additional reduction in alertness and impairment of CNS performance and should be avoided). Products include:
Libritabs Tablets 2177
Limbitrol 2180

Chlordiazepoxide Hydrochloride (Co-administration may result in additional reduction in alertness and impairment of CNS performance and should be avoided). Products include:
Librax Capsules 2176
Librium Capsules........ 2178
Librium Injectable 2179

Chlorpromazine (Co-administration may result in additional reduction in alertness and impairment of CNS performance and should be avoided). Products include:
Thorazine Suppositories........ 2523

Chlorpromazine Hydrochloride (Co-administration may result in additional reduction in alertness and impairment of CNS performance and should be avoided). Products include:
Thorazine 2523

Chlorprothixene (Co-administration may result in additional reduction in alertness and impairment of CNS performance and should be avoided).
No products indexed under this heading.

Chlorprothixene Hydrochloride (Co-administration may result in additional reduction in alertness and impairment of CNS performance and should be avoided).
No products indexed under this heading.

Clorazepate Dipotassium (Co-administration may result in additional reduction in alertness and impairment of CNS performance and should be avoided). Products include:
Tranxene 451

Clozapine (Co-administration may result in additional reduction in alertness and impairment of CNS performance and should be avoided). Products include:
Clozaril Tablets........ 2252

Codeine Phosphate (Co-administration may result in additional reduction in alertness and impairment of CNS performance and should be avoided). Products include:
Actifed with Codeine Cough Syrup.. 1067
Brontex 1981
Deconsal C Expectorant Syrup 456
Deconsal Pediatric Syrup........ 457
Dimetane-DC Cough Syrup 2059
Empirin with Codeine Tablets........ 1093
Fioricet with Codeine Capsules 2260
Fiorinal with Codeine Capsules 2262
Isoclor Expectorant........ 990
Novahistine DH........ 2462
Novahistine Expectorant........ 2463
Nucofed 2051
Phenergan with Codeine........ 2777
Phenergan VC with Codeine 2781
Robitussin A-C Syrup 2073
Robitussin-DAC Syrup 2074
Ryna .... ▣ 841
Soma Compound w/Codeine Tablets 2676
Tussi-Organidin NR Liquid and S NR Liquid 2677
Tylenol with Codeine 1583

Cryptenamine Preparations (Reduced antihypertensive effects of drugs that interfere with sympathetic activity).

Deserpidine (Reduced antihypertensive effects of drugs that interfere with sympathetic activity).
No products indexed under this heading.

Desflurane (Co-administration may result in additional reduction in alertness and impairment of CNS performance and should be avoided). Products include:
Suprane 1813

Dezocine (Co-administration may result in additional reduction in alertness and impairment of CNS performance and should be avoided). Products include:
Dalgan Injection 538

Diazepam (Co-administration may result in additional reduction in alertness and impairment of CNS performance and should be avoided). Products include:
Dizac 1809
Valium Injectable 2182
Valium Tablets 2183
Valrelease Capsules 2169

(▣ Described in PDR For Nonprescription Drugs) (⊙ Described in PDR For Ophthalmology)

Dobutamine Hydrochloride (Beta-adrenergic agonists (other sympathomimetics) increase the effects of pseudoephedrine and combined effects on cardiovascular system may be harmful). Products include:

Dobutrex Solution Vials........................ 1439

Dopamine Hydrochloride (Beta-adrenergic agonists (other sympathomimetics) increase the effects of pseudoephedrine and combined effects on cardiovascular system may be harmful).

No products indexed under this heading.

Droperidol (Co-administration may result in additional reduction in alertness and impairment of CNS performance and should be avoided). Products include:

Inapsine Injection................................... 1296

Enflurane (Co-administration may result in additional reduction in alertness and impairment of CNS performance and should be avoided).

No products indexed under this heading.

Ephedrine Hydrochloride (Beta-adrenergic agonists (other sympathomimetics) increase the effects of pseudoephedrine and combined effects on cardiovascular system may be harmful). Products include:

Primatene Dual Action Formula...... ⊕ 872
Primatene Tablets .... ⊕ 873
Quadrinal Tablets 1350

Ephedrine Sulfate (Beta-adrenergic agonists (other sympathomimetics) increase the effects of pseudoephedrine and combined effects on cardiovascular system may be harmful). Products include:

Bronkaid Caplets .... ⊕ 717
Marax Tablets & DF Syrup.................. 2200

Ephedrine Tannate (Beta-adrenergic agonists (other sympathomimetics) increase the effects of pseudoephedrine and combined effects on cardiovascular system may be harmful). Products include:

Rynatuss 2673

Epinephrine (Beta-adrenergic agonists (other sympathomimetics) increase the effects of pseudoephedrine and combined effects on cardiovascular system may be harmful). Products include:

Bronkaid Mist .... ⊕ 717
EPIFRIN .... ⓒ 239
EpiPen 790
Marcaine Hydrochloride with Epinephrine 1:200,000 2316
Primatene Mist .... ⊕ 873
Sensorcaine with Epinephrine Injection.. 559
Sus-Phrine Injection 1019
Xylocaine with Epinephrine Injections.. 567

Epinephrine Bitartrate (Beta-adrenergic agonists (other sympathomimetics) increase the effects of pseudoephedrine and combined effects on cardiovascular system may be harmful). Products include:

Bronkaid Mist Suspension .... ⊕ 718
Sensorcaine-MPF with Epinephrine Injection 559

Epinephrine Hydrochloride (Beta-adrenergic agonists (other sympathomimetics) increase the effects of pseudoephedrine and combined effects on cardiovascular system may be harmful). Products include:

Ana-Kit Anaphylaxis Emergency Treatment Kit 617

Estazolam (Co-administration may result in additional reduction in alertness and impairment of CNS performance and should be avoided). Products include:

ProSom Tablets 449

Ethchlorvynol (Co-administration may result in additional reduction in alertness and impairment of CNS performance and should be avoided). Products include:

Placidyl Capsules................................... 448

Ethinamate (Co-administration may result in additional reduction in alertness and impairment of CNS performance and should be avoided).

No products indexed under this heading.

Fentanyl (Co-administration may result in additional reduction in alertness and impairment of CNS performance and should be avoided). Products include:

Duragesic Transdermal System........ 1288

Fentanyl Citrate (Co-administration may result in additional reduction in alertness and impairment of CNS performance and should be avoided). Products include:

Sublimaze Injection................................ 1307

Fluphenazine Decanoate (Co-administration may result in additional reduction in alertness and impairment of CNS performance and should be avoided). Products include:

Prolixin Decanoate 509

Fluphenazine Enanthate (Co-administration may result in additional reduction in alertness and impairment of CNS performance and should be avoided). Products include:

Prolixin Enanthate 509

Fluphenazine Hydrochloride (Co-administration may result in additional reduction in alertness and impairment of CNS performance and should be avoided). Products include:

Prolixin 509

Flurazepam Hydrochloride (Co-administration may result in additional reduction in alertness and impairment of CNS performance and should be avoided). Products include:

Dalmane Capsules.................................. 2173

Furazolidone (Increases the effects of sympathomimetics; potential for hypertensive crisis; concurrent and/or sequential use is contraindicated for two weeks). Products include:

Furoxone 2046

Glutethimide (Co-administration may result in additional reduction in alertness and impairment of CNS performance and should be avoided).

No products indexed under this heading.

Guanethidine Monosulfate (Reduced antihypertensive effects of drugs that interfere with sympathetic activity). Products include:

Esimil Tablets 822
Ismelin Tablets 827

Haloperidol (Co-administration may result in additional reduction in alertness and impairment of CNS performance and should be avoided). Products include:

Haldol Injection, Tablets and Concentrate 1575

Haloperidol Decanoate (Co-administration may result in additional reduction in alertness and impairment of CNS performance and should be avoided). Products include:

Haldol Decanoate................................... 1577

Hydrocodone Bitartrate (Co-administration may result in additional reduction in alertness and impairment of CNS performance and should be avoided). Products include:

Anexsia 5/500 Elixir 1781
Anexia Tablets... 1782
Codiclear DH Syrup 791
Deconamine CX Cough and Cold Liquid and Tablets................................. 1319
Duratuss HD Elixir................................. 2565
Hycodan Tablets and Syrup 930
Hycomine Compound Tablets 932
Hycomine 931
Hycotuss Expectorant Syrup 933
Hydrocet Capsules 782
Lorcet 10/650... 1018
Lortab 2566
Tussend 1783
Tussend Expectorant 1785
Vicodin Tablets....................................... 1356
Vicodin ES Tablets 1357
Vicodin Tuss Expectorant 1358
Zydone Capsules 949

Hydrocodone Polistirex (Co-administration may result in additional reduction in alertness and impairment of CNS performance and should be avoided). Products include:

Tussionex Pennkinetic Extended-Release Suspension 998

Hydroxyzine Hydrochloride (Co-administration may result in additional reduction in alertness and impairment of CNS performance and should be avoided). Products include:

Atarax Tablets & Syrup........................ 2185
Marax Tablets & DF Syrup.................. 2200
Vistaril Intramuscular Solution.......... 2216

Isocarboxazid (Increases the effects of sympathomimetics; potential for hypertensive crisis; concurrent and/or sequential use is contraindicated for two weeks).

No products indexed under this heading.

Isoflurane (Co-administration may result in additional reduction in alertness and impairment of CNS performance and should be avoided).

No products indexed under this heading.

Isoproterenol Hydrochloride (Beta-adrenergic agonists (other sympathomimetics) increase the effects of pseudoephedrine and combined effects on cardiovascular system may be harmful). Products include:

Isuprel Hydrochloride Injection 1:5000 2311
Isuprel Hydrochloride Solution 1:200 & 1:100 2313
Isuprel Mistometer 2312

Ketamine Hydrochloride (Co-administration may result in additional reduction in alertness and impairment of CNS performance and should be avoided).

No products indexed under this heading.

Levomethadyl Acetate Hydrochloride (Co-administration may result in additional reduction in alertness and impairment of CNS performance and should be avoided). Products include:

Orlaam 2239

Levorphanol Tartrate (Co-administration may result in additional reduction in alertness and impairment of CNS performance and should be avoided). Products include:

Levo-Dromoran 2129

Lorazepam (Co-administration may result in additional reduction in alertness and impairment of CNS performance and should be avoided). Products include:

Ativan Injection....................................... 2698
Ativan Tablets 2700

Loxapine Hydrochloride (Co-administration may result in additional reduction in alertness and impairment of CNS performance and should be avoided). Products include:

Loxitane 1378

Loxapine Succinate (Co-administration may result in additional reduction in alertness and impairment of CNS performance and should be avoided). Products include:

Loxitane Capsules 1378

Mecamylamine Hydrochloride (Reduced antihypertensive effects of drugs that interfere with sympathetic activity). Products include:

Inversine Tablets 1686

Meperidine Hydrochloride (Co-administration may result in additional reduction in alertness and impairment of CNS performance and should be avoided). Products include:

Demerol 2308
Mepergan Injection 2753

Mephobarbital (Co-administration may result in additional reduction in alertness and impairment of CNS performance and should be avoided). Products include:

Mebaral Tablets 2322

Meprobamate (Co-administration may result in additional reduction in alertness and impairment of CNS performance and should be avoided). Products include:

Miltown Tablets 2672
PMB 200 and PMB 400 2783

Mesoridazine (Co-administration may result in additional reduction in alertness and impairment of CNS performance and should be avoided).

Metaproterenol Sulfate (Beta-adrenergic agonists (other sympathomimetics) increase the effects of pseudoephedrine and combined effects on cardiovascular system may be harmful). Products include:

Alupent.. 669
Metaproterenol Sulfate Inhalation Solution, USP, Arm-a-Med 552

Metaraminol Bitartrate (Beta-adrenergic agonists (other sympathomimetics) increase the effects of pseudoephedrine and combined effects on cardiovascular system may be harmful). Products include:

Aramine Injection................................... 1609

Methadone Hydrochloride (Co-administration may result in additional reduction in alertness and impairment of CNS performance and should be avoided). Products include:

Methadone Hydrochloride Oral Concentrate 2233
Methadone Hydrochloride Oral Solution & Tablets................................. 2235

IMPORTANT NOTE: Always consult each drug listing in the patient's regimen for possible interactions.

Semprex-D

Methohexital Sodium (Co-administration may result in additional reduction in alertness and impairment of CNS performance and should be avoided). Products include:

Brevital Sodium Vials 1429

Methotrimeprazine (Co-administration may result in additional reduction in alertness and impairment of CNS performance and should be avoided). Products include:

Levoprome 1274

Methoxamine Hydrochloride (Beta-adrenergic agonists (other sympathomimetics) increase the effects of pseudoephedrine and combined effects on cardiovascular system may be harmful). Products include:

Vasoxyl Injection 1196

Methoxyflurane (Co-administration may result in additional reduction in alertness and impairment of CNS performance and should be avoided).

No products indexed under this heading.

Methyldopa (Reduced antihypertensive effects of drugs that interfere with sympathetic activity). Products include:

Aldoclor Tablets 1598
Aldomet Oral 1600
Aldoril Tablets 1604

Methyldopate Hydrochloride (Reduced antihypertensive effects of drugs that interfere with sympathetic activity). Products include:

Aldomet Ester HCl Injection 1602

Midazolam Hydrochloride (Co-administration may result in additional reduction in alertness and impairment of CNS performance and should be avoided). Products include:

Versed Injection 2170

Molindone Hydrochloride (Co-administration may result in additional reduction in alertness and impairment of CNS performance and should be avoided). Products include:

Moban Tablets and Concentrate 1048

Morphine Sulfate (Co-administration may result in additional reduction in alertness and impairment of CNS performance and should be avoided). Products include:

Astramorph/PF Injection, USP (Preservative-Free) 535
Duramorph 962
Infumorph 200 and Infumorph 500 Sterile Solutions 965
MS Contin Tablets 1994
MSIR 1997
Oramorph SR (Morphine Sulfate Sustained Release Tablets) 2236
RMS Suppositories 2657
Roxanol 2243

Norepinephrine Bitartrate (Beta-adrenergic agonists (other sympathomimetics) increase the effects of pseudoephedrine and combined effects on cardiovascular system may be harmful). Products include:

Levophed Bitartrate Injection 2315

Opium Alkaloids (Co-administration may result in additional reduction in alertness and impairment of CNS performance and should be avoided).

No products indexed under this heading.

Oxazepam (Co-administration may result in additional reduction in alertness and impairment of CNS performance and should be avoided). Products include:

Serax Capsules 2810
Serax Tablets 2810

Oxycodone Hydrochloride (Co-administration may result in additional reduction in alertness and impairment of CNS performance and should be avoided). Products include:

Percocet Tablets 938
Percodan Tablets 939
Percodan-Demi Tablets 940
Roxicodone Tablets, Oral Solution & Intensol (Oxycodone) 2244
Tylox Capsules 1584

Pentobarbital Sodium (Co-administration may result in additional reduction in alertness and impairment of CNS performance and should be avoided). Products include:

Nembutal Sodium Capsules 436
Nembutal Sodium Solution 438
Nembutal Sodium Suppositories 440

Perphenazine (Co-administration may result in additional reduction in alertness and impairment of CNS performance and should be avoided). Products include:

Etrafon 2355
Triavil Tablets 1757
Trilafon 2389

Phenelzine Sulfate (Increases the effects of sympathomimetics; potential for hypertensive crisis; concurrent and/or sequential use is contraindicated for two weeks). Products include:

Nardil 1920

Phenobarbital (Co-administration may result in additional reduction in alertness and impairment of CNS performance and should be avoided). Products include:

Arco-Lase Plus Tablets 512
Bellergal-S Tablets 2250
Donnatal 2060
Donnatal Extentabs 2061
Donnatal Tablets 2060
Phenobarbital Elixir and Tablets 1469
Quadrinal Tablets 1350

Phenylephrine Bitartrate (Beta-adrenergic agonists (other sympathomimetics) increase the effects of pseudoephedrine and combined effects on cardiovascular system may be harmful).

No products indexed under this heading.

Phenylephrine Hydrochloride (Beta-adrenergic agonists (other sympathomimetics) increase the effects of pseudoephedrine and combined effects on cardiovascular system may be harmful). Products include:

Atrohist Plus Tablets 454
Cerose DM .... ⊕D 878
Comhist 2038
D.A. Chewable Tablets 951
Deconsal Pediatric Capsules 454
Dura-Vent/DA Tablets 953
Entex Capsules 1986
Entex Liquid 1986
Extendryl 1005
4-Way Fast Acting Nasal Spray (regular & mentholated) .... ⊕D 621
Hemorid For Women .... ⊕D 834
Hycomine Compound Tablets 932
Neo-Synephrine Hydrochloride 1 % Carpuject 2324
Neo-Synephrine Hydrochloride 1 % Injection 2324
Neo-Synephrine Hydrochloride (Ophthalmic) 2325
Neo-Synephrine .... ⊕D 726
Nōstril .... ⊕D 644
Novahistine Elixir .... ⊕D 823
Phenergan VC 2779

Phenergan VC with Codeine 2781
Preparation H .... ⊕D 871
Tympagesic Ear Drops 2342
Vasosulf .... ◎ 271
Vicks Sinex Nasal Spray and Ultra Fine Mist .... ⊕D 765

Phenylephrine Tannate (Beta-adrenergic agonists (other sympathomimetics) increase the effects of pseudoephedrine and combined effects on cardiovascular system may be harmful). Products include:

Atrohist Pediatric Suspension 454
Ricobid-D Pediatric Suspension 2038
Ricobid Tablets and Pediatric Suspension 2038
Rynatan 2673
Rynatuss 2673

Phenylpropanolamine Hydrochloride (Beta-adrenergic agonists (other sympathomimetics) increase the effects of pseudoephedrine and combined effects on cardiovascular system may be harmful). Products include:

Acutrim .... ⊕D 628
Allerest Children's Chewable Tablets .... ⊕D 627
Allerest 12 Hour Caplets .... ⊕D 627
Atrohist Plus Tablets 454
BC Cold Powder Multi-Symptom Formula (Cold-Sinus-Allergy) ...... ⊕D 609
BC Cold Powder Non-Drowsy Formula (Cold-Sinus) .... ⊕D 609
Cheracol Plus Head Cold/Cough Formula .... ⊕D 769
Comtrex Multi-Symptom Non-Drowsy Liqui-gels .... ⊕D 618
Contac Continuous Action Nasal Decongestant/Antihistamine 12 Hour Capsules .... ⊕D 813
Contac Maximum Strength Continuous Action Decongestant/ Antihistamine 12 Hour Caplets .. ⊕D 813
Contac Severe Cold and Flu Formula Caplets .... ⊕D 814
Coricidin 'D' Decongestant Tablets .... ⊕D 800
Dexatrim .... ⊕D 832
Dexatrim Plus Vitamins Caplets .... ⊕D 832
Dimetane-DC Cough Syrup 2059
Dimetapp Elixir .... ⊕D 773
Dimetapp Extentabs .... ⊕D 774
Dimetapp Tablets/Liqui-Gels .... ⊕D 775
Dimetapp Cold & Allergy Chewable Tablets .... ⊕D 773
Dimetapp DM Elixir .... ⊕D 774
Dura-Vent Tablets 952
Entex Capsules 1986
Entex LA Tablets 1987
Entex Liquid 1986
Exgest LA Tablets 782
Hycomine 931
Isoclor Timesule Capsules .... ⊕D 637
Nolamine Timed-Release Tablets 785
Ornade Spansule Capsules 2502
Propagest Tablets 786
Pyrroxate Caplets .... ⊕D 772
Robitussin-CF .... ⊕D 777
Sinulin Tablets 787
Tavist-D 12 Hour Relief Tablets .... ⊕D 787
Teldrin 12 Hour Antihistamine/ Nasal Decongestant Allergy Relief Capsules .... ⊕D 826
Triaminic Allergy Tablets .... ⊕D 789
Triaminic Cold Tablets .... ⊕D 790
Triaminic Expectorant .... ⊕D 790
Triaminic Syrup .... ⊕D 792
Triaminic-12 Tablets .... ⊕D 792
Triaminic-DM Syrup .... ⊕D 792
Triaminicin Tablets .... ⊕D 793
Triaminicol Multi-Symptom Cold Tablets .... ⊕D 793
Triaminicol Multi-Symptom Relief ⊕D 794
Vicks DayQuil Allergy Relief 12-Hour Extended Release Tablets .. ⊕D 760
Vicks DayQuil Allergy Relief 4-Hour Tablets .... ⊕D 760
Vicks DayQuil SINUS Pressure & CONGESTION Relief .... ⊕D 761

Pirbuterol Acetate (Beta-adrenergic agonists (other sympathomimetics) increase the effects of pseudoephedrine and combined effects on cardiovascular system may be harmful). Products include:

Maxair Autohaler 1492
Maxair Inhaler 1494

Prazepam (Co-administration may result in additional reduction in alertness and impairment of CNS performance and should be avoided).

No products indexed under this heading.

Prochlorperazine (Co-administration may result in additional reduction in alertness and impairment of CNS performance and should be avoided). Products include:

Compazine 2470

Promethazine Hydrochloride (Co-administration may result in additional reduction in alertness and impairment of CNS performance and should be avoided). Products include:

Mepergan Injection 2753
Phenergan with Codeine 2777
Phenergan with Dextromethorphan 2778
Phenergan Injection 2773
Phenergan Suppositories 2775
Phenergan Syrup 2774
Phenergan Tablets 2775
Phenergan VC 2779
Phenergan VC with Codeine 2781

Propofol (Co-administration may result in additional reduction in alertness and impairment of CNS performance and should be avoided). Products include:

Diprivan Injection 2833

Propoxyphene Hydrochloride (Co-administration may result in additional reduction in alertness and impairment of CNS performance and should be avoided). Products include:

Darvon 1435
Wygesic Tablets 2827

Propoxyphene Napsylate (Co-administration may result in additional reduction in alertness and impairment of CNS performance and should be avoided). Products include:

Darvon-N/Darvocet-N 1433

Pseudoephedrine Sulfate (Beta-adrenergic agonists (other sympathomimetics) increase the effects of pseudoephedrine and combined effects on cardiovascular system may be harmful). Products include:

Cheracol Sinus .... ⊕D 768
Chlor-Trimeton Allergy Decongestant Tablets .... ⊕D 799
Claritin-D 2350
Drixoral Cold and Allergy Sustained-Action Tablets .... ⊕D 802
Drixoral Cold and Flu Extended-Release Tablets .... ⊕D 803
Drixoral Non-Drowsy Formula Extended-Release Tablets .... ⊕D 803
Drixoral Allergy/Sinus Extended Release Tablets .... ⊕D 804
Trinalin Repetabs Tablets 1330

Quazepam (Co-administration may result in additional reduction in alertness and impairment of CNS performance and should be avoided). Products include:

Doral Tablets 2664

Rauwolfia Serpentina (Reduced antihypertensive effects of drugs that interfere with sympathetic activity).

No products indexed under this heading.

Rescinnamine (Reduced antihypertensive effects of drugs that interfere with sympathetic activity).

No products indexed under this heading.

Reserpine (Reduced antihypertensive effects of drugs that interfere with sympathetic activity). Products include:

Diupres Tablets 1650
Hydropres Tablets 1675
Ser-Ap-Es Tablets 849

(⊕D Described in PDR For Nonprescription Drugs) (◎ Described in PDR For Ophthalmology)

Risperidone (Co-administration may result in additional reduction in alertness and impairment of CNS performance and should be avoided). Products include:

Risperdal 1301

Salmeterol Xinafoate (Beta-adrenergic agonists (other sympathomimetics) increase the effects of pseudoephedrine and combined effects on cardiovascular system may be harmful). Products include:

Serevent Inhalation Aerosol................ 1176

Secobarbital Sodium (Co-administration may result in additional reduction in alertness and impairment of CNS performance and should be avoided). Products include:

Seconal Sodium Pulvules 1474

Selegiline Hydrochloride (Increases the effects of sympathomimetics; potential for hypertensive crisis; concurrent and/or sequential use is contraindicated for two weeks). Products include:

Eldepryl Tablets 2550

Sufentanil Citrate (Co-administration may result in additional reduction in alertness and impairment of CNS performance and should be avoided). Products include:

Sufenta Injection 1309

Temazepam (Co-administration may result in additional reduction in alertness and impairment of CNS performance and should be avoided). Products include:

Restoril Capsules 2284

Terbutaline Sulfate (Beta-adrenergic agonists (other sympathomimetics) increase the effects of pseudoephedrine and combined effects on cardiovascular system may be harmful). Products include:

Brethaire Inhaler 813
Brethine Ampuls 815
Brethine Tablets 814
Bricanyl Subcutaneous Injection...... 1502
Bricanyl Tablets 1503

Thiamylal Sodium (Co-administration may result in additional reduction in alertness and impairment of CNS performance and should be avoided).

No products indexed under this heading.

Thioridazine Hydrochloride (Co-administration may result in additional reduction in alertness and impairment of CNS performance and should be avoided). Products include:

Mellaril 2269

Thiothixene (Co-administration may result in additional reduction in alertness and impairment of CNS performance and should be avoided). Products include:

Navane Capsules and Concentrate 2201
Navane Intramuscular 2202

Tranylcypromine Sulfate (Increases the effects of sympathomimetics; potential for hypertensive crisis; concurrent and/or sequential use is contraindicated for two weeks). Products include:

Parnate Tablets 2503

Triazolam (Co-administration may result in additional reduction in alertness and impairment of CNS performance and should be avoided). Products include:

Halcion Tablets...................................... 2611

Trifluoperazine Hydrochloride (Co-administration may result in additional reduction in alertness and impairment of CNS performance and should be avoided). Products include:

Stelazine 2514

Zolpidem Tartrate (Co-administration may result in additional reduction in alertness and impairment of CNS performance and should be avoided). Products include:

Ambien Tablets...................................... 2416

Food Interactions

Alcohol (Co-administration may result in additional reduction in alertness and impairment of CNS performance and should be avoided).

SEMPREX-D CAPSULES

(Acrivastine, Pseudoephedrine Hydrochloride) 1167

May interact with monoamine oxidase inhibitors, sympathomimetics, central nervous system depressants, catecholamine depleting drugs, veratrum alkaloids, and certain other agents. Compounds in these categories include:

Albuterol (Beta-adrenergic agonists (other sympathomimetics) increase the effects of pseudoephedrine and combined effects on cardiovascular system may be harmful). Products include:

Proventil Inhalation Aerosol 2382
Ventolin Inhalation Aerosol and Refill 1197

Albuterol Sulfate (Beta-adrenergic agonists (other sympathomimetics) increase the effects of pseudoephedrine and combined effects on cardiovascular system may be harmful). Products include:

Airet Solution for Inhalation 452
Proventil Inhalation Solution 0.083% 2384
Proventil Repetabs Tablets 2386
Proventil Solution for Inhalation 0.5% 2383
Proventil Syrup 2385
Proventil Tablets 2386
Ventolin Inhalation Solution................ 1198
Ventolin Nebules Inhalation Solution 1199
Ventolin Rotacaps for Inhalation 1200
Ventolin Syrup....................................... 1202
Ventolin Tablets..................................... 1203
Volmax Extended-Release Tablets .. 1788

Alfentanil Hydrochloride (Co-administration may result in additional reduction in alertness and impairment of CNS performance and should be avoided). Products include:

Alfenta Injection 1286

Alprazolam (Co-administration may result in additional reduction in alertness and impairment of CNS performance and should be avoided). Products include:

Xanax Tablets 2649

Aprobarbital (Co-administration may result in additional reduction in alertness and impairment of CNS performance and should be avoided).

No products indexed under this heading.

Buprenorphine (Co-administration may result in additional reduction in alertness and impairment of CNS performance and should be avoided). Products include:

Buprenex Injectable 2006

Buspirone Hydrochloride (Co-administration may result in additional reduction in alertness and impairment of CNS performance and should be avoided). Products include:

BuSpar 737

Butabarbital (Co-administration may result in additional reduction in alertness and impairment of CNS performance and should be avoided).

No products indexed under this heading.

Butalbital (Co-administration may result in additional reduction in alertness and impairment of CNS performance and should be avoided). Products include:

Esgic-plus Tablets 1013
Fioricet Tablets...................................... 2258
Fioricet with Codeine Capsules 2260
Fiorinal Capsules 2261
Fiorinal with Codeine Capsules 2262
Fiorinal Tablets 2261
Phrenilin 785
Sedapap Tablets 50 mg/650 mg .. 1543

Chlordiazepoxide (Co-administration may result in additional reduction in alertness and impairment of CNS performance and should be avoided). Products include:

Libritabs Tablets 2177
Limbitrol 2180

Chlordiazepoxide Hydrochloride (Co-administration may result in additional reduction in alertness and impairment of CNS performance and should be avoided). Products include:

Librax Capsules 2176
Librium Capsules.................................. 2178
Librium Injectable................................. 2179

Chlorpromazine (Co-administration may result in additional reduction in alertness and impairment of CNS performance and should be avoided). Products include:

Thorazine Suppositories...................... 2523

Chlorpromazine Hydrochloride (Co-administration may result in additional reduction in alertness and impairment of CNS performance and should be avoided). Products include:

Thorazine 2523

Chlorprothixene (Co-administration may result in additional reduction in alertness and impairment of CNS performance and should be avoided).

No products indexed under this heading.

Chlorprothixene Hydrochloride (Co-administration may result in additional reduction in alertness and impairment of CNS performance and should be avoided).

No products indexed under this heading.

Clorazepate Dipotassium (Co-administration may result in additional reduction in alertness and impairment of CNS performance and should be avoided). Products include:

Tranxene 451

Clozapine (Co-administration may result in additional reduction in alertness and impairment of CNS performance and should be avoided). Products include:

Clozaril Tablets...................................... 2252

Codeine Phosphate (Co-administration may result in additional reduction in alertness and impairment of CNS performance and should be avoided). Products include:

Actifed with Codeine Cough Syrup.. 1067

Brontex 1981
Deconsal C Expectorant Syrup 456
Deconsal Pediatric Syrup 457
Dimetane-DC Cough Syrup 2059
Empirin with Codeine Tablets............ 1093
Fioricet with Codeine Capsules 2260
Fiorinal with Codeine Capsules 2262
Isoclor Expectorant.............................. 990
Novahistine DH..................................... 2462
Novahistine Expectorant..................... 2463
Nucofed 2051
Phenergan with Codeine..................... 2777
Phenergan VC with Codeine 2781
Robitussin A-C Syrup........................... 2073
Robitussin-DAC Syrup.......................... 2074
Ryna ....**◆D** 841
Soma Compound w/Codeine Tablets 2676
Tussi-Organidin NR Liquid and S NR Liquid 2677
Tylenol with Codeine 1583

Cryptenamine Preparations (Reduced antihypertensive effects of drugs that interfere with sympathetic activity).

Deserpidine (Reduced antihypertensive effects of drugs that interfere with sympathetic activity).

No products indexed under this heading.

Desflurane (Co-administration may result in additional reduction in alertness and impairment of CNS performance and should be avoided). Products include:

Suprane 1813

Dezocine (Co-administration may result in additional reduction in alertness and impairment of CNS performance and should be avoided). Products include:

Dalgan Injection 538

Diazepam (Co-administration may result in additional reduction in alertness and impairment of CNS performance and should be avoided). Products include:

Dizac 1809
Valium Injectable 2182
Valium Tablets 2183
Valrelease Capsules 2169

Dobutamine Hydrochloride (Beta-adrenergic agonists (other sympathomimetics) increase the effects of pseudoephedrine and combined effects on cardiovascular system may be harmful). Products include:

Dobutrex Solution Vials....................... 1439

Dopamine Hydrochloride (Beta-adrenergic agonists (other sympathomimetics) increase the effects of pseudoephedrine and combined effects on cardiovascular system may be harmful).

No products indexed under this heading.

Droperidol (Co-administration may result in additional reduction in alertness and impairment of CNS performance and should be avoided). Products include:

Inapsine Injection................................. 1296

Enflurane (Co-administration may result in additional reduction in alertness and impairment of CNS performance and should be avoided).

No products indexed under this heading.

Ephedrine Hydrochloride (Beta-adrenergic agonists (other sympathomimetics) increase the effects of pseudoephedrine and combined effects on cardiovascular system may be harmful). Products include:

Primatene Dual Action Formula......**◆D** 872
Primatene Tablets ....**◆D** 873
Quadrinal Tablets 1350

IMPORTANT NOTE: Always consult each drug listing in the patient's regimen for possible interactions.

Semprex-D

Ephedrine Sulfate (Beta-adrenergic agonists (other sympathomimetics) increase the effects of pseudoephedrine and combined effects on cardiovascular system may be harmful). Products include:

Bronkaid Caplets .... ⊕◻ 717
Marax Tablets & DF Syrup................... 2200

Ephedrine Tannate (Beta-adrenergic agonists (other sympathomimetics) increase the effects of pseudoephedrine and combined effects on cardiovascular system may be harmful). Products include:

Rynatuss 2673

Epinephrine (Beta-adrenergic agonists (other sympathomimetics) increase the effects of pseudoephedrine and combined effects on cardiovascular system may be harmful). Products include:

Bronkaid Mist .... ⊕◻ 717
EPIFRIN .... ◎ 239
EpiPen 790
Marcaine Hydrochloride with Epinephrine 1:200,000 2316
Primatene Mist .... ⊕◻ 873
Sensorcaine with Epinephrine Injection 559
Sus-Phrine Injection 1019
Xylocaine with Epinephrine Injections 567

Epinephrine Bitartrate (Beta-adrenergic agonists (other sympathomimetics) increase the effects of pseudoephedrine and combined effects on cardiovascular system may be harmful). Products include:

Bronkaid Mist Suspension .... ⊕◻ 718
Sensorcaine-MPF with Epinephrine Injection 559

Epinephrine Hydrochloride (Beta-adrenergic agonists (other sympathomimetics) increase the effects of pseudoephedrine and combined effects on cardiovascular system may be harmful). Products include:

Ana-Kit Anaphylaxis Emergency Treatment Kit 617

Estazolam (Co-administration may result in additional reduction in alertness and impairment of CNS performance and should be avoided). Products include:

ProSom Tablets 449

Ethchlorvynol (Co-administration may result in additional reduction in alertness and impairment of CNS performance and should be avoided). Products include:

Placidyl Capsules 448

Ethinamate (Co-administration may result in additional reduction in alertness and impairment of CNS performance and should be avoided).

No products indexed under this heading.

Fentanyl (Co-administration may result in additional reduction in alertness and impairment of CNS performance and should be avoided). Products include:

Duragesic Transdermal System........ 1288

Fentanyl Citrate (Co-administration may result in additional reduction in alertness and impairment of CNS performance and should be avoided). Products include:

Sublimaze Injection.............................. 1307

Fluphenazine Decanoate (Co-administration may result in additional reduction in alertness and impairment of CNS performance and should be avoided). Products include:

Prolixin Decanoate 509

Fluphenazine Enanthate (Co-administration may result in additional reduction in alertness and impairment of CNS performance and should be avoided). Products include:

Prolixin Enanthate 509

Fluphenazine Hydrochloride (Co-administration may result in additional reduction in alertness and impairment of CNS performance and should be avoided). Products include:

Prolixin 509

Flurazepam Hydrochloride (Co-administration may result in additional reduction in alertness and impairment of CNS performance and should be avoided). Products include:

Dalmane Capsules 2173

Furazolidone (Increases the effects of sympathomimetics; potential for hypertensive crisis; concurrent and/or sequential use is contraindicated for two weeks). Products include:

Furoxone 2046

Glutethimide (Co-administration may result in additional reduction in alertness and impairment of CNS performance and should be avoided).

No products indexed under this heading.

Guanethidine Monosulfate (Reduced antihypertensive effects of drugs that interfere with sympathetic activity). Products include:

Esimil Tablets 822
Ismelin Tablets 827

Haloperidol (Co-administration may result in additional reduction in alertness and impairment of CNS performance and should be avoided). Products include:

Haldol Injection, Tablets and Concentrate 1575

Haloperidol Decanoate (Co-administration may result in additional reduction in alertness and impairment of CNS performance and should be avoided). Products include:

Haldol Decanoate.................................. 1577

Hydrocodone Bitartrate (Co-administration may result in additional reduction in alertness and impairment of CNS performance and should be avoided). Products include:

Anexsia 5/500 Elixir 1781
Anexia Tablets....................................... 1782
Codiclear DH Syrup 791
Deconamine CX Cough and Cold Liquid and Tablets............................... 1319
Duratuss HD Elixir................................ 2565
Hycodan Tablets and Syrup 930
Hycomine Compound Tablets 932
Hycomine 931
Hycotuss Expectorant Syrup 933
Hydrocet Capsules 782
Lorcet 10/650....................................... 1018
Lortab 2566
Tussend 1783
Tussend Expectorant 1785
Vicodin Tablets..................................... 1356
Vicodin ES Tablets 1357
Vicodin Tuss Expectorant 1358
Zydone Capsules 949

Hydrocodone Polistirex (Co-administration may result in additional reduction in alertness and impairment of CNS performance and should be avoided). Products include:

Tussionex Pennkinetic Extended-Release Suspension 998

Hydroxyzine Hydrochloride (Co-administration may result in additional reduction in alertness and impairment of CNS performance and should be avoided). Products include:

Atarax Tablets & Syrup........................ 2185
Marax Tablets & DF Syrup................... 2200
Vistaril Intramuscular Solution.......... 2216

Isocarboxazid (Increases the effects of sympathomimetics; potential for hypertensive crisis; concurrent and/or sequential use is contraindicated for two weeks).

No products indexed under this heading.

Isoflurane (Co-administration may result in additional reduction in alertness and impairment of CNS performance and should be avoided).

No products indexed under this heading.

Isoproterenol Hydrochloride (Beta-adrenergic agonists (other sympathomimetics) increase the effects of pseudoephedrine and combined effects on cardiovascular system may be harmful). Products include:

Isuprel Hydrochloride Injection 1:5000 2311
Isuprel Hydrochloride Solution 1:200 & 1:100 2313
Isuprel Mistometer 2312

Isoproterenol Sulfate (Beta-adrenergic agonists (other sympathomimetics) increase the effects of pseudoephedrine and combined effects on cardiovascular system may be harmful). Products include:

Norisodrine with Calcium Iodide Syrup.. 442

Ketamine Hydrochloride (Co-administration may result in additional reduction in alertness and impairment of CNS performance and should be avoided).

No products indexed under this heading.

Levomethadyl Acetate Hydrochloride (Co-administration may result in additional reduction in alertness and impairment of CNS performance and should be avoided). Products include:

Orlaam 2239

Levorphanol Tartrate (Co-administration may result in additional reduction in alertness and impairment of CNS performance and should be avoided). Products include:

Levo-Dromoran 2129

Lorazepam (Co-administration may result in additional reduction in alertness and impairment of CNS performance and should be avoided). Products include:

Ativan Injection 2698
Ativan Tablets 2700

Loxapine Hydrochloride (Co-administration may result in additional reduction in alertness and impairment of CNS performance and should be avoided). Products include:

Loxitane 1378

Loxapine Succinate (Co-administration may result in additional reduction in alertness and impairment of CNS performance and should be avoided). Products include:

Loxitane Capsules 1378

Mecamylamine Hydrochloride (Reduced antihypertensive effects of drugs that interfere with sympathetic activity). Products include:

Inversine Tablets 1686

Meperidine Hydrochloride (Co-administration may result in additional reduction in alertness and impairment of CNS performance and should be avoided). Products include:

Demerol 2308
Mepergan Injection 2753

Mephobarbital (Co-administration may result in additional reduction in alertness and impairment of CNS performance and should be avoided). Products include:

Mebaral Tablets 2322

Meprobamate (Co-administration may result in additional reduction in alertness and impairment of CNS performance and should be avoided). Products include:

Miltown Tablets 2672
PMB 200 and PMB 400 2783

Mesoridazine (Co-administration may result in additional reduction in alertness and impairment of CNS performance and should be avoided).

Metaproterenol Sulfate (Beta-adrenergic agonists (other sympathomimetics) increase the effects of pseudoephedrine and combined effects on cardiovascular system may be harmful). Products include:

Alupent.. 669
Metaproterenol Sulfate Inhalation Solution, USP, Arm-a-Med 552

Metaraminol Bitartrate (Beta-adrenergic agonists (other sympathomimetics) increase the effects of pseudoephedrine and combined effects on cardiovascular system may be harmful). Products include:

Aramine Injection.................................. 1609

Methadone Hydrochloride (Co-administration may result in additional reduction in alertness and impairment of CNS performance and should be avoided). Products include:

Methadone Hydrochloride Oral Concentrate 2233
Methadone Hydrochloride Oral Solution & Tablets................................ 2235

Methohexital Sodium (Co-administration may result in additional reduction in alertness and impairment of CNS performance and should be avoided). Products include:

Brevital Sodium Vials........................... 1429

Methotrimeprazine (Co-administration may result in additional reduction in alertness and impairment of CNS performance and should be avoided). Products include:

Levoprome 1274

Methoxamine Hydrochloride (Beta-adrenergic agonists (other sympathomimetics) increase the effects of pseudoephedrine and combined effects on cardiovascular system may be harmful). Products include:

Vasoxyl Injection 1196

Methoxyflurane (Co-administration may result in additional reduction in alertness and impairment of CNS performance and should be avoided).

No products indexed under this heading.

Methyldopa (Reduced antihypertensive effects of drugs that interfere with sympathetic activity). Products include:

Aldoclor Tablets 1598
Aldomet Oral 1600
Aldoril Tablets 1604

(⊕◻ Described in PDR For Nonprescription Drugs) (◎ Described in PDR For Ophthalmology)

Methyldopate Hydrochloride (Reduced antihypertensive effects of drugs that interfere with sympathetic activity). Products include:

Aldomet Ester HCl Injection 1602

Midazolam Hydrochloride (Co-administration may result in additional reduction in alertness and impairment of CNS performance and should be avoided). Products include:

Versed Injection 2170

Molindone Hydrochloride (Co-administration may result in additional reduction in alertness and impairment of CNS performance and should be avoided). Products include:

Moban Tablets and Concentrate 1048

Morphine Sulfate (Co-administration may result in additional reduction in alertness and impairment of CNS performance and should be avoided). Products include:

Astramorph/PF Injection, USP (Preservative-Free) .... 535 Duramorph .... 962 Infumorph 200 and Infumorph 500 Sterile Solutions .... 965 MS Contin Tablets .... 1994 MSIR .... 1997 Oramorph SR (Morphine Sulfate Sustained Release Tablets) .... 2236 RMS Suppositories .... 2657 Roxanol 2243

Norepinephrine Bitartrate (Beta-adrenergic agonists (other sympathomimetics) increase the effects of pseudoephedrine and combined effects on cardiovascular system may be harmful). Products include:

Levophed Bitartrate Injection 2315

Opium Alkaloids (Co-administration may result in additional reduction in alertness and impairment of CNS performance and should be avoided).

No products indexed under this heading.

Oxazepam (Co-administration may result in additional reduction in alertness and impairment of CNS performance and should be avoided). Products include:

Serax Capsules .... 2810 Serax Tablets 2810

Oxycodone Hydrochloride (Co-administration may result in additional reduction in alertness and impairment of CNS performance and should be avoided). Products include:

Percocet Tablets .... 938 Percodan Tablets .... 939 Percodan-Demi Tablets .... 940 Roxicodone Tablets, Oral Solution & Intensol (Oxycodone) .... 2244 Tylox Capsules 1584

Pentobarbital Sodium (Co-administration may result in additional reduction in alertness and impairment of CNS performance and should be avoided). Products include:

Nembutal Sodium Capsules .... 436 Nembutal Sodium Solution .... 438 Nembutal Sodium Suppositories 440

Perphenazine (Co-administration may result in additional reduction in alertness and impairment of CNS performance and should be avoided). Products include:

Etrafon .... 2355 Triavil Tablets .... 1757 Trilafon 2389

Phenelzine Sulfate (Increases the effects of sympathomimetics; potential for hypertensive crisis; concurrent and/or sequential use is contraindicated for two weeks). Products include:

Nardil 1920

Phenobarbital (Co-administration may result in additional reduction in alertness and impairment of CNS performance and should be avoided). Products include:

Arco-Lase Plus Tablets .... 512 Bellergal-S Tablets .... 2250 Donnatal .... 2060 Donnatal Extentabs .... 2061 Donnatal Tablets .... 2060 Phenobarbital Elixir and Tablets ...... 1469 Quadrinal Tablets 1350

Phenylephrine Bitartrate (Beta-adrenergic agonists (other sympathomimetics) increase the effects of pseudoephedrine and combined effects on cardiovascular system may be harmful).

No products indexed under this heading.

Phenylephrine Hydrochloride (Beta-adrenergic agonists (other sympathomimetics) increase the effects of pseudoephedrine and combined effects on cardiovascular system may be harmful). Products include:

Atrohist Plus Tablets .... 454 Cerose DM .... ⓢⓓ 878 Comhist .... 2038 D.A. Chewable Tablets .... 951 Deconsal Pediatric Capsules .... 454 Dura-Vent/DA Tablets .... 953 Entex Capsules .... 1986 Entex Liquid .... 1986 Extendryl .... 1005 4-Way Fast Acting Nasal Spray (regular & mentholated) .... ⓢⓓ 621 Hemorrhoid For Women .... ⓢⓓ 834 Hycomine Compound Tablets .... 932 Neo-Synephrine Hydrochloride 1% Carpuject .... 2324 Neo-Synephrine Hydrochloride 1% Injection .... 2324 Neo-Synephrine Hydrochloride (Ophthalmic) .... 2325 Neo-Synephrine .... ⓢⓓ 726 Nōstril .... ⓢⓓ 644 Novahistine Elixir .... ⓢⓓ 823 Phenergan VC .... 2779 Phenergan VC with Codeine .... 2781 Preparation H .... ⓢⓓ 871 Tympagesic Ear Drops .... 2342 Vasosulf .... ⓒ 271 Vicks Sinex Nasal Spray and Ultra Fine Mist .... ⓢⓓ 765

Phenylephrine Tannate (Beta-adrenergic agonists (other sympathomimetics) increase the effects of pseudoephedrine and combined effects on cardiovascular system may be harmful). Products include:

Atrohist Pediatric Suspension .... 454 Ricobid-D Pediatric Suspension .... 2038 Ricobid Tablets and Pediatric Suspension .... 2038 Rynatan .... 2673 Rynatuss 2673

Phenylpropanolamine Hydrochloride (Beta-adrenergic agonists (other sympathomimetics) increase the effects of pseudoephedrine and combined effects on cardiovascular system may be harmful). Products include:

Acutrim .... ⓢⓓ 628 Allerest Children's Chewable Tablets .... ⓢⓓ 627 Allerest 12 Hour Caplets .... ⓢⓓ 627 Atrohist Plus Tablets .... 454 BC Cold Powder Multi-Symptom Formula (Cold-Sinus-Allergy) .... ⓢⓓ 609 BC Cold Powder Non-Drowsy Formula (Cold-Sinus) .... ⓢⓓ 609 Cheracol Plus Head Cold/Cough Formula .... ⓢⓓ 769

Comtrex Multi-Symptom Non-Drowsy Liqui-gels .... ⓢⓓ 618 Contac Continuous Action Nasal Decongestant/Antihistamine 12 Hour Capsules .... ⓢⓓ 813 Contac Maximum Strength Continuous Action Decongestant/ Antihistamine 12 Hour Caplets .. ⓢⓓ 813 Contac Severe Cold and Flu Formula Caplets .... ⓢⓓ 814 Coricidin 'D' Decongestant Tablets .... ⓢⓓ 800 Dexatrim .... ⓢⓓ 832 Dexatrim Plus Vitamins Caplets ..... ⓢⓓ 832 Dimetane-DC Cough Syrup .... 2059 Dimetapp Elixir .... ⓢⓓ 773 Dimetapp Extentabs .... ⓢⓓ 774 Dimetapp Tablets/Liqui-Gels .... ⓢⓓ 775 Dimetapp Cold & Allergy Chewable Tablets .... ⓢⓓ 773 Dimetapp DM Elixir .... ⓢⓓ 774 Dura-Vent Tablets .... 952 Entex Capsules .... 1986 Entex LA Tablets .... 1987 Entex Liquid .... 1986 Exgest LA Tablets .... 782 Hycomine .... 931 Isoclor Timesule Capsules .... ⓢⓓ 637 Nolamine Timed-Release Tablets .... 785 Ornade Spansule Capsules .... 2502 Propagest Tablets .... 786 Pyrroxate Caplets .... ⓢⓓ 772 Robitussin-CF .... ⓢⓓ 777 Sinulin Tablets .... 787 Tavist-D 12 Hour Relief Tablets .... ⓢⓓ 787 Teldrin 12 Hour Antihistamine/ Nasal Decongestant Allergy Relief Capsules .... ⓢⓓ 826 Triaminic Allergy Tablets .... ⓢⓓ 789 Triaminic Cold Tablets .... ⓢⓓ 790 Triaminic Expectorant .... ⓢⓓ 790 Triaminic Syrup .... ⓢⓓ 792 Triaminic-12 Tablets .... ⓢⓓ 792 Triaminic-DM Syrup .... ⓢⓓ 792 Triaminicin Tablets .... ⓢⓓ 793 Triaminicol Multi-Symptom Cold Tablets .... ⓢⓓ 793 Triaminicol Multi-Symptom Relief ⓢⓓ 794 Vicks DayQuil Allergy Relief 12-Hour Extended Release Tablets .. ⓢⓓ 760 Vicks DayQuil Allergy Relief 4-Hour Tablets .... ⓢⓓ 760 Vicks DayQuil SINUS Pressure & CONGESTION Relief .... ⓢⓓ 761

Pirbuterol Acetate (Beta-adrenergic agonists (other sympathomimetics) increase the effects of pseudoephedrine and combined effects on cardiovascular system may be harmful). Products include:

Maxair Autohaler .... 1492 Maxair Inhaler 1494

Prazepam (Co-administration may result in additional reduction in alertness and impairment of CNS performance and should be avoided).

No products indexed under this heading.

Prochlorperazine (Co-administration may result in additional reduction in alertness and impairment of CNS performance and should be avoided). Products include:

Compazine 2470

Promethazine Hydrochloride (Co-administration may result in additional reduction in alertness and impairment of CNS performance and should be avoided). Products include:

Mepergan Injection .... 2753 Phenergan with Codeine .... 2777 Phenergan with Dextromethorphan 2778 Phenergan Injection .... 2773 Phenergan Suppositories .... 2775 Phenergan Syrup .... 2774 Phenergan Tablets .... 2775 Phenergan VC .... 2779 Phenergan VC with Codeine 2781

Propofol (Co-administration may result in additional reduction in alertness and impairment of CNS performance and should be avoided). Products include:

Diprivan Injection 2833

Propoxyphene Hydrochloride (Co-administration may result in additional reduction in alertness and impairment of CNS performance and should be avoided). Products include:

Darvon .... 1435 Wygesic Tablets 2827

Propoxyphene Napsylate (Co-administration may result in additional reduction in alertness and impairment of CNS performance and should be avoided). Products include:

Darvon-N/Darvocet-N 1433

Pseudoephedrine Sulfate (Beta-adrenergic agonists (other sympathomimetics) increase the effects of pseudoephedrine and combined effects on cardiovascular system may be harmful). Products include:

Cheracol Sinus .... ⓢⓓ 768 Chlor-Trimeton Allergy Decongestant Tablets .... ⓢⓓ 799 Claritin-D .... 2350 Drixoral Cold and Allergy Sustained-Action Tablets .... ⓢⓓ 802 Drixoral Cold and Flu Extended-Release Tablets .... ⓢⓓ 803 Drixoral Non-Drowsy Formula Extended-Release Tablets .... ⓢⓓ 803 Drixoral Allergy/Sinus Extended Release Tablets .... ⓢⓓ 804 Trinalin Repetabs Tablets 1330

Quazepam (Co-administration may result in additional reduction in alertness and impairment of CNS performance and should be avoided). Products include:

Doral Tablets 2664

Rauwolfia Serpentina (Reduced antihypertensive effects of drugs that interfere with sympathetic activity).

No products indexed under this heading.

Rescinnamine (Reduced antihypertensive effects of drugs that interfere with sympathetic activity).

No products indexed under this heading.

Reserpine (Reduced antihypertensive effects of drugs that interfere with sympathetic activity). Products include:

Diupres Tablets .... 1650 Hydropres Tablets .... 1675 Ser-Ap-Es Tablets 849

Risperidone (Co-administration may result in additional reduction in alertness and impairment of CNS performance and should be avoided). Products include:

Risperdal 1301

Salmeterol Xinafoate (Beta-adrenergic agonists (other sympathomimetics) increase the effects of pseudoephedrine and combined effects on cardiovascular system may be harmful). Products include:

Serevent Inhalation Aerosol 1176

Secobarbital Sodium (Co-administration may result in additional reduction in alertness and impairment of CNS performance and should be avoided). Products include:

Seconal Sodium Pulvules 1474

Selegiline Hydrochloride (Increases the effects of sympathomimetics; potential for hypertensive crisis; concurrent and/or sequential use is contraindicated for two weeks). Products include:

Eldepryl Tablets 2550

IMPORTANT NOTE: Always consult each drug listing in the patient's regimen for possible interactions.

Sufentanil Citrate (Co-administration may result in additional reduction in alertness and impairment of CNS performance and should be avoided). Products include:

Sufenta Injection 1309

Temazepam (Co-administration may result in additional reduction in alertness and impairment of CNS performance and should be avoided). Products include:

Restoril Capsules 2284

Terbutaline Sulfate (Beta-adrenergic agonists (other sympathomimetics) increase the effects of pseudoephedrine and combined effects on cardiovascular system may be harmful). Products include:

Brethaire Inhaler 813
Brethine Ampuls 815
Brethine Tablets 814
Bricanyl Subcutaneous Injection 1502
Bricanyl Tablets 1503

Thiamylal Sodium (Co-administration may result in additional reduction in alertness and impairment of CNS performance and should be avoided).

No products indexed under this heading.

Thioridazine Hydrochloride (Co-administration may result in additional reduction in alertness and impairment of CNS performance and should be avoided). Products include:

Mellaril 2269

Thiothixene (Co-administration may result in additional reduction in alertness and impairment of CNS performance and should be avoided). Products include:

Navane Capsules and Concentrate 2201
Navane Intramuscular 2202

Tranylcypromine Sulfate (Increases the effects of sympathomimetics; potential for hypertensive crisis; concurrent and/or sequential use is contraindicated for two weeks). Products include:

Parnate Tablets 2503

Triazolam (Co-administration may result in additional reduction in alertness and impairment of CNS performance and should be avoided). Products include:

Halcion Tablets 2611

Trifluoperazine Hydrochloride (Co-administration may result in additional reduction in alertness and impairment of CNS performance and should be avoided). Products include:

Stelazine 2514

Zolpidem Tartrate (Co-administration may result in additional reduction in alertness and impairment of CNS performance and should be avoided). Products include:

Ambien Tablets 2416

Food Interactions

Alcohol (Co-administration may result in additional reduction in alertness and impairment of CNS performance and should be avoided).

SENNA X-PREP BOWEL EVACUANT LIQUID

(Senna Concentrates) 1230
None cited in PDR database.

SENOKOT CHILDREN'S SYRUP

(Senna) 1999
None cited in PDR database.

SENOKOT GRANULES

(Senna Concentrates) 1999
None cited in PDR database.

SENOKOT SYRUP

(Senna Concentrates) 1999
None cited in PDR database.

SENOKOT TABLETS

(Senna Concentrates) 1999
None cited in PDR database.

SENOKOTXTRA TABLETS

(Senna Concentrates) 1999
None cited in PDR database.

SENOKOT-S TABLETS

(Senna Concentrates, Docusate Sodium) 1999
None cited in PDR database.

COOL GEL SENSODYNE

(Potassium Nitrate, Sodium Fluoride) .... ▣ 611
None cited in PDR database.

FRESH MINT SENSODYNE TOOTHPASTE

(Potassium Nitrate, Sodium Monofluorophosphate) .... ▣ 611
None cited in PDR database.

ORIGINAL FORMULA SENSODYNE-SC TOOTHPASTE

(Strontium Chloride Hexahydrate) .. ▣ 611
None cited in PDR database.

SENSODYNE WITH BAKING SODA

(Potassium Nitrate, Sodium Fluoride) .... ▣ 611
None cited in PDR database.

SENSORCAINE WITH EPINEPHRINE INJECTION

(Bupivacaine Hydrochloride, Epinephrine Bitartrate) 559

May interact with phenothiazines, butyrophenones, inhalant anesthetics, monoamine oxidase inhibitors, tricyclic antidepressants, vasopressors, ergot-type oxytocic drugs, and certain other agents. Compounds in these categories include:

Amitriptyline Hydrochloride (May produce severe and prolonged hypertension). Products include:

Elavil 2838
Endep Tablets 2174
Etrafon 2355
Limbitrol 2180
Triavil Tablets 1757

Amoxapine (May produce severe and prolonged hypertension). Products include:

Asendin Tablets 1369

Chlorpromazine (Reduces or reverses the pressor effect of epinephrine). Products include:

Thorazine Suppositories 2523

Clomipramine Hydrochloride (May produce severe and prolonged hypertension). Products include:

Anafranil Capsules 803

Desflurane (Concurrent use may produce serious dose-related cardiac arrhythmias). Products include:

Suprane 1813

Desipramine Hydrochloride (May produce severe and prolonged hypertension). Products include:

Norpramin Tablets 1526

Dopamine Hydrochloride (May produce severe and prolonged hypertension or cerebrovascular accidents).

No products indexed under this heading.

Doxepin Hydrochloride (May produce severe and prolonged hypertension). Products include:

Sinequan 2205
Zonalon Cream 1055

Enflurane (Concurrent use may produce serious dose-related cardiac arrhythmias).

No products indexed under this heading.

Epinephrine Hydrochloride (May produce severe and prolonged hypertension or cerebrovascular accidents). Products include:

Ana-Kit Anaphylaxis Emergency Treatment Kit 617

Fluphenazine Decanoate (Reduces or reverses the pressor effect of epinephrine). Products include:

Prolixin Decanoate 509

Fluphenazine Enanthate (Reduces or reverses the pressor effect of epinephrine). Products include:

Prolixin Enanthate 509

Fluphenazine Hydrochloride (Reduces or reverses the pressor effect of epinephrine). Products include:

Prolixin 509

Furazolidone (May produce severe and prolonged hypertension). Products include:

Furoxone 2046

Haloperidol (Reduces or reverses the pressor effect of epinephrine). Products include:

Haldol Injection, Tablets and Concentrate 1575

Haloperidol Decanoate (Reduces or reverses the pressor effect of epinephrine). Products include:

Haldol Decanoate 1577

Halothane (Concurrent use may produce serious dose-related cardiac arrhythmias). Products include:

Fluothane 2724

Imipramine Hydrochloride (May produce severe and prolonged hypertension). Products include:

Tofranil Ampuls 854
Tofranil Tablets 856

Imipramine Pamoate (May produce severe and prolonged hypertension). Products include:

Tofranil-PM Capsules 857

Isocarboxazid (May produce severe and prolonged hypertension).

No products indexed under this heading.

Isoflurane (Concurrent use may produce serious dose-related cardiac arrhythmias).

No products indexed under this heading.

Maprotiline Hydrochloride (May produce severe and prolonged hypertension). Products include:

Ludiomil Tablets 843

Mesoridazine Besylate (Reduces or reverses the pressor effect of epinephrine). Products include:

Serentil 684

Metaraminol Bitartrate (May produce severe and prolonged hypertension or cerebrovascular accidents). Products include:

Aramine Injection 1609

Methotrimeprazine (Reduces or reverses the pressor effect of epinephrine). Products include:

Levoprome 1274

Methoxamine Hydrochloride (May produce severe and prolonged hypertension or cerebrovascular accidents). Products include:

Vasoxyl Injection 1196

Methoxyflurane (Concurrent use may produce serious dose-related cardiac arrhythmias).

No products indexed under this heading.

Methylergonovine Maleate (May produce severe and prolonged hypertension or cerebrovascular accidents). Products include:

Methergine 2272

Norepinephrine Bitartrate (May produce severe and prolonged hypertension or cerebrovascular accidents). Products include:

Levophed Bitartrate Injection 2315

Nortriptyline Hydrochloride (May produce severe and prolonged hypertension). Products include:

Pamelor 2280

Perphenazine (Reduces or reverses the pressor effect of epinephrine). Products include:

Etrafon 2355
Triavil Tablets 1757
Trilafon 2389

Phenelzine Sulfate (May produce severe and prolonged hypertension). Products include:

Nardil 1920

Phenylephrine Hydrochloride (May produce severe and prolonged hypertension or cerebrovascular accidents). Products include:

Atrohist Plus Tablets 454
Cerose DM .... ▣ 878
Comhist 2038
D.A. Chewable Tablets 951
Deconsal Pediatric Capsules 454
Dura-Vent/DA Tablets 953
Entex Capsules 1986
Entex Liquid 1986
Extendryl 1005
4-Way Fast Acting Nasal Spray (regular & mentholated) .... ▣ 621
Hemorid For Women .... ▣ 834
Hycomine Compound Tablets 932
Neo-Synephrine Hydrochloride 1% Carpuject 2324
Neo-Synephrine Hydrochloride 1% Injection 2324
Neo-Synephrine Hydrochloride (Ophthalmic) 2325
Neo-Synephrine .... ▣ 726
Nōstril .... ▣ 644
Novahistine Elixir .... ▣ 823
Phenergan VC 2779
Phenergan VC with Codeine 2781
Preparation H .... ▣ 871
Tympagesic Ear Drops 2342
Vasosulf .... ⊙ 271
Vicks Sinex Nasal Spray and Ultra Fine Mist .... ▣ 765

Prochlorperazine (Reduces or reverses the pressor effect of epinephrine). Products include:

Compazine 2470

Promethazine Hydrochloride (Reduces or reverses the pressor effect of epinephrine). Products include:

Mepergan Injection 2753
Phenergan with Codeine 2777
Phenergan with Dextromethorphan 2778
Phenergan Injection 2773
Phenergan Suppositories 2775
Phenergan Syrup 2774
Phenergan Tablets 2775
Phenergan VC 2779
Phenergan VC with Codeine 2781

Protriptyline Hydrochloride (May produce severe and prolonged hypertension). Products include:

Vivactil Tablets 1774

Selegiline Hydrochloride (May produce severe and prolonged hypertension). Products include:

Eldepryl Tablets 2550

939 Interactions Index Ser-Ap-Es

Thioridazine Hydrochloride (Reduces or reverses the pressor effect of epinephrine). Products include:
- Mellaril 2269

Tranylcypromine Sulfate (May produce severe and prolonged hypertension). Products include:
- Parnate Tablets 2503

Trifluoperazine Hydrochloride (Reduces or reverses the pressor effect of epinephrine). Products include:
- Stelazine 2514

Trimipramine Maleate (May produce severe and prolonged hypertension). Products include:
- Surmontil Capsules 2811

SENSORCAINE INJECTION
(Bupivacaine Hydrochloride) 559
See **Sensorcaine with Epinephrine Injection**

SENSORCAINE-MPF WITH EPINEPHRINE INJECTION
(Bupivacaine Hydrochloride, Epinephrine Bitartrate) 559
See **Sensorcaine with Epinephrine Injection**

SENSORCAINE-MPF INJECTION
(Bupivacaine Hydrochloride) 559
See **Sensorcaine with Epinephrine Injection**

SEPTRA DS TABLETS
(Trimethoprim, Sulfamethoxazole) 1174
May interact with thiazides, oral anticoagulants, and certain other agents. Compounds in these categories include:

Bendroflumethiazide (Potential for thrombocytopenia with purpura in elderly).
No products indexed under this heading.

Chlorothiazide (Potential for thrombocytopenia with purpura in elderly). Products include:
- Aldoclor Tablets 1598
- Diupres Tablets 1650
- Diuril Oral 1653

Chlorothiazide Sodium (Potential for thrombocytopenia with purpura in elderly). Products include:
- Diuril Sodium Intravenous 1652

Dicumarol (Septra prolongs prothrombin time in patients on anticoagulant).
No products indexed under this heading.

Hydrochlorothiazide (Potential for thrombocytopenia with purpura in elderly). Products include:
- Aldactazide 2413
- Aldoril Tablets 1604
- Apresazide Capsules 808
- Capozide 742
- Dyazide 2479
- Esidrix Tablets 821
- Esimil Tablets 822
- HydroDIURIL Tablets 1674
- Hydropres Tablets 1675
- Hyzaar Tablets 1677
- Inderide Tablets 2732
- Inderide LA Long Acting Capsules .. 2734
- Lopressor HCT Tablets 832
- Lotensin HCT 837
- Maxzide 1380
- Moduretic Tablets 1705
- Oretic Tablets 443
- Prinzide Tablets 1737
- Ser-Ap-Es Tablets 849
- Timolide Tablets 1748
- Vaseretic Tablets 1765
- Zestoretic 2850
- Ziac 1415

Hydroflumethiazide (Potential for thrombocytopenia with purpura in elderly). Products include:
- Diucardin Tablets 2718

Methotrexate Sodium (Increased free methotrexate concentrations). Products include:
- Methotrexate Sodium Tablets, Injection, for Injection and LPF Injection 1275

Methyclothiazide (Potential for thrombocytopenia with purpura in elderly). Products include:
- Enduron Tablets 420

Phenytoin (Decreased hepatic metabolism of phenytoin). Products include:
- Dilantin Infatabs 1908
- Dilantin-125 Suspension 1911

Phenytoin Sodium (Decreased hepatic metabolism of phenytoin). Products include:
- Dilantin Kapseals 1906
- Dilantin Parenteral 1910

Polythiazide (Potential for thrombocytopenia with purpura in elderly). Products include:
- Minizide Capsules 1938

Warfarin Sodium (Prolongs prothrombin time). Products include:
- Coumadin 926

SEPTRA GRAPE SUSPENSION
(Trimethoprim, Sulfamethoxazole) 1174
See **Septra DS Tablets**

SEPTRA I.V. INFUSION
(Trimethoprim, Sulfamethoxazole) 1169
May interact with thiazides and certain other agents. Compounds in these categories include:

Bendroflumethiazide (Potential for thrombocytopenia with purpura in elderly).
No products indexed under this heading.

Chlorothiazide (Potential for thrombocytopenia with purpura in elderly patients). Products include:
- Aldoclor Tablets 1598
- Diupres Tablets 1650
- Diuril Oral 1653

Chlorothiazide Sodium (Potential for thrombocytopenia with purpura in elderly). Products include:
- Diuril Sodium Intravenous 1652

Hydrochlorothiazide (Potential for thrombocytopenia with purpura in elderly). Products include:
- Aldactazide 2413
- Aldoril Tablets 1604
- Apresazide Capsules 808
- Capozide 742
- Dyazide 2479
- Esidrix Tablets 821
- Esimil Tablets 822
- HydroDIURIL Tablets 1674
- Hydropres Tablets 1675
- Hyzaar Tablets 1677
- Inderide Tablets 2732
- Inderide LA Long Acting Capsules .. 2734
- Lopressor HCT Tablets 832
- Lotensin HCT 837
- Maxzide 1380
- Moduretic Tablets 1705
- Oretic Tablets 443
- Prinzide Tablets 1737
- Ser-Ap-Es Tablets 849
- Timolide Tablets 1748
- Vaseretic Tablets 1765
- Zestoretic 2850
- Ziac 1415

Hydroflumethiazide (Potential for thrombocytopenia with purpura in elderly). Products include:
- Diucardin Tablets 2718

Methotrexate Sodium (Increased free methotrexate concentrations). Products include:
- Methotrexate Sodium Tablets, Injection, for Injection and LPF Injection 1275

Methyclothiazide (Potential for thrombocytopenia with purpura in elderly). Products include:
- Enduron Tablets 420

Phenytoin (Decreased metabolism of phenytoin). Products include:
- Dilantin Infatabs 1908
- Dilantin-125 Suspension 1911

Phenytoin Sodium (Decreased metabolism of phenytoin). Products include:
- Dilantin Kapseals 1906
- Dilantin Parenteral 1910

Polythiazide (Potential for thrombocytopenia with purpura in elderly). Products include:
- Minizide Capsules 1938

Warfarin Sodium (Prolonged prothrombin time). Products include:
- Coumadin 926

SEPTRA I.V. INFUSION ADD-VANTAGE VIALS
(Trimethoprim, Sulfamethoxazole) 1171
May interact with thiazides and certain other agents. Compounds in these categories include:

Bendroflumethiazide (Potential for thrombocytopenia with purpura in elderly).
No products indexed under this heading.

Chlorothiazide (Potential for thrombocytopenia with purpura in elderly). Products include:
- Aldoclor Tablets 1598
- Diupres Tablets 1650
- Diuril Oral 1653

Chlorothiazide Sodium (Potential for thrombocytopenia with purpura in elderly). Products include:
- Diuril Sodium Intravenous 1652

Hydrochlorothiazide (Potential for thrombocytopenia with purpura in elderly). Products include:
- Aldactazide 2413
- Aldoril Tablets 1604
- Apresazide Capsules 808
- Capozide 742
- Dyazide 2479
- Esidrix Tablets 821
- Esimil Tablets 822
- HydroDIURIL Tablets 1674
- Hydropres Tablets 1675
- Hyzaar Tablets 1677
- Inderide Tablets 2732
- Inderide LA Long Acting Capsules .. 2734
- Lopressor HCT Tablets 832
- Lotensin HCT 837
- Maxzide 1380
- Moduretic Tablets 1705
- Oretic Tablets 443
- Prinzide Tablets 1737
- Ser-Ap-Es Tablets 849
- Timolide Tablets 1748
- Vaseretic Tablets 1765
- Zestoretic 2850
- Ziac 1415

Hydroflumethiazide (Potential for thrombocytopenia with purpura in elderly). Products include:
- Diucardin Tablets 2718

Methotrexate Sodium (Increased free methotrexate concentrations). Products include:
- Methotrexate Sodium Tablets, Injection, for Injection and LPF Injection 1275

Methyclothiazide (Potential for thrombocytopenia with purpura in elderly). Products include:
- Enduron Tablets 420

Phenytoin (Decreased metabolism of phenytoin). Products include:
- Dilantin Infatabs 1908
- Dilantin-125 Suspension 1911

Phenytoin Sodium (Decreased metabolism of phenytoin). Products include:
- Dilantin Kapseals 1906
- Dilantin Parenteral 1910

Polythiazide (Potential for thrombocytopenia with purpura in elderly). Products include:
- Minizide Capsules 1938

Warfarin Sodium (Prolonged prothrombin time). Products include:
- Coumadin 926

SEPTRA SUSPENSION
(Trimethoprim, Sulfamethoxazole) 1174
See **Septra DS Tablets**

SEPTRA TABLETS
(Trimethoprim, Sulfamethoxazole) 1174
See **Septra DS Tablets**

SER-AP-ES TABLETS
(Hydralazine Hydrochloride, Hydrochlorothiazide, Reserpine) 849
May interact with corticosteroids, lithium preparations, antihypertensives, monoamine oxidase inhibitors, insulin, cardiac glycosides, barbiturates, narcotic analgesics, non-steroidal anti-inflammatory agents, tricyclic antidepressants, direct-acting sympathomimetic amines, indirect-acting sympathomimetic amines, and certain other agents. Compounds in these categories include:

Acebutolol Hydrochloride (Additive or potentiated action). Products include:
- Sectral Capsules 2807

ACTH (Hypokalemia).
No products indexed under this heading.

Alfentanil Hydrochloride (Orthostatic hypotension). Products include:
- Alfenta Injection 1286

Amitriptyline Hydrochloride (Decreases the antihypertensive effect of reserpine). Products include:
- Elavil 2838
- Endep Tablets 2174
- Etrafon 2355
- Limbitrol 2180
- Triavil Tablets 1757

Amlodipine Besylate (Additive or potentiated action). Products include:
- Lotrel Capsules 840
- Norvasc Tablets 1940

Amoxapine (Decreases the antihypertensive effect of reserpine). Products include:
- Asendin Tablets 1369

Amphetamine Resins (The action of indirect-acting sympathomimetic amines is inhibited). Products include:
- Biphetamine Capsules 983

Aprobarbital (Orthostatic hypotension).
No products indexed under this heading.

Atenolol (Additive or potentiated action). Products include:
- Tenoretic Tablets 2845
- Tenormin Tablets and I.V. Injection 2847

Benazepril Hydrochloride (Additive or potentiated action). Products include:
- Lotensin Tablets 834
- Lotensin HCT 837
- Lotrel Capsules 840

IMPORTANT NOTE: Always consult each drug listing in the patient's regimen for possible interactions.

Ser-Ap-Es Interactions Index 940

Bendroflumethiazide (Additive or potentiated action).
No products indexed under this heading.

Betamethasone Acetate (Hypokalemia). Products include:
Celestone Soluspan Suspension 2347

Betamethasone Sodium Phosphate (Hypokalemia). Products include:
Celestone Soluspan Suspension 2347

Betaxolol Hydrochloride (Additive or potentiated action). Products include:
Betoptic Ophthalmic Solution 469
Betoptic S Ophthalmic Suspension 471
Kerlone Tablets 2436

Bisoprolol Fumarate (Additive or potentiated action). Products include:
Zebeta Tablets 1413
Ziac 1415

Buprenorphine (Orthostatic hypotension). Products include:
Buprenex Injectable 2006

Butabarbital (Orthostatic hypotension).
No products indexed under this heading.

Butalbital (Orthostatic hypotension). Products include:
Esgic-plus Tablets 1013
Fioricet Tablets 2258
Fioricet with Codeine Capsules 2260
Fiorinal Capsules 2261
Fiorinal with Codeine Capsules 2262
Fiorinal Tablets 2261
Phrenilin 785
Sedapap Tablets 50 mg/650 mg .. 1543

Captopril (Additive or potentiated action). Products include:
Capoten 739
Capozide 742

Carteolol Hydrochloride (Additive or potentiated action). Products include:
Cartrol Tablets 410
Ocupress Ophthalmic Solution, 1% Sterile .... ⊙ 309

Chlorothiazide (Additive or potentiated action). Products include:
Aldoclor Tablets 1598
Diupres Tablets 1650
Diuril Oral 1653

Chlorothiazide Sodium (Additive or potentiated action). Products include:
Diuril Sodium Intravenous 1652

Chlorthalidone (Additive or potentiated action). Products include:
Combipres Tablets 677
Tenoretic Tablets 2845
Thalitone 1245

Cholestyramine (Impairs the oral absorption of hydrochlorothiazide from gastrointestinal tract by up to 85%). Products include:
Questran Light 769
Questran Powder 770

Clomipramine Hydrochloride (Decreases the antihypertensive effect of reserpine). Products include:
Anafranil Capsules 803

Clonidine (Additive or potentiated action). Products include:
Catapres-TTS 675

Clonidine Hydrochloride (Additive or potentiated action). Products include:
Catapres Tablets 674
Combipres Tablets 677

Codeine Phosphate (Orthostatic hypotension). Products include:
Actifed with Codeine Cough Syrup.. 1067
Brontex 1981
Deconsal C Expectorant Syrup 456
Deconsal Pediatric Syrup 457
Dimetane-DC Cough Syrup 2059
Empirin with Codeine Tablets............ 1093
Fioricet with Codeine Capsules 2260
Fiorinal with Codeine Capsules 2262
Isoclor Expectorant 990
Novahistine DH 2462
Novahistine Expectorant 2463
Nucofed 2051
Phenergan with Codeine 2777
Phenergan VC with Codeine 2781
Robitussin A-C Syrup 2073
Robitussin-DAC Syrup 2074
Ryna .... ▣ 841
Soma Compound w/Codeine Tablets 2676
Tussi-Organidin NR Liquid and S NR Liquid 2677
Tylenol with Codeine 1583

Colestipol Hydrochloride (Impairs the oral absorption of hydrochlorothiazide from gastrointestinal tract by up to 43%). Products include:
Colestid Tablets 2591

Cortisone Acetate (Hypokalemia). Products include:
Cortone Acetate Sterile Suspension 1623
Cortone Acetate Tablets 1624

Deserpidine (Additive or potentiated action).
No products indexed under this heading.

Desipramine Hydrochloride (Decreases the antihypertensive effect of reserpine). Products include:
Norpramin Tablets 1526

Deslanoside (Cardiac arrhythmia).
No products indexed under this heading.

Dexamethasone (Hypokalemia). Products include:
AK-Trol Ointment & Suspension .... ⊙ 205
Decadron Elixir 1633
Decadron Tablets 1635
Decaspray Topical Aerosol 1648
Dexacidin Ointment .... ⊙ 263
Maxitrol Ophthalmic Ointment and Suspension .... ⊙ 224
TobraDex Ophthalmic Suspension and Ointment 473

Dexamethasone Acetate (Hypokalemia). Products include:
Dalalone D.P. Injectable 1011
Decadron-LA Sterile Suspension 1646

Dexamethasone Sodium Phosphate (Hypokalemia). Products include:
Decadron Phosphate Injection 1637
Decadron Phosphate Respihaler 1642
Decadron Phosphate Sterile Ophthalmic Ointment 1641
Decadron Phosphate Sterile Ophthalmic Solution 1642
Decadron Phosphate Topical Cream 1644
Decadron Phosphate Turbinaire 1645
Decadron Phosphate with Xylocaine Injection, Sterile 1639
Dexacort Phosphate in Respihaler .. 458
Dexacort Phosphate in Turbinaire .. 459
NeoDecadron Sterile Ophthalmic Ointment 1712
NeoDecadron Sterile Ophthalmic Solution 1713
NeoDecadron Topical Cream 1714

Dextroamphetamine Sulfate (The action of indirect-acting sympathomimetic amines is inhibited). Products include:
Dexedrine 2474
DextroStat Dextroamphetamine Tablets 2036

Dezocine (Orthostatic hypotension). Products include:
Dalgan Injection 538

Diazoxide (Hypotension; additive or potentiated action). Products include:
Hyperstat I.V. Injection 2363
Proglycem 580

Diclofenac Potassium (May reduce the diuretic, natriuretic, and antihypertensive effects of thiazide diuretics). Products include:
Cataflam 816

Diclofenac Sodium (May reduce the diuretic, natriuretic, and antihypertensive effects of thiazide diuretics). Products include:
Voltaren Ophthalmic Sterile Ophthalmic Solution .... ⊙ 272
Voltaren Tablets 861

Digitoxin (Cardiac arrhythmia). Products include:
Crystodigin Tablets 1433

Digoxin (Cardiac arrhythmia). Products include:
Lanoxicaps 1117
Lanoxin Elixir Pediatric 1120
Lanoxin Injection 1123
Lanoxin Injection Pediatric 1126
Lanoxin Tablets 1128

Diltiazem Hydrochloride (Additive or potentiated action). Products include:
Cardizem CD Capsules 1506
Cardizem SR Capsules 1510
Cardizem Injectable 1508
Cardizem Tablets 1512
Dilacor XR Extended-release Capsules 2018

Doxazosin Mesylate (Additive or potentiated action). Products include:
Cardura Tablets 2186

Doxepin Hydrochloride (Decreases the antihypertensive effect of reserpine). Products include:
Sinequan 2205
Zonalon Cream 1055

Enalapril Maleate (Additive or potentiated action). Products include:
Vaseretic Tablets 1765
Vasotec Tablets 1771

Enalaprilat (Additive or potentiated action). Products include:
Vasotec I.V. 1768

Ephedrine Hydrochloride (The action of indirect-acting sympathomimetic amines is inhibited). Products include:
Primatene Dual Action Formula....▣ 872
Primatene Tablets .... ▣ 873
Quadrinal Tablets 1350

Ephedrine Sulfate (The action of indirect-acting sympathomimetic amines is inhibited). Products include:
Bronkaid Caplets .... ▣ 717
Marax Tablets & DF Syrup 2200

Ephedrine Tannate (The action of indirect-acting sympathomimetic amines is inhibited). Products include:
Rynatuss 2673

Epinephrine Hydrochloride (The action of direct-acting sympathomimetic amines may be prolonged). Products include:
Ana-Kit Anaphylaxis Emergency Treatment Kit 617

Esmolol Hydrochloride (Additive or potentiated action). Products include:
Brevibloc Injection 1808

Etodolac (May reduce the diuretic, natriuretic, and antihypertensive effects of thiazide diuretics). Products include:
Lodine Capsules and Tablets 2743

Felodipine (Additive or potentiated action). Products include:
Plendil Extended-Release Tablets.... 527

Fenoprofen Calcium (May reduce the diuretic, natriuretic, and antihypertensive effects of thiazide diuretics). Products include:
Nalfon 200 Pulvules & Nalfon Tablets 917

Fentanyl (Orthostatic hypotension). Products include:
Duragesic Transdermal System........ 1288

Fentanyl Citrate (Orthostatic hypotension). Products include:
Sublimaze Injection 1307

Fludrocortisone Acetate (Hypokalemia). Products include:
Florinef Acetate Tablets 505

Flurbiprofen (May reduce the diuretic, natriuretic, and antihypertensive effects of thiazide diuretics). Products include:
Ansaid Tablets 2579

Fosinopril Sodium (Additive or potentiated action). Products include:
Monopril Tablets 757

Furazolidone (Concurrent administration of MAOI should be avoided). Products include:
Furoxone 2046

Furosemide (Additive or potentiated action). Products include:
Lasix Injection, Oral Solution and Tablets 1240

Guanabenz Acetate (Additive or potentiated action).
No products indexed under this heading.

Guanethidine Monosulfate (Additive or potentiated action). Products include:
Esimil Tablets 822
Ismelin Tablets 827

Hydrocodone Bitartrate (Orthostatic hypotension). Products include:
Anexsia 5/500 Elixir 1781
Anexia Tablets 1782
Codiclear DH Syrup 791
Deconamine CX Cough and Cold Liquid and Tablets 1319
Duratuss HD Elixir 2565
Hycodan Tablets and Syrup 930
Hycomine Compound Tablets 932
Hycomine 931
Hycotuss Expectorant Syrup 933
Hydrocet Capsules 782
Lorcet 10/650 1018
Lortab 2566
Tussend 1783
Tussend Expectorant 1785
Vicodin Tablets 1356
Vicodin ES Tablets 1357
Vicodin Tuss Expectorant 1358
Zydone Capsules 949

Hydrocodone Polistirex (Orthostatic hypotension). Products include:
Tussionex Pennkinetic Extended-Release Suspension 998

Hydrocortisone (Hypokalemia). Products include:
Anusol-HC Cream 2.5% 1896
Aquanil HC Lotion 1931
Bactine Hydrocortisone Anti-Itch Cream .... ▣ 709
Caldecort Anti-Itch Hydrocortisone Spray .... ▣ 631
Cortaid .... ▣ 836
CORTENEMA 2535
Cortisporin Ointment 1085
Cortisporin Ophthalmic Ointment Sterile 1085
Cortisporin Ophthalmic Suspension Sterile 1086
Cortisporin Otic Solution Sterile 1087
Cortisporin Otic Suspension Sterile 1088
Cortizone-5 .... ▣ 831
Cortizone-10 .... ▣ 831
Hydrocortone Tablets 1672
Hytone 907
Massengill Medicated Soft Cloth Towelettes 2458
PediOtic Suspension Sterile 1153

(▣ Described in PDR For Nonprescription Drugs) (⊙ Described in PDR For Ophthalmology)

941 **Interactions Index** **Ser-Ap-Es**

Preparation H Hydrocortisone 1% Cream .... PD 872
ProctoCream-HC 2.5% 2408
VōSoL HC Otic Solution 2678

Hydrocortisone Acetate (Hypokalemia). Products include:
Analpram-HC Rectal Cream 1% and 2.5% 977
Anusol HC-1 Anti-Itch Hydrocortisone Ointment .... PD 847
Anusol-HC Suppositories 1897
Caldecort .... PD 631
Carmol HC 924
Coly-Mycin S Otic w/Neomycin & Hydrocortisone 1906
Cortaid .... PD 836
Cortifoam 2396
Cortisporin Cream 1084
Epifoam 2399
Hydrocortone Acetate Sterile Suspension 1669
Mantadil Cream 1135
Nupercainal Hydrocortisone 1% Cream .... PD 645
Ophthocort .... ⊙ 311
Pramosone Cream, Lotion & Ointment 978
ProctoCream-HC 2408
ProctoFoam-HC 2409
Terra-Cortril Ophthalmic Suspension 2210

Hydrocortisone Sodium Phosphate (Hypokalemia). Products include:
Hydrocortone Phosphate Injection, Sterile 1670

Hydrocortisone Sodium Succinate (Hypokalemia). Products include:
Solu-Cortef Sterile Powder 2641

Hydroflumethiazide (Additive or potentiated action). Products include:
Diucardin Tablets 2718

Ibuprofen (May reduce the diuretic, natriuretic, and antihypertensive effects of thiazide diuretics). Products include:
Advil Cold and Sinus Caplets and Tablets (formerly CoAdvil) .... PD 870
Advil Ibuprofen Tablets and Caplets .... PD 870
Children's Advil Suspension 2692
Arthritis Foundation Ibuprofen Tablets .... PD 674
Bayer Select Ibuprofen Pain Relief Formula .... PD 715
Cramp End Tablets .... PD 735
Dimetapp Sinus Caplets .... PD 775
Haltran Tablets .... PD 771
IBU Tablets 1342
Ibuprohm .... PD 735
Children's Motrin Ibuprofen Oral Suspension 1546
Motrin Tablets 2625
Motrin IB Caplets, Tablets, and Geltabs .... PD 838
Motrin IB Sinus .... PD 838
Motrin Ibuprofen Suspension, Oral Drops, Chewable Tablets, Caplets 1546
Nuprin Ibuprofen/Analgesic Tablets & Caplets .... PD 622
Sine-Aid IB Caplets 1554
Vicks DayQuil SINUS Pressure & PAIN Relief with IBUPROFEN .... PD 762

Imipramine Hydrochloride (Decreases the antihypertensive effect of reserpine). Products include:
Tofranil Ampuls 854
Tofranil Tablets 856

Imipramine Pamoate (Decreases the antihypertensive effect of reserpine). Products include:
Tofranil-PM Capsules 857

Indapamide (Additive or potentiated action). Products include:
Lozol Tablets 2022

Indomethacin (May reduce the diuretic, natriuretic, and antihypertensive effects of thiazide diuretics). Products include:
Indocin 1680

Indomethacin Sodium Trihydrate (May reduce the diuretic, natriuretic, and antihypertensive effects of thiazide diuretics). Products include:
Indocin I.V. 1684

Insulin, Human (Altered insulin requirements).
No products indexed under this heading.

Insulin, Human Isophane Suspension (Altered insulin requirements). Products include:
Novolin N Human Insulin 10 ml Vials 1795

Insulin, Human NPH (Altered insulin requirements). Products include:
Humulin N, 100 Units 1448
Novolin N PenFill Cartridges Durable Insulin Delivery System 1798
Novolin N Prefilled Syringe Disposable Insulin Delivery System 1798

Insulin, Human Regular (Altered insulin requirements). Products include:
Humulin R, 100 Units 1449
Novolin R Human Insulin 10 ml Vials 1795
Novolin R PenFill Cartridges Durable Insulin Delivery System 1798
Novolin R Prefilled Syringe Disposable Insulin Delivery System 1798
Velosulin BR Human Insulin 10 ml Vials 1795

Insulin, Human, Zinc Suspension (Altered insulin requirements). Products include:
Humulin L, 100 Units 1446
Humulin U, 100 Units 1450
Novolin L Human Insulin 10 ml Vials 1795

Insulin, NPH (Altered insulin requirements). Products include:
NPH, 100 Units 1450
Pork NPH, 100 Units 1452
Purified Pork NPH Isophane Insulin 1801

Insulin, Regular (Altered insulin requirements). Products include:
Regular, 100 Units 1450
Pork Regular, 100 Units 1452
Pork Regular (Concentrated), 500 Units 1453
Purified Pork Regular Insulin 1801

Insulin, Zinc Crystals (Altered insulin requirements). Products include:
NPH, 100 Units 1450

Insulin, Zinc Suspension (Altered insulin requirements). Products include:
Iletin I 1450
Lente, 100 Units 1450
Iletin II 1452
Pork Lente, 100 Units 1452
Purified Pork Lente Insulin 1801

Isocarboxazid (Concurrent administration of MAOI should be avoided).
No products indexed under this heading.

Isoproterenol Hydrochloride (The action of direct-acting sympathomimetic amines may be prolonged). Products include:
Isuprel Hydrochloride Injection 1:5000 2311
Isuprel Hydrochloride Solution 1:200 & 1:100 2313
Isuprel Mistometer 2312

Isoproterenol Sulfate (The action of direct-acting sympathomimetic amines may be prolonged). Products include:
Norisodrine with Calcium Iodide Syrup 442

Isradipine (Additive or potentiated action). Products include:
DynaCirc Capsules 2256

Ketoprofen (May reduce the diuretic, natriuretic, and antihypertensive effects of thiazide diuretics). Products include:
Orudis Capsules 2766
Oruvail Capsules 2766

Ketorolac Tromethamine (May reduce the diuretic, natriuretic, and antihypertensive effects of thiazide diuretics). Products include:
Acular 474
Acular .... ⊙ 277
Toradol 2159

Labetalol Hydrochloride (Additive or potentiated action). Products include:
Normodyne Injection 2377
Normodyne Tablets 2379
Trandate 1185

Levorphanol Tartrate (Orthostatic hypotension). Products include:
Levo-Dromoran 2129

Lisinopril (Additive or potentiated action). Products include:
Prinivil Tablets 1733
Prinzide Tablets 1737
Zestoretic 2850
Zestril Tablets 2854

Lithium Carbonate (Reduced renal clearance and increased risk of lithium toxicity). Products include:
Eskalith 2485
Lithium Carbonate Capsules & Tablets 2230
Lithonate/Lithotabs/Lithobid 2543

Lithium Citrate (Reduced renal clearance and increased risk of lithium toxicity).
No products indexed under this heading.

Losartan Potassium (Additive or potentiated action). Products include:
Cozaar Tablets 1628
Hyzaar Tablets 1677

Maprotiline Hydrochloride (Decreases the antihypertensive effect of reserpine). Products include:
Ludiomil Tablets 843

Mecamylamine Hydrochloride (Additive or potentiated action). Products include:
Inversine Tablets 1686

Meclofenamate Sodium (May reduce the diuretic, natriuretic, and antihypertensive effects of thiazide diuretics).
No products indexed under this heading.

Mefenamic Acid (May reduce the diuretic, natriuretic, and antihypertensive effects of thiazide diuretics). Products include:
Ponstel 1925

Meperidine Hydrochloride (Orthostatic hypotension). Products include:
Demerol 2308
Mepergan Injection 2753

Mephobarbital (Orthostatic hypotension). Products include:
Mebaral Tablets 2322

Metaraminol Bitartrate (The action of direct-acting sympathomimetic amines may be prolonged). Products include:
Aramine Injection 1609

Methadone Hydrochloride (Orthostatic hypotension). Products include:
Methadone Hydrochloride Oral Concentrate 2233
Methadone Hydrochloride Oral Solution & Tablets 2235

Methyclothiazide (Additive or potentiated action). Products include:
Enduron Tablets 420

Methyldopa (Hemolytic anemia; additive or potentiated action). Products include:
Aldoclor Tablets 1598
Aldomet Oral 1600
Aldoril Tablets 1604

Methyldopate Hydrochloride (Hemolytic anemia; additive or potentiated action). Products include:
Aldomet Ester HCl Injection 1602

Methylprednisolone Acetate (Hypokalemia). Products include:
Depo-Medrol Single-Dose Vial 2600
Depo-Medrol Sterile Aqueous Suspension 2597

Methylprednisolone Sodium Succinate (Hypokalemia). Products include:
Solu-Medrol Sterile Powder 2643

Metolazone (Additive or potentiated action). Products include:
Mykrox Tablets 993
Zaroxolyn Tablets 1000

Metoprolol Succinate (Additive or potentiated action). Products include:
Toprol-XL Tablets 565

Metoprolol Tartrate (Additive or potentiated action). Products include:
Lopressor Ampuls 830
Lopressor HCT Tablets 832
Lopressor Tablets 830

Metyrosine (Additive or potentiated action). Products include:
Demser Capsules 1649

Minoxidil (Additive or potentiated action). Products include:
Loniten Tablets 2618
Rogaine Topical Solution 2637

Moexipril Hydrochloride (Additive or potentiated action). Products include:
Univasc Tablets 2410

Morphine Sulfate (Orthostatic hypotension). Products include:
Astramorph/PF Injection, USP (Preservative-Free) 535
Duramorph 962
Infumorph 200 and Infumorph 500 Sterile Solutions 965
MS Contin Tablets 1994
MSIR 1997
Oramorph SR (Morphine Sulfate Sustained Release Tablets) 2236
RMS Suppositories 2657
Roxanol 2243

Nabumetone (May reduce the diuretic, natriuretic, and antihypertensive effects of thiazide diuretics). Products include:
Relafen Tablets 2510

Nadolol (Additive or potentiated action).
No products indexed under this heading.

Naproxen (May reduce the diuretic, natriuretic, and antihypertensive effects of thiazide diuretics). Products include:
Anaprox/Naprosyn 2117

Naproxen Sodium (May reduce the diuretic, natriuretic, and antihypertensive effects of thiazide diuretics). Products include:
Aleve 1975
Anaprox/Naprosyn 2117

Nicardipine Hydrochloride (Additive or potentiated action). Products include:
Cardene Capsules 2095
Cardene I.V. 2709
Cardene SR Capsules 2097

Nifedipine (Additive or potentiated action). Products include:
Adalat Capsules (10 mg and 20 mg) 587
Adalat CC 589
Procardia Capsules 1971

IMPORTANT NOTE: Always consult each drug listing in the patient's regimen for possible interactions.

Procardia XL Extended Release Tablets ... 1972

Nisoldipine (Additive or potentiated action).

No products indexed under this heading.

Nitroglycerin (Additive or potentiated action). Products include:

Deponit NTG Transdermal Delivery System ... 2397
Nitro-Bid IV ... 1523
Nitro-Bid Ointment ... 1524
Nitrodisc ... 2047
Nitro-Dur (nitroglycerin) Transdermal Infusion System ... 1326
Nitrolingual Spray ... 2027
Nitrostat Tablets ... 1925
Transderm-Nitro Transdermal Therapeutic System ... 859

Norepinephrine Bitartrate (Decreased arterial responsiveness to norepinephrine). Products include:

Levophed Bitartrate Injection ... 2315

Norepinephrine Hydrochloride (The action of direct-acting sympathomimetic amines may be prolonged).

Nortriptyline Hydrochloride (Decreases the antihypertensive effect of reserpine). Products include:

Pamelor ... 2280

Opium Alkaloids (Orthostatic hypotension).

No products indexed under this heading.

Oxaprozin (May reduce the diuretic, natriuretic, and antihypertensive effects of thiazide diuretics). Products include:

Daypro Caplets ... 2426

Oxycodone Hydrochloride (Orthostatic hypotension). Products include:

Percocet Tablets ... 938
Percodan Tablets ... 939
Percodan-Demi Tablets ... 940
Roxicodone Tablets, Oral Solution & Intensol (Oxycodone) ... 2244
Tylox Capsules ... 1584

Penbutolol Sulfate (Additive or potentiated action). Products include:

Levatol ... 2403

Pentobarbital Sodium (Orthostatic hypotension). Products include:

Nembutal Sodium Capsules ... 436
Nembutal Sodium Solution ... 438
Nembutal Sodium Suppositories ... 440

Phenelzine Sulfate (Concurrent administration of MAOI should be avoided). Products include:

Nardil ... 1920

Phenobarbital (Orthostatic hypotension). Products include:

Arco-Lase Plus Tablets ... 512
Bellergal-S Tablets ... 2250
Donnatal ... 2060
Donnatal Extentabs ... 2061
Donnatal Tablets ... 2060
Phenobarbital Elixir and Tablets ... 1469
Quadrinal Tablets ... 1350

Phenoxybenzamine Hydrochloride (Additive or potentiated action). Products include:

Dibenzyline Capsules ... 2476

Phentolamine Mesylate (Additive or potentiated action). Products include:

Regitine ... 846

Phenylbutazone (May reduce the diuretic, natriuretic, and antihypertensive effects of thiazide diuretics).

No products indexed under this heading.

Phenylephrine Hydrochloride (The action of direct-acting sympathomimetic amines may be prolonged). Products include:

Atrohist Plus Tablets ... 454
Cerose DM ... ▣ 878
Comhist ... 2038
D.A. Chewable Tablets ... 951
Deconsal Pediatric Capsules ... 454
Dura-Vent/DA Tablets ... 953
Entex Capsules ... 1986
Entex Liquid ... 1986
Extendryl ... 1005
4-Way Fast Acting Nasal Spray (regular & mentholated) ... ▣ 621
Hemorid For Women ... ▣ 834
Hycomine Compound Tablets ... 932
Neo-Synephrine Hydrochloride 1% Carpuject ... 2324
Neo-Synephrine Hydrochloride 1% Injection ... 2324
Neo-Synephrine Hydrochloride (Ophthalmic) ... 2325
Neo-Synephrine ... ▣ 726
Nōstril ... ▣ 644
Novahistine Elixir ... ▣ 823
Phenergan VC ... 2779
Phenergan VC with Codeine ... 2781
Preparation H ... ▣ 871
Tympagesic Ear Drops ... 2342
Vasosulf ... ⊙ 271
Vicks Sinex Nasal Spray and Ultra Fine Mist ... ▣ 765

Phenylephrine Tannate (The action of direct-acting sympathomimetic amines may be prolonged). Products include:

Atrohist Pediatric Suspension ... 454
Ricobid-D Pediatric Suspension ... 2038
Ricobid Tablets and Pediatric Suspension ... 2038
Rynatan ... 2673
Rynatuss ... 2673

Pindolol (Additive or potentiated action). Products include:

Visken Tablets ... 2299

Piroxicam (May reduce the diuretic, natriuretic, and antihypertensive effects of thiazide diuretics). Products include:

Feldene Capsules ... 1965

Polythiazide (Additive or potentiated action). Products include:

Minizide Capsules ... 1938

Prazosin Hydrochloride (Additive or potentiated action). Products include:

Minipress Capsules ... 1937
Minizide Capsules ... 1938

Prednisolone Acetate (Hypokalemia). Products include:

AK-CIDE ... ⊙ 202
AK-CIDE Ointment ... ⊙ 202
Blephamide Liquifilm Sterile Ophthalmic Suspension ... 476
Blephamide Ointment ... ⊙ 237
Econopred & Econopred Plus Ophthalmic Suspensions ... ⊙ 217
Poly-Pred Liquifilm ... ⊙ 248
Pred Forte ... ⊙ 250
Pred Mild ... ⊙ 253
Pred-G Liquifilm Sterile Ophthalmic Suspension ... ⊙ 251
Pred-G S.O.P. Sterile Ophthalmic Ointment ... ⊙ 252
Vasocidin Ointment ... ⊙ 268

Prednisolone Sodium Phosphate (Hypokalemia). Products include:

AK-Pred ... ⊙ 204
Hydeltrasol Injection, Sterile ... 1665
Inflamase ... ⊙ 265
Pediapred Oral Liquid ... 995
Vasocidin Ophthalmic Solution ... ⊙ 270

Prednisolone Tebutate (Hypokalemia). Products include:

Hydeltra-T.B.A. Sterile Suspension 1667

Prednisone (Hypokalemia). Products include:

Deltasone Tablets ... 2595

Propoxyphene Hydrochloride (Orthostatic hypotension). Products include:

Darvon ... 1435
Wygesic Tablets ... 2827

Propoxyphene Napsylate (Orthostatic hypotension). Products include:

Darvon-N/Darvocet-N ... 1433

Propranolol Hydrochloride (Additive or potentiated action). Products include:

Inderal ... 2728
Inderal LA Long Acting Capsules ... 2730
Inderide Tablets ... 2732
Inderide LA Long Acting Capsules .. 2734

Protriptyline Hydrochloride (Decreases the antihypertensive effect of reserpine). Products include:

Vivactil Tablets ... 1774

Quinapril Hydrochloride (Additive or potentiated action). Products include:

Accupril Tablets ... 1893

Quinidine Gluconate (Potential for arrhythmias). Products include:

Quinaglute Dura-Tabs Tablets ... 649

Quinidine Polygalacturonate (Potential for arrhythmias).

No products indexed under this heading.

Quinidine Sulfate (Potential for arrhythmias). Products include:

Quinidex Extentabs ... 2067

Ramipril (Additive or potentiated action). Products include:

Altace Capsules ... 1232

Rauwolfia Serpentina (Additive or potentiated action).

No products indexed under this heading.

Rescinnamine (Additive or potentiated action).

No products indexed under this heading.

Secobarbital Sodium (Orthostatic hypotension). Products include:

Seconal Sodium Pulvules ... 1474

Selegiline Hydrochloride (Concurrent administration of MAOI should be avoided). Products include:

Eldepryl Tablets ... 2550

Sodium Nitroprusside (Additive or potentiated action).

No products indexed under this heading.

Sotalol Hydrochloride (Additive or potentiated action). Products include:

Betapace Tablets ... 641

Spirapril Hydrochloride (Additive or potentiated action).

No products indexed under this heading.

Sufentanil Citrate (Orthostatic hypotension). Products include:

Sufenta Injection ... 1309

Sulindac (May reduce the diuretic, natriuretic, and antihypertensive effects of thiazide diuretics). Products include:

Clinoril Tablets ... 1618

Terazosin Hydrochloride (Additive or potentiated action). Products include:

Hytrin Capsules ... 430

Thiamylal Sodium (Orthostatic hypotension).

No products indexed under this heading.

Timolol Maleate (Additive or potentiated action). Products include:

Blocadren Tablets ... 1614
Timolide Tablets ... 1748
Timoptic in Ocudose ... 1753
Timoptic Sterile Ophthalmic Solution ... 1751
Timoptic-XE ... 1755

Tolmetin Sodium (May reduce the diuretic, natriuretic, and antihypertensive effects of thiazide diuretics). Products include:

Tolectin (200, 400 and 600 mg) .. 1581

Torsemide (Additive or potentiated action). Products include:

Demadex Tablets and Injection ... 686

Tranylcypromine Sulfate (Concurrent administration of MAOI should be avoided). Products include:

Parnate Tablets ... 2503

Triamcinolone (Hypokalemia). Products include:

Aristocort Tablets ... 1022

Triamcinolone Acetonide (Hypokalemia). Products include:

Aristocort A 0.025% Cream ... 1027
Aristocort A 0.5% Cream ... 1031
Aristocort A 0.1% Cream ... 1029
Aristocort A 0.1% Ointment ... 1030
Azmacort Oral Inhaler ... 2011
Nasacort Nasal Inhaler ... 2024

Triamcinolone Diacetate (Hypokalemia). Products include:

Aristocort Suspension (Forte Parenteral) ... 1027
Aristocort Suspension (Intralesional) ... 1025

Triamcinolone Hexacetonide (Hypokalemia). Products include:

Aristospan Suspension (Intra-articular) ... 1033
Aristospan Suspension (Intralesional) ... 1032

Trimethaphan Camsylate (Additive or potentiated action). Products include:

Arfonad Ampuls ... 2080

Trimipramine Maleate (Decreases the antihypertensive effect of reserpine). Products include:

Surmontil Capsules ... 2811

Tubocurarine Chloride (Increased responsiveness to tubocurarine).

No products indexed under this heading.

Tyramine (The action of indirect-acting sympathomimetic amines is inhibited).

Verapamil Hydrochloride (Additive or potentiated action). Products include:

Calan SR Caplets ... 2422
Calan Tablets ... 2419
Isoptin Injectable ... 1344
Isoptin Oral Tablets ... 1346
Isoptin SR Tablets ... 1348
Verelan Capsules ... 1410
Verelan Capsules ... 2824

Food Interactions

Alcohol (Orthostatic hypotension).

Food, unspecified (Concomitant administration enhances gastrointestinal absorption of hydrochlorothiazide and results in higher plasma levels of hydralazine).

SERAX CAPSULES

(Oxazepam) ... 2810

May interact with central nervous system depressants and certain other agents. Compounds in these categories include:

Alfentanil Hydrochloride (Effects may be additive). Products include:

Alfenta Injection ... 1286

Alprazolam (Effects may be additive). Products include:

Xanax Tablets ... 2649

Aprobarbital (Effects may be additive).

No products indexed under this heading.

(▣ Described in PDR For Nonprescription Drugs) (⊙ Described in PDR For Ophthalmology)

Buprenorphine (Effects may be additive). Products include:
- Buprenex Injectable ... 2006

Buspirone Hydrochloride (Effects may be additive). Products include:
- BuSpar ... 737

Butabarbital (Effects may be additive).
- No products indexed under this heading.

Butalbital (Effects may be additive). Products include:
- Esgic-plus Tablets ... 1013
- Fioricet Tablets ... 2258
- Fioricet with Codeine Capsules ... 2260
- Fiorinal Capsules ... 2261
- Fiorinal with Codeine Capsules ... 2262
- Fiorinal Tablets ... 2261
- Phrenilin ... 785
- Sedapap Tablets 50 mg/650 mg .. 1543

Chlordiazepoxide (Effects may be additive). Products include:
- Libritabs Tablets ... 2177
- Limbitrol ... 2180

Chlordiazepoxide Hydrochloride (Effects may be additive). Products include:
- Librax Capsules ... 2176
- Librium Capsules ... 2178
- Librium Injectable ... 2179

Chlorpromazine (Effects may be additive). Products include:
- Thorazine Suppositories ... 2523

Chlorprothixene (Effects may be additive).
- No products indexed under this heading.

Chlorprothixene Hydrochloride (Effects may be additive).
- No products indexed under this heading.

Clorazepate Dipotassium (Effects may be additive). Products include:
- Tranxene ... 451

Clozapine (Effects may be additive). Products include:
- Clozaril Tablets ... 2252

Codeine Phosphate (Effects may be additive). Products include:
- Actifed with Codeine Cough Syrup.. 1067
- Brontex ... 1981
- Deconsal C Expectorant Syrup ... 456
- Deconsal Pediatric Syrup ... 457
- Dimetane-DC Cough Syrup ... 2059
- Empirin with Codeine Tablets ... 1093
- Fioricet with Codeine Capsules ... 2260
- Fiorinal with Codeine Capsules ... 2262
- Isoclor Expectorant ... 990
- Novahistine DH ... 2462
- Novahistine Expectorant ... 2463
- Nucofed ... 2051
- Phenergan with Codeine ... 2777
- Phenergan VC with Codeine ... 2781
- Robitussin A-C Syrup ... 2073
- Robitussin-DAC Syrup ... 2074
- Ryna ... 841
- Soma Compound w/Codeine Tablets ... 2676
- Tussi-Organidin NR Liquid and S NR Liquid ... 2677
- Tylenol with Codeine ... 1583

Desflurane (Effects may be additive). Products include:
- Suprane ... 1813

Dezocine (Effects may be additive). Products include:
- Dalgan Injection ... 538

Diazepam (Effects may be additive). Products include:
- Dizac ... 1809
- Valium Injectable ... 2182
- Valium Tablets ... 2183
- Valrelease Capsules ... 2169

Droperidol (Effects may be additive). Products include:
- Inapsine Injection ... 1296

Enflurane (Effects may be additive).
- No products indexed under this heading.

Estazolam (Effects may be additive). Products include:
- ProSom Tablets ... 449

Ethchlorvynol (Effects may be additive). Products include:
- Placidyl Capsules ... 448

Ethinamate (Effects may be additive).
- No products indexed under this heading.

Fentanyl (Effects may be additive). Products include:
- Duragesic Transdermal System ... 1288

Fentanyl Citrate (Effects may be additive). Products include:
- Sublimaze Injection ... 1307

Fluphenazine Decanoate (Effects may be additive). Products include:
- Prolixin Decanoate ... 509

Fluphenazine Enanthate (Effects may be additive). Products include:
- Prolixin Enanthate ... 509

Fluphenazine Hydrochloride (Effects may be additive). Products include:
- Prolixin ... 509

Flurazepam Hydrochloride (Effects may be additive). Products include:
- Dalmane Capsules ... 2173

Glutethimide (Effects may be additive).
- No products indexed under this heading.

Haloperidol (Effects may be additive). Products include:
- Haldol Injection, Tablets and Concentrate ... 1575

Haloperidol Decanoate (Effects may be additive). Products include:
- Haldol Decanoate ... 1577

Hydrocodone Bitartrate (Effects may be additive). Products include:
- Anexsia 5/500 Elixir ... 1781
- Anexia Tablets ... 1782
- Codiclear DH Syrup ... 791
- Deconamine CX Cough and Cold Liquid and Tablets ... 1319
- Duratuss HD Elixir ... 2565
- Hycodan Tablets and Syrup ... 930
- Hycomine Compound Tablets ... 932
- Hycomine ... 931
- Hycotuss Expectorant Syrup ... 933
- Hydrocet Capsules ... 782
- Lorcet 10/650 ... 1018
- Lortab ... 2566
- Tussend ... 1783
- Tussend Expectorant ... 1785
- Vicodin Tablets ... 1356
- Vicodin ES Tablets ... 1357
- Vicodin Tuss Expectorant ... 1358
- Zydone Capsules ... 949

Hydrocodone Polistirex (Effects may be additive). Products include:
- Tussionex Pennkinetic Extended-Release Suspension ... 998

Hydroxyzine Hydrochloride (Effects may be additive). Products include:
- Atarax Tablets & Syrup ... 2185
- Marax Tablets & DF Syrup ... 2200
- Vistaril Intramuscular Solution ... 2216

Isoflurane (Effects may be additive).
- No products indexed under this heading.

Ketamine Hydrochloride (Effects may be additive).
- No products indexed under this heading.

Levomethadyl Acetate Hydrochloride (Effects may be additive). Products include:
- Orlamm ... 2239

Levorphanol Tartrate (Effects may be additive). Products include:
- Levo-Dromoran ... 2129

Lorazepam (Effects may be additive). Products include:
- Ativan Injection ... 2698
- Ativan Tablets ... 2700

Loxapine Hydrochloride (Effects may be additive). Products include:
- Loxitane ... 1378

Loxapine Succinate (Effects may be additive). Products include:
- Loxitane Capsules ... 1378

Meperidine Hydrochloride (Effects may be additive). Products include:
- Demerol ... 2308
- Mepergan Injection ... 2753

Mephobarbital (Effects may be additive). Products include:
- Mebaral Tablets ... 2322

Meprobamate (Effects may be additive). Products include:
- Miltown Tablets ... 2672
- PMB 200 and PMB 400 ... 2783

Mesoridazine Besylate (Effects may be additive). Products include:
- Serentil ... 684

Methadone Hydrochloride (Effects may be additive). Products include:
- Methadone Hydrochloride Oral Concentrate ... 2233
- Methadone Hydrochloride Oral Solution & Tablets ... 2235

Methohexital Sodium (Effects may be additive). Products include:
- Brevital Sodium Vials ... 1429

Methotrimeprazine (Effects may be additive). Products include:
- Levoprome ... 1274

Methoxyflurane (Effects may be additive).
- No products indexed under this heading.

Midazolam Hydrochloride (Effects may be additive). Products include:
- Versed Injection ... 2170

Molindone Hydrochloride (Effects may be additive). Products include:
- Moban Tablets and Concentrate ... 1048

Morphine Sulfate (Effects may be additive). Products include:
- Astramorph/PF Injection, USP (Preservative-Free) ... 535
- Duramorph ... 962
- Infumorph 200 and Infumorph 500 Sterile Solutions ... 965
- MS Contin Tablets ... 1994
- MSIR ... 1997
- Oramorph SR (Morphine Sulfate Sustained Release Tablets) ... 2236
- RMS Suppositories ... 2657
- Roxanol ... 2243

Opium Alkaloids (Effects may be additive).
- No products indexed under this heading.

Oxycodone Hydrochloride (Effects may be additive). Products include:
- Percocet Tablets ... 938
- Percodan Tablets ... 939
- Percodan-Demi Tablets ... 940
- Roxicodone Tablets, Oral Solution & Intensol (Oxycodone) ... 2244
- Tylox Capsules ... 1584

Pentobarbital Sodium (Effects may be additive). Products include:
- Nembutal Sodium Capsules ... 436
- Nembutal Sodium Solution ... 438
- Nembutal Sodium Suppositories ... 440

Perphenazine (Effects may be additive). Products include:
- Etrafon ... 2355
- Triavil Tablets ... 1757
- Trilafon ... 2389

Phenobarbital (Effects may be additive). Products include:
- Arco-Lase Plus Tablets ... 512
- Bellergal-S Tablets ... 2250
- Donnatal ... 2060
- Donnatal Extentabs ... 2061
- Donnatal Tablets ... 2060
- Phenobarbital Elixir and Tablets ... 1469
- Quadrinal Tablets ... 1350

Prazepam (Effects may be additive).
- No products indexed under this heading.

Prochlorperazine (Effects may be additive). Products include:
- Compazine ... 2470

Promethazine Hydrochloride (Effects may be additive). Products include:
- Mepergan Injection ... 2753
- Phenergan with Codeine ... 2777
- Phenergan with Dextromethorphan 2778
- Phenergan Injection ... 2773
- Phenergan Suppositories ... 2775
- Phenergan Syrup ... 2774
- Phenergan Tablets ... 2775
- Phenergan VC ... 2779
- Phenergan VC with Codeine ... 2781

Propofol (Effects may be additive). Products include:
- Diprivan Injection ... 2833

Propoxyphene Hydrochloride (Effects may be additive). Products include:
- Darvon ... 1435
- Wygesic Tablets ... 2827

Propoxyphene Napsylate (Effects may be additive). Products include:
- Darvon-N/Darvocet-N ... 1433

Quazepam (Effects may be additive). Products include:
- Doral Tablets ... 2664

Risperidone (Effects may be additive). Products include:
- Risperdal ... 1301

Secobarbital Sodium (Effects may be additive). Products include:
- Seconal Sodium Pulvules ... 1474

Sufentanil Citrate (Effects may be additive). Products include:
- Sufenta Injection ... 1309

Temazepam (Effects may be additive). Products include:
- Restoril Capsules ... 2284

Thiamylal Sodium (Effects may be additive).
- No products indexed under this heading.

Thioridazine Hydrochloride (Effects may be additive). Products include:
- Mellaril ... 2269

Thiothixene (Effects may be additive). Products include:
- Navane Capsules and Concentrate ... 2201
- Navane Intramuscular ... 2202

Triazolam (Effects may be additive). Products include:
- Halcion Tablets ... 2611

Trifluoperazine Hydrochloride (Effects may be additive). Products include:
- Stelazine ... 2514

Zolpidem Tartrate (Effects may be additive). Products include:
- Ambien Tablets ... 2416

Food Interactions

Alcohol (Effects may be additive).

SERAX TABLETS

(Oxazepam) ... 2810

See **Serax Capsules**

SERENTIL AMPULS

(Mesoridazine Besylate) ... 684

May interact with central nervous system depressants, barbiturates, general anesthetics, narcotic analge-

IMPORTANT NOTE: Always consult each drug listing in the patient's regimen for possible interactions.

sics, and certain other agents. Compounds in these categories include:

Alfentanil Hydrochloride (Potentiation of central nervous system depressant). Products include:
- Alfenta Injection 1286

Alprazolam (Potentiation of central nervous system depressant). Products include:
- Xanax Tablets 2649

Aprobarbital (Potentiation of central nervous system depressant).
- No products indexed under this heading.

Atropine Sulfate (Potentiation of central nervous system depressant). Products include:
- Arco-Lase Plus Tablets 512
- Atrohist Plus Tablets 454
- Atropine Sulfate Sterile Ophthalmic Solution .... ◉ 233
- Donnatal 2060
- Donnatal Extentabs 2061
- Donnatal Tablets 2060
- Lomotil 2439
- Motofen Tablets 784
- Urised Tablets 1964

Buprenorphine (Potentiation of central nervous system depressant). Products include:
- Buprenex Injectable 2006

Buspirone Hydrochloride (Potentiation of central nervous system depressant). Products include:
- BuSpar 737

Butabarbital (Potentiation of central nervous system depressant).
- No products indexed under this heading.

Butalbital (Potentiation of central nervous system depressant). Products include:
- Esgic-plus Tablets 1013
- Fioricet Tablets 2258
- Fioricet with Codeine Capsules 2260
- Fiorinal Capsules 2261
- Fiorinal with Codeine Capsules 2262
- Fiorinal Tablets 2261
- Phrenilin 785
- Sedapap Tablets 50 mg/650 mg .. 1543

Chlordiazepoxide (Potentiation of central nervous system depressant). Products include:
- Libritabs Tablets 2177
- Limbitrol 2180

Chlordiazepoxide Hydrochloride (Potentiation of central nervous system depressant). Products include:
- Librax Capsules 2176
- Librium Capsules 2178
- Librium Injectable 2179

Chlorpromazine (Potentiation of central nervous system depressant). Products include:
- Thorazine Suppositories 2523

Chlorpromazine Hydrochloride (Potentiation of central nervous system depressant). Products include:
- Thorazine 2523

Chlorprothixene (Potentiation of central nervous system depressant).
- No products indexed under this heading.

Chlorprothixene Hydrochloride (Potentiation of central nervous system depressant).
- No products indexed under this heading.

Clorazepate Dipotassium (Potentiation of central nervous system depressant). Products include:
- Tranxene 451

Clozapine (Potentiation of central nervous system depressant). Products include:
- Clozaril Tablets 2252

Codeine Phosphate (Potentiation of central nervous system depressant). Products include:
- Actifed with Codeine Cough Syrup.. 1067
- Brontex 1981
- Deconsal C Expectorant Syrup 456
- Deconsal Pediatric Syrup 457
- Dimetane-DC Cough Syrup 2059
- Empirin with Codeine Tablets 1093
- Fioricet with Codeine Capsules 2260
- Fiorinal with Codeine Capsules 2262
- Isoclor Expectorant 990
- Novahistine DH 2462
- Novahistine Expectorant 2463
- Nucofed 2051
- Phenergan with Codeine 2777
- Phenergan VC with Codeine 2781
- Robitussin A-C Syrup 2073
- Robitussin-DAC Syrup 2074
- Ryna .... ▣ 841
- Soma Compound w/Codeine Tablets 2676
- Tussi-Organidin NR Liquid and S NR Liquid 2677
- Tylenol with Codeine 1583

Desflurane (Potentiation of central nervous system depressant). Products include:
- Suprane 1813

Dezocine (Potentiation of central nervous system depressant). Products include:
- Dalgan Injection 538

Diazepam (Potentiation of central nervous system depressant). Products include:
- Dizac 1809
- Valium Injectable 2182
- Valium Tablets 2183
- Valrelease Capsules 2169

Droperidol (Potentiation of central nervous system depressant). Products include:
- Inapsine Injection 1296

Enflurane (Potentiation of central nervous system depressant).
- No products indexed under this heading.

Estazolam (Potentiation of central nervous system depressant). Products include:
- ProSom Tablets 449

Ethchlorvynol (Potentiation of central nervous system depressant). Products include:
- Placidyl Capsules 448

Ethinamate (Potentiation of central nervous system depressant).
- No products indexed under this heading.

Fentanyl (Potentiation of central nervous system depressant). Products include:
- Duragesic Transdermal System 1288

Fentanyl Citrate (Potentiation of central nervous system depressant). Products include:
- Sublimaze Injection 1307

Fluphenazine Decanoate (Potentiation of central nervous system depressant). Products include:
- Prolixin Decanoate 509

Fluphenazine Enanthate (Potentiation of central nervous system depressant). Products include:
- Prolixin Enanthate 509

Fluphenazine Hydrochloride (Potentiation of central nervous system depressant). Products include:
- Prolixin 509

Flurazepam Hydrochloride (Potentiation of central nervous system depressant). Products include:
- Dalmane Capsules 2173

Glutethimide (Potentiation of central nervous system depressant).
- No products indexed under this heading.

Haloperidol (Potentiation of central nervous system depressant). Products include:
- Haldol Injection, Tablets and Concentrate 1575

Haloperidol Decanoate (Potentiation of central nervous system depressant). Products include:
- Haldol Decanoate 1577

Hydrocodone Bitartrate (Potentiation of central nervous system depressant). Products include:
- Anexsia 5/500 Elixir 1781
- Anexia Tablets 1782
- Codiclear DH Syrup 791
- Deconamine CX Cough and Cold Liquid and Tablets 1319
- Duratuss HD Elixir 2565
- Hycodan Tablets and Syrup 930
- Hycomine Compound Tablets 932
- Hycomine 931
- Hycotuss Expectorant Syrup 933
- Hydrocet Capsules 782
- Lorcet 10/650 1018
- Lortab 2566
- Tussend 1783
- Tussend Expectorant 1785
- Vicodin Tablets 1356
- Vicodin ES Tablets 1357
- Vicodin Tuss Expectorant 1358
- Zydone Capsules 949

Hydrocodone Polistirex (Potentiation of central nervous system depressant). Products include:
- Tussionex Pennkinetic Extended-Release Suspension 998

Hydroxyzine Hydrochloride (Potentiation of central nervous system depressant). Products include:
- Atarax Tablets & Syrup 2185
- Marax Tablets & DF Syrup 2200
- Vistaril Intramuscular Solution 2216

Isoflurane (Potentiation of central nervous system depressant).
- No products indexed under this heading.

Ketamine Hydrochloride (Potentiation of central nervous system depressant).
- No products indexed under this heading.

Levomethadyl Acetate Hydrochloride (Potentiation of central nervous system depressant). Products include:
- Orlamm 2239

Levorphanol Tartrate (Potentiation of central nervous system depressant). Products include:
- Levo-Dromoran 2129

Lorazepam (Potentiation of central nervous system depressant). Products include:
- Ativan Injection 2698
- Ativan Tablets 2700

Loxapine Hydrochloride (Potentiation of central nervous system depressant). Products include:
- Loxitane 1378

Loxapine Succinate (Potentiation of central nervous system depressant). Products include:
- Loxitane Capsules 1378

Meperidine Hydrochloride (Potentiation of central nervous system depressant). Products include:
- Demerol 2308
- Mepergan Injection 2753

Mephobarbital (Potentiation of central nervous system depressant). Products include:
- Mebaral Tablets 2322

Meprobamate (Potentiation of central nervous system depressant). Products include:
- Miltown Tablets 2672
- PMB 200 and PMB 400 2783

Mesoridazine (Potentiation of central nervous system depressant).

Methadone Hydrochloride (Potentiation of central nervous system depressant). Products include:
- Methadone Hydrochloride Oral Concentrate 2233
- Methadone Hydrochloride Oral Solution & Tablets 2235

Methohexital Sodium (Potentiation of central nervous system depressant). Products include:
- Brevital Sodium Vials 1429

Methotrimeprazine (Potentiation of central nervous system depressant). Products include:
- Levoprome 1274

Methoxyflurane (Potentiation of central nervous system depressant).
- No products indexed under this heading.

Midazolam Hydrochloride (Potentiation of central nervous system depressant). Products include:
- Versed Injection 2170

Molindone Hydrochloride (Potentiation of central nervous system depressant). Products include:
- Moban Tablets and Concentrate 1048

Morphine Sulfate (Potentiation of central nervous system depressant). Products include:
- Astramorph/PF Injection, USP (Preservative-Free) 535
- Duramorph 962
- Infumorph 200 and Infumorph 500 Sterile Solutions 965
- MS Contin Tablets 1994
- MSIR 1997
- Oramorph SR (Morphine Sulfate Sustained Release Tablets) 2236
- RMS Suppositories 2657
- Roxanol 2243

Opium Alkaloids (Potentiation of central nervous system depressant).
- No products indexed under this heading.

Oxazepam (Potentiation of central nervous system depressant). Products include:
- Serax Capsules 2810
- Serax Tablets 2810

Oxycodone Hydrochloride (Potentiation of central nervous system depressant). Products include:
- Percocet Tablets 938
- Percodan Tablets 939
- Percodan-Demi Tablets 940
- Roxicodone Tablets, Oral Solution & Intensol (Oxycodone) 2244
- Tylox Capsules 1584

Pentobarbital Sodium (Potentiation of central nervous system depressant). Products include:
- Nembutal Sodium Capsules 436
- Nembutal Sodium Solution 438
- Nembutal Sodium Suppositories 440

Perphenazine (Potentiation of central nervous system depressant). Products include:
- Etrafon 2355
- Triavil Tablets 1757
- Trilafon 2389

Phenobarbital (Potentiation of central nervous system depressant). Products include:
- Arco-Lase Plus Tablets 512
- Bellergal-S Tablets 2250
- Donnatal 2060
- Donnatal Extentabs 2061
- Donnatal Tablets 2060
- Phenobarbital Elixir and Tablets 1469
- Quadrinal Tablets 1350

Prazepam (Potentiation of central nervous system depressant).
- No products indexed under this heading.

Prochlorperazine (Potentiation of central nervous system depressant). Products include:
- Compazine 2470

(▣ Described in PDR For Nonprescription Drugs) (◉ Described in PDR For Ophthalmology)

945 Interactions Index Serzone

Promethazine Hydrochloride (Potentiation of central nervous system depressant). Products include:
Mepergan Injection ... 2753
Phenergan with Codeine ... 2777
Phenergan with Dextromethorphan 2778
Phenergan Injection ... 2773
Phenergan Suppositories ... 2775
Phenergan Syrup ... 2774
Phenergan Tablets ... 2775
Phenergan VC ... 2779
Phenergan VC with Codeine ... 2781

Propofol (Potentiation of central nervous system depressant). Products include:
Diprivan Injection ... 2833

Propoxyphene Hydrochloride (Potentiation of central nervous system depressant). Products include:
Darvon ... 1435
Wygesic Tablets ... 2827

Propoxyphene Napsylate (Potentiation of central nervous system depressant). Products include:
Darvon-N/Darvocet-N ... 1433

Quazepam (Potentiation of central nervous system depressant). Products include:
Doral Tablets ... 2664

Risperidone (Potentiation of central nervous system depressant). Products include:
Risperdal ... 1301

Secobarbital Sodium (Potentiation of central nervous system depressant). Products include:
Seconal Sodium Pulvules ... 1474

Sufentanil Citrate (Potentiation of central nervous system depressant). Products include:
Sufenta Injection ... 1309

Temazepam (Potentiation of central nervous system depressant). Products include:
Restoril Capsules ... 2284

Thiamylal Sodium (Potentiation of central nervous system depressant).
No products indexed under this heading.

Thioridazine Hydrochloride (Potentiation of central nervous system depressant). Products include:
Mellaril ... 2269

Thiothixene (Potentiation of central nervous system depressant). Products include:
Navane Capsules and Concentrate 2201
Navane Intramuscular ... 2202

Triazolam (Potentiation of central nervous system depressant). Products include:
Halcion Tablets ... 2611

Trifluoperazine Hydrochloride (Potentiation of central nervous system depressant). Products include:
Stelazine ... 2514

Zolpidem Tartrate (Potentiation of central nervous system depressant). Products include:
Ambien Tablets ... 2416

Food Interactions

Alcohol (Potentiation of central nervous system depressant).

SERENTIL CONCENTRATE
(Mesoridazine Besylate) ... 684
See **Serentil Ampuls**

SERENTIL TABLETS
(Mesoridazine Besylate) ... 684
See **Serentil Ampuls**

SEREVENT INHALATION AEROSOL
(Salmeterol Xinafoate) ... 1176
May interact with monoamine oxidase inhibitors and tricyclic antidepressants. Compounds in these categories include:

Amitriptyline Hydrochloride (The action of salmeterol on the vascular system may be potentiated by tricyclic antidepressant). Products include:
Elavil ... 2838
Endep Tablets ... 2174
Etrafon ... 2355
Limbitrol ... 2180
Triavil Tablets ... 1757

Amoxapine (The action of salmeterol on the vascular system may be potentiated by tricyclic antidepressant). Products include:
Asendin Tablets ... 1369

Clomipramine Hydrochloride (The action of salmeterol on the vascular system may be potentiated by tricyclic antidepressant). Products include:
Anafranil Capsules ... 803

Desipramine Hydrochloride (The action of salmeterol on the vascular system may be potentiated by tricyclic antidepressant). Products include:
Norpramin Tablets ... 1526

Doxepin Hydrochloride (The action of salmeterol on the vascular system may be potentiated by tricyclic antidepressant). Products include:
Sinequan ... 2205
Zonalon Cream ... 1055

Furazolidone (The action of salmeterol on the vascular system may be potentiated by MAO inhibitor). Products include:
Furoxone ... 2046

Imipramine Hydrochloride (The action of salmeterol on the vascular system may be potentiated by tricyclic antidepressant). Products include:
Tofranil Ampuls ... 854
Tofranil Tablets ... 856

Imipramine Pamoate (The action of salmeterol on the vascular system may be potentiated by tricyclic antidepressant). Products include:
Tofranil-PM Capsules ... 857

Isocarboxazid (The action of salmeterol on the vascular system may be potentiated by MAO inhibitor).
No products indexed under this heading.

Maprotiline Hydrochloride (The action of salmeterol on the vascular system may be potentiated by tricyclic antidepressant). Products include:
Ludiomil Tablets ... 843

Nortriptyline Hydrochloride (The action of salmeterol on the vascular system may be potentiated by tricyclic antidepressant). Products include:
Pamelor ... 2280

Phenelzine Sulfate (The action of salmeterol on the vascular system may be potentiated by MAO inhibitor). Products include:
Nardil ... 1920

Protriptyline Hydrochloride (The action of salmeterol on the vascular system may be potentiated by tricyclic antidepressant). Products include:
Vivactil Tablets ... 1774

Selegiline Hydrochloride (The action of salmeterol on the vascular system may be potentiated by MAO inhibitor). Products include:
Eldepryl Tablets ... 2550

Tranylcypromine Sulfate (The action of salmeterol on the vascular system may be potentiated by MAO inhibitor). Products include:
Parnate Tablets ... 2503

Trimipramine Maleate (The action of salmeterol on the vascular system may be potentiated by tricyclic antidepressant). Products include:
Surmontil Capsules ... 2811

SEROMYCIN PULVULES
(Cycloserine) ... 1476
May interact with antituberculosis drugs and certain other agents. Compounds in these categories include:

Aminosalicylic Acid (Concurrent use with other antituberculosis drugs may result in vitamin B_{12} and/or folic acid deficiency). Products include:
PASER Granules ... 1285

p-Aminosalicylic Acid (Concurrent use with other antituberculosis drugs may result in vitamin B_{12} and/or folic acid deficiency).
No products indexed under this heading.

Ethambutol Hydrochloride (Concurrent use with other antituberculosis drugs may result in vitamin B_{12} and/or folic acid deficiency). Products include:
Myambutol Tablets ... 1386

Ethionamide (Neurotoxic side effects potentiated). Products include:
Trecator-SC Tablets ... 2814

Isoniazid (Concurrent use with other antituberculosis drugs may result in vitamin B_{12} and/or folic acid deficiency; increased incidence of CNS effects, such as dizziness or drowsiness; dosage adjustment may be necessary). Products include:
Nydrazid Injection ... 508
Rifamate Capsules ... 1530
Rifater ... 1532

Pyrazinamide (Concurrent use with other antituberculosis drugs may result in vitamin B_{12} and/or folic acid deficiency). Products include:
Pyrazinamide Tablets ... 1398
Rifater ... 1532

Rifampin (Concurrent use with other antituberculosis drugs may result in vitamin B_{12} and/or folic acid deficiency). Products include:
Rifadin ... 1528
Rifamate Capsules ... 1530
Rifater ... 1532
Rimactane Capsules ... 847

Food Interactions

Alcohol (Increases risk of epileptic episodes).

SEROPHENE (CLOMIPHENE CITRATE TABLETS, USP)
(Clomiphene Citrate) ... 2451
None cited in PDR database.

SERZONE TABLETS
(Nefazodone Hydrochloride) ... 771
May interact with monoamine oxidase inhibitors, triazolobenzodiazepines, highly protein bound drugs (selected), and certain other agents. Compounds in these categories include:

Alprazolam (Co-administration may increase steady-state peak concentrations, AUC and half-life values; potentiated effects on psychomotor performance tests; reduction in initial dosage of triazolobenzodiazepines is required). Products include:
Xanax Tablets ... 2649

Amiodarone Hydrochloride (Nefazodone is highly bound to the plasma protein hence co-administration with another drug that is highly protein bound may cause increased free concentrations of other drug, potentially resulting in adverse events). Products include:
Cordarone Intravenous ... 2715
Cordarone Tablets ... 2712

Amitriptyline Hydrochloride (Nefazodone is highly bound to the plasma protein hence co-administration with another drug that is highly protein bound may cause increased free concentrations of other drug, potentially resulting in adverse events). Products include:
Elavil ... 2838
Endep Tablets ... 2174
Etrafon ... 2355
Limbitrol ... 2180
Triavil Tablets ... 1757

Astemizole (Nefazodone has been shown *in vitro* to be inhibitor of cytochrome $P_{450}IIIA_4$ resulting in the potential for increased plasma concentration of astemizole leading to QT prolongation and rare cases of serious cardiovascular toxicity; concurrent use is contraindicated). Products include:
Hismanal Tablets ... 1293

Atovaquone (Nefazodone is highly bound to the plasma protein hence co-administration with another drug that is highly protein bound may cause increased free concentrations of other drug, potentially resulting in adverse events). Products include:
Mepron Suspension ... 1135

Cefonicid Sodium (Nefazodone is highly bound to the plasma protein hence co-administration with another drug that is highly protein bound may cause increased free concentrations of other drug, potentially resulting in adverse events). Products include:
Monocid Injection ... 2497

Chlordiazepoxide (Nefazodone is highly bound to the plasma protein hence co-administration with another drug that is highly protein bound may cause increased free concentrations of other drug, potentially resulting in adverse events). Products include:
Libritabs Tablets ... 2177
Limbitrol ... 2180

Chlordiazepoxide Hydrochloride (Nefazodone is highly bound to the plasma protein hence co-administration with another drug that is highly protein bound may cause increased free concentrations of other drug, potentially resulting in adverse events). Products include:
Librax Capsules ... 2176
Librium Capsules ... 2178
Librium Injectable ... 2179

Chlorpromazine (Nefazodone is highly bound to the plasma protein hence co-administration with another drug that is highly protein bound may cause increased free concentrations of other drug, potentially resulting in adverse events). Products include:
Thorazine Suppositories ... 2523

IMPORTANT NOTE: Always consult each drug listing in the patient's regimen for possible interactions.

Serzone | Interactions Index | 946

Chlorpromazine Hydrochloride (Nefazodone is highly bound to the plasma protein hence co-administration with another drug that is highly protein bound may cause increased free concentrations of other drug, potentially resulting in adverse events). Products include:
- Thorazine 2523

Clomipramine Hydrochloride (Nefazodone is highly bound to the plasma protein hence co-administration with another drug that is highly protein bound may cause increased free concentrations of other drug, potentially resulting in adverse events). Products include:
- Anafranil Capsules 803

Clozapine (Nefazodone is highly bound to the plasma protein hence co-administration with another drug that is highly protein bound may cause increased free concentrations of other drug, potentially resulting in adverse events). Products include:
- Clozaril Tablets 2252

Cyclosporine (Nefazodone is highly bound to the plasma protein hence co-administration with another drug that is highly protein bound may cause increased free concentrations of other drug, potentially resulting in adverse events). Products include:
- Neoral 2276
- Sandimmune 2286

Diazepam (Nefazodone is highly bound to the plasma protein hence co-administration with another drug that is highly protein bound may cause increased free concentrations of other drug, potentially resulting in adverse events). Products include:
- Dizac 1809
- Valium Injectable 2182
- Valium Tablets 2183
- Valrelease Capsules 2169

Diclofenac Potassium (Nefazodone is highly bound to the plasma protein hence co-administration with another drug that is highly protein bound may cause increased free concentrations of other drug, potentially resulting in adverse events). Products include:
- Cataflam 816

Diclofenac Sodium (Nefazodone is highly bound to the plasma protein hence co-administration with another drug that is highly protein bound may cause increased free concentrations of other drug, potentially resulting in adverse events). Products include:
- Voltaren Ophthalmic Sterile Ophthalmic Solution .... ⊙ 272
- Voltaren Tablets 861

Digoxin (Potential for increased digoxin C_{max}, C_{min}, and AUC by 29%, 27%, and 15% respectively; caution should be exercised if used concurrently). Products include:
- Lanoxicaps 1117
- Lanoxin Elixir Pediatric 1120
- Lanoxin Injection 1123
- Lanoxin Injection Pediatric 1126
- Lanoxin Tablets 1128

Dipyridamole (Nefazodone is highly bound to the plasma protein hence co-administration with another drug that is highly protein bound may cause increased free concentrations of other drug, potentially resulting in adverse events). Products include:
- Persantine Tablets 681

Fenoprofen Calcium (Nefazodone is highly bound to the plasma protein hence co-administration with another drug that is highly protein bound may cause increased free concentrations of other drug, potentially resulting in adverse events). Products include:
- Nalfon 200 Pulvules & Nalfon Tablets 917

Flurazepam Hydrochloride (Nefazodone is highly bound to the plasma protein hence co-administration with another drug that is highly protein bound may cause increased free concentrations of other drug, potentially resulting in adverse events). Products include:
- Dalmane Capsules 2173

Flurbiprofen (Nefazodone is highly bound to the plasma protein hence co-administration with another drug that is highly protein bound may cause increased free concentrations of other drug, potentially resulting in adverse events). Products include:
- Ansaid Tablets 2579

Furazolidone (Potential for serious, sometimes fatal, reactions including hyperthermia, rigidity, myoclonus, extreme agitation progressing to delirium and coma; concurrent and/or sequential use is contraindicated). Products include:
- Furoxone 2046

Glipizide (Nefazodone is highly bound to the plasma protein hence co-administration with another drug that is highly protein bound may cause increased free concentrations of other drug, potentially resulting in adverse events). Products include:
- Glucotrol Tablets 1967
- Glucotrol XL Extended Release Tablets 1968

Haloperidol (Decreased haloperidol apparent clearance by 35% with no significant increase in peak plasma levels or time to peak; dosage adjustment may be required). Products include:
- Haldol Injection, Tablets and Concentrate 1575

Haloperidol Decanoate (Decreased haloperidol apparent clearance by 35% with no significant increase in peak plasma levels or time to peak; dosage adjustment may be required). Products include:
- Haldol Decanoate 1577

Ibuprofen (Nefazodone is highly bound to the plasma protein hence co-administration with another drug that is highly protein bound may cause increased free concentrations of other drug, potentially resulting in adverse events). Products include:
- Advil Cold and Sinus Caplets and Tablets (formerly CoAdvil) .... ▣ 870
- Advil Ibuprofen Tablets and Caplets .... ▣ 870
- Children's Advil Suspension 2692
- Arthritis Foundation Ibuprofen Tablets .... ▣ 674
- Bayer Select Ibuprofen Pain Relief Formula .... ▣ 715
- Cramp End Tablets .... ▣ 735
- Dimetapp Sinus Caplets .... ▣ 775
- Haltran Tablets .... ▣ 771
- IBU Tablets 1342
- Ibuprohm .... ▣ 735
- Children's Motrin Ibuprofen Oral Suspension 1546
- Motrin Tablets 2625
- Motrin IB Caplets, Tablets, and Geltabs .... ▣ 838
- Motrin IB Sinus .... ▣ 838
- Motrin Ibuprofen Suspension, Oral Drops, Chewable Tablets, Caplets 1546
- Nuprin Ibuprofen/Analgesic Tablets & Caplets .... ▣ 622
- Sine-Aid IB Caplets 1554
- Vicks DayQuil SINUS Pressure & PAIN Relief with IBUPROFEN .... ▣ 762

Imipramine Hydrochloride (Nefazodone is highly bound to the plasma protein hence co-administration with another drug that is highly protein bound may cause increased free concentrations of other drug, potentially resulting in adverse events). Products include:
- Tofranil Ampuls 854
- Tofranil Tablets 856

Imipramine Pamoate (Nefazodone is highly bound to the plasma protein hence co-administration with another drug that is highly protein bound may cause increased free concentrations of other drug, potentially resulting in adverse events). Products include:
- Tofranil-PM Capsules 857

Indomethacin (Nefazodone is highly bound to the plasma protein hence co-administration with another drug that is highly protein bound may cause increased free concentrations of other drug, potentially resulting in adverse events). Products include:
- Indocin 1680

Indomethacin Sodium Trihydrate (Nefazodone is highly bound to the plasma protein hence co-administration with another drug that is highly protein bound may cause increased free concentrations of other drug, potentially resulting in adverse events). Products include:
- Indocin I.V. 1684

Isocarboxazid (Potential for serious, sometimes fatal, reactions including hyperthermia, rigidity, myoclonus, extreme agitation progressing to delirium and coma; concurrent and/or sequential use is contraindicated).
- No products indexed under this heading.

Ketoprofen (Nefazodone is highly bound to the plasma protein hence co-administration with another drug that is highly protein bound may cause increased free concentrations of other drug, potentially resulting in adverse events). Products include:
- Orudis Capsules 2766
- Oruvail Capsules 2766

Ketorolac Tromethamine (Nefazodone is highly bound to the plasma protein hence co-administration with another drug that is highly protein bound may cause increased free concentrations of other drug, potentially resulting in adverse events). Products include:
- Acular 474
- Acular .... ⊙ 277
- Toradol 2159

Meclofenamate Sodium (Nefazodone is highly bound to the plasma protein hence co-administration with another drug that is highly protein bound may cause increased free concentrations of other drug, potentially resulting in adverse events).
- No products indexed under this heading.

Mefenamic Acid (Nefazodone is highly bound to the plasma protein hence co-administration with another drug that is highly protein bound may cause increased free concentrations of other drug, potentially resulting in adverse events). Products include:
- Ponstel 1925

Midazolam Hydrochloride (Nefazodone is highly bound to the plasma protein hence co-administration with another drug that is highly protein bound may cause increased free concentrations of other drug, potentially resulting in adverse events). Products include:
- Versed Injection 2170

Naproxen (Nefazodone is highly bound to the plasma protein hence co-administration with another drug that is highly protein bound may cause increased free concentrations of other drug, potentially resulting in adverse events). Products include:
- Anaprox/Naprosyn 2117

Naproxen Sodium (Nefazodone is highly bound to the plasma protein hence co-administration with another drug that is highly protein bound may cause increased free concentrations of other drug, potentially resulting in adverse events). Products include:
- Aleve 1975
- Anaprox/Naprosyn 2117

Nortriptyline Hydrochloride (Nefazodone is highly bound to the plasma protein hence co-administration with another drug that is highly protein bound may cause increased free concentrations of other drug, potentially resulting in adverse events). Products include:
- Pamelor 2280

Oxaprozin (Nefazodone is highly bound to the plasma protein hence co-administration with another drug that is highly protein bound may cause increased free concentrations of other drug, potentially resulting in adverse events). Products include:
- Daypro Caplets 2426

Oxazepam (Nefazodone is highly bound to the plasma protein hence co-administration with another drug that is highly protein bound may cause increased free concentrations of other drug, potentially resulting in adverse events). Products include:
- Serax Capsules 2810
- Serax Tablets 2810

Phenelzine Sulfate (Potential for serious, sometimes fatal, reactions including hyperthermia, rigidity, myoclonus, extreme agitation progressing to delirium and coma; concurrent and/or sequential use is contraindicated). Products include:
- Nardil 1920

Phenylbutazone (Nefazodone is highly bound to the plasma protein hence co-administration with another drug that is highly protein bound may cause increased free concentrations of other drug, potentially resulting in adverse events).
- No products indexed under this heading.

Piroxicam (Nefazodone is highly bound to the plasma protein hence co-administration with another drug that is highly protein bound may cause increased free concentrations of other drug, potentially resulting in adverse events). Products include:
- Feldene Capsules 1965

(▣ Described in PDR For Nonprescription Drugs) (⊙ Described in PDR For Ophthalmology)

Propranolol Hydrochloride (Potential for reduction in C_{max} and AUC of propranolol with no significant change in clinical outcome). Products include:

Inderal 2728
Inderal LA Long Acting Capsules 2730
Inderide Tablets 2732
Inderide LA Long Acting Capsules .. 2734

Selegiline Hydrochloride (Potential for serious, sometimes fatal, reactions including hyperthermia, rigidity, myoclonus, extreme agitation progressing to delirium and coma; concurrent and/or sequential use is contraindicated). Products include:

Eldepryl Tablets 2550

Sulindac (Nefazodone is highly bound to the plasma protein hence co-administration with another drug that is highly protein bound may cause increased free concentrations of other drug, potentially resulting in adverse events). Products include:

Clinoril Tablets 1618

Temazepam (Nefazodone is highly bound to the plasma protein hence co-administration with another drug that is highly protein bound may cause increased free concentrations of other drug, potentially resulting in adverse events). Products include:

Restoril Capsules 2284

Terfenadine (Nefazodone has been shown *in vitro* to be inhibitor of cytochrome P_{450}IIIA$_4$ resulting in the potential for increased plasma concentration of terfenadine leading to QT prolongation and rare cases of serious cardiovascular toxicity; concurrent use is contraindicated). Products include:

Seldane Tablets 1536
Seldane-D Extended-Release Tablets 1538

Tolbutamide (Nefazodone is highly bound to the plasma protein hence co-administration with another drug that is highly protein bound may cause increased free concentrations of other drug, potentially resulting in adverse events).

No products indexed under this heading.

Tolmetin Sodium (Nefazodone is highly bound to the plasma protein hence co-administration with another drug that is highly protein bound may cause increased free concentrations of other drug, potentially resulting in adverse events). Products include:

Tolectin (200, 400 and 600 mg) .. 1581

Tranylcypromine Sulfate (Potential for serious, sometimes fatal, reactions including hyperthermia, rigidity, myoclonus, extreme agitation progressing to delirium and coma; concurrent and/or sequential use is contraindicated). Products include:

Parnate Tablets 2503

Triazolam (Co-administration may increase steady-state peak concentrations, AUC and half-life values; potentiated effects on psychomotor performance tests; reduction in initial dosage of triazolobenzodiazepines is required). Products include:

Halcion Tablets 2611

Trimipramine Maleate (Nefazodone is highly bound to the plasma protein hence co-administration with another drug that is highly protein bound may cause increased free concentrations of other drug, potentially resulting in adverse events). Products include:

Surmontil Capsules 2811

Warfarin Sodium (Nefazodone is highly bound to the plasma protein hence co-administration with another drug that is highly protein bound may cause increased free concentrations of other drug, potentially resulting in adverse events). Products include:

Coumadin 926

Food Interactions

Alcohol (Concomitant use should be avoided).

Food, unspecified (Food delays the absorption of nefazodone and decreases the bioavailability by approximately 20%).

SHADE GEL SPF 30 SUNBLOCK

(Ethylhexyl p-Methoxycinnamate, Oxybenzone, Homosalate) .... ▣ 807
None cited in PDR database.

SHADE LOTION SPF 45 SUNBLOCK

(Ethylhexyl p-Methoxycinnamate, Oxybenzone, 2-Ethylhexyl Salicylate) .... ▣ 807
None cited in PDR database.

SHADE UVAGUARD SPF 15 SUNCREEN LOTION

(Octyl Methoxycinnamate, Avobenzone, Oxybenzone) .... ▣ 808
None cited in PDR database.

SIGTAB TABLETS

(Vitamins with Minerals) .... ▣ 772
None cited in PDR database.

SIGTAB-M TABLETS

(Vitamins with Minerals) .... ▣ 772
None cited in PDR database.

SILVADENE CREAM 1%

(Silver Sulfadiazine) 1540
May interact with:

Cimetidine (An increased incidence of leukopenia has been reported in patients treated concurrently with cimetidine). Products include:

Tagamet Tablets 2516

Cimetidine Hydrochloride (An increased incidence of leukopenia has been reported in patients treated concurrently with cimetidine). Products include:

Tagamet 2516

Proteolytic Enzymes (Concomitant use of topical proteolytic enzymes with silver sulfadiazine may result in inactivation of enzyme by silver). Products include:

Arco-Lase Tablets 512
Bromase 667
Cotazym 1817
Kutrase Capsules 2402
Ku-Zyme Capsules 2402
Ku-Zyme HP Capsules 2402
Panafil Ointment 2246
Panafil-White Ointment 2247
Travase Ointment 1356

SIMILAC TODDLER'S BEST MILK-BASED NUTRITIONAL BEVERAGE

(Nutritional Beverage) .... ▣ 784
None cited in PDR database.

SIMILASAN EYE DROPS #1

(Homeopathic Medications) .... ◉ 317
None cited in PDR database.

SIMILASAN EYE DROPS #2

(Homeopathic Medications) .... ◉ 317
None cited in PDR database.

SINAREST TABLETS

(Acetaminophen, Chlorpheniramine Maleate, Pseudoephedrine Hydrochloride) .... ▣ 648
May interact with central nervous system depressants, antidepressant drugs, antihypertensives, and certain other agents. Compounds in these categories include:

Acebutolol Hydrochloride (Effect not specified). Products include:

Sectral Capsules 2807

Alfentanil Hydrochloride (Concurrent use produces additive effects). Products include:

Alfenta Injection 1286

Alprazolam (Concurrent use produces additive effects). Products include:

Xanax Tablets 2649

Amitriptyline Hydrochloride (Effect not specified). Products include:

Elavil 2838
Endep Tablets 2174
Etrafon 2355
Limbitrol 2180
Triavil Tablets 1757

Amlodipine Besylate (Effect not specified). Products include:

Lotrel Capsules 840
Norvasc Tablets 1940

Amoxapine (Effect not specified). Products include:

Asendin Tablets 1369

Aprobarbital (Concurrent use produces additive effects).

No products indexed under this heading.

Atenolol (Effect not specified). Products include:

Tenoretic Tablets 2845
Tenormin Tablets and I.V. Injection 2847

Benazepril Hydrochloride (Effect not specified). Products include:

Lotensin Tablets 834
Lotensin HCT 837
Lotrel Capsules 840

Bendroflumethiazide (Effect not specified).

No products indexed under this heading.

Betaxolol Hydrochloride (Effect not specified). Products include:

Betoptic Ophthalmic Solution 469
Betoptic S Ophthalmic Suspension 471
Kerlone Tablets 2436

Bisoprolol Fumarate (Effect not specified). Products include:

Zebeta Tablets 1413
Ziac 1415

Buprenorphine (Concurrent use produces additive effects). Products include:

Buprenex Injectable 2006

Bupropion Hydrochloride (Effect not specified). Products include:

Wellbutrin Tablets 1204

Buspirone Hydrochloride (Concurrent use produces additive effects). Products include:

BuSpar 737

Butabarbital (Concurrent use produces additive effects).

No products indexed under this heading.

Butalbital (Concurrent use produces additive effects). Products include:

Esgic-plus Tablets 1013
Fioricet Tablets 2258
Fioricet with Codeine Capsules 2260
Fiorinal Capsules 2261
Fiorinal with Codeine Capsules 2262
Fiorinal Tablets 2261
Phrenilin 785
Sedapap Tablets 50 mg/650 mg .. 1543

Captopril (Effect not specified). Products include:

Capoten 739
Capozide 742

Carteolol Hydrochloride (Effect not specified). Products include:

Cartrol Tablets 410
Ocupress Ophthalmic Solution, 1% Sterile .... ◉ 309

Chlordiazepoxide (Concurrent use produces additive effects). Products include:

Libritabs Tablets 2177
Limbitrol 2180

Chlordiazepoxide Hydrochloride (Concurrent use produces additive effects). Products include:

Librax Capsules 2176
Librium Capsules 2178
Librium Injectable 2179

Chlorothiazide (Effect not specified). Products include:

Aldoclor Tablets 1598
Diupres Tablets 1650
Diuril Oral 1653

Chlorothiazide Sodium (Effect not specified). Products include:

Diuril Sodium Intravenous 1652

Chlorpromazine (Concurrent use produces additive effects). Products include:

Thorazine Suppositories 2523

Chlorprothixene (Concurrent use produces additive effects).

No products indexed under this heading.

Chlorprothixene Hydrochloride (Concurrent use produces additive effects).

No products indexed under this heading.

Chlorthalidone (Effect not specified). Products include:

Combipres Tablets 677
Tenoretic Tablets 2845
Thalitone 1245

Clonidine (Effect not specified). Products include:

Catapres-TTS 675

Clonidine Hydrochloride (Effect not specified). Products include:

Catapres Tablets 674
Combipres Tablets 677

Clorazepate Dipotassium (Concurrent use produces additive effects). Products include:

Tranxene 451

Clozapine (Concurrent use produces additive effects). Products include:

Clozaril Tablets 2252

Codeine Phosphate (Concurrent use produces additive effects). Products include:

Actifed with Codeine Cough Syrup .. 1067
Brontex 1981
Deconsal C Expectorant Syrup 456
Deconsal Pediatric Syrup 457
Dimetane-DC Cough Syrup 2059
Empirin with Codeine Tablets 1093
Fioricet with Codeine Capsules 2260
Fiorinal with Codeine Capsules 2262
Isoclor Expectorant 990
Novahistine DH 2462
Novahistine Expectorant 2463
Nucofed 2051
Phenergan with Codeine 2777
Phenergan VC with Codeine 2781
Robitussin A-C Syrup 2073
Robitussin-DAC Syrup 2074

IMPORTANT NOTE: Always consult each drug listing in the patient's regimen for possible interactions.

Sinarest Interactions Index 948

Ryna ■ 841
Soma Compound w/Codeine Tablets 2676
Tussi-Organidin NR Liquid and S NR Liquid 2677
Tylenol with Codeine 1583

Deserpidine (Effect not specified).
No products indexed under this heading.

Desflurane (Concurrent use produces additive effects). Products include:
Suprane 1813

Desipramine Hydrochloride (Effect not specified). Products include:
Norpramin Tablets 1526

Dezocine (Concurrent use produces additive effects). Products include:
Dalgan Injection 538

Diazepam (Concurrent use produces additive effects). Products include:
Dizac 1809
Valium Injectable 2182
Valium Tablets 2183
Valrelease Capsules 2169

Diazoxide (Effect not specified). Products include:
Hyperstat I.V. Injection 2363
Proglycem 580

Diltiazem Hydrochloride (Effect not specified). Products include:
Cardizem CD Capsules 1506
Cardizem SR Capsules 1510
Cardizem Injectable 1508
Cardizem Tablets 1512
Dilacor XR Extended-release Capsules 2018

Doxazosin Mesylate (Effect not specified). Products include:
Cardura Tablets 2186

Doxepin Hydrochloride (Effect not specified). Products include:
Sinequan 2205
Zonalon Cream 1055

Droperidol (Concurrent use produces additive effects). Products include:
Inapsine Injection 1296

Enalapril Maleate (Effect not specified). Products include:
Vaseretic Tablets 1765
Vasotec Tablets 1771

Enalaprilat (Effect not specified). Products include:
Vasotec I.V. 1768

Enflurane (Concurrent use produces additive effects).
No products indexed under this heading.

Esmolol Hydrochloride (Effect not specified). Products include:
Brevibloc Injection 1808

Estazolam (Concurrent use produces additive effects). Products include:
ProSom Tablets 449

Ethchlorvynol (Concurrent use produces additive effects). Products include:
Placidyl Capsules 448

Ethinamate (Concurrent use produces additive effects).
No products indexed under this heading.

Felodipine (Effect not specified). Products include:
Plendil Extended-Release Tablets 527

Fentanyl (Concurrent use produces additive effects). Products include:
Duragesic Transdermal System 1288

Fentanyl Citrate (Concurrent use produces additive effects). Products include:
Sublimaze Injection 1307

Fluoxetine Hydrochloride (Effect not specified). Products include:
Prozac Pulvules & Liquid, Oral Solution 919

Fluphenazine Decanoate (Concurrent use produces additive effects). Products include:
Prolixin Decanoate 509

Fluphenazine Enanthate (Concurrent use produces additive effects). Products include:
Prolixin Enanthate 509

Fluphenazine Hydrochloride (Concurrent use produces additive effects). Products include:
Prolixin 509

Flurazepam Hydrochloride (Concurrent use produces additive effects). Products include:
Dalmane Capsules 2173

Fosinopril Sodium (Effect not specified). Products include:
Monopril Tablets 757

Furosemide (Effect not specified). Products include:
Lasix Injection, Oral Solution and Tablets 1240

Glutethimide (Concurrent use produces additive effects).
No products indexed under this heading.

Guanabenz Acetate (Effect not specified).
No products indexed under this heading.

Guanethidine Monosulfate (Effect not specified). Products include:
Esimil Tablets 822
Ismelin Tablets 827

Haloperidol (Concurrent use produces additive effects). Products include:
Haldol Injection, Tablets and Concentrate 1575

Haloperidol Decanoate (Concurrent use produces additive effects). Products include:
Haldol Decanoate 1577

Hydralazine Hydrochloride (Effect not specified). Products include:
Apresazide Capsules 808
Apresoline Hydrochloride Tablets 809
Ser-Ap-Es Tablets 849

Hydrochlorothiazide (Effect not specified). Products include:
Aldactazide 2413
Aldoril Tablets 1604
Apresazide Capsules 808
Capozide 742
Dyazide 2479
Esidrix Tablets 821
Esimil Tablets 822
HydroDIURIL Tablets 1674
Hydropres Tablets 1675
Hyzaar Tablets 1677
Inderide Tablets 2732
Inderide LA Long Acting Capsules 2734
Lopressor HCT Tablets 832
Lotensin HCT 837
Maxzide 1380
Moduretic Tablets 1705
Oretic Tablets 443
Prinzide Tablets 1737
Ser-Ap-Es Tablets 849
Timolide Tablets 1748
Vaseretic Tablets 1765
Zestoretic 2850
Ziac 1415

Hydrocodone Bitartrate (Concurrent use produces additive effects). Products include:
Anexsia 5/500 Elixir 1781
Anexia Tablets 1782
Codiclear DH Syrup 791
Deconamine CX Cough and Cold Liquid and Tablets 1319
Duratuss HD Elixir 2565
Hycodan Tablets and Syrup 930
Hycomine Compound Tablets 932
Hycomine 931
Hycotuss Expectorant Syrup 933
Hydrocet Capsules 782
Lorcet 10/650 1018
Lortab 2566
Tussend 1783
Tussend Expectorant 1785
Vicodin Tablets 1356
Vicodin ES Tablets 1357
Vicodin Tuss Expectorant 1358
Zydone Capsules 949

Hydrocodone Polistirex (Concurrent use produces additive effects). Products include:
Tussionex Pennkinetic Extended-Release Suspension 998

Hydroflumethiazide (Effect not specified). Products include:
Diucardin Tablets 2718

Hydroxyzine Hydrochloride (Concurrent use produces additive effects). Products include:
Atarax Tablets & Syrup 2185
Marax Tablets & DF Syrup 2200
Vistaril Intramuscular Solution 2216

Imipramine Hydrochloride (Effect not specified). Products include:
Tofranil Ampuls 854
Tofranil Tablets 856

Imipramine Pamoate (Effect not specified). Products include:
Tofranil-PM Capsules 857

Indapamide (Effect not specified). Products include:
Lozol Tablets 2022

Isocarboxazid (Effect not specified).
No products indexed under this heading.

Isoflurane (Concurrent use produces additive effects).
No products indexed under this heading.

Isradipine (Effect not specified). Products include:
DynaCirc Capsules 2256

Ketamine Hydrochloride (Concurrent use produces additive effects).
No products indexed under this heading.

Labetalol Hydrochloride (Effect not specified). Products include:
Normodyne Injection 2377
Normodyne Tablets 2379
Trandate 1185

Levomethadyl Acetate Hydrochloride (Concurrent use produces additive effects). Products include:
Orlamm 2239

Levorphanol Tartrate (Concurrent use produces additive effects). Products include:
Levo-Dromoran 2129

Lisinopril (Effect not specified). Products include:
Prinivil Tablets 1733
Prinzide Tablets 1737
Zestoretic 2850
Zestril Tablets 2854

Lorazepam (Concurrent use produces additive effects). Products include:
Ativan Injection 2698
Ativan Tablets 2700

Losartan Potassium (Effect not specified). Products include:
Cozaar Tablets 1628
Hyzaar Tablets 1677

Loxapine Hydrochloride (Concurrent use produces additive effects). Products include:
Loxitane 1378

Loxapine Succinate (Concurrent use produces additive effects). Products include:
Loxitane Capsules 1378

Maprotiline Hydrochloride (Effect not specified). Products include:
Ludiomil Tablets 843

Mecamylamine Hydrochloride (Effect not specified). Products include:
Inversine Tablets 1686

Meperidine Hydrochloride (Concurrent use produces additive effects). Products include:
Demerol 2308
Mepergan Injection 2753

Mephobarbital (Concurrent use produces additive effects). Products include:
Mebaral Tablets 2322

Meprobamate (Concurrent use produces additive effects). Products include:
Miltown Tablets 2672
PMB 200 and PMB 400 2783

Mesoridazine Besylate (Concurrent use produces additive effects). Products include:
Serentil 684

Methadone Hydrochloride (Concurrent use produces additive effects). Products include:
Methadone Hydrochloride Oral Concentrate 2233
Methadone Hydrochloride Oral Solution & Tablets 2235

Methohexital Sodium (Concurrent use produces additive effects). Products include:
Brevital Sodium Vials 1429

Methotrimeprazine (Concurrent use produces additive effects). Products include:
Levoprome 1274

Methoxyflurane (Concurrent use produces additive effects).
No products indexed under this heading.

Methyclothiazide (Effect not specified). Products include:
Enduron Tablets 420

Methyldopa (Effect not specified). Products include:
Aldoclor Tablets 1598
Aldomet Oral 1600
Aldoril Tablets 1604

Methyldopate Hydrochloride (Effect not specified). Products include:
Aldomet Ester HCl Injection 1602

Metolazone (Effect not specified). Products include:
Mykrox Tablets 993
Zaroxolyn Tablets 1000

Metoprolol Succinate (Effect not specified). Products include:
Toprol-XL Tablets 565

Metoprolol Tartrate (Effect not specified). Products include:
Lopressor Ampuls 830
Lopressor HCT Tablets 832
Lopressor Tablets 830

Metyrosine (Effect not specified). Products include:
Demser Capsules 1649

Midazolam Hydrochloride (Concurrent use produces additive effects). Products include:
Versed Injection 2170

Minoxidil (Effect not specified). Products include:
Loniten Tablets 2618
Rogaine Topical Solution 2637

Moexipril Hydrochloride (Effect not specified). Products include:
Univasc Tablets 2410

Molindone Hydrochloride (Concurrent use produces additive effects). Products include:
Moban Tablets and Concentrate 1048

Morphine Sulfate (Concurrent use produces additive effects). Products include:
Astramorph/PF Injection, USP (Preservative-Free) 535

(■ Described in PDR For Nonprescription Drugs) (◉ Described in PDR For Ophthalmology)

949 **Interactions Index** **Sine-Aid Maximum Strength**

Duramorph 962
Infumorph 200 and Infumorph 500 Sterile Solutions 965
MS Contin Tablets 1994
MSIR 1997
Oramorph SR (Morphine Sulfate Sustained Release Tablets) 2236
RMS Suppositories 2657
Roxanol 2243

Nadolol (Effect not specified).
No products indexed under this heading.

Nefazodone Hydrochloride (Effect not specified). Products include:
Serzone Tablets 771

Nicardipine Hydrochloride (Effect not specified). Products include:
Cardene Capsules 2095
Cardene I.V. 2709
Cardene SR Capsules 2097

Nifedipine (Effect not specified). Products include:
Adalat Capsules (10 mg and 20 mg) 587
Adalat CC 589
Procardia Capsules 1971
Procardia XL Extended Release Tablets 1972

Nisoldipine (Effect not specified).
No products indexed under this heading.

Nitroglycerin (Effect not specified). Products include:
Deponit NTG Transdermal Delivery System 2397
Nitro-Bid IV 1523
Nitro-Bid Ointment 1524
Nitrodisc 2047
Nitro-Dur (nitroglycerin) Transdermal Infusion System 1326
Nitrolingual Spray 2027
Nitrostat Tablets 1925
Transderm-Nitro Transdermal Therapeutic System 859

Nortriptyline Hydrochloride (Effect not specified). Products include:
Pamelor 2280

Opium Alkaloids (Concurrent use produces additive effects).
No products indexed under this heading.

Oxazepam (Concurrent use produces additive effects). Products include:
Serax Capsules 2810
Serax Tablets 2810

Oxycodone Hydrochloride (Concurrent use produces additive effects). Products include:
Percocet Tablets 938
Percodan Tablets 939
Percodan-Demi Tablets 940
Roxicodone Tablets, Oral Solution & Intensol (Oxycodone) 2244
Tylox Capsules 1584

Paroxetine Hydrochloride (Effect not specified). Products include:
Paxil Tablets 2505

Penbutolol Sulfate (Effect not specified). Products include:
Levatol 2403

Pentobarbital Sodium (Concurrent use produces additive effects). Products include:
Nembutal Sodium Capsules 436
Nembutal Sodium Solution 438
Nembutal Sodium Suppositories 440

Perphenazine (Concurrent use produces additive effects). Products include:
Etrafon 2355
Triavil Tablets 1757
Trilafon 2389

Phenelzine Sulfate (Effect not specified). Products include:
Nardil 1920

Phenobarbital (Concurrent use produces additive effects). Products include:
Arco-Lase Plus Tablets 512
Bellergal-S Tablets 2250
Donnatal 2060
Donnatal Extentabs 2061
Donnatal Tablets 2060
Phenobarbital Elixir and Tablets 1469
Quadrinal Tablets 1350

Phenoxybenzamine Hydrochloride (Effect not specified). Products include:
Dibenzyline Capsules 2476

Phentolamine Mesylate (Effect not specified). Products include:
Regitine 846

Pindolol (Effect not specified). Products include:
Visken Tablets 2299

Polythiazide (Effect not specified). Products include:
Minizide Capsules 1938

Prazepam (Concurrent use produces additive effects).
No products indexed under this heading.

Prazosin Hydrochloride (Effect not specified). Products include:
Minipress Capsules 1937
Minizide Capsules 1938

Prochlorperazine (Concurrent use produces additive effects). Products include:
Compazine 2470

Promethazine Hydrochloride (Concurrent use produces additive effects). Products include:
Mepergan Injection 2753
Phenergan with Codeine 2777
Phenergan with Dextromethorphan 2778
Phenergan Injection 2773
Phenergan Suppositories 2775
Phenergan Syrup 2774
Phenergan Tablets 2775
Phenergan VC 2779
Phenergan VC with Codeine 2781

Propofol (Concurrent use produces additive effects). Products include:
Diprivan Injection 2833

Propoxyphene Hydrochloride (Concurrent use produces additive effects). Products include:
Darvon 1435
Wygesic Tablets 2827

Propoxyphene Napsylate (Concurrent use produces additive effects). Products include:
Darvon-N/Darvocet-N 1433

Propranolol Hydrochloride (Effect not specified). Products include:
Inderal 2728
Inderal LA Long Acting Capsules 2730
Inderide Tablets 2732
Inderide LA Long Acting Capsules .. 2734

Protriptyline Hydrochloride (Effect not specified). Products include:
Vivactil Tablets 1774

Quazepam (Concurrent use produces additive effects). Products include:
Doral Tablets 2664

Quinapril Hydrochloride (Effect not specified). Products include:
Accupril Tablets 1893

Ramipril (Effect not specified). Products include:
Altace Capsules 1232

Rauwolfia Serpentina (Effect not specified).
No products indexed under this heading.

Rescinnamine (Effect not specified).
No products indexed under this heading.

Reserpine (Effect not specified). Products include:
Diupres Tablets 1650
Hydropres Tablets 1675
Ser-Ap-Es Tablets 849

Risperidone (Concurrent use produces additive effects). Products include:
Risperdal 1301

Secobarbital Sodium (Concurrent use produces additive effects). Products include:
Seconal Sodium Pulvules 1474

Sertraline Hydrochloride (Effect not specified). Products include:
Zoloft Tablets 2217

Sodium Nitroprusside (Effect not specified).
No products indexed under this heading.

Sotalol Hydrochloride (Effect not specified). Products include:
Betapace Tablets 641

Spirapril Hydrochloride (Effect not specified).
No products indexed under this heading.

Sufentanil Citrate (Concurrent use produces additive effects). Products include:
Sufenta Injection 1309

Temazepam (Concurrent use produces additive effects). Products include:
Restoril Capsules 2284

Terazosin Hydrochloride (Effect not specified). Products include:
Hytrin Capsules 430

Thiamylal Sodium (Concurrent use produces additive effects).
No products indexed under this heading.

Thioridazine Hydrochloride (Concurrent use produces additive effects). Products include:
Mellaril 2269

Thiothixene (Concurrent use produces additive effects). Products include:
Navane Capsules and Concentrate 2201
Navane Intramuscular 2202

Timolol Maleate (Effect not specified). Products include:
Blocadren Tablets 1614
Timolide Tablets 1748
Timoptic in Ocudose 1753
Timoptic Sterile Ophthalmic Solution 1751
Timoptic-XE 1755

Torsemide (Effect not specified). Products include:
Demadex Tablets and Injection 686

Tranylcypromine Sulfate (Effect not specified). Products include:
Parnate Tablets 2503

Trazodone Hydrochloride (Effect not specified). Products include:
Desyrel and Desyrel Dividose 503

Triazolam (Concurrent use produces additive effects). Products include:
Halcion Tablets 2611

Trifluoperazine Hydrochloride (Concurrent use produces additive effects). Products include:
Stelazine 2514

Trimethaphan Camsylate (Effect not specified). Products include:
Arfonad Ampuls 2080

Trimipramine Maleate (Effect not specified). Products include:
Surmontil Capsules 2811

Venlafaxine Hydrochloride (Effect not specified). Products include:
Effexor 2719

Verapamil Hydrochloride (Effect not specified). Products include:
Calan SR Caplets 2422
Calan Tablets 2419
Isoptin Injectable 1344
Isoptin Oral Tablets 1346
Isoptin SR Tablets 1348
Verelan Capsules 1410
Verelan Capsules 2824

Zolpidem Tartrate (Concurrent use produces additive effects). Products include:
Ambien Tablets 2416

Food Interactions

Alcohol (Concurrent use produces additive effects).

SINAREST EXTRA STRENGTH TABLETS
(Acetaminophen, Chlorpheniramine Maleate, Pseudoephedrine Hydrochloride) 648
See **Sinarest Tablets**

SINAREST NO DROWSINESS TABLETS
(Acetaminophen, Pseudoephedrine Hydrochloride) 648
See **Sinarest Tablets**

SINE-AID IB CAPLETS
(Ibuprofen, Pseudoephedrine Hydrochloride) 1554
May interact with monoamine oxidase inhibitors and certain other agents. Compounds in these categories include:

Furazolidone (Concurrent and/or sequential use is not recommended). Products include:
Furoxone 2046

Isocarboxazid (Concurrent and/or sequential use is not recommended).
No products indexed under this heading.

Phenelzine Sulfate (Concurrent and/or sequential use is not recommended). Products include:
Nardil 1920

Selegiline Hydrochloride (Concurrent and/or sequential use is not recommended). Products include:
Eldepryl Tablets 2550

Tranylcypromine Sulfate (Concurrent and/or sequential use is not recommended). Products include:
Parnate Tablets 2503

Food Interactions

Alcohol (Chronic heavy alcohol abusers, 3 or more drinks per day, may be at increased risk of liver toxicity from acetaminophen use).

SINE-AID MAXIMUM STRENGTH SINUS MEDICATION GELCAPS, CAPLETS AND TABLETS
(Acetaminophen, Pseudoephedrine Hydrochloride) 1554
May interact with monoamine oxidase inhibitors and certain other agents. Compounds in these categories include:

Furazolidone (Concurrent and/or sequential use is contraindicated). Products include:
Furoxone 2046

Isocarboxazid (Concurrent and/or sequential use is contraindicated).
No products indexed under this heading.

Phenelzine Sulfate (Concurrent and/or sequential use is contraindicated). Products include:
Nardil 1920

Selegiline Hydrochloride (Concurrent and/or sequential use is contraindicated). Products include:
Eldepryl Tablets 2550

Tranylcypromine Sulfate (Concurrent and/or sequential use is contraindicated). Products include:
Parnate Tablets 2503

IMPORTANT NOTE: Always consult each drug listing in the patient's regimen for possible interactions.

Sine-Aid Maximum Strength — Interactions Index — 950

Food Interactions

Alcohol (Chronic heavy alcohol abusers, 3 or more drinks per day, may be at increased risk of liver toxicity from acetaminophen use).

SINE-OFF NO DROWSINESS FORMULA CAPLETS

(Acetaminophen, Pseudoephedrine Hydrochloride) .... ◘ 824

May interact with monoamine oxidase inhibitors. Compounds in this category include:

Furazolidone (Concurrent and/or sequential use is not recommended). Products include:
- Furoxone 2046

Isocarboxazid (Concurrent and/or sequential use is not recommended).
- No products indexed under this heading.

Phenelzine Sulfate (Concurrent and/or sequential use is not recommended). Products include:
- Nardil 1920

Selegiline Hydrochloride (Concurrent and/or sequential use is not recommended). Products include:
- Eldepryl Tablets 2550

Tranylcypromine Sulfate (Concurrent and/or sequential use is not recommended). Products include:
- Parnate Tablets 2503

SINE-OFF SINUS MEDICINE

(Aspirin, Chlorpheniramine Maleate, Phenylpropanolamine Hydrochloride) .... ◘ 825

May interact with phenylpropanolamine containing anorectics and certain other agents. Compounds in these categories include:

Phenylpropanolamine Containing Anorectics (Effect not specified).

Food Interactions

Alcohol (Do not use concomitantly).

SINEMET TABLETS

(Carbidopa, Levodopa) 943

May interact with monoamine oxidase inhibitors, antihypertensives, tricyclic antidepressants, phenothiazines, butyrophenones, and certain other agents. Compounds in these categories include:

Acebutolol Hydrochloride (Symptomatic postural hypotension). Products include:
- Sectral Capsules 2807

Amitriptyline Hydrochloride (Potential for rare adverse reactions, including hypertension and dyskinesia). Products include:
- Elavil 2838
- Endep Tablets 2174
- Etrafon 2355
- Limbitrol 2180
- Triavil Tablets 1757

Amlodipine Besylate (Symptomatic postural hypotension). Products include:
- Lotrel Capsules 840
- Norvasc Tablets 1940

Amoxapine (Potential for rare adverse reactions, including hypertension and dyskinesia). Products include:
- Asendin Tablets 1369

Atenolol (Symptomatic postural hypotension). Products include:
- Tenoretic Tablets 2845
- Tenormin Tablets and I.V. Injection 2847

Benazepril Hydrochloride (Symptomatic postural hypotension). Products include:
- Lotensin Tablets 834
- Lotensin HCT 837
- Lotrel Capsules 840

Bendroflumethiazide (Symptomatic postural hypotension).
- No products indexed under this heading.

Betaxolol Hydrochloride (Symptomatic postural hypotension). Products include:
- Betoptic Ophthalmic Solution 469
- Betoptic S Ophthalmic Suspension 471
- Kerlone Tablets 2436

Bisoprolol Fumarate (Symptomatic postural hypotension). Products include:
- Zebeta Tablets 1413
- Ziac 1415

Captopril (Symptomatic postural hypotension). Products include:
- Capoten 739
- Capozide 742

Carteolol Hydrochloride (Symptomatic postural hypotension). Products include:
- Cartrol Tablets 410
- Ocupress Ophthalmic Solution, 1% Sterile .... ⊙ 309

Chlorothiazide (Symptomatic postural hypotension). Products include:
- Aldoclor Tablets 1598
- Diupres Tablets 1650
- Diuril Oral 1653

Chlorothiazide Sodium (Symptomatic postural hypotension). Products include:
- Diuril Sodium Intravenous 1652

Chlorpromazine (Reduced therapeutic effects of levodopa). Products include:
- Thorazine Suppositories 2523

Chlorthalidone (Symptomatic postural hypotension). Products include:
- Combipres Tablets 677
- Tenoretic Tablets 2845
- Thalitone 1245

Clomipramine Hydrochloride (Potential for rare adverse reactions, including hypertension and dyskinesia). Products include:
- Anafranil Capsules 803

Clonidine (Symptomatic postural hypotension). Products include:
- Catapres-TTS 675

Clonidine Hydrochloride (Symptomatic postural hypotension). Products include:
- Catapres Tablets 674
- Combipres Tablets 677

Deserpidine (Symptomatic postural hypotension).
- No products indexed under this heading.

Desipramine Hydrochloride (Potential for rare adverse reactions, including hypertension and dyskinesia). Products include:
- Norpramin Tablets 1526

Diazoxide (Symptomatic postural hypotension). Products include:
- Hyperstat I.V. Injection 2363
- Proglycem 580

Diltiazem Hydrochloride (Symptomatic postural hypotension). Products include:
- Cardizem CD Capsules 1506
- Cardizem SR Capsules 1510
- Cardizem Injectable 1508
- Cardizem Tablets 1512
- Dilacor XR Extended-release Capsules 2018

Doxazosin Mesylate (Symptomatic postural hypotension). Products include:
- Cardura Tablets 2186

Doxepin Hydrochloride (Potential for rare adverse reactions, including hypertension and dyskinesia). Products include:
- Sinequan 2205
- Zonalon Cream 1055

Enalapril Maleate (Symptomatic postural hypotension). Products include:
- Vaseretic Tablets 1765
- Vasotec Tablets 1771

Enalaprilat (Symptomatic postural hypotension). Products include:
- Vasotec I.V. 1768

Esmolol Hydrochloride (Symptomatic postural hypotension). Products include:
- Brevibloc Injection 1808

Felodipine (Symptomatic postural hypotension). Products include:
- Plendil Extended-Release Tablets 527

Fluphenazine Decanoate (Reduced therapeutic effects of levodopa). Products include:
- Prolixin Decanoate 509

Fluphenazine Enanthate (Reduced therapeutic effects of levodopa). Products include:
- Prolixin Enanthate 509

Fluphenazine Hydrochloride (Reduced therapeutic effects of levodopa). Products include:
- Prolixin 509

Fosinopril Sodium (Symptomatic postural hypotension). Products include:
- Monopril Tablets 757

Furazolidone (Contraindication). Products include:
- Furoxone 2046

Furosemide (Symptomatic postural hypotension). Products include:
- Lasix Injection, Oral Solution and Tablets 1240

Guanabenz Acetate (Symptomatic postural hypotension).
- No products indexed under this heading.

Guanethidine Monosulfate (Symptomatic postural hypotension). Products include:
- Esimil Tablets 822
- Ismelin Tablets 827

Haloperidol (Reduced therapeutic effects of levodopa). Products include:
- Haldol Injection, Tablets and Concentrate 1575

Haloperidol Decanoate (Reduced therapeutic effects of levodopa). Products include:
- Haldol Decanoate 1577

Hydralazine Hydrochloride (Symptomatic postural hypotension). Products include:
- Apresazide Capsules 808
- Apresoline Hydrochloride Tablets 809
- Ser-Ap-Es Tablets 849

Hydrochlorothiazide (Symptomatic postural hypotension). Products include:
- Aldactazide 2413
- Aldoril Tablets 1604
- Apresazide Capsules 808
- Capozide 742
- Dyazide 2479
- Esidrix Tablets 821
- Esimil Tablets 822
- HydroDIURIL Tablets 1674
- Hydropres Tablets 1675
- Hyzaar Tablets 1677
- Inderide Tablets 2732
- Inderide LA Long Acting Capsules 2734
- Lopressor HCT Tablets 832
- Lotensin HCT 837
- Maxzide 1380
- Moduretic Tablets 1705
- Oretic Tablets 443
- Prinzide Tablets 1737
- Ser-Ap-Es Tablets 849
- Timolide Tablets 1748
- Vaseretic Tablets 1765
- Zestoretic 2850
- Ziac 1415

Hydroflumethiazide (Symptomatic postural hypotension). Products include:
- Diucardin Tablets 2718

Imipramine Hydrochloride (Potential for rare adverse reactions, including hypertension and dyskinesia). Products include:
- Tofranil Ampuls 854
- Tofranil Tablets 856

Imipramine Pamoate (Potential for rare adverse reactions, including hypertension and dyskinesia). Products include:
- Tofranil-PM Capsules 857

Indapamide (Symptomatic postural hypotension). Products include:
- Lozol Tablets 2022

Isocarboxazid (Contraindication).
- No products indexed under this heading.

Isradipine (Symptomatic postural hypotension). Products include:
- DynaCirc Capsules 2256

Labetalol Hydrochloride (Symptomatic postural hypotension). Products include:
- Normodyne Injection 2377
- Normodyne Tablets 2379
- Trandate 1185

Lisinopril (Symptomatic postural hypotension). Products include:
- Prinivil Tablets 1733
- Prinzide Tablets 1737
- Zestoretic 2850
- Zestril Tablets 2854

Losartan Potassium (Symptomatic postural hypotension). Products include:
- Cozaar Tablets 1628
- Hyzaar Tablets 1677

Maprotiline Hydrochloride (Potential for rare adverse reactions, including hypertension and dyskinesia). Products include:
- Ludiomil Tablets 843

Mecamylamine Hydrochloride (Symptomatic postural hypotension). Products include:
- Inversine Tablets 1686

Mesoridazine Besylate (Reduced therapeutic effects of levodopa). Products include:
- Serentil 684

Methotrimeprazine (Reduced therapeutic effects of levodopa). Products include:
- Levoprome 1274

Methyclothiazide (Symptomatic postural hypotension). Products include:
- Enduron Tablets 420

Methyldopa (Symptomatic postural hypotension). Products include:
- Aldoclor Tablets 1598
- Aldomet Oral 1600
- Aldoril Tablets 1604

Methyldopate Hydrochloride (Symptomatic postural hypotension). Products include:
- Aldomet Ester HCl Injection 1602

Metolazone (Symptomatic postural hypotension). Products include:
- Mykrox Tablets 993
- Zaroxolyn Tablets 1000

Metoprolol Succinate (Symptomatic postural hypotension). Products include:
- Toprol-XL Tablets 565

(◘ Described in PDR For Nonprescription Drugs) (⊙ Described in PDR For Ophthalmology)

Metoprolol Tartrate (Symptomatic postural hypotension). Products include:
Lopressor Ampuls ... 830
Lopressor HCT Tablets ... 832
Lopressor Tablets ... 830
Metyrosine (Symptomatic postural hypotension). Products include:
Demser Capsules ... 1649
Minoxidil (Symptomatic postural hypotension). Products include:
Loniten Tablets ... 2618
Rogaine Topical Solution ... 2637
Moexipril Hydrochloride (Symptomatic postural hypotension). Products include:
Univasc Tablets ... 2410
Nadolol (Symptomatic postural hypotension).
No products indexed under this heading.
Nicardipine Hydrochloride (Symptomatic postural hypotension). Products include:
Cardene Capsules ... 2095
Cardene I.V. ... 2709
Cardene SR Capsules ... 2097
Nifedipine (Symptomatic postural hypotension). Products include:
Adalat Capsules (10 mg and 20 mg) ... 587
Adalat CC ... 589
Procardia Capsules ... 1971
Procardia XL Extended Release Tablets ... 1972
Nisoldipine (Symptomatic postural hypotension).
No products indexed under this heading.
Nitroglycerin (Symptomatic postural hypotension). Products include:
Deponit NTG Transdermal Delivery System ... 2397
Nitro-Bid IV ... 1523
Nitro-Bid Ointment ... 1524
Nitrodisc ... 2047
Nitro-Dur (nitroglycerin) Transdermal Infusion System ... 1326
Nitrolingual Spray ... 2027
Nitrostat Tablets ... 1925
Transderm-Nitro Transdermal Therapeutic System ... 859
Nortriptyline Hydrochloride (Potential for rare adverse reactions, including hypertension and dyskinesia). Products include:
Pamelor ... 2280
Papaverine Hydrochloride (Beneficial effects of levodopa reversed in Parkinson's Disease). Products include:
Papaverine Hydrochloride Vials and Ampoules ... 1468
Penbutolol Sulfate (Symptomatic postural hypotension). Products include:
Levatol ... 2403
Perphenazine (Reduced therapeutic effects of levodopa). Products include:
Etrafon ... 2355
Triavil Tablets ... 1757
Trilafon ... 2389
Phenelzine Sulfate (Contraindication). Products include:
Nardil ... 1920
Phenoxybenzamine Hydrochloride (Symptomatic postural hypotension). Products include:
Dibenzyline Capsules ... 2476
Phentolamine Mesylate (Symptomatic postural hypotension). Products include:
Regitine ... 846
Phenytoin (Beneficial effects of levodopa reversed in Parkinson's Disease). Products include:
Dilantin Infatabs ... 1908
Dilantin-125 Suspension ... 1911
Phenytoin Sodium (Beneficial effects of levodopa reversed in Parkinson's Disease). Products include:
Dilantin Kapseals ... 1906
Dilantin Parenteral ... 1910
Pindolol (Symptomatic postural hypotension). Products include:
Visken Tablets ... 2299
Polythiazide (Symptomatic postural hypotension). Products include:
Minizide Capsules ... 1938
Prazosin Hydrochloride (Symptomatic postural hypotension). Products include:
Minipress Capsules ... 1937
Minizide Capsules ... 1938
Prochlorperazine (Reduced therapeutic effects of levodopa). Products include:
Compazine ... 2470
Promethazine Hydrochloride (Reduced therapeutic effects of levodopa). Products include:
Mepergan Injection ... 2753
Phenergan with Codeine ... 2777
Phenergan with Dextromethorphan 2778
Phenergan Injection ... 2773
Phenergan Suppositories ... 2775
Phenergan Syrup ... 2774
Phenergan Tablets ... 2775
Phenergan VC ... 2779
Phenergan VC with Codeine ... 2781
Propranolol Hydrochloride (Symptomatic postural hypotension). Products include:
Inderal ... 2728
Inderal LA Long Acting Capsules ... 2730
Inderide Tablets ... 2732
Inderide LA Long Acting Capsules .. 2734
Protriptyline Hydrochloride (Potential for rare adverse reactions, including hypertension and dyskinesia). Products include:
Vivactil Tablets ... 1774
Quinapril Hydrochloride (Symptomatic postural hypotension). Products include:
Accupril Tablets ... 1893
Ramipril (Symptomatic postural hypotension). Products include:
Altace Capsules ... 1232
Rauwolfia Serpentina (Symptomatic postural hypotension).
No products indexed under this heading.
Rescinnamine (Symptomatic postural hypotension).
No products indexed under this heading.
Reserpine (Symptomatic postural hypotension). Products include:
Diupres Tablets ... 1650
Hydropres Tablets ... 1675
Ser-Ap-Es Tablets ... 849
Sodium Nitroprusside (Symptomatic postural hypotension).
No products indexed under this heading.
Sotalol Hydrochloride (Symptomatic postural hypotension). Products include:
Betapace Tablets ... 641
Spirapril Hydrochloride (Symptomatic postural hypotension).
No products indexed under this heading.
Terazosin Hydrochloride (Symptomatic postural hypotension). Products include:
Hytrin Capsules ... 430
Thioridazine Hydrochloride (Reduced therapeutic effects of levodopa). Products include:
Mellaril ... 2269
Timolol Maleate (Symptomatic postural hypotension). Products include:
Blocadren Tablets ... 1614
Timolide Tablets ... 1748
Timoptic in Ocudose ... 1753
Timoptic Sterile Ophthalmic Solution ... 1751
Timoptic-XE ... 1755
Torsemide (Symptomatic postural hypotension). Products include:
Demadex Tablets and Injection ... 686
Tranylcypromine Sulfate (Contraindication). Products include:
Parnate Tablets ... 2503
Trifluoperazine Hydrochloride (Reduced therapeutic effects of levodopa). Products include:
Stelazine ... 2514
Trimethaphan Camsylate (Symptomatic postural hypotension). Products include:
Arfonad Ampuls ... 2080
Trimipramine Maleate (Potential for rare adverse reactions, including hypertension and dyskinesia). Products include:
Surmontil Capsules ... 2811
Verapamil Hydrochloride (Symptomatic postural hypotension). Products include:
Calan SR Caplets ... 2422
Calan Tablets ... 2419
Isoptin Injectable ... 1344
Isoptin Oral Tablets ... 1346
Isoptin SR Tablets ... 1348
Verelan Capsules ... 1410
Verelan Capsules ... 2824

Food Interactions

Diet high in protein (Levodopa competes with certain amino acids, the absorption of levodopa may be impaired in some patients on a high protein diet).

SINEMET CR TABLETS

(Carbidopa, Levodopa) ... 944
May interact with antihypertensives, monoamine oxidase inhibitors, tricyclic antidepressants, phenothiazines, butyrophenones, and certain other agents. Compounds in these categories include:
Acebutolol Hydrochloride (Potential for postural hypertension). Products include:
Sectral Capsules ... 2807
Amitriptyline Hydrochloride (Potential for hypertension and dyskinesia). Products include:
Elavil ... 2838
Endep Tablets ... 2174
Etrafon ... 2355
Limbitrol ... 2180
Triavil Tablets ... 1757
Amlodipine Besylate (Potential for postural hypertension). Products include:
Lotrel Capsules ... 840
Norvasc Tablets ... 1940
Amoxapine (Potential for hypertension and dyskinesia). Products include:
Asendin Tablets ... 1369
Atenolol (Potential for postural hypertension). Products include:
Tenoretic Tablets ... 2845
Tenormin Tablets and I.V. Injection 2847
Benazepril Hydrochloride (Potential for postural hypertension). Products include:
Lotensin Tablets ... 834
Lotensin HCT ... 837
Lotrel Capsules ... 840
Bendroflumethiazide (Potential for postural hypertension).
No products indexed under this heading.
Betaxolol Hydrochloride (Potential for postural hypertension). Products include:
Betoptic Ophthalmic Solution ... 469
Betoptic S Ophthalmic Suspension 471
Kerlone Tablets ... 2436
Bisoprolol Fumarate (Potential for postural hypertension). Products include:
Zebeta Tablets ... 1413
Ziac ... 1415
Captopril (Potential for postural hypertension). Products include:
Capoten ... 739
Capozide ... 742
Carteolol Hydrochloride (Potential for postural hypertension). Products include:
Cartrol Tablets ... 410
Ocupress Ophthalmic Solution, 1% Sterile ... ⊙ 309
Chlorothiazide (Potential for postural hypertension). Products include:
Aldoclor Tablets ... 1598
Diupres Tablets ... 1650
Diuril Oral ... 1653
Chlorothiazide Sodium (Potential for postural hypertension). Products include:
Diuril Sodium intravenous ... 1652
Chlorpromazine (Reduces the therapeutic effects). Products include:
Thorazine Suppositories ... 2523
Chlorthalidone (Potential for postural hypertension). Products include:
Combipres Tablets ... 677
Tenoretic Tablets ... 2845
Thalitone ... 1245
Clomipramine Hydrochloride (Potential for hypertension and dyskinesia). Products include:
Anafranil Capsules ... 803
Clonidine (Potential for postural hypertension). Products include:
Catapres-TTS ... 675
Clonidine Hydrochloride (Potential for postural hypertension). Products include:
Catapres Tablets ... 674
Combipres Tablets ... 677
Deserpidine (Potential for postural hypertension).
No products indexed under this heading.
Desipramine Hydrochloride (Potential for hypertension and dyskinesia). Products include:
Norpramin Tablets ... 1526
Diazoxide (Potential for postural hypertension). Products include:
Hyperstat I.V. Injection ... 2363
Proglycem ... 580
Diltiazem Hydrochloride (Potential for postural hypertension). Products include:
Cardizem CD Capsules ... 1506
Cardizem SR Capsules ... 1510
Cardizem Injectable ... 1508
Cardizem Tablets ... 1512
Dilacor XR Extended-release Capsules ... 2018
Doxazosin Mesylate (Potential for postural hypertension). Products include:
Cardura Tablets ... 2186
Doxepin Hydrochloride (Potential for hypertension and dyskinesia). Products include:
Sinequan ... 2205
Zonalon Cream ... 1055
Enalapril Maleate (Potential for postural hypertension). Products include:
Vaseretic Tablets ... 1765
Vasotec Tablets ... 1771
Enalaprilat (Potential for postural hypertension). Products include:
Vasotec I.V. ... 1768
Esmolol Hydrochloride (Potential for postural hypertension). Products include:
Brevibloc Injection ... 1808

IMPORTANT NOTE: Always consult each drug listing in the patient's regimen for possible interactions.

Sinemet CR Interactions Index 952

Felodipine (Potential for postural hypertension). Products include:
- Plendil Extended-Release Tablets 527

Fluphenazine Decanoate (Reduces the therapeutic effects). Products include:
- Prolixin Decanoate 509

Fluphenazine Enanthate (Reduces the therapeutic effects). Products include:
- Prolixin Enanthate 509

Fluphenazine Hydrochloride (Reduces the therapeutic effects). Products include:
- Prolixin 509

Fosinopril Sodium (Potential for postural hypertension). Products include:
- Monopril Tablets 757

Furazolidone (Concurrent administration is contraindicated). Products include:
- Furoxone 2046

Furosemide (Potential for postural hypertension). Products include:
- Lasix Injection, Oral Solution and Tablets 1240

Guanabenz Acetate (Potential for postural hypertension).
- No products indexed under this heading.

Guanethidine Monosulfate (Potential for postural hypertension). Products include:
- Esimil Tablets 822
- Ismelin Tablets 827

Haloperidol (Reduces the therapeutic effects). Products include:
- Haldol Injection, Tablets and Concentrate 1575

Haloperidol Decanoate (Reduces the therapeutic effects). Products include:
- Haldol Decanoate 1577

Hydralazine Hydrochloride (Potential for postural hypertension). Products include:
- Apresazide Capsules 808
- Apresoline Hydrochloride Tablets 809
- Ser-Ap-Es Tablets 849

Hydrochlorothiazide (Potential for postural hypertension). Products include:
- Aldactazide 2413
- Aldoril Tablets 1604
- Apresazide Capsules 808
- Capozide 742
- Dyazide 2479
- Esidrix Tablets 821
- Esimil Tablets 822
- HydroDIURIL Tablets 1674
- Hydropres Tablets 1675
- Hyzaar Tablets 1677
- Inderide Tablets 2732
- Inderide LA Long Acting Capsules 2734
- Lopressor HCT Tablets 832
- Lotensin HCT 837
- Maxzide 1380
- Moduretic Tablets 1705
- Oretic Tablets 443
- Prinzide Tablets 1737
- Ser-Ap-Es Tablets 849
- Timolide Tablets 1748
- Vaseretic Tablets 1765
- Zestoretic 2850
- Ziac 1415

Hydroflumethiazide (Potential for postural hypertension). Products include:
- Diucardin Tablets 2718

Imipramine Hydrochloride (Potential for hypertension and dyskinesia). Products include:
- Tofranil Ampuls 854
- Tofranil Tablets 856

Imipramine Pamoate (Potential for hypertension and dyskinesia). Products include:
- Tofranil-PM Capsules 857

Indapamide (Potential for postural hypertension). Products include:
- Lozol Tablets 2022

Isocarboxazid (Concurrent administration is contraindicated).
- No products indexed under this heading.

Isradipine (Potential for postural hypertension). Products include:
- DynaCirc Capsules 2256

Labetalol Hydrochloride (Potential for postural hypertension). Products include:
- Normodyne Injection 2377
- Normodyne Tablets 2379
- Trandate 1185

Lisinopril (Potential for postural hypertension). Products include:
- Prinivil Tablets 1733
- Prinzide Tablets 1737
- Zestoretic 2850
- Zestril Tablets 2854

Losartan Potassium (Potential for postural hypertension). Products include:
- Cozaar Tablets 1628
- Hyzaar Tablets 1677

Maprotiline Hydrochloride (Potential for hypertension and dyskinesia). Products include:
- Ludiomil Tablets 843

Mecamylamine Hydrochloride (Potential for postural hypertension). Products include:
- Inversine Tablets 1686

Mesoridazine Besylate (Reduces the therapeutic effects). Products include:
- Serentil 684

Methotrimeprazine (Reduces the therapeutic effects). Products include:
- Levoprome 1274

Methyclothiazide (Potential for postural hypertension). Products include:
- Enduron Tablets 420

Methyldopa (Potential for postural hypertension). Products include:
- Aldoclor Tablets 1598
- Aldomet Oral 1600
- Aldoril Tablets 1604

Methyldopate Hydrochloride (Potential for postural hypertension). Products include:
- Aldomet Ester HCl Injection 1602

Metolazone (Potential for postural hypertension). Products include:
- Mykrox Tablets 993
- Zaroxolyn Tablets 1000

Metoprolol Succinate (Potential for postural hypertension). Products include:
- Toprol-XL Tablets 565

Metoprolol Tartrate (Potential for postural hypertension). Products include:
- Lopressor Ampuls 830
- Lopressor HCT Tablets 832
- Lopressor Tablets 830

Metyrosine (Potential for postural hypertension). Products include:
- Demser Capsules 1649

Minoxidil (Potential for postural hypertension). Products include:
- Loniten Tablets 2618
- Rogaine Topical Solution 2637

Moexipril Hydrochloride (Potential for postural hypertension). Products include:
- Univasc Tablets 2410

Nadolol (Potential for postural hypertension).
- No products indexed under this heading.

Nicardipine Hydrochloride (Potential for postural hypertension). Products include:
- Cardene Capsules 2095
- Cardene I.V. 2709
- Cardene SR Capsules 2097

Nifedipine (Potential for postural hypertension). Products include:
- Adalat Capsules (10 mg and 20 mg) 587
- Adalat CC 589
- Procardia Capsules 1971
- Procardia XL Extended Release Tablets 1972

Nisoldipine (Potential for postural hypertension).
- No products indexed under this heading.

Nitroglycerin (Potential for postural hypertension). Products include:
- Deponit NTG Transdermal Delivery System 2397
- Nitro-Bid IV 1523
- Nitro-Bid Ointment 1524
- Nitrodisc 2047
- Nitro-Dur (nitroglycerin) Transdermal Infusion System 1326
- Nitrolingual Spray 2027
- Nitrostat Tablets 1925
- Transderm-Nitro Transdermal Therapeutic System 859

Nortriptyline Hydrochloride (Potential for hypertension and dyskinesia). Products include:
- Pamelor 2280

Papaverine Hydrochloride (Reverses beneficial effects of levodopa). Products include:
- Papaverine Hydrochloride Vials and Ampoules 1468

Penbutolol Sulfate (Potential for postural hypertension). Products include:
- Levatol 2403

Perphenazine (Reduces the therapeutic effects). Products include:
- Etrafon 2355
- Triavil Tablets 1757
- Trilafon 2389

Phenelzine Sulfate (Concurrent administration is contraindicated). Products include:
- Nardil 1920

Phenoxybenzamine Hydrochloride (Potential for postural hypertension). Products include:
- Dibenzyline Capsules 2476

Phentolamine Mesylate (Potential for postural hypertension). Products include:
- Regitine 846

Phenytoin (Reverses beneficial effects of levodopa). Products include:
- Dilantin Infatabs 1908
- Dilantin-125 Suspension 1911

Phenytoin Sodium (Reverses beneficial effects of levodopa). Products include:
- Dilantin Kapseals 1906
- Dilantin Parenteral 1910

Pindolol (Potential for postural hypertension). Products include:
- Visken Tablets 2299

Polythiazide (Potential for postural hypertension). Products include:
- Minizide Capsules 1938

Prazosin Hydrochloride (Potential for postural hypertension). Products include:
- Minipress Capsules 1937
- Minizide Capsules 1938

Prochlorperazine (Reduces the therapeutic effects). Products include:
- Compazine 2470

Promethazine Hydrochloride (Reduces the therapeutic effects). Products include:
- Mepergan Injection 2753
- Phenergan with Codeine 2777
- Phenergan with Dextromethorphan 2778
- Phenergan Injection 2773
- Phenergan Suppositories 2775
- Phenergan Syrup 2774
- Phenergan Tablets 2775
- Phenergan VC 2779
- Phenergan VC with Codeine 2781

Propranolol Hydrochloride (Potential for postural hypertension). Products include:
- Inderal 2728
- Inderal LA Long Acting Capsules 2730
- Inderide Tablets 2732
- Inderide LA Long Acting Capsules 2734

Protriptyline Hydrochloride (Potential for hypertension and dyskinesia). Products include:
- Vivactil Tablets 1774

Quinapril Hydrochloride (Potential for postural hypertension). Products include:
- Accupril Tablets 1893

Ramipril (Potential for postural hypertension). Products include:
- Altace Capsules 1232

Rauwolfia Serpentina (Potential for postural hypertension).
- No products indexed under this heading.

Rescinnamine (Potential for postural hypertension).
- No products indexed under this heading.

Reserpine (Potential for postural hypertension). Products include:
- Diupres Tablets 1650
- Hydropres Tablets 1675
- Ser-Ap-Es Tablets 849

Sodium Nitroprusside (Potential for postural hypertension).
- No products indexed under this heading.

Sotalol Hydrochloride (Potential for postural hypertension). Products include:
- Betapace Tablets 641

Spirapril Hydrochloride (Potential for postural hypertension).
- No products indexed under this heading.

Terazosin Hydrochloride (Potential for postural hypertension). Products include:
- Hytrin Capsules 430

Thioridazine Hydrochloride (Reduces the therapeutic effects). Products include:
- Mellaril 2269

Timolol Maleate (Potential for postural hypertension). Products include:
- Blocadren Tablets 1614
- Timolide Tablets 1748
- Timoptic in Ocudose 1753
- Timoptic Sterile Ophthalmic Solution 1751
- Timoptic-XE 1755

Torsemide (Potential for postural hypertension). Products include:
- Demadex Tablets and Injection 686

Tranylcypromine Sulfate (Concurrent administration is contraindicated). Products include:
- Parnate Tablets 2503

Trifluoperazine Hydrochloride (Reduces the therapeutic effects). Products include:
- Stelazine 2514

Trimethaphan Camsylate (Potential for postural hypertension). Products include:
- Arfonad Ampuls 2080

Trimipramine Maleate (Potential for hypertension and dyskinesia). Products include:
- Surmontil Capsules 2811

(▭ Described in PDR For Nonprescription Drugs) (⊙ Described in PDR For Ophthalmology)

953 **Interactions Index** **Sinequan**

Verapamil Hydrochloride (Potential for postural hypertension). Products include:

Calan SR Caplets 2422
Calan Tablets 2419
Isoptin Injectable 1344
Isoptin Oral Tablets 1346
Isoptin SR Tablets 1348
Verelan Capsules 1410
Verelan Capsules 2824

Food Interactions

Food, unspecified (Increases the extent of availability and peak concentrations of levodopa).

SINEQUAN CAPSULES

(Doxepin Hydrochloride) 2205

May interact with monoamine oxidase inhibitors, drugs that inhibit cytochrome p450iid6, antidepressant drugs, phenothiazines, selective serotonin reuptake inhibitors, and certain other agents. Compounds in these categories include:

Amitriptyline Hydrochloride (Concurrent use with drugs that are substrate for cytochrome $P_{450}IID_6$ may make normal metabolizer resemble poor metabolizer leading to higher than expected plasma concentrations of TCA with resultant toxicity). Products include:

Elavil 2838
Endep Tablets 2174
Etrafon 2355
Limbitrol 2180
Triavil Tablets 1757

Amoxapine (Concurrent use with drugs that are substrate for cytochrome $P_{450}IID_6$ may make normal metabolizer resemble poor metabolizer leading to higher than expected plasma concentrations of TCA with resultant toxicity). Products include:

Asendin Tablets 1369

Bupropion Hydrochloride (Concurrent use with drugs that are substrate for cytochrome $P_{450}IID_6$ may make normal metabolizer resemble poor metabolizer leading to higher than expected plasma concentrations of TCA with resultant toxicity). Products include:

Wellbutrin Tablets 1204

Chlorpromazine (Concurrent use with drugs that are substrate for cytochrome $P_{450}IID_6$ may make normal metabolizer resemble poor metabolizer leading to higher than expected plasma concentrations of TCA with resultant toxicity). Products include:

Thorazine Suppositories 2523

Chlorpromazine Hydrochloride (Concurrent use with drugs that are substrate for cytochrome $P_{450}IID_6$ may make normal metabolizer resemble poor metabolizer leading to higher than expected plasma concentrations of TCA with resultant toxicity). Products include:

Thorazine 2523

Cimetidine (Produces clinically significant fluctuations in steady-state serum concentrations of various tricyclic antidepressants resulting in frequency and severity of side effects, particularly anticholinergic). Products include:

Tagamet Tablets 2516

Cimetidine Hydrochloride (Produces clinically significant fluctuations in steady-state serum concentrations of various tricyclic antidepressants resulting in frequency and severity of side effects, particularly anticholinergic). Products include:

Tagamet 2516

Desipramine Hydrochloride (Concurrent use with drugs that are substrate for cytochrome $P_{450}IID_6$ may make normal metabolizer resemble poor metabolizer leading to higher than expected plasma concentrations of TCA with resultant toxicity). Products include:

Norpramin Tablets 1526

Flecainide Acetate (Concurrent use with drugs that are substrate for cytochrome $P_{450}IID_6$ may make normal metabolizer resemble poor metabolizer leading to higher than expected plasma concentrations of TCA with resultant toxicity). Products include:

Tambocor Tablets 1497

Fluoxetine Hydrochloride (Concurrent use with drugs that are substrate for cytochrome $P_{450}IID_6$ may make normal metabolizer resemble poor metabolizer leading to higher than expected plasma concentrations of TCA with resultant toxicity; due to variation in the extent of inhibition of $P_{450}IID_6$ and long half-life of the parent (fluoxetine) and active metabolite sufficient time must elapse, at least 5 weeks before switching to TCA). Products include:

Prozac Pulvules & Liquid, Oral Solution 919

Fluphenazine Decanoate (Concurrent use with drugs that are substrate for cytochrome $P_{450}IID_6$ may make normal metabolizer resemble poor metabolizer leading to higher than expected plasma concentrations of TCA with resultant toxicity). Products include:

Prolixin Decanoate 509

Fluphenazine Enanthate (Concurrent use with drugs that are substrate for cytochrome $P_{450}IID_6$ may make normal metabolizer resemble poor metabolizer leading to higher than expected plasma concentrations of TCA with resultant toxicity). Products include:

Prolixin Enanthate 509

Fluphenazine Hydrochloride (Concurrent use with drugs that are substrate for cytochrome $P_{450}IID_6$ may make normal metabolizer resemble poor metabolizer leading to higher than expected plasma concentrations of TCA with resultant toxicity). Products include:

Prolixin 509

Fluvoxamine Maleate (Concurrent use with drugs that are substrate for cytochrome $P_{450}IID_6$ may make normal metabolizer resemble poor metabolizer leading to higher than expected plasma concentrations of TCA with resultant toxicity; due to variation in the extent of inhibition of $P_{450}IID_6$ caution is indicated if co-administered). Products include:

Luvox Tablets 2544

Furazolidone (Concurrent use is not recommended; potential for serious adverse effects). Products include:

Furoxone 2046

Guanethidine Monosulfate (Antihypertensive effect blocked by doxepin at dosage above 150 mg per day). Products include:

Esimil Tablets 822
Ismelin Tablets 827

Imipramine Hydrochloride (Concurrent use with drugs that are substrate for cytochrome $P_{450}IID_6$ may make normal metabolizer resemble poor metabolizer leading to higher than expected plasma concentrations of TCA with resultant toxicity). Products include:

Tofranil Ampuls 854
Tofranil Tablets 856

Imipramine Pamoate (Concurrent use with drugs that are substrate for cytochrome $P_{450}IID_6$ may make normal metabolizer resemble poor metabolizer leading to higher than expected plasma concentrations of TCA with resultant toxicity). Products include:

Tofranil-PM Capsules 857

Isocarboxazid (Concurrent use is not recommended; potential for serious adverse effects).

No products indexed under this heading.

Maprotiline Hydrochloride (Concurrent use with drugs that are substrate for cytochrome $P_{450}IID_6$ may make normal metabolizer resemble poor metabolizer leading to higher than expected plasma concentrations of TCA with resultant toxicity). Products include:

Ludiomil Tablets 843

Mesoridazine Besylate (Concurrent use with drugs that are substrate for cytochrome $P_{450}IID_6$ may make normal metabolizer resemble poor metabolizer leading to higher than expected plasma concentrations of TCA with resultant toxicity). Products include:

Serentil 684

Methotrimeprazine (Concurrent use with drugs that are substrate for cytochrome $P_{450}IID_6$ may make normal metabolizer resemble poor metabolizer leading to higher than expected plasma concentrations of TCA with resultant toxicity). Products include:

Levoprome 1274

Nefazodone Hydrochloride (Concurrent use with drugs that are substrate for cytochrome $P_{450}IID_6$ may make normal metabolizer resemble poor metabolizer leading to higher than expected plasma concentrations of TCA with resultant toxicity). Products include:

Serzone Tablets 771

Nortriptyline Hydrochloride (Concurrent use with drugs that are substrate for cytochrome $P_{450}IID_6$ may make normal metabolizer resemble poor metabolizer leading to higher than expected plasma concentrations of TCA with resultant toxicity). Products include:

Pamelor 2280

Paroxetine Hydrochloride (Concurrent use with drugs that are substrate for cytochrome $P_{450}IID_6$ may make normal metabolizer resemble poor metabolizer leading to higher than expected plasma concentrations of TCA with resultant toxicity; due to variation in the extent of inhibition of $P_{450}IID_6$ caution is indicated if co-administered). Products include:

Paxil Tablets 2505

Perphenazine (Concurrent use with drugs that are substrate for cytochrome $P_{450}IID_6$ may make normal metabolizer resemble poor metabolizer leading to higher than expected plasma concentrations of TCA with resultant toxicity). Products include:

Etrafon 2355
Triavil Tablets 1757
Trilafon 2389

Phenelzine Sulfate (Concurrent use is not recommended; potential for serious adverse effects). Products include:

Nardil 1920

Prochlorperazine (Concurrent use with drugs that are substrate for cytochrome $P_{450}IID_6$ may make normal metabolizer resemble poor metabolizer leading to higher than expected plasma concentrations of TCA with resultant toxicity). Products include:

Compazine 2470

Promethazine Hydrochloride (Concurrent use with drugs that are substrate for cytochrome $P_{450}IID_6$ may make normal metabolizer resemble poor metabolizer leading to higher than expected plasma concentrations of TCA with resultant toxicity). Products include:

Mepergan Injection 2753
Phenergan with Codeine 2777
Phenergan with Dextromethorphan 2778
Phenergan Injection 2773
Phenergan Suppositories 2775
Phenergan Syrup 2774
Phenergan Tablets 2775
Phenergan VC 2779
Phenergan VC with Codeine 2781

Propafenone Hydrochloride (Concurrent use with drugs that are substrate for cytochrome $P_{450}IID_6$ may make normal metabolizer resemble poor metabolizer leading to higher than expected plasma concentrations of TCA with resultant toxicity). Products include:

Rythmol Tablets–150mg, 225mg, 300mg 1352

Protriptyline Hydrochloride (Concurrent use with drugs that are substrate for cytochrome $P_{450}IID_6$ may make normal metabolizer resemble poor metabolizer leading to higher than expected plasma concentrations of TCA with resultant toxicity). Products include:

Vivactil Tablets 1774

Quinidine Gluconate (Concurrent use with drugs that inhibit cytochrome $P_{450}IID_6$ may make normal metabolizer resemble poor metabolizer leading to higher than expected plasma concentrations of TCA with resultant toxicity). Products include:

Quinaglute Dura-Tabs Tablets 649

Quinidine Polygalacturonate (Concurrent use with drugs that inhibit cytochrome $P_{450}IID_6$ may make normal metabolizer resemble poor metabolizer leading to higher than expected plasma concentrations of TCA with resultant toxicity).

No products indexed under this heading.

Quinidine Sulfate (Concurrent use with drugs that inhibit cytochrome $P_{450}IID_6$ may make normal metabolizer resemble poor metabolizer leading to higher than expected plasma concentrations of TCA with resultant toxicity). Products include:

Quinidex Extentabs 2067

IMPORTANT NOTE: Always consult each drug listing in the patient's regimen for possible interactions.

Selegiline Hydrochloride (Concurrent use is not recommended; potential for serious adverse effects). Products include:
- Eldepryl Tablets ... 2550

Sertraline Hydrochloride (Concurrent use with drugs that are substrate for cytochrome $P_{450}IID_6$ may make normal metabolizer resemble poor metabolizer leading to higher than expected plasma concentrations of TCA with resultant toxicity; due to variation in the extent of inhibition of $P_{450}IID_6$ caution is indicated if co-administered sufficient time must elapse). Products include:
- Zoloft Tablets ... 2217

Thioridazine Hydrochloride (Concurrent use with drugs that are substrate for cytochrome $P_{450}IID_6$ may make normal metabolizer resemble poor metabolizer leading to higher than expected plasma concentrations of TCA with resultant toxicity). Products include:
- Mellaril ... 2269

Tolazamide (A case of severe hypoglycemia has been reported in a type II diabetic patient maintained on tolazamide (1 gm/day) 11 days after the addition of doxepin (75 mg/day)).
- No products indexed under this heading.

Tranylcypromine Sulfate (Concurrent use is not recommended; potential for serious adverse effects). Products include:
- Parnate Tablets ... 2503

Trazodone Hydrochloride (Concurrent use with drugs that are substrate for cytochrome $P_{450}IID_6$ may make normal metabolizer resemble poor metabolizer leading to higher than expected plasma concentrations of TCA with resultant toxicity). Products include:
- Desyrel and Desyrel Dividose ... 503

Trifluoperazine Hydrochloride (Concurrent use with drugs that are substrate for cytochrome $P_{450}IID_6$ may make normal metabolizer resemble poor metabolizer leading to higher than expected plasma concentrations of TCA with resultant toxicity). Products include:
- Stelazine ... 2514

Trimipramine Maleate (Concurrent use with drugs that are substrate for cytochrome $P_{450}IID_6$ may make normal metabolizer resemble poor metabolizer leading to higher than expected plasma concentrations of TCA with resultant toxicity). Products include:
- Surmontil Capsules ... 2811

Venlafaxine Hydrochloride (Concurrent use with drugs that are substrate for cytochrome $P_{450}IID_6$ may make normal metabolizer resemble poor metabolizer leading to higher than expected plasma concentrations of TCA with resultant toxicity; due to variation in the extent of inhibition of $P_{450}IID_6$ caution is indicated if co-administered). Products include:
- Effexor ... 2719

Food Interactions

Alcohol (Doxepin may enhance the response to alcohol).

SINEQUAN ORAL CONCENTRATE
(Doxepin Hydrochloride) ... 2205
See **Sinequan Capsules**

SINGLET TABLETS
(Acetaminophen, Chlorpheniramine Maleate, Pseudoephedrine Hydrochloride) ... ▣ 825

May interact with hypnotics and sedatives, tranquilizers, antihypertensives, antidepressant drugs, and certain other agents. Compounds in these categories include:

Acebutolol Hydrochloride (Effect not specified). Products include:
- Sectral Capsules ... 2807

Alprazolam (Increases drowsiness effect). Products include:
- Xanax Tablets ... 2649

Amitriptyline Hydrochloride (Effect not specified). Products include:
- Elavil ... 2838
- Endep Tablets ... 2174
- Etrafon ... 2355
- Limbitrol ... 2180
- Triavil Tablets ... 1757

Amlodipine Besylate (Effect not specified). Products include:
- Lotrel Capsules ... 840
- Norvasc Tablets ... 1940

Amoxapine (Effect not specified). Products include:
- Asendin Tablets ... 1369

Atenolol (Effect not specified). Products include:
- Tenoretic Tablets ... 2845
- Tenormin Tablets and I.V. Injection 2847

Benazepril Hydrochloride (Effect not specified). Products include:
- Lotensin Tablets ... 834
- Lotensin HCT ... 837
- Lotrel Capsules ... 840

Betaxolol Hydrochloride (Effect not specified). Products include:
- Betoptic Ophthalmic Solution ... 469
- Betoptic S Ophthalmic Suspension 471
- Kerlone Tablets ... 2436

Bisoprolol Fumarate (Effect not specified). Products include:
- Zebeta Tablets ... 1413
- Ziac ... 1415

Bupropion Hydrochloride (Effect not specified). Products include:
- Wellbutrin Tablets ... 1204

Buspirone Hydrochloride (Increases drowsiness effect). Products include:
- BuSpar ... 737

Captopril (Effect not specified). Products include:
- Capoten ... 739
- Capozide ... 742

Carteolol Hydrochloride (Effect not specified). Products include:
- Cartrol Tablets ... 410
- Ocupress Ophthalmic Solution, 1% Sterile ... ⊙ 309

Chlordiazepoxide (Increases drowsiness effect). Products include:
- Libritabs Tablets ... 2177
- Limbitrol ... 2180

Chlordiazepoxide Hydrochloride (Increases drowsiness effect). Products include:
- Librax Capsules ... 2176
- Librium Capsules ... 2178
- Librium Injectable ... 2179

Chlorpromazine (Increases drowsiness effect). Products include:
- Thorazine Suppositories ... 2523

Chlorprothixene (Increases drowsiness effect).
- No products indexed under this heading.

Chlorprothixene Hydrochloride (Increases drowsiness effect).
- No products indexed under this heading.

Clonidine (Effect not specified). Products include:
- Catapres-TTS ... 675

Clonidine Hydrochloride (Effect not specified). Products include:
- Catapres Tablets ... 674
- Combipres Tablets ... 677

Clorazepate Dipotassium (Increases drowsiness effect). Products include:
- Tranxene ... 451

Deserpidine (Effect not specified).
- No products indexed under this heading.

Desipramine Hydrochloride (Effect not specified). Products include:
- Norpramin Tablets ... 1526

Diazepam (Increases drowsiness effect). Products include:
- Dizac ... 1809
- Valium Injectable ... 2182
- Valium Tablets ... 2183
- Valrelease Capsules ... 2169

Diazoxide (Effect not specified). Products include:
- Hyperstat I.V. Injection ... 2363
- Proglycem ... 580

Diltiazem Hydrochloride (Effect not specified). Products include:
- Cardizem CD Capsules ... 1506
- Cardizem SR Capsules ... 1510
- Cardizem Injectable ... 1508
- Cardizem Tablets ... 1512
- Dilacor XR Extended-release Capsules ... 2018

Doxazosin Mesylate (Effect not specified). Products include:
- Cardura Tablets ... 2186

Doxepin Hydrochloride (Effect not specified). Products include:
- Sinequan ... 2205
- Zonalon Cream ... 1055

Droperidol (Increases drowsiness effect). Products include:
- Inapsine Injection ... 1296

Enalapril Maleate (Effect not specified). Products include:
- Vaseretic Tablets ... 1765
- Vasotec Tablets ... 1771

Enalaprilat (Effect not specified). Products include:
- Vasotec I.V. ... 1768

Esmolol Hydrochloride (Effect not specified). Products include:
- Brevibloc Injection ... 1808

Estazolam (Increases drowsiness effect). Products include:
- ProSom Tablets ... 449

Ethchlorvynol (Increases drowsiness effect). Products include:
- Placidyl Capsules ... 448

Ethinamate (Increases drowsiness effect).
- No products indexed under this heading.

Felodipine (Effect not specified). Products include:
- Plendil Extended-Release Tablets ... 527

Fluoxetine Hydrochloride (Effect not specified). Products include:
- Prozac Pulvules & Liquid, Oral Solution ... 919

Fluphenazine Decanoate (Increases drowsiness effect). Products include:
- Prolixin Decanoate ... 509

Fluphenazine Enanthate (Increases drowsiness effect). Products include:
- Prolixin Enanthate ... 509

Fluphenazine Hydrochloride (Increases drowsiness effect). Products include:
- Prolixin ... 509

Flurazepam Hydrochloride (Increases drowsiness effect). Products include:
- Dalmane Capsules ... 2173

Fosinopril Sodium (Effect not specified). Products include:
- Monopril Tablets ... 757

Glutethimide (Increases drowsiness effect).
- No products indexed under this heading.

Guanabenz Acetate (Effect not specified).
- No products indexed under this heading.

Guanethidine Monosulfate (Effect not specified). Products include:
- Esimil Tablets ... 822
- Ismelin Tablets ... 827

Haloperidol (Increases drowsiness effect). Products include:
- Haldol Injection, Tablets and Concentrate ... 1575

Haloperidol Decanoate (Increases drowsiness effect). Products include:
- Haldol Decanoate ... 1577

Hydralazine Hydrochloride (Effect not specified). Products include:
- Apresazide Capsules ... 808
- Apresoline Hydrochloride Tablets .. 809
- Ser-Ap-Es Tablets ... 849

Hydroxyzine Hydrochloride (Increases drowsiness effect). Products include:
- Atarax Tablets & Syrup ... 2185
- Marax Tablets & DF Syrup ... 2200
- Vistaril Intramuscular Solution ... 2216

Imipramine Hydrochloride (Effect not specified). Products include:
- Tofranil Ampuls ... 854
- Tofranil Tablets ... 856

Imipramine Pamoate (Effect not specified). Products include:
- Tofranil-PM Capsules ... 857

Isocarboxazid (Effect not specified).
- No products indexed under this heading.

Isradipine (Effect not specified). Products include:
- DynaCirc Capsules ... 2256

Labetalol Hydrochloride (Effect not specified). Products include:
- Normodyne Injection ... 2377
- Normodyne Tablets ... 2379
- Trandate ... 1185

Lisinopril (Effect not specified). Products include:
- Prinivil Tablets ... 1733
- Prinzide Tablets ... 1737
- Zestoretic ... 2850
- Zestril Tablets ... 2854

Lorazepam (Increases drowsiness effect). Products include:
- Ativan Injection ... 2698
- Ativan Tablets ... 2700

Losartan Potassium (Effect not specified). Products include:
- Cozaar Tablets ... 1628
- Hyzaar Tablets ... 1677

Loxapine Hydrochloride (Increases drowsiness effect). Products include:
- Loxitane ... 1378

Loxapine Succinate (Increases drowsiness effect). Products include:
- Loxitane Capsules ... 1378

Maprotiline Hydrochloride (Effect not specified). Products include:
- Ludiomil Tablets ... 843

Mecamylamine Hydrochloride (Effect not specified). Products include:
- Inversine Tablets ... 1686

Meprobamate (Increases drowsiness effect). Products include:
- Miltown Tablets ... 2672
- PMB 200 and PMB 400 ... 2783

(▣ Described in PDR For Nonprescription Drugs) (⊙ Described in PDR For Ophthalmology)

955 **Interactions Index** **Sinulin**

Mesoridazine Besylate (Increases drowsiness effect). Products include:
Serentil ... 684
Methyldopa (Effect not specified). Products include:
Aldoclor Tablets ... 1598
Aldomet Oral ... 1600
Aldoril Tablets ... 1604
Methyldopate Hydrochloride (Effect not specified). Products include:
Aldomet Ester HCl Injection ... 1602
Metolazone (Effect not specified). Products include:
Mykrox Tablets ... 993
Zaroxolyn Tablets ... 1000
Metoprolol Succinate (Effect not specified). Products include:
Toprol-XL Tablets ... 565
Metoprolol Tartrate (Effect not specified). Products include:
Lopressor Ampuls ... 830
Lopressor HCT Tablets ... 832
Lopressor Tablets ... 830
Metyrosine (Effect not specified). Products include:
Demser Capsules ... 1649
Midazolam Hydrochloride (Increases drowsiness effect). Products include:
Versed Injection ... 2170
Minoxidil (Effect not specified). Products include:
Loniten Tablets ... 2618
Rogaine Topical Solution ... 2637
Moexipril Hydrochloride (Effect not specified). Products include:
Univasc Tablets ... 2410
Molindone Hydrochloride (Increases drowsiness effect). Products include:
Moban Tablets and Concentrate ... 1048
Nadolol (Effect not specified).
No products indexed under this heading.
Nefazodone Hydrochloride (Effect not specified). Products include:
Serzone Tablets ... 771
Nicardipine Hydrochloride (Effect not specified). Products include:
Cardene Capsules ... 2095
Cardene I.V. ... 2709
Cardene SR Capsules ... 2097
Nifedipine (Effect not specified). Products include:
Adalat Capsules (10 mg and 20 mg) ... 587
Adalat CC ... 589
Procardia Capsules ... 1971
Procardia XL Extended Release Tablets ... 1972
Nisoldipine (Effect not specified).
No products indexed under this heading.
Nitroglycerin (Effect not specified). Products include:
Deponit NTG Transdermal Delivery System ... 2397
Nitro-Bid IV ... 1523
Nitro-Bid Ointment ... 1524
Nitrodisc ... 2047
Nitro-Dur (nitroglycerin) Transdermal Infusion System ... 1326
Nitrolingual Spray ... 2027
Nitrostat Tablets ... 1925
Transderm-Nitro Transdermal Therapeutic System ... 859
Nortriptyline Hydrochloride (Effect not specified). Products include:
Pamelor ... 2280
Oxazepam (Increases drowsiness effect). Products include:
Serax Capsules ... 2810
Serax Tablets ... 2810
Paroxetine Hydrochloride (Effect not specified). Products include:
Paxil Tablets ... 2505
Penbutolol Sulfate (Effect not specified). Products include:
Levatol ... 2403
Perphenazine (Increases drowsiness effect). Products include:
Etrafon ... 2355
Triavil Tablets ... 1757
Trilafon ... 2389
Phenelzine Sulfate (Effect not specified). Products include:
Nardil ... 1920
Phenoxybenzamine Hydrochloride (Effect not specified). Products include:
Dibenzyline Capsules ... 2476
Phentolamine Mesylate (Effect not specified). Products include:
Regitine ... 846
Pindolol (Effect not specified). Products include:
Visken Tablets ... 2299
Prazepam (Increases drowsiness effect).
No products indexed under this heading.
Prazosin Hydrochloride (Effect not specified). Products include:
Minipress Capsules ... 1937
Minizide Capsules ... 1938
Prochlorperazine (Increases drowsiness effect). Products include:
Compazine ... 2470
Promethazine Hydrochloride (Increases drowsiness effect). Products include:
Mepergan Injection ... 2753
Phenergan with Codeine ... 2777
Phenergan with Dextromethorphan 2778
Phenergan Injection ... 2773
Phenergan Suppositories ... 2775
Phenergan Syrup ... 2774
Phenergan Tablets ... 2775
Phenergan VC ... 2779
Phenergan VC with Codeine ... 2781
Propofol (Increases drowsiness effect). Products include:
Diprivan Injection ... 2833
Propranolol Hydrochloride (Effect not specified). Products include:
Inderal ... 2728
Inderal LA Long Acting Capsules ... 2730
Inderide Tablets ... 2732
Inderide LA Long Acting Capsules .. 2734
Protriptyline Hydrochloride (Effect not specified). Products include:
Vivactil Tablets ... 1774
Quazepam (Increases drowsiness effect). Products include:
Doral Tablets ... 2664
Quinapril Hydrochloride (Effect not specified). Products include:
Accupril Tablets ... 1893
Ramipril (Effect not specified). Products include:
Altace Capsules ... 1232
Rauwolfia Serpentina (Effect not specified).
No products indexed under this heading.
Rescinnamine (Effect not specified).
No products indexed under this heading.
Reserpine (Effect not specified). Products include:
Diupres Tablets ... 1650
Hydropres Tablets ... 1675
Ser-Ap-Es Tablets ... 849
Secobarbital Sodium (Increases drowsiness effect). Products include:
Seconal Sodium Pulvules ... 1474
Sertraline Hydrochloride (Effect not specified). Products include:
Zoloft Tablets ... 2217
Sodium Nitroprusside (Effect not specified).
No products indexed under this heading.
Sotalol Hydrochloride (Effect not specified). Products include:
Betapace Tablets ... 641
Spirapril Hydrochloride (Effect not specified).
No products indexed under this heading.
Temazepam (Increases drowsiness effect). Products include:
Restoril Capsules ... 2284
Terazosin Hydrochloride (Effect not specified). Products include:
Hytrin Capsules ... 430
Thioridazine Hydrochloride (Increases drowsiness effect). Products include:
Mellaril ... 2269
Thiothixene (Increases drowsiness effect). Products include:
Navane Capsules and Concentrate 2201
Navane Intramuscular ... 2202
Timolol Maleate (Effect not specified). Products include:
Blocadren Tablets ... 1614
Timolide Tablets ... 1748
Timoptic in Ocudose ... 1753
Timoptic Sterile Ophthalmic Solution ... 1751
Timoptic-XE ... 1755
Torsemide (Effect not specified). Products include:
Demadex Tablets and Injection ... 686
Tranylcypromine Sulfate (Effect not specified). Products include:
Parnate Tablets ... 2503
Trazodone Hydrochloride (Effect not specified). Products include:
Desyrel and Desyrel Dividose ... 503
Triazolam (Increases drowsiness effect). Products include:
Halcion Tablets ... 2611
Trifluoperazine Hydrochloride (Increases drowsiness effect). Products include:
Stelazine ... 2514
Trimethaphan Camsylate (Effect not specified). Products include:
Arfonad Ampuls ... 2080
Trimipramine Maleate (Effect not specified). Products include:
Surmontil Capsules ... 2811
Venlafaxine Hydrochloride (Effect not specified). Products include:
Effexor ... 2719
Verapamil Hydrochloride (Effect not specified). Products include:
Calan SR Caplets ... 2422
Calan Tablets ... 2419
Isoptin Injectable ... 1344
Isoptin Oral Tablets ... 1346
Isoptin SR Tablets ... 1348
Verelan Capsules ... 1410
Verelan Capsules ... 2824
Zolpidem Tartrate (Increases drowsiness effect). Products include:
Ambien Tablets ... 2416

Food Interactions

Alcohol (Increases drowsiness effect).

SINULIN TABLETS (Acetaminophen, Phenylpropanolamine Hydrochloride, Chlorpheniramine Maleate) ... 787
May interact with antihypertensives, antidepressant drugs, tranquilizers, hypnotics and sedatives, and certain other agents. Compounds in these categories include:
Acebutolol Hydrochloride (Effects not specified). Products include:
Sectral Capsules ... 2807
Alprazolam (May increase drowsiness effect). Products include:
Xanax Tablets ... 2649
Amitriptyline Hydrochloride (Effects not specified). Products include:
Elavil ... 2838
Endep Tablets ... 2174
Etrafon ... 2355
Limbitrol ... 2180
Triavil Tablets ... 1757
Amlodipine Besylate (Effects not specified). Products include:
Lotrel Capsules ... 840
Norvasc Tablets ... 1940
Amoxapine (Effects not specified). Products include:
Asendin Tablets ... 1369
Atenolol (Effects not specified). Products include:
Tenoretic Tablets ... 2845
Tenormin Tablets and I.V. Injection 2847
Benazepril Hydrochloride (Effects not specified). Products include:
Lotensin Tablets ... 834
Lotensin HCT ... 837
Lotrel Capsules ... 840
Betaxolol Hydrochloride (Effects not specified). Products include:
Betoptic Ophthalmic Solution ... 469
Betoptic S Ophthalmic Suspension 471
Kerlone Tablets ... 2436
Bisoprolol Fumarate (Effects not specified). Products include:
Zebeta Tablets ... 1413
Ziac ... 1415
Bupropion Hydrochloride (Effects not specified). Products include:
Wellbutrin Tablets ... 1204
Buspirone Hydrochloride (May increase drowsiness effect). Products include:
BuSpar ... 737
Captopril (Effects not specified). Products include:
Capoten ... 739
Capozide ... 742
Carteolol Hydrochloride (Effects not specified). Products include:
Cartrol Tablets ... 410
Ocupress Ophthalmic Solution, 1% Sterile ... ⊛ 309
Chlordiazepoxide (May increase drowsiness effect). Products include:
Libritabs Tablets ... 2177
Limbitrol ... 2180
Chlordiazepoxide Hydrochloride (May increase drowsiness effect). Products include:
Librax Capsules ... 2176
Librium Capsules ... 2178
Librium Injectable ... 2179
Chlorpromazine (May increase drowsiness effect). Products include:
Thorazine Suppositories ... 2523
Chlorpromazine Hydrochloride (May increase drowsiness effect). Products include:
Thorazine ... 2523
Chlorprothixene (May increase drowsiness effect).
No products indexed under this heading.
Chlorprothixene Hydrochloride (May increase drowsiness effect).
No products indexed under this heading.
Clonidine (Effects not specified). Products include:
Catapres-TTS ... 675
Clonidine Hydrochloride (Effects not specified). Products include:
Catapres Tablets ... 674
Combipres Tablets ... 677

IMPORTANT NOTE: Always consult each drug listing in the patient's regimen for possible interactions.

Sinulin Interactions Index 956

Clorazepate Dipotassium (May increase drowsiness effect). Products include:
Tranxene ... 451

Deserpidine (Effects not specified).
No products indexed under this heading.

Desipramine Hydrochloride (Effects not specified). Products include:
Norpramin Tablets ... 1526

Diazepam (May increase drowsiness effect). Products include:
Dizac ... 1809
Valium Injectable ... 2182
Valium Tablets ... 2183
Valrelease Capsules ... 2169

Diazoxide (Effects not specified). Products include:
Hyperstat I.V. Injection ... 2363
Proglycem ... 580

Diltiazem Hydrochloride (Effects not specified). Products include:
Cardizem CD Capsules ... 1506
Cardizem SR Capsules ... 1510
Cardizem Injectable ... 1508
Cardizem Tablets ... 1512
Dilacor XR Extended-release Capsules ... 2018

Doxazosin Mesylate (Effects not specified). Products include:
Cardura Tablets ... 2186

Doxepin Hydrochloride (Effects not specified). Products include:
Sinequan ... 2205
Zonalon Cream ... 1055

Droperidol (May increase drowsiness effect). Products include:
Inapsine Injection ... 1296

Enalapril Maleate (Effects not specified). Products include:
Vaseretic Tablets ... 1765
Vasotec Tablets ... 1771

Enalaprilat (Effects not specified). Products include:
Vasotec I.V. ... 1768

Esmolol Hydrochloride (Effects not specified). Products include:
Brevibloc Injection ... 1808

Estazolam (May increase drowsiness effect). Products include:
ProSom Tablets ... 449

Ethchlorvynol (May increase drowsiness effect). Products include:
Placidyl Capsules ... 448

Ethinamate (May increase drowsiness effect).
No products indexed under this heading.

Felodipine (Effects not specified). Products include:
Plendil Extended-Release Tablets ... 527

Fluoxetine Hydrochloride (Effects not specified). Products include:
Prozac Pulvules & Liquid, Oral Solution ... 919

Fluphenazine Decanoate (May increase drowsiness effect). Products include:
Prolixin Decanoate ... 509

Fluphenazine Enanthate (May increase drowsiness effect). Products include:
Prolixin Enanthate ... 509

Fluphenazine Hydrochloride (May increase drowsiness effect). Products include:
Prolixin ... 509

Flurazepam Hydrochloride (May increase drowsiness effect). Products include:
Dalmane Capsules ... 2173

Fosinopril Sodium (Effects not specified). Products include:
Monopril Tablets ... 757

Glutethimide (May increase drowsiness effect).
No products indexed under this heading.

Guanabenz Acetate (Effects not specified).
No products indexed under this heading.

Guanethidine Monosulfate (Effects not specified). Products include:
Esimil Tablets ... 822
Ismelin Tablets ... 827

Haloperidol (May increase drowsiness effect). Products include:
Haldol Injection, Tablets and Concentrate ... 1575

Haloperidol Decanoate (May increase drowsiness effect). Products include:
Haldol Decanoate ... 1577

Hydralazine Hydrochloride (Effects not specified). Products include:
Apresazide Capsules ... 808
Apresoline Hydrochloride Tablets ... 809
Ser-Ap-Es Tablets ... 849

Hydroxyzine Hydrochloride (May increase drowsiness effect). Products include:
Atarax Tablets & Syrup ... 2185
Marax Tablets & DF Syrup ... 2200
Vistaril Intramuscular Solution ... 2216

Imipramine Hydrochloride (Effects not specified). Products include:
Tofranil Ampuls ... 854
Tofranil Tablets ... 856

Imipramine Pamoate (Effects not specified). Products include:
Tofranil-PM Capsules ... 857

Indapamide (Effects not specified). Products include:
Lozol Tablets ... 2022

Isocarboxazid (Effects not specified).
No products indexed under this heading.

Isradipine (Effects not specified). Products include:
DynaCirc Capsules ... 2256

Labetalol Hydrochloride (Effects not specified). Products include:
Normodyne Injection ... 2377
Normodyne Tablets ... 2379
Trandate ... 1185

Lisinopril (Effects not specified). Products include:
Prinivil Tablets ... 1733
Prinzide Tablets ... 1737
Zestoretic ... 2850
Zestril Tablets ... 2854

Lorazepam (May increase drowsiness effect). Products include:
Ativan Injection ... 2698
Ativan Tablets ... 2700

Losartan Potassium (Effects not specified). Products include:
Cozaar Tablets ... 1628
Hyzaar Tablets ... 1677

Loxapine Hydrochloride (May increase drowsiness effect). Products include:
Loxitane ... 1378

Loxapine Succinate (May increase drowsiness effect). Products include:
Loxitane Capsules ... 1378

Maprotiline Hydrochloride (Effects not specified). Products include:
Ludiomil Tablets ... 843

Mecamylamine Hydrochloride (Effects not specified). Products include:
Inversine Tablets ... 1686

Meprobamate (May increase drowsiness effect). Products include:
Miltown Tablets ... 2672
PMB 200 and PMB 400 ... 2783

Mesoridazine Besylate (May increase drowsiness effect). Products include:
Serentil ... 684

Methyclothiazide (Effects not specified). Products include:
Enduron Tablets ... 420

Methyldopa (Effects not specified). Products include:
Aldoclor Tablets ... 1598
Aldomet Oral ... 1600
Aldoril Tablets ... 1604

Methyldopate Hydrochloride (Effects not specified). Products include:
Aldomet Ester HCl Injection ... 1602

Metolazone (Effects not specified). Products include:
Mykrox Tablets ... 993
Zaroxolyn Tablets ... 1000

Metoprolol Succinate (Effects not specified). Products include:
Toprol-XL Tablets ... 565

Metoprolol Tartrate (Effects not specified). Products include:
Lopressor Ampuls ... 830
Lopressor HCT Tablets ... 832
Lopressor Tablets ... 830

Metyrosine (Effects not specified). Products include:
Demser Capsules ... 1649

Midazolam Hydrochloride (May increase drowsiness effect). Products include:
Versed Injection ... 2170

Minoxidil (Effects not specified). Products include:
Loniten Tablets ... 2618
Rogaine Topical Solution ... 2637

Moexipril Hydrochloride (Effects not specified). Products include:
Univasc Tablets ... 2410

Molindone Hydrochloride (May increase drowsiness effect). Products include:
Moban Tablets and Concentrate ... 1048

Nadolol (Effects not specified).
No products indexed under this heading.

Nefazodone Hydrochloride (Effects not specified). Products include:
Serzone Tablets ... 771

Nicardipine Hydrochloride (Effects not specified). Products include:
Cardene Capsules ... 2095
Cardene I.V. ... 2709
Cardene SR Capsules ... 2097

Nifedipine (Effects not specified). Products include:
Adalat Capsules (10 mg and 20 mg) ... 587
Adalat CC ... 589
Procardia Capsules ... 1971
Procardia XL Extended Release Tablets ... 1972

Nisoldipine (Effects not specified).
No products indexed under this heading.

Nitroglycerin (Effects not specified). Products include:
Deponit NTG Transdermal Delivery System ... 2397
Nitro-Bid IV ... 1523
Nitro-Bid Ointment ... 1524
Nitrodisc ... 2047
Nitro-Dur (nitroglycerin) Transdermal Infusion System ... 1326
Nitrolingual Spray ... 2027
Nitrostat Tablets ... 1925
Transderm-Nitro Transdermal Therapeutic System ... 859

Nortriptyline Hydrochloride (Effects not specified). Products include:
Pamelor ... 2280

Oxazepam (May increase drowsiness effect). Products include:
Serax Capsules ... 2810
Serax Tablets ... 2810

Paroxetine Hydrochloride (Effects not specified). Products include:
Paxil Tablets ... 2505

Penbutolol Sulfate (Effects not specified). Products include:
Levatol ... 2403

Perphenazine (May increase drowsiness effect). Products include:
Etrafon ... 2355
Triavil Tablets ... 1757
Trilafon ... 2389

Phenelzine Sulfate (Effects not specified). Products include:
Nardil ... 1920

Phenoxybenzamine Hydrochloride (Effects not specified). Products include:
Dibenzyline Capsules ... 2476

Phentolamine Mesylate (Effects not specified). Products include:
Regitine ... 846

Pindolol (Effects not specified). Products include:
Visken Tablets ... 2299

Prazepam (May increase drowsiness effect).
No products indexed under this heading.

Prazosin Hydrochloride (Effects not specified). Products include:
Minipress Capsules ... 1937
Minizide Capsules ... 1938

Prochlorperazine (May increase drowsiness effect). Products include:
Compazine ... 2470

Promethazine Hydrochloride (May increase drowsiness effect). Products include:
Mepergan Injection ... 2753
Phenergan with Codeine ... 2777
Phenergan with Dextromethorphan ... 2778
Phenergan Injection ... 2773
Phenergan Suppositories ... 2775
Phenergan Syrup ... 2774
Phenergan Tablets ... 2775
Phenergan VC ... 2779
Phenergan VC with Codeine ... 2781

Propofol (May increase drowsiness effect). Products include:
Diprivan Injection ... 2833

Propranolol Hydrochloride (Effects not specified). Products include:
Inderal ... 2728
Inderal LA Long Acting Capsules ... 2730
Inderide Tablets ... 2732
Inderide LA Long Acting Capsules ... 2734

Protriptyline Hydrochloride (Effects not specified). Products include:
Vivactil Tablets ... 1774

Quazepam (May increase drowsiness effect). Products include:
Doral Tablets ... 2664

Quinapril Hydrochloride (Effects not specified). Products include:
Accupril Tablets ... 1893

Ramipril (Effects not specified). Products include:
Altace Capsules ... 1232

Rauwolfia Serpentina (Effects not specified).
No products indexed under this heading.

Rescinnamine (Effects not specified).
No products indexed under this heading.

(▣ Described in PDR For Nonprescription Drugs) (◉ Described in PDR For Ophthalmology)

Reserpine (Effects not specified). Products include:

Diupres Tablets 1650
Hydropres Tablets............................... 1675
Ser-Ap-Es Tablets 849

Secobarbital Sodium (May increase drowsiness effect). Products include:

Seconal Sodium Pulvules 1474

Sertraline Hydrochloride (Effects not specified). Products include:

Zoloft Tablets 2217

Sodium Nitroprusside (Effects not specified).

No products indexed under this heading.

Sotalol Hydrochloride (Effects not specified). Products include:

Betapace Tablets 641

Spirapril Hydrochloride (Effects not specified).

No products indexed under this heading.

Temazepam (May increase drowsiness effect). Products include:

Restoril Capsules 2284

Terazosin Hydrochloride (Effects not specified). Products include:

Hytrin Capsules 430

Thioridazine Hydrochloride (May increase drowsiness effect). Products include:

Mellaril 2269

Thiothixene (May increase drowsiness effect). Products include:

Navane Capsules and Concentrate 2201
Navane Intramuscular 2202

Timolol Maleate (Effects not specified). Products include:

Blocadren Tablets 1614
Timolide Tablets.................................. 1748
Timoptic in Ocudose 1753
Timoptic Sterile Ophthalmic Solution.. 1751
Timoptic-XE 1755

Torsemide (Effects not specified). Products include:

Demadex Tablets and Injection 686

Tranylcypromine Sulfate (Effects not specified). Products include:

Parnate Tablets 2503

Trazodone Hydrochloride (Effects not specified). Products include:

Desyrel and Desyrel Dividose 503

Triazolam (May increase drowsiness effect). Products include:

Halcion Tablets................................... 2611

Trifluoperazine Hydrochloride (May increase drowsiness effect). Products include:

Stelazine 2514

Trimethaphan Camsylate (Effects not specified). Products include:

Arfonad Ampuls 2080

Trimipramine Maleate (Effects not specified). Products include:

Surmontil Capsules 2811

Venlafaxine Hydrochloride (Effects not specified). Products include:

Effexor 2719

Verapamil Hydrochloride (Effects not specified). Products include:

Calan SR Caplets 2422
Calan Tablets...................................... 2419
Isoptin Injectable 1344
Isoptin Oral Tablets 1346
Isoptin SR Tablets 1348
Verelan Capsules 1410
Verelan Capsules 2824

Zolpidem Tartrate (May increase drowsiness effect). Products include:

Ambien Tablets................................... 2416

Food Interactions

Alcohol (Increased drowsiness).

SINUTAB NON-DRYING LIQUID CAPS

(Pseudoephedrine Hydrochloride, Guaifenesin)...◆◻ 859

May interact with monoamine oxidase inhibitors. Compounds in this category include:

Furazolidone (Concurrent and/or sequential use not recommended). Products include:

Furoxone 2046

Isocarboxazid (Concurrent and/or sequential use not recommended).

No products indexed under this heading.

Phenelzine Sulfate (Concurrent and/or sequential use not recommended). Products include:

Nardil 1920

Selegiline Hydrochloride (Concurrent and/or sequential use not recommended). Products include:

Eldepryl Tablets 2550

Tranylcypromine Sulfate (Concurrent and/or sequential use not recommended). Products include:

Parnate Tablets 2503

SINUTAB SINUS ALLERGY MEDICATION, MAXIMUM STRENGTH TABLETS AND CAPLETS

(Acetaminophen, Chlorpheniramine Maleate, Pseudoephedrine Hydrochloride)...................................◆◻ 860

May interact with antihypertensives, antidepressant drugs, and certain other agents. Compounds in these categories include:

Acebutolol Hydrochloride (Do not use concomitantly). Products include:

Sectral Capsules 2807

Amitriptyline Hydrochloride (Do not use concomitantly). Products include:

Elavil 2838
Endep Tablets 2174
Etrafon 2355
Limbitrol 2180
Triavil Tablets 1757

Amlodipine Besylate (Do not use concomitantly). Products include:

Lotrel Capsules 840
Norvasc Tablets 1940

Amoxapine (Do not use concomitantly). Products include:

Asendin Tablets 1369

Atenolol (Do not use concomitantly). Products include:

Tenoretic Tablets 2845
Tenormin Tablets and I.V. Injection 2847

Benazepril Hydrochloride (Do not use concomitantly). Products include:

Lotensin Tablets 834
Lotensin HCT...................................... 837
Lotrel Capsules................................... 840

Betaxolol Hydrochloride (Do not use concomitantly). Products include:

Betoptic Ophthalmic Solution............ 469
Betoptic S Ophthalmic Suspension 471
Kerlone Tablets................................... 2436

Bisoprolol Fumarate (Do not use concomitantly). Products include:

Zebeta Tablets 1413
Ziac 1415

Bupropion Hydrochloride (Do not use concomitantly). Products include:

Wellbutrin Tablets 1204

Captopril (Do not use concomitantly). Products include:

Capoten 739
Capozide 742

Carteolol Hydrochloride (Do not use concomitantly). Products include:

Cartrol Tablets 410
Ocupress Ophthalmic Solution, 1% Sterile.. ◉ 309

Clonidine (Do not use concomitantly). Products include:

Catapres-TTS...................................... 675

Clonidine Hydrochloride (Do not use concomitantly). Products include:

Catapres Tablets 674
Combipres Tablets 677

Deserpidine (Do not use concomitantly).

No products indexed under this heading.

Desipramine Hydrochloride (Do not use concomitantly). Products include:

Norpramin Tablets 1526

Diazoxide (Do not use concomitantly). Products include:

Hyperstat I.V. Injection 2363
Proglycem... 580

Diltiazem Hydrochloride (Do not use concomitantly). Products include:

Cardizem CD Capsules 1506
Cardizem SR Capsules 1510
Cardizem Injectable 1508
Cardizem Tablets................................ 1512
Dilacor XR Extended-release Capsules 2018

Doxazosin Mesylate (Do not use concomitantly). Products include:

Cardura Tablets 2186

Doxepin Hydrochloride (Do not use concomitantly). Products include:

Sinequan 2205
Zonalon Cream 1055

Enalapril Maleate (Do not use concomitantly). Products include:

Vaseretic Tablets 1765
Vasotec Tablets 1771

Enalaprilat (Do not use concomitantly). Products include:

Vasotec I.V.. 1768

Esmolol Hydrochloride (Do not use concomitantly). Products include:

Brevibloc Injection.............................. 1808

Felodipine (Do not use concomitantly). Products include:

Plendil Extended-Release Tablets..... 527

Fluoxetine Hydrochloride (Do not use concomitantly). Products include:

Prozac Pulvules & Liquid, Oral Solution 919

Fosinopril Sodium (Do not use concomitantly). Products include:

Monopril Tablets 757

Furosemide (Do not use concomitantly). Products include:

Lasix Injection, Oral Solution and Tablets 1240

Guanabenz Acetate (Do not use concomitantly).

No products indexed under this heading.

Guanethidine Monosulfate (Do not use concomitantly). Products include:

Esimil Tablets 822
Ismelin Tablets 827

Hydralazine Hydrochloride (Do not use concomitantly). Products include:

Apresazide Capsules 808
Apresoline Hydrochloride Tablets .. 809
Ser-Ap-Es Tablets 849

Imipramine Hydrochloride (Do not use concomitantly). Products include:

Tofranil Ampuls 854
Tofranil Tablets 856

Imipramine Pamoate (Do not use concomitantly). Products include:

Tofranil-PM Capsules.......................... 857

Isocarboxazid (Do not use concomitantly).

No products indexed under this heading.

Isradipine (Do not use concomitantly). Products include:

DynaCirc Capsules 2256

Labetalol Hydrochloride (Do not use concomitantly). Products include:

Normodyne Injection 2377
Normodyne Tablets 2379
Trandate 1185

Lisinopril (Do not use concomitantly). Products include:

Prinivil Tablets 1733
Prinzide Tablets 1737
Zestoretic 2850
Zestril Tablets 2854

Losartan Potassium (Do not use concomitantly). Products include:

Cozaar Tablets 1628
Hyzaar Tablets 1677

Maprotiline Hydrochloride (Do not use concomitantly). Products include:

Ludiomil Tablets.................................. 843

Mecamylamine Hydrochloride (Do not use concomitantly). Products include:

Inversine Tablets 1686

Methyldopa (Do not use concomitantly). Products include:

Aldoclor Tablets.................................. 1598
Aldomet Oral 1600
Aldoril Tablets..................................... 1604

Methyldopate Hydrochloride (Do not use concomitantly). Products include:

Aldomet Ester HCl Injection 1602

Metolazone (Do not use concomitantly). Products include:

Mykrox Tablets 993
Zaroxolyn Tablets 1000

Metoprolol Succinate (Do not use concomitantly). Products include:

Toprol-XL Tablets 565

Metoprolol Tartrate (Do not use concomitantly). Products include:

Lopressor Ampuls 830
Lopressor HCT Tablets 832
Lopressor Tablets 830

Metyrosine (Do not use concomitantly). Products include:

Demser Capsules................................. 1649

Minoxidil (Do not use concomitantly). Products include:

Loniten Tablets 2618
Rogaine Topical Solution 2637

Moexipril Hydrochloride (Do not use concomitantly). Products include:

Univasc Tablets 2410

Nadolol (Do not use concomitantly).

No products indexed under this heading.

Nefazodone Hydrochloride (Do not use concomitantly). Products include:

Serzone Tablets 771

IMPORTANT NOTE: Always consult each drug listing in the patient's regimen for possible interactions.

Sinutab Allergy Interactions Index 958

Nicardipine Hydrochloride (Do not use concomitantly). Products include:
- Cardene Capsules 2095
- Cardene I.V. 2709
- Cardene SR Capsules 2097

Nifedipine (Do not use concomitantly). Products include:
- Adalat Capsules (10 mg and 20 mg) 587
- Adalat CC 589
- Procardia Capsules 1971
- Procardia XL Extended Release Tablets 1972

Nisoldipine (Do not use concomitantly).
- No products indexed under this heading.

Nitroglycerin (Do not use concomitantly). Products include:
- Deponit NTG Transdermal Delivery System 2397
- Nitro-Bid IV 1523
- Nitro-Bid Ointment 1524
- Nitrodisc 2047
- Nitro-Dur (nitroglycerin) Transdermal Infusion System 1326
- Nitrolingual Spray 2027
- Nitrostat Tablets 1925
- Transderm-Nitro Transdermal Therapeutic System 859

Nortriptyline Hydrochloride (Do not use concomitantly). Products include:
- Pamelor 2280

Paroxetine Hydrochloride (Do not use concomitantly). Products include:
- Paxil Tablets 2505

Penbutolol Sulfate (Do not use concomitantly). Products include:
- Levatol 2403

Phenelzine Sulfate (Do not use concomitantly). Products include:
- Nardil 1920

Phenoxybenzamine Hydrochloride (Do not use concomitantly). Products include:
- Dibenzyline Capsules 2476

Phentolamine Mesylate (Do not use concomitantly). Products include:
- Regitine 846

Pindolol (Do not use concomitantly). Products include:
- Visken Tablets 2299

Prazosin Hydrochloride (Do not use concomitantly). Products include:
- Minipress Capsules 1937
- Minizide Capsules 1938

Propranolol Hydrochloride (Do not use concomitantly). Products include:
- Inderal 2728
- Inderal LA Long Acting Capsules 2730
- Inderide Tablets 2732
- Inderide LA Long Acting Capsules 2734

Protriptyline Hydrochloride (Do not use concomitantly). Products include:
- Vivactil Tablets 1774

Quinapril Hydrochloride (Do not use concomitantly). Products include:
- Accupril Tablets 1893

Ramipril (Do not use concomitantly). Products include:
- Altace Capsules 1232

Rauwolfia Serpentina (Do not use concomitantly).
- No products indexed under this heading.

Rescinnamine (Do not use concomitantly).
- No products indexed under this heading.

Reserpine (Do not use concomitantly). Products include:
- Diupres Tablets 1650
- Hydropres Tablets 1675
- Ser-Ap-Es Tablets 849

Sertraline Hydrochloride (Do not use concomitantly). Products include:
- Zoloft Tablets 2217

Sodium Nitroprusside (Do not use concomitantly).
- No products indexed under this heading.

Sotalol Hydrochloride (Do not use concomitantly). Products include:
- Betapace Tablets 641

Spirapril Hydrochloride (Do not use concomitantly).
- No products indexed under this heading.

Terazosin Hydrochloride (Do not use concomitantly). Products include:
- Hytrin Capsules 430

Timolol Maleate (Do not use concomitantly). Products include:
- Blocadren Tablets 1614
- Timolide Tablets 1748
- Timoptic in Ocudose 1753
- Timoptic Sterile Ophthalmic Solution 1751
- Timoptic-XE 1755

Torsemide (Do not use concomitantly). Products include:
- Demadex Tablets and Injection 686

Tranylcypromine Sulfate (Do not use concomitantly). Products include:
- Parnate Tablets 2503

Trazodone Hydrochloride (Do not use concomitantly). Products include:
- Desyrel and Desyrel Dividose 503

Trimethaphan Camsylate (Do not use concomitantly). Products include:
- Arfonad Ampuls 2080

Trimipramine Maleate (Do not use concomitantly). Products include:
- Surmontil Capsules 2811

Venlafaxine Hydrochloride (Do not use concomitantly). Products include:
- Effexor 2719

Verapamil Hydrochloride (Do not use concomitantly). Products include:
- Calan SR Caplets 2422
- Calan Tablets 2419
- Isoptin Injectable 1344
- Isoptin Oral Tablets 1346
- Isoptin SR Tablets 1348
- Verelan Capsules 1410
- Verelan Capsules 2824

Food Interactions

Alcohol (Do not use concomitantly).

SINUTAB SINUS MEDICATION, MAXIMUM STRENGTH WITHOUT DROWSINESS FORMULA, TABLETS & CAPLETS

(Acetaminophen, Pseudoephedrine Hydrochloride) .... ◙ 860

May interact with antihypertensives and antidepressant drugs. Compounds in these categories include:

Acebutolol Hydrochloride (Concurrent use not recommended). Products include:
- Sectral Capsules 2807

Amitriptyline Hydrochloride (Concurrent use not recommended). Products include:
- Elavil 2838
- Endep Tablets 2174
- Etrafon 2355
- Limbitrol 2180
- Triavil Tablets 1757

Amlodipine Besylate (Concurrent use not recommended). Products include:
- Lotrel Capsules 840
- Norvasc Tablets 1940

Amoxapine (Concurrent use not recommended). Products include:
- Asendin Tablets 1369

Atenolol (Concurrent use not recommended). Products include:
- Tenoretic Tablets 2845
- Tenormin Tablets and I.V. Injection 2847

Benazepril Hydrochloride (Concurrent use not recommended). Products include:
- Lotensin Tablets 834
- Lotensin HCT 837
- Lotrel Capsules 840

Betaxolol Hydrochloride (Concurrent use not recommended). Products include:
- Betoptic Ophthalmic Solution 469
- Betoptic S Ophthalmic Suspension 471
- Kerlone Tablets 2436

Bisoprolol Fumarate (Concurrent use not recommended). Products include:
- Zebeta Tablets 1413
- Ziac 1415

Bupropion Hydrochloride (Concurrent use not recommended). Products include:
- Wellbutrin Tablets 1204

Captopril (Concurrent use not recommended). Products include:
- Capoten 739
- Capozide 742

Carteolol Hydrochloride (Concurrent use not recommended). Products include:
- Cartrol Tablets 410
- Ocupress Ophthalmic Solution, 1% Sterile .... ⊙ 309

Clonidine (Concurrent use not recommended). Products include:
- Catapres-TTS 675

Clonidine Hydrochloride (Concurrent use not recommended). Products include:
- Catapres Tablets 674
- Combipres Tablets 677

Deserpidine (Concurrent use not recommended).
- No products indexed under this heading.

Desipramine Hydrochloride (Concurrent use not recommended). Products include:
- Norpramin Tablets 1526

Diazoxide (Concurrent use not recommended). Products include:
- Hyperstat I.V. Injection 2363
- Proglycem 580

Diltiazem Hydrochloride (Concurrent use not recommended). Products include:
- Cardizem CD Capsules 1506
- Cardizem SR Capsules 1510
- Cardizem Injectable 1508
- Cardizem Tablets 1512
- Dilacor XR Extended-release Capsules 2018

Doxazosin Mesylate (Concurrent use not recommended). Products include:
- Cardura Tablets 2186

Doxepin Hydrochloride (Concurrent use not recommended). Products include:
- Sinequan 2205
- Zonalon Cream 1055

Enalapril Maleate (Concurrent use not recommended). Products include:
- Vaseretic Tablets 1765
- Vasotec Tablets 1771

Enalaprilat (Concurrent use not recommended). Products include:
- Vasotec I.V. 1768

Esmolol Hydrochloride (Concurrent use not recommended). Products include:
- Brevibloc Injection 1808

Felodipine (Concurrent use not recommended). Products include:
- Plendil Extended-Release Tablets 527

Fluoxetine Hydrochloride (Concurrent use not recommended). Products include:
- Prozac Pulvules & Liquid, Oral Solution 919

Fosinopril Sodium (Concurrent use not recommended). Products include:
- Monopril Tablets 757

Guanabenz Acetate (Concurrent use not recommended).
- No products indexed under this heading.

Guanethidine Monosulfate (Concurrent use not recommended). Products include:
- Esimil Tablets 822
- Ismelin Tablets 827

Hydralazine Hydrochloride (Concurrent use not recommended). Products include:
- Apresazide Capsules 808
- Apresoline Hydrochloride Tablets 809
- Ser-Ap-Es Tablets 849

Imipramine Hydrochloride (Concurrent use not recommended). Products include:
- Tofranil Ampuls 854
- Tofranil Tablets 856

Imipramine Pamoate (Concurrent use not recommended). Products include:
- Tofranil-PM Capsules 857

Indapamide (Concurrent use not recommended). Products include:
- Lozol Tablets 2022

Isocarboxazid (Concurrent use not recommended).
- No products indexed under this heading.

Isradipine (Concurrent use not recommended). Products include:
- DynaCirc Capsules 2256

Labetalol Hydrochloride (Concurrent use not recommended). Products include:
- Normodyne Injection 2377
- Normodyne Tablets 2379
- Trandate 1185

Lisinopril (Concurrent use not recommended). Products include:
- Prinivil Tablets 1733
- Prinzide Tablets 1737
- Zestoretic 2850
- Zestril Tablets 2854

Losartan Potassium (Concurrent use not recommended). Products include:
- Cozaar Tablets 1628
- Hyzaar Tablets 1677

Maprotiline Hydrochloride (Concurrent use not recommended). Products include:
- Ludiomil Tablets 843

Mecamylamine Hydrochloride (Concurrent use not recommended). Products include:
- Inversine Tablets 1686

Methyldopa (Concurrent use not recommended). Products include:
- Aldoclor Tablets 1598
- Aldomet Oral 1600
- Aldoril Tablets 1604

Methyldopate Hydrochloride (Concurrent use not recommended). Products include:
- Aldomet Ester HCl Injection 1602

(◙ Described in PDR For Nonprescription Drugs) (⊙ Described in PDR For Ophthalmology)

959 **Interactions Index** **Sinutab Sinus Medication**

Metoprolol Succinate (Concurrent use not recommended). Products include:
Toprol-XL Tablets ... 565

Metoprolol Tartrate (Concurrent use not recommended). Products include:
Lopressor Ampuls ... 830
Lopressor HCT Tablets ... 832
Lopressor Tablets ... 830

Metyrosine (Concurrent use not recommended). Products include:
Demser Capsules ... 1649

Minoxidil (Concurrent use not recommended). Products include:
Loniten Tablets ... 2618
Rogaine Topical Solution ... 2637

Moexipril Hydrochloride (Concurrent use not recommended). Products include:
Univasc Tablets ... 2410

Nadolol (Concurrent use not recommended).
No products indexed under this heading.

Nefazodone Hydrochloride (Concurrent use not recommended). Products include:
Serzone Tablets ... 771

Nicardipine Hydrochloride (Concurrent use not recommended). Products include:
Cardene Capsules ... 2095
Cardene I.V. ... 2709
Cardene SR Capsules ... 2097

Nifedipine (Concurrent use not recommended). Products include:
Adalat Capsules (10 mg and 20 mg) ... 587
Adalat CC ... 589
Procardia Capsules ... 1971
Procardia XL Extended Release Tablets ... 1972

Nisoldipine (Concurrent use not recommended).
No products indexed under this heading.

Nitroglycerin (Concurrent use not recommended). Products include:
Deponit NTG Transdermal Delivery System ... 2397
Nitro-Bid IV ... 1523
Nitro-Bid Ointment ... 1524
Nitrodisc ... 2047
Nitro-Dur (nitroglycerin) Transdermal Infusion System ... 1326
Nitrolingual Spray ... 2027
Nitrostat Tablets ... 1925
Transderm-Nitro Transdermal Therapeutic System ... 859

Nortriptyline Hydrochloride (Concurrent use not recommended). Products include:
Pamelor ... 2280

Paroxetine Hydrochloride (Concurrent use not recommended). Products include:
Paxil Tablets ... 2505

Penbutolol Sulfate (Concurrent use not recommended). Products include:
Levatol ... 2403

Phenelzine Sulfate (Concurrent use not recommended). Products include:
Nardil ... 1920

Phenoxybenzamine Hydrochloride (Concurrent use not recommended). Products include:
Dibenzyline Capsules ... 2476

Phentolamine Mesylate (Concurrent use not recommended). Products include:
Regitine ... 846

Pindolol (Concurrent use not recommended). Products include:
Visken Tablets ... 2299

Prazosin Hydrochloride (Concurrent use not recommended). Products include:
Minipress Capsules ... 1937
Minizide Capsules ... 1938

Propranolol Hydrochloride (Concurrent use not recommended). Products include:
Inderal ... 2728
Inderal LA Long Acting Capsules ... 2730
Inderide Tablets ... 2732
Inderide LA Long Acting Capsules ... 2734

Protriptyline Hydrochloride (Concurrent use not recommended). Products include:
Vivactil Tablets ... 1774

Quinapril Hydrochloride (Concurrent use not recommended). Products include:
Accupril Tablets ... 1893

Ramipril (Concurrent use not recommended). Products include:
Altace Capsules ... 1232

Rauwolfia Serpentina (Concurrent use not recommended).
No products indexed under this heading.

Rescinnamine (Concurrent use not recommended).
No products indexed under this heading.

Reserpine (Concurrent use not recommended). Products include:
Diupres Tablets ... 1650
Hydropres Tablets ... 1675
Ser-Ap-Es Tablets ... 849

Sertraline Hydrochloride (Concurrent use not recommended). Products include:
Zoloft Tablets ... 2217

Sodium Nitroprusside (Concurrent use not recommended).
No products indexed under this heading.

Sotalol Hydrochloride (Concurrent use not recommended). Products include:
Betapace Tablets ... 641

Spirapril Hydrochloride (Concurrent use not recommended).
No products indexed under this heading.

Terazosin Hydrochloride (Concurrent use not recommended). Products include:
Hytrin Capsules ... 430

Timolol Maleate (Concurrent use not recommended). Products include:
Blocadren Tablets ... 1614
Timolide Tablets ... 1748
Timoptic in Ocudose ... 1753
Timoptic Sterile Ophthalmic Solution ... 1751
Timoptic-XE ... 1755

Torsemide (Concurrent use not recommended). Products include:
Demadex Tablets and Injection ... 686

Tranylcypromine Sulfate (Concurrent use not recommended). Products include:
Parnate Tablets ... 2503

Trazodone Hydrochloride (Concurrent use not recommended). Products include:
Desyrel and Desyrel Dividose ... 503

Trimethaphan Camsylate (Concurrent use not recommended). Products include:
Arfonad Ampuls ... 2080

Trimipramine Maleate (Concurrent use not recommended). Products include:
Surmontil Capsules ... 2811

Venlafaxine Hydrochloride (Concurrent use not recommended). Products include:
Effexor ... 2719

Verapamil Hydrochloride (Concurrent use not recommended). Products include:
Calan SR Caplets ... 2422
Calan Tablets ... 2419
Isoptin Injectable ... 1344
Isoptin Oral Tablets ... 1346
Isoptin SR Tablets ... 1348
Verelan Capsules ... 1410
Verelan Capsules ... 2824

SINUTAB SINUS MEDICATION, REGULAR STRENGTH WITHOUT DROWSINESS FORMULA
(Acetaminophen, Pseudoephedrine Hydrochloride) ... ▣ 859
May interact with antihypertensives, antidepressant drugs, and certain other agents. Compounds in these categories include:

Acebutolol Hydrochloride (Concurrent use not recommended). Products include:
Sectral Capsules ... 2807

Amitriptyline Hydrochloride (Concurrent use not recommended). Products include:
Elavil ... 2838
Endep Tablets ... 2174
Etrafon ... 2355
Limbitrol ... 2180
Triavil Tablets ... 1757

Amlodipine Besylate (Concurrent use not recommended). Products include:
Lotrel Capsules ... 840
Norvasc Tablets ... 1940

Amoxapine (Concurrent use not recommended). Products include:
Asendin Tablets ... 1369

Atenolol (Concurrent use not recommended). Products include:
Tenoretic Tablets ... 2845
Tenormin Tablets and I.V. Injection ... 2847

Benazepril Hydrochloride (Concurrent use not recommended). Products include:
Lotensin Tablets ... 834
Lotensin HCT ... 837
Lotrel Capsules ... 840

Betaxolol Hydrochloride (Concurrent use not recommended). Products include:
Betoptic Ophthalmic Solution ... 469
Betoptic S Ophthalmic Suspension ... 471
Kerlone Tablets ... 2436

Bisoprolol Fumarate (Concurrent use not recommended). Products include:
Zebeta Tablets ... 1413
Ziac ... 1415

Bupropion Hydrochloride (Concurrent use not recommended). Products include:
Wellbutrin Tablets ... 1204

Captopril (Concurrent use not recommended). Products include:
Capoten ... 739
Capozide ... 742

Carteolol Hydrochloride (Concurrent use not recommended). Products include:
Cartrol Tablets ... 410
Ocupress Ophthalmic Solution, 1% Sterile ... ⊙ 309

Clonidine (Concurrent use not recommended). Products include:
Catapres-TTS ... 675

Clonidine Hydrochloride (Concurrent use not recommended). Products include:
Catapres Tablets ... 674
Combipres Tablets ... 677

Deserpidine (Concurrent use not recommended).
No products indexed under this heading.

Desipramine Hydrochloride (Concurrent use not recommended). Products include:
Norpramin Tablets ... 1526

Diazoxide (Concurrent use not recommended). Products include:
Hyperstat I.V. Injection ... 2363
Proglycem ... 580

Diltiazem Hydrochloride (Concurrent use not recommended). Products include:
Cardizem CD Capsules ... 1506
Cardizem SR Capsules ... 1510
Cardizem Injectable ... 1508
Cardizem Tablets ... 1512
Dilacor XR Extended-release Capsules ... 2018

Doxazosin Mesylate (Concurrent use not recommended). Products include:
Cardura Tablets ... 2186

Doxepin Hydrochloride (Concurrent use not recommended). Products include:
Sinequan ... 2205
Zonalon Cream ... 1055

Enalapril Maleate (Concurrent use not recommended). Products include:
Vaseretic Tablets ... 1765
Vasotec Tablets ... 1771

Enalaprilat (Concurrent use not recommended). Products include:
Vasotec I.V. ... 1768

Esmolol Hydrochloride (Concurrent use not recommended). Products include:
Brevibloc Injection ... 1808

Felodipine (Concurrent use not recommended). Products include:
Plendil Extended-Release Tablets ... 527

Fluoxetine Hydrochloride (Concurrent use not recommended). Products include:
Prozac Pulvules & Liquid, Oral Solution ... 919

Fosinopril Sodium (Concurrent use not recommended). Products include:
Monopril Tablets ... 757

Guanabenz Acetate (Concurrent use not recommended).
No products indexed under this heading.

Guanethidine Monosulfate (Concurrent use not recommended). Products include:
Esimil Tablets ... 822
Ismelin Tablets ... 827

Hydralazine Hydrochloride (Concurrent use not recommended). Products include:
Apresazide Capsules ... 808
Apresoline Hydrochloride Tablets ... 809
Ser-Ap-Es Tablets ... 849

Imipramine Hydrochloride (Concurrent use not recommended). Products include:
Tofranil Ampuls ... 854
Tofranil Tablets ... 856

Imipramine Pamoate (Concurrent use not recommended). Products include:
Tofranil-PM Capsules ... 857

Indapamide (Concurrent use not recommended). Products include:
Lozol Tablets ... 2022

Isocarboxazid (Concurrent use not recommended).
No products indexed under this heading.

Isradipine (Concurrent use not recommended). Products include:
DynaCirc Capsules ... 2256

Labetalol Hydrochloride (Concurrent use not recommended). Products include:
Normodyne Injection ... 2377
Normodyne Tablets ... 2379

IMPORTANT NOTE: Always consult each drug listing in the patient's regimen for possible interactions.

Sinutab Sinus Medication — Interactions Index — 960

Trandate 1185

Lisinopril (Concurrent use not recommended). Products include:
- Prinivil Tablets 1733
- Prinzide Tablets 1737
- Zestoretic 2850
- Zestril Tablets 2854

Losartan Potassium (Concurrent use not recommended). Products include:
- Cozaar Tablets 1628
- Hyzaar Tablets 1677

Maprotiline Hydrochloride (Concurrent use not recommended). Products include:
- Ludiomil Tablets 843

Mecamylamine Hydrochloride (Concurrent use not recommended). Products include:
- Inversine Tablets 1686

Methyldopa (Concurrent use not recommended). Products include:
- Aldoclor Tablets 1598
- Aldomet Oral 1600
- Aldoril Tablets 1604

Methyldopate Hydrochloride (Concurrent use not recommended). Products include:
- Aldomet Ester HCl Injection 1602

Metoprolol Succinate (Concurrent use not recommended). Products include:
- Toprol-XL Tablets 565

Metoprolol Tartrate (Concurrent use not recommended). Products include:
- Lopressor Ampuls 830
- Lopressor HCT Tablets 832
- Lopressor Tablets 830

Metyrosine (Concurrent use not recommended). Products include:
- Demser Capsules 1649

Minoxidil (Concurrent use not recommended). Products include:
- Loniten Tablets 2618
- Rogaine Topical Solution 2637

Moexipril Hydrochloride (Concurrent use not recommended). Products include:
- Univasc Tablets 2410

Nadolol (Concurrent use not recommended).
- No products indexed under this heading.

Nefazodone Hydrochloride (Concurrent use not recommended). Products include:
- Serzone Tablets 771

Nicardipine Hydrochloride (Concurrent use not recommended). Products include:
- Cardene Capsules 2095
- Cardene I.V. 2709
- Cardene SR Capsules 2097

Nifedipine (Concurrent use not recommended). Products include:
- Adalat Capsules (10 mg and 20 mg) 587
- Adalat CC 589
- Procardia Capsules 1971
- Procardia XL Extended Release Tablets 1972

Nisoldipine (Concurrent use not recommended).
- No products indexed under this heading.

Nitroglycerin (Concurrent use not recommended). Products include:
- Deponit NTG Transdermal Delivery System 2397
- Nitro-Bid IV 1523
- Nitro-Bid Ointment 1524
- Nitrodisc 2047
- Nitro-Dur (nitroglycerin) Transdermal Infusion System 1326
- Nitrolingual Spray 2027
- Nitrostat Tablets 1925
- Transderm-Nitro Transdermal Therapeutic System 859

Nortriptyline Hydrochloride (Concurrent use not recommended). Products include:
- Pamelor 2280

Paroxetine Hydrochloride (Concurrent use not recommended). Products include:
- Paxil Tablets 2505

Penbutolol Sulfate (Concurrent use not recommended). Products include:
- Levatol 2403

Phenelzine Sulfate (Concurrent use not recommended). Products include:
- Nardil 1920

Phenoxybenzamine Hydrochloride (Concurrent use not recommended). Products include:
- Dibenzyline Capsules 2476

Phentolamine Mesylate (Concurrent use not recommended). Products include:
- Regitine 846

Pindolol (Concurrent use not recommended). Products include:
- Visken Tablets 2299

Prazosin Hydrochloride (Concurrent use not recommended). Products include:
- Minipress Capsules 1937
- Minizide Capsules 1938

Propranolol Hydrochloride (Concurrent use not recommended). Products include:
- Inderal 2728
- Inderal LA Long Acting Capsules 2730
- Inderide Tablets 2732
- Inderide LA Long Acting Capsules .. 2734

Protriptyline Hydrochloride (Concurrent use not recommended). Products include:
- Vivactil Tablets 1774

Quinapril Hydrochloride (Concurrent use not recommended). Products include:
- Accupril Tablets 1893

Ramipril (Concurrent use not recommended). Products include:
- Altace Capsules 1232

Rauwolfia Serpentina (Concurrent use not recommended).
- No products indexed under this heading.

Rescinnamine (Concurrent use not recommended).
- No products indexed under this heading.

Reserpine (Concurrent use not recommended). Products include:
- Diupres Tablets 1650
- Hydropres Tablets 1675
- Ser-Ap-Es Tablets 849

Sertraline Hydrochloride (Concurrent use not recommended). Products include:
- Zoloft Tablets 2217

Sodium Nitroprusside (Concurrent use not recommended).
- No products indexed under this heading.

Sotalol Hydrochloride (Concurrent use not recommended). Products include:
- Betapace Tablets 641

Spirapril Hydrochloride (Concurrent use not recommended).
- No products indexed under this heading.

Terazosin Hydrochloride (Concurrent use not recommended). Products include:
- Hytrin Capsules 430

Timolol Maleate (Concurrent use not recommended). Products include:
- Blocadren Tablets 1614
- Timolide Tablets 1748
- Timoptic in Ocudose 1753
- Timoptic Sterile Ophthalmic Solution 1751
- Timoptic-XE 1755

Torsemide (Concurrent use not recommended). Products include:
- Demadex Tablets and Injection 686

Tranylcypromine Sulfate (Concurrent use not recommended). Products include:
- Parnate Tablets 2503

Trazodone Hydrochloride (Concurrent use not recommended). Products include:
- Desyrel and Desyrel Dividose 503

Trimethaphan Camsylate (Concurrent use not recommended). Products include:
- Arfonad Ampuls 2080

Trimipramine Maleate (Concurrent use not recommended). Products include:
- Surmontil Capsules 2811

Venlafaxine Hydrochloride (Concurrent use not recommended). Products include:
- Effexor 2719

Verapamil Hydrochloride (Concurrent use not recommended). Products include:
- Calan SR Caplets 2422
- Calan Tablets 2419
- Isoptin Injectable 1344
- Isoptin Oral Tablets 1346
- Isoptin SR Tablets 1348
- Verelan Capsules 1410
- Verelan Capsules 2824

SKELAXIN TABLETS

(Metaxalone) 788

None cited in PDR database.

SLEEPINAL NIGHT-TIME SLEEP AID CAPSULES AND SOFTGELS

(Diphenhydramine Hydrochloride) .. ▣ 834

May interact with hypnotics and sedatives, tranquilizers, and certain other agents. Compounds in these categories include:

Alprazolam (Concomitant use is not recommended). Products include:
- Xanax Tablets 2649

Buspirone Hydrochloride (Concomitant use is not recommended). Products include:
- BuSpar 737

Chlordiazepoxide (Concomitant use is not recommended). Products include:
- Libritabs Tablets 2177
- Limbitrol 2180

Chlordiazepoxide Hydrochloride (Concomitant use is not recommended). Products include:
- Librax Capsules 2176
- Librium Capsules 2178
- Librium Injectable 2179

Chlorpromazine (Concomitant use is not recommended). Products include:
- Thorazine Suppositories 2523

Chlorprothixene (Concomitant use is not recommended).
- No products indexed under this heading.

Chlorprothixene Hydrochloride (Concomitant use is not recommended).
- No products indexed under this heading.

Clorazepate Dipotassium (Concomitant use is not recommended). Products include:
- Tranxene 451

Diazepam (Concomitant use is not recommended). Products include:
- Dizac 1809
- Valium Injectable 2182
- Valium Tablets 2183
- Valrelease Capsules 2169

Droperidol (Concomitant use is not recommended). Products include:
- Inapsine Injection 1296

Estazolam (Concomitant use is not recommended). Products include:
- ProSom Tablets 449

Ethchlorvynol (Concomitant use is not recommended). Products include:
- Placidyl Capsules 448

Ethinamate (Concomitant use is not recommended).
- No products indexed under this heading.

Fluphenazine Decanoate (Concomitant use is not recommended). Products include:
- Prolixin Decanoate 509

Fluphenazine Enanthate (Concomitant use is not recommended). Products include:
- Prolixin Enanthate 509

Fluphenazine Hydrochloride (Concomitant use is not recommended). Products include:
- Prolixin 509

Flurazepam Hydrochloride (Concomitant use is not recommended). Products include:
- Dalmane Capsules 2173

Glutethimide (Concomitant use is not recommended).
- No products indexed under this heading.

Haloperidol (Concomitant use is not recommended). Products include:
- Haldol Injection, Tablets and Concentrate 1575

Haloperidol Decanoate (Concomitant use is not recommended). Products include:
- Haldol Decanoate 1577

Hydroxyzine Hydrochloride (Concomitant use is not recommended). Products include:
- Atarax Tablets & Syrup 2185
- Marax Tablets & DF Syrup 2200
- Vistaril Intramuscular Solution 2216

Lorazepam (Concomitant use is not recommended). Products include:
- Ativan Injection 2698
- Ativan Tablets 2700

Loxapine Hydrochloride (Concomitant use is not recommended). Products include:
- Loxitane 1378

Loxapine Succinate (Concomitant use is not recommended). Products include:
- Loxitane Capsules 1378

Meprobamate (Concomitant use is not recommended). Products include:
- Miltown Tablets 2672
- PMB 200 and PMB 400 2783

Mesoridazine Besylate (Concomitant use is not recommended). Products include:
- Serentil 684

Midazolam Hydrochloride (Concomitant use is not recommended). Products include:
- Versed Injection 2170

Molindone Hydrochloride (Concomitant use is not recommended). Products include:
- Moban Tablets and Concentrate 1048

Interactions Index

Oxazepam (Concomitant use is not recommended). Products include:

Serax Capsules 2810
Serax Tablets 2810

Perphenazine (Concomitant use is not recommended). Products include:

Etrafon 2355
Triavil Tablets 1757
Trilafon 2389

Prazepam (Concomitant use is not recommended).

No products indexed under this heading.

Prochlorperazine (Concomitant use is not recommended). Products include:

Compazine 2470

Promethazine Hydrochloride (Concomitant use is not recommended). Products include:

Mepergan Injection 2753
Phenergan with Codeine 2777
Phenergan with Dextromethorphan 2778
Phenergan Injection 2773
Phenergan Suppositories 2775
Phenergan Syrup 2774
Phenergan Tablets 2775
Phenergan VC 2779
Phenergan VC with Codeine 2781

Propofol (Concomitant use is not recommended). Products include:

Diprivan Injection 2833

Quazepam (Concomitant use is not recommended). Products include:

Doral Tablets 2664

Secobarbital Sodium (Concomitant use is not recommended). Products include:

Seconal Sodium Pulvules 1474

Temazepam (Concomitant use is not recommended). Products include:

Restoril Capsules 2284

Thioridazine Hydrochloride (Concomitant use is not recommended). Products include:

Mellaril 2269

Thiothixene (Concomitant use is not recommended). Products include:

Navane Capsules and Concentrate 2201
Navane Intramuscular 2202

Triazolam (Concomitant use is not recommended). Products include:

Halcion Tablets 2611

Trifluoperazine Hydrochloride (Concomitant use is not recommended). Products include:

Stelazine 2514

Zolpidem Tartrate (Concomitant use is not recommended). Products include:

Ambien Tablets 2416

Food Interactions

Alcohol (Avoid alcoholic beverages).

SLO-BID GYROCAPS

(Theophylline Anhydrous) 2033

May interact with sympathomimetic bronchodilators, macrolide antibiotics, oral contraceptives, corticosteroids, thiazides, $beta_2$ agonists, and certain other agents. Compounds in these categories include:

Albuterol (Possible toxic synergism; xanthines can potentiate hypokalemia resulting from $beta_2$ agonist therapy). Products include:

Proventil Inhalation Aerosol 2382
Ventolin Inhalation Aerosol and Refill 1197

Albuterol Sulfate (Possible toxic synergism; xanthines can potentiate hypokalemia resulting from $beta_2$ agonist therapy). Products include:

Airet Solution for Inhalation 452
Proventil Inhalation Solution 0.083% 2384
Proventil Repetabs Tablets 2386
Proventil Solution for Inhalation 0.5% 2383
Proventil Syrup 2385
Proventil Tablets 2386
Ventolin Inhalation Solution 1198
Ventolin Nebules Inhalation Solution 1199
Ventolin Rotacaps for Inhalation 1200
Ventolin Syrup 1202
Ventolin Tablets 1203
Volmax Extended-Release Tablets .. 1788

Allopurinol (Allopurinol in high doses increases serum theophylline levels). Products include:

Zyloprim Tablets 1226

Azithromycin (Increased theophylline serum concentrations). Products include:

Zithromax 1944

Bendroflumethiazide (Xanthines can potentiate hypokalemic effects).

No products indexed under this heading.

Betamethasone Acetate (Xanthines can potentiate hypokalemic effects). Products include:

Celestone Soluspan Suspension 2347

Betamethasone Sodium Phosphate (Xanthines can potentiate hypokalemic effects). Products include:

Celestone Soluspan Suspension 2347

Bitolterol Mesylate (Possible toxic synergism; xanthines can potentiate hypokalemia resulting from $beta_2$ agonist therapy). Products include:

Tornalate Solution for Inhalation, 0.2% 956
Tornalate Metered Dose Inhaler 957

Chlorothiazide (Xanthines can potentiate hypokalemic effects). Products include:

Aldoclor Tablets 1598
Diupres Tablets 1650
Diuril Oral 1653

Chlorothiazide Sodium (Xanthines can potentiate hypokalemic effects). Products include:

Diuril Sodium Intravenous 1652

Cimetidine (Increased theophylline serum concentrations). Products include:

Tagamet Tablets 2516

Cimetidine Hydrochloride (Increased theophylline serum concentrations). Products include:

Tagamet 2516

Ciprofloxacin (Increased serum theophylline levels). Products include:

Cipro I.V. 595
Cipro I.V. Pharmacy Bulk Package.. 597

Ciprofloxacin Hydrochloride (Increased serum theophylline levels). Products include:

Ciloxan Ophthalmic Solution 472
Cipro Tablets 592

Clarithromycin (Increased theophylline serum concentrations). Products include:

Biaxin 405

Cortisone Acetate (Xanthines can potentiate hypokalemic effects). Products include:

Cortone Acetate Sterile Suspension 1623
Cortone Acetate Tablets 1624

Desogestrel (Increased serum theophylline levels). Products include:

Desogen Tablets 1817
Ortho-Cept 1851

Dexamethasone (Xanthines can potentiate hypokalemic effects). Products include:

AK-Trol Ointment & Suspension .... ◎ 205
Decadron Elixir 1633
Decadron Tablets 1635
Decaspray Topical Aerosol 1648
Dexacidin Ointment .... ◎ 263
Maxitrol Ophthalmic Ointment and Suspension .... ◎ 224
TobraDex Ophthalmic Suspension and Ointment 473

Dexamethasone Acetate (Xanthines can potentiate hypokalemic effects). Products include:

Dalalone D.P. Injectable 1011
Decadron-LA Sterile Suspension 1646

Dexamethasone Sodium Phosphate (Xanthines can potentiate hypokalemic effects). Products include:

Decadron Phosphate Injection 1637
Decadron Phosphate Respihaler 1642
Decadron Phosphate Sterile Ophthalmic Ointment 1641
Decadron Phosphate Sterile Ophthalmic Solution 1642
Decadron Phosphate Topical Cream 1644
Decadron Phosphate Turbinaire 1645
Decadron Phosphate with Xylocaine Injection, Sterile 1639
Dexacort Phosphate in Respihaler .. 458
Dexacort Phosphate in Turbinaire .. 459
NeoDecadron Sterile Ophthalmic Ointment 1712
NeoDecadron Sterile Ophthalmic Solution 1713
NeoDecadron Topical Cream 1714

Ephedrine Hydrochloride (Possible toxic synergism; xanthines can potentiate hypokalemia resulting from $beta_2$ agonist therapy). Products include:

Primatene Dual Action Formula ...... ◉ 872
Primatene Tablets .... ◉ 873
Quadrinal Tablets 1350

Ephedrine Sulfate (Possible toxic synergism; xanthines can potentiate hypokalemia resulting from $beta_2$ agonist therapy). Products include:

Bronkaid Caplets .... ◉ 717
Marax Tablets & DF Syrup 2200

Ephedrine Tannate (Possible toxic synergism; xanthines can potentiate hypokalemia resulting from $beta_2$ agonist therapy). Products include:

Rynatuss 2673

Epinephrine (Possible toxic synergism; xanthines can potentiate hypokalemia resulting from $beta_2$ agonist therapy). Products include:

Bronkaid Mist .... ◉ 717
EPIFRIN .... ◎ 239
EpiPen 790
Marcaine Hydrochloride with Epinephrine 1:200,000 2316
Primatene Mist .... ◉ 873
Sensorcaine with Epinephrine Injection 559
Sus-Phrine Injection 1019
Xylocaine with Epinephrine Injections 567

Epinephrine Hydrochloride (Possible toxic synergism; xanthines can potentiate hypokalemia resulting from $beta_2$ agonist therapy). Products include:

Ana-Kit Anaphylaxis Emergency Treatment Kit 617

Erythromycin (Increased theophylline serum concentrations). Products include:

A/T/S 2% Acne Topical Gel and Solution 1234
Benzamycin Topical Gel 905
E-Mycin Tablets 1341
Emgel 2% Topical Gel 1093
ERYC 1915
Erycette (erythromycin 2%) Topical Solution 1888
Ery-Tab Tablets 422
Erythromycin Base Filmtab 426
Erythromycin Delayed-Release Capsules, USP 427
Ilotycin Ophthalmic Ointment 912
PCE Dispertab Tablets 444
T-Stat 2.0% Topical Solution and Pads 2688
Theramycin Z Topical Solution 2% 1592

Erythromycin Estolate (Increased theophylline serum concentrations). Products include:

Ilosone 911

Erythromycin Ethylsuccinate (Increased theophylline serum concentrations). Products include:

E.E.S. 424
EryPed 421

Erythromycin Gluceptate (Increased theophylline serum concentrations). Products include:

Ilotycin Gluceptate, IV, Vials 913

Erythromycin Stearate (Increased theophylline serum concentrations). Products include:

Erythrocin Stearate Filmtab 425

Ethinyl Estradiol (Increased serum theophylline levels). Products include:

Brevicon 2088
Demulen 2428
Desogen Tablets 1817
Levlen/Tri-Levlen 651
Lo/Ovral Tablets 2746
Lo/Ovral-28 Tablets 2751
Modicon 1872
Nordette-21 Tablets 2755
Nordette-28 Tablets 2758
Norinyl 2088
Ortho-Cept 1851
Ortho-Cyclen/Ortho-Tri-Cyclen 1858
Ortho-Novum 1872
Ortho-Cyclen/Ortho Tri-Cyclen 1858
Ovcon 760
Ovral Tablets 2770
Ovral-28 Tablets 2770
Levlen/Tri-Levlen 651
Tri-Norinyl 2164
Triphasil-21 Tablets 2814
Triphasil-28 Tablets 2819

Ethylnorepinephrine Hydrochloride (Possible toxic synergism; xanthines can potentiate hypokalemia resulting from $beta_2$ agonist therapy).

No products indexed under this heading.

Ethynodiol Diacetate (Increased serum theophylline levels). Products include:

Demulen 2428

Fludrocortisone Acetate (Xanthines can potentiate hypokalemic effects). Products include:

Florinef Acetate Tablets 505

Hydrochlorothiazide (Xanthines can potentiate hypokalemic effects). Products include:

Aldactazide 2413
Aldoril Tablets 1604
Apresazide Capsules 808
Capozide 742
Dyazide 2479
Esidrix Tablets 821
Esimil Tablets 822
HydroDIURIL Tablets 1674
Hydropres Tablets 1675
Hyzaar Tablets 1677
Inderide Tablets 2732
Inderide LA Long Acting Capsules .. 2734
Lopressor HCT Tablets 832
Lotensin HCT 837
Maxzide 1380
Moduretic Tablets 1705
Oretic Tablets 443
Prinzide Tablets 1737
Ser-Ap-Es Tablets 849
Timolide Tablets 1748
Vaseretic Tablets 1765
Zestoretic 2850
Ziac 1415

Hydrocortisone (Xanthines can potentiate hypokalemic effects). Products include:

Anusol-HC Cream 2.5% 1896
Aquanil HC Lotion 1931
Bactine Hydrocortisone Anti-Itch Cream .... ◉ 709
Caldecort Anti-Itch Hydrocortisone Spray .... ◉ 631

IMPORTANT NOTE: Always consult each drug listing in the patient's regimen for possible interactions.

Cortaid ◘ 836
CORTENEMA 2535
Cortisporin Ointment 1085
Cortisporin Ophthalmic Ointment Sterile 1085
Cortisporin Ophthalmic Suspension Sterile 1086
Cortisporin Otic Solution Sterile 1087
Cortisporin Otic Suspension Sterile 1088
Cortizone-5 ◘ 831
Cortizone-10 ◘ 831
Hydrocortone Tablets 1672
Hytone 907
Massengill Medicated Soft Cloth Towelettes 2458
PediOtic Suspension Sterile 1153
Preparation H Hydrocortisone 1% Cream ◘ 872
ProctoCream-HC 2.5% 2408
VōSoL HC Otic Solution 2678

Hydrocortisone Acetate (Xanthines can potentiate hypokalemic effects). Products include:
Analpram-HC Rectal Cream 1% and 2.5% 977
Anusol HC-1 Anti-Itch Hydrocortisone Ointment ◘ 847
Anusol-HC Suppositories 1897
Caldecort ◘ 631
Carmol HC 924
Coly-Mycin S Otic w/Neomycin & Hydrocortisone 1906
Cortaid ◘ 836
Cortifoam 2396
Cortisporin Cream 1084
Epifoam 2399
Hydrocortone Acetate Sterile Suspension 1669
Mantadil Cream 1135
Nupercainal Hydrocortisone 1% Cream ◘ 645
Ophthocort ⊙ 311
Pramosone Cream, Lotion & Ointment 978
ProctoCream-HC 2408
ProctoFoam-HC 2409
Terra-Cortril Ophthalmic Suspension 2210

Hydrocortisone Sodium Phosphate (Xanthines can potentiate hypokalemic effects). Products include:
Hydrocortone Phosphate Injection, Sterile 1670

Hydrocortisone Sodium Succinate (Xanthines can potentiate hypokalemic effects). Products include:
Solu-Cortef Sterile Powder 2641

Hydroflumethiazide (Xanthines can potentiate hypokalemic effects). Products include:
Diucardin Tablets 2718

Influenza Virus Vaccine (Decreases theophylline clearance). Products include:
Fluvirin 460
Influenza Virus Vaccine, Trivalent, Types A and B (chromatograph- and filter-purified subviron antigen) FluShield, 1995-1996 Formula 2736

Isoetharine (Possible toxic synergism; xanthines can potentiate hypokalemia resulting from beta$_2$ agonist therapy). Products include:
Bronkometer Aerosol 2302
Bronkosol Solution 2302
Isoetharine Inhalation Solution, USP, Arm-a-Med 551

Isoproterenol Hydrochloride (Possible toxic synergism; xanthines can potentiate hypokalemia resulting from beta$_2$ agonist therapy). Products include:
Isuprel Hydrochloride Injection 1:5000 2311
Isuprel Hydrochloride Solution 1:200 & 1:100 2313
Isuprel Mistometer 2312

Isoproterenol Sulfate (Possible toxic synergism; xanthines can potentiate hypokalemia resulting from beta$_2$ agonist therapy). Products include:
Norisodrine with Calcium Iodide Syrup 442

Levonorgestrel (Increased serum theophylline levels). Products include:
Levlen/Tri-Levlen 651
Nordette-21 Tablets 2755
Nordette-28 Tablets 2758
Norplant System 2759
Levlen/Tri-Levlen 651
Triphasil-21 Tablets 2814
Triphasil-28 Tablets 2819

Lithium Carbonate (Increased excretion of lithium carbonate). Products include:
Eskalith 2485
Lithium Carbonate Capsules & Tablets 2230
Lithonate/Lithotabs/Lithobid 2543

Mestranol (Increased serum theophylline levels). Products include:
Norinyl 2088
Ortho-Novum 1872

Metaproterenol Sulfate (Possible toxic synergism; xanthines can potentiate hypokalemia resulting from beta$_2$ agonist therapy). Products include:
Alupent 669
Metaproterenol Sulfate Inhalation Solution, USP, Arm-a-Med 552

Methyclothiazide (Xanthines can potentiate hypokalemic effects). Products include:
Enduron Tablets 420

Methylprednisolone Acetate (Xanthines can potentiate hypokalemic effects). Products include:
Depo-Medrol Single-Dose Vial 2600
Depo-Medrol Sterile Aqueous Suspension 2597

Methylprednisolone Sodium Succinate (Xanthines can potentiate hypokalemic effects). Products include:
Solu-Medrol Sterile Powder 2643

Norethindrone (Increased serum theophylline levels). Products include:
Brevicon 2088
Micronor Tablets 1872
Modicon 1872
Norinyl 2088
Nor-Q D Tablets 2135
Ortho-Novum 1872
Ovcon 760
Tri-Norinyl 2164

Norethynodrel (Increased serum theophylline levels).
No products indexed under this heading.

Norgestimate (Increased serum theophylline levels). Products include:
Ortho-Cyclen/Ortho-Tri-Cyclen 1858
Ortho-Cyclen/Ortho Tri-Cyclen 1858

Norgestrel (Increased serum theophylline levels). Products include:
Lo/Ovral Tablets 2746
Lo/Ovral-28 Tablets 2751
Ovral Tablets 2770
Ovral-28 Tablets 2770
Ovrette Tablets 2771

Phenytoin (Serum levels of both drugs decreased). Products include:
Dilantin Infatabs 1908
Dilantin-125 Suspension 1911

Phenytoin Sodium (Serum levels of both drugs decreased). Products include:
Dilantin Kapseals 1906
Dilantin Parenteral 1910

Pirbuterol Acetate (Possible toxic synergism; xanthines can potentiate hypokalemia resulting from beta$_2$ agonist therapy). Products include:
Maxair Autohaler 1492
Maxair Inhaler 1494

Polythiazide (Xanthines can potentiate hypokalemic effects). Products include:
Minizide Capsules 1938

Prednisolone Acetate (Xanthines can potentiate hypokalemic effects). Products include:
AK-CIDE ⊙ 202
AK-CIDE Ointment ⊙ 202
Blephamide Liquifilm Sterile Ophthalmic Suspension 476
Blephamide Ointment ⊙ 237
Econopred & Econopred Plus Ophthalmic Suspensions ⊙ 217
Poly-Pred Liquifilm ⊙ 248
Pred Forte ⊙ 250
Pred Mild ⊙ 253
Pred-G Liquifilm Sterile Ophthalmic Suspension ⊙ 251
Pred-G S.O.P. Sterile Ophthalmic Ointment ⊙ 252
Vasocidin Ointment ⊙ 268

Prednisolone Sodium Phosphate (Xanthines can potentiate hypokalemic effects). Products include:
AK-Pred ⊙ 204
Hydeltrasol Injection, Sterile 1665
Inflamase ⊙ 265
Pediapred Oral Liquid 995
Vasocidin Ophthalmic Solution ⊙ 270

Prednisolone Tebutate (Xanthines can potentiate hypokalemic effects). Products include:
Hydeltra-T.B.A. Sterile Suspension 1667

Prednisone (Xanthines can potentiate hypokalemic effects). Products include:
Deltasone Tablets 2595

Propranolol Hydrochloride (Increased theophylline levels). Products include:
Inderal 2728
Inderal LA Long Acting Capsules 2730
Inderide Tablets 2732
Inderide LA Long Acting Capsules 2734

Rifampin (Decreased serum theophylline levels). Products include:
Rifadin 1528
Rifamate Capsules 1530
Rifater 1532
Rimactane Capsules 847

Salmeterol Xinafoate (Possible toxic synergism; xanthines can potentiate hypokalemia resulting from beta$_2$ agonist therapy). Products include:
Serevent Inhalation Aerosol 1176

Terbutaline Sulfate (Possible toxic synergism; xanthines can potentiate hypokalemia resulting from beta$_2$ agonist therapy). Products include:
Brethaire Inhaler 813
Brethine Ampuls 815
Brethine Tablets 814
Bricanyl Subcutaneous Injection 1502
Bricanyl Tablets 1503

Triamcinolone (Xanthines can potentiate hypokalemic effects). Products include:
Aristocort Tablets 1022

Triamcinolone Acetonide (Xanthines can potentiate hypokalemic effects). Products include:
Aristocort A 0.025% Cream 1027
Aristocort A 0.5% Cream 1031
Aristocort A 0.1% Cream 1029
Aristocort A 0.1% Ointment 1030
Azmacort Oral Inhaler 2011
Nasacort Nasal Inhaler 2024

Triamcinolone Diacetate (Xanthines can potentiate hypokalemic effects). Products include:
Aristocort Suspension (Forte Parenteral) 1027
Aristocort Suspension (Intralesional) 1025

Triamcinolone Hexacetonide (Xanthines can potentiate hypokalemic effects). Products include:
Aristospan Suspension (Intra-articular) 1033
Aristospan Suspension (Intralesional) 1032

Troleandomycin (Increased theophylline serum concentrations). Products include:
Tao Capsules 2209

Food Interactions

Diet, high-lipid (Decreases in the rate of absorption, but with no significant difference in the extent of absorption).

SLO-NIACIN TABLETS
(Niacin) 2659
May interact with antihypertensives and lipid-lowering drugs. Compounds in these categories include:

Acebutolol Hydrochloride (Persons taking antihypertensives should contact their physicians before taking niacin because of unspecified interactions). Products include:
Sectral Capsules 2807

Amlodipine Besylate (Persons taking antihypertensives should contact their physicians before taking niacin because of unspecified interactions). Products include:
Lotrel Capsules 840
Norvasc Tablets 1940

Atenolol (Persons taking antihypertensives should contact their physicians before taking niacin because of unspecified interactions). Products include:
Tenoretic Tablets 2845
Tenormin Tablets and I.V. Injection 2847

Benazepril Hydrochloride (Persons taking antihypertensives should contact their physicians before taking niacin because of unspecified interactions). Products include:
Lotensin Tablets 834
Lotensin HCT 837
Lotrel Capsules 840

Bendroflumethiazide (Persons taking antihypertensives should contact their physicians before taking niacin because of unspecified interactions).
No products indexed under this heading.

Betaxolol Hydrochloride (Persons taking antihypertensives should contact their physicians before taking niacin because of unspecified interactions). Products include:
Betoptic Ophthalmic Solution 469
Betoptic S Ophthalmic Suspension 471
Kerlone Tablets 2436

Bisoprolol Fumarate (Persons taking antihypertensives should contact their physicians before taking niacin because of unspecified interactions). Products include:
Zebeta Tablets 1413
Ziac 1415

Captopril (Persons taking antihypertensives should contact their physicians before taking niacin because of unspecified interactions). Products include:
Capoten 739
Capozide 742

Carteolol Hydrochloride (Persons taking antihypertensives should contact their physicians before taking niacin because of unspecified interactions). Products include:
Cartrol Tablets 410
Ocupress Ophthalmic Solution, 1% Sterile ⊙ 309

(◘ Described in PDR For Nonprescription Drugs) (⊙ Described in PDR For Ophthalmology)

Interactions Index — Slo-Niacin

Chlorothiazide (Persons taking antihypertensives should contact their physicians before taking niacin because of unspecified interactions). Products include:

Aldoclor Tablets 1598
Diupres Tablets 1650
Diuril Oral 1653

Chlorothiazide Sodium (Persons taking antihypertensives should contact their physicians before taking niacin because of unspecified interactions). Products include:

Diuril Sodium Intravenous 1652

Chlorthalidone (Persons taking antihypertensives should contact their physicians before taking niacin because of unspecified interactions). Products include:

Combipres Tablets 677
Tenoretic Tablets...................................... 2845
Thalitone 1245

Cholestyramine (Persons taking cholesterol-lowering drugs should contact their physicians before taking niacin because of unspecified interactions). Products include:

Questran Light 769
Questran Powder 770

Clofibrate (Persons taking cholesterol-lowering drugs should contact their physicians before taking niacin because of unspecified interactions). Products include:

Atromid-S Capsules 2701

Clonidine (Persons taking antihypertensives should contact their physicians before taking niacin because of unspecified interactions). Products include:

Catapres-TTS... 675

Clonidine Hydrochloride (Persons taking antihypertensives should contact their physicians before taking niacin because of unspecified interactions). Products include:

Catapres Tablets 674
Combipres Tablets 677

Colestipol Hydrochloride (Persons taking cholesterol-lowering drugs should contact their physicians before taking niacin because of unspecified interactions). Products include:

Colestid Tablets 2591

Deserpidine (Persons taking antihypertensives should contact their physicians before taking niacin because of unspecified interactions).

No products indexed under this heading.

Diazoxide (Persons taking antihypertensives should contact their physicians before taking niacin because of unspecified interactions). Products include:

Hyperstat I.V. Injection 2363
Proglycem... 580

Diltiazem Hydrochloride (Persons taking antihypertensives should contact their physicians before taking niacin because of unspecified interactions). Products include:

Cardizem CD Capsules 1506
Cardizem SR Capsules 1510
Cardizem Injectable 1508
Cardizem Tablets...................................... 1512
Dilacor XR Extended-release Capsules 2018

Doxazosin Mesylate (Persons taking antihypertensives should contact their physicians before taking niacin because of unspecified interactions). Products include:

Cardura Tablets 2186

Enalapril Maleate (Persons taking antihypertensives should contact their physicians before taking niacin because of unspecified interactions). Products include:

Vaseretic Tablets 1765
Vasotec Tablets 1771

Enalaprilat (Persons taking antihypertensives should contact their physicians before taking niacin because of unspecified interactions). Products include:

Vasotec I.V... 1768

Esmolol Hydrochloride (Persons taking antihypertensives should contact their physicians before taking niacin because of unspecified interactions). Products include:

Brevibloc Injection................................... 1808

Felodipine (Persons taking antihypertensives should contact their physicians before taking niacin because of unspecified interactions). Products include:

Plendil Extended-Release Tablets.... 527

Fluvastatin Sodium (Persons taking cholesterol-lowering drugs should contact their physicians before taking niacin because of unspecified interactions). Products include:

Lescol Capsules 2267

Fosinopril Sodium (Persons taking antihypertensives should contact their physicians before taking niacin because of unspecified interactions). Products include:

Monopril Tablets 757

Furosemide (Persons taking antihypertensives should contact their physicians before taking niacin because of unspecified interactions). Products include:

Lasix Injection, Oral Solution and Tablets 1240

Gemfibrozil (Persons taking cholesterol-lowering drugs should contact their physicians before taking niacin because of unspecified interactions). Products include:

Lopid Tablets.. 1917

Guanabenz Acetate (Persons taking antihypertensives should contact their physicians before taking niacin because of unspecified interactions).

No products indexed under this heading.

Guanethidine Monosulfate (Persons taking antihypertensives should contact their physicians before taking niacin because of unspecified interactions). Products include:

Esimil Tablets 822
Ismelin Tablets 827

Hydralazine Hydrochloride (Persons taking antihypertensives should contact their physicians before taking niacin because of unspecified interactions). Products include:

Apresazide Capsules 808
Apresoline Hydrochloride Tablets .. 809
Ser-Ap-Es Tablets 849

Hydrochlorothiazide (Persons taking antihypertensives should contact their physicians before taking niacin because of unspecified interactions). Products include:

Aldactazide... 2413
Aldoril Tablets.. 1604
Apresazide Capsules 808
Capozide 742
Dyazide 2479
Esidrix Tablets 821
Esimil Tablets 822
HydroDIURIL Tablets 1674

Hydropres Tablets.................................... 1675
Hyzaar Tablets 1677
Inderide Tablets 2732
Inderide LA Long Acting Capsules .. 2734
Lopressor HCT Tablets 832
Lotensin HCT... 837
Maxzide 1380
Moduretic Tablets 1705
Oretic Tablets 443
Prinzide Tablets 1737
Ser-Ap-Es Tablets 849
Timolide Tablets....................................... 1748
Vaseretic Tablets 1765
Zestoretic 2850
Ziac 1415

Hydroflumethiazide (Persons taking antihypertensives should contact their physicians before taking niacin because of unspecified interactions). Products include:

Diucardin Tablets..................................... 2718

Indapamide (Persons taking antihypertensives should contact their physicians before taking niacin because of unspecified interactions). Products include:

Lozol Tablets 2022

Isradipine (Persons taking antihypertensives should contact their physicians before taking niacin because of unspecified interactions). Products include:

DynaCirc Capsules 2256

Labetalol Hydrochloride (Persons taking antihypertensives should contact their physicians before taking niacin because of unspecified interactions). Products include:

Normodyne Injection 2377
Normodyne Tablets 2379
Trandate 1185

Levobunolol Hydrochloride (Persons taking antihypertensives should contact their physicians before taking niacin because of unspecified interactions). Products include:

Betagan .... ◉ 233

Lisinopril (Persons taking antihypertensives should contact their physicians before taking niacin because of unspecified interactions). Products include:

Prinivil Tablets 1733
Prinzide Tablets 1737
Zestoretic 2850
Zestril Tablets... 2854

Losartan Potassium (Persons taking antihypertensives should contact their physicians before taking niacin because of unspecified interactions). Products include:

Cozaar Tablets 1628
Hyzaar Tablets 1677

Lovastatin (Persons taking cholesterol-lowering drugs should contact their physicians before taking niacin because of unspecified interactions). Products include:

Mevacor Tablets....................................... 1699

Mecamylamine Hydrochloride (Persons taking antihypertensives should contact their physicians before taking niacin because of unspecified interactions). Products include:

Inversine Tablets 1686

Methyclothiazide (Persons taking antihypertensives should contact their physicians before taking niacin because of unspecified interactions). Products include:

Enduron Tablets....................................... 420

Methyldopa (Persons taking antihypertensives should contact their physicians before taking niacin because of unspecified interactions). Products include:

Aldoclor Tablets 1598
Aldomet Oral 1600
Aldoril Tablets.. 1604

Methyldopate Hydrochloride (Persons taking antihypertensives should contact their physicians before taking niacin because of unspecified interactions). Products include:

Aldomet Ester HCl Injection 1602

Metipranolol Hydrochloride (Persons taking antihypertensives should contact their physicians before taking niacin because of unspecified interactions). Products include:

OptiPranolol (Metipranolol 0.3%) Sterile Ophthalmic Solution.......... ◉ 258

Metolazone (Persons taking antihypertensives should contact their physicians before taking niacin because of unspecified interactions). Products include:

Mykrox Tablets 993
Zaroxolyn Tablets 1000

Metoprolol Succinate (Persons taking antihypertensives should contact their physicians before taking niacin because of unspecified interactions). Products include:

Toprol-XL Tablets 565

Metoprolol Tartrate (Persons taking antihypertensives should contact their physicians before taking niacin because of unspecified interactions). Products include:

Lopressor Ampuls..................................... 830
Lopressor HCT Tablets 832
Lopressor Tablets 830

Metyrosine (Persons taking antihypertensives should contact their physicians before taking niacin because of unspecified interactions). Products include:

Demser Capsules...................................... 1649

Minoxidil (Persons taking antihypertensives should contact their physicians before taking niacin because of unspecified interactions). Products include:

Loniten Tablets... 2618
Rogaine Topical Solution 2637

Moexipril Hydrochloride (Persons taking antihypertensives should contact their physicians before taking niacin because of unspecified interactions). Products include:

Univasc Tablets 2410

Nadolol (Persons taking antihypertensives should contact their physicians before taking niacin because of unspecified interactions).

No products indexed under this heading.

Nicardipine Hydrochloride (Persons taking antihypertensives should contact their physicians before taking niacin because of unspecified interactions). Products include:

Cardene Capsules 2095
Cardene I.V. 2709
Cardene SR Capsules............................... 2097

Nifedipine (Persons taking antihypertensives should contact their physicians before taking niacin because of unspecified interactions). Products include:

Adalat Capsules (10 mg and 20 mg) 587
Adalat CC 589
Procardia Capsules................................... 1971
Procardia XL Extended Release Tablets 1972

Nisoldipine (Persons taking antihypertensives should contact their physicians before taking niacin because of unspecified interactions).

No products indexed under this heading.

IMPORTANT NOTE: Always consult each drug listing in the patient's regimen for possible interactions.

Slo-Niacin Interactions Index 964

Nitroglycerin (Persons taking antihypertensives should contact their physicians before taking niacin because of unspecified interactions). Products include:
Deponit NTG Transdermal Delivery System ... 2397
Nitro-Bid IV ... 1523
Nitro-Bid Ointment ... 1524
Nitrodisc ... 2047
Nitro-Dur (nitroglycerin) Transdermal Infusion System ... 1326
Nitrolingual Spray ... 2027
Nitrostat Tablets ... 1925
Transderm-Nitro Transdermal Therapeutic System ... 859

Penbutolol Sulfate (Persons taking antihypertensives should contact their physicians before taking niacin because of unspecified interactions). Products include:
Levatol ... 2403

Phenoxybenzamine Hydrochloride (Persons taking antihypertensives should contact their physicians before taking niacin because of unspecified interactions). Products include:
Dibenzyline Capsules ... 2476

Phentolamine Mesylate (Persons taking antihypertensives should contact their physicians before taking niacin because of unspecified interactions). Products include:
Regitine ... 846

Pindolol (Persons taking antihypertensives should contact their physicians before taking niacin because of unspecified interactions). Products include:
Visken Tablets ... 2299

Polythiazide (Persons taking antihypertensives should contact their physicians before taking niacin because of unspecified interactions). Products include:
Minizide Capsules ... 1938

Pravastatin Sodium (Persons taking cholesterol-lowering drugs should contact their physicians before taking niacin because of unspecified interactions). Products include:
Pravachol ... 765

Prazosin Hydrochloride (Persons taking antihypertensives should contact their physicians before taking niacin because of unspecified interactions). Products include:
Minipress Capsules ... 1937
Minizide Capsules ... 1938

Probucol (Persons taking cholesterol-lowering drugs should contact their physicians before taking niacin because of unspecified interactions). Products include:
Lorelco Tablets ... 1517

Propranolol Hydrochloride (Persons taking antihypertensives should contact their physicians before taking niacin because of unspecified interactions). Products include:
Inderal ... 2728
Inderal LA Long Acting Capsules ... 2730
Inderide Tablets ... 2732
Inderide LA Long Acting Capsules ... 2734

Quinapril Hydrochloride (Persons taking antihypertensives should contact their physicians before taking niacin because of unspecified interactions). Products include:
Accupril Tablets ... 1893

Ramipril (Persons taking antihypertensives should contact their physicians before taking niacin because of unspecified interactions). Products include:
Altace Capsules ... 1232

Rauwolfia Serpentina (Persons taking antihypertensives should contact their physicians before taking niacin because of unspecified interactions).
No products indexed under this heading.

Rescinnamine (Persons taking antihypertensives should contact their physicians before taking niacin because of unspecified interactions).
No products indexed under this heading.

Reserpine (Persons taking antihypertensives should contact their physicians before taking niacin because of unspecified interactions). Products include:
Diupres Tablets ... 1650
Hydropres Tablets ... 1675
Ser-Ap-Es Tablets ... 849

Simvastatin (Persons taking cholesterol-lowering drugs should contact their physicians before taking niacin because of unspecified interactions). Products include:
Zocor Tablets ... 1775

Sodium Nitroprusside (Persons taking antihypertensives should contact their physicians before taking niacin because of unspecified interactions).
No products indexed under this heading.

Sotalol Hydrochloride (Persons taking antihypertensives should contact their physicians before taking niacin because of unspecified interactions). Products include:
Betapace Tablets ... 641

Spirapril Hydrochloride (Persons taking antihypertensives should contact their physicians before taking niacin because of unspecified interactions).
No products indexed under this heading.

Terazosin Hydrochloride (Persons taking antihypertensives should contact their physicians before taking niacin because of unspecified interactions). Products include:
Hytrin Capsules ... 430

Timolol Maleate (Persons taking antihypertensives should contact their physicians before taking niacin because of unspecified interactions). Products include:
Blocadren Tablets ... 1614
Timolide Tablets ... 1748
Timoptic in Ocudose ... 1753
Timoptic Sterile Ophthalmic Solution ... 1751
Timoptic-XE ... 1755

Torsemide (Persons taking antihypertensives should contact their physicians before taking niacin because of unspecified interactions). Products include:
Demadex Tablets and Injection ... 686

Trimethaphan Camsylate (Persons taking antihypertensives should contact their physicians before taking niacin because of unspecified interactions). Products include:
Arfonad Ampuls ... 2080

Verapamil Hydrochloride (Persons taking antihypertensives should contact their physicians before taking niacin because of unspecified interactions). Products include:
Calan SR Caplets ... 2422
Calan Tablets ... 2419
Isoptin Injectable ... 1344
Isoptin Oral Tablets ... 1346
Isoptin SR Tablets ... 1348
Verelan Capsules ... 1410
Verelan Capsules ... 2824

SLOW FE TABLETS

(Ferrous Sulfate) ... 869
May interact with tetracyclines. Compounds in this category include:

Demeclocycline Hydrochloride (Absorption of oral tetracycline impaired). Products include:
Declomycin Tablets ... 1371

Doxycycline Calcium (Absorption of oral tetracycline impaired). Products include:
Vibramycin Calcium Oral Suspension Syrup ... 1941

Doxycycline Hyclate (Absorption of oral tetracycline impaired). Products include:
Doryx Capsules ... 1913
Vibramycin Hyclate Capsules ... 1941
Vibramycin Hyclate Intravenous ... 2215
Vibra-Tabs Film Coated Tablets ... 1941

Doxycycline Monohydrate (Absorption of oral tetracycline impaired). Products include:
Monodox Capsules ... 1805
Vibramycin Monohydrate for Oral Suspension ... 1941

Methacycline Hydrochloride (Absorption of oral tetracycline impaired).
No products indexed under this heading.

Minocycline Hydrochloride (Absorption of oral tetracycline impaired). Products include:
Dynacin Capsules ... 1590
Minocin Intravenous ... 1382
Minocin Oral Suspension ... 1385
Minocin Pellet-Filled Capsules ... 1383

Oxytetracycline (Absorption of oral tetracycline impaired). Products include:
Terramycin Intramuscular Solution 2210

Oxytetracycline Hydrochloride (Absorption of oral tetracycline impaired). Products include:
TERAK Ointment ... ⊙ 209
Terra-Cortril Ophthalmic Suspension ... 2210
Terramycin with Polymyxin B Sulfate Ophthalmic Ointment ... 2211
Urobiotic-250 Capsules ... 2214

Tetracycline Hydrochloride (Absorption of oral tetracycline impaired). Products include:
Achromycin V Capsules ... 1367

SLOW FE WITH FOLIC ACID

(Ferrous Sulfate, Folic Acid) ... 869
May interact with tetracyclines. Compounds in this category include:

Demeclocycline Hydrochloride (Oral iron products interfere with oral absorption of tetracycline; do not take within two hours of each other). Products include:
Declomycin Tablets ... 1371

Doxycycline Calcium (Oral iron products interfere with oral absorption of tetracycline; do not take within two hours of each other). Products include:
Vibramycin Calcium Oral Suspension Syrup ... 1941

Doxycycline Hyclate (Oral iron products interfere with oral absorption of tetracycline; do not take within two hours of each other). Products include:
Doryx Capsules ... 1913
Vibramycin Hyclate Capsules ... 1941
Vibramycin Hyclate Intravenous ... 2215
Vibra-Tabs Film Coated Tablets ... 1941

Doxycycline Monohydrate (Oral iron products interfere with oral absorption of tetracycline; do not take within two hours of each other). Products include:
Monodox Capsules ... 1805
Vibramycin Monohydrate for Oral Suspension ... 1941

Methacycline Hydrochloride (Oral iron products interfere with oral absorption of tetracycline; do not take within two hours of each other).
No products indexed under this heading.

Minocycline Hydrochloride (Oral iron products interfere with oral absorption of tetracycline; do not take within two hours of each other). Products include:
Dynacin Capsules ... 1590
Minocin Intravenous ... 1382
Minocin Oral Suspension ... 1385
Minocin Pellet-Filled Capsules ... 1383

Oxytetracycline Hydrochloride (Oral iron products interfere with oral absorption of tetracycline; do not take within two hours of each other). Products include:
TERAK Ointment ... ⊙ 209
Terra-Cortril Ophthalmic Suspension ... 2210
Terramycin with Polymyxin B Sulfate Ophthalmic Ointment ... 2211
Urobiotic-250 Capsules ... 2214

Tetracycline Hydrochloride (Oral iron products interfere with oral absorption of tetracycline; do not take within two hours of each other). Products include:
Achromycin V Capsules ... 1367

SLOW-K EXTENDED-RELEASE TABLETS

(Potassium Chloride) ... 851
May interact with potassium sparing diuretics. Compounds in this category include:

Amiloride Hydrochloride (Hyperkalemia). Products include:
Midamor Tablets ... 1703
Moduretic Tablets ... 1705

Spironolactone (Hyperkalemia). Products include:
Aldactazide ... 2413
Aldactone ... 2414

Triamterene (Hyperkalemia). Products include:
Dyazide ... 2479
Dyrenium Capsules ... 2481
Maxzide ... 1380

SODIUM CHLORIDE AND STERILE WATER FOR INHALATION, ARM-A-VIAL

(Sodium Chloride) ... 562
None cited in PDR database.

SODIUM POLYSTYRENE SULFONATE SUSPENSION

(Sodium Polystyrene Sulfonate) ... 2244
May interact with cardiac glycosides, antacids containing aluminium, calcium and magnesium, and certain other agents. Compounds in these categories include:

Aluminum Carbonate Gel (Potential for systemic alkalosis). Products include:
Basaljel ... 2703

Aluminum Hydroxide (Potential for systemic alkalosis). Products include:
ALternaGEL Liquid ... 1316
Maximum Strength Ascriptin ... ▣ 630
Cama Arthritis Pain Reliever ... ▣ 785
Gaviscon Extra Strength Relief Formula Antacid Tablets ... ▣ 819
Gaviscon Extra Strength Relief Formula Liquid Antacid ... ▣ 819
Gaviscon Liquid Antacid ... ▣ 820
Gelusil Liquid & Tablets ... ▣ 855
Maalox Heartburn Relief Suspension ... ▣ 642
Maalox Heartburn Relief Tablets ... ▣ 641

(▣ Described in PDR For Nonprescription Drugs) (⊙ Described in PDR For Ophthalmology)

Maalox Magnesia and Alumina Oral Suspension ....ⓐⓓ 642
Maalox Plus Tablets .... ⓐⓓ 643
Extra Strength Maalox Antacid Plus Antigas Liquid and Tablets ⓐⓓ 638
Tempo Soft Antacid .... ⓐⓓ 835

Aluminum Hydroxide Gel (Potential for systemic alkalosis). Products include:

ALternaGEL Liquid .... ⓐⓓ 659
Aludrox Oral Suspension 2695
Amphojel Suspension 2695
Amphojel Suspension without Flavor 2695
Amphojel Tablets 2695
Arthritis Pain Ascriptin .... ⓐⓓ 631
Regular Strength Ascriptin Tablets .... ⓐⓓ 629
Gaviscon Antacid Tablets...................... ⓐⓓ 819
Gaviscon-2 Antacid Tablets .... ⓐⓓ 820
Mylanta Liquid 1317
Mylanta Tablets .... ⓐⓓ 660
Mylanta Double Strength Liquid 1317
Mylanta Double Strength Tablets . ⓐⓓ 660
Nephrox Suspension .... ⓐⓓ 655

Aluminum Hydroxide Gel, Dried (Potential for systemic alkalosis).

Deslanoside (Potential for digitalis toxicity exaggerated by hypokalemia).

No products indexed under this heading.

Digitoxin (Potential for digitalis toxicity exaggerated by hypokalemia). Products include:

Crystodigin Tablets 1433

Digoxin (Potential for digitalis toxicity exaggerated by hypokalemia). Products include:

Lanoxicaps 1117
Lanoxin Elixir Pediatric 1120
Lanoxin Injection 1123
Lanoxin Injection Pediatric................... 1126
Lanoxin Tablets 1128

Dihydroxyaluminum Sodium Carbonate (Potential for systemic alkalosis).

No products indexed under this heading.

Magaldrate (Potential for systemic alkalosis).

No products indexed under this heading.

Magnesium Hydroxide (Should not be administered concomitantly; potential for systemic alkalosis; one case of grand mal seizure has been reported). Products include:

Aludrox Oral Suspension 2695
Arthritis Pain Ascriptin .... ⓐⓓ 631
Maximum Strength Ascriptin .... ⓐⓓ 630
Regular Strength Ascriptin Tablets .... ⓐⓓ 629
Di-Gel Antacid/Anti-Gas .... ⓐⓓ 801
Gelusil Liquid & Tablets .... ⓐⓓ 855
Maalox Magnesia and Alumina Oral Suspension .... ⓐⓓ 642
Maalox Plus Tablets .... ⓐⓓ 643
Extra Strength Maalox Antacid Plus Antigas Liquid and Tablets ⓐⓓ 638
Mylanta Calcium Carbonate and Magnesium Hydroxide Tablets....... 1318
Mylanta Liquid 1317
Mylanta Tablets .... ⓐⓓ 660
Mylanta Double Strength Liquid 1317
Mylanta Double Strength Tablets.. ⓐⓓ 660
Phillips' Milk of Magnesia Liquid.. ⓐⓓ 729
Rolaids Tablets .... ⓐⓓ 843
Tempo Soft Antacid .... ⓐⓓ 835

Magnesium Oxide (Potential for systemic alkalosis). Products include:

Beelith Tablets 639
Bufferin Analgesic Tablets and Caplets .... ⓐⓓ 613
Caltrate PLUS .... ⓐⓓ 665
Cama Arthritis Pain Reliever................ ⓐⓓ 785
Mag-Ox 400 668
Uro-Mag... 668

SODIUM SULAMYD OPHTHALMIC OINTMENT 10%-STERILE

(Sulfacetamide Sodium) 2387
None cited in PDR database.

SODIUM SULAMYD OPHTHALMIC SOLUTION 10%-STERILE

(Sulfacetamide Sodium) 2387
None cited in PDR database.

SODIUM SULAMYD OPHTHALMIC SOLUTION 30%-STERILE

(Sulfacetamide Sodium) 2387
None cited in PDR database.

SOLAQUIN FORTE 4% CREAM

(Hydroquinone) 1252
None cited in PDR database.

SOLAQUIN FORTE 4% GEL

(Hydroquinone) 1252
None cited in PDR database.

SOLATENE CAPSULES

(Beta Carotene) 2150
May interact with:

Vitamin A (Patients should avoid supplementary Vitamin A intake). Products include:

Aquasol A Vitamin A Capsules, USP 534
Aquasol A Parenteral 534
Materna Tablets 1379
Megadose 512
Nature Made Antioxidant Formula ⓐⓓ 748
One-A-Day Extras Antioxidant .... ⓐⓓ 728
Theragran Antioxidant........................... ⓐⓓ 623
Zymacap Capsules .... ⓐⓓ 772

SOLBAR PF 15 CREAM (PABA FREE)

(Octyl Methoxycinnamate, Oxybenzone)..1932
None cited in PDR database.

SOLBAR PF 15 LIQUID (PABA FREE)

(Octyl Methoxycinnamate, Oxybenzone)..1932
None cited in PDR database.

SOLBAR PF ULTRA CREAM SPF 50 (PABA FREE)

(Oxybenzone)..1932
None cited in PDR database.

SOLBAR PF ULTRA LIQUID SPF 30

(Octyl Methoxycinnamate, Oxybenzone)..1932
None cited in PDR database.

SOLGANAL SUSPENSION

(Aurothioglucose) 2388
May interact with antimalarials, immunosuppressive agents, and certain other agents. Compounds in these categories include:

Azathioprine (Safety of coadministration has not been established). Products include:

Imuran 1110

Chloroquine Hydrochloride (Concurrent use is contraindicated). Products include:

Aralen Hydrochloride Injection 2301

Chloroquine Phosphate (Concurrent use is contraindicated). Products include:

Aralen Phosphate Tablets 2301

Cyclosporine (Safety of coadministration has not been established). Products include:

Neoral 2276
Sandimmune 2286

Immune Globulin (Human) (Safety of coadministration has not been established).

No products indexed under this heading.

Immune Globulin Intravenous (Human) (Safety of coadministration has not been established).

Mefloquine Hydrochloride (Concurrent use is contraindicated). Products include:

Lariam Tablets 2128

Muromonab-CD3 (Safety of coadministration has not been established). Products include:

Orthoclone OKT3 Sterile Solution .. 1837

Mycophenolate Mofetil (Safety of coadministration has not been established). Products include:

CellCept Capsules 2099

Penicillamine (Concurrent use is contraindicated). Products include:

Cuprimine Capsules 1630
Depen Titratable Tablets 2662

Pyrimethamine (Concurrent use is contraindicated). Products include:

Daraprim Tablets..................................... 1090
Fansidar Tablets...................................... 2114

Tacrolimus (Safety of coadministration has not been established). Products include:

Prograf 1042

SOLU-CORTEF STERILE POWDER

(Hydrocortisone Sodium Succinate) ..2641
May interact with oral anticoagulants and certain other agents. Compounds in these categories include:

Aspirin (Increased clearance of chronic high dose aspirin leading to decreased salicylate serum levels or increase the risk of salicylate toxicity when corticosteroid is withdrawn). Products include:

Alka-Seltzer Effervescent Antacid and Pain Reliever .... ⓐⓓ 701
Alka-Seltzer Extra Strength Effervescent Antacid and Pain Reliever .... ⓐⓓ 703
Alka-Seltzer Lemon Lime Effervescent Antacid and Pain Reliever .... ⓐⓓ 703
Alka-Seltzer Plus Cold Medicine .... ⓐⓓ 705
Alka-Seltzer Plus Cold & Cough Medicine .... ⓐⓓ 708
Alka-Seltzer Plus Night-Time Cold Medicine .... ⓐⓓ 707
Alka Seltzer Plus Sinus Medicine .. ⓐⓓ 707
Arthritis Foundation Safety Coated Aspirin Tablets .... ⓐⓓ 675
Arthritis Pain Ascriptin .... ⓐⓓ 631
Maximum Strength Ascriptin .... ⓐⓓ 630
Regular Strength Ascriptin Tablets .... ⓐⓓ 629
Arthritis Strength BC Powder........... ⓐⓓ 609
BC Cold Powder Multi-Symptom Formula (Cold-Sinus-Allergy) ...... ⓐⓓ 609
BC Cold Powder Non-Drowsy Formula (Cold-Sinus) .... ⓐⓓ 609
BC Powder .... ⓐⓓ 609
Bayer Children's Chewable Aspirin .... ⓐⓓ 711
Genuine Bayer Aspirin Tablets & Caplets .... ⓐⓓ 713
Extra Strength Bayer Arthritis Pain Regimen Formula .... ⓐⓓ 711
Extra Strength Bayer Aspirin Caplets & Tablets .... ⓐⓓ 712
Extended-Release Bayer 8-Hour Aspirin .... ⓐⓓ 712
Extra Strength Bayer Plus Aspirin Caplets .... ⓐⓓ 713
Extra Strength Bayer PM Aspirin .. ⓐⓓ 713
Bayer Enteric Aspirin .... ⓐⓓ 709
Bufferin Analgesic Tablets and Caplets .... ⓐⓓ 613
Arthritis Strength Bufferin Analgesic Caplets .... ⓐⓓ 614
Extra Strength Bufferin Analgesic Tablets .... ⓐⓓ 615
Cama Arthritis Pain Reliever............... ⓐⓓ 785
Darvon Compound-65 Pulvules 1435
Easprin 1914
Ecotrin 2455
Ecotrin Enteric Coated Aspirin Maximum Strength Tablets and Caplets .... ⓐⓓ 816
Ecotrin Enteric Coated Aspirin Regular Strength Tablets 2455
Empirin Aspirin Tablets .... ⓐⓓ 854
Empirin with Codeine Tablets............. 1093
Excedrin Extra-Strength Analgesic Tablets & Caplets 732
Fiorinal Capsules 2261
Fiorinal with Codeine Capsules 2262
Fiorinal Tablets 2261
Halfprin 1362
Healthprin Aspirin 2455
Norgesic... 1496
Percodan Tablets..................................... 939
Percodan-Demi Tablets.......................... 940
Robaxisal Tablets.................................... 2071
Soma Compound w/Codeine Tablets 2676
Soma Compound Tablets...................... 2675
St. Joseph Adult Chewable Aspirin (81 mg.) .... ⓐⓓ 808
Talwin Compound 2335
Ursinus Inlay-Tabs.................................. ⓐⓓ 794
Vanquish Analgesic Caplets .... ⓐⓓ 731

Dicumarol (Potential for variable effect; concurrent use may result in enhanced as well as diminished effects of anticoagulant).

No products indexed under this heading.

Immunization (Possible neurological complications; lack of antibody response).

Ketoconazole (May inhibit the metabolism of corticosteroid and thus decrease its clearance; the dose of corticosteroid should be titrated to avoid toxicity). Products include:

Nizoral 2% Cream 1297
Nizoral 2% Shampoo.............................. 1298
Nizoral Tablets 1298

Phenobarbital (Increases clearance of corticosteroid and may require increase in dose of corticosteroid to achieve the desired response). Products include:

Arco-Lase Plus Tablets 512
Bellergal-S Tablets 2250
Donnatal 2060
Donnatal Extentabs................................. 2061
Donnatal Tablets 2060
Phenobarbital Elixir and Tablets 1469
Quadrinal Tablets 1350

Phenytoin (Increases clearance of corticosteroid and may require increase in dose of corticosteroid to achieve the desired response). Products include:

Dilantin Infatabs 1908
Dilantin-125 Suspension 1911

Phenytoin Sodium (Increases clearance of corticosteroid and may require increase in dose of corticosteroid to achieve the desired response). Products include:

Dilantin Kapseals 1906
Dilantin Parenteral 1910

Rifampin (Increases clearance of corticosteroid and may require increase in dose of corticosteroid to achieve the desired response). Products include:

Rifadin 1528
Rifamate Capsules 1530
Rifater.. 1532
Rimactane Capsules 847

Smallpox Vaccine (Possible neurological complications; lack of antibody response).

IMPORTANT NOTE: Always consult each drug listing in the patient's regimen for possible interactions.

Solu-Cortef Interactions Index 966

Troleandomycin (May inhibit the metabolism of corticosteroid and thus decrease its clearance; the dose of corticosteroid should be titrated to avoid toxicity). Products include:
Tao Capsules 2209
Warfarin Sodium (Potential for variable effect; concurrent use may result in enhanced as well as diminished effects of anticoagulant). Products include:
Coumadin 926

SOLU-MEDROL STERILE POWDER
(Methylprednisolone Sodium Succinate) 2643
May interact with:

Aspirin (Increased clearance of chronic high dose aspirin leading to decreased salicylate serum levels or increase the risk of salicylate toxicity when methylprednisolone is withdrawn). Products include:
Alka-Seltzer Effervescent Antacid and Pain Reliever .... ◘ 701
Alka-Seltzer Extra Strength Effervescent Antacid and Pain Reliever .... ◘ 703
Alka-Seltzer Lemon Lime Effervescent Antacid and Pain Reliever .... ◘ 703
Alka-Seltzer Plus Cold Medicine .... ◘ 705
Alka-Seltzer Plus Cold & Cough Medicine .... ◘ 708
Alka-Seltzer Plus Night-Time Cold Medicine .... ◘ 707
Alka Seltzer Plus Sinus Medicine .... ◘ 707
Arthritis Foundation Safety Coated Aspirin Tablets .... ◘ 675
Arthritis Pain Ascriptin .... ◘ 631
Maximum Strength Ascriptin .... ◘ 630
Regular Strength Ascriptin Tablets .... ◘ 629
Arthritis Strength BC Powder .... ◘ 609
BC Cold Powder Multi-Symptom Formula (Cold-Sinus-Allergy) .... ◘ 609
BC Cold Powder Non-Drowsy Formula (Cold-Sinus) .... ◘ 609
BC Powder .... ◘ 609
Bayer Children's Chewable Aspirin .... ◘ 711
Genuine Bayer Aspirin Tablets & Caplets .... ◘ 713
Extra Strength Bayer Arthritis Pain Regimen Formula .... ◘ 711
Extra Strength Bayer Aspirin Caplets & Tablets .... ◘ 712
Extended-Release Bayer 8-Hour Aspirin .... ◘ 712
Extra Strength Bayer Plus Aspirin Caplets .... ◘ 713
Extra Strength Bayer PM Aspirin .... ◘ 713
Bayer Enteric Aspirin .... ◘ 709
Bufferin Analgesic Tablets and Caplets .... ◘ 613
Arthritis Strength Bufferin Analgesic Caplets .... ◘ 614
Extra Strength Bufferin Analgesic Tablets .... ◘ 615
Cama Arthritis Pain Reliever .... ◘ 785
Darvon Compound-65 Pulvules 1435
Easprin 1914
Ecotrin 2455
Ecotrin Enteric Coated Aspirin Maximum Strength Tablets and Caplets .... ◘ 816
Ecotrin Enteric Coated Aspirin Regular Strength Tablets 2455
Empirin Aspirin Tablets .... ◘ 854
Empirin with Codeine Tablets 1093
Excedrin Extra-Strength Analgesic Tablets & Caplets 732
Fiorinal Capsules 2261
Fiorinal with Codeine Capsules 2262
Fiorinal Tablets 2261
Halfprin 1362
Healthprin Aspirin 2455
Norgesic 1496
Percodan Tablets 939
Percodan-Demi Tablets 940
Robaxisal Tablets 2071
Soma Compound w/Codeine Tablets 2676
Soma Compound Tablets 2675
St. Joseph Adult Chewable Aspirin (81 mg.) .... ◘ 808
Talwin Compound 2335
Ursinus Inlay-Tabs .... ◘ 794
Vanquish Analgesic Caplets .... ◘ 731
Cyclosporine (Potential for convulsions; mutual inhibition of metabolism). Products include:
Neoral 2276
Sandimmune 2286
Dicumarol (Potential for variable effect; concurrent use may result in enhanced as well as diminished effects of anticoagulant).
No products indexed under this heading.
Immunization (Possible neurological complications; lack of antibody response).
Ketoconazole (May inhibit the metabolism of methylprednisolone and thus decrease its clearance; the dose of methylprednisolone should be titrated to avoid toxicity). Products include:
Nizoral 2% Cream 1297
Nizoral 2% Shampoo 1298
Nizoral Tablets 1298
Phenobarbital (Increases clearance of methylprednisolone and may require increase in dose of methylprednisolone to achieve the desired response). Products include:
Arco-Lase Plus Tablets 512
Bellergal-S Tablets 2250
Donnatal 2060
Donnatal Extentabs 2061
Donnatal Tablets 2060
Phenobarbital Elixir and Tablets 1469
Quadrinal Tablets 1350
Phenytoin (Increases clearance of methylprednisolone and may require increase in dose of methylprednisolone to achieve the desired response). Products include:
Dilantin Infatabs 1908
Dilantin-125 Suspension 1911
Phenytoin Sodium (Increases clearance of methylprednisolone and may require increase in dose of methylprednisolone to achieve the desired response). Products include:
Dilantin Kapseals 1906
Dilantin Parenteral 1910
Rifampin (Increases clearance of methylprednisolone and may require increase in dose of methylprednisolone to achieve the desired response). Products include:
Rifadin 1528
Rifamate Capsules 1530
Rifater 1532
Rimactane Capsules 847
Smallpox Vaccine (Possible neurological complications; lack of antibody response).
Troleandomycin (May inhibit the metabolism of methylprednisolone and thus decrease its clearance; the dose of methylprednisolone should be titrated to avoid toxicity). Products include:
Tao Capsules 2209
Warfarin Sodium (Potential for variable effect; concurrent use may result in enhanced as well as diminished effects of anticoagulant). Products include:
Coumadin 926

SOMA COMPOUND W/CODEINE TABLETS
(Carisoprodol, Aspirin, Codeine Phosphate) 2676
May interact with central nervous system depressants, psychotropics, oral anticoagulants, oral hypoglycemic agents, antacids, corticosteroids, and certain other agents. Compounds in these categories include:

Acarbose (Possible enhancement of hypoglycemia).
No products indexed under this heading.
Alfentanil Hydrochloride (Additive effects). Products include:
Alfenta Injection 1286
Alprazolam (Additive effects). Products include:
Xanax Tablets 2649
Aluminum Carbonate Gel (May substantially decrease plasma salicylate concentration). Products include:
Basaljel 2703
Aluminum Hydroxide (May substantially decrease plasma salicylate concentration). Products include:
ALternaGEL Liquid 1316
Maximum Strength Ascriptin .... ◘ 630
Cama Arthritis Pain Reliever .... ◘ 785
Gaviscon Extra Strength Relief Formula Antacid Tablets .... ◘ 819
Gaviscon Extra Strength Relief Formula Liquid Antacid .... ◘ 819
Gaviscon Liquid Antacid .... ◘ 820
Gelusil Liquid & Tablets .... ◘ 855
Maalox Heartburn Relief Suspension .... ◘ 642
Maalox Heartburn Relief Tablets .... ◘ 641
Maalox Magnesia and Alumina Oral Suspension .... ◘ 642
Maalox Plus Tablets .... ◘ 643
Extra Strength Maalox Antacid Plus Antigas Liquid and Tablets .... ◘ 638
Tempo Soft Antacid .... ◘ 835
Aluminum Hydroxide Gel (May substantially decrease plasma salicylate concentration). Products include:
ALternaGEL Liquid .... ◘ 659
Aludrox Oral Suspension 2695
Amphojel Suspension 2695
Amphojel Suspension without Flavor 2695
Amphojel Tablets 2695
Arthritis Pain Ascriptin .... ◘ 631
Regular Strength Ascriptin Tablets .... ◘ 629
Gaviscon Antacid Tablets .... ◘ 819
Gaviscon-2 Antacid Tablets .... ◘ 820
Mylanta Liquid 1317
Mylanta Tablets .... ◘ 660
Mylanta Double Strength Liquid 1317
Mylanta Double Strength Tablets .... ◘ 660
Nephrox Suspension .... ◘ 655
Aluminum Hydroxide Gel, Dried (May substantially decrease plasma salicylate concentration).
Amitriptyline Hydrochloride (Additive effects). Products include:
Elavil 2838
Endep Tablets 2174
Etrafon 2355
Limbitrol 2180
Triavil Tablets 1757
Ammonium Chloride (Elevated plasma salicylate concentrations).
No products indexed under this heading.
Amoxapine (Additive effects). Products include:
Asendin Tablets 1369
Aprobarbital (Additive effects).
No products indexed under this heading.
Betamethasone Acetate (May decrease salicylate plasma levels). Products include:
Celestone Soluspan Suspension 2347
Betamethasone Sodium Phosphate (May decrease salicylate plasma levels). Products include:
Celestone Soluspan Suspension 2347
Buprenorphine (Additive effects). Products include:
Buprenex Injectable 2006
Buspirone Hydrochloride (Additive effects). Products include:
BuSpar 737
Butabarbital (Additive effects).
No products indexed under this heading.
Butalbital (Additive effects). Products include:
Esgic-plus Tablets 1013
Fioricet Tablets 2258
Fioricet with Codeine Capsules 2260
Fiorinal Capsules 2261
Fiorinal with Codeine Capsules 2262
Fiorinal Tablets 2261
Phrenilin 785
Sedapap Tablets 50 mg/650 mg 1543
Chlordiazepoxide (Additive effects). Products include:
Libritabs Tablets 2177
Limbitrol 2180
Chlordiazepoxide Hydrochloride (Additive effects). Products include:
Librax Capsules 2176
Librium Capsules 2178
Librium Injectable 2179
Chlorpromazine (Additive effects). Products include:
Thorazine Suppositories 2523
Chlorpropamide (Possible enhancement of hypoglycemia). Products include:
Diabinese Tablets 1935
Chlorprothixene (Additive effects).
No products indexed under this heading.
Chlorprothixene Hydrochloride (Additive effects).
No products indexed under this heading.
Clorazepate Dipotassium (Additive effects). Products include:
Tranxene 451
Clozapine (Additive effects). Products include:
Clozaril Tablets 2252
Cortisone Acetate (May decrease salicylate plasma levels). Products include:
Cortone Acetate Sterile Suspension 1623
Cortone Acetate Tablets 1624
Desflurane (Additive effects). Products include:
Suprane 1813
Desipramine Hydrochloride (Additive effects). Products include:
Norpramin Tablets 1526
Dexamethasone (May decrease salicylate plasma levels). Products include:
AK-Trol Ointment & Suspension .... ⊙ 205
Decadron Elixir 1633
Decadron Tablets 1635
Decaspray Topical Aerosol 1648
Dexacidin Ointment .... ⊙ 263
Maxitrol Ophthalmic Ointment and Suspension .... ⊙ 224
TobraDex Ophthalmic Suspension and Ointment 473
Dexamethasone Acetate (May decrease salicylate plasma levels). Products include:
Dalalone D.P. Injectable 1011
Decadron-LA Sterile Suspension 1646
Dexamethasone Sodium Phosphate (May decrease salicylate plasma levels). Products include:
Decadron Phosphate Injection 1637
Decadron Phosphate Respihaler 1642
Decadron Phosphate Sterile Ophthalmic Ointment 1641
Decadron Phosphate Sterile Ophthalmic Solution 1642
Decadron Phosphate Topical Cream 1644
Decadron Phosphate Turbinaire 1645
Decadron Phosphate with Xylocaine Injection, Sterile 1639
Dexacort Phosphate in Respihaler 458

(◘ Described in PDR For Nonprescription Drugs) (⊙ Described in PDR For Ophthalmology)

967 **Interactions Index** **Soma Compound with Codeine**

Dexacort Phosphate in Turbinaire .. 459
NeoDecadron Sterile Ophthalmic Ointment ... 1712
NeoDecadron Sterile Ophthalmic Solution ... 1713
NeoDecadron Topical Cream ... 1714

Dezocine (Additive effects). Products include:
Dalgan Injection ... 538

Diazepam (Additive effects). Products include:
Dizac ... 1809
Valium Injectable ... 2182
Valium Tablets ... 2183
Valrelease Capsules ... 2169

Dicumarol (Enhanced potential for bleeding).
No products indexed under this heading.

Dihydroxyaluminum Sodium Carbonate (May substantially decrease plasma salicylate concentration).
No products indexed under this heading.

Doxepin Hydrochloride (Additive effects). Products include:
Sinequan ... 2205
Zonalon Cream ... 1055

Droperidol (Additive effects). Products include:
Inapsine Injection ... 1296

Enflurane (Additive effects).
No products indexed under this heading.

Estazolam (Additive effects). Products include:
ProSom Tablets ... 449

Ethchlorvynol (Additive effects). Products include:
Placidyl Capsules ... 448

Ethinamate (Additive effects).
No products indexed under this heading.

Fentanyl (Additive effects). Products include:
Duragesic Transdermal System ... 1288

Fentanyl Citrate (Additive effects). Products include:
Sublimaze Injection ... 1307

Fludrocortisone Acetate (May decrease salicylate plasma levels). Products include:
Florinef Acetate Tablets ... 505

Fluphenazine Decanoate (Additive effects). Products include:
Prolixin Decanoate ... 509

Fluphenazine Enanthate (Additive effects). Products include:
Prolixin Enanthate ... 509

Fluphenazine Hydrochloride (Additive effects). Products include:
Prolixin ... 509

Flurazepam Hydrochloride (Additive effects). Products include:
Dalmane Capsules ... 2173

Glipizide (Possible enhancement of hypoglycemia). Products include:
Glucotrol Tablets ... 1967
Glucotrol XL Extended Release Tablets ... 1968

Glutethimide (Additive effects).
No products indexed under this heading.

Glyburide (Possible enhancement of hypoglycemia). Products include:
DiaBeta Tablets ... 1239
Glynase PresTab Tablets ... 2609
Micronase Tablets ... 2623

Haloperidol (Additive effects). Products include:
Haldol Injection, Tablets and Concentrate ... 1575

Haloperidol Decanoate (Additive effects). Products include:
Haldol Decanoate ... 1577

Hydrocodone Bitartrate (Additive effects). Products include:
Anexsia 5/500 Elixir ... 1781
Anexia Tablets ... 1782
Codiclear DH Syrup ... 791
Deconamine CX Cough and Cold Liquid and Tablets ... 1319
Duratuss HD Elixir ... 2565
Hycodan Tablets and Syrup ... 930
Hycomine Compound Tablets ... 932
Hycomine ... 931
Hycotuss Expectorant Syrup ... 933
Hydrocet Capsules ... 782
Lorcet 10/650 ... 1018
Lortab ... 2566
Tussend ... 1783
Tussend Expectorant ... 1785
Vicodin Tablets ... 1356
Vicodin ES Tablets ... 1357
Vicodin Tuss Expectorant ... 1358
Zydone Capsules ... 949

Hydrocodone Polistirex (Additive effects). Products include:
Tussionex Pennkinetic Extended-Release Suspension ... 998

Hydrocortisone (May decrease salicylate plasma levels). Products include:
Anusol-HC Cream 2.5% ... 1896
Aquanil HC Lotion ... 1931
Bactine Hydrocortisone Anti-Itch Cream ... ⊡ 709
Caldecort Anti-Itch Hydrocortisone Spray ... ⊡ 631
Cortaid ... ⊡ 836
CORTENEMA ... 2535
Cortisporin Ointment ... 1085
Cortisporin Ophthalmic Ointment Sterile ... 1085
Cortisporin Ophthalmic Suspension Sterile ... 1086
Cortisporin Otic Solution Sterile ... 1087
Cortisporin Otic Suspension Sterile ... 1088
Cortizone-5 ... ⊡ 831
Cortizone-10 ... ⊡ 831
Hydrocortone Tablets ... 1672
Hytone ... 907
Massengill Medicated Soft Cloth Towelettes ... 2458
PediOtic Suspension Sterile ... 1153
Preparation H Hydrocortisone 1% Cream ... ⊡ 872
ProctoCream-HC 2.5% ... 2408
VōSoL HC Otic Solution ... 2678

Hydrocortisone Acetate (May decrease salicylate plasma levels). Products include:
Analpram-HC Rectal Cream 1% and 2.5% ... 977
Anusol HC-1 Anti-Itch Hydrocortisone Ointment ... ⊡ 847
Anusol-HC Suppositories ... 1897
Caldecort ... ⊡ 631
Carmol HC ... 924
Coly-Mycin S Otic w/Neomycin & Hydrocortisone ... 1906
Cortaid ... ⊡ 836
Cortifoam ... 2396
Cortisporin Cream ... 1084
Epifoam ... 2399
Hydrocortone Acetate Sterile Suspension ... 1669
Mantadil Cream ... 1135
Nupercainal Hydrocortisone 1% Cream ... ⊡ 645
Ophthocort ... ⊙ 311
Pramosone Cream, Lotion & Ointment ... 978
ProctoCream-HC ... 2408
ProctoFoam-HC ... 2409
Terra-Cortril Ophthalmic Suspension ... 2210

Hydrocortisone Sodium Phosphate (May decrease salicylate plasma levels). Products include:
Hydrocortone Phosphate Injection, Sterile ... 1670

Hydrocortisone Sodium Succinate (May decrease salicylate plasma levels). Products include:
Solu-Cortef Sterile Powder ... 2641

Hydroxyzine Hydrochloride (Additive effects). Products include:
Atarax Tablets & Syrup ... 2185
Marax Tablets & DF Syrup ... 2200
Vistaril Intramuscular Solution ... 2216

Imipramine Hydrochloride (Additive effects). Products include:
Tofranil Ampuls ... 854
Tofranil Tablets ... 856

Imipramine Pamoate (Additive effects). Products include:
Tofranil-PM Capsules ... 857

Isocarboxazid (Additive effects).
No products indexed under this heading.

Isoflurane (Additive effects).
No products indexed under this heading.

Ketamine Hydrochloride (Additive effects).
No products indexed under this heading.

Levomethadyl Acetate Hydrochloride (Additive effects). Products include:
Orlamm ... 2239

Levorphanol Tartrate (Additive effects). Products include:
Levo-Dromoran ... 2129

Lithium Carbonate (Additive effects). Products include:
Eskalith ... 2485
Lithium Carbonate Capsules & Tablets ... 2230
Lithonate/Lithotabs/Lithobid ... 2543

Lithium Citrate (Additive effects).
No products indexed under this heading.

Lorazepam (Additive effects). Products include:
Ativan Injection ... 2698
Ativan Tablets ... 2700

Loxapine Hydrochloride (Additive effects). Products include:
Loxitane ... 1378

Loxapine Succinate (Additive effects). Products include:
Loxitane Capsules ... 1378

Magaldrate (May substantially decrease plasma salicylate concentration).
No products indexed under this heading.

Magnesium Hydroxide (May substantially decrease plasma salicylate concentration). Products include:
Aludrox Oral Suspension ... 2695
Arthritis Pain Ascriptin ... ⊡ 631
Maximum Strength Ascriptin ... ⊡ 630
Regular Strength Ascriptin Tablets ... ⊡ 629
Di-Gel Antacid/Anti-Gas ... ⊡ 801
Gelusil Liquid & Tablets ... ⊡ 855
Maalox Magnesia and Alumina Oral Suspension ... ⊡ 642
Maalox Plus Tablets ... ⊡ 643
Extra Strength Maalox Antacid Plus Antigas Liquid and Tablets ⊡ 638
Mylanta Calcium Carbonate and Magnesium Hydroxide Tablets ... 1318
Mylanta Liquid ... 1317
Mylanta Tablets ... ⊡ 660
Mylanta Double Strength Liquid ... 1317
Mylanta Double Strength Tablets .. ⊡ 660
Phillips' Milk of Magnesia Liquid ... ⊡ 729
Rolaids Tablets ... ⊡ 843
Tempo Soft Antacid ... ⊡ 835

Magnesium Oxide (May substantially decrease plasma salicylate concentration). Products include:
Beelith Tablets ... 639
Bufferin Analgesic Tablets and Caplets ... ⊡ 613
Caltrate PLUS ... ⊡ 665
Cama Arthritis Pain Reliever ... ⊡ 785
Mag-Ox 400 ... 668
Uro-Mag ... 668

Maprotiline Hydrochloride (Additive effects). Products include:
Ludiomil Tablets ... 843

Meperidine Hydrochloride (Additive effects). Products include:
Demerol ... 2308
Mepergan Injection ... 2753

Mephobarbital (Additive effects). Products include:
Mebaral Tablets ... 2322

Meprobamate (Additive effects). Products include:
Miltown Tablets ... 2672
PMB 200 and PMB 400 ... 2783

Mesoridazine Besylate (Additive effects). Products include:
Serentil ... 684

Metformin Hydrochloride (Possible enhancement of hypoglycemia). Products include:
Glucophage ... 752

Methadone Hydrochloride (Additive effects). Products include:
Methadone Hydrochloride Oral Concentrate ... 2233
Methadone Hydrochloride Oral Solution & Tablets ... 2235

Methohexital Sodium (Additive effects). Products include:
Brevital Sodium Vials ... 1429

Methotrexate Sodium (Toxic effects of methotrexate enhanced). Products include:
Methotrexate Sodium Tablets, Injection, for Injection and LPF Injection ... 1275

Methotrimeprazine (Additive effects). Products include:
Levoprome ... 1274

Methoxyflurane (Additive effects).
No products indexed under this heading.

Methylprednisolone Acetate (May decrease salicylate plasma levels). Products include:
Depo-Medrol Single-Dose Vial ... 2600
Depo-Medrol Sterile Aqueous Suspension ... 2597

Methylprednisolone Sodium Succinate (May decrease salicylate plasma levels). Products include:
Solu-Medrol Sterile Powder ... 2643

Midazolam Hydrochloride (Additive effects). Products include:
Versed Injection ... 2170

Molindone Hydrochloride (Additive effects). Products include:
Moban Tablets and Concentrate ... 1048

Morphine Sulfate (Additive effects). Products include:
Astramorph/PF Injection, USP (Preservative-Free) ... 535
Duramorph ... 962
Infumorph 200 and Infumorph 500 Sterile Solutions ... 965
MS Contin Tablets ... 1994
MSIR ... 1997
Oramorph SR (Morphine Sulfate Sustained Release Tablets) ... 2236
RMS Suppositories ... 2657
Roxanol ... 2243

Nortriptyline Hydrochloride (Additive effects). Products include:
Pamelor ... 2280

Opium Alkaloids (Additive effects).
No products indexed under this heading.

Oxazepam (Additive effects). Products include:
Serax Capsules ... 2810
Serax Tablets ... 2810

Oxycodone Hydrochloride (Additive effects). Products include:
Percocet Tablets ... 938
Percodan Tablets ... 939
Percodan-Demi Tablets ... 940
Roxicodone Tablets, Oral Solution & Intensol (Oxycodone) ... 2244
Tylox Capsules ... 1584

Pentobarbital Sodium (Additive effects). Products include:
Nembutal Sodium Capsules ... 436
Nembutal Sodium Solution ... 438
Nembutal Sodium Suppositories ... 440

IMPORTANT NOTE: Always consult each drug listing in the patient's regimen for possible interactions.

Soma Compound with Codeine | Interactions Index | 968

Perphenazine (Additive effects). Products include:
Etrafon ... 2355
Triavil Tablets ... 1757
Trilafon ... 2389

Phenelzine Sulfate (Additive effects). Products include:
Nardil ... 1920

Phenobarbital (Additive effects). Products include:
Arco-Lase Plus Tablets ... 512
Bellergal-S Tablets ... 2250
Donnatal ... 2060
Donnatal Extentabs ... 2061
Donnatal Tablets ... 2060
Phenobarbital Elixir and Tablets ... 1469
Quadrinal Tablets ... 1350

Potassium Acid Phosphate (Elevated plasma salicylate concentrations). Products include:
K-Phos Original Formula 'Sodium Free' Tablets ... 639

Prazepam (Additive effects).
No products indexed under this heading.

Prednisolone Acetate (May decrease salicylate plasma levels). Products include:
AK-CIDE ... ⊙ 202
AK-CIDE Ointment ... ⊙ 202
Blephamide Liquifilm Sterile Ophthalmic Suspension ... 476
Blephamide Ointment ... ⊙ 237
Econopred & Econopred Plus Ophthalmic Suspensions ... ⊙ 217
Poly-Pred Liquifilm ... ⊙ 248
Pred Forte ... ⊙ 250
Pred Mild ... ⊙ 253
Pred-G Liquifilm Sterile Ophthalmic Suspension ... ⊙ 251
Pred-G S.O.P. Sterile Ophthalmic Ointment ... ⊙ 252
Vasocidin Ointment ... ⊙ 268

Prednisolone Sodium Phosphate (May decrease salicylate plasma levels). Products include:
AK-Pred ... ⊙ 204
Hydeltrasol Injection, Sterile ... 1665
Inflamase ... ⊙ 265
Pediapred Oral Liquid ... 995
Vasocidin Ophthalmic Solution ... ⊙ 270

Prednisolone Tebutate (May decrease salicylate plasma levels). Products include:
Hydeltra-T.B.A. Sterile Suspension 1667

Prednisone (May decrease salicylate plasma levels). Products include:
Deltasone Tablets ... 2595

Probenecid (Possible reduced renal excretion of salicylate). Products include:
Benemid Tablets ... 1611
ColBENEMID Tablets ... 1622

Prochlorperazine (Additive effects). Products include:
Compazine ... 2470

Promethazine Hydrochloride (Additive effects). Products include:
Mepergan Injection ... 2753
Phenergan with Codeine ... 2777
Phenergan with Dextromethorphan 2778
Phenergan Injection ... 2773
Phenergan Suppositories ... 2775
Phenergan Syrup ... 2774
Phenergan Tablets ... 2775
Phenergan VC ... 2779
Phenergan VC with Codeine ... 2781

Propofol (Additive effects). Products include:
Diprivan Injection ... 2833

Propoxyphene Hydrochloride (Additive effects). Products include:
Darvon ... 1435
Wygesic Tablets ... 2827

Propoxyphene Napsylate (Additive effects). Products include:
Darvon-N/Darvocet-N ... 1433

Protriptyline Hydrochloride (Additive effects). Products include:
Vivactil Tablets ... 1774

Quazepam (Additive effects). Products include:
Doral Tablets ... 2664

Risperidone (Additive effects). Products include:
Risperdal ... 1301

Secobarbital Sodium (Additive effects). Products include:
Seconal Sodium Pulvules ... 1474

Sodium Acid Phosphate (Elevated plasma salicylate concentrations). Products include:
Uroqid-Acid No. 2 Tablets ... 640

Sodium Bicarbonate (May substantially decrease plasma salicylate concentration). Products include:
Alka-Seltzer Effervescent Antacid and Pain Reliever ... ▣ 701
Alka-Seltzer Extra Strength Effervescent Antacid and Pain Reliever ... ▣ 703
Alka-Seltzer Gold Effervescent Antacid ... ▣ 703
Alka-Seltzer Lemon Lime Effervescent Antacid and Pain Reliever ... ▣ 703
Arm & Hammer Pure Baking Soda ... ▣ 627
Ceo-Two Rectal Suppositories ... 666
Citrocarbonate Antacid ... ▣ 770
Massengill Disposable Douches ... ▣ 820
Massengill Liquid Concentrate ... ▣ 820
NuLYTELY ... 689
Cherry Flavor NuLYTELY ... 689

Sufentanil Citrate (Additive effects). Products include:
Sufenta Injection ... 1309

Sulfinpyrazone (Reduced uricosuric effect of both drugs; possible reduced renal excretion of salicylate). Products include:
Anturane ... 807

Temazepam (Additive effects). Products include:
Restoril Capsules ... 2284

Thiamylal Sodium (Additive effects).
No products indexed under this heading.

Thioridazine Hydrochloride (Additive effects). Products include:
Mellaril ... 2269

Thiothixene (Additive effects). Products include:
Navane Capsules and Concentrate 2201
Navane Intramuscular ... 2202

Tolazamide (Possible enhancement of hypoglycemia).
No products indexed under this heading.

Tolbutamide (Possible enhancement of hypoglycemia).
No products indexed under this heading.

Tranylcypromine Sulfate (Additive effects). Products include:
Parnate Tablets ... 2503

Triamcinolone (May decrease salicylate plasma levels). Products include:
Aristocort Tablets ... 1022

Triamcinolone Acetonide (May decrease salicylate plasma levels). Products include:
Aristocort A 0.025% Cream ... 1027
Aristocort A 0.5% Cream ... 1031
Aristocort A 0.1% Cream ... 1029
Aristocort A 0.1% Ointment ... 1030
Azmacort Oral Inhaler ... 2011
Nasacort Nasal Inhaler ... 2024

Triamcinolone Diacetate (May decrease salicylate plasma levels). Products include:
Aristocort Suspension (Forte Parenteral) ... 1027
Aristocort Suspension (Intralesional) ... 1025

Triamcinolone Hexacetonide (May decrease salicylate plasma levels). Products include:
Aristospan Suspension (Intra-articular) ... 1033
Aristospan Suspension (Intralesional) ... 1032

Triazolam (Additive effects). Products include:
Halcion Tablets ... 2611

Trifluoperazine Hydrochloride (Additive effects). Products include:
Stelazine ... 2514

Trimipramine Maleate (Additive effects). Products include:
Surmontil Capsules ... 2811

Warfarin Sodium (Enhanced potential for bleeding). Products include:
Coumadin ... 926

Zolpidem Tartrate (Additive effects). Products include:
Ambien Tablets ... 2416

Food Interactions

Alcohol (Additive effects including gastrointestinal bleeding).

SOMA COMPOUND TABLETS

(Carisoprodol, Aspirin) ... 2675
May interact with central nervous system depressants, psychotropics, oral anticoagulants, oral hypoglycemic agents, antacids, corticosteroids, and certain other agents. Compounds in these categories include:

Acarbose (Possible enhancement of hypoglycemia).
No products indexed under this heading.

Alfentanil Hydrochloride (Additive effects). Products include:
Alfenta Injection ... 1286

Alprazolam (Additive effects). Products include:
Xanax Tablets ... 2649

Aluminum Carbonate Gel (May substantially decrease plasma salicylate concentration). Products include:
Basaljel ... 2703

Aluminum Hydroxide (May substantially decrease plasma salicylate concentration). Products include:
ALternaGEL Liquid ... 1316
Maximum Strength Ascriptin ... ▣ 630
Cama Arthritis Pain Reliever ... ▣ 785
Gaviscon Extra Strength Relief Formula Antacid Tablets ... ▣ 819
Gaviscon Extra Strength Relief Formula Liquid Antacid ... ▣ 819
Gaviscon Liquid Antacid ... ▣ 820
Gelusil Liquid & Tablets ... ▣ 855
Maalox Heartburn Relief Suspension ... ▣ 642
Maalox Heartburn Relief Tablets ... ▣ 641
Maalox Magnesia and Alumina Oral Suspension ... ▣ 642
Maalox Plus Tablets ... ▣ 643
Extra Strength Maalox Antacid Plus Antigas Liquid and Tablets ▣ 638
Tempo Soft Antacid ... ▣ 835

Aluminum Hydroxide Gel (May substantially decrease plasma salicylate concentration). Products include:
ALternaGEL Liquid ... ▣ 659
Aludrox Oral Suspension ... 2695
Amphojel Suspension ... 2695
Amphojel Suspension without Flavor ... 2695
Amphojel Tablets ... 2695
Arthritis Pain Ascriptin ... ▣ 631
Regular Strength Ascriptin Tablets ... ▣ 629
Gaviscon Antacid Tablets ... ▣ 819
Gaviscon-2 Antacid Tablets ... ▣ 820
Mylanta Liquid ... 1317
Mylanta Tablets ... ▣ 660
Mylanta Double Strength Liquid ... 1317
Mylanta Double Strength Tablets ... ▣ 660
Nephrox Suspension ... ▣ 655

Amitriptyline Hydrochloride (Additive effects). Products include:
Elavil ... 2838
Endep Tablets ... 2174
Etrafon ... 2355
Limbitrol ... 2180
Triavil Tablets ... 1757

Ammonium Chloride (Elevated plasma salicylate concentrations).
No products indexed under this heading.

Amoxapine (Additive effects). Products include:
Asendin Tablets ... 1369

Aprobarbital (Additive effects).
No products indexed under this heading.

Betamethasone Acetate (May decrease salicylate plasma levels). Products include:
Celestone Soluspan Suspension ... 2347

Betamethasone Sodium Phosphate (May decrease salicylate plasma levels). Products include:
Celestone Soluspan Suspension ... 2347

Buprenorphine (Additive effects). Products include:
Buprenex Injectable ... 2006

Buspirone Hydrochloride (Additive effects). Products include:
BuSpar ... 737

Butabarbital (Additive effects).
No products indexed under this heading.

Butalbital (Additive effects). Products include:
Esgic-plus Tablets ... 1013
Fioricet Tablets ... 2258
Fioricet with Codeine Capsules ... 2260
Fiorinal Capsules ... 2261
Fiorinal with Codeine Capsules ... 2262
Fiorinal Tablets ... 2261
Phrenilin ... 785
Sedapap Tablets 50 mg/650 mg ... 1543

Chlordiazepoxide (Additive effects). Products include:
Libritabs Tablets ... 2177
Limbitrol ... 2180

Chlordiazepoxide Hydrochloride (Additive effects). Products include:
Librax Capsules ... 2176
Librium Capsules ... 2178
Librium Injectable ... 2179

Chlorpromazine (Additive effects). Products include:
Thorazine Suppositories ... 2523

Chlorpromazine Hydrochloride (Additive effects). Products include:
Thorazine ... 2523

Chlorpropamide (Possible enhancement of hypoglycemia). Products include:
Diabinese Tablets ... 1935

Chlorprothixene (Additive effects).
No products indexed under this heading.

Chlorprothixene Hydrochloride (Additive effects).
No products indexed under this heading.

Clorazepate Dipotassium (Additive effects). Products include:
Tranxene ... 451

Clozapine (Additive effects). Products include:
Clozaril Tablets ... 2252

Codeine Phosphate (Additive effects). Products include:
Actifed with Codeine Cough Syrup .. 1067
Brontex ... 1981
Deconsal C Expectorant Syrup ... 456
Deconsal Pediatric Syrup ... 457
Dimetane-DC Cough Syrup ... 2059
Empirin with Codeine Tablets ... 1093
Fioricet with Codeine Capsules ... 2260
Fiorinal with Codeine Capsules ... 2262
Isoclor Expectorant ... 990

(▣ Described in PDR For Nonprescription Drugs) (⊙ Described in PDR For Ophthalmology)

Interactions Index — Soma Compound

Novahistine DH 2462
Novahistine Expectorant 2463
Nucofed 2051
Phenergan with Codeine 2777
Phenergan VC with Codeine 2781
Robitussin A-C Syrup 2073
Robitussin-DAC Syrup 2074
Ryna .... ⊕ 841
Soma Compound w/Codeine Tablets 2676
Tussi-Organidin NR Liquid and S NR Liquid 2677
Tylenol with Codeine 1583

Cortisone Acetate (May decrease salicylate plasma levels). Products include:

Cortone Acetate Sterile Suspension 1623
Cortone Acetate Tablets 1624

Desflurane (Additive effects). Products include:

Suprane 1813

Desipramine Hydrochloride (Additive effects). Products include:

Norpramin Tablets 1526

Dexamethasone (May decrease salicylate plasma levels). Products include:

AK-Trol Ointment & Suspension .... ⊙ 205
Decadron Elixir 1633
Decadron Tablets 1635
Decaspray Topical Aerosol 1648
Dexacidin Ointment .... ⊙ 263
Maxitrol Ophthalmic Ointment and Suspension .... ⊙ 224
TobraDex Ophthalmic Suspension and Ointment 473

Dexamethasone Acetate (May decrease salicylate plasma levels). Products include:

Dalalone D.P. Injectable 1011
Decadron-LA Sterile Suspension 1646

Dexamethasone Sodium Phosphate (May decrease salicylate plasma levels). Products include:

Decadron Phosphate Injection 1637
Decadron Phosphate Respihaler 1642
Decadron Phosphate Sterile Ophthalmic Ointment 1641
Decadron Phosphate Sterile Ophthalmic Solution 1642
Decadron Phosphate Topical Cream 1644
Decadron Phosphate Turbinaire 1645
Decadron Phosphate with Xylocaine Injection, Sterile 1639
Dexacort Phosphate in Respihaler.. 458
Dexacort Phosphate in Turbinaire .. 459
NeoDecadron Sterile Ophthalmic Ointment 1712
NeoDecadron Sterile Ophthalmic Solution 1713
NeoDecadron Topical Cream 1714

Dezocine (Additive effects). Products include:

Dalgan Injection 538

Diazepam (Additive effects). Products include:

Dizac 1809
Valium Injectable 2182
Valium Tablets 2183
Valrelease Capsules 2169

Dicumarol (Enhanced potential for bleeding).

No products indexed under this heading.

Dihydroxyaluminum Sodium Carbonate (May substantially decrease plasma salicylate concentration).

No products indexed under this heading.

Doxepin Hydrochloride (Additive effects). Products include:

Sinequan 2205
Zonalon Cream 1055

Droperidol (Additive effects). Products include:

Inapsine Injection 1296

Enflurane (Additive effects).

No products indexed under this heading.

Estazolam (Additive effects). Products include:

ProSom Tablets 449

Ethchlorvynol (Additive effects). Products include:

Placidyl Capsules 448

Ethinamate (Additive effects).

No products indexed under this heading.

Fentanyl (Additive effects). Products include:

Duragesic Transdermal System 1288

Fentanyl Citrate (Additive effects). Products include:

Sublimaze Injection 1307

Fludrocortisone Acetate (May decrease salicylate plasma levels). Products include:

Florinef Acetate Tablets 505

Fluphenazine Decanoate (Additive effects). Products include:

Prolixin Decanoate 509

Fluphenazine Enanthate (Additive effects). Products include:

Prolixin Enanthate 509

Fluphenazine Hydrochloride (Additive effects). Products include:

Prolixin 509

Flurazepam Hydrochloride (Additive effects). Products include:

Dalmane Capsules 2173

Glipizide (Possible enhancement of hypoglycemia). Products include:

Glucotrol Tablets 1967
Glucotrol XL Extended Release Tablets 1968

Glutethimide (Additive effects).

No products indexed under this heading.

Glyburide (Possible enhancement of hypoglycemia). Products include:

DiaBeta Tablets 1239
Glynase PresTab Tablets 2609
Micronase Tablets 2623

Haloperidol (Additive effects). Products include:

Haldol Injection, Tablets and Concentrate 1575

Haloperidol Decanoate (Additive effects). Products include:

Haldol Decanoate 1577

Hydrocodone Bitartrate (Additive effects). Products include:

Anexsia 5/500 Elixir 1781
Anexia Tablets 1782
Codiclear DH Syrup 791
Deconamine CX Cough and Cold Liquid and Tablets 1319
Duratuss HD Elixir 2565
Hycodan Tablets and Syrup 930
Hycomine Compound Tablets 932
Hycomine 931
Hycotuss Expectorant Syrup 933
Hydrocet Capsules 782
Lorcet 10/650 1018
Lortab 2566
Tussend 1783
Tussend Expectorant 1785
Vicodin Tablets 1356
Vicodin ES Tablets 1357
Vicodin Tuss Expectorant 1358
Zydone Capsules 949

Hydrocodone Polistirex (Additive effects). Products include:

Tussionex Pennkinetic Extended-Release Suspension 998

Hydrocortisone (May decrease salicylate plasma levels). Products include:

Anusol-HC Cream 2.5% 1896
Aquanil HC Lotion 1931
Bactine Hydrocortisone Anti-Itch Cream .... ⊕ 709
Caldecort Anti-Itch Hydrocortisone Spray .... ⊕ 631
Cortaid .... ⊕ 836
CORTENEMA 2535
Cortisporin Ointment 1085
Cortisporin Ophthalmic Ointment Sterile 1085

Cortisporin Ophthalmic Suspension Sterile 1086
Cortisporin Otic Solution Sterile 1087
Cortisporin Otic Suspension Sterile 1088
Cortizone-5 .... ⊕ 831
Cortizone-10 .... ⊕ 831
Hydrocortone Tablets 1672
Hytone 907
Massengill Medicated Soft Cloth Towelettes 2458
PediOtic Suspension Sterile 1153
Preparation H Hydrocortisone 1% Cream .... ⊕ 872
ProctoCream-HC 2.5% 2408
VoSoL HC Otic Solution 2678

Hydrocortisone Acetate (May decrease salicylate plasma levels). Products include:

Analpram-HC Rectal Cream 1% and 2.5% 977
Anusol HC-1 Anti-Itch Hydrocortisone Ointment .... ⊕ 847
Anusol-HC Suppositories 1897
Caldecort .... ⊕ 631
Carmol HC 924
Coly-Mycin S Otic w/Neomycin & Hydrocortisone 1906
Cortaid .... ⊕ 836
Cortifoam 2396
Cortisporin Cream 1084
Epifoam 2399
Hydrocortone Acetate Sterile Suspension 1669
Mantadil Cream 1135
Nupercainal Hydrocortisone 1% Cream .... ⊕ 645
Ophthocort .... ⊙ 311
Pramosone Cream, Lotion & Ointment 978
ProctoCream-HC 2408
ProctoFoam-HC 2409
Terra-Cortril Ophthalmic Suspension 2210

Hydrocortisone Sodium Phosphate (May decrease salicylate plasma levels). Products include:

Hydrocortone Phosphate Injection, Sterile 1670

Hydrocortisone Sodium Succinate (May decrease salicylate plasma levels). Products include:

Solu-Cortef Sterile Powder 2641

Hydroxyzine Hydrochloride (Additive effects). Products include:

Atarax Tablets & Syrup 2185
Marax Tablets & DF Syrup 2200
Vistaril Intramuscular Solution 2216

Imipramine Hydrochloride (Additive effects). Products include:

Tofranil Ampuls 854
Tofranil Tablets 856

Imipramine Pamoate (Additive effects). Products include:

Tofranil-PM Capsules 857

Isocarboxazid (Additive effects).

No products indexed under this heading.

Isoflurane (Additive effects).

No products indexed under this heading.

Ketamine Hydrochloride (Additive effects).

No products indexed under this heading.

Levomethadyl Acetate Hydrochloride (Additive effects). Products include:

Orlamm 2239

Levorphanol Tartrate (Additive effects). Products include:

Levo-Dromoran 2129

Lithium Carbonate (Additive effects). Products include:

Eskalith 2485
Lithium Carbonate Capsules & Tablets 2230
Lithonate/Lithotabs/Lithobid 2543

Lithium Citrate (Additive effects).

No products indexed under this heading.

Lorazepam (Additive effects). Products include:

Ativan Injection 2698
Ativan Tablets 2700

Loxapine Hydrochloride (Additive effects). Products include:

Loxitane 1378

Loxapine Succinate (Additive effects). Products include:

Loxitane Capsules 1378

Magaldrate (May substantially decrease plasma salicylate concentration).

No products indexed under this heading.

Magnesium Hydroxide (May substantially decrease plasma salicylate concentration). Products include:

Aludrox Oral Suspension 2695
Arthritis Pain Ascriptin .... ⊕ 631
Maximum Strength Ascriptin .... ⊕ 630
Regular Strength Ascriptin Tablets .... ⊕ 629
Di-Gel Antacid/Anti-Gas .... ⊕ 801
Gelusil Liquid & Tablets .... ⊕ 855
Maalox Magnesia and Alumina Oral Suspension .... ⊕ 642
Maalox Plus Tablets .... ⊕ 643
Extra Strength Maalox Antacid Plus Antigas Liquid and Tablets ⊕ 638
Mylanta Calcium Carbonate and Magnesium Hydroxide Tablets 1318
Mylanta Liquid 1317
Mylanta Tablets .... ⊕ 660
Mylanta Double Strength Liquid 1317
Mylanta Double Strength Tablets .. ⊕ 660
Phillips' Milk of Magnesia Liquid .... ⊕ 729
Rolaids Tablets .... ⊕ 843
Tempo Soft Antacid .... ⊕ 835

Magnesium Oxide (May substantially decrease plasma salicylate concentration). Products include:

Beelith Tablets 639
Bufferin Analgesic Tablets and Caplets .... ⊕ 613
Caltrate PLUS .... ⊕ 665
Cama Arthritis Pain Reliever .... ⊕ 785
Mag-Ox 400 668
Uro-Mag 668

Maprotiline Hydrochloride (Additive effects). Products include:

Ludiomil Tablets 843

Meperidine Hydrochloride (Additive effects). Products include:

Demerol 2308
Mepergan Injection 2753

Mephobarbital (Additive effects). Products include:

Mebaral Tablets 2322

Meprobamate (Additive effects). Products include:

Miltown Tablets 2672
PMB 200 and PMB 400 2783

Mesoridazine Besylate (Additive effects). Products include:

Serentil 684

Metformin Hydrochloride (Possible enhancement of hypoglycemia). Products include:

Glucophage 752

Methadone Hydrochloride (Additive effects). Products include:

Methadone Hydrochloride Oral Concentrate 2233
Methadone Hydrochloride Oral Solution & Tablets 2235

Methohexital Sodium (Additive effects). Products include:

Brevital Sodium Vials 1429

Methotrexate Sodium (Toxic effects of metotrexate enhanced). Products include:

Methotrexate Sodium Tablets, Injection, for Injection and LPF Injection 1275

Methotrimeprazine (Additive effects). Products include:

Levoprome 1274

Methoxyflurane (Additive effects).

No products indexed under this heading.

IMPORTANT NOTE: Always consult each drug listing in the patient's regimen for possible interactions.

Soma Compound **Interactions Index** **970**

Methylprednisolone Acetate (May decrease salicylate plasma levels). Products include:
- Depo-Medrol Single-Dose Vial 2600
- Depo-Medrol Sterile Aqueous Suspension 2597

Methylprednisolone Sodium Succinate (May decrease salicylate plasma levels). Products include:
- Solu-Medrol Sterile Powder 2643

Midazolam Hydrochloride (Additive effects). Products include:
- Versed Injection 2170

Molindone Hydrochloride (Additive effects). Products include:
- Moban Tablets and Concentrate 1048

Morphine Sulfate (Additive effects). Products include:
- Astramorph/PF Injection, USP (Preservative-Free) 535
- Duramorph 962
- Infumorph 200 and Infumorph 500 Sterile Solutions 965
- MS Contin Tablets 1994
- MSIR 1997
- Oramorph SR (Morphine Sulfate Sustained Release Tablets) 2236
- RMS Suppositories 2657
- Roxanol 2243

Nortriptyline Hydrochloride (Additive effects). Products include:
- Pamelor 2280

Opium Alkaloids (Additive effects).
- No products indexed under this heading.

Oxazepam (Additive effects). Products include:
- Serax Capsules 2810
- Serax Tablets 2810

Oxycodone Hydrochloride (Additive effects). Products include:
- Percocet Tablets 938
- Percodan Tablets 939
- Percodan-Demi Tablets 940
- Roxicodone Tablets, Oral Solution & Intensol (Oxycodone) 2244
- Tylox Capsules 1584

Pentobarbital Sodium (Additive effects). Products include:
- Nembutal Sodium Capsules 436
- Nembutal Sodium Solution 438
- Nembutal Sodium Suppositories 440

Perphenazine (Additive effects). Products include:
- Etrafon 2355
- Triavil Tablets 1757
- Trilafon 2389

Phenelzine Sulfate (Additive effects). Products include:
- Nardil 1920

Phenobarbital (Additive effects). Products include:
- Arco-Lase Plus Tablets 512
- Bellergal-S Tablets 2250
- Donnatal 2060
- Donnatal Extentabs 2061
- Donnatal Tablets 2060
- Phenobarbital Elixir and Tablets 1469
- Quadrinal Tablets 1350

Potassium Acid Phosphate (Elevated plasma salicylate concentrations). Products include:
- K-Phos Original Formula 'Sodium Free' Tablets 639

Prazepam (Additive effects).
- No products indexed under this heading.

Prednisolone Acetate (May decrease salicylate plasma levels). Products include:
- AK-CIDE .... ⊙ 202
- AK-CIDE Ointment .... ⊙ 202
- Blephamide Liquifilm Sterile Ophthalmic Suspension 476
- Blephamide Ointment .... ⊙ 237
- Econopred & Econopred Plus Ophthalmic Suspensions .... ⊙ 217
- Poly-Pred Liquifilm .... ⊙ 248
- Pred Forte .... ⊙ 250
- Pred Mild .... ⊙ 253
- Pred-G Liquifilm Sterile Ophthalmic Suspension .... ⊙ 251
- Pred-G S.O.P. Sterile Ophthalmic Ointment .... ⊙ 252
- Vasocidin Ointment .... ⊙ 268

Prednisolone Sodium Phosphate (May decrease salicylate plasma levels). Products include:
- AK-Pred .... ⊙ 204
- Hydeltrasol Injection, Sterile 1665
- Inflamase .... ⊙ 265
- Pediapred Oral Liquid 995
- Vasocidin Ophthalmic Solution .... ⊙ 270

Prednisolone Tebutate (May decrease salicylate plasma levels). Products include:
- Hydeltra-T.B.A. Sterile Suspension 1667

Prednisone (May decrease salicylate plasma levels). Products include:
- Deltasone Tablets 2595

Probenecid (Reduced uricosuric effect of both drugs; possible reduced renal excretion of salicylate). Products include:
- Benemid Tablets 1611
- ColBENEMID Tablets 1622

Prochlorperazine (Additive effects). Products include:
- Compazine 2470

Promethazine Hydrochloride (Additive effects). Products include:
- Mepergan Injection 2753
- Phenergan with Codeine 2777
- Phenergan with Dextromethorphan 2778
- Phenergan Injection 2773
- Phenergan Suppositories 2775
- Phenergan Syrup 2774
- Phenergan Tablets 2775
- Phenergan VC 2779
- Phenergan VC with Codeine 2781

Propofol (Additive effects). Products include:
- Diprivan Injection 2833

Propoxyphene Hydrochloride (Additive effects). Products include:
- Darvon 1435
- Wygesic Tablets 2827

Propoxyphene Napsylate (Additive effects). Products include:
- Darvon-N/Darvocet-N 1433

Protriptyline Hydrochloride (Additive effects). Products include:
- Vivactil Tablets 1774

Quazepam (Additive effects). Products include:
- Doral Tablets 2664

Risperidone (Additive effects). Products include:
- Risperdal 1301

Secobarbital Sodium (Additive effects). Products include:
- Seconal Sodium Pulvules 1474

Sodium Acid Phosphate (Elevated plasma salicylate concentrations). Products include:
- Uroqid-Acid No. 2 Tablets 640

Sodium Bicarbonate (May substantially decrease plasma salicylate concentration). Products include:
- Alka-Seltzer Effervescent Antacid and Pain Reliever .... ▭ 701
- Alka-Seltzer Extra Strength Effervescent Antacid and Pain Reliever .... ▭ 703
- Alka-Seltzer Gold Effervescent Antacid .... ▭ 703
- Alka-Seltzer Lemon Lime Effervescent Antacid and Pain Reliever .... ▭ 703
- Arm & Hammer Pure Baking Soda .... ▭ 627
- Ceo-Two Rectal Suppositories 666
- Citrocarbonate Antacid .... ▭ 770
- Massengill Disposable Douches .... ▭ 820
- Massengill Liquid Concentrate .... ▭ 820
- NuLYTELY 689
- Cherry Flavor NuLYTELY 689

Sufentanil Citrate (Additive effects). Products include:
- Sufenta Injection 1309

Sulfinpyrazone (Reduced uricosuric effect of both drugs; possible reduced renal excretion of salicylate). Products include:
- Anturane 807

Temazepam (Additive effects). Products include:
- Restoril Capsules 2284

Thiamylal Sodium (Additive effects).
- No products indexed under this heading.

Thioridazine Hydrochloride (Additive effects). Products include:
- Mellaril 2269

Thiothixene (Additive effects). Products include:
- Navane Capsules and Concentrate 2201
- Navane Intramuscular 2202

Tolazamide (Possible enhancement of hypoglycemia).
- No products indexed under this heading.

Tolbutamide (Possible enhancement of hypoglycemia).
- No products indexed under this heading.

Tranylcypromine Sulfate (Additive effects). Products include:
- Parnate Tablets 2503

Triamcinolone (May decrease salicylate plasma levels). Products include:
- Aristocort Tablets 1022

Triamcinolone Acetonide (May decrease salicylate plasma levels). Products include:
- Aristocort A 0.025% Cream 1027
- Aristocort A 0.5% Cream 1031
- Aristocort A 0.1% Cream 1029
- Aristocort A 0.1% Ointment 1030
- Azmacort Oral Inhaler 2011
- Nasacort Nasal Inhaler 2024

Triamcinolone Diacetate (May decrease salicylate plasma levels). Products include:
- Aristocort Suspension (Forte Parenteral) 1027
- Aristocort Suspension (Intralesional) 1025

Triamcinolone Hexacetonide (May decrease salicylate plasma levels). Products include:
- Aristospan Suspension (Intra-articular) 1033
- Aristospan Suspension (Intralesional) 1032

Triazolam (Additive effects). Products include:
- Halcion Tablets 2611

Trifluoperazine Hydrochloride (Additive effects). Products include:
- Stelazine 2514

Trimipramine Maleate (Additive effects). Products include:
- Surmontil Capsules 2811

Warfarin Sodium (Enhanced potential for bleeding). Products include:
- Coumadin 926

Zolpidem Tartrate (Additive effects). Products include:
- Ambien Tablets 2416

Food Interactions

Alcohol (Additive effects including enhanced aspirin-induced fecal blood loss).

SOMA TABLETS

(Carisoprodol) 2674

May interact with central nervous system depressants and psychotropics. Compounds in these categories include:

Alfentanil Hydrochloride (Additive effects). Products include:
- Alfenta Injection 1286

Alprazolam (Additive effects). Products include:
- Xanax Tablets 2649

Amitriptyline Hydrochloride (Additive effects). Products include:
- Elavil 2838
- Endep Tablets 2174
- Etrafon 2355
- Limbitrol 2180
- Triavil Tablets 1757

Amoxapine (Additive effects). Products include:
- Asendin Tablets 1369

Aprobarbital (Additive effects).
- No products indexed under this heading.

Buprenorphine (Additive effects). Products include:
- Buprenex Injectable 2006

Buspirone Hydrochloride (Additive effects). Products include:
- BuSpar 737

Butabarbital (Additive effects).
- No products indexed under this heading.

Butalbital (Additive effects). Products include:
- Esgic-plus Tablets 1013
- Fioricet Tablets 2258
- Fioricet with Codeine Capsules 2260
- Fiorinal Capsules 2261
- Fiorinal with Codeine Capsules 2262
- Fiorinal Tablets 2261
- Phrenilin 785
- Sedapap Tablets 50 mg/650 mg 1543

Chlordiazepoxide (Additive effects). Products include:
- Libritabs Tablets 2177
- Limbitrol 2180

Chlordiazepoxide Hydrochloride (Additive effects). Products include:
- Librax Capsules 2176
- Librium Capsules 2178
- Librium Injectable 2179

Chlorpromazine (Additive effects). Products include:
- Thorazine Suppositories 2523

Chlorprothixene (Additive effects).
- No products indexed under this heading.

Chlorprothixene Hydrochloride (Additive effects).
- No products indexed under this heading.

Clorazepate Dipotassium (Additive effects). Products include:
- Tranxene 451

Clozapine (Additive effects). Products include:
- Clozaril Tablets 2252

Codeine Phosphate (Additive effects). Products include:
- Actifed with Codeine Cough Syrup 1067
- Brontex 1981
- Deconsal C Expectorant Syrup 456
- Deconsal Pediatric Syrup 457
- Dimetane-DC Cough Syrup 2059
- Empirin with Codeine Tablets 1093
- Fioricet with Codeine Capsules 2260
- Fiorinal with Codeine Capsules 2262
- Isoclor Expectorant 990
- Novahistine DH 2462
- Novahistine Expectorant 2463
- Nucofed 2051
- Phenergan with Codeine 2777
- Phenergan VC with Codeine 2781
- Robitussin A-C Syrup 2073
- Robitussin-DAC Syrup 2074
- Ryna .... ▭ 841
- Soma Compound w/Codeine Tablets 2676
- Tussi-Organidin NR Liquid and S NR Liquid 2677
- Tylenol with Codeine 1583

Desflurane (Additive effects). Products include:
- Suprane 1813

Desipramine Hydrochloride (Additive effects). Products include:
- Norpramin Tablets 1526

(▭ Described in PDR For Nonprescription Drugs) (⊙ Described in PDR For Ophthalmology)

Dezocine (Additive effects). Products include:

Dalgan Injection 538

Diazepam (Additive effects). Products include:

Dizac 1809
Valium Injectable 2182
Valium Tablets 2183
Valrelease Capsules 2169

Doxepin Hydrochloride (Additive effects). Products include:

Sinequan 2205
Zonalon Cream 1055

Droperidol (Additive effects). Products include:

Inapsine Injection................................... 1296

Enflurane (Additive effects).

No products indexed under this heading.

Estazolam (Additive effects). Products include:

ProSom Tablets 449

Ethchlorvynol (Additive effects). Products include:

Placidyl Capsules................................... 448

Ethinamate (Additive effects).

No products indexed under this heading.

Fentanyl (Additive effects). Products include:

Duragesic Transdermal System....... 1288

Fentanyl Citrate (Additive effects). Products include:

Sublimaze Injection................................ 1307

Fluphenazine Decanoate (Additive effects). Products include:

Prolixin Decanoate 509

Fluphenazine Enanthate (Additive effects). Products include:

Prolixin Enanthate.................................. 509

Fluphenazine Hydrochloride (Additive effects). Products include:

Prolixin 509

Flurazepam Hydrochloride (Additive effects). Products include:

Dalmane Capsules.................................. 2173

Glutethimide (Additive effects).

No products indexed under this heading.

Haloperidol (Additive effects). Products include:

Haldol Injection, Tablets and Concentrate 1575

Haloperidol Decanoate (Additive effects). Products include:

Haldol Decanoate.................................... 1577

Hydrocodone Bitartrate (Additive effects). Products include:

Anexsia 5/500 Elixir 1781
Anexia Tablets... 1782
Codiclear DH Syrup 791
Deconamine CX Cough and Cold Liquid and Tablets................................... 1319
Duratuss HD Elixir.................................. 2565
Hycodan Tablets and Syrup 930
Hycomine Compound Tablets 932
Hycomine 931
Hycotuss Expectorant Syrup 933
Hydrocet Capsules 782
Lorcet 10/650... 1018
Lortab 2566
Tussend 1783
Tussend Expectorant 1785
Vicodin Tablets 1356
Vicodin ES Tablets 1357
Vicodin Tuss Expectorant 1358
Zydone Capsules 949

Hydrocodone Polistirex (Additive effects). Products include:

Tussionex Pennkinetic Extended-Release Suspension 998

Hydroxyzine Hydrochloride (Additive effects). Products include:

Atarax Tablets & Syrup.......................... 2185
Marax Tablets & DF Syrup.................... 2200
Vistaril Intramuscular Solution.......... 2216

Imipramine Hydrochloride (Additive effects). Products include:

Tofranil Ampuls 854
Tofranil Tablets 856

Imipramine Pamoate (Additive effects). Products include:

Tofranil-PM Capsules............................. 857

Isocarboxazid (Additive effects).

No products indexed under this heading.

Isoflurane (Additive effects).

No products indexed under this heading.

Ketamine Hydrochloride (Additive effects).

No products indexed under this heading.

Levomethadyl Acetate Hydrochloride (Additive effects). Products include:

Orlaam 2239

Levorphanol Tartrate (Additive effects). Products include:

Levo-Dromoran.. 2129

Lithium Carbonate (Additive effects). Products include:

Eskalith 2485
Lithium Carbonate Capsules & Tablets 2230
Lithonate/Lithotabs/Lithobid 2543

Lithium Citrate (Additive effects).

No products indexed under this heading.

Lorazepam (Additive effects). Products include:

Ativan Injection....................................... 2698
Ativan Tablets 2700

Loxapine Hydrochloride (Additive effects). Products include:

Loxitane.. 1378

Loxapine Succinate (Additive effects). Products include:

Loxitane Capsules 1378

Maprotiline Hydrochloride (Additive effects). Products include:

Ludiomil Tablets...................................... 843

Meperidine Hydrochloride (Additive effects). Products include:

Demerol 2308
Mepergan Injection 2753

Mephobarbital (Additive effects). Products include:

Mebaral Tablets 2322

Meprobamate (Additive effects). Products include:

Miltown Tablets 2672
PMB 200 and PMB 400 2783

Mesoridazine Besylate (Additive effects). Products include:

Serentil.. 684

Methadone Hydrochloride (Additive effects). Products include:

Methadone Hydrochloride Oral Concentrate 2233
Methadone Hydrochloride Oral Solution & Tablets.................................... 2235

Methohexital Sodium (Additive effects). Products include:

Brevital Sodium Vials............................. 1429

Methotrimeprazine (Additive effects). Products include:

Levoprome 1274

Methoxyflurane (Additive effects).

No products indexed under this heading.

Midazolam Hydrochloride (Additive effects). Products include:

Versed Injection 2170

Molindone Hydrochloride (Additive effects). Products include:

Moban Tablets and Concentrate...... 1048

Morphine Sulfate (Additive effects). Products include:

Astramorph/PF Injection, USP (Preservative-Free) 535
Duramorph 962
Infumorph 200 and Infumorph 500 Sterile Solutions............................. 965
MS Contin Tablets................................... 1994
MSIR 1997
Oramorph SR (Morphine Sulfate Sustained Release Tablets) 2236
RMS Suppositories 2657
Roxanol 2243

Nortriptyline Hydrochloride (Additive effects). Products include:

Pamelor 2280

Opium Alkaloids (Additive effects).

No products indexed under this heading.

Oxazepam (Additive effects). Products include:

Serax Capsules.. 2810
Serax Tablets... 2810

Oxycodone Hydrochloride (Additive effects). Products include:

Percocet Tablets 938
Percodan Tablets.................................... 939
Percodan-Demi Tablets.......................... 940
Roxicodone Tablets, Oral Solution & Intensol (Oxycodone) 2244
Tylox Capsules 1584

Pentobarbital Sodium (Additive effects). Products include:

Nembutal Sodium Capsules 436
Nembutal Sodium Solution 438
Nembutal Sodium Suppositories...... 440

Perphenazine (Additive effects). Products include:

Etrafon 2355
Triavil Tablets 1757
Trilafon.. 2389

Phenelzine Sulfate (Additive effects). Products include:

Nardil 1920

Phenobarbital (Additive effects). Products include:

Arco-Lase Plus Tablets 512
Bellergal-S Tablets 2250
Donnatal 2060
Donnatal Extentabs................................ 2061
Donnatal Tablets..................................... 2060
Phenobarbital Elixir and Tablets 1469
Quadrinal Tablets 1350

Prazepam (Additive effects).

No products indexed under this heading.

Prochlorperazine (Additive effects). Products include:

Compazine 2470

Promethazine Hydrochloride (Additive effects). Products include:

Mepergan Injection 2753
Phenergan with Codeine....................... 2777
Phenergan with Dextromethorphan 2778
Phenergan Injection 2773
Phenergan Suppositories...................... 2775
Phenergan Syrup 2774
Phenergan Tablets 2775
Phenergan VC 2779
Phenergan VC with Codeine 2781

Propofol (Additive effects). Products include:

Diprivan Injection.................................... 2833

Propoxyphene Hydrochloride (Additive effects). Products include:

Darvon 1435
Wygesic Tablets 2827

Propoxyphene Napsylate (Additive effects). Products include:

Darvon-N/Darvocet-N 1433

Protriptyline Hydrochloride (Additive effects). Products include:

Vivactil Tablets 1774

Quazepam (Additive effects). Products include:

Doral Tablets 2664

Risperidone (Additive effects). Products include:

Risperdal 1301

Secobarbital Sodium (Additive effects). Products include:

Seconal Sodium Pulvules 1474

Sufentanil Citrate (Additive effects). Products include:

Sufenta Injection 1309

Temazepam (Additive effects). Products include:

Restoril Capsules 2284

Thiamylal Sodium (Additive effects).

No products indexed under this heading.

Thioridazine Hydrochloride (Additive effects). Products include:

Mellaril 2269

Thiothixene (Additive effects). Products include:

Navane Capsules and Concentrate 2201
Navane Intramuscular 2202

Tranylcypromine Sulfate (Additive effects). Products include:

Parnate Tablets 2503

Triazolam (Additive effects). Products include:

Halcion Tablets.. 2611

Trifluoperazine Hydrochloride (Additive effects). Products include:

Stelazine 2514

Trimipramine Maleate (Additive effects). Products include:

Surmontil Capsules................................ 2811

Zolpidem Tartrate (Additive effects). Products include:

Ambien Tablets.. 2416

Food Interactions

Alcohol (Additive effects).

SORBITRATE CHEWABLE TABLETS

(Isosorbide Dinitrate) 2843

May interact with calcium channel blockers and certain other agents. Compounds in these categories include:

Amlodipine Besylate (Combination therapy of calcium channel blockers and organic nitrates may result in marked symptomatic orthostatic hypotension; dose adjustment of either class of agent may be necessary). Products include:

Lotrel Capsules 840
Norvasc Tablets 1940

Bepridil Hydrochloride (Combination therapy of calcium channel blockers and organic nitrates may result in marked symptomatic orthostatic hypotension; dose adjustment of either class of agent may be necessary). Products include:

Vascor (200, 300 and 400 mg) Tablets 1587

Diltiazem Hydrochloride (Combination therapy of calcium channel blockers and organic nitrates may result in marked symptomatic orthostatic hypotension; dose adjustment of either class of agent may be necessary). Products include:

Cardizem CD Capsules 1506
Cardizem SR Capsules 1510
Cardizem Injectable 1508
Cardizem Tablets.................................... 1512
Dilacor XR Extended-release Capsules 2018

Drugs Depending On Vascular Smooth Muscle (Possible decreased or increased effect depending on the agent that depends on vascular smooth muscle as the final common path).

Felodipine (Combination therapy of calcium channel blockers and organic nitrates may result in marked symptomatic orthostatic hypotension; dose adjustment of either class of agent may be necessary). Products include:

Plendil Extended-Release Tablets.... 527

IMPORTANT NOTE: Always consult each drug listing in the patient's regimen for possible interactions.

Isradipine (Combination therapy of calcium channel blockers and organic nitrates may result in marked symptomatic orthostatic hypotension; dose adjustment of either class of agent may be necessary). Products include:

DynaCirc Capsules ... 2256

Nicardipine Hydrochloride (Combination therapy of calcium channel blockers and organic nitrates may result in marked symptomatic orthostatic hypotension; dose adjustment of either class of agent may be necessary). Products include:

Cardene Capsules ... 2095
Cardene I.V. ... 2709
Cardene SR Capsules ... 2097

Nifedipine (Combination therapy of calcium channel blockers and organic nitrates may result in marked symptomatic orthostatic hypotension; dose adjustment of either class of agent may be necessary). Products include:

Adalat Capsules (10 mg and 20 mg) ... 587
Adalat CC ... 589
Procardia Capsules ... 1971
Procardia XL Extended Release Tablets ... 1972

Nimodipine (Combination therapy of calcium channel blockers and organic nitrates may result in marked symptomatic orthostatic hypotension; dose adjustment of either class of agent may be necessary). Products include:

Nimotop Capsules ... 610

Nisoldipine (Combination therapy of calcium channel blockers and organic nitrates may result in marked symptomatic orthostatic hypotension; dose adjustment of either class of agent may be necessary).

No products indexed under this heading.

Verapamil Hydrochloride (Combination therapy of calcium channel blockers and organic nitrates may result in marked symptomatic orthostatic hypotension; dose adjustment of either class of agent may be necessary). Products include:

Calan SR Caplets ... 2422
Calan Tablets ... 2419
Isoptin Injectable ... 1344
Isoptin Oral Tablets ... 1346
Isoptin SR Tablets ... 1348
Verelan Capsules ... 1410
Verelan Capsules ... 2824

Food Interactions

Alcohol (Enhances sensitivity to hypotensive activity of nitrates).

SORBITRATE ORAL TABLETS

(Isosorbide Dinitrate) ... 2843
See **Sorbitrate Chewable Tablets**

SORBITRATE SUBLINGUAL TABLETS

(Isosorbide Dinitrate) ... 2843
See **Sorbitrate Chewable Tablets**

SOTRADECOL (SODIUM TETRADECYL SULFATE INJECTION)

(Sodium Tetradecyl Sulfate) ... 967
May interact with oral contraceptives and certain other agents. Compounds in these categories include:

Desogestrel (Use caution prior to initiating treatment with Sotradecol). Products include:

Desogen Tablets ... 1817
Ortho-Cept ... 1851

Ethinyl Estradiol (Use caution prior to initiating treatment with Sotradecol). Products include:

Brevicon ... 2088
Demulen ... 2428
Desogen Tablets ... 1817
Levlen/Tri-Levlen ... 651
Lo/Ovral Tablets ... 2746
Lo/Ovral-28 Tablets ... 2751
Modicon ... 1872
Nordette-21 Tablets ... 2755
Nordette-28 Tablets ... 2758
Norinyl ... 2088
Ortho-Cept ... 1851
Ortho-Cyclen/Ortho-Tri-Cyclen ... 1858
Ortho-Novum ... 1872
Ortho-Cyclen/Ortho Tri-Cyclen ... 1858
Ovcon ... 760
Ovral Tablets ... 2770
Ovral-28 Tablets ... 2770
Levlen/Tri-Levlen ... 651
Tri-Norinyl ... 2164
Triphasil-21 Tablets ... 2814
Triphasil-28 Tablets ... 2819

Ethynodiol Diacetate (Use caution prior to initiating treatment with Sotradecol). Products include:

Demulen ... 2428

Heparin Calcium (*In Vitro* incompatibilities).

No products indexed under this heading.

Heparin Sodium (*In Vitro* incompatibilities). Products include:

Heparin Lock Flush Solution ... 2725
Heparin Sodium Injection ... 2726
Heparin Sodium Injection, USP, Sterile Solution ... 2615
Heparin Sodium Vials ... 1441

Levonorgestrel (Use caution prior to initiating treatment with Sotradecol). Products include:

Levlen/Tri-Levlen ... 651
Nordette-21 Tablets ... 2755
Nordette-28 Tablets ... 2758
Norplant System ... 2759
Levlen/Tri-Levlen ... 651
Triphasil-21 Tablets ... 2814
Triphasil-28 Tablets ... 2819

Mestranol (Use caution prior to initiating treatment with Sotradecol). Products include:

Norinyl ... 2088
Ortho-Novum ... 1872

Norethindrone (Use caution prior to initiating treatment with Sotradecol). Products include:

Brevicon ... 2088
Micronor Tablets ... 1872
Modicon ... 1872
Norinyl ... 2088
Nor-Q D Tablets ... 2135
Ortho-Novum ... 1872
Ovcon ... 760
Tri-Norinyl ... 2164

Norethynodrel (Use caution prior to initiating treatment with Sotradecol).

No products indexed under this heading.

Norgestimate (Use caution prior to initiating treatment with Sotradecol). Products include:

Ortho-Cyclen/Ortho-Tri-Cyclen ... 1858
Ortho-Cyclen/Ortho Tri-Cyclen ... 1858

Norgestrel (Use caution prior to initiating treatment with Sotradecol). Products include:

Lo/Ovral Tablets ... 2746
Lo/Ovral-28 Tablets ... 2751
Ovral Tablets ... 2770
Ovral-28 Tablets ... 2770
Ovrette Tablets ... 2771

SPECTAZOLE (ECONAZOLE NITRATE 1%) CREAM

(Econazole Nitrate) ... 1890
None cited in PDR database.

SPECTROBID TABLETS

(Bacampicillin Hydrochloride) ... 2206
May interact with:

Allopurinol (Increased incidence of rashes). Products include:

Zyloprim Tablets ... 1226

Disulfiram (Spectrobid should not be co-administered). Products include:

Antabuse Tablets ... 2695

SPORANOX CAPSULES

(Itraconazole) ... 1305
May interact with oral anticoagulants, oral hypoglycemic agents, histamine h2-receptor antagonists, dihydropyridine calcium channel blockers, antacids, proton pump inhibitor, and certain other agents. Compounds in these categories include:

Acarbose (Potential for severe hypoglycemia).

No products indexed under this heading.

Aluminum Carbonate Gel (Absorption of itraconazole is impaired when gastric acidity is decreased; antacid should not be administered for at least two hours after itraconazole administration). Products include:

Basaljel ... 2703

Aluminum Hydroxide (Absorption of itraconazole is impaired when gastric acidity is decreased; antacid should not be administered for at least two hours after itraconazole administration). Products include:

ALternaGEL Liquid ... 1316
Maximum Strength Ascriptin ... ⊡ 630
Cama Arthritis Pain Reliever ... ⊡ 785
Gaviscon Extra Strength Relief Formula Antacid Tablets ... ⊡ 819
Gaviscon Extra Strength Relief Formula Liquid Antacid ... ⊡ 819
Gaviscon Liquid Antacid ... ⊡ 820
Gelusil Liquid & Tablets ... ⊡ 855
Maalox Heartburn Relief Suspension ... ⊡ 642
Maalox Heartburn Relief Tablets ... ⊡ 641
Maalox Magnesia and Alumina Oral Suspension ... ⊡ 642
Maalox Plus Tablets ... ⊡ 643
Extra Strength Maalox Antacid Plus Antigas Liquid and Tablets ⊡ 638
Tempo Soft Antacid ... ⊡ 835

Aluminum Hydroxide Gel (Absorption of itraconazole is impaired when gastric acidity is decreased; antacid should not be administered for at least two hours after itraconazole administration). Products include:

ALternaGEL Liquid ... ⊡ 659
Aludrox Oral Suspension ... 2695
Amphojel Suspension ... 2695
Amphojel Suspension without Flavor ... 2695
Amphojel Tablets ... 2695
Arthritis Pain Ascriptin ... ⊡ 631
Regular Strength Ascriptin Tablets ... ⊡ 629
Gaviscon Antacid Tablets ... ⊡ 819
Gaviscon-2 Antacid Tablets ... ⊡ 820
Mylanta Liquid ... 1317
Mylanta Tablets ... ⊡ 660
Mylanta Double Strength Liquid ... 1317
Mylanta Double Strength Tablets ... ⊡ 660
Nephrox Suspension ... ⊡ 655

Amlodipine Besylate (Co-administration with dihydropyridine calcium channel blockers may result in edema). Products include:

Lotrel Capsules ... 840
Norvasc Tablets ... 1940

Amphotericin B (In vivo studies suggest that the activity of amphotericin B may be suppressed by azole antifungal therapy; clinical significance of this interaction is unknown). Products include:

Fungizone Intravenous ... 506

Astemizole (Co-administration is contraindicated; potential for prolonged QT intervals). Products include:

Hismanal Tablets ... 1293

Chlorpropamide (Potential for severe hypoglycemia). Products include:

Diabinese Tablets ... 1935

Cimetidine (Potential for reduced plasma levels of itraconazole; absorption of oral itraconazole is enhanced when administered with a cola beverage in patients taking acid suppressors, e.g., H_2 inhibitors). Products include:

Tagamet Tablets ... 2516

Cimetidine Hydrochloride (Potential for reduced plasma levels of itraconazole; absorption of oral itraconazole is enhanced when administered with a cola beverage in patients taking acid suppressors, e.g., H_2 inhibitors). Products include:

Tagamet ... 2516

Cisapride (Itraconazole is expected to markedly raise cisapride plasma concentrations due to its chemical similarities to ketoconazole; potential for prolonged QT interval, ventricular arrhythmias and torsades de pointes; concurrent use is contraindicated). Products include:

Propulsid ... 1300

Cyclosporine (Co-administration results in increased plasma concentration of cyclosporine; dosage of cyclosporine may have to be reduced; very rare reports of rhabdomyolysis involving renal transplant patients on concurrent therapy with HMG-CoA, cyclosporine and itraconazole). Products include:

Neoral ... 2276
Sandimmune ... 2286

Dicumarol (Enhanced anticoagulant effect).

No products indexed under this heading.

Digoxin (Elevated plasma concentrations of digoxin; monitor digoxin concentration and, if needed, reduce the dosage accordingly). Products include:

Lanoxicaps ... 1117
Lanoxin Elixir Pediatric ... 1120
Lanoxin Injection ... 1123
Lanoxin Injection Pediatric ... 1126
Lanoxin Tablets ... 1128

Dihydroxyaluminum Sodium Carbonate (Absorption of itraconazole is impaired when gastric acidity is decreased; antacid should not be administered for at least two hours after itraconazole administration).

No products indexed under this heading.

Famotidine (Potential for reduced plasma levels of itraconazole; absorption of oral itraconazole is enhanced when administered with a cola beverage in patients taking acid suppressors, e.g., H_2 inhibitors). Products include:

Pepcid AC ... 1319
Pepcid Injection ... 1722
Pepcid ... 1720

Felodipine (Co-administration with dihydropyridine calcium channel blockers may result in edema). Products include:

Plendil Extended-Release Tablets ... 527

Glipizide (Potential for severe hypoglycemia). Products include:

Glucotrol Tablets ... 1967
Glucotrol XL Extended Release Tablets ... 1968

Glyburide (Potential for severe hypoglycemia). Products include:

DiaBeta Tablets 1239
Glynase PresTab Tablets 2609
Micronase Tablets 2623

Isoniazid (Co-administration may reduce plasma levels of azole antifungal agents). Products include:

Nydrazid Injection 508
Rifamate Capsules 1530
Rifater 1532

Isradipine (Co-administration with dihydropyridine calcium channel blockers may result in edema). Products include:

DynaCirc Capsules 2256

Lansoprazole (Absorption of oral itraconazole is enhanced when administered with a cola beverage in patients taking acid suppressors, e.g., proton pump inhibitors). Products include:

PREVACID Delayed-Release Capsules 2562

Lovastatin (Very rare reports of rhabdomyolysis involving renal transplant patients on concurrent therapy with simvastatin, cyclosporine and itraconazole). Products include:

Mevacor Tablets 1699

Magaldrate (Absorption of itraconazole is impaired when gastric acidity is decreased; antacid should not be administered for at least two hours after itraconazole administration).

No products indexed under this heading.

Magnesium Hydroxide (Absorption of itraconazole is impaired when gastric acidity is decreased; antacid should not be administered for at least two hours after itraconazole administration). Products include:

Aludrox Oral Suspension 2695
Arthritis Pain Ascriptin .... ⊕D 631
Maximum Strength Ascriptin .... ⊕D 630
Regular Strength Ascriptin Tablets .... ⊕D 629
Di-Gel Antacid/Anti-Gas .... ⊕D 801
Gelusil Liquid & Tablets .... ⊕D 855
Maalox Magnesia and Alumina Oral Suspension .... ⊕D 642
Maalox Plus Tablets .... ⊕D 643
Extra Strength Maalox Antacid Plus Antigas Liquid and Tablets ⊕D 638
Mylanta Calcium Carbonate and Magnesium Hydroxide Tablets...... 1318
Mylanta Liquid 1317
Mylanta Tablets .... ⊕D 660
Mylanta Double Strength Liquid 1317
Mylanta Double Strength Tablets .. ⊕D 660
Phillips' Milk of Magnesia Liquid.... ⊕D 729
Rolaids Tablets .... ⊕D 843
Tempo Soft Antacid .... ⊕D 835

Magnesium Oxide (Absorption of itraconazole is impaired when gastric acidity is decreased; antacid should not be administered for at least two hours after itraconazole administration). Products include:

Beelith Tablets 639
Bufferin Analgesic Tablets and Caplets .... ⊕D 613
Caltrate PLUS .... ⊕D 665
Cama Arthritis Pain Reliever........... ⊕D 785
Mag-Ox 400 668
Uro-Mag 668

Metformin Hydrochloride (Potential for severe hypoglycemia). Products include:

Glucophage 752

Midazolam Hydrochloride (Co-administration with oral midazolam has resulted in elevated plasma concentration of midazolam resulting in prolonged hypnotic and sedative effects; concurrent oral use should be avoided). Products include:

Versed Injection 2170

Nicardipine Hydrochloride (Co-administration with dihydropyridine calcium channel blockers may result in edema). Products include:

Cardene Capsules 2095
Cardene I.V. 2709
Cardene SR Capsules 2097

Nifedipine (Co-administration with dihydropyridine calcium channel blockers may result in edema). Products include:

Adalat Capsules (10 mg and 20 mg) 587
Adalat CC 589
Procardia Capsules 1971
Procardia XL Extended Release Tablets 1972

Nimodipine (Co-administration with dihydropyridine calcium channel blockers may result in edema). Products include:

Nimotop Capsules 610

Nizatidine (Potential for reduced plasma levels of itraconazole; absorption of oral itraconazole is enhanced when administered with a cola beverage in patients taking acid suppressors, e.g., H_2 inhibitors). Products include:

Axid Pulvules 1427

Omeprazole (Absorption of oral itraconazole is enhanced when administered with a cola beverage in patients taking acid suppressors, e.g., proton pump inhibitors). Products include:

Prilosec Delayed-Release Capsules 529

Phenytoin (Potential for reduced plasma levels of itraconazole; coadministration may alter the metabolism of phenytoin). Products include:

Dilantin Infatabs 1908
Dilantin-125 Suspension 1911

Phenytoin Sodium (Potential for reduced plasma levels of itraconazole; coadministration may alter the metabolism of phenytoin). Products include:

Dilantin Kapseals 1906
Dilantin Parenteral 1910

Quinidine Gluconate (Potential for tinnitus and decreased hearing when used concurrently). Products include:

Quinaglute Dura-Tabs Tablets 649

Quinidine Polygalacturonate (Potential for tinnitus and decreased hearing when used concurrently).

No products indexed under this heading.

Quinidine Sulfate (Potential for tinnitus and decreased hearing when used concurrently). Products include:

Quinidex Extentabs 2067

Ranitidine Hydrochloride (Potential for reduced plasma levels of itraconazole; absorption of oral itraconazole is enhanced when administered with a cola beverage in patients taking acid suppressors, e.g., H_2 inhibitors). Products include:

Zantac 1209
Zantac Injection 1207
Zantac Syrup 1209

Rifampin (Potential for reduced plasma levels of itraconazole). Products include:

Rifadin 1528
Rifamate Capsules 1530
Rifater 1532
Rimactane Capsules 847

Simvastatin (Very rare reports of rhabdomyolysis involving renal transplant patients on concurrent therapy with simvastatin, cyclosporine and itraconazole). Products include:

Zocor Tablets 1775

Sodium Bicarbonate (Absorption of itraconazole is impaired when gastric acidity is decreased; antacid should not be administered for at least two hours after itraconazole administration). Products include:

Alka-Seltzer Effervescent Antacid and Pain Reliever .... ⊕D 701
Alka-Seltzer Extra Strength Effervescent Antacid and Pain Reliever .... ⊕D 703
Alka-Seltzer Gold Effervescent Antacid .... ⊕D 703
Alka-Seltzer Lemon Lime Effervescent Antacid and Pain Reliever .... ⊕D 703
Arm & Hammer Pure Baking Soda .... ⊕D 627
Ceo-Two Rectal Suppositories 666
Citrocarbonate Antacid .... ⊕D 770
Massengill Disposable Douches...... ⊕D 820
Massengill Liquid Concentrate .... ⊕D 820
NuLYTELY 689
Cherry Flavor NuLYTELY 689

Tacrolimus (Co-administration results in increased plasma concentration of tacrolimus, dosage of tacrolimus may have to be adjusted). Products include:

Prograf 1042

Terfenadine (Co-administration is contraindicated; potential for serious cardiovascular adverse events, including death, cardiac dysrhythmias, ventricular tachycardia and torsades de pointes). Products include:

Seldane Tablets 1536
Seldane-D Extended-Release Tablets 1538

Tolazamide (Potential for severe hypoglycemia).

No products indexed under this heading.

Tolbutamide (Potential for severe hypoglycemia).

No products indexed under this heading.

Triazolam (Co-administration has resulted in elevated plasma concentration of triazolam resulting in prolonged hypnotic and sedative effects; concurrent use with oral triazolam is contraindicated). Products include:

Halcion Tablets 2611

Warfarin Sodium (Enhanced anticoagulant effect). Products include:

Coumadin 926

Food Interactions

Cola (Absorption of oral itraconazole is enhanced when administered with a cola beverage in patients with achlorhydria, such as AIDS or patients taking acid suppressors, e.g., H_2 inhibitors and proton pump inhibitors).

Food, unspecified (The oral bioavailability of itraconazole is maximal when taken with food).

SPORTSCREME EXTERNAL ANALGESIC RUB CREAM & LOTION

(Trolamine Salicylate) .... ⊕D 834
None cited in PDR database.

ST. JOSEPH ADULT CHEWABLE ASPIRIN (81 MG.)

(Aspirin) .... ⊕D 808
None cited in PDR database.

STADOL INJECTION

(Butorphanol Tartrate) 775
See Stadol NS Nasal Spray

STADOL NS NASAL SPRAY

(Butorphanol Tartrate) 775
May interact with barbiturates, tranquilizers, central nervous system depressants, antihistamines, xanthine bronchodilators, and certain other agents. Compounds in these categories include:

Acrivastine (Potential for increased CNS depressant effect). Products include:

Semprex-D Capsules 463
Semprex-D Capsules 1167

Alfentanil Hydrochloride (Potential for increased CNS depressant effect). Products include:

Alfenta Injection 1286

Alprazolam (Potential for increased CNS depressant effect). Products include:

Xanax Tablets 2649

Aminophylline (Possibility of smaller initial dose and longer intervals between doses may be needed).

No products indexed under this heading.

Aprobarbital (Potential for increased CNS depressant effect).

No products indexed under this heading.

Astemizole (Potential for increased CNS depressant effect). Products include:

Hismanal Tablets 1293

Azatadine Maleate (Potential for increased CNS depressant effect). Products include:

Trinalin Repetabs Tablets 1330

Bromodiphenhydramine Hydrochloride (Potential for increased CNS depressant effect).

No products indexed under this heading.

Brompheniramine Maleate (Potential for increased CNS depressant effect). Products include:

Alka Seltzer Plus Sinus Medicine .. ⊕D 707
Bromfed Capsules (Extended-Release) 1785
Bromfed Syrup .... ⊕D 733
Bromfed Tablets 1785
Bromfed-DM Cough Syrup................... 1786
Bromfed-PD Capsules (Extended-Release) 1785
Dimetane-DC Cough Syrup 2059
Dimetane-DX Cough Syrup 2059
Dimetapp Elixir .... ⊕D 773
Dimetapp Extentabs .... ⊕D 774
Dimetapp Tablets/Liqui-Gels .... ⊕D 775
Dimetapp Cold & Allergy Chewable Tablets .... ⊕D 773
Dimetapp DM Elixir .... ⊕D 774
Vicks DayQuil Allergy Relief 12-Hour Extended Release Tablets.. ⊕D 760
Vicks DayQuil Allergy Relief 4-Hour Tablets .... ⊕D 760

Buprenorphine (Potential for increased CNS depressant effect). Products include:

Buprenex Injectable 2006

Buspirone Hydrochloride (Potential for increased CNS depressant effect). Products include:

BuSpar 737

Butabarbital (Potential for increased CNS depressant effect).

No products indexed under this heading.

Butalbital (Potential for increased CNS depressant effect). Products include:

Esgic-plus Tablets 1013
Fioricet Tablets 2258
Fioricet with Codeine Capsules 2260
Fiorinal Capsules 2261
Fiorinal with Codeine Capsules 2262
Fiorinal Tablets 2261
Phrenilin 785
Sedapap Tablets 50 mg/650 mg .. 1543

Chlordiazepoxide (Potential for increased CNS depressant effect). Products include:

Libritabs Tablets 2177
Limbitrol 2180

IMPORTANT NOTE: Always consult each drug listing in the patient's regimen for possible interactions.

Stadol **Interactions Index** **974**

Chlordiazepoxide Hydrochloride (Potential for increased CNS depressant effect). Products include:
Librax Capsules 2176
Librium Capsules 2178
Librium Injectable 2179

Chlorpheniramine Maleate (Potential for increased CNS depressant effect). Products include:
Alka-Seltzer Plus Cold Medicine ▣ 705
Alka-Seltzer Plus Cold Medicine Liqui-Gels ▣ 706
Alka-Seltzer Plus Cold & Cough Medicine ▣ 708
Alka-Seltzer Plus Cold & Cough Medicine Liqui-Gels ▣ 705
Allerest Children's Chewable Tablets ▣ 627
Allerest Headache Strength Tablets ▣ 627
Allerest Maximum Strength Tablets ▣ 627
Allerest Sinus Pain Formula ▣ 627
Allerest 12 Hour Caplets ▣ 627
Ana-Kit Anaphylaxis Emergency Treatment Kit 617
Atrohist Pediatric Capsules 453
Atrohist Plus Tablets 454
BC Cold Powder Multi-Symptom Formula (Cold-Sinus-Allergy) ▣ 609
Cerose DM ▣ 878
Cheracol Plus Head Cold/Cough Formula ▣ 769
Children's Vicks DayQuil Allergy Relief ▣ 757
Children's Vicks NyQuil Cold/Cough Relief ▣ 758
Chlor-Trimeton Allergy Decongestant Tablets ▣ 799
Chlor-Trimeton Allergy Tablets ▣ 798
Comhist 2038
Comtrex Multi-Symptom Cold Reliever Tablets/Caplets/Liqui-Gels/Liquid ▣ 615
Allergy-Sinus Comtrex Multi-Symptom Allergy-Sinus Formula Tablets ▣ 617
Contac Continuous Action Nasal Decongestant/Antihistamine 12 Hour Capsules ▣ 813
Contac Maximum Strength Continuous Action Decongestant/Antihistamine 12 Hour Caplets ▣ 813
Contac Severe Cold and Flu Formula Caplets ▣ 814
Coricidin 'D' Decongestant Tablets ▣ 800
Coricidin Tablets ▣ 800
D.A. Chewable Tablets 951
Deconamine 1320
Dura-Tap/PD Capsules 2867
Dura-Vent/DA Tablets 953
Extendryl 1005
Fedahist Gyrocaps 2401
Fedahist Timecaps 2401
Hycomine Compound Tablets 932
Isoclor Timesule Capsules ▣ 637
Kronofed-A 977
Nolamine Timed-Release Tablets 785
Novahistine DH 2462
Novahistine Elixir ▣ 823
Ornade Spansule Capsules 2502
PediaCare Cold Allergy Chewable Tablets ▣ 677
PediaCare Cough-Cold Chewable Tablets 1553
PediaCare Cough-Cold Liquid 1553
PediaCare NightRest Cough-Cold Liquid 1553
Pediatric Vicks 44m Cough & Cold Relief ▣ 764
Pyrroxate Caplets ▣ 772
Ryna ▣ 841
Sinarest Tablets ▣ 648
Sinarest Extra Strength Tablets ▣ 648
Sine-Off Sinus Medicine ▣ 825
Singlet Tablets ▣ 825
Sinulin Tablets 787
Sinutab Sinus Allergy Medication, Maximum Strength Tablets and Caplets ▣ 860
Sudafed Plus Liquid ▣ 862
Sudafed Plus Tablets ▣ 863
Teldrin 12 Hour Antihistamine/Nasal Decongestant Allergy Relief Capsules ▣ 826
TheraFlu ▣ 787
TheraFlu Maximum Strength Nighttime Flu, Cold & Cough Medicine ▣ 788
Triaminic Allergy Tablets ▣ 789
Triaminic Cold Tablets ▣ 790
Triaminic Nite Light ▣ 791
Triaminic Syrup ▣ 792
Triaminic-12 Tablets ▣ 792
Triaminicin Tablets ▣ 793
Triaminicol Multi-Symptom Cold Tablets ▣ 793
Triaminicol Multi-Symptom Relief ▣ 794
Tussend 1783
Children's TYLENOL Cold Multi-Symptom Liquid Formula and Chewable Tablets 1561
Children's TYLENOL Cold Plus Cough Multi Symptom Tablets and Liquid ▣ 681
TYLENOL Maximum Strength Allergy Sinus Medication Gelcaps and Caplets 1563
TYLENOL Cold Multi-Symptom Formula Medication Tablets and Caplets 1561
TYLENOL Cold Multi-Symptom Hot Medication Liquid Packets 1557
Vicks 44 LiquiCaps Cough, Cold & Flu Relief ▣ 755
Vicks 44M Cough, Cold & Flu Relief ▣ 756

Chlorpheniramine Polistirex (Potential for increased CNS depressant effect). Products include:
Tussionex Pennkinetic Extended-Release Suspension 998

Chlorpheniramine Tannate (Potential for increased CNS depressant effect). Products include:
Atrohist Pediatric Suspension 454
Ricobid Tablets and Pediatric Suspension 2038
Rynatan 2673
Rynatuss 2673

Chlorpromazine (Potential for increased CNS depressant effect). Products include:
Thorazine Suppositories 2523

Chlorpromazine Hydrochloride (Potential for increased CNS depressant effect). Products include:
Thorazine 2523

Chlorprothixene (Potential for increased CNS depressant effect).
No products indexed under this heading.

Chlorprothixene Hydrochloride (Potential for increased CNS depressant effect).
No products indexed under this heading.

Clemastine Fumarate (Potential for increased CNS depressant effect). Products include:
Tavist Syrup 2297
Tavist Tablets 2298
Tavist-1 12 Hour Relief Tablets ▣ 787
Tavist-D 12 Hour Relief Tablets ▣ 787

Clorazepate Dipotassium (Potential for increased CNS depressant effect). Products include:
Tranxene 451

Clozapine (Potential for increased CNS depressant effect). Products include:
Clozaril Tablets 2252

Codeine Phosphate (Potential for increased CNS depressant effect). Products include:
Actifed with Codeine Cough Syrup 1067
Brontex 1981
Deconsal C Expectorant Syrup 456
Deconsal Pediatric Syrup 457
Dimetane-DC Cough Syrup 2059
Empirin with Codeine Tablets 1093
Fioricet with Codeine Capsules 2260
Fiorinal with Codeine Capsules 2262
Isoclor Expectorant 990
Novahistine DH 2462
Novahistine Expectorant 2463
Nucofed 2051
Phenergan with Codeine 2777
Phenergan VC with Codeine 2781
Robitussin A-C Syrup 2073
Robitussin-DAC Syrup 2074
Ryna ▣ 841
Soma Compound w/Codeine Tablets 2676
Tussi-Organidin NR Liquid and S NR Liquid 2677
Tylenol with Codeine 1583

Cyproheptadine Hydrochloride (Potential for increased CNS depressant effect). Products include:
Periactin 1724

Desflurane (Potential for increased CNS depressant effect). Products include:
Suprane 1813

Dexchlorpheniramine Maleate (Potential for increased CNS depressant effect).
No products indexed under this heading.

Dezocine (Potential for increased CNS depressant effect). Products include:
Dalgan Injection 538

Diazepam (Potential for increased CNS depressant effect). Products include:
Dizac 1809
Valium Injectable 2182
Valium Tablets 2183
Valrelease Capsules 2169

Diphenhydramine Citrate (Potential for increased CNS depressant effect). Products include:
Excedrin P.M. Analgesic/Sleeping Aid Tablets, Caplets, Liquigels 733

Diphenhydramine Hydrochloride (Potential for increased CNS depressant effect). Products include:
Actifed Allergy Daytime/Nighttime Caplets ▣ 844
Actifed Sinus Daytime/Nighttime Tablets and Caplets ▣ 846
Arthritis Foundation NightTime Caplets ▣ 674
Extra Strength Bayer PM Aspirin ▣ 713
Bayer Select Night Time Pain Relief Formula ▣ 716
Benadryl Allergy Decongestant Liquid Medication ▣ 848
Benadryl Allergy Decongestant Tablets ▣ 848
Benadryl Allergy Liquid Medication ▣ 849
Benadryl Allergy ▣ 848
Benadryl Allergy Sinus Headache Formula Caplets ▣ 849
Benadryl Capsules 1898
Benadryl Dye-Free Allergy Liqui-gel Softgels ▣ 850
Benadryl Dye-Free Allergy Liquid Medication ▣ 850
Benadryl Itch Relief Cream, Children's Formula and Maximum Strength 2% ▣ 851
Benadryl Itch Relief Spray, Children's Formula and Maximum Strength 2% ▣ 851
Benadryl Itch Relief Stick Maximum Strength 2% ▣ 850
Benadryl Itch Stopping Gel, Children's Formula and Maximum Strength 2% ▣ 851
Benadryl Kapseals 1898
Benadryl Injection 1898
Contac Day & Night Cold/Flu Night Caplets ▣ 812
Contac Night Allergy/Sinus Caplets ▣ 812
Extra Strength Doan's P.M. ▣ 633
Legatrin PM ▣ 651
Miles Nervine Nighttime Sleep-Aid ▣ 723
Nytol QuickCaps Caplets ▣ 610
Sleepinal Night-time Sleep Aid Capsules and Softgels ▣ 834
TYLENOL Maximum Strength Allergy Sinus NightTime Medication Caplets 1555
TYLENOL Flu NightTime, Maximum Strength, Gelcaps 1566
TYLENOL Maximum Strength Flu NightTime Hot Medication Packets 1562
TYLENOL PM, Extra Strength Pain Reliever/Sleep Aid Caplets, Geltabs, Gelcaps 1560
TYLENOL Severe Allergy Medication Caplets 1564
Maximum Strength Unisom Sleepgels 1934
Unisom With Pain Relief-Nighttime Sleep Aid and Pain Reliever 1934

Diphenylpyraline Hydrochloride (Potential for increased CNS depressant effect).
No products indexed under this heading.

Droperidol (Potential for increased CNS depressant effect). Products include:
Inapsine Injection 1296

Dyphylline (Possibility of smaller initial dose and longer intervals between doses may be needed). Products include:
Lufyllin & Lufyllin-400 Tablets 2670
Lufyllin-GG Elixir & Tablets 2671

Enflurane (Potential for increased CNS depressant effect).
No products indexed under this heading.

Estazolam (Potential for increased CNS depressant effect). Products include:
ProSom Tablets 449

Ethchlorvynol (Potential for increased CNS depressant effect). Products include:
Placidyl Capsules 448

Ethinamate (Potential for increased CNS depressant effect).
No products indexed under this heading.

Fentanyl (Potential for increased CNS depressant effect). Products include:
Duragesic Transdermal System 1288

Fentanyl Citrate (Potential for increased CNS depressant effect). Products include:
Sublimaze Injection 1307

Fluphenazine Decanoate (Potential for increased CNS depressant effect). Products include:
Prolixin Decanoate 509

Fluphenazine Enanthate (Potential for increased CNS depressant effect). Products include:
Prolixin Enanthate 509

Fluphenazine Hydrochloride (Potential for increased CNS depressant effect). Products include:
Prolixin 509

Flurazepam Hydrochloride (Potential for increased CNS depressant effect). Products include:
Dalmane Capsules 2173

Glutethimide (Potential for increased CNS depressant effect).
No products indexed under this heading.

Haloperidol (Potential for increased CNS depressant effect). Products include:
Haldol Injection, Tablets and Concentrate 1575

Haloperidol Decanoate (Potential for increased CNS depressant effect). Products include:
Haldol Decanoate 1577

Hydrocodone Bitartrate (Potential for increased CNS depressant effect). Products include:
Anexsia 5/500 Elixir 1781
Anexia Tablets 1782
Codiclear DH Syrup 791
Deconamine CX Cough and Cold Liquid and Tablets 1319
Duratuss HD Elixir 2565
Hycodan Tablets and Syrup 930
Hycomine Compound Tablets 932
Hycomine 931
Hycotuss Expectorant Syrup 933
Hydrocet Capsules 782
Lorcet 10/650 1018
Lortab 2566
Tussend 1783
Tussend Expectorant 1785
Vicodin Tablets 1356
Vicodin ES Tablets 1357

(▣ Described in PDR For Nonprescription Drugs) (◉ Described in PDR For Ophthalmology)

Vicodin Tuss Expectorant 1358
Zydone Capsules 949

Hydrocodone Polistirex (Potential for increased CNS depressant effect). Products include:

Tussionex Pennkinetic Extended-Release Suspension 998

Hydroxyzine Hydrochloride (Potential for increased CNS depressant effect). Products include:

Atarax Tablets & Syrup......................... 2185
Marax Tablets & DF Syrup................... 2200
Vistaril Intramuscular Solution.......... 2216

Isoflurane (Potential for increased CNS depressant effect).

No products indexed under this heading.

Ketamine Hydrochloride (Potential for increased CNS depressant effect).

No products indexed under this heading.

Levomethadyl Acetate Hydrochloride (Potential for increased CNS depressant effect). Products include:

Orlamm 2239

Levorphanol Tartrate (Potential for increased CNS depressant effect). Products include:

Levo-Dromoran...................................... 2129

Loratadine (Potential for increased CNS depressant effect). Products include:

Claritin 2349
Claritin-D 2350

Lorazepam (Potential for increased CNS depressant effect). Products include:

Ativan Injection...................................... 2698
Ativan Tablets 2700

Loxapine Hydrochloride (Potential for increased CNS depressant effect). Products include:

Loxitane 1378

Loxapine Succinate (Potential for increased CNS depressant effect). Products include:

Loxitane Capsules 1378

Meperidine Hydrochloride (Potential for increased CNS depressant effect). Products include:

Demerol 2308
Mepergan Injection 2753

Mephobarbital (Potential for increased CNS depressant effect). Products include:

Mebaral Tablets 2322

Meprobamate (Potential for increased CNS depressant effect). Products include:

Miltown Tablets 2672
PMB 200 and PMB 400 2783

Mesoridazine (Potential for increased CNS depressant effect).

Mesoridazine Besylate (Potential for increased CNS depressant effect). Products include:

Serentil.. 684

Methadone Hydrochloride (Potential for increased CNS depressant effect). Products include:

Methadone Hydrochloride Oral Concentrate 2233
Methadone Hydrochloride Oral Solution & Tablets................................ 2235

Methdilazine Hydrochloride (Potential for increased CNS depressant effect).

No products indexed under this heading.

Methohexital Sodium (Potential for increased CNS depressant effect). Products include:

Brevital Sodium Vials 1429

Methotrimeprazine (Potential for increased CNS depressant effect). Products include:

Levoprome 1274

Methoxyflurane (Potential for increased CNS depressant effect).

No products indexed under this heading.

Midazolam Hydrochloride (Potential for increased CNS depressant effect). Products include:

Versed Injection 2170

Molindone Hydrochloride (Potential for increased CNS depressant effect). Products include:

Moban Tablets and Concentrate 1048

Morphine Sulfate (Potential for increased CNS depressant effect). Products include:

Astramorph/PF Injection, USP (Preservative-Free) 535
Duramorph 962
Infumorph 200 and Infumorph 500 Sterile Solutions........................... 965
MS Contin Tablets................................. 1994
MSIR 1997
Oramorph SR (Morphine Sulfate Sustained Release Tablets) 2236
RMS Suppositories 2657
Roxanol 2243

Opium Alkaloids (Potential for increased CNS depressant effect).

No products indexed under this heading.

Oxazepam (Potential for increased CNS depressant effect). Products include:

Serax Capsules 2810
Serax Tablets.. 2810

Oxycodone Hydrochloride (Potential for increased CNS depressant effect). Products include:

Percocet Tablets 938
Percodan Tablets................................... 939
Percodan-Demi Tablets........................ 940
Roxicodone Tablets, Oral Solution & Intensol (Oxycodone) 2244
Tylox Capsules 1584

Pentobarbital Sodium (Potential for increased CNS depressant effect). Products include:

Nembutal Sodium Capsules 436
Nembutal Sodium Solution 438
Nembutal Sodium Suppositories...... 440

Perphenazine (Potential for increased CNS depressant effect). Products include:

Etrafon 2355
Triavil Tablets 1757
Trilafon.. 2389

Phenobarbital (Potential for increased CNS depressant effect). Products include:

Arco-Lase Plus Tablets 512
Bellergal-S Tablets 2250
Donnatal 2060
Donnatal Extentabs............................... 2061
Donnatal Tablets 2060
Phenobarbital Elixir and Tablets 1469
Quadrinal Tablets 1350

Prazepam (Potential for increased CNS depressant effect).

No products indexed under this heading.

Prochlorperazine (Potential for increased CNS depressant effect). Products include:

Compazine 2470

Promethazine Hydrochloride (Potential for increased CNS depressant effect). Products include:

Mepergan Injection 2753
Phenergan with Codeine 2777
Phenergan with Dextromethorphan 2778
Phenergan Injection 2773
Phenergan Suppositories 2775
Phenergan Syrup 2774
Phenergan Tablets 2775
Phenergan VC 2779

Phenergan VC with Codeine 2781

Propofol (Potential for increased CNS depressant effect). Products include:

Diprivan Injection.................................. 2833

Propoxyphene Hydrochloride (Potential for increased CNS depressant effect). Products include:

Darvon 1435
Wygesic Tablets 2827

Propoxyphene Napsylate (Potential for increased CNS depressant effect). Products include:

Darvon-N/Darvocet-N 1433

Pyrilamine Maleate (Potential for increased CNS depressant effect). Products include:

4-Way Fast Acting Nasal Spray (regular & mentholated)................. ◙ 621
Maximum Strength Multi-Symptom Formula Midol .... ◙ 722
PMS Multi-Symptom Formula Midol .... ◙ 723

Pyrilamine Tannate (Potential for increased CNS depressant effect). Products include:

Atrohist Pediatric Suspension 454
Rynatan 2673

Quazepam (Potential for increased CNS depressant effect). Products include:

Doral Tablets 2664

Risperidone (Potential for increased CNS depressant effect). Products include:

Risperdal... 1301

Secobarbital Sodium (Potential for increased CNS depressant effect). Products include:

Seconal Sodium Pulvules 1474

Sufentanil Citrate (Potential for increased CNS depressant effect). Products include:

Sufenta Injection 1309

Temazepam (Potential for increased CNS depressant effect). Products include:

Restoril Capsules 2284

Terfenadine (Potential for increased CNS depressant effect). Products include:

Seldane Tablets 1536
Seldane-D Extended-Release Tablets 1538

Theophylline (Possibility of smaller initial dose and longer intervals between doses may be needed). Products include:

Marax Tablets & DF Syrup................... 2200
Quibron 2053

Theophylline Anhydrous (Possibility of smaller initial dose and longer intervals between doses may be needed). Products include:

Aerolate 1004
Primatene Dual Action Formula...... ◙ 872
Primatene Tablets .... ◙ 873
Respbid Tablets 682
Slo-bid Gyrocaps 2033
Theo-24 Extended Release Capsules 2568
Theo-Dur Extended-Release Tablets 1327
Theo-X Extended-Release Tablets .. 788
Uni-Dur Extended-Release Tablets.. 1331
Uniphyl 400 mg Tablets....................... 2001

Theophylline Calcium Salicylate (Possibility of smaller initial dose and longer intervals between doses may be needed). Products include:

Quadrinal Tablets 1350

Theophylline Sodium Glycinate (Possibility of smaller initial dose and longer intervals between doses may be needed).

No products indexed under this heading.

Thiamylal Sodium (Potential for increased CNS depressant effect).

No products indexed under this heading.

Thioridazine Hydrochloride (Potential for increased CNS depressant effect). Products include:

Mellaril 2269

Thiothixene (Potential for increased CNS depressant effect). Products include:

Navane Capsules and Concentrate 2201
Navane Intramuscular 2202

Triazolam (Potential for increased CNS depressant effect). Products include:

Halcion Tablets....................................... 2611

Trifluoperazine Hydrochloride (Potential for increased CNS depressant effect). Products include:

Stelazine 2514

Trimeprazine Tartrate (Potential for increased CNS depressant effect). Products include:

Temaril Tablets, Syrup and Spansule Extended-Release Capsules.. 483

Tripelennamine Hydrochloride (Potential for increased CNS depressant effect). Products include:

PBZ Tablets 845
PBZ-SR Tablets...................................... 844

Triprolidine Hydrochloride (Potential for increased CNS depressant effect). Products include:

Actifed Plus Caplets .... ◙ 845
Actifed Plus Tablets .... ◙ 845
Actifed with Codeine Cough Syrup.. 1067
Actifed Syrup.. ◙ 846
Actifed Tablets .... ◙ 844

Zolpidem Tartrate (Potential for increased CNS depressant effect). Products include:

Ambien Tablets....................................... 2416

Food Interactions

Alcohol (Potential for increased CNS depressant effect).

STAR-OTIC EAR SOLUTION

(Acetic Acid, Boric Acid, Burow's Solution) .... ◙ 830

None cited in PDR database.

STELAZINE CONCENTRATE

(Trifluoperazine Hydrochloride) 2514

May interact with vasopressors, oral anticoagulants, thiazides, anticonvulsants, central nervous system depressants, and certain other agents. Compounds in these categories include:

Alfentanil Hydrochloride (Additive depressant effects). Products include:

Alfenta Injection 1286

Alprazolam (Additive depressant effects). Products include:

Xanax Tablets 2649

Aprobarbital (Additive depressant effects).

No products indexed under this heading.

Bendroflumethiazide (Orthostatic hypotension that occurs with phenothiazines may be accentuated).

No products indexed under this heading.

Buprenorphine (Additive depressant effects). Products include:

Buprenex Injectable 2006

Buspirone Hydrochloride (Additive depressant effects). Products include:

BuSpar 737

IMPORTANT NOTE: Always consult each drug listing in the patient's regimen for possible interactions.

Stelazine

Butabarbital (Additive depressant effects).

No products indexed under this heading.

Butalbital (Additive depressant effects). Products include:

Esgic-plus Tablets	1013
Fioricet Tablets	2258
Fioricet with Codeine Capsules	2260
Fiorinal Capsules	2261
Fiorinal with Codeine Capsules	2262
Fiorinal Tablets	2261
Phrenilin	785
Sedapap Tablets 50 mg/650 mg	1543

Carbamazepine (Stelazine may lower convulsive thresholds; dosage adjustments of anticonvulsants may be necessary). Products include:

Atretol Tablets	573
Tegretol Chewable Tablets	852
Tegretol Suspension	852
Tegretol Tablets	852

Chlordiazepoxide (Additive depressant effects). Products include:

Libritabs Tablets	2177
Limbitrol	2180

Chlordiazepoxide Hydrochloride (Additive depressant effects). Products include:

Librax Capsules	2176
Librium Capsules	2178
Librium Injectable	2179

Chlorothiazide (Orthostatic hypotension that occurs with phenothiazines may be accentuated). Products include:

Aldoclor Tablets	1598
Diupres Tablets	1650
Diuril Oral	1653

Chlorothiazide Sodium (Orthostatic hypotension that occurs with phenothiazines may be accentuated). Products include:

Diuril Sodium Intravenous	1652

Chlorpromazine (Additive depressant effects). Products include:

Thorazine Suppositories	2523

Chlorprothixene (Additive depressant effects).

No products indexed under this heading.

Chlorprothixene Hydrochloride (Additive depressant effects).

No products indexed under this heading.

Clorazepate Dipotassium (Additive depressant effects). Products include:

Tranxene	451

Clozapine (Additive depressant effects). Products include:

Clozaril Tablets	2252

Codeine Phosphate (Additive depressant effects). Products include:

Actifed with Codeine Cough Syrup	1067
Brontex	1981
Deconsal C Expectorant Syrup	456
Deconsal Pediatric Syrup	457
Dimetane-DC Cough Syrup	2059
Empirin with Codeine Tablets	1093
Fioricet with Codeine Capsules	2260
Fiorinal with Codeine Capsules	2262
Isoclor Expectorant	990
Novahistine DH	2462
Novahistine Expectorant	2463
Nucofed	2051
Phenergan with Codeine	2777
Phenergan VC with Codeine	2781
Robitussin A-C Syrup	2073
Robitussin-DAC Syrup	2074
Ryna	◼ 841
Soma Compound w/Codeine Tablets	2676
Tussi-Organidin NR Liquid and S NR Liquid	2677
Tylenol with Codeine	1583

Desflurane (Additive depressant effects). Products include:

Suprane	1813

Dezocine (Additive depressant effects). Products include:

Dalgan Injection	538

Diazepam (Additive depressant effects). Products include:

Dizac	1809
Valium Injectable	2182
Valium Tablets	2183
Valrelease Capsules	2169

Dicumarol (Effect may be diminished).

No products indexed under this heading.

Divalproex Sodium (Stelazine may lower convulsive thresholds; dosage adjustments of anticonvulsants may be necessary). Products include:

Depakote Tablets	415

Dopamine Hydrochloride (May cause a paradoxical further lowering of blood pressure).

No products indexed under this heading.

Droperidol (Additive depressant effects). Products include:

Inapsine Injection	1296

Enflurane (Additive depressant effects).

No products indexed under this heading.

Epinephrine Bitartrate (Reversed epinephrine effect; may cause a paradoxical further lowering of blood pressure). Products include:

Bronkaid Mist Suspension	◼ 718
Sensorcaine-MPF with Epinephrine Injection	559

Epinephrine Hydrochloride (Reversed epinephrine effect; may cause a paradoxical further lowering of blood pressure). Products include:

Ana-Kit Anaphylaxis Emergency Treatment Kit	617

Estazolam (Additive depressant effects). Products include:

ProSom Tablets	449

Ethchlorvynol (Additive depressant effects). Products include:

Placidyl Capsules	448

Ethinamate (Additive depressant effects).

No products indexed under this heading.

Ethosuximide (Stelazine may lower convulsive thresholds; dosage adjustments of anticonvulsants may be necessary). Products include:

Zarontin Capsules	1928
Zarontin Syrup	1929

Ethotoin (Stelazine may lower convulsive thresholds; dosage adjustments of anticonvulsants may be necessary). Products include:

Peganone Tablets	446

Felbamate (Stelazine may lower convulsive thresholds; dosage adjustments of anticonvulsants may be necessary). Products include:

Felbatol	2666

Fentanyl (Additive depressant effects). Products include:

Duragesic Transdermal System	1288

Fentanyl Citrate (Additive depressant effects). Products include:

Sublimaze Injection	1307

Fluphenazine Decanoate (Additive depressant effects). Products include:

Prolixin Decanoate	509

Fluphenazine Enanthate (Additive depressant effects). Products include:

Prolixin Enanthate	509

Fluphenazine Hydrochloride (Additive depressant effects). Products include:

Prolixin	509

Flurazepam Hydrochloride (Additive depressant effects). Products include:

Dalmane Capsules	2173

Glutethimide (Additive depressant effects).

No products indexed under this heading.

Guanethidine Monosulfate (Antihypertensive effects of guanethidine and related compounds may be counteracted when used concurrently). Products include:

Esimil Tablets	822
Ismelin Tablets	827

Haloperidol (Additive depressant effects). Products include:

Haldol Injection, Tablets and Concentrate	1575

Haloperidol Decanoate (Additive depressant effects). Products include:

Haldol Decanoate	1577

Hydrochlorothiazide (Orthostatic hypotension that occurs with Stelazine may be accentuated). Products include:

Aldactazide	2413
Aldoril Tablets	1604
Apresazide Capsules	808
Capozide	742
Dyazide	2479
Esidrix Tablets	821
Esimil Tablets	822
HydroDIURIL Tablets	1674
Hydropres Tablets	1675
Hyzaar Tablets	1677
Inderide Tablets	2732
Inderide LA Long Acting Capsules	2734
Lopressor HCT Tablets	832
Lotensin HCT	837
Maxzide	1380
Moduretic Tablets	1705
Oretic Tablets	443
Prinzide Tablets	1737
Ser-Ap-Es Tablets	849
Timolide Tablets	1748
Vaseretic Tablets	1765
Zestoretic	2850
Ziac	1415

Hydrocodone Bitartrate (Additive depressant effects). Products include:

Anexsia 5/500 Elixir	1781
Anexia Tablets	1782
Codiclear DH Syrup	791
Deconamine CX Cough and Cold Liquid and Tablets	1319
Duratuss HD Elixir	2565
Hycodan Tablets and Syrup	930
Hycomine Compound Tablets	932
Hycomine	931
Hycotuss Expectorant Syrup	933
Hydrocet Capsules	782
Lorcet 10/650	1018
Lortab	2566
Tussend	1783
Tussend Expectorant	1785
Vicodin Tablets	1356
Vicodin ES Tablets	1357
Vicodin Tuss Expectorant	1358
Zydone Capsules	949

Hydrocodone Polistirex (Additive depressant effects). Products include:

Tussionex Pennkinetic Extended-Release Suspension	998

Hydroflumethiazide (Orthostatic hypotension that occurs with Stelazine may be accentuated). Products include:

Diucardin Tablets	2718

Hydroxyzine Hydrochloride (Additive depressant effects). Products include:

Atarax Tablets & Syrup	2185
Marax Tablets & DF Syrup	2200
Vistaril Intramuscular Solution	2216

Isoflurane (Additive depressant effects).

No products indexed under this heading.

Ketamine Hydrochloride (Additive depressant effects).

No products indexed under this heading.

Lamotrigine (Stelazine may lower convulsive thresholds; dosage adjustments of anticonvulsants may be necessary). Products include:

Lamictal Tablets	1112

Levomethadyl Acetate Hydrochloride (Additive depressant effects). Products include:

Orlaam	2239

Levorphanol Tartrate (Additive depressant effects). Products include:

Levo-Dromoran	2129

Lorazepam (Additive depressant effects). Products include:

Ativan Injection	2698
Ativan Tablets	2700

Loxapine Hydrochloride (Additive depressant effects). Products include:

Loxitane	1378

Loxapine Succinate (Additive depressant effects). Products include:

Loxitane Capsules	1378

Meperidine Hydrochloride (Additive depressant effects). Products include:

Demerol	2308
Mepergan Injection	2753

Mephenytoin (Stelazine may lower convulsive thresholds; dosage adjustments of anticonvulsants may be necessary). Products include:

Mesantoin Tablets	2272

Mephobarbital (Additive depressant effects). Products include:

Mebaral Tablets	2322

Meprobamate (Additive depressant effects). Products include:

Miltown Tablets	2672
PMB 200 and PMB 400	2783

Mesoridazine Besylate (Additive depressant effects). Products include:

Serentil	684

Metaraminol Bitartrate (May cause a paradoxical further lowering of blood pressure). Products include:

Aramine Injection	1609

Methadone Hydrochloride (Additive depressant effects). Products include:

Methadone Hydrochloride Oral Concentrate	2233
Methadone Hydrochloride Oral Solution & Tablets	2235

Methohexital Sodium (Additive depressant effects). Products include:

Brevital Sodium Vials	1429

Methotrimeprazine (Additive depressant effects). Products include:

Levoprome	1274

Methoxamine Hydrochloride (May cause a paradoxical further lowering of blood pressure). Products include:

Vasoxyl Injection	1196

Methoxyflurane (Additive depressant effects).

No products indexed under this heading.

Methsuximide (Stelazine may lower convulsive thresholds; dosage adjustments of anticonvulsants may be necessary). Products include:

Celontin Kapseals	1899

(◼ Described in PDR For Nonprescription Drugs) (◉ Described in PDR For Ophthalmology)

Interactions Index

Methyclothiazide (Orthostatic hypotension that occurs with Stelazine may be accentuated). Products include:

Enduron Tablets....................................... 420

Metrizamide (Stelazine may lower the seizure threshold; do not use concurrently).

Midazolam Hydrochloride (Additive depressant effects). Products include:

Versed Injection....................................... 2170

Molindone Hydrochloride (Additive depressant effects). Products include:

Moban Tablets and Concentrate...... 1048

Morphine Sulfate (Additive depressant effects). Products include:

Astramorph/PF Injection, USP (Preservative-Free).............................. 535 Duramorph.. 962 Infumorph 200 and Infumorph 500 Sterile Solutions........................ 965 MS Contin Tablets................................... 1994 MSIR.. 1997 Oramorph SR (Morphine Sulfate Sustained Release Tablets)............ 2236 RMS Suppositories................................. 2657 Roxanol... 2243

Norepinephrine Bitartrate (May cause a paradoxical further lowering of blood pressure). Products include:

Levophed Bitartrate Injection............ 2315

Opium Alkaloids (Additive depressant effects).

No products indexed under this heading.

Oxazepam (Additive depressant effects). Products include:

Serax Capsules... 2810 Serax Tablets... 2810

Oxycodone Hydrochloride (Additive depressant effects). Products include:

Percocet Tablets...................................... 938 Percodan Tablets..................................... 939 Percodan-Demi Tablets......................... 940 Roxicodone Tablets, Oral Solution & Intensol (Oxycodone).................. 2244 Tylox Capsules... 1584

Paramethadione (Stelazine may lower convulsive thresholds; dosage adjustments of anticonvulsants may be necessary).

No products indexed under this heading.

Pentobarbital Sodium (Additive depressant effects). Products include:

Nembutal Sodium Capsules............... 436 Nembutal Sodium Solution................. 438 Nembutal Sodium Suppositories...... 440

Perphenazine (Additive depressant effects). Products include:

Etrafon... 2355 Triavil Tablets... 1757 Trilafon... 2389

Phenacemide (Stelazine may lower convulsive thresholds; dosage adjustments of anticonvulsants may be necessary). Products include:

Phenurone Tablets.................................. 447

Phenobarbital (Additive depressant effects). Products include:

Arco-Lase Plus Tablets.......................... 512 Bellergal-S Tablets.................................. 2250 Donnatal... 2060 Donnatal Extentabs................................ 2061 Donnatal Tablets...................................... 2060 Phenobarbital Elixir and Tablets...... 1469 Quadrinal Tablets.................................... 1350

Phensuximide (Phenothiazines may lower convulsive thresholds; dosage adjustments of anticonvulsants may be necessary). Products include:

Milontin Kapseals................................... 1920

Phenytoin (Phenytoin toxicity may be precipitated; Stelazine may lower convulsive thresholds; dosage adjustments of anticonvulsants may be necessary). Products include:

Dilantin Infatabs..................................... 1908 Dilantin-125 Suspension...................... 1911

Phenytoin Sodium (Phenytoin toxicity may be precipitated; Stelazine may lower convulsive thresholds; dosage adjustments of anticonvulsants may be necessary). Products include:

Dilantin Kapseals.................................... 1906 Dilantin Parenteral................................. 1910

Polythiazide (Orthostatic hypotension that occurs with Stelazine may be accentuated). Products include:

Minizide Capsules.................................. 1938

Prazepam (Additive depressant effects).

No products indexed under this heading.

Primidone (Stelazine may lower convulsive thresholds; dosage adjustments of anticonvulsants may be necessary). Products include:

Mysoline... 2754

Prochlorperazine (Additive depressant effects). Products include:

Compazine... 2470

Promethazine Hydrochloride (Additive depressant effects). Products include:

Mepergan Injection................................ 2753 Phenergan with Codeine...................... 2777 Phenergan with Dextromethorphan 2778 Phenergan Injection............................... 2773 Phenergan Suppositories..................... 2775 Phenergan Syrup..................................... 2774 Phenergan Tablets.................................. 2775 Phenergan VC... 2779 Phenergan VC with Codeine.............. 2781

Propofol (Additive depressant effects). Products include:

Diprivan Injection................................... 2833

Propoxyphene Hydrochloride (Additive depressant effects). Products include:

Darvon... 1435 Wygesic Tablets....................................... 2827

Propoxyphene Napsylate (Additive depressant effects). Products include:

Darvon-N/Darvocet-N.......................... 1433

Propranolol Hydrochloride (Concomitant administration results in increased plasma levels of both drugs). Products include:

Inderal... 2728 Inderal LA Long Acting Capsules.... 2730 Inderide Tablets....................................... 2732 Inderide LA Long Acting Capsules.. 2734

Quazepam (Additive depressant effects). Products include:

Doral Tablets... 2664

Risperidone (Additive depressant effects). Products include:

Risperdal.. 1301

Secobarbital Sodium (Additive depressant effects). Products include:

Seconal Sodium Pulvules..................... 1474

Sufentanil Citrate (Additive depressant effects). Products include:

Sufenta Injection..................................... 1309

Temazepam (Additive depressant effects). Products include:

Restoril Capsules..................................... 2284

Thiamylal Sodium (Additive depressant effects).

No products indexed under this heading.

Thioridazine Hydrochloride (Additive depressant effects). Products include:

Mellaril.. 2269

Thiothixene (Additive depressant effects). Products include:

Navane Capsules and Concentrate 2201 Navane Intramuscular........................... 2202

Triazolam (Additive depressant effects). Products include:

Halcion Tablets.. 2611

Trimethadione (Stelazine may lower convulsive thresholds; dosage adjustments of anticonvulsants may be necessary).

No products indexed under this heading.

Valproic Acid (Stelazine may lower convulsive thresholds; dosage adjustments of anticonvulsants may be necessary). Products include:

Depakene.. 413

Warfarin Sodium (Effect may be diminished). Products include:

Coumadin... 926

Zolpidem Tartrate (Additive depressant effects). Products include:

Ambien Tablets.. 2416

Food Interactions

Alcohol (Additive depressant effects).

STELAZINE INJECTION

(Trifluoperazine Hydrochloride)........2514 See Stelazine Concentrate

STELAZINE MULTI-DOSE VIALS

(Trifluoperazine Hydrochloride)........2514 See Stelazine Concentrate

STELAZINE TABLETS

(Trifluoperazine Hydrochloride)........2514 See Stelazine Concentrate

STEPHAN BIO-NUTRITIONAL DAYTIME HYDRATING CREME

(Chamomile).......................................ᴾᴰ 867 None cited in PDR database.

STEPHAN BIO-NUTRITIONAL EYE-FIRMING CONCENTRATE

(Chamomile).......................................ᴾᴰ 868 None cited in PDR database.

STEPHAN BIO-NUTRITIONAL NIGHTIME MOISTURE CREME

(Moisturizing formula).....................ᴾᴰ 868 None cited in PDR database.

STEPHAN BIO-NUTRITIONAL REFRESHING MOISTURE GEL

(Moisturizing formula).....................ᴾᴰ 868 None cited in PDR database.

STEPHAN BIO-NUTRITIONAL ULTRA HYDRATING FLUID

(Moisturizing formula).....................ᴾᴰ 868 None cited in PDR database.

STEPHAN CLARITY

(Nutritional Supplement)................ᴾᴰ 868 None cited in PDR database.

STEPHAN ELASTICITY

(Nutritional Supplement)................ᴾᴰ 868 None cited in PDR database.

STEPHAN ELIXIR

(Nutritional Supplement)................ᴾᴰ 869 None cited in PDR database.

STEPHAN ESSENTIAL

(Nutritional Supplement)................ᴾᴰ 869 None cited in PDR database.

STEPHAN FEMININE

(Nutritional Supplement)................ᴾᴰ 869 None cited in PDR database.

STEPHAN FLEXIBILITY

(Nutritional Supplement)................ᴾᴰ 869 None cited in PDR database.

STEPHAN LOVPIL

(Nutritional Supplement)................ᴾᴰ 869 None cited in PDR database.

STEPHAN MASCULINE

(Nutritional Supplement)................ᴾᴰ 869 None cited in PDR database.

STEPHAN PROTECTOR

(Nutritional Supplement)................ᴾᴰ 869 None cited in PDR database.

STEPHAN RELIEF

(Nutritional Supplement)................ᴾᴰ 869 None cited in PDR database.

STEPHAN TRANQUILITY

(Nutritional Supplement)................ᴾᴰ 870 None cited in PDR database.

STILPHOSTROL TABLETS AND AMPULS

(Diethylstilbestrol Diphosphate)........ 612 None cited in PDR database.

STIMATE, (DESMOPRESSIN ACETATE) NASAL SPRAY, 1.5 MG/ML

(Desmopressin Acetate)........................ 525 May interact with vasopressors. Compounds in this category include:

Dopamine Hydrochloride (Concurrent use requires caution).

No products indexed under this heading.

Epinephrine Bitartrate (Concurrent use requires caution). Products include:

Bronkaid Mist Suspension.................ᴾᴰ 718 Sensorcaine-MPF with Epinephrine Injection.. 559

Epinephrine Hydrochloride (Concurrent use requires caution). Products include:

Ana-Kit Anaphylaxis Emergency Treatment Kit...................................... 617

Metaraminol Bitartrate (Concurrent use requires caution). Products include:

Aramine Injection................................... 1609

Methoxamine Hydrochloride (Concurrent use requires caution). Products include:

Vasoxyl Injection..................................... 1196

Norepinephrine Bitartrate (Concurrent use requires caution). Products include:

Levophed Bitartrate Injection............ 2315

Phenylephrine Hydrochloride (Concurrent use requires caution). Products include:

Atrohist Plus Tablets............................. 454 Cerose DM..ᴾᴰ 878 Comhist... 2038 D.A. Chewable Tablets.......................... 951 Deconsal Pediatric Capsules.............. 454 Dura-Vent/DA Tablets........................... 953 Entex Capsules... 1986 Entex Liquid... 1986 Extendryl... 1005 4-Way Fast Acting Nasal Spray (regular & mentholated)................ᴾᴰ 621 Hemorid For Women.............................ᴾᴰ 834 Hycomine Compound Tablets........... 932 Neo-Synephrine Hydrochloride 1% Carpuject.. 2324

IMPORTANT NOTE: Always consult each drug listing in the patient's regimen for possible interactions.

Stimate | Interactions Index | 978

Neo-Synephrine Hydrochloride 1% Injection 2324
Neo-Synephrine Hydrochloride (Ophthalmic) 2325
Neo-Synephrine .... ▣ 726
Nōstril .... ▣ 644
Novahistine Elixir .... ▣ 823
Phenergan VC 2779
Phenergan VC with Codeine 2781
Preparation H .... ▣ 871
Tympagesic Ear Drops 2342
Vasosulf .... ⊙ 271
Vicks Sinex Nasal Spray and Ultra Fine Mist .... ▣ 765

STREPTASE FOR INFUSION

(Streptokinase) 562

May interact with platelet inhibitors and anticoagulants. Compounds in these categories include:

Aspirin (Streptokinase, alone or in combination with antiplatelet and anticoagulants, may cause bleeding complications). Products include:

Alka-Seltzer Effervescent Antacid and Pain Reliever .... ▣ 701
Alka-Seltzer Extra Strength Effervescent Antacid and Pain Reliever .... ▣ 703
Alka-Seltzer Lemon Lime Effervescent Antacid and Pain Reliever .... ▣ 703
Alka-Seltzer Plus Cold Medicine .... ▣ 705
Alka-Seltzer Plus Cold & Cough Medicine .... ▣ 708
Alka-Seltzer Plus Night-Time Cold Medicine .... ▣ 707
Alka Seltzer Plus Sinus Medicine .... ▣ 707
Arthritis Foundation Safety Coated Aspirin Tablets .... ▣ 675
Arthritis Pain Ascriptin .... ▣ 631
Maximum Strength Ascriptin .... ▣ 630
Regular Strength Ascriptin Tablets .... ▣ 629
Arthritis Strength BC Powder .... ▣ 609
BC Cold Powder Multi-Symptom Formula (Cold-Sinus-Allergy) .... ▣ 609
BC Cold Powder Non-Drowsy Formula (Cold-Sinus) .... ▣ 609
BC Powder .... ▣ 609
Bayer Children's Chewable Aspirin .... ▣ 711
Genuine Bayer Aspirin Tablets & Caplets .... ▣ 713
Extra Strength Bayer Arthritis Pain Regimen Formula .... ▣ 711
Extra Strength Bayer Aspirin Caplets & Tablets .... ▣ 712
Extended-Release Bayer 8-Hour Aspirin .... ▣ 712
Extra Strength Bayer Plus Aspirin Caplets .... ▣ 713
Extra Strength Bayer PM Aspirin .... ▣ 713
Bayer Enteric Aspirin .... ▣ 709
Bufferin Analgesic Tablets and Caplets .... ▣ 613
Arthritis Strength Bufferin Analgesic Caplets .... ▣ 614
Extra Strength Bufferin Analgesic Tablets .... ▣ 615
Cama Arthritis Pain Reliever .... ▣ 785
Darvon Compound-65 Pulvules 1435
Easprin 1914
Ecotrin 2455
Ecotrin Enteric Coated Aspirin Maximum Strength Tablets and Caplets .... ▣ 816
Ecotrin Enteric Coated Aspirin Regular Strength Tablets 2455
Empirin Aspirin Tablets .... ▣ 854
Empirin with Codeine Tablets 1093
Excedrin Extra-Strength Analgesic Tablets & Caplets 732
Fiorinal Capsules 2261
Fiorinal with Codeine Capsules 2262
Fiorinal Tablets 2261
Halfprin 1362
Healthprin Aspirin 2455
Norgesic 1496
Percodan Tablets 939
Percodan-Demi Tablets 940
Robaxisal Tablets 2071
Soma Compound w/Codeine Tablets 2676
Soma Compound Tablets 2675
St. Joseph Adult Chewable Aspirin (81 mg.) .... ▣ 808
Talwin Compound 2335
Ursinus Inlay-Tabs .... ▣ 794
Vanquish Analgesic Caplets .... ▣ 731

Azlocillin Sodium (Streptokinase, alone or in combination with antiplatelet and anticoagulants, may cause bleeding complications).

No products indexed under this heading.

Carbenicillin Indanyl Sodium (Streptokinase, alone or in combination with antiplatelet and anticoagulants, may cause bleeding complications). Products include:

Geocillin Tablets 2199

Choline Magnesium Trisalicylate (Streptokinase, alone or in combination with antiplatelet and anticoagulants, may cause bleeding complications). Products include:

Trilisate 2000

Dalteparin Sodium (Streptokinase, alone or in combination with antiplatelet and anticoagulants, may cause bleeding complications). Products include:

Fragmin 1954

Diclofenac Potassium (Streptokinase, alone or in combination with antiplatelet and anticoagulants, may cause bleeding complications). Products include:

Cataflam 816

Diclofenac Sodium (Streptokinase, alone or in combination with antiplatelet and anticoagulants, may cause bleeding complications). Products include:

Voltaren Ophthalmic Sterile Ophthalmic Solution .... ⊙ 272
Voltaren Tablets 861

Dicumarol (Streptokinase, alone or in combination with antiplatelet and anticoagulants, may cause bleeding complications).

No products indexed under this heading.

Diflunisal (Streptokinase, alone or in combination with antiplatelet and anticoagulants, may cause bleeding complications). Products include:

Dolobid Tablets 1654

Dipyridamole (Streptokinase, alone or in combination with antiplatelet and anticoagulants, may cause bleeding complications). Products include:

Persantine Tablets 681

Enoxaparin (Streptokinase, alone or in combination with antiplatelet and anticoagulants, may cause bleeding complications). Products include:

Lovenox Injection 2020

Fenoprofen Calcium (Streptokinase, alone or in combination with antiplatelet and anticoagulants, may cause bleeding complications). Products include:

Nalfon 200 Pulvules & Nalfon Tablets 917

Flurbiprofen (Streptokinase, alone or in combination with antiplatelet and anticoagulants, may cause bleeding complications). Products include:

Ansaid Tablets 2579

Heparin Calcium (Streptokinase, alone or in combination with antiplatelet and anticoagulants, may cause bleeding complications).

No products indexed under this heading.

Heparin Sodium (Streptokinase, alone or in combination with antiplatelet and anticoagulants, may cause bleeding complications). Products include:

Heparin Lock Flush Solution 2725
Heparin Sodium Injection 2726
Heparin Sodium Injection, USP, Sterile Solution 2615
Heparin Sodium Vials 1441

Ibuprofen (Streptokinase, alone or in combination with antiplatelet and anticoagulants, may cause bleeding complications). Products include:

Advil Cold and Sinus Caplets and Tablets (formerly CoAdvil) .... ▣ 870
Advil Ibuprofen Tablets and Caplets .... ▣ 870
Children's Advil Suspension 2692
Arthritis Foundation Ibuprofen Tablets .... ▣ 674
Bayer Select Ibuprofen Pain Relief Formula .... ▣ 715
Cramp End Tablets .... ▣ 735
Dimetapp Sinus Caplets .... ▣ 775
Haltran Tablets .... ▣ 771
IBU Tablets 1342
Ibuprohm .... ▣ 735
Children's Motrin Ibuprofen Oral Suspension 1546
Motrin Tablets 2625
Motrin IB Caplets, Tablets, and Geltabs .... ▣ 838
Motrin IB Sinus .... ▣ 838
Motrin Ibuprofen Suspension, Oral Drops, Chewable Tablets, Caplets 1546
Nuprin Ibuprofen/Analgesic Tablets & Caplets .... ▣ 622
Sine-Aid IB Caplets 1554
Vicks DayQuil SINUS Pressure & PAIN Relief with IBUPROFEN .... ▣ 762

Indomethacin (Streptokinase, alone or in combination with antiplatelet and anticoagulants, may cause bleeding complications). Products include:

Indocin 1680

Indomethacin Sodium Trihydrate (Streptokinase, alone or in combination with antiplatelet and anticoagulants, may cause bleeding complications). Products include:

Indocin I.V. 1684

Ketoprofen (Streptokinase, alone or in combination with antiplatelet and anticoagulants, may cause bleeding complications). Products include:

Orudis Capsules 2766
Oruvail Capsules 2766

Magnesium Salicylate (Streptokinase, alone or in combination with antiplatelet and anticoagulants, may cause bleeding complications). Products include:

Backache Caplets .... ▣ 613
Bayer Select Backache Pain Relief Formula .... ▣ 715
Doan's Extra-Strength Analgesic .... ▣ 633
Extra Strength Doan's P.M. .... ▣ 633
Doan's Regular Strength Analgesic .... ▣ 634
Mobigesic Tablets .... ▣ 602

Meclofenamate Sodium (Streptokinase, alone or in combination with antiplatelet and anticoagulants, may cause bleeding complications).

No products indexed under this heading.

Mefenamic Acid (Streptokinase, alone or in combination with antiplatelet and anticoagulants, may cause bleeding complications). Products include:

Ponstel 1925

Mezlocillin Sodium (Streptokinase, alone or in combination with antiplatelet and anticoagulants, may cause bleeding complications). Products include:

Mezlin 601
Mezlin Pharmacy Bulk Package 604

Nafcillin Sodium (Streptokinase, alone or in combination with antiplatelet and anticoagulants, may cause bleeding complications).

No products indexed under this heading.

Naproxen (Streptokinase, alone or in combination with antiplatelet and anticoagulants, may cause bleeding complications). Products include:

Anaprox/Naprosyn 2117

Naproxen Sodium (Streptokinase, alone or in combination with antiplatelet and anticoagulants, may cause bleeding complications). Products include:

Aleve 1975
Anaprox/Naprosyn 2117

Penicillin G Benzathine (Streptokinase, alone or in combination with antiplatelet and anticoagulants, may cause bleeding complications). Products include:

Bicillin C-R Injection 2704
Bicillin C-R 900/300 Injection 2706
Bicillin L-A Injection 2707

Penicillin G Procaine (Streptokinase, alone or in combination with antiplatelet and anticoagulants, may cause bleeding complications). Products include:

Bicillin C-R Injection 2704
Bicillin C-R 900/300 Injection 2706

Phenylbutazone (Streptokinase, alone or in combination with antiplatelet and anticoagulants, may cause bleeding complications).

No products indexed under this heading.

Piroxicam (Streptokinase, alone or in combination with antiplatelet and anticoagulants, may cause bleeding complications). Products include:

Feldene Capsules 1965

Salsalate (Streptokinase, alone or in combination with antiplatelet and anticoagulants, may cause bleeding complications). Products include:

Mono-Gesic Tablets 792
Salflex Tablets 786

Sulindac (Streptokinase, alone or in combination with antiplatelet and anticoagulants, may cause bleeding complications). Products include:

Clinoril Tablets 1618

Ticarcillin Disodium (Streptokinase, alone or in combination with antiplatelet and anticoagulants, may cause bleeding complications). Products include:

Ticar for Injection 2526
Timentin for Injection 2528

Ticlopidine Hydrochloride (Streptokinase, alone or in combination with antiplatelet and anticoagulants, may cause bleeding complications). Products include:

Ticlid Tablets 2156

Tolmetin Sodium (Streptokinase, alone or in combination with antiplatelet and anticoagulants, may cause bleeding complications). Products include:

Tolectin (200, 400 and 600 mg) 1581

Warfarin Sodium (Streptokinase, alone or in combination with antiplatelet and anticoagulants, may cause bleeding complications). Products include:

Coumadin 926

STREPTOMYCIN SULFATE INJECTION

(Streptomycin Sulfate) 2208

May interact with anesthetics, muscle relaxants, diuretics, and certain

(▣ Described in PDR For Nonprescription Drugs) (⊙ Described in PDR For Ophthalmology)

979 **Interactions Index** **Streptomycin**

other agents. Compounds in these categories include:

Alfentanil Hydrochloride (Potential for respiratory paralysis from neuromuscular blockage due to neurotoxicity, especially when given soon after the use of anesthesia). Products include:

Alfenta Injection 1286

Amiloride Hydrochloride (Interaction with furosemide is extrapolated to other diuretic where co-administration may possibly result in the potentiation of ototoxic effects). Products include:

Midamor Tablets 1703
Moduretic Tablets 1705

Atracurium Besylate (Potential for respiratory paralysis from neuromuscular blockage due to neurotoxicity, especially when given soon after the use of muscle relaxants). Products include:

Tracrium Injection 1183

Baclofen (Potential for respiratory paralysis from neuromuscular blockage due to neurotoxicity, especially when given soon after the use of muscle relaxants). Products include:

Lioresal Intrathecal 1596
Lioresal Tablets 829

Bendroflumethiazide (Interaction with furosemide is extrapolated to other diuretic where co-administration may possibly result in the potentiation of ototoxic effects).

No products indexed under this heading.

Bumetanide (Interaction with furosemide is extrapolated to other diuretic where co-administration may possibly result in the potentiation of ototoxic effects). Products include:

Bumex 2093

Carisoprodol (Potential for respiratory paralysis from neuromuscular blockage due to neurotoxicity, especially when given soon after the use of muscle relaxants). Products include:

Soma Compound w/Codeine Tablets 2676
Soma Compound Tablets 2675
Soma Tablets 2674

Cephaloridine (Concurrent and/or sequential use may increase the potential for increased toxicity; co-administration should be avoided).

Chlorothiazide (Interaction with furosemide is extrapolated to other diuretic where co-administration may possibly result in the potentiation of ototoxic effects). Products include:

Aldoclor Tablets 1598
Diupres Tablets 1650
Diuril Oral 1653

Chlorothiazide Sodium (Interaction with furosemide is extrapolated to other diuretic where co-administration may possibly result in the potentiation of ototoxic effects). Products include:

Diuril Sodium Intravenous 1652

Chlorthalidone (Interaction with furosemide is extrapolated to other diuretic where co-administration may possibly result in the potentiation of ototoxic effects). Products include:

Combipres Tablets 677
Tenoretic Tablets 2845
Thalitone 1245

Chlorzoxazone (Potential for respiratory paralysis from neuromuscular blockage due to neurotoxicity, especially when given soon after the use of muscle relaxants). Products include:

Paraflex Caplets 1580
Parafon Forte DSC Caplets 1581

Colistin Sulfate (Concurrent and/or sequential use may increase the potential for increased toxicity; co-administration should be avoided). Products include:

Coly-Mycin S Otic w/Neomycin & Hydrocortisone 1906

Cyclobenzaprine Hydrochloride (Potential for respiratory paralysis from neuromuscular blockage due to neurotoxicity, especially when given soon after the use of muscle relaxants). Products include:

Flexeril Tablets 1661

Cyclosporine (Concurrent and/or sequential use may increase the potential for increased toxicity; co-administration should be avoided). Products include:

Neoral 2276
Sandimmune 2286

Dantrolene Sodium (Potential for respiratory paralysis from neuromuscular blockage due to neurotoxicity, especially when given soon after the use of muscle relaxants). Products include:

Dantrium Capsules 1982
Dantrium Intravenous 1983

Doxacurium Chloride (Potential for respiratory paralysis from neuromuscular blockage due to neurotoxicity, especially when given soon after the use of muscle relaxants). Products include:

Nuromax Injection 1149

Enflurane (Potential for respiratory paralysis from neuromuscular blockage due to neurotoxicity, especially when given soon after the use of anesthesia).

No products indexed under this heading.

Ethacrynic Acid (Co-administration results in the potentiation of ototoxic effects). Products include:

Edecrin Tablets 1657

Fentanyl Citrate (Potential for respiratory paralysis from neuromuscular blockage due to neurotoxicity, especially when given soon after the use of anesthesia). Products include:

Sublimaze Injection 1307

Furosemide (Co-administration results in the potentiation of ototoxic effects). Products include:

Lasix Injection, Oral Solution and Tablets 1240

Gentamicin Sulfate (Concurrent and/or sequential use may increase the potential for increased toxicity; co-administration should be avoided). Products include:

Garamycin Injectable 2360
Genoptic Sterile Ophthalmic Solution .... ⊙ 243
Genoptic Sterile Ophthalmic Ointment .... ⊙ 243
Gentacidin Ointment .... ⊙ 264
Gentacidin Solution .... ⊙ 264
Gentak .... ⊙ 208
Pred-G Liquifilm Sterile Ophthalmic Suspension .... ⊙ 251
Pred-G S.O.P. Sterile Ophthalmic Ointment .... ⊙ 252

Halothane (Potential for respiratory paralysis from neuromuscular blockage due to neurotoxicity, especially when given soon after the use of anesthesia). Products include:

Fluothane 2724

Hydrochlorothiazide (Interaction with furosemide is extrapolated to other diuretic where co-administration may possibly result in the potentiation of ototoxic effects). Products include:

Aldactazide 2413
Aldoril Tablets 1604
Apresazide Capsules 808
Capozide 742
Dyazide 2479
Esidrix Tablets 821
Esimil Tablets 822
HydroDIURIL Tablets 1674
Hydropres Tablets 1675
Hyzaar Tablets 1677
Inderide Tablets 2732
Inderide LA Long Acting Capsules .. 2734
Lopressor HCT Tablets 832
Lotensin HCT 837
Maxzide 1380
Moduretic Tablets 1705
Oretic Tablets 443
Prinzide Tablets 1737
Ser-Ap-Es Tablets 849
Timolide Tablets 1748
Vaseretic Tablets 1765
Zestoretic 2850
Ziac 1415

Hydroflumethiazide (Interaction with furosemide is extrapolated to other diuretic where co-administration may possibly result in the potentiation of ototoxic effects). Products include:

Diucardin Tablets 2718

Indapamide (Interaction with furosemide is extrapolated to other diuretic where co-administration may possibly result in the potentiation of ototoxic effects). Products include:

Lozol Tablets 2022

Isoflurane (Potential for respiratory paralysis from neuromuscular blockage due to neurotoxicity, especially when given soon after the use of anesthesia).

No products indexed under this heading.

Kanamycin Sulfate (Concurrent and/or sequential use may increase the potential for increased toxicity; co-administration should be avoided).

No products indexed under this heading.

Ketamine Hydrochloride (Potential for respiratory paralysis from neuromuscular blockage due to neurotoxicity, especially when given soon after the use of anesthesia).

No products indexed under this heading.

Mannitol (Co-administration results in the potentiation of ototoxic effects).

No products indexed under this heading.

Metaxalone (Potential for respiratory paralysis from neuromuscular blockage due to neurotoxicity, especially when given soon after the use of muscle relaxants). Products include:

Skelaxin Tablets 788

Methocarbamol (Potential for respiratory paralysis from neuromuscular blockage due to neurotoxicity, especially when given soon after the use of muscle relaxants). Products include:

Robaxin Injectable 2070
Robaxin Tablets 2071
Robaxisal Tablets 2071

Methohexital Sodium (Potential for respiratory paralysis from neuromuscular blockage due to neurotoxicity, especially when given soon after the use of anesthesia). Products include:

Brevital Sodium Vials 1429

Methyclothiazide (Interaction with furosemide is extrapolated to other diuretic where co-administration may possibly result in the potentiation of ototoxic effects). Products include:

Enduron Tablets 420

Metocurine Iodide (Potential for respiratory paralysis from neuromuscular blockage due to neurotoxicity, especially when given soon after the use of muscle relaxants). Products include:

Metubine Iodide Vials 916

Metolazone (Interaction with furosemide is extrapolated to other diuretic where co-administration may possibly result in the potentiation of ototoxic effects). Products include:

Mykrox Tablets 993
Zaroxolyn Tablets 1000

Midazolam Hydrochloride (Potential for respiratory paralysis from neuromuscular blockage due to neurotoxicity, especially when given soon after the use of anesthesia). Products include:

Versed Injection 2170

Mivacurium Chloride (Potential for respiratory paralysis from neuromuscular blockage due to neurotoxicity, especially when given soon after the use of muscle relaxants). Products include:

Mivacron 1138

Neomycin Sulfate (Concurrent and/or sequential use may increase the potential for increased toxicity; co-administration should be avoided). Products include:

AK-Spore .... ⊙ 204
AK-Trol Ointment & Suspension .... ⊙ 205
Bactine First Aid Antibiotic Plus Anesthetic Ointment .... ▣ 708
Campho-Phenique Maximum Strength First Aid Antibiotic Plus Pain Reliever Ointment .... ▣ 719
Coly-Mycin S Otic w/Neomycin & Hydrocortisone 1906
Cortisporin Cream 1084
Cortisporin Ointment 1085
Cortisporin Ophthalmic Ointment Sterile 1085
Cortisporin Ophthalmic Suspension Sterile 1086
Cortisporin Otic Solution Sterile 1087
Cortisporin Otic Suspension Sterile 1088
Dexacidin Ointment .... ⊙ 263
Maxitrol Ophthalmic Ointment and Suspension .... ⊙ 224
Mycitracin .... ▣ 839
NeoDecadron Sterile Ophthalmic Ointment 1712
NeoDecadron Sterile Ophthalmic Solution 1713
NeoDecadron Topical Cream 1714
Neosporin G.U. Irrigant Sterile 1148
Neosporin Ointment .... ▣ 857
Neosporin Plus Maximum Strength Cream .... ▣ 858
Neosporin Plus Maximum Strength Ointment .... ▣ 858
Neosporin Ophthalmic Ointment Sterile 1148
Neosporin Ophthalmic Solution Sterile 1149
PediOtic Suspension Sterile 1153
Poly-Pred Liquifilm .... ⊙ 248

Neomycin, oral (Concurrent and/or sequential use may increase the potential for increased toxicity; co-administration should be avoided).

Orphenadrine Citrate (Potential for respiratory paralysis from neuromuscular blockage due to neurotoxicity, especially when given soon after the use of muscle relaxants). Products include:

Norflex 1496
Norgesic 1496

IMPORTANT NOTE: Always consult each drug listing in the patient's regimen for possible interactions.

Pancuronium Bromide Injection (Potential for respiratory paralysis from neuromuscular blockage due to neurotoxicity, especially when given soon after the use of muscle relaxants).
No products indexed under this heading.

Paromomycin Sulfate (Concurrent and/or sequential use may increase the potential for increased toxicity; co-administration should be avoided).
No products indexed under this heading.

Polymyxin B Sulfate (Concurrent and/or sequential use may increase the potential for increased toxicity; co-administration should be avoided). Products include:
AK-Spore ⊙ 204
AK-Trol Ointment & Suspension ⊙ 205
Bactine First Aid Antibiotic Plus Anesthetic Ointment ▣ 708
Betadine Brand First Aid Antibiotics & Moisturizer Ointment 1991
Campho-Phenique Maximum Strength First Aid Antibiotic Plus Pain Reliever Ointment ▣ 719
Cortisporin Cream 1084
Cortisporin Ointment 1085
Cortisporin Ophthalmic Ointment Sterile 1085
Cortisporin Ophthalmic Suspension Sterile 1086
Cortisporin Otic Solution Sterile 1087
Cortisporin Otic Suspension Sterile 1088
Dexacidin Ointment ⊙ 263
Maxitrol Ophthalmic Ointment and Suspension ⊙ 224
Mycitracin ▣ 839
Neosporin G.U. Irrigant Sterile 1148
Neosporin Ointment ▣ 857
Neosporin Plus Maximum Strength Cream ▣ 858
Neosporin Plus Maximum Strength Ointment ▣ 858
Neosporin Ophthalmic Ointment Sterile 1148
Neosporin Ophthalmic Solution Sterile 1149
Ophthocort ⊙ 311
PediOtic Suspension Sterile 1153
Polymyxin B Sulfate, Aerosporin Brand Sterile Powder 1154
Poly-Pred Liquifilm ⊙ 248
Polysporin Ointment ▣ 858
Polysporin Ophthalmic Ointment Sterile 1154
Polysporin Powder ▣ 859
Polytrim Ophthalmic Solution Sterile 482
TERAK Ointment ⊙ 209
Terramycin with Polymyxin B Sulfate Ophthalmic Ointment 2211

Polythiazide (Interaction with furosemide is extrapolated to other diuretic where co-administration may possibly result in the potentiation of ototoxic effects). Products include:
Minizide Capsules 1938

Propofol (Potential for respiratory paralysis from neuromuscular blockage due to neurotoxicity, especially when given soon after the use of anesthesia). Products include:
Diprivan Injection 2833

Rocuronium Bromide (Potential for respiratory paralysis from neuromuscular blockage due to neurotoxicity, especially when given soon after the use of muscle relaxants). Products include:
Zemuron 1830

Spironolactone (Interaction with furosemide is extrapolated to other diuretic where co-administration may possibly result in the potentiation of ototoxic effects). Products include:
Aldactazide 2413
Aldactone 2414

Succinylcholine Chloride (Potential for respiratory paralysis from neuromuscular blockage due to neurotoxicity, especially when given soon after the use of muscle relaxants). Products include:
Anectine 1073

Sufentanil Citrate (Potential for respiratory paralysis from neuromuscular blockage due to neurotoxicity, especially when given soon after the use of anesthesia). Products include:
Sufenta Injection 1309

Thiamylal Sodium (Potential for respiratory paralysis from neuromuscular blockage due to neurotoxicity, especially when given soon after the use of anesthesia).
No products indexed under this heading.

Tobramycin (Concurrent and/or sequential use may increase the potential for increased toxicity; co-administration should be avoided). Products include:
AKTOB ⊙ 206
TobraDex Ophthalmic Suspension and Ointment 473
Tobrex Ophthalmic Ointment and Solution ⊙ 229

Tobramycin Sulfate (Concurrent and/or sequential use may increase the potential for increased toxicity; co-administration should be avoided). Products include:
Nebcin Vials, Hyporets & ADD-Vantage 1464
Tobramycin Sulfate Injection 968

Torsemide (Interaction with furosemide is extrapolated to other diuretic where co-administration may possibly result in the potentiation of ototoxic effects). Products include:
Demadex Tablets and Injection 686

Triamterene (Interaction with furosemide is extrapolated to other diuretic where co-administration may possibly result in the potentiation of ototoxic effects). Products include:
Dyazide 2479
Dyrenium Capsules 2481
Maxzide 1380

Vecuronium Bromide (Potential for respiratory paralysis from neuromuscular blockage due to neurotoxicity, especially when given soon after the use of muscle relaxants). Products include:
Norcuron 1826

Viomycin (Concurrent and/or sequential use may increase the potential for increased toxicity; co-administration should be avoided).

STRESSTABS
(Vitamin B Complex With Vitamin C) ▣ 671
None cited in PDR database.

STRESSTABS + IRON
(Vitamins with Iron) ▣ 671
None cited in PDR database.

STRESSTABS + ZINC
(Vitamins with Minerals) ▣ 671
None cited in PDR database.

STRI-DEX ANTIBACTERIAL CLEANSING BAR
(Triclosan) ▣ 730
None cited in PDR database.

STRI-DEX ANTIBACTERIAL FACE WASH
(Triclosan) ▣ 730
None cited in PDR database.

STRI-DEX CLEAR GEL
(Salicylic Acid) ▣ 730
None cited in PDR database.

STRI-DEX MAXIMUM STRENGTH PADS
(Salicylic Acid) ▣ 730
May interact with:

Concomitant Topical Acne Therapy (May increase dryness or irritation of the skin).

STRI-DEX REGULAR STRENGTH PADS
(Salicylic Acid) ▣ 730
See **Stri-Dex Maximum Strength Pads**

STRI-DEX SENSITIVE SKIN PADS
(Salicylic Acid) ▣ 730
See **Stri-Dex Regular Strength Pads**

STRI-DEX DUAL TEXTURED MAXIMUM STRENGTH PADS
(Salicylic Acid) ▣ 730
See **Stri-Dex Regular Strength Pads**

STRI-DEX SUPER SCRUB PADS—OIL FIGHTING FORMULA
(Salicylic Acid) ▣ 730
See **Stri-Dex Regular Strength Pads**

STUART PRENATAL TABLETS
(Multivitamins with Minerals) ▣ 881
None cited in PDR database.

THE STUART FORMULA TABLETS
(Vitamins with Minerals) ▣ 663
None cited in PDR database.

SUBLIMAZE INJECTION
(Fentanyl Citrate) 1307
May interact with central nervous system depressants and certain other agents. Compounds in these categories include:

Alfentanil Hydrochloride (Additive or potentiating effects). Products include:
Alfenta Injection 1286

Alprazolam (Additive or potentiating effects). Products include:
Xanax Tablets 2649

Aprobarbital (Additive or potentiating effects).
No products indexed under this heading.

Buprenorphine (Additive or potentiating effects). Products include:
Buprenex Injectable 2006

Buspirone Hydrochloride (Additive or potentiating effects). Products include:
BuSpar 737

Butabarbital (Additive or potentiating effects).
No products indexed under this heading.

Butalbital (Additive or potentiating effects). Products include:
Esgic-plus Tablets 1013
Fioricet Tablets 2258
Fioricet with Codeine Capsules 2260
Fiorinal Capsules 2261
Fiorinal with Codeine Capsules 2262
Fiorinal Tablets 2261
Phrenilin 785
Sedapap Tablets 50 mg/650 mg 1543

Chlordiazepoxide (Additive or potentiating effects). Products include:
Libritabs Tablets 2177
Limbitrol 2180

Chlordiazepoxide Hydrochloride (Additive or potentiating effects). Products include:
Librax Capsules 2176
Librium Capsules 2178
Librium Injectable 2179

Chlorpromazine (Additive or potentiating effects). Products include:
Thorazine Suppositories 2523

Chlorprothixene (Additive or potentiating effects).
No products indexed under this heading.

Chlorprothixene Hydrochloride (Additive or potentiating effects).
No products indexed under this heading.

Clorazepate Dipotassium (Additive or potentiating effects). Products include:
Tranxene 451

Clozapine (Additive or potentiating effects). Products include:
Clozaril Tablets 2252

Codeine Phosphate (Additive or potentiating effects). Products include:
Actifed with Codeine Cough Syrup 1067
Brontex 1981
Deconsal C Expectorant Syrup 456
Deconsal Pediatric Syrup 457
Dimetane-DC Cough Syrup 2059
Empirin with Codeine Tablets 1093
Fioricet with Codeine Capsules 2260
Fiorinal with Codeine Capsules 2262
Isoclor Expectorant 990
Novahistine DH 2462
Novahistine Expectorant 2463
Nucofed 2051
Phenergan with Codeine 2777
Phenergan VC with Codeine 2781
Robitussin A-C Syrup 2073
Robitussin-DAC Syrup 2074
Ryna ▣ 841
Soma Compound w/Codeine Tablets 2676
Tussi-Organidin NR Liquid and S NR Liquid 2677
Tylenol with Codeine 1583

Desflurane (Additive or potentiating effects). Products include:
Suprane 1813

Dezocine (Additive or potentiating effects). Products include:
Dalgan Injection 538

Diazepam (Additive or potentiating effects; cardiovascular depression). Products include:
Dizac 1809
Valium Injectable 2182
Valium Tablets 2183
Valrelease Capsules 2169

Droperidol (Decreased pulmonary arterial pressure; additive or potentiating effects). Products include:
Inapsine Injection 1296

Enflurane (Additive or potentiating effects).
No products indexed under this heading.

Estazolam (Additive or potentiating effects). Products include:
ProSom Tablets 449

Ethchlorvynol (Additive or potentiating effects). Products include:
Placidyl Capsules 448

Ethinamate (Additive or potentiating effects).
No products indexed under this heading.

Fentanyl (Additive or potentiating effects). Products include:
Duragesic Transdermal System 1288

(▣ Described in PDR For Nonprescription Drugs) (⊙ Described in PDR For Ophthalmology)

981 **Interactions Index** **Sudafed Liquid**

Fluphenazine Decanoate (Additive or potentiating effects). Products include:
Prolixin Decanoate ... 509
Fluphenazine Enanthate (Additive or potentiating effects). Products include:
Prolixin Enanthate ... 509
Fluphenazine Hydrochloride (Additive or potentiating effects). Products include:
Prolixin ... 509
Flurazepam Hydrochloride (Additive or potentiating effects). Products include:
Dalmane Capsules ... 2173
Glutethimide (Additive or potentiating effects).
No products indexed under this heading.
Haloperidol (Additive or potentiating effects). Products include:
Haldol Injection, Tablets and Concentrate ... 1575
Haloperidol Decanoate (Additive or potentiating effects). Products include:
Haldol Decanoate ... 1577
Hydrocodone Bitartrate (Additive or potentiating effects). Products include:
Anexsia 5/500 Elixir ... 1781
Anexia Tablets ... 1782
Codiclear DH Syrup ... 791
Deconamine CX Cough and Cold Liquid and Tablets ... 1319
Duratuss HD Elixir ... 2565
Hycodan Tablets and Syrup ... 930
Hycomine Compound Tablets ... 932
Hycomine ... 931
Hycotuss Expectorant Syrup ... 933
Hydrocet Capsules ... 782
Lorcet 10/650 ... 1018
Lortab ... 2566
Tussend ... 1783
Tussend Expectorant ... 1785
Vicodin Tablets ... 1356
Vicodin ES Tablets ... 1357
Vicodin Tuss Expectorant ... 1358
Zydone Capsules ... 949
Hydrocodone Polistirex (Additive or potentiating effects). Products include:
Tussionex Pennkinetic Extended-Release Suspension ... 998
Hydroxyzine Hydrochloride (Additive or potentiating effects). Products include:
Atarax Tablets & Syrup ... 2185
Marax Tablets & DF Syrup ... 2200
Vistaril Intramuscular Solution ... 2216
Isoflurane (Additive or potentiating effects).
No products indexed under this heading.
Ketamine Hydrochloride (Additive or potentiating effects).
No products indexed under this heading.
Levomethadyl Acetate Hydrochloride (Additive or potentiating effects). Products include:
Orlamm ... 2239
Levorphanol Tartrate (Additive or potentiating effects). Products include:
Levo-Dromoran ... 2129
Lorazepam (Additive or potentiating effects). Products include:
Ativan Injection ... 2698
Ativan Tablets ... 2700
Loxapine Hydrochloride (Additive or potentiating effects). Products include:
Loxitane ... 1378
Loxapine Succinate (Additive or potentiating effects). Products include:
Loxitane Capsules ... 1378
Meperidine Hydrochloride (Additive or potentiating effects). Products include:
Demerol ... 2308
Mepergan Injection ... 2753
Mephobarbital (Additive or potentiating effects). Products include:
Mebaral Tablets ... 2322
Meprobamate (Additive or potentiating effects). Products include:
Miltown Tablets ... 2672
PMB 200 and PMB 400 ... 2783
Mesoridazine Besylate (Additive or potentiating effects). Products include:
Serentil ... 684
Methadone Hydrochloride (Additive or potentiating effects). Products include:
Methadone Hydrochloride Oral Concentrate ... 2233
Methadone Hydrochloride Oral Solution & Tablets ... 2235
Methohexital Sodium (Additive or potentiating effects). Products include:
Brevital Sodium Vials ... 1429
Methotrimeprazine (Additive or potentiating effects). Products include:
Levoprome ... 1274
Methoxyflurane (Additive or potentiating effects).
No products indexed under this heading.
Midazolam Hydrochloride (Additive of potentiating effects). Products include:
Versed Injection ... 2170
Molindone Hydrochloride (Additive or potentiating effects). Products include:
Moban Tablets and Concentrate ... 1048
Morphine Sulfate (Additive or potentiating effects). Products include:
Astramorph/PF Injection, USP (Preservative-Free) ... 535
Duramorph ... 962
Infumorph 200 and Infumorph 500 Sterile Solutions ... 965
MS Contin Tablets ... 1994
MSIR ... 1997
Oramorph SR (Morphine Sulfate Sustained Release Tablets) ... 2236
RMS Suppositories ... 2657
Roxanol ... 2243
Nitrous Oxide (Cardiovascular depression).
Opium Alkaloids (Additive or potentiating effects).
No products indexed under this heading.
Oxazepam (Additive or potentiating effects). Products include:
Serax Capsules ... 2810
Serax Tablets ... 2810
Oxycodone Hydrochloride (Additive or potentiating effects). Products include:
Percocet Tablets ... 938
Percodan Tablets ... 939
Percodan-Demi Tablets ... 940
Roxicodone Tablets, Oral Solution & Intensol (Oxycodone) ... 2244
Tylox Capsules ... 1584
Pentobarbital Sodium (Additive or potentiating effects). Products include:
Nembutal Sodium Capsules ... 436
Nembutal Sodium Solution ... 438
Nembutal Sodium Suppositories ... 440
Perphenazine (Additive or potentiating effects). Products include:
Etrafon ... 2355
Triavil Tablets ... 1757
Trilafon ... 2389
Phenobarbital (Additive or potentiating effects). Products include:
Arco-Lase Plus Tablets ... 512
Bellergal-S Tablets ... 2250
Donnatal ... 2060
Donnatal Extentabs ... 2061
Donnatal Tablets ... 2060
Phenobarbital Elixir and Tablets ... 1469
Quadrinal Tablets ... 1350
Prazepam (Additive or potentiating effects).
No products indexed under this heading.
Prochlorperazine (Additive or potentiating effects). Products include:
Compazine ... 2470
Promethazine Hydrochloride (Additive or potentiating effects). Products include:
Mepergan Injection ... 2753
Phenergan with Codeine ... 2777
Phenergan with Dextromethorphan ... 2778
Phenergan Injection ... 2773
Phenergan Suppositories ... 2775
Phenergan Syrup ... 2774
Phenergan Tablets ... 2775
Phenergan VC ... 2779
Phenergan VC with Codeine ... 2781
Propofol (Additive or potentiating effects). Products include:
Diprivan Injection ... 2833
Propoxyphene Hydrochloride (Additive or potentiating effects). Products include:
Darvon ... 1435
Wygesic Tablets ... 2827
Propoxyphene Napsylate (Additive or potentiating effects). Products include:
Darvon-N/Darvocet-N ... 1433
Quazepam (Additive or potentiating effects). Products include:
Doral Tablets ... 2664
Risperidone (Additive or potentiating effects). Products include:
Risperdal ... 1301
Secobarbital Sodium (Additive or potentiating effects). Products include:
Seconal Sodium Pulvules ... 1474
Sufentanil Citrate (Additive or potentiating effects). Products include:
Sufenta Injection ... 1309
Temazepam (Additive or potentiating effects). Products include:
Restoril Capsules ... 2284
Thiamylal Sodium (Additive or potentiating effects).
No products indexed under this heading.
Thioridazine Hydrochloride (Additive or potentiating effects). Products include:
Mellaril ... 2269
Thiothixene (Additive or potentiating effects). Products include:
Navane Capsules and Concentrate ... 2201
Navane Intramuscular ... 2202
Triazolam (Additive or potentiating effects). Products include:
Halcion Tablets ... 2611
Trifluoperazine Hydrochloride (Additive or potentiating effects). Products include:
Stelazine ... 2514
Zolpidem Tartrate (Additive or potentiating effects). Products include:
Ambien Tablets ... 2416

SUCRETS CHILDREN'S CHERRY FLAVORED SORE THROAT LOZENGES
(Dyclonine Hydrochloride) ... 826
None cited in PDR database.

SUCRETS MAXIMUM STRENGTH WINTERGREEN AND SUCRETS WILD CHERRY (REGULAR STRENGTH) SORE THROAT LOZENGES
(Dyclonine Hydrochloride) ... 826
None cited in PDR database.

SUCRETS 4-HOUR COUGH SUPPRESSANT
(Dextromethorphan Hydrobromide) ... 826
May interact with monoamine oxidase inhibitors. Compounds in this category include:
Furazolidone (Concurrent and/or sequential use is not recommended). Products include:
Furoxone ... 2046
Isocarboxazid (Concurrent and/or sequential use is not recommended).
No products indexed under this heading.
Phenelzine Sulfate (Concurrent and/or sequential use is not recommended). Products include:
Nardil ... 1920
Selegiline Hydrochloride (Concurrent and/or sequential use is not recommended). Products include:
Eldepryl Tablets ... 2550
Tranylcypromine Sulfate (Concurrent and/or sequential use is not recommended). Products include:
Parnate Tablets ... 2503

SUDAFED CHILDREN'S LIQUID
(Pseudoephedrine Hydrochloride) .. 861
May interact with antihypertensives and antidepressant drugs. Compounds in these categories include:
Acebutolol Hydrochloride (Concurrent use not recommended). Products include:
Sectral Capsules ... 2807
Amitriptyline Hydrochloride (Concurrent use not recommended). Products include:
Elavil ... 2838
Endep Tablets ... 2174
Etrafon ... 2355
Limbitrol ... 2180
Triavil Tablets ... 1757
Amlodipine Besylate (Concurrent use not recommended). Products include:
Lotrel Capsules ... 840
Norvasc Tablets ... 1940
Amoxapine (Concurrent use not recommended). Products include:
Asendin Tablets ... 1369
Atenolol (Concurrent use not recommended). Products include:
Tenoretic Tablets ... 2845
Tenormin Tablets and I.V. Injection ... 2847
Benazepril Hydrochloride (Concurrent use not recommended). Products include:
Lotensin Tablets ... 834
Lotensin HCT ... 837
Lotrel Capsules ... 840
Betaxolol Hydrochloride (Concurrent use not recommended). Products include:
Betoptic Ophthalmic Solution ... 469
Betoptic S Ophthalmic Suspension ... 471
Kerlone Tablets ... 2436
Bisoprolol Fumarate (Concurrent use not recommended). Products include:
Zebeta Tablets ... 1413
Ziac ... 1415
Bupropion Hydrochloride (Concurrent use not recommended). Products include:
Wellbutrin Tablets ... 1204
Captopril (Concurrent use not recommended). Products include:
Capoten ... 739
Capozide ... 742

IMPORTANT NOTE: Always consult each drug listing in the patient's regimen for possible interactions.

Sudafed Liquid Interactions Index 982

Carteolol Hydrochloride (Concurrent use not recommended). Products include:
Cartrol Tablets ... 410
Ocupress Ophthalmic Solution, 1% Sterile ... ◉ 309

Clonidine (Concurrent use not recommended). Products include:
Catapres-TTS ... 675

Clonidine Hydrochloride (Concurrent use not recommended). Products include:
Catapres Tablets ... 674
Combipres Tablets ... 677

Deserpidine (Concurrent use not recommended).
No products indexed under this heading.

Desipramine Hydrochloride (Concurrent use not recommended). Products include:
Norpramin Tablets ... 1526

Diazoxide (Concurrent use not recommended). Products include:
Hyperstat I.V. Injection ... 2363
Proglycem ... 580

Diltiazem Hydrochloride (Concurrent use not recommended). Products include:
Cardizem CD Capsules ... 1506
Cardizem SR Capsules ... 1510
Cardizem Injectable ... 1508
Cardizem Tablets ... 1512
Dilacor XR Extended-release Capsules ... 2018

Doxazosin Mesylate (Concurrent use not recommended). Products include:
Cardura Tablets ... 2186

Doxepin Hydrochloride (Concurrent use not recommended). Products include:
Sinequan ... 2205
Zonalon Cream ... 1055

Enalapril Maleate (Concurrent use not recommended). Products include:
Vaseretic Tablets ... 1765
Vasotec Tablets ... 1771

Enalaprilat (Concurrent use not recommended). Products include:
Vasotec I.V. ... 1768

Esmolol Hydrochloride (Concurrent use not recommended). Products include:
Brevibloc Injection ... 1808

Felodipine (Concurrent use not recommended). Products include:
Plendil Extended-Release Tablets ... 527

Fluoxetine Hydrochloride (Concurrent use not recommended). Products include:
Prozac Pulvules & Liquid, Oral Solution ... 919

Fosinopril Sodium (Concurrent use not recommended). Products include:
Monopril Tablets ... 757

Guanabenz Acetate (Concurrent use not recommended).
No products indexed under this heading.

Guanethidine Monosulfate (Concurrent use not recommended). Products include:
Esimil Tablets ... 822
Ismelin Tablets ... 827

Hydralazine Hydrochloride (Concurrent use not recommended). Products include:
Apresazide Capsules ... 808
Apresoline Hydrochloride Tablets ... 809
Ser-Ap-Es Tablets ... 849

Imipramine Hydrochloride (Concurrent use not recommended). Products include:
Tofranil Ampuls ... 854
Tofranil Tablets ... 856

Imipramine Pamoate (Concurrent use not recommended). Products include:
Tofranil-PM Capsules ... 857

Indapamide (Concurrent use not recommended). Products include:
Lozol Tablets ... 2022

Isocarboxazid (Concurrent use not recommended).
No products indexed under this heading.

Isradipine (Concurrent use not recommended). Products include:
DynaCirc Capsules ... 2256

Labetalol Hydrochloride (Concurrent use not recommended). Products include:
Normodyne Injection ... 2377
Normodyne Tablets ... 2379
Trandate ... 1185

Lisinopril (Concurrent use not recommended). Products include:
Prinivil Tablets ... 1733
Prinzide Tablets ... 1737
Zestoretic ... 2850
Zestril Tablets ... 2854

Losartan Potassium (Concurrent use not recommended). Products include:
Cozaar Tablets ... 1628
Hyzaar Tablets ... 1677

Maprotiline Hydrochloride (Concurrent use not recommended). Products include:
Ludiomil Tablets ... 843

Mecamylamine Hydrochloride (Concurrent use not recommended). Products include:
Inversine Tablets ... 1686

Methyldopa (Concurrent use not recommended). Products include:
Aldoclor Tablets ... 1598
Aldomet Oral ... 1600
Aldoril Tablets ... 1604

Methyldopate Hydrochloride (Concurrent use not recommended). Products include:
Aldomet Ester HCI Injection ... 1602

Metoprolol Succinate (Concurrent use not recommended). Products include:
Toprol-XL Tablets ... 565

Metoprolol Tartrate (Concurrent use not recommended). Products include:
Lopressor Ampuls ... 830
Lopressor HCT Tablets ... 832
Lopressor Tablets ... 830

Metyrosine (Concurrent use not recommended). Products include:
Demser Capsules ... 1649

Minoxidil (Concurrent use not recommended). Products include:
Loniten Tablets ... 2618
Rogaine Topical Solution ... 2637

Moexipril Hydrochloride (Concurrent use not recommended). Products include:
Univasc Tablets ... 2410

Nadolol (Concurrent use not recommended).
No products indexed under this heading.

Nefazodone Hydrochloride (Concurrent use not recommended). Products include:
Serzone Tablets ... 771

Nicardipine Hydrochloride (Concurrent use not recommended). Products include:
Cardene Capsules ... 2095
Cardene I.V. ... 2709
Cardene SR Capsules ... 2097

Nifedipine (Concurrent use not recommended). Products include:
Adalat Capsules (10 mg and 20 mg) ... 587
Adalat CC ... 589
Procardia Capsules ... 1971
Procardia XL Extended Release Tablets ... 1972

Nisoldipine (Concurrent use not recommended).
No products indexed under this heading.

Nitroglycerin (Concurrent use not recommended). Products include:
Deponit NTG Transdermal Delivery System ... 2397
Nitro-Bid IV ... 1523
Nitro-Bid Ointment ... 1524
Nitrodisc ... 2047
Nitro-Dur (nitroglycerin) Transdermal Infusion System ... 1326
Nitrolingual Spray ... 2027
Nitrostat Tablets ... 1925
Transderm-Nitro Transdermal Therapeutic System ... 859

Nortriptyline Hydrochloride (Concurrent use not recommended). Products include:
Pamelor ... 2280

Paroxetine Hydrochloride (Concurrent use not recommended). Products include:
Paxil Tablets ... 2505

Penbutolol Sulfate (Concurrent use not recommended). Products include:
Levatol ... 2403

Phenelzine Sulfate (Concurrent use not recommended). Products include:
Nardil ... 1920

Phenoxybenzamine Hydrochloride (Concurrent use not recommended). Products include:
Dibenzyline Capsules ... 2476

Phentolamine Mesylate (Concurrent use not recommended). Products include:
Regitine ... 846

Pindolol (Concurrent use not recommended). Products include:
Visken Tablets ... 2299

Prazosin Hydrochloride (Concurrent use not recommended). Products include:
Minipress Capsules ... 1937
Minizide Capsules ... 1938

Propranolol Hydrochloride (Concurrent use not recommended). Products include:
Inderal ... 2728
Inderal LA Long Acting Capsules ... 2730
Inderide Tablets ... 2732
Inderide LA Long Acting Capsules ... 2734

Protriptyline Hydrochloride (Concurrent use not recommended). Products include:
Vivactil Tablets ... 1774

Quinapril Hydrochloride (Concurrent use not recommended). Products include:
Accupril Tablets ... 1893

Ramipril (Concurrent use not recommended). Products include:
Altace Capsules ... 1232

Rauwolfia Serpentina (Concurrent use not recommended).
No products indexed under this heading.

Rescinnamine (Concurrent use not recommended).
No products indexed under this heading.

Reserpine (Concurrent use not recommended). Products include:
Diupres Tablets ... 1650
Hydropres Tablets ... 1675
Ser-Ap-Es Tablets ... 849

Sertraline Hydrochloride (Concurrent use not recommended). Products include:
Zoloft Tablets ... 2217

Sodium Nitroprusside (Concurrent use not recommended).
No products indexed under this heading.

Sotalol Hydrochloride (Concurrent use not recommended). Products include:
Betapace Tablets ... 641

Spirapril Hydrochloride (Concurrent use not recommended).
No products indexed under this heading.

Terazosin Hydrochloride (Concurrent use not recommended). Products include:
Hytrin Capsules ... 430

Timolol Maleate (Concurrent use not recommended). Products include:
Blocadren Tablets ... 1614
Timolide Tablets ... 1748
Timoptic in Ocudose ... 1753
Timoptic Sterile Ophthalmic Solution ... 1751
Timoptic-XE ... 1755

Torsemide (Concurrent use not recommended). Products include:
Demadex Tablets and Injection ... 686

Tranylcypromine Sulfate (Concurrent use not recommended). Products include:
Parnate Tablets ... 2503

Trazodone Hydrochloride (Concurrent use not recommended). Products include:
Desyrel and Desyrel Dividose ... 503

Trimethaphan Camsylate (Concurrent use not recommended). Products include:
Arfonad Ampuls ... 2080

Trimipramine Maleate (Concurrent use not recommended). Products include:
Surmontil Capsules ... 2811

Venlafaxine Hydrochloride (Concurrent use not recommended). Products include:
Effexor ... 2719

Verapamil Hydrochloride (Concurrent use not recommended). Products include:
Calan SR Caplets ... 2422
Calan Tablets ... 2419
Isoptin Injectable ... 1344
Isoptin Oral Tablets ... 1346
Isoptin SR Tablets ... 1348
Verelan Capsules ... 1410
Verelan Capsules ... 2824

SUDAFED COLD AND COUGH LIQUIDCAPS
(Acetaminophen, Dextromethorphan Hydrobromide, Guaifenesin, Pseudoephedrine Hydrochloride) ... ▣ 862
May interact with monoamine oxidase inhibitors. Compounds in this category include:

Furazolidone (Concurrent and/or sequential use should be avoided). Products include:
Furoxone ... 2046

Isocarboxazid (Concurrent and/or sequential use should be avoided).
No products indexed under this heading.

Phenelzine Sulfate (Concurrent and/or sequential use should be avoided). Products include:
Nardil ... 1920

Selegiline Hydrochloride (Concurrent and/or sequential use should be avoided). Products include:
Eldepryl Tablets ... 2550

Tranylcypromine Sulfate (Concurrent and/or sequential use should be avoided). Products include:
Parnate Tablets ... 2503

(▣ Described in PDR For Nonprescription Drugs) (◉ Described in PDR For Ophthalmology)

983 Interactions Index Sudafed Plus Tablets

SUDAFED COUGH SYRUP
(Dextromethorphan Hydrobromide, Guaifenesin, Pseudoephedrine Hydrochloride) 862
May interact with monoamine oxidase inhibitors. Compounds in this category include:

Furazolidone (Concurrent administration is not recommended). Products include:
Furoxone 2046
Isocarboxazid (Concurrent administration is not recommended).
No products indexed under this heading.
Phenelzine Sulfate (Concurrent administration is not recommended). Products include:
Nardil 1920
Selegiline Hydrochloride (Concurrent administration is not recommended). Products include:
Eldepryl Tablets 2550
Tranylcypromine Sulfate (Concurrent administration is not recommended). Products include:
Parnate Tablets 2503

SUDAFED PLUS LIQUID
(Chlorpheniramine Maleate, Pseudoephedrine Hydrochloride) 862
May interact with monoamine oxidase inhibitors, hypnotics and sedatives, tranquilizers, and certain other agents. Compounds in these categories include:

Alprazolam (Increases drowsiness effect). Products include:
Xanax Tablets 2649
Buspirone Hydrochloride (Increases drowsiness effect). Products include:
BuSpar 737
Chlordiazepoxide (Increases drowsiness effect). Products include:
Libritabs Tablets 2177
Limbitrol 2180
Chlordiazepoxide Hydrochloride (Increases drowsiness effect). Products include:
Librax Capsules 2176
Librium Capsules 2178
Librium Injectable 2179
Chlorpromazine (Increases drowsiness effect). Products include:
Thorazine Suppositories 2523
Chlorpromazine Hydrochloride (Increases drowsiness effect). Products include:
Thorazine 2523
Chlorprothixene (Increases drowsiness effect).
No products indexed under this heading.
Chlorprothixene Hydrochloride (Increases drowsiness effect).
No products indexed under this heading.
Clorazepate Dipotassium (Increases drowsiness effect). Products include:
Tranxene 451
Diazepam (Increases drowsiness effect). Products include:
Dizac 1809
Valium Injectable 2182
Valium Tablets 2183
Valrelease Capsules 2169
Droperidol (Increases drowsiness effect). Products include:
Inapsine Injection 1296
Estazolam (Increases drowsiness effect). Products include:
ProSom Tablets 449
Ethchlorvynol (Increases drowsiness effect). Products include:
Placidyl Capsules 448
Ethinamate (Increases drowsiness effect).
No products indexed under this heading.
Fluphenazine Decanoate (Increases drowsiness effect). Products include:
Prolixin Decanoate 509
Fluphenazine Enanthate (Increases drowsiness effect). Products include:
Prolixin Enanthate 509
Fluphenazine Hydrochloride (Increases drowsiness effect). Products include:
Prolixin 509
Flurazepam Hydrochloride (Increases drowsiness effect). Products include:
Dalmane Capsules 2173
Furazolidone (Concurrent administration is not recommended). Products include:
Furoxone 2046
Glutethimide (Increases drowsiness effect).
No products indexed under this heading.
Haloperidol (Increases drowsiness effect). Products include:
Haldol Injection, Tablets and Concentrate 1575
Haloperidol Decanoate (Increases drowsiness effect). Products include:
Haldol Decanoate 1577
Hydroxyzine Hydrochloride (Increases drowsiness effect). Products include:
Atarax Tablets & Syrup 2185
Marax Tablets & DF Syrup 2200
Vistaril Intramuscular Solution 2216
Isocarboxazid (Concurrent administration is not recommended).
No products indexed under this heading.
Lorazepam (Increases drowsiness effect). Products include:
Ativan Injection 2698
Ativan Tablets 2700
Loxapine Hydrochloride (Increases drowsiness effect). Products include:
Loxitane 1378
Loxapine Succinate (Increases drowsiness effect). Products include:
Loxitane Capsules 1378
Meprobamate (Increases drowsiness effect). Products include:
Miltown Tablets 2672
PMB 200 and PMB 400 2783
Mesoridazine Besylate (Increases drowsiness effect). Products include:
Serentil 684
Midazolam Hydrochloride (Increases drowsiness effect). Products include:
Versed Injection 2170
Molindone Hydrochloride (Increases drowsiness effect). Products include:
Moban Tablets and Concentrate 1048
Oxazepam (Increases drowsiness effect). Products include:
Serax Capsules 2810
Serax Tablets 2810
Perphenazine (Increases drowsiness effect). Products include:
Etrafon 2355
Triavil Tablets 1757
Trilafon 2389
Phenelzine Sulfate (Concurrent administration is not recommended). Products include:
Nardil 1920
Prazepam (Increases drowsiness effect).
No products indexed under this heading.
Prochlorperazine (Increases drowsiness effect). Products include:
Compazine 2470
Promethazine Hydrochloride (Increases drowsiness effect). Products include:
Mepergan Injection 2753
Phenergan with Codeine 2777
Phenergan with Dextromethorphan 2778
Phenergan Injection 2773
Phenergan Suppositories 2775
Phenergan Syrup 2774
Phenergan Tablets 2775
Phenergan VC 2779
Phenergan VC with Codeine 2781
Propofol (Increases drowsiness effect). Products include:
Diprivan Injection 2833
Quazepam (Increases drowsiness effect). Products include:
Doral Tablets 2664
Secobarbital Sodium (Increases drowsiness effect). Products include:
Seconal Sodium Pulvules 1474
Selegiline Hydrochloride (Concurrent administration is not recommended). Products include:
Eldepryl Tablets 2550
Temazepam (Increases drowsiness effect). Products include:
Restoril Capsules 2284
Thioridazine Hydrochloride (Increases drowsiness effect). Products include:
Mellaril 2269
Thiothixene (Increases drowsiness effect). Products include:
Navane Capsules and Concentrate 2201
Navane Intramuscular 2202
Tranylcypromine Sulfate (Concurrent administration is not recommended). Products include:
Parnate Tablets 2503
Triazolam (Increases drowsiness effect). Products include:
Halcion Tablets 2611
Trifluoperazine Hydrochloride (Increases drowsiness effect). Products include:
Stelazine 2514
Zolpidem Tartrate (Increases drowsiness effect). Products include:
Ambien Tablets 2416

Food Interactions
Alcohol (Increases drowsiness effect).

SUDAFED PLUS TABLETS
(Chlorpheniramine Maleate, Pseudoephedrine Hydrochloride) 863
May interact with monoamine oxidase inhibitors, hypnotics and sedatives, tranquilizers, and certain other agents. Compounds in these categories include:

Alprazolam (Increases drowsiness effect). Products include:
Xanax Tablets 2649
Buspirone Hydrochloride (Increases drowsiness effect). Products include:
BuSpar 737
Chlordiazepoxide (Increases drowsiness effect). Products include:
Libritabs Tablets 2177
Limbitrol 2180
Chlordiazepoxide Hydrochloride (Increases drowsiness effect). Products include:
Librax Capsules 2176
Librium Capsules 2178
Librium Injectable 2179
Chlorpromazine (Increases drowsiness effect). Products include:
Thorazine Suppositories 2523
Chlorpromazine Hydrochloride (Increases drowsiness effect). Products include:
Thorazine 2523
Chlorprothixene (Increases drowsiness effect).
No products indexed under this heading.
Chlorprothixene Hydrochloride (Increases drowsiness effect).
No products indexed under this heading.
Clorazepate Dipotassium (Increases drowsiness effect). Products include:
Tranxene 451
Diazepam (Increases drowsiness effect). Products include:
Dizac 1809
Valium Injectable 2182
Valium Tablets 2183
Valrelease Capsules 2169
Droperidol (Increases drowsiness effect). Products include:
Inapsine Injection 1296
Estazolam (Increases drowsiness effect). Products include:
ProSom Tablets 449
Ethchlorvynol (Increases drowsiness effect). Products include:
Placidyl Capsules 448
Ethinamate (Increases drowsiness effect).
No products indexed under this heading.
Fluphenazine Decanoate (Increases drowsiness effect). Products include:
Prolixin Decanoate 509
Fluphenazine Enanthate (Increases drowsiness effect). Products include:
Prolixin Enanthate 509
Fluphenazine Hydrochloride (Increases drowsiness effect). Products include:
Prolixin 509
Flurazepam Hydrochloride (Increases drowsiness effect). Products include:
Dalmane Capsules 2173
Furazolidone (Concurrent administration is not recommended). Products include:
Furoxone 2046
Glutethimide (Increases drowsiness effect).
No products indexed under this heading.
Haloperidol (Increases drowsiness effect). Products include:
Haldol Injection, Tablets and Concentrate 1575
Haloperidol Decanoate (Increases drowsiness effect). Products include:
Haldol Decanoate 1577
Hydroxyzine Hydrochloride (Increases drowsiness effect). Products include:
Atarax Tablets & Syrup 2185
Marax Tablets & DF Syrup 2200
Vistaril Intramuscular Solution 2216
Isocarboxazid (Concurrent administration is not recommended).
No products indexed under this heading.
Lorazepam (Increases drowsiness effect). Products include:
Ativan Injection 2698
Ativan Tablets 2700
Loxapine Hydrochloride (Increases drowsiness effect). Products include:
Loxitane 1378

IMPORTANT NOTE: Always consult each drug listing in the patient's regimen for possible interactions.

Loxapine Succinate (Increases drowsiness effect). Products include:
- Loxitane Capsules ... 1378

Meprobamate (Increases drowsiness effect). Products include:
- Miltown Tablets ... 2672
- PMB 200 and PMB 400 ... 2783

Mesoridazine Besylate (Increases drowsiness effect). Products include:
- Serentil ... 684

Midazolam Hydrochloride (Increases drowsiness effect). Products include:
- Versed Injection ... 2170

Molindone Hydrochloride (Increases drowsiness effect). Products include:
- Moban Tablets and Concentrate ... 1048

Oxazepam (Increases drowsiness effect). Products include:
- Serax Capsules ... 2810
- Serax Tablets ... 2810

Perphenazine (Increases drowsiness effect). Products include:
- Etrafon ... 2355
- Triavil Tablets ... 1757
- Trilafon ... 2389

Phenelzine Sulfate (Concurrent administration is not recommended). Products include:
- Nardil ... 1920

Prazepam (Increases drowsiness effect).
- No products indexed under this heading.

Prochlorperazine (Increases drowsiness effect). Products include:
- Compazine ... 2470

Promethazine Hydrochloride (Increases drowsiness effect). Products include:
- Mepergan Injection ... 2753
- Phenergan with Codeine ... 2777
- Phenergan with Dextromethorphan 2778
- Phenergan Injection ... 2773
- Phenergan Suppositories ... 2775
- Phenergan Syrup ... 2774
- Phenergan Tablets ... 2775
- Phenergan VC ... 2779
- Phenergan VC with Codeine ... 2781

Propofol (Increases drowsiness effect). Products include:
- Diprivan Injection ... 2833

Quazepam (Increases drowsiness effect). Products include:
- Doral Tablets ... 2664

Secobarbital Sodium (Increases drowsiness effect). Products include:
- Seconal Sodium Pulvules ... 1474

Selegiline Hydrochloride (Concurrent administration is not recommended). Products include:
- Eldepryl Tablets ... 2550

Temazepam (Increases drowsiness effect). Products include:
- Restoril Capsules ... 2284

Thioridazine Hydrochloride (Increases drowsiness effect). Products include:
- Mellaril ... 2269

Thiothixene (Increases drowsiness effect). Products include:
- Navane Capsules and Concentrate 2201
- Navane Intramuscular ... 2202

Tranylcypromine Sulfate (Concurrent administration is not recommended). Products include:
- Parnate Tablets ... 2503

Triazolam (Increases drowsiness effect). Products include:
- Halcion Tablets ... 2611

Trifluoperazine Hydrochloride (Increases drowsiness effect). Products include:
- Stelazine ... 2514

Zolpidem Tartrate (Increases drowsiness effect). Products include:
- Ambien Tablets ... 2416

Food Interactions

Alcohol (Increases drowsiness effect).

SUDAFED SEVERE COLD FORMULA CAPLETS

(Acetaminophen, Dextromethorphan Hydrobromide, Pseudoephedrine Hydrochloride) .... ▣ 863

May interact with monoamine oxidase inhibitors. Compounds in this category include:

Furazolidone (Concurrent and/or sequential use should be avoided). Products include:
- Furoxone ... 2046

Isocarboxazid (Concurrent and/or sequential use should be avoided).
- No products indexed under this heading.

Phenelzine Sulfate (Concurrent and/or sequential use should be avoided). Products include:
- Nardil ... 1920

Selegiline Hydrochloride (Concurrent and/or sequential use should be avoided). Products include:
- Eldepryl Tablets ... 2550

Tranylcypromine Sulfate (Concurrent and/or sequential use should be avoided). Products include:
- Parnate Tablets ... 2503

SUDAFED SEVERE COLD FORMULA TABLETS

(Acetaminophen, Dextromethorphan Hydrobromide, Pseudoephedrine Hydrochloride) .... ▣ 864

May interact with monoamine oxidase inhibitors. Compounds in this category include:

Furazolidone (Concurrent and/or sequential use should be avoided). Products include:
- Furoxone ... 2046

Isocarboxazid (Concurrent and/or sequential use should be avoided).
- No products indexed under this heading.

Phenelzine Sulfate (Concurrent and/or sequential use should be avoided). Products include:
- Nardil ... 1920

Selegiline Hydrochloride (Concurrent and/or sequential use should be avoided). Products include:
- Eldepryl Tablets ... 2550

Tranylcypromine Sulfate (Concurrent and/or sequential use should be avoided). Products include:
- Parnate Tablets ... 2503

SUDAFED SINUS CAPLETS

(Acetaminophen, Pseudoephedrine Hydrochloride) ... ▣ 864

May interact with monoamine oxidase inhibitors. Compounds in this category include:

Furazolidone (Concurrent administration is not recommended). Products include:
- Furoxone ... 2046

Isocarboxazid (Concurrent administration is not recommended).
- No products indexed under this heading.

Phenelzine Sulfate (Concurrent administration is not recommended). Products include:
- Nardil ... 1920

Selegiline Hydrochloride (Concurrent administration is not recommended). Products include:
- Eldepryl Tablets ... 2550

Tranylcypromine Sulfate (Concurrent administration is not recommended). Products include:
- Parnate Tablets ... 2503

SUDAFED SINUS TABLETS

(Acetaminophen, Pseudoephedrine Hydrochloride) ... ▣ 864

May interact with monoamine oxidase inhibitors. Compounds in this category include:

Furazolidone (Concurrent administration is not recommended). Products include:
- Furoxone ... 2046

Isocarboxazid (Concurrent administration is not recommended).
- No products indexed under this heading.

Phenelzine Sulfate (Concurrent administration is not recommended). Products include:
- Nardil ... 1920

Selegiline Hydrochloride (Concurrent administration is not recommended). Products include:
- Eldepryl Tablets ... 2550

Tranylcypromine Sulfate (Concurrent administration is not recommended). Products include:
- Parnate Tablets ... 2503

SUDAFED TABLETS, 30 MG

(Pseudoephedrine Hydrochloride) .. ▣ 861

May interact with monoamine oxidase inhibitors. Compounds in this category include:

Furazolidone (Concurrent administration is not recommended). Products include:
- Furoxone ... 2046

Isocarboxazid (Concurrent administration is not recommended).
- No products indexed under this heading.

Phenelzine Sulfate (Concurrent administration is not recommended). Products include:
- Nardil ... 1920

Selegiline Hydrochloride (Concurrent administration is not recommended). Products include:
- Eldepryl Tablets ... 2550

Tranylcypromine Sulfate (Concurrent administration is not recommended). Products include:
- Parnate Tablets ... 2503

SUDAFED TABLETS, 60 MG

(Pseudoephedrine Hydrochloride) .. ▣ 861

May interact with monoamine oxidase inhibitors. Compounds in this category include:

Furazolidone (Concurrent administration is not recommended). Products include:
- Furoxone ... 2046

Isocarboxazid (Concurrent administration is not recommended).
- No products indexed under this heading.

Phenelzine Sulfate (Concurrent administration is not recommended). Products include:
- Nardil ... 1920

Selegiline Hydrochloride (Concurrent administration is not recommended). Products include:
- Eldepryl Tablets ... 2550

Tranylcypromine Sulfate (Concurrent administration is not recommended). Products include:
- Parnate Tablets ... 2503

SUDAFED 12 HOUR CAPLETS

(Pseudoephedrine Hydrochloride) .. ▣ 861

May interact with:

Antidepressant Medications, unspecified (Effect not specified).

Antihypertensive agents, unspecified (Effect not specified).

SUFENTA INJECTION

(Sufentanil Citrate) ... 1309

May interact with central nervous system depressants, barbiturates, tranquilizers, narcotic analgesics, neuromuscular blocking agents, calcium channel blockers, beta blockers, benzodiazepines, and certain other agents. Compounds in these categories include:

Acebutolol Hydrochloride (The incidence and degree of bradycardia and hypotension during Sufenta-oxygen anesthesia may be greater in patients on chronic beta blocker therapy). Products include:
- Sectral Capsules ... 2807

Alfentanil Hydrochloride (Enhanced magnitude and duration of CNS/cardiovascular effects; respiratory depression may be enhanced). Products include:
- Alfenta Injection ... 1286

Alprazolam (Enhanced magnitude and duration of CNS/cardiovascular effects; respiratory depression may be enhanced; the use of benzodiazepines with Sufenta during induction may result in a decrease in mean arterial pressure and systemic vascular resistance). Products include:
- Xanax Tablets ... 2649

Amlodipine Besylate (The incidence and degree of bradycardia and hypotension during Sufenta-oxygen anesthesia may be greater in patients on chronic calcium channel blocker therapy). Products include:
- Lotrel Capsules ... 840
- Norvasc Tablets ... 1940

Aprobarbital (Enhanced magnitude and duration of CNS/cardiovascular effects; respiratory depression may be enhanced).
- No products indexed under this heading.

Atenolol (The incidence and degree of bradycardia and hypotension during Sufenta-oxygen anesthesia may be greater in patients on chronic beta blocker therapy). Products include:
- Tenoretic Tablets ... 2845
- Tenormin Tablets and I.V. Injection 2847

Atracurium Besylate (May produce bradycardia and hypotension; effect may be pronounced in the presence of calcium channel and/or beta-blockers). Products include:
- Tracrium Injection ... 1183

Bepridil Hydrochloride (The incidence and degree of bradycardia and hypotension during Sufenta-oxygen anesthesia may be greater in patients on chronic calcium channel blocker therapy). Products include:
- Vascor (200, 300 and 400 mg) Tablets ... 1587

Betaxolol Hydrochloride (The incidence and degree of bradycardia and hypotension during Sufenta-oxygen anesthesia may be greater in patients on chronic beta blocker therapy). Products include:
- Betoptic Ophthalmic Solution ... 469
- Betoptic S Ophthalmic Suspension 471
- Kerlone Tablets ... 2436

(▣ Described in PDR For Nonprescription Drugs) (⊙ Described in PDR For Ophthalmology)

985 **Interactions Index** **Sufenta**

Bisoprolol Fumarate (The incidence and degree of bradycardia and hypotension during Sufenta-oxygen anesthesia may be greater in patients on chronic beta blocker therapy). Products include:
Zebeta Tablets 1413
Ziac 1415

Buprenorphine (Enhanced magnitude and duration of CNS/cardiovascular effects; respiratory depression may be enhanced). Products include:
Buprenex Injectable 2006

Buspirone Hydrochloride (Enhanced magnitude and duration of CNS/cardiovascular effects; respiratory depression may be enhanced). Products include:
BuSpar 737

Butabarbital (Enhanced magnitude and duration of CNS/cardiovascular effects; respiratory depression may be enhanced).
No products indexed under this heading.

Butalbital (Enhanced magnitude and duration of CNS/cardiovascular effects; respiratory depression may be enhanced). Products include:
Esgic-plus Tablets 1013
Fioricet Tablets 2258
Fioricet with Codeine Capsules 2260
Fiorinal Capsules 2261
Fiorinal with Codeine Capsules 2262
Fiorinal Tablets 2261
Phrenilin 785
Sedapap Tablets 50 mg/650 mg .. 1543

Carteolol Hydrochloride (The incidence and degree of bradycardia and hypotension during Sufenta-oxygen anesthesia may be greater in patients on chronic beta blocker therapy). Products include:
Cartrol Tablets 410
Ocupress Ophthalmic Solution, 1% Sterile .... ⊙ 309

Chlordiazepoxide (Enhanced magnitude and duration of CNS/cardiovascular effects; respiratory depression may be enhanced; the use of benzodiazepines with Sufenta during induction may result in a decrease in mean arterial pressure and systemic vascular resistance). Products include:
Libritabs Tablets 2177
Limbitrol 2180

Chlordiazepoxide Hydrochloride (Enhanced magnitude and duration of CNS/cardiovascular effects; respiratory depression may be enhanced; the use of benzodiazepines with Sufenta during induction may result in a decrease in mean arterial pressure and systemic vascular resistance). Products include:
Librax Capsules 2176
Librium Capsules 2178
Librium Injectable 2179

Chlorpromazine (Enhanced magnitude and duration of CNS/cardiovascular effects; respiratory depression may be enhanced). Products include:
Thorazine Suppositories 2523

Chlorprothixene (Enhanced magnitude and duration of CNS/cardiovascular effects; respiratory depression may be enhanced).
No products indexed under this heading.

Chlorprothixene Hydrochloride (Enhanced magnitude and duration of CNS/cardiovascular effects; respiratory depression may be enhanced).
No products indexed under this heading.

Clorazepate Dipotassium (Enhanced magnitude and duration of CNS/cardiovascular effects; respiratory depression may be enhanced; the use of benzodiazepines with Sufenta during induction may result in a decrease in mean arterial pressure and systemic vascular resistance). Products include:
Tranxene 451

Clozapine (Enhanced magnitude and duration of CNS/cardiovascular effects; respiratory depression may be enhanced). Products include:
Clozaril Tablets 2252

Codeine Phosphate (Enhanced magnitude and duration of CNS/cardiovascular effects; respiratory depression may be enhanced). Products include:
Actifed with Codeine Cough Syrup.. 1067
Brontex 1981
Deconsal C Expectorant Syrup 456
Deconsal Pediatric Syrup 457
Dimetane-DC Cough Syrup 2059
Empirin with Codeine Tablets 1093
Fioricet with Codeine Capsules 2260
Fiorinal with Codeine Capsules 2262
Isoclor Expectorant 990
Novahistine DH 2462
Novahistine Expectorant 2463
Nucofed 2051
Phenergan with Codeine 2777
Phenergan VC with Codeine 2781
Robitussin A-C Syrup 2073
Robitussin-DAC Syrup 2074
Ryna .... ▣ 841
Soma Compound w/Codeine Tablets 2676
Tussi-Organidin NR Liquid and S NR Liquid 2677
Tylenol with Codeine 1583

Desflurane (Enhanced magnitude and duration of CNS/cardiovascular effects; respiratory depression may be enhanced). Products include:
Suprane 1813

Dezocine (Enhanced magnitude and duration of CNS/cardiovascular effects; respiratory depression may be enhanced). Products include:
Dalgan Injection 538

Diazepam (Enhanced magnitude and duration of CNS/cardiovascular effects; respiratory depression may be enhanced; the use of benzodiazepines with Sufenta during induction may result in a decrease in mean arterial pressure and systemic vascular resistance). Products include:
Dizac 1809
Valium Injectable 2182
Valium Tablets 2183
Valrelease Capsules 2169

Diltiazem Hydrochloride (The incidence and degree of bradycardia and hypotension during Sufenta-oxygen anesthesia may be greater in patients on chronic calcium channel blocker therapy). Products include:
Cardizem CD Capsules 1506
Cardizem SR Capsules 1510
Cardizem Injectable 1508
Cardizem Tablets 1512
Dilacor XR Extended-release Capsules 2018

Doxacurium Chloride (May produce bradycardia and hypotension; effect may be pronounced in the presence of calcium channel and/or beta-blockers). Products include:
Nuromax Injection 1149

Droperidol (Enhanced magnitude and duration of CNS/cardiovascular effects; respiratory depression may be enhanced). Products include:
Inapsine Injection 1296

Enflurane (Enhanced magnitude and duration of CNS/cardiovascular effects; respiratory depression may be enhanced).
No products indexed under this heading.

Esmolol Hydrochloride (The incidence and degree of bradycardia and hypotension during Sufenta-oxygen anesthesia may be greater in patients on chronic beta blocker therapy). Products include:
Brevibloc Injection 1808

Estazolam (Enhanced magnitude and duration of CNS/cardiovascular effects; respiratory depression may be enhanced; the use of benzodiazepines with Sufenta during induction may result in a decrease in mean arterial pressure and systemic vascular resistance). Products include:
ProSom Tablets 449

Ethchlorvynol (Enhanced magnitude and duration of CNS/cardiovascular effects; respiratory depression may be enhanced). Products include:
Placidyl Capsules 448

Ethinamate (Enhanced magnitude and duration of CNS/cardiovascular effects; respiratory depression may be enhanced).
No products indexed under this heading.

Felodipine (The incidence and degree of bradycardia and hypotension during Sufenta-oxygen anesthesia may be greater in patients on chronic calcium channel blocker therapy). Products include:
Plendil Extended-Release Tablets.... 527

Fentanyl (Enhanced magnitude and duration of CNS/cardiovascular effects; respiratory depression may be enhanced). Products include:
Duragesic Transdermal System 1288

Fentanyl Citrate (Enhanced magnitude and duration of CNS/cardiovascular effects; respiratory depression may be enhanced). Products include:
Sublimaze Injection 1307

Fluphenazine Decanoate (Enhanced magnitude and duration of CNS/cardiovascular effects; respiratory depression may be enhanced). Products include:
Prolixin Decanoate 509

Fluphenazine Enanthate (Enhanced magnitude and duration of CNS/cardiovascular effects; respiratory depression may be enhanced). Products include:
Prolixin Enanthate 509

Fluphenazine Hydrochloride (Enhanced magnitude and duration of CNS/cardiovascular effects; respiratory depression may be enhanced). Products include:
Prolixin 509

Flurazepam Hydrochloride (Enhanced magnitude and duration of CNS/cardiovascular effects; respiratory depression may be enhanced). Products include:
Dalmane Capsules 2173

Glutethimide (Enhanced magnitude and duration of CNS/cardiovascular effects; respiratory depression may be enhanced).
No products indexed under this heading.

Halazepam (Enhanced magnitude and duration of CNS/cardiovascular effects; respiratory depression may be enhanced; the use of benzodiazepines with Sufenta during induction may result in a decrease in mean arterial pressure and systemic vascular resistance).
No products indexed under this heading.

Haloperidol (Enhanced magnitude and duration of CNS/cardiovascular effects; respiratory depression may be enhanced). Products include:
Haldol Injection, Tablets and Concentrate 1575

Haloperidol Decanoate (Enhanced magnitude and duration of CNS/cardiovascular effects; respiratory depression may be enhanced). Products include:
Haldol Decanoate 1577

Hydrocodone Bitartrate (Enhanced magnitude and duration of CNS/cardiovascular effects; respiratory depression may be enhanced). Products include:
Anexsia 5/500 Elixir 1781
Anexia Tablets 1782
Codiclear DH Syrup 791
Deconamine CX Cough and Cold Liquid and Tablets 1319
Duratuss HD Elixir 2565
Hycodan Tablets and Syrup 930
Hycomine Compound Tablets 932
Hycomine 931
Hycotuss Expectorant Syrup 933
Hydrocet Capsules 782
Lorcet 10/650 1018
Lortab 2566
Tussend 1783
Tussend Expectorant 1785
Vicodin Tablets 1356
Vicodin ES Tablets 1357
Vicodin Tuss Expectorant 1358
Zydone Capsules 949

Hydrocodone Polistirex (Enhanced magnitude and duration of CNS/cardiovascular effects; respiratory depression may be enhanced). Products include:
Tussionex Pennkinetic Extended-Release Suspension 998

Hydroxyzine Hydrochloride (Enhanced magnitude and duration of CNS/cardiovascular effects; respiratory depression may be enhanced). Products include:
Atarax Tablets & Syrup 2185
Marax Tablets & DF Syrup 2200
Vistaril Intramuscular Solution 2216

Isoflurane (Enhanced magnitude and duration of CNS/cardiovascular effects; respiratory depression may be enhanced).
No products indexed under this heading.

Isradipine (The incidence and degree of bradycardia and hypotension during Sufenta-oxygen anesthesia may be greater in patients on chronic calcium channel blocker therapy). Products include:
DynaCirc Capsules 2256

Ketamine Hydrochloride (Enhanced magnitude and duration of CNS/cardiovascular effects; respiratory depression may be enhanced).
No products indexed under this heading.

Labetalol Hydrochloride (The incidence and degree of bradycardia and hypotension during Sufenta-oxygen anesthesia may be greater in patients on chronic beta blocker therapy). Products include:
Normodyne Injection 2377
Normodyne Tablets 2379
Trandate 1185

IMPORTANT NOTE: Always consult each drug listing in the patient's regimen for possible interactions.

Sufenta

Levobunolol Hydrochloride (The incidence and degree of bradycardia and hypotension during Sufenta-oxygen anesthesia may be greater in patients on chronic beta blocker therapy). Products include:

Betagan .... ◉ 233

Levomethadyl Acetate Hydrochloride (Enhanced magnitude and duration of CNS/cardiovascular effects; respiratory depression may be enhanced). Products include:

Orlaam 2239

Levorphanol Tartrate (Enhanced magnitude and duration of CNS/cardiovascular effects; respiratory depression may be enhanced). Products include:

Levo-Dromoran 2129

Lorazepam (Enhanced magnitude and duration of CNS/cardiovascular effects; respiratory depression may be enhanced; the use of benzodiazepines with Sufenta during induction may result in a decrease in mean arterial pressure and systemic vascular resistance). Products include:

Ativan Injection 2698
Ativan Tablets 2700

Loxapine Hydrochloride (Enhanced magnitude and duration of CNS/cardiovascular effects; respiratory depression may be enhanced). Products include:

Loxitane 1378

Loxapine Succinate (Enhanced magnitude and duration of CNS/cardiovascular effects; respiratory depression may be enhanced). Products include:

Loxitane Capsules 1378

Meperidine Hydrochloride (Enhanced magnitude and duration of CNS/cardiovascular effects; respiratory depression may be enhanced). Products include:

Demerol 2308
Mepergan Injection 2753

Mephobarbital (Enhanced magnitude and duration of CNS/cardiovascular effects; respiratory depression may be enhanced). Products include:

Mebaral Tablets 2322

Meprobamate (Enhanced magnitude and duration of CNS/cardiovascular effects; respiratory depression may be enhanced). Products include:

Miltown Tablets 2672
PMB 200 and PMB 400 2783

Mesoridazine Besylate (Enhanced magnitude and duration of CNS/cardiovascular effects; respiratory depression may be enhanced). Products include:

Serentil 684

Methadone Hydrochloride (Enhanced magnitude and duration of CNS/cardiovascular effects; respiratory depression may be enhanced). Products include:

Methadone Hydrochloride Oral Concentrate 2233
Methadone Hydrochloride Oral Solution & Tablets 2235

Methohexital Sodium (Enhanced magnitude and duration of CNS/cardiovascular effects; respiratory depression may be enhanced). Products include:

Brevital Sodium Vials 1429

Methotrimeprazine (Enhanced magnitude and duration of CNS/cardiovascular effects; respiratory depression may be enhanced). Products include:

Levoprome 1274

Methoxyflurane (Enhanced magnitude and duration of CNS/cardiovascular effects; respiratory depression may be enhanced).

No products indexed under this heading.

Metipranolol Hydrochloride (The incidence and degree of bradycardia and hypotension during Sufenta-oxygen anesthesia may be greater in patients on chronic beta blocker therapy). Products include:

OptiPranolol (Metipranolol 0.3%)
Sterile Ophthalmic Solution .... ◉ 258

Metocurine Iodide (May produce bradycardia and hypotension; effect may be pronounced in the presence of calcium channel and/or beta-blockers). Products include:

Metubine Iodide Vials 916

Metoprolol Succinate (The incidence and degree of bradycardia and hypotension during Sufenta-oxygen anesthesia may be greater in patients on chronic beta blocker therapy). Products include:

Toprol-XL Tablets 565

Metoprolol Tartrate (The incidence and degree of bradycardia and hypotension during Sufenta-oxygen anesthesia may be greater in patients on chronic beta blocker therapy). Products include:

Lopressor Ampuls 830
Lopressor HCT Tablets 832
Lopressor Tablets 830

Midazolam Hydrochloride (Enhanced magnitude and duration of CNS/cardiovascular effects; respiratory depression may be enhanced; the use of benzodiazepines with Sufenta during induction may result in a decrease in mean arterial pressure and systemic vascular resistance). Products include:

Versed Injection 2170

Mivacurium Chloride (May produce bradycardia and hypotension; effect may be pronounced in the presence of calcium channel and/or beta-blockers). Products include:

Mivacron 1138

Molindone Hydrochloride (Enhanced magnitude and duration of CNS/cardiovascular effects; respiratory depression may be enhanced). Products include:

Moban Tablets and Concentrate 1048

Morphine Sulfate (Enhanced magnitude and duration of CNS/cardiovascular effects; respiratory depression may be enhanced). Products include:

Astramorph/PF Injection, USP (Preservative-Free) 535
Duramorph 962
Infumorph 200 and Infumorph 500 Sterile Solutions 965
MS Contin Tablets 1994
MSIR 1997
Oramorph SR (Morphine Sulfate Sustained Release Tablets) 2236
RMS Suppositories 2657
Roxanol 2243

Nadolol (The incidence and degree of bradycardia and hypotension during Sufenta-oxygen anesthesia may be greater in patients on chronic beta blocker therapy).

No products indexed under this heading.

Nicardipine Hydrochloride (The incidence and degree of bradycardia and hypotension during Sufenta-oxygen anesthesia may be greater in patients on chronic calcium channel blocker therapy). Products include:

Cardene Capsules 2095
Cardene I.V. 2709

Cardene SR Capsules 2097

Nifedipine (The incidence and degree of bradycardia and hypotension during Sufenta-oxygen anesthesia may be greater in patients on chronic calcium channel blocker therapy). Products include:

Adalat Capsules (10 mg and 20 mg) 587
Adalat CC 589
Procardia Capsules 1971
Procardia XL Extended Release Tablets 1972

Nimodipine (The incidence and degree of bradycardia and hypotension during Sufenta-oxygen anesthesia may be greater in patients on chronic calcium channel blocker therapy). Products include:

Nimotop Capsules 610

Nisoldipine (The incidence and degree of bradycardia and hypotension during Sufenta-oxygen anesthesia may be greater in patients on chronic calcium channel blocker therapy).

No products indexed under this heading.

Nitrous Oxide (Possible cardiovascular depression).

Opium Alkaloids (Additive or potentiating effects; respiratory depression may be enhanced).

No products indexed under this heading.

Oxazepam (Enhanced magnitude and duration of CNS/cardiovascular effects; respiratory depression may be enhanced; the use of benzodiazepines with Sufenta during induction may result in a decrease in mean arterial pressure and systemic vascular resistance). Products include:

Serax Capsules 2810
Serax Tablets 2810

Oxycodone Hydrochloride (Enhanced magnitude and duration of CNS/cardiovascular effects; respiratory depression may be enhanced). Products include:

Percocet Tablets 938
Percodan Tablets 939
Percodan-Demi Tablets 940
Roxicodone Tablets, Oral Solution & Intensol (Oxycodone) 2244
Tylox Capsules 1584

Pancuronium Bromide Injection (Elevated heart rate; may produce bradycardia and hypotension; effect may be pronounced in the presence of calcium channel and/or beta-blockers).

No products indexed under this heading.

Penbutolol Sulfate (The incidence and degree of bradycardia and hypotension during Sufenta-oxygen anesthesia may be greater in patients on chronic beta blocker therapy). Products include:

Levatol 2403

Pentobarbital Sodium (Enhanced magnitude and duration of CNS/cardiovascular effects; respiratory depression may be enhanced). Products include:

Nembutal Sodium Capsules 436
Nembutal Sodium Solution 438
Nembutal Sodium Suppositories 440

Perphenazine (Enhanced magnitude and duration of CNS/cardiovascular effects; respiratory depression may be enhanced). Products include:

Etrafon 2355
Triavil Tablets 1757
Trilafon 2389

Phenobarbital (Enhanced magnitude and duration of CNS/cardiovascular effects; respiratory depression may be enhanced). Products include:

Arco-Lase Plus Tablets 512
Bellergal-S Tablets 2250
Donnatal 2060
Donnatal Extentabs 2061
Donnatal Tablets 2060
Phenobarbital Elixir and Tablets 1469
Quadrinal Tablets 1350

Pindolol (The incidence and degree of bradycardia and hypotension during Sufenta-oxygen anesthesia may be greater in patients on chronic beta blocker therapy). Products include:

Visken Tablets 2299

Prazepam (Enhanced magnitude and duration of CNS/cardiovascular effects; respiratory depression may be enhanced; the use of benzodiazepines with Sufenta during induction may result in a decrease in mean arterial pressure and systemic vascular resistance).

No products indexed under this heading.

Prochlorperazine (Enhanced magnitude and duration of CNS/cardiovascular effects; respiratory depression may be enhanced). Products include:

Compazine 2470

Promethazine Hydrochloride (Enhanced magnitude and duration of CNS/cardiovascular effects; respiratory depression may be enhanced). Products include:

Mepergan Injection 2753
Phenergan with Codeine 2777
Phenergan with Dextromethorphan 2778
Phenergan Injection 2773
Phenergan Suppositories 2775
Phenergan Syrup 2774
Phenergan Tablets 2775
Phenergan VC 2779
Phenergan VC with Codeine 2781

Propofol (Enhanced magnitude and duration of CNS/cardiovascular effects; respiratory depression may be enhanced). Products include:

Diprivan Injection 2833

Propoxyphene Hydrochloride (Enhanced magnitude and duration of CNS/cardiovascular effects; respiratory depression may be enhanced). Products include:

Darvon 1435
Wygesic Tablets 2827

Propoxyphene Napsylate (Enhanced magnitude and duration of CNS/cardiovascular effects; respiratory depression may be enhanced). Products include:

Darvon-N/Darvocet-N 1433

Propranolol Hydrochloride (The incidence and degree of bradycardia and hypotension during Sufenta-oxygen anesthesia may be greater in patients on chronic beta blocker therapy). Products include:

Inderal 2728
Inderal LA Long Acting Capsules 2730
Inderide Tablets 2732
Inderide LA Long Acting Capsules .. 2734

Quazepam (Enhanced magnitude and duration of CNS/cardiovascular effects; respiratory depression may be enhanced; the use of benzodiazepines with Sufenta during induction may result in a decrease in mean arterial pressure and systemic vascular resistance). Products include:

Doral Tablets 2664

Risperidone (Enhanced magnitude and duration of CNS/cardiovascular effects; respiratory depression may be enhanced). Products include:

Risperdal 1301

Rocuronium Bromide (May produce bradycardia and hypotension; effect may be pronounced in the presence of calcium channel and/or beta-blockers). Products include:

Zemuron 1830

Secobarbital Sodium (Enhanced magnitude and duration of CNS/cardiovascular effects; respiratory depression may be enhanced). Products include:

Seconal Sodium Pulvules 1474

Sotalol Hydrochloride (The incidence and degree of bradycardia and hypotension during Sufenta-oxygen anesthesia may be greater in patients on chronic beta blocker therapy). Products include:

Betapace Tablets 641

Succinylcholine Chloride (May produce bradycardia and hypotension; effect may be pronounced in the presence of calcium channel and/or beta-blockers). Products include:

Anectine.. 1073

Temazepam (Enhanced magnitude and duration of CNS/cardiovascular effects; respiratory depression may be enhanced). Products include:

Restoril Capsules 2284

Thiamylal Sodium (Enhanced magnitude and duration of CNS/cardiovascular effects; respiratory depression may be enhanced).

No products indexed under this heading.

Thioridazine Hydrochloride (Enhanced magnitude and duration of CNS/cardiovascular effects; respiratory depression may be enhanced). Products include:

Mellaril 2269

Thiothixene (Enhanced magnitude and duration of CNS/cardiovascular effects; respiratory depression may be enhanced). Products include:

Navane Capsules and Concentrate 2201
Navane Intramuscular 2202

Timolol Hemihydrate (The incidence and degree of bradycardia and hypotension during Sufenta-oxygen anesthesia may be greater in patients on chronic beta blocker therapy). Products include:

Betimol 0.25%, 0.5% .... ◊ 261

Timolol Maleate (The incidence and degree of bradycardia and hypotension during Sufenta-oxygen anesthesia may be greater in patients on chronic beta blocker therapy). Products include:

Blocadren Tablets 1614
Timolide Tablets.................................... 1748
Timoptic in Ocudose 1753
Timoptic Sterile Ophthalmic Solution... 1751
Timoptic-XE 1755

Triazolam (Enhanced magnitude and duration of CNS/cardiovascular effects; respiratory depression may be enhanced). Products include:

Halcion Tablets...................................... 2611

Trifluoperazine Hydrochloride (Enhanced magnitude and duration of CNS/cardiovascular effects; respiratory depression may be enhanced). Products include:

Stelazine 2514

Vecuronium Bromide (May produce bradycardia and hypotension; effect may be pronounced in the presence of calcium channel and/or beta-blockers). Products include:

Norcuron 1826

Verapamil Hydrochloride (The incidence and degree of bradycardia and hypotension during Sufenta-oxygen anesthesia may be greater in patients on chronic calcium channel blocker therapy). Products include:

Calan SR Caplets 2422
Calan Tablets... 2419
Isoptin Injectable 1344
Isoptin Oral Tablets 1346
Isoptin SR Tablets 1348
Verelan Capsules 1410
Verelan Capsules 2824

Zolpidem Tartrate (Enhanced magnitude and duration of CNS/cardiovascular effects; respiratory depression may be enhanced). Products include:

Ambien Tablets...................................... 2416

SULFACET-R MVL LOTION
(Sodium Sulfacetamide, Sulfur).......... 909
None cited in PDR database.

SULFAMYLON CREAM
(Mafenide Acetate) 925
None cited in PDR database.

SULTRIN TRIPLE SULFA CREAM
(Sulfathiazole, Sulfacetamide, Sulfabenzamide) 1885
None cited in PDR database.

SULTRIN TRIPLE SULFA VAGINAL TABLETS
(Sulfathiazole, Sulfacetamide, Sulfabenzamide) 1885
None cited in PDR database.

SUNKIST CHILDREN'S CHEWABLE MULTIVITAMINS - COMPLETE
(Vitamins with Minerals) ....ᵃᵈ 649
None cited in PDR database.

SUNKIST CHILDREN'S CHEWABLE MULTIVITAMINS - PLUS EXTRA C
(Vitamins with Minerals) ....ᵃᵈ 649
None cited in PDR database.

SUNKIST CHILDREN'S CHEWABLE MULTIVITAMINS - PLUS IRON
(Vitamins with Iron) ....ᵃᵈ 649
None cited in PDR database.

SUNKIST CHILDREN'S CHEWABLE MULTIVITAMINS - REGULAR
(Vitamins with Minerals) ....ᵃᵈ 649
None cited in PDR database.

SUNKIST VITAMIN C - CHEWABLE
(Vitamin C)..ᵃᵈ 649
None cited in PDR database.

SUNKIST VITAMIN C - EASY TO SWALLOW
(Vitamin C)..ᵃᵈ 649
None cited in PDR database.

SUPER EPA
(Docosahexaenoic Acid (DHA)) 468
None cited in PDR database.

SUPLENA SPECIALIZED LIQUID NUTRITION
(Nutritional Supplement) 2226
None cited in PDR database.

SUPPRELIN INJECTION
(Histrelin Acetate) 2056
None cited in PDR database.

SUPRANE
(Desflurane) 1813
May interact with benzodiazepines, narcotic analgesics, antipsychotic agents, and certain other agents. Compounds in these categories include:

Alfentanil Hydrochloride (Decreases the maximum alveolar concentration (MAC) of desflurane). Products include:

Alfenta Injection 1286

Alprazolam (Decreases the maximum alveolar concentration (MAC) of desflurane). Products include:

Xanax Tablets 2649

Buprenorphine (Decreases the maximum alveolar concentration (MAC) of desflurane). Products include:

Buprenex Injectable 2006

Chlordiazepoxide (Decreases the maximum alveolar concentration (MAC) of desflurane). Products include:

Libritabs Tablets 2177
Limbitrol 2180

Chlordiazepoxide Hydrochloride (Decreases the maximum alveolar concentration (MAC) of desflurane). Products include:

Librax Capsules 2176
Librium Capsules.................................. 2178
Librium Injectable 2179

Chlorpromazine (Decreases the doses of neuromuscular blocking agents required; potential for delayed onset of conditions suitable for muscle relaxation). Products include:

Thorazine Suppositories....................... 2523

Chlorpromazine Hydrochloride (Decreases the doses of neuromuscular blocking agents required; potential for delayed onset of conditions suitable for muscle relaxation). Products include:

. Thorazine 2523

Chlorprothixene (Decreases the doses of neuromuscular blocking agents required; potential for delayed onset of conditions suitable for muscle relaxation).

No products indexed under this heading.

Chlorprothixene Hydrochloride (Decreases the doses of neuromuscular blocking agents required; potential for delayed onset of conditions suitable for muscle relaxation).

No products indexed under this heading.

Clorazepate Dipotassium (Decreases the maximum alveolar concentration (MAC) of desflurane). Products include:

Tranxene 451

Clozapine (Decreases the doses of neuromuscular blocking agents required; potential for delayed onset of conditions suitable for muscle relaxation). Products include:

Clozaril Tablets...................................... 2252

Codeine Phosphate (Decreases the maximum alveolar concentration (MAC) of desflurane). Products include:

Actifed with Codeine Cough Syrup.. 1067
Brontex 1981
Deconsal C Expectorant Syrup 456
Deconsal Pediatric Syrup 457
Dimetane-DC Cough Syrup 2059
Empirin with Codeine Tablets............ 1093
Fioricet with Codeine Capsules 2260
Fiorinal with Codeine Capsules 2262
Isoclor Expectorant 990

Novahistine DH..................................... 2462
Novahistine Expectorant..................... 2463
Nucofed 2051
Phenergan with Codeine 2777
Phenergan VC with Codeine 2781
Robitussin A-C Syrup........................... 2073
Robitussin-DAC Syrup 2074
Ryna ....ᵃᵈ 841
Soma Compound w/Codeine Tablets 2676
Tussi-Organidin NR Liquid and S NR Liquid 2677
Tylenol with Codeine 1583

Dezocine (Decreases the maximum alveolar concentration (MAC) of desflurane). Products include:

Dalgan Injection 538

Diazepam (Decreases the maximum alveolar concentration (MAC) of desflurane). Products include:

Dizac 1809
Valium Injectable 2182
Valium Tablets 2183
Valrelease Capsules 2169

Estazolam (Decreases the maximum alveolar concentration (MAC) of desflurane). Products include:

ProSom Tablets 449

Fentanyl (Decreases the maximum alveolar concentration (MAC) of desflurane). Products include:

Duragesic Transdermal System........ 1288

Fentanyl Citrate (Decreases the maximum alveolar concentration (MAC) of desflurane). Products include:

Sublimaze Injection............................... 1307

Fluphenazine Decanoate (Decreases the doses of neuromuscular blocking agents required; potential for delayed onset of conditions suitable for muscle relaxation). Products include:

Prolixin Decanoate 509

Fluphenazine Enanthate (Decreases the doses of neuromuscular blocking agents required; potential for delayed onset of conditions suitable for muscle relaxation). Products include:

Prolixin Enanthate 509

Fluphenazine Hydrochloride (Decreases the doses of neuromuscular blocking agents required; potential for delayed onset of conditions suitable for muscle relaxation). Products include:

Prolixin 509

Flurazepam Hydrochloride (Decreases the maximum alveolar concentration (MAC) of desflurane). Products include:

Dalmane Capsules 2173

Halazepam (Decreases the maximum alveolar concentration (MAC) of desflurane).

No products indexed under this heading.

Haloperidol (Decreases the doses of neuromuscular blocking agents required; potential for delayed onset of conditions suitable for muscle relaxation). Products include:

Haldol Injection, Tablets and Concentrate 1575

Haloperidol Decanoate (Decreases the doses of neuromuscular blocking agents required; potential for delayed onset of conditions suitable for muscle relaxation). Products include:

Haldol Decanoate.................................. 1577

Hydrocodone Bitartrate (Decreases the maximum alveolar concentration (MAC) of desflurane). Products include:

Anexsia 5/500 Elixir 1781
Anexia Tablets....................................... 1782
Codiclear DH Syrup 791

IMPORTANT NOTE: Always consult each drug listing in the patient's regimen for possible interactions.

Deconamine CX Cough and Cold Liquid and Tablets 1319
Duratuss HD Elixir 2565
Hycodan Tablets and Syrup 930
Hycomine Compound Tablets 932
Hycomine 931
Hycotuss Expectorant Syrup 933
Hydrocet Capsules 782
Lorcet 10/650 1018
Lortab 2566
Tussend 1783
Tussend Expectorant 1785
Vicodin Tablets 1356
Vicodin ES Tablets 1357
Vicodin Tuss Expectorant 1358
Zydone Capsules 949

Hydrocodone Polistirex (Decreases the maximum alveolar concentration (MAC) of desflurane). Products include:
Tussionex Pennkinetic Extended-Release Suspension 998

Levorphanol Tartrate (Decreases the maximum alveolar concentration (MAC) of desflurane). Products include:
Levo-Dromoran 2129

Lithium Carbonate (Decreases the doses of neuromuscular blocking agents required; potential for delayed onset of conditions suitable for muscle relaxation). Products include:
Eskalith 2485
Lithium Carbonate Capsules & Tablets 2230
Lithonate/Lithotabs/Lithobid 2543

Lithium Citrate (Decreases the doses of neuromuscular blocking agents required; potential for delayed onset of conditions suitable for muscle relaxation).
No products indexed under this heading.

Lorazepam (Decreases the maximum alveolar concentration (MAC) of desflurane). Products include:
Ativan Injection 2698
Ativan Tablets 2700

Loxapine Hydrochloride (Decreases the doses of neuromuscular blocking agents required; potential for delayed onset of conditions suitable for muscle relaxation). Products include:
Loxitane 1378

Loxapine Succinate (Decreases the doses of neuromuscular blocking agents required; potential for delayed onset of conditions suitable for muscle relaxation). Products include:
Loxitane Capsules 1378

Meperidine Hydrochloride (Decreases the maximum alveolar concentration (MAC) of desflurane). Products include:
Demerol 2308
Mepergan Injection 2753

Methadone Hydrochloride (Decreases the maximum alveolar concentration (MAC) of desflurane). Products include:
Methadone Hydrochloride Oral Concentrate 2233
Methadone Hydrochloride Oral Solution & Tablets 2235

Midazolam Hydrochloride (Decreases the maximum alveolar concentration (MAC) of desflurane). Products include:
Versed Injection 2170

Molindone Hydrochloride (Decreases the doses of neuromuscular blocking agents required; potential for delayed onset of conditions suitable for muscle relaxation). Products include:
Moban Tablets and Concentrate 1048

Morphine Sulfate (Decreases the maximum alveolar concentration (MAC) of desflurane). Products include:
Astramorph/PF Injection, USP (Preservative-Free) 535
Duramorph 962
Infumorph 200 and Infumorph 500 Sterile Solutions 965
MS Contin Tablets 1994
MSIR 1997
Oramorph SR (Morphine Sulfate Sustained Release Tablets) 2236
RMS Suppositories 2657
Roxanol 2243

Opium Alkaloids (Decreases the maximum alveolar concentration (MAC) of desflurane).
No products indexed under this heading.

Oxazepam (Decreases the maximum alveolar concentration (MAC) of desflurane). Products include:
Serax Capsules 2810
Serax Tablets 2810

Oxycodone Hydrochloride (Decreases the maximum alveolar concentration (MAC) of desflurane). Products include:
Percocet Tablets 938
Percodan Tablets 939
Percodan-Demi Tablets 940
Roxicodone Tablets, Oral Solution & Intensol (Oxycodone) 2244
Tylox Capsules 1584

Perphenazine (Decreases the doses of neuromuscular blocking agents required; potential for delayed onset of conditions suitable for muscle relaxation). Products include:
Etrafon 2355
Triavil Tablets 1757
Trilafon 2389

Pimozide (Decreases the doses of neuromuscular blocking agents required; potential for delayed onset of conditions suitable for muscle relaxation). Products include:
Orap Tablets 1050

Prazepam (Decreases the maximum alveolar concentration (MAC) of desflurane).
No products indexed under this heading.

Prochlorperazine (Decreases the doses of neuromuscular blocking agents required; potential for delayed onset of conditions suitable for muscle relaxation). Products include:
Compazine 2470

Promethazine Hydrochloride (Decreases the doses of neuromuscular blocking agents required; potential for delayed onset of conditions suitable for muscle relaxation). Products include:
Mepergan Injection 2753
Phenergan with Codeine 2777
Phenergan with Dextromethorphan 2778
Phenergan Injection 2773
Phenergan Suppositories 2775
Phenergan Syrup 2774
Phenergan Tablets 2775
Phenergan VC 2779
Phenergan VC with Codeine 2781

Propoxyphene Hydrochloride (Decreases the maximum alveolar concentration (MAC) of desflurane). Products include:
Darvon 1435
Wygesic Tablets 2827

Propoxyphene Napsylate (Decreases the maximum alveolar concentration (MAC) of desflurane). Products include:
Darvon-N/Darvocet-N 1433

Quazepam (Decreases the maximum alveolar concentration (MAC) of desflurane). Products include:
Doral Tablets 2664

Risperidone (Decreases the doses of neuromuscular blocking agents required; potential for delayed onset of conditions suitable for muscle relaxation). Products include:
Risperdal 1301

Sufentanil Citrate (Decreases the maximum alveolar concentration (MAC) of desflurane). Products include:
Sufenta Injection 1309

Temazepam (Decreases the maximum alveolar concentration (MAC) of desflurane). Products include:
Restoril Capsules 2284

Thioridazine Hydrochloride (Decreases the doses of neuromuscular blocking agents required; potential for delayed onset of conditions suitable for muscle relaxation). Products include:
Mellaril 2269

Thiothixene (Decreases the doses of neuromuscular blocking agents required; potential for delayed onset of conditions suitable for muscle relaxation). Products include:
Navane Capsules and Concentrate 2201
Navane Intramuscular 2202

Triazolam (Decreases the maximum alveolar concentration (MAC) of desflurane). Products include:
Halcion Tablets 2611

Trifluoperazine Hydrochloride (Decreases the doses of neuromuscular blocking agents required; potential for delayed onset of conditions suitable for muscle relaxation). Products include:
Stelazine 2514

SUPRAX FOR ORAL SUSPENSION
(Cefixime) 1399
None cited in PDR database.

SUPRAX TABLETS
(Cefixime) 1399

Food Interactions

Food, unspecified (Increases time to maximal absorption approximately 0.8 hour).

SURFAK LIQUI-GELS
(Docusate Calcium) .... ▣ 839
None cited in PDR database.

SURGICEL* ABSORBABLE HEMOSTAT
(Oxidized Regenerated Cellulose) 1314
May interact with escharotic chemicals. Compounds in this category include:

Silver Nitrate (Absorption of Surgicel could be prevented in chemically cauterized areas; its use should not be preceded by application of escharotic chemicals).
No products indexed under this heading.

SURGICEL* NU-KNIT ABSORBABLE HEMOSTAT
(Oxidized Regenerated Cellulose) 1314
See **SURGICEL* Absorbable Hemostat**

SURMONTIL CAPSULES
(Trimipramine Maleate) 2811
May interact with anticholinergics, sympathomimetics, monoamine oxidase inhibitors, thyroid preparations, antidepressant drugs, phenothiazines, selective serotonin reuptake inhibitors, drugs that inhibit cytochrome p450iid6, and certain other agents. Compounds in these categories include:

Albuterol (Potentiated effects of catecholamines; careful adjustment of dosage and close supervision are required). Products include:
Proventil Inhalation Aerosol 2382
Ventolin Inhalation Aerosol and Refill 1197

Albuterol Sulfate (Potentiated effects of catecholamines; careful adjustment of dosage and close supervision are required). Products include:
Airet Solution for Inhalation 452
Proventil Inhalation Solution 0.083% 2384
Proventil Repetabs Tablets 2386
Proventil Solution for Inhalation 0.5% 2383
Proventil Syrup 2385
Proventil Tablets 2386
Ventolin Inhalation Solution 1198
Ventolin Nebules Inhalation Solution 1199
Ventolin Rotacaps for Inhalation 1200
Ventolin Syrup 1202
Ventolin Tablets 1203
Volmax Extended-Release Tablets .. 1788

Amitriptyline Hydrochloride (Concurrent use with drugs that are substrate for cytochrome $P_{450}IID_6$ may make normal metabolizer resemble poor metabolizer leading to higher than expected plasma concentrations of TCA with resultant toxicity). Products include:
Elavil 2838
Endep Tablets 2174
Etrafon 2355
Limbitrol 2180
Triavil Tablets 1757

Amoxapine (Concurrent use with drugs that are substrate for cytochrome $P_{450}IID_6$ may make normal metabolizer resemble poor metabolizer leading to higher than expected plasma concentrations of TCA with resultant toxicity). Products include:
Asendin Tablets 1369

Atropine Sulfate (Concurrent use may result in pronounced atropine-like effects). Products include:
Arco-Lase Plus Tablets 512
Atrohist Plus Tablets 454
Atropine Sulfate Sterile Ophthalmic Solution .... ⊙ 233
Donnatal 2060
Donnatal Extentabs 2061
Donnatal Tablets 2060
Lomotil 2439
Motofen Tablets 784
Urised Tablets 1964

Belladonna Alkaloids (Concurrent use may result in pronounced atropinelike effects). Products include:
Bellergal-S Tablets 2250
Hyland's Bed Wetting Tablets .... ▣ 828
Hyland's EnurAid Tablets .... ▣ 829
Hyland's Teething Tablets .... ▣ 830

Benztropine Mesylate (Concurrent use may result in pronounced atropinelike effects). Products include:
Cogentin 1621

Biperiden Hydrochloride (Concurrent use may result in pronounced atropinelike effects). Products include:
Akineton 1333

Bupropion Hydrochloride (Concurrent use with drugs that are substrate for cytochrome $P_{450}IID_6$ may make normal metabolizer resemble poor metabolizer leading to higher than expected plasma concentrations of TCA with resultant toxicity). Products include:
Wellbutrin Tablets 1204

(▣ Described in PDR For Nonprescription Drugs) (⊙ Described in PDR For Ophthalmology)

Interactions Index — Surmontil

Chlorpromazine (Concurrent use with drugs that are substrate for cytochrome $P_{450}IID_6$ may make normal metabolizer resemble poor metabolizer leading to higher than expected plasma concentrations of TCA with resultant toxicity). Products include:

Thorazine Suppositories 2523

Chlorpromazine Hydrochloride (Concurrent use with drugs that are substrate for cytochrome $P_{450}IID_6$ may make normal metabolizer resemble poor metabolizer leading to higher than expected plasma concentrations of TCA with resultant toxicity). Products include:

Thorazine 2523

Cimetidine (Inhibits the elimination of tricyclic antidepressants; downward adjustment of Surmontil dosage may be required if cimetine therapy is initiated; upward adjustment if cimetidine therapy is discontinued). Products include:

Tagamet Tablets 2516

Cimetidine Hydrochloride (Inhibits the elimination of tricyclic antidepressants; downward adjustment of Surmontil dosage may be required if cimetidine therapy is initiated; upward adjustment if cimetidine therapy is discontinued). Products include:

Tagamet.. 2516

Clidinium Bromide (Concurrent use may result in pronounced atropinelike effects). Products include:

Librax Capsules 2176
Quarzan Capsules 2181

Desipramine Hydrochloride (Concurrent use with drugs that are substrate for cytochrome $P_{450}IID_6$ may make normal metabolizer resemble poor metabolizer leading to higher than expected plasma concentrations of TCA with resultant toxicity). Products include:

Norpramin Tablets 1526

Dicyclomine Hydrochloride (Concurrent use may result in pronounced atropinelike effects). Products include:

Bentyl 1501

Dobutamine Hydrochloride (Potentiated effects of catecholamines; careful adjustment of dosage and close supervision are required). Products include:

Dobutrex Solution Vials.......................... 1439

Dopamine Hydrochloride (Potentiated effects of catecholamines; careful adjustment of dosage and close supervision are required).

No products indexed under this heading.

Doxepin Hydrochloride (Concurrent use with drugs that are substrate for cytochrome $P_{450}IID_6$ may make normal metabolizer resemble poor metabolizer leading to higher than expected plasma concentrations of TCA with resultant toxicity). Products include:

Sinequan 2205
Zonalon Cream 1055

Ephedrine Hydrochloride (Potentiated effects of catecholamines; careful adjustment of dosage and close supervision are required). Products include:

Primatene Dual Action Formula...... ⊕ 872
Primatene Tablets .... ⊕ 873
Quadrinal Tablets 1350

Ephedrine Sulfate (Potentiated effects of catecholamines; careful adjustment of dosage and close supervision are required). Products include:

Bronkaid Caplets .... ⊕ 717
Marax Tablets & DF Syrup.................... 2200

Ephedrine Tannate (Potentiated effects of catecholamines; careful adjustment of dosage and close supervision are required). Products include:

Rynatuss 2673

Epinephrine (Potentiated effects of catecholamines; careful adjustment of dosage and close supervision are required). Products include:

Bronkaid Mist .... ⊕ 717
EPIFRIN .... © 239
EpiPen 790
Marcaine Hydrochloride with Epinephrine 1:200,000 2316
Primatene Mist .... ⊕ 873
Sensorcaine with Epinephrine Injection.. 559
Sus-Phrine Injection 1019
Xylocaine with Epinephrine Injections.. 567

Epinephrine Bitartrate (Potentiated effects of catecholamines; careful adjustment of dosage and close supervision are required). Products include:

Bronkaid Mist Suspension .... ⊕ 718
Sensorcaine-MPF with Epinephrine Injection 559

Epinephrine Hydrochloride (Potentiated effects of catecholamines; careful adjustment of dosage and close supervision are required). Products include:

Ana-Kit Anaphylaxis Emergency Treatment Kit 617

Flecainide Acetate (Concurrent use with drugs that are substrate for cytochrome $P_{450}IID_6$ may make normal metabolizer resemble poor metabolizer leading to higher than expected plasma concentrations of TCA with resultant toxicity). Products include:

Tambocor Tablets 1497

Fluoxetine Hydrochloride (Concurrent use with drugs that are substrate for cytochrome $P_{450}IID_6$ may make normal metabolizer resemble poor metabolizer leading to higher than expected plasma concentrations of TCA with resultant toxicity; due to variation in the extent of inhibition of P450 IID_6 and long half-life of the parent (fluoxetine) and active metabolite sufficient time should/ must elapse, at least 5 weeks before switching to TCA). Products include:

Prozac Pulvules & Liquid, Oral Solution 919

Fluphenazine Decanoate (Concurrent use with drugs that are substrate for cytochrome $P_{450}IID_6$ may make normal metabolizer resemble poor metabolizer leading to higher than expected plasma concentrations of TCA with resultant toxicity). Products include:

Prolixin Decanoate 509

Fluphenazine Enanthate (Concurrent use with drugs that are substrate for cytochrome $P_{450}IID_6$ may make normal metabolizer resemble poor metabolizer leading to higher than expected plasma concentrations of TCA with resultant toxicity). Products include:

Prolixin Enanthate 509

Fluphenazine Hydrochloride (Concurrent use with drugs that are substrate for cytochrome $P_{450}IID_6$ may make normal metabolizer resemble poor metabolizer leading to higher than expected plasma concentrations of TCA with resultant toxicity). Products include:

Prolixin 509

Fluvoxamine Maleate (Due to variation in the extent of inhibition of $P_{450}IID_6$ caution is indicated if coadministered sufficient time should/ must elapse). Products include:

Luvox Tablets 2544

Furazolidone (Potential for hyperpyretic crises, severe convulsions, and deaths; concurrent and/or sequential use is contraindicated). Products include:

Furoxone 2046

Glycopyrrolate (Concurrent use may result in pronounced atropinelike effects). Products include:

Robinul Forte Tablets.............................. 2072
Robinul Injectable 2072
Robinul Tablets....................................... 2072

Guanadrel Sulfate (Trimipramine may block the antihypertensive effect). Products include:

Hylorel Tablets 985

Guanethidine Monosulfate (Trimipramine may block the antihypertensive effect of guanethidine or similarly acting compounds). Products include:

Esimil Tablets 822
Ismelin Tablets 827

Hyoscyamine (Concurrent use may result in pronounced atropinelike effects). Products include:

Cystospaz Tablets 1963
Urised Tablets... 1964

Hyoscyamine Sulfate (Concurrent use may result in pronounced atropinelike effects). Products include:

Arco-Lase Plus Tablets 512
Atrohist Plus Tablets 454
Cystospaz-M Capsules 1963
Donnatal 2060
Donnatal Extentabs................................ 2061
Donnatal Tablets 2060
Kutrase Capsules.................................... 2402
Levsin/Levsinex/Levbid 2405

Imipramine Hydrochloride (Concurrent use with drugs that are substrate for cytochrome $P_{450}IID_6$ may make normal metabolizer resemble poor metabolizer leading to higher than expected plasma concentrations of TCA with resultant toxicity). Products include:

Tofranil Ampuls 854
Tofranil Tablets 856

Imipramine Pamoate (Concurrent use with drugs that are substrate for cytochrome $P_{450}IID_6$ may make normal metabolizer resemble poor metabolizer leading to higher than expected plasma concentrations of TCA with resultant toxicity). Products include:

Tofranil-PM Capsules............................. 857

Ipratropium Bromide (Concurrent use may result in pronounced atropinelike effects). Products include:

Atrovent Inhalation Aerosol.................. 671
Atrovent Inhalation Solution 673

Isocarboxazid (Potential for hyperpyretic crises, severe convulsions, and deaths; concurrent and/or sequential use is contraindicated).

No products indexed under this heading.

Isoproterenol Hydrochloride (Potentiated effects of catecholamines; careful adjustment of dosage and close supervision are required). Products include:

Isuprel Hydrochloride Injection 1:5000 2311
Isuprel Hydrochloride Solution 1:200 & 1:100 2313
Isuprel Mistometer 2312

Isoproterenol Sulfate (Potentiated effects of catecholamines; careful adjustment of dosage and close supervision are required). Products include:

Norisodrine with Calcium Iodide Syrup... 442

Levothyroxine Sodium (Potential for cardiovascular toxicity). Products include:

Levothroid Tablets 1016
Levoxyl Tablets....................................... 903
Synthroid... 1359

Liothyronine Sodium (Potential for cardiovascular toxicity). Products include:

Cytomel Tablets 2473
Triostat Injection 2530

Liotrix (Potential for cardiovascular toxicity).

No products indexed under this heading.

Maprotiline Hydrochloride (Concurrent use with drugs that are substrate for cytochrome $P_{450}IID_6$ may make normal metabolizer resemble poor metabolizer leading to higher than expected plasma concentrations of TCA with resultant toxicity). Products include:

Ludiomil Tablets..................................... 843

Mepenzolate Bromide (Concurrent use may result in pronounced atropinelike effects).

No products indexed under this heading.

Mesoridazine Besylate (Concurrent use with drugs that are substrate for cytochrome $P_{450}IID_6$ may make normal metabolizer resemble poor metabolizer leading to higher than expected plasma concentrations of TCA with resultant toxicity). Products include:

Serentil.. 684

Metaproterenol Sulfate (Potentiated effects of catecholamines; careful adjustment of dosage and close supervision are required). Products include:

Alupent.. 669
Metaproterenol Sulfate Inhalation Solution, USP, Arm-a-Med 552

Metaraminol Bitartrate (Potentiated effects of catecholamines; careful adjustment of dosage and close supervision are required). Products include:

Aramine Injection................................... 1609

Methotrimeprazine (Concurrent use with drugs that are substrate for cytochrome $P_{450}IID_6$ may make normal metabolizer resemble poor metabolizer leading to higher than expected plasma concentrations of TCA with resultant toxicity). Products include:

Levoprome 1274

Methoxamine Hydrochloride (Potentiated effects of catecholamines; careful adjustment of dosage and close supervision are required). Products include:

Vasoxyl Injection 1196

IMPORTANT NOTE: Always consult each drug listing in the patient's regimen for possible interactions.

Surmontil **Interactions Index** **990**

Nefazodone Hydrochloride (Concurrent use with drugs that are substrate for cytochrome $P_{450}IID_6$ may make normal metabolizer leading to higher than expected plasma concentrations of TCA with resultant toxicity). Products include:
- Serzone Tablets ... 771

Norepinephrine Bitartrate (Potentiated effects of catecholamines; careful adjustment of dosage and close supervision are required). Products include:
- Levophed Bitartrate Injection ... 2315

Nortriptyline Hydrochloride (Concurrent use with drugs that are substrate for cytochrome $P_{450}IID_6$ may make normal metabolizer resemble poor metabolizer leading to higher than expected plasma concentrations of TCA with resultant toxicity). Products include:
- Pamelor ... 2280

Oxybutynin Chloride (Concurrent use may result in pronounced atropinelike effects). Products include:
- Ditropan ... 1516

Paroxetine Hydrochloride (Concurrent use with drugs that are substrate for cytochrome $P_{450}IID_6$ may make normal metabolizer resemble poor metabolizer leading to higher than expected plasma concentrations of TCA with resultant toxicity; due to variation in the extent of inhibition of $P_{450}IID_6$ caution is indicated; if co-administered sufficient time should/must elapse). Products include:
- Paxil Tablets ... 2505

Perphenazine (Concurrent use with drugs that are substrate for cytochrome $P_{450}IID_6$ may make normal metabolizer resemble poor metabolizer leading to higher than expected plasma concentrations of TCA with resultant toxicity). Products include:
- Etrafon ... 2355
- Triavil Tablets ... 1757
- Trilafon ... 2389

Phenelzine Sulfate (Potential for hyperpyretic crises, severe convulsions, and deaths; concurrent and/or sequential use is contraindicated). Products include:
- Nardil ... 1920

Phenylephrine Bitartrate (Potentiated effects of catecholamines; careful adjustment of dosage and close supervision are required).
- No products indexed under this heading.

Phenylephrine Hydrochloride (Potentiated effects of catecholamines; careful adjustment of dosage and close supervision are required). Products include:
- Atrohist Plus Tablets ... 454
- Cerose DM ... ■ 878
- Comhist ... 2038
- D.A. Chewable Tablets ... 951
- Deconsal Pediatric Capsules ... 454
- Dura-Vent/DA Tablets ... 953
- Entex Capsules ... 1986
- Entex Liquid ... 1986
- Extendryl ... 1005
- 4-Way Fast Acting Nasal Spray (regular & mentholated) ... ■ 621
- Hemorid For Women ... ■ 834
- Hycomine Compound Tablets ... 932
- Neo-Synephrine Hydrochloride 1% Carpuject ... 2324
- Neo-Synephrine Hydrochloride 1% Injection ... 2324
- Neo-Synephrine Hydrochloride (Ophthalmic) ... 2325
- Neo-Synephrine ... ■ 726
- Nōstril ... ■ 644
- Novahistine Elixir ... ■ 823
- Phenergan VC ... 2779
- Phenergan VC with Codeine ... 2781
- Preparation H ... ■ 871
- Tympagesic Ear Drops ... 2342
- Vasosulf ... ⊙ 271
- Vicks Sinex Nasal Spray and Ultra Fine Mist ... ■ 765

Phenylephrine Tannate (Potentiated effects of catecholamines; careful adjustment of dosage and close supervision are required). Products include:
- Atrohist Pediatric Suspension ... 454
- Ricobid-D Pediatric Suspension ... 2038
- Ricobid Tablets and Pediatric Suspension ... 2038
- Rynatan ... 2673
- Rynatuss ... 2673

Phenylpropanolamine Hydrochloride (Potentiated effects of catecholamines; careful adjustment of dosage and close supervision are required). Products include:
- Acutrim ... ■ 628
- Allerest Children's Chewable Tablets ... ■ 627
- Allerest 12 Hour Caplets ... ■ 627
- Atrohist Plus Tablets ... 454
- BC Cold Powder Multi-Symptom Formula (Cold-Sinus-Allergy) ... ■ 609
- BC Cold Powder Non-Drowsy Formula (Cold-Sinus) ... ■ 609
- Cheracol Plus Head Cold/Cough Formula ... ■ 769
- Comtrex Multi-Symptom Non-Drowsy Liqui-gels ... ■ 618
- Contac Continuous Action Nasal Decongestant/Antihistamine 12 Hour Capsules ... ■ 813
- Contac Maximum Strength Continuous Action Decongestant/Antihistamine 12 Hour Caplets ... ■ 813
- Contac Severe Cold and Flu Formula Caplets ... ■ 814
- Coricidin 'D' Decongestant Tablets ... ■ 800
- Dexatrim ... ■ 832
- Dexatrim Plus Vitamins Caplets ... ■ 832
- Dimetane-DC Cough Syrup ... 2059
- Dimetapp Elixir ... ■ 773
- Dimetapp Extentabs ... ■ 774
- Dimetapp Tablets/Liqui-Gels ... ■ 775
- Dimetapp Cold & Allergy Chewable Tablets ... ■ 773
- Dimetapp DM Elixir ... ■ 774
- Dura-Vent Tablets ... 952
- Entex Capsules ... 1986
- Entex LA Tablets ... 1987
- Entex Liquid ... 1986
- Exgest LA Tablets ... 782
- Hycomine ... 931
- Isoclor Timesule Capsules ... ■ 637
- Nolamine Timed-Release Tablets ... 785
- Ornade Spansule Capsules ... 2502
- Propagest Tablets ... 786
- Pyrroxate Caplets ... ■ 772
- Robitussin-CF ... ■ 777
- Sinulin Tablets ... 787
- Tavist-D 12 Hour Relief Tablets ... ■ 787
- Teldrin 12 Hour Antihistamine/Nasal Decongestant Allergy Relief Capsules ... ■ 826
- Triaminic Allergy Tablets ... ■ 789
- Triaminic Cold Tablets ... ■ 790
- Triaminic Expectorant ... ■ 790
- Triaminic Syrup ... ■ 792
- Triaminic-12 Tablets ... ■ 792
- Triaminic-DM Syrup ... ■ 792
- Triaminicin Tablets ... ■ 793
- Triaminicol Multi-Symptom Cold Tablets ... ■ 793
- Triaminicol Multi-Symptom Relief ... ■ 794
- Vicks DayQuil Allergy Relief 12-Hour Extended Release Tablets ... ■ 760
- Vicks DayQuil Allergy Relief 4-Hour Tablets ... ■ 760
- Vicks DayQuil SINUS Pressure & CONGESTION Relief ... ■ 761

Pirbuterol Acetate (Potentiated effects of catecholamines; careful adjustment of dosage and close supervision are required). Products include:
- Maxair Autohaler ... 1492
- Maxair Inhaler ... 1494

Prochlorperazine (Concurrent use with drugs that are substrate for cytochrome $P_{450}IID_6$ may make normal metabolizer resemble poor metabolizer leading to higher than expected plasma concentrations of TCA with resultant toxicity). Products include:
- Compazine ... 2470

Procyclidine Hydrochloride (Concurrent use may result in pronounced atropinelike effects). Products include:
- Kemadrin Tablets ... 1112

Promethazine Hydrochloride (Concurrent use with drugs that are substrate for cytochrome $P_{450}IID_6$ may make normal metabolizer resemble poor metabolizer leading to higher than expected plasma concentrations of TCA with resultant toxicity). Products include:
- Mepergan Injection ... 2753
- Phenergan with Codeine ... 2777
- Phenergan with Dextromethorphan ... 2778
- Phenergan Injection ... 2773
- Phenergan Suppositories ... 2775
- Phenergan Syrup ... 2774
- Phenergan Tablets ... 2775
- Phenergan VC ... 2779
- Phenergan VC with Codeine ... 2781

Propafenone Hydrochloride (Concurrent use with drugs that are substrate for cytochrome $P_{450}IID_6$ may make normal metabolizer resemble poor metabolizer leading to higher than expected plasma concentrations of TCA with resultant toxicity). Products include:
- Rythmol Tablets–150mg, 225mg, 300mg ... 1352

Propantheline Bromide (Concurrent use may result in pronounced atropinelike effects). Products include:
- Pro-Banthine Tablets ... 2052

Protriptyline Hydrochloride (Concurrent use with drugs that are substrate for cytochrome $P_{450}IID_6$ may make normal metabolizer resemble poor metabolizer leading to higher than expected plasma concentrations of TCA with resultant toxicity). Products include:
- Vivactil Tablets ... 1774

Pseudoephedrine Hydrochloride (Potentiated effects of catecholamines; careful adjustment of dosage and close supervision are required). Products include:
- Actifed Allergy Daytime/Nighttime Caplets ... ■ 844
- Actifed Plus Caplets ... ■ 845
- Actifed Plus Tablets ... ■ 845
- Actifed with Codeine Cough Syrup ... 1067
- Actifed Sinus Daytime/Nighttime Tablets and Caplets ... ■ 846
- Actifed Syrup ... ■ 846
- Actifed Tablets ... ■ 844
- Advil Cold and Sinus Caplets and Tablets (formerly CoAdvil) ... ■ 870
- Alka-Seltzer Plus Cold Medicine Liqui-Gels ... ■ 706
- Alka-Seltzer Plus Cold & Cough Medicine Liqui-Gels ... ■ 705
- Alka-Seltzer Plus Night-Time Cold Medicine Liqui-Gels ... ■ 706
- Allerest Headache Strength Tablets ... ■ 627
- Allerest Maximum Strength Tablets ... ■ 627
- Allerest No Drowsiness Tablets ... ■ 627
- Allerest Sinus Pain Formula ... ■ 627
- Anatuss LA Tablets ... 1542
- Atrohist Pediatric Capsules ... 453
- Bayer Select Sinus Pain Relief Formula ... ■ 717
- Benadryl Allergy Decongestant Liquid Medication ... ■ 848
- Benadryl Allergy Decongestant Tablets ... ■ 848
- Benadryl Allergy Sinus Headache Formula Caplets ... ■ 849
- Benylin Multisymptom ... ■ 852
- Bromfed Capsules (Extended-Release) ... 1785
- Bromfed Syrup ... ■ 733
- Bromfed Tablets ... 1785
- Bromfed-DM Cough Syrup ... 1786
- Bromfed-PD Capsules (Extended-Release) ... 1785
- Children's Vicks DayQuil Allergy Relief ... ■ 757
- Children's Vicks NyQuil Cold/Cough Relief ... ■ 758
- Comtrex Multi-Symptom Cold Reliever Tablets/Caplets/Liqui-Gels/Liquid ... ■ 615
- Allergy-Sinus Comtrex Multi-Symptom Allergy-Sinus Formula Tablets ... ■ 617
- Comtrex Multi-Symptom Non-Drowsy Caplets ... ■ 618
- Congess ... 1004
- Contac Day Allergy/Sinus Caplets ■ 812
- Contac Day & Night ... ■ 812
- Contac Night Allergy/Sinus Caplets ... ■ 812
- Contac Severe Cold & Flu Non-Drowsy ... ■ 815
- Deconamine Chewable Tablets ... 1320
- Deconamine CX Cough and Cold Liquid and Tablets ... 1319
- Deconamine ... 1320
- Deconsal C Expectorant Syrup ... 456
- Deconsal Pediatric Syrup ... 457
- Deconsal II Tablets ... 454
- Dimetane-DX Cough Syrup ... 2059
- Dimetapp Sinus Caplets ... ■ 775
- Dorcol Children's Cough Syrup ... ■ 785
- Drixoral Cough + Congestion Liquid Caps ... ■ 802
- Dura-Tap/PD Capsules ... 2867
- Duratuss Tablets ... 2565
- Duratuss HD Elixir ... 2565
- Efidac/24 ... ■ 635
- Entex PSE Tablets ... 1987
- Fedahist Gyrocaps ... 2401
- Fedahist Timecaps ... 2401
- Guaifed ... 1787
- Guaifed Syrup ... ■ 734
- Guaimax-D Tablets ... 792
- Guaitab Tablets ... ■ 734
- Isoclor Expectorant ... 990
- Kronofed-A ... 977
- Motrin IB Sinus ... ■ 838
- Novahistine DH ... 2462
- Novahistine DMX ... ■ 822
- Novahistine Expectorant ... 2463
- Nucofed ... 2051
- PediaCare Cold Allergy Chewable Tablets ... ■ 677
- PediaCare Cough-Cold Chewable Tablets ... 1553
- PediaCare ... 1553
- PediaCare Infants' Decongestant Drops ... ■ 677
- PediCare Infant's Drops Decongestant Plus Cough ... 1553
- PediaCare NightRest Cough-Cold Liquid ... 1553
- Pediatric Vicks 44d Dry Hacking Cough & Head Congestion ... ■ 763
- Pediatric Vicks 44m Cough & Cold Relief ... ■ 764
- Robitussin Cold & Cough Liqui-Gels ... ■ 776
- Robitussin Maximum Strength Cough & Cold ... ■ 778
- Robitussin Pediatric Cough & Cold Formula ... ■ 779
- Robitussin Severe Congestion Liqui-Gels ... ■ 776
- Robitussin-DAC Syrup ... 2074
- Robitussin-PE ... ■ 778
- Rondec Oral Drops ... 953
- Rondec Syrup ... 953
- Rondec Tablet ... 953
- Rondec-DM Oral Drops ... 954
- Rondec-DM Syrup ... 954
- Rondec-TR Tablet ... 953
- Ryna ... ■ 841
- Seldane-D Extended-Release Tablets ... 1538
- Semprex-D Capsules ... 463
- Semprex-D Capsules ... 1167
- Sinarest Tablets ... ■ 648
- Sinarest Extra Strength Tablets ... ■ 648
- Sinarest No Drowsiness Tablets ... ■ 648
- Sine-Aid IB Caplets ... 1554
- Sine-Aid Maximum Strength Sinus Medication Gelcaps, Caplets and Tablets ... 1554
- Sine-Off No Drowsiness Formula Caplets ... ■ 824

(■ Described in PDR For Nonprescription Drugs) (⊙ Described in PDR For Ophthalmology)

Interactions Index Sus-Phrine

Sine-Off Sinus Medicine .... ⊕ 825
Singlet Tablets .... ⊕ 825
Sinutab Non-Drying Liquid Caps .... ⊕ 859
Sinutab Sinus Allergy Medication, Maximum Strength Tablets and Caplets .... ⊕ 860
Sinutab Sinus Medication, Maximum Strength Without Drowsiness Formula, Tablets & Caplets .... ⊕ 860
Sinutab Sinus Medication, Regular Strength Without Drowsiness Formula .... ⊕ 859
Sudafed Children's Liquid .... ⊕ 861
Sudafed Cold and Cough Liquidcaps .... ⊕ 862
Sudafed Cough Syrup .... ⊕ 862
Sudafed Plus Liquid .... ⊕ 862
Sudafed Plus Tablets .... ⊕ 863
Sudafed Severe Cold Formula Caplets .... ⊕ 863
Sudafed Severe Cold Formula Tablets .... ⊕ 864
Sudafed Sinus Caplets .... ⊕ 864
Sudafed Sinus Tablets .... ⊕ 864
Sudafed Tablets, 30 mg .... ⊕ 861
Sudafed Tablets, 60 mg .... ⊕ 861
Sudafed 12 Hour Caplets .... ⊕ 861
Syn-Rx Tablets 465
Syn-Rx DM Tablets 466
TheraFlu .... ⊕ 787
TheraFlu Maximum Strength Nighttime Flu, Cold & Cough Medicine .... ⊕ 788
TheraFlu Maximum Strength Non-Drowsy Formula Flu, Cold & Cough Medicine .... ⊕ 788
Thera Flu Maximum Strength, Non-Drowsy Formula Flu, Cold and Cough Caplets .... ⊕ 789
Triaminic AM Cough and Decongestant Formula .... ⊕ 789
Triaminic AM Decongestant Formula .... ⊕ 790
Triaminic Nite Light .... ⊕ 791
Triaminic Sore Throat Formula ..... ⊕ 791
Tussend 1783
Tussend Expectorant 1785
Children's TYLENOL Cold Multi-Symptom Liquid Formula and Chewable Tablets 1561
Children's TYLENOL Cold Plus Cough Multi Symptom Tablets and Liquid .... ⊕ 681
Infants' TYLENOL Cold Decongestant & Fever-Reducer Drops 1556
TYLENOL Maximum Strength Allergy Sinus Medication Gelcaps and Caplets 1563
TYLENOL Maximum Strength Allergy Sinus NightTime Medication Caplets 1555
TYLENOL Flu Maximum Strength Gelcaps 1565
TYLENOL Flu NightTime, Maximum Strength, Gelcaps 1566
TYLENOL Maximum Strength Flu NightTime Hot Medication Packets 1562
TYLENOL, Maximum Strength, Sinus Medication Geltabs, Gelcaps, Caplets and Tablets 1566
TYLENOL Cold Multi-Symptom Formula Medication Tablets and Caplets 1561
TYLENOL Cold Medication No Drowsiness Formula Gelcaps and Caplets 1562
TYLENOL Cold Multi-Symptom Hot Medication Liquid Packets 1557
TYLENOL Cough Multi-Symptom Medication with Decongestant 1565
Ursinus Inlay-Tabs .... ⊕ 794
Vicks 44 LiquiCaps Cough, Cold & Flu Relief .... ⊕ 755
Vicks 44 LiquiCaps Non-Drowsy Cough & Cold Relief .... ⊕ 756
Vicks 44D Dry Hacking Cough & Head Congestion .... ⊕ 755
Vicks 44M Cough, Cold & Flu Relief .... ⊕ 756
Vicks DayQuil .... ⊕ 761
Vicks DayQuil SINUS Pressure & PAIN Relief with IBUPROFEN ...... ⊕ 762
Vicks Nyquil Hot Therapy .... ⊕ 762
Vicks NyQuil LiquiCaps Multi-Symptom Cold/Flu Relief .... ⊕ 763
Vicks NyQuil Multi-Symptom Cold/Flu Relief - (Original & Cherry Flavor) .... ⊕ 763

Pseudoephedrine Sulfate (Potentiated effects of catecholamines; careful adjustment of dosage and close supervision are required). Products include:

Cheracol Sinus .... ⊕ 768
Chlor-Trimeton Allergy Decongestant Tablets .... ⊕ 799
Claritin-D 2350
Drixoral Cold and Allergy Sustained-Action Tablets .... ⊕ 802
Drixoral Cold and Flu Extended-Release Tablets .... ⊕ 803
Drixoral Non-Drowsy Formula Extended-Release Tablets .... ⊕ 803
Drixoral Allergy/Sinus Extended Release Tablets .... ⊕ 804
Trinalin Repetabs Tablets 1330

Quinidine Gluconate (Concurrent use with drugs that inhibit cytochrome $P_{450}IID_6$ may make normal metabolizer resemble poor metabolizer leading to higher than expected plasma concentrations of TCA with resultant toxicity). Products include:

Quinaglute Dura-Tabs Tablets 649

Quinidine Polygalacturonate (Concurrent use with drugs that inhibit cytochrome $P_{450}IID_6$ may make normal metabolizer resemble poor metabolizer leading to higher than expected plasma concentrations of TCA with resultant toxicity).

No products indexed under this heading.

Quinidine Sulfate (Concurrent use with drugs that inhibit cytochrome $P_{450}IID_6$ may make normal metabolizer resemble poor metabolizer leading to higher than expected plasma concentrations of TCA with resultant toxicity). Products include:

Quinidex Extentabs 2067

Salmeterol Xinafoate (Potentiated effects of catecholamines; careful adjustment of dosage and close supervision are required). Products include:

Serevent Inhalation Aerosol 1176

Scopolamine (Concurrent use may result in pronounced atropinelike effects). Products include:

Transderm Scōp Transdermal Therapeutic System 869

Scopolamine Hydrobromide (Concurrent use may result in pronounced atropinelike effects). Products include:

Atrohist Plus Tablets 454
Donnatal 2060
Donnatal Extentabs 2061
Donnatal Tablets 2060

Selegiline Hydrochloride (Potential for hyperpyretic crises, severe convulsions, and deaths; concurrent and/or sequential use is contraindicated). Products include:

Eldepryl Tablets 2550

Sertraline Hydrochloride (Concurrent use with drugs that are substrate for cytochrome $P_{450}IID_6$ may make normal metabolizer resemble poor metabolizer leading to higher than expected plasma concentrations of TCA with resultant toxicity; due to variation in the extent of inhibition of $P_{450}IID_6$ caution is indicated; if co-administered sufficient time should/must elapse). Products include:

Zoloft Tablets 2217

Terbutaline Sulfate (Potentiated effects of catecholamines; careful adjustment of dosage and close supervision are required). Products include:

Brethaire Inhaler 813
Brethine Ampuls 815
Brethine Tablets 814
Bricanyl Subcutaneous Injection 1502

Bricanyl Tablets 1503

Thioridazine Hydrochloride (Concurrent use with drugs that are substrate for cytochrome $P_{450}IID_6$ may make normal metabolizer resemble poor metabolizer leading to higher than expected plasma concentrations of TCA with resultant toxicity). Products include:

Mellaril 2269

Thyroglobulin (Potential for cardio-ovascular toxicity).

No products indexed under this heading.

Thyroid (Potential for cardiovascular toxicity).

No products indexed under this heading.

Thyroxine (Potential for cardiovascular toxicity).

No products indexed under this heading.

Thyroxine Sodium (Potential for cardiovascular toxicity).

No products indexed under this heading.

Tranylcypromine Sulfate (Potential for hyperpyretic crises, severe convulsions, and deaths; concurrent and/or sequential use is contraindicated). Products include:

Parnate Tablets 2503

Trazodone Hydrochloride (Concurrent use with drugs that are substrate for cytochrome $P_{450}IID_6$ may make normal metabolizer leading to higher than expected plasma concentrations of TCA with resultant toxicity). Products include:

Desyrel and Desyrel Dividose 503

Tridihexethyl Chloride (Concurrent use may result in pronounced atropinelike effects).

No products indexed under this heading.

Trifluoperazine Hydrochloride (Concurrent use with drugs that are substrate for cytochrome $P_{450}IID_6$ may make normal metabolizer resemble poor metabolizer leading to higher than expected plasma concentrations of TCA with resultant toxicity). Products include:

Stelazine 2514

Trihexyphenidyl Hydrochloride (Concurrent use may result in pronounced atropinelike effects). Products include:

Artane 1368

Venlafaxine Hydrochloride (Concurrent use with drugs that are substrate for cytochrome $P_{450}IID_6$ may make normal metabolizer resemble poor metabolizer leading to higher than expected plasma concentrations of TCA with resultant toxicity; due to variation in the extent of inhibition of $P_{450}IID_6$ caution is indicated; if co-administered sufficient time should/must elapse). Products include:

Effexor 2719

Food Interactions

Alcohol (Concomitant use of alcoholic beverages and trimipramine may be associated with exaggerated effects).

SURVANTA BERACTANT INTRATRACHEAL SUSPENSION

(Beractant) 2226
None cited in PDR database.

SUS-PHRINE INJECTION

(Epinephrine) 1019
May interact with tricyclic antidepressants, cardiac glycosides, sympathomimetics, and certain other

agents. Compounds in these categories include:

Albuterol (Combined effects on cardiovascular system may be deleterious). Products include:

Proventil Inhalation Aerosol 2382
Ventolin Inhalation Aerosol ,and Refill 1197

Albuterol Sulfate (Combined effects on cardiovascular system may be deleterious). Products include:

Airet Solution for Inhalation 452
Proventil Inhalation Solution 0.083% 2384
Proventil Repetabs Tablets 2386
Proventil Solution for Inhalation 0.5% 2383
Proventil Syrup 2385
Proventil Tablets 2386
Ventolin Inhalation Solution 1198
Ventolin Nebules Inhalation Solution 1199
Ventolin Rotacaps for Inhalation 1200
Ventolin Syrup 1202
Ventolin Tablets 1203
Volmax Extended-Release Tablets .. 1788

Amitriptyline Hydrochloride (Epinephrine effects may be potentiated). Products include:

Elavil 2838
Endep Tablets 2174
Etrafon 2355
Limbitrol 2180
Triavil Tablets 1757

Amoxapine (Epinephrine effects may be potentiated). Products include:

Asendin Tablets 1369

Chlorpheniramine (Epinephrine effects may be potentiated).

Chlorpheniramine Maleate (Epinephrine effects may be potentiated). Products include:

Alka-Seltzer Plus Cold Medicine .... ⊕ 705
Alka-Seltzer Plus Cold Medicine Liqui-Gels .... ⊕ 706
Alka-Seltzer Plus Cold & Cough Medicine .... ⊕ 708
Alka-Seltzer Plus Cold & Cough Medicine Liqui-Gels .... ⊕ 705
Allerest Children's Chewable Tablets .... ⊕ 627
Allerest Headache Strength Tablets .... ⊕ 627
Allerest Maximum Strength Tablets .... ⊕ 627
Allerest Sinus Pain Formula .... ⊕ 627
Allerest 12 Hour Caplets .... ⊕ 627
Ana-Kit Anaphylaxis Emergency Treatment Kit 617
Atrohist Pediatric Capsules 453
Atrohist Plus Tablets 454
BC Cold Powder Multi-Symptom Formula (Cold-Sinus-Allergy) ...... ⊕ 609
Cerose DM .... ⊕ 878
Cheracol Plus Head Cold/Cough Formula .... ⊕ 769
Children's Vicks DayQuil Allergy Relief .... ⊕ 757
Children's Vicks NyQuil Cold/ Cough Relief .... ⊕ 758
Chlor-Trimeton Allergy Decongestant Tablets .... ⊕ 799
Chlor-Trimeton Allergy Tablets ...... ⊕ 798
Comhist 2038
Comtrex Multi-Symptom Cold Reliever Tablets/Caplets/Liqui-Gels/Liquid .... ⊕ 615
Allergy-Sinus Comtrex Multi-Symptom Allergy-Sinus Formula Tablets .... ⊕ 617
Contac Continuous Action Nasal Decongestant/Antihistamine 12 Hour Capsules .... ⊕ 813
Contac Maximum Strength Continuous Action Decongestant/ Antihistamine 12 Hour Caplets .. ⊕ 813
Contac Severe Cold and Flu Formula Caplets .... ⊕ 814
Coricidin 'D' Decongestant Tablets .... ⊕ 800
Coricidin Tablets .... ⊕ 800
D.A. Chewable Tablets 951
Deconamine 1320
Dura-Tap/PD Capsules 2867
Dura-Vent/DA Tablets 953

IMPORTANT NOTE: Always consult each drug listing in the patient's regimen for possible interactions.

Sus-Phrine **Interactions Index** 992

Extendryl ... 1005
Fedahist Gyrocaps ... 2401
Fedahist Timecaps ... 2401
Hycomine Compound Tablets ... 932
Isoclor Timesule Capsules ... ◘ 637
Kronofed-A ... 977
Nolamine Timed-Release Tablets ... 785
Novahistine DH ... 2462
Novahistine Elixir ... ◘ 823
Ornade Spansule Capsules ... 2502
PediaCare Cold Allergy Chewable Tablets ... ◘ 677
PediaCare Cough-Cold Chewable Tablets ... 1553
PediaCare Cough-Cold Liquid ... 1553
PediaCare NightRest Cough-Cold Liquid ... 1553
Pediatric Vicks 44m Cough & Cold Relief ... ◘ 764
Pyrroxate Caplets ... ◘ 772
Ryna ... ◘ 841
Sinarest Tablets ... ◘ 648
Sinarest Extra Strength Tablets ... ◘ 648
Sine-Off Sinus Medicine ... ◘ 825
Singlet Tablets ... ◘ 825
Sinulin Tablets ... 787
Sinutab Sinus Allergy Medication, Maximum Strength Tablets and Caplets ... ◘ 860
Sudafed Plus Liquid ... ◘ 862
Sudafed Plus Tablets ... ◘ 863
Teldrin 12 Hour Antihistamine/Nasal Decongestant Allergy Relief Capsules ... ◘ 826
TheraFlu ... ◘ 787
TheraFlu Maximum Strength Nighttime Flu, Cold & Cough Medicine ... ◘ 788
Triaminic Allergy Tablets ... ◘ 789
Triaminic Cold Tablets ... ◘ 790
Triaminic Nite Light ... ◘ 791
Triaminic Syrup ... ◘ 792
Triaminic-12 Tablets ... ◘ 792
Triaminicin Tablets ... ◘ 793
Triaminicol Multi-Symptom Cold Tablets ... ◘ 793
Triaminicol Multi-Symptom Relief ◘ 794
Tussend ... 1783
Children's TYLENOL Cold Multi-Symptom Liquid Formula and Chewable Tablets ... 1561
Children's TYLENOL Cold Plus Cough Multi Symptom Tablets and Liquid ... ◘ 681
TYLENOL Maximum Strength Allergy Sinus Medication Gelcaps and Caplets ... 1563
TYLENOL Cold Multi-Symptom Formula Medication Tablets and Caplets ... 1561
TYLENOL Cold Multi-Symptom Hot Medication Liquid Packets ... 1557
Vicks 44 LiquiCaps Cough, Cold & Flu Relief ... ◘ 755
Vicks 44M Cough, Cold & Flu Relief ... ◘ 756

Chlorpheniramine Polistirex (Epinephrine effects may be potentiated). Products include:
Tussionex Pennkinetic Extended-Release Suspension ... 998

Chlorpheniramine Preparations (Epinephrine effects may be potentiated).

Chlorpheniramine Tannate (Epinephrine effects may be potentiated). Products include:
Atrohist Pediatric Suspension ... 454
Ricobid Tablets and Pediatric Suspension ... 2038
Rynatan ... 2673
Rynatuss ... 2673

Clomipramine Hydrochloride (Epinephrine effects may be potentiated). Products include:
Anafranil Capsules ... 803

Desipramine Hydrochloride (Epinephrine effects may be potentiated). Products include:
Norpramin Tablets ... 1526

Deslanoside (Potential for arrhythmias).
No products indexed under this heading.

Digitoxin (Potential for arrhythmias). Products include:
Crystodigin Tablets ... 1433

Digoxin (Potential for arrhythmias). Products include:
Lanoxicaps ... 1117
Lanoxin Elixir Pediatric ... 1120
Lanoxin Injection ... 1123
Lanoxin Injection Pediatric ... 1126
Lanoxin Tablets ... 1128

Diphenhydramine (Epinephrine effects may be potentiated).
No products indexed under this heading.

Diphenhydramine Citrate (Epinephrine effects may be potentiated). Products include:
Excedrin P.M. Analgesic/Sleeping Aid Tablets, Caplets, Liquigels ... 733

Diphenhydramine Hydrochloride (Epinephrine effects may be potentiated). Products include:
Actifed Allergy Daytime/Nighttime Caplets ... ◘ 844
Actifed Sinus Daytime/Nighttime Tablets and Caplets ... ◘ 846
Arthritis Foundation NightTime Caplets ... ◘ 674
Extra Strength Bayer PM Aspirin .. ◘ 713
Bayer Select Night Time Pain Relief Formula ... ◘ 716
Benadryl Allergy Decongestant Liquid Medication ... ◘ 848
Benadryl Allergy Decongestant Tablets ... ◘ 848
Benadryl Allergy Liquid Medication ... ◘ 849
Benadryl Allergy ... ◘ 848
Benadryl Allergy Sinus Headache Formula Caplets ... ◘ 849
Benadryl Capsules ... 1898
Benadryl Dye-Free Allergy Liquigel Softgels ... ◘ 850
Benadryl Dye-Free Allergy Liquid Medication ... ◘ 850
Benadryl Itch Relief Cream, Children's Formula and Maximum Strength 2% ... ◘ 851
Benadryl Itch Relief Spray, Children's Formula and Maximum Strength 2% ... ◘ 851
Benadryl Itch Relief Stick Maximum Strength 2% ... ◘ 850
Benadryl Itch Stopping Gel, Children's Formula and Maximum Strength 2% ... ◘ 851
Benadryl Kapseals ... 1898
Benadryl Injection ... 1898
Contac Day & Night Cold/Flu Night Caplets ... ◘ 812
Contac Night Allergy/Sinus Caplets ... ◘ 812
Extra Strength Doan's P.M. ... ◘ 633
Legatrin PM ... ◘ 651
Miles Nervine Nighttime Sleep-Aid ◘ 723
Nytol QuickCaps Caplets ... ◘ 610
Sleepinal Night-time Sleep Aid Capsules and Softgels ... ◘ 834
TYLENOL Maximum Strength Allergy Sinus NightTime Medication Caplets ... 1555
TYLENOL Flu NightTime, Maximum Strength, Gelcaps ... 1566
TYLENOL Maximum Strength Flu NightTime Hot Medication Packets ... 1562
TYLENOL PM, Extra Strength Pain Reliever/Sleep Aid Caplets, Geltabs, Gelcaps ... 1560
TYLENOL Severe Allergy Medication Caplets ... 1564
Maximum Strength Unisom Sleepgels ... 1934
Unisom With Pain Relief-Nighttime Sleep Aid and Pain Reliever ... 1934

Dobutamine Hydrochloride (Combined effects on cardiovascular system may be deleterious). Products include:
Dobutrex Solution Vials ... 1439

Dopamine Hydrochloride (Combined effects on cardiovascular system may be deleterious).
No products indexed under this heading.

Doxepin Hydrochloride (Epinephrine effects may be potentiated). Products include:
Sinequan ... 2205

Zonalon Cream ... 1055

Ephedrine Hydrochloride (Combined effects on cardiovascular system may be deleterious). Products include:
Primatene Dual Action Formula ... ◘ 872
Primatene Tablets ... ◘ 873
Quadrinal Tablets ... 1350

Ephedrine Sulfate (Combined effects on cardiovascular system may be deleterious). Products include:
Bronkaid Caplets ... ◘ 717
Marax Tablets & DF Syrup ... 2200

Ephedrine Tannate (Combined effects on cardiovascular system may be deleterious). Products include:
Rynatuss ... 2673

Epinephrine Bitartrate (Combined effects on cardiovascular system may be deleterious). Products include:
Bronkaid Mist Suspension ... ◘ 718
Sensorcaine-MPF with Epinephrine Injection ... 559

Epinephrine Hydrochloride (Combined effects on cardiovascular system may be deleterious). Products include:
Ana-Kit Anaphylaxis Emergency Treatment Kit ... 617

Imipramine Hydrochloride (Epinephrine effects may be potentiated). Products include:
Tofranil Ampuls ... 854
Tofranil Tablets ... 856

Imipramine Pamoate (Epinephrine effects may be potentiated). Products include:
Tofranil-PM Capsules ... 857

Isoproterenol Hydrochloride (Combined effects on cardiovascular system may be deleterious). Products include:
Isuprel Hydrochloride Injection 1:5000 ... 2311
Isuprel Hydrochloride Solution 1:200 & 1:100 ... 2313
Isuprel Mistometer ... 2312

Isoproterenol Sulfate (Combined effects on cardiovascular system may be deleterious). Products include:
Norisodrine with Calcium Iodide Syrup ... 442

Maprotiline Hydrochloride (Epinephrine effects may be potentiated). Products include:
Ludiomil Tablets ... 843

Metaproterenol Sulfate (Combined effects on cardiovascular system may be deleterious). Products include:
Alupent ... 669
Metaproterenol Sulfate Inhalation Solution, USP, Arm-a-Med ... 552

Metaraminol Bitartrate (Combined effects on cardiovascular system may be deleterious). Products include:
Aramine Injection ... 1609

Norepinephrine Bitartrate (Combined effects on cardiovascular system may be deleterious). Products include:
Levophed Bitartrate Injection ... 2315

Nortriptyline Hydrochloride (Epinephrine effects may be potentiated). Products include:
Pamelor ... 2280

Phenylephrine Bitartrate (Combined effects on cardiovascular system may be deleterious).
No products indexed under this heading.

Phenylephrine Hydrochloride (Combined effects on cardiovascular system may be deleterious). Products include:
Atrohist Plus Tablets ... 454
Cerose DM ... ◘ 878
Comhist ... 2038
D.A. Chewable Tablets ... 951
Deconsal Pediatric Capsules ... 454
Dura-Vent/DA Tablets ... 953
Entex Capsules ... 1986
Entex Liquid ... 1986
Extendryl ... 1005
4-Way Fast Acting Nasal Spray (regular & mentholated) ... ◘ 621
Hemorid For Women ... ◘ 834
Hycomine Compound Tablets ... 932
Neo-Synephrine Hydrochloride 1% Carpuject ... 2324
Neo-Synephrine Hydrochloride 1% Injection ... 2324
Neo-Synephrine Hydrochloride (Ophthalmic) ... 2325
Neo-Synephrine ... ◘ 726
Nōstril ... ◘ 644
Novahistine Elixir ... ◘ 823
Phenergan VC ... 2779
Phenergan VC with Codeine ... 2781
Preparation H ... ◘ 871
Tympagesic Ear Drops ... 2342
Vasosulf ... ⊙ 271
Vicks Sinex Nasal Spray and Ultra Fine Mist ... ◘ 765

Phenylephrine Tannate (Combined effects on cardiovascular system may be deleterious). Products include:
Atrohist Pediatric Suspension ... 454
Ricobid-D Pediatric Suspension ... 2038
Ricobid Tablets and Pediatric Suspension ... 2038
Rynatan ... 2673
Rynatuss ... 2673

Phenylpropanolamine Hydrochloride (Combined effects on cardiovascular system may be deleterious). Products include:
Acutrim ... ◘ 628
Allerest Children's Chewable Tablets ... ◘ 627
Allerest 12 Hour Caplets ... ◘ 627
Atrohist Plus Tablets ... 454
BC Cold Powder Multi-Symptom Formula (Cold-Sinus-Allergy) ... ◘ 609
BC Cold Powder Non-Drowsy Formula (Cold-Sinus) ... ◘ 609
Cheracol Plus Head Cold/Cough Formula ... ◘ 769
Comtrex Multi-Symptom Non-Drowsy Liqui-gels ... ◘ 618
Contac Continuous Action Nasal Decongestant/Antihistamine 12 Hour Capsules ... ◘ 813
Contac Maximum Strength Continuous Action Decongestant/Antihistamine 12 Hour Caplets .. ◘ 813
Contac Severe Cold and Flu Formula Caplets ... ◘ 814
Coricidin 'D' Decongestant Tablets ... ◘ 800
Dexatrim ... ◘ 832
Dexatrim Plus Vitamins Caplets ... ◘ 832
Dimetane-DC Cough Syrup ... 2059
Dimetapp Elixir ... ◘ 773
Dimetapp Extentabs ... ◘ 774
Dimetapp Tablets/Liqui-Gels ... ◘ 775
Dimetapp Cold & Allergy Chewable Tablets ... ◘ 773
Dimetapp DM Elixir ... ◘ 774
Dura-Vent Tablets ... 952
Entex Capsules ... 1986
Entex LA Tablets ... 1987
Entex Liquid ... 1986
Exgest LA Tablets ... 782
Hycomine ... 931
Isoclor Timesule Capsules ... ◘ 637
Nolamine Timed-Release Tablets ... 785
Ornade Spansule Capsules ... 2502
Propagest Tablets ... 786
Pyrroxate Caplets ... ◘ 772
Robitussin-CF ... ◘ 777
Sinulin Tablets ... 787
Tavist-D 12 Hour Relief Tablets ... ◘ 787
Teldrin 12 Hour Antihistamine/Nasal Decongestant Allergy Relief Capsules ... ◘ 826
Triaminic Allergy Tablets ... ◘ 789
Triaminic Cold Tablets ... ◘ 790
Triaminic Expectorant ... ◘ 790

(◘ Described in PDR For Nonprescription Drugs) (⊙ Described in PDR For Ophthalmology)

Triaminic Syrup .... ⊕ 792
Triaminic-12 Tablets .... ⊕ 792
Triaminic-DM Syrup .... ⊕ 792
Triaminicin Tablets .... ⊕ 793
Triaminicol Multi-Symptom Cold Tablets .... ⊕ 793
Triaminicol Multi-Symptom Relief ⊕ 794
Vicks DayQuil Allergy Relief 12-Hour Extended Release Tablets.. ⊕ 760
Vicks DayQuil Allergy Relief 4-Hour Tablets .... ⊕ 760
Vicks DayQuil SINUS Pressure & CONGESTION Relief........................ ⊕ 761

Pirbuterol Acetate (Combined effects on cardiovascular system may be deleterious). Products include:

Maxair Autohaler 1492
Maxair Inhaler 1494

Protriptyline Hydrochloride (Epinephrine effects may be potentiated). Products include:

Vivactil Tablets 1774

Pseudoephedrine Hydrochloride (Combined effects on cardiovascular system may be deleterious). Products include:

Actifed Allergy Daytime/Nighttime Caplets.. ⊕ 844
Actifed Plus Caplets .... ⊕ 845
Actifed Plus Tablets .... ⊕ 845
Actifed with Codeine Cough Syrup.. 1067
Actifed Sinus Daytime/Nighttime Tablets and Caplets .... ⊕ 846
Actifed Syrup.. ⊕ 846
Actifed Tablets .... ⊕ 844
Advil Cold and Sinus Caplets and Tablets (formerly CoAdvil) .... ⊕ 870
Alka-Seltzer Plus Cold Medicine Liqui-Gels .... ⊕ 706
Alka-Seltzer Plus Cold & Cough Medicine Liqui-Gels.......................... ⊕ 705
Alka-Seltzer Plus Night-Time Cold Medicine Liqui-Gels.......................... ⊕ 706
Allerest Headache Strength Tablets .... ⊕ 627
Allerest Maximum Strength Tablets .... ⊕ 627
Allerest No Drowsiness Tablets...... ⊕ 627
Allerest Sinus Pain Formula .... ⊕ 627
Anatuss LA Tablets................................ 1542
Atrohist Pediatric Capsules................ 453
Bayer Select Sinus Pain Relief Formula .... ⊕ 717
Benadryl Allergy Decongestant Liquid Medication .... ⊕ 848
Benadryl Allergy Decongestant Tablets .... ⊕ 848
Benadryl Allergy Sinus Headache Formula Caplets .... ⊕ 849
Benylin Multisymptom........................ ⊕ 852
Bromfed Capsules (Extended-Release) 1785
Bromfed Syrup .... ⊕ 733
Bromfed Tablets 1785
Bromfed-DM Cough Syrup.................. 1786
Bromfed-PD Capsules (Extended-Release) 1785
Children's Vicks DayQuil Allergy Relief .... ⊕ 757
Children's Vicks NyQuil Cold/Cough Relief.. ⊕ 758
Comtrex Multi-Symptom Cold Reliever Tablets/Caplets/Liqui-Gels/Liquid.. ⊕ 615
Allergy-Sinus Comtrex Multi-Symptom Allergy-Sinus Formula Tablets .... ⊕ 617
Comtrex Multi-Symptom Non-Drowsy Caplets.................................. ⊕ 618
Congess 1004
Contac Day Allergy/Sinus Caplets ⊕ 812
Contac Day & Night .... ⊕ 812
Contac Night Allergy/Sinus Caplets .... ⊕ 812
Contac Severe Cold & Flu Non-Drowsy .... ⊕ 815
Deconamine Chewable Tablets 1320
Deconamine CX Cough and Cold Liquid and Tablets................................ 1319
Deconamine 1320
Deconsal C Expectorant Syrup 456
Deconsal Pediatric Syrup 457
Deconsal II Tablets 454
Dimetane-DX Cough Syrup 2059
Dimetapp Sinus Caplets .... ⊕ 775
Dorcol Children's Cough Syrup ...... ⊕ 785
Drixoral Cough + Congestion Liquid Caps .... ⊕ 802
Dura-Tap/PD Capsules 2867
Duratuss Tablets 2565
Duratuss HD Elixir.................................. 2565
Efidac/24 .... ⊕ 635
Entex PSE Tablets 1987
Fedahist Gyrocaps.................................. 2401
Fedahist Timecaps 2401
Guaifed.. 1787
Guaifed Syrup .... ⊕ 734
Guaimax-D Tablets 792
Guaitab Tablets .... ⊕ 734
Isoclor Expectorant................................ 990
Kronofed-A... 977
Motrin IB Sinus .... ⊕ 838
Novahistine DH.. 2462
Novahistine DMX .... ⊕ 822
Novahistine Expectorant...................... 2463
Nucofed 2051
PediaCare Cold Allergy Chewable Tablets .... ⊕ 677
PediaCare Cough-Cold Chewable Tablets.. 1553
PediaCare 1553
PediaCare Infants' Decongestant Drops .... ⊕ 677
PediCare Infant's Drops Decongestant Plus Cough 1553
PediaCare NightRest Cough-Cold Liquid 1553
Pediatric Vicks 44d Dry Hacking Cough & Head Congestion.............. ⊕ 763
Pediatric Vicks 44m Cough & Cold Relief .... ⊕ 764
Robitussin Cold & Cough Liqui-Gels .... ⊕ 776
Robitussin Maximum Strength Cough & Cold .... ⊕ 778
Robitussin Pediatric Cough & Cold Formula .... ⊕ 779
Robitussin Severe Congestion Liqui-Gels .... ⊕ 776
Robitussin-DAC Syrup 2074
Robitussin-PE .... ⊕ 778
Rondec Oral Drops 953
Rondec Syrup 953
Rondec Tablet 953
Rondec-DM Oral Drops 954
Rondec-DM Syrup 954
Rondec-TR Tablet 953
Ryna .... ⊕ 841
Seldane-D Extended-Release Tablets 1538
Semprex-D Capsules 463
Semprex-D Capsules 1167
Sinarest Tablets .... ⊕ 648
Sinarest Extra Strength Tablets...... ⊕ 648
Sinarest No Drowsiness Tablets .... ⊕ 648
Sine-Aid IB Caplets 1554
Sine-Aid Maximum Strength Sinus Medication Gelcaps, Caplets and Tablets 1554
Sine-Off No Drowsiness Formula Caplets .... ⊕ 824
Sine-Off Sinus Medicine .... ⊕ 825
Singlet Tablets .... ⊕ 825
Sinutab Non-Drying Liquid Caps .... ⊕ 859
Sinutab Sinus Allergy Medication, Maximum Strength Tablets and Caplets .... ⊕ 860
Sinutab Sinus Medication, Maximum Strength Without Drowsiness Formula, Tablets & Caplets .... ⊕ 860
Sinutab Sinus Medication, Regular Strength Without Drowsiness Formula .... ⊕ 859
Sudafed Children's Liquid .... ⊕ 861
Sudafed Cold and Cough Liquidcaps... ⊕ 862
Sudafed Cough Syrup .... ⊕ 862
Sudafed Plus Liquid .... ⊕ 862
Sudafed Plus Tablets .... ⊕ 863
Sudafed Severe Cold Formula Caplets .... ⊕ 863
Sudafed Severe Cold Formula Tablets .... ⊕ 864
Sudafed Sinus Caplets.......................... ⊕ 864
Sudafed Sinus Tablets.......................... ⊕ 864
Sudafed Tablets, 30 mg....................... ⊕ 861
Sudafed Tablets, 60 mg....................... ⊕ 861
Sudafed 12 Hour Caplets .... ⊕ 861
Syn-Rx Tablets 465
Syn-Rx DM Tablets 466
TheraFlu.. ⊕ 787
TheraFlu Maximum Strength Nighttime Flu, Cold & Cough Medicine .... ⊕ 788
TheraFlu Maximum Strength Non-Drowsy Formula Flu, Cold & Cough Medicine .... ⊕ 788
Thera Flu Maximum Strength, Non-Drowsy Formula Flu, Cold and Cough Caplets .... ⊕ 789
Triaminic AM Cough and Decongestant Formula .... ⊕ 789
Triaminic AM Decongestant Formula .... ⊕ 790
Triaminic Nite Light .... ⊕ 791
Triaminic Sore Throat Formula ...... ⊕ 791
Tussend 1783
Tussend Expectorant 1785
Children's TYLENOL Cold Multi-Symptom Liquid Formula and Chewable Tablets................................. 1561
Children's TYLENOL Cold Plus Cough Multi Symptom Tablets and Liquid.. ⊕ 681
Infants' TYLENOL Cold Decongestant & Fever-Reducer Drops 1556
TYLENOL Maximum Strength Allergy Sinus Medication Gelcaps and Caplets 1563
TYLENOL Maximum Strength Allergy Sinus NightTime Medication Caplets 1555
TYLENOL Flu Maximum Strength Gelcaps 1565
TYLENOL Flu NightTime, Maximum Strength, Gelcaps 1566
TYLENOL Maximum Strength Flu NightTime Hot Medication Packets 1562
TYLENOL, Maximum Strength, Sinus Medication Geltabs, Gelcaps, Caplets and Tablets 1566
TYLENOL Cold Multi-Symptom Formula Medication Tablets and Caplets 1561
TYLENOL Cold Medication No Drowsiness Formula Gelcaps and Caplets 1562
TYLENOL Cold Multi-Symptom Hot Medication Liquid Packets.............. 1557
TYLENOL Cough Multi-Symptom Medication with Decongestant...... 1565
Ursinus Inlay-Tabs.................................. ⊕ 794
Vicks 44 LiquiCaps Cough, Cold & Flu Relief.. ⊕ 755
Vicks 44 LiquiCaps Non-Drowsy Cough & Cold Relief .... ⊕ 756
Vicks 44D Dry Hacking Cough & Head Congestion .... ⊕ 755
Vicks 44M Cough, Cold & Flu Relief.. ⊕ 756
Vicks DayQuil .... ⊕ 761
Vicks DayQuil SINUS Pressure & PAIN Relief with IBUPROFEN .... ⊕ 762
Vicks Nyquil Hot Therapy.................... ⊕ 762
Vicks NyQuil LiquiCaps Multi-Symptom Cold/Flu Relief.............. ⊕ 763
Vicks NyQuil Multi-Symptom Cold/Flu Relief - (Original & Cherry Flavor)....................................... ⊕ 763

Pseudoephedrine Sulfate (Combined effects on cardiovascular system may be deleterious). Products include:

Cheracol Sinus .... ⊕ 768
Chlor-Trimeton Allergy Decongestant Tablets .... ⊕ 799
Claritin-D 2350
Drixoral Cold and Allergy Sustained-Action Tablets..................... ⊕ 802
Drixoral Cold and Flu Extended-Release Tablets.................................. ⊕ 803
Drixoral Non-Drowsy Formula Extended-Release Tablets .... ⊕ 803
Drixoral Allergy/Sinus Extended Release Tablets................................... ⊕ 804
Trinalin Repetabs Tablets 1330

Salmeterol Xinafoate (Combined effects on cardiovascular system may be deleterious). Products include:

Serevent Inhalation Aerosol................ 1176

Terbutaline Sulfate (Combined effects on cardiovascular system may be deleterious). Products include:

Brethaire Inhaler 813
Brethine Ampuls 815
Brethine Tablets...................................... 814
Bricanyl Subcutaneous Injection 1502
Bricanyl Tablets 1503

Thyroxine Sodium (Epinephrine effects may be potentiated).

No products indexed under this heading.

Trimipramine Maleate (Epinephrine effects may be potentiated). Products include:

Surmontil Capsules................................ 2811

Tripelennamine Hydrochloride (Epinephrine effects may be potentiated). Products include:

PBZ Tablets 845
PBZ-SR Tablets.. 844

SWEEN CREAM

(Benzethonium Chloride, Lanolin Oil) 2554
None cited in PDR database.

SYMMETREL CAPSULES AND SYRUP

(Amantadine Hydrochloride) 946
May interact with central nervous system stimulants. Compounds in this category include:

Amphetamine Resins (Interaction not specified; careful observation required). Products include:

Biphetamine Capsules........................... 983

Dextroamphetamine Sulfate (Interaction not specified; careful observation required). Products include:

Dexedrine 2474
DextroStat Dextroamphetamine Tablets 2036

Methamphetamine Hydrochloride (Interaction not specified; careful observation required). Products include:

Desoxyn Gradumet Tablets 419

Methylphenidate Hydrochloride (Interaction not specified; careful observation required). Products include:

Ritalin 848

Pemoline (Interaction not specified; careful observation required). Products include:

Cylert Tablets 412

SYNALAR CREAMS 0.025%, 0.01%

(Fluocinolone Acetonide) 2130
None cited in PDR database.

SYNALAR OINTMENT 0.025%

(Fluocinolone Acetonide) 2130
None cited in PDR database.

SYNALAR TOPICAL SOLUTION 0.01%

(Fluocinolone Acetonide) 2130
None cited in PDR database.

SYNAREL NASAL SOLUTION FOR CENTRAL PRECOCIOUS PUBERTY

(Nafarelin Acetate) 2151
None cited in PDR database.

SYNAREL NASAL SOLUTION FOR ENDOMETRIOSIS

(Nafarelin Acetate) 2152
None cited in PDR database.

SYNEMOL CREAM 0.025%

(Fluocinolone Acetonide) 2130
None cited in PDR database.

SYN-RX TABLETS

(Pseudoephedrine Hydrochloride, Guaifenesin) 465
May interact with monoamine oxidase inhibitors, beta blockers, cardiac glycosides, tricyclic antidepressants, and certain other agents. Compounds in these categories include:

Acebutolol Hydrochloride (Po-

IMPORTANT NOTE: Always consult each drug listing in the patient's regimen for possible interactions.

tentiates the pressor effect). Products include:

Sectral Capsules ... 2807

Amitriptyline Hydrochloride (May antagonize the effects of pseudoephedrine). Products include:

Elavil ... 2838
Endep Tablets ... 2174
Etrafon ... 2355
Limbitrol ... 2180
Triavil Tablets ... 1757

Amoxapine (May antagonize the effects of pseudoephedrine). Products include:

Asendin Tablets ... 1369

Atenolol (Potentiates the pressor effect). Products include:

Tenoretic Tablets ... 2845
Tenormin Tablets and I.V. Injection 2847

Betaxolol Hydrochloride (Potentiates the pressor effect). Products include:

Betoptic Ophthalmic Solution ... 469
Betoptic S Ophthalmic Suspension 471
Kerlone Tablets ... 2436

Bisoprolol Fumarate (Potentiates the pressor effect). Products include:

Zebeta Tablets ... 1413
Ziac ... 1415

Carteolol Hydrochloride (Potentiates the pressor effect). Products include:

Cartrol Tablets ... 410
Ocupress Ophthalmic Solution, 1% Sterile ... ⊙ 309

Clomipramine Hydrochloride (May antagonize the effects of pseudoephedrine). Products include:

Anafranil Capsules ... 803

Desipramine Hydrochloride (May antagonize the effects of pseudoephedrine). Products include:

Norpramin Tablets ... 1526

Deslanoside (May increase the possiblity of cardiac arrhythmia).

No products indexed under this heading.

Digitoxin (May increase the possiblity of cardiac arrhythmia). Products include:

Crystodigin Tablets ... 1433

Digoxin (May increase the possiblity of cardiac arrhythmia). Products include:

Lanoxicaps ... 1117
Lanoxin Elixir Pediatric ... 1120
Lanoxin Injection ... 1123
Lanoxin Injection Pediatric ... 1126
Lanoxin Tablets ... 1128

Doxepin Hydrochloride (May antagonize the effects of pseudoephedrine). Products include:

Sinequan ... 2205
Zonalon Cream ... 1055

Esmolol Hydrochloride (Potentiates the pressor effect). Products include:

Brevibloc Injection ... 1808

Furazolidone (Concurrent and/or sequential use may lead to hypertensive crisis; co-administration is contraindicated). Products include:

Furoxone ... 2046

Guanethidine Monosulfate (Reduced hypotensive effect). Products include:

Esimil Tablets ... 822
Ismelin Tablets ... 827

Imipramine Hydrochloride (May antagonize the effects of pseudoephedrine). Products include:

Tofranil Ampuls ... 854
Tofranil Tablets ... 856

Imipramine Pamoate (May antagonize the effects of pseudoephedrine). Products include:

Tofranil-PM Capsules ... 857

Isocarboxazid (Concurrent and/or sequential use may lead to hypertensive crisis; co-administration is contraindicated).

No products indexed under this heading.

Labetalol Hydrochloride (Potentiates the pressor effect). Products include:

Normodyne Injection ... 2377
Normodyne Tablets ... 2379
Trandate ... 1185

Levobunolol Hydrochloride (Potentiates the pressor effect). Products include:

Betagan ... ⊙ 233

Maprotiline Hydrochloride (May antagonize the effects of pseudoephedrine). Products include:

Ludiomil Tablets ... 843

Mecamylamine Hydrochloride (Reduced hypotensive effect). Products include:

Inversine Tablets ... 1686

Methyldopa (Reduced hypotensive effect). Products include:

Aldoclor Tablets ... 1598
Aldomet Oral ... 1600
Aldoril Tablets ... 1604

Methyldopate Hydrochloride (Reduced hypotensive effect). Products include:

Aldomet Ester HCl Injection ... 1602

Metipranolol Hydrochloride (Potentiates the pressor effect). Products include:

OptiPranolol (Metipranolol 0.3%) Sterile Ophthalmic Solution ... ⊙ 258

Metoprolol Succinate (Potentiates the pressor effect). Products include:

Toprol-XL Tablets ... 565

Metoprolol Tartrate (Potentiates the pressor effect). Products include:

Lopressor Ampuls ... 830
Lopressor HCT Tablets ... 832
Lopressor Tablets ... 830

Nadolol (Potentiates the pressor effect).

No products indexed under this heading.

Nortriptyline Hydrochloride (May antagonize the effects of pseudoephedrine). Products include:

Pamelor ... 2280

Penbutolol Sulfate (Potentiates the pressor effect). Products include:

Levatol ... 2403

Phenelzine Sulfate (Concurrent and/or sequential use may lead to hypertensive crisis; co-administration is contraindicated). Products include:

Nardil ... 1920

Pindolol (Potentiates the pressor effect). Products include:

Visken Tablets ... 2299

Propranolol Hydrochloride (Potentiates the pressor effect). Products include:

Inderal ... 2728
Inderal LA Long Acting Capsules ... 2730
Inderide Tablets ... 2732
Inderide LA Long Acting Capsules .. 2734

Protriptyline Hydrochloride (May antagonize the effects of pseudoephedrine). Products include:

Vivactil Tablets ... 1774

Reserpine (Reduced hypotensive effect). Products include:

Diupres Tablets ... 1650
Hydropres Tablets ... 1675
Ser-Ap-Es Tablets ... 849

Selegiline Hydrochloride (Concurrent and/or sequential use may lead to hypertensive crisis; co-administration is contraindicated). Products include:

Eldepryl Tablets ... 2550

Sotalol Hydrochloride (Potentiates the pressor effect). Products include:

Betapace Tablets ... 641

Timolol Hemihydrate (Potentiates the pressor effect). Products include:

Betimol 0.25%, 0.5% ... ⊙ 261

Timolol Maleate (Potentiates the pressor effect). Products include:

Blocadren Tablets ... 1614
Timolide Tablets ... 1748
Timoptic in Ocudose ... 1753
Timoptic Sterile Ophthalmic Solution ... 1751
Timoptic-XE ... 1755

Tranylcypromine Sulfate (Concurrent and/or sequential use may lead to hypertensive crisis; co-administration is contraindicated). Products include:

Parnate Tablets ... 2503

Trimipramine Maleate (May antagonize the effects of pseudoephedrine). Products include:

Surmontil Capsules ... 2811

SYN-RX DM TABLETS

(Guaifenesin, Pseudoephedrine Hydrochloride, Dextromethorphan Hydrobromide) ... **466**

May interact with monoamine oxidase inhibitors, beta blockers, veratrum alkaloids, tricyclic antidepressants, and certain other agents. Compounds in these categories include:

Acebutolol Hydrochloride (Potentiates the pressor effects of pseudoephedrine). Products include:

Sectral Capsules ... 2807

Amitriptyline Hydrochloride (May antagonize the effects of pseudoephedrine). Products include:

Elavil ... 2838
Endep Tablets ... 2174
Etrafon ... 2355
Limbitrol ... 2180
Triavil Tablets ... 1757

Amoxapine (May antagonize the effects of pseudoephedrine). Products include:

Asendin Tablets ... 1369

Atenolol (Potentiates the pressor effects of pseudoephedrine). Products include:

Tenoretic Tablets ... 2845
Tenormin Tablets and I.V. Injection 2847

Betaxolol Hydrochloride (Potentiates the pressor effects of pseudoephedrine). Products include:

Betoptic Ophthalmic Solution ... 469
Betoptic S Ophthalmic Suspension 471
Kerlone Tablets ... 2436

Bisoprolol Fumarate (Potentiates the pressor effects of pseudoephedrine). Products include:

Zebeta Tablets ... 1413
Ziac ... 1415

Carteolol Hydrochloride (Potentiates the pressor effects of pseudoephedrine). Products include:

Cartrol Tablets ... 410
Ocupress Ophthalmic Solution, 1% Sterile ... ⊙ 309

Clomipramine Hydrochloride (May antagonize the effects of pseudoephedrine). Products include:

Anafranil Capsules ... 803

Cryptenamine Preparations (Sympathomimetic may reduce the antihypertensive effects of veratrum alkaloids).

Desipramine Hydrochloride (May antagonize the effects of pseudoephedrine). Products include:

Norpramin Tablets ... 1526

Doxepin Hydrochloride (May antagonize the effects of pseudoephedrine). Products include:

Sinequan ... 2205
Zonalon Cream ... 1055

Esmolol Hydrochloride (Potentiates the pressor effects of pseudoephedrine). Products include:

Brevibloc Injection ... 1808

Furazolidone (Potential for hypertensive crises; concurrent and/or sequential use is contraindicated; potentiates the pressor effects of pseudoephedrine). Products include:

Furoxone ... 2046

Imipramine Hydrochloride (May antagonize the effects of pseudoephedrine). Products include:

Tofranil Ampuls ... 854
Tofranil Tablets ... 856

Imipramine Pamoate (May antagonize the effects of pseudoephedrine). Products include:

Tofranil-PM Capsules ... 857

Isocarboxazid (Potential for hypertensive crises; concurrent and/or sequential use is contraindicated; potentiates the pressor effects of pseudoephedrine).

No products indexed under this heading.

Labetalol Hydrochloride (Potentiates the pressor effects of pseudoephedrine). Products include:

Normodyne Injection ... 2377
Normodyne Tablets ... 2379
Trandate ... 1185

Levobunolol Hydrochloride (Potentiates the pressor effects of pseudoephedrine). Products include:

Betagan ... ⊙ 233

Maprotiline Hydrochloride (May antagonize the effects of pseudoephedrine). Products include:

Ludiomil Tablets ... 843

Mecamylamine Hydrochloride (Sympathomimetic may reduce the antihypertensive effects). Products include:

Inversine Tablets ... 1686

Methyldopa (Sympathomimetic may reduce the antihypertensive effects). Products include:

Aldoclor Tablets ... 1598
Aldomet Oral ... 1600
Aldoril Tablets ... 1604

Methyldopate Hydrochloride (Sympathomimetic may reduce the antihypertensive effects). Products include:

Aldomet Ester HCl Injection ... 1602

Metipranolol Hydrochloride (Potentiates the pressor effects of pseudoephedrine). Products include:

OptiPranolol (Metipranolol 0.3%) Sterile Ophthalmic Solution ... ⊙ 258

Metoprolol Succinate (Potentiates the pressor effects of pseudoephedrine). Products include:

Toprol-XL Tablets ... 565

Metoprolol Tartrate (Potentiates the pressor effects of pseudoephedrine). Products include:

Lopressor Ampuls ... 830
Lopressor HCT Tablets ... 832
Lopressor Tablets ... 830

Nadolol (Potentiates the pressor effects of pseudoephedrine).

No products indexed under this heading.

Nortriptyline Hydrochloride (May antagonize the effects of pseudoephedrine). Products include:

Pamelor ... 2280

995 **Interactions Index** **Synthroid**

Penbutolol Sulfate (Potentiates the pressor effects of pseudoephedrine). Products include:
- Levatol ... 2403

Phenelzine Sulfate (Potential for hypertensive crises; concurrent and/or sequential use is contraindicated; potentiates the pressor effects of pseudoephedrine). Products include:
- Nardil ... 1920

Pindolol (Potentiates the pressor effects of pseudoephedrine). Products include:
- Visken Tablets ... 2299

Propranolol Hydrochloride (Potentiates the pressor effects of pseudoephedrine). Products include:
- Inderal ... 2728
- Inderal LA Long Acting Capsules ... 2730
- Inderide Tablets ... 2732
- Inderide LA Long Acting Capsules .. 2734

Protriptyline Hydrochloride (May antagonize the effects of pseudoephedrine). Products include:
- Vivactil Tablets ... 1774

Reserpine (Sympathomimetic may reduce the antihypertensive effects). Products include:
- Diupres Tablets ... 1650
- Hydropres Tablets ... 1675
- Ser-Ap-Es Tablets ... 849

Selegiline Hydrochloride (Potential for hypertensive crises; concurrent and/or sequential use is contraindicated; potentiates the pressor effects of pseudoephedrine). Products include:
- Eldepryl Tablets ... 2550

Sotalol Hydrochloride (Potentiates the pressor effects of pseudoephedrine). Products include:
- Betapace Tablets ... 641

Timolol Hemihydrate (Potentiates the pressor effects of pseudoephedrine). Products include:
- Betimol 0.25%, 0.5% ... ⊙ 261

Timolol Maleate (Potentiates the pressor effects of pseudoephedrine). Products include:
- Blocadren Tablets ... 1614
- Timolide Tablets ... 1748
- Timoptic in Ocudose ... 1753
- Timoptic Sterile Ophthalmic Solution ... 1751
- Timoptic-XE ... 1755

Tranylcypromine Sulfate (Potential for hypertensive crises; concurrent and/or sequential use is contraindicated; potentiates the pressor effects of pseudoephedrine). Products include:
- Parnate Tablets ... 2503

Trimipramine Maleate (May antagonize the effects of pseudoephedrine). Products include:
- Surmontil Capsules ... 2811

SYNTHROID TABLETS

(Levothyroxine Sodium) ... 1359

May interact with androgens, hepatic microsomal emzyme inducers, estrogens, glucocorticoids, salicylates, beta blockers, tricyclic antidepressants, sympathomimetics, xanthine bronchodilators, cardiac glycosides, insulin, oral hypoglycemic agents, oral anticoagulants, antithyroid agents, dopamine agonists, lithium preparations, sulfonylureas, thiazides, sulfonamides, cytokines, radiographic iodinated contrast media, and certain other agents. Compounds in these categories include:

Acarbose (Requirements of oral antidiabetic agents may be reduced in hypothyroid patients with diabetes and may be subsequently increased with initiation of thyroid hormone therapy).
- No products indexed under this heading.

Acebutolol Hydrochloride (Alters thyroid hormone or TSH levels; actions of some beta blockers may be impaired when hypothyroid patients become euthyroid). Products include:
- Sectral Capsules ... 2807

Albuterol (Possible increased risk of coronary insufficiency in patients with coronary artery disease). Products include:
- Proventil Inhalation Aerosol ... 2382
- Ventolin Inhalation Aerosol and Refill ... 1197

Albuterol Sulfate (Possible increased risk of coronary insufficiency in patients with coronary artery disease). Products include:
- Airet Solution for Inhalation ... 452
- Proventil Inhalation Solution 0.083% ... 2384
- Proventil Repetabs Tablets ... 2386
- Proventil Solution for Inhalation 0.5% ... 2383
- Proventil Syrup ... 2385
- Proventil Tablets ... 2386
- Ventolin Inhalation Solution ... 1198
- Ventolin Nebules Inhalation Solution ... 1199
- Ventolin Rotacaps for Inhalation ... 1200
- Ventolin Syrup ... 1202
- Ventolin Tablets ... 1203
- Volmax Extended-Release Tablets .. 1788

Aldesleukin (Cytokines have been reported to induce both hyperthyroidism or hypothyroidism; dosage adjustment may be necessary). Products include:
- Proleukin for Injection ... 797

Aluminum Hydroxide (Binds and decreases absorption of levothyroxine sodium from the gastrointestinal tract). Products include:
- ALternaGEL Liquid ... 1316
- Maximum Strength Ascriptin ... ▣ 630
- Cama Arthritis Pain Reliever ... ▣ 785
- Gaviscon Extra Strength Relief Formula Antacid Tablets ... ▣ 819
- Gaviscon Extra Strength Relief Formula Liquid Antacid ... ▣ 819
- Gaviscon Liquid Antacid ... ▣ 820
- Gelusil Liquid & Tablets ... ▣ 855
- Maalox Heartburn Relief Suspension ... ▣ 642
- Maalox Heartburn Relief Tablets ... ▣ 641
- Maalox Magnesia and Alumina Oral Suspension ... ▣ 642
- Maalox Plus Tablets ... ▣ 643
- Extra Strength Maalox Antacid Plus Antigas Liquid and Tablets ▣ 638
- Tempo Soft Antacid ... ▣ 835

Aluminum Hydroxide Gel (Binds and decreases absorption of levothyroxine sodium from the gastrointestinal tract). Products include:
- ALternaGEL Liquid ... ▣ 659
- Aludrox Oral Suspension ... 2695
- Amphojel Suspension ... 2695
- Amphojel Suspension without Flavor ... 2695
- Amphojel Tablets ... 2695
- Arthritis Pain Ascriptin ... ▣ 631
- Regular Strength Ascriptin Tablets ... ▣ 629
- Gaviscon Antacid Tablets ... ▣ 819
- Gaviscon-2 Antacid Tablets ... ▣ 820
- Mylanta Liquid ... 1317
- Mylanta Tablets ... ▣ 660
- Mylanta Double Strength Liquid ... 1317
- Mylanta Double Strength Tablets .. ▣ 660
- Nephrox Suspension ... ▣ 655

Aminoglutethimide (Alters thyroid hormone or TSH levels). Products include:
- Cytadren Tablets ... 819

Aminophylline (Theophylline clearance may be decreased in hypothyroid patients and return toward normal when euthyroid state is achieved).
- No products indexed under this heading.

p-Aminosalicylic Acid (Alters thyroid hormone or TSH levels).
- No products indexed under this heading.

Amiodarone Hydrochloride (Alters thyroid hormone or TSH levels; amiodarone therapy alone can cause hypothyroidism or hyperthyroidism). Products include:
- Cordarone Intravenous ... 2715
- Cordarone Tablets ... 2712

Amitriptyline Hydrochloride (Concurrent use may increase the therapeutic and toxic effects of both drugs; onset of action of tricyclics may be accelerated). Products include:
- Elavil ... 2838
- Endep Tablets ... 2174
- Etrafon ... 2355
- Limbitrol ... 2180
- Triavil Tablets ... 1757

Amoxapine (Concurrent use may increase the therapeutic and toxic effects of both drugs; onset of action of tricyclics may be accelerated). Products include:
- Asendin Tablets ... 1369

Asparaginase (May inhibit levothyroxine sodium binding to serum proteins or alter the concentrations of serum proteins). Products include:
- Elspar ... 1659

Aspirin (May inhibit levothyroxine sodium binding to serum proteins or alter the concentrations of serum proteins). Products include:
- Alka-Seltzer Effervescent Antacid and Pain Reliever ... ▣ 701
- Alka-Seltzer Extra Strength Effervescent Antacid and Pain Reliever ... ▣ 703
- Alka-Seltzer Lemon Lime Effervescent Antacid and Pain Reliever ... ▣ 703
- Alka-Seltzer Plus Cold Medicine ... ▣ 705
- Alka-Seltzer Plus Cold & Cough Medicine ... ▣ 708
- Alka-Seltzer Plus Night-Time Cold Medicine ... ▣ 707
- Alka Seltzer Plus Sinus Medicine .. ▣ 707
- Arthritis Foundation Safety Coated Aspirin Tablets ... ▣ 675
- Arthritis Pain Ascriptin ... ▣ 631
- Maximum Strength Ascriptin ... ▣ 630
- Regular Strength Ascriptin Tablets ... ▣ 629
- Arthritis Strength BC Powder ... ▣ 609
- BC Cold Powder Multi-Symptom Formula (Cold-Sinus-Allergy) ... ▣ 609
- BC Cold Powder Non-Drowsy Formula (Cold-Sinus) ... ▣ 609
- BC Powder ... ▣ 609
- Bayer Children's Chewable Aspirin ... ▣ 711
- Genuine Bayer Aspirin Tablets & Caplets ... ▣ 713
- Extra Strength Bayer Arthritis Pain Regimen Formula ... ▣ 711
- Extra Strength Bayer Aspirin Caplets & Tablets ... ▣ 712
- Extended-Release Bayer 8-Hour Aspirin ... ▣ 712
- Extra Strength Bayer Plus Aspirin Caplets ... ▣ 713
- Extra Strength Bayer PM Aspirin .. ▣ 713
- Bayer Enteric Aspirin ... ▣ 709
- Bufferin Analgesic Tablets and Caplets ... ▣ 613
- Arthritis Strength Bufferin Analgesic Caplets ... ▣ 614
- Extra Strength Bufferin Analgesic Tablets ... ▣ 615
- Cama Arthritis Pain Reliever ... ▣ 785
- Darvon Compound-65 Pulvules ... 1435
- Easprin ... 1914
- Ecotrin ... 2455
- Ecotrin Enteric Coated Aspirin Maximum Strength Tablets and Caplets ... ▣ 816
- Ecotrin Enteric Coated Aspirin Regular Strength Tablets ... 2455
- Empirin Aspirin Tablets ... ▣ 854
- Empirin with Codeine Tablets ... 1093
- Excedrin Extra-Strength Analgesic Tablets & Caplets ... 732
- Fiorinal Capsules ... 2261
- Fiorinal with Codeine Capsules ... 2262
- Fiorinal Tablets ... 2261
- Halfprin ... 1362
- Healthprin Aspirin ... 2455
- Norgesic ... 1496
- Percodan Tablets ... 939
- Percodan-Demi Tablets ... 940
- Robaxisal Tablets ... 2071
- Soma Compound w/Codeine Tablets ... 2676
- Soma Compound Tablets ... 2675
- St. Joseph Adult Chewable Aspirin (81 mg.) ... ▣ 808
- Talwin Compound ... 2335
- Ursinus Inlay-Tabs ... ▣ 794
- Vanquish Analgesic Caplets ... ▣ 731

Atenolol (Alters thyroid hormone or TSH levels; actions of some beta blockers may be impaired when hypothyroid patients become euthyroid). Products include:
- Tenoretic Tablets ... 2845
- Tenormin Tablets and I.V. Injection 2847

Bendroflumethiazide (Alters thyroid hormone or TSH levels).
- No products indexed under this heading.

Betamethasone Acetate (May inhibit levothyroxine sodium binding to serum proteins or alter the concentrations of serum proteins). Products include:
- Celestone Soluspan Suspension ... 2347

Betamethasone Sodium Phosphate (May inhibit levothyroxine sodium binding to serum proteins or alter the concentrations of serum proteins). Products include:
- Celestone Soluspan Suspension ... 2347

Betaxolol Hydrochloride (Alters thyroid hormone or TSH levels; actions of some beta blockers may be impaired when hypothyroid patients become euthyroid). Products include:
- Betoptic Ophthalmic Solution ... 469
- Betoptic S Ophthalmic Suspension 471
- Kerlone Tablets ... 2436

Bisoprolol Fumarate (Alters thyroid hormone or TSH levels; actions of some beta blockers may be impaired when hypothyroid patients become euthyroid). Products include:
- Zebeta Tablets ... 1413
- Ziac ... 1415

Bromocriptine Mesylate (Alters thyroid hormone or TSH levels). Products include:
- Parlodel ... 2281

Carbamazepine (Alters thyroid hormone or TSH levels). Products include:
- Atretol Tablets ... 573
- Tegretol Chewable Tablets ... 852
- Tegretol Suspension ... 852
- Tegretol Tablets ... 852

Carteolol Hydrochloride (Alters thyroid hormone or TSH levels; actions of some beta blockers may be impaired when hypothyroid patients become euthyroid). Products include:
- Cartrol Tablets ... 410
- Ocupress Ophthalmic Solution, 1% Sterile ... ⊙ 309

IMPORTANT NOTE: Always consult each drug listing in the patient's regimen for possible interactions.

Chloral Hydrate (Alters thyroid hormone or TSH levels).
- No products indexed under this heading.

Chlorothiazide (Alters thyroid hormone or TSH levels). Products include:
- Aldoclor Tablets ... 1598
- Diupres Tablets ... 1650
- Diuril Oral ... 1653

Chlorothiazide Sodium (Alters thyroid hormone or TSH levels). Products include:
- Diuril Sodium Intravenous ... 1652

Chlorotrianisene (Estrogens or estrogen-containing compounds may inhibit levothyroxine sodium binding to serum proteins or alter the concentrations of serum proteins).
- No products indexed under this heading.

Chlorpropamide (Alters thyroid hormone or TSH levels; requirements of oral antidiabetic agents may be reduced in hypothyroid patients with diabetes and may be subsequently increased with initiation of thyroid hormone therapy). Products include:
- Diabinese Tablets ... 1935

Cholestyramine (Binds and decreases absorption of levothyroxine sodium from the gastrointestinal tract). Products include:
- Questran Light ... 769
- Questran Powder ... 770

Choline Magnesium Trisalicylate (May inhibit levothyroxine sodium binding to serum proteins or alter the concentrations of serum proteins). Products include:
- Trilisate ... 2000

Clofibrate (May inhibit levothyroxine sodium binding to serum proteins or alter the concentrations of serum proteins). Products include:
- Atromid-S Capsules ... 2701

Clomipramine Hydrochloride (Concurrent use may increase the therapeutic and toxic effects of both drugs; onset of action of tricyclics may be accelerated). Products include:
- Anafranil Capsules ... 803

Colestipol Hydrochloride (Binds and decreases absorption of levothyroxine sodium from the gastrointestinal tract). Products include:
- Colestid Tablets ... 2591

Cortisone Acetate (May inhibit levothyroxine sodium binding to serum proteins or alter the concentrations of serum proteins). Products include:
- Cortone Acetate Sterile Suspension ... 1623
- Cortone Acetate Tablets ... 1624

Desipramine Hydrochloride (Concurrent use may increase the therapeutic and toxic effects of both drugs; onset of action of tricyclics may be accelerated). Products include:
- Norpramin Tablets ... 1526

Deslanoside (Therapeutic effects of digitalis glycosides may be reduced; serum digitalis levels may be decreased in hyperthyroidism or when a hypothyroid patient becomes euthyroid).
- No products indexed under this heading.

Dexamethasone (May inhibit levothyroxine sodium binding to serum proteins or alter the concentrations of serum proteins). Products include:
- AK-Trol Ointment & Suspension ... ⊙ 205
- Decadron Elixir ... 1633
- Decadron Tablets ... 1635
- Decaspray Topical Aerosol ... 1648
- Dexacidin Ointment ... ⊙ 263
- Maxitrol Ophthalmic Ointment and Suspension ... ⊙ 224
- TobraDex Ophthalmic Suspension and Ointment ... 473

Dexamethasone Acetate (May inhibit levothyroxine sodium binding to serum proteins or alter the concentrations of serum proteins). Products include:
- Dalalone D.P. Injectable ... 1011
- Decadron-LA Sterile Suspension ... 1646

Dexamethasone Sodium Phosphate (May inhibit levothyroxine sodium binding to serum proteins or alter the concentrations of serum proteins). Products include:
- Decadron Phosphate Injection ... 1637
- Decadron Phosphate Respihaler ... 1642
- Decadron Phosphate Sterile Ophthalmic Ointment ... 1641
- Decadron Phosphate Sterile Ophthalmic Solution ... 1642
- Decadron Phosphate Topical Cream ... 1644
- Decadron Phosphate Turbinaire ... 1645
- Decadron Phosphate with Xylocaine Injection, Sterile ... 1639
- Dexacort Phosphate in Respihaler .. 458
- Dexacort Phosphate in Turbinaire .. 459
- NeoDecadron Sterile Ophthalmic Ointment ... 1712
- NeoDecadron Sterile Ophthalmic Solution ... 1713
- NeoDecadron Topical Cream ... 1714

Diatrizoate Meglumine (Alters thyroid hormone or TSH levels).

Diatrizoate Sodium (Alters thyroid hormone or TSH levels).

Diazepam (Alters thyroid hormone or TSH levels). Products include:
- Dizac ... 1809
- Valium Injectable ... 2182
- Valium Tablets ... 2183
- Valrelease Capsules ... 2169

Dicumarol (The hypoprothrombinemic effect of anticoagulants may be potentiated).
- No products indexed under this heading.

Dienestrol (Estrogens or estrogen-containing compounds may inhibit levothyroxine sodium binding to serum proteins or alter the concentrations of serum proteins). Products include:
- Ortho Dienestrol Cream ... 1866

Diethylstilbestrol (Estrogens or estrogen-containing compounds may inhibit levothyroxine sodium binding to serum proteins or alter the concentrations of serum proteins). Products include:
- Diethylstilbestrol Tablets ... 1437

Diflunisal (May inhibit levothyroxine sodium binding to serum proteins or alter the concentrations of serum proteins). Products include:
- Dolobid Tablets ... 1654

Digitoxin (Therapeutic effects of digitalis glycosides may be reduced; serum digitalis levels may be decreased in hyperthyroidism or when a hypothyroid patient becomes euthyroid). Products include:
- Crystodigin Tablets ... 1433

Digoxin (Therapeutic effects of digitalis glycosides may be reduced; serum digitalis levels may be decreased in hyperthyroidism or when a hypothyroid patient becomes euthyroid). Products include:
- Lanoxicaps ... 1117
- Lanoxin Elixir Pediatric ... 1120
- Lanoxin Injection ... 1123
- Lanoxin Injection Pediatric ... 1126
- Lanoxin Tablets ... 1128

Dobutamine Hydrochloride (Possible increased risk of coronary insufficiency in patients with coronary artery disease). Products include:
- Dobutrex Solution Vials ... 1439

Dopamine Hydrochloride (Alters thyroid hormone or TSH levels).
- No products indexed under this heading.

Doxepin Hydrochloride (Concurrent use may increase the therapeutic and toxic effects of both drugs; onset of action of tricyclics may be accelerated). Products include:
- Sinequan ... 2205
- Zonalon Cream ... 1055

Dyphylline (Theophylline clearance may be decreased in hypothyroid patients and return toward normal when euthyroid state is achieved). Products include:
- Lufyllin & Lufyllin-400 Tablets ... 2670
- Lufyllin-GG Elixir & Tablets ... 2671

Ephedrine Hydrochloride (Possible increased risk of coronary insufficiency in patients with coronary artery disease). Products include:
- Primatene Dual Action Formula ... ◘ 872
- Primatene Tablets ... ◘ 873
- Quadrinal Tablets ... 1350

Ephedrine Sulfate (Possible increased risk of coronary insufficiency in patients with coronary artery disease). Products include:
- Bronkaid Caplets ... ◘ 717
- Marax Tablets & DF Syrup ... 2200

Ephedrine Tannate (Possible increased risk of coronary insufficiency in patients with coronary artery disease). Products include:
- Rynatuss ... 2673

Epinephrine (Possible increased risk of coronary insufficiency in patients with coronary artery disease). Products include:
- Bronkaid Mist ... ◘ 717
- EPIFRIN ... ⊙ 239
- EpiPen ... 790
- Marcaine Hydrochloride with Epinephrine 1:200,000 ... 2316
- Primatene Mist ... ◘ 873
- Sensorcaine with Epinephrine Injection ... 559
- Sus-Phrine Injection ... 1019
- Xylocaine with Epinephrine Injections ... 567

Epinephrine Bitartrate (Possible increased risk of coronary insufficiency in patients with coronary artery disease). Products include:
- Bronkaid Mist Suspension ... ◘ 718
- Sensorcaine-MPF with Epinephrine Injection ... 559

Epinephrine Hydrochloride (Possible increased risk of coronary insufficiency in patients with coronary artery disease). Products include:
- Ana-Kit Anaphylaxis Emergency Treatment Kit ... 617

Esmolol Hydrochloride (Alters thyroid hormone or TSH levels; actions of some beta blockers may be impaired when hypothyroid patients become euthyroid). Products include:
- Brevibloc Injection ... 1808

Estradiol (Estrogens or estrogen-containing compounds may inhibit levothyroxine sodium binding to serum proteins or alter the concentrations of serum proteins). Products include:
- Climara Transdermal System ... 645
- Estrace Cream and Tablets ... 749
- Estraderm Transdermal System ... 824

Estrogens, Conjugated (Estrogens or estrogen-containing compounds may inhibit levothyroxine sodium binding to serum proteins or alter the concentrations of serum proteins). Products include:
- PMB 200 and PMB 400 ... 2783
- Premarin Intravenous ... 2787
- Premarin with Methyltestosterone .. 2794
- Premarin Tablets ... 2789
- Premarin Vaginal Cream ... 2791
- Premphase ... 2797
- Prempro ... 2801

Estrogens, Esterified (Estrogens or estrogen-containing compounds may inhibit levothyroxine sodium binding to serum proteins or alter the concentrations of serum proteins). Products include:
- ESTRATAB Tablets (0.3, 0.625, 1.25, 2.5 mg) ... 2536
- Estratest ... 2539
- Menest Tablets ... 2494

Estropipate (Estrogens or estrogen-containing compounds may inhibit levothyroxine sodium binding to serum proteins or alter the concentrations of serum proteins). Products include:
- Ogen Tablets ... 2627
- Ogen Vaginal Cream ... 2630
- Ortho-Est ... 1869

Ethinyl Estradiol (Estrogens or estrogen-containing compounds may inhibit levothyroxine sodium binding to serum proteins or alter the concentrations of serum proteins). Products include:
- Brevicon ... 2088
- Demulen ... 2428
- Desogen Tablets ... 1817
- Levlen/Tri-Levlen ... 651
- Lo/Ovral Tablets ... 2746
- Lo/Ovral-28 Tablets ... 2751
- Modicon ... 1872
- Nordette-21 Tablets ... 2755
- Nordette-28 Tablets ... 2758
- Norinyl ... 2088
- Ortho-Cept ... 1851
- Ortho-Cyclen/Ortho-Tri-Cyclen ... 1858
- Ortho-Novum ... 1872
- Ortho-Cyclen/Ortho Tri-Cyclen ... 1858
- Ovcon ... 760
- Ovral Tablets ... 2770
- Ovral-28 Tablets ... 2770
- Levlen/Tri-Levlen ... 651
- Tri-Norinyl ... 2164
- Triphasil-21 Tablets ... 2814
- Triphasil-28 Tablets ... 2819

Ethiodized Oil (Alters thyroid hormone or TSH levels).
- No products indexed under this heading.

Ethionamide (Alters thyroid hormone or TSH levels). Products include:
- Trecator-SC Tablets ... 2814

Ferrous Sulfate (Binds and decreases absorption of levothyroxine sodium from the gastrointestinal tract). Products include:
- Feosol Capsules ... 2456
- Feosol Elixir ... 2456
- Feosol Tablets ... 2457
- Fero-Folic-500 Filmtab ... 429
- Fero-Grad-500 Filmtab ... 429
- Fero-Gradumet Filmtab ... 429
- Iberet Tablets ... 433
- Iberet-500 Liquid ... 433
- Iberet-Folic-500 Filmtab ... 429
- Iberet-Liquid ... 433
- Irospan ... 982
- Slow Fe Tablets ... 869
- Slow Fe with Folic Acid ... 869

Fludrocortisone Acetate (May inhibit levothyroxine sodium binding to serum proteins or alter the concentrations of serum proteins). Products include:
- Florinef Acetate Tablets ... 505

(◘ Described in PDR For Nonprescription Drugs) (⊙ Described in PDR For Ophthalmology)

Interactions Index — Synthroid

Fluorouracil (May inhibit levothyroxine sodium binding to serum proteins or alter the concentrations of serum proteins). Products include:

Efudex 2113
Fluoroplex Topical Solution & Cream 1% 479
Fluorouracil Injection 2116

Fluoxymesterone (May inhibit levothyroxine sodium binding to serum proteins or alter the concentrations of serum proteins; alters TSH or thyroid hormone levels). Products include:

Halotestin Tablets 2614

Furosemide (May inhibit levothyroxine sodium binding to serum proteins or alter the concentrations of serum proteins). Products include:

Lasix Injection, Oral Solution and Tablets 1240

Gadopentetate Dimeglumine (Alters thyroid hormone or TSH levels).

No products indexed under this heading.

Glipizide (Alters thyroid hormone or TSH levels; requirements of oral antidiabetic agents may be reduced in hypothyroid patients with diabetes and may be subsequently increased with initiation of thyroid hormone therapy). Products include:

Glucotrol Tablets 1967
Glucotrol XL Extended Release Tablets 1968

Glyburide (Alters thyroid hormone or TSH levels; requirements of oral antidiabetic agents may be reduced in hypothyroid patients with diabetes and may be subsequently increased with initiation of thyroid hormone therapy). Products include:

DiaBeta Tablets 1239
Glynase PresTab Tablets 2609
Micronase Tablets 2623

Heparin Sodium (Alters thyroid hormone or TSH levels). Products include:

Heparin Lock Flush Solution 2725
Heparin Sodium Injection 2726
Heparin Sodium Injection, USP, Sterile Solution 2615
Heparin Sodium Vials........................... 1441

Hydrochlorothiazide (Alters thyroid hormone or TSH levels). Products include:

Aldactazide... 2413
Aldoril Tablets 1604
Apresazide Capsules 808
Capozide 742
Dyazide 2479
Esidrix Tablets 821
Esimil Tablets 822
HydroDIURIL Tablets 1674
Hydropres Tablets................................ 1675
Hyzaar Tablets 1677
Inderide Tablets 2732
Inderide LA Long Acting Capsules .. 2734
Lopressor HCT Tablets 832
Lotensin HCT....................................... 837
Maxzide 1380
Moduretic Tablets 1705
Oretic Tablets 443
Prinzide Tablets 1737
Ser-Ap-Es Tablets 849
Timolide Tablets................................... 1748
Vaseretic Tablets.................................. 1765
Zestoretic 2850
Ziac 1415

Hydrocortisone (May inhibit levothyroxine sodium binding to serum proteins or alter the concentrations of serum proteins). Products include:

Anusol-HC Cream 2.5% 1896
Aquanil HC Lotion 1931
Bactine Hydrocortisone Anti-Itch Cream .... ◆□ 709
Caldecort Anti-Itch Hydrocortisone Spray .... ◆□ 631
Cortaid .... ◆□ 836
CORTENEMA.. 2535
Cortisporin Ointment 1085
Cortisporin Ophthalmic Ointment Sterile 1085
Cortisporin Ophthalmic Suspension Sterile 1086
Cortisporin Otic Solution Sterile 1087
Cortisporin Otic Suspension Sterile 1088
Cortizone-5 .... ◆□ 831
Cortizone-10 .... ◆□ 831
Hydrocortone Tablets 1672
Hytone 907
Massengill Medicated Soft Cloth Towelettes.. 2458
PediOtic Suspension Sterile 1153
Preparation H Hydrocortisone 1% Cream .... ◆□ 872
ProctoCream-HC 2.5% 2408
VōSoL HC Otic Solution....................... 2678

Hydrocortisone Acetate (May inhibit levothyroxine sodium binding to serum proteins or alter the concentrations of serum proteins). Products include:

Analpram-HC Rectal Cream 1% and 2.5% 977
Anusol HC-1 Anti-Itch Hydrocortisone Ointment.................................... ◆□ 847
Anusol-HC Suppositories 1897
Caldecort... ◆□ 631
Carmol HC 924
Coly-Mycin S Otic w/Neomycin & Hydrocortisone 1906
Cortaid .... ◆□ 836
Cortifoam 2396
Cortisporin Cream................................ 1084
Epifoam 2399
Hydrocortone Acetate Sterile Suspension.. 1669
Mantadil Cream 1135
Nupercainal Hydrocortisone 1% Cream .... ◆□ 645
Ophthocort .... ⊙ 311
Pramosone Cream, Lotion & Ointment 978
ProctoCream-HC 2408
ProctoFoam-HC 2409
Terra-Cortril Ophthalmic Suspension 2210

Hydrocortisone Sodium Phosphate (May inhibit levothyroxine sodium binding to serum proteins or alter the concentrations of serum proteins). Products include:

Hydrocortone Phosphate Injection, Sterile 1670

Hydrocortisone Sodium Succinate (May inhibit levothyroxine sodium binding to serum proteins or alter the concentrations of serum proteins). Products include:

Solu-Cortef Sterile Powder.................. 2641

Hydroflumethiazide (Alters thyroid hormone or TSH levels). Products include:

Diucardin Tablets................................. 2718

Imipramine Hydrochloride (Concurrent use may increase the therapeutic and toxic effects of both drugs; onset of action of tricyclics may be accelerated). Products include:

Tofranil Ampuls 854
Tofranil Tablets 856

Imipramine Pamoate (Concurrent use may increase the therapeutic and toxic effects of both drugs; onset of action of tricyclics may be accelerated). Products include:

Tofranil-PM Capsules........................... 857

Insulin, Human (Requirements of insulin may be reduced in hypothyroid patients with diabetes and may be subsequently increased with initiation of thyroid hormone therapy).

No products indexed under this heading.

Insulin, Human Isophane Suspension (Requirements of insulin may be reduced in hypothyroid patients with diabetes and may be subsequently increased with initiation of thyroid hormone therapy). Products include:

Novolin N Human Insulin 10 ml Vials 1795

Insulin, Human NPH (Requirements of insulin may be reduced in hypothyroid patients with diabetes and may be subsequently increased with initiation of thyroid hormone therapy). Products include:

Humulin N, 100 Units 1448
Novolin N PenFill Cartridges Durable Insulin Delivery System 1798
Novolin N Prefilled Syringe Disposable Insulin Delivery System 1798

Insulin, Human Regular (Requirements of insulin may be reduced in hypothyroid patients with diabetes and may be subsequently increased with initiation of thyroid hormone therapy). Products include:

Humulin R, 100 Units 1449
Novolin R Human Insulin 10 ml Vials 1795
Novolin R PenFill Cartridges Durable Insulin Delivery System 1798
Novolin R Prefilled Syringe Disposable Insulin Delivery System 1798
Velosulin BR Human Insulin 10 ml Vials 1795

Insulin, Human, Zinc Suspension (Requirements of insulin may be reduced in hypothyroid patients with diabetes and may be subsequently increased with initiation of thyroid hormone therapy). Products include:

Humulin L, 100 Units 1446
Humulin U, 100 Units 1450
Novolin L Human Insulin 10 ml Vials 1795

Insulin, NPH (Requirements of insulin may be reduced in hypothyroid patients with diabetes and may be subsequently increased with initiation of thyroid hormone therapy). Products include:

NPH, 100 Units 1450
Pork NPH, 100 Units........................... 1452
Purified Pork NPH Isophane Insulin 1801

Insulin, Regular (Requirements of insulin may be reduced in hypothyroid patients with diabetes and may be subsequently increased with initiation of thyroid hormone therapy). Products include:

Regular, 100 Units 1450
Pork Regular, 100 Units 1452
Pork Regular (Concentrated), 500 Units 1453
Purified Pork Regular Insulin 1801

Insulin, Zinc Crystals (Requirements of insulin may be reduced in hypothyroid patients with diabetes and may be subsequently increased with initiation of thyroid hormone therapy). Products include:

NPH, 100 Units 1450

Insulin, Zinc Suspension (Requirements of insulin may be reduced in hypothyroid patients with diabetes and may be subsequently increase with initiation of thyroid hormone therapy). Products include:

Iletin I 1450
Lente, 100 Units 1450
Iletin II.. 1452
Pork Lente, 100 Units.......................... 1452
Purified Pork Lente Insulin 1801

Interferon alfa-2A, Recombinant (Cytokines have been reported to induce both hyperthyroidism or hypothyroidism; dosage adjustment may be necessary). Products include:

Roferon-A Injection 2145

Interferon alfa-2B, Recombinant (Cytokines have been reported to induce both hyperthyroidism or hypothyroidism; dosage adjustment may be necessary). Products include:

Intron A 2364

Interferon Alfa-N3 (Human Leukocyte Derived) (Cytokines have been reported to induce both hyperthyroidism or hypothyroidism; dosage adjustment may be necessary).

No products indexed under this heading.

Interferon Beta-1b (Cytokines have been reported to induce both hyperthyroidism or hypothyroidism; dosage adjustment may be necessary). Products include:

Betaseron for SC Injection................... 658

Interferon Gamma-1B (Cytokines have been reported to induce both hyperthyroidism or hypothyroidism; dosage adjustment may be necessary). Products include:

Actimmune 1056

Iodamide Meglumine (Alters thyroid hormone or TSH levels).

No products indexed under this heading.

Iodinated Glycerol (Alters thyroid hormone or TSH levels).

No products indexed under this heading.

Iodine, radiolabeled (Uptake of radiolabeled ions may be decreased).

Iohexol (Alters thyroid hormone or TSH levels).

No products indexed under this heading.

Iopamidol (Alters thyroid hormone or TSH levels).

No products indexed under this heading.

Iothalamate Meglumine (Alters thyroid hormone or TSH levels).

No products indexed under this heading.

Iopanoic Acid (Alters thyroid hormone or TSH levels).

Ioxaglate Meglumine (Alters thyroid hormone or TSH levels).

No products indexed under this heading.

Ioxaglate Sodium (Alters thyroid hormone or TSH levels).

No products indexed under this heading.

Isoproterenol Hydrochloride (Possible increased risk of coronary insufficiency in patients with coronary artery disease). Products include:

Isuprel Hydrochloride Injection 1:5000 2311
Isuprel Hydrochloride Solution 1:200 & 1:100 2313
Isuprel Mistometer 2312

Isoproterenol Sulfate (Possible increased risk of coronary insufficiency in patients with coronary artery disease). Products include:

Norisodrine with Calcium Iodide Syrup... 442

Ketamine Hydrochloride (Co-administration produces marked hypertension and tachycardia).

No products indexed under this heading.

IMPORTANT NOTE: Always consult each drug listing in the patient's regimen for possible interactions.

Synthroid Interactions Index 998

Labetalol Hydrochloride (Alters thyroid hormone or TSH levels; actions of some beta blockers may be impaired when hypothyroid patients become euthyroid). Products include:
- Normodyne Injection ... 2377
- Normodyne Tablets ... 2379
- Trandate ... 1185

Levobunolol Hydrochloride (Alters thyroid hormone or TSH levels; actions of some beta blockers may be impaired when hypothyroid patients become euthyroid). Products include:
- Betagan ... ⊙ 233

Levodopa (Alters thyroid hormone or TSH levels). Products include:
- Atamet ... 572
- Larodopa Tablets ... 2129
- Sinemet Tablets ... 943
- Sinemet CR Tablets ... 944

Lithium Carbonate (Alters thyroid hormone or TSH levels). Products include:
- Eskalith ... 2485
- Lithium Carbonate Capsules & Tablets ... 2230
- Lithonate/Lithotabs/Lithobid ... 2543

Lithium Citrate (Alters thyroid hormone or TSH levels).
- No products indexed under this heading.

Lovastatin (Alters thyroid hormone or TSH levels). Products include:
- Mevacor Tablets ... 1699

Magnesium Salicylate (May inhibit levothyroxine sodium binding to serum proteins or alter the concentrations of serum proteins). Products include:
- Backache Caplets ... ▣ 613
- Bayer Select Backache Pain Relief Formula ... ▣ 715
- Doan's Extra-Strength Analgesic ... ▣ 633
- Extra Strength Doan's P.M. ... ▣ 633
- Doan's Regular Strength Analgesic ... ▣ 634
- Mobigesic Tablets ... ▣ 602

Maprotiline Hydrochloride (Concurrent use may increase the therapeutic and toxic effects of both drugs; onset of action of tricyclics may be acelerated; risk of cardiac arrhythmias may increase). Products include:
- Ludiomil Tablets ... 843

Meclofenamate Sodium (Meclofenamic acid may inhibit levothyroxine sodium binding to serum proteins or alter the concentrations of serum proteins).
- No products indexed under this heading.

Mefenamic Acid (May inhibit levothyroxine sodium binding to serum proteins or alter the concentrations of serum proteins). Products include:
- Ponstel ... 1925

Mercaptopurine (Alters thyroid hormone or TSH levels). Products include:
- Purinethol Tablets ... 1156

Metaproterenol Sulfate (Possible increased risk of coronary insufficiency in patients with coronary artery disease). Products include:
- Alupent ... 669
- Metaproterenol Sulfate Inhalation Solution, USP, Arm-a-Med ... 552

Metaraminol Bitartrate (Possible increased risk of coronary insufficiency in patients with coronary artery disease). Products include:
- Aramine Injection ... 1609

Metformin Hydrochloride (Requirements of oral antidiabetic agents may be reduced in hypothyroid patients with diabetes and may be subsequently increased with initiation of thyroid hormone therapy). Products include:
- Glucophage ... 752

Methadone Hydrochloride (May inhibit levothyroxine sodium binding to serum proteins or alter the concentrations of serum proteins). Products include:
- Methadone Hydrochloride Oral Concentrate ... 2233
- Methadone Hydrochloride Oral Solution & Tablets ... 2235

Methimazole (Alters thyroid hormone or TSH levels). Products include:
- Tapazole Tablets ... 1477

Methoxamine Hydrochloride (Possible increased risk of coronary insufficiency in patients with coronary artery disease). Products include:
- Vasoxyl Injection ... 1196

Methyclothiazide (Alters thyroid hormone or TSH levels). Products include:
- Enduron Tablets ... 420

Methylprednisolone Acetate (May inhibit levothyroxine sodium binding to serum proteins or alter the concentrations of serum proteins). Products include:
- Depo-Medrol Single-Dose Vial ... 2600
- Depo-Medrol Sterile Aqueous Suspension ... 2597

Methylprednisolone Sodium Succinate (May inhibit levothyroxine sodium binding to serum proteins or alter the concentrations of serum proteins). Products include:
- Solu-Medrol Sterile Powder ... 2643

Methyltestosterone (May inhibit levothyroxine sodium binding to serum proteins or alter the concentrations of serum proteins; alters TSH or thyroid hormone levels). Products include:
- Android Capsules, 10 mg ... 1250
- Android ... 1251
- Estratest ... 2539
- Oreton Methyl ... 1255
- Premarin with Methyltestosterone ... 2794
- Testred Capsules ... 1262

Metipranolol Hydrochloride (Alters thyroid hormone or TSH levels; actions of some beta blockers may be impaired when hypothyroid patients become euthyroid). Products include:
- OptiPranolol (Metipranolol 0.3%) Sterile Ophthalmic Solution ... ⊙ 258

Metoclopramide Hydrochloride (Alters thyroid hormone or TSH levels). Products include:
- Reglan ... 2068

Metoprolol Succinate (Alters thyroid hormone or TSH levels; actions of some beta blockers may be impaired when hypothyroid patients become euthyroid). Products include:
- Toprol-XL Tablets ... 565

Metoprolol Tartrate (Alters thyroid hormone or TSH levels; actions of some beta blockers may be impaired when hypothyroid patients become euthyroid). Products include:
- Lopressor Ampuls ... 830
- Lopressor HCT Tablets ... 832
- Lopressor Tablets ... 830

Mitotane (Alters thyroid hormone or TSH levels). Products include:
- Lysodren ... 698

Nadolol (Alters thyroid hormone or TSH levels; actions of some beta blockers may be impaired when hypothyroid patients become euthyroid).
- No products indexed under this heading.

Norepinephrine Bitartrate (Possible increased risk of coronary insufficiency in patients with coronary artery disease). Products include:
- Levophed Bitartrate Injection ... 2315

Nortriptyline Hydrochloride (Concurrent use may increase the therapeutic and toxic effects of both drugs; onset of action of tricyclics may be accelerated). Products include:
- Pamelor ... 2280

Octreotide Acetate (Alters thyroid hormone or TSH levels). Products include:
- Sandostatin Injection ... 2292

Oxandrolone (May inhibit levothyroxine sodium binding to serum proteins or alter the concentrations of serum proteins; alters TSH or thyroid hormone levels). Products include:
- Oxandrin ... 2862

Oxymetholone (May inhibit levothyroxine sodium binding to serum proteins or alter the concentrations of serum proteins; alters TSH or thyroid hormone levels).
- No products indexed under this heading.

Penbutolol Sulfate (Alters thyroid hormone or TSH levels; actions of some beta blockers may be impaired when hypothyroid patients become euthyroid). Products include:
- Levatol ... 2403

Pergolide Mesylate (Alters thyroid hormone or TSH levels). Products include:
- Permax Tablets ... 575

Perphenazine (May inhibit levothyroxine sodium binding to serum proteins or alter the concentrations of serum proteins). Products include:
- Etrafon ... 2355
- Triavil Tablets ... 1757
- Trilafon ... 2389

Phenobarbital (Alters thyroid hormone or TSH levels). Products include:
- Arco-Lase Plus Tablets ... 512
- Bellergal-S Tablets ... 2250
- Donnatal ... 2060
- Donnatal Extentabs ... 2061
- Donnatal Tablets ... 2060
- Phenobarbital Elixir and Tablets ... 1469
- Quadrinal Tablets ... 1350

Phenylbutazone (May inhibit levothyroxine sodium binding to serum proteins or alter the concentrations of serum proteins).
- No products indexed under this heading.

Phenylephrine Bitartrate (Possible increased risk of coronary insufficiency in patients with coronary artery disease).
- No products indexed under this heading.

Phenylephrine Hydrochloride (Possible increased risk of coronary insufficiency in patients with coronary artery disease). Products include:
- Atrohist Plus Tablets ... 454
- Cerose DM ... ▣ 878
- Comhist ... 2038
- D.A. Chewable Tablets ... 951
- Deconsal Pediatric Capsules ... 454
- Dura-Vent/DA Tablets ... 953
- Entex Capsules ... 1986
- Entex Liquid ... 1986
- Extendryl ... 1005
- 4-Way Fast Acting Nasal Spray (regular & mentholated) ... ▣ 621
- Hemorid For Women ... ▣ 834
- Hycomine Compound Tablets ... 932
- Neo-Synephrine Hydrochloride 1% Carpuject ... 2324
- Neo-Synephrine Hydrochloride 1% Injection ... 2324
- Neo-Synephrine Hydrochloride (Ophthalmic) ... 2325
- Neo-Synephrine ... ▣ 726
- Nōstril ... ▣ 644
- Novahistine Elixir ... ▣ 823
- Phenergan VC ... 2779
- Phenergan VC with Codeine ... 2781
- Preparation H ... ▣ 871
- Tympagesic Ear Drops ... 2342
- Vasosulf ... ⊙ 271
- Vicks Sinex Nasal Spray and Ultra Fine Mist ... ▣ 765

Phenylephrine Tannate (Possible increased risk of coronary insufficiency in patients with coronary artery disease). Products include:
- Atrohist Pediatric Suspension ... 454
- Ricobid-D Pediatric Suspension ... 2038
- Ricobid Tablets and Pediatric Suspension ... 2038
- Rynatan ... 2673
- Rynatuss ... 2673

Phenylpropanolamine Hydrochloride (Possible increased risk of coronary insufficiency in patients with coronary artery disease). Products include:
- Acutrim ... ▣ 628
- Allerest Children's Chewable Tablets ... ▣ 627
- Allerest 12 Hour Caplets ... ▣ 627
- Atrohist Plus Tablets ... 454
- BC Cold Powder Multi-Symptom Formula (Cold-Sinus-Allergy) ... ▣ 609
- BC Cold Powder Non-Drowsy Formula (Cold-Sinus) ... ▣ 609
- Cheracol Plus Head Cold/Cough Formula ... ▣ 769
- Comtrex Multi-Symptom Non-Drowsy Liqui-gels ... ▣ 618
- Contac Continuous Action Nasal Decongestant/Antihistamine 12 Hour Capsules ... ▣ 813
- Contac Maximum Strength Continuous Action Decongestant/Antihistamine 12 Hour Caplets ... ▣ 813
- Contac Severe Cold and Flu Formula Caplets ... ▣ 814
- Coricidin 'D' Decongestant Tablets ... ▣ 800
- Dexatrim ... ▣ 832
- Dexatrim Plus Vitamins Caplets ... ▣ 832
- Dimetane-DC Cough Syrup ... 2059
- Dimetapp Elixir ... ▣ 773
- Dimetapp Extentabs ... ▣ 774
- Dimetapp Tablets/Liqui-Gels ... ▣ 775
- Dimetapp Cold & Allergy Chewable Tablets ... ▣ 773
- Dimetapp DM Elixir ... ▣ 774
- Dura-Vent Tablets ... 952
- Entex Capsules ... 1986
- Entex LA Tablets ... 1987
- Entex Liquid ... 1986
- Exgest LA Tablets ... 782
- Hycomine ... 931
- Isoclor Timesule Capsules ... ▣ 637
- Nolamine Timed-Release Tablets ... 785
- Ornade Spansule Capsules ... 2502
- Propagest Tablets ... 786
- Pyrroxate Caplets ... ▣ 772
- Robitussin-CF ... ▣ 777
- Sinulin Tablets ... 787
- Tavist-D 12 Hour Relief Tablets ... ▣ 787
- Teldrin 12 Hour Antihistamine/Nasal Decongestant Allergy Relief Capsules ... ▣ 826
- Triaminic Allergy Tablets ... ▣ 789
- Triaminic Cold Tablets ... ▣ 790
- Triaminic Expectorant ... ▣ 790
- Triaminic Syrup ... ▣ 792
- Triaminic-12 Tablets ... ▣ 792
- Triaminic-DM Syrup ... ▣ 792
- Triaminicin Tablets ... ▣ 793
- Triaminicol Multi-Symptom Cold Tablets ... ▣ 793
- Triaminicol Multi-Symptom Relief ▣ 794
- Vicks DayQuil Allergy Relief 12-Hour Extended Release Tablets ... ▣ 760
- Vicks DayQuil Allergy Relief 4-Hour Tablets ... ▣ 760

(▣ Described in PDR For Nonprescription Drugs) (⊙ Described in PDR For Ophthalmology)

Interactions Index — Synthroid

Vicks DayQuil SINUS Pressure & CONGESTION Relief .... ✦◆ 761

Phenytoin (May inhibit levothyroxine sodium binding to serum proteins or alter the concentrations of serum proteins; alters thyroid hormone or TSH levels). Products include:

Dilantin Infatabs 1908
Dilantin-125 Suspension 1911

Phenytoin Sodium (May inhibit levothyroxine sodium binding to serum proteins or alter the concentrations of serum proteins; alters thyroid hormone or TSH levels). Products include:

Dilantin Kapseals 1906
Dilantin Parenteral 1910

Pindolol (Alters thyroid hormone or TSH levels; actions of some beta blockers may be impaired when hypothyroid patients become euthyroid). Products include:

Visken Tablets 2299

Pirbuterol Acetate (Possible increased risk of coronary insufficiency in patients with coronary artery disease). Products include:

Maxair Autohaler 1492
Maxair Inhaler 1494

Polyestradiol Phosphate (Estrogens or estrogen-containing compounds may inhibit levothyroxine sodium binding to serum proteins or alter the concentrations of serum proteins).

No products indexed under this heading.

Polythiazide (Alters thyroid hormone or TSH levels). Products include:

Minizide Capsules 1938

Prednisolone Acetate (May inhibit levothyroxine sodium binding to serum proteins or alter the concentrations of serum proteins). Products include:

AK-CIDE .... ◉ 202
AK-CIDE Ointment .... ◉ 202
Blephamide Liquifilm Sterile Ophthalmic Suspension 476
Blephamide Ointment .... ◉ 237
Econopred & Econopred Plus Ophthalmic Suspensions .... ◉ 217
Poly-Pred Liquifilm .... ◉ 248
Pred Forte .... ◉ 250
Pred Mild .... ◉ 253
Pred-G Liquifilm Sterile Ophthalmic Suspension .... ◉ 251
Pred-G S.O.P. Sterile Ophthalmic Ointment .... ◉ 252
Vasocidin Ointment .... ◉ 268

Prednisolone Sodium Phosphate (May inhibit levothyroxine sodium binding to serum proteins or alter the concentrations of serum proteins). Products include:

AK-Pred .... ◉ 204
Hydeltrasol Injection, Sterile 1665
Inflamase .... ◉ 265
Pediapred Oral Liquid 995
Vasocidin Ophthalmic Solution ...... ◉ 270

Prednisolone Tebutate (May inhibit levothyroxine sodium binding to serum proteins or alter the concentrations of serum proteins). Products include:

Hydeltra-T.B.A. Sterile Suspension 1667

Prednisone (May inhibit levothyroxine sodium binding to serum proteins or alter the concentrations of serum proteins). Products include:

Deltasone Tablets 2595

Propranolol Hydrochloride (Alters thyroid hormone or TSH levels; actions of some beta blockers may be impaired when hypothyroid patients become euthyroid). Products include:

Inderal 2728
Inderal LA Long Acting Capsules 2730
Inderide Tablets 2732
Inderide LA Long Acting Capsules .. 2734

Protriptyline Hydrochloride (Concurrent use may increase the therapeutic and toxic effects of both drugs; onset of action of tricyclics may be accelerated). Products include:

Vivactil Tablets 1774

Pseudoephedrine Hydrochloride (Possible increased risk of coronary insufficiency in patients with coronary artery disease). Products include:

Actifed Allergy Daytime/Nighttime Caplets .... ✦◆ 844
Actifed Plus Caplets .... ✦◆ 845
Actifed Plus Tablets .... ✦◆ 845
Actifed with Codeine Cough Syrup.. 1067
Actifed Sinus Daytime/Nighttime Tablets and Caplets .... ✦◆ 846
Actifed Syrup .... ✦◆ 846
Actifed Tablets .... ✦◆ 844
Advil Cold and Sinus Caplets and Tablets (formerly CoAdvil) .... ✦◆ 870
Alka-Seltzer Plus Cold Medicine Liqui-Gels .... ✦◆ 706
Alka-Seltzer Plus Cold & Cough Medicine Liqui-Gels .... ✦◆ 705
Alka-Seltzer Plus Night-Time Cold Medicine Liqui-Gels .... ✦◆ 706
Allerest Headache Strength Tablets .... ✦◆ 627
Allerest Maximum Strength Tablets .... ✦◆ 627
Allerest No Drowsiness Tablets ...... ✦◆ 627
Allerest Sinus Pain Formula .... ✦◆ 627
Anatuss LA Tablets 1542
Atrohist Pediatric Capsules 453
Bayer Select Sinus Pain Relief Formula .... ✦◆ 717
Benadryl Allergy Decongestant Liquid Medication .... ✦◆ 848
Benadryl Allergy Decongestant Tablets .... ✦◆ 848
Benadryl Allergy Sinus Headache Formula Caplets .... ✦◆ 849
Benylin Multisymptom .... ✦◆ 852
Bromfed Capsules (Extended-Release) 1785
Bromfed Syrup .... ✦◆ 733
Bromfed Tablets 1785
Bromfed-DM Cough Syrup 1786
Bromfed-PD Capsules (Extended-Release) 1785
Children's Vicks DayQuil Allergy Relief .... ✦◆ 757
Children's Vicks NyQuil Cold/ Cough Relief .... ✦◆ 758
Comtrex Multi-Symptom Cold Reliever Tablets/Caplets/Liqui-Gels/Liquid .... ✦◆ 615
Allergy-Sinus Comtrex Multi-Symptom Allergy-Sinus Formula Tablets .... ✦◆ 617
Comtrex Multi-Symptom Non-Drowsy Caplets .... ✦◆ 618
Congess 1004
Contac Day Allergy/Sinus Caplets ✦◆ 812
Contac Day & Night .... ✦◆ 812
Contac Night Allergy/Sinus Caplets .... ✦◆ 812
Contac Severe Cold & Flu Non-Drowsy .... ✦◆ 815
Deconamine Chewable Tablets 1320
Deconamine CX Cough and Cold Liquid and Tablets 1319
Deconamine 1320
Deconsal C Expectorant Syrup 456
Deconsal Pediatric Syrup 457
Deconsal II Tablets 454
Dimetane-DX Cough Syrup 2059
Dimetapp Sinus Caplets .... ✦◆ 775
Dorcol Children's Cough Syrup ...... ✦◆ 785
Drixoral Cough + Congestion Liquid Caps .... ✦◆ 802
Dura-Tap/PD Capsules 2867
Duratuss Tablets 2565
Duratuss HD Elixir 2565
Efidac/24 .... ✦◆ 635

Entex PSE Tablets 1987
Fedahist Gyrocaps 2401
Fedahist Timecaps 2401
Guaifed 1787
Guaifed Syrup .... ✦◆ 734
Guaimax-D Tablets 792
Guaitab Tablets .... ✦◆ 734
Isoclor Expectorant 990
Kronofed-A 977
Motrin IB Sinus .... ✦◆ 838
Novahistine DH 2462
Novahistine DMX .... ✦◆ 822
Novahistine Expectorant 2463
Nucofed 2051
PediaCare Cold Allergy Chewable Tablets .... ✦◆ 677
PediaCare Cough-Cold Chewable Tablets 1553
PediaCare 1553
PediaCare Infants' Decongestant Drops .... ✦◆ 677
PediCare Infant's Drops Decongestant Plus Cough 1553
PediaCare NightRest Cough-Cold Liquid 1553
Pediatric Vicks 44d Dry Hacking Cough & Head Congestion .... ✦◆ 763
Pediatric Vicks 44m Cough & Cold Relief .... ✦◆ 764
Robitussin Cold & Cough Liqui-Gels .... ✦◆ 776
Robitussin Maximum Strength Cough & Cold .... ✦◆ 778
Robitussin Pediatric Cough & Cold Formula .... ✦◆ 779
Robitussin Severe Congestion Liqui-Gels .... ✦◆ 776
Robitussin-DAC Syrup 2074
Robitussin-PE .... ✦◆ 778
Rondec Oral Drops 953
Rondec Syrup 953
Rondec Tablet 953
Rondec-DM Oral Drops 954
Rondec-DM Syrup 954
Rondec-TR Tablet 953
Ryna .... ✦◆ 841
Seldane-D Extended-Release Tablets 1538
Semprex-D Capsules 463
Semprex-D Capsules 1167
Sinarest Tablets .... ✦◆ 648
Sinarest Extra Strength Tablets .... ✦◆ 648
Sinarest No Drowsiness Tablets .... ✦◆ 648
Sine-Aid IB Caplets 1554
Sine-Aid Maximum Strength Sinus Medication Gelcaps, Caplets and Tablets 1554
Sine-Off No Drowsiness Formula Caplets .... ✦◆ 824
Sine-Off Sinus Medicine .... ✦◆ 825
Singlet Tablets .... ✦◆ 825
Sinutab Non-Drying Liquid Caps .... ✦◆ 859
Sinutab Sinus Allergy Medication, Maximum Strength Tablets and Caplets .... ✦◆ 860
Sinutab Sinus Medication, Maximum Strength Without Drowsiness Formula, Tablets & Caplets .... ✦◆ 860
Sinutab Sinus Medication, Regular Strength Without Drowsiness Formula .... ✦◆ 859
Sudafed Children's Liquid .... ✦◆ 861
Sudafed Cold and Cough Liquidcaps .... ✦◆ 862
Sudafed Cough Syrup .... ✦◆ 862
Sudafed Plus Liquid .... ✦◆ 862
Sudafed Plus Tablets .... ✦◆ 863
Sudafed Severe Cold Formula Caplets .... ✦◆ 863
Sudafed Severe Cold Formula Tablets .... ✦◆ 864
Sudafed Sinus Caplets .... ✦◆ 864
Sudafed Sinus Tablets .... ✦◆ 864
Sudafed Tablets, 30 mg .... ✦◆ 861
Sudafed Tablets, 60 mg .... ✦◆ 861
Sudafed 12 Hour Caplets .... ✦◆ 861
Syn-Rx Tablets 465
Syn-Rx DM Tablets 466
TheraFlu .... ✦◆ 787
TheraFlu Maximum Strength Nighttime Flu, Cold & Cough Medicine .... ✦◆ 788
TheraFlu Maximum Strength Non-Drowsy Formula Flu, Cold & Cough Medicine .... ✦◆ 788
Thera Flu Maximum Strength, Non-Drowsy Formula Flu, Cold and Cough Caplets .... ✦◆ 789
Triaminic AM Cough and Decongestant Formula .... ✦◆ 789

Triaminic AM Decongestant Formula .... ✦◆ 790
Triaminic Nite Light .... ✦◆ 791
Triaminic Sore Throat Formula ...... ✦◆ 791
Tussend 1783
Tussend Expectorant 1785
Children's TYLENOL Cold Multi-Symptom Liquid Formula and Chewable Tablets 1561
Children's TYLENOL Cold Plus Cough Multi Symptom Tablets and Liquid .... ✦◆ 681
Infants' TYLENOL Cold Decongestant & Fever-Reducer Drops 1556
TYLENOL Maximum Strength Allergy Sinus Medication Gelcaps and Caplets 1563
TYLENOL Maximum Strength Allergy Sinus NightTime Medication Caplets 1555
TYLENOL Flu Maximum Strength Gelcaps 1565
TYLENOL Flu NightTime, Maximum Strength, Gelcaps 1566
TYLENOL Maximum Strength Flu NightTime Hot Medication Packets 1562
TYLENOL, Maximum Strength, Sinus Medication Geltabs, Gelcaps, Caplets and Tablets 1566
TYLENOL Cold Multi-Symptom Formula Medication Tablets and Caplets 1561
TYLENOL Cold Medication No Drowsiness Formula Gelcaps and Caplets 1562
TYLENOL Cold Multi-Symptom Hot Medication Liquid Packets 1557
TYLENOL Cough Multi-Symptom Medication with Decongestant 1565
Ursinus Inlay-Tabs .... ✦◆ 794
Vicks 44 LiquiCaps Cough, Cold & Flu Relief .... ✦◆ 755
Vicks 44 LiquiCaps Non-Drowsy Cough & Cold Relief .... ✦◆ 756
Vicks 44D Dry Hacking Cough & Head Congestion .... ✦◆ 755
Vicks 44M Cough, Cold & Flu Relief .... ✦◆ 756
Vicks DayQuil .... ✦◆ 761
Vicks DayQuil SINUS Pressure & PAIN Relief with IBUPROFEN ...... ✦◆ 762
Vicks Nyquil Hot Therapy .... ✦◆ 762
Vicks NyQuil LiquiCaps Multi-Symptom Cold/Flu Relief .... ✦◆ 763
Vicks NyQuil Multi-Symptom Cold/Flu Relief - (Original & Cherry Flavor) .... ✦◆ 763

Pseudoephedrine Sulfate (Possible increased risk of coronary insufficiency in patients with coronary artery disease). Products include:

Cheracol Sinus .... ✦◆ 768
Chlor-Trimeton Allergy Decongestant Tablets .... ✦◆ 799
Claritin-D 2350
Drixoral Cold and Allergy Sustained-Action Tablets .... ✦◆ 802
Drixoral Cold and Flu Extended-Release Tablets .... ✦◆ 803
Drixoral Non-Drowsy Formula Extended-Release Tablets .... ✦◆ 803
Drixoral Allergy/Sinus Extended Release Tablets .... ✦◆ 804
Trinalin Repetabs Tablets 1330

Quinestrol (Estrogens or estrogen-containing compounds may inhibit levothyroxine sodium binding to serum proteins or alter the concentrations of serum proteins).

No products indexed under this heading.

Resorcinol (Alters thyroid hormone or TSH levels). Products include:

BiCozene Creme .... ✦◆ 785

Rifampin (Alters thyroid hormone or TSH levels). Products include:

Rifadin 1528
Rifamate Capsules 1530
Rifater 1532
Rimactane Capsules 847

Salmeterol Xinafoate (Possible increased risk of coronary insufficiency in patients with coronary artery disease). Products include:

Serevent Inhalation Aerosol 1176

IMPORTANT NOTE: Always consult each drug listing in the patient's regimen for possible interactions.

Salsalate (May inhibit levothyroxine sodium binding to serum proteins or alter the concentrations of serum proteins). Products include:

Mono-Gesic Tablets 792
Salflex Tablets 786

Sodium Iodide I 123 (Uptake of radiolabeled ions may be decreased).

Sodium Iodide I 131 (Uptake of radiolabeled ions may be decreased).

Sodium Nitroprusside (Alters thyroid hormone or TSH levels).

No products indexed under this heading.

Sodium Pertechnetate (Alters thyroid hormone or TSH levels).

Sodium Polystyrene Sulfonate (Binds and decreases absorption of levothyroxine sodium from the gastrointestinal tract). Products include:

Kayexalate 2314
Sodium Polystyrene Sulfonate Suspension 2244

Somatrem (Excessive concurrent use of thyroid hormone may accelerate epiphyseal closure; untreated hypothyroidism may interfere with the growth response to somatrem). Products include:

Protropin 1063

Somatropin (Excessive concurrent use of thyroid hormone may accelerate epiphyseal closure; untreated hypothyroidism may interfere with the growth response to somatrem). Products include:

Genotropin 006
Humatrope Vials 1443
Nutropin 1061

Sotalol Hydrochloride (Alters thyroid hormone or TSH levels; actions of some beta blockers may be impaired when hypothyroid patients become euthyroid). Products include:

Betapace Tablets 641

Stanozolol (May inhibit levothyroxine sodium binding to serum proteins or alter the concentrations of serum proteins; alters TSH or thyroid hormone levels). Products include:

Winstrol Tablets 2337

Sucralfate (Binds and decreases absorption of levothyroxine sodium from the gastrointestinal tract). Products include:

Carafate Suspension 1505
Carafate Tablets 1504

Sulfacytine (Alters thyroid hormone or TSH levels).

Sulfamethizole (Alters thyroid hormone or TSH levels). Products include:

Urobiotic-250 Capsules 2214

Sulfamethoxazole (Alters thyroid hormone or TSH levels). Products include:

Azo Gantanol Tablets 2080
Bactrim DS Tablets 2084
Bactrim I.V. Infusion 2082
Bactrim 2084
Gantanol Tablets 2119
Septra 1174
Septra I.V. Infusion 1169
Septra I.V. Infusion ADD-Vantage Vials 1171
Septra 1174

Sulfasalazine (Alters thyroid hormone or TSH levels). Products include:

Azulfidine 1949

Sulfinpyrazone (Alters thyroid hormone or TSH levels). Products include:

Anturane 807

Sulfisoxazole (Alters thyroid hormone or TSH levels). Products include:

Azo Gantrisin Tablets 2081
Gantrisin Tablets 2120

Sulfisoxazole Diolamine (Alters thyroid hormone or TSH levels).

No products indexed under this heading.

Tamoxifen Citrate (May inhibit levothyroxine sodium binding to serum proteins or alter the concentrations of serum proteins). Products include:

Nolvadex Tablets 2841

Terbutaline Sulfate (Possible increased risk of coronary insufficiency in patients with coronary artery disease). Products include:

Brethaire Inhaler 813
Brethine Ampuls 815
Brethine Tablets 814
Bricanyl Subcutaneous Injection 1502
Bricanyl Tablets 1503

Theophylline (Theophylline clearance may be decreased in hypothyroid patients and return toward normal when euthyroid state is achieved). Products include:

Marax Tablets & DF Syrup 2200
Quibron 2053

Theophylline Anhydrous (Theophylline clearance may be decreased in hypothyroid patients and return toward normal when euthyroid state is achieved). Products include:

Aerolate 1004
Primatene Dual Action Formula .... ▣ 872
Primatene Tablets .... ▣ 873
Respbid Tablets 682
Slo-bid Gyrocaps 2033
Theo-24 Extended Release Capsules 2568
Theo-Dur Extended-Release Tablets 1327
Theo-X Extended-Release Tablets .. 788
Uni-Dur Extended-Release Tablets .. 1331
Uniphyl 400 mg Tablets 2001

Theophylline Calcium Salicylate (Theophylline clearance may be decreased in hypothyroid patients and return toward normal when euthyroid state is achieved). Products include:

Quadrinal Tablets 1350

Theophylline Sodium Glycinate (Theophylline clearance may be decreased in hypothyroid patients and return toward normal when euthyroid state is achieved).

No products indexed under this heading.

Timolol Hemihydrate (Alters thyroid hormone or TSH levels; actions of some beta blockers may be impaired when hypothyroid patients become euthyroid). Products include:

Betimol 0.25%, 0.5% .... ⊙ 261

Timolol Maleate (Alters thyroid hormone or TSH levels; actions of some beta blockers may be impaired when hypothyroid patients become euthyroid). Products include:

Blocadren Tablets 1614
Timolide Tablets 1748
Timoptic in Ocudose 1753
Timoptic Sterile Ophthalmic Solution 1751
Timoptic-XE 1755

Tolazamide (Alters thyroid hormone or TSH levels; requirements of oral antidiabetic agents may be reduced in hypothyroid patients with diabetes and may be subsequently increased with initiation of thyroid hormone therapy).

No products indexed under this heading.

Tolbutamide (Alters thyroid hormone or TSH levels; requirements of oral antidiabetic agents may be reduced in hypothyroid patients with diabetes and may be subsequently increased with initiation of thyroid hormone therapy).

No products indexed under this heading.

Triamcinolone (May inhibit levothyroxine sodium binding to serum proteins or alter the concentrations of serum proteins). Products include:

Aristocort Tablets 1022

Triamcinolone Acetonide (May inhibit levothyroxine sodium binding to serum proteins or alter the concentrations of serum proteins). Products include:

Aristocort A 0.025% Cream 1027
Aristocort A 0.5% Cream 1031
Aristocort A 0.1% Cream 1029
Aristocort A 0.1% Ointment 1030
Azmacort Oral Inhaler 2011
Nasacort Nasal Inhaler 2024

Triamcinolone Diacetate (May inhibit levothyroxine sodium binding to serum proteins or alter the concentrations of serum proteins). Products include:

Aristocort Suspension (Forte Parenteral) 1027
Aristocort Suspension (Intralesional) 1025

Triamcinolone Hexacetonide (May inhibit levothyroxine sodium binding to serum proteins or alter the concentrations of serum proteins). Products include:

Aristospan Suspension (Intra-articular) 1033
Aristospan Suspension (Intralesional) 1032

Trimipramine Maleate (Concurrent use may increase the therapeutic and toxic effects of both drugs; onset of action of tricyclics may be accelerated). Products include:

Surmontil Capsules 2811

Tyropanoate Sodium (Alters thyroid hormone or TSH levels).

No products indexed under this heading.

Warfarin Sodium (The hypoprothrombinemic effect of anticoagulants may be potentiated). Products include:

Coumadin 926

Food Interactions

Soybean formula, children's (Binds and decreases absorption of levothyroxine sodium from the gastrointestinal tract).

SYNTOCINON INJECTION

(Oxytocin) 2296

May interact with vasopressors and certain other agents. Compounds in these categories include:

Cyclopropane (Modifies cardiovascular effects resulting in hypotension).

Dopamine Hydrochloride (Potential for severe hypertension following prophylactic administration of a vasoconstrictor in conjunction with caudal block anesthesia).

No products indexed under this heading.

Epinephrine Hydrochloride (Potential for severe hypertension following prophylactic administration of a vasoconstrictor in conjunction with caudal block anesthesia). Products include:

Ana-Kit Anaphylaxis Emergency Treatment Kit 617

Metaraminol Bitartrate (Potential for severe hypertension following prophylactic administration of a vasoconstrictor in conjunction with caudal block anesthesia). Products include:

Aramine Injection 1609

Methoxamine Hydrochloride (Potential for severe hypertension following prophylactic administration of a vasoconstrictor in conjunction with caudal block anesthesia). Products include:

Vasoxyl Injection 1196

Norepinephrine Bitartrate (Potential for severe hypertension following prophylactic administration of a vasoconstrictor in conjunction with caudal block anesthesia). Products include:

Levophed Bitartrate Injection 2315

Phenylephrine Hydrochloride (Potential for severe hypertension following prophylactic administration of a vasoconstrictor in conjunction with caudal block anesthesia). Products include:

Atrohist Plus Tablets 454
Cerose DM .... ▣ 878
Comhist 2038
D.A. Chewable Tablets 951
Deconsal Pediatric Capsules 454
Dura-Vent/DA Tablets 953
Entex Capsules 1986
Entex Liquid 1986
Extendryl 1005
4-Way Fast Acting Nasal Spray (regular & mentholated) .... ▣ 621
Hemorid For Women .... ▣ 834
Hycomine Compound Tablets 932
Neo-Synephrine Hydrochloride 1% Carpuject 2324
Neo-Synephrine Hydrochloride 1% Injection 2324
Neo-Synephrine Hydrochloride (Ophthalmic) 2325
Neo-Synephrine .... ▣ 726
Nōstril .... ▣ 644
Novahistine Elixir .... ▣ 823
Phenergan VC 2779
Phenergan VC with Codeine 2781
Preparation H .... ▣ 871
Tympagesic Ear Drops 2342
Vasosulf .... ⊙ 271
Vicks Sinex Nasal Spray and Ultra Fine Mist .... ▣ 765

SYPRINE CAPSULES

(Trientine Hydrochloride) 1747

None cited in PDR database.

T-STAT 2.0% TOPICAL SOLUTION AND PADS

(Erythromycin) 2688

May interact with:

Concomitant Topical Acne Therapy (Possible cumulative irritant effect).

TAGAMET INJECTION

(Cimetidine Hydrochloride) 2516

See **Tagamet Tablets**

TAGAMET LIQUID

(Cimetidine Hydrochloride) 2516

See **Tagamet Tablets**

TAGAMET TABLETS

(Cimetidine) 2516

May interact with oral anticoagulants, antacids, tricyclic antidepressants, xanthine bronchodilators, and certain other agents. Compounds in these categories include:

Aluminum Carbonate Gel (Simultaneous administration is not recommended since antacids may interfere with the absorption of cimetidine). Products include:

Basaljel 2703

Interactions Index — Tagamet

Aluminum Hydroxide (Simultaneous administration is not recommended since antacids may interfere with the absorption of cimetidine). Products include:

ALternaGEL Liquid 1316
Maximum Strength Ascriptin .... ◆D 630
Cama Arthritis Pain Reliever............ ◆D 785
Gaviscon Extra Strength Relief Formula Antacid Tablets.................. ◆D 819
Gaviscon Extra Strength Relief Formula Liquid Antacid................... ◆D 819
Gaviscon Liquid Antacid .... ◆D 820
Gelusil Liquid & Tablets .... ◆D 855
Maalox Heartburn Relief Suspension .... ◆D 642
Maalox Heartburn Relief Tablets.... ◆D 641
Maalox Magnesia and Alumina Oral Suspension .... ◆D 642
Maalox Plus Tablets .... ◆D 643
Extra Strength Maalox Antacid Plus Antigas Liquid and Tablets ◆D 638
Tempo Soft Antacid .... ◆D 835

Aluminum Hydroxide Gel (Simultaneous administration is not recommended since antacids may interfere with the absorption of cimetidine). Products include:

ALternaGEL Liquid .... ◆D 659
Aludrox Oral Suspension 2695
Amphojel Suspension 2695
Amphojel Suspension without Flavor 2695
Amphojel Tablets................................... 2695
Arthritis Pain Ascriptin .... ◆D 631
Regular Strength Ascriptin Tablets .... ◆D 629
Gaviscon Antacid Tablets.................... ◆D 819
Gaviscon-2 Antacid Tablets .... ◆D 820
Mylanta Liquid 1317
Mylanta Tablets .... ◆D 660
Mylanta Double Strength Liquid 1317
Mylanta Double Strength Tablets .. ◆D 660
Nephrox Suspension .... ◆D 655

Aminophylline (Reduces hepatic metabolism of theophylline resulting in delayed elimination and increased blood levels of theophylline).

No products indexed under this heading.

Amitriptyline Hydrochloride (Reduces hepatic metabolism of certain unspecified tricyclic antidepressants resulting in delayed elimination and increased blood levels of these drugs). Products include:

Elavil 2838
Endep Tablets 2174
Etrafon 2355
Limbitrol 2180
Triavil Tablets 1757

Amoxapine (Reduces hepatic metabolism of certain unspecified tricyclic antidepressants resulting in delayed elimination and increased blood levels of these drugs). Products include:

Asendin Tablets 1369

Chlordiazepoxide (Reduces hepatic metabolism of chlordiazepoxide resulting in delayed elimination and increased blood levels of chlordiazepoxide). Products include:

Libritabs Tablets 2177
Limbitrol 2180

Chlordiazepoxide Hydrochloride (Reduces hepatic metabolism of chlordiazepoxide resulting in delayed elimination and increased blood levels of chlordiazepoxide). Products include:

Librax Capsules 2176
Librium Capsules................................... 2178
Librium Injectable 2179

Clomipramine Hydrochloride (Reduces hepatic metabolism of certain unspecified tricyclic antidepressants resulting in delayed elimination and increased blood levels of these drugs). Products include:

Anafranil Capsules 803

Desipramine Hydrochloride (Reduces hepatic metabolism of certain unspecified tricyclic antidepressants resulting in delayed elimination and increased blood levels of these drugs). Products include:

Norpramin Tablets 1526

Diazepam (Reduces hepatic metabolism of diazepam resulting in delayed elimination and increased blood levels of diazepam). Products include:

Dizac 1809
Valium Injectable 2182
Valium Tablets 2183
Valrelease Capsules 2169

Dicumarol (Reduces hepatic metabolism of warfarin-type anticoagulants resulting in clinically significant effects; close monitoring of prothrombin time of these recommended).

No products indexed under this heading.

Dihydroxyaluminum Sodium Carbonate (Simultaneous administration is not recommended since antacids may interfere with the absorption of cimetidine).

No products indexed under this heading.

Doxepin Hydrochloride (Reduces hepatic metabolism of certain unspecified tricyclic antidepressants resulting in delayed elimination and increased blood levels of these drugs). Products include:

Sinequan 2205
Zonalon Cream 1055

Dyphylline (Reduces hepatic metabolism of theophylline resulting in delayed elimination and increased blood levels of theophylline). Products include:

Lufyllin & Lufyllin-400 Tablets 2670
Lufyllin-GG Elixir & Tablets 2671

Imipramine Hydrochloride (Reduces hepatic metabolism of certain unspecified tricyclic antidepressants resulting in delayed elimination and increased blood levels of these drugs). Products include:

Tofranil Ampuls 854
Tofranil Tablets 856

Imipramine Pamoate (Reduces hepatic metabolism of certain unspecified tricyclic antidepressants resulting in delayed elimination and increased blood levels of these drugs). Products include:

Tofranil-PM Capsules........................... 857

Ketoconazole (Alteration of pH may affect absorption of ketoconazole; administer oral ketoconazole at least 2 hours before cimetidine). Products include:

Nizoral 2% Cream 1297
Nizoral 2% Shampoo............................ 1298
Nizoral Tablets 1298

Lidocaine Hydrochloride (Reduces hepatic metabolism of lidocaine resulting in delayed elimination and increased blood levels of lidocaine). Products include:

Bactine Antiseptic/Anesthetic First Aid Liquid .... ◆D 708
Campho-Phenique Maximum Strength First Aid Antibiotic Plus Pain Reliever Ointment .... ◆D 719
Decadron Phosphate with Xylocaine Injection, Sterile 1639
Xylocaine Injections 567

Magaldrate (Simultaneous administration is not recommended since antacids may interfere with the absorption of cimetidine).

No products indexed under this heading.

Magnesium Hydroxide (Simultaneous administration is not recommended since antacids may interfere with the absorption of cimetidine). Products include:

Aludrox Oral Suspension 2695
Arthritis Pain Ascriptin .... ◆D 631
Maximum Strength Ascriptin .... ◆D 630
Regular Strength Ascriptin Tablets .... ◆D 629
Di-Gel Antacid/Anti-Gas .... ◆D 801
Gelusil Liquid & Tablets .... ◆D 855
Maalox Magnesia and Alumina Oral Suspension .... ◆D 642
Maalox Plus Tablets .... ◆D 643
Extra Strength Maalox Antacid Plus Antigas Liquid and Tablets ◆D 638
Mylanta Calcium Carbonate and Magnesium Hydroxide Tablets...... 1318
Mylanta Liquid 1317
Mylanta Tablets .... ◆D 660
Mylanta Double Strength Liquid 1317
Mylanta Double Strength Tablets .. ◆D 660
Phillips' Milk of Magnesia Liquid.... ◆D 729
Rolaids Tablets .... ◆D 843
Tempo Soft Antacid .... ◆D 835

Magnesium Oxide (Simultaneous administration is not recommended since antacids may interfere with the absorption of cimetidine). Products include:

Beelith Tablets 639
Bufferin Analgesic Tablets and Caplets .... ◆D 613
Caltrate PLUS .... ◆D 665
Cama Arthritis Pain Reliever............. ◆D 785
Mag-Ox 400 668
Uro-Mag... 668

Maprotiline Hydrochloride (Reduces hepatic metabolism of certain unspecified tricyclic antidepressants resulting in delayed elimination and increased blood levels of these drugs). Products include:

Ludiomil Tablets..................................... 843

Metronidazole (Reduces hepatic metabolism of metronidazole resulting in delayed elimination and increased blood levels of metronidazole). Products include:

Flagyl 375 Capsules.............................. 2434
Flagyl I.V. RTU.. 2247
MetroGel 1047
MetroGel-Vaginal 902
Protostat Tablets 1883

Metronidazole Hydrochloride (Reduces hepatic metabolism of metronidazole resulting in delayed elimination and increased blood levels of metronidazole). Products include:

Flagyl I.V. 2247

Nifedipine (Reduces hepatic metabolism of nifedipine resulting in delayed elimination and increased blood levels of nifedipine). Products include:

Adalat Capsules (10 mg and 20 mg) 587
Adalat CC 589
Procardia Capsules 1971
Procardia XL Extended Release Tablets 1972

Nortriptyline Hydrochloride (Reduces hepatic metabolism of certain unspecified tricyclic antidepressants resulting in delayed elimination and increased blood levels of these drugs). Products include:

Pamelor 2280

Phenytoin (Reduces hepatic metabolism of phenytoin resulting in delayed elimination and increased blood levels of phenytoin). Products include:

Dilantin Infatabs 1908
Dilantin-125 Suspension 1911

Phenytoin Sodium (Reduces hepatic metabolism of phenytoin resulting in delayed elimination and increased blood levels of phenytoin). Products include:

Dilantin Kapseals 1906
Dilantin Parenteral 1910

Propranolol Hydrochloride (Reduces hepatic metabolism of propranolol resulting in delayed elimination and increased blood levels of propranolol). Products include:

Inderal 2728
Inderal LA Long Acting Capsules 2730
Inderide Tablets 2732
Inderide LA Long Acting Capsules .. 2734

Protriptyline Hydrochloride (Reduces hepatic metabolism of certain unspecified tricyclic antidepressants resulting in delayed elimination and increased blood levels of these drugs). Products include:

Vivactil Tablets 1774

Sodium Bicarbonate (Simultaneous administration is not recommended since antacids may interfere with the absorption of cimetidine). Products include:

Alka-Seltzer Effervescent Antacid and Pain Reliever................................ ◆D 701
Alka-Seltzer Extra Strength Effervescent Antacid and Pain Reliever .... ◆D 703
Alka-Seltzer Gold Effervescent Antacid.. ◆D 703
Alka-Seltzer Lemon Lime Effervescent Antacid and Pain Reliever .... ◆D 703
Arm & Hammer Pure Baking Soda .... ◆D 627
Ceo-Two Rectal Suppositories 666
Citrocarbonate Antacid .... ◆D 770
Massengill Disposable Douches...... ◆D 820
Massengill Liquid Concentrate......... ◆D 820
NuLYTELY.. 689
Cherry Flavor NuLYTELY 689

Theophylline (Reduces hepatic metabolism of theophylline resulting in delayed elimination and increased blood levels of theophylline). Products include:

Marax Tablets & DF Syrup................... 2200
Quibron 2053

Theophylline Anhydrous (Reduces hepatic metabolism of theophylline resulting in delayed elimination and increased blood levels of theophylline). Products include:

Aerolate 1004
Primatene Dual Action Formula....... ◆D 872
Primatene Tablets .... ◆D 873
Respbid Tablets 682
Slo-bid Gyrocaps 2033
Theo-24 Extended Release Capsules 2568
Theo-Dur Extended-Release Tablets 1327
Theo-X Extended-Release Tablets .. 788
Uni-Dur Extended-Release Tablets .. 1331
Uniphyl 400 mg Tablets....................... 2001

Theophylline Calcium Salicylate (Reduces hepatic metabolism of theophylline resulting in delayed elimination and increased blood levels of theophylline). Products include:

Quadrinal Tablets 1350

Theophylline Sodium Glycinate (Reduces hepatic metabolism of theophylline resulting in delayed elimination and increased blood levels of theophylline).

No products indexed under this heading.

Trimipramine Maleate (Reduces hepatic metabolism of certain unspecified tricyclic antidepressants resulting in delayed elimination and increased blood levels of these drugs). Products include:

Surmontil Capsules............................... 2811

IMPORTANT NOTE: Always consult each drug listing in the patient's regimen for possible interactions.

Warfarin Sodium (Reduces hepatic metabolism of warfarin-type anticoagulants resulting in clinically significant effects; close monitoring of prothrombin time is recommended). Products include:
Coumadin ... 926

TALACEN
(Pentazocine Hydrochloride) ... 2333
May interact with narcotic analgesics, central nervous system depressants, and certain other agents. Compounds in these categories include:

Alfentanil Hydrochloride (Potential for withdrawal symptoms; additive CNS depressant effects). Products include:
Alfenta Injection ... 1286

Alprazolam (Additive CNS depressant effects). Products include:
Xanax Tablets ... 2649

Aprobarbital (Additive CNS depressant effects).
No products indexed under this heading.

Buprenorphine (Potential for withdrawal symptoms; additive CNS depressant effects). Products include:
Buprenex Injectable ... 2006

Buspirone Hydrochloride (Additive CNS depressant effects). Products include:
BuSpar ... 737

Butabarbital (Additive CNS depressant effects).
No products indexed under this heading.

Butalbital (Additive CNS depressant effects). Products include:
Esgic-plus Tablets ... 1013
Fioricet Tablets ... 2258
Fioricet with Codeine Capsules ... 2260
Fiorinal Capsules ... 2261
Fiorinal with Codeine Capsules ... 2262
Fiorinal Tablets ... 2261
Phrenilin ... 785
Sedapap Tablets 50 mg/650 mg ... 1543

Chlordiazepoxide (Additive CNS depressant effects). Products include:
Libritabs Tablets ... 2177
Limbitrol ... 2180

Chlordiazepoxide Hydrochloride (Additive CNS depressant effects). Products include:
Librax Capsules ... 2176
Librium Capsules ... 2178
Librium Injectable ... 2179

Chlorpromazine (Additive CNS depressant effects). Products include:
Thorazine Suppositories ... 2523

Chlorprothixene (Additive CNS depressant effects).
No products indexed under this heading.

Chlorprothixene Hydrochloride (Additive CNS depressant effects).
No products indexed under this heading.

Clorazepate Dipotassium (Additive CNS depressant effects). Products include:
Tranxene ... 451

Clozapine (Potential for withdrawal symptoms; additive CNS depressant effects). Products include:
Clozaril Tablets ... 2252

Codeine Phosphate (Potential for withdrawal symptoms; additive CNS depressant effects). Products include:
Actifed with Codeine Cough Syrup ... 1067
Brontex ... 1981
Deconsal C Expectorant Syrup ... 456
Deconsal Pediatric Syrup ... 457
Dimetane-DC Cough Syrup ... 2059
Empirin with Codeine Tablets ... 1093
Fioricet with Codeine Capsules ... 2260
Fiorinal with Codeine Capsules ... 2262
Isoclor Expectorant ... 990
Novahistine DH ... 2462
Novahistine Expectorant ... 2463
Nucofed ... 2051
Phenergan with Codeine ... 2777
Phenergan VC with Codeine ... 2781
Robitussin A-C Syrup ... 2073
Robitussin-DAC Syrup ... 2074
Ryna ... ◘ 841
Soma Compound w/Codeine Tablets ... 2676
Tussi-Organidin NR Liquid and S NR Liquid ... 2677
Tylenol with Codeine ... 1583

Desflurane (Potential for withdrawal symptoms; additive CNS depressant effects). Products include:
Suprane ... 1813

Dezocine (Potential for withdrawal symptoms). Products include:
Dalgan Injection ... 538

Diazepam (Additive CNS depressant effects). Products include:
Dizac ... 1809
Valium Injectable ... 2182
Valium Tablets ... 2183
Valrelease Capsules ... 2169

Diphenoxylate Hydrochloride (Potential for withdrawal symptoms). Products include:
Lomotil ... 2439

Droperidol (Additive CNS depressant effects). Products include:
Inapsine Injection ... 1296

Enflurane (Additive CNS depressant effects).
No products indexed under this heading.

Estazolam (Potential for withdrawal symptoms; additive CNS depressant effects). Products include:
ProSom Tablets ... 449

Ethchlorvynol (Additive CNS depressant effects). Products include:
Placidyl Capsules ... 448

Ethinamate (Additive CNS depressant effects).
No products indexed under this heading.

Fentanyl (Potential for withdrawal symptoms). Products include:
Duragesic Transdermal System ... 1288

Fentanyl Citrate (Potential for withdrawal symptoms; additive CNS depressant effects). Products include:
Sublimaze Injection ... 1307

Fluphenazine Decanoate (Additive CNS depressant effects). Products include:
Prolixin Decanoate ... 509

Fluphenazine Enanthate (Additive CNS depressant effects). Products include:
Prolixin Enanthate ... 509

Fluphenazine Hydrochloride (Additive CNS depressant effects). Products include:
Prolixin ... 509

Flurazepam Hydrochloride (Additive CNS depressant effects). Products include:
Dalmane Capsules ... 2173

Glutethimide (Additive CNS depressant effects).
No products indexed under this heading.

Haloperidol (Additive CNS depressant effects). Products include:
Haldol Injection, Tablets and Concentrate ... 1575

Haloperidol Decanoate (Additive CNS depressant effects). Products include:
Haldol Decanoate ... 1577

Hydrocodone Bitartrate (Potential for withdrawal symptoms; additive CNS depressant effects). Products include:
Anexsia 5/500 Elixir ... 1781
Anexia Tablets ... 1782
Codiclear DH Syrup ... 791
Deconamine CX Cough and Cold Liquid and Tablets ... 1319
Duratuss HD Elixir ... 2565
Hycodan Tablets and Syrup ... 930
Hycomine Compound Tablets ... 932
Hycomine ... 931
Hycotuss Expectorant Syrup ... 933
Hydrocet Capsules ... 782
Lorcet 10/650 ... 1018
Lortab ... 2566
Tussend ... 1783
Tussend Expectorant ... 1785
Vicodin Tablets ... 1356
Vicodin ES Tablets ... 1357
Vicodin Tuss Expectorant ... 1358
Zydone Capsules ... 949

Hydrocodone Polistirex (Potential for withdrawal symptoms; additive CNS depressant effects). Products include:
Tussionex Pennkinetic Extended-Release Suspension ... 998

Hydroxyzine Hydrochloride (Additive CNS depressant effects). Products include:
Atarax Tablets & Syrup ... 2185
Marax Tablets & DF Syrup ... 2200
Vistaril Intramuscular Solution ... 2216

Isoflurane (Additive CNS depressant effects).
No products indexed under this heading.

Ketamine Hydrochloride (Additive CNS depressant effects).
No products indexed under this heading.

Levomethadyl Acetate Hydrochloride (Potential for withdrawal symptoms; additive CNS depressant effects). Products include:
Orlamm ... 2239

Levorphanol Tartrate (Potential for withdrawal symptoms; additive CNS depressant effects). Products include:
Levo-Dromoran ... 2129

Lorazepam (Additive CNS depressant effects). Products include:
Ativan Injection ... 2698
Ativan Tablets ... 2700

Loxapine Hydrochloride (Additive CNS depressant effects). Products include:
Loxitane ... 1378

Loxapine Succinate (Additive CNS depressant effects). Products include:
Loxitane Capsules ... 1378

Meperidine Hydrochloride (Potential for withdrawal symptoms; additive CNS depressant effects). Products include:
Demerol ... 2308
Mepergan Injection ... 2753

Mephobarbital (Additive CNS depressant effects). Products include:
Mebaral Tablets ... 2322

Meprobamate (Additive CNS depressant effects). Products include:
Miltown Tablets ... 2672
PMB 200 and PMB 400 ... 2783

Mesoridazine Besylate (Additive CNS depressant effects). Products include:
Serentil ... 684

Methadone Hydrochloride (Potential for withdrawal symptoms; additive CNS depressant effects). Products include:
Methadone Hydrochloride Oral Concentrate ... 2233
Methadone Hydrochloride Oral Solution & Tablets ... 2235

Methohexital Sodium (Additive CNS depressant effects). Products include:
Brevital Sodium Vials ... 1429

Methotrimeprazine (Potential for withdrawal symptoms; additive CNS depressant effects). Products include:
Levoprome ... 1274

Methoxyflurane (Additive CNS depressant effects).
No products indexed under this heading.

Midazolam Hydrochloride (Additive CNS depressant effects). Products include:
Versed Injection ... 2170

Molindone Hydrochloride (Additive CNS depressant effects). Products include:
Moban Tablets and Concentrate ... 1048

Morphine Sulfate (Potential for withdrawal symptoms; additive CNS depressant effects). Products include:
Astramorph/PF Injection, USP (Preservative-Free) ... 535
Duramorph ... 962
Infumorph 200 and Infumorph 500 Sterile Solutions ... 965
MS Contin Tablets ... 1994
MSIR ... 1997
Oramorph SR (Morphine Sulfate Sustained Release Tablets) ... 2236
RMS Suppositories ... 2657
Roxanol ... 2243

Opium Alkaloids (Potential for withdrawal symptoms; additive CNS depressant effects).
No products indexed under this heading.

Oxazepam (Additive CNS depressant effects). Products include:
Serax Capsules ... 2810
Serax Tablets ... 2810

Oxycodone Hydrochloride (Potential for withdrawal symptoms; additive CNS depressant effects). Products include:
Percocet Tablets ... 938
Percodan Tablets ... 939
Percodan-Demi Tablets ... 940
Roxicodone Tablets, Oral Solution & Intensol (Oxycodone) ... 2244
Tylox Capsules ... 1584

Paregoric (Potential for withdrawal symptoms).
No products indexed under this heading.

Pentobarbital Sodium (Additive CNS depressant effects). Products include:
Nembutal Sodium Capsules ... 436
Nembutal Sodium Solution ... 438
Nembutal Sodium Suppositories ... 440

Perphenazine (Additive CNS depressant effects). Products include:
Etrafon ... 2355
Triavil Tablets ... 1757
Trilafon ... 2389

Phenobarbital (Additive CNS depressant effects). Products include:
Arco-Lase Plus Tablets ... 512
Bellergal-S Tablets ... 2250
Donnatal ... 2060
Donnatal Extentabs ... 2061
Donnatal Tablets ... 2060
Phenobarbital Elixir and Tablets ... 1469
Quadrinal Tablets ... 1350

Prazepam (Additive CNS depressant effects).
No products indexed under this heading.

(◘ Described in PDR For Nonprescription Drugs) (◉ Described in PDR For Ophthalmology)

1003 Interactions Index Talwin Injection

Prochlorperazine (Additive CNS depressant effects). Products include:
- Compazine 2470

Promethazine Hydrochloride (Potential for withdrawal symptoms; additive CNS depressant effects). Products include:
- Mepergan Injection 2753
- Phenergan with Codeine 2777
- Phenergan with Dextromethorphan 2778
- Phenergan Injection 2773
- Phenergan Suppositories 2775
- Phenergan Syrup 2774
- Phenergan Tablets 2775
- Phenergan VC 2779
- Phenergan VC with Codeine 2781

Propofol (Additive CNS depressant effects). Products include:
- Diprivan Injection 2833

Propoxyphene Hydrochloride (Potential for withdrawal symptoms; additive CNS depressant effects). Products include:
- Darvon 1435
- Wygesic Tablets 2827

Propoxyphene Napsylate (Potential for withdrawal symptoms; additive CNS depressant effects). Products include:
- Darvon-N/Darvocet-N 1433

Quazepam (Additive CNS depressant effects). Products include:
- Doral Tablets 2664

Risperidone (Potential for withdrawal symptoms; additive CNS depressant effects). Products include:
- Risperdal 1301

Secobarbital Sodium (Potential for withdrawal symptoms; additive CNS depressant effects). Products include:
- Seconal Sodium Pulvules 1474

Sufentanil Citrate (Potential for withdrawal symptoms; additive CNS depressant effects). Products include:
- Sufenta Injection 1309

Temazepam (Potential for withdrawal symptoms; additive CNS depressant effects). Products include:
- Restoril Capsules 2284

Thiamylal Sodium (Potential for withdrawal symptoms; additive CNS depressant effects).
- No products indexed under this heading.

Thioridazine Hydrochloride (Potential for withdrawal symptoms; additive CNS depressant effects). Products include:
- Mellaril 2269

Thiothixene (Potential for withdrawal symptoms; additive CNS depressant effects). Products include:
- Navane Capsules and Concentrate 2201
- Navane Intramuscular 2202

Triazolam (Potential for withdrawal symptoms; additive CNS depressant effects). Products include:
- Halcion Tablets 2611

Trifluoperazine Hydrochloride (Potential for withdrawal symptoms; additive CNS depressant effects). Products include:
- Stelazine 2514

Zolpidem Tartrate (Potential for withdrawal symptoms; additive CNS depressant effects). Products include:
- Ambien Tablets 2416

Food Interactions

Alcohol (Potential for increased CNS depressant effects).

TALWIN AMPULS

(Pentazocine Lactate) 2334

May interact with narcotic analgesics, general anesthetics, preanesthetic medications, central nervous system depressants, and certain other agents. Compounds in these categories include:

Alfentanil Hydrochloride (Potential for withdrawal symptoms; may produce additive CNS depression). Products include:
- Alfenta Injection 1286

Alprazolam (May produce additive CNS depression). Products include:
- Xanax Tablets 2649

Aprobarbital (May produce additive CNS depression).
- No products indexed under this heading.

Buprenorphine (Potential for withdrawal symptoms; may produce additive CNS depression). Products include:
- Buprenex Injectable 2006

Buspirone Hydrochloride (May produce additive CNS depression). Products include:
- BuSpar 737

Butabarbital (May produce additive CNS depression).
- No products indexed under this heading.

Butalbital (May produce additive CNS depression). Products include:
- Esgic-plus Tablets 1013
- Fioricet Tablets 2258
- Fioricet with Codeine Capsules 2260
- Fiorinal Capsules 2261
- Fiorinal with Codeine Capsules 2262
- Fiorinal Tablets 2261
- Phrenilin 785
- Sedapap Tablets 50 mg/650 mg 1543

Chlordiazepoxide (May produce additive CNS depression). Products include:
- Libritabs Tablets 2177
- Limbitrol 2180

Chlordiazepoxide Hydrochloride (May produce additive CNS depression). Products include:
- Librax Capsules 2176
- Librium Capsules 2178
- Librium Injectable 2179

Chlorpromazine (May produce additive CNS depression). Products include:
- Thorazine Suppositories 2523

Chlorprothixene (May produce additive CNS depression).
- No products indexed under this heading.

Chlorprothixene Hydrochloride (May produce additive CNS depression).
- No products indexed under this heading.

Clorazepate Dipotassium (May produce additive CNS depression). Products include:
- Tranxene 451

Clozapine (Potential for withdrawal symptoms; may produce additive CNS depression). Products include:
- Clozaril Tablets 2252

Codeine Phosphate (Potential for withdrawal symptoms; may produce additive CNS depression). Products include:
- Actifed with Codeine Cough Syrup 1067
- Brontex 1981
- Deconsal C Expectorant Syrup 456
- Deconsal Pediatric Syrup 457
- Dimetane-DC Cough Syrup 2059
- Empirin with Codeine Tablets 1093
- Fioricet with Codeine Capsules 2260
- Fiorinal with Codeine Capsules 2262
- Isoclor Expectorant 990
- Novahistine DH 2462
- Novahistine Expectorant 2463
- Nucofed 2051
- Phenergan with Codeine 2777
- Phenergan VC with Codeine 2781
- Robitussin A-C Syrup 2073
- Robitussin-DAC Syrup 2074
- Ryna 841
- Soma Compound w/Codeine Tablets 2676
- Tussi-Organidin NR Liquid and S NR Liquid 2677
- Tylenol with Codeine 1583

Desflurane (Potential for withdrawal symptoms; may produce additive CNS depression). Products include:
- Suprane 1813

Dezocine (Potential for withdrawal symptoms). Products include:
- Dalgan Injection 538

Diazepam (May produce additive CNS depressant effects). Products include:
- Dizac 1809
- Valium Injectable 2182
- Valium Tablets 2183
- Valrelease Capsules 2169

Droperidol (May produce additive CNS depressant effects). Products include:
- Inapsine Injection 1296

Enflurane (May produce additive CNS depressant effects).
- No products indexed under this heading.

Estazolam (Potential for withdrawal symptoms; may produce additive CNS depression). Products include:
- ProSom Tablets 449

Ethchlorvynol (May produce additive CNS depression). Products include:
- Placidyl Capsules 448

Ethinamate (May produce additive CNS depression).
- No products indexed under this heading.

Fentanyl (Potential for withdrawal symptoms). Products include:
- Duragesic Transdermal System 1288

Fentanyl Citrate (Potential for withdrawal symptoms; may produce additive CNS depressant effects). Products include:
- Sublimaze Injection 1307

Fluphenazine Decanoate (May produce additive CNS depression). Products include:
- Prolixin Decanoate 509

Fluphenazine Enanthate (May produce additive CNS depression). Products include:
- Prolixin Enanthate 509

Fluphenazine Hydrochloride (May produce additive CNS depression). Products include:
- Prolixin 509

Flurazepam Hydrochloride (May produce additive CNS depression). Products include:
- Dalmane Capsules 2173

Glutethimide (May produce additive CNS depression).
- No products indexed under this heading.

Haloperidol (May produce additive CNS depression). Products include:
- Haldol Injection, Tablets and Concentrate 1575

Haloperidol Decanoate (May produce additive CNS depression). Products include:
- Haldol Decanoate 1577

Hydrocodone Bitartrate (Potential for withdrawal symptoms; may produce additive CNS depression). Products include:
- Anexsia 5/500 Elixir 1781
- Anexia Tablets 1782
- Codiclear DH Syrup 791
- Deconamine CX Cough and Cold Liquid and Tablets 1319
- Duratuss HD Elixir 2565
- Hycodan Tablets and Syrup 930
- Hycomine Compound Tablets 932
- Hycomine 931
- Hycotuss Expectorant Syrup 933
- Hydrocet Capsules 782
- Lorcet 10/650 1018
- Lortab 2566
- Tussend 1783
- Tussend Expectorant 1785
- Vicodin Tablets 1356
- Vicodin ES Tablets 1357
- Vicodin Tuss Expectorant 1358
- Zydone Capsules 949

Hydrocodone Polistirex (Potential for withdrawal symptoms; may produce additive CNS depression). Products include:
- Tussionex Pennkinetic Extended-Release Suspension 998

Hydroxyzine Hydrochloride (May produce additive CNS depressant effects). Products include:
- Atarax Tablets & Syrup 2185
- Marax Tablets & DF Syrup 2200
- Vistaril Intramuscular Solution 2216

Isoflurane (May produce additive CNS depressant effects).
- No products indexed under this heading.

Ketamine Hydrochloride (May produce additive CNS depressant effects).
- No products indexed under this heading.

Levomethadyl Acetate Hydrochloride (Potential for withdrawal symptoms; may produce additive CNS depression). Products include:
- Orlamm 2239

Levorphanol Tartrate (Potential for withdrawal symptoms; may produce additive CNS depression). Products include:
- Levo-Dromoran 2129

Lorazepam (May produce additive CNS depressant effects). Products include:
- Ativan Injection 2698
- Ativan Tablets 2700

Loxapine Hydrochloride (May produce additive CNS depression). Products include:
- Loxitane 1378

Loxapine Succinate (May produce additive CNS depression). Products include:
- Loxitane Capsules 1378

Meperidine Hydrochloride (Potential for withdrawal symptoms; may produce additive CNS depressant effects). Products include:
- Demerol 2308
- Mepergan Injection 2753

Mephobarbital (May produce additive CNS depression). Products include:
- Mebaral Tablets 2322

Meprobamate (May produce additive CNS depression). Products include:
- Miltown Tablets 2672
- PMB 200 and PMB 400 2783

Mesoridazine Besylate (May produce additive CNS depression). Products include:
- Serentil 684

Methadone Hydrochloride (Potential for withdrawal symptoms; may produce additive CNS depression). Products include:
- Methadone Hydrochloride Oral Concentrate 2233
- Methadone Hydrochloride Oral Solution & Tablets 2235

IMPORTANT NOTE: Always consult each drug listing in the patient's regimen for possible interactions.

Talwin Injection — Interactions Index — 1004

Methohexital Sodium (May produce additive CNS depressant effects). Products include:
Brevital Sodium Vials 1429
Methotrimeprazine (Potential for withdrawal symptoms; may produce additive CNS depression). Products include:
Levoprome 1274
Methoxyflurane (Potential for withdrawal symptoms; may produce additive CNS depression).
No products indexed under this heading.
Midazolam Hydrochloride (May produce additive CNS depression). Products include:
Versed Injection 2170
Molindone Hydrochloride (May produce additive CNS depression). Products include:
Moban Tablets and Concentrate 1048
Morphine Sulfate (Potential for withdrawal symptoms; may produce additive CNS depressant effects). Products include:
Astramorph/PF Injection, USP (Preservative-Free) 535
Duramorph 962
Infumorph 200 and Infumorph 500 Sterile Solutions 965
MS Contin Tablets 1994
MSIR 1997
Oramorph SR (Morphine Sulfate Sustained Release Tablets) 2236
RMS Suppositories 2657
Roxanol 2243
Opium Alkaloids (Potential for withdrawal symptoms; may produce additive CNS depressant effects).
No products indexed under this heading.
Oxazepam (May produce additive CNS depression). Products include:
Serax Capsules 2810
Serax Tablets 2810
Oxycodone Hydrochloride (Potential for withdrawal symptoms; may produce additive CNS depression). Products include:
Percocet Tablets 938
Percodan Tablets 939
Percodan-Demi Tablets 940
Roxicodone Tablets, Oral Solution & Intensol (Oxycodone) 2244
Tylox Capsules 1584
Pentobarbital Sodium (Potential for withdrawal symptoms; may produce additive CNS depression). Products include:
Nembutal Sodium Capsules 436
Nembutal Sodium Solution 438
Nembutal Sodium Suppositories 440
Perphenazine (May produce additive CNS depression). Products include:
Etrafon 2355
Triavil Tablets 1757
Trilafon 2389
Phenobarbital (May produce additive CNS depression). Products include:
Arco-Lase Plus Tablets 512
Bellergal-S Tablets 2250
Donnatal 2060
Donnatal Extentabs 2061
Donnatal Tablets 2060
Phenobarbital Elixir and Tablets 1469
Quadrinal Tablets 1350
Prazepam (May produce additive CNS depression).
No products indexed under this heading.
Prochlorperazine (May produce additive CNS depression). Products include:
Compazine 2470
Promethazine Hydrochloride (May produce additive CNS depressant effects). Products include:
Mepergan Injection 2753
Phenergan with Codeine 2777
Phenergan with Dextromethorphan 2778
Phenergan Injection 2773
Phenergan Suppositories 2775
Phenergan Syrup 2774
Phenergan Tablets 2775
Phenergan VC 2779
Phenergan VC with Codeine 2781
Propofol (May produce additive CNS depressant effects). Products include:
Diprivan Injection 2833
Propoxyphene Hydrochloride (Potential for withdrawal symptoms; may produce additive CNS depressant effects). Products include:
Darvon 1435
Wygesic Tablets 2827
Propoxyphene Napsylate (Potential for withdrawal symptoms; may produce additive CNS depressant effects). Products include:
Darvon-N/Darvocet-N 1433
Risperidone (Potential for withdrawal symptoms; may produce additive CNS depression). Products include:
Risperdal 1301
Secobarbital Sodium (May produce additive CNS depressant effects). Products include:
Seconal Sodium Pulvules 1474
Sufentanil Citrate (Potential for withdrawal symptoms; may produce additive CNS depressant effects). Products include:
Sufenta Injection 1309
Temazepam (May produce additive CNS depressant effects). Products include:
Restoril Capsules 2284
Thiamylal Sodium (Potential for withdrawal symptoms; may produce additive CNS depressant effects).
No products indexed under this heading.
Thioridazine Hydrochloride (May produce additive CNS depressant effects). Products include:
Mellaril 2269
Thiothixene (May produce additive CNS depressant effects). Products include:
Navane Capsules and Concentrate 2201
Navane Intramuscular 2202
Triazolam (May produce additive CNS depressant effects). Products include:
Halcion Tablets 2611
Trifluoperazine Hydrochloride (May produce additive CNS depressant effects). Products include:
Stelazine 2514
Zolpidem Tartrate (Potential for withdrawal symptoms; may produce additive CNS depression). Products include:
Ambien Tablets 2416

Food Interactions

Alcohol (Potential for increased CNS depressant effects).

TALWIN CARPUJECT
(Pentazocine Lactate) 2334
See **Talwin Ampuls**

TALWIN COMPOUND
(Pentazocine Hydrochloride, Aspirin) 2335
May interact with narcotic analgesics, oral anticoagulants, and certain other agents. Compounds in these categories include:

Alfentanil Hydrochloride (Potential for withdrawal symptoms). Products include:
Alfenta Injection 1286
Buprenorphine (Potential for withdrawal symptoms). Products include:
Buprenex Injectable 2006
Codeine Phosphate (Potential for withdrawal symptoms). Products include:
Actifed with Codeine Cough Syrup.. 1067
Brontex 1981
Deconsal C Expectorant Syrup 456
Deconsal Pediatric Syrup 457
Dimetane-DC Cough Syrup 2059
Empirin with Codeine Tablets 1093
Fioricet with Codeine Capsules 2260
Fiorinal with Codeine Capsules 2262
Isoclor Expectorant 990
Novahistine DH 2462
Novahistine Expectorant 2463
Nucofed 2051
Phenergan with Codeine 2777
Phenergan VC with Codeine 2781
Robitussin A-C Syrup 2073
Robitussin-DAC Syrup 2074
Ryna .... ▣ 841
Soma Compound w/Codeine Tablets 2676
Tussi-Organidin NR Liquid and S NR Liquid 2677
Tylenol with Codeine 1583
Dezocine (Potential for withdrawal symptoms). Products include:
Dalgan Injection 538
Dicumarol (Effects of aspirin may be deleterious in conjunction with anticoagulant therapy).
No products indexed under this heading.
Fentanyl (Potential for withdrawal symptoms). Products include:
Duragesic Transdermal System 1288
Fentanyl Citrate (Potential for withdrawal symptoms). Products include:
Sublimaze Injection 1307
Hydrocodone Bitartrate (Potential for withdrawal symptoms). Products include:
Anexsia 5/500 Elixir 1781
Anexia Tablets 1782
Codiclear DH Syrup 791
Deconamine CX Cough and Cold Liquid and Tablets 1319
Duratuss HD Elixir 2565
Hycodan Tablets and Syrup 930
Hycomine Compound Tablets 932
Hycomine 931
Hycotuss Expectorant Syrup 933
Hydrocet Capsules 782
Lorcet 10/650 1018
Lortab 2566
Tussend 1783
Tussend Expectorant 1785
Vicodin Tablets 1356
Vicodin ES Tablets 1357
Vicodin Tuss Expectorant 1358
Zydone Capsules 949
Hydrocodone Polistirex (Potential for withdrawal symptoms). Products include:
Tussionex Pennkinetic Extended-Release Suspension 998
Levorphanol Tartrate (Potential for withdrawal symptoms). Products include:
Levo-Dromoran 2129
Meperidine Hydrochloride (Potential for withdrawal symptoms). Products include:
Demerol 2308
Mepergan Injection 2753
Methadone Hydrochloride (Potential for withdrawal symptoms). Products include:
Methadone Hydrochloride Oral Concentrate 2233
Methadone Hydrochloride Oral Solution & Tablets 2235
Morphine Sulfate (Potential for withdrawal symptoms). Products include:
Astramorph/PF Injection, USP (Preservative-Free) 535
Duramorph 962
Infumorph 200 and Infumorph 500 Sterile Solutions 965
MS Contin Tablets 1994
MSIR 1997
Oramorph SR (Morphine Sulfate Sustained Release Tablets) 2236
RMS Suppositories 2657
Roxanol 2243
Opium Alkaloids (Potential for withdrawal symptoms).
No products indexed under this heading.
Oxycodone Hydrochloride (Potential for withdrawal symptoms). Products include:
Percocet Tablets 938
Percodan Tablets 939
Percodan-Demi Tablets 940
Roxicodone Tablets, Oral Solution & Intensol (Oxycodone) 2244
Tylox Capsules 1584
Propoxyphene Hydrochloride (Potential for withdrawal symptoms). Products include:
Darvon 1435
Wygesic Tablets 2827
Propoxyphene Napsylate (Potential for withdrawal symptoms). Products include:
Darvon-N/Darvocet-N 1433
Sufentanil Citrate (Potential for withdrawal symptoms). Products include:
Sufenta Injection 1309
Warfarin Sodium (Effects of aspirin may be deleterious in conjunction with anticoagulant therapy). Products include:
Coumadin 926

Food Interactions

Alcohol (Potential for increased CNS depressant effects).

TALWIN INJECTION
(Pentazocine Lactate) 2334
See **Talwin Ampuls**

TALWIN NX
(Pentazocine Hydrochloride, Naloxone Hydrochloride) 2336
May interact with narcotic analgesics, central nervous system depressants, and certain other agents. Compounds in these categories include:

Alfentanil Hydrochloride (Potential for withdrawal symptoms). Products include:
Alfenta Injection 1286
Alprazolam (Additive CNS depressant properties). Products include:
Xanax Tablets 2649
Aprobarbital (Additive CNS depressant properties).
No products indexed under this heading.
Buprenorphine (Potential for withdrawal symptoms). Products include:
Buprenex Injectable 2006
Buspirone Hydrochloride (Additive CNS depressant properties). Products include:
BuSpar 737
Butabarbital (Additive CNS depressant properties).
No products indexed under this heading.
Butalbital (Additive CNS depressant properties). Products include:
Esgic-plus Tablets 1013
Fioricet Tablets 2258
Fioricet with Codeine Capsules 2260
Fiorinal Capsules 2261
Fiorinal with Codeine Capsules 2262
Fiorinal Tablets 2261
Phrenilin 785
Sedapap Tablets 50 mg/650 mg .. 1543

(▣ Described in PDR For Nonprescription Drugs) (⊙ Described in PDR For Ophthalmology)

1005 **Interactions Index** **Talwin Nx**

Chlordiazepoxide (Additive CNS depressant properties). Products include:
Libritabs Tablets 2177
Limbitrol 2180

Chlordiazepoxide Hydrochloride (Additive CNS depressant properties). Products include:
Librax Capsules 2176
Librium Capsules 2178
Librium Injectable 2179

Chlorpromazine (Additive CNS depressant properties). Products include:
Thorazine Suppositories 2523

Chlorprothixene (Additive CNS depressant properties).
No products indexed under this heading.

Chlorprothixene Hydrochloride (Additive CNS depressant properties).
No products indexed under this heading.

Clorazepate Dipotassium (Additive CNS depressant properties). Products include:
Tranxene 451

Clozapine (Potential for withdrawal symptoms). Products include:
Clozaril Tablets 2252

Codeine Phosphate (Potential for withdrawal symptoms). Products include:
Actifed with Codeine Cough Syrup 1067
Brontex 1981
Deconsal C Expectorant Syrup 456
Deconsal Pediatric Syrup 457
Dimetane-DC Cough Syrup 2059
Empirin with Codeine Tablets 1093
Fioricet with Codeine Capsules 2260
Fiorinal with Codeine Capsules 2262
Isoclor Expectorant 990
Novahistine DH 2462
Novahistine Expectorant 2463
Nucofed 2051
Phenergan with Codeine 2777
Phenergan VC with Codeine 2781
Robitussin A-C Syrup 2073
Robitussin-DAC Syrup 2074
Ryna 841
Soma Compound w/Codeine Tablets 2676
Tussi-Organidin NR Liquid and S NR Liquid 2677
Tylenol with Codeine 1583

Desflurane (Potential for withdrawal symptoms). Products include:
Suprane 1813

Dezocine (Potential for withdrawal symptoms). Products include:
Dalgan Injection 538

Diazepam (Additive CNS depressant properties). Products include:
Dizac 1809
Valium Injectable 2182
Valium Tablets 2183
Valrelease Capsules 2169

Droperidol (Additive CNS depressant properties). Products include:
Inapsine Injection 1296

Enflurane (Additive CNS depressant properties).
No products indexed under this heading.

Estazolam (Potential for withdrawal symptoms). Products include:
ProSom Tablets 449

Ethchlorvynol (Additive CNS depressant properties). Products include:
Placidyl Capsules 448

Ethinamate (Additive CNS depressant properties).
No products indexed under this heading.

Fentanyl (Potential for withdrawal symptoms). Products include:
Duragesic Transdermal System 1288

Fentanyl Citrate (Potential for withdrawal symptoms). Products include:
Sublimaze Injection 1307

Fluphenazine Decanoate (Additive CNS depressant properties). Products include:
Prolixin Decanoate 509

Fluphenazine Enanthate (Additive CNS depressant properties). Products include:
Prolixin Enanthate 509

Fluphenazine Hydrochloride (Additive CNS depressant properties). Products include:
Prolixin 509

Flurazepam Hydrochloride (Additive CNS depressant properties). Products include:
Dalmane Capsules 2173

Glutethimide (Additive CNS depressant properties).
No products indexed under this heading.

Haloperidol (Additive CNS depressant properties). Products include:
Haldol Injection, Tablets and Concentrate 1575

Haloperidol Decanoate (Additive CNS depressant properties). Products include:
Haldol Decanoate 1577

Hydrocodone Bitartrate (Potential for withdrawal symptoms). Products include:
Anexsia 5/500 Elixir 1781
Anexia Tablets 1782
Codiclear DH Syrup 791
Deconamine CX Cough and Cold Liquid and Tablets 1319
Duratuss HD Elixir 2565
Hycodan Tablets and Syrup 930
Hycomine Compound Tablets 932
Hycomine 931
Hycotuss Expectorant Syrup 933
Hydrocet Capsules 782
Lorcet 10/650 1018
Lortab 2566
Tussend 1783
Tussend Expectorant 1785
Vicodin Tablets 1356
Vicodin ES Tablets 1357
Vicodin Tuss Expectorant 1358
Zydone Capsules 949

Hydrocodone Polistirex (Potential for withdrawal symptoms). Products include:
Tussionex Pennkinetic Extended-Release Suspension 998

Hydroxyzine Hydrochloride (Additive CNS depressant properties). Products include:
Atarax Tablets & Syrup 2185
Marax Tablets & DF Syrup 2200
Vistaril Intramuscular Solution 2216

Isoflurane (Additive CNS depressant properties).
No products indexed under this heading.

Ketamine Hydrochloride (Additive CNS depressant properties).
No products indexed under this heading.

Levomethadyl Acetate Hydrochloride (Potential for withdrawal symptoms). Products include:
Orlamm 2239

Levorphanol Tartrate (Potential for withdrawal symptoms). Products include:
Levo-Dromoran 2129

Lorazepam (Additive CNS depressant properties). Products include:
Ativan Injection 2698
Ativan Tablets 2700

Loxapine Hydrochloride (Additive CNS depressant properties). Products include:
Loxitane 1378

Loxapine Succinate (Additive CNS depressant properties). Products include:
Loxitane Capsules 1378

Meperidine Hydrochloride (Potential for withdrawal symptoms). Products include:
Demerol 2308
Mepergan Injection 2753

Mephobarbital (Additive CNS depressant properties). Products include:
Mebaral Tablets 2322

Meprobamate (Additive CNS depressant properties). Products include:
Miltown Tablets 2672
PMB 200 and PMB 400 2783

Mesoridazine Besylate (Additive CNS depressant properties). Products include:
Serentil 684

Methadone Hydrochloride (Potential for withdrawal symptoms). Products include:
Methadone Hydrochloride Oral Concentrate 2233
Methadone Hydrochloride Oral Solution & Tablets 2235

Methohexital Sodium (Additive CNS depressant properties). Products include:
Brevital Sodium Vials 1429

Methotrimeprazine (Potential for withdrawal symptoms). Products include:
Levoprome 1274

Methoxyflurane (Additive CNS depressant properties).
No products indexed under this heading.

Midazolam Hydrochloride (Additive CNS depressant properties). Products include:
Versed Injection 2170

Molindone Hydrochloride (Additive CNS depressant properties). Products include:
Moban Tablets and Concentrate 1048

Morphine Sulfate (Potential for withdrawal symptoms). Products include:
Astramorph/PF Injection, USP (Preservative-Free) 535
Duramorph 962
Infumorph 200 and Infumorph 500 Sterile Solutions 965
MS Contin Tablets 1994
MSIR 1997
Oramorph SR (Morphine Sulfate Sustained Release Tablets) 2236
RMS Suppositories 2657
Roxanol 2243

Opium Alkaloids (Potential for withdrawal symptoms).
No products indexed under this heading.

Oxazepam (Additive CNS depressant properties). Products include:
Serax Capsules 2810
Serax Tablets 2810

Oxycodone Hydrochloride (Potential for withdrawal symptoms). Products include:
Percocet Tablets 938
Percodan Tablets 939
Percodan-Demi Tablets 940
Roxicodone Tablets, Oral Solution & Intensol (Oxycodone) 2244
Tylox Capsules 1584

Pentobarbital Sodium (Additive CNS depressant properties). Products include:
Nembutal Sodium Capsules 436
Nembutal Sodium Solution 438
Nembutal Sodium Suppositories 440

Perphenazine (Additive CNS depressant properties). Products include:
Etrafon 2355
Triavil Tablets 1757
Trilafon 2389

Phenobarbital (Additive CNS depressant properties). Products include:
Arco-Lase Plus Tablets 512
Bellergal-S Tablets 2250
Donnatal 2060
Donnatal Extentabs 2061
Donnatal Tablets 2060
Phenobarbital Elixir and Tablets 1469
Quadrinal Tablets 1350

Prazepam (Additive CNS depressant properties).
No products indexed under this heading.

Prochlorperazine (Additive CNS depressant properties). Products include:
Compazine 2470

Promethazine Hydrochloride (Additive CNS depressant properties). Products include:
Mepergan Injection 2753
Phenergan with Codeine 2777
Phenergan with Dextromethorphan 2778
Phenergan Injection 2773
Phenergan Suppositories 2775
Phenergan Syrup 2774
Phenergan Tablets 2775
Phenergan VC 2779
Phenergan VC with Codeine 2781

Propofol (Potential for withdrawal symptoms). Products include:
Diprivan Injection 2833

Propoxyphene Hydrochloride (Potential for withdrawal symptoms). Products include:
Darvon 1435
Wygesic Tablets 2827

Propoxyphene Napsylate (Potential for withdrawal symptoms). Products include:
Darvon-N/Darvocet-N 1433

Quazepam (Potential for withdrawal symptoms). Products include:
Doral Tablets 2664

Risperidone (Potential for withdrawal symptoms). Products include:
Risperdal 1301

Secobarbital Sodium (Potential for withdrawal symptoms). Products include:
Seconal Sodium Pulvules 1474

Sufentanil Citrate (Potential for withdrawal symptoms). Products include:
Sufenta Injection 1309

Temazepam (Additive CNS depressant properties). Products include:
Restoril Capsules 2284

Thiamylal Sodium (Additive CNS depressant properties).
No products indexed under this heading.

Thioridazine Hydrochloride (Additive CNS depressant properties). Products include:
Mellaril 2269

Thiothixene (Additive CNS depressant properties). Products include:
Navane Capsules and Concentrate 2201
Navane Intramuscular 2202

Triazolam (Additive CNS depressant properties). Products include:
Halcion Tablets 2611

Trifluoperazine Hydrochloride (Additive CNS depressant properties). Products include:
Stelazine 2514

Zolpidem Tartrate (Potential for withdrawal symptoms). Products include:
Ambien Tablets 2416

Food Interactions

Alcohol (May increase CNS depression).

IMPORTANT NOTE: Always consult each drug listing in the patient's regimen for possible interactions.

TAMBOCOR TABLETS
(Flecainide Acetate) 1497
May interact with beta blockers and certain other agents. Compounds in these categories include:

Acebutolol Hydrochloride (Possibility of additive negative inotropic effects). Products include:
Sectral Capsules 2807

Amiodarone Hydrochloride (Increases plasma levels by two-fold or more; reduction of flecainide dose by 50% is recommended). Products include:
Cordarone Intravenous 2715
Cordarone Tablets 2712

Atenolol (Possibility of additive negative inotropic effects). Products include:
Tenoretic Tablets 2845
Tenormin Tablets and I.V. Injection 2847

Betaxolol Hydrochloride (Possibility of additive negative inotropic effects). Products include:
Betoptic Ophthalmic Solution 469
Betoptic S Ophthalmic Suspension 471
Kerlone Tablets 2436

Bisoprolol Fumarate (Possibility of additive negative inotropic effects). Products include:
Zebeta Tablets 1413
Ziac 1415

Carbamazepine (A 30% increase in the rate of flecainide elimination). Products include:
Atretol Tablets 573
Tegretol Chewable Tablets 852
Tegretol Suspension 852
Tegretol Tablets 852

Carteolol Hydrochloride (Possibility of additive negative inotropic effects). Products include:
Cartrol Tablets 410
Ocupress Ophthalmic Solution, 1% Sterile .... ⊙ 309

Cimetidine (Increases flecainide plasma levels and half-life). Products include:
Tagamet Tablets 2516

Cimetidine Hydrochloride (Increases flecainide plasma levels and half-life). Products include:
Tagamet 2516

Digoxin (Concurrent administration increases plasma digoxin levels by a 13% +/−19%). Products include:
Lanoxicaps 1117
Lanoxin Elixir Pediatric 1120
Lanoxin Injection 1123
Lanoxin Injection Pediatric 1126
Lanoxin Tablets 1128

Disopyramide Phosphate (Concurrent administration is not recommended due to negative inotropic properties). Products include:
Norpace 2444

Esmolol Hydrochloride (Possibility of additive negative inotropic effects). Products include:
Brevibloc Injection 1808

Labetalol Hydrochloride (Possibility of additive negative inotropic effects). Products include:
Normodyne Injection 2377
Normodyne Tablets 2379
Trandate 1185

Levobunolol Hydrochloride (Possibility of additive negative inotropic effects). Products include:
Betagan .... ⊙ 233

Metipranolol Hydrochloride (Possibility of additive negative inotropic effects). Products include:
OptiPranolol (Metipranolol 0.3%) Sterile Ophthalmic Solution .... ⊙ 258

Metoprolol Succinate (Possibility of additive negative inotropic effects). Products include:
Toprol-XL Tablets 565

Metoprolol Tartrate (Possibility of additive negative inotropic effects). Products include:
Lopressor Ampuls 830
Lopressor HCT Tablets 832
Lopressor Tablets 830

Nadolol (Possibility of additive negative inotropic effects).
No products indexed under this heading.

Penbutolol Sulfate (Possibility of additive negative inotropic effects). Products include:
Levatol 2403

Phenobarbital (A 30% increase in the rate of flecainide elimination). Products include:
Arco-Lase Plus Tablets 512
Bellergal-S Tablets 2250
Donnatal 2060
Donnatal Extentabs 2061
Donnatal Tablets 2060
Phenobarbital Elixir and Tablets 1469
Quadrinal Tablets 1350

Phenytoin (A 30% increase in the rate of flecainide elimination). Products include:
Dilantin Infatabs 1908
Dilantin-125 Suspension 1911

Phenytoin Sodium (A 30% increase in the rate of flecainide elimination). Products include:
Dilantin Kapseals 1906
Dilantin Parenteral 1910

Pindolol (Possibility of additive negative inotropic effects). Products include:
Visken Tablets 2299

Propranolol Hydrochloride (Increases plasma flecainide levels by 20% and propranolol levels were increased by 30%; additive negative inotropic effects). Products include:
Inderal 2728
Inderal LA Long Acting Capsules 2730
Inderide Tablets 2732
Inderide LA Long Acting Capsules .. 2734

Sotalol Hydrochloride (Possibility of additive negative inotropic effects). Products include:
Betapace Tablets 641

Timolol Hemihydrate (Possibility of additive negative inotropic effects). Products include:
Betimol 0.25%, 0.5% .... ⊙ 261

Timolol Maleate (Possibility of additive negative inotropic effects). Products include:
Blocadren Tablets 1614
Timolide Tablets 1748
Timoptic in Ocudose 1753
Timoptic Sterile Ophthalmic Solution 1751
Timoptic-XE 1755

Verapamil Hydrochloride (Concurrent administration is not recommended due to negative inotropic properties). Products include:
Calan SR Caplets 2422
Calan Tablets 2419
Isoptin Injectable 1344
Isoptin Oral Tablets 1346
Isoptin SR Tablets 1348
Verelan Capsules 1410
Verelan Capsules 2824

TANAC MEDICATED GEL
(Dyclonine Hydrochloride, Allantoin) .... ▣ 653
None cited in PDR database.

TANAC NO STING LIQUID
(Benzocaine, Benzalkonium Chloride) .... ▣ 653
None cited in PDR database.

TAO CAPSULES
(Troleandomycin) 2209
May interact with antimigraine drugs, xanthine bronchodilators, and certain other agents. Compounds in these categories include:

Aminophylline (Elevated serum concentrations of theophylline).
No products indexed under this heading.

Dihydroergotamine Mesylate (May induce ischemic reactions). Products include:
D.H.E. 45 Injection 2255

Dyphylline (Elevated serum concentrations of theophylline). Products include:
Lufyllin & Lufyllin-400 Tablets 2670
Lufyllin-GG Elixir & Tablets 2671

Ergotamine Tartrate (May induce ischemic reactions). Products include:
Bellergal-S Tablets 2250
Cafergot 2251
Ergomar 1486
Wigraine Tablets & Suppositories .. 1829

Metoclopramide Hydrochloride (May induce ischemic reactions). Products include:
Reglan 2068

Theophylline (Elevated serum concentrations of theophylline). Products include:
Marax Tablets & DF Syrup 2200
Quibron 2053

Theophylline Anhydrous (Elevated serum concentrations of theophylline). Products include:
Aerolate 1004
Primatene Dual Action Formula .... ▣ 872
Primatene Tablets .... ▣ 873
Respbid Tablets 682
Slo-bid Gyrocaps 2033
Theo-24 Extended Release Capsules 2568
Theo-Dur Extended-Release Tablets 1327
Theo-X Extended-Release Tablets .. 788
Uni-Dur Extended-Release Tablets .. 1331
Uniphyl 400 mg Tablets 2001

Theophylline Calcium Salicylate (Elevated serum concentrations of theophylline). Products include:
Quadrinal Tablets 1350

Theophylline Sodium Glycinate (Elevated serum concentrations of theophylline).
No products indexed under this heading.

TAPAZOLE TABLETS
(Methimazole) 1477
May interact with anticoagulants. Compounds in this category include:

Dalteparin Sodium (Activity of anticoagulant may be potentiated). Products include:
Fragmin 1954

Dicumarol (Activity of anticoagulant may be potentiated).
No products indexed under this heading.

Enoxaparin (Activity of anticoagulant may be potentiated). Products include:
Lovenox Injection 2020

Heparin Calcium (Activity of anticoagulant may be potentiated).
No products indexed under this heading.

Heparin Sodium (Activity of anticoagulant may be potentiated). Products include:
Heparin Lock Flush Solution 2725
Heparin Sodium Injection 2726
Heparin Sodium Injection, USP, Sterile Solution 2615
Heparin Sodium Vials 1441

Warfarin Sodium (Activity of anticoagulant may be potentiated). Products include:
Coumadin 926

TAVIST SYRUP
(Clemastine Fumarate) 2297
May interact with central nervous system depressants, hypnotics and sedatives, tranquilizers, monoamine oxidase inhibitors, and certain other agents. Compounds in these categories include:

Alfentanil Hydrochloride (Additive effects). Products include:
Alfenta Injection 1286

Alprazolam (Additive effects). Products include:
Xanax Tablets 2649

Aprobarbital (Additive effects).
No products indexed under this heading.

Buprenorphine (Additive effects). Products include:
Buprenex Injectable 2006

Buspirone Hydrochloride (Additive effects). Products include:
BuSpar 737

Butabarbital (Additive effects).
No products indexed under this heading.

Butalbital (Additive effects). Products include:
Esgic-plus Tablets 1013
Fioricet Tablets 2258
Fioricet with Codeine Capsules 2260
Fiorinal Capsules 2261
Fiorinal with Codeine Capsules 2262
Fiorinal Tablets 2261
Phrenilin 785
Sedapap Tablets 50 mg/650 mg .. 1543

Chlordiazepoxide (Additive effects). Products include:
Libritabs Tablets 2177
Limbitrol 2180

Chlordiazepoxide Hydrochloride (Additive effects). Products include:
Librax Capsules 2176
Librium Capsules 2178
Librium Injectable 2179

Chlorpromazine (Additive effects). Products include:
Thorazine Suppositories 2523

Chlorprothixene (Additive effects).
No products indexed under this heading.

Chlorprothixene Hydrochloride (Additive effects).
No products indexed under this heading.

Chlorprothixene Lactate (Additive effects).
No products indexed under this heading.

Clorazepate Dipotassium (Additive effects). Products include:
Tranxene 451

Clozapine (Additive effects). Products include:
Clozaril Tablets 2252

Codeine Phosphate (Additive effects). Products include:
Actifed with Codeine Cough Syrup.. 1067
Brontex 1981
Deconsal C Expectorant Syrup 456
Deconsal Pediatric Syrup 457
Dimetane-DC Cough Syrup 2059
Empirin with Codeine Tablets 1093
Fioricet with Codeine Capsules 2260
Fiorinal with Codeine Capsules 2262
Isoclor Expectorant 990
Novahistine DH 2462
Novahistine Expectorant 2463
Nucofed 2051
Phenergan with Codeine 2777
Phenergan VC with Codeine 2781
Robitussin A-C Syrup 2073
Robitussin-DAC Syrup 2074
Ryna .... ▣ 841
Soma Compound w/Codeine Tablets 2676
Tussi-Organidin NR Liquid and S NR Liquid 2677
Tylenol with Codeine 1583

(▣ Described in PDR For Nonprescription Drugs) (⊙ Described in PDR For Ophthalmology)

1007 Interactions Index Tavist Tablets

Desflurane (Additive effects). Products include:
Suprane ... 1813
Dezocine (Additive effects). Products include:
Dalgan Injection ... 538
Diazepam (Additive effects). Products include:
Dizac ... 1809
Valium Injectable ... 2182
Valium Tablets ... 2183
Valrelease Capsules ... 2169
Droperidol (Additive effects). Products include:
Inapsine Injection ... 1296
Enflurane (Additive effects).
No products indexed under this heading.
Estazolam (Additive effects). Products include:
ProSom Tablets ... 449
Ethchlorvynol (Additive effects). Products include:
Placidyl Capsules ... 448
Ethinamate (Additive effects).
No products indexed under this heading.
Fentanyl (Additive effects). Products include:
Duragesic Transdermal System ... 1288
Fentanyl Citrate (Additive effects). Products include:
Sublimaze Injection ... 1307
Fluphenazine Decanoate (Additive effects). Products include:
Prolixin Decanoate ... 509
Fluphenazine Enanthate (Additive effects). Products include:
Prolixin Enanthate ... 509
Fluphenazine Hydrochloride (Additive effects). Products include:
Prolixin ... 509
Flurazepam Hydrochloride (Additive effects). Products include:
Dalmane Capsules ... 2173
Furazolidone (Prolongs anticholinergic effects of Tavist). Products include:
Furoxone ... 2046
Glutethimide (Additive effects).
No products indexed under this heading.
Haloperidol (Additive effects). Products include:
Haldol Injection, Tablets and Concentrate ... 1575
Haloperidol Decanoate (Additive effects). Products include:
Haldol Decanoate ... 1577
Hydrocodone Bitartrate (Additive effects). Products include:
Anexsia 5/500 Elixir ... 1781
Anexia Tablets ... 1782
Codiclear DH Syrup ... 791
Deconamine CX Cough and Cold Liquid and Tablets ... 1319
Duratuss HD Elixir ... 2565
Hycodan Tablets and Syrup ... 930
Hycomine Compound Tablets ... 932
Hycomine ... 931
Hycotuss Expectorant Syrup ... 933
Hydrocet Capsules ... 782
Lorcet 10/650 ... 1018
Lortab ... 2566
Tussend ... 1783
Tussend Expectorant ... 1785
Vicodin Tablets ... 1356
Vicodin ES Tablets ... 1357
Vicodin Tuss Expectorant ... 1358
Zydone Capsules ... 949
Hydrocodone Polistirex (Additive effects). Products include:
Tussionex Pennkinetic Extended-Release Suspension ... 998
Hydroxyzine Hydrochloride (Additive effects). Products include:
Atarax Tablets & Syrup ... 2185
Marax Tablets & DF Syrup ... 2200
Vistaril Intramuscular Solution ... 2216
Isocarboxazid (Prolongs anticholinergic effects of Tavist).
No products indexed under this heading.
Isoflurane (Additive effects).
No products indexed under this heading.
Ketamine Hydrochloride (Additive effects).
No products indexed under this heading.
Levomethadyl Acetate Hydrochloride (Additive effects). Products include:
Orlamm ... 2239
Levorphanol Tartrate (Additive effects). Products include:
Levo-Dromoran ... 2129
Lorazepam (Additive effects). Products include:
Ativan Injection ... 2698
Ativan Tablets ... 2700
Loxapine Hydrochloride (Additive effects). Products include:
Loxitane ... 1378
Loxapine Succinate (Additive effects). Products include:
Loxitane Capsules ... 1378
Meperidine Hydrochloride (Additive effects). Products include:
Demerol ... 2308
Mepergan Injection ... 2753
Mephobarbital (Additive effects). Products include:
Mebaral Tablets ... 2322
Meprobamate (Additive effects). Products include:
Miltown Tablets ... 2672
PMB 200 and PMB 400 ... 2783
Mesoridazine Besylate (Additive effects). Products include:
Serentil ... 684
Methadone Hydrochloride (Additive effects). Products include:
Methadone Hydrochloride Oral Concentrate ... 2233
Methadone Hydrochloride Oral Solution & Tablets ... 2235
Methohexital Sodium (Additive effects). Products include:
Brevital Sodium Vials ... 1429
Methotrimeprazine (Additive effects). Products include:
Levoprome ... 1274
Methoxyflurane (Additive effects).
No products indexed under this heading.
Midazolam Hydrochloride (Additive effects). Products include:
Versed Injection ... 2170
Molindone Hydrochloride (Additive effects). Products include:
Moban Tablets and Concentrate ... 1048
Morphine Sulfate (Additive effects). Products include:
Astramorph/PF Injection, USP (Preservative-Free) ... 535
Duramorph ... 962
Infumorph 200 and Infumorph 500 Sterile Solutions ... 965
MS Contin Tablets ... 1994
MSIR ... 1997
Oramorph SR (Morphine Sulfate Sustained Release Tablets) ... 2236
RMS Suppositories ... 2657
Roxanol ... 2243
Opium Alkaloids (Additive effects).
No products indexed under this heading.
Oxazepam (Additive effects). Products include:
Serax Capsules ... 2810
Serax Tablets ... 2810
Oxycodone Hydrochloride (Additive effects). Products include:
Percocet Tablets ... 938
Percodan Tablets ... 939
Percodan-Demi Tablets ... 940
Roxicodone Tablets, Oral Solution & Intensol (Oxycodone) ... 2244
Tylox Capsules ... 1584
Pentobarbital Sodium (Additive effects). Products include:
Nembutal Sodium Capsules ... 436
Nembutal Sodium Solution ... 438
Nembutal Sodium Suppositories ... 440
Perphenazine (Additive effects). Products include:
Etrafon ... 2355
Triavil Tablets ... 1757
Trilafon ... 2389
Phenelzine Sulfate (Prolongs anticholinergic effects of Tavist). Products include:
Nardil ... 1920
Phenobarbital (Additive effects). Products include:
Arco-Lase Plus Tablets ... 512
Bellergal-S Tablets ... 2250
Donnatal ... 2060
Donnatal Extentabs ... 2061
Donnatal Tablets ... 2060
Phenobarbital Elixir and Tablets ... 1469
Quadrinal Tablets ... 1350
Prazepam (Additive effects).
No products indexed under this heading.
Prochlorperazine (Additive effects). Products include:
Compazine ... 2470
Promethazine Hydrochloride (Additive effects). Products include:
Mepergan Injection ... 2753
Phenergan with Codeine ... 2777
Phenergan with Dextromethorphan ... 2778
Phenergan Injection ... 2773
Phenergan Suppositories ... 2775
Phenergan Syrup ... 2774
Phenergan Tablets ... 2775
Phenergan VC ... 2779
Phenergan VC with Codeine ... 2781
Propofol (Additive effects). Products include:
Diprivan Injection ... 2833
Propoxyphene Hydrochloride (Additive effects). Products include:
Darvon ... 1435
Wygesic Tablets ... 2827
Propoxyphene Napsylate (Additive effects). Products include:
Darvon-N/Darvocet-N ... 1433
Quazepam (Additive effects). Products include:
Doral Tablets ... 2664
Risperidone (Additive effects). Products include:
Risperdal ... 1301
Secobarbital Sodium (Additive effects). Products include:
Seconal Sodium Pulvules ... 1474
Selegiline Hydrochloride (Prolongs anticholinergic effects of Tavist). Products include:
Eldepryl Tablets ... 2550
Sufentanil Citrate (Additive effects). Products include:
Sufenta Injection ... 1309
Temazepam (Additive effects). Products include:
Restoril Capsules ... 2284
Thiamylal Sodium (Additive effects).
No products indexed under this heading.
Thioridazine Hydrochloride (Additive effects). Products include:
Mellaril ... 2269
Thiothixene (Additive effects). Products include:
Navane Capsules and Concentrate ... 2201
Navane Intramuscular ... 2202
Tranylcypromine Sulfate (Prolongs anticholinergic effects of Tavist). Products include:
Parnate Tablets ... 2503
Triazolam (Additive effects). Products include:
Halcion Tablets ... 2611
Trifluoperazine Hydrochloride (Additive effects). Products include:
Stelazine ... 2514
Zolpidem Tartrate (Additive effects). Products include:
Ambien Tablets ... 2416

Food Interactions

Alcohol (Additive effects).

TAVIST TABLETS
(Clemastine Fumarate) ... 2298
May interact with monoamine oxidase inhibitors, central nervous system depressants, hypnotics and sedatives, tranquilizers, and certain other agents. Compounds in these categories include:

Alfentanil Hydrochloride (Additive effects). Products include:
Alfenta Injection ... 1286
Alprazolam (Additive effects). Products include:
Xanax Tablets ... 2649
Aprobarbital (Additive effects).
No products indexed under this heading.
Buprenorphine (Additive effects). Products include:
Buprenex Injectable ... 2006
Buspirone Hydrochloride (Additive effects). Products include:
BuSpar ... 737
Butabarbital (Additive effects).
No products indexed under this heading.
Butalbital (Additive effects). Products include:
Esgic-plus Tablets ... 1013
Fioricet Tablets ... 2258
Fioricet with Codeine Capsules ... 2260
Fiorinal Capsules ... 2261
Fiorinal with Codeine Capsules ... 2262
Fiorinal Tablets ... 2261
Phrenilin ... 785
Sedapap Tablets 50 mg/650 mg ... 1543
Chlordiazepoxide (Additive effects). Products include:
Libritabs Tablets ... 2177
Limbitrol ... 2180
Chlordiazepoxide Hydrochloride (Additive effects). Products include:
Librax Capsules ... 2176
Librium Capsules ... 2178
Librium Injectable ... 2179
Chlorpromazine (Additive effects). Products include:
Thorazine Suppositories ... 2523
Chlorprothixene (Additive effects).
No products indexed under this heading.
Chlorprothixene Hydrochloride (Additive effects).
No products indexed under this heading.
Chlorprothixene Lactate (Additive effects).
No products indexed under this heading.
Clorazepate Dipotassium (Additive effects). Products include:
Tranxene ... 451
Clozapine (Additive effects). Products include:
Clozaril Tablets ... 2252
Codeine Phosphate (Additive effects). Products include:
Actifed with Codeine Cough Syrup ... 1067
Brontex ... 1981
Deconsal C Expectorant Syrup ... 456
Deconsal Pediatric Syrup ... 457
Dimetane-DC Cough Syrup ... 2059
Empirin with Codeine Tablets ... 1093
Fioricet with Codeine Capsules ... 2260
Fiorinal with Codeine Capsules ... 2262
Isoclor Expectorant ... 990
Novahistine DH ... 2462
Novahistine Expectorant ... 2463

IMPORTANT NOTE: Always consult each drug listing in the patient's regimen for possible interactions.

Tavist Tablets — Interactions Index — 1008

Nucofed ... 2051
Phenergan with Codeine ... 2777
Phenergan VC with Codeine ... 2781
Robitussin A-C Syrup ... 2073
Robitussin-DAC Syrup ... 2074
Ryna ... ◘ 841
Soma Compound w/Codeine Tablets ... 2676
Tussi-Organidin NR Liquid and S NR Liquid ... 2677
Tylenol with Codeine ... 1583

Desflurane (Additive effects). Products include:
Suprane ... 1813

Dezocine (Additive effects). Products include:
Dalgan Injection ... 538

Diazepam (Additive effects). Products include:
Dizac ... 1809
Valium Injectable ... 2182
Valium Tablets ... 2183
Valrelease Capsules ... 2169

Droperidol (Additive effects). Products include:
Inapsine Injection ... 1296

Enflurane (Additive effects).
No products indexed under this heading.

Estazolam (Additive effects). Products include:
ProSom Tablets ... 449

Ethchlorvynol (Additive effects). Products include:
Placidyl Capsules ... 448

Ethinamate (Additive effects).
No products indexed under this heading.

Fentanyl (Additive effects). Products include:
Duragesic Transdermal System ... 1288

Fentanyl Citrate (Additive effects). Products include:
Sublimaze Injection ... 1307

Fluphenazine Decanoate (Additive effects). Products include:
Prolixin Decanoate ... 509

Fluphenazine Enanthate (Additive effects). Products include:
Prolixin Enanthate ... 509

Fluphenazine Hydrochloride (Additive effects). Products include:
Prolixin ... 509

Flurazepam Hydrochloride (Additive effects). Products include:
Dalmane Capsules ... 2173

Furazolidone (Prolongs anticholinergic effects of Tavist; concurrent use is contraindicated). Products include:
Furoxone ... 2046

Glutethimide (Additive effects).
No products indexed under this heading.

Haloperidol (Additive effects). Products include:
Haldol Injection, Tablets and Concentrate ... 1575

Haloperidol Decanoate (Additive effects). Products include:
Haldol Decanoate ... 1577

Hydrocodone Bitartrate (Additive effects). Products include:
Anexsia 5/500 Elixir ... 1781
Anexia Tablets ... 1782
Codiclear DH Syrup ... 791
Deconamine CX Cough and Cold Liquid and Tablets ... 1319
Duratuss HD Elixir ... 2565
Hycodan Tablets and Syrup ... 930
Hycomine Compound Tablets ... 932
Hycomine ... 931
Hycotuss Expectorant Syrup ... 933
Hydrocet Capsules ... 782
Lorcet 10/650 ... 1018
Lortab ... 2566
Tussend ... 1783
Tussend Expectorant ... 1785
Vicodin Tablets ... 1356
Vicodin ES Tablets ... 1357
Vicodin Tuss Expectorant ... 1358
Zydone Capsules ... 949

Hydrocodone Polistirex (Additive effects). Products include:
Tussionex Pennkinetic Extended-Release Suspension ... 998

Hydroxyzine Hydrochloride (Additive effects). Products include:
Atarax Tablets & Syrup ... 2185
Marax Tablets & DF Syrup ... 2200
Vistaril Intramuscular Solution ... 2216

Isocarboxazid (Prolongs anticholinergic effects of Tavist; concurrent use is contraindicated).
No products indexed under this heading.

Isoflurane (Additive effects).
No products indexed under this heading.

Ketamine Hydrochloride (Additive effects).
No products indexed under this heading.

Levomethadyl Acetate Hydrochloride (Additive effects). Products include:
Orlamm ... 2239

Levorphanol Tartrate (Additive effects). Products include:
Levo-Dromoran ... 2129

Lorazepam (Additive effects). Products include:
Ativan Injection ... 2698
Ativan Tablets ... 2700

Loxapine Hydrochloride (Additive effects). Products include:
Loxitane ... 1378

Loxapine Succinate (Additive effects). Products include:
Loxitane Capsules ... 1378

Meperidine Hydrochloride (Additive effects). Products include:
Demerol ... 2308
Mepergan Injection ... 2753

Mephobarbital (Additive effects). Products include:
Mebaral Tablets ... 2322

Meprobamate (Additive effects). Products include:
Miltown Tablets ... 2672
PMB 200 and PMB 400 ... 2783

Mesoridazine Besylate (Additive effects). Products include:
Serentil ... 684

Methadone Hydrochloride (Additive effects). Products include:
Methadone Hydrochloride Oral Concentrate ... 2233
Methadone Hydrochloride Oral Solution & Tablets ... 2235

Methohexital Sodium (Additive effects). Products include:
Brevital Sodium Vials ... 1429

Methotrimeprazine (Additive effects). Products include:
Levoprome ... 1274

Methoxyflurane (Additive effects).
No products indexed under this heading.

Midazolam Hydrochloride (Additive effects). Products include:
Versed Injection ... 2170

Molindone Hydrochloride (Additive effects). Products include:
Moban Tablets and Concentrate ... 1048

Morphine Sulfate (Additive effects). Products include:
Astramorph/PF Injection, USP (Preservative-Free) ... 535
Duramorph ... 962
Infumorph 200 and Infumorph 500 Sterile Solutions ... 965
MS Contin Tablets ... 1994
MSIR ... 1997
Oramorph SR (Morphine Sulfate Sustained Release Tablets) ... 2236
RMS Suppositories ... 2657
Roxanol ... 2243

Opium Alkaloids (Additive effects).
No products indexed under this heading.

Oxazepam (Additive effects). Products include:
Serax Capsules ... 2810
Serax Tablets ... 2810

Oxycodone Hydrochloride (Additive effects). Products include:
Percocet Tablets ... 938
Percodan Tablets ... 939
Percodan-Demi Tablets ... 940
Roxicodone Tablets, Oral Solution & Intensol (Oxycodone) ... 2244
Tylox Capsules ... 1584

Pentobarbital Sodium (Additive effects). Products include:
Nembutal Sodium Capsules ... 436
Nembutal Sodium Solution ... 438
Nembutal Sodium Suppositories ... 440

Perphenazine (Additive effects). Products include:
Etrafon ... 2355
Triavil Tablets ... 1757
Trilafon ... 2389

Phenelzine Sulfate (Prolongs anticholinergic effects of Tavist; concurrent use is contraindicated). Products include:
Nardil ... 1920

Phenobarbital (Additive effects). Products include:
Arco-Lase Plus Tablets ... 512
Bellergal-S Tablets ... 2250
Donnatal ... 2060
Donnatal Extentabs ... 2061
Donnatal Tablets ... 2060
Phenobarbital Elixir and Tablets ... 1469
Quadrinal Tablets ... 1350

Prazepam (Additive effects).
No products indexed under this heading.

Prochlorperazine (Additive effects). Products include:
Compazine ... 2470

Promethazine Hydrochloride (Additive effects). Products include:
Mepergan Injection ... 2753
Phenergan with Codeine ... 2777
Phenergan with Dextromethorphan ... 2778
Phenergan Injection ... 2773
Phenergan Suppositories ... 2775
Phenergan Syrup ... 2774
Phenergan Tablets ... 2775
Phenergan VC ... 2779
Phenergan VC with Codeine ... 2781

Propofol (Additive effects). Products include:
Diprivan Injection ... 2833

Propoxyphene Hydrochloride (Additive effects). Products include:
Darvon ... 1435
Wygesic Tablets ... 2827

Propoxyphene Napsylate (Additive effects). Products include:
Darvon-N/Darvocet-N ... 1433

Quazepam (Additive effects). Products include:
Doral Tablets ... 2664

Risperidone (Additive effects). Products include:
Risperdal ... 1301

Secobarbital Sodium (Additive effects). Products include:
Seconal Sodium Pulvules ... 1474

Selegiline Hydrochloride (Prolongs anticholinergic effects of Tavist; concurrent use is contraindicated). Products include:
Eldepryl Tablets ... 2550

Sufentanil Citrate (Additive effects). Products include:
Sufenta Injection ... 1309

Temazepam (Additive effects). Products include:
Restoril Capsules ... 2284

Thiamylal Sodium (Additive effects).
No products indexed under this heading.

Thioridazine Hydrochloride (Additive effects). Products include:
Mellaril ... 2269

Thiothixene (Additive effects). Products include:
Navane Capsules and Concentrate ... 2201
Navane Intramuscular ... 2202

Tranylcypromine Sulfate (Prolongs anticholinergic effects of Tavist; concurrent use is contraindicated). Products include:
Parnate Tablets ... 2503

Triazolam (Additive effects). Products include:
Halcion Tablets ... 2611

Trifluoperazine Hydrochloride (Additive effects). Products include:
Stelazine ... 2514

Zolpidem Tartrate (Additive effects). Products include:
Ambien Tablets ... 2416

Food Interactions

Alcohol (Additive effects).

TAVIST-D 12 HOUR RELIEF TABLETS
(Clemastine Fumarate, Phenylpropanolamine Hydrochloride) ... ◘ 787
May interact with hypnotics and sedatives, tranquilizers, antidepressant drugs, antihypertensives, and certain other agents. Compounds in these categories include:

Acebutolol Hydrochloride (Effect of concurrent use not specified). Products include:
Sectral Capsules ... 2807

Alprazolam (Increases drowsiness effect). Products include:
Xanax Tablets ... 2649

Amitriptyline Hydrochloride (Effect of concurrent use not specified). Products include:
Elavil ... 2838
Endep Tablets ... 2174
Etrafon ... 2355
Limbitrol ... 2180
Triavil Tablets ... 1757

Amlodipine Besylate (Effect of concurrent use not specified). Products include:
Lotrel Capsules ... 840
Norvasc Tablets ... 1940

Amoxapine (Effect of concurrent use not specified). Products include:
Asendin Tablets ... 1369

Atenolol (Effect of concurrent use not specified). Products include:
Tenoretic Tablets ... 2845
Tenormin Tablets and I.V. Injection ... 2847

Benazepril Hydrochloride (Effect of concurrent use not specified). Products include:
Lotensin Tablets ... 834
Lotensin HCT ... 837
Lotrel Capsules ... 840

Bendroflumethiazide (Effect of concurrent use not specified).
No products indexed under this heading.

Betaxolol Hydrochloride (Effect of concurrent use not specified). Products include:
Betoptic Ophthalmic Solution ... 469
Betoptic S Ophthalmic Suspension ... 471
Kerlone Tablets ... 2436

Bisoprolol Fumarate (Effect of concurrent use not specified). Products include:
Zebeta Tablets ... 1413
Ziac ... 1415

(◘ Described in PDR For Nonprescription Drugs) (⊙ Described in PDR For Ophthalmology)

1009 Interactions Index Tavist-D

Bupropion Hydrochloride (Effect of concurrent use not specified). Products include:
Wellbutrin Tablets 1204
Buspirone Hydrochloride (Increases drowsiness effect). Products include:
BuSpar 737
Captopril (Effect of concurrent use not specified). Products include:
Capoten 739
Capozide 742
Carteolol Hydrochloride (Effect of concurrent use not specified). Products include:
Cartrol Tablets 410
Ocupress Ophthalmic Solution, 1% Sterile ⊚ 309
Chlordiazepoxide (Increases drowsiness effect). Products include:
Libritabs Tablets 2177
Limbitrol 2180
Chlordiazepoxide Hydrochloride (Increases drowsiness effect). Products include:
Librax Capsules 2176
Librium Capsules 2178
Librium Injectable 2179
Chlorothiazide (Effect of concurrent use not specified). Products include:
Aldoclor Tablets 1598
Diupres Tablets 1650
Diuril Oral 1653
Chlorothiazide Sodium (Effect of concurrent use not specified). Products include:
Diuril Sodium Intravenous 1652
Chlorpromazine (Increases drowsiness effect). Products include:
Thorazine Suppositories 2523
Chlorpromazine Hydrochloride (Increases drowsiness effect). Products include:
Thorazine 2523
Chlorprothixene (Increases drowsiness effect).
No products indexed under this heading.
Chlorprothixene Hydrochloride (Increases drowsiness effect).
No products indexed under this heading.
Chlorthalidone (Effect of concurrent use not specified). Products include:
Combipres Tablets 677
Tenoretic Tablets 2845
Thalitone 1245
Clonidine (Effect of concurrent use not specified). Products include:
Catapres-TTS 675
Clonidine Hydrochloride (Effect of concurrent use not specified). Products include:
Catapres Tablets 674
Combipres Tablets 677
Clorazepate Dipotassium (Increases drowsiness effect). Products include:
Tranxene 451
Deserpidine (Effect of concurrent use not specified).
No products indexed under this heading.
Desipramine Hydrochloride (Effect of concurrent use not specified). Products include:
Norpramin Tablets 1526
Diazepam (Increases drowsiness effect). Products include:
Dizac 1809
Valium Injectable 2182
Valium Tablets 2183
Valrelease Capsules 2169
Diazoxide (Effect of concurrent use not specified). Products include:
Hyperstat I.V. Injection 2363
Proglycem 580
Diltiazem Hydrochloride (Effect of concurrent use not specified). Products include:
Cardizem CD Capsules 1506
Cardizem SR Capsules 1510
Cardizem Injectable 1508
Cardizem Tablets 1512
Dilacor XR Extended-release Capsules 2018
Doxazosin Mesylate (Effect of concurrent use not specified). Products include:
Cardura Tablets 2186
Doxepin Hydrochloride (Effect of concurrent use not specified). Products include:
Sinequan 2205
Zonalon Cream 1055
Droperidol (Increases drowsiness effect). Products include:
Inapsine Injection 1296
Enalapril Maleate (Effect of concurrent use not specified). Products include:
Vaseretic Tablets 1765
Vasotec Tablets 1771
Enalaprilat (Effect of concurrent use not specified). Products include:
Vasotec I.V. 1768
Esmolol Hydrochloride (Effect of concurrent use not specified). Products include:
Brevibloc Injection 1808
Estazolam (Increases drowsiness effect). Products include:
ProSom Tablets 449
Ethchlorvynol (Increases drowsiness effect). Products include:
Placidyl Capsules 448
Ethinamate (Increases drowsiness effect).
No products indexed under this heading.
Felodipine (Effect of concurrent use not specified). Products include:
Plendil Extended-Release Tablets 527
Fluoxetine Hydrochloride (Effect of concurrent use not specified). Products include:
Prozac Pulvules & Liquid, Oral Solution 919
Fluphenazine Decanoate (Increases drowsiness effect). Products include:
Prolixin Decanoate 509
Fluphenazine Enanthate (Increases drowsiness effect). Products include:
Prolixin Enanthate 509
Fluphenazine Hydrochloride (Increases drowsiness effect). Products include:
Prolixin 509
Flurazepam Hydrochloride (Increases drowsiness effect). Products include:
Dalmane Capsules 2173
Fosinopril Sodium (Effect of concurrent use not specified). Products include:
Monopril Tablets 757
Furosemide (Effect of concurrent use not specified). Products include:
Lasix Injection, Oral Solution and Tablets 1240
Glutethimide (Increases drowsiness effect).
No products indexed under this heading.
Guanabenz Acetate (Effect of concurrent use not specified).
No products indexed under this heading.
Guanethidine Monosulfate (Effect of concurrent use not specified). Products include:
Esimil Tablets 822
Ismelin Tablets 827
Haloperidol (Increases drowsiness effect). Products include:
Haldol Injection, Tablets and Concentrate 1575
Haloperidol Decanoate (Increases drowsiness effect). Products include:
Haldol Decanoate 1577
Hydralazine Hydrochloride (Effect of concurrent use not specified). Products include:
Apresazide Capsules 808
Apresoline Hydrochloride Tablets 809
Ser-Ap-Es Tablets 849
Hydrochlorothiazide (Effect of concurrent use not specified). Products include:
Aldactazide 2413
Aldoril Tablets 1604
Apresazide Capsules 808
Capozide 742
Dyazide 2479
Esidrix Tablets 821
Esimil Tablets 822
HydroDIURIL Tablets 1674
Hydropres Tablets 1675
Hyzaar Tablets 1677
Inderide Tablets 2732
Inderide LA Long Acting Capsules 2734
Lopressor HCT Tablets 832
Lotensin HCT 837
Maxzide 1380
Moduretic Tablets 1705
Oretic Tablets 443
Prinzide Tablets 1737
Ser-Ap-Es Tablets 849
Timolide Tablets 1748
Vaseretic Tablets 1765
Zestoretic 2850
Ziac 1415
Hydroflumethiazide (Effect of concurrent use not specified). Products include:
Diucardin Tablets 2718
Hydroxyzine Hydrochloride (Increases drowsiness effect). Products include:
Atarax Tablets & Syrup 2185
Marax Tablets & DF Syrup 2200
Vistaril Intramuscular Solution 2216
Imipramine Hydrochloride (Effect of concurrent use not specified). Products include:
Tofranil Ampuls 854
Tofranil Tablets 856
Imipramine Pamoate (Effect of concurrent use not specified). Products include:
Tofranil-PM Capsules 857
Indapamide (Effect of concurrent use not specified). Products include:
Lozol Tablets 2022
Isocarboxazid (Effect of concurrent use not specified).
No products indexed under this heading.
Isradipine (Effect of concurrent use not specified). Products include:
DynaCirc Capsules 2256
Labetalol Hydrochloride (Effect of concurrent use not specified). Products include:
Normodyne Injection 2377
Normodyne Tablets 2379
Trandate 1185
Lisinopril (Effect of concurrent use not specified). Products include:
Prinivil Tablets 1733
Prinzide Tablets 1737
Zestoretic 2850
Zestril Tablets 2854
Lorazepam (Increases drowsiness effect). Products include:
Ativan Injection 2698
Ativan Tablets 2700
Losartan Potassium (Effect of concurrent use not specified). Products include:
Cozaar Tablets 1628
Hyzaar Tablets 1677
Loxapine Hydrochloride (Increases drowsiness effect). Products include:
Loxitane 1378
Loxapine Succinate (Increases drowsiness effect). Products include:
Loxitane Capsules 1378
Maprotiline Hydrochloride (Effect of concurrent use not specified). Products include:
Ludiomil Tablets 843
Mecamylamine Hydrochloride (Effect of concurrent use not specified). Products include:
Inversine Tablets 1686
Meprobamate (Increases drowsiness effect). Products include:
Miltown Tablets 2672
PMB 200 and PMB 400 2783
Mesoridazine Besylate (Increases drowsiness effect). Products include:
Serentil 684
Methyclothiazide (Effect of concurrent use not specified). Products include:
Enduron Tablets 420
Methyldopa (Effect of concurrent use not specified). Products include:
Aldoclor Tablets 1598
Aldomet Oral 1600
Aldoril Tablets 1604
Methyldopate Hydrochloride (Effect of concurrent use not specified). Products include:
Aldomet Ester HCl Injection 1602
Metolazone (Effect of concurrent use not specified). Products include:
Mykrox Tablets 993
Zaroxolyn Tablets 1000
Metoprolol Succinate (Effect of concurrent use not specified). Products include:
Toprol-XL Tablets 565
Metoprolol Tartrate (Effect of concurrent use not specified). Products include:
Lopressor Ampuls 830
Lopressor HCT Tablets 832
Lopressor Tablets 830
Metyrosine (Effect of concurrent use not specified). Products include:
Demser Capsules 1649
Midazolam Hydrochloride (Increases drowsiness effect). Products include:
Versed Injection 2170
Minoxidil (Effect of concurrent use not specified). Products include:
Loniten Tablets 2618
Rogaine Topical Solution 2637
Moexipril Hydrochloride (Effect of concurrent use not specified). Products include:
Univasc Tablets 2410
Molindone Hydrochloride (Increases drowsiness effect). Products include:
Moban Tablets and Concentrate 1048
Nadolol (Effect of concurrent use not specified).
No products indexed under this heading.
Nefazodone Hydrochloride (Effect of concurrent use not specified). Products include:
Serzone Tablets 771
Nicardipine Hydrochloride (Effect of concurrent use not specified). Products include:
Cardene Capsules 2095
Cardene I.V. 2709
Cardene SR Capsules 2097
Nifedipine (Effect of concurrent use not specified). Products include:
Adalat Capsules (10 mg and 20 mg) 587
Adalat CC 589

IMPORTANT NOTE: Always consult each drug listing in the patient's regimen for possible interactions.

Tavist-D Interactions Index 1010

Procardia Capsules ... 1971
Procardia XL Extended Release Tablets ... 1972

Nisoldipine (Effect of concurrent use not specified).
No products indexed under this heading.

Nitroglycerin (Effect of concurrent use not specified). Products include:
Deponit NTG Transdermal Delivery System ... 2397
Nitro-Bid IV ... 1523
Nitro-Bid Ointment ... 1524
Nitrodisc ... 2047
Nitro-Dur (nitroglycerin) Transdermal Infusion System ... 1326
Nitrolingual Spray ... 2027
Nitrostat Tablets ... 1925
Transderm-Nitro Transdermal Therapeutic System ... 859

Nortriptyline Hydrochloride (Effect of concurrent use not specified). Products include:
Pamelor ... 2280

Oxazepam (Increases drowsiness effect). Products include:
Serax Capsules ... 2810
Serax Tablets ... 2810

Paroxetine Hydrochloride (Effect of concurrent use not specified). Products include:
Paxil Tablets ... 2505

Penbutolol Sulfate (Effect of concurrent use not specified). Products include:
Levatol ... 2403

Perphenazine (Increases drowsiness effect). Products include:
Etrafon ... 2355
Triavil Tablets ... 1757
Trilafon ... 2389

Phenelzine Sulfate (Effect of concurrent use not specified). Products include:
Nardil ... 1920

Phenoxybenzamine Hydrochloride (Effect of concurrent use not specified). Products include:
Dibenzyline Capsules ... 2476

Phentolamine Mesylate (Effect of concurrent use not specified). Products include:
Regitine ... 846

Phenylephrine Hydrochloride (Effect of concurrent use not specified). Products include:
Atrohist Plus Tablets ... 454
Cerose DM ... ▣ 878
Comhist ... 2038
D.A. Chewable Tablets ... 951
Deconsal Pediatric Capsules ... 454
Dura-Vent/DA Tablets ... 953
Entex Capsules ... 1986
Entex Liquid ... 1986
Extendryl ... 1005
4-Way Fast Acting Nasal Spray (regular & mentholated) ... ▣ 621
Hemorid For Women ... ▣ 834
Hycomine Compound Tablets ... 932
Neo-Synephrine Hydrochloride 1% Carpuject ... 2324
Neo-Synephrine Hydrochloride 1% Injection ... 2324
Neo-Synephrine Hydrochloride (Ophthalmic) ... 2325
Neo-Synephrine ... ▣ 726
Nōstril ... ▣ 644
Novahistine Elixir ... ▣ 823
Phenergan VC ... 2779
Phenergan VC with Codeine ... 2781
Preparation H ... ▣ 871
Tympagesic Ear Drops ... 2342
Vasosulf ... ⊙ 271
Vicks Sinex Nasal Spray and Ultra Fine Mist ... ▣ 765

Pindolol (Effect of concurrent use not specified). Products include:
Visken Tablets ... 2299

Polythiazide (Effect of concurrent use not specified). Products include:
Minizide Capsules ... 1938

Prazepam (Increases drowsiness effect).
No products indexed under this heading.

Prazosin Hydrochloride (Effect of concurrent use not specified). Products include:
Minipress Capsules ... 1937
Minizide Capsules ... 1938

Prochlorperazine (Increases drowsiness effect). Products include:
Compazine ... 2470

Promethazine Hydrochloride (Increases drowsiness effect). Products include:
Mepergan Injection ... 2753
Phenergan with Codeine ... 2777
Phenergan with Dextromethorphan ... 2778
Phenergan Injection ... 2773
Phenergan Suppositories ... 2775
Phenergan Syrup ... 2774
Phenergan Tablets ... 2775
Phenergan VC ... 2779
Phenergan VC with Codeine ... 2781

Propofol (Increases drowsiness effect). Products include:
Diprivan Injection ... 2833

Propranolol Hydrochloride (Effect of concurrent use not specified). Products include:
Inderal ... 2728
Inderal LA Long Acting Capsules ... 2730
Inderide Tablets ... 2732
Inderide LA Long Acting Capsules ... 2734

Protriptyline Hydrochloride (Effect of concurrent use not specified). Products include:
Vivactil Tablets ... 1774

Pseudoephedrine Hydrochloride (Effect of concurrent use not specified). Products include:
Actifed Allergy Daytime/Nighttime Caplets ... ▣ 844
Actifed Plus Caplets ... ▣ 845
Actifed Plus Tablets ... ▣ 845
Actifed with Codeine Cough Syrup ... 1067
Actifed Sinus Daytime/Nighttime Tablets and Caplets ... ▣ 846
Actifed Syrup ... ▣ 846
Actifed Tablets ... ▣ 844
Advil Cold and Sinus Caplets and Tablets (formerly CoAdvil) ... ▣ 870
Alka-Seltzer Plus Cold Medicine Liqui-Gels ... ▣ 706
Alka-Seltzer Plus Cold & Cough Medicine Liqui-Gels ... ▣ 705
Alka-Seltzer Plus Night-Time Cold Medicine Liqui-Gels ... ▣ 706
Allerest Headache Strength Tablets ... ▣ 627
Allerest Maximum Strength Tablets ... ▣ 627
Allerest No Drowsiness Tablets ... ▣ 627
Allerest Sinus Pain Formula ... ▣ 627
Anatuss LA Tablets ... 1542
Atrohist Pediatric Capsules ... 453
Bayer Select Sinus Pain Relief Formula ... ▣ 717
Benadryl Allergy Decongestant Liquid Medication ... ▣ 848
Benadryl Allergy Decongestant Tablets ... ▣ 848
Benadryl Allergy Sinus Headache Formula Caplets ... ▣ 849
Benylin Multisymptom ... ▣ 852
Bromfed Capsules (Extended-Release) ... 1785
Bromfed Syrup ... ▣ 733
Bromfed Tablets ... 1785
Bromfed-DM Cough Syrup ... 1786
Bromfed-PD Capsules (Extended-Release) ... 1785
Children's Vicks DayQuil Allergy Relief ... ▣ 757
Children's Vicks NyQuil Cold/Cough Relief ... ▣ 758
Comtrex Multi-Symptom Cold Reliever Tablets/Caplets/Liqui-Gels/Liquid ... ▣ 615
Allergy-Sinus Comtrex Multi-Symptom Allergy-Sinus Formula Tablets ... ▣ 617
Comtrex Multi-Symptom Non-Drowsy Caplets ... ▣ 618
Congess ... 1004
Contac Day Allergy/Sinus Caplets ... ▣ 812
Contac Day & Night ... ▣ 812
Contac Night Allergy/Sinus Caplets ... ▣ 812
Contac Severe Cold & Flu Non-Drowsy ... ▣ 815
Deconamine Chewable Tablets ... 1320
Deconamine CX Cough and Cold Liquid and Tablets ... 1319
Deconamine ... 1320
Deconsal C Expectorant Syrup ... 456
Deconsal Pediatric Syrup ... 457
Deconsal II Tablets ... 454
Dimetane-DX Cough Syrup ... 2059
Dimetapp Sinus Caplets ... ▣ 775
Dorcol Children's Cough Syrup ... ▣ 785
Drixoral Cough + Congestion Liquid Caps ... ▣ 802
Dura-Tap/PD Capsules ... 2867
Duratuss Tablets ... 2565
Duratuss HD Elixir ... 2565
Efidac/24 ... ▣ 635
Entex PSE Tablets ... 1987
Fedahist Gyrocaps ... 2401
Fedahist Timecaps ... 2401
Guaifed ... 1787
Guaifed Syrup ... ▣ 734
Guaimax-D Tablets ... 792
Guaitab Tablets ... ▣ 734
Isoclor Expectorant ... 990
Kronofed-A ... 977
Motrin IB Sinus ... ▣ 838
Novahistine DH ... 2462
Novahistine DMX ... ▣ 822
Novahistine Expectorant ... 2463
Nucofed ... 2051
PediaCare Cold Allergy Chewable Tablets ... ▣ 677
PediaCare Cough-Cold Chewable Tablets ... 1553
PediaCare ... 1553
PediaCare Infants' Decongestant Drops ... ▣ 677
PediCare Infant's Drops Decongestant Plus Cough ... 1553
PediaCare NightRest Cough-Cold Liquid ... 1553
Pediatric Vicks 44d Dry Hacking Cough & Head Congestion ... ▣ 763
Pediatric Vicks 44m Cough & Cold Relief ... ▣ 764
Robitussin Cold & Cough Liqui-Gels ... ▣ 776
Robitussin Maximum Strength Cough & Cold ... ▣ 778
Robitussin Pediatric Cough & Cold Formula ... ▣ 779
Robitussin Severe Congestion Liqui-Gels ... ▣ 776
Robitussin-DAC Syrup ... 2074
Robitussin-PE ... ▣ 778
Rondec Oral Drops ... 953
Rondec Syrup ... 953
Rondec Tablet ... 953
Rondec-DM Oral Drops ... 954
Rondec-DM Syrup ... 954
Rondec-TR Tablet ... 953
Ryna ... ▣ 841
Seldane-D Extended-Release Tablets ... 1538
Semprex-D Capsules ... 463
Semprex-D Capsules ... 1167
Sinarest Tablets ... ▣ 648
Sinarest Extra Strength Tablets ... ▣ 648
Sinarest No Drowsiness Tablets ... ▣ 648
Sine-Aid IB Caplets ... 1554
Sine-Aid Maximum Strength Sinus Medication Gelcaps, Caplets and Tablets ... 1554
Sine-Off No Drowsiness Formula Caplets ... ▣ 824
Sine-Off Sinus Medicine ... ▣ 825
Singlet Tablets ... ▣ 825
Sinutab Non-Drying Liquid Caps ... ▣ 859
Sinutab Sinus Allergy Medication, Maximum Strength Tablets and Caplets ... ▣ 860
Sinutab Sinus Medication, Maximum Strength Without Drowsiness Formula, Tablets & Caplets ... ▣ 860
Sinutab Sinus Medication, Regular Strength Without Drowsiness Formula ... ▣ 859
Sudafed Children's Liquid ... ▣ 861
Sudafed Cold and Cough Liquidcaps ... ▣ 862
Sudafed Cough Syrup ... ▣ 862
Sudafed Plus Liquid ... ▣ 862
Sudafed Plus Tablets ... ▣ 863
Sudafed Severe Cold Formula Caplets ... ▣ 863
Sudafed Severe Cold Formula Tablets ... ▣ 864
Sudafed Sinus Caplets ... ▣ 864
Sudafed Sinus Tablets ... ▣ 864
Sudafed Tablets, 30 mg ... ▣ 861
Sudafed Tablets, 60 mg ... ▣ 861
Sudafed 12 Hour Caplets ... ▣ 861
Syn-Rx Tablets ... 465
Syn-Rx DM Tablets ... 466
TheraFlu ... ▣ 787
TheraFlu Maximum Strength Nighttime Flu, Cold & Cough Medicine ... ▣ 788
TheraFlu Maximum Strength Non-Drowsy Formula Flu, Cold & Cough Medicine ... ▣ 788
Thera Flu Maximum Strength, Non-Drowsy Formula Flu, Cold and Cough Caplets ... ▣ 789
Triaminic AM Cough and Decongestant Formula ... ▣ 789
Triaminic AM Decongestant Formula ... ▣ 790
Triaminic Nite Light ... ▣ 791
Triaminic Sore Throat Formula ... ▣ 791
Tussend ... 1783
Tussend Expectorant ... 1785
Children's TYLENOL Cold Multi-Symptom Liquid Formula and Chewable Tablets ... 1561
Children's TYLENOL Cold Plus Cough Multi Symptom Tablets and Liquid ... ▣ 681
Infants' TYLENOL Cold Decongestant & Fever-Reducer Drops ... 1556
TYLENOL Maximum Strength Allergy Sinus Medication Gelcaps and Caplets ... 1563
TYLENOL Maximum Strength Allergy Sinus NightTime Medication Caplets ... 1555
TYLENOL Flu Maximum Strength Gelcaps ... 1565
TYLENOL Flu NightTime, Maximum Strength, Gelcaps ... 1566
TYLENOL Maximum Strength Flu NightTime Hot Medication Packets ... 1562
TYLENOL, Maximum Strength, Sinus Medication Geltabs, Gelcaps, Caplets and Tablets ... 1566
TYLENOL Cold Multi-Symptom Formula Medication Tablets and Caplets ... 1561
TYLENOL Cold Medication No Drowsiness Formula Gelcaps and Caplets ... 1562
TYLENOL Cold Multi-Symptom Hot Medication Liquid Packets ... 1557
TYLENOL Cough Multi-Symptom Medication with Decongestant ... 1565
Ursinus Inlay-Tabs ... ▣ 794
Vicks 44 LiquiCaps Cough, Cold & Flu Relief ... ▣ 755
Vicks 44 LiquiCaps Non-Drowsy Cough & Cold Relief ... ▣ 756
Vicks 44D Dry Hacking Cough & Head Congestion ... ▣ 755
Vicks 44M Cough, Cold & Flu Relief ... ▣ 756
Vicks DayQuil ... ▣ 761
Vicks DayQuil SINUS Pressure & PAIN Relief with IBUPROFEN ... ▣ 762
Vicks Nyquil Hot Therapy ... ▣ 762
Vicks NyQuil LiquiCaps Multi-Symptom Cold/Flu Relief ... ▣ 763
Vicks NyQuil Multi-Symptom Cold/Flu Relief - (Original & Cherry Flavor) ... ▣ 763

Pseudoephedrine Sulfate (Effect of concurrent use not specified). Products include:
Cheracol Sinus ... ▣ 768
Chlor-Trimeton Allergy Decongestant Tablets ... ▣ 799
Claritin-D ... 2350
Drixoral Cold and Allergy Sustained-Action Tablets ... ▣ 802
Drixoral Cold and Flu Extended-Release Tablets ... ▣ 803
Drixoral Non-Drowsy Formula Extended-Release Tablets ... ▣ 803
Drixoral Allergy/Sinus Extended Release Tablets ... ▣ 804
Trinalin Repetabs Tablets ... 1330

Quazepam (Increases drowsiness effect). Products include:
Doral Tablets ... 2664

(▣ Described in PDR For Nonprescription Drugs) (⊙ Described in PDR For Ophthalmology)

1011 **Interactions Index** **Tegretol**

Quinapril Hydrochloride (Effect of concurrent use not specified). Products include:
Accupril Tablets ... 1893
Ramipril (Effect of concurrent use not specified). Products include:
Altace Capsules ... 1232
Rauwolfia Serpentina (Effect of concurrent use not specified).
No products indexed under this heading.
Rescinnamine (Effect of concurrent use not specified).
No products indexed under this heading.
Reserpine (Effect of concurrent use not specified). Products include:
Diupres Tablets ... 1650
Hydropres Tablets ... 1675
Ser-Ap-Es Tablets ... 849
Secobarbital Sodium (Increases drowsiness effect). Products include:
Seconal Sodium Pulvules ... 1474
Sertraline Hydrochloride (Effect of concurrent use not specified). Products include:
Zoloft Tablets ... 2217
Sodium Nitroprusside (Effect of concurrent use not specified).
No products indexed under this heading.
Sotalol Hydrochloride (Effect of concurrent use not specified). Products include:
Betapace Tablets ... 641
Spirapril Hydrochloride (Effect of concurrent use not specified).
No products indexed under this heading.
Temazepam (Increases drowsiness effect). Products include:
Restoril Capsules ... 2284
Terazosin Hydrochloride (Effect of concurrent use not specified). Products include:
Hytrin Capsules ... 430
Thioridazine Hydrochloride (Increases drowsiness effect). Products include:
Mellaril ... 2269
Thiothixene (Increases drowsiness effect). Products include:
Navane Capsules and Concentrate 2201
Navane Intramuscular 2202
Timolol Maleate (Effect of concurrent use not specified). Products include:
Blocadren Tablets ... 1614
Timolide Tablets ... 1748
Timoptic in Ocudose ... 1753
Timoptic Sterile Ophthalmic Solution ... 1751
Timoptic-XE ... 1755
Torsemide (Effect of concurrent use not specified). Products include:
Demadex Tablets and Injection ... 686
Tranylcypromine Sulfate (Effect of concurrent use not specified). Products include:
Parnate Tablets ... 2503
Trazodone Hydrochloride (Effect of concurrent use not specified). Products include:
Desyrel and Desyrel Dividose ... 503
Triazolam (Increases drowsiness effect). Products include:
Halcion Tablets ... 2611
Trifluoperazine Hydrochloride (Increases drowsiness effect). Products include:
Stelazine ... 2514
Trimethaphan Camsylate (Effect of concurrent use not specified). Products include:
Arfonad Ampuls ... 2080
Trimipramine Maleate (Effect of concurrent use not specified). Products include:
Surmontil Capsules ... 2811
Venlafaxine Hydrochloride (Effect of concurrent use not specified). Products include:
Effexor ... 2719
Verapamil Hydrochloride (Effect of concurrent use not specified). Products include:
Calan SR Caplets ... 2422
Calan Tablets ... 2419
Isoptin Injectable ... 1344
Isoptin Oral Tablets ... 1346
Isoptin SR Tablets ... 1348
Verelan Capsules ... 1410
Verelan Capsules ... 2824
Zolpidem Tartrate (Increases drowsiness effect). Products include:
Ambien Tablets ... 2416

Food Interactions
Alcohol (Increases drowsiness effect).

TAXOL
(Paclitaxel) ... 714
May interact with:

Cisplatin (Decreases paclitaxel clearance approximately 33% when Taxol is administered following cisplatin; concurrent administration given as sequential infusion results in profound myelosuppression when Taxol is given after cisplatin.). Products include:
Platinol ... 708
Platinol-AQ Injection ... 710
Ketoconazole (Possibility of an inhibition of Taxol metabolism based on *in vitro* data). Products include:
Nizoral 2% Cream ... 1297
Nizoral 2% Shampoo ... 1298
Nizoral Tablets ... 1298

TAZICEF FOR INJECTION
(Ceftazidime) ... 2519
May interact with aminoglycosides and certain other agents. Compounds in these categories include:

Amikacin Sulfate (Concomitant administration may result in nephrotoxicity). Products include:
Amikacin Sulfate Injection, USP ... 960
Amikin Injectable ... 501
Chloramphenicol (Chloramphenicol in combination with cephalosporins, including ceftazidime, has been shown to be antagonistic *in vitro;* due to possibility of antagonism *in vivo,* this combination should be avoided). Products include:
Chloromycetin Ophthalmic Ointment, 1% ... ⊙ 310
Chloromycetin Ophthalmic Solution ... ⊙ 310
Chloroptic S.O.P. ... ⊙ 239
Chloroptic Sterile Ophthalmic Solution ... ⊙ 239
Elase-Chloromycetin Ointment ... 1040
Ophthocort ... ⊙ 311
Chloramphenicol Palmitate (Chloramphenicol in combination with cephalosporins, including ceftazidime, has been shown to be antagonistic *in vitro;* due to possibility of antagonism *in vivo,* this combination should be avoided).
No products indexed under this heading.
Chloramphenicol Sodium Succinate (Chloramphenicol in combination with cephalosporins, including ceftazidime, has been shown to be antagonistic *in vitro;* due to possibility of antagonism *in vivo,* this combination should be avoided). Products include:
Chloromycetin Sodium Succinate ... 1900
Furosemide (Concomitant administration may result in nephrotoxicity). Products include:
Lasix Injection, Oral Solution and Tablets ... 1240
Gentamicin Sulfate (Concomitant administration may result in nephrotoxicity). Products include:
Garamycin Injectable ... 2360
Genoptic Sterile Ophthalmic Solution ... ⊙ 243
Genoptic Sterile Ophthalmic Ointment ... ⊙ 243
Gentacidin Ointment ... ⊙ 264
Gentacidin Solution ... ⊙ 264
Gentak ... ⊙ 208
Pred-G Liquifilm Sterile Ophthalmic Suspension ... ⊙ 251
Pred-G S.O.P. Sterile Ophthalmic Ointment ... ⊙ 252
Kanamycin Sulfate (Concomitant administration may result in nephrotoxicity).
No products indexed under this heading.
Streptomycin Sulfate (Concomitant administration may result in nephrotoxicity). Products include:
Streptomycin Sulfate Injection ... 2208
Tobramycin (Concomitant administration may result in nephrotoxicity). Products include:
AKTOB ... ⊙ 206
TobraDex Ophthalmic Suspension and Ointment ... 473
Tobrex Ophthalmic Ointment and Solution ... ⊙ 229
Tobramycin Sulfate (Concomitant administration may result in nephrotoxicity). Products include:
Nebcin Vials, Hyporets & ADD-Vantage ... 1464
Tobramycin Sulfate Injection ... 968

TAZIDIME VIALS, FASPAK & ADD-VANTAGE
(Ceftazidime) ... 1478
May interact with aminoglycosides and certain other agents. Compounds in these categories include:

Amikacin Sulfate (Potential for nephrotoxicity and ototoxicity; monitor renal function). Products include:
Amikacin Sulfate Injection, USP ... 960
Amikin Injectable ... 501
Furosemide (Nephrotoxicity). Products include:
Lasix Injection, Oral Solution and Tablets ... 1240
Gentamicin Sulfate (Potential for nephrotoxicity and ototoxicity; monitor renal function). Products include:
Garamycin Injectable ... 2360
Genoptic Sterile Ophthalmic Solution ... ⊙ 243
Genoptic Sterile Ophthalmic Ointment ... ⊙ 243
Gentacidin Ointment ... ⊙ 264
Gentacidin Solution ... ⊙ 264
Gentak ... ⊙ 208
Pred-G Liquifilm Sterile Ophthalmic Suspension ... ⊙ 251
Pred-G S.O.P. Sterile Ophthalmic Ointment ... ⊙ 252
Kanamycin Sulfate (Potential for nephrotoxicity and ototoxicity; monitor renal function).
No products indexed under this heading.
Streptomycin Sulfate (Potential for nephrotoxicity and ototoxicity; monitor renal function). Products include:
Streptomycin Sulfate Injection ... 2208
Tobramycin (Potential for nephrotoxicity and ototoxicity; monitor renal function). Products include:
AKTOB ... ⊙ 206
TobraDex Ophthalmic Suspension and Ointment ... 473
Tobrex Ophthalmic Ointment and Solution ... ⊙ 229
Tobramycin Sulfate (Potential for nephrotoxicity and ototoxicity; monitor renal function). Products include:
Nebcin Vials, Hyporets & ADD-Vantage ... 1464
Tobramycin Sulfate Injection ... 968

TEARS NATURALE II LUBRICANT EYE DROPS
(Dextran 70, Hydroxypropyl Methylcellulose) ... 473
None cited in PDR database.

TEARS NATURALE FREE
(Dextran 70, Hydroxypropyl Methylcellulose) ... 473
None cited in PDR database.

TEARS RENEWED OINTMENT
(Petrolatum, White) ... ⊙ 209
None cited in PDR database.

TECHNI-CARE SURGICAL SCRUB AND WOUND CLEANSER
(Chloroxylenol) ... ▣ 625
None cited in PDR database.

TEGISON CAPSULES
(Etretinate) ... 2154
May interact with:

Vitamin A (Additive toxic effects). Products include:
Aquasol A Vitamin A Capsules, USP ... 534
Aquasol A Parenteral ... 534
Materna Tablets ... 1379
Megadose ... 512
Nature Made Antioxidant Formula ▣ 748
One-A-Day Extras Antioxidant ... ▣ 728
Theragran Antioxidant ... ▣ 623
Zymacap Capsules ... ▣ 772

Food Interactions
Dairy products (Increases absorption of etretinate).
Diet, high-lipid (Increases absorption of etretinate).

TEGRETOL CHEWABLE TABLETS
(Carbamazepine) ... 852
See **Tegretol Tablets**

TEGRETOL SUSPENSION
(Carbamazepine) ... 852
See **Tegretol Tablets**

TEGRETOL TABLETS
(Carbamazepine) ... 852
May interact with calcium channel blockers, anticonvulsants, oral contraceptives, lithium preparations, monoamine oxidase inhibitors, and certain other agents. Compounds in these categories include:

Aminophylline (Half-life significantly shortened when administered concurrently with Tegretol).
No products indexed under this heading.
Amlodipine Besylate (Elevated plasma levels of carbamazepine). Products include:
Lotrel Capsules ... 840
Norvasc Tablets ... 1940
Bepridil Hydrochloride (Elevated plasma levels of carbamazepine). Products include:
Vascor (200, 300 and 400 mg) Tablets ... 1587
Cimetidine (Elevated plasma levels of total and/or free carbamazepine). Products include:
Tagamet Tablets ... 2516

IMPORTANT NOTE: Always consult each drug listing in the patient's regimen for possible interactions.

Tegretol Interactions Index 1012

Cimetidine Hydrochloride (Elevated plasma levels of total and/or free carbamazepine). Products include:
- Tagamet ... 2516

Desogestrel (Breakthrough bleeding may occur). Products include:
- Desogen Tablets ... 1817
- Ortho-Cept ... 1851

Diltiazem Hydrochloride (Elevated plasma levels of carbamazepine). Products include:
- Cardizem CD Capsules ... 1506
- Cardizem SR Capsules ... 1510
- Cardizem Injectable ... 1508
- Cardizem Tablets ... 1512
- Dilacor XR Extended-release Capsules ... 2018

Divalproex Sodium (Alterations of thyroid function; valproic acid serum levels may be reduced). Products include:
- Depakote Tablets ... 415

Doxycycline Calcium (Half-life significantly shortened when administered concurrently with Tegretol). Products include:
- Vibramycin Calcium Oral Suspension Syrup ... 1941

Doxycycline Hyclate (Half-life significantly shortened when administered concurrently with Tegretol). Products include:
- Doryx Capsules ... 1913
- Vibramycin Hyclate Capsules ... 1941
- Vibramycin Hyclate Intravenous ... 2215
- Vibra-Tabs Film Coated Tablets ... 1941

Doxycycline Monohydrate (Half-life significantly shortened when administered concurrently with Tegretol). Products include:
- Monodox Capsules ... 1805
- Vibramycin Monohydrate for Oral Suspension ... 1941

Dyphylline (Half-life significantly shortened when administered concurrently with Tegretol). Products include:
- Lufyllin & Lufyllin-400 Tablets ... 2670
- Lufyllin-GG Elixir & Tablets ... 2671

Erythromycin (Elevated plasma levels of total and/or free carbamazepine). Products include:
- A/T/S 2% Acne Topical Gel and Solution ... 1234
- Benzamycin Topical Gel ... 905
- E-Mycin Tablets ... 1341
- Emgel 2% Topical Gel ... 1093
- ERYC ... 1915
- Erycette (erythromycin 2%) Topical Solution ... 1888
- Ery-Tab Tablets ... 422
- Erythromycin Base Filmtab ... 426
- Erythromycin Delayed-Release Capsules, USP ... 427
- Ilotycin Ophthalmic Ointment ... 912
- PCE Dispertab Tablets ... 444
- T-Stat 2.0% Topical Solution and Pads ... 2688
- Theramycin Z Topical Solution 2% 1592

Erythromycin Estolate (Elevated plasma levels of total and/or free carbamazepine). Products include:
- Ilosone ... 911

Erythromycin Ethylsuccinate (Elevated plasma levels of total and/or free carbamazepine). Products include:
- E.E.S. ... 424
- EryPed ... 421

Erythromycin Gluceptate (Elevated plasma levels of total and/or free carbamazepine). Products include:
- Ilotycin Gluceptate, IV, Vials ... 913

Erythromycin Lactobionate (Elevated plasma levels of total and/or free carbamazepine).
- No products indexed under this heading.

Erythromycin Stearate (Elevated plasma levels of total and/or free carbamazepine). Products include:
- Erythrocin Stearate Filmtab ... 425

Ethinyl Estradiol (Breakthrough bleeding may occur). Products include:
- Brevicon ... 2088
- Demulen ... 2428
- Desogen Tablets ... 1817
- Levlen/Tri-Levlen ... 651
- Lo/Ovral Tablets ... 2746
- Lo/Ovral-28 Tablets ... 2751
- Modicon ... 1872
- Nordette-21 Tablets ... 2755
- Nordette-28 Tablets ... 2758
- Norinyl ... 2088
- Ortho-Cept ... 1851
- Ortho-Cyclen/Ortho-Tri-Cyclen ... 1858
- Ortho-Novum ... 1872
- Ortho-Cyclen/Ortho Tri-Cyclen ... 1858
- Ovcon ... 760
- Ovral Tablets ... 2770
- Ovral-28 Tablets ... 2770
- Levlen/Tri-Levlen ... 651
- Tri-Norinyl ... 2164
- Triphasil-21 Tablets ... 2814
- Triphasil-28 Tablets ... 2819

Ethosuximide (Alterations of thyroid function). Products include:
- Zarontin Capsules ... 1928
- Zarontin Syrup ... 1929

Ethotoin (Alterations of thyroid function). Products include:
- Peganone Tablets ... 446

Ethynodiol Diacetate (Breakthrough bleeding may occur). Products include:
- Demulen ... 2428

Felbamate (Alterations of thyroid function; valproic acid serum levels may be reduced). Products include:
- Felbatol ... 2666

Felodipine (Elevated plasma levels of carbamazepine). Products include:
- Plendil Extended-Release Tablets ... 527

Fluoxetine Hydrochloride (Elevated plasma levels of total and/or free carbamazepine). Products include:
- Prozac Pulvules & Liquid, Oral Solution ... 919

Furazolidone (Concurrent use is contraindicated). Products include:
- Furoxone ... 2046

Haloperidol (Haloperidol serum levels may be reduced when administered with Tegretol). Products include:
- Haldol Injection, Tablets and Concentrate ... 1575

Haloperidol Decanoate (Haloperidol serum levels may be reduced when administered with Tegretol). Products include:
- Haldol Decanoate ... 1577

Isocarboxazid (Concurrent use is contraindicated).
- No products indexed under this heading.

Isoniazid (Elevated plasma levels of carbamazepine). Products include:
- Nydrazid Injection ... 508
- Rifamate Capsules ... 1530
- Rifater ... 1532

Isradipine (Elevated plasma levels of carbamazepine). Products include:
- DynaCirc Capsules ... 2256

Lamotrigine (Alterations of thyroid function; valproic acid serum levels may be reduced). Products include:
- Lamictal Tablets ... 1112

Levonorgestrel (Breakthrough bleeding may occur). Products include:
- Levlen/Tri-Levlen ... 651
- Nordette-21 Tablets ... 2755
- Nordette-28 Tablets ... 2758
- Norplant System ... 2759
- Levlen/Tri-Levlen ... 651
- Triphasil-21 Tablets ... 2814
- Triphasil-28 Tablets ... 2819

Lithium Carbonate (Increased risk of neurotoxic effects). Products include:
- Eskalith ... 2485
- Lithium Carbonate Capsules & Tablets ... 2230
- Lithonate/Lithotabs/Lithobid ... 2543

Lithium Citrate (Increased risk of neurotoxic effects).
- No products indexed under this heading.

Mephenytoin (Alterations of thyroid function). Products include:
- Mesantoin Tablets ... 2272

Mestranol (Breakthrough bleeding may occur). Products include:
- Norinyl ... 2088
- Ortho-Novum ... 1872

Methsuximide (Alterations of thyroid function). Products include:
- Celontin Kapseals ... 1899

Nicardipine Hydrochloride (Elevated plasma levels of carbamazepine). Products include:
- Cardene Capsules ... 2095
- Cardene I.V. ... 2709
- Cardene SR Capsules ... 2097

Nifedipine (Elevated plasma levels of carbamazepine). Products include:
- Adalat Capsules (10 mg and 20 mg) ... 587
- Adalat CC ... 589
- Procardia Capsules ... 1971
- Procardia XL Extended Release Tablets ... 1972

Nimodipine (Elevated plasma levels of carbamazepine). Products include:
- Nimotop Capsules ... 610

Nisoldipine (Elevated plasma levels of carbamazepine).
- No products indexed under this heading.

Norethindrone (Breakthrough bleeding may occur). Products include:
- Brevicon ... 2088
- Micronor Tablets ... 1872
- Modicon ... 1872
- Norinyl ... 2088
- Nor-Q D Tablets ... 2135
- Ortho-Novum ... 1872
- Ovcon ... 760
- Tri-Norinyl ... 2164

Norethindrone Acetate (Breakthrough bleeding may occur). Products include:
- Aygestin Tablets ... 974

Norethynodrel (Breakthrough bleeding may occur).
- No products indexed under this heading.

Norgestimate (Breakthrough bleeding may occur). Products include:
- Ortho-Cyclen/Ortho-Tri-Cyclen ... 1858
- Ortho-Cyclen/Ortho Tri-Cyclen ... 1858

Norgestrel (Breakthrough bleeding may occur). Products include:
- Lo/Ovral Tablets ... 2746
- Lo/Ovral-28 Tablets ... 2751
- Ovral Tablets ... 2770
- Ovral-28 Tablets ... 2770
- Ovrette Tablets ... 2771

Paramethadione (Alterations of thyroid function).
- No products indexed under this heading.

Phenacemide (Alterations of thyroid function). Products include:
- Phenurone Tablets ... 447

Phenelzine Sulfate (Concurrent use is contraindicated). Products include:
- Nardil ... 1920

Phenobarbital (Marked lowering of serum levels of Tegretol; alterations of thyroid function). Products include:
- Arco-Lase Plus Tablets ... 512
- Bellergal-S Tablets ... 2250
- Donnatal ... 2060
- Donnatal Extentabs ... 2061
- Donnatal Tablets ... 2060
- Phenobarbital Elixir and Tablets ... 1469
- Quadrinal Tablets ... 1350

Phensuximide (Alterations of thyroid function). Products include:
- Milontin Kapseals ... 1920

Phenytoin (Marked lowering of serum levels of Tegretol; half life of phenytoin significantly shortened when administered concurrently with Tegretol; alterations of thyroid function). Products include:
- Dilantin Infatabs ... 1908
- Dilantin-125 Suspension ... 1911

Phenytoin Sodium (Marked lowering of serum levels of Tegretol; half-life of phenytoin significantly shortened when administered concurrently with Tegretol; alterations of thyroid function). Products include:
- Dilantin Kapseals ... 1906
- Dilantin Parenteral ... 1910

Primidone (Marked lowering of serum levels of Tegretol; alterations of thyroid function). Products include:
- Mysoline ... 2754

Propoxyphene Hydrochloride (Elevated plasma levels of total and/or free carbamazepine). Products include:
- Darvon ... 1435
- Wygesic Tablets ... 2827

Propoxyphene Napsylate (Elevated plasma levels of total and/or free carbamazepine). Products include:
- Darvon-N/Darvocet-N ... 1433

Selegiline Hydrochloride (Concurrent use is contraindicated). Products include:
- Eldepryl Tablets ... 2550

Terfenadine (Elevated plasma levels of total and/or free carbamazepine resulting in toxicity in some cases). Products include:
- Seldane Tablets ... 1536
- Seldane-D Extended-Release Tablets ... 1538

Theophylline (Half-life significantly shortened when administered concurrently with Tegretol). Products include:
- Marax Tablets & DF Syrup ... 2200
- Quibron ... 2053

Theophylline Anhydrous (Half-life significantly shortened when administered concurrently with Tegretol). Products include:
- Aerolate ... 1004
- Primatene Dual Action Formula ... ⊞ 872
- Primatene Tablets ... ⊞ 873
- Respbid Tablets ... 682
- Slo-bid Gyrocaps ... 2033
- Theo-24 Extended Release Capsules ... 2568
- Theo-Dur Extended-Release Tablets ... 1327
- Theo-X Extended-Release Tablets ... 788
- Uni-Dur Extended-Release Tablets ... 1331
- Uniphyl 400 mg Tablets ... 2001

Theophylline Calcium Salicylate (Half-life significantly shortened when administered concurrently with Tegretol). Products include:
- Quadrinal Tablets ... 1350

Theophylline Sodium Glycinate (Half-life significantly shortened when administered concurrently with Tegretol).
- No products indexed under this heading.

Interactions Index

Temaril

Tranylcypromine Sulfate (Concurrent use is contraindicated). Products include:

Parnate Tablets 2503

Trimethadione (Alterations of thyroid function).

No products indexed under this heading.

Valproic Acid (Alterations of thyroid function; valproic acid serum levels may be reduced). Products include:

Depakene 413

Verapamil Hydrochloride (Elevated plasma levels of carbamazepine). Products include:

Calan SR Caplets	2422
Calan Tablets	2419
Isoptin Injectable	1344
Isoptin Oral Tablets	1346
Isoptin SR Tablets	1348
Verelan Capsules	1410
Verelan Capsules	2824

Warfarin Sodium (Half-life significantly shortened when administered concurrently with Tegretol). Products include:

Coumadin 926

TEGRIN DANDRUFF SHAMPOO

(Coal Tar) .... ℞ 611

None cited in PDR database.

TEGRIN SKIN CREAM & TEGRIN MEDICATED SOAP

(Coal Tar) .... ℞ 611

None cited in PDR database.

TELDRIN 12 HOUR ANTIHISTAMINE/NASAL DECONGESTANT ALLERGY RELIEF CAPSULES

(Chlorpheniramine Maleate, Phenylpropanolamine Hydrochloride) .... ℞ 826

May interact with hypnotics and sedatives, tranquilizers, monoamine oxidase inhibitors, and certain other agents. Compounds in these categories include:

Alprazolam (May increase drowsiness effect; consult your doctor). Products include:

Xanax Tablets 2649

Buspirone Hydrochloride (May increase drowsiness effect; consult your doctor). Products include:

BuSpar 737

Chlordiazepoxide (May increase drowsiness effect; consult your doctor). Products include:

Libritabs Tablets .... 2177 Limbitrol 2180

Chlordiazepoxide Hydrochloride (May increase drowsiness effect; consult your doctor). Products include:

Librax Capsules .... 2176 Librium Capsules .... 2178 Librium Injectable 2179

Chlorpromazine (May increase drowsiness effect; consult your doctor). Products include:

Thorazine Suppositories 2523

Chlorpromazine Hydrochloride (May increase drowsiness effect; consult your doctor). Products include:

Thorazine 2523

Chlorprothixene (May increase drowsiness effect; consult your doctor).

No products indexed under this heading.

Chlorprothixene Hydrochloride (May increase drowsiness effect; consult your doctor).

No products indexed under this heading.

Clorazepate Dipotassium (May increase drowsiness effect; consult your doctor). Products include:

Tranxene 451

Diazepam (May increase drowsiness effect; consult your doctor). Products include:

Dizac	1809
Valium Injectable	2182
Valium Tablets	2183
Valrelease Capsules	2169

Droperidol (May increase drowsiness effect; consult your doctor). Products include:

Inapsine Injection 1296

Estazolam (May increase drowsiness effect; consult your doctor). Products include:

ProSom Tablets 449

Ethchlorvynol (May increase drowsiness effect; consult your doctor). Products include:

Placidyl Capsules 448

Ethinamate (May increase drowsiness effect; consult your doctor).

No products indexed under this heading.

Fluphenazine Decanoate (May increase drowsiness effect; consult your doctor). Products include:

Prolixin Decanoate 509

Fluphenazine Enanthate (May increase drowsiness effect; consult your doctor). Products include:

Prolixin Enanthate 509

Fluphenazine Hydrochloride (May increase drowsiness effect; consult your doctor). Products include:

Prolixin 509

Flurazepam Hydrochloride (May increase drowsiness effect; consult your doctor). Products include:

Dalmane Capsules 2173

Furazolidone (Concurrent and/or sequential use is not recommended). Products include:

Furoxone 2046

Glutethimide (May increase drowsiness effect; consult your doctor).

No products indexed under this heading.

Haloperidol (May increase drowsiness effect; consult your doctor). Products include:

Haldol Injection, Tablets and Concentrate 1575

Haloperidol Decanoate (May increase drowsiness effect; consult your doctor). Products include:

Haldol Decanoate 1577

Hydroxyzine Hydrochloride (May increase drowsiness effect; consult your doctor). Products include:

Atarax Tablets & Syrup	2185
Marax Tablets & DF Syrup	2200
Vistaril Intramuscular Solution	2216

Isocarboxazid (Concurrent and/or sequential use is not recommended).

No products indexed under this heading.

Lorazepam (May increase drowsiness effect; consult your doctor). Products include:

Ativan Injection .... 2698 Ativan Tablets 2700

Loxapine Hydrochloride (May increase drowsiness effect; consult your doctor). Products include:

Loxitane 1378

Loxapine Succinate (May increase drowsiness effect; consult your doctor). Products include:

Loxitane Capsules 1378

Meprobamate (May increase drowsiness effect; consult your doctor). Products include:

Miltown Tablets .... 2672 PMB 200 and PMB 400 2783

Mesoridazine Besylate (May increase drowsiness effect; consult your doctor). Products include:

Serentil 684

Midazolam Hydrochloride (May increase drowsiness effect; consult your doctor). Products include:

Versed Injection 2170

Molindone Hydrochloride (May increase drowsiness effect; consult your doctor). Products include:

Moban Tablets and Concentrate 1048

Oxazepam (May increase drowsiness effect; consult your doctor). Products include:

Serax Capsules .... 2810 Serax Tablets 2810

Perphenazine (May increase drowsiness effect; consult your doctor). Products include:

Etrafon	2355
Triavil Tablets	1757
Trilafon	2389

Phenelzine Sulfate (Concurrent and/or sequential use is not recommended). Products include:

Nardil 1920

Prazepam (May increase drowsiness effect; consult your doctor).

No products indexed under this heading.

Prochlorperazine (May increase drowsiness effect; consult your doctor). Products include:

Compazine 2470

Promethazine Hydrochloride (May increase drowsiness effect; consult your doctor). Products include:

Mepergan Injection	2753
Phenergan with Codeine	2777
Phenergan with Dextromethorphan	2778
Phenergan Injection	2773
Phenergan Suppositories	2775
Phenergan Syrup	2774
Phenergan Tablets	2775
Phenergan VC	2779
Phenergan VC with Codeine	2781

Propofol (May increase drowsiness effect; consult your doctor). Products include:

Diprivan Injection 2833

Quazepam (May increase drowsiness effect; consult your doctor). Products include:

Doral Tablets 2664

Secobarbital Sodium (May increase drowsiness effect; consult your doctor). Products include:

Seconal Sodium Pulvules 1474

Selegiline Hydrochloride (Concurrent and/or sequential use is not recommended). Products include:

Eldepryl Tablets 2550

Temazepam (May increase drowsiness effect; consult your doctor). Products include:

Restoril Capsules 2284

Thioridazine Hydrochloride (May increase drowsiness effect; consult your doctor). Products include:

Mellaril 2269

Thiothixene (May increase drowsiness effect; consult your doctor). Products include:

Navane Capsules and Concentrate 2201 Navane Intramuscular 2202

Tranylcypromine Sulfate (Concurrent and/or sequential use is not recommended). Products include:

Parnate Tablets 2503

Triazolam (May increase drowsiness effect; consult your doctor). Products include:

Halcion Tablets 2611

Trifluoperazine Hydrochloride (May increase drowsiness effect; consult your doctor). Products include:

Stelazine 2514

Zolpidem Tartrate (May increase drowsiness effect; consult your doctor). Products include:

Ambien Tablets 2416

Food Interactions

Alcohol (May increase drowsiness effect; avoid concurrent use).

TEMARIL TABLETS, SYRUP AND SPANSULE EXTENDED-RELEASE CAPSULES

(Trimeprazine Tartrate) 483

May interact with monoamine oxidase inhibitors, thiazides, narcotic analgesics, oral contraceptives, central nervous system depressants, and certain other agents. Compounds in these categories include:

Alfentanil Hydrochloride (CNS depressant and analgesic effects potentiated). Products include:

Alfenta Injection 1286

Alprazolam (Additive CNS depressant effect). Products include:

Xanax Tablets 2649

Aprobarbital (Additive CNS depressant effect).

No products indexed under this heading.

Atropine Nitrate, Methyl (Action of atropine intensified and prolonged).

No products indexed under this heading.

Atropine Sulfate (Action of atropine intensified and prolonged). Products include:

Arco-Lase Plus Tablets	512
Atrohist Plus Tablets	454
Atropine Sulfate Sterile Ophthalmic Solution	⊙ 233
Donnatal	2060
Donnatal Extentabs	2061
Donnatal Tablets	2060
Lomotil	2439
Motofen Tablets	784
Urised Tablets	1964

Bendroflumethiazide (Anticholinergic effects of Temaril prolonged and intensified).

No products indexed under this heading.

Buprenorphine (CNS depressant and analgesic effects potentiated). Products include:

Buprenex Injectable 2006

Buspirone Hydrochloride (Additive CNS depressant effect). Products include:

BuSpar 737

Butabarbital (Additive CNS depressant effect).

No products indexed under this heading.

Butalbital (Additive CNS depressant effect). Products include:

Esgic-plus Tablets	1013
Fioricet Tablets	2258
Fioricet with Codeine Capsules	2260
Fiorinal Capsules	2261
Fiorinal with Codeine Capsules	2262
Fiorinal Tablets	2261
Phrenilin	785
Sedapap Tablets 50 mg/650 mg	1543

IMPORTANT NOTE: Always consult each drug listing in the patient's regimen for possible interactions.

Temaril

Interactions Index

Chlordiazepoxide (Additive CNS depressant effect). Products include:
- Libritabs Tablets 2177
- Limbitrol 2180

Chlordiazepoxide Hydrochloride (Additive CNS depressant effect). Products include:
- Librax Capsules 2176
- Librium Capsules 2178
- Librium Injectable 2179

Chlorothiazide (Anticholinergic effects of Temaril prolonged and intensified). Products include:
- Aldoclor Tablets 1598
- Diupres Tablets 1650
- Diuril Oral 1653

Chlorothiazide Sodium (Anticholinergic effects of Temaril prolonged and intensified). Products include:
- Diuril Sodium Intravenous 1652

Chlorpromazine (Additive CNS depressant effect). Products include:
- Thorazine Suppositories 2523

Chlorprothixene (Additive CNS depressant effect).
No products indexed under this heading.

Chlorprothixene Hydrochloride (Additive CNS depressant effect).
No products indexed under this heading.

Chlorprothixene Lactate (Additive CNS depressant effect).
No products indexed under this heading.

Clorazepate Dipotassium (Additive CNS depressant effect). Products include:
- Tranxene 451

Clozapine (CNS depressant and analgesic effects potentiated). Products include:
- Clozaril Tablets 2252

Codeine Phosphate (CNS depressant and analgesic effects potentiated). Products include:
- Actifed with Codeine Cough Syrup.. 1067
- Brontex 1981
- Deconsal C Expectorant Syrup 456
- Deconsal Pediatric Syrup 457
- Dimetane-DC Cough Syrup 2059
- Empirin with Codeine Tablets 1093
- Fioricet with Codeine Capsules 2260
- Fiorinal with Codeine Capsules 2262
- Isoclor Expectorant 990
- Novahistine DH 2462
- Novahistine Expectorant 2463
- Nucofed 2051
- Phenergan with Codeine 2777
- Phenergan VC with Codeine 2781
- Robitussin A-C Syrup 2073
- Robitussin-DAC Syrup 2074
- Ryna .... ✦◻ 841
- Soma Compound w/Codeine Tablets 2676
- Tussi-Organidin NR Liquid and S NR Liquid 2677
- Tylenol with Codeine 1583

Desflurane (CNS depressant and analgesic effects potentiated). Products include:
- Suprane 1813

Desogestrel (Potentiates phenothiazine effects). Products include:
- Desogen Tablets 1817
- Ortho-Cept 1851

Dezocine (CNS depressant and analgesic effects potentiated). Products include:
- Dalgan Injection 538

Diazepam (Additive CNS depressant effect). Products include:
- Dizac 1809
- Valium Injectable 2182
- Valium Tablets 2183
- Valrelease Capsules 2169

Droperidol (Additive CNS depressant effect). Products include:
- Inapsine Injection 1296

Enflurane (Additive CNS depressant effect).
No products indexed under this heading.

Epinephrine (Possible blockage or reversal of pressor effect). Products include:
- Bronkaid Mist .... ✦◻ 717
- EPIFRIN .... ◉ 239
- EpiPen 790
- Marcaine Hydrochloride with Epinephrine 1:200,000 2316
- Primatene Mist .... ✦◻ 873
- Sensorcaine with Epinephrine Injection 559
- Sus-Phrine Injection 1019
- Xylocaine with Epinephrine Injections 567

Estazolam (CNS depressant and analgesic effects potentiated). Products include:
- ProSom Tablets 449

Ethchlorvynol (Additive CNS depressant effect). Products include:
- Placidyl Capsules 448

Ethinamate (Additive CNS depressant effect).
No products indexed under this heading.

Ethinyl Estradiol (Potentiates phenothiazine effects). Products include:
- Brevicon 2088
- Demulen 2428
- Desogen Tablets 1817
- Levlen/Tri-Levlen 651
- Lo/Ovral Tablets 2746
- Lo/Ovral-28 Tablets 2751
- Modicon 1872
- Nordette-21 Tablets 2755
- Nordette-28 Tablets 2758
- Norinyl 2088
- Ortho-Cept 1851
- Ortho-Cyclen/Ortho-Tri-Cyclen 1858
- Ortho-Novum 1872
- Ortho-Cyclen/Ortho Tri-Cyclen 1858
- Ovcon 760
- Ovral Tablets 2770
- Ovral-28 Tablets 2770
- Levlen/Tri-Levlen 651
- Tri-Norinyl 2164
- Triphasil-21 Tablets 2814
- Triphasil-28 Tablets 2819

Ethynodiol Diacetate (Potentiates phenothiazine effects). Products include:
- Demulen 2428

Fentanyl (CNS depressant and analgesic effects potentiated). Products include:
- Duragesic Transdermal System 1288

Fentanyl Citrate (CNS depressant and analgesic effects potentiated). Products include:
- Sublimaze Injection 1307

Fluphenazine Decanoate (Additive CNS depressant effect). Products include:
- Prolixin Decanoate 509

Fluphenazine Enanthate (Additive CNS depressant effect). Products include:
- Prolixin Enanthate 509

Fluphenazine Hydrochloride (Additive CNS depressant effect). Products include:
- Prolixin 509

Flurazepam Hydrochloride (Additive CNS depressant effect). Products include:
- Dalmane Capsules 2173

Furazolidone (Anticholinergic effects of Temaril prolonged and intensified; hypertension and extrapyramidal reactions). Products include:
- Furoxone 2046

Glutethimide (Additive CNS depressant effect).
No products indexed under this heading.

Haloperidol (Additive CNS depressant effect). Products include:
- Haldol Injection, Tablets and Concentrate 1575

Haloperidol Decanoate (Additive CNS depressant effect). Products include:
- Haldol Decanoate 1577

Hydrochlorothiazide (Anticholinergic effects of Temaril prolonged and intensified). Products include:
- Aldactazide 2413
- Aldoril Tablets 1604
- Apresazide Capsules 808
- Capozide 742
- Dyazide 2479
- Esidrix Tablets 821
- Esimil Tablets 822
- HydroDIURIL Tablets 1674
- Hydropres Tablets 1675
- Hyzaar Tablets 1677
- Inderide Tablets 2732
- Inderide LA Long Acting Capsules.. 2734
- Lopressor HCT Tablets 832
- Lotensin HCT 837
- Maxzide 1380
- Moduretic Tablets 1705
- Oretic Tablets 443
- Prinzide Tablets 1737
- Ser-Ap-Es Tablets 849
- Timolide Tablets 1748
- Vaseretic Tablets 1765
- Zestoretic 2850
- Ziac 1415

Hydrocodone Bitartrate (CNS depressant and analgesic effects potentiated). Products include:
- Anexsia 5/500 Elixir 1781
- Anexia Tablets 1782
- Codiclear DH Syrup 791
- Deconamine CX Cough and Cold Liquid and Tablets 1319
- Duratuss HD Elixir 2565
- Hycodan Tablets and Syrup 930
- Hycomine Compound Tablets 932
- Hycomine 931
- Hycotuss Expectorant Syrup 933
- Hydrocet Capsules 782
- Lorcet 10/650 1018
- Lortab 2566
- Tussend 1783
- Tussend Expectorant 1785
- Vicodin Tablets 1356
- Vicodin ES Tablets 1357
- Vicodin Tuss Expectorant 1358
- Zydone Capsules 949

Hydrocodone Polistirex (CNS depressant and analgesic effects potentiated). Products include:
- Tussionex Pennkinetic Extended-Release Suspension 998

Hydroflumethiazide (Anticholinergic effects of Temaril prolonged and intensified). Products include:
- Diucardin Tablets 2718

Hydroxyzine Hydrochloride (Additive CNS depressant effect). Products include:
- Atarax Tablets & Syrup 2185
- Marax Tablets & DF Syrup 2200
- Vistaril Intramuscular Solution 2216

Isocarboxazid (Anticholinergic effects of Temaril prolonged and intensified; hypertension and extrapyramidal reactions).
No products indexed under this heading.

Isoflurane (Additive CNS depressant effect).
No products indexed under this heading.

Ketamine Hydrochloride (CNS depressant and analgesic effects potentiated).
No products indexed under this heading.

Levomethadyl Acetate Hydrochloride (CNS depressant and analgesic effects potentiated). Products include:
- Orlaam 2239

Levonorgestrel (Potentiates phenothiazine effects). Products include:
- Levlen/Tri-Levlen 651
- Nordette-21 Tablets 2755
- Nordette-28 Tablets 2758
- Norplant System 2759
- Levlen/Tri-Levlen 651
- Triphasil-21 Tablets 2814
- Triphasil-28 Tablets 2819

Levorphanol Tartrate (CNS depressant and analgesic effects potentiated). Products include:
- Levo-Dromoran 2129

Lorazepam (Additive CNS depressant effect). Products include:
- Ativan Injection 2698
- Ativan Tablets 2700

Loxapine Hydrochloride (Additive CNS depressant effect). Products include:
- Loxitane 1378

Loxapine Succinate (CNS depressant and analgesic effects potentiated). Products include:
- Loxitane Capsules 1378

Meperidine Hydrochloride (CNS depressant and analgesic effects potentiated). Products include:
- Demerol 2308
- Mepergan Injection 2753

Mephobarbital (Additive CNS depressant effect). Products include:
- Mebaral Tablets 2322

Meprobamate (Additive CNS depressant effect). Products include:
- Miltown Tablets 2672
- PMB 200 and PMB 400 2783

Mesoridazine Besylate (Additive CNS depressant effect). Products include:
- Serentil 684

Mestranol (Potentiates phenothiazine effects). Products include:
- Norinyl 2088
- Ortho-Novum 1872

Methadone Hydrochloride (CNS depressant and analgesic effects potentiated). Products include:
- Methadone Hydrochloride Oral Concentrate 2233
- Methadone Hydrochloride Oral Solution & Tablets 2235

Methohexital Sodium (Additive CNS depressant effect). Products include:
- Brevital Sodium Vials 1429

Methotrimeprazine (CNS depressant and analgesic effects potentiated). Products include:
- Levoprome 1274

Methoxyflurane (Additive CNS depressant effect).
No products indexed under this heading.

Methyclothiazide (Anticholinergic effects of Temaril prolonged and intensified). Products include:
- Enduron Tablets 420

Midazolam Hydrochloride (Additive CNS depressant effect). Products include:
- Versed Injection 2170

Molindone Hydrochloride (Additive CNS depressant effect). Products include:
- Moban Tablets and Concentrate 1048

Morphine Sulfate (CNS depressant and analgesic effects potentiated). Products include:
- Astramorph/PF Injection, USP (Preservative-Free) 535
- Duramorph 962
- Infumorph 200 and Infumorph 500 Sterile Solutions 965
- MS Contin Tablets 1994
- MSIR 1997
- Oramorph SR (Morphine Sulfate Sustained Release Tablets) 2236
- RMS Suppositories 2657

(✦◻ Described in PDR For Nonprescription Drugs) (◉ Described in PDR For Ophthalmology)

Roxanol 2243

Norethindrone (Potentiates phenothiazine effects). Products include:
- Brevicon 2088
- Micronor Tablets 1872
- Modicon 1872
- Norinyl 2088
- Nor-Q D Tablets 2135
- Ortho-Novum 1872
- Ovcon 760
- Tri-Norinyl 2164

Norethynodrel (Potentiates phenothiazine effects).
No products indexed under this heading.

Norgestimate (Potentiates phenothiazine effects). Products include:
- Ortho-Cyclen/Ortho-Tri-Cyclen 1858
- Ortho-Cyclen/Ortho Tri-Cyclen 1858

Norgestrel (Potentiates phenothiazine effects). Products include:
- Lo/Ovral Tablets 2746
- Lo/Ovral-28 Tablets 2751
- Ovral Tablets 2770
- Ovral-28 Tablets 2770
- Ovrette Tablets 2771

Nylidrin Hydrochloride (Potentiates phenothiazine effects).
No products indexed under this heading.

Opium Alkaloids (CNS depressant and analgesic effects potentiated).
No products indexed under this heading.

Oxazepam (Additive CNS depressant effect). Products include:
- Serax Capsules 2810
- Serax Tablets 2810

Oxycodone Hydrochloride (CNS depressant and analgesic effects potentiated). Products include:
- Percocet Tablets 938
- Percodan Tablets 939
- Percodan-Demi Tablets 940
- Roxicodone Tablets, Oral Solution & Intensol (Oxycodone) 2244
- Tylox Capsules 1584

Pentobarbital Sodium (Additive CNS depressant effect). Products include:
- Nembutal Sodium Capsules 436
- Nembutal Sodium Solution 438
- Nembutal Sodium Suppositories 440

Perphenazine (Additive CNS depressant effect). Products include:
- Etrafon 2355
- Triavil Tablets 1757
- Trilafon 2389

Phenelzine Sulfate (Anticholinergic effects of Temaril prolonged and intensified; hypertension and extrapyramidal reactions). Products include:
- Nardil 1920

Phenobarbital (Additive CNS depressant effect). Products include:
- Arco-Lase Plus Tablets 512
- Bellergal-S Tablets 2250
- Donnatal 2060
- Donnatal Extentabs 2061
- Donnatal Tablets 2060
- Phenobarbital Elixir and Tablets 1469
- Quadrinal Tablets 1350

Polythiazide (Anticholinergic effects of Temaril prolonged and intensified). Products include:
- Minizide Capsules 1938

Prazepam (Additive CNS depressant effect).
No products indexed under this heading.

Prochlorperazine (Additive CNS depressant effect). Products include:
- Compazine 2470

Progesterone (Potentiates phenothiazine effects).
No products indexed under this heading.

Promethazine Hydrochloride (Additive CNS depressant effect). Products include:
- Mepergan Injection 2753
- Phenergan with Codeine 2777
- Phenergan with Dextromethorphan 2778
- Phenergan Injection 2773
- Phenergan Suppositories 2775
- Phenergan Syrup 2774
- Phenergan Tablets 2775
- Phenergan VC 2779
- Phenergan VC with Codeine 2781

Propofol (CNS depressant and analgesic effects potentiated). Products include:
- Diprivan Injection 2833

Propoxyphene Hydrochloride (CNS depressant and analgesic effects potentiated). Products include:
- Darvon 1435
- Wygesic Tablets 2827

Propoxyphene Napsylate (CNS depressant and analgesic effects potentiated). Products include:
- Darvon-N/Darvocet-N 1433

Quazepam (CNS depressant and analgesic effects potentiated). Products include:
- Doral Tablets 2664

Reserpine (Potentiates phenothiazine effects). Products include:
- Diupres Tablets 1650
- Hydropres Tablets 1675
- Ser-Ap-Es Tablets 849

Risperidone (CNS depressant and analgesic effects potentiated). Products include:
- Risperdal 1301

Secobarbital Sodium (CNS depressant and analgesic effects potentiated). Products include:
- Seconal Sodium Pulvules 1474

Selegiline Hydrochloride (Anticholinergic effects of Temaril prolonged and intensified; hypertension and extrapyramidal reactions). Products include:
- Eldepryl Tablets 2550

Sufentanil Citrate (CNS depressant and analgesic effects potentiated). Products include:
- Sufenta Injection 1309

Temazepam (Additive CNS depressant effect). Products include:
- Restoril Capsules 2284

Thiamylal Sodium (Additive CNS depressant effect).
No products indexed under this heading.

Thioridazine Hydrochloride (Additive CNS depressant effect). Products include:
- Mellaril 2269

Thiothixene (Additive CNS depressant effect). Products include:
- Navane Capsules and Concentrate 2201
- Navane Intramuscular 2202

Tranylcypromine Sulfate (Anticholinergic effects of Temaril prolonged and intensified; hypertension and extrapyramidal reactions). Products include:
- Parnate Tablets 2503

Triazolam (Additive CNS depressant effect). Products include:
- Halcion Tablets 2611

Trifluoperazine Hydrochloride (Additive CNS depressant effect). Products include:
- Stelazine 2514

Zolpidem Tartrate (CNS depressant and analgesic effects potentiated). Products include:
- Ambien Tablets 2416

Food Interactions

Alcohol (Additive CNS depressant effect).

TEMOVATE CREAM (Clobetasol Propionate) 1179
None cited in PDR database.

TEMOVATE EMOLLIENT CREAM (Clobetasol Propionate) 1179
None cited in PDR database.

TEMOVATE GEL (Clobetasol Propionate) 1179
None cited in PDR database.

TEMOVATE OINTMENT (Clobetasol Propionate) 1179
None cited in PDR database.

TEMOVATE SCALP APPLICATION (Clobetasol Propionate) 1179
None cited in PDR database.

TEMPO SOFT ANTACID (Calcium Carbonate, Aluminum Hydroxide, Magnesium Hydroxide, Simethicone) ..... ▣ 835
May interact with:

Drugs, Oral, unspecified (Antacids may interact with certain unspecified drugs).

TENEX TABLETS (Guanfacine Hydrochloride) 2074
May interact with central nervous system depressants and certain other agents. Compounds in these categories include:

Alfentanil Hydrochloride (Potential for increased sedation). Products include:
- Alfenta Injection 1286

Alprazolam (Potential for increased sedation). Products include:
- Xanax Tablets 2649

Aprobarbital (Potential for increased sedation).
No products indexed under this heading.

Buprenorphine (Potential for increased sedation). Products include:
- Buprenex Injectable 2006

Buspirone Hydrochloride (Potential for increased sedation). Products include:
- BuSpar 737

Butabarbital (Potential for increased sedation).
No products indexed under this heading.

Butalbital (Potential for increased sedation). Products include:
- Esgic-plus Tablets 1013
- Fioricet Tablets 2258
- Fioricet with Codeine Capsules 2260
- Fiorinal Capsules 2261
- Fiorinal with Codeine Capsules 2262
- Fiorinal Tablets 2261
- Phrenilin 785
- Sedapap Tablets 50 mg/650 mg 1543

Chlordiazepoxide (Potential for increased sedation). Products include:
- Libritabs Tablets 2177
- Limbitrol 2180

Chlordiazepoxide Hydrochloride (Potential for increased sedation). Products include:
- Librax Capsules 2176
- Librium Capsules 2178
- Librium Injectable 2179

Chlorpromazine (Potential for increased sedation). Products include:
- Thorazine Suppositories 2523

Chlorprothixene (Potential for increased sedation).
No products indexed under this heading.

Chlorprothixene Hydrochloride (Potential for increased sedation).
No products indexed under this heading.

Clorazepate Dipotassium (Potential for increased sedation). Products include:
- Tranxene 451

Clozapine (Potential for increased sedation). Products include:
- Clozaril Tablets 2252

Codeine Phosphate (Potential for increased sedation). Products include:
- Actifed with Codeine Cough Syrup 1067
- Brontex 1981
- Deconsal C Expectorant Syrup 456
- Deconsal Pediatric Syrup 457
- Dimetane-DC Cough Syrup 2059
- Empirin with Codeine Tablets 1093
- Fioricet with Codeine Capsules 2260
- Fiorinal with Codeine Capsules 2262
- Isoclor Expectorant 990
- Novahistine DH 2462
- Novahistine Expectorant 2463
- Nucofed 2051
- Phenergan with Codeine 2777
- Phenergan VC with Codeine 2781
- Robitussin A-C Syrup 2073
- Robitussin-DAC Syrup 2074
- Ryna ..... ▣ 841
- Soma Compound w/Codeine Tablets 2676
- Tussi-Organidin NR Liquid and S NR Liquid 2677
- Tylenol with Codeine 1583

Desflurane (Potential for increased sedation). Products include:
- Suprane 1813

Dezocine (Potential for increased sedation). Products include:
- Dalgan Injection 538

Diazepam (Potential for increased sedation). Products include:
- Dizac 1809
- Valium Injectable 2182
- Valium Tablets 2183
- Valrelease Capsules 2169

Droperidol (Potential for increased sedation). Products include:
- Inapsine Injection 1296

Enflurane (Potential for increased sedation).
No products indexed under this heading.

Estazolam (Potential for increased sedation). Products include:
- ProSom Tablets 449

Ethchlorvynol (Potential for increased sedation). Products include:
- Placidyl Capsules 448

Ethinamate (Potential for increased sedation).
No products indexed under this heading.

Fentanyl (Potential for increased sedation). Products include:
- Duragesic Transdermal System 1288

Fentanyl Citrate (Potential for increased sedation). Products include:
- Sublimaze Injection 1307

Fluphenazine Decanoate (Potential for increased sedation). Products include:
- Prolixin Decanoate 509

Fluphenazine Enanthate (Potential for increased sedation). Products include:
- Prolixin Enanthate 509

Fluphenazine Hydrochloride (Potential for increased sedation). Products include:
- Prolixin 509

Flurazepam Hydrochloride (Potential for increased sedation). Products include:
- Dalmane Capsules 2173

IMPORTANT NOTE: Always consult each drug listing in the patient's regimen for possible interactions.

Glutethimide (Potential for increased sedation).
- No products indexed under this heading.

Haloperidol (Potential for increased sedation). Products include:
- Haldol Injection, Tablets and Concentrate ... 1575

Haloperidol Decanoate (Potential for increased sedation). Products include:
- Haldol Decanoate ... 1577

Hydrocodone Bitartrate (Potential for increased sedation). Products include:
- Anexsia 5/500 Elixir ... 1781
- Anexsia Tablets ... 1782
- Codiclear DH Syrup ... 791
- Deconamine CX Cough and Cold Liquid and Tablets ... 1319
- Duratuss HD Elixir ... 2565
- Hycodan Tablets and Syrup ... 930
- Hycomine Compound Tablets ... 932
- Hycomine ... 931
- Hycotuss Expectorant Syrup ... 933
- Hydrocet Capsules ... 782
- Lorcet 10/650 ... 1018
- Lortab ... 2566
- Tussend ... 1783
- Tussend Expectorant ... 1785
- Vicodin Tablets ... 1356
- Vicodin ES Tablets ... 1357
- Vicodin Tuss Expectorant ... 1358
- Zydone Capsules ... 949

Hydrocodone Polistirex (Potential for increased sedation). Products include:
- Tussionex Pennkinetic Extended-Release Suspension ... 998

Hydroxyzine Hydrochloride (Potential for increased sedation). Products include:
- Atarax Tablets & Syrup ... 2185
- Marax Tablets & DF Syrup ... 2200
- Vistaril Intramuscular Solution ... 2216

Isoflurane (Potential for increased sedation).
- No products indexed under this heading.

Ketamine Hydrochloride (Potential for increased sedation).
- No products indexed under this heading.

Levomethadyl Acetate Hydrochloride (Potential for increased sedation). Products include:
- Orlamm ... 2239

Levorphanol Tartrate (Potential for increased sedation). Products include:
- Levo-Dromoran ... 2129

Lorazepam (Potential for increased sedation). Products include:
- Ativan Injection ... 2698
- Ativan Tablets ... 2700

Loxapine Hydrochloride (Potential for increased sedation). Products include:
- Loxitane ... 1378

Loxapine Succinate (Potential for increased sedation). Products include:
- Loxitane Capsules ... 1378

Meperidine Hydrochloride (Potential for increased sedation). Products include:
- Demerol ... 2308
- Mepergan Injection ... 2753

Mephobarbital (Potential for increased sedation). Products include:
- Mebaral Tablets ... 2322

Meprobamate (Potential for increased sedation). Products include:
- Miltown Tablets ... 2672
- PMB 200 and PMB 400 ... 2783

Mesoridazine Besylate (Potential for increased sedation). Products include:
- Serentil ... 684

Methadone Hydrochloride (Potential for increased sedation). Products include:
- Methadone Hydrochloride Oral Concentrate ... 2233
- Methadone Hydrochloride Oral Solution & Tablets ... 2235

Methohexital Sodium (Potential for increased sedation). Products include:
- Brevital Sodium Vials ... 1429

Methotrimeprazine (Potential for increased sedation). Products include:
- Levoprome ... 1274

Methoxyflurane (Potential for increased sedation).
- No products indexed under this heading.

Midazolam Hydrochloride (Potential for increased sedation). Products include:
- Versed Injection ... 2170

Molindone Hydrochloride (Potential for increased sedation). Products include:
- Moban Tablets and Concentrate ... 1048

Morphine Sulfate (Potential for increased sedation). Products include:
- Astramorph/PF Injection, USP (Preservative-Free) ... 535
- Duramorph ... 962
- Infumorph 200 and Infumorph 500 Sterile Solutions ... 965
- MS Contin Tablets ... 1994
- MSIR ... 1997
- Oramorph SR (Morphine Sulfate Sustained Release Tablets) ... 2236
- RMS Suppositories ... 2657
- Roxanol ... 2243

Opium Alkaloids (Potential for increased sedation).
- No products indexed under this heading.

Oxazepam (Potential for increased sedation). Products include:
- Serax Capsules ... 2810
- Serax Tablets ... 2810

Oxycodone Hydrochloride (Potential for increased sedation). Products include:
- Percocet Tablets ... 938
- Percodan Tablets ... 939
- Percodan-Demi Tablets ... 940
- Roxicodone Tablets, Oral Solution & Intensol (Oxycodone) ... 2244
- Tylox Capsules ... 1584

Pentobarbital Sodium (Potential for increased sedation). Products include:
- Nembutal Sodium Capsules ... 436
- Nembutal Sodium Solution ... 438
- Nembutal Sodium Suppositories ... 440

Perphenazine (Potential for increased sedation). Products include:
- Etrafon ... 2355
- Triavil Tablets ... 1757
- Trilafon ... 2389

Phenobarbital (Potential for increased sedation; concurrent administration may result in significant reductions in elimination half-life and plasma concentration). Products include:
- Arco-Lase Plus Tablets ... 512
- Bellergal-S Tablets ... 2250
- Donnatal ... 2060
- Donnatal Extentabs ... 2061
- Donnatal Tablets ... 2060
- Phenobarbital Elixir and Tablets ... 1469
- Quadrinal Tablets ... 1350

Phenytoin (Concurrent administration may result in significant reductions in elimination half-life and plasma concentration). Products include:
- Dilantin Infatabs ... 1908
- Dilantin-125 Suspension ... 1911

Phenytoin Sodium (Concurrent administration may result in significant reductions in elimination half-life and plasma concentration). Products include:
- Dilantin Kapseals ... 1906
- Dilantin Parenteral ... 1910

Prazepam (Potential for increased sedation).
- No products indexed under this heading.

Prochlorperazine (Potential for increased sedation). Products include:
- Compazine ... 2470

Promethazine Hydrochloride (Potential for increased sedation). Products include:
- Mepergan Injection ... 2753
- Phenergan with Codeine ... 2777
- Phenergan with Dextromethorphan ... 2778
- Phenergan Injection ... 2773
- Phenergan Suppositories ... 2775
- Phenergan Syrup ... 2774
- Phenergan Tablets ... 2775
- Phenergan VC ... 2779
- Phenergan VC with Codeine ... 2781

Propofol (Potential for increased sedation). Products include:
- Diprivan Injection ... 2833

Propoxyphene Hydrochloride (Potential for increased sedation). Products include:
- Darvon ... 1435
- Wygesic Tablets ... 2827

Propoxyphene Napsylate (Potential for increased sedation). Products include:
- Darvon-N/Darvocet-N ... 1433

Quazepam (Potential for increased sedation). Products include:
- Doral Tablets ... 2664

Risperidone (Potential for increased sedation). Products include:
- Risperdal ... 1301

Secobarbital Sodium (Potential for increased sedation). Products include:
- Seconal Sodium Pulvules ... 1474

Sufentanil Citrate (Potential for increased sedation). Products include:
- Sufenta Injection ... 1309

Temazepam (Potential for increased sedation). Products include:
- Restoril Capsules ... 2284

Thiamylal Sodium (Potential for increased sedation).
- No products indexed under this heading.

Thioridazine Hydrochloride (Potential for increased sedation). Products include:
- Mellaril ... 2269

Thiothixene (Potential for increased sedation). Products include:
- Navane Capsules and Concentrate ... 2201
- Navane Intramuscular ... 2202

Triazolam (Potential for increased sedation). Products include:
- Halcion Tablets ... 2611

Trifluoperazine Hydrochloride (Potential for increased sedation). Products include:
- Stelazine ... 2514

Zolpidem Tartrate (Potential for increased sedation). Products include:
- Ambien Tablets ... 2416

TENORETIC TABLETS

(Atenolol, Chlorthalidone) ... 2845

May interact with antihypertensives, catecholamine depleting drugs, calcium channel blockers, lithium preparations, insulin, corticosteroids, cardiac glycosides, and certain other agents. Compounds in these categories include:

Acebutolol Hydrochloride (Concurrent administration may potentiate the action of other antihypertensive agent). Products include:
- Sectral Capsules ... 2807

Amlodipine Besylate (Calcium channel blockers may have an additive effect when given with Tenoretic; potential for bradycardia and heart block). Products include:
- Lotrel Capsules ... 840
- Norvasc Tablets ... 1940

Benazepril Hydrochloride (Concurrent administration may potentiate the action of other antihypertensive agent). Products include:
- Lotensin Tablets ... 834
- Lotensin HCT ... 837
- Lotrel Capsules ... 840

Bendroflumethiazide (Concurrent administration may potentiate the action of other antihypertensive agent).
- No products indexed under this heading.

Bepridil Hydrochloride (Calcium channel blockers may have an additive effect when given with Tenoretic; potential for bradycardia and heart block). Products include:
- Vascor (200, 300 and 400 mg) Tablets ... 1587

Betamethasone Acetate (Potential for hypokalemia). Products include:
- Celestone Soluspan Suspension ... 2347

Betamethasone Sodium Phosphate (Potential for hypokalemia). Products include:
- Celestone Soluspan Suspension ... 2347

Betaxolol Hydrochloride (Concurrent administration may potentiate the action of other antihypertensive agent). Products include:
- Betoptic Ophthalmic Solution ... 469
- Betoptic S Ophthalmic Suspension ... 471
- Kerlone Tablets ... 2436

Bisoprolol Fumarate (Concurrent administration may potentiate the action of other antihypertensive agent). Products include:
- Zebeta Tablets ... 1413
- Ziac ... 1415

Captopril (Concurrent administration may potentiate the action of other antihypertensive agent). Products include:
- Capoten ... 739
- Capozide ... 742

Carteolol Hydrochloride (Concurrent administration may potentiate the action of other antihypertensive agent). Products include:
- Cartrol Tablets ... 410
- Ocupress Ophthalmic Solution, 1% Sterile ... ⊙ 309

Chlorothiazide (Concurrent administration may potentiate the action of other antihypertensive agent). Products include:
- Aldoclor Tablets ... 1598
- Diupres Tablets ... 1650
- Diuril Oral ... 1653

Chlorothiazide Sodium (Concurrent administration may potentiate the action of other antihypertensive agent). Products include:
- Diuril Sodium Intravenous ... 1652

Clonidine (Potential for exacerbation of rebound hypertension; Tenoretic should be discontinued several days before the gradual withdrawal of clonidine). Products include:
- Catapres-TTS ... 675

(▭ Described in PDR For Nonprescription Drugs) (⊙ Described in PDR For Ophthalmology)

1017 **Interactions Index** **Tenoretic**

Clonidine Hydrochloride (Potential for exacerbation of rebound hypertension; Tenoretic should be discontinued several days before the gradual withdrawal of clonidine). Products include:
Catapres Tablets 674
Combipres Tablets 677

Cortisone Acetate (Potential for hypokalemia). Products include:
Cortone Acetate Sterile Suspension 1623
Cortone Acetate Tablets 1624

Deserpidine (Potential for hypotension and/or marked bradycardia which may produce vertigo, syncope or postural hypotension).
No products indexed under this heading.

Deslanoside (Hypokalemia induced by Tenoretic therapy can sensitize or exaggerate the response of the heart to the toxic effects of digitalis).
No products indexed under this heading.

Dexamethasone (Potential for hypokalemia). Products include:
AK-Trol Ointment & Suspension .... ⊙ 205
Decadron Elixir 1633
Decadron Tablets 1635
Decaspray Topical Aerosol 1648
Dexacidin Ointment .... ⊙ 263
Maxitrol Ophthalmic Ointment and Suspension .... ⊙ 224
TobraDex Ophthalmic Suspension and Ointment 473

Dexamethasone Acetate (Potential for hypokalemia). Products include:
Dalalone D.P. Injectable 1011
Decadron-LA Sterile Suspension 1646

Dexamethasone Sodium Phosphate (Potential for hypokalemia). Products include:
Decadron Phosphate Injection 1637
Decadron Phosphate Respihaler 1642
Decadron Phosphate Sterile Ophthalmic Ointment 1641
Decadron Phosphate Sterile Ophthalmic Solution 1642
Decadron Phosphate Topical Cream 1644
Decadron Phosphate Turbinaire 1645
Decadron Phosphate with Xylocaine Injection, Sterile 1639
Dexacort Phosphate in Respihaler .. 458
Dexacort Phosphate in Turbinaire .. 459
NeoDecadron Sterile Ophthalmic Ointment 1712
NeoDecadron Sterile Ophthalmic Solution 1713
NeoDecadron Topical Cream 1714

Diazoxide (Concurrent administration may potentiate the action of other antihypertensive agent). Products include:
Hyperstat I.V. Injection 2363
Proglycem 580

Digitoxin (Hypokalemia induced by Tenoretic therapy can sensitize or exaggerate the response of the heart to the toxic effects of digitalis). Products include:
Crystodigin Tablets 1433

Digoxin (Hypokalemia induced by Tenoretic therapy can sensitize or exaggerate the response of the heart to the toxic effects of digitalis). Products include:
Lanoxicaps 1117
Lanoxin Elixir Pediatric 1120
Lanoxin Injection 1123
Lanoxin Injection Pediatric 1126
Lanoxin Tablets 1128

Diltiazem Hydrochloride (Calcium channel blockers may have an additive effect when given with Tenoretic; potential for bradycardia and heart block). Products include:
Cardizem CD Capsules 1506
Cardizem SR Capsules 1510
Cardizem Injectable 1508
Cardizem Tablets 1512
Dilacor XR Extended-release Capsules 2018

Doxazosin Mesylate (Concurrent administration may potentiate the action of other antihypertensive agent). Products include:
Cardura Tablets 2186

Enalapril Maleate (Concurrent administration may potentiate the action of other antihypertensive agent). Products include:
Vaseretic Tablets 1765
Vasotec Tablets 1771

Enalaprilat (Concurrent administration may potentiate the action of other antihypertensive agent). Products include:
Vasotec I.V. 1768

Epinephrine (Patients with a history of anaphylactic reaction may be unresponsive to the usual dose of epinephrine). Products include:
Bronkaid Mist .... ▣ 717
EPIFRIN .... ⊙ 239
EpiPen 790
Marcaine Hydrochloride with Epinephrine 1:200,000 2316
Primatene Mist .... ▣ 873
Sensorcaine with Epinephrine Injection 559
Sus-Phrine Injection 1019
Xylocaine with Epinephrine Injections 567

Epinephrine Hydrochloride (Patients with a history of anaphylactic reaction may be unresponsive to the usual dose of epinephrine). Products include:
Ana-Kit Anaphylaxis Emergency Treatment Kit 617

Esmolol Hydrochloride (Concurrent administration may potentiate the action of other antihypertensive agent). Products include:
Brevibloc Injection 1808

Felodipine (Calcium channel blockers may have an additive effect when given with Tenoretic; potential for bradycardia and heart block). Products include:
Plendil Extended-Release Tablets 527

Fludrocortisone Acetate (Potential for hypokalemia). Products include:
Florinef Acetate Tablets 505

Fosinopril Sodium (Concurrent administration may potentiate the action of other antihypertensive agent). Products include:
Monopril Tablets 757

Furosemide (Concurrent administration may potentiate the action of other antihypertensive agent). Products include:
Lasix Injection, Oral Solution and Tablets 1240

Guanabenz Acetate (Concurrent administration may potentiate the action of other antihypertensive agent).
No products indexed under this heading.

Guanethidine Monosulfate (Potential for hypotension and/or marked bradycardia which may produce vertigo, syncope or postural hypotension). Products include:
Esimil Tablets 822
Ismelin Tablets 827

Hydralazine Hydrochloride (Concurrent administration may potentiate the action of other antihypertensive agent). Products include:
Apresazide Capsules 808
Apresoline Hydrochloride Tablets .. 809
Ser-Ap-Es Tablets 849

Hydrochlorothiazide (Concurrent administration may potentiate the action of other antihypertensive agent). Products include:
Aldactazide 2413
Aldoril Tablets 1604
Apresazide Capsules 808
Capozide 742
Dyazide 2479
Esidrix Tablets 821
Esimil Tablets 822
HydroDIURIL Tablets 1674
Hydropres Tablets 1675
Hyzaar Tablets 1677
Inderide Tablets 2732
Inderide LA Long Acting Capsules .. 2734
Lopressor HCT Tablets 832
Lotensin HCT 837
Maxzide 1380
Moduretic Tablets 1705
Oretic Tablets 443
Prinzide Tablets 1737
Ser-Ap-Es Tablets 849
Timolide Tablets 1748
Vaseretic Tablets 1765
Zestoretic 2850
Ziac 1415

Hydrocortisone (Potential for hypokalemia). Products include:
Anusol-HC Cream 2.5% 1896
Aquanil HC Lotion 1931
Bactine Hydrocortisone Anti-Itch Cream .... ▣ 709
Caldecort Anti-Itch Hydrocortisone Spray .... ▣ 631
Cortaid .... ▣ 836
CORTENEMA 2535
Cortisporin Ointment 1085
Cortisporin Ophthalmic Ointment Sterile 1085
Cortisporin Ophthalmic Suspension Sterile 1086
Cortisporin Otic Solution Sterile 1087
Cortisporin Otic Suspension Sterile 1088
Cortizone-5 .... ▣ 831
Cortizone-10 .... ▣ 831
Hydrocortone Tablets 1672
Hytone 907
Massengill Medicated Soft Cloth Towelettes 2458
PediOtic Suspension Sterile 1153
Preparation H Hydrocortisone 1% Cream .... ▣ 872
ProctoCream-HC 2.5% 2408
VōSoL HC Otic Solution 2678

Hydrocortisone Acetate (Potential for hypokalemia). Products include:
Analpram-HC Rectal Cream 1% and 2.5% 977
Anusol HC-1 Anti-Itch Hydrocortisone Ointment .... ▣ 847
Anusol-HC Suppositories 1897
Caldecort .... ▣ 631
Carmol HC 924
Coly-Mycin S Otic w/Neomycin & Hydrocortisone 1906
Cortaid .... ▣ 836
Cortifoam 2396
Cortisporin Cream 1084
Epifoam 2399
Hydrocortone Acetate Sterile Suspension 1669
Mantadil Cream 1135
Nupercainal Hydrocortisone 1% Cream .... ▣ 645
Ophthocort .... ⊙ 311
Pramosone Cream, Lotion & Ointment 978
ProctoCream-HC 2408
ProctoFoam-HC 2409
Terra-Cortril Ophthalmic Suspension 2210

Hydrocortisone Sodium Phosphate (Potential for hypokalemia). Products include:
Hydrocortone Phosphate Injection, Sterile 1670

Hydrocortisone Sodium Succinate (Potential for hypokalemia). Products include:
Solu-Cortef Sterile Powder 2641

Hydroflumethiazide (Concurrent administration may potentiate the action of other antihypertensive agent). Products include:
Diucardin Tablets 2718

Indapamide (Concurrent administration may potentiate the action of other antihypertensive agent). Products include:
Lozol Tablets 2022

Insulin, Human (Insulin requirements in diabetic patients may be altered).
No products indexed under this heading.

Insulin, Human Isophane Suspension (Insulin requirements in diabetic patients may be altered). Products include:
Novolin N Human Insulin 10 ml Vials 1795

Insulin, Human NPH (Insulin requirements in diabetic patients may be altered). Products include:
Humulin N, 100 Units 1448
Novolin N PenFill Cartridges Durable Insulin Delivery System 1798
Novolin N Prefilled Syringe Disposable Insulin Delivery System 1798

Insulin, Human Regular (Insulin requirements in diabetic patients may be altered). Products include:
Humulin R, 100 Units 1449
Novolin R Human Insulin 10 ml Vials 1795
Novolin R PenFill Cartridges Durable Insulin Delivery System 1798
Novolin R Prefilled Syringe Disposable Insulin Delivery System 1798
Velosulin BR Human Insulin 10 ml Vials 1795

Insulin, Human, Zinc Suspension (Insulin requirements in diabetic patients may be altered). Products include:
Humulin L, 100 Units 1446
Humulin U, 100 Units 1450
Novolin L Human Insulin 10 ml Vials 1795

Insulin, NPH (Insulin requirements in diabetic patients may be altered). Products include:
NPH, 100 Units 1450
Pork NPH, 100 Units 1452
Purified Pork NPH Isophane Insulin 1801

Insulin, Regular (Insulin requirements in diabetic patients may be altered). Products include:
Regular, 100 Units 1450
Pork Regular, 100 Units 1452
Pork Regular (Concentrated), 500 Units 1453
Purified Pork Regular Insulin 1801

Insulin, Zinc Crystals (Insulin requirements in diabetic patients may be altered). Products include:
NPH, 100 Units 1450

Insulin, Zinc Suspension (Insulin requirements in diabetic patients may be altered). Products include:
Iletin I 1450
Lente, 100 Units 1450
Iletin II 1452
Pork Lente, 100 Units 1452
Purified Pork Lente Insulin 1801

Isradipine (Calcium channel blockers may have an additive effect when given with Tenoretic; potential for bradycardia and heart block). Products include:
DynaCirc Capsules 2256

Labetalol Hydrochloride (Concurrent administration may potentiate the action of other antihypertensive agent). Products include:
Normodyne Injection 2377
Normodyne Tablets 2379
Trandate 1185

Lisinopril (Concurrent administration may potentiate the action of other antihypertensive agent). Products include:
Prinivil Tablets 1733
Prinzide Tablets 1737
Zestoretic 2850

IMPORTANT NOTE: Always consult each drug listing in the patient's regimen for possible interactions.

Zestril Tablets 2854

Lithium Carbonate (Reduced renal clearance; lithium toxicity). Products include:

Eskalith 2485
Lithium Carbonate Capsules & Tablets 2230
Lithonate/Lithotabs/Lithobid 2543

Lithium Citrate (Reduced renal clearance; lithium toxicity).

No products indexed under this heading.

Losartan Potassium (Calcium channel blockers may have an additive effect when given with Tenoretic; potential for bradycardia and heart block). Products include:

Cozaar Tablets 1628
Hyzaar Tablets 1677

Mecamylamine Hydrochloride (Concurrent administration may potentiate the action of other antihypertensive agent). Products include:

Inversine Tablets 1686

Methyclothiazide (Concurrent administration may potentiate the action of other antihypertensive agent). Products include:

Enduron Tablets 420

Methyldopa (Concurrent administration may potentiate the action of other antihypertensive agent). Products include:

Aldoclor Tablets 1598
Aldomet Oral 1600
Aldoril Tablets 1604

Methyldopate Hydrochloride (Concurrent administration may potentiate the action of other antihypertensive agent). Products include:

Aldomet Ester HCl Injection 1602

Methylprednisolone Acetate (Potential for hypokalemia). Products include:

Depo-Medrol Single-Dose Vial 2600
Depo-Medrol Sterile Aqueous Suspension 2597

Methylprednisolone Sodium Succinate (Potential for hypokalemia). Products include:

Solu-Medrol Sterile Powder 2643

Metolazone (Concurrent administration may potentiate the action of other antihypertensive agent). Products include:

Mykrox Tablets 993
Zaroxolyn Tablets 1000

Metoprolol Succinate (Concurrent administration may potentiate the action of other antihypertensive agent). Products include:

Toprol-XL Tablets 565

Metoprolol Tartrate (Concurrent administration may potentiate the action of other antihypertensive agent). Products include:

Lopressor Ampuls 830
Lopressor HCT Tablets 832
Lopressor Tablets 830

Metyrosine (Concurrent administration may potentiate the action of other antihypertensive agent). Products include:

Demser Capsules 1649

Minoxidil (Concurrent administration may potentiate the action of other antihypertensive agent). Products include:

Loniten Tablets 2618
Rogaine Topical Solution 2637

Moexipril Hydrochloride (Calcium channel blockers may have an additive effect when given with Tenoretic; potential for bradycardia and heart block). Products include:

Univasc Tablets 2410

Nadolol (Concurrent administration may potentiate the action of other antihypertensive agent).

No products indexed under this heading.

Nicardipine Hydrochloride (Calcium channel blockers may have an additive effect when given with Tenoretic; potential for bradycardia and heart block). Products include:

Cardene Capsules 2095
Cardene I.V. 2709
Cardene SR Capsules 2097

Nifedipine (Calcium channel blockers may have an additive effect when given with Tenoretic; potential for bradycardia and heart block). Products include:

Adalat Capsules (10 mg and 20 mg) 587
Adalat CC 589
Procardia Capsules 1971
Procardia XL Extended Release Tablets 1972

Nimodipine (Calcium channel blockers may have an additive effect when given with Tenoretic; potential for bradycardia and heart block). Products include:

Nimotop Capsules 610

Nisoldipine (Calcium channel blockers may have an additive effect when given with Tenoretic; potential for bradycardia and heart block).

No products indexed under this heading.

Nitroglycerin (Concurrent administration may potentiate the action of other antihypertensive agent). Products include:

Deponit NTG Transdermal Delivery System 2397
Nitro-Bid IV 1523
Nitro-Bid Ointment 1524
Nitrodisc 2047
Nitro-Dur (nitroglycerin) Transdermal Infusion System 1326
Nitrolingual Spray 2027
Nitrostat Tablets 1925
Transderm-Nitro Transdermal Therapeutic System 859

Norepinephrine Bitartrate (Decreased arterial responsiveness to norepinephrine). Products include:

Levophed Bitartrate Injection 2315

Penbutolol Sulfate (Concurrent administration may potentiate the action of other antihypertensive agent). Products include:

Levatol 2403

Phenoxybenzamine Hydrochloride (Concurrent administration may potentiate the action of other antihypertensive agent). Products include:

Dibenzyline Capsules 2476

Phentolamine Mesylate (Concurrent administration may potentiate the action of other antihypertensive agent). Products include:

Regitine 846

Pindolol (Concurrent administration may potentiate the action of other antihypertensive agent). Products include:

Visken Tablets 2299

Polythiazide (Concurrent administration may potentiate the action of other antihypertensive agent). Products include:

Minizide Capsules 1938

Prazosin Hydrochloride (Concurrent administration may potentiate the action of other antihypertensive agent). Products include:

Minipress Capsules 1937
Minizide Capsules 1938

Prednisolone Acetate (Potential for hypokalemia). Products include:

AK-CIDE .... ◎ 202
AK-CIDE Ointment .... ◎ 202
Blephamide Liquifilm Sterile Ophthalmic Suspension 476
Blephamide Ointment .... ◎ 237
Econopred & Econopred Plus Ophthalmic Suspensions .... ◎ 217
Poly-Pred Liquifilm .... ◎ 248
Pred Forte .... ◎ 250
Pred Mild .... ◎ 253
Pred-G Liquifilm Sterile Ophthalmic Suspension .... ◎ 251
Pred-G S.O.P. Sterile Ophthalmic Ointment .... ◎ 252
Vasocidin Ointment .... ◎ 268

Prednisolone Sodium Phosphate (Potential for hypokalemia). Products include:

AK-Pred .... ◎ 204
Hydeltrasol Injection, Sterile 1665
Inflamase .... ◎ 265
Pediapred Oral Liquid 995
Vasocidin Ophthalmic Solution .... ◎ 270

Prednisolone Tebutate (Potential for hypokalemia). Products include:

Hydeltra-T.B.A. Sterile Suspension 1667

Prednisone (Potential for hypokalemia). Products include:

Deltasone Tablets 2595

Propranolol Hydrochloride (Concurrent administration may potentiate the action of other antihypertensive agent). Products include:

Inderal 2728
Inderal LA Long Acting Capsules 2730
Inderide Tablets 2732
Inderide LA Long Acting Capsules 2734

Quinapril Hydrochloride (Concurrent administration may potentiate the action of other antihypertensive agent). Products include:

Accupril Tablets 1893

Ramipril (Concurrent administration may potentiate the action of other antihypertensive agent). Products include:

Altace Capsules 1232

Rauwolfia Serpentina (Potential for hypotension and/or marked bradycardia which may produce vertigo, syncope or postural hypotension).

No products indexed under this heading.

Rescinnamine (Potential for hypotension and/or marked bradycardia which may produce vertigo, syncope or postural hypotension).

No products indexed under this heading.

Reserpine (Potential for hypotension and/or marked bradycardia which may produce vertigo, syncope or postural hypotension). Products include:

Diupres Tablets 1650
Hydropres Tablets 1675
Ser-Ap-Es Tablets 849

Sodium Nitroprusside (Concurrent administration may potentiate the action of other antihypertensive agent).

No products indexed under this heading.

Sotalol Hydrochloride (Concurrent administration may potentiate the action of other antihypertensive agent). Products include:

Betapace Tablets 641

Spirapril Hydrochloride (Calcium channel blockers may have an additive effect when given with Tenoretic; potential for bradycardia and heart block).

No products indexed under this heading.

Terazosin Hydrochloride (Concurrent administration may potentiate the action of other antihypertensive agent). Products include:

Hytrin Capsules 430

Timolol Maleate (Concurrent administration may potentiate the action of other antihypertensive agent). Products include:

Blocadren Tablets 1614
Timolide Tablets 1748
Timoptic in Ocudose 1753
Timoptic Sterile Ophthalmic Solution 1751
Timoptic-XE 1755

Torsemide (Calcium channel blockers may have an additive effect when given with Tenoretic; potential for bradycardia and heart block). Products include:

Demadex Tablets and Injection 686

Triamcinolone (Potential for hypokalemia). Products include:

Aristocort Tablets 1022

Triamcinolone Acetonide (Potential for hypokalemia). Products include:

Aristocort A 0.025% Cream 1027
Aristocort A 0.5% Cream 1031
Aristocort A 0.1% Cream 1029
Aristocort A 0.1% Ointment 1030
Azmacort Oral Inhaler 2011
Nasacort Nasal Inhaler 2024

Triamcinolone Diacetate (Potential for hypokalemia). Products include:

Aristocort Suspension (Forte Parenteral) 1027
Aristocort Suspension (Intralesional) 1025

Triamcinolone Hexacetonide (Potential for hypokalemia). Products include:

Aristospan Suspension (Intra-articular) 1033
Aristospan Suspension (Intralesional) 1032

Trimethaphan Camsylate (Concurrent administration may potentiate the action of other antihypertensive agent). Products include:

Arfonad Ampuls 2080

Tubocurarine Chloride (Increased responsiveness to tubocurarine).

No products indexed under this heading.

Verapamil Hydrochloride (Calcium channel blockers may have an additive effect when given with Tenoretic; potential for bradycardia and heart block). Products include:

Calan SR Caplets 2422
Calan Tablets 2419
Isoptin Injectable 1344
Isoptin Oral Tablets 1346
Isoptin SR Tablets 1348
Verelan Capsules 1410
Verelan Capsules 2824

TENORMIN TABLETS AND I.V. INJECTION

(Atenolol) 2847

May interact with catecholamine depleting drugs, calcium channel blockers, and certain other agents. Compounds in these categories include:

Amlodipine Besylate (Coadministration may result in bradycardia and heart block; potential for an additive effect). Products include:

Lotrel Capsules 840
Norvasc Tablets 1940

Bepridil Hydrochloride (Coadministration may result in bradycardia and heart block; potential for an additive effect). Products include:

Vascor (200, 300 and 400 mg) Tablets 1587

(■ Described in PDR For Nonprescription Drugs) (◎ Described in PDR For Ophthalmology)

Clonidine (Beta blockers may exacerbate the rebound hypertension which can follow the withdrawal of clonidine). Products include:

Catapres-TTS 675

Clonidine Hydrochloride (Beta blockers may exacerbate the rebound hypertension which can follow the withdrawal of clonidine). Products include:

Catapres Tablets 674
Combipres Tablets 677

Deserpidine (Potential for additive effect; hypotension and/or marked bradycardia which may produce vertigo, syncope or postural hypotension).

No products indexed under this heading.

Diltiazem Hydrochloride (Coadministration may result in bradycardia and heart block; potential for an additive effect). Products include:

Cardizem CD Capsules 1506
Cardizem SR Capsules 1510
Cardizem Injectable 1508
Cardizem Tablets.................................. 1512
Dilacor XR Extended-release Capsules 2018

Epinephrine Hydrochloride (Potential for unresponsiveness to the usual dose of epinephrine to treat allergic reaction). Products include:

Ana-Kit Anaphylaxis Emergency Treatment Kit 617

Felodipine (Coadministration may result in bradycardia and heart block; potential for an additive effect). Products include:

Plendil Extended-Release Tablets 527

Guanethidine Monosulfate (Potential for additive effect; hypotension and/or marked bradycardia which may produce vertigo, syncope or postural hypotension). Products include:

Esimil Tablets 822
Ismelin Tablets 827

Isradipine (Coadministration may result in bradycardia and heart block; potential for an additive effect). Products include:

DynaCirc Capsules 2256

Nicardipine Hydrochloride (Coadministration may result in bradycardia and heart block; potential for an additive effect). Products include:

Cardene Capsules 2095
Cardene I.V. 2709
Cardene SR Capsules............................ 2097

Nifedipine (Coadministration may result in bradycardia and heart block; potential for an additive effect). Products include:

Adalat Capsules (10 mg and 20 mg) 587
Adalat CC 589
Procardia Capsules............................... 1971
Procardia XL Extended Release Tablets 1972

Nimodipine (Coadministration may result in bradycardia and heart block; potential for an additive effect). Products include:

Nimotop Capsules 610

Nisoldipine (Coadministration may result in bradycardia and heart block; potential for an additive effect).

No products indexed under this heading.

Rauwolfia Serpentina (Potential for additive effect; hypotension and/or marked bradycardia which may produce vertigo, syncope or postural hypotension).

No products indexed under this heading.

Rescinnamine (Potential for additive effect; hypotension and/or marked bradycardia which may produce vertigo, syncope or postural hypotension).

No products indexed under this heading.

Reserpine (Potential for additive effect; hypotension and/or marked bradycardia which may produce vertigo, syncope or postural hypotension). Products include:

Diupres Tablets 1650
Hydropres Tablets................................. 1675
Ser-Ap-Es Tablets 849

Verapamil Hydrochloride (Coadministration may result in bradycardia and heart block; potential for an additive effect). Products include:

Calan SR Caplets 2422
Calan Tablets... 2419
Isoptin Injectable 1344
Isoptin Oral Tablets 1346
Isoptin SR Tablets 1348
Verelan Capsules 1410
Verelan Capsules 2824

TENSILON INJECTABLE

(Edrophonium Chloride) 1261
None cited in PDR database.

TERAK OINTMENT

(Oxytetracycline Hydrochloride, Polymyxin B Sulfate) .... ⊕ 209
None cited in PDR database.

TERAZOL 3 VAGINAL CREAM

(Terconazole) 1886
None cited in PDR database.

TERAZOL 3 VAGINAL SUPPOSITORIES

(Terconazole) 1886
None cited in PDR database.

TERAZOL 7 VAGINAL CREAM

(Terconazole) 1887
None cited in PDR database.

TERRA-CORTRIL OPHTHALMIC SUSPENSION

(Oxytetracycline Hydrochloride, Hydrocortisone Acetate) 2210
None cited in PDR database.

TERRAMYCIN INTRAMUSCULAR SOLUTION

(Oxytetracycline) 2210
May interact with anticoagulants, penicillins, and certain other agents. Compounds in these categories include:

Amoxicillin Trihydrate (Interference with penicillin's bactericidal action). Products include:

Amoxil.. 2464
Augmentin 2468

Ampicillin Sodium (Interference with penicillin's bactericidal action). Products include:

Unasyn 2212

Azlocillin Sodium (Interference with penicillin's bactericidal action).

No products indexed under this heading.

Bacampicillin Hydrochloride (Interference with penicillin's bactericidal action). Products include:

Spectrobid Tablets 2206

Carbenicillin Disodium (Interference with penicillin's bactericidal action).

No products indexed under this heading.

Carbenicillin Indanyl Sodium (Interference with penicillin's bactericidal action). Products include:

Geocillin Tablets.................................... 2199

Dalteparin Sodium (Depressed plasma prothrombin activity; downward adjustment of anticoagulant dosage may be necessary). Products include:

Fragmin 1954

Dicloxacillin Sodium (Interference with penicillin's bactericidal action).

No products indexed under this heading.

Dicumarol (Depressed plasma prothrombin activity; downward adjustment of anticoagulant dosage may be necessary).

No products indexed under this heading.

Enoxaparin (Depressed plasma prothrombin activity; downward adjustment of anticoagulant dosage may be necessary). Products include:

Lovenox Injection 2020

Heparin Calcium (Depressed plasma prothrombin activity; downward adjustment of anticoagulant dosage may be necessary).

No products indexed under this heading.

Heparin Sodium (Depressed plasma prothrombin activity; downward adjustment of anticoagulant dosage may be necessary). Products include:

Heparin Lock Flush Solution............... 2725
Heparin Sodium Injection.................... 2726
Heparin Sodium Injection, USP, Sterile Solution 2615
Heparin Sodium Vials........................... 1441

Mezlocillin Sodium (Interference with penicillin's bactericidal action). Products include:

Mezlin 601
Mezlin Pharmacy Bulk Package......... 604

Nafcillin Sodium (Interference with penicillin's bactericidal action).

No products indexed under this heading.

Other Potentially Hepatotoxic Drugs (Should not be prescribed concomitantly).

Penicillin G Benzathine (Interference with penicillin's bactericidal action). Products include:

Bicillin C-R Injection 2704
Bicillin C-R 900/300 Injection 2706
Bicillin L-A Injection 2707

Penicillin G Potassium (Interference with penicillin's bactericidal action). Products include:

Pfizerpen for Injection 2203

Penicillin G Procaine (Interference with penicillin's bactericidal action). Products include:

Bicillin C-R Injection 2704
Bicillin C-R 900/300 Injection 2706

Penicillin G Sodium (Interference with penicillin's bactericidal action).

No products indexed under this heading.

Penicillin V Potassium (Interference with penicillin's bactericidal action). Products include:

Pen•Vee K.. 2772

Ticarcillin Disodium (Interference with penicillin's bactericidal action). Products include:

Ticar for Injection 2526

Timentin for Injection........................... 2528

Warfarin Sodium (Depressed plasma prothrombin activity; downward adjustment of anticoagulant dosage may be necessary). Products include:

Coumadin 926

TERRAMYCIN WITH POLYMYXIN B SULFATE OPHTHALMIC OINTMENT

(Oxytetracycline Hydrochloride, Polymyxin B Sulfate) 2211
None cited in PDR database.

TESLAC

(Testolactone) 717
May interact with oral anticoagulants. Compounds in this category include:

Dicumarol (Increased effects of oral anticoagulant).

No products indexed under this heading.

Warfarin Sodium (Increased effects of oral anticoagulant). Products include:

Coumadin 926

TESSALON PERLES

(Benzonatate) 1020
None cited in PDR database.

TESTODERM TESTOSTERONE TRANSDERMAL SYSTEM

(Testosterone) 486
May interact with oral anticoagulants, insulin, and certain other agents. Compounds in these categories include:

Dicumarol (Potential for decreased requirements of oral anticoagulants).

No products indexed under this heading.

Insulin, Human (Possible decrease in insulin requirements).

No products indexed under this heading.

Insulin, Human Isophane Suspension (Possible decrease in insulin requirements). Products include:

Novolin N Human Insulin 10 ml Vials... 1795

Insulin, Human NPH (Possible decrease in insulin requirements). Products include:

Humulin N, 100 Units........................... 1448
Novolin N PenFill Cartridges Durable Insulin Delivery System 1798
Novolin N Prefilled Syringe Disposable Insulin Delivery System 1798

Insulin, Human Regular (Possible decrease in insulin requirements). Products include:

Humulin R, 100 Units 1449
Novolin R Human Insulin 10 ml Vials... 1795
Novolin R PenFill Cartridges Durable Insulin Delivery System 1798
Novolin R Prefilled Syringe Disposable Insulin Delivery System 1798
Velosulin BR Human Insulin 10 ml Vials... 1795

Insulin, Human, Zinc Suspension (Possible decrease in insulin requirements). Products include:

Humulin L, 100 Units 1446
Humulin U, 100 Units 1450
Novolin L Human Insulin 10 ml Vials... 1795

Insulin, NPH (Possible decrease in insulin requirements). Products include:

NPH, 100 Units 1450
Pork NPH, 100 Units........................... 1452
Purified Pork NPH Isophane Insulin 1801

IMPORTANT NOTE: Always consult each drug listing in the patient's regimen for possible interactions.

Testoderm Interactions Index 1020

Insulin, Regular (Possible decrease in insulin requirements). Products include:
- Regular, 100 Units 1450
- Pork Regular, 100 Units 1452
- Pork Regular (Concentrated), 500 Units 1453
- Purified Pork Regular Insulin 1801

Insulin, Zinc Crystals (Possible decrease in insulin requirements). Products include:
- NPH, 100 Units 1450

Insulin, Zinc Suspension (Possible decrease in insulin requirements). Products include:
- Iletin I 1450
- Lente, 100 Units 1450
- Iletin II 1452
- Pork Lente, 100 Units 1452
- Purified Pork Lente Insulin 1801

Oxyphenbutazone (Concurrent administration may result in elevated serum levels of oxyphenbutazone).

Warfarin Sodium (Potential for decreased requirements of oral anticoagulants). Products include:
- Coumadin 926

TESTRED CAPSULES
(Methyltestosterone) 1262

May interact with oral anticoagulants, insulin, and certain other agents. Compounds in these categories include:

Dicumarol (Decreased need for anticoagulants).
No products indexed under this heading.

Insulin, Human (Possibly decreased insulin requirements).
No products indexed under this heading.

Insulin, Human Isophane Suspension (Possibly decreased insulin requirements). Products include:
- Novolin N Human Insulin 10 ml Vials 1795

Insulin, Human NPH (Possibly decreased insulin requirements). Products include:
- Humulin N, 100 Units 1448
- Novolin N PenFill Cartridges Durable Insulin Delivery System 1798
- Novolin N Prefilled Syringe Disposable Insulin Delivery System 1798

Insulin, Human Regular (Possibly decreased insulin requirements). Products include:
- Humulin R, 100 Units 1449
- Novolin R Human Insulin 10 ml Vials 1795
- Novolin R PenFill Cartridges Durable Insulin Delivery System 1798
- Novolin R Prefilled Syringe Disposable Insulin Delivery System 1798
- Velosulin BR Human Insulin 10 ml Vials 1795

Insulin, Human, Zinc Suspension (Possibly decreased insulin requirements). Products include:
- Humulin L, 100 Units 1446
- Humulin U, 100 Units 1450
- Novolin L Human Insulin 10 ml Vials 1795

Insulin, NPH (Possibly decreased insulin requirements). Products include:
- NPH, 100 Units 1450
- Pork NPH, 100 Units 1452
- Purified Pork NPH Isophane Insulin 1801

Insulin, Regular (Possibly decreased insulin requirements). Products include:
- Regular, 100 Units 1450
- Pork Regular, 100 Units 1452
- Pork Regular (Concentrated), 500 Units 1453
- Purified Pork Regular Insulin 1801

Insulin, Zinc Crystals (Possibly decreased insulin requirements). Products include:
- NPH, 100 Units 1450

Insulin, Zinc Suspension (Possibly decreased insulin requirements). Products include:
- Iletin I 1450
- Lente, 100 Units 1450
- Iletin II 1452
- Pork Lente, 100 Units 1452
- Purified Pork Lente Insulin 1801

Oxyphenbutazone (Elevated serum levels of oxyphenbutazone).

Warfarin Sodium (Decreased need for anticoagulants). Products include:
- Coumadin 926

TETANUS & DIPHTHERIA TOXOIDS ADSORBED PUROGENATED
(Tetanus & Diphtheria Toxoids Adsorbed (For Adult Use)) 1401

None cited in PDR database.

TETANUS TOXOID ADSORBED PUROGENATED
(Tetanus Toxoid, Adsorbed) 1403

May interact with immunosuppressive agents and certain other agents. Compounds in these categories include:

Azathioprine (Concurrent use should be avoided). Products include:
- Imuran 1110

Cyclosporine (Concurrent use should be avoided). Products include:
- Neoral 2276
- Sandimmune 2286

Immune Globulin (Human) (Concurrent use should be avoided).
No products indexed under this heading.

Immune Globulin Intravenous (Human) (Concurrent use should be avoided).

Muromonab-CD3 (Concurrent use should be avoided). Products include:
- Orthoclone OKT3 Sterile Solution 1837

Mycophenolate Mofetil (Concurrent use should be avoided). Products include:
- CellCept Capsules 2099

Tacrolimus (Concurrent use should be avoided). Products include:
- Prograf 1042

TETRAMUNE
(Diphtheria & Tetanus Toxoids and Pertussis Vaccine Adsorbed with Hemophilus B Conjugate Vaccine (Diphtheria-CRM Protein Conjugate)) 1404

May interact with immunosuppressive agents, anticoagulants, and certain other agents. Compounds in these categories include:

Azathioprine (Reduces the response to active immunization procedures). Products include:
- Imuran 1110

Cyclosporine (Reduces the response to active immunization procedures). Products include:
- Neoral 2276
- Sandimmune 2286

Dalteparin Sodium (Caution should be exercised if children are on anticoagulant therapy and are given IM injection of Tetramune). Products include:
- Fragmin 1954

Dicumarol (Caution should be exercised if children are on anticoagulant therapy and are given IM injection of Tetramune).
No products indexed under this heading.

Enoxaparin (Caution should be exercised if children are on anticoagulant therapy and are given IM injection of Tetramune). Products include:
- Lovenox Injection 2020

Heparin Calcium (Caution should be exercised if children are on anticoagulant therapy and are given IM injection of Tetramune).
No products indexed under this heading.

Heparin Sodium (Caution should be exercised if children are on anticoagulant therapy and are given IM injection of Tetramune). Products include:
- Heparin Lock Flush Solution 2725
- Heparin Sodium Injection 2726
- Heparin Sodium Injection, USP, Sterile Solution 2615
- Heparin Sodium Vials 1441

Immune Globulin (Human) (Reduces the response to active immunization procedures).
No products indexed under this heading.

Immune Globulin Intravenous (Human) (Reduces the response to active immunization procedures).

Influenza Virus Vaccine (Potential for increased febrile reactions; influenza virus vaccine should not be administered within 3 days of immunization with a pertussis-containing vaccine). Products include:
- Fluvirin 460
- Influenza Virus Vaccine, Trivalent, Types A and B (chromatograph- and filter-purified subviron antigen) FluShield, 1995-1996 Formula 2736

Muromonab-CD3 (Reduces the response to active immunization procedures). Products include:
- Orthoclone OKT3 Sterile Solution 1837

Mycophenolate Mofetil (Reduces the response to active immunization procedures). Products include:
- CellCept Capsules 2099

Tacrolimus (Reduces the response to active immunization procedures). Products include:
- Prograf 1042

Warfarin Sodium (Caution should be exercised if children are on anticoagulant therapy and are given IM injection of Tetramune). Products include:
- Coumadin 926

THALITONE
(Chlorthalidone) 1245

May interact with antihypertensives, insulin, oral hypoglycemic agents, lithium preparations, barbiturates, narcotic analgesics, and certain other agents. Compounds in these categories include:

Acarbose (Increase in serum glucose level; higher dosage of oral hypoglycemic agents may be necessary).
No products indexed under this heading.

Acebutolol Hydrochloride (Chlorthalidone may add to or potentiate the action of other antihypertensive drugs). Products include:
- Sectral Capsules 2807

Alfentanil Hydrochloride (Aggravates orthostatic hypotension). Products include:
- Alfenta Injection 1286

Amlodipine Besylate (Chlorthalidone may add to or potentiate the action of other antihypertensive drugs). Products include:
- Lotrel Capsules 840
- Norvasc Tablets 1940

Aprobarbital (Aggravates orthostatic hypotension).
No products indexed under this heading.

Atenolol (Chlorthalidone may add to or potentiate the action of other antihypertensive drugs). Products include:
- Tenoretic Tablets 2845
- Tenormin Tablets and I.V. Injection 2847

Benazepril Hydrochloride (Chlorthalidone may add to or potentiate the action of other antihypertensive drugs). Products include:
- Lotensin Tablets 834
- Lotensin HCT 837
- Lotrel Capsules 840

Bendroflumethiazide (Chlorthalidone may add to or potentiate the action of other antihypertensive drugs).
No products indexed under this heading.

Betaxolol Hydrochloride (Chlorthalidone may add to or potentiate the action of other antihypertensive drugs). Products include:
- Betoptic Ophthalmic Solution 469
- Betoptic S Ophthalmic Suspension 471
- Kerlone Tablets 2436

Bisoprolol Fumarate (Chlorthalidone may add to or potentiate the action of other antihypertensive drugs). Products include:
- Zebeta Tablets 1413
- Ziac 1415

Buprenorphine (Aggravates orthostatic hypotension). Products include:
- Buprenex Injectable 2006

Butabarbital (Aggravates orthostatic hypotension).
No products indexed under this heading.

Butalbital (Aggravates orthostatic hypotension). Products include:
- Esgic-plus Tablets 1013
- Fioricet Tablets 2258
- Fioricet with Codeine Capsules 2260
- Fiorinal Capsules 2261
- Fiorinal with Codeine Capsules 2262
- Fiorinal Tablets 2261
- Phrenilin 785
- Sedapap Tablets 50 mg/650 mg .. 1543

Captopril (Chlorthalidone may add to or potentiate the action of other antihypertensive drugs). Products include:
- Capoten 739
- Capozide 742

Carteolol Hydrochloride (Chlorthalidone may add to or potentiate the action of other antihypertensive drugs). Products include:
- Cartrol Tablets 410
- Ocupress Ophthalmic Solution, 1% Sterile .... ⊙ 309

Chlorothiazide (Chlorthalidone may add to or potentiate the action of other antihypertensive drugs). Products include:
- Aldoclor Tablets 1598
- Diupres Tablets 1650
- Diuril Oral 1653

Chlorothiazide Sodium (Chlorthalidone may add to or potentiate the action of other antihypertensive drugs). Products include:
- Diuril Sodium Intravenous 1652

(▭ Described in PDR For Nonprescription Drugs) (⊙ Described in PDR For Ophthalmology)

Interactions Index

Chlorpropamide (Increase in serum glucose level; higher dosage of oral hypoglycemic agents may be necessary). Products include:

Diabinese Tablets 1935

Clonidine (Chlorthalidone may add to or potentiate the action of other antihypertensive drugs). Products include:

Catapres-TTS 675

Clonidine Hydrochloride (Chlorthalidone may add to or potentiate the action of other antihypertensive drugs). Products include:

Catapres Tablets 674
Combipres Tablets 677

Codeine Phosphate (Aggravates orthostatic hypotension). Products include:

Actifed with Codeine Cough Syrup.. 1067
Brontex 1981
Deconsal C Expectorant Syrup 456
Deconsal Pediatric Syrup 457
Dimetane-DC Cough Syrup 2059
Empirin with Codeine Tablets............ 1093
Fioricet with Codeine Capsules 2260
Fiorinal with Codeine Capsules 2262
Isoclor Expectorant 990
Novahistine DH 2462
Novahistine Expectorant...................... 2463
Nucofed 2051
Phenergan with Codeine 2777
Phenergan VC with Codeine 2781
Robitussin A-C Syrup 2073
Robitussin-DAC Syrup 2074
Ryna .... ◆□ 841
Soma Compound w/Codeine Tablets 2676
Tussi-Organidin NR Liquid and S NR Liquid 2677
Tylenol with Codeine 1583

Deserpidine (Chlorthalidone may add to or potentiate the action of other antihypertensive drugs).

No products indexed under this heading.

Dezocine (Aggravates orthostatic hypotension). Products include:

Dalgan Injection 538

Diazoxide (Chlorthalidone may add to or potentiate the action of other antihypertensive drugs). Products include:

Hyperstat I.V. Injection 2363
Proglycem 580

Diltiazem Hydrochloride (Chlorthalidone may add to or potentiate the action of other antihypertensive drugs). Products include:

Cardizem CD Capsules 1506
Cardizem SR Capsules 1510
Cardizem Injectable 1508
Cardizem Tablets................................... 1512
Dilacor XR Extended-release Capsules 2018

Doxazosin Mesylate (Chlorthalidone may add to or potentiate the action of other antihypertensive drugs). Products include:

Cardura Tablets 2186

Enalapril Maleate (Chlorthalidone may add to or potentiate the action of other antihypertensive drugs). Products include:

Vaseretic Tablets 1765
Vasotec Tablets 1771

Enalaprilat (Chlorthalidone may add to or potentiate the action of other antihypertensive drugs). Products include:

Vasotec I.V. 1768

Esmolol Hydrochloride (Chlorthalidone may add to or potentiate the action of other antihypertensive drugs). Products include:

Brevibloc Injection 1808

Felodipine (Chlorthalidone may add to or potentiate the action of other antihypertensive drugs). Products include:

Plendil Extended-Release Tablets 527

Fentanyl (Aggravates orthostatic hypotension). Products include:

Duragesic Transdermal System........ 1288

Fentanyl Citrate (Aggravates orthostatic hypotension). Products include:

Sublimaze Injection............................... 1307

Fosinopril Sodium (Chlorthalidone may add to or potentiate the action of other antihypertensive drugs). Products include:

Monopril Tablets 757

Furosemide (Chlorthalidone may add to or potentiate the action of other antihypertensive drugs). Products include:

Lasix Injection, Oral Solution and Tablets 1240

Glipizide (Increase in serum glucose level; higher dosage of oral hypoglycemic agents may be necessary). Products include:

Glucotrol Tablets 1967
Glucotrol XL Extended Release Tablets 1968

Glyburide (Increase in serum glucose level; higher dosage of oral hypoglycemic agents may be necessary). Products include:

DiaBeta Tablets 1239
Glynase PresTab Tablets 2609
Micronase Tablets 2623

Guanabenz Acetate (Chlorthalidone may add to or potentiate the action of other antihypertensive drugs).

No products indexed under this heading.

Guanethidine Monosulfate (Chlorthalidone may add to or potentiate the action of other antihypertensive drugs). Products include:

Esimil Tablets 822
Ismelin Tablets 827

Hydralazine Hydrochloride (Chlorthalidone may add to or potentiate the action of other antihypertensive drugs). Products include:

Apresazide Capsules............................. 808
Apresoline Hydrochloride Tablets .. 809
Ser-Ap-Es Tablets 849

Hydrochlorothiazide (Chlorthalidone may add to or potentiate the action of other antihypertensive drugs). Products include:

Aldactazide... 2413
Aldoril Tablets... 1604
Apresazide Capsules 808
Capozide 742
Dyazide 2479
Esidrix Tablets 821
Esimil Tablets 822
HydroDIURIL Tablets 1674
Hydropres Tablets.................................. 1675
Hyzaar Tablets 1677
Inderide Tablets 2732
Inderide LA Long Acting Capsules .. 2734
Lopressor HCT Tablets 832
Lotensin HCT 837
Maxzide 1380
Moduretic Tablets 1705
Oretic Tablets 443
Prinzide Tablets 1737
Ser-Ap-Es Tablets 849
Timolide Tablets...................................... 1748
Vaseretic Tablets 1765
Zestoretic 2850
Ziac 1415

Hydrocodone Bitartrate (Aggravates orthostatic hypotension). Products include:

Anexsia 5/500 Elixir 1781
Anexia Tablets... 1782
Codiclear DH Syrup 791
Deconamine CX Cough and Cold Liquid and Tablets................................ 1319
Duratuss HD Elixir 2565
Hycodan Tablets and Syrup 930
Hycomine Compound Tablets 932
Hycomine 931
Hycotuss Expectorant Syrup 933

Hydrocet Capsules 782
Lorcet 10/650 1018
Lortab 2566
Tussend 1783
Tussend Expectorant 1785
Vicodin Tablets 1356
Vicodin ES Tablets 1357
Vicodin Tuss Expectorant 1358
Zydone Capsules 949

Hydrocodone Polistirex (Aggravates orthostatic hypotension). Products include:

Tussionex Pennkinetic Extended-Release Suspension 998

Hydroflumethiazide (Chlorthalidone may add to or potentiate the action of other antihypertensive drugs). Products include:

Diucardin Tablets................................... 2718

Indapamide (Chlorthalidone may add to or potentiate the action of other antihypertensive drugs). Products include:

Lozol Tablets 2022

Insulin, Human (Increase in serum glucose level; insulin requirements in diabetic patients may be increased, decreased or unchanged).

No products indexed under this heading.

Insulin, Human Isophane Suspension (Increase in serum glucose level; insulin requirements in diabetic patients may be increased, decreased or unchanged). Products include:

Novolin N Human Insulin 10 ml Vials.. 1795

Insulin, Human NPH (Increase in serum glucose level; insulin requirements in diabetic patients may be increased, decreased or unchanged). Products include:

Humulin N, 100 Units 1448
Novolin N PenFill Cartridges Durable Insulin Delivery System 1798
Novolin N Prefilled Syringe Disposable Insulin Delivery System 1798

Insulin, Human Regular (Increase in serum glucose level; insulin requirements in diabetic patients may be increased, decreased or unchanged). Products include:

Humulin R, 100 Units 1449
Novolin R Human Insulin 10 ml Vials.. 1795
Novolin R PenFill Cartridges Durable Insulin Delivery System 1798
Novolin R Prefilled Syringe Disposable Insulin Delivery System 1798
Velosulin BR Human Insulin 10 ml Vials.. 1795

Insulin, Human, Zinc Suspension (Increase in serum glucose level; insulin requirements in diabetic patients may be increased, decreased or unchanged). Products include:

Humulin L, 100 Units 1446
Humulin U, 100 Units 1450
Novolin L Human Insulin 10 ml Vials.. 1795

Insulin, NPH (Increase in serum glucose level; insulin requirements in diabetic patients may be increased, decreased or unchanged). Products include:

NPH, 100 Units 1450
Pork NPH, 100 Units............................ 1452
Purified Pork NPH Isophane Insulin 1801

Insulin, Regular (Increase in serum glucose level; insulin requirements in diabetic patients may be increased, decreased or unchanged). Products include:

Regular, 100 Units 1450
Pork Regular, 100 Units 1452
Pork Regular (Concentrated), 500 Units 1453

Purified Pork Regular Insulin 1801

Insulin, Zinc Crystals (Increase in serum glucose level; insulin requirements in diabetic patients may be increased, decreased or unchanged). Products include:

NPH, 100 Units 1450

Insulin, Zinc Suspension (Increase in serum glucose level; insulin requirements in diabetic patients may be increased, decreased or unchanged). Products include:

Iletin I 1450
Lente, 100 Units 1450
Iletin II 1452
Pork Lente, 100 Units.......................... 1452
Purified Pork Lente Insulin 1801

Isradipine (Chlorthalidone may add to or potentiate the action of other antihypertensive drugs). Products include:

DynaCirc Capsules 2256

Labetalol Hydrochloride (Chlorthalidone may add to or potentiate the action of other antihypertensive drugs). Products include:

Normodyne Injection 2377
Normodyne Tablets 2379
Trandate 1185

Levorphanol Tartrate (Aggravates orthostatic hypotension). Products include:

Levo-Dromoran 2129

Lisinopril (Chlorthalidone may add to or potentiate the action of other antihypertensive drugs). Products include:

Prinivil Tablets 1733
Prinzide Tablets 1737
Zestoretic 2850
Zestril Tablets 2854

Lithium Carbonate (Reduced lithium renal clearance and increased risk of lithium toxicity). Products include:

Eskalith 2485
Lithium Carbonate Capsules & Tablets.. 2230
Lithonate/Lithotabs/Lithobid 2543

Lithium Citrate (Reduced lithium renal clearance and increased risk of lithium toxicity).

No products indexed under this heading.

Losartan Potassium (Chlorthalidone may add to or potentiate the action of other antihypertensive drugs). Products include:

Cozaar Tablets 1628
Hyzaar Tablets 1677

Mecamylamine Hydrochloride (Chlorthalidone may add to or potentiate the action of other antihypertensive drugs). Products include:

Inversine Tablets 1686

Meperidine Hydrochloride (Aggravates orthostatic hypotension). Products include:

Demerol 2308
Mepergan Injection 2753

Mephobarbital (Aggravates orthostatic hypotension). Products include:

Mebaral Tablets 2322

Metformin Hydrochloride (Increase in serum glucose level; higher dosage of oral hypoglycemic agents may be necessary). Products include:

Glucophage 752

Methadone Hydrochloride (Aggravates orthostatic hypotension). Products include:

Methadone Hydrochloride Oral Concentrate 2233
Methadone Hydrochloride Oral Solution & Tablets................................ 2235

IMPORTANT NOTE: Always consult each drug listing in the patient's regimen for possible interactions.

Methyclothiazide (Chlorthalidone may add to or potentiate the action of other antihypertensive drugs). Products include:
- Enduron Tablets ... 420

Methyldopa (Chlorthalidone may add to or potentiate the action of other antihypertensive drugs). Products include:
- Aldoclor Tablets ... 1598
- Aldomet Oral ... 1600
- Aldoril Tablets ... 1604

Methyldopate Hydrochloride (Chlorthalidone may add to or potentiate the action of other antihypertensive drugs). Products include:
- Aldomet Ester HCl Injection ... 1602

Metolazone (Chlorthalidone may add to or potentiate the action of other antihypertensive drugs). Products include:
- Mykrox Tablets ... 993
- Zaroxolyn Tablets ... 1000

Metoprolol Succinate (Chlorthalidone may add to or potentiate the action of other antihypertensive drugs). Products include:
- Toprol-XL Tablets ... 565

Metoprolol Tartrate (Chlorthalidone may add to or potentiate the action of other antihypertensive drugs). Products include:
- Lopressor Ampuls ... 830
- Lopressor HCT Tablets ... 832
- Lopressor Tablets ... 830

Metyrosine (Chlorthalidone may add to or potentiate the action of other antihypertensive drugs). Products include:
- Demser Capsules ... 1649

Minoxidil (Chlorthalidone may add to or potentiate the action of other antihypertensive drugs). Products include:
- Loniten Tablets ... 2618
- Rogaine Topical Solution ... 2637

Moexipril Hydrochloride (Chlorthalidone may add to or potentiate the action of other antihypertensive drugs). Products include:
- Univasc Tablets ... 2410

Morphine Sulfate (Aggravates orthostatic hypotension). Products include:
- Astramorph/PF Injection, USP (Preservative-Free) ... 535
- Duramorph ... 962
- Infumorph 200 and Infumorph 500 Sterile Solutions ... 965
- MS Contin Tablets ... 1994
- MSIR ... 1997
- Oramorph SR (Morphine Sulfate Sustained Release Tablets) ... 2236
- RMS Suppositories ... 2657
- Roxanol ... 2243

Nadolol (Chlorthalidone may add to or potentiate the action of other antihypertensive drugs).
- No products indexed under this heading.

Nicardipine Hydrochloride (Chlorthalidone may add to or potentiate the action of other antihypertensive drugs). Products include:
- Cardene Capsules ... 2095
- Cardene I.V. ... 2709
- Cardene SR Capsules ... 2097

Nifedipine (Chlorthalidone may add to or potentiate the action of other antihypertensive drugs). Products include:
- Adalat Capsules (10 mg and 20 mg) ... 587
- Adalat CC ... 589
- Procardia Capsules ... 1971
- Procardia XL Extended Release Tablets ... 1972

Nisoldipine (Chlorthalidone may add to or potentiate the action of other antihypertensive drugs).
- No products indexed under this heading.

Nitroglycerin (Chlorthalidone may add to or potentiate the action of other antihypertensive drugs). Products include:
- Deponit NTG Transdermal Delivery System ... 2397
- Nitro-Bid IV ... 1523
- Nitro-Bid Ointment ... 1524
- Nitrodisc ... 2047
- Nitro-Dur (nitroglycerin) Transdermal Infusion System ... 1326
- Nitrolingual Spray ... 2027
- Nitrostat Tablets ... 1925
- Transderm-Nitro Transdermal Therapeutic System ... 859

Norepinephrine Bitartrate (Decreased arterial responsiveness). Products include:
- Levophed Bitartrate Injection ... 2315

Opium Alkaloids (Aggravates orthostatic hypotension).
- No products indexed under this heading.

Oxycodone Hydrochloride (Aggravates orthostatic hypotension). Products include:
- Percocet Tablets ... 938
- Percodan Tablets ... 939
- Percodan-Demi Tablets ... 940
- Roxicodone Tablets, Oral Solution & Intensol (Oxycodone) ... 2244
- Tylox Capsules ... 1584

Penbutolol Sulfate (Chlorthalidone may add to or potentiate the action of other antihypertensive drugs). Products include:
- Levatol ... 2403

Pentobarbital Sodium (Aggravates orthostatic hypotension). Products include:
- Nembutal Sodium Capsules ... 436
- Nembutal Sodium Solution ... 438
- Nembutal Sodium Suppositories ... 440

Phenobarbital (Aggravates orthostatic hypotension). Products include:
- Arco-Lase Plus Tablets ... 512
- Bellergal-S Tablets ... 2250
- Donnatal ... 2060
- Donnatal Extentabs ... 2061
- Donnatal Tablets ... 2060
- Phenobarbital Elixir and Tablets ... 1469
- Quadrinal Tablets ... 1350

Phenoxybenzamine Hydrochloride (Chlorthalidone may add to or potentiate the action of other antihypertensive drugs). Products include:
- Dibenzyline Capsules ... 2476

Phentolamine Mesylate (Chlorthalidone may add to or potentiate the action of other antihypertensive drugs). Products include:
- Regitine ... 846

Pindolol (Chlorthalidone may add to or potentiate the action of other antihypertensive drugs). Products include:
- Visken Tablets ... 2299

Polythiazide (Chlorthalidone may add to or potentiate the action of other antihypertensive drugs). Products include:
- Minizide Capsules ... 1938

Prazosin Hydrochloride (Chlorthalidone may add to or potentiate the action of other antihypertensive drugs). Products include:
- Minipress Capsules ... 1937
- Minizide Capsules ... 1938

Propoxyphene Hydrochloride (Aggravates orthostatic hypotension). Products include:
- Darvon ... 1435
- Wygesic Tablets ... 2827

Propoxyphene Napsylate (Aggravates orthostatic hypotension). Products include:
- Darvon-N/Darvocet-N ... 1433

Propranolol Hydrochloride (Chlorthalidone may add to or potentiate the action of other antihypertensive drugs). Products include:
- Inderal ... 2728
- Inderal LA Long Acting Capsules ... 2730
- Inderide Tablets ... 2732
- Inderide LA Long Acting Capsules ... 2734

Quinapril Hydrochloride (Chlorthalidone may add to or potentiate the action of other antihypertensive drugs). Products include:
- Accupril Tablets ... 1893

Ramipril (Chlorthalidone may add to or potentiate the action of other antihypertensive drugs). Products include:
- Altace Capsules ... 1232

Rauwolfia Serpentina (Chlorthalidone may add to or potentiate the action of other antihypertensive drugs).
- No products indexed under this heading.

Rescinnamine (Chlorthalidone may add to or potentiate the action of other antihypertensive drugs).
- No products indexed under this heading.

Reserpine (Chlorthalidone may add to or potentiate the action of other antihypertensive drugs). Products include:
- Diupres Tablets ... 1650
- Hydropres Tablets ... 1675
- Ser-Ap-Es Tablets ... 849

Secobarbital Sodium (Aggravates orthostatic hypotension). Products include:
- Seconal Sodium Pulvules ... 1474

Sodium Nitroprusside (Chlorthalidone may add to or potentiate the action of other antihypertensive drugs).
- No products indexed under this heading.

Sotalol Hydrochloride (Chlorthalidone may add to or potentiate the action of other antihypertensive drugs). Products include:
- Betapace Tablets ... 641

Spirapril Hydrochloride (Chlorthalidone may add to or potentiate the action of other antihypertensive drugs).
- No products indexed under this heading.

Sufentanil Citrate (Aggravates orthostatic hypotension). Products include:
- Sufenta Injection ... 1309

Terazosin Hydrochloride (Chlorthalidone may add to or potentiate the action of other antihypertensive drugs). Products include:
- Hytrin Capsules ... 430

Thiamylal Sodium (Aggravates orthostatic hypotension).
- No products indexed under this heading.

Timolol Maleate (Chlorthalidone may add to or potentiate the action of other antihypertensive drugs). Products include:
- Blocadren Tablets ... 1614
- Timolide Tablets ... 1748
- Timoptic in Ocudose ... 1753
- Timoptic Sterile Ophthalmic Solution ... 1751
- Timoptic-XE ... 1755

Tolazamide (Increase in serum glucose level; higher dosage of oral hypoglycemic agents may be necessary).
- No products indexed under this heading.

Tolbutamide (Increase in serum glucose level; higher dosage of oral hypoglycemic agents may be necessary).
- No products indexed under this heading.

Torsemide (Chlorthalidone may add to or potentiate the action of other antihypertensive drugs). Products include:
- Demadex Tablets and Injection ... 686

Trimethaphan Camsylate (Chlorthalidone may add to or potentiate the action of other antihypertensive drugs). Products include:
- Arfonad Ampuls ... 2080

Tubocurarine Chloride (Increased responsiveness to tubocurarine).
- No products indexed under this heading.

Verapamil Hydrochloride (Chlorthalidone may add to or potentiate the action of other antihypertensive drugs). Products include:
- Calan SR Caplets ... 2422
- Calan Tablets ... 2419
- Isoptin Injectable ... 1344
- Isoptin Oral Tablets ... 1346
- Isoptin SR Tablets ... 1348
- Verelan Capsules ... 1410
- Verelan Capsules ... 2824

Food Interactions

Alcohol (Aggravates orthostatic hypotension).

THEO-24 EXTENDED RELEASE CAPSULES

(Theophylline Anhydrous) ... 2568

May interact with macrolide antibiotics, sympathomimetic bronchodilators, oral contraceptives, and certain other agents. Compounds in these categories include:

Albuterol (Potential for toxic synergism). Products include:
- Proventil Inhalation Aerosol ... 2382
- Ventolin Inhalation Aerosol and Refill ... 1197

Albuterol Sulfate (Potential for toxic synergism). Products include:
- Airet Solution for Inhalation ... 452
- Proventil Inhalation Solution 0.083% ... 2384
- Proventil Repetabs Tablets ... 2386
- Proventil Solution for Inhalation 0.5% ... 2383
- Proventil Syrup ... 2385
- Proventil Tablets ... 2386
- Ventolin Inhalation Solution ... 1198
- Ventolin Nebules Inhalation Solution ... 1199
- Ventolin Rotacaps for Inhalation ... 1200
- Ventolin Syrup ... 1202
- Ventolin Tablets ... 1203
- Volmax Extended-Release Tablets .. 1788

Allopurinol (Elevated theophylline serum levels with high dose of allopurinol). Products include:
- Zyloprim Tablets ... 1226

Azithromycin (Elevated theophylline serum levels). Products include:
- Zithromax ... 1944

Bitolterol Mesylate (Potential for toxic synergism). Products include:
- Tornalate Solution for Inhalation, 0.2% ... 956
- Tornalate Metered Dose Inhaler ... 957

Carbamazepine (Decreases serum theophylline levels). Products include:
- Atretol Tablets ... 573
- Tegretol Chewable Tablets ... 852
- Tegretol Suspension ... 852

Interactions Index

Tegretol Tablets 852

Cimetidine (Elevated theophylline serum levels). Products include:

Tagamet Tablets 2516

Cimetidine Hydrochloride (Elevated theophylline serum levels). Products include:

Tagamet.. 2516

Ciprofloxacin Hydrochloride (Increases serum theophylline levels). Products include:

Ciloxan Ophthalmic Solution.............. 472
Cipro Tablets... 592

Clarithromycin (Elevated theophylline serum levels). Products include:

Biaxin 405

Desogestrel (Elevated theophylline serum levels). Products include:

Desogen Tablets...................................... 1817
Ortho-Cept 1851

Ephedrine Hydrochloride (Potential for toxic synergism). Products include:

Primatene Dual Action Formula...... ◆D 872
Primatene Tablets .... ◆D 873
Quadrinal Tablets 1350

Ephedrine Sulfate (Potential for toxic synergism). Products include:

Bronkaid Caplets .... ◆D 717
Marax Tablets & DF Syrup.................. 2200

Ephedrine Tannate (Potential for toxic synergism). Products include:

Rynatuss 2673

Epinephrine (Potential for toxic synergism). Products include:

Bronkaid Mist .... ◆D 717
EPIFRIN .... © 239
EpiPen 790
Marcaine Hydrochloride with Epinephrine 1:200,000 2316
Primatene Mist .... ◆D 873
Sensorcaine with Epinephrine Injection.. 559
Sus-Phrine Injection 1019
Xylocaine with Epinephrine Injections.. 567

Epinephrine Bitartrate (Increased toxicity). Products include:

Bronkaid Mist Suspension .... ◆D 718
Sensorcaine-MPF with Epinephrine Injection 559

Epinephrine Hydrochloride (Potential for toxic synergism). Products include:

Ana-Kit Anaphylaxis Emergency Treatment Kit 617

Erythromycin (Elevated theophylline serum levels). Products include:

A/T/S 2% Acne Topical Gel and Solution 1234
Benzamycin Topical Gel 905
E-Mycin Tablets 1341
Emgel 2% Topical Gel........................... 1093
ERYC... 1915
Erycette (erythromycin 2%) Topical Solution... 1888
Ery-Tab Tablets 422
Erythromycin Base Filmtab 426
Erythromycin Delayed-Release Capsules, USP..................................... 427
Ilotycin Ophthalmic Ointment............ 912
PCE Dispertab Tablets 444
T-Stat 2.0% Topical Solution and Pads 2688
Theramycin Z Topical Solution 2% 1592

Erythromycin Estolate (Elevated theophylline serum levels). Products include:

Ilosone 911

Erythromycin Ethylsuccinate (Elevated theophylline serum levels). Products include:

E.E.S.. 424
EryPed 421

Erythromycin Gluceptate (Elevated theophylline serum levels). Products include:

Ilotycin Gluceptate, IV, Vials 913

Erythromycin Stearate (Elevated theophylline serum levels). Products include:

Erythrocin Stearate Filmtab 425

Ethinyl Estradiol (Elevated theophylline serum levels). Products include:

Brevicon.. 2088
Demulen 2428
Desogen Tablets...................................... 1817
Levlen/Tri-Levlen 651
Lo/Ovral Tablets 2746
Lo/Ovral-28 Tablets............................... 2751
Modicon.. 1872
Nordette-21 Tablets 2755
Nordette-28 Tablets................................ 2758
Norinyl 2088
Ortho-Cept 1851
Ortho-Cyclen/Ortho-Tri-Cyclen 1858
Ortho-Novum.. 1872
Ortho-Cyclen/Ortho Tri-Cyclen 1858
Ovcon 760
Ovral Tablets 2770
Ovral-28 Tablets 2770
Levlen/Tri-Levlen 651
Tri-Norinyl... 2164
Triphasil-21 Tablets............................... 2814
Triphasil-28 Tablets............................... 2819

Ethylnorepinephrine Hydrochloride (Potential for toxic synergism).

No products indexed under this heading.

Ethynodiol Diacetate (Elevated theophylline serum levels). Products include:

Demulen 2428

Halothane (May produce sinus tachycardia or ventricular arrhythmias). Products include:

Fluothane 2724

Isoetharine (Potential for toxic synergism). Products include:

Bronkometer Aerosol............................ 2302
Bronkosol Solution 2302
Isoetharine Inhalation Solution, USP, Arm-a-Med.................................. 551

Isoproterenol Hydrochloride (Potential for toxic synergism). Products include:

Isuprel Hydrochloride Injection 1:5000 2311
Isuprel Hydrochloride Solution 1:200 & 1:100 2313
Isuprel Mistometer 2312

Isoproterenol Sulfate (Potential for toxic synergism). Products include:

Norisodrine with Calcium Iodide Syrup.. 442

Levonorgestrel (Elevated theophylline serum levels). Products include:

Levlen/Tri-Levlen 651
Nordette-21 Tablets 2755
Nordette-28 Tablets................................ 2758
Norplant System 2759
Levlen/Tri-Levlen 651
Triphasil-21 Tablets............................... 2814
Triphasil-28 Tablets............................... 2819

Lithium Carbonate (Increased renal excretion of lithium carbonate). Products include:

Eskalith 2485
Lithium Carbonate Capsules & Tablets 2230
Lithonate/Lithotabs/Lithobid 2543

Mestranol (Elevated theophylline serum levels). Products include:

Norinyl 2088
Ortho-Novum.. 1872

Metaproterenol Sulfate (Potential for toxic synergism). Products include:

Alupent... 669
Metaproterenol Sulfate Inhalation Solution, USP, Arm-a-Med 552

Norethindrone (Elevated theophylline serum levels). Products include:

Brevicon.. 2088
Micronor Tablets 1872
Modicon.. 1872

Norinyl 2088
Nor-Q D Tablets 2135
Ortho-Novum.. 1872
Ovcon 760
Tri-Norinyl... 2164

Norethynodrel (Elevated theophylline serum levels).

No products indexed under this heading.

Norgestimate (Elevated theophylline serum levels). Products include:

Ortho-Cyclen/Ortho-Tri-Cyclen 1858
Ortho-Cyclen/Ortho Tri-Cyclen 1858

Norgestrel (Elevated theophylline serum levels). Products include:

Lo/Ovral Tablets 2746
Lo/Ovral-28 Tablets............................... 2751
Ovral Tablets 2770
Ovral-28 Tablets 2770
Ovrette Tablets....................................... 2771

Phenobarbital (Decreases serum theophylline levels). Products include:

Arco-Lase Plus Tablets 512
Bellergal-S Tablets 2250
Donnatal 2060
Donnatal Extentabs............................... 2061
Donnatal Tablets 2060
Phenobarbital Elixir and Tablets 1469
Quadrinal Tablets 1350

Phenytoin (Decreased theophylline and phenytoin serum levels). Products include:

Dilantin Infatabs.................................... 1908
Dilantin-125 Suspension 1911

Phenytoin Sodium (Decreased theophylline and phenytoin serum levels). Products include:

Dilantin Kapseals 1906
Dilantin Parenteral 1910

Pirbuterol Acetate (Potential for toxic synergism). Products include:

Maxair Autohaler 1492
Maxair Inhaler 1494

Propranolol Hydrochloride (Increased serum theophylline levels). Products include:

Inderal 2728
Inderal LA Long Acting Capsules 2730
Inderide Tablets 2732
Inderide LA Long Acting Capsules .. 2734

Rifampin (Decreased serum theophylline levels). Products include:

Rifadin 1528
Rifamate Capsules 1530
Rifater... 1532
Rimactane Capsules 847

Salmeterol Xinafoate (Potential for toxic synergism). Products include:

Serevent Inhalation Aerosol................ 1176

Terbutaline Sulfate (Potential for toxic synergism). Products include:

Brethaire Inhaler 813
Brethine Ampuls 815
Brethine Tablets..................................... 814
Bricanyl Subcutaneous Injection 1502
Bricanyl Tablets 1503

Troleandomycin (Elevated theophylline serum levels). Products include:

Tao Capsules... 2209

Food Interactions

Diet, high-lipid (May result in a significant increase in peak serum level).

THEO-DUR EXTENDED-RELEASE TABLETS

(Theophylline Anhydrous)....................1327

May interact with macrolide antibiotics, oral contraceptives, sympathomimetic bronchodilators, and certain other agents. Compounds in these categories include:

Albuterol (Potential for toxic synergism). Products include:

Proventil Inhalation Aerosol 2382
Ventolin Inhalation Aerosol and Refill 1197

Albuterol Sulfate (Potential for toxic synergism). Products include:

Airet Solution for Inhalation 452
Proventil Inhalation Solution 0.083%.. 2384
Proventil Repetabs Tablets 2386
Proventil Solution for Inhalation 0.5%.. 2383
Proventil Syrup....................................... 2385
Proventil Tablets 2386
Ventolin Inhalation Solution................ 1198
Ventolin Nebules Inhalation Solution.. 1199
Ventolin Rotacaps for Inhalation 1200
Ventolin Syrup.. 1202
Ventolin Tablets 1203
Volmax Extended-Release Tablets .. 1788

Allopurinol (Increased serum theophylline levels at high dose of allopurinol). Products include:

Zyloprim Tablets 1226

Azithromycin (Increases serum theophylline levels). Products include:

Zithromax 1944

Bitolterol Mesylate (Potential for toxic synergism). Products include:

Tornalate Solution for Inhalation, 0.2%.. 956
Tornalate Metered Dose Inhaler 957

Cimetidine (Increases serum theophylline levels). Products include:

Tagamet Tablets 2516

Cimetidine Hydrochloride (Increases serum theophylline levels). Products include:

Tagamet.. 2516

Ciprofloxacin Hydrochloride (Increases serum theophylline levels). Products include:

Ciloxan Ophthalmic Solution.............. 472
Cipro Tablets... 592

Clarithromycin (Increases serum theophylline levels). Products include:

Biaxin 405

Desogestrel (Increases serum theophylline levels). Products include:

Desogen Tablets...................................... 1817
Ortho-Cept 1851

Ephedrine Hydrochloride (Potential for toxic synergism). Products include:

Primatene Dual Action Formula...... ◆D 872
Primatene Tablets .... ◆D 873
Quadrinal Tablets 1350

Ephedrine Sulfate (Potential for toxic synergism). Products include:

Bronkaid Caplets .... ◆D 717
Marax Tablets & DF Syrup.................. 2200

Ephedrine Tannate (Potential for toxic synergism). Products include:

Rynatuss 2673

Epinephrine (Potential for toxic synergism). Products include:

Bronkaid Mist .... ◆D 717
EPIFRIN .... © 239
EpiPen 790
Marcaine Hydrochloride with Epinephrine 1:200,000 2316
Primatene Mist .... ◆D 873
Sensorcaine with Epinephrine Injection.. 559
Sus-Phrine Injection 1019
Xylocaine with Epinephrine Injections.. 567

Epinephrine Hydrochloride (Potential for toxic synergism). Products include:

Ana-Kit Anaphylaxis Emergency Treatment Kit 617

Erythromycin (Increases serum theophylline levels). Products include:

A/T/S 2% Acne Topical Gel and Solution 1234
Benzamycin Topical Gel 905
E-Mycin Tablets 1341
Emgel 2% Topical Gel........................... 1093
ERYC... 1915

IMPORTANT NOTE: Always consult each drug listing in the patient's regimen for possible interactions.

Erycette (erythromycin 2%) Topical Solution ... 1888
Ery-Tab Tablets ... 422
Erythromycin Base Filmtab ... 426
Erythromycin Delayed-Release Capsules, USP ... 427
Ilotycin Ophthalmic Ointment ... 912
PCE Dispertab Tablets ... 444
T-Stat 2.0% Topical Solution and Pads ... 2688
Theramycin Z Topical Solution 2% ... 1592

Erythromycin Estolate (Increases serum theophylline levels). Products include:
Ilosone ... 911

Erythromycin Ethylsuccinate (Increases serum theophylline levels). Products include:
E.E.S. ... 424
EryPed ... 421

Erythromycin Gluceptate (Increases serum theophylline levels). Products include:
Ilotycin Gluceptate, IV, Vials ... 913

Erythromycin Stearate (Increases serum theophylline levels). Products include:
Erythrocin Stearate Filmtab ... 425

Ethinyl Estradiol (Increases serum theophylline levels). Products include:
Brevicon ... 2088
Demulen ... 2428
Desogen Tablets ... 1817
Levlen/Tri-Levlen ... 651
Lo/Ovral Tablets ... 2746
Lo/Ovral-28 Tablets ... 2751
Modicon ... 1872
Nordette-21 Tablets ... 2755
Nordette-28 Tablets ... 2758
Norinyl ... 2088
Ortho-Cept ... 1851
Ortho-Cyclen/Ortho-Tri-Cyclen ... 1858
Ortho-Novum ... 1872
Ortho-Cyclen/Ortho Tri-Cyclen ... 1858
Ovcon ... 760
Ovral Tablets ... 2770
Ovral-28 Tablets ... 2770
Levlen/Tri-Levlen ... 651
Tri-Norinyl ... 2164
Triphasil-21 Tablets ... 2814
Triphasil-28 Tablets ... 2819

Ethylnorepinephrine Hydrochloride (Potential for toxic synergism).
No products indexed under this heading.

Ethynodiol Diacetate (Increases serum theophylline levels). Products include:
Demulen ... 2428

Isoetharine (Potential for toxic synergism). Products include:
Bronkometer Aerosol ... 2302
Bronkosol Solution ... 2302
Isoetharine Inhalation Solution, USP, Arm-a-Med ... 551

Isoproterenol Hydrochloride (Potential for toxic synergism). Products include:
Isuprel Hydrochloride Injection 1:5000 ... 2311
Isuprel Hydrochloride Solution 1:200 & 1:100 ... 2313
Isuprel Mistometer ... 2312

Isoproterenol Sulfate (Potential for toxic synergism). Products include:
Norisodrine with Calcium Iodide Syrup ... 442

Levonorgestrel (Increases serum theophylline levels). Products include:
Levlen/Tri-Levlen ... 651
Nordette-21 Tablets ... 2755
Nordette-28 Tablets ... 2758
Norplant System ... 2759
Levlen/Tri-Levlen ... 651
Triphasil-21 Tablets ... 2814
Triphasil-28 Tablets ... 2819

Lithium Carbonate (Increased renal excretion of lithium). Products include:
Eskalith ... 2485
Lithium Carbonate Capsules & Tablets ... 2230
Lithonate/Lithotabs/Lithobid ... 2543

Mestranol (Increases serum theophylline levels). Products include:
Norinyl ... 2088
Ortho-Novum ... 1872

Metaproterenol Sulfate (Potential for toxic synergism). Products include:
Alupent ... 669
Metaproterenol Sulfate Inhalation Solution, USP, Arm-a-Med ... 552

Norethindrone (Increases serum theophylline levels). Products include:
Brevicon ... 2088
Micronor Tablets ... 1872
Modicon ... 1872
Norinyl ... 2088
Nor-Q D Tablets ... 2135
Ortho-Novum ... 1872
Ovcon ... 760
Tri-Norinyl ... 2164

Norethynodrel (Increases serum theophylline levels).
No products indexed under this heading.

Norfloxacin (Increases serum theophylline levels). Products include:
Chibroxin Sterile Ophthalmic Solution ... 1617
Noroxin Tablets ... 1715
Noroxin Tablets ... 2048

Norgestimate (Increases serum theophylline levels). Products include:
Ortho-Cyclen/Ortho-Tri-Cyclen ... 1858
Ortho-Cyclen/Ortho Tri-Cyclen ... 1858

Norgestrel (Increases serum theophylline levels). Products include:
Lo/Ovral Tablets ... 2746
Lo/Ovral-28 Tablets ... 2751
Ovral Tablets ... 2770
Ovral-28 Tablets ... 2770
Ovrette Tablets ... 2771

Phenytoin (Decreased theophylline and phenytoin levels). Products include:
Dilantin Infatabs ... 1908
Dilantin-125 Suspension ... 1911

Phenytoin Sodium (Decreased theophylline and phenytoin levels). Products include:
Dilantin Kapseals ... 1906
Dilantin Parenteral ... 1910

Pirbuterol Acetate (Potential for toxic synergism). Products include:
Maxair Autohaler ... 1492
Maxair Inhaler ... 1494

Propranolol Hydrochloride (Increases serum theophylline levels). Products include:
Inderal ... 2728
Inderal LA Long Acting Capsules ... 2730
Inderide Tablets ... 2732
Inderide LA Long Acting Capsules ... 2734

Rifampin (Decreased serum theophylline levels). Products include:
Rifadin ... 1528
Rifamate Capsules ... 1530
Rifater ... 1532
Rimactane Capsules ... 847

Salmeterol Xinafoate (Potential for toxic synergism). Products include:
Serevent Inhalation Aerosol ... 1176

Sucralfate (Reduces absorption of theophylline). Products include:
Carafate Suspension ... 1505
Carafate Tablets ... 1504

Terbutaline Sulfate (Potential for toxic synergism). Products include:
Brethaire Inhaler ... 813
Brethine Ampuls ... 815
Brethine Tablets ... 814
Bricanyl Subcutaneous Injection ... 1502
Bricanyl Tablets ... 1503

Troleandomycin (Increases serum theophylline levels). Products include:
Tao Capsules ... 2209

Food Interactions

Food, unspecified (May influence absorption of theophylline from a 100 mg dosage form).

THEO-X EXTENDED-RELEASE TABLETS

(Theophylline Anhydrous) ... 788
May interact with macrolide antibiotics, oral contraceptives, sympathomimetic bronchodilators, and certain other agents. Compounds in these categories include:

Albuterol (Potential for toxic synergism). Products include:
Proventil Inhalation Aerosol ... 2382
Ventolin Inhalation Aerosol and Refill ... 1197

Albuterol Sulfate (Potential for toxic synergism). Products include:
Airet Solution for Inhalation ... 452
Proventil Inhalation Solution 0.083% ... 2384
Proventil Repetabs Tablets ... 2386
Proventil Solution for Inhalation 0.5% ... 2383
Proventil Syrup ... 2385
Proventil Tablets ... 2386
Ventolin Inhalation Solution ... 1198
Ventolin Nebules Inhalation Solution ... 1199
Ventolin Rotacaps for Inhalation ... 1200
Ventolin Syrup ... 1202
Ventolin Tablets ... 1203
Volmax Extended-Release Tablets ... 1788

Allopurinol (Increased serum theophylline levels at high dose of allopurinol). Products include:
Zyloprim Tablets ... 1226

Azithromycin (Increases serum theophylline levels). Products include:
Zithromax ... 1944

Bitolterol Mesylate (Potential for toxic synergism). Products include:
Tornalate Solution for Inhalation, 0.2% ... 956
Tornalate Metered Dose Inhaler ... 957

Cimetidine (Increases serum theophylline levels). Products include:
Tagamet Tablets ... 2516

Cimetidine Hydrochloride (Increases serum theophylline levels). Products include:
Tagamet ... 2516

Ciprofloxacin (Increases serum theophylline levels). Products include:
Cipro I.V. ... 595
Cipro I.V. Pharmacy Bulk Package ... 597

Ciprofloxacin Hydrochloride (Increases serum theophylline levels). Products include:
Ciloxan Ophthalmic Solution ... 472
Cipro Tablets ... 592

Clarithromycin (Increases serum theophylline levels). Products include:
Biaxin ... 405

Desogestrel (Increases serum theophylline levels). Products include:
Desogen Tablets ... 1817
Ortho-Cept ... 1851

Ephedrine Hydrochloride (Potential for toxic synergism). Products include:
Primatene Dual Action Formula ... ▣ 872
Primatene Tablets ... ▣ 873
Quadrinal Tablets ... 1350

Ephedrine Sulfate (Potential for toxic synergism). Products include:
Bronkaid Caplets ... ▣ 717
Marax Tablets & DF Syrup ... 2200

Ephedrine Tannate (Potential for toxic synergism). Products include:
Rynatuss ... 2673

Epinephrine (Potential for toxic synergism). Products include:
Bronkaid Mist ... ▣ 717
EPIFRIN ... ⊙ 239
EpiPen ... 790
Marcaine Hydrochloride with Epinephrine 1:200,000 ... 2316
Primatene Mist ... ▣ 873
Sensorcaine with Epinephrine Injection ... 559
Sus-Phrine Injection ... 1019
Xylocaine with Epinephrine Injections ... 567

Epinephrine Hydrochloride (Potential for toxic synergism). Products include:
Ana-Kit Anaphylaxis Emergency Treatment Kit ... 617

Erythromycin (Increases serum theophylline levels). Products include:
A/T/S 2% Acne Topical Gel and Solution ... 1234
Benzamycin Topical Gel ... 905
E-Mycin Tablets ... 1341
Emgel 2% Topical Gel ... 1093
ERYC ... 1915
Erycette (erythromycin 2%) Topical Solution ... 1888
Ery-Tab Tablets ... 422
Erythromycin Base Filmtab ... 426
Erythromycin Delayed-Release Capsules, USP ... 427
Ilotycin Ophthalmic Ointment ... 912
PCE Dispertab Tablets ... 444
T-Stat 2.0% Topical Solution and Pads ... 2688
Theramycin Z Topical Solution 2% ... 1592

Erythromycin Estolate (Increases serum theophylline levels). Products include:
Ilosone ... 911

Erythromycin Ethylsuccinate (Increases serum theophylline levels). Products include:
E.E.S. ... 424
EryPed ... 421

Erythromycin Gluceptate (Increases serum theophylline levels). Products include:
Ilotycin Gluceptate, IV, Vials ... 913

Erythromycin Stearate (Increases serum theophylline levels). Products include:
Erythrocin Stearate Filmtab ... 425

Ethinyl Estradiol (Increases serum theophylline levels). Products include:
Brevicon ... 2088
Demulen ... 2428
Desogen Tablets ... 1817
Levlen/Tri-Levlen ... 651
Lo/Ovral Tablets ... 2746
Lo/Ovral-28 Tablets ... 2751
Modicon ... 1872
Nordette-21 Tablets ... 2755
Nordette-28 Tablets ... 2758
Norinyl ... 2088
Ortho-Cept ... 1851
Ortho-Cyclen/Ortho-Tri-Cyclen ... 1858
Ortho-Novum ... 1872
Ortho-Cyclen/Ortho Tri-Cyclen ... 1858
Ovcon ... 760
Ovral Tablets ... 2770
Ovral-28 Tablets ... 2770
Levlen/Tri-Levlen ... 651
Tri-Norinyl ... 2164
Triphasil-21 Tablets ... 2814
Triphasil-28 Tablets ... 2819

Ethylnorepinephrine Hydrochloride (Potential for toxic synergism).
No products indexed under this heading.

(▣ Described in PDR For Nonprescription Drugs) (⊙ Described in PDR For Ophthalmology)

Ethynodiol Diacetate (Increases serum theophylline levels). Products include:

Demulen ... 2428

Isoetharine (Potential for toxic synergism). Products include:

Bronkometer Aerosol ... 2302
Bronkosol Solution ... 2302
Isoetharine Inhalation Solution, USP, Arm-a-Med ... 551

Isoproterenol Hydrochloride (Potential for toxic synergism). Products include:

Isuprel Hydrochloride Injection 1:5000 ... 2311
Isuprel Hydrochloride Solution 1:200 & 1:100 ... 2313
Isuprel Mistometer ... 2312

Isoproterenol Sulfate (Potential for toxic synergism). Products include:

Norisodrine with Calcium Iodide Syrup ... 442

Levonorgestrel (Increases serum theophylline levels). Products include:

Levlen/Tri-Levlen ... 651
Nordette-21 Tablets ... 2755
Nordette-28 Tablets ... 2758
Norplant System ... 2759
Levlen/Tri-Levlen ... 651
Triphasil-21 Tablets ... 2814
Triphasil-28 Tablets ... 2819

Lithium Carbonate (Increased renal excretion of lithium). Products include:

Eskalith ... 2485
Lithium Carbonate Capsules & Tablets ... 2230
Lithonate/Lithotabs/Lithobid ... 2543

Mestranol (Increases serum theophylline levels). Products include:

Norinyl ... 2088
Ortho-Novum ... 1872

Metaproterenol Sulfate (Potential for toxic synergism). Products include:

Alupent ... 669
Metaproterenol Sulfate Inhalation Solution, USP, Arm-a-Med ... 552

Norethindrone (Increases serum theophylline levels). Products include:

Brevicon ... 2088
Micronor Tablets ... 1872
Modicon ... 1872
Norinyl ... 2088
Nor-Q D Tablets ... 2135
Ortho-Novum ... 1872
Ovcon ... 760
Tri-Norinyl ... 2164

Norethynodrel (Increases serum theophylline levels).

No products indexed under this heading.

Norgestimate (Increases serum theophylline levels). Products include:

Ortho-Cyclen/Ortho-Tri-Cyclen ... 1858
Ortho-Cyclen/Ortho Tri-Cyclen ... 1858

Norgestrel (Increases serum theophylline levels). Products include:

Lo/Ovral Tablets ... 2746
Lo/Ovral-28 Tablets ... 2751
Ovral Tablets ... 2770
Ovral-28 Tablets ... 2770
Ovrette Tablets ... 2771

Phenytoin (Decreased theophylline and phenytoin levels). Products include:

Dilantin Infatabs ... 1908
Dilantin-125 Suspension ... 1911

Phenytoin Sodium (Decreased theophylline and phenytoin levels). Products include:

Dilantin Kapseals ... 1906
Dilantin Parenteral ... 1910

Pirbuterol Acetate (Potential for toxic synergism). Products include:

Maxair Autohaler ... 1492
Maxair Inhaler ... 1494

Propranolol Hydrochloride (Increases serum theophylline levels). Products include:

Inderal ... 2728
Inderal LA Long Acting Capsules ... 2730
Inderide Tablets ... 2732
Inderide LA Long Acting Capsules ... 2734

Rifampin (Decreased serum theophylline levels). Products include:

Rifadin ... 1528
Rifamate Capsules ... 1530
Rifater ... 1532
Rimactane Capsules ... 847

Salmeterol Xinafoate (Potential for toxic synergism). Products include:

Serevent Inhalation Aerosol ... 1176

Terbutaline Sulfate (Potential for toxic synergism). Products include:

Brethaire Inhaler ... 813
Brethine Ampuls ... 815
Brethine Tablets ... 814
Bricanyl Subcutaneous Injection ... 1502
Bricanyl Tablets ... 1503

Troleandomycin (Increases serum theophylline levels). Products include:

Tao Capsules ... 2209

Food Interactions

Diet, high-lipid (May result in a somewhat higher C_{max} and delayed T_{max}, and a somewhat greater extent of absorption when compared to taking in the fasting state).

THERACYS BCG LIVE (INTRAVESICAL)

(BCG, Live (Intravesical)) ... 897

May interact with immunosuppressive agents and certain other agents. Compounds in these categories include:

Azathioprine (May impair the response to TheraCys or increase the risk of osteomyelitis or disseminated BCG infection). Products include:

Imuran ... 1110

Bone Marrow Depressants, unspecified (May impair the response to TheraCys or increase the risk of osteomyelitis or disseminated BCG infection).

Cyclosporine (May impair the response to TheraCys or increase the risk of osteomyelitis or disseminated BCG infection). Products include:

Neoral ... 2276
Sandimmune ... 2286

Immune Globulin (Human) (May impair the response to TheraCys or increase the risk of osteomyelitis or disseminated BCG infection).

No products indexed under this heading.

Immune Globulin Intravenous (Human) (May impair the response to TheraCys or increase the risk of osteomyelitis or disseminated BCG infection).

Muromonab-CD3 (May impair the response to TheraCys or increase the risk of osteomyelitis or disseminated BCG infection). Products include:

Orthoclone OKT3 Sterile Solution ... 1837

Mycophenolate Mofetil (May impair the response to TheraCys or increase the risk of osteomyelitis or disseminated BCG infection). Products include:

CellCept Capsules ... 2099

Tacrolimus (May impair the response to TheraCys or increase the risk of osteomyelitis or disseminated BCG infection). Products include:

Prograf ... 1042

THERAFLU FLU AND COLD MEDICINE

(Acetaminophen, Chlorpheniramine Maleate, Pseudoephedrine Hydrochloride) ... ▣ 787

May interact with hypnotics and sedatives, tranquilizers, monoamine oxidase inhibitors, and certain other agents. Compounds in these categories include:

Alprazolam (May increase drowsiness effect). Products include:

Xanax Tablets ... 2649

Buspirone Hydrochloride (May increase drowsiness effect). Products include:

BuSpar ... 737

Chlordiazepoxide (May increase drowsiness effect). Products include:

Libritabs Tablets ... 2177
Limbitrol ... 2180

Chlordiazepoxide Hydrochloride (May increase drowsiness effect). Products include:

Librax Capsules ... 2176
Librium Capsules ... 2178
Librium Injectable ... 2179

Chlorpromazine (May increase drowsiness effect). Products include:

Thorazine Suppositories ... 2523

Chlorpromazine Hydrochloride (May increase drowsiness effect). Products include:

Thorazine ... 2523

Chlorprothixene (May increase drowsiness effect).

No products indexed under this heading.

Chlorprothixene Hydrochloride (May increase drowsiness effect).

No products indexed under this heading.

Clorazepate Dipotassium (May increase drowsiness effect). Products include:

Tranxene ... 451

Diazepam (May increase drowsiness effect). Products include:

Dizac ... 1809
Valium Injectable ... 2182
Valium Tablets ... 2183
Valrelease Capsules ... 2169

Droperidol (May increase drowsiness effect). Products include:

Inapsine Injection ... 1296

Estazolam (May increase drowsiness effect). Products include:

ProSom Tablets ... 449

Ethchlorvynol (May increase drowsiness effect). Products include:

Placidyl Capsules ... 448

Ethinamate (May increase drowsiness effect).

No products indexed under this heading.

Fluphenazine Decanoate (May increase drowsiness effect). Products include:

Prolixin Decanoate ... 509

Fluphenazine Enanthate (May increase drowsiness effect). Products include:

Prolixin Enanthate ... 509

Fluphenazine Hydrochloride (May increase drowsiness effect). Products include:

Prolixin ... 509

Flurazepam Hydrochloride (May increase drowsiness effect). Products include:

Dalmane Capsules ... 2173

Furazolidone (Concurrent and/or sequential use is not recommended). Products include:

Furoxone ... 2046

Glutethimide (May increase drowsiness effect).

No products indexed under this heading.

Haloperidol (May increase drowsiness effect). Products include:

Haldol Injection, Tablets and Concentrate ... 1575

Haloperidol Decanoate (May increase drowsiness effect). Products include:

Haldol Decanoate ... 1577

Hydroxyzine Hydrochloride (May increase drowsiness effect). Products include:

Atarax Tablets & Syrup ... 2185
Marax Tablets & DF Syrup ... 2200
Vistaril Intramuscular Solution ... 2216

Isocarboxazid (Concurrent and/or sequential use is not recommended).

No products indexed under this heading.

Lorazepam (May increase drowsiness effect). Products include:

Ativan Injection ... 2698
Ativan Tablets ... 2700

Loxapine Hydrochloride (May increase drowsiness effect). Products include:

Loxitane ... 1378

Loxapine Succinate (May increase drowsiness effect). Products include:

Loxitane Capsules ... 1378

Meprobamate (May increase drowsiness effect). Products include:

Miltown Tablets ... 2672
PMB 200 and PMB 400 ... 2783

Mesoridazine Besylate (May increase drowsiness effect). Products include:

Serentil ... 684

Midazolam Hydrochloride (May increase drowsiness effect). Products include:

Versed Injection ... 2170

Molindone Hydrochloride (May increase drowsiness effect). Products include:

Moban Tablets and Concentrate ... 1048

Oxazepam (May increase drowsiness effect). Products include:

Serax Capsules ... 2810
Serax Tablets ... 2810

Perphenazine (May increase drowsiness effect). Products include:

Etrafon ... 2355
Triavil Tablets ... 1757
Trilafon ... 2389

Phenelzine Sulfate (Concurrent and/or sequential use is not recommended). Products include:

Nardil ... 1920

Prazepam (May increase drowsiness effect).

No products indexed under this heading.

Prochlorperazine (May increase drowsiness effect). Products include:

Compazine ... 2470

Promethazine Hydrochloride (May increase drowsiness effect). Products include:

Mepergan Injection ... 2753
Phenergan with Codeine ... 2777
Phenergan with Dextromethorphan 2778
Phenergan Injection ... 2773
Phenergan Suppositories ... 2775
Phenergan Syrup ... 2774
Phenergan Tablets ... 2775
Phenergan VC ... 2779
Phenergan VC with Codeine ... 2781

Propofol (May increase drowsiness effect). Products include:

Diprivan Injection ... 2833

Quazepam (May increase drowsiness effect). Products include:

Doral Tablets ... 2664

IMPORTANT NOTE: Always consult each drug listing in the patient's regimen for possible interactions.

Secobarbital Sodium (May increase drowsiness effect). Products include:
Seconal Sodium Pulvules 1474

Selegiline Hydrochloride (Concurrent and/or sequential use is not recommended). Products include:
Eldepryl Tablets 2550

Temazepam (May increase drowsiness effect). Products include:
Restoril Capsules 2284

Thioridazine Hydrochloride (May increase drowsiness effect). Products include:
Mellaril 2269

Thiothixene (May increase drowsiness effect). Products include:
Navane Capsules and Concentrate 2201
Navane Intramuscular 2202

Tranylcypromine Sulfate (Concurrent and/or sequential use is not recommended). Products include:
Parnate Tablets 2503

Triazolam (May increase drowsiness effect). Products include:
Halcion Tablets 2611

Trifluoperazine Hydrochloride (May increase drowsiness effect). Products include:
Stelazine 2514

Zolpidem Tartrate (May increase drowsiness effect). Products include:
Ambien Tablets 2416

Food Interactions

Alcohol (May increase drowsiness effect.).

THERAFLU FLU, COLD AND COUGH MEDICINE

(Acetaminophen, Pseudoephedrine Hydrochloride, Chlorpheniramine Maleate, Dextromethorphan Hydrobromide) .... ◘ 787
See **TheraFlu Flu and Cold Medicine**

THERAFLU MAXIMUM STRENGTH NIGHTTIME FLU, COLD & COUGH MEDICINE

(Acetaminophen, Dextromethorphan Hydrobromide, Pseudoephedrine Hydrochloride, Chlorpheniramine Maleate) .... ◘ 788
May interact with hypnotics and sedatives, tranquilizers, monoamine oxidase inhibitors, and certain other agents. Compounds in these categories include:

Alprazolam (May increase drowsiness effect). Products include:
Xanax Tablets 2649

Buspirone Hydrochloride (May increase drowsiness effect). Products include:
BuSpar 737

Chlordiazepoxide (May increase drowsiness effect). Products include:
Libritabs Tablets 2177
Limbitrol 2180

Chlordiazepoxide Hydrochloride (May increase drowsiness effect). Products include:
Librax Capsules 2176
Librium Capsules 2178
Librium Injectable 2179

Chlorpromazine (May increase drowsiness effect). Products include:
Thorazine Suppositories 2523

Chlorpromazine Hydrochloride (May increase drowsiness effect). Products include:
Thorazine 2523

Chlorprothixene (May increase drowsiness effect).
No products indexed under this heading.

Chlorprothixene Hydrochloride (May increase drowsiness effect).
No products indexed under this heading.

Clorazepate Dipotassium (May increase drowsiness effect). Products include:
Tranxene 451

Diazepam (May increase drowsiness effect). Products include:
Dizac 1809
Valium Injectable 2182
Valium Tablets 2183
Valrelease Capsules 2169

Droperidol (May increase drowsiness effect). Products include:
Inapsine Injection 1296

Estazolam (May increase drowsiness effect). Products include:
ProSom Tablets 449

Ethchlorvynol (May increase drowsiness effect). Products include:
Placidyl Capsules 448

Ethinamate (May increase drowsiness effect).
No products indexed under this heading.

Fluphenazine Decanoate (May increase drowsiness effect). Products include:
Prolixin Decanoate 509

Fluphenazine Enanthate (May increase drowsiness effect). Products include:
Prolixin Enanthate 509

Fluphenazine Hydrochloride (May increase drowsiness effect). Products include:
Prolixin 509

Flurazepam Hydrochloride (May increase drowsiness effect). Products include:
Dalmane Capsules 2173

Furazolidone (Concurrent and/or sequential use is not recommended). Products include:
Furoxone 2046

Glutethimide (May increase drowsiness effect).
No products indexed under this heading.

Haloperidol (May increase drowsiness effect). Products include:
Haldol Injection, Tablets and Concentrate 1575

Haloperidol Decanoate (May increase drowsiness effect). Products include:
Haldol Decanoate 1577

Hydroxyzine Hydrochloride (May increase drowsiness effect). Products include:
Atarax Tablets & Syrup 2185
Marax Tablets & DF Syrup 2200
Vistaril Intramuscular Solution 2216

Isocarboxazid (Concurrent and/or sequential use is not recommended).
No products indexed under this heading.

Lorazepam (May increase drowsiness effect). Products include:
Ativan Injection 2698
Ativan Tablets 2700

Loxapine Hydrochloride (May increase drowsiness effect). Products include:
Loxitane 1378

Loxapine Succinate (May increase drowsiness effect). Products include:
Loxitane Capsules 1378

Meprobamate (May increase drowsiness effect). Products include:
Miltown Tablets 2672
PMB 200 and PMB 400 2783

Mesoridazine Besylate (May increase drowsiness effect). Products include:
Serentil 684

Midazolam Hydrochloride (May increase drowsiness effect). Products include:
Versed Injection 2170

Molindone Hydrochloride (May increase drowsiness effect). Products include:
Moban Tablets and Concentrate 1048

Oxazepam (May increase drowsiness effect). Products include:
Serax Capsules 2810
Serax Tablets 2810

Perphenazine (May increase drowsiness effect). Products include:
Etrafon 2355
Triavil Tablets 1757
Trilafon 2389

Phenelzine Sulfate (Concurrent and/or sequential use is not recommended). Products include:
Nardil 1920

Prazepam (May increase drowsiness effect).
No products indexed under this heading.

Prochlorperazine (May increase drowsiness effect). Products include:
Compazine 2470

Promethazine Hydrochloride (May increase drowsiness effect). Products include:
Mepergan Injection 2753
Phenergan with Codeine 2777
Phenergan with Dextromethorphan 2778
Phenergan Injection 2773
Phenergan Suppositories 2775
Phenergan Syrup 2774
Phenergan Tablets 2775
Phenergan VC 2779
Phenergan VC with Codeine 2781

Propofol (May increase drowsiness effect). Products include:
Diprivan Injection 2833

Quazepam (May increase drowsiness effect). Products include:
Doral Tablets 2664

Secobarbital Sodium (May increase drowsiness effect). Products include:
Seconal Sodium Pulvules 1474

Selegiline Hydrochloride (Concurrent and/or sequential use is not recommended). Products include:
Eldepryl Tablets 2550

Temazepam (May increase drowsiness effect). Products include:
Restoril Capsules 2284

Thioridazine Hydrochloride (May increase drowsiness effect). Products include:
Mellaril 2269

Thiothixene (May increase drowsiness effect). Products include:
Navane Capsules and Concentrate 2201
Navane Intramuscular 2202

Tranylcypromine Sulfate (Concurrent and/or sequential use is not recommended). Products include:
Parnate Tablets 2503

Triazolam (May increase drowsiness effect). Products include:
Halcion Tablets 2611

Trifluoperazine Hydrochloride (May increase drowsiness effect). Products include:
Stelazine 2514

Zolpidem Tartrate (May increase drowsiness effect). Products include:
Ambien Tablets 2416

Food Interactions

Alcohol (May increase drowsiness effect.).

THERAFLU MAXIMUM STRENGTH NON-DROWSY FORMULA FLU, COLD & COUGH MEDICINE

(Acetaminophen, Dextromethorphan Hydrobromide, Pseudoephedrine Hydrochloride) .... ◘ 788
May interact with monoamine oxidase inhibitors. Compounds in this category include:

Furazolidone (Concurrent and/or sequential use is not recommended). Products include:
Furoxone 2046

Isocarboxazid (Concurrent and/or sequential use is not recommended).
No products indexed under this heading.

Phenelzine Sulfate (Concurrent and/or sequential use is not recommended). Products include:
Nardil 1920

Selegiline Hydrochloride (Concurrent and/or sequential use is not recommended). Products include:
Eldepryl Tablets 2550

Tranylcypromine Sulfate (Concurrent and/or sequential use is not recommended). Products include:
Parnate Tablets 2503

THERA FLU MAXIMUM STRENGTH, NON-DROWSY FORMULA FLU, COLD AND COUGH CAPLETS

(Acetaminophen, Dextromethorphan Hydrobromide, Pseudoephedrine Hydrochloride) .... ◘ 789
May interact with monoamine oxidase inhibitors. Compounds in this category include:

Furazolidone (Concurrent use not recommended; consult your doctor). Products include:
Furoxone 2046

Isocarboxazid (Concurrent use not recommended; consult your doctor).
No products indexed under this heading.

Phenelzine Sulfate (Concurrent use not recommended; consult your doctor). Products include:
Nardil 1920

Selegiline Hydrochloride (Concurrent use not recommended; consult your doctor). Products include:
Eldepryl Tablets 2550

Tranylcypromine Sulfate (Concurrent use not recommended; consult your doctor). Products include:
Parnate Tablets 2503

THERA-GESIC

(Methyl Salicylate, Menthol) 1781
None cited in PDR database.

THERAGRAN ANTIOXIDANT

(Vitamins with Minerals) .... ◘ 623
None cited in PDR database.

THERAGRAN TABLETS

(Vitamin B Complex With Vitamin C, Vitamins with Minerals) .... ◘ 623
None cited in PDR database.

THERAGRAN-M TABLETS WITH BETA CAROTENE

(Beta Carotene, Vitamin B Complex With Vitamin C, Vitamins with Minerals) .... ◘ 623
None cited in PDR database.

THERAMYCIN Z TOPICAL SOLUTION 2%

(Erythromycin) 1592
None cited in PDR database.

(◘ Described in PDR For Nonprescription Drugs) (⊙ Described in PDR For Ophthalmology)

1027 **Interactions Index** **Thorazine**

THERAPEUTIC MINERAL ICE, PAIN RELIEVING GEL
(Menthol) 623
None cited in PDR database.

THIOGUANINE TABLETS, TABLOID BRAND
(Thioguanine) 1181
May interact with cytotoxic drugs and certain other agents. Compounds in these categories include:

Bleomycin Sulfate (Combination therapy may produce hepatic disease). Products include:
Blenoxane 692

Busulfan (Potential for esophageal varices associated with abnormal liver function tests). Products include:
Myleran Tablets 1143

Daunorubicin Hydrochloride (Combination therapy may produce hepatic disease). Products include:
Cerubidine 795

Doxorubicin Hydrochloride (Combination therapy may produce hepatic disease). Products include:
Adriamycin PFS 1947
Adriamycin RDF 1947
Doxorubicin Astra 540
Rubex 712

Fluorouracil (Combination therapy may produce hepatic disease). Products include:
Efudex 2113
Fluoroplex Topical Solution & Cream 1% 479
Fluorouracil Injection 2116

Hydroxyurea (Combination therapy may produce hepatic disease). Products include:
Hydrea Capsules 696

Mercaptopurine (Complete cross-resistance). Products include:
Purinethol Tablets 1156

Methotrexate Sodium (Combination therapy may produce hepatic disease). Products include:
Methotrexate Sodium Tablets, Injection, for Injection and LPF Injection 1275

Mitotane (Combination therapy may produce hepatic disease). Products include:
Lysodren 698

Mitoxantrone Hydrochloride (Combination therapy may produce hepatic disease). Products include:
Novantrone 1279

Procarbazine Hydrochloride (Combination therapy may produce hepatic disease). Products include:
Matulane Capsules 2131

Tamoxifen Citrate (Combination therapy may produce hepatic disease). Products include:
Nolvadex Tablets 2841

Vincristine Sulfate (Combination therapy may produce hepatic disease). Products include:
Oncovin Solution Vials & Hyporets 1466

THIOPLEX (THIOTEPA FOR INJECTION)
(Thiotepa) 1281
May interact with nitrogen-mustard-type alkylating agents and certain other agents. Compounds in these categories include:

Bone Marrow Depressants, unspecified (Avoid concurrent use).

Chlorambucil (Intensified toxicity). Products include:
Leukeran Tablets 1133

Cyclophosphamide (Intensified toxicity). Products include:
Cytoxan 694
NEOSAR Lyophilized/Neosar 1959

Estramustine Phosphate Sodium (Intensified toxicity). Products include:
Emcyt Capsules 1953

Mechlorethamine Hydrochloride (Intensified toxicity). Products include:
Mustargen 1709

Melphalan (Intensified toxicity). Products include:
Alkeran Tablets 1071

Succinylcholine Chloride (Prolonged apnea after succinylcholine administration to patients receiving thiotepa and other cancer drugs). Products include:
Anectine 1073

THORAZINE AMPULS
(Chlorpromazine Hydrochloride) 2523
See **Thorazine Concentrate**

THORAZINE CONCENTRATE
(Chlorpromazine Hydrochloride) 2523
May interact with central nervous system depressants, oral anticoagulants, anticonvulsants, thiazides, and certain other agents. Compounds in these categories include:

Alfentanil Hydrochloride (Prolonged and intensified action of CNS depressants). Products include:
Alfenta Injection 1286

Alprazolam (Prolonged and intensified action of CNS depressants). Products include:
Xanax Tablets 2649

Aprobarbital (Prolonged and intensified action of CNS depressants).
No products indexed under this heading.

Atropine Nitrate, Methyl (Use with caution).
No products indexed under this heading.

Atropine Sulfate (Use with caution). Products include:
Arco-Lase Plus Tablets 512
Atrohist Plus Tablets 454
Atropine Sulfate Sterile Ophthalmic Solution .... ◉ 233
Donnatal 2060
Donnatal Extentabs 2061
Donnatal Tablets 2060
Lomotil 2439
Motofen Tablets 784
Urised Tablets 1964

Bendroflumethiazide (Orthostatic hypotension that may occur with chlorpromazine may be accentuated).
No products indexed under this heading.

Buprenorphine (Prolonged and intensified action of CNS depressants). Products include:
Buprenex Injectable 2006

Buspirone Hydrochloride (Prolonged and intensified action of CNS depressants). Products include:
BuSpar 737

Butabarbital (Prolonged and intensified action of CNS depressants).
No products indexed under this heading.

Butalbital (Prolonged and intensified action of CNS depressants). Products include:
Esgic-plus Tablets 1013
Fioricet Tablets 2258
Fioricet with Codeine Capsules 2260
Fiorinal Capsules 2261
Fiorinal with Codeine Capsules 2262
Fiorinal Tablets 2261
Phrenilin 785
Sedapap Tablets 50 mg/650 mg .. 1543

Carbamazepine (Chlorpromazine may lower convulsive threshold; dosage adjustments of anticonvulsants may be necessary). Products include:
Atretol Tablets 573
Tegretol Chewable Tablets 852
Tegretol Suspension 852
Tegretol Tablets 852

Carmustine (BCNU) (Antiemetic action of chlorpromazine may obscure vomiting as a sign of toxicity). Products include:
BiCNU 691

Chlordiazepoxide (Prolonged and intensified action of CNS depressants). Products include:
Libritabs Tablets 2177
Limbitrol 2180

Chlordiazepoxide Hydrochloride (Prolonged and intensified action of CNS depressants). Products include:
Librax Capsules 2176
Librium Capsules 2178
Librium Injectable 2179

Chlorothiazide (Orthostatic hypotension that may occur with chlorpromazine may be accentuated). Products include:
Aldoclor Tablets 1598
Diupres Tablets 1650
Diuril Oral 1653

Chlorothiazide Sodium (Orthostatic hypotension that may occur with chlorpromazine may be accentuated). Products include:
Diuril Sodium Intravenous 1652

Chlorpromazine (Prolonged and intensified action of CNS depressants). Products include:
Thorazine Suppositories 2523

Chlorprothixene (Prolonged and intensified action of CNS depressants).
No products indexed under this heading.

Chlorprothixene Hydrochloride (Prolonged and intensified action of CNS depressants).
No products indexed under this heading.

Clorazepate Dipotassium (Prolonged and intensified action of CNS depressants). Products include:
Tranxene 451

Clozapine (Prolonged and intensified action of CNS depressants). Products include:
Clozaril Tablets 2252

Codeine Phosphate (Prolonged and intensified action of CNS depressants). Products include:
Actifed with Codeine Cough Syrup.. 1067
Brontex 1981
Deconsal C Expectorant Syrup 456
Deconsal Pediatric Syrup 457
Dimetane-DC Cough Syrup 2059
Empirin with Codeine Tablets 1093
Fioricet with Codeine Capsules 2260
Fiorinal with Codeine Capsules 2262
Isoclor Expectorant 990
Novahistine DH 2462
Novahistine Expectorant 2463
Nucofed 2051
Phenergan with Codeine 2777
Phenergan VC with Codeine 2781
Robitussin A-C Syrup 2073
Robitussin-DAC Syrup 2074
Ryna 841
Soma Compound w/Codeine Tablets 2676
Tussi-Organidin NR Liquid and S NR Liquid 2677
Tylenol with Codeine 1583

Desflurane (Prolonged and intensified action of CNS depressants). Products include:
Suprane 1813

Dezocine (Prolonged and intensified action of CNS depressants). Products include:
Dalgan Injection 538

Diazepam (Prolonged and intensified action of CNS depressants). Products include:
Dizac 1809
Valium Injectable 2182
Valium Tablets 2183
Valrelease Capsules 2169

Dicumarol (Effects diminished).
No products indexed under this heading.

Divalproex Sodium (Chlorpromazine may lower convulsive threshold; dosage adjustments of anticonvulsants may be necessary). Products include:
Depakote Tablets 415

Droperidol (Prolonged and intensified action of CNS depressants). Products include:
Inapsine Injection 1296

Enflurane (Prolonged and intensified action of CNS depressants).
No products indexed under this heading.

Estazolam (Prolonged and intensified action of CNS depressants). Products include:
ProSom Tablets 449

Estramustine Phosphate Sodium (Antiemetic action of chlorpromazine may obscure vomiting as a sign of toxicity). Products include:
Emcyt Capsules 1953

Ethchlorvynol (Prolonged and intensified action of CNS depressants). Products include:
Placidyl Capsules 448

Ethinamate (Prolonged and intensified action of CNS depressants).
No products indexed under this heading.

Ethosuximide (Chlorpromazine may lower convulsive threshold; dosage adjustments of anticonvulsants may be necessary). Products include:
Zarontin Capsules 1928
Zarontin Syrup 1929

Ethotoin (Chlorpromazine may lower convulsive threshold; dosage adjustments of anticonvulsants may be necessary). Products include:
Peganone Tablets 446

Felbamate (Chlorpromazine may lower convulsive threshold; dosage adjustments of anticonvulsants may be necessary). Products include:
Felbatol 2666

Fentanyl (Prolonged and intensified action of CNS depressants). Products include:
Duragesic Transdermal System 1288

Fentanyl Citrate (Prolonged and intensified action of CNS depressants). Products include:
Sublimaze Injection 1307

Fluphenazine Decanoate (Prolonged and intensified action of CNS depressants). Products include:
Prolixin Decanoate 509

Fluphenazine Enanthate (Prolonged and intesnified action of CNS depressants). Products include:
Prolixin Enanthate 509

Fluphenazine Hydrochloride (Prolonged and intensified action of CNS depressants). Products include:
Prolixin 509

Flurazepam Hydrochloride (Prolonged and intensified action of CNS depressants). Products include:
Dalmane Capsules 2173

IMPORTANT NOTE: Always consult each drug listing in the patient's regimen for possible interactions.

Thorazine Interactions Index 1028

Glutethimide (Prolonged and intensified action of CNS depressants).
No products indexed under this heading.

Guanethidine Monosulfate (Antihypertensive effect of guanethidine and related compounds may be counteracted). Products include:
Esimil Tablets 822
Ismelin Tablets 827

Haloperidol (Prolonged and intensified action of CNS depressants). Products include:
Haldol Injection, Tablets and Concentrate 1575

Haloperidol Decanoate (Prolonged and intensified action of CNS depressants). Products include:
Haldol Decanoate 1577

Hydrochlorothiazide (Orthostatic hypotension that may occur with chlorpromazine may be accentuated). Products include:
Aldactazide 2413
Aldoril Tablets 1604
Apresazide Capsules 808
Capozide 742
Dyazide 2479
Esidrix Tablets 821
Esimil Tablets 822
HydroDIURIL Tablets 1674
Hydropres Tablets 1675
Hyzaar Tablets 1677
Inderide Tablets 2732
Inderide LA Long Acting Capsules 2734
Lopressor HCT Tablets 832
Lotensin HCT 837
Maxzide 1380
Moduretic Tablets 1705
Oretic Tablets 443
Prinzide Tablets 1737
Ser-Ap-Es Tablets 849
Timolide Tablets 1748
Vaseretic Tablets 1765
Zestoretic 2850
Ziac 1415

Hydrocodone Bitartrate (Prolonged and intensified action of CNS depressants). Products include:
Anexsia 5/500 Elixir 1781
Anexia Tablets 1782
Codiclear DH Syrup 791
Deconamine CX Cough and Cold Liquid and Tablets 1319
Duratuss HD Elixir 2565
Hycodan Tablets and Syrup 930
Hycomine Compound Tablets 932
Hycomine 931
Hycotuss Expectorant Syrup 933
Hydrocet Capsules 782
Lorcet 10/650 1018
Lortab 2566
Tussend 1783
Tussend Expectorant 1785
Vicodin Tablets 1356
Vicodin ES Tablets 1357
Vicodin Tuss Expectorant 1358
Zydone Capsules 949

Hydrocodone Polistirex (Prolonged and intensified action of CNS depressants). Products include:
Tussionex Pennkinetic Extended-Release Suspension 998

Hydroflumethiazide (Orthostatic hypotension that may occur with chlorpromazine may be accentuated). Products include:
Diucardin Tablets 2718

Hydroxyurea (Antiemetic action of chlorpromazine may obscure vomiting as a sign of toxicity). Products include:
Hydrea Capsules 696

Hydroxyzine Hydrochloride (Prolonged and intensified action of CNS depressants). Products include:
Atarax Tablets & Syrup 2185
Marax Tablets & DF Syrup 2200
Vistaril Intramuscular Solution 2216

Isoflurane (Prolonged and intensified action of CNS depressants).
No products indexed under this heading.

Ketamine Hydrochloride (Prolonged and intensified action of CNS depressants).
No products indexed under this heading.

Lamotrigine (Chlorpromazine may lower convulsive threshold; dosage adjustments of anticonvulsants may be necessary). Products include:
Lamictal Tablets 1112

Levomethadyl Acetate Hydrochloride (Prolonged and intensified action of CNS depressants). Products include:
Orlamm 2239

Levorphanol Tartrate (Prolonged and intensified action of CNS depressants). Products include:
Levo-Dromoran 2129

Lorazepam (Prolonged and intensified action of CNS depressants). Products include:
Ativan Injection 2698
Ativan Tablets 2700

Loxapine Hydrochloride (Prolonged and intensified action of CNS depressants). Products include:
Loxitane 1378

Loxapine Succinate (Prolonged and intensified action of CNS depressants). Products include:
Loxitane Capsules 1378

Mechlorethamine Hydrochloride (Antiemetic action of chlorpromazine may obscure vomiting as a sign of toxicity). Products include:
Mustargen 1709

Melphalan (Antiemetic action of chlorpromazine may obscure vomiting as a sign of toxicity). Products include:
Alkeran Tablets 1071

Meperidine Hydrochloride (Prolonged and intensified action of CNS depressants). Products include:
Demerol 2308
Mepergan Injection 2753

Mephenytoin (Chlorpromazine may lower convulsive threshold; dosage adjustments of anticonvulsants may be necessary). Products include:
Mesantoin Tablets 2272

Mephobarbital (Prolonged and intensified action of CNS depressants). Products include:
Mebaral Tablets 2322

Meprobamate (Prolonged and intensified action of CNS depressants). Products include:
Miltown Tablets 2672
PMB 200 and PMB 400 2783

Mesoridazine Besylate (Prolonged and intensified action of CNS depressants). Products include:
Serentil 684

Methadone Hydrochloride (Prolonged and intensified action of CNS depressants). Products include:
Methadone Hydrochloride Oral Concentrate 2233
Methadone Hydrochloride Oral Solution & Tablets 2235

Methohexital Sodium (Prolonged and intensified action of CNS depressants). Products include:
Brevital Sodium Vials 1429

Methotrimeprazine (Prolonged and intensified action of CNS depressants). Products include:
Levoprome 1274

Methoxyflurane (Prolonged and intensified action of CNS depressants).
No products indexed under this heading.

Methsuximide (Chlorpromazine may lower convulsive threshold; dosage adjustments of anticonvulsants may be necessary). Products include:
Celontin Kapseals 1899

Methyclothiazide (Orthostatic hypotension that may occur with chlorpromazine may be accentuated). Products include:
Enduron Tablets 420

Metrizamide (Chlorpromazine may lower convulsive threshold; avoid concurrent use).

Midazolam Hydrochloride (Prolonged and intensified action of CNS depressants). Products include:
Versed Injection 2170

Molindone Hydrochloride (Prolonged and intensified action of CNS depressants). Products include:
Moban Tablets and Concentrate 1048

Morphine Sulfate (Prolonged and intensified action of CNS depressants). Products include:
Astramorph/PF Injection, USP (Preservative-Free) 535
Duramorph 962
Infumorph 200 and Infumorph 500 Sterile Solutions 965
MS Contin Tablets 1994
MSIR 1997
Oramorph SR (Morphine Sulfate Sustained Release Tablets) 2236
RMS Suppositories 2657
Roxanol 2243

Opium Alkaloids (Prolonged and intensified action of CNS depressants).
No products indexed under this heading.

Oxazepam (Prolonged and intensified action of CNS depressants). Products include:
Serax Capsules 2810
Serax Tablets 2810

Oxycodone Hydrochloride (Prolonged and intensified action of CNS depressants). Products include:
Percocet Tablets 938
Percodan Tablets 939
Percodan-Demi Tablets 940
Roxicodone Tablets, Oral Solution & Intensol (Oxycodone) 2244
Tylox Capsules 1584

Paramethadione (Chlorpromazine may lower convulsive threshold; dosage adjustments of anticonvulsants may be necessary).
No products indexed under this heading.

Pentobarbital Sodium (Prolonged and intensified action of CNS depressants). Products include:
Nembutal Sodium Capsules 436
Nembutal Sodium Solution 438
Nembutal Sodium Suppositories 440

Perphenazine (Prolonged and intensified action of CNS depressants). Products include:
Etrafon 2355
Triavil Tablets 1757
Trilafon 2389

Phenacemide (Chlorpromazine may lower convulsive threshold; dosage adjustments of anticonvulsants may be necessary). Products include:
Phenurone Tablets 447

Phenobarbital (Chlorpromazine may lower convulsive threshold and does not potentiate anticonvulsant action of barbiturates). Products include:
Arco-Lase Plus Tablets 512
Bellergal-S Tablets 2250
Donnatal 2060
Donnatal Extentabs 2061
Donnatal Tablets 2060
Phenobarbital Elixir and Tablets 1469
Quadrinal Tablets 1350

Phensuximide (Chlorpromazine may lower convulsive threshold; dosage adjustments of anticonvulsants may be necessary). Products include:
Milontin Kapseals 1920

Phenytoin (Phenytoin toxicity may be precipitated). Products include:
Dilantin Infatabs 1908
Dilantin-125 Suspension 1911

Phenytoin Sodium (Phenytoin toxicity may be precipitated). Products include:
Dilantin Kapseals 1906
Dilantin Parenteral 1910

Polythiazide (Orthostatic hypotension that may occur with chlorpromazine may be accentuated). Products include:
Minizide Capsules 1938

Prazepam (Prolonged and intensified action of CNS depressants).
No products indexed under this heading.

Primidone (Chlorpromazine may lower convulsive threshold; dosage adjustments of anticonvulsants may be necessary). Products include:
Mysoline 2754

Prochlorperazine (Prolonged and intensified action of CNS depressants). Products include:
Compazine 2470

Promethazine Hydrochloride (Prolonged and intensified action of CNS depressants). Products include:
Mepergan Injection 2753
Phenergan with Codeine 2777
Phenergan with Dextromethorphan 2778
Phenergan Injection 2773
Phenergan Suppositories 2775
Phenergan Syrup 2774
Phenergan Tablets 2775
Phenergan VC 2779
Phenergan VC with Codeine 2781

Propofol (Prolonged and intensified action of CNS depressants). Products include:
Diprivan Injection 2833

Propoxyphene Hydrochloride (Prolonged and intensified action of CNS depressants). Products include:
Darvon 1435
Wygesic Tablets 2827

Propoxyphene Napsylate (Prolonged and intensified action of CNS depressants). Products include:
Darvon-N/Darvocet-N 1433

Propranolol Hydrochloride (Concomitant administration results in increased plasma levels of both drugs). Products include:
Inderal 2728
Inderal LA Long Acting Capsules 2730
Inderide Tablets 2732
Inderide LA Long Acting Capsules 2734

Risperidone (Prolonged and intensified action of CNS depressants). Products include:
Risperdal 1301

Secobarbital Sodium (Prolonged and intensified action of CNS depressants). Products include:
Seconal Sodium Pulvules 1474

Sufentanil Citrate (Prolonged and intensified action of CNS depressants). Products include:
Sufenta Injection 1309

Temazepam (Prolonged and intensified action of CNS depressants). Products include:
Restoril Capsules 2284

Thiamylal Sodium (Prolonged and intensified action of CNS depressants).
No products indexed under this heading.

(Described in PDR For Nonprescription Drugs) (Described in PDR For Ophthalmology)

1029 Interactions Index THYREL TRH

Thioridazine Hydrochloride (Prolonged and intensified action of CNS depressants). Products include:
Mellaril ... 2269
Thiothixene (Prolonged and intensified action of CNS depressants). Products include:
Navane Capsules and Concentrate 2201
Navane Intramuscular ... 2202
Triazolam (Prolonged and intensified action of CNS depressants). Products include:
Halcion Tablets ... 2611
Trifluoperazine Hydrochloride (Prolonged and intensified action of CNS depressants). Products include:
Stelazine ... 2514
Trimethadione (Chlorpromazine may lower convulsive threshold; dosage adjustments of anticonvulsants may be necessary).
No products indexed under this heading.
Valproic Acid (Chlorpromazine may lower convulsive threshold; dosage adjustments of anticonvulsants may be necessary). Products include:
Depakene ... 413
Warfarin Sodium (Effect of oral anticoagulants diminished). Products include:
Coumadin ... 926
Zolpidem Tartrate (Prolonged and intensified action of CNS depressants). Products include:
Ambien Tablets ... 2416

THORAZINE MULTI-DOSE VIALS
(Chlorpromazine Hydrochloride) ... 2523
See **Thorazine Concentrate**

THORAZINE SPANSULE CAPSULES
(Chlorpromazine Hydrochloride) ... 2523
See **Thorazine Concentrate**

THORAZINE SUPPOSITORIES
(Chlorpromazine) ... 2523
See **Thorazine Concentrate**

THORAZINE SYRUP
(Chlorpromazine Hydrochloride) ... 2523
See **Thorazine Concentrate**

THORAZINE TABLETS
(Chlorpromazine Hydrochloride) ... 2523
See **Thorazine Concentrate**

THROMBATE III ANTITHROMBIN III (HUMAN)
(Antithrombin III) ... 637
May interact with:

Heparin Calcium (The anticoagulant effect of heparin is enhanced by concurrent treatment with antithrombin III; reduced dosage of heparin may be required).
No products indexed under this heading.
Heparin Sodium (The anticoagulant effect of heparin is enhanced by concurrent treatment with antithrombin III; reduced dosage of heparin may be required). Products include:
Heparin Lock Flush Solution ... 2725
Heparin Sodium Injection ... 2726
Heparin Sodium Injection, USP, Sterile Solution ... 2615
Heparin Sodium Vials ... 1441

THROMBOGEN* TOPICAL THROMBIN, USP WITH DILUENT AND TRANSFER NEEDLE
(Thrombin) ... 1315
None cited in PDR database.

THROMBOGEN* TOPICAL THROMBIN, USP, SPRAY KIT
(Thrombin) ... 1315
None cited in PDR database.

THYREL TRH
(Protirelin) ... 2873
May interact with thyroid preparations, glucocorticoids, and certain other agents. Compounds in these categories include:

Aspirin (Inhibits the TSH response to protirelin when aspirin is given at 2 to 3 g/day). Products include:
Alka-Seltzer Effervescent Antacid and Pain Reliever ... ◙ 701
Alka-Seltzer Extra Strength Effervescent Antacid and Pain Reliever ... ◙ 703
Alka-Seltzer Lemon Lime Effervescent Antacid and Pain Reliever ... ◙ 703
Alka-Seltzer Plus Cold Medicine ... ◙ 705
Alka-Seltzer Plus Cold & Cough Medicine ... ◙ 708
Alka-Seltzer Plus Night-Time Cold Medicine ... ◙ 707
Alka Seltzer Plus Sinus Medicine ... ◙ 707
Arthritis Foundation Safety Coated Aspirin Tablets ... ◙ 675
Arthritis Pain Ascriptin ... ◙ 631
Maximum Strength Ascriptin ... ◙ 630
Regular Strength Ascriptin Tablets ... ◙ 629
Arthritis Strength BC Powder ... ◙ 609
BC Cold Powder Multi-Symptom Formula (Cold-Sinus-Allergy) ... ◙ 609
BC Cold Powder Non-Drowsy Formula (Cold-Sinus) ... ◙ 609
BC Powder ... ◙ 609
Bayer Children's Chewable Aspirin ... ◙ 711
Genuine Bayer Aspirin Tablets & Caplets ... ◙ 713
Extra Strength Bayer Arthritis Pain Regimen Formula ... ◙ 711
Extra Strength Bayer Aspirin Caplets & Tablets ... ◙ 712
Extended-Release Bayer 8-Hour Aspirin ... ◙ 712
Extra Strength Bayer Plus Aspirin Caplets ... ◙ 713
Extra Strength Bayer PM Aspirin ... ◙ 713
Bayer Enteric Aspirin ... ◙ 709
Bufferin Analgesic Tablets and Caplets ... ◙ 613
Arthritis Strength Bufferin Analgesic Caplets ... ◙ 614
Extra Strength Bufferin Analgesic Tablets ... ◙ 615
Cama Arthritis Pain Reliever ... ◙ 785
Darvon Compound-65 Pulvules ... 1435
Easprin ... 1914
Ecotrin ... 2455
Ecotrin Enteric Coated Aspirin Maximum Strength Tablets and Caplets ... ◙ 816
Ecotrin Enteric Coated Aspirin Regular Strength Tablets ... 2455
Empirin Aspirin Tablets ... ◙ 854
Empirin with Codeine Tablets ... 1093
Excedrin Extra-Strength Analgesic Tablets & Caplets ... 732
Fiorinal Capsules ... 2261
Fiorinal with Codeine Capsules ... 2262
Fiorinal Tablets ... 2261
Halfprin ... 1362
Healthprin Aspirin ... 2455
Norgesic ... 1496
Percodan Tablets ... 939
Percodan-Demi Tablets ... 940
Robaxisal Tablets ... 2071
Soma Compound w/Codeine Tablets ... 2676
Soma Compound Tablets ... 2675
St. Joseph Adult Chewable Aspirin (81 mg.) ... ◙ 808
Talwin Compound ... 2335
Ursinus Inlay-Tabs ... ◙ 794
Vanquish Analgesic Caplets ... ◙ 731
Betamethasone Acetate (Pharmacologic doses of steroids reduce the TSH response). Products include:
Celestone Soluspan Suspension ... 2347
Betamethasone Sodium Phosphate (Pharmacologic doses of steroids reduce the TSH response). Products include:
Celestone Soluspan Suspension ... 2347
Cortisone Acetate (Pharmacologic doses of steroids reduce the TSH response). Products include:
Cortone Acetate Sterile Suspension ... 1623
Cortone Acetate Tablets ... 1624
Dexamethasone (Pharmacologic doses of steroids reduce the TSH response). Products include:
AK-Trol Ointment & Suspension ... ⊙ 205
Decadron Elixir ... 1633
Decadron Tablets ... 1635
Decaspray Topical Aerosol ... 1648
Dexacidin Ointment ... ⊙ 263
Maxitrol Ophthalmic Ointment and Suspension ... ⊙ 224
TobraDex Ophthalmic Suspension and Ointment ... 473
Dexamethasone Acetate (Pharmacologic doses of steroids reduce the TSH response). Products include:
Dalalone D.P. Injectable ... 1011
Decadron-LA Sterile Suspension ... 1646
Dexamethasone Sodium Phosphate (Pharmacologic doses of steroids reduce the TSH response). Products include:
Decadron Phosphate Injection ... 1637
Decadron Phosphate Respihaler ... 1642
Decadron Phosphate Sterile Ophthalmic Ointment ... 1641
Decadron Phosphate Sterile Ophthalmic Solution ... 1642
Decadron Phosphate Topical Cream ... 1644
Decadron Phosphate Turbinaire ... 1645
Decadron Phosphate with Xylocaine Injection, Sterile ... 1639
Dexacort Phosphate in Respihaler ... 458
Dexacort Phosphate in Turbinaire ... 459
NeoDecadron Sterile Ophthalmic Ointment ... 1712
NeoDecadron Sterile Ophthalmic Solution ... 1713
NeoDecadron Topical Cream ... 1714
Fludrocortisone Acetate (Pharmacologic doses of steroids reduce the TSH response). Products include:
Florinef Acetate Tablets ... 505
Hydrocortisone (Pharmacologic doses of steroids reduce the TSH response). Products include:
Anusol-HC Cream 2.5% ... 1896
Aquanil HC Lotion ... 1931
Bactine Hydrocortisone Anti-Itch Cream ... ◙ 709
Caldecort Anti-Itch Hydrocortisone Spray ... ◙ 631
Cortaid ... ◙ 836
CORTENEMA ... 2535
Cortisporin Ointment ... 1085
Cortisporin Ophthalmic Ointment Sterile ... 1085
Cortisporin Ophthalmic Suspension Sterile ... 1086
Cortisporin Otic Solution Sterile ... 1087
Cortisporin Otic Suspension Sterile 1088
Cortizone-5 ... ◙ 831
Cortizone-10 ... ◙ 831
Hydrocortone Tablets ... 1672
Hytone ... 907
Massengill Medicated Soft Cloth Towelettes ... 2458
PediOtic Suspension Sterile ... 1153
Preparation H Hydrocortisone 1% Cream ... ◙ 872
ProctoCream-HC 2.5% ... 2408
VōSoL HC Otic Solution ... 2678
Hydrocortisone Acetate (Pharmacologic doses of steroids reduce the TSH response). Products include:
Analpram-HC Rectal Cream 1% and 2.5% ... 977
Anusol HC-1 Anti-Itch Hydrocortisone Ointment ... ◙ 847
Anusol-HC Suppositories ... 1897
Caldecort ... ◙ 631
Carmol HC ... 924
Coly-Mycin S Otic w/Neomycin & Hydrocortisone ... 1906
Cortaid ... ◙ 836
Cortifoam ... 2396
Cortisporin Cream ... 1084
Epifoam ... 2399
Hydrocortone Acetate Sterile Suspension ... 1669
Mantadil Cream ... 1135
Nupercainal Hydrocortisone 1% Cream ... ◙ 645
Ophthocort ... ⊙ 311
Pramosone Cream, Lotion & Ointment ... 978
ProctoCream-HC ... 2408
ProctoFoam-HC ... 2409
Terra-Cortril Ophthalmic Suspension ... 2210
Hydrocortisone Sodium Phosphate (Pharmacologic doses of steroids reduce the TSH response). Products include:
Hydrocortone Phosphate Injection, Sterile ... 1670
Hydrocortisone Sodium Succinate (Pharmacologic doses of steroids reduce the TSH response). Products include:
Solu-Cortef Sterile Powder ... 2641
Levodopa (Chronic administration of levodopa inhibits the TSH response). Products include:
Atamet ... 572
Larodopa Tablets ... 2129
Sinemet Tablets ... 943
Sinemet CR Tablets ... 944
Levothyroxine Sodium (Thyroid hormones reduce the TSH response). Products include:
Levothroid Tablets ... 1016
Levoxyl Tablets ... 903
Synthroid ... 1359
Liothyronine Sodium (Thyroid hormones reduce the TSH response). Products include:
Cytomel Tablets ... 2473
Triostat Injection ... 2530
Liotrix (Thyroid hormones reduce the TSH response).
No products indexed under this heading.
Methylprednisolone Acetate (Pharmacologic doses of steroids reduce the TSH response). Products include:
Depo-Medrol Single-Dose Vial ... 2600
Depo-Medrol Sterile Aqueous Suspension ... 2597
Methylprednisolone Sodium Succinate (Pharmacologic doses of steroids reduce the TSH response). Products include:
Solu-Medrol Sterile Powder ... 2643
Prednisolone Acetate (Pharmacologic doses of steroids reduce the TSH response). Products include:
AK-CIDE ... ⊙ 202
AK-CIDE Ointment ... ⊙ 202
Blephamide Liquifilm Sterile Ophthalmic Suspension ... 476
Blephamide Ointment ... ⊙ 237
Econopred & Econopred Plus Ophthalmic Suspensions ... ⊙ 217
Poly-Pred Liquifilm ... ⊙ 248
Pred Forte ... ⊙ 250
Pred Mild ... ⊙ 253
Pred-G Liquifilm Sterile Ophthalmic Suspension ... ⊙ 251
Pred-G S.O.P. Sterile Ophthalmic Ointment ... ⊙ 252
Vasocidin Ointment ... ⊙ 268

IMPORTANT NOTE: Always consult each drug listing in the patient's regimen for possible interactions.

Prednisolone Sodium Phosphate (Pharmacologic doses of steroids reduce the TSH response). Products include:
- AK-Pred .... ⊙ 204
- Hydeltrasol Injection, Sterile 1665
- Inflamase .... ⊙ 265
- Pediapred Oral Liquid 995
- Vasocidin Ophthalmic Solution .... ⊙ 270

Prednisolone Tebutate (Pharmacologic doses of steroids reduce the TSH response). Products include:
- Hydeltra-T.B.A. Sterile Suspension 1667

Prednisone (Pharmacologic doses of steroids reduce the TSH response). Products include:
- Deltasone Tablets 2595

Thyroglobulin (Thyroid hormones reduce the TSH response).
- No products indexed under this heading.

Thyroid (Thyroid hormones reduce the TSH response).
- No products indexed under this heading.

Thyroxine (Thyroid hormones reduce the TSH response).
- No products indexed under this heading.

Thyroxine Sodium (Thyroid hormones reduce the TSH response).
- No products indexed under this heading.

Triamcinolone (Pharmacologic doses of steroids reduce the TSH response). Products include:
- Aristocort Tablets 1022

Triamcinolone Acetonide (Pharmacologic doses of steroids reduce the TSH response). Products include:
- Aristocort A 0.025% Cream 1027
- Aristocort A 0.5% Cream 1031
- Aristocort A 0.1% Cream 1029
- Aristocort A 0.1% Ointment 1030
- Azmacort Oral Inhaler 2011
- Nasacort Nasal Inhaler 2024

Triamcinolone Diacetate (Pharmacologic doses of steroids reduce the TSH response). Products include:
- Aristocort Suspension (Forte Parenteral) 1027
- Aristocort Suspension (Intralesional) 1025

Triamcinolone Hexacetonide (Pharmacologic doses of steroids reduce the TSH response). Products include:
- Aristospan Suspension (Intra-articular) 1033
- Aristospan Suspension (Intralesional) 1032

TICAR FOR INJECTION
(Ticarcillin Disodium) 2526
May interact with:

Probenecid (Concurrent administration prolongs serum levels of ticarcillin). Products include:
- Benemid Tablets 1611
- ColBENEMID Tablets 1622

TICLID TABLETS
(Ticlopidine Hydrochloride) 2156
May interact with xanthine bronchodilators, antacids, non-steroidal anti-inflammatory agents, anticoagulants, and certain other agents. Compounds in these categories include:

Aluminum Carbonate Gel (18% decrease in plasma levels of ticlopidine when administered after antacids). Products include:
- Basaljel 2703

Aluminum Hydroxide (18% decrease in plasma levels of ticlopidine when administered after antacids). Products include:
- ALternaGEL Liquid 1316
- Maximum Strength Ascriptin .... ▣ 630
- Cama Arthritis Pain Reliever .... ▣ 785
- Gaviscon Extra Strength Relief Formula Antacid Tablets .... ▣ 819
- Gaviscon Extra Strength Relief Formula Liquid Antacid .... ▣ 819
- Gaviscon Liquid Antacid .... ▣ 820
- Gelusil Liquid & Tablets .... ▣ 855
- Maalox Heartburn Relief Suspension .... ▣ 642
- Maalox Heartburn Relief Tablets .... ▣ 641
- Maalox Magnesia and Alumina Oral Suspension .... ▣ 642
- Maalox Plus Tablets .... ▣ 643
- Extra Strength Maalox Antacid Plus Antigas Liquid and Tablets ▣ 638
- Tempo Soft Antacid .... ▣ 835

Aluminum Hydroxide Gel (18% decrease in plasma levels of ticlopidine when administered after antacids). Products include:
- ALternaGEL Liquid .... ▣ 659
- Aludrox Oral Suspension 2695
- Amphojel Suspension 2695
- Amphojel Suspension without Flavor 2695
- Amphojel Tablets 2695
- Arthritis Pain Ascriptin .... ▣ 631
- Regular Strength Ascriptin Tablets .... ▣ 629
- Gaviscon Antacid Tablets .... ▣ 819
- Gaviscon-2 Antacid Tablets .... ▣ 820
- Mylanta Liquid 1317
- Mylanta Tablets .... ▣ 660
- Mylanta Double Strength Liquid 1317
- Mylanta Double Strength Tablets .... ▣ 660
- Nephrox Suspension .... ▣ 655

Aminophylline (Co-administration may result in significant increase in the theophylline elimination half-life and a comparable reduction in total plasma clearance of theophylline).
- No products indexed under this heading.

Aspirin (Ticlopidine potentiates the effect of aspirin on collagen-induced platelet aggregation; concurrent use is not recommended). Products include:
- Alka-Seltzer Effervescent Antacid and Pain Reliever .... ▣ 701
- Alka-Seltzer Extra Strength Effervescent Antacid and Pain Reliever .... ▣ 703
- Alka-Seltzer Lemon Lime Effervescent Antacid and Pain Reliever .... ▣ 703
- Alka-Seltzer Plus Cold Medicine .... ▣ 705
- Alka-Seltzer Plus Cold & Cough Medicine .... ▣ 708
- Alka-Seltzer Plus Night-Time Cold Medicine .... ▣ 707
- Alka Seltzer Plus Sinus Medicine .... ▣ 707
- Arthritis Foundation Safety Coated Aspirin Tablets .... ▣ 675
- Arthritis Pain Ascriptin .... ▣ 631
- Maximum Strength Ascriptin .... ▣ 630
- Regular Strength Ascriptin Tablets .... ▣ 629
- Arthritis Strength BC Powder .... ▣ 609
- BC Cold Powder Multi-Symptom Formula (Cold-Sinus-Allergy) .... ▣ 609
- BC Cold Powder Non-Drowsy Formula (Cold-Sinus) .... ▣ 609
- BC Powder .... ▣ 609
- Bayer Children's Chewable Aspirin .... ▣ 711
- Genuine Bayer Aspirin Tablets & Caplets .... ▣ 713
- Extra Strength Bayer Arthritis Pain Regimen Formula .... ▣ 711
- Extra Strength Bayer Aspirin Caplets & Tablets .... ▣ 712
- Extended-Release Bayer 8-Hour Aspirin .... ▣ 712
- Extra Strength Bayer Plus Aspirin Caplets .... ▣ 713
- Extra Strength Bayer PM Aspirin .... ▣ 713
- Bayer Enteric Aspirin .... ▣ 709
- Bufferin Analgesic Tablets and Caplets .... ▣ 613
- Arthritis Strength Bufferin Analgesic Caplets .... ▣ 614
- Extra Strength Bufferin Analgesic Tablets .... ▣ 615
- Cama Arthritis Pain Reliever .... ▣ 785
- Darvon Compound-65 Pulvules 1435
- Easprin 1914
- Ecotrin 2455
- Ecotrin Enteric Coated Aspirin Maximum Strength Tablets and Caplets .... ▣ 816
- Ecotrin Enteric Coated Aspirin Regular Strength Tablets 2455
- Empirin Aspirin Tablets .... ▣ 854
- Empirin with Codeine Tablets 1093
- Excedrin Extra-Strength Analgesic Tablets & Caplets 732
- Fiorinal Capsules 2261
- Fiorinal with Codeine Capsules 2262
- Fiorinal Tablets 2261
- Halfprin 1362
- Healthprin Aspirin 2455
- Norgesic 1496
- Percodan Tablets 939
- Percodan-Demi Tablets 940
- Robaxisal Tablets 2071
- Soma Compound w/Codeine Tablets 2676
- Soma Compound Tablets 2675
- St. Joseph Adult Chewable Aspirin (81 mg.) .... ▣ 808
- Talwin Compound 2335
- Ursinus Inlay-Tabs .... ▣ 794
- Vanquish Analgesic Caplets .... ▣ 731

Cimetidine (Chronic administration of cimetidine reduces the clearance of a single dose of ticlopidine by 50%). Products include:
- Tagamet Tablets 2516

Cimetidine Hydrochloride (Chronic administration of cimetidine reduces the clearance of a single dose of ticlopidine by 50%). Products include:
- Tagamet 2516

Dalteparin Sodium (The tolerance and safety of co-administration has not been established; anticoagulant should be discontinued prior to Ticlid administration). Products include:
- Fragmin 1954

Diclofenac Potassium (Ticlopidine potentiates the effect of NSAIDS on platelet aggregation). Products include:
- Cataflam 816

Diclofenac Sodium (Ticlopidine potentiates the effect of NSAIDS on platelet aggregation). Products include:
- Voltaren Ophthalmic Sterile Ophthalmic Solution .... ⊙ 272
- Voltaren Tablets 861

Dicumarol (The tolerance and safety of co-administration has not been established; anticoagulant should be discontinued prior to Ticlid administration).
- No products indexed under this heading.

Digoxin (Co-administration resulted in slight decrease in digoxin plasma levels. Little or no change in efficacy of digoxin). Products include:
- Lanoxicaps 1117
- Lanoxin Elixir Pediatric 1120
- Lanoxin Injection 1123
- Lanoxin Injection Pediatric 1126
- Lanoxin Tablets 1128

Dihydroxyaluminum Sodium Carbonate (18% decrease in plasma levels of ticlopidine when administered after antacids).
- No products indexed under this heading.

Dyphylline (Co-administration may result in significant increase in the theophylline elimination half-life and a comparable reduction in total plasma clearance of theophylline). Products include:
- Lufyllin & Lufyllin-400 Tablets 2670
- Lufyllin-GG Elixir & Tablets 2671

Enoxaparin (The tolerance and safety of co-administration has not been established; anticoagulant should be discontinued prior to Ticlid administration). Products include:
- Lovenox Injection 2020

Etodolac (Ticlopidine potentiates the effect of NSAIDS on platelet aggregation). Products include:
- Lodine Capsules and Tablets 2743

Fenoprofen Calcium (Ticlopidine potentiates the effect of NSAIDS on platelet aggregation). Products include:
- Nalfon 200 Pulvules & Nalfon Tablets 917

Flurbiprofen (Ticlopidine potentiates the effect of NSAIDS on platelet aggregation). Products include:
- Ansaid Tablets 2579

Heparin Calcium (The tolerance and safety of co-administration has not been established; anticoagulant should be discontinued prior to Ticlid administration).
- No products indexed under this heading.

Heparin Sodium (The tolerance and safety of co-administration has not been established; anticoagulant should be discontinued prior to Ticlid administration). Products include:
- Heparin Lock Flush Solution 2725
- Heparin Sodium Injection 2726
- Heparin Sodium Injection, USP, Sterile Solution 2615
- Heparin Sodium Vials 1441

Ibuprofen (Ticlopidine potentiates the effect of NSAIDS on platelet aggregation). Products include:
- Advil Cold and Sinus Caplets and Tablets (formerly CoAdvil) .... ▣ 870
- Advil Ibuprofen Tablets and Caplets .... ▣ 870
- Children's Advil Suspension 2692
- Arthritis Foundation Ibuprofen Tablets .... ▣ 674
- Bayer Select Ibuprofen Pain Relief Formula .... ▣ 715
- Cramp End Tablets .... ▣ 735
- Dimetapp Sinus Caplets .... ▣ 775
- Haltran Tablets .... ▣ 771
- IBU Tablets 1342
- Ibuprohm .... ▣ 735
- Children's Motrin Ibuprofen Oral Suspension 1546
- Motrin Tablets 2625
- Motrin IB Caplets, Tablets, and Geltabs .... ▣ 838
- Motrin IB Sinus .... ▣ 838
- Motrin Ibuprofen Suspension, Oral Drops, Chewable Tablets, Caplets 1546
- Nuprin Ibuprofen/Analgesic Tablets & Caplets .... ▣ 622
- Sine-Aid IB Caplets 1554
- Vicks DayQuil SINUS Pressure & PAIN Relief with IBUPROFEN .... ▣ 762

Indomethacin (Ticlopidine potentiates the effect of NSAIDS on platelet aggregation). Products include:
- Indocin 1680

Indomethacin Sodium Trihydrate (Ticlopidine potentiates the effect of NSAIDS on platelet aggregation). Products include:
- Indocin I.V. 1684

Ketoprofen (Ticlopidine potentiates the effect of NSAIDS on platelet aggregation). Products include:
- Orudis Capsules 2766
- Oruvail Capsules 2766

Ketorolac Tromethamine (Ticlopidine potentiates the effect of NSAIDS on platelet aggregation). Products include:
- Acular 474
- Acular .... ⊙ 277
- Toradol 2159

(▣ Described in PDR For Nonprescription Drugs) (⊙ Described in PDR For Ophthalmology)

Magaldrate (18% decrease in plasma levels of ticlopidine when administered after antacids).

No products indexed under this heading.

Magnesium Hydroxide (18% decrease in plasma levels of ticlopidine when administered after antacids). Products include:

Aludrox Oral Suspension 2695
Arthritis Pain Ascriptin .... ⊕ 631
Maximum Strength Ascriptin .... ⊕ 630
Regular Strength Ascriptin Tablets .... ⊕ 629
Di-Gel Antacid/Anti-Gas .... ⊕ 801
Gelusil Liquid & Tablets .... ⊕ 855
Maalox Magnesia and Alumina Oral Suspension .... ⊕ 642
Maalox Plus Tablets .... ⊕ 643
Extra Strength Maalox Antacid Plus Antigas Liquid and Tablets ⊕ 638
Mylanta Calcium Carbonate and Magnesium Hydroxide Tablets...... 1318
Mylanta Liquid 1317
Mylanta Tablets .... ⊕ 660
Mylanta Double Strength Liquid 1317
Mylanta Double Strength Tablets .. ⊕ 660
Phillips' Milk of Magnesia Liquid.... ⊕ 729
Rolaids Tablets .... ⊕ 843
Tempo Soft Antacid .... ⊕ 835

Magnesium Oxide (18% decrease in plasma levels of ticlopidine when administered after antacids). Products include:

Beelith Tablets 639
Bufferin Analgesic Tablets and Caplets .... ⊕ 613
Caltrate PLUS .... ⊕ 665
Cama Arthritis Pain Reliever............ ⊕ 785
Mag-Ox 400 668
Uro-Mag... 668

Meclofenamate Sodium (Ticlopidine potentiates the effect of NSAIDS on platelet aggregation).

No products indexed under this heading.

Mefenamic Acid (Ticlopidine potentiates the effect of NSAIDS on platelet aggregation). Products include:

Ponstel 1925

Nabumetone (Ticlopidine potentiates the effect of NSAIDS on platelet aggregation). Products include:

Relafen Tablets...................................... 2510

Naproxen (Ticlopidine potentiates the effect of NSAIDS on platelet aggregation). Products include:

Anaprox/Naprosyn 2117

Naproxen Sodium (Ticlopidine potentiates the effect of NSAIDS on platelet aggregation). Products include:

Aleve 1975
Anaprox/Naprosyn 2117

Oxaprozin (Ticlopidine potentiates the effect of NSAIDS on platelet aggregation). Products include:

Daypro Caplets 2426

Phenylbutazone (Ticlopidine potentiates the effect of NSAIDS on platelet aggregation).

No products indexed under this heading.

Phenytoin (Potential for elevated phenytoin plasma levels with associated somnolence and lethargy; exercise caution if coadministered). Products include:

Dilantin Infatabs 1908
Dilantin-125 Suspension 1911

Phenytoin Sodium (Potential for elevated phenytoin plasma levels with associated somnolence and lethargy; exercise caution if coadministered). Products include:

Dilantin Kapseals 1906
Dilantin Parenteral 1910

Piroxicam (Ticlopidine potentiates the effect of NSAIDS on platelet aggregation). Products include:

Feldene Capsules................................... 1965

Propranolol Hydrochloride (Exercise caution if co-administered; *in vitro* studies indicate no alteration of plasma protein binding of propranolol). Products include:

Inderal 2728
Inderal LA Long Acting Capsules 2730
Inderide Tablets 2732
Inderide LA Long Acting Capsules.. 2734

Sulindac (Ticlopidine potentiates the effect of NSAIDS on platelet aggregation). Products include:

Clinoril Tablets 1618

Theophylline (Co-administration may result in significant increase in the theophylline elimination half-life and a comparable reduction in total plasma clearance of theophylline). Products include:

Marax Tablets & DF Syrup.................. 2200
Quibron 2053

Theophylline Anhydrous (Co-administration may result in significant increase in the theophylline elimination half-life and a comparable reduction in total plasma clearance of theophylline). Products include:

Aerolate 1004
Primatene Dual Action Formula...... ⊕ 872
Primatene Tablets .... ⊕ 873
Respbid Tablets 682
Slo-bid Gyrocaps 2033
Theo-24 Extended Release Capsules 2568
Theo-Dur Extended-Release Tablets 1327
Theo-X Extended-Release Tablets .. 788
Uni-Dur Extended-Release Tablets.. 1331
Uniphyl 400 mg Tablets...................... 2001

Theophylline Calcium Salicylate (Co-administration may result in significant increase in the theophylline elimination half-life and a comparable reduction in total plasma clearance of theophylline). Products include:

Quadrinal Tablets 1350

Theophylline Sodium Glycinate (Co-administration may result in significant increase in the theophylline elimination half-life and a comparable reduction in total plasma clearance of theophylline).

No products indexed under this heading.

Tolmetin Sodium (Ticlopidine potentiates the effect of NSAIDS on platelet aggregation). Products include:

Tolectin (200, 400 and 600 mg) .. 1581

Warfarin Sodium (The tolerance and safety of co-administration has not been established; anticoagulant should be discontinued prior to Ticlid administration). Products include:

Coumadin 926

Food Interactions

Meal, unspecified (Administration after meals results in a 20% increase in the AUC of ticlopidine).

TIGAN CAPSULES

(Trimethobenzamide Hydrochloride) **2057**

May interact with phenothiazines, barbiturates, belladona products, and certain other agents. Compounds in these categories include:

Aprobarbital (Exercise caution in recent recipients of barbiturates).

No products indexed under this heading.

Atropine Sulfate (Exercise caution in recent recipients of belladonna derivatives). Products include:

Arco-Lase Plus Tablets 512
Atrohist Plus Tablets 454
Atropine Sulfate Sterile Ophthalmic Solution .... ⊙ 233
Donnatal 2060
Donnatal Extentabs.............................. 2061
Donnatal Tablets 2060
Lomotil 2439
Motofen Tablets 784
Urised Tablets.. 1964

Belladonna Alkaloids (Exercise caution in recent recipients of belladonna derivatives). Products include:

Bellergal-S Tablets 2250
Hyland's Bed Wetting Tablets .... ⊕ 828
Hyland's EnurAid Tablets................... ⊕ 829
Hyland's Teething Tablets.................. ⊕ 830

Butabarbital (Exercise caution in recent recipients of barbiturates).

No products indexed under this heading.

Butalbital (Exercise caution in recent recipients of barbiturates). Products include:

Esgic-plus Tablets 1013
Fioricet Tablets...................................... 2258
Fioricet with Codeine Capsules 2260
Fiorinal Capsules 2261
Fiorinal with Codeine Capsules 2262
Fiorinal Tablets 2261
Phrenilin 785
Sedapap Tablets 50 mg/650 mg .. 1543

Chlorpromazine (Exercise caution in recent recipients of phenothiazines). Products include:

Thorazine Suppositories..................... 2523

Chlorpromazine Hydrochloride (Exercise caution in recent recipients of phenothiazines). Products include:

Thorazine 2523

Fluphenazine Decanoate (Exercise caution in recent recipients of phenothiazines). Products include:

Prolixin Decanoate 509

Fluphenazine Enanthate (Exercise caution in recent recipients of phenothiazines). Products include:

Prolixin Enanthate 509

Fluphenazine Hydrochloride (Exercise caution in recent recipients of phenothiazines). Products include:

Prolixin 509

Hyoscyamine (Exercise caution in recent recipients of belladonna derivatives). Products include:

Cystospaz Tablets 1963
Urised Tablets.. 1964

Hyoscyamine Sulfate (Exercise caution in recent recipients of belladonna derivatives). Products include:

Arco-Lase Plus Tablets 512
Atrohist Plus Tablets 454
Cystospaz-M Capsules 1963
Donnatal 2060
Donnatal Extentabs.............................. 2061
Donnatal Tablets 2060
Kutrase Capsules.................................. 2402
Levsin/Levsinex/Levbid 2405

Mephobarbital (Exercise caution in recent recipients of barbiturates). Products include:

Mebaral Tablets 2322

Mesoridazine Besylate (Exercise caution in recent recipients of phenothiazines). Products include:

Serentil 684

Methotrimeprazine (Exercise caution in recent recipients of phenothiazines). Products include:

Levoprome 1274

Pentobarbital Sodium (Exercise caution in recent recipients of barbiturates). Products include:

Nembutal Sodium Capsules 436
Nembutal Sodium Solution 438
Nembutal Sodium Suppositories..... 440

Perphenazine (Exercise caution in recent recipients of phenothiazines). Products include:

Etrafon 2355
Triavil Tablets 1757
Trilafon... 2389

Phenobarbital (Exercise caution in recent recipients of barbiturates). Products include:

Arco-Lase Plus Tablets 512
Bellergal-S Tablets 2250
Donnatal 2060
Donnatal Extentabs.............................. 2061
Donnatal Tablets 2060
Phenobarbital Elixir and Tablets 1469
Quadrinal Tablets 1350

Prochlorperazine (Exercise caution in recent recipients of phenothiazines). Products include:

Compazine 2470

Promethazine Hydrochloride (Exercise caution in recent recipients of phenothiazines). Products include:

Mepergan Injection 2753
Phenergan with Codeine..................... 2777
Phenergan with Dextromethorphan 2778
Phenergan Injection 2773
Phenergan Suppositories 2775
Phenergan Syrup 2774
Phenergan Tablets 2775
Phenergan VC 2779
Phenergan VC with Codeine 2781

Scopolamine (Exercise caution in recent recipients of belladonna derivatives). Products include:

Transderm Scōp Transdermal Therapeutic System 869

Scopolamine Hydrobromide (Exercise caution in recent recipients of belladonna derivatives). Products include:

Atrohist Plus Tablets 454
Donnatal 2060
Donnatal Extentabs.............................. 2061
Donnatal Tablets 2060

Secobarbital Sodium (Exercise caution in recent recipients of barbiturates). Products include:

Seconal Sodium Pulvules 1474

Thiamylal Sodium (Exercise caution in recent recipients of barbiturates).

No products indexed under this heading.

Thioridazine Hydrochloride (Exercise caution in recent recipients of phenothiazines). Products include:

Mellaril 2269

Trifluoperazine Hydrochloride (Exercise caution in recent recipients of phenothiazines). Products include:

Stelazine 2514

Food Interactions

Alcohol (May result in an adverse drug interaction).

TIGAN INJECTABLE

(Trimethobenzamide Hydrochloride) **2057**

See **Tigan Capsules**

TIGAN SUPPOSITORIES

(Trimethobenzamide Hydrochloride) **2057**

See **Tigan Capsules**

TILADE

(Nedocromil Sodium) **996**

None cited in PDR database.

TIMENTIN FOR INJECTION

(Ticarcillin Disodium, Clavulanate Potassium) **2528**

May interact with:

Probenecid (Increases serum concentration and prolongs half-life of ticarcillin). Products include:

Benemid Tablets 1611
ColBENEMID Tablets 1622

IMPORTANT NOTE: Always consult each drug listing in the patient's regimen for possible interactions.

Timolide

TIMOLIDE TABLETS (Timolol Maleate, Hydrochlorothiazide) ....1748 May interact with insulin, corticosteroids, antihypertensives, catecholamine depleting drugs, non-steroidal anti-inflammatory agents, lithium preparations, cardiac glycosides, and certain other agents. Compounds in these categories include:

Acebutolol Hydrochloride (Potentiated). Products include:

Sectral Capsules 2807

ACTH (Hypokalemia).

No products indexed under this heading.

Amlodipine Besylate (Potentiated). Products include:

Lotrel Capsules	840
Norvasc Tablets	1940

Atenolol (Potentiated). Products include:

Tenoretic Tablets	2845
Tenormin Tablets and I.V. Injection	2847

Benazepril Hydrochloride (Potentiated). Products include:

Lotensin Tablets	834
Lotensin HCT	837
Lotrel Capsules	840

Bendroflumethiazide (Potentiated).

No products indexed under this heading.

Betamethasone Acetate (Hypokalemia). Products include:

Celestone Soluspan Suspension 2347

Betamethasone Sodium Phosphate (Hypokalemia). Products include:

Celestone Soluspan Suspension 2347

Betaxolol Hydrochloride (Potentiated). Products include:

Betoptic Ophthalmic Solution	469
Betoptic S Ophthalmic Suspension	471
Kerlone Tablets	2436

Bisoprolol Fumarate (Potentiated). Products include:

Zebeta Tablets	1413
Ziac	1415

Captopril (Potentiated). Products include:

Capoten	739
Capozide	742

Carteolol Hydrochloride (Potentiated). Products include:

Cartrol Tablets	410
Ocupress Ophthalmic Solution, 1% Sterile	◎ 309

Chlorothiazide (Potentiated). Products include:

Aldoclor Tablets	1598
Diupres Tablets	1650
Diuril Oral	1653

Chlorothiazide Sodium (Potentiated). Products include:

Diuril Sodium Intravenous 1652

Chlorthalidone (Potentiated). Products include:

Combipres Tablets	677
Tenoretic Tablets	2845
Thalitone	1245

Cholestyramine (Cholestyramine resin has potential of binding hydrochlorothiazide and reducing its absorption from the GI tract by up to 85%). Products include:

Questran Light	769
Questran Powder	770

Clonidine (Potentiated). Products include:

Catapres-TTS.. 675

Clonidine Hydrochloride (Potentiated). Products include:

Catapres Tablets	674
Combipres Tablets	677

Colestipol Hydrochloride (Colestipol resin has potential of binding hydrochlorothiazide and reducing its absorption from the GI tract by up to 43%). Products include:

Colestid Tablets 2591

Cortisone Acetate (Hypokalemia). Products include:

Cortone Acetate Sterile Suspension	1623
Cortone Acetate Tablets	1624

Deslanoside (Hypokalemia can lead to increased cardiac toxicity of digitalis).

No products indexed under this heading.

Dexamethasone (Hypokalemia). Products include:

AK-Trol Ointment & Suspension	◎ 205
Decadron Elixir	1633
Decadron Tablets	1635
Decaspray Topical Aerosol	1648
Dexacidin Ointment	◎ 263
Maxitrol Ophthalmic Ointment and Suspension	◎ 224
TobraDex Ophthalmic Suspension and Ointment	473

Dexamethasone Acetate (Hypokalemia). Products include:

Dalalone D.P. Injectable	1011
Decadron-LA Sterile Suspension	1646

Dexamethasone Sodium Phosphate (Hypokalemia). Products include:

Decadron Phosphate Injection	1637
Decadron Phosphate Respihaler	1642
Decadron Phosphate Sterile Ophthalmic Ointment	1641
Decadron Phosphate Sterile Ophthalmic Solution	1642
Decadron Phosphate Topical Cream	1644
Decadron Phosphate Turbinaire	1645
Decadron Phosphate with Xylocaine Injection, Sterile	1639
Dexacort Phosphate in Respihaler	458
Dexacort Phosphate in Turbinaire	459
NeoDecadron Sterile Ophthalmic Ointment	1712
NeoDecadron Sterile Ophthalmic Solution	1713
NeoDecadron Topical Cream	1714

Diazoxide (Potentiated). Products include:

Hyperstat I.V. Injection	2363
Proglycem	580

Diclofenac Potassium (Reduced diuretic, natriuretic, and antihypertensive effects of Timolide). Products include:

Cataflam 816

Diclofenac Sodium (Reduced diuretic, natriuretic, and antihypertensive effects of Timolide). Products include:

Voltaren Ophthalmic Sterile Ophthalmic Solution	◎ 272
Voltaren Tablets	861

Digitoxin (Hypokalemia can lead to increased cardiac toxicity of digitalis). Products include:

Crystodigin Tablets................................ 1433

Digoxin (Hypokalemia can lead to increased cardiac toxicity of digitalis). Products include:

Lanoxicaps	1117
Lanoxin Elixir Pediatric	1120
Lanoxin Injection	1123
Lanoxin Injection Pediatric	1126
Lanoxin Tablets	1128

Diltiazem Hydrochloride (Left ventricular failure and AV conduction disturbances). Products include:

Cardizem CD Capsules	1506
Cardizem SR Capsules	1510
Cardizem Injectable	1508
Cardizem Tablets	1512
Dilacor XR Extended-release Capsules	2018

Doxazosin Mesylate (Potentiated). Products include:

Cardura Tablets 2186

Enalapril Maleate (Potentiated). Products include:

Vaseretic Tablets	1765
Vasotec Tablets	1771

Enalaprilat (Potentiated). Products include:

Vasotec I.V. 1768

Esmolol Hydrochloride (Potentiated). Products include:

Brevibloc Injection................................. 1808

Etodolac (Reduced diuretic, natriuretic, and antihypertensive effects of Timolide). Products include:

Lodine Capsules and Tablets 2743

Felodipine (Potentiated). Products include:

Plendil Extended-Release Tablets.... 527

Fenoprofen Calcium (Reduced diuretic, natriuretic, and antihypertensive effects of Timolide). Products include:

Nalfon 200 Pulvules & Nalfon Tablets 917

Fludrocortisone Acetate (Hypokalemia). Products include:

Florinef Acetate Tablets 505

Flurbiprofen (Reduced diuretic, natriuretic, and antihypertensive effects of Timolide). Products include:

Ansaid Tablets 2579

Fosinopril Sodium (Potentiated). Products include:

Monopril Tablets 757

Furosemide (Potentiated). Products include:

Lasix Injection, Oral Solution and Tablets 1240

Guanabenz Acetate (Potentiated).

No products indexed under this heading.

Guanethidine Monosulfate (Potentiated). Products include:

Esimil Tablets	822
Ismelin Tablets	827

Hydralazine Hydrochloride (Potentiated). Products include:

Apresazide Capsules	808
Apresoline Hydrochloride Tablets	809
Ser-Ap-Es Tablets	849

Hydrocortisone (Hypokalemia). Products include:

Anusol-HC Cream 2.5%	1896
Aquanil HC Lotion	1931
Bactine Hydrocortisone Anti-Itch Cream	⊕D 709
Caldecort Anti-Itch Hydrocortisone Spray	⊕D 631
Cortaid	⊕D 836
CORTENEMA	2535
Cortisporin Ointment	1085
Cortisporin Ophthalmic Ointment Sterile	1085
Cortisporin Ophthalmic Suspension Sterile	1086
Cortisporin Otic Solution Sterile	1087
Cortisporin Otic Suspension Sterile	1088
Cortizone-5	⊕D 831
Cortizone-10	⊕D 831
Hydrocortone Tablets	1672
Hytone	907
Massengill Medicated Soft Cloth Towelettes	2458
PediOtic Suspension Sterile	1153
Preparation H Hydrocortisone 1% Cream	⊕D 872
ProctoCream-HC 2.5%	2408
VōSoL HC Otic Solution	2678

Hydrocortisone Acetate (Hypokalemia). Products include:

Analpram-HC Rectal Cream 1% and 2.5%	977
Anusol HC-1 Anti-Itch Hydrocortisone Ointment	⊕D 847
Anusol-HC Suppositories	1897
Caldecort	⊕D 631
Carmol HC	924
Coly-Mycin S Otic w/Neomycin & Hydrocortisone	1906
Cortaid	⊕D 836
Cortifoam	2396
Cortisporin Cream	1084
Epifoam	2399
Hydrocortone Acetate Sterile Suspension	1669
Mantadil Cream	1135
Nupercainal Hydrocortisone 1% Cream	⊕D 645
Ophthocort	◎ 311
Pramosone Cream, Lotion & Ointment	978
ProctoCream-HC	2408
ProctoFoam-HC	2409
Terra-Cortril Ophthalmic Suspension	2210

Hydrocortisone Sodium Phosphate (Hypokalemia). Products include:

Hydrocortone Phosphate Injection, Sterile 1670

Hydrocortisone Sodium Succinate (Hypokalemia). Products include:

Solu-Cortef Sterile Powder................. 2641

Hydroflumethiazide (Potentiated). Products include:

Diucardin Tablets................................... 2718

Ibuprofen (Reduced diuretic, natriuretic, and antihypertensive effects of Timolide). Products include:

Advil Cold and Sinus Caplets and Tablets (formerly CoAdvil)	⊕D 870
Advil Ibuprofen Tablets and Caplets	⊕D 870
Children's Advil Suspension	2692
Arthritis Foundation Ibuprofen Tablets	⊕D 674
Bayer Select Ibuprofen Pain Relief Formula	⊕D 715
Cramp End Tablets	⊕D 735
Dimetapp Sinus Caplets	⊕D 775
Haltran Tablets	⊕D 771
IBU Tablets	1342
Ibuprohm	⊕D 735
Children's Motrin Ibuprofen Oral Suspension	1546
Motrin Tablets	2625
Motrin IB Caplets, Tablets, and Geltabs	⊕D 838
Motrin IB Sinus	⊕D 838
Motrin Ibuprofen Suspension, Oral Drops, Chewable Tablets, Caplets	1546
Nuprin Ibuprofen/Analgesic Tablets & Caplets	⊕D 622
Sine-Aid IB Caplets	1554
Vicks DayQuil SINUS Pressure & PAIN Relief with IBUPROFEN	⊕D 762

Indapamide (Potentiated). Products include:

Lozol Tablets 2022

Indomethacin (Reduced diuretic, natriuretic, and antihypertensive effects of Timolide). Products include:

Indocin 1680

Indomethacin Sodium Trihydrate (Reduced diuretic, natriuretic, and antihypertensive effects of Timolide). Products include:

Indocin I.V. 1684

Insulin, Human (Insulin requirements may be altered).

No products indexed under this heading.

Insulin, Human Isophane Suspension (Insulin requirements may be altered). Products include:

Novolin N Human Insulin 10 ml Vials.. 1795

Insulin, Human NPH (Insulin requirements may be altered). Products include:

Humulin N, 100 Units	1448
Novolin N PenFill Cartridges Durable Insulin Delivery System	1798
Novolin N Prefilled Syringe Disposable Insulin Delivery System	1798

(⊕D Described in PDR For Nonprescription Drugs)

(◎ Described in PDR For Ophthalmology)

1033 **Interactions Index** **Timoptic in Ocudose**

Insulin, Human Regular (Insulin requirements may be altered). Products include:
Humulin R, 100 Units ... 1449
Novolin R Human Insulin 10 ml Vials ... 1795
Novolin R PenFill Cartridges Durable Insulin Delivery System ... 1798
Novolin R Prefilled Syringe Disposable Insulin Delivery System ... 1798
Velosulin BR Human Insulin 10 ml Vials ... 1795

Insulin, Human, Zinc Suspension (Insulin requirements may be altered). Products include:
Humulin L, 100 Units ... 1446
Humulin U, 100 Units ... 1450
Novolin L Human Insulin 10 ml Vials ... 1795

Insulin, NPH (Insulin requirements may be altered). Products include:
NPH, 100 Units ... 1450
Pork NPH, 100 Units ... 1452
Purified Pork NPH Isophane Insulin ... 1801

Insulin, Regular (Insulin requirements may be altered). Products include:
Regular, 100 Units ... 1450
Pork Regular, 100 Units ... 1452
Pork Regular (Concentrated), 500 Units ... 1453
Purified Pork Regular Insulin ... 1801

Insulin, Zinc Crystals (Insulin requirements may be altered). Products include:
NPH, 100 Units ... 1450

Insulin, Zinc Suspension (Insulin requirements may be altered). Products include:
Iletin I ... 1450
Lente, 100 Units ... 1450
Iletin II ... 1452
Pork Lente, 100 Units ... 1452
Purified Pork Lente Insulin ... 1801

Isradipine (Potentiated). Products include:
DynaCirc Capsules ... 2256

Ketoprofen (Reduced diuretic, natriuretic, and antihypertensive effects of Timolide). Products include:
Orudis Capsules ... 2766
Oruvail Capsules ... 2766

Ketorolac Tromethamine (Reduced diuretic, natriuretic, and antihypertensive effects of Timolide). Products include:
Acular ... 474
Acular ... ◎ 277
Toradol ... 2159

Labetalol Hydrochloride (Potentiated). Products include:
Normodyne Injection ... 2377
Normodyne Tablets ... 2379
Trandate ... 1185

Lisinopril (Potentiated). Products include:
Prinivil Tablets ... 1733
Prinzide Tablets ... 1737
Zestoretic ... 2850
Zestril Tablets ... 2854

Lithium Carbonate (High risk of lithium toxicity). Products include:
Eskalith ... 2485
Lithium Carbonate Capsules & Tablets ... 2230
Lithonate/Lithotabs/Lithobid ... 2543

Lithium Citrate (High risk of lithium toxicity).
No products indexed under this heading.

Losartan Potassium (Potentiated). Products include:
Cozaar Tablets ... 1628
Hyzaar Tablets ... 1677

Mecamylamine Hydrochloride (Potentiated). Products include:
Inversine Tablets ... 1686

Meclofenamate Sodium (Reduced diuretic, natriuretic, and antihypertensive effects of Timolide).
No products indexed under this heading.

Mefenamic Acid (Reduced diuretic, natriuretic, and antihypertensive effects of Timolide). Products include:
Ponstel ... 1925

Methyclothiazide (Potentiated). Products include:
Enduron Tablets ... 420

Methyldopa (Potentiated). Products include:
Aldoclor Tablets ... 1598
Aldomet Oral ... 1600
Aldoril Tablets ... 1604

Methyldopate Hydrochloride (Potentiated). Products include:
Aldomet Ester HCl Injection ... 1602

Methylprednisolone (Hypokalemia). Products include:
Medrol ... 2621

Methylprednisolone Acetate (Hypokalemia). Products include:
Depo-Medrol Single-Dose Vial ... 2600
Depo-Medrol Sterile Aqueous Suspension ... 2597

Methylprednisolone Sodium Succinate (Hypokalemia). Products include:
Solu-Medrol Sterile Powder ... 2643

Metolazone (Potentiated). Products include:
Mykrox Tablets ... 993
Zaroxolyn Tablets ... 1000

Metoprolol Succinate (Potentiated). Products include:
Toprol-XL Tablets ... 565

Metoprolol Tartrate (Potentiated). Products include:
Lopressor Ampuls ... 830
Lopressor HCT Tablets ... 832
Lopressor Tablets ... 830

Metyrosine (Potentiated). Products include:
Demser Capsules ... 1649

Minoxidil (Potentiated). Products include:
Loniten Tablets ... 2618
Rogaine Topical Solution ... 2637

Moexipril Hydrochloride (Potentiated). Products include:
Univasc Tablets ... 2410

Nabumetone (Reduced diuretic, natriuretic, and antihypertensive effects of Timolide). Products include:
Relafen Tablets ... 2510

Nadolol (Potentiated).
No products indexed under this heading.

Naproxen (Reduced diuretic, natriuretic, and antihypertensive effects of Timolide). Products include:
Anaprox/Naprosyn ... 2117

Naproxen Sodium (Reduced diuretic, natriuretic, and antihypertensive effects of Timolide). Products include:
Aleve ... 1975
Anaprox/Naprosyn ... 2117

Nicardipine Hydrochloride (Potentiated). Products include:
Cardene Capsules ... 2095
Cardene I.V. ... 2709
Cardene SR Capsules ... 2097

Nifedipine (Potentiated). Products include:
Adalat Capsules (10 mg and 20 mg) ... 587
Adalat CC ... 589
Procardia Capsules ... 1971
Procardia XL Extended Release Tablets ... 1972

Nisoldipine (Potentiated).
No products indexed under this heading.

Nitroglycerin (Potentiated). Products include:
Deponit NTG Transdermal Delivery System ... 2397
Nitro-Bid IV ... 1523
Nitro-Bid Ointment ... 1524
Nitrodisc ... 2047
Nitro-Dur (nitroglycerin) Transdermal Infusion System ... 1326
Nitrolingual Spray ... 2027
Nitrostat Tablets ... 1925
Transderm-Nitro Transdermal Therapeutic System ... 859

Norepinephrine Bitartrate (Decreased arterial responsiveness to norepinephrine). Products include:
Levophed Bitartrate Injection ... 2315

Oxaprozin (Reduced diuretic, natriuretic, and antihypertensive effects of Timolide). Products include:
Daypro Caplets ... 2426

Penbutolol Sulfate (Potentiated). Products include:
Levatol ... 2403

Phenoxybenzamine Hydrochloride (Potentiated). Products include:
Dibenzyline Capsules ... 2476

Phentolamine Mesylate (Potentiated). Products include:
Regitine ... 846

Phenylbutazone (Reduced diuretic, natriuretic, and antihypertensive effects of Timolide).
No products indexed under this heading.

Pindolol (Potentiated). Products include:
Visken Tablets ... 2299

Piroxicam (Reduced diuretic, natriuretic, and antihypertensive effects of Timolide). Products include:
Feldene Capsules ... 1965

Polythiazide (Potentiated). Products include:
Minizide Capsules ... 1938

Prazosin Hydrochloride (Potentiated). Products include:
Minipress Capsules ... 1937
Minizide Capsules ... 1938

Prednisolone Acetate (Hypokalemia). Products include:
AK-CIDE ... ◎ 202
AK-CIDE Ointment ... ◎ 202
Blephamide Liquifilm Sterile Ophthalmic Suspension ... 476
Blephamide Ointment ... ◎ 237
Econopred & Econopred Plus Ophthalmic Suspensions ... ◎ 217
Poly-Pred Liquifilm ... ◎ 248
Pred Forte ... ◎ 250
Pred Mild ... ◎ 253
Pred-G Liquifilm Sterile Ophthalmic Suspension ... ◎ 251
Pred-G S.O.P. Sterile Ophthalmic Ointment ... ◎ 252
Vasocidin Ointment ... ◎ 268

Prednisolone Sodium Phosphate (Hypokalemia). Products include:
AK-Pred ... ◎ 204
Hydeltrasol Injection, Sterile ... 1665
Inflamase ... ◎ 265
Pediapred Oral Liquid ... 995
Vasocidin Ophthalmic Solution ... ◎ 270

Prednisolone Tebutate (Hypokalemia). Products include:
Hydeltra-T.B.A. Sterile Suspension 1667

Prednisone (Hypokalemia). Products include:
Deltasone Tablets ... 2595

Propranolol Hydrochloride (Potentiated). Products include:
Inderal ... 2728
Inderal LA Long Acting Capsules ... 2730
Inderide Tablets ... 2732
Inderide LA Long Acting Capsules .. 2734

Quinapril Hydrochloride (Potentiated). Products include:
Accupril Tablets ... 1893

Ramipril (Potentiated). Products include:
Altace Capsules ... 1232

Rauwolfia Serpentina (Potentiated; hypotension; marked bradycardia).
No products indexed under this heading.

Rescinnamine (Potentiated; hypotension; marked bradycardia).
No products indexed under this heading.

Reserpine (Potentiated; hypotension; marked bradycardia). Products include:
Diupres Tablets ... 1650
Hydropres Tablets ... 1675
Ser-Ap-Es Tablets ... 849

Sodium Nitroprusside (Potentiated).
No products indexed under this heading.

Sotalol Hydrochloride (Potentiated). Products include:
Betapace Tablets ... 641

Spirapril Hydrochloride (Potentiated).
No products indexed under this heading.

Sulindac (Reduced diuretic, natriuretic, and antihypertensive effects of Timolide). Products include:
Clinoril Tablets ... 1618

Terazosin Hydrochloride (Potentiation of other antihypertensives). Products include:
Hytrin Capsules ... 430

Tolmetin Sodium (Reduced diuretic, natriuretic, and antihypertensive effects of Timolide). Products include:
Tolectin (200, 400 and 600 mg) .. 1581

Torsemide (Potentiated). Products include:
Demadex Tablets and Injection ... 686

Triamcinolone (Hypokalemia). Products include:
Aristocort Tablets ... 1022

Triamcinolone Acetonide (Hypokalemia). Products include:
Aristocort A 0.025% Cream ... 1027
Aristocort A 0.5% Cream ... 1031
Aristocort A 0.1% Cream ... 1029
Aristocort A 0.1% Ointment ... 1030
Azmacort Oral Inhaler ... 2011
Nasacort Nasal Inhaler ... 2024

Triamcinolone Diacetate (Hypokalemia). Products include:
Aristocort Suspension (Forte Parenteral) ... 1027
Aristocort Suspension (Intralesional) ... 1025

Triamcinolone Hexacetonide (Hypokalemia). Products include:
Aristospan Suspension (Intra-articular) ... 1033
Aristospan Suspension (Intralesional) ... 1032

Trimethaphan Camsylate (Potentiated). Products include:
Arfonad Ampuls ... 2080

Tubocurarine Chloride (Increased responsiveness to tubocurarine).
No products indexed under this heading.

Verapamil Hydrochloride (Left ventricular failure and AV conduction disturbances). Products include:
Calan SR Caplets ... 2422
Calan Tablets ... 2419
Isoptin Injectable ... 1344
Isoptin Oral Tablets ... 1346
Isoptin SR Tablets ... 1348
Verelan Capsules ... 1410
Verelan Capsules ... 2824

TIMOPTIC IN OCUDOSE
(Timolol Maleate) ... 1753
May interact with beta blockers,

IMPORTANT NOTE: Always consult each drug listing in the patient's regimen for possible interactions.

calcium channel blockers, catecholamine depleting drugs, cardiac glycosides, insulin, oral hypoglycemic agents, and certain other agents. Compounds in these categories include:

Acarbose (Beta blocking agents, usually systemic, may mask the sign and symptoms of acute hypoglycemia).
No products indexed under this heading.

Acebutolol Hydrochloride (Concurrent use with systemic beta blocker may have additive effects of beta blockade, both systemic and on intraocular pressure). Products include:
Sectral Capsules ... 2807

Amlodipine Besylate (Possible atrioventricular conduction disturbances, left ventricular failure, or hypotension when used concurrently). Products include:
Lotrel Capsules ... 840
Norvasc Tablets ... 1940

Atenolol (Concurrent use with systemic beta blocker may have additive effects of beta blockade, both systemic and on intraocular pressure). Products include:
Tenoretic Tablets ... 2845
Tenormin Tablets and I.V. Injection 2847

Bepridil Hydrochloride (Possible atrioventricular conduction disturbances, left ventricular failure, or hypotension when used concurrently). Products include:
Vascor (200, 300 and 400 mg) Tablets ... 1587

Betaxolol Hydrochloride (Concurrent use with systemic beta blocker may have additive effects of beta blockade, both systemic and on intraocular pressure; concurrent use of two ophthalmic beta blockers is not recommended). Products include:
Betoptic Ophthalmic Solution ... 469
Betoptic S Ophthalmic Suspension 471
Kerlone Tablets ... 2436

Bisoprolol Fumarate (Concurrent use with systemic beta blocker may have additive effects of beta blockade, both systemic and on intraocular pressure). Products include:
Zebeta Tablets ... 1413
Ziac ... 1415

Carteolol Hydrochloride (Concurrent use with systemic beta blocker may have additive effects of beta blockade, both systemic and on intraocular pressure; concurrent use of two ophthalmic beta blockers is not recommended). Products include:
Cartrol Tablets ... 410
Ocupress Ophthalmic Solution, 1% Sterile ... ⊙ 309

Chlorpropamide (Beta blocking agents, usually systemic, may mask the sign and symptoms of acute hypoglycemia). Products include:
Diabinese Tablets ... 1935

Deserpidine (Possible additive effects and the production of hypotension and/or bradycardia).
No products indexed under this heading.

Deslanoside (Coadministration with digitalis and calcium antagonists may have additive effects in prolonging atrioventricular conduction time).
No products indexed under this heading.

Digitoxin (Coadministration with digitalis and calcium antagonists may have additive effects in prolonging atrioventricular conduction time). Products include:
Crystodigin Tablets ... 1433

Digoxin (Coadministration with digitalis and calcium antagonists may have additive effects in prolonging atrioventricular conduction time). Products include:
Lanoxicaps ... 1117
Lanoxin Elixir Pediatric ... 1120
Lanoxin Injection ... 1123
Lanoxin Injection Pediatric ... 1126
Lanoxin Tablets ... 1128

Diltiazem Hydrochloride (Possible atrioventricular conduction disturbances, left ventricular failure, or hypotension when used concurrently). Products include:
Cardizem CD Capsules ... 1506
Cardizem SR Capsules ... 1510
Cardizem Injectable ... 1508
Cardizem Tablets ... 1512
Dilacor XR Extended-release Capsules ... 2018

Epinephrine (Patients with a history of atopy or anaphylactic reactions to a variety of allergens may be unresponsive to the usual dose of injectable epinephrine used to treat allergic reactions). Products include:
Bronkaid Mist ... ▣ 717
EPIFRIN ... ⊙ 239
EpiPen ... 790
Marcaine Hydrochloride with Epinephrine 1:200,000 ... 2316
Primatene Mist ... ▣ 873
Sensorcaine with Epinephrine Injection ... 559
Sus-Phrine Injection ... 1019
Xylocaine with Epinephrine Injections ... 567

Epinephrine Bitartrate (Patients with a history of atopy or anaphylactic reactions to a variety of allergens may be unresponsive to the usual dose of injectable epinephrine used to treat allergic reactions). Products include:
Bronkaid Mist Suspension ... ▣ 718
Sensorcaine-MPF with Epinephrine Injection ... 559

Esmolol Hydrochloride (Concurrent use with systemic beta blocker may have additive effects of beta blockade, both systemic and on intraocular pressure). Products include:
Brevibloc Injection ... 1808

Felodipine (Possible atrioventricular conduction disturbances, left ventricular failure, or hypotension when used concurrently). Products include:
Plendil Extended-Release Tablets ... 527

Glipizide (Beta blocking agents, usually systemic, may mask the sign and symptoms of acute hypoglycemia). Products include:
Glucotrol Tablets ... 1967
Glucotrol XL Extended Release Tablets ... 1968

Glyburide (Beta blocking agents, usually systemic, may mask the sign and symptoms of acute hypoglycemia). Products include:
DiaBeta Tablets ... 1239
Glynase PresTab Tablets ... 2609
Micronase Tablets ... 2623

Guanethidine Monosulfate (Possible additive effects and the production of hypotension and/or bradycardia). Products include:
Esimil Tablets ... 822
Ismelin Tablets ... 827

Insulin, Human (Beta blocking agents, usually systemic, may mask the sign and symptoms of acute hypoglycemia).
No products indexed under this heading.

Insulin, Human Isophane Suspension (Beta blocking agents, usually systemic, may mask the sign and symptoms of acute hypoglycemia). Products include:
Novolin N Human Insulin 10 ml Vials ... 1795

Insulin, Human NPH (Beta blocking agents, usually systemic, may mask the sign and symptoms of acute hypoglycemia). Products include:
Humulin N, 100 Units ... 1448
Novolin N PenFill Cartridges Durable Insulin Delivery System ... 1798
Novolin N Prefilled Syringe Disposable Insulin Delivery System ... 1798

Insulin, Human Regular (Beta blocking agents, usually systemic, may mask the sign and symptoms of acute hypoglycemia). Products include:
Humulin R, 100 Units ... 1449
Novolin R Human Insulin 10 ml Vials ... 1795
Novolin R PenFill Cartridges Durable Insulin Delivery System ... 1798
Novolin R Prefilled Syringe Disposable Insulin Delivery System ... 1798
Velosulin BR Human Insulin 10 ml Vials ... 1795

Insulin, Human, Zinc Suspension (Beta blocking agents, usually systemic, may mask the sign and symptoms of acute hypoglycemia). Products include:
Humulin L, 100 Units ... 1446
Humulin U, 100 Units ... 1450
Novolin L Human Insulin 10 ml Vials ... 1795

Insulin, NPH (Beta blocking agents, usually systemic, may mask the sign and symptoms of acute hypoglycemia). Products include:
NPH, 100 Units ... 1450
Pork NPH, 100 Units ... 1452
Purified Pork NPH Isophane Insulin ... 1801

Insulin, Regular (Beta blocking agents, usually systemic, may mask the sign and symptoms of acute hypoglycemia). Products include:
Regular, 100 Units ... 1450
Pork Regular, 100 Units ... 1452
Pork Regular (Concentrated), 500 Units ... 1453
Purified Pork Regular Insulin ... 1801

Insulin, Zinc Crystals (Beta blocking agents, usually systemic, may mask the sign and symptoms of acute hypoglycemia). Products include:
NPH, 100 Units ... 1450

Insulin, Zinc Suspension (Beta blocking agents, usually systemic, may mask the sign and symptoms of acute hypoglycemia). Products include:
Iletin I ... 1450
Lente, 100 Units ... 1450
Iletin II ... 1452
Pork Lente, 100 Units ... 1452
Purified Pork Lente Insulin ... 1801

Isradipine (Possible atrioventricular conduction disturbances, left ventricular failure, or hypotension when used concurrently). Products include:
DynaCirc Capsules ... 2256

Labetalol Hydrochloride (Concurrent use with systemic beta blocker may have additive effects of beta blockade, both systemic and on intraocular pressure). Products include:
Normodyne Injection ... 2377
Normodyne Tablets ... 2379
Trandate ... 1185

Levobunolol Hydrochloride (Concurrent use of two ophthalmic beta blockers is not recommended). Products include:
Betagan ... ⊙ 233

Metformin Hydrochloride (Beta blocking agents, usually systemic, may mask the sign and symptoms of acute hypoglycemia). Products include:
Glucophage ... 752

Metipranolol Hydrochloride (Concurrent use of two ophthalmic beta blockers is not recommended). Products include:
OptiPranolol (Metipranolol 0.3%) Sterile Ophthalmic Solution ... ⊙ 258

Metoprolol Succinate (Concurrent use with systemic beta blocker may have additive effects of beta blockade, both systemic and on intraocular pressure). Products include:
Toprol-XL Tablets ... 565

Metoprolol Tartrate (Concurrent use with systemic beta blocker may have additive effects of beta blockade, both systemic and on intraocular pressure). Products include:
Lopressor Ampuls ... 830
Lopressor HCT Tablets ... 832
Lopressor Tablets ... 830

Nadolol (Concurrent use with systemic beta blocker may have additive effects of beta blockade, both systemic and on intraocular pressure).
No products indexed under this heading.

Nicardipine Hydrochloride (Possible atrioventricular conduction disturbances, left ventricular failure, or hypotension when used concurrently). Products include:
Cardene Capsules ... 2095
Cardene I.V. ... 2709
Cardene SR Capsules ... 2097

Nifedipine (Possible atrioventricular conduction disturbances, left ventricular failure, or hypotension when used concurrently). Products include:
Adalat Capsules (10 mg and 20 mg) ... 587
Adalat CC ... 589
Procardia Capsules ... 1971
Procardia XL Extended Release Tablets ... 1972

Nimodipine (Possible atrioventricular conduction disturbances, left ventricular failure, or hypotension when used concurrently). Products include:
Nimotop Capsules ... 610

Nisoldipine (Possible atrioventricular conduction disturbances, left ventricular failure, or hypotension when used concurrently).
No products indexed under this heading.

Penbutolol Sulfate (Concurrent use with systemic beta blocker may have additive effects of beta blockade, both systemic and on intraocular pressure). Products include:
Levatol ... 2403

(▣ Described in PDR For Nonprescription Drugs) (⊙ Described in PDR For Ophthalmology)

1035 **Interactions Index** **Timoptic**

Pindolol (Concurrent use with systemic beta blocker may have additive effects of beta blockade, both systemic and on intraocular pressure). Products include:

Visken Tablets 2299

Propranolol Hydrochloride (Concurrent use with systemic beta blocker may have additive effects of beta blockade, both systemic and on intraocular pressure). Products include:

Inderal 2728
Inderal LA Long Acting Capsules 2730
Inderide Tablets 2732
Inderide LA Long Acting Capsules .. 2734

Rauwolfia Serpentina (Possible additive effects and the production of hypotension and/or bradycardia).

No products indexed under this heading.

Rescinnamine (Possible additive effects and the production of hypotension and/or bradycardia).

No products indexed under this heading.

Reserpine (Possible additive effects and the production of hypotension and/or bradycardia). Products include:

Diupres Tablets 1650
Hydropres Tablets 1675
Ser-Ap-Es Tablets 849

Sotalol Hydrochloride (Concurrent use with systemic beta blocker may have additive effects of beta blockade, both systemic and on intraocular pressure). Products include:

Betapace Tablets 641

Timolol Hemihydrate (Concurrent use with systemic beta blocker may have additive effects of beta blockade, both systemic and on intraocular pressure). Products include:

Betimol 0.25%, 0.5% .... ◉ 261

Tolazamide (Beta blocking agents, usually systemic, may mask the sign and symptoms of acute hypoglycemia).

No products indexed under this heading.

Tolbutamide (Beta blocking agents, usually systemic, may mask the sign and symptoms of acute hypoglycemia).

No products indexed under this heading.

Verapamil Hydrochloride (Possible atrioventricular conduction disturbances, left ventricular failure, or hypotension when used concurrently). Products include:

Calan SR Caplets 2422
Calan Tablets 2419
Isoptin Injectable 1344
Isoptin Oral Tablets 1346
Isoptin SR Tablets 1348
Verelan Capsules 1410
Verelan Capsules 2824

TIMOPTIC STERILE OPHTHALMIC SOLUTION

(Timolol Maleate) 1751

May interact with general anesthetics, beta blockers, catecholamine depleting drugs, calcium channel blockers, cardiac glycosides, and certain other agents. Compounds in these categories include:

Acebutolol Hydrochloride (Concurrent use with systemic beta blocker may have additive effects of beta blockade, both systemic and on intraocular pressure). Products include:

Sectral Capsules 2807

Amlodipine Besylate (Possible atrioventricular conduction disturbances, left ventricular failure, or hypotension when used concurrently). Products include:

Lotrel Capsules 840
Norvasc Tablets 1940

Atenolol (Concurrent use with systemic beta blocker may have additive effects of beta blockade, both systemic and on intraocular pressure). Products include:

Tenoretic Tablets 2845
Tenormin Tablets and I.V. Injection 2847

Bepridil Hydrochloride (Possible atrioventricular conduction disturbances, left ventricular failure, or hypotension when used concurrently). Products include:

Vascor (200, 300 and 400 mg) Tablets 1587

Betaxolol Hydrochloride (Concurrent use with systemic beta blocker may have additive effects of beta blockade, both systemic and on intraocular pressure; concurrent use of two ophthalmic beta blockers is not recommended). Products include:

Betoptic Ophthalmic Solution 469
Betoptic S Ophthalmic Suspension 471
Kerlone Tablets 2436

Bisoprolol Fumarate (Concurrent use with systemic beta blocker may have additive effects of beta blockade, both systemic and on intraocular pressure). Products include:

Zebeta Tablets 1413
Ziac 1415

Carteolol Hydrochloride (Concurrent use with systemic beta blocker may have additive effects of beta blockade, both systemic and on intraocular pressure; concurrent use of two ophthalmic beta blockers is not recommended). Products include:

Cartrol Tablets 410
Ocupress Ophthalmic Solution, 1% Sterile .... ◉ 309

Chlorpropamide (Beta blocking agents, usually systemic, may mask the sign and symptoms of acute hypoglycemia). Products include:

Diabinese Tablets 1935

Deserpidine (Possible additive effects and the production of hypotension and/or bradycardia).

No products indexed under this heading.

Deslanoside (Coadministration with digitalis and calcium antagonists may have additive effects in prolonging atrioventricular conduction time).

No products indexed under this heading.

Digitoxin (Coadministration with digitalis and calcium antagonists may have additive effects in prolonging atrioventricular conduction time). Products include:

Crystodigin Tablets 1433

Digoxin (Coadministration with digitalis and calcium antagonists may have additive effects in prolonging atrioventricular conduction time). Products include:

Lanoxicaps 1117
Lanoxin Elixir Pediatric 1120
Lanoxin Injection 1123
Lanoxin Injection Pediatric 1126
Lanoxin Tablets 1128

Diltiazem Hydrochloride (Possible atrioventricular conduction disturbances, left ventricular failure, or hypotension when used concurrently). Products include:

Cardizem CD Capsules 1506
Cardizem SR Capsules 1510
Cardizem Injectable 1508
Cardizem Tablets 1512
Dilacor XR Extended-release Capsules 2018

Epinephrine (Patients with a history of atopy or anaphylactic reactions to a variety of allergens may be unresponsive to the usual dose of injectable epinephrine used to treat allergic reactions). Products include:

Bronkaid Mist .... ▣ 717
EPIFRIN .... ◉ 239
EpiPen 790
Marcaine Hydrochloride with Epinephrine 1:200,000 2316
Primatene Mist .... ▣ 873
Sensorcaine with Epinephrine Injection 559
Sus-Phrine Injection 1019
Xylocaine with Epinephrine Injections 567

Epinephrine Bitartrate (Patients with a history of atopy or anaphylactic reactions to a variety of allergens may be unresponsive to the usual dose of injectable epinephrine used to treat allergic reactions). Products include:

Bronkaid Mist Suspension .... ▣ 718
Sensorcaine-MPF with Epinephrine Injection 559

Esmolol Hydrochloride (Concurrent use with systemic beta blocker may have additive effects of beta blockade, both systemic and on intraocular pressure). Products include:

Brevibloc Injection 1808

Felodipine (Possible atrioventricular conduction disturbances, left ventricular failure, or hypotension when used concurrently). Products include:

Plendil Extended-Release Tablets 527

Glipizide (Beta blocking agents, usually systemic, may mask the sign and symptoms of acute hypoglycemia). Products include:

Glucotrol Tablets 1967
Glucotrol XL Extended Release Tablets 1968

Glyburide (Beta blocking agents, usually systemic, may mask the sign and symptoms of acute hypoglycemia). Products include:

DiaBeta Tablets 1239
Glynase PresTab Tablets 2609
Micronase Tablets 2623

Guanethidine Monosulfate (Possible additive effects and the production of hypotension and/or bradycardia). Products include:

Esimil Tablets 822
Ismelin Tablets 827

Insulin, Human (Beta blocking agents, usually systemic, may mask the sign and symptoms of acute hypoglycemia).

No products indexed under this heading.

Insulin, Human Isophane Suspension (Beta blocking agents, usually systemic, may mask the sign and symptoms of acute hypoglycemia). Products include:

Novolin N Human Insulin 10 ml Vials 1795

Insulin, Human NPH (Beta blocking agents, usually systemic, may mask the sign and symptoms of acute hypoglycemia). Products include:

Humulin N, 100 Units 1448
Novolin N PenFill Cartridges Durable Insulin Delivery System 1798
Novolin N Prefilled Syringe Disposable Insulin Delivery System 1798

Insulin, Human Regular (Beta blocking agents, usually systemic, may mask the sign and symptoms of acute hypoglycemia). Products include:

Humulin R, 100 Units 1449
Novolin R Human Insulin 10 ml Vials 1795
Novolin R PenFill Cartridges Durable Insulin Delivery System 1798
Novolin R Prefilled Syringe Disposable Insulin Delivery System 1798
Velosulin BR Human Insulin 10 ml Vials 1795

Insulin, Human, Zinc Suspension (Beta blocking agents, usually systemic, may mask the sign and symptoms of acute hypoglycemia). Products include:

Humulin L, 100 Units 1446
Humulin U, 100 Units 1450
Novolin L Human Insulin 10 ml Vials 1795

Insulin, NPH (Beta blocking agents, usually systemic, may mask the sign and symptoms of acute hypoglycemia). Products include:

NPH, 100 Units 1450
Pork NPH, 100 Units 1452
Purified Pork NPH Isophane Insulin 1801

Insulin, Regular (Beta blocking agents, usually systemic, may mask the sign and symptoms of acute hypoglycemia). Products include:

Regular, 100 Units 1450
Pork Regular, 100 Units 1452
Pork Regular (Concentrated), 500 Units 1453
Purified Pork Regular Insulin 1801

Insulin, Zinc Crystals (Beta blocking agents, usually systemic, may mask the sign and symptoms of acute hypoglycemia). Products include:

NPH, 100 Units 1450

Insulin, Zinc Suspension (Beta blocking agents, usually systemic, may mask the sign and symptoms of acute hypoglycemia). Products include:

Iletin I 1450
Lente, 100 Units 1450
Iletin II 1452
Pork Lente, 100 Units 1452
Purified Pork Lente Insulin 1801

Isradipine (Possible atrioventricular conduction disturbances, left ventricular failure, or hypotension when used concurrently). Products include:

DynaCirc Capsules 2256

Labetalol Hydrochloride (Concurrent use with systemic beta blocker may have additive effects of beta blockade, both systemic and on intraocular pressure). Products include:

Normodyne Injection 2377
Normodyne Tablets 2379
Trandate 1185

Levobunolol Hydrochloride (Concurrent use of two ophthalmic beta blockers is not recommended). Products include:

Betagan .... ◉ 233

Metipranolol Hydrochloride (Concurrent use of two ophthalmic beta blockers is not recommended). Products include:

OptiPranolol (Metipranolol 0.3%) Sterile Ophthalmic Solution .... ◉ 258

Metoprolol Succinate (Concurrent use with systemic beta blocker may have additive effects of beta blockade, both systemic and on intraocular pressure). Products include:

Toprol-XL Tablets 565

IMPORTANT NOTE: Always consult each drug listing in the patient's regimen for possible interactions.

Metoprolol Tartrate (Concurrent use with systemic beta blocker may have additive effects of beta blockade, both systemic and on intraocular pressure). Products include:

Lopressor Ampuls 830
Lopressor HCT Tablets 832
Lopressor Tablets 830

Nadolol (Concurrent use with systemic beta blocker may have additive effects of beta blockade, both systemic and on intraocular pressure).

No products indexed under this heading.

Nicardipine Hydrochloride (Possible atrioventricular conduction disturbances, left ventricular failure, or hypotension when used concurrently). Products include:

Cardene Capsules 2095
Cardene I.V. 2709
Cardene SR Capsules 2097

Nifedipine (Possible atrioventricular conduction disturbances, left ventricular failure, or hypotension when used concurrently). Products include:

Adalat Capsules (10 mg and 20 mg) 587
Adalat CC 589
Procardia Capsules 1971
Procardia XL Extended Release Tablets 1972

Nimodipine (Possible atrioventricular conduction disturbances, left ventricular failure, or hypotension when used concurrently). Products include:

Nimotop Capsules 610

Nisoldipine (Possible atrioventricular conduction disturbances, left ventricular failure, or hypotension when used concurrently).

No products indexed under this heading.

Penbutolol Sulfate (Concurrent use with systemic beta blocker may have additive effects of beta blockade, both systemic and on intraocular pressure). Products include:

Levatol 2403

Pindolol (Concurrent use with systemic beta blocker may have additive effects of beta blockade, both systemic and on intraocular pressure). Products include:

Visken Tablets 2299

Propranolol Hydrochloride (Concurrent use with systemic beta blocker may have additive effects of beta blockade, both systemic and on intraocular pressure). Products include:

Inderal 2728
Inderal LA Long Acting Capsules 2730
Inderide Tablets 2732
Inderide LA Long Acting Capsules 2734

Rauwolfia Serpentina (Possible additive effects and the production of hypotension and/or bradycardia).

No products indexed under this heading.

Rescinnamine (Possible additive effects and the production of hypotension and/or bradycardia).

No products indexed under this heading.

Reserpine (Possible additive effects and the production of hypotension and/or bradycardia). Products include:

Diupres Tablets 1650
Hydropres Tablets 1675
Ser-Ap-Es Tablets 849

Sotalol Hydrochloride (Concurrent use with systemic beta blocker may have additive effects of beta blockade, both systemic and on intraocular pressure). Products include:

Betapace Tablets 641

Timolol Hemihydrate (Concurrent use with systemic beta blocker may have additive effects of beta blockade, both systemic and on intraocular pressure). Products include:

Betimol 0.25%, 0.5% .... ◉ 261

Tolazamide (Beta blocking agents, usually systemic, may mask the sign and symptoms of acute hypoglycemia).

No products indexed under this heading.

Tolbutamide (Beta blocking agents, usually systemic, may mask the sign and symptoms of acute hypoglycemia).

No products indexed under this heading.

Verapamil Hydrochloride (Possible atrioventricular conduction disturbances, left ventricular failure, or hypotension when used concurrently). Products include:

Calan SR Caplets 2422
Calan Tablets 2419
Isoptin Injectable 1344
Isoptin Oral Tablets 1346
Isoptin SR Tablets 1348
Verelan Capsules 1410
Verelan Capsules 2824

TIMOPTIC-XE

(Timolol Maleate) 1755

May interact with beta blockers, calcium channel blockers, catecholamine depleting drugs, cardiac glycosides, insulin, oral hypoglycemic agents, and certain other agents. Compounds in these categories include:

Acarbose (Beta blocking agents, usually systemic, may mask the sign and symptoms of acute hypoglycemia).

No products indexed under this heading.

Acebutolol Hydrochloride (Concurrent use with systemic beta blocker may have additive effects of beta blockade, both systemic and on intraocular pressure). Products include:

Sectral Capsules 2807

Amlodipine Besylate (Possible atrioventricular conduction disturbances, left ventricular failure, or hypotension when used concurrently). Products include:

Lotrel Capsules 840
Norvasc Tablets 1940

Atenolol (Concurrent use with systemic beta blocker may have additive effects of beta blockade, both systemic and on intraocular pressure). Products include:

Tenoretic Tablets 2845
Tenormin Tablets and I.V. Injection 2847

Bepridil Hydrochloride (Possible atrioventricular conduction disturbances, left ventricular failure, or hypotension when used concurrently). Products include:

Vascor (200, 300 and 400 mg) Tablets 1587

Betaxolol Hydrochloride (Concurrent use with systemic beta blocker may have additive effects of beta blockade, both systemic and on intraocular pressure; concurrent use of two ophthalmic beta blockers is not recommended). Products include:

Betoptic Ophthalmic Solution 469
Betoptic S Ophthalmic Suspension 471
Kerlone Tablets 2436

Bisoprolol Fumarate (Concurrent use with systemic beta blocker may have additive effects of beta blockade, both systemic and on intraocular pressure). Products include:

Zebeta Tablets 1413
Ziac 1415

Carteolol Hydrochloride (Concurrent use with systemic beta blocker may have additive effects of beta blockade, both systemic and on intraocular pressure; concurrent use of two ophthalmic beta blockers is not recommended). Products include:

Cartrol Tablets 410
Ocupress Ophthalmic Solution, 1% Sterile .... ◉ 309

Chlorpropamide (Beta blocking agents, usually systemic, may mask the sign and symptoms of acute hypoglycemia). Products include:

Diabinese Tablets 1935

Deserpidine (Possible additive effects and the production of hypotension and/or bradycardia).

No products indexed under this heading.

Deslanoside (Coadministration with digitalis and calcium antagonists may have additive effects in prolonging atrioventricular conduction time).

No products indexed under this heading.

Digitoxin (Coadministration with digitalis and calcium antagonists may have additive effects in prolonging atrioventricular conduction time). Products include:

Crystodigin Tablets 1433

Digoxin (Coadministration with digitalis and calcium antagonists may have additive effects in prolonging atrioventricular conduction time). Products include:

Lanoxicaps 1117
Lanoxin Elixir Pediatric 1120
Lanoxin Injection 1123
Lanoxin Injection Pediatric 1126
Lanoxin Tablets 1128

Diltiazem Hydrochloride (Possible atrioventricular conduction disturbances, left ventricular failure, or hypotension when used concurrently). Products include:

Cardizem CD Capsules 1506
Cardizem SR Capsules 1510
Cardizem Injectable 1508
Cardizem Tablets 1512
Dilacor XR Extended-release Capsules 2018

Epinephrine (Patients with a history of atopy or anaphylactic reactions to a variety of allergens may be unresponsive to the usual dose of injectable epinephrine used to treat allergic reactions). Products include:

Bronkaid Mist .... ▣ 717
EPIFRIN .... ◉ 239
EpiPen 790
Marcaine Hydrochloride with Epinephrine 1:200,000 2316
Primatene Mist .... ▣ 873
Sensorcaine with Epinephrine Injection 559
Sus-Phrine Injection 1019
Xylocaine with Epinephrine Injections 567

Epinephrine Bitartrate (Patients with a history of atopy or anaphylactic reactions to a variety of allergens may be unresponsive to the usual dose of injectable epinephrine used to treat allergic reactions). Products include:

Bronkaid Mist Suspension .... ▣ 718
Sensorcaine-MPF with Epinephrine Injection 559

Esmolol Hydrochloride (Concurrent use with systemic beta blocker may have additive effects of beta blockade, both systemic and on intraocular pressure). Products include:

Brevibloc Injection 1808

Felodipine (Possible atrioventricular conduction disturbances, left ventricular failure, or hypotension when used concurrently). Products include:

Plendil Extended-Release Tablets 527

Glipizide (Beta blocking agents, usually systemic, may mask the sign and symptoms of acute hypoglycemia). Products include:

Glucotrol Tablets 1967
Glucotrol XL Extended Release Tablets 1968

Glyburide (Beta blocking agents, usually systemic, may mask the sign and symptoms of acute hypoglycemia). Products include:

DiaBeta Tablets 1239
Glynase PresTab Tablets 2609
Micronase Tablets 2623

Guanethidine Monosulfate (Possible additive effects and the production of hypotension and/or bradycardia). Products include:

Esimil Tablets 822
Ismelin Tablets 827

Insulin, Human (Beta blocking agents, usually systemic, may mask the sign and symptoms of acute hypoglycemia).

No products indexed under this heading.

Insulin, Human Isophane Suspension (Beta blocking agents, usually systemic, may mask the sign and symptoms of acute hypoglycemia). Products include:

Novolin N Human Insulin 10 ml Vials 1795

Insulin, Human NPH (Beta blocking agents, usually systemic, may mask the sign and symptoms of acute hypoglycemia). Products include:

Humulin N, 100 Units 1448
Novolin N PenFill Cartridges Durable Insulin Delivery System 1798
Novolin N Prefilled Syringe Disposable Insulin Delivery System 1798

Insulin, Human Regular (Beta blocking agents, usually systemic, may mask the sign and symptoms of acute hypoglycemia). Products include:

Humulin R, 100 Units 1449
Novolin R Human Insulin 10 ml Vials 1795
Novolin R PenFill Cartridges Durable Insulin Delivery System 1798
Novolin R Prefilled Syringe Disposable Insulin Delivery System 1798
Velosulin BR Human Insulin 10 ml Vials 1795

Insulin, Human, Zinc Suspension (Beta blocking agents, usually systemic, may mask the sign and symptoms of acute hypoglycemia). Products include:

Humulin L, 100 Units 1446
Humulin U, 100 Units 1450
Novolin L Human Insulin 10 ml Vials 1795

(▣ Described in PDR For Nonprescription Drugs) (◉ Described in PDR For Ophthalmology)

1037 Interactions Index Tobramycin Sulfate

Insulin, NPH (Beta blocking agents, usually systemic, may mask the sign and symptoms of acute hypoglycemia). Products include:
NPH, 100 Units 1450
Pork NPH, 100 Units 1452
Purified Pork NPH Isophane Insulin 1801
Insulin, Regular (Beta blocking agents, usually systemic, may mask the sign and symptoms of acute hypoglycemia). Products include:
Regular, 100 Units 1450
Pork Regular, 100 Units 1452
Pork Regular (Concentrated), 500 Units 1453
Purified Pork Regular Insulin 1801
Insulin, Zinc Crystals (Beta blocking agents, usually systemic, may mask the sign and symptoms of acute hypoglycemia). Products include:
NPH, 100 Units 1450
Insulin, Zinc Suspension (Beta blocking agents, usually systemic, may mask the sign and symptoms of acute hypoglycemia). Products include:
Iletin I 1450
Lente, 100 Units 1450
Iletin II 1452
Pork Lente, 100 Units 1452
Purified Pork Lente Insulin 1801
Isradipine (Possible atrioventricular conduction disturbances, left ventricular failure, or hypotension when used concurrently). Products include:
DynaCirc Capsules 2256
Labetalol Hydrochloride (Concurrent use with systemic beta blocker may have additive effects of beta blockade, both systemic and on intraocular pressure). Products include:
Normodyne Injection 2377
Normodyne Tablets 2379
Trandate 1185
Levobunolol Hydrochloride (Concurrent use of two ophthalmic beta blockers is not recommended). Products include:
Betagan .... ◉ 233
Metformin Hydrochloride (Beta blocking agents, usually systemic, may mask the sign and symptoms of acute hypoglycemia). Products include:
Glucophage 752
Metipranolol Hydrochloride (Concurrent use of two ophthalmic beta blockers is not recommended). Products include:
OptiPranolol (Metipranolol 0.3%) Sterile Ophthalmic Solution .... ◉ 258
Metoprolol Succinate (Concurrent use with systemic beta blocker may have additive effects of beta blockade, both systemic and on intraocular pressure). Products include:
Toprol-XL Tablets 565
Metoprolol Tartrate (Concurrent use with systemic beta blocker may have additive effects of beta blockade, both systemic and on intraocular pressure). Products include:
Lopressor Ampuls 830
Lopressor HCT Tablets 832
Lopressor Tablets 830
Nadolol (Concurrent use with systemic beta blocker may have additive effects of beta blockade, both systemic and on intraocular pressure).
No products indexed under this heading.
Nicardipine Hydrochloride (Possible atrioventricular conduction disturbances, left ventricular failure, or hypotension when used concurrently). Products include:
Cardene Capsules 2095
Cardene I.V. 2709
Cardene SR Capsules 2097
Nifedipine (Possible atrioventricular conduction disturbances, left ventricular failure, or hypotension when used concurrently). Products include:
Adalat Capsules (10 mg and 20 mg) 587
Adalat CC 589
Procardia Capsules 1971
Procardia XL Extended Release Tablets 1972
Nimodipine (Possible atrioventricular conduction disturbances, left ventricular failure, or hypotension when used concurrently). Products include:
Nimotop Capsules 610
Nisoldipine (Possible atrioventricular conduction disturbances, left ventricular failure, or hypotension when used concurrently).
No products indexed under this heading.
Penbutolol Sulfate (Concurrent use with systemic beta blocker may have additive effects of beta blockade, both systemic and on intraocular pressure). Products include:
Levatol 2403
Pindolol (Concurrent use with systemic beta blocker may have additive effects of beta blockade, both systemic and on intraocular pressure). Products include:
Visken Tablets 2299
Propranolol Hydrochloride (Concurrent use with systemic beta blocker may have additive effects of beta blockade, both systemic and on intraocular pressure). Products include:
Inderal 2728
Inderal LA Long Acting Capsules 2730
Inderide Tablets 2732
Inderide LA Long Acting Capsules 2734
Rauwolfia Serpentina (Possible additive effects and the production of hypotension and/or bradycardia).
No products indexed under this heading.
Rescinnamine (Possible additive effects and the production of hypotension and/or bradycardia).
No products indexed under this heading.
Reserpine (Possible additive effects and the production of hypotension and/or bradycardia). Products include:
Diupres Tablets 1650
Hydropres Tablets 1675
Ser-Ap-Es Tablets 849
Sotalol Hydrochloride (Concurrent use with systemic beta blocker may have additive effects of beta blockade, both systemic and on intraocular pressure). Products include:
Betapace Tablets 641
Timolol Hemihydrate (Concurrent use with systemic beta blocker may have additive effects of beta blockade, both systemic and on intraocular pressure). Products include:
Betimol 0.25%, 0.5% .... ◉ 261
Tolazamide (Beta blocking agents, usually systemic, may mask the sign and symptoms of acute hypoglycemia).
No products indexed under this heading.
Tolbutamide (Beta blocking agents, usually systemic, may mask the sign and symptoms of acute hypoglycemia).
No products indexed under this heading.
Verapamil Hydrochloride (Possible atrioventricular conduction disturbances, left ventricular failure, or hypotension when used concurrently). Products include:
Calan SR Caplets 2422
Calan Tablets 2419
Isoptin Injectable 1344
Isoptin Oral Tablets 1346
Isoptin SR Tablets 1348
Verelan Capsules 1410
Verelan Capsules 2824

TINACTIN AEROSOL LIQUID 1%
(Tolnaftate) .... ▣ 809
None cited in PDR database.

TINACTIN AEROSOL POWDER 1%
(Tolnaftate) .... ▣ 809
None cited in PDR database.

TINACTIN ANTIFUNGAL CREAM, SOLUTION & POWDER 1%
(Tolnaftate) .... ▣ 809
None cited in PDR database.

TINACTIN DEODORANT POWDER AEROSOL 1%
(Tolnaftate) .... ▣ 809
None cited in PDR database.

TINACTIN JOCK ITCH CREAM 1%
(Tolnaftate) .... ▣ 809
None cited in PDR database.

TINACTIN JOCK ITCH SPRAY POWDER 1%
(Tolnaftate) .... ▣ 809
None cited in PDR database.

TING ANTIFUNGAL CREAM
(Tolnaftate) .... ▣ 650
None cited in PDR database.

TING ANTIFUNGAL POWDER
(Tolnaftate) .... ▣ 650
None cited in PDR database.

TING ANTIFUNGAL SPRAY LIQUID
(Tolnaftate) .... ▣ 650
None cited in PDR database.

TING ANTIFUNGAL SPRAY POWDER
(Tolnaftate) .... ▣ 650
None cited in PDR database.

TITRALAC ANTACID REGULAR
(Calcium Carbonate) .... ▣ 672
None cited in PDR database.

TITRALAC ANTACID EXTRA STRENGTH
(Calcium Carbonate) .... ▣ 672
None cited in PDR database.

TITRALAC PLUS LIQUID
(Calcium Carbonate, Simethicone) .. ▣ 672
None cited in PDR database.

TITRALAC PLUS TABLETS
(Calcium Carbonate, Simethicone) .. ▣ 672
None cited in PDR database.

TOBRADEX OPHTHALMIC SUSPENSION AND OINTMENT
(Dexamethasone, Tobramycin) 473
May interact with aminoglycosides. Compounds in this category include:

Amikacin Sulfate (Monitor the total serum concentration if administered with systemic aminoglycoside). Products include:
Amikacin Sulfate Injection, USP 960
Amikin Injectable 501
Gentamicin Sulfate (Monitor the total serum concentration if administered with systemic aminoglycoside). Products include:
Garamycin Injectable 2360
Genoptic Sterile Ophthalmic Solution .... ◉ 243
Genoptic Sterile Ophthalmic Ointment .... ◉ 243
Gentacidin Ointment .... ◉ 264
Gentacidin Solution .... ◉ 264
Gentak .... ◉ 208
Pred-G Liquifilm Sterile Ophthalmic Suspension .... ◉ 251
Pred-G S.O.P. Sterile Ophthalmic Ointment .... ◉ 252
Kanamycin Sulfate (Monitor the total serum concentration if administered with systemic aminoglycoside).
No products indexed under this heading.
Streptomycin Sulfate (Monitor the total serum concentration if administered with systemic aminoglycoside). Products include:
Streptomycin Sulfate Injection 2208
Tobramycin Sulfate (Monitor the total serum concentration if administered with systemic aminoglycoside). Products include:
Nebcin Vials, Hyporets & ADD-Vantage 1464
Tobramycin Sulfate Injection 968

TOBRAMYCIN SULFATE INJECTION
(Tobramycin Sulfate) 968
May interact with cephalosporins, aminoglycosides, and certain other agents. Compounds in these categories include:

Amikacin Sulfate (Concurrent and sequential use should be avoided because of increased potential for neurotoxicity and/or nephrotoxicity). Products include:
Amikacin Sulfate Injection, USP 960
Amikin Injectable 501
Bumetanide (Enhances toxicity of aminoglycosides; concurrent administration is not recommended). Products include:
Bumex 2093
Cefaclor (Concomitant administration may increase the incidence of nephrotoxicity). Products include:
Ceclor Pulvules & Suspension 1431
Cefadroxil Monohydrate (Concomitant administration may increase the incidence of nephrotoxicity). Products include:
Duricef 748
Cefamandole Nafate (Concomitant administration may increase the incidence of nephrotoxicity). Products include:
Mandol Vials, Faspak & ADD-Vantage 1461

IMPORTANT NOTE: Always consult each drug listing in the patient's regimen for possible interactions.

Tobramycin Sulfate — Interactions Index — 1038

Cefazolin Sodium (Concomitant administration may increase the incidence of nephrotoxicity). Products include:
Ancef Injection 2465
Kefzol Vials, Faspak & ADD-Vantage 1456

Cefixime (Concomitant administration may increase the incidence of nephrotoxicity). Products include:
Suprax 1399

Cefmetazole Sodium (Concomitant administration may increase the incidence of nephrotoxicity). Products include:
Zefazone 2654

Cefonicid Sodium (Concomitant administration may increase the incidence of nephrotoxicity). Products include:
Monocid Injection 2497

Cefoperazone Sodium (Concomitant administration may increase the incidence of nephrotoxicity). Products include:
Cefobid Intravenous/Intramuscular 2189
Cefobid Pharmacy Bulk Package - Not for Direct Infusion 2192

Ceforanide (Concomitant administration may increase the incidence of nephrotoxicity).
No products indexed under this heading.

Cefotaxime Sodium (Concomitant administration may increase the incidence of nephrotoxicity). Products include:
Claforan Sterile and Injection 1235

Cefotetan (Concomitant administration may increase the incidence of nephrotoxicity). Products include:
Cefotan 2829

Cefoxitin Sodium (Concomitant administration may increase the incidence of nephrotoxicity). Products include:
Mefoxin 1691
Mefoxin Premixed Intravenous Solution 1694

Cefpodoxime Proxetil (Concomitant administration may increase the incidence of nephrotoxicity). Products include:
Vantin for Oral Suspension and Vantin Tablets 2646

Cefprozil (Concomitant administration may increase the incidence of nephrotoxicity). Products include:
Cefzil Tablets and Oral Suspension 746

Ceftazidime (Concomitant administration may increase the incidence of nephrotoxicity). Products include:
Ceptaz 1081
Fortaz 1100
Tazicef for Injection 2519
Tazidime Vials, Faspak & ADD-Vantage 1478

Ceftizoxime Sodium (Concomitant administration may increase the incidence of nephrotoxicity). Products include:
Cefizox for Intramuscular or Intravenous Use 1034

Ceftriaxone Sodium (Concomitant administration may increase the incidence of nephrotoxicity). Products include:
Rocephin Injectable Vials, ADD-Vantage, Galaxy Container 2142

Cefuroxime Axetil (Concomitant administration may increase the incidence of nephrotoxicity). Products include:
Ceftin 1078

Cefuroxime Sodium (Concomitant administration may increase the incidence of nephrotoxicity). Products include:
Kefurox Vials, Faspak & ADD-Vantage 1454
Zinacef 1211

Cephalexin (Concomitant administration may increase the incidence of nephrotoxicity). Products include:
Keflex Pulvules & Oral Suspension 914

Cephaloridine (Concurrent and sequential use should be avoided because of increased potential for neurotoxicity and/or nephrotoxicity).

Cephalothin Sodium (Concomitant administration may increase the incidence of nephrotoxicity).

Cephapirin Sodium (Concomitant administration may increase the incidence of nephrotoxicity).
No products indexed under this heading.

Cephradine (Concomitant administration may increase the incidence of nephrotoxicity).
No products indexed under this heading.

Cisplatin (Concurrent and sequential use should be avoided because of increased potential for neurotoxicity and/or nephrotoxicity). Products include:
Platinol 708
Platinol-AQ Injection 710

Colistin Sulfate (Concurrent and sequential use should be avoided because of increased potential for neurotoxicity and/or nephrotoxicity). Products include:
Coly-Mycin S Otic w/Neomycin & Hydrocortisone 1906

Ethacrynic Acid (Enhances toxicity of aminoglycosides; concurrent administration is not recommended). Products include:
Edecrin Tablets 1657

Furosemide (Enhances toxicity of aminoglycosides; concurrent administration is not recommended). Products include:
Lasix Injection, Oral Solution and Tablets 1240

Gentamicin Sulfate (Concurrent and sequential use should be avoided because of increased potential for neurotoxicity and/or nephrotoxicity). Products include:
Garamycin Injectable 2360
Genoptic Sterile Ophthalmic Solution .... ⊙ 243
Genoptic Sterile Ophthalmic Ointment .... ⊙ 243
Gentacidin Ointment .... ⊙ 264
Gentacidin Solution .... ⊙ 264
Gentak .... ⊙ 208
Pred-G Liquifilm Sterile Ophthalmic Suspension .... ⊙ 251
Pred-G S.O.P. Sterile Ophthalmic Ointment .... ⊙ 252

Kanamycin Sulfate (Concurrent and sequential use should be avoided because of increased potential for neurotoxicity and/or nephrotoxicity).
No products indexed under this heading.

Loracarbef (Concomitant administration may increase the incidence of nephrotoxicity). Products include:
Lorabid Suspension and Pulvules 1459

Polymyxin Preparations (Concurrent and sequential use should be avoided because of increased potential for neurotoxicity and/or nephrotoxicity).

Streptomycin Sulfate (Concurrent and sequential use should be avoided because of increased potential for neurotoxicity and/or nephrotoxicity). Products include:
Streptomycin Sulfate Injection 2208

Tobramycin (Concurrent and sequential use should be avoided because of increased potential for neurotoxicity and/or nephrotoxicity). Products include:
AKTOB .... ⊙ 206
TobraDex Ophthalmic Suspension and Ointment 473
Tobrex Ophthalmic Ointment and Solution .... ⊙ 229

Vancomycin Hydrochloride (Concurrent and sequential use should be avoided because of increased potential for neurotoxicity and/or nephrotoxicity). Products include:
Vancocin HCl, Oral Solution & Pulvules 1483
Vancocin HCl, Vials & ADD-Vantage 1481

Viomycin (Concurrent and sequential use should be avoided because of increased potential for neurotoxicity and/or nephrotoxicity).

TOBREX OPHTHALMIC OINTMENT AND SOLUTION
(Tobramycin) .... ⊙ 229
May interact with aminoglycosides. Compounds in this category include:

Amikacin Sulfate (If topical ocular tobramycin is administered concomitantly with systemic aminoglycosides, care should be taken to monitor the total serum concentration). Products include:
Amikacin Sulfate Injection, USP 960
Amikin Injectable 501

Gentamicin Sulfate (If topical ocular tobramycin is administered concomitantly with systemic aminoglycosides, care should be taken to monitor the total serum concentration). Products include:
Garamycin Injectable 2360
Genoptic Sterile Ophthalmic Solution .... ⊙ 243
Genoptic Sterile Ophthalmic Ointment .... ⊙ 243
Gentacidin Ointment .... ⊙ 264
Gentacidin Solution .... ⊙ 264
Gentak .... ⊙ 208
Pred-G Liquifilm Sterile Ophthalmic Suspension .... ⊙ 251
Pred-G S.O.P. Sterile Ophthalmic Ointment .... ⊙ 252

Kanamycin Sulfate (If topical ocular tobramycin is administered concomitantly with systemic aminoglycosides, care should be taken to monitor the total serum concentration).
No products indexed under this heading.

Streptomycin Sulfate (If topical ocular tobramycin is administered concomitantly with systemic aminoglycosides, care should be taken to monitor the total serum concentration). Products include:
Streptomycin Sulfate Injection 2208

TODAY VAGINAL CONTRACEPTIVE SPONGE
(Nonoxynol-9) .... ▣ 874
None cited in PDR database.

TOFRANIL AMPULS
(Imipramine Hydrochloride) 854
May interact with central nervous system depressants, anticholinergics, sympathomimetics, barbiturates, monoamine oxidase inhibitors, thyroid preparations, drugs that inhibit cytochrome p450iid6, antidepressant drugs, phenothiazines, selective serotonin reuptake inhibitors, and certain other agents. Compounds in these categories include:

Albuterol (Avoid concurrent use since tricyclic antidepressants can potentiate the effects of catecholamines). Products include:
Proventil Inhalation Aerosol 2382
Ventolin Inhalation Aerosol and Refill 1197

Albuterol Sulfate (Avoid concurrent use since tricyclic antidepressants can potentiate the effects of catecholamines). Products include:
Airet Solution for Inhalation 452
Proventil Inhalation Solution 0.083% 2384
Proventil Repetabs Tablets 2386
Proventil Solution for Inhalation 0.5% 2383
Proventil Syrup 2385
Proventil Tablets 2386
Ventolin Inhalation Solution 1198
Ventolin Nebules Inhalation Solution 1199
Ventolin Rotacaps for Inhalation 1200
Ventolin Syrup 1202
Ventolin Tablets 1203
Volmax Extended-Release Tablets .. 1788

Alfentanil Hydrochloride (Imipramine may potentiate the effects of CNS depressant drugs). Products include:
Alfenta Injection 1286

Alprazolam (Imipramine may potentiate the effects of CNS depressant drugs). Products include:
Xanax Tablets 2649

Amitriptyline Hydrochloride (Concurrent use with drugs that are substrate for cytochrome $P_{450}IID_6$ may make normal metabolizer resemble poor metabolizer leading to higher than expected plasma concentrations of TCA with resultant toxicity). Products include:
Elavil 2838
Endep Tablets 2174
Etrafon 2355
Limbitrol 2180
Triavil Tablets 1757

Amoxapine (Concurrent use with drugs that are substrate for cytochrome $P_{450}IID_6$ may make normal metabolizer resemble poor metabolizer leading to higher than expected plasma concentrations of TCA with resultant toxicity). Products include:
Asendin Tablets 1369

Aprobarbital (The plasma concentration of imipramine may decrease when the drug is given with barbiturates, a hepatic enzyme inducer; dosage of imipramine may need to be adjusted; imipramine may potentiate the effects of CNS depressant drugs).
No products indexed under this heading.

Atropine Sulfate (Concurrent use may result in pronounced atropine-like effects e.g., paralytic ileus). Products include:
Arco-Lase Plus Tablets 512
Atrohist Plus Tablets 454
Atropine Sulfate Sterile Ophthalmic Solution .... ⊙ 233
Donnatal 2060
Donnatal Extentabs 2061
Donnatal Tablets 2060
Lomotil 2439
Motofen Tablets 784
Urised Tablets 1964

Belladonna Alkaloids (Concurrent use may result in pronounced atropine-like effects e.g., paralytic ileus). Products include:
Bellergal-S Tablets 2250
Hyland's Bed Wetting Tablets .... ▣ 828
Hyland's EnurAid Tablets .... ▣ 829

(▣ Described in PDR For Nonprescription Drugs) (⊙ Described in PDR For Ophthalmology)

Hyland's Teething Tablets .... ⓔⓓ 830

Benztropine Mesylate (Concurrent use may result in pronounced atropine-like effects e.g., paralytic ileus). Products include:

Cogentin 1621

Biperiden Hydrochloride (Concurrent use may result in pronounced atropine-like effects e.g., paralytic ileus). Products include:

Akineton 1333

Buprenorphine (Imipramine may potentiate the effects of CNS depressant drugs). Products include:

Buprenex Injectable 2006

Bupropion Hydrochloride (Concurrent use with drugs that are substrate for cytochrome $P_{450}IID_6$ may make normal metabolizer resemble poor metabolizer leading to higher than expected plasma concentrations of TCA with resultant toxicity). Products include:

Wellbutrin Tablets 1204

Buspirone Hydrochloride (Imipramine may potentiate the effects of CNS depressant drugs). Products include:

BuSpar 737

Butabarbital (The plasma concentration of imipramine may decrease when the drug is given with barbiturates, a hepatic enzyme inducer; dosage of imipramine may need to be adjusted; imipramine may potentiate the effects of CNS depressant drugs).

No products indexed under this heading.

Butalbital (The plasma concentration of imipramine may decrease when the drug is given with barbiturates, a hepatic enzyme inducer; dosage of imipramine may need to be adjusted; imipramine may potentiate the effects of CNS depressant drugs). Products include:

Esgic-plus Tablets 1013
Fioricet Tablets 2258
Fioricet with Codeine Capsules 2260
Fiorinal Capsules 2261
Fiorinal with Codeine Capsules 2262
Fiorinal Tablets 2261
Phrenilin 785
Sedapap Tablets 50 mg/650 mg .. 1543

Chlordiazepoxide (Imipramine may potentiate the effects of CNS depressant drugs). Products include:

Libritabs Tablets 2177
Limbitrol 2180

Chlordiazepoxide Hydrochloride (Imipramine may potentiate the effects of CNS depressant drugs). Products include:

Librax Capsules 2176
Librium Capsules 2178
Librium Injectable 2179

Chlorpromazine (Concurrent use with drugs that are substrate for cytochrome $P_{450}IID_6$ may make normal metabolizer resemble poor metabolizer leading to higher than expected plasma concentrations of TCA with resultant toxicity; imipramine may potentiate the effects of CNS depressant drugs). Products include:

Thorazine Suppositories 2523

Chlorpromazine Hydrochloride (Concurrent use with drugs that are substrate for cytochrome $P_{450}IID_6$ may make normal metabolizer resemble poor metabolizer leading to higher than expected plasma concentrations of TCA with resultant toxicity; imipramine may potentiate the effects of CNS depressant drugs). Products include:

Thorazine 2523

Chlorprothixene (Imipramine may potentiate the effects of CNS depressant drugs).

No products indexed under this heading.

Chlorprothixene Hydrochloride (Imipramine may potentiate the effects of CNS depressant drugs).

No products indexed under this heading.

Cimetidine (The plasma concentration of imipramine may increase when the drug is given with cimetidine, a hepatic enzyme inhibitor; dosage of imipramine may need to be adjusted). Products include:

Tagamet Tablets 2516

Cimetidine Hydrochloride (The plasma concentration of imipramine may increase when the drug is given with cimetidine, a hepatic enzyme inhibitor; dosage of imipramine may need to be adjusted). Products include:

Tagamet 2516

Clidinium Bromide (Concurrent use may result in pronounced atropine-like effects e.g., paralytic ileus). Products include:

Librax Capsules 2176
Quarzan Capsules 2181

Clonidine (Imipramine may block the antihypertensive effect). Products include:

Catapres-TTS 675

Clonidine Hydrochloride (Imipramine may block the antihypertensive effect). Products include:

Catapres Tablets 674
Combipres Tablets 677

Clorazepate Dipotassium (Imipramine may potentiate the effects of CNS depressant drugs). Products include:

Tranxene 451

Clozapine (Imipramine may potentiate the effects of CNS depressant drugs). Products include:

Clozaril Tablets 2252

Codeine Phosphate (Imipramine may potentiate the effects of CNS depressant drugs). Products include:

Actifed with Codeine Cough Syrup.. 1067
Brontex 1981
Deconsal C Expectorant Syrup 456
Deconsal Pediatric Syrup 457
Dimetane-DC Cough Syrup 2059
Empirin with Codeine Tablets............ 1093
Fioricet with Codeine Capsules 2260
Fiorinal with Codeine Capsules 2262
Isoclor Expectorant 990
Novahistine DH 2462
Novahistine Expectorant 2463
Nucofed 2051
Phenergan with Codeine 2777
Phenergan VC with Codeine 2781
Robitussin A-C Syrup 2073
Robitussin-DAC Syrup 2074
Ryna .... ⓔⓓ 841
Soma Compound w/Codeine Tablets 2676
Tussi-Organidin NR Liquid and S NR Liquid 2677
Tylenol with Codeine 1583

Desflurane (Imipramine may potentiate the effects of CNS depressant drugs). Products include:

Suprane 1813

Desipramine Hydrochloride (Concurrent use with drugs that are substrate for cytochrome $P_{450}IID_6$ may make normal metabolizer resemble poor metabolizer leading to higher than expected plasma concentrations of TCA with resultant toxicity). Products include:

Norpramin Tablets 1526

Dezocine (Imipramine may potentiate the effects of CNS depressant drugs). Products include:

Dalgan Injection 538

Diazepam (Imipramine may potentiate the effects of CNS depressant drugs). Products include:

Dizac 1809
Valium Injectable 2182
Valium Tablets 2183
Valrelease Capsules 2169

Dicyclomine Hydrochloride (Concurrent use may result in pronounced atropine-like effects e.g., paralytic ileus). Products include:

Bentyl 1501

Dobutamine Hydrochloride (Avoid concurrent use since tricyclic antidepressants can potentiate the effects of catecholamines). Products include:

Dobutrex Solution Vials 1439

Dopamine Hydrochloride (Avoid concurrent use since tricyclic antidepressants can potentiate the effects of catecholamines).

No products indexed under this heading.

Doxepin Hydrochloride (Concurrent use with drugs that are substrate for cytochrome $P_{450}IID_6$ may make normal metabolizer resemble poor metabolizer leading to higher than expected plasma concentrations of TCA with resultant toxicity). Products include:

Sinequan 2205
Zonalon Cream 1055

Droperidol (Imipramine may potentiate the effects of CNS depressant drugs). Products include:

Inapsine Injection 1296

Enflurane (Imipramine may potentiate the effects of CNS depressant drugs).

No products indexed under this heading.

Ephedrine Hydrochloride (Avoid concurrent use since tricyclic antidepressants can potentiate the effects of catecholamines). Products include:

Primatene Dual Action Formula....... ⓔⓓ 872
Primatene Tablets .... ⓔⓓ 873
Quadrinal Tablets 1350

Ephedrine Sulfate (Avoid concurrent use since tricyclic antidepressants can potentiate the effects of catecholamines). Products include:

Bronkaid Caplets .... ⓔⓓ 717
Marax Tablets & DF Syrup.................. 2200

Ephedrine Tannate (Avoid concurrent use since tricyclic antidepressants can potentiate the effects of catecholamines). Products include:

Rynatuss 2673

Epinephrine (Avoid concurrent use since tricyclic antidepressants can potentiate the effects of catecholamines). Products include:

Bronkaid Mist .... ⓔⓓ 717
EPIFRIN .... ⓒ 239
EpiPen 790
Marcaine Hydrochloride with Epinephrine 1:200,000 2316
Primatene Mist .... ⓔⓓ 873
Sensorcaine with Epinephrine Injection 559
Sus-Phrine Injection 1019
Xylocaine with Epinephrine Injections 567

Epinephrine Bitartrate (Avoid concurrent use since tricyclic antidepressants can potentiate the effects of catecholamines). Products include:

Bronkaid Mist Suspension .... ⓔⓓ 718

Sensorcaine-MPF with Epinephrine Injection 559

Epinephrine Hydrochloride (Avoid concurrent use since tricyclic antidepressants can potentiate the effects of catecholamines). Products include:

Ana-Kit Anaphylaxis Emergency Treatment Kit 617

Estazolam (Imipramine may potentiate the effects of CNS depressant drugs). Products include:

ProSom Tablets 449

Ethchlorvynol (Imipramine may potentiate the effects of CNS depressant drugs). Products include:

Placidyl Capsules 448

Ethinamate (Imipramine may potentiate the effects of CNS depressant drugs).

No products indexed under this heading.

Fentanyl (Imipramine may potentiate the effects of CNS depressant drugs). Products include:

Duragesic Transdermal System......... 1288

Fentanyl Citrate (Imipramine may potentiate the effects of CNS depressant drugs). Products include:

Sublimaze Injection 1307

Flecainide Acetate (Concurrent use with drugs that are substrate for cytochrome $P_{450}IID_6$ may make normal metabolizer resemble poor metabolizer leading to higher than expected plasma concentrations of TCA with resultant toxicity). Products include:

Tambocor Tablets 1497

Fluoxetine Hydrochloride (Concurrent use with drugs that are substrate for cytochrome P450 IID_6 may make normal metabolizer resemble poor metabolizer leading to higher than expected plasma concentrations of TCA with resultant toxicity; due to variation in the extent of inhibition of $P_{450}IID_6$ and long half-life of the parent (fluoxetine) and active must sufficient time must elapse, at least 5 weeks before switching to TCA). Products include:

Prozac Pulvules & Liquid, Oral Solution 919

Fluphenazine Decanoate (Concurrent use with drugs that are substrate for cytochrome $P_{450}IID_6$ may make normal metabolizer resemble poor metabolizer leading to higher than expected plasma concentrations of TCA with resultant toxicity; imipramine may potentiate the effects of CNS depressant drugs). Products include:

Prolixin Decanoate 509

Fluphenazine Enanthate (Concurrent use with drugs that are substrate for cytochrome $P_{450}IID_6$ may make normal metabolizer resemble poor metabolizer leading to higher than expected plasma concentrations of TCA with resultant toxicity; imipramine may potentiate the effects of CNS depressant drugs). Products include:

Prolixin Enanthate 509

Fluphenazine Hydrochloride (Concurrent use with drugs that are substrate for cytochrome $P_{450}IID_6$ may make normal metabolizer resemble poor metabolizer leading to higher than expected plasma concentrations of TCA with resultant toxicity; imipramine may potentiate the effects of CNS depressant drugs). Products include:

Prolixin 509

IMPORTANT NOTE: Always consult each drug listing in the patient's regimen for possible interactions.

Tofranil

Flurazepam Hydrochloride (Imipramine may potentiate the effects of CNS depressant drugs). Products include:

Dalmane Capsules..............................2173

Fluvoxamine Maleate (Concurrent use with drugs that are substrate for cytochrome $P_{450}IID_6$ may make normal metabolizer resemble poor metabolizer leading to higher than expected plasma concentrations of TCA with resultant toxicity; due to variation in the extent of inhibition of $P_{450}IID_6$ caution is indicated if co-administered sufficient time must elapse). Products include:

Luvox Tablets..2544

Furazolidone (Potential for hyperpyretic crises, severe convulsions, and deaths; concurrent and/or sequential use is contraindicated). Products include:

Furoxone..2046

Glutethimide (Imipramine may potentiate the effects of CNS depressant drugs).

No products indexed under this heading.

Glycopyrrolate (Concurrent use may result in pronounced atropine-like effects e.g., paralytic ileus). Products include:

Robinul Forte Tablets............................2072
Robinul Injectable..................................2072
Robinul Tablets.......................................2072

Guanadrel Sulfate (Imipramine may block the antihypertensive effect). Products include:

Hylorel Tablets..985

Guanethidine Monosulfate (Imipramine may block the antihypertensive effect of guanethidine or similarly acting compounds). Products include:

Esimil Tablets..822
Ismelin Tablets..827

Haloperidol (Imipramine may potentiate the effects of CNS depressant drugs). Products include:

Haldol Injection, Tablets and Concentrate..1575

Haloperidol Decanoate (Imipramine may potentiate the effects of CNS depressant drugs). Products include:

Haldol Decanoate...................................1577

Hydrocodone Bitartrate (Imipramine may potentiate the effects of CNS depressant drugs). Products include:

Anexsia 5/500 Elixir..............................1781
Anexia Tablets...1782
Codiclear DH Syrup...............................791
Deconamine CX Cough and Cold Liquid and Tablets................................1319
Duratuss HD Elixir..................................2565
Hycodan Tablets and Syrup.................930
Hycomine Compound Tablets.............932
Hycomine..931
Hycotuss Expectorant Syrup...............933
Hydrocet Capsules.................................782
Lorcet 10/650..1018
Lortab..2566
Tussend...1783
Tussend Expectorant.............................1785
Vicodin Tablets..1356
Vicodin ES Tablets..................................1357
Vicodin Tuss Expectorant....................1358
Zydone Capsules....................................949

Hydrocodone Polistirex (Imipramine may potentiate the effects of CNS depressant drugs). Products include:

Tussionex Pennkinetic Extended-Release Suspension..............................998

Hydroxyzine Hydrochloride (Imipramine may potentiate the effects of CNS depressant drugs). Products include:

Atarax Tablets & Syrup.........................2185

Marax Tablets & DF Syrup...................2200
Vistaril Intramuscular Solution..........2216

Hyoscyamine (Concurrent use may result in pronounced atropine-like effects e.g., paralytic ileus). Products include:

Cystospaz Tablets..................................1963
Urised Tablets..1964

Hyoscyamine Sulfate (Concurrent use may result in pronounced atropine-like effects e.g., paralytic ileus). Products include:

Arco-Lase Plus Tablets.........................512
Atrohist Plus Tablets.............................454
Cystospaz-M Capsules.........................1963
Donnatal...2060
Donnatal Extentabs...............................2061
Donnatal Tablets.....................................2060
Kutrase Capsules...................................2402
Levsin/Levsinex/Levbid.......................2405

Imipramine Pamoate (Concurrent use with drugs that are substrate for cytochrome $P_{450}IID_6$ may make normal metabolizer resemble poor metabolizer leading to higher than expected plasma concentrations of TCA with resultant toxicity). Products include:

Tofranil-PM Capsules............................857

Ipratropium Bromide (Concurrent use may result in pronounced atropine-like effects e.g., paralytic ileus). Products include:

Atrovent Inhalation Aerosol................671
Atrovent Inhalation Solution...............673

Isocarboxazid (Potential for hyperpyretic crises; severe convulsions, and deaths; concurrent and/or sequential use is contraindicated).

No products indexed under this heading.

Isoflurane (Imipramine may potentiate the effects of CNS depressant drugs).

No products indexed under this heading.

Isoproterenol Hydrochloride (Avoid concurrent use since tricyclic antidepressants can potentiate the effects of catecholamines). Products include:

Isuprel Hydrochloride Injection 1:5000..2311
Isuprel Hydrochloride Solution 1:200 & 1:100.....................................2313
Isuprel Mistometer.................................2312

Isoproterenol Sulfate (Avoid concurrent use since tricyclic antidepressants can potentiate the effects of catecholamines). Products include:

Norisodrine with Calcium Iodide Syrup...442

Ketamine Hydrochloride (Imipramine may potentiate the effects of CNS depressant drugs).

No products indexed under this heading.

Levomethadyl Acetate Hydrochloride (Imipramine may potentiate the effects of CNS depressant drugs). Products include:

Orlaam..2239

Levorphanol Tartrate (Imipramine may potentiate the effects of CNS depressant drugs). Products include:

Levo-Dromoran.......................................2129

Levothyroxine Sodium (Co-administration may produce cardiovascular toxicity). Products include:

Levothroid Tablets..................................1016
Levoxyl Tablets.......................................903
Synthroid..1359

Liothyronine Sodium (Co-administration may produce cardiovascular toxicity). Products include:

Cytomel Tablets......................................2473
Triostat Injection....................................2530

Liotrix (Co-administration may produce cardiovascular toxicity).

No products indexed under this heading.

Lorazepam (Imipramine may potentiate the effects of CNS depressant drugs). Products include:

Ativan Injection.......................................2698
Ativan Tablets..2700

Loxapine Hydrochloride (Imipramine may potentiate the effects of CNS depressant drugs). Products include:

Loxitane..1378

Loxapine Succinate (Imipramine may potentiate the effects of CNS depressant drugs). Products include:

Loxitane Capsules..................................1378

Maprotiline Hydrochloride (Concurrent use with drugs that are substrate for cytochrome $P_{450}IID_6$ may make normal metabolizer resemble poor metabolizer leading to higher than expected plasma concentrations of TCA with resultant toxicity). Products include:

Ludiomil Tablets.....................................843

Mepenzolate Bromide (Concurrent use may result in pronounced atropine-like effects e.g., paralytic ileus).

No products indexed under this heading.

Meperidine Hydrochloride (Imipramine may potentiate the effects of CNS depressant drugs). Products include:

Demerol..2308
Mepergan Injection................................2753

Mephobarbital (The plasma concentration of imipramine may decrease when the drug is given with barbiturates, a hepatic enzyme inducer; dosage of imipramine may need to be adjusted; imipramine may potentiate the effects of CNS depressant drugs). Products include:

Mebaral Tablets......................................2322

Meprobamate (Imipramine may potentiate the effects of CNS depressant drugs). Products include:

Miltown Tablets.......................................2672
PMB 200 and PMB 400........................2783

Mesoridazine (Imipramine may potentiate the effects of CNS depressant drugs).

Mesoridazine Besylate (Concurrent use with drugs that are substrate for cytochrome $P_{450}IID_6$ may make normal metabolizer resemble poor metabolizer leading to higher than expected plasma concentrations of TCA with resultant toxicity; imipramine may potentiate the effects of CNS depressant drugs). Products include:

Serentil...684

Metaproterenol Sulfate (Avoid concurrent use since tricyclic antidepressants can potentiate the effects of catecholamines). Products include:

Alupent...669
Metaproterenol Sulfate Inhalation Solution, USP, Arm-a-Med.................552

Metaraminol Bitartrate (Avoid concurrent use since tricyclic antidepressants can potentiate the effects of catecholamines). Products include:

Aramine Injection...................................1609

Methadone Hydrochloride (Imipramine may potentiate the effects of CNS depressant drugs). Products include:

Methadone Hydrochloride Oral Concentrate..2233

Methadone Hydrochloride Oral Solution & Tablets.................................2235

Methohexital Sodium (Imipramine may potentiate the effects of CNS depressant drugs). Products include:

Brevital Sodium Vials............................1429

Methotrimeprazine (Concurrent use with drugs that are substrate for cytochrome $P_{450}IID_6$ may make normal metabolizer resemble poor metabolizer leading to higher than expected plasma concentrations of TCA with resultant toxicity; imipramine may potentiate the effects of CNS depressant drugs). Products include:

Levoprome..1274

Methoxamine Hydrochloride (Avoid concurrent use since tricyclic antidepressants can potentiate the effects of catecholamines). Products include:

Vasoxyl Injection....................................1196

Methoxyflurane (Imipramine may potentiate the effects of CNS depressant drugs).

No products indexed under this heading.

Methylphenidate Hydrochloride (May inhibit the metabolism of imipramine; downward dosage adjustments of imipramine may be required when given concomitantly). Products include:

Ritalin...848

Midazolam Hydrochloride (Imipramine may potentiate the effects of CNS depressant drugs). Products include:

Versed Injection......................................2170

Molindone Hydrochloride (Imipramine may potentiate the effects of CNS depressant drugs). Products include:

Moban Tablets and Concentrate.......1048

Morphine Sulfate (Imipramine may potentiate the effects of CNS depressant drugs). Products include:

Astramorph/PF Injection, USP (Preservative-Free)...............................535
Duramorph..962
Infumorph 200 and Infumorph 500 Sterile Solutions...............................965
MS Contin Tablets..................................1994
MSIR..1997
Oramorph SR (Morphine Sulfate Sustained Release Tablets)..............2236
RMS Suppositories.................................2657
Roxanol..2243

Nefazodone Hydrochloride (Concurrent use with drugs that are substrate for cytochrome $P_{450}IID_6$ may make normal metabolizer resemble poor metabolizer leading to higher than expected plasma concentrations of TCA with resultant toxicity). Products include:

Serzone Tablets.......................................771

Norepinephrine Bitartrate (Avoid concurrent use since tricyclic antidepressants can potentiate the effects of catecholamines). Products include:

Levophed Bitartrate Injection.............2315

Nortriptyline Hydrochloride (Concurrent use with drugs that are substrate for cytochrome $P_{450}IID_6$ may make normal metabolizer resemble poor metabolizer leading to higher than expected plasma concentrations of TCA with resultant toxicity). Products include:

Pamelor...2280

Opium Alkaloids (Imipramine may potentiate the effects of CNS depressant drugs).

No products indexed under this heading.

(◆□ Described in PDR For Nonprescription Drugs)   (◉ Described in PDR For Ophthalmology)

Interactions Index — Tofranil

Oxazepam (Imipramine may potentiate the effects of CNS depressant drugs). Products include:

Serax Capsules 2810
Serax Tablets 2810

Oxybutynin Chloride (Concurrent use may result in pronounced atropine-like effects e.g., paralytic ileus). Products include:

Ditropan 1516

Oxycodone Hydrochloride (Imipramine may potentiate the effects of CNS depressant drugs). Products include:

Percocet Tablets 938
Percodan Tablets 939
Percodan-Demi Tablets 940
Roxicodone Tablets, Oral Solution & Intensol (Oxycodone) 2244
Tylox Capsules 1584

Paroxetine Hydrochloride (Concurrent use with drugs that are substrate for cytochrome $P_{450}IID_6$ may make normal metabolizer resemble poor metabolizer leading to higher than expected plasma concentrations of TCA with resultant toxicity; due to variation in the extent of inhibition of $P_{450}IID_6$ caution is indicated if co-administered sufficient time must elapse). Products include:

Paxil Tablets 2505

Pentobarbital Sodium (The plasma concentration of imipramine may decrease when the drug is given with barbiturates, a hepatic enzyme inducer; dosage of imipramine may need to be adjusted; imipramine may potentiate the effects of CNS depressant drugs). Products include:

Nembutal Sodium Capsules 436
Nembutal Sodium Solution 438
Nembutal Sodium Suppositories 440

Perphenazine (Concurrent use with drugs that are substrate for cytochrome $P_{450}IID_6$ may make normal metabolizer resemble poor metabolizer leading to higher than expected plasma concentrations of TCA with resultant toxicity; imipramine may potentiate the effects of CNS depressant drugs). Products include:

Etrafon 2355
Triavil Tablets 1757
Trilafon 2389

Phenelzine Sulfate (Potential for hyperpyretic crises, severe convulsions, and deaths; concurrent and/or sequential use is contraindicated). Products include:

Nardil 1920

Phenobarbital (The plasma concentration of imipramine may decrease when the drug is given with barbiturates, a hepatic enzyme inducer; dosage of imipramine may need to be adjusted; imipramine may potentiate the effects of CNS depressant drugs). Products include:

Arco-Lase Plus Tablets 512
Bellergal-S Tablets 2250
Donnatal 2060
Donnatal Extentabs 2061
Donnatal Tablets 2060
Phenobarbital Elixir and Tablets 1469
Quadrinal Tablets 1350

Phenylephrine Bitartrate (Avoid concurrent use since tricyclic antidepressants can potentiate the effects of catecholamines).

No products indexed under this heading.

Phenylephrine Hydrochloride (Avoid concurrent use since tricyclic antidepressants can potentiate the effects of catecholamines). Products include:

Atrohist Plus Tablets 454
Cerose DM .... ᴾᴰ 878
Comhist 2038
D.A. Chewable Tablets 951
Deconsal Pediatric Capsules 454
Dura-Vent/DA Tablets 953
Entex Capsules 1986
Entex Liquid 1986
Extendryl 1005
4-Way Fast Acting Nasal Spray (regular & mentholated) .... ᴾᴰ 621
Hemorid For Women .... ᴾᴰ 834
Hycomine Compound Tablets 932
Neo-Synephrine Hydrochloride 1% Carpuject 2324
Neo-Synephrine Hydrochloride 1% Injection 2324
Neo-Synephrine Hydrochloride (Ophthalmic) 2325
Neo-Synephrine .... ᴾᴰ 726
Nōstril .... ᴾᴰ 644
Novahistine Elixir .... ᴾᴰ 823
Phenergan VC 2779
Phenergan VC with Codeine 2781
Preparation H .... ᴾᴰ 871
Tympagesic Ear Drops 2342
Vasosulf .... © 271
Vicks Sinex Nasal Spray and Ultra Fine Mist .... ᴾᴰ 765

Phenylephrine Tannate (Avoid concurrent use since tricyclic antidepressants can potentiate the effects of catecholamines). Products include:

Atrohist Pediatric Suspension 454
Ricobid-D Pediatric Suspension 2038
Ricobid Tablets and Pediatric Suspension 2038
Rynatan 2673
Rynatuss 2673

Phenylpropanolamine Hydrochloride (Avoid concurrent use since tricyclic antidepressants can potentiate the effects of catecholamines). Products include:

Acutrim .... ᴾᴰ 628
Allerest Children's Chewable Tablets .... ᴾᴰ 627
Allerest 12 Hour Caplets .... ᴾᴰ 627
Atrohist Plus Tablets 454
BC Cold Powder Multi-Symptom Formula (Cold-Sinus-Allergy) .... ᴾᴰ 609
BC Cold Powder Non-Drowsy Formula (Cold-Sinus) .... ᴾᴰ 609
Cheracol Plus Head Cold/Cough Formula .... ᴾᴰ 769
Comtrex Multi-Symptom Non-Drowsy Liqui-gels .... ᴾᴰ 618
Contac Continuous Action Nasal Decongestant/Antihistamine 12 Hour Capsules .... ᴾᴰ 813
Contac Maximum Strength Continuous Action Decongestant/Antihistamine 12 Hour Caplets .. ᴾᴰ 813
Contac Severe Cold and Flu Formula Caplets .... ᴾᴰ 814
Coricidin 'D' Decongestant Tablets .... ᴾᴰ 800
Dexatrim .... ᴾᴰ 832
Dexatrim Plus Vitamins Caplets .... ᴾᴰ 832
Dimetane-DC Cough Syrup 2059
Dimetapp Elixir .... ᴾᴰ 773
Dimetapp Extentabs .... ᴾᴰ 774
Dimetapp Tablets/Liqui-Gels .... ᴾᴰ 775
Dimetapp Cold & Allergy Chewable Tablets .... ᴾᴰ 773
Dimetapp DM Elixir .... ᴾᴰ 774
Dura-Vent Tablets 952
Entex Capsules 1986
Entex LA Tablets 1987
Entex Liquid 1986
Exgest LA Tablets 782
Hycomine 931
Isoclor Timesule Capsules .... ᴾᴰ 637
Nolamine Timed-Release Tablets 785
Ornade Spansule Capsules 2502
Propagest Tablets 786
Pyrroxate Caplets .... ᴾᴰ 772
Robitussin-CF .... ᴾᴰ 777
Sinulin Tablets 787
Tavist-D 12 Hour Relief Tablets .... ᴾᴰ 787
Teldrin 12 Hour Antihistamine/Nasal Decongestant Allergy Relief Capsules .... ᴾᴰ 826
Triaminic Allergy Tablets .... ᴾᴰ 789
Triaminic Cold Tablets .... ᴾᴰ 790
Triaminic Expectorant .... ᴾᴰ 790
Triaminic Syrup .... ᴾᴰ 792
Triaminic-12 Tablets .... ᴾᴰ 792
Triaminic-DM Syrup .... ᴾᴰ 792
Triaminicin Tablets .... ᴾᴰ 793
Triaminicol Multi-Symptom Cold Tablets .... ᴾᴰ 793
Triaminicol Multi-Symptom Relief .... ᴾᴰ 794
Vicks DayQuil Allergy Relief 12-Hour Extended Release Tablets .. ᴾᴰ 760
Vicks DayQuil Allergy Relief 4-Hour Tablets .... ᴾᴰ 760
Vicks DayQuil SINUS Pressure & CONGESTION Relief .... ᴾᴰ 761

Phenytoin (The plasma concentration of imipramine may decrease when the drug is given with phenytoin, a hepatic enzyme inducer; dosage of imipramine may need to be adjusted). Products include:

Dilantin Infatabs 1908
Dilantin-125 Suspension 1911

Phenytoin Sodium (The plasma concentration of imipramine may decrease when the drug is given with phenytoin, a hepatic enzyme inducer; dosage of imipramine may need to be adjusted). Products include:

Dilantin Kapseals 1906
Dilantin Parenteral 1910

Pirbuterol Acetate (Avoid concurrent use since tricyclic antidepressants can potentiate the effects of catecholamines). Products include:

Maxair Autohaler 1492
Maxair Inhaler 1494

Prazepam (Imipramine may potentiate the effects of CNS depressant drugs).

No products indexed under this heading.

Prochlorperazine (Concurrent use with drugs that are substrate for cytochrome $P_{450}IID_6$ may make normal metabolizer resemble poor metabolizer leading to higher than expected plasma concentrations of TCA with resultant toxicity; imipramine may potentiate the effects of CNS depressant drugs). Products include:

Compazine 2470

Procyclidine Hydrochloride (Concurrent use may result in pronounced atropine-like effects e.g., paralytic ileus). Products include:

Kemadrin Tablets 1112

Promethazine Hydrochloride (Concurrent use with drugs that are substrate for cytochrome $P_{450}IID_6$ may make normal metabolizer resemble poor metabolizer leading to higher than expected plasma concentrations of TCA with resultant toxicity; imipramine may potentiate the effects of CNS depressant drugs). Products include:

Mepergan Injection 2753
Phenergan with Codeine 2777
Phenergan with Dextromethorphan 2778
Phenergan Injection 2773
Phenergan Suppositories 2775
Phenergan Syrup 2774
Phenergan Tablets 2775
Phenergan VC 2779
Phenergan VC with Codeine 2781

Propafenone Hydrochloride (Concurrent use with drugs that are substrate for cytochrome $P_{450}IID_6$ may make normal metabolizer resemble poor metabolizer leading to higher than expected plasma concentrations of TCA with resultant toxicity). Products include:

Rythmol Tablets–150mg, 225mg, 300mg 1352

Propantheline Bromide (Concurrent use may result in pronounced atropine-like effects e.g., paralytic ileus). Products include:

Pro-Banthine Tablets 2052

Propofol (Imipramine may potentiate the effects of CNS depressant drugs). Products include:

Diprivan Injection 2833

Propoxyphene Hydrochloride (Imipramine may potentiate the effects of CNS depressant drugs). Products include:

Darvon 1435
Wygesic Tablets 2827

Propoxyphene Napsylate (Imipramine may potentiate the effects of CNS depressant drugs). Products include:

Darvon-N/Darvocet-N 1433

Protriptyline Hydrochloride (Concurrent use with drugs that are substrate for cytochrome $P_{450}IID_6$ may make normal metabolizer resemble poor metabolizer leading to higher than expected plasma concentrations of TCA with resultant toxicity). Products include:

Vivactil Tablets 1774

Pseudoephedrine Hydrochloride (Avoid concurrent use since tricyclic antidepressants can potentiate the effects of catecholamines). Products include:

Actifed Allergy Daytime/Nighttime Caplets .... ᴾᴰ 844
Actifed Plus Caplets .... ᴾᴰ 845
Actifed Plus Tablets .... ᴾᴰ 845
Actifed with Codeine Cough Syrup .. 1067
Actifed Sinus Daytime/Nighttime Tablets and Caplets .... ᴾᴰ 846
Actifed Syrup .... ᴾᴰ 846
Actifed Tablets .... ᴾᴰ 844
Advil Cold and Sinus Caplets and Tablets (formerly CoAdvil) .... ᴾᴰ 870
Alka-Seltzer Plus Cold Medicine Liqui-Gels .... ᴾᴰ 706
Alka-Seltzer Plus Cold & Cough Medicine Liqui-Gels .... ᴾᴰ 705
Alka-Seltzer Plus Night-Time Cold Medicine Liqui-Gels .... ᴾᴰ 706
Allerest Headache Strength Tablets .... ᴾᴰ 627
Allerest Maximum Strength Tablets .... ᴾᴰ 627
Allerest No Drowsiness Tablets .... ᴾᴰ 627
Allerest Sinus Pain Formula .... ᴾᴰ 627
Anatuss LA Tablets 1542
Atrohist Pediatric Capsules 453
Bayer Select Sinus Pain Relief Formula .... ᴾᴰ 717
Benadryl Allergy Decongestant Liquid Medication .... ᴾᴰ 848
Benadryl Allergy Decongestant Tablets .... ᴾᴰ 848
Benadryl Allergy Sinus Headache Formula Caplets .... ᴾᴰ 849
Benylin Multisymptom .... ᴾᴰ 852
Bromfed Capsules (Extended-Release) 1785
Bromfed Syrup .... ᴾᴰ 733
Bromfed Tablets 1785
Bromfed-DM Cough Syrup 1786
Bromfed-PD Capsules (Extended-Release) 1785
Children's Vicks DayQuil Allergy Relief .... ᴾᴰ 757
Children's Vicks NyQuil Cold/Cough Relief .... ᴾᴰ 758
Comtrex Multi-Symptom Cold Reliever Tablets/Caplets/Liqui-Gels/Liquid .... ᴾᴰ 615
Allergy-Sinus Comtrex Multi-Symptom Allergy-Sinus Formula Tablets .... ᴾᴰ 617
Comtrex Multi-Symptom Non-Drowsy Caplets .... ᴾᴰ 618
Congess 1004
Contac Day Allergy/Sinus Caplets ᴾᴰ 812
Contac Day & Night .... ᴾᴰ 812
Contac Night Allergy/Sinus Caplets .... ᴾᴰ 812
Contac Severe Cold & Flu Non-Drowsy .... ᴾᴰ 815
Deconamine Chewable Tablets 1320
Deconamine CX Cough and Cold Liquid and Tablets 1319
Deconamine 1320
Deconsal C Expectorant Syrup 456
Deconsal Pediatric Syrup 457
Deconsal II Tablets 454
Dimetane-DX Cough Syrup 2059
Dimetapp Sinus Caplets .... ᴾᴰ 775
Dorcol Children's Cough Syrup .... ᴾᴰ 785
Drixoral Cough + Congestion Liquid Caps .... ᴾᴰ 802
Dura-Tap/PD Capsules 2867

IMPORTANT NOTE: Always consult each drug listing in the patient's regimen for possible interactions.

Tofranil **Interactions Index** 1042

Duratuss Tablets 2565
Duratuss HD Elixir 2565
Efidac/24 .... ▣ 635
Entex PSE Tablets 1987
Fedahist Gyrocaps 2401
Fedahist Timecaps 2401
Guaifed 1787
Guaifed Syrup .... ▣ 734
Guaimax-D Tablets 792
Guaitab Tablets .... ▣ 734
Isoclor Expectorant 990
Kronofed-A 977
Motrin IB Sinus .... ▣ 838
Novahistine DH 2462
Novahistine DMX .... ▣ 822
Novahistine Expectorant 2463
Nucofed 2051
PediaCare Cold Allergy Chewable Tablets .... ▣ 677
PediaCare Cough-Cold Chewable Tablets 1553
PediaCare 1553
PediaCare Infants' Decongestant Drops .... ▣ 677
PediCare Infant's Drops Decongestant Plus Cough 1553
PediaCare NightRest Cough-Cold Liquid 1553
Pediatric Vicks 44d Dry Hacking Cough & Head Congestion .... ▣ 763
Pediatric Vicks 44m Cough & Cold Relief .... ▣ 764
Robitussin Cold & Cough Liqui-Gels .... ▣ 776
Robitussin Maximum Strength Cough & Cold .... ▣ 778
Robitussin Pediatric Cough & Cold Formula .... ▣ 779
Robitussin Severe Congestion Liqui-Gels .... ▣ 776
Robitussin-DAC Syrup 2074
Robitussin-PE .... ▣ 778
Rondec Oral Drops 953
Rondec Syrup 953
Rondec Tablet 953
Rondec-DM Oral Drops 954
Rondec-DM Syrup 954
Rondec-TR Tablet 953
Ryna .... ▣ 841
Seldane-D Extended-Release Tablets 1538
Semprex-D Capsules 463
Semprex-D Capsules 1167
Sinarest Tablets .... ▣ 648
Sinarest Extra Strength Tablets .... ▣ 648
Sinarest No Drowsiness Tablets .... ▣ 648
Sine-Aid IB Caplets 1554
Sine-Aid Maximum Strength Sinus Medication Gelcaps, Caplets and Tablets 1554
Sine-Off No Drowsiness Formula Caplets .... ▣ 824
Sine-Off Sinus Medicine .... ▣ 825
Singlet Tablets .... ▣ 825
Sinutab Non-Drying Liquid Caps .... ▣ 859
Sinutab Sinus Allergy Medication, Maximum Strength Tablets and Caplets .... ▣ 860
Sinutab Sinus Medication, Maximum Strength Without Drowsiness Formula, Tablets & Caplets .... ▣ 860
Sinutab Sinus Medication, Regular Strength Without Drowsiness Formula .... ▣ 859
Sudafed Children's Liquid .... ▣ 861
Sudafed Cold and Cough Liquidcaps .... ▣ 862
Sudafed Cough Syrup .... ▣ 862
Sudafed Plus Liquid .... ▣ 862
Sudafed Plus Tablets .... ▣ 863
Sudafed Severe Cold Formula Caplets .... ▣ 863
Sudafed Severe Cold Formula Tablets .... ▣ 864
Sudafed Sinus Caplets .... ▣ 864
Sudafed Sinus Tablets .... ▣ 864
Sudafed Tablets, 30 mg .... ▣ 861
Sudafed Tablets, 60 mg .... ▣ 861
Sudafed 12 Hour Caplets .... ▣ 861
Syn-Rx Tablets 465
Syn-Rx DM Tablets 466
TheraFlu .... ▣ 787
TheraFlu Maximum Strength Nighttime Flu, Cold & Cough Medicine .... ▣ 788
TheraFlu Maximum Strength Non-Drowsy Formula Flu, Cold & Cough Medicine .... ▣ 788
Thera Flu Maximum Strength, Non-Drowsy Formula Flu, Cold and Cough Caplets .... ▣ 789
Triaminic AM Cough and Decongestant Formula .... ▣ 789
Triaminic AM Decongestant Formula .... ▣ 790
Triaminic Nite Light .... ▣ 791
Triaminic Sore Throat Formula .... ▣ 791
Tussend 1783
Tussend Expectorant 1785
Children's TYLENOL Cold Multi-Symptom Liquid Formula and Chewable Tablets 1561
Children's TYLENOL Cold Plus Cough Multi Symptom Tablets and Liquid .... ▣ 681
Infants' TYLENOL Cold Decongestant & Fever-Reducer Drops 1556
TYLENOL Maximum Strength Allergy Sinus Medication Gelcaps and Caplets 1563
TYLENOL Maximum Strength Allergy Sinus NightTime Medication Caplets 1555
TYLENOL Flu Maximum Strength Gelcaps 1565
TYLENOL Flu NightTime, Maximum Strength, Gelcaps 1566
TYLENOL Maximum Strength Flu NightTime Hot Medication Packets 1562
TYLENOL, Maximum Strength, Sinus Medication Geltabs, Gelcaps, Caplets and Tablets 1566
TYLENOL Cold Multi-Symptom Formula Medication Tablets and Caplets 1561
TYLENOL Cold Medication No Drowsiness Formula Gelcaps and Caplets 1562
TYLENOL Cold Multi-Symptom Hot Medication Liquid Packets 1557
TYLENOL Cough Multi-Symptom Medication with Decongestant 1565
Ursinus Inlay-Tabs .... ▣ 794
Vicks 44 LiquiCaps Cough, Cold & Flu Relief .... ▣ 755
Vicks 44 LiquiCaps Non-Drowsy Cough & Cold Relief .... ▣ 756
Vicks 44D Dry Hacking Cough & Head Congestion .... ▣ 755
Vicks 44M Cough, Cold & Flu Relief .... ▣ 756
Vicks DayQuil .... ▣ 761
Vicks DayQuil SINUS Pressure & PAIN Relief with IBUPROFEN .... ▣ 762
Vicks Nyquil Hot Therapy .... ▣ 762
Vicks NyQuil LiquiCaps Multi-Symptom Cold/Flu Relief .... ▣ 763
Vicks NyQuil Multi-Symptom Cold/Flu Relief - (Original & Cherry Flavor) .... ▣ 763

Pseudoephedrine Sulfate (Avoid concurrent use since tricyclic antidepressants can potentiate the effects of catecholamines). Products include:
Cheracol Sinus .... ▣ 768
Chlor-Trimeton Allergy Decongestant Tablets .... ▣ 799
Claritin-D 2350
Drixoral Cold and Allergy Sustained-Action Tablets .... ▣ 802
Drixoral Cold and Flu Extended-Release Tablets .... ▣ 803
Drixoral Non-Drowsy Formula Extended-Release Tablets .... ▣ 803
Drixoral Allergy/Sinus Extended Release Tablets .... ▣ 804
Trinalin Repetabs Tablets 1330

Quazepam (Imipramine may potentiate the effects of CNS depressant drugs). Products include:
Doral Tablets 2664

Quinidine Gluconate (Concurrent use with drugs that inhibit cytochrome $P_{450}IID_6$ may make normal metabolizer resemble poor metabolizer leading to higher than expected plasma concentrations of TCA with resultant toxicity). Products include:
Quinaglute Dura-Tabs Tablets 649

Quinidine Polygalacturonate (Concurrent use with drugs that inhibit cytochrome $P_{450}IID_6$ may make normal metabolizer resemble poor metabolizer leading to higher than expected plasma concentrations of TCA with resultant toxicity).
No products indexed under this heading.

Quinidine Sulfate (Concurrent use with drugs that inhibit cytochrome $P_{450}IID_6$ may make normal metabolizer resemble poor metabolizer leading to higher than expected plasma concentrations of TCA with resultant toxicity). Products include:
Quinidex Extentabs 2067

Risperidone (Imipramine may potentiate the effects of CNS depressant drugs). Products include:
Risperdal 1301

Salmeterol Xinafoate (Avoid concurrent use since tricyclic antidepressants can potentiate the effects of catecholamines). Products include:
Serevent Inhalation Aerosol 1176

Scopolamine (Concurrent use may result in pronounced atropine-like effects e.g., paralytic ileus). Products include:
Transderm Scōp Transdermal Therapeutic System 869

Scopolamine Hydrobromide (Concurrent use may result in pronounced atropine-like effects e.g., paralytic ileus). Products include:
Atrohist Plus Tablets 454
Donnatal 2060
Donnatal Extentabs 2061
Donnatal Tablets 2060

Secobarbital Sodium (The plasma concentration of imipramine may decrease when the drug is given with barbiturates, a hepatic enzyme inducer; dosage of imipramine may need to be adjusted; imipramine may potentiate the effects of CNS depressant drugs). Products include:
Seconal Sodium Pulvules 1474

Selegiline Hydrochloride (Potential for hyperpyretic crises, severe convulsions, and deaths; concurrent and/or sequential use is contraindicated). Products include:
Eldepryl Tablets 2550

Sertraline Hydrochloride (Concurrent use with drugs that are substrate for cytochrome $P_{450}IID_6$ may make normal metabolizer resemble poor metabolizer leading to higher than expected plasma concentrations of TCA with resultant toxicity; due to variation in the extent of inhibition of $P_{450}IID_6$ caution is indicated if co-administered sufficient time must elapse). Products include:
Zoloft Tablets 2217

Sufentanil Citrate (Imipramine may potentiate the effects of CNS depressant drugs). Products include:
Sufenta Injection 1309

Temazepam (Imipramine may potentiate the effects of CNS depressant drugs). Products include:
Restoril Capsules 2284

Terbutaline Sulfate (Avoid concurrent use since tricyclic antidepressants can potentiate the effects of catecholamines). Products include:
Brethaire Inhaler 813
Brethine Ampuls 815
Brethine Tablets 814
Bricanyl Subcutaneous Injection 1502
Bricanyl Tablets 1503

Thiamylal Sodium (The plasma concentration of imipramine may decrease when the drug is given with barbiturates, a hepatic enzyme inducer; dosage of imipramine may need to be adjusted; imipramine may potentiate the effects of CNS depressant drugs).
No products indexed under this heading.

Thioridazine Hydrochloride (Concurrent use with drugs that are substrate for cytochrome $P_{450}IID_6$ may make normal metabolizer resemble poor metabolizer leading to higher than expected plasma concentrations of TCA with resultant toxicity; imipramine may potentiate the effects of CNS depressant drugs). Products include:
Mellaril 2269

Thiothixene (Imipramine may potentiate the effects of CNS depressant drugs). Products include:
Navane Capsules and Concentrate 2201
Navane Intramuscular 2202

Thyroglobulin (Co-administration may produce cardiovascular toxicity).
No products indexed under this heading.

Thyroid (Co-administration may produce cardiovascular toxicity).
No products indexed under this heading.

Thyroxine (Co-administration may produce cardiovascular toxicity).
No products indexed under this heading.

Thyroxine Sodium (Co-administration may produce cardiovascular toxicity).
No products indexed under this heading.

Tranylcypromine Sulfate (Potential for hyperpyretic crises, severe convulsions, and deaths; concurrent and/or sequential use is contraindicated). Products include:
Parnate Tablets 2503

Trazodone Hydrochloride (Concurrent use with drugs that are substrate for cytochrome $P_{450}IID_6$ may make normal metabolizer resemble poor metabolizer leading to higher than expected plasma concentrations of TCA with resultant toxicity). Products include:
Desyrel and Desyrel Dividose 503

Triazolam (Imipramine may potentiate the effects of CNS depressant drugs). Products include:
Halcion Tablets 2611

Tridihexethyl Chloride (Concurrent use may result in pronounced atropine-like effects e.g., paralytic ileus).
No products indexed under this heading.

Trifluoperazine Hydrochloride (Concurrent use with drugs that are substrate for cytochrome $P_{450}IID_6$ may make normal metabolizer resemble poor metabolizer leading to higher than expected plasma concentrations of TCA with resultant toxicity; imipramine may potentiate the effects of CNS depressant drugs). Products include:
Stelazine 2514

Trihexyphenidyl Hydrochloride (Concurrent use may result in pronounced atropine-like effects e.g., paralytic ileus). Products include:
Artane 1368

(▣ Described in PDR For Nonprescription Drugs) (◉ Described in PDR For Ophthalmology)

Trimipramine Maleate (Concurrent use with drugs that are substrate for cytochrome $P_{450}IID_6$ may make normal metabolizer resemble poor metabolizer leading to higher than expected plasma concentrations of TCA with resultant toxicity). Products include:

Surmontil Capsules 2811

Venlafaxine Hydrochloride (Concurrent use with drugs that are substrate for cytochrome $P_{450}IID_6$ may make normal metabolizer resemble poor metabolizer leading to higher than expected plasma concentrations of TCA with resultant toxicity; due to variation in the extent of inhibition of $P_{450}IID_6$ caution is indicated if co-administered sufficient time must elapse). Products include:

Effexor 2719

Zolpidem Tartrate (Imipramine may potentiate the effects of CNS depressant drugs). Products include:

Ambien Tablets..................................... 2416

Food Interactions

Alcohol (Imipramine may enhance the CNS depressant effects of alcohol).

TOFRANIL TABLETS

(Imipramine Hydrochloride) .... 856 May interact with central nervous system depressants, anticholinergics, sympathomimetics, barbiturates, monoamine oxidase inhibitors, thyroid preparations, drugs that inhibit cytochrome p450iid6, antidepressant drugs, phenothiazines, selective serotonin reuptake inhibitors, and certain other agents. Compounds in these categories include:

Albuterol (Avoid concurrent use since tricyclic antidepressants can potentiate the effects of catecholamines). Products include:

Proventil Inhalation Aerosol .... 2382 Ventolin Inhalation Aerosol and Refill 1197

Albuterol Sulfate (Avoid concurrent use since tricyclic antidepressants can potentiate the effects of catecholamines). Products include:

Airet Solution for Inhalation .... 452 Proventil Inhalation Solution 0.083% .... 2384 Proventil Repetabs Tablets .... 2386 Proventil Solution for Inhalation 0.5% .... 2383 Proventil Syrup .... 2385 Proventil Tablets .... 2386 Ventolin Inhalation Solution.............. 1198 Ventolin Nebules Inhalation Solution .... 1199 Ventolin Rotacaps for Inhalation ..... 1200 Ventolin Syrup .... 1202 Ventolin Tablets .... 1203 Volmax Extended-Release Tablets .. 1788

Alfentanil Hydrochloride (Imipramine may potentiate the effects of CNS depressant drugs). Products include:

Alfenta Injection 1286

Alprazolam (Imipramine may potentiate the effects of CNS depressant drugs). Products include:

Xanax Tablets 2649

Amitriptyline Hydrochloride (Concurrent use with drugs that are substrate for cytochrome $P_{450}IID_6$ may make normal metabolizer resemble poor metabolizer leading to higher than expected plasma concentrations of TCA with resultant toxicity). Products include:

Elavil .... 2838 Endep Tablets .... 2174 Etrafon .... 2355 Limbitrol .... 2180 Triavil Tablets 1757

Amoxapine (Concurrent use with drugs that are substrate for cytochrome $P_{450}IID_6$ may make normal metabolizer resemble poor metabolizer leading to higher than expected plasma concentrations of TCA with resultant toxicity). Products include:

Asendin Tablets 1369

Aprobarbital (The plasma concentration of imipramine may decrease when the drug is given with barbiturates, a hepatic enzyme inducers; dosage of imipramine may need to be adjusted; imipramine may potentiate the effects of CNS depressant drugs).

No products indexed under this heading.

Atropine Sulfate (Concurrent use may result in pronounced atropine-like effects, e.g., paralytic ileus). Products include:

Arco-Lase Plus Tablets .... 512 Atrohist Plus Tablets .... 454 Atropine Sulfate Sterile Ophthalmic Solution .... ◆ 233 Donnatal .... 2060 Donnatal Extentabs........................... 2061 Donnatal Tablets .... 2060 Lomotil .... 2439 Motofen Tablets................................. 784 Urised Tablets................................... 1964

Belladonna Alkaloids (Concurrent use may result in pronounced atropine-like effects, e.g., paralytic ileus). Products include:

Bellergal-S Tablets .... 2250 Hyland's Bed Wetting Tablets .... ◆D 828 Hyland's EnurAid Tablets.................. ◆D 829 Hyland's Teething Tablets .... ◆D 830

Benztropine Mesylate (Concurrent use may result in pronounced atropine-like effects, e.g., paralytic ileus). Products include:

Cogentin 1621

Biperiden Hydrochloride (Concurrent use may result in pronounced atropine-like effects, e.g., paralytic ileus). Products include:

Akineton 1333

Buprenorphine (Imipramine may potentiate the effects of CNS depressant drugs). Products include:

Buprenex Injectable 2006

Bupropion Hydrochloride (Concurrent use with drugs that are substrate for cytochrome $P_{450}IID_6$ may make normal metabolizer resemble poor metabolizer leading to higher than expected plasma concentrations of TCA with resultant toxicity). Products include:

Wellbutrin Tablets 1204

Buspirone Hydrochloride (Imipramine may potentiate the effects of CNS depressant drugs). Products include:

BuSpar 737

Butabarbital (The plasma concentration of imipramine may decrease when the drug is given with barbiturates, a hepatic enzyme inducers; dosage of imipramine may need to be adjusted; imipramine may potentiate the effects of CNS depressant drugs).

No products indexed under this heading.

Butalbital (The plasma concentration of imipramine may decrease when the drug is given with barbiturates, a hepatic enzyme inducers; dosage of imipramine may need to be adjusted; imipramine may potentiate the effects of CNS depressant drugs). Products include:

Esgic-plus Tablets .... 1013 Fioricet Tablets .... 2258 Fioricet with Codeine Capsules 2260

Fiorinal Capsules .... 2261 Fiorinal with Codeine Capsules .... 2262 Fiorinal Tablets .... 2261 Phrenilin .... 785 Sedapap Tablets 50 mg/650 mg .. 1543

Chlordiazepoxide (Imipramine may potentiate the effects of CNS depressant drugs). Products include:

Libritabs Tablets .... 2177 Limbitrol 2180

Chlordiazepoxide Hydrochloride (Imipramine may potentiate the effects of CNS depressant drugs). Products include:

Librax Capsules .... 2176 Librium Capsules .... 2178 Librium Injectable 2179

Chlorpromazine (Concurrent use with drugs that are substrate for cytochrome $P_{450}IID_6$ may make normal metabolizer resemble poor metabolizer leading to higher than expected plasma concentrations of TCA with resultant toxicity; imipramine may potentiate the effects of CNS depressant drugs). Products include:

Thorazine Suppositories................... 2523

Chlorpromazine Hydrochloride (Concurrent use with drugs that are substrate for cytochrome $P_{450}IID_6$ may make normal metabolizer resemble poor metabolizer leading to higher than expected plasma concentrations of TCA with resultant toxicity; imipramine may potentiate the effects of CNS depressant drugs). Products include:

Thorazine 2523

Chlorprothixene (Imipramine may potentiate the effects of CNS depressant drugs).

No products indexed under this heading.

Chlorprothixene Hydrochloride (Imipramine may potentiate the effects of CNS depressant drugs).

No products indexed under this heading.

Cimetidine (The plasma concentration of imipramine may increase when the drug is given with cimetidine, a hepatic enzyme inhibitor; dosage of imipramine may need to be adjusted). Products include:

Tagamet Tablets 2516

Cimetidine Hydrochloride (The plasma concentration of imipramine may increase when the drug is given with cimetidine, a hepatic enzyme inhibitor; dosage of imipramine may need to be adjusted). Products include:

Tagamet... 2516

Clidinium Bromide (Concurrent use may result in pronounced atropine-like effects, e.g., paralytic ileus). Products include:

Librax Capsules .... 2176 Quarzan Capsules 2181

Clonidine (Imipramine may block the antihypertensive effect). Products include:

Catapres-TTS.................................... 675

Clonidine Hydrochloride (Imipramine may block the antihypertensive effect). Products include:

Catapres Tablets .... 674 Combipres Tablets 677

Clorazepate Dipotassium (Imipramine may potentiate the effects of CNS depressant drugs). Products include:

Tranxene 451

Clozapine (Imipramine may potentiate the effects of CNS depressant drugs). Products include:

Clozaril Tablets.................................. 2252

Codeine Phosphate (Imipramine may potentiate the effects of CNS depressant drugs). Products include:

Actifed with Codeine Cough Syrup.. 1067 Brontex .... 1981 Deconsal C Expectorant Syrup .... 456 Deconsal Pediatric Syrup .... 457 Dimetane-DC Cough Syrup .... 2059 Empirin with Codeine Tablets........... 1093 Fioricet with Codeine Capsules .... 2260 Fiorinal with Codeine Capsules .... 2262 Isoclor Expectorant .... 990 Novahistine DH.................................. 2462 Novahistine Expectorant................... 2463 Nucofed .... 2051 Phenergan with Codeine................... 2777 Phenergan VC with Codeine .... 2781 Robitussin A-C Syrup .... 2073 Robitussin-DAC Syrup .... 2074 Ryna .... ◆D 841 Soma Compound w/Codeine Tablets .... 2676 Tussi-Organidin NR Liquid and S NR Liquid .... 2677 Tylenol with Codeine 1583

Desflurane (Imipramine may potentiate the effects of CNS depressant drugs). Products include:

Suprane 1813

Desipramine Hydrochloride (Concurrent use with drugs that are substrate for cytochrome $P_{450}IID_6$ may make normal metabolizer resemble poor metabolizer leading to higher than expected plasma concentrations of TCA with resultant toxicity). Products include:

Norpramin Tablets 1526

Dezocine (Imipramine may potentiate the effects of CNS depressant drugs). Products include:

Dalgan Injection 538

Diazepam (Imipramine may potentiate the effects of CNS depressant drugs). Products include:

Dizac.. 1809 Valium Injectable .... 2182 Valium Tablets .... 2183 Valrelease Capsules 2169

Dicyclomine Hydrochloride (Concurrent use may result in pronounced atropine-like effects, e.g., paralytic ileus). Products include:

Bentyl 1501

Dobutamine Hydrochloride (Avoid concurrent use since tricyclic antidepressants can potentiate the effects of catecholamines). Products include:

Dobutrex Solution Vials.................... 1439

Dopamine Hydrochloride (Avoid concurrent use since tricyclic antidepressants can potentiate the effects of catecholamines).

No products indexed under this heading.

Doxepin Hydrochloride (Concurrent use with drugs that are substrate for cytochrome $P_{450}IID_6$ may make normal metabolizer resemble poor metabolizer leading to higher than expected plasma concentrations of TCA with resultant toxicity). Products include:

Sinequan .... 2205 Zonalon Cream 1055

Droperidol (Imipramine may potentiate the effects of CNS depressant drugs). Products include:

Inapsine Injection 1296

Enflurane (Imipramine may potentiate the effects of CNS depressant drugs).

No products indexed under this heading.

Ephedrine Hydrochloride (Avoid concurrent use since tricyclic antidepressants can potentiate the effects of catecholamines). Products include:

Primatene Dual Action Formula...... ◆D 872

IMPORTANT NOTE: Always consult each drug listing in the patient's regimen for possible interactions.

Tofranil Tablets — Interactions Index — 1044

Primatene Tablets .... ◘ 873
Quadrinal Tablets 1350

Ephedrine Sulfate (Avoid concurrent use since tricyclic antidepressants can potentiate the effects of catecholamines). Products include:
Bronkaid Caplets .... ◘ 717
Marax Tablets & DF Syrup 2200

Ephedrine Tannate (Avoid concurrent use since tricyclic antidepressants can potentiate the effects of catecholamines). Products include:
Rynatuss 2673

Epinephrine (Avoid concurrent use since tricyclic antidepressants can potentiate the effects of catecholamines). Products include:
Bronkaid Mist .... ◘ 717
EPIFRIN .... ◉ 239
EpiPen 790
Marcaine Hydrochloride with Epinephrine 1:200,000 2316
Primatene Mist .... ◘ 873
Sensorcaine with Epinephrine Injection 559
Sus-Phrine Injection 1019
Xylocaine with Epinephrine Injections 567

Epinephrine Bitartrate (Avoid concurrent use since tricyclic antidepressants can potentiate the effects of catecholamines). Products include:
Bronkaid Mist Suspension .... ◘ 718
Sensorcaine-MPF with Epinephrine Injection 559

Epinephrine Hydrochloride (Avoid concurrent use since tricyclic antidepressants can potentiate the effects of catecholamines). Products include:
Ana-Kit Anaphylaxis Emergency Treatment Kit 617

Estazolam (Imipramine may potentiate the effects of CNS depressant drugs). Products include:
ProSom Tablets 449

Ethchlorvynol (Imipramine may potentiate the effects of CNS depressant drugs). Products include:
Placidyl Capsules 448

Ethinamate (Imipramine may potentiate the effects of CNS depressant drugs).
No products indexed under this heading.

Fentanyl (Imipramine may potentiate the effects of CNS depressant drugs). Products include:
Duragesic Transdermal System 1288

Fentanyl Citrate (Imipramine may potentiate the effects of CNS depressant drugs). Products include:
Sublimaze Injection 1307

Flecainide Acetate (Concurrent use with drugs that are substrate for cytochrome $P_{450}IID_6$ may make normal metabolizer resemble poor metabolizer leading to higher than expected plasma concentrations of TCA with resultant toxicity). Products include:
Tambocor Tablets 1497

Fluoxetine Hydrochloride (Concurrent use with drugs that are substrate for cytochrome $P_{450}IID_6$ may make normal metabolizer resemble poor metabolizer leading to higher than expected plasma concentrations of TCA with resultant toxicity; due to variation in the extent of inhibition of $P_{450}IID_6$ and long half-life of the parent (fluoxetine) and active metabolite sufficient time must elapse, at least 5 weeks before switching to TCA). Products include:
Prozac Pulvules & Liquid, Oral Solution 919

Fluphenazine Decanoate (Concurrent use with drugs that are substrate for cytochrome $P_{450}IID_6$ may make normal metabolizer resemble poor metabolizer leading to higher than expected plasma concentrations of TCA with resultant toxicity; imipramine may potentiate the effects of CNS depressant drugs). Products include:
Prolixin Decanoate 509

Fluphenazine Enanthate (Concurrent use with drugs that are substrate for cytochrome $P_{450}IID_6$ may make normal metabolizer resemble poor metabolizer leading to higher than expected plasma concentrations of TCA with resultant toxicity; imipramine may potentiate the effects of CNS depressant drugs). Products include:
Prolixin Enanthate 509

Fluphenazine Hydrochloride (Concurrent use with drugs that are substrate for cytochrome $P_{450}IID_6$ may make normal metabolizer resemble poor metabolizer leading to higher than expected plasma concentrations of TCA with resultant toxicity; imipramine may potentiate the effects of CNS depressant drugs). Products include:
Prolixin 509

Flurazepam Hydrochloride (Imipramine may potentiate the effects of CNS depressant drugs). Products include:
Dalmane Capsules 2173

Fluvoxamine Maleate (Concurrent use with drugs that are substrate for cytochrome $P_{450}IID_6$ may make normal metabolizer resemble poor metabolizer leading to higher than expected plasma concentrations of TCA with resultant toxicity; due to variation in the extent of inhibition of $P_{450}IID_6$ caution is indicated if co-administered sufficient time must elapse). Products include:
Luvox Tablets 2544

Furazolidone (Potential for hyperpyretic crises, severe convulsions, and deaths; concurrent and/or sequential use is contraindicated). Products include:
Furoxone 2046

Glutethimide (Imipramine may potentiate the effects of CNS depressant drugs).
No products indexed under this heading.

Glycopyrrolate (Concurrent use may result in pronounced atropine-like effects, e.g., paralytic ileus). Products include:
Robinul Forte Tablets 2072
Robinul Injectable 2072
Robinul Tablets 2072

Guanadrel Sulfate (Imipramine may block the antihypertensive effect). Products include:
Hylorel Tablets 985

Guanethidine Monosulfate (Imipramine may block the antihypertensive effect of guanethidine or similarly acting compounds). Products include:
Esimil Tablets 822
Ismelin Tablets 827

Haloperidol (Imipramine may potentiate the effects of CNS depressant drugs). Products include:
Haldol Injection, Tablets and Concentrate 1575

Haloperidol Decanoate (Imipramine may potentiate the effects of CNS depressant drugs). Products include:
Haldol Decanoate 1577

Hydrocodone Bitartrate (Imipramine may potentiate the effects of CNS depressant drugs). Products include:
Anexsia 5/500 Elixir 1781
Anexia Tablets 1782
Codiclear DH Syrup 791
Deconamine CX Cough and Cold Liquid and Tablets 1319
Duratuss HD Elixir 2565
Hycodan Tablets and Syrup 930
Hycomine Compound Tablets 932
Hycomine 931
Hycotuss Expectorant Syrup 933
Hydrocet Capsules 782
Lorcet 10/650 1018
Lortab 2566
Tussend 1783
Tussend Expectorant 1785
Vicodin Tablets 1356
Vicodin ES Tablets 1357
Vicodin Tuss Expectorant 1358
Zydone Capsules 949

Hydrocodone Polistirex (Imipramine may potentiate the effects of CNS depressant drugs). Products include:
Tussionex Pennkinetic Extended-Release Suspension 998

Hydroxyzine Hydrochloride (Imipramine may potentiate the effects of CNS depressant drugs). Products include:
Atarax Tablets & Syrup 2185
Marax Tablets & DF Syrup 2200
Vistaril Intramuscular Solution 2216

Hyoscyamine (Concurrent use may result in pronounced atropine-like effects, e.g., paralytic ileus). Products include:
Cystospaz Tablets 1963
Urised Tablets 1964

Hyoscyamine Sulfate (Concurrent use may result in pronounced atropine-like effects, e.g., paralytic ileus). Products include:
Arco-Lase Plus Tablets 512
Atrohist Plus Tablets 454
Cystospaz-M Capsules 1963
Donnatal 2060
Donnatal Extentabs 2061
Donnatal Tablets 2060
Kutrase Capsules 2402
Levsin/Levsinex/Levbid 2405

Imipramine Pamoate (Concurrent use with drugs that are substrate for cytochrome $P_{450}IID_6$ may make normal metabolizer resemble poor metabolizer leading to higher than expected plasma concentrations of TCA with resultant toxicity). Products include:
Tofranil-PM Capsules 857

Ipratropium Bromide (Concurrent use may result in pronounced atropine-like effects, e.g., paralytic ileus). Products include:
Atrovent Inhalation Aerosol 671
Atrovent Inhalation Solution 673

Isocarboxazid (Potential for hyperpyretic crises; severe convulsions, and deaths; concurrent and/or sequential use is contraindicated).
No products indexed under this heading.

Isoflurane (Imipramine may potentiate the effects of CNS depressant drugs).
No products indexed under this heading.

Isoproterenol Hydrochloride (Avoid concurrent use since tricyclic antidepressants can potentiate the effects of catecholamines). Products include:
Isuprel Hydrochloride Injection 1:5000 2311
Isuprel Hydrochloride Solution 1:200 & 1:100 2313
Isuprel Mistometer 2312

Isoproterenol Sulfate (Avoid concurrent use since tricyclic antidepressants can potentiate the effects of catecholamines). Products include:
Norisodrine with Calcium Iodide Syrup 442

Ketamine Hydrochloride (Imipramine may potentiate the effects of CNS depressant drugs).
No products indexed under this heading.

Levomethadyl Acetate Hydrochloride (Imipramine may potentiate the effects of CNS depressant drugs). Products include:
Orlamm 2239

Levorphanol Tartrate (Imipramine may potentiate the effects of CNS depressant drugs). Products include:
Levo-Dromoran 2129

Levothyroxine Sodium (Co-administration may produce cardiovascular toxicity). Products include:
Levothroid Tablets 1016
Levoxyl Tablets 903
Synthroid 1359

Liothyronine Sodium (Co-administration may produce cardiovascular toxicity). Products include:
Cytomel Tablets 2473
Triostat Injection 2530

Liotrix (Co-administration may produce cardiovascular toxicity).
No products indexed under this heading.

Lorazepam (Imipramine may potentiate the effects of CNS depressant drugs). Products include:
Ativan Injection 2698
Ativan Tablets 2700

Loxapine Hydrochloride (Imipramine may potentiate the effects of CNS depressant drugs). Products include:
Loxitane 1378

Loxapine Succinate (Imipramine may potentiate the effects of CNS depressant drugs). Products include:
Loxitane Capsules 1378

Maprotiline Hydrochloride (Concurrent use with drugs that are substrate for cytochrome $P_{450}IID_6$ may make normal metabolizer resemble poor metabolizer leading to higher than expected plasma concentrations of TCA with resultant toxicity). Products include:
Ludiomil Tablets 843

Mepenzolate Bromide (Concurrent use may result in pronounced atropine-like effects, e.g., paralytic ileus).
No products indexed under this heading.

Meperidine Hydrochloride (Imipramine may potentiate the effects of CNS depressant drugs). Products include:
Demerol 2308
Mepergan Injection 2753

Mephobarbital (The plasma concentration of imipramine may decrease when the drug is given with barbiturates, a hepatic enzyme inducers; dosage of imipramine may need to be adjusted; imipramine may potentiate the effects of CNS depressant drugs). Products include:
Mebaral Tablets 2322

Meprobamate (Imipramine may potentiate the effects of CNS depressant drugs). Products include:
Miltown Tablets 2672
PMB 200 and PMB 400 2783

Interactions Index — Tofranil Tablets

Mesoridazine (Imipramine may potentiate the effects of CNS depressant drugs).

Mesoridazine Besylate (Concurrent use with drugs that are substrate for cytochrome $P_{450}IID_6$ may make normal metabolizer resemble poor metabolizer leading to higher than expected plasma concentrations of TCA with resultant toxicity; imipramine may potentiate the effects of CNS depressant drugs). Products include:

Serentil 684

Metaproterenol Sulfate (Avoid concurrent use since tricyclic antidepressants can potentiate the effects of catecholamines). Products include:

Alupent 669
Metaproterenol Sulfate Inhalation Solution, USP, Arm-a-Med 552

Metaraminol Bitartrate (Avoid concurrent use since tricyclic antidepressants can potentiate the effects of catecholamines). Products include:

Aramine Injection 1609

Methadone Hydrochloride (Imipramine may potentiate the effects of CNS depressant drugs). Products include:

Methadone Hydrochloride Oral Concentrate 2233
Methadone Hydrochloride Oral Solution & Tablets 2235

Methohexital Sodium (Imipramine may potentiate the effects of CNS depressant drugs). Products include:

Brevital Sodium Vials 1429

Methotrimeprazine (Concurrent use with drugs that are substrate for cytochrome $P_{450}IID_6$ may make normal metabolizer resemble poor metabolizer leading to higher than expected plasma concentrations of TCA with resultant toxicity; imipramine may potentiate the effects of CNS depressant drugs). Products include:

Levoprome 1274

Methoxamine Hydrochloride (Avoid concurrent use since tricyclic antidepressants can potentiate the effects of catecholamines). Products include:

Vasoxyl Injection 1196

Methoxyflurane (Imipramine may potentiate the effects of CNS depressant drugs).

No products indexed under this heading.

Methylphenidate Hydrochloride (May inhibit the metabolism of imipramine; downward dosage adjustments of imipramine may be required when given concomitantly). Products include:

Ritalin 848

Midazolam Hydrochloride (Imipramine may potentiate the effects of CNS depressant drugs). Products include:

Versed Injection 2170

Molindone Hydrochloride (Imipramine may potentiate the effects of CNS depressant drugs). Products include:

Moban Tablets and Concentrate 1048

Morphine Sulfate (Imipramine may potentiate the effects of CNS depressant drugs). Products include:

Astramorph/PF Injection, USP (Preservative-Free) 535
Duramorph 962
Infumorph 200 and Infumorph 500 Sterile Solutions 965
MS Contin Tablets 1994
MSIR 1997
Oramorph SR (Morphine Sulfate Sustained Release Tablets) 2236
RMS Suppositories 2657
Roxanol 2243

Nefazodone Hydrochloride (Concurrent use with drugs that are substrate for cytochrome $P_{450}IID_6$ may make normal metabolizer resemble poor metabolizer leading to higher than expected plasma concentrations of TCA with resultant toxicity). Products include:

Serzone Tablets 771

Norepinephrine Bitartrate (Avoid concurrent use since tricyclic antidepressants can potentiate the effects of catecholamines). Products include:

Levophed Bitartrate Injection 2315

Nortriptyline Hydrochloride (Concurrent use with drugs that are substrate for cytochrome $P_{450}IID_6$ may make normal metabolizer resemble poor metabolizer leading to higher than expected plasma concentrations of TCA with resultant toxicity). Products include:

Pamelor 2280

Opium Alkaloids (Imipramine may potentiate the effects of CNS depressant drugs).

No products indexed under this heading.

Oxazepam (Imipramine may potentiate the effects of CNS depressant drugs). Products include:

Serax Capsules 2810
Serax Tablets 2810

Oxybutynin Chloride (Concurrent use may result in pronounced atropine-like effects, e.g., paralytic ileus). Products include:

Ditropan 1516

Oxycodone Hydrochloride (Imipramine may potentiate the effects of CNS depressant drugs). Products include:

Percocet Tablets 938
Percodan Tablets 939
Percodan-Demi Tablets 940
Roxicodone Tablets, Oral Solution & Intensol (Oxycodone) 2244
Tylox Capsules 1584

Paroxetine Hydrochloride (Concurrent use with drugs that are substrate for cytochrome $P_{450}IID_6$ may make normal metabolizer resemble poor metabolizer leading to higher than expected plasma concentrations of TCA with resultant toxicity; due to variation in the extent of inhibition of $P_{450}IID_6$ and long half-life of the parent (fluoxetine) and active metabolite sufficient time must elapse, at least 5 weeks before switching to TCA). Products include:

Paxil Tablets 2505

Pentobarbital Sodium (The plasma concentration of imipramine may decrease when the drug is given with barbiturates, a hepatic enzyme inducer; dosage of imipramine may need to be adjusted; imipramine may potentiate the effects of CNS depressant drugs). Products include:

Nembutal Sodium Capsules 436
Nembutal Sodium Solution 438
Nembutal Sodium Suppositories 440

Perphenazine (Concurrent use with drugs that are substrate for cytochrome $P_{450}IID_6$ may make normal metabolizer resemble poor metabolizer leading to higher than expected plasma concentrations of TCA with resultant toxicity; imipramine may potentiate the effects of CNS depressant drugs). Products include:

Etrafon 2355
Triavil Tablets 1757
Trilafon 2389

Phenelzine Sulfate (Potential for hyperpyretic crises, severe convulsions, and deaths; concurrent and/or sequential use is contraindicated). Products include:

Nardil 1920

Phenobarbital (The plasma concentration of imipramine may decrease when the drug is given with barbiturates, a hepatic enzyme inducer; dosage of imipramine may need to be adjusted; imipramine may potentiate the effects of CNS depressant drugs). Products include:

Arco-Lase Plus Tablets 512
Bellergal-S Tablets 2250
Donnatal 2060
Donnatal Extentabs 2061
Donnatal Tablets 2060
Phenobarbital Elixir and Tablets 1469
Quadrinal Tablets 1350

Phenylephrine Bitartrate (Avoid concurrent use since tricyclic antidepressants can potentiate the effects of catecholamines).

No products indexed under this heading.

Phenylephrine Hydrochloride (Avoid concurrent use since tricyclic antidepressants can potentiate the effects of catecholamines). Products include:

Atrohist Plus Tablets 454
Cerose DM .... ⊕ 878
Comhist 2038
D.A. Chewable Tablets 951
Deconsal Pediatric Capsules 454
Dura-Vent/DA Tablets 953
Entex Capsules 1986
Entex Liquid 1986
Extendryl 1005
4-Way Fast Acting Nasal Spray (regular & mentholated) .... ⊕ 621
Hemorid For Women .... ⊕ 834
Hycomine Compound Tablets 932
Neo-Synephrine Hydrochloride 1% Carpuject 2324
Neo-Synephrine Hydrochloride 1% Injection 2324
Neo-Synephrine Hydrochloride (Ophthalmic) 2325
Neo-Synephrine .... ⊕ 726
Nöstril .... ⊕ 644
Novahistine Elixir .... ⊕ 823
Phenergan VC 2779
Phenergan VC with Codeine 2781
Preparation H .... ⊕ 871
Tympagesic Ear Drops 2342
Vasosulf .... © 271
Vicks Sinex Nasal Spray and Ultra Fine Mist .... ⊕ 765

Phenylephrine Tannate (Avoid concurrent use since tricyclic antidepressants can potentiate the effects of catecholamines). Products include:

Atrohist Pediatric Suspension 454
Ricobid-D Pediatric Suspension 2038
Ricobid Tablets and Pediatric Suspension 2038
Rynatan 2673
Rynatuss 2673

Phenylpropanolamine Hydrochloride (Avoid concurrent use since tricyclic antidepressants can potentiate the effects of catecholamines). Products include:

Acutrim .... ⊕ 628
Allerest Children's Chewable Tablets .... ⊕ 627
Allerest 12 Hour Caplets .... ⊕ 627
Atrohist Plus Tablets 454
BC Cold Powder Multi-Symptom Formula (Cold-Sinus-Allergy) ...... ⊕ 609
BC Cold Powder Non-Drowsy Formula (Cold-Sinus) .... ⊕ 609
Cheracol Plus Head Cold/Cough Formula .... ⊕ 769
Comtrex Multi-Symptom Non-Drowsy Liqui-gels .... ⊕ 618
Contac Continuous Action Nasal Decongestant/Antihistamine 12 Hour Capsules .... ⊕ 813
Contac Maximum Strength Continuous Action Decongestant/Antihistamine 12 Hour Caplets .. ⊕ 813
Contac Severe Cold and Flu Formula Caplets .... ⊕ 814
Coricidin 'D' Decongestant Tablets .... ⊕ 800
Dexatrim .... ⊕ 832
Dexatrim Plus Vitamins Caplets .... ⊕ 832
Dimetane-DC Cough Syrup 2059
Dimetapp Elixir .... ⊕ 773
Dimetapp Extentabs .... ⊕ 774
Dimetapp Tablets/Liqui-Gels .... ⊕ 775
Dimetapp Cold & Allergy Chewable Tablets .... ⊕ 773
Dimetapp DM Elixir .... ⊕ 774
Dura-Vent Tablets 952
Entex Capsules 1986
Entex LA Tablets 1987
Entex Liquid 1986
Exgest LA Tablets 782
Hycomine 931
Isoclor Timesule Capsules .... ⊕ 637
Nolamine Timed-Release Tablets 785
Ornade Spansule Capsules 2502
Propagest Tablets 786
Pyrroxate Caplets .... ⊕ 772
Robitussin-CF .... ⊕ 777
Sinulin Tablets 787
Tavist-D 12 Hour Relief Tablets .... ⊕ 787
Teldrin 12 Hour Antihistamine/Nasal Decongestant Allergy Relief Capsules .... ⊕ 826
Triaminic Allergy Tablets .... ⊕ 789
Triaminic Cold Tablets .... ⊕ 790
Triaminic Expectorant .... ⊕ 790
Triaminic Syrup .... ⊕ 792
Triaminic-12 Tablets .... ⊕ 792
Triaminic-DM Syrup .... ⊕ 792
Triaminicin Tablets .... ⊕ 793
Triaminicol Multi-Symptom Cold Tablets .... ⊕ 793
Triaminicol Multi-Symptom Relief ⊕ 794
Vicks DayQuil Allergy Relief 12-Hour Extended Release Tablets .. ⊕ 760
Vicks DayQuil Allergy Relief 4-Hour Tablets .... ⊕ 760
Vicks DayQuil SINUS Pressure & CONGESTION Relief .... ⊕ 761

Phenytoin (The plamsa concentration of imipramine may decrease when the drug is given with phenytoin, a hepatic enzyme inducer; dosage of imipramine may need to be adjusted). Products include:

Dilantin Infatabs 1908
Dilantin-125 Suspension 1911

Phenytoin Sodium (The plamsa concentration of imipramine may decrease when the drug is given with phenytoin, a hepatic enzyme inducer; dosage of imipramine may need to be adjusted). Products include:

Dilantin Kapseals 1906
Dilantin Parenteral 1910

Pirbuterol Acetate (Avoid concurrent use since tricyclic antidepressants can potentiate the effects of catecholamines). Products include:

Maxair Autohaler 1492
Maxair Inhaler 1494

Prazepam (Imipramine may potentiate the effects of CNS depressant drugs).

No products indexed under this heading.

Prochlorperazine (Concurrent use with drugs that are substrate for cytochrome $P_{450}IID_6$ may make normal metabolizer resemble poor metabolizer leading to higher than expected plasma concentrations of TCA with resultant toxicity; imipramine may potentiate the effects of CNS depressant drugs). Products include:

Compazine 2470

Procyclidine Hydrochloride (Concurrent use may result in pronounced atropine-like effects, e.g., paralytic ileus). Products include:

Kemadrin Tablets 1112

IMPORTANT NOTE: Always consult each drug listing in the patient's regimen for possible interactions.

Promethazine Hydrochloride (Concurrent use with drugs that are substrate for cytochrome $P_{450}IID_6$ may make normal metabolizer resemble poor metabolizer leading to higher than expected plasma concentrations of TCA with resultant toxicity; imipramine may potentiate the effects of CNS depressant drugs). Products include:

Mepergan Injection ... 2753
Phenergan with Codeine ... 2777
Phenergan with Dextromethorphan 2778
Phenergan Injection ... 2773
Phenergan Suppositories ... 2775
Phenergan Syrup ... 2774
Phenergan Tablets ... 2775
Phenergan VC ... 2779
Phenergan VC with Codeine ... 2781

Propafenone Hydrochloride (Concurrent use with drugs that are substrate for cytochrome $P_{450}IID_6$ may make normal metabolizer resemble poor metabolizer leading to higher than expected plasma concentrations of TCA with resultant toxicity). Products include:

Rythmol Tablets–150mg, 225mg, 300mg ... 1352

Propantheline Bromide (Concurrent use may result in pronounced atropine-like effects, e.g., paralytic ileus). Products include:

Pro-Banthīne Tablets ... 2052

Propofol (Imipramine may potentiate the effects of CNS depressant drugs). Products include:

Diprivan Injection ... 2833

Propoxyphene Hydrochloride (Imipramine may potentiate the effects of CNS depressant drugs). Products include:

Darvon ... 1435
Wygesic Tablets ... 2827

Propoxyphene Napsylate (Imipramine may potentiate the effects of CNS depressant drugs). Products include:

Darvon-N/Darvocet-N ... 1433

Protriptyline Hydrochloride (Concurrent use with drugs that are substrate for cytochrome $P_{450}IID_6$ may make normal metabolizer resemble poor metabolizer leading to higher than expected plasma concentrations of TCA with resultant toxicity). Products include:

Vivactil Tablets ... 1774

Pseudoephedrine Hydrochloride (Avoid concurrent use since tricyclic antidepressants can potentiate the effects of catecholamines). Products include:

Actifed Allergy Daytime/Nighttime Caplets ... ▣ 844
Actifed Plus Caplets ... ▣ 845
Actifed Plus Tablets ... ▣ 845
Actifed with Codeine Cough Syrup .. 1067
Actifed Sinus Daytime/Nighttime Tablets and Caplets ... ▣ 846
Actifed Syrup ... ▣ 846
Actifed Tablets ... ▣ 844
Advil Cold and Sinus Caplets and Tablets (formerly CoAdvil) ... ▣ 870
Alka-Seltzer Plus Cold Medicine Liqui-Gels ... ▣ 706
Alka-Seltzer Plus Cold & Cough Medicine Liqui-Gels ... ▣ 705
Alka-Seltzer Plus Night-Time Cold Medicine Liqui-Gels ... ▣ 706
Allerest Headache Strength Tablets ... ▣ 627
Allerest Maximum Strength Tablets ... ▣ 627
Allerest No Drowsiness Tablets ... ▣ 627
Allerest Sinus Pain Formula ... ▣ 627
Anatuss LA Tablets ... 1542
Atrohist Pediatric Capsules ... 453
Bayer Select Sinus Pain Relief Formula ... ▣ 717
Benadryl Allergy Decongestant Liquid Medication ... ▣ 848
Benadryl Allergy Decongestant Tablets ... ▣ 848
Benadryl Allergy Sinus Headache Formula Caplets ... ▣ 849
Benylin Multisymptom ... ▣ 852
Bromfed Capsules (Extended-Release) ... 1785
Bromfed Syrup ... ▣ 733
Bromfed Tablets ... 1785
Bromfed-DM Cough Syrup ... 1786
Bromfed-PD Capsules (Extended-Release) ... 1785
Children's Vicks DayQuil Allergy Relief ... ▣ 757
Children's Vicks NyQuil Cold/Cough Relief ... ▣ 758
Comtrex Multi-Symptom Cold Reliever Tablets/Caplets/Liqui-Gels/Liquid ... ▣ 615
Allergy-Sinus Comtrex Multi-Symptom Allergy-Sinus Formula Tablets ... ▣ 617
Comtrex Multi-Symptom Non-Drowsy Caplets ... ▣ 618
Congess ... 1004
Contac Day Allergy/Sinus Caplets ▣ 812
Contac Day & Night ... ▣ 812
Contac Night Allergy/Sinus Caplets ... ▣ 812
Contac Severe Cold & Flu Non-Drowsy ... ▣ 815
Deconamine Chewable Tablets ... 1320
Deconamine CX Cough and Cold Liquid and Tablets ... 1319
Deconamine ... 1320
Deconsal C Expectorant Syrup ... 456
Deconsal Pediatric Syrup ... 457
Deconsal II Tablets ... 454
Dimetane-DX Cough Syrup ... 2059
Dimetapp Sinus Caplets ... ▣ 775
Dorcol Children's Cough Syrup ... ▣ 785
Drixoral Cough + Congestion Liquid Caps ... ▣ 802
Dura-Tap/PD Capsules ... 2867
Duratuss Tablets ... 2565
Duratuss HD Elixir ... 2565
Efidac/24 ... ▣ 635
Entex PSE Tablets ... 1987
Fedahist Gyrocaps ... 2401
Fedahist Timecaps ... 2401
Guaifed ... 1787
Guaifed Syrup ... ▣ 734
Guaimax-D Tablets ... 792
Guaitab Tablets ... ▣ 734
Isoclor Expectorant ... 990
Kronofed-A ... 977
Motrin IB Sinus ... ▣ 838
Novahistine DH ... 2462
Novahistine DMX ... ▣ 822
Novahistine Expectorant ... 2463
Nucofed ... 2051
PediaCare Cold Allergy Chewable Tablets ... ▣ 677
PediaCare Cough-Cold Chewable Tablets ... 1553
PediaCare ... 1553
PediaCare Infants' Decongestant Drops ... ▣ 677
PediCare Infant's Drops Decongestant Plus Cough ... 1553
PediaCare NightRest Cough-Cold Liquid ... 1553
Pediatric Vicks 44d Dry Hacking Cough & Head Congestion ... ▣ 763
Pediatric Vicks 44m Cough & Cold Relief ... ▣ 764
Robitussin Cold & Cough Liqui-Gels ... ▣ 776
Robitussin Maximum Strength Cough & Cold ... ▣ 778
Robitussin Pediatric Cough & Cold Formula ... ▣ 779
Robitussin Severe Congestion Liqui-Gels ... ▣ 776
Robitussin-DAC Syrup ... 2074
Robitussin-PE ... ▣ 778
Rondec Oral Drops ... 953
Rondec Syrup ... 953
Rondec Tablet ... 953
Rondec-DM Oral Drops ... 954
Rondec-DM Syrup ... 954
Rondec-TR Tablet ... 953
Ryna ... ▣ 841
Seldane-D Extended-Release Tablets ... 1538
Semprex-D Capsules ... 463
Semprex-D Capsules ... 1167
Sinarest Tablets ... ▣ 648
Sinarest Extra Strength Tablets ... ▣ 648
Sinarest No Drowsiness Tablets ... ▣ 648
Sine-Aid IB Caplets ... 1554
Sine-Aid Maximum Strength Sinus Medication Gelcaps, Caplets and Tablets ... 1554
Sine-Off No Drowsiness Formula Caplets ... ▣ 824
Sine-Off Sinus Medicine ... ▣ 825
Singlet Tablets ... ▣ 825
Sinutab Non-Drying Liquid Caps ... ▣ 859
Sinutab Sinus Allergy Medication, Maximum Strength Tablets and Caplets ... ▣ 860
Sinutab Sinus Medication, Maximum Strength Without Drowsiness Formula, Tablets & Caplets ... ▣ 860
Sinutab Sinus Medication, Regular Strength Without Drowsiness Formula ... ▣ 859
Sudafed Children's Liquid ... ▣ 861
Sudafed Cold and Cough Liquidcaps ... ▣ 862
Sudafed Cough Syrup ... ▣ 862
Sudafed Plus Liquid ... ▣ 862
Sudafed Plus Tablets ... ▣ 863
Sudafed Severe Cold Formula Caplets ... ▣ 863
Sudafed Severe Cold Formula Tablets ... ▣ 864
Sudafed Sinus Caplets ... ▣ 864
Sudafed Sinus Tablets ... ▣ 864
Sudafed Tablets, 30 mg ... ▣ 861
Sudafed Tablets, 60 mg ... ▣ 861
Sudafed 12 Hour Caplets ... ▣ 861
Syn-Rx Tablets ... 465
Syn-Rx DM Tablets ... 466
TheraFlu ... ▣ 787
TheraFlu Maximum Strength Nighttime Flu, Cold & Cough Medicine ... ▣ 788
TheraFlu Maximum Strength Non-Drowsy Formula Flu, Cold & Cough Medicine ... ▣ 788
Thera Flu Maximum Strength, Non-Drowsy Formula Flu, Cold and Cough Caplets ... ▣ 789
Triaminic AM Cough and Decongestant Formula ... ▣ 789
Triaminic AM Decongestant Formula ... ▣ 790
Triaminic Nite Light ... ▣ 791
Triaminic Sore Throat Formula ... ▣ 791
Tussend ... 1783
Tussend Expectorant ... 1785
Children's TYLENOL Cold Multi-Symptom Liquid Formula and Chewable Tablets ... 1561
Children's TYLENOL Cold Plus Cough Multi Symptom Tablets and Liquid ... ▣ 681
Infants' TYLENOL Cold Decongestant & Fever-Reducer Drops ... 1556
TYLENOL Maximum Strength Allergy Sinus Medication Gelcaps and Caplets ... 1563
TYLENOL Maximum Strength Allergy Sinus NightTime Medication Caplets ... 1555
TYLENOL Flu Maximum Strength Gelcaps ... 1565
TYLENOL Flu NightTime, Maximum Strength, Gelcaps ... 1566
TYLENOL Maximum Strength Flu NightTime Hot Medication Packets ... 1562
TYLENOL, Maximum Strength, Sinus Medication Geltabs, Gelcaps, Caplets and Tablets ... 1566
TYLENOL Cold Multi-Symptom Formula Medication Tablets and Caplets ... 1561
TYLENOL Cold Medication No Drowsiness Formula Gelcaps and Caplets ... 1562
TYLENOL Cold Multi-Symptom Hot Medication Liquid Packets ... 1557
TYLENOL Cough Multi-Symptom Medication with Decongestant ... 1565
Ursinus Inlay-Tabs ... ▣ 794
Vicks 44 LiquiCaps Cough, Cold & Flu Relief ... ▣ 755
Vicks 44 LiquiCaps Non-Drowsy Cough & Cold Relief ... ▣ 756
Vicks 44D Dry Hacking Cough & Head Congestion ... ▣ 755
Vicks 44M Cough, Cold & Flu Relief ... ▣ 756
Vicks DayQuil ... ▣ 761
Vicks DayQuil SINUS Pressure & PAIN Relief with IBUPROFEN ... ▣ 762
Vicks Nyquil Hot Therapy ... ▣ 762
Vicks NyQuil LiquiCaps Multi-Symptom Cold/Flu Relief ... ▣ 763
Vicks NyQuil Multi-Symptom Cold/Flu Relief - (Original & Cherry Flavor) ... ▣ 763

Pseudoephedrine Sulfate (Avoid concurrent use since tricyclic antidepressants can potentiate the effects of catecholamines). Products include:

Cheracol Sinus ... ▣ 768
Chlor-Trimeton Allergy Decongestant Tablets ... ▣ 799
Claritin-D ... 2350
Drixoral Cold and Allergy Sustained-Action Tablets ... ▣ 802
Drixoral Cold and Flu Extended-Release Tablets ... ▣ 803
Drixoral Non-Drowsy Formula Extended-Release Tablets ... ▣ 803
Drixoral Allergy/Sinus Extended Release Tablets ... ▣ 804
Trinalin Repetabs Tablets ... 1330

Quazepam (Imipramine may potentiate the effects of CNS depressant drugs). Products include:

Doral Tablets ... 2664

Quinidine Gluconate (Concurrent use with drugs that inhibit cytochrome $P_{450}IID_6$ may make normal metabolizer resemble poor metabolizer leading to higher than expected plasma concentrations of TCA with resultant toxicity). Products include:

Quinaglute Dura-Tabs Tablets ... 649

Quinidine Polygalacturonate (Concurrent use with drugs that inhibit cytochrome $P_{450}IID_6$ may make normal metabolizer resemble poor metabolizer leading to higher than expected plasma concentrations of TCA with resultant toxicity).

No products indexed under this heading.

Quinidine Sulfate (Concurrent use with drugs that inhibit cytochrome $P_{450}IID_6$ may make normal metabolizer resemble poor metabolizer leading to higher than expected plasma concentrations of TCA with resultant toxicity). Products include:

Quinidex Extentabs ... 2067

Risperidone (Imipramine may potentiate the effects of CNS depressant drugs). Products include:

Risperdal ... 1301

Salmeterol Xinafoate (Avoid concurrent use since tricyclic antidepressants can potentiate the effects of catecholamines). Products include:

Serevent Inhalation Aerosol ... 1176

Scopolamine (Concurrent use may result in pronounced atropine-like effects, e.g., paralytic ileus). Products include:

Transderm Scōp Transdermal Therapeutic System ... 869

Scopolamine Hydrobromide (Concurrent use may result in pronounced atropine-like effects, e.g., paralytic ileus). Products include:

Atrohist Plus Tablets ... 454
Donnatal ... 2060
Donnatal Extentabs ... 2061
Donnatal Tablets ... 2060

Secobarbital Sodium (The plasma concentration of imipramine may decrease when the drug is given with barbiturates, a hepatic enzyme inducers; dosage of imipramine may need to be adjusted; imipramine may potentiate the effects of CNS depressant drugs). Products include:

Seconal Sodium Pulvules ... 1474

(▣ Described in PDR For Nonprescription Drugs) (◉ Described in PDR For Ophthalmology)

Selegiline Hydrochloride (Potential for hyperpyretic crises, severe convulsions, and deaths; concurrent and/or sequential use is contraindicated). Products include:

Eldepryl Tablets 2550

Sertraline Hydrochloride (Concurrent use with drugs that are substrate for cytochrome $P_{450}IID_6$ may make normal metabolizer resemble poor metabolizer leading to higher than expected plasma concentrations of TCA with resultant toxicity; due to variation in the extent of inhibition of $P_{450}IID_6$ sufficient time must elapse, at least 5 weeks before switching to TCA). Products include:

Zoloft Tablets 2217

Sufentanil Citrate (Imipramine may potentiate the effects of CNS depressant drugs). Products include:

Sufenta Injection 1309

Temazepam (Imipramine may potentiate the effects of CNS depressant drugs). Products include:

Restoril Capsules 2284

Terbutaline Sulfate (Avoid concurrent use since tricyclic antidepressants can potentiate the effects of catecholamines). Products include:

Brethaire Inhaler 813
Brethine Ampuls 815
Brethine Tablets 814
Bricanyl Subcutaneous Injection 1502
Bricanyl Tablets 1503

Thiamylal Sodium (The plasma concentration of imipramine may decrease when the drug is given with barbiturates, a hepatic enzyme inducer; dosage of imipramine may need to be adjusted; imipramine may potentiate the effects of CNS depressant drugs).

No products indexed under this heading.

Thioridazine Hydrochloride (Concurrent use with drugs that are substrate for cytochrome $P_{450}IID_6$ may make normal metabolizer resemble poor metabolizer leading to higher than expected plasma concentrations of TCA with resultant toxicity; imipramine may potentiate the effects of CNS depressant drugs). Products include:

Mellaril 2269

Thiothixene (Imipramine may potentiate the effects of CNS depressant drugs). Products include:

Navane Capsules and Concentrate 2201
Navane Intramuscular 2202

Thyroglobulin (Co-administration may produce cardiovascular toxicity).

No products indexed under this heading.

Thyroid (Co-administration may produce cardiovascular toxicity).

No products indexed under this heading.

Thyroxine (Co-administration may produce cardiovascular toxicity).

No products indexed under this heading.

Thyroxine Sodium (Co-administration may produce cardiovascular toxicity).

No products indexed under this heading.

Tranylcypromine Sulfate (Potential for hyperpyretic crises, severe convulsions, and deaths; concurrent and/or sequential use is contraindicated). Products include:

Parnate Tablets 2503

Trazodone Hydrochloride (Concurrent use with drugs that are substrate for cytochrome $P_{450}IID_6$ may make normal metabolizer resemble poor metabolizer leading to higher than expected plasma concentrations of TCA with resultant toxicity). Products include:

Desyrel and Desyrel Dividose 503

Triazolam (Imipramine may potentiate the effects of CNS depressant drugs). Products include:

Halcion Tablets 2611

Tridihexethyl Chloride (Concurrent use may result in pronounced atropine-like effects, e.g., paralytic ileus).

No products indexed under this heading.

Trifluoperazine Hydrochloride (Concurrent use with drugs that are substrate for cytochrome $P_{450}IID_6$ may make normal metabolizer resemble poor metabolizer leading to higher than expected plasma concentrations of TCA with resultant toxicity; imipramine may potentiate the effects of CNS depressant drugs). Products include:

Stelazine 2514

Trihexyphenidyl Hydrochloride (Concurrent use may result in pronounced atropine-like effects, e.g., paralytic ileus). Products include:

Artane 1368

Trimipramine Maleate (Concurrent use with drugs that are substrate for cytochrome $P_{450}IID_6$ may make normal metabolizer resemble poor metabolizer leading to higher than expected plasma concentrations of TCA with resultant toxicity). Products include:

Surmontil Capsules 2811

Venlafaxine Hydrochloride (Concurrent use with drugs that are substrate for cytochrome $P_{450}IID_6$ may make normal metabolizer resemble poor metabolizer leading to higher than expected plasma concentrations of TCA with resultant toxicity; due to variation in the extent of inhibition of $P_{450}IID_6$ sufficient time must elapse, at least 5 weeks before switching to TCA). Products include:

Effexor 2719

Zolpidem Tartrate (Imipramine may potentiate the effects of CNS depressant drugs). Products include:

Ambien Tablets 2416

Food Interactions

Alcohol (Imipramine may enhance the CNS depressant effects of alcohol).

TOFRANIL-PM CAPSULES

(Imipramine Pamoate) 857

May interact with central nervous system depressants, anticholinergics, sympathomimetics, barbiturates, monoamine oxidase inhibitors, thyroid preparations, drugs that inhibit cytochrome p450iid6, antidepressant drugs, phenothiazines, selective serotonin reuptake inhibitors, and certain other agents. Compounds in these categories include:

Albuterol (Avoid concurrent use since tricyclic antidepressants can potentiate the effects of catecholamines). Products include:

Proventil Inhalation Aerosol 2382
Ventolin Inhalation Aerosol and Refill 1197

Albuterol Sulfate (Avoid concurrent use since tricyclic antidepressants can potentiate the effects of catecholamines). Products include:

Airet Solution for Inhalation 452
Proventil Inhalation Solution 0.083% 2384
Proventil Repetabs Tablets 2386
Proventil Solution for Inhalation 0.5% 2383
Proventil Syrup 2385
Proventil Tablets 2386
Ventolin Inhalation Solution 1198
Ventolin Nebules Inhalation Solution 1199
Ventolin Rotacaps for Inhalation 1200
Ventolin Syrup 1202
Ventolin Tablets 1203
Volmax Extended-Release Tablets .. 1788

Alfentanil Hydrochloride (Imipramine may potentiate the effects of CNS depressant drugs). Products include:

Alfenta Injection 1286

Alprazolam (Imipramine may potentiate the effects of CNS depressant drugs). Products include:

Xanax Tablets 2649

Amitriptyline Hydrochloride (Concurrent use with drugs that are substrate for cytochrome $P_{450}IID_6$ may make normal metabolizer resemble poor metabolizer leading to higher than expected plasma concentrations of TCA with resultant toxicity). Products include:

Elavil 2838
Endep Tablets 2174
Etrafon 2355
Limbitrol 2180
Triavil Tablets 1757

Amoxapine (Concurrent use with drugs that are substrate for cytochrome $P_{450}IID_6$ may make normal metabolizer resemble poor metabolizer leading to higher than expected plasma concentrations of TCA with resultant toxicity). Products include:

Asendin Tablets 1369

Aprobarbital (The plasma concentration of imipramine may decrease when the drug is given with barbiturates, a hepatic enzyme inducer; dosage of imipramine may need to be adjusted; imipramine may potentiate the effects of CNS depressant drugs).

No products indexed under this heading.

Atropine Sulfate (Concurrent use may result in pronounced atropine-like effects, e.g., paralytic ileus). Products include:

Arco-Lase Plus Tablets 512
Atrohist Plus Tablets 454
Atropine Sulfate Sterile Ophthalmic Solution .... ⊙ 233
Donnatal 2060
Donnatal Extentabs 2061
Donnatal Tablets 2060
Lomotil 2439
Motofen Tablets 784
Urised Tablets 1964

Belladonna Alkaloids (Concurrent use may result in pronounced atropine-like effects, e.g., paralytic ileus). Products include:

Bellergal-S Tablets 2250
Hyland's Bed Wetting Tablets .... ▣ 828
Hyland's EnurAid Tablets .... ▣ 829
Hyland's Teething Tablets .... ▣ 830

Benztropine Mesylate (Concurrent use may result in pronounced atropine-like effects, e.g., paralytic ileus). Products include:

Cogentin 1621

Biperiden Hydrochloride (Concurrent use may result in pronounced atropine-like effects, e.g., paralytic ileus). Products include:

Akineton 1333

Buprenorphine (Imipramine may potentiate the effects of CNS depressant drugs). Products include:

Buprenex Injectable 2006

Bupropion Hydrochloride (Concurrent use with drugs that are substrate for cytochrome $P_{450}IID_6$ may make normal metabolizer resemble poor metabolizer leading to higher than expected plasma concentrations of TCA with resultant toxicity). Products include:

Wellbutrin Tablets 1204

Buspirone Hydrochloride (Imipramine may potentiate the effects of CNS depressant drugs). Products include:

BuSpar 737

Butabarbital (The plasma concentration of imipramine may decrease when the drug is given with barbiturates, a hepatic enzyme inducer; dosage of imipramine may need to be adjusted; imipramine may potentiate the effects of CNS depressant drugs).

No products indexed under this heading.

Butalbital (The plasma concentration of imipramine may decrease when the drug is given with barbiturates, a hepatic enzyme inducer; dosage of imipramine may need to be adjusted; imipramine may potentiate the effects of CNS depressant drugs). Products include:

Esgic-plus Tablets 1013
Fioricet Tablets 2258
Fioricet with Codeine Capsules 2260
Fiorinal Capsules 2261
Fiorinal with Codeine Capsules 2262
Fiorinal Tablets 2261
Phrenilin 785
Sedapap Tablets 50 mg/650 mg .. 1543

Chlordiazepoxide (Imipramine may potentiate the effects of CNS depressant drugs). Products include:

Libritabs Tablets 2177
Limbitrol 2180

Chlordiazepoxide Hydrochloride (Imipramine may potentiate the effects of CNS depressant drugs). Products include:

Librax Capsules 2176
Librium Capsules 2178
Librium Injectable 2179

Chlorpromazine (Concurrent use with drugs that are substrate for cytochrome $P_{450}IID_6$ may make normal metabolizer resemble poor metabolizer leading to higher than expected plasma concentrations of TCA with resultant toxicity; imipramine may potentiate the effects of CNS depressant drugs). Products include:

Thorazine Suppositories 2523

Chlorpromazine Hydrochloride (Concurrent use with drugs that are substrate for cytochrome $P_{450}IID_6$ may make normal metabolizer resemble poor metabolizer leading to higher than expected plasma concentrations of TCA with resultant toxicity; imipramine may potentiate the effects of CNS depressant drugs). Products include:

Thorazine 2523

Chlorprothixene (Imipramine may potentiate the effects of CNS depressant drugs).

No products indexed under this heading.

Chlorprothixene Hydrochloride (Imipramine may potentiate the effects of CNS depressant drugs).

No products indexed under this heading.

IMPORTANT NOTE: Always consult each drug listing in the patient's regimen for possible interactions.

Tofranil-PM — Interactions Index — 1048

Cimetidine (The plasma concentration of imipramine may increase when the drug is given with cimetidine, a hepatic enzyme inhibitor; dosage of imipramine may need to be adjusted). Products include:
- Tagamet Tablets ... 2516

Cimetidine Hydrochloride (The plasma concentration of imipramine may increase when the drug is given with cimetidine, a hepatic enzyme inhibitor; dosage of imipramine may need to be adjusted). Products include:
- Tagamet ... 2516

Clidinium Bromide (Concurrent use may result in pronounced atropine-like effects, e.g., paralytic ileus). Products include:
- Librax Capsules ... 2176
- Quarzan Capsules ... 2181

Clonidine (Imipramine may block the antihypertensive effect). Products include:
- Catapres-TTS ... 675

Clonidine Hydrochloride (Imipramine may block the antihypertensive effect). Products include:
- Catapres Tablets ... 674
- Combipres Tablets ... 677

Clorazepate Dipotassium (Imipramine may potentiate the effects of CNS depressant drugs). Products include:
- Tranxene ... 451

Clozapine (Imipramine may potentiate the effects of CNS depressant drugs). Products include:
- Clozaril Tablets ... 2252

Codeine Phosphate (Imipramine may potentiate the effects of CNS depressant drugs). Products include:
- Actifed with Codeine Cough Syrup.. 1067
- Brontex ... 1981
- Deconsal C Expectorant Syrup ... 456
- Deconsal Pediatric Syrup ... 457
- Dimetane-DC Cough Syrup ... 2059
- Empirin with Codeine Tablets ... 1093
- Fioricet with Codeine Capsules ... 2260
- Fiorinal with Codeine Capsules ... 2262
- Isoclor Expectorant ... 990
- Novahistine DH ... 2462
- Novahistine Expectorant ... 2463
- Nucofed ... 2051
- Phenergan with Codeine ... 2777
- Phenergan VC with Codeine ... 2781
- Robitussin A-C Syrup ... 2073
- Robitussin-DAC Syrup ... 2074
- Ryna ... ▣ 841
- Soma Compound w/Codeine Tablets ... 2676
- Tussi-Organidin NR Liquid and S NR Liquid ... 2677
- Tylenol with Codeine ... 1583

Desflurane (Imipramine may potentiate the effects of CNS depressant drugs). Products include:
- Suprane ... 1813

Desipramine Hydrochloride (Concurrent use with drugs that are substrate for cytochrome $P_{450}IID_6$ may make normal metabolizer resemble poor metabolizer leading to higher than expected plasma concentrations of TCA with resultant toxicity). Products include:
- Norpramin Tablets ... 1526

Dezocine (Imipramine may potentiate the effects of CNS depressant drugs). Products include:
- Dalgan Injection ... 538

Diazepam (Imipramine may potentiate the effects of CNS depressant drugs). Products include:
- Dizac ... 1809
- Valium Injectable ... 2182
- Valium Tablets ... 2183
- Valrelease Capsules ... 2169

Dicyclomine Hydrochloride (Concurrent use may result in pronounced atropine-like effects, e.g., paralytic ileus). Products include:
- Bentyl ... 1501

Dobutamine Hydrochloride (Avoid concurrent use since tricyclic antidepressants can potentiate the effects of catecholamines). Products include:
- Dobutrex Solution Vials ... 1439

Dopamine Hydrochloride (Avoid concurrent use since tricyclic antidepressants can potentiate the effects of catecholamines).
- No products indexed under this heading.

Doxepin Hydrochloride (Concurrent use with drugs that are substrate for cytochrome $P_{450}IID_6$ may make normal metabolizer resemble poor metabolizer leading to higher than expected plasma concentrations of TCA with resultant toxicity). Products include:
- Sinequan ... 2205
- Zonalon Cream ... 1055

Droperidol (Imipramine may potentiate the effects of CNS depressant drugs). Products include:
- Inapsine Injection ... 1296

Enflurane (Imipramine may potentiate the effects of CNS depressant drugs).
- No products indexed under this heading.

Ephedrine Hydrochloride (Avoid concurrent use since tricyclic antidepressants can potentiate the effects of catecholamines). Products include:
- Primatene Dual Action Formula ... ▣ 872
- Primatene Tablets ... ▣ 873
- Quadrinal Tablets ... 1350

Ephedrine Sulfate (Avoid concurrent use since tricyclic antidepressants can potentiate the effects of catecholamines). Products include:
- Bronkaid Caplets ... ▣ 717
- Marax Tablets & DF Syrup ... 2200

Ephedrine Tannate (Avoid concurrent use since tricyclic antidepressants can potentiate the effects of catecholamines). Products include:
- Rynatuss ... 2673

Epinephrine (Avoid concurrent use since tricyclic antidepressants can potentiate the effects of catecholamines). Products include:
- Bronkaid Mist ... ▣ 717
- EPIFRIN ... ⊙ 239
- EpiPen ... 790
- Marcaine Hydrochloride with Epinephrine 1:200,000 ... 2316
- Primatene Mist ... ▣ 873
- Sensorcaine with Epinephrine Injection ... 559
- Sus-Phrine Injection ... 1019
- Xylocaine with Epinephrine Injections ... 567

Epinephrine Bitartrate (Avoid concurrent use since tricyclic antidepressants can potentiate the effects of catecholamines). Products include:
- Bronkaid Mist Suspension ... ▣ 718
- Sensorcaine-MPF with Epinephrine Injection ... 559

Epinephrine Hydrochloride (Avoid concurrent use since tricyclic antidepressants can potentiate the effects of catecholamines). Products include:
- Ana-Kit Anaphylaxis Emergency Treatment Kit ... 617

Estazolam (Imipramine may potentiate the effects of CNS depressant drugs). Products include:
- ProSom Tablets ... 449

Ethchlorvynol (Imipramine may potentiate the effects of CNS depressant drugs). Products include:
- Placidyl Capsules ... 448

Ethinamate (Imipramine may potentiate the effects of CNS depressant drugs).
- No products indexed under this heading.

Fentanyl (Imipramine may potentiate the effects of CNS depressant drugs). Products include:
- Duragesic Transdermal System ... 1288

Fentanyl Citrate (Imipramine may potentiate the effects of CNS depressant drugs). Products include:
- Sublimaze Injection ... 1307

Flecainide Acetate (Concurent use with drugs that are substrate for cytochrome $P_{450}IID_6$ may make normal metabolizer resemble poor metabolizer leading to higher than expected plasma concentrations of TCA with resultant toxicity). Products include:
- Tambocor Tablets ... 1497

Fluoxetine Hydrochloride (Concurrent use with drugs that are substrate for cytochrome $P_{450}IID_6$ may make normal metabolizer resemble poor metabolizer leading to higher than expected plasma concentrations of TCA with resultant toxicity; due to variation in the extent of inhibition of $P_{450}IID_6$ and long half-life of the parent (fluoxetine) and active metabolite sufficient time must elapse, at least 5 weeks before switching to TCA). Products include:
- Prozac Pulvules & Liquid, Oral Solution ... 919

Fluphenazine Decanoate (Concurrent use with drugs that are substrate for cytochrome $P_{450}IID_6$ may make normal metabolizer resemble poor metabolizer leading to higher than expected plasma concentrations of TCA with resultant toxicity; imipramine may potentiate the effects of CNS depressant drugs). Products include:
- Prolixin Decanoate ... 509

Fluphenazine Enanthate (Concurrent use with drugs that are substrate for cytochrome $P_{450}IID_6$ may make normal metabolizer resemble poor metabolizer leading to higher than expected plasma concentrations of TCA with resultant toxicity; imipramine may potentiate the effects of CNS depressant drugs). Products include:
- Prolixin Enanthate ... 509

Fluphenazine Hydrochloride (Concurrent use with drugs that are substrate for cytochrome $P_{450}IID_6$ may make normal metabolizer resemble poor metabolizer leading to higher than expected plasma concentrations of TCA with resultant toxicity; imipramine may potentiate the effects of CNS depressant drugs). Products include:
- Prolixin ... 509

Flurazepam Hydrochloride (Imipramine may potentiate the effects of CNS depressant drugs). Products include:
- Dalmane Capsules ... 2173

Fluvoxamine Maleate (Concurrent use with drugs that are substrate for cytochrome $P_{450}IID_6$ may make normal metabolizer resemble poor metabolizer leading to higher than expected plasma concentrations of TCA with resultant toxicity; due to variation in the extent of inhibition of $P_{450}IID_6$ caution is indicated if co-administered sufficient time must elapse). Products include:
- Luvox Tablets ... 2544

Furazolidone (Potential for hyperpyretic crises, severe convulsions, and deaths; concurrent and/or sequential use is contraindicated). Products include:
- Furoxone ... 2046

Glutethimide (Imipramine may potentiate the effects of CNS depressant drugs).
- No products indexed under this heading.

Glycopyrrolate (Concurrent use may result in pronounced atropine-like effects, e.g., paralytic ileus). Products include:
- Robinul Forte Tablets ... 2072
- Robinul Injectable ... 2072
- Robinul Tablets ... 2072

Guanadrel Sulfate (Imipramine may block the antihypertensive effect). Products include:
- Hylorel Tablets ... 985

Guanethidine Monosulfate (Imipramine may block the antihypertensive effect of guanethidine or similarly acting compounds). Products include:
- Esimil Tablets ... 822
- Ismelin Tablets ... 827

Haloperidol (Imipramine may potentiate the effects of CNS depressant drugs). Products include:
- Haldol Injection, Tablets and Concentrate ... 1575

Haloperidol Decanoate (Imipramine may potentiate the effects of CNS depressant drugs). Products include:
- Haldol Decanoate ... 1577

Hydrocodone Bitartrate (Imipramine may potentiate the effects of CNS depressant drugs). Products include:
- Anexsia 5/500 Elixir ... 1781
- Anexia Tablets ... 1782
- Codiclear DH Syrup ... 791
- Deconamine CX Cough and Cold Liquid and Tablets ... 1319
- Duratuss HD Elixir ... 2565
- Hycodan Tablets and Syrup ... 930
- Hycomine Compound Tablets ... 932
- Hycomine ... 931
- Hycotuss Expectorant Syrup ... 933
- Hydrocet Capsules ... 782
- Lorcet 10/650 ... 1018
- Lortab ... 2566
- Tussend ... 1783
- Tussend Expectorant ... 1785
- Vicodin Tablets ... 1356
- Vicodin ES Tablets ... 1357
- Vicodin Tuss Expectorant ... 1358
- Zydone Capsules ... 949

Hydrocodone Polistirex (Imipramine may potentiate the effects of CNS depressant drugs). Products include:
- Tussionex Pennkinetic Extended-Release Suspension ... 998

Hydroxyzine Hydrochloride (Imipramine may potentiate the effects of CNS depressant drugs). Products include:
- Atarax Tablets & Syrup ... 2185
- Marax Tablets & DF Syrup ... 2200
- Vistaril Intramuscular Solution ... 2216

(▣ Described in PDR For Nonprescription Drugs) (⊙ Described in PDR For Ophthalmology)

Hyoscyamine (Concurrent use may result in pronounced atropine-like effects, e.g., paralytic ileus). Products include:

Cystospaz Tablets 1963
Urised Tablets 1964

Hyoscyamine Sulfate (Concurrent use may result in pronounced atropine-like effects, e.g., paralytic ileus). Products include:

Arco-Lase Plus Tablets 512
Atrohist Plus Tablets 454
Cystospaz-M Capsules 1963
Donnatal 2060
Donnatal Extentabs 2061
Donnatal Tablets 2060
Kutrase Capsules 2402
Levsin/Levsinex/Levbid 2405

Imipramine Hydrochloride (Concurrent use with drugs that are substrate for cytochrome $P_{450}IID_6$ may make normal metabolizer resemble poor metabolizer leading to higher than expected plasma concentrations of TCA with resultant toxicity). Products include:

Tofranil Ampuls 854
Tofranil Tablets 856

Ipratropium Bromide (Concurrent use may result in pronounced atropine-like effects, e.g., paralytic ileus). Products include:

Atrovent Inhalation Aerosol 671
Atrovent Inhalation Solution 673

Isocarboxazid (Potential for hyperpyretic crises; severe convulsions, and deaths; concurrent and/or sequential use is contraindicated).

No products indexed under this heading.

Isoflurane (Imipramine may potentiate the effects of CNS depressant drugs).

No products indexed under this heading.

Isoproterenol Hydrochloride (Avoid concurrent use since tricyclic antidepressants can potentiate the effects of catecholamines). Products include:

Isuprel Hydrochloride Injection 1:5000 2311
Isuprel Hydrochloride Solution 1:200 & 1:100 2313
Isuprel Mistometer 2312

Isoproterenol Sulfate (Avoid concurrent use since tricyclic antidepressants can potentiate the effects of catecholamines). Products include:

Norisodrine with Calcium Iodide Syrup 442

Ketamine Hydrochloride (Imipramine may potentiate the effects of CNS depressant drugs).

No products indexed under this heading.

Levomethadyl Acetate Hydrochloride (Imipramine may potentiate the effects of CNS depressant drugs). Products include:

Orlamm 2239

Levorphanol Tartrate (Imipramine may potentiate the effects of CNS depressant drugs). Products include:

Levo-Dromoran 2129

Levothyroxine Sodium (Co-administration may produce cardiovascular toxicity). Products include:

Levothroid Tablets 1016
Levoxyl Tablets 903
Synthroid 1359

Liothyronine Sodium (Co-administration may produce cardiovascular toxicity). Products include:

Cytomel Tablets 2473
Triostat Injection 2530

Liotrix (Co-administration may produce cardiovascular toxicity).

No products indexed under this heading.

Lorazepam (Imipramine may potentiate the effects of CNS depressant drugs). Products include:

Ativan Injection 2698
Ativan Tablets 2700

Loxapine Hydrochloride (Imipramine may potentiate the effects of CNS depressant drugs). Products include:

Loxitane 1378

Loxapine Succinate (Imipramine may potentiate the effects of CNS depressant drugs). Products include:

Loxitane Capsules 1378

Maprotiline Hydrochloride (Concurrent use with drugs that are substrate for cytochrome $P_{450}IID_6$ may make normal metabolizer resemble poor metabolizer leading to higher than expected plasma concentrations of TCA with resultant toxicity). Products include:

Ludiomil Tablets 843

Mepenzolate Bromide (Concurrent use may result in pronounced atropine-like effects, e.g., paralytic ileus).

No products indexed under this heading.

Meperidine Hydrochloride (Imipramine may potentiate the effects of CNS depressant drugs). Products include:

Demerol 2308
Mepergan Injection 2753

Mephobarbital (The plasma concentration of imipramine may decrease when the drug is given with barbiturates, a hepatic enzyme inducer; dosage of imipramine may need to be adjusted; imipramine may potentiate the effects of CNS depressant drugs). Products include:

Mebaral Tablets 2322

Meprobamate (Imipramine may potentiate the effects of CNS depressant drugs). Products include:

Miltown Tablets 2672
PMB 200 and PMB 400 2783

Mesoridazine (Imipramine may potentiate the effects of CNS depressant drugs).

Mesoridazine Besylate (Concurrent use with drugs that are substrate for cytochrome $P_{450}IID_6$ may make normal metabolizer resemble poor metabolizer leading to higher than expected plasma concentrations of TCA with resultant toxicity). Products include:

Serentil 684

Metaproterenol Sulfate (Avoid concurrent use since tricyclic antidepressants can potentiate the effects of catecholamines). Products include:

Alupent 669
Metaproterenol Sulfate Inhalation Solution, USP, Arm-a-Med 552

Metaraminol Bitartrate (Avoid concurrent use since tricyclic antidepressants can potentiate the effects of catecholamines). Products include:

Aramine Injection 1609

Methadone Hydrochloride (Imipramine may potentiate the effects of CNS depressant drugs). Products include:

Methadone Hydrochloride Oral Concentrate 2233
Methadone Hydrochloride Oral Solution & Tablets 2235

Methohexital Sodium (Imipramine may potentiate the effects of CNS depressant drugs). Products include:

Brevital Sodium Vials 1429

Methotrimeprazine (Concurrent use with drugs that are substrate for cytochrome $P_{450}IID_6$ may make normal metabolizer resemble poor metabolizer leading to higher than expected plasma concentrations of TCA with resultant toxicity; imipramine may potentiate the effects of CNS depressant drugs). Products include:

Levoprome 1274

Methoxamine Hydrochloride (Avoid concurrent use since tricyclic antidepressants can potentiate the effects of catecholamines). Products include:

Vasoxyl Injection 1196

Methoxyflurane (Imipramine may potentiate the effects of CNS depressant drugs).

No products indexed under this heading.

Methylphenidate Hydrochloride (May inhibit the metabolism of imipramine; downward dosage adjustments of imipramine may be required when given concomitantly). Products include:

Ritalin 848

Midazolam Hydrochloride (Imipramine may potentiate the effects of CNS depressant drugs). Products include:

Versed Injection 2170

Molindone Hydrochloride (Imipramine may potentiate the effects of CNS depressant drugs). Products include:

Moban Tablets and Concentrate 1048

Morphine Sulfate (Imipramine may potentiate the effects of CNS depressant drugs). Products include:

Astramorph/PF Injection, USP (Preservative-Free) 535
Duramorph 962
Infumorph 200 and Infumorph 500 Sterile Solutions 965
MS Contin Tablets 1994
MSIR 1997
Oramorph SR (Morphine Sulfate Sustained Release Tablets) 2236
RMS Suppositories 2657
Roxanol 2243

Nefazodone Hydrochloride (Concurrent use with drugs that are substrate for cytochrome $P_{450}IID_6$ may make normal metabolizer resemble poor metabolizer leading to higher than expected plasma concentrations of TCA with resultant toxicity). Products include:

Serzone Tablets 771

Norepinephrine Bitartrate (Avoid concurrent use since tricyclic antidepressants can potentiate the effects of catecholamines). Products include:

Levophed Bitartrate Injection 2315

Nortriptyline Hydrochloride (Concurrent use with drugs that are substrate for cytochrome $P_{450}IID_6$ may make normal metabolizer resemble poor metabolizer leading to higher than expected plasma concentrations of TCA with resultant toxicity). Products include:

Pamelor 2280

Opium Alkaloids (Imipramine may potentiate the effects of CNS depressant drugs).

No products indexed under this heading.

Oxazepam (Imipramine may potentiate the effects of CNS depressant drugs). Products include:

Serax Capsules 2810
Serax Tablets 2810

Oxybutynin Chloride (Concurrent use may result in pronounced atropine-like effects, e.g., paralytic ileus). Products include:

Ditropan 1516

Oxycodone Hydrochloride (Imipramine may potentiate the effects of CNS depressant drugs). Products include:

Percocet Tablets 938
Percodan Tablets 939
Percodan-Demi Tablets 940
Roxicodone Tablets, Oral Solution & Intensol (Oxycodone) 2244
Tylox Capsules 1584

Paroxetine Hydrochloride (Concurrent use with drugs that are substrate for cytochrome $P_{450}IID_6$ may make normal metabolizer resemble poor metabolizer leading to higher than expected plasma concentrations of TCA with resultant toxicity; due to variation in the extent of inhibition of $P_{450}IID_6$ caution is indicated if co-administered sufficient time must elapse). Products include:

Paxil Tablets 2505

Pentobarbital Sodium (The plasma concentration of imipramine may decrease when the drug is given with barbiturates, a hepatic enzyme inducer; dosage of imipramine may need to be adjusted; imipramine may potentiate the effects of CNS depressant drugs). Products include:

Nembutal Sodium Capsules 436
Nembutal Sodium Solution 438
Nembutal Sodium Suppositories 440

Perphenazine (Concurrent use with drugs that are substrate for cytochrome $P_{450}IID_6$ may make normal metabolizer resemble poor metabolizer leading to higher than expected plasma concentrations of TCA with resultant toxicity; imipramine may potentiate the effects of CNS depressant drugs). Products include:

Etrafon 2355
Triavil Tablets 1757
Trilafon 2389

Phenelzine Sulfate (Potential for hyperpyretic crises, severe convulsions, and deaths; concurrent and/or sequential use is contraindicated). Products include:

Nardil 1920

Phenobarbital (The plasma concentration of imipramine may decrease when the drug is given with barbiturates, a hepatic enzyme inducer; dosage of imipramine may need to be adjusted; imipramine may potentiate the effects of CNS depressant drugs). Products include:

Arco-Lase Plus Tablets 512
Bellergal-S Tablets 2250
Donnatal 2060
Donnatal Extentabs 2061
Donnatal Tablets 2060
Phenobarbital Elixir and Tablets 1469
Quadrinal Tablets 1350

Phenylephrine Bitartrate (Avoid concurrent use since tricyclic antidepressants can potentiate the effects of catecholamines).

No products indexed under this heading.

Phenylephrine Hydrochloride (Avoid concurrent use since tricyclic antidepressants can potentiate the effects of catecholamines). Products include:

Atrohist Plus Tablets 454
Cerose DM .... ◾◻ 878

IMPORTANT NOTE: Always consult each drug listing in the patient's regimen for possible interactions.

Comhist 2038
D.A. Chewable Tablets 951
Deconsal Pediatric Capsules 454
Dura-Vent/DA Tablets 953
Entex Capsules 1986
Entex Liquid 1986
Extendryl 1005
4-Way Fast Acting Nasal Spray (regular & mentholated) ▣ 621
Hemorid For Women ▣ 834
Hycomine Compound Tablets 932
Neo-Synephrine Hydrochloride 1% Carpuject 2324
Neo-Synephrine Hydrochloride 1% Injection 2324
Neo-Synephrine Hydrochloride (Ophthalmic) 2325
Neo-Synephrine ▣ 726
Nōstril ▣ 644
Novahistine Elixir ▣ 823
Phenergan VC 2779
Phenergan VC with Codeine 2781
Preparation H ▣ 871
Tympagesic Ear Drops 2342
Vasosulf ⊙ 271
Vicks Sinex Nasal Spray and Ultra Fine Mist ▣ 765

Phenylephrine Tannate (Avoid concurrent use since tricyclic antidepressants can potentiate the effects of catecholamines). Products include:

Atrohist Pediatric Suspension 454
Ricobid-D Pediatric Suspension 2038
Ricobid Tablets and Pediatric Suspension 2038
Rynatan 2673
Rynatuss 2673

Phenylpropanolamine Hydrochloride (Avoid concurrent use since tricyclic antidepressants can potentiate the effects of catecholamines). Products include:

Acutrim ▣ 628
Allerest Children's Chewable Tablets ▣ 627
Allerest 12 Hour Caplets ▣ 627
Atrohist Plus Tablets 454
BC Cold Powder Multi-Symptom Formula (Cold-Sinus-Allergy) ▣ 609
BC Cold Powder Non-Drowsy Formula (Cold-Sinus) ▣ 609
Cheracol Plus Head Cold/Cough Formula ▣ 769
Comtrex Multi-Symptom Non-Drowsy Liqui-gels ▣ 618
Contac Continuous Action Nasal Decongestant/Antihistamine 12 Hour Capsules ▣ 813
Contac Maximum Strength Continuous Action Decongestant/Antihistamine 12 Hour Caplets ▣ 813
Contac Severe Cold and Flu Formula Caplets ▣ 814
Coricidin 'D' Decongestant Tablets ▣ 800
Dexatrim ▣ 832
Dexatrim Plus Vitamins Caplets ▣ 832
Dimetane-DC Cough Syrup 2059
Dimetapp Elixir ▣ 773
Dimetapp Extentabs ▣ 774
Dimetapp Tablets/Liqui-Gels ▣ 775
Dimetapp Cold & Allergy Chewable Tablets ▣ 773
Dimetapp DM Elixir ▣ 774
Dura-Vent Tablets 952
Entex Capsules 1986
Entex LA Tablets 1987
Entex Liquid 1986
Exgest LA Tablets 782
Hycomine 931
Isoclor Timesule Capsules ▣ 637
Nolamine Timed-Release Tablets 785
Ornade Spansule Capsules 2502
Propagest Tablets 786
Pyrroxate Caplets ▣ 772
Robitussin-CF ▣ 777
Sinulin Tablets 787
Tavist-D 12 Hour Relief Tablets ▣ 787
Teldrin 12 Hour Antihistamine/Nasal Decongestant Allergy Relief Capsules ▣ 826
Triaminic Allergy Tablets ▣ 789
Triaminic Cold Tablets ▣ 790
Triaminic Expectorant ▣ 790
Triaminic Syrup ▣ 792
Triaminic-12 Tablets ▣ 792
Triaminic-DM Syrup ▣ 792
Triaminicin Tablets ▣ 793
Triaminicol Multi-Symptom Cold Tablets ▣ 793
Triaminicol Multi-Symptom Relief ▣ 794
Vicks DayQuil Allergy Relief 12-Hour Extended Release Tablets ▣ 760
Vicks DayQuil Allergy Relief 4-Hour Tablets ▣ 760
Vicks DayQuil SINUS Pressure & CONGESTION Relief ▣ 761

Phenytoin (The plamsa concentration of imipramine may decrease when the drug is given with phenytoin, a hepatic enzyme inducer; dosage of imipramine may need to be adjusted). Products include:

Dilantin Infatabs 1908
Dilantin-125 Suspension 1911

Phenytoin Sodium (The plamsa concentration of imipramine may decrease when the drug is given with phenytoin, a hepatic enzyme inducer; dosage of imipramine may need to be adjusted). Products include:

Dilantin Kapseals 1906
Dilantin Parenteral 1910

Pirbuterol Acetate (Avoid concurrent use since tricyclic antidepressants can potentiate the effects of catecholamines). Products include:

Maxair Autohaler 1492
Maxair Inhaler 1494

Prazepam (Imipramine may potentiate the effects of CNS depressant drugs).

No products indexed under this heading.

Prochlorperazine (Concurrent use with drugs that are substrate for cytochrome $P_{450}IID_6$ may make normal metabolizer resemble poor metabolizer leading to higher than expected plasma concentrations of TCA with resultant toxicity; imipramine may potentiate the effects of CNS depressant drugs). Products include:

Compazine 2470

Procyclidine Hydrochloride (Concurrent use may result in pronounced atropine-like effects, e.g., paralytic ileus). Products include:

Kemadrin Tablets 1112

Promethazine Hydrochloride (Concurrent use with drugs that are substrate for cytochrome $P_{450}IID_6$ may make normal metabolizer resemble poor metabolizer leading to higher than expected plasma concentrations of TCA with resultant toxicity; imipramine may potentiate the effects of CNS depressant drugs). Products include:

Mepergan Injection 2753
Phenergan with Codeine 2777
Phenergan with Dextromethorphan 2778
Phenergan Injection 2773
Phenergan Suppositories 2775
Phenergan Syrup 2774
Phenergan Tablets 2775
Phenergan VC 2779
Phenergan VC with Codeine 2781

Propafenone Hydrochloride (Concurent use with drugs that are substrate for cytochrome $P_{450}IID_6$ may make normal metabolizer resemble poor metabolizer leading to higher than expected plasma concentrations of TCA with resultant toxicity). Products include:

Rythmol Tablets–150mg, 225mg, 300mg 1352

Propantheline Bromide (Concurrent use may result in pronounced atropine-like effects, e.g., paralytic ileus). Products include:

Pro-Banthīne Tablets 2052

Propofol (Imipramine may potentiate the effects of CNS depressant drugs). Products include:

Diprivan Injection 2833

Propoxyphene Hydrochloride (Imipramine may potentiate the effects of CNS depressant drugs). Products include:

Darvon 1435
Wygesic Tablets 2827

Propoxyphene Napsylate (Imipramine may potentiate the effects of CNS depressant drugs). Products include:

Darvon-N/Darvocet-N 1433

Protriptyline Hydrochloride (Concurrent use with drugs that are substrate for cytochrome $P_{450}IID_6$ may make normal metabolizer resemble poor metabolizer leading to higher than expected plasma concentrations of TCA with resultant toxicity). Products include:

Vivactil Tablets 1774

Pseudoephedrine Hydrochloride (Avoid concurrent use since tricyclic antidepressants can potentiate the effects of catecholamines). Products include:

Actifed Allergy Daytime/Nighttime Caplets ▣ 844
Actifed Plus Caplets ▣ 845
Actifed Plus Tablets ▣ 845
Actifed with Codeine Cough Syrup 1067
Actifed Sinus Daytime/Nighttime Tablets and Caplets ▣ 846
Actifed Syrup ▣ 846
Actifed Tablets ▣ 844
Advil Cold and Sinus Caplets and Tablets (formerly CoAdvil) ▣ 870
Alka-Seltzer Plus Cold Medicine Liqui-Gels ▣ 706
Alka-Seltzer Plus Cold & Cough Medicine Liqui-Gels ▣ 705
Alka-Seltzer Plus Night-Time Cold Medicine Liqui-Gels ▣ 706
Allerest Headache Strength Tablets ▣ 627
Allerest Maximum Strength Tablets ▣ 627
Allerest No Drowsiness Tablets ▣ 627
Allerest Sinus Pain Formula ▣ 627
Anatuss LA Tablets 1542
Atrohist Pediatric Capsules 453
Bayer Select Sinus Pain Relief Formula ▣ 717
Benadryl Allergy Decongestant Liquid Medication ▣ 848
Benadryl Allergy Decongestant Tablets ▣ 848
Benadryl Allergy Sinus Headache Formula Caplets ▣ 849
Benylin Multisymptom ▣ 852
Bromfed Capsules (Extended-Release) 1785
Bromfed Syrup ▣ 733
Bromfed Tablets 1785
Bromfed-DM Cough Syrup 1786
Bromfed-PD Capsules (Extended-Release) 1785
Children's Vicks DayQuil Allergy Relief ▣ 757
Children's Vicks NyQuil Cold/Cough Relief ▣ 758
Comtrex Multi-Symptom Cold Reliever Tablets/Caplets/Liqui-Gels/Liquid ▣ 615
Allergy-Sinus Comtrex Multi-Symptom Allergy-Sinus Formula Tablets ▣ 617
Comtrex Multi-Symptom Non-Drowsy Caplets ▣ 618
Congess 1004
Contac Day Allergy/Sinus Caplets ▣ 812
Contac Day & Night ▣ 812
Contac Night Allergy/Sinus Caplets ▣ 812
Contac Severe Cold & Flu Non-Drowsy ▣ 815
Deconamine Chewable Tablets 1320
Deconamine CX Cough and Cold Liquid and Tablets 1319
Deconamine 1320
Deconsal C Expectorant Syrup 456
Deconsal Pediatric Syrup 457
Deconsal II Tablets 454
Dimetane-DX Cough Syrup 2059
Dimetapp Sinus Caplets ▣ 775
Dorcol Children's Cough Syrup ▣ 785
Drixoral Cough + Congestion Liquid Caps ▣ 802
Dura-Tap/PD Capsules 2867
Duratuss Tablets 2565
Duratuss HD Elixir 2565
Efidac/24 ▣ 635
Entex PSE Tablets 1987
Fedahist Gyrocaps 2401
Fedahist Timecaps 2401
Guaifed 1787
Guaifed Syrup ▣ 734
Guaimax-D Tablets 792
Guaitab Tablets ▣ 734
Isoclor Expectorant 990
Kronofed-A 977
Motrin IB Sinus ▣ 838
Novahistine DH 2462
Novahistine DMX ▣ 822
Novahistine Expectorant 2463
Nucofed 2051
PediaCare Cold Allergy Chewable Tablets ▣ 677
PediaCare Cough-Cold Chewable Tablets 1553
PediaCare 1553
PediaCare Infants' Decongestant Drops ▣ 677
PediCare Infant's Drops Decongestant Plus Cough 1553
PediaCare NightRest Cough-Cold Liquid 1553
Pediatric Vicks 44d Dry Hacking Cough & Head Congestion ▣ 763
Pediatric Vicks 44m Cough & Cold Relief ▣ 764
Robitussin Cold & Cough Liqui-Gels ▣ 776
Robitussin Maximum Strength Cough & Cold ▣ 778
Robitussin Pediatric Cough & Cold Formula ▣ 779
Robitussin Severe Congestion Liqui-Gels ▣ 776
Robitussin-DAC Syrup 2074
Robitussin-PE ▣ 778
Rondec Oral Drops 953
Rondec Syrup 953
Rondec Tablet 953
Rondec-DM Oral Drops 954
Rondec-DM Syrup 954
Rondec-TR Tablet 953
Ryna ▣ 841
Seldane-D Extended-Release Tablets 1538
Semprex-D Capsules 463
Semprex-D Capsules 1167
Sinarest Tablets ▣ 648
Sinarest Extra Strength Tablets ▣ 648
Sinarest No Drowsiness Tablets ▣ 648
Sine-Aid IB Caplets 1554
Sine-Aid Maximum Strength Sinus Medication Gelcaps, Caplets and Tablets 1554
Sine-Off No Drowsiness Formula Caplets ▣ 824
Sine-Off Sinus Medicine ▣ 825
Singlet Tablets ▣ 825
Sinutab Non-Drying Liquid Caps ▣ 859
Sinutab Sinus Allergy Medication, Maximum Strength Tablets and Caplets ▣ 860
Sinutab Sinus Medication, Maximum Strength Without Drowsiness Formula, Tablets & Caplets ▣ 860
Sinutab Sinus Medication, Regular Strength Without Drowsiness Formula ▣ 859
Sudafed Children's Liquid ▣ 861
Sudafed Cold and Cough Liquidcaps ▣ 862
Sudafed Cough Syrup ▣ 862
Sudafed Plus Liquid ▣ 862
Sudafed Plus Tablets ▣ 863
Sudafed Severe Cold Formula Caplets ▣ 863
Sudafed Severe Cold Formula Tablets ▣ 864
Sudafed Sinus Caplets ▣ 864
Sudafed Sinus Tablets ▣ 864
Sudafed Tablets, 30 mg ▣ 861
Sudafed Tablets, 60 mg ▣ 861
Sudafed 12 Hour Caplets ▣ 861
Syn-Rx Tablets 465
Syn-Rx DM Tablets 466
TheraFlu ▣ 787
TheraFlu Maximum Strength Nighttime Flu, Cold & Cough Medicine ▣ 788
TheraFlu Maximum Strength Non-Drowsy Formula Flu, Cold & Cough Medicine ▣ 788

(▣ Described in PDR For Nonprescription Drugs) (⊙ Described in PDR For Ophthalmology)

Interactions Index

Topical Analgesic Ointment

Thera Flu Maximum Strength, Non-Drowsy Formula Flu, Cold and Cough Caplets .... ✦ 789

Triaminic AM Cough and Decongestant Formula .... ✦ 789

Triaminic AM Decongestant Formula .... ✦ 790

Triaminic Nite Light .... ✦ 791

Triaminic Sore Throat Formula ...... ✦ 791

Tussend 1783

Tussend Expectorant 1785

Children's TYLENOL Cold Multi-Symptom Liquid Formula and Chewable Tablets.............................. 1561

Children's TYLENOL Cold Plus Cough Multi Symptom Tablets and Liquid .... ✦ 681

Infants' TYLENOL Cold Decongestant & Fever-Reducer Drops 1556

TYLENOL Maximum Strength Allergy Sinus Medication Gelcaps and Caplets 1563

TYLENOL Maximum Strength Allergy Sinus NightTime Medication Caplets 1555

TYLENOL Flu Maximum Strength Gelcaps 1565

TYLENOL Flu NightTime, Maximum Strength, Gelcaps 1566

TYLENOL Maximum Strength Flu NightTime Hot Medication Packets 1562

TYLENOL, Maximum Strength, Sinus Medication Geltabs, Gelcaps, Caplets and Tablets 1566

TYLENOL Cold Multi-Symptom Formula Medication Tablets and Caplets... 1561

TYLENOL Cold Medication No Drowsiness Formula Gelcaps and Caplets... 1562

TYLENOL Cold Multi-Symptom Hot Medication Liquid Packets......... 1557

TYLENOL Cough Multi-Symptom Medication with Decongestant 1565

Ursinus Inlay-Tabs............................ ✦ 794

Vicks 44 LiquiCaps Cough, Cold & Flu Relief .... ✦ 755

Vicks 44 LiquiCaps Non-Drowsy Cough & Cold Relief .... ✦ 756

Vicks 44D Dry Hacking Cough & Head Congestion .... ✦ 755

Vicks 44M Cough, Cold & Flu Relief .... ✦ 756

Vicks DayQuil .... ✦ 761

Vicks DayQuil SINUS Pressure & PAIN Relief with IBUPROFEN ..... ✦ 762

Vicks Nyquil Hot Therapy................. ✦ 762

Vicks NyQuil LiquiCaps Multi-Symptom Cold/Flu Relief .... ✦ 763

Vicks NyQuil Multi-Symptom Cold/Flu Relief - (Original & Cherry Flavor) .... ✦ 763

Pseudoephedrine Sulfate (Avoid concurrent use since tricyclic antidepressants can potentiate the effects of catecholamines). Products include:

Cheracol Sinus .... ✦ 768

Chlor-Trimeton Allergy Decongestant Tablets .... ✦ 799

Claritin-D 2350

Drixoral Cold and Allergy Sustained-Action Tablets .... ✦ 802

Drixoral Cold and Flu Extended-Release Tablets................................. ✦ 803

Drixoral Non-Drowsy Formula Extended-Release Tablets .... ✦ 803

Drixoral Allergy/Sinus Extended Release Tablets................................ ✦ 804

Trinalin Repetabs Tablets 1330

Quazepam (Imipramine may potentiate the effects of CNS depressant drugs). Products include:

Doral Tablets 2664

Quinidine Gluconate (Concurrent use with drugs that inhibit cytochrome $P_{450}IID_6$ may make normal metabolizer resemble poor metabolizer leading to higher than expected plasma concentrations of TCA with resultant toxicity). Products include:

Quinaglute Dura-Tabs Tablets 649

Quinidine Polygalacturonate (Concurrent use with drugs that inhibit cytochrome $P_{450}IID_6$ may make normal metabolizer resemble poor metabolizer leading to higher than expected plasma concentrations of TCA with resultant toxicity).

No products indexed under this heading.

Quinidine Sulfate (Concurrent use with drugs that inhibit cytochrome $P_{450}IID_6$ may make normal metabolizer resemble poor metabolizer leading to higher than expected plasma concentrations of TCA with resultant toxicity). Products include:

Quinidex Extentabs 2067

Risperidone (Imipramine may potentiate the effects of CNS depressant drugs). Products include:

Risperdal 1301

Salmeterol Xinafoate (Avoid concurrent use since tricyclic antidepressants can potentiate the effects of catecholamines). Products include:

Serevent Inhalation Aerosol................. 1176

Scopolamine (Concurrent use may result in pronounced atropine-like effects, e.g., paralytic ileus). Products include:

Transderm Scōp Transdermal Therapeutic System 869

Scopolamine Hydrobromide (Concurrent use may result in pronounced atropine-like effects, e.g., paralytic ileus). Products include:

Atrohist Plus Tablets 454

Donnatal 2060

Donnatal Extentabs........................... 2061

Donnatal Tablets 2060

Secobarbital Sodium (The plasma concentration of imipramine may decrease when the drug is given with barbiturates, a hepatic enzyme inducer; dosage of imipramine may need to be adjusted; imipramine may potentiate the effects of CNS depressant drugs). Products include:

Seconal Sodium Pulvules 1474

Selegiline Hydrochloride (Potential for hyperpyretic crises, severe convulsions, and deaths; concurrent and/or sequential use is contraindicated). Products include:

Eldepryl Tablets 2550

Sertraline Hydrochloride (Concurrent use with drugs that are substrate for cytochrome $P_{450}IID_6$ may make normal metabolizer resemble poor metabolizer leading to higher than expected plasma concentrations of TCA with resultant toxicity; due to variation in the extent of inhibition of $P_{450}IID_6$ caution is indicated if co-administered sufficient time must elapse). Products include:

Zoloft Tablets 2217

Sufentanil Citrate (Imipramine may potentiate the effects of CNS depressant drugs). Products include:

Sufenta Injection 1309

Temazepam (Imipramine may potentiate the effects of CNS depressant drugs). Products include:

Restoril Capsules 2284

Terbutaline Sulfate (Avoid concurrent use since tricyclic antidepressants can potentiate the effects of catecholamines). Products include:

Brethaire Inhaler 813

Brethine Ampuls 815

Brethine Tablets 814

Bricanyl Subcutaneous Injection 1502

Bricanyl Tablets 1503

Thiamylal Sodium (The plasma concentration of imipramine may decrease when the drug is given with barbiturates, a hepatic enzyme inducer; dosage of imipramine may need to be adjusted; imipramine may potentiate the effects of CNS depressant drugs).

No products indexed under this heading.

Thioridazine Hydrochloride (Concurrent use with drugs that are substrate for cytochrome $P_{450}IID_6$ may make normal metabolizer resemble poor metabolizer leading to higher than expected plasma concentrations of TCA with resultant toxicity; imipramine may potentiate the effects of CNS depressant drugs). Products include:

Mellaril 2269

Thiothixene (Imipramine may potentiate the effects of CNS depressant drugs). Products include:

Navane Capsules and Concentrate 2201

Navane Intramuscular 2202

Thyroglobulin (Co-administration may produce cardiovascular toxicity).

No products indexed under this heading.

Thyroid (Co-administration may produce cardiovascular toxicity).

No products indexed under this heading.

Thyroxine (Co-administration may produce cardiovascular toxicity).

No products indexed under this heading.

Thyroxine Sodium (Co-administration may produce cardiovascular toxicity).

No products indexed under this heading.

Tranylcypromine Sulfate (Potential for hyperpyretic crises, severe convulsions, and deaths; concurrent and/or sequential use is contraindicated). Products include:

Parnate Tablets 2503

Trazodone Hydrochloride (Concurrent use with drugs that are substrate for cytochrome $P_{450}IID_6$ may make normal metabolizer resemble poor metabolizer leading to higher than expected plasma concentrations of TCA with resultant toxicity). Products include:

Desyrel and Desyrel Dividose 503

Triazolam (Imipramine may potentiate the effects of CNS depressant drugs). Products include:

Halcion Tablets 2611

Tridihexethyl Chloride (Concurrent use may result in pronounced atropine-like effects, e.g., paralytic ileus).

No products indexed under this heading.

Trifluoperazine Hydrochloride (Concurrent use with drugs that are substrate for cytochrome $P_{450}IID_6$ may make normal metabolizer resemble poor metabolizer leading to higher than expected plasma concentrations of TCA with resultant toxicity; imipramine may potentiate the effects of CNS depressant drugs). Products include:

Stelazine 2514

Trihexyphenidyl Hydrochloride (Concurrent use may result in pronounced atropine-like effects, e.g., paralytic ileus). Products include:

Artane 1368

Trimipramine Maleate (Concurrent use with drugs that are substrate for cytochrome $P_{450}IID_6$ may make normal metabolizer resemble poor metabolizer leading to higher than expected plasma concentrations of TCA with resultant toxicity). Products include:

Surmontil Capsules........................... 2811

Venlafaxine Hydrochloride (Concurrent use with drugs that are substrate for cytochrome $P_{450}IID_6$ may make normal metabolizer resemble poor metabolizer leading to higher than expected plasma concentrations of TCA with resultant toxicity; due to variation in the extent of inhibition of $P_{450}IID_6$ caution is indicated if co-administered sufficient time must elapse). Products include:

Effexor 2719

Zolpidem Tartrate (Imipramine may potentiate the effects of CNS depressant drugs). Products include:

Ambien Tablets.................................. 2416

Food Interactions

Alcohol (Imipramine may enhance the CNS depressant effects of alcohol).

TOLECTIN (200, 400 AND 600 MG)

(Tolmetin Sodium) 1581

May interact with oral anticoagulants and certain other agents. Compounds in these categories include:

Dicumarol (Increased prothrombin time and bleeding).

No products indexed under this heading.

Methotrexate Sodium (Reduced tubular secretion of methotrexate in an animal model). Products include:

Methotrexate Sodium Tablets, Injection, for Injection and LPF Injection 1275

Warfarin Sodium (Increased prothrombin time and bleeding). Products include:

Coumadin 926

Food Interactions

Dairy products (Decreases total tolmetin bioavailability by 16%).

Meal, unspecified (Decreases total tolmetin bioavailability by 16%; reduces peak plasma concentrations by 50%).

TONOCARD TABLETS

(Tocainide Hydrochloride) 531

May interact with:

Lidocaine Hydrochloride (Increased incidence of adverse reactions such as seizure). Products include:

Bactine Antiseptic/Anesthetic First Aid Liquid .... ✦ 708

Campho-Phenique Maximum Strength First Aid Antibiotic Plus Pain Reliever Ointment .... ✦ 719

Decadron Phosphate with Xylocaine Injection, Sterile 1639

Xylocaine Injections 567

Metoprolol Tartrate (Additive effects on wedge pressure and cardiac index). Products include:

Lopressor Ampuls 830

Lopressor HCT Tablets 832

Lopressor Tablets 830

TOPICAL ANALGESIC OINTMENT

(Ammonia Solution, Strong) .... ✦ 835

None cited in PDR database.

IMPORTANT NOTE: Always consult each drug listing in the patient's regimen for possible interactions.

TOPICORT EMOLLIENT CREAM 0.25%
(Desoximetasone) 1243
None cited in PDR database.

TOPICORT GEL 0.05%
(Desoximetasone) 1243
None cited in PDR database.

TOPICORT LP EMOLLIENT CREAM 0.05%
(Desoximetasone) 1243
None cited in PDR database.

TOPICORT OINTMENT 0.25%
(Desoximetasone) 1243
None cited in PDR database.

TOPROL-XL TABLETS
(Metoprolol Succinate) 565
May interact with catecholamine depleting drugs, cardiac glycosides, and certain other agents. Compounds in these categories include:

Deserpidine (Potential for additive effect; hypotension or marked bradycardia).
No products indexed under this heading.

Deslanoside (Metoprolol should be used cautiously in patients with hypertension and angina who have congestive heart failure and are on digitalis and diuretics since both digitalis and metoprolol slow AV conduction).
No products indexed under this heading.

Digitoxin (Metoprolol should be used cautiously in patients with hypertension and angina who have congestive heart failure and are on digitalis and diuretics since both digitalis and metoprolol slow AV conduction). Products include:
Crystodigin Tablets 1433

Digoxin (Metoprolol should be used cautiously in patients with hypertension and angina who have congestive heart failure and are on digitalis and diuretics since both digitalis and metoprolol slow AV conduction). Products include:
Lanoxicaps 1117
Lanoxin Elixir Pediatric 1120
Lanoxin Injection 1123
Lanoxin Injection Pediatric 1126
Lanoxin Tablets 1128

Epinephrine Hydrochloride (Potential unresponsiveness to the usual dose of epinephrine to treat allergic reactions in certain patients). Products include:
Ana-Kit Anaphylaxis Emergency Treatment Kit 617

Guanethidine Monosulfate (Potential for additive effect; hypotension or marked bradycardia). Products include:
Esimil Tablets 822
Ismelin Tablets 827

Rauwolfia Serpentina (Potential for additive effect; hypotension or marked bradycardia).
No products indexed under this heading.

Rescinnamine (Potential for additive effect; hypotension or marked bradycardia).
No products indexed under this heading.

Reserpine (Potential for additive effect; hypotension or marked bradycardia). Products include:
Diupres Tablets 1650
Hydropres Tablets 1675
Ser-Ap-Es Tablets 849

TORADOL IM INJECTION, IV INJECTION
(Ketorolac Tromethamine) 2159
See **Toradol Tablets**

TORADOL TABLETS
(Ketorolac Tromethamine) 2159
May interact with non-steroidal anti-inflammatory agents, lithium preparations, ACE inhibitors, nondepolarizing neuromuscular blocking agents, salicylates, and certain other agents. Compounds in these categories include:

Alprazolam (Concurrent use may produce hallucinations). Products include:
Xanax Tablets 2649

Aspirin (Concurrent use is contraindicated because of the cumulative risk of inducing serious NSAID-related side effects). Products include:
Alka-Seltzer Effervescent Antacid and Pain Reliever .... ▣ 701
Alka-Seltzer Extra Strength Effervescent Antacid and Pain Reliever .... ▣ 703
Alka-Seltzer Lemon Lime Effervescent Antacid and Pain Reliever .... ▣ 703
Alka-Seltzer Plus Cold Medicine .... ▣ 705
Alka-Seltzer Plus Cold & Cough Medicine .... ▣ 708
Alka-Seltzer Plus Night-Time Cold Medicine .... ▣ 707
Alka Seltzer Plus Sinus Medicine .... ▣ 707
Arthritis Foundation Safety Coated Aspirin Tablets .... ▣ 675
Arthritis Pain Ascriptin .... ▣ 631
Maximum Strength Ascriptin .... ▣ 630
Regular Strength Ascriptin Tablets .... ▣ 629
Arthritis Strength BC Powder .... ▣ 609
BC Cold Powder Multi-Symptom Formula (Cold-Sinus-Allergy) .... ▣ 609
BC Cold Powder Non-Drowsy Formula (Cold-Sinus) .... ▣ 609
BC Powder .... ▣ 609
Bayer Children's Chewable Aspirin .... ▣ 711
Genuine Bayer Aspirin Tablets & Caplets .... ▣ 713
Extra Strength Bayer Arthritis Pain Regimen Formula .... ▣ 711
Extra Strength Bayer Aspirin Caplets & Tablets .... ▣ 712
Extended-Release Bayer 8-Hour Aspirin .... ▣ 712
Extra Strength Bayer Plus Aspirin Caplets .... ▣ 713
Extra Strength Bayer PM Aspirin .... ▣ 713
Bayer Enteric Aspirin .... ▣ 709
Bufferin Analgesic Tablets and Caplets .... ▣ 613
Arthritis Strength Bufferin Analgesic Caplets .... ▣ 614
Extra Strength Bufferin Analgesic Tablets .... ▣ 615
Cama Arthritis Pain Reliever .... ▣ 785
Darvon Compound-65 Pulvules 1435
Easprin 1914
Ecotrin 2455
Ecotrin Enteric Coated Aspirin Maximum Strength Tablets and Caplets .... ▣ 816
Ecotrin Enteric Coated Aspirin Regular Strength Tablets 2455
Empirin Aspirin Tablets .... ▣ 854
Empirin with Codeine Tablets 1093
Excedrin Extra-Strength Analgesic Tablets & Caplets 732
Fiorinal Capsules 2261
Fiorinal with Codeine Capsules 2262
Fiorinal Tablets 2261
Halfprin 1362
Healthprin Aspirin 2455
Norgesic 1496
Percodan Tablets 939
Percodan-Demi Tablets 940
Robaxisal Tablets 2071
Soma Compound w/Codeine Tablets 2676
Soma Compound Tablets 2675
St. Joseph Adult Chewable Aspirin (81 mg.) .... ▣ 808
Talwin Compound 2335
Ursinus Inlay-Tabs .... ▣ 794
Vanquish Analgesic Caplets .... ▣ 731

Atracurium Besylate (Concurrent use with parenteral form of Toradol has resulted in apnea). Products include:
Tracrium Injection 1183

Benazepril Hydrochloride (Concomitant use may increase the risk of renal impairment, particularly in volume-depleted patients). Products include:
Lotensin Tablets 834
Lotensin HCT 837
Lotrel Capsules 840

Captopril (Concomitant use may increase the risk of renal impairment, particularly in volume-depleted patients). Products include:
Capoten 739
Capozide 742

Carbamazepine (Concomitant use has resulted in sporadic cases of seizures). Products include:
Atretol Tablets 573
Tegretol Chewable Tablets 852
Tegretol Suspension 852
Tegretol Tablets 852

Choline Magnesium Trisalicylate (*In Vitro* studies indicate that, at therapeutic concentrations of salicylates, the binding of ketorolac was reduced from approximately 99.2% to 97.5%, representing a potential 2-fold increase in unbound ketorolac plasma levels). Products include:
Trilisate 2000

Diclofenac Potassium (Concurrent use is contraindicated because of the cumulative risk of inducing serious NSAID-related side effects). Products include:
Cataflam 816

Diclofenac Sodium (Concurrent use is contraindicated because of the cumulative risk of inducing serious NSAID-related side effects). Products include:
Voltaren Ophthalmic Sterile Ophthalmic Solution .... ⊙ 272
Voltaren Tablets 861

Diflunisal (*In Vitro* studies indicate that, at therapeutic concentrations of salicylates, the binding of ketorolac was reduced from approximately 99.2% to 97.5%, representing a potential 2-fold increase in unbound ketorolac plasma levels). Products include:
Dolobid Tablets 1654

Enalapril Maleate (Concomitant use may increase the risk of renal impairment, particularly in volume-depleted patients). Products include:
Vaseretic Tablets 1765
Vasotec Tablets 1771

Enalaprilat (Concomitant use may increase the risk of renal impairment, particularly in volume-depleted patients). Products include:
Vasotec I.V. 1768

Etodolac (Concurrent use is contraindicated because of the cumulative risk of inducing serious NSAID-related side effects). Products include:
Lodine Capsules and Tablets 2743

Fenoprofen Calcium (Concurrent use is contraindicated because of the cumulative risk of inducing serious NSAID-related side effects). Products include:
Nalfon 200 Pulvules & Nalfon Tablets 917

Fluoxetine Hydrochloride (Concurrent use may produce hallucinations). Products include:
Prozac Pulvules & Liquid, Oral Solution 919

Flurbiprofen (Concurrent use is contraindicated because of the cumulative risk of inducing serious NSAID-related side effects). Products include:
Ansaid Tablets 2579

Fosinopril Sodium (Concomitant use may increase the risk of renal impairment, particularly in volume-depleted patients). Products include:
Monopril Tablets 757

Furosemide (Potential for reduced diuretic response in normovolemic healthy subjects by 20%). Products include:
Lasix Injection, Oral Solution and Tablets 1240

Heparin Sodium (Co-administration results in mean template bleeding time of 6.4 minutes compared to 6.0 minutes, however extreme caution and close monitoring is recommended). Products include:
Heparin Lock Flush Solution 2725
Heparin Sodium Injection 2726
Heparin Sodium Injection, USP, Sterile Solution 2615
Heparin Sodium Vials 1441

Ibuprofen (Concurrent use is contraindicated because of the cumulative risk of inducing serious NSAID-related side effects). Products include:
Advil Cold and Sinus Caplets and Tablets (formerly CoAdvil) .... ▣ 870
Advil Ibuprofen Tablets and Caplets .... ▣ 870
Children's Advil Suspension 2692
Arthritis Foundation Ibuprofen Tablets .... ▣ 674
Bayer Select Ibuprofen Pain Relief Formula .... ▣ 715
Cramp End Tablets .... ▣ 735
Dimetapp Sinus Caplets .... ▣ 775
Haltran Tablets .... ▣ 771
IBU Tablets 1342
Ibuprohm .... ▣ 735
Children's Motrin Ibuprofen Oral Suspension 1546
Motrin Tablets 2625
Motrin IB Caplets, Tablets, and Geltabs .... ▣ 838
Motrin IB Sinus .... ▣ 838
Motrin Ibuprofen Suspension, Oral Drops, Chewable Tablets, Caplets 1546
Nuprin Ibuprofen/Analgesic Tablets & Caplets .... ▣ 622
Sine-Aid IB Caplets 1554
Vicks DayQuil SINUS Pressure & PAIN Relief with IBUPROFEN .... ▣ 762

Indomethacin (Concurrent use is contraindicated because of the cumulative risk of inducing serious NSAID-related side effects). Products include:
Indocin 1680

Indomethacin Sodium Trihydrate (Concurrent use is contraindicated because of the cumulative risk of inducing serious NSAID-related side effects). Products include:
Indocin I.V. 1684

Ketoprofen (Concurrent use is contraindicated because of the cumulative risk of inducing serious NSAID-related side effects). Products include:
Orudis Capsules 2766
Oruvail Capsules 2766

Lisinopril (Concomitant use may increase the risk of renal impairment, particularly in volume-depleted patients). Products include:
Prinivil Tablets 1733
Prinzide Tablets 1737
Zestoretic 2850
Zestril Tablets 2854

Lithium Carbonate (Potential for increased lithium plasma levels). Products include:
Eskalith 2485

(▣ Described in PDR For Nonprescription Drugs) (⊙ Described in PDR For Ophthalmology)

Lithium Carbonate Capsules & Tablets 2230
Lithonate/Lithotabs/Lithobid 2543

Lithium Citrate (Potential for increased lithium plasma levels).

No products indexed under this heading.

Magnesium Salicylate (*In Vitro* studies indicate that, at therapeutic concentrations of salicylates, the binding of ketorolac was reduced from approximately 99.2% to 97.5%, representing a potential 2-fold increase in unbound ketorolac plasma levels). Products include:

Backache Caplets .... ◉ 613
Bayer Select Backache Pain Relief Formula .... ◉ 715
Doan's Extra-Strength Analgesic.... ◉ 633
Extra Strength Doan's P.M. .... ◉ 633
Doan's Regular Strength Analgesic .... ◉ 634
Mobigesic Tablets .... ◉ 602

Meclofenamate Sodium (Current use is contraindicated because of the cumulative risk of inducing serious NSAID-related side effects).

No products indexed under this heading.

Mefenamic Acid (Concurrent use is contraindicated because of the cumulative risk of inducing serious NSAID-related side effects). Products include:

Ponstel 1925

Methotrexate Sodium (Co-administration may result in reduced clearance of methotrexate thereby enhancing the toxicity). Products include:

Methotrexate Sodium Tablets, Injection, for Injection and LPF Injection 1275

Metocurine Iodide (Concurrent use with parenteral form of Toradol has resulted in apnea). Products include:

Metubine Iodide Vials.......................... 916

Mivacurium Chloride (Concurrent use with parenteral form of Toradol has resulted in apnea). Products include:

Mivacron 1138

Moexipril Hydrochloride (Concomitant use may increase the risk of renal impairment, particularly in volume-depleted patients). Products include:

Univasc Tablets 2410

Nabumetone (Concurrent use is contraindicated because of the cumulative risk of inducing serious NSAID-related side effects). Products include:

Relafen Tablets 2510

Naproxen (Concurrent use is contraindicated because of the cumulative risk of inducing serious NSAID-related side effects). Products include:

Anaprox/Naprosyn 2117

Naproxen Sodium (Concurrent use is contraindicated because of the cumulative risk of inducing serious NSAID-related side effects). Products include:

Aleve 1975
Anaprox/Naprosyn 2117

Oxaprozin (Concurrent use is contraindicated because of the cumulative risk of inducing serious NSAID-related side effects). Products include:

Daypro Caplets 2426

Pancuronium Bromide Injection (Concurrent use with parenteral form of Toradol has resulted in apnea).

No products indexed under this heading.

Phenylbutazone (Concurrent use is contraindicated because of the cumulative risk of inducing serious NSAID-related side effects).

No products indexed under this heading.

Phenytoin (Concomitant use has resulted in sporadic cases of seizures). Products include:

Dilantin Infatabs 1908
Dilantin-125 Suspension 1911

Phenytoin Sodium (Concomitant use has resulted in sporadic cases of seizures). Products include:

Dilantin Kapseals 1906
Dilantin Parenteral 1910

Piroxicam (Concurrent use is contraindicated because of the cumulative risk of inducing serious NSAID-related side effects). Products include:

Feldene Capsules 1965

Probenecid (Co-administration decreases clearance of ketorolac and significant increase in plasma levels, total AUC increases from 5.4 to 17.8 mcgm/h/uL and terminal half-life increases approximately 2-fold; concurrent use is contraindicated). Products include:

Benemid Tablets 1611
ColBENEMID Tablets 1622

Quinapril Hydrochloride (Concomitant use may increase the risk of renal impairment, particularly in volume-depleted patients). Products include:

Accupril Tablets 1893

Ramipril (Concomitant use may increase the risk of renal impairment, particularly in volume-depleted patients). Products include:

Altace Capsules 1232

Rocuronium Bromide (Concurrent use with parenteral form of Toradol has resulted in apnea). Products include:

Zemuron 1830

Salsalate (*In Vitro* studies indicate that, at therapeutic concentrations of salicylates, the binding of ketorolac was reduced from approximately 99.2% to 97.5%, representing a potential 2-fold increase in unbound ketorolac plasma levels). Products include:

Mono-Gesic Tablets 792
Salflex Tablets 786

Spirapril Hydrochloride (Concomitant use may increase the risk of renal impairment, particularly in volume-depleted patients).

No products indexed under this heading.

Sulindac (Concurrent use is contraindicated because of the cumulative risk of inducing serious NSAID-related side effects). Products include:

Clinoril Tablets 1618

Thiothixene (Concurrent use may produce hallucinations). Products include:

Navane Capsules and Concentrate 2201
Navane Intramuscular 2202

Thiothixene Hydrochloride (Concurrent use may produce hallucinations).

No products indexed under this heading.

Tolmetin Sodium (Concurrent use is contraindicated because of the cumulative risk of inducing serious NSAID-related side effects). Products include:

Tolectin (200, 400 and 600 mg) .. 1581

Vecuronium Bromide (Concurrent use with parenteral form of Toradol has resulted in apnea). Products include:

Norcuron 1826

Warfarin Sodium (*In Vitro* binding of warfarin to plasma proteins is slightly reduced by ketorolac; extreme caution and close monitoring is recommended). Products include:

Coumadin 926

Food Interactions

Diet, high-lipid (Oral administration of Toradol after a high-fat meal resulted in decreased peak and delayed time-to-peak concentrations of Toradol by about 1 hour).

TORECAN INJECTION

(Thiethylperazine Malate)....................2245

May interact with central nervous system depressants, narcotic analgesics, barbiturates, general anesthetics, and certain other agents. Compounds in these categories include:

Alfentanil Hydrochloride (Phenothiazines are capable of potentiating CNS depressants). Products include:

Alfenta Injection 1286

Alprazolam (Phenothiazines are capable of potentiating CNS depressants). Products include:

Xanax Tablets 2649

Aprobarbital (Phenothiazines are capable of potentiating CNS depressants).

No products indexed under this heading.

Atropine Sulfate (Phenothiazines are capabale of potentiating atropine). Products include:

Arco-Lase Plus Tablets 512
Atrohist Plus Tablets 454
Atropine Sulfate Sterile Ophthalmic Solution .... ◉ 233
Donnatal 2060
Donnatal Extentabs.............................. 2061
Donnatal Tablets 2060
Lomotil 2439
Motofen Tablets 784
Urised Tablets 1964

Buprenorphine (Phenothiazines are capable of potentiating CNS depressants). Products include:

Buprenex Injectable 2006

Buspirone Hydrochloride (Phenothiazines are capable of potentiating CNS depressants). Products include:

BuSpar 737

Butabarbital (Phenothiazines are capable of potentiating CNS depressants).

No products indexed under this heading.

Butalbital (Phenothiazines are capable of potentiating CNS depressants). Products include:

Esgic-plus Tablets 1013
Fioricet Tablets 2258
Fioricet with Codeine Capsules 2260
Fiorinal Capsules 2261
Fiorinal with Codeine Capsules 2262
Fiorinal Tablets 2261
Phrenilin 785
Sedapap Tablets 50 mg/650 mg .. 1543

Chlordiazepoxide (Phenothiazines are capable of potentiating CNS depressants). Products include:

Libritabs Tablets 2177

Limbitrol 2180

Chlordiazepoxide Hydrochloride (Phenothiazines are capable of potentiating CNS depressants). Products include:

Librax Capsules 2176
Librium Capsules 2178
Librium Injectable 2179

Chlorpromazine (Phenothiazines are capable of potentiating CNS depressants). Products include:

Thorazine Suppositories 2523

Chlorpromazine Hydrochloride (Phenothiazines are capable of potentiating CNS depressants). Products include:

Thorazine 2523

Chlorprothixene (Phenothiazines are capable of potentiating CNS depressants).

No products indexed under this heading.

Chlorprothixene Hydrochloride (Phenothiazines are capable of potentiating CNS depressants).

No products indexed under this heading.

Clorazepate Dipotassium (Phenothiazines are capable of potentiating CNS depressants). Products include:

Tranxene 451

Clozapine (Phenothiazines are capable of potentiating CNS depressants). Products include:

Clozaril Tablets 2252

Codeine Phosphate (Phenothiazines are capable of potentiating CNS depressants). Products include:

Actifed with Codeine Cough Syrup.. 1067
Brontex 1981
Deconsal C Expectorant Syrup 456
Deconsal Pediatric Syrup 457
Dimetane-DC Cough Syrup 2059
Empirin with Codeine Tablets............ 1093
Fioricet with Codeine Capsules 2260
Fiorinal with Codeine Capsules 2262
Isoclor Expectorant.............................. 990
Novahistine DH..................................... 2462
Novahistine Expectorant..................... 2463
Nucofed 2051
Phenergan with Codeine..................... 2777
Phenergan VC with Codeine 2781
Robitussin A-C Syrup........................... 2073
Robitussin-DAC Syrup 2074
Ryna .... ◉ 841
Soma Compound w/Codeine Tablets 2676
Tussi-Organidin NR Liquid and S NR Liquid 2677
Tylenol with Codeine 1583

Desflurane (Phenothiazines are capable of potentiating CNS depressants). Products include:

Suprane 1813

Dezocine (Phenothiazines are capable of potentiating CNS depressants). Products include:

Dalgan Injection 538

Diazepam (Phenothiazines are capable of potentiating CNS depressants). Products include:

Dizac 1809
Valium Injectable 2182
Valium Tablets 2183
Valrelease Capsules 2169

Droperidol (Phenothiazines are capable of potentiating CNS depressants). Products include:

Inapsine Injection................................. 1296

Enflurane (Phenothiazines are capable of potentiating CNS depressants).

No products indexed under this heading.

Estazolam (Phenothiazines are capable of potentiating CNS depressants). Products include:

ProSom Tablets 449

IMPORTANT NOTE: Always consult each drug listing in the patient's regimen for possible interactions.

Ethchlorvynol (Phenothiazines are capable of potentiating CNS depressants). Products include:
- Placidyl Capsules ... 448

Ethinamate (Phenothiazines are capable of potentiating CNS depressants).
- No products indexed under this heading.

Fentanyl (Phenothiazines are capable of potentiating CNS depressants). Products include:
- Duragesic Transdermal System ... 1288

Fentanyl Citrate (Phenothiazines are capable of potentiating CNS depressants). Products include:
- Sublimaze Injection ... 1307

Fluphenazine Decanoate (Phenothiazines are capable of potentiating CNS depressants). Products include:
- Prolixin Decanoate ... 509

Fluphenazine Enanthate (Phenothiazines are capable of potentiating CNS depressants). Products include:
- Prolixin Enanthate ... 509

Fluphenazine Hydrochloride (Phenothiazines are capable of potentiating CNS depressants). Products include:
- Prolixin ... 509

Flurazepam Hydrochloride (Phenothiazines are capable of potentiating CNS depressants). Products include:
- Dalmane Capsules ... 2173

Glutethimide (Phenothiazines are capable of potentiating CNS depressants).
- No products indexed under this heading.

Haloperidol (Phenothiazines are capable of potentiating CNS depressants). Products include:
- Haldol Injection, Tablets and Concentrate ... 1575

Haloperidol Decanoate (Phenothiazines are capable of potentiating CNS depressants). Products include:
- Haldol Decanoate ... 1577

Hydrocodone Bitartrate (Phenothiazines are capable of potentiating CNS depressants). Products include:
- Anexsia 5/500 Elixir ... 1781
- Anexia Tablets ... 1782
- Codiclear DH Syrup ... 791
- Deconamine CX Cough and Cold Liquid and Tablets ... 1319
- Duratuss HD Elixir ... 2565
- Hycodan Tablets and Syrup ... 930
- Hycomine Compound Tablets ... 932
- Hycomine ... 931
- Hycotuss Expectorant Syrup ... 933
- Hydrocet Capsules ... 782
- Lorcet 10/650 ... 1018
- Lortab ... 2566
- Tussend ... 1783
- Tussend Expectorant ... 1785
- Vicodin Tablets ... 1356
- Vicodin ES Tablets ... 1357
- Vicodin Tuss Expectorant ... 1358
- Zydone Capsules ... 949

Hydrocodone Polistirex (Phenothiazines are capable of potentiating CNS depressants). Products include:
- Tussionex Pennkinetic Extended-Release Suspension ... 998

Hydroxyzine Hydrochloride (Phenothiazines are capable of potentiating CNS depressants). Products include:
- Atarax Tablets & Syrup ... 2185
- Marax Tablets & DF Syrup ... 2200
- Vistaril Intramuscular Solution ... 2216

Isoflurane (Phenothiazines are capable of potentiating CNS depressants).
- No products indexed under this heading.

Ketamine Hydrochloride (Phenothiazines are capable of potentiating CNS depressants).
- No products indexed under this heading.

Levomethadyl Acetate Hydrochloride (Phenothiazines are capable of potentiating CNS depressants). Products include:
- Orlamm ... 2239

Levorphanol Tartrate (Phenothiazines are capable of potentiating CNS depressants). Products include:
- Levo-Dromoran ... 2129

Lorazepam (Phenothiazines are capable of potentiating CNS depressants). Products include:
- Ativan Injection ... 2698
- Ativan Tablets ... 2700

Loxapine Hydrochloride (Phenothiazines are capable of potentiating CNS depressants). Products include:
- Loxitane ... 1378

Loxapine Succinate (Phenothiazines are capable of potentiating CNS depressants). Products include:
- Loxitane Capsules ... 1378

Meperidine Hydrochloride (Phenothiazines are capable of potentiating CNS depressants). Products include:
- Demerol ... 2308
- Mepergan Injection ... 2753

Mephobarbital (Phenothiazines are capable of potentiating CNS depressants). Products include:
- Mebaral Tablets ... 2322

Meprobamate (Phenothiazines are capable of potentiating CNS depressants). Products include:
- Miltown Tablets ... 2672
- PMB 200 and PMB 400 ... 2783

Mesoridazine (Phenothiazines are capable of potentiating CNS depressants).

Methadone Hydrochloride (Phenothiazines are capable of potentiating CNS depressants). Products include:
- Methadone Hydrochloride Oral Concentrate ... 2233
- Methadone Hydrochloride Oral Solution & Tablets ... 2235

Methohexital Sodium (Phenothiazines are capable of potentiating CNS depressants). Products include:
- Brevital Sodium Vials ... 1429

Methotrimeprazine (Phenothiazines are capable of potentiating CNS depressants). Products include:
- Levoprome ... 1274

Methoxyflurane (Phenothiazines are capable of potentiating CNS depressants).
- No products indexed under this heading.

Midazolam Hydrochloride (Phenothiazines are capable of potentiating CNS depressants). Products include:
- Versed Injection ... 2170

Molindone Hydrochloride (Phenothiazines are capable of potentiating CNS depressants). Products include:
- Moban Tablets and Concentrate ... 1048

Morphine Sulfate (Phenothiazines are capable of potentiating CNS depressants). Products include:
- Astramorph/PF Injection, USP (Preservative-Free) ... 535
- Duramorph ... 962
- Infumorph 200 and Infumorph 500 Sterile Solutions ... 965
- MS Contin Tablets ... 1994
- MSIR ... 1997
- Oramorph SR (Morphine Sulfate Sustained Release Tablets) ... 2236
- RMS Suppositories ... 2657
- Roxanol ... 2243

Opium Alkaloids (Phenothiazines are capable of potentiating CNS depressants).
- No products indexed under this heading.

Oxazepam (Phenothiazines are capable of potentiating CNS depressants). Products include:
- Serax Capsules ... 2810
- Serax Tablets ... 2810

Oxycodone Hydrochloride (Phenothiazines are capable of potentiating CNS depressants). Products include:
- Percocet Tablets ... 938
- Percodan Tablets ... 939
- Percodan-Demi Tablets ... 940
- Roxicodone Tablets, Oral Solution & Intensol (Oxycodone) ... 2244
- Tylox Capsules ... 1584

Pentobarbital Sodium (Phenothiazines are capable of potentiating CNS depressants). Products include:
- Nembutal Sodium Capsules ... 436
- Nembutal Sodium Solution ... 438
- Nembutal Sodium Suppositories ... 440

Perphenazine (Phenothiazines are capable of potentiating CNS depressants). Products include:
- Etrafon ... 2355
- Triavil Tablets ... 1757
- Trilafon ... 2389

Phenobarbital (Phenothiazines are capable of potentiating CNS depressants). Products include:
- Arco-Lase Plus Tablets ... 512
- Bellergal-S Tablets ... 2250
- Donnatal ... 2060
- Donnatal Extentabs ... 2061
- Donnatal Tablets ... 2060
- Phenobarbital Elixir and Tablets ... 1469
- Quadrinal Tablets ... 1350

Prazepam (Phenothiazines are capable of potentiating CNS depressants).
- No products indexed under this heading.

Prochlorperazine (Phenothiazines are capable of potentiating CNS depressants). Products include:
- Compazine ... 2470

Promethazine Hydrochloride (Phenothiazines are capable of potentiating CNS depressants). Products include:
- Mepergan Injection ... 2753
- Phenergan with Codeine ... 2777
- Phenergan with Dextromethorphan ... 2778
- Phenergan Injection ... 2773
- Phenergan Suppositories ... 2775
- Phenergan Syrup ... 2774
- Phenergan Tablets ... 2775
- Phenergan VC ... 2779
- Phenergan VC with Codeine ... 2781

Propofol (Phenothiazines are capable of potentiating CNS depressants). Products include:
- Diprivan Injection ... 2833

Propoxyphene Hydrochloride (Phenothiazines are capable of potentiating CNS depressants). Products include:
- Darvon ... 1435
- Wygesic Tablets ... 2827

Propoxyphene Napsylate (Phenothiazines are capable of potentiating CNS depressants). Products include:
- Darvon-N/Darvocet-N ... 1433

Quazepam (Phenothiazines are capable of potentiating CNS depressants). Products include:
- Doral Tablets ... 2664

Risperidone (Phenothiazines are capable of potentiating CNS depressants). Products include:
- Risperdal ... 1301

Secobarbital Sodium (Phenothiazines are capable of potentiating CNS depressants). Products include:
- Seconal Sodium Pulvules ... 1474

Sufentanil Citrate (Phenothiazines are capable of potentiating CNS depressants). Products include:
- Sufenta Injection ... 1309

Temazepam (Phenothiazines are capable of potentiating CNS depressants). Products include:
- Restoril Capsules ... 2284

Thiamylal Sodium (Phenothiazines are capable of potentiating CNS depressants).
- No products indexed under this heading.

Thioridazine Hydrochloride (Phenothiazines are capable of potentiating CNS depressants). Products include:
- Mellaril ... 2269

Thiothixene (Phenothiazines are capable of potentiating CNS depressants). Products include:
- Navane Capsules and Concentrate ... 2201
- Navane Intramuscular ... 2202

Triazolam (Phenothiazines are capable of potentiating CNS depressants). Products include:
- Halcion Tablets ... 2611

Trifluoperazine Hydrochloride (Phenothiazines are capable of potentiating CNS depressants). Products include:
- Stelazine ... 2514

Zolpidem Tartrate (Phenothiazines are capable of potentiating CNS depressants). Products include:
- Ambien Tablets ... 2416

Food Interactions

Alcohol (Phenothiazines are capable of potentiating CNS depressants).

TORECAN TABLETS

(Thiethylperazine Maleate) ... 2245

See **Torecan Injection**

TORNALATE SOLUTION FOR INHALATION, 0.2%

(Bitolterol Mesylate) ... 956

May interact with sympathomimetic bronchodilators, monoamine oxidase inhibitors, and tricyclic antidepressants. Compounds in these categories include:

Albuterol (Potential for additive effects). Products include:
- Proventil Inhalation Aerosol ... 2382
- Ventolin Inhalation Aerosol and Refill ... 1197

Albuterol Sulfate (Potential for additive effects). Products include:
- Airet Solution for Inhalation ... 452
- Proventil Inhalation Solution 0.083% ... 2384
- Proventil Repetabs Tablets ... 2386
- Proventil Solution for Inhalation 0.5% ... 2383
- Proventil Syrup ... 2385
- Proventil Tablets ... 2386
- Ventolin Inhalation Solution ... 1198
- Ventolin Nebules Inhalation Solution ... 1199
- Ventolin Rotacaps for Inhalation ... 1200
- Ventolin Syrup ... 1202
- Ventolin Tablets ... 1203
- Volmax Extended-Release Tablets ... 1788

Amitriptyline Hydrochloride (Action of bitolterol on the vascular system may be potentiated). Products include:
- Elavil ... 2838
- Endep Tablets ... 2174
- Etrafon ... 2355
- Limbitrol ... 2180
- Triavil Tablets ... 1757

(Described in PDR For Nonprescription Drugs) (◉ Described in PDR For Ophthalmology)

Amoxapine (Action of bitolterol on the vascular system may be potentiated). Products include:

Asendin Tablets ... 1369

Clomipramine Hydrochloride (Action of bitolterol on the vascular system may be potentiated). Products include:

Anafranil Capsules ... 803

Desipramine Hydrochloride (Action of bitolterol on the vascular system may be potentiated). Products include:

Norpramin Tablets ... 1526

Doxepin Hydrochloride (Action of bitolterol on the vascular system may be potentiated). Products include:

Sinequan ... 2205
Zonalon Cream ... 1055

Ephedrine Hydrochloride (Potential for additive effects). Products include:

Primatene Dual Action Formula ... ▣ 872
Primatene Tablets ... ▣ 873
Quadrinal Tablets ... 1350

Ephedrine Sulfate (Potential for additive effects). Products include:

Bronkaid Caplets ... ▣ 717
Marax Tablets & DF Syrup ... 2200

Ephedrine Tannate (Potential for additive effects). Products include:

Rynatuss ... 2673

Epinephrine (Potential for additive effects). Products include:

Bronkaid Mist ... ▣ 717
EPIFRIN ... ⊙ 239
EpiPen ... 790
Marcaine Hydrochloride with Epinephrine 1:200,000 ... 2316
Primatene Mist ... ▣ 873
Sensorcaine with Epinephrine Injection ... 559
Sus-Phrine Injection ... 1019
Xylocaine with Epinephrine Injections ... 567

Epinephrine Hydrochloride (Potential for additive effects). Products include:

Ana-Kit Anaphylaxis Emergency Treatment Kit ... 617

Ethylnorepinephrine Hydrochloride (Potential for additive effects).

No products indexed under this heading.

Furazolidone (Action of bitolterol on the vascular system may be potentiated). Products include:

Furoxone ... 2046

Imipramine Hydrochloride (Action of bitolterol on the vascular system may be potentiated). Products include:

Tofranil Ampuls ... 854
Tofranil Tablets ... 856

Imipramine Pamoate (Action of bitolterol on the vascular system may be potentiated). Products include:

Tofranil-PM Capsules ... 857

Isocarboxazid (Action of bitolterol on the vascular system may be potentiated).

No products indexed under this heading.

Isoetharine (Potential for additive effects). Products include:

Bronkometer Aerosol ... 2302
Bronkosol Solution ... 2302
Isoetharine Inhalation Solution, USP, Arm-a-Med ... 551

Isoproterenol Hydrochloride (Potential for additive effects). Products include:

Isuprel Hydrochloride Injection 1:5000 ... 2311
Isuprel Hydrochloride Solution 1:200 & 1:100 ... 2313
Isuprel Mistometer ... 2312

Isoproterenol Sulfate (Potential for additive effects). Products include:

Norisodrine with Calcium Iodide Syrup ... 442

Maprotiline Hydrochloride (Action of bitolterol on the vascular system may be potentiated). Products include:

Ludiomil Tablets ... 843

Metaproterenol Sulfate (Potential for additive effects). Products include:

Alupent ... 669
Metaproterenol Sulfate Inhalation Solution, USP, Arm-a-Med ... 552

Nortriptyline Hydrochloride (Action of bitolterol on the vascular system may be potentiated). Products include:

Pamelor ... 2280

Phenelzine Sulfate (Action of bitolterol on the vascular system may be potentiated). Products include:

Nardil ... 1920

Pirbuterol Acetate (Potential for additive effects). Products include:

Maxair Autohaler ... 1492
Maxair Inhaler ... 1494

Protriptyline Hydrochloride (Action of bitolterol on the vascular system may be potentiated). Products include:

Vivactil Tablets ... 1774

Salmeterol Xinafoate (Potential for additive effects). Products include:

Serevent Inhalation Aerosol ... 1176

Selegiline Hydrochloride (Action of bitolterol on the vascular system may be potentiated). Products include:

Eldepryl Tablets ... 2550

Terbutaline Sulfate (Potential for additive effects). Products include:

Brethaire Inhaler ... 813
Brethine Ampuls ... 815
Brethine Tablets ... 814
Bricanyl Subcutaneous Injection ... 1502
Bricanyl Tablets ... 1503

Tranylcypromine Sulfate (Action of bitolterol on the vascular system may be potentiated). Products include:

Parnate Tablets ... 2503

Trimipramine Maleate (Action of bitolterol on the vascular system may be potentiated). Products include:

Surmontil Capsules ... 2811

TORNALATE METERED DOSE INHALER

(Bitolterol Mesylate) ... 957

May interact with sympathomimetic aerosol bronchodilators and sympathomimetic bronchodilators. Compounds in these categories include:

Albuterol (Concurrent use should be avoided to prevent deleterious cardiovascular effects). Products include:

Proventil Inhalation Aerosol ... 2382
Ventolin Inhalation Aerosol and Refill ... 1197

Albuterol Sulfate (Concurrent use should be avoided to prevent deleterious cardiovascular effects). Products include:

Airet Solution for Inhalation ... 452
Proventil Inhalation Solution 0.083% ... 2384
Proventil Repetabs Tablets ... 2386
Proventil Solution for Inhalation 0.5% ... 2383
Proventil Syrup ... 2385
Proventil Tablets ... 2386
Ventolin Inhalation Solution ... 1198
Ventolin Nebules Inhalation Solution ... 1199
Ventolin Rotacaps for Inhalation ... 1200
Ventolin Syrup ... 1202
Ventolin Tablets ... 1203
Volmax Extended-Release Tablets .. 1788

Ephedrine Hydrochloride (Concurrent use should be avoided to prevent deleterious cardiovascular effects). Products include:

Primatene Dual Action Formula ... ▣ 872
Primatene Tablets ... ▣ 873
Quadrinal Tablets ... 1350

Ephedrine Sulfate (Concurrent use should be avoided to prevent deleterious cardiovascular effects). Products include:

Bronkaid Caplets ... ▣ 717
Marax Tablets & DF Syrup ... 2200

Ephedrine Tannate (Concurrent use should be avoided to prevent deleterious cardiovascular effects). Products include:

Rynatuss ... 2673

Epinephrine (Concurrent use should be avoided to prevent deleterious cardiovascular effects). Products include:

Bronkaid Mist ... ▣ 717
EPIFRIN ... ⊙ 239
EpiPen ... 790
Marcaine Hydrochloride with Epinephrine 1:200,000 ... 2316
Primatene Mist ... ▣ 873
Sensorcaine with Epinephrine Injection ... 559
Sus-Phrine Injection ... 1019
Xylocaine with Epinephrine Injections ... 567

Epinephrine Hydrochloride (Concurrent use should be avoided to prevent deleterious cardiovascular effects). Products include:

Ana-Kit Anaphylaxis Emergency Treatment Kit ... 617

Ethylnorepinephrine Hydrochloride (Concurrent use should be avoided to prevent deleterious cardiovascular effects).

No products indexed under this heading.

Isoetharine (Concurrent use should be avoided to prevent deleterious cardiovascular effects). Products include:

Bronkometer Aerosol ... 2302
Bronkosol Solution ... 2302
Isoetharine Inhalation Solution, USP, Arm-a-Med ... 551

Isoproterenol Hydrochloride (Concurrent use should be avoided to prevent deleterious cardiovascular effects). Products include:

Isuprel Hydrochloride Injection 1:5000 ... 2311
Isuprel Hydrochloride Solution 1:200 & 1:100 ... 2313
Isuprel Mistometer ... 2312

Isoproterenol Sulfate (Concurrent use should be avoided to prevent deleterious cardiovascular effects). Products include:

Norisodrine with Calcium Iodide Syrup ... 442

Metaproterenol Sulfate (Concurrent use should be avoided to prevent deleterious cardiovascular effects). Products include:

Alupent ... 669
Metaproterenol Sulfate Inhalation Solution, USP, Arm-a-Med ... 552

Pirbuterol Acetate (Concurrent use should be avoided to prevent deleterious cardiovascular effects). Products include:

Maxair Autohaler ... 1492
Maxair Inhaler ... 1494

Salmeterol Xinafoate (Concurrent use should be avoided to prevent deleterious cardiovascular effects). Products include:

Serevent Inhalation Aerosol ... 1176

Terbutaline Sulfate (Concurrent use should be avoided to prevent deleterious cardiovascular effects). Products include:

Brethaire Inhaler ... 813
Brethine Ampuls ... 815
Brethine Tablets ... 814
Bricanyl Subcutaneous Injection ... 1502
Bricanyl Tablets ... 1503

TRACRIUM INJECTION

(Atracurium Besylate) ... 1183

May interact with aminoglycosides, muscle relaxants, and certain other agents. Compounds in these categories include:

Amikacin Sulfate (Enhances neuromuscular blocking action of Tracrium). Products include:

Amikacin Sulfate Injection, USP ... 960
Amikin Injectable ... 501

Baclofen (Synergistic or antagonist effect). Products include:

Lioresal Intrathecal ... 1596
Lioresal Tablets ... 829

Carisoprodol (Synergistic or antagonist effect). Products include:

Soma Compound w/Codeine Tablets ... 2676
Soma Compound Tablets ... 2675
Soma Tablets ... 2674

Chlorzoxazone (Synergistic or antagonist effect). Products include:

Paraflex Caplets ... 1580
Parafon Forte DSC Caplets ... 1581

Cyclobenzaprine Hydrochloride (Synergistic or antagonist effect). Products include:

Flexeril Tablets ... 1661

Dantrolene Sodium (Synergistic or antagonist effect). Products include:

Dantrium Capsules ... 1982
Dantrium Intravenous ... 1983

Doxacurium Chloride (Synergistic or antagonist effect). Products include:

Nuromax Injection ... 1149

Enflurane (Enhances neuromuscular blocking action of Tracrium).

No products indexed under this heading.

Gentamicin Sulfate (Enhances neuromuscular blocking action of Tracrium). Products include:

Garamycin Injectable ... 2360
Genoptic Sterile Ophthalmic Solution ... ⊙ 243
Genoptic Sterile Ophthalmic Ointment ... ⊙ 243
Gentacidin Ointment ... ⊙ 264
Gentacidin Solution ... ⊙ 264
Gentak ... ⊙ 208
Pred-G Liquifilm Sterile Ophthalmic Suspension ... ⊙ 251
Pred-G S.O.P. Sterile Ophthalmic Ointment ... ⊙ 252

Halothane (Enhances neuromuscular blocking action of Tracrium). Products include:

Fluothane ... 2724

Isoflurane (Enhances neuromuscular blocking action of Tracrium).

No products indexed under this heading.

Kanamycin Sulfate (Enhances neuromuscular blocking action of Tracrium).

No products indexed under this heading.

Lithium Carbonate (Enhances neuromuscular blocking action of Tracrium). Products include:

Eskalith ... 2485

IMPORTANT NOTE: Always consult each drug listing in the patient's regimen for possible interactions.

Tracrium Injection — Interactions Index — 1056

Lithium Carbonate Capsules & Tablets 2230
Lithonate/Lithotabs/Lithobid 2543

Lithium Citrate (Enhances neuromuscular blocking action of Tracrium).
No products indexed under this heading.

Magnesium Salts (Enhances neuromuscular blocking action of Tracrium).

Metaxalone (Synergistic or antagonist effect). Products include:
Skelaxin Tablets 788

Methocarbamol (Synergistic or antagonist effect). Products include:
Robaxin Injectable 2070
Robaxin Tablets 2071
Robaxisal Tablets 2071

Metocurine Iodide (Synergistic or antagonist effect). Products include:
Metubine Iodide Vials 916

Orphenadrine Citrate (Synergistic or antagonist effect). Products include:
Norflex 1496
Norgesic 1496

Pancuronium Bromide Injection (Synergistic or antagonist effect).
No products indexed under this heading.

Polymyxin Preparations (Enhances neuromuscular blocking action of Tracrium).

Procainamide (Enhances neuromuscular blocking action of Tracrium).

Quinidine Gluconate (Enhances neuromuscular blocking action of Tracrium). Products include:
Quinaglute Dura-Tabs Tablets 649

Quinidine Polygalacturonate (Enhances neuromuscular blocking action of Tracrium).
No products indexed under this heading.

Quinidine Sulfate (Enhances neuromuscular blocking action of Tracrium). Products include:
Quinidex Extentabs 2067

Rocuronium Bromide (Synergistic or antagonist effect). Products include:
Zemuron 1830

Streptomycin Sulfate (Enhances neuromuscular blocking action of Tracrium). Products include:
Streptomycin Sulfate Injection 2208

Succinylcholine Chloride (Increases neuromuscular blockade induced by Tracrium). Products include:
Anectine 1073

Tobramycin (Enhances neuromuscular blocking action of Tracrium). Products include:
AKTOB ..... ⊙ 206
TobraDex Ophthalmic Suspension and Ointment 473
Tobrex Ophthalmic Ointment and Solution ..... ⊙ 229

Tobramycin Sulfate (Enhances neuromuscular blocking action of Tracrium). Products include:
Nebcin Vials, Hyporets & ADD-Vantage 1464
Tobramycin Sulfate Injection 968

Vecuronium Bromide (Synergistic or antagonist effect). Products include:
Norcuron 1826

TRANCOPAL CAPLETS
(Chlormezanone) 2337
May interact with central nervous system depressants and certain other agents. Compounds in these categories include:

Alfentanil Hydrochloride (Possible additive effects). Products include:
Alfenta Injection 1286

Alprazolam (Possible additive effects). Products include:
Xanax Tablets 2649

Aprobarbital (Possible additive effects).
No products indexed under this heading.

Buprenorphine (Possible additive effects). Products include:
Buprenex Injectable 2006

Buspirone Hydrochloride (Possible additive effects). Products include:
BuSpar 737

Butabarbital (Possible additive effects).
No products indexed under this heading.

Butalbital (Possible additive effects). Products include:
Esgic-plus Tablets 1013
Fioricet Tablets 2258
Fioricet with Codeine Capsules 2260
Fiorinal Capsules 2261
Fiorinal with Codeine Capsules 2262
Fiorinal Tablets 2261
Phrenilin 785
Sedapap Tablets 50 mg/650 mg 1543

Chlordiazepoxide (Possible additive effects). Products include:
Libritabs Tablets 2177
Limbitrol 2180

Chlordiazepoxide Hydrochloride (Possible additive effects). Products include:
Librax Capsules 2176
Librium Capsules 2178
Librium Injectable 2179

Chlorpromazine (Possible additive effects). Products include:
Thorazine Suppositories 2523

Chlorprothixene (Possible additive effects).
No products indexed under this heading.

Chlorprothixene Hydrochloride (Possible additive effects).
No products indexed under this heading.

Clorazepate Dipotassium (Possible additive effects). Products include:
Tranxene 451

Clozapine (Possible additive effects). Products include:
Clozaril Tablets 2252

Codeine Phosphate (Possible additive effects). Products include:
Actifed with Codeine Cough Syrup 1067
Brontex 1981
Deconsal C Expectorant Syrup 456
Deconsal Pediatric Syrup 457
Dimetane-DC Cough Syrup 2059
Empirin with Codeine Tablets 1093
Fioricet with Codeine Capsules 2260
Fiorinal with Codeine Capsules 2262
Isoclor Expectorant 990
Novahistine DH 2462
Novahistine Expectorant 2463
Nucofed 2051
Phenergan with Codeine 2777
Phenergan VC with Codeine 2781
Robitussin A-C Syrup 2073
Robitussin-DAC Syrup 2074
Ryna ..... ◘ 841
Soma Compound w/Codeine Tablets 2676
Tussi-Organidin NR Liquid and S NR Liquid 2677
Tylenol with Codeine 1583

Desflurane (Possible additive effects). Products include:
Suprane 1813

Dezocine (Possible additive effects). Products include:
Dalgan Injection 538

Diazepam (Possible additive effects). Products include:
Dizac 1809
Valium Injectable 2182
Valium Tablets 2183
Valrelease Capsules 2169

Droperidol (Possible additive effects). Products include:
Inapsine Injection 1296

Enflurane (Possible additive effects).
No products indexed under this heading.

Estazolam (Possible additive effects). Products include:
ProSom Tablets 449

Ethchlorvynol (Possible additive effects). Products include:
Placidyl Capsules 448

Ethinamate (Possible additive effects).
No products indexed under this heading.

Fentanyl (Possible additive effects). Products include:
Duragesic Transdermal System 1288

Fentanyl Citrate (Possible additive effects). Products include:
Sublimaze Injection 1307

Fluphenazine Decanoate (Possible additive effects). Products include:
Prolixin Decanoate 509

Fluphenazine Enanthate (Possible additive effects). Products include:
Prolixin Enanthate 509

Fluphenazine Hydrochloride (Possible additive effects). Products include:
Prolixin 509

Flurazepam Hydrochloride (Possible additive effects). Products include:
Dalmane Capsules 2173

Glutethimide (Possible additive effects).
No products indexed under this heading.

Haloperidol (Possible additive effects). Products include:
Haldol Injection, Tablets and Concentrate 1575

Haloperidol Decanoate (Possible additive effects). Products include:
Haldol Decanoate 1577

Hydrocodone Bitartrate (Possible additive effects). Products include:
Anexsia 5/500 Elixir 1781
Anexia Tablets 1782
Codiclear DH Syrup 791
Deconamine CX Cough and Cold Liquid and Tablets 1319
Duratuss HD Elixir 2565
Hycodan Tablets and Syrup 930
Hycomine Compound Tablets 932
Hycomine 931
Hycotuss Expectorant Syrup 933
Hydrocet Capsules 782
Lorcet 10/650 1018
Lortab 2566
Tussend 1783
Tussend Expectorant 1785
Vicodin Tablets 1356
Vicodin ES Tablets 1357
Vicodin Tuss Expectorant 1358
Zydone Capsules 949

Hydrocodone Polistirex (Possible additive effects). Products include:
Tussionex Pennkinetic Extended-Release Suspension 998

Hydroxyzine Hydrochloride (Possible additive effects). Products include:
Atarax Tablets & Syrup 2185
Marax Tablets & DF Syrup 2200
Vistaril Intramuscular Solution 2216

Isoflurane (Possible additive effects).
No products indexed under this heading.

Ketamine Hydrochloride (Possible additive effects).
No products indexed under this heading.

Levomethadyl Acetate Hydrochloride (Possible additive effects). Products include:
Orlamm 2239

Levorphanol Tartrate (Possible additive effects). Products include:
Levo-Dromoran 2129

Lorazepam (Possible additive effects). Products include:
Ativan Injection 2698
Ativan Tablets 2700

Loxapine Hydrochloride (Possible additive effects). Products include:
Loxitane 1378

Loxapine Succinate (Possible additive effects). Products include:
Loxitane Capsules 1378

Meperidine Hydrochloride (Possible additive effects). Products include:
Demerol 2308
Mepergan Injection 2753

Mephobarbital (Possible additive effects). Products include:
Mebaral Tablets 2322

Meprobamate (Possible additive effects). Products include:
Miltown Tablets 2672
PMB 200 and PMB 400 2783

Mesoridazine Besylate (Possible additive effects). Products include:
Serentil 684

Methadone Hydrochloride (Possible additive effects). Products include:
Methadone Hydrochloride Oral Concentrate 2233
Methadone Hydrochloride Oral Solution & Tablets 2235

Methohexital Sodium (Possible additive effects). Products include:
Brevital Sodium Vials 1429

Methotrimeprazine (Possible additive effects). Products include:
Levoprome 1274

Methoxyflurane (Possible additive effects).
No products indexed under this heading.

Midazolam Hydrochloride (Possible additive effects). Products include:
Versed Injection 2170

Molindone Hydrochloride (Possible additive effects). Products include:
Moban Tablets and Concentrate 1048

Morphine Sulfate (Possible additive effects). Products include:
Astramorph/PF Injection, USP (Preservative-Free) 535
Duramorph 962
Infumorph 200 and Infumorph 500 Sterile Solutions 965
MS Contin Tablets 1994
MSIR 1997
Oramorph SR (Morphine Sulfate Sustained Release Tablets) 2236
RMS Suppositories 2657
Roxanol 2243

Opium Alkaloids (Possible additive effects).
No products indexed under this heading.

(◘ Described in PDR For Nonprescription Drugs) (⊙ Described in PDR For Ophthalmology)

Oxazepam (Possible additive effects). Products include:

Serax Capsules 2810
Serax Tablets... 2810

Oxycodone Hydrochloride (Possible additive effects). Products include:

Percocet Tablets 938
Percodan Tablets..................................... 939
Percodan-Demi Tablets........................... 940
Roxicodone Tablets, Oral Solution & Intensol (Oxycodone) 2244
Tylox Capsules 1584

Pentobarbital Sodium (Possible additive effects). Products include:

Nembutal Sodium Capsules 436
Nembutal Sodium Solution 438
Nembutal Sodium Suppositories...... 440

Perphenazine (Possible additive effects). Products include:

Etrafon 2355
Triavil Tablets 1757
Trilafon... 2389

Phenobarbital (Possible additive effects). Products include:

Arco-Lase Plus Tablets 512
Bellergal-S Tablets 2250
Donnatal 2060
Donnatal Extentabs................................ 2061
Donnatal Tablets 2060
Phenobarbital Elixir and Tablets 1469
Quadrinal Tablets 1350

Prazepam (Possible additive effects).

No products indexed under this heading.

Prochlorperazine (Possible additive effects). Products include:

Compazine 2470

Promethazine Hydrochloride (Possible additive effects). Products include:

Mepergan Injection 2753
Phenergan with Codeine 2777
Phenergan with Dextromethorphan 2778
Phenergan Injection 2773
Phenergan Suppositories 2775
Phenergan Syrup 2774
Phenergan Tablets 2775
Phenergan VC.. 2779
Phenergan VC with Codeine 2781

Propofol (Possible additive effects). Products include:

Diprivan Injection................................... 2833

Propoxyphene Hydrochloride (Possible additive effects). Products include:

Darvon 1435
Wygesic Tablets 2827

Propoxyphene Napsylate (Possible additive effects). Products include:

Darvon-N/Darvocet-N 1433

Quazepam (Possible additive effects). Products include:

Doral Tablets 2664

Risperidone (Possible additive effects). Products include:

Risperdal 1301

Secobarbital Sodium (Possible additive effects). Products include:

Seconal Sodium Pulvules 1474

Sufentanil Citrate (Possible additive effects). Products include:

Sufenta Injection 1309

Temazepam (Possible additive effects). Products include:

Restoril Capsules 2284

Thiamylal Sodium (Possible additive effects).

No products indexed under this heading.

Thioridazine Hydrochloride (Possible additive effects). Products include:

Mellaril 2269

Thiothixene (Possible additive effects). Products include:

Navane Capsules and Concentrate 2201
Navane Intramuscular 2202

Triazolam (Possible additive effects). Products include:

Halcion Tablets.. 2611

Trifluoperazine Hydrochloride (Possible additive effects). Products include:

Stelazine 2514

Zolpidem Tartrate (Possible additive effects). Products include:

Ambien Tablets.. 2416

Food Interactions

Alcohol (Possible additive effects).

TRANDATE INJECTION

(Labetalol Hydrochloride).....................1185
See Trandate Tablets

TRANDATE TABLETS

(Labetalol Hydrochloride).....................1185
May interact with tricyclic antidepressants, $beta_2$ agonists, insulin, oral hypoglycemic agents, and certain other agents. Compounds in these categories include:

Acarbose (Beta-blockade may prevent the appearance of premonitory signs and symptoms of acute hypoglycemia; reduces the release of insulin in response to hyperglycemia).

No products indexed under this heading.

Albuterol (Beta-blocker can blunt the bronchodilator effect of beta-receptor agonists in patients with bronchospasm; greater than normal anti-asthmatic dose of beta-agonist may be required). Products include:

Proventil Inhalation Aerosol 2382
Ventolin Inhalation Aerosol and Refill 1197

Albuterol Sulfate (Beta-blocker can blunt the bronchodilator effect of beta-receptor agonists in patients with bronchospasm; greater than normal anti-asthmatic dose of beta-agonist may be required). Products include:

Airet Solution for Inhalation 452
Proventil Inhalation Solution 0.083% 2384
Proventil Repetabs Tablets 2386
Proventil Solution for Inhalation 0.5% 2383
Proventil Syrup....................................... 2385
Proventil Tablets 2386
Ventolin Inhalation Solution................ 1198
Ventolin Nebules Inhalation Solution 1199
Ventolin Rotacaps for Inhalation....... 1200
Ventolin Syrup... 1202
Ventolin Tablets 1203
Volmax Extended-Release Tablets .. 1788

Amitriptyline Hydrochloride (Potential for increase in tremors). Products include:

Elavil 2838
Endep Tablets 2174
Etrafon 2355
Limbitrol 2180
Triavil Tablets 1757

Amoxapine (Potential for increase in tremors). Products include:

Asendin Tablets 1369

Bitolterol Mesylate (Beta-blocker can blunt the bronchodilator effect of beta-receptor agonists in patients with bronchospasm; greater than normal anti-asthmatic dose of beta-agonist may be required). Products include:

Tornalate Solution for Inhalation, 0.2% 956

Tornalate Metered Dose Inhaler 957

Chlorpropamide (Beta-blockade may prevent the appearance of premonitory signs and symptoms of acute hypoglycemia; reduces the release of insulin in response to hyperglycemia). Products include:

Diabinese Tablets 1935

Cimetidine (Increases bioavailability of oral labetalol). Products include:

Tagamet Tablets 2516

Cimetidine Hydrochloride (Increases bioavailability of oral labetalol). Products include:

Tagamet.. 2516

Clomipramine Hydrochloride (Potential for increase in tremors). Products include:

Anafranil Capsules 803

Desipramine Hydrochloride (Potential for increase in tremors). Products include:

Norpramin Tablets 1526

Doxepin Hydrochloride (Potential for increase in tremors). Products include:

Sinequan 2205
Zonalon Cream 1055

Ephedrine Hydrochloride (Beta-blocker can blunt the bronchodilator effect of beta-receptor agonists in patients with bronchospasm; greater than normal anti-asthmatic dose of beta-agonist may be required). Products include:

Primatene Dual Action Formula...... ◼◻ 872
Primatene Tablets .... ◼◻ 873
Quadrinal Tablets 1350

Ephedrine Sulfate (Beta-blocker can blunt the bronchodilator effect of beta-receptor agonists in patients with bronchospasm; greater than normal anti-asthmatic dose of beta-agonist may be required). Products include:

Bronkaid Caplets .... ◼◻ 717
Marax Tablets & DF Syrup................... 2200

Ephedrine Tannate (Beta-blocker can blunt the bronchodilator effect of beta-receptor agonists in patients with bronchospasm; greater than normal anti-asthmatic dose of beta-agonist may be required). Products include:

Rynatuss 2673

Epinephrine (Beta-blocker can blunt the bronchodilator effect of beta-receptor agonists in patients with bronchospasm; greater than normal anti-asthmatic dose of beta-agonist may be required). Products include:

Bronkaid Mist .... ◼◻ 717
EPIFRIN .... ◎ 239
EpiPen 790
Marcaine Hydrochloride with Epinephrine 1:200,000 2316
Primatene Mist .... ◼◻ 873
Sensorcaine with Epinephrine Injection 559
Sus-Phrine Injection 1019
Xylocaine with Epinephrine Injections... 567

Epinephrine Hydrochloride (Beta-blocker can blunt the bronchodilator effect of beta-receptor agonists in patients with bronchospasm; greater than normal anti-asthmatic dose of beta-agonist may be required). Products include:

Ana-Kit Anaphylaxis Emergency Treatment Kit 617

Ethylnorepinephrine Hydrochloride (Beta-blocker can blunt the bronchodilator effect of beta-receptor agonists in patients with bronchospasm; greater than normal anti-asthmatic dose of beta-agonist may be required).

No products indexed under this heading.

Glipizide (Beta-blockade may prevent the appearance of premonitory signs and symptoms of acute hypoglycemia; reduces the release of insulin in response to hyperglycemia). Products include:

Glucotrol Tablets 1967
Glucotrol XL Extended Release Tablets 1968

Glyburide (Beta-blockade may prevent the appearance of premonitory signs and symptoms of acute hypoglycemia; reduces the release of insulin in response to hyperglycemia). Products include:

DiaBeta Tablets 1239
Glynase PresTab Tablets 2609
Micronase Tablets 2623

Halothane (Synergism has been reported between labetalol I.V. and halothane anesthesia; potential increased hypotensive effect, reduction in cardiac output and increased central venous pressure). Products include:

Fluothane 2724

Imipramine Hydrochloride (Potential for increase in tremors). Products include:

Tofranil Ampuls 854
Tofranil Tablets 856

Imipramine Pamoate (Potential for increase in tremors). Products include:

Tofranil-PM Capsules............................ 857

Insulin, Human (Beta-blockade may prevent the appearance of premonitory signs and symptoms of acute hypoglycemia; reduces the release of insulin in response to hyperglycemia).

No products indexed under this heading.

Insulin, Human Isophane Suspension (Beta-blockade may prevent the appearance of premonitory signs and symptoms of acute hypoglycemia; reduces the release of insulin in response to hyperglycemia). Products include:

Novolin N Human Insulin 10 ml Vials.. 1795

Insulin, Human NPH (Beta-blockade may prevent the appearance of premonitory signs and symptoms of acute hypoglycemia; reduces the release of insulin in response to hyperglycemia). Products include:

Humulin N, 100 Units 1448
Novolin N PenFill Cartridges Durable Insulin Delivery System 1798
Novolin N Prefilled Syringe Disposable Insulin Delivery System 1798

Insulin, Human Regular (Beta-blockade may prevent the appearance of premonitory signs and symptoms of acute hypoglycemia; reduces the release of insulin in response to hyperglycemia). Products include:

Humulin R, 100 Units 1449
Novolin R Human Insulin 10 ml Vials.. 1795
Novolin R PenFill Cartridges Durable Insulin Delivery System 1798
Novolin R Prefilled Syringe Disposable Insulin Delivery System 1798
Velosulin BR Human Insulin 10 ml Vials.. 1795

IMPORTANT NOTE: Always consult each drug listing in the patient's regimen for possible interactions.

Trandate | Interactions Index | 1058

Insulin, Human, Zinc Suspension (Beta-blockade may prevent the appearance of premonitory signs and symptoms of acute hypoglycemia; reduces the release of insulin in response to hyperglycemia). Products include:

Humulin L, 100 Units 1446
Humulin U, 100 Units 1450
Novolin L Human Insulin 10 ml Vials 1795

Insulin, NPH (Beta-blockade may prevent the appearance of premonitory signs and symptoms of acute hypoglycemia; reduces the release of insulin in response to hyperglycemia). Products include:

NPH, 100 Units 1450
Pork NPH, 100 Units 1452
Purified Pork NPH Isophane Insulin 1801

Insulin, Regular (Beta-blockade may prevent the appearance of premonitory signs and symptoms of acute hypoglycemia; reduces the release of insulin in response to hyperglycemia). Products include:

Regular, 100 Units 1450
Pork Regular, 100 Units 1452
Pork Regular (Concentrated), 500 Units 1453
Purified Pork Regular Insulin 1801

Insulin, Zinc Crystals (Beta-blockade may prevent the appearance of premonitory signs and symptoms of acute hypoglycemia; reduces the release of insulin in response to hyperglycemia). Products include:

NPH, 100 Units 1450

Insulin, Zinc Suspension (Beta-blockade may prevent the appearance of premonitory signs and symptoms of acute hypoglycemia; reduces the release of insulin in response to hyperglycemia). Products include:

Iletin I 1450
Lente, 100 Units 1450
Iletin II 1452
Pork Lente, 100 Units 1452
Purified Pork Lente Insulin 1801

Isoetharine (Beta-blocker can blunt the bronchodilator effect of beta-receptor agonists in patients with bronchospasm; greater than normal anti-asthmatic dose of beta-agonist may be required). Products include:

Bronkometer Aerosol 2302
Bronkosol Solution 2302
Isoetharine Inhalation Solution, USP, Arm-a-Med 551

Isoproterenol Hydrochloride (Beta-blocker can blunt the bronchodilator effect of beta-receptor agonists in patients with bronchospasm; greater than normal anti-asthmatic dose of beta-agonist may be required). Products include:

Isuprel Hydrochloride Injection 1:5000 2311
Isuprel Hydrochloride Solution 1:200 & 1:100 2313
Isuprel Mistometer 2312

Isoproterenol Sulfate (Beta-blocker can blunt the bronchodilator effect of beta-receptor agonists in patients with bronchospasm; greater than normal anti-asthmatic dose of beta-agonist may be required). Products include:

Norisodrine with Calcium Iodide Syrup 442

Maprotiline Hydrochloride (Potential for increase in tremors). Products include:

Ludiomil Tablets 843

Metaproterenol Sulfate (Beta-blocker can blunt the bronchodilator effect of beta-receptor agonists in patients with bronchospasm; greater than normal anti-asthmatic dose of beta-agonist may be required). Products include:

Alupent 669
Metaproterenol Sulfate Inhalation Solution, USP, Arm-a-Med 552

Metformin Hydrochloride (Beta-blockade may prevent the appearance of premonitory signs and symptoms of acute hypoglycemia; reduces the release of insulin in response to hyperglycemia). Products include:

Glucophage 752

Nitroglycerin (Potential for additional antihypertensive effect). Products include:

Deponit NTG Transdermal Delivery System 2397
Nitro-Bid IV 1523
Nitro-Bid Ointment 1524
Nitrodisc 2047
Nitro-Dur (nitroglycerin) Transdermal Infusion System 1326
Nitrolingual Spray 2027
Nitrostat Tablets 1925
Transderm-Nitro Transdermal Therapeutic System 859

Nortriptyline Hydrochloride (Potential for increase in tremors). Products include:

Pamelor 2280

Pirbuterol Acetate (Beta-blocker can blunt the bronchodilator effect of beta-receptor agonists in patients with bronchospasm; greater than normal anti-asthmatic dose of beta-agonist may be required). Products include:

Maxair Autohaler 1492
Maxair Inhaler 1494

Protriptyline Hydrochloride (Potential for increase in tremors). Products include:

Vivactil Tablets 1774

Salmeterol Xinafoate (Beta-blocker can blunt the bronchodilator effect of beta-receptor agonists in patients with bronchospasm; greater than normal anti-asthmatic dose of beta-agonist may be required). Products include:

Serevent Inhalation Aerosol 1176

Terbutaline Sulfate (Beta-blocker can blunt the bronchodilator effect of beta-receptor agonists in patients with bronchospasm; greater than normal anti-asthmatic dose of beta-agonist may be required). Products include:

Brethaire Inhaler 813
Brethine Ampuls 815
Brethine Tablets 814
Bricanyl Subcutaneous Injection 1502
Bricanyl Tablets 1503

Tolazamide (Beta-blockade may prevent the appearance of premonitory signs and symptoms of acute hypoglycemia; reduces the release of insulin in response to hyperglycemia).

No products indexed under this heading.

Tolbutamide (Beta-blockade may prevent the appearance of premonitory signs and symptoms of acute hypoglycemia; reduces the release of insulin in response to hyperglycemia).

No products indexed under this heading.

Trimipramine Maleate (Potential for increase in tremors). Products include:

Surmontil Capsules 2811

Verapamil Hydrochloride (Care should be taken if co-administered; effects of concomitant use not specified). Products include:

Calan SR Caplets 2422
Calan Tablets 2419
Isoptin Injectable 1344
Isoptin Oral Tablets 1346
Isoptin SR Tablets 1348
Verelan Capsules 1410
Verelan Capsules 2824

Food Interactions

Food, unspecified (The absolute bioavailability of labetalol is increased when administered with food).

TRANSDERM SCōP TRANSDERMAL THERAPEUTIC SYSTEM

(Scopolamine) 869

May interact with anticholinergics, belladona products, antihistamines, tricyclic antidepressants, and certain other agents. Compounds in these categories include:

Acrivastine (Effect unspecified). Products include:

Semprex-D Capsules 463
Semprex-D Capsules 1167

Amitriptyline Hydrochloride (Effect unspecified). Products include:

Elavil 2838
Endep Tablets 2174
Etrafon 2355
Limbitrol 2180
Triavil Tablets 1757

Amoxapine (Effect unspecified). Products include:

Asendin Tablets 1369

Astemizole (Effect unspecified). Products include:

Hismanal Tablets 1293

Atropine Sulfate (Effect unspecified). Products include:

Arco-Lase Plus Tablets 512
Atrohist Plus Tablets 454
Atropine Sulfate Sterile Ophthalmic Solution .... ⊙ 233
Donnatal 2060
Donnatal Extentabs 2061
Donnatal Tablets 2060
Lomotil 2439
Motofen Tablets 784
Urised Tablets 1964

Azatadine Maleate (Effect unspecified). Products include:

Trinalin Repetabs Tablets 1330

Benztropine Mesylate (Effect unspecified). Products include:

Cogentin 1621

Biperiden Hydrochloride (Effect unspecified). Products include:

Akineton 1333

Bromodiphenhydramine Hydrochloride (Effect unspecified).

No products indexed under this heading.

Brompheniramine Maleate (Effect unspecified). Products include:

Alka Seltzer Plus Sinus Medicine .... ▣ 707
Bromfed Capsules (Extended-Release) 1785
Bromfed Syrup .... ▣ 733
Bromfed Tablets 1785
Bromfed-DM Cough Syrup 1786
Bromfed-PD Capsules (Extended-Release) 1785
Dimetane-DC Cough Syrup 2059
Dimetane-DX Cough Syrup 2059
Dimetapp Elixir .... ▣ 773
Dimetapp Extentabs .... ▣ 774
Dimetapp Tablets/Liqui-Gels .... ▣ 775
Dimetapp Cold & Allergy Chewable Tablets .... ▣ 773
Dimetapp DM Elixir .... ▣ 774
Vicks DayQuil Allergy Relief 12-Hour Extended Release Tablets .... ▣ 760
Vicks DayQuil Allergy Relief 4-Hour Tablets .... ▣ 760

Chlorpheniramine Maleate (Effect unspecified). Products include:

Alka-Seltzer Plus Cold Medicine .... ▣ 705
Alka-Seltzer Plus Cold Medicine Liqui-Gels .... ▣ 706
Alka-Seltzer Plus Cold & Cough Medicine .... ▣ 708
Alka-Seltzer Plus Cold & Cough Medicine Liqui-Gels .... ▣ 705
Allerest Children's Chewable Tablets .... ▣ 627
Allerest Headache Strength Tablets .... ▣ 627
Allerest Maximum Strength Tablets .... ▣ 627
Allerest Sinus Pain Formula .... ▣ 627
Allerest 12 Hour Caplets .... ▣ 627
Ana-Kit Anaphylaxis Emergency Treatment Kit 617
Atrohist Pediatric Capsules 453
Atrohist Plus Tablets 454
BC Cold Powder Multi-Symptom Formula (Cold-Sinus-Allergy) .... ▣ 609
Cerose DM .... ▣ 878
Cheracol Plus Head Cold/Cough Formula .... ▣ 769
Children's Vicks DayQuil Allergy Relief .... ▣ 757
Children's Vicks NyQuil Cold/Cough Relief .... ▣ 758
Chlor-Trimeton Allergy Decongestant Tablets .... ▣ 799
Chlor-Trimeton Allergy Tablets .... ▣ 798
Comhist 2038
Comtrex Multi-Symptom Cold Reliever Tablets/Caplets/Liqui-Gels/Liquid .... ▣ 615
Allergy-Sinus Comtrex Multi-Symptom Allergy-Sinus Formula Tablets .... ▣ 617
Contac Continuous Action Nasal Decongestant/Antihistamine 12 Hour Capsules .... ▣ 813
Contac Maximum Strength Continuous Action Decongestant/Antihistamine 12 Hour Caplets .... ▣ 813
Contac Severe Cold and Flu Formula Caplets .... ▣ 814
Coricidin 'D' Decongestant Tablets .... ▣ 800
Coricidin Tablets .... ▣ 800
D.A. Chewable Tablets 951
Deconamine 1320
Dura-Tap/PD Capsules 2867
Dura-Vent/DA Tablets 953
Extendryl 1005
Fedahist Gyrocaps 2401
Fedahist Timecaps 2401
Hycomine Compound Tablets 932
Isoclor Timesule Capsules .... ▣ 637
Kronofed-A 977
Nolamine Timed-Release Tablets 785
Novahistine DH 2462
Novahistine Elixir .... ▣ 823
Ornade Spansule Capsules 2502
PediaCare Cold Allergy Chewable Tablets .... ▣ 677
PediaCare Cough-Cold Chewable Tablets 1553
PediaCare Cough-Cold Liquid 1553
PediaCare NightRest Cough-Cold Liquid 1553
Pediatric Vicks 44m Cough & Cold Relief .... ▣ 764
Pyrroxate Caplets .... ▣ 772
Ryna .... ▣ 841
Sinarest Tablets .... ▣ 648
Sinarest Extra Strength Tablets .... ▣ 648
Sine-Off Sinus Medicine .... ▣ 825
Singlet Tablets .... ▣ 825
Sinulin Tablets 787
Sinutab Sinus Allergy Medication, Maximum Strength Tablets and Caplets .... ▣ 860
Sudafed Plus Liquid .... ▣ 862
Sudafed Plus Tablets .... ▣ 863
Teldrin 12 Hour Antihistamine/Nasal Decongestant Allergy Relief Capsules .... ▣ 826
TheraFlu .... ▣ 787
TheraFlu Maximum Strength Nighttime Flu, Cold & Cough Medicine .... ▣ 788
Triaminic Allergy Tablets .... ▣ 789
Triaminic Cold Tablets .... ▣ 790
Triaminic Nite Light .... ▣ 791
Triaminic Syrup .... ▣ 792
Triaminic-12 Tablets .... ▣ 792
Triaminicin Tablets .... ▣ 793

(▣ Described in PDR For Nonprescription Drugs) (⊙ Described in PDR For Ophthalmology)

Triaminicol Multi-Symptom Cold Tablets .... ⊕D 793
Triaminicol Multi-Symptom Relief ⊕D 794
Tussend 1783
Children's TYLENOL Cold Multi-Symptom Liquid Formula and Chewable Tablets................................ 1561
Children's TYLENOL Cold Plus Cough Multi Symptom Tablets and Liquid .... ⊕D 681
TYLENOL Maximum Strength Allergy Sinus Medication Gelcaps and Caplets 1563
TYLENOL Cold Multi-Symptom Formula Medication Tablets and Caplets 1561
TYLENOL Cold Multi-Symptom Hot Medication Liquid Packets.............. 1557
Vicks 44 LiquiCaps Cough, Cold & Flu Relief.. ⊕D 755
Vicks 44M Cough, Cold & Flu Relief .... ⊕D 756

Chlorpheniramine Polistirex (Effect unspecified). Products include:

Tussionex Pennkinetic Extended-Release Suspension 998

Chlorpheniramine Tannate (Effect unspecified). Products include:

Atrohist Pediatric Suspension 454
Ricobid Tablets and Pediatric Suspension.. 2038
Rynatan 2673
Rynatuss 2673

Clemastine Fumarate (Effect unspecified). Products include:

Tavist Syrup.. 2297
Tavist Tablets 2298
Tavist-1 12 Hour Relief Tablets ....⊕D 787
Tavist-D 12 Hour Relief Tablets ....⊕D 787

Clidinium Bromide (Effect unspecified). Products include:

Librax Capsules 2176
Quarzan Capsules 2181

Clomipramine Hydrochloride (Effect unspecified). Products include:

Anafranil Capsules 803

Cyproheptadine Hydrochloride (Effect unspecified). Products include:

Periactin 1724

Desipramine Hydrochloride (Effect unspecified). Products include:

Norpramin Tablets 1526

Dexchlorpheniramine Maleate (Effect unspecified).

No products indexed under this heading.

Dicyclomine Hydrochloride (Effect unspecified). Products include:

Bentyl 1501

Diphenhydramine Citrate (Effect unspecified). Products include:

Excedrin P.M. Analgesic/Sleeping Aid Tablets, Caplets, Liquigels...... 733

Diphenylpyraline Hydrochloride (Effect unspecified).

No products indexed under this heading.

Doxepin Hydrochloride (Effect unspecified). Products include:

Sinequan 2205
Zonalon Cream 1055

Glycopyrrolate (Effect unspecified). Products include:

Robinul Forte Tablets.............................. 2072
Robinul Injectable 2072
Robinul Tablets.. 2072

Hyoscyamine (Effect unspecified). Products include:

Cystospaz Tablets.................................. 1963
Urised Tablets.. 1964

Hyoscyamine Sulfate (Effect unspecified). Products include:

Arco-Lase Plus Tablets 512
Atrohist Plus Tablets 454
Cystospaz-M Capsules 1963
Donnatal 2060

Donnatal Extentabs................................ 2061
Donnatal Tablets 2060
Kutrase Capsules.................................... 2402
Levsin/Levsinex/Levbid 2405

Imipramine Hydrochloride (Effect unspecified). Products include:

Tofranil Ampuls 854
Tofranil Tablets 856

Imipramine Pamoate (Effect unspecified). Products include:

Tofranil-PM Capsules.............................. 857

Ipratropium Bromide (Effect unspecified). Products include:

Atrovent Inhalation Aerosol.................. 671
Atrovent Inhalation Solution 673

Loratadine (Effect unspecified). Products include:

Claritin 2349
Claritin-D 2350

Maprotiline Hydrochloride (Effect unspecified). Products include:

Ludiomil Tablets.. 843

Meclizine Hydrochloride (Effect unspecified). Products include:

Antivert, Antivert/25 Tablets, &
Antivert/50 Tablets 2185
Bonine Tablets 1933
Dramamine II Tablets............................ ⊕D 837

Mepenzolate Bromide (Effect unspecified).

No products indexed under this heading.

Methdilazine Hydrochloride (Effect unspecified).

No products indexed under this heading.

Nortriptyline Hydrochloride (Effect unspecified). Products include:

Pamelor 2280

Oxybutynin Chloride (Effect unspecified). Products include:

Ditropan.. 1516

Procyclidine Hydrochloride (Effect unspecified). Products include:

Kemadrin Tablets 1112

Promethazine Hydrochloride (Effect unspecified). Products include:

Mepergan Injection 2753
Phenergan with Codeine...................... 2777
Phenergan with Dextromethorphan 2778
Phenergan Injection 2773
Phenergan Suppositories 2775
Phenergan Syrup 2774
Phenergan Tablets 2775
Phenergan VC 2779
Phenergan VC with Codeine 2781

Propantheline Bromide (Effect unspecified). Products include:

Pro-Banthine Tablets 2052

Protriptyline Hydrochloride (Effect unspecified). Products include:

Vivactil Tablets 1774

Pyrilamine Maleate (Effect unspecified). Products include:

4-Way Fast Acting Nasal Spray (regular & mentholated)................ ⊕D 621
Maximum Strength Multi-Symptom Formula Midol .... ⊕D 722
PMS Multi-Symptom Formula Midol .... ⊕D 723

Pyrilamine Tannate (Effect unspecified). Products include:

Atrohist Pediatric Suspension 454
Rynatan 2673

Terfenadine (Effect unspecified). Products include:

Seldane Tablets 1536
Seldane-D Extended-Release Tablets 1538

Tridihexethyl Chloride (Effect unspecified).

No products indexed under this heading.

Trihexyphenidyl Hydrochloride (Effect unspecified). Products include:

Artane.. 1368

Trimeprazine Tartrate (Effect unspecified). Products include:

Temaril Tablets, Syrup and Spansule Extended-Release Capsules.. 483

Trimipramine Maleate (Effect unspecified). Products include:

Surmontil Capsules................................ 2811

Tripelennamine Hydrochloride (Effect unspecified). Products include:

PBZ Tablets 845
PBZ-SR Tablets.. 844

Triprolidine Hydrochloride (Effect unspecified). Products include:

Actifed Plus Caplets .... ⊕D 845
Actifed Plus Tablets .... ⊕D 845
Actifed with Codeine Cough Syrup.. 1067
Actifed Syrup.. ⊕D 846
Actifed Tablets .... ⊕D 844

Food Interactions

Alcohol (Effect unspecified).

TRANSDERM-NITRO TRANSDERMAL THERAPEUTIC SYSTEM

(Nitroglycerin) 859

May interact with calcium channel blockers, vasodilators, and certain other agents. Compounds in these categories include:

Amlodipine Besylate (Potential for marked symptomatic hypotension). Products include:

Lotrel Capsules.. 840
Norvasc Tablets 1940

Bepridil Hydrochloride (Potential for marked symptomatic hypotension). Products include:

Vascor (200, 300 and 400 mg) Tablets 1587

Diazoxide (Additive vasodilating effects). Products include:

Hyperstat I.V. Injection 2363
Proglycem.. 580

Diltiazem Hydrochloride (Potential for marked symptomatic hypotension). Products include:

Cardizem CD Capsules 1506
Cardizem SR Capsules 1510
Cardizem Injectable 1508
Cardizem Tablets.................................... 1512
Dilacor XR Extended-release Capsules 2018

Felodipine (Potential for marked symptomatic hypotension). Products include:

Plendil Extended-Release Tablets.... 527

Hydralazine Hydrochloride (Additive vasodilating effects). Products include:

Apresazide Capsules 808
Apresoline Hydrochloride Tablets .. 809
Ser-Ap-Es Tablets 849

Isradipine (Potential for marked symptomatic hypotension). Products include:

DynaCirc Capsules 2256

Minoxidil (Additive vasodilating effects). Products include:

Loniten Tablets.. 2618
Rogaine Topical Solution 2637

Nicardipine Hydrochloride (Potential for marked symptomatic hypotension). Products include:

Cardene Capsules 2095
Cardene I.V. 2709
Cardene SR Capsules.............................. 2097

Nifedipine (Potential for marked symptomatic hypotension). Products include:

Adalat Capsules (10 mg and 20 mg) 587
Adalat CC 589
Procardia Capsules 1971

Procardia XL Extended Release Tablets 1972

Nimodipine (Potential for marked symptomatic hypotension). Products include:

Nimotop Capsules.................................... 610

Nisoldipine (Potential for marked symptomatic hypotension).

No products indexed under this heading.

Verapamil Hydrochloride (Potential for marked symptomatic hypotension). Products include:

Calan SR Caplets 2422
Calan Tablets.. 2419
Isoptin Injectable 1344
Isoptin Oral Tablets 1346
Isoptin SR Tablets.................................... 1348
Verelan Capsules 1410
Verelan Capsules 2824

Food Interactions

Alcohol (Additive vasodilating effects).

TRANXENE T-TAB TABLETS

(Clorazepate Dipotassium).................. 451

May interact with central nervous system depressants, monoamine oxidase inhibitors, antidepressant drugs, narcotic analgesics, barbiturates, phenothiazines, and certain other agents. Compounds in these categories include:

Alfentanil Hydrochloride (Increased effects, prolonged sleeping time, potentiates action). Products include:

Alfenta Injection 1286

Alprazolam (Increased effects, prolonged sleeping time). Products include:

Xanax Tablets 2649

Amitriptyline Hydrochloride (Potentiates action). Products include:

Elavil 2838
Endep Tablets 2174
Etrafon 2355
Limbitrol 2180
Triavil Tablets 1757

Amoxapine (Potentiates action). Products include:

Asendin Tablets 1369

Aprobarbital (Increased effects, prolonged sleeping time).

No products indexed under this heading.

Buprenorphine (Increased effects, prolonged sleeping time, potentiates action). Products include:

Buprenex Injectable 2006

Bupropion Hydrochloride (Potentiates action). Products include:

Wellbutrin Tablets.................................... 1204

Buspirone Hydrochloride (Increased effects, prolonged sleeping time). Products include:

BuSpar 737

Butabarbital (Increased effects, prolonged sleeping time).

No products indexed under this heading.

Butalbital (Increased effects, prolonged sleeping time). Products include:

Esgic-plus Tablets 1013
Fioricet Tablets.. 2258
Fioricet with Codeine Capsules 2260
Fiorinal Capsules 2261
Fiorinal with Codeine Capsules 2262
Fiorinal Tablets.. 2261
Phrenilin 785
Sedapap Tablets 50 mg/650 mg .. 1543

Chlordiazepoxide (Increased effects, prolonged sleeping time). Products include:

Libritabs Tablets 2177
Limbitrol 2180

IMPORTANT NOTE: Always consult each drug listing in the patient's regimen for possible interactions.

Tranxene Interactions Index 1060

Chlordiazepoxide Hydrochloride (Increased effects, prolonged sleeping time). Products include:
Librax Capsules ... 2176
Librium Capsules ... 2178
Librium Injectable ... 2179
Chlorpromazine (Increased inhibitory effects). Products include:
Thorazine Suppositories ... 2523
Chlorpromazine Hydrochloride (Increased inhibitory effects). Products include:
Thorazine ... 2523
Chlorprothixene (Increased effects, prolonged sleeping time, potentiates action).
No products indexed under this heading.
Chlorprothixene Hydrochloride (Increased effects, prolonged sleeping time, potentiates action).
No products indexed under this heading.
Clozapine (Increased effects, prolonged sleeping time, potentiates action). Products include:
Clozaril Tablets ... 2252
Codeine Phosphate (Increased effects, prolonged sleeping time, potentiates action). Products include:
Actifed with Codeine Cough Syrup.. 1067
Brontex ... 1981
Deconsal C Expectorant Syrup ... 456
Deconsal Pediatric Syrup ... 457
Dimetane-DC Cough Syrup ... 2059
Empirin with Codeine Tablets ... 1093
Fioricet with Codeine Capsules ... 2260
Fiorinal with Codeine Capsules ... 2262
Isoclor Expectorant ... 990
Novahistine DH ... 2462
Novahistine Expectorant ... 2463
Nucofed ... 2051
Phenergan with Codeine ... 2777
Phenergan VC with Codeine ... 2781
Robitussin A-C Syrup ... 2073
Robitussin-DAC Syrup ... 2074
Ryna ... ◘ 841
Soma Compound w/Codeine Tablets ... 2676
Tussi-Organidin NR Liquid and S NR Liquid ... 2677
Tylenol with Codeine ... 1583
Desflurane (Increased effects, prolonged sleeping time, potentiates action). Products include:
Suprane ... 1813
Desipramine Hydrochloride (Potentiates action). Products include:
Norpramin Tablets ... 1526
Dezocine (Increased effects, prolonged sleeping time, potentiates action). Products include:
Dalgan Injection ... 538
Diazepam (Increased effects, prolonged sleeping time). Products include:
Dizac ... 1809
Valium Injectable ... 2182
Valium Tablets ... 2183
Valrelease Capsules ... 2169
Doxepin Hydrochloride (Potentiates action). Products include:
Sinequan ... 2205
Zonalon Cream ... 1055
Droperidol (Increased effects, prolonged sleeping time). Products include:
Inapsine Injection ... 1296
Enflurane (Increased effects, prolonged sleeping time).
No products indexed under this heading.
Estazolam (Increased effects, prolonged sleeping time, potentiates action). Products include:
ProSom Tablets ... 449
Ethchlorvynol (Increased effects, prolonged sleeping time). Products include:
Placidyl Capsules ... 448
Ethinamate (Increased effects, prolonged sleeping time).
No products indexed under this heading.
Fentanyl (Increased effects, prolonged sleeping time, potentiates action). Products include:
Duragesic Transdermal System ... 1288
Fentanyl Citrate (Increased effects, prolonged sleeping time, potentiates action). Products include:
Sublimaze Injection ... 1307
Fluoxetine Hydrochloride (Potentiates action). Products include:
Prozac Pulvules & Liquid, Oral Solution ... 919
Fluphenazine Decanoate (Increased effects, prolonged sleeping time). Products include:
Prolixin Decanoate ... 509
Fluphenazine Enanthate (Increased effects, prolonged sleeping time). Products include:
Prolixin Enanthate ... 509
Fluphenazine Hydrochloride (Increased effects, prolonged sleeping time). Products include:
Prolixin ... 509
Flurazepam Hydrochloride (Increased effects, prolonged sleeping time). Products include:
Dalmane Capsules ... 2173
Furazolidone (Potentiates action). Products include:
Furoxone ... 2046
Glutethimide (Increased effects, prolonged sleeping time).
No products indexed under this heading.
Haloperidol (Increased effects, prolonged sleeping time). Products include:
Haldol Injection, Tablets and Concentrate ... 1575
Haloperidol Decanoate (Increased effects, prolonged sleeping time). Products include:
Haldol Decanoate ... 1577
Hydrocodone Bitartrate (Increased effects, prolonged sleeping time, potentiates action). Products include:
Anexsia 5/500 Elixir ... 1781
Anexia Tablets ... 1782
Codiclear DH Syrup ... 791
Deconamine CX Cough and Cold Liquid and Tablets ... 1319
Duratuss HD Elixir ... 2565
Hycodan Tablets and Syrup ... 930
Hycomine Compound Tablets ... 932
Hycomine ... 931
Hycotuss Expectorant Syrup ... 933
Hydrocet Capsules ... 782
Lorcet 10/650 ... 1018
Lortab ... 2566
Tussend ... 1783
Tussend Expectorant ... 1785
Vicodin Tablets ... 1356
Vicodin ES Tablets ... 1357
Vicodin Tuss Expectorant ... 1358
Zydone Capsules ... 949
Hydrocodone Polistirex (Increased effects, prolonged sleeping time, potentiates action). Products include:
Tussionex Pennkinetic Extended-Release Suspension ... 998
Hydroxyzine Hydrochloride (Increased effects, prolonged sleeping time). Products include:
Atarax Tablets & Syrup ... 2185
Marax Tablets & DF Syrup ... 2200
Vistaril Intramuscular Solution ... 2216
Imipramine Hydrochloride (Potentiates action). Products include:
Tofranil Ampuls ... 854
Tofranil Tablets ... 856
Imipramine Pamoate (Potentiates action). Products include:
Tofranil-PM Capsules ... 857
Isocarboxazid (Potentiates action).
No products indexed under this heading.
Isoflurane (Increased effects, prolonged sleeping time).
No products indexed under this heading.
Ketamine Hydrochloride (Increased effects, prolonged sleeping time, potentiates action).
No products indexed under this heading.
Levomethadyl Acetate Hydrochloride (Increased effects, prolonged sleeping time, potentiates action). Products include:
Orlamm ... 2239
Levorphanol Tartrate (Increased effects, prolonged sleeping time, potentiates action). Products include:
Levo-Dromoran ... 2129
Lorazepam (Increased effects, prolonged sleeping time). Products include:
Ativan Injection ... 2698
Ativan Tablets ... 2700
Loxapine Hydrochloride (Increased effects, prolonged sleeping time). Products include:
Loxitane ... 1378
Loxapine Succinate (Increased effects, prolonged sleeping time, potentiates action). Products include:
Loxitane Capsules ... 1378
Maprotiline Hydrochloride (Potentiates action). Products include:
Ludiomil Tablets ... 843
Meperidine Hydrochloride (Increased effects, prolonged sleeping time, potentiates action). Products include:
Demerol ... 2308
Mepergan Injection ... 2753
Mephobarbital (Increased effects, prolonged sleeping time). Products include:
Mebaral Tablets ... 2322
Meprobamate (Increased effects, prolonged sleeping time). Products include:
Miltown Tablets ... 2672
PMB 200 and PMB 400 ... 2783
Mesoridazine Besylate (Increased effects, prolonged sleeping time). Products include:
Serentil ... 684
Methadone Hydrochloride (Increased effects, prolonged sleeping time, potentiates action). Products include:
Methadone Hydrochloride Oral Concentrate ... 2233
Methadone Hydrochloride Oral Solution & Tablets ... 2235
Methohexital Sodium (Increased effects, prolonged sleeping time). Products include:
Brevital Sodium Vials ... 1429
Methotrimeprazine (Increased effects, prolonged sleeping time, potentiates action). Products include:
Levoprome ... 1274
Methoxyflurane (Increased effects, prolonged sleeping time).
No products indexed under this heading.
Midazolam Hydrochloride (Increased effects, prolonged sleeping time). Products include:
Versed Injection ... 2170
Molindone Hydrochloride (Increased effects, prolonged sleeping time). Products include:
Moban Tablets and Concentrate ... 1048
Morphine Sulfate (Increased effects, prolonged sleeping time, potentiates action). Products include:
Astramorph/PF Injection, USP (Preservative-Free) ... 535
Duramorph ... 962
Infumorph 200 and Infumorph 500 Sterile Solutions ... 965
MS Contin Tablets ... 1994
MSIR ... 1997
Oramorph SR (Morphine Sulfate Sustained Release Tablets) ... 2236
RMS Suppositories ... 2657
Roxanol ... 2243
Nefazodone Hydrochloride (Potentiates action). Products include:
Serzone Tablets ... 771
Nortriptyline Hydrochloride (Potentiates action). Products include:
Pamelor ... 2280
Opium Alkaloids (Increased effects, prolonged sleeping time, potentiates action).
No products indexed under this heading.
Oxazepam (Increased effects, prolonged sleeping time). Products include:
Serax Capsules ... 2810
Serax Tablets ... 2810
Oxycodone Hydrochloride (Increased effects, prolonged sleeping time, potentiates action). Products include:
Percocet Tablets ... 938
Percodan Tablets ... 939
Percodan-Demi Tablets ... 940
Roxicodone Tablets, Oral Solution & Intensol (Oxycodone) ... 2244
Tylox Capsules ... 1584
Paroxetine Hydrochloride (Potentiates action). Products include:
Paxil Tablets ... 2505
Pentobarbital Sodium (Increased effects, prolonged sleeping time). Products include:
Nembutal Sodium Capsules ... 436
Nembutal Sodium Solution ... 438
Nembutal Sodium Suppositories ... 440
Perphenazine (Increased effects, prolonged sleeping time). Products include:
Etrafon ... 2355
Triavil Tablets ... 1757
Trilafon ... 2389
Phenelzine Sulfate (Potentiates action). Products include:
Nardil ... 1920
Phenobarbital (Increased effects, prolonged sleeping time). Products include:
Arco-Lase Plus Tablets ... 512
Bellergal-S Tablets ... 2250
Donnatal ... 2060
Donnatal Extentabs ... 2061
Donnatal Tablets ... 2060
Phenobarbital Elixir and Tablets ... 1469
Quadrinal Tablets ... 1350
Phenothiazine Derivatives (Potentiates action).
Prazepam (Increased effects, prolonged sleeping time).
No products indexed under this heading.
Prochlorperazine (Increased inhibitory effects). Products include:
Compazine ... 2470
Promethazine Hydrochloride (Increased effects, prolonged sleeping time). Products include:
Mepergan Injection ... 2753
Phenergan with Codeine ... 2777
Phenergan with Dextromethorphan 2778
Phenergan Injection ... 2773
Phenergan Suppositories ... 2775

(◘ Described in PDR For Nonprescription Drugs) (⊙ Described in PDR For Ophthalmology)

Phenergan Syrup 2774
Phenergan Tablets 2775
Phenergan VC 2779
Phenergan VC with Codeine 2781

Propofol (Increased effects, prolonged sleeping time, potentiates action). Products include:
Diprivan Injection 2833

Propoxyphene Hydrochloride (Increased effects, prolonged sleeping time, potentiates action). Products include:
Darvon 1435
Wygesic Tablets 2827

Propoxyphene Napsylate (Increased effects, prolonged sleeping time, potentiates action). Products include:
Darvon-N/Darvocet-N 1433

Protriptyline Hydrochloride (Potentiates action). Products include:
Vivactil Tablets 1774

Quazepam (Increased effects, prolonged sleeping time, potentiates action). Products include:
Doral Tablets 2664

Risperidone (Increased effects, prolonged sleeping time, potentiates action). Products include:
Risperdal 1301

Secobarbital Sodium (Increased effects, prolonged sleeping time, potentiates action). Products include:
Seconal Sodium Pulvules 1474

Selegiline Hydrochloride (Potentiates action). Products include:
Eldepryl Tablets 2550

Sertraline Hydrochloride (Potentiates action). Products include:
Zoloft Tablets 2217

Sufentanil Citrate (Increased effects, prolonged sleeping time, potentiates action). Products include:
Sufenta Injection 1309

Temazepam (Increased effects, prolonged sleeping time). Products include:
Restoril Capsules 2284

Thiamylal Sodium (Increased effects, prolonged sleeping time). No products indexed under this heading.

Thioridazine Hydrochloride (Increased effects, prolonged sleeping time). Products include:
Mellaril 2269

Thiothixene (Increased effects, prolonged sleeping time). Products include:
Navane Capsules and Concentrate 2201
Navane Intramuscular 2202

Tranylcypromine Sulfate (Potentiates action). Products include:
Parnate Tablets 2503

Trazodone Hydrochloride (Potentiates action). Products include:
Desyrel and Desyrel Dividose 503

Triazolam (Increased effects, prolonged sleeping time). Products include:
Halcion Tablets 2611

Trifluoperazine Hydrochloride (Increased effects, prolonged sleeping time). Products include:
Stelazine 2514

Trimipramine Maleate (Potentiates action). Products include:
Surmontil Capsules 2811

Venlafaxine Hydrochloride (Potentiates action). Products include:
Effexor 2719

Zolpidem Tartrate (Increased effects, prolonged sleeping time, potentiates action). Products include:
Ambien Tablets 2416

Food Interactions

Alcohol (Increased effects, prolonged sleeping time).

TRANXENE-SD HALF STRENGTH TABLETS

(Clorazepate Dipotassium) 451
See Tranxene T-TAB Tablets

TRANXENE-SD TABLETS

(Clorazepate Dipotassium) 451
See Tranxene T-TAB Tablets

TRASYLOL

(Aprotinin) 613
May interact with fibrinolytic agents and certain other agents. Compounds in these categories include:

Alteplase, Recombinant (Aprotinin may inhibit the effects of fibrinolytic agents). Products include:
Activase 1058

Anistreplase (Aprotinin may inhibit the effects of fibrinolytic agents). Products include:
Eminase 2039

Captopril (Aprotinin may block the acute hypotensive effects of captopril). Products include:
Capoten 739
Capozide 742

Heparin Calcium (Aprotinin, in the presence of heparin, has been found to prolong the activated clotting time (ACT) as measured by surface activation methods).
No products indexed under this heading.

Heparin Sodium (Aprotinin, in the presence of heparin, has been found to prolong the activated clotting time (ACT) as measured by surface activation methods). Products include:
Heparin Lock Flush Solution 2725
Heparin Sodium Injection 2726
Heparin Sodium Injection, USP, Sterile Solution 2615
Heparin Sodium Vials 1441

Streptokinase (Aprotinin may inhibit the effects of fibrinolytic agents). Products include:
Streptase for Infusion 562

Urokinase (Aprotinin may inhibit the effects of fibrinolytic agents). Products include:
Abbokinase 403
Abbokinase Open-Cath 405

TRAVASE OINTMENT

(Sutilains) 1356
May interact with:

Benzalkonium Chloride (May render substrate indifferent to enzyme activity in vitro). Products include:
Amino-Cerv 1779
Bactine Antiseptic/Anesthetic First Aid Liquid .... ᵐᵈ 708
Enuclene Cleaning, Lubricating Solution for Artificial Eyes .... © 218
Orajel Mouth-Aid for Canker and Cold Sores .... ᵐᵈ 652
Tanac No Sting Liquid .... ᵐᵈ 653
Total All-in-One Hard Contact Lens Solution .... © 342
Wet-N-Soak Plus Wetting and Soaking Solution .... © 345
Zephiran .... ᵐᵈ 795

Hexachlorophene (May render substrate indifferent to enzyme activity in vitro). Products include:
pHisoHex 2327

Iodine Preparations (May render substrate indifferent to enzyme activity in vitro). Products include:
Ethiodol 2340
Pima Syrup 1005
Ponaris Nasal Mucosal Emollient .. ᵐᵈ 658
The Stuart Formula Tablets .... ᵐᵈ 663

Nitrofurazone (May render substrate indifferent to enzyme activity in vitro). Products include:
Furacin Soluble Dressing 2045
Furacin Topical Cream 2045

Thimerosal (Interferes directly with enzyme activity to a slight degree in vitro).
No products indexed under this heading.

TRECATOR-SC TABLETS

(Ethionamide) 2814
May interact with antituberculosis drugs. Compounds in this category include:

Aminosalicylic Acid (Convulsions; the adverse effects of other antituberculous drugs intensified). Products include:
PASER Granules 1285

p-Aminosalicylic Acid (Convulsions; the adverse effects of other antituberculous drugs intensified).
No products indexed under this heading.

Cycloserine (Convulsions; the adverse effects of other antituberculous drugs intensified). Products include:
Seromycin Pulvules 1476

Ethambutol Hydrochloride (The adverse effects of other antituberculous drugs intensified). Products include:
Myambutol Tablets 1386

Isoniazid (The adverse effects of other antituberculous drugs intensified). Products include:
Nydrazid Injection 508
Rifamate Capsules 1530
Rifater 1532

Pyrazinamide (Convulsions; the adverse effects of other antituberculous drugs intensified). Products include:
Pyrazinamide Tablets 1398
Rifater 1532

Rifampin (The adverse effects of other antituberculous drugs intensified). Products include:
Rifadin 1528
Rifamate Capsules 1530
Rifater 1532
Rimactane Capsules 847

TRENTAL TABLETS

(Pentoxifylline) 1244
May interact with anticoagulants, antihypertensives, platelet inhibitors, xanthine bronchodilators, and certain other agents. Compounds in these categories include:

Acebutolol Hydrochloride (May require reduction in the dosage of antihypertensive). Products include:
Sectral Capsules 2807

Aminophylline (Concomitant administration leads to increased theophylline levels and theophylline toxicity).
No products indexed under this heading.

Amlodipine Besylate (May require reduction in the dosage of antihypertensive). Products include:
Lotrel Capsules 840
Norvasc Tablets 1940

Aspirin (Potential for bleeding and/or prolonged prothrombin time in patients treated with Trental with or without platelet aggregation inhibitors). Products include:
Alka-Seltzer Effervescent Antacid and Pain Reliever .... ᵐᵈ 701
Alka-Seltzer Extra Strength Effervescent Antacid and Pain Reliever .... ᵐᵈ 703
Alka-Seltzer Lemon Lime Effervescent Antacid and Pain Reliever .... ᵐᵈ 703
Alka-Seltzer Plus Cold Medicine .... ᵐᵈ 705
Alka-Seltzer Plus Cold & Cough Medicine .... ᵐᵈ 708
Alka-Seltzer Plus Night-Time Cold Medicine .... ᵐᵈ 707
Alka Seltzer Plus Sinus Medicine .. ᵐᵈ 707
Arthritis Foundation Safety Coated Aspirin Tablets .... ᵐᵈ 675
Arthritis Pain Ascriptin .... ᵐᵈ 631
Maximum Strength Ascriptin .... ᵐᵈ 630
Regular Strength Ascriptin Tablets .... ᵐᵈ 629
Arthritis Strength BC Powder .... ᵐᵈ 609
BC Cold Powder Multi-Symptom Formula (Cold-Sinus-Allergy) ..... ᵐᵈ 609
BC Cold Powder Non-Drowsy Formula (Cold-Sinus) .... ᵐᵈ 609
BC Powder .... ᵐᵈ 609
Bayer Children's Chewable Aspirin .... ᵐᵈ 711
Genuine Bayer Aspirin Tablets & Caplets .... ᵐᵈ 713
Extra Strength Bayer Arthritis Pain Regimen Formula .... ᵐᵈ 711
Extra Strength Bayer Aspirin Caplets & Tablets .... ᵐᵈ 712
Extended-Release Bayer 8-Hour Aspirin .... ᵐᵈ 712
Extra Strength Bayer Plus Aspirin Caplets .... ᵐᵈ 713
Extra Strength Bayer PM Aspirin .. ᵐᵈ 713
Bayer Enteric Aspirin .... ᵐᵈ 709
Bufferin Analgesic Tablets and Caplets .... ᵐᵈ 613
Arthritis Strength Bufferin Analgesic Caplets .... ᵐᵈ 614
Extra Strength Bufferin Analgesic Tablets .... ᵐᵈ 615
Cama Arthritis Pain Reliever .... ᵐᵈ 785
Darvon Compound-65 Pulvules 1435
Easprin 1914
Ecotrin 2455
Ecotrin Enteric Coated Aspirin Maximum Strength Tablets and Caplets .... ᵐᵈ 816
Ecotrin Enteric Coated Aspirin Regular Strength Tablets 2455
Empirin Aspirin Tablets .... ᵐᵈ 854
Empirin with Codeine Tablets 1093
Excedrin Extra-Strength Analgesic Tablets & Caplets 732
Fiorinal Capsules 2261
Fiorinal with Codeine Capsules 2262
Fiorinal Tablets 2261
Halfprin 1362
Healthprin Aspirin 2455
Norgescic 1496
Percodan Tablets 939
Percodan-Demi Tablets 940
Robaxisal Tablets 2071
Soma Compound w/Codeine Tablets 2676
Soma Compound Tablets 2675
St. Joseph Adult Chewable Aspirin (81 mg.) .... ᵐᵈ 808
Talwin Compound 2335
Ursinus Inlay-Tabs .... ᵐᵈ 794
Vanquish Analgesic Caplets .... ᵐᵈ 731

Atenolol (May require reduction in the dosage of antihypertensive). Products include:
Tenoretic Tablets 2845
Tenormin Tablets and I.V. Injection 2847

Azlocillin Sodium (Potential for bleeding and/or prolonged prothrombin time in patients treated with Trental with or without platelet aggregation inhibitors).
No products indexed under this heading.

Benazepril Hydrochloride (May require reduction in the dosage of antihypertensive). Products include:
Lotensin Tablets 834
Lotensin HCT 837

IMPORTANT NOTE: Always consult each drug listing in the patient's regimen for possible interactions.

Lotrel Capsules 840

Bendroflumethiazide (May require reduction in the dosage of antihypertensive).

No products indexed under this heading.

Betaxolol Hydrochloride (May require reduction in the dosage of antihypertensive). Products include:

Betoptic Ophthalmic Solution 469
Betoptic S Ophthalmic Suspension 471
Kerlone Tablets 2436

Bisoprolol Fumarate (May require reduction in the dosage of antihypertensive). Products include:

Zebeta Tablets 1413
Ziac 1415

Captopril (May require reduction in the dosage of antihypertensive). Products include:

Capoten 739
Capozide 742

Carbenicillin Indanyl Sodium (Potential for bleeding and/or prolonged prothrombin time in patients treated with Trental with or without platelet aggregation inhibitors). Products include:

Geocillin Tablets 2199

Carteolol Hydrochloride (May require reduction in the dosage of antihypertensive). Products include:

Cartrol Tablets 410
Ocupress Ophthalmic Solution, 1% Sterile .... ⊙ 309

Chlorothiazide (May require reduction in the dosage of antihypertensive). Products include:

Aldoclor Tablets 1598
Diupres Tablets 1650
Diuril Oral 1653

Chlorothiazide Sodium (May require reduction in the dosage of antihypertensive). Products include:

Diuril Sodium Intravenous 1652

Chlorthalidone (May require reduction in the dosage of antihypertensive). Products include:

Combipres Tablets 677
Tenoretic Tablets 2845
Thalitone 1245

Choline Magnesium Trisalicylate (Potential for bleeding and/or prolonged prothrombin time in patients treated with Trental with or without platelet aggregation inhibitors). Products include:

Trilisate 2000

Clonidine (May require reduction in the dosage of antihypertensive). Products include:

Catapres-TTS 675

Clonidine Hydrochloride (May require reduction in the dosage of antihypertensive). Products include:

Catapres Tablets 674
Combipres Tablets 677

Dalteparin Sodium (Potential for bleeding and/or prolonged prothrombin time in patients treated with Trental with or without platelet aggregation inhibitors). Products include:

Fragmin 1954

Deserpidine (May require reduction in the dosage of antihypertensive).

No products indexed under this heading.

Diazoxide (May require reduction in the dosage of antihypertensive). Products include:

Hyperstat I.V. Injection 2363
Proglycem 580

Diclofenac Potassium (Potential for bleeding and/or prolonged prothrombin time in patients treated with Trental with or without platelet aggregation inhibitors). Products include:

Cataflam 816

Diclofenac Sodium (Potential for bleeding and/or prolonged prothrombin time in patients treated with Trental with or without platelet aggregation inhibitors). Products include:

Voltaren Ophthalmic Sterile Ophthalmic Solution .... ⊙ 272
Voltaren Tablets 861

Dicumarol (Potential for bleeding and/or prolonged prothrombin time in patients treated with Trental with or without platelet aggregation inhibitors).

No products indexed under this heading.

Diflunisal (Potential for bleeding and/or prolonged prothrombin time in patients treated with Trental with or without platelet aggregation inhibitors). Products include:

Dolobid Tablets 1654

Diltiazem Hydrochloride (May require reduction in the dosage of antihypertensive). Products include:

Cardizem CD Capsules 1506
Cardizem SR Capsules 1510
Cardizem Injectable 1508
Cardizem Tablets 1512
Dilacor XR Extended-release Capsules 2018

Dipyridamole (Potential for bleeding and/or prolonged prothrombin time in patients treated with Trental with or without platelet aggregation inhibitors). Products include:

Persantine Tablets 681

Doxazosin Mesylate (May require reduction in the dosage of antihypertensive). Products include:

Cardura Tablets 2186

Dyphylline (Concomitant administration leads to increased theophylline levels and theophylline toxicity). Products include:

Lufyllin & Lufyllin-400 Tablets 2670
Lufyllin-GG Elixir & Tablets 2671

Enalapril Maleate (May require reduction in the dosage of antihypertensive). Products include:

Vaseretic Tablets 1765
Vasotec Tablets 1771

Enalaprilat (May require reduction in the dosage of antihypertensive). Products include:

Vasotec I.V. 1768

Enoxaparin (Potential for bleeding and/or prolonged prothrombin time in patients treated with Trental with or without platelet aggregation inhibitors). Products include:

Lovenox Injection 2020

Esmolol Hydrochloride (May require reduction in the dosage of antihypertensive). Products include:

Brevibloc Injection 1808

Felodipine (May require reduction in the dosage of antihypertensive). Products include:

Plendil Extended-Release Tablets 527

Fenoprofen Calcium (Potential for bleeding and/or prolonged prothrombin time in patients treated with Trental with or without platelet aggregation inhibitors). Products include:

Nalfon 200 Pulvules & Nalfon Tablets 917

Flurbiprofen (Potential for bleeding and/or prolonged prothrombin time in patients treated with Trental with or without platelet aggregation inhibitors). Products include:

Ansaid Tablets 2579

Fosinopril Sodium (May require reduction in the dosage of antihypertensive). Products include:

Monopril Tablets 757

Furosemide (May require reduction in the dosage of antihypertensive). Products include:

Lasix Injection, Oral Solution and Tablets 1240

Guanabenz Acetate (May require reduction in the dosage of antihypertensive).

No products indexed under this heading.

Guanethidine Monosulfate (May require reduction in the dosage of antihypertensive). Products include:

Esimil Tablets 822
Ismelin Tablets 827

Heparin Calcium (Potential for bleeding and/or prolonged prothrombin time in patients treated with Trental with or without platelet aggregation inhibitors).

No products indexed under this heading.

Heparin Sodium (Potential for bleeding and/or prolonged prothrombin time in patients treated with Trental with or without platelet aggregation inhibitors). Products include:

Heparin Lock Flush Solution 2725
Heparin Sodium Injection 2726
Heparin Sodium Injection, USP, Sterile Solution 2615
Heparin Sodium Vials 1441

Hydralazine Hydrochloride (May require reduction in the dosage of antihypertensive). Products include:

Apresazide Capsules 808
Apresoline Hydrochloride Tablets .. 809
Ser-Ap-Es Tablets 849

Hydrochlorothiazide (May require reduction in the dosage of antihypertensive). Products include:

Aldactazide 2413
Aldoril Tablets 1604
Apresazide Capsules 808
Capozide 742
Dyazide 2479
Esidrix Tablets 821
Esimil Tablets 822
HydroDIURIL Tablets 1674
Hydropres Tablets 1675
Hyzaar Tablets 1677
Inderide Tablets 2732
Inderide LA Long Acting Capsules .. 2734
Lopressor HCT Tablets 832
Lotensin HCT 837
Maxzide 1380
Moduretic Tablets 1705
Oretic Tablets 443
Prinzide Tablets 1737
Ser-Ap-Es Tablets 849
Timolide Tablets 1748
Vaseretic Tablets 1765
Zestoretic 2850
Ziac 1415

Hydroflumethiazide (May require reduction in the dosage of antihypertensive). Products include:

Diucardin Tablets 2718

Ibuprofen (Potential for bleeding and/or prolonged prothrombin time in patients treated with Trental with or without platelet aggregation inhibitors). Products include:

Advil Cold and Sinus Caplets and Tablets (formerly CoAdvil) .... ▣ 870
Advil Ibuprofen Tablets and Caplets .... ▣ 870
Children's Advil Suspension 2692
Arthritis Foundation Ibuprofen Tablets .... ▣ 674
Bayer Select Ibuprofen Pain Relief Formula .... ▣ 715
Cramp End Tablets .... ▣ 735
Dimetapp Sinus Caplets .... ▣ 775
Haltran Tablets .... ▣ 771
IBU Tablets 1342
Ibuprohm .... ▣ 735
Children's Motrin Ibuprofen Oral Suspension 1546
Motrin Tablets 2625
Motrin IB Caplets, Tablets, and Geltabs .... ▣ 838
Motrin IB Sinus .... ▣ 838
Motrin Ibuprofen Suspension, Oral Drops, Chewable Tablets, Caplets 1546
Nuprin Ibuprofen/Analgesic Tablets & Caplets .... ▣ 622
Sine-Aid IB Caplets 1554
Vicks DayQuil SINUS Pressure & PAIN Relief with IBUPROFEN .... ▣ 762

Indapamide (May require reduction in the dosage of antihypertensive). Products include:

Lozol Tablets 2022

Indomethacin (Potential for bleeding and/or prolonged prothrombin time in patients treated with Trental with or without platelet aggregation inhibitors). Products include:

Indocin 1680

Indomethacin Sodium Trihydrate (Potential for bleeding and/or prolonged prothrombin time in patients treated with Trental with or without platelet aggregation inhibitors). Products include:

Indocin I.V. 1684

Isradipine (May require reduction in the dosage of antihypertensive). Products include:

DynaCirc Capsules 2256

Ketoprofen (Potential for bleeding and/or prolonged prothrombin time in patients treated with Trental with or without platelet aggregation inhibitors). Products include:

Orudis Capsules 2766
Oruvail Capsules 2766

Labetalol Hydrochloride (May require reduction in the dosage of antihypertensive). Products include:

Normodyne Injection 2377
Normodyne Tablets 2379
Trandate 1185

Levobunolol Hydrochloride (May require reduction in the dosage of antihypertensive). Products include:

Betagan .... ⊙ 233

Lisinopril (May require reduction in the dosage of antihypertensive). Products include:

Prinivil Tablets 1733
Prinzide Tablets 1737
Zestoretic 2850
Zestril Tablets 2854

Losartan Potassium (May require reduction in the dosage of antihypertensive). Products include:

Cozaar Tablets 1628
Hyzaar Tablets 1677

Magnesium Salicylate (Potential for bleeding and/or prolonged prothrombin time in patients treated with Trental with or without platelet aggregation inhibitors). Products include:

Backache Caplets .... ▣ 613
Bayer Select Backache Pain Relief Formula .... ▣ 715
Doan's Extra-Strength Analgesic .... ▣ 633
Extra Strength Doan's P.M. .... ▣ 633
Doan's Regular Strength Analgesic .... ▣ 634
Mobigesic Tablets .... ▣ 602

Mecamylamine Hydrochloride (May require reduction in the dosage of antihypertensive). Products include:

Inversine Tablets 1686

(▣ Described in PDR For Nonprescription Drugs) (⊙ Described in PDR For Ophthalmology)

Interactions Index

Meclofenamate Sodium (Potential for bleeding and/or prolonged prothrombin time in patients treated with Trental with or without platelet aggregation inhibitors).

No products indexed under this heading.

Mefenamic Acid (Potential for bleeding and/or prolonged prothrombin time in patients treated with Trental with or without platelet aggregation inhibitors). Products include:

Ponstel 1925

Methyclothiazide (May require reduction in the dosage of antihypertensive). Products include:

Enduron Tablets...................................... 420

Methyldopa (May require reduction in the dosage of antihypertensive). Products include:

Aldoclor Tablets 1598
Aldomet Oral 1600
Aldoril Tablets... 1604

Methyldopate Hydrochloride (May require reduction in the dosage of antihypertensive). Products include:

Aldomet Ester HCl Injection 1602

Metolazone (May require reduction in the dosage of antihypertensive). Products include:

Mykrox Tablets....................................... 993
Zaroxolyn Tablets 1000

Metoprolol Succinate (May require reduction in the dosage of antihypertensive). Products include:

Toprol-XL Tablets 565

Metoprolol Tartrate (May require reduction in the dosage of antihypertensive). Products include:

Lopressor Ampuls 830
Lopressor HCT Tablets 832
Lopressor Tablets 830

Metyrosine (May require reduction in the dosage of antihypertensive). Products include:

Demser Capsules.................................... 1649

Mezlocillin Sodium (Potential for bleeding and/or prolonged prothrombin time in patients treated with Trental with or without platelet aggregation inhibitors). Products include:

Mezlin 601
Mezlin Pharmacy Bulk Package......... 604

Minoxidil (May require reduction in the dosage of antihypertensive). Products include:

Loniten Tablets....................................... 2618
Rogaine Topical Solution 2637

Moexipril Hydrochloride (May require reduction in the dosage of antihypertensive). Products include:

Univasc Tablets 2410

Nadolol (May require reduction in the dosage of antihypertensive).

No products indexed under this heading.

Nafcillin Sodium (Potential for bleeding and/or prolonged prothrombin time in patients treated with Trental with or without platelet aggregation inhibitors).

No products indexed under this heading.

Naproxen (Potential for bleeding and/or prolonged prothrombin time in patients treated with Trental with or without platelet aggregation inhibitors). Products include:

Anaprox/Naprosyn 2117

Naproxen Sodium (Potential for bleeding and/or prolonged prothrombin time in patients treated with Trental with or without platelet aggregation inhibitors). Products include:

Aleve 1975
Anaprox/Naprosyn 2117

Nicardipine Hydrochloride (May require reduction in the dosage of antihypertensive). Products include:

Cardene Capsules 2095
Cardene I.V. 2709
Cardene SR Capsules............................. 2097

Nifedipine (May require reduction in the dosage of antihypertensive). Products include:

Adalat Capsules (10 mg and 20 mg) 587
Adalat CC 589
Procardia Capsules................................ 1971
Procardia XL Extended Release Tablets 1972

Nisoldipine (May require reduction in the dosage of antihypertensive).

No products indexed under this heading.

Nitroglycerin (May require reduction in the dosage of antihypertensive). Products include:

Deponit NTG Transdermal Delivery System 2397
Nitro-Bid IV.. 1523
Nitro-Bid Ointment 1524
Nitrodisc 2047
Nitro-Dur (nitroglycerin) Transdermal Infusion System 1326
Nitrolingual Spray 2027
Nitrostat Tablets 1925
Transderm-Nitro Transdermal Therapeutic System 859

Penbutolol Sulfate (May require reduction in the dosage of antihypertensive). Products include:

Levatol 2403

Penicillin G Benzathine (Potential for bleeding and/or prolonged prothrombin time in patients treated with Trental with or without platelet aggregation inhibitors). Products include:

Bicillin C-R Injection 2704
Bicillin C-R 900/300 Injection 2706
Bicillin L-A Injection 2707

Penicillin G Procaine (Potential for bleeding and/or prolonged prothrombin time in patients treated with Trental with or without platelet aggregation inhibitors). Products include:

Bicillin C-R Injection 2704
Bicillin C-R 900/300 Injection 2706

Phenoxybenzamine Hydrochloride (May require reduction in the dosage of antihypertensive). Products include:

Dibenzyline Capsules 2476

Phentolamine Mesylate (May require reduction in the dosage of antihypertensive). Products include:

Regitine 846

Phenylbutazone (Potential for bleeding and/or prolonged prothrombin time in patients treated with Trental with or without platelet aggregation inhibitors).

No products indexed under this heading.

Pindolol (May require reduction in the dosage of antihypertensive). Products include:

Visken Tablets... 2299

Piroxicam (Potential for bleeding and/or prolonged prothrombin time in patients treated with Trental with or without platelet aggregation inhibitors). Products include:

Feldene Capsules.................................... 1965

Polythiazide (May require reduction in the dosage of antihypertensive). Products include:

Minizide Capsules 1938

Prazosin Hydrochloride (May require reduction in the dosage of antihypertensive). Products include:

Minipress Capsules................................ 1937
Minizide Capsules 1938

Propranolol Hydrochloride (May require reduction in the dosage of antihypertensive). Products include:

Inderal 2728
Inderal LA Long Acting Capsules 2730
Inderide Tablets 2732
Inderide LA Long Acting Capsules .. 2734

Quinapril Hydrochloride (May require reduction in the dosage of antihypertensive). Products include:

Accupril Tablets 1893

Ramipril (May require reduction in the dosage of antihypertensive). Products include:

Altace Capsules 1232

Rauwolfia Serpentina (May require reduction in the dosage of antihypertensive).

No products indexed under this heading.

Rescinnamine (May require reduction in the dosage of antihypertensive).

No products indexed under this heading.

Reserpine (May require reduction in the dosage of antihypertensive). Products include:

Diupres Tablets 1650
Hydropres Tablets.................................. 1675
Ser-Ap-Es Tablets 849

Salsalate (Potential for bleeding and/or prolonged prothrombin time in patients treated with Trental with or without platelet aggregation inhibitors). Products include:

Mono-Gesic Tablets 792
Salflex Tablets... 786

Sodium Nitroprusside (May require reduction in the dosage of antihypertensive).

No products indexed under this heading.

Sotalol Hydrochloride (May require reduction in the dosage of antihypertensive). Products include:

Betapace Tablets 641

Spirapril Hydrochloride (May require reduction in the dosage of antihypertensive).

No products indexed under this heading.

Sulindac (Potential for bleeding and/or prolonged prothrombin time in patients treated with Trental with or without platelet aggregation inhibitors). Products include:

Clinoril Tablets 1618

Terazosin Hydrochloride (May require reduction in the dosage of antihypertensive). Products include:

Hytrin Capsules 430

Theophylline (Concomitant administration leads to increased theophylline levels and theophylline toxicity). Products include:

Marax Tablets & DF Syrup.................... 2200
Quibron 2053

Theophylline Anhydrous (Concomitant administration leads to increased theophylline levels and theophylline toxicity). Products include:

Aerolate 1004
Primatene Dual Action Formula...... ◙ 872
Primatene Tablets .... ◙ 873
Respbid Tablets 682
Slo-bid Gyrocaps 2033

Theo-24 Extended Release Capsules 2568
Theo-Dur Extended-Release Tablets 1327
Theo-X Extended-Release Tablets .. 788
Uni-Dur Extended-Release Tablets.. 1331
Uniphyl 400 mg Tablets........................ 2001

Theophylline Calcium Salicylate (Concomitant administration leads to increased theophylline levels and theophylline toxicity). Products include:

Quadrinal Tablets 1350

Theophylline Sodium Glycinate (Concomitant administration leads to increased theophylline levels and theophylline toxicity).

No products indexed under this heading.

Ticarcillin Disodium (Potential for bleeding and/or prolonged prothrombin time in patients treated with Trental with or without platelet aggregation inhibitors). Products include:

Ticar for Injection 2526
Timentin for Injection............................ 2528

Ticlopidine Hydrochloride (Potential for bleeding and/or prolonged prothrombin time in patients treated with Trental with or without platelet aggregation inhibitors). Products include:

Ticlid Tablets 2156

Timolol Maleate (May require reduction in the dosage of antihypertensive). Products include:

Blocadren Tablets 1614
Timolide Tablets..................................... 1748
Timoptic in Ocudose 1753
Timoptic Sterile Ophthalmic Solution... 1751
Timoptic-XE 1755

Tolmetin Sodium (Potential for bleeding and/or prolonged prothrombin time in patients treated with Trental with or without platelet aggregation inhibitors). Products include:

Tolectin (200, 400 and 600 mg) .. 1581

Torsemide (May require reduction in the dosage of antihypertensive). Products include:

Demadex Tablets and Injection 686

Trimethaphan Camsylate (May require reduction in the dosage of antihypertensive). Products include:

Arfonad Ampuls...................................... 2080

Verapamil Hydrochloride (May require reduction in the dosage of antihypertensive). Products include:

Calan SR Caplets 2422
Calan Tablets... 2419
Isoptin Injectable 1344
Isoptin Oral Tablets 1346
Isoptin SR Tablets 1348
Verelan Capsules 1410
Verelan Capsules 2824

Warfarin Sodium (Potential for bleeding and/or prolonged prothrombin time in patients treated with Trental with or without platelet aggregation inhibitors; frequent monitoring of prothrombin time is recommended). Products include:

Coumadin 926

Food Interactions

Food, unspecified (Delays absorption but does not affect total absorption).

TRIAD, HYDROPHILIC WOUND DRESSING

(Zinc Oxide) 2554
None cited in PDR database.

TRIAMINIC ALLERGY TABLETS

(Chlorpheniramine Maleate,

IMPORTANT NOTE: Always consult each drug listing in the patient's regimen for possible interactions.

Phenylpropanolamine Hydrochloride)........▣ 789
May interact with monoamine oxidase inhibitors, hypnotics and sedatives, tranquilizers, and certain other agents. Compounds in these categories include:

Alprazolam (May increase drowsiness effect). Products include:
- Xanax Tablets 2649

Buspirone Hydrochloride (May increase drowsiness effect). Products include:
- BuSpar 737

Chlordiazepoxide (May increase drowsiness effect). Products include:
- Libritabs Tablets 2177
- Limbitrol 2180

Chlordiazepoxide Hydrochloride (May increase drowsiness effect). Products include:
- Librax Capsules 2176
- Librium Capsules 2178
- Librium Injectable 2179

Chlorpromazine (May increase drowsiness effect). Products include:
- Thorazine Suppositories 2523

Chlorpromazine Hydrochloride (May increase drowsiness effect). Products include:
- Thorazine 2523

Chlorprothixene (May increase drowsiness effect).
- No products indexed under this heading.

Chlorprothixene Hydrochloride (May increase drowsiness effect).
- No products indexed under this heading.

Clorazepate Dipotassium (May increase drowsiness effect). Products include:
- Tranxene 451

Diazepam (May increase drowsiness effect). Products include:
- Dizac 1809
- Valium Injectable 2182
- Valium Tablets 2183
- Valrelease Capsules 2169

Droperidol (May increase drowsiness effect). Products include:
- Inapsine Injection 1296

Estazolam (May increase drowsiness effect). Products include:
- ProSom Tablets 449

Ethchlorvynol (May increase drowsiness effect). Products include:
- Placidyl Capsules 448

Ethinamate (May increase drowsiness effect).
- No products indexed under this heading.

Fluphenazine Decanoate (May increase drowsiness effect). Products include:
- Prolixin Decanoate 509

Fluphenazine Enanthate (May increase drowsiness effect). Products include:
- Prolixin Enanthate 509

Fluphenazine Hydrochloride (May increase drowsiness effect). Products include:
- Prolixin 509

Flurazepam Hydrochloride (May increase drowsiness effect). Products include:
- Dalmane Capsules 2173

Furazolidone (Concurrent and/or sequential use is not recommended). Products include:
- Furoxone 2046

Glutethimide (May increase drowsiness effect).
- No products indexed under this heading.

Haloperidol (May increase drowsiness effect). Products include:
- Haldol Injection, Tablets and Concentrate 1575

Haloperidol Decanoate (May increase drowsiness effect). Products include:
- Haldol Decanoate 1577

Hydroxyzine Hydrochloride (May increase drowsiness effect). Products include:
- Atarax Tablets & Syrup 2185
- Marax Tablets & DF Syrup 2200
- Vistaril Intramuscular Solution 2216

Isocarboxazid (Concurrent and/or sequential use is not recommended).
- No products indexed under this heading.

Lorazepam (May increase drowsiness effect). Products include:
- Ativan Injection 2698
- Ativan Tablets 2700

Loxapine Hydrochloride (May increase drowsiness effect). Products include:
- Loxitane 1378

Loxapine Succinate (May increase drowsiness effect). Products include:
- Loxitane Capsules 1378

Meprobamate (May increase drowsiness effect). Products include:
- Miltown Tablets 2672
- PMB 200 and PMB 400 2783

Mesoridazine Besylate (May increase drowsiness effect). Products include:
- Serentil 684

Midazolam Hydrochloride (May increase drowsiness effect). Products include:
- Versed Injection 2170

Molindone Hydrochloride (May increase drowsiness effect). Products include:
- Moban Tablets and Concentrate 1048

Oxazepam (May increase drowsiness effect). Products include:
- Serax Capsules 2810
- Serax Tablets 2810

Perphenazine (May increase drowsiness effect). Products include:
- Etrafon 2355
- Triavil Tablets 1757
- Trilafon 2389

Phenelzine Sulfate (Concurrent and/or sequential use is not recommended). Products include:
- Nardil 1920

Prazepam (May increase drowsiness effect).
- No products indexed under this heading.

Prochlorperazine (May increase drowsiness effect). Products include:
- Compazine 2470

Promethazine Hydrochloride (May increase drowsiness effect). Products include:
- Mepergan Injection 2753
- Phenergan with Codeine 2777
- Phenergan with Dextromethorphan 2778
- Phenergan Injection 2773
- Phenergan Suppositories 2775
- Phenergan Syrup 2774
- Phenergan Tablets 2775
- Phenergan VC 2779
- Phenergan VC with Codeine 2781

Propofol (May increase drowsiness effect). Products include:
- Diprivan Injection 2833

Quazepam (May increase drowsiness effect). Products include:
- Doral Tablets 2664

Secobarbital Sodium (May increase drowsiness effect). Products include:
- Seconal Sodium Pulvules 1474

Selegiline Hydrochloride (Concurrent and/or sequential use is not recommended). Products include:
- Eldepryl Tablets 2550

Temazepam (May increase drowsiness effect). Products include:
- Restoril Capsules 2284

Thioridazine Hydrochloride (May increase drowsiness effect). Products include:
- Mellaril 2269

Thiothixene (May increase drowsiness effect). Products include:
- Navane Capsules and Concentrate 2201
- Navane Intramuscular 2202

Tranylcypromine Sulfate (Concurrent and/or sequential use is not recommended). Products include:
- Parnate Tablets 2503

Triazolam (May increase drowsiness effect). Products include:
- Halcion Tablets 2611

Trifluoperazine Hydrochloride (May increase drowsiness effect). Products include:
- Stelazine 2514

Zolpidem Tartrate (May increase drowsiness effect). Products include:
- Ambien Tablets 2416

Food Interactions

Alcohol (May increase drowsiness effect).

TRIAMINIC AM COUGH AND DECONGESTANT FORMULA

(Dextromethorphan Hydrobromide, Pseudoephedrine Hydrochloride)....▣ 789
May interact with monoamine oxidase inhibitors. Compounds in this category include:

Furazolidone (Concurrent use not recommended; consult your doctor). Products include:
- Furoxone 2046

Isocarboxazid (Concurrent use not recommended; consult your doctor).
- No products indexed under this heading.

Phenelzine Sulfate (Concurrent use not recommended; consult your doctor). Products include:
- Nardil 1920

Selegiline Hydrochloride (Concurrent use not recommended; consult your doctor). Products include:
- Eldepryl Tablets 2550

Tranylcypromine Sulfate (Concurrent use not recommended; consult your doctor). Products include:
- Parnate Tablets 2503

TRIAMINIC AM DECONGESTANT FORMULA

(Pseudoephedrine Hydrochloride) ..▣ 790
May interact with monoamine oxidase inhibitors. Compounds in this category include:

Furazolidone (Concurrent use not recommended; consult your doctor). Products include:
- Furoxone 2046

Isocarboxazid (Concurrent use not recommended; consult your doctor).
- No products indexed under this heading.

Phenelzine Sulfate (Concurrent use not recommended; consult your doctor). Products include:
- Nardil 1920

Selegiline Hydrochloride (Concurrent use not recommended; consult your doctor). Products include:
- Eldepryl Tablets 2550

Tranylcypromine Sulfate (Concurrent use not recommended; consult your doctor). Products include:
- Parnate Tablets 2503

TRIAMINIC COLD TABLETS

(Phenylpropanolamine Hydrochloride, Chlorpheniramine Maleate) ....▣ 790
May interact with monoamine oxidase inhibitors, hypnotics and sedatives, tranquilizers, and certain other agents. Compounds in these categories include:

Alprazolam (May increase drowsiness effect). Products include:
- Xanax Tablets 2649

Buspirone Hydrochloride (May increase drowsiness effect). Products include:
- BuSpar 737

Chlordiazepoxide (May increase drowsiness effect). Products include:
- Libritabs Tablets 2177
- Limbitrol 2180

Chlordiazepoxide Hydrochloride (May increase drowsiness effect). Products include:
- Librax Capsules 2176
- Librium Capsules 2178
- Librium Injectable 2179

Chlorpromazine (May increase drowsiness effect). Products include:
- Thorazine Suppositories 2523

Chlorpromazine Hydrochloride (May increase drowsiness effect). Products include:
- Thorazine 2523

Chlorprothixene (May increase drowsiness effect).
- No products indexed under this heading.

Chlorprothixene Hydrochloride (May increase drowsiness effect).
- No products indexed under this heading.

Clorazepate Dipotassium (May increase drowsiness effect). Products include:
- Tranxene 451

Diazepam (May increase drowsiness effect). Products include:
- Dizac 1809
- Valium Injectable 2182
- Valium Tablets 2183
- Valrelease Capsules 2169

Droperidol (May increase drowsiness effect). Products include:
- Inapsine Injection 1296

Estazolam (May increase drowsiness effect). Products include:
- ProSom Tablets 449

Ethchlorvynol (May increase drowsiness effect). Products include:
- Placidyl Capsules 448

Ethinamate (May increase drowsiness effect).
- No products indexed under this heading.

Fluphenazine Decanoate (May increase drowsiness effect). Products include:
- Prolixin Decanoate 509

Fluphenazine Enanthate (May increase drowsiness effect). Products include:
- Prolixin Enanthate 509

Fluphenazine Hydrochloride (May increase drowsiness effect). Products include:
- Prolixin 509

Interactions Index

Flurazepam Hydrochloride (May increase drowsiness effect). Products include:

Dalmane Capsules................................. 2173

Furazolidone (Concurrent and/or sequential use is not recommended). Products include:

Furoxone 2046

Glutethimide (May increase drowsiness effect).

No products indexed under this heading.

Haloperidol (May increase drowsiness effect). Products include:

Haldol Injection, Tablets and Concentrate 1575

Haloperidol Decanoate (May increase drowsiness effect). Products include:

Haldol Decanoate................................... 1577

Hydroxyzine Hydrochloride (May increase drowsiness effect). Products include:

Atarax Tablets & Syrup......................... 2185
Marax Tablets & DF Syrup................... 2200
Vistaril Intramuscular Solution.......... 2216

Isocarboxazid (Concurrent and/or sequential use is not recommended).

No products indexed under this heading.

Lorazepam (May increase drowsiness effect). Products include:

Ativan Injection..................................... 2698
Ativan Tablets.. 2700

Loxapine Hydrochloride (May increase drowsiness effect). Products include:

Loxitane 1378

Loxapine Succinate (May increase drowsiness effect). Products include:

Loxitane Capsules 1378

Meprobamate (May increase drowsiness effect). Products include:

Miltown Tablets 2672
PMB 200 and PMB 400 2783

Mesoridazine Besylate (May increase drowsiness effect). Products include:

Serentil.. 684

Midazolam Hydrochloride (May increase drowsiness effect). Products include:

Versed Injection 2170

Molindone Hydrochloride (May increase drowsiness effect). Products include:

Moban Tablets and Concentrate...... 1048

Oxazepam (May increase drowsiness effect). Products include:

Serax Capsules 2810
Serax Tablets.. 2810

Perphenazine (May increase drowsiness effect). Products include:

Etrafon 2355
Triavil Tablets 1757
Trilafon.. 2389

Phenelzine Sulfate (Concurrent and/or sequential use is not recommended). Products include:

Nardil 1920

Prazepam (May increase drowsiness effect).

No products indexed under this heading.

Prochlorperazine (May increase drowsiness effect). Products include:

Compazine 2470

Promethazine Hydrochloride (May increase drowsiness effect). Products include:

Mepergan Injection 2753
Phenergan with Codeine....................... 2777
Phenergan with Dextromethorphan 2778
Phenergan Injection 2773
Phenergan Suppositories 2775
Phenergan Syrup 2774
Phenergan Tablets 2775
Phenergan VC 2779
Phenergan VC with Codeine 2781

Propofol (May increase drowsiness effect). Products include:

Diprivan Injection.................................. 2833

Quazepam (May increase drowsiness effect). Products include:

Doral Tablets 2664

Secobarbital Sodium (May increase drowsiness effect). Products include:

Seconal Sodium Pulvules 1474

Selegiline Hydrochloride (Concurrent and/or sequential use is not recommended). Products include:

Eldepryl Tablets 2550

Temazepam (May increase drowsiness effect). Products include:

Restoril Capsules 2284

Thioridazine Hydrochloride (May increase drowsiness effect). Products include:

Mellaril 2269

Thiothixene (May increase drowsiness effect). Products include:

Navane Capsules and Concentrate 2201
Navane Intramuscular 2202

Tranylcypromine Sulfate (Concurrent and/or sequential use is not recommended). Products include:

Parnate Tablets 2503

Triazolam (May increase drowsiness effect). Products include:

Halcion Tablets....................................... 2611

Trifluoperazine Hydrochloride (May increase drowsiness effect). Products include:

Stelazine 2514

Zolpidem Tartrate (May increase drowsiness effect). Products include:

Ambien Tablets....................................... 2416

Food Interactions

Alcohol (May increase drowsiness effect).

TRIAMINIC EXPECTORANT

(Phenylpropanolamine Hydrochloride, Guaifenesin) ....◾ 790

May interact with monoamine oxidase inhibitors. Compounds in this category include:

Furazolidone (Concurrent and/or sequential use is not recommended). Products include:

Furoxone 2046

Isocarboxazid (Concurrent and/or sequential use is not recommended).

No products indexed under this heading.

Phenelzine Sulfate (Concurrent and/or sequential use is not recommended). Products include:

Nardil 1920

Selegiline Hydrochloride (Concurrent and/or sequential use is not recommended). Products include:

Eldepryl Tablets 2550

Tranylcypromine Sulfate (Concurrent and/or sequential use is not recommended). Products include:

Parnate Tablets 2503

TRIAMINIC NITE LIGHT

(Chlorpheniramine Maleate, Dextromethorphan Hydrobromide, Pseudoephedrine Hydrochloride) ....◾ 791

May interact with hypnotics and sedatives, tranquilizers, monoamine oxidase inhibitors, and certain other agents. Compounds in these categories include:

Alprazolam (May increase drowsiness effect). Products include:

Xanax Tablets 2649

Buspirone Hydrochloride (May increase drowsiness effect). Products include:

BuSpar 737

Chlordiazepoxide (May increase drowsiness effect). Products include:

Libritabs Tablets 2177
Limbitrol 2180

Chlordiazepoxide Hydrochloride (May increase drowsiness effect). Products include:

Librax Capsules 2176
Librium Capsules................................... 2178
Librium Injectable 2179

Chlorpromazine (May increase drowsiness effect). Products include:

Thorazine Suppositories....................... 2523

Chlorpromazine Hydrochloride (May increase drowsiness effect). Products include:

Thorazine 2523

Chlorprothixene (May increase drowsiness effect).

No products indexed under this heading.

Chlorprothixene Hydrochloride (May increase drowsiness effect).

No products indexed under this heading.

Clorazepate Dipotassium (May increase drowsiness effect). Products include:

Tranxene 451

Diazepam (May increase drowsiness effect). Products include:

Dizac 1809
Valium Injectable 2182
Valium Tablets 2183
Valrelease Capsules 2169

Droperidol (May increase drowsiness effect). Products include:

Inapsine Injection.................................. 1296

Estazolam (May increase drowsiness effect). Products include:

ProSom Tablets 449

Ethchlorvynol (May increase drowsiness effect). Products include:

Placidyl Capsules................................... 448

Ethinamate (May increase drowsiness effect).

No products indexed under this heading.

Fluphenazine Decanoate (May increase drowsiness effect). Products include:

Prolixin Decanoate 509

Fluphenazine Enanthate (May increase drowsiness effect). Products include:

Prolixin Enanthate 509

Fluphenazine Hydrochloride (May increase drowsiness effect). Products include:

Prolixin 509

Flurazepam Hydrochloride (May increase drowsiness effect). Products include:

Dalmane Capsules.................................. 2173

Furazolidone (Concurrent and/or sequential use is not recommended). Products include:

Furoxone 2046

Glutethimide (May increase drowsiness effect).

No products indexed under this heading.

Haloperidol (May increase drowsiness effect). Products include:

Haldol Injection, Tablets and Concentrate 1575

Haloperidol Decanoate (May increase drowsiness effect). Products include:

Haldol Decanoate................................... 1577

Hydroxyzine Hydrochloride (May increase drowsiness effect). Products include:

Atarax Tablets & Syrup......................... 2185

Marax Tablets & DF Syrup................... 2200
Vistaril Intramuscular Solution.......... 2216

Isocarboxazid (Concurrent and/or sequential use is not recommended).

No products indexed under this heading.

Lorazepam (May increase drowsiness effect). Products include:

Ativan Injection...................................... 2698
Ativan Tablets... 2700

Loxapine Hydrochloride (May increase drowsiness effect). Products include:

Loxitane 1378

Loxapine Succinate (May increase drowsiness effect). Products include:

Loxitane Capsules 1378

Meprobamate (May increase drowsiness effect). Products include:

Miltown Tablets 2672
PMB 200 and PMB 400 2783

Mesoridazine Besylate (May increase drowsiness effect). Products include:

Serentil.. 684

Midazolam Hydrochloride (May increase drowsiness effect). Products include:

Versed Injection 2170

Molindone Hydrochloride (May increase drowsiness effect). Products include:

Moban Tablets and Concentrate...... 1048

Oxazepam (May increase drowsiness effect). Products include:

Serax Capsules 2810
Serax Tablets.. 2810

Perphenazine (May increase drowsiness effect). Products include:

Etrafon 2355
Triavil Tablets 1757
Trilafon.. 2389

Phenelzine Sulfate (Concurrent and/or sequential use is not recommended). Products include:

Nardil 1920

Prazepam (May increase drowsiness effect).

No products indexed under this heading.

Prochlorperazine (May increase drowsiness effect). Products include:

Compazine 2470

Promethazine Hydrochloride (May increase drowsiness effect). Products include:

Mepergan Injection 2753
Phenergan with Codeine....................... 2777
Phenergan with Dextromethorphan 2778
Phenergan Injection 2773
Phenergan Suppositories 2775
Phenergan Syrup 2774
Phenergan Tablets 2775
Phenergan VC 2779
Phenergan VC with Codeine 2781

Propofol (May increase drowsiness effect). Products include:

Diprivan Injection.................................. 2833

Quazepam (May increase drowsiness effect). Products include:

Doral Tablets 2664

Secobarbital Sodium (May increase drowsiness effect). Products include:

Seconal Sodium Pulvules 1474

Selegiline Hydrochloride (Concurrent and/or sequential use is not recommended). Products include:

Eldepryl Tablets 2550

Temazepam (May increase drowsiness effect). Products include:

Restoril Capsules................................... 2284

Thioridazine Hydrochloride (May increase drowsiness effect). Products include:

Mellaril 2269

IMPORTANT NOTE: Always consult each drug listing in the patient's regimen for possible interactions.

Triaminic Nite Light — Interactions Index — 1066

Thiothixene (May increase drowsiness effect). Products include:
Navane Capsules and Concentrate 2201
Navane Intramuscular 2202
Tranylcypromine Sulfate (Concurrent and/or sequential use is not recommended). Products include:
Parnate Tablets 2503
Triazolam (May increase drowsiness effect). Products include:
Halcion Tablets 2611
Trifluoperazine Hydrochloride (May increase drowsiness effect). Products include:
Stelazine 2514
Zolpidem Tartrate (May increase drowsiness effect). Products include:
Ambien Tablets 2416

Food Interactions
Alcohol (May increase drowsiness effect).

TRIAMINIC SORE THROAT FORMULA
(Acetaminophen, Dextromethorphan Hydrobromide, Pseudoephedrine Hydrochloride) ◘ 791
May interact with monoamine oxidase inhibitors. Compounds in this category include:

Furazolidone (Concurrent and/or sequential use is not recommended). Products include:
Furoxone 2046
Isocarboxazid (Concurrent and/or sequential use is not recommended).
No products indexed under this heading.
Phenelzine Sulfate (Concurrent and/or sequential use is not recommended). Products include:
Nardil 1920
Selegiline Hydrochloride (Concurrent and/or sequential use is not recommended). Products include:
Eldepryl Tablets 2550
Tranylcypromine Sulfate (Concurrent and/or sequential use is not recommended). Products include:
Parnate Tablets 2503

TRIAMINIC SYRUP
(Phenylpropanolamine Hydrochloride, Chlorpheniramine Maleate) ◘ 792
May interact with hypnotics and sedatives, tranquilizers, monoamine oxidase inhibitors, and certain other agents. Compounds in these categories include:

Alprazolam (May increase drowsiness). Products include:
Xanax Tablets 2649
Buspirone Hydrochloride (May increase drowsiness). Products include:
BuSpar 737
Chlordiazepoxide (May increase drowsiness). Products include:
Libritabs Tablets 2177
Limbitrol 2180
Chlordiazepoxide Hydrochloride (May increase drowsiness). Products include:
Librax Capsules 2176
Librium Capsules 2178
Librium Injectable 2179
Chlorpromazine (May increase drowsiness). Products include:
Thorazine Suppositories 2523
Chlorpromazine Hydrochloride (May increase drowsiness). Products include:
Thorazine 2523
Chlorprothixene (May increase drowsiness).
No products indexed under this heading.
Chlorprothixene Hydrochloride (May increase drowsiness).
No products indexed under this heading.
Clorazepate Dipotassium (May increase drowsiness). Products include:
Tranxene 451
Diazepam (May increase drowsiness). Products include:
Dizac 1809
Valium Injectable 2182
Valium Tablets 2183
Valrelease Capsules 2169
Droperidol (May increase drowsiness). Products include:
Inapsine Injection 1296
Estazolam (May increase drowsiness). Products include:
ProSom Tablets 449
Ethchlorvynol (May increase drowsiness). Products include:
Placidyl Capsules 448
Ethinamate (May increase drowsiness).
No products indexed under this heading.
Fluphenazine Decanoate (May increase drowsiness). Products include:
Prolixin Decanoate 509
Fluphenazine Enanthate (May increase drowsiness). Products include:
Prolixin Enanthate 509
Fluphenazine Hydrochloride (May increase drowsiness). Products include:
Prolixin 509
Flurazepam Hydrochloride (May increase drowsiness). Products include:
Dalmane Capsules 2173
Furazolidone (Concurrent and/or sequential use is not recommended). Products include:
Furoxone 2046
Glutethimide (May increase drowsiness).
No products indexed under this heading.
Haloperidol (May increase drowsiness). Products include:
Haldol Injection, Tablets and Concentrate 1575
Haloperidol Decanoate (May increase drowsiness). Products include:
Haldol Decanoate 1577
Hydroxyzine Hydrochloride (May increase drowsiness). Products include:
Atarax Tablets & Syrup 2185
Marax Tablets & DF Syrup 2200
Vistaril Intramuscular Solution 2216
Isocarboxazid (Concurrent and/or sequential use is not recommended).
No products indexed under this heading.
Lorazepam (May increase drowsiness). Products include:
Ativan Injection 2698
Ativan Tablets 2700
Loxapine Hydrochloride (May increase drowsiness). Products include:
Loxitane 1378
Loxapine Succinate (May increase drowsiness). Products include:
Loxitane Capsules 1378
Meprobamate (May increase drowsiness). Products include:
Miltown Tablets 2672
PMB 200 and PMB 400 2783
Mesoridazine Besylate (May increase drowsiness). Products include:
Serentil 684
Midazolam Hydrochloride (May increase drowsiness). Products include:
Versed Injection 2170
Molindone Hydrochloride (May increase drowsiness). Products include:
Moban Tablets and Concentrate 1048
Oxazepam (May increase drowsiness). Products include:
Serax Capsules 2810
Serax Tablets 2810
Perphenazine (May increase drowsiness). Products include:
Etrafon 2355
Triavil Tablets 1757
Trilafon 2389
Phenelzine Sulfate (Concurrent and/or sequential use is not recommended). Products include:
Nardil 1920
Prazepam (May increase drowsiness).
No products indexed under this heading.
Prochlorperazine (May increase drowsiness). Products include:
Compazine 2470
Promethazine Hydrochloride (May increase drowsiness). Products include:
Mepergan Injection 2753
Phenergan with Codeine 2777
Phenergan with Dextromethorphan 2778
Phenergan Injection 2773
Phenergan Suppositories 2775
Phenergan Syrup 2774
Phenergan Tablets 2775
Phenergan VC 2779
Phenergan VC with Codeine 2781
Propofol (May increase drowsiness). Products include:
Diprivan Injection 2833
Quazepam (May increase drowsiness). Products include:
Doral Tablets 2664
Secobarbital Sodium (May increase drowsiness). Products include:
Seconal Sodium Pulvules 1474
Selegiline Hydrochloride (Concurrent and/or sequential use is not recommended). Products include:
Eldepryl Tablets 2550
Temazepam (May increase drowsiness). Products include:
Restoril Capsules 2284
Thioridazine Hydrochloride (May increase drowsiness). Products include:
Mellaril 2269
Thiothixene (May increase drowsiness). Products include:
Navane Capsules and Concentrate 2201
Navane Intramuscular 2202
Tranylcypromine Sulfate (Concurrent and/or sequential use is not recommended). Products include:
Parnate Tablets 2503
Triazolam (May increase drowsiness). Products include:
Halcion Tablets 2611
Trifluoperazine Hydrochloride (May increase drowsiness). Products include:
Stelazine 2514
Zolpidem Tartrate (May increase drowsiness). Products include:
Ambien Tablets 2416

Food Interactions
Alcohol (May increase drowsiness effect).

TRIAMINIC-12 TABLETS
(Phenylpropanolamine Hydrochloride, Chlorpheniramine Maleate) ◘ 792
May interact with monoamine oxidase inhibitors, hypnotics and sedatives, tranquilizers, and certain other agents. Compounds in these categories include:

Alprazolam (May increase drowsiness effect). Products include:
Xanax Tablets 2649
Buspirone Hydrochloride (May increase drowsiness effect). Products include:
BuSpar 737
Chlordiazepoxide (May increase drowsiness effect). Products include:
Libritabs Tablets 2177
Limbitrol 2180
Chlordiazepoxide Hydrochloride (May increase drowsiness effect). Products include:
Librax Capsules 2176
Librium Capsules 2178
Librium Injectable 2179
Chlorpromazine (May increase drowsiness effect). Products include:
Thorazine Suppositories 2523
Chlorpromazine Hydrochloride (May increase drowsiness effect). Products include:
Thorazine 2523
Chlorprothixene (May increase drowsiness effect).
No products indexed under this heading.
Chlorprothixene Hydrochloride (May increase drowsiness effect).
No products indexed under this heading.
Clorazepate Dipotassium (May increase drowsiness effect). Products include:
Tranxene 451
Diazepam (May increase drowsiness effect). Products include:
Dizac 1809
Valium Injectable 2182
Valium Tablets 2183
Valrelease Capsules 2169
Droperidol (May increase drowsiness effect). Products include:
Inapsine Injection 1296
Estazolam (May increase drowsiness effect). Products include:
ProSom Tablets 449
Ethchlorvynol (May increase drowsiness effect). Products include:
Placidyl Capsules 448
Ethinamate (May increase drowsiness effect).
No products indexed under this heading.
Fluphenazine Decanoate (May increase drowsiness effect). Products include:
Prolixin Decanoate 509
Fluphenazine Enanthate (May increase drowsiness effect). Products include:
Prolixin Enanthate 509
Fluphenazine Hydrochloride (May increase drowsiness effect). Products include:
Prolixin 509
Flurazepam Hydrochloride (May increase drowsiness effect). Products include:
Dalmane Capsules 2173
Furazolidone (Concurrent and/or sequential use is not recommended). Products include:
Furoxone 2046
Glutethimide (May increase drowsiness effect).
No products indexed under this heading.

(◘ Described in PDR For Nonprescription Drugs) (◉ Described in PDR For Ophthalmology)

Interactions Index — Triaminicin

Haloperidol (May increase drowsiness effect). Products include:
- Haldol Injection, Tablets and Concentrate 1575

Haloperidol Decanoate (May increase drowsiness effect). Products include:
- Haldol Decanoate 1577

Hydroxyzine Hydrochloride (May increase drowsiness effect). Products include:
- Atarax Tablets & Syrup 2185
- Marax Tablets & DF Syrup 2200
- Vistaril Intramuscular Solution 2216

Isocarboxazid (Concurrent and/or sequential use is not recommended).
- No products indexed under this heading.

Lorazepam (May increase drowsiness effect). Products include:
- Ativan Injection 2698
- Ativan Tablets 2700

Loxapine Hydrochloride (May increase drowsiness effect). Products include:
- Loxitane 1378

Loxapine Succinate (May increase drowsiness effect). Products include:
- Loxitane Capsules 1378

Meprobamate (May increase drowsiness effect). Products include:
- Miltown Tablets 2672
- PMB 200 and PMB 400 2783

Mesoridazine Besylate (May increase drowsiness effect). Products include:
- Serentil 684

Midazolam Hydrochloride (May increase drowsiness effect). Products include:
- Versed Injection 2170

Molindone Hydrochloride (May increase drowsiness effect). Products include:
- Moban Tablets and Concentrate 1048

Oxazepam (May increase drowsiness effect). Products include:
- Serax Capsules 2810
- Serax Tablets 2810

Perphenazine (May increase drowsiness effect). Products include:
- Etrafon 2355
- Triavil Tablets 1757
- Trilafon 2389

Phenelzine Sulfate (Concurrent and/or sequential use is not recommended). Products include:
- Nardil 1920

Prazepam (May increase drowsiness effect).
- No products indexed under this heading.

Prochlorperazine (May increase drowsiness effect). Products include:
- Compazine 2470

Promethazine Hydrochloride (May increase drowsiness effect). Products include:
- Mepergan Injection 2753
- Phenergan with Codeine 2777
- Phenergan with Dextromethorphan 2778
- Phenergan Injection 2773
- Phenergan Suppositories 2775
- Phenergan Syrup 2774
- Phenergan Tablets 2775
- Phenergan VC 2779
- Phenergan VC with Codeine 2781

Propofol (May increase drowsiness effect). Products include:
- Diprivan Injection 2833

Quazepam (May increase drowsiness effect). Products include:
- Doral Tablets 2664

Secobarbital Sodium (May increase drowsiness effect). Products include:
- Seconal Sodium Pulvules 1474

Selegiline Hydrochloride (Concurrent and/or sequential use is not recommended). Products include:
- Eldepryl Tablets 2550

Temazepam (May increase drowsiness effect). Products include:
- Restoril Capsules 2284

Thioridazine Hydrochloride (May increase drowsiness effect). Products include:
- Mellaril 2269

Thiothixene (May increase drowsiness effect). Products include:
- Navane Capsules and Concentrate 2201
- Navane Intramuscular 2202

Tranylcypromine Sulfate (Concurrent and/or sequential use is not recommended). Products include:
- Parnate Tablets 2503

Triazolam (May increase drowsiness effect). Products include:
- Halcion Tablets 2611

Trifluoperazine Hydrochloride (May increase drowsiness effect). Products include:
- Stelazine 2514

Zolpidem Tartrate (May increase drowsiness effect). Products include:
- Ambien Tablets 2416

Food Interactions

Alcohol (May increase drowsiness effect).

TRIAMINIC-DM SYRUP

(Phenylpropanolamine Hydrochloride, Dextromethorphan Hydrobromide) .... ◆D 792

May interact with monoamine oxidase inhibitors. Compounds in this category include:

Furazolidone (Concurrent and/or sequential use is not recommended). Products include:
- Furoxone 2046

Isocarboxazid (Concurrent and/or sequential use is not recommended).
- No products indexed under this heading.

Phenelzine Sulfate (Concurrent and/or sequential use is not recommended). Products include:
- Nardil 1920

Selegiline Hydrochloride (Concurrent and/or sequential use is not recommended). Products include:
- Eldepryl Tablets 2550

Tranylcypromine Sulfate (Concurrent and/or sequential use is not recommended). Products include:
- Parnate Tablets 2503

TRIAMINICIN TABLETS

(Acetaminophen, Chlorpheniramine Maleate, Phenylpropanolamine Hydrochloride) .... ◆D 793

May interact with tranquilizers, hypnotics and sedatives, and certain other agents. Compounds in these categories include:

Alprazolam (May increase the drowsiness effect). Products include:
- Xanax Tablets 2649

Buspirone Hydrochloride (May increase the drowsiness effect). Products include:
- BuSpar 737

Chlordiazepoxide (May increase the drowsiness effect). Products include:
- Libritabs Tablets 2177
- Limbitrol 2180

Chlordiazepoxide Hydrochloride (May increase the drowsiness effect). Products include:
- Librax Capsules 2176
- Librium Capsules 2178
- Librium Injectable 2179

Chlorpromazine (May increase the drowsiness effect). Products include:
- Thorazine Suppositories 2523

Chlorpromazine Hydrochloride (May increase the drowsiness effect). Products include:
- Thorazine 2523

Chlorprothixene (May increase the drowsiness effect).
- No products indexed under this heading.

Chlorprothixene Hydrochloride (May increase the drowsiness effect).
- No products indexed under this heading.

Clorazepate Dipotassium (May increase the drowsiness effect). Products include:
- Tranxene 451

Diazepam (May increase the drowsiness effect). Products include:
- Dizac 1809
- Valium Injectable 2182
- Valium Tablets 2183
- Valrelease Capsules 2169

Droperidol (May increase the drowsiness effect). Products include:
- Inapsine Injection 1296

Estazolam (May increase the drowsiness effect). Products include:
- ProSom Tablets 449

Ethchlorvynol (May increase the drowsiness effect). Products include:
- Placidyl Capsules 448

Ethinamate (May increase the drowsiness effect).
- No products indexed under this heading.

Fluphenazine Decanoate (May increase the drowsiness effect). Products include:
- Prolixin Decanoate 509

Fluphenazine Enanthate (May increase the drowsiness effect). Products include:
- Prolixin Enanthate 509

Fluphenazine Hydrochloride (May increase the drowsiness effect). Products include:
- Prolixin 509

Flurazepam Hydrochloride (May increase the drowsiness effect). Products include:
- Dalmane Capsules 2173

Furazolidone (Concurrent and/or sequential use is not recommended). Products include:
- Furoxone 2046

Glutethimide (May increase the drowsiness effect).
- No products indexed under this heading.

Haloperidol (May increase the drowsiness effect). Products include:
- Haldol Injection, Tablets and Concentrate 1575

Haloperidol Decanoate (May increase the drowsiness effect). Products include:
- Haldol Decanoate 1577

Hydroxyzine Hydrochloride (May increase the drowsiness effect). Products include:
- Atarax Tablets & Syrup 2185
- Marax Tablets & DF Syrup 2200
- Vistaril Intramuscular Solution 2216

Isocarboxazid (Concurrent and/or sequential use is not recommended).
- No products indexed under this heading.

Lorazepam (May increase the drowsiness effect). Products include:
- Ativan Injection 2698
- Ativan Tablets 2700

Loxapine Hydrochloride (May increase the drowsiness effect). Products include:
- Loxitane 1378

Loxapine Succinate (May increase the drowsiness effect). Products include:
- Loxitane Capsules 1378

Meprobamate (May increase the drowsiness effect). Products include:
- Miltown Tablets 2672
- PMB 200 and PMB 400 2783

Mesoridazine Besylate (May increase the drowsiness effect). Products include:
- Serentil 684

Midazolam Hydrochloride (May increase the drowsiness effect). Products include:
- Versed Injection 2170

Molindone Hydrochloride (May increase the drowsiness effect). Products include:
- Moban Tablets and Concentrate 1048

Oxazepam (May increase the drowsiness effect). Products include:
- Serax Capsules 2810
- Serax Tablets 2810

Perphenazine (May increase the drowsiness effect). Products include:
- Etrafon 2355
- Triavil Tablets 1757
- Trilafon 2389

Phenelzine Sulfate (Concurrent and/or sequential use is not recommended). Products include:
- Nardil 1920

Prazepam (May increase the drowsiness effect).
- No products indexed under this heading.

Prochlorperazine (May increase the drowsiness effect). Products include:
- Compazine 2470

Promethazine Hydrochloride (May increase the drowsiness effect). Products include:
- Mepergan Injection 2753
- Phenergan with Codeine 2777
- Phenergan with Dextromethorphan 2778
- Phenergan Injection 2773
- Phenergan Suppositories 2775
- Phenergan Syrup 2774
- Phenergan Tablets 2775
- Phenergan VC 2779
- Phenergan VC with Codeine 2781

Propofol (May increase the drowsiness effect). Products include:
- Diprivan Injection 2833

Quazepam (May increase the drowsiness effect). Products include:
- Doral Tablets 2664

Secobarbital Sodium (May increase the drowsiness effect). Products include:
- Seconal Sodium Pulvules 1474

Selegiline Hydrochloride (Concurrent and/or sequential use is not recommended). Products include:
- Eldepryl Tablets 2550

Temazepam (May increase the drowsiness effect). Products include:
- Restoril Capsules 2284

Thioridazine Hydrochloride (May increase the drowsiness effect). Products include:
- Mellaril 2269

Thiothixene (May increase the drowsiness effect). Products include:
- Navane Capsules and Concentrate 2201
- Navane Intramuscular 2202

Tranylcypromine Sulfate (Concurrent and/or sequential use is not recommended). Products include:
- Parnate Tablets 2503

IMPORTANT NOTE: Always consult each drug listing in the patient's regimen for possible interactions.

Triaminicin Interactions Index 1068

Triazolam (May increase the drowsiness effect). Products include:
Halcion Tablets 2611
Trifluoperazine Hydrochloride (May increase the drowsiness effect). Products include:
Stelazine 2514
Zolpidem Tartrate (May increase the drowsiness effect). Products include:
Ambien Tablets 2416

Food Interactions

Alcohol (May increase drowsiness; avoid concurrent use).

TRIAMINICOL MULTI-SYMPTOM COLD TABLETS

(Phenylpropanolamine Hydrochloride, Chlorpheniramine Maleate, Dextromethorphan Hydrobromide) ..... ⊞ 793
May interact with hypnotics and sedatives, tranquilizers, and certain other agents. Compounds in these categories include:

Alprazolam (May increase drowsiness effect). Products include:
Xanax Tablets 2649
Buspirone Hydrochloride (May increase drowsiness effect). Products include:
BuSpar 737
Chlordiazepoxide (May increase drowsiness effect). Products include:
Libritabs Tablets 2177
Limbitrol 2180
Chlordiazepoxide Hydrochloride (May increase drowsiness effect). Products include:
Librax Capsules 2176
Librium Capsules 2178
Librium Injectable 2179
Chlorpromazine (May increase drowsiness effect). Products include:
Thorazine Suppositories 2523
Chlorpromazine Hydrochloride (May increase drowsiness effect). Products include:
Thorazine 2523
Chlorprothixene (May increase drowsiness effect).
No products indexed under this heading.
Chlorprothixene Hydrochloride (May increase drowsiness effect).
No products indexed under this heading.
Clorazepate Dipotassium (May increase drowsiness effect). Products include:
Tranxene 451
Diazepam (May increase drowsiness effect). Products include:
Dizac 1809
Valium Injectable 2182
Valium Tablets 2183
Valrelease Capsules 2169
Droperidol (May increase drowsiness effect). Products include:
Inapsine Injection 1296
Estazolam (May increase drowsiness effect). Products include:
ProSom Tablets 449
Ethchlorvynol (May increase drowsiness effect). Products include:
Placidyl Capsules 448
Ethinamate (May increase drowsiness effect).
No products indexed under this heading.
Fluphenazine Decanoate (May increase drowsiness effect). Products include:
Prolixin Decanoate 509
Fluphenazine Enanthate (May increase drowsiness effect). Products include:
Prolixin Enanthate 509
Fluphenazine Hydrochloride (May increase drowsiness effect). Products include:
Prolixin 509
Flurazepam Hydrochloride (May increase drowsiness effect). Products include:
Dalmane Capsules 2173
Furazolidone (Concurrent and/or sequential use is not recommended). Products include:
Furoxone 2046
Glutethimide (May increase drowsiness effect).
No products indexed under this heading.
Haloperidol (May increase drowsiness effect). Products include:
Haldol Injection, Tablets and Concentrate 1575
Haloperidol Decanoate (May increase drowsiness effect). Products include:
Haldol Decanoate 1577
Hydroxyzine Hydrochloride (May increase drowsiness effect). Products include:
Atarax Tablets & Syrup 2185
Marax Tablets & DF Syrup 2200
Vistaril Intramuscular Solution 2216
Isocarboxazid (Concurrent and/or sequential use is not recommended).
No products indexed under this heading.
Lorazepam (May increase drowsiness effect). Products include:
Ativan Injection 2698
Ativan Tablets 2700
Loxapine Hydrochloride (May increase drowsiness effect). Products include:
Loxitane 1378
Loxapine Succinate (May increase drowsiness effect). Products include:
Loxitane Capsules 1378
Meprobamate (May increase drowsiness effect). Products include:
Miltown Tablets 2672
PMB 200 and PMB 400 2783
Mesoridazine Besylate (May increase drowsiness effect). Products include:
Serentil 684
Midazolam Hydrochloride (May increase drowsiness effect). Products include:
Versed Injection 2170
Molindone Hydrochloride (May increase drowsiness effect). Products include:
Moban Tablets and Concentrate 1048
Oxazepam (May increase drowsiness effect). Products include:
Serax Capsules 2810
Serax Tablets 2810
Perphenazine (May increase drowsiness effect). Products include:
Etrafon 2355
Triavil Tablets 1757
Trilafon 2389
Phenelzine Sulfate (Concurrent and/or sequential use is not recommended). Products include:
Nardil 1920
Prazepam (May increase drowsiness effect).
No products indexed under this heading.
Prochlorperazine (May increase drowsiness effect). Products include:
Compazine 2470
Promethazine Hydrochloride (May increase drowsiness effect). Products include:
Mepergan Injection 2753
Phenergan with Codeine 2777
Phenergan with Dextromethorphan 2778
Phenergan Injection 2773
Phenergan Suppositories 2775
Phenergan Syrup 2774
Phenergan Tablets 2775
Phenergan VC 2779
Phenergan VC with Codeine 2781
Propofol (May increase drowsiness effect). Products include:
Diprivan Injection 2833
Quazepam (May increase drowsiness effect). Products include:
Doral Tablets 2664
Secobarbital Sodium (May increase drowsiness effect). Products include:
Seconal Sodium Pulvules 1474
Selegiline Hydrochloride (Concurrent and/or sequential use is not recommended). Products include:
Eldepryl Tablets 2550
Temazepam (May increase drowsiness effect). Products include:
Restoril Capsules 2284
Thioridazine Hydrochloride (May increase drowsiness effect). Products include:
Mellaril 2269
Thiothixene (May increase drowsiness effect). Products include:
Navane Capsules and Concentrate 2201
Navane Intramuscular 2202
Tranylcypromine Sulfate (Concurrent and/or sequential use is not recommended). Products include:
Parnate Tablets 2503
Triazolam (May increase drowsiness effect). Products include:
Halcion Tablets 2611
Trifluoperazine Hydrochloride (May increase drowsiness effect). Products include:
Stelazine 2514
Zolpidem Tartrate (May increase drowsiness effect). Products include:
Ambien Tablets 2416

Food Interactions

Alcohol (May increase drowsiness effect).

TRIAMINICOL MULTI-SYMPTOM RELIEF

(Phenylpropanolamine Hydrochloride, Chlorpheniramine Maleate, Dextromethorphan Hydrobromide) ..... ⊞ 794
May interact with hypnotics and sedatives, tranquilizers, monoamine oxidase inhibitors, and certain other agents. Compounds in these categories include:

Alprazolam (May increase drowsiness effect). Products include:
Xanax Tablets 2649
Buspirone Hydrochloride (May increase drowsiness effect). Products include:
BuSpar 737
Chlordiazepoxide (May increase drowsiness effect). Products include:
Libritabs Tablets 2177
Limbitrol 2180
Chlordiazepoxide Hydrochloride (May increase drowsiness effect). Products include:
Librax Capsules 2176
Librium Capsules 2178
Librium Injectable 2179
Chlorpromazine (May increase drowsiness effect). Products include:
Thorazine Suppositories 2523
Chlorpromazine Hydrochloride (May increase drowsiness effect). Products include:
Thorazine 2523
Chlorprothixene (May increase drowsiness effect).
No products indexed under this heading.
Chlorprothixene Hydrochloride (May increase drowsiness effect).
No products indexed under this heading.
Clorazepate Dipotassium (May increase drowsiness effect). Products include:
Tranxene 451
Diazepam (May increase drowsiness effect). Products include:
Dizac 1809
Valium Injectable 2182
Valium Tablets 2183
Valrelease Capsules 2169
Droperidol (May increase drowsiness effect). Products include:
Inapsine Injection 1296
Estazolam (May increase drowsiness effect). Products include:
ProSom Tablets 449
Ethchlorvynol (May increase drowsiness effect). Products include:
Placidyl Capsules 448
Ethinamate (May increase drowsiness effect).
No products indexed under this heading.
Fluphenazine Decanoate (May increase drowsiness effect). Products include:
Prolixin Decanoate 509
Fluphenazine Enanthate (May increase drowsiness effect). Products include:
Prolixin Enanthate 509
Fluphenazine Hydrochloride (May increase drowsiness effect). Products include:
Prolixin 509
Flurazepam Hydrochloride (May increase drowsiness effect). Products include:
Dalmane Capsules 2173
Furazolidone (Concurrent and/or sequential use is not recommended). Products include:
Furoxone 2046
Glutethimide (May increase drowsiness effect).
No products indexed under this heading.
Haloperidol (May increase drowsiness effect). Products include:
Haldol Injection, Tablets and Concentrate 1575
Haloperidol Decanoate (May increase drowsiness effect). Products include:
Haldol Decanoate 1577
Hydroxyzine Hydrochloride (May increase drowsiness effect). Products include:
Atarax Tablets & Syrup 2185
Marax Tablets & DF Syrup 2200
Vistaril Intramuscular Solution 2216
Isocarboxazid (Concurrent and/or sequential use is not recommended).
No products indexed under this heading.
Lorazepam (May increase drowsiness effect). Products include:
Ativan Injection 2698
Ativan Tablets 2700
Loxapine Hydrochloride (May increase drowsiness effect). Products include:
Loxitane 1378

(⊞ Described in PDR For Nonprescription Drugs) (⊙ Described in PDR For Ophthalmology)

Interactions Index

Triavil

Loxapine Succinate (May increase drowsiness effect). Products include:

Loxitane Capsules 1378

Meprobamate (May increase drowsiness effect). Products include:

Miltown Tablets 2672
PMB 200 and PMB 400 2783

Mesoridazine Besylate (May increase drowsiness effect). Products include:

Serentil 684

Midazolam Hydrochloride (May increase drowsiness effect). Products include:

Versed Injection 2170

Molindone Hydrochloride (May increase drowsiness effect). Products include:

Moban Tablets and Concentrate 1048

Oxazepam (May increase drowsiness effect). Products include:

Serax Capsules 2810
Serax Tablets 2810

Perphenazine (May increase drowsiness effect). Products include:

Etrafon 2355
Triavil Tablets 1757
Trilafon 2389

Phenelzine Sulfate (Concurrent and/or sequential use is not recommended). Products include:

Nardil 1920

Prazepam (May increase drowsiness effect).

No products indexed under this heading.

Prochlorperazine (May increase drowsiness effect). Products include:

Compazine 2470

Promethazine Hydrochloride (May increase drowsiness effect). Products include:

Mepergan Injection 2753
Phenergan with Codeine 2777
Phenergan with Dextromethorphan 2778
Phenergan Injection 2773
Phenergan Suppositories 2775
Phenergan Syrup 2774
Phenergan Tablets 2775
Phenergan VC 2779
Phenergan VC with Codeine 2781

Propofol (May increase drowsiness effect). Products include:

Diprivan Injection 2833

Quazepam (May increase drowsiness effect). Products include:

Doral Tablets 2664

Secobarbital Sodium (May increase drowsiness effect). Products include:

Seconal Sodium Pulvules 1474

Selegiline Hydrochloride (Concurrent and/or sequential use is not recommended). Products include:

Eldepryl Tablets 2550

Temazepam (May increase drowsiness effect). Products include:

Restoril Capsules 2284

Thioridazine Hydrochloride (May increase drowsiness effect). Products include:

Mellaril 2269

Thiothixene (May increase drowsiness effect). Products include:

Navane Capsules and Concentrate 2201
Navane Intramuscular 2202

Tranylcypromine Sulfate (Concurrent and/or sequential use is not recommended). Products include:

Parnate Tablets 2503

Triazolam (May increase drowsiness effect). Products include:

Halcion Tablets 2611

Trifluoperazine Hydrochloride (May increase drowsiness effect). Products include:

Stelazine 2514

Zolpidem Tartrate (May increase drowsiness effect). Products include:

Ambien Tablets 2416

Food Interactions

Alcohol (May increase drowsiness effect).

TRIAVIL TABLETS

(Perphenazine, Amitriptyline Hydrochloride) 1757

May interact with thyroid preparations, antihistamines, monoamine oxidase inhibitors, peripheral adrenergic blockers, anticonvulsants, central nervous system depressants, anticholinergics, sympathomimetics, antipsychotic agents, barbiturates, and certain other agents. Compounds in these categories include:

Acrivastine (Potentiated). Products include:

Semprex-D Capsules 463
Semprex-D Capsules 1167

Albuterol (Close supervision and careful dosage adjustment required). Products include:

Proventil Inhalation Aerosol 2382
Ventolin Inhalation Aerosol and Refill 1197

Albuterol Sulfate (Close supervision and careful dosage adjustment required). Products include:

Airet Solution for Inhalation 452
Proventil Inhalation Solution 0.083% 2384
Proventil Repetabs Tablets 2386
Proventil Solution for Inhalation 0.5% 2383
Proventil Syrup 2385
Proventil Tablets 2386
Ventolin Inhalation Solution 1198
Ventolin Nebules Inhalation Solution 1199
Ventolin Rotacaps for Inhalation 1200
Ventolin Syrup 1202
Ventolin Tablets 1203
Volmax Extended-Release Tablets .. 1788

Alfentanil Hydrochloride (Potentiated). Products include:

Alfenta Injection 1286

Alprazolam (Potentiated). Products include:

Xanax Tablets 2649

Aprobarbital (Potentiated).

No products indexed under this heading.

Astemizole (Potentiated). Products include:

Hismanal Tablets 1293

Atropine Sulfate (Potentiated; hyperpyrexia; paralytic ileus). Products include:

Arco-Lase Plus Tablets 512
Atrohist Plus Tablets 454
Atropine Sulfate Sterile Ophthalmic Solution .... ◉ 233
Donnatal 2060
Donnatal Extentabs 2061
Donnatal Tablets 2060
Lomotil 2439
Motofen Tablets 784
Urised Tablets 1964

Azatadine Maleate (Potentiated). Products include:

Trinalin Repetabs Tablets 1330

Belladonna Alkaloids (Hyperpyrexia; paralytic ileus). Products include:

Bellergal-S Tablets 2250
Hyland's Bed Wetting Tablets .... ◈ 828
Hyland's EnurAid Tablets .... ◈ 829
Hyland's Teething Tablets .... ◈ 830

Benztropine Mesylate (Hyperpyrexia; paralytic ileus). Products include:

Cogentin 1621

Biperiden Hydrochloride (Hyperpyrexia; paralytic ileus). Products include:

Akineton 1333

Bromodiphenhydramine Hydrochloride (Potentiated).

No products indexed under this heading.

Brompheniramine Maleate (Potentiated). Products include:

Alka Seltzer Plus Sinus Medicine .. ◈ 707
Bromfed Capsules (Extended-Release) 1785
Bromfed Syrup .... ◈ 733
Bromfed Tablets 1785
Bromfed-DM Cough Syrup 1786
Bromfed-PD Capsules (Extended-Release) 1785
Dimetane-DC Cough Syrup 2059
Dimetane-DX Cough Syrup 2059
Dimetapp Elixir .... ◈ 773
Dimetapp Extentabs .... ◈ 774
Dimetapp Tablets/Liqui-Gels .... ◈ 775
Dimetapp Cold & Allergy Chewable Tablets .... ◈ 773
Dimetapp DM Elixir .... ◈ 774
Vicks DayQuil Allergy Relief 12-Hour Extended Release Tablets .. ◈ 760
Vicks DayQuil Allergy Relief 4-Hour Tablets .... ◈ 760

Buprenorphine (Potentiated). Products include:

Buprenex Injectable 2006

Buspirone Hydrochloride (Potentiated). Products include:

BuSpar 737

Butabarbital (Potentiated).

No products indexed under this heading.

Butalbital (Potentiated). Products include:

Esgic-plus Tablets 1013
Fioricet Tablets 2258
Fioricet with Codeine Capsules 2260
Fiorinal Capsules 2261
Fiorinal with Codeine Capsules 2262
Fiorinal Tablets 2261
Phrenilin 785
Sedapap Tablets 50 mg/650 mg .. 1543

Carbamazepine (Increased anticonvulsant dosage may be necessary). Products include:

Atretol Tablets 573
Tegretol Chewable Tablets 852
Tegretol Suspension 852
Tegretol Tablets 852

Chlordiazepoxide (Potentiated). Products include:

Libritabs Tablets 2177
Limbitrol 2180

Chlordiazepoxide Hydrochloride (Potentiated). Products include:

Librax Capsules 2176
Librium Capsules 2178
Librium Injectable 2179

Chlorpheniramine Maleate (Potentiated). Products include:

Alka-Seltzer Plus Cold Medicine .... ◈ 705
Alka-Seltzer Plus Cold Medicine Liqui-Gels .... ◈ 706
Alka-Seltzer Plus Cold & Cough Medicine .... ◈ 708
Alka-Seltzer Plus Cold & Cough Medicine Liqui-Gels .... ◈ 705
Allerest Children's Chewable Tablets .... ◈ 627
Allerest Headache Strength Tablets .... ◈ 627
Allerest Maximum Strength Tablets .... ◈ 627
Allerest Sinus Pain Formula .... ◈ 627
Allerest 12 Hour Caplets .... ◈ 627
Ana-Kit Anaphylaxis Emergency Treatment Kit 617
Atrohist Pediatric Capsules 453
Atrohist Plus Tablets 454
BC Cold Powder Multi-Symptom Formula (Cold-Sinus-Allergy) ...... ◈ 609
Cerose DM .... ◈ 878
Cheracol Plus Head Cold/Cough Formula .... ◈ 769
Children's Vicks DayQuil Allergy Relief .... ◈ 757
Children's Vicks NyQuil Cold/ Cough Relief .... ◈ 758
Chlor-Trimeton Allergy Decongestant Tablets .... ◈ 799
Chlor-Trimeton Allergy Tablets ...... ◈ 798
Comhist 2038
Comtrex Multi-Symptom Cold Reliever Tablets/Caplets/Liqui-Gels/Liquid .... ◈ 615
Allergy-Sinus Comtrex Multi-Symptom Allergy-Sinus Formula Tablets .... ◈ 617
Contac Continuous Action Nasal Decongestant/Antihistamine 12 Hour Capsules .... ◈ 813
Contac Maximum Strength Continuous Action Decongestant/ Antihistamine 12 Hour Caplets .. ◈ 813
Contac Severe Cold and Flu Formula Caplets .... ◈ 814
Coricidin 'D' Decongestant Tablets .... ◈ 800
Coricidin Tablets .... ◈ 800
D.A. Chewable Tablets 951
Deconamine 1320
Dura-Tap/PD Capsules 2867
Dura-Vent/DA Tablets 953
Extendryl 1005
Fedahist Gyrocaps 2401
Fedahist Timecaps 2401
Hycomine Compound Tablets 932
Isoclor Timesule Capsules .... ◈ 637
Kronofed-A 977
Nolamine Timed-Release Tablets 785
Novahistine DH 2462
Novahistine Elixir .... ◈ 823
Ornade Spansule Capsules 2502
PediaCare Cold Allergy Chewable Tablets .... ◈ 677
PediaCare Cough-Cold Chewable Tablets 1553
PediaCare Cough-Cold Liquid 1553
PediaCare NightRest Cough-Cold Liquid 1553
Pediatric Vicks 44m Cough & Cold Relief .... ◈ 764
Pyrroxate Caplets .... ◈ 772
Ryna .... ◈ 841
Sinarest Tablets .... ◈ 648
Sinarest Extra Strength Tablets ...... ◈ 648
Sine-Off Sinus Medicine .... ◈ 825
Singlet Tablets .... ◈ 825
Sinulin Tablets 787
Sinutab Sinus Allergy Medication, Maximum Strength Tablets and Caplets .... ◈ 860
Sudafed Plus Liquid .... ◈ 862
Sudafed Plus Tablets .... ◈ 863
Teldrin 12 Hour Antihistamine/ Nasal Decongestant Allergy Relief Capsules .... ◈ 826
TheraFlu .... ◈ 787
TheraFlu Maximum Strength Nighttime Flu, Cold & Cough Medicine .... ◈ 788
Triaminic Allergy Tablets .... ◈ 789
Triaminic Cold Tablets .... ◈ 790
Triaminic Nite Light .... ◈ 791
Triaminic Syrup .... ◈ 792
Triaminic-12 Tablets .... ◈ 792
Triaminicin Tablets .... ◈ 793
Triaminicol Multi-Symptom Cold Tablets .... ◈ 793
Triaminicol Multi-Symptom Relief ◈ 794
Tussend 1783
Children's TYLENOL Cold Multi-Symptom Liquid Formula and Chewable Tablets 1561
Children's TYLENOL Cold Plus Cough Multi Symptom Tablets and Liquid .... ◈ 681
TYLENOL Maximum Strength Allergy Sinus Medication Gelcaps and Caplets 1563
TYLENOL Cold Multi-Symptom Formula Medication Tablets and Caplets 1561
TYLENOL Cold Multi-Symptom Hot Medication Liquid Packets 1557
Vicks 44 LiquiCaps Cough, Cold & Flu Relief .... ◈ 755
Vicks 44M Cough, Cold & Flu Relief .... ◈ 756

Chlorpheniramine Polistirex (Potentiated). Products include:

Tussionex Pennkinetic Extended-Release Suspension 998

Chlorpheniramine Tannate (Potentiated). Products include:

Atrohist Pediatric Suspension 454
Ricobid Tablets and Pediatric Suspension 2038
Rynatan 2673
Rynatuss 2673

IMPORTANT NOTE: Always consult each drug listing in the patient's regimen for possible interactions.

Triavil **Interactions Index** **1070**

Chlorpromazine (Potentiated; hyperpyrexia). Products include:
Thorazine Suppositories 2523

Chlorprothixene (Potentiated; hyperpyrexia).
No products indexed under this heading.

Chlorprothixene Hydrochloride (Potentiated; hyperpyrexia).
No products indexed under this heading.

Cimetidine (Increased frequency and severity of side effects). Products include:
Tagamet Tablets 2516

Cimetidine Hydrochloride (Increased frequency and severity of side effects). Products include:
Tagamet 2516

Clemastine Fumarate (Potentiated). Products include:
Tavist Syrup 2297
Tavist Tablets 2298
Tavist-1 12 Hour Relief Tablets ..... ▣ 787
Tavist-D 12 Hour Relief Tablets ..... ▣ 787

Clidinium Bromide (Hyperpyrexia; paralytic ileus). Products include:
Librax Capsules 2176
Quarzan Capsules 2181

Clorazepate Dipotassium (Potentiated). Products include:
Tranxene 451

Clozapine (Potentiated; hyperpyrexia). Products include:
Clozaril Tablets 2252

Codeine Phosphate (Potentiated). Products include:
Actifed with Codeine Cough Syrup .. 1067
Brontex 1981
Deconsal C Expectorant Syrup 456
Deconsal Pediatric Syrup 457
Dimetane-DC Cough Syrup 2059
Empirin with Codeine Tablets 1093
Fioricet with Codeine Capsules 2260
Fiorinal with Codeine Capsules 2262
Isoclor Expectorant 990
Novahistine DH 2462
Novahistine Expectorant 2463
Nucofed 2051
Phenergan with Codeine 2777
Phenergan VC with Codeine 2781
Robitussin A-C Syrup 2073
Robitussin-DAC Syrup 2074
Ryna ..... ▣ 841
Soma Compound w/Codeine Tablets 2676
Tussi-Organidin NR Liquid and S NR Liquid 2677
Tylenol with Codeine 1583

Cyproheptadine Hydrochloride (Potentiated). Products include:
Periactin 1724

Deserpidine (Antihypertensive effect of deserpidine blocked).
No products indexed under this heading.

Desflurane (Potentiated). Products include:
Suprane 1813

Dexchlorpheniramine Maleate (Potentiated).
No products indexed under this heading.

Dezocine (Potentiated). Products include:
Dalgan Injection 538

Diazepam (Potentiated). Products include:
Dizac 1809
Valium Injectable 2182
Valium Tablets 2183
Valrelease Capsules 2169

Dicyclomine Hydrochloride (Hyperpyrexia; paralytic ileus). Products include:
Bentyl 1501

Diphenhydramine Citrate (Potentiated). Products include:
Excedrin P.M. Analgesic/Sleeping Aid Tablets, Caplets, Liquigels 733

Diphenhydramine Hydrochloride (Potentiated). Products include:
Actifed Allergy Daytime/Nighttime Caplets ..... ▣ 844
Actifed Sinus Daytime/Nighttime Tablets and Caplets ..... ▣ 846
Arthritis Foundation NightTime Caplets ..... ▣ 674
Extra Strength Bayer PM Aspirin .. ▣ 713
Bayer Select Night Time Pain Relief Formula ..... ▣ 716
Benadryl Allergy Decongestant Liquid Medication ..... ▣ 848
Benadryl Allergy Decongestant Tablets ..... ▣ 848
Benadryl Allergy Liquid Medication ..... ▣ 849
Benadryl Allergy ..... ▣ 848
Benadryl Allergy Sinus Headache Formula Caplets ..... ▣ 849
Benadryl Capsules 1898
Benadryl Dye-Free Allergy Liquigel Softgels ..... ▣ 850
Benadryl Dye-Free Allergy Liquid Medication ..... ▣ 850
Benadryl Itch Relief Cream, Children's Formula and Maximum Strength 2% ..... ▣ 851
Benadryl Itch Relief Spray, Children's Formula and Maximum Strength 2% ..... ▣ 851
Benadryl Itch Relief Stick Maximum Strength 2% ..... ▣ 850
Benadryl Itch Stopping Gel, Children's Formula and Maximum Strength 2% ..... ▣ 851
Benadryl Kapseals 1898
Benadryl Injection 1898
Contac Day & Night Cold/Flu Night Caplets ..... ▣ 812
Contac Night Allergy/Sinus Caplets ..... ▣ 812
Extra Strength Doan's P.M. ..... ▣ 633
Legatrin PM ..... ▣ 651
Miles Nervine Nighttime Sleep-Aid ▣ 723
Nytol QuickCaps Caplets ..... ▣ 610
Sleepinal Night-time Sleep Aid Capsules and Softgels ..... ▣ 834
TYLENOL Maximum Strength Allergy Sinus NightTime Medication Caplets 1555
TYLENOL Flu NightTime, Maximum Strength, Gelcaps 1566
TYLENOL Maximum Strength Flu NightTime Hot Medication Packets 1562
TYLENOL PM, Extra Strength Pain Reliever/Sleep Aid Caplets, Geltabs, Gelcaps 1560
TYLENOL Severe Allergy Medication Caplets 1564
Maximum Strength Unisom Sleepgels 1934
Unisom With Pain Relief-Nighttime Sleep Aid and Pain Reliever 1934

Diphenylpyraline Hydrochloride (Potentiated).
No products indexed under this heading.

Disulfiram (Delirium). Products include:
Antabuse Tablets 2695

Divalproex Sodium (Increased anticonvulsant dosage may be necessary). Products include:
Depakote Tablets 415

Dobutamine Hydrochloride (Close supervision and careful dosage adjustment required). Products include:
Dobutrex Solution Vials 1439

Dopamine Hydrochloride (Close supervision and careful dosage adjustment required).
No products indexed under this heading.

Droperidol (Potentiated). Products include:
Inapsine Injection 1296

Enflurane (Potentiated).
No products indexed under this heading.

Ephedrine (Close supervision and careful dosage adjustment required).

Ephedrine Hydrochloride (Close supervision and careful dosage adjustment required). Products include:
Primatene Dual Action Formula ..... ▣ 872
Primatene Tablets ..... ▣ 873
Quadrinal Tablets 1350

Ephedrine Sulfate (Close supervision and careful dosage adjustment required). Products include:
Bronkaid Caplets ..... ▣ 717
Marax Tablets & DF Syrup 2200

Ephedrine Tannate (Close supervision and careful dosage adjustment required). Products include:
Rynatuss 2673

Epinephrine (Close supervision and careful dosage adjustment required). Products include:
Bronkaid Mist ..... ▣ 717
EPIFRIN ..... ◉ 239
EpiPen 790
Marcaine Hydrochloride with Epinephrine 1:200,000 2316
Primatene Mist ..... ▣ 873
Sensorcaine with Epinephrine Injection 559
Sus-Phrine Injection 1019
Xylocaine with Epinephrine Injections 567

Epinephrine Bitartrate (Close supervision and careful dosage adjustment required). Products include:
Bronkaid Mist Suspension ..... ▣ 718
Sensorcaine-MPF with Epinephrine Injection 559

Epinephrine Hydrochloride (Close supervision and careful dosage adjustment required). Products include:
Ana-Kit Anaphylaxis Emergency Treatment Kit 617

Estazolam (Potentiated). Products include:
ProSom Tablets 449

Ethchlorvynol (Potentiated; transient delirium). Products include:
Placidyl Capsules 448

Ethinamate (Potentiated).
No products indexed under this heading.

Ethopropazine Hydrochloride (Hyperpyrexia; paralytic ileus).

Ethosuximide (Increased anticonvulsant dosage may be necessary). Products include:
Zarontin Capsules 1928
Zarontin Syrup 1929

Ethotoin (Increased anticonvulsant dosage may be necessary). Products include:
Peganone Tablets 446

Felbamate (Increased anticonvulsant dosage may be necessary). Products include:
Felbatol 2666

Fentanyl (Potentiated). Products include:
Duragesic Transdermal System 1288

Fentanyl Citrate (Potentiated). Products include:
Sublimaze Injection 1307

Fluphenazine Decanoate (Potentiated; hyperpyrexia). Products include:
Prolixin Decanoate 509

Fluphenazine Enanthate (Potentiated; hyperpyrexia). Products include:
Prolixin Enanthate 509

Fluphenazine Hydrochloride (Potentiated; hyperpyrexia). Products include:
Prolixin 509

Flurazepam Hydrochloride (Potentiated). Products include:
Dalmane Capsules 2173

Furazolidone (Concomitant administration is contraindicated; hyperpyretic crises and severe convulsions have occurred). Products include:
Furoxone 2046

Glutethimide (Potentiated).
No products indexed under this heading.

Glycopyrrolate (Hyperpyrexia; paralytic ileus). Products include:
Robinul Forte Tablets 2072
Robinul Injectable 2072
Robinul Tablets 2072

Guanethidine Monosulfate (Antihypertensive effect of guanethidine). Products include:
Esimil Tablets 822
Ismelin Tablets 827

Haloperidol (Potentiated; hyperpyrexia). Products include:
Haldol Injection, Tablets and Concentrate 1575

Haloperidol Decanoate (Potentiated; hyperpyrexia). Products include:
Haldol Decanoate 1577

Hydrocodone Bitartrate (Potentiated). Products include:
Anexsia 5/500 Elixir 1781
Anexia Tablets 1782
Codiclear DH Syrup 791
Deconamine CX Cough and Cold Liquid and Tablets 1319
Duratuss HD Elixir 2565
Hycodan Tablets and Syrup 930
Hycomine Compound Tablets 932
Hycomine 931
Hycotuss Expectorant Syrup 933
Hydrocet Capsules 782
Lorcet 10/650 1018
Lortab 2566
Tussend 1783
Tussend Expectorant 1785
Vicodin Tablets 1356
Vicodin ES Tablets 1357
Vicodin Tuss Expectorant 1358
Zydone Capsules 949

Hydrocodone Polistirex (Potentiated). Products include:
Tussionex Pennkinetic Extended-Release Suspension 998

Hydroxyzine Hydrochloride (Potentiated). Products include:
Atarax Tablets & Syrup 2185
Marax Tablets & DF Syrup 2200
Vistaril Intramuscular Solution 2216

Hyoscyamine (Hyperpyrexia; paralytic ileus). Products include:
Cystospaz Tablets 1963
Urised Tablets 1964

Hyoscyamine Sulfate (Hyperpyrexia; paralytic ileus). Products include:
Arco-Lase Plus Tablets 512
Atrohist Plus Tablets 454
Cystospaz-M Capsules 1963
Donnatal 2060
Donnatal Extentabs 2061
Donnatal Tablets 2060
Kutrase Capsules 2402
Levsin/Levsinex/Levbid 2405

Ipratropium Bromide (Hyperpyrexia; paralytic ileus). Products include:
Atrovent Inhalation Aerosol 671
Atrovent Inhalation Solution 673

Isocarboxazid (Concomitant administration is contraindicated; hyperpyretic crises and severe convulsions have occurred).
No products indexed under this heading.

Isoflurane (Potentiated; contraindication).
No products indexed under this heading.

Isoproterenol Hydrochloride (Close supervision and careful dosage adjustment required). Products include:
Isuprel Hydrochloride Injection 1:5000 2311
Isuprel Hydrochloride Solution 1:200 & 1:100 2313
Isuprel Mistometer 2312

Isoproterenol Sulfate (Close supervision and careful dosage adjustment required). Products include:
Norisodrine with Calcium Iodide Syrup 442

Ketamine Hydrochloride (Potentiated).
No products indexed under this heading.

Lamotrigine (Increased anticonvulsant dosage may be necessary). Products include:
Lamictal Tablets 1112

Levomethadyl Acetate Hydrochloride (Potentiated). Products include:
Orlamm 2239

Levorphanol Tartrate (Potentiated). Products include:
Levo-Dromoran 2129

Levothyroxine Sodium (Close supervision is indicated). Products include:
Levothroid Tablets 1016
Levoxyl Tablets 903
Synthroid 1359

Liothyronine Sodium (Close supervision is indicated). Products include:
Cytomel Tablets 2473
Triostat Injection 2530

Lithium Carbonate (Hyperpyrexia). Products include:
Eskalith 2485
Lithium Carbonate Capsules & Tablets 2230
Lithonate/Lithotabs/Lithobid 2543

Lithium Citrate (Hyperpyrexia).
No products indexed under this heading.

Loratadine (Potentiated). Products include:
Claritin 2349
Claritin-D 2350

Lorazepam (Potentiated; contraindication). Products include:
Ativan Injection 2698
Ativan Tablets 2700

Loxapine Hydrochloride (Potentiated; hyperpyrexia). Products include:
Loxitane 1378

Loxapine Succinate (Potentiated). Products include:
Loxitane Capsules 1378

Mepenzolate Bromide (Hyperpyrexia; paralytic ileus).
No products indexed under this heading.

Meperidine Hydrochloride (Potentiated). Products include:
Demerol 2308
Mepergan Injection 2753

Mephenytoin (Increased anticonvulsant dosage may be necessary). Products include:
Mesantoin Tablets 2272

Mephobarbital (Potentiated). Products include:
Mebaral Tablets 2322

Meprobamate (Potentiated). Products include:
Miltown Tablets 2672
PMB 200 and PMB 400 2783

Mesoridazine Besylate (Potentiated; hyperpyrexia; contraindication). Products include:
Serentil 684

Metaproterenol Sulfate (Close supervision and careful dosage adjustment required). Products include:
Alupent 669
Metaproterenol Sulfate Inhalation Solution, USP, Arm-a-Med 552

Metaraminol Bitartrate (Close supervision and careful dosage adjustment required). Products include:
Aramine Injection 1609

Methadone Hydrochloride (Potentiated). Products include:
Methadone Hydrochloride Oral Concentrate 2233
Methadone Hydrochloride Oral Solution & Tablets 2235

Methdilazine Hydrochloride (Potentiated).
No products indexed under this heading.

Methohexital Sodium (Potentiated). Products include:
Brevital Sodium Vials 1429

Methotrimeprazine (Potentiated). Products include:
Levoprome 1274

Methoxamine Hydrochloride (Close supervision and careful dosage adjustment required). Products include:
Vasoxyl Injection 1196

Methoxyflurane (Potentiated).
No products indexed under this heading.

Methsuximide (Increased anticonvulsant dosage may be necessary). Products include:
Celontin Kapseals 1899

Midazolam Hydrochloride (Potentiated). Products include:
Versed Injection 2170

Molindone Hydrochloride (Potentiated; hyperpyrexia). Products include:
Moban Tablets and Concentrate 1048

Morphine Sulfate (Potentiated). Products include:
Astramorph/PF Injection, USP (Preservative-Free) 535
Duramorph 962
Infumorph 200 and Infumorph 500 Sterile Solutions 965
MS Contin Tablets 1994
MSIR 1997
Oramorph SR (Morphine Sulfate Sustained Release Tablets) 2236
RMS Suppositories 2657
Roxanol 2243

Norepinephrine Bitartrate (Close supervision and careful dosage adjustment required). Products include:
Levophed Bitartrate Injection 2315

Opium Alkaloids (Potentiated).
No products indexed under this heading.

Oxazepam (Potentiated). Products include:
Serax Capsules 2810
Serax Tablets 2810

Oxybutynin Chloride (Hyperpyrexia; paralytic ileus). Products include:
Ditropan 1516

Oxycodone Hydrochloride (Potentiated). Products include:
Percocet Tablets 938
Percodan Tablets 939
Percodan-Demi Tablets 940
Roxicodone Tablets, Oral Solution & Intensol (Oxycodone) 2244
Tylox Capsules 1584

Paramethadione (Increased anticonvulsant dosage may be necessary).
No products indexed under this heading.

Pentobarbital Sodium (Potentiated). Products include:
Nembutal Sodium Capsules 436
Nembutal Sodium Solution 438
Nembutal Sodium Suppositories 440

Phenacemide (Increased anticonvulsant dosage may be necessary). Products include:
Phenurone Tablets 447

Phenelzine Sulfate (Concomitant administration is contraindicated; hyperpyretic crises and severe convulsions have occurred). Products include:
Nardil 1920

Phenobarbital (Potentiated; increased anticonvulsant dosage may be necessary). Products include:
Arco-Lase Plus Tablets 512
Bellergal-S Tablets 2250
Donnatal 2060
Donnatal Extentabs 2061
Donnatal Tablets 2060
Phenobarbital Elixir and Tablets 1469
Quadrinal Tablets 1350

Phensuximide (Increased anticonvulsant dosage may be necessary). Products include:
Milontin Kapseals 1920

Phenylephrine Bitartrate (Close supervision and careful dosage adjustment required).
No products indexed under this heading.

Phenylephrine Hydrochloride (Close supervision and careful dosage adjustment required). Products include:
Atrohist Plus Tablets 454
Cerose DM .... ▣ 878
Comhist 2038
D.A. Chewable Tablets 951
Deconsal Pediatric Capsules 454
Dura-Vent/DA Tablets 953
Entex Capsules 1986
Entex Liquid 1986
Extendryl 1005
4-Way Fast Acting Nasal Spray (regular & mentholated) .... ▣ 621
Hemorid For Women .... ▣ 834
Hycomine Compound Tablets 932
Neo-Synephrine Hydrochloride 1% Carpuject 2324
Neo-Synephrine Hydrochloride 1% Injection 2324
Neo-Synephrine Hydrochloride (Ophthalmic) 2325
Neo-Synephrine .... ▣ 726
Nostril .... ▣ 644
Novahistine Elixir .... ▣ 823
Phenergan VC 2779
Phenergan VC with Codeine 2781
Preparation H .... ▣ 871
Tympagesic Ear Drops 2342
Vasosulf .... ⊙ 271
Vicks Sinex Nasal Spray and Ultra Fine Mist .... ▣ 765

Phenylephrine Tannate (Close supervision and careful dosage adjustment required). Products include:
Atrohist Pediatric Suspension 454
Ricobid-D Pediatric Suspension 2038
Ricobid Tablets and Pediatric Suspension 2038
Rynatan 2673
Rynatuss 2673

Phenylpropanolamine Hydrochloride (Close supervision and careful dosage adjustment required). Products include:
Acutrim .... ▣ 628
Allerest Children's Chewable Tablets .... ▣ 627
Allerest 12 Hour Caplets .... ▣ 627
Atrohist Plus Tablets 454
BC Cold Powder Multi-Symptom Formula (Cold-Sinus-Allergy) .... ▣ 609
BC Cold Powder Non-Drowsy Formula (Cold-Sinus) .... ▣ 609
Cheracol Plus Head Cold/Cough Formula .... ▣ 769
Comtrex Multi-Symptom Non-Drowsy Liqui-gels .... ▣ 618
Contac Continuous Action Nasal Decongestant/Antihistamine 12 Hour Capsules .... ▣ 813
Contac Maximum Strength Continuous Action Decongestant/Antihistamine 12 Hour Caplets .... ▣ 813
Contac Severe Cold and Flu Formula Caplets .... ▣ 814
Coricidin 'D' Decongestant Tablets .... ▣ 800
Dexatrim .... ▣ 832
Dexatrim Plus Vitamins Caplets .... ▣ 832
Dimetane-DC Cough Syrup 2059
Dimetapp Elixir .... ▣ 773
Dimetapp Extentabs .... ▣ 774
Dimetapp Tablets/Liqui-Gels .... ▣ 775
Dimetapp Cold & Allergy Chewable Tablets .... ▣ 773
Dimetapp DM Elixir .... ▣ 774
Dura-Vent Tablets 952
Entex Capsules 1986
Entex LA Tablets 1987
Entex Liquid 1986
Exgest LA Tablets 782
Hycomine 931
Isoclor Timesule Capsules .... ▣ 637
Nolamine Timed-Release Tablets 785
Ornade Spansule Capsules 2502
Propagest Tablets 786
Pyrroxate Caplets .... ▣ 772
Robitussin-CF .... ▣ 777
Sinulin Tablets 787
Tavist-D 12 Hour Relief Tablets .... ▣ 787
Teldrin 12 Hour Antihistamine/Nasal Decongestant Allergy Relief Capsules .... ▣ 826
Triaminic Allergy Tablets .... ▣ 789
Triaminic Cold Tablets .... ▣ 790
Triaminic Expectorant .... ▣ 790
Triaminic Syrup .... ▣ 792
Triaminic-12 Tablets .... ▣ 792
Triaminic-DM Syrup .... ▣ 792
Triaminicin Tablets .... ▣ 793
Triaminicol Multi-Symptom Cold Tablets .... ▣ 793
Triaminicol Multi-Symptom Relief ▣ 794
Vicks DayQuil Allergy Relief 12-Hour Extended Release Tablets .... ▣ 760
Vicks DayQuil Allergy Relief 4-Hour Tablets .... ▣ 760
Vicks DayQuil SINUS Pressure & CONGESTION Relief .... ▣ 761

Phenytoin (Increased anticonvulsant dosage may be necessary). Products include:
Dilantin Infatabs 1908
Dilantin-125 Suspension 1911

Phenytoin Sodium (Increased anticonvulsant dosage may be necessary). Products include:
Dilantin Kapseals 1906
Dilantin Parenteral 1910

Pimozide (Hyperpyrexia). Products include:
Orap Tablets 1050

Pirbuterol Acetate (Close supervision and careful dosage adjustment required). Products include:
Maxair Autohaler 1492
Maxair Inhaler 1494

Prazepam (Potentiated).
No products indexed under this heading.

Prazosin Hydrochloride (Antihypertensive effect of prazosin blocked). Products include:
Minipress Capsules 1937
Minizide Capsules 1938

Primidone (Increased anticonvulsant dosage may be necessary). Products include:
Mysoline 2754

Prochlorperazine (Potentiated; hyperpyrexia). Products include:
Compazine 2470

Procyclidine Hydrochloride (Hyperpyrexia; paralytic ileus). Products include:
Kemadrin Tablets 1112

Promethazine Hydrochloride (Potentiated; hyperpyrexia). Products include:
Mepergan Injection 2753
Phenergan with Codeine 2777
Phenergan with Dextromethorphan 2778

IMPORTANT NOTE: Always consult each drug listing in the patient's regimen for possible interactions.

Triavil **Interactions Index** 1072

Phenergan Injection ... 2773
Phenergan Suppositories ... 2775
Phenergan Syrup ... 2774
Phenergan Tablets ... 2775
Phenergan VC ... 2779
Phenergan VC with Codeine ... 2781

Propantheline Bromide (Hyperpyrexia; paralytic ileus). Products include:
Pro-Banthine Tablets ... 2052

Propofol (Potentiated). Products include:
Diprivan Injection ... 2833

Propoxyphene Hydrochloride (Potentiated). Products include:
Darvon ... 1435
Wygesic Tablets ... 2827

Propoxyphene Napsylate (Potentiated). Products include:
Darvon-N/Darvocet-N ... 1433

Pseudoephedrine Hydrochloride (Close supervision and careful dosage adjustment required). Products include:
Actifed Allergy Daytime/Nighttime Caplets ... ▣ 844
Actifed Plus Caplets ... ▣ 845
Actifed Plus Tablets ... ▣ 845
Actifed with Codeine Cough Syrup .. 1067
Actifed Sinus Daytime/Nighttime Tablets and Caplets ... ▣ 846
Actifed Syrup ... ▣ 846
Actifed Tablets ... ▣ 844
Advil Cold and Sinus Caplets and Tablets (formerly CoAdvil) ... ▣ 870
Alka-Seltzer Plus Cold Medicine Liqui-Gels ... ▣ 706
Alka-Seltzer Plus Cold & Cough Medicine Liqui-Gels ... ▣ 705
Alka-Seltzer Plus Night-Time Cold Medicine Liqui-Gels ... ▣ 706
Allerest Headache Strength Tablets ... ▣ 627
Allerest Maximum Strength Tablets ... ▣ 627
Allerest No Drowsiness Tablets ... ▣ 627
Allerest Sinus Pain Formula ... ▣ 627
Anatuss LA Tablets ... 1542
Atrohist Pediatric Capsules ... 453
Bayer Select Sinus Pain Relief Formula ... ▣ 717
Benadryl Allergy Decongestant Liquid Medication ... ▣ 848
Benadryl Allergy Decongestant Tablets ... ▣ 848
Benadryl Allergy Sinus Headache Formula Caplets ... ▣ 849
Benylin Multisymptom ... ▣ 852
Bromfed Capsules (Extended-Release) ... 1785
Bromfed Syrup ... ▣ 733
Bromfed Tablets ... 1785
Bromfed-DM Cough Syrup ... 1786
Bromfed-PD Capsules (Extended-Release) ... 1785
Children's Vicks DayQuil Allergy Relief ... ▣ 757
Children's Vicks NyQuil Cold/Cough Relief ... ▣ 758
Comtrex Multi-Symptom Cold Reliever Tablets/Caplets/Liqui-Gels/Liquid ... ▣ 615
Allergy-Sinus Comtrex Multi-Symptom Allergy-Sinus Formula Tablets ... ▣ 617
Comtrex Multi-Symptom Non-Drowsy Caplets ... ▣ 618
Congess ... 1004
Contac Day Allergy/Sinus Caplets ▣ 812
Contac Day & Night ... ▣ 812
Contac Night Allergy/Sinus Caplets ... ▣ 812
Contac Severe Cold & Flu Non-Drowsy ... ▣ 815
Deconamine Chewable Tablets ... 1320
Deconamine CX Cough and Cold Liquid and Tablets ... 1319
Deconamine ... 1320
Deconsal C Expectorant Syrup ... 456
Deconsal Pediatric Syrup ... 457
Deconsal II Tablets ... 454
Dimetane-DX Cough Syrup ... 2059
Dimetapp Sinus Caplets ... ▣ 775
Dorcol Children's Cough Syrup ... ▣ 785
Drixoral Cough + Congestion Liquid Caps ... ▣ 802
Dura-Tap/PD Capsules ... 2867
Duratuss Tablets ... 2565
Duratuss HD Elixir ... 2565
Efidac/24 ... ▣ 635
Entex PSE Tablets ... 1987
Fedahist Gyrocaps ... 2401
Fedahist Timecaps ... 2401
Guaifed ... 1787
Guaifed Syrup ... ▣ 734
Guaimax-D Tablets ... 792
Guaitab Tablets ... ▣ 734
Isoclor Expectorant ... 990
Kronofed-A ... 977
Motrin IB Sinus ... ▣ 838
Novahistine DH ... 2462
Novahistine DMX ... ▣ 822
Novahistine Expectorant ... 2463
Nucofed ... 2051
PediaCare Cold Allergy Chewable Tablets ... ▣ 677
PediaCare Cough-Cold Chewable Tablets ... 1553
PediaCare ... 1553
PediaCare Infants' Decongestant Drops ... ▣ 677
PediCare Infant's Drops Decongestant Plus Cough ... 1553
PediaCare NightRest Cough-Cold Liquid ... 1553
Pediatric Vicks 44d Dry Hacking Cough & Head Congestion ... ▣ 763
Pediatric Vicks 44m Cough & Cold Relief ... ▣ 764
Robitussin Cold & Cough Liqui-Gels ... ▣ 776
Robitussin Maximum Strength Cough & Cold ... ▣ 778
Robitussin Pediatric Cough & Cold Formula ... ▣ 779
Robitussin Severe Congestion Liqui-Gels ... ▣ 776
Robitussin-DAC Syrup ... 2074
Robitussin-PE ... ▣ 778
Rondec Oral Drops ... 953
Rondec Syrup ... 953
Rondec Tablet ... 953
Rondec-DM Oral Drops ... 954
Rondec-DM Syrup ... 954
Rondec-TR Tablet ... 953
Ryna ... ▣ 841
Seldane-D Extended-Release Tablets ... 1538
Semprex-D Capsules ... 463
Semprex-D Capsules ... 1167
Sinarest Tablets ... ▣ 648
Sinarest Extra Strength Tablets ... ▣ 648
Sinarest No Drowsiness Tablets ... ▣ 648
Sine-Aid IB Caplets ... 1554
Sine-Aid Maximum Strength Sinus Medication Gelcaps, Caplets and Tablets ... 1554
Sine-Off No Drowsiness Formula Caplets ... ▣ 824
Sine-Off Sinus Medicine ... ▣ 825
Singlet Tablets ... ▣ 825
Sinutab Non-Drying Liquid Caps ... ▣ 859
Sinutab Sinus Allergy Medication, Maximum Strength Tablets and Caplets ... ▣ 860
Sinutab Sinus Medication, Maximum Strength Without Drowsiness Formula, Tablets & Caplets ... ▣ 860
Sinutab Sinus Medication, Regular Strength Without Drowsiness Formula ... ▣ 859
Sudafed Children's Liquid ... ▣ 861
Sudafed Cold and Cough Liquidcaps ... ▣ 862
Sudafed Cough Syrup ... ▣ 862
Sudafed Plus Liquid ... ▣ 862
Sudafed Plus Tablets ... ▣ 863
Sudafed Severe Cold Formula Caplets ... ▣ 863
Sudafed Severe Cold Formula Tablets ... ▣ 864
Sudafed Sinus Caplets ... ▣ 864
Sudafed Sinus Tablets ... ▣ 864
Sudafed Tablets, 30 mg ... ▣ 861
Sudafed Tablets, 60 mg ... ▣ 861
Sudafed 12 Hour Caplets ... ▣ 861
Syn-Rx Tablets ... 465
Syn-Rx DM Tablets ... 466
TheraFlu ... ▣ 787
TheraFlu Maximum Strength Nighttime Flu, Cold & Cough Medicine ... ▣ 788
TheraFlu Maximum Strength Non-Drowsy Formula Flu, Cold & Cough Medicine ... ▣ 788
Thera Flu Maximum Strength, Non-Drowsy Formula Flu, Cold and Cough Caplets ... ▣ 789
Triaminic AM Cough and Decongestant Formula ... ▣ 789
Triaminic AM Decongestant Formula ... ▣ 790
Triaminic Nite Light ... ▣ 791
Triaminic Sore Throat Formula ... ▣ 791
Tussend ... 1783
Tussend Expectorant ... 1785
Children's TYLENOL Cold Multi-Symptom Liquid Formula and Chewable Tablets ... 1561
Children's TYLENOL Cold Plus Cough Multi Symptom Tablets and Liquid ... ▣ 681
Infants' TYLENOL Cold Decongestant & Fever-Reducer Drops ... 1556
TYLENOL Maximum Strength Allergy Sinus Medication Gelcaps and Caplets ... 1563
TYLENOL Maximum Strength Allergy Sinus NightTime Medication Caplets ... 1555
TYLENOL Flu Maximum Strength Gelcaps ... 1565
TYLENOL Flu NightTime, Maximum Strength, Gelcaps ... 1566
TYLENOL Maximum Strength Flu NightTime Hot Medication Packets ... 1562
TYLENOL, Maximum Strength, Sinus Medication Geltabs, Gelcaps, Caplets and Tablets ... 1566
TYLENOL Cold Multi-Symptom Formula Medication Tablets and Caplets ... 1561
TYLENOL Cold Medication No Drowsiness Formula Gelcaps and Caplets ... 1562
TYLENOL Cold Multi-Symptom Hot Medication Liquid Packets ... 1557
TYLENOL Cough Multi-Symptom Medication with Decongestant ... 1565
Ursinus Inlay-Tabs ... ▣ 794
Vicks 44 LiquiCaps Cough, Cold & Flu Relief ... ▣ 755
Vicks 44 LiquiCaps Non-Drowsy Cough & Cold Relief ... ▣ 756
Vicks 44D Dry Hacking Cough & Head Congestion ... ▣ 755
Vicks 44M Cough, Cold & Flu Relief ... ▣ 756
Vicks DayQuil ... ▣ 761
Vicks DayQuil SINUS Pressure & PAIN Relief with IBUPROFEN ... ▣ 762
Vicks Nyquil Hot Therapy ... ▣ 762
Vicks NyQuil LiquiCaps Multi-Symptom Cold/Flu Relief ... ▣ 763
Vicks NyQuil Multi-Symptom Cold/Flu Relief - (Original & Cherry Flavor) ... ▣ 763

Pseudoephedrine Sulfate (Close supervision and careful dosage adjustment required). Products include:
Cheracol Sinus ... ▣ 768
Chlor-Trimeton Allergy Decongestant Tablets ... ▣ 799
Claritin-D ... 2350
Drixoral Cold and Allergy Sustained-Action Tablets ... ▣ 802
Drixoral Cold and Flu Extended-Release Tablets ... ▣ 803
Drixoral Non-Drowsy Formula Extended-Release Tablets ... ▣ 803
Drixoral Allergy/Sinus Extended Release Tablets ... ▣ 804
Trinalin Repetabs Tablets ... 1330

Pyrilamine Maleate (Potentiated). Products include:
4-Way Fast Acting Nasal Spray (regular & mentholated) ... ▣ 621
Maximum Strength Multi-Symptom Formula Midol ... ▣ 722
PMS Multi-Symptom Formula Midol ... ▣ 723

Pyrilamine Tannate (Potentiated). Products include:
Atrohist Pediatric Suspension ... 454
Rynatan ... 2673

Quazepam (Potentiated). Products include:
Doral Tablets ... 2664

Rauwolfia Serpentina (Antihypertensive effect of rauwolfia serpentina blocked).
No products indexed under this heading.

Rescinnamine (Antihypertensive effect of rescinnamine blocked).
No products indexed under this heading.

Reserpine (Antihypertensive effect of reserpine blocked). Products include:
Diupres Tablets ... 1650
Hydropres Tablets ... 1675
Ser-Ap-Es Tablets ... 849

Risperidone (Potentiated). Products include:
Risperdal ... 1301

Salmeterol Xinafoate (Close supervision and careful dosage adjustment required). Products include:
Serevent Inhalation Aerosol ... 1176

Scopolamine (Hyperpyrexia; paralytic ileus). Products include:
Transderm Scōp Transdermal Therapeutic System ... 869

Scopolamine Hydrobromide (Hyperpyrexia; paralytic ileus). Products include:
Atrohist Plus Tablets ... 454
Donnatal ... 2060
Donnatal Extentabs ... 2061
Donnatal Tablets ... 2060

Secobarbital Sodium (Potentiated). Products include:
Seconal Sodium Pulvules ... 1474

Selegiline Hydrochloride (Concomitant administration is contraindicated; hyperpyretic crises and severe convulsions have occurred). Products include:
Eldepryl Tablets ... 2550

Sufentanil Citrate (Potentiated). Products include:
Sufenta Injection ... 1309

Temazepam (Potentiated). Products include:
Restoril Capsules ... 2284

Terazosin Hydrochloride (Antihypertensive effect of terazosin blocked). Products include:
Hytrin Capsules ... 430

Terbutaline Sulfate (Close supervision and careful dosage adjustment required). Products include:
Brethaire Inhaler ... 813
Brethine Ampuls ... 815
Brethine Tablets ... 814
Bricanyl Subcutaneous Injection ... 1502
Bricanyl Tablets ... 1503

Terfenadine (Potentiated). Products include:
Seldane Tablets ... 1536
Seldane-D Extended-Release Tablets ... 1538

Thiamylal Sodium (Potentiated).
No products indexed under this heading.

Thioridazine Hydrochloride (Potentiated; hyperpyrexia). Products include:
Mellaril ... 2269

Thiothixene (Potentiated; hyperpyrexia). Products include:
Navane Capsules and Concentrate 2201
Navane Intramuscular ... 2202

Thyroid (Close supervision is indicated).
No products indexed under this heading.

Thyroxine (Close supervision is indicated).
No products indexed under this heading.

Thyroxine Sodium (Close supervision is indicated).
No products indexed under this heading.

(▣ Described in PDR For Nonprescription Drugs) (⊙ Described in PDR For Ophthalmology)

Tranylcypromine Sulfate (Concomitant administration is contraindicated; hyperpyretic crises and severe convulsions have occurred). Products include:

Parnate Tablets 2503

Triazolam (Potentiated). Products include:

Halcion Tablets 2611

Tridihexethyl Chloride (Hyperpyrexia; paralytic ileus).

No products indexed under this heading.

Trifluoperazine Hydrochloride (Potentiated; hyperpyrexia). Products include:

Stelazine 2514

Trihexyphenidyl Hydrochloride (Hyperpyrexia; paralytic ileus). Products include:

Artane 1368

Trimeprazine Tartrate (Potentiated). Products include:

Temaril Tablets, Syrup and Spansule Extended-Release Capsules .. 483

Trimethadione (Increased anticonvulsant dosage may be necessary).

No products indexed under this heading.

Tripelennamine Hydrochloride (Potentiated). Products include:

PBZ Tablets 845
PBZ-SR Tablets 844

Triprolidine Hydrochloride (Potentiated). Products include:

Actifed Plus Caplets .... ◆□ 845
Actifed Plus Tablets .... ◆□ 845
Actifed with Codeine Cough Syrup.. 1067
Actifed Syrup .... ◆□ 846
Actifed Tablets .... ◆□ 844

Valproic Acid (Increased anticonvulsant dosage may be necessary). Products include:

Depakene 413

Zolpidem Tartrate (Potentiated). Products include:

Ambien Tablets 2416

Food Interactions

Alcohol (Potentiated; contraindication).

TRIAZ 6% AND 10% GELS AND 10% CLEANER

(Benzoyl Peroxide) 1592
None cited in PDR database.

TRIDESILON CREAM 0.05%

(Desonide) 615
None cited in PDR database.

TRIDESILON OINTMENT 0.05%

(Desonide) 616
None cited in PDR database.

TRI-IMMUNOL ADSORBED

(Diphtheria & Tetanus Toxoids w/Pertussis Vaccine Combined, Aluminum Phosphate Adsorbed) 1408
May interact with corticosteroids, antineoplastics, and cytotoxic drugs. Compounds in these categories include:

Altretamine (Aberrant responses to active immunization procedures). Products include:

Hexalen Capsules 2571

Asparaginase (Aberrant responses to active immunization procedures). Products include:

Elspar 1659

Betamethasone Acetate (Aberrant responses to active immunization procedures). Products include:

Celestone Soluspan Suspension 2347

Betamethasone Sodium Phosphate (Aberrant responses to active immunization procedures). Products include:

Celestone Soluspan Suspension 2347

Bleomycin Sulfate (Aberrant responses to active immunization procedures). Products include:

Blenoxane 692

Busulfan (Aberrant responses to active immunization procedures). Products include:

Myleran Tablets 1143

Carboplatin (Aberrant responses to active immunization procedures). Products include:

Paraplatin for Injection 705

Carmustine (BCNU) (Aberrant responses to active immunization procedures). Products include:

BiCNU 691

Chlorambucil (Aberrant responses to active immunization procedures). Products include:

Leukeran Tablets 1133

Cisplatin (Aberrant responses to active immunization procedures). Products include:

Platinol 708
Platinol-AQ Injection 710

Cortisone Acetate (Aberrant responses to active immunization procedures). Products include:

Cortone Acetate Sterile Suspension 1623
Cortone Acetate Tablets 1624

Cyclophosphamide (Aberrant responses to active immunization procedures). Products include:

Cytoxan 694
NEOSAR Lyophilized/Neosar 1959

Dacarbazine (Aberrant responses to active immunization procedures). Products include:

DTIC-Dome 600

Daunorubicin Hydrochloride (Aberrant responses to active immunization procedures). Products include:

Cerubidine 795

Dexamethasone (Aberrant responses to active immunization procedures). Products include:

AK-Trol Ointment & Suspension .... ◎ 205
Decadron Elixir 1633
Decadron Tablets 1635
Decaspray Topical Aerosol 1648
Dexacidin Ointment .... ◎ 263
Maxitrol Ophthalmic Ointment and Suspension .... ◎ 224
TobraDex Ophthalmic Suspension and Ointment 473

Dexamethasone Acetate (Aberrant responses to active immunization procedures). Products include:

Dalalone D.P. Injectable 1011
Decadron-LA Sterile Suspension 1646

Dexamethasone Sodium Phosphate (Aberrant responses to active immunization procedures). Products include:

Decadron Phosphate Injection 1637
Decadron Phosphate Respihaler 1642
Decadron Phosphate Sterile Ophthalmic Ointment 1641
Decadron Phosphate Sterile Ophthalmic Solution 1642
Decadron Phosphate Topical Cream 1644
Decadron Phosphate Turbinaire 1645
Decadron Phosphate with Xylocaine Injection, Sterile 1639
Dexacort Phosphate in Respihaler .. 458
Dexacort Phosphate in Turbinaire .. 459
NeoDecadron Sterile Ophthalmic Ointment 1712
NeoDecadron Sterile Ophthalmic Solution 1713
NeoDecadron Topical Cream 1714

Doxorubicin Hydrochloride (Aberrant responses to active immunization procedures). Products include:

Adriamycin PFS 1947
Adriamycin RDF 1947
Doxorubicin Astra 540
Rubex 712

Estramustine Phosphate Sodium (Aberrant responses to active immunization procedures). Products include:

Emcyt Capsules 1953

Etoposide (Aberrant responses to active immunization procedures). Products include:

VePesid Capsules and Injection 718

Floxuridine (Aberrant responses to active immunization procedures). Products include:

Sterile FUDR 2118

Fludrocortisone Acetate (Aberrant responses to active immunization procedures). Products include:

Florinef Acetate Tablets 505

Fluorouracil (Aberrant responses to active immunization procedures). Products include:

Efudex 2113
Fluoroplex Topical Solution & Cream 1% 479
Fluorouracil Injection 2116

Flutamide (Abberrant responses to active immunization procedures). Products include:

Eulexin Capsules 2358

Hydrocortisone (Aberrant responses to active immunization procedures). Products include:

Anusol-HC Cream 2.5% 1896
Aquanil HC Lotion 1931
Bactine Hydrocortisone Anti-Itch Cream .... ◆□ 709
Caldecort Anti-Itch Hydrocortisone Spray .... ◆□ 631
Cortaid .... ◆□ 836
CORTENEMA 2535
Cortisporin Ointment 1085
Cortisporin Ophthalmic Ointment Sterile 1085
Cortisporin Ophthalmic Suspension Sterile 1086
Cortisporin Otic Solution Sterile 1087
Cortisporin Otic Suspension Sterile 1088
Cortizone-5 .... ◆□ 831
Cortizone-10 .... ◆□ 831
Hydrocortone Tablets 1672
Hytone 907
Massengill Medicated Soft Cloth Towelettes 2458
PediOtic Suspension Sterile 1153
Preparation H Hydrocortisone 1% Cream .... ◆□ 872
ProctoCream-HC 2.5% 2408
VoSoL HC Otic Solution 2678

Hydrocortisone Acetate (Aberrant responses to active immunization procedures). Products include:

Analpram-HC Rectal Cream 1% and 2.5% 977
Anusol HC-1 Anti-Itch Hydrocortisone Ointment .... ◆□ 847
Anusol-HC Suppositories 1897
Caldecort .... ◆□ 631
Carmol HC 924
Coly-Mycin S Otic w/Neomycin & Hydrocortisone 1906
Cortaid .... ◆□ 836
Cortifoam 2396
Cortisporin Cream 1084
Epifoam 2399
Hydrocortone Acetate Sterile Suspension 1669
Mantadil Cream 1135
Nupercainal Hydrocortisone 1% Cream .... ◆□ 645
Ophthocort .... ◎ 311
Pramosone Cream, Lotion & Ointment 978
ProctoCream-HC 2408
ProctoFoam-HC 2409
Terra-Cortril Ophthalmic Suspension 2210

Hydrocortisone Sodium Phosphate (Aberrant responses to active immunization procedures). Products include:

Hydrocortone Phosphate Injection, Sterile 1670

Hydrocortisone Sodium Succinate (Aberrant responses to active immunization procedures). Products include:

Solu-Cortef Sterile Powder 2641

Hydroxyurea (Aberrant responses to active immunization procedures). Products include:

Hydrea Capsules 696

Idarubicin Hydrochloride (Aberrant responses to active immunization procedures). Products include:

Idamycin 1955

Ifosfamide (Aberrant responses to active immunization procedures). Products include:

IFEX 697

Interferon alfa-2A, Recombinant (Aberrant responses to active immunization procedures). Products include:

Roferon-A Injection 2145

Interferon alfa-2B, Recombinant (Aberrant responses to active immunization procedures). Products include:

Intron A 2364

Levamisole Hydrochloride (Aberrant responses to active immunization procedures). Products include:

Ergamisol Tablets 1292

Lomustine (CCNU) (Aberrant responses to active immunization procedures). Products include:

CeeNU 693

Mechlorethamine Hydrochloride (Aberrant responses to active immunization procedures). Products include:

Mustargen 1709

Megestrol Acetate (Aberrant responses to active immunization procedures). Products include:

Megace Oral Suspension 699
Megace Tablets 701

Melphalan (Aberrant responses to active immunization procedures). Products include:

Alkeran Tablets 1071

Mercaptopurine (Aberrant responses to active immunization procedures). Products include:

Purinethol Tablets 1156

Methotrexate Sodium (Aberrant responses to active immunization procedures) Products include:

Methotrexate Sodium Tablets, Injection, for Injection and LPF Injection 1275

Methylprednisolone Acetate (Aberrant responses to active immunization procedures). Products include:

Depo-Medrol Single-Dose Vial 2600
Depo-Medrol Sterile Aqueous Suspension 2597

Methylprednisolone Sodium Succinate (Aberrant responses to active immunization procedures). Products include:

Solu-Medrol Sterile Powder 2643

Mitomycin (Mitomycin-C) (Aberrant responses to active immunization procedures). Products include:

Mutamycin 703

Mitotane (Aberrant responses to active immunization procedures). Products include:

Lysodren 698

IMPORTANT NOTE: Always consult each drug listing in the patient's regimen for possible interactions.

Tri-Immunol | Interactions Index | 1074

Mitoxantrone Hydrochloride (Aberrant responses to active immunization procedures). Products include:
Novantrone ... 1279

Paclitaxel (Aberrant responses to active immunization procedures). Products include:
Taxol ... 714

Prednisolone Acetate (Aberrant responses to active immunization procedures). Products include:
AK-CIDE ... ⊙ 202
AK-CIDE Ointment ... ⊙ 202
Blephamide Liquifilm Sterile Ophthalmic Suspension ... 476
Blephamide Ointment ... ⊙ 237
Econopred & Econopred Plus Ophthalmic Suspensions ... ⊙ 217
Poly-Pred Liquifilm ... ⊙ 248
Pred Forte ... ⊙ 250
Pred Mild ... ⊙ 253
Pred-G Liquifilm Sterile Ophthalmic Suspension ... ⊙ 251
Pred-G S.O.P. Sterile Ophthalmic Ointment ... ⊙ 252
Vasocidin Ointment ... ⊙ 268

Prednisolone Sodium Phosphate (Aberrant responses to active immunization procedures). Products include:
AK-Pred ... ⊙ 204
Hydeltrasol Injection, Sterile ... 1665
Inflamase ... ⊙ 265
Pediapred Oral Liquid ... 995
Vasocidin Ophthalmic Solution ... ⊙ 270

Prednisolone Tebutate (Aberrant responses to active immunization procedures). Products include:
Hydeltra-T.B.A. Sterile Suspension 1667

Prednisone (Aberrant responses to active immunization procedures). Products include:
Deltasone Tablets ... 2595

Procarbazine Hydrochloride (Aberrant responses to active immunization procedures). Products include:
Matulane Capsules ... 2131

Streptozocin (Aberrant responses to active immunization procedures). Products include:
Zanosar Sterile Powder ... 2653

Tamoxifen Citrate (Aberrant responses to active immunization procedures). Products include:
Nolvadex Tablets ... 2841

Teniposide (Aberrant responses to active immunization procedures). Products include:
Vumon ... 727

Thioguanine (Aberrant responses to active immunization procedures). Products include:
Thioguanine Tablets, Tabloid Brand ... 1181

Thiotepa (Aberrant responses to active immunization procedures). Products include:
Thioplex (Thiotepa For Injection) ... 1281

Triamcinolone (Aberrant responses to active immunization procedures). Products include:
Aristocort Tablets ... 1022

Triamcinolone Acetonide (Aberrant responses to active immunization procedures). Products include:
Aristocort A 0.025% Cream ... 1027
Aristocort A 0.5% Cream ... 1031
Aristocort A 0.1% Cream ... 1029
Aristocort A 0.1% Ointment ... 1030
Azmacort Oral Inhaler ... 2011
Nasacort Nasal Inhaler ... 2024

Triamcinolone Diacetate (Aberrant responses to active immunization procedures). Products include:
Aristocort Suspension (Forte Parenteral) ... 1027
Aristocort Suspension (Intralesional) ... 1025

Triamcinolone Hexacetonide (Aberrant responses to active immunization procedures). Products include:
Aristospan Suspension (Intra-articular) ... 1033
Aristospan Suspension (Intralesional) ... 1032

Vincristine Sulfate (Aberrant responses to active immunization procedures). Products include:
Oncovin Solution Vials & Hyporets 1466

Vinorelbine Tartrate (Aberrant responses to active immunization procedures). Products include:
Navelbine Injection ... 1145

TRILAFON CONCENTRATE
(Perphenazine) ... 2389
May interact with central nervous system depressants, anticonvulsants, and certain other agents. Compounds in these categories include:

Alfentanil Hydrochloride (Potentiation of both drugs). Products include:
Alfenta Injection ... 1286

Alprazolam (Potentiation of both drugs). Products include:
Xanax Tablets ... 2649

Aprobarbital (Potentiation of both drugs).
No products indexed under this heading.

Atropine Sulfate (Additive anticholinergic effects). Products include:
Arco-Lase Plus Tablets ... 512
Atrohist Plus Tablets ... 454
Atropine Sulfate Sterile Ophthalmic Solution ... ⊙ 233
Donnatal ... 2060
Donnatal Extentabs ... 2061
Donnatal Tablets ... 2060
Lomotil ... 2439
Motofen Tablets ... 784
Urised Tablets ... 1964

Buprenorphine (Potentiation of both drugs). Products include:
Buprenex Injectable ... 2006

Buspirone Hydrochloride (Potentiation of both drugs). Products include:
BuSpar ... 737

Butabarbital (Potentiation of both drugs).
No products indexed under this heading.

Butalbital (Potentiation of both drugs). Products include:
Esgic-plus Tablets ... 1013
Fioricet Tablets ... 2258
Fioricet with Codeine Capsules ... 2260
Fiorinal Capsules ... 2261
Fiorinal with Codeine Capsules ... 2262
Fiorinal Tablets ... 2261
Phrenilin ... 785
Sedapap Tablets 50 mg/650 mg ... 1543

Carbamazepine (Increased dosage of anticonvulsant may be required). Products include:
Atretol Tablets ... 573
Tegretol Chewable Tablets ... 852
Tegretol Suspension ... 852
Tegretol Tablets ... 852

Chlordiazepoxide (Potentiation of both drugs). Products include:
Libritabs Tablets ... 2177
Limbitrol ... 2180

Chlordiazepoxide Hydrochloride (Potentiation of both drugs). Products include:
Librax Capsules ... 2176
Librium Capsules ... 2178
Librium Injectable ... 2179

Chlorpromazine (Potentiation of both drugs). Products include:
Thorazine Suppositories ... 2523

Chlorprothixene (Potentiation of both drugs).
No products indexed under this heading.

Chlorprothixene Hydrochloride (Potentiation of both drugs).
No products indexed under this heading.

Clorazepate Dipotassium (Potentiation of both drugs). Products include:
Tranxene ... 451

Clozapine (Potentiation of both drugs). Products include:
Clozaril Tablets ... 2252

Codeine Phosphate (Potentiation of both drugs). Products include:
Actifed with Codeine Cough Syrup .. 1067
Brontex ... 1981
Deconsal C Expectorant Syrup ... 456
Deconsal Pediatric Syrup ... 457
Dimetane-DC Cough Syrup ... 2059
Empirin with Codeine Tablets ... 1093
Fioricet with Codeine Capsules ... 2260
Fiorinal with Codeine Capsules ... 2262
Isoclor Expectorant ... 990
Novahistine DH ... 2462
Novahistine Expectorant ... 2463
Nucofed ... 2051
Phenergan with Codeine ... 2777
Phenergan VC with Codeine ... 2781
Robitussin A-C Syrup ... 2073
Robitussin-DAC Syrup ... 2074
Ryna ... ▣ 841
Soma Compound w/Codeine Tablets ... 2676
Tussi-Organidin NR Liquid and S NR Liquid ... 2677
Tylenol with Codeine ... 1583

Desflurane (Potentiation of both drugs). Products include:
Suprane ... 1813

Dezocine (Potentiation of both drugs). Products include:
Dalgan Injection ... 538

Diazepam (Potentiation of both drugs). Products include:
Dizac ... 1809
Valium Injectable ... 2182
Valium Tablets ... 2183
Valrelease Capsules ... 2169

Divalproex Sodium (Increased dosage of anticonvulsant may be required). Products include:
Depakote Tablets ... 415

Droperidol (Potentiation of both drugs). Products include:
Inapsine Injection ... 1296

Enflurane (Potentiation of both drugs).
No products indexed under this heading.

Epinephrine (Action of epinephrine blocked and partially reversed). Products include:
Bronkaid Mist ... ▣ 717
EPIFRIN ... ⊙ 239
EpiPen ... 790
Marcaine Hydrochloride with Epinephrine 1:200,000 ... 2316
Primatene Mist ... ▣ 873
Sensorcaine with Epinephrine Injection ... 559
Sus-Phrine Injection ... 1019
Xylocaine with Epinephrine Injections ... 567

Epinephrine Bitartrate (Action of epinephrine blocked and partially reversed). Products include:
Bronkaid Mist Suspension ... ▣ 718
Sensorcaine-MPF with Epinephrine Injection ... 559

Estazolam (Potentiation of both drugs). Products include:
ProSom Tablets ... 449

Ethchlorvynol (Potentiation of both drugs). Products include:
Placidyl Capsules ... 448

Ethinamate (Potentiation of both drugs).
No products indexed under this heading.

Ethosuximide (Increased dosage of anticonvulsant may be required). Products include:
Zarontin Capsules ... 1928
Zarontin Syrup ... 1929

Ethotoin (Increased dosage of anticonvulsant may be required). Products include:
Peganone Tablets ... 446

Felbamate (Increased dosage of anticonvulsant may be required). Products include:
Felbatol ... 2666

Fentanyl (Potentiation of both drugs). Products include:
Duragesic Transdermal System ... 1288

Fentanyl Citrate (Potentiation of both drugs). Products include:
Sublimaze Injection ... 1307

Fluphenazine Decanoate (Potentiation of both drugs). Products include:
Prolixin Decanoate ... 509

Fluphenazine Enanthate (Potentiation of both drugs). Products include:
Prolixin Enanthate ... 509

Fluphenazine Hydrochloride (Potentiation of both drugs). Products include:
Prolixin ... 509

Flurazepam Hydrochloride (Potentiation of both drugs). Products include:
Dalmane Capsules ... 2173

Glutethimide (Potentiation of both drugs).
No products indexed under this heading.

Haloperidol (Potentiation of both drugs). Products include:
Haldol Injection, Tablets and Concentrate ... 1575

Haloperidol Decanoate (Potentiation of both drugs). Products include:
Haldol Decanoate ... 1577

Hydrocodone Bitartrate (Potentiation of both drugs). Products include:
Anexsia 5/500 Elixir ... 1781
Anexia Tablets ... 1782
Codiclear DH Syrup ... 791
Deconamine CX Cough and Cold Liquid and Tablets ... 1319
Duratuss HD Elixir ... 2565
Hycodan Tablets and Syrup ... 930
Hycomine Compound Tablets ... 932
Hycomine ... 931
Hycotuss Expectorant Syrup ... 933
Hydrocet Capsules ... 782
Lorcet 10/650 ... 1018
Lortab ... 2566
Tussend ... 1783
Tussend Expectorant ... 1785
Vicodin Tablets ... 1356
Vicodin ES Tablets ... 1357
Vicodin Tuss Expectorant ... 1358
Zydone Capsules ... 949

Hydrocodone Polistirex (Potentiation of both drugs). Products include:
Tussionex Pennkinetic Extended-Release Suspension ... 998

Hydroxyzine Hydrochloride (Potentiation of both drugs). Products include:
Atarax Tablets & Syrup ... 2185
Marax Tablets & DF Syrup ... 2200
Vistaril Intramuscular Solution ... 2216

Isoflurane (Potentiation of both drugs).
No products indexed under this heading.

Ketamine Hydrochloride (Potentiation of both drugs).
No products indexed under this heading.

(▣ Described in PDR For Nonprescription Drugs) (⊙ Described in PDR For Ophthalmology)

Interactions Index — Trilisate

Lamotrigine (Increased dosage of anticonvulsant may be required). Products include:

Lamictal Tablets 1112

Levomethadyl Acetate Hydrochloride (Potentiation of both drugs). Products include:

Orlaam 2239

Levorphanol Tartrate (Potentiation of both drugs). Products include:

Levo-Dromoran 2129

Lorazepam (Potentiation of both drugs). Products include:

Ativan Injection 2698
Ativan Tablets 2700

Loxapine Hydrochloride (Potentiation of both drugs). Products include:

Loxitane 1378

Loxapine Succinate (Potentiation of both drugs). Products include:

Loxitane Capsules 1378

Meperidine Hydrochloride (Potentiation of both drugs). Products include:

Demerol 2308
Mepergan Injection 2753

Mephenytoin (Increased dosage of anticonvulsant may be required). Products include:

Mesantoin Tablets 2272

Mephobarbital (Potentiation of both drugs). Products include:

Mebaral Tablets 2322

Meprobamate (Potentiation of both drugs). Products include:

Miltown Tablets 2672
PMB 200 and PMB 400 2783

Mesoridazine Besylate (Potentiation of both drugs). Products include:

Serentil 684

Methadone Hydrochloride (Potentiation of both drugs). Products include:

Methadone Hydrochloride Oral Concentrate 2233
Methadone Hydrochloride Oral Solution & Tablets 2235

Methohexital Sodium (Potentiation of both drugs). Products include:

Brevital Sodium Vials 1429

Methotrimeprazine (Potentiation of both drugs). Products include:

Levoprome 1274

Methoxyflurane (Potentiation of both drugs).

No products indexed under this heading.

Methsuximide (Increased dosage of anticonvulsant may be required). Products include:

Celontin Kapseals 1899

Midazolam Hydrochloride (Potentiation of both drugs). Products include:

Versed Injection 2170

Molindone Hydrochloride (Potentiation of both drugs). Products include:

Moban Tablets and Concentrate 1048

Morphine Sulfate (Potentiation of both drugs). Products include:

Astramorph/PF Injection, USP (Preservative-Free) 535
Duramorph 962
Infumorph 200 and Infumorph 500 Sterile Solutions 965
MS Contin Tablets 1994
MSIR 1997
Oramorph SR (Morphine Sulfate Sustained Release Tablets) 2236
RMS Suppositories 2657
Roxanol 2243

Opium Alkaloids (Potentiation of both drugs).

No products indexed under this heading.

Oxazepam (Potentiation of both drugs). Products include:

Serax Capsules 2810
Serax Tablets 2810

Oxycodone Hydrochloride (Potentiation of both drugs). Products include:

Percocet Tablets 938
Percodan Tablets 939
Percodan-Demi Tablets 940
Roxicodone Tablets, Oral Solution & Intensol (Oxycodone) 2244
Tylox Capsules 1584

Paramethadione (Increased dosage of anticonvulsant may be required).

No products indexed under this heading.

Pentobarbital Sodium (Potentiation of both drugs). Products include:

Nembutal Sodium Capsules 436
Nembutal Sodium Solution 438
Nembutal Sodium Suppositories...... 440

Phenacemide (Increased dosage of anticonvulsant may be required). Products include:

Phenurone Tablets 447

Phenobarbital (Increased dosage of anticonvulsant may be required; potentiation of both drugs). Products include:

Arco-Lase Plus Tablets 512
Bellergal-S Tablets 2250
Donnatal 2060
Donnatal Extentabs 2061
Donnatal Tablets 2060
Phenobarbital Elixir and Tablets ... 1469
Quadrinal Tablets 1350

Phensuximide (Increased dosage of anticonvulsant may be required). Products include:

Milontin Kapseals 1920

Phenytoin (Increased dosage of anticonvulsant may be required). Products include:

Dilantin Infatabs 1908
Dilantin-125 Suspension 1911

Phenytoin Sodium (Increased dosage of anticonvulsant may be required). Products include:

Dilantin Kapseals 1906
Dilantin Parenteral 1910

Prazepam (Potentiation of both drugs).

No products indexed under this heading.

Primidone (Increased dosage of anticonvulsant may be required). Products include:

Mysoline 2754

Prochlorperazine (Potentiation of both drugs). Products include:

Compazine 2470

Promethazine Hydrochloride (Potentiation of both drugs). Products include:

Mepergan Injection 2753
Phenergan with Codeine 2777
Phenergan with Dextromethorphan 2778
Phenergan Injection 2773
Phenergan Suppositories 2775
Phenergan Syrup 2774
Phenergan Tablets 2775
Phenergan VC 2779
Phenergan VC with Codeine 2781

Propofol (Potentiation of both drugs). Products include:

Diprivan Injection 2833

Propoxyphene Hydrochloride (Potentiation of both drugs). Products include:

Darvon 1435
Wygesic Tablets 2827

Propoxyphene Napsylate (Potentiation of both drugs). Products include:

Darvon-N/Darvocet-N 1433

Quazepam (Potentiation of both drugs). Products include:

Doral Tablets 2664

Risperidone (Potentiation of both drugs). Products include:

Risperdal 1301

Secobarbital Sodium (Potentiation of both drugs). Products include:

Seconal Sodium Pulvules 1474

Sufentanil Citrate (Potentiation of both drugs). Products include:

Sufenta Injection 1309

Temazepam (Potentiation of both drugs). Products include:

Restoril Capsules 2284

Thiamylal Sodium (Potentiation of both drugs).

No products indexed under this heading.

Thioridazine Hydrochloride (Potentiation of both drugs). Products include:

Mellaril 2269

Thiothixene (Potentiation of both drugs). Products include:

Navane Capsules and Concentrate 2201
Navane Intramuscular 2202

Triazolam (Potentiation of both drugs). Products include:

Halcion Tablets 2611

Trifluoperazine Hydrochloride (Potentiation of both drugs). Products include:

Stelazine 2514

Trimethadione (Increased dosage of anticonvulsant may be required).

No products indexed under this heading.

Valproic Acid (Increased dosage of anticonvulsant may be required). Products include:

Depakene 413

Zolpidem Tartrate (Potentiation of both drugs). Products include:

Ambien Tablets 2416

Food Interactions

Alcohol (Additive effects; hypotension).

TRILAFON INJECTION
(Perphenazine) **2389**
See Trilafon Concentrate

TRILAFON TABLETS
(Perphenazine) **2389**
See Trilafon Concentrate

TRI-LEVLEN 21 TABLETS
(Levonorgestrel, Ethinyl Estradiol) **651**
See Levlen 21 Tablets

TRI-LEVLEN 28 TABLETS
(Levonorgestrel, Ethinyl Estradiol) **651**
See Levlen 21 Tablets

TRILISATE LIQUID
(Choline Magnesium Trisalicylate) **2000**
May interact with corticosteroids, oral anticoagulants, oral hypoglycemic agents, insulin, carbonic anhydrase inhibitors, and certain other agents. Compounds in these categories include:

Acarbose (Enhanced hypoglycemic effect).

No products indexed under this heading.

Acetazolamide (Competition for protein binding sites). Products include:

Diamox Sequels (Sustained Release) 1373

Diamox Sequels (Sustained Release) .... ◉ 319
Diamox Tablets 1372
Diamox Tablets .... ◉ 317

Allopurinol (Decreased efficacy of uricosuric agents). Products include:

Zyloprim Tablets 1226

Betamethasone Acetate (Reduces plasma salicylate levels by increasing renal elimination). Products include:

Celestone Soluspan Suspension 2347

Betamethasone Sodium Phosphate (Reduces plasma salicylate levels by increasing renal elimination). Products include:

Celestone Soluspan Suspension 2347

Chlorpropamide (Enhanced hypoglycemic effect). Products include:

Diabinese Tablets 1935

Cortisone Acetate (Reduces plasma salicylate levels by increasing renal elimination). Products include:

Cortone Acetate Sterile Suspension 1623
Cortone Acetate Tablets 1624

Dexamethasone (Reduces plasma salicylate levels by increasing renal elimination). Products include:

AK-Trol Ointment & Suspension .... ◉ 205
Decadron Elixir 1633
Decadron Tablets 1635
Decaspray Topical Aerosol 1648
Dexacidin Ointment .... ◉ 263
Maxitrol Ophthalmic Ointment and Suspension .... ◉ 224
TobraDex Ophthalmic Suspension and Ointment 473

Dexamethasone Acetate (Reduces plasma salicylate levels by increasing renal elimination). Products include:

Dalalone D.P. Injectable 1011
Decadron-LA Sterile Suspension 1646

Dexamethasone Sodium Phosphate (Reduces plasma salicylate levels by increasing renal elimination). Products include:

Decadron Phosphate Injection 1637
Decadron Phosphate Respihaler 1642
Decadron Phosphate Sterile Ophthalmic Ointment 1641
Decadron Phosphate Sterile Ophthalmic Solution 1642
Decadron Phosphate Topical Cream 1644
Decadron Phosphate Turbinaire 1645
Decadron Phosphate with Xylocaine Injection, Sterile 1639
Dexacort Phosphate in Respihaler.. 458
Dexacort Phosphate in Turbinaire .. 459
NeoDecadron Sterile Ophthalmic Ointment 1712
NeoDecadron Sterile Ophthalmic Solution 1713
NeoDecadron Topical Cream 1714

Dichlorphenamide (Competition for protein binding sites). Products include:

Daranide Tablets 1633

Dicumarol (Potential exists for increased levels of unbound anticoagulant with the concurrent use).

No products indexed under this heading.

Divalproex Sodium (Competition for protein binding sites). Products include:

Depakote Tablets 415

Dorzolamide Hydrochloride (Competition for protein binding sites). Products include:

Trusopt Sterile Ophthalmic Solution 1760

Fludrocortisone Acetate (Reduces plasma salicylate levels by increasing renal elimination). Products include:

Florinef Acetate Tablets 505

IMPORTANT NOTE: Always consult each drug listing in the patient's regimen for possible interactions.

Glipizide (Enhanced hypoglycemic effect). Products include:
- Glucotrol Tablets 1967
- Glucotrol XL Extended Release Tablets 1968

Glyburide (Enhanced hypoglycemic effect). Products include:
- DiaBeta Tablets 1239
- Glynase PresTab Tablets 2609
- Micronase Tablets 2623

Heparin Calcium (Use cautiously).
- No products indexed under this heading.

Heparin Sodium (Use cautiously). Products include:
- Heparin Lock Flush Solution 2725
- Heparin Sodium Injection 2726
- Heparin Sodium Injection, USP, Sterile Solution 2615
- Heparin Sodium Vials 1441

Hydrocortisone (Reduces plasma salicylate levels by increasing renal elimination). Products include:
- Anusol-HC Cream 2.5% 1896
- Aquanil HC Lotion 1931
- Bactine Hydrocortisone Anti-Itch Cream ..... ▣ 709
- Caldecort Anti-Itch Hydrocortisone Spray ..... ▣ 631
- Cortaid ..... ▣ 836
- CORTENEMA 2535
- Cortisporin Ointment 1085
- Cortisporin Ophthalmic Ointment Sterile 1085
- Cortisporin Ophthalmic Suspension Sterile 1086
- Cortisporin Otic Solution Sterile 1087
- Cortisporin Otic Suspension Sterile 1088
- Cortizone-5 ..... ▣ 831
- Cortizone-10 ..... ▣ 831
- Hydrocortone Tablets 1672
- Hytone 907
- Massengill Medicated Soft Cloth Towelettes 2458
- PediOtic Suspension Sterile 1153
- Preparation H Hydrocortisone 1% Cream ..... ▣ 872
- ProctoCream-HC 2.5% 2408
- VōSoL HC Otic Solution 2678

Hydrocortisone Acetate (Reduces plasma salicylate levels by increasing renal elimination). Products include:
- Analpram-HC Rectal Cream 1% and 2.5% 977
- Anusol HC-1 Anti-Itch Hydrocortisone Ointment ..... ▣ 847
- Anusol-HC Suppositories 1897
- Caldecort ..... ▣ 631
- Carmol HC 924
- Coly-Mycin S Otic w/Neomycin & Hydrocortisone 1906
- Cortaid ..... ▣ 836
- Cortifoam 2396
- Cortisporin Cream 1084
- Epifoam 2399
- Hydrocortone Acetate Sterile Suspension 1669
- Mantadil Cream 1135
- Nupercainal Hydrocortisone 1% Cream ..... ▣ 645
- Ophthocort ..... ⊙ 311
- Pramosone Cream, Lotion & Ointment 978
- ProctoCream-HC 2408
- ProctoFoam-HC 2409
- Terra-Cortril Ophthalmic Suspension 2210

Hydrocortisone Sodium Phosphate (Reduces plasma salicylate levels by increasing renal elimination). Products include:
- Hydrocortone Phosphate Injection, Sterile 1670

Hydrocortisone Sodium Succinate (Reduces plasma salicylate levels by increasing renal elimination). Products include:
- Solu-Cortef Sterile Powder 2641

Insulin, Human (Insulin-treated diabetics on high doses of salicylates should be monitored for enhanced hypoglycemic response).
- No products indexed under this heading.

Insulin, Human Isophane Suspension (Insulin-treated diabetics on high doses of salicylates should be monitored for enhanced hypoglycemic response). Products include:
- Novolin N Human Insulin 10 ml Vials 1795

Insulin, Human NPH (Insulin-treated diabetics on high doses of salicylates should be monitored for enhanced hypoglycemic response). Products include:
- Humulin N, 100 Units 1448
- Novolin N PenFill Cartridges Durable Insulin Delivery System 1798
- Novolin N Prefilled Syringe Disposable Insulin Delivery System 1798

Insulin, Human Regular (Insulin-treated diabetics on high doses of salicylates should be monitored for enhanced hypoglycemic response). Products include:
- Humulin R, 100 Units 1449
- Novolin R Human Insulin 10 ml Vials 1795
- Novolin R PenFill Cartridges Durable Insulin Delivery System 1798
- Novolin R Prefilled Syringe Disposable Insulin Delivery System 1798
- Velosulin BR Human Insulin 10 ml Vials 1795

Insulin, Human, Zinc Suspension (Insulin-treated diabetics on high doses of salicylates should be monitored for enhanced hypoglycemic response). Products include:
- Humulin L, 100 Units 1446
- Humulin U, 100 Units 1450
- Novolin L Human Insulin 10 ml Vials 1795

Insulin, NPH (Insulin-treated diabetics on high doses of salicylates should be monitored for enhanced hypoglycemic response). Products include:
- NPH, 100 Units 1450
- Pork NPH, 100 Units 1452
- Purified Pork NPH Isophane Insulin 1801

Insulin, Regular (Insulin-treated diabetics on high doses of salicylates should be monitored for enhanced hypoglycemic response). Products include:
- Regular, 100 Units 1450
- Pork Regular, 100 Units 1452
- Pork Regular (Concentrated), 500 Units 1453
- Purified Pork Regular Insulin 1801

Insulin, Zinc Crystals (Insulin-treated diabetics on high doses of salicylates should be monitored for enhanced hypoglycemic response). Products include:
- NPH, 100 Units 1450

Insulin, Zinc Suspension (Insulin-treated diabetics on high doses of salicylates should be monitored for enhanced hypoglycemic response). Products include:
- Iletin I 1450
- Lente, 100 Units 1450
- Iletin II 1452
- Pork Lente, 100 Units 1452
- Purified Pork Lente Insulin 1801

Metformin Hydrochloride (Enhanced hypoglycemic effect). Products include:
- Glucophage 752

Methazolamide (Competition for protein binding sites). Products include:
- Glauctabs ..... ⊙ 208
- MZM ..... ⊙ 267
- Neptazane Tablets 1388
- Neptazane Tablets ..... ⊙ 320

Methotrexate Sodium (Increased methotrexate effects). Products include:
- Methotrexate Sodium Tablets, Injection, for Injection and LPF Injection 1275

Methylprednisolone (Increased risk of gastrointestinal ulceration). Products include:
- Medrol 2621

Methylprednisolone Acetate (Reduces plasma salicylate levels by increasing renal elimination). Products include:
- Depo-Medrol Single-Dose Vial 2600
- Depo-Medrol Sterile Aqueous Suspension 2597

Methylprednisolone Sodium Succinate (Reduces plasma salicylate levels by increasing renal elimination). Products include:
- Solu-Medrol Sterile Powder 2643

Phenylbutazone (Increased risk of gastrointestinal ulceration).
- No products indexed under this heading.

Phenytoin (Competition for protein binding sites). Products include:
- Dilantin Infatabs 1908
- Dilantin-125 Suspension 1911

Phenytoin Sodium (Competition for protein binding sites). Products include:
- Dilantin Kapseals 1906
- Dilantin Parenteral 1910

Prednisolone Acetate (Reduces plasma salicylate levels by increasing renal elimination). Products include:
- AK-CIDE ..... ⊙ 202
- AK-CIDE Ointment ..... ⊙ 202
- Blephamide Liquifilm Sterile Ophthalmic Suspension 476
- Blephamide Ointment ..... ⊙ 237
- Econopred & Econopred Plus Ophthalmic Suspensions ..... ⊙ 217
- Poly-Pred Liquifilm ..... ⊙ 248
- Pred Forte ..... ⊙ 250
- Pred Mild ..... ⊙ 253
- Pred-G Liquifilm Sterile Ophthalmic Suspension ..... ⊙ 251
- Pred-G S.O.P. Sterile Ophthalmic Ointment ..... ⊙ 252
- Vasocidin Ointment ..... ⊙ 268

Prednisolone Sodium Phosphate (Reduces plasma salicylate levels by increasing renal elimination). Products include:
- AK-Pred ..... ⊙ 204
- Hydeltrasol Injection, Sterile 1665
- Inflamase ..... ⊙ 265
- Pediapred Oral Liquid 995
- Vasocidin Ophthalmic Solution ..... ⊙ 270

Prednisolone Tebutate (Reduces plasma salicylate levels by increasing renal elimination). Products include:
- Hydeltra-T.B.A. Sterile Suspension 1667

Prednisone (Reduces plasma salicylate levels by increasing renal elimination). Products include:
- Deltasone Tablets 2595

Probenecid (Decreased efficacy of uricosuric agents). Products include:
- Benemid Tablets 1611
- ColBENEMID Tablets 1622

Sulfinpyrazone (Decreased efficacy of uricosuric agents). Products include:
- Anturane 807

Tolazamide (Enhanced hypoglycemic effect).
- No products indexed under this heading.

Tolbutamide (Enhanced hypoglycemic effect).
- No products indexed under this heading.

Triamcinolone (Reduces plasma salicylate levels by increasing renal elimination). Products include:
- Aristocort Tablets 1022

Triamcinolone Acetonide (Reduces plasma salicylate levels by increasing renal elimination). Products include:
- Aristocort A 0.025% Cream 1027
- Aristocort A 0.5% Cream 1031
- Aristocort A 0.1% Cream 1029
- Aristocort A 0.1% Ointment 1030
- Azmacort Oral Inhaler 2011
- Nasacort Nasal Inhaler 2024

Triamcinolone Diacetate (Reduces plasma salicylate levels by increasing renal elimination). Products include:
- Aristocort Suspension (Forte Parenteral) 1027
- Aristocort Suspension (Intralesional) 1025

Triamcinolone Hexacetonide (Reduces plasma salicylate levels by increasing renal elimination). Products include:
- Aristospan Suspension (Intra-articular) 1033
- Aristospan Suspension (Intralesional) 1032

Valproic Acid (Competition for protein binding sites). Products include:
- Depakene 413

Warfarin Sodium (Potential exists for increased levels of unbound anticoagulant with the concurrent use). Products include:
- Coumadin 926

Food Interactions

Alcohol (Increased risk of gastrointestinal ulceration).

Food that lowers urinary pH (Decreases urinary salicylate excretion & increases plasma levels).

Food that raises urinary pH (Enhances renal salicylate clearance & diminishes plasma salicylate concentration).

TRILISATE TABLETS

(Choline Magnesium Trisalicylate) 2000

See **Trilisate Liquid**

TRIMPEX TABLETS

(Trimethoprim) 2163

May interact with:

Phenytoin (Possible excessive phenytoin effect). Products include:
- Dilantin Infatabs 1908
- Dilantin-125 Suspension 1911

Phenytoin Sodium (Possible excessive phenytoin effect). Products include:
- Dilantin Kapseals 1906
- Dilantin Parenteral 1910

TRINALIN REPETABS TABLETS

(Azatadine Maleate, Pseudoephedrine Sulfate) 1330

May interact with monoamine oxidase inhibitors, tricyclic antidepressants, barbiturates, central nervous system depressants, veratrum alkaloids, antacids, oral anticoagulants, beta blockers, and certain other agents. Compounds in these categories include:

Acebutolol Hydrochloride (Effect not specified). Products include:
- Sectral Capsules 2807

Alfentanil Hydrochloride (Additive effect). Products include:
- Alfenta Injection 1286

Alprazolam (Additive effect). Products include:
- Xanax Tablets 2649

(▣ Described in PDR For Nonprescription Drugs) (⊙ Described in PDR For Ophthalmology)

Interactions Index

Aluminum Carbonate Gel (Increased rate of absorption of pseudoephedrine). Products include:

Basaljel 2703

Aluminum Hydroxide (Increased rate of absorption of pseudoephedrine). Products include:

ALternaGEL Liquid 1316
Maximum Strength Ascriptin .... ⊕ 630
Cama Arthritis Pain Reliever .... ⊕ 785
Gaviscon Extra Strength Relief Formula Antacid Tablets .... ⊕ 819
Gaviscon Extra Strength Relief Formula Liquid Antacid .... ⊕ 819
Gaviscon Liquid Antacid .... ⊕ 820
Gelusil Liquid & Tablets .... ⊕ 855
Maalox Heartburn Relief Suspension .... ⊕ 642
Maalox Heartburn Relief Tablets .... ⊕ 641
Maalox Magnesia and Alumina Oral Suspension .... ⊕ 642
Maalox Plus Tablets .... ⊕ 643
Extra Strength Maalox Antacid Plus Antigas Liquid and Tablets ⊕ 638
Tempo Soft Antacid .... ⊕ 835

Aluminum Hydroxide Gel (Increased rate of absorption of pseudoephedrine). Products include:

ALternaGEL Liquid .... ⊕ 659
Aludrox Oral Suspension 2695
Amphojel Suspension 2695
Amphojel Suspension without Flavor 2695
Amphojel Tablets 2695
Arthritis Pain Ascriptin .... ⊕ 631
Regular Strength Ascriptin Tablets .... ⊕ 629
Gaviscon Antacid Tablets .... ⊕ 819
Gaviscon-2 Antacid Tablets .... ⊕ 820
Mylanta Liquid 1317
Mylanta Tablets .... ⊕ 660
Mylanta Double Strength Liquid 1317
Mylanta Double Strength Tablets .. ⊕ 660
Nephrox Suspension .... ⊕ 655

Aluminum Hydroxide Gel, Dried (Increased rate of absorption of pseudoephedrine).

Amitriptyline Hydrochloride (Additive effect). Products include:

Elavil 2838
Endep Tablets 2174
Etrafon 2355
Limbitrol 2180
Triavil Tablets 1757

Amoxapine (Additive effect). Products include:

Asendin Tablets 1369

Aprobarbital (Additive effect).

No products indexed under this heading.

Atenolol (Effect not specified). Products include:

Tenoretic Tablets 2845
Tenormin Tablets and I.V. Injection 2847

Betaxolol Hydrochloride (Effect not specified). Products include:

Betoptic Ophthalmic Solution 469
Betoptic S Ophthalmic Suspension 471
Kerlone Tablets 2436

Bisoprolol Fumarate (Effect not specified). Products include:

Zebeta Tablets 1413
Ziac 1415

Buprenorphine (Additive effect). Products include:

Buprenex Injectable 2006

Buspirone Hydrochloride (Additive effect). Products include:

BuSpar 737

Butabarbital (Additive effect).

No products indexed under this heading.

Butalbital (Additive effect). Products include:

Esgic-plus Tablets 1013
Fioricet Tablets 2258
Fioricet with Codeine Capsules 2260
Fiorinal Capsules 2261
Fiorinal with Codeine Capsules 2262
Fiorinal Tablets 2261
Phrenilin 785
Sedapap Tablets 50 mg/650 mg .. 1543

Carteolol Hydrochloride (Effect not specified). Products include:

Cartrol Tablets 410
Ocupress Ophthalmic Solution, 1 % Sterile .... ⊙ 309

Chlordiazepoxide (Additive effect). Products include:

Libritabs Tablets 2177
Limbitrol 2180

Chlordiazepoxide Hydrochloride (Additive effect). Products include:

Librax Capsules 2176
Librium Capsules 2178
Librium Injectable 2179

Chlorpromazine (Additive effect). Products include:

Thorazine Suppositories 2523

Chlorprothixene (Additive effect).

No products indexed under this heading.

Chlorprothixene Hydrochloride (Additive effect).

No products indexed under this heading.

Clomipramine Hydrochloride (Additive effect). Products include:

Anafranil Capsules 803

Clorazepate Dipotassium (Additive effect). Products include:

Tranxene 451

Clozapine (Additive effect). Products include:

Clozaril Tablets 2252

Codeine Phosphate (Additive effect). Products include:

Actifed with Codeine Cough Syrup.. 1067
Brontex 1981
Deconsal C Expectorant Syrup 456
Deconsal Pediatric Syrup 457
Dimetane-DC Cough Syrup 2059
Empirin with Codeine Tablets 1093
Fioricet with Codeine Capsules 2260
Fiorinal with Codeine Capsules 2262
Isoclor Expectorant 990
Novahistine DH 2462
Novahistine Expectorant 2463
Nucofed 2051
Phenergan with Codeine 2777
Phenergan VC with Codeine 2781
Robitussin A-C Syrup 2073
Robitussin-DAC Syrup 2074
Ryna .... ⊕ 841
Soma Compound w/Codeine Tablets 2676
Tussi-Organidin NR Liquid and S NR Liquid 2677
Tylenol with Codeine 1583

Cryptenamine Preparations (Antihypertensive effects of veratrum alkaloids reduced).

Desflurane (Additive effect). Products include:

Suprane 1813

Desipramine Hydrochloride (Additive effect). Products include:

Norpramin Tablets 1526

Deslanoside (Increased ectopic pacemaker activity).

No products indexed under this heading.

Dezocine (Additive effect). Products include:

Dalgan Injection 538

Diazepam (Additive effect). Products include:

Dizac 1809
Valium Injectable 2182
Valium Tablets 2183
Valrelease Capsules 2169

Dicumarol (Action of oral anticoagulants inhibited).

No products indexed under this heading.

Digitoxin (Increased ectopic pacemaker activity). Products include:

Crystodigin Tablets 1433

Digoxin (Increased ectopic pacemaker activity). Products include:

Lanoxicaps 1117

Lanoxin Elixir Pediatric 1120
Lanoxin Injection 1123
Lanoxin Injection Pediatric 1126
Lanoxin Tablets 1128

Dihydroxyaluminum Sodium Carbonate (Increased rate of absorption of pseudoephedrine).

No products indexed under this heading.

Doxepin Hydrochloride (Additive effect). Products include:

Sinequan 2205
Zonalon Cream 1055

Droperidol (Additive effect). Products include:

Inapsine Injection 1296

Enflurane (Additive effect).

No products indexed under this heading.

Esmolol Hydrochloride (Effect not specified). Products include:

Brevibloc Injection 1808

Estazolam (Additive effect). Products include:

ProSom Tablets 449

Ethchlorvynol (Additive effect). Products include:

Placidyl Capsules 448

Ethinamate (Additive effect).

No products indexed under this heading.

Fentanyl (Additive effect). Products include:

Duragesic Transdermal System 1288

Fentanyl Citrate (Additive effect). Products include:

Sublimaze Injection 1307

Fluphenazine Decanoate (Additive effect). Products include:

Prolixin Decanoate 509

Fluphenazine Enanthate (Additive effect). Products include:

Prolixin Enanthate 509

Fluphenazine Hydrochloride (Additive effect). Products include:

Prolixin 509

Flurazepam Hydrochloride (Additive effect). Products include:

Dalmane Capsules 2173

Furazolidone (Hypertensive crisis; effects of antihistamines prolonged and intensified; concurrent use is contraindicated). Products include:

Furoxone 2046

Glutethimide (Additive effect).

No products indexed under this heading.

Haloperidol (Additive effect). Products include:

Haldol Injection, Tablets and Concentrate 1575

Haloperidol Decanoate (Additive effect). Products include:

Haldol Decanoate 1577

Hydrocodone Bitartrate (Additive effect). Products include:

Anexsia 5/500 Elixir 1781
Anexia Tablets 1782
Codiclear DH Syrup 791
Deconamine CX Cough and Cold Liquid and Tablets 1319
Duratuss HD Elixir 2565
Hycodan Tablets and Syrup 930
Hycomine Compound Tablets 932
Hycomine 931
Hycotuss Expectorant Syrup 933
Hydrocet Capsules 782
Lorcet 10/650 1018
Lortab 2566
Tussend 1783
Tussend Expectorant 1785
Vicodin Tablets 1356
Vicodin ES Tablets 1357
Vicodin Tuss Expectorant 1358
Zydone Capsules 949

Hydrocodone Polistirex (Additive effect). Products include:

Tussionex Pennkinetic Extended-Release Suspension 998

Hydroxyzine Hydrochloride (Additive effect). Products include:

Atarax Tablets & Syrup 2185
Marax Tablets & DF Syrup 2200
Vistaril Intramuscular Solution 2216

Imipramine Hydrochloride (Additive effect). Products include:

Tofranil Ampuls 854
Tofranil Tablets 856

Imipramine Pamoate (Additive effect). Products include:

Tofranil-PM Capsules 857

Isocarboxazid (Hypertensive crisis; effects of antihistamines prolonged and intensified; concurrent use is contraindicated).

No products indexed under this heading.

Isoflurane (Additive effect).

No products indexed under this heading.

Kaolin (Decreased rate of absorption of pseudoephedrine).

No products indexed under this heading.

Ketamine Hydrochloride (Additive effect).

No products indexed under this heading.

Labetalol Hydrochloride (Effect not specified). Products include:

Normodyne Injection 2377
Normodyne Tablets 2379
Trandate 1185

Levobunolol Hydrochloride (Effect not specified). Products include:

Betagan .... ⊙ 233

Levomethadyl Acetate Hydrochloride (Additive effect). Products include:

Orlamm 2239

Levorphanol Tartrate (Additive effect). Products include:

Levo-Dromoran 2129

Lorazepam (Additive effect). Products include:

Ativan Injection 2698
Ativan Tablets 2700

Loxapine Hydrochloride (Additive effect). Products include:

Loxitane 1378

Loxapine Succinate (Additive effect). Products include:

Loxitane Capsules 1378

Magaldrate (Increased rate of absorption of pseudoephedrine).

No products indexed under this heading.

Magnesium Hydroxide (Increased rate of absorption of pseudoephedrine). Products include:

Aludrox Oral Suspension 2695
Arthritis Pain Ascriptin .... ⊕ 631
Maximum Strength Ascriptin .... ⊕ 630
Regular Strength Ascriptin Tablets .... ⊕ 629
Di-Gel Antacid/Anti-Gas .... ⊕ 801
Gelusil Liquid & Tablets .... ⊕ 855
Maalox Magnesia and Alumina Oral Suspension .... ⊕ 642
Maalox Plus Tablets .... ⊕ 643
Extra Strength Maalox Antacid Plus Antigas Liquid and Tablets ⊕ 638
Mylanta Calcium Carbonate and Magnesium Hydroxide Tablets 1318
Mylanta Liquid 1317
Mylanta Tablets .... ⊕ 660
Mylanta Double Strength Liquid 1317
Mylanta Double Strength Tablets .. ⊕ 660
Phillips' Milk of Magnesia Liquid .... ⊕ 729
Rolaids Tablets .... ⊕ 843
Tempo Soft Antacid .... ⊕ 835

Magnesium Oxide (Increased rate of absorption of pseudoephedrine). Products include:

Beelith Tablets 639
Bufferin Analgesic Tablets and Caplets .... ⊕ 613
Caltrate PLUS .... ⊕ 665
Cama Arthritis Pain Reliever .... ⊕ 785

IMPORTANT NOTE: Always consult each drug listing in the patient's regimen for possible interactions.

Trinalin Interactions Index 1078

Mag-Ox 400 ... 668
Uro-Mag ... 668

Maprotiline Hydrochloride (Additive effect). Products include:
Ludiomil Tablets ... 843

Mecamylamine Hydrochloride (Antihypertensive effects of mecamylamine reduced). Products include:
Inversine Tablets ... 1686

Meperidine Hydrochloride (Additive effect). Products include:
Demerol ... 2308
Mepergan Injection ... 2753

Mephobarbital (Additive effect). Products include:
Mebaral Tablets ... 2322

Meprobamate (Additive effect). Products include:
Miltown Tablets ... 2672
PMB 200 and PMB 400 ... 2783

Mesoridazine Besylate (Additive effect). Products include:
Serentil ... 684

Methadone Hydrochloride (Additive effect). Products include:
Methadone Hydrochloride Oral Concentrate ... 2233
Methadone Hydrochloride Oral Solution & Tablets ... 2235

Methohexital Sodium (Additive effect). Products include:
Brevital Sodium Vials ... 1429

Methotrimeprazine (Additive effect). Products include:
Levoprome ... 1274

Methoxyflurane (Additive effect).
No products indexed under this heading.

Methyldopa (Antihypertensive effects of methyldopa reduced). Products include:
Aldoclor Tablets ... 1598
Aldomet Oral ... 1600
Aldoril Tablets ... 1604

Methyldopate Hydrochloride (Antihypertensive effects of methyldopa reduced). Products include:
Aldomet Ester HCl Injection ... 1602

Metipranolol Hydrochloride (Effect not specified). Products include:
OptiPranolol (Metipranolol 0.3%) Sterile Ophthalmic Solution ... ⊙ 258

Metoprolol Succinate (Effect not specified). Products include:
Toprol-XL Tablets ... 565

Metoprolol Tartrate (Not specified). Products include:
Lopressor Ampuls ... 830
Lopressor HCT Tablets ... 832
Lopressor Tablets ... 830

Midazolam Hydrochloride (Additive effect). Products include:
Versed Injection ... 2170

Molindone Hydrochloride (Additive effect). Products include:
Moban Tablets and Concentrate ... 1048

Morphine Sulfate (Additive effect). Products include:
Astramorph/PF Injection, USP (Preservative-Free) ... 535
Duramorph ... 962
Infumorph 200 and Infumorph 500 Sterile Solutions ... 965
MS Contin Tablets ... 1994
MSIR ... 1997
Oramorph SR (Morphine Sulfate Sustained Release Tablets) ... 2236
RMS Suppositories ... 2657
Roxanol ... 2243

Nadolol (Effect not specified).
No products indexed under this heading.

Nortriptyline Hydrochloride (Additive effect). Products include:
Pamelor ... 2280

Opium Alkaloids (Additive effect).
No products indexed under this heading.

Oxazepam (Additive effect). Products include:
Serax Capsules ... 2810
Serax Tablets ... 2810

Oxycodone Hydrochloride (Additive effect). Products include:
Percocet Tablets ... 938
Percodan Tablets ... 939
Percodan-Demi Tablets ... 940
Roxicodone Tablets, Oral Solution & Intensol (Oxycodone) ... 2244
Tylox Capsules ... 1584

Penbutolol Sulfate (Effect not specified). Products include:
Levatol ... 2403

Pentobarbital Sodium (Additive effect). Products include:
Nembutal Sodium Capsules ... 436
Nembutal Sodium Solution ... 438
Nembutal Sodium Suppositories ... 440

Perphenazine (Additive effect). Products include:
Etrafon ... 2355
Triavil Tablets ... 1757
Trilafon ... 2389

Phenelzine Sulfate (Hypertensive crisis; effects of antihistamines prolonged and intensified; concurrent use is contraindicated). Products include:
Nardil ... 1920

Phenobarbital (Additive effect). Products include:
Arco-Lase Plus Tablets ... 512
Bellergal-S Tablets ... 2250
Donnatal ... 2060
Donnatal Extentabs ... 2061
Donnatal Tablets ... 2060
Phenobarbital Elixir and Tablets ... 1469
Quadrinal Tablets ... 1350

Pindolol (Effect not specified). Products include:
Visken Tablets ... 2299

Prazepam (Additive effect).
No products indexed under this heading.

Prochlorperazine (Additive effect). Products include:
Compazine ... 2470

Promethazine Hydrochloride (Additive effect). Products include:
Mepergan Injection ... 2753
Phenergan with Codeine ... 2777
Phenergan with Dextromethorphan ... 2778
Phenergan Injection ... 2773
Phenergan Suppositories ... 2775
Phenergan Syrup ... 2774
Phenergan Tablets ... 2775
Phenergan VC ... 2779
Phenergan VC with Codeine ... 2781

Propofol (Additive effect). Products include:
Diprivan Injection ... 2833

Propoxyphene Hydrochloride (Additive effect). Products include:
Darvon ... 1435
Wygesic Tablets ... 2827

Propoxyphene Napsylate (Additive effect). Products include:
Darvon-N/Darvocet-N ... 1433

Propranolol Hydrochloride (Effect not specified). Products include:
Inderal ... 2728
Inderal LA Long Acting Capsules ... 2730
Inderide Tablets ... 2732
Inderide LA Long Acting Capsules ... 2734

Protriptyline Hydrochloride (Additive effect). Products include:
Vivactil Tablets ... 1774

Quazepam (Additive effect). Products include:
Doral Tablets ... 2664

Reserpine (Antihypertensive effects of reserpine reduced). Products include:
Diupres Tablets ... 1650
Hydropres Tablets ... 1675
Ser-Ap-Es Tablets ... 849

Risperidone (Additive effect). Products include:
Risperdal ... 1301

Secobarbital Sodium (Additive effect). Products include:
Seconal Sodium Pulvules ... 1474

Selegiline Hydrochloride (Hypertensive crisis; effects of antihistamines prolonged and intensified; concurrent use is contraindicated). Products include:
Eldepryl Tablets ... 2550

Sotalol Hydrochloride (Effect not specified). Products include:
Betapace Tablets ... 641

Sufentanil Citrate (Additive effect). Products include:
Sufenta Injection ... 1309

Temazepam (Additive effect). Products include:
Restoril Capsules ... 2284

Thiamylal Sodium (Additive effect).
No products indexed under this heading.

Thioridazine Hydrochloride (Additive effect). Products include:
Mellaril ... 2269

Thiothixene (Additive effect). Products include:
Navane Capsules and Concentrate ... 2201
Navane Intramuscular ... 2202

Timolol Hemihydrate (Effect not specified). Products include:
Betimol 0.25%, 0.5% ... ⊙ 261

Timolol Maleate (Effect not specified). Products include:
Blocadren Tablets ... 1614
Timolide Tablets ... 1748
Timoptic in Ocudose ... 1753
Timoptic Sterile Ophthalmic Solution ... 1751
Timoptic-XE ... 1755

Tranylcypromine Sulfate (Hypertensive crisis; effects of antihistamines prolonged and intensified; concurrent use is contraindicated). Products include:
Parnate Tablets ... 2503

Triazolam (Additive effect). Products include:
Halcion Tablets ... 2611

Trifluoperazine Hydrochloride (Additive effect). Products include:
Stelazine ... 2514

Trimipramine Maleate (Additive effect). Products include:
Surmontil Capsules ... 2811

Warfarin Sodium (Action of oral anticoagulants inhibited). Products include:
Coumadin ... 926

Zolpidem Tartrate (Additive effect). Products include:
Ambien Tablets ... 2416

Food Interactions

Alcohol (Additive effect).

TRI-NORINYL 21-DAY TABLETS
(Norethindrone, Ethinyl Estradiol) ... 2164
See **Brevicon 21-Day Tablets**

TRI-NORINYL 28-DAY TABLETS
(Norethindrone, Ethinyl Estradiol) ... 2164
See **Brevicon 21-Day Tablets**

TRINSICON CAPSULES
(Vitamins with Iron) ... 2570
None cited in PDR database.

TRIOSTAT INJECTION
(Liothyronine Sodium) ... 2530
May interact with oral anticoagulants, insulin, oral hypoglycemic agents, estrogens, oral contraceptives, tricyclic antidepressants, cardiac glycosides, vasopressors, and certain other agents. Compounds in these categories include:

Acarbose (Potential for increased oral hypoglycemic requirements).
No products indexed under this heading.

Amitriptyline Hydrochloride (Increased receptor sensitivity and enhanced antidepressant activity). Products include:
Elavil ... 2838
Endep Tablets ... 2174
Etrafon ... 2355
Limbitrol ... 2180
Triavil Tablets ... 1757

Amoxapine (Increased receptor sensitivity and enhanced antidepressant activity). Products include:
Asendin Tablets ... 1369

Chlorotrianisene (Increases serum thyroxine-binding globulin).
No products indexed under this heading.

Chlorpropamide (Potential for increased oral hypoglycemic requirements). Products include:
Diabinese Tablets ... 1935

Clomipramine Hydrochloride (Increased receptor sensitivity and enhanced antidepressant activity). Products include:
Anafranil Capsules ... 803

Desipramine Hydrochloride (Increased receptor sensitivity and enhanced antidepressant activity). Products include:
Norpramin Tablets ... 1526

Deslanoside (Toxic effects of digitalis potentiated).
No products indexed under this heading.

Desogestrel (Increases serum thyroxine-binding globulin). Products include:
Desogen Tablets ... 1817
Ortho-Cept ... 1851

Dicumarol (Increased catabolism of vitamin k-dependent clotting factors).
No products indexed under this heading.

Dienestrol (Increases serum thyroxine-binding globulin). Products include:
Ortho Dienestrol Cream ... 1866

Diethylstilbestrol (Increases serum thyroxine-binding globulin). Products include:
Diethylstilbestrol Tablets ... 1437

Digitoxin (Toxic effects of digitalis potentiated). Products include:
Crystodigin Tablets ... 1433

Digoxin (Toxic effects of digitalis potentiated). Products include:
Lanoxicaps ... 1117
Lanoxin Elixir Pediatric ... 1120
Lanoxin Injection ... 1123
Lanoxin Injection Pediatric ... 1126
Lanoxin Tablets ... 1128

Dopamine Hydrochloride (Increased adrenergic effect).
No products indexed under this heading.

Doxepin Hydrochloride (Increased receptor sensitivity and enhanced antidepressant activity). Products include:
Sinequan ... 2205
Zonalon Cream ... 1055

Epinephrine Bitartrate (Increased adrenergic effect). Products include:
Bronkaid Mist Suspension ... ▣ 718
Sensorcaine-MPF with Epinephrine Injection ... 559

(▣ Described in PDR For Nonprescription Drugs) (⊙ Described in PDR For Ophthalmology)

Interactions Index

Epinephrine Hydrochloride (Increased adrenergic effect). Products include:

Ana-Kit Anaphylaxis Emergency Treatment Kit 617

Estradiol (Increases serum thyroxine-binding globulin). Products include:

Climara Transdermal System 645
Estrace Cream and Tablets 749
Estraderm Transdermal System 824

Estrogens, Conjugated (Increases serum thyroxine-binding globulin). Products include:

PMB 200 and PMB 400 2783
Premarin Intravenous 2787
Premarin with Methyltestosterone.. 2794
Premarin Tablets 2789
Premarin Vaginal Cream.................. 2791
Premphase 2797
Prempro 2801

Estrogens, Esterified (Increases serum thyroxine-binding globulin). Products include:

ESTRATAB Tablets (0.3, 0.625, 1.25, 2.5 mg) 2536
Estratest 2539
Menest Tablets 2494

Estropipate (Increases serum thyroxine-binding globulin). Products include:

Ogen Tablets 2627
Ogen Vaginal Cream.......................... 2630
Ortho-Est 1869

Ethinyl Estradiol (Increases serum thyroxine-binding globulin). Products include:

Brevicon.. 2088
Demulen 2428
Desogen Tablets.................................. 1817
Levlen/Tri-Levlen............................... 651
Lo/Ovral Tablets 2746
Lo/Ovral-28 Tablets........................... 2751
Modicon 1872
Nordette-21 Tablets............................ 2755
Nordette-28 Tablets............................ 2758
Norinyl 2088
Ortho-Cept 1851
Ortho-Cyclen/Ortho-Tri-Cyclen 1858
Ortho-Novum....................................... 1872
Ortho-Cyclen/Ortho Tri-Cyclen 1858
Ovcon 760
Ovral Tablets 2770
Ovral-28 Tablets 2770
Levlen/Tri-Levlen............................... 651
Tri-Norinyl... 2164
Triphasil-21 Tablets........................... 2814
Triphasil-28 Tablets........................... 2819

Ethynodiol Diacetate (Increases serum thyroxine-binding globulin). Products include:

Demulen 2428

Glipizide (Potential for increased oral hypoglycemic requirements). Products include:

Glucotrol Tablets 1967
Glucotrol XL Extended Release Tablets 1968

Glyburide (Potential for increased oral hypoglycemic requirements). Products include:

DiaBeta Tablets 1239
Glynase PresTab Tablets 2609
Micronase Tablets 2623

Imipramine Hydrochloride (Increased receptor sensitivity and enhanced antidepressant activity). Products include:

Tofranil Ampuls 854
Tofranil Tablets 856

Imipramine Pamoate (Increased receptor sensitivity and enhanced antidepressant activity). Products include:

Tofranil-PM Capsules........................ 857

Insulin, Human (Potential for increased insulin requirements).

No products indexed under this heading.

Insulin, Human Isophane Suspension (Potential for increased insulin requirements). Products include:

Novolin N Human Insulin 10 ml Vials.. 1795

Insulin, Human NPH (Potential for increased insulin requirements). Products include:

Humulin N, 100 Units 1448
Novolin N PenFill Cartridges Durable Insulin Delivery System 1798
Novolin N Prefilled Syringe Disposable Insulin Delivery System 1798

Insulin, Human Regular (Potential for increased insulin requirements). Products include:

Humulin R, 100 Units 1449
Novolin R Human Insulin 10 ml Vials.. 1795
Novolin R PenFill Cartridges Durable Insulin Delivery System 1798
Novolin R Prefilled Syringe Disposable Insulin Delivery System 1798
Velosulin BR Human Insulin 10 ml Vials.. 1795

Insulin, Human, Zinc Suspension (Potential for increased insulin requirements). Products include:

Humulin L, 100 Units 1446
Humulin U, 100 Units....................... 1450
Novolin L Human Insulin 10 ml Vials.. 1795

Insulin, NPH (Potential for increased insulin requirements). Products include:

NPH, 100 Units 1450
Pork NPH, 100 Units......................... 1452
Purified Pork NPH Isophane Insulin 1801

Insulin, Regular (Potential for increased insulin requirements). Products include:

Regular, 100 Units 1450
Pork Regular, 100 Units 1452
Pork Regular (Concentrated), 500 Units 1453
Purified Pork Regular Insulin 1801

Insulin, Zinc Crystals (Potential for increased insulin requirements). Products include:

NPH, 100 Units 1450

Insulin, Zinc Suspension (Potential for increased insulin requirements). Products include:

Iletin I 1450
Lente, 100 Units 1450
Iletin II.. 1452
Pork Lente, 100 Units....................... 1452
Purified Pork Lente Insulin 1801

Ketamine Hydrochloride (Potential for hypertension and tachycardia).

No products indexed under this heading.

Levonorgestrel (Increases serum thyroxine-binding globulin). Products include:

Levlen/Tri-Levlen............................... 651
Nordette-21 Tablets............................ 2755
Nordette-28 Tablets............................ 2758
Norplant System 2759
Levlen/Tri-Levlen............................... 651
Triphasil-21 Tablets........................... 2814
Triphasil-28 Tablets........................... 2819

Maprotiline Hydrochloride (Increased receptor sensitivity and enhanced antidepressant activity). Products include:

Ludiomil Tablets................................. 843

Mestranol (Increases serum thyroxine-binding globulin). Products include:

Norinyl 2088
Ortho-Novum....................................... 1872

Metaraminol Bitartrate (Increased adrenergic effect). Products include:

Aramine Injection............................... 1609

Metformin Hydrochloride (Potential for increased oral hypoglycemic requirements). Products include:

Glucophage 752

Methoxamine Hydrochloride (Increased adrenergic effect). Products include:

Vasoxyl Injection 1196

Norepinephrine Bitartrate (Increased adrenergic effect). Products include:

Levophed Bitartrate Injection........... 2315

Norethindrone (Increases serum thyroxine-binding globulin). Products include:

Brevicon.. 2088
Micronor Tablets 1872
Modicon 1872
Norinyl 2088
Nor-Q D Tablets 2135
Ortho-Novum....................................... 1872
Ovcon 760
Tri-Norinyl... 2164

Norethynodrel (Increases serum thyroxine-binding globulin).

No products indexed under this heading.

Norgestimate (Increases serum thyroxine-binding globulin). Products include:

Ortho-Cyclen/Ortho-Tri-Cyclen 1858
Ortho-Cyclen/Ortho Tri-Cyclen 1858

Norgestrel (Increases serum thyroxine-binding globulin). Products include:

Lo/Ovral Tablets 2746
Lo/Ovral-28 Tablets........................... 2751
Ovral Tablets 2770
Ovral-28 Tablets 2770
Ovrette Tablets................................... 2771

Nortriptyline Hydrochloride (Increased receptor sensitivity and enhanced antidepressant activity). Products include:

Pamelor 2280

Phenylephrine Hydrochloride (Increased adrenergic effect). Products include:

Atrohist Plus Tablets 454
Cerose DM .... ◆◻ 878
Comhist 2038
D.A. Chewable Tablets....................... 951
Deconsal Pediatric Capsules............. 454
Dura-Vent/DA Tablets 953
Entex Capsules 1986
Entex Liquid 1986
Extendryl 1005
4-Way Fast Acting Nasal Spray (regular & mentholated) .... ◆◻ 621
Hemorid For Women .... ◆◻ 834
Hycomine Compound Tablets 932
Neo-Synephrine Hydrochloride 1 % Carpuject.. 2324
Neo-Synephrine Hydrochloride 1 % Injection 2324
Neo-Synephrine Hydrochloride (Ophthalmic) 2325
Neo-Synephrine .... ◆◻ 726
Nōstril .... ◆◻ 644
Novahistine Elixir .... ◆◻ 823
Phenergan VC 2779
Phenergan VC with Codeine 2781
Preparation H .... ◆◻ 871
Tympagesic Ear Drops 2342
Vasosulf .... ⊙ 271
Vicks Sinex Nasal Spray and Ultra Fine Mist .... ◆◻ 765

Polyestradiol Phosphate (Increases serum thyroxine-binding globulin).

No products indexed under this heading.

Protriptyline Hydrochloride (Increased receptor sensitivity and enhanced antidepressant activity). Products include:

Vivactil Tablets 1774

Quinestrol (Increases serum thyroxine-binding globulin).

No products indexed under this heading.

Tolazamide (Potential for increased oral hypoglycemic requirements).

No products indexed under this heading.

Tolbutamide (Potential for increased oral hypoglycemic requirements).

No products indexed under this heading.

Trimipramine Maleate (Increased receptor sensitivity and enhanced antidepressant activity). Products include:

Surmontil Capsules............................. 2811

Warfarin Sodium (Increased catabolism of vitamin k-dependent clotting factors). Products include:

Coumadin 926

TRIPEDIA

(Diphtheria & Tetanus Toxoids w/Pertussis Vaccine Combined, Aluminum Potassium Sulfate Adsorbed) 892

May interact with anticoagulants, alkylating agents, cytotoxic drugs, corticosteroids, and immunosuppressive agents. Compounds in these categories include:

Azathioprine (An adequate immunologic response may not be obtained if used concurrently). Products include:

Imuran 1110

Betamethasone Acetate (Corticosteroids, used in greater than physiologic doses, may reduce the immune response to vaccine). Products include:

Celestone Soluspan Suspension 2347

Betamethasone Sodium Phosphate (Corticosteroids, used in greater than physiologic doses, may reduce the immune response to vaccine). Products include:

Celestone Soluspan Suspension 2347

Bleomycin Sulfate (May reduce the immune response to vaccine). Products include:

Blenoxane 692

Busulfan (May reduce the immune response to vaccine). Products include:

Myleran Tablets 1143

Carmustine (BCNU) (May reduce the immune response to vaccine). Products include:

BiCNU.. 691

Chlorambucil (May reduce the immune response to vaccine). Products include:

Leukeran Tablets 1133

Cortisone Acetate (Corticosteroids, used in greater than physiologic doses, may reduce the immune response to vaccine). Products include:

Cortone Acetate Sterile Suspension 1623
Cortone Acetate Tablets..................... 1624

Cyclophosphamide (May reduce the immune response to vaccine). Products include:

Cytoxan 694
NEOSAR Lyophilized/Neosar 1959

Cyclosporine (An adequate immunologic response may not be obtained if used concurrently). Products include:

Neoral.. 2276
Sandimmune 2286

Cytarabine (May reduce the immune response to vaccine). Products include:

Cytosar-U Sterile Powder 2592

IMPORTANT NOTE: Always consult each drug listing in the patient's regimen for possible interactions.

Tripedia | **Interactions Index** | **1080**

Dacarbazine (May reduce the immune response to vaccine). Products include:
- DTIC-Dome ... 600

Dalteparin Sodium (Concurrent use requires caution). Products include:
- Fragmin ... 1954

Daunorubicin Hydrochloride (May reduce the immune response to vaccine). Products include:
- Cerubidine ... 795

Dexamethasone (Corticosteroids, used in greater than physiologic doses, may reduce the immune response to vaccine). Products include:
- AK-Trol Ointment & Suspension ... ⊙ 205
- Decadron Elixir ... 1633
- Decadron Tablets ... 1635
- Decaspray Topical Aerosol ... 1648
- Dexacidin Ointment ... ⊙ 263
- Maxitrol Ophthalmic Ointment and Suspension ... ⊙ 224
- TobraDex Ophthalmic Suspension and Ointment ... 473

Dexamethasone Acetate (Corticosteroids, used in greater than physiologic doses, may reduce the immune response to vaccine). Products include:
- Dalalone D.P. Injectable ... 1011
- Decadron-LA Sterile Suspension ... 1646

Dexamethasone Sodium Phosphate (Corticosteroids, used in greater than physiologic doses, may reduce the immune response to vaccine). Products include:
- Decadron Phosphate Injection ... 1637
- Decadron Phosphate Respihaler ... 1642
- Decadron Phosphate Sterile Ophthalmic Ointment ... 1641
- Decadron Phosphate Sterile Ophthalmic Solution ... 1642
- Decadron Phosphate Topical Cream ... 1644
- Decadron Phosphate Turbinaire ... 1645
- Decadron Phosphate with Xylocaine Injection, Sterile ... 1639
- Dexacort Phosphate in Respihaler .. 458
- Dexacort Phosphate in Turbinaire .. 459
- NeoDecadron Sterile Ophthalmic Ointment ... 1712
- NeoDecadron Sterile Ophthalmic Solution ... 1713
- NeoDecadron Topical Cream ... 1714

Dicumarol (Concurrent use requires caution).
- No products indexed under this heading.

Doxorubicin Hydrochloride (May reduce the immune response to vaccine). Products include:
- Adriamycin PFS ... 1947
- Adriamycin RDF ... 1947
- Doxorubicin Astra ... 540
- Rubex ... 712

Enoxaparin (Concurrent use requires caution). Products include:
- Lovenox Injection ... 2020

Floxuridine (May reduce the immune response to vaccine). Products include:
- Sterile FUDR ... 2118

Fludarabine Phosphate (May reduce the immune response to vaccine). Products include:
- Fludara for Injection ... 663

Fludrocortisone Acetate (Corticosteroids, used in greater than physiologic doses, may reduce the immune response to vaccine). Products include:
- Florinef Acetate Tablets ... 505

Fluorouracil (May reduce the immune response to vaccine). Products include:
- Efudex ... 2113
- Fluoroplex Topical Solution & Cream 1% ... 479
- Fluorouracil Injection ... 2116

Heparin Calcium (Concurrent use requires caution).
- No products indexed under this heading.

Heparin Sodium (Concurrent use requires caution). Products include:
- Heparin Lock Flush Solution ... 2725
- Heparin Sodium Injection ... 2726
- Heparin Sodium Injection, USP, Sterile Solution ... 2615
- Heparin Sodium Vials ... 1441

Hydrocortisone (Corticosteroids, used in greater than physiologic doses, may reduce the immune response to vaccine). Products include:
- Anusol-HC Cream 2.5% ... 1896
- Aquanil HC Lotion ... 1931
- Bactine Hydrocortisone Anti-Itch Cream ... ▣ 709
- Caldecort Anti-Itch Hydrocortisone Spray ... ▣ 631
- Cortaid ... ▣ 836
- CORTENEMA ... 2535
- Cortisporin Ointment ... 1085
- Cortisporin Ophthalmic Ointment Sterile ... 1085
- Cortisporin Ophthalmic Suspension Sterile ... 1086
- Cortisporin Otic Solution Sterile ... 1087
- Cortisporin Otic Suspension Sterile 1088
- Cortizone-5 ... ▣ 831
- Cortizone-10 ... ▣ 831
- Hydrocortone Tablets ... 1672
- Hytone ... 907
- Massengill Medicated Soft Cloth Towelettes ... 2458
- PediOtic Suspension Sterile ... 1153
- Preparation H Hydrocortisone 1% Cream ... ▣ 872
- ProctoCream-HC 2.5% ... 2408
- VōSoL HC Otic Solution ... 2678

Hydrocortisone Acetate (Corticosteroids, used in greater than physiologic doses, may reduce the immune response to vaccine). Products include:
- Analpram-HC Rectal Cream 1% and 2.5% ... 977
- Anusol HC-1 Anti-Itch Hydrocortisone Ointment ... ▣ 847
- Anusol-HC Suppositories ... 1897
- Caldecort ... ▣ 631
- Carmol HC ... 924
- Coly-Mycin S Otic w/Neomycin & Hydrocortisone ... 1906
- Cortaid ... ▣ 836
- Cortifoam ... 2396
- Cortisporin Cream ... 1084
- Epifoam ... 2399
- Hydrocortone Acetate Sterile Suspension ... 1669
- Mantadil Cream ... 1135
- Nupercainal Hydrocortisone 1% Cream ... ▣ 645
- Ophthocort ... ⊙ 311
- Pramosone Cream, Lotion & Ointment ... 978
- ProctoCream-HC ... 2408
- ProctoFoam-HC ... 2409
- Terra-Cortril Ophthalmic Suspension ... 2210

Hydrocortisone Sodium Phosphate (Corticosteroids, used in greater than physiologic doses, may reduce the immune response to vaccine). Products include:
- Hydrocortone Phosphate Injection, Sterile ... 1670

Hydrocortisone Sodium Succinate (Corticosteroids, used in greater than physiologic doses, may reduce the immune response to vaccine). Products include:
- Solu-Cortef Sterile Powder ... 2641

Hydroxyurea (May reduce the immune response to vaccine). Products include:
- Hydrea Capsules ... 696

Immune Globulin (Human) (An adequate immunologic response may not be obtained if used concurrently).
- No products indexed under this heading.

Immune Globulin Intravenous (Human) (An adequate immunologic response may not be obtained if used concurrently).

Influenza Virus Vaccine (Influenza Virus Vaccine should not be given within three days of the administration of Tripedia). Products include:
- Fluvirin ... 460
- Influenza Virus Vaccine, Trivalent, Types A and B (chromatograph- and filter-purified subviron antigen) FluShield, 1995-1996 Formula ... 2736

Lomustine (CCNU) (May reduce the immune response to vaccine). Products include:
- CeeNU ... 693

Mechlorethamine Hydrochloride (May reduce the immune response to vaccine). Products include:
- Mustargen ... 1709

Melphalan (May reduce the immune response to vaccine). Products include:
- Alkeran Tablets ... 1071

Methotrexate Sodium (May reduce the immune response to vaccine). Products include:
- Methotrexate Sodium Tablets, Injection, for Injection and LPF Injection ... 1275

Methylprednisolone Acetate (Corticosteroids, used in greater than physiologic doses, may reduce the immune response to vaccine). Products include:
- Depo-Medrol Single-Dose Vial ... 2600
- Depo-Medrol Sterile Aqueous Suspension ... 2597

Methylprednisolone Sodium Succinate (Corticosteroids, used in greater than physiologic doses, may reduce the immune response to vaccine). Products include:
- Solu-Medrol Sterile Powder ... 2643

Mitotane (May reduce the immune response to vaccine). Products include:
- Lysodren ... 698

Mitoxantrone Hydrochloride (May reduce the immune response to vaccine). Products include:
- Novantrone ... 1279

Muromonab-CD3 (An adequate immunologic response may not be obtained if used concurrently). Products include:
- Orthoclone OKT3 Sterile Solution .. 1837

Mycophenolate Mofetil (An adequate immunologic response may not be obtained if used concurrently). Products include:
- CellCept Capsules ... 2099

Prednisolone Acetate (Corticosteroids, used in greater than physiologic doses, may reduce the immune response to vaccine). Products include:
- AK-CIDE ... ⊙ 202
- AK-CIDE Ointment ... ⊙ 202
- Blephamide Liquifilm Sterile Ophthalmic Suspension ... 476
- Blephamide Ointment ... ⊙ 237
- Econopred & Econopred Plus Ophthalmic Suspensions ... ⊙ 217
- Poly-Pred Liquifilm ... ⊙ 248
- Pred Forte ... ⊙ 250
- Pred Mild ... ⊙ 253
- Pred-G Liquifilm Sterile Ophthalmic Suspension ... ⊙ 251
- Pred-G S.O.P. Sterile Ophthalmic Ointment ... ⊙ 252
- Vasocidin Ointment ... ⊙ 268

Prednisolone Sodium Phosphate (Corticosteroids, used in greater than physiologic doses, may reduce the immune response to vaccine). Products include:
- AK-Pred ... ⊙ 204
- Hydeltrasol Injection, Sterile ... 1665
- Inflamase ... ⊙ 265
- Pediapred Oral Liquid ... 995
- Vasocidin Ophthalmic Solution ... ⊙ 270

Prednisolone Tebutate (Corticosteroids, used in greater than physiologic doses, may reduce the immune response to vaccine). Products include:
- Hydeltra-T.B.A. Sterile Suspension 1667

Prednisone (Corticosteroids, used in greater than physiologic doses, may reduce the immune response to vaccine). Products include:
- Deltasone Tablets ... 2595

Procarbazine Hydrochloride (May reduce the immune response to vaccine). Products include:
- Matulane Capsules ... 2131

Tacrolimus (An adequate immunologic response may not be obtained if used concurrently). Products include:
- Prograf ... 1042

Tamoxifen Citrate (May reduce the immune response to vaccine). Products include:
- Nolvadex Tablets ... 2841

Thioguanine (May reduce the immune response to vaccine). Products include:
- Thioguanine Tablets, Tabloid Brand ... 1181

Thiotepa (May reduce the immune response to vaccine). Products include:
- Thioplex (Thiotepa For Injection) 1281

Triamcinolone (Corticosteroids, used in greater than physiologic doses, may reduce the immune response to vaccine). Products include:
- Aristocort Tablets ... 1022

Triamcinolone Acetonide (Corticosteroids, used in greater than physiologic doses, may reduce the immune response to vaccine). Products include:
- Aristocort A 0.025% Cream ... 1027
- Aristocort A 0.5% Cream ... 1031
- Aristocort A 0.1% Cream ... 1029
- Aristocort A 0.1% Ointment ... 1030
- Azmacort Oral Inhaler ... 2011
- Nasacort Nasal Inhaler ... 2024

Triamcinolone Diacetate (Corticosteroids, used in greater than physiologic doses, may reduce the immune response to vaccine). Products include:
- Aristocort Suspension (Forte Parenteral) ... 1027
- Aristocort Suspension (Intralesional) ... 1025

Triamcinolone Hexacetonide (Corticosteroids, used in greater than physiologic doses, may reduce the immune response to vaccine). Products include:
- Aristospan Suspension (Intra-articular) ... 1033
- Aristospan Suspension (Intralesional) ... 1032

Vincristine Sulfate (May reduce the immune response to vaccine). Products include:
- Oncovin Solution Vials & Hyporets 1466

Warfarin Sodium (Concurrent use requires caution). Products include:
- Coumadin ... 926

TRIPHASIL-21 TABLETS (Levonorgestrel, Ethinyl Estradiol) 2814
May interact with barbiturates and

(▣ Described in PDR For Nonprescription Drugs) (⊙ Described in PDR For Ophthalmology)

1081 Interactions Index Tuberculin, Old

certain other agents. Compounds in these categories include:

Ampicillin Sodium (Reduced efficacy; increased incidence of breakthrough bleeding). Products include:
- Unasyn 2212

Aprobarbital (Reduced efficacy; increased incidence of breakthrough bleeding).
- No products indexed under this heading.

Butabarbital (Reduced efficacy; increased incidence of breakthrough bleeding).
- No products indexed under this heading.

Butalbital (Reduced efficacy; increased incidence of breakthrough bleeding). Products include:
- Esgic-plus Tablets 1013
- Fioricet Tablets 2258
- Fioricet with Codeine Capsules 2260
- Fiorinal Capsules 2261
- Fiorinal with Codeine Capsules 2262
- Fiorinal Tablets 2261
- Phrenilin 785
- Sedapap Tablets 50 mg/650 mg 1543

Mephobarbital (Reduced efficacy; increased incidence of breakthrough bleeding). Products include:
- Mebaral Tablets 2322

Oxytetracycline (Reduced efficacy; increased incidence of breakthrough bleeding). Products include:
- Terramycin Intramuscular Solution 2210

Oxytetracycline Hydrochloride (Reduced efficacy; increased incidence of breakthrough bleeding). Products include:
- TERAK Ointment ..... ◉ 209
- Terra-Cortril Ophthalmic Suspension 2210
- Terramycin with Polymyxin B Sulfate Ophthalmic Ointment 2211
- Urobiotic-250 Capsules 2214

Pentobarbital Sodium (Reduced efficacy; increased incidence of breakthroughbleeding). Products include:
- Nembutal Sodium Capsules 436
- Nembutal Sodium Solution 438
- Nembutal Sodium Suppositories..... 440

Phenobarbital (Reduced efficacy; increased incidence of breakthrough bleeding). Products include:
- Arco-Lase Plus Tablets 512
- Bellergal-S Tablets 2250
- Donnatal 2060
- Donnatal Extentabs..... 2061
- Donnatal Tablets 2060
- Phenobarbital Elixir and Tablets 1469
- Quadrinal Tablets 1350

Phenylbutazone (Reduced efficacy; increased incidence of breakthrough bleeding).
- No products indexed under this heading.

Phenytoin Sodium (Reduced efficacy; increased incidence of breakthrough bleeding). Products include:
- Dilantin Kapseals 1906
- Dilantin Parenteral 1910

Rifampin (Reduced efficacy; increased incidence of breakthrough bleeding). Products include:
- Rifadin 1528
- Rifamate Capsules 1530
- Rifater..... 1532
- Rimactane Capsules 847

Secobarbital Sodium (Reduced efficacy; increased incidence of breakthrough bleeding). Products include:
- Seconal Sodium Pulvules 1474

Tetracycline Hydrochloride (Reduced efficacy; increased incidence of breakthrough bleeding). Products include:
- Achromycin V Capsules 1367

Thiamylal Sodium (Reduced efficacy; increased incidence of breakthrough bleeding).
- No products indexed under this heading.

TRIPHASIL-28 TABLETS
(Levonorgestrel, Ethinyl Estradiol) 2819
See **Triphasil-21 Tablets**

TRISORALEN TABLETS
(Trioxsalen)..... 1264

Food Interactions

Food, furocoumarin-containing (Potential for severe reactions).

TROBICIN STERILE POWDER
(Spectinomycin Hydrochloride) 2645
None cited in PDR database.

TRONOLANE ANESTHETIC CREAM FOR HEMORRHOIDS
(Pramoxine Hydrochloride) ..... ▣ 784
None cited in PDR database.

TRONOLANE HEMORRHOIDAL SUPPOSITORIES
(Fat, Hard, Zinc Oxide)..... ▣ 784
None cited in PDR database.

TRUSOPT STERILE OPHTHALMIC SOLUTION
(Dorzolamide Hydrochloride).....1760
May interact with carbonic anhydrase inhibitors and certain other agents. Compounds in these categories include:

Acetazolamide (Potential for an additive effect on the known systemic effects of carbonic anhydrase inhibition in patients receiving an oral carbonic anhydrase inhibitor and Trusopt). Products include:
- Diamox Sequels (Sustained Release) 1373
- Diamox Sequels (Sustained Release) ..... ◉ 319
- Diamox Tablets..... 1372
- Diamox Tablets..... ◉ 317

Aspirin (Potential for acid-base and electrolyte disturbances with concomitant use; these disturbances have been reported with oral agent and have not been reported during clinical trials with Trusopt). Products include:
- Alka-Seltzer Effervescent Antacid and Pain Reliever ..... ▣ 701
- Alka-Seltzer Extra Strength Effervescent Antacid and Pain Reliever ..... ▣ 703
- Alka-Seltzer Lemon Lime Effervescent Antacid and Pain Reliever ..... ▣ 703
- Alka-Seltzer Plus Cold Medicine ..... ▣ 705
- Alka-Seltzer Plus Cold & Cough Medicine ..... ▣ 708
- Alka-Seltzer Plus Night-Time Cold Medicine ..... ▣ 707
- Alka Seltzer Plus Sinus Medicine ..... ▣ 707
- Arthritis Foundation Safety Coated Aspirin Tablets ..... ▣ 675
- Arthritis Pain Ascriptin ..... ▣ 631
- Maximum Strength Ascriptin ..... ▣ 630
- Regular Strength Ascriptin Tablets ..... ▣ 629
- Arthritis Strength BC Powder..... ▣ 609
- BC Cold Powder Multi-Symptom Formula (Cold-Sinus-Allergy) ..... ▣ 609
- BC Cold Powder Non-Drowsy Formula (Cold-Sinus) ..... ▣ 609
- BC Powder ..... ▣ 609
- Bayer Children's Chewable Aspirin ..... ▣ 711
- Genuine Bayer Aspirin Tablets & Caplets ..... ▣ 713
- Extra Strength Bayer Arthritis Pain Regimen Formula ..... ▣ 711
- Extra Strength Bayer Aspirin Caplets & Tablets ..... ▣ 712
- Extended-Release Bayer 8-Hour Aspirin ..... ▣ 712
- Extra Strength Bayer Plus Aspirin Caplets ..... ▣ 713
- Extra Strength Bayer PM Aspirin ..... ▣ 713
- Bayer Enteric Aspirin ..... ▣ 709
- Bufferin Analgesic Tablets and Caplets ..... ▣ 613
- Arthritis Strength Bufferin Analgesic Caplets ..... ▣ 614
- Extra Strength Bufferin Analgesic Tablets ..... ▣ 615
- Cama Arthritis Pain Reliever..... ▣ 785
- Darvon Compound-65 Pulvules 1435
- Easprin 1914
- Ecotrin 2455
- Ecotrin Enteric Coated Aspirin Maximum Strength Tablets and Caplets ..... ▣ 816
- Ecotrin Enteric Coated Aspirin Regular Strength Tablets 2455
- Empirin Aspirin Tablets ..... ▣ 854
- Empirin with Codeine Tablets..... 1093
- Excedrin Extra-Strength Analgesic Tablets & Caplets 732
- Fiorinal Capsules 2261
- Fiorinal with Codeine Capsules 2262
- Fiorinal Tablets 2261
- Halfprin 1362
- Healthprin Aspirin 2455
- Norgesic..... 1496
- Percodan Tablets..... 939
- Percodan-Demi Tablets..... 940
- Robaxisal Tablets..... 2071
- Soma Compound w/Codeine Tablets 2676
- Soma Compound Tablets..... 2675
- St. Joseph Adult Chewable Aspirin (81 mg.) ..... ▣ 808
- Talwin Compound 2335
- Ursinus Inlay-Tabs..... ▣ 794
- Vanquish Analgesic Caplets ..... ▣ 731

Dichlorphenamide (Potential for an additive effect on the known systemic effects of carbonic anhydrase inhibition in patients receiving an oral carbonic anhydrase inhibitor and Trusopt). Products include:
- Daranide Tablets 1633

Methazolamide (Potential for an additive effect on the known systemic effects of carbonic anhydrase inhibition in patients receiving an oral carbonic anhydrase inhibitor and Trusopt). Products include:
- Glauctabs ..... ◉ 208
- MZM ..... ◉ 267
- Neptazane Tablets 1388
- Neptazane Tablets ..... ◉ 320

T.R.U.E. TEST
(Allergens).....1189
None cited in PDR database.

TUBERCULIN, OLD, TINE TEST
(Tuberculin, Old) 2875
May interact with corticosteroids and immunosuppressive agents. Compounds in these categories include:

Azathioprine (Reactivity to the test may be suppressed). Products include:
- Imuran 1110

Betamethasone Acetate (Reactivity to the test may be suppressed). Products include:
- Celestone Soluspan Suspension 2347

Betamethasone Sodium Phosphate (Reactivity to the test may be suppressed). Products include:
- Celestone Soluspan Suspension 2347

Cortisone Acetate (Reactivity to the test may be suppressed). Products include:
- Cortone Acetate Sterile Suspension 1623
- Cortone Acetate Tablets..... 1624

Cyclosporine (Reactivity to the test may be suppressed). Products include:
- Neoral 2276
- Sandimmune 2286

Desoximetasone (Reactivity to the test may be suppressed). Products include:
- Topicort 1243

Dexamethasone Acetate (Reactivity to the test may be suppressed). Products include:
- Dalalone D.P. Injectable 1011
- Decadron-LA Sterile Suspension..... 1646

Dexamethasone Sodium Phosphate (Reactivity to the test may be suppressed). Products include:
- Decadron Phosphate Injection 1637
- Decadron Phosphate Respihaler 1642
- Decadron Phosphate Sterile Ophthalmic Ointment 1641
- Decadron Phosphate Sterile Ophthalmic Solution 1642
- Decadron Phosphate Topical Cream 1644
- Decadron Phosphate Turbinaire 1645
- Decadron Phosphate with Xylocaine Injection, Sterile 1639
- Dexacort Phosphate in Respihaler 458
- Dexacort Phosphate in Turbinaire 459
- NeoDecadron Sterile Ophthalmic Ointment 1712
- NeoDecadron Sterile Ophthalmic Solution 1713
- NeoDecadron Topical Cream 1714

Fludrocortisone Acetate (Reactivity to the test may be suppressed). Products include:
- Florinef Acetate Tablets 505

Hydrocortisone (Reactivity to the test may be suppressed). Products include:
- Anusol-HC Cream 2.5% 1896
- Aquanil HC Lotion 1931
- Bactine Hydrocortisone Anti-Itch Cream ..... ▣ 709
- Caldecort Anti-Itch Hydrocortisone Spray ..... ▣ 631
- Cortaid ..... ▣ 836
- CORTENEMA..... 2535
- Cortisporin Ointment 1085
- Cortisporin Ophthalmic Ointment Sterile 1085
- Cortisporin Ophthalmic Suspension Sterile 1086
- Cortisporin Otic Solution Sterile 1087
- Cortisporin Otic Suspension Sterile 1088
- Cortizone-5 ..... ▣ 831
- Cortizone-10 ..... ▣ 831
- Hydrocortone Tablets 1672
- Hytone 907
- Massengill Medicated Soft Cloth Towelettes..... 2458
- PediOtic Suspension Sterile 1153
- Preparation H Hydrocortisone 1% Cream ..... ▣ 872
- ProctoCream-HC 2.5%..... 2408
- VōSoL HC Otic Solution..... 2678

Hydrocortisone Acetate (Reactivity to the test may be suppressed). Products include:
- Analpram-HC Rectal Cream 1% and 2.5% 977
- Anusol HC-1 Anti-Itch Hydrocortisone Ointment..... ▣ 847
- Anusol-HC Suppositories 1897
- Caldecort..... ▣ 631
- Carmol HC 924
- Coly-Mycin S Otic w/Neomycin & Hydrocortisone..... 1906
- Cortaid..... ▣ 836
- Cortifoam 2396
- Cortisporin Cream..... 1084
- Epifoam 2399
- Hydrocortone Acetate Sterile Suspension..... 1669
- Mantadil Cream 1135
- Nupercainal Hydrocortisone 1% Cream ..... ▣ 645
- Ophthocort..... ◉ 311

IMPORTANT NOTE: Always consult each drug listing in the patient's regimen for possible interactions.

Tuberculin, Old | Interactions Index | 1082

Pramosone Cream, Lotion & Ointment 978
ProctoCream-HC 2408
ProctoFoam-HC 2409
Terra-Cortril Ophthalmic Suspension 2210

Hydrocortisone Sodium Phosphate (Reactivity to the test may be suppressed). Products include:
Hydrocortone Phosphate Injection, Sterile 1670

Hydrocortisone Sodium Succinate (Reactivity to the test may be suppressed). Products include:
Solu-Cortef Sterile Powder 2641

Immune Globulin (Human) (Reactivity to the test may be suppressed).
No products indexed under this heading.

Immune Globulin Intravenous (Human) (Reactivity to the test may be suppressed).

Methylprednisolone Acetate (Reactivity to the test may be suppressed). Products include:
Depo-Medrol Single-Dose Vial 2600
Depo-Medrol Sterile Aqueous Suspension 2597

Methylprednisolone Sodium Succinate (Reactivity to the test may be suppressed). Products include:
Solu-Medrol Sterile Powder 2643

Muromonab-CD3 (Reactivity to the test may be suppressed). Products include:
Orthoclone OKT3 Sterile Solution .. 1837

Mycophenolate Mofetil (Reactivity to the test may be suppressed). Products include:
CellCept Capsules 2099

Prednisolone Acetate (Reactivity to the test may be suppressed). Products include:
AK-CIDE .... ◉ 202
AK-CIDE Ointment .... ◉ 202
Blephamide Liquifilm Sterile Ophthalmic Suspension 476
Blephamide Ointment .... ◉ 237
Econopred & Econopred Plus Ophthalmic Suspensions .... ◉ 217
Poly-Pred Liquifilm .... ◉ 248
Pred Forte .... ◉ 250
Pred Mild .... ◉ 253
Pred-G Liquifilm Sterile Ophthalmic Suspension .... ◉ 251
Pred-G S.O.P. Sterile Ophthalmic Ointment .... ◉ 252
Vasocidin Ointment .... ◉ 268

Prednisolone Sodium Phosphate (Reactivity to the test may be suppressed). Products include:
AK-Pred .... ◉ 204
Hydeltrasol Injection, Sterile 1665
Inflamase .... ◉ 265
Pediapred Oral Liquid 995
Vasocidin Ophthalmic Solution .... ◉ 270

Prednisolone Tebutate (Reactivity to the test may be suppressed). Products include:
Hydeltra-T.B.A. Sterile Suspension 1667

Prednisone (Reactivity to the test may be suppressed). Products include:
Deltasone Tablets 2595

Tacrolimus (Reactivity to the test may be suppressed). Products include:
Prograf 1042

Triamcinolone (Reactivity to the test may be suppressed). Products include:
Aristocort Tablets 1022

Triamcinolone Acetonide (Reactivity to the test may be suppressed). Products include:
Aristocort A 0.025% Cream 1027
Aristocort A 0.5% Cream 1031
Aristocort A 0.1% Cream 1029
Aristocort A 0.1% Ointment 1030
Azmacort Oral Inhaler 2011
Nasacort Nasal Inhaler 2024

Triamcinolone Diacetate (Reactivity to the test may be suppressed). Products include:
Aristocort Suspension (Forte Parenteral) 1027
Aristocort Suspension (Intralesional) 1025

Triamcinolone Hexacetonide (Reactivity to the test may be suppressed). Products include:
Aristospan Suspension (Intra-articular) 1033
Aristospan Suspension (Intralesional) 1032

TUBERSOL (TUBERCULIN PURIFIED PROTEIN DERIVATIVE [MANTOUX])
(Tuberculin, Purified Protein Derivative For Mantoux Test) 2872
May interact with corticosteroids, immunosuppressive agents, and certain other agents. Compounds in these categories include:

Azathioprine (Reactivity to the test may be suppressed or depressed). Products include:
Imuran 1110

Betamethasone Acetate (Reactivity to the test may be suppressed or depressed). Products include:
Celestone Soluspan Suspension 2347

Betamethasone Sodium Phosphate (Reactivity to the test may be suppressed or depressed). Products include:
Celestone Soluspan Suspension 2347

Cortisone Acetate (Reactivity to the test may be suppressed or depressed). Products include:
Cortone Acetate Sterile Suspension 1623
Cortone Acetate Tablets 1624

Cyclosporine (Reactivity to the test may be suppressed or depressed). Products include:
Neoral 2276
Sandimmune 2286

Dexamethasone (Reactivity to the test may be suppressed or depressed). Products include:
AK-Trol Ointment & Suspension .... ◉ 205
Decadron Elixir 1633
Decadron Tablets 1635
Decaspray Topical Aerosol 1648
Dexacidin Ointment .... ◉ 263
Maxitrol Ophthalmic Ointment and Suspension .... ◉ 224
TobraDex Ophthalmic Suspension and Ointment 473

Dexamethasone Acetate (Reactivity to the test may be suppressed or depressed). Products include:
Dalalone D.P. Injectable 1011
Decadron-LA Sterile Suspension 1646

Dexamethasone Sodium Phosphate (Reactivity to the test may be suppressed or depressed). Products include:
Decadron Phosphate Injection 1637
Decadron Phosphate Respihaler 1642
Decadron Phosphate Sterile Ophthalmic Ointment 1641
Decadron Phosphate Sterile Ophthalmic Solution 1642
Decadron Phosphate Topical Cream 1644
Decadron Phosphate Turbinaire 1645
Decadron Phosphate with Xylocaine Injection, Sterile 1639
Dexacort Phosphate in Respihaler .. 458
Dexacort Phosphate in Turbinaire .. 459
NeoDecadron Sterile Ophthalmic Ointment 1712
NeoDecadron Sterile Ophthalmic Solution 1713
NeoDecadron Topical Cream 1714

Fludrocortisone Acetate (Reactivity to the test may be suppressed or depressed). Products include:
Florinef Acetate Tablets 505

Hydrocortisone (Reactivity to the test may be suppressed or depressed). Products include:
Anusol-HC Cream 2.5% 1896
Aquanil HC Lotion 1931
Bactine Hydrocortisone Anti-Itch Cream .... ▣ 709
Caldecort Anti-Itch Hydrocortisone Spray .... ▣ 631
Cortaid .... ▣ 836
CORTENEMA 2535
Cortisporin Ointment 1085
Cortisporin Ophthalmic Ointment Sterile 1085
Cortisporin Ophthalmic Suspension Sterile 1086
Cortisporin Otic Solution Sterile 1087
Cortisporin Otic Suspension Sterile 1088
Cortizone-5 .... ▣ 831
Cortizone-10 .... ▣ 831
Hydrocortone Tablets 1672
Hytone 907
Massengill Medicated Soft Cloth Towelettes 2458
PediOtic Suspension Sterile 1153
Preparation H Hydrocortisone 1% Cream .... ▣ 872
ProctoCream-HC 2.5% 2408
VōSoL HC Otic Solution 2678

Hydrocortisone Acetate (Reactivity to the test may be suppressed or depressed). Products include:
Analpram-HC Rectal Cream 1% and 2.5% 977
Anusol HC-1 Anti-Itch Hydrocortisone Ointment .... ▣ 847
Anusol-HC Suppositories 1897
Caldecort .... ▣ 631
Carmol HC 924
Coly-Mycin S Otic w/Neomycin & Hydrocortisone 1906
Cortaid .... ▣ 836
Cortifoam 2396
Cortisporin Cream 1084
Epifoam 2399
Hydrocortone Acetate Sterile Suspension 1669
Mantadil Cream 1135
Nupercainal Hydrocortisone 1% Cream .... ▣ 645
Ophthocort .... ◉ 311
Pramosone Cream, Lotion & Ointment 978
ProctoCream-HC 2408
ProctoFoam-HC 2409
Terra-Cortril Ophthalmic Suspension 2210

Hydrocortisone Sodium Phosphate (Reactivity to the test may be suppressed or depressed). Products include:
Hydrocortone Phosphate Injection, Sterile 1670

Hydrocortisone Sodium Succinate (Reactivity to the test may be suppressed or depressed). Products include:
Solu-Cortef Sterile Powder 2641

Immune Globulin (Human) (Reactivity to the test may be suppressed or depressed).
No products indexed under this heading.

Measles, Mumps & Rubella Virus Vaccine Live (Reactivity to the test may be temporarily depressed). Products include:
M-M-R II 1687

Methylprednisolone Acetate (Reactivity to the test may be suppressed or depressed). Products include:
Depo-Medrol Single-Dose Vial 2600
Depo-Medrol Sterile Aqueous Suspension 2597

Methylprednisolone Sodium Succinate (Reactivity to the test may be suppressed or depressed). Products include:
Solu-Medrol Sterile Powder 2643

Muromonab-CD3 (Reactivity to the test may be suppressed or depressed). Products include:
Orthoclone OKT3 Sterile Solution .. 1837

Mycophenolate Mofetil (Reactivity to the test may be suppressed or depressed). Products include:
CellCept Capsules 2099

Prednisolone Acetate (Reactivity to the test may be suppressed or depressed). Products include:
AK-CIDE .... ◉ 202
AK-CIDE Ointment .... ◉ 202
Blephamide Liquifilm Sterile Ophthalmic Suspension 476
Blephamide Ointment .... ◉ 237
Econopred & Econopred Plus Ophthalmic Suspensions .... ◉ 217
Poly-Pred Liquifilm .... ◉ 248
Pred Forte .... ◉ 250
Pred Mild .... ◉ 253
Pred-G Liquifilm Sterile Ophthalmic Suspension .... ◉ 251
Pred-G S.O.P. Sterile Ophthalmic Ointment .... ◉ 252
Vasocidin Ointment .... ◉ 268

Prednisolone Sodium Phosphate (Reactivity to the test may be suppressed or depressed). Products include:
AK-Pred .... ◉ 204
Hydeltrasol Injection, Sterile 1665
Inflamase .... ◉ 265
Pediapred Oral Liquid 995
Vasocidin Ophthalmic Solution .... ◉ 270

Prednisolone Tebutate (Reactivity to the test may be suppressed or depressed). Products include:
Hydeltra-T.B.A. Sterile Suspension 1667

Prednisone (Reactivity to the test may be suppressed or depressed). Products include:
Deltasone Tablets 2595

Tacrolimus (Reactivity to the test may be suppressed or depressed). Products include:
Prograf 1042

Triamcinolone (Reactivity to the test may be suppressed or depressed). Products include:
Aristocort Tablets 1022

Triamcinolone Acetonide (Reactivity to the test may be suppressed or depressed). Products include:
Aristocort A 0.025% Cream 1027
Aristocort A 0.5% Cream 1031
Aristocort A 0.1% Cream 1029
Aristocort A 0.1% Ointment 1030
Azmacort Oral Inhaler 2011
Nasacort Nasal Inhaler 2024

Triamcinolone Diacetate (Reactivity to the test may be suppressed or depressed). Products include:
Aristocort Suspension (Forte Parenteral) 1027
Aristocort Suspension (Intralesional) 1025

Triamcinolone Hexacetonide (Reactivity to the test may be suppressed or depressed). Products include:
Aristospan Suspension (Intra-articular) 1033
Aristospan Suspension (Intralesional) 1032

TUCKS CLEAR HEMORRHOIDAL GEL
(Witch Hazel, Glycerin) .... ▣ 865
None cited in PDR database.

TUCKS PREMOISTENED HEMORRHOIDAL/VAGINAL PADS
(Witch Hazel) .... ▣ 865
None cited in PDR database.

TUCKS TAKE-ALONGS
(Witch Hazel) .... ▣ 865
None cited in PDR database.

(▣ Described in PDR For Nonprescription Drugs) (◉ Described in PDR For Ophthalmology)

TUMS ANTACID TABLETS

(Calcium Carbonate) .... RD 827

May interact with:

Drugs, Oral, unspecified (Antacids may interact with certain unspecified prescription drugs).

TUMS ANTI-GAS/ANTACID FORMULA TABLETS, ASSORTED FRUIT

(Calcium Carbonate, Simethicone).. RD 827

May interact with:

Prescription Drugs, unspecified (Antacids may interact with certain unspecified prescription drugs; consult your doctor).

TUMS E-X ANTACID TABLETS

(Calcium Carbonate) .... RD 827

See Tums Antacid Tablets

TUMS 500 CALCIUM SUPPLEMENT

(Calcium Carbonate) .... RD 828

None cited in PDR database.

TUMS ULTRA ANTACID TABLETS

(Calcium Carbonate) .... RD 827

See Tums Antacid Tablets

TUSSEND

(Hydrocodone Bitartrate, Pseudoephedrine Hydrochloride, Chlorpheniramine Maleate) 1783

May interact with narcotic analgesics, antipsychotic agents, tranquilizers, central nervous system depressants, tricyclic antidepressants, monoamine oxidase inhibitors, beta blockers, veratrum alkaloids, anticholinergics, cardiac glycosides, and certain other agents. Compounds in these categories include:

Acebutolol Hydrochloride (Potentiates the sympathomimetic effects of pseudoephedrine; hypertensive crises can occur with concurrent use). Products include:

Sectral Capsules 2807

Alfentanil Hydrochloride (Concomitant use may exhibit additive CNS depression). Products include:

Alfenta Injection 1286

Alprazolam (Concomitant use may exhibit additive CNS depression). Products include:

Xanax Tablets 2649

Amitriptyline Hydrochloride (Concomitant use may increase the effects of either the antidepressant or hydrocodone; may antagonize the effects of pseudoephedrine). Products include:

Elavil 2838
Endep Tablets 2174
Etrafon 2355
Limbitrol 2180
Triavil Tablets 1757

Amoxapine (Concomitant use may increase the effects of either the antidepressant or hydrocodone; may antagonize the effects of pseudoephedrine). Products include:

Asendin Tablets 1369

Aprobarbital (Concomitant use may exhibit additive CNS depression).

No products indexed under this heading.

Atenolol (Potentiates the sympathomimetic effects of pseudoephedrine; hypertensive crises can occur with concurrent use). Products include:

Tenoretic Tablets 2845

Tenormin Tablets and I.V. Injection 2847

Atropine Sulfate (Concurrent use of anticholinergics and hydrocodone may produce paralytic ileus). Products include:

Arco-Lase Plus Tablets 512
Atrohist Plus Tablets 454
Atropine Sulfate Sterile Ophthalmic Solution .... ◊ 233
Donnatal 2060
Donnatal Extentabs............................. 2061
Donnatal Tablets 2060
Lomotil 2439
Motofen Tablets 784
Urised Tablets....................................... 1964

Belladonna Alkaloids (Concurrent use of anticholinergics and hydrocodone may produce paralytic ileus). Products include:

Bellergal-S Tablets 2250
Hyland's Bed Wetting Tablets .... RD 828
Hyland's EnurAid Tablets.................. RD 829
Hyland's Teething Tablets .... RD 830

Benztropine Mesylate (Concurrent use of anticholinergics and hydrocodone may produce paralytic ileus). Products include:

Cogentin 1621

Betaxolol Hydrochloride (Potentiates the sympathomimetic effects of pseudoephedrine; hypertensive crises can occur with concurrent use). Products include:

Betoptic Ophthalmic Solution........... 469
Betopic S Ophthalmic Suspension 471
Kerlone Tablets.................................... 2436

Biperiden Hydrochloride (Concurrent use of anticholinergics and hydrocodone may produce paralytic ileus). Products include:

Akineton 1333

Bisoprolol Fumarate (Potentiates the sympathomimetic effects of pseudoephedrine; hypertensive crises can occur with concurrent use). Products include:

Zebeta Tablets 1413
Ziac 1415

Buprenorphine (Concomitant use may exhibit additive CNS depression). Products include:

Buprenex Injectable 2006

Buspirone Hydrochloride (Concomitant use may exhibit additive CNS depression). Products include:

BuSpar 737

Butabarbital (Concomitant use may exhibit additive CNS depression).

No products indexed under this heading.

Butalbital (Concomitant use may exhibit additive CNS depression). Products include:

Esgic-plus Tablets 1013
Fioricet Tablets..................................... 2258
Fioricet with Codeine Capsules 2260
Fiorinal Capsules 2261
Fiorinal with Codeine Capsules 2262
Fiorinal Tablets 2261
Phrenilin 785
Sedapap Tablets 50 mg/650 mg .. 1543

Carteolol Hydrochloride (Potentiates the sympathomimetic effects of pseudoephedrine; hypertensive crises can occur with concurrent use). Products include:

Cartrol Tablets 410
Ocupress Ophthalmic Solution, 1% Sterile... ◊ 309

Chlordiazepoxide (Concomitant use may exhibit additive CNS depression). Products include:

Libritabs Tablets 2177
Limbitrol 2180

Chlordiazepoxide Hydrochloride (Concomitant use may exhibit additive CNS depression). Products include:

Librax Capsules 2176

Librium Capsules 2178
Librium Injectable 2179

Chlorpromazine (Concomitant use may exhibit additive CNS depression). Products include:

Thorazine Suppositories 2523

Chlorpromazine Hydrochloride (Concomitant use may exhibit additive CNS depression). Products include:

Thorazine 2523

Chlorprothixene (Concomitant use may exhibit additive CNS depression).

No products indexed under this heading.

Chlorprothixene Hydrochloride (Concomitant use may exhibit additive CNS depression).

No products indexed under this heading.

Clidinium Bromide (Concurrent use of anticholinergics and hydrocodone may produce paralytic ileus). Products include:

Librax Capsules 2176
Quarzan Capsules 2181

Clomipramine Hydrochloride (Concomitant use may increase the effects of either the antidepressant or hydrocodone; may antagonize the effects of pseudoephedrine). Products include:

Anafranil Capsules 803

Clorazepate Dipotassium (Concomitant use may exhibit additive CNS depression). Products include:

Tranxene 451

Clozapine (Concomitant use may exhibit additive CNS depression). Products include:

Clozaril Tablets..................................... 2252

Codeine Phosphate (Concomitant use may exhibit additive CNS depression). Products include:

Actifed with Codeine Cough Syrup.. 1067
Brontex 1981
Deconsal C Expectorant Syrup 456
Deconsal Pediatric Syrup................... 457
Dimetane-DC Cough Syrup 2059
Empirin with Codeine Tablets........... 1093
Fioricet with Codeine Capsules 2260
Fiorinal with Codeine Capsules 2262
Isoclor Expectorant............................. 990
Novahistine DH.................................... 2462
Novahistine Expectorant.................... 2463
Nucofed 2051
Phenergan with Codeine.................... 2777
Phenergan VC with Codeine 2781
Robitussin A-C Syrup.......................... 2073
Robitussin-DAC Syrup 2074
Ryna .... RD 841
Soma Compound w/Codeine Tablets 2676
Tussi-Organidin NR Liquid and S NR Liquid 2677
Tylenol with Codeine 1583

Cryptenamine Preparations (Sympathomimetic may reduce the antihypertensive effects of veratrum alkaloids).

Desflurane (Concomitant use may exhibit additive CNS depression). Products include:

Suprane 1813

Desipramine Hydrochloride (Concomitant use may increase the effects of either the antidepressant or hydrocodone; may antagonize the effects of pseudoephedrine). Products include:

Norpramin Tablets 1526

Deslanoside (Concurrent use of digitalis glycoside may increase the possibility of cardiac arrhythmias).

No products indexed under this heading.

Dezocine (Concomitant use may exhibit additive CNS depression). Products include:

Dalgan Injection 538

Diazepam (Concomitant use may exhibit additive CNS depression). Products include:

Dizac 1809
Valium Injectable 2182
Valium Tablets 2183
Valrelease Capsules 2169

Dicyclomine Hydrochloride (Concurrent use of anticholinergics and hydrocodone may produce paralytic ileus). Products include:

Bentyl 1501

Digitoxin (Concurrent use of digitalis glycoside may increase the possibility of cardiac arrhythmias). Products include:

Crystodigin Tablets.............................. 1433

Digoxin (Concurrent use of digitalis glycoside may increase the possibility of cardiac arrhythmias). Products include:

Lanoxicaps 1117
Lanoxin Elixir Pediatric 1120
Lanoxin Injection 1123
Lanoxin Injection Pediatric................ 1126
Lanoxin Tablets 1128

Doxepin Hydrochloride (Concomitant use may increase the effects of either the antidepressant or hydrocodone; may antagonize the effects of pseudoephedrine). Products include:

Sinequan 2205
Zonalon Cream 1055

Droperidol (Concomitant use may exhibit additive CNS depression). Products include:

Inapsine Injection................................ 1296

Enflurane (Concomitant use may exhibit additive CNS depression).

No products indexed under this heading.

Esmolol Hydrochloride (Potentiates the sympathomimetic effects of pseudoephedrine; hypertensive crises can occur with concurrent use). Products include:

Brevibloc Injection............................... 1808

Estazolam (Concomitant use may exhibit additive CNS depression). Products include:

ProSom Tablets 449

Ethchlorvynol (Concomitant use may exhibit additive CNS depression). Products include:

Placidyl Capsules................................. 448

Ethinamate (Concomitant use may exhibit additive CNS depression).

No products indexed under this heading.

Fentanyl (Concomitant use may exhibit additive CNS depression). Products include:

Duragesic Transdermal System........ 1288

Fentanyl Citrate (Concomitant use may exhibit additive CNS depression). Products include:

Sublimaze Injection............................. 1307

Fluphenazine Decanoate (Concomitant use may exhibit additive CNS depression). Products include:

Prolixin Decanoate 509

Fluphenazine Enanthate (Concomitant use may exhibit additive CNS depression). Products include:

Prolixin Enanthate 509

Fluphenazine Hydrochloride (Concomitant use may exhibit additive CNS depression). Products include:

Prolixin 509

Flurazepam Hydrochloride (Concomitant use may exhibit additive CNS depression). Products include:

Dalmane Capsules................................ 2173

IMPORTANT NOTE: Always consult each drug listing in the patient's regimen for possible interactions.

Tussend

Furazolidone (Potentiates the sympathomimetic effects of pseudoephedrine and may result in hypertensive crisis; concurrent use is contraindicated). Products include:

Furoxone 2046

Glutethimide (Concomitant use may exhibit additive CNS depression).

No products indexed under this heading.

Glycopyrrolate (Concurrent use of anticholinergics and hydrocodone may produce paralytic ileus). Products include:

Robinul Forte Tablets............................ 2072
Robinul Injectable 2072
Robinul Tablets....................................... 2072

Guanethidine Monosulfate (Sympathomimetic may reduce the antihypertensive effects). Products include:

Esimil Tablets 822
Ismelin Tablets 827

Haloperidol (Concomitant use may exhibit additive CNS depression). Products include:

Haldol Injection, Tablets and Concentrate 1575

Haloperidol Decanoate (Concomitant use may exhibit additive CNS depression). Products include:

Haldol Decanoate.................................... 1577

Hydrocodone Polistirex (Concomitant use may exhibit additive CNS depression). Products include:

Tussionex Pennkinetic Extended-Release Suspension 998

Hydroxyzine Hydrochloride (Concomitant use may exhibit additive CNS depression). Products include:

Atarax Tablets & Syrup.......................... 2185
Marax Tablets & DF Syrup.................... 2200
Vistaril Intramuscular Solution......... 2216

Hyoscyamine (Concurrent use of anticholinergics and hydrocodone may produce paralytic ileus). Products include:

Cystospaz Tablets 1963
Urised Tablets... 1964

Hyoscyamine Sulfate (Concurrent use of anticholinergics and hydrocodone may produce paralytic ileus). Products include:

Arco-Lase Plus Tablets 512
Atrohist Plus Tablets 454
Cystospaz-M Capsules 1963
Donnatal 2060
Donnatal Extentabs................................ 2061
Donnatal Tablets 2060
Kutrase Capsules.................................... 2402
Levsin/Levsinex/Levbid 2405

Imipramine Hydrochloride (Concomitant use may increase the effects of either the antidepressant or hydrocodone; may antagonize the effects of pseudoephedrine). Products include:

Tofranil Ampuls 854
Tofranil Tablets 856

Imipramine Pamoate (Concomitant use may increase the effects of either the antidepressant or hydrocodone; may antagonize the effects of pseudoephedrine). Products include:

Tofranil-PM Capsules............................. 857

Indomethacin (Hypertensive crises can occur with concurrent use). Products include:

Indocin 1680

Indomethacin Sodium Trihydrate (Hypertensive crises can occur with concurrent use). Products include:

Indocin I.V. 1684

Ipratropium Bromide (Concurrent use of anticholinergics and hydrocodone may produce paralytic ileus). Products include:

Atrovent Inhalation Aerosol................. 671
Atrovent Inhalation Solution 673

Isocarboxazid (Potentiates the sympathomimetic effects of pseudoephedrine and may result in hypertensive crisis; concurrent use is contraindicated).

No products indexed under this heading.

Isoflurane (Concomitant use may exhibit additive CNS depression).

No products indexed under this heading.

Ketamine Hydrochloride (Concomitant use may exhibit additive CNS depression).

No products indexed under this heading.

Labetalol Hydrochloride (Potentiates the sympathomimetic effects of pseudoephedrine; hypertensive crises can occur with concurrent use). Products include:

Normodyne Injection 2377
Normodyne Tablets 2379
Trandate 1185

Levobunolol Hydrochloride (Potentiates the sympathomimetic effects of pseudoephedrine; hypertensive crises can occur with concurrent use). Products include:

Betagan .... ◉ 233

Levomethadyl Acetate Hydrochloride (Concomitant use may exhibit additive CNS depression). Products include:

Orlaam 2239

Levorphanol Tartrate (Concomitant use may exhibit additive CNS depression). Products include:

Levo-Dromoran 2129

Lithium Carbonate (Concomitant use may exhibit additive CNS depression). Products include:

Eskalith 2485
Lithium Carbonate Capsules & Tablets 2230
Lithonate/Lithotabs/Lithobid 2543

Lithium Citrate (Concomitant use may exhibit additive CNS depression).

No products indexed under this heading.

Lorazepam (Concomitant use may exhibit additive CNS depression). Products include:

Ativan Injection....................................... 2698
Ativan Tablets 2700

Loxapine Hydrochloride (Concomitant use may exhibit additive CNS depression). Products include:

Loxitane 1378

Loxapine Succinate (Concomitant use may exhibit additive CNS depression). Products include:

Loxitane Capsules 1378

Maprotiline Hydrochloride (Concomitant use may increase the effects of either the antidepressant or hydrocodone; may antagonize the effects of pseudoephedrine). Products include:

Ludiomil Tablets..................................... 843

Mecamylamine Hydrochloride (Sympathomimetic may reduce the antihypertensive effects). Products include:

Inversine Tablets 1686

Mepenzolate Bromide (Concurrent use of anticholinergics and hydrocodone may produce paralytic ileus).

No products indexed under this heading.

Meperidine Hydrochloride (Concomitant use may exhibit additive CNS depression). Products include:

Demerol 2308
Mepergan Injection 2753

Mephobarbital (Concomitant use may exhibit additive CNS depression). Products include:

Mebaral Tablets 2322

Meprobamate (Concomitant use may exhibit additive CNS depression). Products include:

Miltown Tablets 2672
PMB 200 and PMB 400 2783

Mesoridazine Besylate (Concomitant use may exhibit additive CNS depression). Products include:

Serentil... 684

Methadone Hydrochloride (Concomitant use may exhibit additive CNS depression). Products include:

Methadone Hydrochloride Oral Concentrate 2233
Methadone Hydrochloride Oral Solution & Tablets................................... 2235

Methohexital Sodium (Concomitant use may exhibit additive CNS depression). Products include:

Brevital Sodium Vials............................ 1429

Methotrimeprazine (Concomitant use may exhibit additive CNS depression). Products include:

Levoprome 1274

Methoxyflurane (Concomitant use may exhibit additive CNS depression).

No products indexed under this heading.

Methyldopa (Sympathomimetic may reduce the antihypertensive effects; hypertensive crises can occur with concurrent use). Products include:

Aldoclor Tablets 1598
Aldomet Oral 1600
Aldoril Tablets... 1604

Methyldopate Hydrochloride (Sympathomimetic may reduce the antihypertensive effects; hypertensive crises can occur with concurrent use). Products include:

Aldomet Ester HCl Injection 1602

Metipranolol Hydrochloride (Potentiates the sympathomimetic effects of pseudoephedrine; hypertensive crises can occur with concurrent use). Products include:

OptiPranolol (Metipranolol 0.3%)
Sterile Ophthalmic Solution........... ◉ 258

Metoprolol Succinate (Potentiates the sympathomimetic effects of pseudoephedrine; hypertensive crises can occur with concurrent use). Products include:

Toprol-XL Tablets 565

Metoprolol Tartrate (Potentiates the sympathomimetic effects of pseudoephedrine; hypertensive crises can occur with concurrent use). Products include:

Lopressor Ampuls................................... 830
Lopressor HCT Tablets 832
Lopressor Tablets 830

Midazolam Hydrochloride (Concomitant use may exhibit additive CNS depression). Products include:

Versed Injection 2170

Molindone Hydrochloride (Concomitant use may exhibit additive CNS depression). Products include:

Moban Tablets and Concentrate...... 1048

Morphine Sulfate (Concomitant use may exhibit additive CNS depression). Products include:

Astramorph/PF Injection, USP (Preservative-Free) 535

Duramorph 962
Infumorph 200 and Infumorph 500 Sterile Solutions............................ 965
MS Contin Tablets................................... 1994
MSIR 1997
Oramorph SR (Morphine Sulfate Sustained Release Tablets) 2236
RMS Suppositories 2657
Roxanol 2243

Nadolol (Potentiates the sympathomimetic effects of pseudoephedrine; hypertensive crises can occur with concurrent use).

No products indexed under this heading.

Nortriptyline Hydrochloride (Concomitant use may increase the effects of either the antidepressant or hydrocodone; may antagonize the effects of pseudoephedrine). Products include:

Pamelor 2280

Opium Alkaloids (Concomitant use may exhibit additive CNS depression).

No products indexed under this heading.

Oxazepam (Concomitant use may exhibit additive CNS depression). Products include:

Serax Capsules 2810
Serax Tablets... 2810

Oxybutynin Chloride (Concurrent use of anticholinergics and hydrocodone may produce paralytic ileus). Products include:

Ditropan.. 1516

Oxycodone Hydrochloride (Concomitant use may exhibit additive CNS depression). Products include:

Percocet Tablets 938
Percodan Tablets.................................... 939
Percodan-Demi Tablets.......................... 940
Roxicodone Tablets, Oral Solution & Intensol (Oxycodone) 2244
Tylox Capsules 1584

Penbutolol Sulfate (Potentiates the sympathomimetic effects of pseudoephedrine; hypertensive crises can occur with concurrent use). Products include:

Levatol 2403

Pentobarbital Sodium (Concomitant use may exhibit additive CNS depression). Products include:

Nembutal Sodium Capsules 436
Nembutal Sodium Solution 438
Nembutal Sodium Suppositories....... 440

Perphenazine (Concomitant use may exhibit additive CNS depression). Products include:

Etrafon 2355
Triavil Tablets 1757
Trilafon.. 2389

Phenelzine Sulfate (Potentiates the sympathomimetic effects of pseudoephedrine and may result in hypertensive crisis; concurrent use is contraindicated). Products include:

Nardil 1920

Phenobarbital (Concomitant use may exhibit additive CNS depression). Products include:

Arco-Lase Plus Tablets 512
Bellergal-S Tablets 2250
Donnatal... 2060
Donnatal Extentabs................................ 2061
Donnatal Tablets..................................... 2060
Phenobarbital Elixir and Tablets 1469
Quadrinal Tablets 1350

Pimozide (Concomitant use may exhibit additive CNS depression). Products include:

Orap Tablets 1050

Pindolol (Potentiates the sympathomimetic effects of pseudoephedrine; hypertensive crises can occur with concurrent use). Products include:

Visken Tablets... 2299

(◈ Described in PDR For Nonprescription Drugs) (◉ Described in PDR For Ophthalmology)

Prazepam (Concomitant use may exhibit additive CNS depression).

No products indexed under this heading.

Prochlorperazine (Concomitant use may exhibit additive CNS depression). Products include:

Compazine 2470

Procyclidine Hydrochloride (Concurrent use of anticholinergics and hydrocodone may produce paralytic ileus). Products include:

Kemadrin Tablets 1112

Promethazine Hydrochloride (Concomitant use may exhibit additive CNS depression). Products include:

Mepergan Injection 2753
Phenergan with Codeine 2777
Phenergan with Dextromethorphan 2778
Phenergan Injection 2773
Phenergan Suppositories 2775
Phenergan Syrup 2774
Phenergan Tablets 2775
Phenergan VC 2779
Phenergan VC with Codeine 2781

Propantheline Bromide (Concurrent use of anticholinergics and hydrocodone may produce paralytic ileus). Products include:

Pro-Banthine Tablets 2052

Propofol (Concomitant use may exhibit additive CNS depression). Products include:

Diprivan Injection 2833

Propoxyphene Hydrochloride (Concomitant use may exhibit additive CNS depression). Products include:

Darvon 1435
Wygesic Tablets 2827

Propoxyphene Napsylate (Concomitant use may exhibit additive CNS depression). Products include:

Darvon-N/Darvocet-N 1433

Propranolol Hydrochloride (Potentiates the sympathomimetic effects of pseudoephedrine; hypertensive crises can occur with concurrent use). Products include:

Inderal 2728
Inderal LA Long Acting Capsules 2730
Inderide Tablets 2732
Inderide LA Long Acting Capsules .. 2734

Protriptyline Hydrochloride (Concomitant use may increase the effects of either the antidepressant or hydrocodone; may antagonize the effects of pseudoephedrine). Products include:

Vivactil Tablets 1774

Quazepam (Concomitant use may exhibit additive CNS depression). Products include:

Doral Tablets 2664

Reserpine (Sympathomimetic may reduce the antihypertensive effects). Products include:

Diupres Tablets 1650
Hydropres Tablets 1675
Ser-Ap-Es Tablets 849

Risperidone (Concomitant use may exhibit additive CNS depression). Products include:

Risperdal 1301

Scopolamine (Concurrent use of anticholinergics and hydrocodone may produce paralytic ileus). Products include:

Transderm Scōp Transdermal Therapeutic System 869

Scopolamine Hydrobromide (Concurrent use of anticholinergics and hydrocodone may produce paralytic ileus). Products include:

Atrohist Plus Tablets 454
Donnatal 2060
Donnatal Extentabs 2061
Donnatal Tablets 2060

Secobarbital Sodium (Concomitant use may exhibit additive CNS depression). Products include:

Seconal Sodium Pulvules 1474

Selegiline Hydrochloride (Potentiates the sympathomimetic effects of pseudoephedrine and may result in hypertensive crisis; concurrent use is contraindicated). Products include:

Eldepryl Tablets 2550

Sotalol Hydrochloride (Potentiates the sympathomimetic effects of pseudoephedrine; hypertensive crises can occur with concurrent use). Products include:

Betapace Tablets 641

Sufentanil Citrate (Concomitant use may exhibit additive CNS depression). Products include:

Sufenta Injection 1309

Temazepam (Concomitant use may exhibit additive CNS depression). Products include:

Restoril Capsules 2284

Thiamylal Sodium (Concomitant use may exhibit additive CNS depression).

No products indexed under this heading.

Thioridazine Hydrochloride (Concomitant use may exhibit additive CNS depression). Products include:

Mellaril 2269

Thiothixene (Concomitant use may exhibit additive CNS depression). Products include:

Navane Capsules and Concentrate 2201
Navane Intramuscular 2202

Timolol Hemihydrate (Potentiates the sympathomimetic effects of pseudoephedrine; hypertensive crises can occur with concurrent use). Products include:

Betimol 0.25%, 0.5% .... ◉ 261

Timolol Maleate (Potentiates the sympathomimetic effects of pseudoephedrine; hypertensive crises can occur with concurrent use). Products include:

Blocadren Tablets 1614
Timolide Tablets 1748
Timoptic in Ocudose 1753
Timoptic Sterile Ophthalmic Solution 1751
Timoptic-XE 1755

Tranylcypromine Sulfate (Potentiates the sympathomimetic effects of pseudoephedrine and may result in hypertensive crisis; concurrent use is contraindicated). Products include:

Parnate Tablets 2503

Triazolam (Concomitant use may exhibit additive CNS depression). Products include:

Halcion Tablets 2611

Tridihexethyl Chloride (Concurrent use of anticholinergics and hydrocodone may produce paralytic ileus).

No products indexed under this heading.

Trifluoperazine Hydrochloride (Concomitant use may exhibit additive CNS depression). Products include:

Stelazine 2514

Trihexyphenidyl Hydrochloride (Concurrent use of anticholinergics and hydrocodone may produce paralytic ileus). Products include:

Artane 1368

Trimipramine Maleate (Concomitant use may increase the effects of either the antidepressant or hydrocodone; may antagonize the effects of pseudoephedrine). Products include:

Surmontil Capsules 2811

Zolpidem Tartrate (Concomitant use may exhibit additive CNS depression). Products include:

Ambien Tablets 2416

Food Interactions

Alcohol (Concomitant use may exhibit additive CNS depression).

TUSSEND EXPECTORANT

(Hydrocodone Bitartrate, Pseudoephedrine Hydrochloride, Guaifenesin) 1785

May interact with narcotic analgesics, general anesthetics, tranquilizers, hypnotics and sedatives, tricyclic antidepressants, central nervous system depressants, monoamine oxidase inhibitors, beta blockers, veratrum alkaloids, and certain other agents. Compounds in these categories include:

Acebutolol Hydrochloride (Potentiates the sympathomimetic effects of pseudoephedrine). Products include:

Sectral Capsules 2807

Alfentanil Hydrochloride (Hydrocodone may potentiate CNS depressant effects). Products include:

Alfenta Injection 1286

Alprazolam (Hydrocodone may potentiate CNS depressant effects). Products include:

Xanax Tablets 2649

Amitriptyline Hydrochloride (Hydrocodone may potentiate CNS depressant effects). Products include:

Elavil 2838
Endep Tablets 2174
Etrafon 2355
Limbitrol 2180
Triavil Tablets 1757

Amoxapine (Hydrocodone may potentiate CNS depressant effects). Products include:

Asendin Tablets 1369

Aprobarbital (Hydrocodone may potentiate CNS depressant effects).

No products indexed under this heading.

Atenolol (Potentiates the sympathomimetic effects of pseudoephedrine). Products include:

Tenoretic Tablets 2845
Tenormin Tablets and I.V. Injection 2847

Betaxolol Hydrochloride (Potentiates the sympathomimetic effects of pseudoephedrine). Products include:

Betoptic Ophthalmic Solution 469
Betoptic S Ophthalmic Suspension 471
Kerlone Tablets 2436

Bisoprolol Fumarate (Potentiates the sympathomimetic effects of pseudoephedrine). Products include:

Zebeta Tablets 1413
Ziac 1415

Buprenorphine (Hydrocodone may potentiate CNS depressant effects). Products include:

Buprenex Injectable 2006

Buspirone Hydrochloride (Hydrocodone may potentiate CNS depressant effects). Products include:

BuSpar 737

Butabarbital (Hydrocodone may potentiate CNS depressant effects).

No products indexed under this heading.

Butalbital (Hydrocodone may potentiate CNS depressant effects). Products include:

Esgic-plus Tablets 1013
Fioricet Tablets 2258
Fioricet with Codeine Capsules 2260
Fiorinal Capsules 2261
Fiorinal with Codeine Capsules 2262
Fiorinal Tablets 2261
Phrenilin 785
Sedapap Tablets 50 mg/650 mg .. 1543

Carteolol Hydrochloride (Potentiates the sympathomimetic effects of pseudoephedrine). Products include:

Cartrol Tablets 410
Ocupress Ophthalmic Solution, 1% Sterile .... ◉ 309

Chlordiazepoxide (Hydrocodone may potentiate CNS depressant effects). Products include:

Libritabs Tablets 2177
Limbitrol 2180

Chlordiazepoxide Hydrochloride (Hydrocodone may potentiate CNS depressant effects). Products include:

Librax Capsules 2176
Librium Capsules 2178
Librium Injectable 2179

Chlorpromazine (Hydrocodone may potentiate CNS depressant effects). Products include:

Thorazine Suppositories 2523

Chlorpromazine Hydrochloride (Hydrocodone may potentiate CNS depressant effects). Products include:

Thorazine 2523

Chlorprothixene (Hydrocodone may potentiate CNS depressant effects).

No products indexed under this heading.

Chlorprothixene Hydrochloride (Hydrocodone may potentiate CNS depressant effects).

No products indexed under this heading.

Clomipramine Hydrochloride (Hydrocodone may potentiate CNS depressant effects). Products include:

Anafranil Capsules 803

Clorazepate Dipotassium (Hydrocodone may potentiate CNS depressant effects). Products include:

Tranxene 451

Clozapine (Hydrocodone may potentiate CNS depressant effects). Products include:

Clozaril Tablets 2252

Codeine Phosphate (Hydrocodone may potentiate CNS depressant effects). Products include:

Actifed with Codeine Cough Syrup.. 1067
Brontex 1981
Deconsal C Expectorant Syrup 456
Deconsal Pediatric Syrup 457
Dimetane-DC Cough Syrup 2059
Empirin with Codeine Tablets 1093
Fioricet with Codeine Capsules 2260
Fiorinal with Codeine Capsules 2262
Isoclor Expectorant 990
Novahistine DH 2462
Novahistine Expectorant 2463
Nucofed 2051
Phenergan with Codeine 2777
Phenergan VC with Codeine 2781
Robitussin A-C Syrup 2073
Robitussin-DAC Syrup 2074
Ryna .... ®◻ 841
Soma Compound w/Codeine Tablets 2676
Tussi-Organidin NR Liquid and S NR Liquid 2677
Tylenol with Codeine 1583

Cryptenamine Preparations (Sympathomimetic may reduce the antihypertensive effects of veratrum alkaloids).

IMPORTANT NOTE: Always consult each drug listing in the patient's regimen for possible interactions.

Tussend Expectorant

Interactions Index

Desflurane (Hydrocodone may potentiate CNS depressant effects). Products include:
Suprane 1813

Desipramine Hydrochloride (Hydrocodone may potentiate CNS depressant effects). Products include:
Norpramin Tablets 1526

Dezocine (Hydrocodone may potentiate CNS depressant effects). Products include:
Dalgan Injection 538

Diazepam (Hydrocodone may potentiate CNS depressant effects). Products include:
Dizac 1809
Valium Injectable 2182
Valium Tablets 2183
Valrelease Capsules 2169

Doxepin Hydrochloride (Hydrocodone may potentiate CNS depressant effects). Products include:
Sinequan 2205
Zonalon Cream 1055

Droperidol (Hydrocodone may potentiate CNS depressant effects). Products include:
Inapsine Injection.................................. 1296

Enflurane (Hydrocodone may potentiate CNS depressant effects).
No products indexed under this heading.

Esmolol Hydrochloride (Potentiates the sympathomimetic effects of pseudoephedrine). Products include:
Brevibloc Injection................................ 1808

Estazolam (Hydrocodone may potentiate CNS depressant effects). Products include:
ProSom Tablets 449

Ethchlorvynol (Hydrocodone may potentiate CNS depressant effects). Products include:
Placidyl Capsules................................... 448

Ethinamate (Hydrocodone may potentiate CNS depressant effects).
No products indexed under this heading.

Fentanyl (Hydrocodone may potentiate CNS depressant effects). Products include:
Duragesic Transdermal System....... 1288

Fentanyl Citrate (Hydrocodone may potentiate CNS depressant effects). Products include:
Sublimaze Injection............................... 1307

Fluphenazine Decanoate (Hydrocodone may potentiate CNS depressant effects). Products include:
Prolixin Decanoate 509

Fluphenazine Enanthate (Hydrocodone may potentiate CNS depressant effects). Products include:
Prolixin Enanthate 509

Fluphenazine Hydrochloride (Hydrocodone may potentiate CNS depressant effects). Products include:
Prolixin 509

Flurazepam Hydrochloride (Hydrocodone may potentiate CNS depressant effects). Products include:
Dalmane Capsules................................. 2173

Furazolidone (Potentiates the sympathomimetic effects of pseudoephedrine; hydrocodone may potentiate CNS depressant effects; concurrent use is contraindicated). Products include:
Furoxone 2046

Glutethimide (Hydrocodone may potentiate CNS depressant effects).
No products indexed under this heading.

Haloperidol (Hydrocodone may potentiate CNS depressant effects). Products include:
Haldol Injection, Tablets and Concentrate 1575

Haloperidol Decanoate (Hydrocodone may potentiate CNS depressant effects). Products include:
Haldol Decanoate................................... 1577

Hydrocodone Polistirex (Hydrocodone may potentiate CNS depressant effects). Products include:
Tussionex Pennkinetic Extended-Release Suspension 998

Hydroxyzine Hydrochloride (Hydrocodone may potentiate CNS depressant effects). Products include:
Atarax Tablets & Syrup......................... 2185
Marax Tablets & DF Syrup.................... 2200
Vistaril Intramuscular Solution......... 2216

Imipramine Hydrochloride (Hydrocodone may potentiate CNS depressant effects). Products include:
Tofranil Ampuls 854
Tofranil Tablets 856

Imipramine Pamoate (Hydrocodone may potentiate CNS depressant effects). Products include:
Tofranil-PM Capsules............................ 857

Isocarboxazid (Potentiates the sympathomimetic effects of pseudoephedrine; hydrocodone may potentiate CNS depressant effects; concurrent use is contraindicated).
No products indexed under this heading.

Isoflurane (Hydrocodone may potentiate CNS depressant effects).
No products indexed under this heading.

Ketamine Hydrochloride (Hydrocodone may potentiate CNS depressant effects).
No products indexed under this heading.

Labetalol Hydrochloride (Potentiates the sympathomimetic effects of pseudoephedrine). Products include:
Normodyne Injection 2377
Normodyne Tablets 2379
Trandate 1185

Levobunolol Hydrochloride (Potentiates the sympathomimetic effects of pseudoephedrine). Products include:
Betagan .... ◉ 233

Levomethadyl Acetate Hydrochloride (Hydrocodone may potentiate CNS depressant effects). Products include:
Orlaam 2239

Levorphanol Tartrate (Hydrocodone may potentiate CNS depressant effects). Products include:
Levo-Dromoran...................................... 2129

Lorazepam (Hydrocodone may potentiate CNS depressant effects). Products include:
Ativan Injection..................................... 2698
Ativan Tablets 2700

Loxapine Hydrochloride (Hydrocodone may potentiate CNS depressant effects). Products include:
Loxitane 1378

Loxapine Succinate (Hydrocodone may potentiate CNS depressant effects). Products include:
Loxitane Capsules 1378

Maprotiline Hydrochloride (Hydrocodone may potentiate CNS depressant effects). Products include:
Ludiomil Tablets.................................... 843

Mecamylamine Hydrochloride (Sympathomimetic may reduce the antihypertensive effects). Products include:
Inversine Tablets 1686

Meperidine Hydrochloride (Hydrocodone may potentiate CNS depressant effects). Products include:
Demerol 2308
Mepergan Injection 2753

Mephobarbital (Hydrocodone may potentiate CNS depressant effects). Products include:
Mebaral Tablets 2322

Meprobamate (Hydrocodone may potentiate CNS depressant effects). Products include:
Miltown Tablets..................................... 2672
PMB 200 and PMB 400 2783

Mesoridazine Besylate (Hydrocodone may potentiate CNS depressant effects). Products include:
Serentil 684

Methadone Hydrochloride (Hydrocodone may potentiate CNS depressant effects). Products include:
Methadone Hydrochloride Oral Concentrate 2233
Methadone Hydrochloride Oral Solution & Tablets.................................. 2235

Methohexital Sodium (Hydrocodone may potentiate CNS depressant effects). Products include:
Brevital Sodium Vials 1429

Methotrimeprazine (Hydrocodone may potentiate CNS depressant effects). Products include:
Levoprome 1274

Methoxyflurane (Hydrocodone may potentiate CNS depressant effects).
No products indexed under this heading.

Methyldopa (Sympathomimetic may reduce the antihypertensive effects). Products include:
Aldoclor Tablets 1598
Aldomet Oral 1600
Aldoril Tablets....................................... 1604

Methyldopate Hydrochloride (Sympathomimetic may reduce the antihypertensive effects). Products include:
Aldomet Ester HCl Injection 1602

Metipranolol Hydrochloride (Potentiates the sympathomimetic effects of pseudoephedrine). Products include:
OptiPranolol (Metipranolol 0.3%) Sterile Ophthalmic Solution.......... ◉ 258

Metoprolol Succinate (Potentiates the sympathomimetic effects of pseudoephedrine). Products include:
Toprol-XL Tablets 565

Metoprolol Tartrate (Potentiates the sympathomimetic effects of pseudoephedrine). Products include:
Lopressor Ampuls.................................. 830
Lopressor HCT Tablets 832
Lopressor Tablets 830

Midazolam Hydrochloride (Hydrocodone may potentiate CNS depressant effects). Products include:
Versed Injection 2170

Molindone Hydrochloride (Hydrocodone may potentiate CNS depressant effects). Products include:
Moban Tablets and Concentrate....... 1048

Morphine Sulfate (Hydrocodone may potentiate CNS depressant effects). Products include:
Astramorph/PF Injection, USP (Preservative-Free) 535
Duramorph 962
Infumorph 200 and Infumorph 500 Sterile Solutions........................... 965
MS Contin Tablets................................. 1994
MSIR 1997

Oramorph SR (Morphine Sulfate Sustained Release Tablets) 2236
RMS Suppositories 2657
Roxanol 2243

Nadolol (Potentiates the sympathomimetic effects of pseudoephedrine).
No products indexed under this heading.

Nortriptyline Hydrochloride (Hydrocodone may potentiate CNS depressant effects). Products include:
Pamelor 2280

Opium Alkaloids (Hydrocodone may potentiate CNS depressant effects).
No products indexed under this heading.

Oxazepam (Hydrocodone may potentiate CNS depressant effects). Products include:
Serax Capsules 2810
Serax Tablets... 2810

Oxycodone Hydrochloride (Hydrocodone may potentiate CNS depressant effects). Products include:
Percocet Tablets 938
Percodan Tablets................................... 939
Percodan-Demi Tablets......................... 940
Roxicodone Tablets, Oral Solution & Intensol (Oxycodone) 2244
Tylox Capsules 1584

Penbutolol Sulfate (Potentiates the sympathomimetic effects of pseudoephedrine). Products include:
Levatol 2403

Pentobarbital Sodium (Hydrocodone may potentiate CNS depressant effects). Products include:
Nembutal Sodium Capsules 436
Nembutal Sodium Solution 438
Nembutal Sodium Suppositories...... 440

Perphenazine (Hydrocodone may potentiate CNS depressant effects). Products include:
Etrafon 2355
Triavil Tablets 1757
Trilafon... 2389

Phenelzine Sulfate (Potentiates the sympathomimetic effects of pseudoephedrine; hydrocodone may potentiate CNS depressant effects; concurrent use is contraindicated). Products include:
Nardil 1920

Phenobarbital (Hydrocodone may potentiate CNS depressant effects). Products include:
Arco-Lase Plus Tablets 512
Bellergal-S Tablets 2250
Donnatal 2060
Donnatal Extentabs............................... 2061
Donnatal Tablets 2060
Phenobarbital Elixir and Tablets 1469
Quadrinal Tablets 1350

Pindolol (Potentiates the sympathomimetic effects of pseudoephedrine). Products include:
Visken Tablets.. 2299

Prazepam (Hydrocodone may potentiate CNS depressant effects).
No products indexed under this heading.

Prochlorperazine (Hydrocodone may potentiate CNS depressant effects). Products include:
Compazine 2470

Promethazine Hydrochloride (Hydrocodone may potentiate CNS depressant effects). Products include:
Mepergan Injection 2753
Phenergan with Codeine....................... 2777
Phenergan with Dextromethorphan 2778
Phenergan Injection 2773
Phenergan Suppositories 2775
Phenergan Syrup................................... 2774
Phenergan Tablets 2775
Phenergan VC 2779
Phenergan VC with Codeine 2781

(◻ Described in PDR For Nonprescription Drugs) (◉ Described in PDR For Ophthalmology)

Interactions Index

Propofol (Hydrocodone may potentiate CNS depressant effects). Products include:

Diprivan Injection 2833

Propoxyphene Hydrochloride (Hydrocodone may potentiate CNS depressant effects). Products include:

Darvon 1435
Wygesic Tablets 2827

Propoxyphene Napsylate (Hydrocodone may potentiate CNS depressant effects). Products include:

Darvon-N/Darvocet-N 1433

Propranolol Hydrochloride (Potentiates the sympathomimetic effects of pseudoephedrine). Products include:

Inderal 2728
Inderal LA Long Acting Capsules 2730
Inderide Tablets 2732
Inderide LA Long Acting Capsules .. 2734

Protriptyline Hydrochloride (Hydrocodone may potentiate CNS depressant effects). Products include:

Vivactil Tablets 1774

Quazepam (Hydrocodone may potentiate CNS depressant effects). Products include:

Doral Tablets 2664

Reserpine (Sympathomimetic may reduce the antihypertensive effects). Products include:

Diupres Tablets 1650
Hydropres Tablets 1675
Ser-Ap-Es Tablets 849

Risperidone (Hydrocodone may potentiate CNS depressant effects). Products include:

Risperdal 1301

Secobarbital Sodium (Hydrocodone may potentiate CNS depressant effects). Products include:

Seconal Sodium Pulvules 1474

Selegiline Hydrochloride (Potentiates the sympathomimetic effects of pseudoephedrine; hydrocodone may potentiate CNS depressant effects; concurrent use is contraindicated). Products include:

Eldepryl Tablets 2550

Sotalol Hydrochloride (Potentiates the sympathomimetic effects of pseudoephedrine). Products include:

Betapace Tablets 641

Sufentanil Citrate (Hydrocodone may potentiate CNS depressant effects). Products include:

Sufenta Injection 1309

Temazepam (Hydrocodone may potentiate CNS depressant effects). Products include:

Restoril Capsules 2284

Thiamylal Sodium (Hydrocodone may potentiate CNS depressant effects).

No products indexed under this heading.

Thioridazine Hydrochloride (Hydrocodone may potentiate CNS depressant effects). Products include:

Mellaril 2269

Thiothixene (Hydrocodone may potentiate CNS depressant effects). Products include:

Navane Capsules and Concentrate 2201
Navane Intramuscular 2202

Timolol Hemihydrate (Potentiates the sympathomimetic effects of pseudoephedrine). Products include:

Betimol 0.25%, 0.5% .... ◉ 261

Timolol Maleate (Potentiates the sympathomimetic effects of pseudoephedrine). Products include:

Blocadren Tablets 1614
Timolide Tablets 1748

Timoptic in Ocudose 1753
Timoptic Sterile Ophthalmic Solution 1751
Timoptic-XE 1755

Tranylcypromine Sulfate (Potentiates the sympathomimetic effects of pseudoephedrine; hydrocodone may potentiate CNS depressant effects; concurrent use is contraindicated). Products include:

Parnate Tablets 2503

Triazolam (Hydrocodone may potentiate CNS depressant effects). Products include:

Halcion Tablets 2611

Trifluoperazine Hydrochloride (Hydrocodone may potentiate CNS depressant effects). Products include:

Stelazine 2514

Trimipramine Maleate (Hydrocodone may potentiate CNS depressant effects). Products include:

Surmontil Capsules 2811

Zolpidem Tartrate (Hydrocodone may potentiate CNS depressant effects). Products include:

Ambien Tablets 2416

Food Interactions

Alcohol (Hydrocodone may potentiate CNS depressant effects).

TUSSIONEX PENNKINETIC EXTENDED-RELEASE SUSPENSION

(Hydrocodone Polistirex, Chlorpheniramine Polistirex) 998

May interact with central nervous system depressants, antihistamines, monoamine oxidase inhibitors, tricyclic antidepressants, anticholinergics, narcotic analgesics, antipsychotic agents, tranquilizers, and certain other agents. Compounds in these categories include:

Acrivastine (Additive CNS depression). Products include:

Semprex-D Capsules 463
Semprex-D Capsules 1167

Alfentanil Hydrochloride (Additive CNS depression). Products include:

Alfenta Injection 1286

Alprazolam (Additive CNS depression). Products include:

Xanax Tablets 2649

Amitriptyline Hydrochloride (Effect of either agent may be increased). Products include:

Elavil 2838
Endep Tablets 2174
Etrafon 2355
Limbitrol 2180
Triavil Tablets 1757

Amoxapine (Effect of either agent may be increased). Products include:

Asendin Tablets 1369

Aprobarbital (Additive CNS depression).

No products indexed under this heading.

Astemizole (Additive CNS depression). Products include:

Hismanal Tablets 1293

Atropine Sulfate (Concurrent use may produce paralytic ileus). Products include:

Arco-Lase Plus Tablets 512
Atrohist Plus Tablets 454
Atropine Sulfate Sterile Ophthalmic Solution .... ◉ 233
Donnatal 2060
Donnatal Extentabs 2061
Donnatal Tablets 2060
Lomotil 2439
Motofen Tablets 784
Urised Tablets 1964

Azatadine Maleate (Additive CNS depression). Products include:

Trinalin Repetabs Tablets 1330

Belladonna Alkaloids (Concurrent use may produce paralytic ileus). Products include:

Bellergal-S Tablets 2250
Hyland's Bed Wetting Tablets .... ⊕D 828
Hyland's EnurAid Tablets .... ⊕D 829
Hyland's Teething Tablets .... ⊕D 830

Benztropine Mesylate (Concurrent use may produce paralytic ileus). Products include:

Cogentin 1621

Biperiden Hydrochloride (Concurrent use may produce paralytic ileus). Products include:

Akineton 1333

Bromodiphenhydramine Hydrochloride (Additive CNS depression).

No products indexed under this heading.

Brompheniramine Maleate (Additive CNS depression). Products include:

Alka Seltzer Plus Sinus Medicine .. ⊕D 707
Bromfed Capsules (Extended-Release) 1785
Bromfed Syrup .... ⊕D 733
Bromfed Tablets 1785
Bromfed-DM Cough Syrup 1786
Bromfed-PD Capsules (Extended-Release) 1785
Dimetane-DC Cough Syrup 2059
Dimetane-DX Cough Syrup 2059
Dimetapp Elixir .... ⊕D 773
Dimetapp Extentabs .... ⊕D 774
Dimetapp Tablets/Liqui-Gels .... ⊕D 775
Dimetapp Cold & Allergy Chewable Tablets .... ⊕D 773
Dimetapp DM Elixir .... ⊕D 774
Vicks DayQuil Allergy Relief 12-Hour Extended Release Tablets.. ⊕D 760
Vicks DayQuil Allergy Relief 4-Hour Tablets .... ⊕D 760

Buprenorphine (Additive CNS depression). Products include:

Buprenex Injectable 2006

Buspirone Hydrochloride (Additive CNS depression). Products include:

BuSpar 737

Butabarbital (Additive CNS depression).

No products indexed under this heading.

Butalbital (Additive CNS depression). Products include:

Esgic-plus Tablets 1013
Fioricet Tablets 2258
Fioricet with Codeine Capsules 2260
Fiorinal Capsules 2261
Fiorinal with Codeine Capsules 2262
Fiorinal Tablets 2261
Phrenilin 785
Sedapap Tablets 50 mg/650 mg .. 1543

Chlordiazepoxide (Additive CNS depression). Products include:

Libritabs Tablets 2177
Limbitrol 2180

Chlordiazepoxide Hydrochloride (Additive CNS depression). Products include:

Librax Capsules 2176
Librium Capsules 2178
Librium Injectable 2179

Chlorpheniramine Maleate (Additive CNS depression). Products include:

Alka-Seltzer Plus Cold Medicine .... ⊕D 705
Alka-Seltzer Plus Cold Medicine Liqui-Gels .... ⊕D 706
Alka-Seltzer Plus Cold & Cough Medicine .... ⊕D 708
Alka-Seltzer Plus Cold & Cough Medicine Liqui-Gels .... ⊕D 705
Allerest Children's Chewable Tablets .... ⊕D 627
Allerest Headache Strength Tablets .... ⊕D 627
Allerest Maximum Strength Tablets .... ⊕D 627

Allerest Sinus Pain Formula .... ⊕D 627
Allerest 12 Hour Caplets .... ⊕D 627
Ana-Kit Anaphylaxis Emergency Treatment Kit 617
Atrohist Pediatric Capsules 453
Atrohist Plus Tablets 454
BC Cold Powder Multi-Symptom Formula (Cold-Sinus-Allergy) ...... ⊕D 609
Cerose DM .... ⊕D 878
Cheracol Plus Head Cold/Cough Formula .... ⊕D 769
Children's Vicks DayQuil Allergy Relief .... ⊕D 757
Children's Vicks NyQuil Cold/Cough Relief .... ⊕D 758
Chlor-Trimeton Allergy Decongestant Tablets .... ⊕D 799
Chlor-Trimeton Allergy Tablets ...... ⊕D 798
Comhist 2038
Comtrex Multi-Symptom Cold Reliever Tablets/Caplets/Liqui-Gels/Liquid .... ⊕D 615
Allergy-Sinus Comtrex Multi-Symptom Allergy-Sinus Formula Tablets .... ⊕D 617
Contac Continuous Action Nasal Decongestant/Antihistamine 12 Hour Capsules .... ⊕D 813
Contac Maximum Strength Continuous Action Decongestant/Antihistamine 12 Hour Caplets.. ⊕D 813
Contac Severe Cold and Flu Formula Caplets .... ⊕D 814
Coricidin 'D' Decongestant Tablets .... ⊕D 800
Coricidin Tablets .... ⊕D 800
D.A. Chewable Tablets 951
Deconamine 1320
Dura-Tap/PD Capsules 2867
Dura-Vent/DA Tablets 953
Extendryl 1005
Fedahist Gyrocaps 2401
Fedahist Timecaps 2401
Hycomine Compound Tablets 932
Isoclor Timesule Capsules .... ⊕D 637
Kronofed-A 977
Nolamine Timed-Release Tablets 785
Novahistine DH 2462
Novahistine Elixir .... ⊕D 823
Ornade Spansule Capsules 2502
PediaCare Cold Allergy Chewable Tablets .... ⊕D 677
PediaCare Cough-Cold Chewable Tablets 1553
PediaCare Cough-Cold Liquid 1553
PediaCare NightRest Cough-Cold Liquid 1553
Pediatric Vicks 44m Cough & Cold Relief .... ⊕D 764
Pyrroxate Caplets .... ⊕D 772
Ryna .... ⊕D 841
Sinarest Tablets .... ⊕D 648
Sinarest Extra Strength Tablets ...... ⊕D 648
Sine-Off Sinus Medicine .... ⊕D 825
Singlet Tablets .... ⊕D 825
Sinulin Tablets 787
Sinutab Sinus Allergy Medication, Maximum Strength Tablets and Caplets .... ⊕D 860
Sudafed Plus Liquid .... ⊕D 862
Sudafed Plus Tablets .... ⊕D 863
Teldrin 12 Hour Antihistamine/Nasal Decongestant Allergy Relief Capsules .... ⊕D 826
TheraFlu .... ⊕D 787
TheraFlu Maximum Strength Nighttime Flu, Cold & Cough Medicine .... ⊕D 788
Triaminic Allergy Tablets .... ⊕D 789
Triaminic Cold Tablets .... ⊕D 790
Triaminic Nite Light .... ⊕D 791
Triaminic Syrup .... ⊕D 792
Triaminic-12 Tablets .... ⊕D 792
Triaminicin Tablets .... ⊕D 793
Triaminicol Multi-Symptom Cold Tablets .... ⊕D 793
Triaminicol Multi-Symptom Relief ⊕D 794
Tussend 1783
Children's TYLENOL Cold Multi-Symptom Liquid Formula and Chewable Tablets 1561
Children's TYLENOL Cold Plus Cough Multi Symptom Tablets and Liquid .... ⊕D 681
TYLENOL Maximum Strength Allergy Sinus Medication Gelcaps and Caplets 1563
TYLENOL Cold Multi-Symptom Formula Medication Tablets and Caplets 1561

IMPORTANT NOTE: Always consult each drug listing in the patient's regimen for possible interactions.

Tussionex

TYLENOL Cold Multi-Symptom Hot Medication Liquid Packets 1557
Vicks 44 LiquiCaps Cough, Cold & Flu Relief .... ◆□ 755
Vicks 44M Cough, Cold & Flu Relief .... ◆□ 756

Chlorpheniramine Tannate (Additive CNS depression). Products include:

Atrohist Pediatric Suspension 454
Ricobid Tablets and Pediatric Suspension 2038
Rynatan 2673
Rynatuss 2673

Chlorpromazine (Additive CNS depression). Products include:

Thorazine Suppositories 2523

Chlorpromazine Hydrochloride (Additive CNS depression). Products include:

Thorazine 2523

Chlorprothixene (Additive CNS depression).

No products indexed under this heading.

Chlorprothixene Hydrochloride (Additive CNS depression).

No products indexed under this heading.

Clemastine Fumarate (Additive CNS depression). Products include:

Tavist Syrup 2297
Tavist Tablets 2298
Tavist-1 12 Hour Relief Tablets .... ◆□ 787
Tavist-D 12 Hour Relief Tablets .... ◆□ 787

Clidinium Bromide (Concurrent use may produce paralytic ileus). Products include:

Librax Capsules 2176
Quarzan Capsules 2181

Clomipramine Hydrochloride (Effect of either agent may be increased). Products include:

Anafranil Capsules 803

Clorazepate Dipotassium (Additive CNS depression). Products include:

Tranxene 451

Clozapine (Additive CNS depression). Products include:

Clozaril Tablets 2252

Codeine Phosphate (Additive CNS depression). Products include:

Actifed with Codeine Cough Syrup.. 1067
Brontex 1981
Deconsal C Expectorant Syrup 456
Deconsal Pediatric Syrup 457
Dimetane-DC Cough Syrup 2059
Empirin with Codeine Tablets 1093
Fioricet with Codeine Capsules 2260
Fiorinal with Codeine Capsules 2262
Isoclor Expectorant 990
Novahistine DH 2462
Novahistine Expectorant 2463
Nucofed 2051
Phenergan with Codeine 2777
Phenergan VC with Codeine 2781
Robitussin A-C Syrup 2073
Robitussin-DAC Syrup 2074
Ryna .... ◆□ 841
Soma Compound w/Codeine Tablets 2676
Tussi-Organidin NR Liquid and S NR Liquid 2677
Tylenol with Codeine 1583

Cyproheptadine Hydrochloride (Additive CNS depression). Products include:

Periactin 1724

Desflurane (Additive CNS depression). Products include:

Suprane 1813

Desipramine Hydrochloride (Effect of either agent may be increased). Products include:

Norpramin Tablets 1526

Dexchlorpheniramine Maleate (Additive CNS depression).

No products indexed under this heading.

Dezocine (Additive CNS depression). Products include:

Dalgan Injection 538

Diazepam (Additive CNS depression). Products include:

Dizac 1809
Valium Injectable 2182
Valium Tablets 2183
Valrelease Capsules 2169

Dicyclomine Hydrochloride (Concurrent use may produce paralytic ileus). Products include:

Bentyl 1501

Diphenhydramine Citrate (Additive CNS depression). Products include:

Excedrin P.M. Analgesic/Sleeping Aid Tablets, Caplets, Liquigels 733

Diphenhydramine Hydrochloride (Additive CNS depression). Products include:

Actifed Allergy Daytime/Nighttime Caplets .... ◆□ 844
Actifed Sinus Daytime/Nighttime Tablets and Caplets .... ◆□ 846
Arthritis Foundation NightTime Caplets .... ◆□ 674
Extra Strength Bayer PM Aspirin .. ◆□ 713
Bayer Select Night Time Pain Relief Formula .... ◆□ 716
Benadryl Allergy Decongestant Liquid Medication .... ◆□ 848
Benadryl Allergy Decongestant Tablets .... ◆□ 848
Benadryl Allergy Liquid Medication .... ◆□ 849
Benadryl Allergy .... ◆□ 848
Benadryl Allergy Sinus Headache Formula Caplets .... ◆□ 849
Benadryl Capsules 1898
Benadryl Dye-Free Allergy Liquigel Softgels .... ◆□ 850
Benadryl Dye-Free Allergy Liquid Medication .... ◆□ 850
Benadryl Itch Relief Cream, Children's Formula and Maximum Strength 2% .... ◆□ 851
Benadryl Itch Relief Spray, Children's Formula and Maximum Strength 2% .... ◆□ 851
Benadryl Itch Relief Stick Maximum Strength 2% .... ◆□ 850
Benadryl Itch Stopping Gel, Children's Formula and Maximum Strength 2% .... ◆□ 851
Benadryl Kapseals 1898
Benadryl Injection 1898
Contac Day & Night Cold/Flu Night Caplets .... ◆□ 812
Contac Night Allergy/Sinus Caplets .... ◆□ 812
Extra Strength Doan's P.M. .... ◆□ 633
Legatrin PM .... ◆□ 651
Miles Nervine Nighttime Sleep-Aid ◆□ 723
Nytol QuickCaps Caplets .... ◆□ 610
Sleepinal Night-time Sleep Aid Capsules and Softgels .... ◆□ 834
TYLENOL Maximum Strength Allergy Sinus NightTime Medication Caplets 1555
TYLENOL Flu NightTime, Maximum Strength, Gelcaps 1566
TYLENOL Maximum Strength Flu NightTime Hot Medication Packets 1562
TYLENOL PM, Extra Strength Pain Reliever/Sleep Aid Caplets, Geltabs, Gelcaps 1560
TYLENOL Severe Allergy Medication Caplets 1564
Maximum Strength Unisom Sleepgels 1934
Unisom With Pain Relief-Nighttime Sleep Aid and Pain Reliever 1934

Diphenylpyraline Hydrochloride (Additive CNS depression).

No products indexed under this heading.

Doxepin Hydrochloride (Effect of either agent may be increased). Products include:

Sinequan 2205
Zonalon Cream 1055

Droperidol (Additive CNS depression). Products include:

Inapsine Injection 1296

Enflurane (Additive CNS depression).

No products indexed under this heading.

Estazolam (Additive CNS depression). Products include:

ProSom Tablets 449

Ethchlorvynol (Additive CNS depression). Products include:

Placidyl Capsules 448

Ethinamate (Additive CNS depression).

No products indexed under this heading.

Fentanyl (Additive CNS depression). Products include:

Duragesic Transdermal System 1288

Fentanyl Citrate (Additive CNS depression). Products include:

Sublimaze Injection 1307

Fluphenazine Decanoate (Additive CNS depression). Products include:

Prolixin Decanoate 509

Fluphenazine Enanthate (Additive CNS depression). Products include:

Prolixin Enanthate 509

Fluphenazine Hydrochloride (Additive CNS depression). Products include:

Prolixin 509

Flurazepam Hydrochloride (Additive CNS depression). Products include:

Dalmane Capsules 2173

Furazolidone (Effect of either agent may be increased). Products include:

Furoxone 2046

Glutethimide (Additive CNS depression).

No products indexed under this heading.

Glycopyrrolate (Concurrent use may produce paralytic ileus). Products include:

Robinul Forte Tablets 2072
Robinul Injectable 2072
Robinul Tablets 2072

Haloperidol (Additive CNS depression). Products include:

Haldol Injection, Tablets and Concentrate 1575

Haloperidol Decanoate (Additive CNS depression). Products include:

Haldol Decanoate 1577

Hydrocodone Bitartrate (Additive CNS depression). Products include:

Anexsia 5/500 Elixir 1781
Anexia Tablets 1782
Codiclear DH Syrup 791
Deconamine CX Cough and Cold Liquid and Tablets 1319
Duratuss HD Elixir 2565
Hycodan Tablets and Syrup 930
Hycomine Compound Tablets 932
Hycomine 931
Hycotuss Expectorant Syrup 933
Hydrocet Capsules 782
Lorcet 10/650 1018
Lortab 2566
Tussend 1783
Tussend Expectorant 1785
Vicodin Tablets 1356
Vicodin ES Tablets 1357
Vicodin Tuss Expectorant 1358
Zydone Capsules 949

Hydroxyzine Hydrochloride (Additive CNS depression). Products include:

Atarax Tablets & Syrup 2185
Marax Tablets & DF Syrup 2200
Vistaril Intramuscular Solution 2216

Hyoscyamine (Concurrent use may produce paralytic ileus). Products include:

Cystospaz Tablets 1963
Urised Tablets 1964

Hyoscyamine Sulfate (Concurrent use may produce paralytic ileus). Products include:

Arco-Lase Plus Tablets 512
Atrohist Plus Tablets 454
Cystospaz-M Capsules 1963
Donnatal 2060
Donnatal Extentabs 2061
Donnatal Tablets 2060
Kutrase Capsules 2402
Levsin/Levsinex/Levbid 2405

Imipramine Hydrochloride (Effect of either agent may be increased). Products include:

Tofranil Ampuls 854
Tofranil Tablets 856

Imipramine Pamoate (Effect of either agent may be increased). Products include:

Tofranil-PM Capsules 857

Ipratropium Bromide (Concurrent use may produce paralytic ileus). Products include:

Atrovent Inhalation Aerosol 671
Atrovent Inhalation Solution 673

Isocarboxazid (Effect of either agent may be increased).

No products indexed under this heading.

Isoflurane (Additive CNS depression).

No products indexed under this heading.

Ketamine Hydrochloride (Additive CNS depression).

No products indexed under this heading.

Levomethadyl Acetate Hydrochloride (Additive CNS depression). Products include:

Orlaam 2239

Levorphanol Tartrate (Additive CNS depression). Products include:

Levo-Dromoran 2129

Lithium Carbonate (Additive CNS depression). Products include:

Eskalith 2485
Lithium Carbonate Capsules & Tablets 2230
Lithonate/Lithotabs/Lithobid 2543

Lithium Citrate (Additive CNS depression).

No products indexed under this heading.

Loratadine (Additive CNS depression). Products include:

Claritin 2349
Claritin-D 2350

Lorazepam (Additive CNS depression). Products include:

Ativan Injection 2698
Ativan Tablets 2700

Loxapine Hydrochloride (Additive CNS depression). Products include:

Loxitane 1378

Loxapine Succinate (Additive CNS depression). Products include:

Loxitane Capsules 1378

Maprotiline Hydrochloride (Effect of either agent may be increased). Products include:

Ludiomil Tablets 843

Mepenzolate Bromide (Concurrent use may produce paralytic ileus).

No products indexed under this heading.

Meperidine Hydrochloride (Additive CNS depression). Products include:

Demerol 2308
Mepergan Injection 2753

Mephobarbital (Additive CNS depression). Products include:

Mebaral Tablets 2322

Meprobamate (Additive CNS depression). Products include:

Miltown Tablets 2672

(◆□ Described in PDR For Nonprescription Drugs) (◉ Described in PDR For Ophthalmology)

Interactions Index

Tussi-Organidin DM NR

PMB 200 and PMB 400 2783

Mesoridazine Besylate (Additive CNS depression). Products include:

Serentil 684

Methadone Hydrochloride (Additive CNS depression). Products include:

Methadone Hydrochloride Oral Concentrate 2233

Methadone Hydrochloride Oral Solution & Tablets 2235

Methdilazine Hydrochloride (Additive CNS depression).

No products indexed under this heading.

Methohexital Sodium (Additive CNS depression). Products include:

Brevital Sodium Vials 1429

Methotrimeprazine (Additive CNS depression). Products include:

Levoprome 1274

Methoxyflurane (Additive CNS depression).

No products indexed under this heading.

Midazolam Hydrochloride (Additive CNS depression). Products include:

Versed Injection 2170

Molindone Hydrochloride (Additive CNS depression). Products include:

Moban Tablets and Concentrate 1048

Morphine Sulfate (Additive CNS depression). Products include:

Astramorph/PF Injection, USP (Preservative-Free) 535

Duramorph 962

Infumorph 200 and Infumorph 500 Sterile Solutions 965

MS Contin Tablets 1994

MSIR 1997

Oramorph SR (Morphine Sulfate Sustained Release Tablets) 2236

RMS Suppositories 2657

Roxanol 2243

Nortriptyline Hydrochloride (Effect of either agent may be increased). Products include:

Pamelor 2280

Opium Alkaloids (Additive CNS depression).

No products indexed under this heading.

Oxazepam (Additive CNS depression). Products include:

Serax Capsules 2810

Serax Tablets 2810

Oxybutynin Chloride (Concurrent use may produce paralytic ileus). Products include:

Ditropan 1516

Oxycodone Hydrochloride (Additive CNS depression). Products include:

Percocet Tablets 938

Percodan Tablets 939

Percodan-Demi Tablets 940

Roxicodone Tablets, Oral Solution & Intensol (Oxycodone) 2244

Tylox Capsules 1584

Pentobarbital Sodium (Additive CNS depression). Products include:

Nembutal Sodium Capsules 436

Nembutal Sodium Solution 438

Nembutal Sodium Suppositories 440

Perphenazine (Additive CNS depression). Products include:

Etrafon 2355

Triavil Tablets 1757

Trilafon 2389

Phenelzine Sulfate (Effect of either agent may be increased). Products include:

Nardil 1920

Phenobarbital (Additive CNS depression). Products include:

Arco-Lase Plus Tablets 512

Bellergal-S Tablets 2250

Donnatal 2060

Donnatal Extentabs 2061

Donnatal Tablets 2060

Phenobarbital Elixir and Tablets 1469

Quadrinal Tablets 1350

Pimozide (Additive CNS depression). Products include:

Orap Tablets 1050

Prazepam (Additive CNS depression).

No products indexed under this heading.

Prochlorperazine (Additive CNS depression). Products include:

Compazine 2470

Procyclidine Hydrochloride (Concurrent use may produce paralytic ileus). Products include:

Kemadrin Tablets 1112

Promethazine Hydrochloride (Additive CNS depression). Products include:

Mepergan Injection 2753

Phenergan with Codeine 2777

Phenergan with Dextromethorphan 2778

Phenergan Injection 2773

Phenergan Suppositories 2775

Phenergan Syrup 2774

Phenergan Tablets 2775

Phenergan VC 2779

Phenergan VC with Codeine 2781

Propantheline Bromide (Concurrent use may produce paralytic ileus). Products include:

Pro-Banthine Tablets 2052

Propofol (Additive CNS depression). Products include:

Diprivan Injection 2833

Propoxyphene Hydrochloride (Additive CNS depression). Products include:

Darvon 1435

Wygesic Tablets 2827

Propoxyphene Napsylate (Additive CNS depression). Products include:

Darvon-N/Darvocet-N 1433

Protriptyline Hydrochloride (Effect of either agent may be increased). Products include:

Vivactil Tablets 1774

Pyrilamine Maleate (Additive CNS depression). Products include:

4-Way Fast Acting Nasal Spray (regular & mentholated) .... ⊕ 621

Maximum Strength Multi-Symptom Formula Midol .... ⊕ 722

PMS Multi-Symptom Formula Midol .... ⊕ 723

Pyrilamine Tannate (Additive CNS depression). Products include:

Atrohist Pediatric Suspension 454

Rynatan 2673

Quazepam (Additive CNS depression). Products include:

Doral Tablets 2664

Risperidone (Additive CNS depression). Products include:

Risperdal 1301

Scopolamine (Concurrent use may produce paralytic ileus). Products include:

Transderm Scōp Transdermal Therapeutic System 869

Scopolamine Hydrobromide (Concurrent use may produce paralytic ileus). Products include:

Atrohist Plus Tablets 454

Donnatal 2060

Donnatal Extentabs 2061

Donnatal Tablets 2060

Secobarbital Sodium (Additive CNS depression). Products include:

Seconal Sodium Pulvules 1474

Selegiline Hydrochloride (Effect of either agent may be increased). Products include:

Eldepryl Tablets 2550

Sufentanil Citrate (Additive CNS depression). Products include:

Sufenta Injection 1309

Temazepam (Additive CNS depression). Products include:

Restoril Capsules 2284

Terfenadine (Additive CNS depression). Products include:

Seldane Tablets 1536

Seldane-D Extended-Release Tablets 1538

Thiamylal Sodium (Additive CNS depression).

No products indexed under this heading.

Thioridazine Hydrochloride (Additive CNS depression). Products include:

Mellaril 2269

Thiothixene (Additive CNS depression). Products include:

Navane Capsules and Concentrate 2201

Navane Intramuscular 2202

Tranylcypromine Sulfate (Effect of either agent may be increased). Products include:

Parnate Tablets 2503

Triazolam (Additive CNS depression). Products include:

Halcion Tablets 2611

Tridihexethyl Chloride (Concurrent use may produce paralytic ileus).

No products indexed under this heading.

Trifluoperazine Hydrochloride (Additive CNS depression). Products include:

Stelazine 2514

Trihexyphenidyl Hydrochloride (Concurrent use may produce paralytic ileus). Products include:

Artane 1368

Trimeprazine Tartrate (Additive CNS depression). Products include:

Temaril Tablets, Syrup and Spansule Extended-Release Capsules .. 483

Trimipramine Maleate (Effect of either agent may be increased). Products include:

Surmontil Capsules 2811

Tripelennamine Hydrochloride (Additive CNS depression). Products include:

PBZ Tablets 845

PBZ-SR Tablets 844

Triprolidine Hydrochloride (Additive CNS depression). Products include:

Actifed Plus Caplets .... ⊕ 845

Actifed Plus Tablets .... ⊕ 845

Actifed with Codeine Cough Syrup.. 1067

Actifed Syrup .... ⊕ 846

Actifed Tablets .... ⊕ 844

Zolpidem Tartrate (Additive CNS depression). Products include:

Ambien Tablets 2416

Food Interactions

Alcohol (Additive CNS depression).

TUSSI-ORGANIDIN DM NR LIQUID AND DM-S NR LIQUID

(Guaifenesin, Dextromethorphan Hydrobromide) 2677

May interact with monoamine oxidase inhibitors, central nervous system depressants, antihistamines, psychotropics, and certain other agents. Compounds in these categories include:

Acrivastine (Potential for additive CNS depressant effects). Products include:

Semprex-D Capsules 463

Semprex-D Capsules 1167

Alfentanil Hydrochloride (Potential for additive CNS depressant effects). Products include:

Alfenta Injection 1286

Alprazolam (Potential for additive CNS depressant effects). Products include:

Xanax Tablets 2649

Amitriptyline Hydrochloride (Potential for additive CNS depressant effects). Products include:

Elavil 2838

Endep Tablets 2174

Etrafon 2355

Limbitrol 2180

Triavil Tablets 1757

Amoxapine (Potential for additive CNS depressant effects). Products include:

Asendin Tablets 1369

Aprobarbital (Potential for additive CNS depressant effects).

No products indexed under this heading.

Astemizole (Potential for additive CNS depressant effects). Products include:

Hismanal Tablets 1293

Azatadine Maleate (Potential for additive CNS depressant effects). Products include:

Trinalin Repetabs Tablets 1330

Bromodiphenhydramine Hydrochloride (Potential for additive CNS depressant effects).

No products indexed under this heading.

Brompheniramine Maleate (Potential for additive CNS depressant effects). Products include:

Alka Seltzer Plus Sinus Medicine .. ⊕ 707

Bromfed Capsules (Extended-Release) 1785

Bromfed Syrup .... ⊕ 733

Bromfed Tablets 1785

Bromfed-DM Cough Syrup 1786

Bromfed-PD Capsules (Extended-Release) 1785

Dimetane-DC Cough Syrup 2059

Dimetane-DX Cough Syrup 2059

Dimetapp Elixir .... ⊕ 773

Dimetapp Extentabs .... ⊕ 774

Dimetapp Tablets/Liqui-Gels .... ⊕ 775

Dimetapp Cold & Allergy Chewable Tablets .... ⊕ 773

Dimetapp DM Elixir .... ⊕ 774

Vicks DayQuil Allergy Relief 12-Hour Extended Release Tablets .. ⊕ 760

Vicks DayQuil Allergy Relief 4-Hour Tablets .... ⊕ 760

Buprenorphine (Potential for additive CNS depressant effects). Products include:

Buprenex Injectable 2006

Buspirone Hydrochloride (Potential for additive CNS depressant effects). Products include:

BuSpar 737

Butabarbital (Potential for additive CNS depressant effects).

No products indexed under this heading.

Butalbital (Potential for additive CNS depressant effects). Products include:

Esgic-plus Tablets 1013

Fioricet Tablets 2258

Fioricet with Codeine Capsules 2260

Fiorinal Capsules 2261

Fiorinal with Codeine Capsules 2262

Fiorinal Tablets 2261

Phrenilin 785

Sedapap Tablets 50 mg/650 mg .. 1543

Chlordiazepoxide (Potential for additive CNS depressant effects). Products include:

Libritabs Tablets 2177

Limbitrol 2180

Chlordiazepoxide Hydrochloride (Potential for additive CNS depressant effects). Products include:

Librax Capsules 2176

Librium Capsules 2178

Librium Injectable 2179

IMPORTANT NOTE: Always consult each drug listing in the patient's regimen for possible interactions.

Tussi-Organidin DM NR Interactions Index 1090

Chlorpheniramine Maleate (Potential for additive CNS depressant effects). Products include:
Alka-Seltzer Plus Cold Medicine .... ▣ 705
Alka-Seltzer Plus Cold Medicine Liqui-Gels .... ▣ 706
Alka-Seltzer Plus Cold & Cough Medicine .... ▣ 708
Alka-Seltzer Plus Cold & Cough Medicine Liqui-Gels .... ▣ 705
Allerest Children's Chewable Tablets .... ▣ 627
Allerest Headache Strength Tablets .... ▣ 627
Allerest Maximum Strength Tablets .... ▣ 627
Allerest Sinus Pain Formula .... ▣ 627
Allerest 12 Hour Caplets .... ▣ 627
Ana-Kit Anaphylaxis Emergency Treatment Kit 617
Atrohist Pediatric Capsules 453
Atrohist Plus Tablets 454
BC Cold Powder Multi-Symptom Formula (Cold-Sinus-Allergy) .... ▣ 609
Cerose DM .... ▣ 878
Cheracol Plus Head Cold/Cough Formula .... ▣ 769
Children's Vicks DayQuil Allergy Relief .... ▣ 757
Children's Vicks NyQuil Cold/Cough Relief .... ▣ 758
Chlor-Trimeton Allergy Decongestant Tablets .... ▣ 799
Chlor-Trimeton Allergy Tablets .... ▣ 798
Comhist 2038
Comtrex Multi-Symptom Cold Reliever Tablets/Caplets/Liqui-Gels/Liquid .... ▣ 615
Allergy-Sinus Comtrex Multi-Symptom Allergy-Sinus Formula Tablets .... ▣ 617
Contac Continuous Action Nasal Decongestant/Antihistamine 12 Hour Capsules .... ▣ 813
Contac Maximum Strength Continuous Action Decongestant/Antihistamine 12 Hour Caplets .. ▣ 813
Contac Severe Cold and Flu Formula Caplets .... ▣ 814
Coricidin 'D' Decongestant Tablets .... ▣ 800
Coricidin Tablets .... ▣ 800
D.A. Chewable Tablets 951
Deconamine 1320
Dura-Tap/PD Capsules 2867
Dura-Vent/DA Tablets 953
Extendryl 1005
Fedahist Gyrocaps 2401
Fedahist Timecaps 2401
Hycomine Compound Tablets 932
Isoclor Timesule Capsules .... ▣ 637
Kronofed-A 977
Nolamine Timed-Release Tablets 785
Novahistine DH 2462
Novahistine Elixir .... ▣ 823
Ornade Spansule Capsules 2502
PediaCare Cold Allergy Chewable Tablets .... ▣ 677
PediaCare Cough-Cold Chewable Tablets 1553
PediaCare Cough-Cold Liquid 1553
PediaCare NightRest Cough-Cold Liquid 1553
Pediatric Vicks 44m Cough & Cold Relief .... ▣ 764
Pyrroxate Caplets .... ▣ 772
Ryna .... ▣ 841
Sinarest Tablets .... ▣ 648
Sinarest Extra Strength Tablets .... ▣ 648
Sine-Off Sinus Medicine .... ▣ 825
Singlet Tablets .... ▣ 825
Sinulin Tablets 787
Sinutab Sinus Allergy Medication, Maximum Strength Tablets and Caplets .... ▣ 860
Sudafed Plus Liquid .... ▣ 862
Sudafed Plus Tablets .... ▣ 863
Teldrin 12 Hour Antihistamine/Nasal Decongestant Allergy Relief Capsules .... ▣ 826
TheraFlu .... ▣ 787
TheraFlu Maximum Strength Nighttime Flu, Cold & Cough Medicine .... ▣ 788
Triaminic Allergy Tablets .... ▣ 789
Triaminic Cold Tablets .... ▣ 790
Triaminic Nite Light .... ▣ 791
Triaminic Syrup .... ▣ 792
Triaminic-12 Tablets .... ▣ 792
Triaminicin Tablets .... ▣ 793
Triaminicol Multi-Symptom Cold Tablets .... ▣ 793
Triaminicol Multi-Symptom Relief ▣ 794
Tussend 1783
Children's TYLENOL Cold Multi-Symptom Liquid Formula and Chewable Tablets 1561
Children's TYLENOL Cold Plus Cough Multi Symptom Tablets and Liquid .... ▣ 681
TYLENOL Maximum Strength Allergy Sinus Medication Gelcaps and Caplets 1563
TYLENOL Cold Multi-Symptom Formula Medication Tablets and Caplets 1561
TYLENOL Cold Multi-Symptom Hot Medication Liquid Packets 1557
Vicks 44 LiquiCaps Cough, Cold & Flu Relief .... ▣ 755
Vicks 44M Cough, Cold & Flu Relief .... ▣ 756

Chlorpheniramine Polistirex (Potential for additive CNS depressant effects). Products include:
Tussionex Pennkinetic Extended-Release Suspension 998

Chlorpheniramine Tannate (Potential for additive CNS depressant effects). Products include:
Atrohist Pediatric Suspension 454
Ricobid Tablets and Pediatric Suspension 2038
Rynatan 2673
Rynatuss 2673

Chlorpromazine (Potential for additive CNS depressant effects). Products include:
Thorazine Suppositories 2523

Chlorpromazine Hydrochloride (Potential for additive CNS depressant effects). Products include:
Thorazine 2523

Chlorprothixene (Potential for additive CNS depressant effects).
No products indexed under this heading.

Chlorprothixene Hydrochloride (Potential for additive CNS depressant effects).
No products indexed under this heading.

Clemastine Fumarate (Potential for additive CNS depressant effects). Products include:
Tavist Syrup 2297
Tavist Tablets 2298
Tavist-1 12 Hour Relief Tablets .... ▣ 787
Tavist-D 12 Hour Relief Tablets .... ▣ 787

Clorazepate Dipotassium (Potential for additive CNS depressant effects). Products include:
Tranxene 451

Clozapine (Potential for additive CNS depressant effects). Products include:
Clozaril Tablets 2252

Codeine Phosphate (Potential for additive CNS depressant effects). Products include:
Actifed with Codeine Cough Syrup .. 1067
Brontex 1981
Deconsal C Expectorant Syrup 456
Deconsal Pediatric Syrup 457
Dimetane-DC Cough Syrup 2059
Empirin with Codeine Tablets 1093
Fioricet with Codeine Capsules 2260
Fiorinal with Codeine Capsules 2262
Isoclor Expectorant 990
Novahistine DH 2462
Novahistine Expectorant 2463
Nucofed 2051
Phenergan with Codeine 2777
Phenergan VC with Codeine 2781
Robitussin A-C Syrup 2073
Robitussin-DAC Syrup 2074
Ryna .... ▣ 841
Soma Compound w/Codeine Tablets 2676
Tussi-Organidin NR Liquid and S NR Liquid 2677
Tylenol with Codeine 1583

Cyproheptadine Hydrochloride (Potential for additive CNS depressant effects). Products include:
Periactin 1724

Desflurane (Potential for additive CNS depressant effects). Products include:
Suprane 1813

Desipramine Hydrochloride (Potential for additive CNS depressant effects). Products include:
Norpramin Tablets 1526

Dexchlorpheniramine Maleate (Potential for additive CNS depressant effects).
No products indexed under this heading.

Dezocine (Potential for additive CNS depressant effects). Products include:
Dalgan Injection 538

Diazepam (Potential for additive CNS depressant effects). Products include:
Dizac 1809
Valium Injectable 2182
Valium Tablets 2183
Valrelease Capsules 2169

Diphenhydramine Citrate (Potential for additive CNS depressant effects). Products include:
Excedrin P.M. Analgesic/Sleeping Aid Tablets, Caplets, Liquigels 733

Diphenhydramine Hydrochloride (Potential for additive CNS depressant effects). Products include:
Actifed Allergy Daytime/Nighttime Caplets .... ▣ 844
Actifed Sinus Daytime/Nighttime Tablets and Caplets .... ▣ 846
Arthritis Foundation NightTime Caplets .... ▣ 674
Extra Strength Bayer PM Aspirin .. ▣ 713
Bayer Select Night Time Pain Relief Formula .... ▣ 716
Benadryl Allergy Decongestant Liquid Medication .... ▣ 848
Benadryl Allergy Decongestant Tablets .... ▣ 848
Benadryl Allergy Liquid Medication .... ▣ 849
Benadryl Allergy .... ▣ 848
Benadryl Allergy Sinus Headache Formula Caplets .... ▣ 849
Benadryl Capsules 1898
Benadryl Dye-Free Allergy Liquigel Softgels .... ▣ 850
Benadryl Dye-Free Allergy Liquid Medication .... ▣ 850
Benadryl Itch Relief Cream, Children's Formula and Maximum Strength 2% .... ▣ 851
Benadryl Itch Relief Spray, Children's Formula and Maximum Strength 2% .... ▣ 851
Benadryl Itch Relief Stick Maximum Strength 2% .... ▣ 850
Benadryl Itch Stopping Gel, Children's Formula and Maximum Strength 2% .... ▣ 851
Benadryl Kapseals 1898
Benadryl Injection 1898
Contac Day & Night Cold/Flu Night Caplets .... ▣ 812
Contac Night Allergy/Sinus Caplets .... ▣ 812
Extra Strength Doan's P.M. .... ▣ 633
Legatrin PM .... ▣ 651
Miles Nervine Nighttime Sleep-Aid ▣ 723
Nytol QuickCaps Caplets .... ▣ 610
Sleepinal Night-time Sleep Aid Capsules and Softgels .... ▣ 834
TYLENOL Maximum Strength Allergy Sinus NightTime Medication Caplets 1555
TYLENOL Flu NightTime, Maximum Strength, Gelcaps 1566
TYLENOL Maximum Strength Flu NightTime Hot Medication Packets 1562
TYLENOL PM, Extra Strength Pain Reliever/Sleep Aid Caplets, Geltabs, Gelcaps 1560
TYLENOL Severe Allergy Medication Caplets 1564
Maximum Strength Unisom Sleepgels 1934
Unisom With Pain Relief-Nighttime Sleep Aid and Pain Reliever 1934

Diphenylpyraline Hydrochloride (Potential for additive CNS depressant effects).
No products indexed under this heading.

Doxepin Hydrochloride (Potential for additive CNS depressant effects). Products include:
Sinequan 2205
Zonalon Cream 1055

Droperidol (Potential for additive CNS depressant effects). Products include:
Inapsine Injection 1296

Enflurane (Potential for additive CNS depressant effects).
No products indexed under this heading.

Estazolam (Potential for additive CNS depressant effects). Products include:
ProSom Tablets 449

Ethchlorvynol (Potential for additive CNS depressant effects). Products include:
Placidyl Capsules 448

Ethinamate (Potential for additive CNS depressant effects).
No products indexed under this heading.

Fentanyl (Potential for additive CNS depressant effects). Products include:
Duragesic Transdermal System 1288

Fentanyl Citrate (Potential for additive CNS depressant effects). Products include:
Sublimaze Injection 1307

Fluphenazine Decanoate (Potential for additive CNS depressant effects). Products include:
Prolixin Decanoate 509

Fluphenazine Enanthate (Potential for additive CNS depressant effects). Products include:
Prolixin Enanthate 509

Fluphenazine Hydrochloride (Potential for additive CNS depressant effects). Products include:
Prolixin 509

Flurazepam Hydrochloride (Potential for additive CNS depressant effects). Products include:
Dalmane Capsules 2173

Furazolidone (Coadministration may result in serious toxicity; concurrent use is contraindicated). Products include:
Furoxone 2046

Glutethimide (Potential for additive CNS depressant effects).
No products indexed under this heading.

Haloperidol (Potential for additive CNS depressant effects). Products include:
Haldol Injection, Tablets and Concentrate 1575

Haloperidol Decanoate (Potential for additive CNS depressant effects). Products include:
Haldol Decanoate 1577

Hydrocodone Bitartrate (Potential for additive CNS depressant effects). Products include:
Anexsia 5/500 Elixir 1781
Anexia Tablets 1782
Codiclear DH Syrup 791
Deconamine CX Cough and Cold Liquid and Tablets 1319
Duratuss HD Elixir 2565
Hycodan Tablets and Syrup 930
Hycomine Compound Tablets 932
Hycomine 931
Hycotuss Expectorant Syrup 933

(▣ Described in PDR For Nonprescription Drugs) (◉ Described in PDR For Ophthalmology)

Interactions Index Tussi-Organidin NR

Hydrocet Capsules 782
Lorcet 10/650................................... 1018
Lortab 2566
Tussend 1783
Tussend Expectorant 1785
Vicodin Tablets 1356
Vicodin ES Tablets 1357
Vicodin Tuss Expectorant 1358
Zydone Capsules 949

Hydrocodone Polistirex (Potential for additive CNS depressant effects). Products include:

Tussionex Pennkinetic Extended-Release Suspension 998

Hydroxyzine Hydrochloride (Potential for additive CNS depressant effects). Products include:

Atarax Tablets & Syrup..................... 2185
Marax Tablets & DF Syrup................ 2200
Vistaril Intramuscular Solution......... 2216

Imipramine Hydrochloride (Potential for additive CNS depressant effects). Products include:

Tofranil Ampuls 854
Tofranil Tablets 856

Imipramine Pamoate (Potential for additive CNS depressant effects). Products include:

Tofranil-PM Capsules........................ 857

Isocarboxazid (Coadministration may result in serious toxicity; concurrent use is contraindicated; potential for additive CNS depressant effects).

No products indexed under this heading.

Isoflurane (Potential for additive CNS depressant effects).

No products indexed under this heading.

Ketamine Hydrochloride (Potential for additive CNS depressant effects).

No products indexed under this heading.

Levomethadyl Acetate Hydrochloride (Potential for additive CNS depressant effects). Products include:

Orlamm 2239

Levorphanol Tartrate (Potential for additive CNS depressant effects). Products include:

Levo-Dromoran.................................. 2129

Lithium Carbonate (Potential for additive CNS depressant effects). Products include:

Eskalith 2485
Lithium Carbonate Capsules & Tablets 2230
Lithonate/Lithotabs/Lithobid 2543

Lithium Citrate (Potential for additive CNS depressant effects).

No products indexed under this heading.

Loratadine (Potential for additive CNS depressant effects). Products include:

Claritin 2349
Claritin-D 2350

Lorazepam (Potential for additive CNS depressant effects). Products include:

Ativan Injection.................................. 2698
Ativan Tablets 2700

Loxapine Hydrochloride (Potential for additive CNS depressant effects). Products include:

Loxitane 1378

Loxapine Succinate (Potential for additive CNS depressant effects). Products include:

Loxitane Capsules 1378

Maprotiline Hydrochloride (Potential for additive CNS depressant effects). Products include:

Ludiomil Tablets................................. 843

Meperidine Hydrochloride (Potential for additive CNS depressant effects). Products include:

Demerol 2308
Mepergan Injection 2753

Mephobarbital (Potential for additive CNS depressant effects). Products include:

Mebaral Tablets 2322

Meprobamate (Potential for additive CNS depressant effects). Products include:

Miltown Tablets 2672
PMB 200 and PMB 400 2783

Mesoridazine (Potential for additive CNS depressant effects).

Mesoridazine Besylate (Potential for additive CNS depressant effects). Products include:

Serentil.. 684

Methadone Hydrochloride (Potential for additive CNS depressant effects). Products include:

Methadone Hydrochloride Oral Concentrate 2233
Methadone Hydrochloride Oral Solution & Tablets.............................. 2235

Methdilazine Hydrochloride (Potential for additive CNS depressant effects).

No products indexed under this heading.

Methohexital Sodium (Potential for additive CNS depressant effects). Products include:

Brevital Sodium Vials 1429

Methotrimeprazine (Potential for additive CNS depressant effects). Products include:

Levoprome 1274

Methoxyflurane (Potential for additive CNS depressant effects).

No products indexed under this heading.

Midazolam Hydrochloride (Potential for additive CNS depressant effects). Products include:

Versed Injection 2170

Molindone Hydrochloride (Potential for additive CNS depressant effects). Products include:

Moban Tablets and Concentrate...... 1048

Morphine Sulfate (Potential for additive CNS depressant effects). Products include:

Astramorph/PF Injection, USP (Preservative-Free) 535
Duramorph 962
Infumorph 200 and Infumorph 500 Sterile Solutions.......................... 965
MS Contin Tablets.............................. 1994
MSIR 1997
Oramorph SR (Morphine Sulfate Sustained Release Tablets) 2236
RMS Suppositories 2657
Roxanol 2243

Nortriptyline Hydrochloride (Potential for additive CNS depressant effects). Products include:

Pamelor 2280

Opium Alkaloids (Potential for additive CNS depressant effects).

No products indexed under this heading.

Oxazepam (Potential for additive CNS depressant effects). Products include:

Serax Capsules 2810
Serax Tablets...................................... 2810

Oxycodone Hydrochloride (Potential for additive CNS depressant effects). Products include:

Percocet Tablets 938
Percodan Tablets................................ 939
Percodan-Demi Tablets...................... 940
Roxicodone Tablets, Oral Solution & Intensol (Oxycodone) 2244
Tylox Capsules 1584

Pentobarbital Sodium (Potential for additive CNS depressant effects). Products include:

Nembutal Sodium Capsules 436
Nembutal Sodium Solution 438
Nembutal Sodium Suppositories...... 440

Perphenazine (Potential for additive CNS depressant effects). Products include:

Etrafon 2355
Triavil Tablets 1757
Trilafon.. 2389

Phenelzine Sulfate (Coadministration may result in serious toxicity; concurrent use is contraindicated; potential for additive CNS depressant effects). Products include:

Nardil 1920

Phenobarbital (Potential for additive CNS depressant effects). Products include:

Arco-Lase Plus Tablets 512
Bellergal-S Tablets 2250
Donnatal 2060
Donnatal Extentabs............................ 2061
Donnatal Tablets 2060
Phenobarbital Elixir and Tablets 1469
Quadrinal Tablets 1350

Prazepam (Potential for additive CNS depressant effects).

No products indexed under this heading.

Prochlorperazine (Potential for additive CNS depressant effects). Products include:

Compazine 2470

Promethazine Hydrochloride (Potential for additive CNS depressant effects). Products include:

Mepergan Injection 2753
Phenergan with Codeine................... 2777
Phenergan with Dextromethorphan 2778
Phenergan Injection 2773
Phenergan Suppositories 2775
Phenergan Syrup................................ 2774
Phenergan Tablets 2775
Phenergan VC 2779
Phenergan VC with Codeine 2781

Propofol (Potential for additive CNS depressant effects). Products include:

Diprivan Injection............................... 2833

Propoxyphene Hydrochloride (Potential for additive CNS depressant effects). Products include:

Darvon 1435
Wygesic Tablets 2827

Propoxyphene Napsylate (Potential for additive CNS depressant effects). Products include:

Darvon-N/Darvocet-N 1433

Protriptyline Hydrochloride (Potential for additive CNS depressant effects). Products include:

Vivactil Tablets 1774

Pyrilamine Maleate (Potential for additive CNS depressant effects). Products include:

4-Way Fast Acting Nasal Spray (regular & mentholated) .... ◆◻ 621
Maximum Strength Multi-Symptom Formula Midol .... ◆◻ 722
PMS Multi-Symptom Formula Midol .... ◆◻ 723

Pyrilamine Tannate (Potential for additive CNS depressant effects). Products include:

Atrohist Pediatric Suspension 454
Rynatan 2673

Quazepam (Potential for additive CNS depressant effects). Products include:

Doral Tablets 2664

Risperidone (Potential for additive CNS depressant effects). Products include:

Risperdal 1301

Secobarbital Sodium (Potential for additive CNS depressant effects). Products include:

Seconal Sodium Pulvules 1474

Selegiline Hydrochloride (Coadministration may result in serious toxicity; concurrent use is contraindicated). Products include:

Eldepryl Tablets 2550

Sufentanil Citrate (Potential for additive CNS depressant effects). Products include:

Sufenta Injection 1309

Temazepam (Potential for additive CNS depressant effects). Products include:

Restoril Capsules 2284

Terfenadine (Potential for additive CNS depressant effects). Products include:

Seldane Tablets 1536
Seldane-D Extended-Release Tablets 1538

Thiamylal Sodium (Potential for additive CNS depressant effects).

No products indexed under this heading.

Thioridazine Hydrochloride (Potential for additive CNS depressant effects). Products include:

Mellaril 2269

Thiothixene (Potential for additive CNS depressant effects). Products include:

Navane Capsules and Concentrate 2201
Navane Intramuscular 2202

Tranylcypromine Sulfate (Coadministration may result in serious toxicity; concurrent use is contraindicated; potential for additive CNS depressant effects). Products include:

Parnate Tablets 2503

Triazolam (Potential for additive CNS depressant effects). Products include:

Halcion Tablets................................... 2611

Trifluoperazine Hydrochloride (Potential for additive CNS depressant effects). Products include:

Stelazine 2514

Trimeprazine Tartrate (Potential for additive CNS depressant effects). Products include:

Temaril Tablets, Syrup and Spansule Extended-Release Capsules.. 483

Trimipramine Maleate (Potential for additive CNS depressant effects). Products include:

Surmontil Capsules............................ 2811

Tripelennamine Hydrochloride (Potential for additive CNS depressant effects). Products include:

PBZ Tablets 845
PBZ-SR Tablets................................... 844

Triprolidine Hydrochloride (Potential for additive CNS depressant effects). Products include:

Actifed Plus Caplets .... ◆◻ 845
Actifed Plus Tablets .... ◆◻ 845
Actifed with Codeine Cough Syrup.. 1067
Actifed Syrup...................................... ◆◻ 846
Actifed Tablets .... ◆◻ 844

Zolpidem Tartrate (Potential for additive CNS depressant effects). Products include:

Ambien Tablets................................... 2416

Food Interactions

Alcohol (Potential for additive CNS depressant effects).

TUSSI-ORGANIDIN NR LIQUID AND S NR LIQUID

(Guaifenesin, Codeine Phosphate) 2677

May interact with central nervous system depressants, antihistamines, psychotropics, and certain other

IMPORTANT NOTE: Always consult each drug listing in the patient's regimen for possible interactions.

agents. Compounds in these categories include:

Acrivastine (Potential for additive CNS depressant effects). Products include:
Semprex-D Capsules 463
Semprex-D Capsules 1167

Alfentanil Hydrochloride (Potential for additive CNS depressant effects). Products include:
Alfenta Injection 1286

Alprazolam (Potential for additive CNS depressant effects). Products include:
Xanax Tablets 2649

Amitriptyline Hydrochloride (Potential for additive CNS depressant effects). Products include:
Elavil 2838
Endep Tablets 2174
Etrafon 2355
Limbitrol 2180
Triavil Tablets 1757

Amoxapine (Potential for additive CNS depressant effects). Products include:
Asendin Tablets 1369

Aprobarbital (Potential for additive CNS depressant effects).
No products indexed under this heading.

Astemizole (Potential for additive CNS depressant effects). Products include:
Hismanal Tablets 1293

Azatadine Maleate (Potential for additive CNS depressant effects). Products include:
Trinalin Repetabs Tablets 1330

Bromodiphenhydramine Hydrochloride (Potential for additive CNS depressant effects).
No products indexed under this heading.

Brompheniramine Maleate (Potential for additive CNS depressant effects). Products include:
Alka Seltzer Plus Sinus Medicine ■ 707
Bromfed Capsules (Extended-Release) 1785
Bromfed Syrup ■ 733
Bromfed Tablets 1785
Bromfed-DM Cough Syrup 1786
Bromfed-PD Capsules (Extended-Release) 1785
Dimetane-DC Cough Syrup 2059
Dimetane-DX Cough Syrup 2059
Dimetapp Elixir ■ 773
Dimetapp Extentabs ■ 774
Dimetapp Tablets/Liqui-Gels ■ 775
Dimetapp Cold & Allergy Chewable Tablets ■ 773
Dimetapp DM Elixir ■ 774
Vicks DayQuil Allergy Relief 12-Hour Extended Release Tablets ■ 760
Vicks DayQuil Allergy Relief 4-Hour Tablets ■ 760

Buprenorphine (Potential for additive CNS depressant effects). Products include:
Buprenex Injectable 2006

Buspirone Hydrochloride (Potential for additive CNS depressant effects). Products include:
BuSpar 737

Butabarbital (Potential for additive CNS depressant effects).
No products indexed under this heading.

Butalbital (Potential for additive CNS depressant effects). Products include:
Esgic-plus Tablets 1013
Fioricet Tablets 2258
Fioricet with Codeine Capsules 2260
Fiorinal Capsules 2261
Fiorinal with Codeine Capsules 2262
Fiorinal Tablets 2261
Phrenilin 785
Sedapap Tablets 50 mg/650 mg 1543

Chlordiazepoxide (Potential for additive CNS depressant effects). Products include:
Libritabs Tablets 2177
Limbitrol 2180

Chlordiazepoxide Hydrochloride (Potential for additive CNS depressant effects). Products include:
Librax Capsules 2176
Librium Capsules 2178
Librium Injectable 2179

Chlorpheniramine Maleate (Potential for additive CNS depressant effects). Products include:
Alka-Seltzer Plus Cold Medicine ■ 705
Alka-Seltzer Plus Cold Medicine Liqui-Gels ■ 706
Alka-Seltzer Plus Cold & Cough Medicine ■ 708
Alka-Seltzer Plus Cold & Cough Medicine Liqui-Gels ■ 705
Allerest Children's Chewable Tablets ■ 627
Allerest Headache Strength Tablets ■ 627
Allerest Maximum Strength Tablets ■ 627
Allerest Sinus Pain Formula ■ 627
Allerest 12 Hour Caplets ■ 627
Ana-Kit Anaphylaxis Emergency Treatment Kit 617
Atrohist Pediatric Capsules 453
Atrohist Plus Tablets 454
BC Cold Powder Multi-Symptom Formula (Cold-Sinus-Allergy) ■ 609
Cerose DM ■ 878
Cheracol Plus Head Cold/Cough Formula ■ 769
Children's Vicks DayQuil Allergy Relief ■ 757
Children's Vicks NyQuil Cold/Cough Relief ■ 758
Chlor-Trimeton Allergy Decongestant Tablets ■ 799
Chlor-Trimeton Allergy Tablets ■ 798
Comhist 2038
Comtrex Multi-Symptom Cold Reliever Tablets/Caplets/Liqui-Gels/Liquid ■ 615
Allergy-Sinus Comtrex Multi-Symptom Allergy-Sinus Formula Tablets ■ 617
Contac Continuous Action Nasal Decongestant/Antihistamine 12 Hour Capsules ■ 813
Contac Maximum Strength Continuous Action Decongestant/Antihistamine 12 Hour Caplets ■ 813
Contac Severe Cold and Flu Formula Caplets ■ 814
Coricidin 'D' Decongestant Tablets ■ 800
Coricidin Tablets ■ 800
D.A. Chewable Tablets 951
Deconamine 1320
Dura-Tap/PD Capsules 2867
Dura-Vent/DA Tablets 953
Extendryl 1005
Fedahist Gyrocaps 2401
Fedahist Timecaps 2401
Hycomine Compound Tablets 932
Isoclor Timesule Capsules ■ 637
Kronofed-A 977
Nolamine Timed-Release Tablets 785
Novahistine DH 2462
Novahistine Elixir ■ 823
Ornade Spansule Capsules 2502
PediaCare Cold Allergy Chewable Tablets ■ 677
PediaCare Cough-Cold Chewable Tablets 1553
PediaCare Cough-Cold Liquid 1553
PediaCare NightRest Cough-Cold Liquid 1553
Pediatric Vicks 44m Cough & Cold Relief ■ 764
Pyrroxate Caplets ■ 772
Ryna ■ 841
Sinarest Tablets ■ 648
Sinarest Extra Strength Tablets ■ 648
Sine-Off Sinus Medicine ■ 825
Singlet Tablets ■ 825
Sinulin Tablets 787
Sinutab Sinus Allergy Medication, Maximum Strength Tablets and Caplets ■ 860
Sudafed Plus Liquid ■ 862
Sudafed Plus Tablets ■ 863
Teldrin 12 Hour Antihistamine/Nasal Decongestant Allergy Relief Capsules ■ 826
TheraFlu ■ 787
TheraFlu Maximum Strength Nighttime Flu, Cold & Cough Medicine ■ 788
Triaminic Allergy Tablets ■ 789
Triaminic Cold Tablets ■ 790
Triaminic Nite Light ■ 791
Triaminic Syrup ■ 792
Triaminic-12 Tablets ■ 792
Triaminicin Tablets ■ 793
Triaminicol Multi-Symptom Cold Tablets ■ 793
Triaminicol Multi-Symptom Relief ■ 794
Tussend 1783
Children's TYLENOL Cold Multi-Symptom Liquid Formula and Chewable Tablets 1561
Children's TYLENOL Cold Plus Cough Multi Symptom Tablets and Liquid ■ 681
TYLENOL Maximum Strength Allergy Sinus Medication Gelcaps and Caplets 1563
TYLENOL Cold Multi-Symptom Formula Medication Tablets and Caplets 1561
TYLENOL Cold Multi-Symptom Hot Medication Liquid Packets 1557
Vicks 44 LiquiCaps Cough, Cold & Flu Relief ■ 755
Vicks 44M Cough, Cold & Flu Relief ■ 756

Chlorpheniramine Polistirex (Potential for additive CNS depressant effects). Products include:
Tussionex Pennkinetic Extended-Release Suspension 998

Chlorpheniramine Tannate (Potential for additive CNS depressant effects). Products include:
Atrohist Pediatric Suspension 454
Ricobid Tablets and Pediatric Suspension 2038
Rynatan 2673
Rynatuss 2673

Chlorpromazine (Potential for additive CNS depressant effects). Products include:
Thorazine Suppositories 2523

Chlorpromazine Hydrochloride (Potential for additive CNS depressant effects). Products include:
Thorazine 2523

Chlorprothixene (Potential for additive CNS depressant effects).
No products indexed under this heading.

Chlorprothixene Hydrochloride (Potential for additive CNS depressant effects).
No products indexed under this heading.

Clemastine Fumarate (Potential for additive CNS depressant effects). Products include:
Tavist Syrup 2297
Tavist Tablets 2298
Tavist-1 12 Hour Relief Tablets ■ 787
Tavist-D 12 Hour Relief Tablets ■ 787

Clorazepate Dipotassium (Potential for additive CNS depressant effects). Products include:
Tranxene 451

Clozapine (Potential for additive CNS depressant effects). Products include:
Clozaril Tablets 2252

Cyproheptadine Hydrochloride (Potential for additive CNS depressant effects). Products include:
Periactin 1724

Desflurane (Potential for additive CNS depressant effects). Products include:
Suprane 1813

Desipramine Hydrochloride (Potential for additive CNS depressant effects). Products include:
Norpramin Tablets 1526

Dexchlorpheniramine Maleate (Potential for additive CNS depressant effects).
No products indexed under this heading.

Dezocine (Potential for additive CNS depressant effects). Products include:
Dalgan Injection 538

Diazepam (Potential for additive CNS depressant effects). Products include:
Dizac 1809
Valium Injectable 2182
Valium Tablets 2183
Valrelease Capsules 2169

Diphenhydramine Citrate (Potential for additive CNS depressant effects). Products include:
Excedrin P.M. Analgesic/Sleeping Aid Tablets, Caplets, Liquigels 733

Diphenhydramine Hydrochloride (Potential for additive CNS depressant effects). Products include:
Actifed Allergy Daytime/Nighttime Caplets ■ 844
Actifed Sinus Daytime/Nighttime Tablets and Caplets ■ 846
Arthritis Foundation NightTime Caplets ■ 674
Extra Strength Bayer PM Aspirin ■ 713
Bayer Select Night Time Pain Relief Formula ■ 716
Benadryl Allergy Decongestant Liquid Medication ■ 848
Benadryl Allergy Decongestant Tablets ■ 848
Benadryl Allergy Liquid Medication ■ 849
Benadryl Allergy ■ 848
Benadryl Allergy Sinus Headache Formula Caplets ■ 849
Benadryl Capsules 1898
Benadryl Dye-Free Allergy Liquigel Softgels ■ 850
Benadryl Dye-Free Allergy Liquid Medication ■ 850
Benadryl Itch Relief Cream, Children's Formula and Maximum Strength 2% ■ 851
Benadryl Itch Relief Spray, Children's Formula and Maximum Strength 2% ■ 851
Benadryl Itch Relief Stick Maximum Strength 2% ■ 850
Benadryl Itch Stopping Gel, Children's Formula and Maximum Strength 2% ■ 851
Benadryl Kapseals 1898
Benadryl Injection 1898
Contac Day & Night Cold/Flu Night Caplets ■ 812
Contac Night Allergy/Sinus Caplets ■ 812
Extra Strength Doan's P.M. ■ 633
Legatrin PM ■ 651
Miles Nervine Nighttime Sleep-Aid ■ 723
Nytol QuickCaps Caplets ■ 610
Sleepinal Night-time Sleep Aid Capsules and Softgels ■ 834
TYLENOL Maximum Strength Allergy Sinus NightTime Medication Caplets 1555
TYLENOL Flu NightTime, Maximum Strength, Gelcaps 1566
TYLENOL Maximum Strength Flu NightTime Hot Medication Packets 1562
TYLENOL PM, Extra Strength Pain Reliever/Sleep Aid Caplets, Geltabs, Gelcaps 1560
TYLENOL Severe Allergy Medication Caplets 1564
Maximum Strength Unisom Sleepgels 1934
Unisom With Pain Relief-Nighttime Sleep Aid and Pain Reliever 1934

Diphenylpyraline Hydrochloride (Potential for additive CNS depressant effects).
No products indexed under this heading.

(■ Described in PDR For Nonprescription Drugs) (⊙ Described in PDR For Ophthalmology)

1093 Interactions Index Tussi-Organidin NR

Doxepin Hydrochloride (Potential for additive CNS depressant effects). Products include:
- Sinequan ... 2205
- Zonalon Cream ... 1055

Droperidol (Potential for additive CNS depressant effects). Products include:
- Inapsine Injection ... 1296

Enflurane (Potential for additive CNS depressant effects).
- No products indexed under this heading.

Estazolam (Potential for additive CNS depressant effects). Products include:
- ProSom Tablets ... 449

Ethchlorvynol (Potential for additive CNS depressant effects). Products include:
- Placidyl Capsules ... 448

Ethinamate (Potential for additive CNS depressant effects).
- No products indexed under this heading.

Fentanyl (Potential for additive CNS depressant effects). Products include:
- Duragesic Transdermal System ... 1288

Fentanyl Citrate (Potential for additive CNS depressant effects). Products include:
- Sublimaze Injection ... 1307

Fluphenazine Decanoate (Potential for additive CNS depressant effects). Products include:
- Prolixin Decanoate ... 509

Fluphenazine Enanthate (Potential for additive CNS depressant effects). Products include:
- Prolixin Enanthate ... 509

Fluphenazine Hydrochloride (Potential for additive CNS depressant effects). Products include:
- Prolixin ... 509

Flurazepam Hydrochloride (Potential for additive CNS depressant effects). Products include:
- Dalmane Capsules ... 2173

Glutethimide (Potential for additive CNS depressant effects).
- No products indexed under this heading.

Haloperidol (Potential for additive CNS depressant effects). Products include:
- Haldol Injection, Tablets and Concentrate ... 1575

Haloperidol Decanoate (Potential for additive CNS depressant effects). Products include:
- Haldol Decanoate ... 1577

Hydrocodone Bitartrate (Potential for additive CNS depressant effects). Products include:
- Anexsia 5/500 Elixir ... 1781
- Anexia Tablets ... 1782
- Codiclear DH Syrup ... 791
- Deconamine CX Cough and Cold Liquid and Tablets ... 1319
- Duratuss HD Elixir ... 2565
- Hycodan Tablets and Syrup ... 930
- Hycomine Compound Tablets ... 932
- Hycomine ... 931
- Hycotuss Expectorant Syrup ... 933
- Hydrocet Capsules ... 782
- Lorcet 10/650 ... 1018
- Lortab ... 2566
- Tussend ... 1783
- Tussend Expectorant ... 1785
- Vicodin Tablets ... 1356
- Vicodin ES Tablets ... 1357
- Vicodin Tuss Expectorant ... 1358
- Zydone Capsules ... 949

Hydrocodone Polistirex (Potential for additive CNS depressant effects). Products include:
- Tussionex Pennkinetic Extended-Release Suspension ... 998

Hydroxyzine Hydrochloride (Potential for additive CNS depressant effects). Products include:
- Atarax Tablets & Syrup ... 2185
- Marax Tablets & DF Syrup ... 2200
- Vistaril Intramuscular Solution ... 2216

Imipramine Hydrochloride (Potential for additive CNS depressant effects). Products include:
- Tofranil Ampuls ... 854
- Tofranil Tablets ... 856

Imipramine Pamoate (Potential for additive CNS depressant effects). Products include:
- Tofranil-PM Capsules ... 857

Isocarboxazid (Potential for additive CNS depressant effects).
- No products indexed under this heading.

Isoflurane (Potential for additive CNS depressant effects).
- No products indexed under this heading.

Ketamine Hydrochloride (Potential for additive CNS depressant effects).
- No products indexed under this heading.

Levomethadyl Acetate Hydrochloride (Potential for additive CNS depressant effects). Products include:
- Orlamm ... 2239

Levorphanol Tartrate (Potential for additive CNS depressant effects). Products include:
- Levo-Dromoran ... 2129

Lithium Carbonate (Potential for additive CNS depressant effects). Products include:
- Eskalith ... 2485
- Lithium Carbonate Capsules & Tablets ... 2230
- Lithonate/Lithotabs/Lithobid ... 2543

Lithium Citrate (Potential for additive CNS depressant effects).
- No products indexed under this heading.

Loratadine (Potential for additive CNS depressant effects). Products include:
- Claritin ... 2349
- Claritin-D ... 2350

Lorazepam (Potential for additive CNS depressant effects). Products include:
- Ativan Injection ... 2698
- Ativan Tablets ... 2700

Loxapine Hydrochloride (Potential for additive CNS depressant effects). Products include:
- Loxitane ... 1378

Loxapine Succinate (Potential for additive CNS depressant effects). Products include:
- Loxitane Capsules ... 1378

Maprotiline Hydrochloride (Potential for additive CNS depressant effects). Products include:
- Ludiomil Tablets ... 843

Meperidine Hydrochloride (Potential for additive CNS depressant effects). Products include:
- Demerol ... 2308
- Mepergan Injection ... 2753

Mephobarbital (Potential for additive CNS depressant effects). Products include:
- Mebaral Tablets ... 2322

Meprobamate (Potential for additive CNS depressant effects). Products include:
- Miltown Tablets ... 2672
- PMB 200 and PMB 400 ... 2783

Mesoridazine (Potential for additive CNS depressant effects).

Mesoridazine Besylate (Potential for additive CNS depressant effects). Products include:
- Serentil ... 684

Methadone Hydrochloride (Potential for additive CNS depressant effects). Products include:
- Methadone Hydrochloride Oral Concentrate ... 2233
- Methadone Hydrochloride Oral Solution & Tablets ... 2235

Methdilazine Hydrochloride (Potential for additive CNS depressant effects).
- No products indexed under this heading.

Methohexital Sodium (Potential for additive CNS depressant effects). Products include:
- Brevital Sodium Vials ... 1429

Methotrimeprazine (Potential for additive CNS depressant effects). Products include:
- Levoprome ... 1274

Methoxyflurane (Potential for additive CNS depressant effects).
- No products indexed under this heading.

Midazolam Hydrochloride (Potential for additive CNS depressant effects). Products include:
- Versed Injection ... 2170

Molindone Hydrochloride (Potential for additive CNS depressant effects). Products include:
- Moban Tablets and Concentrate ... 1048

Morphine Sulfate (Potential for additive CNS depressant effects). Products include:
- Astramorph/PF Injection, USP (Preservative-Free) ... 535
- Duramorph ... 962
- Infumorph 200 and Infumorph 500 Sterile Solutions ... 965
- MS Contin Tablets ... 1994
- MSIR ... 1997
- Oramorph SR (Morphine Sulfate Sustained Release Tablets) ... 2236
- RMS Suppositories ... 2657
- Roxanol ... 2243

Nortriptyline Hydrochloride (Potential for additive CNS depressant effects). Products include:
- Pamelor ... 2280

Opium Alkaloids (Potential for additive CNS depressant effects).
- No products indexed under this heading.

Oxazepam (Potential for additive CNS depressant effects). Products include:
- Serax Capsules ... 2810
- Serax Tablets ... 2810

Oxycodone Hydrochloride (Potential for additive CNS depressant effects). Products include:
- Percocet Tablets ... 938
- Percodan Tablets ... 939
- Percodan-Demi Tablets ... 940
- Roxicodone Tablets, Oral Solution & Intensol (Oxycodone) ... 2244
- Tylox Capsules ... 1584

Pentobarbital Sodium (Potential for additive CNS depressant effects). Products include:
- Nembutal Sodium Capsules ... 436
- Nembutal Sodium Solution ... 438
- Nembutal Sodium Suppositories ... 440

Perphenazine (Potential for additive CNS depressant effects). Products include:
- Etrafon ... 2355
- Triavil Tablets ... 1757
- Trilafon ... 2389

Phenelzine Sulfate (Potential for additive CNS depressant effects). Products include:
- Nardil ... 1920

Phenobarbital (Potential for additive CNS depressant effects). Products include:
- Arco-Lase Plus Tablets ... 512
- Bellergal-S Tablets ... 2250
- Donnatal ... 2060
- Donnatal Extentabs ... 2061
- Donnatal Tablets ... 2060
- Phenobarbital Elixir and Tablets ... 1469
- Quadrinal Tablets ... 1350

Prazepam (Potential for additive CNS depressant effects).
- No products indexed under this heading.

Prochlorperazine (Potential for additive CNS depressant effects). Products include:
- Compazine ... 2470

Promethazine Hydrochloride (Potential for additive CNS depressant effects). Products include:
- Mepergan Injection ... 2753
- Phenergan with Codeine ... 2777
- Phenergan with Dextromethorphan 2778
- Phenergan Injection ... 2773
- Phenergan Suppositories ... 2775
- Phenergan Syrup ... 2774
- Phenergan Tablets ... 2775
- Phenergan VC ... 2779
- Phenergan VC with Codeine ... 2781

Propofol (Potential for additive CNS depressant effects). Products include:
- Diprivan Injection ... 2833

Propoxyphene Hydrochloride (Potential for additive CNS depressant effects). Products include:
- Darvon ... 1435
- Wygesic Tablets ... 2827

Propoxyphene Napsylate (Potential for additive CNS depressant effects). Products include:
- Darvon-N/Darvocet-N ... 1433

Protriptyline Hydrochloride (Potential for additive CNS depressant effects). Products include:
- Vivactil Tablets ... 1774

Pyrilamine Maleate (Potential for additive CNS depressant effects). Products include:
- 4-Way Fast Acting Nasal Spray (regular & mentholated) ... ◘ 621
- Maximum Strength Multi-Symptom Formula Midol ... ◘ 722
- PMS Multi-Symptom Formula Midol ... ◘ 723

Pyrilamine Tannate (Potential for additive CNS depressant effects). Products include:
- Atrohist Pediatric Suspension ... 454
- Rynatan ... 2673

Quazepam (Potential for additive CNS depressant effects). Products include:
- Doral Tablets ... 2664

Risperidone (Potential for additive CNS depressant effects). Products include:
- Risperdal ... 1301

Secobarbital Sodium (Potential for additive CNS depressant effects). Products include:
- Seconal Sodium Pulvules ... 1474

Sufentanil Citrate (Potential for additive CNS depressant effects). Products include:
- Sufenta Injection ... 1309

Temazepam (Potential for additive CNS depressant effects). Products include:
- Restoril Capsules ... 2284

Terfenadine (Potential for additive CNS depressant effects). Products include:
- Seldane Tablets ... 1536
- Seldane-D Extended-Release Tablets ... 1538

IMPORTANT NOTE: Always consult each drug listing in the patient's regimen for possible interactions.

Tussi-Organidin NR

Thiamylal Sodium (Potential for additive CNS depressant effects).

No products indexed under this heading.

Thioridazine Hydrochloride (Potential for additive CNS depressant effects). Products include:

Mellaril 2269

Thiothixene (Potential for additive CNS depressant effects). Products include:

Navane Capsules and Concentrate 2201 Navane Intramuscular 2202

Tranylcypromine Sulfate (Potential for additive CNS depressant effects). Products include:

Parnate Tablets 2503

Triazolam (Potential for additive CNS depressant effects). Products include:

Halcion Tablets... 2611

Trifluoperazine Hydrochloride (Potential for additive CNS depressant effects). Products include:

Stelazine 2514

Trimeprazine Tartrate (Potential for additive CNS depressant effects). Products include:

Temaril Tablets, Syrup and Spansule Extended-Release Capsules.. 483

Trimipramine Maleate (Potential for additive CNS depressant effects). Products include:

Surmontil Capsules................................. 2811

Tripelennamine Hydrochloride (Potential for additive CNS depressant effects). Products include:

PBZ Tablets .... 845 PBZ-SR Tablets... 844

Triprolidine Hydrochloride (Potential for additive CNS depressant effects). Products include:

Actifed Plus Caplets .... ◆D 845 Actifed Plus Tablets .... ◆D 845 Actifed with Codeine Cough Syrup.. 1067 Actifed Syrup.. ◆D 846 Actifed Tablets .... ◆D 844

Zolpidem Tartrate (Potential for additive CNS depressant effects). Products include:

Ambien Tablets... 2416

Food Interactions

Alcohol (Potential for additive CNS depressant effects).

CHILDREN'S TYLENOL ACETAMINOPHEN CHEWABLE TABLETS, ELIXIR, SUSPENSION LIQUID

(Acetaminophen) ....1555 None cited in PDR database.

CHILDREN'S TYLENOL COLD MULTI-SYMPTOM LIQUID FORMULA AND CHEWABLE TABLETS

(Acetaminophen, Chlorpheniramine Maleate, Pseudoephedrine Hydrochloride) ....1561 May interact with hypnotics and sedatives, tranquilizers, and monoamine oxidase inhibitors. Compounds in these categories include:

Alprazolam (Increases drowsiness effect). Products include:

Xanax Tablets 2649

Buspirone Hydrochloride (Increases drowsiness effect). Products include:

BuSpar 737

Chlordiazepoxide (Increases drowsiness effect). Products include:

Libritabs Tablets .... 2177 Limbitrol 2180

Chlordiazepoxide Hydrochloride (Increases drowsiness effect). Products include:

Librax Capsules .... 2176 Librium Capsules..................................... 2178 Librium Injectable 2179

Chlorpromazine (Increases drowsiness effect). Products include:

Thorazine Suppositories 2523

Chlorpromazine Hydrochloride (Increases drowsiness effect). Products include:

Thorazine 2523

Chlorprothixene (Increases drowsiness effect).

No products indexed under this heading.

Chlorprothixene Hydrochloride (Increases drowsiness effect).

No products indexed under this heading.

Clorazepate Dipotassium (Increases drowsiness effect). Products include:

Tranxene 451

Diazepam (Increases drowsiness effect). Products include:

Dizac .... 1809 Valium Injectable .... 2182 Valium Tablets .... 2183 Valrelease Capsules 2169

Droperidol (Increases drowsiness effect). Products include:

Inapsine Injection.................................... 1296

Estazolam (Increases drowsiness effect). Products include:

ProSom Tablets 449

Ethchlorvynol (Increases drowsiness effect). Products include:

Placidyl Capsules..................................... 448

Ethinamate (Increases drowsiness effect).

No products indexed under this heading.

Fluphenazine Decanoate (Increases drowsiness effect). Products include:

Prolixin Decanoate 509

Fluphenazine Enanthate (Increases drowsiness effect). Products include:

Prolixin Enanthate 509

Fluphenazine Hydrochloride (Increases drowsiness effect). Products include:

Prolixin 509

Flurazepam Hydrochloride (Increases drowsiness effect). Products include:

Dalmane Capsules................................... 2173

Furazolidone (Concurrent and/or sequential administration is not recommended). Products include:

Furoxone 2046

Glutethimide (Increases drowsiness effect).

No products indexed under this heading.

Haloperidol (Increases drowsiness effect). Products include:

Haldol Injection, Tablets and Concentrate 1575

Haloperidol Decanoate (Increases drowsiness effect). Products include:

Haldol Decanoate..................................... 1577

Hydroxyzine Hydrochloride (Increases drowsiness effect). Products include:

Atarax Tablets & Syrup.......................... 2185 Marax Tablets & DF Syrup.................... 2200 Vistaril Intramuscular Solution.......... 2216

Isocarboxazid (Concurrent and/or sequential administration is not recommended).

No products indexed under this heading.

Lorazepam (Increases drowsiness effect). Products include:

Ativan Injection.. 2698 Ativan Tablets... 2700

Loxapine Hydrochloride (Increases drowsiness effect). Products include:

Loxitane 1378

Loxapine Succinate (Increases drowsiness effect). Products include:

Loxitane Capsules 1378

Meprobamate (Increases drowsiness effect). Products include:

Miltown Tablets .... 2672 PMB 200 and PMB 400 2783

Mesoridazine Besylate (Increases drowsiness effect). Products include:

Serentil.. 684

Midazolam Hydrochloride (Increases drowsiness effect). Products include:

Versed Injection 2170

Molindone Hydrochloride (Increases drowsiness effect). Products include:

Moban Tablets and Concentrate...... 1048

Oxazepam (Increases drowsiness effect). Products include:

Serax Capsules .... 2810 Serax Tablets... 2810

Perphenazine (Increases drowsiness effect). Products include:

Etrafon... 2355 Triavil Tablets .... 1757 Trilafon... 2389

Phenelzine Sulfate (Concurrent and/or sequential administration is not recommended). Products include:

Nardil 1920

Prazepam (Increases drowsiness effect).

No products indexed under this heading.

Prochlorperazine (Increases drowsiness effect). Products include:

Compazine 2470

Promethazine Hydrochloride (Increases drowsiness effect). Products include:

Mepergan Injection .... 2753 Phenergan with Codeine....................... 2777 Phenergan with Dextromethorphan 2778 Phenergan Injection .... 2773 Phenergan Suppositories .... 2775 Phenergan Syrup .... 2774 Phenergan Tablets .... 2775 Phenergan VC .... 2779 Phenergan VC with Codeine 2781

Propofol (Increases drowsiness effect). Products include:

Diprivan Injection.................................... 2833

Quazepam (Increases drowsiness effect). Products include:

Doral Tablets 2664

Secobarbital Sodium (Increases drowsiness effect). Products include:

Seconal Sodium Pulvules 1474

Selegiline Hydrochloride (Concurrent and/or sequential administration is not recommended). Products include:

Eldepryl Tablets 2550

Temazepam (Increases drowsiness effect). Products include:

Restoril Capsules 2284

Thioridazine Hydrochloride (Increases drowsiness effect). Products include:

Mellaril 2269

Thiothixene (Increases drowsiness effect). Products include:

Navane Capsules and Concentrate 2201 Navane Intramuscular 2202

Tranylcypromine Sulfate (Concurrent and/or sequential administration is not recommended). Products include:

Parnate Tablets 2503

Triazolam (Increases drowsiness effect). Products include:

Halcion Tablets... 2611

Trifluoperazine Hydrochloride (Increases drowsiness effect). Products include:

Stelazine 2514

Zolpidem Tartrate (Increases drowsiness effect). Products include:

Ambien Tablets... 2416

INFANTS' TYLENOL ACETAMINOPHEN DROPS AND SUSPENSION DROPS

(Acetaminophen) ....1555 None cited in PDR database.

INFANTS' TYLENOL COLD DECONGESTANT & FEVER-REDUCER DROPS

(Acetaminophen, Pseudoephedrine Hydrochloride) ....1556 May interact with monoamine oxidase inhibitors. Compounds in this category include:

Furazolidone (Concurrent and/or sequential use is not recommended). Products include:

Furoxone 2046

Isocarboxazid (Concurrent and/or sequential use is not recommended).

No products indexed under this heading.

Phenelzine Sulfate (Concurrent and/or sequential use is not recommended). Products include:

Nardil 1920

Selegiline Hydrochloride (Concurrent and/or sequential use is not recommended). Products include:

Eldepryl Tablets 2550

Tranylcypromine Sulfate (Concurrent and/or sequential use is not recommended). Products include:

Parnate Tablets 2503

TYLENOL EXTENDED RELIEF CAPLETS

(Acetaminophen) 1558

Food Interactions

Alcohol (Chronic heavy alcohol abusers, 3 or more drinks per day, may be at increased risk of liver toxicity from acetaminophen use).

TYLENOL, EXTRA STRENGTH, ACETAMINOPHEN ADULT LIQUID PAIN RELIEVER

(Acetaminophen) 1560

Food Interactions

Alcohol (Patients consuming 3 or more alcohol-containing drinks per day should consult their physician for advice on when and how they should take acetaminophen containing products).

TYLENOL, EXTRA STRENGTH, ACETAMINOPHEN GELCAPS, GELTABS, CAPLETS, TABLETS

(Acetaminophen) 1559

Food Interactions

Alcohol (Chronic heavy alcohol abusers, 3 or more drinks per day, may be at increased risk of liver toxicity from acetaminophen use).

(◆D Described in PDR For Nonprescription Drugs) (◆ Described in PDR For Ophthalmology)

TYLENOL, EXTRA STRENGTH, HEADACHE PLUS PAIN RELIEVER WITH ANTACID CAPLETS
(Acetaminophen, Calcium Carbonate) 1559
May interact with:

Prescription Drugs, unspecified (Antacid present in this product may interact with certain unspecified prescription drugs).

Food Interactions

Alcohol (Chronic heavy alcohol abusers, 3 or more drinks per day, may be at increased risk of liver toxicity from acetaminophen use).

TYLENOL, JUNIOR STRENGTH, ACETAMINOPHEN COATED CAPLETS, GRAPE AND FRUIT CHEWABLE TABLETS
(Acetaminophen) 1557
None cited in PDR database.

TYLENOL MAXIMUM STRENGTH ALLERGY SINUS MEDICATION GELCAPS AND CAPLETS
(Acetaminophen, Chlorpheniramine Maleate, Pseudoephedrine Hydrochloride) 1563
May interact with hypnotics and sedatives, tranquilizers, monoamine oxidase inhibitors, and certain other agents. Compounds in these categories include:

Alprazolam (May increase drowsiness). Products include:
Xanax Tablets 2649
Buspirone Hydrochloride (May increase drowsiness). Products include:
BuSpar 737
Chlordiazepoxide (May increase drowsiness). Products include:
Libritabs Tablets 2177
Limbitrol 2180
Chlordiazepoxide Hydrochloride (May increase drowsiness). Products include:
Librax Capsules 2176
Librium Capsules 2178
Librium Injectable 2179
Chlorpromazine (May increase drowsiness). Products include:
Thorazine Suppositories 2523
Chlorpromazine Hydrochloride (May increase drowsiness). Products include:
Thorazine 2523
Chlorprothixene (May increase drowsiness).
No products indexed under this heading.
Chlorprothixene Hydrochloride (May increase drowsiness).
No products indexed under this heading.
Clorazepate Dipotassium (May increase drowsiness). Products include:
Tranxene 451
Diazepam (May increase drowsiness). Products include:
Dizac 1809
Valium Injectable 2182
Valium Tablets 2183
Valrelease Capsules 2169
Droperidol (May increase drowsiness). Products include:
Inapsine Injection 1296
Estazolam (May increase drowsiness). Products include:
ProSom Tablets 449
Ethchlorvynol (May increase drowsiness). Products include:
Placidyl Capsules 448
Ethinamate (May increase drowsiness).
No products indexed under this heading.
Fluphenazine Decanoate (May increase drowsiness). Products include:
Prolixin Decanoate 509
Fluphenazine Enanthate (May increase drowsiness). Products include:
Prolixin Enanthate 509
Fluphenazine Hydrochloride (May increase drowsiness). Products include:
Prolixin 509
Flurazepam Hydrochloride (May increase drowsiness). Products include:
Dalmane Capsules 2173
Furazolidone (Concurrent and/or sequential use is contraindicated). Products include:
Furoxone 2046
Glutethimide (May increase drowsiness).
No products indexed under this heading.
Haloperidol (May increase drowsiness). Products include:
Haldol Injection, Tablets and Concentrate 1575
Haloperidol Decanoate (May increase drowsiness). Products include:
Haldol Decanoate 1577
Hydroxyzine Hydrochloride (May increase drowsiness). Products include:
Atarax Tablets & Syrup 2185
Marax Tablets & DF Syrup 2200
Vistaril Intramuscular Solution 2216
Isocarboxazid (Concurrent and/or sequential use is contraindicated).
No products indexed under this heading.
Lorazepam (May increase drowsiness). Products include:
Ativan Injection 2698
Ativan Tablets 2700
Loxapine Hydrochloride (May increase drowsiness). Products include:
Loxitane 1378
Loxapine Succinate (May increase drowsiness). Products include:
Loxitane Capsules 1378
Meprobamate (May increase drowsiness). Products include:
Miltown Tablets 2672
PMB 200 and PMB 400 2783
Mesoridazine Besylate (May increase drowsiness). Products include:
Serentil 684
Midazolam Hydrochloride (May increase drowsiness). Products include:
Versed Injection 2170
Molindone Hydrochloride (May increase drowsiness). Products include:
Moban Tablets and Concentrate 1048
Oxazepam (May increase drowsiness). Products include:
Serax Capsules 2810
Serax Tablets 2810
Perphenazine (May increase drowsiness). Products include:
Etrafon 2355
Triavil Tablets 1757
Trilafon 2389
Phenelzine Sulfate (Concurrent and/or sequential use is contraindicated). Products include:
Nardil 1920
Prazepam (May increase drowsiness).
No products indexed under this heading.
Prochlorperazine (May increase drowsiness). Products include:
Compazine 2470
Promethazine Hydrochloride (May increase drowsiness). Products include:
Mepergan Injection 2753
Phenergan with Codeine 2777
Phenergan with Dextromethorphan 2778
Phenergan Injection 2773
Phenergan Suppositories 2775
Phenergan Syrup 2774
Phenergan Tablets 2775
Phenergan VC 2779
Phenergan VC with Codeine 2781
Propofol (May increase drowsiness). Products include:
Diprivan Injection 2833
Quazepam (May increase drowsiness). Products include:
Doral Tablets 2664
Quinapril Hydrochloride (Effects not specified). Products include:
Accupril Tablets 1893
Secobarbital Sodium (May increase drowsiness). Products include:
Seconal Sodium Pulvules 1474
Selegiline Hydrochloride (Concurrent and/or sequential use is contraindicated). Products include:
Eldepryl Tablets 2550
Temazepam (May increase drowsiness). Products include:
Restoril Capsules 2284
Thioridazine Hydrochloride (May increase drowsiness). Products include:
Mellaril 2269
Thiothixene (May increase drowsiness). Products include:
Navane Capsules and Concentrate 2201
Navane Intramuscular 2202
Tranylcypromine Sulfate (Concurrent and/or sequential use is contraindicated). Products include:
Parnate Tablets 2503
Triazolam (May increase drowsiness). Products include:
Halcion Tablets 2611
Trifluoperazine Hydrochloride (May increase drowsiness). Products include:
Stelazine 2514
Zolpidem Tartrate (May increase drowsiness). Products include:
Ambien Tablets 2416

Food Interactions

Alcohol (May increase drowsiness; chronic heavy alcohol abusers, 3 or more drinks per day, may be at increased risk of liver toxicity from acetaminophen use).

TYLENOL MAXIMUM STRENGTH ALLERGY SINUS NIGHTTIME MEDICATION CAPLETS
(Acetaminophen, Pseudoephedrine Hydrochloride, Diphenhydramine Hydrochloride) 1555
May interact with hypnotics and sedatives, tranquilizers, antidepressant drugs, antihypertensives, and certain other agents. Compounds in these categories include:

Acebutolol Hydrochloride (Concurrent use is not recommended). Products include:
Sectral Capsules 2807
Alprazolam (May increase the drowsiness effect). Products include:
Xanax Tablets 2649
Amitriptyline Hydrochloride (Concurrent use is not recommended). Products include:
Elavil 2838
Endep Tablets 2174
Etrafon 2355
Limbitrol 2180
Triavil Tablets 1757
Amlodipine Besylate (Concurrent use is not recommended). Products include:
Lotrel Capsules 840
Norvasc Tablets 1940
Amoxapine (Concurrent use is not recommended). Products include:
Asendin Tablets 1369
Atenolol (Concurrent use is not recommended). Products include:
Tenoretic Tablets 2845
Tenormin Tablets and I.V. Injection 2847
Benazepril Hydrochloride (Concurrent use is not recommended). Products include:
Lotensin Tablets 834
Lotensin HCT 837
Lotrel Capsules 840
Bendroflumethiazide (Concurrent use is not recommended).
No products indexed under this heading.
Betaxolol Hydrochloride (Concurrent use is not recommended). Products include:
Betoptic Ophthalmic Solution 469
Betoptic S Ophthalmic Suspension 471
Kerlone Tablets 2436
Bisoprolol Fumarate (Concurrent use is not recommended). Products include:
Zebeta Tablets 1413
Ziac 1415
Bupropion Hydrochloride (Concurrent use is not recommended). Products include:
Wellbutrin Tablets 1204
Buspirone Hydrochloride (May increase the drowsiness effect). Products include:
BuSpar 737
Captopril (Concurrent use is not recommended). Products include:
Capoten 739
Capozide 742
Carteolol Hydrochloride (Concurrent use is not recommended). Products include:
Cartrol Tablets 410
Ocupress Ophthalmic Solution, 1% Sterile .... ⊙ 309
Chlordiazepoxide (May increase the drowsiness effect). Products include:
Libritabs Tablets 2177
Limbitrol 2180
Chlordiazepoxide Hydrochloride (May increase the drowsiness effect). Products include:
Librax Capsules 2176
Librium Capsules 2178
Librium Injectable 2179
Chlorothiazide (Concurrent use is not recommended). Products include:
Aldoclor Tablets 1598
Diupres Tablets 1650
Diuril Oral 1653
Chlorothiazide Sodium (Concurrent use is not recommended). Products include:
Diuril Sodium Intravenous 1652
Chlorpromazine (May increase the drowsiness effect). Products include:
Thorazine Suppositories 2523

IMPORTANT NOTE: Always consult each drug listing in the patient's regimen for possible interactions.

Tylenol Allergy Sinus | Interactions Index | 1096

Chlorpromazine Hydrochloride (May increase the drowsiness effect). Products include:
Thorazine ... 2523

Chlorprothixene (May increase the drowsiness effect).
No products indexed under this heading.

Chlorprothixene Hydrochloride (May increase the drowsiness effect).
No products indexed under this heading.

Chlorthalidone (Concurrent use is not recommended). Products include:
Combipres Tablets ... 677
Tenoretic Tablets ... 2845
Thalitone ... 1245

Clonidine (Concurrent use is not recommended). Products include:
Catapres-TTS ... 675

Clonidine Hydrochloride (Concurrent use is not recommended). Products include:
Catapres Tablets ... 674
Combipres Tablets ... 677

Clorazepate Dipotassium (May increase the drowsiness effect). Products include:
Tranxene ... 451

Deserpidine (Concurrent use is not recommended).
No products indexed under this heading.

Desipramine Hydrochloride (Concurrent use is not recommended). Products include:
Norpramin Tablets ... 1526

Diazepam (May increase the drowsiness effect). Products include:
Dizac ... 1809
Valium Injectable ... 2182
Valium Tablets ... 2183
Valrelease Capsules ... 2169

Diazoxide (Concurrent use is not recommended). Products include:
Hyperstat I.V. Injection ... 2363
Proglycem ... 580

Diltiazem Hydrochloride (Concurrent use is not recommended). Products include:
Cardizem CD Capsules ... 1506
Cardizem SR Capsules ... 1510
Cardizem Injectable ... 1508
Cardizem Tablets ... 1512
Dilacor XR Extended-release Capsules ... 2018

Doxazosin Mesylate (Concurrent use is not recommended). Products include:
Cardura Tablets ... 2186

Doxepin Hydrochloride (Concurrent use is not recommended). Products include:
Sinequan ... 2205
Zonalon Cream ... 1055

Droperidol (May increase the drowsiness effect). Products include:
Inapsine Injection ... 1296

Enalapril Maleate (Concurrent use is not recommended). Products include:
Vaseretic Tablets ... 1765
Vasotec Tablets ... 1771

Enalaprilat (Concurrent use is not recommended). Products include:
Vasotec I.V. ... 1768

Esmolol Hydrochloride (Concurrent use is not recommended). Products include:
Brevibloc Injection ... 1808

Estazolam (May increase the drowsiness effect). Products include:
ProSom Tablets ... 449

Ethchlorvynol (May increase the drowsiness effect). Products include:
Placidyl Capsules ... 448

Ethinamate (May increase the drowsiness effect).
No products indexed under this heading.

Felodipine (Concurrent use is not recommended). Products include:
Plendil Extended-Release Tablets ... 527

Fluoxetine Hydrochloride (Concurrent use is not recommended). Products include:
Prozac Pulvules & Liquid, Oral Solution ... 919

Fluphenazine Decanoate (May increase the drowsiness effect). Products include:
Prolixin Decanoate ... 509

Fluphenazine Enanthate (May increase the drowsiness effect). Products include:
Prolixin Enanthate ... 509

Fluphenazine Hydrochloride (May increase the drowsiness effect). Products include:
Prolixin ... 509

Flurazepam Hydrochloride (May increase the drowsiness effect). Products include:
Dalmane Capsules ... 2173

Fosinopril Sodium (Concurrent use is not recommended). Products include:
Monopril Tablets ... 757

Furosemide (Concurrent use is not recommended). Products include:
Lasix Injection, Oral Solution and Tablets ... 1240

Glutethimide (May increase the drowsiness effect).
No products indexed under this heading.

Guanabenz Acetate (Concurrent use is not recommended).
No products indexed under this heading.

Guanethidine Monosulfate (Concurrent use is not recommended). Products include:
Esimil Tablets ... 822
Ismelin Tablets ... 827

Haloperidol (May increase the drowsiness effect). Products include:
Haldol Injection, Tablets and Concentrate ... 1575

Haloperidol Decanoate (May increase the drowsiness effect). Products include:
Haldol Decanoate ... 1577

Hydralazine Hydrochloride (Concurrent use is not recommended). Products include:
Apresazide Capsules ... 808
Apresoline Hydrochloride Tablets ... 809
Ser-Ap-Es Tablets ... 849

Hydrochlorothiazide (Concurrent use is not recommended). Products include:
Aldactazide ... 2413
Aldoril Tablets ... 1604
Apresazide Capsules ... 808
Capozide ... 742
Dyazide ... 2479
Esidrix Tablets ... 821
Esimil Tablets ... 822
HydroDIURIL Tablets ... 1674
Hydropres Tablets ... 1675
Hyzaar Tablets ... 1677
Inderide Tablets ... 2732
Inderide LA Long Acting Capsules ... 2734
Lopressor HCT Tablets ... 832
Lotensin HCT ... 837
Maxzide ... 1380
Moduretic Tablets ... 1705
Oretic Tablets ... 443
Prinzide Tablets ... 1737
Ser-Ap-Es Tablets ... 849
Timolide Tablets ... 1748
Vaseretic Tablets ... 1765
Zestoretic ... 2850
Ziac ... 1415

Hydroflumethiazide (Concurrent use is not recommended). Products include:
Diucardin Tablets ... 2718

Hydroxyzine Hydrochloride (May increase the drowsiness effect). Products include:
Atarax Tablets & Syrup ... 2185
Marax Tablets & DF Syrup ... 2200
Vistaril Intramuscular Solution ... 2216

Imipramine Hydrochloride (Concurrent use is not recommended). Products include:
Tofranil Ampuls ... 854
Tofranil Tablets ... 856

Imipramine Pamoate (Concurrent use is not recommended). Products include:
Tofranil-PM Capsules ... 857

Indapamide (Concurrent use is not recommended). Products include:
Lozol Tablets ... 2022

Isocarboxazid (Concurrent use is not recommended).
No products indexed under this heading.

Isradipine (Concurrent use is not recommended). Products include:
DynaCirc Capsules ... 2256

Labetalol Hydrochloride (Concurrent use is not recommended). Products include:
Normodyne Injection ... 2377
Normodyne Tablets ... 2379
Trandate ... 1185

Lisinopril (Concurrent use is not recommended). Products include:
Prinivil Tablets ... 1733
Prinzide Tablets ... 1737
Zestoretic ... 2850
Zestril Tablets ... 2854

Lorazepam (May increase the drowsiness effect). Products include:
Ativan Injection ... 2698
Ativan Tablets ... 2700

Losartan Potassium (Concurrent use is not recommended). Products include:
Cozaar Tablets ... 1628
Hyzaar Tablets ... 1677

Loxapine Hydrochloride (May increase the drowsiness effect). Products include:
Loxitane ... 1378

Loxapine Succinate (May increase the drowsiness effect). Products include:
Loxitane Capsules ... 1378

Maprotiline Hydrochloride (Concurrent use is not recommended). Products include:
Ludiomil Tablets ... 843

Mecamylamine Hydrochloride (Concurrent use is not recommended). Products include:
Inversine Tablets ... 1686

Meprobamate (May increase the drowsiness effect). Products include:
Miltown Tablets ... 2672
PMB 200 and PMB 400 ... 2783

Mesoridazine Besylate (May increase the drowsiness effect). Products include:
Serentil ... 684

Methyclothiazide (Concurrent use is not recommended). Products include:
Enduron Tablets ... 420

Methyldopa (Concurrent use is not recommended). Products include:
Aldoclor Tablets ... 1598
Aldomet Oral ... 1600
Aldoril Tablets ... 1604

Methyldopate Hydrochloride (Concurrent use is not recommended). Products include:
Aldomet Ester HCl Injection ... 1602

Metolazone (Concurrent use is not recommended). Products include:
Mykrox Tablets ... 993
Zaroxolyn Tablets ... 1000

Metoprolol Succinate (Concurrent use is not recommended). Products include:
Toprol-XL Tablets ... 565

Metoprolol Tartrate (Concurrent use is not recommended). Products include:
Lopressor Ampuls ... 830
Lopressor HCT Tablets ... 832
Lopressor Tablets ... 830

Metyrosine (Concurrent use is not recommended). Products include:
Demser Capsules ... 1649

Midazolam Hydrochloride (May increase the drowsiness effect). Products include:
Versed Injection ... 2170

Minoxidil (Concurrent use is not recommended). Products include:
Loniten Tablets ... 2618
Rogaine Topical Solution ... 2637

Moexipril Hydrochloride (Concurrent use is not recommended). Products include:
Univasc Tablets ... 2410

Molindone Hydrochloride (May increase the drowsiness effect). Products include:
Moban Tablets and Concentrate ... 1048

Nadolol (Concurrent use is not recommended).
No products indexed under this heading.

Nefazodone Hydrochloride (Concurrent use is not recommended). Products include:
Serzone Tablets ... 771

Nicardipine Hydrochloride (Concurrent use is not recommended). Products include:
Cardene Capsules ... 2095
Cardene I.V. ... 2709
Cardene SR Capsules ... 2097

Nifedipine (Concurrent use is not recommended). Products include:
Adalat Capsules (10 mg and 20 mg) ... 587
Adalat CC ... 589
Procardia Capsules ... 1971
Procardia XL Extended Release Tablets ... 1972

Nisoldipine (Concurrent use is not recommended).
No products indexed under this heading.

Nitroglycerin (Concurrent use is not recommended). Products include:
Deponit NTG Transdermal Delivery System ... 2397
Nitro-Bid IV ... 1523
Nitro-Bid Ointment ... 1524
Nitrodisc ... 2047
Nitro-Dur (nitroglycerin) Transdermal Infusion System ... 1326
Nitrolingual Spray ... 2027
Nitrostat Tablets ... 1925
Transderm-Nitro Transdermal Therapeutic System ... 859

Nortriptyline Hydrochloride (Concurrent use is not recommended). Products include:
Pamelor ... 2280

Oxazepam (May increase the drowsiness effect). Products include:
Serax Capsules ... 2810
Serax Tablets ... 2810

Paroxetine Hydrochloride (Concurrent use is not recommended). Products include:
Paxil Tablets ... 2505

Penbutolol Sulfate (Concurrent use is not recommended). Products include:
Levatol ... 2403

(▭ Described in PDR For Nonprescription Drugs) (◉ Described in PDR For Ophthalmology)

1097 Interactions Index Tylenol Flu Nighttime

Perphenazine (May increase the drowsiness effect). Products include:
- Etrafon 2355
- Triavil Tablets 1757
- Trilafon 2389

Phenelzine Sulfate (Concurrent use is not recommended). Products include:
- Nardil 1920

Phenoxybenzamine Hydrochloride (Concurrent use is not recommended). Products include:
- Dibenzyline Capsules 2476

Phentolamine Mesylate (Concurrent use is not recommended). Products include:
- Regitine 846

Pindolol (Concurrent use is not recommended). Products include:
- Visken Tablets 2299

Polythiazide (Concurrent use is not recommended). Products include:
- Minizide Capsules 1938

Prazepam (May increase the drowsiness effect).
- No products indexed under this heading.

Prazosin Hydrochloride (Concurrent use is not recommended). Products include:
- Minipress Capsules 1937
- Minizide Capsules 1938

Prochlorperazine (May increase the drowsiness effect). Products include:
- Compazine 2470

Promethazine Hydrochloride (May increase the drowsiness effect). Products include:
- Mepergan Injection 2753
- Phenergan with Codeine 2777
- Phenergan with Dextromethorphan 2778
- Phenergan Injection 2773
- Phenergan Suppositories 2775
- Phenergan Syrup 2774
- Phenergan Tablets 2775
- Phenergan VC 2779
- Phenergan VC with Codeine 2781

Propofol (May increase the drowsiness effect). Products include:
- Diprivan Injection 2833

Propranolol Hydrochloride (Concurrent use is not recommended). Products include:
- Inderal 2728
- Inderal LA Long Acting Capsules 2730
- Inderide Tablets 2732
- Inderide LA Long Acting Capsules 2734

Protriptyline Hydrochloride (Concurrent use is not recommended). Products include:
- Vivactil Tablets 1774

Quazepam (May increase the drowsiness effect). Products include:
- Doral Tablets 2664

Quinapril Hydrochloride (Concurrent use is not recommended). Products include:
- Accupril Tablets 1893

Ramipril (Concurrent use is not recommended). Products include:
- Altace Capsules 1232

Rauwolfia Serpentina (Concurrent use is not recommended).
- No products indexed under this heading.

Rescinnamine (Concurrent use is not recommended).
- No products indexed under this heading.

Reserpine (Concurrent use is not recommended). Products include:
- Diupres Tablets 1650
- Hydropres Tablets 1675
- Ser-Ap-Es Tablets 849

Secobarbital Sodium (May increase the drowsiness effect). Products include:
- Seconal Sodium Pulvules 1474

Sertraline Hydrochloride (Concurrent use is not recommended). Products include:
- Zoloft Tablets 2217

Sodium Nitroprusside (Concurrent use is not recommended).
- No products indexed under this heading.

Sotalol Hydrochloride (Concurrent use is not recommended). Products include:
- Betapace Tablets 641

Spirapril Hydrochloride (Concurrent use is not recommended).
- No products indexed under this heading.

Temazepam (May increase the drowsiness effect). Products include:
- Restoril Capsules 2284

Terazosin Hydrochloride (Concurrent use is not recommended). Products include:
- Hytrin Capsules 430

Thioridazine Hydrochloride (May increase the drowsiness effect). Products include:
- Mellaril 2269

Thiothixene (May increase the drowsiness effect). Products include:
- Navane Capsules and Concentrate 2201
- Navane Intramuscular 2202

Timolol Maleate (Concurrent use is not recommended). Products include:
- Blocadren Tablets 1614
- Timolide Tablets 1748
- Timoptic in Ocudose 1753
- Timoptic Sterile Ophthalmic Solution 1751
- Timoptic-XE 1755

Torsemide (Concurrent use is not recommended). Products include:
- Demadex Tablets and Injection 686

Tranylcypromine Sulfate (Concurrent use is not recommended). Products include:
- Parnate Tablets 2503

Trazodone Hydrochloride (Concurrent use is not recommended). Products include:
- Desyrel and Desyrel Dividose 503

Triazolam (May increase the drowsiness effect). Products include:
- Halcion Tablets 2611

Trifluoperazine Hydrochloride (May increase the drowsiness effect). Products include:
- Stelazine 2514

Trimethaphan Camsylate (Concurrent use is not recommended). Products include:
- Arfonad Ampuls 2080

Trimipramine Maleate (Concurrent use is not recommended). Products include:
- Surmontil Capsules 2811

Venlafaxine Hydrochloride (Concurrent use is not recommended). Products include:
- Effexor 2719

Verapamil Hydrochloride (Concurrent use is not recommended). Products include:
- Calan SR Caplets 2422
- Calan Tablets 2419
- Isoptin Injectable 1344
- Isoptin Oral Tablets 1346
- Isoptin SR Tablets 1348
- Verelan Capsules 1410
- Verelan Capsules 2824

Zolpidem Tartrate (May increase the drowsiness effect). Products include:
- Ambien Tablets 2416

Food Interactions

Alcohol (May increase drowsiness effect; chronic heavy alcohol abusers, 3 or more drinks per day, may be at increased risk of liver toxicity from acetaminophen use).

TYLENOL FLU MAXIMUM STRENGTH GELCAPS

(Acetaminophen, Dextromethorphan Hydrobromide, Pseudoephedrine Hydrochloride) 1565

May interact with monoamine oxidase inhibitors and certain other agents. Compounds in these categories include:

Furazolidone (Concurrent and/or sequential use is not recommended). Products include:
- Furoxone 2046

Isocarboxazid (Concurrent and/or sequential use is not recommended).
- No products indexed under this heading.

Phenelzine Sulfate (Concurrent and/or sequential use is not recommended). Products include:
- Nardil 1920

Selegiline Hydrochloride (Concurrent and/or sequential use is not recommended). Products include:
- Eldepryl Tablets 2550

Tranylcypromine Sulfate (Concurrent and/or sequential use is not recommended). Products include:
- Parnate Tablets 2503

Verapamil Hydrochloride (Concurrent use is not recommended). Products include:
- Calan SR Caplets 2422
- Calan Tablets 2419
- Isoptin Injectable 1344
- Isoptin Oral Tablets 1346
- Isoptin SR Tablets 1348
- Verelan Capsules 1410
- Verelan Capsules 2824

Food Interactions

Alcohol (Chronic heavy alcohol abusers, 3 or more drinks per day, may be at increased risk of liver toxicity from acetaminophen use).

TYLENOL FLU NIGHTTIME, MAXIMUM STRENGTH, GELCAPS

(Acetaminophen, Pseudoephedrine Hydrochloride, Diphenhydramine Hydrochloride) 1566

May interact with hypnotics and sedatives, tranquilizers, antidepressant drugs, antihypertensives, and certain other agents. Compounds in these categories include:

Acebutolol Hydrochloride (Concurrent use should be avoided). Products include:
- Sectral Capsules 2807

Alprazolam (May increase drowsiness effect). Products include:
- Xanax Tablets 2649

Amitriptyline Hydrochloride (Concurrent use should be avoided). Products include:
- Elavil 2838
- Endep Tablets 2174
- Etrafon 2355
- Limbitrol 2180
- Triavil Tablets 1757

Amlodipine Besylate (Concurrent use should be avoided). Products include:
- Lotrel Capsules 840
- Norvasc Tablets 1940

Amoxapine (Concurrent use should be avoided). Products include:
- Asendin Tablets 1369

Atenolol (Concurrent use should be avoided). Products include:
- Tenoretic Tablets 2845
- Tenormin Tablets and I.V. Injection 2847

Benazepril Hydrochloride (Concurrent use should be avoided). Products include:
- Lotensin Tablets 834
- Lotensin HCT 837
- Lotrel Capsules 840

Bendroflumethiazide (Concurrent use should be avoided).
- No products indexed under this heading.

Betaxolol Hydrochloride (Concurrent use should be avoided). Products include:
- Betoptic Ophthalmic Solution 469
- Betoptic S Ophthalmic Suspension 471
- Kerlone Tablets 2436

Bisoprolol Fumarate (Concurrent use should be avoided). Products include:
- Zebeta Tablets 1413
- Ziac 1415

Bupropion Hydrochloride (Concurrent use should be avoided). Products include:
- Wellbutrin Tablets 1204

Buspirone Hydrochloride (May increase drowsiness effect). Products include:
- BuSpar 737

Captopril (Concurrent use should be avoided). Products include:
- Capoten 739
- Capozide 742

Carteolol Hydrochloride (Concurrent use should be avoided). Products include:
- Cartrol Tablets 410
- Ocupress Ophthalmic Solution, 1% Sterile .... ⊙ 309

Chlordiazepoxide (May increase drowsiness effect). Products include:
- Libritabs Tablets 2177
- Limbitrol 2180

Chlordiazepoxide Hydrochloride (May increase drowsiness effect). Products include:
- Librax Capsules 2176
- Librium Capsules 2178
- Librium Injectable 2179

Chlorothiazide (Concurrent use should be avoided). Products include:
- Aldoclor Tablets 1598
- Diupres Tablets 1650
- Diuril Oral 1653

Chlorothiazide Sodium (Concurrent use should be avoided). Products include:
- Diuril Sodium Intravenous 1652

Chlorpromazine (May increase drowsiness effect). Products include:
- Thorazine Suppositories 2523

Chlorpromazine Hydrochloride (May increase drowsiness effect). Products include:
- Thorazine 2523

Chlorprothixene (May increase drowsiness effect).
- No products indexed under this heading.

Chlorprothixene Hydrochloride (May increase drowsiness effect).
- No products indexed under this heading.

Chlorthalidone (Concurrent use should be avoided). Products include:
- Combipres Tablets 677
- Tenoretic Tablets 2845
- Thalitone 1245

Clonidine (Concurrent use should be avoided). Products include:
- Catapres-TTS 675

IMPORTANT NOTE: Always consult each drug listing in the patient's regimen for possible interactions.

Tylenol Flu Nighttime | Interactions Index | 1098

Clonidine Hydrochloride (Concurrent use should be avoided). Products include:
- Catapres Tablets ... 674
- Combipres Tablets ... 677

Clorazepate Dipotassium (May increase drowsiness effect). Products include:
- Tranxene ... 451

Deserpidine (Concurrent use should be avoided).
- No products indexed under this heading.

Desipramine Hydrochloride (Concurrent use should be avoided). Products include:
- Norpramin Tablets ... 1526

Diazepam (May increase drowsiness effect). Products include:
- Dizac ... 1809
- Valium Injectable ... 2182
- Valium Tablets ... 2183
- Valrelease Capsules ... 2169

Diazoxide (Concurrent use should be avoided). Products include:
- Hyperstat I.V. Injection ... 2363
- Proglycem ... 580

Diltiazem Hydrochloride (Concurrent use should be avoided). Products include:
- Cardizem CD Capsules ... 1506
- Cardizem SR Capsules ... 1510
- Cardizem Injectable ... 1508
- Cardizem Tablets ... 1512
- Dilacor XR Extended-release Capsules ... 2018

Doxazosin Mesylate (Concurrent use should be avoided). Products include:
- Cardura Tablets ... 2186

Doxepin Hydrochloride (Concurrent use should be avoided). Products include:
- Sinequan ... 2205
- Zonalon Cream ... 1055

Droperidol (May increase drowsiness effect). Products include:
- Inapsine Injection ... 1296

Enalapril Maleate (Concurrent use should be avoided). Products include:
- Vaseretic Tablets ... 1765
- Vasotec Tablets ... 1771

Enalaprilat (Concurrent use should be avoided). Products include:
- Vasotec I.V. ... 1768

Esmolol Hydrochloride (Concurrent use should be avoided). Products include:
- Brevibloc Injection ... 1808

Estazolam (May increase drowsiness effect). Products include:
- ProSom Tablets ... 449

Ethchlorvynol (May increase drowsiness effect). Products include:
- Placidyl Capsules ... 448

Ethinamate (May increase drowsiness effect).
- No products indexed under this heading.

Felodipine (Concurrent use should be avoided). Products include:
- Plendil Extended-Release Tablets ... 527

Fluoxetine Hydrochloride (Concurrent use should be avoided). Products include:
- Prozac Pulvules & Liquid, Oral Solution ... 919

Fluphenazine Decanoate (May increase drowsiness effect). Products include:
- Prolixin Decanoate ... 509

Fluphenazine Enanthate (May increase drowsiness effect). Products include:
- Prolixin Enanthate ... 509

Fluphenazine Hydrochloride (May increase drowsiness effect). Products include:
- Prolixin ... 509

Flurazepam Hydrochloride (May increase drowsiness effect). Products include:
- Dalmane Capsules ... 2173

Fosinopril Sodium (Concurrent use should be avoided). Products include:
- Monopril Tablets ... 757

Furosemide (Concurrent use should be avoided). Products include:
- Lasix Injection, Oral Solution and Tablets ... 1240

Glutethimide (May increase drowsiness effect).
- No products indexed under this heading.

Guanabenz Acetate (Concurrent use should be avoided).
- No products indexed under this heading.

Guanethidine Monosulfate (Concurrent use should be avoided). Products include:
- Esimil Tablets ... 822
- Ismelin Tablets ... 827

Haloperidol (May increase drowsiness effect). Products include:
- Haldol Injection, Tablets and Concentrate ... 1575

Haloperidol Decanoate (May increase drowsiness effect). Products include:
- Haldol Decanoate ... 1577

Hydralazine Hydrochloride (Concurrent use should be avoided). Products include:
- Apresazide Capsules ... 808
- Apresoline Hydrochloride Tablets ... 809
- Ser-Ap-Es Tablets ... 849

Hydrochlorothiazide (Concurrent use should be avoided). Products include:
- Aldactazide ... 2413
- Aldoril Tablets ... 1604
- Apresazide Capsules ... 808
- Capozide ... 742
- Dyazide ... 2479
- Esidrix Tablets ... 821
- Esimil Tablets ... 822
- HydroDIURIL Tablets ... 1674
- Hydropres Tablets ... 1675
- Hyzaar Tablets ... 1677
- Inderide Tablets ... 2732
- Inderide LA Long Acting Capsules ... 2734
- Lopressor HCT Tablets ... 832
- Lotensin HCT ... 837
- Maxzide ... 1380
- Moduretic Tablets ... 1705
- Oretic Tablets ... 443
- Prinzide Tablets ... 1737
- Ser-Ap-Es Tablets ... 849
- Timolide Tablets ... 1748
- Vaseretic Tablets ... 1765
- Zestoretic ... 2850
- Ziac ... 1415

Hydroflumethiazide (Concurrent use should be avoided). Products include:
- Diucardin Tablets ... 2718

Hydroxyzine Hydrochloride (May increase drowsiness effect). Products include:
- Atarax Tablets & Syrup ... 2185
- Marax Tablets & DF Syrup ... 2200
- Vistaril Intramuscular Solution ... 2216

Imipramine Hydrochloride (Concurrent use should be avoided). Products include:
- Tofranil Ampuls ... 854
- Tofranil Tablets ... 856

Imipramine Pamoate (Concurrent use should be avoided). Products include:
- Tofranil-PM Capsules ... 857

Indapamide (Concurrent use should be avoided). Products include:
- Lozol Tablets ... 2022

Isocarboxazid (Concurrent use should be avoided).
- No products indexed under this heading.

Isradipine (Concurrent use should be avoided). Products include:
- DynaCirc Capsules ... 2256

Labetalol Hydrochloride (Concurrent use should be avoided). Products include:
- Normodyne Injection ... 2377
- Normodyne Tablets ... 2379
- Trandate ... 1185

Levobunolol Hydrochloride (Concurrent use should be avoided). Products include:
- Betagan ... ◉ 233

Lisinopril (Concurrent use should be avoided). Products include:
- Prinivil Tablets ... 1733
- Prinzide Tablets ... 1737
- Zestoretic ... 2850
- Zestril Tablets ... 2854

Lorazepam (May increase drowsiness effect). Products include:
- Ativan Injection ... 2698
- Ativan Tablets ... 2700

Losartan Potassium (Concurrent use should be avoided). Products include:
- Cozaar Tablets ... 1628
- Hyzaar Tablets ... 1677

Loxapine Hydrochloride (May increase drowsiness effect). Products include:
- Loxitane ... 1378

Loxapine Succinate (May increase drowsiness effect). Products include:
- Loxitane Capsules ... 1378

Maprotiline Hydrochloride (Concurrent use should be avoided). Products include:
- Ludiomil Tablets ... 843

Mecamylamine Hydrochloride (Concurrent use should be avoided). Products include:
- Inversine Tablets ... 1686

Meprobamate (May increase drowsiness effect). Products include:
- Miltown Tablets ... 2672
- PMB 200 and PMB 400 ... 2783

Mesoridazine Besylate (May increase drowsiness effect). Products include:
- Serentil ... 684

Methyclothiazide (Concurrent use should be avoided). Products include:
- Enduron Tablets ... 420

Methyldopa (Concurrent use should be avoided). Products include:
- Aldoclor Tablets ... 1598
- Aldomet Oral ... 1600
- Aldoril Tablets ... 1604

Methyldopate Hydrochloride (Concurrent use should be avoided). Products include:
- Aldomet Ester HCl Injection ... 1602

Metipranolol Hydrochloride (Concurrent use should be avoided). Products include:
- OptiPranolol (Metipranolol 0.3%) Sterile Ophthalmic Solution ... ◉ 258

Metolazone (Concurrent use should be avoided). Products include:
- Mykrox Tablets ... 993
- Zaroxolyn Tablets ... 1000

Metoprolol Succinate (Concurrent use should be avoided). Products include:
- Toprol-XL Tablets ... 565

Metoprolol Tartrate (Concurrent use should be avoided). Products include:
- Lopressor Ampuls ... 830
- Lopressor HCT Tablets ... 832
- Lopressor Tablets ... 830

Metyrosine (Concurrent use should be avoided). Products include:
- Demser Capsules ... 1649

Midazolam Hydrochloride (May increase drowsiness effect). Products include:
- Versed Injection ... 2170

Minoxidil (Concurrent use should be avoided). Products include:
- Loniten Tablets ... 2618
- Rogaine Topical Solution ... 2637

Moexipril Hydrochloride (Concurrent use should be avoided). Products include:
- Univasc Tablets ... 2410

Molindone Hydrochloride (May increase drowsiness effect). Products include:
- Moban Tablets and Concentrate ... 1048

Nadolol (Concurrent use should be avoided).
- No products indexed under this heading.

Nefazodone Hydrochloride (Concurrent use should be avoided). Products include:
- Serzone Tablets ... 771

Nicardipine Hydrochloride (Concurrent use should be avoided). Products include:
- Cardene Capsules ... 2095
- Cardene I.V. ... 2709
- Cardene SR Capsules ... 2097

Nifedipine (Concurrent use should be avoided). Products include:
- Adalat Capsules (10 mg and 20 mg) ... 587
- Adalat CC ... 589
- Procardia Capsules ... 1971
- Procardia XL Extended Release Tablets ... 1972

Nisoldipine (Concurrent use should be avoided).
- No products indexed under this heading.

Nitroglycerin (Concurrent use should be avoided). Products include:
- Deponit NTG Transdermal Delivery System ... 2397
- Nitro-Bid IV ... 1523
- Nitro-Bid Ointment ... 1524
- Nitrodisc ... 2047
- Nitro-Dur (nitroglycerin) Transdermal Infusion System ... 1326
- Nitrolingual Spray ... 2027
- Nitrostat Tablets ... 1925
- Transderm-Nitro Transdermal Therapeutic System ... 859

Nortriptyline Hydrochloride (Concurrent use should be avoided). Products include:
- Pamelor ... 2280

Oxazepam (May increase drowsiness effect). Products include:
- Serax Capsules ... 2810
- Serax Tablets ... 2810

Paroxetine Hydrochloride (Concurrent use should be avoided). Products include:
- Paxil Tablets ... 2505

Penbutolol Sulfate (Concurrent use should be avoided). Products include:
- Levatol ... 2403

Perphenazine (May increase drowsiness effect). Products include:
- Etrafon ... 2355
- Triavil Tablets ... 1757
- Trilafon ... 2389

(▭ Described in PDR For Nonprescription Drugs) (◉ Described in PDR For Ophthalmology)

1099 **Interactions Index** **Tylenol Cold & Flu**

Phenelzine Sulfate (Concurrent use should be avoided). Products include:
Nardil ... 1920
Phenoxybenzamine Hydrochloride (Concurrent use should be avoided). Products include:
Dibenzyline Capsules ... 2476
Phentolamine Mesylate (Concurrent use should be avoided). Products include:
Regitine ... 846
Pindolol (Concurrent use should be avoided). Products include:
Visken Tablets ... 2299
Polythiazide (Concurrent use should be avoided). Products include:
Minizide Capsules ... 1938
Prazepam (May increase drowsiness effect).
No products indexed under this heading.
Prazosin Hydrochloride (Concurrent use should be avoided). Products include:
Minipress Capsules ... 1937
Minizide Capsules ... 1938
Prochlorperazine (May increase drowsiness effect). Products include:
Compazine ... 2470
Promethazine Hydrochloride (May increase drowsiness effect). Products include:
Mepergan Injection ... 2753
Phenergan with Codeine ... 2777
Phenergan with Dextromethorphan 2778
Phenergan Injection ... 2773
Phenergan Suppositories ... 2775
Phenergan Syrup ... 2774
Phenergan Tablets ... 2775
Phenergan VC ... 2779
Phenergan VC with Codeine ... 2781
Propofol (May increase drowsiness effect). Products include:
Diprivan Injection ... 2833
Propranolol Hydrochloride (Concurrent use should be avoided). Products include:
Inderal ... 2728
Inderal LA Long Acting Capsules ... 2730
Inderide Tablets ... 2732
Inderide LA Long Acting Capsules .. 2734
Protriptyline Hydrochloride (Concurrent use should be avoided). Products include:
Vivactil Tablets ... 1774
Quazepam (May increase drowsiness effect). Products include:
Doral Tablets ... 2664
Quinapril Hydrochloride (Concurrent use should be avoided). Products include:
Accupril Tablets ... 1893
Ramipril (Concurrent use should be avoided). Products include:
Altace Capsules ... 1232
Rauwolfia Serpentina (Concurrent use should be avoided).
No products indexed under this heading.
Rescinnamine (Concurrent use should be avoided).
No products indexed under this heading.
Reserpine (Concurrent use should be avoided). Products include:
Diupres Tablets ... 1650
Hydropres Tablets ... 1675
Ser-Ap-Es Tablets ... 849
Secobarbital Sodium (May increase drowsiness effect). Products include:
Seconal Sodium Pulvules ... 1474
Sertraline Hydrochloride (Concurrent use should be avoided). Products include:
Zoloft Tablets ... 2217
Sodium Nitroprusside (Concurrent use should be avoided).
No products indexed under this heading.
Sotalol Hydrochloride (Concurrent use should be avoided). Products include:
Betapace Tablets ... 641
Spirapril Hydrochloride (Concurrent use should be avoided).
No products indexed under this heading.
Temazepam (May increase drowsiness effect). Products include:
Restoril Capsules ... 2284
Terazosin Hydrochloride (Concurrent use should be avoided). Products include:
Hytrin Capsules ... 430
Thioridazine Hydrochloride (May increase drowsiness effect). Products include:
Mellaril ... 2269
Thiothixene (May increase drowsiness effect). Products include:
Navane Capsules and Concentrate 2201
Navane Intramuscular ... 2202
Timolol Maleate (Concurrent use should be avoided). Products include:
Blocadren Tablets ... 1614
Timolide Tablets ... 1748
Timoptic in Ocudose ... 1753
Timoptic Sterile Ophthalmic Solution ... 1751
Timoptic-XE ... 1755
Torsemide (Concurrent use should be avoided). Products include:
Demadex Tablets and Injection ... 686
Tranylcypromine Sulfate (Concurrent use should be avoided). Products include:
Parnate Tablets ... 2503
Trazodone Hydrochloride (Concurrent use should be avoided). Products include:
Desyrel and Desyrel Dividose ... 503
Triazolam (May increase drowsiness effect). Products include:
Halcion Tablets ... 2611
Trifluoperazine Hydrochloride (May increase drowsiness effect). Products include:
Stelazine ... 2514
Trimethaphan Camsylate (Concurrent use should be avoided). Products include:
Arfonad Ampuls ... 2080
Trimipramine Maleate (Concurrent use should be avoided). Products include:
Surmontil Capsules ... 2811
Venlafaxine Hydrochloride (Concurrent use should be avoided). Products include:
Effexor ... 2719
Verapamil Hydrochloride (Concurrent use should be avoided). Products include:
Calan SR Caplets ... 2422
Calan Tablets ... 2419
Isoptin Injectable ... 1344
Isoptin Oral Tablets ... 1346
Isoptin SR Tablets ... 1348
Verelan Capsules ... 1410
Verelan Capsules ... 2824
Zolpidem Tartrate (May increase drowsiness effect). Products include:
Ambien Tablets ... 2416

Food Interactions

Alcohol (May increase drowsiness effect; chronic heavy alcohol abusers, 3 or more drinks per day, may be at increased risk of liver toxicity from acetaminophen use).

TYLENOL MAXIMUM STRENGTH FLU NIGHTTIME HOT MEDICATION PACKETS
(Acetaminophen, Dextromethorphan Hydrobromide, Pseudoephedrine Hydrochloride) ... 1562
May interact with hypnotics and sedatives, tranquilizers, antidepressant drugs, antihypertensives, and certain other agents. Compounds in these categories include:

Acebutolol Hydrochloride (Concurrent use is not recommended). Products include:
Sectral Capsules ... 2807
Alprazolam (May increase drowsiness effect). Products include:
Xanax Tablets ... 2649
Amitriptyline Hydrochloride (Concurrent use is not recommended). Products include:
Elavil ... 2838
Endep Tablets ... 2174
Etrafon ... 2355
Limbitrol ... 2180
Triavil Tablets ... 1757
Amlodipine Besylate (Concurrent use is not recommended). Products include:
Lotrel Capsules ... 840
Norvasc Tablets ... 1940
Amoxapine (Concurrent use is not recommended). Products include:
Asendin Tablets ... 1369
Atenolol (Concurrent use is not recommended). Products include:
Tenoretic Tablets ... 2845
Tenormin Tablets and I.V. Injection 2847
Benazepril Hydrochloride (Concurrent use is not recommended). Products include:
Lotensin Tablets ... 834
Lotensin HCT ... 837
Lotrel Capsules ... 840
Bendroflumethiazide (Concurrent use is not recommended).
No products indexed under this heading.
Betaxolol Hydrochloride (Concurrent use is not recommended). Products include:
Betoptic Ophthalmic Solution ... 469
Betoptic S Ophthalmic Suspension 471
Kerlone Tablets ... 2436
Bisoprolol Fumarate (Concurrent use is not recommended). Products include:
Zebeta Tablets ... 1413
Ziac ... 1415
Bupropion Hydrochloride (Concurrent use is not recommended). Products include:
Wellbutrin Tablets ... 1204
Buspirone Hydrochloride (May increase drowsiness effect). Products include:
BuSpar ... 737
Captopril (Concurrent use is not recommended). Products include:
Capoten ... 739
Capozide ... 742
Carteolol Hydrochloride (Concurrent use is not recommended). Products include:
Cartrol Tablets ... 410
Ocupress Ophthalmic Solution, 1% Sterile ... ◉ 309
Chlordiazepoxide (May increase drowsiness effect). Products include:
Libritabs Tablets ... 2177
Limbitrol ... 2180
Chlordiazepoxide Hydrochloride (May increase drowsiness effect). Products include:
Librax Capsules ... 2176
Librium Capsules ... 2178
Librium Injectable ... 2179
Chlorothiazide (Concurrent use is not recommended). Products include:
Aldoclor Tablets ... 1598
Diupres Tablets ... 1650
Diuril Oral ... 1653
Chlorothiazide Sodium (Concurrent use is not recommended). Products include:
Diuril Sodium Intravenous ... 1652
Chlorpromazine (May increase drowsiness effect). Products include:
Thorazine Suppositories ... 2523
Chlorpromazine Hydrochloride (May increase drowsiness effect). Products include:
Thorazine ... 2523
Chlorprothixene (May increase drowsiness effect).
No products indexed under this heading.
Chlorprothixene Hydrochloride (May increase drowsiness effect).
No products indexed under this heading.
Chlorthalidone (Concurrent use is not recommended). Products include:
Combipres Tablets ... 677
Tenoretic Tablets ... 2845
Thalitone ... 1245
Clonidine (Concurrent use is not recommended). Products include:
Catapres-TTS ... 675
Clonidine Hydrochloride (Concurrent use is not recommended). Products include:
Catapres Tablets ... 674
Combipres Tablets ... 677
Clorazepate Dipotassium (May increase drowsiness effect). Products include:
Tranxene ... 451
Deserpidine (Concurrent use is not recommended).
No products indexed under this heading.
Desipramine Hydrochloride (Concurrent use is not recommended). Products include:
Norpramin Tablets ... 1526
Diazepam (May increase drowsiness effect). Products include:
Dizac ... 1809
Valium Injectable ... 2182
Valium Tablets ... 2183
Valrelease Capsules ... 2169
Diazoxide (Concurrent use is not recommended). Products include:
Hyperstat I.V. Injection ... 2363
Proglycem ... 580
Diltiazem Hydrochloride (Concurrent use is not recommended). Products include:
Cardizem CD Capsules ... 1506
Cardizem SR Capsules ... 1510
Cardizem Injectable ... 1508
Cardizem Tablets ... 1512
Dilacor XR Extended-release Capsules ... 2018
Doxazosin Mesylate (Concurrent use is not recommended). Products include:
Cardura Tablets ... 2186
Doxepin Hydrochloride (Concurrent use is not recommended). Products include:
Sinequan ... 2205
Zonalon Cream ... 1055
Droperidol (May increase drowsiness effect). Products include:
Inapsine Injection ... 1296
Enalapril Maleate (Concurrent use is not recommended). Products include:
Vaseretic Tablets ... 1765
Vasotec Tablets ... 1771

IMPORTANT NOTE: Always consult each drug listing in the patient's regimen for possible interactions.

Tylenol Cold & Flu Interactions Index 1100

Enalaprilat (Concurrent use is not recommended). Products include:
Vasotec I.V. ... 1768
Esmolol Hydrochloride (Concurrent use is not recommended). Products include:
Brevibloc Injection ... 1808
Estazolam (May increase drowsiness effect). Products include:
ProSom Tablets ... 449
Ethchlorvynol (May increase drowsiness effect). Products include:
Placidyl Capsules ... 448
Ethinamate (May increase drowsiness effect).
No products indexed under this heading.
Felodipine (Concurrent use is not recommended). Products include:
Plendil Extended-Release Tablets ... 527
Fluoxetine Hydrochloride (Concurrent use is not recommended). Products include:
Prozac Pulvules & Liquid, Oral Solution ... 919
Fluphenazine Decanoate (May increase drowsiness effect). Products include:
Prolixin Decanoate ... 509
Fluphenazine Enanthate (May increase drowsiness effect). Products include:
Prolixin Enanthate ... 509
Fluphenazine Hydrochloride (May increase drowsiness effect). Products include:
Prolixin ... 509
Flurazepam Hydrochloride (May increase drowsiness effect). Products include:
Dalmane Capsules ... 2173
Fosinopril Sodium (Concurrent use is not recommended). Products include:
Monopril Tablets ... 757
Furosemide (Concurrent use is not recommended). Products include:
Lasix Injection, Oral Solution and Tablets ... 1240
Glutethimide (May increase drowsiness effect).
No products indexed under this heading.
Guanabenz Acetate (Concurrent use is not recommended).
No products indexed under this heading.
Guanethidine Monosulfate (Concurrent use is not recommended). Products include:
Esimil Tablets ... 822
Ismelin Tablets ... 827
Haloperidol (May increase drowsiness effect). Products include:
Haldol Injection, Tablets and Concentrate ... 1575
Haloperidol Decanoate (May increase drowsiness effect). Products include:
Haldol Decanoate ... 1577
Hydralazine Hydrochloride (Concurrent use is not recommended). Products include:
Apresazide Capsules ... 808
Apresoline Hydrochloride Tablets ... 809
Ser-Ap-Es Tablets ... 849
Hydrochlorothiazide (Concurrent use is not recommended). Products include:
Aldactazide ... 2413
Aldoril Tablets ... 1604
Apresazide Capsules ... 808
Capozide ... 742
Dyazide ... 2479
Esidrix Tablets ... 821
Esimil Tablets ... 822
HydroDIURIL Tablets ... 1674
Hydropres Tablets ... 1675
Hyzaar Tablets ... 1677
Inderide Tablets ... 2732
Inderide LA Long Acting Capsules ... 2734
Lopressor HCT Tablets ... 832
Lotensin HCT ... 837
Maxzide ... 1380
Moduretic Tablets ... 1705
Oretic Tablets ... 443
Prinzide Tablets ... 1737
Ser-Ap-Es Tablets ... 849
Timolide Tablets ... 1748
Vaseretic Tablets ... 1765
Zestoretic ... 2850
Ziac ... 1415
Hydroflumethiazide (Concurrent use is not recommended). Products include:
Diucardin Tablets ... 2718
Hydroxyzine Hydrochloride (May increase drowsiness effect). Products include:
Atarax Tablets & Syrup ... 2185
Marax Tablets & DF Syrup ... 2200
Vistaril Intramuscular Solution ... 2216
Imipramine Hydrochloride (Concurrent use is not recommended). Products include:
Tofranil Ampuls ... 854
Tofranil Tablets ... 856
Imipramine Pamoate (Concurrent use is not recommended). Products include:
Tofranil-PM Capsules ... 857
Indapamide (Concurrent use is not recommended). Products include:
Lozol Tablets ... 2022
Isocarboxazid (Concurrent use is not recommended).
No products indexed under this heading.
Isradipine (Concurrent use is not recommended). Products include:
DynaCirc Capsules ... 2256
Labetalol Hydrochloride (Concurrent use is not recommended). Products include:
Normodyne Injection ... 2377
Normodyne Tablets ... 2379
Trandate ... 1185
Levobunolol Hydrochloride (Concurrent use is not recommended). Products include:
Betagan ... ⊙ 233
Lisinopril (Concurrent use is not recommended). Products include:
Prinivil Tablets ... 1733
Prinzide Tablets ... 1737
Zestoretic ... 2850
Zestril Tablets ... 2854
Lorazepam (May increase drowsiness effect). Products include:
Ativan Injection ... 2698
Ativan Tablets ... 2700
Losartan Potassium (Concurrent use is not recommended). Products include:
Cozaar Tablets ... 1628
Hyzaar Tablets ... 1677
Loxapine Hydrochloride (May increase drowsiness effect). Products include:
Loxitane ... 1378
Loxapine Succinate (May increase drowsiness effect). Products include:
Loxitane Capsules ... 1378
Maprotiline Hydrochloride (Concurrent use is not recommended). Products include:
Ludiomil Tablets ... 843
Mecamylamine Hydrochloride (Concurrent use is not recommended). Products include:
Inversine Tablets ... 1686
Meprobamate (May increase drowsiness effect). Products include:
Miltown Tablets ... 2672
PMB 200 and PMB 400 ... 2783
Mesoridazine Besylate (May increase drowsiness effect). Products include:
Serentil ... 684
Methyclothiazide (Concurrent use is not recommended). Products include:
Enduron Tablets ... 420
Methyldopa (Concurrent use is not recommended). Products include:
Aldoclor Tablets ... 1598
Aldomet Oral ... 1600
Aldoril Tablets ... 1604
Methyldopate Hydrochloride (Concurrent use is not recommended). Products include:
Aldomet Ester HCl Injection ... 1602
Metipranolol Hydrochloride (Concurrent use is not recommended). Products include:
OptiPranolol (Metipranolol 0.3%) Sterile Ophthalmic Solution ... ⊙ 258
Metolazone (Concurrent use is not recommended). Products include:
Mykrox Tablets ... 993
Zaroxolyn Tablets ... 1000
Metoprolol Succinate (Concurrent use is not recommended). Products include:
Toprol-XL Tablets ... 565
Metoprolol Tartrate (Concurrent use is not recommended). Products include:
Lopressor Ampuls ... 830
Lopressor HCT Tablets ... 832
Lopressor Tablets ... 830
Metyrosine (Concurrent use is not recommended). Products include:
Demser Capsules ... 1649
Midazolam Hydrochloride (May increase drowsiness effect). Products include:
Versed Injection ... 2170
Minoxidil (Concurrent use is not recommended). Products include:
Loniten Tablets ... 2618
Rogaine Topical Solution ... 2637
Moexipril Hydrochloride (Concurrent use is not recommended). Products include:
Univasc Tablets ... 2410
Molindone Hydrochloride (May increase drowsiness effect). Products include:
Moban Tablets and Concentrate ... 1048
Nadolol (Concurrent use is not recommended).
No products indexed under this heading.
Nefazodone Hydrochloride (Concurrent use is not recommended). Products include:
Serzone Tablets ... 771
Nicardipine Hydrochloride (Concurrent use is not recommended). Products include:
Cardene Capsules ... 2095
Cardene I.V. ... 2709
Cardene SR Capsules ... 2097
Nifedipine (Concurrent use is not recommended). Products include:
Adalat Capsules (10 mg and 20 mg) ... 587
Adalat CC ... 589
Procardia Capsules ... 1971
Procardia XL Extended Release Tablets ... 1972
Nisoldipine (Concurrent use is not recommended).
No products indexed under this heading.
Nitroglycerin (Concurrent use is not recommended). Products include:
Deponit NTG Transdermal Delivery System ... 2397
Nitro-Bid IV ... 1523
Nitro-Bid Ointment ... 1524
Nitrodisc ... 2047
Nitro-Dur (nitroglycerin) Transdermal Infusion System ... 1326
Nitrolingual Spray ... 2027
Nitrostat Tablets ... 1925
Transderm-Nitro Transdermal Therapeutic System ... 859
Nortriptyline Hydrochloride (Concurrent use is not recommended). Products include:
Pamelor ... 2280
Oxazepam (May increase drowsiness effect). Products include:
Serax Capsules ... 2810
Serax Tablets ... 2810
Paroxetine Hydrochloride (Concurrent use is not recommended). Products include:
Paxil Tablets ... 2505
Penbutolol Sulfate (Concurrent use is not recommended). Products include:
Levatol ... 2403
Perphenazine (May increase drowsiness effect). Products include:
Etrafon ... 2355
Triavil Tablets ... 1757
Trilafon ... 2389
Phenelzine Sulfate (Concurrent use is not recommended). Products include:
Nardil ... 1920
Phenoxybenzamine Hydrochloride (Concurrent use is not recommended). Products include:
Dibenzyline Capsules ... 2476
Phentolamine Mesylate (Concurrent use is not recommended). Products include:
Regitine ... 846
Pindolol (Concurrent use is not recommended). Products include:
Visken Tablets ... 2299
Polythiazide (Concurrent use is not recommended). Products include:
Minizide Capsules ... 1938
Prazepam (May increase drowsiness effect).
No products indexed under this heading.
Prazosin Hydrochloride (Concurrent use is not recommended). Products include:
Minipress Capsules ... 1937
Minizide Capsules ... 1938
Prochlorperazine (May increase drowsiness effect). Products include:
Compazine ... 2470
Promethazine Hydrochloride (May increase drowsiness effect). Products include:
Mepergan Injection ... 2753
Phenergan with Codeine ... 2777
Phenergan with Dextromethorphan ... 2778
Phenergan Injection ... 2773
Phenergan Suppositories ... 2775
Phenergan Syrup ... 2774
Phenergan Tablets ... 2775
Phenergan VC ... 2779
Phenergan VC with Codeine ... 2781
Propofol (May increase drowsiness effect). Products include:
Diprivan Injection ... 2833
Propranolol Hydrochloride (Concurrent use is not recommended). Products include:
Inderal ... 2728
Inderal LA Long Acting Capsules ... 2730
Inderide Tablets ... 2732
Inderide LA Long Acting Capsules ... 2734
Protriptyline Hydrochloride (Concurrent use is not recommended). Products include:
Vivactil Tablets ... 1774
Quazepam (May increase drowsiness effect). Products include:
Doral Tablets ... 2664

(▭ Described in PDR For Nonprescription Drugs) (⊙ Described in PDR For Ophthalmology)

Quinapril Hydrochloride (Concurrent use is not recommended). Products include:
- Accupril Tablets ... 1893

Ramipril (Concurrent use is not recommended). Products include:
- Altace Capsules ... 1232

Rauwolfia Serpentina (Concurrent use is not recommended).
- No products indexed under this heading.

Rescinnamine (Concurrent use is not recommended).
- No products indexed under this heading.

Reserpine (Concurrent use is not recommended). Products include:
- Diupres Tablets ... 1650
- Hydropres Tablets ... 1675
- Ser-Ap-Es Tablets ... 849

Secobarbital Sodium (May increase drowsiness effect). Products include:
- Seconal Sodium Pulvules ... 1474

Sertraline Hydrochloride (Concurrent use is not recommended). Products include:
- Zoloft Tablets ... 2217

Sodium Nitroprusside (Concurrent use is not recommended).
- No products indexed under this heading.

Sotalol Hydrochloride (Concurrent use is not recommended). Products include:
- Betapace Tablets ... 641

Spirapril Hydrochloride (Concurrent use is not recommended).
- No products indexed under this heading.

Temazepam (May increase drowsiness effect). Products include:
- Restoril Capsules ... 2284

Terazosin Hydrochloride (Concurrent use is not recommended). Products include:
- Hytrin Capsules ... 430

Thioridazine Hydrochloride (May increase drowsiness effect). Products include:
- Mellaril ... 2269

Thiothixene (May increase drowsiness effect). Products include:
- Navane Capsules and Concentrate ... 2201
- Navane Intramuscular ... 2202

Timolol Maleate (Concurrent use is not recommended). Products include:
- Blocadren Tablets ... 1614
- Timolide Tablets ... 1748
- Timoptic in Ocudose ... 1753
- Timoptic Sterile Ophthalmic Solution ... 1751
- Timoptic-XE ... 1755

Torsemide (Concurrent use is not recommended). Products include:
- Demadex Tablets and Injection ... 686

Tranylcypromine Sulfate (Concurrent use is not recommended). Products include:
- Parnate Tablets ... 2503

Trazodone Hydrochloride (Concurrent use is not recommended). Products include:
- Desyrel and Desyrel Dividose ... 503

Triazolam (May increase drowsiness effect). Products include:
- Halcion Tablets ... 2611

Trifluoperazine Hydrochloride (May increase drowsiness effect). Products include:
- Stelazine ... 2514

Trimethaphan Camsylate (Concurrent use is not recommended). Products include:
- Arfonad Ampuls ... 2080

Trimipramine Maleate (Concurrent use is not recommended). Products include:
- Surmontil Capsules ... 2811

Venlafaxine Hydrochloride (Concurrent use is not recommended). Products include:
- Effexor ... 2719

Verapamil Hydrochloride (Concurrent use is not recommended). Products include:
- Calan SR Caplets ... 2422
- Calan Tablets ... 2419
- Isoptin Injectable ... 1344
- Isoptin Oral Tablets ... 1346
- Isoptin SR Tablets ... 1348
- Verelan Capsules ... 1410
- Verelan Capsules ... 2824

Zolpidem Tartrate (May increase drowsiness effect). Products include:
- Ambien Tablets ... 2416

Food Interactions

Alcohol (May increase drowsiness effect; chronic heavy alcohol abusers, 3 or more drinks per day, may be at increased risk of liver toxicity from acetaminophen use).

TYLENOL, MAXIMUM STRENGTH, SINUS MEDICATION GELTABS, GELCAPS, CAPLETS AND TABLETS

(Acetaminophen, Pseudoephedrine Hydrochloride) ... 1566

May interact with antidepressant drugs, antihypertensives, and certain other agents. Compounds in these categories include:

Acebutolol Hydrochloride (Concurrent use is not recommended). Products include:
- Sectral Capsules ... 2807

Amitriptyline Hydrochloride (Concurrent use is not recommended). Products include:
- Elavil ... 2838
- Endep Tablets ... 2174
- Etrafon ... 2355
- Limbitrol ... 2180
- Triavil Tablets ... 1757

Amlodipine Besylate (Concurrent use is not recommended). Products include:
- Lotrel Capsules ... 840
- Norvasc Tablets ... 1940

Amoxapine (Concurrent use is not recommended). Products include:
- Asendin Tablets ... 1369

Atenolol (Concurrent use is not recommended). Products include:
- Tenoretic Tablets ... 2845
- Tenormin Tablets and I.V. Injection ... 2847

Benazepril Hydrochloride (Concurrent use is not recommended). Products include:
- Lotensin Tablets ... 834
- Lotensin HCT ... 837
- Lotrel Capsules ... 840

Bendroflumethiazide (Concurrent use is not recommended).
- No products indexed under this heading.

Betaxolol Hydrochloride (Concurrent use is not recommended). Products include:
- Betoptic Ophthalmic Solution ... 469
- Betoptic S Ophthalmic Suspension ... 471
- Kerlone Tablets ... 2436

Bisoprolol Fumarate (Concurrent use is not recommended). Products include:
- Zebeta Tablets ... 1413
- Ziac ... 1415

Bupropion Hydrochloride (Concurrent use is not recommended). Products include:
- Wellbutrin Tablets ... 1204

Captopril (Concurrent use is not recommended). Products include:
- Capoten ... 739
- Capozide ... 742

Carteolol Hydrochloride (Concurrent use is not recommended). Products include:
- Cartrol Tablets ... 410
- Ocupress Ophthalmic Solution, 1% Sterile ... ⊙ 309

Chlorothiazide (Concurrent use is not recommended). Products include:
- Aldoclor Tablets ... 1598
- Diupres Tablets ... 1650
- Diuril Oral ... 1653

Chlorothiazide Sodium (Concurrent use is not recommended). Products include:
- Diuril Sodium Intravenous ... 1652

Chlorthalidone (Concurrent use is not recommended). Products include:
- Combipres Tablets ... 677
- Tenoretic Tablets ... 2845
- Thalitone ... 1245

Clonidine (Concurrent use is not recommended). Products include:
- Catapres-TTS ... 675

Clonidine Hydrochloride (Concurrent use is not recommended). Products include:
- Catapres Tablets ... 674
- Combipres Tablets ... 677

Deserpidine (Concurrent use is not recommended).
- No products indexed under this heading.

Desipramine Hydrochloride (Concurrent use is not recommended). Products include:
- Norpramin Tablets ... 1526

Diazoxide (Concurrent use is not recommended). Products include:
- Hyperstat I.V. Injection ... 2363
- Proglycem ... 580

Diltiazem Hydrochloride (Concurrent use is not recommended). Products include:
- Cardizem CD Capsules ... 1506
- Cardizem SR Capsules ... 1510
- Cardizem Injectable ... 1508
- Cardizem Tablets ... 1512
- Dilacor XR Extended-release Capsules ... 2018

Doxazosin Mesylate (Concurrent use is not recommended). Products include:
- Cardura Tablets ... 2186

Doxepin Hydrochloride (Concurrent use is not recommended). Products include:
- Sinequan ... 2205
- Zonalon Cream ... 1055

Enalapril Maleate (Concurrent use is not recommended). Products include:
- Vaseretic Tablets ... 1765
- Vasotec Tablets ... 1771

Enalaprilat (Concurrent use is not recommended). Products include:
- Vasotec I.V. ... 1768

Esmolol Hydrochloride (Concurrent use is not recommended). Products include:
- Brevibloc Injection ... 1808

Felodipine (Concurrent use is not recommended). Products include:
- Plendil Extended-Release Tablets ... 527

Fluoxetine Hydrochloride (Concurrent use is not recommended). Products include:
- Prozac Pulvules & Liquid, Oral Solution ... 919

Fosinopril Sodium (Concurrent use is not recommended). Products include:
- Monopril Tablets ... 757

Furosemide (Concurrent use is not recommended). Products include:
- Lasix Injection, Oral Solution and Tablets ... 1240

Guanabenz Acetate (Concurrent use is not recommended).
- No products indexed under this heading.

Guanethidine Monosulfate (Concurrent use is not recommended). Products include:
- Esimil Tablets ... 822
- Ismelin Tablets ... 827

Hydralazine Hydrochloride (Concurrent use is not recommended). Products include:
- Apresazide Capsules ... 808
- Apresoline Hydrochloride Tablets ... 809
- Ser-Ap-Es Tablets ... 849

Hydrochlorothiazide (Concurrent use is not recommended). Products include:
- Aldactazide ... 2413
- Aldoril Tablets ... 1604
- Apresazide Capsules ... 808
- Capozide ... 742
- Dyazide ... 2479
- Esidrix Tablets ... 821
- Esimil Tablets ... 822
- HydroDIURIL Tablets ... 1674
- Hydropres Tablets ... 1675
- Hyzaar Tablets ... 1677
- Inderide Tablets ... 2732
- Inderide LA Long Acting Capsules ... 2734
- Lopressor HCT Tablets ... 832
- Lotensin HCT ... 837
- Maxzide ... 1380
- Moduretic Tablets ... 1705
- Oretic Tablets ... 443
- Prinzide Tablets ... 1737
- Ser-Ap-Es Tablets ... 849
- Timolide Tablets ... 1748
- Vaseretic Tablets ... 1765
- Zestoretic ... 2850
- Ziac ... 1415

Hydroflumethiazide (Concurrent use is not recommended). Products include:
- Diucardin Tablets ... 2718

Imipramine Hydrochloride (Concurrent use is not recommended). Products include:
- Tofranil Ampuls ... 854
- Tofranil Tablets ... 856

Imipramine Pamoate (Concurrent use is not recommended). Products include:
- Tofranil-PM Capsules ... 857

Indapamide (Concurrent use is not recommended). Products include:
- Lozol Tablets ... 2022

Isocarboxazid (Concurrent use is not recommended).
- No products indexed under this heading.

Isradipine (Concurrent use is not recommended). Products include:
- DynaCirc Capsules ... 2256

Labetalol Hydrochloride (Concurrent use is not recommended). Products include:
- Normodyne Injection ... 2377
- Normodyne Tablets ... 2379
- Trandate ... 1185

Levobunolol Hydrochloride (Concurrent use is not recommended). Products include:
- Betagan ... ⊙ 233

Lisinopril (Concurrent use is not recommended). Products include:
- Prinivil Tablets ... 1733
- Prinzide Tablets ... 1737
- Zestoretic ... 2850
- Zestril Tablets ... 2854

Losartan Potassium (Concurrent use is not recommended). Products include:
- Cozaar Tablets ... 1628
- Hyzaar Tablets ... 1677

IMPORTANT NOTE: Always consult each drug listing in the patient's regimen for possible interactions.

Tylenol, Maximum Strength — Interactions Index — 1102

Maprotiline Hydrochloride (Concurrent use is not recommended). Products include:
Ludiomil Tablets ... 843

Mecamylamine Hydrochloride (Concurrent use is not recommended). Products include:
Inversine Tablets ... 1686

Methyclothiazide (Concurrent use is not recommended). Products include:
Enduron Tablets ... 420

Methyldopa (Concurrent use is not recommended). Products include:
Aldoclor Tablets ... 1598
Aldomet Oral ... 1600
Aldoril Tablets ... 1604

Methyldopate Hydrochloride (Concurrent use is not recommended). Products include:
Aldomet Ester HCl Injection ... 1602

Metipranolol Hydrochloride (Concurrent use is not recommended). Products include:
OptiPranolol (Metipranolol 0.3%) Sterile Ophthalmic Solution ... ⊙ 258

Metolazone (Concurrent use is not recommended). Products include:
Mykrox Tablets ... 993
Zaroxolyn Tablets ... 1000

Metoprolol Succinate (Concurrent use is not recommended). Products include:
Toprol-XL Tablets ... 565

Metoprolol Tartrate (Concurrent use is not recommended). Products include:
Lopressor Ampuls ... 830
Lopressor HCT Tablets ... 832
Lopressor Tablets ... 830

Metyrosine (Concurrent use is not recommended). Products include:
Demser Capsules ... 1649

Minoxidil (Concurrent use is not recommended). Products include:
Loniten Tablets ... 2618
Rogaine Topical Solution ... 2637

Moexipril Hydrochloride (Concurrent use is not recommended). Products include:
Univasc Tablets ... 2410

Nadolol (Concurrent use is not recommended).
No products indexed under this heading.

Nefazodone Hydrochloride (Concurrent use is not recommended). Products include:
Serzone Tablets ... 771

Nicardipine Hydrochloride (Concurrent use is not recommended). Products include:
Cardene Capsules ... 2095
Cardene I.V. ... 2709
Cardene SR Capsules ... 2097

Nifedipine (Concurrent use is not recommended). Products include:
Adalat Capsules (10 mg and 20 mg) ... 587
Adalat CC ... 589
Procardia Capsules ... 1971
Procardia XL Extended Release Tablets ... 1972

Nisoldipine (Concurrent use is not recommended).
No products indexed under this heading.

Nitroglycerin (Concurrent use is not recommended). Products include:
Deponit NTG Transdermal Delivery System ... 2397
Nitro-Bid IV ... 1523
Nitro-Bid Ointment ... 1524
Nitrodisc ... 2047
Nitro-Dur (nitroglycerin) Transdermal Infusion System ... 1326
Nitrolingual Spray ... 2027
Nitrostat Tablets ... 1925
Transderm-Nitro Transdermal Therapeutic System ... 859

Nortriptyline Hydrochloride (Concurrent use is not recommended). Products include:
Pamelor ... 2280

Paroxetine Hydrochloride (Concurrent use is not recommended). Products include:
Paxil Tablets ... 2505

Penbutolol Sulfate (Concurrent use is not recommended). Products include:
Levatol ... 2403

Phenelzine Sulfate (Concurrent use is not recommended). Products include:
Nardil ... 1920

Phenoxybenzamine Hydrochloride (Concurrent use is not recommended). Products include:
Dibenzyline Capsules ... 2476

Phentolamine Mesylate (Concurrent use is not recommended). Products include:
Regitine ... 846

Pindolol (Concurrent use is not recommended). Products include:
Visken Tablets ... 2299

Polythiazide (Concurrent use is not recommended). Products include:
Minizide Capsules ... 1938

Prazosin Hydrochloride (Concurrent use is not recommended). Products include:
Minipress Capsules ... 1937
Minizide Capsules ... 1938

Propranolol Hydrochloride (Concurrent use is not recommended). Products include:
Inderal ... 2728
Inderal LA Long Acting Capsules ... 2730
Inderide Tablets ... 2732
Inderide LA Long Acting Capsules ... 2734

Protriptyline Hydrochloride (Concurrent use is not recommended). Products include:
Vivactil Tablets ... 1774

Quinapril Hydrochloride (Concurrent use is not recommended). Products include:
Accupril Tablets ... 1893

Ramipril (Concurrent use is not recommended). Products include:
Altace Capsules ... 1232

Rauwolfia Serpentina (Concurrent use is not recommended).
No products indexed under this heading.

Rescinnamine (Concurrent use is not recommended).
No products indexed under this heading.

Reserpine (Concurrent use is not recommended). Products include:
Diupres Tablets ... 1650
Hydropres Tablets ... 1675
Ser-Ap-Es Tablets ... 849

Sertraline Hydrochloride (Concurrent use is not recommended). Products include:
Zoloft Tablets ... 2217

Sodium Nitroprusside (Concurrent use is not recommended).
No products indexed under this heading.

Sotalol Hydrochloride (Concurrent use is not recommended). Products include:
Betapace Tablets ... 641

Spirapril Hydrochloride (Concurrent use is not recommended).
No products indexed under this heading.

Terazosin Hydrochloride (Concurrent use is not recommended). Products include:
Hytrin Capsules ... 430

Timolol Maleate (Concurrent use is not recommended). Products include:
Blocadren Tablets ... 1614
Timolide Tablets ... 1748
Timoptic in Ocudose ... 1753
Timoptic Sterile Ophthalmic Solution ... 1751
Timoptic-XE ... 1755

Torsemide (Concurrent use is not recommended). Products include:
Demadex Tablets and Injection ... 686

Tranylcypromine Sulfate (Concurrent use is not recommended). Products include:
Parnate Tablets ... 2503

Trazodone Hydrochloride (Concurrent use is not recommended). Products include:
Desyrel and Desyrel Dividose ... 503

Trimethaphan Camsylate (Concurrent use is not recommended). Products include:
Arfonad Ampuls ... 2080

Trimipramine Maleate (Concurrent use is not recommended). Products include:
Surmontil Capsules ... 2811

Venlafaxine Hydrochloride (Concurrent use is not recommended). Products include:
Effexor ... 2719

Verapamil Hydrochloride (Concurrent use is not recommended). Products include:
Calan SR Caplets ... 2422
Calan Tablets ... 2419
Isoptin Injectable ... 1344
Isoptin Oral Tablets ... 1346
Isoptin SR Tablets ... 1348
Verelan Capsules ... 1410
Verelan Capsules ... 2824

Food Interactions

Alcohol (Chronic heavy alcohol abusers, 3 or more drinks per day, may be at increased risk of liver toxicity from acetaminophen use).

TYLENOL COLD MULTI-SYMPTOM FORMULA MEDICATION TABLETS AND CAPLETS

(Acetaminophen, Chlorpheniramine Maleate, Pseudoephedrine Hydrochloride, Dextromethorphan Hydrobromide) ... 1561

May interact with hypnotics and sedatives, tranquilizers, monoamine oxidase inhibitors, and certain other agents. Compounds in these categories include:

Alprazolam (May increase drowsiness). Products include:
Xanax Tablets ... 2649

Antidepressant Medications, unspecified (Effect not specified).

Antihypertensive agents, unspecified (Effect not specified).

Buspirone Hydrochloride (May increase drowsiness). Products include:
BuSpar ... 737

Chlordiazepoxide (May increase drowsiness). Products include:
Libritabs Tablets ... 2177
Limbitrol ... 2180

Chlordiazepoxide Hydrochloride (May increase drowsiness). Products include:
Librax Capsules ... 2176
Librium Capsules ... 2178
Librium Injectable ... 2179

Chlorpromazine (May increase drowsiness). Products include:
Thorazine Suppositories ... 2523

Chlorpromazine Hydrochloride (May increase drowsiness). Products include:
Thorazine ... 2523

Chlorprothixene (May increase drowsiness).
No products indexed under this heading.

Chlorprothixene Hydrochloride (May increase drowsiness).
No products indexed under this heading.

Clorazepate Dipotassium (May increase drowsiness). Products include:
Tranxene ... 451

Diazepam (May increase drowsiness). Products include:
Dizac ... 1809
Valium Injectable ... 2182
Valium Tablets ... 2183
Valrelease Capsules ... 2169

Droperidol (May increase drowsiness). Products include:
Inapsine Injection ... 1296

Estazolam (May increase drowsiness). Products include:
ProSom Tablets ... 449

Ethchlorvynol (May increase drowsiness). Products include:
Placidyl Capsules ... 448

Ethinamate (May increase drowsiness).
No products indexed under this heading.

Fluphenazine Decanoate (May increase drowsiness). Products include:
Prolixin Decanoate ... 509

Fluphenazine Enanthate (May increase drowsiness). Products include:
Prolixin Enanthate ... 509

Fluphenazine Hydrochloride (May increase drowsiness). Products include:
Prolixin ... 509

Flurazepam Hydrochloride (May increase drowsiness). Products include:
Dalmane Capsules ... 2173

Furazolidone (Concurrent and/or sequential use is not recommended). Products include:
Furoxone ... 2046

Glutethimide (May increase drowsiness).
No products indexed under this heading.

Haloperidol (May increase drowsiness). Products include:
Haldol Injection, Tablets and Concentrate ... 1575

Haloperidol Decanoate (May increase drowsiness). Products include:
Haldol Decanoate ... 1577

Hydroxyzine Hydrochloride (May increase drowsiness). Products include:
Atarax Tablets & Syrup ... 2185
Marax Tablets & DF Syrup ... 2200
Vistaril Intramuscular Solution ... 2216

Isocarboxazid (Concurrent and/or sequential use is not recommended).
No products indexed under this heading.

Lorazepam (May increase drowsiness). Products include:
Ativan Injection ... 2698
Ativan Tablets ... 2700

Loxapine Hydrochloride (May increase drowsiness). Products include:
Loxitane ... 1378

(▣ Described in PDR For Nonprescription Drugs) (⊙ Described in PDR For Ophthalmology)

Loxapine Succinate (May increase drowsiness). Products include:
Loxitane Capsules ... 1378
Meprobamate (May increase drowsiness). Products include:
Miltown Tablets ... 2672
PMB 200 and PMB 400 ... 2783
Mesoridazine Besylate (May increase drowsiness). Products include:
Serentil ... 684
Midazolam Hydrochloride (May increase drowsiness). Products include:
Versed Injection ... 2170
Molindone Hydrochloride (May increase drowsiness). Products include:
Moban Tablets and Concentrate ... 1048
Oxazepam (May increase drowsiness). Products include:
Serax Capsules ... 2810
Serax Tablets ... 2810
Perphenazine (May increase drowsiness). Products include:
Etrafon ... 2355
Triavil Tablets ... 1757
Trilafon ... 2389
Phenelzine Sulfate (Concurrent and/or sequential use is not recommended). Products include:
Nardil ... 1920
Prazepam (May increase drowsiness).
No products indexed under this heading.
Prochlorperazine (May increase drowsiness). Products include:
Compazine ... 2470
Promethazine Hydrochloride (May increase drowsiness). Products include:
Mepergan Injection ... 2753
Phenergan with Codeine ... 2777
Phenergan with Dextromethorphan 2778
Phenergan Injection ... 2773
Phenergan Suppositories ... 2775
Phenergan Syrup ... 2774
Phenergan Tablets ... 2775
Phenergan VC ... 2779
Phenergan VC with Codeine ... 2781
Propofol (May increase drowsiness). Products include:
Diprivan Injection ... 2833
Quazepam (May increase drowsiness). Products include:
Doral Tablets ... 2664
Secobarbital Sodium (May increase drowsiness). Products include:
Seconal Sodium Pulvules ... 1474
Selegiline Hydrochloride (Concurrent and/or sequential use is not recommended). Products include:
Eldepryl Tablets ... 2550
Temazepam (May increase drowsiness). Products include:
Restoril Capsules ... 2284
Thioridazine Hydrochloride (May increase drowsiness). Products include:
Mellaril ... 2269
Thiothixene (May increase drowsiness). Products include:
Navane Capsules and Concentrate 2201
Navane Intramuscular ... 2202
Tranylcypromine Sulfate (Concurrent and/or sequential use is not recommended). Products include:
Parnate Tablets ... 2503
Triazolam (May increase drowsiness). Products include:
Halcion Tablets ... 2611
Trifluoperazine Hydrochloride (May increase drowsiness). Products include:
Stelazine ... 2514
Zolpidem Tartrate (May increase drowsiness). Products include:
Ambien Tablets ... 2416

Food Interactions

Alcohol (May increase drowsiness; chronic heavy alcohol abusers, 3 or more drinks per day, may be at increased risk of liver toxicity from acetaminophen use).

TYLENOL COLD MEDICATION NO DROWSINESS FORMULA GELCAPS AND CAPLETS

(Acetaminophen, Pseudoephedrine Hydrochloride, Dextromethorphan Hydrobromide) ... 1562
May interact with monoamine oxidase inhibitors and certain other agents. Compounds in these categories include:

Furazolidone (Concurrent and/or sequential use is not recommended). Products include:
Furoxone ... 2046
Isocarboxazid (Concurrent and/or sequential use is not recommended).
No products indexed under this heading.
Phenelzine Sulfate (Concurrent and/or sequential use is not recommended). Products include:
Nardil ... 1920
Selegiline Hydrochloride (Concurrent and/or sequential use is not recommended). Products include:
Eldepryl Tablets ... 2550
Tranylcypromine Sulfate (Concurrent and/or sequential use is not recommended). Products include:
Parnate Tablets ... 2503

Food Interactions

Alcohol (Chronic heavy alcohol abusers, 3 or more drinks per day, may be at increased risk of liver toxicity from acetaminophen use).

TYLENOL COLD MULTI-SYMPTOM HOT MEDICATION LIQUID PACKETS

(Acetaminophen, Chlorpheniramine Maleate, Pseudoephedrine Hydrochloride, Dextromethorphan Hydrobromide) ... 1557
May interact with hypnotics and sedatives, tranquilizers, monoamine oxidase inhibitors, and certain other agents. Compounds in these categories include:

Alprazolam (Increases drowsiness effect). Products include:
Xanax Tablets ... 2649
Buspirone Hydrochloride (Increases drowsiness effect). Products include:
BuSpar ... 737
Chlordiazepoxide (Increases drowsiness effect). Products include:
Libritabs Tablets ... 2177
Limbitrol ... 2180
Chlordiazepoxide Hydrochloride (Increases drowsiness effect). Products include:
Librax Capsules ... 2176
Librium Capsules ... 2178
Librium Injectable ... 2179
Chlorpromazine (Increases drowsiness effect). Products include:
Thorazine Suppositories ... 2523
Chlorpromazine Hydrochloride (Increases drowsiness effect). Products include:
Thorazine ... 2523
Chlorprothixene (Increases drowsiness effect).
No products indexed under this heading.
Chlorprothixene Hydrochloride (Increases drowsiness effect).
No products indexed under this heading.
Clorazepate Dipotassium (Increases drowsiness effect). Products include:
Tranxene ... 451
Diazepam (Increases drowsiness effect). Products include:
Dizac ... 1809
Valium Injectable ... 2182
Valium Tablets ... 2183
Valrelease Capsules ... 2169
Droperidol (Increases drowsiness effect). Products include:
Inapsine Injection ... 1296
Estazolam (Increases drowsiness effect). Products include:
ProSom Tablets ... 449
Ethchlorvynol (Increases drowsiness effect). Products include:
Placidyl Capsules ... 448
Ethinamate (Increases drowsiness effect).
No products indexed under this heading.
Fluphenazine Decanoate (Increases drowsiness effect). Products include:
Prolixin Decanoate ... 509
Fluphenazine Enanthate (Increases drowsiness effect). Products include:
Prolixin Enanthate ... 509
Fluphenazine Hydrochloride (Increases drowsiness effect). Products include:
Prolixin ... 509
Flurazepam Hydrochloride (Increases drowsiness effect). Products include:
Dalmane Capsules ... 2173
Furazolidone (Concurrent and/or sequential use is not recommended). Products include:
Furoxone ... 2046
Glutethimide (Increases drowsiness effect).
No products indexed under this heading.
Haloperidol (Increases drowsiness effect). Products include:
Haldol Injection, Tablets and Concentrate ... 1575
Haloperidol Decanoate (Increases drowsiness effect). Products include:
Haldol Decanoate ... 1577
Hydroxyzine Hydrochloride (Increases drowsiness effect). Products include:
Atarax Tablets & Syrup ... 2185
Marax Tablets & DF Syrup ... 2200
Vistaril Intramuscular Solution ... 2216
Isocarboxazid (Concurrent and/or sequential use is not recommended).
No products indexed under this heading.
Lorazepam (Increases drowsiness effect). Products include:
Ativan Injection ... 2698
Ativan Tablets ... 2700
Loxapine Hydrochloride (Increases drowsiness effect). Products include:
Loxitane ... 1378
Loxapine Succinate (Increases drowsiness effect). Products include:
Loxitane Capsules ... 1378
Meprobamate (Increases drowsiness effect). Products include:
Miltown Tablets ... 2672
PMB 200 and PMB 400 ... 2783
Mesoridazine Besylate (Increases drowsiness effect). Products include:
Serentil ... 684
Midazolam Hydrochloride (Increases drowsiness effect). Products include:
Versed Injection ... 2170
Molindone Hydrochloride (Increases drowsiness effect). Products include:
Moban Tablets and Concentrate ... 1048
Oxazepam (Increases drowsiness effect). Products include:
Serax Capsules ... 2810
Serax Tablets ... 2810
Perphenazine (Increases drowsiness effect). Products include:
Etrafon ... 2355
Triavil Tablets ... 1757
Trilafon ... 2389
Phenelzine Sulfate (Concurrent and/or sequential use is not recommended). Products include:
Nardil ... 1920
Prazepam (Increases drowsiness effect).
No products indexed under this heading.
Prochlorperazine (Increases drowsiness effect). Products include:
Compazine ... 2470
Promethazine Hydrochloride (Increases drowsiness effect). Products include:
Mepergan Injection ... 2753
Phenergan with Codeine ... 2777
Phenergan with Dextromethorphan 2778
Phenergan Injection ... 2773
Phenergan Suppositories ... 2775
Phenergan Syrup ... 2774
Phenergan Tablets ... 2775
Phenergan VC ... 2779
Phenergan VC with Codeine ... 2781
Propofol (Increases drowsiness effect). Products include:
Diprivan Injection ... 2833
Quazepam (Increases drowsiness effect). Products include:
Doral Tablets ... 2664
Secobarbital Sodium (Increases drowsiness effect). Products include:
Seconal Sodium Pulvules ... 1474
Selegiline Hydrochloride (Concurrent and/or sequential use is not recommended). Products include:
Eldepryl Tablets ... 2550
Temazepam (Increases drowsiness effect). Products include:
Restoril Capsules ... 2284
Thioridazine Hydrochloride (Increases drowsiness effect). Products include:
Mellaril ... 2269
Thiothixene (Increases drowsiness effect). Products include:
Navane Capsules and Concentrate 2201
Navane Intramuscular ... 2202
Tranylcypromine Sulfate (Concurrent and/or sequential use is not recommended). Products include:
Parnate Tablets ... 2503
Triazolam (Increases drowsiness effect). Products include:
Halcion Tablets ... 2611
Trifluoperazine Hydrochloride (Increases drowsiness effect). Products include:
Stelazine ... 2514
Zolpidem Tartrate (Increases drowsiness effect). Products include:
Ambien Tablets ... 2416

Food Interactions

Alcohol (Increases drowsiness effect; chronic heavy alcohol abusers, 3 or more drinks per day, may be at increased risk of liver toxicity from acetaminophen use).

IMPORTANT NOTE: Always consult each drug listing in the patient's regimen for possible interactions.

TYLENOL COUGH MULTI-SYMPTOM MEDICATION
(Dextromethorphan Hydrobromide, Acetaminophen) 1564
May interact with monoamine oxidase inhibitors and certain other agents. Compounds in these categories include:

Furazolidone (Concurrent and/or sequential use is not recommended). Products include:
Furoxone 2046
Isocarboxazid (Concurrent and/or sequential use is not recommended).
No products indexed under this heading.
Phenelzine Sulfate (Concurrent and/or sequential use is not recommended). Products include:
Nardil 1920
Selegiline Hydrochloride (Concurrent and/or sequential use is not recommended). Products include:
Eldepryl Tablets 2550
Tranylcypromine Sulfate (Concurrent and/or sequential use is not recommended). Products include:
Parnate Tablets 2503

Food Interactions
Alcohol (Chronic heavy alcohol abusers, 3 or more drinks per day, may be at increased risk of liver toxicity from acetaminophen use).

TYLENOL COUGH MULTI-SYMPTOM MEDICATION WITH DECONGESTANT
(Dextromethorphan Hydrobromide, Acetaminophen, Pseudoephedrine Hydrochloride) 1565
May interact with monoamine oxidase inhibitors and certain other agents. Compounds in these categories include:

Furazolidone (Concurrent and/or sequential use is not recommended). Products include:
Furoxone 2046
Isocarboxazid (Concurrent and/or sequential use is not recommended).
No products indexed under this heading.
Phenelzine Sulfate (Concurrent and/or sequential use is not recommended). Products include:
Nardil 1920
Selegiline Hydrochloride (Concurrent and/or sequential use is not recommended). Products include:
Eldepryl Tablets 2550
Tranylcypromine Sulfate (Concurrent and/or sequential use is not recommended). Products include:
Parnate Tablets 2503

Food Interactions
Alcohol (Chronic heavy alcohol abusers, 3 or more drinks per day, may be at increased risk of liver toxicity from acetaminophen use).

TYLENOL, REGULAR STRENGTH, ACETAMINOPHEN CAPLETS AND TABLETS
(Acetaminophen) 1558

Food Interactions
Alcohol (Chronic heavy alcohol abusers, 3 or more drinks per day, may be at increased risk of liver toxicity from acetaminophen use).

TYLENOL PM, EXTRA STRENGTH PAIN RELIEVER/SLEEP AID CAPLETS, GELTABS, GELCAPS
(Acetaminophen, Diphenhydramine Hydrochloride) 1560
May interact with hypnotics and sedatives, tranquilizers, and certain other agents. Compounds in these categories include:

Alprazolam (Effect not specified). Products include:
Xanax Tablets 2649
Buspirone Hydrochloride (Effect not specified). Products include:
BuSpar 737
Chlordiazepoxide (Effect not specified). Products include:
Libritabs Tablets 2177
Limbitrol 2180
Chlordiazepoxide Hydrochloride (Effect not specified). Products include:
Librax Capsules 2176
Librium Capsules 2178
Librium Injectable 2179
Chlorpromazine (Effect not specified). Products include:
Thorazine Suppositories 2523
Chlorprothixene (Effect not specified).
No products indexed under this heading.
Chlorprothixene Hydrochloride (Effect not specified).
No products indexed under this heading.
Clorazepate Dipotassium (Effect not specified). Products include:
Tranxene 451
Diazepam (Effect not specified). Products include:
Dizac 1809
Valium Injectable 2182
Valium Tablets 2183
Valrelease Capsules 2169
Droperidol (Effect not specified). Products include:
Inapsine Injection 1296
Estazolam (Effect not specified). Products include:
ProSom Tablets 449
Ethchlorvynol (Effect not specified). Products include:
Placidyl Capsules 448
Ethinamate (Effect not specified).
No products indexed under this heading.
Fluphenazine Decanoate (Effect not specified). Products include:
Prolixin Decanoate 509
Fluphenazine Enanthate (Effect not specified). Products include:
Prolixin Enanthate 509
Fluphenazine Hydrochloride (Effect not specified). Products include:
Prolixin 509
Flurazepam Hydrochloride (Effect not specified). Products include:
Dalmane Capsules 2173
Glutethimide (Effect not specified).
No products indexed under this heading.
Haloperidol (Effect not specified). Products include:
Haldol Injection, Tablets and Concentrate 1575
Haloperidol Decanoate (Effect not specified). Products include:
Haldol Decanoate 1577
Hydroxyzine Hydrochloride (Effect not specified). Products include:
Atarax Tablets & Syrup 2185
Marax Tablets & DF Syrup 2200
Vistaril Intramuscular Solution 2216
Lorazepam (Effect not specified). Products include:
Ativan Injection 2698
Ativan Tablets 2700
Loxapine Hydrochloride (Effect not specified). Products include:
Loxitane 1378
Loxapine Succinate (Effect not specified). Products include:
Loxitane Capsules 1378
Meprobamate (Effect not specified). Products include:
Miltown Tablets 2672
PMB 200 and PMB 400 2783
Mesoridazine Besylate (Effect not specified). Products include:
Serentil 684
Midazolam Hydrochloride (Effect not specified). Products include:
Versed Injection 2170
Molindone Hydrochloride (Effect not specified). Products include:
Moban Tablets and Concentrate 1048
Oxazepam (Effect not specified). Products include:
Serax Capsules 2810
Serax Tablets 2810
Perphenazine (Effect not specified). Products include:
Etrafon 2355
Triavil Tablets 1757
Trilafon 2389
Prazepam (Effect not specified).
No products indexed under this heading.
Prochlorperazine (Effect not specified). Products include:
Compazine 2470
Promethazine Hydrochloride (Effect not specified). Products include:
Mepergan Injection 2753
Phenergan with Codeine 2777
Phenergan with Dextromethorphan 2778
Phenergan Injection 2773
Phenergan Suppositories 2775
Phenergan Syrup 2774
Phenergan Tablets 2775
Phenergan VC 2779
Phenergan VC with Codeine 2781
Propofol (Effect not specified). Products include:
Diprivan Injection 2833
Quazepam (Effect not specified). Products include:
Doral Tablets 2664
Secobarbital Sodium (Effect not specified). Products include:
Seconal Sodium Pulvules 1474
Temazepam (Effect not specified). Products include:
Restoril Capsules 2284
Thioridazine Hydrochloride (Effect not specified). Products include:
Mellaril 2269
Thiothixene (Effect not specified). Products include:
Navane Capsules and Concentrate 2201
Navane Intramuscular 2202
Triazolam (Effect not specified). Products include:
Halcion Tablets 2611
Trifluoperazine Hydrochloride (Effect not specified). Products include:
Stelazine 2514
Zolpidem Tartrate (Effect not specified). Products include:
Ambien Tablets 2416

Food Interactions
Alcohol (Avoid concurrent use; chronic heavy alcohol abusers, 3 or more drinks per day, may be at increased risk of liver toxicity from acetaminophen use).

TYLENOL SEVERE ALLERGY MEDICATION CAPLETS
(Acetaminophen, Diphenhydramine Hydrochloride) 1564
May interact with hypnotics and sedatives, tranquilizers, and certain other agents. Compounds in these categories include:

Alprazolam (May increase the drowsiness effect; consult your doctor). Products include:
Xanax Tablets 2649
Buspirone Hydrochloride (May increase the drowsiness effect; consult your doctor). Products include:
BuSpar 737
Chlordiazepoxide (May increase the drowsiness effect; consult your doctor). Products include:
Libritabs Tablets 2177
Limbitrol 2180
Chlordiazepoxide Hydrochloride (May increase the drowsiness effect; consult your doctor). Products include:
Librax Capsules 2176
Librium Capsules 2178
Librium Injectable 2179
Chlorpromazine (May increase the drowsiness effect; consult your doctor). Products include:
Thorazine Suppositories 2523
Chlorpromazine Hydrochloride (May increase the drowsiness effect; consult your doctor). Products include:
Thorazine 2523
Chlorprothixene (May increase the drowsiness effect; consult your doctor).
No products indexed under this heading.
Chlorprothixene Hydrochloride (May increase the drowsiness effect; consult your doctor).
No products indexed under this heading.
Clorazepate Dipotassium (May increase the drowsiness effect; consult your doctor). Products include:
Tranxene 451
Diazepam (May increase the drowsiness effect; consult your doctor). Products include:
Dizac 1809
Valium Injectable 2182
Valium Tablets 2183
Valrelease Capsules 2169
Droperidol (May increase the drowsiness effect; consult your doctor). Products include:
Inapsine Injection 1296
Estazolam (May increase the drowsiness effect; consult your doctor). Products include:
ProSom Tablets 449
Ethchlorvynol (May increase the drowsiness effect; consult your doctor). Products include:
Placidyl Capsules 448
Ethinamate (May increase the drowsiness effect; consult your doctor).
No products indexed under this heading.
Fluphenazine Decanoate (May increase the drowsiness effect; consult your doctor). Products include:
Prolixin Decanoate 509
Fluphenazine Enanthate (May increase the drowsiness effect; consult your doctor). Products include:
Prolixin Enanthate 509

(▣ Described in PDR For Nonprescription Drugs) (⊙ Described in PDR For Ophthalmology)

Interactions Index — Tylenol with Codeine

Fluphenazine Hydrochloride (May increase the drowsiness effect; consult your doctor). Products include:

Prolixin 509

Flurazepam Hydrochloride (May increase the drowsiness effect; consult your doctor). Products include:

Dalmane Capsules 2173

Glutethimide (May increase the drowsiness effect; consult your doctor).

No products indexed under this heading.

Haloperidol (May increase the drowsiness effect; consult your doctor). Products include:

Haldol Injection, Tablets and Concentrate 1575

Haloperidol Decanoate (May increase the drowsiness effect; consult your doctor). Products include:

Haldol Decanoate 1577

Hydroxyzine Hydrochloride (May increase the drowsiness effect; consult your doctor). Products include:

Atarax Tablets & Syrup 2185
Marax Tablets & DF Syrup 2200
Vistaril Intramuscular Solution 2216

Lorazepam (May increase the drowsiness effect; consult your doctor). Products include:

Ativan Injection 2698
Ativan Tablets 2700

Loxapine Hydrochloride (May increase the drowsiness effect; consult your doctor). Products include:

Loxitane 1378

Loxapine Succinate (May increase the drowsiness effect; consult your doctor). Products include:

Loxitane Capsules 1378

Meprobamate (May increase the drowsiness effect; consult your doctor). Products include:

Miltown Tablets 2672
PMB 200 and PMB 400 2783

Mesoridazine Besylate (May increase the drowsiness effect; consult your doctor). Products include:

Serentil 684

Midazolam Hydrochloride (May increase the drowsiness effect; consult your doctor). Products include:

Versed Injection 2170

Molindone Hydrochloride (May increase the drowsiness effect; consult your doctor). Products include:

Moban Tablets and Concentrate 1048

Oxazepam (May increase the drowsiness effect; consult your doctor). Products include:

Serax Capsules 2810
Serax Tablets 2810

Perphenazine (May increase the drowsiness effect; consult your doctor). Products include:

Etrafon 2355
Triavil Tablets 1757
Trilafon 2389

Prazepam (May increase the drowsiness effect; consult your doctor).

No products indexed under this heading.

Prochlorperazine (May increase the drowsiness effect; consult your doctor). Products include:

Compazine 2470

Promethazine Hydrochloride (May increase the drowsiness effect; consult your doctor). Products include:

Mepergan Injection 2753
Phenergan with Codeine 2777
Phenergan with Dextromethorphan 2778
Phenergan Injection 2773
Phenergan Suppositories 2775
Phenergan Syrup 2774
Phenergan Tablets 2775
Phenergan VC 2779
Phenergan VC with Codeine 2781

Propofol (May increase the drowsiness effect; consult your doctor). Products include:

Diprivan Injection 2833

Quazepam (May increase the drowsiness effect; consult your doctor). Products include:

Doral Tablets 2664

Secobarbital Sodium (May increase the drowsiness effect; consult your doctor). Products include:

Seconal Sodium Pulvules 1474

Temazepam (May increase the drowsiness effect; consult your doctor). Products include:

Restoril Capsules 2284

Thioridazine Hydrochloride (May increase the drowsiness effect; consult your doctor). Products include:

Mellaril 2269

Thiothixene (May increase the drowsiness effect; consult your doctor). Products include:

Navane Capsules and Concentrate 2201
Navane Intramuscular 2202

Triazolam (May increase the drowsiness effect; consult your doctor). Products include:

Halcion Tablets 2611

Trifluoperazine Hydrochloride (May increase the drowsiness effect; consult your doctor). Products include:

Stelazine 2514

Zolpidem Tartrate (May increase the drowsiness effect; consult your doctor). Products include:

Ambien Tablets 2416

Food Interactions

Alcohol (Chronic heavy alcohol abusers, 3 or more drinks per day, may be at increased risk of liver toxicity from acetaminophen use).

TYLENOL WITH CODEINE ELIXIR

(Acetaminophen, Codeine Phosphate) 1583

May interact with central nervous system depressants, anticholinergics, antipsychotic agents, narcotic analgesics, and certain other agents. Compounds in these categories include:

Alfentanil Hydrochloride (Additive CNS depression). Products include:

Alfenta Injection 1286

Alprazolam (Additive CNS depression). Products include:

Xanax Tablets 2649

Aprobarbital (Additive CNS depression).

No products indexed under this heading.

Atropine Sulfate (May produce paralytic ileus). Products include:

Arco-Lase Plus Tablets 512
Atrohist Plus Tablets 454
Atropine Sulfate Sterile Ophthalmic Solution .... ◆ 233
Donnatal 2060
Donnatal Extentabs 2061
Donnatal Tablets 2060
Lomotil 2439
Motofen Tablets 784
Urised Tablets 1964

Belladonna Alkaloids (May produce paralytic ileus). Products include:

Bellergal-S Tablets 2250
Hyland's Bed Wetting Tablets .... ⊕ 828
Hyland's EnurAid Tablets .... ⊕ 829
Hyland's Teething Tablets .... ⊕ 830

Benztropine Mesylate (May produce paralytic ileus). Products include:

Cogentin 1621

Biperiden Hydrochloride (May produce paralytic ileus). Products include:

Akineton 1333

Buprenorphine (Additive CNS depression). Products include:

Buprenex Injectable 2006

Buspirone Hydrochloride (Additive CNS depression). Products include:

BuSpar 737

Butabarbital (Additive CNS depression).

No products indexed under this heading.

Butalbital (Additive CNS depression). Products include:

Esgic-plus Tablets 1013
Fioricet Tablets 2258
Fioricet with Codeine Capsules 2260
Fiorinal Capsules 2261
Fiorinal with Codeine Capsules 2262
Fiorinal Tablets 2261
Phrenilin 785
Sedapap Tablets 50 mg/650 mg .. 1543

Chlordiazepoxide (Additive CNS depression). Products include:

Libritabs Tablets 2177
Limbitrol 2180

Chlordiazepoxide Hydrochloride (Additive CNS depression). Products include:

Librax Capsules 2176
Librium Capsules 2178
Librium Injectable 2179

Chlorpromazine (Additive CNS depression). Products include:

Thorazine Suppositories 2523

Chlorprothixene (Additive CNS depression).

No products indexed under this heading.

Chlorprothixene Hydrochloride (Additive CNS depression).

No products indexed under this heading.

Clidinium Bromide (May produce paralytic ileus). Products include:

Librax Capsules 2176
Quarzan Capsules 2181

Clorazepate Dipotassium (Additive CNS depression). Products include:

Tranxene 451

Clozapine (Additive CNS depression). Products include:

Clozaril Tablets 2252

Desflurane (Additive CNS depression). Products include:

Suprane 1813

Dezocine (Additive CNS depression). Products include:

Dalgan Injection 538

Diazepam (Additive CNS depression). Products include:

Dizac 1809
Valium Injectable 2182
Valium Tablets 2183
Valrelease Capsules 2169

Dicyclomine Hydrochloride (May produce paralytic ileus). Products include:

Bentyl 1501

Droperidol (Additive CNS depression). Products include:

Inapsine Injection 1296

Enflurane (Additive CNS depression).

No products indexed under this heading.

Estazolam (Additive CNS depression). Products include:

ProSom Tablets 449

Ethchlorvynol (Additive CNS depression). Products include:

Placidyl Capsules 448

Ethinamate (Additive CNS depression).

No products indexed under this heading.

Ethopropazine Hydrochloride (May produce paralytic ileus).

Fentanyl (Additive CNS depression). Products include:

Duragesic Transdermal System 1288

Fentanyl Citrate (Additive CNS depression). Products include:

Sublimaze Injection 1307

Fluphenazine Decanoate (Additive CNS depression). Products include:

Prolixin Decanoate 509

Fluphenazine Enanthate (Additive CNS depression). Products include:

Prolixin Enanthate 509

Fluphenazine Hydrochloride (Additive CNS depression). Products include:

Prolixin 509

Flurazepam Hydrochloride (Additive CNS depression). Products include:

Dalmane Capsules 2173

Glutethimide (Additive CNS depression).

No products indexed under this heading.

Glycopyrrolate (May produce paralytic ileus). Products include:

Robinul Forte Tablets 2072
Robinul Injectable 2072
Robinul Tablets 2072

Haloperidol (Additive CNS depression). Products include:

Haldol Injection, Tablets and Concentrate 1575

Haloperidol Decanoate (Additive CNS depression). Products include:

Haldol Decanoate 1577

Hydrocodone Bitartrate (Additive CNS depression). Products include:

Anexsia 5/500 Elixir 1781
Anexia Tablets 1782
Codiclear DH Syrup 791
Deconamine CX Cough and Cold Liquid and Tablets 1319
Duratuss HD Elixir 2565
Hycodan Tablets and Syrup 930
Hycomine Compound Tablets 932
Hycomine 931
Hycotuss Expectorant Syrup 933
Hydrocet Capsules 782
Lorcet 10/650 1018
Lortab 2566
Tussend 1783
Tussend Expectorant 1785
Vicodin Tablets 1356
Vicodin ES Tablets 1357
Vicodin Tuss Expectorant 1358
Zydone Capsules 949

Hydrocodone Polistirex (Additive CNS depression). Products include:

Tussionex Pennkinetic Extended-Release Suspension 998

Hydroxyzine Hydrochloride (Additive CNS depression). Products include:

Atarax Tablets & Syrup 2185
Marax Tablets & DF Syrup 2200
Vistaril Intramuscular Solution 2216

Hyoscyamine (May produce paralytic ileus). Products include:

Cystospaz Tablets 1963
Urised Tablets 1964

Hyoscyamine Sulfate (May produce paralytic ileus). Products include:

Arco-Lase Plus Tablets 512
Atrohist Plus Tablets 454
Cystospaz-M Capsules 1963

IMPORTANT NOTE: Always consult each drug listing in the patient's regimen for possible interactions.

Tylenol with Codeine | Interactions Index | 1106

Donnatal 2060
Donnatal Extentabs 2061
Donnatal Tablets 2060
Kutrase Capsules 2402
Levsin/Levsinex/Levbid 2405

Ipratropium Bromide (May produce paralytic ileus). Products include:
Atrovent Inhalation Aerosol 671
Atrovent Inhalation Solution 673

Isoflurane (Additive CNS depression).
No products indexed under this heading.

Ketamine Hydrochloride (Additive CNS depression).
No products indexed under this heading.

Levomethadyl Acetate Hydrochloride (Additive CNS depression). Products include:
Orlamm 2239

Levorphanol Tartrate (Additive CNS depression). Products include:
Levo-Dromoran 2129

Lithium Carbonate (Additive CNS depression). Products include:
Eskalith 2485
Lithium Carbonate Capsules & Tablets 2230
Lithonate/Lithotabs/Lithobid 2543

Lithium Citrate (Additive CNS depression).
No products indexed under this heading.

Lorazepam (Additive CNS depression). Products include:
Ativan Injection 2698
Ativan Tablets 2700

Loxapine Hydrochloride (Additive CNS depression). Products include:
Loxitane 1378

Loxapine Succinate (Additive CNS depression). Products include:
Loxitane Capsules 1378

Maprotiline Hydrochloride (May result in increased effects). Products include:
Ludiomil Tablets 843

Mepenzolate Bromide (May produce paralytic ileus).
No products indexed under this heading.

Meperidine Hydrochloride (Additive CNS depression). Products include:
Demerol 2308
Mepergan Injection 2753

Mephobarbital (Additive CNS depression). Products include:
Mebaral Tablets 2322

Meprobamate (Additive CNS depression). Products include:
Miltown Tablets 2672
PMB 200 and PMB 400 2783

Mesoridazine Besylate (Additive CNS depression). Products include:
Serentil 684

Methadone Hydrochloride (Additive CNS depression). Products include:
Methadone Hydrochloride Oral Concentrate 2233
Methadone Hydrochloride Oral Solution & Tablets 2235

Methohexital Sodium (Additive CNS depression). Products include:
Brevital Sodium Vials 1429

Methotrimeprazine (Additive CNS depression). Products include:
Levoprome 1274

Methoxyflurane (Additive CNS depression).
No products indexed under this heading.

Midazolam Hydrochloride (Additive CNS depression). Products include:
Versed Injection 2170

Molindone Hydrochloride (Additive CNS depression). Products include:
Moban Tablets and Concentrate 1048

Morphine Sulfate (Additive CNS depression). Products include:
Astramorph/PF Injection, USP (Preservative-Free) 535
Duramorph 962
Infumorph 200 and Infumorph 500 Sterile Solutions 965
MS Contin Tablets 1994
MSIR 1997
Oramorph SR (Morphine Sulfate Sustained Release Tablets) 2236
RMS Suppositories 2657
Roxanol 2243

Opium Alkaloids (Additive CNS depression).
No products indexed under this heading.

Oxazepam (Additive CNS depression). Products include:
Serax Capsules 2810
Serax Tablets 2810

Oxybutynin Chloride (May produce paralytic ileus). Products include:
Ditropan 1516

Oxycodone Hydrochloride (Additive CNS depression). Products include:
Percocet Tablets 938
Percodan Tablets 939
Percodan-Demi Tablets 940
Roxicodone Tablets, Oral Solution & Intensol (Oxycodone) 2244
Tylox Capsules 1584

Oxyphenonium Bromide (May produce paralytic ileus).

Pentobarbital Sodium (Additive CNS depression). Products include:
Nembutal Sodium Capsules 436
Nembutal Sodium Solution 438
Nembutal Sodium Suppositories 440

Perphenazine (Additive CNS depression). Products include:
Etrafon 2355
Triavil Tablets 1757
Trilafon 2389

Phenobarbital (Additive CNS depression). Products include:
Arco-Lase Plus Tablets 512
Bellergal-S Tablets 2250
Donnatal 2060
Donnatal Extentabs 2061
Donnatal Tablets 2060
Phenobarbital Elixir and Tablets 1469
Quadrinal Tablets 1350

Pimozide (Additive CNS depression). Products include:
Orap Tablets 1050

Prazepam (Additive CNS depression).
No products indexed under this heading.

Prochlorperazine (Additive CNS depression). Products include:
Compazine 2470

Procyclidine Hydrochloride (May produce paralytic ileus). Products include:
Kemadrin Tablets 1112

Promethazine Hydrochloride (Additive CNS depression). Products include:
Mepergan Injection 2753
Phenergan with Codeine 2777
Phenergan with Dextromethorphan 2778
Phenergan Injection 2773
Phenergan Suppositories 2775
Phenergan Syrup 2774
Phenergan Tablets 2775
Phenergan VC 2779
Phenergan VC with Codeine 2781

Propantheline Bromide (May produce paralytic ileus). Products include:
Pro-Banthīne Tablets 2052

Propofol (Additive CNS depression). Products include:
Diprivan Injection 2833

Propoxyphene Hydrochloride (Additive CNS depression). Products include:
Darvon 1435
Wygesic Tablets 2827

Propoxyphene Napsylate (Additive CNS depression). Products include:
Darvon-N/Darvocet-N 1433

Quazepam (Additive CNS depression). Products include:
Doral Tablets 2664

Risperidone (Additive CNS depression). Products include:
Risperdal 1301

Scopolamine (May produce paralytic ileus). Products include:
Transderm Scōp Transdermal Therapeutic System 869

Scopolamine Hydrobromide (May produce paralytic ileus). Products include:
Atrohist Plus Tablets 454
Donnatal 2060
Donnatal Extentabs 2061
Donnatal Tablets 2060

Secobarbital Sodium (Additive CNS depression). Products include:
Seconal Sodium Pulvules 1474

Sufentanil Citrate (Additive CNS depression). Products include:
Sufenta Injection 1309

Temazepam (Additive CNS depression). Products include:
Restoril Capsules 2284

Thiamylal Sodium (Additive CNS depression).
No products indexed under this heading.

Thioridazine Hydrochloride (Additive CNS depression). Products include:
Mellaril 2269

Thiothixene (Additive CNS depression). Products include:
Navane Capsules and Concentrate 2201
Navane Intramuscular 2202

Triazolam (Additive CNS depression). Products include:
Halcion Tablets 2611

Tridihexethyl Chloride (May produce paralytic ileus).
No products indexed under this heading.

Trifluoperazine Hydrochloride (Additive CNS depression). Products include:
Stelazine 2514

Trihexyphenidyl Hydrochloride (May produce paralytic ileus). Products include:
Artane 1368

Zolpidem Tartrate (Additive CNS depression). Products include:
Ambien Tablets 2416

Food Interactions

Alcohol (Additive CNS depression).

TYLENOL WITH CODEINE PHOSPHATE TABLETS
(Acetaminophen, Codeine Phosphate) 1583
See **Tylenol with Codeine Elixir**

TYLOX CAPSULES
(Oxycodone Hydrochloride, Acetaminophen) 1584
May interact with anticholinergics, central nervous system depressants, antipsychotic agents, narcotic analgesics, phenothiazines, general anesthetics, hypnotics and sedatives, tranquilizers, and certain other agents. Compounds in these categories include:

Alfentanil Hydrochloride (Additive CNS depression). Products include:
Alfenta Injection 1286

Alprazolam (Additive CNS depression). Products include:
Xanax Tablets 2649

Aprobarbital (Additive CNS depression).
No products indexed under this heading.

Atropine Sulfate (May produce paralytic ileus). Products include:
Arco-Lase Plus Tablets 512
Atrohist Plus Tablets 454
Atropine Sulfate Sterile Ophthalmic Solution ⊙ 233
Donnatal 2060
Donnatal Extentabs 2061
Donnatal Tablets 2060
Lomotil 2439
Motofen Tablets 784
Urised Tablets 1964

Belladonna Alkaloids (May produce paralytic ileus). Products include:
Bellergal-S Tablets 2250
Hyland's Bed Wetting Tablets ▣ 828
Hyland's EnurAid Tablets ▣ 829
Hyland's Teething Tablets ▣ 830

Benztropine Mesylate (May produce paralytic ileus). Products include:
Cogentin 1621

Biperiden Hydrochloride (May produce paralytic ileus). Products include:
Akineton 1333

Buprenorphine (Additive CNS depression). Products include:
Buprenex Injectable 2006

Buspirone Hydrochloride (Additive CNS depression). Products include:
BuSpar 737

Butabarbital (Additive CNS depression).
No products indexed under this heading.

Butalbital (Additive CNS depression). Products include:
Esgic-plus Tablets 1013
Fioricet Tablets 2258
Fioricet with Codeine Capsules 2260
Fiorinal Capsules 2261
Fiorinal with Codeine Capsules 2262
Fiorinal Tablets 2261
Phrenilin 785
Sedapap Tablets 50 mg/650 mg 1543

Chlordiazepoxide (Additive CNS depression). Products include:
Libritabs Tablets 2177
Limbitrol 2180

Chlordiazepoxide Hydrochloride (Additive CNS depression). Products include:
Librax Capsules 2176
Librium Capsules 2178
Librium Injectable 2179

Chlorpromazine (Additive CNS depression). Products include:
Thorazine Suppositories 2523

Chlorprothixene (Additive CNS depression).
No products indexed under this heading.

Chlorprothixene Hydrochloride (Additive CNS depression).
No products indexed under this heading.

Chlorprothixene Lactate (Additive CNS depression).
No products indexed under this heading.

(▣ Described in PDR For Nonprescription Drugs) (⊙ Described in PDR For Ophthalmology)

1107 **Interactions Index** **Tylox**

Clidinium Bromide (May produce paralytic ileus). Products include:
- Librax Capsules 2176
- Quarzan Capsules 2181

Clorazepate Dipotassium (Additive CNS depression). Products include:
- Tranxene 451

Clozapine (Additive CNS depression). Products include:
- Clozaril Tablets 2252

Codeine Phosphate (Additive CNS depression). Products include:
- Actifed with Codeine Cough Syrup 1067
- Brontex 1981
- Deconsal C Expectorant Syrup 456
- Deconsal Pediatric Syrup 457
- Dimetane-DC Cough Syrup 2059
- Empirin with Codeine Tablets 1093
- Fioricet with Codeine Capsules 2260
- Fiorinal with Codeine Capsules 2262
- Isoclor Expectorant 990
- Novahistine DH 2462
- Novahistine Expectorant 2463
- Nucofed 2051
- Phenergan with Codeine 2777
- Phenergan VC with Codeine 2781
- Robitussin A-C Syrup 2073
- Robitussin-DAC Syrup 2074
- Ryna 841
- Soma Compound w/Codeine Tablets 2676
- Tussi-Organidin NR Liquid and S NR Liquid 2677
- Tylenol with Codeine 1583

Desflurane (Additive CNS depression). Products include:
- Suprane 1813

Dezocine (Additive CNS depression). Products include:
- Dalgan Injection 538

Diazepam (Additive CNS depression). Products include:
- Dizac 1809
- Valium Injectable 2182
- Valium Tablets 2183
- Valrelease Capsules 2169

Dicyclomine Hydrochloride (May produce paralytic ileus). Products include:
- Bentyl 1501

Droperidol (Additive CNS depression). Products include:
- Inapsine Injection 1296

Enflurane (Additive CNS depression).
- No products indexed under this heading.

Estazolam (Additive CNS depression). Products include:
- ProSom Tablets 449

Ethchlorvynol (Additive CNS depression). Products include:
- Placidyl Capsules 448

Ethinamate (Additive CNS depression).
- No products indexed under this heading.

Fentanyl (Additive CNS depression). Products include:
- Duragesic Transdermal System 1288

Fentanyl Citrate (Additive CNS depression). Products include:
- Sublimaze Injection 1307

Fluphenazine Decanoate (Additive CNS depression). Products include:
- Prolixin Decanoate 509

Fluphenazine Enanthate (Additive CNS depression). Products include:
- Prolixin Enanthate 509

Fluphenazine Hydrochloride (Additive CNS depression). Products include:
- Prolixin 509

Flurazepam Hydrochloride (Additive CNS depression). Products include:
- Dalmane Capsules 2173

Glutethimide (Additive CNS depression).
- No products indexed under this heading.

Glycopyrrolate (May produce paralytic ileus). Products include:
- Robinul Forte Tablets 2072
- Robinul Injectable 2072
- Robinul Tablets 2072

Haloperidol (Additive CNS depression). Products include:
- Haldol Injection, Tablets and Concentrate 1575

Haloperidol Decanoate (Additive CNS depression). Products include:
- Haldol Decanoate 1577

Hydrocodone Bitartrate (Additive CNS depression). Products include:
- Anexsia 5/500 Elixir 1781
- Anexia Tablets 1782
- Codiclear DH Syrup 791
- Deconamine CX Cough and Cold Liquid and Tablets 1319
- Duratuss HD Elixir 2565
- Hycodan Tablets and Syrup 930
- Hycomine Compound Tablets 932
- Hycomine 931
- Hycotuss Expectorant Syrup 933
- Hydrocet Capsules 782
- Lorcet 10/650 1018
- Lortab 2566
- Tussend 1783
- Tussend Expectorant 1785
- Vicodin Tablets 1356
- Vicodin ES Tablets 1357
- Vicodin Tuss Expectorant 1358
- Zydone Capsules 949

Hydrocodone Polistirex (Additive CNS depression). Products include:
- Tussionex Pennkinetic Extended-Release Suspension 998

Hydroxyzine Hydrochloride (Additive CNS depression). Products include:
- Atarax Tablets & Syrup 2185
- Marax Tablets & DF Syrup 2200
- Vistaril Intramuscular Solution 2216

Hyoscyamine (May produce paralytic ileus). Products include:
- Cystospaz Tablets 1963
- Urised Tablets 1964

Hyoscyamine Sulfate (May produce paralytic ileus). Products include:
- Arco-Lase Plus Tablets 512
- Atrohist Plus Tablets 454
- Cystospaz-M Capsules 1963
- Donnatal 2060
- Donnatal Extentabs 2061
- Donnatal Tablets 2060
- Kutrase Capsules 2402
- Levsin/Levsinex/Levbid 2405

Ipratropium Bromide (May produce paralytic ileus). Products include:
- Atrovent Inhalation Aerosol 671
- Atrovent Inhalation Solution 673

Isoflurane (Additive CNS depression).
- No products indexed under this heading.

Ketamine Hydrochloride (Additive CNS depression).
- No products indexed under this heading.

Levomethadyl Acetate Hydrochloride (Additive CNS depression). Products include:
- Orlamm 2239

Levorphanol Tartrate (Additive CNS depression). Products include:
- Levo-Dromoran 2129

Lithium Carbonate (Additive CNS depression). Products include:
- Eskalith 2485
- Lithium Carbonate Capsules & Tablets 2230
- Lithonate/Lithotabs/Lithobid 2543

Lithium Citrate (Additive CNS depression).
- No products indexed under this heading.

Lorazepam (Additive CNS depression). Products include:
- Ativan Injection 2698
- Ativan Tablets 2700

Loxapine Hydrochloride (Additive CNS depression). Products include:
- Loxitane 1378

Loxapine Succinate (Additive CNS depression). Products include:
- Loxitane Capsules 1378

Mepenzolate Bromide (May produce paralytic ileus).
- No products indexed under this heading.

Meperidine Hydrochloride (Additive CNS depression). Products include:
- Demerol 2308
- Mepergan Injection 2753

Mephobarbital (Additive CNS depression). Products include:
- Mebaral Tablets 2322

Meprobamate (Additive CNS depression). Products include:
- Miltown Tablets 2672
- PMB 200 and PMB 400 2783

Mesoridazine Besylate (Additive CNS depression). Products include:
- Serentil 684

Methadone Hydrochloride (Additive CNS depression). Products include:
- Methadone Hydrochloride Oral Concentrate 2233
- Methadone Hydrochloride Oral Solution & Tablets 2235

Methohexital Sodium (Additive CNS depression). Products include:
- Brevital Sodium Vials 1429

Methotrimeprazine (Additive CNS depression). Products include:
- Levoprome 1274

Methoxyflurane (Additive CNS depression).
- No products indexed under this heading.

Midazolam Hydrochloride (Additive CNS depression). Products include:
- Versed Injection 2170

Molindone Hydrochloride (Additive CNS depression). Products include:
- Moban Tablets and Concentrate 1048

Morphine Sulfate (Additive CNS depression). Products include:
- Astramorph/PF Injection, USP (Preservative-Free) 535
- Duramorph 962
- Infumorph 200 and Infumorph 500 Sterile Solutions 965
- MS Contin Tablets 1994
- MSIR 1997
- Oramorph SR (Morphine Sulfate Sustained Release Tablets) 2236
- RMS Suppositories 2657
- Roxanol 2243

Opium Alkaloids (Additive CNS depression).
- No products indexed under this heading.

Oxazepam (Additive CNS depression). Products include:
- Serax Capsules 2810
- Serax Tablets 2810

Oxybutynin Chloride (May produce paralytic ileus). Products include:
- Ditropan 1516

Pentobarbital Sodium (Additive CNS depression). Products include:
- Nembutal Sodium Capsules 436
- Nembutal Sodium Solution 438
- Nembutal Sodium Suppositories 440

Perphenazine (Additive CNS depression). Products include:
- Etrafon 2355
- Triavil Tablets 1757
- Trilafon 2389

Phenobarbital (Additive CNS depression). Products include:
- Arco-Lase Plus Tablets 512
- Bellergal-S Tablets 2250
- Donnatal 2060
- Donnatal Extentabs 2061
- Donnatal Tablets 2060
- Phenobarbital Elixir and Tablets 1469
- Quadrinal Tablets 1350

Pimozide (Additive CNS depression). Products include:
- Orap Tablets 1050

Prazepam (Additive CNS depression).
- No products indexed under this heading.

Prochlorperazine (Additive CNS depression). Products include:
- Compazine 2470

Procyclidine Hydrochloride (May produce paralytic ileus). Products include:
- Kemadrin Tablets 1112

Promethazine Hydrochloride (Additive CNS depression). Products include:
- Mepergan Injection 2753
- Phenergan with Codeine 2777
- Phenergan with Dextromethorphan 2778
- Phenergan Injection 2773
- Phenergan Suppositories 2775
- Phenergan Syrup 2774
- Phenergan Tablets 2775
- Phenergan VC 2779
- Phenergan VC with Codeine 2781

Propantheline Bromide (May produce paralytic ileus). Products include:
- Pro-Banthine Tablets 2052

Propofol (Additive CNS depression). Products include:
- Diprivan Injection 2833

Propoxyphene Hydrochloride (Additive CNS depression). Products include:
- Darvon 1435
- Wygesic Tablets 2827

Propoxyphene Napsylate (Additive CNS depression). Products include:
- Darvon-N/Darvocet-N 1433

Quazepam (Additive CNS depression). Products include:
- Doral Tablets 2664

Risperidone (Additive CNS depression). Products include:
- Risperdal 1301

Scopolamine (May produce paralytic ileus). Products include:
- Transderm Scōp Transdermal Therapeutic System 869

Scopolamine Hydrobromide (May produce paralytic ileus). Products include:
- Atrohist Plus Tablets 454
- Donnatal 2060
- Donnatal Extentabs 2061
- Donnatal Tablets 2060

Secobarbital Sodium (Additive CNS depression). Products include:
- Seconal Sodium Pulvules 1474

Sufentanil Citrate (Additive CNS depression). Products include:
- Sufenta Injection 1309

Temazepam (Additive CNS depression). Products include:
- Restoril Capsules 2284

Thiamylal Sodium (Additive CNS depression).
- No products indexed under this heading.

Thioridazine Hydrochloride (Additive CNS depression). Products include:
- Mellaril 2269

IMPORTANT NOTE: Always consult each drug listing in the patient's regimen for possible interactions.

Tylox **Interactions Index** 1108

Thiothixene (Additive CNS depression). Products include:
Navane Capsules and Concentrate 2201
Navane Intramuscular 2202

Triazolam (Additive CNS depression). Products include:
Halcion Tablets 2611

Tridihexethyl Chloride (May produce paralytic ileus).
No products indexed under this heading.

Trifluoperazine Hydrochloride (Additive CNS depression). Products include:
Stelazine 2514

Trihexyphenidyl Hydrochloride (May produce paralytic ileus). Products include:
Artane 1368

Zolpidem Tartrate (Additive CNS depression). Products include:
Ambien Tablets 2416

Food Interactions

Alcohol (Additive CNS depression).

TYMPAGESIC EAR DROPS
(Antipyrine, Benzocaine, Phenylephrine Hydrochloride) 2342
None cited in PDR database.

TYPHIM VI
(Typhoid Vi Polysaccharide Vaccine) 899
May interact with anticoagulants, alkylating agents, corticosteroids, and immunosuppressive agents. Compounds in these categories include:

Azathioprine (The expected immune response may not be obtained in individuals whose immune system has been compromised by treatment with corticosteroids). Products include:
Imuran 1110

Betamethasone Acetate (The expected immune response may not be obtained in individuals whose immune system has been compromised by treatment with corticosteroids). Products include:
Celestone Soluspan Suspension 2347

Betamethasone Sodium Phosphate (The expected immune response may not be obtained in individuals whose immune system has been compromised by treatment with corticosteroids). Products include:
Celestone Soluspan Suspension 2347

Busulfan (The expected immune response may not be obtained in individuals whose immune system has been compromised by treatment with alkylating drugs). Products include:
Myleran Tablets 1143

Carmustine (BCNU) (The expected immune response may not be obtained in individuals whose immune system has been compromised by treatment with alkylating drugs). Products include:
BiCNU 691

Chlorambucil (The expected immune response may not be obtained in individuals whose immune system has been compromised by treatment with alkylating drugs). Products include:
Leukeran Tablets 1133

Cortisone Acetate (The expected immune response may not be obtained in individuals whose immune system has been compromised by treatment with corticosteroids). Products include:
Cortone Acetate Sterile Suspension 1623
Cortone Acetate Tablets 1624

Cyclophosphamide (The expected immune response may not be obtained in individuals whose immune system has been compromised by treatment with alkylating drugs). Products include:
Cytoxan 694
NEOSAR Lyophilized/Neosar 1959

Cyclosporine (The expected immune response may not be obtained in individuals whose immune system has been compromised by treatment with corticosteroids). Products include:
Neoral 2276
Sandimmune 2286

Dacarbazine (The expected immune response may not be obtained in individuals whose immune system has been compromised by treatment with alkylating drugs). Products include:
DTIC-Dome 600

Dalteparin Sodium (Typhim VI should be given with caution to individuals on anticoagulant therapy). Products include:
Fragmin 1954

Dexamethasone (The expected immune response may not be obtained in individuals whose immune system has been compromised by treatment with corticosteroids). Products include:
AK-Trol Ointment & Suspension ⊙ 205
Decadron Elixir 1633
Decadron Tablets 1635
Decaspray Topical Aerosol 1648
Dexacidin Ointment ⊙ 263
Maxitrol Ophthalmic Ointment and Suspension ⊙ 224
TobraDex Ophthalmic Suspension and Ointment 473

Dexamethasone Acetate (The expected immune response may not be obtained in individuals whose immune system has been compromised by treatment with corticosteroids). Products include:
Dalalone D.P. Injectable 1011
Decadron-LA Sterile Suspension 1646

Dexamethasone Sodium Phosphate (The expected immune response may not be obtained in individuals whose immune system has been compromised by treatment with corticosteroids). Products include:
Decadron Phosphate Injection 1637
Decadron Phosphate Respihaler 1642
Decadron Phosphate Sterile Ophthalmic Ointment 1641
Decadron Phosphate Sterile Ophthalmic Solution 1642
Decadron Phosphate Topical Cream 1644
Decadron Phosphate Turbinaire 1645
Decadron Phosphate with Xylocaine Injection, Sterile 1639
Dexacort Phosphate in Respihaler 458
Dexacort Phosphate in Turbinaire 459
NeoDecadron Sterile Ophthalmic Ointment 1712
NeoDecadron Sterile Ophthalmic Solution 1713
NeoDecadron Topical Cream 1714

Dicumarol (Typhim VI should be given with caution to individuals on anticoagulant therapy).
No products indexed under this heading.

Enoxaparin (Typhim VI should be given with caution to individuals on anticoagulant therapy). Products include:
Lovenox Injection 2020

Fludrocortisone Acetate (The expected immune response may not be obtained in individuals whose immune system has been compromised by treatment with corticosteroids). Products include:
Florinef Acetate Tablets 505

Heparin Calcium (Typhim VI should be given with caution to individuals on anticoagulant therapy).
No products indexed under this heading.

Heparin Sodium (Typhim VI should be given with caution to individuals on anticoagulant therapy). Products include:
Heparin Lock Flush Solution 2725
Heparin Sodium Injection 2726
Heparin Sodium Injection, USP, Sterile Solution 2615
Heparin Sodium Vials 1441

Hydrocortisone (The expected immune response may not be obtained in individuals whose immune system has been compromised by treatment with corticosteroids). Products include:
Anusol-HC Cream 2.5% 1896
Aquanil HC Lotion 1931
Bactine Hydrocortisone Anti-Itch Cream ▣ 709
Caldecort Anti-Itch Hydrocortisone Spray ▣ 631
Cortaid ▣ 836
CORTENEMA 2535
Cortisporin Ointment 1085
Cortisporin Ophthalmic Ointment Sterile 1085
Cortisporin Ophthalmic Suspension Sterile 1086
Cortisporin Otic Solution Sterile 1087
Cortisporin Otic Suspension Sterile 1088
Cortizone-5 ▣ 831
Cortizone-10 ▣ 831
Hydrocortone Tablets 1672
Hytone 907
Massengill Medicated Soft Cloth Towelettes 2458
PediOtic Suspension Sterile 1153
Preparation H Hydrocortisone 1% Cream ▣ 872
ProctoCream-HC 2.5% 2408
VōSoL HC Otic Solution 2678

Hydrocortisone Acetate (The expected immune response may not be obtained in individuals whose immune system has been compromised by treatment with corticosteroids). Products include:
Analpram-HC Rectal Cream 1% and 2.5% 977
Anusol HC-1 Anti-Itch Hydrocortisone Ointment ▣ 847
Anusol-HC Suppositories 1897
Caldecort ▣ 631
Carmol HC 924
Coly-Mycin S Otic w/Neomycin & Hydrocortisone 1906
Cortaid ▣ 836
Cortifoam 2396
Cortisporin Cream 1084
Epifoam 2399
Hydrocortone Acetate Sterile Suspension 1669
Mantadil Cream 1135
Nupercainal Hydrocortisone 1% Cream ▣ 645
Ophthocort ⊙ 311
Pramosone Cream, Lotion & Ointment 978
ProctoCream-HC 2408
ProctoFoam-HC 2409
Terra-Cortril Ophthalmic Suspension 2210

Hydrocortisone Sodium Phosphate (The expected immune response may not be obtained in individuals whose immune system has been compromised by treatment with corticosteroids). Products include:
Hydrocortone Phosphate Injection, Sterile 1670

Hydrocortisone Sodium Succinate (The expected immune response may not be obtained in individuals whose immune system has been compromised by treatment with corticosteroids). Products include:
Solu-Cortef Sterile Powder 2641

Immune Globulin (Human) (The expected immune response may not be obtained in individuals whose immune system has been compromised by treatment with corticosteroids).
No products indexed under this heading.

Lomustine (CCNU) (The expected immune response may not be obtained in individuals whose immune system has been compromised by treatment with alkylating drugs). Products include:
CeeNU 693

Mechlorethamine Hydrochloride (The expected immune response may not be obtained in individuals whose immune system has been compromised by treatment with alkylating drugs). Products include:
Mustargen 1709

Melphalan (The expected immune response may not be obtained in individuals whose immune system has been compromised by treatment with alkylating drugs). Products include:
Alkeran Tablets 1071

Methylprednisolone Acetate (The expected immune response may not be obtained in individuals whose immune system has been compromised by treatment with corticosteroids). Products include:
Depo-Medrol Single-Dose Vial 2600
Depo-Medrol Sterile Aqueous Suspension 2597

Methylprednisolone Sodium Succinate (The expected immune response may not be obtained in individuals whose immune system has been compromised by treatment with corticosteroids). Products include:
Solu-Medrol Sterile Powder 2643

Muromonab-CD3 (The expected immune response may not be obtained in individuals whose immune system has been compromised by treatment with corticosteroids). Products include:
Orthoclone OKT3 Sterile Solution 1837

Mycophenolate Mofetil (The expected immune response may not be obtained in individuals whose immune system has been compromised by treatment with corticosteroids). Products include:
CellCept Capsules 2099

Prednisolone Acetate (The expected immune response may not be obtained in individuals whose immune system has been compromised by treatment with corticosteroids). Products include:
AK-CIDE ⊙ 202
AK-CIDE Ointment ⊙ 202
Blephamide Liquifilm Sterile Ophthalmic Suspension 476

(▣ Described in PDR For Nonprescription Drugs) (⊙ Described in PDR For Ophthalmology)

Blephamide Ointment ◉ 237
Econopred & Econopred Plus Ophthalmic Suspensions ◉ 217
Poly-Pred Liquifilm ◉ 248
Pred Forte ◉ 250
Pred Mild ◉ 253
Pred-G Liquifilm Sterile Ophthalmic Suspension ◉ 251
Pred-G S.O.P. Sterile Ophthalmic Ointment ◉ 252
Vasocidin Ointment ◉ 268

Prednisolone Sodium Phosphate (The expected immune response may not be obtained in individuals whose immune system has been compromised by treatment with corticosteroids). Products include:
AK-Pred ◉ 204
Hydeltrasol Injection, Sterile 1665
Inflamase ◉ 265
Pediapred Oral Liquid 995
Vasocidin Ophthalmic Solution ◉ 270

Prednisolone Tebutate (The expected immune response may not be obtained in individuals whose immune system has been compromised by treatment with corticosteroids). Products include:
Hydeltra-T.B.A. Sterile Suspension 1667

Prednisone (The expected immune response may not be obtained in individuals whose immune system has been compromised by treatment with corticosteroids). Products include:
Deltasone Tablets 2595

Tacrolimus (The expected immune response may not be obtained in individuals whose immune system has been compromised by treatment with corticosteroids). Products include:
Prograf 1042

Thiotepa (The expected immune response may not be obtained in individuals whose immune system has been compromised by treatment with alkylating drugs). Products include:
Thioplex (Thiotepa For Injection) 1281

Triamcinolone (The expected immune response may not be obtained in individuals whose immune system has been compromised by treatment with corticosteroids). Products include:
Aristocort Tablets 1022

Triamcinolone Acetonide (The expected immune response may not be obtained in individuals whose immune system has been compromised by treatment with corticosteroids). Products include:
Aristocort A 0.025% Cream 1027
Aristocort A 0.5% Cream 1031
Aristocort A 0.1% Cream 1029
Aristocort A 0.1% Ointment 1030
Azmacort Oral Inhaler 2011
Nasacort Nasal Inhaler 2024

Triamcinolone Diacetate (The expected immune response may not be obtained in individuals whose immune system has been compromised by treatment with corticosteroids). Products include:
Aristocort Suspension (Forte Parenteral) 1027
Aristocort Suspension (Intralesional) 1025

Triamcinolone Hexacetonide (The expected immune response may not be obtained in individuals whose immune system has been compromised by treatment with corticosteroids). Products include:
Aristospan Suspension (Intra-articular) 1033
Aristospan Suspension (Intralesional) 1032

Warfarin Sodium (Typhim Vi should be given with caution to individuals on anticoagulant therapy). Products include:
Coumadin 926

TYPHOID VACCINE
(Typhoid Vaccine) 2823
None cited in PDR database.

ULTRA DERM MOISTURIZER
(Propylene Glycol, Mineral Oil) 🅾 605
None cited in PDR database.

ULTRAM TABLETS (50 MG)
(Tramadol Hydrochloride) 1585
May interact with monoamine oxidase inhibitors, narcotic analgesics, phenothiazines, hypnotics and sedatives, tranquilizers, anesthetics, and certain other agents. Compounds in these categories include:

Alfentanil Hydrochloride (Effect of concurrent use not specified; use with caution and in reduced dosages). Products include:
Alfenta Injection 1286

Alprazolam (Effect of concurrent use not specified; use with caution and in reduced dosages). Products include:
Xanax Tablets 2649

Buprenorphine (Effect of concurrent use not specified; use with caution and in reduced dosages). Products include:
Buprenex Injectable 2006

Buspirone Hydrochloride (Effect of concurrent use not specified; use with caution and in reduced dosages). Products include:
BuSpar 737

Carbamazepine (Causes significant increase in tramadol metabolism, presumably through metabolic induction; patients on chronic carbamazepine may require higher than recommended dose of tramadol). Products include:
Atretol Tablets 573
Tegretol Chewable Tablets 852
Tegretol Suspension 852
Tegretol Tablets 852

Chlordiazepoxide (Effect of concurrent use not specified; use with caution and in reduced dosages). Products include:
Libritabs Tablets 2177
Limbitrol 2180

Chlordiazepoxide Hydrochloride (Effect of concurrent use not specified; use with caution and in reduced dosages). Products include:
Librax Capsules 2176
Librium Capsules 2178
Librium Injectable 2179

Chlorpromazine (Effect of concurrent use not specified; use with caution and in reduced dosages). Products include:
Thorazine Suppositories 2523

Chlorpromazine Hydrochloride (Effect of concurrent use not specified; use with caution and in reduced dosages). Products include:
Thorazine 2523

Chlorprothixene (Effect of concurrent use not specified; use with caution and in reduced dosages).
No products indexed under this heading.

Chlorprothixene Hydrochloride (Effect of concurrent use not specified; use with caution and in reduced dosages).
No products indexed under this heading.

Clorazepate Dipotassium (Effect of concurrent use not specified; use with caution and in reduced dosages). Products include:
Tranxene 451

Codeine Phosphate (Effect of concurrent use not specified; use with caution and in reduced dosages). Products include:
Actifed with Codeine Cough Syrup 1067
Brontex 1981
Deconsal C Expectorant Syrup 456
Deconsal Pediatric Syrup 457
Dimetane-DC Cough Syrup 2059
Empirin with Codeine Tablets 1093
Fioricet with Codeine Capsules 2260
Fiorinal with Codeine Capsules 2262
Isoclor Expectorant 990
Novahistine DH 2462
Novahistine Expectorant 2463
Nucofed 2051
Phenergan with Codeine 2777
Phenergan VC with Codeine 2781
Robitussin A-C Syrup 2073
Robitussin-DAC Syrup 2074
Ryna 🅾 841
Soma Compound w/Codeine Tablets 2676
Tussi-Organidin NR Liquid and S NR Liquid 2677
Tylenol with Codeine 1583

Dezocine (Effect of concurrent use not specified; use with caution and in reduced dosages). Products include:
Dalgan Injection 538

Diazepam (Effect of concurrent use not specified; use with caution and in reduced dosages). Products include:
Dizac 1809
Valium Injectable 2182
Valium Tablets 2183
Valrelease Capsules 2169

Droperidol (Effect of concurrent use not specified; use with caution and in reduced dosages). Products include:
Inapsine Injection 1296

Enflurane (Effect of concurrent use not specified; use with caution and in reduced dosages).
No products indexed under this heading.

Estazolam (Effect of concurrent use not specified; use with caution and in reduced dosages). Products include:
ProSom Tablets 449

Ethchlorvynol (Effect of concurrent use not specified; use with caution and in reduced dosages). Products include:
Placidyl Capsules 448

Ethinamate (Effect of concurrent use not specified; use with caution and in reduced dosages).
No products indexed under this heading.

Fentanyl (Effect of concurrent use not specified; use with caution and in reduced dosages). Products include:
Duragesic Transdermal System 1288

Fentanyl Citrate (Effect of concurrent use not specified; use with caution and in reduced dosages). Products include:
Sublimaze Injection 1307

Fluphenazine Decanoate (Effect of concurrent use not specified; use with caution and in reduced dosages). Products include:
Prolixin Decanoate 509

Fluphenazine Enanthate (Effect of concurrent use not specified; use with caution and in reduced dosages). Products include:
Prolixin Enanthate 509

Fluphenazine Hydrochloride (Effect of concurrent use not specified; use with caution and in reduced dosages). Products include:
Prolixin 509

Flurazepam Hydrochloride (Effect of concurrent use not specified; use with caution and in reduced dosages). Products include:
Dalmane Capsules 2173

Furazolidone (Tramadol inhibits the uptake of norepinephrine and serotonin; concurrent use requires great caution). Products include:
Furoxone 2046

Glutethimide (Effect of concurrent use not specified; use with caution and in reduced dosages).
No products indexed under this heading.

Haloperidol (Effect of concurrent use not specified; use with caution and in reduced dosages). Products include:
Haldol Injection, Tablets and Concentrate 1575

Haloperidol Decanoate (Effect of concurrent use not specified; use with caution and in reduced dosages). Products include:
Haldol Decanoate 1577

Halothane (Effect of concurrent use not specified; use with caution and in reduced dosages). Products include:
Fluothane 2724

Hydrocodone Bitartrate (Effect of concurrent use not specified; use with caution and in reduced dosages). Products include:
Anexsia 5/500 Elixir 1781
Anexia Tablets 1782
Codiclear DH Syrup 791
Deconamine CX Cough and Cold Liquid and Tablets 1319
Duratuss HD Elixir 2565
Hycodan Tablets and Syrup 930
Hycomine Compound Tablets 932
Hycomine 931
Hycotuss Expectorant Syrup 933
Hydrocet Capsules 782
Lorcet 10/650 1018
Lortab 2566
Tussend 1783
Tussend Expectorant 1785
Vicodin Tablets 1356
Vicodin ES Tablets 1357
Vicodin Tuss Expectorant 1358
Zydone Capsules 949

Hydrocodone Polistirex (Effect of concurrent use not specified; use with caution and in reduced dosages). Products include:
Tussionex Pennkinetic Extended-Release Suspension 998

Hydroxyzine Hydrochloride (Effect of concurrent use not specified; use with caution and in reduced dosages). Products include:
Atarax Tablets & Syrup 2185
Marax Tablets & DF Syrup 2200
Vistaril Intramuscular Solution 2216

Isocarboxazid (Tramadol inhibits the uptake of norepinephrine and serotonin; concurrent use requires great caution).
No products indexed under this heading.

Isoflurane (Effect of concurrent use not specified; use with caution and in reduced dosages).
No products indexed under this heading.

IMPORTANT NOTE: Always consult each drug listing in the patient's regimen for possible interactions.

Ultram | Interactions Index | 1110

Ketamine Hydrochloride (Effect of concurrent use not specified; use with caution and in reduced dosages).
No products indexed under this heading.

Levorphanol Tartrate (Effect of concurrent use not specified; use with caution and in reduced dosages). Products include:
Levo-Dromoran ... 2129

Lorazepam (Effect of concurrent use not specified; use with caution and in reduced dosages). Products include:
Ativan Injection ... 2698
Ativan Tablets ... 2700

Loxapine Hydrochloride (Effect of concurrent use not specified; use with caution and in reduced dosages). Products include:
Loxitane ... 1378

Loxapine Succinate (Effect of concurrent use not specified; use with caution and in reduced dosages). Products include:
Loxitane Capsules ... 1378

Meperidine Hydrochloride (Effect of concurrent use not specified; use with caution and in reduced dosages). Products include:
Demerol ... 2308
Mepergan Injection ... 2753

Meprobamate (Effect of concurrent use not specified; use with caution and in reduced dosages). Products include:
Miltown Tablets ... 2672
PMB 200 and PMB 400 ... 2783

Mesoridazine Besylate (Effect of concurrent use not specified; use with caution and in reduced dosages). Products include:
Serentil ... 684

Methadone Hydrochloride (Effect of concurrent use not specified; use with caution and in reduced dosages). Products include:
Methadone Hydrochloride Oral Concentrate ... 2233
Methadone Hydrochloride Oral Solution & Tablets ... 2235

Methohexital Sodium (Effect of concurrent use not specified; use with caution and in reduced dosages). Products include:
Brevital Sodium Vials ... 1429

Methotrimeprazine (Effect of concurrent use not specified; use with caution and in reduced dosages). Products include:
Levoprome ... 1274

Midazolam Hydrochloride (Effect of concurrent use not specified; use with caution and in reduced dosages). Products include:
Versed Injection ... 2170

Molindone Hydrochloride (Effect of concurrent use not specified; use with caution and in reduced dosages). Products include:
Moban Tablets and Concentrate ... 1048

Morphine Sulfate (Effect of concurrent use not specified; use with caution and in reduced dosages). Products include:
Astramorph/PF Injection, USP (Preservative-Free) ... 535
Duramorph ... 962
Infumorph 200 and Infumorph 500 Sterile Solutions ... 965
MS Contin Tablets ... 1994
MSIR ... 1997
Oramorph SR (Morphine Sulfate Sustained Release Tablets) ... 2236
RMS Suppositories ... 2657
Roxanol ... 2243

Opium Alkaloids (Effect of concurrent use not specified; use with caution and in reduced dosages).
No products indexed under this heading.

Oxazepam (Effect of concurrent use not specified; use with caution and in reduced dosages). Products include:
Serax Capsules ... 2810
Serax Tablets ... 2810

Oxycodone Hydrochloride (Effect of concurrent use not specified; use with caution and in reduced dosages). Products include:
Percocet Tablets ... 938
Percodan Tablets ... 939
Percodan-Demi Tablets ... 940
Roxicodone Tablets, Oral Solution & Intensol (Oxycodone) ... 2244
Tylox Capsules ... 1584

Perphenazine (Effect of concurrent use not specified; use with caution and in reduced dosages). Products include:
Etrafon ... 2355
Triavil Tablets ... 1757
Trilafon ... 2389

Phenelzine Sulfate (Tramadol inhibits the uptake of norepinephrine and serotonin; concurrent use requires great caution). Products include:
Nardil ... 1920

Prazepam (Effect of concurrent use not specified; use with caution and in reduced dosages).
No products indexed under this heading.

Prochlorperazine (Effect of concurrent use not specified; use with caution and in reduced dosages). Products include:
Compazine ... 2470

Promethazine Hydrochloride (Effect of concurrent use not specified; use with caution and in reduced dosages). Products include:
Mepergan Injection ... 2753
Phenergan with Codeine ... 2777
Phenergan with Dextromethorphan 2778
Phenergan Injection ... 2773
Phenergan Suppositories ... 2775
Phenergan Syrup ... 2774
Phenergan Tablets ... 2775
Phenergan VC ... 2779
Phenergan VC with Codeine ... 2781

Propofol (Effect of concurrent use not specified; use with caution and in reduced dosages). Products include:
Diprivan Injection ... 2833

Propoxyphene Hydrochloride (Effect of concurrent use not specified; use with caution and in reduced dosages). Products include:
Darvon ... 1435
Wygesic Tablets ... 2827

Propoxyphene Napsylate (Effect of concurrent use not specified; use with caution and in reduced dosages). Products include:
Darvon-N/Darvocet-N ... 1433

Quazepam (Effect of concurrent use not specified; use with caution and in reduced dosages). Products include:
Doral Tablets ... 2664

Quinidine Gluconate (Concomitant use results in increased concentrations of tramadol and reduced concentration of M1). Products include:
Quinaglute Dura-Tabs Tablets ... 649

Quinidine Polygalacturonate (Concomitant use results in increased concentrations of tramadol and reduced concentration of M1).
No products indexed under this heading.

Quinidine Sulfate (Concomitant use results in increased concentrations of tramadol and reduced concentration of M1). Products include:
Quinidex Extentabs ... 2067

Secobarbital Sodium (Effect of concurrent use not specified; use with caution and in reduced dosages). Products include:
Seconal Sodium Pulvules ... 1474

Selegiline Hydrochloride (Tramadol inhibits the uptake of norepinephrine and serotonin; concurrent use requires great caution). Products include:
Eldepryl Tablets ... 2550

Sufentanil Citrate (Effect of concurrent use not specified; use with caution and in reduced dosages). Products include:
Sufenta Injection ... 1309

Temazepam (Effect of concurrent use not specified; use with caution and in reduced dosages). Products include:
Restoril Capsules ... 2284

Thiamylal Sodium (Effect of concurrent use not specified; use with caution and in reduced dosages).
No products indexed under this heading.

Thioridazine Hydrochloride (Effect of concurrent use not specified; use with caution and in reduced dosages). Products include:
Mellaril ... 2269

Thiothixene (Effect of concurrent use not specified; use with caution and in reduced dosages). Products include:
Navane Capsules and Concentrate 2201
Navane Intramuscular ... 2202

Tranylcypromine Sulfate (Tramadol inhibits the uptake of norepinephrine and serotonin; concurrent use requires great caution). Products include:
Parnate Tablets ... 2503

Triazolam (Effect of concurrent use not specified; use with caution and in reduced dosages). Products include:
Halcion Tablets ... 2611

Trifluoperazine Hydrochloride (Effect of concurrent use not specified; use with caution and in reduced dosages). Products include:
Stelazine ... 2514

Zolpidem Tartrate (Effect of concurrent use not specified; use with caution and in reduced dosages). Products include:
Ambien Tablets ... 2416

Food Interactions

Alcohol (Effect of concurrent use not specified; use with caution and in reduced dosages).

ULTRA MIDE 25 EXTRA STRENGTH MOISTURIZER
(Urea, Mineral Oil) ... ⊡ 605
None cited in PDR database.

ULTRA MIDE 25 LOTION
(Urea, Mineral Oil, Glycerin) ... ⊡ 605
None cited in PDR database.

ULTRASE CAPSULES
(Pancrelipase) ... 2343

Food Interactions

Food having a pH greater than 5.5 (Can dissolve the protective coating resulting in early release of enzymes, irritation of oral mucosa, and/or loss of enzyme activity).

ULTRASE MT CAPSULES
(Pancrelipase) ... 2344

Food Interactions

Food having a pH greater than 5.5 (Can dissolve the protective enteric shell).

ULTRAVATE CREAM 0.05%
(Halobetasol Propionate) ... 2689
None cited in PDR database.

ULTRAVATE OINTMENT 0.05%
(Halobetasol Propionate) ... 2690
None cited in PDR database.

UNASYN
(Ampicillin Sodium, Sulbactam Sodium) ... 2212
May interact with aminoglycosides and certain other agents. Compounds in these categories include:

Allopurinol (Increased incidence of rash). Products include:
Zyloprim Tablets ... 1226

Amikacin Sulfate (In vitro inactivation of aminoglycosides when reconstituted with Unasyn). Products include:
Amikacin Sulfate Injection, USP ... 960
Amikin Injectable ... 501

Gentamicin Sulfate (In vitro inactivation of aminoglycosides when reconstituted with Unasyn). Products include:
Garamycin Injectable ... 2360
Genoptic Sterile Ophthalmic Solution ... ⊙ 243
Genoptic Sterile Ophthalmic Ointment ... ⊙ 243
Gentacidin Ointment ... ⊙ 264
Gentacidin Solution ... ⊙ 264
Gentak ... ⊙ 208
Pred-G Liquifilm Sterile Ophthalmic Suspension ... ⊙ 251
Pred-G S.O.P. Sterile Ophthalmic Ointment ... ⊙ 252

Kanamycin Sulfate (In vitro inactivation of aminoglycosides when reconstituted with Unasyn).
No products indexed under this heading.

Probenecid (Increased and prolonged blood levels of ampicillin and sulbactam). Products include:
Benemid Tablets ... 1611
ColBENEMID Tablets ... 1622

Streptomycin Sulfate (In vitro inactivation of aminoglycosides when reconstituted with Unasyn). Products include:
Streptomycin Sulfate Injection ... 2208

Tobramycin Sulfate (In vitro inactivation of aminoglycosides when reconstituted with Unasyn). Products include:
Nebcin Vials, Hyporets & ADD-Vantage ... 1464
Tobramycin Sulfate Injection ... 968

UNI-DUR EXTENDED-RELEASE TABLETS
(Theophylline Anhydrous) ... 1331
May interact with sympathomimetic bronchodilators, oral contraceptives, and certain other agents. Compounds in these categories include:

Albuterol (Toxic synergism has been reported with ephedrine and may occur with some other sympathomimetic bronchodilators). Products include:
Proventil Inhalation Aerosol ... 2382
Ventolin Inhalation Aerosol and Refill ... 1197

Interactions Index

Albuterol Sulfate (Toxic synergism has been reported with ephedrine and may occur with some other sympathomimetic bronchodilators). Products include:

Airet Solution for Inhalation 452
Proventil Inhalation Solution 0.083% 2384
Proventil Repetabs Tablets 2386
Proventil Solution for Inhalation 0.5% 2383
Proventil Syrup 2385
Proventil Tablets 2386
Ventolin Inhalation Solution.............. 1198
Ventolin Nebules Inhalation Solution 1199
Ventolin Rotacaps for Inhalation 1200
Ventolin Syrup.................................... 1202
Ventolin Tablets 1203
Volmax Extended-Release Tablets .. 1788

Allopurinol (High dose of allopurinol increases serum theophylline levels). Products include:

Zyloprim Tablets 1226

Bitolterol Mesylate (Toxic synergism has been reported with ephedrine and may occur with some other sympathomimetic bronchodilators). Products include:

Tornalate Solution for Inhalation, 0.2% 956
Tornalate Metered Dose Inhaler 957

Cimetidine (Increases serum theophylline levels). Products include:

Tagamet Tablets 2516

Cimetidine Hydrochloride (Increases serum theophylline levels). Products include:

Tagamet 2516

Ciprofloxacin Hydrochloride (Increases serum theophylline levels). Products include:

Ciloxan Ophthalmic Solution............. 472
Cipro Tablets 592

Desogestrel (Increases serum theophylline levels). Products include:

Desogen Tablets 1817
Ortho-Cept 1851

Ephedrine Hydrochloride (Toxic synergism has been reported with ephedrine and may occur with some other sympathomimetic bronchodilators). Products include:

Primatene Dual Action Formula.... ◉◻ 872
Primatene Tablets .... ◉◻ 873
Quadrinal Tablets 1350

Ephedrine Sulfate (Toxic synergism has been reported with ephedrine and may occur with some other sympathomimetic bronchodilators). Products include:

Bronkaid Caplets .... ◉◻ 717
Marax Tablets & DF Syrup................. 2200

Ephedrine Tannate (Toxic synergism has been reported with ephedrine and may occur with some other sympathomimetic bronchodilators). Products include:

Rynatuss 2673

Epinephrine (Toxic synergism has been reported with ephedrine and may occur with some other sympathomimetic bronchodilators). Products include:

Bronkaid Mist .... ◉◻ 717
EPIFRIN .... ◎ 239
EpiPen 790
Marcaine Hydrochloride with Epinephrine 1:200,000 2316
Primatene Mist .... ◉◻ 873
Sensorcaine with Epinephrine Injection 559
Sus-Phrine Injection 1019
Xylocaine with Epinephrine Injections 567

Epinephrine Hydrochloride (Toxic synergism has been reported with ephedrine and may occur with some other sympathomimetic bronchodilators). Products include:

Ana-Kit Anaphylaxis Emergency Treatment Kit 617

Erythromycin (Increases serum theophylline levels). Products include:

A/T/S 2% Acne Topical Gel and Solution 1234
Benzamycin Topical Gel 905
E-Mycin Tablets 1341
Emgel 2% Topical Gel......................... 1093
ERYC... 1915
Erycette (erythromycin 2%) Topical Solution.. 1888
Ery-Tab Tablets 422
Erythromycin Base Filmtab 426
Erythromycin Delayed-Release Capsules, USP..................................... 427
Ilotycin Ophthalmic Ointment........... 912
PCE Dispertab Tablets 444
T-Stat 2.0% Topical Solution and Pads 2688
Theramycin Z Topical Solution 2% 1592

Erythromycin Estolate (Increases serum theophylline levels). Products include:

Ilosone 911

Erythromycin Ethylsuccinate (Increases serum theophylline levels). Products include:

E.E.S. 424
EryPed 421

Erythromycin Gluceptate (Increases serum theophylline levels). Products include:

Ilotycin Gluceptate, IV, Vials 913

Erythromycin Stearate (Increases serum theophylline levels). Products include:

Erythrocin Stearate Filmtab 425

Ethinyl Estradiol (Increases serum theophylline levels). Products include:

Brevicon.. 2088
Demulen 2428
Desogen Tablets.................................. 1817
Levlen/Tri-Levlen................................ 651
Lo/Oval Tablets 2746
Lo/Oval-28 Tablets.............................. 2751
Modicon 1872
Nordette-21 Tablets............................. 2755
Nordette-28 Tablets............................. 2758
Norinyl 2088
Ortho-Cept 1851
Ortho-Cyclen/Ortho-Tri-Cyclen 1858
Ortho-Novum.. 1872
Ortho-Cyclen/Ortho Tri-Cyclen 1858
Ovcon 760
Ovral Tablets 2770
Ovral-28 Tablets 2770
Levlen/Tri-Levlen................................ 651
Tri-Norinyl.. 2164
Triphasil-21 Tablets............................. 2814
Triphasil-28 Tablets............................. 2819

Ethylnorepinephrine Hydrochloride (Toxic synergism has been reported with ephedrine and may occur with some other sympathomimetic bronchodilators).

No products indexed under this heading.

Ethynodiol Diacetate (Increases serum theophylline levels). Products include:

Demulen 2428

Isoetharine (Toxic synergism has been reported with ephedrine and may occur with some other sympathomimetic bronchodilators). Products include:

Bronkometer Aerosol........................... 2302
Bronkosol Solution 2302
Isoetharine Inhalation Solution, USP, Arm-a-Med.................................. 551

Isoproterenol Hydrochloride (Toxic synergism has been reported with ephedrine and may occur with some other sympathomimetic bronchodilators). Products include:

Isuprel Hydrochloride Injection 1:5000 2311
Isuprel Hydrochloride Solution 1:200 & 1:100 2313
Isuprel Mistometer 2312

Isoproterenol Sulfate (Toxic synergism has been reported with ephedrine and may occur with some other sympathomimetic bronchodilators). Products include:

Norisodrine with Calcium Iodide Syrup.. 442

Levonorgestrel (Increases serum theophylline levels). Products include:

Levlen/Tri-Levlen................................ 651
Nordette-21 Tablets............................. 2755
Nordette-28 Tablets............................. 2758
Norplant System 2759
Levlen/Tri-Levlen................................ 651
Triphasil-21 Tablets 2814
Triphasil-28 Tablets 2819

Lithium Carbonate (Increased renal excretion of lithium). Products include:

Eskalith 2485
Lithium Carbonate Capsules & Tablets 2230
Lithonate/Lithotabs/Lithobid 2543

Mestranol (Increases serum theophylline levels). Products include:

Norinyl 2088
Ortho-Novum.. 1872

Metaproterenol Sulfate (Toxic synergism has been reported with ephedrine and may occur with some other sympathomimetic bronchodilators). Products include:

Alupent.. 669
Metaproterenol Sulfate Inhalation Solution, USP, Arm-a-Med 552

Norethindrone (Increases serum theophylline levels). Products include:

Brevicon... 2088
Micronor Tablets 1872
Modicon 1872
Norinyl 2088
Nor-Q D Tablets................................... 2135
Ortho-Novum.. 1872
Ovcon 760
Tri-Norinyl.. 2164

Norethynodrel (Increases serum theophylline levels).

No products indexed under this heading.

Norfloxacin (Increases serum theophylline levels). Products include:

Chibroxin Sterile Ophthalmic Solution 1617
Noroxin Tablets 1715
Noroxin Tablets 2048

Norgestimate (Increases serum theophylline levels). Products include:

Ortho-Cyclen/Ortho-Tri-Cyclen 1858
Ortho-Cyclen/Ortho Tri-Cyclen 1858

Norgestrel (Increases serum theophylline levels). Products include:

Lo/Ovral Tablets 2746
Lo/Ovral-28 Tablets............................. 2751
Ovral Tablets 2770
Ovral-28 Tablets 2770
Ovrette Tablets..................................... 2771

Phenytoin (Decreased theophylline and phenytoin serum levels). Products include:

Dilantin Infatabs 1908
Dilantin-125 Suspension 1911

Phenytoin Sodium (Decreased theophylline and phenytoin serum levels). Products include:

Dilantin Kapseals 1906
Dilantin Parenteral 1910

Pirbuterol Acetate (Toxic synergism has been reported with ephedrine and may occur with some other sympathomimetic bronchodilators). Products include:

Maxair Autohaler 1492
Maxair Inhaler 1494

Propranolol Hydrochloride (Increases serum theophylline levels). Products include:

Inderal 2728
Inderal LA Long Acting Capsules 2730
Inderide Tablets 2732
Inderide LA Long Acting Capsules .. 2734

Rifampin (Decreases serum theophylline levels). Products include:

Rifadin 1528
Rifamate Capsules 1530
Rifater.. 1532
Rimactane Capsules 847

Salmeterol Xinafoate (Toxic synergism has been reported with ephedrine and may occur with some other sympathomimetic bronchodilators). Products include:

Serevent Inhalation Aerosol............... 1176

Sucralfate (Reduced absorption of theophylline). Products include:

Carafate Suspension 1505
Carafate Tablets................................... 1504

Terbutaline Sulfate (Toxic synergism has been reported with ephedrine and may occur with some other sympathomimetic bronchodilators). Products include:

Brethaire Inhaler 813
Brethine Ampuls 815
Brethine Tablets................................... 814
Bricanyl Subcutaneous Injection 1502
Bricanyl Tablets 1503

Troleandomycin (Increases serum theophylline levels). Products include:

Tao Capsules 2209

Food Interactions

Food, unspecified (Prolongs the time to peak concentration but does not affect the extent of absorption).

UNIPHYL 400 MG TABLETS

(Theophylline Anhydrous)....................2001

May interact with macrolide antibiotics, sympathomimetic bronchodilators, oral contraceptives, and certain other agents. Compounds in these categories include:

Albuterol (Toxic synergism). Products include:

Proventil Inhalation Aerosol 2382
Ventolin Inhalation Aerosol and Refill 1197

Albuterol Sulfate (Toxic synergism). Products include:

Airet Solution for Inhalation 452
Proventil Inhalation Solution 0.083% 2384
Proventil Repetabs Tablets 2386
Proventil Solution for Inhalation 0.5% 2383
Proventil Syrup.................................... 2385
Proventil Tablets 2386
Ventolin Inhalation Solution............... 1198
Ventolin Nebules Inhalation Solution 1199
Ventolin Rotacaps for Inhalation 1200
Ventolin Syrup...................................... 1202
Ventolin Tablets 1203
Volmax Extended-Release Tablets .. 1788

Allopurinol (Increased serum theophylline levels with high doses of allopurinol). Products include:

Zyloprim Tablets 1226

Azithromycin (Increases serum theophylline levels). Products include:

Zithromax 1944

IMPORTANT NOTE: Always consult each drug listing in the patient's regimen for possible interactions.

Uniphyl 400

Bitolterol Mesylate (Toxic synergism). Products include:

Tornalate Solution for Inhalation, 0.2% 956
Tornalate Metered Dose Inhaler 957

Cimetidine (Increases serum theophylline levels). Products include:

Tagamet Tablets 2516

Cimetidine Hydrochloride (Increases serum theophylline levels). Products include:

Tagamet 2516

Ciprofloxacin Hydrochloride (Increases serum theophylline levels). Products include:

Ciloxan Ophthalmic Solution 472
Cipro Tablets 592

Clarithromycin (Increases serum theophylline levels). Products include:

Biaxin 405

Desogestrel (Increases serum theophylline levels). Products include:

Desogen Tablets 1817
Ortho-Cept 1851

Ephedrine Hydrochloride (Toxic synergism). Products include:

Primatene Dual Action Formula ...... ᴹᴰ 872
Primatene Tablets ...... ᴹᴰ 873
Quadrinal Tablets 1350

Ephedrine Sulfate (Toxic synergism). Products include:

Bronkaid Caplets ...... ᴹᴰ 717
Marax Tablets & DF Syrup 2200

Ephedrine Tannate (Toxic synergism). Products include:

Rynatuss 2673

Epinephrine (Toxic synergism). Products include:

Bronkaid Mist ...... ᴹᴰ 717
EPIFRIN ...... ◉ 239
EpiPen 790
Marcaine Hydrochloride with Epinephrine 1:200,000 2316
Primatene Mist ...... ᴹᴰ 873
Sensorcaine with Epinephrine Injection 559
Sus-Phrine Injection 1019
Xylocaine with Epinephrine Injections 567

Epinephrine Hydrochloride (Toxic synergism). Products include:

Ana-Kit Anaphylaxis Emergency Treatment Kit 617

Erythromycin (Increases serum theophylline levels). Products include:

A/T/S 2% Acne Topical Gel and Solution 1234
Benzamycin Topical Gel 905
E-Mycin Tablets 1341
Emgel 2% Topical Gel 1093
ERYC 1915
Erycette (erythromycin 2%) Topical Solution 1888
Ery-Tab Tablets 422
Erythromycin Base Filmtab 426
Erythromycin Delayed-Release Capsules, USP 427
Ilotycin Ophthalmic Ointment 912
PCE Dispertab Tablets 444
T-Stat 2.0% Topical Solution and Pads 2688
Theramycin Z Topical Solution 2% 1592

Erythromycin Estolate (Increases serum theophylline levels). Products include:

Ilosone 911

Erythromycin Ethylsuccinate (Increases serum theophylline levels). Products include:

E.E.S. 424
EryPed 421

Erythromycin Gluceptate (Increases serum theophylline levels). Products include:

Ilotycin Gluceptate, IV, Vials 913

Erythromycin Stearate (Increases serum theophylline levels). Products include:

Erythrocin Stearate Filmtab 425

Ethinyl Estradiol (Increases serum theophylline levels). Products include:

Brevicon 2088
Demulen 2428
Desogen Tablets 1817
Levlen/Tri-Levlen 651
Lo/Ovral Tablets 2746
Lo/Ovral-28 Tablets 2751
Modicon 1872
Nordette-21 Tablets 2755
Nordette-28 Tablets 2758
Norinyl 2088
Ortho-Cept 1851
Ortho-Cyclen/Ortho-Tri-Cyclen 1858
Ortho-Novum 1872
Ortho-Cyclen/Ortho Tri-Cyclen 1858
Ovcon 760
Ovral Tablets 2770
Ovral-28 Tablets 2770
Levlen/Tri-Levlen 651
Tri-Norinyl 2164
Triphasil-21 Tablets 2814
Triphasil-28 Tablets 2819

Ethylnorepinephrine Hydrochloride (Toxic synergism).

No products indexed under this heading.

Ethynodiol Diacetate (Increases serum theophylline levels). Products include:

Demulen 2428

Influenza Virus Vaccine (Decreased theophylline clearance). Products include:

Fluvirin 460
Influenza Virus Vaccine, Trivalent, Types A and B (chromatograph- and filter-purified subvirion antigen) FluShield, 1995-1996 Formula 2736

Isoetharine (Toxic synergism). Products include:

Bronkometer Aerosol 2302
Bronkosol Solution 2302
Isoetharine Inhalation Solution, USP, Arm-a-Med 551

Isoproterenol Hydrochloride (Toxic synergism). Products include:

Isuprel Hydrochloride Injection 1:5000 2311
Isuprel Hydrochloride Solution 1:200 & 1:100 2313
Isuprel Mistometer 2312

Isoproterenol Sulfate (Toxic synergism). Products include:

Norisodrine with Calcium Iodide Syrup 442

Levonorgestrel (Increases serum theophylline levels). Products include:

Levlen/Tri-Levlen 651
Nordette-21 Tablets 2755
Nordette-28 Tablets 2758
Norplant System 2759
Levlen/Tri-Levlen 651
Triphasil-21 Tablets 2814
Triphasil-28 Tablets 2819

Lithium Carbonate (Increased renal excretion of lithium). Products include:

Eskalith 2485
Lithium Carbonate Capsules & Tablets 2230
Lithonate/Lithotabs/Lithobid 2543

Mestranol (Increases serum theophylline levels). Products include:

Norinyl 2088
Ortho-Novum 1872

Metaproterenol Sulfate (Toxic synergism). Products include:

Alupent 669
Metaproterenol Sulfate Inhalation Solution, USP, Arm-a-Med 552

Norethindrone (Increases serum theophylline levels). Products include:

Brevicon 2088
Micronor Tablets 1872

Modicon 1872
Norinyl 2088
Nor-Q D Tablets 2135
Ortho-Novum 1872
Ovcon 760
Tri-Norinyl 2164

Norethynodrel (Increases serum theophylline levels).

No products indexed under this heading.

Norfloxacin (Increased serum theophylline levels). Products include:

Chibroxin Sterile Ophthalmic Solution 1617
Noroxin Tablets 1715
Noroxin Tablets 2048

Norgestimate (Increases serum theophylline levels). Products include:

Ortho-Cyclen/Ortho-Tri-Cyclen 1858
Ortho-Cyclen/Ortho Tri-Cyclen 1858

Norgestrel (Increases serum theophylline levels). Products include:

Lo/Ovral Tablets 2746
Lo/Ovral-28 Tablets 2751
Ovral Tablets 2770
Ovral-28 Tablets 2770
Ovrette Tablets 2771

Phenytoin (Decreased theophylline and phenytoin serum levels). Products include:

Dilantin Infatabs 1908
Dilantin-125 Suspension 1911

Phenytoin Sodium (Decreased theophylline and phenytoin serum levels). Products include:

Dilantin Kapseals 1906
Dilantin Parenteral 1910

Pirbuterol Acetate (Toxic synergism). Products include:

Maxair Autohaler 1492
Maxair Inhaler 1494

Propranolol Hydrochloride (Increased serum theophylline levels). Products include:

Inderal 2728
Inderal LA Long Acting Capsules 2730
Inderide Tablets 2732
Inderide LA Long Acting Capsules .. 2734

Rifampin (Decreases serum theophylline levels). Products include:

Rifadin 1528
Rifamate Capsules 1530
Rifater 1532
Rimactane Capsules 847

Salmeterol Xinafoate (Toxic synergism). Products include:

Serevent Inhalation Aerosol 1176

Terbutaline Sulfate (Toxic synergism). Products include:

Brethaire Inhaler 813
Brethine Ampuls 815
Brethine Tablets 814
Bricanyl Subcutaneous Injection 1502
Bricanyl Tablets 1503

Troleandomycin (Increases serum theophylline levels). Products include:

Tao Capsules 2209

Food Interactions

Diet, high-lipid (Affects the bioavailability of theophylline).

UNIQUE E VITAMIN E CAPSULES

(Vitamin E) ...... ᴹᴰ 656

None cited in PDR database.

MAXIMUM STRENGTH UNISOM SLEEPGELS

(Diphenhydramine Hydrochloride) 1934

May interact with monoamine oxidase inhibitors, central nervous system depressants, hypnotics and sedatives, tranquilizers, and certain other agents. Compounds in these categories include:

Alfentanil Hydrochloride

(Heightens the CNS depressant effect). Products include:

Alfenta Injection 1286

Alprazolam (Heightens the CNS depressant effect). Products include:

Xanax Tablets 2649

Aprobarbital (Heightens the CNS depressant effect).

No products indexed under this heading.

Buprenorphine (Heightens the CNS depressant effect). Products include:

Buprenex Injectable 2006

Buspirone Hydrochloride (Heightens the CNS depressant effect). Products include:

BuSpar 737

Butabarbital (Heightens the CNS depressant effect).

No products indexed under this heading.

Butalbital (Heightens the CNS depressant effect). Products include:

Esgic-plus Tablets 1013
Fioricet Tablets 2258
Fioricet with Codeine Capsules 2260
Fiorinal Capsules 2261
Fiorinal with Codeine Capsules 2262
Fiorinal Tablets 2261
Phrenilin 785
Sedapap Tablets 50 mg/650 mg .. 1543

Chlordiazepoxide (Heightens the CNS depressant effect). Products include:

Libritabs Tablets 2177
Limbitrol 2180

Chlordiazepoxide Hydrochloride (Heightens the CNS depressant effect). Products include:

Librax Capsules 2176
Librium Capsules 2178
Librium Injectable 2179

Chlorpromazine (Heightens the CNS depressant effect). Products include:

Thorazine Suppositories 2523

Chlorpromazine Hydrochloride (Heightens the CNS depressant effect). Products include:

Thorazine 2523

Chlorprothixene (Heightens the CNS depressant effect).

No products indexed under this heading.

Chlorprothixene Hydrochloride (Heightens the CNS depressant effect).

No products indexed under this heading.

Clorazepate Dipotassium (Heightens the CNS depressant effect). Products include:

Tranxene 451

Clozapine (Heightens the CNS depressant effect). Products include:

Clozaril Tablets 2252

Codeine Phosphate (Heightens the CNS depressant effect). Products include:

Actifed with Codeine Cough Syrup.. 1067
Brontex 1981
Deconsal C Expectorant Syrup 456
Deconsal Pediatric Syrup 457
Dimetane-DC Cough Syrup 2059
Empirin with Codeine Tablets 1093
Fioricet with Codeine Capsules 2260
Fiorinal with Codeine Capsules 2262
Isoclor Expectorant 990
Novahistine DH 2462
Novahistine Expectorant 2463
Nucofed 2051
Phenergan with Codeine 2777
Phenergan VC with Codeine 2781
Robitussin A-C Syrup 2073
Robitussin-DAC Syrup 2074
Ryna ...... ᴹᴰ 841
Soma Compound w/Codeine Tablets 2676
Tussi-Organidin NR Liquid and S NR Liquid 2677
Tylenol with Codeine 1583

(ᴹᴰ Described in PDR For Nonprescription Drugs) (◉ Described in PDR For Ophthalmology)

1113 Interactions Index Unisom With Pain Relief

Desflurane (Heightens the CNS depressant effect). Products include:
Suprane ... 1813
Dezocine (Heightens the CNS depressant effect). Products include:
Dalgan Injection ... 538
Diazepam (Heightens the CNS depressant effect). Products include:
Dizac ... 1809
Valium Injectable ... 2182
Valium Tablets ... 2183
Valrelease Capsules ... 2169
Droperidol (Heightens the CNS depressant effect). Products include:
Inapsine Injection ... 1296
Enflurane (Heightens the CNS depressant effect).
No products indexed under this heading.
Estazolam (Heightens the CNS depressant effect). Products include:
ProSom Tablets ... 449
Ethchlorvynol (Heightens the CNS depressant effect). Products include:
Placidyl Capsules ... 448
Ethinamate (Heightens the CNS depressant effect).
No products indexed under this heading.
Fentanyl (Heightens the CNS depressant effect). Products include:
Duragesic Transdermal System ... 1288
Fentanyl Citrate (Heightens the CNS depressant effect). Products include:
Sublimaze Injection ... 1307
Fluphenazine Decanoate (Heightens the CNS depressant effect). Products include:
Prolixin Decanoate ... 509
Fluphenazine Enanthate (Heightens the CNS depressant effect). Products include:
Prolixin Enanthate ... 509
Fluphenazine Hydrochloride (Heightens the CNS depressant effect). Products include:
Prolixin ... 509
Flurazepam Hydrochloride (Heightens the CNS depressant effect). Products include:
Dalmane Capsules ... 2173
Furazolidone (Prolongs and intensifies the anticholinergic effects of antihistamines). Products include:
Furoxone ... 2046
Glutethimide (Heightens the CNS depressant effect).
No products indexed under this heading.
Haloperidol (Heightens the CNS depressant effect). Products include:
Haldol Injection, Tablets and Concentrate ... 1575
Haloperidol Decanoate (Heightens the CNS depressant effect). Products include:
Haldol Decanoate ... 1577
Hydrocodone Bitartrate (Heightens the CNS depressant effect). Products include:
Anexsia 5/500 Elixir ... 1781
Anexia Tablets ... 1782
Codiclear DH Syrup ... 791
Deconamine CX Cough and Cold Liquid and Tablets ... 1319
Duratuss HD Elixir ... 2565
Hycodan Tablets and Syrup ... 930
Hycomine Compound Tablets ... 932
Hycomine ... 931
Hycotuss Expectorant Syrup ... 933
Hydrocet Capsules ... 782
Lorcet 10/650 ... 1018
Lortab ... 2566
Tussend ... 1783
Tussend Expectorant ... 1785
Vicodin Tablets ... 1356
Vicodin ES Tablets ... 1357
Vicodin Tuss Expectorant ... 1358
Zydone Capsules ... 949
Hydrocodone Polistirex (Heightens the CNS depressant effect). Products include:
Tussionex Pennkinetic Extended-Release Suspension ... 998
Hydroxyzine Hydrochloride (Heightens the CNS depressant effect). Products include:
Atarax Tablets & Syrup ... 2185
Marax Tablets & DF Syrup ... 2200
Vistaril Intramuscular Solution ... 2216
Isocarboxazid (Prolongs and intensifies the anticholinergic effects of antihistamines).
No products indexed under this heading.
Isoflurane (Heightens the CNS depressant effect).
No products indexed under this heading.
Ketamine Hydrochloride (Heightens the CNS depressant effect).
No products indexed under this heading.
Levomethadyl Acetate Hydrochloride (Heightens the CNS depressant effect). Products include:
Orlamm ... 2239
Levorphanol Tartrate (Heightens the CNS depressant effect). Products include:
Levo-Dromoran ... 2129
Lorazepam (Heightens the CNS depressant effect). Products include:
Ativan Injection ... 2698
Ativan Tablets ... 2700
Loxapine Hydrochloride (Heightens the CNS depressant effect). Products include:
Loxitane ... 1378
Loxapine Succinate (Heightens the CNS depressant effect). Products include:
Loxitane Capsules ... 1378
Meperidine Hydrochloride (Heightens the CNS depressant effect). Products include:
Demerol ... 2308
Mepergan Injection ... 2753
Mephobarbital (Heightens the CNS depressant effect). Products include:
Mebaral Tablets ... 2322
Meprobamate (Heightens the CNS depressant effect). Products include:
Miltown Tablets ... 2672
PMB 200 and PMB 400 ... 2783
Mesoridazine (Heightens the CNS depressant effect).
Mesoridazine Besylate (Heightens the CNS depressant effect). Products include:
Serentil ... 684
Methadone Hydrochloride (Heightens the CNS depressant effect). Products include:
Methadone Hydrochloride Oral Concentrate ... 2233
Methadone Hydrochloride Oral Solution & Tablets ... 2235
Methohexital Sodium (Heightens the CNS depressant effect). Products include:
Brevital Sodium Vials ... 1429
Methotrimeprazine (Heightens the CNS depressant effect). Products include:
Levoprome ... 1274
Methoxyflurane (Heightens the CNS depressant effect).
No products indexed under this heading.
Midazolam Hydrochloride (Heightens the CNS depressant effect). Products include:
Versed Injection ... 2170
Molindone Hydrochloride (Heightens the CNS depressant effect). Products include:
Moban Tablets and Concentrate ... 1048
Morphine Sulfate (Heightens the CNS depressant effect). Products include:
Astramorph/PF Injection, USP (Preservative-Free) ... 535
Duramorph ... 962
Infumorph 200 and Infumorph 500 Sterile Solutions ... 965
MS Contin Tablets ... 1994
MSIR ... 1997
Oramorph SR (Morphine Sulfate Sustained Release Tablets) ... 2236
RMS Suppositories ... 2657
Roxanol ... 2243
Opium Alkaloids (Heightens the CNS depressant effect).
No products indexed under this heading.
Oxazepam (Heightens the CNS depressant effect). Products include:
Serax Capsules ... 2810
Serax Tablets ... 2810
Oxycodone Hydrochloride (Heightens the CNS depressant effect). Products include:
Percocet Tablets ... 938
Percodan Tablets ... 939
Percodan-Demi Tablets ... 940
Roxicodone Tablets, Oral Solution & Intensol (Oxycodone) ... 2244
Tylox Capsules ... 1584
Pentobarbital Sodium (Heightens the CNS depressant effect). Products include:
Nembutal Sodium Capsules ... 436
Nembutal Sodium Solution ... 438
Nembutal Sodium Suppositories ... 440
Perphenazine (Heightens the CNS depressant effect). Products include:
Etrafon ... 2355
Triavil Tablets ... 1757
Trilafon ... 2389
Phenelzine Sulfate (Prolongs and intensifies the anticholinergic effects of antihistamines). Products include:
Nardil ... 1920
Phenobarbital (Heightens the CNS depressant effect). Products include:
Arco-Lase Plus Tablets ... 512
Bellergal-S Tablets ... 2250
Donnatal ... 2060
Donnatal Extentabs ... 2061
Donnatal Tablets ... 2060
Phenobarbital Elixir and Tablets ... 1469
Quadrinal Tablets ... 1350
Prazepam (Heightens the CNS depressant effect).
No products indexed under this heading.
Prochlorperazine (Heightens the CNS depressant effect). Products include:
Compazine ... 2470
Promethazine Hydrochloride (Heightens the CNS depressant effect). Products include:
Mepergan Injection ... 2753
Phenergan with Codeine ... 2777
Phenergan with Dextromethorphan 2778
Phenergan Injection ... 2773
Phenergan Suppositories ... 2775
Phenergan Syrup ... 2774
Phenergan Tablets ... 2775
Phenergan VC ... 2779
Phenergan VC with Codeine ... 2781
Propofol (Heightens the CNS depressant effect). Products include:
Diprivan Injection ... 2833
Propoxyphene Hydrochloride (Heightens the CNS depressant effect). Products include:
Darvon ... 1435
Wygesic Tablets ... 2827
Propoxyphene Napsylate (Heightens the CNS depressant effect). Products include:
Darvon-N/Darvocet-N ... 1433
Quazepam (Heightens the CNS depressant effect). Products include:
Doral Tablets ... 2664
Risperidone (Heightens the CNS depressant effect). Products include:
Risperdal ... 1301
Secobarbital Sodium (Heightens the CNS depressant effect). Products include:
Seconal Sodium Pulvules ... 1474
Selegiline Hydrochloride (Prolongs and intensifies the anticholinergic effects of antihistamines). Products include:
Eldepryl Tablets ... 2550
Sufentanil Citrate (Heightens the CNS depressant effect). Products include:
Sufenta Injection ... 1309
Temazepam (Heightens the CNS depressant effect). Products include:
Restoril Capsules ... 2284
Thiamylal Sodium (Heightens the CNS depressant effect).
No products indexed under this heading.
Thioridazine Hydrochloride (Heightens the CNS depressant effect). Products include:
Mellaril ... 2269
Thiothixene (Heightens the CNS depressant effect). Products include:
Navane Capsules and Concentrate 2201
Navane Intramuscular ... 2202
Tranylcypromine Sulfate (Prolongs and intensifies the anticholinergic effects of antihistamines). Products include:
Parnate Tablets ... 2503
Triazolam (Heightens the CNS depressant effect). Products include:
Halcion Tablets ... 2611
Trifluoperazine Hydrochloride (Heightens the CNS depressant effect). Products include:
Stelazine ... 2514
Zolpidem Tartrate (Heightens the CNS depressant effect). Products include:
Ambien Tablets ... 2416

Food Interactions

Alcohol (Heightens the CNS depressant effect).

UNISOM NIGHTTIME SLEEP AID
(Doxylamine Succinate) ... 1934

Food Interactions

Alcohol (Use Unisom cautiously).

UNISOM WITH PAIN RELIEF-NIGHTTIME SLEEP AID AND PAIN RELIEVER
(Diphenhydramine Hydrochloride, Acetaminophen) ... 1934
May interact with monoamine oxidase inhibitors, central nervous system depressants, and certain other agents. Compounds in these categories include:

Alfentanil Hydrochloride (Heightened CNS depressant effect of antihistamines). Products include:
Alfenta Injection ... 1286
Alprazolam (Heightened CNS depressant effect of antihistamines). Products include:
Xanax Tablets ... 2649
Aprobarbital (Heightened CNS depressant effect of antihistamines).
No products indexed under this heading.

IMPORTANT NOTE: Always consult each drug listing in the patient's regimen for possible interactions.

Unisom With Pain Relief

Buprenorphine (Heightened CNS depressant effect of antihistamines). Products include:

Buprenex Injectable 2006

Buspirone Hydrochloride (Heightened CNS depressant effect of antihistamines). Products include:

BuSpar 737

Butabarbital (Heightened CNS depressant effect of antihistamines).

No products indexed under this heading.

Butalbital (Heightened CNS depressant effect of antihistamines). Products include:

Esgic-plus Tablets 1013
Fioricet Tablets....................................... 2258
Fioricet with Codeine Capsules 2260
Fiorinal Capsules 2261
Fiorinal with Codeine Capsules 2262
Fiorinal Tablets....................................... 2261
Phrenilin 785
Sedapap Tablets 50 mg/650 mg .. 1543

Chlordiazepoxide (Heightened CNS depressant effect of antihistamines). Products include:

Libritabs Tablets 2177
Limbitrol 2180

Chlordiazepoxide Hydrochloride (Heightened CNS depressant effect of antihistamines). Products include:

Librax Capsules 2176
Librium Capsules................................... 2178
Librium Injectable 2179

Chlorpromazine (Heightened CNS depressant effect of antihistamines). Products include:

Thorazine Suppositories 2523

Chlorpromazine Hydrochloride (Heightened CNS depressant effect of antihistamines). Products include:

Thorazine 2523

Chlorprothixene (Heightened CNS depressant effect of antihistamines).

No products indexed under this heading.

Chlorprothixene Hydrochloride (Heightened CNS depressant effect of antihistamines).

No products indexed under this heading.

Clorazepate Dipotassium (Heightened CNS depressant effect of antihistamines). Products include:

Tranxene 451

Clozapine (Heightened CNS depressant effect of antihistamines). Products include:

Clozaril Tablets....................................... 2252

Codeine Phosphate (Heightened CNS depressant effect of antihistamines). Products include:

Actifed with Codeine Cough Syrup.. 1067
Brontex 1981
Deconsal C Expectorant Syrup 456
Deconsal Pediatric Syrup 457
Dimetane-DC Cough Syrup 2059
Empirin with Codeine Tablets............ 1093
Fioricet with Codeine Capsules 2260
Fiorinal with Codeine Capsules 2262
Isoclor Expectorant............................... 990
Novahistine DH..................................... 2462
Novahistine Expectorant...................... 2463
Nucofed 2051
Phenergan with Codeine 2777
Phenergan VC with Codeine 2781
Robitussin A-C Syrup 2073
Robitussin-DAC Syrup 2074
Ryna .... ◾◻ 841
Soma Compound w/Codeine Tablets 2676
Tussi-Organidin NR Liquid and S NR Liquid 2677
Tylenol with Codeine 1583

Desflurane (Heightened CNS depressant effect of antihistamines). Products include:

Suprane 1813

Dezocine (Heightened CNS depressant effect of antihistamines). Products include:

Dalgan Injection 538

Diazepam (Heightened CNS depressant effect of antihistamines). Products include:

Dizac 1809
Valium Injectable 2182
Valium Tablets 2183
Valrelease Capsules 2169

Droperidol (Heightened CNS depressant effect of antihistamines). Products include:

Inapsine Injection.................................. 1296

Enflurane (Heightened CNS depressant effect of antihistamines).

No products indexed under this heading.

Estazolam (Heightened CNS depressant effect of antihistamines). Products include:

ProSom Tablets 449

Ethchlorvynol (Heightened CNS depressant effect of antihistamines). Products include:

Placidyl Capsules................................... 448

Ethinamate (Heightened CNS depressant effect of antihistamines).

No products indexed under this heading.

Fentanyl (Heightened CNS depressant effect of antihistamines). Products include:

Duragesic Transdermal System........ 1288

Fentanyl Citrate (Heightened CNS depressant effect of antihistamines). Products include:

Sublimaze Injection 1307

Fluphenazine Decanoate (Heightened CNS depressant effect of antihistamines). Products include:

Prolixin Decanoate 509

Fluphenazine Enanthate (Heightened CNS depressant effect of antihistamines). Products include:

Prolixin Enanthate 509

Fluphenazine Hydrochloride (Heightened CNS depressant effect of antihistamines). Products include:

Prolixin 509

Flurazepam Hydrochloride (Heightened CNS depressant effect of antihistamines). Products include:

Dalmane Capsules................................. 2173

Furazolidone (Prolonged and intensified anticholinergic effects of antihistamines). Products include:

Furoxone 2046

Glutethimide (Heightened CNS depressant effect of antihistamines).

No products indexed under this heading.

Haloperidol (Heightened CNS depressant effect of antihistamines). Products include:

Haldol Injection, Tablets and Concentrate 1575

Haloperidol Decanoate (Heightened CNS depressant effect of antihistamines). Products include:

Haldol Decanoate................................... 1577

Hydrocodone Bitartrate (Heightened CNS depressant effect of antihistamines). Products include:

Anexsia 5/500 Elixir 1781
Anexia Tablets.. 1782
Codiclear DH Syrup 791
Deconamine CX Cough and Cold Liquid and Tablets............................. 1319
Duratuss HD Elixir................................. 2565
Hycodan Tablets and Syrup 930
Hycomine Compound Tablets 932
Hycomine 931
Hycotuss Expectorant Syrup 933
Hydrocet Capsules 782
Lorcet 10/650.. 1018
Lortab 2566
Tussend 1783

Tussend Expectorant 1785
Vicodin Tablets....................................... 1356
Vicodin ES Tablets 1357
Vicodin Tuss Expectorant 1358
Zydone Capsules 949

Hydrocodone Polistirex (Heightened CNS depressant effect of antihistamines). Products include:

Tussionex Pennkinetic Extended-Release Suspension 998

Hydroxyzine Hydrochloride (Heightened CNS depressant effect of antihistamines). Products include:

Atarax Tablets & Syrup........................ 2185
Marax Tablets & DF Syrup................... 2200
Vistaril Intramuscular Solution......... 2216

Isocarboxazid (Prolonged and intensified anticholinergic effects of antihistamines).

No products indexed under this heading.

Isoflurane (Heightened CNS depressant effect of antihistamines).

No products indexed under this heading.

Ketamine Hydrochloride (Heightened CNS depressant effect of antihistamines).

No products indexed under this heading.

Levomethadyl Acetate Hydrochloride (Heightened CNS depressant effect of antihistamines). Products include:

Orlaam 2239

Levorphanol Tartrate (Heightened CNS depressant effect of antihistamines). Products include:

Levo-Dromoran 2129

Lorazepam (Heightened CNS depressant effect of antihistamines). Products include:

Ativan Injection 2698
Ativan Tablets 2700

Loxapine Hydrochloride (Heightened CNS depressant effect of antihistamines). Products include:

Loxitane 1378

Loxapine Succinate (Heightened CNS depressant effect of antihistamines). Products include:

Loxitane Capsules 1378

Meperidine Hydrochloride (Heightened CNS depressant effect of antihistamines). Products include:

Demerol 2308
Mepergan Injection 2753

Mephobarbital (Heightened CNS depressant effect of antihistamines). Products include:

Mebaral Tablets 2322

Meprobamate (Heightened CNS depressant effect of antihistamines). Products include:

Miltown Tablets 2672
PMB 200 and PMB 400 2783

Mesoridazine (Heightened CNS depressant effect of antihistamines).

Methadone Hydrochloride (Heightened CNS depressant effect of antihistamines). Products include:

Methadone Hydrochloride Oral Concentrate 2233
Methadone Hydrochloride Oral Solution & Tablets............................... 2235

Methohexital Sodium (Heightened CNS depressant effect of antihistamines). Products include:

Brevital Sodium Vials............................ 1429

Methotrimeprazine (Heightened CNS depressant effect of antihistamines). Products include:

Levoprome 1274

Methoxyflurane (Heightened CNS depressant effect of antihistamines).

No products indexed under this heading.

Midazolam Hydrochloride (Heightened CNS depressant effect of antihistamines). Products include:

Versed Injection 2170

Molindone Hydrochloride (Heightened CNS depressant effect of antihistamines). Products include:

Moban Tablets and Concentrate...... 1048

Morphine Sulfate (Heightened CNS depressant effect of antihistamines). Products include:

Astramorph/PF Injection, USP (Preservative-Free) 535
Duramorph 962
Infumorph 200 and Infumorph 500 Sterile Solutions........................... 965
MS Contin Tablets.................................. 1994
MSIR 1997
Oramorph SR (Morphine Sulfate Sustained Release Tablets).............. 2236
RMS Suppositories 2657
Roxanol 2243

Opium Alkaloids (Heightened CNS depressant effect of antihistamines).

No products indexed under this heading.

Oxazepam (Heightened CNS depressant effect of antihistamines). Products include:

Serax Capsules 2810
Serax Tablets.. 2810

Oxycodone Hydrochloride (Heightened CNS depressant effect of antihistamines). Products include:

Percocet Tablets 938
Percodan Tablets................................... 939
Percodan-Demi Tablets........................ 940
Roxicodone Tablets, Oral Solution & Intensol (Oxycodone) 2244
Tylox Capsules 1584

Pentobarbital Sodium (Heightened CNS depressant effect of antihistamines). Products include:

Nembutal Sodium Capsules 436
Nembutal Sodium Solution 438
Nembutal Sodium Suppositories...... 440

Perphenazine (Heightened CNS depressant effect of antihistamines). Products include:

Etrafon 2355
Triavil Tablets 1757
Trilafon... 2389

Phenelzine Sulfate (Prolonged and intensified anticholinergic effects of antihistamines). Products include:

Nardil 1920

Phenobarbital (Heightened CNS depressant effect of antihistamines). Products include:

Arco-Lase Plus Tablets 512
Bellergal-S Tablets 2250
Donnatal 2060
Donnatal Extentabs............................... 2061
Donnatal Tablets 2060
Phenobarbital Elixir and Tablets...... 1469
Quadrinal Tablets 1350

Prazepam (Heightened CNS depressant effect of antihistamines).

No products indexed under this heading.

Prochlorperazine (Heightened CNS depressant effect of antihistamines). Products include:

Compazine 2470

Promethazine Hydrochloride (Heightened CNS depressant effect of antihistamines). Products include:

Mepergan Injection 2753
Phenergan with Codeine 2777
Phenergan with Dextromethorphan 2778
Phenergan Injection 2773
Phenergan Suppositories 2775
Phenergan Syrup 2774
Phenergan Tablets 2775
Phenergan VC 2779
Phenergan VC with Codeine 2781

Propofol (Heightened CNS depressant effect of antihistamines). Products include:

Diprivan Injection................................... 2833

(◾◻ Described in PDR For Nonprescription Drugs) (◉ Described in PDR For Ophthalmology)

Propoxyphene Hydrochloride (Heightened CNS depressant effect of antihistamines). Products include:

Darvon 1435
Wygesic Tablets 2827

Propoxyphene Napsylate (Heightened CNS depressant effect of antihistamines). Products include:

Darvon-N/Darvocet-N 1433

Quazepam (Heightened CNS depressant effect of antihistamines). Products include:

Doral Tablets 2664

Risperidone (Heightened CNS depressant effect of antihistamines). Products include:

Risperdal 1301

Secobarbital Sodium (Heightened CNS depressant effect of antihistamines). Products include:

Seconal Sodium Pulvules 1474

Selegiline Hydrochloride (Prolonged and intensified anticholinergic effects of antihistamines). Products include:

Eldepryl Tablets 2550

Sufentanil Citrate (Heightened CNS depressant effect of antihistamines). Products include:

Sufenta Injection 1309

Temazepam (Heightened CNS depressant effect of antihistamines). Products include:

Restoril Capsules 2284

Thiamylal Sodium (Heightened CNS depressant effect of antihistamines).

No products indexed under this heading.

Thioridazine Hydrochloride (Heightened CNS depressant effect of antihistamines). Products include:

Mellaril 2269

Thiothixene (Heightened CNS depressant effect of antihistamines). Products include:

Navane Capsules and Concentrate 2201
Navane Intramuscular 2202

Tranylcypromine Sulfate (Prolonged and intensified anticholinergic effects of antihistamines). Products include:

Parnate Tablets 2503

Triazolam (Heightened CNS depressant effect of antihistamines). Products include:

Halcion Tablets 2611

Trifluoperazine Hydrochloride (Heightened CNS depressant effect of antihistamines). Products include:

Stelazine 2514

Zolpidem Tartrate (Heightened CNS depressant effect of antihistamines). Products include:

Ambien Tablets... 2416

Food Interactions

Alcohol (Heightened CNS depressant effect of antihistamines).

UNIVASC TABLETS

(Moexipril Hydrochloride)....................2410

May interact with diuretics, potassium sparing diuretics, potassium preparations, lithium preparations, and certain other agents. Compounds in these categories include:

Amiloride Hydrochloride (ACE inhibitors can increase the risk of hyperkalemia with concomitant use). Products include:

Midamor Tablets 1703
Moduretic Tablets 1705

Bendroflumethiazide (Excessive reduction in blood pressure may occur in patients on diuretic therapy when ACE inhibitors are started).

No products indexed under this heading.

Bumetanide (Excessive reduction in blood pressure may occur in patients on diuretic therapy when ACE inhibitors are started). Products include:

Bumex 2093

Chlorothiazide (Excessive reduction in blood pressure may occur in patients on diuretic therapy when ACE inhibitors are started). Products include:

Aldoclor Tablets 1598
Diupres Tablets 1650
Diuril Oral 1653

Chlorothiazide Sodium (Excessive reduction in blood pressure may occur in patients on diuretic therapy when ACE inhibitors are started). Products include:

Diuril Sodium Intravenous 1652

Chlorthalidone (Excessive reduction in blood pressure may occur in patients on diuretic therapy when ACE inhibitors are started). Products include:

Combipres Tablets 677
Tenoretic Tablets....................................... 2845
Thalitone 1245

Ethacrynic Acid (Excessive reduction in blood pressure may occur in patients on diuretic therapy when ACE inhibitors are started). Products include:

Edecrin Tablets... 1657

Furosemide (Excessive reduction in blood pressure may occur in patients on diuretic therapy when ACE inhibitors are started). Products include:

Lasix Injection, Oral Solution and Tablets 1240

Hydrochlorothiazide (Excessive reduction in blood pressure may occur in patients on diuretic therapy when ACE inhibitors are started). Products include:

Aldactazide... 2413
Aldoril Tablets.. 1604
Apresazide Capsules 808
Capozide 742
Dyazide 2479
Esidrix Tablets 821
Esimil Tablets 822
HydroDIURIL Tablets 1674
Hydropres Tablets..................................... 1675
Hyzaar Tablets 1677
Inderide Tablets 2732
Inderide LA Long Acting Capsules .. 2734
Lopressor HCT Tablets 832
Lotensin HCT.. 837
Maxzide 1380
Moduretic Tablets 1705
Oretic Tablets 443
Prinzide Tablets 1737
Ser-Ap-Es Tablets 849
Timolide Tablets... 1748
Vaseretic Tablets 1765
Zestoretic 2850
Ziac 1415

Hydroflumethiazide (Excessive reduction in blood pressure may occur in patients on diuretic therapy when ACE inhibitors are started). Products include:

Diucardin Tablets...................................... 2718

Indapamide (Excessive reduction in blood pressure may occur in patients on diuretic therapy when ACE inhibitors are started). Products include:

Lozol Tablets 2022

Lithium Carbonate (Potential for increased serum lithium levels and risk of lithium toxicity). Products include:

Eskalith 2485
Lithium Carbonate Capsules & Tablets 2230
Lithonate/Lithotabs/Lithobid 2543

Lithium Citrate (Potential for increased serum lithium levels and risk of lithium toxicity).

No products indexed under this heading.

Methyclothiazide (Excessive reduction in blood pressure may occur in patients on diuretic therapy when ACE inhibitors are started). Products include:

Enduron Tablets... 420

Metolazone (Excessive reduction in blood pressure may occur in patients on diuretic therapy when ACE inhibitors are started). Products include:

Mykrox Tablets 993
Zaroxolyn Tablets 1000

Polythiazide (Excessive reduction in blood pressure may occur in patients on diuretic therapy when ACE inhibitors are started). Products include:

Minizide Capsules 1938

Potassium Acid Phosphate (ACE inhibitors can increase the risk of hyperkalemia with concomitant use). Products include:

K-Phos Original Formula 'Sodium Free' Tablets 639

Potassium Bicarbonate (ACE inhibitors can increase the risk of hyperkalemia with concomitant use). Products include:

Alka-Seltzer Gold Effervescent Antacid... ◆◻ 703

Potassium Chloride (ACE inhibitors can increase the risk of hyperkalemia with concomitant use). Products include:

Chlor-3 Condiment 1004
K-Dur Microburst Release System (potassium chloride, USP) E.R. Tablets 1325
K-Lor Powder Packets 434
K-Norm Extended-Release Capsules 991
K-Tab Filmtab 434
Kolyum Liquid 992
Micro-K... 2063
Micro-K LS Packets.................................. 2064
NuLYTELY... 689
Cherry Flavor NuLYTELY 689
Rum-K Syrup 1005
Slow-K Extended-Release Tablets.... 851

Potassium Citrate (ACE inhibitors can increase the risk of hyperkalemia with concomitant use). Products include:

Polycitra Syrup 578
Polycitra-K Crystals 579
Polycitra-K Oral Solution 579
Polycitra-LC 578

Potassium Gluconate (ACE inhibitors can increase the risk of hyperkalemia with concomitant use). Products include:

Kolyum Liquid 992

Potassium Phosphate, Dibasic (ACE inhibitors can increase the risk of hyperkalemia with concomitant use).

No products indexed under this heading.

Potassium Phosphate, Monobasic (ACE inhibitors can increase the risk of hyperkalemia with concomitant use). Products include:

K-Phos Neutral Tablets 639
K-Phos Original Formula 'Sodium Free' Tablets 639

Spironolactone (ACE inhibitors can increase the risk of hyperkalemia with concomitant use). Products include:

Aldactazide... 2413
Aldactone 2414

Torsemide (Excessive reduction in blood pressure may occur in patients on diuretic therapy when ACE inhibitors are started). Products include:

Demadex Tablets and Injection 686

Triamterene (ACE inhibitors can increase the risk of hyperkalemia with concomitant use). Products include:

Dyazide 2479
Dyrenium Capsules.................................. 2481
Maxzide 1380

Food Interactions

Food, unspecified (Food reduces C_{max} and AUC by about 70% and 40% respectively after ingestion of a low-fat breakfast or by 80% and 50% respectively after the ingestion of high-fat breakfast).

URECHOLINE INJECTION

(Bethanechol Chloride) 1761

See **Urecholine Tablets**

URECHOLINE TABLETS

(Bethanechol Chloride) 1761

May interact with ganglionic blocking agents. Compounds in this category include:

Mecamylamine Hydrochloride (Critical fall in blood pressure). Products include:

Inversine Tablets 1686

Trimethaphan Camsylate (Critical fall in blood pressure). Products include:

Arfonad Ampuls 2080

URISED TABLETS

(Atropine Sulfate, Hyoscyamine, Methenamine, Phenyl Salicylate) 1964

May interact with sulfonamides, urinary alkalizing agents, and certain other agents. Compounds in these categories include:

Potassium Citrate (Methenamine has therapeutic activity in acidic urine; concurrent use with drugs which produce an alkaline urine should be restricted). Products include:

Polycitra Syrup 578
Polycitra-K Crystals 579
Polycitra-K Oral Solution 579
Polycitra-LC 578

Sodium Citrate (Methenamine has therapeutic activity in acidic urine; concurrent use with drugs which produce an alkaline urine should be restricted). Products include:

Bicitra 578
Citrocarbonate Antacid .... ◆◻ 770
Polycitra... 578
Salix SST Lozenges Saliva Stimulant.. ◆◻ 797

Sulfamethizole (Mutual antagonism; concurrent use should be avoided since insoluble precipitate may form in the urine). Products include:

Urobiotic-250 Capsules 2214

Sulfamethoxazole (Mutual antagonism; concurrent use should be avoided since insoluble precipitate may form in the urine). Products include:

Azo Gantanol Tablets.............................. 2080
Bactrim DS Tablets................................... 2084
Bactrim I.V. Infusion............................... 2082
Bactrim 2084
Gantanol Tablets 2119
Septra... 1174
Septra I.V. Infusion 1169

IMPORTANT NOTE: Always consult each drug listing in the patient's regimen for possible interactions.

Septra I.V. Infusion ADD-Vantage Vials ... 1171
Septra ... 1174

Sulfasalazine (Mutual antagonism; concurrent use should be avoided since insoluble precipitate may form in the urine). Products include:
Azulfidine ... 1949

Sulfinpyrazone (Mutual antagonism; concurrent use should be avoided since insoluble precipitate may form in the urine). Products include:
Anturane ... 807

Sulfisoxazole (Mutual antagonism; concurrent use should be avoided since insoluble precipitate may form in the urine). Products include:
Azo Gantrisin Tablets ... 2081
Gantrisin Tablets ... 2120

Sulfisoxazole Diolamine (Mutual antagonism; concurrent use should be avoided since insoluble precipitate may form in the urine).
No products indexed under this heading.

Food Interactions

Food that raises urinary pH (Methenamine has therapeutic activity in acidic urine; concurrent use with foods which produce an alkaline urine should be restricted).

URISPAS TABLETS
(Flavoxate Hydrochloride) ... 2532
None cited in PDR database.

UROBIOTIC-250 CAPSULES
(Oxytetracycline Hydrochloride, Sulfamethizole, Phenazopyridine Hydrochloride) ... 2214
May interact with:

Aluminum Hydroxide (Decreases absorption of Urobiotic). Products include:
ALternaGEL Liquid ... 1316
Maximum Strength Ascriptin ... ⊡ 630
Cama Arthritis Pain Reliever ... ⊡ 785
Gaviscon Extra Strength Relief Formula Antacid Tablets ... ⊡ 819
Gaviscon Extra Strength Relief Formula Liquid Antacid ... ⊡ 819
Gaviscon Liquid Antacid ... ⊡ 820
Gelusil Liquid & Tablets ... ⊡ 855
Maalox Heartburn Relief Suspension ... ⊡ 642
Maalox Heartburn Relief Tablets ... ⊡ 641
Maalox Magnesia and Alumina Oral Suspension ... ⊡ 642
Maalox Plus Tablets ... ⊡ 643
Extra Strength Maalox Antacid Plus Antigas Liquid and Tablets ⊡ 638
Tempo Soft Antacid ... ⊡ 835

Aluminum Hydroxide Gel (Decreases absorption of Urobiotic). Products include:
ALternaGEL Liquid ... ⊡ 659
Aludrox Oral Suspension ... 2695
Amphojel Suspension ... 2695
Amphojel Suspension without Flavor ... 2695
Amphojel Tablets ... 2695
Arthritis Pain Ascriptin ... ⊡ 631
Regular Strength Ascriptin Tablets ... ⊡ 629
Gaviscon Antacid Tablets ... ⊡ 819
Gaviscon-2 Antacid Tablets ... ⊡ 820
Mylanta Liquid ... 1317
Mylanta Tablets ... ⊡ 660
Mylanta Double Strength Liquid ... 1317
Mylanta Double Strength Tablets .. ⊡ 660
Nephrox Suspension ... ⊡ 655

Aluminum Hydroxide Gel, Dried (Decreases absorption of Urobiotic).

URO-MAG
(Magnesium Oxide) ... 668
None cited in PDR database.

UROQID-ACID NO. 2 TABLETS
(Methenamine Mandelate, Sodium Acid Phosphate) ... 640
May interact with:

Acetazolamide (Reduces the effectiveness of methenamine by causing urine to become alkaline). Products include:
Diamox Sequels (Sustained Release) ... 1373
Diamox Sequels (Sustained Release) ... ⊙ 319
Diamox Tablets ... 1372
Diamox Tablets ... ⊙ 317

ACTH (Concurrent use with sodium phosphate may result in hypernatremia).
No products indexed under this heading.

Aluminum Carbonate Gel (Reduces the effectiveness of methenamine by causing urine to become alkaline). Products include:
Basaljel ... 2703

Aluminum Hydroxide (Reduces the effectiveness of methenamine by causing urine to become alkaline). Products include:
ALternaGEL Liquid ... 1316
Maximum Strength Ascriptin ... ⊡ 630
Cama Arthritis Pain Reliever ... ⊡ 785
Gaviscon Extra Strength Relief Formula Antacid Tablets ... ⊡ 819
Gaviscon Extra Strength Relief Formula Liquid Antacid ... ⊡ 819
Gaviscon Liquid Antacid ... ⊡ 820
Gelusil Liquid & Tablets ... ⊡ 855
Maalox Heartburn Relief Suspension ... ⊡ 642
Maalox Heartburn Relief Tablets ... ⊡ 641
Maalox Magnesia and Alumina Oral Suspension ... ⊡ 642
Maalox Plus Tablets ... ⊡ 643
Extra Strength Maalox Antacid Plus Antigas Liquid and Tablets ⊡ 638
Tempo Soft Antacid ... ⊡ 835

Aluminum Hydroxide Gel (Reduces the effectiveness of methenamine by causing urine to become alkaline). Products include:
ALternaGEL Liquid ... ⊡ 659
Aludrox Oral Suspension ... 2695
Amphojel Suspension ... 2695
Amphojel Suspension without Flavor ... 2695
Amphojel Tablets ... 2695
Arthritis Pain Ascriptin ... ⊡ 631
Regular Strength Ascriptin Tablets ... ⊡ 629
Gaviscon Antacid Tablets ... ⊡ 819
Gaviscon-2 Antacid Tablets ... ⊡ 820
Mylanta Liquid ... 1317
Mylanta Tablets ... ⊡ 660
Mylanta Double Strength Liquid ... 1317
Mylanta Double Strength Tablets .. ⊡ 660
Nephrox Suspension ... ⊡ 655

Aspirin (Concurrent use may lead to increased serum salicylate levels since excretion of salicylates is reduced in acidic urine). Products include:
Alka-Seltzer Effervescent Antacid and Pain Reliever ... ⊡ 701
Alka-Seltzer Extra Strength Effervescent Antacid and Pain Reliever ... ⊡ 703
Alka-Seltzer Lemon Lime Effervescent Antacid and Pain Reliever ... ⊡ 703
Alka-Seltzer Plus Cold Medicine ... ⊡ 705
Alka-Seltzer Plus Cold & Cough Medicine ... ⊡ 708
Alka-Seltzer Plus Night-Time Cold Medicine ... ⊡ 707
Alka Seltzer Plus Sinus Medicine .. ⊡ 707
Arthritis Foundation Safety Coated Aspirin Tablets ... ⊡ 675
Arthritis Pain Ascriptin ... ⊡ 631
Maximum Strength Ascriptin ... ⊡ 630
Regular Strength Ascriptin Tablets ... ⊡ 629
Arthritis Strength BC Powder ... ⊡ 609
BC Cold Powder Multi-Symptom Formula (Cold-Sinus-Allergy) ... ⊡ 609
BC Cold Powder Non-Drowsy Formula (Cold-Sinus) ... ⊡ 609
BC Powder ... ⊡ 609
Bayer Children's Chewable Aspirin ... ⊡ 711
Genuine Bayer Aspirin Tablets & Caplets ... ⊡ 713
Extra Strength Bayer Arthritis Pain Regimen Formula ... ⊡ 711
Extra Strength Bayer Aspirin Caplets & Tablets ... ⊡ 712
Extended-Release Bayer 8-Hour Aspirin ... ⊡ 712
Extra Strength Bayer Plus Aspirin Caplets ... ⊡ 713
Extra Strength Bayer PM Aspirin .. ⊡ 713
Bayer Enteric Aspirin ... ⊡ 709
Bufferin Analgesic Tablets and Caplets ... ⊡ 613
Arthritis Strength Bufferin Analgesic Caplets ... ⊡ 614
Extra Strength Bufferin Analgesic Tablets ... ⊡ 615
Cama Arthritis Pain Reliever ... ⊡ 785
Darvon Compound-65 Pulvules ... 1435
Easprin ... 1914
Ecotrin ... 2455
Ecotrin Enteric Coated Aspirin Maximum Strength Tablets and Caplets ... ⊡ 816
Ecotrin Enteric Coated Aspirin Regular Strength Tablets ... 2455
Empirin Aspirin Tablets ... ⊡ 854
Empirin with Codeine Tablets ... 1093
Excedrin Extra-Strength Analgesic Tablets & Caplets ... 732
Fiorinal Capsules ... 2261
Fiorinal with Codeine Capsules ... 2262
Fiorinal Tablets ... 2261
Halfprin ... 1362
Healthprin Aspirin ... 2455
Norgesic ... 1496
Percodan Tablets ... 939
Percodan-Demi Tablets ... 940
Robaxisal Tablets ... 2071
Soma Compound w/Codeine Tablets ... 2676
Soma Compound Tablets ... 2675
St. Joseph Adult Chewable Aspirin (81 mg.) ... ⊡ 808
Talwin Compound ... 2335
Ursinus Inlay-Tabs ... ⊡ 794
Vanquish Analgesic Caplets ... ⊡ 731

Bendroflumethiazide (Reduces the effectiveness of methenamine by causing urine to become alkaline).
No products indexed under this heading.

Betamethasone Acetate (Concurrent use with sodium phosphate may result in hypernatremia). Products include:
Celestone Soluspan Suspension ... 2347

Betamethasone Sodium Phosphate (Concurrent use with sodium phosphate may result in hypernatremia). Products include:
Celestone Soluspan Suspension ... 2347

Chlorothiazide (Reduces the effectiveness of methenamine by causing urine to become alkaline). Products include:
Aldoclor Tablets ... 1598
Diupres Tablets ... 1650
Diuril Oral ... 1653

Chlorothiazide Sodium (Reduces the effectiveness of methenamine by causing urine to become alkaline). Products include:
Diuril Sodium Intravenous ... 1652

Choline Magnesium Trisalicylate (Concurrent use may lead to increased serum salicylate levels since excretion of salicylates is reduced in acidic urine). Products include:
Trilisate ... 2000

Cortisone Acetate (Concurrent use with sodium phosphate may result in hypernatremia). Products include:
Cortone Acetate Sterile Suspension ... 1623
Cortone Acetate Tablets ... 1624

Deserpidine (Concurrent use with sodium phosphate may result in hypernatremia).
No products indexed under this heading.

Desoxycorticosterone Acetate (Concurrent use with sodium phosphate may result in hypernatremia).

Desoxycorticosterone Pivalate (Concurrent use with sodium phosphate may result in hypernatremia).

Dexamethasone (Concurrent use with sodium phosphate may result in hypernatremia). Products include:
AK-Trol Ointment & Suspension ... ⊙ 205
Decadron Elixir ... 1633
Decadron Tablets ... 1635
Decaspray Topical Aerosol ... 1648
Dexacidin Ointment ... ⊙ 263
Maxitrol Ophthalmic Ointment and Suspension ... ⊙ 224
TobraDex Ophthalmic Suspension and Ointment ... 473

Dexamethasone Acetate (Concurrent use with sodium phosphate may result in hypernatremia). Products include:
Dalalone D.P. Injectable ... 1011
Decadron-LA Sterile Suspension ... 1646

Dexamethasone Sodium Phosphate (Concurrent use with sodium phosphate may result in hypernatremia). Products include:
Decadron Phosphate Injection ... 1637
Decadron Phosphate Respihaler ... 1642
Decadron Phosphate Sterile Ophthalmic Ointment ... 1641
Decadron Phosphate Sterile Ophthalmic Solution ... 1642
Decadron Phosphate Topical Cream ... 1644
Decadron Phosphate Turbinaire ... 1645
Decadron Phosphate with Xylocaine Injection, Sterile ... 1639
Dexacort Phosphate in Respihaler .. 458
Dexacort Phosphate in Turbinaire .. 459
NeoDecadron Sterile Ophthalmic Ointment ... 1712
NeoDecadron Sterile Ophthalmic Solution ... 1713
NeoDecadron Topical Cream ... 1714

Diazoxide (Concurrant use with sodium phosphate may result in hypernatremia). Products include:
Hyperstat I.V. Injection ... 2363
Proglycem ... 580

Dichlorphenamide (Reduces the effectiveness of methenamine by causing urine to become alkaline). Products include:
Daranide Tablets ... 1633

Diflunisal (Concurrent use may lead to increased serum salicylate levels since excretion of salicylates is reduced in acidic urine). Products include:
Dolobid Tablets ... 1654

Dihydroxyaluminum Sodium Carbonate (Reduces the effectiveness of methenamine by causing urine to become alkaline).
No products indexed under this heading.

Fludrocortisone Acetate (Concurrent use with sodium phosphate may result in hypernatremia). Products include:
Florinef Acetate Tablets ... 505

Guanethidine Monosulfate (Concurrent use with sodium phosphate may result in hypernatremia). Products include:
Esimil Tablets ... 822
Ismelin Tablets ... 827

Hydralazine Hydrochloride (Concurrent use with sodium phosphate may result in hypernatremia). Products include:
Apresazide Capsules ... 808
Apresoline Hydrochloride Tablets .. 809
Ser-Ap-Es Tablets ... 849

(⊡ Described in PDR For Nonprescription Drugs) (⊙ Described in PDR For Ophthalmology)

Hydrochlorothiazide (Reduces the effectiveness of methenamine by causing urine to become alkaline). Products include:

Aldactazide 2413
Aldoril Tablets 1604
Apresazide Capsules 808
Capozide 742
Dyazide 2479
Esidrix Tablets 821
Esimil Tablets 822
HydroDIURIL Tablets 1674
Hydropres Tablets 1675
Hyzaar Tablets 1677
Inderide Tablets 2732
Inderide LA Long Acting Capsules .. 2734
Lopressor HCT Tablets 832
Lotensin HCT 837
Maxzide 1380
Moduretic Tablets 1705
Oretic Tablets 443
Prinzide Tablets 1737
Ser-Ap-Es Tablets 849
Timolide Tablets 1748
Vaseretic Tablets 1765
Zestoretic 2850
Ziac 1415

Hydrocortisone (Concurrent use with sodium phosphate may result in hypernatremia). Products include:

Anusol-HC Cream 2.5% 1896
Aquanil HC Lotion 1931
Bactine Hydrocortisone Anti-Itch Cream ..... ◘ 709
Caldecort Anti-Itch Hydrocortisone Spray ..... ◘ 631
Cortaid ..... ◘ 836
CORTENEMA 2535
Cortisporin Ointment 1085
Cortisporin Ophthalmic Ointment Sterile 1085
Cortisporin Ophthalmic Suspension Sterile 1086
Cortisporin Otic Solution Sterile 1087
Cortisporin Otic Suspension Sterile 1088
Cortizone-5 ..... ◘ 831
Cortizone-10 ..... ◘ 831
Hydrocortone Tablets 1672
Hytone 907
Massengill Medicated Soft Cloth Towelettes 2458
PediOtic Suspension Sterile 1153
Preparation H Hydrocortisone 1% Cream ..... ◘ 872
ProctoCream-HC 2.5% 2408
VōSoL HC Otic Solution 2678

Hydrocortisone Acetate (Concurrent use with sodium phosphate may result in hypernatremia). Products include:

Analpram-HC Rectal Cream 1% and 2.5% 977
Anusol HC-1 Anti-Itch Hydrocortisone Ointment ..... ◘ 847
Anusol-HC Suppositories 1897
Caldecort ..... ◘ 631
Carmol HC 924
Coly-Mycin S Otic w/Neomycin & Hydrocortisone 1906
Cortaid ..... ◘ 836
Cortifoam 2396
Cortisporin Cream 1084
Epifoam 2399
Hydrocortone Acetate Sterile Suspension 1669
Mantadil Cream 1135
Nupercainal Hydrocortisone 1% Cream ..... ◘ 645
Ophthocort ..... ⊙ 311
Pramosone Cream, Lotion & Ointment 978
ProctoCream-HC 2408
ProctoFoam-HC 2409
Terra-Cortril Ophthalmic Suspension 2210

Hydrocortisone Sodium Phosphate (Concurrent use with sodium phosphate may result in hypernatremia). Products include:

Hydrocortone Phosphate Injection, Sterile 1670

Hydrocortisone Sodium Succinate (Concurrent use with sodium phosphate may result in hypernatremia). Products include:

Solu-Cortef Sterile Powder 2641

Hydroflumethiazide (Reduces the effectiveness of methenamine by causing urine to become alkaline). Products include:

Diucardin Tablets 2718

Magaldrate (Reduces the effectiveness of methenamine by causing urine to become alkaline).

No products indexed under this heading.

Magnesium Hydroxide (Reduces the effectiveness of methenamine by causing urine to become alkaline). Products include:

Aludrox Oral Suspension 2695
Arthritis Pain Ascriptin ..... ◘ 631
Maximum Strength Ascriptin ..... ◘ 630
Regular Strength Ascriptin Tablets ..... ◘ 629
Di-Gel Antacid/Anti-Gas ..... ◘ 801
Gelusil Liquid & Tablets ..... ◘ 855
Maalox Magnesia and Alumina Oral Suspension ..... ◘ 642
Maalox Plus Tablets ..... ◘ 643
Extra Strength Maalox Antacid Plus Antigas Liquid and Tablets ◘ 638
Mylanta Calcium Carbonate and Magnesium Hydroxide Tablets 1318
Mylanta Liquid 1317
Mylanta Tablets ..... ◘ 660
Mylanta Double Strength Liquid 1317
Mylanta Double Strength Tablets .. ◘ 660
Phillips' Milk of Magnesia Liquid .... ◘ 729
Rolaids Tablets ..... ◘ 843
Tempo Soft Antacid ..... ◘ 835

Magnesium Oxide (Reduces the effectiveness of methenamine by causing urine to become alkaline). Products include:

Beelith Tablets 639
Bufferin Analgesic Tablets and Caplets ..... ◘ 613
Caltrate PLUS ..... ◘ 665
Cama Arthritis Pain Reliever ..... ◘ 785
Mag-Ox 400 668
Uro-Mag 668

Magnesium Salicylate (Concurrent use may lead to increased serum salicylate levels since excretion of salicylates is reduced in acidic urine). Products include:

Backache Caplets ..... ◘ 613
Bayer Select Backache Pain Relief Formula ..... ◘ 715
Doan's Extra-Strength Analgesic .... ◘ 633
Extra Strength Doan's P.M. ..... ◘ 633
Doan's Regular Strength Analgesic ..... ◘ 634
Mobigesic Tablets ..... ◘ 602

Methazolamide (Reduces the effectiveness of methenamine by causing urine to become alkaline). Products include:

Glauctabs ..... ⊙ 208
MZM ..... ⊙ 267
Neptazane Tablets 1388
Neptazane Tablets ..... ⊙ 320

Methyclothiazide (Reduces the effectiveness of methenamine by causing urine to become alkaline). Products include:

Enduron Tablets 420

Methyldopa (Concurrent use with sodium phosphate may result in hypernatremia). Products include:

Aldoclor Tablets 1598
Aldomet Oral 1600
Aldoril Tablets 1604

Methylprednisolone Acetate (Concurrent use with sodium phosphate may result in hypernatremia). Products include:

Depo-Medrol Single-Dose Vial 2600
Depo-Medrol Sterile Aqueous Suspension 2597

Methylprednisolone Sodium Succinate (Concurrent use with sodium phosphate may result in hypernatremia). Products include:

Solu-Medrol Sterile Powder 2643

Polythiazide (Reduces the effectiveness of methenamine by causing urine to become alkaline). Products include:

Minizide Capsules 1938

Potassium Citrate (Reduces the effectiveness of methenamine by causing urine to become alkaline). Products include:

Polycitra Syrup 578
Polycitra-K Crystals 579
Polycitra-K Oral Solution 579
Polycitra-LC 578

Prednisolone Acetate (Concurrent use with sodium phosphate may result in hypernatremia). Products include:

AK-CIDE ..... ⊙ 202
AK-CIDE Ointment ..... ⊙ 202
Blephamide Liquifilm Sterile Ophthalmic Suspension 476
Blephamide Ointment ..... ⊙ 237
Econopred & Econopred Plus Ophthalmic Suspensions ..... ⊙ 217
Poly-Pred Liquifilm ..... ⊙ 248
Pred Forte ..... ⊙ 250
Pred Mild ..... ⊙ 253
Pred-G Liquifilm Sterile Ophthalmic Suspension ..... ⊙ 251
Pred-G S.O.P. Sterile Ophthalmic Ointment ..... ⊙ 252
Vasocidin Ointment ..... ⊙ 268

Prednisolone Sodium Phosphate (Concurrent use with sodium phosphate may result in hypernatremia). Products include:

AK-Pred ..... ⊙ 204
Hydeltrasol Injection, Sterile 1665
Inflamase ..... ⊙ 265
Pediapred Oral Liquid 995
Vasocidin Ophthalmic Solution ..... ⊙ 270

Prednisolone Tebutate (Concurrent use with sodium phosphate may result in hypernatremia). Products include:

Hydeltra-T.B.A. Sterile Suspension 1667

Prednisone (Concurrent use with sodium phosphate may result in hypernatremia). Products include:

Deltasone Tablets 2595

Rauwolfia Serpentina (Concurrent use with sodium phosphate may result in hypernatremia).

No products indexed under this heading.

Rescinnamine (Concurrent use with sodium phosphate may result in hypernatremia).

No products indexed under this heading.

Reserpine (Concurrent use with sodium phosphate may result in hypernatremia). Products include:

Diupres Tablets 1650
Hydropres Tablets 1675
Ser-Ap-Es Tablets 849

Salsalate (Concurrent use may lead to increased serum salicylate levels since excretion of salicylates is reduced in acidic urine). Products include:

Mono-Gesic Tablets 792
Salflex Tablets 786

Sodium Bicarbonate (Reduces the effectiveness of methenamine by causing urine to become alkaline). Products include:

Alka-Seltzer Effervescent Antacid and Pain Reliever ..... ◘ 701
Alka-Seltzer Extra Strength Effervescent Antacid and Pain Reliever ..... ◘ 703
Alka-Seltzer Gold Effervescent Antacid ..... ◘ 703
Alka-Seltzer Lemon Lime Effervescent Antacid and Pain Reliever ..... ◘ 703
Arm & Hammer Pure Baking Soda ..... ◘ 627
Ceo-Two Rectal Suppositories 666
Citrocarbonate Antacid ..... ◘ 770
Massengill Disposable Douches ..... ◘ 820
Massengill Liquid Concentrate ..... ◘ 820
NuLYTELY 689
Cherry Flavor NuLYTELY 689

Sodium Citrate (Reduces the effectiveness of methenamine by causing urine to become alkaline). Products include:

Bicitra 578
Citrocarbonate Antacid ..... ◘ 770
Polycitra 578
Salix SST Lozenges Saliva Stimulant ..... ◘ 797

Sulfamethizole (Concurrent use with sulfamethizole and formaldehyde forms an insoluble precipitate in acid urine and increases the risk of crystaluria). Products include:

Urobiotic-250 Capsules 2214

Triamcinolone (Concurrent use with sodium phosphate may result in hypernatremia). Products include:

Aristocort Tablets 1022

Triamcinolone Acetonide (Concurrent use with sodium phosphate may result in hypernatremia). Products include:

Aristocort A 0.025% Cream 1027
Aristocort A 0.5% Cream 1031
Aristocort A 0.1% Cream 1029
Aristocort A 0.1% Ointment 1030
Azmacort Oral Inhaler 2011
Nasacort Nasal Inhaler 2024

Triamcinolone Diacetate (Concurrent use with sodium phosphate may result in hypernatremia). Products include:

Aristocort Suspension (Forte Parenteral) 1027
Aristocort Suspension (Intralesional) 1025

Triamcinolone Hexacetonide (Concurrent use with sodium phosphate may result in hypernatremia). Products include:

Aristospan Suspension (Intra-articular) 1033
Aristospan Suspension (Intralesional) 1032

URSINUS INLAY-TABS

(Aspirin, Pseudoephedrine Hydrochloride) ..... ◘ 794

May interact with oral anticoagulants, monoamine oxidase inhibitors, and certain other agents. Compounds in these categories include:

Antiarthritic Drugs, unspecified (Effect not specified).

Antidiabetic Drugs, unspecified (Effect not specified).

Antigout Drugs, unspecified (Effect not specified).

Dicumarol (Effect not specified).

No products indexed under this heading.

Furazolidone (Concurrent and/or sequential use is not recommended). Products include:

Furoxone 2046

Isocarboxazid (Concurrent and/or sequential use is not recommended).

No products indexed under this heading.

Phenelzine Sulfate (Concurrent and/or sequential use is not recommended). Products include:

Nardil 1920

Selegiline Hydrochloride (Concurrent and/or sequential use is not recommended). Products include:

Eldepryl Tablets 2550

Tranylcypromine Sulfate (Concurrent and/or sequential use is not recommended). Products include:

Parnate Tablets 2503

Warfarin Sodium (Effect not specified). Products include:

Coumadin 926

IMPORTANT NOTE: Always consult each drug listing in the patient's regimen for possible interactions.

VAGISTAT-1

(Tioconazole) 778

May interact with:

Rubber or latex products (The Vagistat ointment base may interact with rubber or latex products, such as condoms or vaginal contraceptive diaphragms; therefore, use of such products within 72 hours following treatment is not recommended).

VALIUM INJECTABLE

(Diazepam) 2182

May interact with barbiturates, anticonvulsants, phenothiazines, narcotic analgesics, monoamine oxidase inhibitors, tricyclic antidepressants, central nervous system depressants, and certain other agents. Compounds in these categories include:

Alfentanil Hydrochloride (Potentiated action of Valium; increased depression/apnea). Products include:

Alfenta Injection 1286

Alprazolam (Increased depression/apnea). Products include:

Xanax Tablets 2649

Amitriptyline Hydrochloride (Potentiated action of Valium). Products include:

Elavil	2838
Endep Tablets	2174
Etrafon	2355
Limbitrol	2180
Triavil Tablets	1757

Amoxapine (Potentiated action of Valium). Products include:

Asendin Tablets 1369

Aprobarbital (Increased depression/apnea; hypotension/muscular weakness; potentiated action of Valium).

No products indexed under this heading.

Buprenorphine (Potentiated action of Valium; increased depression/apnea). Products include:

Buprenex Injectable 2006

Buspirone Hydrochloride (Increased depression/apnea). Products include:

BuSpar 737

Butabarbital (Increased depression/apnea; hypotension/muscular weakness; potentiated action of Valium).

No products indexed under this heading.

Butalbital (Increased depression/apnea; hypotension/muscular weakness; potentiated action of Valium). Products include:

Esgic-plus Tablets	1013
Fioricet Tablets	2258
Fioricet with Codeine Capsules	2260
Fiorinal Capsules	2261
Fiorinal with Codeine Capsules	2262
Fiorinal Tablets	2261
Phrenilin	785
Sedapap Tablets 50 mg/650 mg	1543

Carbamazepine (Potentiated action of Valium). Products include:

Atretol Tablets	573
Tegretol Chewable Tablets	852
Tegretol Suspension	852
Tegretol Tablets	852

Chlordiazepoxide (Potentiated action of Valium; increased depression/apnea). Products include:

Libritabs Tablets	2177
Limbitrol	2180

Chlordiazepoxide Hydrochloride (Potentiated action of Valium; increased depression/apnea). Products include:

Librax Capsules	2176
Librium Capsules	2178
Librium Injectable	2179

Chlorpromazine (Potentiated action of Valium; increased depression/apnea). Products include:

Thorazine Suppositories 2523

Chlorprothixene (Potentiated action of Valium; increased depression/apnea).

No products indexed under this heading.

Chlorprothixene Hydrochloride (Potentiated action of Valium; increased depression/apnea).

No products indexed under this heading.

Cimetidine (Delayed Valium clearance). Products include:

Tagamet Tablets 2516

Cimetidine Hydrochloride (Delayed Valium clearance). Products include:

Tagamet.. 2516

Clomipramine Hydrochloride (Potentiated action of Valium). Products include:

Anafranil Capsules 803

Clorazepate Dipotassium (Increased depression/apnea). Products include:

Tranxene 451

Clozapine (Potentiated action of Valium; increased depression/apnea). Products include:

Clozaril Tablets..................................... 2252

Codeine Phosphate (Potentiated action of Valium; increased depression/apnea). Products include:

Actifed with Codeine Cough Syrup..	1067
Brontex	1981
Deconsal C Expectorant Syrup	456
Deconsal Pediatric Syrup	457
Dimetane-DC Cough Syrup	2059
Empirin with Codeine Tablets	1093
Fioricet with Codeine Capsules	2260
Fiorinal with Codeine Capsules	2262
Isoclor Expectorant	990
Novahistine DH	2462
Novahistine Expectorant	2463
Nucofed	2051
Phenergan with Codeine	2777
Phenergan VC with Codeine	2781
Robitussin A-C Syrup	2073
Robitussin-DAC Syrup	2074
Ryna	◆D 841
Soma Compound w/Codeine Tablets	2676
Tussi-Organidin NR Liquid and S NR Liquid	2677
Tylenol with Codeine	1583

Desflurane (Potentiated action of Valium; increased depression/apnea). Products include:

Suprane 1813

Desipramine Hydrochloride (Potentiated action of Valium). Products include:

Norpramin Tablets 1526

Dezocine (Potentiated action of Valium; increased depression/apnea). Products include:

Dalgan Injection 538

Divalproex Sodium (Potentiated action of Valium). Products include:

Depakote Tablets.................................. 415

Doxepin Hydrochloride (Potentiated action of Valium). Products include:

Sinequan	2205
Zonalon Cream	1055

Droperidol (Increased depression/apnea). Products include:

Inapsine Injection................................. 1296

Enflurane (Increased depression/apnea).

No products indexed under this heading.

Estazolam (Potentiated action of Valium; increased depression/apnea). Products include:

ProSom Tablets 449

Ethchlorvynol (Increased depression/apnea). Products include:

Placidyl Capsules.................................. 448

Ethinamate (Increased depression/apnea).

No products indexed under this heading.

Ethosuximide (Potentiated action of Valium). Products include:

Zarontin Capsules	1928
Zarontin Syrup	1929

Ethotoin (Potentiated action of Valium). Products include:

Peganone Tablets 446

Felbamate (Potentiated action of Valium). Products include:

Felbatol 2666

Fentanyl (Potentiated action of Valium; increased depression/apnea). Products include:

Duragesic Transdermal System......... 1288

Fentanyl Citrate (Potentiated action of Valium; increased depression/apnea). Products include:

Sublimaze Injection.............................. 1307

Fluphenazine Decanoate (Potentiated action of Valium; increased depression/apnea). Products include:

Prolixin Decanoate 509

Fluphenazine Enanthate (Potentiated action of Valium; increased depression/apnea). Products include:

Prolixin Enanthate 509

Fluphenazine Hydrochloride (Potentiated action of Valium; increased depression/apnea). Products include:

Prolixin 509

Flurazepam Hydrochloride (Increased depression/apnea). Products include:

Dalmane Capsules................................ 2173

Furazolidone (Potentiated action of Valium). Products include:

Furoxone 2046

Glutethimide (Increased depression/apnea).

No products indexed under this heading.

Haloperidol (Increased depression/apnea). Products include:

Haldol Injection, Tablets and Concentrate 1575

Haloperidol Decanoate (Increased depression/apnea). Products include:

Haldol Decanoate................................. 1577

Hydrocodone Bitartrate (Potentiated action of Valium; increased depression/apnea). Products include:

Anexsia 5/500 Elixir	1781
Anexia Tablets	1782
Codiclear DH Syrup	791
Deconamine CX Cough and Cold Liquid and Tablets	1319
Duratuss HD Elixir	2565
Hycodan Tablets and Syrup	930
Hycomine Compound Tablets	932
Hycomine	931
Hycotuss Expectorant Syrup	933
Hydrocet Capsules	782
Lorcet 10/650	1018
Lortab	2566
Tussend	1783
Tussend Expectorant	1785
Vicodin Tablets	1356
Vicodin ES Tablets	1357
Vicodin Tuss Expectorant	1358
Zydone Capsules	949

Hydrocodone Polistirex (Potentiated action of Valium; increased depression/apnea). Products include:

Tussionex Pennkinetic Extended-Release Suspension 998

Hydroxyzine Hydrochloride (Increased depression/apnea). Products include:

Atarax Tablets & Syrup	2185
Marax Tablets & DF Syrup	2200
Vistaril Intramuscular Solution	2216

Imipramine Hydrochloride (Potentiated action of Valium). Products include:

Tofranil Ampuls	854
Tofranil Tablets	856

Imipramine Pamoate (Potentiated action of Valium). Products include:

Tofranil-PM Capsules........................... 857

Isocarboxazid (Potentiated action of Valium).

No products indexed under this heading.

Isoflurane (Increased depression/apnea).

No products indexed under this heading.

Ketamine Hydrochloride (Potentiated action of Valium; increased depression/apnea).

No products indexed under this heading.

Lamotrigine (Potentiated action of Valium). Products include:

Lamictal Tablets.................................... 1112

Levomethadyl Acetate Hydrochloride (Potentiated action of Valium; increased depression/apnea). Products include:

Orlamm 2239

Levorphanol Tartrate (Potentiated action of Valium; increased depression/apnea). Products include:

Levo-Dromoran 2129

Lorazepam (Increased depression/apnea). Products include:

Ativan Injection	2698
Ativan Tablets	2700

Loxapine Hydrochloride (Increased depression/apnea). Products include:

Loxitane 1378

Loxapine Succinate (Potentiated action of Valium; increased depression/apnea). Products include:

Loxitane Capsules 1378

Maprotiline Hydrochloride (Potentiated action of Valium). Products include:

Ludiomil Tablets................................... 843

Meperidine Hydrochloride (Potentiated action of Valium; increased depression/apnea). Products include:

Demerol	2308
Mepergan Injection	2753

Mephenytoin (Potentiated action of Valium). Products include:

Mesantoin Tablets................................. 2272

Mephobarbital (Increased depression/apnea; hypotension/muscular weakness; potentiated action of Valium). Products include:

Mebaral Tablets 2322

Meprobamate (Increased depression/apnea). Products include:

Miltown Tablets	2672
PMB 200 and PMB 400	2783

Mesoridazine Besylate (Potentiated action of Valium; increased depression/apnea). Products include:

Serentil 684

Methadone Hydrochloride (Potentiated action of Valium; increased depression/apnea). Products include:

Methadone Hydrochloride Oral Concentrate	2233
Methadone Hydrochloride Oral Solution & Tablets	2235

Interactions Index — Valium Tablets

Methohexital Sodium (Increased depression/apnea). Products include:

Brevital Sodium Vials 1429

Methotrimeprazine (Potentiated action of Valium; increased depression/apnea). Products include:

Levoprome 1274

Methoxyflurane (Increased depression/apnea).

No products indexed under this heading.

Methsuximide (Potentiated action of Valium). Products include:

Celontin Kapseals 1899

Midazolam Hydrochloride (Increased depression/apnea; potentiated action of Valium). Products include:

Versed Injection 2170

Molindone Hydrochloride (Increased depression/apnea). Products include:

Moban Tablets and Concentrate 1048

Morphine Sulfate (Potentiated action of Valium; increased depression/apnea). Products include:

Astramorph/PF Injection, USP (Preservative-Free) 535

Duramorph 962

Infumorph 200 and Infumorph 500 Sterile Solutions 965

MS Contin Tablets 1994

MSIR 1997

Oramorph SR (Morphine Sulfate Sustained Release Tablets) 2236

RMS Suppositories 2657

Roxanol 2243

Nortriptyline Hydrochloride (Potentiated action of Valium). Products include:

Pamelor 2280

Opium Alkaloids (Potentiated action of Valium; increased depression/apnea).

No products indexed under this heading.

Oxazepam (Increased depression/apnea). Products include:

Serax Capsules 2810

Serax Tablets 2810

Oxycodone Hydrochloride (Potentiated action of Valium; increased depression/apnea). Products include:

Percocet Tablets 938

Percodan Tablets 939

Percodan-Demi Tablets 940

Roxicodone Tablets, Oral Solution & Intensol (Oxycodone) 2244

Tylox Capsules 1584

Paramethadione (Potentiated action of Valium).

No products indexed under this heading.

Pentobarbital Sodium (Increased depression/apnea; hypotension/muscular weakness; potentiated action of Valium). Products include:

Nembutal Sodium Capsules 436

Nembutal Sodium Solution 438

Nembutal Sodium Suppositories 440

Perphenazine (Potentiated action of Valium; increased depression/apnea). Products include:

Etrafon 2355

Triavil Tablets 1757

Trilafon 2389

Phenacemide (Potentiated action of Valium). Products include:

Phenurone Tablets 447

Phenelzine Sulfate (Potentiated action of Valium). Products include:

Nardil 1920

Phenobarbital (Increased depression/apnea; hypotension/muscular weakness; potentiated action of Valium). Products include:

Arco-Lase Plus Tablets 512

Bellergal-S Tablets 2250

Donnatal 2060

Donnatal Extentabs 2061

Donnatal Tablets 2060

Phenobarbital Elixir and Tablets 1469

Quadrinal Tablets 1350

Phensuximide (Potentiated action of Valium). Products include:

Milontin Kapseals 1920

Phenytoin (Potentiated action of Valium). Products include:

Dilantin Infatabs 1908

Dilantin-125 Suspension 1911

Phenytoin Sodium (Potentiated action of Valium). Products include:

Dilantin Kapseals 1906

Dilantin Parenteral 1910

Prazepam (Increased depression/apnea).

No products indexed under this heading.

Primidone (Potentiated action of Valium). Products include:

Mysoline 2754

Prochlorperazine (Potentiated action of Valium; increased depression/apnea). Products include:

Compazine 2470

Promethazine Hydrochloride (Potentiated action of Valium; increased depression/apnea). Products include:

Mepergan Injection 2753

Phenergan with Codeine 2777

Phenergan with Dextromethorphan 2778

Phenergan Injection 2773

Phenergan Suppositories 2775

Phenergan Syrup 2774

Phenergan Tablets 2775

Phenergan VC 2779

Phenergan VC with Codeine 2781

Propofol (Potentiated action of Valium; increased depression/apnea). Products include:

Diprivan Injection 2833

Propoxyphene Hydrochloride (Potentiated action of Valium; increased depression/apnea). Products include:

Darvon 1435

Wygesic Tablets 2827

Propoxyphene Napsylate (Potentiated action of Valium; increased depression/apnea). Products include:

Darvon-N/Darvocet-N 1433

Protriptyline Hydrochloride (Potentiated action of Valium). Products include:

Vivactil Tablets 1774

Quazepam (Potentiated action of Valium; increased depression/apnea). Products include:

Doral Tablets 2664

Risperidone (Potentiated action of Valium; increased depression/apnea). Products include:

Risperdal 1301

Secobarbital Sodium (Increased depression/apnea; hypotension/muscular weakness; potentiated action of Valium). Products include:

Seconal Sodium Pulvules 1474

Selegiline Hydrochloride (Potentiated action of Valium). Products include:

Eldepryl Tablets 2550

Sufentanil Citrate (Potentiated action of Valium; increased depression/apnea). Products include:

Sufenta Injection 1309

Temazepam (Increased depression/apnea). Products include:

Restoril Capsules 2284

Thiamylal Sodium (Increased depression/apnea; hypotension/muscular weakness; potentiated action of Valium).

No products indexed under this heading.

Thioridazine Hydrochloride (Potentiated action of Valium; increased depression/apnea). Products include:

Mellaril 2269

Thiothixene (Increased depression/apnea). Products include:

Navane Capsules and Concentrate 2201

Navane Intramuscular 2202

Tranylcypromine Sulfate (Potentiated action of Valium). Products include:

Parnate Tablets 2503

Triazolam (Increased depression/apnea). Products include:

Halcion Tablets 2611

Trifluoperazine Hydrochloride (Potentiated action of Valium; increased depression/apnea). Products include:

Stelazine 2514

Trimethadione (Potentiated action of Valium).

No products indexed under this heading.

Trimipramine Maleate (Potentiated action of Valium). Products include:

Surmontil Capsules 2811

Valproic Acid (Potentiated action of Valium). Products include:

Depakene 413

Zolpidem Tartrate (Potentiated action of Valium; increased depression/apnea). Products include:

Ambien Tablets 2416

Food Interactions

Alcohol (Increased depression/apnea; hypotension/muscular weakness).

VALIUM TABLETS

(Diazepam) 2183

May interact with anticonvulsants, phenothiazines, narcotic analgesics, barbiturates, monoamine oxidase inhibitors, tricyclic antidepressants, central nervous system depressants, and certain other agents. Compounds in these categories include:

Alfentanil Hydrochloride (Potentiated action of Valium; concurrent use not recommended). Products include:

Alfenta Injection 1286

Alprazolam (Concurrent use not recommended). Products include:

Xanax Tablets 2649

Amitriptyline Hydrochloride (Potentiated action of Valium). Products include:

Elavil 2838

Endep Tablets 2174

Etrafon 2355

Limbitrol 2180

Triavil Tablets 1757

Amoxapine (Potentiated action of Valium). Products include:

Asendin Tablets 1369

Aprobarbital (Potentiated action of Valium; concurrent use not recommended).

No products indexed under this heading.

Buprenorphine (Potentiated action of Valium; concurrent use not recommended). Products include:

Buprenex Injectable 2006

Buspirone Hydrochloride (Concurrent use not recommended). Products include:

BuSpar 737

Butabarbital (Potentiated action of Valium; concurrent use not recommended).

No products indexed under this heading.

Butalbital (Potentiated action of Valium; concurrent use not recommended). Products include:

Esgic-plus Tablets 1013

Fioricet Tablets 2258

Fioricet with Codeine Capsules 2260

Fiorinal Capsules 2261

Fiorinal with Codeine Capsules 2262

Fiorinal Tablets 2261

Phrenilin 785

Sedapap Tablets 50 mg/650 mg .. 1543

Carbamazepine (Increase in dosage may be required). Products include:

Atretol Tablets 573

Tegretol Chewable Tablets 852

Tegretol Suspension 852

Tegretol Tablets 852

Chlordiazepoxide (Potentiated action of Valium; concurrent use not recommended). Products include:

Libritabs Tablets 2177

Limbitrol 2180

Chlordiazepoxide Hydrochloride (Potentiated action of Valium; concurrent use not recommended). Products include:

Librax Capsules 2176

Librium Capsules 2178

Librium Injectable 2179

Chlorpromazine (Potentiated action of Valium; concurrent use not recommended). Products include:

Thorazine Suppositories 2523

Chlorprothixene (Concurrent use not recommended).

No products indexed under this heading.

Chlorprothixene Hydrochloride (Concurrent use not recommended).

No products indexed under this heading.

Cimetidine (Delayed Valium clearance). Products include:

Tagamet Tablets 2516

Cimetidine Hydrochloride (Delayed Valium clearance). Products include:

Tagamet 2516

Clomipramine Hydrochloride (Potentiated action of Valium). Products include:

Anafranil Capsules 803

Clorazepate Dipotassium (Concurrent use not recommended). Products include:

Tranxene 451

Clozapine (Potentiated action of Valium; concurrent use not recommended). Products include:

Clozaril Tablets 2252

Codeine Phosphate (Potentiated action of Valium; concurrent use not recommended). Products include:

Actifed with Codeine Cough Syrup.. 1067

Brontex 1981

Deconsal C Expectorant Syrup 456

Deconsal Pediatric Syrup 457

Dimetane-DC Cough Syrup 2059

Empirin with Codeine Tablets 1093

Fioricet with Codeine Capsules 2260

Fiorinal with Codeine Capsules 2262

Isoclor Expectorant 990

Novahistine DH 2462

Novahistine Expectorant 2463

Nucofed 2051

Phenergan with Codeine 2777

Phenergan VC with Codeine 2781

Robitussin A-C Syrup 2073

Robitussin-DAC Syrup 2074

Ryna .... ◆◻ 841

Soma Compound w/Codeine Tablets 2676

Tussi-Organidin NR Liquid and S NR Liquid 2677

Tylenol with Codeine 1583

Desflurane (Potentiated action of Valium; concurrent use not recommended). Products include:

Suprane 1813

IMPORTANT NOTE: Always consult each drug listing in the patient's regimen for possible interactions.

Valium Tablets

Interactions Index

Desipramine Hydrochloride (Potentiated action of Valium). Products include:

Norpramin Tablets 1526

Dezocine (Potentiated action of Valium; concurrent use not recommended). Products include:

Dalgan Injection 538

Divalproex Sodium (Increase in dosage may be required). Products include:

Depakote Tablets..................................... 415

Doxepin Hydrochloride (Potentiated action of Valium). Products include:

Sinequan 2205
Zonalon Cream 1055

Droperidol (Concurrent use not recommended). Products include:

Inapsine Injection.................................... 1296

Enflurane (Concurrent use not recommended).

No products indexed under this heading.

Estazolam (Potentiated action of Valium; concurrent use not recommended). Products include:

ProSom Tablets 449

Ethchlorvynol (Concurrent use not recommended). Products include:

Placidyl Capsules.................................... 448

Ethinamate (Concurrent use not recommended).

No products indexed under this heading.

Ethosuximide (Increase in dosage may be required). Products include:

Zarontin Capsules 1928
Zarontin Syrup 1929

Ethotoin (Increase in dosage may be required). Products include:

Peganone Tablets 446

Felbamate (Increase in dosage may be required). Products include:

Felbatol 2666

Fentanyl (Potentiated action of Valium; concurrent use not recommended). Products include:

Duragesic Transdermal System........ 1288

Fentanyl Citrate (Potentiated action of Valium; concurrent use not recommended). Products include:

Sublimaze Injection................................. 1307

Fluphenazine Decanoate (Potentiated action of Valium; concurrent use not recommended). Products include:

Prolixin Decanoate 509

Fluphenazine Enanthate (Potentiated action of Valium; concurrent use not recommended). Products include:

Prolixin Enanthate 509

Fluphenazine Hydrochloride (Potentiated action of Valium; concurrent use not recommended). Products include:

Prolixin 509

Flurazepam Hydrochloride (Concurrent use not recommended). Products include:

Dalmane Capsules................................... 2173

Furazolidone (Potentiated action of Valium). Products include:

Furoxone 2046

Glutethimide (Concurrent use not recommended).

No products indexed under this heading.

Haloperidol (Concurrent use not recommended). Products include:

Haldol Injection, Tablets and Concentrate 1575

Haloperidol Decanoate (Concurrent use not recommended). Products include:

Haldol Decanoate.................................... 1577

Hydrocodone Bitartrate (Potentiated action of Valium; concurrent use not recommended). Products include:

Anexsia 5/500 Elixir 1781
Anexia Tablets... 1782
Codiclear DH Syrup 791
Deconamine CX Cough and Cold Liquid and Tablets.................................... 1319
Duratuss HD Elixir 2565
Hycodan Tablets and Syrup 930
Hycomine Compound Tablets 932
Hycomine 931
Hycotuss Expectorant Syrup 933
Hydrocet Capsules 782
Lorcet 10/650.. 1018
Lortab 2566
Tussend 1783
Tussend Expectorant 1785
Vicodin Tablets.. 1356
Vicodin ES Tablets 1357
Vicodin Tuss Expectorant 1358
Zydone Capsules 949

Hydrocodone Polistirex (Potentiated action of Valium; concurrent use not recommended). Products include:

Tussionex Pennkinetic Extended-Release Suspension 998

Hydroxyzine Hydrochloride (Concurrent use not recommended). Products include:

Atarax Tablets & Syrup........................... 2185
Marax Tablets & DF Syrup...................... 2200
Vistaril Intramuscular Solution......... 2216

Imipramine Hydrochloride (Potentiated action of Valium). Products include:

Tofranil Ampuls 854
Tofranil Tablets 856

Imipramine Pamoate (Potentiated action of Valium). Products include:

Tofranil-PM Capsules.............................. 857

Isocarboxazid (Potentiated action of Valium).

No products indexed under this heading.

Isoflurane (Concurrent use not recommended).

No products indexed under this heading.

Ketamine Hydrochloride (Potentiated action of Valium; concurrent use not recommended).

No products indexed under this heading.

Lamotrigine (Increase in dosage may be required). Products include:

Lamictal Tablets 1112

Levomethadyl Acetate Hydrochloride (Potentiated action of Valium; concurrent use not recommended). Products include:

Orlaam 2239

Levorphanol Tartrate (Potentiated action of Valium; concurrent use not recommended). Products include:

Levo-Dromoran.. 2129

Lorazepam (Potentiated action of Valium; concurrent use not recommended). Products include:

Ativan Injection....................................... 2698
Ativan Tablets 2700

Loxapine Hydrochloride (Potentiated action of Valium; concurrent use not recommended). Products include:

Loxitane 1378

Loxapine Succinate (Potentiated action of Valium; concurrent use not recommended). Products include:

Loxitane Capsules 1378

Maprotiline Hydrochloride (Potentiated action of Valium). Products include:

Ludiomil Tablets...................................... 843

Meperidine Hydrochloride (Potentiated action of Valium; concurrent use not recommended). Products include:

Demerol 2308
Mepergan Injection 2753

Mephenytoin (Increase in dosage may be required). Products include:

Mesantoin Tablets.................................... 2272

Mephobarbital (Potentiated action of Valium; concurrent use not recommended). Products include:

Mebaral Tablets 2322

Meprobamate (Concurrent use not recommended). Products include:

Miltown Tablets 2672
PMB 200 and PMB 400 2783

Mesoridazine Besylate (Potentiated action of Valium; concurrent use not recommended). Products include:

Serentil 684

Methadone Hydrochloride (Potentiated action of Valium; concurrent use not recommended). Products include:

Methadone Hydrochloride Oral Concentrate 2233
Methadone Hydrochloride Oral Solution & Tablets.................................... 2235

Methohexital Sodium (Concurrent use not recommended). Products include:

Brevital Sodium Vials.............................. 1429

Methotrimeprazine (Potentiated action of Valium; concurrent use not recommended). Products include:

Levoprome 1274

Methoxyflurane (Concurrent use not recommended).

No products indexed under this heading.

Methsuximide (Increase in dosage may be required). Products include:

Celontin Kapseals 1899

Midazolam Hydrochloride (Potentiated action of Valium; concurrent use not recommended). Products include:

Versed Injection 2170

Molindone Hydrochloride (Concurrent use not recommended). Products include:

Moban Tablets and Concentrate...... 1048

Morphine Sulfate (Potentiated action of Valium; concurrent use not recommended). Products include:

Astramorph/PF Injection, USP (Preservative-Free) 535
Duramorph... 962
Infumorph 200 and Infumorph 500 Sterile Solutions.......................... 965
MS Contin Tablets................................... 1994
MSIR 1997
Oramorph SR (Morphine Sulfate Sustained Release Tablets) 2236
RMS Suppositories 2657
Roxanol 2243

Nortriptyline Hydrochloride (Potentiated action of Valium). Products include:

Pamelor 2280

Opium Alkaloids (Potentiated action of Valium; concurrent use not recommended).

No products indexed under this heading.

Oxazepam (Concurrent use not recommended). Products include:

Serax Capsules 2810
Serax Tablets... 2810

Oxycodone Hydrochloride (Potentiated action of Valium; concurrent use not recommended). Products include:

Percocet Tablets 938
Percodan Tablets..................................... 939
Percodan-Demi Tablets........................... 940
Roxicodone Tablets, Oral Solution & Intensol (Oxycodone) 2244
Tylox Capsules 1584

Paramethadione (Increase in dosage may be required).

No products indexed under this heading.

Pentobarbital Sodium (Potentiated action of Valium; concurrent use not recommended). Products include:

Nembutal Sodium Capsules 436
Nembutal Sodium Solution 438
Nembutal Sodium Suppositories...... 440

Perphenazine (Potentiated action of Valium; concurrent use not recommended). Products include:

Etrafon 2355
Triavil Tablets 1757
Trilafon... 2389

Phenacemide (Increase in dosage may be required). Products include:

Phenurone Tablets 447

Phenelzine Sulfate (Potentiated action of Valium). Products include:

Nardil 1920

Phenobarbital (Increase in dosage may be required; concurrent use not recommended). Products include:

Arco-Lase Plus Tablets 512
Bellergal-S Tablets 2250
Donnatal 2060
Donnatal Extentabs................................. 2061
Donnatal Tablets 2060
Phenobarbital Elixir and Tablets 1469
Quadrinal Tablets 1350

Phensuximide (Increase in dosage may be required). Products include:

Milontin Kapseals.................................... 1920

Phenytoin (Increase in dosage may be required). Products include:

Dilantin Infatabs...................................... 1908
Dilantin-125 Suspension 1911

Phenytoin Sodium (Increase in dosage may be required). Products include:

Dilantin Kapseals 1906
Dilantin Parenteral 1910

Prazepam (Concurrent use not recommended).

No products indexed under this heading.

Primidone (Increase in dosage may be required). Products include:

Mysoline... 2754

Prochlorperazine (Potentiated action of Valium; concurrent use not recommended). Products include:

Compazine 2470

Promethazine Hydrochloride (Potentiated action of Valium; concurrent use not recommended). Products include:

Mepergan Injection 2753
Phenergan with Codeine......................... 2777
Phenergan with Dextromethorphan 2778
Phenergan Injection 2773
Phenergan Suppositories 2775
Phenergan Syrup 2774
Phenergan Tablets 2775
Phenergan VC 2779
Phenergan VC with Codeine 2781

Propofol (Potentiated action of Valium; concurrent use not recommended). Products include:

Diprivan Injection.................................... 2833

Propoxyphene Hydrochloride (Potentiated action of Valium; concurrent use not recommended). Products include:

Darvon 1435
Wygesic Tablets 2827

Propoxyphene Napsylate (Potentiated action of Valium; concurrent use not recommended). Products include:

Darvon-N/Darvocet-N 1433

Interactions Index

Valrelease

Protriptyline Hydrochloride (Potentiated action of Valium). Products include:

Vivactil Tablets 1774

Quazepam (Potentiated action of Valium; concurrent use not recommended). Products include:

Doral Tablets 2664

Risperidone (Potentiated action of Valium; concurrent use not recommended). Products include:

Risperdal 1301

Secobarbital Sodium (Potentiated action of Valium; concurrent use not recommended). Products include:

Seconal Sodium Pulvules 1474

Selegiline Hydrochloride (Potentiated action of Valium). Products include:

Eldepryl Tablets 2550

Sufentanil Citrate (Potentiated action of Valium; concurrent use not recommended). Products include:

Sufenta Injection 1309

Temazepam (Concurrent use not recommended). Products include:

Restoril Capsules 2284

Thiamylal Sodium (Potentiated action of Valium; concurrent use not recommended).

No products indexed under this heading.

Thioridazine Hydrochloride (Potentiated action of Valium; concurrent use not recommended). Products include:

Mellaril 2269

Thiothixene (Concurrent use not recommended). Products include:

Navane Capsules and Concentrate 2201
Navane Intramuscular 2202

Tranylcypromine Sulfate (Potentiated action of Valium). Products include:

Parnate Tablets 2503

Triazolam (Concurrent use not recommended). Products include:

Halcion Tablets.................................. 2611

Trifluoperazine Hydrochloride (Potentiated action of Valium; concurrent use not recommended). Products include:

Stelazine 2514

Trimethadione (Increase in dosage may be required).

No products indexed under this heading.

Trimipramine Maleate (Potentiated action of Valium). Products include:

Surmontil Capsules........................... 2811

Valproic Acid (Increase in dosage may be required). Products include:

Depakene 413

Zolpidem Tartrate (Potentiated action of Valium; concurrent use not recommended). Products include:

Ambien Tablets.................................. 2416

Food Interactions

Alcohol (Simultaneous use of alcohol not recommended).

VALRELEASE CAPSULES

(Diazepam) 2169

May interact with phenothiazines, narcotic analgesics, barbiturates, monoamine oxidase inhibitors, tricyclic antidepressants, and certain other agents. Compounds in these categories include:

Alfentanil Hydrochloride (Potentiates action of diazepam). Products include:

Alfenta Injection 1286

Amitriptyline Hydrochloride (Potentiates action of diazepam). Products include:

Elavil 2838
Endep Tablets 2174
Etrafon 2355
Limbitrol 2180
Triavil Tablets 1757

Amoxapine (Potentiates action of diazepam). Products include:

Asendin Tablets 1369

Aprobarbital (Potentiates action of diazepam).

No products indexed under this heading.

Buprenorphine (Potentiates action of diazepam). Products include:

Buprenex Injectable 2006

Butabarbital (Potentiates action of diazepam).

No products indexed under this heading.

Butalbital (Potentiates action of diazepam). Products include:

Esgic-plus Tablets 1013
Fioricet Tablets 2258
Fioricet with Codeine Capsules 2260
Fiorinal Capsules 2261
Fiorinal with Codeine Capsules 2262
Fiorinal Tablets 2261
Phrenilin 785
Sedapap Tablets 50 mg/650 mg .. 1543

Chlorpromazine (Potentiates action of diazepam). Products include:

Thorazine Suppositories 2523

Cimetidine (Delays clearance of diazepam). Products include:

Tagamet Tablets 2516

Cimetidine Hydrochloride (Delays clearance of diazepam). Products include:

Tagamet.. 2516

Clomipramine Hydrochloride (Potentiates action of diazepam). Products include:

Anafranil Capsules 803

Codeine Phosphate (Potentiates action of diazepam). Products include:

Actifed with Codeine Cough Syrup.. 1067
Brontex 1981
Deconsal C Expectorant Syrup 456
Deconsal Pediatric Syrup 457
Dimetane-DC Cough Syrup 2059
Empirin with Codeine Tablets........... 1093
Fioricet with Codeine Capsules 2260
Fiorinal with Codeine Capsules 2262
Isoclor Expectorant........................... 990
Novahistine DH................................. 2462
Novahistine Expectorant................... 2463
Nucofed 2051
Phenergan with Codeine................... 2777
Phenergan VC with Codeine 2781
Robitussin A-C Syrup........................ 2073
Robitussin-DAC Syrup 2074
Ryna .... ◆□ 841
Soma Compound w/Codeine Tablets 2676
Tussi-Organidin NR Liquid and S NR Liquid 2677
Tylenol with Codeine 1583

Desipramine Hydrochloride (Potentiates action of diazepam). Products include:

Norpramin Tablets 1526

Dezocine (Potentiates action of diazepam). Products include:

Dalgan Injection 538

Doxepin Hydrochloride (Potentiates action of diazepam). Products include:

Sinequan 2205
Zonalon Cream 1055

Fentanyl (Potentiates action of diazepam). Products include:

Duragesic Transdermal System........ 1288

Fentanyl Citrate (Potentiates action of diazepam). Products include:

Sublimaze Injection........................... 1307

Fluphenazine Decanoate (Potentiates action of diazepam). Products include:

Prolixin Decanoate 509

Fluphenazine Enanthate (Potentiates action of diazepam). Products include:

Prolixin Enanthate 509

Fluphenazine Hydrochloride (Potentiates action of diazepam). Products include:

Prolixin 509

Furazolidone (Potentiates action of diazepam). Products include:

Furoxone 2046

Hydrocodone Bitartrate (Potentiates action of diazepam). Products include:

Anexsia 5/500 Elixir 1781
Anexia Tablets................................... 1782
Codiclear DH Syrup 791
Deconamine CX Cough and Cold Liquid and Tablets............................. 1319
Duratuss HD Elixir............................ 2565
Hycodan Tablets and Syrup 930
Hycomine Compound Tablets 932
Hycomine 931
Hycotuss Expectorant Syrup 933
Hydrocet Capsules 782
Lorcet 10/650................................... 1018
Lortab 2566
Tussend 1783
Tussend Expectorant 1785
Vicodin Tablets.................................. 1356
Vicodin ES Tablets 1357
Vicodin Tuss Expectorant 1358
Zydone Capsules 949

Hydrocodone Polistirex (Potentiates action of diazepam). Products include:

Tussionex Pennkinetic Extended-Release Suspension 998

Imipramine Hydrochloride (Potentiates action of diazepam). Products include:

Tofranil Ampuls 854
Tofranil Tablets 856

Imipramine Pamoate (Potentiates action of diazepam). Products include:

Tofranil-PM Capsules........................ 857

Isocarboxazid (Potentiates action of diazepam).

No products indexed under this heading.

Levorphanol Tartrate (Potentiates action of diazepam). Products include:

Levo-Dromoran.................................. 2129

Maprotiline Hydrochloride (Potentiates action of diazepam). Products include:

Ludiomil Tablets................................ 843

Meperidine Hydrochloride (Potentiates action of diazepam). Products include:

Demerol 2308
Mepergan Injection 2753

Mephobarbital (Potentiates action of diazepam). Products include:

Mebaral Tablets 2322

Mesoridazine Besylate (Potentiates action of diazepam). Products include:

Serentil 684

Methadone Hydrochloride (Potentiates action of diazepam). Products include:

Methadone Hydrochloride Oral Concentrate 2233
Methadone Hydrochloride Oral Solution & Tablets.............................. 2235

Methotrimeprazine (Potentiates action of diazepam). Products include:

Levoprome 1274

Morphine Sulfate (Potentiates action of diazepam). Products include:

Astramorph/PF Injection, USP (Preservative-Free) 535
Duramorph 962
Infumorph 200 and Infumorph 500 Sterile Solutions......................... 965
MS Contin Tablets.............................. 1994
MSIR 1997
Oramorph SR (Morphine Sulfate Sustained Release Tablets) 2236
RMS Suppositories 2657
Roxanol 2243

Nortriptyline Hydrochloride (Potentiates action of diazepam). Products include:

Pamelor 2280

Opium Alkaloids (Potentiates action of diazepam).

No products indexed under this heading.

Oxycodone Hydrochloride (Potentiates action of diazepam). Products include:

Percocet Tablets 938
Percodan Tablets............................... 939
Percodan-Demi Tablets...................... 940
Roxicodone Tablets, Oral Solution & Intensol (Oxycodone) 2244
Tylox Capsules 1584

Pentobarbital Sodium (Potentiates action of diazepam). Products include:

Nembutal Sodium Capsules 436
Nembutal Sodium Solution 438
Nembutal Sodium Suppositories...... 440

Perphenazine (Potentiates action of diazepam). Products include:

Etrafon 2355
Triavil Tablets 1757
Trilafon.. 2389

Phenelzine Sulfate (Potentiates action of diazepam). Products include:

Nardil 1920

Phenobarbital (Potentiates action of diazepam). Products include:

Arco-Lase Plus Tablets 512
Bellergal-S Tablets 2250
Donnatal 2060
Donnatal Extentabs........................... 2061
Donnatal Tablets 2060
Phenobarbital Elixir and Tablets 1469
Quadrinal Tablets 1350

Prochlorperazine (Potentiates action of diazepam). Products include:

Compazine 2470

Promethazine Hydrochloride (Potentiates action of diazepam). Products include:

Mepergan Injection 2753
Phenergan with Codeine................... 2777
Phenergan with Dextromethorphan 2778
Phenergan Injection 2773
Phenergan Suppositories 2775
Phenergan Syrup............................... 2774
Phenergan Tablets 2775
Phenergan VC 2779
Phenergan VC with Codeine 2781

Propoxyphene Hydrochloride (Potentiates action of diazepam). Products include:

Darvon 1435
Wygesic Tablets 2827

Propoxyphene Napsylate (Potentiates action of diazepam). Products include:

Darvon-N/Darvocet-N 1433

Protriptyline Hydrochloride (Potentiates action of diazepam). Products include:

Vivactil Tablets 1774

Secobarbital Sodium (Potentiates action of diazepam). Products include:

Seconal Sodium Pulvules 1474

Selegiline Hydrochloride (Potentiates action of diazepam). Products include:

Eldepryl Tablets 2550

IMPORTANT NOTE: Always consult each drug listing in the patient's regimen for possible interactions.

Sufentanil Citrate (Potentiates action of diazepam). Products include:

Sufenta Injection 1309

Thiamylal Sodium (Potentiates action of diazepam).

No products indexed under this heading.

Thioridazine Hydrochloride (Potentiates action of diazepam). Products include:

Mellaril 2269

Tranylcypromine Sulfate (Potentiates action of diazepam). Products include:

Parnate Tablets 2503

Trifluoperazine Hydrochloride (Potentiates action of diazepam). Products include:

Stelazine 2514

Trimipramine Maleate (Potentiates action of diazepam). Products include:

Surmontil Capsules 2811

Food Interactions

Alcohol (Potentiates action of diazepam).

VALTREX CAPLETS

(Valacyclovir Hydrochloride) 1194

May interact with:

Cimetidine (Co-administration reduces the rate but not the extent of conversion of valacyclovir to acyclovir; additive increase in acyclovir AUC and C_{max}). Products include:

Tagamet Tablets 2516

Cimetidine Hydrochloride (Co-administration reduces the rate but not the extent of conversion of valacyclovir to acyclovir; additive increase in acyclovir AUC and C_{max}). Products include:

Tagamet 2516

Probenecid (Co-administration reduces the rate but not the extent of conversion of valacyclovir to acyclovir; additive increase in acyclovir AUC and C_{max}). Products include:

Benemid Tablets 1611
ColBENEMID Tablets 1622

VANCENASE AQ NASAL SPRAY 0.042%

(Beclomethasone Dipropionate) 2393

None cited in PDR database.

VANCENASE POCKETHALER NASAL INHALER

(Beclomethasone Dipropionate) 2391

May interact with:

Prednisone (Increased likelihood of HPA suppression). Products include:

Deltasone Tablets 2595

VANCERIL INHALER

(Beclomethasone Dipropionate) 2394

None cited in PDR database.

VANCOCIN HCL, ORAL SOLUTION & PULVULES

(Vancomycin Hydrochloride) 1483

May interact with aminoglycosides and ototoxic drugs. Compounds in these categories include:

Amikacin Sulfate (Concurrent use may result in increased ototoxicity and/or nephrotoxicity). Products include:

Amikacin Sulfate Injection, USP 960
Amikin Injectable 501

Cisplatin (Concurrent use may result in increased ototoxicity and/or nephrotoxicity). Products include:

Platinol 708
Platinol-AQ Injection 710

Gentamicin Sulfate (Concurrent use may result in increased ototoxicity and/or nephrotoxicity). Products include:

Garamycin Injectable 2360
Genoptic Sterile Ophthalmic Solution .... ⊙ 243
Genoptic Sterile Ophthalmic Ointment .... ⊙ 243
Gentacidin Ointment .... ⊙ 264
Gentacidin Solution .... ⊙ 264
Gentak .... ⊙ 208
Pred-G Liquifilm Sterile Ophthalmic Suspension .... ⊙ 251
Pred-G S.O.P. Sterile Ophthalmic Ointment .... ⊙ 252

Kanamycin Sulfate (Concurrent use may result in increased ototoxicity and/or nephrotoxicity).

No products indexed under this heading.

Streptomycin Sulfate (Concurrent use may result in increased ototoxicity and/or nephrotoxicity). Products include:

Streptomycin Sulfate Injection 2208

Tobramycin Sulfate (Concurrent use may result in increased ototoxicity and/or nephrotoxicity). Products include:

Nebcin Vials, Hyporets & ADD-Vantage 1464
Tobramycin Sulfate Injection 968

VANCOCIN HCL, VIALS & ADD-VANTAGE

(Vancomycin Hydrochloride) 1481

May interact with aminoglycosides, general anesthetics, and certain other agents. Compounds in these categories include:

Amikacin Sulfate (Concurrent use may result in increased ototoxicity). Products include:

Amikacin Sulfate Injection, USP 960
Amikin Injectable 501

Amphotericin B (Concurrent and/or sequential use requires careful monitoring due to increased potential for nephrotoxicity and/or neurotoxicity). Products include:

Fungizone Intravenous 506

Bacitracin Zinc (Concurrent and/or sequential use requires careful monitoring due to increased potential for nephrotoxicity and/or neurotoxicity). Products include:

AK-Spore Ointment .... ⊙ 204
Bactine First Aid Antibiotic Plus Anesthetic Ointment .... ▣ 708
Betadine Brand First Aid Antibiotics & Moisturizer Ointment 1991
Campho-Phenique Maximum Strength First Aid Antibiotic Plus Pain Reliever Ointment .... ▣ 719
Cortisporin Ointment 1085
Cortisporin Ophthalmic Ointment Sterile 1085
Neosporin Ointment .... ▣ 857
Neosporin Plus Maximum Strength Ointment .... ▣ 858
Neosporin Ophthalmic Ointment Sterile 1148
Polysporin Ointment .... ▣ 858
Polysporin Ophthalmic Ointment Sterile 1154
Polysporin Powder .... ▣ 859

Cisplatin (Concurrent and/or sequential use requires careful monitoring due to increased potential for nephrotoxicity and/or neurotoxicity). Products include:

Platinol 708
Platinol-AQ Injection 710

Colistin Sulfate (Concurrent and/or sequential use requires careful monitoring due to increased potential for nephrotoxicity and/or neurotoxicity). Products include:

Coly-Mycin S Otic w/Neomycin & Hydrocortisone 1906

Enflurane (Concomitant administration has been associated with erythema and histamine-like flushing).

No products indexed under this heading.

Gentamicin Sulfate (Concurrent use may result in increased ototoxicity). Products include:

Garamycin Injectable 2360
Genoptic Sterile Ophthalmic Solution .... ⊙ 243
Genoptic Sterile Ophthalmic Ointment .... ⊙ 243
Gentacidin Ointment .... ⊙ 264
Gentacidin Solution .... ⊙ 264
Gentak .... ⊙ 208
Pred-G Liquifilm Sterile Ophthalmic Suspension .... ⊙ 251
Pred-G S.O.P. Sterile Ophthalmic Ointment .... ⊙ 252

Isoflurane (Concomitant administration has been associated with erythema and histamine-like flushing).

No products indexed under this heading.

Kanamycin Sulfate (Concurrent use may result in increased ototoxicity).

No products indexed under this heading.

Ketamine Hydrochloride (Concomitant administration has been associated with erythema and histamine-like flushing).

No products indexed under this heading.

Methohexital Sodium (Concomitant administration has been associated with erythema and histamine-like flushing). Products include:

Brevital Sodium Vials 1429

Methoxyflurane (Concomitant administration has been associated with erythema and histamine-like flushing).

No products indexed under this heading.

Polymyxin B Sulfate (Concurrent and/or sequential use requires careful monitoring due to increased potential for nephrotoxicity and/or neurotoxicity). Products include:

AK-Spore .... ⊙ 204
AK-Trol Ointment & Suspension .... ⊙ 205
Bactine First Aid Antibiotic Plus Anesthetic Ointment .... ▣ 708
Betadine Brand First Aid Antibiotics & Moisturizer Ointment 1991
Campho-Phenique Maximum Strength First Aid Antibiotic Plus Pain Reliever Ointment .... ▣ 719
Cortisporin Cream 1084
Cortisporin Ointment 1085
Cortisporin Ophthalmic Ointment Sterile 1085
Cortisporin Ophthalmic Suspension Sterile 1086
Cortisporin Otic Solution Sterile 1087
Cortisporin Otic Suspension Sterile 1088
Dexacidin Ointment .... ⊙ 263
Maxitrol Ophthalmic Ointment and Suspension .... ⊙ 224
Mycitracin .... ▣ 839
Neosporin G.U. Irrigant Sterile 1148
Neosporin Ointment .... ▣ 857
Neosporin Plus Maximum Strength Cream .... ▣ 858
Neosporin Plus Maximum Strength Ointment .... ▣ 858
Neosporin Ophthalmic Ointment Sterile 1148
Neosporin Ophthalmic Solution Sterile 1149
Ophthocort .... ⊙ 311
PediOtic Suspension Sterile 1153
Polymyxin B Sulfate, Aerosporin Brand Sterile Powder 1154
Poly-Pred Liquifilm .... ⊙ 248
Polysporin Ointment .... ▣ 858
Polysporin Ophthalmic Ointment Sterile 1154
Polysporin Powder .... ▣ 859
Polytrim Ophthalmic Solution Sterile 482
TERAK Ointment .... ⊙ 209
Terramycin with Polymyxin B Sulfate Ophthalmic Ointment 2211

Propofol (Concomitant administration has been associated with erythema and histamine-like flushing). Products include:

Diprivan Injection 2833

Streptomycin Sulfate (Concurrent use may result in increased ototoxicity). Products include:

Streptomycin Sulfate Injection 2208

Tobramycin (Concurrent use may result in increased ototoxicity). Products include:

AKTOB .... ⊙ 206
TobraDex Ophthalmic Suspension and Ointment 473
Tobrex Ophthalmic Ointment and Solution .... ⊙ 229

Tobramycin Sulfate (Concurrent use may result in increased ototoxicity). Products include:

Nebcin Vials, Hyporets & ADD-Vantage 1464
Tobramycin Sulfate Injection 968

VANQUISH ANALGESIC CAPLETS

(Acetaminophen, Aspirin, Caffeine, Aluminum Hydroxide Gel, Magnesium Hydroxide) .... ▣ 731

May interact with oral anticoagulants and certain other agents. Compounds in these categories include:

Antiarthritic Drugs, unspecified (Effect not specified).

Antidiabetic Drugs, unspecified (Effect not specified).

Antigout Drugs, unspecified (Effect not specified).

Dicumarol (Concurrent use requires caution).

No products indexed under this heading.

Warfarin Sodium (Concurrent use requires caution). Products include:

Coumadin 926

VANTIN FOR ORAL SUSPENSION AND VANTIN TABLETS

(Cefpodoxime Proxetil) 2646

May interact with antacids, histamine h2-receptor antagonists, anticholinergics, and certain other agents. Compounds in these categories include:

Aluminum Carbonate Gel (High doses of antacids reduces peak plasma levels by 24% and the extent of absorption by 27%; the rate of absorption is not altered). Products include:

Basaljel 2703

Aluminum Hydroxide (High doses of antacids reduces peak plasma levels by 24% and the extent of absorption by 27%; the rate of absorption is not altered). Products include:

ALternaGEL Liquid 1316
Maximum Strength Ascriptin .... ▣ 630
Cama Arthritis Pain Reliever .... ▣ 785
Gaviscon Extra Strength Relief Formula Antacid Tablets .... ▣ 819
Gaviscon Extra Strength Relief Formula Liquid Antacid .... ▣ 819
Gaviscon Liquid Antacid .... ▣ 820
Gelusil Liquid & Tablets .... ▣ 855

(▣ Described in PDR For Nonprescription Drugs) (⊙ Described in PDR For Ophthalmology)

Interactions Index

Maalox Heartburn Relief Suspension .... ◆D 642
Maalox Heartburn Relief Tablets.... ◆D 641
Maalox Magnesia and Alumina Oral Suspension .... ◆D 642
Maalox Plus Tablets .... ◆D 643
Extra Strength Maalox Antacid Plus Antigas Liquid and Tablets ◆D 638
Tempo Soft Antacid .... ◆D 835

Aluminum Hydroxide Gel (High doses of antacids reduces peak plasma levels by 24% and the extent of absorption by 27%; the rate of absorption is not altered). Products include:

ALternaGEL Liquid .... ◆D 659
Aludrox Oral Suspension 2695
Amphojel Suspension 2695
Amphojel Suspension without Flavor 2695
Amphojel Tablets.................................. 2695
Arthritis Pain Ascriptin .... ◆D 631
Regular Strength Ascriptin Tablets .... ◆D 629
Gaviscon Antacid Tablets................... ◆D 819
Gaviscon-2 Antacid Tablets .... ◆D 820
Mylanta Liquid 1317
Mylanta Tablets .... ◆D 660
Mylanta Double Strength Liquid 1317
Mylanta Double Strength Tablets .. ◆D 660
Nephrox Suspension .... ◆D 655

Atropine Sulfate (Oral anti-cholinergics delay peak plasma levels but do not affect the extent of absorption). Products include:

Arco-Lase Plus Tablets 512
Atrohist Plus Tablets 454
Atropine Sulfate Sterile Ophthalmic Solution .... ◉ 233
Donnatal 2060
Donnatal Extentabs 2061
Donnatal Tablets 2060
Lomotil 2439
Motofen Tablets 784
Urised Tablets.. 1964

Belladonna Alkaloids (Oral anti-cholinergics delay peak plasma levels but do not affect the extent of absorption). Products include:

Bellergal-S Tablets 2250
Hyland's Bed Wetting Tablets .... ◆D 828
Hyland's EnurAid Tablets.................. ◆D 829
Hyland's Teething Tablets .... ◆D 830

Benztropine Mesylate (Oral anti-cholinergics delay peak plasma levels but do not affect the extent of absorption). Products include:

Cogentin 1621

Biperiden Hydrochloride (Oral anti-cholinergics delay peak plasma levels but do not affect the extent of absorption). Products include:

Akineton 1333

Cimetidine (High doses of H_2 blockers reduces peak plasma levels by 42% and the extent of absorption by 32%; the rate of absorption is not altered). Products include:

Tagamet Tablets 2516

Cimetidine Hydrochloride (High doses of H_2 blockers reduces peak plasma levels by 42% and the extent of absorption by 32%; the rate of absorption is not altered). Products include:

Tagamet... 2516

Clidinium Bromide (Oral anti-cholinergics delay peak plasma levels but do not affect the extent of absorption). Products include:

Librax Capsules 2176
Quarzan Capsules................................. 2181

Dicyclomine Hydrochloride (Oral anti-cholinergics delay peak plasma levels but do not affect the extent of absorption). Products include:

Bentyl 1501

Dihydroxyaluminum Sodium Carbonate (High doses of antacids reduces peak plasma levels by 24% and the extent of absorption by 27%; the rate of absorption is not altered).

No products indexed under this heading.

Famotidine (High doses of H_2 blockers reduces peak plasma levels by 42% and the extent of absorption by 32%; the rate of absorption is not altered). Products include:

Pepcid AC 1319
Pepcid Injection 1722
Pepcid.. 1720

Glycopyrrolate (Oral anti-cholinergics delay peak plasma levels but do not affect the extent of absorption). Products include:

Robinul Forte Tablets........................... 2072
Robinul Injectable 2072
Robinul Tablets...................................... 2072

Hyoscyamine (Oral anti-cholinergics delay peak plasma levels but do not affect the extent of absorption). Products include:

Cystospaz Tablets 1963
Urised Tablets... 1964

Hyoscyamine Sulfate (Oral anti-cholinergics delay peak plasma levels but do not affect the extent of absorption). Products include:

Arco-Lase Plus Tablets 512
Atrohist Plus Tablets 454
Cystospaz-M Capsules 1963
Donnatal 2060
Donnatal Extentabs.............................. 2061
Donnatal Tablets 2060
Kutrase Capsules.................................. 2402
Levsin/Levsinex/Levbid 2405

Ipratropium Bromide (Oral anti-cholinergics delay peak plasma levels but do not affect the extent of absorption). Products include:

Atrovent Inhalation Aerosol............... 671
Atrovent Inhalation Solution.............. 673

Magaldrate (High doses of antacids reduces peak plasma levels by 24% and the extent of absorption by 27%; the rate of absorption is not altered).

No products indexed under this heading.

Magnesium Hydroxide (High doses of antacids reduces peak plasma levels by 24% and the extent of absorption by 27%; the rate of absorption is not altered). Products include:

Aludrox Oral Suspension 2695
Arthritis Pain Ascriptin .... ◆D 631
Maximum Strength Ascriptin .... ◆D 630
Regular Strength Ascriptin Tablets .... ◆D 629
Di-Gel Antacid/Anti-Gas .... ◆D 801
Gelusil Liquid & Tablets .... ◆D 855
Maalox Magnesia and Alumina Oral Suspension................................... ◆D 642
Maalox Plus Tablets............................. ◆D 643
Extra Strength Maalox Antacid Plus Antigas Liquid and Tablets ◆D 638
Mylanta Calcium Carbonate and Magnesium Hydroxide Tablets...... 1318
Mylanta Liquid 1317
Mylanta Tablets .... ◆D 660
Mylanta Double Strength Liquid 1317
Mylanta Double Strength Tablets.. ◆D 660
Phillips' Milk of Magnesia Liquid.... ◆D 729
Rolaids Tablets....................................... ◆D 843
Tempo Soft Antacid .... ◆D 835

Magnesium Oxide (High doses of antacids reduces peak plasma levels by 24% and the extent of absorption by 27%; the rate of absorption is not altered). Products include:

Beelith Tablets 639
Bufferin Analgesic Tablets and Caplets.. ◆D 613
Caltrate PLUS .... ◆D 665
Cama Arthritis Pain Reliever............ ◆D 785
Mag-Ox 400 668
Uro-Mag.. 668

Mepenzolate Bromide (Oral anti-cholinergics delay peak plasma levels but do not affect the extent of absorption).

No products indexed under this heading.

Nephrotoxic Drugs (Close monitoring of renal function is required when co-administered with compounds of known nephrotoxicity potential).

Nizatidine (High doses of H_2 blockers reduces peak plasma levels by 42% and the extent of absorption by 32%; the rate of absorption is not altered). Products include:

Axid Pulvules 1427

Oxybutynin Chloride (Oral anti-cholinergics delay peak plasma levels but do not affect the extent of absorption). Products include:

Ditropan... 1516

Probenecid (Renal excretion of cefpodoxime is inhibited by probenecid and resulting in an approximately 31% increase in AUC and 20% increase in peak plasma levels). Products include:

Benemid Tablets 1611
ColBENEMID Tablets 1622

Procyclidine Hydrochloride (Oral anti-cholinergics delay peak plasma levels but do not affect the extent of absorption). Products include:

Kemadrin Tablets 1112

Propantheline Bromide (Oral anti-cholinergics delay peak plasma levels but do not affect the extent of absorption). Products include:

Pro-Banthine Tablets............................ 2052

Ranitidine Hydrochloride (High doses of H_2 blockers reduces peak plasma levels by 42% and the extent of absorption by 32%; the rate of absorption is not altered). Products include:

Zantac.. 1209
Zantac Injection 1207
Zantac Syrup 1209

Scopolamine (Oral anti-cholinergics delay peak plasma levels but do not affect the extent of absorption). Products include:

Transderm Scōp Transdermal Therapeutic System 869

Scopolamine Hydrobromide (Oral anti-cholinergics delay peak plasma levels but do not affect the extent of absorption). Products include:

Atrohist Plus Tablets 454
Donnatal 2060
Donnatal Extentabs.............................. 2061
Donnatal Tablets 2060

Sodium Bicarbonate (High doses of antacids reduces peak plasma levels by 24% and the extent of absorption by 27%; the rate of absorption is not altered). Products include:

Alka-Seltzer Effervescent Antacid and Pain Reliever .... ◆D 701
Alka-Seltzer Extra Strength Effervescent Antacid and Pain Reliever .... ◆D 703
Alka-Seltzer Gold Effervescent Antacid.. ◆D 703
Alka-Seltzer Lemon Lime Effervescent Antacid and Pain Reliever .... ◆D 703
Arm & Hammer Pure Baking Soda .... ◆D 627
Ceo-Two Rectal Suppositories 666
Citrocarbonate Antacid .... ◆D 770
Massengill Disposable Douches...... ◆D 820
Massengill Liquid Concentrate........ ◆D 820
NuLYTELY.. 689
Cherry Flavor NuLYTELY 689

Tridihexethyl Chloride (Oral anti-cholinergics delay peak plasma levels but do not affect the extent of absorption).

No products indexed under this heading.

Trihexyphenidyl Hydrochloride (Oral anti-cholinergics delay peak plasma levels but do not affect the extent of absorption). Products include:

Artane.. 1368

Food Interactions

Food, unspecified (The extent of absorption and the mean peak plasma concentration increased when film-coated tablets were administered with food).

VARIVAX

(Varicella Virus Vaccine Live)..............1762

May interact with salicylates, immunosuppressive agents, and certain other agents. Compounds in these categories include:

Aspirin (Vaccine recipients should avoid use of salicylates for 6 weeks after vaccination with Varivax because of the potential for Reye's syndrome). Products include:

Alka-Seltzer Effervescent Antacid and Pain Reliever .... ◆D 701
Alka-Seltzer Extra Strength Effervescent Antacid and Pain Reliever .... ◆D 703
Alka-Seltzer Lemon Lime Effervescent Antacid and Pain Reliever .... ◆D 703
Alka-Seltzer Plus Cold Medicine .... ◆D 705
Alka-Seltzer Plus Cold & Cough Medicine .... ◆D 708
Alka-Seltzer Plus Night-Time Cold Medicine .... ◆D 707
Alka Seltzer Plus Sinus Medicine .. ◆D 707
Arthritis Foundation Safety Coated Aspirin Tablets .... ◆D 675
Arthritis Pain Ascriptin .... ◆D 631
Maximum Strength Ascriptin .... ◆D 630
Regular Strength Ascriptin Tablets .... ◆D 629
Arthritis Strength BC Powder.......... ◆D 609
BC Cold Powder Multi-Symptom Formula (Cold-Sinus-Allergy) ...... ◆D 609
BC Cold Powder Non-Drowsy Formula (Cold-Sinus)......................... ◆D 609
BC Powder .... ◆D 609
Bayer Children's Chewable Aspirin .... ◆D 711
Genuine Bayer Aspirin Tablets & Caplets.. ◆D 713
Extra Strength Bayer Arthritis Pain Regimen Formula .... ◆D 711
Extra Strength Bayer Aspirin Caplets & Tablets .... ◆D 712
Extended-Release Bayer 8-Hour Aspirin .... ◆D 712
Extra Strength Bayer Plus Aspirin Caplets.. ◆D 713
Extra Strength Bayer PM Aspirin .. ◆D 713
Bayer Enteric Aspirin .... ◆D 709
Bufferin Analgesic Tablets and Caplets.. ◆D 613
Arthritis Strength Bufferin Analgesic Caplets .... ◆D 614
Extra Strength Bufferin Analgesic Tablets .... ◆D 615
Cama Arthritis Pain Reliever............ ◆D 785
Darvon Compound-65 Pulvules 1435
Easprin 1914
Ecotrin 2455
Ecotrin Enteric Coated Aspirin Maximum Strength Tablets and Caplets.. ◆D 816
Ecotrin Enteric Coated Aspirin Regular Strength Tablets 2455
Empirin Aspirin Tablets .... ◆D 854
Empirin with Codeine Tablets........... 1093
Excedrin Extra-Strength Analgesic Tablets & Caplets 732
Fiorinal Capsules 2261
Fiorinal with Codeine Capsules 2262
Fiorinal Tablets...................................... 2261
Halfprin 1362
Healthprin Aspirin 2455
Norgesic.. 1496
Percodan Tablets................................... 939
Percodan-Demi Tablets........................ 940

IMPORTANT NOTE: Always consult each drug listing in the patient's regimen for possible interactions.

Varivax Interactions Index 1124

Robaxisal Tablets 2071
Soma Compound w/Codeine Tablets 2676
Soma Compound Tablets 2675
St. Joseph Adult Chewable Aspirin (81 mg.) .... ⊡ 808
Talwin Compound 2335
Ursinus Inlay-Tabs .... ⊡ 794
Vanquish Analgesic Caplets .... ⊡ 731

Azathioprine (Concurrent use is contraindicated). Products include:
Imuran 1110

Choline Magnesium Trisalicylate (Vaccine recipients should avoid use of salicylates for 6 weeks after vaccination with Varivax because of the potential for Reye's syndrome). Products include:
Trilisate 2000

Cyclosporine (Concurrent use is contraindicated). Products include:
Neoral 2276
Sandimmune 2286

Diflunisal (Vaccine recipients should avoid use of salicylates for 6 weeks after vaccination with Varivax because of the potential for Reye's syndrome). Products include:
Dolobid Tablets 1654

Globulin, Immune (Human) (Vaccination should be deferred for at least 5 months following immune globulin administration; following administration of Varivax, immune globulin should not be given for 2 months). Products include:
Gamimune N, 5% Immune Globulin Intravenous (Human), 5% 619
Gamimune N, 10% Immune Globulin Intravenous (Human), 10% 621
Gammagard S/D, Immune Globulin, Intravenous (Human) 585
Gammar, Immune Globulin (Human) U.S.P. 515
Gammar I.V., Immune Globulin Intravenous (Human), Lyophilized 516
Hyper-Tet Tetanus Immune Globulin (Human) 627
HypRho-D Full Dose Rho (D) Immune Globulin (Human) 629
HypRho-D Mini-Dose Rho (D) Immune Globulin (Human) 628
MICRhoGAM Rh_0(D) Immune Globulin (Human) 1847
RhoGAM Rh_0(D) Immune Globulin (Human) 1847
Sandoglobulin I.V. 2290

Immune Globulin (Human) (Concurrent use is contraindicated).
No products indexed under this heading.

Magnesium Salicylate (Vaccine recipients should avoid use of salicylates for 6 weeks after vaccination with Varivax because of the potential for Reye's syndrome). Products include:
Backache Caplets .... ⊡ 613
Bayer Select Backache Pain Relief Formula .... ⊡ 715
Doan's Extra-Strength Analgesic .... ⊡ 633
Extra Strength Doan's P.M. .... ⊡ 633
Doan's Regular Strength Analgesic .... ⊡ 634
Mobigesic Tablets .... ⊡ 602

Muromonab-CD3 (Concurrent use is contraindicated). Products include:
Orthoclone OKT3 Sterile Solution 1837

Mycophenolate Mofetil (Concurrent use is contraindicated). Products include:
CellCept Capsules 2099

Salsalate (Vaccine recipients should avoid use of salicylates for 6 weeks after vaccination with Varivax because of the potential for Reye's syndrome). Products include:
Mono-Gesic Tablets 792
Salflex Tablets 786

Tacrolimus (Concurrent use is contraindicated). Products include:
Prograf 1042

VASCOR (200, 300 AND 400 MG) TABLETS

(Bepridil Hydrochloride) 1587

May interact with type 1 antiarrhythmic drugs, tricyclic antidepressants, cardiac glycosides, beta blockers, and certain other agents. Compounds in these categories include:

Acebutolol Hydrochloride (Available data are not sufficient to predict the effects of concomitant medication on patients with impaired ventricular function or cardiac conduction abnormalities). Products include:
Sectral Capsules 2807

Amitriptyline Hydrochloride (Potential for exaggeration of the QT interval prolongation). Products include:
Elavil 2838
Endep Tablets 2174
Etrafon 2355
Limbitrol 2180
Triavil Tablets 1757

Amoxapine (Potential for exaggeration of the QT interval prolongation). Products include:
Asendin Tablets 1369

Atenolol (Available data are not sufficient to predict the effects of concomitant medication on patients with impaired ventricular function or cardiac conduction abnormalities). Products include:
Tenoretic Tablets 2845
Tenormin Tablets and I.V. Injection 2847

Betaxolol Hydrochloride (Available data are not sufficient to predict the effects of concomitant medication on patients with impaired ventricular function or cardiac conduction abnormalities). Products include:
Betoptic Ophthalmic Solution 469
Betoptic S Ophthalmic Suspension 471
Kerlone Tablets 2436

Bisoprolol Fumarate (Available data are not sufficient to predict the effects of concomitant medication on patients with impaired ventricular function or cardiac conduction abnormalities). Products include:
Zebeta Tablets 1413
Ziac 1415

Carteolol Hydrochloride (Available data are not sufficient to predict the effects of concomitant medication on patients with impaired ventricular function or cardiac conduction abnormalities). Products include:
Cartrol Tablets 410
Ocupress Ophthalmic Solution, 1% Sterile .... ⊙ 309

Clomipramine Hydrochloride (Potential for exaggeration of the QT interval prolongation). Products include:
Anafranil Capsules 803

Desipramine Hydrochloride (Potential for exaggeration of the QT interval prolongation). Products include:
Norpramin Tablets 1526

Deslanoside (Cardiac glycosides could exaggerate the depression of AV nodal conduction).
No products indexed under this heading.

Digitoxin (Cardiac glycosides could exaggerate the depression of AV nodal conduction). Products include:
Crystodigin Tablets 1433

Digoxin (May be associated with modest increases in steady-state serum digoxin concentrations; cardiac glycosides could exaggerate the depression of AV nodal conduction). Products include:
Lanoxicaps 1117
Lanoxin Elixir Pediatric 1120
Lanoxin Injection 1123
Lanoxin Injection Pediatric 1126
Lanoxin Tablets 1128

Disopyramide Phosphate (Potential for exaggeration of the QT interval prolongation). Products include:
Norpace 2444

Doxepin Hydrochloride (Potential for exaggeration of the QT interval prolongation). Products include:
Sinequan 2205
Zonalon Cream 1055

Esmolol Hydrochloride (Available data are not sufficient to predict the effects of concomitant medication on patients with impaired ventricular function or cardiac conduction abnormalities). Products include:
Brevibloc Injection 1808

Imipramine Hydrochloride (Potential for exaggeration of the QT interval prolongation). Products include:
Tofranil Ampuls 854
Tofranil Tablets 856

Imipramine Pamoate (Potential for exaggeration of the QT interval prolongation). Products include:
Tofranil-PM Capsules 857

Labetalol Hydrochloride (Available data are not sufficient to predict the effects of concomitant medication on patients with impaired ventricular function or cardiac conduction abnormalities). Products include:
Normodyne Injection 2377
Normodyne Tablets 2379
Trandate 1185

Levobunolol Hydrochloride (Available data are not sufficient to predict the effects of concomitant medication on patients with impaired ventricular function or cardiac conduction abnormalities). Products include:
Betagan .... ⊙ 233

Maprotiline Hydrochloride (Potential for exaggeration of the QT interval prolongation). Products include:
Ludiomil Tablets 843

Metipranolol Hydrochloride (Available data are not sufficient to predict the effects of concomitant medication on patients with impaired ventricular function or cardiac conduction abnormalities). Products include:
OptiPranolol (Metipranolol 0.3%) Sterile Ophthalmic Solution .... ⊙ 258

Metoprolol Succinate (Available data are not sufficient to predict the effects of concomitant medication on patients with impaired ventricular function or cardiac conduction abnormalities). Products include:
Toprol-XL Tablets 565

Metoprolol Tartrate (Available data are not sufficient to predict the effects of concomitant medication on patients with impaired ventricular function or cardiac conduction abnormalities). Products include:
Lopressor Ampuls 830
Lopressor HCT Tablets 832
Lopressor Tablets 830

Moricizine Hydrochloride (Potential for exaggeration of the QT interval prolongation). Products include:
Ethmozine Tablets 2041

Nadolol (Available data are not sufficient to predict the effects of concomitant medication on patients with impaired ventricular function or cardiac conduction abnormalities).
No products indexed under this heading.

Nortriptyline Hydrochloride (Potential for exaggeration of the QT interval prolongation). Products include:
Pamelor 2280

Penbutolol Sulfate (Available data are not sufficient to predict the effects of concomitant medication on patients with impaired ventricular function or cardiac conduction abnormalities). Products include:
Levatol 2403

Pindolol (Available data are not sufficient to predict the effects of concomitant medication on patients with impaired ventricular function or cardiac conduction abnormalities). Products include:
Visken Tablets 2299

Procainamide Hydrochloride (Potential for exaggeration of the QT interval prolongation). Products include:
Procan SR Tablets 1926

Propafenone Hydrochloride (Potential for exaggeration of the QT interval prolongation). Products include:
Rythmol Tablets–150mg, 225mg, 300mg 1352

Propranolol Hydrochloride (Available data are not sufficient to predict the effects of concomitant medication on patients with impaired ventricular function or cardiac conduction abnormalities). Products include:
Inderal 2728
Inderal LA Long Acting Capsules 2730
Inderide Tablets 2732
Inderide LA Long Acting Capsules 2734

Protriptyline Hydrochloride (Potential for exaggeration of the QT interval prolongation). Products include:
Vivactil Tablets 1774

Quinidine Gluconate (Potential for exaggeration of the QT interval prolongation). Products include:
Quinaglute Dura-Tabs Tablets 649

Quinidine Polygalacturonate (Potential for exaggeration of the QT interval prolongation).
No products indexed under this heading.

Quinidine Sulfate (Potential for exaggeration of the QT interval prolongation). Products include:
Quinidex Extentabs 2067

Sotalol Hydrochloride (Available data are not sufficient to predict the effects of concomitant medication on patients with impaired ventricular function or cardiac conduction abnormalities). Products include:
Betapace Tablets 641

Timolol Hemihydrate (Available data are not sufficient to predict the effects of concomitant medication on patients with impaired ventricular function or cardiac conduction abnormalities). Products include:
Betimol 0.25%, 0.5% .... ⊙ 261

Timolol Maleate (Available data are not sufficient to predict the effects of concomitant medication on patients with impaired ventricular function or cardiac conduction abnormalities). Products include:
- Blocadren Tablets ... 1614
- Timolide Tablets ... 1748
- Timoptic in Ocudose ... 1753
- Timoptic Sterile Ophthalmic Solution ... 1751
- Timoptic-XE ... 1755

Trimipramine Maleate (Potential for exaggeration of the QT interval prolongation). Products include:
- Surmontil Capsules ... 2811

Food Interactions

Meal, unspecified (May result in a clinically insignificant delay in time to peak concentration, but neither peak plasma levels nor the extent of absorption was changed).

VASERETIC TABLETS

(Enalapril Maleate, Hydrochlorothiazide) ... 1765

May interact with insulin, potassium preparations, diuretics, potassium sparing diuretics, barbiturates, narcotic analgesics, oral hypoglycemic agents, antihypertensives, corticosteroids, nondepolarizing neuromuscular blocking agents, lithium preparations, non-steroidal anti-inflammatory agents, cardiac glycosides, and certain other agents. Compounds in these categories include:

Acarbose (Dosage adjustment of hypoglycemic may be required).
- No products indexed under this heading.

Acebutolol Hydrochloride (Additive effect or potentiation). Products include:
- Sectral Capsules ... 2807

ACTH (Intensifed electrolyte depletion, particularly hypokalemia).
- No products indexed under this heading.

Alfentanil Hydrochloride (Potentiation of orthostatic hypotension may occur). Products include:
- Alfenta Injection ... 1286

Amiloride Hydrochloride (Significant increases in serum potassium; excessive hypotension). Products include:
- Midamor Tablets ... 1703
- Moduretic Tablets ... 1705

Amlodipine Besylate (Additive effect or potentiation). Products include:
- Lotrel Capsules ... 840
- Norvasc Tablets ... 1940

Aprobarbital (Potentiation of orthostatic hypotension may occur).
- No products indexed under this heading.

Atenolol (Additive effect or potentiation). Products include:
- Tenoretic Tablets ... 2845
- Tenormin Tablets and I.V. Injection ... 2847

Atracurium Besylate (Increased responsiveness to muscle relaxant). Products include:
- Tracrium Injection ... 1183

Benazepril Hydrochloride (Additive effect or potentiation). Products include:
- Lotensin Tablets ... 834
- Lotensin HCT ... 837
- Lotrel Capsules ... 840

Bendroflumethiazide (Additive effect or potentiation; excessive hypotension).
- No products indexed under this heading.

Betamethasone Acetate (Intensified electrolyte depletion, particularly hypokalemia). Products include:
- Celestone Soluspan Suspension ... 2347

Betamethasone Sodium Phosphate (Intensified electrolyte depletion, particularly hypokalemia). Products include:
- Celestone Soluspan Suspension ... 2347

Betaxolol Hydrochloride (Additive effect or potentiation). Products include:
- Betoptic Ophthalmic Solution ... 469
- Betoptic S Ophthalmic Suspension ... 471
- Kerlone Tablets ... 2436

Bisoprolol Fumarate (Additive effect or potentiation). Products include:
- Zebeta Tablets ... 1413
- Ziac ... 1415

Bumetanide (Excessive hypotension). Products include:
- Bumex ... 2093

Buprenorphine (Potentiation of orthostatic hypotension may occur). Products include:
- Buprenex Injectable ... 2006

Butabarbital (Potentiation of orthostatic hypotension may occur).
- No products indexed under this heading.

Butalbital (Potentiation of orthostatic hypotension may occur). Products include:
- Esgic-plus Tablets ... 1013
- Fioricet Tablets ... 2258
- Fioricet with Codeine Capsules ... 2260
- Fiorinal Capsules ... 2261
- Fiorinal with Codeine Capsules ... 2262
- Fiorinal Tablets ... 2261
- Phrenilin ... 785
- Sedapap Tablets 50 mg/650 mg ... 1543

Captopril (Additive effect or potentiation). Products include:
- Capoten ... 739
- Capozide ... 742

Carteolol Hydrochloride (Additive effect or potentiation). Products include:
- Cartrol Tablets ... 410
- Ocupress Ophthalmic Solution, 1% Sterile ... ⊙ 309

Chlorothiazide (Additive effect or potentiation; excessive hypotension). Products include:
- Aldoclor Tablets ... 1598
- Diupres Tablets ... 1650
- Diuril Oral ... 1653

Chlorothiazide Sodium (Additive effect or potentiation; excessive hypotension). Products include:
- Diuril Sodium Intravenous ... 1652

Chlorpropamide (Dosage adjustment of hypoglycemic may be required). Products include:
- Diabinese Tablets ... 1935

Chlorthalidone (Additive effect or potentiation; significant increases in serum potassium; excessive hypotension). Products include:
- Combipres Tablets ... 677
- Tenoretic Tablets ... 2845
- Thalitone ... 1245

Cholestyramine (Binds the hydrochlorothiazide and reduces its absorption from gastrointestinal tract by up to 85%). Products include:
- Questran Light ... 769
- Questran Powder ... 770

Clonidine (Additive effect or potentiation). Products include:
- Catapres-TTS ... 675

Clonidine Hydrochloride (Additive effect or potentiation). Products include:
- Catapres Tablets ... 674
- Combipres Tablets ... 677

Codeine Phosphate (Potentiation of orthostatic hypotension may occur). Products include:
- Actifed with Codeine Cough Syrup ... 1067
- Brontex ... 1981
- Deconsal C Expectorant Syrup ... 456
- Deconsal Pediatric Syrup ... 457
- Dimetane-DC Cough Syrup ... 2059
- Empirin with Codeine Tablets ... 1093
- Fioricet with Codeine Capsules ... 2260
- Fiorinal with Codeine Capsules ... 2262
- Isoclor Expectorant ... 990
- Novahistine DH ... 2462
- Novahistine Expectorant ... 2463
- Nucofed ... 2051
- Phenergan with Codeine ... 2777
- Phenergan VC with Codeine ... 2781
- Robitussin A-C Syrup ... 2073
- Robitussin-DAC Syrup ... 2074
- Ryna ... ⊞ 841
- Soma Compound w/Codeine Tablets ... 2676
- Tussi-Organidin NR Liquid and S NR Liquid ... 2677
- Tylenol with Codeine ... 1583

Colestipol Hydrochloride (Binds the hydrochlorothiazide and reduces its absorption from gastrointestinal tract by up to 43%). Products include:
- Colestid Tablets ... 2591

Cortisone Acetate (Intensified electrolyte depletion, particularly hypokalemia). Products include:
- Cortone Acetate Sterile Suspension ... 1623
- Cortone Acetate Tablets ... 1624

Deserpidine (Additive effect or potentiation).
- No products indexed under this heading.

Deslanoside (Hypokalemia produced by hydrochlorothiazide may exaggerate the response of the heart to the digitalis toxicity).
- No products indexed under this heading.

Dexamethasone (Intensified electrolyte depletion, particularly hypokalemia). Products include:
- AK-Trol Ointment & Suspension ... ⊙ 205
- Decadron Elixir ... 1633
- Decadron Tablets ... 1635
- Decaspray Topical Aerosol ... 1648
- Dexacidin Ointment ... ⊙ 263
- Maxitrol Ophthalmic Ointment and Suspension ... ⊙ 224
- TobraDex Ophthalmic Suspension and Ointment ... 473

Dexamethasone Acetate (Intensified electrolyte depletion, particularly hypokalemia). Products include:
- Dalalone D.P. Injectable ... 1011
- Decadron-LA Sterile Suspension ... 1646

Dexamethasone Sodium Phosphate (Intensified electrolyte depletion, particularly hypokalemia). Products include:
- Decadron Phosphate Injection ... 1637
- Decadron Phosphate Respihaler ... 1642
- Decadron Phosphate Sterile Ophthalmic Ointment ... 1641
- Decadron Phosphate Sterile Ophthalmic Solution ... 1642
- Decadron Phosphate Topical Cream ... 1644
- Decadron Phosphate Turbinaire ... 1645
- Decadron Phosphate with Xylocaine Injection, Sterile ... 1639
- Dexacort Phosphate in Respihaler ... 458
- Dexacort Phosphate in Turbinaire ... 459
- NeoDecadron Sterile Ophthalmic Ointment ... 1712
- NeoDecadron Sterile Ophthalmic Solution ... 1713
- NeoDecadron Topical Cream ... 1714

Dezocine (Potentiation of orthostatic hypotension may occur). Products include:
- Dalgan Injection ... 538

Diazoxide (Additive effect or potentiation). Products include:
- Hyperstat I.V. Injection ... 2363
- Proglycem ... 580

Diclofenac Potassium (Reduced diuretic, natriuretic, and antihypertensive effects of Vaseretic). Products include:
- Cataflam ... 816

Diclofenac Sodium (Reduced diuretic, natriuretic, and antihypertensive effects of Vaseretic). Products include:
- Voltaren Ophthalmic Sterile Ophthalmic Solution ... ⊙ 272
- Voltaren Tablets ... 861

Digitoxin (Hypokalemia produced by hydrochlorothiazide may exaggerate the response of the heart to the digitalis toxicity). Products include:
- Crystodigin Tablets ... 1433

Digoxin (Hypokalemia produced by hydrochlorothiazide may exaggerate the response of the heart to the digitalis toxicity). Products include:
- Lanoxicaps ... 1117
- Lanoxin Elixir Pediatric ... 1120
- Lanoxin Injection ... 1123
- Lanoxin Injection Pediatric ... 1126
- Lanoxin Tablets ... 1128

Diltiazem Hydrochloride (Additive effect or potentiation). Products include:
- Cardizem CD Capsules ... 1506
- Cardizem SR Capsules ... 1510
- Cardizem Injectable ... 1508
- Cardizem Tablets ... 1512
- Dilacor XR Extended-release Capsules ... 2018

Doxazosin Mesylate (Additive effect or potentiation). Products include:
- Cardura Tablets ... 2186

Enalaprilat (Additive effect or potentiation). Products include:
- Vasotec I.V. ... 1768

Esmolol Hydrochloride (Additive effect or potentiation). Products include:
- Brevibloc Injection ... 1808

Ethacrynic Acid (Excessive hypotension). Products include:
- Edecrin Tablets ... 1657

Etodolac (Reduced diuretic, natriuretic, and antihypertensive effects of Vaseretic). Products include:
- Lodine Capsules and Tablets ... 2743

Felodipine (Additive effect or potentiation). Products include:
- Plendil Extended-Release Tablets ... 527

Fenoprofen Calcium (Reduced diuretic, natriuretic, and antihypertensive effects of Vaseretic). Products include:
- Nalfon 200 Pulvules & Nalfon Tablets ... 917

Fentanyl (Potentiation of orthostatic hypotension may occur). Products include:
- Duragesic Transdermal System ... 1288

Fentanyl Citrate (Potentiation of orthostatic hypotension may occur). Products include:
- Sublimaze Injection ... 1307

Fludrocortisone Acetate (Intensified electrolyte depletion, particularly hypokalemia). Products include:
- Florinef Acetate Tablets ... 505

Flurbiprofen (Reduced diuretic, natriuretic, and antihypertensive effects of Vaseretic). Products include:
- Ansaid Tablets ... 2579

Fosinopril Sodium (Additive effect or potentiation). Products include:
- Monopril Tablets ... 757

Furosemide (Additive effect or potentiation; excessive hypotension). Products include:
- Lasix Injection, Oral Solution and Tablets ... 1240

Vaseretic Interactions Index 1126

Glipizide (Dosage adjustment of hypoglycemic may be required). Products include:
Glucotrol Tablets ... 1967
Glucotrol XL Extended Release Tablets ... 1968

Glyburide (Dosage adjustment of hypoglycemic may be required). Products include:
DiaBeta Tablets ... 1239
Glynase PresTab Tablets ... 2609
Micronase Tablets ... 2623

Guanabenz Acetate (Additive effect or potentiation).
No products indexed under this heading.

Guanethidine Monosulfate (Additive effect or potentiation). Products include:
Esimil Tablets ... 822
Ismelin Tablets ... 827

Hydralazine Hydrochloride (Additive effect or potentiation). Products include:
Apresazide Capsules ... 808
Apresoline Hydrochloride Tablets ... 809
Ser-Ap-Es Tablets ... 849

Hydrocodone Bitartrate (Potentiation of orthostatic hypotension may occur). Products include:
Anexsia 5/500 Elixir ... 1781
Anexia Tablets ... 1782
Codiclear DH Syrup ... 791
Deconamine CX Cough and Cold Liquid and Tablets ... 1319
Duratuss HD Elixir ... 2565
Hycodan Tablets and Syrup ... 930
Hycomine Compound Tablets ... 932
Hycomine ... 931
Hycotuss Expectorant Syrup ... 933
Hydrocet Capsules ... 782
Lorcet 10/650 ... 1018
Lortab ... 2566
Tussend ... 1783
Tussend Expectorant ... 1785
Vicodin Tablets ... 1356
Vicodin ES Tablets ... 1357
Vicodin Tuss Expectorant ... 1358
Zydone Capsules ... 949

Hydrocodone Polistirex (Potentiation of orthostatic hypotension may occur). Products include:
Tussionex Pennkinetic Extended-Release Suspension ... 998

Hydrocortisone (Intensified electrolyte depletion, particularly hypokalemia). Products include:
Anusol-HC Cream 2.5% ... 1896
Aquanil HC Lotion ... 1931
Bactine Hydrocortisone Anti-Itch Cream ... ▣ 709
Caldecort Anti-Itch Hydrocortisone Spray ... ▣ 631
Cortaid ... ▣ 836
CORTENEMA ... 2535
Cortisporin Ointment ... 1085
Cortisporin Ophthalmic Ointment Sterile ... 1085
Cortisporin Ophthalmic Suspension Sterile ... 1086
Cortisporin Otic Solution Sterile ... 1087
Cortisporin Otic Suspension Sterile ... 1088
Cortizone-5 ... ▣ 831
Cortizone-10 ... ▣ 831
Hydrocortone Tablets ... 1672
Hytone ... 907
Massengill Medicated Soft Cloth Towelettes ... 2458
PediOtic Suspension Sterile ... 1153
Preparation H Hydrocortisone 1% Cream ... ▣ 872
ProctoCream-HC 2.5% ... 2408
VōSoL HC Otic Solution ... 2678

Hydrocortisone Acetate (Intensified electrolyte depletion, particularly hypokalemia). Products include:
Analpram-HC Rectal Cream 1% and 2.5% ... 977
Anusol HC-1 Anti-Itch Hydrocortisone Ointment ... ▣ 847
Anusol-HC Suppositories ... 1897
Caldecort ... ▣ 631
Carmol HC ... 924
Coly-Mycin S Otic w/Neomycin & Hydrocortisone ... 1906
Cortaid ... ▣ 836
Cortifoam ... 2396
Cortisporin Cream ... 1084
Epifoam ... 2399
Hydrocortone Acetate Sterile Suspension ... 1669
Mantadil Cream ... 1135
Nupercainal Hydrocortisone 1% Cream ... ▣ 645
Ophthocort ... ⊙ 311
Pramosone Cream, Lotion & Ointment ... 978
ProctoCream-HC ... 2408
ProctoFoam-HC ... 2409
Terra-Cortril Ophthalmic Suspension ... 2210

Hydrocortisone Sodium Phosphate (Intensified electrolyte depletion, particularly hypokalemia). Products include:
Hydrocortone Phosphate Injection, Sterile ... 1670

Hydrocortisone Sodium Succinate (Intensified electrolyte depletion, particularly hypokalemia). Products include:
Solu-Cortef Sterile Powder ... 2641

Hydroflumethiazide (Additive effect or potentiation; excessive hypotension). Products include:
Diucardin Tablets ... 2718

Ibuprofen (Reduced diuretic, natriuretic, and antihypertensive effects of Vaseretic). Products include:
Advil Cold and Sinus Caplets and Tablets (formerly CoAdvil) ... ▣ 870
Advil Ibuprofen Tablets and Caplets ... ▣ 870
Children's Advil Suspension ... 2692
Arthritis Foundation Ibuprofen Tablets ... ▣ 674
Bayer Select Ibuprofen Pain Relief Formula ... ▣ 715
Cramp End Tablets ... ▣ 735
Dimetapp Sinus Caplets ... ▣ 775
Haltran Tablets ... ▣ 771
IBU Tablets ... 1342
Ibuprohm ... ▣ 735
Children's Motrin Ibuprofen Oral Suspension ... 1546
Motrin Tablets ... 2625
Motrin IB Caplets, Tablets, and Geltabs ... ▣ 838
Motrin IB Sinus ... ▣ 838
Motrin Ibuprofen Suspension, Oral Drops, Chewable Tablets, Caplets ... 1546
Nuprin Ibuprofen/Analgesic Tablets & Caplets ... ▣ 622
Sine-Aid IB Caplets ... 1554
Vicks DayQuil SINUS Pressure & PAIN Relief with IBUPROFEN ... ▣ 762

Indapamide (Additive effect or potentiation; excessive hypotension). Products include:
Lozol Tablets ... 2022

Indomethacin (Reduced diuretic, natriuretic, and antihypertensive effects of Vaseretic). Products include:
Indocin ... 1680

Indomethacin Sodium Trihydrate (Reduced diuretic, natriuretic, and antihypertensive effects of Vaseretic). Products include:
Indocin I.V. ... 1684

Insulin, Human (Dosage adjustments of insulin may be required).
No products indexed under this heading.

Insulin, Human Isophane Suspension (Dosage adjustments of insulin may be required). Products include:
Novolin N Human Insulin 10 ml Vials ... 1795

Insulin, Human NPH (Dosage adjustments of insulin may be required). Products include:
Humulin N, 100 Units ... 1448
Novolin N PenFill Cartridges Durable Insulin Delivery System ... 1798
Novolin N Prefilled Syringe Disposable Insulin Delivery System ... 1798

Insulin, Human Regular (Dosage adjustments of insulin may be required). Products include:
Humulin R, 100 Units ... 1449
Novolin R Human Insulin 10 ml Vials ... 1795
Novolin R PenFill Cartridges Durable Insulin Delivery System ... 1798
Novolin R Prefilled Syringe Disposable Insulin Delivery System ... 1798
Velosulin BR Human Insulin 10 ml Vials ... 1795

Insulin, Human, Zinc Suspension (Dosage adjustments of insulin may be required). Products include:
Humulin L, 100 Units ... 1446
Humulin U, 100 Units ... 1450
Novolin L Human Insulin 10 ml Vials ... 1795

Insulin, NPH (Dosage adjustments of insulin may be required). Products include:
NPH, 100 Units ... 1450
Pork NPH, 100 Units ... 1452
Purified Pork NPH Isophane Insulin ... 1801

Insulin, Regular (Dosage adjustments of insulin may be required). Products include:
Regular, 100 Units ... 1450
Pork Regular, 100 Units ... 1452
Pork Regular (Concentrated), 500 Units ... 1453
Purified Pork Regular Insulin ... 1801

Insulin, Zinc Crystals (Dosage adjustments of insulin may be required). Products include:
NPH, 100 Units ... 1450

Insulin, Zinc Suspension (Dosage adjustments of insulin may be required). Products include:
Iletin I ... 1450
Lente, 100 Units ... 1450
Iletin II ... 1452
Pork Lente, 100 Units ... 1452
Purified Pork Lente Insulin ... 1801

Isradipine (Additive effect or potentiation). Products include:
DynaCirc Capsules ... 2256

Ketoprofen (Reduced diuretic, natriuretic, and antihypertensive effects of Vaseretic). Products include:
Orudis Capsules ... 2766
Oruvail Capsules ... 2766

Ketorolac Tromethamine (Reduced diuretic, natriuretic, and antihypertensive effects of Vaseretic). Products include:
Acular ... 474
Acular ... ⊙ 277
Toradol ... 2159

Labetalol Hydrochloride (Additive effect or potentiation). Products include:
Normodyne Injection ... 2377
Normodyne Tablets ... 2379
Trandate ... 1185

Levobunolol Hydrochloride (Additive effect or potentiation). Products include:
Betagan ... ⊙ 233

Levorphanol Tartrate (Potentiation of orthostatic hypotension may occur). Products include:
Levo-Dromoran ... 2129

Lisinopril (Additive effect or potentiation). Products include:
Prinivil Tablets ... 1733
Prinzide Tablets ... 1737
Zestoretic ... 2850
Zestril Tablets ... 2854

Lithium Carbonate (High risk of lithium toxicity; frequent monitoring of lithium serum levels is recommended). Products include:
Eskalith ... 2485
Lithium Carbonate Capsules & Tablets ... 2230
Lithonate/Lithotabs/Lithobid ... 2543

Lithium Citrate (High risk of lithium toxicity; frequent monitoring of lithium serum levels is recommended).
No products indexed under this heading.

Losartan Potassium (Additive effect or potentiation). Products include:
Cozaar Tablets ... 1628
Hyzaar Tablets ... 1677

Mecamylamine Hydrochloride (Additive effect or potentiation). Products include:
Inversine Tablets ... 1686

Meclofenamate Sodium (Reduced diuretic, natriuretic, and antihypertensive effects of Vaseretic).
No products indexed under this heading.

Mefenamic Acid (Reduced diuretic, natriuretic, and antihypertensive effects of Vaseretic). Products include:
Ponstel ... 1925

Meperidine Hydrochloride (Potentiation of orthostatic hypotension may occur). Products include:
Demerol ... 2308
Mepergan Injection ... 2753

Mephobarbital (Potentiation of orthostatic hypotension may occur). Products include:
Mebaral Tablets ... 2322

Metformin Hydrochloride (Dosage adjustment of hypoglycemic may be required). Products include:
Glucophage ... 752

Methadone Hydrochloride (Potentiation of orthostatic hypotension may occur). Products include:
Methadone Hydrochloride Oral Concentrate ... 2233
Methadone Hydrochloride Oral Solution & Tablets ... 2235

Methyclothiazide (Additive effect or potentiation; excessive hypotension). Products include:
Enduron Tablets ... 420

Methyldopa (Additive effect or potentiation). Products include:
Aldoclor Tablets ... 1598
Aldomet Oral ... 1600
Aldoril Tablets ... 1604

Methyldopate Hydrochloride (Additive effect or potentiation). Products include:
Aldomet Ester HCl Injection ... 1602

Methylprednisolone Acetate (Intensified electrolyte depletion, particularly hypokalemia). Products include:
Depo-Medrol Single-Dose Vial ... 2600
Depo-Medrol Sterile Aqueous Suspension ... 2597

Methylprednisolone Sodium Succinate (Intensified electrolyte depletion, particularly hypokalemia). Products include:
Solu-Medrol Sterile Powder ... 2643

Metipranolol Hydrochloride (Additive effect or potentiation). Products include:
OptiPranolol (Metipranolol 0.3%) Sterile Ophthalmic Solution ... ⊙ 258

Metocurine Iodide (Increased responsiveness to muscle relaxant). Products include:
Metubine Iodide Vials ... 916

Metolazone (Additive effect or potentiation; excessive hypotension). Products include:
Mykrox Tablets ... 993
Zaroxolyn Tablets ... 1000

Metoprolol Succinate (Additive effect or potentiation). Products include:
Toprol-XL Tablets ... 565

(▣ Described in PDR For Nonprescription Drugs) (⊙ Described in PDR For Ophthalmology)

1127 **Interactions Index** **Vaseretic**

Metoprolol Tartrate (Additive effect or potentiation). Products include:
Lopressor Ampuls 830
Lopressor HCT Tablets 832
Lopressor Tablets 830

Metyrosine (Additive effect or potentiation). Products include:
Demser Capsules 1649

Minoxidil (Additive effect or potentiation). Products include:
Loniten Tablets 2618
Rogaine Topical Solution 2637

Mivacurium Chloride (Increased responsiveness to muscle relaxant). Products include:
Mivacron 1138

Moexipril Hydrochloride (Additive effect or potentiation). Products include:
Univasc Tablets 2410

Morphine Sulfate (Potentiation of orthostatic hypotension may occur). Products include:
Astramorph/PF Injection, USP (Preservative-Free) 535
Duramorph 962
Infumorph 200 and Infumorph 500 Sterile Solutions 965
MS Contin Tablets 1994
MSIR 1997
Oramorph SR (Morphine Sulfate Sustained Release Tablets) 2236
RMS Suppositories 2657
Roxanol 2243

Nabumetone (Reduced diuretic, natriuretic, and antihypertensive effects of Vaseretic). Products include:
Relafen Tablets 2510

Nadolol (Additive effect or potentiation).
No products indexed under this heading.

Naproxen (Reduced diuretic, natriuretic, and antihypertensive effects of Vaseretic). Products include:
Anaprox/Naprosyn 2117

Naproxen Sodium (Reduced diuretic, natriuretic, and antihypertensive effects of Vaseretic). Products include:
Aleve 1975
Anaprox/Naprosyn 2117

Nicardipine Hydrochloride (Additive effect or potentiation). Products include:
Cardene Capsules 2095
Cardene I.V. 2709
Cardene SR Capsules 2097

Nifedipine (Additive effect or potentiation). Products include:
Adalat Capsules (10 mg and 20 mg) 587
Adalat CC 589
Procardia Capsules 1971
Procardia XL Extended Release Tablets 1972

Nisoldipine (Additive effect or potentiation).
No products indexed under this heading.

Nitroglycerin (Additive effect or potentiation). Products include:
Deponit NTG Transdermal Delivery System 2397
Nitro-Bid IV 1523
Nitro-Bid Ointment 1524
Nitrodisc 2047
Nitro-Dur (nitroglycerin) Transdermal Infusion System 1326
Nitrolingual Spray 2027
Nitrostat Tablets 1925
Transderm-Nitro Transdermal Therapeutic System 859

Norepinephrine Bitartrate (Decreased reponse to pressor amines). Products include:
Levophed Bitartrate Injection 2315

Opium Alkaloids (Potentiation of orthostatic hypotension may occur).
No products indexed under this heading.

Oxaprozin (Reduced diuretic, natriuretic, and antihypertensive effects of Vaseretic). Products include:
Daypro Caplets 2426

Oxycodone Hydrochloride (Potentiation of orthostatic hypotension may occur). Products include:
Percocet Tablets 938
Percodan Tablets 939
Percodan-Demi Tablets 940
Roxicodone Tablets, Oral Solution & Intensol (Oxycodone) 2244
Tylox Capsules 1584

Pancuronium Bromide Injection (Increased responsiveness to muscle relaxant).
No products indexed under this heading.

Penbutolol Sulfate (Additive effect or potentiation). Products include:
Levatol 2403

Pentobarbital Sodium (Potentiation of orthostatic hypotension may occur). Products include:
Nembutal Sodium Capsules 436
Nembutal Sodium Solution 438
Nembutal Sodium Suppositories 440

Phenobarbital (Potentiation of orthostatic hypotension may occur). Products include:
Arco-Lase Plus Tablets 512
Bellergal-S Tablets 2250
Donnatal 2060
Donnatal Extentabs 2061
Donnatal Tablets 2060
Phenobarbital Elixir and Tablets 1469
Quadrinal Tablets 1350

Phenoxybenzamine Hydrochloride (Additive effect or potentiation). Products include:
Dibenzyline Capsules 2476

Phentolamine Mesylate (Additive effect or potentiation). Products include:
Regitine 846

Phenylbutazone (Reduced diuretic, natriuretic, and antihypertensive effects of Vaseretic).
No products indexed under this heading.

Pindolol (Additive effect or potentiation). Products include:
Visken Tablets 2299

Piroxicam (Reduced diuretic, natriuretic, and antihypertensive effects of Vaseretic). Products include:
Feldene Capsules 1965

Polythiazide (Additive effect or potentiation; excessive hypotension). Products include:
Minizide Capsules 1938

Potassium Acid Phosphate (Significant increases in serum potassium). Products include:
K-Phos Original Formula 'Sodium Free' Tablets 639

Potassium Bicarbonate (Significant increases in serum potassium). Products include:
Alka-Seltzer Gold Effervescent Antacid ▣ 703

Potassium Chloride (Significant increases in serum potassium). Products include:
Chlor-3 Condiment 1004
K-Dur Microburst Release System (potassium chloride, USP) E.R. Tablets 1325
K-Lor Powder Packets 434
K-Norm Extended-Release Capsules 991
K-Tab Filmtab 434
Kolyum Liquid 992
Micro-K 2063
Micro-K LS Packets 2064
NuLYTELY 689
Cherry Flavor NuLYTELY 689
Rum-K Syrup 1005
Slow-K Extended-Release Tablets 851

Potassium Citrate (Significant increases in serum potassium). Products include:
Polycitra Syrup 578
Polycitra-K Crystals 579
Polycitra-K Oral Solution 579
Polycitra-LC 578

Potassium Gluconate (Significant increases in serum potassium). Products include:
Kolyum Liquid 992

Potassium Phosphate, Dibasic (Significant increases in serum potassium).
No products indexed under this heading.

Potassium Phosphate, Monobasic (Significant increases in serum potassium). Products include:
K-Phos Neutral Tablets 639
K-Phos Original Formula 'Sodium Free' Tablets 639

Prazosin Hydrochloride (Additive effect or potentiation). Products include:
Minipress Capsules 1937
Minizide Capsules 1938

Prednisolone Acetate (Intensified electrolyte depletion, particularly hypokalemia). Products include:
AK-CIDE ⊙ 202
AK-CIDE Ointment ⊙ 202
Blephamide Liquifilm Sterile Ophthalmic Suspension 476
Blephamide Ointment ⊙ 237
Econopred & Econopred Plus Ophthalmic Suspensions ⊙ 217
Poly-Pred Liquifilm ⊙ 248
Pred Forte ⊙ 250
Pred Mild ⊙ 253
Pred-G Liquifilm Sterile Ophthalmic Suspension ⊙ 251
Pred-G S.O.P. Sterile Ophthalmic Ointment ⊙ 252
Vasocidin Ointment ⊙ 268

Prednisolone Sodium Phosphate (Intensified electrolyte depletion, particularly hypokalemia). Products include:
AK-Pred ⊙ 204
Hydeltrasol Injection, Sterile 1665
Inflamase ⊙ 265
Pediapred Oral Liquid 995
Vasocidin Ophthalmic Solution ⊙ 270

Prednisolone Tebutate (Intensified electrolyte depletion, particularly hypokalemia). Products include:
Hydeltra-T.B.A. Sterile Suspension 1667

Prednisone (Intensified electrolyte depletion, particularly hypokalemia). Products include:
Deltasone Tablets 2595

Propoxyphene Hydrochloride (Potentiation of orthostatic hypotension may occur). Products include:
Darvon 1435
Wygesic Tablets 2827

Propoxyphene Napsylate (Potentiation of orthostatic hypotension may occur). Products include:
Darvon-N/Darvocet-N 1433

Propranolol Hydrochloride (Additive effect or potentiation). Products include:
Inderal 2728
Inderal LA Long Acting Capsules 2730
Inderide Tablets 2732
Inderide LA Long Acting Capsules 2734

Quinapril Hydrochloride (Additive effect or potentiation). Products include:
Accupril Tablets 1893

Ramipril (Additive effect or potentiation). Products include:
Altace Capsules 1232

Rauwolfia Serpentina (Additive effect or potentiation).
No products indexed under this heading.

Rescinnamine (Additive effect or potentiation).
No products indexed under this heading.

Reserpine (Additive effect or potentiation). Products include:
Diupres Tablets 1650
Hydropres Tablets 1675
Ser-Ap-Es Tablets 849

Rocuronium Bromide (Increased responsiveness to muscle relaxant). Products include:
Zemuron 1830

Secobarbital Sodium (Potentiation of orthostatic hypotension may occur). Products include:
Seconal Sodium Pulvules 1474

Sodium Nitroprusside (Additive effect or potentiation).
No products indexed under this heading.

Sotalol Hydrochloride (Additive effect or potentiation). Products include:
Betapace Tablets 641

Spirapril Hydrochloride (Additive effect or potentiation).
No products indexed under this heading.

Spironolactone (Significant increases in serum potassium; excessive hypotension). Products include:
Aldactazide 2413
Aldactone 2414

Sufentanil Citrate (Potentiation of orthostatic hypotension may occur). Products include:
Sufenta Injection 1309

Sulindac (Reduced diuretic, natriuretic, and antihypertensive effects of Vaseretic). Products include:
Clinoril Tablets 1618

Terazosin Hydrochloride (Additive effect or potentiation). Products include:
Hytrin Capsules 430

Thiamylal Sodium (Potentiation of orthostatic hypotension may occur).
No products indexed under this heading.

Timolol Maleate (Additive effect or potentiation). Products include:
Blocadren Tablets 1614
Timolide Tablets 1748
Timoptic in Ocudose 1753
Timoptic Sterile Ophthalmic Solution 1751
Timoptic-XE 1755

Tolazamide (Dosage adjustment of hypoglycemic may be required).
No products indexed under this heading.

Tolbutamide (Dosage adjustment of hypoglycemic may be required).
No products indexed under this heading.

Tolmetin Sodium (Reduced diuretic, natriuretic, and antihypertensive effects of Vaseretic). Products include:
Tolectin (200, 400 and 600 mg) 1581

Torsemide (Additive effect or potentiation). Products include:
Demadex Tablets and Injection 686

Triamcinolone (Intensified electrolyte depletion, particularly hypokalemia). Products include:
Aristocort Tablets 1022

Triamcinolone Acetonide (Intensified electrolyte depletion, particularly hypokalemia). Products include:
Aristocort A 0.025% Cream 1027

IMPORTANT NOTE: Always consult each drug listing in the patient's regimen for possible interactions.

Vaseretic **Interactions Index** **1128**

Aristocort A 0.5% Cream 1031
Aristocort A 0.1% Cream 1029
Aristocort A 0.1% Ointment 1030
Azmacort Oral Inhaler 2011
Nasacort Nasal Inhaler 2024

Triamcinolone Diacetate (Intensified electrolyte depletion, particularly hypokalemia). Products include:
Aristocort Suspension (Forte Parenteral) 1027
Aristocort Suspension (Intralesional) 1025

Triamcinolone Hexacetonide (Intensified electrolyte depletion, particularly hypokalemia). Products include:
Aristospan Suspension (Intra-articular) 1033
Aristospan Suspension (Intralesional) 1032

Triamterene (Significant increases potentiation; excessive hypotension). Products include:
Dyazide 2479
Dyrenium Capsules 2481
Maxzide 1380

Trimethaphan Camsylate (Additive effect or potentiation). Products include:
Arfonad Ampuls 2080

Vecuronium Bromide (Increased responsiveness to muscle relaxant). Products include:
Norcuron 1826

Verapamil Hydrochloride (Additive effect or potentiation). Products include:
Calan SR Caplets 2422
Calan Tablets 2419
Isoptin Injectable 1344
Isoptin Oral Tablets 1346
Isoptin SR Tablets 1348
Verelan Capsules 1410
Verelan Capsules 2824

Food Interactions

Alcohol (Potentiation of orthostatic hypotension may occur).

VASOCIDIN OINTMENT
(Prednisolone Acetate, Sulfacetamide Sodium) .... ◉ 268
None cited in PDR database.

VASOCIDIN OPHTHALMIC SOLUTION
(Prednisolone Sodium Phosphate, Sulfacetamide Sodium) .... ◉ 270
May interact with silver preparations and para-aminobenzoic acid based local anesthetics. Compounds in these categories include:

Procaine Hydrochloride (May antagonize the actions of sulfonamides). Products include:
Novocain Hydrochloride for Spinal Anesthesia 2326

Silver Nitrate (Incompatible).
No products indexed under this heading.

Tetracaine Hydrochloride (May antagonize the actions of sulfonamides). Products include:
Cetacaine Topical Anesthetic 794
Pontocaine Hydrochloride for Spinal Anesthesia 2330

VASOCON-A
(Antazoline Phosphate, Naphazoline Hydrochloride) .... ◉ 271
None cited in PDR database.

VASOSULF
(Phenylephrine Hydrochloride, Sulfacetamide Sodium) .... ◉ 271
May interact with silver preparations. Compounds in this category include:

Silver Nitrate (Incompatible).
No products indexed under this heading.

VASOTEC I.V.
(Enalaprilat) 1768
May interact with diuretics, potassium sparing diuretics, potassium preparations, lithium preparations, and certain other agents. Compounds in these categories include:

Amiloride Hydrochloride (Potential for excessive hypotension and significant hyperkalemia). Products include:
Midamor Tablets 1703
Moduretic Tablets 1705

Bendroflumethiazide (Potential for excessive hypotension).
No products indexed under this heading.

Bumetanide (Potential for excessive hypotension). Products include:
Bumex 2093

Chlorothiazide (Potential for excessive hypotension). Products include:
Aldoclor Tablets 1598
Diupres Tablets 1650
Diuril Oral 1653

Chlorothiazide Sodium (Potential for excessive hypotension). Products include:
Diuril Sodium Intravenous 1652

Chlorthalidone (Potential for excessive hypotension). Products include:
Combipres Tablets 677
Tenoretic Tablets 2845
Thalitone 1245

Ethacrynic Acid (Potential for excessive hypotension). Products include:
Edecrin Tablets 1657

Furosemide (Potential for excessive hypotension). Products include:
Lasix Injection, Oral Solution and Tablets 1240

Hydrochlorothiazide (Potential for excessive hypotension). Products include:
Aldactazide 2413
Aldoril Tablets 1604
Apresazide Capsules 808
Capozide 742
Dyazide 2479
Esidrix Tablets 821
Esimil Tablets 822
HydroDIURIL Tablets 1674
Hydropres Tablets 1675
Hyzaar Tablets 1677
Inderide Tablets 2732
Inderide LA Long Acting Capsules .. 2734
Lopressor HCT Tablets 832
Lotensin HCT 837
Maxzide 1380
Moduretic Tablets 1705
Oretic Tablets 443
Prinzide Tablets 1737
Ser-Ap-Es Tablets 849
Timolide Tablets 1748
Vaseretic Tablets 1765
Zestoretic 2850
Ziac 1415

Hydroflumethiazide (Potential for excessive hypotension). Products include:
Diucardin Tablets 2718

Indapamide (Potential for excessive hypotension). Products include:
Lozol Tablets 2022

Lithium Carbonate (Potential for reversible lithium toxicity; monitor lithium levels frequently). Products include:
Eskalith 2485
Lithium Carbonate Capsules & Tablets 2230
Lithonate/Lithotabs/Lithobid 2543

Lithium Citrate (Potential for reversible lithium toxicity; monitor lithium levels frequently).
No products indexed under this heading.

Methyclothiazide (Potential for excessive hypotension). Products include:
Enduron Tablets 420

Metolazone (Potential for excessive hypotension). Products include:
Mykrox Tablets 993
Zaroxolyn Tablets 1000

Polythiazide (Potential for excessive hypotension). Products include:
Minizide Capsules 1938

Potassium Acid Phosphate (Potential for significant hyperkalemia). Products include:
K-Phos Original Formula 'Sodium Free' Tablets 639

Potassium Bicarbonate (Potential for significant hyperkalemia). Products include:
Alka-Seltzer Gold Effervescent Antacid .... ▣ 703

Potassium Chloride (Potential for significant hyperkalemia). Products include:
Chlor-3 Condiment 1004
K-Dur Microburst Release System (potassium chloride, USP) E.R. Tablets 1325
K-Lor Powder Packets 434
K-Norm Extended-Release Capsules 991
K-Tab Filmtab 434
Kolyum Liquid 992
Micro-K 2063
Micro-K LS Packets 2064
NuLYTELY 689
Cherry Flavor NuLYTELY 689
Rum-K Syrup 1005
Slow-K Extended-Release Tablets 851

Potassium Citrate (Potential for significant hyperkalemia). Products include:
Polycitra Syrup 578
Polycitra-K Crystals 579
Polycitra-K Oral Solution 579
Polycitra-LC 578

Potassium Gluconate (Potential for significant hyperkalemia). Products include:
Kolyum Liquid 992

Potassium Phosphate, Dibasic (Potential for significant hyperkalemia).
No products indexed under this heading.

Potassium Phosphate, Monobasic (Potential for significant hyperkalemia). Products include:
K-Phos Neutral Tablets 639
K-Phos Original Formula 'Sodium Free' Tablets 639

Spironolactone (Potential for excessive hypotension and significant hyperkalemia). Products include:
Aldactazide 2413
Aldactone 2414

Torsemide (Potential for excessive hypotension). Products include:
Demadex Tablets and Injection 686

Triamterene (Potential for excessive hypotension and significant hyperkalemia). Products include:
Dyazide 2479
Dyrenium Capsules 2481
Maxzide 1380

VASOTEC TABLETS
(Enalapril Maleate) 1771
May interact with diuretics, thiazides, potassium preparations, lithium preparations, potassium sparing diuretics, and certain other agents. Compounds in these categories include:

Amiloride Hydrochloride (Significant increases in serum potassium; excessive hypotension). Products include:
Midamor Tablets 1703
Moduretic Tablets 1705

Bendroflumethiazide (Attenuated potassium loss; excessive hypotension).
No products indexed under this heading.

Bumetanide (Excessive hypotension). Products include:
Bumex 2093

Chlorothiazide (Attenuated potassium loss; excessive hypotension). Products include:
Aldoclor Tablets 1598
Diupres Tablets 1650
Diuril Oral 1653

Chlorothiazide Sodium (Attenuated potassium loss; excessive hypotension). Products include:
Diuril Sodium Intravenous 1652

Chlorthalidone (Significant increases in serum potassium; excessive hypotension). Products include:
Combipres Tablets 677
Tenoretic Tablets 2845
Thalitone 1245

Ethacrynic Acid (Excessive hypotension). Products include:
Edecrin Tablets 1657

Furosemide (Excessive hypotension). Products include:
Lasix Injection, Oral Solution and Tablets 1240

Hydrochlorothiazide (Attenuated potassium loss; excessive hypotension). Products include:
Aldactazide 2413
Aldoril Tablets 1604
Apresazide Capsules 808
Capozide 742
Dyazide 2479
Esidrix Tablets 821
Esimil Tablets 822
HydroDIURIL Tablets 1674
Hydropres Tablets 1675
Hyzaar Tablets 1677
Inderide Tablets 2732
Inderide LA Long Acting Capsules .. 2734
Lopressor HCT Tablets 832
Lotensin HCT 837
Maxzide 1380
Moduretic Tablets 1705
Oretic Tablets 443
Prinzide Tablets 1737
Ser-Ap-Es Tablets 849
Timolide Tablets 1748
Vaseretic Tablets 1765
Zestoretic 2850
Ziac 1415

Hydroflumethiazide (Attenuated potassium loss; excessive hypotension). Products include:
Diucardin Tablets 2718

Indapamide (Excessive hypotension). Products include:
Lozol Tablets 2022

Lithium Carbonate (Potential for reversible lithium toxicity; frequent monitoring of serum lithium levels is recommended). Products include:
Eskalith 2485
Lithium Carbonate Capsules & Tablets 2230
Lithonate/Lithotabs/Lithobid 2543

Lithium Citrate (Potential for reversible lithium toxicity; frequent monitoring of serum lithium levels is recommended).
No products indexed under this heading.

Methyclothiazide (Attenuated potassium loss; excessive hypotension). Products include:
Enduron Tablets 420

Metolazone (Excessive hypotension). Products include:
Mykrox Tablets 993
Zaroxolyn Tablets 1000

Polythiazide (Attenuated potassium loss; excessive hypotension). Products include:
Minizide Capsules 1938

1129 Interactions Index Ventolin Inhalation Aerosol

Potassium Acid Phosphate (Significant increases in serum potassium). Products include:
K-Phos Original Formula 'Sodium Free' Tablets ... 639

Potassium Bicarbonate (Significant increases in serum potassium). Products include:
Alka-Seltzer Gold Effervescent Antacid ... ▣ 703

Potassium Chloride (Significant increases in serum potassium). Products include:
Chlor-3 Condiment ... 1004
K-Dur Microburst Release System (potassium chloride, USP) E.R. Tablets ... 1325
K-Lor Powder Packets ... 434
K-Norm Extended-Release Capsules ... 991
K-Tab Filmtab ... 434
Kolyum Liquid ... 992
Micro-K ... 2063
Micro-K LS Packets ... 2064
NuLYTELY ... 689
Cherry Flavor NuLYTELY ... 689
Rum-K Syrup ... 1005
Slow-K Extended-Release Tablets ... 851

Potassium Citrate (Significant increases in serum potassium). Products include:
Polycitra Syrup ... 578
Polycitra-K Crystals ... 579
Polycitra-K Oral Solution ... 579
Polycitra-LC ... 578

Potassium Gluconate (Significant increases in serum potassium). Products include:
Kolyum Liquid ... 992

Potassium Phosphate, Dibasic (Significant increases in serum potassium).
No products indexed under this heading.

Potassium Phosphate, Monobasic (Significant increases in serum potassium). Products include:
K-Phos Neutral Tablets ... 639
K-Phos Original Formula 'Sodium Free' Tablets ... 639

Spironolactone (Significant increases in serum potassium; excessive hypotension). Products include:
Aldactazide ... 2413
Aldactone ... 2414

Torsemide (Excessive hypotension). Products include:
Demadex Tablets and Injection ... 686

Triamterene (Significant increases in serum potassium; excessive hypotension). Products include:
Dyazide ... 2479
Dyrenium Capsules ... 2481
Maxzide ... 1380

VASOXYL INJECTION
(Methoxamine Hydrochloride) ... 1196
May interact with monoamine oxidase inhibitors, tricyclic antidepressants, and certain other agents. Compounds in these categories include:

Amitriptyline Hydrochloride (Potentiation of pressor effect). Products include:
Elavil ... 2838
Endep Tablets ... 2174
Etrafon ... 2355
Limbitrol ... 2180
Triavil Tablets ... 1757

Amoxapine (Potentiation of pressor effect). Products include:
Asendin Tablets ... 1369

Clomipramine Hydrochloride (Potentiation of pressor effect). Products include:
Anafranil Capsules ... 803

Desipramine Hydrochloride (Potentiation of pressor effect). Products include:
Norpramin Tablets ... 1526

Doxepin Hydrochloride (Potentiation of pressor effect). Products include:
Sinequan ... 2205
Zonalon Cream ... 1055

Ergonovine Maleate (Potentiation of pressor effect).
No products indexed under this heading.

Ergot Alkaloids (Hydrogenated) (Potentiation of pressor effect).

Ergotamine Tartrate (Potentiation of pressor effect). Products include:
Bellergal-S Tablets ... 2250
Cafergot ... 2251
Ergomar ... 1486
Wigraine Tablets & Suppositories ... 1829

Furazolidone (Potentiation of pressor effect). Products include:
Furoxone ... 2046

Imipramine Hydrochloride (Potentiation of pressor effect). Products include:
Tofranil Ampuls ... 854
Tofranil Tablets ... 856

Imipramine Pamoate (Potentiation of pressor effect). Products include:
Tofranil-PM Capsules ... 857

Isocarboxazid (Potentiation of pressor effect).
No products indexed under this heading.

Maprotiline Hydrochloride (Potentiation of pressor effect). Products include:
Ludiomil Tablets ... 843

Methylergonovine Maleate (Potentiation of pressor effect). Products include:
Methergine ... 2272

Nortriptyline Hydrochloride (Potentiation of pressor effect). Products include:
Pamelor ... 2280

Phenelzine Sulfate (Potentiation of pressor effect). Products include:
Nardil ... 1920

Protriptyline Hydrochloride (Potentiation of pressor effect). Products include:
Vivactil Tablets ... 1774

Selegiline Hydrochloride (Potentiation of pressor effect). Products include:
Eldepryl Tablets ... 2550

Tranylcypromine Sulfate (Potentiation of pressor effect). Products include:
Parnate Tablets ... 2503

Trimipramine Maleate (Potentiation of pressor effect). Products include:
Surmontil Capsules ... 2811

Vasopressin (Potentiation of pressor effect).
No products indexed under this heading.

VELBAN VIALS
(Vinblastine Sulfate) ... 1484
May interact with:

Mitomycin (Mitomycin-C) (Acute shortness of breath; severe bronchospasm). Products include:
Mutamycin ... 703

Phenytoin (Reduced blood levels of phenytoin and increased seizure activity). Products include:
Dilantin Infatabs ... 1908
Dilantin-125 Suspension ... 1911

Phenytoin Sodium (Reduced blood levels of phenytoin and increased seizure activity). Products include:
Dilantin Kapseals ... 1906
Dilantin Parenteral ... 1910

VELOSULIN BR HUMAN INSULIN 10 ML VIALS
(Insulin, Human Regular) ... 1795
None cited in PDR database.

VENTOLIN INHALATION AEROSOL AND REFILL
(Albuterol) ... 1197
May interact with sympathomimetic bronchodilators, monoamine oxidase inhibitors, tricyclic antidepressants, beta blockers, and certain other agents. Compounds in these categories include:

Acebutolol Hydrochloride (Beta receptor blocking agents and albuterol inhibit effect of each other). Products include:
Sectral Capsules ... 2807

Amitriptyline Hydrochloride (Action of albuterol on vascular system may be potentiated). Products include:
Elavil ... 2838
Endep Tablets ... 2174
Etrafon ... 2355
Limbitrol ... 2180
Triavil Tablets ... 1757

Amoxapine (Action of albuterol on vascular system may be potentiated). Products include:
Asendin Tablets ... 1369

Atenolol (Beta receptor blocking agents and albuterol inhibit effect of each other). Products include:
Tenoretic Tablets ... 2845
Tenormin Tablets and I.V. Injection ... 2847

Betaxolol Hydrochloride (Beta receptor blocking agents and albuterol inhibit effect of each other). Products include:
Betoptic Ophthalmic Solution ... 469
Betoptic S Ophthalmic Suspension ... 471
Kerlone Tablets ... 2436

Bisoprolol Fumarate (Beta receptor blocking agents and albuterol inhibit effect of each other). Products include:
Zebeta Tablets ... 1413
Ziac ... 1415

Bitolterol Mesylate (Sympathomimetic aerosol bronchodilators should not be used concomitantly with albuterol, may have additive effects). Products include:
Tornalate Solution for Inhalation, 0.2% ... 956
Tornalate Metered Dose Inhaler ... 957

Carteolol Hydrochloride (Beta receptor blocking agents and albuterol inhibit effect of each other). Products include:
Cartrol Tablets ... 410
Ocupress Ophthalmic Solution, 1% Sterile ... ⊙ 309

Clomipramine Hydrochloride (Action of albuterol on vascular system may be potentiated). Products include:
Anafranil Capsules ... 803

Desipramine Hydrochloride (Action of albuterol on vascular system may be potentiated). Products include:
Norpramin Tablets ... 1526

Doxepin Hydrochloride (Action of albuterol on vascular system may be potentiated). Products include:
Sinequan ... 2205
Zonalon Cream ... 1055

Ephedrine Hydrochloride (Sympathomimetic aerosol bronchodilators should not be used concomitantly with albuterol, may have additive effects). Products include:
Primatene Dual Action Formula ... ▣ 872
Primatene Tablets ... ▣ 873
Quadrinal Tablets ... 1350

Ephedrine Sulfate (Sympathomimetic aerosol bronchodilators should not be used concomitantly with albuterol, may have additive effects). Products include:
Bronkaid Caplets ... ▣ 717
Marax Tablets & DF Syrup ... 2200

Ephedrine Tannate (Sympathomimetic aerosol bronchodilators should not be used concomitantly with albuterol, may have additive effects). Products include:
Rynatuss ... 2673

Epinephrine (Sympathomimetic aerosol bronchodilators should not be used concomitantly with albuterol, may have additive effects). Products include:
Bronkaid Mist ... ▣ 717
EPIFRIN ... ⊙ 239
EpiPen ... 790
Marcaine Hydrochloride with Epinephrine 1:200,000 ... 2316
Primatene Mist ... ▣ 873
Sensorcaine with Epinephrine Injection ... 559
Sus-Phrine Injection ... 1019
Xylocaine with Epinephrine Injections ... 567

Epinephrine Hydrochloride (Sympathomimetic aerosol bronchodilators should not be used concomitantly with albuterol). Products include:
Ana-Kit Anaphylaxis Emergency Treatment Kit ... 617

Esmolol Hydrochloride (Beta receptor blocking agents and albuterol inhibit effect of each other). Products include:
Brevibloc Injection ... 1808

Ethylnorepinephrine Hydrochloride (Sympathomimetic aerosol bronchodilators should not be used concomitantly with albuterol, may have additive effects).
No products indexed under this heading.

Furazolidone (Action of albuterol on vascular system may be potentiated). Products include:
Furoxone ... 2046

Imipramine Hydrochloride (Action of albuterol on vascular system may be potentiated). Products include:
Tofranil Ampuls ... 854
Tofranil Tablets ... 856

Imipramine Pamoate (Action of albuterol on vascular system may be potentiated). Products include:
Tofranil-PM Capsules ... 857

Isocarboxazid (Action of albuterol on vascular system may be potentiated).
No products indexed under this heading.

Isoetharine (Sympathomimetic aerosol bronchodilators should not be used concomitantly with albuterol, may have additive effects). Products include:
Bronkometer Aerosol ... 2302
Bronkosol Solution ... 2302
Isoetharine Inhalation Solution, USP, Arm-a-Med ... 551

IMPORTANT NOTE: Always consult each drug listing in the patient's regimen for possible interactions.

Ventolin Inhalation Aerosol — Interactions Index — 1130

Isoproterenol Hydrochloride (Sympathomimetic aerosol bronchodilators should not be used concomitantly with albuterol, may have additive effects). Products include:
Isuprel Hydrochloride Injection 1:5000 2311
Isuprel Hydrochloride Solution 1:200 & 1:100 2313
Isuprel Mistometer 2312

Isoproterenol Sulfate (Sympathomimetic aerosol bronchodilators should not be used concomitantly with albuterol, may have additive effects). Products include:
Norisodrine with Calcium Iodide Syrup........ 442

Labetalol Hydrochloride (Beta receptor blocking agents and albuterol inhibit effect of each other). Products include:
Normodyne Injection 2377
Normodyne Tablets 2379
Trandate 1185

Levobunolol Hydrochloride (Beta receptor blocking agents and albuterol inhibit effect of each other). Products include:
Betagan .... ◉ 233

Maprotiline Hydrochloride (Action of albuterol on vascular system may be potentiated). Products include:
Ludiomil Tablets........ 843

Metaproterenol Sulfate (Sympathomimetic aerosol bronchodilators should not be used concomitantly with albuterol, may have additive effects). Products include:
Alupent........ 669
Metaproterenol Sulfate Inhalation Solution, USP, Arm-a-Med 552

Metipranolol Hydrochloride (Beta receptor blocking agents and albuterol inhibit effect of each other). Products include:
OptiPranolol (Metipranolol 0.3%) Sterile Ophthalmic Solution........ ◉ 258

Metoprolol Succinate (Beta receptor blocking agents and albuterol inhibit effect of each other). Products include:
Toprol-XL Tablets 565

Metoprolol Tartrate (Beta receptor blocking agents and albuterol inhibit effect of each other). Products include:
Lopressor Ampuls........ 830
Lopressor HCT Tablets........ 832
Lopressor Tablets 830

Nadolol (Beta receptor blocking agents and albuterol inhibit effect of each other).
No products indexed under this heading.

Nortriptyline Hydrochloride (Action of albuterol on vascular system may be potentiated). Products include:
Pamelor 2280

Penbutolol Sulfate (Beta receptor blocking agents and albuterol inhibit effect of each other). Products include:
Levatol 2403

Phenelzine Sulfate (Action of albuterol on vascular system may be potentiated). Products include:
Nardil 1920

Pindolol (Beta receptor blocking agents and albuterol inhibit effect of each other). Products include:
Visken Tablets........ 2299

Pirbuterol Acetate (Sympathomimetic aerosol bronchodilators should not be used concomitantly with albuterol, may have additive effects). Products include:
Maxair Autohaler 1492
Maxair Inhaler 1494

Propranolol Hydrochloride (Beta receptor blocking agents and albuterol inhibit effect of each other). Products include:
Inderal 2728
Inderal LA Long Acting Capsules 2730
Inderide Tablets 2732
Inderide LA Long Acting Capsules 2734

Protriptyline Hydrochloride (Action of albuterol on vascular system may be potentiated). Products include:
Vivactil Tablets 1774

Salmeterol Xinafoate (Sympathomimetic aerosol bronchodilators should not be used concomitantly with albuterol, may have additive effects). Products include:
Serevent Inhalation Aerosol........ 1176

Selegiline Hydrochloride (Action of albuterol on vascular system may be potentiated). Products include:
Eldepryl Tablets 2550

Sotàlol Hydrochloride (Beta receptor blocking agents and albuterol inhibit effect of each other). Products include:
Betapace Tablets 641

Terbutaline Sulfate (Sympathomimetic aerosol bronchodilators should not be used concomitantly with albuterol, may have additive effects). Products include:
Brethaire Inhaler 813
Brethine Ampuls 815
Brethine Tablets........ 814
Bricanyl Subcutaneous Injection........ 1502
Bricanyl Tablets 1503

Timolol Hemihydrate (Beta receptor blocking agents and albuterol inhibit effect of each other). Products include:
Betimol 0.25%, 0.5% .... ◉ 261

Timolol Maleate (Beta receptor blocking agents and albuterol inhibit effect of each other). Products include:
Blocadren Tablets 1614
Timolide Tablets........ 1748
Timoptic in Ocudose 1753
Timoptic Sterile Ophthalmic Solution........ 1751
Timoptic-XE 1755

Tranylcypromine Sulfate (Action of albuterol on vascular system may be potentiated). Products include:
Parnate Tablets 2503

Trimipramine Maleate (Action of albuterol on vascular system may be potentiated). Products include:
Surmontil Capsules........ 2811

VENTOLIN INHALATION SOLUTION

(Albuterol Sulfate) 1198
May interact with sympathomimetics, monoamine oxidase inhibitors, beta blockers, and tricyclic antidepressants. Compounds in these categories include:

Acebutolol Hydrochloride (Beta-receptor blocking agents and albuterol inhibit effect of each other). Products include:
Sectral Capsules 2807

Amitriptyline Hydrochloride (Action of albuterol on the vascular system may be potentiated). Products include:
Elavil 2838
Endep Tablets 2174
Etrafon 2355
Limbitrol 2180
Triavil Tablets 1757

Amoxapine (Action of albuterol on the vascular system may be potentiated). Products include:
Asendin Tablets 1369

Atenolol (Beta-receptor blocking agents and albuterol inhibit effect of each other). Products include:
Tenoretic Tablets........ 2845
Tenormin Tablets and I.V. Injection 2847

Betaxolol Hydrochloride (Beta-receptor blocking agents and albuterol inhibit effect of each other). Products include:
Betoptic Ophthalmic Solution........ 469
Betoptic S Ophthalmic Suspension 471
Kerlone Tablets........ 2436

Bisoprolol Fumarate (Beta-receptor blocking agents and albuterol inhibit effect of each other). Products include:
Zebeta Tablets 1413
Ziac 1415

Carteolol Hydrochloride (Beta-receptor blocking agents and albuterol inhibit effect of each other). Products include:
Cartrol Tablets 410
Ocupress Ophthalmic Solution, 1% Sterile........ ◉ 309

Clomipramine Hydrochloride (Action of albuterol on the vascular system may be potentiated). Products include:
Anafranil Capsules 803

Desipramine Hydrochloride (Action of albuterol on the vascular system may be potentiated). Products include:
Norpramin Tablets 1526

Doxepin Hydrochloride (Action of albuterol on the vascular system may be potentiated). Products include:
Sinequan 2205
Zonalon Cream 1055

Ephedrine Hydrochloride (Concomitant use of albuterol with oral sympathomimetic agents is not recommended due to potential for cardiovascular toxicity). Products include:
Primatene Dual Action Formula........ ▣ 872
Primatene Tablets .... ▣ 873
Quadrinal Tablets 1350

Ephedrine Sulfate (Concomitant use of albuterol with oral sympathomimetic agents is not recommended due to potential for cardiovascular toxicity). Products include:
Bronkaid Caplets .... ▣ 717
Marax Tablets & DF Syrup........ 2200

Ephedrine Tannate (Concomitant use of albuterol with oral sympathomimetic agents is not recommended due to potential for cardiovascular toxicity). Products include:
Rynatuss 2673

Esmolol Hydrochloride (Beta-receptor blocking agents and albuterol inhibit effect of each other). Products include:
Brevibloc Injection........ 1808

Furazolidone (Action of albuterol on the vascular system may be potentiated). Products include:
Furoxone 2046

Imipramine Hydrochloride (Action of albuterol on the vascular system may be potentiated). Products include:
Tofranil Ampuls 854
Tofranil Tablets 856

Imipramine Pamoate (Action of albuterol on the vascular system may be potentiated). Products include:
Tofranil-PM Capsules........ 857

Isocarboxazid (Action of albuterol on the vascular system may be potentiated).
No products indexed under this heading.

Labetalol Hydrochloride (Beta-receptor blocking agents and albuterol inhibit effect of each other). Products include:
Normodyne Injection 2377
Normodyne Tablets 2379
Trandate 1185

Levobunolol Hydrochloride (Beta-receptor blocking agents and albuterol inhibit effect of each other). Products include:
Betagan .... ◉ 233

Maprotiline Hydrochloride (Action of albuterol on the vascular system may be potentiated). Products include:
Ludiomil Tablets........ 843

Metaproterenol Sulfate (Concomitant use of albuterol with oral sympathomimetic agents is not recommended due to potential for cardiovascular toxicity). Products include:
Alupent........ 669
Metaproterenol Sulfate Inhalation Solution, USP, Arm-a-Med 552

Metipranolol Hydrochloride (Beta-receptor blocking agents and albuterol inhibit effect of each other). Products include:
OptiPranolol (Metipranolol 0.3%) Sterile Ophthalmic Solution........ ◉ 258

Metoprolol Succinate (Beta-receptor blocking agents and albuterol inhibit effect of each other). Products include:
Toprol-XL Tablets 565

Metoprolol Tartrate (Beta-receptor blocking agents and albuterol inhibit effect of each other). Products include:
Lopressor Ampuls........ 830
Lopressor HCT Tablets........ 832
Lopressor Tablets 830

Nadolol (Beta-receptor blocking agents and albuterol inhibit effect of each other).
No products indexed under this heading.

Norepinephrine Bitartrate (Concomitant use of albuterol with oral sympathomimetic agents is not recommended due to potential for cardiovascular toxicity). Products include:
Levophed Bitartrate Injection........ 2315

Nortriptyline Hydrochloride (Action of albuterol on the vascular system may be potentiated). Products include:
Pamelor 2280

Penbutolol Sulfate (Beta-receptor blocking agents and albuterol inhibit effect of each other). Products include:
Levatol 2403

Phenelzine Sulfate (Action of albuterol on the vascular system may be potentiated). Products include:
Nardil 1920

Phenylephrine Bitartrate (Concomitant use of albuterol with oral sympathomimetic agents is not recommended due to potential for cardiovascular toxicity).
No products indexed under this heading.

(▣ Described in PDR For Nonprescription Drugs) (◉ Described in PDR For Ophthalmology)

Interactions Index

Ventolin Inhalation Solution

Phenylephrine Hydrochloride (Concomitant use of albuterol with oral sympathomimetic agents is not recommended due to potential for cardiovascular toxicity). Products include:

Atrohist Plus Tablets 454
Cerose DM .... ⊕ 878
Comhist 2038
D.A. Chewable Tablets........................... 951
Deconsal Pediatric Capsules................ 454
Dura-Vent/DA Tablets 953
Entex Capsules 1986
Entex Liquid 1986
Extendryl 1005
4-Way Fast Acting Nasal Spray (regular & mentholated) .... ⊕ 621
Hemorid For Women .... ⊕ 834
Hycomine Compound Tablets 932
Neo-Synephrine Hydrochloride 1% Carpuject.. 2324
Neo-Synephrine Hydrochloride 1% Injection 2324
Neo-Synephrine Hydrochloride (Ophthalmic) 2325
Neo-Synephrine .... ⊕ 726
Nōstril .... ⊕ 644
Novahistine Elixir .... ⊕ 823
Phenergan VC 2779
Phenergan VC with Codeine 2781
Preparation H .... ⊕ 871
Tympagesic Ear Drops 2342
Vasosulf .... © 271
Vicks Sinex Nasal Spray and Ultra Fine Mist .... ⊕ 765

Phenylephrine Tannate (Concomitant use of albuterol with oral sympathomimetic agents is not recommended due to potential for cardiovascular toxicity). Products include:

Atrohist Pediatric Suspension 454
Ricobid-D Pediatric Suspension........ 2038
Ricobid Tablets and Pediatric Suspension.. 2038
Rynatan 2673
Rynatuss 2673

Phenylpropanolamine Hydrochloride (Concomitant use of albuterol with oral sympathomimetic agents is not recommended due to potential for cardiovascular toxicity). Products include:

Acutrim .... ⊕ 628
Allerest Children's Chewable Tablets .... ⊕ 627
Allerest 12 Hour Caplets .... ⊕ 627
Atrohist Plus Tablets 454
BC Cold Powder Multi-Symptom Formula (Cold-Sinus-Allergy) .... ⊕ 609
BC Cold Powder Non-Drowsy Formula (Cold-Sinus) .... ⊕ 609
Cheracol Plus Head Cold/Cough Formula .... ⊕ 769
Comtrex Multi-Symptom Non-Drowsy Liqui-gels................................... ⊕ 618
Contac Continuous Action Nasal Decongestant/Antihistamine 12 Hour Capsules... ⊕ 813
Contac Maximum Strength Continuous Action Decongestant/Antihistamine 12 Hour Caplets.. ⊕ 813
Contac Severe Cold and Flu Formula Caplets .... ⊕ 814
Coricidin 'D' Decongestant Tablets .... ⊕ 800
Dexatrim .... ⊕ 832
Dexatrim Plus Vitamins Caplets .... ⊕ 832
Dimetane-DC Cough Syrup 2059
Dimetapp Elixir .... ⊕ 773
Dimetapp Extentabs .... ⊕ 774
Dimetapp Tablets/Liqui-Gels .... ⊕ 775
Dimetapp Cold & Allergy Chewable Tablets .... ⊕ 773
Dimetapp DM Elixir .... ⊕ 774
Dura-Vent Tablets 952
Entex Capsules 1986
Entex LA Tablets 1987
Entex Liquid 1986
Exgest LA Tablets 782
Hycomine 931
Isoclor Timesule Capsules .... ⊕ 637
Nolamine Timed-Release Tablets 785
Ornade Spansule Capsules 2502
Propagest Tablets 786
Pyrroxate Caplets .... ⊕ 772
Robitussin-CF .... ⊕ 777

Sinulin Tablets 787
Tavist-D 12 Hour Relief Tablets .... ⊕ 787
Teldrin 12 Hour Antihistamine/Nasal Decongestant Allergy Relief Capsules .... ⊕ 826
Triaminic Allergy Tablets .... ⊕ 789
Triaminic Cold Tablets .... ⊕ 790
Triaminic Expectorant .... ⊕ 790
Triaminic Syrup .... ⊕ 792
Triaminic-12 Tablets .... ⊕ 792
Triaminic-DM Syrup .... ⊕ 792
Triaminicin Tablets .... ⊕ 793
Triaminicol Multi-Symptom Cold Tablets .... ⊕ 793
Triaminicol Multi-Symptom Relief ⊕ 794
Vicks DayQuil Allergy Relief 12-Hour Extended Release Tablets.. ⊕ 760
Vicks DayQuil Allergy Relief 4-Hour Tablets .... ⊕ 760
Vicks DayQuil SINUS Pressure & CONGESTION Relief.......................... ⊕ 761

Pindolol (Beta-receptor blocking agents and albuterol inhibit effect of each other). Products include:

Visken Tablets... 2299

Pirbuterol Acetate (Concomitant use of albuterol with oral sympathomimetic agents is not recommended due to potential for cardiovascular toxicity). Products include:

Maxair Autohaler 1492
Maxair Inhaler 1494

Propranolol Hydrochloride (Beta-receptor blocking agents and albuterol inhibit effect of each other). Products include:

Inderal 2728
Inderal LA Long Acting Capsules 2730
Inderide Tablets 2732
Inderide LA Long Acting Capsules .. 2734

Protriptyline Hydrochloride (Action of albuterol on the vascular system may be potentiated). Products include:

Vivactil Tablets 1774

Pseudoephedrine Hydrochloride (Concomitant use of albuterol with oral sympathomimetic agents is not recommended due to potential for cardiovascular toxicity). Products include:

Actifed Allergy Daytime/Nighttime Caplets... ⊕ 844
Actifed Plus Caplets .... ⊕ 845
Actifed Plus Tablets .... ⊕ 845
Actifed with Codeine Cough Syrup.. 1067
Actifed Sinus Daytime/Nighttime Tablets and Caplets .... ⊕ 846
Actifed Syrup... ⊕ 846
Actifed Tablets .... ⊕ 844
Advil Cold and Sinus Caplets and Tablets (formerly CoAdvil) .... ⊕ 870
Alka-Seltzer Plus Cold Medicine Liqui-Gels .... ⊕ 706
Alka-Seltzer Plus Cold & Cough Medicine Liqui-Gels............................... ⊕ 705
Alka-Seltzer Plus Night-Time Cold Medicine Liqui-Gels.............................. ⊕ 706
Allerest Headache Strength Tablets .... ⊕ 627
Allerest Maximum Strength Tablets .... ⊕ 627
Allerest No Drowsiness Tablets......... ⊕ 627
Allerest Sinus Pain Formula .... ⊕ 627
Anatuss LA Tablets................................. 1542
Atrohist Pediatric Capsules................. 453
Bayer Select Sinus Pain Relief Formula .... ⊕ 717
Benadryl Allergy Decongestant Liquid Medication .... ⊕ 848
Benadryl Allergy Decongestant Tablets .... ⊕ 848
Benadryl Allergy Sinus Headache Formula Caplets .... ⊕ 849
Benylin Multisymptom.......................... ⊕ 852
Bromfed Capsules (Extended-Release) 1785
Bromfed Syrup .... ⊕ 733
Bromfed Tablets 1785
Bromfed-DM Cough Syrup.................. 1786
Bromfed-PD Capsules (Extended-Release).. 1785
Children's Vicks DayQuil Allergy Relief... ⊕ 757
Children's Vicks NyQuil Cold/Cough Relief... ⊕ 758

Comtrex Multi-Symptom Cold Reliever Tablets/Caplets/Liqui-Gels/Liquid... ⊕ 615
Allergy-Sinus Comtrex Multi-Symptom Allergy-Sinus Formula Tablets .... ⊕ 617
Comtrex Multi-Symptom Non-Drowsy Caplets...................................... ⊕ 618
Congess 1004
Contac Day Allergy/Sinus Caplets ⊕ 812
Contac Day & Night .... ⊕ 812
Contac Night Allergy/Sinus Caplets .... ⊕ 812
Contac Severe Cold & Flu Non-Drowsy .... ⊕ 815
Deconamine Chewable Tablets 1320
Deconamine CX Cough and Cold Liquid and Tablets.................................. 1319
Deconamine 1320
Deconsal C Expectorant Syrup 456
Deconsal Pediatric Syrup 457
Deconsal II Tablets 454
Dimetane-DX Cough Syrup 2059
Dimetapp Sinus Caplets .... ⊕ 775
Dorcol Children's Cough Syrup .... ⊕ 785
Drixoral Cough + Congestion Liquid Caps .... ⊕ 802
Dura-Tap/PD Capsules 2867
Duratuss Tablets 2565
Duratuss HD Elixir.................................. 2565
Efidac/24 .... ⊕ 635
Entex PSE Tablets................................... 1987
Fedahist Gyrocaps................................. 2401
Fedahist Timecaps 2401
Guaifed.. 1787
Guaifed Syrup .... ⊕ 734
Guaimax-D Tablets 792
Guaitab Tablets .... ⊕ 734
Isoclor Expectorant................................ 990
Kronofed-A 977
Motrin IB Sinus....................................... ⊕ 838
Novahistine DH....................................... 2462
Novahistine DMX .... ⊕ 822
Novahistine Expectorant...................... 2463
Nucofed 2051
PediaCare Cold Allergy Chewable Tablets .... ⊕ 677
PediaCare Cough-Cold Chewable Tablets 1553
PediaCare 1553
PediaCare Infants' Decongestant Drops .... ⊕ 677
PediCare Infant's Drops Decongestant Plus Cough 1553
PediaCare NightRest Cough-Cold Liquid 1553
Pediatric Vicks 44d Dry Hacking Cough & Head Congestion.............. ⊕ 763
Pediatric Vicks 44m Cough & Cold Relief .... ⊕ 764
Robitussin Cold & Cough Liqui-Gels .... ⊕ 776
Robitussin Maximum Strength Cough & Cold .... ⊕ 778
Robitussin Pediatric Cough & Cold Formula... ⊕ 779
Robitussin Severe Congestion Liqui-Gels .... ⊕ 776
Robitussin-DAC Syrup........................... 2074
Robitussin-PE .... ⊕ 778
Rondec Oral Drops 953
Rondec Syrup 953
Rondec Tablet.. 953
Rondec-DM Oral Drops 954
Rondec-DM Syrup 954
Rondec-TR Tablet 953
Ryna .... ⊕ 841
Seldane-D Extended-Release Tablets 1538
Semprex-D Capsules 463
Semprex-D Capsules 1167
Sinarest Tablets .... ⊕ 648
Sinarest Extra Strength Tablets......... ⊕ 648
Sinarest No Drowsiness Tablets .... ⊕ 648
Sine-Aid IB Caplets 1554
Sine-Aid Maximum Strength Sinus Medication Gelcaps, Caplets and Tablets 1554
Sine-Off No Drowsiness Formula Caplets .... ⊕ 824
Sine-Off Sinus Medicine .... ⊕ 825
Singlet Tablets .... ⊕ 825
Sinutab Non-Drying Liquid Caps........ ⊕ 859
Sinutab Sinus Allergy Medication, Maximum Strength Tablets and Caplets .... ⊕ 860
Sinutab Sinus Medication, Maximum Strength Without Drowsiness Formula, Tablets & Caplets .... ⊕ 860

Sinutab Sinus Medication, Regular Strength Without Drowsiness Formula .... ⊕ 859
Sudafed Children's Liquid .... ⊕ 861
Sudafed Cold and Cough Liquidcaps .... ⊕ 862
Sudafed Cough Syrup .... ⊕ 862
Sudafed Plus Liquid .... ⊕ 862
Sudafed Plus Tablets .... ⊕ 863
Sudafed Severe Cold Formula Caplets .... ⊕ 863
Sudafed Severe Cold Formula Tablets .... ⊕ 864
Sudafed Sinus Caplets.......................... ⊕ 864
Sudafed Sinus Tablets........................... ⊕ 864
Sudafed Tablets, 30 mg........................ ⊕ 861
Sudafed Tablets, 60 mg........................ ⊕ 861
Sudafed 12 Hour Caplets .... ⊕ 861
Syn-Rx Tablets 465
Syn-Rx DM Tablets 466
TheraFlu.. ⊕ 787
TheraFlu Maximum Strength Nighttime Flu, Cold & Cough Medicine .... ⊕ 788
TheraFlu Maximum Strength Non-Drowsy Formula Flu, Cold & Cough Medicine .... ⊕ 788
Thera Flu Maximum Strength, Non-Drowsy Formula Flu, Cold and Cough Caplets .... ⊕ 789
Triaminic AM Cough and Decongestant Formula .... ⊕ 789
Triaminic AM Decongestant Formula .... ⊕ 790
Triaminic Nite Light .... ⊕ 791
Triaminic Sore Throat Formula .... ⊕ 791
Tussend 1783
Tussend Expectorant 1785
Children's TYLENOL Cold Multi-Symptom Liquid Formula and Chewable Tablets.................................... 1561
Children's TYLENOL Cold Plus Cough Multi Symptom Tablets and Liquid .... ⊕ 681
Infants' TYLENOL Cold Decongestant & Fever-Reducer Drops.......... 1556
TYLENOL Maximum Strength Allergy Sinus Medication Gelcaps and Caplets 1563
TYLENOL Maximum Strength Allergy Sinus NightTime Medication Caplets 1555
TYLENOL Flu Maximum Strength Gelcaps 1565
TYLENOL Flu NightTime, Maximum Strength, Gelcaps 1566
TYLENOL Maximum Strength Flu NightTime Hot Medication Packets 1562
TYLENOL, Maximum Strength, Sinus Medication Geltabs, Gelcaps, Caplets and Tablets 1566
TYLENOL Cold Multi-Symptom Formula Medication Tablets and Caplets 1561
TYLENOL Cold Medication No Drowsiness Formula Gelcaps and Caplets 1562
TYLENOL Cold Multi-Symptom Hot Medication Liquid Packets.................. 1557
TYLENOL Cough Multi-Symptom Medication with Decongestant 1565
Ursinus Inlay-Tabs.................................. ⊕ 794
Vicks 44 LiquiCaps Cough, Cold & Flu Relief .... ⊕ 755
Vicks 44 LiquiCaps Non-Drowsy Cough & Cold Relief .... ⊕ 756
Vicks 44D Dry Hacking Cough & Head Congestion .... ⊕ 755
Vicks 44M Cough, Cold & Flu Relief .... ⊕ 756
Vicks DayQuil .... ⊕ 761
Vicks DayQuil SINUS Pressure & PAIN Relief with IBUPROFEN .... ⊕ 762
Vicks Nyquil Hot Therapy..................... ⊕ 762
Vicks NyQuil LiquiCaps Multi-Symptom Cold/Flu Relief .... ⊕ 763
Vicks NyQuil Multi-Symptom Cold/Flu Relief - (Original & Cherry Flavor)... ⊕ 763

Pseudoephedrine Sulfate (Concomitant use of albuterol with oral sympathomimetic agents is not recommended due to potential for cardiovascular toxicity). Products include:

Cheracol Sinus .... ⊕ 768
Chlor-Trimeton Allergy Decongestant Tablets .... ⊕ 799
Claritin-D 2350

IMPORTANT NOTE: Always consult each drug listing in the patient's regimen for possible interactions.

Ventolin Inhalation Solution — Interactions Index — 1132

Drixoral Cold and Allergy Sustained-Action Tablets ⊡ 802
Drixoral Cold and Flu Extended-Release Tablets ⊡ 803
Drixoral Non-Drowsy Formula Extended-Release Tablets ⊡ 803
Drixoral Allergy/Sinus Extended Release Tablets ⊡ 804
Trinalin Repetabs Tablets 1330

Salmeterol Xinafoate (Concomitant use of albuterol with oral sympathomimetic agents is not recommended due to potential for cardiovascular toxicity). Products include:
Serevent Inhalation Aerosol 1176

Selegiline Hydrochloride (Action of albuterol on the vascular system may be potentiated). Products include:
Eldepryl Tablets 2550

Sotalol Hydrochloride (Beta-receptor blocking agents and albuterol inhibit effect of each other). Products include:
Betapace Tablets 641

Terbutaline Sulfate (Concomitant use of albuterol with oral sympathomimetic agents is not recommended due to potential for cardiovascular toxicity). Products include:
Brethaire Inhaler 813
Brethine Ampuls 815
Brethine Tablets 814
Bricanyl Subcutaneous Injection 1502
Bricanyl Tablets 1503

Timolol Hemihydrate (Beta-receptor blocking agents and albuterol inhibit effect of each other). Products include:
Betimol 0.25%, 0.5% ⊙ 261

Timolol Maleate (Beta-receptor blocking agents and albuterol inhibit effect of each other). Products include:
Blocadren Tablets 1614
Timolide Tablets 1748
Timoptic in Ocudose 1753
Timoptic Sterile Ophthalmic Solution 1751
Timoptic-XE 1755

Tranylcypromine Sulfate (Action of albuterol on the vascular system may be potentiated). Products include:
Parnate Tablets 2503

Trimipramine Maleate (Action of albuterol on the vascular system may be potentiated). Products include:
Surmontil Capsules 2811

VENTOLIN NEBULES INHALATION SOLUTION

(Albuterol Sulfate) 1199
May interact with sympathomimetic bronchodilators, monoamine oxidase inhibitors, beta blockers, and tricyclic antidepressants. Compounds in these categories include:

Acebutolol Hydrochloride (Beta-receptor blocking agents and albuterol inhibit effect of each other). Products include:
Sectral Capsules 2807

Amitriptyline Hydrochloride (Action of albuterol on the vascular system may be potentiated). Products include:
Elavil 2838
Endep Tablets 2174
Etrafon 2355
Limbitrol 2180
Triavil Tablets 1757

Amoxapine (Action of albuterol on the vascular system may be potentiated). Products include:
Asendin Tablets 1369

Atenolol (Beta-receptor blocking agents and albuterol inhibit effect of each other). Products include:
Tenoretic Tablets 2845
Tenormin Tablets and I.V. Injection 2847

Betaxolol Hydrochloride (Beta-receptor blocking agents and albuterol inhibit effect of each other). Products include:
Betoptic Ophthalmic Solution 469
Betoptic S Ophthalmic Suspension 471
Kerlone Tablets 2436

Bisoprolol Fumarate (Beta-receptor blocking agents and albuterol inhibit effect of each other). Products include:
Zebeta Tablets 1413
Ziac 1415

Bitolterol Mesylate (Concomitant use with other sympathomimetic aerosol bronchodilators is not recommended). Products include:
Tornalate Solution for Inhalation, 0.2% 956
Tornalate Metered Dose Inhaler 957

Carteolol Hydrochloride (Beta-receptor blocking agents and albuterol inhibit effect of each other). Products include:
Cartrol Tablets 410
Ocupress Ophthalmic Solution, 1% Sterile ⊙ 309

Clomipramine Hydrochloride (Action of albuterol on the vascular system may be potentiated). Products include:
Anafranil Capsules 803

Desipramine Hydrochloride (Action of albuterol on the vascular system may be potentiated). Products include:
Norpramin Tablets 1526

Doxepin Hydrochloride (Action of albuterol on the vascular system may be potentiated). Products include:
Sinequan 2205
Zonalon Cream 1055

Ephedrine Hydrochloride (Concomitant use with other sympathomimetic aerosol bronchodilators is not recommended). Products include:
Primatene Dual Action Formula ⊡ 872
Primatene Tablets ⊡ 873
Quadrinal Tablets 1350

Ephedrine Sulfate (Concomitant use with other sympathomimetic aerosol bronchodilators is not recommended). Products include:
Bronkaid Caplets ⊡ 717
Marax Tablets & DF Syrup 2200

Ephedrine Tannate (Concomitant use with other sympathomimetic aerosol bronchodilators is not recommended). Products include:
Rynatuss 2673

Epinephrine (Concomitant use with other sympathomimetic aerosol bronchodilators is not recommended). Products include:
Bronkaid Mist ⊡ 717
EPIFRIN ⊙ 239
EpiPen 790
Marcaine Hydrochloride with Epinephrine 1:200,000 2316
Primatene Mist ⊡ 873
Sensorcaine with Epinephrine Injection 559
Sus-Phrine Injection 1019
Xylocaine with Epinephrine Injections 567

Epinephrine Hydrochloride (Concomitant use with other sympathomimetic aerosol bronchodilators is not recommended). Products include:
Ana-Kit Anaphylaxis Emergency Treatment Kit 617

Esmolol Hydrochloride (Beta-receptor blocking agents and albuterol inhibit effect of each other). Products include:
Brevibloc Injection 1808

Ethylnorepinephrine Hydrochloride (Concomitant use with other sympathomimetic aerosol bronchodilators is not recommended).
No products indexed under this heading.

Furazolidone (Action of albuterol on the vascular system may be potentiated). Products include:
Furoxone 2046

Imipramine Hydrochloride (Action of albuterol on the vascular system may be potentiated). Products include:
Tofranil Ampuls 854
Tofranil Tablets 856

Imipramine Pamoate (Action of albuterol on the vascular system may be potentiated). Products include:
Tofranil-PM Capsules 857

Isocarboxazid (Action of albuterol on the vascular system may be potentiated).
No products indexed under this heading.

Isoetharine (Concomitant use with other sympathomimetic aerosol bronchodilators is not recommended). Products include:
Bronkometer Aerosol 2302
Bronkosol Solution 2302
Isoetharine Inhalation Solution, USP, Arm-a-Med 551

Isoproterenol Hydrochloride (Concomitant use with other sympathomimetic aerosol bronchodilators is not recommended). Products include:
Isuprel Hydrochloride Injection 1:5000 2311
Isuprel Hydrochloride Solution 1:200 & 1:100 2313
Isuprel Mistometer 2312

Isoproterenol Sulfate (Concomitant use with other sympathomimetic aerosol bronchodilators is not recommended). Products include:
Norisodrine with Calcium Iodide Syrup 442

Labetalol Hydrochloride (Beta-receptor blocking agents and albuterol inhibit effect of each other). Products include:
Normodyne Injection 2377
Normodyne Tablets 2379
Trandate 1185

Levobunolol Hydrochloride (Beta-receptor blocking agents and albuterol inhibit effect of each other). Products include:
Betagan ⊙ 233

Maprotiline Hydrochloride (Action of albuterol on the vascular system may be potentiated). Products include:
Ludiomil Tablets 843

Metaproterenol Sulfate (Concomitant use with other sympathomimetic aerosol bronchodilators is not recommended). Products include:
Alupent 669
Metaproterenol Sulfate Inhalation Solution, USP, Arm-a-Med 552

Metipranolol Hydrochloride (Beta-receptor blocking agents and albuterol inhibit effect of each other). Products include:
OptiPranolol (Metipranolol 0.3%) Sterile Ophthalmic Solution ⊙ 258

Metoprolol Succinate (Beta-receptor blocking agents and albuterol inhibit effect of each other). Products include:
Toprol-XL Tablets 565

Metoprolol Tartrate (Beta-receptor blocking agents and albuterol inhibit effect of each other). Products include:
Lopressor Ampuls 830
Lopressor HCT Tablets 832
Lopressor Tablets 830

Nadolol (Beta-receptor blocking agents and albuterol inhibit effect of each other).
No products indexed under this heading.

Nortriptyline Hydrochloride (Action of albuterol on the vascular system may be potentiated). Products include:
Pamelor 2280

Penbutolol Sulfate (Beta-receptor blocking agents and albuterol inhibit effect of each other). Products include:
Levatol 2403

Phenelzine Sulfate (Action of albuterol on the vascular system may be potentiated). Products include:
Nardil 1920

Pindolol (Beta-receptor blocking agents and albuterol inhibit effect of each other). Products include:
Visken Tablets 2299

Pirbuterol Acetate (Concomitant use with other sympathomimetic aerosol bronchodilators is not recommended). Products include:
Maxair Autohaler 1492
Maxair Inhaler 1494

Propranolol Hydrochloride (Beta-receptor blocking agents and albuterol inhibit effect of each other). Products include:
Inderal 2728
Inderal LA Long Acting Capsules 2730
Inderide Tablets 2732
Inderide LA Long Acting Capsules 2734

Protriptyline Hydrochloride (Action of albuterol on the vascular system may be potentiated). Products include:
Vivactil Tablets 1774

Salmeterol Xinafoate (Concomitant use with other sympathomimetic aerosol bronchodilators is not recommended). Products include:
Serevent Inhalation Aerosol 1176

Selegiline Hydrochloride (Action of albuterol on the vascular system may be potentiated). Products include:
Eldepryl Tablets 2550

Sotalol Hydrochloride (Beta-receptor blocking agents and albuterol inhibit effect of each other). Products include:
Betapace Tablets 641

Terbutaline Sulfate (Concomitant use with other sympathomimetic aerosol bronchodilators is not recommended). Products include:
Brethaire Inhaler 813
Brethine Ampuls 815
Brethine Tablets 814
Bricanyl Subcutaneous Injection 1502
Bricanyl Tablets 1503

Timolol Hemihydrate (Beta-receptor blocking agents and albuterol inhibit effect of each other). Products include:
Betimol 0.25%, 0.5% ⊙ 261

(⊡ Described in PDR For Nonprescription Drugs) (⊙ Described in PDR For Ophthalmology)

1133 **Interactions Index** **Ventolin Syrup**

Timolol Maleate (Beta-receptor blocking agents and albuterol inhibit effect of each other). Products include:
- Blocadren Tablets ... 1614
- Timolide Tablets ... 1748
- Timoptic in Ocudose ... 1753
- Timoptic Sterile Ophthalmic Solution ... 1751
- Timoptic-XE ... 1755

Tranylcypromine Sulfate (Action of albuterol on the vascular system may be potentiated). Products include:
- Parnate Tablets ... 2503

Trimipramine Maleate (Action of albuterol on the vascular system may be potentiated). Products include:
- Surmontil Capsules ... 2811

VENTOLIN ROTACAPS FOR INHALATION

(Albuterol Sulfate) ... 1200

May interact with sympathomimetic bronchodilators, monoamine oxidase inhibitors, beta blockers, and tricyclic antidepressants. Compounds in these categories include:

Acebutolol Hydrochloride (Beta-receptor blocking agents and albuterol inhibit effect of each other). Products include:
- Sectral Capsules ... 2807

Amitriptyline Hydrochloride (Action of albuterol on the vascular system may be potentiated). Products include:
- Elavil ... 2838
- Endep Tablets ... 2174
- Etrafon ... 2355
- Limbitrol ... 2180
- Triavil Tablets ... 1757

Amoxapine (Action of albuterol on the vascular system may be potentiated). Products include:
- Asendin Tablets ... 1369

Atenolol (Beta-receptor blocking agents and albuterol inhibit effect of each other). Products include:
- Tenoretic Tablets ... 2845
- Tenormin Tablets and I.V. Injection 2847

Betaxolol Hydrochloride (Beta-receptor blocking agents and albuterol inhibit effect of each other). Products include:
- Betoptic Ophthalmic Solution ... 469
- Betoptic S Ophthalmic Suspension 471
- Kerlone Tablets ... 2436

Bisoprolol Fumarate (Beta-receptor blocking agents and albuterol inhibit effect of each other). Products include:
- Zebeta Tablets ... 1413
- Ziac ... 1415

Bitolterol Mesylate (Concomitant use with other sympathomimetic aerosol bronchodilators is not recommended). Products include:
- Tornalate Solution for Inhalation, 0.2% ... 956
- Tornalate Metered Dose Inhaler ... 957

Carteolol Hydrochloride (Beta-receptor blocking agents and albuterol inhibit effect of each other). Products include:
- Cartrol Tablets ... 410
- Ocupress Ophthalmic Solution, 1% Sterile ... ⊙ 309

Clomipramine Hydrochloride (Action of albuterol on the vascular system may be potentiated). Products include:
- Anafranil Capsules ... 803

Desipramine Hydrochloride (Action of albuterol on the vascular system may be potentiated). Products include:
- Norpramin Tablets ... 1526

Doxepin Hydrochloride (Action of albuterol on the vascular system may be potentiated). Products include:
- Sinequan ... 2205
- Zonalon Cream ... 1055

Ephedrine Hydrochloride (Concomitant use with other sympathomimetic aerosol bronchodilators is not recommended). Products include:
- Primatene Dual Action Formula ... ⊡ 872
- Primatene Tablets ... ⊡ 873
- Quadrinal Tablets ... 1350

Ephedrine Sulfate (Concomitant use with other sympathomimetic aerosol bronchodilators is not recommended). Products include:
- Bronkaid Caplets ... ⊡ 717
- Marax Tablets & DF Syrup ... 2200

Ephedrine Tannate (Concomitant use with other sympathomimetic aerosol bronchodilators is not recommended). Products include:
- Rynatuss ... 2673

Epinephrine (Concomitant use with other sympathomimetic aerosol bronchodilators is not recommended). Products include:
- Bronkaid Mist ... ⊡ 717
- EPIFRIN ... ⊙ 239
- EpiPen ... 790
- Marcaine Hydrochloride with Epinephrine 1:200,000 ... 2316
- Primatene Mist ... ⊡ 873
- Sensorcaine with Epinephrine Injection ... 559
- Sus-Phrine Injection ... 1019
- Xylocaine with Epinephrine Injections ... 567

Epinephrine Hydrochloride (Concomitant use with other sympathomimetic aerosol bronchodilators is not recommended). Products include:
- Ana-Kit Anaphylaxis Emergency Treatment Kit ... 617

Esmolol Hydrochloride (Beta-receptor blocking agents and albuterol inhibit effect of each other). Products include:
- Brevibloc Injection ... 1808

Ethylnorepinephrine Hydrochloride (Concomitant use with other sympathomimetic aerosol bronchodilators is not recommended).
- No products indexed under this heading.

Furazolidone (Action of albuterol on the vascular system may be potentiated). Products include:
- Furoxone ... 2046

Imipramine Hydrochloride (Action of albuterol on the vascular system may be potentiated). Products include:
- Tofranil Ampuls ... 854
- Tofranil Tablets ... 856

Imipramine Pamoate (Action of albuterol on the vascular system may be potentiated). Products include:
- Tofranil-PM Capsules ... 857

Isocarboxazid (Action of albuterol on the vascular system may be potentiated).
- No products indexed under this heading.

Isoetharine (Concomitant use with other sympathomimetic aerosol bronchodilators is not recommended). Products include:
- Bronkometer Aerosol ... 2302
- Bronkosol Solution ... 2302
- Isoetharine Inhalation Solution, USP, Arm-a-Med ... 551

Isoproterenol Hydrochloride (Concomitant use with other sympathomimetic aerosol bronchodilators is not recommended). Products include:
- Isuprel Hydrochloride Injection 1:5000 ... 2311
- Isuprel Hydrochloride Solution 1:200 & 1:100 ... 2313
- Isuprel Mistometer ... 2312

Isoproterenol Sulfate (Concomitant use with other sympathomimetic aerosol bronchodilators is not recommended). Products include:
- Norisodrine with Calcium Iodide Syrup ... 442

Labetalol Hydrochloride (Beta-receptor blocking agents and albuterol inhibit effect of each other). Products include:
- Normodyne Injection ... 2377
- Normodyne Tablets ... 2379
- Trandate ... 1185

Levobunolol Hydrochloride (Beta-receptor blocking agents and albuterol inhibit effect of each other). Products include:
- Betagan ... ⊙ 233

Maprotiline Hydrochloride (Action of albuterol on the vascular system may be potentiated). Products include:
- Ludiomil Tablets ... 843

Metaproterenol Sulfate (Concomitant use with other sympathomimetic aerosol bronchodilators is not recommended). Products include:
- Alupent ... 669
- Metaproterenol Sulfate Inhalation Solution, USP, Arm-a-Med ... 552

Metipranolol Hydrochloride (Beta-receptor blocking agents and albuterol inhibit effect of each other). Products include:
- OptiPranolol (Metipranolol 0.3%) Sterile Ophthalmic Solution ... ⊙ 258

Metoprolol Succinate (Beta-receptor blocking agents and albuterol inhibit effect of each other). Products include:
- Toprol-XL Tablets ... 565

Metoprolol Tartrate (Beta-receptor blocking agents and albuterol inhibit effect of each other). Products include:
- Lopressor Ampuls ... 830
- Lopressor HCT Tablets ... 832
- Lopressor Tablets ... 830

Nadolol (Beta-receptor blocking agents and albuterol inhibit effect of each other).
- No products indexed under this heading.

Nortriptyline Hydrochloride (Action of albuterol on the vascular system may be potentiated). Products include:
- Pamelor ... 2280

Penbutolol Sulfate (Beta-receptor blocking agents and albuterol inhibit effect of each other). Products include:
- Levatol ... 2403

Phenelzine Sulfate (Action of albuterol on the vascular system may be potentiated). Products include:
- Nardil ... 1920

Pindolol (Beta-receptor blocking agents and albuterol inhibit effect of each other). Products include:
- Visken Tablets ... 2299

Pirbuterol Acetate (Concomitant use with other sympathomimetic aerosol bronchodilators is not recommended). Products include:
- Maxair Autohaler ... 1492
- Maxair Inhaler ... 1494

Propranolol Hydrochloride (Beta-receptor blocking agents and albuterol inhibit effect of each other). Products include:
- Inderal ... 2728
- Inderal LA Long Acting Capsules ... 2730
- Inderide Tablets ... 2732
- Inderide LA Long Acting Capsules .. 2734

Protriptyline Hydrochloride (Action of albuterol on the vascular system may be potentiated). Products include:
- Vivactil Tablets ... 1774

Salmeterol Xinafoate (Concomitant use with other sympathomimetic aerosol bronchodilators is not recommended). Products include:
- Serevent Inhalation Aerosol ... 1176

Selegiline Hydrochloride (Action of albuterol on the vascular system may be potentiated). Products include:
- Eldepryl Tablets ... 2550

Sotalol Hydrochloride (Beta-receptor blocking agents and albuterol inhibit effect of each other). Products include:
- Betapace Tablets ... 641

Terbutaline Sulfate (Concomitant use with other sympathomimetic aerosol bronchodilators is not recommended). Products include:
- Brethaire Inhaler ... 813
- Brethine Ampuls ... 815
- Brethine Tablets ... 814
- Bricanyl Subcutaneous Injection ... 1502
- Bricanyl Tablets ... 1503

Timolol Hemihydrate (Beta-receptor blocking agents and albuterol inhibit effect of each other). Products include:
- Betimol 0.25%, 0.5% ... ⊙ 261

Timolol Maleate (Beta-receptor blocking agents and albuterol inhibit effect of each other). Products include:
- Blocadren Tablets ... 1614
- Timolide Tablets ... 1748
- Timoptic in Ocudose ... 1753
- Timoptic Sterile Ophthalmic Solution ... 1751
- Timoptic-XE ... 1755

Tranylcypromine Sulfate (Action of albuterol on the vascular system may be potentiated). Products include:
- Parnate Tablets ... 2503

Trimipramine Maleate (Action of albuterol on the vascular system may be potentiated). Products include:
- Surmontil Capsules ... 2811

VENTOLIN SYRUP

(Albuterol Sulfate) ... 1202

May interact with monoamine oxidase inhibitors, beta blockers, tricyclic antidepressants, sympathomimetics, and certain other agents. Compounds in these categories include:

Acebutolol Hydrochloride (Beta receptor blocking agents and albuterol inhibit effect of each other). Products include:
- Sectral Capsules ... 2807

Albuterol (Concomitant use of albuterol with oral sympathomimetic agents is not recommended due to potential for cardiovascular toxicity). Products include:
- Proventil Inhalation Aerosol ... 2382
- Ventolin Inhalation Aerosol and Refill ... 1197

Amitriptyline Hydrochloride (Action of albuterol on vascular system may be potentiated). Products include:
- Elavil ... 2838

IMPORTANT NOTE: Always consult each drug listing in the patient's regimen for possible interactions.

Ventolin Syrup | Interactions Index | 1134

Endep Tablets ... 2174
Etrafon ... 2355
Limbitrol ... 2180
Triavil Tablets ... 1757

Amoxapine (Action of albuterol on vascular system may be potentiated). Products include:
Asendin Tablets ... 1369

Atenolol (Beta receptor blocking agents and albuterol inhibit effect of each other). Products include:
Tenoretic Tablets ... 2845
Tenormin Tablets and I.V. Injection 2847

Betaxolol Hydrochloride (Beta receptor blocking agents and albuterol inhibit effect of each other). Products include:
Betoptic Ophthalmic Solution ... 469
Betoptic S Ophthalmic Suspension 471
Kerlone Tablets ... 2436

Bisoprolol Fumarate (Beta receptor blocking agents and albuterol inhibit effect of each other). Products include:
Zebeta Tablets ... 1413
Ziac ... 1415

Carteolol Hydrochloride (Beta receptor blocking agents and albuterol inhibit effect of each other). Products include:
Cartrol Tablets ... 410
Ocupress Ophthalmic Solution, 1% Sterile ... ⊙ 309

Clomipramine Hydrochloride (Action of albuterol on vascular system may be potentiated). Products include:
Anafranil Capsules ... 803

Desipramine Hydrochloride (Action of albuterol on vascular system may be potentiated). Products include:
Norpramin Tablets ... 1526

Dopamine Hydrochloride (Concomitant use of albuterol with oral sympathomimetic agents is not recommended due to potential for cardiovascular toxicity).
No products indexed under this heading.

Doxepin Hydrochloride (Action of albuterol on vascular system may be potentiated). Products include:
Sinequan ... 2205
Zonalon Cream ... 1055

Ephedrine Hydrochloride (Concomitant use of albuterol with oral sympathomimetic agents is not recommended due to potential for cardiovascular toxicity). Products include:
Primatene Dual Action Formula ... ▣ 872
Primatene Tablets ... ▣ 873
Quadrinal Tablets ... 1350

Ephedrine Sulfate (Concomitant use of albuterol with oral sympathomimetic agents is not recommended due to potential for cardiovascular toxicity). Products include:
Bronkaid Caplets ... ▣ 717
Marax Tablets & DF Syrup ... 2200

Ephedrine Tannate (Concomitant use of albuterol with oral sympathomimetic agents is not recommended due to potential for cardiovascular toxicity). Products include:
Rynatuss ... 2673

Esmolol Hydrochloride (Beta receptor blocking agents and albuterol inhibit effect of each other). Products include:
Brevibloc Injection ... 1808

Furazolidone (Action of albuterol on vascular system may be potentiated). Products include:
Furoxone ... 2046

Imipramine Hydrochloride (Action of albuterol on vascular system may be potentiated). Products include:
Tofranil Ampuls ... 854
Tofranil Tablets ... 856

Imipramine Pamoate (Action of albuterol on vascular system may be potentiated). Products include:
Tofranil-PM Capsules ... 857

Isocarboxazid (Action of albuterol on vascular system may be potentiated).
No products indexed under this heading.

Labetalol Hydrochloride (Beta receptor blocking agents and albuterol inhibit effect of each other). Products include:
Normodyne Injection ... 2377
Normodyne Tablets ... 2379
Trandate ... 1185

Levobunolol Hydrochloride (Beta receptor blocking agents and albuterol inhibit effect of each other). Products include:
Betagan ... ⊙ 233

Maprotiline Hydrochloride (Action of albuterol on vascular system may be potentiated). Products include:
Ludiomil Tablets ... 843

Metaproterenol Sulfate (Concomitant use of albuterol with oral sympathomimetic agents is not recommended due to potential for cardiovascular toxicity). Products include:
Alupent ... 669
Metaproterenol Sulfate Inhalation Solution, USP, Arm-a-Med ... 552

Metipranolol Hydrochloride (Beta receptor blocking agents and albuterol inhibit effect of each other). Products include:
OptiPranolol (Metipranolol 0.3%) Sterile Ophthalmic Solution ... ⊙ 258

Metoprolol Succinate (Beta receptor blocking agents and albuterol inhibit effect of each other). Products include:
Toprol-XL Tablets ... 565

Metoprolol Tartrate (Beta receptor blocking agents and albuterol inhibit effect of each other). Products include:
Lopressor Ampuls ... 830
Lopressor HCT Tablets ... 832
Lopressor Tablets ... 830

Nadolol (Beta receptor blocking agents and albuterol inhibit effect of each other).
No products indexed under this heading.

Nortriptyline Hydrochloride (Action of albuterol on vascular system may be potentiated). Products include:
Pamelor ... 2280

Penbutolol Sulfate (Beta receptor blocking agents and albuterol inhibit effect of each other). Products include:
Levatol ... 2403

Phenelzine Sulfate (Action of albuterol on vascular system may be potentiated). Products include:
Nardil ... 1920

Phenylephrine Bitartrate (Concomitant use of albuterol with oral sympathomimetic agents is not recommended due to potential for cardiovascular toxicity).
No products indexed under this heading.

Phenylephrine Hydrochloride (Concomitant use of albuterol with oral sympathomimetic agents is not recommended due to potential for cardiovascular toxicity). Products include:
Atrohist Plus Tablets ... 454
Cerose DM ... ▣ 878
Comhist ... 2038
D.A. Chewable Tablets ... 951
Deconsal Pediatric Capsules ... 454
Dura-Vent/DA Tablets ... 953
Entex Capsules ... 1986
Entex Liquid ... 1986
Extendryl ... 1005
4-Way Fast Acting Nasal Spray (regular & mentholated) ... ▣ 621
Hemorid For Women ... ▣ 834
Hycomine Compound Tablets ... 932
Neo-Synephrine Hydrochloride 1% Carpuject ... 2324
Neo-Synephrine Hydrochloride 1% Injection ... 2324
Neo-Synephrine Hydrochloride (Ophthalmic) ... 2325
Neo-Synephrine ... ▣ 726
Nōstril ... ▣ 644
Novahistine Elixir ... ▣ 823
Phenergan VC ... 2779
Phenergan VC with Codeine ... 2781
Preparation H ... ▣ 871
Tympagesic Ear Drops ... 2342
Vasosulf ... ⊙ 271
Vicks Sinex Nasal Spray and Ultra Fine Mist ... ▣ 765

Phenylephrine Tannate (Concomitant use of albuterol with oral sympathomimetic agents is not recommended due to potential for cardiovascular toxicity). Products include:
Atrohist Pediatric Suspension ... 454
Ricobid-D Pediatric Suspension ... 2038
Ricobid Tablets and Pediatric Suspension ... 2038
Rynatan ... 2673
Rynatuss ... 2673

Phenylpropanolamine Hydrochloride (Concomitant use of albuterol with oral sympathomimetic agents is not recommended due to potential for cardiovascular toxicity). Products include:
Acutrim ... ▣ 628
Allerest Children's Chewable Tablets ... ▣ 627
Allerest 12 Hour Caplets ... ▣ 627
Atrohist Plus Tablets ... 454
BC Cold Powder Multi-Symptom Formula (Cold-Sinus-Allergy) ... ▣ 609
BC Cold Powder Non-Drowsy Formula (Cold-Sinus) ... ▣ 609
Cheracol Plus Head Cold/Cough Formula ... ▣ 769
Comtrex Multi-Symptom Non-Drowsy Liqui-gels ... ▣ 618
Contac Continuous Action Nasal Decongestant/Antihistamine 12 Hour Capsules ... ▣ 813
Contac Maximum Strength Continuous Action Decongestant/Antihistamine 12 Hour Caplets ... ▣ 813
Contac Severe Cold and Flu Formula Caplets ... ▣ 814
Coricidin 'D' Decongestant Tablets ... ▣ 800
Dexatrim ... ▣ 832
Dexatrim Plus Vitamins Caplets ... ▣ 832
Dimetane-DC Cough Syrup ... 2059
Dimetapp Elixir ... ▣ 773
Dimetapp Extentabs ... ▣ 774
Dimetapp Tablets/Liqui-Gels ... ▣ 775
Dimetapp Cold & Allergy Chewable Tablets ... ▣ 773
Dimetapp DM Elixir ... ▣ 774
Dura-Vent Tablets ... 952
Entex Capsules ... 1986
Entex LA Tablets ... 1987
Entex Liquid ... 1986
Exgest LA Tablets ... 782
Hycomine ... 931
Isoclor Timesule Capsules ... ▣ 637
Nolamine Timed-Release Tablets ... 785
Ornade Spansule Capsules ... 2502
Propagest Tablets ... 786
Pyrroxate Caplets ... ▣ 772
Robitussin-CF ... ▣ 777
Sinulin Tablets ... 787
Tavist-D 12 Hour Relief Tablets ... ▣ 787
Teldrin 12 Hour Antihistamine/Nasal Decongestant Allergy Relief Capsules ... ▣ 826
Triaminic Allergy Tablets ... ▣ 789
Triaminic Cold Tablets ... ▣ 790
Triaminic Expectorant ... ▣ 790
Triaminic Syrup ... ▣ 792
Triaminic-12 Tablets ... ▣ 792
Triaminic-DM Syrup ... ▣ 792
Triaminicin Tablets ... ▣ 793
Triaminicol Multi-Symptom Cold Tablets ... ▣ 793
Triaminicol Multi-Symptom Relief ▣ 794
Vicks DayQuil Allergy Relief 12-Hour Extended Release Tablets ... ▣ 760
Vicks DayQuil Allergy Relief 4-Hour Tablets ... ▣ 760
Vicks DayQuil SINUS Pressure & CONGESTION Relief ... ▣ 761

Pindolol (Beta receptor blocking agents and albuterol inhibit effect of each other). Products include:
Visken Tablets ... 2299

Pirbuterol Acetate (Concomitant use of albuterol with oral sympathomimetic agents is not recommended due to potential for cardiovascular toxicity). Products include:
Maxair Autohaler ... 1492
Maxair Inhaler ... 1494

Propranolol Hydrochloride (Beta receptor blocking agents and albuterol inhibit effect of each other). Products include:
Inderal ... 2728
Inderal LA Long Acting Capsules ... 2730
Inderide Tablets ... 2732
Inderide LA Long Acting Capsules ... 2734

Protriptyline Hydrochloride (Action of albuterol on vascular system may be potentiated). Products include:
Vivactil Tablets ... 1774

Pseudoephedrine Hydrochloride (Concomitant use of albuterol with oral sympathomimetic agents is not recommended due to potential for cardiovascular toxicity). Products include:
Actifed Allergy Daytime/Nighttime Caplets ... ▣ 844
Actifed Plus Caplets ... ▣ 845
Actifed Plus Tablets ... ▣ 845
Actifed with Codeine Cough Syrup ... 1067
Actifed Sinus Daytime/Nighttime Tablets and Caplets ... ▣ 846
Actifed Syrup ... ▣ 846
Actifed Tablets ... ▣ 844
Advil Cold and Sinus Caplets and Tablets (formerly CoAdvil) ... ▣ 870
Alka-Seltzer Plus Cold Medicine Liqui-Gels ... ▣ 706
Alka-Seltzer Plus Cold & Cough Medicine Liqui-Gels ... ▣ 705
Alka-Seltzer Plus Night-Time Cold Medicine Liqui-Gels ... ▣ 706
Allerest Headache Strength Tablets ... ▣ 627
Allerest Maximum Strength Tablets ... ▣ 627
Allerest No Drowsiness Tablets ... ▣ 627
Allerest Sinus Pain Formula ... ▣ 627
Anatuss LA Tablets ... 1542
Atrohist Pediatric Capsules ... 453
Bayer Select Sinus Pain Relief Formula ... ▣ 717
Benadryl Allergy Decongestant Liquid Medication ... ▣ 848
Benadryl Allergy Decongestant Tablets ... ▣ 848
Benadryl Allergy Sinus Headache Formula Caplets ... ▣ 849
Benylin Multisymptom ... ▣ 852
Bromfed Capsules (Extended-Release) ... 1785
Bromfed Syrup ... ▣ 733
Bromfed Tablets ... 1785
Bromfed-DM Cough Syrup ... 1786
Bromfed-PD Capsules (Extended-Release) ... 1785
Children's Vicks DayQuil Allergy Relief ... ▣ 757
Children's Vicks NyQuil Cold/Cough Relief ... ▣ 758

(▣ Described in PDR For Nonprescription Drugs) (⊙ Described in PDR For Ophthalmology)

Interactions Index

Ventolin Tablets

Comtrex Multi-Symptom Cold Reliever Tablets/Caplets/Liqui-Gels/Liquid................................. ✦D 615

Allergy-Sinus Comtrex Multi-Symptom Allergy-Sinus Formula Tablets .... ✦D 617

Comtrex Multi-Symptom Non-Drowsy Caplets.............................. ✦D 618

Congess 1004

Contac Day Allergy/Sinus Caplets ✦D 812

Contac Day & Night .... ✦D 812

Contac Night Allergy/Sinus Caplets .... ✦D 812

Contac Severe Cold & Flu Non-Drowsy .... ✦D 815

Deconamine Chewable Tablets 1320

Deconamine CX Cough and Cold Liquid and Tablets............................. 1319

Deconamine 1320

Deconsal C Expectorant Syrup 456

Deconsal Pediatric Syrup 457

Deconsal II Tablets 454

Dimetane-DX Cough Syrup 2059

Dimetapp Sinus Caplets .... ✦D 775

Dorcol Children's Cough Syrup ..... ✦D 785

Drixoral Cough + Congestion Liquid Caps .... ✦D 802

Dura-Tap/PD Capsules 2867

Duratuss Tablets 2565

Duratuss HD Elixir 2565

Efidac/24 .... ✦D 635

Entex PSE Tablets 1987

Fedahist Gyrocaps............................. 2401

Fedahist Timecaps 2401

Guaifed... 1787

Guaifed Syrup .... ✦D 734

Guaimax-D Tablets 792

Guaitab Tablets .... ✦D 734

Isoclor Expectorant............................ 990

Kronofed-A 977

Motrin IB Sinus................................... ✦D 838

Novahistine DH................................... 2462

Novahistine DMX .... ✦D 822

Novahistine Expectorant................... 2463

Nucofed 2051

PediaCare Cold Allergy Chewable Tablets .... ✦D 677

PediaCare Cough-Cold Chewable Tablets 1553

PediaCare 1553

PediaCare Infants' Decongestant Drops .... ✦D 677

PediCare Infant's Drops Decongestant Plus Cough 1553

PediaCare NightRest Cough-Cold Liquid 1553

Pediatric Vicks 44d Dry Hacking Cough & Head Congestion.............. ✦D 763

Pediatric Vicks 44m Cough & Cold Relief .... ✦D 764

Robitussin Cold & Cough Liqui-Gels .... ✦D 776

Robitussin Maximum Strength Cough & Cold .... ✦D 778

Robitussin Pediatric Cough & Cold Formula .... ✦D 779

Robitussin Severe Congestion Liqui-Gels .... ✦D 776

Robitussin-DAC Syrup 2074

Robitussin-PE .... ✦D 778

Rondec Oral Drops 953

Rondec Syrup 953

Rondec Tablet...................................... 953

Rondec-DM Oral Drops...................... 954

Rondec-DM Syrup 954

Rondec-TR Tablet 953

Ryna .... ✦D 841

Seldane-D Extended-Release Tablets 1538

Semprex-D Capsules 463

Semprex-D Capsules 1167

Sinarest Tablets .... ✦D 648

Sinarest Extra Strength Tablets...... ✦D 648

Sinarest No Drowsiness Tablets .... ✦D 648

Sine-Aid IB Caplets 1554

Sine-Aid Maximum Strength Sinus Medication Gelcaps, Caplets and Tablets 1554

Sine-Off No Drowsiness Formula Caplets .... ✦D 824

Sine-Off Sinus Medicine .... ✦D 825

Singlet Tablets .... ✦D 825

Sinutab Non-Drying Liquid Caps.... ✦D 859

Sinutab Sinus Allergy Medication, Maximum Strength Tablets and Caplets .... ✦D 860

Sinutab Sinus Medication, Maximum Strength Without Drowsiness Formula, Tablets & Caplets .... ✦D 860

Sinutab Sinus Medication, Regular Strength Without Drowsiness Formula .... ✦D 859

Sudafed Children's Liquid .... ✦D 861

Sudafed Cold and Cough Liquidcaps .... ✦D 862

Sudafed Cough Syrup .... ✦D 862

Sudafed Plus Liquid .... ✦D 862

Sudafed Plus Tablets .... ✦D 863

Sudafed Severe Cold Formula Caplets .... ✦D 863

Sudafed Severe Cold Formula Tablets .... ✦D 864

Sudafed Sinus Caplets...................... ✦D 864

Sudafed Sinus Tablets....................... ✦D 864

Sudafed Tablets, 30 mg.................... ✦D 861

Sudafed Tablets, 60 mg.................... ✦D 861

Sudafed 12 Hour Caplets .... ✦D 861

Syn-Rx Tablets 465

Syn-Rx DM Tablets 466

TheraFlu.. ✦D 787

TheraFlu Maximum Strength Nighttime Flu, Cold & Cough Medicine .... ✦D 788

TheraFlu Maximum Strength Non-Drowsy Formula Flu, Cold & Cough Medicine .... ✦D 788

Thera Flu Maximum Strength, Non-Drowsy Formula Flu, Cold and Cough Caplets .... ✦D 789

Triaminic AM Cough and Decongestant Formula .... ✦D 789

Triaminic AM Decongestant Formula .... ✦D 790

Triaminic Nite Light .... ✦D 791

Triaminic Sore Throat Formula ...... ✦D 791

Tussend 1783

Tussend Expectorant 1785

Children's TYLENOL Cold Multi-Symptom Liquid Formula and Chewable Tablets................................ 1561

Children's TYLENOL Cold Plus Cough Multi Symptom Tablets and Liquid .... ✦D 681

Infants' TYLENOL Cold Decongestant & Fever-Reducer Drops 1556

TYLENOL Maximum Strength Allergy Sinus Medication Gelcaps and Caplets 1563

TYLENOL Maximum Strength Allergy Sinus NightTime Medication Caplets 1555

TYLENOL Flu Maximum Strength Gelcaps 1565

TYLENOL Flu NightTime, Maximum Strength, Gelcaps 1566

TYLENOL Maximum Strength Flu NightTime Hot Medication Packets 1562

TYLENOL, Maximum Strength, Sinus Medication Geltabs, Gelcaps, Caplets and Tablets 1566

TYLENOL Cold Multi-Symptom Formula Medication Tablets and Caplets 1561

TYLENOL Cold Medication No Drowsiness Formula Gelcaps and Caplets 1562

TYLENOL Cold Multi-Symptom Hot Medication Liquid Packets.............. 1557

TYLENOL Cough Multi-Symptom Medication with Decongestant...... 1565

Ursinus Inlay-Tabs.............................. ✦D 794

Vicks 44 LiquiCaps Cough, Cold & Flu Relief.. ✦D 755

Vicks 44 LiquiCaps Non-Drowsy Cough & Cold Relief.......................... ✦D 756

Vicks 44D Dry Hacking Cough & Head Congestion .... ✦D 755

Vicks 44M Cough, Cold & Flu Relief .... ✦D 756

Vicks DayQuil .... ✦D 761

Vicks DayQuil SINUS Pressure & PAIN Relief with IBUPROFEN ...... ✦D 762

Vicks Nyquil Hot Therapy.................. ✦D 762

Vicks NyQuil LiquiCaps Multi-Symptom Cold/Flu Relief .... ✦D 763

Vicks NyQuil Multi-Symptom Cold/Flu Relief - (Original & Cherry Flavor) .... ✦D 763

Pseudoephedrine Sulfate (Concomitant use of albuterol with oral sympathomimetic agents is not recommended due to potential for cardiovascular toxicity). Products include:

Cheracol Sinus .... ✦D 768

Chlor-Trimeton Allergy Decongestant Tablets .... ✦D 799

Claritin-D 2350

Drixoral Cold and Allergy Sustained-Action Tablets .... ✦D 802

Drixoral Cold and Flu Extended-Release Tablets................................... ✦D 803

Drixoral Non-Drowsy Formula Extended-Release Tablets .... ✦D 803

Drixoral Allergy/Sinus Extended Release Tablets.................................. ✦D 804

Trinalin Repetabs Tablets 1330

Salmeterol Xinafoate (Concomitant use of albuterol with oral sympathomimetic agents is not recommended due to potential for cardiovascular toxicity). Products include:

Serevent Inhalation Aerosol.............. 1176

Selegiline Hydrochloride (Action of albuterol on vascular system may be potentiated). Products include:

Eldepryl Tablets 2550

Sotalol Hydrochloride (Beta receptor blocking agents and albuterol inhibit effect of each other). Products include:

Betapace Tablets 641

Terbutaline Sulfate (Concomitant use of albuterol with oral sympathomimetic agents is not recommended due to potential for cardiovascular toxicity). Products include:

Brethaire Inhaler 813

Brethine Ampuls 815

Brethine Tablets.................................. 814

Bricanyl Subcutaneous Injection..... 1502

Bricanyl Tablets 1503

Timolol Hemihydrate (Beta receptor blocking agents and albuterol inhibit effect of each other). Products include:

Betimol 0.25%, 0.5% .... ◎ 261

Timolol Maleate (Beta receptor blocking agents and albuterol inhibit effect of each other). Products include:

Blocadren Tablets 1614

Timolide Tablets.................................. 1748

Timoptic in Ocudose 1753

Timoptic Sterile Ophthalmic Solution.. 1751

Timoptic-XE 1755

Tranylcypromine Sulfate (Action of albuterol on vascular system may be potentiated). Products include:

Parnate Tablets 2503

Trimipramine Maleate (Action of albuterol on vascular system may be potentiated). Products include:

Surmontil Capsules............................. 2811

VENTOLIN TABLETS

(Albuterol Sulfate) 1203

May interact with sympathomimetics, monoamine oxidase inhibitors, beta blockers, and tricyclic antidepressants. Compounds in these categories include:

Acebutolol Hydrochloride (Beta-receptor blocking agents and albuterol inhibit effect of each other). Products include:

Sectral Capsules 2807

Amitriptyline Hydrochloride (Action of albuterol on the vascular system may be potentiated). Products include:

Elavil 2838

Endep Tablets 2174

Etrafon 2355

Limbitrol 2180

Triavil Tablets 1757

Amoxapine (Action of albuterol on the vascular system may be potentiated). Products include:

Asendin Tablets 1369

Atenolol (Beta-receptor blocking agents and albuterol inhibit effect of each other). Products include:

Tenoretic Tablets................................. 2845

Tenormin Tablets and I.V. Injection 2847

Betaxolol Hydrochloride (Beta-receptor blocking agents and albuterol inhibit effect of each other). Products include:

Betoptic Ophthalmic Solution........... 469

Betoptic S Ophthalmic Suspension 471

Kerlone Tablets.................................... 2436

Bisoprolol Fumarate (Beta-receptor blocking agents and albuterol inhibit effect of each other). Products include:

Zebeta Tablets 1413

Ziac 1415

Carteolol Hydrochloride (Beta-receptor blocking agents and albuterol inhibit effect of each other). Products include:

Cartrol Tablets 410

Ocupress Ophthalmic Solution, 1% Sterile.. ◎ 309

Clomipramine Hydrochloride (Action of albuterol on the vascular system may be potentiated). Products include:

Anafranil Capsules 803

Desipramine Hydrochloride (Action of albuterol on the vascular system may be potentiated). Products include:

Norpramin Tablets 1526

Dobutamine Hydrochloride (Concomitant use of albuterol with oral sympathomimetic agents is not recommended due to potential for cardiovascular toxicity). Products include:

Dobutrex Solution Vials..................... 1439

Dopamine Hydrochloride (Concomitant use of albuterol with oral sympathomimetic agents is not recommended due to potential for cardiovascular toxicity).

No products indexed under this heading.

Doxepin Hydrochloride (Action of albuterol on the vascular system may be potentiated). Products include:

Sinequan 2205

Zonalon Cream.................................... 1055

Ephedrine Hydrochloride (Concomitant use of albuterol with oral sympathomimetic agents is not recommended due to potential for cardiovascular toxicity). Products include:

Primatene Dual Action Formula...... ✦D 872

Primatene Tablets .... ✦D 873

Quadrinal Tablets 1350

Ephedrine Sulfate (Concomitant use of albuterol with oral sympathomimetic agents is not recommended due to potential for cardiovascular toxicity). Products include:

Bronkaid Caplets .... ✦D 717

Marax Tablets & DF Syrup................ 2200

Ephedrine Tannate (Concomitant use of albuterol with oral sympathomimetic agents is not recommended due to potential for cardiovascular toxicity). Products include:

Rynatuss 2673

Esmolol Hydrochloride (Beta-receptor blocking agents and albuterol inhibit effect of each other). Products include:

Brevibloc Injection............................... 1808

Furazolidone (Action of albuterol on the vascular system may be potentiated). Products include:

Furoxone 2046

Imipramine Hydrochloride (Action of albuterol on the vascular system may be potentiated). Products include:

Tofranil Ampuls 854

Tofranil Tablets 856

IMPORTANT NOTE: Always consult each drug listing in the patient's regimen for possible interactions.

Ventolin Tablets

Interactions Index

Imipramine Pamoate (Action of albuterol on the vascular system may be potentiated). Products include:

Tofranil-PM Capsules............................ 857

Isocarboxazid (Action of albuterol on the vascular system may be potentiated).

No products indexed under this heading.

Labetalol Hydrochloride (Beta-receptor blocking agents and albuterol inhibit effect of each other). Products include:

Normodyne Injection 2377
Normodyne Tablets 2379
Trandate 1185

Levobunolol Hydrochloride (Beta-receptor blocking agents and albuterol inhibit effect of each other). Products include:

Betagan .... ◉ 233

Maprotiline Hydrochloride (Action of albuterol on the vascular system may be potentiated). Products include:

Ludiomil Tablets.................................... 843

Metaproterenol Sulfate (Concomitant use of albuterol with oral sympathomimetic agents is not recommended due to potential for cardiovascular toxicity). Products include:

Alupent.. 669
Metaproterenol Sulfate Inhalation Solution, USP, Arm-a-Med 552

Metaraminol Bitartrate (Concomitant use of albuterol with oral sympathomimetic agents is not recommended due to potential for cardiovascular toxicity). Products include:

Aramine Injection.................................. 1609

Metipranolol Hydrochloride (Beta-receptor blocking agents and albuterol inhibit effect of each other). Products include:

OptiPranolol (Metipranolol 0.3%)
Sterile Ophthalmic Solution.......... ◉ 258

Metoprolol Succinate (Beta-receptor blocking agents and albuterol inhibit effect of each other). Products include:

Toprol-XL Tablets 565

Metoprolol Tartrate (Beta-receptor blocking agents and albuterol inhibit effect of each other). Products include:

Lopressor Ampuls 830
Lopressor HCT Tablets 832
Lopressor Tablets 830

Nadolol (Beta-receptor blocking agents and albuterol inhibit effect of each other).

No products indexed under this heading.

Nortriptyline Hydrochloride (Action of albuterol on the vascular system may be potentiated). Products include:

Pamelor 2280

Penbutolol Sulfate (Beta-receptor blocking agents and albuterol inhibit effect of each other). Products include:

Levatol 2403

Phenelzine Sulfate (Action of albuterol on the vascular system may be potentiated). Products include:

Nardil 1920

Phenylephrine Bitartrate (Concomitant use of albuterol with oral sympathomimetic agents is not recommended due to potential for cardiovascular toxicity).

No products indexed under this heading.

Phenylephrine Hydrochloride (Concomitant use of albuterol with oral sympathomimetic agents is not recommended due to potential for cardiovascular toxicity). Products include:

Atrohist Plus Tablets 454
Cerose DM .... ᴹᴰ 878
Comhist 2038
D.A. Chewable Tablets........................... 951
Deconsal Pediatric Capsules.................. 454
Dura-Vent/DA Tablets............................ 953
Entex Capsules 1986
Entex Liquid 1986
Extendryl 1005
4-Way Fast Acting Nasal Spray
(regular & mentholated).................. ᴹᴰ 621
Hemorid For Women .... ᴹᴰ 834
Hycomine Compound Tablets 932
Neo-Synephrine Hydrochloride 1%
Carpuject... 2324
Neo-Synephrine Hydrochloride 1%
Injection 2324
Neo-Synephrine Hydrochloride
(Ophthalmic) 2325
Neo-Synephrine .... ᴹᴰ 726
Nōstril .... ᴹᴰ 644
Novahistine Elixir .... ᴹᴰ 823
Phenergan VC 2779
Phenergan VC with Codeine 2781
Preparation H .... ᴹᴰ 871
Tympagesic Ear Drops 2342
Vasosulf.. ◉ 271
Vicks Sinex Nasal Spray and Ultra
Fine Mist .... ᴹᴰ 765

Phenylephrine Tannate (Concomitant use of albuterol with oral sympathomimetic agents is not recommended due to potential for cardiovascular toxicity). Products include:

Atrohist Pediatric Suspension 454
Ricobid-D Pediatric Suspension....... 2038
Ricobid Tablets and Pediatric Suspension.. 2038
Rynatan 2673
Rynatuss 2673

Phenylpropanolamine Hydrochloride (Concomitant use of albuterol with oral sympathomimetic agents is not recommended due to potential for cardiovascular toxicity). Products include:

Acutrim .... ᴹᴰ 628
Allerest Children's Chewable Tablets.. ᴹᴰ 627
Allerest 12 Hour Caplets .... ᴹᴰ 627
Atrohist Plus Tablets 454
BC Cold Powder Multi-Symptom
Formula (Cold-Sinus-Allergy) .... ᴹᴰ 609
BC Cold Powder Non-Drowsy
Formula (Cold-Sinus)..................... ᴹᴰ 609
Cheracol Plus Head Cold/Cough
Formula .... ᴹᴰ 769
Comtrex Multi-Symptom Non-
Drowsy Liqui-gels............................. ᴹᴰ 618
Contac Continuous Action Nasal
Decongestant/Antihistamine 12
Hour Capsules................................... ᴹᴰ 813
Contac Maximum Strength Continuous Action Decongestant/
Antihistamine 12 Hour Caplets.. ᴹᴰ 813
Contac Severe Cold and Flu Formula Caplets .... ᴹᴰ 814
Coricidin 'D' Decongestant Tablets.. ᴹᴰ 800
Dexatrim .... ᴹᴰ 832
Dexatrim Plus Vitamins Caplets .... ᴹᴰ 832
Dimetane-DC Cough Syrup 2059
Dimetapp Elixir .... ᴹᴰ 773
Dimetapp Extentabs .... ᴹᴰ 774
Dimetapp Tablets/Liqui-Gels .... ᴹᴰ 775
Dimetapp Cold & Allergy Chewable Tablets .... ᴹᴰ 773
Dimetapp DM Elixir.............................. ᴹᴰ 774
Dura-Vent Tablets 952
Entex Capsules 1986
Entex LA Tablets 1987
Entex Liquid 1986
Exgest LA Tablets 782
Hycomine 931
Isoclor Timesule Capsules.................... ᴹᴰ 637
Nolamine Timed-Release Tablets 785
Ornade Spansule Capsules 2502
Propagest Tablets 786
Pyrroxate Caplets .... ᴹᴰ 772
Robitussin-CF .... ᴹᴰ 777

Sinulin Tablets 787
Tavist-D 12 Hour Relief Tablets .... ᴹᴰ 787
Teldrin 12 Hour Antihistamine/
Nasal Decongestant Allergy
Relief Capsules .... ᴹᴰ 826
Triaminic Allergy Tablets .... ᴹᴰ 789
Triaminic Cold Tablets .... ᴹᴰ 790
Triaminic Expectorant .... ᴹᴰ 790
Triaminic Syrup .... ᴹᴰ 792
Triaminic-12 Tablets .... ᴹᴰ 792
Triaminic-DM Syrup .... ᴹᴰ 792
Triaminicin Tablets .... ᴹᴰ 793
Triaminicol Multi-Symptom Cold
Tablets.. ᴹᴰ 793
Triaminicol Multi-Symptom Relief ᴹᴰ 794
Vicks DayQuil Allergy Relief 12-
Hour Extended Release Tablets.. ᴹᴰ 760
Vicks DayQuil Allergy Relief 4-
Hour Tablets .... ᴹᴰ 760
Vicks DayQuil SINUS Pressure &
CONGESTION Relief........................ ᴹᴰ 761

Pindolol (Beta-receptor blocking agents and albuterol inhibit effect of each other). Products include:

Visken Tablets.. 2299

Pirbuterol Acetate (Concomitant use of albuterol with oral sympathomimetic agents is not recommended due to potential for cardiovascular toxicity). Products include:

Maxair Autohaler 1492
Maxair Inhaler 1494

Propranolol Hydrochloride (Beta-receptor blocking agents and albuterol inhibit effect of each other). Products include:

Inderal 2728
Inderal LA Long Acting Capsules 2730
Inderide Tablets 2732
Inderide LA Long Acting Capsules .. 2734

Protriptyline Hydrochloride (Action of albuterol on the vascular system may be potentiated). Products include:

Vivactil Tablets 1774

Pseudoephedrine Hydrochloride (Concomitant use of albuterol with oral sympathomimetic agents is not recommended due to potential for cardiovascular toxicity). Products include:

Actifed Allergy Daytime/Nighttime Caplets....................................... ᴹᴰ 844
Actifed Plus Caplets .... ᴹᴰ 845
Actifed Plus Tablets .... ᴹᴰ 845
Actifed with Codeine Cough Syrup.. 1067
Actifed Sinus Daytime/Nighttime
Tablets and Caplets .... ᴹᴰ 846
Actifed Syrup... ᴹᴰ 846
Actifed Tablets .... ᴹᴰ 844
Advil Cold and Sinus Caplets and
Tablets (formerly CoAdvil) .... ᴹᴰ 870
Alka-Seltzer Plus Cold Medicine
Liqui-Gels .... ᴹᴰ 706
Alka-Seltzer Plus Cold & Cough
Medicine Liqui-Gels.......................... ᴹᴰ 705
Alka-Seltzer Plus Night-Time Cold
Medicine Liqui-Gels.......................... ᴹᴰ 706
Allerest Headache Strength Tablets.. ᴹᴰ 627
Allerest Maximum Strength Tablets.. ᴹᴰ 627
Allerest No Drowsiness Tablets ...... ᴹᴰ 627
Allerest Sinus Pain Formula .... ᴹᴰ 627
Anatuss LA Tablets................................ 1542
Atrohist Pediatric Capsules.................. 453
Bayer Select Sinus Pain Relief
Formula .... ᴹᴰ 717
Benadryl Allergy Decongestant
Liquid Medication .... ᴹᴰ 848
Benadryl Allergy Decongestant
Tablets.. ᴹᴰ 848
Benadryl Allergy Sinus Headache
Formula Caplets .... ᴹᴰ 849
Benylin Multisymptom.......................... ᴹᴰ 852
Bromfed Capsules (Extended-Release) 1785
Bromfed Syrup .... ᴹᴰ 733
Bromfed Tablets 1785
Bromfed-DM Cough Syrup................... 1786
Bromfed-PD Capsules (Extended-
Release)... 1785
Children's Vicks DayQuil Allergy
Relief... ᴹᴰ 757
Children's Vicks NyQuil Cold/
Cough Relief....................................... ᴹᴰ 758

Comtrex Multi-Symptom Cold
Reliever Tablets/Caplets/Liqui-
Gels/Liquid... ᴹᴰ 615
Allergy-Sinus Comtrex Multi-
Symptom Allergy-Sinus Formula
Tablets .... ᴹᴰ 617
Comtrex Multi-Symptom Non-
Drowsy Caplets.................................. ᴹᴰ 618
Congress 1004
Contac Day Allergy/Sinus Caplets ᴹᴰ 812
Contac Day & Night .... ᴹᴰ 812
Contac Night Allergy/Sinus Caplets.. ᴹᴰ 812
Contac Severe Cold & Flu Non-
Drowsy .... ᴹᴰ 815
Deconamine Chewable Tablets 1320
Deconamine CX Cough and Cold
Liquid and Tablets.............................. 1319
Deconamine 1320
Deconsal C Expectorant Syrup 456
Deconsal Pediatric Syrup 457
Deconsal II Tablets 454
Dimetane-DX Cough Syrup 2059
Dimetapp Sinus Caplets .... ᴹᴰ 775
Dorcol Children's Cough Syrup ...... ᴹᴰ 785
Drixoral Cough + Congestion
Liquid Caps .... ᴹᴰ 802
Dura-Tap/PD Capsules 2867
Duratuss Tablets 2565
Duratuss HD Elixir................................. 2565
Efidac/24 .... ᴹᴰ 635
Entex PSE Tablets 1987
Fedahist Gyrocaps................................. 2401
Fedahist Timecaps................................. 2401
Guaifed... 1787
Guaifed Syrup .... ᴹᴰ 734
Guaimax-D Tablets 792
Guaitab Tablets .... ᴹᴰ 734
Isoclor Expectorant............................... 990
Kronofe-A 977
Motrin IB Sinus...................................... ᴹᴰ 838
Novahistine DH...................................... 2462
Novahistine DMX .... ᴹᴰ 822
Novahistine Expectorant....................... 2463
Nucofed 2051
PediaCare Cold Allergy Chewable
Tablets... ᴹᴰ 677
PediaCare Cough-Cold Chewable
Tablets... 1553
PediaCare 1553
PediaCare Infants' Decongestant
Drops .... ᴹᴰ 677
PediCare Infant's Drops Decongestant Plus Cough 1553
PediaCare NightRest Cough-Cold
Liquid 1553
Pediatric Vicks 44d Dry Hacking
Cough & Head Congestion.............. ᴹᴰ 763
Pediatric Vicks 44m Cough &
Cold Relief .... ᴹᴰ 764
Robitussin Cold & Cough Liqui-
Gels .... ᴹᴰ 776
Robitussin Maximum Strength
Cough & Cold .... ᴹᴰ 778
Robitussin Pediatric Cough &
Cold Formula .... ᴹᴰ 779
Robitussin Severe Congestion
Liqui-Gels .... ᴹᴰ 776
Robitussin-DAC Syrup 2074
Robitussin-PE .... ᴹᴰ 778
Rondec Oral Drops 953
Rondec Syrup 953
Rondec Tablet 953
Rondec-DM Oral Drops 954
Rondec-DM Syrup 954
Rondec-TR Tablet 953
Ryna .... ᴹᴰ 841
Seldane-D Extended-Release Tablets.. 1538
Semprex-D Capsules 463
Semprex-D Capsules 1167
Sinarest Tablets .... ᴹᴰ 648
Sinarest Extra Strength Tablets...... ᴹᴰ 648
Sinarest No Drowsiness Tablets .... ᴹᴰ 648
Sine-Aid IB Caplets 1554
Sine-Aid Maximum Strength Sinus
Medication Gelcaps, Caplets and
Tablets... 1554
Sine-Off No Drowsiness Formula
Caplets.. ᴹᴰ 824
Sine-Off Sinus Medicine .... ᴹᴰ 825
Singlet Tablets .... ᴹᴰ 825
Sinutab Non-Drying Liquid Caps ... ᴹᴰ 859
Sinutab Sinus Allergy Medication,
Maximum Strength Tablets and
Caplets.. ᴹᴰ 860
Sinutab Sinus Medication, Maximum Strength Without Drowsiness Formula, Tablets & Caplets.. ᴹᴰ 860

(ᴹᴰ Described in PDR For Nonprescription Drugs) (◉ Described in PDR For Ophthalmology)

Interactions Index

Sinutab Sinus Medication, Regular Strength Without Drowsiness Formula .... ✦D 859
Sudafed Children's Liquid .... ✦D 861
Sudafed Cold and Cough Liquidcaps .... ✦D 862
Sudafed Cough Syrup .... ✦D 862
Sudafed Plus Liquid .... ✦D 862
Sudafed Plus Tablets .... ✦D 863
Sudafed Severe Cold Formula Caplets .... ✦D 863
Sudafed Severe Cold Formula Tablets .... ✦D 864
Sudafed Sinus Caplets...................... ✦D 864
Sudafed Sinus Tablets .... ✦D 864
Sudafed Tablets, 30 mg.................... ✦D 861
Sudafed Tablets, 60 mg.................... ✦D 861
Sudafed 12 Hour Caplets .... ✦D 861
Syn-Rx Tablets 465
Syn-Rx DM Tablets 466
TheraFlu.. ✦D 787
TheraFlu Maximum Strength Nighttime Flu, Cold & Cough Medicine .... ✦D 788
TheraFlu Maximum Strength Non-Drowsy Formula Flu, Cold & Cough Medicine .... ✦D 788
Thera Flu Maximum Strength, Non-Drowsy Formula Flu, Cold and Cough Caplets .... ✦D 789
Triaminic AM Cough and Decongestant Formula .... ✦D 789
Triaminic AM Decongestant Formula .... ✦D 790
Triaminic Nite Light .... ✦D 791
Triaminic Sore Throat Formula ...... ✦D 791
Tussend 1783
Tussend Expectorant 1785
Children's TYLENOL Cold Multi-Symptom Liquid Formula and Chewable Tablets................................. 1561
Children's TYLENOL Cold Plus Cough Multi Symptom Tablets and Liquid .... ✦D 681
Infants' TYLENOL Cold Decongestant & Fever-Reducer Drops 1556
TYLENOL Maximum Strength Allergy Sinus Medication Gelcaps and Caplets 1563
TYLENOL Maximum Strength Allergy Sinus NightTime Medication Caplets 1555
TYLENOL Flu Maximum Strength Gelcaps 1565
TYLENOL Flu NightTime, Maximum Strength, Gelcaps 1566
TYLENOL Maximum Strength Flu NightTime Hot Medication Packets 1562
TYLENOL, Maximum Strength, Sinus Medication Geltabs, Gelcaps, Caplets and Tablets 1566
TYLENOL Cold Multi-Symptom Formula Medication Tablets and Caplets 1561
TYLENOL Cold Medication No Drowsiness Formula Gelcaps and Caplets 1562
TYLENOL Cold Multi-Symptom Hot Medication Liquid Packets.............. 1557
TYLENOL Cough Multi-Symptom Medication with Decongestant 1565
Ursinus Inlay-Tabs................................ ✦D 794
Vicks 44 LiquiCaps Cough, Cold & Flu Relief .... ✦D 755
Vicks 44 LiquiCaps Non-Drowsy Cough & Cold Relief .... ✦D 756
Vicks 44D Dry Hacking Cough & Head Congestion .... ✦D 755
Vicks 44M Cough, Cold & Flu Relief .... ✦D 756
Vicks DayQuil .... ✦D 761
Vicks DayQuil SINUS Pressure & PAIN Relief with IBUPROFEN ...... ✦D 762
Vicks Nyquil Hot Therapy................... ✦D 762
Vicks NyQuil LiquiCaps Multi-Symptom Cold/Flu Relief .... ✦D 763
Vicks NyQuil Multi-Symptom Cold/Flu Relief - (Original & Cherry Flavor) .... ✦D 763

Pseudoephedrine Sulfate (Concomitant use of albuterol with oral sympathomimetic agents is not recommended due to potential for cardiovascular toxicity). Products include:

Cheracol Sinus .... ✦D 768
Chlor-Trimeton Allergy Decongestant Tablets .... ✦D 799
Claritin-D 2350
Drixoral Cold and Allergy Sustained-Action Tablets .... ✦D 802
Drixoral Cold and Flu Extended-Release Tablets................................... ✦D 803
Drixoral Non-Drowsy Formula Extended-Release Tablets .... ✦D 803
Drixoral Allergy/Sinus Extended Release Tablets................................... ✦D 804
Trinalin Repetabs Tablets 1330

Salmeterol Xinafoate (Concomitant use of albuterol with oral sympathomimetic agents is not recommended due to potential for cardiovascular toxicity). Products include:

Serevent Inhalation Aerosol................ 1176

Selegiline Hydrochloride (Action of albuterol on the vascular system may be potentiated). Products include:

Eldepryl Tablets 2550

Sotalol Hydrochloride (Beta-receptor blocking agents and albuterol inhibit effect of each other). Products include:

Betapace Tablets 641

Terbutaline Sulfate (Concomitant use of albuterol with oral sympathomimetic agents is not recommended due to potential for cardiovascular toxicity). Products include:

Brethaire Inhaler 813
Brethine Ampuls 815
Brethine Tablets 814
Bricanyl Subcutaneous Injection 1502
Bricanyl Tablets 1503

Timolol Hemihydrate (Beta-receptor blocking agents and albuterol inhibit effect of each other). Products include:

Betimol 0.25%, 0.5% .... © 261

Timolol Maleate (Beta-receptor blocking agents and albuterol inhibit effect of each other). Products include:

Blocadren Tablets 1614
Timolide Tablets..................................... 1748
Timoptic in Ocudose 1753
Timoptic Sterile Ophthalmic Solution.. 1751
Timoptic-XE 1755

Tranylcypromine Sulfate (Action of albuterol on the vascular system may be potentiated). Products include:

Parnate Tablets 2503

Trimipramine Maleate (Action of albuterol on the vascular system may be potentiated). Products include:

Surmontil Capsules................................ 2811

VEPESID CAPSULES AND INJECTION

(Etoposide) 718
May interact with antineoplastics. Compounds in this category include:

Altretamine (Concomitant administration may result rarely in leukemia). Products include:

Hexalen Capsules 2571

Asparaginase (Concomitant administration may result rarely in leukemia). Products include:

Elspar 1659

Bleomycin Sulfate (Concomitant administration may result rarely in leukemia). Products include:

Blenoxane 692

Busulfan (Concomitant administration may result rarely in leukemia). Products include:

Myleran Tablets 1143

Carboplatin (Concomitant administration may result rarely in leukemia). Products include:

Paraplatin for Injection 705

Carmustine (BCNU) (Concomitant administration may result rarely in leukemia). Products include:

BiCNU 691

Chlorambucil (Concomitant administration may result rarely in leukemia). Products include:

Leukeran Tablets 1133

Cisplatin (Concomitant administration may result rarely in leukemia). Products include:

Platinol 708
Platinol-AQ Injection 710

Cyclophosphamide (Concomitant administration may result rarely in leukemia). Products include:

Cytoxan 694
NEOSAR Lyophilized/Neosar 1959

Dacarbazine (Concomitant administration may result rarely in leukemia). Products include:

DTIC-Dome 600

Daunorubicin Hydrochloride (Concomitant administration may result rarely in leukemia). Products include:

Cerubidine 795

Doxorubicin Hydrochloride (Concomitant administration may result rarely in leukemia). Products include:

Adriamycin PFS 1947
Adriamycin RDF 1947
Doxorubicin Astra 540
Rubex 712

Estramustine Phosphate Sodium (Concomitant administration may result rarely in leukemia). Products include:

Emcyt Capsules 1953

Floxuridine (Concomitant administration may result rarely in leukemia). Products include:

Sterile FUDR 2118

Fluorouracil (Concomitant administration may result rarely in leukemia). Products include:

Efudex 2113
Fluoroplex Topical Solution & Cream 1% 479
Fluorouracil Injection 2116

Flutamide (Concomitant administration may result rarely in leukemia). Products include:

Eulexin Capsules 2358

Hydroxyurea (Concomitant administration may result rarely in leukemia). Products include:

Hydrea Capsules 696

Idarubicin Hydrochloride (Concomitant administration may result rarely in leukemia). Products include:

Idamycin 1955

Ifosfamide (Concomitant administration may result rarely in leukemia). Products include:

IFEX 697

Interferon alfa-2A, Recombinant (Concomitant administration may result rarely in leukemia). Products include:

Roferon-A Injection 2145

Interferon alfa-2B, Recombinant (Concomitant administration may result rarely in leukemia). Products include:

Intron A 2364

Levamisole Hydrochloride (Concomitant administration may result rarely in leukemia). Products include:

Ergamisol Tablets 1292

Lomustine (CCNU) (Concomitant administration may result rarely in leukemia). Products include:

CeeNU 693

Mechlorethamine Hydrochloride (Concomitant administration may result rarely in leukemia). Products include:

Mustargen... 1709

Megestrol Acetate (Concomitant administration may result rarely in leukemia). Products include:

Megace Oral Suspension 699
Megace Tablets 701

Melphalan (Concomitant administration may result rarely in leukemia). Products include:

Alkeran Tablets... 1071

Mercaptopurine (Concomitant administration may result rarely in leukemia). Products include:

Purinethol Tablets 1156

Methotrexate Sodium (Concomitant administration may result rarely in leukemia). Products include:

Methotrexate Sodium Tablets, Injection, for Injection and LPF Injection 1275

Mitomycin (Mitomycin-C) (Concomitant administration may result rarely in leukemia). Products include:

Mutamycin 703

Mitotane (Concomitant administration may result rarely in leukemia). Products include:

Lysodren 698

Mitoxantrone Hydrochloride (Concomitant administration may result rarely in leukemia). Products include:

Novantrone.. 1279

Paclitaxel (Concomitant administration may result rarely in leukemia). Products include:

Taxol 714

Procarbazine Hydrochloride (Concomitant administration may result rarely in leukemia). Products include:

Matulane Capsules 2131

Streptozocin (Concomitant administration may result rarely in leukemia). Products include:

Zanosar Sterile Powder 2653

Tamoxifen Citrate (Concomitant administration may result rarely in leukemia). Products include:

Nolvadex Tablets 2841

Teniposide (Concomitant administration may result rarely in leukemia). Products include:

Vumon 727

Thioguanine (Concomitant administration may result rarely in leukemia). Products include:

Thioguanine Tablets, Tabloid Brand 1181

Thiotepa (Concomitant administration may result rarely in leukemia). Products include:

Thioplex (Thiotepa For Injection) 1281

Vincristine Sulfate (Concomitant administration may result rarely in leukemia). Products include:

Oncovin Solution Vials & Hyporets 1466

Vinorelbine Tartrate (Concomitant administration may result rarely in leukemia). Products include:

Navelbine Injection 1145

VERELAN CAPSULES

(Verapamil Hydrochloride) 1410
May interact with antihypertensives, beta blockers, diuretics, inhalant anesthetics, nondepolarizing neuromuscular blocking agents, vasodilators, ACE inhibitors, lithium preparations, alpha adrenergic blockers, cardiac glycosides, and certain other

IMPORTANT NOTE: Always consult each drug listing in the patient's regimen for possible interactions.

Verelan Interactions Index 1138

agents. Compounds in these categories include:

Acebutolol Hydrochloride (Additive negative effects on heart rate, AV conduction and/or cardiac contractility). Products include:
Sectral Capsules 2807

Amiloride Hydrochloride (Additive effect on lowering blood pressure). Products include:
Midamor Tablets 1703
Moduretic Tablets 1705

Amlodipine Besylate (Additive effect on lowering blood pressure). Products include:
Lotrel Capsules 840
Norvasc Tablets 1940

Atenolol (Additive negative effects on heart rate, AV conduction and/or cardiac contractility). Products include:
Tenoretic Tablets 2845
Tenormin Tablets and I.V. Injection 2847

Atracurium Besylate (Verapamil may potentiate the activity of neuromuscular blocking agents). Products include:
Tracrium Injection 1183

Benazepril Hydrochloride (Additive effect on lowering blood pressure). Products include:
Lotensin Tablets 834
Lotensin HCT 837
Lotrel Capsules 840

Bendroflumethiazide (Additive effect on lowering blood pressure).
No products indexed under this heading.

Betaxolol Hydrochloride (Additive effect on lowering blood pressure). Products include:
Betoptic Ophthalmic Solution 469
Betoptic S Ophthalmic Suspension 471
Kerlone Tablets 2436

Bisoprolol Fumarate (Additive negative effects on heart rate, AV conduction and/or cardiac contractility). Products include:
Zebeta Tablets 1413
Ziac 1415

Bumetanide (Additive effect on lowering blood pressure). Products include:
Bumex 2093

Captopril (Additive effect on lowering blood pressure). Products include:
Capoten 739
Capozide 742

Carbamazepine (Increased carbamazepine concentrations). Products include:
Atretol Tablets 573
Tegretol Chewable Tablets 852
Tegretol Suspension 852
Tegretol Tablets 852

Carteolol Hydrochloride (Additive negative effects on heart rate, AV conduction and/or cardiac contractility). Products include:
Cartrol Tablets 410
Ocupress Ophthalmic Solution, 1% Sterile .... ◉ 309

Chlorothiazide (Additive effect on lowering blood pressure). Products include:
Aldoclor Tablets 1598
Diupres Tablets 1650
Diuril Oral 1653

Chlorothiazide Sodium (Additive effect on lowering blood pressure). Products include:
Diuril Sodium Intravenous 1652

Chlorthalidone (Additive effect on lowering blood pressure). Products include:
Combipres Tablets 677
Tenoretic Tablets 2845

Thalitone 1245

Cimetidine (Possible reduced verapamil clearance). Products include:
Tagamet Tablets 2516

Cimetidine Hydrochloride (Possible reduced verapamil clearance). Products include:
Tagamet 2516

Clonidine (Additive effect on lowering blood pressure). Products include:
Catapres-TTS 675

Clonidine Hydrochloride (Additive effect on lowering blood pressure;). Products include:
Catapres Tablets 674
Combipres Tablets 677

Cyclosporine (Increased serum levels of cyclosporine). Products include:
Neoral 2276
Sandimmune 2286

Deserpidine (Additive effect on lowering blood pressure).
No products indexed under this heading.

Desflurane (Potential for excessive cardiovascular depression). Products include:
Suprane 1813

Deslanoside (Chronic verapamil treatment can increase serum digoxin levels and this can result in digitalis toxicity).
No products indexed under this heading.

Diazoxide (Additive effects on lowering of blood pressure). Products include:
Hyperstat I.V. Injection 2363
Proglycem 580

Digitoxin (Chronic verapamil treatment can increase serum digoxin levels and this can result in digitalis toxicity). Products include:
Crystodigin Tablets 1433

Digoxin (Chronic verapamil treatment can increase serum digoxin levels and this can result in digitalis toxicity). Products include:
Lanoxicaps 1117
Lanoxin Elixir Pediatric 1120
Lanoxin Injection 1123
Lanoxin Injection Pediatric 1126
Lanoxin Tablets 1128

Diltiazem Hydrochloride (Additive effect on lowering blood pressure). Products include:
Cardizem CD Capsules 1506
Cardizem SR Capsules 1510
Cardizem Injectable 1508
Cardizem Tablets 1512
Dilacor XR Extended-release Capsules 2018

Disopyramide Phosphate (Should not be administered within 48 hours before or 24 hours after verapamil administration). Products include:
Norpace 2444

Doxazosin Mesylate (May result in a reduction in blood pressure that is excessive in some patients). Products include:
Cardura Tablets 2186

Enalapril Maleate (Additive effect on lowering blood pressure). Products include:
Vaseretic Tablets 1765
Vasotec Tablets 1771

Enalaprilat (Additive effect on lowering blood pressure). Products include:
Vasotec I.V. 1768

Enflurane (Potential for excessive cardiovascular depression).
No products indexed under this heading.

Esmolol Hydrochloride (Additive negative effects on heart rate, AV conduction and/or cardiac contractility). Products include:
Brevibloc Injection 1808

Ethacrynic Acid (Additive effect on lowering blood pressure). Products include:
Edecrin Tablets 1657

Felodipine (Additive effect on lowering blood pressure). Products include:
Plendil Extended-Release Tablets 527

Flecainide Acetate (Additive effects on myocardial contractility, AV conduction, and repolarization). Products include:
Tambocor Tablets 1497

Fosinopril Sodium (Additive effect on lowering blood pressure). Products include:
Monopril Tablets 757

Furosemide (Additive effect on lowering blood pressure). Products include:
Lasix Injection, Oral Solution and Tablets 1240

Guanabenz Acetate (Additive effect on lowering blood pressure).
No products indexed under this heading.

Guanethidine Monosulfate (Additive effect on lowering blood pressure). Products include:
Esimil Tablets 822
Ismelin Tablets 827

Halothane (Potential for excessive cardiovascular depression). Products include:
Fluothane 2724

Hydralazine Hydrochloride (Additive effect on lowering blood pressure;). Products include:
Apresazide Capsules 808
Apresoline Hydrochloride Tablets .. 809
Ser-Ap-Es Tablets 849

Hydrochlorothiazide (Additive effect on lowering blood pressure). Products include:
Aldactazide 2413
Aldoril Tablets 1604
Apresazide Capsules 808
Capozide 742
Dyazide 2479
Esidrix Tablets 821
Esimil Tablets 822
HydroDIURIL Tablets 1674
Hydropres Tablets 1675
Hyzaar Tablets 1677
Inderide Tablets 2732
Inderide LA Long Acting Capsules .. 2734
Lopressor HCT Tablets 832
Lotensin HCT 837
Maxzide 1380
Moduretic Tablets 1705
Oretic Tablets 443
Prinzide Tablets 1737
Ser-Ap-Es Tablets 849
Timolide Tablets 1748
Vaseretic Tablets 1765
Zestoretic 2850
Ziac 1415

Hydroflumethiazide (Additive effect on lowering blood pressure). Products include:
Diucardin Tablets 2718

Indapamide (Additive effect on lowering blood pressure). Products include:
Lozol Tablets 2022

Isoflurane (Potential for excessive cardiovascular depression).
No products indexed under this heading.

Isradipine (Additive effect on lowering blood pressure). Products include:
DynaCirc Capsules 2256

Labetalol Hydrochloride (Additive negative effects on heart rate, AV conduction and/or cardiac contractility). Products include:
Normodyne Injection 2377
Normodyne Tablets 2379
Trandate 1185

Levobunolol Hydrochloride (Additive negative effects on heart rate, AV conduction and/or cardiac contractility). Products include:
Betagan .... ◉ 233

Lisinopril (Additive effect on lowering blood pressure). Products include:
Prinivil Tablets 1733
Prinzide Tablets 1737
Zestoretic 2850
Zestril Tablets 2854

Lithium Carbonate (May result in lowering of serum lithium levels and increased sensitivity to the effects of lithium). Products include:
Eskalith 2485
Lithium Carbonate Capsules & Tablets 2230
Lithonate/Lithotabs/Lithobid 2543

Lithium Citrate (May result in lowering of serum lithium levels and increased sensitivity to the effects of lithium).
No products indexed under this heading.

Losartan Potassium (Additive effect on lowering blood pressure). Products include:
Cozaar Tablets 1628
Hyzaar Tablets 1677

Mecamylamine Hydrochloride (Additive effect on lowering blood pressure). Products include:
Inversine Tablets 1686

Methoxyflurane (Potential for excessive cardiovascular depression).
No products indexed under this heading.

Methyclothiazide (Additive effect on lowering blood pressure). Products include:
Enduron Tablets 420

Methyldopa (Additive effect on lowering blood pressure). Products include:
Aldoclor Tablets 1598
Aldomet Oral 1600
Aldoril Tablets 1604

Methyldopate Hydrochloride (Additive effect on lowering blood pressure). Products include:
Aldomet Ester HCl Injection 1602

Metipranolol Hydrochloride (Additive negative effects on heart rate, AV conduction and/or cardiac contractility). Products include:
OptiPranolol (Metipranolol 0.3%) Sterile Ophthalmic Solution .... ◉ 258

Metocurine Iodide (Verapamil may potentiate the activity of neuromuscular blocking agents). Products include:
Metubine Iodide Vials 916

Metolazone (Additive effect on lowering blood pressure). Products include:
Mykrox Tablets 993
Zaroxolyn Tablets 1000

Metoprolol Succinate (Additive negative effects on heart rate, AV conduction and/or cardiac contractility; a decrease in metoprolol clearance). Products include:
Toprol-XL Tablets 565

Metoprolol Tartrate (Additive negative effects on heart rate, AV conduction and/or cardiac contractility; a decrease in metoprolol clearance). Products include:
Lopressor Ampuls 830

(◘ Described in PDR For Nonprescription Drugs) (◉ Described in PDR For Ophthalmology)

Lopressor HCT Tablets 832
Lopressor Tablets 830

Metyrosine (Additive effect on lowering blood pressure). Products include:
Demser Capsules 1649

Minoxidil (Additive effect on lowering blood pressure). Products include:
Loniten Tablets 2618
Rogaine Topical Solution 2637

Mivacurium Chloride (Verapamil may potentiate the activity of neuromuscular blocking agents). Products include:
Mivacron 1138

Moexipril Hydrochloride (Additive effect on lowering blood pressure). Products include:
Univasc Tablets 2410

Nadolol (Additive negative effects on heart rate, AV conduction and/or cardiac contractility).
No products indexed under this heading.

Nicardipine Hydrochloride (Additive effect on lowering blood pressure). Products include:
Cardene Capsules 2095
Cardene I.V. 2709
Cardene SR Capsules 2097

Nifedipine (Additive effect on lowering blood pressure). Products include:
Adalat Capsules (10 mg and 20 mg) 587
Adalat CC 589
Procardia Capsules 1971
Procardia XL Extended Release Tablets 1972

Nisoldipine (Additive effect on lowering blood pressure).
No products indexed under this heading.

Nitroglycerin (Additive effect on lowering blood pressure). Products include:
Deponit NTG Transdermal Delivery System 2397
Nitro-Bid IV 1523
Nitro-Bid Ointment 1524
Nitrodisc 2047
Nitro-Dur (nitroglycerin) Transdermal Infusion System 1326
Nitrolingual Spray 2027
Nitrostat Tablets 1925
Transderm-Nitro Transdermal Therapeutic System 859

Pancuronium Bromide Injection (Verapamil may potentiate the activity of neuromuscular blocking agents).
No products indexed under this heading.

Penbutolol Sulfate (Additive negative effects on heart rate, AV conduction and/or cardiac contractility). Products include:
Levatol 2403

Phenobarbital (Increases verapamil clearance). Products include:
Arco-Lase Plus Tablets 512
Bellergal-S Tablets 2250
Donnatal 2060
Donnatal Extentabs 2061
Donnatal Tablets 2060
Phenobarbital Elixir and Tablets 1469
Quadrinal Tablets 1350

Phenoxybenzamine Hydrochloride (Additive effect on lowering blood pressure). Products include:
Dibenzyline Capsules 2476

Phentolamine Mesylate (Additive effect on lowering blood pressure). Products include:
Regitine 846

Pindolol (Additive negative effects on heart rate, AV conduction and/or cardiac contractility). Products include:
Visken Tablets 2299

Polythiazide (Additive effect on lowering blood pressure). Products include:
Minizide Capsules 1938

Prazosin Hydrochloride (May result in a reduction in blood pressure that is excessive in some patients). Products include:
Minipress Capsules 1937
Minizide Capsules 1938

Propranolol Hydrochloride (Additive negative effects on heart rate, AV conduction and/or cardiac contractility). Products include:
Inderal 2728
Inderal LA Long Acting Capsules 2730
Inderide Tablets 2732
Inderide LA Long Acting Capsules 2734

Quinapril Hydrochloride (Additive effect on lowering blood pressure). Products include:
Accupril Tablets 1893

Quinidine Gluconate (Hypotension (in patients with hypertrophic cardiomyopathy); increased quinidine levels). Products include:
Quinaglute Dura-Tabs Tablets 649

Quinidine Polygalacturonate (Hypotension (in patients with hypertrophic cardiomyopathy); increased quinidine levels).
No products indexed under this heading.

Quinidine Sulfate (Hypotension (in patients with hypertrophic cardiomyopathy); increased quinidine levels). Products include:
Quinidex Extentabs 2067

Ramipril (Additive effect on lowering blood pressure). Products include:
Altace Capsules 1232

Rauwolfia Serpentina (Additive effect on lowering blood pressure).
No products indexed under this heading.

Rescinnamine (Additive effect on lowering blood pressure).
No products indexed under this heading.

Reserpine (Additive effect on lowering blood pressure). Products include:
Diupres Tablets 1650
Hydropres Tablets 1675
Ser-Ap-Es Tablets 849

Rifampin (Reduced verapamil bioavailability). Products include:
Rifadin 1528
Rifamate Capsules 1530
Rifater 1532
Rimactane Capsules 847

Rocuronium Bromide (Verapamil may potentiate the activity of neuromuscular blocking agents). Products include:
Zemuron 1830

Sodium Nitroprusside (Additive effect on lowering blood pressure).
No products indexed under this heading.

Sotalol Hydrochloride (Additive negative effects on heart rate, AV conduction and/or cardiac contractility). Products include:
Betapace Tablets 641

Spirapril Hydrochloride (Additive effect on lowering blood pressure).
No products indexed under this heading.

Spironolactone (Additive effect on lowering blood pressure). Products include:
Aldactazide 2413
Aldactone 2414

Succinylcholine Chloride (Verapamil may potentiate the activity of neuromuscular blocking agents). Products include:
Anectine 1073

Terazosin Hydrochloride (May result in a reduction in blood preesure that is excessive in some patients). Products include:
Hytrin Capsules 430

Timolol Hemihydrate (Additive negative effects on heart rate, AV conduction and/or cardiac contractility). Products include:
Betimol 0.25%, 0.5% ⊙ 261

Timolol Maleate (Additive negative effects on heart rate, AV conduction and/or cardiac contractility). Products include:
Blocadren Tablets 1614
Timolide Tablets 1748
Timoptic in Ocudose 1753
Timoptic Sterile Ophthalmic Solution 1751
Timoptic-XE 1755

Torsemide (Additive effect on lowering blood pressure). Products include:
Demadex Tablets and Injection 686

Triamterene (Additive effect on lowering blood pressure). Products include:
Dyazide 2479
Dyrenium Capsules 2481
Maxzide 1380

Trimethaphan Camsylate (Additive effect on lowering blood pressure). Products include:
Arfonad Ampuls 2080

Vecuronium Bromide (Verapamil may potentiate the activity of neuromuscular blocking agents). Products include:
Norcuron 1826

Food Interactions

Alcohol (Verapamil has been found to significantly inhibit ethanol elimination resulting in elevated blood ethanol concentration that may prolong the intoxicating effects of alcohol).

VERELAN CAPSULES

(Verapamil Hydrochloride) 2824
May interact with antihypertensives, beta blockers, diuretics, inhalant anesthetics, nondepolarizing neuromuscular blocking agents, vasodilators, ACE inhibitors, lithium preparations, alpha adrenergic blockers, cardiac glycosides, and certain other agents. Compounds in these categories include:

Acebutolol Hydrochloride (Additive negative effects on heart rate, AV conduction and/or cardiac contractility). Products include:
Sectral Capsules 2807

Amiloride Hydrochloride (Additive effect on lowering blood pressure). Products include:
Midamor Tablets 1703
Moduretic Tablets 1705

Amlodipine Besylate (Additive negative effects on heart rate, AV conduction and/or cardiac contractility). Products include:
Lotrel Capsules 840
Norvasc Tablets 1940

Atenolol (Additive negative effects on heart rate, AV conduction and/or cardiac contractility). Products include:
Tenoretic Tablets 2845
Tenormin Tablets and I.V. Injection 2847

Atracurium Besylate (Verapamil may potentiate the activity of neuromuscular blocking agents). Products include:
Tracrium Injection 1183

Benazepril Hydrochloride (Additive effect on lowering blood pressure). Products include:
Lotensin Tablets 834
Lotensin HCT 837
Lotrel Capsules 840

Bendroflumethiazide (Additive effect on lowering blood pressure).
No products indexed under this heading.

Betaxolol Hydrochloride (Additive negative effects on heart rate, AV conduction and/or cardiac contractility). Products include:
Betoptic Ophthalmic Solution 469
Betoptic S Ophthalmic Suspension 471
Kerlone Tablets 2436

Bisoprolol Fumarate (Additive negative effects on heart rate, AV conduction and/or cardiac contractility). Products include:
Zebeta Tablets 1413
Ziac 1415

Bumetanide (Additive effect on lowering blood pressure). Products include:
Bumex 2093

Captopril (Additive effect on lowering blood pressure). Products include:
Capoten 739
Capozide 742

Carbamazepine (Increased carbamazepine concentrations). Products include:
Atretol Tablets 573
Tegretol Chewable Tablets 852
Tegretol Suspension 852
Tegretol Tablets 852

Carteolol Hydrochloride (Additive negative effects on heart rate, AV conduction and/or cardiac contractility). Products include:
Cartrol Tablets 410
Ocupress Ophthalmic Solution, 1% Sterile ⊙ 309

Chlorothiazide (Additive effect on lowering blood pressure). Products include:
Aldoclor Tablets 1598
Diupres Tablets 1650
Diuril Oral 1653

Chlorothiazide Sodium (Additive effect on lowering blood pressure). Products include:
Diuril Sodium Intravenous 1652

Chlorthalidone (Additive effect on lowering blood pressure). Products include:
Combipres Tablets 677
Tenoretic Tablets 2845
Thalitone 1245

Cimetidine (Possible reduced verapamil clearance). Products include:
Tagamet Tablets 2516

Cimetidine Hydrochloride (Possible reduced verapamil clearance). Products include:
Tagamet 2516

Clonidine (Additive effect on lowering blood pressure). Products include:
Catapres-TTS 675

Clonidine Hydrochloride (Additive effect on lowering blood pressure). Products include:
Catapres Tablets 674
Combipres Tablets 677

Deserpidine (Additive effect on lowering blood pressure).
No products indexed under this heading.

IMPORTANT NOTE: Always consult each drug listing in the patient's regimen for possible interactions.

Verelan Interactions Index 1140

Desflurane (Potential for excessive cardiovascular depression). Products include:
Suprane ... 1813
Deslanoside (Chronic verapamil treatment can increase serum digoxin levels and this can result in digitalis toxicity).
No products indexed under this heading.
Diazoxide (Additive negative effects on heart rate, AV conduction and/or cardiac contractility). Products include:
Hyperstat I.V. Injection ... 2363
Proglycem ... 580
Digitoxin (Chronic verapamil treatment can increase serum digoxin levels and this can result in digitalis toxicity). Products include:
Crystodigin Tablets ... 1433
Digoxin (Chronic verapamil treatment can increase serum digoxin levels and this can result in digitalis toxicity). Products include:
Lanoxicaps ... 1117
Lanoxin Elixir Pediatric ... 1120
Lanoxin Injection ... 1123
Lanoxin Injection Pediatric ... 1126
Lanoxin Tablets ... 1128
Diltiazem Hydrochloride (Additive effect on lowering blood pressure). Products include:
Cardizem CD Capsules ... 1506
Cardizem SR Capsules ... 1510
Cardizem Injectable ... 1508
Cardizem Tablets ... 1512
Dilacor XR Extended-release Capsules ... 2018
Disopyramide Phosphate (Should not be administered within 48 hours before or 24 hours after verapamil administration). Products include:
Norpace ... 2444
Doxazosin Mesylate (May result in a reduction in blood pressure that is excessive in some patients). Products include:
Cardura Tablets ... 2186
Enalapril Maleate (Additive effect on lowering blood pressure). Products include:
Vaseretic Tablets ... 1765
Vasotec Tablets ... 1771
Enalaprilat (Additive effect on lowering blood pressure). Products include:
Vasotec I.V. ... 1768
Enflurane (Potential for excessive cardiovascular depression).
No products indexed under this heading.
Esmolol Hydrochloride (Additive negative effects on heart rate, AV conduction and/or cardiac contractility). Products include:
Brevibloc Injection ... 1808
Ethacrynic Acid (Additive effect on lowering blood pressure). Products include:
Edecrin Tablets ... 1657
Felodipine (Additive effect on lowering blood pressure). Products include:
Plendil Extended-Release Tablets ... 527
Flecainide Acetate (Additive effects on myocardial contractility, AV conduction, and repolarization). Products include:
Tambocor Tablets ... 1497
Fosinopril Sodium (Additive effect on lowering blood pressure). Products include:
Monopril Tablets ... 757
Furosemide (Additive effect on lowering blood pressure). Products include:
Lasix Injection, Oral Solution and Tablets ... 1240
Guanabenz Acetate (Additive effect on lowering blood pressure).
No products indexed under this heading.
Guanethidine Monosulfate (Additive effect on lowering blood pressure). Products include:
Esimil Tablets ... 822
Ismelin Tablets ... 827
Halothane (Potential for excessive cardiovascular depression). Products include:
Fluothane ... 2724
Hydralazine Hydrochloride (Additive effect on lowering blood pressure; adverse effects on cardiac function). Products include:
Apresazide Capsules ... 808
Apresoline Hydrochloride Tablets .. 809
Ser-Ap-Es Tablets ... 849
Hydrochlorothiazide (Additive effect on lowering blood pressure). Products include:
Aldactazide ... 2413
Aldoril Tablets ... 1604
Apresazide Capsules ... 808
Capozide ... 742
Dyazide ... 2479
Esidrix Tablets ... 821
Esimil Tablets ... 822
HydroDIURIL Tablets ... 1674
Hydropres Tablets ... 1675
Hyzaar Tablets ... 1677
Inderide Tablets ... 2732
Inderide LA Long Acting Capsules .. 2734
Lopressor HCT Tablets ... 832
Lotensin HCT ... 837
Maxzide ... 1380
Moduretic Tablets ... 1705
Oretic Tablets ... 443
Prinzide Tablets ... 1737
Ser-Ap-Es Tablets ... 849
Timolide Tablets ... 1748
Vaseretic Tablets ... 1765
Zestoretic ... 2850
Ziac ... 1415
Hydroflumethiazide (Additive effect on lowering blood pressure). Products include:
Diucardin Tablets ... 2718
Indapamide (Additive effect on lowering blood pressure). Products include:
Lozol Tablets ... 2022
Isoflurane (Potential for excessive cardiovascular depression).
No products indexed under this heading.
Isradipine (Additive effect on lowering blood pressure). Products include:
DynaCirc Capsules ... 2256
Labetalol Hydrochloride (Additive negative effects on heart rate, AV conduction and/or cardiac contractility). Products include:
Normodyne Injection ... 2377
Normodyne Tablets ... 2379
Trandate ... 1185
Levobunolol Hydrochloride (Additive negative effects on heart rate, AV conduction and/or cardiac contractility). Products include:
Betagan ... ⊙ 233
Lisinopril (Additive effect on lowering blood pressure). Products include:
Prinivil Tablets ... 1733
Prinzide Tablets ... 1737
Zestoretic ... 2850
Zestril Tablets ... 2854
Lithium Carbonate (May result in lowering of serum lithium levels and increased sensitivity to the effects of lithium). Products include:
Eskalith ... 2485
Lithium Carbonate Capsules & Tablets ... 2230
Lithonate/Lithotabs/Lithobid ... 2543
Lithium Citrate (May result in lowering of serum lithium levels and increased sensitivity to the effects of lithium).
No products indexed under this heading.
Losartan Potassium (Additive negative effects on heart rate, AV conduction and/or cardiac contractility). Products include:
Cozaar Tablets ... 1628
Hyzaar Tablets ... 1677
Mecamylamine Hydrochloride (Additive effect on lowering blood pressure). Products include:
Inversine Tablets ... 1686
Methoxyflurane (Potential for excessive cardiovascular depression).
No products indexed under this heading.
Methyclothiazide (Additive effect on lowering blood pressure). Products include:
Enduron Tablets ... 420
Methyldopa (Additive effect on lowering blood pressure). Products include:
Aldoclor Tablets ... 1598
Aldomet Oral ... 1600
Aldoril Tablets ... 1604
Methyldopate Hydrochloride (Additive effect on lowering blood pressure). Products include:
Aldomet Ester HCl Injection ... 1602
Metipranolol Hydrochloride (Additive negative effects on heart rate, AV conduction and/or cardiac contractility). Products include:
OptiPranolol (Metipranolol 0.3%) Sterile Ophthalmic Solution ... ⊙ 258
Metocurine Iodide (Verapamil may potentiate the activity of neuromuscular blocking agents). Products include:
Metubine Iodide Vials ... 916
Metolazone (Additive effect on lowering blood pressure). Products include:
Mykrox Tablets ... 993
Zaroxolyn Tablets ... 1000
Metoprolol Succinate (Additive effect on lowering blood pressure). Products include:
Toprol-XL Tablets ... 565
Metoprolol Tartrate (Additive negative effects on heart rate, AV conduction and/or cardiac contractility). Products include:
Lopressor Ampuls ... 830
Lopressor HCT Tablets ... 832
Lopressor Tablets ... 830
Metyrosine (Additive effect on lowering blood pressure). Products include:
Demser Capsules ... 1649
Minoxidil (Additive effect on lowering blood pressure). Products include:
Loniten Tablets ... 2618
Rogaine Topical Solution ... 2637
Mivacurium Chloride (Verapamil may potentiate the activity of neuromuscular blocking agents). Products include:
Mivacron ... 1138
Moexipril Hydrochloride (Additive effect on lowering blood pressure). Products include:
Univasc Tablets ... 2410
Nadolol (Additive negative effects on heart rate, AV conduction and/or cardiac contractility).
No products indexed under this heading.
Nicardipine Hydrochloride (Additive effect on lowering blood pressure). Products include:
Cardene Capsules ... 2095
Cardene I.V. ... 2709
Cardene SR Capsules ... 2097
Nifedipine (Additive effect on lowering blood pressure). Products include:
Adalat Capsules (10 mg and 20 mg) ... 587
Adalat CC ... 589
Procardia Capsules ... 1971
Procardia XL Extended Release Tablets ... 1972
Nisoldipine (Additive effect on lowering blood pressure).
No products indexed under this heading.
Pancuronium Bromide Injection (Verapamil may potentiate the activity of neuromuscular blocking agents).
No products indexed under this heading.
Penbutolol Sulfate (Additive negative effects on heart rate, AV conduction and/or cardiac contractility). Products include:
Levatol ... 2403
Phenobarbital (Increases verapamil clearance). Products include:
Arco-Lase Plus Tablets ... 512
Bellergal-S Tablets ... 2250
Donnatal ... 2060
Donnatal Extentabs ... 2061
Donnatal Tablets ... 2060
Phenobarbital Elixir and Tablets ... 1469
Quadrinal Tablets ... 1350
Phenoxybenzamine Hydrochloride (Additive effect on lowering blood pressure). Products include:
Dibenzyline Capsules ... 2476
Phentolamine Mesylate (Additive effect on lowering blood pressure). Products include:
Regitine ... 846
Pindolol (Additive negative effects on heart rate, AV conduction and/or cardiac contractility). Products include:
Visken Tablets ... 2299
Polythiazide (Additive effect on lowering blood pressure). Products include:
Minizide Capsules ... 1938
Prazosin Hydrochloride (May result in a reduction in blood pressure that is excessive in some patients). Products include:
Minipress Capsules ... 1937
Minizide Capsules ... 1938
Propranolol Hydrochloride (Additive negative effects on heart rate, AV conduction and/or cardiac contractility). Products include:
Inderal ... 2728
Inderal LA Long Acting Capsules ... 2730
Inderide Tablets ... 2732
Inderide LA Long Acting Capsules .. 2734
Quinapril Hydrochloride (Additive effect on lowering blood pressure). Products include:
Accupril Tablets ... 1893
Quinidine Gluconate (Hypotension (in patients with hypertrophic cardiomyopathy); increased quinidine levels). Products include:
Quinaglute Dura-Tabs Tablets ... 649
Quinidine Polygalacturonate (Hypotension (in patients with hypertrophic cardiomyopathy); increased quinidine levels).
No products indexed under this heading.

(▭ Described in PDR For Nonprescription Drugs) (⊙ Described in PDR For Ophthalmology)

1141 **Interactions Index** **Versed**

Quinidine Sulfate (Hypotension (in patients with hypertrophic cardiomyopathy); increased quinidine levels). Products include:
Quinidex Extentabs ... 2067
Ramipril (Additive effect on lowering blood pressure). Products include:
Altace Capsules ... 1232
Rauwolfia Serpentina (Additive effect on lowering blood pressure).
No products indexed under this heading.
Rescinnamine (Additive effect on lowering blood pressure).
No products indexed under this heading.
Reserpine (Additive effect on lowering blood pressure). Products include:
Diupres Tablets ... 1650
Hydropres Tablets ... 1675
Ser-Ap-Es Tablets ... 849
Rocuronium Bromide (Verapamil may potentiate the activity of neuromuscular blocking agents). Products include:
Zemuron ... 1830
Sodium Nitroprusside (Additive effect on lowering blood pressure).
No products indexed under this heading.
Sotalol Hydrochloride (Additive negative effects on heart rate, AV conduction and/or cardiac contractility). Products include:
Betapace Tablets ... 641
Spirapril Hydrochloride (Additive effect on lowering blood pressure).
No products indexed under this heading.
Spironolactone (Additive effect on lowering blood pressure). Products include:
Aldactazide ... 2413
Aldactone ... 2414
Succinylcholine Chloride (Verapamil may potentiate the activity of neuromuscular blocking agents). Products include:
Anectine ... 1073
Terazosin Hydrochloride (May result in a reduction in blood pressure that is excessive in some patients). Products include:
Hytrin Capsules ... 430
Timolol Hemihydrate (Additive negative effects on heart rate, AV conduction and/or cardiac contractility). Products include:
Betimol 0.25%, 0.5% ... ◉ 261
Timolol Maleate (Additive negative effects on heart rate, AV conduction and/or cardiac contractility). Products include:
Blocadren Tablets ... 1614
Timolide Tablets ... 1748
Timoptic in Ocudose ... 1753
Timoptic Sterile Ophthalmic Solution ... 1751
Timoptic-XE ... 1755
Torsemide (Additive effect on lowering blood pressure). Products include:
Demadex Tablets and Injection ... 686
Triamterene (Additive effect on lowering blood pressure). Products include:
Dyazide ... 2479
Dyrenium Capsules ... 2481
Maxzide ... 1380
Trimethaphan Camsylate (Additive effect on lowering blood pressure). Products include:
Arfonad Ampuls ... 2080
Vecuronium Bromide (Verapamil prolongs receovry from the neuromuscular blockade; may potentiate the activity of neuromuscular blocking agents). Products include:
Norcuron ... 1826

Food Interactions

Alcohol (Verapamil has been found to significantly inhibit ethanol elimination resulting in elevated blood ethanol concentration that may prolong the intoxicating effects of alcohol).

VERMOX CHEWABLE TABLETS
(Mebendazole) ... 1312
May interact with:

Cimetidine (Inhibits mebendazole metabolism and may result in an increase in plasma concentrations of mebendazole). Products include:
Tagamet Tablets ... 2516
Cimetidine Hydrochloride (Inhibits mebendazole metabolism and may result in an increase in plasma concentrations of mebendazole). Products include:
Tagamet ... 2516

VERSED INJECTION
(Midazolam Hydrochloride) ... 2170
May interact with narcotic analgesics, barbiturates, tranquilizers, central nervous system depressants, and certain other agents. Compounds in these categories include:

Alfentanil Hydrochloride (Increases the risk of underventilation or apnea; accentuates the sedative effect of Versed). Products include:
Alfenta Injection ... 1286
Alprazolam (Increases the risk of underventilation or apnea). Products include:
Xanax Tablets ... 2649
Aprobarbital (Increases the risk of underventilation or apnea).
No products indexed under this heading.
Buprenorphine (Increases the risk of underventilation or apnea; accentuates the sedative effect of Versed). Products include:
Buprenex Injectable ... 2006
Buspirone Hydrochloride (Increases the risk of underventilation or apnea). Products include:
BuSpar ... 737
Butabarbital (Increases the risk of underventilation or apnea).
No products indexed under this heading.
Butalbital (Increases the risk of underventilation or apnea). Products include:
Esgic-plus Tablets ... 1013
Fioricet Tablets ... 2258
Fioricet with Codeine Capsules ... 2260
Fiorinal Capsules ... 2261
Fiorinal with Codeine Capsules ... 2262
Fiorinal Tablets ... 2261
Phrenilin ... 785
Sedapap Tablets 50 mg/650 mg .. 1543
Chlordiazepoxide (Increases the risk of underventilation or apnea). Products include:
Libritabs Tablets ... 2177
Limbitrol ... 2180
Chlordiazepoxide Hydrochloride (Increases the risk of underventilation or apnea). Products include:
Librax Capsules ... 2176
Librium Capsules ... 2178
Librium Injectable ... 2179
Chlorpromazine (Increases the risk of underventilation or apnea). Products include:
Thorazine Suppositories ... 2523
Chlorprothixene (Increases the risk of underventilation or apnea).
No products indexed under this heading.
Chlorprothixene Hydrochloride (Increases the risk of underventilation or apnea).
No products indexed under this heading.
Cimetidine (May delay the clearance of cimetidine). Products include:
Tagamet Tablets ... 2516
Cimetidine Hydrochloride (May delay the clearance of cimetidine). Products include:
Tagamet ... 2516
Clorazepate Dipotassium (Increases the risk of underventilation or apnea). Products include:
Tranxene ... 451
Clozapine (Increases the risk of underventilation or apnea; accentuates the sedative effect of Versed). Products include:
Clozaril Tablets ... 2252
Codeine Phosphate (Increases the risk of underventilation or apnea; accentuates the sedative effect of Versed). Products include:
Actifed with Codeine Cough Syrup.. 1067
Brontex ... 1981
Deconsal C Expectorant Syrup ... 456
Deconsal Pediatric Syrup ... 457
Dimetane-DC Cough Syrup ... 2059
Empirin with Codeine Tablets ... 1093
Fioricet with Codeine Capsules ... 2260
Fiorinal with Codeine Capsules ... 2262
Isoclor Expectorant ... 990
Novahistine DH ... 2462
Novahistine Expectorant ... 2463
Nucofed ... 2051
Phenergan with Codeine ... 2777
Phenergan VC with Codeine ... 2781
Robitussin A-C Syrup ... 2073
Robitussin-DAC Syrup ... 2074
Ryna ... ▣ 841
Soma Compound w/Codeine Tablets ... 2676
Tussi-Organidin NR Liquid and S NR Liquid ... 2677
Tylenol with Codeine ... 1583
Desflurane (Increases the risk of underventilation or apnea; accentuates the sedative effect of Versed). Products include:
Suprane ... 1813
Dezocine (Increases the risk of underventilation or apnea; accentuates the sedative effect of Versed). Products include:
Dalgan Injection ... 538
Diazepam (Increases the risk of underventilation or apnea). Products include:
Dizac ... 1809
Valium Injectable ... 2182
Valium Tablets ... 2183
Valrelease Capsules ... 2169
Droperidol (Increases the risk of underventilation or apnea). Products include:
Inapsine Injection ... 1296
Enflurane (Increases the risk of underventilation or apnea).
No products indexed under this heading.
Erythromycin (Concurrent use may result in a decrease in the plasma clearance of midazolam). Products include:
A/T/S 2% Acne Topical Gel and Solution ... 1234
Benzamycin Topical Gel ... 905
E-Mycin Tablets ... 1341
Emgel 2% Topical Gel ... 1093
ERYC ... 1915
Erycette (erythromycin 2%) Topical Solution ... 1888
Ery-Tab Tablets ... 422
Erythromycin Base Filmtab ... 426
Erythromycin Delayed-Release Capsules, USP ... 427
Ilotycin Ophthalmic Ointment ... 912
PCE Dispertab Tablets ... 444
T-Stat 2.0% Topical Solution and Pads ... 2688
Theramycin Z Topical Solution 2% 1592
Erythromycin Estolate (Concurrent use may result in a decrease in the plasma clearance of midazolam). Products include:
Ilosone ... 911
Erythromycin Ethylsuccinate (Concurrent use may result in a decrease in the plasma clearance of midazolam). Products include:
E.E.S. ... 424
EryPed ... 421
Erythromycin Gluceptate (Concurrent use may result in a decrease in the plasma clearance of midazolam). Products include:
Ilotycin Gluceptate, IV, Vials ... 913
Erythromycin Stearate (Concurrent use may result in a decrease in the plasma clearance of midazolam). Products include:
Erythrocin Stearate Filmtab ... 425
Estazolam (Increases the risk of underventilation or apnea). Products include:
ProSom Tablets ... 449
Ethchlorvynol (Increases the risk of underventilation or apnea). Products include:
Placidyl Capsules ... 448
Ethinamate (Increases the risk of underventilation or apnea).
No products indexed under this heading.
Fentanyl (Increases the risk of underventilation or apnea; accentuates the sedative effect of Versed). Products include:
Duragesic Transdermal System ... 1288
Fentanyl Citrate (Increases the risk of underventilation or apnea; accentuates the sedative effect of Versed). Products include:
Sublimaze Injection ... 1307
Fluphenazine Decanoate (Increases the risk of underventilation or apnea). Products include:
Prolixin Decanoate ... 509
Fluphenazine Enanthate (Increases the risk of underventilation or apnea). Products include:
Prolixin Enanthate ... 509
Fluphenazine Hydrochloride (Increases the risk of underventilation or apnea). Products include:
Prolixin ... 509
Flurazepam Hydrochloride (Increases the risk of underventilation or apnea). Products include:
Dalmane Capsules ... 2173
Glutethimide (Increases the risk of underventilation or apnea).
No products indexed under this heading.
Haloperidol (Increases the risk of underventilation or apnea). Products include:
Haldol Injection, Tablets and Concentrate ... 1575
Haloperidol Decanoate (Increases the risk of underventilation or apnea). Products include:
Haldol Decanoate ... 1577
Halothane (Reduced amount of inhalant required). Products include:
Fluothane ... 2724

IMPORTANT NOTE: Always consult each drug listing in the patient's regimen for possible interactions.

Versed Interactions Index 1142

Hydrocodone Bitartrate (Increases the risk of underventilation or apnea; accentuates the sedative effect of Versed). Products include:

Anexsia 5/500 Elixir 1781
Anexia Tablets 1782
Codiclear DH Syrup 791
Deconamine CX Cough and Cold Liquid and Tablets 1319
Duratuss HD Elixir 2565
Hycodan Tablets and Syrup 930
Hycomine Compound Tablets 932
Hycomine 931
Hycotuss Expectorant Syrup 933
Hydrocet Capsules 782
Lorcet 10/650 1018
Lortab 2566
Tussend 1783
Tussend Expectorant 1785
Vicodin Tablets 1356
Vicodin ES Tablets 1357
Vicodin Tuss Expectorant 1358
Zydone Capsules 949

Hydrocodone Polistirex (Increases the risk of underventilation or apnea; accentuates the sedative effect of Versed). Products include:

Tussionex Pennkinetic Extended-Release Suspension 998

Hydroxyzine Hydrochloride (Increases the risk of underventilation or apnea). Products include:

Atarax Tablets & Syrup 2185
Marax Tablets & DF Syrup 2200
Vistaril Intramuscular Solution 2216

Isoflurane (Increases the risk of underventilation or apnea).

No products indexed under this heading.

Ketamine Hydrochloride (Increases the risk of underventilation or apnea).

No products indexed under this heading.

Levomethadyl Acetate Hydrochloride (Increases the risk of underventilation or apnea; accentuates the sedative effect of Versed). Products include:

Orlamm 2239

Levorphanol Tartrate (Increases the risk of underventilation or apnea; accentuates the sedative effect of Versed). Products include:

Levo-Dromoran 2129

Lorazepam (Increases the risk of underventilation or apnea). Products include:

Ativan Injection 2698
Ativan Tablets 2700

Loxapine Hydrochloride (Increases the risk of underventilation or apnea). Products include:

Loxitane 1378

Loxapine Succinate (Increases the risk of underventilation or apnea). Products include:

Loxitane Capsules 1378

Meperidine Hydrochloride (Increases the risk of underventilation or apnea; accentuates the sedative effect of Versed). Products include:

Demerol 2308
Mepergan Injection 2753

Mephobarbital (Increases the risk of underventilation or apnea). Products include:

Mebaral Tablets 2322

Meprobamate (Increases the risk of underventilation or apnea). Products include:

Miltown Tablets 2672
PMB 200 and PMB 400 2783

Mesoridazine Besylate (Increases the risk of underventilation or apnea). Products include:

Serentil 684

Methadone Hydrochloride (Increases the risk of underventilation or apnea; accentuates the sedative effect of Versed). Products include:

Methadone Hydrochloride Oral Concentrate 2233
Methadone Hydrochloride Oral Solution & Tablets 2235

Methohexital Sodium (Increases the risk of underventilation or apnea). Products include:

Brevital Sodium Vials 1429

Methotrimeprazine (Increases the risk of underventilation or apnea; accentuates the sedative effect of Versed). Products include:

Levoprome 1274

Methoxyflurane (Increases the risk of underventilation or apnea).

No products indexed under this heading.

Molindone Hydrochloride (Increases the risk of underventilation or apnea). Products include:

Moban Tablets and Concentrate 1048

Morphine Sulfate (Increases the risk of underventilation or apnea; accentuates the sedative effect of Versed). Products include:

Astramorph/PF Injection, USP (Preservative-Free) 535
Duramorph 962
Infumorph 200 and Infumorph 500 Sterile Solutions 965
MS Contin Tablets 1994
MSIR 1997
Oramorph SR (Morphine Sulfate Sustained Release Tablets) 2236
RMS Suppositories 2657
Roxanol 2243

Opium Alkaloids (Increases the risk of underventilation or apnea; accentuates the sedative effect of Versed).

No products indexed under this heading.

Oxazepam (Increases the risk of underventilation or apnea). Products include:

Serax Capsules 2810
Serax Tablets 2810

Oxycodone Hydrochloride (Increases the risk of underventilation or apnea; accentuates the sedative effect of Versed). Products include:

Percocet Tablets 938
Percodan Tablets 939
Percodan-Demi Tablets 940
Roxicodone Tablets, Oral Solution & Intensol (Oxycodone) 2244
Tylox Capsules 1584

Pentobarbital Sodium (Increases the risk of underventilation or apnea). Products include:

Nembutal Sodium Capsules 436
Nembutal Sodium Solution 438
Nembutal Sodium Suppositories 440

Perphenazine (Increases the risk of underventilation or apnea). Products include:

Etrafon 2355
Triavil Tablets 1757
Trilafon 2389

Phenobarbital (Increases the risk of underventilation or apnea). Products include:

Arco-Lase Plus Tablets 512
Bellergal-S Tablets 2250
Donnatal 2060
Donnatal Extentabs 2061
Donnatal Tablets 2060
Phenobarbital Elixir and Tablets 1469
Quadrinal Tablets 1350

Prazepam (Increases the risk of underventilation or apnea).

No products indexed under this heading.

Prochlorperazine (Increases the risk of underventilation or apnea). Products include:

Compazine 2470

Promethazine Hydrochloride (Increases the risk of underventilation or apnea). Products include:

Mepergan Injection 2753
Phenergan with Codeine 2777
Phenergan with Dextromethorphan 2778
Phenergan Injection 2773
Phenergan Suppositories 2775
Phenergan Syrup 2774
Phenergan Tablets 2775
Phenergan VC 2779
Phenergan VC with Codeine 2781

Propofol (Increases the risk of underventilation or apnea). Products include:

Diprivan Injection 2833

Propoxyphene Hydrochloride (Increases the risk of underventilation or apnea; accentuates the sedative effect of Versed). Products include:

Darvon 1435
Wygesic Tablets 2827

Propoxyphene Napsylate (Increases the risk of underventilation or apnea; accentuates the sedative effect of Versed). Products include:

Darvon-N/Darvocet-N 1433

Quazepam (Increases the risk of underventilation or apnea). Products include:

Doral Tablets 2664

Risperidone (Increases the risk of underventilation or apnea; accentuates the sedative effect of Versed). Products include:

Risperdal 1301

Secobarbital Sodium (Increases the risk of underventilation or apnea). Products include:

Seconal Sodium Pulvules 1474

Sufentanil Citrate (Increases the risk of underventilation or apnea; accentuates the sedative effect of Versed). Products include:

Sufenta Injection 1309

Temazepam (Increases the risk of underventilation or apnea). Products include:

Restoril Capsules 2284

Thiamylal Sodium (Increases the risk of underventilation or apnea).

No products indexed under this heading.

Thioridazine Hydrochloride (Increases the risk of underventilation or apnea). Products include:

Mellaril 2269

Thiothixene (Increases the risk of underventilation or apnea). Products include:

Navane Capsules and Concentrate 2201
Navane Intramuscular 2202

Triazolam (Increases the risk of underventilation or apnea). Products include:

Halcion Tablets 2611

Trifluoperazine Hydrochloride (Increases the risk of underventilation or apnea). Products include:

Stelazine 2514

Zolpidem Tartrate (Increases the risk of underventilation or apnea; accentuates the sedative effect of Versed). Products include:

Ambien Tablets 2416

Food Interactions

Alcohol (May increase risk of underventilation and prolong drug effect).

VEXOL 1% OPHTHALMIC SUSPENSION

(Rimexolone) .... ◉ 230
None cited in PDR database.

VIBRAMYCIN CALCIUM ORAL SUSPENSION SYRUP

(Doxycycline Calcium) 1941
See **Vibramycin Hyclate Capsules**

VIBRAMYCIN HYCLATE CAPSULES

(Doxycycline Hyclate) 1941
May interact with oral anticoagulants, penicillins, antacids containing aluminium, calcium and magnesium, barbiturates, oral contraceptives, and certain other agents. Compounds in these categories include:

Aluminum Carbonate Gel (Concomitant therapy may impair oral absorption of tetracycline). Products include:

Basaljel 2703

Aluminum Hydroxide (Concomitant therapy may impair oral absorption of tetracycline). Products include:

ALternaGEL Liquid 1316
Maximum Strength Ascriptin .... ▣ 630
Cama Arthritis Pain Reliever .... ▣ 785
Gaviscon Extra Strength Relief Formula Antacid Tablets .... ▣ 819
Gaviscon Extra Strength Relief Formula Liquid Antacid .... ▣ 819
Gaviscon Liquid Antacid .... ▣ 820
Gelusil Liquid & Tablets .... ▣ 855
Maalox Heartburn Relief Suspension .... ▣ 642
Maalox Heartburn Relief Tablets .... ▣ 641
Maalox Magnesia and Alumina Oral Suspension .... ▣ 642
Maalox Plus Tablets .... ▣ 643
Extra Strength Maalox Antacid Plus Antigas Liquid and Tablets ▣ 638
Tempo Soft Antacid .... ▣ 835

Aluminum Hydroxide Gel (Concomitant therapy may impair oral absorption of tetracycline). Products include:

ALternaGEL Liquid .... ▣ 659
Aludrox Oral Suspension 2695
Amphojel Suspension 2695
Amphojel Suspension without Flavor 2695
Amphojel Tablets 2695
Arthritis Pain Ascriptin .... ▣ 631
Regular Strength Ascriptin Tablets .... ▣ 629
Gaviscon Antacid Tablets .... ▣ 819
Gaviscon-2 Antacid Tablets .... ▣ 820
Mylanta Liquid 1317
Mylanta Tablets .... ▣ 660
Mylanta Double Strength Liquid 1317
Mylanta Double Strength Tablets .... ▣ 660
Nephrox Suspension .... ▣ 655

Aluminum Hydroxide Gel, Dried (Concomitant therapy may impair oral absorption of tetracycline).

Amoxicillin Trihydrate (Bacteriostatic drugs may interfere with bactericidal action of penicillin). Products include:

Amoxil 2464
Augmentin 2468

Ampicillin Sodium (Bacteriostatic drugs may interfere with bactericidal action of penicillin). Products include:

Unasyn 2212

Aprobarbital (Decreases the half-life of doxycycline).

No products indexed under this heading.

Azlocillin Sodium (Bacteriostatic drugs may interfere with bactericidal action of penicillin).

No products indexed under this heading.

Bacampicillin Hydrochloride (Bacteriostatic drugs may interfere with bactericidal action of penicillin). Products include:

Spectrobid Tablets 2206

(▣ Described in PDR For Nonprescription Drugs) (◉ Described in PDR For Ophthalmology)

Interactions Index

Vibramycin Hyclate

Bismuth Subsalicylate (Absorption of tetracyclines is impaired by bismuth subsalicylate). Products include:

Maximum Strength Pepto-Bismol Liquid .... ◽ 753

Pepto-Bismol Original Liquid, Original and Cherry Tablets and Easy-To-Swallow Caplets 1976

Pepto-Bismol Maximum Strength Liquid 1976

Butabarbital (Decreases the half-life of doxycycline).

No products indexed under this heading.

Butalbital (Decreases the half-life of doxycycline). Products include:

Esgic-plus Tablets 1013

Fioricet Tablets 2258

Fioricet with Codeine Capsules 2260

Fiorinal Capsules 2261

Fiorinal with Codeine Capsules 2262

Fiorinal Tablets 2261

Phrenilin 785

Sedapap Tablets 50 mg/650 mg .. 1543

Carbamazepine (Decreases the half-life of doxycycline). Products include:

Atretol Tablets 573

Tegretol Chewable Tablets 852

Tegretol Suspension 852

Tegretol Tablets 852

Carbenicillin Disodium (Bacteriostatic drugs may interfere with bactericidal action of penicillin).

No products indexed under this heading.

Carbenicillin Indanyl Sodium (Bacteriostatic drugs may interfere with bactericidal action of penicillin). Products include:

Geocillin Tablets 2199

Desogestrel (Concurrent use may render oral contraceptive less effective). Products include:

Desogen Tablets 1817

Ortho-Cept 1851

Dicloxacillin Sodium (Bacteriostatic drugs may interfere with bactericidal action of penicillin).

No products indexed under this heading.

Dicumarol (Depressed plasma prothrombin activity; may require downward adjustment of the anticoagulant dosage).

No products indexed under this heading.

Dihydroxyaluminum Sodium Carbonate (Concomitant therapy may impair oral absorption of tetracycline).

No products indexed under this heading.

Ethinyl Estradiol (Concurrent use may render oral contraceptive less effective). Products include:

Brevicon 2088

Demulen 2428

Desogen Tablets 1817

Levlen/Tri-Levlen 651

Lo/Ovral Tablets 2746

Lo/Ovral-28 Tablets 2751

Modicon 1872

Nordette-21 Tablets 2755

Nordette-28 Tablets 2758

Norinyl 2088

Ortho-Cept 1851

Ortho-Cyclen/Ortho-Tri-Cyclen 1858

Ortho-Novum 1872

Ortho-Cyclen/Ortho Tri-Cyclen 1858

Ovcon 760

Ovral Tablets 2770

Ovral-28 Tablets 2770

Levlen/Tri-Levlen 651

Tri-Norinyl 2164

Triphasil-21 Tablets 2814

Triphasil-28 Tablets 2819

Ethynodiol Diacetate (Concurrent use may render oral contraceptive less effective). Products include:

Demulen 2428

Levonorgestrel (Concurrent use may render oral contraceptive less effective). Products include:

Levlen/Tri-Levlen 651

Nordette-21 Tablets 2755

Nordette-28 Tablets 2758

Norplant System 2759

Levlen/Tri-Levlen 651

Triphasil-21 Tablets 2814

Triphasil-28 Tablets 2819

Magaldrate (Concomitant therapy may impair oral absorption of tetracycline).

No products indexed under this heading.

Magnesium Hydroxide (Concomitant therapy may impair oral absorption of tetracycline). Products include:

Aludrox Oral Suspension 2695

Arthritis Pain Ascriptin .... ◽ 631

Maximum Strength Ascriptin .... ◽ 630

Regular Strength Ascriptin Tablets .... ◽ 629

Di-Gel Antacid/Anti-Gas .... ◽ 801

Gelusil Liquid & Tablets .... ◽ 855

Maalox Magnesia and Alumina Oral Suspension .... ◽ 642

Maalox Plus Tablets .... ◽ 643

Extra Strength Maalox Antacid Plus Antigas Liquid and Tablets ◽ 638

Mylanta Calcium Carbonate and Magnesium Hydroxide Tablets 1318

Mylanta Liquid 1317

Mylanta Tablets .... ◽ 660

Mylanta Double Strength Liquid 1317

Mylanta Double Strength Tablets .. ◽ 660

Phillips' Milk of Magnesia Liquid .... ◽ 729

Rolaids Tablets .... ◽ 843

Tempo Soft Antacid .... ◽ 835

Magnesium Oxide (Concomitant therapy may impair oral absorption of tetracycline). Products include:

Beelith Tablets 639

Bufferin Analgesic Tablets and Caplets .... ◽ 613

Caltrate PLUS .... ◽ 665

Cama Arthritis Pain Reliever .... ◽ 785

Mag-Ox 400 668

Uro-Mag 668

Mephobarbital (Decreases the half-life of doxycycline). Products include:

Mebaral Tablets 2322

Mestranol (Concurrent use may render oral contraceptive less effective). Products include:

Norinyl 2088

Ortho-Novum 1872

Methoxyflurane (Potential for fatal renal toxicity).

No products indexed under this heading.

Mezlocillin Sodium (Bacteriostatic drugs may interfere with bactericidal action of penicillin). Products include:

Mezlin 601

Mezlin Pharmacy Bulk Package 604

Nafcillin Sodium (Bacteriostatic drugs may interfere with bactericidal action of penicillin).

No products indexed under this heading.

Norethindrone (Concurrent use may render oral contraceptive less effective). Products include:

Brevicon 2088

Micronor Tablets 1872

Modicon 1872

Norinyl 2088

Nor-Q D Tablets 2135

Ortho-Novum 1872

Ovcon 760

Tri-Norinyl 2164

Norethynodrel (Concurrent use may render oral contraceptive less effective).

No products indexed under this heading.

Norgestimate (Concurrent use may render oral contraceptive less effective). Products include:

Ortho-Cyclen/Ortho-Tri-Cyclen 1858

Ortho-Cyclen/Ortho Tri-Cyclen 1858

Norgestrel (Concurrent use may render oral contraceptive less effective). Products include:

Lo/Ovral Tablets 2746

Lo/Ovral-28 Tablets 2751

Ovral Tablets 2770

Ovral-28 Tablets 2770

Ovrette Tablets 2771

Penicillin G Benzathine (Bacteriostatic drugs may interfere with bactericidal action of penicillin). Products include:

Bicillin C-R Injection 2704

Bicillin C-R 900/300 Injection 2706

Bicillin L-A Injection 2707

Penicillin G Potassium (Bacteriostatic drugs may interfere with bactericidal action of penicillin). Products include:

Pfizerpen for Injection 2203

Penicillin G Procaine (Bacteriostatic drugs may interfere with bactericidal action of penicillin). Products include:

Bicillin C-R Injection 2704

Bicillin C-R 900/300 Injection 2706

Penicillin G Sodium (Bacteriostatic drugs may interfere with bactericidal action of penicillin).

No products indexed under this heading.

Penicillin V Potassium (Bacteriostatic drugs may interfere with bactericidal action of penicillin). Products include:

Pen•Vee K 2772

Pentobarbital Sodium (Decreases the half-life of doxycycline). Products include:

Nembutal Sodium Capsules 436

Nembutal Sodium Solution 438

Nembutal Sodium Suppositories 440

Phenobarbital (Decreases the half-life of doxycycline). Products include:

Arco-Lase Plus Tablets 512

Bellergal-S Tablets 2250

Donnatal 2060

Donnatal Extentabs 2061

Donnatal Tablets 2060

Phenobarbital Elixir and Tablets 1469

Quadrinal Tablets 1350

Phenytoin (Decreases the half-life of doxycycline). Products include:

Dilantin Infatabs 1908

Dilantin-125 Suspension 1911

Phenytoin Sodium (Decreases the half-life of doxycycline). Products include:

Dilantin Kapseals 1906

Dilantin Parenteral 1910

Secobarbital Sodium (Decreases the half-life of doxycycline). Products include:

Seconal Sodium Pulvules 1474

Thiamylal Sodium (Decreases the half-life of doxycycline).

No products indexed under this heading.

Ticarcillin Disodium (Bacteriostatic drugs may interfere with bactericidal action of penicillin). Products include:

Ticar for Injection 2526

Timentin for Injection 2528

Warfarin Sodium (Depressed plasma prothrombin activity; may require downward adjustment of the anticoagulant dosage). Products include:

Coumadin 926

Food Interactions

Dairy products (Absorption of doxycycline is not markedly influenced by simultaneous ingestion of milk).

Food, unspecified (Absorption of doxycycline is not markedly influenced by simultaneous ingestion of food).

VIBRAMYCIN HYCLATE INTRAVENOUS

(Doxycycline Hyclate) 2215

May interact with anticoagulants and penicillins. Compounds in these categories include:

Amoxicillin Trihydrate (Interference with bactericidal action of penicillin). Products include:

Amoxil 2464

Augmentin 2468

Ampicillin Sodium (Interference with bactericidal action of penicillin). Products include:

Unasyn 2212

Azlocillin Sodium (Interference with bactericidal action of penicillin).

No products indexed under this heading.

Bacampicillin Hydrochloride (Interference with bactericidal action of penicillin). Products include:

Spectrobid Tablets 2206

Carbenicillin Disodium (Interference with bactericidal action of penicillin).

No products indexed under this heading.

Carbenicillin Indanyl Sodium (Interference with bactericidal action of penicillin). Products include:

Geocillin Tablets 2199

Dalteparin Sodium (Depressed plasma prothrombin activity; downward adjustment of anticoagulant dosage may be necessary). Products include:

Fragmin 1954

Dicloxacillin Sodium (Interference with bactericidal action of penicillin).

No products indexed under this heading.

Dicumarol (Depressed plasma prothrombin activity; downward adjustment of anticoagulant dosage may be necessary).

No products indexed under this heading.

Enoxaparin (Depressed plasma prothrombin activity; downward adjustment of anticoagulant dosage may be necessary). Products include:

Lovenox Injection 2020

Heparin Calcium (Depressed plasma prothrombin activity; downward adjustment of anticoagulant dosage may be necessary).

No products indexed under this heading.

Heparin Sodium (Depressed plasma prothrombin activity; downward adjustment of anticoagulant dosage may be necessary). Products include:

Heparin Lock Flush Solution 2725

Heparin Sodium Injection 2726

Heparin Sodium Injection, USP, Sterile Solution 2615

Heparin Sodium Vials 1441

Mezlocillin Sodium (Interference with bactericidal action of penicillin). Products include:

Mezlin 601

Mezlin Pharmacy Bulk Package 604

Nafcillin Sodium (Interference with bactericidal action of penicillin).

No products indexed under this heading.

IMPORTANT NOTE: Always consult each drug listing in the patient's regimen for possible interactions.

Vibramycin Hyclate | Interactions Index | 1144

Penicillin G Benzathine (Interference with bactericidal action of penicillin). Products include:
- Bicillin C-R Injection ... 2704
- Bicillin C-R 900/300 Injection ... 2706
- Bicillin L-A Injection ... 2707

Penicillin G Potassium (Interference with bactericidal action of penicillin). Products include:
- Pfizerpen for Injection ... 2203

Penicillin G Procaine (Interference with bactericidal action of penicillin). Products include:
- Bicillin C-R Injection ... 2704
- Bicillin C-R 900/300 Injection ... 2706

Penicillin G Sodium (Interference with bactericidal action of penicillin).
- No products indexed under this heading.

Penicillin V Potassium (Interference with bactericidal action of penicillin). Products include:
- Pen•Vee K ... 2772

Ticarcillin Disodium (Interference with bactericidal action of penicillin). Products include:
- Ticar for Injection ... 2526
- Timentin for Injection ... 2528

Warfarin Sodium (Depressed plasma prothrombin activity; downward adjustment of anticoagulant dosage may be necessary). Products include:
- Coumadin ... 926

VIBRAMYCIN MONOHYDRATE FOR ORAL SUSPENSION
(Doxycycline Monohydrate) ... 1941
See **Vibramycin Hyclate Capsules**

VIBRA-TABS FILM COATED TABLETS
(Doxycycline Hyclate) ... 1941
See **Vibramycin Hyclate Capsules**

VICKS 44 DRY HACKING COUGH
(Dextromethorphan Hydrobromide) ... ◘ 755
May interact with monoamine oxidase inhibitors. Compounds in this category include:

Furazolidone (Concurrent or sequential use not recommended). Products include:
- Furoxone ... 2046

Isocarboxazid (Concurrent or sequential use not recommended).
- No products indexed under this heading.

Phenelzine Sulfate (Concurrent or sequential use not recommended). Products include:
- Nardil ... 1920

Selegiline Hydrochloride (Concurrent or sequential use not recommended). Products include:
- Eldepryl Tablets ... 2550

Tranylcypromine Sulfate (Concurrent or sequential use not recommended). Products include:
- Parnate Tablets ... 2503

VICKS 44 LIQUICAPS COUGH, COLD & FLU RELIEF
(Dextromethorphan Hydrobromide, Pseudoephedrine Hydrochloride, Chlorpheniramine Maleate, Acetaminophen) ... ◘ 755
May interact with monoamine oxidase inhibitors, hypnotics and sedatives, tranquilizers, and certain other agents. Compounds in these categories include:

Alprazolam (May increase the drowsiness effect). Products include:
- Xanax Tablets ... 2649

Buspirone Hydrochloride (May increase the drowsiness effect). Products include:
- BuSpar ... 737

Chlordiazepoxide (May increase the drowsiness effect). Products include:
- Libritabs Tablets ... 2177
- Limbitrol ... 2180

Chlordiazepoxide Hydrochloride (May increase the drowsiness effect). Products include:
- Librax Capsules ... 2176
- Librium Capsules ... 2178
- Librium Injectable ... 2179

Chlorpromazine (May increase the drowsiness effect). Products include:
- Thorazine Suppositories ... 2523

Chlorpromazine Hydrochloride (May increase the drowsiness effect). Products include:
- Thorazine ... 2523

Chlorprothixene (May increase the drowsiness effect).
- No products indexed under this heading.

Chlorprothixene Hydrochloride (May increase the drowsiness effect).
- No products indexed under this heading.

Clorazepate Dipotassium (May increase the drowsiness effect). Products include:
- Tranxene ... 451

Diazepam (May increase the drowsiness effect). Products include:
- Dizac ... 1809
- Valium Injectable ... 2182
- Valium Tablets ... 2183
- Valrelease Capsules ... 2169

Droperidol (May increase the drowsiness effect). Products include:
- Inapsine Injection ... 1296

Estazolam (May increase the drowsiness effect). Products include:
- ProSom Tablets ... 449

Ethchlorvynol (May increase the drowsiness effect). Products include:
- Placidyl Capsules ... 448

Ethinamate (May increase the drowsiness effect).
- No products indexed under this heading.

Fluphenazine Decanoate (May increase the drowsiness effect). Products include:
- Prolixin Decanoate ... 509

Fluphenazine Enanthate (May increase the drowsiness effect). Products include:
- Prolixin Enanthate ... 509

Fluphenazine Hydrochloride (May increase the drowsiness effect). Products include:
- Prolixin ... 509

Flurazepam Hydrochloride (May increase the drowsiness effect). Products include:
- Dalmane Capsules ... 2173

Furazolidone (Concomitant and/or sequential use not recommended). Products include:
- Furoxone ... 2046

Glutethimide (May increase the drowsiness effect).
- No products indexed under this heading.

Haloperidol (May increase the drowsiness effect). Products include:
- Haldol Injection, Tablets and Concentrate ... 1575

Haloperidol Decanoate (May increase the drowsiness effect). Products include:
- Haldol Decanoate ... 1577

Hydroxyzine Hydrochloride (May increase the drowsiness effect). Products include:
- Atarax Tablets & Syrup ... 2185
- Marax Tablets & DF Syrup ... 2200
- Vistaril Intramuscular Solution ... 2216

Isocarboxazid (Concomitant and/or sequential use not recommended).
- No products indexed under this heading.

Lorazepam (May increase the drowsiness effect). Products include:
- Ativan Injection ... 2698
- Ativan Tablets ... 2700

Loxapine Hydrochloride (May increase the drowsiness effect). Products include:
- Loxitane ... 1378

Loxapine Succinate (May increase the drowsiness effect). Products include:
- Loxitane Capsules ... 1378

Meprobamate (May increase the drowsiness effect). Products include:
- Miltown Tablets ... 2672
- PMB 200 and PMB 400 ... 2783

Mesoridazine Besylate (May increase the drowsiness effect). Products include:
- Serentil ... 684

Midazolam Hydrochloride (May increase the drowsiness effect). Products include:
- Versed Injection ... 2170

Molindone Hydrochloride (May increase the drowsiness effect). Products include:
- Moban Tablets and Concentrate ... 1048

Oxazepam (May increase the drowsiness effect). Products include:
- Serax Capsules ... 2810
- Serax Tablets ... 2810

Perphenazine (May increase the drowsiness effect). Products include:
- Etrafon ... 2355
- Triavil Tablets ... 1757
- Trilafon ... 2389

Phenelzine Sulfate (Concomitant and/or sequential use not recommended). Products include:
- Nardil ... 1920

Prazepam (May increase the drowsiness effect).
- No products indexed under this heading.

Prochlorperazine (May increase the drowsiness effect). Products include:
- Compazine ... 2470

Promethazine Hydrochloride (May increase the drowsiness effect). Products include:
- Mepergan Injection ... 2753
- Phenergan with Codeine ... 2777
- Phenergan with Dextromethorphan ... 2778
- Phenergan Injection ... 2773
- Phenergan Suppositories ... 2775
- Phenergan Syrup ... 2774
- Phenergan Tablets ... 2775
- Phenergan VC ... 2779
- Phenergan VC with Codeine ... 2781

Propofol (May increase the drowsiness effect). Products include:
- Diprivan Injection ... 2833

Quazepam (May increase the drowsiness effect). Products include:
- Doral Tablets ... 2664

Secobarbital Sodium (May increase the drowsiness effect). Products include:
- Seconal Sodium Pulvules ... 1474

Selegiline Hydrochloride (Concomitant and/or sequential use not recommended). Products include:
- Eldepryl Tablets ... 2550

Temazepam (May increase the drowsiness effect). Products include:
- Restoril Capsules ... 2284

Thioridazine Hydrochloride (May increase the drowsiness effect). Products include:
- Mellaril ... 2269

Thiothixene (May increase the drowsiness effect). Products include:
- Navane Capsules and Concentrate ... 2201
- Navane Intramuscular ... 2202

Tranylcypromine Sulfate (Concomitant and/or sequential use not recommended). Products include:
- Parnate Tablets ... 2503

Triazolam (May increase the drowsiness effect). Products include:
- Halcion Tablets ... 2611

Trifluoperazine Hydrochloride (May increase the drowsiness effect). Products include:
- Stelazine ... 2514

Zolpidem Tartrate (May increase the drowsiness effect). Products include:
- Ambien Tablets ... 2416

Food Interactions

Alcohol (May increase the drowsiness effect).

VICKS 44 LIQUICAPS NON-DROWSY COUGH & COLD RELIEF
(Dextromethorphan Hydrobromide, Pseudoephedrine Hydrochloride) ... ◘ 756
May interact with monoamine oxidase inhibitors. Compounds in this category include:

Furazolidone (Concurrent and/or sequential use is not recommended). Products include:
- Furoxone ... 2046

Isocarboxazid (Concurrent and/or sequential use is not recommended).
- No products indexed under this heading.

Phenelzine Sulfate (Concurrent and/or sequential use is not recommended). Products include:
- Nardil ... 1920

Selegiline Hydrochloride (Concurrent and/or sequential use is not recommended). Products include:
- Eldepryl Tablets ... 2550

Tranylcypromine Sulfate (Concurrent and/or sequential use is not recommended). Products include:
- Parnate Tablets ... 2503

VICKS 44D DRY HACKING COUGH & HEAD CONGESTION
(Dextromethorphan Hydrobromide, Pseudoephedrine Hydrochloride) ... ◘ 755
May interact with monoamine oxidase inhibitors. Compounds in this category include:

Furazolidone (Concurrent and/or sequential use is not recommended). Products include:
- Furoxone ... 2046

Isocarboxazid (Concurrent and/or sequential use is not recommended).
- No products indexed under this heading.

Phenelzine Sulfate (Concurrent and/or sequential use is not recommended). Products include:

Nardil 1920

Selegiline Hydrochloride (Concurrent and/or sequential use is not recommended). Products include:

Eldepryl Tablets 2550

Tranylcypromine Sulfate (Concurrent and/or sequential use is not recommended). Products include:

Parnate Tablets 2503

VICKS 44E CHEST COUGH & CHEST CONGESTION

(Dextromethorphan Hydrobromide, Guaifenesin) .... ☞ 756

May interact with monoamine oxidase inhibitors. Compounds in this category include:

Furazolidone (Concurrent and/or sequential use is not recommended). Products include:

Furoxone 2046

Isocarboxazid (Concurrent and/or sequential use is not recommended).

No products indexed under this heading.

Phenelzine Sulfate (Concurrent and/or sequential use is not recommended). Products include:

Nardil 1920

Selegiline Hydrochloride (Concurrent and/or sequential use is not recommended). Products include:

Eldepryl Tablets 2550

Tranylcypromine Sulfate (Concurrent and/or sequential use is not recommended). Products include:

Parnate Tablets 2503

VICKS 44M COUGH, COLD & FLU RELIEF

(Acetaminophen, Dextromethorphan Hydrobromide, Chlorpheniramine Maleate, Pseudoephedrine Hydrochloride) .... ☞ 756

May interact with hypnotics and sedatives, tranquilizers, monoamine oxidase inhibitors, and certain other agents. Compounds in these categories include:

Alprazolam (May increase drowsiness effect). Products include:

Xanax Tablets 2649

Buspirone Hydrochloride (May increase drowsiness effect). Products include:

BuSpar 737

Chlordiazepoxide (May increase drowsiness effect). Products include:

Libritabs Tablets .... 2177 Limbitrol 2180

Chlordiazepoxide Hydrochloride (May increase drowsiness effect). Products include:

Librax Capsules .... 2176 Librium Capsules .... 2178 Librium Injectable 2179

Chlorpromazine (May increase drowsiness effect). Products include:

Thorazine Suppositories 2523

Chlorpromazine Hydrochloride (May increase drowsiness effect). Products include:

Thorazine 2523

Chlorprothixene (May increase drowsiness effect).

No products indexed under this heading.

Chlorprothixene Hydrochloride (May increase drowsiness effect).

No products indexed under this heading.

Clorazepate Dipotassium (May increase drowsiness effect). Products include:

Tranxene 451

Diazepam (May increase drowsiness effect). Products include:

Dizac .... 1809 Valium Injectable .... 2182 Valium Tablets .... 2183 Valrelease Capsules 2169

Droperidol (May increase drowsiness effect). Products include:

Inapsine Injection................................ 1296

Estazolam (May increase drowsiness effect). Products include:

ProSom Tablets 449

Ethchlorvynol (May increase drowsiness effect). Products include:

Placidyl Capsules 448

Ethinamate (May increase drowsiness effect).

No products indexed under this heading.

Fluphenazine Decanoate (May increase drowsiness effect). Products include:

Prolixin Decanoate 509

Fluphenazine Enanthate (May increase drowsiness effect). Products include:

Prolixin Enanthate 509

Fluphenazine Hydrochloride (May increase drowsiness effect). Products include:

Prolixin 509

Flurazepam Hydrochloride (May increase drowsiness effect). Products include:

Dalmane Capsules 2173

Furazolidone (Concurrent and/or sequential use is not recommended). Products include:

Furoxone 2046

Glutethimide (May increase drowsiness effect).

No products indexed under this heading.

Haloperidol (May increase drowsiness effect). Products include:

Haldol Injection, Tablets and Concentrate 1575

Haloperidol Decanoate (May increase drowsiness effect). Products include:

Haldol Decanoate 1577

Hydroxyzine Hydrochloride (May increase drowsiness effect). Products include:

Atarax Tablets & Syrup....................... 2185 Marax Tablets & DF Syrup.................. 2200 Vistaril Intramuscular Solution........... 2216

Isocarboxazid (Concurrent and/or sequential use is not recommended).

No products indexed under this heading.

Lorazepam (May increase drowsiness effect). Products include:

Ativan Injection .... 2698 Ativan Tablets 2700

Loxapine Hydrochloride (May increase drowsiness effect). Products include:

Loxitane 1378

Loxapine Succinate (May increase drowsiness effect). Products include:

Loxitane Capsules 1378

Meprobamate (May increase drowsiness effect). Products include:

Miltown Tablets .... 2672 PMB 200 and PMB 400 2783

Mesoridazine Besylate (May increase drowsiness effect). Products include:

Serentil 684

Midazolam Hydrochloride (May increase drowsiness effect). Products include:

Versed Injection 2170

Molindone Hydrochloride (May increase drowsiness effect). Products include:

Moban Tablets and Concentrate 1048

Oxazepam (May increase drowsiness effect). Products include:

Serax Capsules .... 2810 Serax Tablets....................................... 2810

Perphenazine (May increase drowsiness effect). Products include:

Etrafon .... 2355 Triavil Tablets .... 1757 Trilafon.. 2389

Phenelzine Sulfate (Concurrent and/or sequential use is not recommended). Products include:

Nardil 1920

Prazepam (May increase drowsiness effect).

No products indexed under this heading.

Prochlorperazine (May increase drowsiness effect). Products include:

Compazine 2470

Promethazine Hydrochloride (May increase drowsiness effect). Products include:

Mepergan Injection .... 2753 Phenergan with Codeine...................... 2777 Phenergan with Dextromethorphan 2778 Phenergan Injection .... 2773 Phenergan Suppositories .... 2775 Phenergan Syrup .... 2774 Phenergan Tablets .... 2775 Phenergan VC .... 2779 Phenergan VC with Codeine 2781

Propofol (May increase drowsiness effect). Products include:

Diprivan Injection................................ 2833

Quazepam (May increase drowsiness effect). Products include:

Doral Tablets 2664

Secobarbital Sodium (May increase drowsiness effect). Products include:

Seconal Sodium Pulvules 1474

Selegiline Hydrochloride (Concurrent and/or sequential use is not recommended). Products include:

Eldepryl Tablets 2550

Temazepam (May increase drowsiness effect). Products include:

Restoril Capsules 2284

Thioridazine Hydrochloride (May increase drowsiness effect). Products include:

Mellaril 2269

Thiothixene (May increase drowsiness effect). Products include:

Navane Capsules and Concentrate 2201 Navane Intramuscular 2202

Tranylcypromine Sulfate (Concurrent and/or sequential use is not recommended). Products include:

Parnate Tablets 2503

Triazolam (May increase drowsiness effect). Products include:

Halcion Tablets.................................... 2611

Trifluoperazine Hydrochloride (May increase drowsiness effect). Products include:

Stelazine 2514

Zolpidem Tartrate (May increase drowsiness effect). Products include:

Ambien Tablets.................................... 2416

Food Interactions

Alcohol (May increase drowsiness effect).

VICKS CHLORASEPTIC COUGH & THROAT DROPS

(Menthol) .... ☞ 759

None cited in PDR database.

VICKS CHLORASEPTIC SORE THROAT LOZENGES

(Benzocaine, Menthol) .... ☞ 759

None cited in PDR database.

VICKS CHLORASEPTIC SORE THROAT SPRAY, AND GARGLE AND MOUTH RINSE

(Phenol) .... ☞ 759

None cited in PDR database.

VICKS COUGH DROPS

(Menthol) .... ☞ 759

None cited in PDR database.

VICKS DAYQUIL ALLERGY RELIEF 12-HOUR EXTENDED RELEASE TABLETS

(Phenylpropanolamine Hydrochloride, Brompheniramine Maleate) .... ☞ 760

May interact with monoamine oxidase inhibitors and certain other agents. Compounds in these categories include:

Furazolidone (Concurrent use is not recommended). Products include:

Furoxone 2046

Isocarboxazid (Concurrent use is not recommended).

No products indexed under this heading.

Phenelzine Sulfate (Concurrent use is not recommended). Products include:

Nardil 1920

Selegiline Hydrochloride (Concurrent use is not recommended). Products include:

Eldepryl Tablets 2550

Tranylcypromine Sulfate (Concurrent use is not recommended). Products include:

Parnate Tablets 2503

Food Interactions

Alcohol (Avoid concurrent use).

VICKS DAYQUIL ALLERGY RELIEF 4-HOUR TABLETS

(Phenylpropanolamine Hydrochloride, Brompheniramine Maleate) .... ☞ 760

May interact with antihypertensives, antidepressant drugs, hypnotics and sedatives, tranquilizers, and certain other agents. Compounds in these categories include:

Acebutolol Hydrochloride (Do not use concomitantly; consult your doctor). Products include:

Sectral Capsules 2807

Alprazolam (May increase the drowsiness effect). Products include:

Xanax Tablets 2649

Amitriptyline Hydrochloride (Do not use concomitantly; consult your doctor). Products include:

Elavil .... 2838 Endep Tablets .... 2174 Etrafon .... 2355 Limbitrol .... 2180 Triavil Tablets...................................... 1757

Amlodipine Besylate (Do not use concomitantly; consult your doctor). Products include:

Lotrel Capsules .... 840 Norvasc Tablets 1940

Amoxapine (Do not use concomitantly; consult your doctor). Products include:

Asendin Tablets 1369

IMPORTANT NOTE: Always consult each drug listing in the patient's regimen for possible interactions.

Vicks DayQuil Allergy — Interactions Index — 1146

Atenolol (Do not use concomitantly; consult your doctor). Products include:
Tenoretic Tablets 2845
Tenormin Tablets and I.V. Injection 2847

Benazepril Hydrochloride (Do not use concomitantly; consult your doctor). Products include:
Lotensin Tablets 834
Lotensin HCT 837
Lotrel Capsules 840

Bendroflumethiazide (Do not use concomitantly; consult your doctor).
No products indexed under this heading.

Betaxolol Hydrochloride (Do not use concomitantly; consult your doctor). Products include:
Betoptic Ophthalmic Solution 469
Betoptic S Ophthalmic Suspension 471
Kerlone Tablets 2436

Bisoprolol Fumarate (Do not use concomitantly; consult your doctor). Products include:
Zebeta Tablets 1413
Ziac 1415

Bupropion Hydrochloride (Do not use concomitantly; consult your doctor). Products include:
Wellbutrin Tablets 1204

Buspirone Hydrochloride (May increase the drowsiness effect). Products include:
BuSpar 737

Captopril (Do not use concomitantly; consult your doctor). Products include:
Capoten 739
Capozide 742

Carteolol Hydrochloride (Do not use concomitantly; consult your doctor). Products include:
Cartrol Tablets 410
Ocupress Ophthalmic Solution, 1% Sterile .... ⊙ 309

Chlordiazepoxide (May increase the drowsiness effect). Products include:
Libritabs Tablets 2177
Limbitrol 2180

Chlordiazepoxide Hydrochloride (May increase the drowsiness effect). Products include:
Librax Capsules 2176
Librium Capsules 2178
Librium Injectable 2179

Chlorothiazide (Do not use concomitantly; consult your doctor). Products include:
Aldoclor Tablets 1598
Diupres Tablets 1650
Diuril Oral 1653

Chlorothiazide Sodium (Do not use concomitantly; consult your doctor). Products include:
Diuril Sodium Intravenous 1652

Chlorpromazine (May increase the drowsiness effect). Products include:
Thorazine Suppositories 2523

Chlorpromazine Hydrochloride (May increase the drowsiness effect). Products include:
Thorazine 2523

Chlorprothixene (May increase the drowsiness effect).
No products indexed under this heading.

Chlorprothixene Hydrochloride (May increase the drowsiness effect).
No products indexed under this heading.

Chlorthalidone (Do not use concomitantly; consult your doctor). Products include:
Combipres Tablets 677
Tenoretic Tablets 2845
Thalitone 1245

Clonidine (Do not use concomitantly; consult your doctor). Products include:
Catapres-TTS 675

Clonidine Hydrochloride (Do not use concomitantly; consult your doctor). Products include:
Catapres Tablets 674
Combipres Tablets 677

Clorazepate Dipotassium (May increase the drowsiness effect). Products include:
Tranxene 451

Deserpidine (Do not use concomitantly; consult your doctor).
No products indexed under this heading.

Desipramine Hydrochloride (Do not use concomitantly; consult your doctor). Products include:
Norpramin Tablets 1526

Diazepam (May increase the drowsiness effect). Products include:
Dizac 1809
Valium Injectable 2182
Valium Tablets 2183
Valrelease Capsules 2169

Diazoxide (Do not use concomitantly; consult your doctor). Products include:
Hyperstat I.V. Injection 2363
Proglycem 580

Diltiazem Hydrochloride (Do not use concomitantly; consult your doctor). Products include:
Cardizem CD Capsules 1506
Cardizem SR Capsules 1510
Cardizem Injectable 1508
Cardizem Tablets 1512
Dilacor XR Extended-release Capsules 2018

Doxazosin Mesylate (Do not use concomitantly; consult your doctor). Products include:
Cardura Tablets 2186

Doxepin Hydrochloride (Do not use concomitantly; consult your doctor). Products include:
Sinequan 2205
Zonalon Cream 1055

Droperidol (May increase the drowsiness effect). Products include:
Inapsine Injection 1296

Enalapril Maleate (Do not use concomitantly; consult your doctor). Products include:
Vaseretic Tablets 1765
Vasotec Tablets 1771

Enalaprilat (Do not use concomitantly; consult your doctor). Products include:
Vasotec I.V. 1768

Esmolol Hydrochloride (Do not use concomitantly; consult your doctor). Products include:
Brevibloc Injection 1808

Estazolam (May increase the drowsiness effect). Products include:
ProSom Tablets 449

Ethchlorvynol (May increase the drowsiness effect). Products include:
Placidyl Capsules 448

Ethinamate (May increase the drowsiness effect).
No products indexed under this heading.

Felodipine (Do not use concomitantly; consult your doctor). Products include:
Plendil Extended-Release Tablets 527

Fluoxetine Hydrochloride (Do not use concomitantly; consult your doctor). Products include:
Prozac Pulvules & Liquid, Oral Solution 919

Fluphenazine Decanoate (May increase the drowsiness effect). Products include:
Prolixin Decanoate 509

Fluphenazine Enanthate (May increase the drowsiness effect). Products include:
Prolixin Enanthate 509

Fluphenazine Hydrochloride (May increase the drowsiness effect). Products include:
Prolixin 509

Flurazepam Hydrochloride (May increase the drowsiness effect). Products include:
Dalmane Capsules 2173

Fosinopril Sodium (Do not use concomitantly; consult your doctor). Products include:
Monopril Tablets 757

Furosemide (Do not use concomitantly; consult your doctor). Products include:
Lasix Injection, Oral Solution and Tablets 1240

Glutethimide (May increase the drowsiness effect).
No products indexed under this heading.

Guanabenz Acetate (Do not use concomitantly; consult your doctor).
No products indexed under this heading.

Guanethidine Monosulfate (Do not use concomitantly; consult your doctor). Products include:
Esimil Tablets 822
Ismelin Tablets 827

Haloperidol (May increase the drowsiness effect). Products include:
Haldol Injection, Tablets and Concentrate 1575

Haloperidol Decanoate (May increase the drowsiness effect). Products include:
Haldol Decanoate 1577

Hydralazine Hydrochloride (Do not use concomitantly; consult your doctor). Products include:
Apresazide Capsules 808
Apresoline Hydrochloride Tablets .. 809
Ser-Ap-Es Tablets 849

Hydrochlorothiazide (Do not use concomitantly; consult your doctor). Products include:
Aldactazide 2413
Aldoril Tablets 1604
Apresazide Capsules 808
Capozide 742
Dyazide 2479
Esidrix Tablets 821
Esimil Tablets 822
HydroDIURIL Tablets 1674
Hydropres Tablets 1675
Hyzaar Tablets 1677
Inderide Tablets 2732
Inderide LA Long Acting Capsules .. 2734
Lopressor HCT Tablets 832
Lotensin HCT 837
Maxzide 1380
Moduretic Tablets 1705
Oretic Tablets 443
Prinzide Tablets 1737
Ser-Ap-Es Tablets 849
Timolide Tablets 1748
Vaseretic Tablets 1765
Zestoretic 2850
Ziac 1415

Hydroflumethiazide (Do not use concomitantly; consult your doctor). Products include:
Diucardin Tablets 2718

Hydroxyzine Hydrochloride (May increase the drowsiness effect). Products include:
Atarax Tablets & Syrup 2185
Marax Tablets & DF Syrup 2200
Vistaril Intramuscular Solution 2216

Imipramine Hydrochloride (Do not use concomitantly; consult your doctor). Products include:
Tofranil Ampuls 854
Tofranil Tablets 856

Imipramine Pamoate (Do not use concomitantly; consult your doctor). Products include:
Tofranil-PM Capsules 857

Indapamide (Do not use concomitantly; consult your doctor). Products include:
Lozol Tablets 2022

Isocarboxazid (Do not use concomitantly; consult your doctor).
No products indexed under this heading.

Isradipine (Do not use concomitantly; consult your doctor). Products include:
DynaCirc Capsules 2256

Labetalol Hydrochloride (Do not use concomitantly; consult your doctor). Products include:
Normodyne Injection 2377
Normodyne Tablets 2379
Trandate 1185

Lisinopril (Do not use concomitantly; consult your doctor). Products include:
Prinivil Tablets 1733
Prinzide Tablets 1737
Zestoretic 2850
Zestril Tablets 2854

Lorazepam (May increase the drowsiness effect). Products include:
Ativan Injection 2698
Ativan Tablets 2700

Losartan Potassium (Do not use concomitantly; consult your doctor). Products include:
Cozaar Tablets 1628
Hyzaar Tablets 1677

Loxapine Hydrochloride (May increase the drowsiness effect). Products include:
Loxitane 1378

Loxapine Succinate (May increase the drowsiness effect). Products include:
Loxitane Capsules 1378

Maprotiline Hydrochloride (Do not use concomitantly; consult your doctor). Products include:
Ludiomil Tablets 843

Mecamylamine Hydrochloride (Do not use concomitantly; consult your doctor). Products include:
Inversine Tablets 1686

Meprobamate (May increase the drowsiness effect). Products include:
Miltown Tablets 2672
PMB 200 and PMB 400 2783

Mesoridazine Besylate (May increase the drowsiness effect). Products include:
Serentil 684

Methyclothiazide (Do not use concomitantly; consult your doctor). Products include:
Enduron Tablets 420

Methyldopa (Do not use concomitantly; consult your doctor). Products include:
Aldoclor Tablets 1598
Aldomet Oral 1600
Aldoril Tablets 1604

Methyldopate Hydrochloride (Do not use concomitantly; consult your doctor). Products include:
Aldomet Ester HCl Injection 1602

Metipranolol Hydrochloride (Do not use concomitantly; consult your doctor). Products include:
OptiPranolol (Metipranolol 0.3%) Sterile Ophthalmic Solution .... ⊙ 258

Interactions Index — Vicks DayQuil Sinus

Metolazone (Do not use concomitantly; consult your doctor). Products include:

Mykrox Tablets 993
Zaroxolyn Tablets 1000

Metoprolol Succinate (Do not use concomitantly; consult your doctor). Products include:

Toprol-XL Tablets 565

Metoprolol Tartrate (Do not use concomitantly; consult your doctor). Products include:

Lopressor Ampuls 830
Lopressor HCT Tablets 832
Lopressor Tablets 830

Metyrosine (Do not use concomitantly; consult your doctor). Products include:

Demser Capsules 1649

Midazolam Hydrochloride (May increase the drowsiness effect). Products include:

Versed Injection 2170

Minoxidil (Do not use concomitantly; consult your doctor). Products include:

Loniten Tablets 2618
Rogaine Topical Solution 2637

Moexipril Hydrochloride (Do not use concomitantly; consult your doctor). Products include:

Univasc Tablets 2410

Molindone Hydrochloride (May increase the drowsiness effect). Products include:

Moban Tablets and Concentrate 1048

Nadolol (Do not use concomitantly; consult your doctor).

No products indexed under this heading.

Nefazodone Hydrochloride (Do not use concomitantly; consult your doctor). Products include:

Serzone Tablets 771

Nicardipine Hydrochloride (Do not use concomitantly; consult your doctor). Products include:

Cardene Capsules 2095
Cardene I.V. 2709
Cardene SR Capsules 2097

Nifedipine (Do not use concomitantly; consult your doctor). Products include:

Adalat Capsules (10 mg and 20 mg) 587
Adalat CC 589
Procardia Capsules 1971
Procardia XL Extended Release Tablets 1972

Nisoldipine (Do not use concomitantly; consult your doctor).

No products indexed under this heading.

Nitroglycerin (Do not use concomitantly; consult your doctor). Products include:

Deponit NTG Transdermal Delivery System 2397
Nitro-Bid IV 1523
Nitro-Bid Ointment 1524
Nitrodisc 2047
Nitro-Dur (nitroglycerin) Transdermal Infusion System 1326
Nitrolingual Spray 2027
Nitrostat Tablets 1925
Transderm-Nitro Transdermal Therapeutic System 859

Nortriptyline Hydrochloride (Do not use concomitantly; consult your doctor). Products include:

Pamelor 2280

Oxazepam (May increase the drowsiness effect). Products include:

Serax Capsules 2810
Serax Tablets 2810

Paroxetine Hydrochloride (Do not use concomitantly; consult your doctor). Products include:

Paxil Tablets 2505

Penbutolol Sulfate (Do not use concomitantly; consult your doctor). Products include:

Levatol 2403

Perphenazine (May increase the drowsiness effect). Products include:

Etrafon 2355
Triavil Tablets 1757
Trilafon 2389

Phenelzine Sulfate (Do not use concomitantly; consult your doctor). Products include:

Nardil 1920

Phenoxybenzamine Hydrochloride (Do not use concomitantly; consult your doctor). Products include:

Dibenzyline Capsules 2476

Phentolamine Mesylate (Do not use concomitantly; consult your doctor). Products include:

Regitine 846

Pindolol (Do not use concomitantly; consult your doctor). Products include:

Visken Tablets 2299

Polythiazide (Do not use concomitantly; consult your doctor). Products include:

Minizide Capsules 1938

Prazepam (May increase the drowsiness effect).

No products indexed under this heading.

Prazosin Hydrochloride (Do not use concomitantly; consult your doctor). Products include:

Minipress Capsules 1937
Minizide Capsules 1938

Prochlorperazine (May increase the drowsiness effect). Products include:

Compazine 2470

Promethazine Hydrochloride (May increase the drowsiness effect). Products include:

Mepergan Injection 2753
Phenergan with Codeine 2777
Phenergan with Dextromethorphan 2778
Phenergan Injection 2773
Phenergan Suppositories 2775
Phenergan Syrup 2774
Phenergan Tablets 2775
Phenergan VC 2779
Phenergan VC with Codeine 2781

Propofol (May increase the drowsiness effect). Products include:

Diprivan Injection 2833

Propranolol Hydrochloride (Do not use concomitantly; consult your doctor). Products include:

Inderal 2728
Inderal LA Long Acting Capsules 2730
Inderide Tablets 2732
Inderide LA Long Acting Capsules .. 2734

Protriptyline Hydrochloride (Do not use concomitantly; consult your doctor). Products include:

Vivactil Tablets 1774

Quazepam (May increase the drowsiness effect). Products include:

Doral Tablets 2664

Quinapril Hydrochloride (Do not use concomitantly; consult your doctor). Products include:

Accupril Tablets 1893

Ramipril (Do not use concomitantly; consult your doctor). Products include:

Altace Capsules 1232

Rauwolfia Serpentina (Do not use concomitantly; consult your doctor).

No products indexed under this heading.

Rescinnamine (Do not use concomitantly; consult your doctor).

No products indexed under this heading.

Reserpine (Do not use concomitantly; consult your doctor). Products include:

Diupres Tablets 1650
Hydropres Tablets 1675
Ser-Ap-Es Tablets 849

Secobarbital Sodium (May increase the drowsiness effect). Products include:

Seconal Sodium Pulvules 1474

Sertraline Hydrochloride (Do not use concomitantly; consult your doctor). Products include:

Zoloft Tablets 2217

Sodium Nitroprusside (Do not use concomitantly; consult your doctor).

No products indexed under this heading.

Sotalol Hydrochloride (Do not use concomitantly; consult your doctor). Products include:

Betapace Tablets 641

Spirapril Hydrochloride (Do not use concomitantly; consult your doctor).

No products indexed under this heading.

Temazepam (May increase the drowsiness effect). Products include:

Restoril Capsules 2284

Terazosin Hydrochloride (Do not use concomitantly; consult your doctor). Products include:

Hytrin Capsules 430

Thioridazine Hydrochloride (May increase the drowsiness effect). Products include:

Mellaril 2269

Thiothixene (May increase the drowsiness effect). Products include:

Navane Capsules and Concentrate 2201
Navane Intramuscular 2202

Timolol Maleate (Do not use concomitantly; consult your doctor). Products include:

Blocadren Tablets 1614
Timolide Tablets 1748
Timoptic in Ocudose 1753
Timoptic Sterile Ophthalmic Solution 1751
Timoptic-XE 1755

Torsemide (Do not use concomitantly; consult your doctor). Products include:

Demadex Tablets and Injection 686

Tranylcypromine Sulfate (Do not use concomitantly; consult your doctor). Products include:

Parnate Tablets 2503

Trazodone Hydrochloride (Do not use concomitantly; consult your doctor). Products include:

Desyrel and Desyrel Dividose 503

Triazolam (May increase the drowsiness effect). Products include:

Halcion Tablets 2611

Trifluoperazine Hydrochloride (May increase the drowsiness effect). Products include:

Stelazine 2514

Trimethaphan Camsylate (Do not use concomitantly; consult your doctor). Products include:

Arfonad Ampuls 2080

Trimipramine Maleate (Do not use concomitantly; consult your doctor). Products include:

Surmontil Capsules 2811

Venlafaxine Hydrochloride (Do not use concomitantly; consult your doctor). Products include:

Effexor 2719

Verapamil Hydrochloride (Do not use concomitantly; consult your doctor). Products include:

Calan SR Caplets 2422
Calan Tablets 2419
Isoptin Injectable 1344
Isoptin Oral Tablets 1346
Isoptin SR Tablets 1348
Verelan Capsules 1410
Verelan Capsules 2824

Zolpidem Tartrate (May increase the drowsiness effect). Products include:

Ambien Tablets 2416

Food Interactions

Alcohol (May increase the drowsiness effect; avoid concurrent use).

VICKS DAYQUIL LIQUICAPS MULTI-SYMPTOM COLD/FLU RELIEF

(Acetaminophen, Dextromethorphan Hydrobromide, Pseudoephedrine Hydrochloride, Guaifenesin) .... ◾ 761

See Vicks DayQuil Multi-Symptom Cold/Flu Relief–(Liquid)

VICKS DAYQUIL MULTI-SYMPTOM COLD/FLU RELIEF–(LIQUID)

(Acetaminophen, Dextromethorphan Hydrobromide, Pseudoephedrine Hydrochloride, Guaifenesin) .... ◾ 761

May interact with monoamine oxidase inhibitors. Compounds in this category include:

Furazolidone (Concurrent and/or sequential use is not recommended). Products include:

Furoxone 2046

Isocarboxazid (Concurrent and/or sequential use is not recommended).

No products indexed under this heading.

Phenelzine Sulfate (Concurrent and/or sequential use is not recommended). Products include:

Nardil 1920

Selegiline Hydrochloride (Concurrent and/or sequential use is not recommended). Products include:

Eldepryl Tablets 2550

Tranylcypromine Sulfate (Concurrent and/or sequential use is not recommended). Products include:

Parnate Tablets 2503

VICKS DAYQUIL SINUS PRESSURE & CONGESTION RELIEF

(Guaifenesin, Phenylpropanolamine Hydrochloride) .... ◾ 761

May interact with monoamine oxidase inhibitors. Compounds in this category include:

Furazolidone (Concurrent and/or sequential use is not recommended). Products include:

Furoxone 2046

Isocarboxazid (Concurrent and/or sequential use is not recommended).

No products indexed under this heading.

Phenelzine Sulfate (Concurrent and/or sequential use is not recommended). Products include:

Nardil 1920

Selegiline Hydrochloride (Concurrent and/or sequential use is not recommended). Products include:

Eldepryl Tablets 2550

Tranylcypromine Sulfate (Concurrent and/or sequential use is not recommended). Products include:

Parnate Tablets 2503

IMPORTANT NOTE: Always consult each drug listing in the patient's regimen for possible interactions.

Vicks DayQuil Sinus | Interactions Index | 1148

VICKS DAYQUIL SINUS PRESSURE & PAIN RELIEF WITH IBUPROFEN
(Ibuprofen, Pseudoephedrine Hydrochloride) ▣ 762
May interact with antidepressant drugs and antihypertensives. Compounds in these categories include:

Acebutolol Hydrochloride (Concurrent use is not recommended). Products include:
Sectral Capsules 2807

Amitriptyline Hydrochloride (Concurrent use is not recommended). Products include:
Elavil 2838
Endep Tablets 2174
Etrafon 2355
Limbitrol 2180
Triavil Tablets 1757

Amlodipine Besylate (Concurrent use is not recommended). Products include:
Lotrel Capsules 840
Norvasc Tablets 1940

Amoxapine (Concurrent use is not recommended). Products include:
Asendin Tablets 1369

Atenolol (Concurrent use is not recommended). Products include:
Tenoretic Tablets 2845
Tenormin Tablets and I.V. Injection 2847

Benazepril Hydrochloride (Concurrent use is not recommended). Products include:
Lotensin Tablets 834
Lotensin HCT 837
Lotrel Capsules 840

Bendroflumethiazide (Concurrent use is not recommended).
No products indexed under this heading.

Betaxolol Hydrochloride (Concurrent use is not recommended). Products include:
Betoptic Ophthalmic Solution 469
Betoptic S Ophthalmic Suspension 471
Kerlone Tablets 2436

Bisoprolol Fumarate (Concurrent use is not recommended). Products include:
Zebeta Tablets 1413
Ziac 1415

Bupropion Hydrochloride (Concurrent use is not recommended). Products include:
Wellbutrin Tablets 1204

Captopril (Concurrent use is not recommended). Products include:
Capoten 739
Capozide 742

Carteolol Hydrochloride (Concurrent use is not recommended). Products include:
Cartrol Tablets 410
Ocupress Ophthalmic Solution, 1% Sterile ◉ 309

Chlorothiazide (Concurrent use is not recommended). Products include:
Aldoclor Tablets 1598
Diupres Tablets 1650
Diuril Oral 1653

Chlorothiazide Sodium (Concurrent use is not recommended). Products include:
Diuril Sodium Intravenous 1652

Chlorthalidone (Concurrent use is not recommended). Products include:
Combipres Tablets 677
Tenoretic Tablets 2845
Thalitone 1245

Clonidine (Concurrent use is not recommended). Products include:
Catapres-TTS 675

Clonidine Hydrochloride (Concurrent use is not recommended). Products include:
Catapres Tablets 674
Combipres Tablets 677

Deserpidine (Concurrent use is not recommended).
No products indexed under this heading.

Desipramine Hydrochloride (Concurrent use is not recommended). Products include:
Norpramin Tablets 1526

Diazoxide (Concurrent use is not recommended). Products include:
Hyperstat I.V. Injection 2363
Proglycem 580

Diltiazem Hydrochloride (Concurrent use is not recommended). Products include:
Cardizem CD Capsules 1506
Cardizem SR Capsules 1510
Cardizem Injectable 1508
Cardizem Tablets 1512
Dilacor XR Extended-release Capsules 2018

Doxazosin Mesylate (Concurrent use is not recommended). Products include:
Cardura Tablets 2186

Doxepin Hydrochloride (Concurrent use is not recommended). Products include:
Sinequan 2205
Zonalon Cream 1055

Enalapril Maleate (Concurrent use is not recommended). Products include:
Vaseretic Tablets 1765
Vasotec Tablets 1771

Enalaprilat (Concurrent use is not recommended). Products include:
Vasotec I.V. 1768

Esmolol Hydrochloride (Concurrent use is not recommended). Products include:
Brevibloc Injection 1808

Felodipine (Concurrent use is not recommended). Products include:
Plendil Extended-Release Tablets 527

Fluoxetine Hydrochloride (Concurrent use is not recommended). Products include:
Prozac Pulvules & Liquid, Oral Solution 919

Fosinopril Sodium (Concurrent use is not recommended). Products include:
Monopril Tablets 757

Furosemide (Concurrent use is not recommended). Products include:
Lasix Injection, Oral Solution and Tablets 1240

Guanabenz Acetate (Concurrent use is not recommended).
No products indexed under this heading.

Guanethidine Monosulfate (Concurrent use is not recommended). Products include:
Esimil Tablets 822
Ismelin Tablets 827

Hydralazine Hydrochloride (Concurrent use is not recommended). Products include:
Apresazide Capsules 808
Apresoline Hydrochloride Tablets 809
Ser-Ap-Es Tablets 849

Hydrochlorothiazide (Concurrent use is not recommended). Products include:
Aldactazide 2413
Aldoril Tablets 1604
Apresazide Capsules 808
Capozide 742
Dyazide 2479
Esidrix Tablets 821
Esimil Tablets 822
HydroDIURIL Tablets 1674
Hydropres Tablets 1675
Hyzaar Tablets 1677
Inderide Tablets 2732
Inderide LA Long Acting Capsules 2734
Lopressor HCT Tablets 832
Lotensin HCT 837
Maxzide 1380
Moduretic Tablets 1705
Oretic Tablets 443
Prinzide Tablets 1737
Ser-Ap-Es Tablets 849
Timolide Tablets 1748
Vaseretic Tablets 1765
Zestoretic 2850
Ziac 1415

Hydroflumethiazide (Concurrent use is not recommended). Products include:
Diucardin Tablets 2718

Imipramine Hydrochloride (Concurrent use is not recommended). Products include:
Tofranil Ampuls 854
Tofranil Tablets 856

Imipramine Pamoate (Concurrent use is not recommended). Products include:
Tofranil-PM Capsules 857

Indapamide (Concurrent use is not recommended). Products include:
Lozol Tablets 2022

Isocarboxazid (Concurrent use is not recommended).
No products indexed under this heading.

Isradipine (Concurrent use is not recommended). Products include:
DynaCirc Capsules 2256

Labetalol Hydrochloride (Concurrent use is not recommended). Products include:
Normodyne Injection 2377
Normodyne Tablets 2379
Trandate 1185

Levobunolol Hydrochloride (Concurrent use is not recommended). Products include:
Betagan ◉ 233

Lisinopril (Concurrent use is not recommended). Products include:
Prinivil Tablets 1733
Prinzide Tablets 1737
Zestoretic 2850
Zestril Tablets 2854

Losartan Potassium (Concurrent use is not recommended). Products include:
Cozaar Tablets 1628
Hyzaar Tablets 1677

Maprotiline Hydrochloride (Concurrent use is not recommended). Products include:
Ludiomil Tablets 843

Mecamylamine Hydrochloride (Concurrent use is not recommended). Products include:
Inversine Tablets 1686

Methyclothiazide (Concurrent use is not recommended). Products include:
Enduron Tablets 420

Methyldopa (Concurrent use is not recommended). Products include:
Aldoclor Tablets 1598
Aldomet Oral 1600
Aldoril Tablets 1604

Methyldopate Hydrochloride (Concurrent use is not recommended). Products include:
Aldomet Ester HCl Injection 1602

Metipranolol Hydrochloride (Concurrent use is not recommended). Products include:
OptiPranolol (Metipranolol 0.3%) Sterile Ophthalmic Solution ◉ 258

Metolazone (Concurrent use is not recommended). Products include:
Mykrox Tablets 993
Zaroxolyn Tablets 1000

Metoprolol Succinate (Concurrent use is not recommended). Products include:
Toprol-XL Tablets 565

Metoprolol Tartrate (Concurrent use is not recommended). Products include:
Lopressor Ampuls 830
Lopressor HCT Tablets 832
Lopressor Tablets 830

Metyrosine (Concurrent use is not recommended). Products include:
Demser Capsules 1649

Minoxidil (Concurrent use is not recommended). Products include:
Loniten Tablets 2618
Rogaine Topical Solution 2637

Moexipril Hydrochloride (Concurrent use is not recommended). Products include:
Univasc Tablets 2410

Nadolol (Concurrent use is not recommended).
No products indexed under this heading.

Nefazodone Hydrochloride (Concurrent use is not recommended). Products include:
Serzone Tablets 771

Nicardipine Hydrochloride (Concurrent use is not recommended). Products include:
Cardene Capsules 2095
Cardene I.V. 2709
Cardene SR Capsules 2097

Nifedipine (Concurrent use is not recommended). Products include:
Adalat Capsules (10 mg and 20 mg) 587
Adalat CC 589
Procardia Capsules 1971
Procardia XL Extended Release Tablets 1972

Nisoldipine (Concurrent use is not recommended).
No products indexed under this heading.

Nitroglycerin (Concurrent use is not recommended). Products include:
Deponit NTG Transdermal Delivery System 2397
Nitro-Bid IV 1523
Nitro-Bid Ointment 1524
Nitrodisc 2047
Nitro-Dur (nitroglycerin) Transdermal Infusion System 1326
Nitrolingual Spray 2027
Nitrostat Tablets 1925
Transderm-Nitro Transdermal Therapeutic System 859

Nortriptyline Hydrochloride (Concurrent use is not recommended). Products include:
Pamelor 2280

Paroxetine Hydrochloride (Concurrent use is not recommended). Products include:
Paxil Tablets 2505

Penbutolol Sulfate (Concurrent use is not recommended). Products include:
Levatol 2403

Phenelzine Sulfate (Concurrent use is not recommended). Products include:
Nardil 1920

Phenoxybenzamine Hydrochloride (Concurrent use is not recommended). Products include:
Dibenzyline Capsules 2476

Phentolamine Mesylate (Concurrent use is not recommended). Products include:
Regitine 846

Pindolol (Concurrent use is not recommended). Products include:
Visken Tablets 2299

(▣ Described in PDR For Nonprescription Drugs) (◉ Described in PDR For Ophthalmology)

1149 Interactions Index Vicks NyQuil LiquiCaps

Polythiazide (Concurrent use is not recommended). Products include:
Minizide Capsules ... 1938
Prazosin Hydrochloride (Concurrent use is not recommended). Products include:
Minipress Capsules ... 1937
Minizide Capsules ... 1938
Propranolol Hydrochloride (Concurrent use is not recommended). Products include:
Inderal ... 2728
Inderal LA Long Acting Capsules ... 2730
Inderide Tablets ... 2732
Inderide LA Long Acting Capsules ... 2734
Protriptyline Hydrochloride (Concurrent use is not recommended). Products include:
Vivactil Tablets ... 1774
Quinapril Hydrochloride (Concurrent use is not recommended). Products include:
Accupril Tablets ... 1893
Ramipril (Concurrent use is not recommended). Products include:
Altace Capsules ... 1232
Rauwolfia Serpentina (Concurrent use is not recommended).
No products indexed under this heading.
Rescinnamine (Concurrent use is not recommended).
No products indexed under this heading.
Reserpine (Concurrent use is not recommended). Products include:
Diupres Tablets ... 1650
Hydropres Tablets ... 1675
Ser-Ap-Es Tablets ... 849
Sertraline Hydrochloride (Concurrent use is not recommended). Products include:
Zoloft Tablets ... 2217
Sodium Nitroprusside (Concurrent use is not recommended).
No products indexed under this heading.
Sotalol Hydrochloride (Concurrent use is not recommended). Products include:
Betapace Tablets ... 641
Spirapril Hydrochloride (Concurrent use is not recommended).
No products indexed under this heading.
Terazosin Hydrochloride (Concurrent use is not recommended). Products include:
Hytrin Capsules ... 430
Timolol Maleate (Concurrent use is not recommended). Products include:
Blocadren Tablets ... 1614
Timolide Tablets ... 1748
Timoptic in Ocudose ... 1753
Timoptic Sterile Ophthalmic Solution ... 1751
Timoptic-XE ... 1755
Torsemide (Concurrent use is not recommended). Products include:
Demadex Tablets and Injection ... 686
Tranylcypromine Sulfate (Concurrent use is not recommended). Products include:
Parnate Tablets ... 2503
Trazodone Hydrochloride (Concurrent use is not recommended). Products include:
Desyrel and Desyrel Dividose ... 503
Trimethaphan Camsylate (Concurrent use is not recommended). Products include:
Arfonad Ampuls ... 2080
Trimipramine Maleate (Concurrent use is not recommended). Products include:
Surmontil Capsules ... 2811
Venlafaxine Hydrochloride (Concurrent use is not recommended). Products include:
Effexor ... 2719
Verapamil Hydrochloride (Concurrent use is not recommended). Products include:
Calan SR Caplets ... 2422
Calan Tablets ... 2419
Isoptin Injectable ... 1344
Isoptin Oral Tablets ... 1346
Isoptin SR Tablets ... 1348
Verelan Capsules ... 1410
Verelan Capsules ... 2824

VICKS NYQUIL HOT THERAPY
(Acetaminophen, Pseudoephedrine Hydrochloride, Dextromethorphan Hydrobromide, Doxylamine Succinate) ... 762
May interact with hypnotics and sedatives, tranquilizers, monoamine oxidase inhibitors, and certain other agents. Compounds in these categories include:
Alprazolam (May increase the drowsiness effect). Products include:
Xanax Tablets ... 2649
Buspirone Hydrochloride (May increase the drowsiness effect). Products include:
BuSpar ... 737
Chlordiazepoxide (May increase the drowsiness effect). Products include:
Libritabs Tablets ... 2177
Limbitrol ... 2180
Chlordiazepoxide Hydrochloride (May increase the drowsiness effect). Products include:
Librax Capsules ... 2176
Librium Capsules ... 2178
Librium Injectable ... 2179
Chlorpromazine (May increase the drowsiness effect). Products include:
Thorazine Suppositories ... 2523
Chlorpromazine Hydrochloride (May increase the drowsiness effect). Products include:
Thorazine ... 2523
Chlorprothixene (May increase the drowsiness effect).
No products indexed under this heading.
Chlorprothixene Hydrochloride (May increase the drowsiness effect).
No products indexed under this heading.
Clorazepate Dipotassium (May increase the drowsiness effect). Products include:
Tranxene ... 451
Diazepam (May increase the drowsiness effect). Products include:
Dizac ... 1809
Valium Injectable ... 2182
Valium Tablets ... 2183
Valrelease Capsules ... 2169
Droperidol (May increase the drowsiness effect). Products include:
Inapsine Injection ... 1296
Estazolam (May increase the drowsiness effect). Products include:
ProSom Tablets ... 449
Ethchlorvynol (May increase the drowsiness effect). Products include:
Placidyl Capsules ... 448
Ethinamate (May increase the drowsiness effect).
No products indexed under this heading.
Fluphenazine Decanoate (May increase the drowsiness effect). Products include:
Prolixin Decanoate ... 509
Fluphenazine Enanthate (May increase the drowsiness effect). Products include:
Prolixin Enanthate ... 509
Fluphenazine Hydrochloride (May increase the drowsiness effect). Products include:
Prolixin ... 509
Flurazepam Hydrochloride (May increase the drowsiness effect). Products include:
Dalmane Capsules ... 2173
Furazolidone (Concurrent and/or sequential use is not recommended). Products include:
Furoxone ... 2046
Glutethimide (May increase the drowsiness effect).
No products indexed under this heading.
Haloperidol (May increase the drowsiness effect). Products include:
Haldol Injection, Tablets and Concentrate ... 1575
Haloperidol Decanoate (May increase the drowsiness effect). Products include:
Haldol Decanoate ... 1577
Hydroxyzine Hydrochloride (May increase the drowsiness effect). Products include:
Atarax Tablets & Syrup ... 2185
Marax Tablets & DF Syrup ... 2200
Vistaril Intramuscular Solution ... 2216
Isocarboxazid (Concurrent and/or sequential use is not recommended).
No products indexed under this heading.
Lorazepam (May increase the drowsiness effect). Products include:
Ativan Injection ... 2698
Ativan Tablets ... 2700
Loxapine Hydrochloride (May increase the drowsiness effect). Products include:
Loxitane ... 1378
Loxapine Succinate (May increase the drowsiness effect). Products include:
Loxitane Capsules ... 1378
Meprobamate (May increase the drowsiness effect). Products include:
Miltown Tablets ... 2672
PMB 200 and PMB 400 ... 2783
Mesoridazine Besylate (May increase the drowsiness effect). Products include:
Serentil ... 684
Midazolam Hydrochloride (May increase the drowsiness effect). Products include:
Versed Injection ... 2170
Molindone Hydrochloride (May increase the drowsiness effect). Products include:
Moban Tablets and Concentrate ... 1048
Oxazepam (May increase the drowsiness effect). Products include:
Serax Capsules ... 2810
Serax Tablets ... 2810
Perphenazine (May increase the drowsiness effect). Products include:
Etrafon ... 2355
Triavil Tablets ... 1757
Trilafon ... 2389
Phenelzine Sulfate (Concurrent and/or sequential use is not recommended). Products include:
Nardil ... 1920
Prazepam (May increase the drowsiness effect).
No products indexed under this heading.
Prochlorperazine (May increase the drowsiness effect). Products include:
Compazine ... 2470
Promethazine Hydrochloride (May increase the drowsiness effect). Products include:
Mepergan Injection ... 2753
Phenergan with Codeine ... 2777
Phenergan with Dextromethorphan ... 2778
Phenergan Injection ... 2773
Phenergan Suppositories ... 2775
Phenergan Syrup ... 2774
Phenergan Tablets ... 2775
Phenergan VC ... 2779
Phenergan VC with Codeine ... 2781
Propofol (May increase the drowsiness effect). Products include:
Diprivan Injection ... 2833
Quazepam (May increase the drowsiness effect). Products include:
Doral Tablets ... 2664
Secobarbital Sodium (May increase the drowsiness effect). Products include:
Seconal Sodium Pulvules ... 1474
Selegiline Hydrochloride (Concurrent and/or sequential use is not recommended). Products include:
Eldepryl Tablets ... 2550
Temazepam (May increase the drowsiness effect). Products include:
Restoril Capsules ... 2284
Thioridazine Hydrochloride (May increase the drowsiness effect). Products include:
Mellaril ... 2269
Thiothixene (May increase the drowsiness effect). Products include:
Navane Capsules and Concentrate ... 2201
Navane Intramuscular ... 2202
Tranylcypromine Sulfate (Concurrent and/or sequential use is not recommended). Products include:
Parnate Tablets ... 2503
Triazolam (May increase the drowsiness effect). Products include:
Halcion Tablets ... 2611
Trifluoperazine Hydrochloride (May increase the drowsiness effect). Products include:
Stelazine ... 2514
Zolpidem Tartrate (May increase the drowsiness effect). Products include:
Ambien Tablets ... 2416

Food Interactions
Alcohol (May increase drowsiness effect).

VICKS NYQUIL LIQUICAPS MULTI-SYMPTOM COLD/FLU RELIEF
(Acetaminophen, Pseudoephedrine Hydrochloride, Dextromethorphan Hydrobromide, Doxylamine Succinate) ... 763
May interact with hypnotics and sedatives, tranquilizers, monoamine oxidase inhibitors, and certain other agents. Compounds in these categories include:
Alprazolam (May increase drowsiness effect). Products include:
Xanax Tablets ... 2649
Buspirone Hydrochloride (May increase drowsiness effect). Products include:
BuSpar ... 737
Chlordiazepoxide (May increase drowsiness effect). Products include:
Libritabs Tablets ... 2177
Limbitrol ... 2180
Chlordiazepoxide Hydrochloride (May increase drowsiness effect). Products include:
Librax Capsules ... 2176
Librium Capsules ... 2178
Librium Injectable ... 2179
Chlorpromazine (May increase drowsiness effect). Products include:
Thorazine Suppositories ... 2523

IMPORTANT NOTE: Always consult each drug listing in the patient's regimen for possible interactions.

Vicks NyQuil LiquiCaps Interactions Index 1150

Chlorpromazine Hydrochloride (May increase drowsiness effect). Products include:
Thorazine ... 2523
Chlorprothixene (May increase drowsiness effect).
No products indexed under this heading.
Chlorprothixene Hydrochloride (May increase drowsiness effect).
No products indexed under this heading.
Clorazepate Dipotassium (May increase drowsiness effect). Products include:
Tranxene ... 451
Diazepam (May increase drowsiness effect). Products include:
Dizac ... 1809
Valium Injectable ... 2182
Valium Tablets ... 2183
Valrelease Capsules ... 2169
Droperidol (May increase drowsiness effect). Products include:
Inapsine Injection ... 1296
Estazolam (May increase drowsiness effect). Products include:
ProSom Tablets ... 449
Ethchlorvynol (May increase drowsiness effect). Products include:
Placidyl Capsules ... 448
Ethinamate (May increase drowsiness effect).
No products indexed under this heading.
Fluphenazine Decanoate (May increase drowsiness effect). Products include:
Prolixin Decanoate ... 509
Fluphenazine Enanthate (May increase drowsiness effect). Products include:
Prolixin Enanthate ... 509
Fluphenazine Hydrochloride (May increase drowsiness effect). Products include:
Prolixin ... 509
Flurazepam Hydrochloride (May increase drowsiness effect). Products include:
Dalmane Capsules ... 2173
Furazolidone (Concurrent and/or sequential use is not recommended). Products include:
Furoxone ... 2046
Glutethimide (May increase drowsiness effect).
No products indexed under this heading.
Haloperidol (May increase drowsiness effect). Products include:
Haldol Injection, Tablets and Concentrate ... 1575
Haloperidol Decanoate (May increase drowsiness effect). Products include:
Haldol Decanoate ... 1577
Hydroxyzine Hydrochloride (May increase drowsiness effect). Products include:
Atarax Tablets & Syrup ... 2185
Marax Tablets & DF Syrup ... 2200
Vistaril Intramuscular Solution ... 2216
Isocarboxazid (Concurrent and/or sequential use is not recommended).
No products indexed under this heading.
Lorazepam (May increase drowsiness effect). Products include:
Ativan Injection ... 2698
Ativan Tablets ... 2700
Loxapine Hydrochloride (May increase drowsiness effect). Products include:
Loxitane ... 1378
Loxapine Succinate (May increase drowsiness effect). Products include:
Loxitane Capsules ... 1378
Meprobamate (May increase drowsiness effect). Products include:
Miltown Tablets ... 2672
PMB 200 and PMB 400 ... 2783
Mesoridazine Besylate (May increase drowsiness effect). Products include:
Serentil ... 684
Midazolam Hydrochloride (May increase drowsiness effect). Products include:
Versed Injection ... 2170
Molindone Hydrochloride (May increase drowsiness effect). Products include:
Moban Tablets and Concentrate ... 1048
Oxazepam (May increase drowsiness effect). Products include:
Serax Capsules ... 2810
Serax Tablets ... 2810
Perphenazine (May increase drowsiness effect). Products include:
Etrafon ... 2355
Triavil Tablets ... 1757
Trilafon ... 2389
Phenelzine Sulfate (Concurrent and/or sequential use is not recommended). Products include:
Nardil ... 1920
Prazepam (May increase drowsiness effect).
No products indexed under this heading.
Prochlorperazine (May increase drowsiness effect). Products include:
Compazine ... 2470
Promethazine Hydrochloride (May increase drowsiness effect). Products include:
Mepergan Injection ... 2753
Phenergan with Codeine ... 2777
Phenergan with Dextromethorphan 2778
Phenergan Injection ... 2773
Phenergan Suppositories ... 2775
Phenergan Syrup ... 2774
Phenergan Tablets ... 2775
Phenergan VC ... 2779
Phenergan VC with Codeine ... 2781
Propofol (May increase drowsiness effect). Products include:
Diprivan Injection ... 2833
Quazepam (May increase drowsiness effect). Products include:
Doral Tablets ... 2664
Secobarbital Sodium (May increase drowsiness effect). Products include:
Seconal Sodium Pulvules ... 1474
Selegiline Hydrochloride (Concurrent and/or sequential use is not recommended). Products include:
Eldepryl Tablets ... 2550
Temazepam (May increase drowsiness effect). Products include:
Restoril Capsules ... 2284
Thioridazine Hydrochloride (May increase drowsiness effect). Products include:
Mellaril ... 2269
Thiothixene (May increase drowsiness effect). Products include:
Navane Capsules and Concentrate 2201
Navane Intramuscular ... 2202
Tranylcypromine Sulfate (Concurrent and/or sequential use is not recommended). Products include:
Parnate Tablets ... 2503
Triazolam (May increase drowsiness effect). Products include:
Halcion Tablets ... 2611
Trifluoperazine Hydrochloride (May increase drowsiness effect). Products include:
Stelazine ... 2514
Zolpidem Tartrate (May increase drowsiness effect). Products include:
Ambien Tablets ... 2416

Food Interactions

Alcohol (May increase drowsiness effect).

VICKS NYQUIL MULTI-SYMPTOM COLD/FLU RELIEF - (ORIGINAL & CHERRY FLAVOR)
(Acetaminophen, Dextromethorphan Hydrobromide, Doxylamine Succinate, Pseudoephedrine Hydrochloride) ... ▣ 763
See **Vicks NyQuil LiquiCaps Multi-Symptom Cold/Flu Relief**

VICKS SINEX 12-HOUR NASAL DECONGESTANT SPRAY AND ULTRA FINE MIST
(Oxymetazoline Hydrochloride) ... ▣ 765
None cited in PDR database.

VICKS SINEX NASAL SPRAY AND ULTRA FINE MIST
(Phenylephrine Hydrochloride) ... ▣ 765
None cited in PDR database.

VICKS VAPOR INHALER
(Desoxyephedrine-Levo) ... ▣ 765
None cited in PDR database.

VICKS VAPORUB CREAM
(Menthol, Camphor, Eucalyptus, Oil of) ... ▣ 766
None cited in PDR database.

VICKS VAPORUB OINTMENT
(Menthol, Camphor, Eucalyptus, Oil of) ... ▣ 766
None cited in PDR database.

VICKS VAPOSTEAM
(Camphor, Eucalyptus, Oil of, Menthol) ... ▣ 766
None cited in PDR database.

VICODIN TABLETS
(Hydrocodone Bitartrate, Acetaminophen) ... 1356
May interact with tricyclic antidepressants, monoamine oxidase inhibitors, anticholinergics, antipsychotic agents, tranquilizers, central nervous system depressants, narcotic analgesics, and certain other agents. Compounds in these categories include:

Alfentanil Hydrochloride (May exhibit an additive CNS depression; the dose of one or both agents should be reduced). Products include:
Alfenta Injection ... 1286
Alprazolam (May exhibit an additive CNS depression; the dose of one or both agents should be reduced). Products include:
Xanax Tablets ... 2649
Amitriptyline Hydrochloride (Co-administration may increase the effect of either drug). Products include:
Elavil ... 2838
Endep Tablets ... 2174
Etrafon ... 2355
Limbitrol ... 2180
Triavil Tablets ... 1757
Amoxapine (Co-administration may increase the effect of either drug). Products include:
Asendin Tablets ... 1369
Aprobarbital (May exhibit an additive CNS depression; the dose of one or both agents should be reduced).
No products indexed under this heading.
Atropine Sulfate (Potential for paralytic ileus). Products include:
Arco-Lase Plus Tablets ... 512
Atrohist Plus Tablets ... 454
Atropine Sulfate Sterile Ophthalmic Solution ... ⊙ 233
Donnatal ... 2060
Donnatal Extentabs ... 2061
Donnatal Tablets ... 2060
Lomotil ... 2439
Motofen Tablets ... 784
Urised Tablets ... 1964
Belladonna Alkaloids (Potential for paralytic ileus). Products include:
Bellergal-S Tablets ... 2250
Hyland's Bed Wetting Tablets ... ▣ 828
Hyland's EnurAid Tablets ... ▣ 829
Hyland's Teething Tablets ... ▣ 830
Benztropine Mesylate (Potential for paralytic ileus). Products include:
Cogentin ... 1621
Biperiden Hydrochloride (Potential for paralytic ileus). Products include:
Akineton ... 1333
Buprenorphine (May exhibit an additive CNS depression; the dose of one or both agents should be reduced). Products include:
Buprenex Injectable ... 2006
Buspirone Hydrochloride (May exhibit an additive CNS depression; the dose of one or both agents should be reduced). Products include:
BuSpar ... 737
Butabarbital (May exhibit an additive CNS depression; the dose of one or both agents should be reduced).
No products indexed under this heading.
Butalbital (May exhibit an additive CNS depression; the dose of one or both agents should be reduced). Products include:
Esgic-plus Tablets ... 1013
Fioricet Tablets ... 2258
Fioricet with Codeine Capsules ... 2260
Fiorinal Capsules ... 2261
Fiorinal with Codeine Capsules ... 2262
Fiorinal Tablets ... 2261
Phrenilin ... 785
Sedapap Tablets 50 mg/650 mg .. 1543
Chlordiazepoxide (May exhibit an additive CNS depression; the dose of one or both agents should be reduced). Products include:
Libritabs Tablets ... 2177
Limbitrol ... 2180
Chlordiazepoxide Hydrochloride (May exhibit an additive CNS depression; the dose of one or both agents should be reduced). Products include:
Librax Capsules ... 2176
Librium Capsules ... 2178
Librium Injectable ... 2179
Chlorpromazine (May exhibit an additive CNS depression; the dose of one or both agents should be reduced). Products include:
Thorazine Suppositories ... 2523
Chlorpromazine Hydrochloride (May exhibit an additive CNS depression; the dose of one or both agents should be reduced). Products include:
Thorazine ... 2523
Chlorprothixene (May exhibit an additive CNS depression; the dose of one or both agents should be reduced).
No products indexed under this heading.

(▣ Described in PDR For Nonprescription Drugs) (⊙ Described in PDR For Ophthalmology)

1151 Interactions Index Vicodin

Chlorprothixene Hydrochloride (May exhibit an additive CNS depression; the dose of one or both agents should be reduced).
No products indexed under this heading.

Clidinium Bromide (Potential for paralytic ileus). Products include:
Librax Capsules ... 2176
Quarzan Capsules ... 2181

Clomipramine Hydrochloride (Co-administration may increase the effect of either drug). Products include:
Anafranil Capsules ... 803

Clorazepate Dipotassium (May exhibit an additive CNS depression; the dose of one or both agents should be reduced). Products include:
Tranxene ... 451

Clozapine (May exhibit an additive CNS depression; the dose of one or both agents should be reduced). Products include:
Clozaril Tablets ... 2252

Codeine Phosphate (May exhibit an additive CNS depression; the dose of one or both agents should be reduced). Products include:
Actifed with Codeine Cough Syrup.. 1067
Brontex ... 1981
Deconsal C Expectorant Syrup ... 456
Deconsal Pediatric Syrup ... 457
Dimetane-DC Cough Syrup ... 2059
Empirin with Codeine Tablets ... 1093
Fioricet with Codeine Capsules ... 2260
Fiorinal with Codeine Capsules ... 2262
Isoclor Expectorant ... 990
Novahistine DH ... 2462
Novahistine Expectorant ... 2463
Nucofed ... 2051
Phenergan with Codeine ... 2777
Phenergan VC with Codeine ... 2781
Robitussin A-C Syrup ... 2073
Robitussin-DAC Syrup ... 2074
Ryna ... 841
Soma Compound w/Codeine Tablets ... 2676
Tussi-Organidin NR Liquid and S NR Liquid ... 2677
Tylenol with Codeine ... 1583

Desflurane (May exhibit an additive CNS depression; the dose of one or both agents should be reduced). Products include:
Suprane ... 1813

Desipramine Hydrochloride (Co-administration may increase the effect of either drug). Products include:
Norpramin Tablets ... 1526

Dezocine (May exhibit an additive CNS depression; the dose of one or both agents should be reduced). Products include:
Dalgan Injection ... 538

Diazepam (May exhibit an additive CNS depression; the dose of one or both agents should be reduced). Products include:
Dizac ... 1809
Valium Injectable ... 2182
Valium Tablets ... 2183
Valrelease Capsules ... 2169

Dicyclomine Hydrochloride (Potential for paralytic ileus). Products include:
Bentyl ... 1501

Doxepin Hydrochloride (Co-administration may increase the effect of either drug). Products include:
Sinequan ... 2205
Zonalon Cream ... 1055

Droperidol (May exhibit an additive CNS depression; the dose of one or both agents should be reduced). Products include:
Inapsine Injection ... 1296

Enflurane (May exhibit an additive CNS depression; the dose of one or both agents should be reduced).
No products indexed under this heading.

Estazolam (May exhibit an additive CNS depression; the dose of one or both agents should be reduced). Products include:
ProSom Tablets ... 449

Ethchlorvynol (May exhibit an additive CNS depression; the dose of one or both agents should be reduced). Products include:
Placidyl Capsules ... 448

Ethinamate (May exhibit an additive CNS depression; the dose of one or both agents should be reduced).
No products indexed under this heading.

Fentanyl (May exhibit an additive CNS depression; the dose of one or both agents should be reduced). Products include:
Duragesic Transdermal System ... 1288

Fentanyl Citrate (May exhibit an additive CNS depression; the dose of one or both agents should be reduced). Products include:
Sublimaze Injection ... 1307

Fluphenazine Decanoate (May exhibit an additive CNS depression; the dose of one or both agents should be reduced). Products include:
Prolixin Decanoate ... 509

Fluphenazine Enanthate (May exhibit an additive CNS depression; the dose of one or both agents should be reduced). Products include:
Prolixin Enanthate ... 509

Fluphenazine Hydrochloride (May exhibit an additive CNS depression; the dose of one or both agents should be reduced). Products include:
Prolixin ... 509

Flurazepam Hydrochloride (May exhibit an additive CNS depression; the dose of one or both agents should be reduced). Products include:
Dalmane Capsules ... 2173

Furazolidone (Co-administration may increase the effect of either drug). Products include:
Furoxone ... 2046

Glutethimide (May exhibit an additive CNS depression; the dose of one or both agents should be reduced).
No products indexed under this heading.

Glycopyrrolate (Potential for paralytic ileus). Products include:
Robinul Forte Tablets ... 2072
Robinul Injectable ... 2072
Robinul Tablets ... 2072

Haloperidol (May exhibit an additive CNS depression; the dose of one or both agents should be reduced). Products include:
Haldol Injection, Tablets and Concentrate ... 1575

Haloperidol Decanoate (May exhibit an additive CNS depression; the dose of one or both agents should be reduced). Products include:
Haldol Decanoate ... 1577

Hydrocodone Polistirex (May exhibit an additive CNS depression; the dose of one or both agents should be reduced). Products include:
Tussionex Pennkinetic Extended-Release Suspension ... 998

Hydroxyzine Hydrochloride (May exhibit an additive CNS depression; the dose of one or both agents should be reduced). Products include:
Atarax Tablets & Syrup ... 2185
Marax Tablets & DF Syrup ... 2200
Vistaril Intramuscular Solution ... 2216

Hyoscyamine (Potential for paralytic ileus). Products include:
Cystospaz Tablets ... 1963
Urised Tablets ... 1964

Hyoscyamine Sulfate (Potential for paralytic ileus). Products include:
Arco-Lase Plus Tablets ... 512
Atrohist Plus Tablets ... 454
Cystospaz-M Capsules ... 1963
Donnatal ... 2060
Donnatal Extentabs ... 2061
Donnatal Tablets ... 2060
Kutrase Capsules ... 2402
Levsin/Levsinex/Levbid ... 2405

Imipramine Hydrochloride (Co-administration may increase the effect of either drug). Products include:
Tofranil Ampuls ... 854
Tofranil Tablets ... 856

Imipramine Pamoate (Co-administration may increase the effect of either drug). Products include:
Tofranil-PM Capsules ... 857

Ipratropium Bromide (Potential for paralytic ileus). Products include:
Atrovent Inhalation Aerosol ... 671
Atrovent Inhalation Solution ... 673

Isocarboxazid (Co-administration may increase the effect of either drug).
No products indexed under this heading.

Isoflurane (May exhibit an additive CNS depression; the dose of one or both agents should be reduced).
No products indexed under this heading.

Ketamine Hydrochloride (May exhibit an additive CNS depression; the dose of one or both agents should be reduced).
No products indexed under this heading.

Levomethadyl Acetate Hydrochloride (May exhibit an additive CNS depression; the dose of one or both agents should be reduced). Products include:
Orlamm ... 2239

Levorphanol Tartrate (May exhibit an additive CNS depression; the dose of one or both agents should be reduced). Products include:
Levo-Dromoran ... 2129

Lithium Carbonate (May exhibit an additive CNS depression; the dose of one or both agents should be reduced). Products include:
Eskalith ... 2485
Lithium Carbonate Capsules & Tablets ... 2230
Lithonate/Lithotabs/Lithobid ... 2543

Lithium Citrate (May exhibit an additive CNS depression; the dose of one or both agents should be reduced).
No products indexed under this heading.

Lorazepam (May exhibit an additive CNS depression; the dose of one or both agents should be reduced). Products include:
Ativan Injection ... 2698
Ativan Tablets ... 2700

Loxapine Hydrochloride (May exhibit an additive CNS depression; the dose of one or both agents should be reduced). Products include:
Loxitane ... 1378

Loxapine Succinate (May exhibit an additive CNS depression; the dose of one or both agents should be reduced). Products include:
Loxitane Capsules ... 1378

Maprotiline Hydrochloride (Co-administration may increase the effect of either drug). Products include:
Ludiomil Tablets ... 843

Mepenzolate Bromide (Potential for paralytic ileus).
No products indexed under this heading.

Meperidine Hydrochloride (May exhibit an additive CNS depression; the dose of one or both agents should be reduced). Products include:
Demerol ... 2308
Mepergan Injection ... 2753

Mephobarbital (May exhibit an additive CNS depression; the dose of one or both agents should be reduced). Products include:
Mebaral Tablets ... 2322

Meprobamate (May exhibit an additive CNS depression; the dose of one or both agents should be reduced). Products include:
Miltown Tablets ... 2672
PMB 200 and PMB 400 ... 2783

Mesoridazine Besylate (May exhibit an additive CNS depression; the dose of one or both agents should be reduced). Products include:
Serentil ... 684

Methadone Hydrochloride (May exhibit an additive CNS depression; the dose of one or both agents should be reduced). Products include:
Methadone Hydrochloride Oral Concentrate ... 2233
Methadone Hydrochloride Oral Solution & Tablets ... 2235

Methohexital Sodium (May exhibit an additive CNS depression; the dose of one or both agents should be reduced). Products include:
Brevital Sodium Vials ... 1429

Methotrimeprazine (May exhibit an additive CNS depression; the dose of one or both agents should be reduced). Products include:
Levoprome ... 1274

Methoxyflurane (May exhibit an additive CNS depression; the dose of one or both agents should be reduced).
No products indexed under this heading.

Midazolam Hydrochloride (May exhibit an additive CNS depression; the dose of one or both agents should be reduced). Products include:
Versed Injection ... 2170

Molindone Hydrochloride (May exhibit an additive CNS depression; the dose of one or both agents should be reduced). Products include:
Moban Tablets and Concentrate ... 1048

Morphine Sulfate (May exhibit an additive CNS depression; the dose of one or both agents should be reduced). Products include:
Astramorph/PF Injection, USP (Preservative-Free) ... 535
Duramorph ... 962
Infumorph 200 and Infumorph 500 Sterile Solutions ... 965
MS Contin Tablets ... 1994
MSIR ... 1997
Oramorph SR (Morphine Sulfate Sustained Release Tablets) ... 2236
RMS Suppositories ... 2657

IMPORTANT NOTE: Always consult each drug listing in the patient's regimen for possible interactions.

Roxanol 2243

Nortriptyline Hydrochloride (Co-administration may increase the effect of either drug). Products include:
- Pamelor 2280

Opium Alkaloids (May exhibit an additive CNS depression; the dose of one or both agents should be reduced).
- No products indexed under this heading.

Oxazepam (May exhibit an additive CNS depression; the dose of one or both agents should be reduced). Products include:
- Serax Capsules 2810
- Serax Tablets 2810

Oxybutynin Chloride (Potential for paralytic ileus). Products include:
- Ditropan 1516

Oxycodone Hydrochloride (May exhibit an additive CNS depression; the dose of one or both agents should be reduced). Products include:
- Percocet Tablets 938
- Percodan Tablets 939
- Percodan-Demi Tablets 940
- Roxicodone Tablets, Oral Solution & Intensol (Oxycodone) 2244
- Tylox Capsules 1584

Pentobarbital Sodium (May exhibit an additive CNS depression; the dose of one or both agents should be reduced). Products include:
- Nembutal Sodium Capsules 436
- Nembutal Sodium Solution 438
- Nembutal Sodium Suppositories 440

Perphenazine (May exhibit an additive CNS depression; the dose of one or both agents should be reduced). Products include:
- Etrafon 2355
- Triavil Tablets 1757
- Trilafon 2389

Phenelzine Sulfate (Co-administration may increase the effect of either drug). Products include:
- Nardil 1920

Phenobarbital (May exhibit an additive CNS depression; the dose of one or both agents should be reduced). Products include:
- Arco-Lase Plus Tablets 512
- Bellergal-S Tablets 2250
- Donnatal 2060
- Donnatal Extentabs 2061
- Donnatal Tablets 2060
- Phenobarbital Elixir and Tablets 1469
- Quadrinal Tablets 1350

Pimozide (May exhibit an additive CNS depression; the dose of one or both agents should be reduced). Products include:
- Orap Tablets 1050

Prazepam (May exhibit an additive CNS depression; the dose of one or both agents should be reduced).
- No products indexed under this heading.

Prochlorperazine (May exhibit an additive CNS depression; the dose of one or both agents should be reduced). Products include:
- Compazine 2470

Procyclidine Hydrochloride (Potential for paralytic ileus). Products include:
- Kemadrin Tablets 1112

Promethazine Hydrochloride (May exhibit an additive CNS depression; the dose of one or both agents should be reduced). Products include:
- Mepergan Injection 2753
- Phenergan with Codeine 2777
- Phenergan with Dextromethorphan 2778
- Phenergan Injection 2773
- Phenergan Suppositories 2775
- Phenergan Syrup 2774
- Phenergan Tablets 2775
- Phenergan VC 2779
- Phenergan VC with Codeine 2781

Propantheline Bromide (Potential for paralytic ileus). Products include:
- Pro-Banthīne Tablets 2052

Propofol (May exhibit an additive CNS depression; the dose of one or both agents should be reduced). Products include:
- Diprivan Injection 2833

Propoxyphene Hydrochloride (May exhibit an additive CNS depression; the dose of one or both agents should be reduced). Products include:
- Darvon 1435
- Wygesic Tablets 2827

Propoxyphene Napsylate (May exhibit an additive CNS depression; the dose of one or both agents should be reduced). Products include:
- Darvon-N/Darvocet-N 1433

Protriptyline Hydrochloride (Co-administration may increase the effect of either drug). Products include:
- Vivactil Tablets 1774

Quazepam (May exhibit an additive CNS depression; the dose of one or both agents should be reduced). Products include:
- Doral Tablets 2664

Risperidone (May exhibit an additive CNS depression; the dose of one or both agents should be reduced). Products include:
- Risperdal 1301

Scopolamine (Potential for paralytic ileus). Products include:
- Transderm Scōp Transdermal Therapeutic System 869

Scopolamine Hydrobromide (Potential for paralytic ileus). Products include:
- Atrohist Plus Tablets 454
- Donnatal 2060
- Donnatal Extentabs 2061
- Donnatal Tablets 2060

Secobarbital Sodium (May exhibit an additive CNS depression; the dose of one or both agents should be reduced). Products include:
- Seconal Sodium Pulvules 1474

Selegiline Hydrochloride (Co-administration may increase the effect of either drug). Products include:
- Eldepryl Tablets 2550

Sufentanil Citrate (May exhibit an additive CNS depression; the dose of one or both agents should be reduced). Products include:
- Sufenta Injection 1309

Temazepam (May exhibit an additive CNS depression; the dose of one or both agents should be reduced). Products include:
- Restoril Capsules 2284

Thiamylal Sodium (May exhibit an additive CNS depression; the dose of one or both agents should be reduced).
- No products indexed under this heading.

Thioridazine Hydrochloride (May exhibit an additive CNS depression; the dose of one or both agents should be reduced). Products include:
- Mellaril 2269

Thiothixene (May exhibit an additive CNS depression; the dose of one or both agents should be reduced). Products include:
- Navane Capsules and Concentrate 2201
- Navane Intramuscular 2202

Tranylcypromine Sulfate (Co-administration may increase the effect of either drug). Products include:
- Parnate Tablets 2503

Triazolam (May exhibit an additive CNS depression; the dose of one or both agents should be reduced). Products include:
- Halcion Tablets 2611

Tridihexethyl Chloride (Potential for paralytic ileus).
- No products indexed under this heading.

Trifluoperazine Hydrochloride (May exhibit an additive CNS depression; the dose of one or both agents should be reduced). Products include:
- Stelazine 2514

Trihexyphenidyl Hydrochloride (Potential for paralytic ileus). Products include:
- Artane 1368

Trimipramine Maleate (Co-administration may increase the effect of either drug). Products include:
- Surmontil Capsules 2811

Zolpidem Tartrate (May exhibit an additive CNS depression; the dose of one or both agents should be reduced). Products include:
- Ambien Tablets 2416

Food Interactions

Alcohol (May exhibit an additive CNS depression).

VICODIN ES TABLETS

(Hydrocodone Bitartrate, Acetaminophen) 1357

May interact with central nervous system depressants, narcotic analgesics, psychotropics, tranquilizers, monoamine oxidase inhibitors, tricyclic antidepressants, anticholinergics, and certain other agents. Compounds in these categories include:

Alfentanil Hydrochloride (Additive CNS depression; the dose of one or both agents should be reduced). Products include:
- Alfenta Injection 1286

Alprazolam (Additive CNS depression; the dose of one or both agents should be reduced). Products include:
- Xanax Tablets 2649

Amitriptyline Hydrochloride (Additive CNS depression; the dose of one or both agents should be reduced; increased effect of either hydrocodone or antidepressant). Products include:
- Elavil 2838
- Endep Tablets 2174
- Etrafon 2355
- Limbitrol 2180
- Triavil Tablets 1757

Amoxapine (Additive CNS depression; the dose of one or both agents should be reduced; increased effect of either hydrocodone or antidepressant). Products include:
- Asendin Tablets 1369

Aprobarbital (Additive CNS depression; the dose of one or both agents should be reduced).
- No products indexed under this heading.

Atropine Sulfate (May produce paralytic ileus). Products include:
- Arco-Lase Plus Tablets 512
- Atrohist Plus Tablets 454
- Atropine Sulfate Sterile Ophthalmic Solution .... ⊙ 233
- Donnatal 2060
- Donnatal Extentabs 2061
- Donnatal Tablets 2060
- Lomotil 2439
- Motofen Tablets 784
- Urised Tablets 1964

Belladonna Alkaloids (May produce paralytic ileus). Products include:
- Bellergal-S Tablets 2250
- Hyland's Bed Wetting Tablets .... ▣ 828
- Hyland's EnurAid Tablets .... ▣ 829
- Hyland's Teething Tablets .... ▣ 830

Benztropine Mesylate (May produce paralytic ileus). Products include:
- Cogentin 1621

Biperiden Hydrochloride (May produce paralytic ileus). Products include:
- Akineton 1333

Buprenorphine (Additive CNS depression; the dose of one or both agents should be reduced). Products include:
- Buprenex Injectable 2006

Buspirone Hydrochloride (Additive CNS depression; the dose of one or both agents should be reduced). Products include:
- BuSpar 737

Butabarbital (Additive CNS depression; the dose of one or both agents should be reduced).
- No products indexed under this heading.

Butalbital (Additive CNS depression; the dose of one or both agents should be reduced). Products include:
- Esgic-plus Tablets 1013
- Fioricet Tablets 2258
- Fioricet with Codeine Capsules 2260
- Fiorinal Capsules 2261
- Fiorinal with Codeine Capsules 2262
- Fiorinal Tablets 2261
- Phrenilin 785
- Sedapap Tablets 50 mg/650 mg 1543

Chlordiazepoxide (Additive CNS depression; the dose of one or both agents should be reduced). Products include:
- Libritabs Tablets 2177
- Limbitrol 2180

Chlordiazepoxide Hydrochloride (Additive CNS depression; the dose of one or both agents should be reduced). Products include:
- Librax Capsules 2176
- Librium Capsules 2178
- Librium Injectable 2179

Chlorpromazine (Additive CNS depression; the dose of one or both agents should be reduced). Products include:
- Thorazine Suppositories 2523

Chlorprothixene (Additive CNS depression; the dose of one or both agents should be reduced).
- No products indexed under this heading.

Chlorprothixene Hydrochloride (Additive CNS depression; the dose of one or both agents should be reduced).
- No products indexed under this heading.

Clidinium Bromide (May produce paralytic ileus). Products include:
- Librax Capsules 2176
- Quarzan Capsules 2181

(▣ Described in PDR For Nonprescription Drugs) (⊙ Described in PDR For Ophthalmology)

1153 **Interactions Index** **Vicodin ES**

Clomipramine Hydrochloride (Additive CNS depression; the dose of one or both agents should be reduced; increased effect of either hydrocodone or antidepressant). Products include:
Anafranil Capsules ... 803
Clorazepate Dipotassium (Additive CNS depression; the dose of one or both agents should be reduced). Products include:
Tranxene ... 451
Clozapine (Additive CNS depression; the dose of one or both agents should be reduced). Products include:
Clozaril Tablets ... 2252
Codeine Phosphate (Additive CNS depression; the dose of one or both agents should be reduced). Products include:
Actifed with Codeine Cough Syrup.. 1067
Brontex ... 1981
Deconsal C Expectorant Syrup ... 456
Deconsal Pediatric Syrup ... 457
Dimetane-DC Cough Syrup ... 2059
Empirin with Codeine Tablets ... 1093
Fioricet with Codeine Capsules ... 2260
Fiorinal with Codeine Capsules ... 2262
Isoclor Expectorant ... 990
Novahistine DH ... 2462
Novahistine Expectorant ... 2463
Nucofed ... 2051
Phenergan with Codeine ... 2777
Phenergan VC with Codeine ... 2781
Robitussin A-C Syrup ... 2073
Robitussin-DAC Syrup ... 2074
Ryna ... 841
Soma Compound w/Codeine Tablets ... 2676
Tussi-Organidin NR Liquid and S NR Liquid ... 2677
Tylenol with Codeine ... 1583
Desflurane (Additive CNS depression; the dose of one or both agents should be reduced). Products include:
Suprane ... 1813
Desipramine Hydrochloride (Additive CNS depression; the dose of one or both agents should be reduced; increased effect of either hydrocodone or antidepressant). Products include:
Norpramin Tablets ... 1526
Dezocine (Additive CNS depression; the dose of one or both agents should be reduced). Products include:
Dalgan Injection ... 538
Diazepam (Additive CNS depression; the dose of one or both agents should be reduced). Products include:
Dizac ... 1809
Valium Injectable ... 2182
Valium Tablets ... 2183
Valrelease Capsules ... 2169
Dicyclomine Hydrochloride (May produce paralytic ileus). Products include:
Bentyl ... 1501
Doxepin Hydrochloride (Additive CNS depression; the dose of one or both agents should be reduced; increased effect of either hydrocodone or antidepressant). Products include:
Sinequan ... 2205
Zonalon Cream ... 1055
Droperidol (Additive CNS depression; the dose of one or both agents should be reduced). Products include:
Inapsine Injection ... 1296
Enflurane (Additive CNS depression; the dose of one or both agents should be reduced).
No products indexed under this heading.
Estazolam (Additive CNS depression; the dose of one or both agents should be reduced). Products include:
ProSom Tablets ... 449
Ethchlorvynol (Additive CNS depression; the dose of one or both agents should be reduced). Products include:
Placidyl Capsules ... 448
Ethinamate (Additive CNS depression; the dose of one or both agents should be reduced).
No products indexed under this heading.
Fentanyl (Additive CNS depression; the dose of one or both agents should be reduced). Products include:
Duragesic Transdermal System ... 1288
Fentanyl Citrate (Additive CNS depression; the dose of one or both agents should be reduced). Products include:
Sublimaze Injection ... 1307
Fluphenazine Decanoate (Additive CNS depression; the dose of one or both agents should be reduced). Products include:
Prolixin Decanoate ... 509
Fluphenazine Enanthate (Additive CNS depression; the dose of one or both agents should be reduced). Products include:
Prolixin Enanthate ... 509
Fluphenazine Hydrochloride (Additive CNS depression; the dose of one or both agents should be reduced). Products include:
Prolixin ... 509
Flurazepam Hydrochloride (Additive CNS depression; the dose of one or both agents should be reduced). Products include:
Dalmane Capsules ... 2173
Furazolidone (Additive CNS depression; the dose of one or both agents should be reduced; increased effect of either hydrocodone or MAO inhibitor). Products include:
Furoxone ... 2046
Glutethimide (Additive CNS depression; the dose of one or both agents should be reduced).
No products indexed under this heading.
Glycopyrrolate (May produce paralytic ileus). Products include:
Robinul Forte Tablets ... 2072
Robinul Injectable ... 2072
Robinul Tablets ... 2072
Haloperidol (Additive CNS depression; the dose of one or both agents should be reduced). Products include:
Haldol Injection, Tablets and Concentrate ... 1575
Haloperidol Decanoate (Additive CNS depression; the dose of one or both agents should be reduced). Products include:
Haldol Decanoate ... 1577
Hydrocodone Polistirex (Additive CNS depression; the dose of one or both agents should be reduced). Products include:
Tussionex Pennkinetic Extended-Release Suspension ... 998
Hydroxyzine Hydrochloride (Additive CNS depression; the dose of one or both agents should be reduced). Products include:
Atarax Tablets & Syrup ... 2185
Marax Tablets & DF Syrup ... 2200
Vistaril Intramuscular Solution ... 2216
Hyoscyamine (May produce paralytic ileus). Products include:
Cystospaz Tablets ... 1963
Urised Tablets ... 1964
Hyoscyamine Sulfate (May produce paralytic ileus). Products include:
Arco-Lase Plus Tablets ... 512
Atrohist Plus Tablets ... 454
Cystospaz-M Capsules ... 1963
Donnatal ... 2060
Donnatal Extentabs ... 2061
Donnatal Tablets ... 2060
Kutrase Capsules ... 2402
Levsin/Levsinex/Levbid ... 2405
Imipramine Hydrochloride (Additive CNS depression; the dose of one or both agents should be reduced; increased effect of either hydrocodone or antidepressant). Products include:
Tofranil Ampuls ... 854
Tofranil Tablets ... 856
Imipramine Pamoate (Additive CNS depression; the dose of one or both agents should be reduced; increased effect of either hydrocodone or antidepressant). Products include:
Tofranil-PM Capsules ... 857
Ipratropium Bromide (May produce paralytic ileus). Products include:
Atrovent Inhalation Aerosol ... 671
Atrovent Inhalation Solution ... 673
Isocarboxazid (Additive CNS depression; the dose of one or both agents should be reduced; increased effect of either hydrocodone or MAO inhibitor).
No products indexed under this heading.
Isoflurane (Additive CNS depression; the dose of one or both agents should be reduced).
No products indexed under this heading.
Ketamine Hydrochloride (Additive CNS depression; the dose of one or both agents should be reduced).
No products indexed under this heading.
Levomethadyl Acetate Hydrochloride (Additive CNS depression; the dose of one or both agents should be reduced). Products include:
Orlamm ... 2239
Levorphanol Tartrate (Additive CNS depression; the dose of one or both agents should be reduced). Products include:
Levo-Dromoran ... 2129
Lithium Carbonate (Additive CNS depression; the dose of one or both agents should be reduced). Products include:
Eskalith ... 2485
Lithium Carbonate Capsules & Tablets ... 2230
Lithonate/Lithotabs/Lithobid ... 2543
Lithium Citrate (Additive CNS depression; the dose of one or both agents should be reduced).
No products indexed under this heading.
Lorazepam (Additive CNS depression; the dose of one or both agents should be reduced). Products include:
Ativan Injection ... 2698
Ativan Tablets ... 2700
Loxapine Hydrochloride (Additive CNS depression; the dose of one or both agents should be reduced). Products include:
Loxitane ... 1378
Loxapine Succinate (Additive CNS depression; the dose of one or both agents should be reduced). Products include:
Loxitane Capsules ... 1378
Maprotiline Hydrochloride (Additive CNS depression; the dose of one or both agents should be reduced; increased effect of either hydrocodone or antidepressant). Products include:
Ludiomil Tablets ... 843
Mepenzolate Bromide (May produce paralytic ileus).
No products indexed under this heading.
Meperidine Hydrochloride (Additive CNS depression; the dose of one or both agents should be reduced). Products include:
Demerol ... 2308
Mepergan Injection ... 2753
Mephobarbital (Additive CNS depression; the dose of one or both agents should be reduced). Products include:
Mebaral Tablets ... 2322
Meprobamate (Additive CNS depression; the dose of one or both agents should be reduced). Products include:
Miltown Tablets ... 2672
PMB 200 and PMB 400 ... 2783
Mesoridazine Besylate (Additive CNS depression; the dose of one or both agents should be reduced). Products include:
Serentil ... 684
Methadone Hydrochloride (Additive CNS depression; the dose of one or both agents should be reduced). Products include:
Methadone Hydrochloride Oral Concentrate ... 2233
Methadone Hydrochloride Oral Solution & Tablets ... 2235
Methohexital Sodium (Additive CNS depression; the dose of one or both agents should be reduced). Products include:
Brevital Sodium Vials ... 1429
Methotrimeprazine (Additive CNS depression; the dose of one or both agents should be reduced). Products include:
Levoprome ... 1274
Methoxyflurane (Additive CNS depression; the dose of one or both agents should be reduced).
No products indexed under this heading.
Midazolam Hydrochloride (Additive CNS depression; the dose of one or both agents should be reduced). Products include:
Versed Injection ... 2170
Molindone Hydrochloride (Additive CNS depression; the dose of one or both agents should be reduced). Products include:
Moban Tablets and Concentrate ... 1048
Morphine Sulfate (Additive CNS depression; the dose of one or both agents should be reduced). Products include:
Astramorph/PF Injection, USP (Preservative-Free) ... 535
Duramorph ... 962
Infumorph 200 and Infumorph 500 Sterile Solutions ... 965
MS Contin Tablets ... 1994
MSIR ... 1997
Oramorph SR (Morphine Sulfate Sustained Release Tablets) ... 2236
RMS Suppositories ... 2657
Roxanol ... 2243
Nortriptyline Hydrochloride (Additive CNS depression; the dose of one or both agents should be reduced; increased effect of either hydrocodone or antidepressant). Products include:
Pamelor ... 2280

IMPORTANT NOTE: Always consult each drug listing in the patient's regimen for possible interactions.

Opium Alkaloids (Additive CNS depression; the dose of one or both agents should be reduced).
No products indexed under this heading.

Oxazepam (Additive CNS depression; the dose of one or both agents should be reduced). Products include:
Serax Capsules ... 2810
Serax Tablets ... 2810

Oxybutynin Chloride (May produce paralytic ileus). Products include:
Ditropan ... 1516

Oxycodone Hydrochloride (Additive CNS depression; the dose of one or both agents should be reduced). Products include:
Percocet Tablets ... 938
Percodan Tablets ... 939
Percodan-Demi Tablets ... 940
Roxicodone Tablets, Oral Solution & Intensol (Oxycodone) ... 2244
Tylox Capsules ... 1584

Pentobarbital Sodium (Additive CNS depression; the dose of one or both agents should be reduced). Products include:
Nembutal Sodium Capsules ... 436
Nembutal Sodium Solution ... 438
Nembutal Sodium Suppositories ... 440

Perphenazine (Additive CNS depression; the dose of one or both agents should be reduced). Products include:
Etrafon ... 2355
Triavil Tablets ... 1757
Trilafon ... 2389

Phenelzine Sulfate (Additive CNS depression; the dose of one or both agents should be reduced; increased effect of either hydrocodone or MAO inhibitor). Products include:
Nardil ... 1920

Phenobarbital (Additive CNS depression; the dose of one or both agents should be reduced). Products include:
Arco-Lase Plus Tablets ... 512
Bellergal-S Tablets ... 2250
Donnatal ... 2060
Donnatal Extentabs ... 2061
Donnatal Tablets ... 2060
Phenobarbital Elixir and Tablets ... 1469
Quadrinal Tablets ... 1350

Prazepam (Additive CNS depression; the dose of one or both agents should be reduced).
No products indexed under this heading.

Prochlorperazine (Additive CNS depression; the dose of one or both agents should be reduced). Products include:
Compazine ... 2470

Procyclidine Hydrochloride (May produce paralytic ileus). Products include:
Kemadrin Tablets ... 1112

Promethazine Hydrochloride (Additive CNS depression; the dose of one or both agents should be reduced). Products include:
Mepergan Injection ... 2753
Phenergan with Codeine ... 2777
Phenergan with Dextromethorphan 2778
Phenergan Injection ... 2773
Phenergan Suppositories ... 2775
Phenergan Syrup ... 2774
Phenergan Tablets ... 2775
Phenergan VC ... 2779
Phenergan VC with Codeine ... 2781

Propantheline Bromide (May produce paralytic ileus). Products include:
Pro-Banthine Tablets ... 2052

Propofol (Additive CNS depression; the dose of one or both agents should be reduced). Products include:
Diprivan Injection ... 2833

Propoxyphene Hydrochloride (Additive CNS depression; the dose of one or both agents should be reduced). Products include:
Darvon ... 1435
Wygesic Tablets ... 2827

Propoxyphene Napsylate (Additive CNS depression; the dose of one or both agents should be reduced). Products include:
Darvon-N/Darvocet-N ... 1433

Protriptyline Hydrochloride (Additive CNS depression; the dose of one or both agents should be reduced; increased effect of either hydrocodone or antidepressant). Products include:
Vivactil Tablets ... 1774

Quazepam (Additive CNS depression; the dose of one or both agents should be reduced). Products include:
Doral Tablets ... 2664

Risperidone (Additive CNS depression; the dose of one or both agents should be reduced). Products include:
Risperdal ... 1301

Scopolamine (May produce paralytic ileus). Products include:
Transderm Scōp Transdermal Therapeutic System ... 869

Scopolamine Hydrobromide (May produce paralytic ileus). Products include:
Atrohist Plus Tablets ... 454
Donnatal ... 2060
Donnatal Extentabs ... 2061
Donnatal Tablets ... 2060

Secobarbital Sodium (Additive CNS depression; the dose of one or both agents should be reduced). Products include:
Seconal Sodium Pulvules ... 1474

Selegiline Hydrochloride (Additive CNS depression; the dose of one or both agents should be reduced; increased effect of either hydrocodone or MAO inhibitor). Products include:
Eldepryl Tablets ... 2550

Sufentanil Citrate (Additive CNS depression; the dose of one or both agents should be reduced). Products include:
Sufenta Injection ... 1309

Temazepam (Additive CNS depression; the dose of one or both agents should be reduced). Products include:
Restoril Capsules ... 2284

Thiamylal Sodium (Additive CNS depression; the dose of one or both agents should be reduced).
No products indexed under this heading.

Thioridazine Hydrochloride (Additive CNS depression; the dose of one or both agents sjould be reduced). Products include:
Mellaril ... 2269

Thiothixene (Additive CNS depression; the dose of one or both agents should be reduced). Products include:
Navane Capsules and Concentrate 2201
Navane Intramuscular ... 2202

Tranylcypromine Sulfate (Additive CNS depression; the dose of one or both agents should be reduced; increased effect of either hydrocodone or MAO inhibitor). Products include:
Parnate Tablets ... 2503

Triazolam (Additive CNS depression; the dose of one or both agents should be reduced). Products include:
Halcion Tablets ... 2611

Tridihexethyl Chloride (May produce paralytic ileus).
No products indexed under this heading.

Trifluoperazine Hydrochloride (Additive CNS depression; the dose of one or both agents should be reduced). Products include:
Stelazine ... 2514

Trihexyphenidyl Hydrochloride (May produce paralytic ileus). Products include:
Artane ... 1368

Trimipramine Maleate (Additive CNS depression; the dose of one or both agents should be reduced; increased effect of either hydrocodone or antidepressant). Products include:
Surmontil Capsules ... 2811

Zolpidem Tartrate (Additive CNS depression; the dose of one or both agents should be reduced). Products include:
Ambien Tablets ... 2416

Food Interactions

Alcohol (Additive CNS depression).

VICODIN TUSS EXPECTORANT

(Hydrocodone Bitartrate, Guaifenesin) ... 1358

May interact with central nervous system depressants, phenothiazines, narcotic analgesics, general anesthetics, tranquilizers, hypnotics and sedatives, and certain other agents. Compounds in these categories include:

Alfentanil Hydrochloride (Co-administration may exhibit an additive CNS depression; the dose of one or both agents should be reduced). Products include:
Alfenta Injection ... 1286

Alprazolam (Co-administration may exhibit an additive CNS depression; the dose of one or both agents should be reduced). Products include:
Xanax Tablets ... 2649

Aprobarbital (Co-administration may exhibit an additive CNS depression; the dose of one or both agents should be reduced).
No products indexed under this heading.

Buprenorphine (Co-administration may exhibit an additive CNS depression; the dose of one or both agents should be reduced). Products include:
Buprenex Injectable ... 2006

Buspirone Hydrochloride (Co-administration may exhibit an additive CNS depression; the dose of one or both agents should be reduced). Products include:
BuSpar ... 737

Butabarbital (Co-administration may exhibit an additive CNS depression; the dose of one or both agents should be reduced).
No products indexed under this heading.

Butalbital (Co-administration may exhibit an additive CNS depression; the dose of one or both agents should be reduced). Products include:
Esgic-plus Tablets ... 1013
Fioricet Tablets ... 2258
Fioricet with Codeine Capsules ... 2260
Fiorinal Capsules ... 2261
Fiorinal with Codeine Capsules ... 2262
Fiorinal Tablets ... 2261
Phrenilin ... 785
Sedapap Tablets 50 mg/650 mg .. 1543

Chlordiazepoxide (Co-administration may exhibit an additive CNS depression; the dose of one or both agents should be reduced). Products include:
Libritabs Tablets ... 2177
Limbitrol ... 2180

Chlordiazepoxide Hydrochloride (Co-administration may exhibit an additive CNS depression; the dose of one or both agents should be reduced). Products include:
Librax Capsules ... 2176
Librium Capsules ... 2178
Librium Injectable ... 2179

Chlorpromazine (Co-administration may exhibit an additive CNS depression; the dose of one or both agents should be reduced). Products include:
Thorazine Suppositories ... 2523

Chlorpromazine Hydrochloride (Co-administration may exhibit an additive CNS depression; the dose of one or both agents should be reduced). Products include:
Thorazine ... 2523

Chlorprothixene (Co-administration may exhibit an additive CNS depression; the dose of one or both agents should be reduced).
No products indexed under this heading.

Chlorprothixene Hydrochloride (Co-administration may exhibit an additive CNS depression; the dose of one or both agents should be reduced).
No products indexed under this heading.

Clorazepate Dipotassium (Co-administration may exhibit an additive CNS depression; the dose of one or both agents should be reduced). Products include:
Tranxene ... 451

Clozapine (Co-administration may exhibit an additive CNS depression; the dose of one or both agents should be reduced). Products include:
Clozaril Tablets ... 2252

Codeine Phosphate (Co-administration may exhibit an additive CNS depression; the dose of one or both agents should be reduced). Products include:
Actifed with Codeine Cough Syrup.. 1067
Brontex ... 1981
Deconsal C Expectorant Syrup ... 456
Deconsal Pediatric Syrup ... 457
Dimetane-DC Cough Syrup ... 2059
Empirin with Codeine Tablets ... 1093
Fioricet with Codeine Capsules ... 2260
Fiorinal with Codeine Capsules ... 2262
Isoclor Expectorant ... 990
Novahistine DH ... 2462
Novahistine Expectorant ... 2463
Nucofed ... 2051
Phenergan with Codeine ... 2777
Phenergan VC with Codeine ... 2781
Robitussin A-C Syrup ... 2073
Robitussin-DAC Syrup ... 2074
Ryna ... ⊞ 841
Soma Compound w/Codeine Tablets ... 2676
Tussi-Organidin NR Liquid and S NR Liquid ... 2677
Tylenol with Codeine ... 1583

(⊞ Described in PDR For Nonprescription Drugs) (⊙ Described in PDR For Ophthalmology)

Desflurane (Co-administration may exhibit an additive CNS depression; the dose of one or both agents should be reduced). Products include:

Suprane 1813

Dezocine (Co-administration may exhibit an additive CNS depression; the dose of one or both agents should be reduced). Products include:

Dalgan Injection 538

Diazepam (Co-administration may exhibit an additive CNS depression; the dose of one or both agents should be reduced). Products include:

Dizac 1809
Valium Injectable 2182
Valium Tablets 2183
Valrelease Capsules 2169

Droperidol (Co-administration may exhibit an additive CNS depression; the dose of one or both agents should be reduced). Products include:

Inapsine Injection 1296

Enflurane (Co-administration may exhibit an additive CNS depression; the dose of one or both agents should be reduced).

No products indexed under this heading.

Estazolam (Co-administration may exhibit an additive CNS depression; the dose of one or both agents should be reduced). Products include:

ProSom Tablets 449

Ethchlorvynol (Co-administration may exhibit an additive CNS depression; the dose of one or both agents should be reduced). Products include:

Placidyl Capsules 448

Ethinamate (Co-administration may exhibit an additive CNS depression; the dose of one or both agents should be reduced).

No products indexed under this heading.

Fentanyl (Co-administration may exhibit an additive CNS depression; the dose of one or both agents should be reduced). Products include:

Duragesic Transdermal System........ 1288

Fentanyl Citrate (Co-administration may exhibit an additive CNS depression; the dose of one or both agents should be reduced). Products include:

Sublimaze Injection 1307

Fluphenazine Decanoate (Co-administration may exhibit an additive CNS depression; the dose of one or both agents should be reduced). Products include:

Prolixin Decanoate 509

Fluphenazine Enanthate (Co-administration may exhibit an additive CNS depression; the dose of one or both agents should be reduced). Products include:

Prolixin Enanthate 509

Fluphenazine Hydrochloride (Co-administration may exhibit an additive CNS depression; the dose of one or both agents should be reduced). Products include:

Prolixin 509

Flurazepam Hydrochloride (Co-administration may exhibit an additive CNS depression; the dose of one or both agents should be reduced). Products include:

Dalmane Capsules 2173

Glutethimide (Co-administration may exhibit an additive CNS depression; the dose of one or both agents should be reduced).

No products indexed under this heading.

Haloperidol (Co-administration may exhibit an additive CNS depression; the dose of one or both agents should be reduced). Products include:

Haldol Injection, Tablets and Concentrate 1575

Haloperidol Decanoate (Co-administration may exhibit an additive CNS depression; the dose of one or both agents should be reduced). Products include:

Haldol Decanoate 1577

Hydrocodone Polistirex (Co-administration may exhibit an additive CNS depression; the dose of one or both agents should be reduced). Products include:

Tussionex Pennkinetic Extended-Release Suspension 998

Hydroxyzine Hydrochloride (Co-administration may exhibit an additive CNS depression; the dose of one or both agents should be reduced). Products include:

Atarax Tablets & Syrup 2185
Marax Tablets & DF Syrup 2200
Vistaril Intramuscular Solution 2216

Isoflurane (Co-administration may exhibit an additive CNS depression; the dose of one or both agents should be reduced).

No products indexed under this heading.

Ketamine Hydrochloride (Co-administration may exhibit an additive CNS depression; the dose of one or both agents should be reduced).

No products indexed under this heading.

Levomethadyl Acetate Hydrochloride (Co-administration may exhibit an additive CNS depression; the dose of one or both agents should be reduced). Products include:

Orlamm 2239

Levorphanol Tartrate (Co-administration may exhibit an additive CNS depression; the dose of one or both agents should be reduced). Products include:

Levo-Dromoran 2129

Lorazepam (Co-administration may exhibit an additive CNS depression; the dose of one or both agents should be reduced). Products include:

Ativan Injection 2698
Ativan Tablets 2700

Loxapine Hydrochloride (Co-administration may exhibit an additive CNS depression; the dose of one or both agents should be reduced). Products include:

Loxitane 1378

Loxapine Succinate (Co-administration may exhibit an additive CNS depression; the dose of one or both agents should be reduced). Products include:

Loxitane Capsules 1378

Meperidine Hydrochloride (Co-administration may exhibit an additive CNS depression; the dose of one or both agents should be reduced). Products include:

Demerol 2308
Mepergan Injection 2753

Mephobarbital (Co-administration may exhibit an additive CNS depression; the dose of one or both agents should be reduced). Products include:

Mebaral Tablets 2322

Meprobamate (Co-administration may exhibit an additive CNS depression; the dose of one or both agents should be reduced). Products include:

Miltown Tablets 2672
PMB 200 and PMB 400 2783

Mesoridazine (Co-administration may exhibit an additive CNS depression; the dose of one or both agents should be reduced).

Mesoridazine Besylate (Co-administration may exhibit an additive CNS depression; the dose of one or both agents should be reduced). Products include:

Serentil 684

Methadone Hydrochloride (Co-administration may exhibit an additive CNS depression; the dose of one or both agents should be reduced). Products include:

Methadone Hydrochloride Oral Concentrate 2233
Methadone Hydrochloride Oral Solution & Tablets 2235

Methohexital Sodium (Co-administration may exhibit an additive CNS depression; the dose of one or both agents should be reduced). Products include:

Brevital Sodium Vials 1429

Methotrimeprazine (Co-administration may exhibit an additive CNS depression; the dose of one or both agents should be reduced). Products include:

Levoprome 1274

Methoxyflurane (Co-administration may exhibit an additive CNS depression; the dose of one or both agents should be reduced).

No products indexed under this heading.

Midazolam Hydrochloride (Co-administration may exhibit an additive CNS depression; the dose of one or both agents should be reduced). Products include:

Versed Injection 2170

Molindone Hydrochloride (Co-administration may exhibit an additive CNS depression; the dose of one or both agents should be reduced). Products include:

Moban Tablets and Concentrate 1048

Morphine Sulfate (Co-administration may exhibit an additive CNS depression; the dose of one or both agents should be reduced). Products include:

Astramorph/PF Injection, USP (Preservative-Free) 535
Duramorph 962
Infumorph 200 and Infumorph 500 Sterile Solutions 965
MS Contin Tablets 1994
MSIR 1997
Oramorph SR (Morphine Sulfate Sustained Release Tablets) 2236
RMS Suppositories 2657
Roxanol 2243

Opium Alkaloids (Co-administration may exhibit an additive CNS depression; the dose of one or both agents should be reduced).

No products indexed under this heading.

Oxazepam (Co-administration may exhibit an additive CNS depression; the dose of one or both agents should be reduced). Products include:

Serax Capsules 2810
Serax Tablets 2810

Oxycodone Hydrochloride (Co-administration may exhibit an additive CNS depression; the dose of one or both agents should be reduced). Products include:

Percocet Tablets 938
Percodan Tablets 939
Percodan-Demi Tablets 940
Roxicodone Tablets, Oral Solution & Intensol (Oxycodone) 2244
Tylox Capsules 1584

Pentobarbital Sodium (Co-administration may exhibit an additive CNS depression; the dose of one or both agents should be reduced). Products include:

Nembutal Sodium Capsules 436
Nembutal Sodium Solution 438
Nembutal Sodium Suppositories 440

Perphenazine (Co-administration may exhibit an additive CNS depression; the dose of one or both agents should be reduced). Products include:

Etrafon 2355
Triavil Tablets 1757
Trilafon 2389

Phenobarbital (Co-administration may exhibit an additive CNS depression; the dose of one or both agents should be reduced). Products include:

Arco-Lase Plus Tablets 512
Bellergal-S Tablets 2250
Donnatal 2060
Donnatal Extentabs 2061
Donnatal Tablets 2060
Phenobarbital Elixir and Tablets 1469
Quadrinal Tablets 1350

Prazepam (Co-administration may exhibit an additive CNS depression; the dose of one or both agents should be reduced).

No products indexed under this heading.

Prochlorperazine (Co-administration may exhibit an additive CNS depression; the dose of one or both agents should be reduced). Products include:

Compazine 2470

Promethazine Hydrochloride (Co-administration may exhibit an additive CNS depression; the dose of one or both agents should be reduced). Products include:

Mepergan Injection 2753
Phenergan with Codeine 2777
Phenergan with Dextromethorphan 2778
Phenergan Injection 2773
Phenergan Suppositories 2775
Phenergan Syrup 2774
Phenergan Tablets 2775
Phenergan VC 2779
Phenergan VC with Codeine 2781

Propofol (Co-administration may exhibit an additive CNS depression; the dose of one or both agents should be reduced). Products include:

Diprivan Injection 2833

Propoxyphene Hydrochloride (Co-administration may exhibit an additive CNS depression; the dose of one or both agents should be reduced). Products include:

Darvon 1435
Wygesic Tablets 2827

Propoxyphene Napsylate (Co-administration may exhibit an additive CNS depression; the dose of one or both agents should be reduced). Products include:

Darvon-N/Darvocet-N 1433

IMPORTANT NOTE: Always consult each drug listing in the patient's regimen for possible interactions.

Quazepam (Co-administration may exhibit an additive CNS depression; the dose of one or both agents should be reduced). Products include:

Doral Tablets 2664

Risperidone (Co-administration may exhibit an additive CNS depression; the dose of one or both agents should be reduced). Products include:

Risperdal 1301

Secobarbital Sodium (Co-administration may exhibit an additive CNS depression; the dose of one or both agents should be reduced). Products include:

Seconal Sodium Pulvules 1474

Sufentanil Citrate (Co-administration may exhibit an additive CNS depression; the dose of one or both agents should be reduced). Products include:

Sufenta Injection 1309

Temazepam (Co-administration may exhibit an additive CNS depression; the dose of one or both agents should be reduced). Products include:

Restoril Capsules 2284

Thiamylal Sodium (Co-administration may exhibit an additive CNS depression; the dose of one or both agents should be reduced).

No products indexed under this heading.

Thioridazine Hydrochloride (Co-administration may exhibit an additive CNS depression; the dose of one or both agents should be reduced). Products include:

Mellaril 2269

Thiothixene (Co-administration may exhibit an additive CNS depression; the dose of one or both agents should be reduced). Products include:

Navane Capsules and Concentrate 2201
Navane Intramuscular 2202

Triazolam (Co-administration may exhibit an additive CNS depression; the dose of one or both agents should be reduced). Products include:

Halcion Tablets 2611

Trifluoperazine Hydrochloride (Co-administration may exhibit an additive CNS depression; the dose of one or both agents should be reduced). Products include:

Stelazine 2514

Zolpidem Tartrate (Co-administration may exhibit an additive CNS depression; the dose of one or both agents should be reduced). Products include:

Ambien Tablets 2416

Food Interactions

Alcohol (Co-administration may exhibit an additive CNS depression).

VICON FORTE CAPSULES

(Vitamins with Minerals) 2571
None cited in PDR database.

VIDEX TABLETS, POWDER FOR ORAL SOLUTION, & PEDIATRIC POWDER FOR ORAL SOLUTION

(Didanosine) 720
May interact with drugs whose absorption can be affected by the level of gastric acidity (selected), drugs that are known to cause peripheral neuropathy and pancreatitis (selected), tetracyclines, antacids, and certain other agents. Compounds in these categories include:

Altretamine (Increased risk of toxicity due to peripheral neuropathy and pancreatitis). Products include:

Hexalen Capsules 2571

Aluminum Carbonate Gel (Potential for adverse effects associated with the antacid components). Products include:

Basaljel 2703

Aluminum Hydroxide (Potential for adverse effects associated with the antacid components). Products include:

ALternaGEL Liquid 1316
Maximum Strength Ascriptin .... ▣ 630
Cama Arthritis Pain Reliever .... ▣ 785
Gaviscon Extra Strength Relief Formula Antacid Tablets .... ▣ 819
Gaviscon Extra Strength Relief Formula Liquid Antacid .... ▣ 819
Gaviscon Liquid Antacid .... ▣ 820
Gelusil Liquid & Tablets .... ▣ 855
Maalox Heartburn Relief Suspension .... ▣ 642
Maalox Heartburn Relief Tablets .... ▣ 641
Maalox Magnesia and Alumina Oral Suspension .... ▣ 642
Maalox Plus Tablets .... ▣ 643
Extra Strength Maalox Antacid Plus Antigas Liquid and Tablets ▣ 638
Tempo Soft Antacid .... ▣ 835

Aluminum Hydroxide Gel (Potential for adverse effects associated with the antacid components). Products include:

ALternaGEL Liquid .... ▣ 659
Aludrox Oral Suspension 2695
Amphojel Suspension 2695
Amphojel Suspension without Flavor 2695
Amphojel Tablets 2695
Arthritis Pain Ascriptin .... ▣ 631
Regular Strength Ascriptin Tablets .... ▣ 629
Gaviscon Antacid Tablets .... ▣ 819
Gaviscon-2 Antacid Tablets .... ▣ 820
Mylanta Liquid 1317
Mylanta Tablets .... ▣ 660
Mylanta Double Strength Liquid 1317
Mylanta Double Strength Tablets .. ▣ 660
Nephrox Suspension .... ▣ 655

Auranofin (Increased risk of toxicity due to peripheral neuropathy and pancreatitis). Products include:

Ridaura Capsules 2513

Carboplatin (Increased risk of toxicity due to peripheral neuropathy and pancreatitis). Products include:

Paraplatin for Injection 705

Chloramphenicol (Increased risk of toxicity due to peripheral neuropathy and pancreatitis). Products include:

Chloromycetin Ophthalmic Ointment, 1% .... ⊙ 310
Chloromycetin Ophthalmic Solution .... ⊙ 310
Chloroptic S.O.P. .... ⊙ 239
Chloroptic Sterile Ophthalmic Solution .... ⊙ 239
Elase-Chloromycetin Ointment 1040
Ophthocort .... ⊙ 311

Chloramphenicol Palmitate (Increased risk of toxicity due to peripheral neuropathy and pancreatitis).

No products indexed under this heading.

Chloramphenicol Sodium Succinate (Increased risk of toxicity due to peripheral neuropathy and pancreatitis). Products include:

Chloromycetin Sodium Succinate 1900

Ciprofloxacin (Potential for decreased plasma concentrations of some quinolone antibiotics). Products include:

Cipro I.V. 595
Cipro I.V. Pharmacy Bulk Package .. 597

Ciprofloxacin Hydrochloride (Potential for decreased plasma concentrations of some quinolone antibiotics). Products include:

Ciloxan Ophthalmic Solution 472
Cipro Tablets 592

Cisplatin (Increased risk of toxicity due to peripheral neuropathy and pancreatitis). Products include:

Platinol 708
Platinol-AQ Injection 710

Dapsone (Increased risk of toxicity due to peripheral neuropathy and pancreatitis; gastric absorption affected by Videx; Dapsone should be administered at least 2 hours prior to dosing with Videx). Products include:

Dapsone Tablets USP 1284

Demeclocycline Hydrochloride (Concurrent administration should be avoided). Products include:

Declomycin Tablets 1371

Dihydroxyaluminum Sodium Carbonate (Potential for adverse effects associated with the antacid components).

No products indexed under this heading.

Disulfiram (Increased risk of toxicity due to peripheral neuropathy and pancreatitis). Products include:

Antabuse Tablets 2695

Doxycycline Calcium (Concurrent administration should be avoided). Products include:

Vibramycin Calcium Oral Suspension Syrup 1941

Doxycycline Hyclate (Concurrent administration should be avoided). Products include:

Doryx Capsules 1913
Vibramycin Hyclate Capsules 1941
Vibramycin Hyclate Intravenous 2215
Vibra-Tabs Film Coated Tablets 1941

Doxycycline Monohydrate (Concurrent administration should be avoided). Products include:

Monodox Capsules 1805
Vibramycin Monohydrate for Oral Suspension 1941

Ethionamide (Increased risk of toxicity due to peripheral neuropathy and pancreatitis). Products include:

Trecator-SC Tablets 2814

Glutethimide (Increased risk of toxicity due to peripheral neuropathy and pancreatitis).

No products indexed under this heading.

Gold Sodium Thiomalate (Increased risk of toxicity due to peripheral neuropathy and pancreatitis). Products include:

Myochrysine Injection 1711

Hydralazine Hydrochloride (Increased risk of toxicity due to peripheral neuropathy and pancreatitis). Products include:

Apresazide Capsules 808
Apresoline Hydrochloride Tablets .. 809
Ser-Ap-Es Tablets 849

Iodoquinol (Increased risk of toxicity due to peripheral neuropathy and pancreatitis). Products include:

Yodoxin 1230

Isoniazid (Increased risk of toxicity due to peripheral neuropathy and pancreatitis). Products include:

Nydrazid Injection 508
Rifamate Capsules 1530
Rifater 1532

Ketoconazole (Gastric absorption affected by Videx; Dapsone should be administered at least 2 hours prior to dosing with Videx). Products include:

Nizoral 2% Cream 1297
Nizoral 2% Shampoo 1298
Nizoral Tablets 1298

Leuprolide Acetate (Increased risk of toxicity due to peripheral neuropathy and pancreatitis). Products include:

Lupron Depot 3.75 mg 2556
Lupron Depot 7.5 mg 2559
Lupron Depot-PED 7.5 mg, 11.25 mg and 15 mg 2560
Lupron Injection 2555

Magaldrate (Potential for adverse effects associated with the antacid components).

No products indexed under this heading.

Magnesium Hydroxide (Potential for adverse effects associated with the antacid components). Products include:

Aludrox Oral Suspension 2695
Arthritis Pain Ascriptin .... ▣ 631
Maximum Strength Ascriptin .... ▣ 630
Regular Strength Ascriptin Tablets .... ▣ 629
Di-Gel Antacid/Anti-Gas .... ▣ 801
Gelusil Liquid & Tablets .... ▣ 855
Maalox Magnesia and Alumina Oral Suspension .... ▣ 642
Maalox Plus Tablets .... ▣ 643
Extra Strength Maalox Antacid Plus Antigas Liquid and Tablets ▣ 638
Mylanta Calcium Carbonate and Magnesium Hydroxide Tablets...... 1318
Mylanta Liquid 1317
Mylanta Tablets .... ▣ 660
Mylanta Double Strength Liquid 1317
Mylanta Double Strength Tablets .. ▣ 660
Phillips' Milk of Magnesia Liquid .... ▣ 729
Rolaids Tablets .... ▣ 843
Tempo Soft Antacid .... ▣ 835

Magnesium Oxide (Potential for adverse effects associated with the antacid components). Products include:

Beelith Tablets 639
Bufferin Analgesic Tablets and Caplets .... ▣ 613
Caltrate PLUS .... ▣ 665
Cama Arthritis Pain Reliever .... ▣ 785
Mag-Ox 400 668
Uro-Mag 668

Methacycline Hydrochloride (Concurrent administration should be avoided).

No products indexed under this heading.

Metronidazole (Increased risk of toxicity due to peripheral neuropathy and pancreatitis). Products include:

Flagyl 375 Capsules 2434
Flagyl I.V. RTU 2247
MetroGel 1047
MetroGel-Vaginal 902
Protostat Tablets 1883

Minocycline Hydrochloride (Concurrent administration should be avoided). Products include:

Dynacin Capsules 1590
Minocin Intravenous 1382
Minocin Oral Suspension 1385
Minocin Pellet-Filled Capsules 1383

Nitrofurantoin (Increased risk of toxicity due to peripheral neuropathy and pancreatitis). Products include:

Macrodantin Capsules 1989

Norfloxacin (Potential for decreased plasma concentrations of some quinolone antibiotics). Products include:

Chibroxin Sterile Ophthalmic Solution 1617
Noroxin Tablets 1715
Noroxin Tablets 2048

Ofloxacin (Potential for decreased plasma concentrations of some quinolone antibiotics). Products include:

Floxin I.V. 1571
Floxin Tablets (200 mg, 300 mg, 400 mg) 1567
Ocuflox 481
Ocuflox .... ⊙ 246

(▣ Described in PDR For Nonprescription Drugs) (⊙ Described in PDR For Ophthalmology)

1157 Interactions Index Visken

Oxytetracycline Hydrochloride (Concurrent administration should be avoided). Products include:
- TERAK Ointment ⊙ 209
- Terra-Cortril Ophthalmic Suspension 2210
- Terramycin with Polymyxin B Sulfate Ophthalmic Ointment 2211
- Urobiotic-250 Capsules 2214

Pentamidine Isethionate (Increased risk of toxicity due to peripheral neuropathy and pancreatitis). Products include:
- NebuPent for Inhalation Solution 1040
- Pentam 300 Injection 1041

Phenytoin (Increased risk of toxicity due to peripheral neuropathy and pancreatitis). Products include:
- Dilantin Infatabs 1908
- Dilantin-125 Suspension 1911

Phenytoin Sodium (Increased risk of toxicity due to peripheral neuropathy and pancreatitis). Products include:
- Dilantin Kapseals 1906
- Dilantin Parenteral 1910

Ribavirin (Increased risk of toxicity due to peripheral neuropathy and pancreatitis). Products include:
- Virazole 1264

Sulfamethoxazole (Increased risk of toxicity due to peripheral neuropathy and pancreatitis). Products include:
- Azo Gantanol Tablets 2080
- Bactrim DS Tablets 2084
- Bactrim I.V. Infusion 2082
- Bactrim 2084
- Gantanol Tablets 2119
- Septra 1174
- Septra I.V. Infusion 1169
- Septra I.V. Infusion ADD-Vantage Vials 1171
- Septra 1174

Tetracycline Hydrochloride (Concurrent administration should be avoided). Products include:
- Achromycin V Capsules 1367

Vincristine Sulfate (Increased risk of toxicity due to peripheral neuropathy and pancreatitis). Products include:
- Oncovin Solution Vials & Hyporets 1466

Food Interactions

Food, unspecified (Reduces the absorption of Videx by 50%; administer Videx on an empty stomach).

VIOKASE POWDER
(Pancrelipase) 2076
None cited in PDR database.

VIOKASE TABLETS
(Pancrelipase) 2076
None cited in PDR database.

VIRA-A OPHTHALMIC OINTMENT, 3%
(Vidarabine) ⊙ 312
None cited in PDR database.

VIRAZOLE
(Ribavirin) 1264
None cited in PDR database.

VIROPTIC OPHTHALMIC SOLUTION, 1% STERILE
(Trifluridine) 1204
None cited in PDR database.

VISINE MAXIMUM STRENGTH ALLERGY RELIEF
(Tetrahydrozoline Hydrochloride) ⊙ 313
None cited in PDR database.

VISINE MOISTURIZING EYE DROPS
(Tetrahydrozoline Hydrochloride) ⊙ 313
None cited in PDR database.

VISINE ORIGINAL EYE DROPS
(Tetrahydrozoline Hydrochloride) ⊙ 314
None cited in PDR database.

VISINE L.R. EYE DROPS
(Oxymetazoline Hydrochloride) ⊙ 313
None cited in PDR database.

VISKEN TABLETS
(Pindolol) 2299
May interact with general anesthetics, insulin, oral hypoglycemic agents, catecholamine depleting drugs, beta$_2$ agonists, and certain other agents. Compounds in these categories include:

Acarbose (Beta-blockade reduces the release of insulin in response to hyperglycemia; adjust the dose of antidiabetic drugs).
- No products indexed under this heading.

Albuterol (Beta-blockade may block bronchodilation produced by exogenous catecholamine stimulation of beta$_2$ receptors). Products include:
- Proventil Inhalation Aerosol 2382
- Ventolin Inhalation Aerosol and Refill 1197

Albuterol Sulfate (Beta-blockade may block bronchodilation produced by exogenous catecholamine stimulation of beta$_2$ receptors). Products include:
- Airet Solution for Inhalation 452
- Proventil Inhalation Solution 0.083% 2384
- Proventil Repetabs Tablets 2386
- Proventil Solution for Inhalation 0.5% 2383
- Proventil Syrup 2385
- Proventil Tablets 2386
- Ventolin Inhalation Solution 1198
- Ventolin Nebules Inhalation Solution 1199
- Ventolin Rotacaps for Inhalation 1200
- Ventolin Syrup 1202
- Ventolin Tablets 1203
- Volmax Extended-Release Tablets 1788

Bitolterol Mesylate (Beta-blockade may block bronchodilation produced by exogenous catecholamine stimulation of beta$_2$ receptors). Products include:
- Tornalate Solution for Inhalation, 0.2% 956
- Tornalate Metered Dose Inhaler 957

Chlorpropamide (Beta-blockade reduces the release of insulin in response to hyperglycemia; adjust the dose of antidiabetic drugs). Products include:
- Diabinese Tablets 1935

Deserpidine (Potential for additive effect; observe patients for evidence of hypotension, and/or bradycardia, vertigo, syncope, or postural hypotension).
- No products indexed under this heading.

Enflurane (Risks of general anesthesia increased).
- No products indexed under this heading.

Ephedrine Hydrochloride (Beta-blockade may block bronchodilation produced by exogenous catecholamine stimulation of beta$_2$ receptors). Products include:
- Primatene Dual Action Formula ▣ 872
- Primatene Tablets ▣ 873
- Quadrinal Tablets 1350

Ephedrine Sulfate (Beta-blockade may block bronchodilation produced by exogenous catecholamine stimulation of beta$_2$ receptors). Products include:
- Bronkaid Caplets ▣ 717
- Marax Tablets & DF Syrup 2200

Ephedrine Tannate (Beta-blockade may block bronchodilation produced by exogenous catecholamine stimulation of beta$_2$ receptors). Products include:
- Rynatuss 2673

Epinephrine (Patients with a history of severe anaphylactic reaction may be unresponsive to the usual dose of epinephrine used to treat allergy; Beta-blockade may block bronchodilation produced by exogenous catecholamine stimulation of beta$_2$ receptors). Products include:
- Bronkaid Mist ▣ 717
- EPIFRIN ⊙ 239
- EpiPen 790
- Marcaine Hydrochloride with Epinephrine 1:200,000 2316
- Primatene Mist ▣ 873
- Sensorcaine with Epinephrine Injection 559
- Sus-Phrine Injection 1019
- Xylocaine with Epinephrine Injections 567

Epinephrine Hydrochloride (Patients with a history of severe anaphylactic reaction may be unresponsive to the usual dose of epinephrine used to treat allergy; Beta-blockade may block bronchodilation produced by exogenous catecholamine stimulation of beta$_2$ receptors). Products include:
- Ana-Kit Anaphylaxis Emergency Treatment Kit 617

Ethylnorepinephrine Hydrochloride (Beta-blockade may block bronchodilation produced by exogenous catecholamine stimulation of beta$_2$ receptors).
- No products indexed under this heading.

Glipizide (Beta-blockade reduces the release of insulin in response to hyperglycemia; adjust the dose of antidiabetic drugs). Products include:
- Glucotrol Tablets 1967
- Glucotrol XL Extended Release Tablets 1968

Glyburide (Beta-blockade reduces the release of insulin in response to hyperglycemia; adjust the dose of antidiabetic drugs). Products include:
- DiaBeta Tablets 1239
- Glynase PresTab Tablets 2609
- Micronase Tablets 2623

Guanethidine Monosulfate (Potential for additive effect; observe patients for evidence of hypotension, and/or bradycardia, vertigo, syncope or postural hypotension). Products include:
- Esimil Tablets 822
- Ismelin Tablets 827

Insulin, Human (Beta-blockade reduces the release of insulin in response to hyperglycemia; adjust the dose of antidiabetic drugs).
- No products indexed under this heading.

Insulin, Human Isophane Suspension (Beta-blockade reduces the release of insulin in response to hyperglycemia; adjust the dose of antidiabetic drugs). Products include:
- Novolin N Human Insulin 10 ml Vials 1795

Insulin, Human NPH (Beta-blockade reduces the release of insulin in response to hyperglycemia; adjust the dose of antidiabetic drugs). Products include:
- Humulin N, 100 Units 1448
- Novolin N PenFill Cartridges Durable Insulin Delivery System 1798
- Novolin N Prefilled Syringe Disposable Insulin Delivery System 1798

Insulin, Human Regular (Beta-blockade reduces the release of insulin in response to hyperglycemia; adjust the dose of antidiabetic drugs). Products include:
- Humulin R, 100 Units 1449
- Novolin R Human Insulin 10 ml Vials 1795
- Novolin R PenFill Cartridges Durable Insulin Delivery System 1798
- Novolin R Prefilled Syringe Disposable Insulin Delivery System 1798
- Velosulin BR Human Insulin 10 ml Vials 1795

Insulin, Human, Zinc Suspension (Beta-blockade reduces the release of insulin in response to hyperglycemia; adjust the dose of antidiabetic drugs). Products include:
- Humulin L, 100 Units 1446
- Humulin U, 100 Units 1450
- Novolin L Human Insulin 10 ml Vials 1795

Insulin, NPH (Beta-blockade reduces the release of insulin in response to hyperglycemia; adjust the dose of antidiabetic drugs). Products include:
- NPH, 100 Units 1450
- Pork NPH, 100 Units 1452
- Purified Pork NPH Isophane Insulin 1801

Insulin, Regular (Beta-blockade reduces the release of insulin in response to hyperglycemia; adjust the dose of antidiabetic drugs). Products include:
- Regular, 100 Units 1450
- Pork Regular, 100 Units 1452
- Pork Regular (Concentrated), 500 Units 1453
- Purified Pork Regular Insulin 1801

Insulin, Zinc Crystals (Beta-blockade reduces the release of insulin in response to hyperglycemia; adjust the dose of antidiabetic drugs). Products include:
- NPH, 100 Units 1450

Insulin, Zinc Suspension (Beta-blockade reduces the release of insulin in response to hyperglycemia; adjust the dose of antidiabetic drugs). Products include:
- Iletin I 1450
- Lente, 100 Units 1450
- Iletin II 1452
- Pork Lente, 100 Units 1452
- Purified Pork Lente Insulin 1801

Isoetharine (Beta-blockade may block bronchodilation produced by exogenous catecholamine stimulation of beta$_2$ receptors). Products include:
- Bronkometer Aerosol 2302
- Bronkosol Solution 2302
- Isoetharine Inhalation Solution, USP, Arm-a-Med 551

Isoflurane (Risks of general anesthesia increased).
- No products indexed under this heading.

Isoproterenol Hydrochloride (Beta-blockade may block bronchodilation produced by exogenous catecholamine stimulation of beta$_2$ receptors). Products include:
- Isuprel Hydrochloride Injection 1:5000 2311
- Isuprel Hydrochloride Solution 1:200 & 1:100 2313
- Isuprel Mistometer 2312

IMPORTANT NOTE: Always consult each drug listing in the patient's regimen for possible interactions.

Visken **Interactions Index** 1158

Isoproterenol Sulfate (Beta-blockade may block bronchodilation produced by exogenous catecholamine stimulation of $beta_2$ receptors). Products include:

Norisodrine with Calcium Iodide Syrup ... 442

Ketamine Hydrochloride (Risks of general anesthesia increased).

No products indexed under this heading.

Metaproterenol Sulfate (Beta-blockade may block bronchodilation produced by exogenous catecholamine stimulation of $beta_2$ receptors). Products include:

Alupent ... 669
Metaproterenol Sulfate Inhalation Solution, USP, Arm-a-Med ... 552

Metformin Hydrochloride (Beta-blockade reduces the release of insulin in response to hyperglycemia; adjust the dose of antidiabetic drugs). Products include:

Glucophage ... 752

Methohexital Sodium (Risks of general anesthesia increased). Products include:

Brevital Sodium Vials ... 1429

Methoxyflurane (Risks of general anesthesia increased).

No products indexed under this heading.

Pirbuterol Acetate (Beta-blockade may block bronchodilation produced by exogenous catecholamine stimulation of $beta_2$ receptors). Products include:

Maxair Autohaler ... 1492
Maxair Inhaler ... 1494

Propofol (Risks of general anesthesia increased). Products include:

Diprivan Injection ... 2833

Rauwolfia Serpentina (Potential for additive effect; observe patients for evidence of hypotension, and/or bradycardia, vertigo, syncope, or postural hypotension).

No products indexed under this heading.

Rescinnamine (Potential for additive effect; observe patients for evidence of hypotension, and/or bradycardia, vertigo, syncope, or postural hypotension).

No products indexed under this heading.

Reserpine (Potential for additive effect; observe patients for evidence of hypotension, and/or bradycardia, vertigo, syncope, or postural hypotension). Products include:

Diupres Tablets ... 1650
Hydropres Tablets ... 1675
Ser-Ap-Es Tablets ... 849

Salmeterol Xinafoate (Beta-blockade may block bronchodilation produced by exogenous catecholamine stimulation of $beta_2$ receptors). Products include:

Serevent Inhalation Aerosol ... 1176

Terbutaline Sulfate (Beta-blockade may block bronchodilation produced by exogenous catecholamine stimulation of $beta_2$ receptors). Products include:

Brethaire Inhaler ... 813
Brethine Ampuls ... 815
Brethine Tablets ... 814
Bricanyl Subcutaneous Injection ... 1502
Bricanyl Tablets ... 1503

Thioridazine Hydrochloride (Increased serum levels of both drugs). Products include:

Mellaril ... 2269

Tolazamide (Beta-blockade reduces the release of insulin in response to hyperglycemia; adjust the dose of antidiabetic drugs).

No products indexed under this heading.

Tolbutamide (Beta-blockade reduces the release of insulin in response to hyperglycemia; adjust the dose of antidiabetic drugs).

No products indexed under this heading.

VISTARIL CAPSULES
(Hydroxyzine Pamoate) ... 1944

May interact with barbiturates, preanesthetic medications, narcotic analgesics, central nervous system depressants, hypnotics and sedatives, benzodiazepines, and certain other agents. Compounds in these categories include:

Alfentanil Hydrochloride (Potentiation of narcotics). Products include:

Alfenta Injection ... 1286

Alprazolam (Potentiation of CNS depression). Products include:

Xanax Tablets ... 2649

Aprobarbital (Potentiation of barbiturates).

No products indexed under this heading.

Buprenorphine (Potentiation of narcotics). Products include:

Buprenex Injectable ... 2006

Buspirone Hydrochloride (Potentiation of CNS depression). Products include:

BuSpar ... 737

Butabarbital (Potentiation of barbiturates).

No products indexed under this heading.

Butalbital (Potentiation of barbiturates). Products include:

Esgic-plus Tablets ... 1013
Fioricet Tablets ... 2258
Fioricet with Codeine Capsules ... 2260
Fiorinal Capsules ... 2261
Fiorinal with Codeine Capsules ... 2262
Fiorinal Tablets ... 2261
Phrenilin ... 785
Sedapap Tablets 50 mg/650 mg ... 1543

Chlordiazepoxide (Potentiation of CNS depression). Products include:

Libritabs Tablets ... 2177
Limbitrol ... 2180

Chlordiazepoxide Hydrochloride (Potentiation of CNS depression). Products include:

Librax Capsules ... 2176
Librium Capsules ... 2178
Librium Injectable ... 2179

Chlorpromazine (Potentiation of CNS depression). Products include:

Thorazine Suppositories ... 2523

Chlorprothixene (Potentiation of CNS depression).

No products indexed under this heading.

Chlorprothixene Hydrochloride (Potentiation of CNS depression).

No products indexed under this heading.

Chlorprothixene Lactate (Potentiation of CNS depression).

No products indexed under this heading.

Clorazepate Dipotassium (Potentiation of CNS depression). Products include:

Tranxene ... 451

Clozapine (Potentiation of narcotics). Products include:

Clozaril Tablets ... 2252

Codeine Phosphate (Potentiation of narcotics). Products include:

Actifed with Codeine Cough Syrup ... 1067
Brontex ... 1981
Deconsal C Expectorant Syrup ... 456
Deconsal Pediatric Syrup ... 457
Dimetane-DC Cough Syrup ... 2059
Empirin with Codeine Tablets ... 1093
Fioricet with Codeine Capsules ... 2260
Fiorinal with Codeine Capsules ... 2262
Isoclor Expectorant ... 990
Novahistine DH ... 2462
Novahistine Expectorant ... 2463
Nucofed ... 2051
Phenergan with Codeine ... 2777
Phenergan VC with Codeine ... 2781
Robitussin A-C Syrup ... 2073
Robitussin-DAC Syrup ... 2074
Ryna ... ⊡ 841
Soma Compound w/Codeine Tablets ... 2676
Tussi-Organidin NR Liquid and S NR Liquid ... 2677
Tylenol with Codeine ... 1583

Desflurane (Potentiation of narcotics). Products include:

Suprane ... 1813

Dezocine (Potentiation of narcotics). Products include:

Dalgan Injection ... 538

Diazepam (Potentiation of CNS depression). Products include:

Dizac ... 1809
Valium Injectable ... 2182
Valium Tablets ... 2183
Valrelease Capsules ... 2169

Droperidol (Potentiation of CNS depression). Products include:

Inapsine Injection ... 1296

Enflurane (Potentiation of CNS depression).

No products indexed under this heading.

Epinephrine (Pressor action counteracted). Products include:

Bronkaid Mist ... ⊡ 717
EPIFRIN ... ⊙ 239
EpiPen ... 790
Marcaine Hydrochloride with Epinephrine 1:200,000 ... 2316
Primatene Mist ... ⊡ 873
Sensorcaine with Epinephrine Injection ... 559
Sus-Phrine Injection ... 1019
Xylocaine with Epinephrine Injections ... 567

Estazolam (Potentiation of CNS depression). Products include:

ProSom Tablets ... 449

Ethchlorvynol (Potentiation of CNS depression). Products include:

Placidyl Capsules ... 448

Ethinamate (Potentiation of CNS depression).

No products indexed under this heading.

Fentanyl (Potentiation of narcotics). Products include:

Duragesic Transdermal System ... 1288

Fentanyl Citrate (Potentiation of narcotics). Products include:

Sublimaze Injection ... 1307

Fluphenazine Decanoate (Potentiation of CNS depression). Products include:

Prolixin Decanoate ... 509

Fluphenazine Enanthate (Potentiation of CNS depression). Products include:

Prolixin Enanthate ... 509

Fluphenazine Hydrochloride (Potentiation of CNS depression). Products include:

Prolixin ... 509

Flurazepam Hydrochloride (Potentiation of CNS depression). Products include:

Dalmane Capsules ... 2173

Glutethimide (Potentiation of CNS depression).

No products indexed under this heading.

Halazepam (Potentiation of CNS depression).

No products indexed under this heading.

Haloperidol (Potentiation of CNS depression). Products include:

Haldol Injection, Tablets and Concentrate ... 1575

Haloperidol Decanoate (Potentiation of CNS depression). Products include:

Haldol Decanoate ... 1577

Hydrocodone Bitartrate (Potentiation of narcotics). Products include:

Anexsia 5/500 Elixir ... 1781
Anexia Tablets ... 1782
Codiclear DH Syrup ... 791
Deconamine CX Cough and Cold Liquid and Tablets ... 1319
Duratuss HD Elixir ... 2565
Hycodan Tablets and Syrup ... 930
Hycomine Compound Tablets ... 932
Hycomine ... 931
Hycotuss Expectorant Syrup ... 933
Hydrocet Capsules ... 782
Lorcet 10/650 ... 1018
Lortab ... 2566
Tussend ... 1783
Tussend Expectorant ... 1785
Vicodin Tablets ... 1356
Vicodin ES Tablets ... 1357
Vicodin Tuss Expectorant ... 1358
Zydone Capsules ... 949

Hydrocodone Polistirex (Potentiation of narcotics). Products include:

Tussionex Pennkinetic Extended-Release Suspension ... 998

Hydroxyzine Hydrochloride (Potentiation of narcotics). Products include:

Atarax Tablets & Syrup ... 2185
Marax Tablets & DF Syrup ... 2200
Vistaril Intramuscular Solution ... 2216

Isoflurane (Potentiation of CNS depression).

No products indexed under this heading.

Ketamine Hydrochloride (Potentiation of CNS depression).

No products indexed under this heading.

Levomethadyl Acetate Hydrochloride (Potentiation of narcotics). Products include:

Orlamm ... 2239

Levorphanol Tartrate (Potentiation of narcotics). Products include:

Levo-Dromoran ... 2129

Lorazepam (Potentiation of CNS depression). Products include:

Ativan Injection ... 2698
Ativan Tablets ... 2700

Loxapine Hydrochloride (Potentiation of CNS depression). Products include:

Loxitane ... 1378

Loxapine Succinate (Potentiation of CNS depression). Products include:

Loxitane Capsules ... 1378

Meperidine Hydrochloride (Potentiation of meperidine). Products include:

Demerol ... 2308
Mepergan Injection ... 2753

Mephobarbital (Potentiation of barbiturates). Products include:

Mebaral Tablets ... 2322

Meprobamate (Potentiation of CNS depression). Products include:

Miltown Tablets ... 2672
PMB 200 and PMB 400 ... 2783

Mesoridazine Besylate (Potentiation of CNS depression). Products include:

Serentil ... 684

(⊡ Described in PDR For Nonprescription Drugs) (⊙ Described in PDR For Ophthalmology)

Interactions Index

Methadone Hydrochloride (Potentiation of narcotics). Products include:

Methadone Hydrochloride Oral Concentrate 2233

Methadone Hydrochloride Oral Solution & Tablets.............................. 2235

Methohexital Sodium (Potentiation of CNS depression). Products include:

Brevital Sodium Vials 1429

Methotrimeprazine (Potentiation of narcotics). Products include:

Levoprome 1274

Methoxyflurane (Potentiation of CNS depression).

No products indexed under this heading.

Midazolam Hydrochloride (Potentiation of CNS depression). Products include:

Versed Injection 2170

Molindone Hydrochloride (Potentiation of CNS depression). Products include:

Moban Tablets and Concentrate...... 1048

Morphine Sulfate (Potentiation of narcotics). Products include:

Astramorph/PF Injection, USP (Preservative-Free) 535

Duramorph 962

Infumorph 200 and Infumorph 500 Sterile Solutions 965

MS Contin Tablets............................... 1994

MSIR 1997

Oramorph SR (Morphine Sulfate Sustained Release Tablets) 2236

RMS Suppositories 2657

Roxanol 2243

Opium Alkaloids (Potentiation of narcotics).

No products indexed under this heading.

Oxazepam (Potentiation of CNS depression). Products include:

Serax Capsules 2810

Serax Tablets.. 2810

Oxycodone Hydrochloride (Potentiation of narcotics). Products include:

Percocet Tablets 938

Percodan Tablets................................. 939

Percodan-Demi Tablets....................... 940

Roxicodone Tablets, Oral Solution & Intensol (Oxycodone) 2244

Tylox Capsules 1584

Pentobarbital Sodium (Potentiation of barbiturates). Products include:

Nembutal Sodium Capsules 436

Nembutal Sodium Solution 438

Nembutal Sodium Suppositories...... 440

Perphenazine (Potentiation of CNS depression). Products include:

Etrafon 2355

Triavil Tablets 1757

Trilafon.. 2389

Phenobarbital (Potentiation of barbiturates). Products include:

Arco-Lase Plus Tablets 512

Bellergal-S Tablets 2250

Donnatal 2060

Donnatal Extentabs............................. 2061

Donnatal Tablets 2060

Phenobarbital Elixir and Tablets...... 1469

Quadrinal Tablets 1350

Prazepam (Potentiation of CNS depression).

No products indexed under this heading.

Prochlorperazine (Potentiation of CNS depression). Products include:

Compazine 2470

Promethazine Hydrochloride (Potentiation of CNS depression). Products include:

Mepergan Injection 2753

Phenergan with Codeine.................... 2777

Phenergan with Dextromethorphan 2778

Phenergan Injection 2773

Phenergan Suppositories 2775

Phenergan Syrup 2774

Phenergan Tablets 2775

Phenergan VC 2779

Phenergan VC with Codeine 2781

Propofol (Potentiation of narcotics). Products include:

Diprivan Injection................................ 2833

Propoxyphene Hydrochloride (Potentiation of narcotics). Products include:

Darvon 1435

Wygesic Tablets 2827

Propoxyphene Napsylate (Potentiation of narcotics). Products include:

Darvon-N/Darvocet-N 1433

Quazepam (Potentiation of CNS depression). Products include:

Doral Tablets 2664

Risperidone (Potentiation of narcotics). Products include:

Risperdal 1301

Secobarbital Sodium (Potentiation of barbiturates). Products include:

Seconal Sodium Pulvules 1474

Sufentanil Citrate (Potentiation of narcotics). Products include:

Sufenta Injection 1309

Temazepam (Potentiation of CNS depression). Products include:

Restoril Capsules 2284

Thiamylal Sodium (Potentiation of barbiturates).

No products indexed under this heading.

Thioridazine Hydrochloride (Potentiation of CNS depression). Products include:

Mellaril 2269

Thiothixene (Potentiation of barbiturates). Products include:

Navane Capsules and Concentrate 2201

Navane Intramuscular 2202

Triazolam (Potentiation of CNS depression). Products include:

Halcion Tablets.................................... 2611

Trifluoperazine Hydrochloride (Potentiation of CNS depression). Products include:

Stelazine 2514

Zolpidem Tartrate (Potentiation of narcotics). Products include:

Ambien Tablets.................................... 2416

Food Interactions

Alcohol (Increased effect of alcohol).

VISTARIL INTRAMUSCULAR SOLUTION

(Hydroxyzine Hydrochloride) 2216

May interact with central nervous system depressants, narcotic analgesics, barbiturates, and certain other agents. Compounds in these categories include:

Alfentanil Hydrochloride (May be potentiated; dosage should be decreased by up to 50%; rare potential for cardiac arrest and death). Products include:

Alfenta Injection 1286

Alprazolam (May be potentiated; dosage should be decreased by up to 50%; rare potential for cardiac arrest and death). Products include:

Xanax Tablets 2649

Aprobarbital (May be potentiated; dosage should be decreased by up to 50%; rare potential for cardiac arrest and death).

No products indexed under this heading.

Buprenorphine (May be potentiated; dosage should be decreased by up to 50%; rare potential for cardiac arrest and death). Products include:

Buprenex Injectable 2006

Buspirone Hydrochloride (May be potentiated; dosage should be decreased by up to 50%; rare potential for cardiac arrest and death). Products include:

BuSpar 737

Butabarbital (May be potentiated; dosage should be decreased by up to 50%; rare potential for cardiac arrest and death).

No products indexed under this heading.

Butalbital (May be potentiated; dosage should be decreased by up to 50%; rare potential for cardiac arrest and death). Products include:

Esgic-plus Tablets 1013

Fioricet Tablets.................................... 2258

Fioricet with Codeine Capsules 2260

Fiorinal Capsules 2261

Fiorinal with Codeine Capsules 2262

Fiorinal Tablets.................................... 2261

Phrenilin 785

Sedapap Tablets 50 mg/650 mg .. 1543

Chlordiazepoxide (May be potentiated; dosage should be decreased by up to 50%; rare potential for cardiac arrest and death). Products include:

Libritabs Tablets 2177

Limbitrol 2180

Chlordiazepoxide Hydrochloride (May be potentiated; dosage should be decreased by up to 50%; rare potential for cardiac arrest and death). Products include:

Librax Capsules 2176

Librium Capsules................................. 2178

Librium Injectable 2179

Chlorpromazine (May be potentiated; dosage should be decreased by up to 50%; rare potential for cardiac arrest and death). Products include:

Thorazine Suppositories..................... 2523

Chlorprothixene (May be potentiated; dosage should be decreased by up to 50%; rare potential for cardiac arrest and death).

No products indexed under this heading.

Chlorprothixene Hydrochloride (May be potentiated; dosage should be decreased by up to 50%; rare potential for cardiac arrest and death).

No products indexed under this heading.

Clorazepate Dipotassium (May be potentiated; dosage should be decreased by up to 50%; rare potential for cardiac arrest and death). Products include:

Tranxene 451

Clozapine (May be potentiated; dosage should be decreased by up to 50%; rare potential for cardiac arrest and death). Products include:

Clozaril Tablets.................................... 2252

Codeine Phosphate (May be potentiated; dosage should be decreased by up to 50%; rare potential for cardiac arrest and death). Products include:

Actifed with Codeine Cough Syrup.. 1067

Brontex 1981

Deconsal C Expectorant Syrup 456

Deconsal Pediatric Syrup 457

Dimetane-DC Cough Syrup 2059

Empirin with Codeine Tablets........... 1093

Fioricet with Codeine Capsules 2260

Fiorinal with Codeine Capsules 2262

Isoclor Expectorant............................. 990

Novahistine DH................................... 2462

Novahistine Expectorant.................... 2463

Nucofed 2051

Phenergan with Codeine.................... 2777

Phenergan VC with Codeine 2781

Robitussin A-C Syrup.......................... 2073

Robitussin-DAC Syrup 2074

Ryna .... ◙ 841

Soma Compound w/Codeine Tablets 2676

Tussi-Organidin NR Liquid and S NR Liquid 2677

Tylenol with Codeine 1583

Desflurane (May be potentiated; dosage should be decreased by up to 50%; rare potential for cardiac arrest and death). Products include:

Suprane 1813

Dezocine (May be potentiated; dosage should be decreased by up to 50%; rare potential for cardiac arrest and death). Products include:

Dalgan Injection 538

Diazepam (May be potentiated; dosage should be decreased by up to 50%; rare potential for cardiac arrest and death). Products include:

Dizac 1809

Valium Injectable 2182

Valium Tablets 2183

Valrelease Capsules 2169

Droperidol (May be potentiated; dosage should be decreased by up to 50%; rare potential for cardiac arrest and death). Products include:

Inapsine Injection................................ 1296

Enflurane (May be potentiated; dosage should be decreased by up to 50%; rare potential for cardiac arrest and death).

No products indexed under this heading.

Estazolam (May be potentiated; dosage should be decreased by up to 50%; rare potential for cardiac arrest and death). Products include:

ProSom Tablets 449

Ethchlorvynol (May be potentiated; dosage should be decreased by up to 50%; rare potential for cardiac arrest and death). Products include:

Placidyl Capsules................................. 448

Ethinamate (May be potentiated; dosage should be decreased by up to 50%; rare potential for cardiac arrest and death).

No products indexed under this heading.

Fentanyl (May be potentiated; dosage should be decreased by up to 50%; rare potential for cardiac arrest and death). Products include:

Duragesic Transdermal System........ 1288

Fentanyl Citrate (May be potentiated; dosage should be decreased by up to 50%; rare potential for cardiac arrest and death). Products include:

Sublimaze Injection............................. 1307

Fluphenazine Decanoate (May be potentiated; dosage should be decreased by up to 50%; rare potential for cardiac arrest and death). Products include:

Prolixin Decanoate 509

Fluphenazine Enanthate (May be potentiated; dosage should be decreased by up to 50%; rare potential for cardiac arrest and death). Products include:

Prolixin Enanthate 509

Fluphenazine Hydrochloride (May be potentiated; dosage should be decreased by up to 50%; rare potential for cardiac arrest and death). Products include:

Prolixin 509

Flurazepam Hydrochloride (May be potentiated; dosage should be decreased by up to 50%; rare potential for cardiac arrest and death). Products include:

Dalmane Capsules............................... 2173

IMPORTANT NOTE: Always consult each drug listing in the patient's regimen for possible interactions.

Glutethimide (May be potentiated; dosage should be decreased by up to 50%; rare potential for cardiac arrest and death).
No products indexed under this heading.

Haloperidol (May be potentiated; dosage should be decreased by up to 50%; rare potential for cardiac arrest and death). Products include:
Haldol Injection, Tablets and Concentrate 1575

Haloperidol Decanoate (May be potentiated; dosage should be decreased by up to 50%; rare potential for cardiac arrest and death). Products include:
Haldol Decanoate 1577

Hydrocodone Bitartrate (May be potentiated; dosage should be decreased by up to 50%; rare potential for cardiac arrest and death). Products include:
Anexsia 5/500 Elixir 1781
Anexia Tablets 1782
Codiclear DH Syrup 791
Deconamine CX Cough and Cold Liquid and Tablets 1319
Duratuss HD Elixir 2565
Hycodan Tablets and Syrup 930
Hycomine Compound Tablets 932
Hycomine 931
Hycotuss Expectorant Syrup 933
Hydrocet Capsules 782
Lorcet 10/650 1018
Lortab 2566
Tussend 1783
Tussend Expectorant 1785
Vicodin Tablets 1356
Vicodin ES Tablets 1357
Vicodin Tuss Expectorant 1358
Zydone Capsules 949

Hydrocodone Polistirex (May be potentiated; dosage should be decreased by up to 50%; rare potential for cardiac arrest and death). Products include:
Tussionex Pennkinetic Extended-Release Suspension 998

Isoflurane (May be potentiated; dosage should be decreased by up to 50%; rare potential for cardiac arrest and death).
No products indexed under this heading.

Ketamine Hydrochloride (May be potentiated; dosage should be decreased by up to 50%; rare potential for cardiac arrest and death).
No products indexed under this heading.

Levomethadyl Acetate Hydrochloride (May be potentiated; dosage should be decreased by up to 50%; rare potential for cardiac arrest and death). Products include:
Orlamm 2239

Levorphanol Tartrate (May be potentiated; dosage should be decreased by up to 50%; rare potential for cardiac arrest and death). Products include:
Levo-Dromoran 2129

Lorazepam (May be potentiated; dosage should be decreased by up to 50%; rare potential for cardiac arrest and death). Products include:
Ativan Injection 2698
Ativan Tablets 2700

Loxapine Hydrochloride (May be potentiated; dosage should be decreased by up to 50%; rare potential for cardiac arrest and death). Products include:
Loxitane 1378

Loxapine Succinate (May be potentiated; dosage should be decreased by up to 50%; rare potential for cardiac arrest and death). Products include:
Loxitane Capsules 1378

Meperidine Hydrochloride (May be potentiated; dosage should be decreased by up to 50%; rare potential for cardiac arrest and death). Products include:
Demerol 2308
Mepergan Injection 2753

Mephobarbital (May be potentiated; dosage should be decreased by up to 50%; rare potential for cardiac arrest and death). Products include:
Mebaral Tablets 2322

Meprobamate (May be potentiated; dosage should be decreased by up to 50%; rare potential for cardiac arrest and death). Products include:
Miltown Tablets 2672
PMB 200 and PMB 400 2783

Mesoridazine Besylate (May be potentiated; dosage should be decreased by up to 50%; rare potential for cardiac arrest and death). Products include:
Serentil 684

Methadone Hydrochloride (May be potentiated; dosage should be decreased by up to 50%; rare potential for cardiac arrest and death). Products include:
Methadone Hydrochloride Oral Concentrate 2233
Methadone Hydrochloride Oral Solution & Tablets 2235

Methohexital Sodium (May be potentiated; dosage should be decreased by up to 50%; rare potential for cardiac arrest and death). Products include:
Brevital Sodium Vials 1429

Methotrimeprazine (May be potentiated; dosage should be decreased by up to 50%; rare potential for cardiac arrest and death). Products include:
Levoprome 1274

Methoxyflurane (May be potentiated; dosage should be decreased by up to 50%; rare potential for cardiac arrest and death).
No products indexed under this heading.

Midazolam Hydrochloride (May be potentiated; dosage should be decreased by up to 50%; rare potential for cardiac arrest and death). Products include:
Versed Injection 2170

Molindone Hydrochloride (May be potentiated; dosage should be decreased by up to 50%; rare potential for cardiac arrest and death). Products include:
Moban Tablets and Concentrate 1048

Morphine Sulfate (May be potentiated; dosage should be decreased by up to 50%; rare potential for cardiac arrest and death). Products include:
Astramorph/PF Injection, USP (Preservative-Free) 535
Duramorph 962
Infumorph 200 and Infumorph 500 Sterile Solutions 965
MS Contin Tablets 1994
MSIR 1997
Oramorph SR (Morphine Sulfate Sustained Release Tablets) 2236
RMS Suppositories 2657
Roxanol 2243

Opium Alkaloids (May be potentiated; dosage should be decreased by up to 50%; rare potential for cardiac arrest and death).
No products indexed under this heading.

Oxazepam (May be potentiated; dosage should be decreased by up to 50%; rare potential for cardiac arrest and death). Products include:
Serax Capsules 2810
Serax Tablets 2810

Oxycodone Hydrochloride (May be potentiated; dosage should be decreased by up to 50%; rare potential for cardiac arrest and death). Products include:
Percocet Tablets 938
Percodan Tablets 939
Percodan-Demi Tablets 940
Roxicodone Tablets, Oral Solution & Intensol (Oxycodone) 2244
Tylox Capsules 1584

Pentobarbital Sodium (May be potentiated; dosage should be decreased by up to 50%; rare potential for cardiac arrest and death). Products include:
Nembutal Sodium Capsules 436
Nembutal Sodium Solution 438
Nembutal Sodium Suppositories 440

Perphenazine (May be potentiated; dosage should be decreased by up to 50%; rare potential for cardiac arrest and death). Products include:
Etrafon 2355
Triavil Tablets 1757
Trilafon 2389

Phenobarbital (May be potentiated; dosage should be decreased by up to 50%; rare potential for cardiac arrest and death). Products include:
Arco-Lase Plus Tablets 512
Bellergal-S Tablets 2250
Donnatal 2060
Donnatal Extentabs 2061
Donnatal Tablets 2060
Phenobarbital Elixir and Tablets 1469
Quadrinal Tablets 1350

Prazepam (May be potentiated; dosage should be decreased by up to 50%; rare potential for cardiac arrest and death).
No products indexed under this heading.

Prochlorperazine (May be potentiated; dosage should be decreased by up to 50%; rare potential for cardiac arrest and death). Products include:
Compazine 2470

Promethazine Hydrochloride (May be potentiated; dosage should be decreased by up to 50%; rare potential for cardiac arrest and death). Products include:
Mepergan Injection 2753
Phenergan with Codeine 2777
Phenergan with Dextromethorphan 2778
Phenergan Injection 2773
Phenergan Suppositories 2775
Phenergan Syrup 2774
Phenergan Tablets 2775
Phenergan VC 2779
Phenergan VC with Codeine 2781

Propofol (May be potentiated; dosage should be decreased by up to 50%; rare potential for cardiac arrest and death). Products include:
Diprivan Injection 2833

Propoxyphene Hydrochloride (May be potentiated; dosage should be decreased by up to 50%; rare potential for cardiac arrest and death). Products include:
Darvon 1435
Wygesic Tablets 2827

Propoxyphene Napsylate (May be potentiated; dosage should be decreased by up to 50%; rare potential for cardiac arrest and death). Products include:
Darvon-N/Darvocet-N 1433

Quazepam (May be potentiated; dosage should be decreased by up to 50%; rare potential for cardiac arrest and death). Products include:
Doral Tablets 2664

Risperidone (May be potentiated; dosage should be decreased by up to 50%; rare potential for cardiac arrest and death). Products include:
Risperdal 1301

Secobarbital Sodium (May be potentiated; dosage should be decreased by up to 50%; rare potential for cardiac arrest and death). Products include:
Seconal Sodium Pulvules 1474

Sufentanil Citrate (May be potentiated; dosage should be decreased by up to 50%; rare potential for cardiac arrest and death). Products include:
Sufenta Injection 1309

Temazepam (May be potentiated; dosage should be decreased by up to 50%; rare potential for cardiac arrest and death). Products include:
Restoril Capsules 2284

Thiamylal Sodium (May be potentiated; dosage should be decreased by up to 50%; rare potential for cardiac arrest and death).
No products indexed under this heading.

Thioridazine Hydrochloride (May be potentiated; dosage should be decreased by up to 50%; rare potential for cardiac arrest and death). Products include:
Mellaril 2269

Thiothixene (May be potentiated; dosage should be decreased by up to 50%; rare potential for cardiac arrest and death). Products include:
Navane Capsules and Concentrate 2201
Navane Intramuscular 2202

Triazolam (May be potentiated; dosage should be decreased by up to 50%; rare potential for cardiac arrest and death). Products include:
Halcion Tablets 2611

Trifluoperazine Hydrochloride (May be potentiated; dosage should be decreased by up to 50%; rare potential for cardiac arrest and death). Products include:
Stelazine 2514

Zolpidem Tartrate (May be potentiated; dosage should be decreased by up to 50%; rare potential for cardiac arrest and death). Products include:
Ambien Tablets 2416

Food Interactions

Alcohol (May be potentiated).

VISTARIL ORAL SUSPENSION
(Hydroxyzine Pamoate) 1944
See **Vistaril Capsules**

VITAL HIGH NITROGEN NUTRITIONALLY COMPLETE PARTIALLY HYDROLYZED DIET
(Nutritional Supplement) 2228
None cited in PDR database.

1161 **Interactions Index** **Vivactil**

VITAMIST INTRA-ORAL SPRAY DIETARY SUPPLEMENTS
(Vitamins with Minerals) 1542
None cited in PDR database.

VITRON-C TABLETS
(Ferrous Fumarate, Vitamin C) .... 🕮 650
May interact with tetracyclines. Compounds in this category include:

Demeclocycline Hydrochloride (Oral iron products interfere with absorption of oral tetracycline antibiotics; should not be taken within 2 hours of each other). Products include:
Declomycin Tablets 1371

Doxycycline Calcium (Oral iron products interfere with absorption of oral tetracycline antibiotics; should not be taken within 2 hours of each other). Products include:
Vibramycin Calcium Oral Suspension Syrup 1941

Doxycycline Hyclate (Oral iron products interfere with absorption of oral tetracycline antibiotics; should not be taken within 2 hours of each other). Products include:
Doryx Capsules 1913
Vibramycin Hyclate Capsules 1941
Vibramycin Hyclate Intravenous 2215
Vibra-Tabs Film Coated Tablets 1941

Doxycycline Monohydrate (Oral iron products interfere with absorption of oral tetracycline antibiotics; should not be taken within 2 hours of each other). Products include:
Monodox Capsules 1805
Vibramycin Monohydrate for Oral Suspension 1941

Methacycline Hydrochloride (Oral iron products interfere with absorption of oral tetracycline antibiotics; should not be taken within 2 hours of each other).
No products indexed under this heading.

Minocycline Hydrochloride (Oral iron products interfere with absorption of oral tetracycline antibiotics; should not be taken within 2 hours of each other). Products include:
Dynacin Capsules 1590
Minocin Intravenous 1382
Minocin Oral Suspension 1385
Minocin Pellet-Filled Capsules 1383

Oxytetracycline Hydrochloride (Oral iron products interfere with absorption of oral tetracycline antibiotics; should not be taken within 2 hours of each other). Products include:
TERAK Ointment .... ◉ 209
Terra-Cortril Ophthalmic Suspension 2210
Terramycin with Polymyxin B Sulfate Ophthalmic Ointment 2211
Urobiotic-250 Capsules 2214

Tetracycline Hydrochloride (Oral iron products interfere with absorption of oral tetracycline antibiotics; should not be taken within 2 hours of each other). Products include:
Achromycin V Capsules 1367

VIVA-DROPS
(Polysorbate 80) .... ◉ 325
None cited in PDR database.

VIVACTIL TABLETS
(Protriptyline Hydrochloride) 1774
May interact with barbiturates, central nervous system depressants, anticholinergics, antipsychotic agents, sympathomimetics, monoamine oxidase inhibitors, thyroid preparations, drugs that inhibit cytochrome p450iid6, antidepressant drugs, phenothiazines, selective serotonin reuptake inhibitors, and certain other agents. Compounds in these categories include:

Albuterol (Effects of concurrent use not specified; careful adjustment of dosage and close supervision are required). Products include:
Proventil Inhalation Aerosol 2382
Ventolin Inhalation Aerosol and Refill 1197

Albuterol Sulfate (Effects of concurrent use not specified; careful adjustment of dosage and close supervision are required). Products include:
Airet Solution for Inhalation 452
Proventil Inhalation Solution 0.083% 2384
Proventil Repetabs Tablets 2386
Proventil Solution for Inhalation 0.5% 2383
Proventil Syrup 2385
Proventil Tablets 2386
Ventolin Inhalation Solution 1198
Ventolin Nebules Inhalation Solution 1199
Ventolin Rotacaps for Inhalation 1200
Ventolin Syrup 1202
Ventolin Tablets 1203
Volmax Extended-Release Tablets .. 1788

Alfentanil Hydrochloride (Protriptyline may enhance the response to CNS depressants). Products include:
Alfenta Injection 1286

Alprazolam (Protriptyline may enhance the response to CNS depressants). Products include:
Xanax Tablets 2649

Amitriptyline Hydrochloride (Concurrent use with drugs that are substrate for cytochrome $P_{450}IID_6$ may make normal metabolizer resemble poor metabolizer leading to higher than expected plasma concentrations of TCA with resultant toxicity). Products include:
Elavil 2838
Endep Tablets 2174
Etrafon 2355
Limbitrol 2180
Triavil Tablets 1757

Amoxapine (Concurrent use with drugs that are substrate for cytochrome $P_{450}IID_6$ may make normal metabolizer resemble poor metabolizer leading to higher than expected plasma concentrations of TCA with resultant toxicity). Products include:
Asendin Tablets 1369

Aprobarbital (Protriptyline may enhance the response to CNS depressants).
No products indexed under this heading.

Atropine Sulfate (Concurrent use may result in hyperpyrexia, particularly in hot weather). Products include:
Arco-Lase Plus Tablets 512
Atrohist Plus Tablets 454
Atropine Sulfate Sterile Ophthalmic Solution .... ◉ 233
Donnatal 2060
Donnatal Extentabs 2061
Donnatal Tablets 2060
Lomotil 2439
Motofen Tablets 784
Urised Tablets 1964

Belladonna Alkaloids (Concurrent use may result in hyperpyrexia, particularly in hot weather). Products include:
Bellergal-S Tablets 2250
Hyland's Bed Wetting Tablets .... 🕮 828
Hyland's EnurAid Tablets .... 🕮 829
Hyland's Teething Tablets .... 🕮 830

Benztropine Mesylate (Concurrent use may result in hyperpyrexia, particularly in hot weather). Products include:
Cogentin 1621

Biperiden Hydrochloride (Concurrent use may result in hyperpyrexia, particularly in hot weather). Products include:
Akineton 1333

Buprenorphine (Protriptyline may enhance the response to CNS depressants). Products include:
Buprenex Injectable 2006

Bupropion Hydrochloride (Concurrent use with drugs that are substrate for cytochrome $P_{450}IID_6$ may make normal metabolizer resemble poor metabolizer leading to higher than expected plasma concentrations of TCA with resultant toxicity). Products include:
Wellbutrin Tablets 1204

Buspirone Hydrochloride (Protriptyline may enhance the response to CNS depressants). Products include:
BuSpar 737

Butabarbital (Protriptyline may enhance the response to CNS depressants).
No products indexed under this heading.

Butalbital (Protriptyline may enhance the response to CNS depressants). Products include:
Esgic-plus Tablets 1013
Fioricet Tablets 2258
Fioricet with Codeine Capsules 2260
Fiorinal Capsules 2261
Fiorinal with Codeine Capsules 2262
Fiorinal Tablets 2261
Phrenilin 785
Sedapap Tablets 50 mg/650 mg .. 1543

Chlordiazepoxide (Protriptyline may enhance the response to CNS depressants). Products include:
Libritabs Tablets 2177
Limbitrol 2180

Chlordiazepoxide Hydrochloride (Protriptyline may enhance the response to CNS depressants). Products include:
Librax Capsules 2176
Librium Capsules 2178
Librium Injectable 2179

Chlorpromazine (Concurrent use with drugs that are substrate for cytochrome $P_{450}IID_6$ may make normal metabolizer resemble poor metabolizer leading to higher than expected plasma; concentrations of TCA with resultant toxicity; potential for hyperpyrexia, particularly in hot weather). Products include:
Thorazine Suppositories 2523

Chlorpromazine Hydrochloride (Concurrent use with drugs that are substrate for cytochrome $P_{450}IID_6$ may make normal metabolizer resemble poor metabolizer leading to higher than expected plasma; concentrations of TCA with resultant toxicity; potential for hyperpyrexia, particularly in hot weather). Products include:
Thorazine 2523

Chlorprothixene (Concurrent use with drugs that are substrate for cytochrome $P_{450}IID_6$ may make normal metabolizer resemble poor metabolizer leading to higher than expected plasma; concentrations of TCA with resultant toxicity; potential for hyperpyrexia, particularly in hot weather).
No products indexed under this heading.

Chlorprothixene Hydrochloride (Concurrent use with drugs that are substrate for cytochrome $P_{450}IID_6$ may make normal metabolizer resemble poor metabolizer leading to higher than expected plasma; concentrations of TCA with resultant toxicity; potential for hyperpyrexia, particularly in hot weather).
No products indexed under this heading.

Cimetidine (Reduces the hepatic metabolism of certain tricyclic antidepressants, thereby delaying elimination and increasing steady-state concentrations resulting in frequency and severity of side effects, particularly anticholinergic). Products include:
Tagamet Tablets 2516

Cimetidine Hydrochloride (Reduces the hepatic metabolism of certain tricyclic antidepressants, thereby delaying elimination and increasing steady-state concentrations resulting in frequency and severity of side effects, particularly anticholinergic). Products include:
Tagamet 2516

Clidinium Bromide (Concurrent use may result in hyperpyrexia, particularly in hot weather). Products include:
Librax Capsules 2176
Quarzan Capsules 2181

Clonidine (Protryptyline may block the antihypertensive effect). Products include:
Catapres-TTS 675

Clonidine Hydrochloride (Protryptyline may block the antihypertensive effect). Products include:
Catapres Tablets 674
Combipres Tablets 677

Clorazepate Dipotassium (Protriptyline may enhance the response to CNS depressants). Products include:
Tranxene 451

Clozapine (Concurrent use with drugs that are substrate for cytochrome $P_{450}IID_6$ may make normal metabolizer resemble poor metabolizer leading to higher than expected plasma; concentrations of TCA with resultant toxicity; potential for hyperpyrexia, particularly in hot weather). Products include:
Clozaril Tablets 2252

Codeine Phosphate (Protriptyline may enhance the response to CNS depressants). Products include:
Actifed with Codeine Cough Syrup .. 1067
Brontex 1981
Deconsal C Expectorant Syrup 456
Deconsal Pediatric Syrup 457
Dimetane-DC Cough Syrup 2059
Empirin with Codeine Tablets 1093
Fioricet with Codeine Capsules 2260
Fiorinal with Codeine Capsules 2262
Isoclor Expectorant 990
Novahistine DH 2462
Novahistine Expectorant 2463
Nucofed 2051
Phenergan with Codeine 2777
Phenergan VC with Codeine 2781
Robitussin A-C Syrup 2073
Robitussin-DAC Syrup 2074
Ryna .... 🕮 841
Soma Compound w/Codeine Tablets 2676
Tussi-Organidin NR Liquid and S NR Liquid 2677
Tylenol with Codeine 1583

Desflurane (Protriptyline may enhance the response to CNS depressants). Products include:
Suprane 1813

IMPORTANT NOTE: Always consult each drug listing in the patient's regimen for possible interactions.

Vivactil **Interactions Index** 1162

Desipramine Hydrochloride (Concurrent use with drugs that are substrate for cytochrome $P_{450}IID_6$ may make normal metabolizer resemble poor metabolizer leading to higher than expected plasma concentrations of TCA with resultant toxicity). Products include:
Norpramin Tablets ... 1526

Dezocine (Protriptyline may enhance the response to CNS depressants). Products include:
Dalgan Injection ... 538

Diazepam (Protriptyline may enhance the response to CNS depressants). Products include:
Dizac ... 1809
Valium Injectable ... 2182
Valium Tablets ... 2183
Valrelease Capsules ... 2169

Dicyclomine Hydrochloride (Concurrent use may result in hyperpyrexia, particularly in hot weather). Products include:
Bentyl ... 1501

Dobutamine Hydrochloride (Effects of concurrent use not specified; careful adjustment of dosage and close supervision are required). Products include:
Dobutrex Solution Vials ... 1439

Dopamine Hydrochloride (Effects of concurrent use not specified; careful adjustment of dosage and close supervision are required).
No products indexed under this heading.

Doxepin Hydrochloride (Concurrent use with drugs that are substrate for cytochrome $P_{450}IID_6$ may make normal metabolizer resemble poor metabolizer leading to higher than expected plasma concentrations of TCA with resultant toxicity). Products include:
Sinequan ... 2205
Zonalon Cream ... 1055

Droperidol (Protriptyline may enhance the response to CNS depressants). Products include:
Inapsine Injection ... 1296

Enflurane (Protriptyline may enhance the response to CNS depressants).
No products indexed under this heading.

Ephedrine Hydrochloride (Effects of concurrent use not specified; careful adjustment of dosage and close supervision are required). Products include:
Primatene Dual Action Formula ... ▣ 872
Primatene Tablets ... ▣ 873
Quadrinal Tablets ... 1350

Ephedrine Sulfate (Effects of concurrent use not specified; careful adjustment of dosage and close supervision are required). Products include:
Bronkaid Caplets ... ▣ 717
Marax Tablets & DF Syrup ... 2200

Ephedrine Tannate (Effects of concurrent use not specified; careful adjustment of dosage and close supervision are required). Products include:
Rynatuss ... 2673

Epinephrine (Effects of concurrent use of epinephrine (combined with local anesthetics) not specified; careful adjustment of dosage and close supervision are required). Products include:
Bronkaid Mist ... ▣ 717
EPIFRIN ... ⊙ 239
EpiPen ... 790
Marcaine Hydrochloride with Epinephrine 1:200,000 ... 2316
Primatene Mist ... ▣ 873
Sensorcaine with Epinephrine Injection ... 559
Sus-Phrine Injection ... 1019
Xylocaine with Epinephrine Injections ... 567

Epinephrine Bitartrate (Effects of concurrent use not specified; careful adjustment of dosage and close supervision are required). Products include:
Bronkaid Mist Suspension ... ▣ 718
Sensorcaine-MPF with Epinephrine Injection ... 559

Epinephrine Hydrochloride (Effects of concurrent use of epinephrine (combined with local anesthetics) not specified; careful adjustment of dosage and close supervision are required). Products include:
Ana-Kit Anaphylaxis Emergency Treatment Kit ... 617

Estazolam (Protriptyline may enhance the response to CNS depressants). Products include:
ProSom Tablets ... 449

Ethchlorvynol (Protriptyline may enhance the response to CNS depressants). Products include:
Placidyl Capsules ... 448

Ethinamate (Protriptyline may enhance the response to CNS depressants).
No products indexed under this heading.

Fentanyl (Protriptyline may enhance the response to CNS depressants). Products include:
Duragesic Transdermal System ... 1288

Fentanyl Citrate (Protriptyline may enhance the response to CNS depressants). Products include:
Sublimaze Injection ... 1307

Flecainide Acetate (Concurrent use with drugs that are substrate for cytochrome $P_{450}IID_6$ may make normal metabolizer resemble poor metabolizer leading to higher than expected plasma concentrations of TCA with resultant toxicity). Products include:
Tambocor Tablets ... 1497

Fluoxetine Hydrochloride (Concurrent use with drugs that are substrate for cytochrome $P_{450}IID_6$ may make normal metabolizer resemble poor metabolizer leading to higher than expected plasma concentrations of TCA with resultant toxicity; due to variation in the extent of inhibition of $P_{450}IID_6$ and long half-life of the parent (fluoxetine) and active metabolite sufficient time should/must elapse, at least 5 weeks before switching to TCA). Products include:
Prozac Pulvules & Liquid, Oral Solution ... 919

Fluphenazine Decanoate (Concurrent use with drugs that are substrate for cytochrome $P_{450}IID_6$ may make normal metabolizer resemble poor metabolizer leading to higher than expected plasma; concentrations of TCA with resultant toxicity; potential for hyperpyrexia, particularly in hot weather). Products include:
Prolixin Decanoate ... 509

Fluphenazine Enanthate (Concurrent use with drugs that are substrate for cytochrome $P_{450}IID_6$ may make normal metabolizer resemble poor metabolizer leading to higher than expected plasma; concentrations of TCA with resultant toxicity; potential for hyperpyrexia, particularly in hot weather). Products include:
Prolixin Enanthate ... 509

Fluphenazine Hydrochloride (Concurrent use with drugs that are substrate for cytochrome $P_{450}IID_6$ may make normal metabolizer resemble poor metabolizer leading to higher than expected plasma; concentrations of TCA with resultant toxicity; potential for hyperpyrexia, particularly in hot weather). Products include:
Prolixin ... 509

Flurazepam Hydrochloride (Protriptyline may enhance the response to CNS depressants). Products include:
Dalmane Capsules ... 2173

Fluvoxamine Maleate (Concurrent use with drugs that are substrate for cytochrome $P_{450}IID_6$ may make normal metabolizer resemble poor metabolizer leading to higher than expected plasma concentrations of TCA with resultant toxicity). Products include:
Luvox Tablets ... 2544

Furazolidone (Potential for hyperpyretic crises, severe convulsions, and deaths; concurrent and/or sequential use is contraindicated). Products include:
Furoxone ... 2046

Glutethimide (Protriptyline may enhance the response to CNS depressants).
No products indexed under this heading.

Glycopyrrolate (Concurrent use may result in hyperpyrexia, particularly in hot weather). Products include:
Robinul Forte Tablets ... 2072
Robinul Injectable ... 2072
Robinul Tablets ... 2072

Guanadrel Sulfate (Protryptyline may block the antihypertensive effect). Products include:
Hylorel Tablets ... 985

Guanethidine Monosulfate (Protryptyline may block the antihypertensive effect of guanethidine or similarly acting compounds). Products include:
Esimil Tablets ... 822
Ismelin Tablets ... 827

Haloperidol (Concurrent use with drugs that are substrate for cytochrome $P_{450}IID_6$ may make normal metabolizer resemble poor metabolizer leading to higher than expected plasma; concentrations of TCA with resultant toxicity; potential for hyperpyrexia, particularly in hot weather). Products include:
Haldol Injection, Tablets and Concentrate ... 1575

Haloperidol Decanoate (Concurrent use with drugs that are substrate for cytochrome $P_{450}IID_6$ may make normal metabolizer resemble poor metabolizer leading to higher than expected plasma; concentrations of TCA with resultant toxicity; potential for hyperpyrexia, particularly in hot weather). Products include:
Haldol Decanoate ... 1577

Hydrocodone Bitartrate (Protriptyline may enhance the response to CNS depressants). Products include:
Anexsia 5/500 Elixir ... 1781
Anexia Tablets ... 1782
Codiclear DH Syrup ... 791
Deconamine CX Cough and Cold Liquid and Tablets ... 1319
Duratuss HD Elixir ... 2565
Hycodan Tablets and Syrup ... 930
Hycomine Compound Tablets ... 932
Hycomine ... 931
Hycotuss Expectorant Syrup ... 933
Hydrocet Capsules ... 782
Lorcet 10/650 ... 1018
Lortab ... 2566
Tussend ... 1783
Tussend Expectorant ... 1785
Vicodin Tablets ... 1356
Vicodin ES Tablets ... 1357
Vicodin Tuss Expectorant ... 1358
Zydone Capsules ... 949

Hydrocodone Polistirex (Protriptyline may enhance the response to CNS depressants). Products include:
Tussionex Pennkinetic Extended-Release Suspension ... 998

Hydroxyzine Hydrochloride (Protriptyline may enhance the response to CNS depressants). Products include:
Atarax Tablets & Syrup ... 2185
Marax Tablets & DF Syrup ... 2200
Vistaril Intramuscular Solution ... 2216

Hyoscyamine (Concurrent use may result in hyperpyrexia, particularly in hot weather). Products include:
Cystospaz Tablets ... 1963
Urised Tablets ... 1964

Hyoscyamine Sulfate (Concurrent use may result in hyperpyrexia, particularly in hot weather). Products include:
Arco-Lase Plus Tablets ... 512
Atrohist Plus Tablets ... 454
Cystospaz-M Capsules ... 1963
Donnatal ... 2060
Donnatal Extentabs ... 2061
Donnatal Tablets ... 2060
Kutrase Capsules ... 2402
Levsin/Levsinex/Levbid ... 2405

Imipramine Hydrochloride (Concurrent use with drugs that are substrate for cytochrome $P_{450}IID_6$ may make normal metabolizer resemble poor metabolizer leading to higher than expected plasma concentrations of TCA with resultant toxicity). Products include:
Tofranil Ampuls ... 854
Tofranil Tablets ... 856

Imipramine Pamoate (Concurrent use with drugs that are substrate for cytochrome $P_{450}IID_6$ may make normal metabolizer resemble poor metabolizer leading to higher than expected plasma concentrations of TCA with resultant toxicity). Products include:
Tofranil-PM Capsules ... 857

Ipratropium Bromide (Concurrent use may result in hyperpyrexia, particularly in hot weather). Products include:
Atrovent Inhalation Aerosol ... 671
Atrovent Inhalation Solution ... 673

Isocarboxazid (Potential for hyperpyretic crises, severe convulsions, and deaths; concurrent and/or sequential use is contraindicated).
No products indexed under this heading.

Isoflurane (Protriptyline may enhance the response to CNS depressants).
No products indexed under this heading.

Isoproterenol Hydrochloride (Effects of concurrent use not specified; careful adjustment of dosage and close supervision are required). Products include:
Isuprel Hydrochloride Injection 1:5000 ... 2311
Isuprel Hydrochloride Solution 1:200 & 1:100 ... 2313
Isuprel Mistometer ... 2312

(▣ Described in PDR For Nonprescription Drugs) (⊙ Described in PDR For Ophthalmology)

1163 **Interactions Index** **Vivactil**

Isoproterenol Sulfate (Effects of concurrent use not specified; careful adjustment of dosage and close supervision are required). Products include:
- Norisodrine with Calcium Iodide Syrup ... 442

Ketamine Hydrochloride (Protriptyline may enhance the response to CNS depressants).
- No products indexed under this heading.

Levomethadyl Acetate Hydrochloride (Protriptyline may enhance the response to CNS depressants). Products include:
- Orlamm ... 2239

Levorphanol Tartrate (Protriptyline may enhance the response to CNS depressants). Products include:
- Levo-Dromoran ... 2129

Levothyroxine Sodium (On rare occasions, co-administration may produce arrhythmias). Products include:
- Levothroid Tablets ... 1016
- Levoxyl Tablets ... 903
- Synthroid ... 1359

Liothyronine Sodium (On rare occasions, co-administration may produce arrhythmias). Products include:
- Cytomel Tablets ... 2473
- Triostat Injection ... 2530

Liotrix (On rare occasions, co-administration may produce arrhythmias).
- No products indexed under this heading.

Lorazepam (Protriptyline may enhance the response to CNS depressants). Products include:
- Ativan Injection ... 2698
- Ativan Tablets ... 2700

Loxapine Hydrochloride (Concurrent use with drugs that are substrate for cytochrome $P_{450}IID_6$ may make normal metabolizer resemble poor metabolizer leading to higher than expected plasma; concentrations of TCA with resultant toxicity; potential for hyperpyrexia, particularly in hot weather). Products include:
- Loxitane ... 1378

Loxapine Succinate (Concurrent use with drugs that are substrate for cytochrome $P_{450}IID_6$ may make normal metabolizer resemble poor metabolizer leading to higher than expected plasma; concentrations of TCA with resultant toxicity; potential for hyperpyrexia, particularly in hot weather). Products include:
- Loxitane Capsules ... 1378

Maprotiline Hydrochloride (Concurrent use with drugs that are substrate for cytochrome $P_{450}IID_6$ may make normal metabolizer resemble poor metabolizer leading to higher than expected plasma concentrations of TCA with resultant toxicity). Products include:
- Ludiomil Tablets ... 843

Mepenzolate Bromide (Concurrent use may result in hyperpyrexia, particularly in hot weather).
- No products indexed under this heading.

Meperidine Hydrochloride (Protriptyline may enhance the response to CNS depressants). Products include:
- Demerol ... 2308
- Mepergan Injection ... 2753

Mephobarbital (Protriptyline may enhance the response to CNS depressants). Products include:
- Mebaral Tablets ... 2322

Meprobamate (Protriptyline may enhance the response to CNS depressants). Products include:
- Miltown Tablets ... 2672
- PMB 200 and PMB 400 ... 2783

Mesoridazine (Protriptyline may enhance the response to CNS depressants).

Mesoridazine Besylate (Concurrent use with drugs that are substrate for cytochrome $P_{450}IID_6$ may make normal metabolizer resemble poor metabolizer leading to higher than expected plasma; concentrations of TCA with resultant toxicity; potential for hyperpyrexia, particularly in hot weather). Products include:
- Serentil ... 684

Metaproterenol Sulfate (Effects of concurrent use not specified; careful adjustment of dosage and close supervision are required). Products include:
- Alupent ... 669
- Metaproterenol Sulfate Inhalation Solution, USP, Arm-a-Med ... 552

Metaraminol Bitartrate (Effects of concurrent use not specified; careful adjustment of dosage and close supervision are required). Products include:
- Aramine Injection ... 1609

Methadone Hydrochloride (Protriptyline may enhance the response to CNS depressants). Products include:
- Methadone Hydrochloride Oral Concentrate ... 2233
- Methadone Hydrochloride Oral Solution & Tablets ... 2235

Methohexital Sodium (Protriptyline may enhance the response to CNS depressants). Products include:
- Brevital Sodium Vials ... 1429

Methotrimeprazine (Concurrent use with drugs that are substrate for cytochrome $P_{450}IID_6$ may make normal metabolizer resemble poor metabolizer leading to higher than expected plasma; concentrations of TCA with resultant toxicity; potential for hyperpyrexia, particularly in hot weather). Products include:
- Levoprome ... 1274

Methoxamine Hydrochloride (Effects of concurrent use not specified; careful adjustment of dosage and close supervision are required). Products include:
- Vasoxyl Injection ... 1196

Methoxyflurane (Protriptyline may enhance the response to CNS depressants).
- No products indexed under this heading.

Midazolam Hydrochloride (Protriptyline may enhance the response to CNS depressants). Products include:
- Versed Injection ... 2170

Molindone Hydrochloride (Concurrent use with drugs that are substrate for cytochrome $P_{450}IID_6$ may make normal metabolizer resemble poor metabolizer leading to higher than expected plasma; concentrations of TCA with resultant toxicity; potential for hyperpyrexia, particularly in hot weather). Products include:
- Moban Tablets and Concentrate ... 1048

Morphine Sulfate (Protriptyline may enhance the response to CNS depressants). Products include:
- Astramorph/PF Injection, USP (Preservative-Free) ... 535
- Duramorph ... 962
- Infumorph 200 and Infumorph 500 Sterile Solutions ... 965
- MS Contin Tablets ... 1994
- MSIR ... 1997
- Oramorph SR (Morphine Sulfate Sustained Release Tablets) ... 2236
- RMS Suppositories ... 2657
- Roxanol ... 2243

Nefazodone Hydrochloride (Concurrent use with drugs that are substrate for cytochrome $P_{450}IID_6$ may make normal metabolizer resemble poor metabolizer leading to higher than expected plasma concentrations of TCA with resultant toxicity). Products include:
- Serzone Tablets ... 771

Norepinephrine Bitartrate (Effects of concurrent use not specified; careful adjustment of dosage and close supervision are required). Products include:
- Levophed Bitartrate Injection ... 2315

Nortriptyline Hydrochloride (Concurrent use with drugs that are substrate for cytochrome $P_{450}IID_6$ may make normal metabolizer resemble poor metabolizer leading to higher than expected plasma concentrations of TCA with resultant toxicity). Products include:
- Pamelor ... 2280

Opium Alkaloids (Protriptyline may enhance the response to CNS depressants).
- No products indexed under this heading.

Oxazepam (Protriptyline may enhance the response to CNS depressants). Products include:
- Serax Capsules ... 2810
- Serax Tablets ... 2810

Oxybutynin Chloride (Concurrent use may result in hyperpyrexia, particularly in hot weather). Products include:
- Ditropan ... 1516

Oxycodone Hydrochloride (Protriptyline may enhance the response to CNS depressants). Products include:
- Percocet Tablets ... 938
- Percodan Tablets ... 939
- Percodan-Demi Tablets ... 940
- Roxicodone Tablets, Oral Solution & Intensol (Oxycodone) ... 2244
- Tylox Capsules ... 1584

Paroxetine Hydrochloride (Concurrent use with drugs that are substrate for cytochrome $P_{450}IID_6$ may make normal metabolizer resemble poor metabolizer leading to higher than expected plasma concentrations of TCA with resultant toxicity; due to variation in the extent of inhibition of $P_{450}IID_6$ caution is indicated; if coadministered sufficient time should must elapse). Products include:
- Paxil Tablets ... 2505

Pentobarbital Sodium (Protriptyline may enhance the response to CNS depressants). Products include:
- Nembutal Sodium Capsules ... 436
- Nembutal Sodium Solution ... 438
- Nembutal Sodium Suppositories ... 440

Perphenazine (Concurrent use with drugs that are substrate for cytochrome $P_{450}IID_6$ may make normal metabolizer resemble poor metabolizer leading to higher than expected plasma; concentrations of TCA with resultant toxicity; potential for hyperpyrexia, particularly in hot weather). Products include:
- Etrafon ... 2355
- Triavil Tablets ... 1757
- Trilafon ... 2389

Phenelzine Sulfate (Potential for hyperpyretic crises, severe convulsions, and deaths; concurrent and/or sequential use is contraindicated). Products include:
- Nardil ... 1920

Phenobarbital (Protriptyline may enhance the response to CNS depressants). Products include:
- Arco-Lase Plus Tablets ... 512
- Bellergal-S Tablets ... 2250
- Donnatal ... 2060
- Donnatal Extentabs ... 2061
- Donnatal Tablets ... 2060
- Phenobarbital Elixir and Tablets ... 1469
- Quadrinal Tablets ... 1350

Phenylephrine Bitartrate (Effects of concurrent use not specified; careful adjustment of dosage and close supervision are required).
- No products indexed under this heading.

Phenylephrine Hydrochloride (Effects of concurrent use not specified; careful adjustment of dosage and close supervision are required). Products include:
- Atrohist Plus Tablets ... 454
- Cerose DM ... ◙ 878
- Comhist ... 2038
- D.A. Chewable Tablets ... 951
- Deconsal Pediatric Capsules ... 454
- Dura-Vent/DA Tablets ... 953
- Entex Capsules ... 1986
- Entex Liquid ... 1986
- Extendryl ... 1005
- 4-Way Fast Acting Nasal Spray (regular & mentholated) ... ◙ 621
- Hemorid For Women ... ◙ 834
- Hycomine Compound Tablets ... 932
- Neo-Synephrine Hydrochloride 1% Carpuject ... 2324
- Neo-Synephrine Hydrochloride 1% Injection ... 2324
- Neo-Synephrine Hydrochloride (Ophthalmic) ... 2325
- Neo-Synephrine ... ◙ 726
- Nōstril ... ◙ 644
- Novahistine Elixir ... ◙ 823
- Phenergan VC ... 2779
- Phenergan VC with Codeine ... 2781
- Preparation H ... ◙ 871
- Tympagesic Ear Drops ... 2342
- Vasosulf ... ⊙ 271
- Vicks Sinex Nasal Spray and Ultra Fine Mist ... ◙ 765

Phenylephrine Tannate (Effects of concurrent use not specified; careful adjustment of dosage and close supervision are required). Products include:
- Atrohist Pediatric Suspension ... 454
- Ricobid-D Pediatric Suspension ... 2038
- Ricobid Tablets and Pediatric Suspension ... 2038
- Rynatan ... 2673
- Rynatuss ... 2673

Phenylpropanolamine Hydrochloride (Effects of concurrent use not specified; careful adjustment of dosage and close supervision are required). Products include:
- Acutrim ... ◙ 628
- Allerest Children's Chewable Tablets ... ◙ 627
- Allerest 12 Hour Caplets ... ◙ 627
- Atrohist Plus Tablets ... 454
- BC Cold Powder Multi-Symptom Formula (Cold-Sinus-Allergy) ... ◙ 609
- BC Cold Powder Non-Drowsy Formula (Cold-Sinus) ... ◙ 609

IMPORTANT NOTE: Always consult each drug listing in the patient's regimen for possible interactions.

Vivactil | Interactions Index | 1164

Cheracol Plus Head Cold/Cough Formula ▣ 769
Comtrex Multi-Symptom Non-Drowsy Liqui-gels ▣ 618
Contac Continuous Action Nasal Decongestant/Antihistamine 12 Hour Capsules ▣ 813
Contac Maximum Strength Continuous Action Decongestant/Antihistamine 12 Hour Caplets ▣ 813
Contac Severe Cold and Flu Formula Caplets ▣ 814
Coricidin 'D' Decongestant Tablets ▣ 800
Dexatrim ▣ 832
Dexatrim Plus Vitamins Caplets ▣ 832
Dimetane-DC Cough Syrup 2059
Dimetapp Elixir ▣ 773
Dimetapp Extentabs ▣ 774
Dimetapp Tablets/Liqui-Gels ▣ 775
Dimetapp Cold & Allergy Chewable Tablets ▣ 773
Dimetapp DM Elixir ▣ 774
Dura-Vent Tablets 952
Entex Capsules 1986
Entex LA Tablets 1987
Entex Liquid 1986
Exgest LA Tablets 782
Hycomine 931
Isoclor Timesule Capsules ▣ 637
Nolamine Timed-Release Tablets 785
Ornade Spansule Capsules 2502
Propagest Tablets 786
Pyrroxate Caplets ▣ 772
Robitussin-CF ▣ 777
Sinulin Tablets 787
Tavist-D 12 Hour Relief Tablets ▣ 787
Teldrin 12 Hour Antihistamine/Nasal Decongestant Allergy Relief Capsules ▣ 826
Triaminic Allergy Tablets ▣ 789
Triaminic Cold Tablets ▣ 790
Triaminic Expectorant ▣ 790
Triaminic Syrup ▣ 792
Triaminic-12 Tablets ▣ 792
Triaminic-DM Syrup ▣ 792
Triaminicin Tablets ▣ 793
Triaminicol Multi-Symptom Cold Tablets ▣ 793
Triaminicol Multi-Symptom Relief ▣ 794
Vicks DayQuil Allergy Relief 12-Hour Extended Release Tablets ▣ 760
Vicks DayQuil Allergy Relief 4-Hour Tablets ▣ 760
Vicks DayQuil SINUS Pressure & CONGESTION Relief ▣ 761

Pimozide (Concurrent use with drugs that are substrate for cytochrome $P_{450}IID_6$ may make normal metabolizer resemble poor metabolizer leading to higher than expected plasma; concentrations of TCA with resultant toxicity; potential for hyperpyrexia, particularly in hot weather). Products include:
Orap Tablets 1050

Pirbuterol Acetate (Effects of concurrent use not specified; careful adjustment of dosage and close supervision are required). Products include:
Maxair Autohaler 1492
Maxair Inhaler 1494

Prazepam (Protriptyline may enhance the response to CNS depressants).
No products indexed under this heading.

Prochlorperazine (Concurrent use with drugs that are substrate for cytochrome $P_{450}IID_6$ may make normal metabolizer resemble poor metabolizer leading to higher than expected plasma; concentrations of TCA with resultant toxicity; potential for hyperpyrexia, particularly in hot weather). Products include:
Compazine 2470

Procyclidine Hydrochloride (Concurrent use may result in hyperpyrexia, particularly in hot weather). Products include:
Kemadrin Tablets 1112

Promethazine Hydrochloride (Concurrent use with drugs that are substrate for cytochrome $P_{450}IID_6$ may make normal metabolizer resemble poor metabolizer leading to higher than expected plasma; concentrations of TCA with resultant toxicity; potential for hyperpyrexia, particularly in hot weather). Products include:
Mepergan Injection 2753
Phenergan with Codeine 2777
Phenergan with Dextromethorphan 2778
Phenergan Injection 2773
Phenergan Suppositories 2775
Phenergan Syrup 2774
Phenergan Tablets 2775
Phenergan VC 2779
Phenergan VC with Codeine 2781

Propafenone Hydrochloride (Concurrent use with drugs that are substrate for cytochrome $P_{450}IID_6$ may make normal metabolizer resemble poor metabolizer leading to higher than expected plasma concentrations of TCA with resultant toxicity). Products include:
Rythmol Tablets–150mg, 225mg, 300mg 1352

Propantheline Bromide (Concurrent use may result in hyperpyrexia, particularly in hot weather). Products include:
Pro-Banthine Tablets 2052

Propofol (Protriptyline may enhance the response to CNS depressants). Products include:
Diprivan Injection 2833

Propoxyphene Hydrochloride (Protriptyline may enhance the response to CNS depressants). Products include:
Darvon 1435
Wygesic Tablets 2827

Propoxyphene Napsylate (Protriptyline may enhance the response to CNS depressants). Products include:
Darvon-N/Darvocet-N 1433

Pseudoephedrine Hydrochloride (Effects of concurrent use not specified; careful adjustment of dosage and close supervision are required). Products include:
Actifed Allergy Daytime/Nighttime Caplets ▣ 844
Actifed Plus Caplets ▣ 845
Actifed Plus Tablets ▣ 845
Actifed with Codeine Cough Syrup 1067
Actifed Sinus Daytime/Nighttime Tablets and Caplets ▣ 846
Actifed Syrup ▣ 846
Actifed Tablets ▣ 844
Advil Cold and Sinus Caplets and Tablets (formerly CoAdvil) ▣ 870
Alka-Seltzer Plus Cold Medicine Liqui-Gels ▣ 706
Alka-Seltzer Plus Cold & Cough Medicine Liqui-Gels ▣ 705
Alka-Seltzer Plus Night-Time Cold Medicine Liqui-Gels ▣ 706
Allerest Headache Strength Tablets ▣ 627
Allerest Maximum Strength Tablets ▣ 627
Allerest No Drowsiness Tablets ▣ 627
Allerest Sinus Pain Formula ▣ 627
Anatuss LA Tablets 1542
Atrohist Pediatric Capsules 453
Bayer Select Sinus Pain Relief Formula ▣ 717
Benadryl Allergy Decongestant Liquid Medication ▣ 848
Benadryl Allergy Decongestant Tablets ▣ 848
Benadryl Allergy Sinus Headache Formula Caplets ▣ 849
Benylin Multisymptom ▣ 852
Bromfed Capsules (Extended-Release) 1785
Bromfed Syrup ▣ 733
Bromfed Tablets 1785
Bromfed-DM Cough Syrup 1786
Bromfed-PD Capsules (Extended-Release) 1785
Children's Vicks DayQuil Allergy Relief ▣ 757
Children's Vicks NyQuil Cold/Cough Relief ▣ 758
Comtrex Multi-Symptom Cold Reliever Tablets/Caplets/Liqui-Gels/Liquid ▣ 615
Allergy-Sinus Comtrex Multi-Symptom Allergy-Sinus Formula Tablets ▣ 617
Comtrex Multi-Symptom Non-Drowsy Caplets ▣ 618
Congess 1004
Contac Day Allergy/Sinus Caplets ▣ 812
Contac Day & Night ▣ 812
Contac Night Allergy/Sinus Caplets ▣ 812
Contac Severe Cold & Flu Non-Drowsy ▣ 815
Deconamine Chewable Tablets 1320
Deconamine CX Cough and Cold Liquid and Tablets 1319
Deconamine 1320
Deconsal C Expectorant Syrup 456
Deconsal Pediatric Syrup 457
Deconsal II Tablets 454
Dimetane-DX Cough Syrup 2059
Dimetapp Sinus Caplets ▣ 775
Dorcol Children's Cough Syrup ▣ 785
Drixoral Cough + Congestion Liquid Caps ▣ 802
Dura-Tap/PD Capsules 2867
Duratuss Tablets 2565
Duratuss HD Elixir 2565
Efidac/24 ▣ 635
Entex PSE Tablets 1987
Fedahist Gyrocaps 2401
Fedahist Timecaps 2401
Guaifed 1787
Guaifed Syrup ▣ 734
Guaimax-D Tablets 792
Guaitab Tablets ▣ 734
Isoclor Expectorant 990
Kronofed-A 977
Motrin IB Sinus ▣ 838
Novahistine DH 2462
Novahistine DMX ▣ 822
Novahistine Expectorant 2463
Nucofed 2051
PediaCare Cold Allergy Chewable Tablets ▣ 677
PediaCare Cough-Cold Chewable Tablets 1553
PediaCare 1553
PediaCare Infants' Decongestant Drops ▣ 677
PediCare Infant's Drops Decongestant Plus Cough 1553
PediaCare NightRest Cough-Cold Liquid 1553
Pediatric Vicks 44d Dry Hacking Cough & Head Congestion ▣ 763
Pediatric Vicks 44m Cough & Cold Relief ▣ 764
Robitussin Cold & Cough Liqui-Gels ▣ 776
Robitussin Maximum Strength Cough & Cold ▣ 778
Robitussin Pediatric Cough & Cold Formula ▣ 779
Robitussin Severe Congestion Liqui-Gels ▣ 776
Robitussin-DAC Syrup 2074
Robitussin-PE ▣ 778
Rondec Oral Drops 953
Rondec Syrup 953
Rondec Tablet 953
Rondec-DM Oral Drops 954
Rondec-DM Syrup 954
Rondec-TR Tablet 953
Ryna ▣ 841
Seldane-D Extended-Release Tablets 1538
Semprex-D Capsules 463
Semprex-D Capsules 1167
Sinarest Tablets ▣ 648
Sinarest Extra Strength Tablets ▣ 648
Sinarest No Drowsiness Tablets ▣ 648
Sine-Aid IB Caplets 1554
Sine-Aid Maximum Strength Sinus Medication Gelcaps, Caplets and Tablets 1554
Sine-Off No Drowsiness Formula Caplets ▣ 824
Sine-Off Sinus Medicine ▣ 825
Singlet Tablets ▣ 825
Sinutab Non-Drying Liquid Caps ▣ 859
Sinutab Sinus Allergy Medication, Maximum Strength Tablets and Caplets ▣ 860
Sinutab Sinus Medication, Maximum Strength Without Drowsiness Formula, Tablets & Caplets ▣ 860
Sinutab Sinus Medication, Regular Strength Without Drowsiness Formula ▣ 859
Sudafed Children's Liquid ▣ 861
Sudafed Cold and Cough Liquidcaps ▣ 862
Sudafed Cough Syrup ▣ 862
Sudafed Plus Liquid ▣ 862
Sudafed Plus Tablets ▣ 863
Sudafed Severe Cold Formula Caplets ▣ 863
Sudafed Severe Cold Formula Tablets ▣ 864
Sudafed Sinus Caplets ▣ 864
Sudafed Sinus Tablets ▣ 864
Sudafed Tablets, 30 mg ▣ 861
Sudafed Tablets, 60 mg ▣ 861
Sudafed 12 Hour Caplets ▣ 861
Syn-Rx Tablets 465
Syn-Rx DM Tablets 466
TheraFlu ▣ 787
TheraFlu Maximum Strength Nighttime Flu, Cold & Cough Medicine ▣ 788
TheraFlu Maximum Strength Non-Drowsy Formula Flu, Cold & Cough Medicine ▣ 788
Thera Flu Maximum Strength, Non-Drowsy Formula Flu, Cold and Cough Caplets ▣ 789
Triaminic AM Cough and Decongestant Formula ▣ 789
Triaminic AM Decongestant Formula ▣ 790
Triaminic Nite Light ▣ 791
Triaminic Sore Throat Formula ▣ 791
Tussend 1783
Tussend Expectorant 1785
Children's TYLENOL Cold Multi-Symptom Liquid Formula and Chewable Tablets 1561
Children's TYLENOL Cold Plus Cough Multi Symptom Tablets and Liquid ▣ 681
Infants' TYLENOL Cold Decongestant & Fever-Reducer Drops 1556
TYLENOL Maximum Strength Allergy Sinus Medication Gelcaps and Caplets 1563
TYLENOL Maximum Strength Allergy Sinus NightTime Medication Caplets 1555
TYLENOL Flu Maximum Strength Gelcaps 1565
TYLENOL Flu NightTime, Maximum Strength, Gelcaps 1566
TYLENOL Maximum Strength Flu NightTime Hot Medication Packets 1562
TYLENOL, Maximum Strength, Sinus Medication Geltabs, Gelcaps, Caplets and Tablets 1566
TYLENOL Cold Multi-Symptom Formula Medication Tablets and Caplets 1561
TYLENOL Cold Medication No Drowsiness Formula Gelcaps and Caplets 1562
TYLENOL Cold Multi-Symptom Hot Medication Liquid Packets 1557
TYLENOL Cough Multi-Symptom Medication with Decongestant 1565
Ursinus Inlay-Tabs ▣ 794
Vicks 44 LiquiCaps Cough, Cold & Flu Relief ▣ 755
Vicks 44 LiquiCaps Non-Drowsy Cough & Cold Relief ▣ 756
Vicks 44D Dry Hacking Cough & Head Congestion ▣ 755
Vicks 44M Cough, Cold & Flu Relief ▣ 756
Vicks DayQuil ▣ 761
Vicks DayQuil SINUS Pressure & PAIN Relief with IBUPROFEN ▣ 762
Vicks Nyquil Hot Therapy ▣ 762
Vicks NyQuil LiquiCaps Multi-Symptom Cold/Flu Relief ▣ 763
Vicks NyQuil Multi-Symptom Cold/Flu Relief - (Original & Cherry Flavor) ▣ 763

(▣ Described in PDR For Nonprescription Drugs) (⊙ Described in PDR For Ophthalmology)

Pseudoephedrine Sulfate (Effects of concurrent use not specified; careful adjustment of dosage and close supervision are required). Products include:

Cheracol Sinus .... ⊕ 768
Chlor-Trimeton Allergy Decongestant Tablets .... ⊕ 799
Claritin-D 2350
Drixoral Cold and Allergy Sustained-Action Tablets .... ⊕ 802
Drixoral Cold and Flu Extended-Release Tablets..................................... ⊕ 803
Drixoral Non-Drowsy Formula Extended-Release Tablets .... ⊕ 803
Drixoral Allergy/Sinus Extended Release Tablets..................................... ⊕ 804
Trinalin Repetabs Tablets 1330

Quazepam (Protriptyline may enhance the response to CNS depressants). Products include:

Doral Tablets 2664

Quinidine Gluconate (Concurrent use with drugs that inhibit cytochrome $P_{450}IID_6$ may make normal metabolizer resemble poor metabolizer leading to higher than expected plasma concentrations of TCA with resultant toxicity). Products include:

Quinaglute Dura-Tabs Tablets 649

Quinidine Polygalacturonate (Concurrent use with drugs that inhibit cytochrome $P_{450}IID_6$ may make normal metabolizer resemble poor metabolizer leading to higher than expected plasma concentrations of TCA with resultant toxicity).

No products indexed under this heading.

Quinidine Sulfate (Concurrent use with drugs that inhibit cytochrome $P_{450}IID_6$ may make normal metabolizer resemble poor metabolizer leading to higher than expected plasma concentrations of TCA with resultant toxicity). Products include:

Quinidex Extentabs 2067

Risperidone (Concurrent use with drugs that are substrate for cytochrome $P_{450}IID_6$ may make normal metabolizer resemble poor metabolizer leading to higher than expected plasma; concentrations of TCA with resultant toxicity; potential for hyperpyrexia, particularly in hot weather). Products include:

Risperdal 1301

Salmeterol Xinafoate (Effects of concurrent use not specified; careful adjustment of dosage and close supervision are required). Products include:

Serevent Inhalation Aerosol................. 1176

Scopolamine (Concurrent use may result in hyperpyrexia, particularly in hot weather). Products include:

Transderm Scōp Transdermal Therapeutic System 869

Scopolamine Hydrobromide (Concurrent use may result in hyperpyrexia, particularly in hot weather). Products include:

Atrohist Plus Tablets 454
Donnatal 2060
Donnatal Extentabs................................. 2061
Donnatal Tablets 2060

Secobarbital Sodium (Protriptyline may enhance the response to CNS depressants). Products include:

Seconal Sodium Pulvules 1474

Selegiline Hydrochloride (Potential for hyperpyretic crises, severe convulsions, and deaths; concurrent and/or sequential use is contraindicated). Products include:

Eldepryl Tablets 2550

Sertraline Hydrochloride (Concurrent use with drugs that are substrate for cytochrome $P_{450}IID_6$ may make normal metabolizer resemble poor metabolizer leading to higher than expected plasma concentrations of TCA with resultant toxicity; due to variation in the extent of inhibition of $P_{450}IID_6$ caution is indicated; if co-administered sufficient time should/must elapse). Products include:

Zoloft Tablets 2217

Sufentanil Citrate (Protriptyline may enhance the response to CNS depressants). Products include:

Sufenta Injection 1309

Temazepam (Protriptyline may enhance the response to CNS depressants). Products include:

Restoril Capsules 2284

Terbutaline Sulfate (Effects of concurrent use not specified; careful adjustment of dosage and close supervision are required). Products include:

Brethaire Inhaler 813
Brethine Ampuls 815
Brethine Tablets....................................... 814
Bricanyl Subcutaneous Injection 1502
Bricanyl Tablets 1503

Thiamylal Sodium (Protriptyline may enhance the response to CNS depressants).

No products indexed under this heading.

Thioridazine Hydrochloride (Concurrent use with drugs that are substrate for cytochrome $P_{450}IID_6$ may make normal metabolizer resemble poor metabolizer leading to higher than expected plasma; concentrations of TCA with resultant toxicity; potential for hyperpyrexia, particularly in hot weather). Products include:

Mellaril 2269

Thiothixene (Concurrent use with drugs that are substrate for cytochrome $P_{450}IID_6$ may make normal metabolizer resemble poor metabolizer leading to higher than expected plasma; concentrations of TCA with resultant toxicity; potential for hyperpyrexia, particularly in hot weather). Products include:

Navane Capsules and Concentrate 2201
Navane Intramuscular 2202

Thyroglobulin (On rare occasions, co-administration may produce arrhythmias).

No products indexed under this heading.

Thyroid (On rare occasions, co-administration may produce arrhythmias).

No products indexed under this heading.

Thyroxine (On rare occasions, co-administration may produce arrhythmias).

No products indexed under this heading.

Thyroxine Sodium (On rare occasions, co-administration may produce arrhythmias).

No products indexed under this heading.

Tranylcypromine Sulfate (Potential for hyperpyretic crises, severe convulsions, and deaths; concurrent and/or sequential use is contraindicated). Products include:

Parnate Tablets 2503

Trazodone Hydrochloride (Concurrent use with drugs that are substrate for cytochrome $P_{450}IID_6$ may make normal metabolizer resemble poor metabolizer leading to higher than expected plasma concentrations of TCA with resultant toxicity). Products include:

Desyrel and Desyrel Dividose 503

Triazolam (Protriptyline may enhance the response to CNS depressants). Products include:

Halcion Tablets... 2611

Tridihexethyl Chloride (Concurrent use may result in hyperpyrexia, particularly in hot weather).

No products indexed under this heading.

Trifluoperazine Hydrochloride (Concurrent use with drugs that are substrate for cytochrome $P_{450}IID_6$ may make normal metabolizer resemble poor metabolizer leading to higher than expected plasma; concentrations of TCA with resultant toxicity; potential for hyperpyrexia, particularly in hot weather). Products include:

Stelazine 2514

Trihexyphenidyl Hydrochloride (Concurrent use may result in hyperpyrexia, particularly in hot weather). Products include:

Artane... 1368

Trimipramine Maleate (Concurrent use with drugs that are substrate for cytochrome $P_{450}IID_6$ may make normal metabolizer resemble poor metabolizer leading to higher than expected plasma concentrations of TCA with resultant toxicity). Products include:

Surmontil Capsules................................. 2811

Venlafaxine Hydrochloride (Concurrent use with drugs that are substrate for cytochrome $P_{450}IID_6$ may make normal metabolizer resemble poor metabolizer leading to higher than expected plasma concentrations of TCA with resultant toxicity; due to variation in the extent of inhibition of $P_{450}IID_6$ caution is indicated; if co-administered sufficient time should/must elapse). Products include:

Effexor 2719

Zolpidem Tartrate (Protriptyline may enhance the response to CNS depressants). Products include:

Ambien Tablets... 2416

Food Interactions

Alcohol (Protriptyline may enhance the response to alcohol).

VIVOTIF BERNA

(Typhoid Vaccine Live Oral TY21a) .. 665
May interact with:

Antibiotics, unspecified (The vaccine should not be administered to individuals receiving unspecified antibiotics and other antibacterial drugs including sulfonamides since these agents may interfere with protective immune response).

VOLMAX EXTENDED-RELEASE TABLETS

(Albuterol Sulfate) 1788
May interact with sympathomimetics, monoamine oxidase inhibitors, tricyclic antidepressants, beta blockers, and certain other agents. Compounds in these categories include:

Acebutolol Hydrochloride (Effect of each other inhibited). Products include:

Sectral Capsules 2807

Albuterol (Potential for deleterious cardiovascular effects with other oral sympathomimetic agents). Products include:

Proventil Inhalation Aerosol 2382
Ventolin Inhalation Aerosol and Refill 1197

Amitriptyline Hydrochloride (Action of albuterol on the vascular system may be potentiated). Products include:

Elavil 2838
Endep Tablets 2174
Etrafon 2355
Limbitrol 2180
Triavil Tablets 1757

Amoxapine (Action of albuterol on the vascular system may be potentiated). Products include:

Asendin Tablets 1369

Atenolol (Effect of each other inhibited). Products include:

Tenoretic Tablets...................................... 2845
Tenormin Tablets and I.V. Injection 2847

Betaxolol Hydrochloride (Effect of each other inhibited). Products include:

Betoptic Ophthalmic Solution............. 469
Betoptic S Ophthalmic Suspension 471
Kerlone Tablets... 2436

Bisoprolol Fumarate (Effect of each other inhibited). Products include:

Zebeta Tablets 1413
Ziac 1415

Carteolol Hydrochloride (Effect of each other inhibited). Products include:

Cartrol Tablets 410
Ocupress Ophthalmic Solution, 1% Sterile... ⊙ 309

Clomipramine Hydrochloride (Action of albuterol on the vascular system may be potentiated). Products include:

Anafranil Capsules 803

Desipramine Hydrochloride (Action of albuterol on the vascular system may be potentiated). Products include:

Norpramin Tablets 1526

Dobutamine Hydrochloride (Potential for deleterious cardiovascular effects with other oral sympathomimetic agents). Products include:

Dobutrex Solution Vials......................... 1439

Dopamine Hydrochloride (Potential for deleterious cardiovascular effects with other oral sympathomimetic agents).

No products indexed under this heading.

Doxepin Hydrochloride (Action of albuterol on the vascular system may be potentiated). Products include:

Sinequan 2205
Zonalon Cream 1055

Ephedrine Hydrochloride (Potential for deleterious cardiovascular effects with other oral sympathomimetic agents). Products include:

Primatene Dual Action Formula...... ⊕ 872
Primatene Tablets .... ⊕ 873
Quadrinal Tablets 1350

Ephedrine Sulfate (Potential for deleterious cardiovascular effects with other oral sympathomimetic agents). Products include:

Bronkaid Caplets .... ⊕ 717
Marax Tablets & DF Syrup................... 2200

IMPORTANT NOTE: Always consult each drug listing in the patient's regimen for possible interactions.

Volmax Interactions Index 1166

Ephedrine Tannate (Potential for deleterious cardiovascular effects with other oral sympathomimetic agents). Products include:
- Rynatuss ... 2673

Epinephrine (Potential for deleterious cardiovascular effects with other oral sympathomimetic agents). Products include:
- Bronkaid Mist ... ▣ 717
- EPIFRIN ... ⊙ 239
- EpiPen ... 790
- Marcaine Hydrochloride with Epinephrine 1:200,000 ... 2316
- Primatene Mist ... ▣ 873
- Sensorcaine with Epinephrine Injection ... 559
- Sus-Phrine Injection ... 1019
- Xylocaine with Epinephrine Injections ... 567

Epinephrine Bitartrate (Potential for deleterious cardiovascular effects with other oral sympathomimetic agents). Products include:
- Bronkaid Mist Suspension ... ▣ 718
- Sensorcaine-MPF with Epinephrine Injection ... 559

Epinephrine Hydrochloride (Potential for deleterious cardiovascular effects with other oral sympathomimetic agents). Products include:
- Ana-Kit Anaphylaxis Emergency Treatment Kit ... 617

Esmolol Hydrochloride (Effect of each other inhibited). Products include:
- Brevibloc Injection ... 1808

Furazolidone (Action of albuterol on the vascular system may be potentiated). Products include:
- Furoxone ... 2046

Imipramine Hydrochloride (Action of albuterol on the vascular system may be potentiated). Products include:
- Tofranil Ampuls ... 854
- Tofranil Tablets ... 856

Imipramine Pamoate (Action of albuterol on the vascular system may be potentiated). Products include:
- Tofranil-PM Capsules ... 857

Isocarboxazid (Action of albuterol on the vascular system may be potentiated).
- No products indexed under this heading.

Isoproterenol Hydrochloride (Potential for deleterious cardiovascular effects with other oral sympathomimetic agents). Products include:
- Isuprel Hydrochloride Injection 1:5000 ... 2311
- Isuprel Hydrochloride Solution 1:200 & 1:100 ... 2313
- Isuprel Mistometer ... 2312

Isoproterenol Sulfate (Potential for deleterious cardiovascular effects with other oral sympathomimetic agents). Products include:
- Norisodrine with Calcium Iodide Syrup ... 442

Labetalol Hydrochloride (Effect of each other inhibited). Products include:
- Normodyne Injection ... 2377
- Normodyne Tablets ... 2379
- Trandate ... 1185

Levobunolol Hydrochloride (Effect of each other inhibited). Products include:
- Betagan ... ⊙ 233

Maprotiline Hydrochloride (Action of albuterol on the vascular system may be potentiated). Products include:
- Ludiomil Tablets ... 843

Metaproterenol Sulfate (Potential for deleterious cardiovascular effects with other oral sympathomimetic agents). Products include:
- Alupent ... 669
- Metaproterenol Sulfate Inhalation Solution, USP, Arm-a-Med ... 552

Metaraminol Bitartrate (Potential for deleterious cardiovascular effects with other oral sympathomimetic agents). Products include:
- Aramine Injection ... 1609

Methoxamine Hydrochloride (Potential for deleterious cardiovascular effects with other oral sympathomimetic agents). Products include:
- Vasoxyl Injection ... 1196

Metipranolol Hydrochloride (Effect of each other inhibited). Products include:
- OptiPranolol (Metipranolol 0.3%) Sterile Ophthalmic Solution ... ⊙ 258

Metoprolol Succinate (Effect of each other inhibited). Products include:
- Toprol-XL Tablets ... 565

Metoprolol Tartrate (Effect of each other inhibited). Products include:
- Lopressor Ampuls ... 830
- Lopressor HCT Tablets ... 832
- Lopressor Tablets ... 830

Nadolol (Effect of each other inhibited).
- No products indexed under this heading.

Norepinephrine Bitartrate (Potential for deleterious cardiovascular effects with other oral sympathomimetic agents). Products include:
- Levophed Bitartrate Injection ... 2315

Nortriptyline Hydrochloride (Action of albuterol on the vascular system may be potentiated). Products include:
- Pamelor ... 2280

Penbutolol Sulfate (Effect of each other inhibited). Products include:
- Levatol ... 2403

Phenelzine Sulfate (Action of albuterol on the vascular system may be potentiated). Products include:
- Nardil ... 1920

Phenylephrine Bitartrate (Potential for deleterious cardiovascular effects with other oral sympathomimetic agents).
- No products indexed under this heading.

Phenylephrine Hydrochloride (Potential for deleterious cardiovascular effects with other oral sympathomimetic agents). Products include:
- Atrohist Plus Tablets ... 454
- Cerose DM ... ▣ 878
- Comhist ... 2038
- D.A. Chewable Tablets ... 951
- Deconsal Pediatric Capsules ... 454
- Dura-Vent/DA Tablets ... 953
- Entex Capsules ... 1986
- Entex Liquid ... 1986
- Extendryl ... 1005
- 4-Way Fast Acting Nasal Spray (regular & mentholated) ... ▣ 621
- Hemorid For Women ... ▣ 834
- Hycomine Compound Tablets ... 932
- Neo-Synephrine Hydrochloride 1% Carpuject ... 2324
- Neo-Synephrine Hydrochloride 1% Injection ... 2324
- Neo-Synephrine Hydrochloride (Ophthalmic) ... 2325
- Neo-Synephrine ... ▣ 726
- Nōstril ... ▣ 644
- Novahistine Elixir ... ▣ 823
- Phenergan VC ... 2779
- Phenergan VC with Codeine ... 2781
- Preparation H ... ▣ 871
- Tympagesic Ear Drops ... 2342
- Vasosulf ... ⊙ 271
- Vicks Sinex Nasal Spray and Ultra Fine Mist ... ▣ 765

Phenylephrine Tannate (Potential for deleterious cardiovascular effects with other oral sympathomimetic agents). Products include:
- Atrohist Pediatric Suspension ... 454
- Ricobid-D Pediatric Suspension ... 2038
- Ricobid Tablets and Pediatric Suspension ... 2038
- Rynatan ... 2673
- Rynatuss ... 2673

Phenylpropanolamine Hydrochloride (Potential for deleterious cardiovascular effects with other oral sympathomimetic agents). Products include:
- Acutrim ... ▣ 628
- Allerest Children's Chewable Tablets ... ▣ 627
- Allerest 12 Hour Caplets ... ▣ 627
- Atrohist Plus Tablets ... 454
- BC Cold Powder Multi-Symptom Formula (Cold-Sinus-Allergy) ... ▣ 609
- BC Cold Powder Non-Drowsy Formula (Cold-Sinus) ... ▣ 609
- Cheracol Plus Head Cold/Cough Formula ... ▣ 769
- Comtrex Multi-Symptom Non-Drowsy Liqui-gels ... ▣ 618
- Contac Continuous Action Nasal Decongestant/Antihistamine 12 Hour Capsules ... ▣ 813
- Contac Maximum Strength Continuous Action Decongestant/Antihistamine 12 Hour Caplets ... ▣ 813
- Contac Severe Cold and Flu Formula Caplets ... ▣ 814
- Coricidin 'D' Decongestant Tablets ... ▣ 800
- Dexatrim ... ▣ 832
- Dexatrim Plus Vitamins Caplets ... ▣ 832
- Dimetane-DC Cough Syrup ... 2059
- Dimetapp Elixir ... ▣ 773
- Dimetapp Extentabs ... ▣ 774
- Dimetapp Tablets/Liqui-Gels ... ▣ 775
- Dimetapp Cold & Allergy Chewable Tablets ... ▣ 773
- Dimetapp DM Elixir ... ▣ 774
- Dura-Vent Tablets ... 952
- Entex Capsules ... 1986
- Entex LA Tablets ... 1987
- Entex Liquid ... 1986
- Exgest LA Tablets ... 782
- Hycomine ... 931
- Isoclor Timesule Capsules ... ▣ 637
- Nolamine Timed-Release Tablets ... 785
- Ornade Spansule Capsules ... 2502
- Propagest Tablets ... 786
- Pyrroxate Caplets ... ▣ 772
- Robitussin-CF ... ▣ 777
- Sinulin Tablets ... 787
- Tavist-D 12 Hour Relief Tablets ... ▣ 787
- Teldrin 12 Hour Antihistamine/Nasal Decongestant Allergy Relief Capsules ... ▣ 826
- Triaminic Allergy Tablets ... ▣ 789
- Triaminic Cold Tablets ... ▣ 790
- Triaminic Expectorant ... ▣ 790
- Triaminic Syrup ... ▣ 792
- Triaminic-12 Tablets ... ▣ 792
- Triaminic-DM Syrup ... ▣ 792
- Triaminicin Tablets ... ▣ 793
- Triaminicol Multi-Symptom Cold Tablets ... ▣ 793
- Triaminicol Multi-Symptom Relief ... ▣ 794
- Vicks DayQuil Allergy Relief 12-Hour Extended Release Tablets ... ▣ 760
- Vicks DayQuil Allergy Relief 4-Hour Tablets ... ▣ 760
- Vicks DayQuil SINUS Pressure & CONGESTION Relief ... ▣ 761

Pindolol (Effect of each other inhibited). Products include:
- Visken Tablets ... 2299

Pirbuterol Acetate (Potential for deleterious cardiovascular effects with other oral sympathomimetic agents). Products include:
- Maxair Autohaler ... 1492
- Maxair Inhaler ... 1494

Propranolol Hydrochloride (Effect of each other inhibited). Products include:
- Inderal ... 2728
- Inderal LA Long Acting Capsules ... 2730
- Inderide Tablets ... 2732
- Inderide LA Long Acting Capsules ... 2734

Protriptyline Hydrochloride (Action of albuterol on the vascular system may be potentiated). Products include:
- Vivactil Tablets ... 1774

Pseudoephedrine Hydrochloride (Potential for deleterious cardiovascular effects with other oral sympathomimetic agents). Products include:
- Actifed Allergy Daytime/Nighttime Caplets ... ▣ 844
- Actifed Plus Caplets ... ▣ 845
- Actifed Plus Tablets ... ▣ 845
- Actifed with Codeine Cough Syrup ... 1067
- Actifed Sinus Daytime/Nighttime Tablets and Caplets ... ▣ 846
- Actifed Syrup ... ▣ 846
- Actifed Tablets ... ▣ 844
- Advil Cold and Sinus Caplets and Tablets (formerly CoAdvil) ... ▣ 870
- Alka-Seltzer Plus Cold Medicine Liqui-Gels ... ▣ 706
- Alka-Seltzer Plus Cold & Cough Medicine Liqui-Gels ... ▣ 705
- Alka-Seltzer Plus Night-Time Cold Medicine Liqui-Gels ... ▣ 706
- Allerest Headache Strength Tablets ... ▣ 627
- Allerest Maximum Strength Tablets ... ▣ 627
- Allerest No Drowsiness Tablets ... ▣ 627
- Allerest Sinus Pain Formula ... ▣ 627
- Anatuss LA Tablets ... 1542
- Atrohist Pediatric Capsules ... 453
- Bayer Select Sinus Pain Relief Formula ... ▣ 717
- Benadryl Allergy Decongestant Liquid Medication ... ▣ 848
- Benadryl Allergy Decongestant Tablets ... ▣ 848
- Benadryl Allergy Sinus Headache Formula Caplets ... ▣ 849
- Benylin Multisymptom ... ▣ 852
- Bromfed Capsules (Extended-Release) ... 1785
- Bromfed Syrup ... ▣ 733
- Bromfed Tablets ... 1785
- Bromfed-DM Cough Syrup ... 1786
- Bromfed-PD Capsules (Extended-Release) ... 1785
- Children's Vicks DayQuil Allergy Relief ... ▣ 757
- Children's Vicks NyQuil Cold/Cough Relief ... ▣ 758
- Comtrex Multi-Symptom Cold Reliever Tablets/Caplets/Liqui-Gels/Liquid ... ▣ 615
- Allergy-Sinus Comtrex Multi-Symptom Allergy-Sinus Formula Tablets ... ▣ 617
- Comtrex Multi-Symptom Non-Drowsy Caplets ... ▣ 618
- Congess ... 1004
- Contac Day Allergy/Sinus Caplets ... ▣ 812
- Contac Day & Night ... ▣ 812
- Contac Night Allergy/Sinus Caplets ... ▣ 812
- Contac Severe Cold & Flu Non-Drowsy ... ▣ 815
- Deconamine Chewable Tablets ... 1320
- Deconamine CX Cough and Cold Liquid and Tablets ... 1319
- Deconamine ... 1320
- Deconsal C Expectorant Syrup ... 456
- Deconsal Pediatric Syrup ... 457
- Deconsal II Tablets ... 454
- Dimetane-DX Cough Syrup ... 2059
- Dimetapp Sinus Caplets ... ▣ 775
- Dorcol Children's Cough Syrup ... ▣ 785
- Drixoral Cough + Congestion Liquid Caps ... ▣ 802
- Dura-Tap/PD Capsules ... 2867
- Duratuss Tablets ... 2565
- Duratuss HD Elixir ... 2565
- Efidac/24 ... ▣ 635
- Entex PSE Tablets ... 1987
- Fedahist Gyrocaps ... 2401
- Fedahist Timecaps ... 2401
- Guaifed ... 1787
- Guaifed Syrup ... ▣ 734
- Guaimax-D Tablets ... 792
- Guaitab Tablets ... ▣ 734
- Isoclor Expectorant ... 990
- Kronofed-A ... 977
- Motrin IB Sinus ... ▣ 838
- Novahistine DH ... 2462

(▣ Described in PDR For Nonprescription Drugs) (⊙ Described in PDR For Ophthalmology)

Interactions Index

Cataflam/Voltaren

Novahistine DMX .... ®◻ 822
Novahistine Expectorant........................ 2463
Nucofed 2051
PediaCare Cold Allergy Chewable Tablets .... ®◻ 677
PediaCare Cough-Cold Chewable Tablets 1553
PediaCare 1553
PediaCare Infants' Decongestant Drops .... ®◻ 677
PediCare Infant's Drops Decongestant Plus Cough 1553
PediaCare NightRest Cough-Cold Liquid 1553
Pediatric Vicks 44d Dry Hacking Cough & Head Congestion.............. ®◻ 763
Pediatric Vicks 44m Cough & Cold Relief .... ®◻ 764
Robitussin Cold & Cough Liqui-Gels .... ®◻ 776
Robitussin Maximum Strength Cough & Cold .... ®◻ 778
Robitussin Pediatric Cough & Cold Formula.. ®◻ 779
Robitussin Severe Congestion Liqui-Gels .... ®◻ 776
Robitussin-DAC Syrup 2074
Robitussin-PE .... ®◻ 778
Rondec Oral Drops 953
Rondec Syrup 953
Rondec Tablet 953
Rondec-DM Oral Drops 954
Rondec-DM Syrup 954
Rondec-TR Tablet 953
Ryna .... ®◻ 841
Seldane-D Extended-Release Tablets 1538
Semprex-D Capsules 463
Semprex-D Capsules 1167
Sinarest Tablets .... ®◻ 648
Sinarest Extra Strength Tablets...... ®◻ 648
Sinarest No Drowsiness Tablets .... ®◻ 648
Sine-Aid IB Caplets 1554
Sine-Aid Maximum Strength Sinus Medication Gelcaps, Caplets and Tablets 1554
Sine-Off No Drowsiness Formula Caplets .... ®◻ 824
Sine-Off Sinus Medicine .... ®◻ 825
Singlet Tablets .... ®◻ 825
Sinutab Non-Drying Liquid Caps .... ®◻ 859
Sinutab Sinus Allergy Medication, Maximum Strength Tablets and Caplets .... ®◻ 860
Sinutab Sinus Medication, Maximum Strength Without Drowsiness Formula, Tablets & Caplets .... ®◻ 860
Sinutab Sinus Medication, Regular Strength Without Drowsiness Formula .... ®◻ 859
Sudafed Children's Liquid .... ®◻ 861
Sudafed Cold and Cough Liquidcaps .... ®◻ 862
Sudafed Cough Syrup .... ®◻ 862
Sudafed Plus Liquid .... ®◻ 862
Sudafed Plus Tablets .... ®◻ 863
Sudafed Severe Cold Formula Caplets .... ®◻ 863
Sudafed Severe Cold Formula Tablets .... ®◻ 864
Sudafed Sinus Caplets.......................... ®◻ 864
Sudafed Sinus Tablets.......................... ®◻ 864
Sudafed Tablets, 30 mg........................ ®◻ 861
Sudafed Tablets, 60 mg........................ ®◻ 861
Sudafed 12 Hour Caplets .... ®◻ 861
Syn-Rx Tablets 465
Syn-Rx DM Tablets 466
TheraFlu... ®◻ 787
TheraFlu Maximum Strength Nighttime Flu, Cold & Cough Medicine .... ®◻ 788
TheraFlu Maximum Strength Non-Drowsy Formula Flu, Cold & Cough Medicine .... ®◻ 788
Thera Flu Maximum Strength, Non-Drowsy Formula Flu, Cold and Cough Caplets .... ®◻ 789
Triaminic AM Cough and Decongestant Formula .... ®◻ 789
Triaminic AM Decongestant Formula .... ®◻ 790
Triaminic Nite Light .... ®◻ 791
Triaminic Sore Throat Formula ...... ®◻ 791
Tussend 1783
Tussend Expectorant 1785
Children's TYLENOL Cold Multi-Symptom Liquid Formula and Chewable Tablets.................................... 1561

Children's TYLENOL Cold Plus Cough Multi Symptom Tablets and Liquid .... ®◻ 681
Infants' TYLENOL Cold Decongestant & Fever-Reducer Drops 1556
TYLENOL Maximum Strength Allergy Sinus Medication Gelcaps and Caplets 1563
TYLENOL Maximum Strength Allergy Sinus NightTime Medication Caplets 1555
TYLENOL Flu Maximum Strength Gelcaps 1565
TYLENOL Flu NightTime, Maximum Strength, Gelcaps 1566
TYLENOL Maximum Strength Flu NightTime Hot Medication Packets 1562
TYLENOL, Maximum Strength, Sinus Medication Geltabs, Gelcaps, Caplets and Tablets 1566
TYLENOL Cold Multi-Symptom Formula Medication Tablets and Caplets 1561
TYLENOL Cold Medication No Drowsiness Formula Gelcaps and Caplets 1562
TYLENOL Cold Multi-Symptom Hot Medication Liquid Packets.............. 1557
TYLENOL Cough Multi-Symptom Medication with Decongestant...... 1565
Ursinus Inlay-Tabs.................................. ®◻ 794
Vicks 44 LiquiCaps Cough, Cold & Flu Relief .... ®◻ 755
Vicks 44 LiquiCaps Non-Drowsy Cough & Cold Relief .... ®◻ 756
Vicks 44D Dry Hacking Cough & Head Congestion .... ®◻ 755
Vicks 44M Cough, Cold & Flu Relief.. ®◻ 756
Vicks DayQuil .... ®◻ 761
Vicks DayQuil SINUS Pressure & PAIN Relief with IBUPROFEN ...... ®◻ 762
Vicks Nyquil Hot Therapy.................... ®◻ 762
Vicks NyQuil LiquiCaps Multi-Symptom Cold/Flu Relief .... ®◻ 763
Vicks NyQuil Multi-Symptom Cold/Flu Relief - (Original & Cherry Flavor) .... ®◻ 763

Pseudoephedrine Sulfate (Potential for deleterious cardiovascular effects with other oral sympathomimetic agents). Products include:

Cheracol Sinus .... ®◻ 768
Chlor-Trimeton Allergy Decongestant Tablets .... ®◻ 799
Claritin-D 2350
Drixoral Cold and Allergy Sustained-Action Tablets .... ®◻ 802
Drixoral Cold and Flu Extended-Release Tablets.................................... ®◻ 803
Drixoral Non-Drowsy Formula Extended-Release Tablets .... ®◻ 803
Drixoral Allergy/Sinus Extended Release Tablets.................................... ®◻ 804
Trinalin Repetabs Tablets 1330

Salmeterol Xinafoate (Potential for deleterious cardiovascular effects with other oral sympathomimetic agents). Products include:

Serevent Inhalation Aerosol.................. 1176

Selegiline Hydrochloride (Action of albuterol on the vascular system may be potentiated). Products include:

Eldepryl Tablets 2550

Sotalol Hydrochloride (Effect of each other inhibited). Products include:

Betapace Tablets 641

Terbutaline Sulfate (Potential for deleterious cardiovascular effects with other oral sympathomimetic agents). Products include:

Brethaire Inhaler 813
Brethine Ampuls 815
Brethine Tablets.. 814
Bricanyl Subcutaneous Injection...... 1502
Bricanyl Tablets 1503

Timolol Hemihydrate (Effect of each other inhibited). Products include:

Betimol 0.25%, 0.5% .... © 261

Timolol Maleate (Effect of each other inhibited). Products include:

Blocadren Tablets 1614

Timolide Tablets.. 1748
Timoptic in Ocudose 1753
Timoptic Sterile Ophthalmic Solution.. 1751
Timoptic-XE 1755

Tranylcypromine Sulfate (Action of albuterol on the vascular system may be potentiated). Products include:

Parnate Tablets 2503

Trimipramine Maleate (Action of albuterol on the vascular system may be potentiated). Products include:

Surmontil Capsules.................................... 2811

Food Interactions

Food, unspecified (Food may decrease the rate of absorption without altering the extent of bioavailability).

VOLTAREN OPHTHALMIC STERILE OPHTHALMIC SOLUTION

(Diclofenac Sodium) .... © 272
None cited in PDR database.

VOLTAREN TABLETS

(Diclofenac Sodium) 861
May interact with oral anticoagulants, oral hypoglycemic agents, diuretics, lithium preparations, potassium sparing diuretics, insulin, and certain other agents. Compounds in these categories include:

Acarbose (Diclofenac may alter a diabetic patient's response to oral hypoglycemic agents).

No products indexed under this heading.

Amiloride Hydrochloride (Potential for increased serum potassium levels; Voltaren can inhibit diuretic activity). Products include:

Midamor Tablets 1703
Moduretic Tablets 1705

Aspirin (Lowers plasma concentrations, peak plasma levels, and AUC values). Products include:

Alka-Seltzer Effervescent Antacid and Pain Reliever................................ ®◻ 701
Alka-Seltzer Extra Strength Effervescent Antacid and Pain Reliever .... ®◻ 703
Alka-Seltzer Lemon Lime Effervescent Antacid and Pain Reliever .... ®◻ 703
Alka-Seltzer Plus Cold Medicine .... ®◻ 705
Alka-Seltzer Plus Cold & Cough Medicine .... ®◻ 708
Alka-Seltzer Plus Night-Time Cold Medicine .... ®◻ 707
Alka Seltzer Plus Sinus Medicine .. ®◻ 707
Arthritis Foundation Safety Coated Aspirin Tablets .... ®◻ 675
Arthritis Pain Ascriptin .... ®◻ 631
Maximum Strength Ascriptin .... ®◻ 630
Regular Strength Ascriptin Tablets .... ®◻ 629
Arthritis Strength BC Powder.......... ®◻ 609
BC Cold Powder Multi-Symptom Formula (Cold-Sinus-Allergy) ...... ®◻ 609
BC Cold Powder Non-Drowsy Formula (Cold-Sinus) .... ®◻ 609
BC Powder .... ®◻ 609
Bayer Children's Chewable Aspirin.. ®◻ 711
Genuine Bayer Aspirin Tablets & Caplets .... ®◻ 713
Extra Strength Bayer Arthritis Pain Regimen Formula .... ®◻ 711
Extra Strength Bayer Aspirin Caplets & Tablets .... ®◻ 712
Extended-Release Bayer 8-Hour Aspirin .... ®◻ 712
Extra Strength Bayer Plus Aspirin Caplets .... ®◻ 713
Extra Strength Bayer PM Aspirin .. ®◻ 713
Bayer Enteric Aspirin .... ®◻ 709
Bufferin Analgesic Tablets and Caplets .... ®◻ 613
Arthritis Strength Bufferin Analgesic Caplets .... ®◻ 614

Extra Strength Bufferin Analgesic Tablets .... ®◻ 615
Cama Arthritis Pain Reliever.............. ®◻ 785
Darvon Compound-65 Pulvules 1435
Easprin.. 1914
Ecotrin 2455
Ecotrin Enteric Coated Aspirin Maximum Strength Tablets and Caplets .... ®◻ 816
Ecotrin Enteric Coated Aspirin Regular Strength Tablets 2455
Empirin Aspirin Tablets .... ®◻ 854
Empirin with Codeine Tablets.............. 1093
Excedrin Extra-Strength Analgesic Tablets & Caplets 732
Fiorinal Capsules 2261
Fiorinal with Codeine Capsules 2262
Fiorinal Tablets.. 2261
Halfprin 1362
Healthprin Aspirin 2455
Norgesic.. 1496
Percodan Tablets.. 939
Percodan-Demi Tablets.............................. 940
Robaxisal Tablets.. 2071
Soma Compound w/Codeine Tablets 2676
Soma Compound Tablets........................ 2675
St. Joseph Adult Chewable Aspirin (81 mg.) .... ®◻ 808
Talwin Compound 2335
Ursinus Inlay-Tabs.................................... ®◻ 794
Vanquish Analgesic Caplets .... ®◻ 731

Bendroflumethiazide (Voltaren can inhibit diuretic activity).

No products indexed under this heading.

Bumetanide (Voltaren can inhibit diuretic activity). Products include:

Bumex 2093

Chlorothiazide (Voltaren can inhibit diuretic activity). Products include:

Aldoclor Tablets 1598
Diupres Tablets 1650
Diuril Oral 1653

Chlorothiazide Sodium (Voltaren can inhibit diuretic activity). Products include:

Diuril Sodium Intravenous 1652

Chlorpropamide (Diclofenac may alter a diabetic patient's response to oral hypoglycemic agents). Products include:

Diabinese Tablets 1935

Chlorthalidone (Voltaren can inhibit diuretic activity). Products include:

Combipres Tablets 677
Tenoretic Tablets.. 2845
Thalitone 1245

Cyclosporine (Voltaren through renal prostaglandins may cause increased toxicity of cyclosporine). Products include:

Neoral.. 2276
Sandimmune 2286

Diclofenac Potassium (Concomitant use with other diclofenac-containing products should be avoided since they also circulate in plasma as diclofenac anion). Products include:

Cataflam 816

Dicumarol (Concurrent therapy requires close monitoring of patients for anticoagulant dosage).

No products indexed under this heading.

Digoxin (Voltaren through renal prostaglandins may cause increased toxicity of digoxin). Products include:

Lanoxicaps 1117
Lanoxin Elixir Pediatric 1120
Lanoxin Injection 1123
Lanoxin Injection Pediatric.................... 1126
Lanoxin Tablets 1128

Ethacrynic Acid (Voltaren can inhibit diuretic activity). Products include:

Edecrin Tablets.. 1657

Furosemide (Voltaren can inhibit diuretic activity). Products include:

Lasix Injection, Oral Solution and Tablets 1240

IMPORTANT NOTE: Always consult each drug listing in the patient's regimen for possible interactions.

Voltaren / Cataflam Interactions Index 1168

Glipizide (Diclofenac may alter a diabetic patient's response to oral hypoglycemic agents). Products include:
Glucotrol Tablets ... 1967
Glucotrol XL Extended Release Tablets ... 1968
Glyburide (Diclofenac may alter a diabetic patient's response to oral hypoglycemic agents). Products include:
DiaBeta Tablets ... 1239
Glynase PresTab Tablets ... 2609
Micronase Tablets ... 2623
Hydrochlorothiazide (Voltaren can inhibit diuretic activity). Products include:
Aldactazide ... 2413
Aldoril Tablets ... 1604
Apresazide Capsules ... 808
Capozide ... 742
Dyazide ... 2479
Esidrix Tablets ... 821
Esimil Tablets ... 822
HydroDIURIL Tablets ... 1674
Hydropres Tablets ... 1675
Hyzaar Tablets ... 1677
Inderide Tablets ... 2732
Inderide LA Long Acting Capsules .. 2734
Lopressor HCT Tablets ... 832
Lotensin HCT ... 837
Maxzide ... 1380
Moduretic Tablets ... 1705
Oretic Tablets ... 443
Prinzide Tablets ... 1737
Ser-Ap-Es Tablets ... 849
Timolide Tablets ... 1748
Vaseretic Tablets ... 1765
Zestoretic ... 2850
Ziac ... 1415
Hydroflumethiazide (Voltaren can inhibit diuretic activity). Products include:
Diucardin Tablets ... 2718
Indapamide (Voltaren can inhibit diuretic activity). Products include:
Lozol Tablets ... 2022
Insulin, Human (Diclofenac may alter a diabetic patient's response to insulin).
No products indexed under this heading.
Insulin, Human Isophane Suspension (Diclofenac may alter a diabetic patient's response to insulin). Products include:
Novolin N Human Insulin 10 ml Vials ... 1795
Insulin, Human NPH (Diclofenac may alter a diabetic patient's response to insulin). Products include:
Humulin N, 100 Units ... 1448
Novolin N PenFill Cartridges Durable Insulin Delivery System ... 1798
Novolin N Prefilled Syringe Disposable Insulin Delivery System ... 1798
Insulin, Human Regular (Diclofenac may alter a diabetic patient's response to insulin). Products include:
Humulin R, 100 Units ... 1449
Novolin R Human Insulin 10 ml Vials ... 1795
Novolin R PenFill Cartridges Durable Insulin Delivery System ... 1798
Novolin R Prefilled Syringe Disposable Insulin Delivery System ... 1798
Velosulin BR Human Insulin 10 ml Vials ... 1795
Insulin, Human, Zinc Suspension (Diclofenac may alter a diabetic patient's response to insulin). Products include:
Humulin L, 100 Units ... 1446
Humulin U, 100 Units ... 1450
Novolin L Human Insulin 10 ml Vials ... 1795
Insulin, NPH (Diclofenac may alter a diabetic patient's response to insulin). Products include:
NPH, 100 Units ... 1450
Pork NPH, 100 Units ... 1452
Purified Pork NPH Isophane Insulin ... 1801
Insulin, Regular (Diclofenac may alter a diabetic patient's response to insulin). Products include:
Regular, 100 Units ... 1450
Pork Regular, 100 Units ... 1452
Pork Regular (Concentrated), 500 Units ... 1453
Purified Pork Regular Insulin ... 1801
Insulin, Zinc Crystals (Diclofenac may alter a diabetic patient's response to insulin). Products include:
NPH, 100 Units ... 1450
Insulin, Zinc Suspension (Diclofenac may alter a diabetic patient's response to insulin). Products include:
Iletin I ... 1450
Lente, 100 Units ... 1450
Iletin II ... 1452
Pork Lente, 100 Units ... 1452
Purified Pork Lente Insulin ... 1801
Lithium Carbonate (Decreased lithium renal clearance and increased lithium plasma levels). Products include:
Eskalith ... 2485
Lithium Carbonate Capsules & Tablets ... 2230
Lithonate/Lithotabs/Lithobid ... 2543
Lithium Citrate (Decreased lithium renal clearance and increased lithium plasma levels).
No products indexed under this heading.
Metformin Hydrochloride (Diclofenac may alter a diabetic patient's response to oral hypoglycemic agents). Products include:
Glucophage ... 752
Methotrexate Sodium (Voltaren through renal prostaglandins may cause increased toxicity of methotrexate). Products include:
Methotrexate Sodium Tablets, Injection, for Injection and LPF Injection ... 1275
Methyclothiazide (Voltaren can inhibit diuretic activity). Products include:
Enduron Tablets ... 420
Metolazone (Voltaren can inhibit diuretic activity). Products include:
Mykrox Tablets ... 993
Zaroxolyn Tablets ... 1000
Polythiazide (Voltaren can inhibit diuretic activity). Products include:
Minizide Capsules ... 1938
Spironolactone (Potential for increased serum potassium levels; Voltaren can inhibit diuretic activity). Products include:
Aldactazide ... 2413
Aldactone ... 2414
Tolazamide (Diclofenac may alter a diabetic patient's response to oral hypoglycemic agents).
No products indexed under this heading.
Tolbutamide (Diclofenac may alter a diabetic patient's response to oral hypoglycemic agents).
No products indexed under this heading.
Torsemide (Voltaren can inhibit diuretic activity). Products include:
Demadex Tablets and Injection ... 686
Triamterene (Potential for increased serum potassium levels; Voltaren can inhibit diuretic activity). Products include:
Dyazide ... 2479
Dyrenium Capsules ... 2481
Maxzide ... 1380
Warfarin Sodium (Concurrent therapy requires close monitoring of patients for anticoagulant dosage). Products include:
Coumadin ... 926

Food Interactions

Food, unspecified (Delays the onset of absorption by 1 to 4.5 hours, with delays as long as 10 hours in some patients and reduction in peak plasma levels by approximately 40%; rate of Cataflam absorption is reduced by food; the extent of absorption is not significantly affected).

VONTROL TABLETS
(Diphenidol) ... 2532
None cited in PDR database.

VōSOL HC OTIC SOLUTION
(Acetic Acid, Hydrocortisone) ... 2678
None cited in PDR database.

VōSOL OTIC SOLUTION
(Acetic Acid) ... 2678
None cited in PDR database.

VUMON
(Teniposide) ... 727
May interact with:

Methotrexate Sodium (Co-administration slightly increases methotrexate clearance; an increase in intracellular levels of methotrexate has been observed *in vitro* in the presence of teniposide). Products include:
Methotrexate Sodium Tablets, Injection, for Injection and LPF Injection ... 1275
Sodium Salicylate (Possible potentiation of drug toxicity due to small decrease in protein binding causing substantial increase in free teniposide).
No products indexed under this heading.
Sulfamethizole (Possible potentiation of drug toxicity due to small decrease in protein binding causing substantial increase in free teniposide). Products include:
Urobiotic-250 Capsules ... 2214
Tolbutamide (Possible potentiation of drug toxicity due to small decrease in protein binding causing substantial increase in free teniposide).
No products indexed under this heading.

WART-OFF WART REMOVER
(Salicylic Acid) ... ▭ 747
None cited in PDR database.

WATER-JEL BURN JEL
(Lidocaine) ... 2682
None cited in PDR database.

WATER-JEL STERILE BURN DRESSINGS
(Dressings, sterile) ... 2682
None cited in PDR database.

WELLBUTRIN TABLETS
(Bupropion Hydrochloride) ... 1204
May interact with drugs affecting hepatic drug metabolizing enzyme systems, monoamine oxidase inhibitors, drugs which lower seizure threshold, and certain other agents. Compounds in these categories include:

Alprazolam (Concurrent therapy should be undertaken with extreme caution). Products include:
Xanax Tablets ... 2649
Amitriptyline Hydrochloride (Concurrent therapy should be undertaken with extreme caution). Products include:
Elavil ... 2838
Endep Tablets ... 2174
Etrafon ... 2355
Limbitrol ... 2180
Triavil Tablets ... 1757
Amoxapine (Concurrent therapy should be undertaken with extreme caution). Products include:
Asendin Tablets ... 1369
Carbamazepine (Concurrent therapy may affect metabolism of bupropion). Products include:
Atretol Tablets ... 573
Tegretol Chewable Tablets ... 852
Tegretol Suspension ... 852
Tegretol Tablets ... 852
Chlordiazepoxide (Concurrent therapy should be undertaken with extreme caution). Products include:
Libritabs Tablets ... 2177
Limbitrol ... 2180
Chlordiazepoxide Hydrochloride (Concurrent therapy should be undertaken with extreme caution). Products include:
Librax Capsules ... 2176
Librium Capsules ... 2178
Librium Injectable ... 2179
Chlorpromazine (Concurrent therapy should be undertaken with extreme caution). Products include:
Thorazine Suppositories ... 2523
Cimetidine (Concurrent therapy may affect metabolism of bupropion). Products include:
Tagamet Tablets ... 2516
Cimetidine Hydrochloride (Concurrent therapy may affect metabolism of bupropion). Products include:
Tagamet ... 2516
Desipramine Hydrochloride (Concurrent therapy should be undertaken with extreme caution). Products include:
Norpramin Tablets ... 1526
Diazepam (Concurrent therapy should be undertaken with extreme caution). Products include:
Dizac ... 1809
Valium Injectable ... 2182
Valium Tablets ... 2183
Valrelease Capsules ... 2169
Doxepin Hydrochloride (Concurrent therapy should be undertaken with extreme caution). Products include:
Sinequan ... 2205
Zonalon Cream ... 1055
Fluoxetine Hydrochloride (Concurrent therapy should be undertaken with extreme caution). Products include:
Prozac Pulvules & Liquid, Oral Solution ... 919
Fluphenazine Decanoate (Concurrent therapy should be undertaken with extreme caution). Products include:
Prolixin Decanoate ... 509
Fluphenazine Enanthate (Concurrent therapy should be undertaken with extreme caution). Products include:
Prolixin Enanthate ... 509
Fluphenazine Hydrochloride (Concurrent therapy should be undertaken with extreme caution). Products include:
Prolixin ... 509
Furazolidone (Concurrent administration is contraindicated). Products include:
Furoxone ... 2046

Interactions Index

Haloperidol (Concurrent therapy should be undertaken with extreme caution). Products include:

Haldol Injection, Tablets and Concentrate 1575

Haloperidol Decanoate (Concurrent therapy should be undertaken with extreme caution). Products include:

Haldol Decanoate.................................. 1577

Imipramine Hydrochloride (Concurrent therapy should be undertaken with extreme caution). Products include:

Tofranil Ampuls 854
Tofranil Tablets 856

Imipramine Pamoate (Concurrent therapy should be undertaken with extreme caution). Products include:

Tofranil-PM Capsules............................ 857

Isocarboxazid (Concurrent administration is contraindicated).

No products indexed under this heading.

Levodopa (Potential for higher incidence of adverse experiences). Products include:

Atamet 572
Larodopa Tablets.................................. 2129
Sinemet Tablets 943
Sinemet CR Tablets 944

Lorazepam (Concurrent therapy should be undertaken with extreme caution). Products include:

Ativan Injection.................................... 2698
Ativan Tablets....................................... 2700

Maprotiline Hydrochloride (Concurrent therapy should be undertaken with extreme caution). Products include:

Ludiomil Tablets................................... 843

Mesoridazine Besylate (Concurrent therapy should be undertaken with extreme caution). Products include:

Serentil... 684

Nortriptyline Hydrochloride (Concurrent therapy should be undertaken with extreme caution). Products include:

Pamelor 2280

Oxazepam (Concurrent therapy should be undertaken with extreme caution). Products include:

Serax Capsules 2810
Serax Tablets.. 2810

Perphenazine (Concurrent therapy should be undertaken with extreme caution). Products include:

Etrafon 2355
Triavil Tablets 1757
Trilafon... 2389

Phenelzine Sulfate (Concurrent administration is contraindicated). Products include:

Nardil 1920

Phenobarbital (Concurrent therapy may affect metabolism of bupropion). Products include:

Arco-Lase Plus Tablets 512
Bellergal-S Tablets 2250
Donnatal 2060
Donnatal Extentabs............................... 2061
Donnatal Tablets 2060
Phenobarbital Elixir and Tablets 1469
Quadrinal Tablets 1350

Phenytoin (Concurrent therapy may affect metabolism of bupropion). Products include:

Dilantin Infatabs................................... 1908
Dilantin-125 Suspension 1911

Phenytoin Sodium (Concurrent therapy may affect metabolism of bupropion). Products include:

Dilantin Kapseals 1906
Dilantin Parenteral 1910

Prazepam (Concurrent therapy should be undertaken with extreme caution).

No products indexed under this heading.

Prochlorperazine (Concurrent therapy should be undertaken with extreme caution). Products include:

Compazine 2470

Promethazine Hydrochloride (Concurrent therapy should be undertaken with extreme caution). Products include:

Mepergan Injection 2753
Phenergan with Codeine....................... 2777
Phenergan with Dextromethorphan 2778
Phenergan Injection 2773
Phenergan Suppositories 2775
Phenergan Syrup 2774
Phenergan Tablets 2775
Phenergan VC....................................... 2779
Phenergan VC with Codeine 2781

Protriptyline Hydrochloride (Concurrent therapy should be undertaken with extreme caution). Products include:

Vivactil Tablets...................................... 1774

Selegiline Hydrochloride (Concurrent administration is contraindicated). Products include:

Eldepryl Tablets 2550

Thioridazine Hydrochloride (Concurrent therapy should be undertaken with extreme caution). Products include:

Mellaril 2269

Tranylcypromine Sulfate (Concurrent administration is contraindicated). Products include:

Parnate Tablets 2503

Trazodone Hydrochloride (Concurrent therapy should be undertaken with extreme caution). Products include:

Desyrel and Desyrel Dividose.............. 503

Trifluoperazine Hydrochloride (Concurrent therapy should be undertaken with extreme caution). Products include:

Stelazine 2514

Trimipramine Maleate (Concurrent therapy should be undertaken with extreme caution). Products include:

Surmontil Capsules............................... 2811

Food Interactions

Alcohol (Concurrent alcohol consumption should be avoided or minimized).

WESTCORT CREAM 0.2%

(Hydrocortisone Valerate) 2690
None cited in PDR database.

WESTCORT OINTMENT 0.2%

(Hydrocortisone Valerate) 2690
None cited in PDR database.

WIGRAINE TABLETS & SUPPOSITORIES

(Ergotamine Tartrate, Caffeine)..........1829
None cited in PDR database.

WINRGY

(Nutritional Beverage) .... ✦ 870
May interact with:

Aluminum Carbonate Gel (Concomitant use with aluminum-containing antacids should be avoided). Products include:

Basaljel... 2703

Aluminum Hydroxide (Concomitant use with aluminum-containing antacids should be avoided). Products include:

ALternaGEL Liquid 1316
Maximum Strength Ascriptin .... ✦ 630

Cama Arthritis Pain Reliever............. ✦ 785
Gaviscon Extra Strength Relief Formula Antacid Tablets.................. ✦ 819
Gaviscon Extra Strength Relief Formula Liquid Antacid................... ✦ 819
Gaviscon Liquid Antacid .... ✦ 820
Gelusil Liquid & Tablets .... ✦ 855
Maalox Heartburn Relief Suspension .... ✦ 642
Maalox Heartburn Relief Tablets.... ✦ 641
Maalox Magnesia and Alumina Oral Suspension .... ✦ 642
Maalox Plus Tablets .... ✦ 643
Extra Strength Maalox Antacid Plus Antigas Liquid and Tablets ✦ 638
Tempo Soft Antacid .... ✦ 835

Aluminum Hydroxide Gel (Concomitant use with aluminum-containing antacids should be avoided). Products include:

ALternaGEL Liquid .... ✦ 659
Aludrox Oral Suspension 2695
Amphojel Suspension 2695
Amphojel Suspension without Flavor 2695
Amphojel Tablets.................................. 2695
Arthritis Pain Ascriptin .... ✦ 631
Regular Strength Ascriptin Tablets .... ✦ 629
Gaviscon Antacid Tablets..................... ✦ 819
Gaviscon-2 Antacid Tablets .... ✦ 820
Mylanta Liquid 1317
Mylanta Tablets .... ✦ 660
Mylanta Double Strength Liquid 1317
Mylanta Double Strength Tablets .. ✦ 660
Nephrox Suspension .... ✦ 655

WINRHO SD

(Immune Globulin Intravenous (Human))..2576
None cited in PDR database.

WINRHO SD

(Globulin, Immune (Human)) 2577
None cited in PDR database.

WINSTROL TABLETS

(Stanozolol)...2337
May interact with oral anticoagulants. Compounds in this category include:

Dicumarol (Increased sensitivity to anticoagulants).

No products indexed under this heading.

Warfarin Sodium (Increased sensitivity to anticoagulants). Products include:

Coumadin 926

WOBENZYM N

(Pancreatin, Trypsin, Chymotrypsin, Bromelains, Papain) ✦ 673
None cited in PDR database.

WOUN'DRES, NATURAL COLLAGEN HYDROGEL WOUND DRESSING

(Allantoin) 2555
None cited in PDR database.

WYANOIDS RELIEF FACTOR HEMORRHOIDAL SUPPOSITORIES

(Liver, Desiccated, Shark Liver Oil) ✦ 881
None cited in PDR database.

WYGESIC TABLETS

(Propoxyphene Hydrochloride, Acetaminophen)......................................2827
May interact with central nervous system depressants, antidepressant drugs, oral anticoagulants, anticonvulsants, tranquilizers, and certain other agents. Compounds in these categories include:

Alfentanil Hydrochloride (Additive effects). Products include:

Alfenta Injection 1286

Alprazolam (Additive effects). Products include:

Xanax Tablets 2649

Amitriptyline Hydrochloride (Propoxyphene may slow the metabolism of antidepressants). Products include:

Elavil 2838
Endep Tablets....................................... 2174
Etrafon 2355
Limbitrol 2180
Triavil Tablets 1757

Amoxapine (Propoxyphene may slow the metabolism of antidepressants). Products include:

Asendin Tablets 1369

Aprobarbital (Additive effects).

No products indexed under this heading.

Buprenorphine (Additive effects). Products include:

Buprenex Injectable 2006

Bupropion Hydrochloride (Propoxyphene may slow the metabolism of antidepressants). Products include:

Wellbutrin Tablets 1204

Buspirone Hydrochloride (Additive effects). Products include:

BuSpar 737

Butabarbital (Additive effects).

No products indexed under this heading.

Butalbital (Additive effects). Products include:

Esgic-plus Tablets 1013
Fioricet Tablets..................................... 2258
Fioricet with Codeine Capsules 2260
Fiorinal Capsules 2261
Fiorinal with Codeine Capsules 2262
Fiorinal Tablets..................................... 2261
Phrenilin 785
Sedapap Tablets 50 mg/650 mg .. 1543

Carbamazepine (Propoxyphene may slow the metabolism of anticonvulsants). Products include:

Atretol Tablets 573
Tegretol Chewable Tablets 852
Tegretol Suspension.............................. 852
Tegretol Tablets 852

Chlordiazepoxide (Additive effects). Products include:

Libritabs Tablets 2177
Limbitrol 2180

Chlordiazepoxide Hydrochloride (Additive effects). Products include:

Librax Capsules 2176
Librium Capsules.................................. 2178
Librium Injectable 2179

Chlorpromazine (Additive effects). Products include:

Thorazine Suppositories....................... 2523

Chlorprothixene (Additive effects).

No products indexed under this heading.

Chlorprothixene Hydrochloride (Additive effects).

No products indexed under this heading.

Clorazepate Dipotassium (Additive effects). Products include:

Tranxene 451

Clozapine (Additive effects). Products include:

Clozaril Tablets..................................... 2252

Codeine Phosphate (Additive effects). Products include:

Actifed with Codeine Cough Syrup.. 1067
Brontex 1981
Deconsal C Expectorant Syrup 456
Deconsal Pediatric Syrup 457
Dimetane-DC Cough Syrup 2059
Empirin with Codeine Tablets............ 1093
Fioricet with Codeine Capsules 2260
Fiorinal with Codeine Capsules 2262
Isoclor Expectorant.............................. 990
Novahistine DH.................................... 2462
Novahistine Expectorant...................... 2463
Nucofed 2051
Phenergan with Codeine...................... 2777
Phenergan VC with Codeine 2781
Robitussin A-C Syrup........................... 2073

IMPORTANT NOTE: Always consult each drug listing in the patient's regimen for possible interactions.

Wygesic

Robitussin-DAC Syrup 2074
Ryna .... ◻ 841
Soma Compound w/Codeine Tablets 2676
Tussi-Organidin NR Liquid and S NR Liquid 2677
Tylenol with Codeine 1583

Desflurane (Additive effects). Products include:

Suprane 1813

Desipramine Hydrochloride (Propoxyphene may slow the metabolism of antidepressants). Products include:

Norpramin Tablets 1526

Dezocine (Additive effects). Products include:

Dalgan Injection 538

Diazepam (Additive effects). Products include:

Dizac 1809
Valium Injectable 2182
Valium Tablets 2183
Valrelease Capsules 2169

Dicumarol (Propoxyphene may slow the metabolism of warfarin-like drug).

No products indexed under this heading.

Divalproex Sodium (Propoxyphene may slow the metabolism of anticonvulsants). Products include:

Depakote Tablets 415

Doxepin Hydrochloride (Propoxyphene may slow the metabolism of antidepressants). Products include:

Sinequan 2205
Zonalon Cream 1055

Droperidol (Additive effects). Products include:

Inapsine Injection 1296

Enflurane (Additive effects).

No products indexed under this heading.

Estazolam (Additive effects). Products include:

ProSom Tablets 449

Ethchlorvynol (Additive effects). Products include:

Placidyl Capsules 448

Ethinamate (Additive effects).

No products indexed under this heading.

Ethosuximide (Propoxyphene may slow the metabolism of anticonvulsants). Products include:

Zarontin Capsules 1928
Zarontin Syrup 1929

Ethotoin (Propoxyphene may slow the metabolism of anticonvulsants). Products include:

Peganone Tablets 446

Felbamate (Propoxyphene may slow the metabolism of anticonvulsants). Products include:

Felbatol 2666

Fentanyl (Additive effects). Products include:

Duragesic Transdermal System 1288

Fentanyl Citrate (Additive effects). Products include:

Sublimaze Injection 1307

Fluoxetine Hydrochloride (Propoxyphene may slow the metabolism of antidepressants). Products include:

Prozac Pulvules & Liquid, Oral Solution 919

Fluphenazine Decanoate (Additive effects). Products include:

Prolixin Decanoate 509

Fluphenazine Enanthate (Additive effects). Products include:

Prolixin Enanthate 509

Fluphenazine Hydrochloride (Additive effects). Products include:

Prolixin 509

Flurazepam Hydrochloride (Additive effects). Products include:

Dalmane Capsules 2173

Glutethimide (Additive effects).

No products indexed under this heading.

Haloperidol (Additive effects). Products include:

Haldol Injection, Tablets and Concentrate 1575

Haloperidol Decanoate (Additive effects). Products include:

Haldol Decanoate 1577

Hydrocodone Bitartrate (Additive effects). Products include:

Anexsia 5/500 Elixir 1781
Anexia Tablets 1782
Codiclear DH Syrup 791
Deconamine CX Cough and Cold ,Liquid and Tablets 1319
Duratuss HD Elixir 2565
Hycodan Tablets and Syrup 930
Hycomine Compound Tablets 932
Hycomine 931
Hycotuss Expectorant Syrup 933
Hydrocet Capsules 782
Lorcet 10/650 1018
Lortab 2566
Tussend 1783
Tussend Expectorant 1785
Vicodin Tablets 1356
Vicodin ES Tablets 1357
Vicodin Tuss Expectorant 1358
Zydone Capsules 949

Hydrocodone Polistirex (Additive effects). Products include:

Tussionex Pennkinetic Extended-Release Suspension 998

Hydroxyzine Hydrochloride (Additive effects). Products include:

Atarax Tablets & Syrup 2185
Marax Tablets & DF Syrup 2200
Vistaril Intramuscular Solution 2216

Imipramine Hydrochloride (Propoxyphene may slow the metabolism of antidepressants). Products include:

Tofranil Ampuls 854
Tofranil Tablets 856

Imipramine Pamoate (Propoxyphene may slow the metabolism of antidepressants). Products include:

Tofranil-PM Capsules 857

Isocarboxazid (Propoxyphene may slow the metabolism of antidepressants).

No products indexed under this heading.

Isoflurane (Additive effects).

No products indexed under this heading.

Ketamine Hydrochloride (Additive effects).

No products indexed under this heading.

Lamotrigine (Propoxyphene may slow the metabolism of anticonvulsants). Products include:

Lamictal Tablets 1112

Levomethadyl Acetate Hydrochloride (Additive effects). Products include:

Orlamm 2239

Levorphanol Tartrate (Additive effects). Products include:

Levo-Dromoran 2129

Lorazepam (Additive effects). Products include:

Ativan Injection 2698
Ativan Tablets 2700

Loxapine Hydrochloride (Additive effects). Products include:

Loxitane 1378

Loxapine Succinate (Additive effects). Products include:

Loxitane Capsules 1378

Maprotiline Hydrochloride (Propoxyphene may slow the metabolism of antidepressants). Products include:

Ludiomil Tablets 843

Meperidine Hydrochloride (Additive effects). Products include:

Demerol 2308
Mepergan Injection 2753

Mephenytoin (Propoxyphene may slow the metabolism of anticonvulsants). Products include:

Mesantoin Tablets 2272

Mephobarbital (Additive effects). Products include:

Mebaral Tablets 2322

Meprobamate (Additive effects). Products include:

Miltown Tablets 2672
PMB 200 and PMB 400 2783

Mesoridazine Besylate (Additive effects). Products include:

Serentil 684

Methadone Hydrochloride (Additive effects). Products include:

Methadone Hydrochloride Oral Concentrate 2233
Methadone Hydrochloride Oral Solution & Tablets 2235

Methohexital Sodium (Additive effects). Products include:

Brevital Sodium Vials 1429

Methotrimeprazine (Additive effects). Products include:

Levoprome 1274

Methoxyflurane (Additive effects).

No products indexed under this heading.

Methsuximide (Propoxyphene may slow the metabolism of anticonvulsants). Products include:

Celontin Kapseals 1899

Midazolam Hydrochloride (Additive effects). Products include:

Versed Injection 2170

Molindone Hydrochloride (Additive effects). Products include:

Moban Tablets and Concentrate 1048

Morphine Sulfate (Additive effects). Products include:

Astramorph/PF Injection, USP (Preservative-Free) 535
Duramorph 962
Infumorph 200 and Infumorph 500 Sterile Solutions 965
MS Contin Tablets 1994
MSIR 1997
Oramorph SR (Morphine Sulfate Sustained Release Tablets) 2236
RMS Suppositories 2657
Roxanol 2243

Nefazodone Hydrochloride (Propoxyphene may slow the metabolism of antidepressants). Products include:

Serzone Tablets 771

Nortriptyline Hydrochloride (Propoxyphene may slow the metabolism of antidepressants). Products include:

Pamelor 2280

Opium Alkaloids (Additive effects).

No products indexed under this heading.

Oxazepam (Additive effects). Products include:

Serax Capsules 2810
Serax Tablets 2810

Oxycodone Hydrochloride (Additive effects). Products include:

Percocet Tablets 938
Percodan Tablets 939
Percodan-Demi Tablets 940
Roxicodone Tablets, Oral Solution & Intensol (Oxycodone) 2244
Tylox Capsules 1584

Paramethadione (Propoxyphene may slow the metabolism of anticonvulsants).

No products indexed under this heading.

Paroxetine Hydrochloride (Propoxyphene may slow the metabolism of antidepressants). Products include:

Paxil Tablets 2505

Pentobarbital Sodium (Additive effects). Products include:

Nembutal Sodium Capsules 436
Nembutal Sodium Solution 438
Nembutal Sodium Suppositories 440

Perphenazine (Additive effects). Products include:

Etrafon 2355
Triavil Tablets 1757
Trilafon 2389

Phenacemide (Propoxyphene may slow the metabolism of anticonvulsants). Products include:

Phenurone Tablets 447

Phenelzine Sulfate (Propoxyphene may slow the metabolism of antidepressants). Products include:

Nardil 1920

Phenobarbital (Additive effects; propoxyphene may slow the metabolism of anticonvulsants). Products include:

Arco-Lase Plus Tablets 512
Bellergal-S Tablets 2250
Donnatal 2060
Donnatal Extentabs 2061
Donnatal Tablets 2060
Phenobarbital Elixir and Tablets 1469
Quadrinal Tablets 1350

Phensuximide (Propoxyphene may slow the metabolism of anticonvulsants). Products include:

Milontin Kapseals 1920

Phenytoin (Propoxyphene may slow the metabolism of anticonvulsants). Products include:

Dilantin Infatabs 1908
Dilantin-125 Suspension 1911

Phenytoin Sodium (Propoxyphene may slow the metabolism of anticonvulsants). Products include:

Dilantin Kapseals 1906
Dilantin Parenteral 1910

Prazepam (Additive effects).

No products indexed under this heading.

Primidone (Propoxyphene may slow the metabolism of anticonvulsants). Products include:

Mysoline 2754

Prochlorperazine (Additive effects). Products include:

Compazine 2470

Promethazine Hydrochloride (Additive effects). Products include:

Mepergan Injection 2753
Phenergan with Codeine 2777
Phenergan with Dextromethorphan 2778
Phenergan Injection 2773
Phenergan Suppositories 2775
Phenergan Syrup 2774
Phenergan Tablets 2775
Phenergan VC 2779
Phenergan VC with Codeine 2781

Propofol (Additive effects). Products include:

Diprivan Injection 2833

Propoxyphene Napsylate (Additive effects). Products include:

Darvon-N/Darvocet-N 1433

Protriptyline Hydrochloride (Propoxyphene may slow the metabolism of antidepressants). Products include:

Vivactil Tablets 1774

Quazepam (Additive effects). Products include:

Doral Tablets 2664

(◻ Described in PDR For Nonprescription Drugs) (◈ Described in PDR For Ophthalmology)

Interactions Index

Risperidone (Additive effects). Products include:

Risperdal 1301

Secobarbital Sodium (Additive effects). Products include:

Seconal Sodium Pulvules 1474

Sertraline Hydrochloride (Propoxyphene may slow the metabolism of antidepressants). Products include:

Zoloft Tablets 2217

Sufentanil Citrate (Additive effects). Products include:

Sufenta Injection 1309

Temazepam (Additive effects). Products include:

Restoril Capsules 2284

Thiamylal Sodium (Additive effects).

No products indexed under this heading.

Thioridazine Hydrochloride (Additive effects). Products include:

Mellaril 2269

Thiothixene (Additive effects). Products include:

Navane Capsules and Concentrate 2201
Navane Intramuscular 2202

Tranylcypromine Sulfate (Propoxyphene may slow the metabolism of antidepressants). Products include:

Parnate Tablets 2503

Trazodone Hydrochloride (Propoxyphene may slow the metabolism of antidepressants). Products include:

Desyrel and Desyrel Dividose 503

Triazolam (Additive effects). Products include:

Halcion Tablets...................................... 2611

Trifluoperazine Hydrochloride (Additive effects). Products include:

Stelazine 2514

Trimethadione (Propoxyphene may slow the metabolism of anticonvulsants).

No products indexed under this heading.

Trimipramine Maleate (Propoxyphene may slow the metabolism of antidepressants). Products include:

Surmontil Capsules............................... 2811

Valproic Acid (Propoxyphene may slow the metabolism of anticonvulsants). Products include:

Depakene 413

Venlafaxine Hydrochloride (Propoxyphene may slow the metabolism of antidepressants). Products include:

Effexor 2719

Warfarin Sodium (Propoxyphene may slow the metabolism of warfarin-like drug). Products include:

Coumadin 926

Zolpidem Tartrate (Additive effects). Products include:

Ambien Tablets....................................... 2416

Food Interactions

Alcohol (Additive effects).

X-SEB SHAMPOO

(Pyrithione Zinc) .... ✽◻ 605

None cited in PDR database.

X-SEB PLUS ANTIDANDRUFF CONDITIONING SHAMPOO

(Pyrithione Zinc) .... ✽◻ 605

None cited in PDR database.

X-SEB T PEARL SHAMPOO

(Coal Tar) .... ✽◻ 606

None cited in PDR database.

X-SEB T PLUS CONDITIONING SHAMPOO

(Coal Tar) .... ✽◻ 606

None cited in PDR database.

XANAX TABLETS

(Alprazolam) 2649

May interact with central nervous system depressants, anticonvulsants, antihistamines, oral contraceptives, and certain other agents. Compounds in these categories include:

Acrivastine (Additive CNS depressant effects). Products include:

Semprex-D Capsules 463
Semprex-D Capsules 1167

Alfentanil Hydrochloride (Additive CNS depressant effects). Products include:

Alfenta Injection 1286

Aprobarbital (Additive CNS depressant effects).

No products indexed under this heading.

Astemizole (Additive CNS depressant effects). Products include:

Hismanal Tablets 1293

Azatadine Maleate (Additive CNS depressant effects). Products include:

Trinalin Repetabs Tablets 1330

Bromodiphenhydramine Hydrochloride (Additive CNS depressant effects).

No products indexed under this heading.

Brompheniramine Maleate (Additive CNS depressant effects). Products include:

Alka Seltzer Plus Sinus Medicine ..✽◻ 707
Bromfed Capsules (Extended-Release) 1785
Bromfed Syrup .... ✽◻ 733
Bromfed Tablets 1785
Bromfed-DM Cough Syrup.................. 1786
Bromfed-PD Capsules (Extended-Release) 1785
Dimetane-DC Cough Syrup 2059
Dimetane-DX Cough Syrup 2059
Dimetapp Elixir .... ✽◻ 773
Dimetapp Extentabs .... ✽◻ 774
Dimetapp Tablets/Liqui-Gels .... ✽◻ 775
Dimetapp Cold & Allergy Chewable Tablets .... ✽◻ 773
Dimetapp DM Elixir............................... ✽◻ 774
Vicks DayQuil Allergy Relief 12-Hour Extended Release Tablets.. ✽◻ 760
Vicks DayQuil Allergy Relief 4-Hour Tablets .... ✽◻ 760

Buprenorphine (Additive CNS depressant effects). Products include:

Buprenex Injectable 2006

Buspirone Hydrochloride (Additive CNS depressant effects). Products include:

BuSpar 737

Butabarbital (Additive CNS depressant effects).

No products indexed under this heading.

Butalbital (Additive CNS depressant effects). Products include:

Esgic-plus Tablets 1013
Fioricet Tablets 2258
Fioricet with Codeine Capsules 2260
Fiorinal Capsules 2261
Fiorinal with Codeine Capsules 2262
Fiorinal Tablets 2261
Phrenlin 785
Sedapap Tablets 50 mg/650 mg .. 1543

Carbamazepine (Additive CNS depressant effects). Products include:

Atretol Tablets 573
Tegretol Chewable Tablets 852
Tegretol Suspension.............................. 852
Tegretol Tablets 852

Chlordiazepoxide (Additive CNS depressant effects). Products include:

Libritabs Tablets 2177
Limbitrol 2180

Chlordiazepoxide Hydrochloride (Additive CNS depressant effects). Products include:

Librax Capsules 2176
Librium Capsules................................... 2178
Librium Injectable 2179

Chlorpheniramine Maleate (Additive CNS depressant effects). Products include:

Alka-Seltzer Plus Cold Medicine .... ✽◻ 705
Alka-Seltzer Plus Cold Medicine Liqui-Gels .... ✽◻ 706
Alka-Seltzer Plus Cold & Cough Medicine .... ✽◻ 708
Alka-Seltzer Plus Cold & Cough Medicine Liqui-Gels........................... ✽◻ 705
Allerest Children's Chewable Tablets .... ✽◻ 627
Allerest Headache Strength Tablets .... ✽◻ 627
Allerest Maximum Strength Tablets .... ✽◻ 627
Allerest Sinus Pain Formula .... ✽◻ 627
Allerest 12 Hour Caplets.................. ✽◻ 627
Ana-Kit Anaphylaxis Emergency Treatment Kit 617
Atrohist Pediatric Capsules.................. 453
Atrohist Plus Tablets 454
BC Cold Powder Multi-Symptom Formula (Cold-Sinus-Allergy) ...... ✽◻ 609
Cerose DM .... ✽◻ 878
Cheracol Plus Head Cold/Cough Formula .... ✽◻ 769
Children's Vicks DayQuil Allergy Relief.. ✽◻ 757
Children's Vicks NyQuil Cold/Cough Relief.. ✽◻ 758
Chlor-Trimeton Allergy Decongestant Tablets .... ✽◻ 799
Chlor-Trimeton Allergy Tablets ...... ✽◻ 798
Comhist 2038
Comtrex Multi-Symptom Cold Reliever Tablets/Caplets/Liqui-Gels/Liquid... ✽◻ 615
Allergy-Sinus Comtrex Multi-Symptom Allergy-Sinus Formula Tablets .... ✽◻ 617
Contac Continuous Action Nasal Decongestant/Antihistamine 12 Hour Capsules.................................... ✽◻ 813
Contac Maximum Strength Continuous Action Decongestant/Antihistamine 12 Hour Caplets.. ✽◻ 813
Contac Severe Cold and Flu Formula Caplets .... ✽◻ 814
Coricidin 'D' Decongestant Tablets .... ✽◻ 800
Coricidin Tablets .... ✽◻ 800
D.A. Chewable Tablets.......................... 951
Deconamine 1320
Dura-Tap/PD Capsules 2867
Dura-Vent/DA Tablets 953
Extendryl... 1005
Fedahist Gyrocaps................................. 2401
Fedahist Timecaps 2401
Hycomine Compound Tablets 932
Isoclor Timesule Capsules .... ✽◻ 637
Kronofed-A 977
Nolamine Timed-Release Tablets 785
Novahistine DH...................................... 2462
Novahistine Elixir .... ✽◻ 823
Ornade Spansule Capsules 2502
PediaCare Cold Allergy Chewable Tablets .... ✽◻ 677
PediaCare Cough-Cold Chewable Tablets 1553
PediaCare Cough-Cold Liquid.............. 1553
PediaCare NightRest Cough-Cold Liquid 1553
Pediatric Vicks 44m Cough & Cold Relief .... ✽◻ 764
Pyrroxate Caplets .... ✽◻ 772
Ryna .... ✽◻ 841
Sinarest Tablets .... ✽◻ 648
Sinarest Extra Strength Tablets...... ✽◻ 648
Sine-Off Sinus Medicine .... ✽◻ 825
Singlet Tablets .... ✽◻ 825
Sinulin Tablets 787
Sinutab Sinus Allergy Medication, Maximum Strength Tablets and Caplets .... ✽◻ 860
Sudafed Plus Liquid .... ✽◻ 862
Sudafed Plus Tablets .... ✽◻ 863

Teldrin 12 Hour Antihistamine/Nasal Decongestant Allergy Relief Capsules .... ✽◻ 826
TheraFlu.. ✽◻ 787
TheraFlu Maximum Strength Nighttime Flu, Cold & Cough Medicine .... ✽◻ 788
Triaminic Allergy Tablets .... ✽◻ 789
Triaminic Cold Tablets .... ✽◻ 790
Triaminic Nite Light .... ✽◻ 791
Triaminic Syrup .... ✽◻ 792
Triaminic-12 Tablets .... ✽◻ 792
Triaminicin Tablets................................ ✽◻ 793
Triaminicol Multi-Symptom Cold Tablets .... ✽◻ 793
Triaminicol Multi-Symptom Relief ✽◻ 794
Tussend 1783
Children's TYLENOL Cold Multi-Symptom Liquid Formula and Chewable Tablets................................ 1561
Children's TYLENOL Cold Plus Cough Multi Symptom Tablets and Liquid... ✽◻ 681
TYLENOL Maximum Strength Allergy Sinus Medication Gelcaps and Caplets 1563
TYLENOL Cold Multi-Symptom Formula Medication Tablets and Caplets 1561
TYLENOL Cold Multi-Symptom Hot Medication Liquid Packets.............. 1557
Vicks 44 LiquiCaps Cough, Cold & Flu Relief... ✽◻ 755
Vicks 44M Cough, Cold & Flu Relief... ✽◻ 756

Chlorpheniramine Polistirex (Additive CNS depressant effects). Products include:

Tussionex Pennkinetic Extended-Release Suspension 998

Chlorpheniramine Tannate (Additive CNS depressant effects). Products include:

Atrohist Pediatric Suspension 454
Ricobid Tablets and Pediatric Suspension... 2038
Rynatan 2673
Rynatuss 2673

Chlorpromazine (Additive CNS depressant effects). Products include:

Thorazine Suppositories....................... 2523

Chlorpromazine Hydrochloride (Additive CNS depressant effects). Products include:

Thorazine 2523

Chlorprothixene (Additive CNS depressant effects).

No products indexed under this heading.

Chlorprothixene Hydrochloride (Additive CNS depressant effects).

No products indexed under this heading.

Cimetidine (Delayed clearance of alprazolam). Products include:

Tagamet Tablets 2516

Cimetidine Hydrochloride (Delayed clearance of alprazolam). Products include:

Tagamet.. 2516

Clemastine Fumarate (Additive CNS depressant effects). Products include:

Tavist Syrup.. 2297
Tavist Tablets 2298
Tavist-1 12 Hour Relief Tablets .... ✽◻ 787
Tavist-D 12 Hour Relief Tablets .... ✽◻ 787

Clorazepate Dipotassium (Additive CNS depressant effects). Products include:

Tranxene 451

Clozapine (Additive CNS depressant effects). Products include:

Clozaril Tablets...................................... 2252

Codeine Phosphate (Additive CNS depressant effects). Products include:

Actifed with Codeine Cough Syrup.. 1067
Brontex 1981
Deconsal C Expectorant Syrup 456
Deconsal Pediatric Syrup 457
Dimetane-DC Cough Syrup 2059
Empirin with Codeine Tablets............ 1093

IMPORTANT NOTE: Always consult each drug listing in the patient's regimen for possible interactions.

Xanax

Fioricet with Codeine Capsules 2260
Fiorinal with Codeine Capsules 2262
Isoclor Expectorant 990
Novahistine DH 2462
Novahistine Expectorant 2463
Nucofed 2051
Phenergan with Codeine 2777
Phenergan VC with Codeine 2781
Robitussin A-C Syrup 2073
Robitussin-DAC Syrup 2074
Ryna .... ◆◻ 841
Soma Compound w/Codeine Tablets 2676
Tussi-Organidin NR Liquid and S NR Liquid 2677
Tylenol with Codeine 1583

Cyproheptadine Hydrochloride (Additive CNS depressant effects). Products include:

Periactin 1724

Desflurane (Additive CNS depressant effects). Products include:

Suprane 1813

Desipramine Hydrochloride (Increased steady state-plasma concentrations of desipramine by 20%). Products include:

Norpramin Tablets 1526

Desogestrel (Delayed clearance of alprazolam). Products include:

Desogen Tablets 1817
Ortho-Cept 1851

Dexchlorpheniramine Maleate (Additive CNS depressant effects).

No products indexed under this heading.

Dezocine (Additive CNS depressant effects). Products include:

Dalgan Injection 538

Diazepam (Additive CNS depressant effects). Products include:

Dizac 1809
Valium Injectable 2182
Valium Tablets 2183
Valrelease Capsules 2169

Diphenhydramine Citrate (Additive CNS depressant effects). Products include:

Excedrin P.M. Analgesic/Sleeping Aid Tablets, Caplets, Liquigels 733

Diphenhydramine Hydrochloride (Additive CNS depressant effects). Products include:

Actifed Allergy Daytime/Nighttime Caplets .... ◆◻ 844
Actifed Sinus Daytime/Nighttime Tablets and Caplets .... ◆◻ 846
Arthritis Foundation NightTime Caplets .... ◆◻ 674
Extra Strength Bayer PM Aspirin .. ◆◻ 713
Bayer Select Night Time Pain Relief Formula .... ◆◻ 716
Benadryl Allergy Decongestant Liquid Medication .... ◆◻ 848
Benadryl Allergy Decongestant Tablets .... ◆◻ 848
Benadryl Allergy Liquid Medication .... ◆◻ 849
Benadryl Allergy .... ◆◻ 848
Benadryl Allergy Sinus Headache Formula Caplets .... ◆◻ 849
Benadryl Capsules 1898
Benadryl Dye-Free Allergy Liqui-gel Softgels .... ◆◻ 850
Benadryl Dye-Free Allergy Liquid Medication .... ◆◻ 850
Benadryl Itch Relief Cream, Children's Formula and Maximum Strength 2% .... ◆◻ 851
Benadryl Itch Relief Spray, Children's Formula and Maximum Strength 2% .... ◆◻ 851
Benadryl Itch Relief Stick Maximum Strength 2% .... ◆◻ 850
Benadryl Itch Stopping Gel, Children's Formula and Maximum Strength 2% .... ◆◻ 851
Benadryl Kapseals 1898
Benadryl Injection 1898
Contac Day & Night Cold/Flu Night Caplets .... ◆◻ 812
Contac Night Allergy/Sinus Caplets .... ◆◻ 812
Extra Strength Doan's P.M. .... ◆◻ 633
Legatrin PM .... ◆◻ 651

Miles Nervine Nighttime Sleep-Aid ◆◻ 723
Nytol QuickCaps Caplets .... ◆◻ 610
Sleepinal Night-time Sleep Aid Capsules and Softgels .... ◆◻ 834
TYLENOL Maximum Strength Allergy Sinus NightTime Medication Caplets 1555
TYLENOL Flu NightTime, Maximum Strength, Gelcaps 1566
TYLENOL Maximum Strength Flu NightTime Hot Medication Packets 1562
TYLENOL PM, Extra Strength Pain Reliever/Sleep Aid Caplets, Geltabs, Gelcaps 1560
TYLENOL Severe Allergy Medication Caplets 1564
Maximum Strength Unisom Sleepgels 1934
Unisom With Pain Relief-Nighttime Sleep Aid and Pain Reliever 1934

Diphenylpyraline Hydrochloride (Additive CNS depressant effects).

No products indexed under this heading.

Divalproex Sodium (Additive CNS depressant effects). Products include:

Depakote Tablets 415

Droperidol (Additive CNS depressant effects). Products include:

Inapsine Injection 1296

Enflurane (Additive CNS depressant effects).

No products indexed under this heading.

Estazolam (Additive CNS depressant effects). Products include:

ProSom Tablets 449

Ethchlorvynol (Additive CNS depressant effects). Products include:

Placidyl Capsules 448

Ethinamate (Additive CNS depressant effects).

No products indexed under this heading.

Ethinyl Estradiol (Delayed clearance of alprazolam). Products include:

Brevicon 2088
Demulen 2428
Desogen Tablets 1817
Levlen/Tri-Levlen 651
Lo/Ovral Tablets 2746
Lo/Ovral-28 Tablets 2751
Modicon 1872
Nordette-21 Tablets 2755
Nordette-28 Tablets 2758
Norinyl 2088
Ortho-Cept 1851
Ortho-Cyclen/Ortho-Tri-Cyclen 1858
Ortho-Novum 1872
Ortho-Cyclen/Ortho Tri-Cyclen 1858
Ovcon 760
Ovral Tablets 2770
Ovral-28 Tablets 2770
Levlen/Tri-Levlen 651
Tri-Norinyl 2164
Triphasil-21 Tablets 2814
Triphasil-28 Tablets 2819

Ethosuximide (Additive CNS depressant effects). Products include:

Zarontin Capsules 1928
Zarontin Syrup 1929

Ethotoin (Additive CNS depressant effects). Products include:

Peganone Tablets 446

Ethynodiol Diacetate (Delayed clearance of alprazolam). Products include:

Demulen 2428

Felbamate (Additive CNS depressant effects). Products include:

Felbatol 2666

Fentanyl (Additive CNS depressant effects). Products include:

Duragesic Transdermal System 1288

Fentanyl Citrate (Additive CNS depressant effects). Products include:

Sublimaze Injection 1307

Fluphenazine Decanoate (Additive CNS depressant effects). Products include:

Prolixin Decanoate 509

Fluphenazine Enanthate (Additive CNS depressant effects). Products include:

Prolixin Enanthate 509

Fluphenazine Hydrochloride (Additive CNS depressant effects). Products include:

Prolixin 509

Flurazepam Hydrochloride (Additive CNS depressant effects). Products include:

Dalmane Capsules 2173

Glutethimide (Additive CNS depressant effects).

No products indexed under this heading.

Haloperidol (Additive CNS depressant effects). Products include:

Haldol Injection, Tablets and Concentrate 1575

Haloperidol Decanoate (Additive CNS depressant effects). Products include:

Haldol Decanoate 1577

Hydrocodone Bitartrate (Additive CNS depressant effects). Products include:

Anexsia 5/500 Elixir 1781
Anexia Tablets 1782
Codiclear DH Syrup 791
Deconamine CX Cough and Cold Liquid and Tablets 1319
Duratuss HD Elixir 2565
Hycodan Tablets and Syrup 930
Hycomine Compound Tablets 932
Hycomine 931
Hycotuss Expectorant Syrup 933
Hydrocet Capsules 782
Lorcet 10/650 1018
Lortab 2566
Tussend 1783
Tussend Expectorant 1785
Vicodin Tablets 1356
Vicodin ES Tablets 1357
Vicodin Tuss Expectorant 1358
Zydone Capsules 949

Hydrocodone Polistirex (Additive CNS depressant effects). Products include:

Tussionex Pennkinetic Extended-Release Suspension 998

Hydroxyzine Hydrochloride (Additive CNS depressant effects). Products include:

Atarax Tablets & Syrup 2185
Marax Tablets & DF Syrup 2200
Vistaril Intramuscular Solution 2216

Imipramine Hydrochloride (Increased steady state-plasma concentrations of imipramine by 31%). Products include:

Tofranil Ampuls 854
Tofranil Tablets 856

Imipramine Pamoate (Increased steady state-plasma concentrations of imipramine by 31%). Products include:

Tofranil-PM Capsules 857

Isoflurane (Additive CNS depressant effects).

No products indexed under this heading.

Ketamine Hydrochloride (Additive CNS depressant effects).

No products indexed under this heading.

Lamotrigine (Additive CNS depressant effects). Products include:

Lamictal Tablets 1112

Levomethadyl Acetate Hydrochloride (Additive CNS depressant effects). Products include:

Orlaam 2239

Levonorgestrel (Delayed clearance of alprazolam). Products include:

Levlen/Tri-Levlen 651
Nordette-21 Tablets 2755
Nordette-28 Tablets 2758
Norplant System 2759
Levlen/Tri-Levlen 651
Triphasil-21 Tablets 2814
Triphasil-28 Tablets 2819

Levorphanol Tartrate (Additive CNS depressant effects). Products include:

Levo-Dromoran 2129

Loratadine (Additive CNS depressant effects). Products include:

Claritin 2349
Claritin-D 2350

Lorazepam (Additive CNS depressant effects). Products include:

Ativan Injection 2698
Ativan Tablets 2700

Loxapine Hydrochloride (Additive CNS depressant effects). Products include:

Loxitane 1378

Loxapine Succinate (Additive CNS depressant effects). Products include:

Loxitane Capsules 1378

Meperidine Hydrochloride (Additive CNS depressant effects). Products include:

Demerol 2308
Mepergan Injection 2753

Mephenytoin (Additive CNS depressant effects). Products include:

Mesantoin Tablets 2272

Mephobarbital (Additive CNS depressant effects). Products include:

Mebaral Tablets 2322

Meprobamate (Additive CNS depressant effects). Products include:

Miltown Tablets 2672
PMB 200 and PMB 400 2783

Mesoridazine Besylate (Additive CNS depressant effects). Products include:

Serentil 684

Mestranol (Delayed clearance of alprazolam). Products include:

Norinyl 2088
Ortho-Novum 1872

Methadone Hydrochloride (Additive CNS depressant effects). Products include:

Methadone Hydrochloride Oral Concentrate 2233
Methadone Hydrochloride Oral Solution & Tablets 2235

Methdilazine Hydrochloride (Additive CNS depressant effects).

No products indexed under this heading.

Methohexital Sodium (Additive CNS depressant effects). Products include:

Brevital Sodium Vials 1429

Methotrimeprazine (Additive CNS depressant effects). Products include:

Levoprome 1274

Methoxyflurane (Additive CNS depressant effects).

No products indexed under this heading.

Methsuximide (Additive CNS depressant effects). Products include:

Celontin Kapseals 1899

Midazolam Hydrochloride (Additive CNS depressant effects). Products include:

Versed Injection 2170

Molindone Hydrochloride (Additive CNS depressant effects). Products include:

Moban Tablets and Concentrate 1048

(◆◻ Described in PDR For Nonprescription Drugs) (◉ Described in PDR For Ophthalmology)

Interactions Index

Morphine Sulfate (Additive CNS depressant effects). Products include:

Astramorph/PF Injection, USP (Preservative-Free) 535
Duramorph 962
Infumorph 200 and Infumorph 500 Sterile Solutions 965
MS Contin Tablets 1994
MSIR 1997
Oramorph SR (Morphine Sulfate Sustained Release Tablets) 2236
RMS Suppositories 2657
Roxanol 2243

Norethindrone (Delayed clearance of alprazolam). Products include:

Brevicon 2088
Micronor Tablets 1872
Modicon 1872
Norinyl 2088
Nor-Q D Tablets 2135
Ortho-Novum 1872
Ovcon 760
Tri-Norinyl 2164

Norethynodrel (Delayed clearance of alprazolam).

No products indexed under this heading.

Norgestimate (Delayed clearance of alprazolam). Products include:

Ortho-Cyclen/Ortho-Tri-Cyclen 1858
Ortho-Cyclen/Ortho Tri-Cyclen 1858

Norgestrel (Delayed clearance of alprazolam). Products include:

Lo/Ovral Tablets 2746
Lo/Ovral-28 Tablets 2751
Ovral Tablets 2770
Ovral-28 Tablets 2770
Ovrette Tablets 2771

Opium Alkaloids (Additive CNS depressant effects).

No products indexed under this heading.

Oxazepam (Additive CNS depressant effects). Products include:

Serax Capsules 2810
Serax Tablets 2810

Oxycodone Hydrochloride (Additive CNS depressant effects). Products include:

Percocet Tablets 938
Percodan Tablets 939
Percodan-Demi Tablets 940
Roxicodone Tablets, Oral Solution & Intensol (Oxycodone) 2244
Tylox Capsules 1584

Paramethadione (Additive CNS depressant effects).

No products indexed under this heading.

Pentobarbital Sodium (Additive CNS depressant effects). Products include:

Nembutal Sodium Capsules 436
Nembutal Sodium Solution 438
Nembutal Sodium Suppositories 440

Perphenazine (Additive CNS depressant effects). Products include:

Etrafon 2355
Triavil Tablets 1757
Trilafon 2389

Phenacemide (Additive CNS depressant effects). Products include:

Phenurone Tablets 447

Phenobarbital (Additive CNS depressant effects). Products include:

Arco-Lase Plus Tablets 512
Bellergal-S Tablets 2250
Donnatal 2060
Donnatal Extentabs 2061
Donnatal Tablets 2060
Phenobarbital Elixir and Tablets 1469
Quadrinal Tablets 1350

Phensuximide (Additive CNS depressant effects). Products include:

Milontin Kapseals 1920

Phenytoin (Additive CNS depressant effects). Products include:

Dilantin Infatabs 1908
Dilantin-125 Suspension 1911

Phenytoin Sodium (Additive CNS depressant effects). Products include:

Dilantin Kapseals 1906
Dilantin Parenteral 1910

Prazepam (Additive CNS depressant effects).

No products indexed under this heading.

Primidone (Additive CNS depressant effects). Products include:

Mysoline 2754

Prochlorperazine (Additive CNS depressant effects). Products include:

Compazine 2470

Promethazine Hydrochloride (Additive CNS depressant effects). Products include:

Mepergan Injection 2753
Phenergan with Codeine 2777
Phenergan with Dextromethorphan 2778
Phenergan Injection 2773
Phenergan Suppositories 2775
Phenergan Syrup 2774
Phenergan Tablets 2775
Phenergan VC 2779
Phenergan VC with Codeine 2781

Propofol (Additive CNS depressant effects). Products include:

Diprivan Injection 2833

Propoxyphene Hydrochloride (Additive CNS depressant effects). Products include:

Darvon 1435
Wygesic Tablets 2827

Propoxyphene Napsylate (Additive CNS depressant effects). Products include:

Darvon-N/Darvocet-N 1433

Pyrilamine Maleate (Additive CNS depressant effects). Products include:

4-Way Fast Acting Nasal Spray (regular & mentholated) .... ✪D 621
Maximum Strength Multi-Symptom Formula Midol .... ✪D 722
PMS Multi-Symptom Formula Midol .... ✪D 723

Pyrilamine Tannate (Additive CNS depressant effects). Products include:

Atrohist Pediatric Suspension 454
Rynatan 2673

Quazepam (Additive CNS depressant effects). Products include:

Doral Tablets 2664

Risperidone (Additive CNS depressant effects). Products include:

Risperdal 1301

Secobarbital Sodium (Additive CNS depressant effects). Products include:

Seconal Sodium Pulvules 1474

Sufentanil Citrate (Additive CNS depressant effects). Products include:

Sufenta Injection 1309

Temazepam (Additive CNS depressant effects). Products include:

Restoril Capsules 2284

Terfenadine (Additive CNS depressant effects). Products include:

Seldane Tablets 1536
Seldane-D Extended-Release Tablets 1538

Thiamylal Sodium (Additive CNS depressant effects).

No products indexed under this heading.

Thioridazine Hydrochloride (Additive CNS depressant effects). Products include:

Mellaril 2269

Thiothixene (Additive CNS depressant effects). Products include:

Navane Capsules and Concentrate 2201
Navane Intramuscular 2202

Triazolam (Additive CNS depressant effects). Products include:

Halcion Tablets 2611

Trifluoperazine Hydrochloride (Additive CNS depressant effects). Products include:

Stelazine 2514

Trimeprazine Tartrate (Additive CNS depressant effects). Products include:

Temaril Tablets, Syrup and Spansule Extended-Release Capsules.. 483

Trimethadione (Additive CNS depressant effects).

No products indexed under this heading.

Tripelennamine Hydrochloride (Additive CNS depressant effects). Products include:

PBZ Tablets 845
PBZ-SR Tablets 844

Triprolidine Hydrochloride (Additive CNS depressant effects). Products include:

Actifed Plus Caplets .... ✪D 845
Actifed Plus Tablets .... ✪D 845
Actifed with Codeine Cough Syrup.. 1067
Actifed Syrup .... ✪D 846
Actifed Tablets .... ✪D 844

Valproic Acid (Additive CNS depressant effects). Products include:

Depakene 413

Zolpidem Tartrate (Additive CNS depressant effects). Products include:

Ambien Tablets 2416

Food Interactions

Alcohol (Additive CNS depressant effects).

XERAC AC

(Aluminum Chloride) 1933

None cited in PDR database.

XYLOCAINE INJECTIONS

(Lidocaine Hydrochloride) 567

See Xylocaine with Epinephrine Injections

XYLOCAINE WITH EPINEPHRINE INJECTIONS

(Lidocaine Hydrochloride, Epinephrine) 567

May interact with monoamine oxidase inhibitors, tricyclic antidepressants, phenothiazines, butyrophenones, and certain other agents. Compounds in these categories include:

Amitriptyline Hydrochloride (Potential for severe, prolonged hypertension). Products include:

Elavil 2838
Endep Tablets 2174
Etrafon 2355
Limbitrol 2180
Triavil Tablets 1757

Amoxapine (Potential for severe, prolonged hypertension). Products include:

Asendin Tablets 1369

Chlorpromazine (Reduces or reverses the pressor effect of epinephrine). Products include:

Thorazine Suppositories 2523

Clomipramine Hydrochloride (Potential for severe, prolonged hypertension). Products include:

Anafranil Capsules 803

Desipramine Hydrochloride (Potential for severe, prolonged hypertension). Products include:

Norpramin Tablets 1526

Doxepin Hydrochloride (Potential for severe, prolonged hypertension). Products include:

Sinequan 2205
Zonalon Cream 1055

Ergonovine Maleate (Potential for severe, persistent hypertension or cerebrovascular accidents).

No products indexed under this heading.

Fluphenazine Decanoate (Reduces or reverses the pressor effect of epinephrine). Products include:

Prolixin Decanoate 509

Fluphenazine Enanthate (Reduces or reverses the pressor effect of epinephrine). Products include:

Prolixin Enanthate 509

Fluphenazine Hydrochloride (Reduces or reverses the pressor effect of epinephrine). Products include:

Prolixin 509

Furazolidone (Potential for severe, prolonged hypertension). Products include:

Furoxone 2046

Haloperidol (Reduces or reverses the pressor effect of epinephrine). Products include:

Haldol Injection, Tablets and Concentrate 1575

Haloperidol Decanoate (Reduces or reverses the pressor effect of epinephrine). Products include:

Haldol Decanoate 1577

Imipramine Hydrochloride (Potential for severe, prolonged hypertension). Products include:

Tofranil Ampuls 854
Tofranil Tablets 856

Imipramine Pamoate (Potential for severe, prolonged hypertension). Products include:

Tofranil-PM Capsules 857

Isocarboxazid (Potential for severe, prolonged hypertension).

No products indexed under this heading.

Maprotiline Hydrochloride (Potential for severe, prolonged hypertension). Products include:

Ludiomil Tablets 843

Mesoridazine Besylate (Reduces or reverses the pressor effect of epinephrine). Products include:

Serentil 684

Methotrimeprazine (Reduces or reverses the pressor effect of epinephrine). Products include:

Levoprome 1274

Methylergonovine Maleate (Potential for severe, persistent hypertension or cerebrovascular accidents). Products include:

Methergine 2272

Nortriptyline Hydrochloride (Potential for severe, prolonged hypertension). Products include:

Pamelor 2280

Perphenazine (Reduces or reverses the pressor effect of epinephrine). Products include:

Etrafon 2355
Triavil Tablets 1757
Trilafon 2389

Phenelzine Sulfate (Potential for severe, prolonged hypertension). Products include:

Nardil 1920

Prochlorperazine (Reduces or reverses the pressor effect of epinephrine). Products include:

Compazine 2470

Promethazine Hydrochloride (Reduces or reverses the pressor effect of epinephrine). Products include:

Mepergan Injection 2753
Phenergan with Codeine 2777
Phenergan with Dextromethorphan 2778
Phenergan Injection 2773
Phenergan Suppositories 2775

IMPORTANT NOTE: Always consult each drug listing in the patient's regimen for possible interactions.

Xylocaine Injections

Phenergan Syrup 2774
Phenergan Tablets 2775
Phenergan VC 2779
Phenergan VC with Codeine 2781

Protriptyline Hydrochloride (Potential for severe, prolonged hypertension). Products include:

Vivactil Tablets 1774

Selegiline Hydrochloride (Potential for severe, prolonged hypertension). Products include:

Eldepryl Tablets 2550

Thioridazine Hydrochloride (Reduces or reverses the pressor effect of epinephrine). Products include:

Mellaril 2269

Tranylcypromine Sulfate (Potential for severe, prolonged hypertension). Products include:

Parnate Tablets 2503

Trifluoperazine Hydrochloride (Reduces or reverses the pressor effect of epinephrine). Products include:

Stelazine 2514

Trimipramine Maleate (Potential for severe, prolonged hypertension). Products include:

Surmontil Capsules................................... 2811

XYLOCAINE OINTMENT 2.5%

(Lidocaine) .... ✪◻ 603
None cited in PDR database.

YOCON

(Yohimbine Hydrochloride) 1892
May interact with antidepressant drugs. Compounds in this category include:

Amitriptyline Hydrochloride (Should not be used together). Products include:

Elavil 2838
Endep Tablets 2174
Etrafon 2355
Limbitrol 2180
Triavil Tablets 1757

Amoxapine (Should not be used together). Products include:

Asendin Tablets 1369

Bupropion Hydrochloride (Should not be used together). Products include:

Wellbutrin Tablets 1204

Clomipramine Hydrochloride (Should not be used together). Products include:

Anafranil Capsules 803

Desipramine Hydrochloride (Should not be used together). Products include:

Norpramin Tablets 1526

Doxepin Hydrochloride (Should not be used together). Products include:

Sinequan 2205
Zonalon Cream 1055

Fluoxetine Hydrochloride (Should not be used together). Products include:

Prozac Pulvules & Liquid, Oral Solution 919

Imipramine Hydrochloride (Should not be used together). Products include:

Tofranil Ampuls 854
Tofranil Tablets 856

Imipramine Pamoate (Should not be used together). Products include:

Tofranil-PM Capsules................................ 857

Isocarboxazid (Should not be used together).

No products indexed under this heading.

Maprotiline Hydrochloride (Should not be used together). Products include:

Ludiomil Tablets.. 843

Nefazodone Hydrochloride (Should not be used together). Products include:

Serzone Tablets 771

Nortriptyline Hydrochloride (Should not be used together). Products include:

Pamelor 2280

Paroxetine Hydrochloride (Should not be used together). Products include:

Paxil Tablets 2505

Phenelzine Sulfate (Should not be used together). Products include:

Nardil 1920

Protriptyline Hydrochloride (Should not be used together). Products include:

Vivactil Tablets 1774

Sertraline Hydrochloride (Should not be used together). Products include:

Zoloft Tablets 2217

Tranylcypromine Sulfate (Should not be used together). Products include:

Parnate Tablets 2503

Trazodone Hydrochloride (Should not be used together). Products include:

Desyrel and Desyrel Dividose 503

Trimipramine Maleate (Should not be used together). Products include:

Surmontil Capsules................................... 2811

Venlafaxine Hydrochloride (Should not be used together). Products include:

Effexor 2719

YODOXIN

(Iodoquinol)..1230
None cited in PDR database.

YOHIMEX TABLETS

(Yohimbine Hydrochloride) 1363
May interact with antidepressant drugs, antipsychotic agents, and certain other agents. Compounds in these categories include:

Amitriptyline Hydrochloride (Do not use concomitantly). Products include:

Elavil 2838
Endep Tablets 2174
Etrafon 2355
Limbitrol 2180
Triavil Tablets 1757

Amoxapine (Do not use concomitantly). Products include:

Asendin Tablets 1369

Bupropion Hydrochloride (Do not use concomitantly). Products include:

Wellbutrin Tablets 1204

Chlorpromazine (Do not use concomitantly). Products include:

Thorazine Suppositories........................... 2523

Chlorprothixene (Do not use concomitantly).

No products indexed under this heading.

Chlorprothixene Hydrochloride (Do not use concomitantly).

No products indexed under this heading.

Clomipramine Hydrochloride (Do not use concomitantly). Products include:

Anafranil Capsules 803

Clozapine (Do not use concomitantly). Products include:

Clozaril Tablets.. 2252

Desipramine Hydrochloride (Do not use concomitantly). Products include:

Norpramin Tablets 1526

Doxepin Hydrochloride (Do not use concomitantly). Products include:

Sinequan 2205
Zonalon Cream 1055

Fluoxetine Hydrochloride (Do not use concomitantly). Products include:

Prozac Pulvules & Liquid, Oral Solution 919

Fluphenazine Decanoate (Do not use concomitantly). Products include:

Prolixin Decanoate 509

Fluphenazine Enanthate (Do not use concomitantly). Products include:

Prolixin Enanthate..................................... 509

Fluphenazine Hydrochloride (Do not use concomitantly). Products include:

Prolixin... 509

Haloperidol (Do not use concomitantly). Products include:

Haldol Injection, Tablets and Concentrate 1575

Haloperidol Decanoate (Do not use concomitantly). Products include:

Haldol Decanoate....................................... 1577

Imipramine Hydrochloride (Do not use concomitantly). Products include:

Tofranil Ampuls 854
Tofranil Tablets 856

Imipramine Pamoate (Do not use concomitantly). Products include:

Tofranil-PM Capsules................................ 857

Isocarboxazid (Do not use concomitantly).

No products indexed under this heading.

Lithium Carbonate (Do not use concomitantly). Products include:

Eskalith 2485
Lithium Carbonate Capsules & Tablets 2230
Lithonate/Lithotabs/Lithobid 2543

Lithium Citrate (Do not use concomitantly).

No products indexed under this heading.

Loxapine Hydrochloride (Do not use concomitantly). Products include:

Loxitane 1378

Loxapine Succinate (Do not use concomitantly). Products include:

Loxitane Capsules 1378

Maprotiline Hydrochloride (Do not use concomitantly). Products include:

Ludiomil Tablets.. 843

Mesoridazine Besylate (Do not use concomitantly). Products include:

Serentil.. 684

Molindone Hydrochloride (Do not use concomitantly). Products include:

Moban Tablets and Concentrate 1048

Nefazodone Hydrochloride (Do not use concomitantly). Products include:

Serzone Tablets 771

Nortriptyline Hydrochloride (Do not use concomitantly). Products include:

Pamelor 2280

Paroxetine Hydrochloride (Do not use concomitantly). Products include:

Paxil Tablets 2505

Perphenazine (Do not use concomitantly). Products include:

Etrafon 2355
Triavil Tablets 1757
Trilafon.. 2389

Phenelzine Sulfate (Do not use concomitantly). Products include:

Nardil 1920

Pimozide (Do not use concomitantly). Products include:

Orap Tablets 1050

Prochlorperazine (Do not use concomitantly). Products include:

Compazine 2470

Promethazine Hydrochloride (Do not use concomitantly). Products include:

Mepergan Injection 2753
Phenergan with Codeine........................... 2777
Phenergan with Dextromethorphan 2778
Phenergan Injection 2773
Phenergan Suppositories.......................... 2775
Phenergan Syrup.. 2774
Phenergan Tablets 2775
Phenergan VC 2779
Phenergan VC with Codeine 2781

Protriptyline Hydrochloride (Do not use concomitantly). Products include:

Vivactil Tablets 1774

Risperidone (Do not use concomitantly). Products include:

Risperdal 1301

Sertraline Hydrochloride (Do not use concomitantly). Products include:

Zoloft Tablets 2217

Thioridazine Hydrochloride (Do not use concomitantly). Products include:

Mellaril 2269

Thiothixene (Do not use concomitantly). Products include:

Navane Capsules and Concentrate 2201
Navane Intramuscular............................... 2202

Tranylcypromine Sulfate (Do not use concomitantly). Products include:

Parnate Tablets 2503

Trazodone Hydrochloride (Do not use concomitantly). Products include:

Desyrel and Desyrel Dividose 503

Trifluoperazine Hydrochloride (Do not use concomitantly). Products include:

Stelazine 2514

Trimipramine Maleate (Do not use concomitantly). Products include:

Surmontil Capsules................................... 2811

Venlafaxine Hydrochloride (Do not use concomitantly). Products include:

Effexor 2719

YUTOPAR INTRAVENOUS INJECTION

(Ritodrine Hydrochloride)..................... 570
May interact with corticosteroids, general anesthetics, anticholinergics, sympathomimetics, beta blockers, and certain other agents. Compounds in these categories include:

Acebutolol Hydrochloride (Inhibition of Yutopar's action). Products include:

Sectral Capsules 2807

Albuterol (Possible additive effects). Products include:

Proventil Inhalation Aerosol 2382
Ventolin Inhalation Aerosol and Refill 1197

Albuterol Sulfate (Possible additive effects). Products include:

Airet Solution for Inhalation 452
Proventil Inhalation Solution 0.083% 2384

(✪◻ Described in PDR For Nonprescription Drugs) (◎ Described in PDR For Ophthalmology)

1175 **Interactions Index** **Yutopar**

Proventil Repetabs Tablets ... 2386
Proventil Solution for Inhalation 0.5% ... 2383
Proventil Syrup ... 2385
Proventil Tablets ... 2386
Ventolin Inhalation Solution ... 1198
Ventolin Nebules Inhalation Solution ... 1199
Ventolin Rotacaps for Inhalation ... 1200
Ventolin Syrup ... 1202
Ventolin Tablets ... 1203
Volmax Extended-Release Tablets .. 1788

Atenolol (Inhibition of Yutopar's action). Products include:
Tenoretic Tablets ... 2845
Tenormin Tablets and I.V. Injection 2847

Atropine Sulfate (Systemic hypertension exaggerated). Products include:
Arco-Lase Plus Tablets ... 512
Atrohist Plus Tablets ... 454
Atropine Sulfate Sterile Ophthalmic Solution ... ⊙ 233
Donnatal ... 2060
Donnatal Extentabs ... 2061
Donnatal Tablets ... 2060
Lomotil ... 2439
Motofen Tablets ... 784
Urised Tablets ... 1964

Belladonna Alkaloids (Systemic hypertension exaggerated). Products include:
Bellergal-S Tablets ... 2250
Hyland's Bed Wetting Tablets ... ▣ 828
Hyland's EnurAid Tablets ... ▣ 829
Hyland's Teething Tablets ... ▣ 830

Benztropine Mesylate (Systemic hypertension exaggerated). Products include:
Cogentin ... 1621

Betamethasone Acetate (Increased risk of pulmonary edema with concomitant use). Products include:
Celestone Soluspan Suspension ... 2347

Betamethasone Sodium Phosphate (Increased risk of pulmonary edema with concomitant use). Products include:
Celestone Soluspan Suspension ... 2347

Betaxolol Hydrochloride (Inhibition of Yutopar's action). Products include:
Betoptic Ophthalmic Solution ... 469
Betoptic S Ophthalmic Suspension 471
Kerlone Tablets ... 2436

Biperiden Hydrochloride (Systemic hypertension exaggerated). Products include:
Akineton ... 1333

Bisoprolol Fumarate (Inhibition of Yutopar's action). Products include:
Zebeta Tablets ... 1413
Ziac ... 1415

Carteolol Hydrochloride (Inhibition of Yutopar's action). Products include:
Cartrol Tablets ... 410
Ocupress Ophthalmic Solution, 1% Sterile ... ⊙ 309

Clidinium Bromide (Systemic hypertension exaggerated). Products include:
Librax Capsules ... 2176
Quarzan Capsules ... 2181

Cortisone Acetate (Increased risk of pulmonary edema with concomitant use). Products include:
Cortone Acetate Sterile Suspension ... 1623
Cortone Acetate Tablets ... 1624

Dexamethasone (Increased risk of pulmonary edema with concomitant use). Products include:
AK-Trol Ointment & Suspension ... ⊙ 205
Decadron Elixir ... 1633
Decadron Tablets ... 1635
Decaspray Topical Aerosol ... 1648
Dexacidin Ointment ... ⊙ 263
Maxitrol Ophthalmic Ointment and Suspension ... ⊙ 224
TobraDex Ophthalmic Suspension and Ointment ... 473

Dexamethasone Acetate (Increased risk of pulmonary edema with concomitant use). Products include:
Dalalone D.P. Injectable ... 1011
Decadron-LA Sterile Suspension ... 1646

Dexamethasone Sodium Phosphate (Increased risk of pulmonary edema with concomitant use). Products include:
Decadron Phosphate Injection ... 1637
Decadron Phosphate Respihaler ... 1642
Decadron Phosphate Sterile Ophthalmic Ointment ... 1641
Decadron Phosphate Sterile Ophthalmic Solution ... 1642
Decadron Phosphate Topical Cream ... 1644
Decadron Phosphate Turbinaire ... 1645
Decadron Phosphate with Xylocaine Injection, Sterile ... 1639
Dexacort Phosphate in Respihaler .. 458
Dexacort Phosphate in Turbinaire .. 459
NeoDecadron Sterile Ophthalmic Ointment ... 1712
NeoDecadron Sterile Ophthalmic Solution ... 1713
NeoDecadron Topical Cream ... 1714

Diazoxide (Potentiates Yutopar's cardiovascular effects, particularly cardiac arrhythmia or hypotension). Products include:
Hyperstat I.V. Injection ... 2363
Proglycem ... 580

Dicyclomine Hydrochloride (Systemic hypertension exaggerated). Products include:
Bentyl ... 1501

Dobutamine Hydrochloride (Possible additive effects). Products include:
Dobutrex Solution Vials ... 1439

Dopamine Hydrochloride (Possible additive effects).
No products indexed under this heading.

Enflurane (Potentiates Yutopar's cardiovascular effects, particularly cardiac arrhythmia or hypotension).
No products indexed under this heading.

Ephedrine Hydrochloride (Possible additive effects). Products include:
Primatene Dual Action Formula ... ▣ 872
Primatene Tablets ... ▣ 873
Quadrinal Tablets ... 1350

Ephedrine Sulfate (Possible additive effects). Products include:
Bronkaid Caplets ... ▣ 717
Marax Tablets & DF Syrup ... 2200

Ephedrine Tannate (Possible additive effects). Products include:
Rynatuss ... 2673

Epinephrine (Possible additive effects). Products include:
Bronkaid Mist ... ▣ 717
EPIFRIN ... ⊙ 239
EpiPen ... 790
Marcaine Hydrochloride with Epinephrine 1:200,000 ... 2316
Primatene Mist ... ▣ 873
Sensorcaine with Epinephrine Injection ... 559
Sus-Phrine Injection ... 1019
Xylocaine with Epinephrine Injections ... 567

Epinephrine Bitartrate (Possible additive effects). Products include:
Bronkaid Mist Suspension ... ▣ 718
Sensorcaine-MPF with Epinephrine Injection ... 559

Epinephrine Hydrochloride (Possible additive effects). Products include:
Ana-Kit Anaphylaxis Emergency Treatment Kit ... 617

Esmolol Hydrochloride (Inhibition of Yotopar's action). Products include:
Brevibloc Injection ... 1808

Fludrocortisone Acetate (Increased risk of pulmonary edema with concomitant use). Products include:
Florinef Acetate Tablets ... 505

Glycopyrrolate (Systemic hypertension exaggerated). Products include:
Robinul Forte Tablets ... 2072
Robinul Injectable ... 2072
Robinul Tablets ... 2072

Hydrocortisone (Increased risk of pulmonary edema with concomitant use). Products include:
Anusol-HC Cream 2.5% ... 1896
Aquanil HC Lotion ... 1931
Bactine Hydrocortisone Anti-Itch Cream ... ▣ 709
Caldecort Anti-Itch Hydrocortisone Spray ... ▣ 631
Cortaid ... ▣ 836
CORTENEMA ... 2535
Cortisporin Ointment ... 1085
Cortisporin Ophthalmic Ointment Sterile ... 1085
Cortisporin Ophthalmic Suspension Sterile ... 1086
Cortisporin Otic Solution Sterile ... 1087
Cortisporin Otic Suspension Sterile 1088
Cortizone-5 ... ▣ 831
Cortizone-10 ... ▣ 831
Hydrocortone Tablets ... 1672
Hytone ... 907
Massengill Medicated Soft Cloth Towelettes ... 2458
PediOtic Suspension Sterile ... 1153
Preparation H Hydrocortisone 1% Cream ... ▣ 872
ProctoCream-HC 2.5% ... 2408
VōSoL HC Otic Solution ... 2678

Hydrocortisone Acetate (Increased risk of pulmonary edema with concomitant use). Products include:
Analpram-HC Rectal Cream 1% and 2.5% ... 977
Anusol HC-1 Anti-Itch Hydrocortisone Ointment ... ▣ 847
Anusol-HC Suppositories ... 1897
Caldecort ... ▣ 631
Carmol HC ... 924
Coly-Mycin S Otic w/Neomycin & Hydrocortisone ... 1906
Cortaid ... ▣ 836
Cortifoam ... 2396
Cortisporin Cream ... 1084
Epifoam ... 2399
Hydrocortone Acetate Sterile Suspension ... 1669
Mantadil Cream ... 1135
Nupercainal Hydrocortisone 1% Cream ... ▣ 645
Ophthocort ... ⊙ 311
Pramosone Cream, Lotion & Ointment ... 978
ProctoCream-HC ... 2408
ProctoFoam-HC ... 2409
Terra-Cortril Ophthalmic Suspension ... 2210

Hydrocortisone Sodium Phosphate (Increased risk of pulmonary edema with concomitant use). Products include:
Hydrocortone Phosphate Injection, Sterile ... 1670

Hydrocortisone Sodium Succinate (Increased risk of pulmonary edema with concomitant use). Products include:
Solu-Cortef Sterile Powder ... 2641

Hyoscyamine (Systemic hypertension exaggerated). Products include:
Cystospaz Tablets ... 1963
Urised Tablets ... 1964

Hyoscyamine Sulfate (Systemic hypertension exaggerated). Products include:
Arco-Lase Plus Tablets ... 512
Atrohist Plus Tablets ... 454
Cystospaz-M Capsules ... 1963
Donnatal ... 2060
Donnatal Extentabs ... 2061
Donnatal Tablets ... 2060
Kutrase Capsules ... 2402
Levsin/Levsinex/Levbid ... 2405

Ipratropium Bromide (Systemic hypertension exaggerated). Products include:
Atrovent Inhalation Aerosol ... 671
Atrovent Inhalation Solution ... 673

Isoflurane (Potentiates Yutopar's cardiovascular effects, particularly cardiac arrhythmia or hypotension).
No products indexed under this heading.

Isoproterenol Hydrochloride (Possible additive effects). Products include:
Isuprel Hydrochloride Injection 1:5000 ... 2311
Isuprel Hydrochloride Solution 1:200 & 1:100 ... 2313
Isuprel Mistometer ... 2312

Isoproterenol Sulfate (Possible additive effects). Products include:
Norisodrine with Calcium Iodide Syrup ... 442

Labetalol Hydrochloride (Inhibition of Yutopar's action). Products include:
Normodyne Injection ... 2377
Normodyne Tablets ... 2379
Trandate ... 1185

Levobunolol Hydrochloride (Inhibition of Yutopar's action). Products include:
Betagan ... ⊙ 233

Magnesium Sulfate (Potentiates Yutopar's cardiovascular effects, particularly cardiac arrhythmia or hypotension hypotension).
No products indexed under this heading.

Mepenzolate Bromide (Systemic hypertension exaggerated).
No products indexed under this heading.

Meperidine Hydrochloride (Potentiates Yutopar's cardiovascular effects, particularly cardiac arrhythmia or hypotension). Products include:
Demerol ... 2308
Mepergan Injection ... 2753

Metaproterenol Sulfate (Possible additive effects). Products include:
Alupent ... 669
Metaproterenol Sulfate Inhalation Solution, USP, Arm-a-Med ... 552

Metaraminol Bitartrate (Possible additive effects). Products include:
Aramine Injection ... 1609

Methohexital Sodium (Potentiates Yutopar's cardiovascular effects, particularly cardiac arrhythmia or hypotension). Products include:
Brevital Sodium Vials ... 1429

Methoxamine Hydrochloride (Possible addictive effects). Products include:
Vasoxyl Injection ... 1196

Methoxyflurane (Potentiates Yutopar's cardiovascular effects, particularly cardiac arrhythmia or hypotension).
No products indexed under this heading.

Methylprednisolone Acetate (Increased risk of pulmonary edema with concomitant use). Products include:
Depo-Medrol Single-Dose Vial ... 2600
Depo-Medrol Sterile Aqueous Suspension ... 2597

Methylprednisolone Sodium Succinate (Increased risk of pulmonary edema with concomitant use). Products include:
Solu-Medrol Sterile Powder ... 2643

IMPORTANT NOTE: Always consult each drug listing in the patient's regimen for possible interactions.

Yutopar Interactions Index 1176

Metipranolol Hydrochloride (Inhibition of Yutopar's action). Products include:
- OptiPranolol (Metipranolol 0.3%) Sterile Ophthalmic Solution ⊙ 258

Metoprolol Succinate (Inhibition of Yutopar's action). Products include:
- Toprol-XL Tablets 565

Metoprolol Tartrate (Inhibition of Yutopar's action). Products include:
- Lopressor Ampuls 830
- Lopressor HCT Tablets 832
- Lopressor Tablets 830

Nadolol (Inhibition of Yutopar's action).
- No products indexed under this heading.

Norepinephrine Bitartrate (Possible additive effects). Products include:
- Levophed Bitartrate Injection 2315

Oxybutynin Chloride (Systemic hypertension exaggerated). Products include:
- Ditropan 1516

Penbutolol Sulfate (Inhibition of Yutopar's action). Products include:
- Levatol 2403

Phenylephrine Bitartrate (Possible additive effects).
- No products indexed under this heading.

Phenylephrine Hydrochloride (Possible additive effects). Products include:
- Atrohist Plus Tablets 454
- Cerose DM ■ 878
- Comhist 2038
- D.A. Chewable Tablets 951
- Deconsal Pediatric Capsules 454
- Dura-Vent/DA Tablets 953
- Entex Capsules 1986
- Entex Liquid 1986
- Extendryl 1005
- 4-Way Fast Acting Nasal Spray (regular & mentholated) ■ 621
- Hemorid For Women ■ 834
- Hycomine Compound Tablets 932
- Neo-Synephrine Hydrochloride 1% Carpuject 2324
- Neo-Synephrine Hydrochloride 1% Injection 2324
- Neo-Synephrine Hydrochloride (Ophthalmic) 2325
- Neo-Synephrine ■ 726
- Nōstril ■ 644
- Novahistine Elixir ■ 823
- Phenergan VC 2779
- Phenergan VC with Codeine 2781
- Preparation H ■ 871
- Tympagesic Ear Drops 2342
- Vasosulf ⊙ 271
- Vicks Sinex Nasal Spray and Ultra Fine Mist ■ 765

Phenylephrine Tannate (Possible additive effects). Products include:
- Atrohist Pediatric Suspension 454
- Ricobid-D Pediatric Suspension 2038
- Ricobid Tablets and Pediatric Suspension 2038
- Rynatan 2673
- Rynatuss 2673

Phenylpropanolamine Hydrochloride (Possible additive effects). Products include:
- Acutrim ■ 628
- Allerest Children's Chewable Tablets ■ 627
- Allerest 12 Hour Caplets ■ 627
- Atrohist Plus Tablets 454
- BC Cold Powder Multi-Symptom Formula (Cold-Sinus-Allergy) ■ 609
- BC Cold Powder Non-Drowsy Formula (Cold-Sinus) ■ 609
- Cheracol Plus Head Cold/Cough Formula ■ 769
- Comtrex Multi-Symptom Non-Drowsy Liqui-gels ■ 618
- Contac Continuous Action Nasal Decongestant/Antihistamine 12 Hour Capsules ■ 813
- Contac Maximum Strength Continuous Action Decongestant/Antihistamine 12 Hour Caplets ■ 813
- Contac Severe Cold and Flu Formula Caplets ■ 814
- Coricidin 'D' Decongestant Tablets ■ 800
- Dexatrim ■ 832
- Dexatrim Plus Vitamins Caplets ■ 832
- Dimetane-DC Cough Syrup 2059
- Dimetapp Elixir ■ 773
- Dimetapp Extentabs ■ 774
- Dimetapp Tablets/Liqui-Gels ■ 775
- Dimetapp Cold & Allergy Chewable Tablets ■ 773
- Dimetapp DM Elixir ■ 774
- Dura-Vent Tablets 952
- Entex Capsules 1986
- Entex LA Tablets 1987
- Entex Liquid 1986
- Exgest LA Tablets 782
- Hycomine 931
- Isoclor Timesule Capsules ■ 637
- Nolamine Timed-Release Tablets 785
- Ornade Spansule Capsules 2502
- Propagest Tablets 786
- Pyrroxate Caplets ■ 772
- Robitussin-CF ■ 777
- Sinulin Tablets 787
- Tavist-D 12 Hour Relief Tablets ■ 787
- Teldrin 12 Hour Antihistamine/Nasal Decongestant Allergy Relief Capsules ■ 826
- Triaminic Allergy Tablets ■ 789
- Triaminic Cold Tablets ■ 790
- Triaminic Expectorant ■ 790
- Triaminic Syrup ■ 792
- Triaminic-12 Tablets ■ 792
- Triaminic-DM Syrup ■ 792
- Triaminicin Tablets ■ 793
- Triaminicol Multi-Symptom Cold Tablets ■ 793
- Triaminicol Multi-Symptom Relief ■ 794
- Vicks DayQuil Allergy Relief 12-Hour Extended Release Tablets ■ 760
- Vicks DayQuil Allergy Relief 4-Hour Tablets ■ 760
- Vicks DayQuil SINUS Pressure & CONGESTION Relief ■ 761

Pindolol (Inhibition of Yutopar's action). Products include:
- Visken Tablets 2299

Pirbuterol Acetate (Possible additive effects). Products include:
- Maxair Autohaler 1492
- Maxair Inhaler 1494

Prednisolone Acetate (Increased risk of pulmonary edema with concomitant use). Products include:
- AK-CIDE ⊙ 202
- AK-CIDE Ointment ⊙ 202
- Blephamide Liquifilm Sterile Ophthalmic Suspension 476
- Blephamide Ointment ⊙ 237
- Econopred & Econopred Plus Ophthalmic Suspensions ⊙ 217
- Poly-Pred Liquifilm ⊙ 248
- Pred Forte ⊙ 250
- Pred Mild ⊙ 253
- Pred-G Liquifilm Sterile Ophthalmic Suspension ⊙ 251
- Pred-G S.O.P. Sterile Ophthalmic Ointment ⊙ 252
- Vasocidin Ointment ⊙ 268

Prednisolone Sodium Phosphate (Increased risk of pulmonary edema with concomitant use). Products include:
- AK-Pred ⊙ 204
- Hydeltrasol Injection, Sterile 1665
- Inflamase ⊙ 265
- Pediapred Oral Liquid 995
- Vasocidin Ophthalmic Solution ⊙ 270

Prednisolone Tebutate (Increased risk of pulmonary edema with concomitant use). Products include:
- Hydeltra-T.B.A. Sterile Suspension 1667

Prednisone (Increased risk of pulmonary edema with concomitant use). Products include:
- Deltasone Tablets 2595

Procyclidine Hydrochloride (Systemic hypertension exaggerated). Products include:
- Kemadrin Tablets 1112

Propantheline Bromide (Systemic hypertension exaggerated). Products include:
- Pro-Banthīne Tablets 2052

Propofol (Potentiates Yutopar's cardiovascular effects, particularly cardiac arrhythmia or hypotension). Products include:
- Diprivan Injection 2833

Propranolol Hydrochloride (Inhibition of Yutopar's action). Products include:
- Inderal 2728
- Inderal LA Long Acting Capsules 2730
- Inderide Tablets 2732
- Inderide LA Long Acting Capsules 2734

Pseudoephedrine Hydrochloride (Possible additive effects). Products include:
- Actifed Allergy Daytime/Nighttime Caplets ■ 844
- Actifed Plus Caplets ■ 845
- Actifed Plus Tablets ■ 845
- Actifed with Codeine Cough Syrup 1067
- Actifed Sinus Daytime/Nighttime Tablets and Caplets ■ 846
- Actifed Syrup ■ 846
- Actifed Tablets ■ 844
- Advil Cold and Sinus Caplets and Tablets (formerly CoAdvil) ■ 870
- Alka-Seltzer Plus Cold Medicine Liqui-Gels ■ 706
- Alka-Seltzer Plus Cold & Cough Medicine Liqui-Gels ■ 705
- Alka-Seltzer Plus Night-Time Cold Medicine Liqui-Gels ■ 706
- Allerest Headache Strength Tablets ■ 627
- Allerest Maximum Strength Tablets ■ 627
- Allerest No Drowsiness Tablets ■ 627
- Allerest Sinus Pain Formula ■ 627
- Anatuss LA Tablets 1542
- Atrohist Pediatric Capsules 453
- Bayer Select Sinus Pain Relief Formula ■ 717
- Benadryl Allergy Decongestant Liquid Medication ■ 848
- Benadryl Allergy Decongestant Tablets ■ 848
- Benadryl Allergy Sinus Headache Formula Caplets ■ 849
- Benylin Multisymptom ■ 852
- Bromfed Capsules (Extended-Release) 1785
- Bromfed Syrup ■ 733
- Bromfed Tablets 1785
- Bromfed-DM Cough Syrup 1786
- Bromfed-PD Capsules (Extended-Release) 1785
- Children's Vicks DayQuil Allergy Relief ■ 757
- Children's Vicks NyQuil Cold/Cough Relief ■ 758
- Comtrex Multi-Symptom Cold Reliever Tablets/Caplets/Liqui-Gels/Liquid ■ 615
- Allergy-Sinus Comtrex Multi-Symptom Allergy-Sinus Formula Tablets ■ 617
- Comtrex Multi-Symptom Non-Drowsy Caplets ■ 618
- Congess 1004
- Contac Day Allergy/Sinus Caplets ■ 812
- Contac Day & Night ■ 812
- Contac Night Allergy/Sinus Caplets ■ 812
- Contac Severe Cold & Flu Non-Drowsy ■ 815
- Deconamine Chewable Tablets 1320
- Deconamine CX Cough and Cold Liquid and Tablets 1319
- Deconamine 1320
- Deconsal C Expectorant Syrup 456
- Deconsal Pediatric Syrup 457
- Deconsal II Tablets 454
- Dimetane-DX Cough Syrup 2059
- Dimetapp Sinus Caplets ■ 775
- Dorcol Children's Cough Syrup ■ 785
- Drixoral Cough + Congestion Liquid Caps ■ 802
- Dura-Tap/PD Capsules 2867
- Duratuss Tablets 2565
- Duratuss HD Elixir 2565
- Efidac/24 ■ 635
- Entex PSE Tablets 1987
- Fedahist Gyrocaps 2401
- Fedahist Timecaps 2401
- Guaifed 1787
- Guaifed Syrup ■ 734
- Guaimax-D Tablets 792
- Guaitab Tablets ■ 734
- Isoclor Expectorant 990
- Kronofed-A 977
- Motrin IB Sinus ■ 838
- Novahistine DH 2462
- Novahistine DMX ■ 822
- Novahistine Expectorant 2463
- Nucofed 2051
- PediaCare Cold Allergy Chewable Tablets ■ 677
- PediaCare Cough-Cold Chewable Tablets 1553
- PediaCare 1553
- PediaCare Infants' Decongestant Drops ■ 677
- PediCare Infant's Drops Decongestant Plus Cough 1553
- PediaCare NightRest Cough-Cold Liquid 1553
- Pediatric Vicks 44d Dry Hacking Cough & Head Congestion ■ 763
- Pediatric Vicks 44m Cough & Cold Relief ■ 764
- Robitussin Cold & Cough Liqui-Gels ■ 776
- Robitussin Maximum Strength Cough & Cold ■ 778
- Robitussin Pediatric Cough & Cold Formula ■ 779
- Robitussin Severe Congestion Liqui-Gels ■ 776
- Robitussin-DAC Syrup 2074
- Robitussin-PE ■ 778
- Rondec Oral Drops 953
- Rondec Syrup 953
- Rondec Tablet 953
- Rondec-DM Oral Drops 954
- Rondec-DM Syrup 954
- Rondec-TR Tablet 953
- Ryna ■ 841
- Seldane-D Extended-Release Tablets 1538
- Semprex-D Capsules 463
- Semprex-D Capsules 1167
- Sinarest Tablets ■ 648
- Sinarest Extra Strength Tablets ■ 648
- Sinarest No Drowsiness Tablets ■ 648
- Sine-Aid IB Caplets 1554
- Sine-Aid Maximum Strength Sinus Medication Gelcaps, Caplets and Tablets 1554
- Sine-Off No Drowsiness Formula Caplets ■ 824
- Sine-Off Sinus Medicine ■ 825
- Singlet Tablets ■ 825
- Sinutab Non-Drying Liquid Caps ■ 859
- Sinutab Sinus Allergy Medication, Maximum Strength Tablets and Caplets ■ 860
- Sinutab Sinus Medication, Maximum Strength Without Drowsiness Formula, Tablets & Caplets ■ 860
- Sinutab Sinus Medication, Regular Strength Without Drowsiness Formula ■ 859
- Sudafed Children's Liquid ■ 861
- Sudafed Cold and Cough Liquidcaps ■ 862
- Sudafed Cough Syrup ■ 862
- Sudafed Plus Liquid ■ 862
- Sudafed Plus Tablets ■ 863
- Sudafed Severe Cold Formula Caplets ■ 863
- Sudafed Severe Cold Formula Tablets ■ 864
- Sudafed Sinus Caplets ■ 864
- Sudafed Sinus Tablets ■ 864
- Sudafed Tablets, 30 mg ■ 861
- Sudafed Tablets, 60 mg ■ 861
- Sudafed 12 Hour Caplets ■ 861
- Syn-Rx Tablets 465
- Syn-Rx DM Tablets 466
- TheraFlu ■ 787
- TheraFlu Maximum Strength Nighttime Flu, Cold & Cough Medicine ■ 788
- TheraFlu Maximum Strength Non-Drowsy Formula Flu, Cold & Cough Medicine ■ 788
- Thera Flu Maximum Strength, Non-Drowsy Formula Flu, Cold and Cough Caplets ■ 789
- Triaminic AM Cough and Decongestant Formula ■ 789
- Triaminic AM Decongestant Formula ■ 790
- Triaminic Nite Light ■ 791
- Triaminic Sore Throat Formula ■ 791

(■ Described in PDR For Nonprescription Drugs) (⊙ Described in PDR For Ophthalmology)

Interactions Index

Tussend 1783
Tussend Expectorant 1785
Children's TYLENOL Cold Multi-Symptom Liquid Formula and Chewable Tablets............................... 1561
Children's TYLENOL Cold Plus Cough Multi Symptom Tablets and Liquid .... ⓢⓓ 681
Infants' TYLENOL Cold Decongestant & Fever-Reducer Drops 1556
TYLENOL Maximum Strength Allergy Sinus Medication Gelcaps and Caplets 1563
TYLENOL Maximum Strength Allergy Sinus NightTime Medication Caplets 1555
TYLENOL Flu Maximum Strength Gelcaps 1565
TYLENOL Flu NightTime, Maximum Strength, Gelcaps 1566
TYLENOL Maximum Strength Flu NightTime Hot Medication Packets 1562
TYLENOL, Maximum Strength, Sinus Medication Geltabs, Gelcaps, Caplets and Tablets 1566
TYLENOL Cold Multi-Symptom Formula Medication Tablets and Caplets 1561
TYLENOL Cold Medication No Drowsiness Formula Gelcaps and Caplets 1562
TYLENOL Cold Multi-Symptom Hot Medication Liquid Packets.............. 1557
TYLENOL Cough Multi-Symptom Medication with Decongestant 1565
Ursinus Inlay-Tabs................................ ⓢⓓ 794
Vicks 44 LiquiCaps Cough, Cold & Flu Relief .... ⓢⓓ 755
Vicks 44 LiquiCaps Non-Drowsy Cough & Cold Relief .... ⓢⓓ 756
Vicks 44D Dry Hacking Cough & Head Congestion .... ⓢⓓ 755
Vicks 44M Cough, Cold & Flu Relief .... ⓢⓓ 756
Vicks DayQuil .... ⓢⓓ 761
Vicks DayQuil SINUS Pressure & PAIN Relief with IBUPROFEN ...... ⓢⓓ 762
Vicks Nyquil Hot Therapy.................... ⓢⓓ 762
Vicks NyQuil LiquiCaps Multi-Symptom Cold/Flu Relief.................. ⓢⓓ 763
Vicks NyQuil Multi-Symptom Cold/Flu Relief - (Original & Cherry Flavor) .... ⓢⓓ 763

Pseudoephedrine Sulfate (Possible additive effects). Products include:

Cheracol Sinus .... ⓢⓓ 768
Chlor-Trimeton Allergy Decongestant Tablets .... ⓢⓓ 799
Claritin-D 2350
Drixoral Cold and Allergy Sustained-Action Tablets .... ⓢⓓ 802
Drixoral Cold and Flu Extended-Release Tablets.................................... ⓢⓓ 803
Drixoral Non-Drowsy Formula Extended-Release Tablets .... ⓢⓓ 803
Drixoral Allergy/Sinus Extended Release Tablets................................... ⓢⓓ 804
Trinalin Repetabs Tablets 1330

Salmeterol Xinafoate (Possible additive effects). Products include:

Serevent Inhalation Aerosol................ 1176

Scopolamine (Systemic hypertension exaggerated). Products include:

Transderm Scōp Transdermal Therapeutic System 869

Scopolamine Hydrobromide (Systemic hypertension exaggerated). Products include:

Atrohist Plus Tablets 454
Donnatal 2060
Donnatal Extentabs.............................. 2061
Donnatal Tablets 2060

Sotalol Hydrochloride (Inhibition of Yutopar's action). Products include:

Betapace Tablets 641

Terbutaline Sulfate (Possible additive effects). Products include:

Brethaire Inhaler 813
Brethine Ampuls 815
Brethine Tablets.................................... 814
Bricanyl Subcutaneous Injection 1502
Bricanyl Tablets 1503

Timolol Hemihydrate (Inhibition of Yutopar's action). Products include:

Betimol 0.25%, 0.5% .... ⓒ 261

Timolol Maleate (Inhibition of Yutopar's action). Products include:

Blocadren Tablets 1614
Timolide Tablets.................................... 1748
Timoptic in Ocudose 1753
Timoptic Sterile Ophthalmic Solution.. 1751
Timoptic-XE 1755

Triamcinolone (Increased risk of pulmonary edema with concomitant use). Products include:

Aristocort Tablets 1022

Triamcinolone Acetonide (Increased risk of pulmonary edema with concomitant use). Products include:

Aristocort A 0.025% Cream 1027
Aristocort A 0.5% Cream 1031
Aristocort A 0.1% Cream 1029
Aristocort A 0.1% Ointment 1030
Azmacort Oral Inhaler 2011
Nasacort Nasal Inhaler 2024

Triamcinolone Diacetate (Increased risk of pulmonary edema with concomitant use). Products include:

Aristocort Suspension (Forte Parenteral).. 1027
Aristocort Suspension (Intralesional) 1025

Triamcinolone Hexacetonide (Increased risk of pulmonary edema with concomitant use). Products include:

Aristospan Suspension (Intra-articular).. 1033
Aristospan Suspension (Intralesional) 1032

Tridihexethyl Chloride (Systemic hypertension exaggerated).

No products indexed under this heading.

Trihexyphenidyl Hydrochloride (Systemic hypertension exaggerated). Products include:

Artane... 1368

ZANOSAR STERILE POWDER

(Streptozocin).......................................2653
May interact with:

Nephrotoxic Drugs (Concomitant or combination use should be avoided).

ZANTAC 150 EFFERDOSE GRANULES

(Ranitidine Hydrochloride) 1209
See Zantac 150 Tablets

ZANTAC 150 EFFERDOSE TABLETS

(Ranitidine Hydrochloride) 1209
See Zantac 150 Tablets

ZANTAC 150 GELDOSE CAPSULES

(Ranitidine Hydrochloride) 1209
See Zantac 150 Tablets

ZANTAC 300 GELDOSE CAPSULES

(Ranitidine Hydrochloride) 1209
See Zantac 150 Tablets

ZANTAC 150 TABLETS

(Ranitidine Hydrochloride) 1209
May interact with:

Warfarin Sodium (Potential for increased or decreased prothrombin time; doses of ranitidine up to 400 mg per day had no effect on prothrombin time or warfarin clearance). Products include:

Coumadin 926

ZANTAC 300 TABLETS

(Ranitidine Hydrochloride) 1209
See Zantac 150 Tablets

ZANTAC INJECTION

(Ranitidine Hydrochloride) 1207
May interact with:

Warfarin Sodium (Potential for increased or decreased prothrombin time; doses of ranitidine up to 400 mg per day had no effect on prothrombin time or warfarin clearance). Products include:

Coumadin 926

ZANTAC INJECTION PREMIXED

(Ranitidine Hydrochloride) 1207
See Zantac Injection

ZANTAC SYRUP

(Ranitidine Hydrochloride) 1209
See Zantac 150 Tablets

ZARONTIN CAPSULES

(Ethosuximide) 1928
May interact with:

Divalproex Sodium (Valproic acid may increase or decrease ethosuximide levels). Products include:

Depakote Tablets................................... 415

Phenytoin (Ethosuximide may elevate phenytoin serum levels). Products include:

Dilantin Infatabs.................................... 1908
Dilantin-125 Suspension 1911

Phenytoin Sodium (Ethosuximide may elevate phenytoin serum levels). Products include:

Dilantin Kapseals 1906
Dilantin Parenteral 1910

Valproic Acid (Valproic acid may increase or decrease ethosuximide levels). Products include:

Depakene 413

ZARONTIN SYRUP

(Ethosuximide) 1929
May interact with:

Divalproex Sodium (Valproic acid may increase or decrease ethosuximide levels). Products include:

Depakote Tablets................................... 415

Phenytoin (Ethosuximide may elevate phenytoin serum levels). Products include:

Dilantin Infatabs.................................... 1908
Dilantin-125 Suspension 1911

Phenytoin Sodium (Ethosuximide may elevate phenytoin serum levels). Products include:

Dilantin Kapseals 1906
Dilantin Parenteral 1910

Valproic Acid (Valproic acid may increase or decrease ethosuximide levels). Products include:

Depakene 413

ZAROXOLYN TABLETS

(Metolazone)...1000
May interact with loop diuretics, antihypertensives, barbiturates, narcotic analgesics, cardiac glycosides, corticosteroids, lithium preparations, salicylates, non-steroidal anti-inflammatory agents, oral hypoglycemic agents, insulin, and certain other agents. Compounds in these categories include:

Acarbose (Blood glucose concentration may be raised).

No products indexed under this heading.

Acebutolol Hydrochloride (Excessive hypotension may result especially during initial therapy). Products include:

Sectral Capsules 2807

ACTH (May increase the risk of hypokalemia and increase salt and water retention).

No products indexed under this heading.

Alfentanil Hydrochloride (Hypotensive effect may be potentiated). Products include:

Alfenta Injection 1286

Amlodipine Besylate (Excessive hypotension may result especially during initial therapy). Products include:

Lotrel Capsules...................................... 840
Norvasc Tablets 1940

Aprobarbital (Hypotensive effect may be potentiated).

No products indexed under this heading.

Aspirin (Increases the antihypertensive effect). Products include:

Alka-Seltzer Effervescent Antacid and Pain Reliever............................... ⓢⓓ 701
Alka-Seltzer Extra Strength Effervescent Antacid and Pain Reliever .... ⓢⓓ 703
Alka-Seltzer Lemon Lime Effervescent Antacid and Pain Reliever .... ⓢⓓ 703
Alka-Seltzer Plus Cold Medicine .... ⓢⓓ 705
Alka-Seltzer Plus Cold & Cough Medicine .... ⓢⓓ 708
Alka-Seltzer Plus Night-Time Cold Medicine .... ⓢⓓ 707
Alka Seltzer Plus Sinus Medicine .. ⓢⓓ 707
Arthritis Foundation Safety Coated Aspirin Tablets .... ⓢⓓ 675
Arthritis Pain Ascriptin .... ⓢⓓ 631
Maximum Strength Ascriptin .... ⓢⓓ 630
Regular Strength Ascriptin Tablets .... ⓢⓓ 629
Arthritis Strength BC Powder......... ⓢⓓ 609
BC Cold Powder Multi-Symptom Formula (Cold-Sinus-Allergy) ...... ⓢⓓ 609
BC Cold Powder Non-Drowsy Formula (Cold-Sinus) .... ⓢⓓ 609
BC Powder .... ⓢⓓ 609
Bayer Children's Chewable Aspirin.. ⓢⓓ 711
Genuine Bayer Aspirin Tablets & Caplets .... ⓢⓓ 713
Extra Strength Bayer Arthritis Pain Regimen Formula .... ⓢⓓ 711
Extra Strength Bayer Aspirin Caplets & Tablets .... ⓢⓓ 712
Extended-Release Bayer 8-Hour Aspirin .... ⓢⓓ 712
Extra Strength Bayer Plus Aspirin Caplets.. ⓢⓓ 713
Extra Strength Bayer PM Aspirin .. ⓢⓓ 713
Bayer Enteric Aspirin .... ⓢⓓ 709
Bufferin Analgesic Tablets and Caplets .... ⓢⓓ 613
Arthritis Strength Bufferin Analgesic Caplets .... ⓢⓓ 614
Extra Strength Bufferin Analgesic Tablets .... ⓢⓓ 615
Cama Arthritis Pain Reliever........... ⓢⓓ 785
Darvon Compound-65 Pulvules 1435
Easprin 1914
Ecotrin 2455
Ecotrin Enteric Coated Aspirin Maximum Strength Tablets and Caplets .... ⓢⓓ 816
Ecotrin Enteric Coated Aspirin Regular Strength Tablets 2455
Empirin Aspirin Tablets .... ⓢⓓ 854
Empirin with Codeine Tablets........... 1093
Excedrin Extra-Strength Analgesic Tablets & Caplets 732
Fiorinal Capsules 2261
Fiorinal with Codeine Capsules 2262
Fiorinal Tablets...................................... 2261

IMPORTANT NOTE: Always consult each drug listing in the patient's regimen for possible interactions.

Zaroxolyn Interactions Index 1178

Halfprin 1362
Healthprin Aspirin 2455
Norgesic 1496
Percodan Tablets 939
Percodan-Demi Tablets 940
Robaxisal Tablets 2071
Soma Compound w/Codeine Tablets 2676
Soma Compound Tablets 2675
St. Joseph Adult Chewable Aspirin (81 mg.) .... ▣ 808
Talwin Compound 2335
Ursinus Inlay-Tabs .... ▣ 794
Vanquish Analgesic Caplets .... ▣ 731

Atenolol (Excessive hypotension may result especially during initial therapy). Products include:
Tenoretic Tablets 2845
Tenormin Tablets and I.V. Injection 2847

Benazepril Hydrochloride (Excessive hypotension may result especially during initial therapy). Products include:
Lotensin Tablets 834
Lotensin HCT 837
Lotrel Capsules 840

Bendroflumethiazide (Excessive hypotension may result especially during initial therapy).
No products indexed under this heading.

Betamethasone Acetate (May increase the risk of hypokalemia and increase salt and water retention). Products include:
Celestone Soluspan Suspension 2347

Betamethasone Sodium Phosphate (May increase the risk of hypokalemia and increase salt and water retention). Products include:
Celestone Soluspan Suspension 2347

Betaxolol Hydrochloride (Excessive hypotension may result especially during initial therapy). Products include:
Betoptic Ophthalmic Solution 469
Betoptic S Ophthalmic Suspension 471
Kerlone Tablets 2436

Bisoprolol Fumarate (Excessive hypotension may result especially during initial therapy). Products include:
Zebeta Tablets 1413
Ziac 1415

Bumetanide (May result in large or prolonged losses of fluids and electrolytes). Products include:
Bumex 2093

Buprenorphine (Hypotensive effect may be potentiated). Products include:
Buprenex Injectable 2006

Butabarbital (Hypotensive effect may be potentiated).
No products indexed under this heading.

Butalbital (Hypotensive effect may be potentiated). Products include:
Esgic-plus Tablets 1013
Fioricet Tablets 2258
Fioricet with Codeine Capsules 2260
Fiorinal Capsules 2261
Fiorinal with Codeine Capsules 2262
Fiorinal Tablets 2261
Phrenilin 785
Sedapap Tablets 50 mg/650 mg .. 1543

Captopril (Excessive hypotension may result especially during initial therapy). Products include:
Capoten 739
Capozide 742

Carteolol Hydrochloride (Excessive hypotension may result especially during initial therapy). Products include:
Cartrol Tablets 410
Ocupress Ophthalmic Solution, 1% Sterile .... ⊙ 309

Chlorothiazide (Excessive hypotension may result especially during initial therapy). Products include:
Aldoclor Tablets 1598
Diupres Tablets 1650
Diuril Oral 1653

Chlorothiazide Sodium (Excessive hypotension may result especially during initial therapy). Products include:
Diuril Sodium Intravenous 1652

Chlorpropamide (Blood glucose concentration may be raised). Products include:
Diabinese Tablets 1935

Chlorthalidone (Excessive hypotension may result especially during initial therapy). Products include:
Combipres Tablets 677
Tenoretic Tablets 2845
Thalitone 1245

Choline Magnesium Trisalicylate (Increases the antihypertensive effect). Products include:
Trilisate 2000

Clonidine (Excessive hypotension may result especially during initial therapy). Products include:
Catapres-TTS 675

Clonidine Hydrochloride (Excessive hypotension may result especially during initial therapy). Products include:
Catapres Tablets 674
Combipres Tablets 677

Codeine Phosphate (Hypotensive effect may be potentiated). Products include:
Actifed with Codeine Cough Syrup.. 1067
Brontex 1981
Deconsal C Expectorant Syrup 456
Deconsal Pediatric Syrup 457
Dimetane-DC Cough Syrup 2059
Empirin with Codeine Tablets 1093
Fioricet with Codeine Capsules 2260
Fiorinal with Codeine Capsules 2262
Isoclor Expectorant 990
Novahistine DH 2462
Novahistine Expectorant 2463
Nucofed 2051
Phenergan with Codeine 2777
Phenergan VC with Codeine 2781
Robitussin A-C Syrup 2073
Robitussin-DAC Syrup 2074
Ryna .... ▣ 841
Soma Compound w/Codeine Tablets 2676
Tussi-Organidin NR Liquid and S NR Liquid 2677
Tylenol with Codeine 1583

Cortisone Acetate (May increase the risk of hypokalemia and increase salt and water retention). Products include:
Cortone Acetate Sterile Suspension 1623
Cortone Acetate Tablets 1624

Deserpidine (Excessive hypotension may result especially during initial therapy).
No products indexed under this heading.

Deslanoside (Hypokalemia induced by diuretic may increase the sensitivity of the myocardium to digitalis therapy).
No products indexed under this heading.

Dexamethasone (May increase the risk of hypokalemia and increase salt and water retention). Products include:
AK-Trol Ointment & Suspension .... ⊙ 205
Decadron Elixir 1633
Decadron Tablets 1635
Decaspray Topical Aerosol 1648
Dexacidin Ointment .... ⊙ 263
Maxitrol Ophthalmic Ointment and Suspension .... ⊙ 224
TobraDex Ophthalmic Suspension and Ointment 473

Dexamethasone Acetate (May increase the risk of hypokalemia and increase salt and water retention). Products include:
Dalalone D.P. Injectable 1011
Decadron-LA Sterile Suspension 1646

Dexamethasone Sodium Phosphate (May increase the risk of hypokalemia and increase salt and water retention). Products include:
Decadron Phosphate Injection 1637
Decadron Phosphate Respihaler 1642
Decadron Phosphate Sterile Ophthalmic Ointment 1641
Decadron Phosphate Sterile Ophthalmic Solution 1642
Decadron Phosphate Topical Cream 1644
Decadron Phosphate Turbinaire 1645
Decadron Phosphate with Xylocaine Injection, Sterile 1639
Dexacort Phosphate in Respihaler .. 458
Dexacort Phosphate in Turbinaire .. 459
NeoDecadron Sterile Ophthalmic Ointment 1712
NeoDecadron Sterile Ophthalmic Solution 1713
NeoDecadron Topical Cream 1714

Dezocine (Hypotensive effect may be potentiated). Products include:
Dalgan Injection 538

Diazoxide (Excessive hypotension may result especially during initial therapy). Products include:
Hyperstat I.V. Injection 2363
Proglycem 580

Diclofenac Potassium (Increases the antihypertensive effect). Products include:
Cataflam 816

Diclofenac Sodium (Increases the antihypertensive effect). Products include:
Voltaren Ophthalmic Sterile Ophthalmic Solution .... ⊙ 272
Voltaren Tablets 861

Dicumarol (May affect the hypoprothrombinemic response to anticoagulants; dosage adjustments may be necessary).
No products indexed under this heading.

Diflunisal (Increases the antihypertensive effect). Products include:
Dolobid Tablets 1654

Digitoxin (Hypokalemia induced by diuretic may increase the sensitivity of the myocardium to digitalis therapy). Products include:
Crystodigin Tablets 1433

Digoxin (Hypokalemia induced by diuretic may increase the sensitivity of the myocardium to digitalis therapy). Products include:
Lanoxicaps 1117
Lanoxin Elixir Pediatric 1120
Lanoxin Injection 1123
Lanoxin Injection Pediatric 1126
Lanoxin Tablets 1128

Diltiazem Hydrochloride (Excessive hypotension may result especially during initial therapy). Products include:
Cardizem CD Capsules 1506
Cardizem SR Capsules 1510
Cardizem Injectable 1508
Cardizem Tablets 1512
Dilacor XR Extended-release Capsules 2018

Doxazosin Mesylate (Excessive hypotension may result especially during initial therapy). Products include:
Cardura Tablets 2186

Enalapril Maleate (Excessive hypotension may result especially during initial therapy). Products include:
Vaseretic Tablets 1765
Vasotec Tablets 1771

Enalaprilat (Excessive hypotension may result especially during initial therapy). Products include:
Vasotec I.V. 1768

Esmolol Hydrochloride (Excessive hypotension may result especially during initial therapy). Products include:
Brevibloc Injection 1808

Ethacrynic Acid (May result in large or prolonged losses of fluids and electrolytes). Products include:
Edecrin Tablets 1657

Etodolac (Increases the antihypertensive effect). Products include:
Lodine Capsules and Tablets 2743

Felodipine (Excessive hypotension may result especially during initial therapy). Products include:
Plendil Extended-Release Tablets 527

Fenoprofen Calcium (Increases the antihypertensive effect). Products include:
Nalfon 200 Pulvules & Nalfon Tablets 917

Fentanyl (Hypotensive effect may be potentiated). Products include:
Duragesic Transdermal System 1288

Fentanyl Citrate (Hypotensive effect may be potentiated). Products include:
Sublimaze Injection 1307

Fludrocortisone Acetate (May increase the risk of hypokalemia and increase salt and water retention). Products include:
Florinef Acetate Tablets 505

Flurbiprofen (Increases the antihypertensive effect). Products include:
Ansaid Tablets 2579

Fosinopril Sodium (Excessive hypotension may result especially during initial therapy). Products include:
Monopril Tablets 757

Furosemide (May result in large or prolonged losses of fluids and electrolytes; excessive hypotension may result especially during initial therapy). Products include:
Lasix Injection, Oral Solution and Tablets 1240

Glipizide (Blood glucose concentration may be raised). Products include:
Glucotrol Tablets 1967
Glucotrol XL Extended Release Tablets 1968

Glyburide (Blood glucose concentration may be raised). Products include:
DiaBeta Tablets 1239
Glynase PresTab Tablets 2609
Micronase Tablets 2623

Guanabenz Acetate (Excessive hypotension may result especially during initial therapy).
No products indexed under this heading.

Guanethidine Monosulfate (Excessive hypotension may result especially during initial therapy). Products include:
Esimil Tablets 822
Ismelin Tablets 827

Hydralazine Hydrochloride (Excessive hypotension may result especially during initial therapy). Products include:
Apresazide Capsules 808
Apresoline Hydrochloride Tablets .. 809
Ser-Ap-Es Tablets 849

Hydrochlorothiazide (Excessive hypotension may result especially during initial therapy). Products include:
Aldactazide 2413
Aldoril Tablets 1604

(▣ Described in PDR For Nonprescription Drugs) (⊙ Described in PDR For Ophthalmology)

1179 **Interactions Index** **Zaroxolyn**

Apresazide Capsules 808
Capozide 742
Dyazide 2479
Esidrix Tablets 821
Esimil Tablets 822
HydroDIURIL Tablets 1674
Hydropres Tablets 1675
Hyzaar Tablets 1677
Inderide Tablets 2732
Inderide LA Long Acting Capsules 2734
Lopressor HCT Tablets 832
Lotensin HCT 837
Maxzide 1380
Moduretic Tablets 1705
Oretic Tablets 443
Prinzide Tablets 1737
Ser-Ap-Es Tablets 849
Timolide Tablets 1748
Vaseretic Tablets 1765
Zestoretic 2850
Ziac 1415

Hydrocodone Bitartrate (Hypotensive effect may be potentiated). Products include:
Anexsia 5/500 Elixir 1781
Anexia Tablets 1782
Codiclear DH Syrup 791
Deconamine CX Cough and Cold Liquid and Tablets 1319
Duratuss HD Elixir 2565
Hycodan Tablets and Syrup 930
Hycomine Compound Tablets 932
Hycomine 931
Hycotuss Expectorant Syrup 933
Hydrocet Capsules 782
Lorcet 10/650 1018
Lortab 2566
Tussend 1783
Tussend Expectorant 1785
Vicodin Tablets 1356
Vicodin ES Tablets 1357
Vicodin Tuss Expectorant 1358
Zydone Capsules 949

Hydrocodone Polistirex (Hypotensive effect may be potentiated). Products include:
Tussionex Pennkinetic Extended-Release Suspension 998

Hydrocortisone (May increase the risk of hypokalemia and increase salt and water retention). Products include:
Anusol-HC Cream 2.5% 1896
Aquanil HC Lotion 1931
Bactine Hydrocortisone Anti-Itch Cream ◘ 709
Caldecort Anti-Itch Hydrocortisone Spray ◘ 631
Cortaid ◘ 836
CORTENEMA 2535
Cortisporin Ointment 1085
Cortisporin Ophthalmic Ointment Sterile 1085
Cortisporin Ophthalmic Suspension Sterile 1086
Cortisporin Otic Solution Sterile 1087
Cortisporin Otic Suspension Sterile 1088
Cortizone-5 ◘ 831
Cortizone-10 ◘ 831
Hydrocortone Tablets 1672
Hytone 907
Massengill Medicated Soft Cloth Towelettes 2458
PediOtic Suspension Sterile 1153
Preparation H Hydrocortisone 1% Cream ◘ 872
ProctoCream-HC 2.5% 2408
VōSoL HC Otic Solution 2678

Hydrocortisone Acetate (May increase the risk of hypokalemia and increase salt and water retention). Products include:
Analpram-HC Rectal Cream 1% and 2.5% 977
Anusol HC-1 Anti-Itch Hydrocortisone Ointment ◘ 847
Anusol-HC Suppositories 1897
Caldecort ◘ 631
Carmol HC 924
Coly-Mycin S Otic w/Neomycin & Hydrocortisone 1906
Cortaid ◘ 836
Cortifoam 2396
Cortisporin Cream 1084
Epifoam 2399
Hydrocortone Acetate Sterile Suspension 1669
Mantadil Cream 1135
Nupercainal Hydrocortisone 1% Cream ◘ 645
Ophthocort ◉ 311
Pramosone Cream, Lotion & Ointment 978
ProctoCream-HC 2408
ProctoFoam-HC 2409
Terra-Cortril Ophthalmic Suspension 2210

Hydrocortisone Sodium Phosphate (May increase the risk of hypokalemia and increase salt and water retention). Products include:
Hydrocortone Phosphate Injection, Sterile 1670

Hydrocortisone Sodium Succinate (May increase the risk of hypokalemia and increase salt and water retention). Products include:
Solu-Cortef Sterile Powder 2641

Hydroflumethiazide (Excessive hypotension may result especially during initial therapy). Products include:
Diucardin Tablets 2718

Ibuprofen (Increases the antihypertensive effect). Products include:
Advil Cold and Sinus Caplets and Tablets (formerly CoAdvil) ◘ 870
Advil Ibuprofen Tablets and Caplets ◘ 870
Children's Advil Suspension 2692
Arthritis Foundation Ibuprofen Tablets ◘ 674
Bayer Select Ibuprofen Pain Relief Formula ◘ 715
Cramp End Tablets ◘ 735
Dimetapp Sinus Caplets ◘ 775
Haltran Tablets ◘ 771
IBU Tablets 1342
Ibuprohm ◘ 735
Children's Motrin Ibuprofen Oral Suspension 1546
Motrin Tablets 2625
Motrin IB Caplets, Tablets, and Geltabs ◘ 838
Motrin IB Sinus ◘ 838
Motrin Ibuprofen Suspension, Oral Drops, Chewable Tablets, Caplets 1546
Nuprin Ibuprofen/Analgesic Tablets & Caplets ◘ 622
Sine-Aid IB Caplets 1554
Vicks DayQuil SINUS Pressure & PAIN Relief with IBUPROFEN ◘ 762

Indapamide (Excessive hypotension may result especially during initial therapy). Products include:
Lozol Tablets 2022

Indomethacin (Increases the antihypertensive effect). Products include:
Indocin 1680

Indomethacin Sodium Trihydrate (Increases the antihypertensive effect). Products include:
Indocin I.V. 1684

Insulin, Human (Blood glucose concentration may be raised).
No products indexed under this heading.

Insulin, Human Isophane Suspension (Blood glucose concentration may be raised). Products include:
Novolin N Human Insulin 10 ml Vials 1795

Insulin, Human NPH (Blood glucose concentration may be raised). Products include:
Humulin N, 100 Units 1448
Novolin N PenFill Cartridges Durable Insulin Delivery System 1798
Novolin N Prefilled Syringe Disposable Insulin Delivery System 1798

Insulin, Human Regular (Blood glucose concentration may be raised). Products include:
Humulin R, 100 Units 1449
Novolin R Human Insulin 10 ml Vials 1795
Novolin R PenFill Cartridges Durable Insulin Delivery System 1798
Novolin R Prefilled Syringe Disposable Insulin Delivery System 1798
Velosulin BR Human Insulin 10 ml Vials 1795

Insulin, Human, Zinc Suspension (Blood glucose concentration may be raised). Products include:
Humulin L, 100 Units 1446
Humulin U, 100 Units 1450
Novolin L Human Insulin 10 ml Vials 1795

Insulin, NPH (Blood glucose concentration may be raised). Products include:
NPH, 100 Units 1450
Pork NPH, 100 Units 1452
Purified Pork NPH Isophane Insulin 1801

Insulin, Regular (Blood glucose concentration may be raised). Products include:
Regular, 100 Units 1450
Pork Regular, 100 Units 1452
Pork Regular (Concentrated), 500 Units 1453
Purified Pork Regular Insulin 1801

Insulin, Zinc Crystals (Blood glucose concentration may be raised). Products include:
NPH, 100 Units 1450

Insulin, Zinc Suspension (Blood glucose concentration may be raised). Products include:
Iletin I 1450
Lente, 100 Units 1450
Iletin II 1452
Pork Lente, 100 Units 1452
Purified Pork Lente Insulin 1801

Isradipine (Excessive hypotension may result especially during initial therapy). Products include:
DynaCirc Capsules 2256

Ketoprofen (Increases the antihypertensive effect). Products include:
Orudis Capsules 2766
Oruvail Capsules 2766

Ketorolac Tromethamine (Increases the antihypertensive effect). Products include:
Acular 474
Acular ◉ 277
Toradol 2159

Labetalol Hydrochloride (Excessive hypotension may result especially during initial therapy). Products include:
Normodyne Injection 2377
Normodyne Tablets 2379
Trandate 1185

Levorphanol Tartrate (Hypotensive effect may be potentiated). Products include:
Levo-Dromoran 2129

Lisinopril (Excessive hypotension may result especially during initial therapy). Products include:
Prinivil Tablets 1733
Prinzide Tablets 1737
Zestoretic 2850
Zestril Tablets 2854

Lithium Carbonate (Serum lithium levels may increase). Products include:
Eskalith 2485
Lithium Carbonate Capsules & Tablets 2230
Lithonate/Lithotabs/Lithobid 2543

Lithium Citrate (Serum lithium levels may increase).
No products indexed under this heading.

Losartan Potassium (Excessive hypotension may result especially during initial therapy). Products include:
Cozaar Tablets 1628
Hyzaar Tablets 1677

Magnesium Salicylate (Increases the antihypertensive effect). Products include:
Backache Caplets ◘ 613
Bayer Select Backache Pain Relief Formula ◘ 715
Doan's Extra-Strength Analgesic ◘ 633
Extra Strength Doan's P.M. ◘ 633
Doan's Regular Strength Analgesic ◘ 634
Mobigesic Tablets ◘ 602

Mecamylamine Hydrochloride (Excessive hypotension may result especially during initial therapy). Products include:
Inversine Tablets 1686

Meclofenamate Sodium (Increases the antihypertensive effect).
No products indexed under this heading.

Mefenamic Acid (Increases the antihypertensive effect). Products include:
Ponstel 1925

Meperidine Hydrochloride (Hypotensive effect may be potentiated). Products include:
Demerol 2308
Mepergan Injection 2753

Mephobarbital (Hypotensive effect may be potentiated). Products include:
Mebaral Tablets 2322

Metformin Hydrochloride (Blood glucose concentration may be raised). Products include:
Glucophage 752

Methadone Hydrochloride (Hypotensive effect may be potentiated). Products include:
Methadone Hydrochloride Oral Concentrate 2233
Methadone Hydrochloride Oral Solution & Tablets 2235

Methenamine (Efficacy of methenamine may be decreased). Products include:
Urised Tablets 1964

Methenamine Hippurate (Efficacy of methenamine may be decreased).
No products indexed under this heading.

Methenamine Mandelate (Efficacy of methenamine may be decreased). Products include:
Uroqid-Acid No. 2 Tablets 640

Methyclothiazide (Excessive hypotension may result especially during initial therapy). Products include:
Enduron Tablets 420

Methyldopa (Excessive hypotension may result especially during initial therapy). Products include:
Aldoclor Tablets 1598
Aldomet Oral 1600
Aldoril Tablets 1604

Methyldopate Hydrochloride (Excessive hypotension may result especially during initial therapy). Products include:
Aldomet Ester HCl Injection 1602

Methylprednisolone Acetate (May increase the risk of hypokalemia and increase salt and water retention). Products include:
Depo-Medrol Single-Dose Vial 2600
Depo-Medrol Sterile Aqueous Suspension 2597

Methylprednisolone Sodium Succinate (May increase the risk of hypokalemia and increase salt and water retention). Products include:
Solu-Medrol Sterile Powder 2643

Metoprolol Succinate (Excessive hypotension may result especially during initial therapy). Products include:
Toprol-XL Tablets 565

IMPORTANT NOTE: Always consult each drug listing in the patient's regimen for possible interactions.

Zaroxolyn **Interactions Index** **1180**

Metoprolol Tartrate (Excessive hypotension may result especially during initial therapy). Products include:

- Lopressor Ampuls 830
- Lopressor HCT Tablets 832
- Lopressor Tablets 830

Metyrosine (Excessive hypotension may result especially during initial therapy). Products include:

- Demser Capsules 1649

Minoxidil (Excessive hypotension may result especially during initial therapy). Products include:

- Loniten Tablets 2618
- Rogaine Topical Solution 2637

Moexipril Hydrochloride (Excessive hypotension may result especially during initial therapy). Products include:

- Univasc Tablets 2410

Morphine Sulfate (Hypotensive effect may be potentiated). Products include:

- Astramorph/PF Injection, USP (Preservative-Free) 535
- Duramorph 962
- Infumorph 200 and Infumorph 500 Sterile Solutions 965
- MS Contin Tablets 1994
- MSIR 1997
- Oramorph SR (Morphine Sulfate Sustained Release Tablets) 2236
- RMS Suppositories 2657
- Roxanol 2243

Nabumetone (Increases the antihypertensive effect). Products include:

- Relafen Tablets 2510

Nadolol (Excessive hypotension may result especially during initial therapy).

- No products indexed under this heading.

Naproxen (Increases the antihypertensive effect). Products include:

- Anaprox/Naprosyn 2117

Naproxen Sodium (Increases the antihypertensive effect). Products include:

- Aleve 1975
- Anaprox/Naprosyn 2117

Nicardipine Hydrochloride (Excessive hypotension may result especially during initial therapy). Products include:

- Cardene Capsules 2095
- Cardene I.V. 2709
- Cardene SR Capsules 2097

Nifedipine (Excessive hypotension may result especially during initial therapy). Products include:

- Adalat Capsules (10 mg and 20 mg) 587
- Adalat CC 589
- Procardia Capsules 1971
- Procardia XL Extended Release Tablets 1972

Nisoldipine (Excessive hypotension may result especially during initial therapy).

- No products indexed under this heading.

Nitroglycerin (Excessive hypotension may result especially during initial therapy). Products include:

- Deponit NTG Transdermal Delivery System 2397
- Nitro-Bid IV 1523
- Nitro-Bid Ointment 1524
- Nitrodisc 2047
- Nitro-Dur (nitroglycerin) Transdermal Infusion System 1326
- Nitrolingual Spray 2027
- Nitrostat Tablets 1925
- Transderm-Nitro Transdermal Therapeutic System 859

Norepinephrine Bitartrate (Arterial responsiveness to norepinephrine may be decreased). Products include:

- Levophed Bitartrate Injection 2315

Opium Alkaloids (Hypotensive effect may be potentiated).

- No products indexed under this heading.

Oxaprozin (Increases the antihypertensive effect). Products include:

- Daypro Caplets 2426

Oxycodone Hydrochloride (Hypotensive effect may be potentiated). Products include:

- Percocet Tablets 938
- Percodan Tablets 939
- Percodan-Demi Tablets 940
- Roxicodone Tablets, Oral Solution & Intensol (Oxycodone) 2244
- Tylox Capsules 1584

Penbutolol Sulfate (Excessive hypotension may result especially during initial therapy). Products include:

- Levatol 2403

Pentobarbital Sodium (Hypotensive effect may be potentiated). Products include:

- Nembutal Sodium Capsules 436
- Nembutal Sodium Solution 438
- Nembutal Sodium Suppositories 440

Phenobarbital (Hypotensive effect may be potentiated). Products include:

- Arco-Lase Plus Tablets 512
- Bellergal-S Tablets 2250
- Donnatal 2060
- Donnatal Extentabs 2061
- Donnatal Tablets 2060
- Phenobarbital Elixir and Tablets 1469
- Quadrinal Tablets 1350

Phenoxybenzamine Hydrochloride (Excessive hypotension may result especially during initial therapy). Products include:

- Dibenzyline Capsules 2476

Phentolamine Mesylate (Excessive hypotension may result especially during initial therapy). Products include:

- Regitine 846

Phenylbutazone (Increases the antihypertensive effect).

- No products indexed under this heading.

Pindolol (Excessive hypotension may result especially during initial therapy). Products include:

- Visken Tablets 2299

Piroxicam (Increases the antihypertensive effect). Products include:

- Feldene Capsules 1965

Polythiazide (Excessive hypotension may result especially during initial therapy). Products include:

- Minizide Capsules 1938

Prazosin Hydrochloride (Excessive hypotension may result especially during initial therapy). Products include:

- Minipress Capsules 1937
- Minizide Capsules 1938

Prednisolone Acetate (May increase the risk of hypokalemia and increase salt and water retention). Products include:

- AK-CIDE .... ◉ 202
- AK-CIDE Ointment .... ◉ 202
- Blephamide Liquifilm Sterile Ophthalmic Suspension 476
- Blephamide Ointment .... ◉ 237
- Econopred & Econopred Plus Ophthalmic Suspensions .... ◉ 217
- Poly-Pred Liquifilm .... ◉ 248
- Pred Forte .... ◉ 250
- Pred Mild .... ◉ 253
- Pred-G Liquifilm Sterile Ophthalmic Suspension .... ◉ 251
- Pred-G S.O.P. Sterile Ophthalmic Ointment .... ◉ 252
- Vasocidin Ointment .... ◉ 268

Prednisolone Sodium Phosphate (May increase the risk of hypokalemia and increase salt and water retention). Products include:

- AK-Pred .... ◉ 204
- Hydeltrasol Injection, Sterile 1665
- Inflamase .... ◉ 265
- Pediapred Oral Liquid 995
- Vasocidin Ophthalmic Solution .... ◉ 270

Prednisolone Tebutate (May increase the risk of hypokalemia and increase salt and water retention). Products include:

- Hydeltra-T.B.A. Sterile Suspension 1667

Prednisone (May increase the risk of hypokalemia and increase salt and water retention). Products include:

- Deltasone Tablets 2595

Propoxyphene Hydrochloride (Hypotensive effect may be potentiated). Products include:

- Darvon 1435
- Wygesic Tablets 2827

Propoxyphene Napsylate (Hypotensive effect may be potentiated). Products include:

- Darvon-N/Darvocet-N 1433

Propranolol Hydrochloride (Excessive hypotension may result especially during initial therapy). Products include:

- Inderal 2728
- Inderal LA Long Acting Capsules 2730
- Inderide Tablets 2732
- Inderide LA Long Acting Capsules 2734

Quinapril Hydrochloride (Excessive hypotension may result especially during initial therapy). Products include:

- Accupril Tablets 1893

Ramipril (Excessive hypotension may result especially during initial therapy). Products include:

- Altace Capsules 1232

Rauwolfia Serpentina (Excessive hypotension may result especially during initial therapy).

- No products indexed under this heading.

Rescinnamine (Excessive hypotension may result especially during initial therapy).

- No products indexed under this heading.

Reserpine (Excessive hypotension may result especially during initial therapy). Products include:

- Diupres Tablets 1650
- Hydropres Tablets 1675
- Ser-Ap-Es Tablets 849

Salsalate (Increases the antihypertensive effect). Products include:

- Mono-Gesic Tablets 792
- Salflex Tablets 786

Secobarbital Sodium (Hypotensive effect may be potentiated). Products include:

- Seconal Sodium Pulvules 1474

Sodium Nitroprusside (Excessive hypotension may result especially during initial therapy).

- No products indexed under this heading.

Sotalol Hydrochloride (Excessive hypotension may result especially during initial therapy). Products include:

- Betapace Tablets 641

Spirapril Hydrochloride (Excessive hypotension may result especially during initial therapy).

- No products indexed under this heading.

Sufentanil Citrate (Hypotensive effect may be potentiated). Products include:

- Sufenta Injection 1309

Sulindac (Increases the antihypertensive effect). Products include:

- Clinoril Tablets 1618

Terazosin Hydrochloride (Excessive hypotension may result especially during initial therapy). Products include:

- Hytrin Capsules 430

Thiamylal Sodium (Hypotensive effect may be potentiated).

- No products indexed under this heading.

Timolol Maleate (Excessive hypotension may result especially during initial therapy). Products include:

- Blocadren Tablets 1614
- Timolide Tablets 1748
- Timoptic in Ocudose 1753
- Timoptic Sterile Ophthalmic Solution 1751
- Timoptic-XE 1755

Tolazamide (Blood glucose concentration may be raised).

- No products indexed under this heading.

Tolbutamide (Blood glucose concentration may be raised).

- No products indexed under this heading.

Tolmetin Sodium (Increases the antihypertensive effect). Products include:

- Tolectin (200, 400 and 600 mg) .. 1581

Torsemide (Excessive hypotension may result especially during initial therapy). Products include:

- Demadex Tablets and Injection 686

Triamcinolone (May increase the risk of hypokalemia and increase salt and water retention). Products include:

- Aristocort Tablets 1022

Triamcinolone Acetonide (May increase the risk of hypokalemia and increase salt and water retention). Products include:

- Aristocort A 0.025% Cream 1027
- Aristocort A 0.5% Cream 1031
- Aristocort A 0.1% Cream 1029
- Aristocort A 0.1% Ointment 1030
- Azmacort Oral Inhaler 2011
- Nasacort Nasal Inhaler 2024

Triamcinolone Diacetate (May increase the risk of hypokalemia and increase salt and water retention). Products include:

- Aristocort Suspension (Forte Parenteral) 1027
- Aristocort Suspension (Intralesional) 1025

Triamcinolone Hexacetonide (May increase the risk of hypokalemia and increase salt and water retention). Products include:

- Aristospan Suspension (Intra-articular) 1033
- Aristospan Suspension (Intralesional) 1032

Trimethaphan Camsylate (Excessive hypotension may result especially during initial therapy). Products include:

- Arfonad Ampuls 2080

Tubocurarine Chloride (Neuromuscular blocking effects of curariform drugs may be enhanced).

- No products indexed under this heading.

Verapamil Hydrochloride (Excessive hypotension may result especially during initial therapy). Products include:

- Calan SR Caplets 2422
- Calan Tablets 2419
- Isoptin Injectable 1344
- Isoptin Oral Tablets 1346

(▣ Described in PDR For Nonprescription Drugs) (◉ Described in PDR For Ophthalmology)

Isoptin SR Tablets ... 1348
Verelan Capsules ... 1410
Verelan Capsules ... 2824

Warfarin Sodium (May affect the hypoprothrombinemic response to anticoagulants; dosage adjustments may be necessary). Products include:
Coumadin ... 926

Food Interactions

Alcohol (Hypotensive effect may be potentiated).

ZEBETA TABLETS

(Bisoprolol Fumarate) ... 1413

May interact with beta blockers, catecholamine depleting drugs, oral hypoglycemic agents, and insulin. Compounds in these categories include:

Acarbose (Possible masking of some of the manifestations of hypoglycemia).
No products indexed under this heading.

Acebutolol Hydrochloride (Zebeta should not be combined with other beta-blocking drugs). Products include:
Sectral Capsules ... 2807

Atenolol (Zebeta should not be combined with other beta-blocking drugs). Products include:
Tenoretic Tablets ... 2845
Tenormin Tablets and I.V. Injection 2847

Betaxolol Hydrochloride (Zebeta should not be combined with other beta-blocking drugs). Products include:
Betoptic Ophthalmic Solution ... 469
Betoptic S Ophthalmic Suspension 471
Kerlone Tablets ... 2436

Carteolol Hydrochloride (Zebeta should not be combined with other beta-blocking drugs). Products include:
Cartrol Tablets ... 410
Ocupress Ophthalmic Solution, 1% Sterile ... ⊙ 309

Chlorpropamide (Possible masking of some of the manifestations of hypoglycemia). Products include:
Diabinese Tablets ... 1935

Clonidine (In patients receiving concurrent clonidine, Zebeta should be discontinued for several days before the withdrawal of clonidine). Products include:
Catapres-TTS ... 675

Clonidine Hydrochloride (In patients receiving concurrent clonidine, Zebeta should be discontinued for several days before the withdrawal of clonidine). Products include:
Catapres Tablets ... 674
Combipres Tablets ... 677

Cyclopropane (Care should be taken when anesthetic agents which depress myocardial function are used with Zebeta).

Deserpidine (Potential for added beta-adrenergic blocking action of Zebeta resulting in excessive reduction of sympathetic activity).
No products indexed under this heading.

Diltiazem Hydrochloride (Potential for additional myocardial depression and/or inhibition of AV conduction). Products include:
Cardizem CD Capsules ... 1506
Cardizem SR Capsules ... 1510
Cardizem Injectable ... 1508
Cardizem Tablets ... 1512
Dilacor XR Extended-release Capsules ... 2018

Disopyramide Phosphate (Potential for additional myocardial depression and/or inhibition of AV conduction). Products include:
Norpace ... 2444

Epinephrine (Patients with a history of anaphylactic reactions to a variety of allergens may be unresponsive to the usual dose of epinephrine used to treat allergic reactions). Products include:
Bronkaid Mist ... ◘ 717
EPIFRIN ... ⊙ 239
EpiPen ... 790
Marcaine Hydrochloride with Epinephrine 1:200,000 ... 2316
Primatene Mist ... ◘ 873
Sensorcaine with Epinephrine Injection ... 559
Sus-Phrine Injection ... 1019
Xylocaine with Epinephrine Injections ... 567

Epinephrine Bitartrate (Patients with a history of anaphylactic reactions to a variety of allergens may be unresponsive to the usual dose of epinephrine used to treat allergic reactions). Products include:
Bronkaid Mist Suspension ... ◘ 718
Sensorcaine-MPF with Epinephrine Injection ... 559

Esmolol Hydrochloride (Zebeta should not be combined with other beta-blocking drugs). Products include:
Brevibloc Injection ... 1808

Ether (Care should be taken when anesthetic agents which depress myocardial function are used with Zebeta).

Glipizide (Possible masking of some of the manifestations of hypoglycemia). Products include:
Glucotrol Tablets ... 1967
Glucotrol XL Extended Release Tablets ... 1968

Glyburide (Possible masking of some of the manifestations of hypoglycemia). Products include:
DiaBeta Tablets ... 1239
Glynase PresTab Tablets ... 2609
Micronase Tablets ... 2623

Guanethidine Monosulfate (Potential for added beta-adrenergic blocking action of Zebeta resulting in excessive reduction of sympathetic activity). Products include:
Esimil Tablets ... 822
Ismelin Tablets ... 827

Insulin, Human (Possible masking of some of the manifestations of hypoglycemia).
No products indexed under this heading.

Insulin, Human Isophane Suspension (Possible masking of some of the manifestations of hypoglycemia). Products include:
Novolin N Human Insulin 10 ml Vials ... 1795

Insulin, Human NPH (Possible masking of some of the manifestations of hypoglycemia). Products include:
Humulin N, 100 Units ... 1448
Novolin N PenFill Cartridges Durable Insulin Delivery System ... 1798
Novolin N Prefilled Syringe Disposable Insulin Delivery System ... 1798

Insulin, Human Regular (Possible masking of some of the manifestations of hypoglycemia). Products include:
Humulin R, 100 Units ... 1449
Novolin R Human Insulin 10 ml Vials ... 1795
Novolin R PenFill Cartridges Durable Insulin Delivery System ... 1798
Novolin R Prefilled Syringe Disposable Insulin Delivery System ... 1798
Velosulin BR Human Insulin 10 ml Vials ... 1795

Insulin, Human, Zinc Suspension (Possible masking of some of the manifestations of hypoglycemia). Products include:
Humulin L, 100 Units ... 1446
Humulin U, 100 Units ... 1450
Novolin L Human Insulin 10 ml Vials ... 1795

Insulin, NPH (Possible masking of some of the manifestations of hypoglycemia). Products include:
NPH, 100 Units ... 1450
Pork NPH, 100 Units ... 1452
Purified Pork NPH Isophane Insulin ... 1801

Insulin, Regular (Possible masking of some of the manifestations of hypoglycemia). Products include:
Regular, 100 Units ... 1450
Pork Regular, 100 Units ... 1452
Pork Regular (Concentrated), 500 Units ... 1453
Purified Pork Regular Insulin ... 1801

Insulin, Zinc Crystals (Possible masking of some of the manifestations of hypoglycemia). Products include:
NPH, 100 Units ... 1450

Insulin, Zinc Suspension (Possible masking of some of the manifestations of hypoglycemia). Products include:
Iletin I ... 1450
Lente, 100 Units ... 1450
Iletin II ... 1452
Pork Lente, 100 Units ... 1452
Purified Pork Lente Insulin ... 1801

Labetalol Hydrochloride (Zebeta should not be combined with other beta-blocking drugs). Products include:
Normodyne Injection ... 2377
Normodyne Tablets ... 2379
Trandate ... 1185

Levobunolol Hydrochloride (Zebeta should not be combined with other beta-blocking drugs). Products include:
Betagan ... ⊙ 233

Metformin Hydrochloride (Possible masking of some of the manifestations of hypoglycemia). Products include:
Glucophage ... 752

Metipranolol Hydrochloride (Zebeta should not be combined with other beta-blocking drugs). Products include:
OptiPranolol (Metipranolol 0.3%) Sterile Ophthalmic Solution ... ⊙ 258

Metoprolol Succinate (Zebeta should not be combined with other beta-blocking drugs). Products include:
Toprol-XL Tablets ... 565

Metoprolol Tartrate (Zebeta should not be combined with other beta-blocking drugs). Products include:
Lopressor Ampuls ... 830
Lopressor HCT Tablets ... 832
Lopressor Tablets ... 830

Nadolol (Zebeta should not be combined with other beta-blocking drugs).
No products indexed under this heading.

Penbutolol Sulfate (Zebeta should not be combined with other beta-blocking drugs). Products include:
Levatol ... 2403

Pindolol (Zebeta should not be combined with other beta-blocking drugs). Products include:
Visken Tablets ... 2299

Propranolol Hydrochloride (Zebeta should not be combined with other beta-blocking drugs). Products include:
Inderal ... 2728
Inderal LA Long Acting Capsules ... 2730
Inderide Tablets ... 2732
Inderide LA Long Acting Capsules .. 2734

Rauwolfia Serpentina (Potential for added beta-adrenergic blocking action of Zebeta resulting in excessive reduction of sympathetic activity).
No products indexed under this heading.

Rescinnamine (Potential for added beta-adrenergic blocking action of Zebeta resulting in excessive reduction of sympathetic activity).
No products indexed under this heading.

Reserpine (Potential for added beta-adrenergic blocking action of Zebeta resulting in excessive reduction of sympathetic activity). Products include:
Diupres Tablets ... 1650
Hydropres Tablets ... 1675
Ser-Ap-Es Tablets ... 849

Rifampin (Concurrent use increases the metabolic clearance of Zebeta, resulting in shortened elimination half-life of Zebeta). Products include:
Rifadin ... 1528
Rifamate Capsules ... 1530
Rifater ... 1532
Rimactane Capsules ... 847

Sotalol Hydrochloride (Zebeta should not be combined with other beta-blocking drugs). Products include:
Betapace Tablets ... 641

Timolol Hemihydrate (Zebeta should not be combined with other beta-blocking drugs). Products include:
Betimol 0.25%, 0.5% ... ⊙ 261

Timolol Maleate (Zebeta should not be combined with other beta-blocking drugs). Products include:
Blocadren Tablets ... 1614
Timolide Tablets ... 1748
Timoptic in Ocudose ... 1753
Timoptic Sterile Ophthalmic Solution ... 1751
Timoptic-XE ... 1755

Tolazamide (Possible masking of some of the manifestations of hypoglycemia).
No products indexed under this heading.

Tolbutamide (Possible masking of some of the manifestations of hypoglycemia).
No products indexed under this heading.

Verapamil Hydrochloride (Potential for additional myocardial depression and/or inhibition of AV conduction). Products include:
Calan SR Caplets ... 2422
Calan Tablets ... 2419
Isoptin Injectable ... 1344
Isoptin Oral Tablets ... 1346
Isoptin SR Tablets ... 1348
Verelan Capsules ... 1410
Verelan Capsules ... 2824

ZEFAZONE I.V. SOLUTION

(Cefmetazole Sodium) ... 2654

See **Zefazone Sterile Powder**

ZEFAZONE STERILE POWDER

(Cefmetazole Sodium) ... 2654

May interact with aminoglycosides

IMPORTANT NOTE: Always consult each drug listing in the patient's regimen for possible interactions.

and certain other agents. Compounds in these categories include:

Amikacin Sulfate (Nephrotoxicity possible with concomitant use). Products include:

Amikacin Sulfate Injection, USP 960
Amikin Injectable 501

Gentamicin Sulfate (Nephrotoxicity possible with concomitant use). Products include:

Garamycin Injectable 2360
Genoptic Sterile Ophthalmic Solution ...... ◉ 243
Genoptic Sterile Ophthalmic Ointment ...... ◉ 243
Gentacidin Ointment ...... ◉ 264
Gentacidin Solution ...... ◉ 264
Gentak ...... ◉ 208
Pred-G Liquifilm Sterile Ophthalmic Suspension ...... ◉ 251
Pred-G S.O.P. Sterile Ophthalmic Ointment ...... ◉ 252

Kanamycin Sulfate (Nephrotoxicity possible with concomitant use).

No products indexed under this heading.

Streptomycin Sulfate (Nephrotoxicity possible with concomitant use). Products include:

Streptomycin Sulfate Injection 2208

Tobramycin (Nephrotoxicity possible with concomitant use). Products include:

AKTOB ...... ◉ 206
TobraDex Ophthalmic Suspension and Ointment 473
Tobrex Ophthalmic Ointment and Solution ...... ◉ 229

Tobramycin Sulfate (Nephrotoxicity possible with concomitant use). Products include:

Nebcin Vials, Hyporets & ADD-Vantage 1464
Tobramycin Sulfate Injection 968

Food Interactions

Alcohol (Disulfiram-like reactions characterized by flushing, sweating, headache, and tachycardia; patients should be advised against the ingestion of alcohol-containing beverages during and for 24 hours after the administration of cefmetazole).

ZEMURON

(Rocuronium Bromide) 1830

May interact with aminoglycosides, tetracyclines, anticonvulsants, inhalant anesthetics, and certain other agents. Compounds in these categories include:

Amikacin Sulfate (Possible prolongation of neuromuscular blockade). Products include:

Amikacin Sulfate Injection, USP 960
Amikin Injectable 501

Bacitracin (Possible prolongation of neuromuscular blockade). Products include:

Mycitracin ...... ▣ 839

Carbamazepine (Potential for apparent resistance to the effects of rocuronium in the form of diminished magnitude of neuromuscular blockade). Products include:

Atretol Tablets 573
Tegretol Chewable Tablets 852
Tegretol Suspension 852
Tegretol Tablets 852

Colistimethate Sodium (Possible prolongation of neuromuscular blockade). Products include:

Coly-Mycin M Parenteral 1905

Colistin Sulfate (Possible prolongation of neuromuscular blockade). Products include:

Coly-Mycin S Otic w/Neomycin & Hydrocortisone 1906

Demeclocycline Hydrochloride (Possible prolongation of neuromuscular blockade). Products include:

Declomycin Tablets 1371

Desflurane (Possible enhanced activity of neuromuscular blocking agent). Products include:

Suprane 1813

Divalproex Sodium (Potential for apparent resistance to the effects of rocuronium in the form of diminished magnitude of neuromuscular blockade). Products include:

Depakote Tablets 415

Doxycycline Calcium (Possible prolongation of neuromuscular blockade). Products include:

Vibramycin Calcium Oral Suspension Syrup 1941

Doxycycline Hyclate (Possible prolongation of neuromuscular blockade). Products include:

Doryx Capsules 1913
Vibramycin Hyclate Capsules 1941
Vibramycin Hyclate Intravenous 2215
Vibra-Tabs Film Coated Tablets 1941

Doxycycline Monohydrate (Possible prolongation of neuromuscular blockade). Products include:

Monodox Capsules 1805
Vibramycin Monohydrate for Oral Suspension 1941

Enflurane (Possible enhanced activity of neuromuscular blocking agent; may prolong the duration of action).

No products indexed under this heading.

Ethosuximide (Potential for apparent resistance to the effects of rocuronium in the form of diminished magnitude of neuromuscular blockade). Products include:

Zarontin Capsules 1928
Zarontin Syrup 1929

Ethotoin (Potential for apparent resistance to the effects of rocuronium in the form of diminished magnitude of neuromuscular blockade). Products include:

Peganone Tablets 446

Felbamate (Potential for apparent resistance to the effects of rocuronium in the form of diminished magnitude of neuromuscular blockade). Products include:

Felbatol 2666

Gentamicin Sulfate (Possible prolongation of neuromuscular blockade). Products include:

Garamycin Injectable 2360
Genoptic Sterile Ophthalmic Solution ...... ◉ 243
Genoptic Sterile Ophthalmic Ointment ...... ◉ 243
Gentacidin Ointment ...... ◉ 264
Gentacidin Solution ...... ◉ 264
Gentak ...... ◉ 208
Pred-G Liquifilm Sterile Ophthalmic Suspension ...... ◉ 251
Pred-G S.O.P. Sterile Ophthalmic Ointment ...... ◉ 252

Halothane (Possible enhanced activity of neuromuscular blocking agent). Products include:

Fluothane 2724

Isoflurane (Possible enhanced activity of neuromuscular blocking agent; may prolong the duration of action).

No products indexed under this heading.

Kanamycin Sulfate (Possible prolongation of neuromuscular blockade).

No products indexed under this heading.

Lamotrigine (Potential for apparent resistance to the effects of rocuronium in the form of diminished magnitude of neuromuscular blockade). Products include:

Lamictal Tablets 1112

Lithium Carbonate (May increase the duration of neuromuscular block). Products include:

Eskalith 2485
Lithium Carbonate Capsules & Tablets 2230
Lithonate/Lithotabs/Lithobid 2543

Lithium Citrate (May increase the duration of neuromuscular block).

No products indexed under this heading.

Magnesium Sulfate Injection (May enhance the neuromuscular blockade).

Mephenytoin (Potential for apparent resistance to the effects of rocuronium in the form of diminished magnitude of neuromuscular blockade). Products include:

Mesantoin Tablets 2272

Methacycline Hydrochloride (Possible prolongation of neuromuscular blockade).

No products indexed under this heading.

Methoxyflurane (Possible enhanced activity of neuromuscular blocking agent).

No products indexed under this heading.

Methsuximide (Potential for apparent resistance to the effects of rocuronium in the form of diminished magnitude of neuromuscular blockade). Products include:

Celontin Kapseals 1899

Minocycline Hydrochloride (Possible prolongation of neuromuscular blockade). Products include:

Dynacin Capsules 1590
Minocin Intravenous 1382
Minocin Oral Suspension 1385
Minocin Pellet-Filled Capsules 1383

Oxytetracycline Hydrochloride (Possible prolongation of neuromuscular blockade). Products include:

TERAK Ointment ...... ◉ 209
Terra-Cortril Ophthalmic Suspension 2210
Terramycin with Polymyxin B Sulfate Ophthalmic Ointment 2211
Urobiotic-250 Capsules 2214

Paramethadione (Potential for apparent resistance to the effects of rocuronium in the form of diminished magnitude of neuromuscular blockade).

No products indexed under this heading.

Phenacemide (Potential for apparent resistance to the effects of rocuronium in the form of diminished magnitude of neuromuscular blockade). Products include:

Phenurone Tablets 447

Phenobarbital (Potential for apparent resistance to the effects of rocuronium in the form of diminished magnitude of neuromuscular blockade). Products include:

Arco-Lase Plus Tablets 512
Bellergal-S Tablets 2250
Donnatal 2060
Donnatal Extentabs 2061
Donnatal Tablets 2060
Phenobarbital Elixir and Tablets 1469
Quadrinal Tablets 1350

Phensuximide (Potential for apparent resistance to the effects of rocuronium in the form of diminished magnitude of neuromuscular blockade). Products include:

Milontin Kapseals 1920

Phenytoin (Potential for apparent resistance to the effects of rocuronium in the form of diminished magnitude of neuromuscular blockade). Products include:

Dilantin Infatabs 1908
Dilantin-125 Suspension 1911

Phenytoin Sodium (Potential for apparent resistance to the effects of rocuronium in the form of diminished magnitude of neuromuscular blockade). Products include:

Dilantin Kapseals 1906
Dilantin Parenteral 1910

Polymyxin B Sulfate (Possible prolongation of neuromuscular blockade). Products include:

AK-Spore ...... ◉ 204
AK-Trol Ointment & Suspension ...... ◉ 205
Bactine First Aid Antibiotic Plus Anesthetic Ointment ...... ▣ 708
Betadine Brand First Aid Antibiotics & Moisturizer Ointment 1991
Campho-Phenique Maximum Strength First Aid Antibiotic Plus Pain Reliever Ointment ...... ▣ 719
Cortisporin Cream 1084
Cortisporin Ointment 1085
Cortisporin Ophthalmic Ointment Sterile 1085
Cortisporin Ophthalmic Suspension Sterile 1086
Cortisporin Otic Solution Sterile 1087
Cortisporin Otic Suspension Sterile 1088
Dexacidin Ointment ...... ◉ 263
Maxitrol Ophthalmic Ointment and Suspension ...... ◉ 224
Mycitracin ...... ▣ 839
Neosporin G.U. Irrigant Sterile 1148
Neosporin Ointment ...... ▣ 857
Neosporin Plus Maximum Strength Cream ...... ▣ 858
Neosporin Plus Maximum Strength Ointment ...... ▣ 858
Neosporin Ophthalmic Ointment Sterile 1148
Neosporin Ophthalmic Solution Sterile 1149
Ophthocort ...... ◉ 311
PediOtic Suspension Sterile 1153
Polymyxin B Sulfate, Aerosporin Brand Sterile Powder 1154
Poly-Pred Liquifilm ...... ◉ 248
Polysporin Ointment ...... ▣ 858
Polysporin Ophthalmic Ointment Sterile 1154
Polysporin Powder ...... ▣ 859
Polytrim Ophthalmic Solution Sterile 482
TERAK Ointment ...... ◉ 209
Terramycin with Polymyxin B Sulfate Ophthalmic Ointment 2211

Primidone (Potential for apparent resistance to the effects of rocuronium in the form of diminished magnitude of neuromuscular blockade). Products include:

Mysoline 2754

Procainamide Hydrochloride (May increase the duration of neuromuscular block). Products include:

Procan SR Tablets 1926

Quinidine Gluconate (Possible recurrent paralysis; increased duration of neuromuscular block). Products include:

Quinaglute Dura-Tabs Tablets 649

Quinidine Polygalacturonate (Possible recurrent paralysis; increased duration of neuromuscular block).

No products indexed under this heading.

Quinidine Sulfate (Possible recurrent paralysis; increased duration of neuromuscular block). Products include:

Quinidex Extentabs 2067

Streptomycin Sulfate (Possible prolongation of neuromuscular blockade). Products include:

Streptomycin Sulfate Injection 2208

(▣ Described in PDR For Nonprescription Drugs) (◉ Described in PDR For Ophthalmology)

1183 Interactions Index Zestoretic

Succinylcholine Chloride (Rocuronium should not be given until recovery from succinylcholine has been observed). Products include:
- Anectine 1073

Tetracycline Hydrochloride (Possible prolongation of neuromuscular blockade). Products include:
- Achromycin V Capsules 1367

Tobramycin (Possible prolongation of neuromuscular blockade). Products include:
- AKTOB .... ⊙ 206
- TobraDex Ophthalmic Suspension and Ointment 473
- Tobrex Ophthalmic Ointment and Solution .... ⊙ 229

Tobramycin Sulfate (Possible prolongation of neuromuscular blockade). Products include:
- Nebcin Vials, Hyporets & ADD-Vantage 1464
- Tobramycin Sulfate Injection 968

Trimethadione (Potential for apparent resistance to the effects of rocuronium in the form of diminished magnitude of neuromuscular blockade).
- No products indexed under this heading.

Valproic Acid (Potential for apparent resistance to the effects of rocuronium in the form of diminished magnitude of neuromuscular blockade). Products include:
- Depakene 413

Vancomycin Hydrochloride (Possible prolongation of neuromuscular blockade). Products include:
- Vancocin HCl, Oral Solution & Pulvules 1483
- Vancocin HCl, Vials & ADD-Vantage 1481

ADVANCED FORMULA ZENATE TABLETS
(Vitamins with Minerals) 2550
None cited in PDR database.

ZEPHIRAN CHLORIDE AQUEOUS SOLUTION
(Benzalkonium Chloride) .... ▣ 795
None cited in PDR database.

ZEPHIRAN CHLORIDE SPRAY
(Benzalkonium Chloride) .... ▣ 795
None cited in PDR database.

ZEPHIRAN CHLORIDE TINTED TINCTURE
(Benzalkonium Chloride) .... ▣ 795
None cited in PDR database.

ZERIT CAPSULES
(Stavudine) 729
May interact with drugs that may exacerbate peripheral neuropathy (selected). Compounds in this category include:

Carboplatin (Concurrent use may exacerbate peripheral neuropathy). Products include:
- Paraplatin for Injection 705

Didanosine (Concurrent use may exacerbate peripheral neuropathy). Products include:
- Videx Tablets, Powder for Oral Solution, & Pediatric Powder for Oral Solution 720

Isoniazid (Concurrent use may exacerbate peripheral neuropathy). Products include:
- Nydrazid Injection 508
- Rifamate Capsules 1530
- Rifater 1532

Paclitaxel (Concurrent use may exacerbate peripheral neuropathy). Products include:
- Taxol 714

Zalcitabine (Concurrent use may exacerbate peripheral neuropathy). Products include:
- Hivid Tablets 2121

Food Interactions

Meal, unspecified (Reduces mean SD C_{max} of stavudine and prolongs the median time to reach C_{max} from 0.6 to 1.5 hours; systemic exposure (AUC) remains unchanged).

ZESTORETIC
(Lisinopril, Hydrochlorothiazide) 2850
May interact with diuretics, non-steroidal anti-inflammatory agents, potassium sparing diuretics, potassium preparations, barbiturates, narcotic analgesics, oral hypoglycemic agents, insulin, antihypertensives, corticosteroids, lithium preparations, nondepolarizing neuromuscular blocking agents, and certain other agents. Compounds in these categories include:

Acarbose (Dosage adjustment of the antidiabetic may be required).
- No products indexed under this heading.

Acebutolol Hydrochloride (Additive effects). Products include:
- Sectral Capsules 2807

ACTH (Intensifies electrolyte depletion).
- No products indexed under this heading.

Alfentanil Hydrochloride (Potentiates orthostatic hypotension). Products include:
- Alfenta Injection 1286

Amiloride Hydrochloride (Additive antihypertensive effects; potential for hyperkalemia). Products include:
- Midamor Tablets 1703
- Moduretic Tablets 1705

Amlodipine Besylate (Additive effects). Products include:
- Lotrel Capsules 840
- Norvasc Tablets 1940

Aprobarbital (Potentiates orthostatic hypotension).
- No products indexed under this heading.

Atenolol (Additive effects). Products include:
- Tenoretic Tablets 2845
- Tenormin Tablets and I.V. Injection 2847

Atracurium Besylate (Possible increased responsiveness to the muscle relaxant). Products include:
- Tracrium Injection 1183

Benazepril Hydrochloride (Additive effects). Products include:
- Lotensin Tablets 834
- Lotensin HCT 837
- Lotrel Capsules 840

Bendroflumethiazide (Additive effects).
- No products indexed under this heading.

Betamethasone Acetate (Intensifies electrolyte depletion). Products include:
- Celestone Soluspan Suspension 2347

Betamethasone Sodium Phosphate (Intensifies electrolyte depletion). Products include:
- Celestone Soluspan Suspension 2347

Betaxolol Hydrochloride (Additive effects). Products include:
- Betoptic Ophthalmic Solution 469
- Betoptic S Ophthalmic Suspension 471
- Kerlone Tablets 2436

Bisoprolol Fumarate (Additive effects). Products include:
- Zebeta Tablets 1413
- Ziac 1415

Bumetanide (Additive effects). Products include:
- Bumex 2093

Buprenorphine (Potentiates orthostatic hypotension). Products include:
- Buprenex Injectable 2006

Butabarbital (Potentiates orthostatic hypotension).
- No products indexed under this heading.

Butalbital (Potentiates orthostatic hypotension). Products include:
- Esgic-plus Tablets 1013
- Fioricet Tablets 2258
- Fioricet with Codeine Capsules 2260
- Fiorinal Capsules 2261
- Fiorinal with Codeine Capsules 2262
- Fiorinal Tablets 2261
- Phrenilin 785
- Sedapap Tablets 50 mg/650 mg 1543

Captopril (Additive effects). Products include:
- Capoten 739
- Capozide 742

Carteolol Hydrochloride (Additive effects). Products include:
- Cartrol Tablets 410
- Ocupress Ophthalmic Solution, 1% Sterile .... ⊙ 309

Chlorothiazide (Additive effects). Products include:
- Aldoclor Tablets 1598
- Diupres Tablets 1650
- Diuril Oral 1653

Chlorothiazide Sodium (Additive effects). Products include:
- Diuril Sodium Intravenous 1652

Chlorpropamide (Dosage adjustment of the antidiabetic may be required). Products include:
- Diabinese Tablets 1935

Chlorthalidone (Additive effects). Products include:
- Combipres Tablets 677
- Tenoretic Tablets 2845
- Thalitone 1245

Cholestyramine (Absorption of hydrochlorothiazide is impaired in the presence of anionic exchange resins, such as cholestyramine; binds hydrochlorothiazide and reduces its absorption from the GI tract by up to 85%). Products include:
- Questran Light 769
- Questran Powder 770

Clonidine (Additive effects). Products include:
- Catapres-TTS 675

Clonidine Hydrochloride (Additive effects). Products include:
- Catapres Tablets 674
- Combipres Tablets 677

Codeine Phosphate (Potentiates orthostatic hypotension). Products include:
- Actifed with Codeine Cough Syrup 1067
- Brontex 1981
- Deconsal C Expectorant Syrup 456
- Deconsal Pediatric Syrup 457
- Dimetane-DC Cough Syrup 2059
- Empirin with Codeine Tablets 1093
- Fioricet with Codeine Capsules 2260
- Fiorinal with Codeine Capsules 2262
- Isoclor Expectorant 990
- Novahistine DH 2462
- Novahistine Expectorant 2463
- Nucofed 2051
- Phenergan with Codeine 2777
- Phenergan VC with Codeine 2781
- Robitussin A-C Syrup 2073
- Robitussin-DAC Syrup 2074
- Ryna .... ▣ 841
- Soma Compound w/Codeine Tablets 2676
- Tussi-Organidin NR Liquid and S NR Liquid 2677
- Tylenol with Codeine 1583

Colestipol Hydrochloride (Absorption of hydrochlorothiazide is impaired in the presence of anionic exchange resins, such as colestipol; binds hydrochlorothiazide and reduces its absorption from the GI tract by up to 43%). Products include:
- Colestid Tablets 2591

Cortisone Acetate (Intensifies electrolyte depletion). Products include:
- Cortone Acetate Sterile Suspension 1623
- Cortone Acetate Tablets 1624

Deserpidine (Additive effects).
- No products indexed under this heading.

Dexamethasone (Intensifies electrolyte depletion). Products include:
- AK-Trol Ointment & Suspension .... ⊙ 205
- Decadron Elixir 1633
- Decadron Tablets 1635
- Decaspray Topical Aerosol 1648
- Dexacidin Ointment .... ⊙ 263
- Maxitrol Ophthalmic Ointment and Suspension .... ⊙ 224
- TobraDex Ophthalmic Suspension and Ointment 473

Dexamethasone Acetate (Intensifies electrolyte depletion). Products include:
- Dalalone D.P. Injectable 1011
- Decadron-LA Sterile Suspension 1646

Dexamethasone Sodium Phosphate (Intensifies electrolyte depletion). Products include:
- Decadron Phosphate Injection 1637
- Decadron Phosphate Respihaler 1642
- Decadron Phosphate Sterile Ophthalmic Ointment 1641
- Decadron Phosphate Sterile Ophthalmic Solution 1642
- Decadron Phosphate Topical Cream 1644
- Decadron Phosphate Turbinaire 1645
- Decadron Phosphate with Xylocaine Injection, Sterile 1639
- Dexacort Phosphate in Respihaler 458
- Dexacort Phosphate in Turbinaire 459
- NeoDecadron Sterile Ophthalmic Ointment 1712
- NeoDecadron Sterile Ophthalmic Solution 1713
- NeoDecadron Topical Cream 1714

Dezocine (Potentiates orthostatic hypotension). Products include:
- Dalgan Injection 538

Diazoxide (Additive effects). Products include:
- Hyperstat I.V. Injection 2363
- Proglycem 580

Diclofenac Potassium (Reduces antihypertensive effects). Products include:
- Cataflam 816

Diclofenac Sodium (Reduces antihypertensive effects). Products include:
- Voltaren Ophthalmic Sterile Ophthalmic Solution .... ⊙ 272
- Voltaren Tablets 861

Diltiazem Hydrochloride (Additive effects). Products include:
- Cardizem CD Capsules 1506
- Cardizem SR Capsules 1510
- Cardizem Injectable 1508
- Cardizem Tablets 1512
- Dilacor XR Extended-release Capsules 2018

Doxazosin Mesylate (Additive effects). Products include:
- Cardura Tablets 2186

Enalapril Maleate (Additive effects). Products include:
- Vaseretic Tablets 1765
- Vasotec Tablets 1771

Enalaprilat (Additive effects). Products include:
- Vasotec I.V. 1768

IMPORTANT NOTE: Always consult each drug listing in the patient's regimen for possible interactions.

Zestoretic

Esmolol Hydrochloride (Additive effects). Products include:

Brevibloc Injection................................. 1808

Ethacrynic Acid (Additive effects). Products include:

Edecrin Tablets.. 1657

Etodolac (Reduces antihypertensive effects). Products include:

Lodine Capsules and Tablets 2743

Felodipine (Additive effects). Products include:

Plendil Extended-Release Tablets.... 527

Fenoprofen Calcium (Reduces antihypertensive effects). Products include:

Nalfon 200 Pulvules & Nalfon Tablets 917

Fentanyl (Potentiates orthostatic hypotension). Products include:

Duragesic Transdermal System........ 1288

Fentanyl Citrate (Potentiates orthostatic hypotension). Products include:

Sublimaze Injection................................ 1307

Fludrocortisone Acetate (Intensifies electrolyte depletion). Products include:

Florinef Acetate Tablets 505

Flurbiprofen (Reduces antihypertensive effects). Products include:

Ansaid Tablets 2579

Fosinopril Sodium (Additive effects). Products include:

Monopril Tablets 757

Furosemide (Additive effects). Products include:

Lasix Injection, Oral Solution and Tablets 1240

Glipizide (Dosage adjustment of the antidiabetic may be required). Products include:

Glucotrol Tablets 1967

Glucotrol XL Extended Release Tablets 1968

Glyburide (Dosage adjustment of the antidiabetic may be required). Products include:

DiaBeta Tablets 1239

Glynase PresTab Tablets 2609

Micronase Tablets 2623

Guanabenz Acetate (Additive effects).

No products indexed under this heading.

Guanethidine Monosulfate (Additive effects). Products include:

Esimil Tablets 822

Ismelin Tablets 827

Hydralazine Hydrochloride (Additive effects). Products include:

Apresazide Capsules 808

Apresoline Hydrochloride Tablets .. 809

Ser-Ap-Es Tablets 849

Hydrocodone Bitartrate (Potentiates orthostatic hypotension). Products include:

Anexsia 5/500 Elixir 1781

Anexia Tablets... 1782

Codiclear DH Syrup 791

Deconamine CX Cough and Cold Liquid and Tablets................................... 1319

Duratuss HD Elixir................................... 2565

Hycodan Tablets and Syrup 930

Hycomine Compound Tablets 932

Hycomine 931

Hycotuss Expectorant Syrup 933

Hydrocet Capsules 782

Lorcet 10/650.. 1018

Lortab 2566

Tussend 1783

Tussend Expectorant 1785

Vicodin Tablets 1356

Vicodin ES Tablets 1357

Vicodin Tuss Expectorant 1358

Zydone Capsules 949

Hydrocodone Polistirex (Potentiates orthostatic hypotension). Products include:

Tussionex Pennkinetic Extended-Release Suspension 998

Hydrocortisone (Intensifies electrolyte depletion). Products include:

Anusol-HC Cream 2.5% 1896

Aquanil HC Lotion 1931

Bactine Hydrocortisone Anti-Itch Cream... �tweaD 709

Caldecort Anti-Itch Hydrocortisone Spray .... ✪D 631

Cortaid .... ✪D 836

CORTENEMA... 2535

Cortisporin Ointment 1085

Cortisporin Ophthalmic Ointment Sterile 1085

Cortisporin Ophthalmic Suspension Sterile 1086

Cortisporin Otic Solution Sterile 1087

Cortisporin Otic Suspension Sterile 1088

Cortizone-5 .... ✪D 831

Cortizone-10 .... ✪D 831

Hydrocortone Tablets 1672

Hytone 907

Massengill Medicated Soft Cloth Towelettes... 2458

PediOtic Suspension Sterile 1153

Preparation H Hydrocortisone 1% Cream .... ✪D 872

ProctoCream-HC 2.5% 2408

VōSoL HC Otic Solution......................... 2678

Hydrocortisone Acetate (Intensifies electrolyte depletion). Products include:

Analpram-HC Rectal Cream 1% and 2.5% 977

Anusol HC-1 Anti-Itch Hydrocortisone Ointment...................................... ✪D 847

Anusol-HC Suppositories 1897

Caldecort.. ✪D 631

Carmol HC 924

Coly-Mycin S Otic w/Neomycin & Hydrocortisone 1906

Cortaid .... ✪D 836

Cortifoam 2396

Cortisporin Cream................................... 1084

Epifoam 2399

Hydrocortone Acetate Sterile Suspension... 1669

Mantadil Cream 1135

Nupercainal Hydrocortisone 1% Cream... ✪D 645

Ophthocort .... ◉ 311

Pramosone Cream, Lotion & Ointment 978

ProctoCream-HC 2408

ProctoFoam-HC 2409

Terra-Cortril Ophthalmic Suspension 2210

Hydrocortisone Sodium Phosphate (Intensifies electrolyte depletion). Products include:

Hydrocortone Phosphate Injection, Sterile 1670

Hydrocortisone Sodium Succinate (Intensifies electrolyte depletion). Products include:

Solu-Cortef Sterile Powder.................. 2641

Hydroflumethiazide (Additive effects). Products include:

Diucardin Tablets..................................... 2718

Ibuprofen (Reduces antihypertensive effects). Products include:

Advil Cold and Sinus Caplets and Tablets (formerly CoAdvil) .... ✪D 870

Advil Ibuprofen Tablets and Caplets .... ✪D 870

Children's Advil Suspension 2692

Arthritis Foundation Ibuprofen Tablets .... ✪D 674

Bayer Select Ibuprofen Pain Relief Formula .... ✪D 715

Cramp End Tablets .... ✪D 735

Dimetapp Sinus Caplets .... ✪D 775

Haltran Tablets.. ✪D 771

IBU Tablets... 1342

Ibuprohm.. ✪D 735

Children's Motrin Ibuprofen Oral Suspension 1546

Motrin Tablets.. 2625

Motrin IB Caplets, Tablets, and Geltabs... ✪D 838

Motrin IB Sinus .... ✪D 838

Motrin Ibuprofen Suspension, Oral Drops, Chewable Tablets, Caplets 1546

Nuprin Ibuprofen/Analgesic Tablets & Caplets .... ✪D 622

Sine-Aid IB Caplets 1554

Vicks DayQuil SINUS Pressure & PAIN Relief with IBUPROFEN ...... ✪D 762

Indapamide (Additive effects). Products include:

Lozol Tablets 2022

Indomethacin (Reduces antihypertensive effects). Products include:

Indocin 1680

Indomethacin Sodium Trihydrate (Reduces antihypertensive effects). Products include:

Indocin I.V. 1684

Insulin, Human (Dosage adjustment of the antidiabetic may be required).

No products indexed under this heading.

Insulin, Human Isophane Suspension (Dosage adjustment of the antidiabetic may be required). Products include:

Novolin N Human Insulin 10 ml Vials.. 1795

Insulin, Human NPH (Dosage adjustment of the antidiabetic may be required). Products include:

Humulin N, 100 Units 1448

Novolin N PenFill Cartridges Durable Insulin Delivery System 1798

Novolin N Prefilled Syringe Disposable Insulin Delivery System 1798

Insulin, Human Regular (Dosage adjustment of the antidiabetic may be required). Products include:

Humulin R, 100 Units 1449

Novolin R Human Insulin 10 ml Vials.. 1795

Novolin R PenFill Cartridges Durable Insulin Delivery System 1798

Novolin R Prefilled Syringe Disposable Insulin Delivery System 1798

Velosulin BR Human Insulin 10 ml Vials.. 1795

Insulin, Human, Zinc Suspension (Dosage adjustment of the antidiabetic may be required). Products include:

Humulin L, 100 Units 1446

Humulin U, 100 Units 1450

Novolin L Human Insulin 10 ml Vials.. 1795

Insulin, NPH (Dosage adjustment of the antidiabetic may be required). Products include:

NPH, 100 Units 1450

Pork NPH, 100 Units.............................. 1452

Purified Pork NPH Isophane Insulin 1801

Insulin, Regular (Dosage adjustment of the antidiabetic may be required). Products include:

Regular, 100 Units 1450

Pork Regular, 100 Units 1452

Pork Regular (Concentrated), 500 Units 1453

Purified Pork Regular Insulin 1801

Insulin, Zinc Crystals (Dosage adjustment of the antidiabetic may be required). Products include:

NPH, 100 Units 1450

Insulin, Zinc Suspension (Dosage adjustment of the antidiabetic may be required). Products include:

Iletin I 1450

Lente, 100 Units 1450

Iletin II... 1452

Pork Lente, 100 Units............................ 1452

Purified Pork Lente Insulin 1801

Isradipine (Additive effects). Products include:

DynaCirc Capsules 2256

Ketoprofen (Reduces antihypertensive effects). Products include:

Orudis Capsules 2766

Oruvail Capsules 2766

Ketorolac Tromethamine (Reduces antihypertensive effects). Products include:

Acular 474

Acular .... ◉ 277

Toradol.. 2159

Labetalol Hydrochloride (Additive effects). Products include:

Normodyne Injection 2377

Normodyne Tablets 2379

Trandate 1185

Levobunolol Hydrochloride (Additive effects). Products include:

Betagan .... ◉ 233

Levorphanol Tartrate (Potentiates orthostatic hypotension). Products include:

Levo-Dromoran.. 2129

Lithium Carbonate (Reduced renal clearance of lithium resulting in lithium toxicity). Products include:

Eskalith 2485

Lithium Carbonate Capsules & Tablets 2230

Lithonate/Lithotabs/Lithobid 2543

Lithium Citrate (Reduced renal clearance of lithium resulting in lithium toxicity).

No products indexed under this heading.

Losartan Potassium (Additive effects). Products include:

Cozaar Tablets 1628

Hyzaar Tablets 1677

Mecamylamine Hydrochloride (Additive effects). Products include:

Inversine Tablets 1686

Meclofenamate Sodium (Reduces antihypertensive effects).

No products indexed under this heading.

Mefenamic Acid (Reduces antihypertensive effects). Products include:

Ponstel 1925

Meperidine Hydrochloride (Potentiates orthostatic hypotension). Products include:

Demerol 2308

Mepergan Injection 2753

Mephobarbital (Potentiates orthostatic hypotension). Products include:

Mebaral Tablets 2322

Metformin Hydrochloride (Dosage adjustment of the antidiabetic may be required). Products include:

Glucophage 752

Methadone Hydrochloride (Potentiates orthostatic hypotension). Products include:

Methadone Hydrochloride Oral Concentrate 2233

Methadone Hydrochloride Oral Solution & Tablets................................. 2235

Methyclothiazide (Additive effects). Products include:

Enduron Tablets... 420

Methyldopa (Additive effects). Products include:

Aldoclor Tablets 1598

Aldomet Oral 1600

Aldoril Tablets 1604

Methyldopate Hydrochloride (Additive effects). Products include:

Aldomet Ester HCl Injection 1602

Methylprednisolone Acetate (Intensifies electrolyte depletion). Products include:

Depo-Medrol Single-Dose Vial 2600

Depo-Medrol Sterile Aqueous Suspension... 2597

Methylprednisolone Sodium Succinate (Intensifies electrolyte depletion). Products include:

Solu-Medrol Sterile Powder 2643

Metipranolol Hydrochloride (Additive effects). Products include:

OptiPranolol (Metipranolol 0.3%) Sterile Ophthalmic Solution.......... ◉ 258

Metocurine Iodide (Possible increased responsiveness to the muscle relaxant). Products include:

Metubine Iodide Vials............................. 916

(✪D Described in PDR For Nonprescription Drugs) (◉ Described in PDR For Ophthalmology)

Metolazone (Additive effects). Products include:

Mykrox Tablets 993
Zaroxolyn Tablets 1000

Metoprolol Succinate (Additive effects). Products include:

Toprol-XL Tablets 565

Metoprolol Tartrate (Additive effects). Products include:

Lopressor Ampuls 830
Lopressor HCT Tablets 832
Lopressor Tablets 830

Metyrosine (Additive effects). Products include:

Demser Capsules 1649

Minoxidil (Additive effects). Products include:

Loniten Tablets 2618
Rogaine Topical Solution 2637

Mivacurium Chloride (Possible increased responsiveness to the muscle relaxant). Products include:

Mivacron 1138

Moexipril Hydrochloride (Additive effects). Products include:

Univasc Tablets 2410

Morphine Sulfate (Potentiates orthostatic hypotension). Products include:

Astramorph/PF Injection, USP (Preservative-Free) 535
Duramorph 962
Infumorph 200 and Infumorph 500 Sterile Solutions 965
MS Contin Tablets 1994
MSIR 1997
Oramorph SR (Morphine Sulfate Sustained Release Tablets) 2236
RMS Suppositories 2657
Roxanol 2243

Nabumetone (Reduces antihypertensive effects). Products include:

Relafen Tablets 2510

Nadolol (Additive effects).

No products indexed under this heading.

Naproxen (Reduces antihypertensive effects). Products include:

Anaprox/Naprosyn 2117

Naproxen Sodium (Reduces antihypertensive effects). Products include:

Aleve 1975
Anaprox/Naprosyn 2117

Nicardipine Hydrochloride (Additive effects). Products include:

Cardene Capsules 2095
Cardene I.V. 2709
Cardene SR Capsules 2097

Nifedipine (Additive effects). Products include:

Adalat Capsules (10 mg and 20 mg) 587
Adalat CC 589
Procardia Capsules 1971
Procardia XL Extended Release Tablets 1972

Nisoldipine (Additive effects).

No products indexed under this heading.

Nitroglycerin (Additive effects). Products include:

Deponit NTG Transdermal Delivery System 2397
Nitro-Bid IV 1523
Nitro-Bid Ointment 1524
Nitrodisc 2047
Nitro-Dur (nitroglycerin) Transdermal Infusion System 1326
Nitrolingual Spray 2027
Nitrostat Tablets 1925
Transderm-Nitro Transdermal Therapeutic System 859

Norepinephrine Bitartrate (Possible decreased response to pressor amines). Products include:

Levophed Bitartrate Injection 2315

Opium Alkaloids (Potentiates orthostatic hypotension).

No products indexed under this heading.

Oxaprozin (Reduces antihypertensive effects). Products include:

Daypro Caplets 2426

Oxycodone Hydrochloride (Potentiates orthostatic hypotension). Products include:

Percocet Tablets 938
Percodan Tablets 939
Percodan-Demi Tablets 940
Roxicodone Tablets, Oral Solution & Intensol (Oxycodone) 2244
Tylox Capsules 1584

Pancuronium Bromide Injection (Possible increased responsiveness to the muscle relaxant).

No products indexed under this heading.

Penbutolol Sulfate (Additive effects). Products include:

Levatol 2403

Pentobarbital Sodium (Potentiates orthostatic hypotension). Products include:

Nembutal Sodium Capsules 436
Nembutal Sodium Solution 438
Nembutal Sodium Suppositories 440

Phenobarbital (Potentiates orthostatic hypotension). Products include:

Arco-Lase Plus Tablets 512
Bellergal-S Tablets 2250
Donnatal 2060
Donnatal Extentabs 2061
Donnatal Tablets 2060
Phenobarbital Elixir and Tablets 1469
Quadrinal Tablets 1350

Phenoxybenzamine Hydrochloride (Additive effects). Products include:

Dibenzyline Capsules 2476

Phentolamine Mesylate (Additive effects). Products include:

Regitine 846

Phenylbutazone (Reduces antihypertensive effects).

No products indexed under this heading.

Pindolol (Additive effects). Products include:

Visken Tablets 2299

Piroxicam (Reduces antihypertensive effects). Products include:

Feldene Capsules 1965

Polythiazide (Additive effects). Products include:

Minizide Capsules 1938

Potassium Acid Phosphate (Potential for hyperkalemia). Products include:

K-Phos Original Formula 'Sodium Free' Tablets 639

Potassium Bicarbonate (Potential for hyperkalemia). Products include:

Alka-Seltzer Gold Effervescent Antacid .... ⊕ 703

Potassium Chloride (Potential for hyperkalemia). Products include:

Chlor-3 Condiment 1004
K-Dur Microburst Release System (potassium chloride, USP) E.R. Tablets 1325
K-Lor Powder Packets 434
K-Norm Extended-Release Capsules 991
K-Tab Filmtab 434
Kolyum Liquid 992
Micro-K 2063
Micro-K LS Packets 2064
NuLYTELY 689
Cherry Flavor NuLYTELY 689
Rum-K Syrup 1005
Slow-K Extended-Release Tablets 851

Potassium Citrate (Potential for hyperkalemia). Products include:

Polycitra Syrup 578
Polycitra-K Crystals 579
Polycitra-K Oral Solution 579
Polycitra-LC 578

Potassium Gluconate (Potential for hyperkalemia). Products include:

Kolyum Liquid 992

Potassium Phosphate, Dibasic (Potential for hyperkalemia).

No products indexed under this heading.

Potassium Phosphate, Monobasic (Potential for hyperkalemia). Products include:

K-Phos Neutral Tablets 639
K-Phos Original Formula 'Sodium Free' Tablets 639

Prazosin Hydrochloride (Additive effects). Products include:

Minipress Capsules 1937
Minizide Capsules 1938

Prednisolone Acetate (Intensifies electrolyte depletion). Products include:

AK-CIDE .... ⊙ 202
AK-CIDE Ointment .... ⊙ 202
Blephamide Liquifilm Sterile Ophthalmic Suspension 476
Blephamide Ointment .... ⊙ 237
Econopred & Econopred Plus Ophthalmic Suspensions .... ⊙ 217
Poly-Pred Liquifilm .... ⊙ 248
Pred Forte .... ⊙ 250
Pred Mild .... ⊙ 253
Pred-G Liquifilm Sterile Ophthalmic Suspension .... ⊙ 251
Pred-G S.O.P. Sterile Ophthalmic Ointment .... ⊙ 252
Vasocidin Ointment .... ⊙ 268

Prednisolone Sodium Phosphate (Intensifies electrolyte depletion). Products include:

AK-Pred .... ⊙ 204
Hydeltrasol Injection, Sterile 1665
Inflamase .... ⊙ 265
Pediapred Oral Liquid 995
Vasocidin Ophthalmic Solution .... ⊙ 270

Prednisolone Tebutate (Intensifies electrolyte depletion). Products include:

Hydeltra-T.B.A. Sterile Suspension 1667

Prednisone (Intensifies electrolyte depletion). Products include:

Deltasone Tablets 2595

Propoxyphene Hydrochloride (Potentiates orthostatic hypotension). Products include:

Darvon 1435
Wygesic Tablets 2827

Propoxyphene Napsylate (Potentiates orthostatic hypotension). Products include:

Darvon-N/Darvocet-N 1433

Propranolol Hydrochloride (Additive effects). Products include:

Inderal 2728
Inderal LA Long Acting Capsules 2730
Inderide Tablets 2732
Inderide LA Long Acting Capsules .. 2734

Quinapril Hydrochloride (Additive effects). Products include:

Accupril Tablets 1893

Ramipril (Additive effects). Products include:

Altace Capsules 1232

Rauwolfia Serpentina (Additive effects).

No products indexed under this heading.

Rescinnamine (Additive effects).

No products indexed under this heading.

Reserpine (Additive effects). Products include:

Diupres Tablets 1650
Hydropres Tablets 1675
Ser-Ap-Es Tablets 849

Rocuronium Bromide (Possible increased responsiveness to the muscle relaxant). Products include:

Zemuron 1830

Secobarbital Sodium (Potentiates orthostatic hypotension). Products include:

Seconal Sodium Pulvules 1474

Sodium Nitroprusside (Additive effects).

No products indexed under this heading.

Sotalol Hydrochloride (Additive effects). Products include:

Betapace Tablets 641

Spirapril Hydrochloride (Additive effects).

No products indexed under this heading.

Spironolactone (Additive antihypertensive effects; potential for hyperkalemia). Products include:

Aldactazide 2413
Aldactone 2414

Sufentanil Citrate (Potentiates orthostatic hypotension). Products include:

Sufenta Injection 1309

Sulindac (Reduces antihypertensive effects). Products include:

Clinoril Tablets 1618

Terazosin Hydrochloride (Additive effects). Products include:

Hytrin Capsules 430

Thiamylal Sodium (Potentiates orthostatic hypotension).

No products indexed under this heading.

Timolol Maleate (Additive effects). Products include:

Blocadren Tablets 1614
Timolide Tablets 1748
Timoptic in Ocudose 1753
Timoptic Sterile Ophthalmic Solution 1751
Timoptic-XE 1755

Tolazamide (Dosage adjustment of the antidiabetic may be required).

No products indexed under this heading.

Tolbutamide (Dosage adjustment of the antidiabetic may be required).

No products indexed under this heading.

Tolmetin Sodium (Reduces antihypertensive effects). Products include:

Tolectin (200, 400 and 600 mg) .. 1581

Torsemide (Additive effects). Products include:

Demadex Tablets and Injection 686

Triamcinolone (Intensifies electrolyte depletion). Products include:

Aristocort Tablets 1022

Triamcinolone Acetonide (Intensifies electrolyte depletion). Products include:

Aristocort A 0.025% Cream 1027
Aristocort A 0.5% Cream 1031
Aristocort A 0.1% Cream 1029
Aristocort A 0.1% Ointment 1030
Azmacort Oral Inhaler 2011
Nasacort Nasal Inhaler 2024

Triamcinolone Diacetate (Intensifies electrolyte depletion). Products include:

Aristocort Suspension (Forte Parenteral) 1027
Aristocort Suspension (Intralesional) 1025

Triamcinolone Hexacetonide (Intensifies electrolyte depletion). Products include:

Aristospan Suspension (Intra-articular) 1033
Aristospan Suspension (Intralesional) 1032

Triamterene (Additive antihypertensive effects; potential for hyperkalemia). Products include:

Dyazide 2479
Dyrenium Capsules 2481
Maxzide 1380

Trimethaphan Camsylate (Additive effects). Products include:

Arfonad Ampuls 2080

IMPORTANT NOTE: Always consult each drug listing in the patient's regimen for possible interactions.

Zestoretic Interactions Index 1186

Tubocurarine Chloride (Possible increased responsiveness to the muscle relaxant).
No products indexed under this heading.

Vecuronium Bromide (Possible increased responsiveness to the muscle relaxant). Products include:
Norcuron ... 1826

Verapamil Hydrochloride (Additive effects). Products include:
Calan SR Caplets ... 2422
Calan Tablets ... 2419
Isoptin Injectable ... 1344
Isoptin Oral Tablets ... 1346
Isoptin SR Tablets ... 1348
Verelan Capsules ... 1410
Verelan Capsules ... 2824

Food Interactions

Alcohol (Potentiates orthostatic hypotension).

ZESTRIL TABLETS

(Lisinopril) ... 2854
May interact with diuretics, potassium sparing diuretics, potassium preparations, thiazides, lithium preparations, and certain other agents. Compounds in these categories include:

Amiloride Hydrochloride (Potential for significant hyperkalemia; possibility of excessive reduction in blood pressure). Products include:
Midamor Tablets ... 1703
Moduretic Tablets ... 1705

Bendroflumethiazide (Thiazide-induced potassium loss attenuated; possibility of excessive reduction in blood pressure).
No products indexed under this heading.

Bumetanide (Possibility of excessive reduction in blood pressure). Products include:
Bumex ... 2093

Chlorothiazide (Thiazide-induced potassium loss attenuated; possibility of excessive reduction in blood pressure). Products include:
Aldoclor Tablets ... 1598
Diupres Tablets ... 1650
Diuril Oral ... 1653

Chlorothiazide Sodium (Thiazide-induced potassium loss attenuated; possibility of excessive reduction in blood pressure). Products include:
Diuril Sodium Intravenous ... 1652

Chlorthalidone (Possibility of excessive reduction in blood pressure). Products include:
Combipres Tablets ... 677
Tenoretic Tablets ... 2845
Thalitone ... 1245

Ethacrynic Acid (Possibility of excessive reduction in blood pressure). Products include:
Edecrin Tablets ... 1657

Furosemide (Possibility of excessive reduction in blood pressure). Products include:
Lasix Injection, Oral Solution and Tablets ... 1240

Hydrochlorothiazide (Thiazide-induced potassium loss attenuated; possibility of excessive reduction in blood pressure). Products include:
Aldactazide ... 2413
Aldoril Tablets ... 1604
Apresazide Capsules ... 808
Capozide ... 742
Dyazide ... 2479
Esidrix Tablets ... 821
Esimil Tablets ... 822
HydroDIURIL Tablets ... 1674
Hydropres Tablets ... 1675
Hyzaar Tablets ... 1677
Inderide Tablets ... 2732
Inderide LA Long Acting Capsules ... 2734
Lopressor HCT Tablets ... 832
Lotensin HCT ... 837
Maxzide ... 1380
Moduretic Tablets ... 1705
Oretic Tablets ... 443
Prinzide Tablets ... 1737
Ser-Ap-Es Tablets ... 849
Timolide Tablets ... 1748
Vaseretic Tablets ... 1765
Zestoretic ... 2850
Ziac ... 1415

Hydroflumethiazide (Thiazide-induced potassium loss attenuated; possibility of excessive reduction in blood pressure). Products include:
Diucardin Tablets ... 2718

Indapamide (Possibility of excessive reduction in blood pressure). Products include:
Lozol Tablets ... 2022

Indomethacin (Reduces antihypertensive effect). Products include:
Indocin ... 1680

Indomethacin Sodium Trihydrate (Reduces antihypertensive effect). Products include:
Indocin I.V. ... 1684

Lithium Carbonate (Possibility of lithium toxicity—serum lithium levels should be monitored frequently). Products include:
Eskalith ... 2485
Lithium Carbonate Capsules & Tablets ... 2230
Lithonate/Lithotabs/Lithobid ... 2543

Lithium Citrate (Possibility of lithium toxicity—serum lithium levels should be monitored frequently).
No products indexed under this heading.

Methyclothiazide (Thiazide-induced potassium loss attenuated; possibility of excessive reduction in blood pressure). Products include:
Enduron Tablets ... 420

Metolazone (Possibility of excessive reduction in blood pressure). Products include:
Mykrox Tablets ... 993
Zaroxolyn Tablets ... 1000

Polythiazide (Thiazide-induced potassium loss attenuated; possibility of excessive reduction in blood pressure). Products include:
Minizide Capsules ... 1938

Potassium Acid Phosphate (Potential for significant hyperkalemia). Products include:
K-Phos Original Formula 'Sodium Free' Tablets ... 639

Potassium Bicarbonate (Potential for significant hyperkalemia). Products include:
Alka-Seltzer Gold Effervescent Antacid ... ▣ 703

Potassium Chloride (Potential for significant hyperkalemia). Products include:
Chlor-3 Condiment ... 1004
K-Dur Microburst Release System (potassium chloride, USP) E.R. Tablets ... 1325
K-Lor Powder Packets ... 434
K-Norm Extended-Release Capsules ... 991
K-Tab Filmtab ... 434
Kolyum Liquid ... 992
Micro-K ... 2063
Micro-K LS Packets ... 2064
NuLYTELY ... 689
Cherry Flavor NuLYTELY ... 689
Rum-K Syrup ... 1005
Slow-K Extended-Release Tablets ... 851

Potassium Citrate (Potential for significant hyperkalemia). Products include:
Polycitra Syrup ... 578
Polycitra-K Crystals ... 579
Polycitra-K Oral Solution ... 579
Polycitra-LC ... 578

Potassium Gluconate (Potential for significant hyperkalemia). Products include:
Kolyum Liquid ... 992

Potassium Phosphate, Dibasic (Potential for significant hyperkalemia).
No products indexed under this heading.

Potassium Phosphate, Monobasic (Potential for significant hyperkalemia). Products include:
K-Phos Neutral Tablets ... 639
K-Phos Original Formula 'Sodium Free' Tablets ... 639

Spironolactone (Potential for significant hyperkalemia; possibility of excessive reduction in blood pressure). Products include:
Aldactazide ... 2413
Aldactone ... 2414

Torsemide (Possibility of excessive reduction in blood pressure). Products include:
Demadex Tablets and Injection ... 686

Triamterene (Potential for significant hyperkalemia; possibility of excessive reduction in blood pressure). Products include:
Dyazide ... 2479
Dyrenium Capsules ... 2481
Maxzide ... 1380

ZIAC

(Bisoprolol Fumarate, Hydrochlorothiazide) ... 1415
May interact with insulin, oral hypoglycemic agents, antihypertensives, catecholamine depleting drugs, barbiturates, narcotic analgesics, corticosteroids, nondepolarizing neuromuscular blocking agents, lithium preparations, non-steroidal anti-inflammatory agents, and certain other agents. Compounds in these categories include:

Acarbose (Beta blockers may mask some of the manifestations of hypoglycemia, particularly tachycardia; dosage adjustment of the antidiabetic drug may be required).
No products indexed under this heading.

Acebutolol Hydrochloride (Ziac may potentiate the action of other antihypertensive agents used concomitantly). Products include:
Sectral Capsules ... 2807

ACTH (Intensifies electrolyte depletion, particularly hypokalemia).
No products indexed under this heading.

Alfentanil Hydrochloride (Potentiation of orthostatic hypotension may occur when thiazide diuretics are used with narcotics). Products include:
Alfenta Injection ... 1286

Amlodipine Besylate (Ziac may potentiate the action of other antihypertensive agents used concomitantly). Products include:
Lotrel Capsules ... 840
Norvasc Tablets ... 1940

Aprobarbital (Potentiation of orthostatic hypotension may occur when thiazide diuretics are used with barbiturates).
No products indexed under this heading.

Atenolol (Ziac may potentiate the action of other antihypertensive agents used concomitantly). Products include:
Tenoretic Tablets ... 2845
Tenormin Tablets and I.V. Injection 2847

Atracurium Besylate (Possible increased responsiveness to the muscle relaxant). Products include:
Tracrium Injection ... 1183

Benazepril Hydrochloride (Ziac may potentiate the action of other antihypertensive agents used concomitantly). Products include:
Lotensin Tablets ... 834
Lotensin HCT ... 837
Lotrel Capsules ... 840

Bendroflumethiazide (Ziac may potentiate the action of other antihypertensive agents used concomitantly).
No products indexed under this heading.

Betamethasone Acetate (Intensifies electrolyte depletion, particularly hypokalemia). Products include:
Celestone Soluspan Suspension ... 2347

Betamethasone Sodium Phosphate (Intensifies electrolyte depletion, particularly hypokalemia). Products include:
Celestone Soluspan Suspension ... 2347

Betaxolol Hydrochloride (Ziac may potentiate the action of other antihypertensive agents used concomitantly). Products include:
Betoptic Ophthalmic Solution ... 469
Betoptic S Ophthalmic Suspension ... 471
Kerlone Tablets ... 2436

Buprenorphine (Potentiation of orthostatic hypotension may occur when thiazide diuretics are used with narcotics). Products include:
Buprenex Injectable ... 2006

Butabarbital (Potentiation of orthostatic hypotension may occur when thiazide diuretics are used with barbiturates).
No products indexed under this heading.

Butalbital (Potentiation of orthostatic hypotension may occur when thiazide diuretics are used with barbiturates). Products include:
Esgic-plus Tablets ... 1013
Fioricet Tablets ... 2258
Fioricet with Codeine Capsules ... 2260
Fiorinal Capsules ... 2261
Fiorinal with Codeine Capsules ... 2262
Fiorinal Tablets ... 2261
Phrenilin ... 785
Sedapap Tablets 50 mg/650 mg ... 1543

Captopril (Ziac may potentiate the action of other antihypertensive agents used concomitantly). Products include:
Capoten ... 739
Capozide ... 742

Carteolol Hydrochloride (Ziac may potentiate the action of other antihypertensive agents used concomitantly). Products include:
Cartrol Tablets ... 410
Ocupress Ophthalmic Solution, 1% Sterile ... ◉ 309

Chlorothiazide (Ziac may potentiate the action of other antihypertensive agents used concomitantly). Products include:
Aldoclor Tablets ... 1598
Diupres Tablets ... 1650
Diuril Oral ... 1653

Chlorothiazide Sodium (Ziac may potentiate the action of other antihypertensive agents used concomitantly). Products include:
Diuril Sodium Intravenous ... 1652

Chlorpropamide (Beta blockers may mask some of the manifestations of hypoglycemia, particularly tachycardia; dosage adjustment of the antidiabetic drug may be required). Products include:
Diabinese Tablets ... 1935

(▣ Described in PDR For Nonprescription Drugs) (◉ Described in PDR For Ophthalmology)

Chlorthalidone (Ziac may potentiate the action of other antihypertensive agents used concomitantly). Products include:
- Combipres Tablets 677
- Tenoretic Tablets 2845
- Thalitone 1245

Cholestyramine (Binds the hydrochlorothiazide and reduces its absorption in the GI tract by up to 85%). Products include:
- Questran Light 769
- Questran Powder 770

Clonidine (Ziac may potentiate the action of other antihypertensive agents used concomitantly). Products include:
- Catapres-TTS 675

Clonidine Hydrochloride (Ziac may potentiate the action of other antihypertensive agents used concomitantly). Products include:
- Catapres Tablets 674
- Combipres Tablets 677

Codeine Phosphate (Potentiation of orthostatic hypotension may occur when thiazide diuretics are used with narcotics). Products include:
- Actifed with Codeine Cough Syrup.. 1067
- Brontex 1981
- Deconsal C Expectorant Syrup 456
- Deconsal Pediatric Syrup 457
- Dimetane-DC Cough Syrup 2059
- Empirin with Codeine Tablets 1093
- Fioricet with Codeine Capsules 2260
- Fiorinal with Codeine Capsules 2262
- Isoclor Expectorant 990
- Novahistine DH 2462
- Novahistine Expectorant 2463
- Nucofed 2051
- Phenergan with Codeine 2777
- Phenergan VC with Codeine 2781
- Robitussin A-C Syrup 2073
- Robitussin-DAC Syrup 2074
- Ryna .... ▣ 841
- Soma Compound w/Codeine Tablets 2676
- Tussi-Organidin NR Liquid and S NR Liquid 2677
- Tylenol with Codeine 1583

Colestipol Hydrochloride (Binds the hydrochlorothiazide and reduces its absorption in the GI tract by up to 43%). Products include:
- Colestid Tablets 2591

Cortisone Acetate (Intensifies electrolyte depletion, particularly hypokalemia). Products include:
- Cortone Acetate Sterile Suspension 1623
- Cortone Acetate Tablets 1624

Cyclopropane (Use with caution when administered with anesthetic agent that depresses myocardial function).

Deserpidine (Concomitant use may produce excessive reduction of sympathetic activity).
- No products indexed under this heading.

Dexamethasone (Intensifies electrolyte depletion, particularly hypokalemia). Products include:
- AK-Trol Ointment & Suspension .... ⊙ 205
- Decadron Elixir 1633
- Decadron Tablets 1635
- Decaspray Topical Aerosol 1648
- Dexacidin Ointment .... ⊙ 263
- Maxitrol Ophthalmic Ointment and Suspension .... ⊙ 224
- TobraDex Ophthalmic Suspension and Ointment 473

Dexamethasone Acetate (Intensifies electrolyte depletion, particularly hypokalemia). Products include:
- Dalalone D.P. Injectable 1011
- Decadron-LA Sterile Suspension 1646

Dexamethasone Sodium Phosphate (Intensifies electrolyte depletion, particularly hypokalemia). Products include:
- Decadron Phosphate Injection 1637
- Decadron Phosphate Respihaler 1642
- Decadron Phosphate Sterile Ophthalmic Ointment 1641
- Decadron Phosphate Sterile Ophthalmic Solution 1642
- Decadron Phosphate Topical Cream 1644
- Decadron Phosphate Turbinaire 1645
- Decadron Phosphate with Xylocaine Injection, Sterile 1639
- Dexacort Phosphate in Respihaler .. 458
- Dexacort Phosphate in Turbinaire .. 459
- NeoDecadron Sterile Ophthalmic Ointment 1712
- NeoDecadron Sterile Ophthalmic Solution 1713
- NeoDecadron Topical Cream 1714

Dezocine (Potentiation of orthostatic hypotension may occur when thiazide diuretics are used with narcotics). Products include:
- Dalgan Injection 538

Diazoxide (Ziac may potentiate the action of other antihypertensive agents used concomitantly). Products include:
- Hyperstat I.V. Injection 2363
- Proglycem 580

Diclofenac Potassium (Reduces the diuretic, natriuretic, and antihypertensive effects of thiazides). Products include:
- Cataflam 816

Diclofenac Sodium (Reduces the diuretic, natriuretic, and antihypertensive effects of thiazides). Products include:
- Voltaren Ophthalmic Sterile Ophthalmic Solution .... ⊙ 272
- Voltaren Tablets 861

Diltiazem Hydrochloride (Ziac should be used with caution when myocardial depressants or inhibitors of AV conduction are used concurrently). Products include:
- Cardizem CD Capsules 1506
- Cardizem SR Capsules 1510
- Cardizem Injectable 1508
- Cardizem Tablets 1512
- Dilacor XR Extended-release Capsules 2018

Disopyramide Phosphate (Ziac should be used with caution when myocardial depressants or inhibitors of AV conduction are used concurrently). Products include:
- Norpace 2444

Doxazosin Mesylate (Ziac may potentiate the action of other antihypertensive agents used concomitantly). Products include:
- Cardura Tablets 2186

Enalapril Maleate (Ziac may potentiate the action of other antihypertensive agents used concomitantly). Products include:
- Vaseretic Tablets 1765
- Vasotec Tablets 1771

Enalaprilat (Ziac may potentiate the action of other antihypertensive agents used concomitantly). Products include:
- Vasotec I.V. 1768

Epinephrine Hydrochloride (Patients with history of severe anaphylactic reaction to variety of allergens may be unresponsive to the usual doses of epinephrine used to treat allergic reactions). Products include:
- Ana-Kit Anaphylaxis Emergency Treatment Kit 617

Esmolol Hydrochloride (Ziac may potentiate the action of other antihypertensive agents used concomitantly). Products include:
- Brevibloc Injection 1808

Ether (Use with caution when administered with anesthetic agent that depresses myocardial function).

Etodolac (Reduces the diuretic, natriuretic, and antihypertensive effects of thiazides). Products include:
- Lodine Capsules and Tablets 2743

Felodipine (Ziac may potentiate the action of other antihypertensive agents used concomitantly). Products include:
- Plendil Extended-Release Tablets 527

Fenoprofen Calcium (Reduces the diuretic, natriuretic, and antihypertensive effects of thiazides). Products include:
- Nalfon 200 Pulvules & Nalfon Tablets 917

Fentanyl (Potentiation of orthostatic hypotension may occur when thiazide diuretics are used with narcotics). Products include:
- Duragesic Transdermal System 1288

Fentanyl Citrate (Potentiation of orthostatic hypotension may occur when thiazide diuretics are used with narcotics). Products include:
- Sublimaze Injection 1307

Fludrocortisone Acetate (Intensifies electrolyte depletion, particularly hypokalemia). Products include:
- Florinef Acetate Tablets 505

Flurbiprofen (Reduces the diuretic, natriuretic, and antihypertensive effects of thiazides). Products include:
- Ansaid Tablets 2579

Fosinopril Sodium (Ziac may potentiate the action of other antihypertensive agents used concomitantly). Products include:
- Monopril Tablets 757

Furosemide (Ziac may potentiate the action of other antihypertensive agents used concomitantly). Products include:
- Lasix Injection, Oral Solution and Tablets 1240

Glipizide (Beta blockers may mask some of the manifestations of hypoglycemia, particularly tachycardia; dosage adjustment of the antidiabetic drug may be required). Products include:
- Glucotrol Tablets 1967
- Glucotrol XL Extended Release Tablets 1968

Glyburide (Beta blockers may mask some of the manifestations of hypoglycemia, particularly tachycardia; dosage adjustment of the antidiabetic drug may be required). Products include:
- DiaBeta Tablets 1239
- Glynase PresTab Tablets 2609
- Micronase Tablets 2623

Guanabenz Acetate (Ziac may potentiate the action of other antihypertensive agents used concomitantly).
- No products indexed under this heading.

Guanethidine Monosulfate (Concomitant use may produce excessive reduction of sympathetic activity). Products include:
- Esimil Tablets 822
- Ismelin Tablets 827

Hydralazine Hydrochloride (Ziac may potentiate the action of other antihypertensive agents used concomitantly). Products include:
- Apresazide Capsules 808
- Apresoline Hydrochloride Tablets .. 809
- Ser-Ap-Es Tablets 849

Hydrocodone Bitartrate (Potentiation of orthostatic hypotension may occur when thiazide diuretics are used with narcotics). Products include:
- Anexsia 5/500 Elixir 1781
- Anexia Tablets 1782
- Codiclear DH Syrup 791
- Deconamine CX Cough and Cold Liquid and Tablets 1319
- Duratuss HD Elixir 2565
- Hycodan Tablets and Syrup 930
- Hycomine Compound Tablets 932
- Hycomine 931
- Hycotuss Expectorant Syrup 933
- Hydrocet Capsules 782
- Lorcet 10/650 1018
- Lortab 2566
- Tussend 1783
- Tussend Expectorant 1785
- Vicodin Tablets 1356
- Vicodin ES Tablets 1357
- Vicodin Tuss Expectorant 1358
- Zydone Capsules 949

Hydrocodone Polistirex (Potentiation of orthostatic hypotension may occur when thiazide diuretics are used with narcotics). Products include:
- Tussionex Pennkinetic Extended-Release Suspension 998

Hydrocortisone (Intensifies electrolyte depletion, particularly hypokalemia). Products include:
- Anusol-HC Cream 2.5% 1896
- Aquanil HC Lotion 1931
- Bactine Hydrocortisone Anti-Itch Cream .... ▣ 709
- Caldecort Anti-Itch Hydrocortisone Spray .... ▣ 631
- Cortaid .... ▣ 836
- CORTENEMA 2535
- Cortisporin Ointment 1085
- Cortisporin Ophthalmic Ointment Sterile 1085
- Cortisporin Ophthalmic Suspension Sterile 1086
- Cortisporin Otic Solution Sterile 1087
- Cortisporin Otic Suspension Sterile 1088
- Cortizone-5 .... ▣ 831
- Cortizone-10 .... ▣ 831
- Hydrocortone Tablets 1672
- Hytone 907
- Massengill Medicated Soft Cloth Towelettes 2458
- PediOtic Suspension Sterile 1153
- Preparation H Hydrocortisone 1% Cream .... ▣ 872
- ProctoCream-HC 2.5% 2408
- VōSoL HC Otic Solution 2678

Hydrocortisone Acetate (Intensifies electrolyte depletion, particularly hypokalemia). Products include:
- Analpram-HC Rectal Cream 1% and 2.5% 977
- Anusol HC-1 Anti-Itch Hydrocortisone Ointment .... ▣ 847
- Anusol-HC Suppositories 1897
- Caldecort .... ▣ 631
- Carmol HC 924
- Coly-Mycin S Otic w/Neomycin & Hydrocortisone 1906
- Cortaid .... ▣ 836
- Cortifoam 2396
- Cortisporin Cream 1084
- Epifoam 2399
- Hydrocortone Acetate Sterile Suspension 1669
- Mantadil Cream 1135
- Nupercainal Hydrocortisone 1% Cream .... ▣ 645
- Ophthocort .... ⊙ 311
- Pramosone Cream, Lotion & Ointment 978
- ProctoCream-HC 2408
- ProctoFoam-HC 2409
- Terra-Cortril Ophthalmic Suspension 2210

Hydrocortisone Sodium Phosphate (Intensifies electrolyte depletion, particularly hypokalemia). Products include:
- Hydrocortone Phosphate Injection, Sterile 1670

IMPORTANT NOTE: Always consult each drug listing in the patient's regimen for possible interactions.

Ziac | Interactions Index | 1188

Hydrocortisone Sodium Succinate (Intensifies electrolyte depletion, particularly hypokalemia). Products include:
Solu-Cortef Sterile Powder 2641

Hydroflumethiazide (Ziac may potentiate the action of other antihypertensive agents used concomitantly). Products include:
Diucardin Tablets 2718

Ibuprofen (Reduces the diuretic, natriuretic, and antihypertensive effects of thiazides). Products include:
Advil Cold and Sinus Caplets and Tablets (formerly CoAdvil) .... ▣ 870
Advil Ibuprofen Tablets and Caplets .... ▣ 870
Children's Advil Suspension 2692
Arthritis Foundation Ibuprofen Tablets .... ▣ 674
Bayer Select Ibuprofen Pain Relief Formula .... ▣ 715
Cramp End Tablets .... ▣ 735
Dimetapp Sinus Caplets .... ▣ 775
Haltran Tablets .... ▣ 771
IBU Tablets 1342
Ibuprohm .... ▣ 735
Children's Motrin Ibuprofen Oral Suspension 1546
Motrin Tablets 2625
Motrin IB Caplets, Tablets, and Geltabs .... ▣ 838
Motrin IB Sinus .... ▣ 838
Motrin Ibuprofen Suspension, Oral Drops, Chewable Tablets, Caplets 1546
Nuprin Ibuprofen/Analgesic Tablets & Caplets .... ▣ 622
Sine-Aid IB Caplets 1554
Vicks DayQuil SINUS Pressure & PAIN Relief with IBUPROFEN .... ▣ 762

Indapamide (Ziac may potentiate the action of other antihypertensive agents used concomitantly). Products include:
Lozol Tablets 2022

Indomethacin (Reduces the diuretic, natriuretic, and antihypertensive effects of thiazides). Products include:
Indocin 1680

Indomethacin Sodium Trihydrate (Reduces the diuretic, natriuretic, and antihypertensive effects of thiazides). Products include:
Indocin I.V. 1684

Insulin, Human (Beta blockers may mask some of the manifestations of hypoglycemia, particularly tachycardia; dosage adjustment of the antidiabetic drug may be required).
No products indexed under this heading.

Insulin, Human Isophane Suspension (Beta blockers may mask some of the manifestations of hypoglycemia, particularly tachycardia; dosage adjustment of the antidiabetic drug may be required). Products include:
Novolin N Human Insulin 10 ml Vials 1795

Insulin, Human NPH (Beta blockers may mask some of the manifestations of hypoglycemia, particularly tachycardia; dosage adjustment of the antidiabetic drug may be required). Products include:
Humulin N, 100 Units 1448
Novolin N PenFill Cartridges Durable Insulin Delivery System 1798
Novolin N Prefilled Syringe Disposable Insulin Delivery System 1798

Insulin, Human Regular (Beta blockers may mask some of the manifestations of hypoglycemia, particularly tachycardia; dosage adjustment of the antidiabetic drug may be required). Products include:
Humulin R, 100 Units 1449
Novolin R Human Insulin 10 ml Vials 1795
Novolin R PenFill Cartridges Durable Insulin Delivery System 1798
Novolin R Prefilled Syringe Disposable Insulin Delivery System 1798
Velosulin BR Human Insulin 10 ml Vials 1795

Insulin, Human, Zinc Suspension (Beta blockers may mask some of the manifestations of hypoglycemia, particularly tachycardia; dosage adjustment of the antidiabetic drug may be required). Products include:
Humulin L, 100 Units 1446
Humulin U, 100 Units 1450
Novolin L Human Insulin 10 ml Vials 1795

Insulin, NPH (Beta blockers may mask some of the manifestations of hypoglycemia, particularly tachycardia; dosage adjustment of the antidiabetic drug may be required). Products include:
NPH, 100 Units 1450
Pork NPH, 100 Units 1452
Purified Pork NPH Isophane Insulin 1801

Insulin, Regular (Beta blockers may mask some of the manifestations of hypoglycemia, particularly tachycardia; dosage adjustment of the antidiabetic drug may be required). Products include:
Regular, 100 Units 1450
Pork Regular, 100 Units 1452
Pork Regular (Concentrated), 500 Units 1453
Purified Pork Regular Insulin 1801

Insulin, Zinc Crystals (Beta blockers may mask some of the manifestations of hypoglycemia, particularly tachycardia; dosage adjustment of the antidiabetic drug may be required). Products include:
NPH, 100 Units 1450

Insulin, Zinc Suspension (Beta blockers may mask some of the manifestations of hypoglycemia, particularly tachycardia; dosage adjustment of the antidiabetic drug may be required). Products include:
Iletin I 1450
Lente, 100 Units 1450
Iletin II 1452
Pork Lente, 100 Units 1452
Purified Pork Lente Insulin 1801

Isradipine (Ziac may potentiate the action of other antihypertensive agents used concomitantly). Products include:
DynaCirc Capsules 2256

Ketoprofen (Reduces the diuretic, natriuretic, and antihypertensive effects of thiazides). Products include:
Orudis Capsules 2766
Oruvail Capsules 2766

Ketorolac Tromethamine (Reduces the diuretic, natriuretic, and antihypertensive effects of thiazides). Products include:
Acular 474
Acular .... ⊙ 277
Toradol 2159

Labetalol Hydrochloride (Ziac may potentiate the action of other antihypertensive agents used concomitantly). Products include:
Normodyne Injection 2377
Normodyne Tablets 2379
Trandate 1185

Levorphanol Tartrate (Potentiation of orthostatic hypotension may occur when thiazide diuretics are used with narcotics). Products include:
Levo-Dromoran 2129

Lisinopril (Ziac may potentiate the action of other antihypertensive agents used concomitantly). Products include:
Prinivil Tablets 1733
Prinzide Tablets 1737
Zestoretic 2850
Zestril Tablets 2854

Lithium Carbonate (Reduced renal clearance of lithium and increased risk of lithium toxicity). Products include:
Eskalith 2485
Lithium Carbonate Capsules & Tablets 2230
Lithonate/Lithotabs/Lithobid 2543

Lithium Citrate (Reduced renal clearance of lithium and increased risk of lithium toxicity).
No products indexed under this heading.

Losartan Potassium (Ziac may potentiate the action of other antihypertensive agents used concomitantly). Products include:
Cozaar Tablets 1628
Hyzaar Tablets 1677

Mecamylamine Hydrochloride (Ziac may potentiate the action of other antihypertensive agents used concomitantly). Products include:
Inversine Tablets 1686

Meclofenamate Sodium (Reduces the diuretic, natriuretic, and antihypertensive effects of thiazides).
No products indexed under this heading.

Mefenamic Acid (Reduces the diuretic, natriuretic, and antihypertensive effects of thiazides). Products include:
Ponstel 1925

Meperidine Hydrochloride (Potentiation of orthostatic hypotension may occur when thiazide diuretics are used with narcotics). Products include:
Demerol 2308
Mepergan Injection 2753

Mephobarbital (Potentiation of orthostatic hypotension may occur when thiazide diuretics are used with barbiturates). Products include:
Mebaral Tablets 2322

Metformin Hydrochloride (Beta blockers may mask some of the manifestations of hypoglycemia, particularly tachycardia; dosage adjustment of the antidiabetic drug may be required). Products include:
Glucophage 752

Methadone Hydrochloride (Potentiation of orthostatic hypotension may occur when thiazide diuretics are used with narcotics). Products include:
Methadone Hydrochloride Oral Concentrate 2233
Methadone Hydrochloride Oral Solution & Tablets 2235

Methyclothiazide (Ziac may potentiate the action of other antihypertensive agents used concomitantly). Products include:
Enduron Tablets 420

Methyldopa (Ziac may potentiate the action of other antihypertensive agents used concomitantly). Products include:
Aldoclor Tablets 1598
Aldomet Oral 1600
Aldoril Tablets 1604

Methyldopate Hydrochloride (Ziac may potentiate the action of other antihypertensive agents used concomitantly). Products include:
Aldomet Ester HCl Injection 1602

Methylprednisolone Acetate (Intensifies electrolyte depletion, particularly hypokalemia). Products include:
Depo-Medrol Single-Dose Vial 2600
Depo-Medrol Sterile Aqueous Suspension 2597

Methylprednisolone Sodium Succinate (Intensifies electrolyte depletion, particularly hypokalemia). Products include:
Solu-Medrol Sterile Powder 2643

Metocurine Iodide (Possible increased responsiveness to the muscle relaxant). Products include:
Metubine Iodide Vials 916

Metolazone (Ziac may potentiate the action of other antihypertensive agents used concomitantly). Products include:
Mykrox Tablets 993
Zaroxolyn Tablets 1000

Metoprolol Succinate (Ziac may potentiate the action of other antihypertensive agents used concomitantly). Products include:
Toprol-XL Tablets 565

Metoprolol Tartrate (Ziac may potentiate the action of other antihypertensive agents used concomitantly). Products include:
Lopressor Ampuls 830
Lopressor HCT Tablets 832
Lopressor Tablets 830

Metyrosine (Ziac may potentiate the action of other antihypertensive agents used concomitantly). Products include:
Demser Capsules 1649

Minoxidil (Ziac may potentiate the action of other antihypertensive agents used concomitantly). Products include:
Loniten Tablets 2618
Rogaine Topical Solution 2637

Mivacurium Chloride (Possible increased responsiveness to the muscle relaxant). Products include:
Mivacron 1138

Moexipril Hydrochloride (Ziac may potentiate the action of other antihypertensive agents used concomitantly). Products include:
Univasc Tablets 2410

Morphine Sulfate (Potentiation of orthostatic hypotension may occur when thiazide diuretics are used with narcotics). Products include:
Astramorph/PF Injection, USP (Preservative-Free) 535
Duramorph 962
Infumorph 200 and Infumorph 500 Sterile Solutions 965
MS Contin Tablets 1994
MSIR 1997
Oramorph SR (Morphine Sulfate Sustained Release Tablets) 2236
RMS Suppositories 2657
Roxanol 2243

Nabumetone (Reduces the diuretic, natriuretic, and antihypertensive effects of thiazides). Products include:
Relafen Tablets 2510

Nadolol (Ziac may potentiate the action of other antihypertensive agents used concomitantly).
No products indexed under this heading.

Naproxen (Reduces the diuretic, natriuretic, and antihypertensive effects of thiazides). Products include:
Anaprox/Naprosyn 2117

Naproxen Sodium (Reduces the diuretic, natriuretic, and antihypertensive effects of thiazides). Products include:
Aleve 1975

(▣ Described in PDR For Nonprescription Drugs) (⊙ Described in PDR For Ophthalmology)

1189 **Interactions Index** **Ziac**

Anaprox/Naprosyn 2117

Nicardipine Hydrochloride (Ziac may potentiate the action of other antihypertensive agents used concomitantly). Products include:

Cardene Capsules 2095
Cardene I.V. 2709
Cardene SR Capsules 2097

Nifedipine (Ziac may potentiate the action of other antihypertensive agents used concomitantly). Products include:

Adalat Capsules (10 mg and 20 mg) 587
Adalat CC 589
Procardia Capsules 1971
Procardia XL Extended Release Tablets 1972

Nisoldipine (Ziac may potentiate the action of other antihypertensive agents used concomitantly).

No products indexed under this heading.

Nitroglycerin (Ziac may potentiate the action of other antihypertensive agents used concomitantly). Products include:

Deponit NTG Transdermal Delivery System 2397
Nitro-Bid IV 1523
Nitro-Bid Ointment 1524
Nitrodisc 2047
Nitro-Dur (nitroglycerin) Transdermal Infusion System 1326
Nitrolingual Spray 2027
Nitrostat Tablets 1925
Transderm-Nitro Transdermal Therapeutic System 859

Norepinephrine Bitartrate (Possible decreased response to pressor amines). Products include:

Levophed Bitartrate Injection 2315

Norepinephrine Hydrochloride (Possible decreased response to pressor amines).

Opium Alkaloids (Potentiation of orthostatic hypotension may occur when thiazide diuretics are used with narcotics).

No products indexed under this heading.

Oxaprozin (Reduces the diuretic, natriuretic, and antihypertensive effects of thiazides). Products include:

Daypro Caplets 2426

Oxycodone Hydrochloride (Potentiation of orthostatic hypotension may occur when thiazide diuretics are used with narcotics). Products include:

Percocet Tablets 938
Percodan Tablets 939
Percodan-Demi Tablets 940
Roxicodone Tablets, Oral Solution & Intensol (Oxycodone) 2244
Tylox Capsules 1584

Pancuronium Bromide Injection (Possible increased responsiveness to the muscle relaxant).

No products indexed under this heading.

Penbutolol Sulfate (Ziac may potentiate the action of other antihypertensive agents used concomitantly). Products include:

Levatol 2403

Pentobarbital Sodium (Potentiation of orthostatic hypotension may occur when thiazide diuretics are used with barbiturates). Products include:

Nembutal Sodium Capsules 436
Nembutal Sodium Solution 438
Nembutal Sodium Suppositories 440

Phenobarbital (Potentiation of orthostatic hypotension may occur when thiazide diuretics are used with barbiturates). Products include:

Arco-Lase Plus Tablets 512
Bellergal-S Tablets 2250
Donnatal 2060
Donnatal Extentabs 2061
Donnatal Tablets 2060
Phenobarbital Elixir and Tablets 1469
Quadrinal Tablets 1350

Phenoxybenzamine Hydrochloride (Ziac may potentiate the action of other antihypertensive agents used concomitantly). Products include:

Dibenzyline Capsules 2476

Phentolamine Mesylate (Ziac may potentiate the action of other antihypertensive agents used concomitantly). Products include:

Regitine 846

Phenylbutazone (Reduces the diuretic, natriuretic, and antihypertensive effects of thiazides).

No products indexed under this heading.

Pindolol (Ziac may potentiate the action of other antihypertensive agents used concomitantly). Products include:

Visken Tablets 2299

Piroxicam (Reduces the diuretic, natriuretic, and antihypertensive effects of thiazides). Products include:

Feldene Capsules 1965

Polythiazide (Ziac may potentiate the action of other antihypertensive agents used concomitantly). Products include:

Minizide Capsules 1938

Prazosin Hydrochloride (Ziac may potentiate the action of other antihypertensive agents used concomitantly). Products include:

Minipress Capsules 1937
Minizide Capsules 1938

Prednisolone Acetate (Intensifies electrolyte depletion, particularly hypokalemia). Products include:

AK-CIDE ..... ⊙ 202
AK-CIDE Ointment ..... ⊙ 202
Blephamide Liquifilm Sterile Ophthalmic Suspension 476
Blephamide Ointment ..... ⊙ 237
Econopred & Econopred Plus Ophthalmic Suspensions ..... ⊙ 217
Poly-Pred Liquifilm ..... ⊙ 248
Pred Forte ..... ⊙ 250
Pred Mild ..... ⊙ 253
Pred-G Liquifilm Sterile Ophthalmic Suspension ..... ⊙ 251
Pred-G S.O.P. Sterile Ophthalmic Ointment ..... ⊙ 252
Vasocidin Ointment ..... ⊙ 268

Prednisolone Sodium Phosphate (Intensifies electrolyte depletion, particularly hypokalemia). Products include:

AK-Pred ..... ⊙ 204
Hydeltrasol Injection, Sterile 1665
Inflamase ..... ⊙ 265
Pediapred Oral Liquid 995
Vasocidin Ophthalmic Solution ..... ⊙ 270

Prednisolone Tebutate (Intensifies electrolyte depletion, particularly hypokalemia). Products include:

Hydeltra-T.B.A. Sterile Suspension 1667

Prednisone (Intensifies electrolyte depletion, particularly hypokalemia). Products include:

Deltasone Tablets 2595

Propoxyphene Hydrochloride (Potentiation of orthostatic hypotension may occur when thiazide diuretics are used with narcotics). Products include:

Darvon 1435
Wygesic Tablets 2827

Propoxyphene Napsylate (Potentiation of orthostatic hypotension may occur when thiazide diuretics are used with narcotics). Products include:

Darvon-N/Darvocet-N 1433

Propranolol Hydrochloride (Ziac may potentiate the action of other antihypertensive agents used concomitantly). Products include:

Inderal 2728
Inderal LA Long Acting Capsules 2730
Inderide Tablets 2732
Inderide LA Long Acting Capsules 2734

Quinapril Hydrochloride (Ziac may potentiate the action of other antihypertensive agents used concomitantly). Products include:

Accupril Tablets 1893

Ramipril (Ziac may potentiate the action of other antihypertensive agents used concomitantly). Products include:

Altace Capsules 1232

Rauwolfia Serpentina (Concomitant use may produce excessive reduction of sympathetic activity).

No products indexed under this heading.

Rescinnamine (Concomitant use may produce excessive reduction of sympathetic activity).

No products indexed under this heading.

Reserpine (Concomitant use may produce excessive reduction of sympathetic activity). Products include:

Diupres Tablets 1650
Hydropres Tablets 1675
Ser-Ap-Es Tablets 849

Rifampin (Increases the metabolic clearance of bisoprolol fumarate and shortening its elimination half-life). Products include:

Rifadin 1528
Rifamate Capsules 1530
Rifater 1532
Rimactane Capsules 847

Rocuronium Bromide (Possible increased responsiveness to the muscle relaxant). Products include:

Zemuron 1830

Secobarbital Sodium (Potentiation of orthostatic hypotension may occur when thiazide diuretics are used with barbiturates). Products include:

Seconal Sodium Pulvules 1474

Sodium Nitroprusside (Ziac may potentiate the action of other antihypertensive agents used concomitantly).

No products indexed under this heading.

Sotalol Hydrochloride (Ziac may potentiate the action of other antihypertensive agents used concomitantly). Products include:

Betapace Tablets 641

Spirapril Hydrochloride (Ziac may potentiate the action of other antihypertensive agents used concomitantly).

No products indexed under this heading.

Sufentanil Citrate (Potentiation of orthostatic hypotension may occur when thiazide diuretics are used with narcotics). Products include:

Sufenta Injection 1309

Sulindac (Reduces the diuretic, natriuretic, and antihypertensive effects of thiazides). Products include:

Clinoril Tablets 1618

Terazosin Hydrochloride (Ziac may potentiate the action of other antihypertensive agents used concomitantly). Products include:

Hytrin Capsules 430

Thiamylal Sodium (Potentiation of orthostatic hypotension may occur when thiazide diuretics are used with barbiturates).

No products indexed under this heading.

Timolol Maleate (Ziac may potentiate the action of other antihypertensive agents used concomitantly). Products include:

Blocadren Tablets 1614
Timolide Tablets 1748
Timoptic in Ocudose 1753
Timoptic Sterile Ophthalmic Solution 1751
Timoptic-XE 1755

Tolazamide (Beta blockers may mask some of the manifestations of hypoglycemia, particularly tachycardia; dosage adjustment of the antidiabetic drug may be required).

No products indexed under this heading.

Tolbutamide (Beta blockers may mask some of the manifestations of hypoglycemia, particularly tachycardia; dosage adjustment of the antidiabetic drug may be required).

No products indexed under this heading.

Tolmetin Sodium (Reduces the diuretic, natriuretic, and antihypertensive effects of thiazides). Products include:

Tolectin (200, 400 and 600 mg) 1581

Torsemide (Ziac may potentiate the action of other antihypertensive agents used concomitantly). Products include:

Demadex Tablets and Injection 686

Triamcinolone (Intensifies electrolyte depletion, particularly hypokalemia). Products include:

Aristocort Tablets 1022

Triamcinolone Acetonide (Intensifies electrolyte depletion, particularly hypokalemia). Products include:

Aristocort A 0.025% Cream 1027
Aristocort A 0.5% Cream 1031
Aristocort A 0.1% Cream 1029
Aristocort A 0.1% Ointment 1030
Azmacort Oral Inhaler 2011
Nasacort Nasal Inhaler 2024

Triamcinolone Diacetate (Intensifies electrolyte depletion, particularly hypokalemia). Products include:

Aristocort Suspension (Forte Parenteral) 1027
Aristocort Suspension (Intralesional) 1025

Triamcinolone Hexacetonide (Intensifies electrolyte depletion, particularly hypokalemia). Products include:

Aristospan Suspension (Intra-articular) 1033
Aristospan Suspension (Intralesional) 1032

Trichloroethylene (Use with caution when administered with anesthetic agent that depresses myocardial function).

No products indexed under this heading.

Trimethaphan Camsylate (Ziac may potentiate the action of other antihypertensive agents used concomitantly). Products include:

Arfonad Ampuls 2080

Tubocurarine Chloride (Possible increased responsiveness to the muscle relaxant).

No products indexed under this heading.

Vecuronium Bromide (Possible increased responsiveness to the muscle relaxant). Products include:

Norcuron 1826

IMPORTANT NOTE: Always consult each drug listing in the patient's regimen for possible interactions.

Verapamil Hydrochloride (Ziac should be used with caution when myocardial depressants or inhibitors of AV conduction are used concurrently). Products include:

Calan SR Caplets ... 2422
Calan Tablets ... 2419
Isoptin Injectable ... 1344
Isoptin Oral Tablets ... 1346
Isoptin SR Tablets ... 1348
Verelan Capsules ... 1410
Verelan Capsules ... 2824

Food Interactions

Alcohol (Potentiation of orthostatic hypotension may occur when thiazide diuretics are used with alcohol).

ZILACTIN MEDICATED GEL
(Benzyl Alcohol) ... ■ 882
None cited in PDR database.

ZILACTIN-B MEDICATED GEL WITH BENZOCAINE
(Benzocaine) ... ■ 882
None cited in PDR database.

ZILACTIN-L LIQUID
(Lidocaine) ... ■ 882
None cited in PDR database.

ZINACEF
(Cefuroxime Sodium) ... 1211
May interact with aminoglycosides and certain other agents. Compounds in these categories include:

Amikacin Sulfate (Concomitant administration may produce nephrotoxicity). Products include:

Amikacin Sulfate Injection, USP ... 960
Amikin Injectable ... 501

Gentamicin Sulfate (Concomitant administration may produce nephrotoxicity). Products include:

Garamycin Injectable ... 2360
Genoptic Sterile Ophthalmic Solution ... ⊙ 243
Genoptic Sterile Ophthalmic Ointment ... ⊙ 243
Gentacidin Ointment ... ⊙ 264
Gentacidin Solution ... ⊙ 264
Gentak ... ⊙ 208
Pred-G Liquifilm Sterile Ophthalmic Suspension ... ⊙ 251
Pred-G S.O.P. Sterile Ophthalmic Ointment ... ⊙ 252

Kanamycin Sulfate (Concomitant administration may produce nephrotoxicity).

No products indexed under this heading.

Probenecid (Concurrent administration of probenecid decreases renal clearance and increases peak serum levels of cefuroxime). Products include:

Benemid Tablets ... 1611
ColBENEMID Tablets ... 1622

Streptomycin Sulfate (Concomitant administration may produce nephrotoxicity). Products include:

Streptomycin Sulfate Injection ... 2208

Tobramycin Sulfate (Concomitant administration may produce nephrotoxicity). Products include:

Nebcin Vials, Hyporets & ADD-Vantage ... 1464
Tobramycin Sulfate Injection ... 968

ZINCON DANDRUFF SHAMPOO
(Pyrithione Zinc) ... ■ 671
None cited in PDR database.

ZINECARD
(Dexrazoxane) ... 1961
May interact with antineoplastics and certain other agents. Compounds in these categories include:

Altretamine (Dexrazoxane may add to the myelosuppression caused by chemotherapeutic agents). Products include:

Hexalen Capsules ... 2571

Asparaginase (Dexrazoxane may add to the myelosuppression caused by chemotherapeutic agents). Products include:

Elspar ... 1659

Bleomycin Sulfate (Dexrazoxane may add to the myelosuppression caused by chemotherapeutic agents). Products include:

Blenoxane ... 692

Busulfan (Dexrazoxane may add to the myelosuppression caused by chemotherapeutic agents). Products include:

Myleran Tablets ... 1143

Carboplatin (Dexrazoxane may add to the myelosuppression caused by chemotherapeutic agents). Products include:

Paraplatin for Injection ... 705

Carmustine (BCNU) (Dexrazoxane may add to the myelosuppression caused by chemotherapeutic agents). Products include:

BiCNU ... 691

Chlorambucil (Dexrazoxane may add to the myelosuppression caused by chemotherapeutic agents). Products include:

Leukeran Tablets ... 1133

Cisplatin (Dexrazoxane may add to the myelosuppression caused by chemotherapeutic agents). Products include:

Platinol ... 708
Platinol-AQ Injection ... 710

Cyclophosphamide (Use of dexrazoxane concurrently with the initiation of fluorouracil, doxorubicin and cyclophosphamide (FAC) therapy may interfere with the antitumor efficacy of the regimen). Products include:

Cytoxan ... 694
NEOSAR Lyophilized/Neosar ... 1959

Dacarbazine (Dexrazoxane may add to the myelosuppression caused by chemotherapeutic agents). Products include:

DTIC-Dome ... 600

Daunorubicin Hydrochloride (Dexrazoxane may add to the myelosuppression caused by chemotherapeutic agents). Products include:

Cerubidine ... 795

Doxorubicin Hydrochloride (Use of dexrazoxane concurrently with the initiation of fluorouracil, doxorubicin and cyclophosphamide (FAC) therapy may interfere with the antitumor efficacy of the regimen). Products include:

Adriamycin PFS ... 1947
Adriamycin RDF ... 1947
Doxorubicin Astra ... 540
Rubex ... 712

Estramustine Phosphate Sodium (Dexrazoxane may add to the myelosuppression caused by chemotherapeutic agents). Products include:

Emcyt Capsules ... 1953

Etoposide (Dexrazoxane may add to the myelosuppression caused by chemotherapeutic agents). Products include:

VePesid Capsules and Injection ... 718

Floxuridine (Dexrazoxane may add to the myelosuppression caused by chemotherapeutic agents). Products include:

Sterile FUDR ... 2118

Fluorouracil (Use of dexrazoxane concurrently with the initiation of fluorouracil, doxorubicin and cyclophosphamide (FAC) therapy may interfere with the antitumor efficacy of the regimen). Products include:

Efudex ... 2113
Fluoroplex Topical Solution & Cream 1% ... 479
Fluorouracil Injection ... 2116

Flutamide (Dexrazoxane may add to the myelosuppression caused by chemotherapeutic agents). Products include:

Eulexin Capsules ... 2358

Hydroxyurea (Dexrazoxane may add to the myelosuppression caused by chemotherapeutic agents). Products include:

Hydrea Capsules ... 696

Idarubicin Hydrochloride (Dexrazoxane may add to the myelosuppression caused by chemotherapeutic agents). Products include:

Idamycin ... 1955

Ifosfamide (Dexrazoxane may add to the myelosuppression caused by chemotherapeutic agents). Products include:

IFEX ... 697

Interferon alfa-2A, Recombinant (Dexrazoxane may add to the myelosuppression caused by chemotherapeutic agents). Products include:

Roferon-A Injection ... 2145

Interferon alfa-2B, Recombinant (Dexrazoxane may add to the myelosuppression caused by chemotherapeutic agents). Products include:

Intron A ... 2364

Levamisole Hydrochloride (Dexrazoxane may add to the myelosuppression caused by chemotherapeutic agents). Products include:

Ergamisol Tablets ... 1292

Lomustine (CCNU) (Dexrazoxane may add to the myelosuppression caused by chemotherapeutic agents). Products include:

CeeNU ... 693

Mechlorethamine Hydrochloride (Dexrazoxane may add to the myelosuppression caused by chemotherapeutic agents). Products include:

Mustargen ... 1709

Megestrol Acetate (Dexrazoxane may add to the myelosuppression caused by chemotherapeutic agents). Products include:

Megace Oral Suspension ... 699
Megace Tablets ... 701

Melphalan (Dexrazoxane may add to the myelosuppression caused by chemotherapeutic agents). Products include:

Alkeran Tablets ... 1071

Mercaptopurine (Dexrazoxane may add to the myelosuppression caused by chemotherapeutic agents). Products include:

Purinethol Tablets ... 1156

Methotrexate Sodium (Dexrazoxane may add to the myelosuppression caused by chemotherapeutic agents). Products include:

Methotrexate Sodium Tablets, Injection, for Injection and LPF Injection ... 1275

Mitomycin (Mitomycin-C) (Dexrazoxane may add to the myelosuppression caused by chemotherapeutic agents). Products include:

Mutamycin ... 703

Mitotane (Dexrazoxane may add to the myelosuppression caused by chemotherapeutic agents). Products include:

Lysodren ... 698

Mitoxantrone Hydrochloride (Dexrazoxane may add to the myelosuppression caused by chemotherapeutic agents). Products include:

Novantrone ... 1279

Paclitaxel (Dexrazoxane may add to the myelosuppression caused by chemotherapeutic agents). Products include:

Taxol ... 714

Procarbazine Hydrochloride (Dexrazoxane may add to the myelosuppression caused by chemotherapeutic agents). Products include:

Matulane Capsules ... 2131

Streptozocin (Dexrazoxane may add to the myelosuppression caused by chemotherapeutic agents). Products include:

Zanosar Sterile Powder ... 2653

Tamoxifen Citrate (Dexrazoxane may add to the myelosuppression caused by chemotherapeutic agents). Products include:

Nolvadex Tablets ... 2841

Teniposide (Dexrazoxane may add to the myelosuppression caused by chemotherapeutic agents). Products include:

Vumon ... 727

Thioguanine (Dexrazoxane may add to the myelosuppression caused by chemotherapeutic agents). Products include:

Thioguanine Tablets, Tabloid Brand ... 1181

Thiotepa (Dexrazoxane may add to the myelosuppression caused by chemotherapeutic agents). Products include:

Thioplex (Thiotepa For Injection) ... 1281

Vincristine Sulfate (Dexrazoxane may add to the myelosuppression caused by chemotherapeutic agents). Products include:

Oncovin Solution Vials & Hyporets 1466

Vinorelbine Tartrate (Dexrazoxane may add to the myelosuppression caused by chemotherapeutic agents). Products include:

Navelbine Injection ... 1145

ZITHROMAX CAPSULES
(Azithromycin) ... 1944
May interact with antacids containing aluminium, calcium and magnesium, xanthine bronchodilators, oral anticoagulants, and certain other agents. Compounds in these categories include:

Aluminum Carbonate Gel (Reduces the peak serum levels but not the AUC). Products include:

Basaljel ... 2703

Aluminum Hydroxide (Reduces the peak serum levels but not the AUC). Products include:

ALternaGEL Liquid ... 1316
Maximum Strength Ascriptin ... ■ 630
Cama Arthritis Pain Reliever ... ■ 785
Gaviscon Extra Strength Relief Formula Antacid Tablets ... ■ 819
Gaviscon Extra Strength Relief Formula Liquid Antacid ... ■ 819
Gaviscon Liquid Antacid ... ■ 820
Gelusil Liquid & Tablets ... ■ 855
Maalox Heartburn Relief Suspension ... ■ 642
Maalox Heartburn Relief Tablets ... ■ 641
Maalox Magnesia and Alumina Oral Suspension ... ■ 642
Maalox Plus Tablets ... ■ 643
Extra Strength Maalox Antacid Plus Antigas Liquid and Tablets ■ 638
Tempo Soft Antacid ... ■ 835

(■ Described in PDR For Nonprescription Drugs) (⊙ Described in PDR For Ophthalmology)

Interactions Index

Zofran Tablets

Aluminum Hydroxide Gel (Reduces the peak serum levels but not the AUC). Products include:

ALternaGEL Liquid	◆D 659
Aludrox Oral Suspension	2695
Amphojel Suspension	2695
Amphojel Suspension without Flavor	2695
Amphojel Tablets	2695
Arthritis Pain Ascriptin	◆D 631
Regular Strength Ascriptin Tablets	◆D 629
Gaviscon Antacid Tablets	◆D 819
Gaviscon-2 Antacid Tablets	◆D 820
Mylanta Liquid	1317
Mylanta Tablets	◆D 660
Mylanta Double Strength Liquid	1317
Mylanta Double Strength Tablets	◆D 660
Nephrox Suspension	◆D 655

Aluminum Hydroxide Gel, Dried (Reduces the peak serum levels but not the AUC).

Aminophylline (Careful monitoring of plasma theophylline levels in patient receiving azithromycin and theophylline concurrently is recommended).

No products indexed under this heading.

Carbamazepine (Potential for elevation of serum carbamazepine levels). Products include:

Atretol Tablets	573
Tegretol Chewable Tablets	852
Tegretol Suspension	852
Tegretol Tablets	852

Cyclosporine (Potential for elevation of serum cyclosporine levels). Products include:

Neoral	2276
Sandimmune	2286

Dicumarol (Concurrent use of macrolides and warfarin in clinical practice has been associated with increased anticoagulant effects).

No products indexed under this heading.

Digoxin (Potential for elevated digoxin levels). Products include:

Lanoxicaps	1117
Lanoxin Elixir Pediatric	1120
Lanoxin Injection	1123
Lanoxin Injection Pediatric	1126
Lanoxin Tablets	1128

Dihydroergotamine Mesylate (Potential for acute ergot toxicity). Products include:

D.H.E. 45 Injection	2255

Dihydroxyaluminum Sodium Carbonate (Reduces the peak serum levels but not the AUC).

No products indexed under this heading.

Dyphylline (Careful monitoring of plasma theophylline levels in patient receiving azithromycin and theophylline concurrently is recommended). Products include:

Lufyllin & Lufyllin-400 Tablets	2670
Lufyllin-GG Elixir & Tablets	2671

Ergotamine Tartrate (Potential for acute ergot toxicity). Products include:

Bellergal-S Tablets	2250
Cafergot	2251
Ergomar	1486
Wigraine Tablets & Suppositories	1829

Hexobarbital (Potential for elevation of serum hexobarbital levels).

Magaldrate (Reduces the peak serum levels but not the AUC).

No products indexed under this heading.

Magnesium Hydroxide (Reduces the peak serum levels but not the AUC). Products include:

Aludrox Oral Suspension	2695
Arthritis Pain Ascriptin	◆D 631
Maximum Strength Ascriptin	◆D 630
Regular Strength Ascriptin Tablets	◆D 629

Di-Gel Antacid/Anti-Gas .... ◆D 801
Gelusil Liquid & Tablets .... ◆D 855
Maalox Magnesia and Alumina Oral Suspension .... ◆D 642
Maalox Plus Tablets .... ◆D 643
Extra Strength Maalox Antacid Plus Antigas Liquid and Tablets ◆D 638
Mylanta Calcium Carbonate and Magnesium Hydroxide Tablets...... 1318
Mylanta Liquid 1317
Mylanta Tablets .... ◆D 660
Mylanta Double Strength Liquid 1317
Mylanta Double Strength Tablets.. ◆D 660
Phillips' Milk of Magnesia Liquid.... ◆D 729
Rolaids Tablets .... ◆D 843
Tempo Soft Antacid .... ◆D 835

Magnesium Oxide (Reduces the peak serum levels but not the AUC). Products include:

Beelith Tablets	639
Bufferin Analgesic Tablets and Caplets	◆D 613
Caltrate PLUS	◆D 665
Cama Arthritis Pain Reliever	◆D 785
Mag-Ox 400	668
Uro-Mag	668

Phenytoin (Potential for elevation of serum phenytoin levels). Products include:

Dilantin Infatabs	1908
Dilantin-125 Suspension	1911

Phenytoin Sodium (Potential for elevation of serum phenytoin levels azithromycin). Products include:

Dilantin Kapseals	1906
Dilantin Parenteral	1910

Theophylline (Careful monitoring of plasma theophylline levels in patient receiving azithromycin and theophylline concurrently is recommended). Products include:

Marax Tablets & DF Syrup	2200
Quibron	2053

Theophylline Anhydrous (Careful monitoring of plasma theophylline levels in patient receiving azithromycin and theophylline concurrently is recommended). Products include:

Aerolate	1004
Primatene Dual Action Formula	◆D 872
Primatene Tablets	◆D 873
Respbid Tablets	682
Slo-bid Gyrocaps	2033
Theo-24 Extended Release Capsules	2568
Theo-Dur Extended-Release Tablets	1327
Theo-X Extended-Release Tablets	788
Uni-Dur Extended-Release Tablets	1331
Uniphyl 400 mg Tablets	2001

Theophylline Calcium Salicylate (Careful monitoring of plasma theophylline levels in patient receiving azithromycin and theophylline concurrently is recommended). Products include:

Quadrinal Tablets	1350

Theophylline Sodium Glycinate (Careful monitoring of plasma theophylline levels in patient receiving azithromycin and theophylline concurrently is recommended).

No products indexed under this heading.

Triazolam (Potential for decreased clearance of triazolam). Products include:

Halcion Tablets	2611

Warfarin Sodium (Concurrent use of macrolides and warfarin in clinical practice has been associated with increased anticoagulant effects). Products include:

Coumadin	926

Food Interactions

Food, unspecified (Reduces the rate of absorption (Cmax) of azithromycin capsules by 52% and the extent of absorption (AUC) by 43%; when oral suspension of azithromycin was administered with food

the Cmax increased by 46% and the AUC by 14%).

ZITHROMAX FOR ORAL SUSPENSION

(Azithromycin) 1944

See Zithromax Capsules

ZOCOR TABLETS

(Simvastatin) 1775

May interact with immunosuppressive agents, fibrates, and certain other agents. Compounds in these categories include:

Azathioprine (Concomitant administration may produce rhabdomyolysis). Products include:

Imuran	1110

Clofibrate (Concomitant administration may produce rhabdomyolysis). Products include:

Atromid-S Capsules	2701

Cyclosporine (Concomitant administration may produce rhabdomyolysis). Products include:

Neoral	2276
Sandimmune	2286

Digoxin (Slight elevation in digoxin plasma levels). Products include:

Lanoxicaps	1117
Lanoxin Elixir Pediatric	1120
Lanoxin Injection	1123
Lanoxin Injection Pediatric	1126
Lanoxin Tablets	1128

Erythromycin (Concomitant administration may produce rhabdomyolysis). Products include:

A/T/S 2% Acne Topical Gel and Solution	1234
Benzamycin Topical Gel	905
E-Mycin Tablets	1341
Emgel 2% Topical Gel	1093
ERYC	1915
Erycette (erythromycin 2%) Topical Solution	1888
Ery-Tab Tablets	422
Erythromycin Base Filmtab	426
Erythromycin Delayed-Release Capsules, USP	427
Ilotycin Ophthalmic Ointment	912
PCE Dispertab Tablets	444
T-Stat 2.0% Topical Solution and Pads	2688
Theramycin Z Topical Solution 2%	1592

Erythromycin Estolate (Concomitant administration may produce rhabdomyolysis). Products include:

Ilosone	911

Erythromycin Ethylsuccinate (Concomitant administration may produce rhabdomyolysis). Products include:

E.E.S.	424
EryPed	421

Erythromycin Gluceptate (Concomitant administration may produce rhabdomyolysis). Products include:

Ilotycin Gluceptate, IV, Vials	913

Erythromycin Stearate (Concomitant administration may produce rhabdomyolysis). Products include:

Erythrocin Stearate Filmtab	425

Gemfibrozil (Concomitant administration may produce rhabdomyolysis). Products include:

Lopid Tablets	1917

Itraconazole (Concomitant administration may produce rhabdomyolysis). Products include:

Sporanox Capsules	1305

Muromonab-CD3 (Concomitant administration may produce rhabdomyolysis). Products include:

Orthoclone OKT3 Sterile Solution	1837

Mycophenolate Mofetil (Concomitant administration may produce rhabdomyolysis). Products include:

CellCept Capsules	2099

Nicotinic Acid (Concomitant administration may produce rhabdomyolysis).

No products indexed under this heading.

Propranolol Hydrochloride (Significant decreases in mean C_{max}, but no change in AUC). Products include:

Inderal	2728
Inderal LA Long Acting Capsules	2730
Inderide Tablets	2732
Inderide LA Long Acting Capsules	2734

Tacrolimus (Concomitant administration may produce rhabdomyolysis). Products include:

Prograf	1042

Warfarin Sodium (Slightly enhanced anticoagulant effect). Products include:

Coumadin	926

ZOFRAN INJECTION

(Ondansetron Hydrochloride) 1214

May interact with drugs affecting hepatic drug metabolizing enzyme systems and certain other agents. Compounds in these categories include:

Carbamazepine (Inducers or inhibitors of these enzymes may change the clearance and hence, the half-life). Products include:

Atretol Tablets	573
Tegretol Chewable Tablets	852
Tegretol Suspension	852
Tegretol Tablets	852

Cimetidine (Inducers or inhibitors of these enzymes may change the clearance and hence, the half-life). Products include:

Tagamet Tablets	2516

Cimetidine Hydrochloride (Inducers or inhibitors of these enzymes may change the clearance and hence, the half-life). Products include:

Tagamet	2516

Phenobarbital (Inducers or inhibitors of these enzymes may change the clearance and hence, the half-life). Products include:

Arco-Lase Plus Tablets	512
Bellergal-S Tablets	2250
Donnatal	2060
Donnatal Extentabs	2061
Donnatal Tablets	2060
Phenobarbital Elixir and Tablets	1469
Quadrinal Tablets	1350

Phenytoin (Inducers or inhibitors of these enzymes may change the clearance and hence, the half-life). Products include:

Dilantin Infatabs	1908
Dilantin-125 Suspension	1911

Phenytoin Sodium (Inducers or inhibitors of these enzymes may change the clearance and hence, the half-life). Products include:

Dilantin Kapseals	1906
Dilantin Parenteral	1910

ZOFRAN INJECTION PREMIXED

(Ondansetron Hydrochloride) 1214

See Zofran Injection

ZOFRAN TABLETS

(Ondansetron Hydrochloride) 1217

May interact with drugs affecting hepatic drug metabolizing enzyme systems and certain other agents. Compounds in these categories include:

Carbamazepine (Inducers or inhibitors of these enzymes may change the clearance and hence, the half-life). Products include:

Atretol Tablets	573

IMPORTANT NOTE: Always consult each drug listing in the patient's regimen for possible interactions.

Tegretol Chewable Tablets 852
Tegretol Suspension 852
Tegretol Tablets 852

Cimetidine (Inducers or inhibitors of these enzymes may change the clearance and hence, the half-life). Products include:

Tagamet Tablets 2516

Cimetidine Hydrochloride (Inducers or inhibitors of these enzymes may change the clearance and hence, the half-life). Products include:

Tagamet 2516

Phenobarbital (Inducers or inhibitors of these enzymes may change the clearance and hence, the half-life). Products include:

Arco-Lase Plus Tablets 512
Bellergal-S Tablets 2250
Donnatal 2060
Donnatal Extentabs 2061
Donnatal Tablets 2060
Phenobarbital Elixir and Tablets 1469
Quadrinal Tablets 1350

Phenytoin (Inducers or inhibitors of these enzymes may change the clearance and hence, the half-life). Products include:

Dilantin Infatabs 1908
Dilantin-125 Suspension 1911

Phenytoin Sodium (Inducers or inhibitors of these enzymes may change the clearance and hence, the half-life). Products include:

Dilantin Kapseals 1906
Dilantin Parenteral 1910

Food Interactions

Food, unspecified (Increases significantly (about 17%) the extent of absorption of ondansetron).

ZOLADEX

(Goserelin Acetate Implant) 2858
None cited in PDR database.

ZOLOFT TABLETS

(Sertraline Hydrochloride) 2217
May interact with oral anticoagulants, antidepressant drugs, lithium preparations, monoamine oxidase inhibitors, highly protein bound drugs (selected), tricyclic antidepressants, and certain other agents. Compounds in these categories include:

Amiodarone Hydrochloride (Co-administration with another drug which is tightly bound to protein may cause a shift in plasma concentrations resulting in an adverse effect). Products include:

Cordarone Intravenous 2715
Cordarone Tablets 2712

Amitriptyline Hydrochloride (Concurrent use of drugs that inhibit the biochemical activity of $P_{450}IID_6$, such as tricyclic antidepressants, may increase plasma concentrations of co-administered drugs that are metabolized by $P_{450}IID_6$; changes in the dosage may be required; the duration of an appropriate washout period which should intervene before switching has not been established). Products include:

Elavil 2838
Endep Tablets 2174
Etrafon 2355
Limbitrol 2180
Triavil Tablets 1757

Amoxapine (Concurrent use of drugs that inhibit the biochemical activity of $P_{450}IID_6$, such as tricyclic antidepressants, may increase plasma concentrations of co-administered drugs that are metabolized by $P_{450}IID_6$; changes in the dosage may be required; the duration of an appropriate washout period which should intervene before switching has not been established). Products include:

Asendin Tablets 1369

Atovaquone (Co-administration with another drug which is tightly bound to protein may cause a shift in plasma concentrations resulting in an adverse effect). Products include:

Mepron Suspension 1135

Cefonicid Sodium (Co-administration with another drug which is tightly bound to protein may cause a shift in plasma concentrations resulting in an adverse effect). Products include:

Monocid Injection 2497

Chlordiazepoxide (Co-administration with another drug which is tightly bound to protein may cause a shift in plasma concentrations resulting in an adverse effect). Products include:

Libritabs Tablets 2177
Limbitrol 2180

Chlordiazepoxide Hydrochloride (Co-administration with another drug which is tightly bound to protein may cause a shift in plasma concentrations resulting in an adverse effect). Products include:

Librax Capsules 2176
Librium Capsules 2178
Librium Injectable 2179

Chlorpromazine (Co-administration with another drug which is tightly bound to protein may cause a shift in plasma concentrations resulting in an adverse effect). Products include:

Thorazine Suppositories 2523

Chlorpromazine Hydrochloride (Co-administration with another drug which is tightly bound to protein may cause a shift in plasma concentrations resulting in an adverse effect). Products include:

Thorazine 2523

Cimetidine (Potential for increase in Zoloft mean AUC (50%), C_{max} (24%) and half-life (26%); clinical significance is unknown). Products include:

Tagamet Tablets 2516

Cimetidine Hydrochloride (Potential for increase in Zoloft mean AUC (50%), C_{max} (24%) and half-life (26%); clinical significance is unknown). Products include:

Tagamet 2516

Clomipramine Hydrochloride (Concurrent use of drugs that inhibit the biochemical activity of $P_{450}IID_6$, such as tricyclic antidepressants, may increase plasma concentrations of co-administered drugs that are metabolized by $P_{450}IID_6$; changes in the dosage may be required; the duration of an appropriate washout period which should intervene before switching has not been established). Products include:

Anafranil Capsules 803

Clozapine (Co-administration with another drug which is tightly bound to protein may cause a shift in plasma concentrations resulting in an adverse effect). Products include:

Clozaril Tablets 2252

CNS-Active Drugs, unspecified (Caution is advised if Zoloft is co-administered with other CNS active drugs).

Cyclosporine (Co-administration with another drug which is tightly bound to protein may cause a shift in plasma concentrations resulting in an adverse effect). Products include:

Neoral 2276
Sandimmune 2286

Desipramine Hydrochloride (Concurrent use of drugs that inhibit the biochemical activity of $P_{450}IID_6$, such as tricyclic antidepressants, may increase plasma concentrations of co-administered drugs that are metabolized by $P_{450}IID_6$; changes in the dosage may be required; the duration of an appropriate washout period which should intervene before switching has not been established). Products include:

Norpramin Tablets 1526

Diazepam (Potential for decrease in diazepam clearance; co-administration with another drug which is tightly bound to protein may cause a shift in plasma concentrations resulting in an adverse effect). Products include:

Dizac 1809
Valium Injectable 2182
Valium Tablets 2183
Valrelease Capsules 2169

Diclofenac Potassium (Co-administration with another drug which is tightly bound to protein may cause a shift in plasma concentrations resulting in an adverse effect). Products include:

Cataflam 816

Diclofenac Sodium (Co-administration with another drug which is tightly bound to protein may cause a shift in plasma concentrations resulting in an adverse effect). Products include:

Voltaren Ophthalmic Sterile Ophthalmic Solution .... ◉ 272
Voltaren Tablets 861

Dicumarol (May cause a shift in plasma concentrations potentially resulting in an adverse effect; prothrombin time should be carefully monitored when Zoloft therapy is initiated or stopped).

No products indexed under this heading.

Digitoxin (May cause shift in plasma concentrations potentially resulting in an adverse effect; in clinical trials, during co-administration, there was no change in serum digoxin levels or plasma digitalis glycoside clearance). Products include:

Crystodigin Tablets 1433

Digoxin (May cause a shift in plasma concentrations potentially resulting in an adverse effect; in clinical trials, during co-administration, there was no change in serum digoxin levels or digoxin clearance). Products include:

Lanoxicaps 1117
Lanoxin Elixir Pediatric 1120
Lanoxin Injection 1123
Lanoxin Injection Pediatric 1126
Lanoxin Tablets 1128

Dipyridamole (Co-administration with another drug which is tightly bound to protein may cause a shift in plasma concentrations resulting in an adverse effect). Products include:

Persantine Tablets 681

Doxepin Hydrochloride (Concurrent use of drugs that inhibit the biochemical activity of $P_{450}IID_6$, such as tricyclic antidepressants, may increase plasma concentrations of co-administered drugs that are metabolized by $P_{450}IID_6$; changes in the dosage may be required; the duration of an appropriate washout period which should intervene before switching has not been established). Products include:

Sinequan 2205
Zonalon Cream 1055

Fenoprofen Calcium (Co-administration with another drug which is tightly bound to protein may cause a shift in plasma concentrations resulting in an adverse effect). Products include:

Nalfon 200 Pulvules & Nalfon Tablets 917

Flecainide Acetate (Concurrent use of drugs that inhibit the biochemical activity of $P_{450}IID_6$, such as flecainide, may increase plasma concentrations of co-administered drugs that are metabolized by $P_{450}IID_6$; changes in the dosage may be required). Products include:

Tambocor Tablets 1497

Fluoxetine Hydrochloride (Concurrent use of drugs that inhibit the biochemical activity of $P_{450}IID_6$, such as SSRIs, may increase plasma concentrations of co-administered drugs that are metabolized by $P_{450}IID_6$; changes in the dosage may be required; the duration of an appropriate washout period which should intervene before switching has not been established). Products include:

Prozac Pulvules & Liquid, Oral Solution 919

Flurazepam Hydrochloride (Co-administration with another drug which is tightly bound to protein may cause a shift in plasma concentrations resulting in an adverse effect). Products include:

Dalmane Capsules 2173

Flurbiprofen (Co-administration with another drug which is tightly bound to protein may cause a shift in plasma concentrations resulting in an adverse effect). Products include:

Ansaid Tablets 2579

Fluvoxamine Maleate (Concurrent use of drugs that inhibit the biochemical activity of $P_{450}IID_6$, such as SSRIs, may increase plasma concentrations of co-administered drugs that are metabolized by $P_{450}IID_6$; changes in the dosage may be required; the duration of an appropriate washout period which should intervene before switching has not been established). Products include:

Luvox Tablets 2544

Furazolidone (Potential for fatal reactions including hyperthermia, rigidity, myoclonus and other serious reactions; concurrent and/or sequential use is contraindicated). Products include:

Furoxone 2046

Glipizide (Co-administration with another drug which is tightly bound to protein may cause a shift in plasma concentrations resulting in an adverse effect). Products include:

Glucotrol Tablets 1967
Glucotrol XL Extended Release Tablets 1968

(▣ Described in PDR For Nonprescription Drugs) (◉ Described in PDR For Ophthalmology)

Interactions Index

Zoloft

Ibuprofen (Co-administration with another drug which is tightly bound to protein may cause a shift in plasma concentrations resulting in an adverse effect). Products include:

Advil Cold and Sinus Caplets and Tablets (formerly CoAdvil) .... ◉ 870

Advil Ibuprofen Tablets and Caplets .... ◉ 870

Children's Advil Suspension 2692

Arthritis Foundation Ibuprofen Tablets .... ◉ 674

Bayer Select Ibuprofen Pain Relief Formula .... ◉ 715

Cramp End Tablets .... ◉ 735

Dimetapp Sinus Caplets .... ◉ 775

Haltran Tablets .... ◉ 771

IBU Tablets 1342

Ibuprohm .... ◉ 735

Children's Motrin Ibuprofen Oral Suspension 1546

Motrin Tablets 2625

Motrin IB Caplets, Tablets, and Geltabs .... ◉ 838

Motrin IB Sinus .... ◉ 838

Motrin Ibuprofen Suspension, Oral Drops, Chewable Tablets, Caplets 1546

Nuprin Ibuprofen/Analgesic Tablets & Caplets .... ◉ 622

Sine-Aid IB Caplets 1554

Vicks DayQuil SINUS Pressure & PAIN Relief with IBUPROFEN .... ◉ 762

Imipramine Hydrochloride (Concurrent use of drugs that inhibit the biochemical activity of $P_{450}IID_6$, such as tricyclic antidepressants, may increase plasma concentrations of co-administered drugs that are metabolized by $P_{450}IID_6$; changes in the dosage may be required; the duration of an appropriate washout period which should intervene before switching has not been established). Products include:

Tofranil Ampuls 854

Tofranil Tablets 856

Imipramine Pamoate (Concurrent use of drugs that inhibit the biochemical activity of $P_{450}IID_6$, such as tricyclic antidepressants, may increase plasma concentrations of co-administered drugs that are metabolized by $P_{450}IID_6$; changes in the dosage may be required; the duration of an appropriate washout period which should intervene before switching has not been established). Products include:

Tofranil-PM Capsules 857

Indomethacin (Co-administration with another drug which is tightly bound to protein may cause a shift in plasma concentrations resulting in an adverse effect). Products include:

Indocin 1680

Indomethacin Sodium Trihydrate (Co-administration with another drug which is tightly bound to protein may cause a shift in plasma concentrations resulting in an adverse effect). Products include:

Indocin I.V. 1684

Isocarboxazid (Potential for fatal reactions including hyperthermia, rigidity, myoclonus and other serious reactions; concurrent and/or sequential use is contraindicated).

No products indexed under this heading.

Ketoprofen (Co-administration with another drug which is tightly bound to protein may cause a shift in plasma concentrations resulting in an adverse effect). Products include:

Orudis Capsules 2766

Oruvail Capsules 2766

Ketorolac Tromethamine (Co-administration with another drug which is tightly bound to protein may cause a shift in plasma concentrations resulting in an adverse effect). Products include:

Acular 474

Acular .... ◉ 277

Toradol 2159

Lithium Carbonate (No significant alteration in plasma lithium levels or renal clearance, nonetheless, plasma lithium levels should be monitored). Products include:

Eskalith 2485

Lithium Carbonate Capsules & Tablets 2230

Lithonate/Lithotabs/Lithobid 2543

Lithium Citrate (No significant alteration in plasma lithium levels or renal clearance, nonetheless, plasma lithium levels should be monitored).

No products indexed under this heading.

Maprotiline Hydrochloride (Concurrent use of drugs that inhibit the biochemical activity of $P_{450}IID_6$, such as tricyclic antidepressants, may increase plasma concentrations of co-administered drugs that are metabolized by $P_{450}IID_6$; changes in the dosage may be required; the duration of an appropriate washout period which should intervene before switching has not been established). Products include:

Ludiomil Tablets 843

Meclofenamate Sodium (Co-administration with another drug which is tightly bound to protein may cause a shift in plasma concentrations resulting in an adverse effect).

No products indexed under this heading.

Mefenamic Acid (Co-administration with another drug which is tightly bound to protein may cause a shift in plasma concentrations resulting in an adverse effect). Products include:

Ponstel 1925

Midazolam Hydrochloride (Co-administration with another drug which is tightly bound to protein may cause a shift in plasma concentrations resulting in an adverse effect). Products include:

Versed Injection 2170

Naproxen (Co-administration with another drug which is tightly bound to protein may cause a shift in plasma concentrations resulting in an adverse effect). Products include:

Anaprox/Naprosyn 2117

Naproxen Sodium (Co-administration with another drug which is tightly bound to protein may cause a shift in plasma concentrations resulting in an adverse effect). Products include:

Aleve 1975

Anaprox/Naprosyn 2117

Nefazodone Hydrochloride (Care and prudent medical judgment should be exercised regarding the optimal timing of switching from another antidepressant to Zoloft; the duration of an appropriate washout period which should intervene before switching has not been established). Products include:

Serzone Tablets 771

Nortriptyline Hydrochloride (Concurrent use of drugs that inhibit the biochemical activity of $P_{450}IID_6$, such as tricyclic antidepressants, may increase plasma concentrations of co-administered drugs that are metabolized by $P_{450}IID_6$; changes in the dosage may be required; the duration of an appropriate washout period which should intervene before switching has not been established). Products include:

Pamelor 2280

Oxaprozin (Co-administration with another drug which is tightly bound to protein may cause a shift in plasma concentrations resulting in an adverse effect). Products include:

Daypro Caplets 2426

Oxazepam (Co-administration with another drug which is tightly bound to protein may cause a shift in plasma concentrations resulting in an adverse effect). Products include:

Serax Capsules 2810

Serax Tablets 2810

Paroxetine Hydrochloride (Concurrent use of drugs that inhibit the biochemical activity of $P_{450}IID_6$, such as SSRIs, may increase plasma concentrations of co-administered drugs that are metabolized by $P_{450}IID_6$; changes in the dosage may be required; the duration of an appropriate washout period which should intervene before switching has not been established). Products include:

Paxil Tablets 2505

Phenelzine Sulfate (Potential for fatal reactions including hyperthermia, rigidity, myoclonus and other serious reactions; concurrent and/or sequential use is contraindicated). Products include:

Nardil 1920

Phenylbutazone (Co-administration with another drug which is tightly bound to protein may cause a shift in plasma concentrations resulting in an adverse effect).

No products indexed under this heading.

Piroxicam (Co-administration with another drug which is tightly bound to protein may cause a shift in plasma concentrations resulting in an adverse effect). Products include:

Feldene Capsules 1965

Propafenone Hydrochloride (Concurrent use of drugs that inhibit the biochemical activity of $P_{450}IID_6$, such as propafenone, may increase plasma concentrations of co-administered drugs that are metabolized by $P_{450}IID_6$; changes in the dosage may be required). Products include:

Rythmol Tablets–150mg, 225mg, 300mg 1352

Propranolol Hydrochloride (Co-administration with another drug which is tightly bound to protein may cause a shift in plasma concentrations resulting in an adverse effect). Products include:

Inderal 2728

Inderal LA Long Acting Capsules 2730

Inderide Tablets 2732

Inderide LA Long Acting Capsules .. 2734

Protriptyline Hydrochloride (Concurrent use of drugs that inhibit the biochemical activity of $P_{450}IID_6$, such as tricyclic antidepressants, may increase plasma concentrations of co-administered drugs that are metabolized by $P_{450}IID_6$; changes in the dosage may be required; the duration of an appropriate washout period which should intervene before switching has not been established). Products include:

Vivactil Tablets 1774

Selegiline Hydrochloride (Potential for fatal reactions including hyperthermia, rigidity, myoclonus and other serious reactions; concurrent and/or sequential use is contraindicated). Products include:

Eldepryl Tablets 2550

Sulindac (Co-administration with another drug which is tightly bound to protein may cause a shift in plasma concentrations resulting in an adverse effect). Products include:

Clinoril Tablets 1618

Temazepam (Co-administration with another drug which is tightly bound to protein may cause a shift in plasma concentrations resulting in an adverse effect). Products include:

Restoril Capsules 2284

Tolbutamide (A statistically significant decrease in tolbutamide clearance due to a change in the metabolism of the drug).

No products indexed under this heading.

Tolmetin Sodium (Co-administration with another drug which is tightly bound to protein may cause a shift in plasma concentrations resulting in an adverse effect). Products include:

Tolectin (200, 400 and 600 mg) .. 1581

Tranylcypromine Sulfate (Potential for fatal reactions including hyperthermia, rigidity, myoclonus and other serious reactions; concurrent and/or sequential use is contraindicated). Products include:

Parnate Tablets 2503

Trimipramine Maleate (Concurrent use of drugs that inhibit the biochemical activity of $P_{450}IID_6$, such as tricyclic antidepressants, may increase plasma concentrations of co-administered drugs that are metabolized by $P_{450}IID_6$; changes in the dosage may be required; the duration of an appropriate washout period which should intervene before switching has not been established). Products include:

Surmontil Capsules 2811

Venlafaxine Hydrochloride (Concurrent use drugs that inhibit the biochemical activity of $P_{450}IID_6$, such as SSRIs, may increase plasma concentrations of co-administered drugs that are metabolized by $P_{450}IID_6$; changes in the dosage may be required; the duration of an appropriate washout period which should intervene before switching has not been established). Products include:

Effexor 2719

Warfarin Sodium (May cause a shift in plasma concentrations potentially resulting in an adverse effect; prothrombin time should be carefully monitored when Zoloft therapy is initiated or stopped). Products include:

Coumadin 926

IMPORTANT NOTE: Always consult each drug listing in the patient's regimen for possible interactions.

Zoloft

Food Interactions

Alcohol (Concomitant use of Zoloft and alcohol in depressed patient is not recommended).

Food, unspecified (AUC was slightly increased when drug was administered with food but the C_{max} was 25% greater).

ZONALON CREAM

(Doxepin Hydrochloride)........................1055

May interact with monoamine oxidase inhibitors, antidepressant drugs, phenothiazines, and certain other agents. Compounds in these categories include:

Amitriptyline Hydrochloride (Concomitant use of doxepin, a tricyclic antidepressant, with other drugs metabolized by cytochrome $P_{450}IID_6$ may require lower than usual doses prescribed for either drug). Products include:

Elavil 2838
Endep Tablets 2174
Etrafon 2355
Limbitrol 2180
Triavil Tablets 1757

Amoxapine (Concomitant use of doxepin, a tricyclic antidepressant, with other drugs metabolized by cytochrome $P_{450}IID_6$ may require lower than usual doses prescribed for either drug). Products include:

Asendin Tablets 1369

Bupropion Hydrochloride (Concomitant use of doxepin, a tricyclic antidepressant, with other drugs metabolized by cytochrome $P_{450}IID_6$ may require lower than usual doses prescribed for either drug). Products include:

Wellbutrin Tablets 1204

Carbamazepine (Concomitant use of doxepin, a tricyclic antidepressant, with other drugs metabolized by cytochrome $P_{450}IID_6$ may require lower than usual doses prescribed for either drug). Products include:

Atretol Tablets 573
Tegretol Chewable Tablets 852
Tegretol Suspension 852
Tegretol Tablets 852

Chlorpromazine (Concomitant use of doxepin, a tricyclic antidepressant, with other drugs metabolized by cytochrome $P_{450}IID_6$ may require lower than usual doses prescribed for either drug). Products include:

Thorazine Suppositories 2523

Chlorpromazine Hydrochloride (Concomitant use of doxepin, a tricyclic antidepressant, with other drugs metabolized by cytochrome $P_{450}IID_6$ may require lower than usual doses prescribed for either drug). Products include:

Thorazine 2523

Cimetidine (Potential for clinically significant fluctuations in steady-state serum concentrations). Products include:

Tagamet Tablets 2516

Cimetidine Hydrochloride (Potential for clinically significant fluctuations in steady-state serum concentrations). Products include:

Tagamet 2516

Desipramine Hydrochloride (Concomitant use of doxepin, a tricyclic antidepressant, with other drugs metabolized by cytochrome $P_{450}IID_6$ may require lower than usual doses prescribed for either drug). Products include:

Norpramin Tablets 1526

Flecainide Acetate (Concomitant use of doxepin, a tricyclic antidepressant, with other drugs metabolized by cytochrome $P_{450}IID_6$ may require lower than usual doses prescribed for either drug). Products include:

Tambocor Tablets 1497

Fluoxetine Hydrochloride (Concomitant use of doxepin, a tricyclic antidepressant, with other drugs metabolized by cytochrome $P_{450}IID_6$ may require lower than usual doses prescribed for either drug). Products include:

Prozac Pulvules & Liquid, Oral Solution 919

Fluphenazine Decanoate (Concomitant use of doxepin, a tricyclic antidepressant, with other drugs metabolized by cytochrome $P_{450}IID_6$ may require lower than usual doses prescribed for either drug). Products include:

Prolixin Decanoate 509

Fluphenazine Enanthate (Concomitant use of doxepin, a tricyclic antidepressant, with other drugs metabolized by cytochrome $P_{450}IID_6$ may require lower than usual doses prescribed for either drug). Products include:

Prolixin Enanthate 509

Fluphenazine Hydrochloride (Concomitant use of doxepin, a tricyclic antidepressant, with other drugs metabolized by cytochrome $P_{450}IID_6$ may require lower than usual doses prescribed for either drug). Products include:

Prolixin 509

Furazolidone (Potential for serious side effects and fatality have been reported with orally administered drugs; plasma levels of doxepin obtained with topical administered doxepin are similar to systemic therapy; concurrent and/or sequential therapy is not recommended). Products include:

Furoxone 2046

Imipramine Hydrochloride (Concomitant use of doxepin, a tricyclic antidepressant, with other drugs metabolized by cytochrome $P_{450}IID_6$ may require lower than usual doses prescribed for either drug). Products include:

Tofranil Ampuls 854
Tofranil Tablets 856

Imipramine Pamoate (Concomitant use of doxepin, a tricyclic antidepressant, with other drugs metabolized by cytochrome $P_{450}IID_6$ may require lower than usual doses prescribed for either drug). Products include:

Tofranil-PM Capsules 857

Isocarboxazid (Potential for serious side effects and fatality have been reported with orally administered drugs; plasma levels of doxepin obtained with topical administered doxepin are similar to systemic therapy; concurrent and/or sequential therapy is not recommended; concomitant use of doxepin, a tricyclic antidepressant, with other drugs metabolized by cytochrome $P_{450}IID_6$ may require lower than usual doses prescribed for either drug).

No products indexed under this heading.

Maprotiline Hydrochloride (Concomitant use of doxepin, a tricyclic antidepressant, with other drugs metabolized by cytochrome $P_{450}IID_6$ may require lower than usual doses prescribed for either drug). Products include:

Ludiomil Tablets 843

Mesoridazine Besylate (Concomitant use of doxepin, a tricyclic antidepressant, with other drugs metabolized by cytochrome $P_{450}IID_6$ may require lower than usual doses prescribed for either drug). Products include:

Serentil 684

Methotrimeprazine (Concomitant use of doxepin, a tricyclic antidepressant, with other drugs metabolized by cytochrome $P_{450}IID_6$ may require lower than usual doses prescribed for either drug). Products include:

Levoprome 1274

Nefazodone Hydrochloride (Concomitant use of doxepin, a tricyclic antidepressant, with other drugs metabolized by cytochrome $P_{450}IID_6$ may require lower than usual doses prescribed for either drug). Products include:

Serzone Tablets 771

Nortriptyline Hydrochloride (Concomitant use of doxepin, a tricyclic antidepressant, with other drugs metabolized by cytochrome $P_{450}IID_6$ may require lower than usual doses prescribed for either drug). Products include:

Pamelor 2280

Paroxetine Hydrochloride (Concomitant use of doxepin, a tricyclic antidepressant, with other drugs metabolized by cytochrome $P_{450}IID_6$ may require lower than usual doses prescribed for either drug). Products include:

Paxil Tablets 2505

Perphenazine (Concomitant use of doxepin, a tricyclic antidepressant, with other drugs metabolized by cytochrome $P_{450}IID_6$ may require lower than usual doses prescribed for either drug). Products include:

Etrafon 2355
Triavil Tablets 1757
Trilafon 2389

Phenelzine Sulfate (Potential for serious side effects and fatality have been reported with orally administered drugs; plasma levels of doxepin obtained with topical administered doxepin are similar to systemic therapy; concurrent and/or sequential therapy is not recommended; concomitant use of doxepin, a tricyclic antidepressant, with other drugs metabolized by cytochrome $P_{450}IID_6$ may require lower than usual doses prescribed for either drug). Products include:

Nardil 1920

Prochlorperazine (Concomitant use of doxepin, a tricyclic antidepressant, with other drugs metabolized by cytochrome $P_{450}IID_6$ may require lower than usual doses prescribed for either drug). Products include:

Compazine 2470

Promethazine Hydrochloride (Concomitant use of doxepin, a tricyclic antidepressant, with other drugs metabolized by cytochrome $P_{450}IID_6$ may require lower than usual doses prescribed for either drug). Products include:

Mepergan Injection 2753

Phenergan with Codeine 2777
Phenergan with Dextromethorphan 2778
Phenergan Injection 2773
Phenergan Suppositories 2775
Phenergan Syrup 2774
Phenergan Tablets 2775
Phenergan VC 2779
Phenergan VC with Codeine 2781

Propafenone Hydrochloride (Concomitant use of doxepin, a tricyclic antidepressant, with other drugs metabolized by cytochrome $P_{450}IID_6$ may require lower than usual doses prescribed for either drug). Products include:

Rythmol Tablets–150mg, 225mg, 300mg 1352

Protriptyline Hydrochloride (Concomitant use of doxepin, a tricyclic antidepressant, with other drugs metabolized by cytochrome $P_{450}IID_6$ may require lower than usual doses prescribed for either drug). Products include:

Vivactil Tablets 1774

Quinidine Gluconate (Concomitant use of doxepin, a tricyclic antidepressant, with quinidine which inhibits cytochrome $P_{450}IID_6$ should be approached with caution). Products include:

Quinaglute Dura-Tabs Tablets 649

Quinidine Polygalacturonate (Concomitant use of doxepin, a tricyclic antidepressant, with quinidine which inhibits cytochrome $P_{450}IID_6$ should be approached with caution).

No products indexed under this heading.

Quinidine Sulfate (Concomitant use of doxepin, a tricyclic antidepressant, with quinidine which inhibits cytochrome $P_{450}IID_6$ should be approached with caution). Products include:

Quinidex Extentabs 2067

Selegiline Hydrochloride (Potential for serious side effects and fatality have been reported with orally administered drugs; plasma levels of doxepin obtained with topical administered doxepin are similar to systemic therapy; concurrent and/or sequential therapy is not recommended). Products include:

Eldepryl Tablets 2550

Sertraline Hydrochloride (Concomitant use of doxepin, a tricyclic antidepressant, with other drugs metabolized by cytochrome $P_{450}IID_6$ may require lower than usual doses prescribed for either drug). Products include:

Zoloft Tablets 2217

Thioridazine Hydrochloride (Concomitant use of doxepin, a tricyclic antidepressant, with other drugs metabolized by cytochrome $P_{450}IID_6$ may require lower than usual doses prescribed for either drug). Products include:

Mellaril 2269

Tranylcypromine Sulfate (Potential for serious side effects and fatality have been reported with orally administered drugs; plasma levels of doxepin obtained with topical administered doxepin are similar to systemic therapy; concurrent and/or sequential therapy is not recommended; concomitant use of doxepin, a tricyclic antidepressant, with other drugs metabolized by cytochrome $P_{450}IID_6$ may require lower than usual doses prescribed for either drug). Products include:

Parnate Tablets 2503

(◙ Described in PDR For Nonprescription Drugs) (◉ Described in PDR For Ophthalmology)

Trazodone Hydrochloride (Concomitant use of doxepin, a tricyclic antidepressant, with other drugs metabolized by cytochrome $P_{450}IID_6$ may require lower than usual doses prescribed for either drug). Products include:

Desyrel and Desyrel Dividose 503

Trifluoperazine Hydrochloride (Concomitant use of doxepin, a tricyclic antidepressant, with other drugs metabolized by cytochrome $P_{450}IID_6$ may require lower than usual doses prescribed for either drug). Products include:

Stelazine 2514

Trimipramine Maleate (Concomitant use of doxepin, a tricyclic antidepressant, with other drugs metabolized by cytochrome $P_{450}IID_6$ may require lower than usual doses prescribed for either drug). Products include:

Surmontil Capsules................................ 2811

Venlafaxine Hydrochloride (Concomitant use of doxepin, a tricyclic antidepressant, with other drugs metabolized by cytochrome $P_{450}IID_6$ may require lower than usual doses prescribed for either drug). Products include:

Effexor 2719

Food Interactions

Alcohol (Alcohol ingestion may exacerbate the potential sedative effects of Zonalon Cream).

ZOSTRIX

(Capsaicin) 1056
None cited in PDR database.

ZOSTRIX-HP TOPICAL ANALGESIC CREAM

(Capsaicin) 1056
None cited in PDR database.

ZOSYN

(Piperacillin Sodium, Tazobactam Sodium) 1419

May interact with aminoglycosides, anticoagulants, nondepolarizing neuromuscular blocking agents, and certain other agents. Compounds in these categories include:

Amikacin Sulfate (Concomitant administration can result in substantial inactivation of the aminoglycoside). Products include:

Amikacin Sulfate Injection, USP 960
Amikin Injectable 501

Atracurium Besylate (Prolongation of the neuromuscular blockade). Products include:

Tracrium Injection 1183

Dalteparin Sodium (Coagulation parameters should be tested more frequently and monitored regularly during simultaneous administration; effect of concurrent use is not specified). Products include:

Fragmin 1954

Dicumarol (Coagulation parameters should be tested more frequently and monitored regularly during simultaneous administration; effect of concurrent use is not specified).

No products indexed under this heading.

Enoxaparin (Coagulation parameters should be tested more frequently and monitored regularly during simultaneous administration; effect of concurrent use is not specified). Products include:

Lovenox Injection 2020

Gentamicin Sulfate (Concomitant administration can result in substantial inactivation of the aminoglycoside). Products include:

Garamycin Injectable 2360
Genoptic Sterile Ophthalmic Solution... ◉ 243
Genoptic Sterile Ophthalmic Ointment .... ◉ 243
Gentacidin Ointment .... ◉ 264
Gentacidin Solution................................ ◉ 264
Gentak .... ◉ 208
Pred-G Liquifilm Sterile Ophthalmic Suspension .... ◉ 251
Pred-G S.O.P. Sterile Ophthalmic Ointment .... ◉ 252

Heparin Calcium (Coagulation parameters should be tested more frequently and monitored regularly during simultaneous administration; effect of concurrent use is not specified).

No products indexed under this heading.

Heparin Sodium (Coagulation parameters should be tested more frequently and monitored regularly during simultaneous administration; effect of concurrent use is not specified). Products include:

Heparin Lock Flush Solution 2725
Heparin Sodium Injection.................... 2726
Heparin Sodium Injection, USP, Sterile Solution 2615
Heparin Sodium Vials........................... 1441

Kanamycin Sulfate (Concomitant administration can result in substantial inactivation of the aminoglycoside).

No products indexed under this heading.

Metocurine Iodide (Prolongation of the neuromuscular blockade). Products include:

Metubine Iodide Vials............................. 916

Mivacurium Chloride (Prolongation of the neuromuscular blockade). Products include:

Mivacron 1138

Pancuronium Bromide Injection (Prolongation of the neuromuscular blockade).

No products indexed under this heading.

Probenecid (Concomitant administration prolongs half-life of piperacillin by 21% and of tazobactam by 71%). Products include:

Benemid Tablets 1611
ColBENEMID Tablets 1622

Rocuronium Bromide (Prolongation of the neuromuscular blockade). Products include:

Zemuron 1830

Streptomycin Sulfate (Concomitant administration can result in substantial inactivation of the aminoglycoside). Products include:

Streptomycin Sulfate Injection 2208

Tobramycin (When co-administration with tobramycin, the area under the curve, renal clearance, and urinary recovery of tobramycin were decreased by 11%, 32% and 38%). Products include:

AKTOB .... ◉ 206
TobraDex Ophthalmic Suspension and Ointment.. 473
Tobrex Ophthalmic Ointment and Solution .... ◉ 229

Tobramycin Sulfate (When co-administration with tobramycin, the area under the curve, renal clearance, and urinary recovery of tobramycin were decreased by 11%, 32% and 38%). Products include:

Nebcin Vials, Hyporets & ADD-Vantage 1464
Tobramycin Sulfate Injection 968

Vecuronium Bromide (Prolongation of the neuromuscular blockade). Products include:

Norcuron 1826

Warfarin Sodium (Coagulation parameters should be tested more frequently and monitored regularly during simultaneous administration; effect of concurrent use is not specified). Products include:

Coumadin 926

ZOSYN PHARMACY BULK PACKAGE

(Piperacillin Sodium, Tazobactam Sodium) 1422

May interact with aminoglycosides, anticoagulants, nondepolarizing neuromuscular blocking agents, and certain other agents. Compounds in these categories include:

Amikacin Sulfate (Concomitant administration can result in substantial inactivation of the aminoglycoside). Products include:

Amikacin Sulfate Injection, USP 960
Amikin Injectable 501

Atracurium Besylate (Prolongation of the neuromuscular blockade). Products include:

Tracrium Injection 1183

Dalteparin Sodium (Coagulation parameters should be tested more frequently and monitored regularly during simultaneous administration; effect of concurrent use is not specified). Products include:

Fragmin 1954

Dicumarol (Coagulation parameters should be tested more frequently and monitored regularly during simultaneous administration; effect of concurrent use is not specified).

No products indexed under this heading.

Enoxaparin (Coagulation parameters should be tested more frequently and monitored regularly during simultaneous administration; effect of concurrent use is not specified). Products include:

Lovenox Injection 2020

Gentamicin Sulfate (Concomitant administration can result in substantial inactivation of the aminoglycoside). Products include:

Garamycin Injectable 2360
Genoptic Sterile Ophthalmic Solution... ◉ 243
Genoptic Sterile Ophthalmic Ointment .... ◉ 243
Gentacidin Ointment .... ◉ 264
Gentacidin Solution................................ ◉ 264
Gentak .... ◉ 208
Pred-G Liquifilm Sterile Ophthalmic Suspension .... ◉ 251
Pred-G S.O.P. Sterile Ophthalmic Ointment .... ◉ 252

Heparin Calcium (Coagulation parameters should be tested more frequently and monitored regularly during simultaneous administration; effect of concurrent use is not specified).

No products indexed under this heading.

Heparin Sodium (Coagulation parameters should be tested more frequently and monitored regularly during simultaneous administration; effect of concurrent use is not specified). Products include:

Heparin Lock Flush Solution 2725
Heparin Sodium Injection.................... 2726
Heparin Sodium Injection, USP, Sterile Solution 2615

Heparin Sodium Vials........................... 1441

Kanamycin Sulfate (Concomitant administration can result in substantial inactivation of the aminoglycoside).

No products indexed under this heading.

Metocurine Iodide (Prolongation of the neuromuscular blockade). Products include:

Metubine Iodide Vials............................. 916

Mivacurium Chloride (Prolongation of the neuromuscular blockade). Products include:

Mivacron 1138

Pancuronium Bromide Injection (Prolongation of the neuromuscular blockade).

No products indexed under this heading.

Probenecid (Concomitant administration prolongs half-life of piperacillin by 21% and of tazobactam by 71%). Products include:

Benemid Tablets 1611
ColBENEMID Tablets 1622

Rocuronium Bromide (Prolongation of the neuromuscular blockade). Products include:

Zemuron 1830

Streptomycin Sulfate (Concomitant administration can result in substantial inactivation of the aminoglycoside). Products include:

Streptomycin Sulfate Injection 2208

Tobramycin (When co-administration with tobramycin, the area under the curve, renal clearance, and urinary recovery of tobramycin were decreased by 11%, 32% and 38%). Products include:

AKTOB .... ◉ 206
TobraDex Ophthalmic Suspension and Ointment.. 473
Tobrex Ophthalmic Ointment and Solution .... ◉ 229

Tobramycin Sulfate (When co-administration with tobramycin, the area under the curve, renal clearance, and urinary recovery of tobramycin were decreased by 11%, 32% and 38%). Products include:

Nebcin Vials, Hyporets & ADD-Vantage 1464
Tobramycin Sulfate Injection 968

Vecuronium Bromide (Prolongation of the neuromuscular blockade). Products include:

Norcuron 1826

Warfarin Sodium (Coagulation parameters should be tested more frequently and monitored regularly during simultaneous administration; effect of concurrent use is not specified). Products include:

Coumadin 926

ZOVIRAX CAPSULES

(Acyclovir)...1219

May interact with:

Nephrotoxic Drugs (Increased risk of renal dysfunction).

Probenecid (Increases mean half-life and the AUC when co-administered with intravenous acyclovir). Products include:

Benemid Tablets 1611
ColBENEMID Tablets 1622

ZOVIRAX OINTMENT 5%

(Acyclovir)...1223
None cited in PDR database.

ZOVIRAX STERILE POWDER

(Acyclovir Sodium) 1223

IMPORTANT NOTE: Always consult each drug listing in the patient's regimen for possible interactions.

Zovirax Sterile Powder — Interactions Index — 1196

May interact with cytotoxic drugs and certain other agents. Compounds in these categories include:

Bleomycin Sulfate (Use with caution in patients who have manifested prior neurologic reactions to cytotoxic drugs). Products include:
Blenoxane ... 692

Daunorubicin Hydrochloride (Use with caution in patients who have manifested prior neurologic reactions to cytotoxic drugs). Products include:
Cerubidine ... 795

Doxorubicin Hydrochloride (Use with caution in patients who have manifested prior neurologic reactions to cytotoxic drugs). Products include:
Adriamycin PFS ... 1947
Adriamycin RDF ... 1947
Doxorubicin Astra ... 540
Rubex ... 712

Fluorouracil (Use with caution in patients who have manifested prior neurologic reactions to cytotoxic drugs). Products include:
Efudex ... 2113
Fluoroplex Topical Solution & Cream 1% ... 479
Fluorouracil Injection ... 2116

Hydroxyurea (Use with caution in patients who have manifested prior neurologic reactions to cytotoxic drugs). Products include:
Hydrea Capsules ... 696

Interferon alfa-2A, Recombinant (Concomitant administration requires caution). Products include:
Roferon-A Injection ... 2145

Interferon alfa-2B, Recombinant (Concomitant administration requires caution). Products include:
Intron A ... 2364

Methotrexate Sodium (Use with caution in patients who have manifested prior neurologic reactions to cytotoxic drugs; use with caution in patients receiving intrathecal methotrexate). Products include;
Methotrexate Sodium Tablets, Injection, for Injection and LPF Injection ... 1275

Mitotane (Use with caution in patients who have manifested prior neurologic reactions to cytotoxic drugs). Products include:
Lysodren ... 698

Mitoxantrone Hydrochloride (Use with caution in patients who have manifested prior neurologic reactions to cytotoxic drugs). Products include:
Novantrone ... 1279

Probenecid (Increases mean half-life of Zovirax). Products include:
Benemid Tablets ... 1611
ColBENEMID Tablets ... 1622

Procarbazine Hydrochloride (Use with caution in patients who have manifested prior neurologic reactions to cytotoxic drugs). Products include:
Matulane Capsules ... 2131

Tamoxifen Citrate (Use with caution in patients who have manifested prior neurologic reactions to cytotoxic drugs). Products include:
Nolvadex Tablets ... 2841

Vincristine Sulfate (Use with caution in patients who have manifested prior neurologic reactions to cytotoxic drugs). Products include:
Oncovin Solution Vials & Hyporets 1466

ZOVIRAX SUSPENSION
(Acyclovir) ... 1219
See **Zovirax Capsules**

ZOVIRAX TABLETS
(Acyclovir) ... 1219
See **Zovirax Capsules**

ZYDONE CAPSULES
(Hydrocodone Bitartrate, Acetaminophen) ... 949
May interact with narcotic analgesics, antipsychotic agents, tranquilizers, central nervous system depressants, monoamine oxidase inhibitors, tricyclic antidepressants, anticholinergics, phenothiazines, and certain other agents. Compounds in these categories include:

Alfentanil Hydrochloride (Additive CNS depression). Products include:
Alfenta Injection ... 1286

Alprazolam (Additive CNS depression). Products include:
Xanax Tablets ... 2649

Amitriptyline Hydrochloride (Increased effect of either drug). Products include:
Elavil ... 2838
Endep Tablets ... 2174
Etrafon ... 2355
Limbitrol ... 2180
Triavil Tablets ... 1757

Amoxapine (Increased effect of either drug). Products include:
Asendin Tablets ... 1369

Aprobarbital (Additive CNS depression).
No products indexed under this heading.

Atropine Sulfate (May produce paralytic). Products include:
Arco-Lase Plus Tablets ... 512
Atrohist Plus Tablets ... 454
Atropine Sulfate Sterile Ophthalmic Solution ... ◉ 233
Donnatal ... 2060
Donnatal Extentabs ... 2061
Donnatal Tablets ... 2060
Lomotil ... 2439
Motofen Tablets ... 784
Urised Tablets ... 1964

Belladonna Alkaloids (May produce paralytic ileus). Products include:
Bellergal-S Tablets ... 2250
Hyland's Bed Wetting Tablets ... ▣ 828
Hyland's EnurAid Tablets ... ▣ 829
Hyland's Teething Tablets ... ▣ 830

Benztropine Mesylate (May produce paralytic ileus). Products include:
Cogentin ... 1621

Biperiden Hydrochloride (May produce paralytic ileus). Products include:
Akineton ... 1333

Buprenorphine (Additive CNS depression). Products include:
Buprenex Injectable ... 2006

Buspirone Hydrochloride (Additive CNS depression). Products include:
BuSpar ... 737

Butabarbital (Additive CNS depression).
No products indexed under this heading.

Butalbital (Additive CNS depression). Products include:
Esgic-plus Tablets ... 1013
Fioricet Tablets ... 2258
Fioricet with Codeine Capsules ... 2260
Fiorinal Capsules ... 2261
Fiorinal with Codeine Capsules ... 2262
Fiorinal Tablets ... 2261
Phrenilin ... 785
Sedapap Tablets 50 mg/650 mg .. 1543

Chlordiazepoxide (Additive CNS depression). Products include:
Libritabs Tablets ... 2177
Limbitrol ... 2180

Chlordiazepoxide Hydrochloride (Additive CNS depression). Products include:
Librax Capsules ... 2176
Librium Capsules ... 2178
Librium Injectable ... 2179

Chlorpromazine (Reduction or increase in amount of narcotic needed for pain relief; additive CNS depression). Products include:
Thorazine Suppositories ... 2523

Chlorpromazine Hydrochloride (Reduction or increase in amount of narcotic needed for pain relief; additive CNS depression). Products include:
Thorazine ... 2523

Chlorprothixene (Additive CNS depression).
No products indexed under this heading.

Chlorprothixene Hydrochloride (Additive CNS depression).
No products indexed under this heading.

Clidinium Bromide (May produce paralytic ileus). Products include:
Librax Capsules ... 2176
Quarzan Capsules ... 2181

Clomipramine Hydrochloride (Increased effect of either drug). Products include:
Anafranil Capsules ... 803

Clorazepate Dipotassium (Additive CNS depression). Products include:
Tranxene ... 451

Clozapine (Additive CNS depression). Products include:
Clozaril Tablets ... 2252

Codeine Phosphate (Additive CNS depression). Products include:
Actifed with Codeine Cough Syrup.. 1067
Brontex ... 1981
Deconsal C Expectorant Syrup ... 456
Deconsal Pediatric Syrup ... 457
Dimetane-DC Cough Syrup ... 2059
Empirin with Codeine Tablets ... 1093
Fioricet with Codeine Capsules ... 2260
Fiorinal with Codeine Capsules ... 2262
Isoclor Expectorant ... 990
Novahistine DH ... 2462
Novahistine Expectorant ... 2463
Nucofed ... 2051
Phenergan with Codeine ... 2777
Phenergan VC with Codeine ... 2781
Robitussin A-C Syrup ... 2073
Robitussin-DAC Syrup ... 2074
Ryna ... ▣ 841
Soma Compound w/Codeine Tablets ... 2676
Tussi-Organidin NR Liquid and S NR Liquid ... 2677
Tylenol with Codeine ... 1583

Desflurane (Additive CNS depression). Products include:
Suprane ... 1813

Desipramine Hydrochloride (Increased effect of either drug). Products include:
Norpramin Tablets ... 1526

Dezocine (Additive CNS depression). Products include:
Dalgan Injection ... 538

Diazepam (Additive CNS depression). Products include:
Dizac ... 1809
Valium Injectable ... 2182
Valium Tablets ... 2183
Valrelease Capsules ... 2169

Dicyclomine Hydrochloride (May produce paralytic ileus). Products include:
Bentyl ... 1501

Doxepin Hydrochloride (Increased effect of either drug). Products include:
Sinequan ... 2205
Zonalon Cream ... 1055

Droperidol (Additive CNS depression). Products include:
Inapsine Injection ... 1296

Enflurane (Additive CNS depression).
No products indexed under this heading.

Estazolam (Additive CNS depression). Products include:
ProSom Tablets ... 449

Ethchlorvynol (Additive CNS depression). Products include:
Placidyl Capsules ... 448

Ethinamate (Additive CNS depression).
No products indexed under this heading.

Fentanyl (Additive CNS depression). Products include:
Duragesic Transdermal System ... 1288

Fentanyl Citrate (Additive CNS depression). Products include:
Sublimaze Injection ... 1307

Fluphenazine Decanoate (Reduction or increase in amount of narcotic needed for pain relief; additive CNS depression). Products include:
Prolixin Decanoate ... 509

Fluphenazine Enanthate (Reduction or increase in amount of narcotic needed for pain relief; additive CNS depression). Products include:
Prolixin Enanthate ... 509

Fluphenazine Hydrochloride (Reduction or increase in amount of narcotic needed for pain relief; additive CNS depression). Products include:
Prolixin ... 509

Flurazepam Hydrochloride (Additive CNS depression). Products include:
Dalmane Capsules ... 2173

Furazolidone (Increased effect of either drug). Products include:
Furoxone ... 2046

Glutethimide (Additive CNS depression).
No products indexed under this heading.

Glycopyrrolate (May produce paralytic ileus). Products include:
Robinul Forte Tablets ... 2072
Robinul Injectable ... 2072
Robinul Tablets ... 2072

Haloperidol (Additive CNS depression). Products include:
Haldol Injection, Tablets and Concentrate ... 1575

Haloperidol Decanoate (Additive CNS depression). Products include:
Haldol Decanoate ... 1577

Hydrocodone Polistirex (Additive CNS depression). Products include:
Tussionex Pennkinetic Extended-Release Suspension ... 998

Hydroxyzine Hydrochloride (Additive CNS depression). Products include:
Atarax Tablets & Syrup ... 2185
Marax Tablets & DF Syrup ... 2200
Vistaril Intramuscular Solution ... 2216

Hyoscyamine (May produce paralytic ileus). Products include:
Cystospaz Tablets ... 1963
Urised Tablets ... 1964

Hyoscyamine Sulfate (May produce paralytic ileus). Products include:
Arco-Lase Plus Tablets ... 512
Atrohist Plus Tablets ... 454
Cystospaz-M Capsules ... 1963
Donnatal ... 2060
Donnatal Extentabs ... 2061
Donnatal Tablets ... 2060
Kutrase Capsules ... 2402
Levsin/Levsinex/Levbid ... 2405

(▣ Described in PDR For Nonprescription Drugs) (◉ Described in PDR For Ophthalmology)

1197 Interactions Index Zyloprim

Imipramine Hydrochloride (Increased effect of either drug). Products include:
Tofranil Ampuls 854
Tofranil Tablets 856
Imipramine Pamoate (Increased effect of either drug). Products include:
Tofranil-PM Capsules 857
Ipratropium Bromide (May produce paralytic ileus). Products include:
Atrovent Inhalation Aerosol 671
Atrovent Inhalation Solution 673
Isocarboxazid (Increased effect of either drug).
No products indexed under this heading.
Isoflurane (Additive CNS depression).
No products indexed under this heading.
Ketamine Hydrochloride (Additive CNS depression).
No products indexed under this heading.
Levomethadyl Acetate Hydrochloride (Additive CNS depression). Products include:
Orlamm 2239
Levorphanol Tartrate (Additive CNS depression). Products include:
Levo-Dromoran 2129
Lithium Carbonate (Additive CNS depression). Products include:
Eskalith 2485
Lithium Carbonate Capsules & Tablets 2230
Lithonate/Lithotabs/Lithobid 2543
Lithium Citrate (Additive CNS depression).
No products indexed under this heading.
Lorazepam (Additive CNS depression). Products include:
Ativan Injection 2698
Ativan Tablets 2700
Loxapine Hydrochloride (Additive CNS depression). Products include:
Loxitane 1378
Loxapine Succinate (Additive CNS depression). Products include:
Loxitane Capsules 1378
Maprotiline Hydrochloride (Increased effect of either drug). Products include:
Ludiomil Tablets 843
Mepenzolate Bromide (May produce paralytic ileus).
No products indexed under this heading.
Meperidine Hydrochloride (Additive CNS depression). Products include:
Demerol 2308
Mepergan Injection 2753
Mephobarbital (Additive CNS depression). Products include:
Mebaral Tablets 2322
Meprobamate (Additive CNS depression). Products include:
Miltown Tablets 2672
PMB 200 and PMB 400 2783
Mesoridazine Besylate (Reduction or increase in amount of narcotic needed for pain relief; additive CNS depression). Products include:
Serentil 684
Methadone Hydrochloride (Additive CNS depression). Products include:
Methadone Hydrochloride Oral Concentrate 2233
Methadone Hydrochloride Oral Solution & Tablets 2235
Methohexital Sodium (Additive CNS depression). Products include:
Brevital Sodium Vials 1429
Methotrimeprazine (Reduction or increase in amount of narcotic needed for pain relief; additive CNS depression). Products include:
Levoprome 1274
Methoxyflurane (Additive CNS depression).
No products indexed under this heading.
Midazolam Hydrochloride (Additive CNS depression). Products include:
Versed Injection 2170
Molindone Hydrochloride (Additive CNS depression). Products include:
Moban Tablets and Concentrate 1048
Morphine Sulfate (Additive CNS depression). Products include:
Astramorph/PF Injection, USP (Preservative-Free) 535
Duramorph 962
Infumorph 200 and Infumorph 500 Sterile Solutions 965
MS Contin Tablets 1994
MSIR 1997
Oramorph SR (Morphine Sulfate Sustained Release Tablets) 2236
RMS Suppositories 2657
Roxanol 2243
Nortriptyline Hydrochloride (Increased effect of either drug). Products include:
Pamelor 2280
Opium Alkaloids (Additive CNS depression).
No products indexed under this heading.
Oxazepam (Additive CNS depression). Products include:
Serax Capsules 2810
Serax Tablets 2810
Oxybutynin Chloride (May produce paralytic ileus). Products include:
Ditropan 1516
Oxycodone Hydrochloride (Additive CNS depression). Products include:
Percocet Tablets 938
Percodan Tablets 939
Percodan-Demi Tablets 940
Roxicodone Tablets, Oral Solution & Intensol (Oxycodone) 2244
Tylox Capsules 1584
Pentobarbital Sodium (Additive CNS depression). Products include:
Nembutal Sodium Capsules 436
Nembutal Sodium Solution 438
Nembutal Sodium Suppositories 440
Perphenazine (Reduction or increase in amount of narcotic needed for pain relief; additive CNS depression). Products include:
Etrafon 2355
Triavil Tablets 1757
Trilafon 2389
Phenelzine Sulfate (Increased effect of either drug). Products include:
Nardil 1920
Phenobarbital (Additive CNS depression). Products include:
Arco-Lase Plus Tablets 512
Bellergal-S Tablets 2250
Donnatal 2060
Donnatal Extentabs 2061
Donnatal Tablets 2060
Phenobarbital Elixir and Tablets 1469
Quadrinal Tablets 1350
Pimozide (Additive CNS depression). Products include:
Orap Tablets 1050
Prazepam (Additive CNS depression).
No products indexed under this heading.
Prochlorperazine (Reduction or increase in amount of narcotic needed for pain relief; additive CNS depression). Products include:
Compazine 2470
Procyclidine Hydrochloride (May produce paralytic ileus). Products include:
Kemadrin Tablets 1112
Promethazine Hydrochloride (Reduction or increase in amount of narcotic needed for pain relief; additive CNS depression). Products include:
Mepergan Injection 2753
Phenergan with Codeine 2777
Phenergan with Dextromethorphan 2778
Phenergan Injection 2773
Phenergan Suppositories 2775
Phenergan Syrup 2774
Phenergan Tablets 2775
Phenergan VC 2779
Phenergan VC with Codeine 2781
Propantheline Bromide (May produce paralytic ileus). Products include:
Pro-Banthīne Tablets 2052
Propofol (Additive CNS depression). Products include:
Diprivan Injection 2833
Propoxyphene Hydrochloride (Additive CNS depression). Products include:
Darvon 1435
Wygesic Tablets 2827
Propoxyphene Napsylate (Additive CNS depression). Products include:
Darvon-N/Darvocet-N 1433
Protriptyline Hydrochloride (Increased effect of either drug). Products include:
Vivactil Tablets 1774
Quazepam (Additive CNS depression). Products include:
Doral Tablets 2664
Risperidone (Additive CNS depression). Products include:
Risperdal 1301
Scopolamine (May produce paralytic ileus). Products include:
Transderm Scōp Transdermal Therapeutic System 869
Scopolamine Hydrobromide (May produce paralytic ileus). Products include:
Atrohist Plus Tablets 454
Donnatal 2060
Donnatal Extentabs 2061
Donnatal Tablets 2060
Secobarbital Sodium (Additive CNS depression). Products include:
Seconal Sodium Pulvules 1474
Selegiline Hydrochloride (Increased effect of either drug). Products include:
Eldepryl Tablets 2550
Sufentanil Citrate (Additive CNS depression). Products include:
Sufenta Injection 1309
Temazepam (Additive CNS depression). Products include:
Restoril Capsules 2284
Thiamylal Sodium (Additive CNS depression).
No products indexed under this heading.
Thioridazine Hydrochloride (Reduction or increase in amount of narcotic needed for pain relief; additive CNS depression). Products include:
Mellaril 2269
Thiothixene (Additive CNS depression). Products include:
Navane Capsules and Concentrate 2201
Navane Intramuscular 2202
Tranylcypromine Sulfate (Increased effect of either drug). Products include:
Parnate Tablets 2503
Triazolam (Additive CNS depression). Products include:
Halcion Tablets 2611
Tridihexethyl Chloride (May produce paralytic ileus).
No products indexed under this heading.
Trifluoperazine Hydrochloride (Additive CNS depression). Products include:
Stelazine 2514
Trihexyphenidyl Hydrochloride (May produce paralytic ileus). Products include:
Artane 1368
Trimipramine Maleate (Increased effect of either drug). Products include:
Surmontil Capsules 2811
Zolpidem Tartrate (Additive CNS depression). Products include:
Ambien Tablets 2416

Food Interactions

Alcohol (Additive CNS depression).

ZYLOPRIM TABLETS
(Allopurinol) 1226
May interact with antigout agents, thiazides, and certain other agents. Compounds in these categories include:

Amoxicillin Trihydrate (Increased frequency of skin rash). Products include:
Amoxil 2464
Augmentin 2468
Ampicillin Sodium (Increased frequency of skin rash). Products include:
Unasyn 2212
Azathioprine (Enhanced therapeutic response). Products include:
Imuran 1110
Bendroflumethiazide (May enhance allopurinol toxicity).
No products indexed under this heading.
Chlorothiazide (May enhance allopurinol toxicity). Products include:
Aldoclor Tablets 1598
Diupres Tablets 1650
Diuril Oral 1653
Chlorothiazide Sodium (May enhance allopurinol toxicity). Products include:
Diuril Sodium Intravenous 1652
Chlorpropamide (Prolonged half-life). Products include:
Diabinese Tablets 1935
Cyclophosphamide (Enhanced bone marrow suppression). Products include:
Cytoxan 694
NEOSAR Lyophilized/Neosar 1959
Cyclosporine (Rare reports indicate that cyclosporine levels may be increased during concomitant treatment with allopurinol). Products include:
Neoral 2276
Sandimmune 2286
Dicumarol (Prolonged half-life).
No products indexed under this heading.
Hydrochlorothiazide (May enhance allopurinol toxicity). Products include:
Aldactazide 2413
Aldoril Tablets 1604
Apresazide Capsules 808
Capozide 742
Dyazide 2479

IMPORTANT NOTE: Always consult each drug listing in the patient's regimen for possible interactions.

Zyloprim

Esidrix Tablets 821
Esimil Tablets 822
HydroDIURIL Tablets 1674
Hydropres Tablets................................... 1675
Hyzaar Tablets 1677
Inderide Tablets 2732
Inderide LA Long Acting Capsules .. 2734
Lopressor HCT Tablets 832
Lotensin HCT... 837
Maxzide 1380
Moduretic Tablets 1705
Oretic Tablets 443
Prinzide Tablets 1737
Ser-Ap-Es Tablets 849
Timolide Tablets..................................... 1748
Vaseretic Tablets 1765
Zestoretic 2850
Ziac 1415

Hydroflumethiazide (May enhance allopurinol toxicity). Products include:

Diucardin Tablets................................... 2718

Mercaptopurine (Enhanced therapeutic response). Products include:

Purinethol Tablets 1156

Methylclothiazide (May enhance allopurinol toxicity). Products include:

Enduron Tablets...................................... 420

Polythiazide (May enhance allopurinol toxicity). Products include:

Minizide Capsules 1938

Probenecid (Decreased excretion of oxypurines and increased excretion of urinary uric acid). Products include:

Benemid Tablets 1611
ColBENEMID Tablets 1622

Sulfinpyrazone (Decreased excretion of oxypurines and increased excretion of urinary uric acid). Products include:

Anturane 807

Tolbutamide (Metabolism of tolbutamide may be affected).

No products indexed under this heading.

ZYMACAP CAPSULES

(Vitamins with Minerals) .... ✦◻ 772
None cited in PDR database.

ZYMASE CAPSULES

(Pancrelipase) 1834
None cited in PDR database.

(✦◻ Described in PDR For Nonprescription Drugs) (◆ Described in PDR For Ophthalmology)

SECTION 2

FOOD INTERACTIONS CROSS-REFERENCE

In this section, drug/food and drug/alcohol interactions listed in the preceding index are cross-referenced by dietary item. Under each entry is an alphabetical list, by brand name, of drugs said to interact with the item. A brief description of the interaction follows each brand, along with the page number of the underlying text. Page numbers refer to the 1996 editions of *PDR* and *PDR For Ophthalmology* and the 1995 edition of

PDR For Nonprescription Drugs, which is published later each year. A key to the symbols denoting the companion volumes appears in the bottom margin.

Entries in this section are limited to drug/food and drug/alcohol interactions cited in official prescribing information as published by *PDR*.

Alcohol

Actifed Allergy Daytime/Nighttime Caplets (Increases drowsiness effect).... **⊞** 844

Actifed Plus Caplets (Increases drowsiness effect)........................... **⊞** 845

Actifed Plus Tablets (Increases drowsiness effect)........................... **⊞** 845

Actifed with Codeine Cough Syrup (Increased CNS depression).......... 1067

Actifed Sinus Daytime/Nighttime Tablets and Caplets (Increases the drowsiness effect).................. **⊞** 846

Actifed Syrup (Increases drowsiness effect)........................... **⊞** 846

Actifed Tablets (Increases drowsiness effect)........................... **⊞** 844

Adipex-P Tablets and Capsules (May result in adverse drug interaction)... 1048

Aldoclor Tablets (Aggravates orthostatic hypotension).................. 1598

Aldoril Tablets (Aggravates orthostatic hypotension).................. 1604

Aleve (Concurrent use should be undertaken with the physician's consultation)... 1975

Alka-Seltzer Plus Cold Medicine (May increase drowsiness effect).. **⊞** 705

Alka-Seltzer Plus Cold Medicine Liqui-Gels (May increase drowsiness effect; consult your doctor).. **⊞** 706

Alka-Seltzer Plus Cold & Cough Medicine (Increases drowsiness effect)........................... **⊞** 708

Alka-Seltzer Plus Cold & Cough Medicine Liqui-Gels (May increase drowsiness effect; consult your doctor)..................... **⊞** 705

Alka-Seltzer Plus Night-Time Cold Medicine (May increase the drowsiness effect; avoid concurrent use)................................ **⊞** 707

Alka-Seltzer Plus Night-Time Cold Medicine Liqui-Gels (May increase drowsiness effect; consult your doctor)..................... **⊞** 706

Alka Seltzer Plus Sinus Medicine (May increase the drowsiness effect; avoid concurrent use).... **⊞** 707

Allerest Maximum Strength Tablets (Concurrent use produces additive effects).......... **⊞** 627

Ambien Tablets (Co-administration produces additive effects on psychomotor performance)............ 2416

Anafranil Capsules (Anafranil may exaggerate patients' response to alcohol).. 803

Anexsia 5/500 Elixir (Exhibits an additive CNS depression)................. 1781

Anexsia 5/500 Tablets (Exhibits an additive CNS depression)....... 1782

Antabuse Tablets (Antabuse plus alcohol, even small amounts, produces flushing, throbbing in head and neck, respiratory difficulty, headache and other serious reactions including convulsions and death; concurrent use is contraindicated)................................ 2695

Antivert, Antivert/25 Tablets, & Antivert/50 Tablets (Concurrent use should be avoided).................... 2185

Apresazide Capsules (May potentiate orthostatic hypotension).. 808

Arthritis Foundation Aspirin Free Caplets (Patients consuming 3 or more drinks per day on a regular basis should consult their physician for advice on when and how they should take acetaminophen-containing products).. **⊞** 673

Arthritis Foundation NightTime Caplets (Patients consuming 3 or more alcohol-containing drinks per day should consult their physician for advice on when and how they should take acetaminophen-containing products).. **⊞** 674

Asendin Tablets (Enhanced response to alcohol)........................ 1369

Astramorph/PF Injection, USP (Preservative-Free) (Potentiation of depressant effects of morphine)... 535

Atarax Tablets & Syrup (Increased effect of alcohol).............................. 2185

Ativan Injection (Additive CNS depressant effects)........................... 2698

Ativan Tablets (Depressant effect) 2700

Atrohist Pediatric Capsules (Potential for additive effects)..... 453

Atrohist Pediatric Suspension (Potential for additive central nervous system effects)..................... 454

Atrohist Plus Tablets (Possible additive drowsiness effects).......... 454

BC Cold Powder Multi-Symptom Formula (Cold-Sinus-Allergy) (Concurrent use not recommended; consult your doctor).. **⊞** 609

Extra Strength Bayer PM Aspirin (Avoid concurrent use)................ **⊞** 713

Bayer Select Night Time Pain Relief Formula (Avoid concurrent use).............................. **⊞** 716

Bellergal-S Tablets (Combined use may result in a potentiation of the depressant action)...................... 2250

Benadryl Allergy Decongestant Liquid Medication (May increase drowsiness effect; avoid concurrent use).................. **⊞** 848

Benadryl Allergy Decongestant Tablets (Increases the drowsiness effect; avoid concomitant use)........................... **⊞** 848

Benadryl Allergy Liquid Medication (Increases drowsiness effect)........................... **⊞** 849

Benadryl Allergy Kapseals (May increase drowsiness effect)........ **⊞** 848

Benadryl Allergy Sinus Headache Formula Caplets (May increase drowsiness effect)........................... **⊞** 849

Benadryl Capsules (Additive effects).. 1898

Benadryl Dye-Free Allergy Liqui-gel Softgels (May increase the drowsiness effect) **⊞** 850

Benadryl Dye-Free Allergy Liquid Medication (May increase the drowsiness effect)........................... **⊞** 850

Benadryl Parenteral (Additive effects).. 1898

Bonine Tablets (May increase drowsiness effect).............................. 1933

Brevital Sodium Vials (Additive effect).. 1429

Bromfed Capsules (Extended-Release) (Additive effects).. 1785

Bromfed Syrup (Effect not specified)... **⊞** 733

Bromfed-DM Cough Syrup (Potential for additive effects)...... 1786

Brontex (Potential for greater sedation).. 1981

Buprenex Injectable (Increased CNS depression).............................. 2006

BuSpar (Concomitant use should be avoided)... 737

Butisol Sodium Elixir & Tablets (Additive CNS depressant effects).. 2660

(**⊞** Described in PDR For Nonprescription Drugs) (◉ Described in PDR For Ophthalmology)

Alcohol **Food Interactions Cross-Reference** 1200

Capozide (Potentation of orthostatic hypotension) 742
Catapres Tablets (Enhanced CNS-depressive effects) 674
Catapres-TTS (Enhanced CNS-depressive effects) 675
Cefobid Intravenous/Intramuscular (When ingested within 72 hours, flushing, sweating, headache, and tachycardia have been reported) 2189
Cefobid Pharmacy Bulk Package - Not for Direct Infusion (A disulfiram-like reaction characterized by flushing, sweating, headache, and tachycardia has been reported when alcohol was ingested within 72 hours after Cefobid administration) 2192
Cefotan (When ingested within 72 hours after Cefotan administration may cause disulfiram-like reactions, including flushing, headache, sweating and tachycardia) 2829
Cerose DM (May increase the drowsiness effect; avoid concurrent use) ▣ 878
Cheracol Sinus (May increase drowsiness effect) ▣ 768
Children's Vicks DayQuil Allergy Relief (May increase drowsiness effect) ▣ 757
Children's Vicks NyQuil Cold/Cough Relief (May increase drowsiness effect) ▣ 758
Chlor-Trimeton Allergy Decongestant Tablets (Increases the drowsiness effect) ▣ 799
Chlor-Trimeton Allergy Tablets (Do not use concomitantly) ▣ 798
Clozaril Tablets (Caution is advised with concomitant use) 2252
Codiclear DH Syrup (Additive CNS depression) 791
Combipres Tablets (Orthostatic hypotension; enhanced CNS-depressive effects) 677
Comhist LA Capsules (Sedative effects additive to CNS depressant effects) 2038
Compazine Tablets (Phenothiazines may intensify or prolong the action of other central nervous system depressants) 2470
Comtrex Multi-Symptom Cold Reliever Tablets/Caplets/Liqui-Gels/Liquid (May increase drowsiness effect) ▣ 615
Allergy-Sinus Comtrex Multi-Symptom Allergy-Sinus Formula Tablets (Increases drowsiness effect) ▣ 617
Contac Continuous Action Nasal Decongestant/Antihistamine 12 Hour Capsules (May increase drowsiness effect; concurrent use should be avoided) ▣ 813
Contac Day & Night Cold/Flu Night Caplets (Increases drowsiness effect) ▣ 812
Contac Maximum Strength Continuous Action Decongestant/Antihistamine 12 Hour Caplets (May increase drowsiness effect; concurrent use should be avoided) ▣ 813
Contac Night Allergy/Sinus Caplets (May increase the drowsiness effect; avoid concurrent use) ▣ 812
Contac Severe Cold and Flu Formula Caplets (May increase drowsiness effect; concurrent use should be avoided) ▣ 814
Coricidin 'D' Decongestant Tablets (May increase drowsiness effect) ▣ 800
Coumadin Tablets (Decreased or increased prothrombin time response) 926
Cytadren Tablets (Effects of alcohol potentiated) 819
D.A. Chewable Tablets (Potential for additive effects) 951
DHCplus Capsules (Potential for additive CNS depression) 1993
Dalgan Injection (Concomitant administration may have an additive effect) 538
Dalmane Capsules (Additive effects; potential for continuation of interaction after discontinuance of flurazepam) 2173
Darvocet-N 50 Tablets (Additive CNS depression) 1433
Darvon Compound-65 Pulvules (Additive CNS-depressant effect) 1435
Deconamine CX Cough and Cold Liquid and Tablets (Hydrocodone may potentiate CNS depressant effects) 1319
Deconamine SR Capsules (Additive effects; potentiates the sedative effects of chlorpheniramine) 1320
Deconsal C Expectorant Syrup (Effects of concurrent use not specified) 456
Deconsal Pediatric Syrup (Potential for unspecified CNS effect) 457
Demerol Hydrochloride Carpuject (Respiratory depression, hypotension, profound sedation or coma) 2308
Demser Capsules (Additive sedative effects) 1649
Depakene Capsules (Depakene may potentiate CNS depressant activity) 413
Depakote Tablets (May result in additive CNS depression) 415
Deponit NTG Transdermal Delivery System (Additive vasodilating effects) 2397
Desyrel and Desyrel Dividose (Enhanced response to alcohol) 503
DiaBeta Tablets (Potential for hypoglycemia) 1239
Diabinese Tablets (Potential for disulfiram-like reaction) 1935
Dilantin Infatabs (Increased phenytoin serum levels with acute alcohol intake; decreased levels with chronic alcohol intake) 1908
Dilantin Kapseals (Increased phenytoin serum levels with acute alcohol intake; decreased levels with chronic alcohol intake) 1906
Dilantin Parenteral (Increased phenytoin levels with acute alcohol intake; decreased levels with chronic alcohol intake) 1910
Dilantin-125 Suspension (Increased phenytoin serum levels with acute alcohol intake; decreased levels with chronic alcohol intake) 1911
Dilatrate-SR (Enhanced hypotensive effects) 2398
Dilaudid Ampules (Additive CNS depression) 1335
Dilaudid Cough Syrup (Additive CNS depression) 1336
Dilaudid-HP Injection (Additive depressant effects) 1337
Dilaudid Oral Liquid (May exhibit an additive CNS depression) 1339
Dimetane-DC Cough Syrup (Additive effects) 2059
Dimetane-DX Cough Syrup (Additive effect) 2059
Dimetapp Elixir (May increase drowsiness effect) ▣ 773
Dimetapp Extentabs (Do not use concomitantly) ▣ 774
Dimetapp Liqui-Gels (Increases drowsiness effect; avoid concurrent use) ▣ 775
Dimetapp DM Elixir (Increases drowsiness effect; avoid concurrent use) ▣ 774
Ditropan Tablets (Enhances the drowsiness effect) 1516
Diupres Tablets (Orthostatic hypotension may be aggravated) 1650
Diuril Oral Suspension (Orthostatic hypotension may be aggravated) 1653
Diuril Sodium Intravenous (Potentiation of orthostatic hypotension) 1652
Dizac (Potentiates the action of diazepam; concomitant use increases depression with increased risk of apnea) 1809
Extra Strength Doan's P.M. (Avoid concomitant use) ▣ 633
Doral Tablets (Additive CNS depressant effects) 2664
Dramamine Tablets (May increase drowsiness effect) ▣ 836
Dramamine II Tablets (May increase drowsiness effect) ▣ 837
Drixoral Cold and Allergy Sustained-Action Tablets (Increases drowsiness effect) ▣ 802
Drixoral Cold and Flu Extended-Release Tablets (Increases drowsiness effect) ▣ 803
Drixoral Allergy/Sinus Extended Release Tablets (May increase the drowsiness effect) ▣ 804
Duragesic Transdermal System (May produce additive depressant effects) 1288
Duramorph (Potentiation of depressant effect) 962
Dura-Tap/PD Capsules (Potential for additive effects) 2867
Dura-Vent/DA Tablets (Potential for additive effects) 953
Duratuss HD Elixir (Potentiation of central nervous system effects) 2565
Easprin (Synergism; gastrointestinal bleeding) 1914
Effexor (Concurrent use should be avoided) 2719
Elavil Injection (Amitriptyline may enhance the response to alcohol) 2838
Empirin with Codeine Tablets (Increased CNS depressant) 1093
Endep Tablets (Increased response) 2174
Enduron Tablets (Potentiates orthostatic hypotension) 420
Ergamisol Tablets (May result in ANTABUSE-like side effects) 1292
Esgic-plus Tablets (May exhibit additive CNS depressant effects) 1013
Esidrix Tablets (May potentiate orthostatic hypotension) 821
Esimil Tablets (Orthostatic hypotension aggravated) 822
Etrafon Tablets (2-25) (Amitriptyline may enhance the response to alcohol; potential for additive effects and hypotension; concurrent use should be avoided) 2355
Excedrin P.M. Analgesic/Sleeping Aid Tablets, Caplets, Liquigels (Effect not specified) 733
Fastin Capsules (Concomitant use may result in adverse drug interaction) 2488
Fedahist Gyrocaps (May have an additive CNS depressant effect) 2401
Fioricet Tablets (Additive CNS depressant effects) 2258
Fioricet with Codeine Capsules (Enhanced effect of central nervous system depressant) 2260
Fiorinal Capsules (Increased CNS depression) 2261
Fiorinal with Codeine Capsules (Increased CNS depression) 2262
Flagyl 375 Capsules (Alcohol should not be consumed during metronidazole therapy and for at least three days afterward because abdominal cramps, nausea, vomiting, headaches, and flushing may occur) 2434
Flagyl I.V. (Potential for abdominal cramps, nausea, vomiting, and headaches, and flushing) 2247
Flexeril Tablets (Enhanced effect of alcohol) 1661
Fulvicin P/G Tablets (Potentiation of effects of alcohol) 2359
Fulvicin P/G 165 & 330 Tablets (Potentiation of effects of alcohol) 2359
Furoxone Liquid (Possible disulfiram-like reaction may occur; alcohol intake should be avoided during or within four days after Furoxone therapy) 2046
Glucophage (Alcohol potentiates the effect of metfomrin on lactate metabolism; patients should be warned against excessive alcohol intake, acute or chronic) 752
Glucotrol Tablets (Potential for hypoglycemia) 1967
Gris-PEG Tablets, 125 mg & 250 mg (The effect of alcohol may be potentiated) 479
Halcion Tablets (Additive CNS depressant effects) 2611
Haldol Decanoate 50 (50 mg/mL) Injection (CNS depressant potentiated) 1577
Haldol Injection, Tablets and Concentrate (CNS depressant potentiated) 1575
Hycodan Tablets and Syrup (Exhibits an additive CNS depression) 930
Hycomine Compound Tablets (Exhibits an additive CNS depression) 932
Hycotuss Expectorant Syrup (Exhibits an additive CNS depression) 933
Hydrocet Capsules (Additive CNS depression) 782
HydroDIURIL Tablets (Potentiation of orthostatic hypotension) 1674
Hydropres Tablets (Potentiation of orthostatic hypotension) 1675
Hylorel Tablets (Exaggerates postural hypotension) 985
Hyzaar Tablets (Potentiation of orthostatic hypotension) 1677
Imdur (Additive vasodilating effects) 1323
Inderal Injectable (Slows the rate of absorption of propranolol) 2728
Inderal LA Long Acting Capsules (Absorption rate of propranolol slowed) 2730
Inderide Tablets (Slows the rate of absorption of propranolol) 2732
Inderide LA Long Acting Capsules (May aggravate orthostatic hypotension) 2734
Infumorph 200 and Infumorph 500 Sterile Solutions (Potentiates CNS depressant effects) 965
Inversine Tablets (Potentiation of Inversine) 1686
Ionamin Capsules (Possibility of adverse interactions) 990
Ismelin Tablets (Aggravates orthostatic hypotensive effects) 827
Ismo Tablets (Additive vasodilating effects) 2738
Isoclor Timesule Capsules (Concurrent use is not recommended) ▣ 637
Isordil Sublingual Tablets (Alcohol exhibits additive vasodilating effects) 2739
Isordil Tembids Capsules (Alcohol exhibits additive vasodilating effects) 2741
Isordil Titradose Tablets (Alcohol exhibits additive vasodilating effects) 2742
Klonopin Tablets (Potentiates CNS-depressant action) 2126
Legatrin PM (Concurrent use not recommended; consult your doctor) ▣ 651
Levatol (Increased number of errors in the eye-hand psychomotor function test) 2403
Levoprome (Potentiation of CNS depression) 1274
Librax Capsules (Additive effects) 2176
Libritabs Tablets (Additive effect) 2177
Librium Injectable (Additive effect) 2179
Limbitrol Tablets (Potential for additive effects leading to harmful level of sedation and CNS depression) 2180
Lioresal Intrathecal (CNS depressant effect of Lioresal Intrathecal may be additive to those of alcohol) 1596
Lioresal Tablets (Additive depressant effect) 829
Lomotil Liquid (Potentiation of alcohol) 2439
Lopressor HCT Tablets (Orthostatic hypotension may be potentiated) 832
Lorcet 10/650 (Potential for additive CNS depression) 1018
Lortab 2.5/500 Tablets (Additive CNS depression) 2566

(▣ Described in PDR For Nonprescription Drugs) (◉ Described in PDR For Ophthalmology)

1201 Food Interactions Cross-Reference Alcohol

Lotensin HCT (Thiazide-induced orthostatic hypotension potentiated by alcohol) ... 837
Ludiomil Tablets (Enhanced response to alcohol) ... 843
Luvox Tablets (Concurrent use should be avoided) ... 2544
MS Contin Tablets (Respiratory depression, hypotension and profound sedation or coma may result) ... 1994
MSIR Oral Solution (Additive depressant effects; potential for respiratory depression, hypotension and profound sedation or coma) ... 1997
Mandol Vials, Faspak & ADD-Vantage (Concurrent ingestion of ethanol may result in nausea, vomiting, vasomotor instability with hypotension and peripheral vasodilation) ... 1461
Marax Tablets & DF Syrup (Potentiated) ... 2200
Marinol (Dronabinol) Capsules (Additive drowsiness and CNS depression) ... 2231
Matulane Capsules (May result in disulfiram-like reaction) ... 2131
Maxzide Tablets (May aggravate orthostatic hypotension) ... 1380
Mellaril Concentrate (Potentiation of central nervous system depressants) ... 2269
Mepergan Injection (Respiratory depression, hypotension, profound sedation or coma) ... 2753
Mesantoin Tablets (Acute alcohol intoxication may increase the anticonvulsant effect; chronic alcohol abuse may decrease anticonvulsant effect) ... 2272
Methadone Hydrochloride Oral Concentrate (Potential for respiratory depression, hypotension, and profound sedation or coma; use caution and reduced dosage in patients who are concurrently receiving these drugs) ... 2233
Methadone Hydrochloride Oral Solution & Tablets (Respiratory depression, hypotension, and profound sedation or coma may result) ... 2235
MetroGel-Vaginal (Possibility of a disulfiram-like reaction) ... 902
Mevacor Tablets (Increased potential for liver dysfunction in patients who consume substantial quantity of alcohol) ... 1699
Maximum Strength Multi-Symptom Formula Midol (May increase drowsiness) ... ▣ 722
PMS Multi-Symptom Formula Midol (May increase drowsiness) ... ▣ 723
Miles Nervine Nighttime Sleep-Aid (Concurrent use not recommended) ... ▣ 723
Miltown Tablets (Additive effects) ... 2672
Minizide Capsules (Orthostatic hypotension) ... 1938
Mobigesic Tablets (Avoid concurrent use; may cause drowsiness) ... ▣ 602
Moduretic Tablets (Potentiation of orthostatic hypotension) ... 1705
Monoket (Additive vasodilating effects) ... 2406
Motofen Tablets (Effects potentiated) ... 784
Mykrox Tablets (Potentiates orthostatic hypotensive effects) ... 993
Nardil (Hypertensive crises) ... 1920
Nicolar Tablets (May increase the side effects of flushing and pruritus) ... 2026
Nitro-Bid Ointment (Exhibits additive vasodilating effects) ... 1524
Nitrodisc (Exhibits additive effects) ... 2047
Nitro-Dur (nitroglycerin) Transdermal Infusion System (Enhances sensitivity to the hypotensive effects) ... 1326
Nitrolingual Spray (Enhanced sensitivity to hypotensive effects) ... 2027
Nitrostat Tablets (Hypotension) ... 1925
Nizoral Tablets (Potential for disulfiram-like reaction to alcohol resulting in flushing, rash, peripheral edema, nausea and headache) ... 1298
Nolahist Tablets (Increased drowsiness) ... 785
Norpramin Tablets (Exaggerated response to alcohol; increased danger of suicide or overdose; induces liver enzyme activity thereby reduces tricyclic antidepressant plasma levels) ... 1526
Novahistine DH (Potentiated effects) ... 2462
Novahistine Elixir (May increase the drowsiness effect; avoid concurrent use) ... ▣ 823
Novahistine Expectorant (Codeine may potentiate CNS depressant effects) ... 2463
Nubain Injection (Additive CNS depression) ... 935
Nucofed Syrup and Capsules (May increase the depressant effects of codeine) ... 2051
Numorphan Injection (Additive CNS depression) ... 936
Numorphan Suppositories (Additive CNS depression) ... 937
Nydrazid Injection (Daily ingestion of alcohol may be associated with a higher incidence of isoniazid hepatitis) ... 508
Maximum Strength Nytol Caplets (When consuming alcohol, use Nytol with caution) ... ▣ 610
Nytol QuickCaps Caplets (Heightens depressant effect) .. ▣ 610
Oramorph SR (Morphine Sulfate Sustained Release Tablets) (CNS depressant effects are potentiated) ... 2236
Orap Tablets (CNS depression potentiated) ... 1050
Oretic Tablets (May aggravate orthostatic hypotension) ... 443
Orlamm (Potential for serious side effects, including respiratory depression, hypotension, profound sedation and coma, if used concurrently) ... 2239
Ornade Spansule Capsules (Potentiated) ... 2502
PBZ Tablets (CNS effects may be additive) ... 845
PBZ-SR Tablets (CNS effects may be additive) ... 844
PMB 200 and PMB 400 (Additive effects) ... 2783
Pamelor Capsules (Excessive consumption of alcohol with nortriptyline may have a potentiating effect and exaggerated response to alcohol) 2280
Paraflex Caplets (May produce additive effect) ... 1580
Parafon Forte DSC Caplets (May produce additive effect) ... 1581
Parnate Tablets (Contraindicated; potentiated) ... 2503
Paxil Tablets (Concurrent use should be avoided) ... 2505
Pediatric Vicks 44m Cough & Cold Relief (May increase drowsiness effect) ... ▣ 764
Percocet Tablets (Additive CNS depression) ... 938
Percodan Tablets (Additive CNS depression) ... 939
Percodan-Demi Tablets (CNS depressant effects of Percodan-Demi may be additive) 940
Percogesic Analgesic Tablets (May increase the drowsiness effect) ... ▣ 754
Periactin Syrup (Additive effects) ... 1724
Phenergan with Codeine (Additive sedative effects) ... 2777
Phenergan with Dextromethorphan (Additive sedative effects) ... 2778
Phenergan Injection (Additive sedative effects) ... 2773
Phenergan Suppositories (Additive sedative effects) ... 2775
Phenergan Syrup Fortis (Additive sedative effects) ... 2774
Phenergan VC (Additive sedative effects) ... 2779
Phenergan VC with Codeine (Additive sedative effects) ... 2781
Phenobarbital Elixir and Tablets (Additive depressant effects) ... 1469
Phrenilin Forte Capsules (Potential for increased CNS depression) ... 785
Prinzide Tablets (Potentiates orthostatic hypotension) ... 1737
Prolixin Decanoate (Potentiation of the effect of alcohol may occur) .. 509
Propulsid (Sedative effects of alcohol may be accelerated) ... 1300
ProSom Tablets (Potentiates the action of benzodiazepines) ... 449
Protostat Tablets (Abdominal cramps, nausea, vomiting, headache, and flushing may occur; alcohol should not be consumed during and for at least one day after therapy) ... 1883
Pyrroxate Caplets (Concurrent use not recommended) ... ▣ 772
Quadrinal Tablets (Increased effects) ... 1350
RMS Suppositories (Additive CNS depressant effect) ... 2657
Reglan Injectable (Increased rate and/or extent of absorption from the small bowel; additive sedative effects) ... 2068
Restoril Capsules (Additive effects) ... 2284
Rifamate Capsules (Increased incidence of Isoniazid hepatitis) .. 1530
Rifater (Daily ingestion of alcohol may be associated with higher incidence of isoniazid hepatitis) .. 1532
Risperdal (Effects not specified; concurrent use should be avoided) ... 1301
Robaxin Injectable (Increased depressant effect) ... 2070
Robaxin Tablets (Increased CNS depressant effect) ... 2071
Robaxisal Tablets (Increased depressant effect) ... 2071
Romazicon (Concurrent use should be avoided) ... 2147
Rondec Oral Drops (Enhanced effects of alcohol) ... 953
Rondec-DM Oral Drops (Enhanced effects of alcohol) ... 954
Roxanol (Morphine Sulfate Concentrated Oral Solution) (Respiratory depression, hypotension, and profound sedation or coma may result; depressant effects of morphine may be enhanced) ... 2243
Roxicodone Tablets, Oral Solution & Intensol (Oxycodone) (Possible additive CNS depression) ... 2244
Ryna-C Liquid (May increase drowsiness effect) ... ▣ 841
Rynatan-S Pediatric Suspension (Additive CNS effects) ... 2673
Rynatuss Pediatric Suspension (Additive CNS effects) ... 2673
Seconal Sodium Pulvules (Concomitant use may produce additive CNS-depressant effects) 1474
Sedapap Tablets 50 mg/650 mg (Additive CNS depression) ... 1543
Semprex-D Capsules (Co-administration may result in additional reduction in alertness and impairment of CNS performance and should be avoided) ... 463
Semprex-D Capsules (Co-administration may result in additional reduction in alertness and impairment of CNS performance and should be avoided) ... 1167
Ser-Ap-Es Tablets (Orthostatic hypotension) ... 849
Serax Capsules (Effects may be additive) ... 2810
Serentil Ampuls (Potentiation of central nervous system depressant) ... 684
Seromycin Pulvules (Increases risk of epileptic episodes) ... 1476
Serzone Tablets (Concomitant use should be avoided) ... 771
Sinarest Tablets (Concurrent use produces additive effects) ... ▣ 648
Sine-Aid IB Caplets (Chronic heavy alcohol abusers, 3 or more drinks per day, may be at increased risk of liver toxicity from acetaminophen use) ... 1554
Sine-Aid Maximum Strength Sinus Medication Gelcaps, Caplets and Tablets (Chronic heavy alcohol abusers, 3 or more drinks per day, may be at increased risk of liver toxicity from acetaminophen use) ... 1554
Sine-Off Sinus Medicine (Do not use concomitantly) ... ▣ 825
Sinequan Capsules (Doxepin may enhance the response to alcohol) 2205
Singlet Tablets (Increases drowsiness effect) ... ▣ 825
Sinulin Tablets (Increased drowsiness) ... 787
Sinutab Sinus Allergy Medication, Maximum Strength Tablets and Caplets (Do not use concomitantly) ... ▣ 860
Sleepinal Night-time Sleep Aid Capsules and Softgels (Avoid alcoholic beverages) ... ▣ 834
Soma Compound w/Codeine Tablets (Additive effects including gastrointestinal bleeding) ... 2676
Soma Compound Tablets (Additive effects including enhanced aspirin-induced fecal blood loss) 2675
Soma Tablets (Additive effects) ... 2674
Sorbitrate Chewable Tablets (Enhances sensitivity to hypotensive activity of nitrates) .. 2843
Stadol NS Nasal Spray (Potential for increased CNS depressant effect) ... 775
Stelazine Concentrate (Additive depressant effects) ... 2514
Sudafed Plus Liquid (Increases drowsiness effect) ... ▣ 862
Sudafed Plus Tablets (Increases drowsiness effect) ... ▣ 863
Surmontil Capsules (Concomitant use of alcoholic beverages and trimipramine may be associated with exaggerated effects) ... 2811
Talacen (Potential for increased CNS depressant effects) ... 2333
Talwin Ampuls (Potential for increased CNS depressant effects) ... 2334
Talwin Compound (Potential for increased CNS depressant effects) ... 2335
Talwin Nx (May increase CNS depression) ... 2336
Tavist Syrup (Additive effects) ... 2297
Tavist Tablets (Additive effects) ... 2298
Tavist-D 12 Hour Relief Tablets (Increases drowsiness effect) ... ▣ 787
Teldrin 12 Hour Antihistamine/Nasal Decongestant Allergy Relief Capsules (May increase drowsiness effect; avoid concurrent use) ... ▣ 826
Temaril Tablets, Syrup and Spansule Extended-Release Capsules (Additive CNS depressant effect) ... 483
Thalitone (Aggravates orthostatic hypotension) ... 1245
TheraFlu Flu and Cold Medicine (May increase drowsiness effect.) ... ▣ 787
TheraFlu Maximum Strength Nighttime Flu, Cold & Cough Medicine (May increase drowsiness effect.) ... ▣ 788
Tigan Capsules (May result in an adverse drug interaction) ... 2057
Tofranil Ampuls (Imipramine may enhance the CNS depressant effects of alcohol) ... 854
Tofranil Tablets (Imipramine may enhance the CNS depressant effects of alcohol) ... 856
Tofranil-PM Capsules (Imipramine may enhance the CNS depressant effects of alcohol) ... 857
Torecan Injection (Phenothiazines are capable of potentiating CNS depressants) ... 2245
Trancopal Caplets (Possible additive effects) ... 2337
Transderm Scōp Transdermal Therapeutic System (Effect unspecified) ... 869
Transderm-Nitro Transdermal Therapeutic System (Additive vasodilating effects) ... 859

(▣ Described in PDR For Nonprescription Drugs) (◉ Described in PDR For Ophthalmology)

Alcohol

Food Interactions Cross-Reference

Tranxene T-TAB Tablets (Increased effects, prolonged sleeping time) 451

Triaminic Allergy Tablets (May increase drowsiness effect)........ ◾️⃞ 789

Triaminic Cold Tablets (May increase drowsiness effect)........ ◾️⃞ 790

Triaminic Nite Light (May increase drowsiness effect)........ ◾️⃞ 791

Triaminic Syrup (May increase drowsiness effect) .... ◾️⃞ 792

Triaminic-12 Tablets (May increase drowsiness effect)........ ◾️⃞ 792

Triaminicin Tablets (May increase drowsiness; avoid concurrent use) .... ◾️⃞ 793

Triaminicol Multi-Symptom Cold Tablets (May increase drowsiness effect) .... ◾️⃞ 793

Triaminicol Multi-Symptom Relief (May increase drowsiness effect) .... ◾️⃞ 794

Triavil Tablets (Potentiated; contraindication) 1757

Trilafon Concentrate (Additive effects; hypotension) 2389

Trilisate Liquid (Increased risk of gastrointestinal ulceration) 2000

Trinalin Repetabs Tablets (Additive effect) 1330

Tussend (Concomitant use may exhibit additive CNS depression) 1783

Tussend Expectorant (Hydrocodone may potentiate CNS depressant effects).................. 1785

Tussionex Pennkinetic Extended-Release Suspension (Additive CNS depression) 998

Tussi-Organidin DM NR Liquid and DM-S NR Liquid (Potential for additive CNS depressant effects) 2677

Tussi-Organidin NR Liquid and S NR Liquid (Potential for additive CNS depressant effects).................. 2677

TYLENOL Extended Relief Caplets (Chronic heavy alcohol abusers, 3 or more drinks per day, may be at increased risk of liver toxicity from acetaminophen use) 1558

TYLENOL, Extra Strength, Acetaminophen Adult Liquid Pain Reliever (Patients consuming 3 or more alcohol-containing drinks per day should consult their physician for advice on when and how they should take acetaminophen containing products) 1560

TYLENOL, Extra Strength, acetaminophen Gelcaps, Geltabs, Caplets, Tablets (Chronic heavy alcohol abusers, 3 or more drinks per day, may be at increased risk of liver toxicity from acetaminophen use) 1559

TYLENOL, Extra Strength, Headache Plus Pain Reliever with Antacid Caplets (Chronic heavy alcohol abusers, 3 or more drinks per day, may be at increased risk of liver toxicity from acetaminophen use) 1559

TYLENOL Maximum Strength Allergy Sinus Medication Gelcaps and Caplets (May increase drowsiness; chronic heavy alcohol abusers, 3 or more drinks per day, may be at increased risk of liver toxicity from acetaminophen use) 1563

TYLENOL Maximum Strength Allergy Sinus NightTime Medication Caplets (May increase drowsiness effect; chronic heavy alcohol abusers, 3 or more drinks per day, may be at increased risk of liver toxicity from acetaminophen use) 1555

TYLENOL Flu Maximum Strength Gelcaps (Chronic heavy alcohol abusers, 3 or more drinks per day, may be at increased risk of liver toxicity from acetaminophen use) 1565

TYLENOL Flu NightTime, Maximum Strength, Gelcaps (May increase drowsiness effect; chronic heavy alcohol abusers, 3 or more drinks per day, may be at increased risk of liver toxicity from acetaminophen use) 1566

TYLENOL Maximum Strength Flu NightTime Hot Medication Packets (May increase drowsiness effect; chronic heavy alcohol abusers, 3 or more drinks per day, may be at increased risk of liver toxicity from acetaminophen use) 1562

TYLENOL, Maximum Strength, Sinus Medication Geltabs, Gelcaps, Caplets and Tablets (Chronic heavy alcohol abusers, 3 or more drinks per day, may be at increased risk of liver toxicity from acetaminophen use) 1566

TYLENOL Cold Multi-Symptom Formula Medication Tablets and Caplets (May increase drowsiness; chronic heavy alcohol abusers, 3 or more drinks per day, may be at increased risk of liver toxicity from acetaminophen use) 1561

TYLENOL Cold Medication No Drowsiness Formula Gelcaps and Caplets (Chronic heavy alcohol abusers, 3 or more drinks per day, may be at increased risk of liver toxicity from acetaminophen use) 1562

TYLENOL Cold Multi-Symptom Hot Medication Liquid Packets (Increases drowsiness effect; chronic heavy alcohol abusers, 3 or more drinks per day, may be at increased risk of liver toxicity from acetaminophen use) 1557

TYLENOL Cold Multi-Symptom Hot Medication Liquid Packets (Increases drowsiness effect; chronic heavy alcohol abusers, 3 or more drinks per day, may be at increased risk of liver toxicity from acetaminophen use) 1557

TYLENOL Cough Multi-Symptom Medication with Decongestant (Chronic heavy alcohol abusers, 3 or more drinks per day, may be at increased risk of liver toxicity from acetaminophen use) 1565

TYLENOL, Regular Strength, acetaminophen Caplets and Tablets (Chronic heavy alcohol abusers, 3 or more drinks per day, may be at increased risk of liver toxicity from acetaminophen use) 1558

TYLENOL PM, Extra Strength Pain Reliever/Sleep Aid Caplets, Geltabs, Gelcaps (Avoid concurrent use; chronic heavy alcohol abusers, 3 or more drinks per day, may be at increased risk of liver toxicity from acetaminophen use) 1560

TYLENOL Severe Allergy Medication Caplets (Chronic heavy alcohol abusers, 3 or more drinks per day, may be at increased risk of liver toxicity from acetaminophen use) 1564

Tylenol with Codeine Elixir (Additive CNS depression) 1583

Tylox Capsules (Additive CNS depression) 1584

Ultram Tablets (50 mg) (Effect of concurrent use not specified; use with caution and in reduced dosages) 1585

Maximum Strength Unisom Sleepgels (Heightens the CNS depressant effect) 1934

Unisom Nighttime Sleep Aid (Use Unisom cautiously) 1934

Unisom With Pain Relief-Nighttime Sleep Aid and Pain Reliever (Heightened CNS depressant effect of antihistamines).................. 1934

Valium Injectable (Increased depression/apnea; hypotension/muscular weakness) 2182

Valium Tablets (Simultaneous use of alcohol not recommended) 2183

Valrelease Capsules (Potentiates action of diazepam) 2169

Vaseretic Tablets (Potentiation of orthostatic hypotension may occur) 1765

Verelan Capsules (Verapamil has been found to significantly inhibit ethanol elimination resulting in elevated blood ethanol concentration that may prolong the intoxicating effects of alcohol) 1410

Verelan Capsules (Verapamil has been found to significantly inhibit ethanol elimination resulting in elevated blood ethanol concentration that may prolong the intoxicating effects of alcohol) 2824

Versed Injection (May increase risk of underventilation and prolong drug effect) 2170

Vicks 44 LiquiCaps Cough, Cold & Flu Relief (May increase the drowsiness effect) .... ◾️⃞ 755

Vicks 44M Cough, Cold & Flu Relief (May increase drowsiness effect) .... ◾️⃞ 756

Vicks DayQuil Allergy Relief 12-Hour Extended Release Tablets (Avoid concurrent use) ◾️⃞ 760

Vicks DayQuil Allergy Relief 4-Hour Tablets (May increase the drowsiness effect; avoid concurrent use) .... ◾️⃞ 760

Vicks Nyquil Hot Therapy (May increase drowsiness effect)........ ◾️⃞ 762

Vicks NyQuil LiquiCaps Multi-Symptom Cold/Flu Relief (May increase drowsiness effect) .... ◾️⃞ 763

Vicodin Tablets (May exhibit an additive CNS depression)................ 1356

Vicodin ES Tablets (Additive CNS depression) 1357

Vicodin Tuss Expectorant (Co-administration may exhibit an additive CNS depression) 1358

Vistaril Capsules (Increased effect of alcohol) 1944

Vistaril Intramuscular Solution (May be potentiated) 2216

Vivactil Tablets (Protriptyline may enhance the response to alcohol) 1774

Wellbutrin Tablets (Concurrent alcohol consumption should be avoided or minimized) 1204

Wygesic Tablets (Additive effects).. 2827

Xanax Tablets (Additive CNS depressant effects) 2649

Zaroxolyn Tablets (Hypotensive effect may be potentiated) 1000

Zefazone Sterile Powder (Disulfiram-like reactions characterized by flushing, sweating, headache, and tachycardia; patients should be advised against the ingestion of alcohol-containing beverages during and for 24 hours after the administration of cefmetazole) 2654

Zestoretic (Potentiates orthostatic hypotension) 2850

Ziac (Potentiation of orthostatic hypotension may occur when thiazide diuretics are used with alcohol) 1415

Zoloft Tablets (Concomitant use of Zoloft and alcohol in depressed patient is not recommended) 2217

Zonalon Cream (Alcohol ingestion may exacerbate the potential sedative effects of Zonalon Cream) 1055

Zydone Capsules (Additive CNS depression) 949

Anchovies

Parnate Tablets (Potential for hypertensive crisis).............................. 2503

Avocados

Parnate Tablets (Potential for hypertensive crisis).............................. 2503

Bananas

Matulane Capsules (Concurrent use should be avoided).................... 2131

Parnate Tablets (Potential for hypertensive crisis).............................. 2503

Beans, broad

Furoxone Liquid (Concurrent and/or sequential intake must be avoided) 2046

Nardil (Concurrent and/or sequential intake must be avoided) 1920

Parnate Tablets (Potential for hypertensive crisis).............................. 2503

Beans, Fava

Nardil (Concurrent and/or sequential intake must be avoided) 1920

Parnate Tablets (Potential for hypertensive crisis).............................. 2503

Beer, alcohol-free

Nardil (Concurrent and/or sequential intake must be avoided) 1920

Parnate Tablets (Potential for hypertensive crisis).............................. 2503

Beer, reduced-alcohol

(see also under Alcohol)

Nardil (Concurrent and/or sequential intake must be avoided) 1920

Beer, unspecified

(see also under Alcohol)

Furoxone Liquid (Concurrent and/or sequential intake must be avoided).

Nardil (Concurrent and/or sequential intake must be avoided) 1920

Parnate Tablets (Potential for hypertensive crisis).............................. 2503

Beverages, acidic

Nicorette (Interferes with buccal absorption of nicotine from Nicorette) 2458

Beverages, alcoholic

(see under Alcohol; Beer, unspecified; Wine products; Wine, Chianti; Wine, unspecified)

Beverages, caffeine-containing

Bayer Select Headache Pain Relief Formula (Concurrent use may cause nervousness, irritability, and occasionally rapid heart beat) .... ◾️⃞ 716

Maximum Strength Multi-Symptom Formula Midol (Concomitant use may cause nervousness, irritability, sleeplessness, and occasionally, rapid heartbeat) .. ◾️⃞ 722

Nardil (Excessive caffeine intake should be avoided) 1920

Nicorette (Interferes with buccal absorption of nicotine from Nicorette) 2458

No Doz Maximum Strength Caplets (May cause sleeplessness, irritability, nervousness and rapid heart beat) .... ◾️⃞ 622

Respbid Tablets (Avoid large quantities; increased side effects) 682

Bologna, Lebanon

Nardil (Concurrent and/or sequential intake must be avoided) 1920

Broccoli

(see under Diet high in vitamin K)

Carrots

(see under Food, furocoumarin-containing)

Celery

(see under Food, furocoumarin-containing)

Caviar

Parnate Tablets (Potential for hypertensive crisis).............................. 2503

(◾️⃞ Described in PDR For Nonprescription Drugs)

(◉ Described in PDR For Ophthalmology)

Cheese, aged
- Matulane Capsules (Concurrent use should be avoided) 2131
- Nardil (Concurrent and/or sequential intake must be avoided) 1920
- Parnate Tablets (Potential for hypertensive crisis) 2503

Cheese, strong, unpasteurized
- Furoxone Liquid (Concurrent and/or sequential intake must be avoided) 2046
- Parnate Tablets (Potential for hypertensive crisis) 2503

Cheese, unspecified
- Nardil (Concurrent and/or sequential intake must be avoided) 1920
- Parnate Tablets (Potential for hypertensive crisis) 2503
- Rifater (Isoniazid has some MAO inhibiting activity, an interaction with tyramine containing food may occur) 1532

Chocolate
- Nardil (Concurrent and/or sequential intake must be avoided) 1920
- Parnate Tablets (Potential for hypertensive crisis) 2503
- Respbid Tablets (Eating large quantity of chocolate increases theophylline side effects) 682

Coffee (see under Beverages, caffeine-containing)

Cola
- Respbid Tablets (Drinking large quantity of cola increases theophylline side effects) 682
- Sporanox Capsules (Absorption of oral itraconazole is enhanced when administered with a cola beverage in patients with achlorhydria, such as AIDS or patients taking acid suppressors, e.g., H_2 inhibitors and proton pump inhibitors) 1305

Cream, sour
- Parnate Tablets (Potential for hypertensive crisis) 2503

Dairy products
- Accutane Capsules (Increases oral absorption of isotretinoin) 2076
- Achromycin V Capsules (Interfers with absorption of oral forms of tetracycline) 1367
- Declomycin Tablets (Interferes with absorption) 1371
- Emcyt Capsules (Impairs the absorption of Emcyt) 1953
- Fero-Folic-500 Filmtab (Ingestion of milk inhibits iron absorption) 429
- Fleet Prep Kits (Concurrent use within one-hour should be avoided) 1003
- Luride Drops 50 ml (Incompatibility of fluoride with dairy) 871
- Luride Lozi-Tabs Tablets (Incompatibility of fluoride with dairy foods results in the formation of poorly absorbed calcium fluoride) 871
- Maalox Antacid Caplets (Concurrent prolonged use with homogenized milk containing Vitamin D may result in the milk-alkali syndrome) ▣ 638
- Minocin Pellet-Filled Capsules (The peak plasma concentrations were slightly decreased (11.2%) and delayed by 1 hour) 1383
- Nalfon 200 Pulvules & Nalfon Tablets (Peak blood levels are delayed and diminished) 917
- Relafen Tablets (Potential for more rapid absorption, however, the total amount of GMNA in the plasma is unchanged) 2510
- Tegison Capsules (Increases absorption of etretinate) 2154
- Tolectin (200, 400 and 600 mg) (Decreases total tolmetin bioavailability by 16%) 1581
- Vibramycin Hyclate Capsules (Absorption of doxycycline is not markedly influenced by simultaneous ingestion of milk) 1941

Diet high in protein
- Atamet (Levodopa competes with certain amino acids, the absorption of levodopa may be impaired in some patients on a high protein diet) 572
- Sinemet Tablets (Levodopa competes with certain amino acids, the absorption of levodopa may be impaired in some patients on a high protein diet) 943

Diet high in vitamin K
- Coumadin Tablets (Decreased prothrombin time) 926

Diet, high-lipid
- Accupril Tablets (Rate and extent of Quinapril absorption are diminished moderately) 1893
- Adalat CC (High fat meal increases peak plasma nifedipine concentrations by 60%, a prolongation in the time to peak concentration, but no significant change in the AUC; administer on an empty stomach) 589
- Cardene SR Capsules (Results in lower C_{max} and AUC; higher trough levels) 2097
- Dilacor XR Extended-release Capsules (Simultaneous administration of Dilacor XR with a high-fat breakfast has a modest effect on diltiazem bioavailability) 2018
- Glucotrol XL Extended Release Tablets (Administration of Glucotrol XL immediately before a high fat breakfast resulted in a 40% increase in the glipizide mean Cmax value; the effect on the AUC was not significant) 1968
- Neoral Soft Gelatin Capsules for Microemulsion (A high fat meal consumed within one-half hour before Neoral administration decreased the AUC by 13% and C_{max} by 33%) 2276
- Respbid Tablets (Reduced plasma concentration levels; delay in time of peak plasma levels) 682
- Salagen Tablets (Decrease in the rate of absorption of pilocarpine when taken with high fat meal) 1489
- Slo-bid Gyrocaps (Decreases in the rate of absorption, but with no significant difference in the extent of absorption) 2033
- Tegison Capsules (Increases absorption of etretinate) 2154
- Theo-24 Extended Release Capsules (May result in a significant increase in peak serum level) 2568
- Theo-X Extended-Release Tablets (May result in a somewhat higher C_{max} and delayed T_{max}, and a somewhat greater extent of absorption when compared to taking in the fasting state) 788
- Theo-X Extended-Release Tablets (May result in a somewhat higher C_{max} and delayed T_{max}, and a somewhat greater extent of absorption when compared to taking in the fasting state) 788
- Uniphyl 400 mg Tablets (Affects the bioavailability of theophylline) 2001

Diet, potassium-rich
- Maxzide Tablets (Concurrent use is contraindicated) 1380
- Midamor Tablets (Potential for rapid increases in serum potassium levels) 1703
- Moduretic Tablets (Potential for rapid increases in serum potassium levels) 1705

Drinks, hot, unspecified
- Nicolar Tablets (May increase the side effects of flushing and pruritus) 2026

Eggs
- Fero-Folic-500 Filmtab (Ingestion of eggs inhibits iron absorption) 429

Figs (see under Food, furocoumarin-containing)

Figs, canned
- Parnate Tablets (Potential for hypertensive crisis) 2503

Fish, smoked
- Nardil (Concurrent and/or sequential intake must be avoided) 1920

Fish, tropical
- Rifater (Isoniazid may inhibit diamine oxidase, causing exaggerated response (headache, sweating, palpitations, flushing, hypotension) to food containing histamine) 1532

Food having a pH greater than 5.5
- CREON 5 Capsules (Can dissolve the protective coating resulting in early release of enzymes, irritation of oral mucosa, and/or loss of enzyme activity) 2536
- Ultrase Capsules (Can dissolve the protective coating resulting in early release of enzymes, irritation of oral mucosa, and/or loss of enzyme activity) 2343
- Ultrase MT Capsules (Can dissolve the protective enteric shell) 2344

Food that lowers urinary pH
- Mono-Gesic Tablets (Decreases urinary excretion and increases plasma levels) 792
- Trilisate Liquid (Decrease urinary salicylate excretion & increases plasma levels) 2000

Food that raises urinary pH
- Mono-Gesic Tablets (Increases renal clearance and urinary excretion of salicylic acid) 792
- Trilisate Liquid (Enhance renal salicylate clearance & diminishes plasma salicylate concentration) 2000
- Urised Tablets (Methenamine has therapeutic activity in acidic urine; concurrent use with foods which produce an alkaline urine should be restricted) 1964

Food with high concentration of dopamine
- Nardil (Concurrent and/or sequential intake must be avoided) 1920

Food with high concentration of tyramine
- Eldepryl Tablets (Potential for "cheese reaction" if attention is not paid to the dose dependent nature of selegine's selectivity) 2550
- Furoxone Liquid (Concurrent and/or sequential intake must be avoided) 2046
- Matulane Capsules (Concurrent use should be avoided) 2131
- Nardil (Concurrent and/or sequential intake must be avoided) 1920
- Parnate Tablets (Potential for hypertensive crisis) 2503
- Rifater (Isoniazid has some MAO inhibiting activity, an interaction with tyramine containing food may occur) 1532

Food, caffeine containing
- Bayer Select Headache Pain Relief Formula (Concurrent use may cause nervousness, irritability, and occasionally rapid heart beat) ▣ 716
- DHCplus Capsules (Concomitant use may result in caffeine accumulation when DHC Plus is consumed with caffeine-containing foods) 1993
- Maximum Strength Multi-Symptom Formula Midol (Concomitant use may cause nervousness, irritability, sleeplessness, and occasionally, rapid heartbeat) ▣ 722
- No Doz Maximum Strength Caplets (May cause sleeplessness, irritability, nervousness and rapid heart beat) ▣ 622

Food, calcium-rich
- Emcyt Capsules (Impairs the absorption of Emcyt) 1953

Food, furocoumarin-containing
- Trisoralen Tablets (Potential for severe reactions) 1264

Food, unspecified
- Accutane Capsules (Increases oral absorption of isotretinoin) 2076
- Achromycin V Capsules (Interferes with absorption of oral forms of tetracycline) 1367
- Children's Advil Suspension (Peak plasma levels are somewhat lower (up to 30%) and the time to reach peak levels is slightly prolonged (up to 30 min.)) 2692
- Altace Capsules (The rate of absorption is reduced, not the extent of absorption) 1232
- Ansaid Tablets (Alters the rate of absorption but does not affect the extent of drug availability) 2579
- Apresazide Capsules (Enhances gastrointestinal absorption of hydrochlorothiazide) 808
- Apresoline Hydrochloride Tablets (Results in higher plasma levels) 809
- BuSpar (Food may decrease presystemic clearance of buspirone) 737
- Calan SR Caplets (Produces decreased bioavailability (AUC) but a narrower peak-to-trough ratio) 2422
- Capoten (Reduces absorption by about 30 to 40%; should be given one hour before meals) 739
- Cardura Tablets (Reduction of 18% in mean maximum plasma concentration and 12% in the AUC occurred when Cardura was administered with food; neither of these differences were statistically or clinically significant) 2186
- Ceftin Tablets (Absorption is greater when taken after food) 1078
- CellCept Capsules (Decreased Cmax of mycophenolate mofetil by 40% in the presence of food; no effect on the extent of absorption) 2099
- Cipro Tablets (Delays the absorption of the drug resulting in peak concentrations that are closer to 2 hours after dosing) 592
- Clinoril Tablets (The peak plasma concentrations of biologically active sulfide metabolite is delayed slightly in the presence of food) 1618
- Cognex Capsules (Food reduces tacrine bioavailability by approximately 30% to 40%; no effect if tacrine is administered at least one hour before meals) 1901
- Cytotec (Diminishes maximum plasma concentrations) 2424
- Daypro Caplets (Reduces the rate of absorption of oxaprozin, but the extent of absorption is unchanged) 2426
- Declomycin Tablets (Interferes with absorption) 1371
- Desyrel and Desyrel Dividose (Total drug absorption may be up to 20% higher when the drug is taken with food rather than on an empty stomach; the risk of dizziness, lightheadedness may

(▣ Described in PDR For Nonprescription Drugs) (◉ Described in PDR For Ophthalmology)

increase under fasting conditions) ... 503
Dyclone 0.5% and 1% Topical Solutions, USP (Topical anesthesia may impair swallowing and thus enhance the danger of aspiration; food should not be ingested for 60 minutes) .. 544
DynaCirc Capsules (Coadministration significantly increases the time to peak by about an hour with no effect on AUC) ... 2256
EC-Naprosyn Delayed-Release Tablets (The presence of food prolonged the time the EC-Naprosyn remained in the stomach, time to first detectable serum naproxen levels, and time to maximal naproxen levels (T_{max}), but did not affect peak naproxen levels (C_{max})) ... 2117
Empirin with Codeine Tablets (The presence of food slightly delays absorption) ... 1093
Erythromycin Delayed-Release Capsules, USP (Lowers the blood levels of systemically available erythromycin) ... 427
Esimil Tablets (Enhances gastrointestinal absorption of hydrochlorothiazide) ... 822
Floxin Tablets (200 mg, 300 mg, 400 mg) (Food does not affect the C_{max} and AUC_{∞} of the drug, but T_{max} is prolonged) ... 1567
Glucophage (Food decreases the extent and slightly delays the absorption of metformin) ... 752
Glucotrol Tablets (Delays the absorption by 40 minutes; total absorption and disposition is unaffected; Glucotrol is more effective when administered about 30 minutes before, rather than with, a meal) ... 1967
GoLYTELY (For best results, no solid food should be consumed during 3 to 4 hour period before drinking solution) ... 688
Hytrin Capsules (Delays the time to peak concentration by about 40 minutes) ... 430
IBU Tablets (Food affects the rate but not the extent of absorption) 1342
Imdur (May decrease the rate (increase in T_{max}) but not the extent (AUC) of absorption) ... 1323
Imitrex Tablets (Delays the T_{max} slightly by about 0.5 hour with no significant effect on the bioavailability) ... 1106
Isoptin SR Tablets (Produces decreased bioavailability (AUC) but a narrower peak to trough ratio) ... 1348
Kytril Tablets (When oral granisetron was administered with food, AUC was decreased by 5% and C_{max} increased by 30% in non-fasted individuals) 2492
Lodine Capsules and Tablets (Reduces the peak concentration reached by approximately one-half and increases the time-to-peak concentration by 1.4 to 3.8 hours) ... 2743
Lorabid Suspension and Pulvules (Delays the peak plasma concentration with no change in the total absorption) ... 1459
Macrobid Capsules (Increases bioavailability by approximately 40%) ... 1988
Macrodantin Capsules (Increases bioavailability of Macrodantin) ... 1989
Maxaquin Tablets (The rate of drug absorption may be delayed by 41%, however, the drug can be taken without regard to meal) 2440
Mepron Suspension (Food enhances absorption by approximately two-fold) ... 1135
Methotrexate Sodium Tablets, Injection, for Injection and LPF Injection (Delays absorption and reduces peak concentration) ... 1275
Monopril Tablets (Rate of absorption may be slowed by the presence of food in the GI tract; the extent of absorption is not affected) ... 757
Children's Motrin Ibuprofen Oral Suspension (The peak levels are somewhat lower (up to 30%) and the time to reach peak levels is slightly prolonged (up to 30 min.) although the extent of absorption is unchanged) ... 1546
Motrin Tablets (A reduction in the rate of absorption but no appreciable decrease in the extent of absorption) ... 2625
Motrin Ibuprofen Suspension, Oral Drops, Chewable Tablets, Caplets (Food affects the rate but not the extent of absorption; T_{max} is delayed by approximately 30 to 60 minutes and peak levels are reduced by approximately 30 to 50%) ... 1546
Neoral Soft Gelatin Capsules for Microemulsion (Administration of food with Neoral decreases the AUC and C_{max}) ... 2276
Noroxin Tablets (The presence of food may decrease the absorption) ... 1715
Noroxin Tablets (The presence of food may decrease the absorption) ... 2048
NuLYTELY (Solid food should not be given for at least two hours before the solution is given) ... 689
Orudis Capsules (Slows rate of absorption resulting in delayed and reduced peak concentrations) ... 2766
Pepcid Oral Suspension (Bioavailability may be slightly increased by antacids) ... 1720
Premphase (Administration with food approximately doubles MPA C_{max} and increases MPA AUC by approximately 30%) ... 2797
Prempro (Administration with food approximately doubles MPA C_{max} and increases MPA AUC by approximately 30%) ... 2801
PREVACID Delayed-Release Capsules (Cmax and AUC are diminished by about 50% if the drug is given 30 minutes after food as opposed to the fasting condition) ... 2562
Procardia XL Extended Release Tablets (Presence of food slightly alters the early rate of drug absorption) ... 1972
Prozac Pulvules & Liquid, Oral Solution (May delay absorption of fluoxetine inconsequentially) 919
Quibron-T/SR Tablets (Food ingestion may influence the absorption characteristics of some or all theophylline controlled-release products) ... 2053
Quinaglute Dura-Tabs Tablets (Increases absorption of quinidine in both rate (27%) and extent (17%)) ... 649
Relafen Tablets (Potential for more rapid absorption, however, the total amount of GMNA in the plasma is unchanged) ... 2510
Retrovir Capsules (Administration of Retrovir Capsules with food decreased peak plasma concentrations by greater than 50%, however, bioavailability as determined by AUC may not be affected) ... 1158
Rythmol Tablets–150mg, 225mg, 300mg (Increased peak blood level and bioavailability in a single dose study) ... 1352
Salflex Tablets (Slows the absorption) ... 786
Sectral Capsules (Slightly decreases absorption and peak concentration) ... 2807
Ser-Ap-Es Tablets (Concomitant administration enhances gastrointestinal absorption of hydrochlorothiazide and results in higher plasma levels of hydralazine) ... 849
Serzone Tablets (Food delays the absorption of nefazodone and decreases the bioavailability by approximately 20%) ... 771
Sinemet CR Tablets (Increases the extent of availability and peak concentrations of levodopa) ... 944
Sporanox Capsules (The oral bioavailability of itraconazole is maximal when taken with food) ... 1305
Suprax Tablets (Increases time to maximal absorption approximately 0.8 hour) ... 1399
Theo-Dur Extended-Release Tablets (May influence absorption of theophylline from a 100 mg dosage form) ... 1327
Trandate Tablets (The absolute bioavailability of labetalol is increased when administered with food) ... 1185
Trental Tablets (Delays absorption but does not affect total absorption) ... 1244
Uni-Dur Extended-Release Tablets (Prolongs the time to peak concentration but does not affect the extent of absorption) 1331
Univasc Tablets (Food reduces C_{max} and AUC by about 70% and 40% respectively after ingestion of a low-fat breakfast or by 80% and 50% respectively after the ingestion of high-fat breakfast) ... 2410
Vantin for Oral Suspension and Vantin Tablets (The extent of absorption and the mean peak plasma concentration increased when film-coated tablets were administered with food) ... 2646
Vibramycin Hyclate Capsules (Absorption of doxycycline is not markedly influenced by simultaneous ingestion of food) .. 1941
Videx Tablets, Powder for Oral Solution, & Pediatric Powder for Oral Solution (Reduces the absorption of Videx by 50%; administer Videx on an empty stomach) ... 720
Volmax Extended-Release Tablets (Food may decrease the rate of absorption without altering the extent of bioavailability) ... 1788
Voltaren Tablets (Delays the onset of absorption by 1 to 4.5 hours, with delays as long as 10 hours in some patients and reduction in peak plasma levels by approximately 40%; rate of Cataflam absorption is reduced by food; the extent of absorption is not significantly affected) ... 861
Zithromax Capsules (Reduces the rate of absorption (Cmax) of azithromycin capsules by 52% and the extent of absorption (AUC) by 43%; when oral suspension of azithromycin was administered with food the Cmax increased by 46% and the AUC by 14%) ... 1944
Zofran Tablets (Increases significantly (about 17%) the extent of absorption of ondansetron) ... 1217
Zoloft Tablets (AUC was slightly increased when drug was administered with food but the C_{max} was 25% greater) ... 2217

Fruit juices, unspecified

Dexedrine Spansule Capsules (Lowers absorption of amphetamines) ... 2474
DextroStat Dextroamphetamine Tablets (Lowers absorption of amphetamines by acting as gastrointestinal acidifying agent) 2036
Nicorette (Interferes with buccal absorption of nictoine from Nicorette) ... 2458

Grapefruit

Neoral Soft Gelatin Capsules for Microemulsion (Affects the metabolism of cyclosporine and should be avoided) ... 2276

Grapefruit Juice

Neoral Soft Gelatin Capsules for Microemulsion (Affects the metabolism of cyclosporine and should be avoided) ... 2276

Grapefruit juice, doubly concentrated

Plendil Extended-Release Tablets (Increases bioavailability more than two-fold) ... 527

Herring, pickled

Furoxone Liquid (Concurrent and/or sequential intake must be avoided) ... 2046
Nardil (Concurrent and/or sequential intake must be avoided) ... 1920
Parnate Tablets (Potential for hypertensive crisis) ... 2503

Limes (see under Food, furocoumarin-containing)

Liqueurs (see also under Alcohol)

Parnate Tablets (Potential for hypertensive crisis) ... 2503

Liver

Nardil (Concurrent and/or sequential intake must be avoided) ... 1920
Parnate Tablets (Potential for hypertensive crisis) ... 2503

Liver, chicken

Furoxone Liquid (Concurrent and/or sequential intake must be avoided) ... 2046

Meal with dairy products

Minocin Pellet-Filled Capsules (The peak plasma concentrations were slightly decreased (11.2%) and delayed by 1 hour) ... 1383

Meal, high in bran fiber

Lanoxicaps (Reduces the amount of digoxin from an oral dose) ... 1117
Lanoxin Tablets (The amount of digoxin from an oral dose may be reduced) ... 1128

Meal, unspecified

Ambien Tablets (Mean AUC and C_{max} decreased by 15% and 25% respectively, while T_{max} was prolonged by 60%; for faster sleep onset, Ambien should not be administered with or immediately after meal) ... 2416
Betapace Tablets (Reduces oral absorption by 20%) ... 641
Claritin (Food increases the AUC by approximately 73%, the time to peak plasma concentration is delayed by one-hour; Claritin should be administered on an empty stomach) ... 2349
Claritin-D (Food increases the AUC of loratadine by approximately 40% and of decarboethoxyloratadine by approximately 15%; the time of peak plasma concentration (T_{max}) of loratadine and decarboethoxyloratadine was delayed by 1 hour with meal) ... 2350
Cozaar Tablets (Meal slows absorption and decreases C_{max} but has minor effects on losartan AUC or on the AUC of the metabolite) ... 1628
Cytovene Capsules (Meal containing 46.5% fat increases the steady-state AUC of oral Cytovene by 22% +/- 22% and significant prolongation of time T_{max} and a higher C_{max}) ... 2103
Depen Titratable Tablets (Potential for reduced absorption and the likelihood of inactivation by metal binding in the GI tract; Depen should be given on an empty stomach) ... 2662
ERYC (Optimum blood levels are obtained on a fasting stomach; administration is preferable one-half hour pre- or two hours post-meal) ... 1915
Ethmozine Tablets (Administration 30 minutes after a meal delays the rate of absorption but the

(▭ Described in PDR For Nonprescription Drugs) (◉ Described in PDR For Ophthalmology)

Food Interactions Cross-Reference

extent of absorption is not altered)... 2041

Famvir (Penciclovir C_{max} decreased approximately 50% and T_{max} was delayed by 1.5 hours when a capsule formulation of famciclovir was administered with food; there is no effect on the extent of availability (AUC) of penciclovir).. 2486

Hismanal Tablets (Reduces the absorption by 60%; patients should be instructed to take Hismanal on an empty stomach, e.g. at least 2 hours after a meal)... 1293

Hyzaar Tablets (Meal slows absorption and decreases C_{max} but has minor effects on losartan AUC or on the AUC of the metabolite)... 1677

Lanoxicaps (The rate of absorption is slowed)... 1117

Lanoxin Tablets (Slows the rate of absorption)... 1128

Lescol Capsules (Administration of fluvastatin with the evening meal results in a two-fold decrease in C_{max} and more than two-fold increase in t_{max} as compared to patients receiving the drug 4 hours after evening meal).............. 2267

Nalfon 200 Pulvules & Nalfon Tablets (Peak blood levels are delayed and diminished).................. 917

Nimotop Capsules (Administration of nimodipine capsules following a standard breakfast resulted in 68% lower peak plasma concentration and 38% lower bioavailability)... 610

PCE Dispertab Tablets (Optimal blood levels are obtained when PCE is given in the fasting state) 444

Prograf (The presence of food reduces the absorption of tacrolimus (decrease in AUC and C_{max} and increase in T_{max}).............. 1042

Ticlid Tablets (Administration after meals results in a 20% increase in the AUC of ticlopidine).................. 2156

Tolectin (200, 400 and 600 mg) (Decreases total tolmetin bioavailability by 16%; reduces peak plasma concentrations by 50%)... 1581

Vascor (200, 300 and 400 mg) Tablets (May result in a clinically insignificant delay in time to peak concentration, but neither peak plasma levels nor the extent of absorption was changed)... 1587

Zerit Capsules (Reduces mean SD C_{max} of stavudine and prolongs the median time to reach C_{max} from 0.6 to 1.5 hours; systemic exposure (AUC) remains unchanged)... 729

Meat extracts

Nardil (Concurrent and/or sequential intake must be avoided).. 1920

Parnate Tablets (Potential for hypertensive crisis)............................ 2503

Meat prepared with tenderizers

Parnate Tablets (Potential for hypertensive crisis)............................ 2503

Meat, unspecified

Nardil (Concurrent and/or sequential intake must be avoided).. 1920

Milk

(see under Dairy products)

Milk products

(see under Dairy products)

Milk, low fat

Dyazide (Concurrent use of low-salt milk with triamterene may result in hyperkalemia, especially in patients with renal insufficiency)... 2479

Milk, low salt

Dyrenium Capsules (Co-administration may promote serum potassium accumulation and possibly resulting in hyperkalemia)... 2481

Mustard

(see under Food, furocoumarin-containing)

Parsley

(see under Food, furocoumarin-containing)

Parsnips

(see under Food, furocoumarin-containing)

Pepperoni

Nardil (Concurrent and/or sequential intake must be avoided).. 1920

Raisins

Parnate Tablets (Potential for hypertensive crisis)............................ 2503

Salami, hard

Nardil (Concurrent and/or sequential intake must be avoided).. 1920

Salami, Genoa

Nardil (Concurrent and/or sequential intake must be avoided).. 1920

Salt substitutes, potassium-containing

Altace Capsules (Increases risk of hyperkalemia)................................... 1232

Sauerkraut

Nardil (Concurrent and/or sequential intake must be avoided).. 1920

Parnate Tablets (Potential for hypertensive crisis)............................ 2503

Sausage, dry

Nardil (Concurrent and/or sequential intake must be avoided).. 1920

Sherry

Parnate Tablets (Potential for hypertensive crisis)............................ 2503

Skipjack fish

Rifater (Isoniazid may inhibit diamine oxidase, causing exaggerated response (headache, sweating, palpitations, flushing, hypotension) to food containing histamine).. 1532

Soy sauce

Parnate Tablets (Potential for hypertensive crisis)............................ 2503

Soybean formula, children's

Synthroid Tablets (Binds and decreases absorption of levothyroxine sodium from the gastrointestinal tract)........................ 1359

Tea

(see under Beverages, caffeine-containing)

Tuna fish

Rifater (Isoniazid may inhibit diamine oxidase, causing exaggerated response (headache, sweating, palpitations, flushing, hypotension) to food containing histamine).. 1532

Vegetables, green leafy

Coumadin Tablets (Large amounts of green leafy vegetables may affect Coumadin therapy).............. 926

Wine products

(see also under Alcohol)

Nardil (Concurrent and/or sequential intake must be avoided).. 1920

Wine, unspecified

(see also under Alcohol)

Furoxone Liquid (Concurrent and/or sequential intake must be avoided).. 2046

Matulane Capsules (Concurrent use should be avoided).................. 2131

Nardil (Concurrent and/or sequential intake must be avoided).. 1920

Nicorette (Interferes with buccal absorption of nicotine from Nicorette)... 2458

Wine, Chianti

(see also under Alcohol)

Parnate Tablets (Potential for hypertensive crisis)............................ 2503

Wine, red

Rifater (Isoniazid has some MAO inhibiting activity, an interaction with tyramine containing food may occur)... 1532

Yeast extract

Furoxone Liquid (Concurrent and/or sequential intake must be avoided).. 2046

Nardil (Concurrent and/or sequential intake must be avoided).. 1920

Parnate Tablets (Potential for hypertensive crisis)............................ 2503

Yeast, brewer's

Nardil (Concurrent and/or sequential intake must be avoided).. 1920

Yogurt

Matulane Capsules (Concurrent use should be avoided).................. 2131

Nardil (Concurrent and/or sequential intake must be avoided).. 1920

Parnate Tablets (Potential for hypertensive crisis)............................ 2503

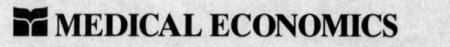

SECTION 3

SIDE EFFECTS INDEX

Presented in this section is an alphabetical list of every side effect reported in the "Adverse Reactions" section of the product descriptions in *PDR* and its companion volumes. Under each side effect is an alphabetical list of brands associated with the reaction. If noted in the underlying text, incidence is shown in parentheses immediately after the brand name. Products reporting an incidence of 3% or more are marked with a ▲ symbol at their left. Page numbers refer to the 1996 editions of *PDR* and *PDR For Ophthalmology* and the 1995 edition of *PDR For Nonprescription Drugs*, which is published later each year. A key to the symbols denoting the companion volumes appears in the bottom margin.

This index lists only side effects noted in official prescribing information as published by *PDR*. Entries are restricted to reactions occurring at recommended dosages in the general patient population. Precautions to be taken under special circumstances are not included, nor are the effects of overdosage.

A

A-V block

Adenocard Injection 1021
Atretol Tablets 573
Blocadren Tablets (Less than 1%) 1614
Brethaire Inhaler 813
Calan SR Caplets (0.8% to 1.2%) 2422
Calan Tablets (0.8% to 1.2%) 2419
Cardene I.V. (Rare) 2709
▲ Cardizem SR Capsules (0.6% to 7.6%) 1510
Cardizem Tablets (Less than 1%) .. 1512
Cartrol Tablets 410
Catapres Tablets (Rare) 674
Catapres-TTS (Rare) 675
Cognex Capsules (Rare) 1901
Combipres Tablets (Rare) 677
Cordarone Intravenous 2715
Dilacor XR Extended-release Capsules 2018
Diprivan Injection (Less than 1%) .. 2833
Ethmozine Tablets................................... 2041
Inderide Tablets 2732
Inderide LA Long Acting Capsules .. 2734
Isoptin Injectable (Rare) 1344
Isoptin Oral Tablets (0.8 to 1.2%) 1346
Isoptin SR Tablets (0.8% to 1.2%) 1348
Kerlone Tablets.. 2436
Kytril Injection (Rare)............................ 2490
Lanoxicaps 1117
Lanoxin Elixir Pediatric (Common).. 1120
Lanoxin Injection 1123
Lanoxin Injection Pediatric (Common)... 1126
Lanoxin Tablets 1128
Levatol 2403
Luvox Tablets (Rare) 2544
Mexitil Capsules (Less than 1% or about 2 in 1,000) 678
Normodyne Tablets 2379
Norpace (Less than 1%) 2444

Pepcid Injection (Infrequent) 1722
Pepcid (Infrequent)................................ 1720
Permax Tablets (Infrequent).............. 575
Prostigmin Injectable 1260
Prostigmin Tablets 1261
Quinidex Extentabs 2067
ReoPro Vials (1.3%) 1471
Risperdal (Infrequent)........................... 1301
Salagen Tablets (Rare) 1489
Sectral Capsules 2807
Serzone Tablets (Rare) 771
Tagamet (Rare) 2516
Tambocor Tablets 1497
Taxol (Two cases) 714
Tegretol Chewable Tablets 852
Tegretol Suspension................................ 852
Tegretol Tablets 852
Timolide Tablets....................................... 1748
Tonocard Tablets (Less than 1%) .. 531
Verelan Capsules (0.8 to 1.2%)...... 1410
Verelan Capsules (0.8 to 1.2%)...... 2824
Zantac (Rare) 1209
Zantac Injection (Rare) 1207
Zantac Syrup (Rare)............................... 1209

A-V block, first-degree

Adenocard Injection 1021
Adenoscan (2.9% to 3%) 1024
Calan SR Caplets (1.2%)...................... 2422
Calan Tablets (1.2%) 2419
Cardizem CD Capsules (2.4% to 3.3%) 1506
▲ Cardizem SR Capsules (1.8% to 7.6%) 1510
Cardizem Injectable (Less than 1%) 1508
Cardizem Tablets (Less than 1%) .. 1512
Dilacor XR Extended-release Capsules (Infrequent) 2018
Effexor (Rare) 2719
Foscavir Injection (Between 1% and 5%) 547
Isoptin Oral Tablets (1.2%) 1346

Isoptin SR Tablets (1.2%).................... 1348
Prozac Pulvules & Liquid, Oral Solution (Rare) 919
▲ Rythmol Tablets–150mg, 225mg, 300mg (0.8 to 4.5%)......................... 1352
Verelan Capsules (1.2%)...................... 1410
Verelan Capsules (1.2%)...................... 2824

A-V block, intensification of

Blocadren Tablets 1614
Cartrol Tablets 410
Inderal 2728
Inderal LA Long Acting Capsules 2730
Inderide Tablets 2732
Inderide LA Long Acting Capsules .. 2734
Levatol 2403
Lopressor HCT Tablets 832
Sectral Capsules 2807
Tenoretic Tablets..................................... 2845
Toprol-XL Tablets 565
Trandate Tablets 1185
Visken Tablets.. 2299

A-V block, second-degree

Adenocard Injection 1021
Adenoscan (2.6% to 3%) 1024
Blocadren Tablets (Less than 1%) 1614
Calan SR Caplets (0.8%) 2422
Calan Tablets (0.8%) 2419
Cardizem CD Capsules (Less than 1%) 1506
Cardizem SR Capsules (0.6%) 1510
Cardizem Injectable (Less than 1%) 1508
Cardizem Tablets (Less than 1%).. 1512
Cozaar Tablets (Less than 1%)......... 1628
Hyzaar Tablets 1677
Isoptin Oral Tablets (0.8%) 1346
Isoptin SR Tablets (0.8%).................... 1348
Rythmol Tablets–150mg, 225mg, 300mg (1.2%) 1352
Tambocor Tablets (Less than 1%) 1497
Verelan Capsules (0.8% to 1.2%) 1410

Verelan Capsules (0.8% to 1.2%) 2824

A-V block, third-degree

Adenocard Injection 1021
Adenoscan (0.8%; less than 1%) .. 1024
Blocadren Tablets (Less than 1%) 1614
Calan SR Caplets (0.8%)...................... 2422
Calan Tablets (0.8%) 2419
Cardizem CD Capsules (Less than 1%) 1506
Cardizem SR Capsules (Less than 1%) 1510
Cardizem Injectable 1508
Cardizem Tablets (Less than 1%) .. 1512
Isoptin Oral Tablets (0.8%) 1346
Isoptin SR Tablets (0.8%).................... 1348
Tambocor Tablets (Less than 1%) 1497
Verelan Capsules (0.8% to 1.2%) 1410
Verelan Capsules (0.8% to 1.2%) 2824

A-V conduction, prolongation

Isoptin Injectable 1344
Sensorcaine 559

A-V conduction changes, unspecified

Elavil 2838
Endep Tablets 2174
Nimotop Capsules 610

A-V fistula, clotted

Atgam Sterile Solution (More than 1% but less than 5%)........................ 2581

A-V shunt, thrombosis of (see under Thrombosis of vascular access)

Abdominal adhesion

Lippes Loop Intrauterine Double-S.. 1848
ParaGard T380A Intrauterine Copper Contraceptive 1880

(**◻** Described in PDR For Nonprescription Drugs) Incidence data in parenthesis; ▲ 3% or more (◎ Described in PDR For Ophthalmology)

Abdominal bloating

AeroBid Inhaler System (Less than 1%) 1005
Aerobid-M Inhaler System (Less than 1%) 1005
Asacol Delayed-Release Tablets 1979
Atromid-S Capsules 2701
Brevicon 2088
Climara Transdermal System 645
▲ Clomid (5.5%) 1514
Colestid Tablets (Less frequent) 2591
▲ Colyte and Colyte-flavored (Among most frequent) 2396
▲ Creon (Among most frequent) 2536
Demulen 2428
DiaBeta Tablets (1.8%) 1239
Estraderm Transdermal System 824
ESTRATAB Tablets (0.3, 0.625, 1.25, 2.5 mg) 2536
Estratest 2539
▲ Glucophage (Among most common) 752
Glynase PresTab Tablets (1.8%) 2609
▲ GoLYTELY (Up to 50%) 688
Hivid Tablets (Less than 1% to less than 3%) 2121
Humegon 1824
Levlen/Tri-Levlen 651
Metrodin (urofollitropin for injection) 2446
Midamor Tablets (Less than or equal to 1%) 1703
Moduretic Tablets (Less than or equal to 1%) 1705
Motrin Ibuprofen Suspension, Oral Drops, Chewable Tablets, Caplets (1% to less than 3%) 1546
Mycelex-G 500 mg Vaginal Tablets (Rare) 609
Mykrox Tablets (Less than 2%) 993
Norinyl 2088
Noroxin Tablets (Less frequent) 1715
Noroxin Tablets (Less frequent) 2048
▲ Norpace (3 to 9%) 2444
Nor-Q D Tablets 2135
▲ NuLYTELY (Up to 50% of patients) 689
▲ Cherry Flavor NuLYTELY (Among most common) 689
Ogen Tablets 2627
Ogen Vaginal Cream 2630
PMB 200 and PMB 400 2783
Pergonal (menotropins for injection, USP) 2448
Premarin Intravenous 2787
Premarin with Methyltestosterone 2794
Premarin Tablets 2789
Premarin Vaginal Cream 2791
Premphase 2797
Prempro 2801
Prilosec Delayed-Release Capsules (Less than 1%) 529
Roferon-A Injection (Less than 1%) 2145
▲ THROMBATE III Antithrombin III (Human) (1 of 17) 637
Ticlid Tablets (0.5% to 1.0%) 2156
Toradol (Greater than 1%) 2159
Trental Tablets (0.6%) 1244
Levlen/Tri-Levlen 651
Tri-Norinyl 2164
Zaroxolyn Tablets 1000

Abdominal discomfort (see also under Distress, gastrointestinal; Distress, abdominal)

Children's Advil Suspension (Less than 3%) 2692
Aquasol A Vitamin A Capsules, USP 534
Aquasol A Parenteral 534
Arfonad Ampuls 2080
Biaxin (2%) 405
Brevibloc Injection (Less than 1%) 1808
BuSpar (2%) 737
Carafate Tablets (Less than 0.5%) 1504
Cipro I.V. (1.7%) 595
Cipro Tablets (0.3% to 1.7%) 592
▲ Clomid (5.5%) 1514
▲ Clozaril Tablets (4%) 2252
Colestid Tablets (Less frequent) 2591
Crystodigin Tablets 1433
Cytoxan (Less frequent) 694
Dalgan Injection (Less than 1%) 538
Desferal Vials 820
Dulcolax 864
Duvoid (Infrequent) 2044
▲ E.E.S. (Most frequent) 424
▲ E-Mycin Tablets (One of the two most frequent) 1341
▲ EryPed 200 & EryPed 400 Granules (Most frequent) 421
Feldene Capsules (Greater than 1%) 1965
Flagyl I.V. 2247
Fleet Bisacodyl Enema 1002
Fleet Prep Kits 1003
Hyperstat I.V. Injection 2363
Imodium Capsules 1295
K-Dur Microburst Release System (potassium chloride, USP) E.R. Tablets 1325
▲ Kolyum Liquid (Among most common) 992
Lomotil 2439
Children's Motrin Ibuprofen Oral Suspension (Greater than 1% but less than 3%) 1546
Motrin Tablets (Less than 3%) 2625
Mykrox Tablets (Less than 2%) 993
Neoral (Up to 7%) 2276
Papaverine Hydrochloride Vials and Ampoules 1468
Parlodel 2281
Pepcid Injection (Infrequent) 1722
Pepcid (Infrequent) 1720
▲ Rowasa (8.10%) 2548
▲ Sandimmune (Less than 1 to 7%) 2286
▲ Serophene (clomiphene citrate tablets, USP) (Approximately 1 in 15 patients) 2451
▲ Slow-K Extended-Release Tablets (Among most common) 851
Tonocard Tablets (Less than 1%) 531
Trental Tablets 1244
▲ Visken Tablets (4%) 2299

Abdominal distention

Children's Advil Suspension (Less than 3%) 2692
Aldoclor Tablets 1598
Aldomet Ester HCl Injection 1602
Aldomet Oral 1600
Aldoril Tablets 1604
Aristocort Suspension (Forte Parenteral) 1027
Aristocort Suspension (Intralesional) 1025
Aristocort Tablets 1022
Aristospan Suspension (Intra-articular) 1033
Aristospan Suspension (Intralesional) 1032
Cataflam (1% to 3%) 816
Celestone Soluspan Suspension 2347
▲ CellCept Capsules (More than or equal to 3%) 2099
Claritin-D (Less frequent) 2350
▲ Clomid (5.5%) 1514
Clozaril Tablets (Less than 1%) 2252
CORTENEMA 2535
Cortone Acetate Sterile Suspension 1623
Cortone Acetate Tablets 1624
Cytovene (1% or less) 2103
Dalalone D.P. Injectable 1011
Decadron Elixir 1633
Decadron Phosphate Injection 1637
Decadron Phosphate Respihaler 1642
Decadron Phosphate Turbinaire 1645
Decadron Phosphate with Xylocaine Injection, Sterile 1639
Decadron Tablets 1635
Decadron-LA Sterile Suspension 1646
Deltasone Tablets 2595
Depo-Medrol Single-Dose Vial 2600
Depo-Medrol Sterile Aqueous Suspension 2597
Dexacort Phosphate in Respihaler 458
Dexacort Phosphate in Turbinaire 459
Duragesic Transdermal System (Less than 1%) 1288
Effexor (Infrequent) 2719
Ensure Plus High Calorie Complete Nutrition 2221
Florinef Acetate Tablets 505
Humegon 1824
Hydeltrasol Injection, Sterile 1665
Hydeltra-T.B.A. Sterile Suspension 1667
Hydrocortone Acetate Sterile Suspension 1669
Hydrocortone Phosphate Injection, Sterile 1670
Hydrocortone Tablets 1672
Imodium Capsules 1295
Indocin I.V. (1% to 3%) 1684
Intron A (Less than 5%) 2364
Lamictal Tablets (Rare) 1112
Medrol 2621
▲ Metrodin (urofollitropin for injection) (Approximately 20%) 2446
Monopril Tablets (0.2% to 1.0%) 757
Motrin Tablets (Less than 3%) 2625
▲ Cherry Flavor NuLYTELY (Among most common) 689
Osmolite HN High Nitrogen Isotonic Liquid Nutrition 2222
Pediapred Oral Liquid 995
Pentasa (Less than 1%) 1527
Pergonal (menotropins for injection, USP) 2448
Permax Tablets (Infrequent) 575
Prelone Syrup 1787
▲ Prograf (Greater than 3%) 1042
Prozac Pulvules & Liquid, Oral Solution (Rare) 919
Risperdal (Rare) 1301
▲ Sandostatin Injection (Less than 10%) 2292
Serophene (clomiphene citrate tablets, USP) 2451
Serzone Tablets (Infrequent) 771
Solu-Cortef Sterile Powder 2641
Solu-Medrol Sterile Powder 2643
Unasyn (Less than 1%) 2212
Voltaren Tablets (1% to 3%) 861
Zoloft Tablets (Rare) 2217

Abdominal mass

Demulen 2428
Estraderm Transdermal System 824
Estratest 2539

Abdominal pain/cramps

Accupril Tablets (1.0%) 1893
Accutane Capsules 2076
Actigall Capsules 802
▲ Actimmune (8%) 1056
Adalat CC (Less than 1.0%) 589
Children's Advil Suspension (Less than 1%) 2692
▲ AeroBid Inhaler System (3-9%) 1005
▲ Aerobid-M Inhaler System (3-9%) 1005
Aldactazide 2413
Aldactone 2414
Aldoclor Tablets 1598
Aldoril Tablets 1604
Altace Capsules (Less than 1%) 1232
Ambien Tablets (2%) 2416
Aminohippurate Sodium Injection 1606
▲ Anafranil Capsules (11% to 13%) 803
▲ Anaprox/Naprosyn (3% to 9%) 2117
Ancef Injection 2465
Ancobon Capsules 2079
▲ Ansaid Tablets (3-9%) 2579
Apresazide Capsules 808
Aralen Hydrochloride Injection 2301
Aralen Phosphate Tablets 2301
▲ Aredia for Injection (Up to at least 15%) 810
▲ Asacol Delayed-Release Tablets (18%) 1979
Asendin Tablets (Less than 1%) 1369
Atamet 572
Atgam Sterile Solution (Less than 5%) 2581
Atretol Tablets 573
▲ Axid Pulvules (7.5%) 1427
Azactam for Injection (Less than 1%) 734
Azo Gantanol Tablets 2080
Azo Gantrisin Tablets 2081
Azulfidine (Rare) 1949
▲ BCG Vaccine, USP (TICE) (1.5% to 4.0%) 1814
Bactrim DS Tablets 2084
Bactrim I.V. Infusion 2082
Bactrim 2084
Bentyl 1501
Betapace Tablets (Less than 1% to 3%) 641
▲ Betaseron for SC Injection (32%) 658
Biaxin (2%) 405
Blocadren Tablets 1614
Brevicon 2088
Brevital Sodium Vials 1429
Bumex (0.2%) 2093
Capoten (About 0.5 to 2%) 739
Capozide (0.5 to 2%) 742
Cardene I.V. (0.7%) 2709
Cardura Tablets (2.4%) 2186
Carnitor Tablets and Solution 2453
Cartrol Tablets (1.3%) 410
▲ Cataflam (3% to 9%) 816
Cefotan 2829
Ceftin (Less than 1% but more than 0.1%) 1078
Cefzil Tablets and Oral Suspension (1%) 746
▲ CellCept Capsules (24.7% to 27.6%; 11.9% to 12.1%) 2099
Celontin Kapseals (Frequent) 1899
Ceptaz (One in 416 patients) 1081
Ceredase 1065
Cervidil (Less than 1%) 1010
▲ CHEMET (succimer) Capsules (5.2 to 15.7%) 1545
Cipro I.V. (1% or less) 595
Cipro I.V. Pharmacy Bulk Package (Less than 1%) 597
Cipro Tablets (1.7%) 592
Claritin-D (Less frequent) 2350
Cleocin Phosphate Injection 2586
Cleocin T Topical 2590
Climara Transdermal System 645
Cleocin Vaginal Cream (Less than 1%) 2589
▲ Clinoril Tablets (10%) 1618
Clomid 1514
▲ Cognex Capsules (8%) 1901
ColBENEMID Tablets 1622
Colestid Tablets (Less frequent) 2591
Colyte and Colyte-flavored 2396
Cordarone Tablets (1 to 3%) 2712
Cosmegen Injection 1626
Coumadin (Infrequent) 926
Cozaar Tablets (1% or greater) 1628
▲ Creon (Among most frequent) 2536
Crystodigin Tablets 1433
Cytosar-U Sterile Powder (Less frequent) 2592
▲ Cytotec (13-20%) 2424
▲ Cytovene (17%) 2103
Cytoxan (Less frequent) 694
DDAVP Injection (Infrequent) 2014
DDAVP Injection 15 mcg/mL (Infrequent) 2015
DDAVP (2%) 2017
Dalgan Injection (Less than 1%) 538
Dalmane Capsules (Rare) 2173
Dantrium Capsules (Less frequent) 1982
Dapsone Tablets USP 1284
Darvon-N/Darvocet-N 1433
Darvon 1435
Darvon-N Suspension & Tablets 1433
Daypro Caplets (Greater than 1% but less than 3%) 2426
Demser Capsules (Infrequent) 1649
Demulen 2428
Depakene 413
▲ Depakote Tablets (9%) 415
▲ Depo-Provera Contraceptive Injection (More than 5%) 2602
Desmopressin Acetate Rhinal Tube (2%) 979
Desogen Tablets 1817
Diethylstilbestrol Tablets 1437
▲ Diflucan Injection, Tablets, and Oral Suspension (1.7% to 6%) 2194
Dilacor XR Extended-release Capsules (1.0%) 2018
Dilaudid-HP Injection (Less frequent) 1337
Dilaudid-HP Lyophilized Powder 250 mg (Less frequent) 1337
▲ Dipentum Capsules (10.1%) 1951
Diprivan Injection (Less than 1%) 2833
Diucardin Tablets 2718
Diuril Sodium Intravenous 1652
Doral Tablets 2664
▲ Duragesic Transdermal System (3% to 10%) 1288
Duricef 748
Duvoid (Infrequent) 2044
Dyazide 2479
▲ E.E.S. (Most frequent) 424
▲ E-Mycin Tablets (One of the most frequent) 1341
▲ EC-Naprosyn Delayed-Release Tablets (3% to 9%) 2117
Edecrin 1657
▲ Effexor (2.2% to 8.0%) 2719
▲ Eldepryl Tablets (4 of 49 patients) 2550
Elspar 1659
Empirin with Codeine Tablets 1093
Enduron Tablets 420
Engerix-B Unit-Dose Vials (Less than 1%) 2482
Ensure Plus High Calorie Complete Nutrition 2221
▲ Ergamisol Tablets (2% to 5%) 1292
▲ ERYC (Among most frequent) 1915
▲ EryPed (Among most frequent) 421
▲ Ery-Tab Tablets (Among most frequent) 422
▲ Erythrocin Stearate Filmtab (Among most frequent) 425
▲ Erythromycin Base Filmtab (Among most frequent) 426
▲ Erythromycin Delayed-Release

(◘ Described in PDR For Nonprescription Drugs) Incidence data in parenthesis; ▲ 3% or more (◉ Described in PDR For Ophthalmology)

1209 Side Effects Index Abdominal pain/cramps

Capsules, USP (Among most frequent) 427
▲ Esgic-plus Tablets (Among most frequent) 1013
Esidrix Tablets 821
Esimil Tablets 822
Eskalith 2485
Estrace Cream and Tablets 749
Estraderm Transdermal System 824
ESTRATAB Tablets (0.3, 0.625, 1.25, 2.5 mg) 2536
Estratest 2539
Ethiodol 2340
▲ Ethmozine Tablets (2% to 5%) 2041
Famvir (1.1%) 2486
Fansidar Tablets 2114
▲ Felbatol (5.3%) 2666
Feldene Capsules (Greater than 1%) 1965
▲ Fioricet Tablets (Among most frequent) 2258
Fioricet with Codeine Capsules (Frequent) 2260
▲ Fiorinal with Codeine Capsules (3.7%) 2262
Flagyl 375 Capsules 2434
Fleet Bisacodyl Enema 1002
Fleet Prep Kits 1003
Floropryl Sterile Ophthalmic Ointment (Rare) 1662
Floxin I.V. (1% to 3%) 1571
Floxin Tablets (200 mg, 300 mg, 400 mg) (1% to 3%) 1567
Flumadine Tablets & Syrup (1.4%) 1015
Fortaz (1 in 416) 1100
▲ Foscavir Injection (5% or greater) 547
Sterile FUDR 2118
▲ Fungizone Intravenous (Among most common) 506
Gamimune N, 5% Immune Globulin Intravenous (Human), 5% 619
Gamimune N, 10% Immune Globulin Intravenous (Human), 10% 621
Gantanol Tablets 2119
Gantrisin 2120
Gastrocrom Capsules (2 of 87 patients) 984
Geocillin Tablets 2199
GoLYTELY (Infrequent) 688
▲ Habitrol Nicotine Transdermal System (3% to 9% of patients) 865
Halcion Tablets (0.9% to 0.5%) 2611
Havrix (Less than 1%) 2489
Hismanal Tablets (1.4%) 1293
Hivid Tablets (Less than 1% to less than 3%) 2121
Humegon 1824
Humorsol Sterile Ophthalmic Solution (Rare) 1664
HydroDIURIL Tablets 1674
Hylorel Tablets (1.7%) 985
Hytrin Capsules (At least 1%) 430
Hyzaar Tablets (1.2%) 1677
IBU Tablets (Greater than 1%) 1342
▲ Idamycin (73%) 1955
▲ Ilosone (One of the two most frequent) 911
Imdur (Less than or equal to 5%) 1323
Imodium Capsules 1295
▲ Imovax Rabies Vaccine (About 20%) 881
Imuran (Rare) 1110
Inderal 2728
Inderal LA Long Acting Capsules 2730
Inderide Tablets 2732
Inderide LA Long Acting Capsules 2734
Indocin (Greater than 1%) 1680
INFeD (Iron Dextran Injection, USP) 2345
Inocor Lactate Injection (0.4%) 2309
▲ Intron A (1% to 21%) 2364
IOPIDINE Sterile Ophthalmic Solution ◉ 219
Ismo Tablets (Fewer than 1%) 2738
Isopto Carbachol Ophthalmic Solution ◉ 223
▲ JE-VAX (Approximately 10%) 886
K-Dur Microburst Release System (potassium chloride, USP) E.R. Tablets 1325
▲ K-Lor Powder Packets (Most common) 434
▲ K-Norm Extended-Release Capsules (Among most common) 991
Keflex Pulvules & Oral Suspension 914
Keftab Tablets 915
▲ Kolyum Liquid (Among most common) 992
Ku-Zyme HP Capsules 2402
▲ Kytril Tablets (6%) 2492
▲ Lamictal Tablets (5.2%) 1112
▲ Lamprene Capsules (40-50%) 828
Lanoxicaps (Very rare) 1117
Lanoxin Elixir Pediatric (Very rare) 1120
Lanoxin Injection (Very rare) 1123
Lanoxin Injection Pediatric (Very rare) 1126
Lanoxin Tablets (Very rare) 1128
▲ Lariam Tablets (Among most frequent) 2128
Larodopa Tablets (Relatively frequent) 2129
Lasix Injection, Oral Solution and Tablets 1240
▲ Lescol Capsules (5.5%) 2267
▲ Leustatin (6%) 1834
Levlen/Tri-Levlen 651
Lioresal Tablets (Rare) 829
Lithonate/Lithotabs/Lithobid 2543
▲ Lodine Capsules and Tablets (3-9%) 2743
Lo/Ovral Tablets 2746
Lo/Ovral-28 Tablets 2751
▲ Lopid Tablets (9.8%) 1917
Lopressor (Less than 1%) 830
Lorabid Suspension and Pulvules (1.4%) 1459
Lorelco Tablets 1517
Lotensin HCT (0.3% to 1.0%) 837
Lotrel Capsules 840
Lozol Tablets (Less than 5%) 2022
Ludiomil Tablets (Rare) 843
Luvox Tablets 2544
MS Contin Tablets (Less frequent) 1994
MSIR (Infrequent) 1997
Macrobid Capsules (Less than 1%) 1988
Macrodantin Capsules (Less common) 1989
Marax Tablets & DF Syrup (Frequent, on empty stomach) 2200
▲ Marinol (Dronabinol) Capsules (3% to 10%) 2231
Massengill Disposable Douche 2457
Massengill Medicated Disposable Douche 2458
Massengill Medicated Liquid Concentrate ⊡ 821
Matulane Capsules 2131
Maxair Autohaler 1492
Maxair Inhaler (Less than 1%) 1494
Maxaquin Tablets (Less than 1%) 2440
Megace Oral Suspension (1% to 3%) 699
Menest Tablets 2494
▲ Mepron Suspension (4% to 10%) 1135
Mestinon Injectable 1253
Mestinon 1254
Methadone Hydrochloride Oral Concentrate 2233
▲ Metrodin (urofollitropin for injection) (Approximately 20%) 2446
MetroGel-Vaginal (Equal to or less than 3.4%) 902
▲ Mevacor Tablets (2.0% to 5.7%) 1699
Mexitil Capsules (1.2%) 678
Miacalcin Injection 2273
Miacalcin Nasal Spray (1% to 3%) 2275
Micro-K 2063
▲ Micro-K LS Packets (Most common) 2064
Micronor Tablets 1872
Midamor Tablets (Between 1% and 3%) 1703
Minipress Capsules (Less than 1%) 1937
Minizide Capsules (Rare) 1938
MIOSTAT Intraocular Solution ◉ 224
Modicon 1872
Moduretic Tablets (Greater than 1%, less than 3%) 1705
Monoket (Up to 2%) 2406
Monopril Tablets (0.2% to 1.0%) 757
Children's Motrin Ibuprofen Oral Suspension (Greater than 1% but less than 3%) 1546
Motrin Tablets (Less than 1%) 2625
Motrin Ibuprofen Suspension, Oral Drops, Chewable Tablets, Caplets (1% to less than 3%) 1546
Myambutol Tablets 1386
Mycelex-G 500 mg Vaginal Tablets (Rare) 609
▲ Mycobutin Capsules (4%) 1957
Mykrox Tablets (Less than 2%) 993
Myochrysine Injection 1711
Nalfon 200 Pulvules & Nalfon Tablets (2%) 917
▲ Anaprox/Naprosyn (3% to 9%) 2117
NebuPent for Inhalation Solution (Greater than 1%, up to 5%) 1040
NegGram 2323
NEOSAR Lyophilized/Neosar (Less frequent) 1959
Neupogen for Injection (Infrequent) 495
Neurontin Capsules (More than 1%) 1922
Nicoderm (nicotine transdermal system) (1% to 3%) 1518
▲ Nicorette (3% to 9% of patients) 2458
Nicotrol Nicotine Transdermal System (1% to 3%) 1550
Nizoral Tablets (1.2%) 1298
Nolvadex Tablets (1%) 2841
Nordette-21 Tablets 2755
Nordette-28 Tablets 2758
Norinyl 2088
Normodyne Tablets 2379
Noroxin Tablets (0.3% to 1.6%) 1715
Noroxin Tablets (0.3% to 1.6%) 2048
▲ Norpace (3 to 9%) 2444
Norpramin Tablets 1526
Nor-Q D Tablets 2135
Norvasc Tablets (1.6%) 1940
▲ Novantrone (9 to 15%) 1279
Nubain Injection (1% or less) 935
NuLYTELY (Less frequent) 689
Cherry Flavor NuLYTELY (Less frequent) 689
Ogen Tablets 2627
Ogen Vaginal Cream 2630
▲ Oncaspar (Greater than 1% but less than 5%) 2028
Oncovin Solution Vials & Hyporets 1466
Oramorph SR (Morphine Sulfate Sustained Release Tablets) (Less frequent) 2236
Oreton Methyl 1255
▲ Orlamm (3% to 9%) 2239
Ornade Spansule Capsules 2502
Ortho-Cept 1851
Ortho-Cyclen/Ortho-Tri-Cyclen 1858
Ortho Dienestrol Cream 1866
Ortho-Est 1869
Ortho-Novum 1872
Ortho-Cyclen/Ortho Tri-Cyclen 1858
Orthoclone OKT3 Sterile Solution 1837
▲ Orudis Capsules (3% to 9%) 2766
▲ Oruvail Capsules (3% to 9%) 2766
Osmolite HN High Nitrogen Isotonic Liquid Nutrition 2222
Ovcon 760
Ovral Tablets 2770
Ovral-28 Tablets 2770
Ovrette Tablets 2771
▲ PCE Dispertab Tablets (Among most frequent) 444
PMB 200 and PMB 400 2783
Pamelor 2280
ParaGard T380A Intrauterine Copper Contraceptive 1880
▲ Parlodel (4%) 2281
Parnate Tablets 2503
▲ PASER Granules (Among most common) 1285
▲ Paxil Tablets (3.1%) 2505
Penetrex Tablets (Less than 1% to 2%) 2031
Pentasa (1.1% to 1.7%) 1527
Peptavlon 2878
Pergonal (menotropins for injection, USP) 2448
Peri-Colace 2052
▲ Permax Tablets (5.8%) 575
▲ Phrenilin (Among most frequent) 785
Plaquenil Sulfate Tablets 2328
Plendil Extended-Release Tablets (0.5% to 1.5%) 527
Pondimin Tablets 2066
Ponstel 1925
▲ Pravachol (2.0% to 5.4%) 765
Premarin Intravenous 2787
Premarin with Methyltestosterone 2794
Premarin Tablets 2789
Premarin Vaginal Cream 2791
Premphase 2797
Prempro 2801
PREVACID Delayed-Release Capsules (1.8%) 2562
▲ Prilosec Delayed-Release Capsules (2.4% to 5.2%) 529
Primaxin I.M. 1727
Primaxin I.V. (Less than 0.2%) 1729
▲ Prinivil Tablets (0.3% to 4.0%) 1733
Prinzide Tablets (0.3 to 1%) 1737
Procan SR Tablets (Common) 1926
Procardia Capsules (2% or less) 1971
Procardia XL Extended Release Tablets (Less than 3%) 1972
Proglycem (Frequent) 580
▲ Prograf (26% to 59%) 1042
▲ Proleukin for Injection (15%) 797
▲ Propulsid (10.2%) 1300
ProSom Tablets (1%) 449
Prostep (nicotine transdermal system) (1% to 3% of patients) 1394
▲ Prostigmin Injectable (Most common) 1260
Prostigmin Tablets 1261
Protostat Tablets (Occasional) 1883
▲ Prozac Pulvules & Liquid, Oral Solution (3.4%) 919
Pulmozyme Inhalation 1064
Questran Light (Less frequent) 769
Questran Powder (Less frequent) 770
▲ Quinidex Extentabs (Among most frequent) 2067
▲ Rabies Vaccine, Imovax Rabies I.D. (About 20%) 883
Recombivax HB (Less than 1%) 1744
▲ Relafen Tablets (12%) 2510
▲ Retrovir Capsules (3.2%) 1158
▲ Retrovir I.V. Infusion (4%) 1163
▲ Retrovir Syrup (3.2%) 1158
▲ ReVia Tablets (More than 10%) 940
Revex 1811
▲ Ridaura Capsules (14%) 2513
Rifadin (Some patients) 1528
Rifater 1532
Rimactane Capsules 847
Risperdal (1% to 4%) 1301
Ritalin 848
Rocephin Injectable Vials, ADD-Vantage, Galaxy Container (Rare) 2142
▲ Roferon-A Injection (15%) 2145
▲ Rowasa (3.0 to 8.10%) 2548
Rythmol Tablets–150mg, 225mg, 300mg (0.8 to 1.9%) 1352
▲ Salagen Tablets (4%) 1489
Salflex Tablets 786
Sansert Tablets 2295
Sectral Capsules (Up to 2%) 2807
▲ Sedapap Tablets 50 mg/650 mg (Among the most frequent) 1543
Septra 1174
Septra I.V. Infusion 1169
Septra I.V. Infusion ADD-Vantage Vials 1171
Septra 1174
Ser-Ap-Es Tablets 849
Serevent Inhalation Aerosol (1% to 3%) 1176
Serophene (clomiphene citrate tablets, USP) 2451
Serzone Tablets 771
Sinemet Tablets 943
Sinemet CR Tablets 944
Solganal Suspension (Rare) 2388
Sporanox Capsules (1.4% to 1.5%) 1305
Stilphostrol Tablets and Ampuls 612
Stimate, (desmopressin acetate) Nasal Spray, 1.5 mg/mL (Infrequent) 525
▲ Supprelin Injection (1% to 12%) 2056
▲ Suprax (3%) 1399
Surmontil Capsules 2811
Talwin Injection (Rare) 2334
▲ Tambocor Tablets (3.3%) 1497
Tao Capsules (Most frequent) 2209
Tazicef for Injection (Less than 2%; 1 in 416 patients) 2519
Tazidime Vials, Faspak & ADD-Vantage (1 in 416) 1478
▲ Tegison Capsules (25-50%) 2154
Tegretol Chewable Tablets 852
Tegretol Suspension 852
Tegretol Tablets 852
Tenex Tablets (3% or less) 2074
Tensilon Injectable 1261
▲ Terazol 3 Vaginal Cream (3.4%) 1886
▲ TheraCys BCG Live (Intravesical) (2.7% to 6.3%) 897
Thioplex (Thiotepa For Injection) 1281
Tilade (1.2%) 996
Tofranil Ampuls 854
Tofranil Tablets 856
Tofranil-PM Capsules 857
▲ Tolectin (200, 400 and 600 mg) (3 to 9%) 1581
Tonocard Tablets (Less than 1%) 531
Levlen/Tri-Levlen 651
Trinalin Repetabs Tablets 1330
Tri-Norinyl 2164
Triphasil-21 Tablets (Occasional) 2814
Triphasil-28 Tablets 2819
Tylenol with Codeine 1583
Typhim Vi 899

(⊡ Described in PDR For Nonprescription Drugs) Incidence data in parenthesis; ▲ 3% or more (◉ Described in PDR For Ophthalmology)

Abdominal pain/cramps — Side Effects Index — 1210

Ultram Tablets (50 mg) (1% to 5%) ... 1585
Ultrase Capsules ... 2343
▲ Ultrase MT Capsules (5.7%) ... 2344
Univasc Tablets (Less than 1%) ... 2410
Urecholine ... 1761
Valtrex Caplets (2% to 3%) ... 1194
Vantin for Oral Suspension and Vantin Tablets (Less than 1% to 1.6%) ... 2646
Varivax (Greater than or equal to 1%) ... 1762
▲ Vascor (200, 300 and 400 mg) Tablets (3.02%) ... 1587
Vaseretic Tablets (0.5% to 2.0%) ... 1765
Vasotec I.V. ... 1768
Vasotec Tablets (1.6%) ... 1771
Velban Vials ... 1484
VePesid Capsules and Injection (Infrequent; up to 2%) ... 718
Vermox Chewable Tablets ... 1312
▲ Videx Tablets, Powder for Oral Solution, & Pediatric Powder for Oral Solution (6% to 35%) ... 720
Vivactil Tablets ... 1774
Vivotif Berna ... 665
▲ Voltaren Tablets (3% to 9%) ... 861
Wygesic Tablets ... 2827
Yodoxin ... 1230
Zantac ... 1209
Zantac Injection ... 1207
Zantac Syrup ... 1209
Zarontin Capsules (Frequent) ... 1928
Zarontin Syrup (Frequent) ... 1929
Zaroxolyn Tablets ... 1000
Zebeta Tablets ... 1413
▲ Zerit Capsules (4% to 26%) ... 729
Zestoretic (0.3 to 1.0%) ... 2850
Zestril Tablets (0.3% to 4.0%) ... 2854
Ziac ... 1415
Zinacef ... 1211
▲ Zithromax (3% to 5%) ... 1944
▲ Zocor Tablets (3.2%) ... 1775
Zofran Tablets (1% to 3%) ... 1217
▲ Zoladex (7%) ... 2858
Zoloft Tablets (2.4%) ... 2217
Zosyn (1.3%) ... 1419
Zosyn Pharmacy Bulk Package (1.3%) ... 1422
Zovirax Capsules (0.6%) ... 1219
Zovirax Sterile Powder (Less than 1%) ... 1223
Zovirax (0.6%) ... 1219
Zyloprim Tablets (Less than 1%) ... 1226

Abdominal symptom complex, acute
Clomid ... 1514
Fiorinal with Codeine Capsules ... 2262
Permax Tablets (Rare) ... 575
Questran Light (One patient) ... 769
Questran Powder (One patient) ... 770

Abortion
Amen Tablets ... 780
Effexor (Rare) ... 2719
Imitrex Tablets (Rare) ... 1106
Methotrexate Sodium Tablets, Injection, for Injection and LPF Injection ... 1275
Metrodin (urofollitropin for injection) (3 reported) ... 2446
Nicorette ... 2458
Paxil Tablets (Infrequent) ... 2505
Permax Tablets (Infrequent) ... 575
Prozac Pulvules & Liquid, Oral Solution (Rare) ... 919

Abortion, septic
Lippes Loop Intrauterine Double-S.. 1848
ParaGard T380A Intrauterine Copper Contraceptive ... 1880

Abortion, spontaneous
Accutane Capsules ... 2076
Depo-Provera Sterile Aqueous Suspension ... 2606
Lippes Loop Intrauterine Double-S.. 1848
Lupron Depot-PED 7.5 mg, 11.25 mg and 15 mg (Possible) ... 2560
Nolvadex Tablets (A small number of reports) ... 2841
ParaGard T380A Intrauterine Copper Contraceptive ... 1880
▲ Parlodel (11.4%) ... 2281
Syntocinon Injection ... 2296
Vermox Chewable Tablets ... 1312

Abscess
Ambien Tablets (Rare) ... 2416
Aramine Injection ... 1609
Aristocort Suspension (Forte Parenteral) ... 1027
Aristocort Suspension (Intralesional) ... 1025
Aristospan Suspension (Intra-articular) ... 1033
Aristospan Suspension (Intralesional) ... 1032
BCG Vaccine, USP (TICE) (1.8%) .. 1814
Betaseron for SC Injection ... 658
Capastat Sulfate Vials ... 2868
Celestone Soluspan Suspension ... 2347
Cortone Acetate Sterile Suspension ... 1623
Cytovene (1% or less) ... 2103
Dalalone D.P. Injectable ... 1011
Decadron Phosphate Injection ... 1637
Decadron Phosphate with Xylocaine Injection, Sterile ... 1639
Decadron-LA Sterile Suspension ... 1646
Depo-Medrol Single-Dose Vial ... 2600
Depo-Medrol Sterile Aqueous Suspension ... 2597
Depo-Provera Sterile Aqueous Suspension (A few instances) ... 2606
Diphtheria and Tetanus Toxoids and Pertussis Vaccine Adsorbed.. 2477
Diphtheria and Tetanus Toxoids and Pertussis Vaccine Adsorbed USP (For Pediatric Use) (6 to 10 per million doses) ... 875
Foscavir Injection (Between 1% and 5%) ... 547
Sterile FUDR ... 2118
Gelfoam Sterile Sponge ... 2608
Hydeltrasol Injection, Sterile ... 1665
Hydeltra-T.B.A. Sterile Suspension ... 1667
Hydrocortone Acetate Sterile Suspension ... 1669
Hydrocortone Phosphate Injection, Sterile ... 1670
INFeD (Iron Dextran Injection, USP) ... 2345
Intron A (Less than 5%) ... 2364
▲ Lupron Depot-PED 7.5 mg, 11.25 mg and 15 mg (5%) ... 2560
▲ Neoral (4.4%) ... 2276
Paxil Tablets (Rare) ... 2505
▲ Pentam 300 Injection (11.1%) ... 1041
Permax Tablets (Infrequent) ... 575
▲ Prograf (Greater than 3%) ... 1042
▲ Sandimmune (4.4 to 5.3%) ... 2286
Solu-Cortef Sterile Powder ... 2641
Solu-Medrol Sterile Powder ... 2643
Videx Tablets, Powder for Oral Solution, & Pediatric Powder for Oral Solution (Less than 1%) ... 720

Abscess at injection site
Ceredase ... 1065
Cleocin Phosphate Injection ... 2586
Cytovene-IV (1% or less) ... 2103
MSTA Mumps Skin Test Antigen ... 890
PedvaxHIB ... 1718

Abscess, periesophageal
Ethamolin (0.1 to 0.4%) ... 2400

Abscess, periodontal
Ansaid Tablets (Less than 1%) ... 2579
Betaseron for SC Injection ... 658
Depakote Tablets (Greater than 1% but not more than 5%) ... 415
Hivid Tablets (Less than 1% to less than 3%) ... 2121
NebuPent for Inhalation Solution (1% or less) ... 1040
Permax Tablets (Infrequent) ... 575
Serzone Tablets (Infrequent) ... 771

Abscess, tubo-ovarian
ParaGard T380A Intrauterine Copper Contraceptive ... 1880

Abuse
Astramorph/PF Injection, USP (Preservative-Free) ... 535
Cafergot ... 2251
Fioricet with Codeine Capsules ... 2260
Fiorinal with Codeine Capsules ... 2262
Miltown Tablets ... 2672
Prozac Pulvules & Liquid, Oral Solution ... 919

Accommodation, impaired
AK-CIDE (Occasional) ... ⊙ 202
AK-CIDE Ointment (Occasional) .. ⊙ 202
Anafranil Capsules (Infrequent) ... 803
Aralen Hydrochloride Injection ... 2301
Aralen Phosphate Tablets ... 2301
Arfonad Ampuls ... 2080
Asendin Tablets (Less than 1%) ... 1369
Atrovent Inhalation Aerosol (About 1 in 100) ... 671
Blephamide Ointment (Occasional) ... ⊙ 237
Clomid ... 1514
DiaBeta Tablets ... 1239
Econopred & Econopred Plus Ophthalmic Suspensions (Occasional) ... ⊙ 217
▲ Effexor (5.6% to 9.1%) ... 2719
Elavil ... 2838
Endep Tablets ... 2174
Etrafon ... 2355
FML Forte Liquifilm (Occasional) ... ⊙ 240
FML Liquifilm (Occasional) ... ⊙ 241
FML S.O.P. (Occasional) ... ⊙ 241
Glynase PresTab Tablets ... 2609
Lamictal Tablets (Infrequent) ... 1112
Limbitrol ... 2180
Lioresal Intrathecal ... 1596
Ludiomil Tablets (Rare) ... 843
Luvox Tablets (Infrequent) ... 2544
Micronase Tablets ... 2623
Neurontin Capsules (Rare) ... 1922
Norpramin Tablets ... 1526
Norvasc Tablets (Less than or equal to 0.1%) ... 1940
▲ Orap Tablets (4 of 20 patients) ... 1050
PMB 200 and PMB 400 ... 2783
Pamelor ... 2280
Paxil Tablets (Infrequent) ... 2505
Plaquenil Sulfate Tablets ... 2328
Protopam Chloride for Injection ... 2806
Risperdal (Infrequent) ... 1301
Serzone Tablets (Infrequent) ... 771
Surmontil Capsules ... 2811
Tofranil Ampuls ... 854
Tofranil Tablets ... 856
Tofranil-PM Capsules ... 857
Transderm Scōp Transdermal Therapeutic System ... 869
Triavil Tablets ... 1757
Urispas Tablets ... 2532
Vasocidin Ointment (Occasional) ... ⊙ 268
Vasocidin Ophthalmic Solution (Occasional) ... ⊙ 270
Vivactil Tablets ... 1774
Zantac (Rare) ... 1209
Zantac Injection (Rare) ... 1207
Zantac Syrup (Rare) ... 1209
Zofran Injection ... 1214
Zoloft Tablets (Infrequent) ... 2217

Accommodation, paresis
Diphtheria and Tetanus Toxoids and Pertussis Vaccine Adsorbed USP (For Pediatric Use) ... 875
Tripedia ... 892

Accommodation, spasm
Pilagan ... ⊙ 248
Tensilon Injectable ... 1261

Aches
Asacol Delayed-Release Tablets ... 1979
Atgam Sterile Solution (Less than 5%) ... 2581
Cartrol Tablets ... 410
Cipro I.V. (1% or less) ... 595
Cipro I.V. Pharmacy Bulk Package (Less than 1%) ... 597
Cipro Tablets (Less than 1%) ... 592
Cytotec (Infrequent) ... 2424
Eldepryl Tablets (1 of 49 patients) ... 2550
Humegon ... 1824
Humorsol Sterile Ophthalmic Solution ... 1664
Hydropres Tablets ... 1675
Inderal ... 2728
Inderal LA Long Acting Capsules ... 2730
Inderide Tablets ... 2732
Inderide LA Long Acting Capsules .. 2734
Kerlone Tablets ... 2436
Levatol ... 2403
Lysodren (Infrequent) ... 698
Methadone Hydrochloride Oral Concentrate ... 2233
Midamor Tablets (Less than or equal to 1%) ... 1703
Normodyne Tablets ... 2379
Orlamm ... 2239
Orthoclone OKT3 Sterile Solution ... 1837
Pergonal (menotropins for injection, USP) ... 2448
Recombivax HB (Less than 1%) ... 1744
Rogaine Topical Solution (2.59%).. 2637
Sectral Capsules ... 2807
Tenoretic Tablets ... 2845
Tenormin Tablets and I.V. Injection ... 2847
Teslac ... 717
Timoptic in Ocudose ... 1753
Timoptic Sterile Ophthalmic Solution ... 1751
Timoptic-XE ... 1755
Toprol-XL Tablets ... 565
Trandate Tablets ... 1185
Trilafon ... 2389
Visken Tablets ... 2299
Ziac ... 1415

Aches, joints (see under Arthralgia)

Acid-base disturbances
Demadex Tablets and Injection ... 686

Acidosis
Abbokinase ... 403
Abbokinase Open-Cath ... 405
Achromycin V Capsules ... 1367
Children's Advil Suspension (Less than 1%) ... 2692
▲ CellCept Capsules (More than or equal to 3%) ... 2099
Cipro I.V. (1% or less) ... 595
Cipro I.V. Pharmacy Bulk Package (Less than 1%) ... 597
Cipro Tablets (Less than 1%) ... 592
Cytovene-IV (Two or more reports) 2103
Dyazide ... 2479
Fleet Enema ... 1002
Floxin I.V. ... 1571
Floxin Tablets (200 mg, 300 mg, 400 mg) ... 1567
Foscavir Injection (Between 1% and 5%) ... 547
IBU Tablets (Less than 1%) ... 1342
IFEX (Rare) ... 697
Indocin I.V. (Less than 3%) ... 1684
Kerlone Tablets (Less than 2%) ... 2436
Maxaquin Tablets ... 2440
Minocin Intravenous ... 1382
Minocin Oral Suspension ... 1385
Minocin Pellet-Filled Capsules ... 1383
Children's Motrin Ibuprofen Oral Suspension (Less than 1%) ... 1546
Motrin Tablets (Less than 1%) ... 2625
Motrin Ibuprofen Suspension, Oral Drops, Chewable Tablets, Caplets (Less than 1%) ... 1546
Permax Tablets (Rare) ... 575
Proglycem (Infrequent) ... 580
▲ Prograf (Greater than 3%) ... 1042
▲ Proleukin for Injection (16%) ... 797
Sulfamylon Cream ... 925
Videx Tablets, Powder for Oral Solution, & Pediatric Powder for Oral Solution (Less than 1%) ... 720

Acidosis, hypochloremic metabolic
Neoral (Occasional) ... 2276
Sandimmune (Occasional) ... 2286

Acidosis, metabolic
Daranide Tablets ... 1633
Diamox Intravenous (Occasional) ... 1372
Diamox Sequels (Sustained Release) ... 1373
Diamox Tablets (Occasional) ... 1372
Diprivan Injection (Less than 1%) .. 2833
Fludara for Injection ... 663
Glauctabs ... ⊙ 208
▲ IFEX (31%) ... 697
MZM ... ⊙ 267
Nardil (Less frequent) ... 1920
NegGram (Rare) ... 2323
Neptazane Tablets ... 1388
Nydrazid Injection ... 508
Oncaspar ... 2028
Rifamate Capsules ... 1530
Rifater ... 1532
Sensorcaine ... 559
VePesid Capsules and Injection ... 718

Acidosis, renal tubular
▲ Fungizone Intravenous (Among most common) ... 506
IFEX (1 episode) ... 697
Zanosar Sterile Powder ... 2653

Acidosis, respiratory, during weaning
Diprivan Injection (Greater than 1%) ... 2833

Acne (see under Acneiform eruptions)

Acne fulminaris
Accutane Capsules ... 2076

(■ Described in PDR For Nonprescription Drugs) — Incidence data in parenthesis; ▲ 3% or more — (⊙ Described in PDR For Ophthalmology)

1211 **Side Effects Index** **Ageusia**

Acne vulgaris

Hyland's ClearAc ▣ 828

Acne, cystic, flare-up

Parnate Tablets 2503

Acne, transient exacerbation of

Accutane Capsules 2076
Oxandrin 2862

Acneiform eruptions

Aclovate Cream 1069
AeroBid Inhaler System (1-3%) 1005
Aerobid-M Inhaler System (1-3%) 1005
Ambien Tablets (Rare) 2416
Amen Tablets (Few cases) 780
Anafranil Capsules (Up to 2%) 803
Analpram-HC Rectal Cream 1% and 2.5% 977
▲ Android Capsules, 10 mg (Among most common) 1250
Android 1251
Antabuse Tablets (Small number of patients) 2695
Anusol-HC Cream 2.5% (Infrequent to frequent) 1896
Aristocort A 0.025% Cream (Infrequent) 1027
Aristocort A 0.5% Cream 1031
Aristocort A 0.1% Cream (Infrequent) 1029
Aristocort A 0.1% Ointment (Infrequent) 1030
Asacol Delayed-Release Tablets (1% to 2%) 1979
Brevicon 2088
BuSpar (Rare) 737
Carmol HC (Infrequent to frequent) 924
▲ CellCept Capsules (9.7% to 10.1%) 2099
Claritin-D (Less frequent) 2350
Clomid 1514
Cognex Capsules (Infrequent) 1901
Cordran Lotion (Infrequent) 1803
Cordran Tape (Infrequent) 1804
Cortifoam 2396
Cortisporin Cream 1084
Cortisporin Ointment 1085
Cortisporin Otic Solution Sterile 1087
Cortisporin Otic Suspension Sterile 1088
Cosmegen Injection 1626
Cutivate Cream 1088
Cutivate Ointment (Infrequent to more frequent) 1089
Cyclocort Topical (Infrequent) 1037
Cycrin Tablets (A few cases) 975
Cytovene (1% or less) 2103
Danocrine Capsules 2307
Dantrium Capsules (Less frequent) 1982
Decadron Phosphate Topical Cream 1644
Decaspray Topical Aerosol 1648
Delatestryl Injection 2860
Demulen 2428
Depo-Provera Contraceptive Injection (1% to 5%) 2602
Depo-Provera Sterile Aqueous Suspension 2606
Dermatop Emollient Cream 0.1% (Infrequent to frequent) 1238
Desogen Tablets 1817
DesOwen Cream, Ointment and Lotion (Infrequent) 1046
Diprolene AF Cream (Infrequent) 2352
Diprolene Gel 0.05% (Infrequent) 2353
Diprolene (Infrequent) 2352
Effexor (Infrequent) 2719
Elocon (Infrequent) 2354
Epifoam (Infrequent) 2399
Eskalith 2485
Estratest 2539
▲ Felbatol (3.4%) 2666
Florinef Acetate Tablets 505
Florone/Florone E 906
Halog (Infrequent) 2686
Halotestin Tablets 2614
Hivid Tablets (Less than 1% to less than 3%) 2121
Hytone 907
Imdur (Less than or equal to 5%) 1323
Intron A (Less than 5%) 2364
Lamictal Tablets (1.3%) 1112
Lamprene Capsules (Less than 1%) 828
Levlen/Tri-Levlen 651
Lidex (Infrequent) 2130
Lithonate/Lithotabs/Lithobid 2543
Lotrisone Cream (Infrequent) 2372
Lupron Depot 3.75 mg 2556
Lupron Depot-PED 7.5 mg, 11.25 mg and 15 mg (2%) 2560
Luvox Tablets (Infrequent) 2544
Mantadil Cream 1135
Methotrexate Sodium Tablets, Injection, for Injection and LPF Injection 1275
Micronor Tablets 1872
Modicon 1872
NeoDecadron Topical Cream 1714
Neoral (1% to 2%) 2276
Neurontin Capsules (More than 1%) 1922
Nimotop Capsules (Up to 1.4%) 610
Norinyl 2088
Norisodrine with Calcium Iodide Syrup 442
Norplant System 2759
Nor-Q D Tablets 2135
Oreton Methyl 1255
Ortho-Cept 1851
Ortho-Cyclen/Ortho-Tri-Cyclen 1858
Ortho-Novum 1872
Ortho-Cyclen/Ortho Tri-Cyclen 1858
Ovcon 760
Oxandrin 2862
Paxil Tablets (Infrequent) 2505
PediOtic Suspension Sterile 1153
Pentasa (0.2%) 1527
Pentaspan Injection 937
Pepcid Injection (Infrequent) 1722
Pepcid (Infrequent) 1720
Permax Tablets (Infrequent) 575
Pramosone Cream, Lotion & Ointment 978
Premarin with Methyltestosterone 2794
Premphase 2797
Prempro 2801
PREVACID Delayed-Release Capsules (Less than 1%) 2562
ProctoCream-HC (Infrequent) 2408
ProctoCream-HC 2.5% (Infrequent to frequent) 2408
ProctoFoam-HC 2409
ProSom Tablets (Rare) 449
Provera Tablets (A few cases) 2636
Prozac Pulvules & Liquid, Oral Solution (2%) 919
Psorcon Cream 0.05% (Infrequent) 909
Psorcon Ointment 0.05% 908
Pyrazinamide Tablets (Rare) 1398
Relafen Tablets (Less than 1%) 2510
Retrovir Capsules 1158
Retrovir I.V. Infusion 1163
Retrovir Syrup 1158
ReVia Tablets (Less than 1%) 940
Rifater (Rare) 1532
Risperdal (Infrequent) 1301
Rowasa (1.2%) 2548
▲ Sandimmune (1 to 6%) 2286
Serzone Tablets (Infrequent) 771
▲ Supprelin Injection (3% to 10%) 2056
Synalar (Infrequent) 2130
▲ Synarel Nasal Solution for Central Precocious Puberty (10%) 2151
▲ Synarel Nasal Solution for Endometriosis (13% of patients) 2152
Synemol Cream 0.025% (Infrequent) 2130
Temovate (Infrequent) 1179
Testoderm Testosterone Transdermal System (Four in 104 patients) 486
Testred Capsules 1262
Topicort (Infrequent) 1243
Tridesilon Cream 0.05% 615
Tridesilon Ointment 0.05% 616
Levlen/Tri-Levlen 651
Tri-Norinyl 2164
Ultravate Cream 0.05% (Infrequent) 2689
Ultravate Ointment 0.05% (Less frequent) 2690
Vantin for Oral Suspension and Vantin Tablets (Less than 1%) 2646
Videx Tablets, Powder for Oral Solution, & Pediatric Powder for Oral Solution (Less than 1%) 720
Wellbutrin Tablets (Rare) 1204
Westcort 2690
Winstrol Tablets 2337
Yodoxin 1230
Zebeta Tablets 1413
Ziac 1415
▲ Zoladex (42%) 2858
Zoloft Tablets (Infrequent) 2217

Acneiform reactions

Elocon Lotion 0.1% (2 in 209 patients) 2354
Foscavir Injection (Less than 1%) 547
Haldol Decanoate 1577
Haldol Injection, Tablets and Concentrate 1575

Adams-Stokes syndrome

Isuprel Hydrochloride Injection 1:5000 2311

Adenitis

Asendin Tablets 1369
Clinoril Tablets 1618
Dolobid Tablets (Less than 1 in 100) 1654
Ludiomil Tablets (Isolated reports) 843
Norpramin Tablets (Rare) 1526
Pamelor (Rare) 2280
Pneumovax 23 (Rare) 1725
Pnu-Imune 23 (Rare) 1393
Surmontil Capsules 2811
Tofranil Ampuls (Rare) 854
Tofranil Tablets (Rare) 856
Tofranil-PM Capsules (Rare) 857
Vivactil Tablets (Rare) 1774

Adenoma, nephrogenic

BCG Vaccine, USP (TICE) (Two cases) 1814

Adenomas, benign

Betaseron for SC Injection 658
Demulen 2428

Adenomas, endocrine system

Permax Tablets (Infrequent) 575

Adenopathy

Atretol Tablets 573
Miltown Tablets 2672
PMB 200 and PMB 400 2783
Tegretol Chewable Tablets 852
Tegretol Suspension 852
Tegretol Tablets 852
Tetanus Toxoid Adsorbed Purogenated 1403

Adenopathy, inguinal

Zovirax (0.3%) 1219

Adhesion

INSTAT* Collagen Absorbable Hemostat 1312
INSTAT* MCH Microfibrillar Collagen Hemostat 1313
Lippes Loop Intrauterine Double-S 1848

Adnexal enlargement

Norplant System 2759

Adnexal torsion, ovarian

Humegon 1824
Metrodin (urofollitropin for injection) 2446
Pergonal (menotropins for injection, USP) 2448
Serophene (clomiphene citrate tablets, USP) 2451

Adrenal insufficiency

Azmacort Oral Inhaler 2011
Beclovent Inhalation Aerosol and Refill 1075
Beconase 1076
Cortifoam 2396
Heparin Lock Flush Solution 2725
Heparin Sodium Injection 2726
Heparin Sodium Injection, USP, Sterile Solution 2615
Heparin Sodium Vials 1441
Megace Tablets (Rare) 701
Motrin Tablets 2625
Nasacort Nasal Inhaler 2024
Sporanox Capsules (Less than 1%) 1305

Adrenergic syndrome, unspecified

Paxil Tablets (Rare) 2505

Adrenocortical suppression

Dermatop Emollient Cream 0.1% 1238
Dexacort Phosphate in Respihaler 458
Dexacort Phosphate in Turbinaire 459
Nasacort Nasal Inhaler 2024
ProctoCream-HC 2.5% 2408

Adrenocortical unresponsiveness, secondary

Aristocort Suspension (Forte Parenteral) 1027
Aristocort Suspension (Intralesional) 1025
Aristocort Tablets 1022
Aristospan Suspension (Intra-articular) 1033
Aristospan Suspension (Intralesional) 1032
Celestone Soluspan Suspension 2347
CORTENEMA 2535
Cortone Acetate Sterile Suspension 1623
Cortone Acetate Tablets 1624
Dalalone D.P. Injectable 1011
Decadron Elixir 1633
Decadron Phosphate Injection 1637
Decadron Phosphate Respihaler 1642
Decadron Phosphate Turbinaire 1645
Decadron Phosphate with Xylocaine Injection, Sterile 1639
Decadron Tablets 1635
Decadron-LA Sterile Suspension 1646
Deltasone Tablets 2595
Depo-Medrol Single-Dose Vial 2600
Depo-Medrol Sterile Aqueous Suspension 2597
Dexacort Phosphate in Respihaler 458
Dexacort Phosphate in Turbinaire 459
Florinef Acetate Tablets 505
Hydeltrasol Injection, Sterile 1665
Hydeltra-T.B.A. Sterile Suspension 1667
Hydrocortone Acetate Sterile Suspension 1669
Hydrocortone Phosphate Injection, Sterile 1670
Hydrocortone Tablets 1672
Medrol 2621
Pediapred Oral Liquid 995
Prelone Syrup 1787
Solu-Cortef Sterile Powder 2641
Solu-Medrol Sterile Powder 2643

Afibrinogenemia

Depakene (One infant) 413
Depakote Tablets (One infant) 415
Oxytocin Injection 2771
Syntocinon Injection 2296

Aftertaste

Antabuse Tablets (Small number of patients) 2695
▲ Nasarel Nasal Solution (8% to 17%) 2133
Placidyl Capsules 448
VePesid Capsules and Injection (Infrequent) 718

Ageusia

▲ AeroBid Inhaler System (3-9%) 1005
▲ Aerobid-M Inhaler System (3-9%) 1005
Anafranil Capsules (Infrequent) 803
Beconase (Rare) 1076
Bentyl 1501
Betaseron for SC Injection 658
Capoten (Approximately 2 to 4 of 100 patients) 739
Capozide (Approximately 2 to 4 of 100 patients) 742
Claritin-D (Less frequent) 2350
Clinoril Tablets (Less than 1 in 100) 1618
▲ Depen Titratable Tablets (12%) 2662
▲ Didronel I.V. Infusion (5%) 1488
Donnatal 2060
Donnatal Extentabs 2061
Donnatal Tablets 2060
Effexor (Infrequent) 2719
Elavil 2838
Endep Tablets 2174
Flexeril Tablets (Less than 1%) 1661
Flumadine Tablets & Syrup (Less than 0.3%) 1015
Hivid Tablets (Less than 1% to less than 3%) 2121
Intron A (Less than 5%) 2364
Kerlone Tablets (Less than 2%) 2436
Lamictal Tablets (Rare) 1112
Levsin/Levsinex/Levbid 2405
Lorelco Tablets 1517
Luvox Tablets (Infrequent) 2544
Nasalide Nasal Solution 0.025% 2110
NebuPent for Inhalation Solution (1% or less) 1040
Neptazane Tablets 1388
Neurontin Capsules (Infrequent) 1922
Nolvadex Tablets (Infrequent) 2841
Paxil Tablets (Infrequent) 2505
Platinol 708
Platinol-AQ Injection 710
Pro-Banthine Tablets 2052
Proglycem (Frequent) 580
Prolixin 509
Prozac Pulvules & Liquid, Oral Solution (Rare) 919

(▣ Described in PDR For Nonprescription Drugs) Incidence data in parenthesis; ▲ 3% or more (◉ Described in PDR For Ophthalmology)

Robinul Forte Tablets 2072
Robinul Injectable 2072
Robinul Tablets 2072
Serzone Tablets (Rare) 771
Tapazole Tablets 1477
Tornalate Solution for Inhalation, 0.2% (Less than 1%) 956
Zyloprim Tablets (Less than 1%) 1226

Aggression

Ambien Tablets (Rare) 2416
Anafranil Capsules (Up to 2%) 803
Celontin Kapseals 1899
Claritin-D (Less frequent) 2350
Depakene 413
Depakote Tablets 415
Felbatol (Frequent) 2666
Floxin I.V. 1571
Floxin Tablets (200 mg, 300 mg, 400 mg) 1567
Foscavir Injection (Between 1% and 5%) 547
Halcion Tablets 2611
Imitrex Tablets (Rare) 1106
Intron A (Less than 5%) 2364
Prilosec Delayed-Release Capsules (Less than 1%) 529
Risperdal (1% to 3%) 1301
Seromycin Pulvules 1476
Ventolin Inhalation Aerosol and Refill (1%) 1197
Xanax Tablets (Rare) 2649
Zarontin Capsules 1928
Zarontin Syrup 1929
Zoloft Tablets (Infrequent) 2217

Agitation

Akineton 1333
Alfenta Injection 1286
Ambien Tablets (Infrequent) 2416
Amoxil (Rare) 2464
Anafranil Capsules (Up to 3%) 803
Artane 1368
Atamet 572
Atgam Sterile Solution (Less than 5%) 2581
Ativan Tablets (Less frequent) 2700
Atretol Tablets 573
Augmentin (Rare) 2468
Betaseron for SC Injection 658
Bontril Slow-Release Capsules 781
Brevibloc Injection (About 2%) 1808
Buprenex Injectable (Rare) 2006
Butisol Sodium Elixir & Tablets (Less than 1 in 100) 2660
Cardura Tablets (0.5% to 1%) 2186
Catapres Tablets (About 3 in 100 patients) 674
Catapres-TTS (Less frequent) 675
Claritin (2% or fewer patients) 2349
Claritin-D (Less frequent) 2350
▲ Clozaril Tablets (4%) 2252
▲ Cognex Capsules (7%) 1901
Combipres Tablets (About 3%) 677
Compazine 2470
Cytovene (1% or less) 2103
Demerol 2308
Depakote Tablets (Greater than 1% but not more than 5%) 415
Desyrel and Desyrel Dividose 503
Dexedrine 2474
Dilaudid-HP Injection (Less frequent) 1337
Dilaudid-HP Lyophilized Powder 250 mg (Less frequent) 1337
Dilaudid Tablets and Liquid (Less frequent) 1339
Diprivan Injection (Less than 1%) 2833
Donnatal (In elderly patients) 2060
Donnatal Extentabs (In elderly patients) 2061
Donnatal Tablets (In elderly patients) 2060
Doral Tablets 2664
Duragesic Transdermal System (1% or greater) 1288
▲ Effexor (2% to 4.5%) 2719
Eldepryl Tablets 2550
Elspar 1659
▲ Eminase (Less than 10%) 2039
Engerix-B Unit-Dose Vials (Less than 1%) 2482
Esgic-plus Tablets (Infrequent) 1013
Ethmozine Tablets (Less than 2%) 2041
Felbatol (Frequent) 2666
Fioricet Tablets (Infrequent) 2258
Fioricet with Codeine Capsules (Infrequent) 2260
Fiorinal with Codeine Capsules (Infrequent) 2262
Flexeril Tablets (Less than 1%) 1661
Floxin I.V. 1571
Floxin Tablets (200 mg, 300 mg, 400 mg) 1567
Fludara for Injection 663
Flumadine Tablets & Syrup (0.3% to 1%) 1015
Foscavir Injection (Between 1% and 5%) 547
Halcion Tablets 2611
Haldol Decanoate 1577
Haldol Injection, Tablets and Concentrate 1575
Hivid Tablets (Less than 1% to less than 3%) 2121
Imitrex Injection (Infrequent) 1103
Imitrex Tablets (Up to 2%) 1106
Intron A (Less than 5%) 2364
Ismo Tablets (Fewer than 1%) 2738
Keflex Pulvules & Oral Suspension 914
Keftab Tablets 915
Kytril Injection (Less than 2%) 2490
Lamictal Tablets (Infrequent) 1112
Larodopa Tablets (Relatively frequent) 2129
Leukeran Tablets (Rare) 1133
Levsin/Levsinex/Levbid 2405
Loxitane 1378
▲ Lozol Tablets (Greater than or equal to 5%) 2022
Ludiomil Tablets (2%) 843
Lufyllin & Lufyllin-400 Tablets 2670
Lufyllin-GG Elixir & Tablets 2671
Luvox Tablets (2%) 2544
MS Contin Tablets (Less frequent) 1994
MSIR (Infrequent) 1997
Maxaquin Tablets (Less than 1%) 2440
Mebaral Tablets (Less than 1 in 100) 2322
Mellaril 2269
Mepergan Injection 2753
Methadone Hydrochloride Oral Concentrate 2233
Methadone Hydrochloride Oral Solution & Tablets 2235
Miacalcin Nasal Spray (Less than 1%) 2275
Nardil (Uncommon) 1920
Navane Capsules and Concentrate 2201
Navane Intramuscular 2202
Nembutal Sodium Capsules (Less than 1%) 436
Nembutal Sodium Solution (Less than 1%) 438
Nembutal Sodium Suppositories (Less than 1%) 440
Neurontin Capsules (Infrequent) 1922
Norflex 1496
Norgesic 1496
Norpramin Tablets 1526
Norvasc Tablets (Less than or equal to 0.1%) 1940
Oramorph SR (Morphine Sulfate Sustained Release Tablets) (Less frequent) 2236
Orthoclone OKT3 Sterile Solution 1837
Pamelor 2280
Parnate Tablets 2503
Paxil Tablets (2.1%) 2505
Penetrex Tablets (Less than 1% but more than or equal to 0.1%) 2031
Pepcid Injection (Infrequent) 1722
Pepcid (Infrequent) 1720
Permax Tablets (Infrequent) 575
Phenobarbital Elixir and Tablets (Less than 1 in 100 patients) 1469
Phrenilin (Infrequent) 785
Placidyl Capsules 448
Pondimin Tablets 2066
PREVACID Delayed-Release Capsules (Less than 1%) 2562
▲ Prograf (Greater than 3%) 1042
Proleukin for Injection 797
ProSom Tablets (Infrequent) 449
Prozac Pulvules & Liquid, Oral Solution (Frequent to 2%) 919
RMS Suppositories 2657
Recombivax HB 1744
Reglan 2068
Relafen Tablets (1%) 2510
Revex (Less than 1%) 1811
▲ Risperdal (22% to 26%) 1301
▲ Romazicon (3% to 9%) 2147
Roxanol 2243
Salagen Tablets (Rare) 1489
Seconal Sodium Pulvules (Less than 1 in 100) 1474
Sedapap Tablets 50 mg/650 mg (Infrequent) 1543
Serentil 684
Serzone Tablets 771
Sinemet Tablets 943
Sinemet CR Tablets 944
Soma Compound w/Codeine Tablets (Infrequent or rare) 2676
Soma Compound Tablets (Very rare to infrequent) 2675
Soma Tablets 2674
Stadol (Less than 1%) 775
Stelazine 2514
Stimate, (desmopressin acetate) Nasal Spray, 1.5 mg/mL 525
Suprane (Less than 1%) 1813
Surmontil Capsules 2811
Symmetrel Capsules and Syrup (1% to 5%) 946
Tagamet 2516
Tegretol Chewable Tablets 852
Tegretol Suspension 852
Tegretol Tablets 852
Tenex Tablets (Less frequent) 2074
Thorazine 2523
Tofranil Ampuls 854
Tofranil Tablets 856
Tofranil-PM Capsules 857
Tonocard Tablets (Less than 1%) 531
Torecan 2245
Trental Tablets 1244
▲ Ultram Tablets (50 mg) (1% to 14%) 1585
Ventolin Inhalation Aerosol and Refill (1%) 1197
Versed Injection (Less than 1%) 2170
Videx Tablets, Powder for Oral Solution, & Pediatric Powder for Oral Solution (Up to 1%) 720
Vivactil Tablets 1774
▲ Wellbutrin Tablets (31.9%) 1204
Xanax Tablets (Rare) 2649
Zantac (Rare) 1209
Zantac Injection 1207
Zantac Syrup (Rare) 1209
Zofran Injection (2%) 1214
▲ Zofran Tablets (6%) 1217
▲ Zoloft Tablets (5.6%) 2217
Zosyn (2.1%) 1419
Zosyn Pharmacy Bulk Package (2.1%) 1422
Zovirax Sterile Powder (Approximately 1%) 1223

Agoraphobia

Luvox Tablets (Infrequent) 2544

Agranulocytopenia

Sterile FUDR (Remote possibility) 2118

Agranulocytosis

Accupril Tablets (Rare) 1893
Actifed with Codeine Cough Syrup 1067
Children's Advil Suspension (Less than 1%) 2692
Aldactazide (A few cases) 2413
Aldactone (A few cases) 2414
Aldoclor Tablets 1598
Aldoril Tablets 1604
Altace Capsules (Rare to more frequent) 1232
Amoxil 2464
Anaprox/Naprosyn (Less than 1%) 2117
Ancobon Capsules 2079
Anexia Tablets 1782
Anturane (Rare) 807
Apresazide Capsules (Less frequent) 808
Apresoline Hydrochloride Tablets (Less frequent) 809
Asacol Delayed-Release Tablets (Rare) 1979
Asendin Tablets (Less than 1%) 1369
Atamet (Rare) 572
Atretol Tablets 573
Atrohist Plus Tablets 454
Atromid-S Capsules 2701
Augmentin 2468
Azo Gantanol Tablets 2080
Azo Gantrisin Tablets 2081
Azulfidine (Rare) 1949
Bactrim DS Tablets (Rare) 2084
Bactrim I.V. Infusion (Rare) 2082
Bactrim (Rare) 2084
Benadryl Capsules 1898
Benadryl Injection 1898
▲ Blephamide Ointment (Among most often) ⊙ 237
Blocadren Tablets 1614
▲ Bromfed-DM Cough Syrup (Among most frequent) 1786
Capoten 739
Capozide 742
Cartrol Tablets 410
Cataflam (Rare) 816
Cefizox for Intramuscular or Intravenous Use 1034
Cefotan 2829
Ceftin 1078
Cefzil Tablets and Oral Suspension 746
Ceptaz (Very rare) 1081
Cipro I.V. 595
Cipro I.V. Pharmacy Bulk Package (Less than 1%) 597
Cipro Tablets 592
Claforan Sterile and Injection (Less than 1%) 1235
Cleocin Phosphate Injection 2586
Cleocin Vaginal Cream 2589
Clinoril Tablets (Less than 1%) 1618
Clozaril Tablets (1%; approximately 1.3%) 2252
ColBENEMID Tablets 1622
Combipres Tablets 677
Comhist 2038
Compazine 2470
Cosmegen Injection 1626
Cuprimine Capsules 1630
▲ Cytadren Tablets (4 out of 27) 819
Dapsone Tablets USP 1284
Daranide Tablets 1633
Deconamine 1320
Depen Titratable Tablets 2662
DiaBeta Tablets 1239
Diabinese Tablets 1935
Diamox Intravenous 1372
Diamox Sequels (Sustained Release) 1373
Diamox Tablets 1372
Didronel Tablets (Rare) 1984
Dilantin Infatabs (Occasional) 1908
Dilantin Kapseals (Occasional) 1906
Dilantin Parenteral (Occasional) 1910
Dilantin-125 Suspension (Occasional) 1911
Dimetane-DC Cough Syrup 2059
Dimetane-DX Cough Syrup 2059
Diucardin Tablets 2718
Diupres Tablets 1650
Diuril Oral Suspension 1653
Diuril Sodium Intravenous 1652
Diuril Tablets 1653
Dolobid Tablets (Less than 1 in 100) 1654
Duricef 748
Dyazide 2479
EC-Naprosyn Delayed-Release Tablets (Less than 1%) 2117
Edecrin 1657
Elavil 2838
Endep Tablets 2174
Enduron Tablets 420
Ergamisol Tablets (One patient) 1292
Esgic-plus Tablets 1013
Esidrix Tablets 821
Esimil Tablets 822
Etrafon 2355
FML-S Liquifilm ⊙ 242
Fansidar Tablets 2114
Felbatol (Rare) 2666
Fioricet Tablets (Infrequent) 2258
Fioricet with Codeine Capsules 2260
Floxin I.V. 1571
Floxin Tablets (200 mg, 300 mg, 400 mg) 1567
Fluorouracil Injection 2116
Fortaz (Very rare) 1100
Fungizone Intravenous 506
Gantanol Tablets 2119
Gantrisin (Rare) 2120
Garamycin Injectable 2360
Glauctabs ⊙ 208
Glucotrol Tablets 1967
Glucotrol XL Extended Release Tablets 1968
Glynase PresTab Tablets 2609
Haldol Decanoate (Rare) 1577
Haldol Injection, Tablets and Concentrate (Rare) 1575
Hydrocet Capsules 782
HydroDIURIL Tablets 1674
Hydropres Tablets 1675
Hyzaar Tablets 1677
IBU Tablets (Less than 1%) 1342
Inderal 2728
Inderal LA Long Acting Capsules 2730
Inderide Tablets 2732
Inderide LA Long Acting Capsules 2734
Indocin Capsules (Less than 1%) 1680
Indocin I.V. (Less than 1%) 1684
Indocin (Less than 1%) 1680
Kefurox Vials, Faspak & ADD-Vantage 1454
Kerlone Tablets 2436
Larodopa Tablets (Rare) 2129

(▣ Described in PDR For Nonprescription Drugs) Incidence data in parenthesis; ▲ 3% or more (⊙ Described in PDR For Ophthalmology)

Lasix Injection, Oral Solution and Tablets (Rare) 1240
Levatol 2403
Levoprome 1274
Librax Capsules (Occasional) 2176
Libritabs Tablets (Occasional) 2177
Librium Capsules (Occasional) 2178
Librium Injectable (Occasional) 2179
Limbitrol 2180
Lincocin 2617
Lodine Capsules and Tablets (Less than 1%) 2743
Lopressor Ampuls (Rare) 830
Lopressor HCT Tablets 832
Lopressor Tablets (Rare) 830
Lorabid Suspension and Pulvules 1459
Lortab 2566
Lotensin Tablets (Rare) 834
Lotensin HCT 837
Lotrel Capsules 840
Loxitane (Rare) 1378
Lozol Tablets 2022
Ludiomil Tablets (Isolated reports) 843
Luvox Tablets 2544
MZM (Common) .... ⊚ 267
Macrobid Capsules 1988
Macrodantin Capsules 1989
Maxaquin Tablets 2440
Maxzide 1380
Mellaril (Infrequent; increased risk in aged) 2269
Mepergan Injection (1 instance) 2753
Mesantoin Tablets 2272
Mexitil Capsules (About 1 in 1,000) 678
Micronase Tablets 2623
Miltown Tablets 2672
Minizide Capsules 1938
Moduretic Tablets 1705
Monopril Tablets 757
Children's Motrin Ibuprofen Oral Suspension (Less than 1%) 1546
Motrin Tablets (Less than 1%) 2625
Motrin Ibuprofen Suspension, Oral Drops, Chewable Tablets, Caplets (Less than 1%) 1546
Mustargen (Relatively infrequent) 1709
Mykrox Tablets 993
Mysoline Suspension 2754
Nalfon 200 Pulvules & Nalfon Tablets (Less than 1%) 917
Anaprox/Naprosyn (Less than 1%) 2117
Navane Capsules and Concentrate 2201
Navane Intramuscular 2202
Neptazane Tablets 1388
Normodyne Tablets 2379
Noroxin Tablets 1715
Noroxin Tablets 2048
Norpace (Rare) 2444
Norpramin Tablets 1526
Nydrazid Injection 508
Omnipen Capsules 2764
Omnipen for Oral Suspension 2765
Oncaspar 2028
Oretic Tablets 443
Ornade Spansule Capsules 2502
Orudis Capsules (Less than 1%) 2766
Oruvail Capsules (Less than 1%) 2766
PBZ Tablets 845
PBZ-SR Tablets 844
PMB 200 and PMB 400 2783
Pamelor 2280
Parnate Tablets 2503
PASER Granules 1285
Penetrex Tablets 2031
Pepcid Injection (Rare) 1722
Pepcid (Rare) 1720
Periactin 1724
Phenergan with Codeine (1 case) 2777
Phenergan with Dextromethorphan (1 case) 2778
Phenergan Injection 2773
Phenergan Suppositories (1 case) 2775
Phenergan Syrup (1 case) 2774
Phenergan Tablets (1 case) 2775
Phenergan VC (1 case) 2779
Phenergan VC with Codeine (1 case) 2781
Phrenilin (Infrequent) 785
Plaquenil Sulfate Tablets 2328
Ponstel (Occasional) 1925
Prilosec Delayed-Release Capsules (Rare) 529
Primaxin I.M. 1727
Primaxin I.V. 1729
Prinivil Tablets (Rare to frequent) 1733
Prinzide Tablets (Rare) 1737
Procan SR Tablets (0.5%) 1926
Prolixin 509
ProSom Tablets (Rare) 449
Quinaglute Dura-Tabs Tablets 649
Quinidex Extentabs 2067
Reglan (A few cases) 2068
Ridaura Capsules (Less than 0.1%) 2513
Rifamate Capsules 1530
Rifater 1532
Rythmol Tablets–150mg, 225mg, 300mg (Less than 1%) 1352
SSD 1355
Sectral Capsules 2807
Sedapap Tablets 50 mg/650 mg 1543
Septra 1174
Septra I.V. Infusion 1169
Septra I.V. Infusion ADD-Vantage Vials (Rare) 1171
Septra 1174
Ser-Ap-Es Tablets 849
Serax Capsules 2810
Serax Tablets 2810
Serentil 684
Silvadene Cream 1% 1540
Sinemet Tablets (Rare) 943
Sinemet CR Tablets 944
Sinequan (Occasional) 2205
Solganal Suspension (Rare) 2388
Spectrobid Tablets 2206
Stelazine 2514
Sultrin (One case) 1885
Suprax 1399
Surmontil Capsules 2811
Tagamet (Approximately 3 per 1,000,000) 2516
Talacen (Rare) 2333
Tapazole Tablets 1477
Tavist Syrup 2297
Tavist Tablets 2298
Tazicef for Injection (Very rare) 2519
Tegretol Chewable Tablets (Very low incidence) 852
Tegretol Suspension (Very low incidence) 852
Tegretol Tablets (Very low incidence) 852
Temaril Tablets, Syrup and Spansule Extended-Release Capsules 483
Tenoretic Tablets 2845
Tenormin Tablets and I.V. Injection 2847
Thalitone 1245
Thorazine 2523
Ticlid Tablets (Rare; 0.8%) 2156
Timolide Tablets 1748
Timoptic in Ocudose 1753
Timoptic Sterile Ophthalmic Solution 1751
Timoptic-XE 1755
Tofranil Ampuls 854
Tofranil Tablets 856
Tofranil-PM Capsules 857
Tolectin (200, 400 and 600 mg) (Less than 1%) 1581
Tonocard Tablets (Less than 1%) 531
Toprol-XL Tablets (Rare) 565
Torecan 2245
Trandate Tablets 1185
Triavil Tablets 1757
Trilafon 2389
Trinalin Repetabs Tablets 1330
Trusopt Sterile Ophthalmic Solution (Rare) 1760
Tussend 1783
Tympagesic Ear Drops 2342
Unasyn 2212
Univasc Tablets (More than 1%) 2410
Urobiotic-250 Capsules 2214
Vancocin HCl, Vials & ADD-Vantage (Rare) 1481
Vantin for Oral Suspension and Vantin Tablets 2646
Vascor (200, 300 and 400 mg) Tablets 1587
Vaseretic Tablets (Rare; several cases) 1765
Vasocidin Ophthalmic Solution .... ⊚ 270
Vasotec I.V. (Rare; several cases) 1768
Vasotec Tablets (Several cases) 1771
Visken Tablets 2299
Vivactil Tablets 1774
Voltaren Tablets (Rare) 861
Yutopar Intravenous Injection 570
Zantac (Rare) 1209
Zantac Injection (Rare) 1207
Zantac Syrup (Rare) 1209
Zarontin Capsules 1928
Zarontin Syrup 1929
Zaroxolyn Tablets 1000
Zebeta Tablets 1413
Zefazone 2654
Zestoretic 2850
Zestril Tablets (Rare) 2854
Ziac 1415
Zinacef 1211
Zyloprim Tablets (Less than 1%) 1226

Airway obstruction

Altace Capsules 1232
Ativan Injection (5 patients) 2698
Capoten 739
Capozide 742
Diprivan Injection (Less than 1%) 2833
Fiorinal with Codeine Capsules 2262
Floxin I.V. 1571
Floxin Tablets (200 mg, 300 mg, 400 mg) 1567
Monopril Tablets 757
Orthoclone OKT3 Sterile Solution 1837
Prinivil Tablets 1733
Prinzide Tablets 1737
Vaseretic Tablets 1765
Vasotec I.V. 1768
Vasotec Tablets 1771
Versed Injection (Less than 1%) 2170
Zestoretic 2850
Zestril Tablets 2854

Airway resistance

Demerol 2308
Isuprel Mistometer (Occasional) 2312

Akathisia

BuSpar (Infrequent) 737
▲ Clozaril Tablets (3%) 2252
Cognex Capsules (Rare) 1901
Compazine 2470
Desyrel and Desyrel Dividose 503
Effexor (Rare) 2719
Ethmozine Tablets (Less than 2%) 2041
Etrafon 2355
Feldene Capsules (Less than 1%) 1965
Haldol Decanoate (Frequent) 1577
Haldol Injection, Tablets and Concentrate 1575
Inapsine Injection 1296
Lamictal Tablets (Infrequent) 1112
Loxitane 1378
Ludiomil Tablets (Rare) 843
Luvox Tablets (Infrequent) 2544
Mellaril 2269
Moban Tablets and Concentrate 1048
Navane Capsules and Concentrate 2201
Navane Intramuscular 2202
▲ Orap Tablets (8 of 20 patients) 1050
Paxil Tablets 2505
Permax Tablets (1.6%) 575
Prolixin 509
Prozac Pulvules & Liquid, Oral Solution (Infrequent) 919
Reglan 2068
▲ Risperdal (17% to 34%) 1301
Serentil 684
Stelazine 2514
Sublimaze Injection 1307
Temaril Tablets, Syrup and Spansule Extended-Release Capsules 483
Torecan 2245
Triavil Tablets 1757
Trilafon 2389
Vascor (200, 300 and 400 mg) Tablets (0.5 to 2.0%) 1587
Wellbutrin Tablets (1.5%) 1204
Xanax Tablets (1.6% to 3.0%) 2649

Akinesia

Cardura Tablets (1%) 2186
▲ Clozaril Tablets (4%) 2252
Effexor (Rare) 2719
Loxitane 1378
Luvox Tablets (Rare) 2544
Mellaril 2269
Moban Tablets and Concentrate 1048
▲ Orap Tablets (8 of 20 patients) 1050
Parnate Tablets 2503
Paxil Tablets (Infrequent) 2505
Permax Tablets (1.1%) 575
Serentil 684
Torecan 2245
▲ Wellbutrin Tablets (8.0%) 1204

Albuminuria

Amikacin Sulfate Injection, USP 960
Amikin Injectable 501
Anafranil Capsules (Rare) 803
Atretol Tablets 573
▲ CellCept Capsules (More than or equal to 3%) 2099
Cipro I.V. (1% or less) 595
Cipro I.V. Pharmacy Bulk Package (Less than 1%) 597
Cipro Tablets 592
Dapsone Tablets USP 1284
Dopram Injectable 2061
Effexor (Infrequent) 2719
Eskalith 2485
Floxin I.V. 1571
Floxin Tablets (200 mg, 300 mg, 400 mg) 1567
Foscavir Injection (Between 1% and 5%) 547
Hivid Tablets (Less than 1% to less than 3%) 2121
Lamprene Capsules (Less than 1%) 828
Lithium Carbonate Capsules & Tablets 2230
Lithonate/Lithotabs/Lithobid 2543
Lufyllin & Lufyllin-400 Tablets 2670
Lufyllin-GG Elixir & Tablets 2671
Lysodren (Infrequent) 698
Maxaquin Tablets 2440
Megace Oral Suspension (1% to 3%) 699
Noroxin Tablets (1.0%) 1715
Noroxin Tablets (1.0%) 2048
Pentasa (Less than 1%) 1527
Polymyxin B Sulfate, Aerosporin Brand Sterile Powder 1154
PREVACID Delayed-Release Capsules (Less than 1%) 2562
Proglycem 580
Prozac Pulvules & Liquid, Oral Solution (Rare) 919
Quadrinal Tablets 1350
Relafen Tablets (Less than 1%) 2510
Rocaltrol Capsules 2141
Solganal Suspension 2388
Sporanox Capsules (0.1% to 1.2%) 1305
Tegretol Chewable Tablets 852
Tegretol Suspension 852
Tegretol Tablets 852
Uroqid-Acid No. 2 Tablets 640
Xanax Tablets (Less than 1%) 2649
Zyloprim Tablets (Less than 1%) 1226

Alcohol abuse

BuSpar (Rare) 737
Effexor (Rare) 2719
Paxil Tablets (Infrequent) 2505

Alcohol, increased sensitivity to

Ativan Injection 2698
Betaseron for SC Injection 658
Catapres Tablets 674
Catapres-TTS 675
Combipres Tablets 677
Effexor (Rare) 2719
Neurontin Capsules (Rare) 1922
Nicotinex Elixir .... ▣ 655
Parlodel (Less than 1%) 2281

Aldosterone synthesis, suppression

Heparin Lock Flush Solution 2725
Heparin Sodium Injection 2726
Heparin Sodium Injection, USP, Sterile Solution 2615
Heparin Sodium Vials 1441

Alkalinuria

Floxin I.V. (More than or equal to 1%) 1571
Floxin Tablets (200 mg, 300 mg, 400 mg) (More than or equal to 1%) 1567

Alkalosis

Ancef Injection 2465
Bicitra 578
CeeNU (Small percentage) 693
Kefurox Vials, Faspak & ADD-Vantage (1 in 50) 1454
Lioresal Tablets 829
Netromycin Injection 100 mg/ml (15 of 1000 patients) 2373
Polycitra Syrup 578
Polycitra-K Crystals 579
Polycitra-K Oral Solution 579
Polycitra-LC 578
▲ Prograf (Greater than 3%) 1042
▲ Proleukin for Injection (4%) 797
▲ Tazidime Vials, Faspak & ADD-Vantage (1 in 23) 1478

Alkalosis, metabolic

Indocin I.V. (Less than 3%) 1684

Allergic contact dermatitis

Aclovate Cream 1069
Analpram-HC Rectal Cream 1% and 2.5% 977
Anusol-HC Cream 2.5% (Infrequent to frequent) 1896

(▣ Described in PDR For Nonprescription Drugs) Incidence data in parenthesis; ▲ 3% or more (⊚ Described in PDR For Ophthalmology)

Anusol-HC Suppositories ... 1897
Aristocort A 0.025% Cream (Infrequent) ... 1027
Aristocort A 0.5% Cream ... 1031
Aristocort A 0.1% Cream (Infrequent) ... 1029
Aristocort A 0.1% Ointment (Infrequent) ... 1030
Benzac ... 1045
Carmol HC (Infrequent to frequent) ... 924
▲Catapres-TTS (About 19 in 100) ... 675
Cerumenex Drops ... 1993
Cordran Lotion (Infrequent) ... 1803
Cordran Tape (Infrequent) ... 1804
Cortisporin Cream ... 1084
Cortisporin Ointment ... 1085
Cortisporin Otic Solution Sterile ... 1087
Cortisporin Otic Suspension Sterile ... 1088
Cutivate Cream ... 1088
Cutivate Ointment (Infrequent to more frequent) ... 1089
Cyclocort Topical (Infrequent) ... 1037
Decadron Phosphate Topical Cream ... 1644
Decaspray Topical Aerosol ... 1648
Dermatop Emollient Cream 0.1% (Less than 1%) ... 1238
DesOwen Cream, Ointment and Lotion (Less than 2%) ... 1046
Diprolene AF Cream (Infrequent) ... 2352
Diprolene Gel 0.05% (Less frequent) ... 2353
Diprolene (Infrequent) ... 2352
▲Efudex (Among most frequent) ... 2113
Elocon Lotion 0.1% ... 2354
Epifoam (Infrequent) ... 2399
Florone/Florone E ... 906
Fluoracaine ... ⊙ 206
Fluoroplex Topical Solution & Cream 1% ... 479
FLURESS ... ⊙ 207
Habitrol Nicotine Transdermal System (3 patients or 2% of patients) ... 865
Hytone ... 907
Locoid Cream, Ointment and Topical Solution (Infrequent) ... 978
Mantadil Cream ... 1135
Monistat Dual-Pak ... 1850
NeoDecadron Topical Cream ... 1714
Ophthetic ... ⊙ 247
Oxistat Cream ... 1152
PediOtic Suspension Sterile ... 1153
Pramosone Cream, Lotion & Ointment ... 978
ProctoCream-HC (Infrequent) ... 2408
ProctoCream-HC 2.5% (Infrequent to frequent) ... 2408
Psorcon Cream 0.05% (Infrequent) ... 909
Psorcon Ointment 0.05% ... 908
Retin-A (tretinoin) Cream/Gel/Liquid (Rare) ... 1889
▲Rogaine Topical Solution (7.36%) ... 2637
Synalar (Infrequent) ... 2130
Temovate (Infrequent) ... 1179
Topicort (Infrequent) ... 1243
Triaz 6% and 10% Gels and 10% Cleaner ... 1592
Ultravate Cream 0.05% (Infrequent) ... 2689
Ultravate Ointment 0.05% (Less frequent) ... 2690
Westcort ... 2690

Allergic reactions

Abbokinase ... 403
Abbokinase Open-Cath ... 405
Activase (Very rare) ... 1058
▲Acular (3%) ... 474
Adipex-P Tablets and Capsules ... 1048
Children's Advil Suspension (Less than 1%) ... 2692
Alkeran for Injection ... 1070
Alkeran Tablets ... 1071
Ambien Tablets (Rare to 4%) ... 2416
Americaine Hemorrhoidal Ointment ... ▣ 629
Amoxil ... 2464
▲Anafranil Capsules (3% to 7%) ... 803
Ancef Injection ... 2465
Anexia Tablets ... 1782
AquaMEPHYTON Injection ... 1608
Aquasol A Parenteral (Rare) ... 534
Atromid-S Capsules ... 2701
Atropine Sulfate Sterile Ophthalmic Solution ... ⊙ 233
Atrovent Inhalation Aerosol ... 671
Attenuvax (Rare) ... 1610
Augmentin ... 2468
Azo Gantrisin Tablets ... 2081
BCG Vaccine, USP (TICE) (2.1%) ... 1814
▲Bactrim DS Tablets (Among most common) ... 2084
▲Bactrim I.V. Infusion (Among most common) ... 2082
▲Bactrim (Among most common) ... 2084
Bayer Select Ibuprofen Pain Relief Formula ... ▣ 715
Benemid Tablets ... 1611
Bentyl ... 1501
Berocca Plus Tablets (Possible) ... 2087
Berocca Tablets ... 2087
Betasept Surgical Scrub ... 1993
Betimol 0.25%, 0.5% (1% to 5%) ... ⊙ 261
Betoptic Ophthalmic Solution (Small numbers of patients) ... 469
Betoptic S Ophthalmic Suspension ... 471
Biavax II ... 1613
Bicillin L-A Injection ... 2707
Brevital Sodium Vials ... 1429
BuSpar (Rare) ... 737
Calcimar Injection, Synthetic (A few cases) ... 2013
Carbocaine Hydrochloride Injection ... 2303
Cardene Capsules (Rare) ... 2095
Carmol HC ... 924
Cataflam ... 816
Catapres Tablets ... 674
▲Catapres-TTS (5 of 101 patients) ... 675
Ceclor Pulvules & Suspension ... 1431
Cefol Filmtab ... 412
Cefotan ... 2829
Ceftin Tablets ... 1078
CellCept Capsules ... 2099
▲Ceptaz (Among most common) ... 1081
Cetacaine Topical Anesthetic ... 794
Chloromycetin Ophthalmic Ointment, 1% ... ⊙ 310
Ciloxan Ophthalmic Solution (Less than 1%) ... 472
Cipro I.V. (1% or less) ... 595
Cipro I.V. Pharmacy Bulk Package (Less than 1%) ... 597
Cipro Tablets ... 592
Claritin (2% or fewer patients) ... 2349
Clomid ... 1514
Cogentin Injection ... 1621
ColBENEMID Tablets ... 1622
Colyte and Colyte-flavored ... 2396
Compazine ... 2470
Cortisporin Cream (Approximately 1%) ... 1084
Cortisporin Ointment (Approximately 1%) ... 1085
Cortisporin Otic Solution Sterile (0.09% to approximately 1%) ... 1087
Cortisporin Otic Suspension Sterile (0.09% to approximately 1%) ... 1088
Creon (Less frequent) ... 2536
Cystospaz ... 1963
Cytadren Tablets (Rare) ... 819
CytoGam (Rare) ... 1593
Cytomel Tablets (Rare) ... 2473
DDAVP Injection (Rare) ... 2014
DDAVP Injection 15 mcg/mL (Rare) ... 2015
DDAVP ... 2017
Danocrine Capsules ... 2307
Deltasone Tablets ... 2595
Depen Titratable Tablets ... 2662
Depo-Medrol Single-Dose Vial ... 2600
Depo-Medrol Sterile Aqueous Suspension ... 2597
Depo-Provera Contraceptive Injection (Fewer than 1%) ... 2602
Deponit NTG Transdermal Delivery System (Uncommon) ... 2397
Desquam-E Gel (10 to 25 patients per 1,000) ... 2684
Desquam-X Gel (10 to 25 patients per 1,000) ... 2684
Desquam-X 10 Bar (10 to 25 patients per 1,000) ... 2684
Desquam-X Wash (10 to 25 patients per 1,000) ... 2684
Desyrel and Desyrel Dividose ... 503
DiaBeta Tablets (1.5%) ... 1239
Didrex Tablets ... 2607
Digibind (Rare) ... 1091
Dilantin-125 Suspension ... 1911
Dilaudid Tablets and Liquid ... 1339
Diphtheria and Tetanus Toxoids and Pertussis Vaccine Adsorbed ... 2477
Diphtheria and Tetanus Toxoids and Pertussis Vaccine Adsorbed USP (For Pediatric Use) ... 875
Donnatal ... 2060
Donnatal Extentabs ... 2061
Donnatal Tablets ... 2060
Drithocreme 0.1%, 0.25%, 0.5%, 1.0% (HP) (Very few instances) ... 905
Dritho-Scalp 0.25%, 0.5% (Very few instances) ... 906
Duranest Injections ... 542
Dyclone 0.5% and 1% Topical Solutions, USP ... 544
E.E.S. ... 424
E-Mycin Tablets ... 1341
Effexor (Infrequent) ... 2719
Elspar ... 1659
Emete-con Intramuscular/Intravenous ... 2198
Eminase (0.2%) ... 2039
Emla Cream ... 545
Empirin with Codeine Tablets ... 1093
EPIFRIN ... ⊙ 239
Epogen for Injection (Rare) ... 489
Ergamisol Tablets ... 1292
ERYC ... 1915
EryPed 200 & EryPed 400 Granules ... 421
Ery-Tab Tablets ... 422
Erythrocin Stearate Filmtab ... 425
Esgic-plus Tablets ... 1013
Estraderm Transdermal System (Rare) ... 824
Eurax Cream & Lotion ... 2685
Felbatol (Rare) ... 2666
Fero-Folic-500 Filmtab ... 429
Fiberall Fiber Wafers - Fruit & Nut ... ▣ 636
Fioricet Tablets (Infrequent) ... 2258
Fioricet with Codeine Capsules (Infrequent) ... 2260
Fiorinal with Codeine Capsules ... 2262
Fluorouracil Injection ... 2116
Fluvirin (Infrequent) ... 460
▲Fortaz (Among most common) ... 1100
Fragmin (Rare) ... 1954
Sterile FUDR (Remote possibility) ... 2118
Fungizone Intravenous ... 506
Gamimune N, 5% Immune Globulin Intravenous (Human), 5% ... 619
Gamimune N, 10% Immune Globulin Intravenous (Human), 10% ... 621
Gammar I.V., Immune Globulin Intravenous (Human), Lyophilized ... 516
Gamulin Rh, Rh_0(D) Immune Globulin (Human) (Infrequent) ... 517
Gantanol Tablets ... 2119
Gantrisin ... 2120
Genoptic Sterile Ophthalmic Solution (Rare) ... ⊙ 243
Genoptic Sterile Ophthalmic Ointment (Rare) ... ⊙ 243
Gentak (Rare) ... ⊙ 208
Geref (sermorelin acetate for injection) (One patient) ... 2876
Glucagon for Injection Vials and Emergency Kit ... 1440
Glynase PresTab Tablets (1.5%) ... 2609
▲Habitrol Nicotine Transdermal System (3% to 9% of patients) ... 865
Halcion Tablets (Rare) ... 2611
Haldol Injection, Tablets and Concentrate ... 1575
Halotestin Tablets ... 2614
Herplex Liquifilm ... ⊙ 244
Hibiclens Antimicrobial Skin Cleanser ... 2840
Hibistat (Very rare) ... 2841
Hivid Tablets (Less than 1% to less than 3%) ... 2121
Humate-P, Antihemophilic Factor (Human), Pasteurized (Rare) ... 520
Humegon ... 1824
Humulin 50/50, 100 Units (Less common to occasional) ... 1444
Humulin 70/30, 100 Units ... 1445
Humulin L, 100 Units ... 1446
Hurricaine (Rare) ... 666
Hurricaine Topical (Rare) ... 666
Hydrocet Capsules ... 782
Hytrin Capsules (Rare) ... 430
IBU Tablets (Less than 1%) ... 1342
Iberet-Folic-500 Filmtab ... 429
IFEX (Less than 1%) ... 697
Regular, 100 Units ... 1450
Pork Regular, 100 Units ... 1452
Ilosone ... 911
Ilotycin Gluceptate, IV, Vials ... 913
Inderide Tablets ... 2732
Influenza Virus Vaccine, Trivalent, Types A and B (chromatograph- and filter-purified subviron antigen) FluShield, 1995-1996 Formula (Rare) ... 2736
INSTAT* Collagen Absorbable Hemostat ... 1312
INSTAT* MCH Microfibrillar Collagen Hemostat ... 1313
IOPIDINE Sterile Ophthalmic Solution ... ⊙ 219
Keflex Pulvules & Oral Suspension ... 914
Keftab Tablets ... 915
Kefzol Vials, Faspak & ADD-Vantage ... 1456
Kerlone Tablets (Less than 2%) ... 2436
Koāte-HP Antihemophilic Factor (Human) ... 630
Konakion Injection ... 2127
Konsyl Powder Sugar Free Unflavored ... ▣ 664
Konsyl-D Powder Unflavored ... ▣ 664
Konsyl-Orange Ultra Fine Powder ... ▣ 664
Kutrase Capsules ... 2402
Kytril Injection (Rare) ... 2490
Lamictal Tablets (Rare) ... 1112
Lescol Capsules (2.6%) ... 2267
Levsin/Levsinex/Levbid ... 2405
Lincocin ... 2617
Lodine Capsules and Tablets (Less than 1%) ... 2743
Loniten Tablets ... 2618
Lorabid Suspension and Pulvules ... 1459
Lortab ... 2566
Lutrepulse for Injection ... 980
Luvox Tablets (Infrequent) ... 2544
M-M-R II ... 1687
M-R-VAX II ... 1689
Maalox Daily Fiber Therapy ... ▣ 641
Marcaine Hydrochloride with Epinephrine 1:200,000 (Rare) ... 2316
Marcaine Hydrochloride Injection (Rare) ... 2316
Marcaine Spinal (Rare) ... 2319
Matulane Capsules ... 2131
Maxaquin Tablets (Less than 1%) ... 2440
May-Vita Elixir ... 1543
Medrol ... 2621
Mefoxin ... 1691
Mefoxin Premixed Intravenous Solution ... 1694
▲Mesnex Injection (17%) ... 702
Metamucil ... 1975
Metubine Iodide Vials ... 916
Mezlin ... 601
Miacalcin Injection (A few cases) ... 2273
Miacalcin Nasal Spray (Less than 1%; a few reports) ... 2275
Micronase Tablets (1.5%) ... 2623
Miltown Tablets ... 2672
Minocin Intravenous (Rare) ... 1382
Minocin Oral Suspension ... 1385
Mivacron ... 1138
8-MOP Capsules ... 1246
Monoclate-P, Factor VIII:C, Pasteurized, Monoclonal Antibody Purified Antihemophilic Factor (Human) ... 521
Monoket (Extremely rare) ... 2406
Mononine, Coagulation Factor IX (Human) ... 523
Children's Motrin Ibuprofen Oral Suspension (Less than 1%) ... 1546
Motrin Tablets (Less than 1%) ... 2625
Mumpsvax (Extremely rare) ... 1708
Myochrysine Injection ... 1711
Natacyn Antifungal Ophthalmic Suspension (One case) ... ⊙ 225
NebuPent for Inhalation Solution (1% or less) ... 1040
Neoral (2% or less) ... 2276
Neosporin G.U. Irrigant Sterile ... 1148
Nescaine/Nescaine MPF (Rare) ... 554
Neupogen for Injection ... 495
Neurontin Capsules (Infrequent) ... 1922
Nicobid ... 2026
Nicorette (1% to 3% of patients) ... 2458
Niferex-PN Tablets ... 794
Nitro-Bid IV (Extremely rare; uncommon) ... 1523
Nitro-Bid Ointment (Uncommon; extremely rare) ... 1524
Nitrodisc (Uncommon) ... 2047
Nitro-Dur (nitroglycerin) Transdermal Infusion System (Uncommon) ... 1326
▲Nizoral 2% Cream (5%) ... 1297
Noroxin Tablets (Less frequent) ... 1715
Noroxin Tablets (Less frequent) ... 2048
Novocain Hydrochloride for Spinal Anesthesia ... 2326
Novolin 70/30 Prefilled Disposable Insulin Delivery System (Rare) ... 1798
Nubain Injection (1% or less) ... 935
NuLYTELY ... 689

(▣ Described in PDR For Nonprescription Drugs) Incidence data in parenthesis; ▲ 3% or more (⊙ Described in PDR For Ophthalmology)

1215 **Side Effects Index** **Alopecia**

Cherry Flavor NuLYTELY (Isolated cases) ... 689
Nutropin ... 1061
Ocusert Pilo-20 and Pilo-40 Ocular Therapeutic Systems (Uncommon) ... ◉ 254
▲ Oncaspar (Greater than 5%) ... 2028
Oncovin Solution Vials & Hyporets (Rare) ... 1466
OptiPranolol (Metipranolol 0.3%) Sterile Ophthalmic Solution (A small number of patients) ... ◉ 258
Orudis Capsules (Less than 1%) ... 2766
Oruvail Capsules (Less than 1%) ... 2766
PBZ Tablets ... 845
PBZ-SR Tablets ... 844
PCE Dispertab Tablets ... 444
PMB 200 and PMB 400 ... 2783
Pamelor ... 2280
Pancrease Capsules (Less frequent) ... 1579
Pancrease MT Capsules (Less frequent) ... 1579
Paraflex Caplets (Rare) ... 1580
ParaGard T380A Intrauterine Copper Contraceptive ... 1880
▲ Paraplatin for Injection (10% to 12%) ... 705
Paremyd ... ◉ 247
Paxil Tablets (Infrequent) ... 2505
PediOtic Suspension Sterile (0.09% to approximately 1%) ... 1153
Peptavlon ... 2878
Perdiem Fiber ... ▣ 646
Perdiem ... ▣ 646
Pergonal (menotropins for injection, USP) ... 2448
Peridex (Rare) ... 1978
Phenergan Injection ... 2773
Phenobarbital Elixir and Tablets ... 1469
PhosLo Tablets ... 690
Phrenilin (Infrequent) ... 785
Polysporin Ophthalmic Ointment Sterile ... 1154
Pontocaine Hydrochloride for Spinal Anesthesia ... 2330
Pred Mild ... ◉ 253
Primaxin I.M. ... 1727
Pro-Banthine Tablets ... 2052
Procrit for Injection (Rare) ... 1841
Profasi (chorionic gonadotropin for injection, USP) ... 2450
Prolastin Alpha$_1$-Proteinase Inhibitor (Human) (Occasional) ... 635
Proleukin for Injection (1%) ... 797
Prolixin Oral Concentrate ... 509
PROPINE with C CAP Compliance Cap (Infrequent) ... ◉ 253
ProSom Tablets (Infrequent) ... 449
Prostigmin Injectable ... 1260
Prostigmin Tablets ... 1261
Protropin ... 1063
Prozac Pulvules & Liquid, Oral Solution (1.2% to 3%) ... 919
Quarzan Capsules ... 2181
Rabies Vaccine Adsorbed ... 2508
ReoPro Vials ... 1471
Risperdal (Rare) ... 1301
Robinul Forte Tablets ... 2072
Robinul Injectable ... 2072
Robinul Tablets ... 2072
Rogaine Topical Solution (1.27%) ... 2637
Rowasa ... 2548
SSD ... 1355
Sandimmune (2% or less) ... 2286
Sandostatin Injection (Less than 1%) ... 2292
Secretin-Ferring ... 2872
Sedapap Tablets 50 mg/650 mg (Infrequent) ... 1543
Selsun Rx 2.5% Selenium Sulfide Lotion, USP ... 2225
Semicid Vaginal Contraceptive Inserts ... ▣ 874
Sensorcaine (Rare) ... 559
▲ Septra (Among most common) ... 1174
▲ Septra I.V. Infusion (Among most common) ... 1169
▲ Septra I.V. Infusion ADD-Vantage Vials (Among most common) ... 1171
▲ Septra (Among most common) ... 1174
Seromycin Pulvules ... 1476
Serzone Tablets (Infrequent) ... 771
Silvadene Cream 1% ... 1540
Sinequan (Occasional) ... 2205
Slo-Niacin Tablets ... 2659
Solu-Cortef Sterile Powder ... 2641
Soma Compound w/Codeine Tablets ... 2676
Soma Compound Tablets ... 2675
Sotradecol (Sodium Tetradecyl Sulfate Injection) ... 967
Stelazine (Occasional) ... 2514
Stimate, (desmopressin acetate) Nasal Spray, 1.5 mg/mL (Rare) ... 525
▲ Streptase for Infusion (Among most common; 1% to 4%) ... 562
Sultrin (Frequent) ... 1885
Suprax ... 1399
Synarel Nasal Solution for Central Precocious Puberty (2.6%) ... 2151
Tagamet (Rare) ... 2516
Talacen ... 2333
▲ Tazicef for Injection (Among most common) ... 2519
TERAK Ointment (Rare) ... ◉ 209
Terra-Cortril Ophthalmic Suspension ... 2210
Terramycin Intramuscular Solution ... 2210
Terramycin with Polymyxin B Sulfate Ophthalmic Ointment (Rare) ... 2211
Thioplex (Thiotepa For Injection) (Rare) ... 1281
Thorazine (Occasional) ... 2523
THROMBOGEN* Topical Thrombin, USP with Diluent and Transfer Needle ... 1315
THROMBOGEN* Topical Thrombin, USP, Spray Kit ... 1315
THYREL TRH (Less frequent) ... 2873
Tigan ... 2057
Today Vaginal Contraceptive Sponge ... ▣ 874
Torecan ... 2245
Tracrium Injection ... 1183
Transderm-Nitro Transdermal Therapeutic System (Uncommon) ... 859
Trasylol (0.3%) ... 613
Trinsicon Capsules ... 2570
Triostat Injection (Rare) ... 2530
Trobicin Sterile Powder ... 2645
Tronolane Anesthetic Cream for Hemorrhoids ... ▣ 784
Tylenol with Codeine ... 1583
Tylox Capsules ... 1584
Tympagesic Ear Drops (Infrequently) ... 2342
Typhim Vi (Rare) ... 899
Ultram Tablets (50 mg) (Less than 1%) ... 1585
Ultrase Capsules (Less frequent) ... 2343
Ultrase MT Capsules (Less frequent) ... 2344
Urobiotic-250 Capsules (Rare) ... 2214
Vantin for Oral Suspension and Vantin Tablets ... 2646
Varivax (Greater than or equal to 1%) ... 1762
Vasocidin Ophthalmic Solution ... ◉ 270
VePesid Capsules and Injection (1% to 2%) ... 718
Versed Injection ... 2170
Vibramycin Hyclate Intravenous ... 2215
Videx Tablets, Powder for Oral Solution, & Pediatric Powder for Oral Solution (1% to 2%) ... 720
Voltaren Tablets ... 861
▲ Xanax Tablets (3.8%) ... 2649
Xylocaine Injections (Extremely rare) ... 567
Zefazone ... 2654
▲ Zerit Capsules (Fewer than 1% to 9%) ... 729
Zinacef ... 1211
Zithromax (Rare) ... 1944
Zoladex (1% or greater) ... 2858
Zosyn ... 1419
Zosyn Pharmacy Bulk Package ... 1422

Allergic sensitization

▲ AK-CIDE (Most often) ... ◉ 202
▲ AK-CIDE Ointment (Most often) ... ◉ 202
▲ AK-Trol Ointment & Suspension (Most often) ... ◉ 205
▲ Blephamide Liquifilm Sterile Ophthalmic Suspension (Most often) ... 476
▲ Blephamide Ointment (Among most often) ... ◉ 237
Cerezyme (A number of patients) ... 1066
Chloroptic S.O.P. ... ◉ 239
Cortisporin Ophthalmic Ointment Sterile ... 1085
Cortisporin Ophthalmic Suspension Sterile ... 1086
▲ Cortisporin Otic Solution Sterile (Most often) ... 1087
▲ Cortisporin Otic Suspension Sterile (Most often) ... 1088
Desquam-E Gel (10 to 25 per 1,000) ... 2684
Desquam-X Gel (10 to 25 per 1,000) ... 2684
Desquam-X 10 Bar (10 to 25 per 1,000) ... 2684
Desquam-X Wash (10 to 25 per 1,000) ... 2684
▲ Dexacidin Ointment (Most often) ... ◉ 263
▲ FML-S Liquifilm (Among most often) ... ◉ 242
Leucovorin Calcium for Injection, Wellcovorin Brand ... 1132
Leucovorin Calcium for Injection ... 1268
Leucovorin Calcium Tablets, Wellcovorin Brand ... 1132
Leucovorin Calcium Tablets ... 1270
▲ Maxitrol Ophthalmic Ointment and Suspension (Most often) ... ◉ 224
NeoDecadron Sterile Ophthalmic Ointment ... 1712
▲ NeoDecadron Sterile Ophthalmic Solution (Most often) ... 1713
Neosporin Ophthalmic Ointment Sterile ... 1148
Neosporin Ophthalmic Solution Sterile ... 1149
Ophthocort ... ◉ 311
▲ PediOtic Suspension Sterile (Most often) ... 1153
▲ Poly-Pred Liquifilm (Most often) ... ◉ 248
▲ Polysporin Ophthalmic Ointment Sterile (Among those occurring most often) ... 1154
Precare Prenatal Multi-Vitamin/Mineral ... 2568
▲ Pred-G Liquifilm Sterile Ophthalmic Suspension (Most often) ... ◉ 251
Pred-G S.O.P. Sterile Ophthalmic Ointment ... ◉ 252
▲ Vasocidin Ointment (Most often) ... ◉ 268
▲ Vasocidin Ophthalmic Solution (Most often) ... ◉ 270
▲ Vasosulf (Most often) ... ◉ 271
Advanced Formula ZENATE Tablets ... 2550

Allergic vasospastic reactions

Heparin Lock Flush Solution ... 2725
Heparin Sodium Injection ... 2726

Allergy (see under Allergic reactions)

Alopecia

Adalat CC (Rare) ... 589
▲ Adriamycin PFS (Most cases) ... 1947
▲ Adriamycin RDF (Most cases) ... 1947
Children's Advil Suspension (Less than 1%) ... 2692
Aldoclor Tablets ... 1598
Aldoril Tablets ... 1604
Alkeran for Injection ... 1070
Alkeran Tablets ... 1071
Amen Tablets (Few cases) ... 780
Anafranil Capsules (Infrequent) ... 803
Anaprox/Naprosyn (Less than 1%) ... 2117
Ansaid Tablets (Less than 1%) ... 2579
Aquasol A Vitamin A Capsules, USP ... 534
Aquasol A Parenteral ... 534
Aralen Phosphate Tablets ... 2301
Asacol Delayed-Release Tablets ... 1979
Asendin Tablets (Very rare) ... 1369
Atamet ... 572
Atretol Tablets ... 573
Atromid-S Capsules (Less frequent) ... 2701
Atrovent Inhalation Aerosol (Less frequent) ... 671
Azulfidine (Rare) ... 1949
Benemid Tablets ... 1611
Betapace Tablets (Rare) ... 641
▲ Betaseron for SC Injection (4%) ... 658
Betimol 0.25%, 0.5% ... ◉ 261
Betoptic Ophthalmic Solution (Rare) ... 469
Betoptic S Ophthalmic Suspension (Rare) ... 471
Blenoxane ... 692
Blocadren Tablets (Less than 1%) ... 1614
Brevicon ... 2088
BuSpar (Infrequent) ... 737
Calan SR Caplets (1% or less) ... 2422
Calan Tablets (1% or less) ... 2419
Capoten (About 0.5 to 2%) ... 739
Capozide (0.5 to 2%) ... 742
Cardizem CD Capsules (Infrequent) ... 1506
Cardizem SR Capsules (Infrequent) ... 1510
Cardizem Injectable ... 1508
Cardizem Tablets (Infrequent) ... 1512
Cardura Tablets (Less than 0.5% of 3960 patients) ... 2186
Cartrol Tablets ... 410
Cataflam (Less than 1%) ... 816
Catapres Tablets ... 674
Catapres-TTS (Less frequent) ... 675
CeeNU (Infrequent) ... 693
▲ CellCept Capsules (More than or equal to 3%) ... 2099
▲ Cerubidine (In most patients) ... 795
Claritin (Rare) ... 2349
Claritin-D ... 2350
Climara Transdermal System ... 645
Clinoril Tablets (Less than 1%) ... 1618
Clomid (Fewer than 1%) ... 1514
Cognex Capsules (Infrequent) ... 1901
ColBENEMID Tablets ... 1622
Combipres Tablets (About 2 in 1,000) ... 677
Cordarone Tablets (Less than 1%) ... 2712
Cosmegen Injection ... 1626
Coumadin (Infrequent) ... 926
Cozaar Tablets (Less than 1%) ... 1628
Cuprimine Capsules (Rare) ... 1630
Cycrin Tablets (A few cases) ... 975
Cytosar-U Sterile Powder (Less frequent) ... 2592
Cytotec (Infrequent) ... 2424
Cytovene (1% or less) ... 2103
Cytoxan (Common) ... 694
DTIC-Dome ... 600
Danocrine Capsules ... 2307
Daypro Caplets (Less than 1%) ... 2426
Demulen ... 2428
Depakene ... 413
Depakote Tablets ... 415
Depen Titratable Tablets (Rare) ... 2662
▲ Depo-Provera Contraceptive Injection (1% to 5%) ... 2602
Depo-Provera Sterile Aqueous Suspension ... 2606
Desogen Tablets ... 1817
Desyrel and Desyrel Dividose ... 503
Didronel Tablets ... 1984
Diethylstilbestrol Tablets ... 1437
Diflucan Injection, Tablets, and Oral Suspension ... 2194
Dipentum Capsules (Rare) ... 1951
Diupres Tablets ... 1650
Diuril Oral Suspension ... 1653
Diuril Sodium Intravenous ... 1652
Diuril Tablets ... 1653
▲ Doxorubicin Astra (Most cases) ... 540
EC-Naprosyn Delayed-Release Tablets (Less than 1%) ... 2117
Effexor (Infrequent) ... 2719
Efudex ... 2113
Elavil ... 2838
Eldepryl Tablets ... 2550
Emcyt Capsules (1%) ... 1953
Endep Tablets ... 2174
Engerix-B Unit-Dose Vials ... 2482
▲ Ergamisol Tablets (3% to 22%) ... 1292
Esimil Tablets ... 822
Eskalith ... 2485
Estrace Cream and Tablets ... 749
ESTRATAB Tablets (0.3, 0.625, 1.25, 2.5 mg) ... 2536
Estratest ... 2539
Etrafon ... 2355
Felbatol ... 2666
Feldene Capsules (Less than 1%) ... 1965
Flexeril Tablets (Rare) ... 1661
Fludara for Injection (Up to 3%) ... 663
Fluorouracil Injection (Substantial number of cases) ... 2116
Foscavir Injection (Less than 1%) ... 547
Sterile FUDR ... 2118
Garamycin Injectable ... 2360
Haldol Decanoate (Isolated cases) ... 1577
Haldol Injection, Tablets and Concentrate (Isolated cases) ... 1575
Heparin Lock Flush Solution ... 2725
Heparin Sodium Injection ... 2726
Heparin Sodium Injection, USP, Sterile Solution ... 2615
Heparin Sodium Vials ... 1441
Hexalen Capsules (Less than 1%) ... 2571
Hivid Tablets (Less than 1% to less than 3%) ... 2121
Hydrea Capsules (Very rare) ... 696
HydroDIURIL Tablets ... 1674
Hydropres Tablets ... 1675
Hyzaar Tablets ... 1677
IBU Tablets (Less than 1%) ... 1342
▲ Idamycin (77%) ... 1955
▲ IFEX (83%) ... 697

(▣ Described in PDR For Nonprescription Drugs) Incidence data in parenthesis; ▲ 3% or more (◉ Described in PDR For Ophthalmology)

Imuran (Less than 1%) 1110
Inderal (Rare) 2728
Inderal LA Long Acting Capsules (Rare) 2730
Inderide Tablets (Rare) 2732
Inderide LA Long Acting Capsules (Rare) 2734
Indocin Capsules (Less than 1%) 1680
Indocin I.V. (Less than 1%) 1684
Indocin (Less than 1%) 1680
▲ Intron A (Up to 38%) 2364
Ismelin Tablets 827
Isoptin Oral Tablets (Less than 1%) 1346
Isoptin SR Tablets (1% or less) 1348
Kerlone Tablets (Less than 2%) 2436
Klonopin Tablets 2126
▲ Kytril Tablets (3%) 2492
Lamictal Tablets (1.3%) 1112
Lariam Tablets (Less than 1%) 2128
Larodopa Tablets (Rare) 2129
Lescol Capsules 2267
▲ Leucovorin Calcium for Injection (5% to 43%) 1268
▲ Leukine for IV Infusion (73%) 1271
Levatol 2403
Levlen/Tri-Levlen 651
Levothroid Tablets 1016
Limbitrol 2180
Lioresal Intrathecal 1596
Lithium Carbonate Capsules & Tablets 2230
Lithonate/Lithotabs/Lithobid 2543
Lodine Capsules and Tablets (Less than 1%) 2743
Lo/Ovral Tablets 2746
Lo/Ovral-28 Tablets 2751
Lopid Tablets 1917
Lopressor Ampuls (Rare) 830
Lopressor HCT Tablets 832
Lopressor Tablets (Rare) 830
Loxitane 1378
Ludiomil Tablets (Rare) 843
▲ Lupron Depot 3.75 mg (Among most frequent) 2556
Lupron Depot 7.5 mg 2559
Lupron Depot-PED 7.5 mg, 11.25 mg and 15 mg (Less than 2%) 2560
Lupron Injection (Less than 5%) 2555
Luvox Tablets (Infrequent) 2544
Macrobid Capsules (Less than 1%) 1988
Macrodantin Capsules 1989
Matulane Capsules 2131
Maxair Autohaler 1492
Maxair Inhaler (Less than 1%) 1494
Megace Oral Suspension (1% to 3%) 699
Megace Tablets 701
Menest Tablets 2494
Mesantoin Tablets 2272
▲ Methotrexate Sodium Tablets, Injection, for Injection and LPF Injection (1 to 10%) 1275
Metrodin (urofollitropin for injection) 2446
Mevacor Tablets (0.5% to 1.0%) 1699
Mexitil Capsules (About 4 in 1,000) 678
Miacalcin Nasal Spray (Less than 1%) 2275
Micronor Tablets 1872
Midamor Tablets (Less than or equal to 1%) 1703
Milontin Kapseals 1920
Minipress Capsules (Less than 1%) 1937
Minizide Capsules (Rare) 1938
Modicon 1872
Moduretic Tablets 1705
Children's Motrin Ibuprofen Oral Suspension (Less than 1%) 1546
Motrin Tablets (Less than 1%) 2625
Motrin Ibuprofen Suspension, Oral Drops, Chewable Tablets, Caplets (Less than 1%) 1546
Mustargen (Infrequent) 1709
▲ Mutamycin (Frequent) 703
Myleran Tablets (Rare) 1143
Myochrysine Injection 1711
Nalfon 200 Pulvules & Nalfon Tablets (Less than 1%) 917
Anaprox/Naprosyn (Less than 1%) 2117
▲ Navelbine Injection (Up to 12%) 1145
NEOSAR Lyophilized/Neosar (Common) 1959
▲ Neupogen for Injection (18%) 495
Neurontin Capsules (Infrequent) 1922
Nizoral 2% Shampoo (Less than 1%) 1298
Nizoral Tablets (Rare) 1298
Nolvadex Tablets (Infrequent) 2841
Nordette-21 Tablets 2755
Nordette-28 Tablets 2758
Norinyl 2088
Normodyne Tablets (Less common) 2379
Norplant System 2759
Norpramin Tablets 1526
Nor-Q D Tablets 2135
Norvasc Tablets (Less than or equal to 0.1%) 1940
▲ Novantrone (22 to 37%) 1279
Ogen Tablets 2627
Ogen Vaginal Cream 2630
Oncaspar 2028
▲ Oncovin Solution Vials & Hyporets (Most common) 1466
Ortho-Cept 1851
Ortho-Cyclen/Ortho-Tri-Cyclen 1858
Ortho Dienestrol Cream 1866
Ortho-Est 1869
Ortho-Novum 1872
Ortho-Cyclen/Ortho Tri-Cyclen 1858
Orudis Capsules (Less than 1%) 2766
Oruvail Capsules (Less than 1%) 2766
Ovcon 760
Ovral Tablets 2770
Ovral-28 Tablets 2770
Ovrette Tablets 2771
PMB 200 and PMB 400 2783
Pamelor 2280
▲ Paraplatin for Injection (2% to 50%) 705
Parlodel (Less than 1%) 2281
Paxil Tablets (Infrequent) 2505
Pentasa (Less than 1%) 1527
Pepcid Injection (Infrequent) 1722
Pepcid (Infrequent) 1720
Permax Tablets (Infrequent) 575
Plaquenil Sulfate Tablets 2328
Platinol 708
Platinol-AQ Injection 710
Pravachol 765
Premarin Intravenous 2787
Premarin with Methyltestosterone 2794
Premarin Tablets 2789
Premarin Vaginal Cream 2791
Premphase 2797
Prempro 2801
Synthroid Injection 1359
PREVACID Delayed-Release Capsules (Less than 1%) 2562
Prilosec Delayed-Release Capsules (Less than 1%) 529
Prinivil Tablets (0.3% to 1.0%) 1733
Prinzide Tablets 1737
Procardia XL Extended Release Tablets (1% or less) 1972
Proglycem 580
▲ Prograf (Greater than 3%) 1042
Proleukin for Injection (1%) 797
Provera Tablets (A few cases) 2636
Prozac Pulvules & Liquid, Oral Solution (Infrequent) 919
Quibron 2053
Relafen Tablets (Less than 1%) 2510
Respbid Tablets 682
ReVia Tablets (Less than 1%) 940
Rhinocort Nasal Inhaler (Rare) 556
Ridaura Capsules (Rare) 2513
Risperdal (Infrequent) 1301
Ritalin (A few instances) 848
▲ Roferon-A Injection (8% to 22%) 2145
Rogaine Topical Solution 2637
Rowasa (0.86%) 2548
▲ Rubex (Most cases) 712
Rythmol Tablets–150mg, 225mg, 300mg (Less than 1%) 1352
Sandostatin Injection (1% to 4%) 2292
Sectral Capsules 2807
Seldane Tablets 1536
Seldane-D Extended-Release Tablets 1538
Selsun Rx 2.5% Selenium Sulfide Lotion, USP 2225
Serophene (clomiphene citrate tablets, USP) (Less than 1 in 100 patients) 2451
Serzone Tablets (Infrequent) 771
Sinemet Tablets 943
Sinemet CR Tablets 944
Sinequan (Occasional) 2205
Slo-bid Gyrocaps 2033
Solganal Suspension 2388
Stilphostrol Tablets and Ampuls 612
Supprelin Injection (1% to 3%) 2056
Surmontil Capsules 2811
Synthroid Tablets 1359
Tagamet (Very rare) 2516
Tambocor Tablets (Less than 1%) 1497
Tapazole Tablets 1477
▲ Taxol (87%) 714
▲ Tegison Capsules (Less than 75%) 2154
Tegretol Chewable Tablets 852
Tegretol Suspension 852
Tegretol Tablets 852
Temovate Scalp Application (1 of 294 patients) 1179
Tenex Tablets (Less frequent) 2074
Tenoretic Tablets 2845
Tenormin Tablets and I.V. Injection 2847
Teslac (Rare) 717
Theo-24 Extended Release Capsules 2568
Theo-Dur Extended-Release Tablets 1327
Theo-X Extended-Release Tablets 788
Thioplex (Thiotepa For Injection) 1281
Timolide Tablets 1748
Timoptic in Ocudose (Less frequent) 1753
Timoptic Sterile Ophthalmic Solution (Less frequent) 1751
Timoptic-XE 1755
Tofranil Ampuls 854
Tofranil Tablets 856
Tofranil-PM Capsules 857
Tonocard Tablets (Less than 1%) 531
Toprol-XL Tablets (Rare) 565
Trandate Tablets (Less common) 1185
Triavil Tablets 1757
Levlen/Tri-Levlen 651
Tri-Norinyl 2164
Triphasil-21 Tablets 2814
Triphasil-28 Tablets 2819
Uni-Dur Extended-Release Tablets 1331
Uniphyl 400 mg Tablets 2001
Vaseretic Tablets 1765
Vasotec I.V. 1768
Vasotec Tablets (0.5% to 1.0%) 1771
▲ Velban Vials (Among most common) 1484
▲ VePesid Capsules and Injection (Up to 66%) 718
Verelan Capsules (1% or less) 1410
Verelan Capsules (Less than 1%) 2824
▲ Videx Tablets, Powder for Oral Solution, & Pediatric Powder for Oral Solution (5% to 7%) 720
Visken Tablets 2299
Vivactil Tablets 1774
Voltaren Tablets (Less than 1%) 861
▲ Vumon (9%) 727
Wellbutrin Tablets (Infrequent) 1204
Winstrol Tablets 2337
Zantac (Rare) 1209
Zantac Injection (Rare) 1207
Zantac Syrup (Rare) 1209
Zebeta Tablets 1413
Zestoretic 2850
Zestril Tablets (0.3% to 1.0%) 2854
Ziac 1415
▲ Zinecard (94% to 100%) 1961
Zocor Tablets 1775
Zoladex (1% or greater) 2858
Zoloft Tablets (Infrequent) 2217
Zovirax 1219
Zyloprim Tablets (Less than 1%) 1226

Alopecia, hereditaria
▲ Android Capsules, 10 mg (Among most common) 1250
Android 1251
Delatestryl Injection 2860
Estratest 2539
Halotestin Tablets 2614
Oreton Methyl 1255
Oxandrin 2862
Testoderm Testosterone Transdermal System 486
Testred Capsules 1262

Alpha-glutamyl transferase, elevation
Eulexin Capsules 2358

Alveolalgia
INSTAT* Collagen Absorbable Hemostat 1312
INSTAT* MCH Microfibrillar Collagen Hemostat 1313

Alveolar infiltrates, interstitial
Cytadren Tablets (Rare) 819

Alveolitis
Cordarone Tablets 2712
Cuprimine Capsules 1630
Prozac Pulvules & Liquid, Oral Solution (Rare) 919

Alveolitis, allergic
Cytadren Tablets (Rare) 819
Depen Titratable Tablets (Rare) 2662
Relafen Tablets (Less than 1%) 2510

Alveolitis, fibrosing
Azulfidine (Rare) 1949
Rowasa 2548
Tonocard Tablets (Less than 1%) 531

Amaurosis
Zofran Injection (One patient) 1214

Amblyopia
Accupril Tablets (0.5% to 1.0%) 1893
Adalat CC (Less than 1.0%) 589
Children's Advil Suspension (Less than 1%) 2692
Axid Pulvules (1.0%) 1427
Buprenex Injectable (Infrequent) 2006
Cardizem CD Capsules (Less than 1%) 1506
Cardizem SR Capsules (Less than 1%) 1510
Cardizem Injectable (Less than 1%) 1508
Cardizem Tablets (Less than 1%) 1512
Cataflam (Less than 1%) 816
▲ CellCept Capsules (More than or equal to 3%) 2099
Cognex Capsules (Infrequent) 1901
Cytovene (1% or less) 2103
Depakote Tablets (Greater than 1% but not more than 5%) 415
Dilacor XR Extended-release Capsules (Infrequent) 2018
Diprivan Injection (Less than 1%) 2833
Ditropan 1516
Duragesic Transdermal System (Less than 1%) 1288
Hytrin Capsules (0.6% to 1.3%) 430
IBU Tablets (Less than 1%) 1342
▲ Luvox Tablets (3%) 2544
Macrobid Capsules (Less than 1%) 1988
Megace Oral Suspension (1% to 3%) 699
Monoket (Fewer than 1%) 2406
Children's Motrin Ibuprofen Oral Suspension (Less than 1%) 1546
Motrin Tablets (Less than 1%) 2625
Motrin Ibuprofen Suspension, Oral Drops, Chewable Tablets, Caplets (Less than 1%) 1546
▲ Neurontin Capsules (4.2%) 1922
Nicolar Tablets 2026
Paxil Tablets (Rare) 2505
Penetrex Tablets (Less than 1% but more than or equal to 0.1%) 2031
Placidyl Capsules 448
PREVACID Delayed-Release Capsules (Less than 1%) 2562
▲ Prograf (Greater than 3%) 1042
Prozac Pulvules & Liquid, Oral Solution (Infrequent to 3%) 919
Retrovir Capsules 1158
Retrovir I.V. Infusion 1163
Retrovir Syrup 1158
▲ Salagen Tablets (4%) 1489
Voltaren Tablets (Less than 1%) 861
Zoladex (1% or greater) 2858
Zyloprim Tablets (Less than 1%) 1226

Amebiasis, precipitation of latent
Dexacort Phosphate in Respihaler 458

Amenorrhea
Aldactazide 2413
Aldactone 2414
Aldoclor Tablets 1598
Aldomet Ester HCl Injection 1602
Aldomet Oral 1600
Aldoril Tablets 1604
Alkeran for Injection 1070
Alkeran Tablets (A significant number of patients) 1071
Amen Tablets 780
Anafranil Capsules (Up to 1%) 803
▲ Android Capsules, 10 mg (Among most common) 1250
▲ Android (Among most common) 1251
Aygestin Tablets 974
Brevicon 2088
BuSpar (Rare) 737
Compazine 2470
Cycrin Tablets 975
Cytoxan (A significant proportion of women) 694
Danocrine Capsules (Occasional) 2307
▲ Delatestryl Injection (One of most common) 2860

(▣ Described in PDR For Nonprescription Drugs) Incidence data in parenthesis; ▲ 3% or more (◉ Described in PDR For Ophthalmology)

1217 Side Effects Index Anaphylactic shock

Demulen 2428
Depakene 413
Depakote Tablets 415
▲ Depo-Provera Contraceptive Injection (Up to 68%) 2602
Depo-Provera Sterile Aqueous Suspension 2606
Desogen Tablets 1817
Diethylstilbestrol Tablets 1437
Effexor (Infrequent) 2719
▲ Estratest (Among most common) 2539
Etrafon 2355
Haldol Decanoate 1577
Haldol Injection, Tablets and Concentrate 1575
Halotestin Tablets 2614
Intron A (Less than 5%) 2364
Lamictal Tablets (1.9%) 1112
Leukeran Tablets 1133
Levlen/Tri-Levlen 651
Lo/Ovral Tablets 2746
Lo/Ovral-28 Tablets 2751
Loxitane (Rare) 1378
Mellaril 2269
Menest Tablets 2494
Micronor Tablets 1872
Moban Tablets and Concentrate (Infrequent) 1048
Modicon 1872
Mustargen 1709
Navane Capsules and Concentrate 2201
Navane Intramuscular 2202
NEOSAR Lyophilized/Neosar (A significant proportion of women) 1959
Neurontin Capsules (Infrequent) 1922
▲ Nolvadex Tablets (16.3%) 2841
Nordette-21 Tablets 2755
Nordette-28 Tablets 2758
Norinyl 2088
▲ Norplant System (9.4%) 2759
Nor-Q D Tablets 2135
▲ Oreton Methyl (Among most common) 1255
Orlamm (Low frequency) 2239
Ortho-Cept 1851
Ortho-Cyclen/Ortho-Tri-Cyclen 1858
Ortho Dienestrol Cream 1866
Ortho-Est 1869
Ortho-Novum 1872
Ortho-Cyclen/Ortho Tri-Cyclen 1858
Ovcon 760
Ovral Tablets 2770
Ovral-28 Tablets 2770
Ovrette Tablets 2771
PMB 200 and PMB 400 2783
ParaGard T380A Intrauterine Copper Contraceptive 1880
Paxil Tablets (Infrequent) 2505
Pentasa (Less than 1%) 1527
Permax Tablets (Rare) 575
Premarin Intravenous 2787
Premarin with Methyltestosterone 2794
Premarin Vaginal Cream 2791
Premphase 2797
Prempro 2801
Prolixin Oral Concentrate 509
Provera Tablets 2636
Prozac Pulvules & Liquid, Oral Solution (Infrequent) 919
Reglan 2068
Risperdal (Infrequent) 1301
Sandostatin Injection (Less than 1%) 2292
Serentil 684
Serzone Tablets (Infrequent) 771
Stelazine 2514
Testred Capsules 1262
Thioplex (Thiotepa For Injection) 1281
Thorazine 2523
Trilafon 2389
Levlen/Tri-Levlen 651
Tri-Norinyl 2164
Triphasil-21 Tablets 2814
Triphasil-28 Tablets 2819
Zoladex (Rare) 2858
Zoloft Tablets (Rare) 2217

Amnesia

Altace Capsules (Less than 1%) 1232
Ambien Tablets (1%) 2416
Ansaid Tablets (1-3%) 2579
Ativan Tablets 2700
Betaseron for SC Injection (2%) 658
Cardizem CD Capsules (Less than 1%) 1506
Cardizem SR Capsules (Less than 1%) 1510
Cardizem Injectable 1508
Cardizem Tablets (Less than 1%) 1512
Cardura Tablets (Less than 0.5% of 3960 patients) 2186
Claritin (2% or fewer patients) 2349
Claritin-D 2350
Clozaril Tablets (Less than 1%) 2252
Cognex Capsules (Infrequent) 1901
Cytovene (1% or less) 2103
Didronel Tablets 1984
Doral Tablets 2664
Duragesic Transdermal System (1% or greater) 1288
Effexor 2719
Ergamisol Tablets (Up to 1%) 1292
Foscavir Injection (Between 1% and 5%) 547
Halcion Tablets 2611
Hivid Tablets (Less than 1% to less than 3%) 2121
▲ Intron A (Up to 14%) 2364
Kerlone Tablets (Less than 2%) 2436
Klonopin Tablets 2126
Lamictal Tablets (Frequent) 1112
Luvox Tablets (Frequent) 2544
Marinol (Dronabinol) Capsules (Greater than 1%) 2231
Neurontin Capsules (2.2%) 1922
Norvasc Tablets (Less than or equal to 0.1%) 1940
Orudis Capsules (Less than 1%) 2766
Oruvail Capsules (Less than 1%) 2766
Paxil Tablets (Frequent) 2505
Penetrex Tablets (Less than 0.1%) 2031
Permax Tablets (Frequent) 575
PREVACID Delayed-Release Capsules (Less than 1%) 2562
ProSom Tablets (Infrequent) 449
Prozac Pulvules & Liquid, Oral Solution (2%) 919
Risperdal (Infrequent) 1301
Roferon-A Injection (Less than 0.5%) 2145
Serax Capsules 2810
Serax Tablets 2810
Symmetrel Capsules and Syrup (0.1% to 1%) 946
Tambocor Tablets (Less than 1%) 1497
Tegison Capsules (Less than 1%) 2154
Tenex Tablets (3% or less) 2074
Ultram Tablets (50 mg) (Less than 1%) 1585
Versed Injection (Less than 1%) 2170
Videx Tablets, Powder for Oral Solution, & Pediatric Powder for Oral Solution (1%) 720
Xanax Tablets 2649
Zoloft Tablets (Infrequent) 2217
Zyloprim Tablets (Less than 1%) 1226

Amnesia, traveler's

Halcion Tablets 2611

Amnionitis

Prepidil Gel 2633

Amputation, gangrene of the extremities-induced

Heparin Lock Flush Solution 2725
Heparin Sodium Injection 2726

Analgesia, reversal

Narcan Injection 934

Anaphylactic reactions

Acel-Imune Diphtheria and Tetanus Toxoids and Acellular Pertussis Vaccine Adsorbed (Rare) 1364
Aldoclor Tablets 1598
Aldoril Tablets 1604
Amoxil 2464
Ancef Injection 2465
Ansaid Tablets (Rare) 2579
Antivenin (Black Widow Spider) 1607
AquaMEPHYTON Injection 1608
Atgam Sterile Solution (Less than 5%) 2581
Atrovent Inhalation Aerosol 671
Augmentin 2468
Azo Gantanol Tablets 2080
Benemid Tablets 1611
Biavax II 1613
Bicillin C-R Injection 2704
Bicillin L-A Injection 2707
Brontex (Rare) 1981
Capozide 742
Carmol HC 924
Cefotan 2829
Chloromycetin Sodium Succinate 1900
Cipro I.V. (1% or less) 595
Cipro I.V. Pharmacy Bulk Package (Less than 1%) 597
Cipro Tablets 592
Cortisporin Otic Solution Sterile 1087
Cytosar-U Sterile Powder (Less frequent) 2592
Cytovene-IV (Two or more reports) 2103
Cytoxan (Rare) 694
Deltasone Tablets 2595
Depo-Medrol Single-Dose Vial 2600
Desferal Vials 820
Diflucan Injection, Tablets, and Oral Suspension (Rare) 2194
Digibind 1091
Dilaudid Tablets and Liquid 1339
Diphtheria and Tetanus Toxoids and Pertussis Vaccine Adsorbed (Rare) 2477
Diphtheria and Tetanus Toxoids and Pertussis Vaccine Adsorbed USP (For Pediatric Use) (Rare) 875
Diucardin Tablets 2718
Diupres Tablets 1650
Diuril Oral Suspension 1653
Diuril Sodium Intravenous 1652
Diuril Tablets 1653
Dobutrex Solution Vials 1439
Dolobid Tablets (Less than 1 in 100) 1654
Dyclone 0.5% and 1% Topical Solutions, USP 544
Easprin 1914
Elspar 1659
Eminase (0.2%) 2039
Enduron Tablets 420
Factrel (Rare) 2877
Floxin I.V. 1571
Floxin Tablets (200 mg, 300 mg, 400 mg) 1567
Gamimune N, 5% Immune Globulin Intravenous (Human), 5% 619
Gamimune N, 10% Immune Globulin Intravenous (Human), 10% 621
Gammagard S/D, Immune Globulin, Intravenous (Human) (A remote possibility) 585
Gammar, Immune Globulin (Human) U.S.P. (Rare) 515
Gammar I.V., Immune Globulin Intravenous (Human), Lyophilized 516
Geocillin Tablets 2199
Heparin Lock Flush Solution 2725
Heparin Sodium Injection 2726
Hep-B-Gammagee (Rare) 1663
Hespan Injection (Rare) 929
HydroDIURIL Tablets 1674
Hydropres Tablets 1675
HyperHep Hepatitis B Immune Globulin (Human) (Rare) 626
Hyskon Hysteroscopy Fluid (Rare) 1595
Hyzaar Tablets 1677
Imogam Rabies Immune Globulin (Human) (Rare) 880
Imovax Rabies Vaccine 881
Inderide Tablets 2732
Inderide LA Long Acting Capsules 2734
INFeD (Iron Dextran Injection, USP) 2345
Isuprel Hydrochloride Solution 1:200 & 1:100 2313
Levatol 2403
Lodine Capsules and Tablets (Less than 1%) 2743
Lozol Tablets 2022
Lupron Injection 2555
Luvox Tablets 2544
M-M-R II 1687
Marcaine Spinal (Rare) 2319
Maxaquin Tablets (Occasional) 2440
Medrol 2621
Mefoxin Premixed Intravenous Solution 1694
Meruvax II 1697
Mesnex Injection 702
Mezlin 601
Mezlin Pharmacy Bulk Package 604
Mintezol 1704
Moduretic Tablets 1705
MSTA Mumps Skin Test Antigen 890
Mykrox Tablets (rare) 993
Nasalcrom Nasal Solution (1 in 430) 994
NEOSAR Lyophilized/Neosar (Rare) 1959
Nescaine/Nescaine MPF 554
Norflex (Rare) 1496
Normodyne Injection 2377
Normodyne Tablets 2379
Noroxin Tablets (Occasional) 1715
Noroxin Tablets (Occasional) 2048
Nubain Injection (1% or less) 935
Omnipen Capsules 2764
▲ Oncaspar (Greater than 1% but less than 5%) 2028
Orthoclone OKT3 Sterile Solution 1837
Orudis Capsules (Less than 1%) 2766
Oruvail Capsules (Less than 1%) 2766
Oxytocin Injection 2771
Paraflex Caplets (Extremely rare) 1580
Parafon Forte DSC Caplets (Extremely rare) 1581
Paraplatin for Injection 705
Pergonal (menotropins for injection, USP) (Some patients) 2448
Pfizerpen for Injection (Occasional) 2203
Phenergan Injection 2773
Pipracil 1390
Platinol (Occasional) 708
Platinol-AQ Injection (Occasional) 710
Premarin with Methyltestosterone (Rare) 2794
Primaxin I.M. 1727
Primaxin I.V. 1729
Prinzide Tablets 1737
Prograf (A few patients) 1042
Protamine Sulfate Ampoules & Vials 1471
Quarzan Capsules 2181
Rabies Vaccine, Imovax Rabies I.D. 883
Ridaura Capsules 2513
Risperdal 1301
Robaxin Injectable 2070
Rowasa 2548
Sandimmune I.V. Ampuls for Infusion (Rare) 2286
Sandoglobulin I.V. 2290
Sensorcaine 559
Septra I.V. Infusion 1169
Septra I.V. Infusion ADD-Vantage Vials 1171
Solu-Cortef Sterile Powder 2641
Solu-Medrol Sterile Powder (Rare) 2643
Soma Compound w/Codeine Tablets 2676
Spectrobid Tablets (Occasional) 2206
Stelazine 2514
Streptase for Infusion (Rare) 562
Streptomycin Sulfate Injection 2208
Syntocinon Injection 2296
Talacen (One instance) 2333
Tao Capsules 2209
Temaril Tablets, Syrup and Spansule Extended-Release Capsules 483
Terramycin Intramuscular Solution 2210
Tetramune (Rare) 1404
Thorazine 2523
Timentin for Injection 2528
Timolide Tablets 1748
Toradol 2159
Tracrium Injection 1183
Trandate Injection 1185
Trasylol (Less than 0.5%) 613
Triavil Tablets 1757
Tri-Immunol Adsorbed (Rare) 1408
Trilafon 2389
Tripedia 892
Tympagesic Ear Drops 2342
Typhim Vi 899
Unasyn (Occasional) 2212
Vaseretic Tablets 1765
VePesid Capsules and Injection 718
Vibramycin Hyclate Intravenous 2215
Vibra-Tabs Film Coated Tablets 1941
Zaroxolyn Tablets 1000
Zestoretic 2850
Ziac 1415
Zosyn (Occasional) 1419
Zosyn Pharmacy Bulk Package (Occasional) 1422

Anaphylactic shock

Actifed with Codeine Cough Syrup 1067
Ambien Tablets (Rare) 2416
Aquasol A Parenteral 534
Benadryl Capsules 1898
Benadryl Injection 1898
Calcimar Injection, Synthetic (A few cases) 2013
CytoGam (A possibility) 1593
Declomycin Tablets 1371
Deconamine 1320
Eminase (0,1%) 2039
Empirin with Codeine Tablets 1093
Ethamolin 2400
Fioricet with Codeine Capsules 2260
Fiorinal with Codeine Capsules 2262
Hep-B-Gammagee 1663
Hyperab Rabies Immune Globulin (Human) (Rare) 624

(Described in PDR For Nonprescription Drugs) Incidence data in parenthesis; ▲ 3% or more (◉ Described in PDR For Ophthalmology)

Hyper-Tet Tetanus Immune Globulin (Human) (Few isolated cases) 627
Miacalcin Injection (A few cases) 2273
Myochrysine Injection 1711
Ornade Spansule Capsules 2502
Orthoclone OKT3 Sterile Solution 1837
PBZ Tablets 845
PBZ-SR Tablets 844
Periactin 1724
Protamine Sulfate Ampoules & Vials 1471
Salflex Tablets 786
Sandostatin Injection (Several patients) 2292
Solganal Suspension 2388
Soma Compound w/Codeine Tablets 2676
Soma Compound Tablets 2675
Soma Tablets 2674
Sotradecol (Sodium Tetradecyl Sulfate Injection) 967
Streptase for Infusion (Very rare) 562
Tavist Syrup 2297
Tavist Tablets 2298
Tetramune (Rare) 1404
Thioplex (Thiotepa For Injection) 1281
Toradol 2159
Trasylol 613
Trinalin Repetabs Tablets 1330
Tripedia 892
Tussend 1783
Vantin for Oral Suspension and Vantin Tablets (Less than 1%) 2646
Yutopar Intravenous Injection (Infrequent) 570

Anaphylactoid reactions

Accupril Tablets 1893
Achromycin V Capsules 1367
Activase (Very rare) 1058
Altace Capsules (Less than 1%) 1232
Amen Tablets 780
Amoxil (occasional) 2464
Anaprox/Naprosyn (Less than 1%) 2117
Android Capsules, 10 mg (Rare) 1250
Android (Rare) 1251
Aquasol A Parenteral (One case) 534
Aristocort Suspension (Forte Parenteral) (Rare) 1027
Aristocort Suspension (Intralesional) (Rare) 1025
Aristocort Tablets (Rare) 1022
Aristospan Suspension (Intra-articular) (Rare) 1033
Aristospan Suspension (Intralesional) (Rare) 1032
Attenuvax 1610
Betaseron for SC Injection 658
Biavax II 1613
Capoten 739
Capozide 742
Carbocaine Hydrochloride Injection (Rare) 2303
Cataflam (Less than 1%) 816
Ceclor Pulvules & Suspension 1431
Celestone Soluspan Suspension (Rare) 2347
Cerubidine (Rare) 795
Chibroxin Sterile Ophthalmic Solution (With oral form) 1617
Cleocin Phosphate Injection (A few cases) 2586
Cleocin Vaginal Cream (A few cases) 2589
Compazine 2470
Cortone Acetate Sterile Suspension 1623
Cycrin Tablets 975
Dalalone D.P. Injectable 1011
Decadron Phosphate Injection 1637
Decadron Phosphate with Xylocaine Injection, Sterile 1639
Decadron-LA Sterile Suspension 1646
Delatestryl Injection (Rare) 2860
Depo-Medrol Single-Dose Vial (Rare) 2600
Depo-Medrol Sterile Aqueous Suspension (Rare) 2597
Depo-Provera Contraceptive Injection 2602
Depo-Provera Sterile Aqueous Suspension 2606
Deponit NTG Transdermal Delivery System 2397
Digibind 1091
Diprivan Injection (Less than 1%) 2833
Duranest Injections 542
EC-Naprosyn Delayed-Release Tablets (Less than 1%) 2117
Eminase (0.2%) 2039
Emla Cream 545
Engerix-B Unit-Dose Vials 2482
Epogen for Injection 489
Estratest (Rare) 2539
Etrafon 2355
Fansidar Tablets 2114
Felbatol (Rare) 2666
Florinef Acetate Tablets 505
Floxin I.V. 1571
Floxin Tablets (200 mg, 300 mg, 400 mg) 1567
Fragmin (A few cases) 1954
Fungizone Intravenous 506
Gamimune N, 5% Immune Globulin Intravenous (Human), 5% (Very rare) 619
Gamimune N, 10% Immune Globulin Intravenous (Human), 10% (Very rare) 621
Gammar I.V., Immune Globulin Intravenous (Human), Lyophilized (Rare) 516
Garamycin Injectable 2360
Halotestin Tablets 2614
Havrix (Rare) 2489
Heparin Sodium Injection, USP, Sterile Solution 2615
Heparin Sodium Vials (Rare) 1441
Hespan Injection 929
Hydeltrasol Injection, Sterile 1665
Hydeltra-T.B.A. Sterile Suspension 1667
Hydrocortone Acetate Sterile Suspension 1669
Hydrocortone Phosphate Injection, Sterile 1670
Imitrex Injection (Rare) 1103
Imitrex Tablets (Rare) 1106
Imogam Rabies Immune Globulin (Human) (Rare) 880
Konakion Injection 2127
Kytril Injection (Rare) 2490
Leucovorin Calcium for Injection 1268
Leucovorin Calcium Tablets 1270
Levoprome 1274
Lotensin Tablets 834
Lotensin HCT (Two patients) 837
Lotrel Capsules 840
M-M-R II 1687
M-R-VAX II 1689
Marcaine Hydrochloride with Epinephrine 1:200,000 2316
Marcaine Hydrochloride Injection 2316
Maxaquin Tablets 2440
Meruvax II 1697
Methotrexate Sodium Tablets, Injection, for Injection and LPF Injection (A few cases) 1275
Mezlin 601
Monocid Injection (Less than 1%) 2497
Monopril Tablets 757
Motrin Ibuprofen Suspension, Oral Drops, Chewable Tablets, Caplets (Less than 1%) 1546
Mumpsvax 1708
Myambutol Tablets 1386
Anaprox/Naprosyn (Less than 1%) 2117
NegGram (Rare) 2323
Neutrexin (One report) 2572
Nitro-Bid IV (A few reports) 1523
Nitro-Bid Ointment (A few reports) 1524
Nitrodisc (A few reports) 2047
Nitro-Dur (nitroglycerin) Transdermal Infusion System (A few reports) 1326
Normodyne Injection (Rare) 2377
Normodyne Tablets (Rare) 2379
Noroxin Tablets (Occasional) 1715
Noroxin Tablets (Occasional) 2048
Novocain Hydrochloride for Spinal Anesthesia 2326
Nubain Injection (1% or less) 935
Oreton Methyl (Rare) 1255
Orthoclone OKT3 Sterile Solution 1837
Pen•Vee K (Occasional) 2772
Pneumovax 23 (Rare) 1725
Pnu-Imune 23 (Rare) 1393
Premphase 2797
Prempro 2801
Prinivil Tablets (0.3% to 1.0%) 1733
Prinzide Tablets 1737
Procrit for Injection 1841
Prolixin 509
Protamine Sulfate Ampoules & Vials 1471
Provera Tablets 2636
Pyridium (One report) 1928
Relafen Tablets (Rarer) 2510
Sandoglobulin I.V. 2290
Sandostatin Injection (Several patients) 2292
Sensorcaine 559
Stelazine Concentrate 2514
Streptase for Infusion (Rare) 562
Testoderm Testosterone Transdermal System (Rare) 486
Testred Capsules (Rare) 1262
Tetanus Toxoid Adsorbed Purogenated 1403
Tolectin (200, 400 and 600 mg) (Less than 1%) 1581
Toradol 2159
Tracrium Injection 1183
Trandate (Rare) 1185
Transderm-Nitro Transdermal Therapeutic System (A few reports) 859
Trental Tablets (Rare) 1244
Trobicin Sterile Powder 2645
Univasc Tablets 2410
Vancocin HCl, Vials & ADD-Vantage 1481
Vaseretic Tablets 1765
Vasotec I.V. 1768
Vasotec Tablets (0.5% to 1.0%) 1771
Versed Injection 2170
Videx Tablets, Powder for Oral Solution, & Pediatric Powder for Oral Solution (Less than 1%) 720
Voltaren Tablets (Less than 1%) 861
Xylocaine Injections (Extremely rare) 567
Zestoretic 2850
Zestril Tablets (0.3% to 1.0%) 2854

Anaphylaxis

Abbokinase (Rare) 403
Abbokinase Open-Cath (Rare) 405
Achromycin V Capsules 1367
Adriamycin PFS 1947
Adriamycin RDF 1947
Children's Advil Suspension (Less than 1%) 2692
Alfenta Injection 1286
Alkeran for Injection (2.4%) 1070
Alkeran Tablets (Rare) 1071
Amen Tablets 780
Amoxil 2464
Ancef Injection 2465
Anectine (Rare) 1073
Antivenin (Crotalidae) Polyvalent 2696
AquaMEPHYTON Injection 1608
Atgam Sterile Solution (Less than 1% to less than 5%) 2581
Atrovent Inhalation Solution (A single case) 673
Attenuvax 1610
Axid Pulvules (Rare) 1427
Azactam for Injection (Less than 1%) 734
Azo Gantrisin Tablets 2081
Azulfidine (Rare) 1949
Bactrim DS Tablets 2084
Bactrim I.V. Infusion 2082
Bactrim 2084
Benemid Tablets 1611
Bentyl 1501
Biavax II 1613
Bicillin C-R Injection 2704
Bicillin C-R 900/300 Injection 2706
Blenoxane 692
Brevital Sodium Vials 1429
Calcimar Injection, Synthetic (One case) 2013
Cataflam (Rare) 816
Ceclor Pulvules & Suspension (Rare) 1431
Cefizox for Intramuscular or Intravenous Use (Rare) 1034
Ceftin 1078
Cefzil Tablets and Oral Suspension (Rare) 746
Ceptaz (Very rare) 1081
Chloromycetin Sodium Succinate 1900
Claforan Sterile and Injection (Less frequent) 1235
Claritin (Rare) 2349
Claritin-D 2350
Clinoril Tablets 1618
ColBENEMID Tablets 1622
Cortisporin Ophthalmic Ointment Sterile (Rare) 1085
Cortisporin Ophthalmic Suspension Sterile (Rare) 1086
Cycrin Tablets 975
CytoGam 1593
Cytosar-U Sterile Powder (One case) 2592
Cytotec (Infrequent) 2424
DDAVP Injection (Rare) 2014
DDAVP Injection 15 mcg/mL (Rare) 2015
Dantrium Capsules (Less frequent) 1982
Dantrium Intravenous (One case) 1983
Daypro Caplets (Less than 1%) 2426
Declomycin Tablets 1371
Depo-Provera Contraceptive Injection 2602
Depo-Provera Sterile Aqueous Suspension 2606
Diamox 1372
Diflucan Injection, Tablets, and Oral Suspension (Rare) 2194
Digibind 1091
Diprivan Injection (Rare; less than 1%) 2833
Donnatal 2060
Donnatal Extentabs 2061
Donnatal Tablets 2060
Doryx Capsules 1913
Doxorubicin Astra 540
Duricef 748
Dyazide 2479
Dynacin Capsules 1590
Dyrenium Capsules 2481
E.E.S. 424
E-Mycin Tablets 1341
Easprin 1914
Elspar 1659
Engerix-B Unit-Dose Vials 2482
Ergamisol Tablets (Less frequent) 1292
ERYC 1915
EryPed 421
Ery-Tab Tablets 422
Erythrocin Stearate Filmtab 425
Erythromycin Base Filmtab 426
Erythromycin Delayed-Release Capsules, USP 427
Ethamolin (Three reports) 2400
Feldene Capsules (Less than 1%) 1965
Flexeril Tablets 1661
Fludara for Injection (Up to 1%) 663
Fluorescite ⊙ 219
Fluorouracil Injection 2116
Fluvirin (Rare) 460
Fortaz (Very rare) 1100
Sterile FUDR (Remote possibility) 2118
Gamimune N, 5% Immune Globulin Intravenous (Human), 5% (Rare) 619
Gammar, Immune Globulin (Human) U.S.P. 515
Gantanol Tablets 2119
Gantrisin 2120
Glauctabs ⊙ 208
Havrix (Rare) 2489
Hep-B-Gammagee 1663
Hytrin Capsules (Rare) 430
IBU Tablets (Less than 1%) 1342
Ilosone 911
Ilotycin Gluceptate, IV, Vials 913
Imitrex Injection (Rare) 1103
Imitrex Tablets (Rare) 1106
Inapsine Injection (Less common) 1296
Indocin Capsules (Less than 1%) 1680
Indocin I.V. (Less than 1%) 1684
Indocin (Less than 1%) 1680
INFeD (Iron Dextran Injection, USP) 2345
Influenza Virus Vaccine, Trivalent, Types A and B (chromatograph- and filter-purified subviron antigen) FluShield, 1995-1996 Formula (Rare) 2736
Intal Capsules (Less than 1 in 100,000 patients) 987
Intal Inhaler (Infrequent) 988
Intal Nebulizer Solution (Rare) 989
Intron A (Rare) 2364
JE-VAX (One episode) 886
Keflex Pulvules & Oral Suspension 914
Keftab Tablets 915
Kefurox Vials, Faspak & ADD-Vantage (Rare) 1454
Kefzol Vials, Faspak & ADD-Vantage 1456
Kytril Injection (Rare) 2490
Kytril Tablets (Rare) 2492
Lescol Capsules (Rare) 2267
Lincocin 2617
Lomotil 2439
Lopid Tablets 1917
Lorabid Suspension and Pulvules (Rare) 1459
Lutrepulse for Injection 980
M-M-R II 1687
M-R-VAX II 1689
MZM (Common) ⊙ 267
Macrobid Capsules 1988
Macrodantin Capsules 1989

(▣ Described in PDR For Nonprescription Drugs) Incidence data in parenthesis; ▲ 3% or more (⊙ Described in PDR For Ophthalmology)

1219 Side Effects Index Anemia

Mandol Vials, Faspak & ADD-Vantage 1461
Maxaquin Tablets 2440
Maxzide 1380
Mefoxin 1691
Mefoxin Premixed Intravenous Solution 1694
Meruvax II 1697
Methergine (Rare isolated reports) 2272
Mevacor Tablets (Rare) 1699
Miltown Tablets (Rare) 2672
Minocin Intravenous 1382
Minocin Oral Suspension 1385
Minocin Pellet-Filled Capsules 1383
Mintezol 1704
Monoclate-P, Factor VIII:C, Pasteurized, Monoclonal Antibody Purified Antihemophilic Factor (Human) 521
Monodox Capsules 1805
Mononine, Coagulation Factor IX (Human) 523
Motofen Tablets 784
Children's Motrin Ibuprofen Oral Suspension (Less than 1%) 1546
Motrin Tablets (Less than 1%) 2625
Motrin Ibuprofen Suspension, Oral Drops, Chewable Tablets, Caplets (Less than 1%) 1546
Mumpsvax 1708
Mustargen 1709
Nalfon 200 Pulvules & Nalfon Tablets (Less than 1%) 917
Nasalcrom Nasal Solution (1 case) 994
Navane Capsules and Concentrate (Rare) 2201
Navane Intramuscular (Rare) 2202
Neosporin Ophthalmic Ointment Sterile (Rare) 1148
Neosporin Ophthalmic Solution Sterile (Rare) 1149
Neptazane Tablets 1388
Nizoral Tablets (Rare) 1298
Omnipen Capsules 2764
Omnipen for Oral Suspension 2765
Oncaspar 2028
Oncovin Solution Vials & Hyporets (Rare) 1466
Orthoclone OKT3 Sterile Solution 1837
Orudis Capsules (Less than 1%) 2766
Oruvail Capsules (Less than 1%) 2766
PCE Dispertab Tablets 444
PMB 200 and PMB 400 2783
Pen•Vee K (Occasional) 2772
Pepcid Injection (Infrequent) 1722
Pepcid (Infrequent) 1720
Pfizerpen for Injection (Severe & occasionally fatal. (See Warnings)) 2203
Polysporin Ophthalmic Ointment Sterile (Rare) 1154
Pontocaine Hydrochloride for Spinal Anesthesia 2330
Pravachol (Rare) 765
Pred Mild ⊙ 253
Premphase 2797
Prempro 2801
Pro-Banthīne Tablets 2052
Prograf (A small percentage of patients) 1042
Proloprim Tablets (Rare) 1155
Prostigmin Injectable 1260
Prostigmin Tablets 1261
Protamine Sulfate Ampoules & Vials 1471
Proventil Syrup (Rare) 2385
Provera Tablets 2636
Quarzan Capsules 2181
Recombivax HB (Less than 1%) 1744
Relafen Tablets (Rarer) 2510
ReoPro Vials 1471
Retrovir Capsules (One patient) 1158
Retrovir I.V. Infusion (One patient) 1163
Retrovir Syrup (One patient) 1158
Robinul Forte Tablets 2072
Robinul Injectable 2072
Robinul Tablets 2072
Rocephin Injectable Vials, ADD-Vantage, Galaxy Container (Rare) 2142
Rubex (Occasional) 712
Seldane Tablets 1536
Seldane-D Extended-Release Tablets 1538
Semprex-D Capsules (Rare) 463
Semprex-D Capsules (Rare) 1167
Septra 1174
Septra I.V. Infusion 1169
Septra I.V. Infusion ADD-Vantage Vials 1171
Septra 1174
Sporanox Capsules (Rare) 1305
Stimate, (desmopressin acetate) Nasal Spray, 1.5 mg/mL (One patient) 525
Sublimaze Injection 1307
Sufenta Injection 1309
Suprax 1399
Tagamet (Rare) 2516
Tao Capsules 2209
Tazicef for Injection (Very rare) 2519
Terramycin Intramuscular Solution 2210
Tetanus Toxoid Adsorbed Purogenated 1403
Tilade (Isolated cases) 996
Toradol 2159
Trasylol 613
Trimpex Tablets (Rare) 2163
Trobicin Sterile Powder (Few cases) 2645
Vancocin HCl, Oral Solution & Pulvules (Infrequent) 1483
Vancocin HCl, Vials & ADD-Vantage (Infrequent) 1481
Velosulin BR Human Insulin 10 ml Vials 1795
Ventolin Inhalation Aerosol and Refill 1197
Ventolin Rotacaps for Inhalation (Rare) 1200
Ventolin Syrup (Rare) 1202
Vibramycin 1941
Voltaren Tablets (Rare) 861
Vumon 727
Zantac (Rare) 1209
Zantac Injection (Rare) 1207
Zantac Syrup (Rare) 1209
Zefazone 2654
Zinacef (Rare) 1211
Zithromax (Rare) 1944
Zocor Tablets (Rare) 1775
Zofran Injection (Rare) 1214
Zofran Tablets (Rare) 1217
Zosyn (1.0% or less) 1419
Zosyn Pharmacy Bulk Package (1.0% or less) 1422
Zovirax Capsules (Rare) 1219
Zovirax Sterile Powder (Rare) 1223
Zovirax (Rare) 1219

Androgen excess, signs or symptoms of

Danocrine Capsules 2307
Lupron Depot 3.75 mg (Less than 5%) 2556

Anemia

(see also under Aplastic anemia; Hypoplastic anemia; Megaloblastic anemia)

Accutane Capsules (Less than 1%) 2076
Adalat Capsules (10 mg and 20 mg) (Less than 0.5%) 587
Adalat CC (Rare) 589
Children's Advil Suspension (Less than 1%) 2692
Alkeran for Injection 1070
Alkeran Tablets 1071
Ambien Tablets (Rare) 2416
Amikacin Sulfate Injection, USP (Rare) 960
Amikin Injectable (Rare) 501
Amoxil 2464
Anafranil Capsules (Up to 2%) 803
Ancobon Capsules 2079
Ansaid Tablets (Rare; common) 2579
Anturane (Rare) 807
▲ Aredia for Injection (Up to at least 15%) 810
Asacol Delayed-Release Tablets 1979
Atamet (Rare) 572
Atgam Sterile Solution (Less than 5%) 2581
Atromid-S Capsules 2701
Augmentin 2468
▲ Axid Pulvules (More frequent) 1427
Azactam for Injection (Less than 1%) 734
Azo Gantrisin Tablets 2081
Azulfidine 1949
BCG Vaccine, USP (TICE) (1.3%) 1814
Benemid Tablets 1611
BiCNU (Less frequent) 691
Capoten 739
Capozide 742
CeeNU 693
Cefizox for Intramuscular or Intravenous Use (Rare) 1034
▲ CellCept Capsules (25.6% to 25.8%) 2099
Cipro Tablets (Less than 1%) 592
Clinoril Tablets (Less than 1%) 1618
Clozaril Tablets (Less than 1%) 2252
Cognex Capsules (Infrequent) 1901
ColBENEMID Tablets 1622
Cosmegen Injection 1626
Cozaar Tablets (Less than 1%) 1628
Cytosar-U Sterile Powder 2592
Cytotec (Infrequent) 2424
▲ Cytovene (19%) 2103
Cytoxan (Occasional) 694
DTIC-Dome 600
Dalgan Injection (Less than 1%) 538
Daypro Caplets (Less than 1%) 2426
Demser Capsules (Rare) 1649
Demulen 2428
Depakene 413
Depakote Tablets 415
Depo-Provera Contraceptive Injection (Fewer than 1%) 2602
Desyrel and Desyrel Dividose 503
Dipentum Capsules (Rare) 1951
Effexor (Infrequent) 2719
Eldepryl Tablets 2550
▲ Ergamisol Tablets (Up to 6%) 1292
Esimil Tablets (A few instances) 822
▲ Eulexin Capsules (6%) 2358
Felbatol 2666
Feldene Capsules (Greater than 1%) 1965
Floxin I.V. (More than or equal to 1%) 1571
Floxin Tablets (200 mg, 300 mg, 400 mg) (More than or equal to 1%) 1567
▲ Fludara for Injection (Among most common) 663
Fluorouracil Injection 2116
▲ Foscavir Injection (5% or greater up to 33%) 547
▲ Sterile FUDR (Among more common) 2118
Ganite 2533
Garamycin Injectable 2360
Geocillin Tablets 2199
Glucophage (Very rare) 752
Haldol Decanoate 1577
Haldol Injection, Tablets and Concentrate 1575
Hivid Tablets (Less than 1% to less than 3%) 2121
Hydrea Capsules (Less often) 696
Hyzaar Tablets 1677
Imitrex Tablets (Rare) 1106
Indocin Capsules (Less than 1%) 1680
Indocin I.V. (Less than 1%) 1684
Indocin (Less than 1%) 1680
Intal Capsules (Less than 1 in 100,000 patients) 987
Intal Inhaler (Rare) 988
Intal Nebulizer Solution (Rare) 989
Intron A (Less than 5%) 2364
Ismelin Tablets 827
Kerlone Tablets (Less than 2%) 2436
Klonopin Tablets 2126
▲ Kytril Tablets (4%) 2492
Lamictal Tablets (Infrequent) 1112
Lamprene Capsules (Less than 1%) 828
Lasix Injection, Oral Solution and Tablets 1240
▲ Leustatin (37%) 1834
Lincocin (Rare) 2617
Lippes Loop Intrauterine Double-S 1848
Lodine Capsules and Tablets (Less than 1%) 2743
Lopid Tablets (Rare) 1917
Lupron Depot 3.75 mg 2556
Lupron Depot 7.5 mg 2559
Lupron Injection 2555
Luvox Tablets (Infrequent) 2544
Macrobid Capsules 1988
Macrodantin Capsules 1989
▲ Matulane Capsules (Frequent) 2131
Maxaquin Tablets (Less than or equal to 0.1%) 2440
Mefoxin 1691
Mefoxin Premixed Intravenous Solution 1694
▲ Megace Oral Suspension (Up to 5%) 699
Mellaril 2269
▲ Mepron Suspension (4% to 6%) 1135
Mesantoin Tablets (Uncommon) 2272
Methotrexate Sodium Tablets, Injection, for Injection and LPF Injection 1275
Miacalcin Nasal Spray (Less than 1%) 2275
Monopril Tablets 757
Motrin Tablets (Less than 1%) 2625
▲ Mycobutin Capsules (6%) 1957
Myleran Tablets 1143
▲ Navelbine Injection (1% to 77%) 1145
Nebcin Vials, Hyporets & ADD-Vantage 1464
NebuPent for Inhalation Solution (Greater than 1%, up to 5%) 1040
Neoral (2% or less) 2276
Netromycin Injection 100 mg/ml (Fewer than 1 per 1000 patients) 2373
▲ Neupogen for Injection (Approximately 10%) 495
Neurontin Capsules (Infrequent) 1922
▲ Neutrexin (7.3%) 2572
Nimotop Capsules (Less than 1%) 610
Nolvadex Tablets 2841
Omnipen Capsules 2764
Omnipen for Oral Suspension 2765
Oncaspar 2028
Oncovin Solution Vials & Hyporets 1466
Orudis Capsules (Less than 1%) 2766
Oruvail Capsules (Less than 1%) 2766
ParaGard T380A Intrauterine Copper Contraceptive 1880
▲ Paraplatin for Injection (8% to 91%) 705
Parnate Tablets 2503
Paxil Tablets (Infrequent) 2505
Pentam 300 Injection (1.2%) 1041
Permax Tablets (1.1%) 575
Platinol 708
Platinol-AQ Injection 710
Plendil Extended-Release Tablets (0.5% to 1.5%) 527
Pravachol 765
PREVACID Delayed-Release Capsules (Less than 1%) 2562
Prilosec Delayed-Release Capsules (Rare) 529
Prinivil Tablets 1733
Procardia Capsules (Less than 0.5%) 1971
▲ Prograf (4% to 47%) 1042
▲ Proleukin for Injection (77%) 797
Prostin VR Pediatric Sterile Solution (Less than 1%) 2635
Prozac Pulvules & Liquid, Oral Solution (Infrequent) 919
Purinethol Tablets (Frequent) 1156
Questran Light 769
Questran Powder 770
Relafen Tablets (Less than 1%) 2510
ReoPro Vials (1.2%) 1471
▲ Retrovir Capsules (1.1% to 29%) 1158
▲ Retrovir I.V. Infusion (1.1% to 29%) 1163
▲ Retrovir Syrup (1.1% to 29%) 1158
Ridaura Capsules (3.1%) 2513
Risperdal (Infrequent) 1301
Ritalin 848
Rocephin Injectable Vials, ADD-Vantage, Galaxy Container (Less than 1%) 2142
Rogaine Topical Solution (0.31%) 2637
Rythmol Tablets–150mg, 225mg, 300mg (Less than 1%) 1352
Sandimmune (2% or less) 2286
Sandostatin Injection (Less than 1%) 2292
Serentil 684
Serzone Tablets (Infrequent) 771
Sinemet Tablets (Rare) 943
Spectrobid Tablets 2206
Stelazine 2514
Supprelin Injection (1%) 2056
▲ Taxol (16% to 78%) 714
▲ TheraCys BCG Live (Intravesical) (Up to 20.5%) 897
Thioguanine Tablets, Tabloid Brand 1181
Thioplex (Thiotepa For Injection) 1281
Ticar for Injection 2526
Tobramycin Sulfate Injection 968
Tonocard Tablets (Less than 1%) 531
Toradol (1% or less) 2159
Vaseretic Tablets 1765
Vasotec I.V. 1768
Vasotec Tablets 1771
Velban Vials 1484
▲ VePesid Capsules and Injection (Up to 33%) 718
Videx Tablets, Powder for Oral Solution, & Pediatric Powder for Oral Solution 720
Virazole 1264
▲ Vumon (88%) 727
Wellbutrin Tablets (Rare) 1204
Zerit Capsules (Up to 3%) 729
Zestoretic 2850

(▭ Described in PDR For Nonprescription Drugs) Incidence data in parenthesis; ▲ 3% or more (⊙ Described in PDR For Ophthalmology)

Anemia Side Effects Index 1220

Zoladex (Greater than 1% but less than 5%) ... 2858
Zoloft Tablets (Rare) ... 2217
Zovirax Sterile Powder (Less than 1%) ... 1223
Zyloprim Tablets (Less than 1%) ... 1226

Anemia, aplastic (see under Aplastic anemia)

Anemia, dilutional
Prolastin Alpha$_1$-Proteinase Inhibitor (Human) ... 635

Anemia, glucose-6-phosphate dehydrogenase deficiency
Macrobid Capsules ... 1988
Macrodantin Capsules ... 1989

Anemia, Heinz-body
Azulfidine (One in every 30 patients or less) ... 1949

Anemia, hemolytic, immune
Fludara for Injection ... 663
Tagamet (Extremely rare) ... 2516
Zantac (Exceedingly rare) ... 1209
Zantac Injection (Exceedingly rare) 1207
Zantac Syrup (Exceedingly rare) ... 1209

Anemia, hemolytic, sideroblastic
Rifamate Capsules ... 1530

Anemia, hypochromic
▲ CellCept Capsules (7.4% to 11.5%) ... 2099
Cytovene (1% or less) ... 2103
Felbatol ... 2666
Foscavir Injection (Less than 1%) .. 547
Imdur (Less than or equal to 5%) .. 1323
Lovenox Injection (2%) ... 2020
▲ Prograf (Greater than 3%) ... 1042
Risperdal (Infrequent) ... 1301

Anemia, hypoplastic (see under Hypoplastic anemia)

Anemia, iron deficiency
Ansaid Tablets (Less than 1%) ... 2579
Empirin with Codeine Tablets (Infrequent) ... 1093
Fiorinal with Codeine Capsules ... 2262
Lamictal Tablets (Rare) ... 1112
Prozac Pulvules & Liquid, Oral Solution (Rare) ... 919

Anemia, microangiopathic hemolytic
Mutamycin ... 703
Sandimmune (Occasional) ... 2286

Anemia, microcytic
Paxil Tablets (Rare) ... 2505

Anemia, nonhemolytic
Sinemet CR Tablets ... 944

Anemia, normochromic
▲ Fungizone Intravenous (Among most common) ... 506

Anemia, normocytic
▲ Fungizone Intravenous (Among most common) ... 506
Paxil Tablets (Rare) ... 2505
Risperdal (Rare) ... 1301

Anemia, sideroblastic
Cuprimine Capsules ... 1630
Depen Titratable Tablets ... 2662
Nydrazid Injection ... 508
Pyrazinamide Tablets (Rare) ... 1398
Rifater (Rare) ... 1532

Anencephaly
Serophene (clomiphene citrate tablets, USP) ... 2451

Anesthesia, local
Zoloft Tablets (Rare) ... 2217

Anesthesia, persistent
Marcaine Hydrochloride with Epinephrine 1:200,000 ... 2316
Marcaine Hydrochloride Injection ... 2316

Anesthetic effect
Lithium Carbonate Capsules & Tablets ... 2230
Sensorcaine ... 559
Tonocard Tablets (Less than 1%) .. 531
Versed Injection ... 2170

Anetoderma
Cuprimine Capsules (Rare) ... 1630
Depen Titratable Tablets (Rare) ... 2662

Aneurysm
Anafranil Capsules (Rare) ... 803
Cognex Capsules (Infrequent) ... 1901
Fludara for Injection (Up to 1%) ... 663
Videx Tablets, Powder for Oral Solution, & Pediatric Powder for Oral Solution (Less than 1%) ... 720

Anger
BuSpar (2%) ... 737
Desyrel and Desyrel Dividose (1.3% to 3.5%) ... 503
Valium Injectable ... 2182
Valrelease Capsules (Infrequent) ... 2169

Angiectases, cutaneous
Adalat CC (Less than 1.0%) ... 589

Angiitis
Esidrix Tablets ... 821
Esimil Tablets ... 822
Indocin Capsules (Less than 1%) ... 1680
Indocin I.V. (Less than 1%) ... 1684
Indocin (Less than 1%) ... 1680
Timolide Tablets ... 1748

Angina
Adalat Capsules (10 mg and 20 mg) (1 in 8 patients) ... 587
Ana-Kit Anaphylaxis Emergency Treatment Kit ... 617
Apresazide Capsules ... 808
Arfonad Ampuls ... 2080
Atromid-S Capsules ... 2701
▲ Cardene Capsules (5.6%) ... 2095
Cardizem CD Capsules (Less than 1%) ... 1506
Cardizem SR Capsules (Less than 1%) ... 1510
Cardizem Tablets (Less than 1%) .. 1512
Clozaril Tablets (1%) ... 2252
Colestid Tablets (Infrequent) ... 2591
Dobutrex Solution Vials (1% to 3%) ... 1439
Ergamisol Tablets ... 1292
Esimil Tablets ... 822
▲ Fludara for Injection (Up to 6%) ... 663
Fluorouracil Injection ... 2116
Sterile FUDR (Remote possibility) .. 2118
Hyperstat I.V. Injection ... 2363
Imitrex Tablets (Rare) ... 1106
Ismelin Tablets ... 827
Isuprel Hydrochloride Injection 1:5000 ... 2311
Isuprel Hydrochloride Solution 1:200 & 1:100 ... 2313
Isuprel Mistometer ... 2312
Lupron Depot 3.75 mg ... 2556
Lupron Depot 7.5 mg (Less than 5%) ... 2559
Lupron Injection (Less than 5%) ... 2555
Mexitil Capsules (1.7% or about 3 in 1,000) ... 678
Monopril Tablets (0.2% to 1.0%) .. 757
Norisodrine with Calcium Iodide Syrup ... 442
Normodyne Tablets ... 2379
Norvasc Tablets ... 1940
OptiPranolol (Metipranolol 0.3%) Sterile Ophthalmic Solution (A small number of patients) ... ⊙ 258
Ornade Spansule Capsules ... 2502
Orthoclone OKT3 Sterile Solution .. 1837
Pravachol (0.1% to 4.0%) ... 765
PREVACID Delayed-Release Capsules (Less than 1%) ... 2562
Prilosec Delayed-Release Capsules (Less than 1%) ... 529
Primacor Injection (1.2%) ... 2331
Proleukin for Injection ... 797
Proventil Inhalation Aerosol ... 2382
Proventil Repetabs Tablets ... 2386
Proventil Syrup ... 2385
Proventil Tablets ... 2386
Relafen Tablets (Less than 1%) ... 2510
Rifater ... 1532
Ritalin ... 848
Rogaine Topical Solution ... 2637
▲ Rythmol Tablets–150mg, 225mg, 300mg (1.2 to 4.6%) ... 1352
Ser-Ap-Es Tablets ... 849
Sus-Phrine Injection ... 1019
Tonocard Tablets (Less than 1%) .. 531
Trandate ... 1185
Trental Tablets (0.3%) ... 1244
Trinalin Repetabs Tablets ... 1330
Triostat Injection (Approximately 1%) ... 2530
Univasc Tablets (Less than 1%) ... 2410
Ventolin Inhalation Aerosol and Refill ... 1197
Ventolin Rotacaps for Inhalation ... 1200
Ventolin Syrup ... 1202
Ventolin Tablets ... 1203
Volmax Extended-Release Tablets .. 1788
Zofran Injection (Rare) ... 1214
Zofran Tablets (Rare) ... 1217

Angina, crescendo
Deponit NTG Transdermal Delivery System (Uncommon) ... 2397
Isordil Sublingual Tablets (Uncommon) ... 2739
Isordil Tembids (Uncommon) ... 2741
Isordil Titradose Tablets (Uncommon) ... 2742
Nitro-Bid IV (Uncommon) ... 1523
Nitro-Bid Ointment (Uncommon) ... 1524
Nitrodisc (Uncommon) ... 2047
Nitro-Dur (nitroglycerin) Transdermal Infusion System (Uncommon) ... 1326
Sorbitrate (Uncommon) ... 2843
Transderm-Nitro Transdermal Therapeutic System (Uncommon) ... 859

Angina, increased
Deponit NTG Transdermal Delivery System (2%) ... 2397
Isordil Sublingual Tablets ... 2739
Isordil Tembids ... 2741
Isordil Titradose Tablets ... 2742
Lotrel Capsules (Rare) ... 840
Nitro-Bid IV ... 1523
Nitrodisc (2%) ... 2047
Procardia Capsules (Rare) ... 1971
Procardia XL Extended Release Tablets (1% or less) ... 1972
Transderm-Nitro Transdermal Therapeutic System (2%) ... 859
▲ Vascor (200, 300 and 400 mg) Tablets (4.5%) ... 1587

Angina, Prinzmetal's, episodes of
Imitrex Injection ... 1103
Respbid Tablets ... 682

Angina pectoris
Accupril Tablets (Rare) ... 1893
Altace Capsules (Less than 1% to 2.9%) ... 1232
Ansaid Tablets (Less than 1%) ... 2579
Apresazide Capsules (Common) ... 808
Apresoline Hydrochloride Tablets (Common) ... 809
Betaseron for SC Injection ... 658
Brethaire Inhaler ... 813
Calan SR Caplets (1% or less) ... 2422
Calan Tablets (1% or less) ... 2419
Capoten (2 to 3 of 1000 patients) 739
Capozide (2 to 3 of 1000 patients) ... 742
Cardene I.V. (Rare) ... 2709
Cardura Tablets (Less than 0.5% of 3960 patients to 0.6%) ... 2186
Cartrol Tablets (Less common) ... 410
▲ CellCept Capsules (More than or equal to 3%) ... 2099
Cipro I.V. (1% or less) ... 595
Cipro I.V. Pharmacy Bulk Package (Less than 1%) ... 597
Cipro Tablets (Less than 1%) ... 592
Cognex Capsules (Infrequent) ... 1901
Cozaar Tablets (Less than 1%) ... 1628
Demulen ... 2428
Dilacor XR Extended-release Capsules ... 2018
Diupres Tablets ... 1650
Dobutrex Solution Vials (1% to 3%) ... 1439
Effexor (Infrequent) ... 2719
Eldepryl Tablets ... 2550
Esimil Tablets ... 822
Hydropres Tablets ... 1675
Hyzaar Tablets ... 1677
Imitrex Injection ... 1103
Imitrex Tablets ... 1106
Ismelin Tablets ... 827
Isoptin Oral Tablets (Less than 1%) ... 1346
Isoptin SR Tablets (1% or less) ... 1348
Kerlone Tablets (Less than 2%) ... 2436
Kytril Tablets (Rare) ... 2492
Lamictal Tablets (Rare) ... 1112
Levlen/Tri-Levlen (Very infrequent) 651
Lotensin Tablets ... 834
Luvox Tablets (Infrequent) ... 2544
Maxaquin Tablets (Less than 1%) .. 2440
Miacalcin Nasal Spray (1% to 3%) 2275
Micronor Tablets ... 1872
Midamor Tablets (Less than or equal to 1%) ... 1703
Modicon ... 1872
Moduretic Tablets (Less than or equal to 1%) ... 1705
Monopril Tablets (1.0% or more) .. 757
Neurontin Capsules (Infrequent) ... 1922
Ortho-Cyclen/Ortho-Tri-Cyclen ... 1858
Ortho-Novum ... 1872
Ortho-Cyclen/Ortho Tri-Cyclen ... 1858
Paxil Tablets (Rare) ... 2505
Permax Tablets (Infrequent) ... 575
Persantine Tablets (Rare) ... 681
Plendil Extended-Release Tablets (0.5% to 1.5%) ... 527
▲ Prinivil Tablets (1.5% to 3.7%) ... 1733
Prinzide Tablets ... 1737
Prozac Pulvules & Liquid, Oral Solution (Infrequent) ... 919
Risperdal (Rare) ... 1301
Ser-Ap-Es Tablets ... 849
Serzone Tablets (Infrequent) ... 771
Tambocor Tablets (Less than 1%) 1497
Timolide Tablets ... 1748
Levlen/Tri-Levlen (Very infrequent) 651
Vaseretic Tablets ... 1765
Vasotec I.V. ... 1768
Vasotec Tablets (1.5%) ... 1771
Verelan Capsules (1% or less) ... 1410
Verelan Capsules (Less than 1%) .. 2824
Videx Tablets, Powder for Oral Solution, & Pediatric Powder for Oral Solution (Less than 1%) ... 720
Zestoretic ... 2850
Zestril Tablets (1.5% to 3.7%) ... 2854

Angina pectoris, aggravation
Aldoclor Tablets ... 1598
Aldomet Ester HCl Injection ... 1602
Aldomet Oral ... 1600
Aldoril Tablets ... 1604
Blocadren Tablets (Less than 1%) 1614
Eldepryl Tablets ... 2550
Feldene Capsules (Less than 1%) . 1965
Imdur (Less than or equal to 5%) .. 1323
Ismo Tablets (Fewer than 1%) ... 2738
Isordil Sublingual Tablets ... 2739
Isordil Tembids ... 2741
Isordil Titradose Tablets ... 2742
Loniten Tablets ... 2618
Nitro-Bid IV ... 1523
Sorbitrate ... 2843
Timoptic in Ocudose (Less frequent) ... 1753
Timoptic Sterile Ophthalmic Solution (Less frequent) ... 1751
Timoptic-XE ... 1755

Angina pectoris, exacerbation of, post-abrupt discontinuation
Cartrol Tablets ... 410
Inderal ... 2728
Inderal LA Long Acting Capsules ... 2730
Normodyne Injection ... 2377
Normodyne Tablets ... 2379
Tenoretic Tablets ... 2845
Tenormin Tablets and I.V. Injection 2847
Toprol-XL Tablets ... 565
Trandate ... 1185
Visken Tablets ... 2299

Angioedema (see also under Edema, angioneurotic)
Children's Advil Suspension (Less than 1%) ... 2692
Bactrim DS Tablets ... 2084
Bactrim I.V. Infusion ... 2082
Bactrim ... 2084
Beclovent Inhalation Aerosol and Refill ... 1075
Beconase (Rare) ... 1076
Butisol Sodium Elixir & Tablets ... 2660
Capoten (Approximately 1 in 1000 patients) ... 739
Capozide (Approximately 1 in 1000 patients) ... 742
Cataflam (Less than 1%) ... 816
Catapres Tablets ... 674
Ceptaz (Very rare) ... 1081
Chloromycetin Sodium Succinate ... 1900
Cipro I.V. (1% or less) ... 595
Cipro Tablets (Less than 1%) ... 592
Didronel Tablets ... 1984
Easprin ... 1914

(▭ Described in PDR For Nonprescription Drugs) Incidence data in parenthesis; ▲ 3% or more (⊙ Described in PDR For Ophthalmology)

1221 **Side Effects Index** **Anorexia**

Eskalith 2485
Feldene Capsules (Less than 1%) 1965
Fortaz (Very rare) 1100
Gammar, Immune Globulin (Human) U.S.P. 515
Hep-B-Gammagee 1663
Indocin (Less than 1%) 1680
Intal Capsules (Less than 1 in 10,000 patients) 987
Intal Inhaler (Infrequent) 988
Keflex Pulvules & Oral Suspension 914
Keftab Tablets 915
Lotrel Capsules (About 0.5%) 840
Macrobid Capsules 1988
Macrodantin Capsules 1989
Mebaral Tablets 2322
Mintezol 1704
Children's Motrin Ibuprofen Oral Suspension (Less than 1%) 1546
Motrin Tablets 2625
Nalfon 200 Pulvules & Nalfon Tablets 917
Nasalcrom Nasal Solution 994
NegGram 2323
Nembutal Sodium Capsules 436
Nembutal Sodium Solution 438
Nembutal Sodium Suppositories (Less than 1%) 440
Noroxin Tablets 1715
Noroxin Tablets 2048
Phenobarbital Elixir and Tablets (Less than 1 in 100 patients) 1469
Prinivil Tablets (0.1%) 1733
Proventil Inhalation Aerosol (Rare) 2382
Quinaglute Dura-Tabs Tablets 649
Quinidex Extentabs 2067
Recombivax HB (Less than 1%) 1744
Reglan (Rare) 2068
Ridaura Capsules 2513
Robaxisal Tablets 2071
Seconal Sodium Pulvules (Less than 1 in 100) 1474
Septra 1174
Septra I.V. Infusion 1169
Septra I.V. Infusion ADD-Vantage Vials 1171
Septra 1174
Soma Compound w/Codeine Tablets 2676
Soma Compound Tablets (Less common) 2675
Trental Tablets (Less than 1%) 1244
Vancenase PocketHaler Nasal Inhaler (Rare) 2391
Vanceril Inhaler 2394
Vaseretic Tablets (0.6%) 1765
Vasotec I.V. (0.5 to 1%) 1768
Vasotec Tablets 1771
Ventolin Inhalation Aerosol and Refill (Rare) 1197
Ventolin Inhalation Solution 1198
Ventolin Syrup 1202
Ventolin Tablets 1203
Voltaren Tablets (Less than 1%) 861
Zestril Tablets (0.1%) 2854
Zithromax (1% or less; rare) 1944

Angioedema, extremities

Accupril Tablets (0.1%) 1893
Altace Capsules 1232
Capoten (Approximately 1 in 1000 patients) 739
Capozide (Approximately 1 in 1000 patients) 742
Lotensin Tablets 834
Lotensin HCT (About 0.5%) 837
Lotrel Capsules 840
Monopril Tablets 757
Prinivil Tablets 1733
Prinzide Tablets (Rare) 1737
Univasc Tablets 2410
Vaseretic Tablets 1765
Vasotec I.V. 1768
Vasotec Tablets 1771
Zestoretic (Rare) 2850
Zestril Tablets 2854

Angioedema, eyes

Accupril Tablets 1893
Capoten 739
Capozide 742
Lotensin HCT 837
Zestoretic 2850
Zestril Tablets 2854

Angioedema, face

Accupril Tablets (0.1%) 1893
Altace Capsules 1232
Atrovent Inhalation Aerosol 671
Capoten (Approximately 1 in 1000 patients) 739
Capozide (Approximately 1 in 1000 patients) 742
Catapres-TTS (2 of 3,539 patients) 675
Hyzaar Tablets 1677
Lotensin Tablets (0.5%) 834
Lotensin HCT (0.3% to about 0.5%) 837
Lotrel Capsules (About 0.5%) 840
Monopril Tablets 757
Prinivil Tablets 1733
Prinzide Tablets (Rare) 1737
Univasc Tablets (Less than 0.5%) 2410
Vaseretic Tablets 1765
Vasotec I.V. 1768
Vasotec Tablets 1771
Zestoretic (Rare) 2850
Zestril Tablets 2854

Angioedema, glottis

Accupril Tablets (0.1%) 1893
Altace Capsules 1232
Capoten (Approximately 1 in 1000 patients) 739
Capozide (Approximately 1 in 1000 patients) 742
Lotensin Tablets 834
Lotensin HCT (About 0.5%) 837
Lotrel Capsules (About 0.5%) 840
Monopril Tablets 757
Prinivil Tablets 1733
Prinzide Tablets (Rare) 1737
Univasc Tablets 2410
Vaseretic Tablets 1765
Vasotec I.V. 1768
Vasotec Tablets 1771
Zestoretic (Rare) 2850
Zestril Tablets 2854

Angioedema, larynx

Accupril Tablets (0.1%) 1893
Altace Capsules 1232
Capoten (Approximately 1 in 1000 patients) 739
Capozide (Approximately 1 in 1000 patients) 742
Floxin Tablets (200 mg, 300 mg, 400 mg) 1567
Lotensin Tablets 834
Lotensin HCT (About 0.5%) 837
Monopril Tablets 757
Prinivil Tablets 1733
Prinzide Tablets (Rare) 1737
Univasc Tablets 2410
Vaseretic Tablets 1765
Vasotec I.V. 1768
Vasotec Tablets 1771
Zestoretic (Rare) 2850
Zestril Tablets 2854

Angioedema, lips

Accupril Tablets (0.1%) 1893
Altace Capsules 1232
Atrovent Inhalation Aerosol 671
Capoten (Approximately 1 in 1000 patients) 739
Capozide (Approximately 1 in 1000 patients) 742
Hyzaar Tablets (1% or greater) 1677
Lotensin Tablets (0.5%) 834
Lotensin HCT (0.3% to about 0.5%) 837
Lotrel Capsules 840
Monopril Tablets 757
Prinivil Tablets 1733
Prinzide Tablets (Rare) 1737
Univasc Tablets 2410
Vaseretic Tablets 1765
Vasotec I.V. 1768
Vasotec Tablets 1771
Zestoretic (Rare) 2850
Zestril Tablets 2854

Angioedema, mucous membranes of the mouth

Capozide (Approximately 1 in 1000 patients) 742

Angioedema, oropharyngeal

Adalat Capsules (10 mg and 20 mg) (Less than 0.5%) 587

Angioedema of tongue

Accupril Tablets (0.1%) 1893
Altace Capsules 1232
Atrovent Inhalation Aerosol 671
Capoten (Approximately 1 in 1000 patients) 739
Capozide (Approximately 1 in 1000 patients) 742
Catapres-TTS (One case) 675
Floxin I.V. 1571
Floxin Tablets (200 mg, 300 mg, 400 mg) 1567
Lotensin Tablets 834
Lotensin HCT (About 0.5%) 837
Lotrel Capsules (About 0.5%) 840
Monopril Tablets 757
Prinivil Tablets 1733
Prinzide Tablets (Rare) 1737
Univasc Tablets 2410
Vaseretic Tablets 1765
Vasotec I.V. 1768
Vasotec Tablets 1771
Zestoretic (Rare) 2850
Zestril Tablets 2854

Angioma, spider

Betaseron for SC Injection 658

Anhidrosis

Cogentin 1621
Kutrase Capsules 2402

Anisocoria

Anafranil Capsules (Up to 2%) 803
Betoptic Ophthalmic Solution (Rare) 469
Betoptic S Ophthalmic Suspension 471

Ankylosing spondylosis

Lupron Depot 7.5 mg 2559
Lupron Injection 2555

Anorexia

Achromycin V Capsules (Rare) 1367
▲ ActHIB (2.2% to 26.1%) 872
Actifed with Codeine Cough Syrup 1067
▲ Actimmune (3%) 1056
Adriamycin PFS (Occasional) 1947
Adriamycin RDF (Occasional) 1947
Aldactazide 2413
Aldoclor Tablets 1598
Aldoril Tablets 1604
Altace Capsules (Less than 1%) 1232
Ambien Tablets (1%) 2416
▲ Anafranil Capsules (12% to 22%) 803
Ancef Injection 2465
Ancobon Capsules 2079
Apresazide Capsules (Common) 808
Apresoline Hydrochloride Tablets (Common) 809
Aquasol A Vitamin A Capsules, USP 534
Aquasol A Parenteral 534
Aralen Hydrochloride Injection 2301
Aralen Phosphate Tablets 2301
▲ Aredia for Injection (1% to at least 15%) 810
Arfonad Ampuls 2080
Asacol Delayed-Release Tablets 1979
Asendin Tablets (Very rare) 1369
Atamet (Less frequent) 572
Atretol Tablets 573
Atrohist Plus Tablets 454
Axid Pulvules (1.2%) 1427
Azo Gantanol Tablets 2080
Azo Gantrisin Tablets 2081
▲ Azulfidine (Approximately one-third of patients) 1949
BCG Vaccine, USP (TICE) (2.2%) 1814
▲ Bactrim DS Tablets (Among most common) 2084
▲ Bactrim I.V. Infusion (Among most common) 2082
▲ Bactrim (Among most common) 2084
Benadryl Capsules 1898
Benadryl Injection 1898
Benemid Tablets 1611
Bentyl 1501
Blenoxane (Common) 692
Brevibloc Injection (Less than 1%) 1808
▲ Bromfed-DM Cough Syrup (Among most frequent) 1786
Bronkaid Caplets ◘ 717
Buprenex Injectable (Rare) 2006
BuSpar (Infrequent) 737
Capoten (About 0.5 to 2%) 739
Capozide (0.5 to 2%) 742
Cardizem CD Capsules (Less than 1%) 1506
Cardizem SR Capsules (Less than 1%) 1510
Cardizem Injectable 1508
Cardizem Tablets (Less than 1%) 1512
Cardura Tablets (Less than 0.5% of 3960 patients) 2186
Catapres Tablets (About 1 in 100 patients) 674
Catapres-TTS (Less frequent) 675
Ceftin (Less than 1% but more than 0.1%) 1078
▲ CellCept Capsules (More than or equal to 3%) 2099
Celontin Kapseals (Frequent) 1899
Cipro I.V. (1% or less) 595
Cipro I.V. Pharmacy Bulk Package (Less than 1%) 597
Cipro Tablets (Less than 1%) 592
Claritin (2% or fewer patients) 2349
Claritin-D (2%) 2350
Clinoril Tablets (Greater than 1%) 1618
Clozaril Tablets (1%) 2252
▲ Cognex Capsules (9%) 1901
ColBENEMID Tablets 1622
Colestid Tablets (Infrequent) 2591
Combipres Tablets (About 1%) 677
Comhist 2038
▲ Cordarone Tablets (4 to 9%) 2712
Cosmegen Injection 1626
Cozaar Tablets (Less than 1%) 1628
Crystodigin Tablets 1433
Cuprimine Capsules 1630
Cylert Tablets 412
▲ Cytadren Tablets (1 in 8) 819
▲ Cytosar-U Sterile Powder (Among most frequent) 2592
▲ Cytovene (15%) 2103
Cytoxan 694
▲ DTIC-Dome (90% with the initial few doses) 600
Dalmane Capsules (Rare) 2173
Dantrium Capsules (Less frequent) 1982
▲ Daranide Tablets (Among the most common effects) 1633
Daraprim Tablets 1090
Daypro Caplets (Greater than 1% but less than 3%) 2426
Declomycin Tablets 1371
Deconamine 1320
Demulen 2428
Depakene 413
Depakote Tablets 415
▲ Depen Titratable Tablets (17%) 2662
Dexedrine 2474
DextroStat Dextroamphetamine Tablets 2036
Diabinese Tablets (Less than 2%) 1935
Diamox Intravenous 1372
Diamox Sequels (Sustained Release) 1373
Diamox Tablets 1372
Dilacor XR Extended-release Capsules (Infrequent) 2018
Dilaudid-HP Injection (Less frequent) 1337
Dilaudid-HP Lyophilized Powder 250 mg (Less frequent) 1337
Dilaudid Tablets and Liquid 1339
Dimetane-DC Cough Syrup 2059
Dimetane-DX Cough Syrup 2059
Dipentum Capsules (1.3%) 1951
Diphtheria and Tetanus Toxoids and Pertussis Vaccine Adsorbed 2477
Diphtheria and Tetanus Toxoids and Pertussis Vaccine Adsorbed USP (For Pediatric Use) (Frequent; 1 in 5 doses) 875
Diucardin Tablets 2718
Diupres Tablets 1650
Diuril Oral Suspension 1653
Diuril Sodium Intravenous 1652
Diuril Tablets 1653
Dolobid Tablets (Less than 1 in 100) 1654
Doral Tablets 2664
Doryx Capsules 1913
Doxorubicin Astra (Occasional) 540
▲ Duragesic Transdermal System (3% to 10%) 1288
Dynacin Capsules 1590
▲ E.E.S. (Among most frequent) 424
Edecrin 1657
▲ Effexor (11% to 17.0%) 2719
Elavil 2838
Eldepryl Tablets 2550
Elspar 1659
▲ Emcyt Capsules (4%) 1953
Emete-con Intramuscular/Intravenous 2198
Endep Tablets 2174
Enduron Tablets 420
Engerix-B Unit-Dose Vials (Less than 1%) 2482
▲ Ergamisol Tablets (2% to 6%) 1292
▲ ERYC (Among most frequent) 1915
▲ EryPed (Among most frequent) 421
▲ Ery-Tab Tablets (Among most frequent) 422
▲ Erythrocin Stearate Filmtab (Among most frequent) 425
▲ Erythromycin Base Filmtab (Among most frequent) 426

(◘ Described in PDR For Nonprescription Drugs) Incidence data in parenthesis; ▲ 3% or more (◉ Described in PDR For Ophthalmology)

▲ Erythromycin Delayed-Release Capsules, USP (Among most frequent) ... 427
Esidrix Tablets ... 821
Esimil Tablets ... 822
Eskalith ... 2485
Ethmozine Tablets (Less than 2%) 2041
Etrafon ... 2355
▲ Eulexin Capsules (4%) ... 2358
Famvir (2.6%) ... 2486
Fedahist Gyrocaps ... 2401
Fedahist Timecaps ... 2401
▲ Felbatol (Among most common; 19.3% to 54.8%) ... 2666
Feldene Capsules (Greater than 1%) ... 1965
Fioricet with Codeine Capsules ... 2260
Fiorinal with Codeine Capsules ... 2262
Flagyl 375 Capsules (Sometimes) .. 2434
Flexeril Tablets (Less than 1%) ... 1661
▲ Fludara for Injection (7% to 34%) 663
Flumadine Tablets & Syrup (1.6%) 1015
Fluorouracil Injection (Common)... 2116
▲ Foscavir Injection (5% or greater).. 547
Sterile FUDR ... 2118
▲ Fungizone Intravenous (Among most common) ... 506
Gantanol Tablets ... 2119
Gantrisin ... 2120
Geocillin Tablets ... 2199
Glauctabs ... ⊙ 208
▲ Glucophage (Among most common) ... 752
Glucotrol XL Extended Release Tablets (Less than 1%) ... 1968
Halcion Tablets ... 2611
Haldol Decanoate ... 1577
Haldol Injection, Tablets and Concentrate ... 1575
▲ Havrix (1% to 10%) ... 2489
Hexalen Capsules (1%) ... 2571
HibTITER ... 1375
▲ Hivid Tablets (Less than 1% to less than 3%) ... 2121
Hydrea Capsules (Less frequent) ... 696
HydroDIURIL Tablets ... 1674
Hydropres Tablets ... 1675
▲ Hylorel Tablets (18.7%) ... 985
Hyperstat I.V. Injection ... 2363
Hyzaar Tablets ... 1677
IFEX (Less than 1%) ... 697
Inderide Tablets ... 2732
Inderide LA Long Acting Capsules .. 2734
Indocin (Less than 1%) ... 1680
Inocor Lactate Injection (0.4%) ... 2309
▲ Intron A (1% to 53%) ... 2364
Inversine Tablets ... 1686
Kayexalate ... 2314
Kefzol Vials, Faspak & ADD-Vantage ... 1456
Kerlone Tablets (Less than 2%) ... 2436
Klonopin Tablets ... 2126
Lamictal Tablets (1.8%) ... 1112
Lamprene Capsules (Less than 1%) ... 828
Lanoxicaps (Common) ... 1117
Lanoxin Elixir Pediatric ... 1120
Lanoxin Injection (Common) ... 1123
Lanoxin Injection Pediatric ... 1126
Lanoxin Tablets (Common) ... 1128
▲ Lariam Tablets (Among most frequent) ... 2128
Larodopa Tablets (Relatively frequent) ... 2129
Lasix Injection, Oral Solution and Tablets ... 1240
Lescol Capsules ... 2267
▲ Leucovorin Calcium for Injection (1% to 22%) ... 1268
▲ Leukine for IV Infusion (54%) ... 1271
Levlen/Tri-Levlen ... 651
Limbitrol ... 2180
Lioresal Tablets (Rare) ... 829
Lithium Carbonate Capsules & Tablets ... 2230
Lithonate/Lithotabs/Lithobid ... 2543
Lodine Capsules and Tablets (Less than 1%) ... 2743
Lomotil ... 2439
Lopressor HCT Tablets (1 in 100 patients) ... 832
Lorabid Suspension and Pulvules (0.3% to 2.3%) ... 1459
Lorelco Tablets ... 1517
Lotensin HCT ... 837
Lozol Tablets (Less than 5%) ... 2022
Lupron Depot 7.5 mg (Less than 5%) ... 2559
▲ Lupron Injection (5% or more) ... 2555
▲ Luvox Tablets (6%) ... 2544
Lysodren ... 698
MS Contin Tablets (Less frequent) 1994
MSIR (Infrequent) ... 1997
▲ MZM (Among reactions occurring most often) ... ⊙ 267
▲ Macrodantin Capsules (Among most often) ... 1989
Marinol (Dronabinol) Capsules (Less than 1%) ... 2231
Maxair Autohaler ... 1492
Maxair Inhaler (Less than 1%) ... 1494
Maxaquin Tablets (Less than 1%).. 2440
Maxzide ... 1380
Mellaril ... 2269
▲ Mepron Suspension (7%) ... 1135
Methadone Hydrochloride Oral Concentrate ... 2233
Methadone Hydrochloride Oral Solution & Tablets ... 2235
Methotrexate Sodium Tablets, Injection, for Injection and LPF Injection (Less common) ... 1275
MetroGel-Vaginal ... 902
Mevacor Tablets (Rare) ... 1699
Miacalcin Nasal Spray (Less than 1%) ... 2275
Micronor Tablets ... 1872
▲ Midamor Tablets (3% to 8%) ... 1703
Milontin Kapseals (Frequent) ... 1920
Minizide Capsules ... 1938
Minocin Intravenous ... 1382
Minocin Oral Suspension ... 1385
Minocin Pellet-Filled Capsules ... 1383
Mintezol ... 1704
Mithracin ... 607
Modicon ... 1872
▲ Moduretic Tablets (3% to 8%) ... 1705
Monodox Capsules ... 1805
Monoket (Fewer than 1%) ... 2406
Motofen Tablets ... 784
Children's Motrin Ibuprofen Oral Suspension ... 1546
MSTA Mumps Skin Test Antigen ... 890
Mustargen ... 1709
▲ Mutamycin (14%) ... 703
Myambutol Tablets ... 1386
Mycobutin Capsules (2%) ... 1957
Mykrox Tablets ... 993
Myleran Tablets ... 1143
Myochrysine Injection ... 1711
Mysoline (Occasional) ... 2754
Nalfon 200 Pulvules & Nalfon Tablets (Less than 1%) ... 917
Navane Capsules and Concentrate 2201
Navane Intramuscular ... 2202
▲ Navelbine Injection (Less than 20%) ... 1145
Neoral (2% or less) ... 2276
NEOSAR Lyophilized/Neosar ... 1959
Neptazane Tablets ... 1388
▲ Neupogen for Injection (9%) ... 495
Neurontin Capsules (Frequent) ... 1922
Nicorette ... 2458
Nizoral Tablets ... 1298
Nolvadex Tablets (1%) ... 2841
Normodyne Injection ... 2377
Normodyne Tablets ... 2379
Noroxin Tablets (Less frequent or 0.3% to 1.0%) ... 1715
Noroxin Tablets (Less frequent or 0.3% to 1.0%) ... 2048
Norpace (1 to 3%) ... 2444
Norpramin Tablets ... 1526
Norvasc Tablets (More than 0.1% to 1%) ... 1940
Novahistine DH ... 2462
Novahistine Elixir ... ■ 823
Nydrazid Injection ... 508
▲ OmniHIB (2.2% t0 15.3%) ... 2499
▲ Oncaspar (Greater than 1% but less than 5%) ... 2028
Oncovin Solution Vials & Hyporets 1466
Oramorph SR (Morphine Sulfate Sustained Release Tablets) (Less frequent) ... 2236
Orap Tablets ... 1050
Oretic Tablets ... 443
Ornade Spansule Capsules ... 2502
Ortho-Cyclen/Ortho-Tri-Cyclen ... 1858
Ortho-Novum ... 1872
Ortho-Cyclen/Ortho Tri-Cyclen ... 1858
Orthoclone OKT3 Sterile Solution .. 1837
Orudis Capsules (Greater than 1%) ... 2766
Oruvail Capsules (Greater than 1%) ... 2766
PBZ Tablets ... 845
PBZ-SR Tablets ... 844
▲ PCE Dispertab Tablets (Among most frequent) ... 444
Pamelor ... 2280
Papaverine Hydrochloride Vials and Ampoules ... 1468
Paraflex Caplets ... 1580
Parafon Forte DSC Caplets ... 1581
▲ Parlodel (4%) ... 2281
Parnate Tablets ... 2503
PASER Granules (Less frequent) ... 1285
▲ Pentam 300 Injection (5.9%) ... 1041
Pentasa (Less than 1% to 1.1%) .. 1527
Pepcid Injection (Infrequent) ... 1722
Pepcid (Infrequent) ... 1720
Periactin ... 1724
▲ Permax Tablets (4.8%) ... 575
▲ Phenurone Tablets (5%) ... 447
PhosLo Tablets ... 690
Placidyl Capsules ... 448
Plaquenil Sulfate Tablets ... 2328
Platinol ... 708
Platinol-AQ Injection ... 710
Ponstel (Less frequent) ... 1925
Potaba (Infrequent) ... 1229
Pravachol (Rare) ... 765
PREVACID Delayed-Release Capsules (Less than 1%) ... 2562
Prilosec Delayed-Release Capsules (Less than 1%) ... 529
Prinivil Tablets (0.7 to 1.5%) ... 1733
Prinzide Tablets ... 1737
▲ Procan SR Tablets (3-4%) ... 1926
Proglycem (Frequent) ... 580
▲ Prograf (6% to 34%) ... 1042
▲ Proleukin for Injection (27%) ... 797
Protostat Tablets ... 1883
Proventil Syrup (Children 2 to 6 years, 1%) ... 2385
▲ Prozac Pulvules & Liquid, Oral Solution (8.7% to 17%) ... 919
Purinethol Tablets (Uncommon) ... 1156
Pyrazinamide Tablets ... 1398
Quadrinal Tablets ... 1350
Questran Light (Less frequent) ... 769
Questran Powder (Less frequent) ... 770
▲ Quinidex Extentabs (Among most frequent) ... 2067
RMS Suppositories ... 2657
Relafen Tablets (1%) ... 2510
Restoril Capsules (1-2%) ... 2284
▲ Retrovir Capsules (11% to 20.1%) ... 1158
▲ Retrovir I.V. Infusion (11% to 20.1%) ... 1163
▲ Retrovir Syrup (11% to 20.1%) ... 1158
▲ ReVia Tablets (Less than 10%) ... 940
▲ Ridaura Capsules (3 to 9%) ... 2513
Rifadin (Some patients) ... 1528
Rifamate Capsules (Some patients) ... 1530
Rifater ... 1532
Rimactane Capsules ... 847
Risperdal (Frequent) ... 1301
Ritalin ... 848
Rocaltrol Capsules ... 2141
▲ Roferon-A Injection (46% to 65%) 2145
Rondec Oral Drops ... 953
Rondec Syrup ... 953
Rondec Tablet ... 953
Rondec-DM Oral Drops ... 954
Rondec-DM Syrup ... 954
Rondec-TR Tablet ... 953
Roxanol ... 2243
Rubex (Occasional) ... 712
Rythmol Tablets–150mg, 225mg, 300mg (0.5 to 1.7%) ... 1352
Salagen Tablets (Less than 1%) ... 1489
Sandimmune (2% or less) ... 2286
Sectral Capsules ... 2807
▲ Seldane-D Extended-Release Tablets (3.7%) ... 1538
▲ Septra (Among most common) ... 1174
▲ Septra I.V. Infusion (Among the most common) ... 1169
▲ Septra I.V. Infusion ADD-Vantage Vials (Among most common) ... 1171
▲ Septra (Among most common) ... 1174
Ser-Ap-Es Tablets ... 849
Serentil ... 684
Serzone Tablets ... 771
Sinemet Tablets (Less frequent) ... 943
Sinemet CR Tablets (1.2%) ... 944
Sinequan ... 2205
Slo-Niacin Tablets ... 2659
Sodium Polystyrene Sulfonate Suspension ... 2244
Solganal Suspension (Rare) ... 2388
Sporanox Capsules (0.3% to 1.2%) ... 1305
▲ Stadol (3% to 9%) ... 775
Stelazine ... 2514
Stilphostrol Tablets and Ampuls ... 612
Surmontil Capsules ... 2811
Symmetrel Capsules and Syrup (1% to 5%) ... 946
Talacen (Rare) ... 2333
Talwin Compound (Rare) ... 2335
Talwin Nx ... 2336
Tambocor Tablets (1% to less than 3%) ... 1497
Tapazole Tablets ... 1477
Tavist Syrup ... 2297
Tavist Tablets ... 2298
Tegretol Chewable Tablets ... 852
Tegretol Suspension ... 852
Tegretol Tablets ... 852
Temaril Tablets, Syrup and Spansule Extended-Release Capsules ... 483
Tenoretic Tablets ... 2845
Terramycin Intramuscular Solution 2210
Teslac ... 717
Tetramune (Up to 4%) ... 1404
Thalitone ... 1245
▲ TheraCys BCG Live (Intravesical) (Up to 10.7%) ... 897
Thioguanine Tablets, Tabloid Brand (Less frequent) ... 1181
Thioplex (Thiotepa For Injection) ... 1281
Ticlid Tablets (1.0%) ... 2156
Timolide Tablets ... 1748
Timoptic in Ocudose (Less frequent) ... 1753
Timoptic Sterile Ophthalmic Solution (Less frequent) ... 1751
Timoptic-XE ... 1755
Tofranil Ampuls ... 854
Tofranil Tablets ... 856
Tofranil-PM Capsules ... 857
▲ Tonocard Tablets (1.2-11.3%) ... 531
Toradol (1% or less) ... 2159
Torecan ... 2245
Trandate ... 1185
Trental Tablets (Less than 1%) ... 1244
Triavil Tablets ... 1757
Tri-Immunol Adsorbed ... 1408
Trilafon (Occasional) ... 2389
Levlen/Tri-Levlen ... 651
Trilisate (Less than 1%) ... 2000
Trinalin Repetabs Tablets ... 1330
▲ Tripedia (1% to 6%) ... 892
Tussend ... 1783
Ultram Tablets (50 mg) (1% to 5%) ... 1585
Valtrex Caplets (Less than 1% to 3%) ... 1194
▲ Vascor (200, 300 and 400 mg) Tablets (3.02 to 6.82%) ... 1587
Vaseretic Tablets ... 1765
Vasotec I.V. ... 1768
Vasotec Tablets (0.5% to 1.0%) ... 1771
Velban Vials ... 1484
Ventolin Syrup (1% of children) ... 1202
▲ VePesid Capsules and Injection (10% to 13%) ... 718
Vibramycin ... 1941
Vibramycin Hyclate Intravenous ... 2215
Vibramycin ... 1941
▲ Videx Tablets, Powder for Oral Solution, & Pediatric Powder for Oral Solution (1% to 52%) ... 720
Vivactil Tablets ... 1774
▲ Wellbutrin Tablets (18.3%) ... 1204
Xanax Tablets ... 2649
Zarontin Capsules (Frequent) ... 1928
Zarontin Syrup (Frequent) ... 1929
Zaroxolyn Tablets ... 1000
▲ Zerit Capsules (Fewer than 1% to 10%) ... 729
Zestoretic ... 2850
Zestril Tablets (0.7% to 1.5%) ... 2854
Ziac ... 1415
▲ Zinecard (27% to 42%) ... 1961
Zocor Tablets ... 1775
Zoladex (1% to 5%) ... 2858
Zoloft Tablets (2.8%) ... 2217
Zovirax Capsules (0.3%) ... 1219
Zovirax Sterile Powder (Less than 1%) ... 1223
Zovirax (0.3%) ... 1219
Zyloprim Tablets (Less than 1%) ... 1226

Anorgasmia

Anafranil Capsules (Rare) ... 803
Depo-Provera Contraceptive Injection (1% to 5%) ... 2602
Effexor (Frequent) ... 2719
Eldepryl Tablets ... 2550
Luvox Tablets (2%) ... 2544
Nardil (Common) ... 1920
Neurontin Capsules (Infrequent) ... 1922
▲ Paxil Tablets (1.8% to 10.0%) ... 2505
Risperdal (Frequent) ... 1301
Serzone Tablets (Rare) ... 771

(■ Described in PDR For Nonprescription Drugs) Incidence data in parenthesis; ▲ 3% or more (⊙ Described in PDR For Ophthalmology)

1223 Side Effects Index Anxiety

Anosmia
▲ AeroBid Inhaler System (3-9%) 1005
▲ Aerobid-M Inhaler System (3-9%).. 1005
Beconase (Rare) 1076
Cipro I.V. (1% or less) 595
Cipro I.V. Pharmacy Bulk Package (Less than 1%) 597
Cipro Tablets 592
Cytovene-IV (One report) 2103
Decadron Phosphate Turbinaire 1645
Dexacort Phosphate in Turbinaire .. 459
Nasalide Nasal Solution 0.025% 2110
NebuPent for Inhalation Solution (1% or less) 1040
Vaseretic Tablets 1765
Vasotec I.V. 1768
Vasotec Tablets (0.5% to 1.0%) 1771

Anotia, fetal
Accutane Capsules 2076

Antibodies development, persistent
Geref (sermorelin acetate for injection) (Approximately 1 in 4 patients) 2876
Humatrope Vials 1443
Protropin (A small percentage of patients) 1063

Anticholinergic syndrome
Anafranil Capsules (Rare) 803
Clozaril Tablets 2252
Serentil 684

Antidiuretic effect
Brontex 1981
Demerol 2308
Dilaudid-HP Injection (Less frequent) 1337
Dilaudid-HP Lyophilized Powder 250 mg (Less frequent) 1337
MS Contin Tablets (Less frequent) 1994
MSIR 1997
Mepergan Injection 2753
Methadone Hydrochloride Oral Concentrate 2233
Oramorph SR (Morphine Sulfate Sustained Release Tablets) (Less frequent) 2236
Phenergan with Codeine 2777
Phenergan VC with Codeine 2781
RMS Suppositories 2657
Risperdal (Rare) 1301
Yohimex Tablets 1363

Antimitochondrial antibodies
Normodyne Tablets (Less common) 2379
Trandate Tablets (Less common) 1185

Antithrombin, decrease
Brevicon 2088
Estrace Cream and Tablets 749
Estratest 2539
Norinyl 2088
Nor-Q D Tablets 2135
Oncaspar 2028
Ortho-Cyclen/Ortho-Tri-Cyclen 1858
Ortho-Cyclen/Ortho Tri-Cyclen 1858
Tri-Norinyl 2164

Anuria
Azo Gantanol Tablets 2080
Azo Gantrisin Tablets 2081
Azulfidine (Rare) 1949
Bactrim DS Tablets 2084
Bactrim I.V. Infusion 2082
Bactrim 2084
Betaseron for SC Injection 658
Calcium Disodium Versenate Injection 1490
Fansidar Tablets 2114
Floxin I.V. 1571
Floxin Tablets (200 mg, 300 mg, 400 mg) 1567
Fungizone Intravenous 506
Gantanol Tablets 2119
Gantrisin 2120
Luvox Tablets (Infrequent) 2544
Maxaquin Tablets (Less than 1%) .. 2440
Miltown Tablets (Rare) 2672
Nalfon 200 Pulvules & Nalfon Tablets (Less than 1%) 917
Neurontin Capsules (Rare) 1922
Orthoclone OKT3 Sterile Solution ... 1837
PMB 200 and PMB 400 (Rare) 2783
Primaxin I.M. 1727
Primaxin I.V. (Less than 0.2%) 1729
Prinivil Tablets (0.3% to 1.0%) 1733
Prinzide Tablets 1737
▲ Proleukin for Injection (76%) 797
Prostin VR Pediatric Sterile Solution (Less than 1%) 2635
Septra 1174
Septra I.V. Infusion 1169
Septra I.V. Infusion ADD-Vantage Vials 1171
Septra 1174
Zanosar Sterile Powder 2653
Zestoretic 2850
Zestril Tablets (0.3% to 1.0%) 2854
Zovirax Sterile Powder (Less than 1%) 1223

Anuria, neonatal
Accupril Tablets 1893
Altace Capsules 1232
Capoten 739
Capozide 742
Cozaar Tablets 1628
Hyzaar Tablets 1677
Lotensin Tablets 834
Lotensin HCT 837
Lotrel Capsules 840
Monopril Tablets 757
Prinivil Tablets 1733
Prinzide Tablets 1737
Univasc Tablets 2410
Vaseretic Tablets 1765
Vasotec I.V. 1768
Vasotec Tablets 1771
Zestoretic 2850
Zestril Tablets 2854

Anxiety
▲ Acel-Imune Diphtheria and Tetanus Toxoids and Acellular Pertussis Vaccine Adsorbed (17% to 20%).. 1364
Actifed with Codeine Cough Syrup.. 1067
Actigall Capsules 802
Adalat CC (Less than 1.0%) 589
AeroBid Inhaler System (1-3%) 1005
Aerobid-M Inhaler System (1-3%) 1005
Altace Capsules (Less than 1%) 1232
Ambien Tablets (1%) 2416
Amoxil (Rare) 2464
▲ Anafranil Capsules (2% to 9%) 803
Ana-Kit Anaphylaxis Emergency Treatment Kit (Common) 617
▲ Android Capsules, 10 mg (Among most common) 1250
Android 1251
Anexsia 5/500 Elixir 1781
Anexia Tablets 1782
Ansaid Tablets (1-3%) 2579
Apresazide Capsules (Less frequent) 808
Apresoline Hydrochloride Tablets (Less frequent) 809
Asacol Delayed-Release Tablets 1979
Asendin Tablets (Less frequent) 1369
Astramorph/PF Injection, USP (Preservative-Free) 535
Atamet 572
Augmentin (Rare) 2468
Axid Pulvules (1.6%) 1427
Azo Gantrisin Tablets 2081
▲ Betapace Tablets (2% to 4%) 641
▲ Betaseron for SC Injection (15%) .. 658
Brethine Ampuls (Less than 0.5%) 815
Brevibloc Injection (Less than 1%) 1808
Brevital Sodium Vials 1429
Bronkometer Aerosol 2302
Bronkosol Solution 2302
Butisol Sodium Elixir & Tablets (Less than 1 in 100) 2660
Carbocaine Hydrochloride Injection 2303
Cardene Capsules (Rare) 2095
Cardura Tablets (1.1%) 2186
Cartrol Tablets (Less common) 410
Cataflam (Less than 1%) 816
Catapres Tablets 674
Catapres-TTS 675
▲ CellCept Capsules (More than or equal to 3%) 2099
Cipro I.V. (1% or less) 595
Cipro I.V. Pharmacy Bulk Package (Less than 1%) 597
Claritin (2% or fewer patients) 2349
Claritin-D (Less frequent) 2350
Clomid 1514
Clozaril Tablets (1%) 2252
▲ Cognex Capsules (3%) 1901
Combipres Tablets 677
Cozaar Tablets (Less than 1%) 1628
Cytotec (Infrequent) 2424
Cytovene (1% or less) 2103
D.A. Chewable Tablets 951
D.H.E. 45 Injection (Occasional) 2255
Dalgan Injection (Less than 1%) 538
Danocrine Capsules (Rare) 2307
Deconamine Chewable Tablets 1320
Deconamine CX Cough and Cold Liquid and Tablets 1319
Deconamine 1320
Deconsal 454
Delatestryl Injection 2860
Demser Capsules 1649
Desyrel and Desyrel Dividose 503
Dilaudid Ampules 1335
Dilaudid Cough Syrup 1336
Dilaudid 1335
Diphtheria and Tetanus Toxoids and Pertussis Vaccine Adsorbed.. 2477
Diphtheria and Tetanus Toxoids and Pertussis Vaccine Adsorbed USP (For Pediatric Use) (Frequent; 1 in 2 doses) 875
Diprivan Injection (Less than 1%) .. 2833
Doral Tablets 2664
▲ Duragesic Transdermal System (3% to 10%) 1288
Duramorph 962
Dura-Tap/PD Capsules 2867
Dura-Vent/DA Tablets 953
Dura-Vent Tablets 952
▲ Effexor (2% to 11.2%) 2719
Elavil 2838
Eldepryl Tablets (1 of 49 patients) 2550
Emcyt Capsules (1%) 1953
Endep Tablets 2174
Entex PSE Tablets 1987
EpiPen 790
Ergamisol Tablets (1%) 1292
Estratest 2539
Ethmozine Tablets (Less than 2%) 2041
Etrafon 2355
Eulexin Capsules (1%) 2358
Fedahist Gyrocaps 2401
Fedahist Timecaps 2401
▲ Felbatol (5.2% to 5.3%) 2666
Fioricet with Codeine Capsules 2260
Fiorinal with Codeine Capsules 2262
Flexeril Tablets (Less than 1%) 1661
Floxin I.V. (Less than 1%) 1571
Floxin Tablets (200 mg, 300 mg, 400 mg) (Less than 1%) 1567
▲ Foscavir Injection (5% or greater).. 547
Gamimune N, 5% Immune Globulin Intravenous (Human), 5% 619
Gamimune N, 10% Immune Globulin Intravenous (Human), 10% 621
Gastrocrom Capsules (Infrequent).. 984
Glucotrol XL Extended Release Tablets (Less than 3%) 1968
Guaimax-D Tablets 792
Haldol Decanoate 1577
Haldol Injection, Tablets and Concentrate 1575
Halotestin Tablets 2614
Hivid Tablets (Less than 1% to less than 3%) 2121
Hycodan Tablets and Syrup 930
Hycomine Compound Tablets 932
Hycomine 931
Hycotuss Expectorant Syrup 933
Hydrocet Capsules 782
Hyperstat I.V. Injection 2363
Hytrin Capsules (At least 1%) 430
Hyzaar Tablets 1677
Imdur (Less than or equal to 5%) .. 1323
Imitrex Injection (1.1%) 1103
Imitrex Tablets 1106
▲ Inapsine Injection (Among most common) 1296
Indocin (Less than 1%) 1680
Infumorph 200 and Infumorph 500 Sterile Solutions 965
▲ Intron A (Up to 5%) 2364
Ismo Tablets (Fewer than 1%) 2738
Isoetharine Inhalation Solution, USP, Arm-a-Med 551
Kytril Injection (Less than 2%) 2490
Kytril Tablets (2%) 2492
▲ Lamictal Tablets (3.8%) 1112
Lariam Tablets 2128
Larodopa Tablets (Relatively frequent) 2129
Lescol Capsules 2267
Levbid Extended-Release Tablets 2405
Levophed Bitartrate Injection 2315
Levsin/Levsinex/Levbid 2405
Lioresal Intrathecal 1596
Lorcet 10/650 1018
Lortab 2566
Lotensin Tablets 834
Lotrel Capsules 840
▲ Lozol Tablets (Greater than or equal to 5%) 2022
▲ Ludiomil Tablets (3%) 843
▲ Lupron Depot 3.75 mg (Among most frequent; less than 5%) 2556
Lupron Depot 7.5 mg 2559
▲ Lupron Injection (Greater than 5%) 2555
▲ Luvox Tablets (5%) 2544
Marcaine Hydrochloride with Epinephrine 1:200,000 2316
Marcaine Hydrochloride Injection.... 2316
Marcaine Spinal 2319
Marinol (Dronabinol) Capsules (Greater than 1%) 2231
Maxair Autohaler 1492
Maxair Inhaler (Less than 1%) 1494
Maxaquin Tablets (Less than 1%).. 2440
Maxzide 1380
Mebaral Tablets (Less than 1 in 100) 2322
▲ Mepron Suspension (7%) 1135
Methadone Hydrochloride Oral Concentrate 2233
Mevacor Tablets (0.5% to 1.0%) .. 1699
Miacalcin Nasal Spray (Less than 1%) 2275
Monoket (Fewer than 1%) 2406
Mykrox Tablets (Less than 2%) 993
Nardil (Less frequent) 1920
NebuPent for Inhalation Solution (1% or less) 1040
Nembutal Sodium Capsules (Less than 1%) 436
Nembutal Sodium Solution (Less than 1%) 438
Nembutal Sodium Suppositories (Less than 1%) 440
Neoral (Rare) 2276
Nescaine/Nescaine MPF 554
Neurontin Capsules (Frequent) 1922
Noroxin Tablets (Less frequent) 1715
Noroxin Tablets (Less frequent) 2048
Norplant System 2759
Norpramin Tablets 1526
Norvasc Tablets (More than 0.1% to 1%) 1940
Novahistine DH 2462
Novahistine DMX ...... ▣ 822
Novahistine Elixir ...... ▣ 823
Novahistine Expectorant 2463
OptiPranolol (Metipranolol 0.3%) Sterile Ophthalmic Solution (A small number of patients) ...... ◉ 258
Oreton Methyl 1255
Orlamm (1% to 3%) 2239
Pamelor 2280
Parlodel 2281
Parnate Tablets 2503
▲ Paxil Tablets (2.0% to 5.9%) 2505
Penetrex Tablets (1%) 2031
Pentaspan Injection 937
Pepcid Injection (Infrequent) 1722
Pepcid (Infrequent) 1720
▲ Permax Tablets (6.4%) 575
Phenergan VC 2779
Phenergan VC with Codeine 2781
Phenobarbital Elixir and Tablets (Less than 1 in 100 patients) 1469
Placidyl Capsules 448
Plendil Extended-Release Tablets (0.5% to 1.5%) 527
Pondimin Tablets 2066
Pravachol 765
Premarin with Methyltestosterone .. 2794
PREVACID Delayed-Release Capsules (Less than 1%) 2562
Prilosec Delayed-Release Capsules (Less than 1%) 529
Procardia XL Extended Release Tablets (1% or less) 1972
Proglycem 580
▲ Prograf (Greater than 3%) 1042
Propulsid (1.4%) 1300
ProSom Tablets (Frequent) 449
▲ Prozac Pulvules & Liquid, Oral Solution (5% to 14%) 919
Questran Light 769
Questran Powder 770
Reglan 2068
Relafen Tablets (1%) 2510
Retrovir Capsules 1158
Retrovir I.V. Infusion 1163
Retrovir Syrup 1158
▲ ReVia Tablets (2% to more than 10%) 940
Rifater 1532
▲ Risperdal (12% to 20%) 1301
Roferon-A Injection (Less than 3%) 2145
Rogaine Topical Solution (0.36%).. 2637
▲ Romazicon (3% to 9%) 2147

(▣ Described in PDR For Nonprescription Drugs) Incidence data in parenthesis; ▲ 3% or more (◉ Described in PDR For Ophthalmology)

Anxiety Side Effects Index 1224

Rythmol Tablets–150mg, 225mg, 300mg (0.7 to 2.0%) 1352
Salagen Tablets (Less than 1%) 1489
Sandimmune (Rare) 2286
Sandostatin Injection (Less than 1%) 2292
Seconal Sodium Pulvules (Less than 1 in 100) 1474
Sectral Capsules (Up to 2%) 2807
Seldane-D Extended-Release Tablets 1538
Sensorcaine 559
Ser-Ap-Es Tablets 849
Serzone Tablets 771
Sinemet Tablets 943
Sinemet CR Tablets 944
Stadol (1% or greater) 775
▲ Supprelin Injection (3% to 10%) 2056
Surmontil Capsules 2811
Sus-Phrine Injection 1019
Symmetrel Capsules and Syrup (1% to 5%) 946
Syn-Rx Tablets 465
Syn-Rx DM Tablets 466
Tagamet 2516
Tambocor Tablets (1% to less than 3%) 1497
Tegison Capsules (Less than 1%) 2154
Tenex Tablets (Less frequent) 2074
Testoderm Testosterone Transdermal System 486
Testred Capsules 1262
THYREL TRH (Less frequent) 2873
Timoptic in Ocudose (Less frequent) 1753
Timoptic Sterile Ophthalmic Solution (Less frequent) 1751
Timoptic-XE 1755
Tofranil Ampuls 854
Tofranil Tablets 856
Tofranil-PM Capsules 857
Tonocard Tablets (1.1-1.5%) 531
Tornalate Solution for Inhalation, 0.2% (Less than 1%) 956
Trental Tablets (Less than 1%) 1244
Triavil Tablets 1757
Trinalin Repetabs Tablets 1330
Tripedia 892
Tussend 1783
Tussend Expectorant 1785
Tussionex Pennkinetic Extended-Release Suspension 998
Tympagesic Ear Drops 2342
▲ Ultram Tablets (50 mg) (1% to 14%) 1585
Univasc Tablets (Less than 1%) 2410
Vantin for Oral Suspension and Vantin Tablets (Less than 1%) 2646
Vascor (200, 300 and 400 mg) Tablets (0.5 to 2.0%) 1587
Vasoxyl Injection 1196
Versed Injection (Less than 1%) 2170
Vicodin Tablets 1356
Vicodin ES Tablets 1357
Vicodin Tuss Expectorant 1358
Videx Tablets, Powder for Oral Solution, & Pediatric Powder for Oral Solution (Up to 1% to 2%) 720
Visken Tablets (2% or fewer patients) 2299
Vivactil Tablets 1774
Voltaren Tablets (Less than 1%) 861
▲ Wellbutrin Tablets (3.1%) 1204
▲ Xanax Tablets (16.6%) 2649
Xylocaine Injections 567
▲ Yutopar Intravenous Injection (5% to 6%) 570
Zebeta Tablets 1413
▲ Zerit Capsules (Fewer than 1% to 22%) 729
Ziac 1415
Zocor Tablets 1775
Zofran Injection (2%) 1214
▲ Zofran Tablets (6%) 1217
▲ Zoladex (Greater than 1% but less than 5%) 2858
Zoloft Tablets (2.6%) 2217
Zonalon Cream (Less than 1%) 1055
Zosyn (1.2%) 1419
Zosyn Pharmacy Bulk Package (1.2%) 1422
Zydone Capsules 949

Anxiety, paradoxical

Diupres Tablets 1650
Dizac (Less frequent) 1809
Halcion Tablets 2611
Hydropres Tablets 1675
Ser-Ap-Es Tablets 849
Valium Injectable 2182
Valium Tablets 2183
Valrelease Capsules 2169
Vivactil Tablets 1774

Apathy

Anafranil Capsules (Infrequent) 803
Bactrim DS Tablets 2084
Bactrim I.V. Infusion 2082
Bactrim 2084
Betaseron for SC Injection 658
BuSpar (Infrequent) 737
Claritin-D (Less frequent) 2350
Cognex Capsules (Infrequent) 1901
Doral Tablets 2664
Effexor (Infrequent) 2719
Eldepryl Tablets 2550
Fansidar Tablets 2114
Gantanol Tablets 2119
Gantrisin 2120
Imitrex Tablets (Rare) 1106
Intron A (Less than 5%) 2364
Lamictal Tablets (Rare) 1112
Lanoxicaps 1117
Lanoxin Elixir Pediatric 1120
Lanoxin Injection 1123
Lanoxin Injection Pediatric 1126
Lanoxin Tablets 1128
Luvox Tablets (Frequent) 2544
Neurontin Capsules (Infrequent) 1922
Norvasc Tablets (Less than or equal to 0.1%) 1940
Permax Tablets (Infrequent) 575
PREVACID Delayed-Release Capsules (Less than 1%) 2562
Prilosec Delayed-Release Capsules (Less than 1%) 529
ProSom Tablets (Infrequent) 449
Prozac Pulvules & Liquid, Oral Solution (Infrequent) 919
Risperdal (Infrequent) 1301
Roferon-A Injection (Less than 1%) 2145
Septra 1174
Septra I.V. Infusion 1169
Septra I.V. Infusion ADD-Vantage Vials 1171
Septra 1174
Serzone Tablets (Infrequent) 771
Tambocor Tablets (Less than 1%) 1497
Zoloft Tablets (Infrequent) 2217

Apgar score, low

Syntocinon Injection 2296

Aphasia

Anafranil Capsules (Rare) 803
Betaseron for SC Injection 658
Cognex Capsules (Infrequent) 1901
Desyrel and Desyrel Dividose 503
Duragesic Transdermal System (Less than 1%) 1288
Effexor (Rare) 2719
Foscavir Injection (Between 1% and 5%) 547
Hivid Tablets (Less than 1% to less than 3%) 2121
Intron A (Less than 5%) 2364
Lamictal Tablets (Infrequent) 1112
Methotrexate Sodium Tablets, Injection, for Injection and LPF Injection 1275
Mycobutin Capsules (More than one patient) 1957
Neurontin Capsules (Infrequent) 1922
Orthoclone OKT3 Sterile Solution 1837
Risperdal (Rare) 1301
Roferon-A Injection (Less than 0.5%) 2145
Videx Tablets, Powder for Oral Solution, & Pediatric Powder for Oral Solution (Up to 1%) 720
Wellbutrin Tablets (Rare) 1204

Aphonia

BuSpar (Rare) 737
Klonopin Tablets 2126
Roferon-A Injection (Less than 0.5%) 2145

Aphthous stomatitis (see under Stomatitis, ulcerative)

Aplasia, red cell

Cuprimine Capsules 1630
Depen Titratable Tablets 2662
Ridaura Capsules (Less than 1%) 2513

Aplasia, unspecified

Atgam Sterile Solution (Less than 5%) 2581

Aplasia cutis, fetal

Tapazole Tablets (Rare) 1477

Aplastic anemia

Aldactazide 2413
Aldoclor Tablets 1598
Aldoril Tablets 1604
Anaprox/Naprosyn (Less than 1%) 2117
Ancobon Capsules 2079
Ansaid Tablets (Rare) 2579
Anturane 807
Apresazide Capsules 808
Atretol Tablets 573
Azo Gantanol Tablets 2080
Azo Gantrisin Tablets 2081
Azulfidine (Rare) 1949
Bactrim DS Tablets (Rare) 2084
Bactrim I.V. Infusion (Rare) 2082
Bactrim (Rare) 2084
▲ Blephamide Ointment (Among most often) ⊙ 237
Capozide 742
Cataflam (Rare) 816
Cefizox for Intramuscular or Intravenous Use 1034
Cefotan 2829
Ceftin 1078
Cefzil Tablets and Oral Suspension 746
Ceptaz 1081
Chloromycetin Ophthalmic Ointment, 1% ⊙ 310
Chloromycetin Ophthalmic Solution ⊙ 310
Chloromycetin Sodium Succinate 1900
Chloroptic Sterile Ophthalmic Solution (Rare) ⊙ 239
Clinoril Tablets (Less than 1 in 100) 1618
Combipres Tablets 677
Compazine 2470
Cosmegen Injection 1626
Cuprimine Capsules 1630
Cylert Tablets (Isolated reports) 412
Dantrium Capsules (Less frequent) 1982
Dantrium Intravenous 1983
Dapsone Tablets USP 1284
Depen Titratable Tablets 2662
DiaBeta Tablets (Occasional) 1239
Diabinese Tablets 1935
Diamox Intravenous 1372
Diamox Sequels (Sustained Release) 1373
Diamox Tablets 1372
Diucardin Tablets 2718
Diupres Tablets 1650
Diuril Oral Suspension 1653
Diuril Sodium Intravenous 1652
Diuril Tablets 1653
Duricef 748
Dyazide 2479
EC-Naprosyn Delayed-Release Tablets (Less than 1%) 2117
Elase-Chloromycetin Ointment 1040
Eminase (Less than 1%) 2039
Enduron Tablets 420
Esidrix Tablets 821
Esimil Tablets 822
FML-S Liquifilm ⊙ 242
Fansidar Tablets 2114
Felbatol (A marked increase (maybe more than 100 fold)) 2666
Feldene Capsules (Less than 1%) 1965
Floxin I.V. 1571
Floxin Tablets (200 mg, 300 mg, 400 mg) 1567
Fortaz 1100
Gantanol Tablets 2119
Gantrisin (Rare) 2120
Glauctabs ⊙ 208
Glucotrol Tablets 1967
Glucotrol XL Extended Release Tablets 1968
Glynase PresTab Tablets 2609
▲ Hexalen Capsules (13% to 33%) 2571
HydroDIURIL Tablets 1674
Hydropres Tablets 1675
Hyzaar Tablets 1677
IBU Tablets (Less than 1%) 1342
Inderide Tablets 2732
Inderide LA Long Acting Capsules 2734
Indocin Capsules (Less than 1%) 1680
Indocin I.V. (Less than 1%) 1684
Indocin (Less than 1%) 1680
Kefurox Vials, Faspak & ADD-Vantage 1454
Lamictal Tablets 1112
Lasix Injection, Oral Solution and Tablets (Rare) 1240
Lopressor HCT Tablets 832
Lorabid Suspension and Pulvules 1459
Lotensin HCT 837
Lozol Tablets 2022
Luvox Tablets 2544
MZM ⊙ 267
Macrobid Capsules (Rare) 1988
Macrodantin Capsules (Rare) 1989
Maxzide 1380
Mellaril 2269
Mesantoin Tablets (Uncommon) 2272
Micronase Tablets 2623
Midamor Tablets (Rare) 1703
Miltown Tablets 2672
Minizide Capsules 1938
Moduretic Tablets 1705
Monopril Tablets 757
Children's Motrin Ibuprofen Oral Suspension (Less than 1%) 1546
Motrin Ibuprofen Suspension, Oral Drops, Chewable Tablets, Caplets (Less than 1%) 1546
Mykrox Tablets 993
Myochrysine Injection 1711
Nalfon 200 Pulvules & Nalfon Tablets (Less than 1%) 917
Anaprox/Naprosyn (Less than 1%) 2117
Neptazane Tablets 1388
Norflex (Very rare) 1496
Norgesic (1 case) 1496
Nydrazid Injection 508
Ophthocort ⊙ 311
Oretic Tablets 443
Orthoclone OKT3 Sterile Solution 1837
PBZ Tablets 845
PBZ-SR Tablets 844
PMB 200 and PMB 400 2783
Phenurone Tablets (2%) 447
Plaquenil Sulfate Tablets 2328
Prinzide Tablets 1737
Propulsid (Rare) 1300
Prozac Pulvules & Liquid, Oral Solution 919
Ridaura Capsules (Less than 0.1%) 2513
Rifamate Capsules 1530
Rifater (Rare) 1532
SSD 1355
Septra 1174
Septra I.V. Infusion 1169
Septra I.V. Infusion ADD-Vantage Vials (Rare) 1171
Septra 1174
Ser-Ap-Es Tablets 849
Serentil 684
Silvadene Cream 1% 1540
Solganal Suspension (Rare) 2388
Stelazine 2514
Suprax 1399
Tagamet (Very rare) 2516
Tapazole Tablets 1477
Tazicef for Injection 2519
Tegretol Chewable Tablets (Very low incidence) 852
Tegretol Suspension (Very low incidence) 852
Tegretol Tablets (Very low incidence) 852
Tenoretic Tablets 2845
Thalitone 1245
Thorazine 2523
Ticlid Tablets (Rare) 2156
Timolide Tablets 1748
Torecan 2245
Trental Tablets (Rare) 1244
Trusopt Sterile Ophthalmic Solution (Rare) 1760
Urobiotic-250 Capsules 2214
Vantin for Oral Suspension and Vantin Tablets 2646
Vaseretic Tablets 1765
Vasocidin Ophthalmic Solution ⊙ 270
Voltaren Tablets (Rare) 861
Zantac (Rare) 1209
Zantac Injection (Rare) 1207
Zantac Syrup (Rare) 1209
Zaroxolyn Tablets 1000
Zefazone 2654
Zestoretic 2850
Zinacef 1211
Zyloprim Tablets (Less than 1%) 1226

Apnea

▲ Alfenta Injection (3% to 9%) 1286
Amikacin Sulfate Injection, USP 960
Amikin Injectable 501
Anectine 1073
▲ Atgam Sterile Solution (5% to 10%) 2581
Bentyl 1501
Betaseron for SC Injection 658
Brevital Sodium Vials 1429

(▣ Described in PDR For Nonprescription Drugs) Incidence data in parenthesis; ▲ 3% or more (⊙ Described in PDR For Ophthalmology)

1225 Side Effects Index Arrhythmias

Buprenex Injectable (Infrequent) 2006
Butisol Sodium Elixir & Tablets (Less than 1 in 100) 2660
Carbocaine Hydrochloride Injection 2303
Coly-Mycin M Parenteral 1905
Demerol 2308
Desyrel and Desyrel Dividose 503
Dilaudid-HP Injection 1337
Dilaudid-HP Lyophilized Powder 250 mg 1337
Dilaudid Tablets and Liquid 1339
Diphtheria and Tetanus Toxoids and Pertussis Vaccine Adsorbed.. 2477
Diphtheria and Tetanus Toxoids and Pertussis Vaccine Adsorbed USP (For Pediatric Use) 875
Diprivan Injection (1% to 3%) 2833
▲ Duragesic Transdermal System (3% to 10%) 1288
Ethmozine Tablets (Less than 2%) 2041
▲ Exosurf Neonatal for Intratracheal Suspension (33% to 73%) 1095
Indocin I.V. (Less than 3%) 1684
Lamictal Tablets 1112
Luvox Tablets (Rare) 2544
MS Contin Tablets 1994
MSIR 1997
Marcaine Hydrochloride with Epinephrine 1:200,000 2316
Marcaine Hydrochloride Injection.... 2316
Mebaral Tablets (Less than 1 in 100) 2322
Metubine Iodide Vials 916
Motrin Ibuprofen Suspension, Oral Drops, Chewable Tablets, Caplets (Less than 1%) 1546
Nembutal Sodium Capsules (Less than 1%) 436
Nembutal Sodium Solution (Less than 1%) 438
Nembutal Sodium Suppositories (Less than 1%) 440
Nescaine/Nescaine MPF 554
Netromycin Injection 100 mg/ml.... 2373
Neurontin Capsules (Infrequent).... 1922
Norcuron 1826
Nuromax Injection 1149
Oramorph SR (Morphine Sulfate Sustained Release Tablets) (Less frequent) 2236
Orthoclone OKT3 Sterile Solution .. 1837
Permax Tablets (Infrequent) 575
Phenobarbital Elixir and Tablets (Less than 1 in 100 patients) 1469
Polymyxin B Sulfate, Aerosporin Brand Sterile Powder 1154
Proleukin for Injection (1%) 797
Prozac Pulvules & Liquid, Oral Solution (Rare) 919
Pulmozyme Inhalation 1064
Rythmol Tablets–150mg, 225mg, 300mg (Less than 1%) 1352
Seconal Sodium Pulvules (Less than 1 in 100) 1474
Sensorcaine 559
Stadol (Less than 1%) 775
▲ Sublimaze Injection (Among most common) 1307
Sufenta Injection (0.3% to 1%) 1309
▲ Suprane (3%-15%) 1813
▲ Survanta Beractant Intratracheal Suspension (46.1 to 65.4%) 2226
Talwin Injection 2334
Tetramune (Rare) 1404
Thioplex (Thiotepa For Injection) 1281
▲ Trasylol (3%) 613
Tri-Immunol Adsorbed (Rare) 1408
VePesid Capsules and Injection (Rare) 718
▲ Versed Injection (15.4%) 2170
Videx Tablets, Powder for Oral Solution, & Pediatric Powder for Oral Solution (Less than 1%) 720
Virazole 1264

Apnea, neonatal

▲ Prostin VR Pediatric Sterile Solution (About 10% to 12%) 2635
Sinequan (One case) 2205
Survanta Beractant Intratracheal Suspension (Less than 1%) 2226

Appendicitis, acute

Effexor (Rare) 2719
Lopid Tablets (1.2%) 1917
Sandostatin Injection (Less than 1%) 2292

Appetite, changes

Children's Advil Suspension (Less than 3%) 2692
Alupent Tablets (0.4%) 669
Amen Tablets 780
Ansaid Tablets (Less than 1%) 2579
Asendin Tablets (Less frequent) 1369
Ativan Tablets (Less frequent) 2700
Betapace Tablets (1% to 3%) 641
Brevicon 2088
Cataflam (Less than 1%) 816
Compazine 2470
Cortone Acetate Sterile Suspension 1623
Cortone Acetate Tablets 1624
Cycrin Tablets 975
Cytotec (Infrequent) 2424
Danocrine Capsules (Rare) 2307
Decadron Elixir 1633
Decadron Phosphate Injection 1637
Decadron Phosphate Respihaler 1642
Decadron Phosphate Turbinaire 1645
Decadron Phosphate with Xylocaine Injection, Sterile 1639
Decadron Tablets 1635
Decadron-LA Sterile Suspension 1646
Demulen 2428
Depo-Provera Contraceptive Injection (Fewer than 1%) 2602
Depo-Provera Sterile Aqueous Suspension 2606
Desogen Tablets 1817
▲ Effexor (1% to 6%) 2719
Eldepryl Tablets 2550
▲ Hismanal Tablets (3.9%) 1293
Hydeltrasol Injection, Sterile 1665
Hydeltra-T.B.A. Sterile Suspension 1667
Hydrocortone Acetate Sterile Suspension 1669
Hydrocortone Phosphate Injection, Sterile 1670
Hydrocortone Tablets 1672
Klonopin Tablets 2126
Levlen/Tri-Levlen 651
Lo/Ovral Tablets 2746
Lo/Ovral-28 Tablets 2751
▲ Lupron Depot 3.75 mg (Among most frequent; less than 5%) 2556
Maxzide 1380
Mexitil Capsules (2.6%) 678
Micronor Tablets 1872
Midamor Tablets (Between 1% and 3%) 1703
Modicon 1872
Moduretic Tablets (Less than or equal to 1%) 1705
Monopril Tablets (0.2% to 1.0%).. 757
Navane Capsules and Concentrate 2201
Navane Intramuscular 2202
Nordette-21 Tablets 2755
Nordette-28 Tablets 2758
Norinyl 2088
Norplant System 2759
Nor-Q D Tablets 2135
Orap Tablets 1050
Ortho-Cept 1851
Ortho-Cyclen/Ortho-Tri-Cyclen 1858
Ortho-Novum 1872
Ortho-Cyclen/Ortho Tri-Cyclen 1858
Ovcon 760
Ovral Tablets 2770
Ovral-28 Tablets 2770
Ovrette Tablets 2771
Premphase 2797
Prempro 2801
Provera Tablets 2636
Quadrinal Tablets 1350
Stelazine (Occasional) 2514
▲ Tegison Capsules (25-50%) 2154
Thorazine (Sometimes) 2523
Trilafon 2389
Levlen/Tri-Levlen 651
Tri-Norinyl 2164
Triphasil-21 Tablets 2814
Triphasil-28 Tablets 2819
Univasc Tablets (Less than 1%) 2410
▲ Videx Tablets, Powder for Oral Solution, & Pediatric Powder for Oral Solution (6% to 10%) 720
Voltaren Tablets (Less than 1%) 861
▲ Wellbutrin Tablets (3.7%) 1204

Appetite, decreased

AeroBid Inhaler System 1005
▲ Aerobid-M Inhaler System (3-9%).. 1005
Desyrel and Desyrel Dividose (Up to 3.5%) 503
Floxin I.V. (1% to 3%) 1571
Floxin Tablets (200 mg, 300 mg, 400 mg) (1% to 3%) 1567
Garamycin Injectable 2360
IBU Tablets (Greater than 1%) 1342
Imitrex Injection (Rare) 1103
Imitrex Tablets (Rare) 1106
IPOL Poliovirus Vaccine Inactivated 885
▲ Kytril Tablets (5%) 2492
▲ Leustatin (17%) 1834
Lioresal Intrathecal 1596
MetroGel-Vaginal (Equal to or less than 2%) 902
Children's Motrin Ibuprofen Oral Suspension (Greater than 1% but less than 3%) 1546
Motrin Tablets (Less than 3%) 2625
▲ NebuPent for Inhalation Solution (53 to 72%) 1040
Oncaspar 2028
▲ Paxil Tablets (2.0% to 6.4%) 2505
▲ Poliovax (More than 5%) 891
ProSom Tablets (Infrequent) 449
Recombivax HB (Less to greater than 1%) 1744
Supprelin Injection (1% to 3%) 2056
Vantin for Oral Suspension and Vantin Tablets (Less than 1%) 2646
▲ Xanax Tablets (27.8%) 2649

Appetite, increased

AeroBid Inhaler System (1-3%) 1005
Aerobid-M Inhaler System (1-3%).. 1005
Ambien Tablets (Rare) 2416
▲ Anafranil Capsules (Up to 11%) 803
Asacol Delayed-Release Tablets 1979
BuSpar (Infrequent) 737
Cardura Tablets (Less than 0.5% of 3960 patients) 2186
Claritin (2% or fewer patients) 2349
Claritin-D (Less frequent) 2350
Clomid (Fewer than 1%) 1514
Clozaril Tablets (Less than 1%) 2252
Cognex Capsules (Infrequent) 1901
Cortifoam 2396
Dalalone D.P. Injectable 1011
Depakene 413
Depakote Tablets 415
Desyrel and Desyrel Dividose 503
Dexacort Phosphate in Respihaler .. 458
Dexacort Phosphate in Turbinaire .. 459
Etrafon 2355
Felbatol (Infrequent) 2666
Fioricet with Codeine Capsules 2260
Fiorinal with Codeine Capsules 2262
Intron A (Less than 5%) 2364
Ismo Tablets (Fewer than 1%) 2738
Kerlone Tablets (Less than 2%) 2436
Lamictal Tablets (Infrequent) 1112
Luvox Tablets 2544
Maxaquin Tablets (Less than 1%).. 2440
Megace Tablets 701
Miacalcin Nasal Spray (Less than 1%) 2275
Neurontin Capsules (1.1%) 1922
Norvasc Tablets (Less than or equal to 0.1%) 1940
Oncaspar (Less than 1%) 2028
Orudis Capsules (Less than 1%) 2766
Oruvail Capsules (Less than 1%).... 2766
Paxil Tablets (1.4%) 2505
Periactin 1724
Permax Tablets (Infrequent) 575
PREVACID Delayed-Release Capsules (Less than 1%) 2562
▲ Prograf (Greater than 3%) 1042
ProSom Tablets (Infrequent) 449
▲ Proventil Syrup (3 of 100 patients) 2385
Prozac Pulvules & Liquid, Oral Solution (Frequent) 919
Relafen Tablets (1%) 2510
ReVia Tablets (Less than 1%) 940
Risperdal (Infrequent) 1301
Salagen Tablets (Less than 1%) 1489
Seldane Tablets (0.5% to 0.6%).... 1536
Seldane-D Extended-Release Tablets 1538
▲ Serzone Tablets (5%) 771
Temaril Tablets, Syrup and Spansule Extended-Release Capsules 483
Toradol (1% or less) 2159
Vascor (200, 300 and 400 mg) Tablets (0.5 to 2.0%) 1587
▲ Ventolin Syrup (3 of 100 patients) 1202
▲ Videx Tablets, Powder for Oral Solution, & Pediatric Powder for Oral Solution (2 to 5%) 720
▲ Xanax Tablets (32.7%) 2649
Zoladex (2%) 2858
Zoloft Tablets (1.3%) 2217

Appetite, loss of (see also under Anorexia)

▲ CHEMET (succimer) Capsules (12 to 20.9%) 1545
HibTITER (23 of 1,118 vaccinations) 1375
Miacalcin Injection 2273
Varivax (Greater than or equal to 1%) 1762

Apprehension

Adenocard Injection (Less than 1%) 1021
Ana-Kit Anaphylaxis Emergency Treatment Kit 617
Antivenin (Crotalidae) Polyvalent 2696
Dalmane Capsules 2173
Dilaudid-HP Injection (Less frequent) 1337
Dilaudid-HP Lyophilized Powder 250 mg (Less frequent) 1337
Dilaudid Tablets and Liquid (Less frequent) 1339
Dopram Injectable 2061
Duranest Injections 542
Dyclone 0.5% and 1% Topical Solutions, USP 544
Edecrin 1657
Emla Cream 545
EpiPen Jr. 790
Hyperstat I.V. Injection 2363
Limbitrol 2180
MS Contin Tablets (Less frequent) 1994
MSIR (Infrequent) 1997
Matulane Capsules 2131
Oramorph SR (Morphine Sulfate Sustained Release Tablets) (Less frequent) 2236
Quinaglute Dura-Tabs Tablets 649
Quinidex Extentabs 2067
▲ Xylocaine Injections (Among most common) 567

Apraxia

Anafranil Capsules (Rare) 803
Cognex Capsules (Rare) 1901
Eldepryl Tablets 2550
Neurontin Capsules (Rare) 1922

Arachnoiditis

Depo-Medrol Single-Dose Vial 2600
Depo-Medrol Sterile Aqueous Suspension 2597
Gelfoam Sterile Sponge 2608
Marcaine Spinal 2319
Methotrexate Sodium Tablets, Injection, for Injection and LPF Injection 1275
Nescaine/Nescaine MPF 554
Novocain Hydrochloride for Spinal Anesthesia 2326
Pontocaine Hydrochloride for Spinal Anesthesia 2330
Streptomycin Sulfate Injection 2208

Areflexia

Cognex Capsules (Infrequent) 1901
Neurontin Capsules (Frequent) 1922
Platinol 708
Platinol-AQ Injection 710

Argumentativeness

Versed Injection (Less than 1%) 2170

Arm, stiffness of

Engerix-B Unit-Dose Vials (Less than 1%) 2482

Arrhythmia, exacerbation of

Cordarone Tablets 2712

Arrhythmias

Abbokinase (Occasional) 403
Activase 1058
Adenocard Injection 1021
Adenoscan (1%) 1024
Adriamycin PFS 1947
Adriamycin RDF 1947
Children's Advil Suspension (Less than 1%) 2692
▲ Alfenta Injection (14%) 1286
Altace Capsules (Less than 1%) 1232
Ambien Tablets (Rare) 2416
Anafranil Capsules (Infrequent) 803
Ana-Kit Anaphylaxis Emergency Treatment Kit 617
Anectine 1073
Ansaid Tablets (Less than 1%) 2579
Aramine Injection 1609
Atgam Sterile Solution (Less than 5%) 2581
Atretol Tablets 573
Atromid-S Capsules 2701
Betagan .... ⊙ 233
Betaseron for SC Injection 658

(▣ Described in PDR For Nonprescription Drugs) Incidence data in parenthesis; ▲ 3% or more (⊙ Described in PDR For Ophthalmology)

Arrhythmias **Side Effects Index** 1226

Betimol 0.25%, 0.5% ◉ 261
Blocadren Tablets (Greater than 1.1%) 1614
▲ Bromfed-DM Cough Syrup (Among most frequent) 1786
Carbocaine Hydrochloride Injection 2303
Cardizem CD Capsules (Less than 1%) 1506
Cardizem SR Capsules (Less than 1%) 1510
Cardizem Injectable (1.0%) 1508
Cardizem Tablets (Less than 1%) 1512
Cardura Tablets (1%) 2186
Cartrol Tablets (Less common) 410
Catapres Tablets (Rare) 674
Catapres-TTS (Rare) 675
CHEMET (succimer) Capsules (Up to 1.8%) 1545
Cipro I.V. (1% or less) 595
Cipro I.V. Pharmacy Bulk Package (Less than 1%) 597
Claforan Sterile and Injection 1235
Claritin-D 2350
Clinoril Tablets (Rare) 1618
Clomid 1514
Clozaril Tablets (Several patients) 2252
Combipres Tablets (Rare) 677
Compazine 2470
Cordarone Tablets (1 to 3%) 2712
Cozaar Tablets (Less than 1%) 1628
Cytotec (Infrequent) 2424
Cytovene (1% or less) 2103
D.A. Chewable Tablets 951
Dalgan Injection (Less than 1%) 538
Deconamine Chewable Tablets 1320
Deconamine CX Cough and Cold Liquid and Tablets 1319
Deconamine 1320
Deconsal 454
Demadex Tablets and Injection 686
Desyrel and Desyrel Dividose 503
Dexatrim ▣ 832
Dexatrim Plus Vitamins Caplets ▣ 832
Dilacor XR Extended-release Capsules (Infrequent) 2018
Dimetane-DC Cough Syrup 2059
Dimetane-DX Cough Syrup 2059
Diprivan Injection (Less than 1%) 2833
Diupres Tablets 1650
Dopram Injectable 2061
Doxorubicin Astra 540
Duragesic Transdermal System (1% or greater) 1288
Dura-Tap/PD Capsules 2867
Dura-Vent/DA Tablets 953
Dura-Vent Tablets 952
Dyazide 2479
E.E.S. (Occasional reports) 424
Effexor (Rare) 2719
Elavil 2838
Eldepryl Tablets 2550
▲ Eminase (38%) 2039
Endep Tablets 2174
EpiPen Jr. 790
EryPed (Occasional reports) 421
Ery-Tab Tablets (Occasional reports) 422
Erythrocin Stearate Filmtab (Occasional reports) 425
Erythromycin Base Filmtab (Occasional reports) 426
Erythromycin Delayed-Release Capsules, USP (Occasional reports) 427
Eskalith 2485
Etrafon 2355
Fedahist Gyrocaps 2401
Fedahist Timecaps 2401
Flexeril Tablets (Less than 1%) 1661
Fludara for Injection (Up to 3%) 663
Fluothane 2724
Foscavir Injection (Less than 1%) 547
Fungizone Intravenous 506
Glucotrol XL Extended Release Tablets (Less than 1%) 1968
Haldol Decanoate 1577
Hivid Tablets (Less than 1% to less than 3%) 2121
Hydropres Tablets 1675
Hytrin Capsules (At least 1%) 430
Hyzaar Tablets 1677
IBU Tablets (Less than 1%) 1342
Idamycin 1955
Imdur (Less than or equal to 5%) 1323
Imitrex Injection (Rare) 1103
Imitrex Tablets (Rare to infrequent) 1106
Indocin Capsules (Less than 1%) 1680
Indocin I.V. (Less than 1%) 1684
Indocin (Less than 1%) 1680
INFeD (Iron Dextran Injection, USP) 2345
▲ Inocor Lactate Injection (3%) 2309
Intron A (Less than 5%) 2364
Iopidine 0.5% (Less than 1%) ◉ 221
Ismo Tablets (Fewer than 1%) 2738
Isopto Carbachol Ophthalmic Solution ◉ 223
Kerlone Tablets (Less than 2%) 2436
Kytril Injection (Rare) 2490
Lanoxicaps 1117
Lanoxin Elixir Pediatric 1120
Lanoxin Injection 1123
Lanoxin Injection Pediatric 1126
Lanoxin Tablets 1128
Lasix Injection, Oral Solution and Tablets 1240
Levo-Dromoran (Infrequent) 2129
Levophed Bitartrate Injection 2315
Limbitrol 2180
Lithium Carbonate Capsules & Tablets 2230
Lithonate/Lithotabs/Lithobid 2543
Lodine Capsules and Tablets (Less than 1%) 2743
Lorelco Tablets 1517
Ludiomil Tablets (Rare) 843
Lufyllin & Lufyllin-400 Tablets 2670
Lufyllin-GG Elixir & Tablets 2671
Lupron Depot 3.75 mg 2556
Lupron Depot 7.5 mg (Less than 5%) 2559
Lupron Injection (Less than 5%) 2555
Marax Tablets & DF Syrup 2200
Maxaquin Tablets (Less than 1%) 2440
Mellaril 2269
Midamor Tablets (Less than or equal to 1%) 1703
Miltown Tablets 2672
Mivacron (Less than 1%) 1138
Moban Tablets and Concentrate 1048
Moduretic Tablets (Greater than 1%, less than 3%) 1705
Monoket (Fewer than 1%) 2406
Monopril Tablets (0.2% to 1.0%) 757
Children's Motrin Ibuprofen Oral Suspension (Less than 1%) 1546
Motrin Tablets (Less than 1%) 2625
Motrin Ibuprofen Suspension, Oral Drops, Chewable Tablets, Caplets (Less than 1%) 1546
Navane Capsules and Concentrate 2201
Navane Intramuscular 2202
Neo-Synephrine Hydrochloride 1% Carpuject (Rare) 2324
Neo-Synephrine Hydrochloride 1% Injection (Rare) 2324
▲ Neupogen for Injection (11 of 375 cancer patients) 495
Nicolar Tablets 2026
Norisodrine with Calcium Iodide Syrup 442
Norpramin Tablets 1526
Norvasc Tablets (More than 0.1% to 1%) 1940
Novahistine DH 2462
Novahistine DMX ▣ 822
Novahistine Elixir ▣ 823
Novahistine Expectorant 2463
▲ Novantrone (3 to 4%) 1279
Ocupress Ophthalmic Solution, 1% Sterile (Occasional) ◉ 309
Orap Tablets 1050
Orthoclone OKT3 Sterile Solution 1837
Orudis Capsules (Rare) 2766
Oruvail Capsules (Rare) 2766
OSM_GLYN Oral Osmotic Agent ◉ 226
Oxytocin Injection 2771
PCE Dispertab Tablets (Rare) 444
PMB 200 and PMB 400 2783
Pamelor 2280
Parlodel (Less than 1%) 2281
Paxil Tablets (Rare) 2505
Pentam 300 Injection 1041
Pepcid Injection (Infrequent) 1722
Pepcid (Infrequent) 1720
Permax Tablets (1.1%) 575
Pfizerpen for Injection 2203
Plendil Extended-Release Tablets (0.5% to 1.5%) 527
Prinivil Tablets (0.3% to 1.0%) 1733
Prinzide Tablets 1737
Priscoline Hydrochloride Ampuls 845
Procardia XL Extended Release Tablets (1% or less) 1972
▲ Proleukin for Injection (22%) 797
Prolixin 509
PROPINE with C CAP Compliance Cap ◉ 253
Propulsid (Rare) 1300
ProSom Tablets (Rare) 449
Prostigmin Injectable 1260
Prostigmin Tablets 1261
Prostin E2 Suppository 2634
Prozac Pulvules & Liquid, Oral Solution (Infrequent) 919
Quibron 2053
▲ Quinaglute Dura-Tabs Tablets (3%) 649
Regitine 846
Relafen Tablets (Less than 1%) 2510
Revex (Less than 1%) 1811
Risperdal 1301
Ritalin 848
Rocaltrol Capsules 2141
Roferon-A Injection (Less than 3%) 2145
Romazicon (Less than 1%) 2147
Rondec Oral Drops 953
Rondec Syrup 953
Rondec Tablet 953
Rondec-DM Oral Drops 954
Rondec-DM Syrup 954
Rondec-TR Tablet 953
Rubex 712
Rum-K Syrup 1005
▲ Sandostatin Injection (9%) 2292
Seldane Tablets 1536
Seldane-D Extended-Release Tablets 1538
Sensorcaine 559
Ser-Ap-Es Tablets 849
Serentil 684
Slo-bid Gyrocaps 2033
Sodium Polystyrene Sulfonate Suspension 2244
Solu-Medrol Sterile Powder 2643
Stelazine 2514
Streptase for Infusion 562
Sufenta Injection (0.3% to 1%) 1309
Suprane (Less than 1%) 1813
Surmontil Capsules 2811
Sus-Phrine Injection 1019
Syn-Rx Tablets 465
Syn-Rx DM Tablets 466
Syntocinon Injection 2296
Tagamet Injection (Rare) 2516
Taxol (Approximately 1%) 714
Tegretol Chewable Tablets 852
Tegretol Suspension 852
Tegretol Tablets 852
Tensilon Injectable 1261
Timolide Tablets (Less than 1%) 1748
Timoptic in Ocudose (Less frequent) 1753
Timoptic Sterile Ophthalmic Solution (Less frequent) 1751
Timoptic-XE 1755
Tofranil Ampuls 854
Tofranil Tablets 856
Tofranil-PM Capsules 857
▲ Trasylol (4%) 613
Trental Tablets (Rare) 1244
Triavil Tablets 1757
Trilafon 2389
Trinalin Repetabs Tablets 1330
▲ Triostat Injection (6%) 2530
Tussend 1783
Tussend Expectorant 1785
Uniphyl 400 mg Tablets 2001
Univasc Tablets (Less than 1%) 2410
Vascor (200, 300 and 400 mg) Tablets (About 2.4%) 1587
Vaseretic Tablets 1765
Vasotec Tablets (0.5% to 1.0%) 1771
Ventolin Inhalation Solution 1198
Ventolin Nebules Inhalation Solution 1199
▲ Videx Tablets, Powder for Oral Solution, & Pediatric Powder for Oral Solution (Less than 1% to 10%) 720
Vivactil Tablets 1774
Vumon 727
▲ Wellbutrin Tablets (5.3%) 1204
Yutopar Intravenous Injection (1% to 2%) 570
Zantac (Rare) 1209
Zantac Injection (Rare) 1207
Zantac Syrup (Rare) 1209
Zaroxolyn Tablets 1000
Zemuron (Less than 1%) 1830
Zestoretic 2850
Zestril Tablets (0.3% to 1.0%) 2854
Ziac (Up to 0.4%) 1415
▲ Zoladex (Greater than 1% but less than 5%) 2858
Zosyn (1.0% or less) 1419
Zosyn Pharmacy Bulk Package (1.0% or less) 1422

Arrhythmias, pre-existing, worsening of

Cordarone Intravenous 2715
Quibron 2053
▲ Rythmol Tablets–150mg, 225mg, 300mg (4.7%) 1352
Slo-bid Gyrocaps 2033

Arrhythmias, junctional

Proleukin for Injection (1%) 797
Tornalate Solution for Inhalation, 0.2% (Less than 1%) 956

Arrhythmias, sinus

Imitrex Injection (Infrequent) 1103

Arrhythmias, supraventricular

Ethmozine Tablets (Less than 2%) 2041
Intron A (Rare) 2364
Primacor Injection 2331
▲ Proleukin for Injection (5%) 797

Arterial carbon dioxide, decrease

Sulfamylon Cream 925

Arterial insufficiency

Blocadren Tablets 1614
Inderal 2728
Inderal LA Long Acting Capsules 2730
Inderide Tablets 2732
Inderide LA Long Acting Capsules 2734
Lopressor Ampuls (1%) 830
Lopressor HCT Tablets 832
Lopressor Tablets (1%) 830
Timolide Tablets 1748
Timoptic in Ocudose 1753
Timoptic Sterile Ophthalmic Solution 1751
Timoptic-XE 1755
Toprol-XL Tablets (About 1 of 100 patients) 565

Arterial occlusion

Humegon 1824
Metrodin (urofollitropin for injection) 2446
Serophene (clomiphene citrate tablets, USP) (Rare) 2451

Arteriospasm

Ceptaz 1081
Fortaz 1100

Arteritis

Ambien Tablets (Rare) 2416
Azo Gantrisin Tablets 2081

Arteritis, temporal

Imitrex Tablets 1106
Orthoclone OKT3 Sterile Solution 1837

Arthralgia

▲ Accutane Capsules (Approximately 16%) 2076
Acel-Imune Diphtheria and Tetanus Toxoids and Acellular Pertussis Vaccine Adsorbed (Rare) 1364
Actigall Capsules 802
Actimmune (2%) 1056
Adalat CC (Less than 1.0%) 589
Aldoclor Tablets 1598
Aldomet Ester HCl Injection 1602
Aldomet Oral 1600
Aldoril Tablets 1604
All-Flex Arcing Spring Diaphragm (See also Ortho Diaphragm Kits) 1865
Altace Capsules (Less than 1%) 1232
▲ Ambien Tablets (4%) 2416
Amikacin Sulfate Injection, USP (Rare) 960
Amikin Injectable (Rare) 501
Anafranil Capsules (Up to 3%) 803
Antivenin (Crotalidae) Polyvalent 2696
Apresazide Capsules (Less frequent) 808
Apresoline Hydrochloride Tablets (Less frequent) 809
▲ Asacol Delayed-Release Tablets (5%) 1979
▲ Atgam Sterile Solution (More than 1% to 10%; 1 in 2 patients) 2581
Atretol Tablets 573
Atromid-S Capsules 2701
Augmentin 2468
Azmacort Oral Inhaler 2011
Azo Gantanol Tablets 2080
Azo Gantrisin Tablets 2081
Azulfidine (Rare) 1949
BCG Vaccine, USP (TICE) 1814
Bactrim DS Tablets 2084
Bactrim I.V. Infusion 2082

(▣ Described in PDR For Nonprescription Drugs) Incidence data in parenthesis; ▲ 3% or more (◉ Described in PDR For Ophthalmology)

1227 Side Effects Index Arthritis

Bactrim 2084
Beconase 1076
Biavax II 1613
Bicillin C-R Injection 2704
Bicillin C-R 900/300 Injection 2706
Bicillin L-A Injection 2707
Blocadren Tablets (Less than 1%) 1614
BuSpar (Infrequent) 737
Calan SR Caplets (1% or less) 2422
Calan Tablets (1% or less) 2419
▲Capoten (About 4 to 7 of 100 patients) 739
Capozide (Sometimes) 742
Cardene Capsules (Rare) 2095
Cardura Tablets (1%) 2186
Cartrol Tablets (1.2%) 410
Catapres Tablets (About 6 in 1,000 patients) 674
Catapres-TTS (Less frequent) 675
Ceclor Pulvules & Suspension 1431
Ceftin for Oral Suspension (Less than 1% but more than 0.1%) 1078
▲CellCept Capsules (More than or equal to 3%) 2099
Chibroxin Sterile Ophthalmic Solution (With oral form) 1617
Cipro I.V. (1% or less) 595
Cipro I.V. Pharmacy Bulk Package (Less than 1%) 597
Cipro Tablets (Less than 1%) 592
Claritin (2% or fewer patients) 2349
Claritin-D (Less frequent) 2350
Clinoril Tablets (Less than 1 in 100) 1618
Clomid 1514
Clozaril Tablets (Less than 1%) 2252
Cognex Capsules (Frequent) 1901
Colestid Tablets 2591
Combipres Tablets (About 6 in 1,000) 677
Coumadin 926
Cozaar Tablets (Less than 1%) 1628
Cuprimine Capsules 1630
CytoGam (Less than 5.0%) 1593
Cytotec (Infrequent) 2424
Danocrine Capsules 2307
Demadex Tablets and Injection (1.8%) 686
Depakote Tablets (Greater than 1% but not more than 5%) 415
Depen Titratable Tablets 2662
Depo-Provera Contraceptive Injection (1% to 5%) 2602
DiaBeta Tablets 1239
Didronel Tablets 1984
Dilacor XR Extended-release Capsules (Infrequent; 1.4%) 2018
Dilantin Infatabs 1908
Dilantin Kapseals 1906
Dilantin-125 Suspension 1911
▲Dipentum Capsules (4.0%) 1951
Diphtheria and Tetanus Toxoids and Pertussis Vaccine Adsorbed 2477
Dolobid Tablets (Less than 1 in 100) 1654
Duricef (Rare) 748
Effexor 2719
Elspar 1659
▲Eminase (Less than 10%) 2039
Engerix-B Unit-Dose Vials (Less than 1%) 2482
▲Epogen for Injection (11%; rare) 489
▲Ergamisol Tablets (4% to 5%) 1292
Eskalith 2485
Famvir (1.5%) 2486
Fansidar Tablets 2114
Felbatol 2666
Feldene Capsules (Occasional) 1965
Flagyl 375 Capsules 2434
Floxin I.V. (Less than 1%) 1571
Floxin Tablets (200 mg, 300 mg, 400 mg) (Less than 1%) 1567
Fludara for Injection (Up to 1%) 663
Foscavir Injection (Between 1% and 5%) 547
▲Fungizone Intravenous (Among most common) 506
Furoxone 2046
Gamimune N, 5% Immune Globulin Intravenous (Human), 5% 619
Gamimune N, 10% Immune Globulin Intravenous (Human), 10% 621
Gantanol Tablets 2119
Gantrisin 2120
Garamycin Injectable 2360
Gastrocrom Capsules (Infrequent) 984
Glucotrol XL Extended Release Tablets (Less than 3%) 1968
Glynase PresTab Tablets 2609
▲Habitrol Nicotine Transdermal System (3% to 9% of patients) 865
Havrix (Less than 1%) 2489
Hismanal Tablets (1.2%) 1293
Hivid Tablets (Less than 1% to less than 3%) 2121
Humegon 1824
Hylorel Tablets (1.7%) 985
Hyskon Hysteroscopy Fluid (Rare) 1595
Hytrin Capsules (At least 1%) 430
Hyzaar Tablets 1677
Imdur (Less than or equal to 5%) 1323
Imitrex Injection (Infrequent) 1103
▲Imovax Rabies Vaccine (Up to 6%) 881
Imuran (Less than 1%) 1110
INFeD (Iron Dextran Injection, USP) 2345
Intal Capsules (Less than 1 in 10,000 patients) 987
Intal Inhaler (Infrequent) 988
Intal Nebulizer Solution 989
▲Intron A (Up to 19%) 2364
Ismo Tablets (Fewer than 1%) 2738
Isoptin Oral Tablets (Less than 1%) 1346
Isoptin SR Tablets (1% or less) 1348
K-Phos Neutral Tablets 639
K-Phos Original Formula 'Sodium Free' Tablets (Less frequent) 639
Keflex Pulvules & Oral Suspension 914
Keftab Tablets 915
▲Kerlone Tablets (3.1%) 2436
Lamictal Tablets (2.0%) 1112
Lescol Capsules 2267
▲Leukine for IV Infusion (21%) 1271
▲Leustatin (5%) 1834
Lithonate/Lithotabs/Lithobid 2543
Lopid Tablets 1917
Lotensin Tablets 834
Lotensin HCT (0.3% to more than 1%) 837
Lupron Depot 7.5 mg 2559
Lupron Injection (Less than 5%) 2555
Luvox Tablets (Infrequent) 2544
M-M-R II 1687
M-R-VAX II 1689
Macrobid Capsules 1988
Macrodantin Capsules 1989
Matulane Capsules 2131
Maxaquin Tablets (Less than 1%) 2440
Meruvax II 1697
Methotrexate Sodium Tablets, Injection, for Injection and LPF Injection (Rare to less common) 1275
Metrodin (urofollitropin for injection) 2446
MetroGel-Vaginal 902
Mevacor Tablets (0.5% to 1.0%; rare) 1699
Mexitil Capsules (1.7%) 678
▲Miacalcin Nasal Spray (3.8%) 2275
Micronase Tablets 2623
Midamor Tablets (Less than or equal to 1%) 1703
Minipress Capsules 1937
Moduretic Tablets (Less than or equal to 1%) 1705
Monopril Tablets (0.2% to 1.0%) 757
Myambutol Tablets 1386
Mycobutin Capsules (Less than 1%) 1957
▲Mykrox Tablets (3.1%) 993
Myochrysine Injection 1711
Nasacort Nasal Inhaler 2024
Nasalcrom Nasal Solution 994
Navelbine Injection (Less than 5%) 1145
NebuPent for Inhalation Solution (1% or less) 1040
NegGram 2323
Neoral (Rare) 2276
Neupogen for Injection (Infrequent) 495
Neurontin Capsules (Frequent) 1922
Nicoderm (nicotine transdermal system) (1% to 3%) 1518
Nicotrol Nicotine Transdermal System (1% to 3%) 1550
Noroxin Tablets 1715
Noroxin Tablets 2048
Norvasc Tablets (More than 0.1% to 1%) 1940
▲Oncaspar (Greater than 1% but less than 5%) 2028
▲Orlamm (3% to 9%) 2239
Ortho Diaphragm Kits—All-Flex Arcing Spring; Ortho Coil Spring; Ortho-White Flat Spring 1865
Ortho Diaphragm Kit 1865
Orthoclone OKT3 Sterile Solution 1837
Paxil Tablets (Infrequent) 2505
Penetrex Tablets (Less than 1% but more than or equal to 0.1%) 2031
Pentasa (Less than 1%) 1527
Pepcid Injection (Infrequent) 1722
Pepcid (Infrequent) 1720
Pergonal (menotropins for injection, USP) 2448
Permax Tablets (1.6%) 575
Pfizerpen for Injection 2203
Phenobarbital Elixir and Tablets (Rare) 1469
Plendil Extended-Release Tablets (0.5% to 1.5%) 527
Pneumovax 23 (Rare) 1725
Pnu-Imune 23 (Rare to infrequent) 1393
Pravachol (Rare) 765
PREVACID Delayed-Release Capsules (Less than 1%) 2562
Prilosec Delayed-Release Capsules (Less than 1%) 529
Prinivil Tablets (0.3% to 1.0%) 1733
Prinzide Tablets 1737
Procan SR Tablets (Common) 1926
Procardia XL Extended Release Tablets (Less than 3%) 1972
▲Procrit for Injection (Rare to 11%) 1841
▲Prograf (Greater than 3%) 1042
▲Proleukin for Injection (6%) 797
Propulsid (1.4%) 1300
ProSom Tablets (Rare) 449
Prostigmin Injectable 1260
Prostigmin Tablets 1261
Prostin E2 Suppository 2634
Protostat Tablets 1883
Prozac Pulvules & Liquid, Oral Solution (1.2% to 3%) 919
Pyrazinamide Tablets (Frequent) 1398
Quadrinal Tablets 1350
Questran Light 769
Questran Powder 770
Quinaglute Dura-Tabs Tablets 649
Quinidex Extentabs 2067
Rabies Vaccine Adsorbed (Less than 1%) 2508
▲Rabies Vaccine, Imovax Rabies I.D. (Less frequent; up to 6%) 883
Recombivax HB (Less than 1%) 1744
Retrovir Capsules 1158
Retrovir I.V. Infusion 1163
Retrovir Syrup 1158
▲ReVia Tablets (More than 10%) 940
Revex 1811
Rhinocort Nasal Inhaler (Less than 1%) 556
Rifater (Frequent) 1532
Risperdal (2% to 3%) 1301
Ritalin 848
▲Roferon-A Injection (5% to 24%) 2145
Rowasa (2.09%) 2548
Rythmol Tablets–150mg, 225mg, 300mg (0.2 to 1.0%) 1352
Sandimmune (Rare) 2286
Sandostatin Injection (1% to 4%) 2292
Sansert Tablets 2295
Sectral Capsules 2807
Septra 1174
Septra I.V. Infusion 1169
Septra I.V. Infusion ADD-Vantage Vials 1171
Septra 1174
Ser-Ap-Es Tablets 849
Serevent Inhalation Aerosol (1% to 3%) 1176
Serzone Tablets (1%) 771
Solatene Capsules (Rare) 2150
Solganal Suspension 2388
Solu-Medrol Sterile Powder 2643
▲Supprelin Injection (3% to 10%) 2056
Synarel Nasal Solution for Endometriosis (Less than 1%) 2152
Tagamet (Rare) 2516
Tambocor Tablets (Less than 1%) 1497
Tapazole Tablets 1477
▲Taxol (8% to 60%) 714
▲Tegison Capsules (50-75%) 2154
Tegretol Chewable Tablets 852
Tegretol Suspension 852
Tegretol Tablets 852
Tenex Tablets (Less frequent) 2074
Tetramune 1404
▲TheraCys BCG Live (Intravesical) (1.0% to 7.1%) 897
Timentin for Injection 2528
Timolide Tablets 1748
Timoptic in Ocudose 1753
Timoptic Sterile Ophthalmic Solution 1751
Timoptic-XE 1755
▲Tonocard Tablets (Less than 1%-4.7%) 531
Tornalate Solution for Inhalation, 0.2% (Less than 1%) 956
Tri-Immunol Adsorbed 1408
Typhim Vi (One report) 899
Univasc Tablets (Less than 1%) 2410
Uroqid-Acid No. 2 Tablets 640
Varivax (Greater than or equal to 1%) 1762
Vaseretic Tablets (0.5% to 2.0%) 1765
Vasotec I.V. 1768
Vasotec Tablets (0.5% to 1.0%) 1771
Verelan Capsules (1% or less) 1410
Verelan Capsules (Less than 1%) 2824
Videx Tablets, Powder for Oral Solution, & Pediatric Powder for Oral Solution (Up to 2%) 720
▲Visken Tablets (7%) 2299
Wellbutrin Tablets 1204
Zantac (Rare) 1209
Zantac Injection (Rare) 1207
Zantac Syrup (Rare) 1209
Zaroxolyn Tablets 1000
Zebeta Tablets (2.2% to 2.7%) 1413
Zefazone 2654
▲Zerit Capsules (Fewer than 1% to 19%) 729
Zestoretic 2850
Zestril Tablets (0.3% to 1.0%) 2854
Ziac 1415
Zocor Tablets 1775
Zoladex (1% or greater) 2858
Zoloft Tablets (Infrequent) 2217
Zosyn (1.0% or less) 1419
Zosyn Pharmacy Bulk Package (1.0% or less) 1422
Zyloprim Tablets (Less than 1%) 1226

Arthralgia, migratory

Aquasol A Vitamin A Capsules, USP 534
Aquasol A Parenteral 534

Arthralgia, monoarticular

Recombivax HB (Less than 1%) 1744

Arthritis

Accutane Capsules (Less than 1%) 2076
Adalat Capsules (10 mg and 20 mg) (Less than 0.5%) 587
Adalat CC (Less than 1.0%) 589
Altace Capsules (Less than 1%) 1232
Ambien Tablets (Infrequent) 2416
Asacol Delayed-Release Tablets (1% to 2%) 1979
Atrovent Inhalation Solution (0.9%) 673
Augmentin 2468
BCG Vaccine, USP (TICE) (2.7%) 1814
Benemid Tablets 1611
Betaseron for SC Injection 658
Biavax II (Rare) 1613
Bumex (0.2%) 2093
Cardura Tablets (1%) 2186
Cartrol Tablets (Less common) 410
Ceclor Pulvules & Suspension 1431
Chibroxin Sterile Ophthalmic Solution (With oral form) 1617
Clinoril Tablets (Less than 1 in 100) 1618
Cognex Capsules (Frequent) 1901
ColBENEMID Tablets 1622
Colestid Tablets 2591
Cozaar Tablets (Less than 1%) 1628
Cytovene-IV (One report) 2103
Demadex Tablets and Injection 686
Didronel Tablets 1984
Dolobid Tablets (Less than 1 in 100) 1654
Effexor (Infrequent) 2719
Engerix-B Unit-Dose Vials 2482
Hivid Tablets (Less than 1% to less than 3%) 2121
Hylorel Tablets (1.7%) 985
Hytrin Capsules (At least 1%) 430
Hyzaar Tablets 1677
▲Imovax Rabies Vaccine (Up to 6%) 881
INFeD (Iron Dextran Injection, USP) 2345
Intron A (Less than 5%) 2364
Keflex Pulvules & Oral Suspension 914
Keftab Tablets 915
Lamictal Tablets (Rare) 1112
Lescol Capsules (Rare) 2267
Lotensin Tablets 834
Lotensin HCT (0.3% or more) 837
Luvox Tablets (Infrequent) 2544
M-M-R II 1687
M-R-VAX II 1689
Meruvax II (Rare) 1697
Mevacor Tablets (Rare) 1699

(▣ Described in PDR For Nonprescription Drugs) Incidence data in parenthesis; ▲ 3% or more (◉ Described in PDR For Ophthalmology)

Arthritis **Side Effects Index** 1228

Miacalcin Nasal Spray (Less than 1%) 2275
Monopril Tablets 757
Neurontin Capsules (Infrequent) 1922
Noroxin Tablets 1715
Noroxin Tablets 2048
OptiPranolol (Metipranolol 0.3%) Sterile Ophthalmic Solution (A small number of patients) ⊙ 258
Orthoclone OKT3 Sterile Solution 1837
Paxil Tablets (Infrequent) 2505
Permax Tablets (Infrequent) 575
Pneumovax 23 1725
Pnu-Imune 23 (Rare) 1393
Pravachol (Rare) 765
PREVACID Delayed-Release Capsules (Less than 1%) 2562
Prinivil Tablets (0.3% to 1.0%) 1733
Prinzide Tablets 1737
Procan SR Tablets (Common) 1926
Procardia Capsules (Less than 0.5%) 1971
Proleukin for Injection (1%) 797
ProSom Tablets (Infrequent) 449
Prostin E2 Suppository 2634
Prozac Pulvules & Liquid, Oral Solution (Infrequent) 919
Questran Light 769
Questran Powder 770
▲ Rabies Vaccine, Imovax Rabies I.D. (Less frequent; up to 6%) 883
Recombivax HB 1744
Risperdal (Rare) 1301
Roferon-A Injection (Rare; less than 3%) 2145
Sandostatin Injection (Less than 1%) 2292
Serzone Tablets (Infrequent) 771
▲ TheraCys BCG Live (Intravesical) (1.0% to 7.1%) 897
Tilade (Less than 1%) 996
▲ Tonocard Tablets (4.7%) 531
Vascor (200, 300 and 400 mg) Tablets (0.5 to 2.0%) 1587
Vaseretic Tablets 1765
Vasotec I.V. 1768
Vasotec Tablets (0.5% to 1.0%) 1771
▲ Videx Tablets, Powder for Oral Solution, & Pediatric Powder for Oral Solution (Less than 1% to 12%) 720
▲ Wellbutrin Tablets (3.1%) 1204
Zefazone 2654
Zestoretic 2850
Zestril Tablets (0.3% to 1.0%) 2854
Zocor Tablets (Rare) 1775

Arthritis, acute gouty, precipitation of
Benemid Tablets 1611
Pyrazinamide Tablets 1398

Arthritis, migratory
Elavil 2838
Endep Tablets 2174

Arthropathy, Charcot-like
Aristocort Suspension (Forte Parenteral) 1027
Aristocort Suspension (Intralesional) 1025
Aristospan Suspension (Intra-articular) 1033
Celestone Soluspan Suspension 2347
Dalalone D.P. Injectable 1011
Decadron Phosphate Injection 1637
Decadron Phosphate with Xylocaine Injection, Sterile 1639
Decadron-LA Sterile Suspension 1646
Depo-Medrol Single-Dose Vial 2600
Depo-Medrol Sterile Aqueous Suspension 2597
Hydeltrasol Injection, Sterile 1665
Hydeltra-T.B.A. Sterile Suspension 1667
Hydrocortone Acetate Sterile Suspension 1669

Arthropathy, unspecified
Didronel Tablets 1984
Hivid Tablets (Less than 1% to less than 3%) 2121
Kerlone Tablets (Less than 2%) 2436
▲ Lescol Capsules (4.0%) 2267
Ticlid Tablets (Rare) 2156

Arthrosis
Ambien Tablets (Rare) 2416
Anafranil Capsules (Infrequent) 803
▲ Aredia for Injection (At least 10%) 810
Betaseron for SC Injection 658
Depakote Tablets (Greater than 1% but not more than 5%) 415
Dilacor XR Extended-release Capsules (1.0%) 2018
Effexor (Infrequent) 2719
Foscavir Injection (Less than 1%) 547
Intron A (Less than 5%) 2364
Luvox Tablets (Rare) 2544
Miacalcin Nasal Spray (1% to 3%) 2275
Norvasc Tablets (More than 0.1% to 1%) 1940
Paxil Tablets (Rare) 2505
Risperdal (Rare) 1301
Zoloft Tablets (Infrequent) 2217

Ascaris, appearance in mouth and nose
Mintezol 1704

Ascites
Betaseron for SC Injection 658
Clomid 1514
Cosmegen Injection 1626
Foscavir Injection (Less than 1%) 547
Humegon 1824
Hyskon Hysteroscopy Fluid (Rare) 1595
Inocor Lactate Injection (1 case) 2309
Lutrepulse for Injection (Rare) 980
Oncaspar 2028
Profasi (chorionic gonadotropin for injection, USP) 2450
▲ Prograf (5% to 27%) 1042
▲ Proleukin for Injection (4%) 797
Risperdal (Rare) 1301
Serophene (clomiphene citrate tablets, USP) 2451

Aseptic meningitis syndrome
Children's Advil Suspension (Less than 1%) 2692
Clinoril Tablets (Less than 1 in 100) 1618
Gamimune N, 5% Immune Globulin Intravenous (Human), 5% (Infrequent) 619
Gamimune N, 10% Immune Globulin Intravenous (Human), 10% (Infrequent) 621
Children's Motrin Ibuprofen Oral Suspension (Less than 1%) 1546
Motrin Tablets (Less than 1%) 2625
Orthoclone OKT3 Sterile Solution 1837
Trimpex Tablets (Rare) 2163

Aseptic necrosis of femoral/humeral heads
Aristocort Suspension (Forte Parenteral) 1027
Aristocort Suspension (Intralesional) 1025
Aristocort Tablets 1022
Aristospan Suspension (Intra-articular) 1033
Aristospan Suspension (Intralesional) 1032
Celestone Soluspan Suspension 2347
CORTENEMA 2535
Cortone Acetate Sterile Suspension 1623
Cortone Acetate Tablets 1624
Dalalone D.P. Injectable 1011
Decadron Elixir 1633
Decadron Phosphate Injection 1637
Decadron Phosphate Respihaler 1642
Decadron Phosphate Turbinaire 1645
Decadron Phosphate with Xylocaine Injection, Sterile 1639
Decadron Tablets 1635
Decadron-LA Sterile Suspension 1646
Deltasone Tablets 2595
Depo-Medrol Single-Dose Vial 2600
Depo-Medrol Sterile Aqueous Suspension 2597
Dexacort Phosphate in Respihaler 458
Dexacort Phosphate in Turbinaire 459
Florinef Acetate Tablets 505
Hydeltrasol Injection, Sterile 1665
Hydeltra-T.B.A. Sterile Suspension 1667
Hydrocortone Acetate Sterile Suspension 1669
Hydrocortone Phosphate Injection, Sterile 1670
Hydrocortone Tablets 1672
Medrol 2621
Pediapred Oral Liquid 995
Prelone Syrup 1787
Solu-Cortef Sterile Powder 2641
Solu-Medrol Sterile Powder 2643

Aspermatogenesis
Velban Vials 1484

Asphyxia
Bentyl 1501
Compazine 2470
Navane Intramuscular 2202
Stelazine 2514
Thorazine 2523

Aspiration
Clozaril Tablets 2252
Compazine 2470
Risperdal (Rare) 1301

Asterixis
Bumex (0.1%) 2093
Ceptaz 1081
Depakene 413
Depakote Tablets 415
Dilantin Infatabs (Rare) 1908
Dilantin Kapseals (Rare) 1906
Dilantin Parenteral (Rare) 1910
Dilantin-125 Suspension (Rare) 1911
Fortaz 1100
Gelfoam Sterile Sponge 2608
Orthoclone OKT3 Sterile Solution 1837

Asthenia
Accutane Capsules 2076
▲ Adalat Capsules (10 mg and 20 mg) (About 10% to 12%) 587
▲ Adalat CC (4%) 589
Adenoscan (Less than 1%) 1024
AeroBid Inhaler System (1-3%) 1005
Aerobid-M Inhaler System (1-3%) 1005
Albalon Solution with Liquifilm ⊙ 231
Aldactazide 2413
Aldoclor Tablets 1598
Aldomet Ester HCl Injection 1602
Aldomet Oral 1600
Aldoril Tablets 1604
All-Flex Arcing Spring Diaphragm (See also Ortho Diaphragm Kits) 1865
Altace Capsules (0.3% to 2.0%) 1232
Alupent Tablets (0.2%) 669
Ambien Tablets (Infrequent) 2416
Amicar Syrup, Tablets, and Injection 1267
Anafranil Capsules (Up to 2%) 803
Ana-Kit Anaphylaxis Emergency Treatment Kit (Common) 617
Anatuss LA Tablets 1542
Ancobon Capsules 2079
Ansaid Tablets (1-3%) 2579
Apresazide Capsules 808
Arfonad Ampuls 2080
Artane 1368
▲ Asacol Delayed-Release Tablets (7%) 1979
Asendin Tablets (Less frequent) 1369
Atamet 572
Atgam Sterile Solution (Less than 1%) 2581
▲ Ativan Tablets (4.2%) 2700
Atromid-S Capsules (Less often) 2701
▲ Axid Pulvules (3.1%) 1427
Azactam for Injection (Less than 1%) 734
Bactrim DS Tablets 2084
Bactrim I.V. Infusion 2082
Bactrim 2084
▲ Bentyl (7%) 1501
Betagan ⊙ 233
▲ Betapace Tablets (4% to 13%) 641
▲ Betaseron for SC Injection (49%) 658
Betimol 0.25%, 0.5% (1% to 5%) ⊙ 261
Blocadren Tablets (0.6%) 1614
Brevibloc Injection (Less than 1%) 1808
▲ Bromfed-DM Cough Syrup (Among most frequent) 1786
Bronkometer Aerosol 2302
Bronkosol Solution 2302
Brontex 1981
Bumex (0.2%) 2093
BuSpar (2%) 737
Cafergot 2251
Capoten 739
Capozide 742
Carbocaine Hydrochloride Injection 2303
▲ Cardene Capsules (4.2-5.8%) 2095
Cardene I.V. (0.7%) 2709
Cardene SR Capsules (0.9%) 2097
Cardizem CD Capsules (1.8% to 2.6%) 1506
▲ Cardizem SR Capsules (2.8% to 5%) 1510
Cardizem Injectable (Less than 1%) 1508
Cardizem Tablets (1.2%) 1512
Cardura Tablets (1%) 2186
▲ Cartrol Tablets (7.1%) 410
Catapres Tablets (About 10 in 100 patients) 674
Catapres-TTS (Less frequent) 675
Caverject (Less than 1%) 2583
Ceclor Pulvules & Suspension 1431
▲ CellCept Capsules (13.7% to 16.1%) 2099
Ceredase 1065
Cipro I.V. (1% or less) 595
Cipro I.V. Pharmacy Bulk Package (Less than 1%) 597
Cipro Tablets (Less than 1%) 592
Claritin (2% or fewer patients) 2349
Claritin-D (Less frequent) 2350
Clinoril Tablets (Less than 1 in 100) 1618
Clomid 1514
Clozaril Tablets (1%) 2252
Cogentin 1621
Cognex Capsules (2%) 1901
ColBENEMID Tablets 1622
Colestid Tablets (Infrequent) 2591
▲ Combipres Tablets (About 10%) 677
Cortone Acetate Sterile Suspension 1623
Cortone Acetate Tablets 1624
Cozaar Tablets (1% or greater) 1628
Cystospaz 1963
Cytotec (Infrequent) 2424
▲ Cytovene (6%) 2103
D.A. Chewable Tablets 951
DDAVP (Up to 2%) 2017
Dalmane Capsules 2173
Danocrine Capsules 2307
▲ Dantrium Capsules (Among most frequent) 1982
Dapsone Tablets USP 1284
Daranide Tablets 1633
Darvon-N/Darvocet-N 1433
Darvon 1435
Darvon-N Suspension & Tablets 1433
Daypro Caplets (Less than 1%) 2426
Decadron Elixir 1633
Decadron Phosphate Respihaler 1642
Decadron Phosphate Turbinaire 1645
Decadron Phosphate with Xylocaine Injection, Sterile 1639
Deconamine Chewable Tablets 1320
Deconamine CX Cough and Cold Liquid and Tablets 1319
Deconamine 1320
Deconsal C Expectorant Syrup 456
Deconsal Pediatric Capsules 454
Deconsal Pediatric Syrup 457
Deconsal II Tablets 454
Demadex Tablets and Injection (2.0%) 686
Demerol 2308
Demulen 2428
Depakene 413
▲ Depakote Tablets (10%) 415
▲ Depo-Provera Contraceptive Injection (More than 5%) 2602
Desmopressin Acetate Rhinal Tube (Up to 2%) 979
Desyrel and Desyrel Dividose 503
Dilacor XR Extended-release Capsules (1.7% to 3.6%) 2018
Dilatrate-SR 2398
Dilaudid-HP Injection (Less frequent) 1337
Dilaudid-HP Lyophilized Powder 250 mg (Less frequent) 1337
Dilaudid Tablets and Liquid (Less frequent) 1339
Dimetane-DC Cough Syrup 2059
Dimetane-DX Cough Syrup 2059
Diprivan Injection (Less than 1%) 2833
Ditropan 1516
Diucardin Tablets 2718
Diupres Tablets 1650
Diuril Oral Suspension 1653
Diuril Sodium Intravenous 1652
Diuril Tablets 1653
Dolobid Tablets (Less than 1 in 100) 1654
Donnatal 2060
Donnatal Extentabs 2061
Donnatal Tablets 2060
Doral Tablets 2664
▲ Duragesic Transdermal System (10% or more) 1288
Dura-Tap/PD Capsules 2867
Dura-Vent/DA Tablets 953
Dura-Vent Tablets 952
Dyazide 2479
DynaCirc Capsules (Up to 1.2%) 2256
Dyrenium Capsules (Rare) 2481
▲ Effexor (2% to 16.9%) 2719
Elavil 2838
Eldepryl Tablets 2550

(▣ Described in PDR For Nonprescription Drugs) Incidence data in parenthesis; ▲ 3% or more (⊙ Described in PDR For Ophthalmology)

1229 **Side Effects Index** **Asthenia**

Emete-con Intramuscular/Intravenous 2198
Empirin with Codeine Tablets (Occasional) 1093
Endep Tablets 2174
Enduron Tablets 420
Engerix-B Unit-Dose Vials (Less than 1%) 2482
Entex PSE Tablets 1987
EpiPen 790
▲ Epogen for Injection (7% to 13%) 489
Ergamisol Tablets (10 out of 463 patients) 1292
Esidrix Tablets 821
Esimil Tablets 822
Eskalith 2485
Estrace Cream and Tablets 749
▲ Ethmozine Tablets (2% to 5%) 2041
Etrafon 2355
Fansidar Tablets 2114
Fedahist Gyrocaps 2401
Fedahist Timecaps 2401
Felbatol (Frequent) 2666
Feldene Capsules (Less than 1%) 1965
Fiorinal with Codeine Capsules 2262
Flagyl 375 Capsules 2434
Flexeril Tablets (Less than 1%) 1661
Floxin I.V. (Less than 1%) 1571
Floxin Tablets (200 mg, 300 mg, 400 mg) (Less than 1%) 1567
▲ Fludara for Injection (9% to 65%) 663
Flumadine Tablets & Syrup (1.4%) 1015
▲ Foscavir Injection (5% or greater) 547
Sterile FUDR 2118
Gantanol Tablets 2119
Gantrisin 2120
▲ Glucotrol XL Extended Release Tablets (10.1%) 1968
Guaimax-D Tablets 792
Halcion Tablets (Rare) 2611
Hivid Tablets (Less than 1% to less than 3%) 2121
Humatrope Vials (Infrequent) 1443
Hydeltrasol Injection, Sterile 1665
HydroDIURIL Tablets 1674
Hydropres Tablets 1675
Hyperstat I.V. Injection (2%) 2363
▲ Hytrin Capsules (At least 1% to 11.3%) 430
Hyzaar Tablets (1% or greater) 1677
Imdur (Less than or equal to 5%) 1323
▲ Imitrex Injection (4.9%) 1103
Imitrex Tablets (Less than 1% to 2%) 1106
Inderal 2728
Inderal LA Long Acting Capsules 2730
Inderide Tablets 2732
Inderide LA Long Acting Capsules 2734
INFeD (Iron Dextran Injection, USP) 2345
▲ Intron A (Less than 5% to 24%) 2364
Inversine Tablets 1686
Iopidine 0.5% (Less than 3%) ⊙ 221
Ismelin Tablets 827
Ismo Tablets (Fewer than 1%) 2738
Isoetharine Inhalation Solution, USP, Arm-a-Med 551
Isuprel Hydrochloride Injection 1:5000 2311
Isuprel Hydrochloride Solution 1:200 & 1:100 2313
Isuprel Mistometer 2312
K-Phos Neutral Tablets 639
▲ Kerlone Tablets (7.1%) 2436
Kutrase Capsules 2402
▲ Kytril Injection (5%) 2490
▲ Kytril Tablets (5% to 14%) 2492
Lamictal Tablets (More than 1%) 1112
Lanoxicaps 1117
Lanoxin Elixir Pediatric 1120
Lanoxin Injection 1123
Lanoxin Injection Pediatric 1126
Lanoxin Tablets 1128
Lariam Tablets (Less than 1%) 2128
Larodopa Tablets (Relatively frequent) 2129
Lasix Injection, Oral Solution and Tablets 1240
Lescol Capsules (Rare) 2267
▲ Leukine for IV Infusion (66%) 1271
▲ Leustatin (9%) 1834
Levatol (1.6%) 2403
Levbid Extended-Release Tablets 2405
Levlen/Tri-Levlen 651
▲ Levoprome (Among the most important) 1274
Levsin/Levsinex/Levbid 2405
Limbitrol 2180
Lioresal Intrathecal (1 to 15 of 214 patients) 1596
▲ Lioresal Tablets (5-15%) 829
Lithonate/Lithotabs/Lithobid 2543
Lodine Capsules and Tablets (More than 1% but less than 3%) 2743
Lopid Tablets 1917
Lopressor HCT Tablets 832
Lotensin Tablets 834
Lotensin HCT (0.3% to more than 1%) 837
Lotrel Capsules 840
Loxitane 1378
▲ Lozol Tablets (Less than or greater than 5%) 2022
▲ Ludiomil Tablets (4%) 843
▲ Lupron Depot 3.75 mg (8.4%) 2556
▲ Lupron Depot 7.5 mg (5.4%) 2559
▲ Lupron Injection (5% or more) 2555
▲ Luvox Tablets (14%) 2544
MS Contin Tablets (Less frequent) 1994
MSIR (Infrequent) 1997
Macrobid Capsules 1988
Macrodantin Capsules 1989
Marcaine Hydrochloride with Epinephrine 1:200,000 2316
Marcaine Hydrochloride Injection 2316
Marcaine Spinal 2319
Marinol (Dronabinol) Capsules (Greater than 1%) 2231
Matulane Capsules 2131
Maxair Autohaler 1492
Maxair Inhaler (Less than 1%) 1494
Maxaquin Tablets (Less than 1%) 2440
Maxzide 1380
▲ Megace Oral Suspension (2% to 6%) 699
Mepergan Injection 2753
▲ Mepron Suspension (8%) 1135
Mestinon Injectable 1253
Mestinon 1254
Methadone Hydrochloride Oral Concentrate 2233
Methadone Hydrochloride Oral Solution & Tablets 2235
Mevacor Tablets (1.2% to 1.7%; rare) 1699
▲ Mexitil Capsules (1.9% to 5%) 678
Micronor Tablets 1872
Midamor Tablets (Between 1% and 3%) 1703
▲ Minipress Capsules (6.5%) 1937
▲ Minizide Capsules (6.5%) 1938
Mithracin 607
Modicon 1872
▲ Moduretic Tablets (3% to 8%) 1705
Monopril Tablets (0.2% to 1.4%) 757
Mustargen 1709
Mycobutin Capsules (1%) 1957
Mykrox Tablets (Less than 2%) 993
Myleran Tablets 1143
Myochrysine Injection 1711
▲ Nalfon 200 Pulvules & Nalfon Tablets (5.4%) 917
Nardil (Common) 1920
Navane Capsules and Concentrate 2201
Navane Intramuscular 2202
▲ Navelbine Injection (Up to 27%) 1145
NegGram 2323
Neoral (Rare) 2276
▲ Neupogen for Injection (4%) 495
Neurontin Capsules (Frequent) 1922
▲ Nicoderm (nicotine transdermal system) (3% to 9%) 1518
Nitrolingual Spray 2027
Nitrostat Tablets (Occasional) 1925
Norflex 1496
Norgesic 1496
Norisodrine with Calcium Iodide Syrup 442
Normodyne Tablets (1%) 2379
Noroxin Tablets (Less frequent or 0.3% to 1.3%) 1715
Noroxin Tablets (Less frequent or 0.3% to 1.3%) 2048
Norpramin Tablets 1526
Norvasc Tablets (Less than 1% to 2%) 1940
Novahistine DH 2462
Novahistine DMX ▣ 822
Novahistine Elixir ▣ 823
Novahistine Expectorant 2463
Nubain Injection (1% or less) 935
Nucofed 2051
Nydrazid Injection 508
Ocupress Ophthalmic Solution, 1% Sterile (Occasional) ⊙ 309
OptiPranolol (Metipranolol 0.3%) Sterile Ophthalmic Solution (A small number of patients) ⊙ 258
Oramorph SR (Morphine Sulfate Sustained Release Tablets) (Less frequent) 2236
Orap Tablets 1050
Oretic Tablets 443
▲ Orlamm (3% to 9%) 2239
Ornade Spansule Capsules 2502
Ortho-Cyclen/Ortho-Tri-Cyclen 1858
Ortho Diaphragm Kits—All-Flex Arcing Spring; Ortho Coil Spring; Ortho-White Flat Spring 1865
Ortho Diaphragm Kit-Coil Spring 1865
Ortho-Est 1869
Ortho-Novum 1872
Ortho-Cyclen/Ortho Tri-Cyclen 1858
Ortho-White Diaphragm Kit-Flat Spring (See also Ortho Diaphragm Kits) 1865
Orthoclone OKT3 Sterile Solution 1837
PMB 200 and PMB 400 2783
Pamelor 2280
▲ Paraplatin for Injection (11% to 43%) 705
Parlodel 2281
Parnate Tablets 2503
▲ Paxil Tablets (2.9% to 15.0%) 2505
Penetrex Tablets (Less than 1% but more than or equal to 0.1%) 2031
Pentasa (Less than 1%) 1527
Pentaspan Injection 937
Pepcid Injection (Infrequent) 1722
Pepcid (Infrequent) 1720
▲ Permax Tablets (4.2%) 575
Phenergan with Codeine 2777
Phenergan VC 2779
Phenergan VC with Codeine 2781
Placidyl Capsules 448
Plaquenil Sulfate Tablets 2328
▲ Plendil Extended-Release Tablets (2.2% to 3.9%) 527
Pneumovax 23 1725
Polycitra Syrup 578
Polycitra-K Crystals 579
Polycitra-K Oral Solution 579
Polycitra-LC 578
Polymyxin B Sulfate, Aerosporin Brand Sterile Powder 1154
Pondimin Tablets 2066
Pravachol (Rare) 765
PREVACID Delayed-Release Capsules (Less than 1%) 2562
Prilosec Delayed-Release Capsules (1.1% to 1.3%) 529
Primaxin I.M. 1727
Primaxin I.V. (Less than 0.2%) 1729
▲ Prinivil Tablets (1.3% to 6.9%) 1733
Prinzide Tablets (1.8%) 1737
Pro-Banthine Tablets 2052
Procan SR Tablets (Occasional) 1926
▲ Procardia Capsules (Approximately 10% to 12%) 1971
▲ Procardia XL Extended Release Tablets (Less than 3% to 12%) 1972
▲ Procrit for Injection (7% to 13%) 1841
Proglycem 580
▲ Prograf (7% to 52%) 1042
▲ Proleukin for Injection (53%) 797
▲ ProSom Tablets (11%) 449
Prostigmin Injectable 1260
Prostigmin Tablets 1261
Prostin E2 Suppository 2634
Protostat Tablets 1883
Proventil Repetabs Tablets (2%) 2386
Proventil Syrup (Less than 1 of 100 patients) 2385
Proventil Tablets (2%) 2386
▲ Prozac Pulvules & Liquid, Oral Solution (4.4% to 15%) 919
Pulmozyme Inhalation 1064
Quadrinal Tablets 1350
Quarzan Capsules 2181
Quinaglute Dura-Tabs Tablets (2%) 649
RMS Suppositories 2657
Recombivax HB (Equal to or greater than 1%) 1744
Regitine 846
Relafen Tablets (1%) 2510
Restoril Capsules (1-2%) 2284
▲ Retrovir Capsules (8.6% to 69%) 1158
▲ Retrovir I.V. Infusion (19% to 69%) 1163
▲ Retrovir Syrup (8.6% to 69%) 1158
Rifamate Capsules 1530
Rifater 1532
Risperdal 1301
Robinul Forte Tablets 2072
Robinul Injectable 2072
Robinul Tablets 2072
Rocaltrol Capsules 2141
Roferon-A Injection (Less than 0.5%) 2145
Romazicon (1% to 3%) 2147
Rondec Oral Drops 953
Rondec Syrup 953
Rondec Tablet 953
Rondec-DM Oral Drops 954
Rondec-DM Syrup 954
Rondec-TR Tablet 953
Rowasa (0.12% to 1.2%) 2548
Roxanol 2243
Rum-K Syrup 1005
Rythmol Tablets–150mg, 225mg, 300mg (0.6 to 2.4%) 1352
▲ Salagen Tablets (6% to 12%) 1489
Sandimmune (Rare) 2286
Sandostatin Injection (1% to 4%) 2292
Sanorex Tablets 2294
Sansert Tablets 2295
Scleromate (Rare) 1891
Seldane Tablets (0.6% to 0.9%) 1536
Seldane-D Extended-Release Tablets 1538
Semprex-D Capsules (2%) 463
Semprex-D Capsules (2%) 1167
Sensorcaine 559
Septra 1174
Septra I.V. Infusion 1169
Septra I.V. Infusion ADD-Vantage Vials 1171
Septra 1174
Ser-Ap-Es Tablets 849
Serentil 684
▲ Serzone Tablets (11%) 771
Sinemet Tablets 943
Sinemet CR Tablets 944
Sinequan (Occasional) 2205
Solganal Suspension (Rare) 2388
Soma Compound w/Codeine Tablets (Very rare) 2676
Soma Compound Tablets (Very rare) 2675
Soma Tablets 2674
Sorbitrate 2843
Stadol (1% or greater) 775
Surmontil Capsules 2811
Sus-Phrine Injection 1019
Symmetrel Capsules and Syrup (0.1% to 1%) 946
Synarel Nasal Solution for Endometriosis (Less than 1%) 2152
Syn-Rx Tablets 465
Syn-Rx DM Tablets 466
Talacen (Infrequent) 2333
Talwin Injection (Infrequent) 2334
Talwin Compound (Infrequent) 2335
Talwin Injection (Infrequent) 2334
Talwin Nx (Infrequent) 2336
▲ Tambocor Tablets (Less than 1% to 4.9%) 1497
▲ Tenex Tablets (Up to 10%) 2074
Tenoretic Tablets 2845
Tensilon Injectable 1261
Thalitone 1245
Thioplex (Thiotepa For Injection) 1281
Ticlid Tablets (0.5% to 1.0%) 2156
Timolide Tablets (1.9%) 1748
Timoptic in Ocudose (Less frequent) 1753
Timoptic Sterile Ophthalmic Solution (Less frequent) 1751
Timoptic-XE 1755
Tofranil Ampuls 854
Tofranil Tablets 856
Tofranil-PM Capsules 857
▲ Tolectin (200, 400 and 600 mg) (3 to 9%) 1581
Tonocard Tablets (Less than 1%) 531
Toradol (1% or less) 2159
Tornalate Solution for Inhalation, 0.2% (Less than 1%) 956
Trancopal Caplets 2337
Trandate Tablets (1%) 1185
Triavil Tablets 1757
Levlen/Tri-Levlen 651
Trinalin Repetabs Tablets 1330
Trusopt Sterile Ophthalmic Solution (Infrequent) 1760
Tussend 1783
Tussend Expectorant 1785
Tympagesic Ear Drops 2342
Uroqid-Acid No. 2 Tablets 640
▲ Valtrex Caplets (3% to 4%) 1194
Vantin for Oral Suspension and Vantin Tablets (Less than 1%) 2646
▲ Vascor (200, 300 and 400 mg) Tablets (0.5 to 13.95%) 1587
Vaseretic Tablets (2.4%) 1765
Vasotec I.V. 1768
Vasotec Tablets (1.1% to 1.6%) 1771
Velban Vials 1484

(▣ Described in PDR For Nonprescription Drugs) Incidence data in parenthesis; ▲ 3% or more (⊙ Described in PDR For Ophthalmology)

Asthenia Side Effects Index 1230

Ventolin Syrup (Less than 1 of 100) 1202
Ventolin Tablets (2 of 100 patients) 1203
Versed Injection (Less than 1%) 2170
▲ Videx Tablets, Powder for Oral Solution, & Pediatric Powder for Oral Solution (4% to 42%) 720
Virazole 1264
▲ Visken Tablets (4%) 2299
Vivactil Tablets 1774
Volmax Extended-Release Tablets 1788
Wygesic Tablets 2827
▲ Xanax Tablets (7.1%) 2649
Yutopar Intravenous Injection (Infrequent) 570
Zaroxolyn Tablets 1000
Zebeta Tablets (0.4% to 1.5%) 1413
▲ Zerit Capsules (2% to 28%) 729
Zestoretic (1.8%) 2850
▲ Zestril Tablets (1.3% to 6.9%) 2854
Ziac 1415
Zocor Tablets (1.6%; rare) 1775
Zofran Tablets (Up to 2%) 1217
▲ Zoladex (11%) 2858
Zoloft Tablets (Frequent) 2217
Zovirax (1.2%) 1219
Zyloprim Tablets (Less than 1%) 1226

Asthma, allergic

Fluvirin (Rare) 460
Influenza Virus Vaccine, Trivalent, Types A and B (chromatograph- and filter-purified subviron antigen) FluShield, 1995-1996 Formula (Rare) 2736

Asthma, bronchial

Ansaid Tablets (Less than 1%) 2579
▲ CellCept Capsules (More than or equal to 3%) 2099
Cuprimine Capsules 1630
Cytovene-IV (One report) 2103
Decadron Phosphate Turbinaire 1645
Depen Titratable Tablets 2662
Dexacort Phosphate in Turbinaire 459
Haldol Injection, Tablets and Concentrate 1575
Halotestin Tablets 2614
Nubain Injection (1% or less) 935
Permax Tablets (Infrequent) 575
PREVACID Delayed-Release Capsules (Less than 1%) 2562
Prolixin 509
Prozac Pulvules & Liquid, Oral Solution (Infrequent) 919
Relafen Tablets (Less than 1%) 2510
Serzone Tablets (Infrequent) 771
Soma Compound Tablets 2675
Toradol 2159
Vaseretic Tablets 1765
Vasotec I.V. 1768
Vasotec Tablets (0.5% to 1.0%) 1771
Zestoretic 2850
Zyloprim Tablets (Less than 1%) 1226

Asthmatic episodes

Alupent (1% to 4%) 669
Betapace Tablets (1% to 2%) 641
Betaseron for SC Injection 658
Betoptic Ophthalmic Solution (Rare) 469
Betoptic S Ophthalmic Suspension (Rare) 471
Carmol HC 924
Cataflam (Less than 1%) 816
Cognex Capsules (Infrequent) 1901
Compazine 2470
Cortisporin Otic Solution Sterile 1087
Depo-Provera Contraceptive Injection (Fewer than 1%) 2602
Dilaudid Tablets and Liquid 1339
Dobutrex Solution Vials 1439
Duragesic Transdermal System (Less than 1%) 1288
Duvoid (Infrequent) 2044
Easprin 1914
Effexor (Infrequent) 2719
Eldepryl Tablets 2550
Empirin with Codeine Tablets 1093
Engerix-B Unit-Dose Vials 2482
Esimil Tablets 822
Estrace Cream and Tablets 749
Ethmozine Tablets (Less than 2%) 2041
Etrafon 2355
Heparin Lock Flush Solution 2725
Heparin Sodium Injection 2726
Heparin Sodium Injection, USP, Sterile Solution 2615
Heparin Sodium Vials (Rare) 1441
Imitrex Tablets (Infrequent) 1106
Indocin Capsules (Less than 1%) 1680
Indocin I.V. (Less than 1%) 1684
Indocin (Less than 1%) 1680
Intal Capsules 987
Iopidine 0.5% (Less than 1%) .... ⊙ 221
Ismelin Tablets 827
Isopto Carbachol Ophthalmic Solution .... ⊙ 223
Isuprel Hydrochloride Solution 1:200 & 1:100 2313
Kutrase Capsules 2402
Levoprome 1274
Lodine Capsules and Tablets (Less than 1%) 2743
Lotensin Tablets 834
Luvox Tablets (Infrequent) 2544
Mellaril 2269
Minocin Oral Suspension 1385
Monoket (Fewer than 1%) 2406
Paxil Tablets (Infrequent) 2505
Phenergan Injection 2773
Phenergan Tablets 2775
Pred Mild .... ⊙ 253
Prinzide Tablets 1737
▲ Prograf (Greater than 3%) 1042
Prolixin 509
ProSom Tablets (Infrequent) 449
Questran Light 769
Questran Powder 770
Quinidex Extentabs 2067
Risperdal (Rare) 1301
Robaxisal Tablets 2071
Rowasa 2548
Scleromate (Rare) 1891
Sensorcaine 559
Septra I.V. Infusion 1169
Septra I.V. Infusion ADD-Vantage Vials 1171
Serentil 684
Soma Compound w/Codeine Tablets (Rare) 2676
Soma Compound Tablets (Less common) 2675
Soma Tablets 2674
Sotradecol (Sodium Tetradecyl Sulfate Injection) 967
Stelazine 2514
Streptomycin Sulfate Injection 2208
Supprelin Injection (2% to 3%) 2056
Suprane (Less than 1%) 1813
Temaril Tablets, Syrup and Spansule Extended-Release Capsules 483
Terramycin Intramuscular Solution 2210
Thioplex (Thiotepa For Injection) 1281
Thorazine 2523
Torecan 2245
▲ Trasylol (3%) 613
Triavil Tablets 1757
Trilafon 2389
Trilisate (Rare) 2000
Urecholine 1761
▲ Videx Tablets, Powder for Oral Solution, & Pediatric Powder for Oral Solution (Less than 1% to 28%) 720
Viokase 2076
Voltaren Tablets (Less than 1%) 861
Zebeta Tablets 1413
Zemuron (Less than 1%) 1830
▲ Zerit Capsules (Fewer than 1% to 2%) 729
Zestril Tablets (0.3% to 1.0%) 2854
Ziac 1415

Asystole

Adenocard Injection 1021
Alfenta Injection 1286
Brevibloc Injection (2 Patients) 1808
Diprivan Injection 2833
Isoptin Injectable (In extreme cases) 1344
Zantac Injection (Rare) 1207

Asystole, ventricular

Procan SR Tablets (Common) 1926

Ataxia

Aldactazide 2413
Aldactone 2414
Ambien Tablets (Frequent) 2416
Anafranil Capsules (Infrequent) 803
Ancobon Capsules 2079
Ansaid Tablets (Less than 1%) 2579
Asendin Tablets (Less frequent) 1369
Atamet 572
Atrohist Plus Tablets 454
Attenuvax (Rare) 1610
Azo Gantanol Tablets 2080
Azo Gantrisin Tablets 2081
Azulfidine (Rare) 1949
Bactrim DS Tablets 2084
Bactrim I.V. Infusion 2082
Bactrim 2084
Bentyl 10 mg Capsules 1501
Betagan (Rare) .... ⊙ 233
Betapace Tablets (Rare) 641
Betaseron for SC Injection 658
▲ Bromfed-DM Cough Syrup (Among most frequent) 1786
Buprenex Injectable (Rare) 2006
BuSpar (1%) 737
Butisol Sodium Elixir & Tablets (Less than 1 in 100) 2660
Capoten 739
Capozide 742
Cardura Tablets (1%) 2186
CeeNU 693
Celontin Kapseals (Frequent) 1899
Chibroxin Sterile Ophthalmic Solution (With oral form) 1617
Cipro I.V. (1% or less) 595
Cipro I.V. Pharmacy Bulk Package (Less than 1%) 597
Cipro Tablets (Less than 1%) 592
Clozaril Tablets (1%) 2252
▲ Cognex Capsules (6%) 1901
▲ Cordarone Tablets (4 to 9%) 2712
Cozaar Tablets (Less than 1%) 1628
Cytovene (1% or less) 2103
Dalalone D.P. Injectable 1011
Dalmane Capsules 2173
Daranide Tablets 1633
Decadron-LA Sterile Suspension (Low) 1646
Demerol 2308
Depakene 413
Depakote Tablets 415
▲ Desyrel and Desyrel Dividose (1.9% to 4.9%) 503
▲ Dilantin Infatabs (Among most common) 1908
▲ Dilantin Kapseals (Among most common) 1906
▲ Dilantin Parenteral (Among most common) 1910
▲ Dilantin-125 Suspension (Among most common) 1911
▲ Dizac (Among most common) 1809
Doral Tablets 2664
Effexor (Infrequent) 2719
Elavil 2838
Endep Tablets 2174
Ergamisol Tablets (Up to 2%) 1292
Eskalith 2485
Ethmozine Tablets (Less than 2%) 2041
Etrafon 2355
Fansidar Tablets 2114
▲ Felbatol (3.5% to 6.5%) 2666
Flagyl 375 Capsules 2434
Flagyl I.V. 2247
Flexeril Tablets (Less than 1%) 1661
Floxin I.V. 1571
Floxin Tablets (200 mg, 300 mg, 400 mg) 1567
Flumadine Tablets & Syrup (0.3% to 1%) 1015
Foscavir Injection (Between 1% and 5%) 547
Gantanol Tablets 2119
Gantrisin 2120
Garamycin Injectable 2360
▲ Halcion Tablets (4.6%) 2611
Hexalen Capsules 2571
Hivid Tablets (Less than 1% to less than 3%) 2121
Hyzaar Tablets 1677
Imitrex Tablets (Infrequent) 1106
Intron A (Less than 5%) 2364
Kerlone Tablets (Less than 2%) 2436
▲ Klonopin Tablets (30%) 2126
▲ Lamictal Tablets (Among most common; 10% to 28%) 1112
Larodopa Tablets (Relatively frequent) 2129
Leukeran Tablets (Rare) 1133
Levsin/Levsinex/Levbid 2405
Librax Capsules 2176
Libritabs Tablets 2177
Librium Capsules (Some patients) 2178
Librium Injectable 2179
Limbitrol 2180
Lioresal Tablets 829
Lithium Carbonate Capsules & Tablets 2230
Lithonate/Lithotabs/Lithobid 2543
Ludiomil Tablets (Rare) 843
Luvox Tablets (Infrequent) 2544
M-M-R II (Rare) 1687
M-R-VAX II (Rare) 1689
Marinol (Dronabinol) Capsules (Greater than 1%) 2231
Matulane Capsules 2131
Maxaquin Tablets 2440
Mebaral Tablets (Less than 1 in 100) 2322
Mepergan Injection 2753
Mesantoin Tablets 2272
Methotrexate Sodium Tablets, Injection, for Injection and LPF Injection 1275
MetroGel-Vaginal 902
Milontin Kapseals 1920
Miltown Tablets 2672
▲ Mysoline (Among most frequent) 2754
Nardil (Less frequent) 1920
Nembutal Sodium Capsules (Less than 1%) 436
Nembutal Sodium Solution (Less than 1%) 438
Nembutal Sodium Suppositories (Less than 1%) 440
▲ Neurontin Capsules (Among most common; 12.5%) 1922
Noroxin Tablets 1715
Noroxin Tablets 2048
Norpramin Tablets 1526
Norvasc Tablets (Less than or equal to 0.1%) 1940
Oncovin Solution Vials & Hyporets 1466
PBZ-SR Tablets 844
PMB 200 and PMB 400 (Rare) 2783
Pamelor 2280
Parlodel 2281
Parnate Tablets 2503
Paxil Tablets (Infrequent) 2505
Peganone Tablets (Rare) 446
Penetrex Tablets (Less than 0.1%) 2031
Permax Tablets (1.6%) 575
Phenergan Injection 2773
Phenergan Tablets 2775
Phenobarbital Elixir and Tablets (Less than 1 in 100 patients) 1469
Placidyl Capsules 448
Plaquenil Sulfate Tablets 2328
Polymyxin B Sulfate, Aerosporin Brand Sterile Powder 1154
Pondimin Tablets 2066
Prinivil Tablets (0.3% to 1.0%) 1733
Prinzide Tablets 1737
Procardia XL Extended Release Tablets (1% or less) 1972
▲ Prograf (Greater than 3%) 1042
ProSom Tablets (Rare) 449
Protostat Tablets 1883
Prozac Pulvules & Liquid, Oral Solution (Infrequent) 919
Quinaglute Dura-Tabs Tablets 649
Quinidex Extentabs 2067
Restoril Capsules (Less than 1%) 2284
Rifadin 1528
Rifamate Capsules 1530
Rifater 1532
Rimactane Capsules 847
▲ Risperdal (17% to 34%) 1301
Robaxin Injectable 2070
Roferon-A Injection (Less than 1%) 2145
▲ Romazicon (10%) 2147
Rythmol Tablets–150mg, 225mg, 300mg (0.3 to 1.6%) 1352
Sansert Tablets 2295
Seconal Sodium Pulvules (Less than 1 in 100) 1474
Septra 1174
Septra I.V. Infusion 1169
Septra I.V. Infusion ADD-Vantage Vials 1171
Septra 1174
Serax Capsules (Rare) 2810
Serax Tablets (Rare) 2810
Serentil 684
Serzone Tablets (2%) 771
Sinemet Tablets 943
Sinequan (Infrequent) 2205
Soma Compound w/Codeine Tablets 2676
Soma Compound Tablets (Very rare to less frequent) 2675
Soma Tablets 2674
Surmontil Capsules 2811
Symmetrel Capsules and Syrup (1% to 5%) 946
Tambocor Tablets (1% to less than 3%) 1497
Taxol (Rare; less than 1%) 714
Temaril Tablets, Syrup and Spansule Extended-Release Capsules 483
Tofranil Ampuls 854
Tofranil Tablets 856
Tofranil-PM Capsules 857
▲ Tonocard Tablets (0.2-10.8%) 531

(Described in PDR For Nonprescription Drugs) Incidence data in parenthesis; ▲ 3% or more (⊙ Described in PDR For Ophthalmology)

1231 Side Effects Index ADH syndrome, inappropriate

Tornalate Solution for Inhalation, 0.2% (Less than 1%) ... 956
Tranxene ... 451
Triavil Tablets ... 1757
Trilafon ... 2389
Tussend ... 1783
▲ Valium Injectable (Among most common) ... 2182
▲ Valium Tablets (Among most common) ... 2183
▲ Valrelease Capsules (Among most common) ... 2169
Vaseretic Tablets ... 1765
Vasotec I.V. ... 1768
Vasotec Tablets (0.5% to 1.0%) ... 1771
Versed Injection (Less than 1%) ... 2170
▲ Videx Tablets, Powder for Oral Solution, & Pediatric Powder for Oral Solution (Less than 1% to 8%) ... 720
Vivactil Tablets ... 1774
Wellbutrin Tablets (Frequent) ... 1204
Xanax Tablets ... 2649
Yohimex Tablets ... 1363
Zarontin Capsules ... 1928
Zarontin Syrup ... 1929
Zestoretic ... 2850
Zestril Tablets (0.3% to 1.0%) ... 2854
Zoloft Tablets (Infrequent) ... 2217

Ataxia, cerebellar
JE-VAX (One case) ... 886

Atelectasis
Betaseron for SC Injection ... 658
Dalgan Injection (Less than 1%) ... 538
Effexor (Rare) ... 2719
Humegon ... 1824
Metrodin (urofollitropin for injection) ... 2446
Pergonal (menotropins for injection, USP) ... 2448
▲ Prograf (5% to 28%) ... 1042
Virazole (Infrequent) ... 1264

Athetosis
Versed Injection (Less than 1%) ... 2170

Atrial arrhythmias
Adalat Capsules (10 mg and 20 mg) (1 in 150 patients) ... 587
Asendin Tablets (Very rare) ... 1369
Felbatol ... 2666
Foscavir Injection (Less than 1%) ... 547
Hyperstat I.V. Injection ... 2363
Imdur (Less than or equal to 5%) ... 1323
Mexitil Capsules (1 in 1,000) ... 678
Monopril Tablets (0.4% to 1.0%) ... 757
▲ Proleukin for Injection (8%) ... 797
Romazicon (Less than 1%) ... 2147
Tornalate Solution for Inhalation, 0.2% (Less than 1%) ... 956
Trasylol (2%) ... 613

Atrial contractions, premature
Adenocard Injection ... 1021
Brethaire Inhaler ... 813
Cognex Capsules (Rare) ... 1901
Diprivan Injection (Less than 1%) ... 2833
Emete-con Intramuscular/Intravenous ... 2198
Neurontin Capsules (Rare) ... 1922
▲ Proleukin for Injection (4%) ... 797
Risperdal (Rare) ... 1301
Sodium Polystyrene Sulfonate Suspension ... 2244
Yutopar Intravenous Injection ... 570

Atrial depression
Dilantin Parenteral ... 1910

Atrial flutter
Anafranil Capsules (Rare) ... 803
Aredia for Injection (Up to 1%) ... 810
Cardizem Injectable (Less than 1%) ... 1508
Cipro Tablets (Less than 1%) ... 592
Cognex Capsules (Infrequent) ... 1901
Ethmozine Tablets (Less than 2%) 2041
▲ ReoPro Vials (3.5%) ... 1471
Rythmol Tablets–150mg, 225mg, 300mg (Less than 1%) ... 1352
Tenormin Tablets and I.V. Injection (1.6%) ... 2847
▲ Trasylol (8%) ... 613

Atrial tachycardia
▲ Lanoxicaps (Among most common) ... 1117
▲ Lanoxin Elixir Pediatric (Among most common) ... 1120
▲ Lanoxin Injection (Among most common) ... 1123
▲ Lanoxin Injection Pediatric (Among most common) ... 1126
▲ Lanoxin Tablets (Among most common) ... 1128
Prinivil Tablets (0.3% to 1.0%) ... 1733
Prinzide Tablets ... 1737
Vaseretic Tablets ... 1765
Vasotec I.V. ... 1768
Vasotec Tablets (0.5% to 1.0%) ... 1771
Zestril Tablets (0.3% to 1.0%) ... 2854

Atrioventricular dissociation
Calan SR Caplets (1% or less) ... 2422
Calan Tablets (1% or less) ... 2419
Isoptin Oral Tablets (Less than 1%) ... 1346
Isoptin SR Tablets (1% or less) ... 1348
Lanoxicaps (Common) ... 1117
Lanoxin Injection (Common) ... 1123
Lanoxin Tablets (Common) ... 1128
Rythmol Tablets–150mg, 225mg, 300mg (Less than 1%) ... 1352
Verelan Capsules (1% or less) ... 1410
Verelan Capsules (Less than 1%) .. 2824

Atrophy
Antivenin (Crotalidae) Polyvalent ... 2696
Cuprimine Capsules ... 1630
Norcuron ... 1826
Nydrazid Injection (Uncommon) ... 508

Atrophy, acute yellow
Solganal Suspension ... 2388

Atrophy, cutaneous
Anusol-HC Cream 2.5% (Infrequent to frequent) ... 1896
Aristocort Suspension (Forte Parenteral) ... 1027
Aristocort Suspension (Intralesional) ... 1025
Aristospan Suspension (Intra-articular) ... 1033
Aristospan Suspension (Intralesional) ... 1032
Celestone Soluspan Suspension ... 2347
▲ Cordran Lotion (More frequent) ... 1803
▲ Cordran Tape (More frequent) ... 1804
Cortone Acetate Sterile Suspension ... 1623
Dalalone D.P. Injectable ... 1011
Decadron Phosphate Injection ... 1637
Decadron Phosphate with Xylocaine Injection, Sterile ... 1639
Decadron-LA Sterile Suspension ... 1646
Depen Titratable Tablets (Rare) ... 2662
Depo-Medrol Single-Dose Vial ... 2600
Depo-Medrol Sterile Aqueous Suspension ... 2597
Hydeltrasol Injection, Sterile ... 1665
Hydeltra-T.B.A. Sterile Suspension 1667
Hydrocortone Acetate Sterile Suspension ... 1669
Hydrocortone Phosphate Injection, Sterile ... 1670
Psorcon Cream 0.05% (Infrequent) ... 909
Solu-Cortef Sterile Powder ... 2641
Solu-Medrol Sterile Powder ... 2643

Atrophy, iris
Healon GV ... ⊚ 315

Atrophy, subcutaneous
Aristocort Suspension (Forte Parenteral) ... 1027
Aristocort Suspension (Intralesional) ... 1025
Aristospan Suspension (Intra-articular) ... 1033
Aristospan Suspension (Intralesional) ... 1032
Celestone Soluspan Suspension ... 2347
Cortone Acetate Sterile Suspension ... 1623
Dalalone D.P. Injectable ... 1011
Decadron Phosphate Injection ... 1637
Decadron Phosphate with Xylocaine Injection, Sterile ... 1639
Decadron-LA Sterile Suspension ... 1646
Depo-Medrol Single-Dose Vial ... 2600
Depo-Medrol Sterile Aqueous Suspension ... 2597
Diphtheria and Tetanus Toxoids and Pertussis Vaccine Adsorbed .. 2477
Garamycin Injectable (Rare) ... 2360
Hydeltrasol Injection, Sterile ... 1665
Hydeltra-T.B.A. Sterile Suspension 1667
Hydrocortone Acetate Sterile Suspension ... 1669
Hydrocortone Phosphate Injection, Sterile ... 1670
Lidex ... 2130
Solu-Cortef Sterile Powder ... 2641
Solu-Medrol Sterile Powder ... 2643
Synalar ... 2130

Atypical measles
Attenuvax ... 1610

Auditory acuity, decrease
▲ Capastat Sulfate Vials (Approximately 11%) ... 2868
Desferal Vials ... 820
Quinidex Extentabs ... 2067

Auditory canals, small or absent, fetal
Accutane Capsules ... 2076

Auditory disturbances
Aralen Hydrochloride Injection ... 2301
Aralen Phosphate Tablets ... 2301
▲ Wellbutrin Tablets (5.3%) ... 1204

Autonomic deficit, persistent
Duranest Injections ... 542
Nescaine/Nescaine MPF ... 554
Stelazine ... 2514
Torecan ... 2245
Xylocaine Injections (Rare) ... 567

Awareness, altered
Diprivan Injection (Less than 1%) .. 2833
Halcion Tablets ... 2611
▲ Tonocard Tablets (1.5-11.0%) ... 531

Awareness, heightened
Demser Capsules ... 1649
Imitrex Tablets (Rare) ... 1106
▲ Marinol (Dronabinol) Capsules (8% to 24%) ... 2231

Axyhemoglobin desaturation
▲ Suprane (Greater than 1%-10%) .. 1813

Azoospermia
ColBENEMID Tablets ... 1622
Cytoxan (Reported in a number of patients) ... 694
Matulane Capsules ... 2131
Mustargen ... 1709
NEOSAR Lyophilized/Neosar ... 1959

Azotemia
Achromycin V Capsules ... 1367
Children's Advil Suspension (Less than 1%) ... 2692
Altace Capsules ... 1232
Amikacin Sulfate Injection, USP ... 960
Amikin Injectable ... 501
Ancobon Capsules ... 2079
Aredia for Injection (Up to 4%) ... 810
Atretol Tablets ... 573
BiCNU ... 691
▲ Bumex (10.6%) ... 2093
Cataflam (Less than 1%) ... 816
CeeNU ... 693
Cleocin Phosphate Injection (Rare) 2586
Cleocin Vaginal Cream (Rare) ... 2589
Daypro Caplets ... 2426
Demadex Tablets and Injection ... 686
Diuril Sodium Intravenous ... 1652
Dyrenium Capsules (Rare) ... 2481
Effexor (Rare) ... 2719
Elspar (Frequent) ... 1659
Esidrix Tablets ... 821
Foscavir Injection (Less than 1%) .. 547
▲ Fungizone Intravenous (Among most common) ... 506
Glucophage ... 752
HydroDIURIL Tablets ... 1674
Hydropres Tablets ... 1675
Hyzaar Tablets ... 1677
IBU Tablets (Less than 1%) ... 1342
▲ Indocin I.V. (41% of infants) ... 1684
Lasix Injection, Oral Solution and Tablets ... 1240
Lincocin (Rare instances) ... 2617
Lotrel Capsules ... 840
Methotrexate Sodium Tablets, Injection, for Injection and LPF Injection ... 1275
Minocin Intravenous ... 1382
Minocin Oral Suspension ... 1385
Minocin Pellet-Filled Capsules ... 1383
Monopril Tablets ... 757
Children's Motrin Ibuprofen Oral Suspension (Less than 1%) ... 1546
Motrin Tablets (Less than 1%) ... 2625
Motrin Ibuprofen Suspension, Oral Drops, Chewable Tablets, Caplets (Less than 1%) ... 1546
Mykrox Tablets ... 993
Nalfon 200 Pulvules & Nalfon Tablets (Less than 1%) ... 917
Oncovin Solution Vials & Hyporets 1466
Polymyxin B Sulfate, Aerosporin Brand Sterile Powder ... 1154
Prinivil Tablets (0.3% to 1.0%) ... 1733
Prinzide Tablets ... 1737
Proglycem ... 580
Relafen Tablets (Less than 1%) ... 2510
Tegretol Chewable Tablets ... 852
Tegretol Suspension ... 852
Tegretol Tablets ... 852
Tenoretic Tablets ... 2845
Toradol ... 2159
Vancocin HCl, Oral Solution & Pulvules ... 1483
Vancocin HCl, Vials & ADD-Vantage ... 1481
Vaseretic Tablets ... 1765
Vasotec I.V. ... 1768
Vasotec Tablets ... 1771
Voltaren Tablets (Less than 1%) ... 861
Zanosar Sterile Powder ... 2653
Zaroxolyn Tablets ... 1000
Zestoretic ... 2850
Zestril Tablets (0.3% to 1.0%) ... 2854
Zyloprim Tablets (Less than 1%) ... 1226

ADH syndrome, inappropriate
Asendin Tablets (Less than 1%) ... 1369
Atretol Tablets ... 573
Betaseron for SC Injection ... 658
Cytovene-IV (One report) ... 2103
Depakene ... 413
Depakote Tablets ... 415
Desyrel and Desyrel Dividose ... 503
DiaBeta Tablets ... 1239
Diabinese Tablets (Rare) ... 1935
Elavil ... 2838
Endep Tablets ... 2174
Etrafon ... 2355
Felbatol ... 2666
Flexeril Tablets (Rare) ... 1661
Foscavir Injection (Less than 1%) .. 547
Glucotrol Tablets ... 1967
Glucotrol XL Extended Release Tablets ... 1968
Glynase PresTab Tablets ... 2609
Limbitrol ... 2180
Lufyllin & Lufyllin-400 Tablets ... 2670
Lufyllin-GG Elixir & Tablets ... 2671
Methadone Hydrochloride Oral Solution & Tablets ... 2235
Micronase Tablets ... 2623
Navelbine Injection (Less than 1%) 1145
Norpramin Tablets ... 1526
Oncovin Solution Vials & Hyporets (Rare) ... 1466
Oretic Tablets ... 443
Pamelor ... 2280
Parnate Tablets ... 2503
Paxil Tablets ... 2505
Permax Tablets (Infrequent) ... 575
Platinol ... 708
Platinol-AQ Injection ... 710
Quadrinal Tablets ... 1350
Quibron ... 2053
Respbid Tablets ... 682
Roxanol ... 2243
Rythmol Tablets–150mg, 225mg, 300mg (Less than 1%) ... 1352
Sinequan ... 2205
Slo-bid Gyrocaps ... 2033
Surmontil Capsules ... 2811
Tegretol Chewable Tablets ... 852
Tegretol Suspension ... 852
Tegretol Tablets ... 852
Theo-24 Extended Release Capsules ... 2568
Theo-Dur Extended-Release Tablets ... 1327
Theo-X Extended-Release Tablets .. 788
Tofranil Ampuls ... 854
Tofranil Tablets ... 856
Tofranil-PM Capsules ... 857
Triavil Tablets ... 1757
Trilafon ... 2389
Uni-Dur Extended-Release Tablets .. 1331
Uniphyl 400 mg Tablets ... 2001
Velban Vials ... 1484
Videx Tablets, Powder for Oral Solution, & Pediatric Powder for Oral Solution (Less than 1%) ... 720
Vivactil Tablets ... 1774
Wellbutrin Tablets ... 1204

(▣ Described in PDR For Nonprescription Drugs) Incidence data in parenthesis; ▲ 3% or more (⊚ Described in PDR For Ophthalmology)

AICD discharge — Side Effects Index — 1232

AICD discharge
Betapace Tablets (Less than 1% to 3%) ... 641

ANA, positive
Adalat Capsules (10 mg and 20 mg) (Less than 0.5%) ... 587
Adalat CC (Rare) ... 589
Aldoclor Tablets ... 1598
Aldomet Ester HCl Injection ... 1602
Aldomet Oral ... 1600
Aldoril Tablets ... 1604
Altace Capsules (Less than 1%) ... 1232
Capoten ... 739
Capozide ... 742
Depen Titratable Tablets (Certain patients) ... 2662
Elavil ... 2838
Endep Tablets ... 2174
Felbatol (Rare) ... 2666
Feldene Capsules (Less than 1%) .. 1965
Lescol Capsules (Rare) ... 2267
Lopid Tablets ... 1917
Mevacor Tablets (Rare) ... 1699
Mexitil Capsules (About 2 in 1,000) ... 678
Minipress Capsules ... 1937
Monopril Tablets ... 757
Normodyne Tablets (Less common) ... 2379
Pravachol (Rare) ... 765
Prinivil Tablets (0.3% to 1.0%) ... 1733
Prinzide Tablets ... 1737
Procan SR Tablets ... 1926
Procardia Capsules (Less than 0.5%) ... 1971
Rythmol Tablets–150mg, 225mg, 300mg (0.7%) ... 1352
Tenoretic Tablets ... 2845
Tenormin Tablets and I.V. Injection 2847
Ticlid Tablets (Rare) ... 2156
Tonocard Tablets (Less than 1%) .. 531
Trandate Tablets (Less common) ... 1185
Vaseretic Tablets ... 1765
Vasotec I.V. ... 1768
Vasotec Tablets (0.5% to 1.0%) ... 1771
Zestoretic ... 2850
Zestril Tablets (0.3% to 1.0%) ... 2854
Zocor Tablets (Rare) ... 1775

B

Babinski's phenomenon, bilateral
Dopram Injectable ... 2061
Neurontin Capsules (Infrequent) ... 1922

Backache
Abbokinase ... 403
Abbokinase Open-Cath ... 405
Accupril Tablets (0.5% to 1.2%) .. 1893
Actigall Capsules ... 802
Actimmune (2%) ... 1056
Adenocard Injection (Less than 1%) ... 1021
Adenoscan (Less than 1%) ... 1024
▲ Ambien Tablets (3%) ... 2416
Amen Tablets ... 780
▲ Anafranil Capsules (Up to 6%) ... 803
▲ Asacol Delayed-Release Tablets (7%) ... 1979
▲ Atgam Sterile Solution (More than 1% to 10%) ... 2581
▲ Atrovent Inhalation Solution (3.2%) ... 673
Axid Pulvules (2.4%) ... 1427
Betapace Tablets (1% to 3%) ... 641
Carafate Suspension (Less than 0.5%) ... 1505
Carafate Tablets (Less than 0.5%) 1504
Carbocaine Hydrochloride Injection 2303
Cardura Tablets (Less than 0.5% of 3960 patients to 1.8%) ... 2186
Cartrol Tablets (2.1%) ... 410
Caverject (1%) ... 2583
▲ CellCept Capsules (11.6% to 12.1%) ... 2099
Ceredase ... 1065
▲ CHEMET (succimer) Capsules (5.2 to 15.7%) ... 1545
Cipro I.V. (1% or less) ... 595
Cipro I.V. Pharmacy Bulk Package (Less than 1%) ... 597
Cipro Tablets (Less than 1%) ... 592
Claritin (2% or fewer patients) ... 2349
Claritin-D (Less frequent) ... 2350
Clomid ... 1514
Clozaril Tablets (1%) ... 2252
Cognex Capsules (2%) ... 1901
Colestid Tablets ... 2591
Cozaar Tablets (1.8%) ... 1628
Cycrin Tablets ... 975
CytoGam (Less than 5%) ... 1593
Cytotec (Infrequent) ... 2424
Cytovene (1% or less) ... 2103
Danocrine Capsules ... 2307
Dantrium Capsules (Less frequent) 1982
Depakote Tablets ... 415
▲ Depo-Provera Contraceptive Injection (1% to 5%) ... 2602
Depo-Provera Sterile Aqueous Suspension ... 2606
Dilacor XR Extended-release Capsules (1.7% to 2.9%) ... 2018
Duranest Injections ... 542
Effexor ... 2719
Eldepryl Tablets (1 of 49 patients) 2550
Engerix-B Unit-Dose Vials (Less than 1%) ... 2482
Famvir (1.5%) ... 2486
Foscavir Injection (Between 1% and 5%) ... 547
Gamimune N, 5% Immune Globulin Intravenous (Human), 5% ... 619
Gamimune N, 10% Immune Globulin Intravenous (Human), 10% ... 621
Gammagard S/D, Immune Globulin, Intravenous (Human) (Occasional) ... 585
Gammar I.V., Immune Globulin Intravenous (Human), Lyophilized ... 516
Gelfoam Sterile Sponge ... 2608
▲ Habitrol Nicotine Transdermal System (3% to 9% of patients) ... 865
Hivid Tablets (Less than 1% to less than 3%) ... 2121
Hylorel Tablets (1.5%) ... 985
Hyperstat I.V. Injection ... 2363
Hytrin Capsules (2.4%) ... 430
Hyzaar Tablets (2.1%) ... 1677
Imdur (Less than or equal to 5%) .. 1323
Imitrex Injection (Rare) ... 1103
INFeD (Iron Dextran Injection, USP) ... 2345
▲ Intron A (Up to 19%) ... 2364
Lamictal Tablets (More than 1%) .. 1112
▲ Lescol Capsules (6.1%) ... 2267
Lippes Loop Intrauterine Double-S.. 1848
Lotensin HCT (More than 1.0%) ... 837
Lotrel Capsules ... 840
Lozol Tablets (Greater than or equal to 5%) ... 2022
Luvox Tablets ... 2544
Marcaine Hydrochloride with Epinephrine 1:200,000 ... 2316
Marcaine Hydrochloride Injection ... 2316
Marcaine Spinal ... 2319
Maxaquin Tablets (Less than 1%) .. 2440
Methotrexate Sodium Tablets, Injection, for Injection and LPF Injection ... 1275
▲ Miacalcin Nasal Spray (5.0%) ... 2275
Midamor Tablets (Less than or equal to 1%) ... 1703
Moduretic Tablets (Less than or equal to 1%) ... 1705
Monoket (Fewer than 1%) ... 2406
Mykrox Tablets (Less than 2%) ... 993
Nescaine/Nescaine MPF ... 554
Neurontin Capsules (1.8%) ... 1922
▲ Nicoderm (nicotine transdermal system) (3% to 9%) ... 1518
▲ Nicorette (3% to 9% of patients) .. 2458
Nicotrol Nicotine Transdermal System (1% to 3%) ... 1550
Noroxin Tablets (0.3% to 1.0%) ... 1715
Noroxin Tablets (0.3% to 1.0%) ... 2048
Norvasc Tablets (More than 0.1% to 1%) ... 1940
Oncovin Solution Vials & Hyporets 1466
Orlamm (1% to 3%) ... 2239
ParaGard T380A Intrauterine Copper Contraceptive ... 1880
Paxil Tablets (1.2%) ... 2505
Penetrex Tablets (Less than 1% but more than or equal to 0.1%) 2031
Permax Tablets (1.6%) ... 575
Plendil Extended-Release Tablets (0.5% to 1.5%) ... 527
Premphase ... 2797
Prempro ... 2801
▲ Prepidil Gel (3.1%) ... 2633
Prilosec Delayed-Release Capsules (1.1%) ... 529
Prinivil Tablets (0.6% to 1.6%) ... 1733
Prinzide Tablets (0.3% to 1%) ... 1737
Procardia XL Extended Release Tablets (1% or less) ... 1972
▲ Prograf (13% to 30%) ... 1042
▲ Proleukin for Injection (9%) ... 797
Propulsid (More than 1%) ... 1300
ProSom Tablets (2%) ... 449
Prostep (nicotine transdermal system) (1% to 3% of patients).. 1394
Prostin E2 Suppository ... 2634
Protamine Sulfate Ampoules & Vials ... 1471
Provera Tablets ... 2636
Prozac Pulvules & Liquid, Oral Solution (2.0%) ... 919
Questran Light ... 769
Questran Powder ... 770
Recombivax HB (Less than 1%) ... 1744
Retrovir Capsules ... 1158
Retrovir I.V. Infusion ... 1163
Retrovir Syrup ... 1158
Risperdal (Up to 2%) ... 1301
Rogaine Topical Solution (2.59%).. 2637
Rowasa (1.35%) ... 2548
Sandostatin Injection (1% to 4%).. 2292
Sansert Tablets ... 2295
Sectral Capsules (Up to 2%) ... 2807
Sensorcaine ... 559
Serevent Inhalation Aerosol (1% to 3%) ... 1176
Serzone Tablets ... 771
Sinemet CR Tablets (1.6%) ... 944
Stilphostrol Tablets and Ampuls ... 612
Vancocin HCl, Vials & ADD-Vantage ... 1481
Vaseretic Tablets (0.5% to 2.0%) 1765
VePesid Capsules and Injection (Sometimes) ... 718
▲ Xylocaine Injections (3%) ... 567
Zebeta Tablets ... 1413
▲ Zerit Capsules (Fewer than 1% to 20%) ... 729
Zestoretic (0.3 to 1%) ... 2850
Zestril Tablets (0.3% to 1.6%) ... 2854
Ziac ... 1415
▲ Zoladex (7%) ... 2858
Zoloft Tablets (1.5%) ... 2217
Zosyn (1.0% or less) ... 1419
Zosyn Pharmacy Bulk Package (1.0% or less) ... 1422

Back strain
Prinzide Tablets (0.3% to 1.0%) .. 1737
Zestoretic (0.3% to 1.0%) ... 2850

Bacteremia
Ethamolin ... 2400
Retrovir Capsules (1.6%) ... 1158
Retrovir I.V. Infusion (2%) ... 1163
Retrovir Syrup (1.6%) ... 1158

Bacteriuria
Primaxin I.M. ... 1727
Sinemet CR Tablets (1% or greater) ... 944

Balance, loss of (see also under Equilibrium, dysfunction)
Adalat Capsules (10 mg and 20 mg) (2% or less) ... 587
Amikacin Sulfate Injection, USP ... 960
Amikin Injectable ... 501
Eldepryl Tablets ... 2550
Rythmol Tablets–150mg, 225mg, 300mg (1.2%) ... 1352
Versed Injection (Less than 1%) ... 2170

Balanitis
Achromycin V Capsules (Rare) ... 1367
Betaseron for SC Injection ... 658
Declomycin Tablets ... 1371
Minocin Intravenous (Rare) ... 1382
Minocin Oral Suspension (Rare) ... 1385
Minocin Pellet-Filled Capsules (Rare) ... 1383
Stimate, (desmopressin acetate) Nasal Spray, 1.5 mg/mL ... 525

Balanoposthitis
Zoloft Tablets (Rare) ... 2217

Baldness, male pattern (see under Alopecia, hereditaria)

Bartter's syndrome
Capastat Sulfate Vials (1 patient) ... 2868

Basophils, increase
Effexor (Rare) ... 2719
Primaxin I.M. ... 1727
Primaxin I.V. ... 1729
Rocephin Injectable Vials, ADD-Vantage, Galaxy Container (Rare) ... 2142
Unasyn ... 2212
Vantin for Oral Suspension and Vantin Tablets ... 2646
Zefazone ... 2654

Behavior, hypochondriacal
Celontin Kapseals ... 1899

Behavior, inappropriate
Artane ... 1368
Ativan Injection (Occasional) ... 2698
Diprivan Injection (Less than 1%) .. 2833
Halcion Tablets ... 2611
Mellaril ... 2269
ProSom Tablets ... 449
Serentil ... 684
Tessalon Perles ... 1020
Xanax Tablets (Rare) ... 2649

Behavior, violent
Prozac Pulvules & Liquid, Oral Solution ... 919

Behavioral changes
Akineton ... 1333
Ambien Tablets ... 2416
Amoxil (Rare) ... 2464
Augmentin (Rare) ... 2468
Catapres Tablets ... 674
Catapres-TTS ... 675
Combipres Tablets ... 677
Cytotec (Infrequent) ... 2424
Eldepryl Tablets ... 2550
Gastrocrom Capsules (Infrequent).. 984
JE-VAX (One case) ... 886
▲ Klonopin Tablets (25%) ... 2126
Methotrexate Sodium Tablets, Injection, for Injection and LPF Injection ... 1275
Monopril Tablets (0.4% to 1.0%).. 757
▲ Orap Tablets (5 of 20 patients) ... 1050
Paremyd ... ◉ 247
Rifadin ... 1528
Rifater ... 1532
Timoptic in Ocudose (Less frequent) ... 1753
Timoptic Sterile Ophthalmic Solution (Less frequent) ... 1751
Timoptic-XE ... 1755
Torecan ... 2245
Vascor (200, 300 and 400 mg) Tablets (0.5 to 2.0%) ... 1587

Behavioral deterioration
Depakene ... 413
Depakote Tablets ... 415

Bell's palsy
Aldoclor Tablets ... 1598
Aldomet Ester HCl Injection ... 1602
Aldomet Oral ... 1600
Aldoril Tablets ... 1604
Cognex Capsules (Rare) ... 1901
Cytovene-IV (One report) ... 2103
Engerix-B Unit-Dose Vials ... 2482
Flexeril Tablets (Rare) ... 1661
Hivid Tablets (Less than 1% to less than 3%) ... 2121
JE-VAX (One case) ... 886
Lescol Capsules ... 2267
Mevacor Tablets (0.5% to 1.0%) .. 1699
Permax Tablets (Rare) ... 575
Pravachol ... 765
Recombivax HB ... 1744
Sandostatin Injection (Less than 1%) ... 2292
Zocor Tablets ... 1775

Benzyl alcohol, sensitivity to
AquaMEPHYTON Injection ... 1608
Cleocin Phosphate Injection ... 2586
Cytosar-U Sterile Powder ... 2592
Depo-Medrol Sterile Aqueous Suspension ... 2597
Heparin Sodium Injection, USP, Sterile Solution ... 2615
Leustatin ... 1834
Lincocin ... 2617
Mesnex Injection ... 702
Mivacron Injection ... 1138
Nuromax Injection ... 1149
Nutropin ... 1061
Procrit for Injection ... 1841
Profasi (chorionic gonadotropin for injection, USP) ... 2450
Protropin ... 1063
Septra I.V. Infusion ... 1169
Septra I.V. Infusion ADD-Vantage Vials ... 1171
Tracrium Injection ... 1183
Trobicin Sterile Powder ... 2645

(▣ Described in PDR For Nonprescription Drugs) Incidence data in parenthesis; ▲ 3% or more (◉ Described in PDR For Ophthalmology)

1233 **Side Effects Index** **Bleeding, dental**

Bezoar
Carafate Suspension ... 1505
Carafate Tablets ... 1504
Ecotrin ... 2455
PREVACID Delayed-Release Capsules (Less than 1%) ... 2562

Bigeminy
Diprivan Injection (Less than 1%) .. 2833
Suprane (Less than 1%) ... 1813
Taxol (Approximately 1%; rare) ... 714
Versed Injection (Less than 1%) ... 2170
Virazole (Infrequent) ... 1264

Bile duct "sludge", presence of metabolites
Clinoril Tablets (Rare) ... 1618

Biliary sclerosis
Sterile FUDR ... 2118

Biliary sludge
▲Sandostatin Injection (22% to 48%) ... 2292

Biliary stasis
Compazine ... 2470
Levoprome ... 1274
Mellaril ... 2269
Serentil ... 684
Stelazine ... 2514
Torecan ... 2245
Triavil Tablets ... 1757
Trilafon ... 2389

Biliary tract abnormalities
▲Sandostatin Injection (52%) ... 2292

Biliary tract spasm
Mepergan Injection ... 2753
Methadone Hydrochloride Oral Concentrate ... 2233

Biliary tree, calcification
Questran Light (Occasional) ... 769
Questran Powder ... 770

Bilirubinemia
Ambien Tablets (Rare) ... 2416
Effexor (Rare) ... 2719
Hivid Tablets (Less than 1% to less than 3%) ... 2121
Intron A (Less than 5%) ... 2364
▲Oncaspar (Greater than 1% but less than 5%) ... 2028
Paxil Tablets (Rare) ... 2505
PREVACID Delayed-Release Capsules (Less than 1%) ... 2562
▲Prograf (Greater than 3%) ... 1042
Rifater ... 1532

Bilirubinuria
Primaxin I.M. ... 1727
Primaxin I.V. ... 1729
Relafen Tablets (Less than 1%) ... 2510
Rifamate Capsules ... 1530
Rifater ... 1532

Birth, premature
Accutane Capsules ... 2076
Sandimmune ... 2286

Birth defects
Aygestin Tablets ... 974
Celontin Kapseals ... 1899
Coumadin ... 926
Cuprimine Capsules ... 1630
Depakene (Multiple reports) ... 413
Depakote Tablets (Multiple reports) ... 415
Depen Titratable Tablets ... 2662
Dilantin Infatabs ... 1908
Dilantin Kapseals ... 1906
Dilantin Parenteral ... 1910
Dilantin-125 Suspension ... 1911
Encare Vaginal Contraceptive Suppositories ... ▣ 833
Humegon (1.7%) ... 1824
Klonopin Tablets ... 2126
Lo/Ovral Tablets ... 2746
Lo/Ovral-28 Tablets ... 2751
Mesantoin Tablets ... 2272
Metrodin (urofollitropin for injection) (4 incidents) ... 2446
Milontin Kapseals ... 1920
Mysoline ... 2754
Nolvadex Tablets (A small number of reports) ... 2841
Nordette-21 Tablets ... 2755
Nordette-28 Tablets ... 2758
Ortho Dienestrol Cream ... 1866
Ortho-Est ... 1869
Ovral Tablets ... 2770
Ovral-28 Tablets ... 2770
Ovrette Tablets ... 2771
▲Parlodel (3.3%) ... 2281
Peganone Tablets (Multiple reports) ... 446
Pergonal (menotropins for injection, USP) (1.7%) ... 2448
Phenurone Tablets (Multiple reports) ... 447
Podocon-25 ... 1891
Premarin Intravenous ... 2787
Premarin with Methyltestosterone .. 2794
Premarin Vaginal Cream ... 2791
Premphase ... 2797
Prempro ... 2801
Quadrinal Tablets ... 1350
Serophene (clomiphene citrate tablets, USP) (2.5%) ... 2451
Triphasil-21 Tablets ... 2814
Triphasil-28 Tablets ... 2819
Zarontin Capsules ... 1928
Zarontin Syrup ... 1929

Birth weight, low
Betapace Tablets ... 641
Cytosar-U Sterile Powder (Five infants) ... 2592
Dexedrine ... 2474
Easprin ... 1914
Nicorette ... 2458
Sandimmune ... 2286
Sectral Capsules ... 2807

Births, multiple
▲Humegon (20%) ... 1824
▲Metrodin (urofollitropin for injection) (17%) ... 2446
▲Pergonal (menotropins for injection, USP) (20%) ... 2448
Profasi (chorionic gonadotropin for injection, USP) ... 2450
▲Serophene (clomiphene citrate tablets, USP) (Less than 1% to 10%) ... 2451

Blackout spells
Eskalith ... 2485
Lithium Carbonate Capsules & Tablets ... 2230
Lithonate/Lithotabs/Lithobid ... 2543
Lupron Depot 3.75 mg ... 2556
Lupron Depot 7.5 mg ... 2559
Lupron Injection (Less than 5%) ... 2555

Bladder, dysfunction
Depo-Medrol Single-Dose Vial ... 2600
Depo-Medrol Sterile Aqueous Suspension ... 2597
Gelfoam Sterile Sponge ... 2608
Lioresal Intrathecal ... 1596
▲TheraCys BCG Live (Intravesical) (Up to 5.4%) ... 897

Bladder, irritability
IFEX ... 697
Oxandrin ... 2862
Winstrol Tablets ... 2337

Bladder, loss of control
Duranest Injections ... 542
Nescaine/Nescaine MPF ... 554
Trilafon ... 2389
Xylocaine Injections ... 567

Bladder, neurogenic
Gelfoam Sterile Sponge ... 2608

Bladder, spasms
Lasix Injection, Oral Solution and Tablets ... 1240
Lioresal Intrathecal ... 1596
Lupron Depot 3.75 mg ... 2556
Lupron Depot 7.5 mg ... 2559
Lupron Injection (Less than 5%) ... 2555
Midamor Tablets (Less than or equal to 1%) ... 1703
Moduretic Tablets ... 1705

Blanching
Catapres-TTS (1 of 101 patients) .. 675
▲Emla Cream (37%) ... 545
Iopidine 0.5% (Less than 3%) ... ◉ 221
Tympagesic Ear Drops ... 2342

Blebs, filtering (ocular)
Blephamide Ointment (Increased incidence) ... ◉ 237
Cortisporin Ophthalmic Ointment Sterile ... 1085
Decadron Phosphate Sterile Ophthalmic Ointment (Rare) ... 1641
Decadron Phosphate Sterile Ophthalmic Solution (Rare) ... 1642
FML Forte Liquifilm ... ◉ 240
FML Liquifilm ... ◉ 241
FML S.O.P. ... ◉ 241
Inflamase (Rare) ... ◉ 265
Vasocidin Ophthalmic Solution ... ◉ 270

Bleeding
Abbokinase ... 403
Abbokinase Open-Cath ... 405
▲Activase (Most common complication) ... 1058
Adriamycin PFS ... 1947
Adriamycin RDF ... 1947
Children's Advil Suspension (Less than 1%) ... 2692
Alka-Seltzer Effervescent Antacid and Pain Reliever ... ▣ 701
Alkeran for Injection ... 1070
Alkeran Tablets ... 1071
Android ... 1251
Betapace Tablets (1% to 2%) ... 641
Betaseron for SC Injection ... 658
BiCNU ... 691
CeeNU ... 693
Cefizox for Intramuscular or Intravenous Use ... 1034
Cefotan ... 2829
Ceftin ... 1078
Cefzil Tablets and Oral Suspension 746
▲CellCept Capsules (More than or equal to 3%) ... 2099
Ceptaz ... 1081
Condylox (Less than 5%) ... 1802
Coumadin ... 926
▲Cytosar-U Sterile Powder (Among most frequent) ... 2592
Cytovene (1% or less) ... 2103
Demadex Tablets and Injection ... 686
Depakene ... 413
Depakote Tablets ... 415
Depen Titratable Tablets ... 2662
Diprivan Injection (Less than 1%) .. 2833
Diupres Tablets ... 1650
Doxorubicin Astra ... 540
Duricef ... 748
Elspar ... 1659
▲Eminase (14.6% to 14.8%) ... 2039
Empirin with Codeine Tablets (Sometimes; occasional) ... 1093
Felbatol ... 2666
Floxin I.V. ... 1571
Floxin Tablets (200 mg, 300 mg, 400 mg) ... 1567
Fludara for Injection (Up to 1%) ... 663
Fluorouracil Injection ... 2116
Fortaz ... 1100
Fragmin ... 1954
Sterile FUDR ... 2118
Halotestin Tablets ... 2614
Heparin Lock Flush Solution ... 2725
Heparin Sodium Injection ... 2726
Heparin Sodium Injection, USP, Sterile Solution ... 2615
Heparin Sodium Vials ... 1441
Hydropres Tablets ... 1675
▲Idamycin (63%) ... 1955
Imuran (2 cases) ... 1110
Lamictal Tablets (Rare) ... 1112
Leukeran Tablets ... 1133
▲Leukine for IV Infusion (23%) ... 1271
Lorabid Suspension and Pulvules ... 1459
▲Lovenox Injection (4%) ... 2020
Children's Motrin Ibuprofen Oral Suspension (Less than 1%) ... 1546
Motrin Tablets (Less than 1%) ... 2625
Motrin Ibuprofen Suspension, Oral Drops, Chewable Tablets, Caplets (Less than 1%) ... 1546
Mustargen ... 1709
▲Novantrone (20 to 37%) ... 1279
Oncaspar ... 2028
PPD Tine Test ... 2874
▲Paraplatin for Injection (6% to 10%) ... 705
Priscoline Hydrochloride Ampuls ... 845
Proglycem ... 580
▲Prograf (Greater than 3%) ... 1042
Prostin VR Pediatric Sterile Solution (Less than 1%) ... 2635
Protamine Sulfate Ampoules & Vials (Some patients) ... 1471
Prozac Pulvules & Liquid, Oral Solution (Infrequent) ... 919
Quadrinal Tablets ... 1350
▲ReoPro Vials (Most common) ... 1471
Risperdal (Rare) ... 1301
Rubex ... 712
Serzone Tablets (Rare) ... 771
Soma Compound w/Codeine Tablets ... 2676
Streptase for Infusion ... 562
Suprane (Less than 1%) ... 1813
Suprax ... 1399
▲Taxol (14%) ... 714
Tazicef for Injection ... 2519
Testred Capsules ... 1262
Thioplex (Thiotepa For Injection) ... 1281
Tonocard Tablets ... 531
Travase Ointment ... 1356
Tuberculin, Old, Tine Test ... 2875
Vantin for Oral Suspension and Vantin Tablets ... 2646
VePesid Capsules and Injection ... 718
▲Videx Tablets, Powder for Oral Solution, & Pediatric Powder for Oral Solution (1% to 10%) ... 720
▲Vumon (5%) ... 727
Winstrol Tablets ... 2337
Zefazone ... 2654
Zinacef ... 1211
Zinecard (2% to 3%) ... 1961
Zoladex (1% or greater) ... 2858
Zosyn (1.0% or less) ... 1419
Zosyn Pharmacy Bulk Package (1.0% or less) ... 1422

Bleeding, at invaded sites
Eminase ... 2039
Streptase for Infusion ... 562

Bleeding, at site of administration
Cytovene (1% or less) ... 2103
Eminase ... 2039
Genotropin (Infrequent) ... 111
Intron A (Less than 5%) ... 2364
ReoPro Vials (1 to 50 events) ... 1471
Streptase for Infusion ... 562
Zefazone (1.4%) ... 2654

Bleeding, breakthrough
Amen Tablets ... 780
Aygestin Tablets ... 974
Brevicon ... 2088
Climara Transdermal System ... 645
Cycrin Tablets ... 975
Demulen ... 2428
Depo-Provera Sterile Aqueous Suspension ... 2606
Desogen Tablets ... 1817
Diethylstilbestrol Tablets ... 1437
Estrace Cream and Tablets ... 749
Estraderm Transdermal System ... 824
ESTRATAB Tablets (0.3, 0.625, 1.25, 2.5 mg) ... 2536
Estratest ... 2539
Levlen/Tri-Levlen ... 651
Lo/Ovral Tablets ... 2746
Lo/Ovral-28 Tablets ... 2751
Megace Oral Suspension ... 699
Megace Tablets ... 701
Menest Tablets ... 2494
Micronor Tablets ... 1872
Modicon ... 1872
Nordette-21 Tablets ... 2755
Nordette-28 Tablets ... 2758
Norinyl ... 2088
Nor-Q D Tablets ... 2135
Ogen Tablets ... 2627
Ogen Vaginal Cream ... 2630
Ortho-Cept ... 1851
Ortho-Cyclen/Ortho-Tri-Cyclen ... 1858
Ortho Dienestrol Cream ... 1866
Ortho-Est ... 1869
Ortho-Novum ... 1872
Ortho-Cyclen/Ortho Tri-Cyclen ... 1858
Ovcon (Sometimes) ... 760
Ovral Tablets ... 2770
Ovral-28 Tablets ... 2770
Ovrette Tablets ... 2771
PMB 200 and PMB 400 ... 2783
Premarin Intravenous ... 2787
Premarin with Methyltestosterone .. 2794
Premarin Tablets ... 2789
Premarin Vaginal Cream ... 2791
Premphase ... 2797
Prempro ... 2801
Provera Tablets ... 2636
Levlen/Tri-Levlen ... 651
Tri-Norinyl ... 2164
Triphasil-21 Tablets ... 2814
Triphasil-28 Tablets ... 2819

Bleeding, dental
Accutane Capsules (Less than 1%) ... 2076
Activase (Less than 1%) ... 1058
Anafranil Capsules (Rare) ... 803
Claritin-D (Less frequent) ... 2350

(▣ Described in PDR For Nonprescription Drugs) Incidence data in parenthesis; ▲ 3% or more (◉ Described in PDR For Ophthalmology)

Bleeding, dental Side Effects Index 1234

Coumadin 926
Danocrine Capsules (Rare) 2307
Effexor (Rare) 2719
Eminase (1%) 2039
Felbatol 2666
Hivid Tablets (Less than 1% to less than 3%) 2121
Intron A (Less than 5%) 2364
Lamictal Tablets (Rare) 1112
Mustargen 1709
Neurontin Capsules (Infrequent) 1922
Nicorette (1%) 2458
Questran Light 769
Questran Powder 770
Retrovir Capsules 1158
Retrovir I.V. Infusion 1163
Retrovir Syrup 1158
Roferon-A Injection (Less than 3%) 2145
▲ Tegison Capsules (1-10%) 2154
Videx Tablets, Powder for Oral Solution, & Pediatric Powder for Oral Solution (Less than 1%) 720

Bleeding, duodenal ulcer

Questran Light 769
Questran Powder 770

Bleeding, gastrointestinal

Abbokinase 403
Abbokinase Open-Cath 405
Accupril Tablets (Rare) 1893
Actimmune (Rare) 1056
▲ Activase (5%) 1058
Adalat CC (Less than 1.0%) 589
Children's Advil Suspension (Less than 1%) 2692
Aldactazide 2413
Aldactone 2414
Anaprox/Naprosyn (Approximately 1% to 4%) 2117
Ancobon Capsules 2079
Ansaid Tablets (Rare; 1-3%) 2579
▲ Aredia for Injection (Up to 6%) 810
Regular Strength Ascriptin Tablets ▣ 629
Atamet (Rare) 572
Atgam Sterile Solution (Less than 5%) 2581
Atromid-S Capsules 2701
Azactam for Injection (Less than 1%) 734
Azo Gantrisin Tablets 2081
Genuine Bayer Aspirin Tablets & Caplets ▣ 713
Aspirin Regimen Bayer Regular Strength 325 mg Caplets ▣ 709
Betaseron for SC Injection 658
Bufferin Analgesic Tablets and Caplets ▣ 613
Cataflam (0.6% to 1.6%) 816
▲ CellCept Capsules (More than or equal to 3%) 2099
Cipro I.V. (Less than 1%) 595
Cipro I.V. Pharmacy Bulk Package (Less than 1%) 597
Cipro Tablets (Less than 1%) 592
Clinoril Tablets (Less than 1%) 1618
Cognex Capsules (Infrequent) 1901
Cortone Acetate Sterile Suspension 1623
Cortone Acetate Tablets 1624
Cytotec (Infrequent) 2424
Dantrium Capsules (Less frequent) 1982
Daypro Caplets (Less than 1%) 2426
Decadron Phosphate Respihaler 1642
Decadron Phosphate Turbinaire 1645
Demadex Tablets and Injection 686
Dilacor XR Extended-release Capsules 2018
Dolobid Tablets (Less than 1 in 100) 1654
Easprin 1914
EC-Naprosyn Delayed-Release Tablets (Approximately 1% to 4%) 2117
Ecotrin 2455
Edecrin 1657
Eldepryl Tablets 2550
Emcyt Capsules (1%) 1953
Eminase (2%) 2039
Empirin with Codeine Tablets (Occasional) 1093
Ergamisol Tablets 1292
Felbatol 2666
Feldene Capsules (Less than 1%) 1965
Floxin I.V. 1571
Floxin Tablets (200 mg, 300 mg, 400 mg) 1567
▲ Fludara for Injection (3% to 13%) 663
Fluorouracil Injection 2116
Sterile FUDR 2118
Fulvicin P/G Tablets (Rare) 2359
Fulvicin P/G 165 & 330 Tablets (Rare) 2359
Glucotrol XL Extended Release Tablets (Rare) 1968
Halfprin 1362
Heparin Lock Flush Solution 2725
Heparin Sodium Injection 2726
Hivid Tablets (Less than 1% to less than 3%) 2121
IBU Tablets (Less than 1%) 1342
Imitrex Tablets (Rare) 1106
Indocin Capsules (Less than 1%) 1680
▲ Indocin I.V. (3% to 9%) 1684
Indocin (Less than 1%) 1680
Intron A (Less than 5%) 2364
K-Dur Microburst Release System (potassium chloride, USP) E.R. Tablets 1325
K-Norm Extended-Release Capsules 991
K-Tab Filmtab 434
Lamictal Tablets (Rare) 1112
Lamprene Capsules (Less than 1%) 828
Larodopa Tablets (Rare) 2129
▲ Leukine for IV Infusion (27%) 1271
Lodine Capsules and Tablets 2743
Lorelco Tablets 1517
Lupron Depot 3.75 mg 2556
Lupron Depot 7.5 mg 2559
Lupron Injection (Less than 5%) 2555
Luvox Tablets (Infrequent) 2544
Maxaquin Tablets (Less than 1%) 2440
Methotrexate Sodium Tablets, Injection, for Injection and LPF Injection 1275
Mexitil Capsules (About 7 in 10,000) 678
Micro-K 2063
Micro-K LS Packets 2064
Midamor Tablets (Less than or equal to 1%) 1703
Moduretic Tablets (Less than or equal to 1%) 1705
Children's Motrin Ibuprofen Oral Suspension (Approximately 1% to 4%) 1546
Motrin Tablets (Less than 1%) 2625
Motrin Ibuprofen Suspension, Oral Drops, Chewable Tablets, Caplets (Approximately 1% to 4%) 1546
Mustargen 1709
Nalfon 200 Pulvules & Nalfon Tablets (Less than 1%) 917
Anaprox/Naprosyn (Approximately 1% to 4%) 2117
Neoral (Rare) 2276
Nimotop Capsules (Less than 1%) 610
Norgesic (Rare) 1496
▲ Novantrone (2 to 16%) 1279
Orthoclone OKT3 Sterile Solution 1837
Orudis Capsules (Less than 1%) 2766
Oruvail Capsules (Less than 1%) 2766
Paraflex Caplets (Rare) 1580
Parafon Forte DSC Caplets (Rare) 1581
Parlodel (Less than 2%) 2281
Pentasa (Less than 1%) 1527
Ponstel 1925
PREVACID Delayed-Release Capsules (Less than 1%) 2562
Priscoline Hydrochloride Ampuls 845
Procardia XL Extended Release Tablets (Less than 1%) 1972
▲ Prograf (Greater than 3%) 1042
▲ Proleukin for Injection (13%) 797
Questran Light 769
Questran Powder 770
Relafen Tablets (1%) 2510
ReoPro Vials (11 events) 1471
Ridaura Capsules (0.1 to 1%) 2513
Risperdal (Rare) 1301
SSKI Solution (Less frequent) 2658
Salflex Tablets 786
Sandimmune (Rare) 2286
Sandostatin Injection (Less than 1%) 2292
Serzone Tablets (Rare) 771
Sinemet Tablets (Rare) 943
Sinemet CR Tablets 944
Slow-K Extended-Release Tablets 851
Soma Compound Tablets 2675
St. Joseph Adult Chewable Aspirin (81 mg.) ▣ 808
Streptase for Infusion 562
Ticlid Tablets 2156
Tolectin (200, 400 and 600 mg) (Less than 1%) 1581
Toradol 2159
Ultram Tablets (50 mg) (Infrequent) 1585
Videx Tablets, Powder for Oral Solution, & Pediatric Powder for Oral Solution (Up to 2%) 720
Voltaren Tablets (0.6% to 1.6%) 861
Wellbutrin Tablets (Rare) 1204
Zyloprim Tablets (Less than 1%) 1226

Bleeding, genitourinary tract

Abbokinase 403
Abbokinase Open-Cath 405
▲ Activase (4%) 1058
Eminase 2039
Premphase 2797
Prempro 2801
ReoPro Vials (5 to 8 events) 1471
Streptase for Infusion 562

Bleeding, gingival (see under Bleeding, dental)

Bleeding, hemorrhoidal

Colestid Tablets (Infrequent) 2591
Daypro Caplets (Less than 1%) 2426
Questran Light 769
Questran Powder 770

Bleeding, in immediate coronary catheterization

▲ Eminase (13.3%) 2039

Bleeding, in patients not undergoing coronary catheterization

▲ Eminase (3%) 2039

Bleeding, intermenstrual

Imitrex Tablets (Infrequent) 1106
Maxaquin Tablets (Less than 1%) 2440
Risperdal (Infrequent) 1301
Zoloft Tablets (Infrequent) 2217

Bleeding, internal

Abbokinase 403
Activase 1058
Eminase 2039
Streptase for Infusion 562

Bleeding, intracerebral

▲ Lopid Tablets (More common) 1917
Streptase for Infusion 562
Ticlid Tablets (Rare) 2156

Bleeding, intracranial

Abbokinase 403
Abbokinase Open-Cath 405
Activase (0.4% to 1.3%) 1058
Cardene I.V. (0.7%) 2709
Elspar 1659
Eminase (1%) 2039
Hespan Injection 929
▲ Indocin I.V. (3% to 9%) 1684
Neurontin Capsules (Infrequent) 1922
ReoPro Vials (1 to 3 events) 1471
▲ Survanta Beractant Intratracheal Suspension (24.1 to 48.1%) 2226
Videx Tablets, Powder for Oral Solution, & Pediatric Powder for Oral Solution (Less than 1%) 720

Bleeding, menstrual, frequent onsets

▲ Norplant System (7.0%) 2759

Bleeding, menstrual, prolonged episodes

▲ Norplant System (27.6%) 2759

Bleeding, menstrual, scanty

▲ Norplant System (5.2%) 2759

Bleeding, mouth

Eminase (1%) 2039
Foscavir Injection (Less than 1%) 547
ReoPro Vials (4 events) 1471

Bleeding, mucosal

Effexor (Rare) 2719
Quadrinal Tablets 1350
Unasyn (Less than 1%) 2212
Vancenase PocketHaler Nasal Inhaler (2 per 100 patients) 2391

Bleeding, nasal (see under Epistaxis)

Bleeding, nonpuncture site

▲ Eminase (10.2%) 2039

Bleeding, otic

ReoPro Vials (9 to 11 events) 1471

Bleeding, pericardial

Activase 1058
Eminase 2039

Bleeding, perioperative

Ticlid Tablets 2156
Toradol IM Injection, IV Injection 2159

Bleeding, postmenopausal

Aldactazide 2413
Aldactone 2414

Bleeding, puncture site

Capastat Sulfate Vials 2868
▲ Eminase (Up to 5.7%) 2039

Bleeding, renal-pelvic

Cipro I.V. (1% or less) 595

Bleeding, retroperitoneal

▲ ReoPro Vials (2 to 12 events) 1471
Streptase for Infusion 562

Bleeding, superficial

Abbokinase 403
Abbokinase Open-Cath 405
Activase 1058
Eminase 2039

Bleeding, Upper GI (see under Bleeding, gastrointestinal)

Bleeding, urethral

Ceftin (Less than 1% but more than 0.1%) 1078
Cipro Tablets (Less than 1%) 592

Bleeding, uterine, irregularities

Clomid (1.3%) 1514
Depo-Provera Contraceptive Injection 2602
ESTRATAB Tablets (0.3, 0.625, 1.25, 2.5 mg) 2536
Lodine Capsules and Tablets (Less than 1%) 2743

Bleeding, uterine

Anafranil Capsules (Infrequent) 803
Ansaid Tablets (Less than 1%) 2579
Climara Transdermal System 645
Clomid 1514
Cytotec 2424
Effexor (Infrequent) 2719
Estrace Cream and Tablets 749
Estratest 2539
Intron A (Less than 5%) 2364
Menest Tablets 2494
Ogen Tablets 2627
Ogen Vaginal Cream 2630
Ortho-Est 1869
PMB 200 and PMB 400 2783
Permax Tablets (Infrequent) 575
Premarin Intravenous 2787
Premarin with Methyltestosterone 2794
Premarin Tablets 2789
Premarin Vaginal Cream 2791
Premphase 2797
Prempro 2801
Prozac Pulvules & Liquid, Oral Solution (Rare) 919
Serophene (clomiphene citrate tablets, USP) (Less than 1 in 100 patients) 2451
Serzone Tablets (Rare) 771

Bleeding, vaginal

Abbokinase 403
Abbokinase Open-Cath 405
Anafranil Capsules (Infrequent) 803
Ansaid Tablets (Less than 1%) 2579
Betaseron for SC Injection 658
Brevicon 2088
Cataflam (Less than 1%) 816
Climara Transdermal System 645
Clinoril Tablets (Less than 1%) 1618
Cognex Capsules (Infrequent) 1901
Coumadin 926
Demulen 2428
▲ Depo-Provera Contraceptive Injection (More than 5%) 2602
Effexor (Infrequent) 2719
Ergamisol Tablets (Less frequent) 1292
Estrace Cream and Tablets 749
Estraderm Transdermal System 824
Estratest 2539
Felbatol 2666
Indocin Capsules (Less than 1%) 1680

(▣ Described in PDR For Nonprescription Drugs) Incidence data in parenthesis; ▲ 3% or more (⊙ Described in PDR For Ophthalmology)

1235 Side Effects Index Blood dyscrasias

Indocin I.V. (Less than 1%) 1684
Indocin (Less than 1%) 1680
Levlen/Tri-Levlen 651
Lo/Ovral Tablets 2746
Lo/Ovral-28 Tablets 2751
Lupron Depot-PED 7.5 mg, 11.25 mg and 15 mg (2%) 2560
Luvox Tablets (Infrequent) 2544
Massengill Disposable Douche 2457
Micronor Tablets 1872
Modicon 1872
Neurontin Capsules (Infrequent) 1922
Nolvadex Tablets (Less frequent; 2%) 2841
Norinyl 2088
Nor-Q D Tablets 2135
Ogen Tablets 2627
Ogen Vaginal Cream 2630
Ortho-Cyclen/Ortho-Tri-Cyclen 1858
Ortho-Novum 1872
Ortho-Cyclen/Ortho Tri-Cyclen 1858
Ovral Tablets 2770
Ovral-28 Tablets 2770
Ovrette Tablets 2771
Permax Tablets (Infrequent) 575
Premarin Tablets 2789
Prozac Pulvules & Liquid, Oral Solution (Rare) 919
Relafen Tablets (Less than 1%) 2510
Risperdal (Infrequent) 1301
Serzone Tablets (Infrequent) 771
▲ Supprelin Injection (22%) 2056
▲ Synarel Nasal Solution for Central Precocious Puberty (8%) 2151
Synarel Nasal Solution for Endometriosis 2152
Levlen/Tri-Levlen 651
Tri-Norinyl 2164
Triphasil-21 Tablets 2814
Triphasil-28 Tablets 2819
Videx Tablets, Powder for Oral Solution, & Pediatric Powder for Oral Solution (Less than 1%) 720
Voltaren Tablets (Less than 1%) 861
Zarontin Capsules 1928
Zarontin Syrup 1929
Zoladex (1% or greater) 2858

Bleeding diathesis
Cipro I.V. (Rare) 595
Cipro Tablets (Less than 0.1%) 592

Bleeding irregularities
BuSpar (Rare) 737
Climara Transdermal System 645
Cycrin Tablets 975
▲ Demulen (Among most common) 2428
Estrace Cream and Tablets 749
Levlen/Tri-Levlen 651
▲ Norplant System (7.6%) 2759
Ogen Tablets 2627
Ortho-Est 1869
Ovcon 760
Premarin Tablets 2789
Premphase 2797
Prempro 2801
Quadrinal Tablets 1350
Levlen/Tri-Levlen 651

Bleeding syndrome
Mithracin 607

Bleeding tendencies due to hypoprothrombinemia
Questran Light (Less frequent) 769
Questran Powder (Less frequent) 770

Bleeding time, prolongation
Children's Advil Suspension 2692
Cardizem CD Capsules (Infrequent) 1506
Cardizem SR Capsules (Less than 1%) 1510
Cardizem Injectable 1508
Cardizem Tablets (Infrequent) 1512
Cefotan 2829
Daypro Caplets 2426
Depakene 413
Easprin 1914
Fiorinal with Codeine Capsules 2262
Hespan Injection 929
Lodine Capsules and Tablets (Less than 1%) 2743
Mithracin 607
Motrin Tablets 2625
Neurontin Capsules (Rare) 1922
Ocufen ⊙ 245
Pentaspan Injection 937
Procardia Capsules (Some patients) 1971
Procardia XL Extended Release Tablets (Some patients) 1972
Prozac Pulvules & Liquid, Oral Solution (Rare) 919
Rythmol Tablets–150mg, 225mg, 300mg (Less than 1%) 1352
Timentin for Injection 2528
Tolectin (200, 400 and 600 mg) 1581
Toradol 2159

Blepharitis
Alomide (Less than 1%) 469
Anafranil Capsules (Rare) 803
Betaseron for SC Injection 658
Betimol 0.25%, 0.5% (1% to 5%) ⊙ 261
Cognex Capsules (Rare) 1901
Effexor (Rare) 2719
Iopidine 0.5% (Less than 3%) ⊙ 221
Kerlone Tablets (Less than 2%) 2436
NebuPent for Inhalation Solution (1% or less) 1040
OptiPranolol (Metipranolol 0.3%) Sterile Ophthalmic Solution (A small number of patients) ⊙ 258
Prozac Pulvules & Liquid, Oral Solution (Rare) 919
Risperdal (Rare) 1301
Timoptic in Ocudose (Less frequent) 1753
Timoptic Sterile Ophthalmic Solution (Less frequent) 1751
Timoptic-XE 1755

Blepharoconjunctivitis
▲ Betagan (About 1 in 20 patients) ⊙ 233
Iopidine 0.5% (Less than 3%) ⊙ 221
Ocupress Ophthalmic Solution, 1% Sterile (Occasional) ⊙ 309

Blepharoptosis (see also under Ptosis, eyelids)
Betagan ⊙ 233
Betimol 0.25%, 0.5% ⊙ 261

Blepharospasm
Anafranil Capsules (Up to 2%) 803
Atamet 572
Claritin (2% or fewer patients) 2349
Claritin-D 2350
Eldepryl Tablets 2550
Larodopa Tablets (Infrequent) 2129
Parlodel 2281
Sinemet Tablets 943
Sinemet CR Tablets 944

Blind spot, enlargement
Eskalith 2485

Blindness
Aristocort Suspension (Forte Parenteral) (Rare) 1027
Aristocort Suspension (Intralesional) (Rare) 1025
Aristospan Suspension (Intra-articular) (Rare) 1033
Aristospan Suspension (Intralesional) (Rare) 1032
Betaseron for SC Injection 658
Celestone Soluspan Suspension (Rare instances) 2347
Cortone Acetate Sterile Suspension 1623
Cytovene (1% or less) 2103
Dalalone D.P. Injectable (Rare) 1011
Decadron Phosphate Injection (Rare) 1637
Decadron Phosphate with Xylocaine Injection, Sterile (Rare) 1639
Decadron-LA Sterile Suspension (Rare) 1646
Depo-Medrol Single-Dose Vial 2600
Depo-Medrol Sterile Aqueous Suspension 2597
Eskalith 2485
Foscavir Injection (Less than 1%) 547
Hydeltrasol Injection, Sterile (Rare) 1665
Hydeltra-T.B.A. Sterile Suspension (Rare) 1667
Hydrocortone Acetate Sterile Suspension (Rare) 1669
Hydrocortone Phosphate Injection, Sterile (Rare) 1670
Micronor Tablets (Rare) 1872
Modicon (Rare) 1872
Neurontin Capsules (Rare) 1922
Oncovin Solution Vials & Hyporets 1466
Ortho-Cyclen/Ortho-Tri-Cyclen (Rare) 1858
Ortho-Novum (Rare) 1872
Ortho-Cyclen/Ortho Tri-Cyclen (Rare) 1858
Orthoclone OKT3 Sterile Solution 1837
Permax Tablets (Rare) 575
Proleukin for Injection (Less than 1%) 797
Surgicel 1314

Blindness, cerebral
Platinol (Infrequent) 708
Platinol-AQ Injection (Infrequent) 710

Blindness, night (see under Nyctalopia)

Blindness, sudden
Factrel 2877

Blindness, transient
Adalat Capsules (10 mg and 20 mg) (Less than 0.5%) 587
Adalat CC (Rare) 589
Proleukin for Injection (Less than 1%) 797
THYREL TRH 2873

Blindness, transient cortical
Oncovin Solution Vials & Hyporets 1466
Procardia Capsules (Less than 0.5%) 1971
VePesid Capsules and Injection (Infrequent) 718

Blistering
BuSpar (Infrequent) 737
Doxorubicin Astra 540
Efudex (Infrequent) 2113
Lotrimin 2371
Lotrisone Cream 2372
Maxaquin Tablets 2440
Norplant System 2759
Retin-A (tretinoin) Cream/Gel/Liquid 1889
Sulfamylon Cream 925
Surgicel 1314

Bloated feeling (see under Bloating)

Bloating
Children's Advil Suspension (Less than 3%) 2692
Bentyl 1501
▲ Colyte and Colyte-flavored (Among most frequent) 2396
▲ CREON 5 Capsules (Among most frequent) 2536
Depo-Provera Contraceptive Injection (1% to 5%) 2602
Desogen Tablets 1817
Dipentum Capsules (1.5%) 1951
Donnatal 2060
Donnatal Extentabs 2061
Donnatal Tablets 2060
Estrace Cream and Tablets 749
▲ GoLYTELY (Up to 50%) 688
IBU Tablets (Greater than 1%) 1342
Indocin Capsules (Less than 1%) 1680
Indocin I.V. (Less than 1%) 1684
Indocin (Less than 1%) 1680
Levsin/Levsinex/Levbid 2405
▲ Limbitrol (Among most frequent) 2180
Lo/Ovral Tablets 2746
Lo/Ovral-28 Tablets 2751
Menest Tablets 2494
Micronor Tablets 1872
Modicon 1872
Children's Motrin Ibuprofen Oral Suspension (Greater than 1% but less than 3%) 1546
Motrin Tablets (Less than 3%) 2625
Nephro-Fer Rx Tablets 2005
Nordette-21 Tablets 2755
Nordette-28 Tablets 2758
▲ Norpace (3 to 9%) 2444
Ortho-Cept 1851
Ortho-Cyclen/Ortho-Tri-Cyclen 1858
Ortho Dienestrol Cream 1866
Ortho-Est 1869
Ortho-Novum 1872
Ortho-Cyclen/Ortho Tri-Cyclen 1858
Ovcon 760
Ovral Tablets 2770
Ovral-28 Tablets 2770
Ovrette Tablets 2771
Premarin Vaginal Cream 2791
Pro-Banthine Tablets 2052
Quarzan Capsules 2181
Robinul Forte Tablets 2072
Robinul Injectable 2072
Robinul Tablets 2072
Rowasa (1.47%) 2548
Stilphostrol Tablets and Ampuls 612
Triphasil-21 Tablets 2814
Triphasil-28 Tablets 2819
Yutopar Intravenous Injection (Infrequent) 570

Blood clotting, mechanisms, disorders of
Estrace Cream and Tablets 749
Ortho-Est 1869
Pyrazinamide Tablets (Rare) 1398
Rifater (Rare) 1532

Blood dyscrasias
Anturane (Rare) 807
Apresazide Capsules (Less frequent) 808
Apresoline Hydrochloride Tablets (Less frequent) 809
Aralen Hydrochloride Injection 2301
Aralen Phosphate Tablets 2301
Azo Gantanol Tablets 2080
Bactrim DS Tablets (Rare) 2084
Bactrim I.V. Infusion (Rare) 2082
Bactrim (Rare) 2084
▲ Blephamide Ointment (Among most often) ⊙ 237
Celontin Kapseals 1899
Chloromycetin Ophthalmic Ointment, 1% ⊙ 310
Chloromycetin Ophthalmic Solution ⊙ 310
Chloromycetin Sodium Succinate 1900
Chloroptic Sterile Ophthalmic Solution (Rare) ⊙ 239
Compazine 2470
Dapsone Tablets USP 1284
Depo-Provera Contraceptive Injection (Fewer than 1%) 2602
Diamox Intravenous 1372
Diamox Sequels (Sustained Release) 1373
Diamox Tablets 1372
Elase-Chloromycetin Ointment 1040
Esimil Tablets (A few instances) 822
Etrafon (Less frequent) 2355
Fansidar Tablets 2114
Gantrisin (Rare) 2120
Glauctabs ⊙ 208
Ismelin Tablets 827
Lasix Injection, Oral Solution and Tablets 1240
▲ Leukine for IV Infusion (25%) 1271
Levoprome 1274
Librax Capsules 2176
Libritabs Tablets (Occasional) 2177
Librium Capsules (Occasional) 2178
MZM ⊙ 267
Mesantoin Tablets 2272
Mexitil Capsules 678
Milontin Kapseals 1920
Myochrysine Injection (Rare) 1711
Neptazane Tablets 1388
Ophthocort ⊙ 311
Phenurone Tablets (2%) 447
Plaquenil Sulfate Tablets 2328
Procan SR Tablets 1926
Prolixin 509
Prozac Pulvules & Liquid, Oral Solution (Rare) 919
Ridaura Capsules 2513
SSD 1355
Septra 1174
Septra I.V. Infusion 1169
Septra I.V. Infusion ADD-Vantage Vials (Rare) 1171
Septra 1174
Ser-Ap-Es Tablets 849
Serax Capsules 2810
Serax Tablets 2810
Silvadene Cream 1% 1540
Solganal Suspension (Rare) 2388
Stelazine 2514
Tambocor Tablets (Extremely rare) 1497
Tigan 2057
Tonocard Tablets 531
Triavil Tablets 1757
Trusopt Sterile Ophthalmic Solution (Rare) 1760
Urobiotic-250 Capsules 2214
Vasocidin Ophthalmic Solution ⊙ 270
Zarontin Capsules 1928
Zarontin Syrup 1929

(Described in PDR For Nonprescription Drugs) Incidence data in parenthesis; ▲ 3% or more (⊙ Described in PDR For Ophthalmology)

Blood glucose, elevation (see under Hyperglycinemia)

Blood glucose, reduction (see under Hypoglycemia)

Blood loss, increase (see under Bleeding)

Blood pressure, changes

Alka-Seltzer Effervescent Antacid and Pain Reliever ▣ 701
Alka-Seltzer Lemon Lime Effervescent Antacid and Pain Reliever ▣ 703
Asendin Tablets 1369
Bronkometer Aerosol 2302
Bronkosol Solution 2302
Bufferin Analgesic Tablets and Caplets ▣ 613
Cartrol Tablets 410
Clozaril Tablets 2252
DDAVP Injection (Infrequent) 2014
DDAVP Injection 15 mcg/mL (Infrequent) 2015
Dantrium Capsules (Less frequent) 1982
Daypro Caplets (Less than 1%) 2426
Desoxyn Gradumet Tablets 419
Haldol Decanoate 1577
Isoetharine Inhalation Solution, USP, Arm-a-Med 551
Isordil Sublingual Tablets 2739
Isordil Tembids 2741
Isordil Titradose Tablets 2742
Loxitane 1378
Mellaril 2269
Moban Tablets and Concentrate 1048
Orap Tablets 1050
Pontocaine Hydrochloride for Spinal Anesthesia 2330
Premphase (Occasional) 2797
Prempro (Occasional) 2801
Prolixin 509
Risperdal 1301
Ritalin 848
Sandimmune 2286
Sensorcaine 559
Serentil 684
Stelazine 2514
Tornalate Metered Dose Inhaler 957
Trilafon 2389
Ventolin Rotacaps for Inhalation 1200
▲ Vumon (Approximately 5%) 727
▲ Yutopar Intravenous Injection (80% to 100%) 570
Zemuron 1830

Blood pressure, elevation (see under Hypertension)

Blood pressure, reduction (see under Hypotension)

Blood urea levels, increase

Ceptaz (Occasional) 1081
Fortaz (Occasional) 1100
Inderide Tablets 2732
Normodyne Tablets (Rare) 2379
▲ Paraplatin for Injection (Up to 17%) 705

Blood urea nitrogen levels, increase (see under BUN levels, elevation)

Blurred vision

Achromycin V Capsules 1367
Actifed with Codeine Cough Syrup 1067
Adalat Capsules (10 mg and 20 mg) (2% or less) 587
Adenocard Injection (Less than 1%) 1021
Adenoscan (Less than 1%) 1024
Children's Advil Suspension (Less than 1%) 2692
AeroBid Inhaler System (1-3%) 1005
Aerobid-M Inhaler System (1-3%) 1005
Akineton 1333
Albalon Solution with Liquifilm ◉ 231
Alfenta Injection (1% to 3%) 1286
▲ Alomide (1% to 5%) 469
Alupent Tablets (0.2%) 669
Ana-Kit Anaphylaxis Emergency Treatment Kit 617
Antivert, Antivert/25 Tablets, & Antivert/50 Tablets (Rare) 2185
Aralen Hydrochloride Injection 2301
Aralen Phosphate Tablets 2301
Arco-Lase Plus Tablets 512
▲ Artane (30% to 50%) 1368
Asacol Delayed-Release Tablets 1979
▲ Asendin Tablets (7%) 1369
Atamet 572
Ativan Injection (Occasional) 2698
Atretol Tablets 573
Atrohist Pediatric Capsules 453
Atrohist Plus Tablets 454
Atromid-S Capsules 2701
Atrovent Inhalation Aerosol (1.2%; about 1 in 100) 671
Bellergal-S Tablets (Rare) 2250
Benadryl Capsules 1898
Benadryl Injection 1898
▲ Bentyl (27%) 1501
Betimol 0.25%, 0.5% (1% to 5%) ◉ 261
Betoptic Ophthalmic Solution 469
Betoptic S Ophthalmic Suspension (Small number of patients) 471
Bonine Tablets (Rare) 1933
Bontril Slow-Release Capsules 781
Bromfed 1785
BuSpar (2%) 737
Calan SR Caplets (1% or less) 2422
Calan Tablets (1% or less) 2419
Capoten 739
Capozide 742
Carbocaine Hydrochloride Injection 2303
Cardene Capsules (Rare) 2095
Cartrol Tablets (Less common) 410
Cataflam (Less than 1%) 816
Catapres Tablets 674
Catapres-TTS 675
Celontin Kapseals 1899
Cipro I.V. (1% or less) 595
Cipro I.V. Pharmacy Bulk Package (Less than 1%) 597
Cipro Tablets (Less than 1%) 592
Claritin (2% or fewer patients) 2349
Claritin-D (Less frequent) 2350
Clinoril Tablets (Less than 1 in 100) 1618
Clomid (Occasional; 1.5%) 1514
Cogentin 1621
Combipres Tablets 677
Comhist 2038
Compazine 2470
Cozaar Tablets (Less than 1%) 1628
Cystospaz 1963
D.A. Chewable Tablets 951
Dalgan Injection (Less than 1%) 538
Dalmane Capsules (Rare) 2173
Dapsone Tablets USP 1284
Daypro Caplets (Less than 1%) 2426
Decadron Phosphate Sterile Ophthalmic Ointment 1641
Decadron Phosphate Sterile Ophthalmic Solution 1642
Decadron Phosphate with Xylocaine Injection, Sterile 1639
Declomycin Tablets 1371
Deconamine 1320
Desferal Vials 820
▲ Desyrel and Desyrel Dividose (6.3% to 14.7%) 503
DiaBeta Tablets 1239
Dilacor XR Extended-release Capsules (Infrequent) 2018
Dilaudid-HP Injection (Less frequent) 1337
Dilaudid-HP Lyophilized Powder 250 mg (Less frequent) 1337
Dilaudid Tablets and Liquid (Less frequent) 1339
Dipentum Capsules (Rare) 1951
Ditropan 1516
Diucardin Tablets 2718
Diupres Tablets 1650
Dizac (Less frequent) 1809
Dolobid Tablets (Less than 1 in 100) 1654
Donnagel Liquid and Donnagel Chewable Tablets (Rare) ▣ 879
Donnatal 2060
Donnatal Extentabs 2061
Donnatal Tablets 2060
Duranest Injections 542
Dura-Tap/PD Capsules 2867
Dura-Vent/DA Tablets 953
Dyclone 0.5% and 1% Topical Solutions, USP 544
Edecrin 1657
▲ Effexor (6%) 2719
Elavil 2838
Eldepryl Tablets 2550
Emete-con Intramuscular/Intravenous 2198
Emla Cream 545
Endep Tablets 2174
Enduron Tablets 420
Ergamisol Tablets (1% to 2%) 1292
Esimil Tablets 822
Eskalith 2485
▲ Ethmozine Tablets (2% to 5%) 2041
Etrafon 2355
Fedahist Gyrocaps 2401
Fedahist Timecaps 2401
Feldene Capsules (Less than 1%) 1965
Flexeril Tablets (1% to 3%) 1661
Floropryl Sterile Ophthalmic Ointment 1662
Floxin I.V. 1571
Floxin Tablets (200 mg, 300 mg, 400 mg) 1567
Glucotrol XL Extended Release Tablets (Less than 3%) 1968
Glynase PresTab Tablets 2609
Haldol Decanoate 1577
Haldol Injection, Tablets and Concentrate 1575
Hivid Tablets (Less than 1% to less than 3%) 2121
Humorsol Sterile Ophthalmic Solution 1664
Hycomine Compound Tablets 932
Hycomine 931
Hycotuss Expectorant Syrup 933
HydroDIURIL Tablets 1674
Hydropres Tablets 1675
Hyperstat I.V. Injection 2363
Hytrin Capsules (0.6% to 1.6%) 430
Hyzaar Tablets 1677
IBU Tablets (Less than 1%) 1342
Indocin (Less than 1%) 1680
Intron A (Less than 5%) 2364
Inversine Tablets 1686
IOPIDINE Sterile Ophthalmic Solution ◉ 219
Iopidine 0.5% (Less than 3%) ◉ 221
Ismelin Tablets 827
Ismo Tablets (Fewer than 1%) 2738
Isoptin Oral Tablets (Less than 1%) 1346
Isoptin SR Tablets (1% or less) 1348
Kemadrin Tablets 1112
Kutrase Capsules 2402
Lacrisert Sterile Ophthalmic Insert 1686
▲ Lamictal Tablets (Among most common; 11% to 25%) 1112
Lanoxicaps 1117
Lanoxin Elixir Pediatric 1120
Lanoxin Injection 1123
Lanoxin Injection Pediatric 1126
Lanoxin Tablets 1128
Larodopa Tablets (Infrequent) 2129
Lasix Injection, Oral Solution and Tablets 1240
Levsin/Levsinex/Levbid 2405
Librax Capsules 2176
Librium Injectable (Isolated instances) 2179
▲ Limbitrol (Among most frequent) 2180
Lioresal Intrathecal (Up to 5 of 214 patients) 1596
Lioresal Tablets 829
Lithium Carbonate Capsules & Tablets 2230
Lithonate/Lithotabs/Lithobid 2543
Lodine Capsules and Tablets (More than 1% but less than 3%) 2743
Lopid Tablets 1917
Lopressor Ampuls 830
Lopressor HCT Tablets (1 in 100 patients) 832
Lopressor Tablets 830
Lorelco Tablets 1517
Lotensin HCT 837
Loxitane 1378
Lozol Tablets (Less than 5%) 2022
▲ Ludiomil Tablets (4%) 843
Lupron Depot 7.5 mg 2559
Lupron Injection (Less than 5%) 2555
▲ Luvox Tablets (3%) 2544
Lysodren (Infrequent) 698
MS Contin Tablets (Less frequent) 1994
MSIR (Infrequent) 1997
Marcaine Hydrochloride with Epinephrine 1:200,000 2316
Marcaine Hydrochloride Injection 2316
Marcaine Spinal 2319
Mellaril 2269
Mepergan Injection (Occasional) 2753
Methotrexate Sodium Tablets, Injection, for Injection and LPF Injection 1275
Mevacor Tablets (0.9% to 1.5%) 1699
▲ Mexitil Capsules (5.7% to 7.5%) 678
Miacalcin Nasal Spray (Less than 1%) 2275
Micronase Tablets 2623
Minipress Capsules (1-4%) 1937
Minizide Capsules 1938
Minocin Intravenous 1382
Minocin Oral Suspension 1385
Minocin Pellet-Filled Capsules 1383
Mintezol 1704
Moban Tablets and Concentrate (Occasional) 1048
Moduretic Tablets 1705
Motofen Tablets (Less frequent) 784
Children's Motrin Ibuprofen Oral Suspension (Less than 1%) 1546
Motrin Tablets (Less than 1%) 2625
Motrin Ibuprofen Suspension, Oral Drops, Chewable Tablets, Caplets (Less than 1%) 1546
Mutamycin 703
Nalfon 200 Pulvules & Nalfon Tablets (2.2%) 917
Nardil (Less common) 1920
Navane Capsules and Concentrate 2201
Navane Intramuscular 2202
NebuPent for Inhalation Solution (1% or less) 1040
Nescaine/Nescaine MPF 554
Netromycin Injection 100 mg/ml (Fewer than 1 of 1000 patients) 2373
Norflex 1496
Norgesic 1496
Noroxin Tablets (Less frequent) 1715
Noroxin Tablets (Less frequent) 2048
▲ Norpace (3 to 9%) 2444
Norpramin Tablets 1526
Novocain Hydrochloride for Spinal Anesthesia 2326
Nubain Injection (1% or less) 935
Ocupress Ophthalmic Solution, 1% Sterile (Occasional) ◉ 309
OptiPranolol (Metipranolol 0.3%) Sterile Ophthalmic Solution (A small number of patients) ◉ 258
Oramorph SR (Morphine Sulfate Sustained Release Tablets) (Less frequent) 2236
Orap Tablets 1050
Orlamm (1% to 3%) 2239
Ornade Spansule Capsules 2502
Orthoclone OKT3 Sterile Solution 1837
PBZ Tablets 845
PBZ-SR Tablets 844
Pamelor 2280
Paremyd ◉ 247
Parnate Tablets 2503
▲ Paxil Tablets (2.0% to 7.8%) 2505
Periactin 1724
Phenergan with Codeine (Occasional) 2777
Phenergan with Dextromethorphan (Occasional) 2778
Phenergan Injection 2773
Phenergan Suppositories (Occasional) 2775
Phenergan Syrup (Occasional) 2774
Phenergan Tablets (Occasional) 2775
Phenergan VC (Occasional) 2779
Phenergan VC with Codeine (Occasional) 2781
Phospholine Iodide ◉ 326
Pilagan ◉ 248
Placidyl Capsules 448
Plaquenil Sulfate Tablets (Fairly common) 2328
Platinol 708
Platinol-AQ Injection 710
Polymyxin B Sulfate, Aerosporin Brand Sterile Powder 1154
Pondimin Tablets 2066
Ponstel 1925
Pontocaine Hydrochloride for Spinal Anesthesia 2330
Prinivil Tablets (0.3% to 1.0%) 1733
Prinzide Tablets (0.3 to 1%) 1737
Pro-Banthine Tablets 2052
Procardia Capsules (2% or less) 1971
Proglycem 580
Prolixin 509
Prostin E2 Suppository 2634
Protopam Chloride for Injection 2806
Quarzan Capsules (Among most frequent) 2181
Quinaglute Dura-Tabs Tablets 649
Quinidex Extentabs 2067
Rēv-Eyes Ophthalmic Eyedrops 0.5% (Less frequently) ◉ 323
ReVia Tablets (Less than 1%) 940
Robaxin Injectable 2070
Robaxin Tablets 2071
Robaxisal Tablets 2071
Robinul Forte Tablets 2072
Robinul Injectable 2072
Robinul Tablets 2072
▲ Romazicon (1% to 9%) 2147

(▣ Described in PDR For Nonprescription Drugs) Incidence data in parenthesis; ▲ 3% or more (◉ Described in PDR For Ophthalmology)

1237 Side Effects Index Bradycardia

▲Rythmol Tablets–150mg, 225mg, 300mg (0.6 to 5.7%) 1352
Sandostatin Injection (1% to 4%) 2292
Sanorex Tablets 2294
Seldane-D Extended-Release Tablets (1.1%) 1538
Sensorcaine 559
Ser-Ap-Es Tablets 849
Serax Capsules 2810
Serax Tablets 2810
Serentil 684
Serophene (clomiphene citrate tablets, USP) (Occasionally) 2451
▲Serzone Tablets (3% to 9%) 771
Sinemet Tablets 943
Sinemet CR Tablets 944
Sinequan 2205
Slo-Niacin Tablets 2659
Stadol (1% or greater) 775
Stelazine 2514
Sublimaze Injection 1307
Surmontil Capsules 2811
Talacen (Infrequent) 2333
Talwin Injection 2334
Talwin Compound (Infrequent) 2335
Talwin Injection 2334
Talwin Nx 2336
Tambocor Tablets 1497
Tavist Syrup 2297
Tavist Tablets 2298
Tegretol Chewable Tablets 852
Tegretol Suspension 852
Tegretol Tablets 852
Temaril Tablets, Syrup and Spansule Extended-Release Capsules 483
Tenex Tablets (Less frequent) 2074
Thioplex (Thiotepa For Injection) 1281
Tigan 2057
Timolide Tablets 1748
Tofranil Ampuls 854
Tofranil Tablets 856
Tofranil-PM Capsules 857
▲Tonocard Tablets (1.3-10.0%) 531
Toprol-XL Tablets 565
Toradol (1% or less) 2159
Torecan 2245
Transderm Scōp Transdermal Therapeutic System 869
Tranxene (Less common) 451
Trental Tablets (Less than 1%) 1244
Triaminic Cold Tablets ▣ 790
Triavil Tablets 1757
Trilafon (Occasional) 2389
Trinalin Repetabs Tablets 1330
Trusopt Sterile Ophthalmic Solution (Approximately 1% to 5%) 1760
Tussend 1783
Urised Tablets 1964
Urispas Tablets 2532
Valium Injectable 2182
Valium Tablets (Infrequent) 2183
Valrelease Capsules (Infrequent) 2169
Vascor (200, 300 and 400 mg) Tablets (0.5 to 2.0%) 1587
Vasosulf ⊙ 271
Vasotec I.V. 1768
Vasotec Tablets (0.5% to 1.0%) 1771
Verelan Capsules (1% or less) 1410
Verelan Capsules (1% or less) 2824
Versed Injection (Less than 1%) 2170
Vexol 1% Ophthalmic Suspension (1% to 5%) ⊙ 230
Vicodin Tuss Expectorant 1358
Videx Tablets, Powder for Oral Solution, & Pediatric Powder for Oral Solution (Up to 2%) 720
Vivactil Tablets 1774
Voltaren Tablets (Less than 1%) 861
Vontrol Tablets 2532
▲Wellbutrin Tablets (14.6%) 1204
▲Xanax Tablets (6.2% to 21%) 2649
▲Xylocaine Injections (Among most common) 567
Zantac (Rare) 1209
Zantac Injection (Rare) 1207
Zantac Syrup (Rare) 1209
Zestoretic (0.3 to 1%) 2850
Zestril Tablets (0.3% to 1.0%) 2854
Ziac 1415
Zofran Injection 1214

Blurred vision, transient (see also under Blurred vision)
Aldoclor Tablets 1598
Aldoril Tablets 1604
Apresazide Capsules 808
Capozide 742
Diucardin Tablets 2718
Diupres Tablets 1650
Diuril Oral Suspension 1653
Diuril Sodium Intravenous 1652
Diuril Tablets 1653
Dyazide 2479
Esidrix Tablets 821
Esimil Tablets 822
HydroDIURIL Tablets 1674
Inderide Tablets 2732
Inderide LA Long Acting Capsules 2734
Lopressor HCT Tablets 832
Maxzide 1380
Mykrox Tablets 993
Peptavlon 2878
Ser-Ap-Es Tablets 849
Vaseretic Tablets 1765
Zaroxolyn Tablets 1000

Body odor
Carnitor Injection (Less frequent) 2452
Carnitor Tablets and Solution 2453
Depo-Provera Contraceptive Injection (Fewer than 1%) 2602
Effexor (Rare) 2719
Felbatol 2666
Lupron Depot 3.75 mg (Less than 5%) 2556
Lupron Depot-PED 7.5 mg, 11.25 mg and 15 mg (Less than 2%) 2560
Retrovir Capsules 1158
Retrovir I.V. Infusion 1163
Retrovir Syrup 1158
Salagen Tablets (Less than 1%) 1489
Supprelin Injection (1% to 3%) 2056
▲Synarel Nasal Solution for Central Precocious Puberty (4%) 2151
Wellbutrin Tablets (Rare) 1204

Bone density, changes
Depo-Provera Contraceptive Injection 2602
▲Lupron Depot 3.75 mg (2.7% to 3.9%) 2556
▲Zoladex (4.3% decrease) 2858

Bone disorders
Accutane Capsules 2076
Clomid 1514
Effexor (Infrequent) 2719
Proglycem Capsules 580
Risperdal (Rare) 1301
Videx Tablets, Powder for Oral Solution, & Pediatric Powder for Oral Solution (Less than 1%) 720

Bone fractures
Didronel Tablets 1984

Bone marrow depression
Accupril Tablets (Rare) 1893
▲Adriamycin PFS (High incidence) 1947
▲Adriamycin RDF (High incidence) 1947
Aldoclor Tablets 1598
Aldomet Ester HCl Injection 1602
Aldomet Oral 1600
Aldoril Tablets 1604
Altace Capsules (Rare to more frequent) 1232
Anafranil Capsules (Rare) 803
Atretol Tablets 573
Bleph-10 Ophthalmic Solution 10% 475
Chloromycetin Sodium Succinate 1900
Chloroptic Sterile Ophthalmic Solution (Three cases) ⊙ 239
Clinoril Tablets (Less than 1%) 1618
Cuprimine Capsules 1630
Depen Titratable Tablets 2662
Diamox 1372
▲Doxorubicin Astra (High incidence) 540
Elavil 2838
Elspar (Rare) 1659
Endep Tablets 2174
FML-S Liquifilm ⊙ 242
Felbatol 2666
Feldene Capsules (Less than 1%) 1965
Flexeril Tablets (Rare) 1661
Floxin I.V. 1571
Floxin Tablets (200 mg, 300 mg, 400 mg) 1567
Glauctabs ⊙ 208
Hydrea Capsules 696
Indocin Capsules (Less than 1%) 1680
Indocin I.V. (Less than 1%) 1684
Indocin (Less than 1%) 1680
Limbitrol 2180
Lotensin Tablets (Rare) 834
Lotensin HCT 837
Lotrel Capsules 840
Ludiomil Tablets (Isolated reports) 843
MZM (Common) ⊙ 267
Mefoxin 1691
Mefoxin Premixed Intravenous Solution 1694
Methotrexate Sodium Tablets, Injection, for Injection and LPF Injection 1275
Neptazane Tablets 1388
Norpramin Tablets 1526
Oncovin Solution Vials & Hyporets 1466
Pamelor 2280
Primaxin I.M. 1727
Primaxin I.V. 1729
Prinivil Tablets (Rare) 1733
Prinzide Tablets (Rare) 1737
Procan SR Tablets 1926
Rubex (A high incidence) 712
Sinequan (Occasional) 2205
Sulfamylon Cream (A single case) 925
Surmontil Capsules 2811
Tegretol Chewable Tablets 852
Tegretol Suspension 852
Tegretol Tablets 852
Thioplex (Thiotepa For Injection) 1281
Ticlid Tablets 2156
Tofranil Ampuls 854
Tofranil Tablets 856
Tofranil-PM Capsules 857
Tonocard Tablets (Less than 1%) 531
Triavil Tablets 1757
Vaseretic Tablets (Rare) 1765
Vasotec I.V. (Rare) 1768
Vasotec Tablets (Rare) 1771
Vivactil Tablets 1774
Zestoretic (Rare) 2850
Zestril Tablets (Rare) 2854

Bone marrow dysplasia
BiCNU 691
CeeNU 693

Bone marrow fibrosis
Fludara for Injection (One patient) 663

Bone marrow hyperplasia
Ponstel (Occasional) 1925

Bone marrow hypoplasia
Capoten 739
Capozide 742
Chloromycetin Ophthalmic Ointment, 1% ⊙ 310
Chloromycetin Ophthalmic Solution ⊙ 310
Elase-Chloromycetin Ointment 1040
Lopid Tablets (Rare) 1917
Ophthocort ⊙ 311
Zantac (Rare) 1209
Zantac Injection (Sometimes) 1207
Zantac Syrup (Rare) 1209

Bone marrow suppression
▲Alkeran for Injection (Most common) 1070
▲Alkeran Tablets (Most common) 1071
▲BiCNU (Most common) 691
▲CeeNU (Most common) 693
Celontin Kapseals 1899
▲Cerubidine (All patients) 795
Chloroptic S.O.P. ⊙ 239
Clozaril Tablets 2252
Cytosar-U Sterile Powder 2592
Depakene 413
Depakote Tablets 415
Dilantin Infatabs 1908
Dilantin Kapseals 1906
Dilantin Parenteral 1910
Dilantin-125 Suspension 1911
Empirin with Codeine Tablets (Occasional) 1093
Etrafon 2355
Fiorinal (Single case) 2261
Fludara for Injection 663
▲Foscavir Injection (7% to 10%) 547
Hydrea Capsules 696
Imuran 1110
Leukeran Tablets (Frequent) 1133
Leustatin (Common) 1834
Milontin Kapseals 1920
Neutrexin 2572
Paraplatin for Injection 705
Purinethol Tablets (Frequent) 1156
▲Septra I.V. Infusion (Among most frequent) 1169
Thioguanine Tablets, Tabloid Brand 1181
VePesid Capsules and Injection 718
Vumon 727
Zarontin Capsules 1928
Zarontin Syrup 1929

Borborygmi
Duvoid (Infrequent) 2044
Peptavlon 2878
Urecholine 1761

Bowel, loss of control
Duranest Injections 542
Nescaine/Nescaine MPF 554
Xylocaine Injections 567

Bowel disease, inflammatory, exacerbation of
Accutane Capsules 2076
Ansaid Tablets (Less than 1%) 2579
Asacol Delayed-Release Tablets 1979

Bowel dysfunction
Depo-Medrol Single-Dose Vial 2600
Depo-Medrol Sterile Aqueous Suspension 2597
Gelfoam Sterile Sponge 2608

Bowel frequency, increase
Esimil Tablets 822
Fluorouracil Injection 2116
Sterile FUDR 2118
▲Hylorel Tablets (4.9%) 985
Ismelin Tablets 827

Bowel habits, changes
▲Seldane Tablets (4.6% to 7.6%) 1536
Seldane-D Extended-Release Tablets 1538

Bowel infarction
Activase 1058
Orthoclone OKT3 Sterile Solution 1837
Proleukin for Injection 797

Bowel strictures, fibrotic
Pancrease MT Capsules 1579

Bowel syndrome, irritable
Anafranil Capsules (Infrequent) 803
Neurontin Capsules (Rare) 1922

Bowels, perforation
Cortone Acetate Sterile Suspension 1623
Cortone Acetate Tablets 1624
Dalalone D.P. Injectable 1011
Decadron Elixir 1633
Decadron Phosphate Injection 1637
Decadron Phosphate Respihaler 1642
Decadron Phosphate Turbinaire 1645
Decadron Phosphate with Xylocaine Injection, Sterile 1639
Decadron Tablets 1635
Decadron-LA Sterile Suspension 1646
Dexacort Phosphate in Respihaler 458
Dexacort Phosphate in Turbinaire 459
Hydeltrasol Injection, Sterile 1665
Hydeltra-T.B.A. Sterile Suspension 1667
Hydrocortone Acetate Sterile Suspension 1669
Hydrocortone Phosphate Injection, Sterile 1670
Hydrocortone Tablets 1672
Indocin I.V. (1% to 3%) 1684
Proleukin for Injection 797

Brachial plexus neuropathies
Diphtheria and Tetanus Toxoids and Pertussis Vaccine Adsorbed USP (For Pediatric Use) 875
Tripedia 892

Bradycardia
Adalat CC (Less than 1.0%) 589
Adenoscan (Less than 1%) 1024
Akineton 1333
Aldoclor Tablets 1598
Aldomet Ester HCl Injection 1602
Aldomet Oral 1600
Aldoril Tablets 1604
▲Alfenta Injection (14%) 1286
Anafranil Capsules (Infrequent) 803
Anectine 1073
Antilirium Injectable 1009
Atgam Sterile Solution (Less than 5%) 2581
Betagan ⊙ 233
▲Betapace Tablets (8% to 16%) 641
Betimol 0.25%, 0.5% ⊙ 261
Betoptic Ophthalmic Solution (Rare) 469
Betoptic S Ophthalmic Suspension (Rare) 471
▲Blocadren Tablets (5% to 9.1%) 1614
Brevibloc Injection (Less than 1%) 1808
Brontex 1981
Buprenex Injectable (Less than 1%) 2006

(▣ Described in PDR For Nonprescription Drugs) Incidence data in parenthesis; ▲ 3% or more (⊙ Described in PDR For Ophthalmology)

BuSpar (Rare) 737
Butisol Sodium Elixir & Tablets (Less than 1 in 100) 2660
Cafergot 2251
Calan SR Caplets (1.4%) 2422
Calan Tablets (1.4%) 2419
Carbocaine Hydrochloride Injection 2303
Cardizem CD Capsules (1.7% to 3.3%) 1506
▲ Cardizem SR Capsules (1.5% to 6%) 1510
Cardizem Injectable (Less than 1%) 1508
Cardizem Tablets (Less than 1%) 1512
Cartrol Tablets (0.0%) 410
Catapres Tablets (About 5 in 1,000 patients) 674
Catapres-TTS (Less frequent) 675
Clozaril Tablets (Less than 1%) 2252
Cognex Capsules (Infrequent) 1901
Combipres Tablets (About 5 in 1,000) 677
▲ Cordarone Intravenous (4.9%) 2715
Cordarone Tablets (Uncommon) 2712
D.H.E. 45 Injection 2255
Decadron Phosphate with Xylocaine Injection, Sterile 1639
Demerol 2308
Desyrel and Desyrel Dividose 503
Dilacor XR Extended-release Capsules (1.4%) 2018
Dilaudid-HP Injection (Less frequent) 1337
Dilaudid-HP Lyophilized Powder 250 mg (Less frequent) 1337
Dilaudid Tablets and Liquid 1339
Diprivan Injection (1% to 3%) 2833
Diupres Tablets 1650
Dizac 1809
Duragesic Transdermal System (Less than 1%) 1288
Duranest Injections 542
Dyclone 0.5% and 1% Topical Solutions, USP 544
Effexor (Rare) 2719
Emla Cream 545
Esimil Tablets 822
Eskalith 2485
Ethmozine Tablets (Less than 2%) 2041
Etrafon 2355
Floropryl Sterile Ophthalmic Ointment (Rare) 1662
Foscavir Injection (Less than 1%) 547
Glucophage 752
Hespan Injection 929
Humorsol Sterile Ophthalmic Solution (Rare) 1664
Hydropres Tablets 1675
Hyperstat I.V. Injection 2363
Imdur (Less than or equal to 5%) 1323
Imitrex Injection (Infrequent) 1103
Imitrex Tablets (Rare) 1106
Inderal 2728
Inderal LA Long Acting Capsules 2730
Inderide Tablets 2732
Inderide LA Long Acting Capsules 2734
Indocin I.V. (Less than 3%) 1684
Intron A (Less than 5%) 2364
IOPIDINE Sterile Ophthalmic Solution ⊙ 219
Ismelin Tablets 827
Isoptin Injectable (1.2%) 1344
Isoptin Oral Tablets (1.4%) 1346
Isoptin SR Tablets (1.4%) 1348
▲ Kerlone Tablets (5.8% to 8.8%) 2436
Lariam Tablets (Less than 1%) 2128
Levophed Bitartrate Injection 2315
Lioresal Intrathecal 1596
Lippes Loop Intrauterine Double-S 1848
Lithonate/Lithotabs/Lithobid 2543
▲ Lopressor Ampuls (3%) 830
▲ Lopressor HCT Tablets (3 to 6 in 100 patients) 832
▲ Lopressor Tablets (3%) 830
Luvox Tablets (Infrequent) 2544
MS Contin Tablets (Less frequent) 1994
MSIR (Infrequent) 1997
Marcaine Hydrochloride with Epinephrine 1:200,000 2316
Marcaine Hydrochloride Injection 2316
Marcaine Spinal 2319
Maxaquin Tablets (Less than 1%) 2440
Mebaral Tablets (Less than 1 in 100) 2322
Mepergan Injection 2753
Methadone Hydrochloride Oral Concentrate 2233
Methadone Hydrochloride Oral Solution & Tablets 2235
Mexitil Capsules (About 4 in 1,000) 678
Midamor Tablets 1703
Miochol-E with Iocare Steri-Tags and Miochol-E System Pak (Rare) ⊙ 273
Mivacron (Less than 1%) 1138
Monoket (Fewer than 1%) 2406
Monopril Tablets (0.4% to 1.0%) 757
Motrin Tablets (Less than 1%) 2625
Myochrysine Injection 1711
Nembutal Sodium Capsules (Less than 1%) 436
Nembutal Sodium Solution (Less than 1%) 438
Nembutal Sodium Suppositories (Less than 1%) 440
Neo-Synephrine Hydrochloride 1% Carpuject 2324
Neo-Synephrine Hydrochloride 1% Injection 2324
Nescaine/Nescaine MPF 554
Neurontin Capsules (Rare) 1922
Nimotop Capsules (Up to 1.0%) 610
Normodyne Injection (Rare) 2377
Normodyne Tablets (Rare) 2379
Norvasc Tablets (More than 0.1% to 1%) 1940
Novocain Hydrochloride for Spinal Anesthesia 2326
Nubain Injection (1% or less) 935
Ocupress Ophthalmic Solution, 1% Sterile ⊙ 309
OptiPranolol (Metipranolol 0.3%) Sterile Ophthalmic Solution (A small number of patients) ⊙ 258
Oramorph SR (Morphine Sulfate Sustained Release Tablets) (Less frequent) 2236
Orthoclone OKT3 Sterile Solution 1837
Oxytocin Injection 2771
ParaGard T380A Intrauterine Copper Contraceptive 1880
Parlodel (Less than 1%) 2281
Paxil Tablets (Infrequent) 2505
Permax Tablets (Infrequent) 575
Phenergan with Codeine 2777
Phenergan Injection 2773
Phenergan Tablets 2775
Phenergan VC with Codeine 2781
Phenobarbital Elixir and Tablets (Less than 1 in 100 patients) 1469
Prilosec Delayed-Release Capsules (Less than 1%) 529
Prinivil Tablets (0.3% to 1.0%) 1733
Prinzide Tablets 1737
▲ Proleukin for Injection (7%) 797
Prostigmin Injectable 1260
Prostigmin Tablets 1261
▲ Prostin VR Pediatric Sterile Solution (About 7%) 2635
Protamine Sulfate Ampoules & Vials 1471
Prozac Pulvules & Liquid, Oral Solution (Rare) 919
RMS Suppositories 2657
Reglan 2068
▲ ReoPro Vials (5.2%) 1471
Revex (Less than 1%) 1811
Risperdal 1301
Robaxin Injectable 2070
Romazicon (Less than 1%) 2147
Roxanol 2243
Rythmol Tablets–150mg, 225mg, 300mg (0.5 to 1.5%) 1352
Salagen Tablets (Less than 1%) 1489
Seconal Sodium Pulvules (Less than 1 in 100) 1474
Sectral Capsules (Up to 2%) 2807
Sensorcaine 559
Ser-Ap-Es Tablets 849
Solganal Suspension 2388
▲ Sublimaze Injection (Among most common) 1307
▲ Sufenta Injection (3% to 9%) 1309
Suprane (Greater than 1%) 1813
Tagamet (Rare) 2516
Tambocor Tablets (Less than 1%) 1497
▲ Taxol (3%) 714
Temaril Tablets, Syrup and Spansule Extended-Release Capsules 483
Tenex Tablets (3% or less) 2074
▲ Tenoretic Tablets (3%) 2845
▲ Tenormin Tablets and I.V. Injection (3% to 18%) 2847
Tensilon Injectable 1261
Timolide Tablets (1.2%) 1748
Timoptic in Ocudose (Less frequent) 1753
Timoptic Sterile Ophthalmic Solution (Less frequent) 1751
Timoptic-XE 1755
Tonocard Tablets (0.4-1.8%) 531
▲ Toprol-XL Tablets (Approximately 3 of 100 patients) 565
Tracrium Injection 1183
Trandate (Rare) 1185
Trilafon 2389
Valium Injectable 2182
Vancocin HCl, Vials & ADD-Vantage (Infrequent) 1481
Vascor (200, 300 and 400 mg) Tablets 1587
Vaseretic Tablets 1765
Vasotec I.V. 1768
Vasotec Tablets (0.5% to 1.0%) 1771
Verelan Capsules (1.4%) 1410
Verelan Capsules (1.4%) 2824
Versed Injection 2170
Virazole (Infrequent) 1264
Visken Tablets (2% or fewer patients) 2299
Xylocaine Injections 567
Zantac (Rare) 1209
Zantac Injection (Rare) 1207
Zantac Syrup (Rare) 1209
Zebeta Tablets (0.4% to 0.5%) 1413
Zestril Tablets (0.3% to 1.0%) 2854
Ziac (0.9% to 1.1%) 1415
Zofran Injection (Rare) 1214
▲ Zofran Tablets (6%) 1217
Zosyn (1.0% or less) 1419
Zosyn Pharmacy Bulk Package (1.0% or less) 1422
Zyloprim Tablets (Less than 1%) 1226

Bradycardia, fetal

Carbocaine Hydrochloride Injection 2303
Duranest Injections 542
Nescaine/Nescaine MPF 554
▲ Prepidil Gel (4.1%) 2633
Sensorcaine 559
Sufenta Injection (One case) 1309
Syntocinon Injection 2296
Vasoxyl Injection 1196
▲ Xylocaine Injections (20% to 30%) 567

Bradycardia, neonatal

Diupres Tablets 1650
Hydropres Tablets 1675
Normodyne Injection 2377
Normodyne Tablets (Rare) 2379
Oxytocin Injection 2771
Syntocinon Injection 2296
Tenoretic Tablets 2845
Tenormin Tablets and I.V. Injection 2847
Trandate 1185

Bradycardia, paradoxical

Ismo Tablets 2738
Isordil Sublingual Tablets 2739
Isordil Tembids 2741
Isordil Titradose Tablets 2742
Nitro-Bid IV 1523
Sorbitrate 2843
Transderm-Nitro Transdermal Therapeutic System 859

Bradycardia, severe

Eskalith 2485

Bradycardia, symptomatic

Kerlone Tablets (0.8% to 1.9%) 2436

Bradycardia, transient

Calan SR Caplets 2422
Calan Tablets 2419
▲ Survanta Beractant Intratracheal Suspension (11.9%) 2226
Wigraine Tablets & Suppositories 1829

Bradycardia with nodal escape rhythms

Isoptin SR Tablets 1348
Verelan Capsules 1410
Verelan Capsules 2824

Bradykinesia

Cognex Capsules (Infrequent) 1901
Effexor (Rare) 2719
Eldepryl Tablets 2550
Paxil Tablets 2505
Reglan 2068
▲ Wellbutrin Tablets (8.0%) 1204

Bradykinetic episodes

Atamet (Less frequent) 572
Larodopa Tablets (Infrequent) 2129
Sinemet Tablets (Less frequent) 943
Sinemet CR Tablets 944

Bradylogia

Imitrex Tablets (Rare) 1106

Bradypnea

Alfenta Injection 1286
Prostin VR Pediatric Sterile Solution (Less than 1%) 2635
Zoloft Tablets (Rare) 2217

Brain, compression

Gelfoam Sterile Sponge 2608

Brain syndrome, acute

Betaseron for SC Injection 658
Permax Tablets (Infrequent) 575
Prozac Pulvules & Liquid, Oral Solution (Infrequent) 919
Videx Tablets, Powder for Oral Solution, & Pediatric Powder for Oral Solution (Less than 1%) 720
Virazole 1264

Brain syndrome, chronic

Betaseron for SC Injection 658
Prozac Pulvules & Liquid, Oral Solution (Rare) 919

Brain syndrome, organic, acute

Garamycin Injectable 2360

Breast abscess

Lamictal Tablets (Rare) 1112

Breast atrophy

Paxil Tablets (Rare) 2505
▲ Zoladex (33%) 2858

Breast carcinoma

Aldactazide 2413
Aldactone 2414
Ambien Tablets (Rare) 2416
Betaseron for SC Injection (2%) 658
Climara Transdermal System (Moderate increased risk) 645
Clomid 1514
Cognex Capsules (Rare) 1901
Demulen 2428
Depo-Provera Contraceptive Injection (Fewer than 1%) 2602
Estratest 2539
Eulexin Capsules (Two reports) 2358
Lamictal Tablets (Rare) 1112
Levlen/Tri-Levlen 651
Ogen Tablets 2627
Ogen Vaginal Cream 2630
Ortho-Cyclen/Ortho-Tri-Cyclen 1858
Ortho-Est 1869
Ortho-Cyclen/Ortho Tri-Cyclen 1858
Paxil Tablets (Rare) 2505
Permax Tablets (Infrequent) 575
Premphase (A moderate increased risk) 2797
Prempro (A moderate increased risk) 2801
Protostat Tablets 1883
Levlen/Tri-Levlen 651

Breast changes, unspecified

Brevicon 2088
Demulen 2428
Desogen Tablets 1817
▲ Emcyt Capsules (10 to 66%) 1953
Lo/Ovral Tablets 2746
Lo/Ovral-28 Tablets 2751
Lupron Depot 3.75 mg (Less than 5%) 2556
Lupron Depot-PED 7.5 mg, 11.25 mg and 15 mg (Less than 2%) 2560
Micronor Tablets 1872
Modicon 1872
Nordette-21 Tablets 2755
Nordette-28 Tablets 2758
Norinyl 2088
Nor-Q D Tablets 2135
Ortho-Cept 1851
Ortho-Cyclen/Ortho-Tri-Cyclen 1858
Ortho-Novum 1872
Ortho-Cyclen/Ortho Tri-Cyclen 1858
Ovral Tablets 2770
Ovral-28 Tablets 2770
Ovrette Tablets 2771
Proglycem 580
Rogaine Topical Solution (0.47%) 2637
Tri-Norinyl 2164
Triphasil-21 Tablets 2814
Triphasil-28 Tablets 2819

Breast engorgement

Adalat CC (Less than 1.0%) 589
Anafranil Capsules (Rare) 803
Betaseron for SC Injection 658

(Described in PDR For Nonprescription Drugs) Incidence data in parenthesis; ▲ 3% or more (⊙ Described in PDR For Ophthalmology)

Desyrel and Desyrel Dividose 503
Effexor (Rare) 2719
Haldol Decanoate 1577
Haldol Injection, Tablets and Concentrate 1575
Mellaril 2269
Permax Tablets (Rare) 575
Ser-Ap-Es Tablets 849
Synarel Nasal Solution for Endometriosis (Less than 1%) 2152
▲ Zoladex (Greater than 1% but less than 5%) 2858

Breast enlargement

Aldoclor Tablets 1598
Aldomet Ester HCl Injection 1602
Aldomet Oral 1600
Aldoril Tablets 1604
Anafranil Capsules (Up to 2%) 803
Asendin Tablets (Less than 1%) 1369
Brevicon 2088
Claritin (Rare) 2349
Claritin-D 2350
Climara Transdermal System 645
Demser Capsules (Infrequent) 1649
Demulen 2428
Depakene 413
Depakote Tablets 415
Desogen Tablets 1817
Desyrel and Desyrel Dividose 503
Diethylstilbestrol Tablets 1437
Effexor (Rare) 2719
Elavil 2838
▲ Emcyt Capsules (60%) 1953
Endep Tablets 2174
Estrace Cream and Tablets 749
Estraderm Transdermal System 824
ESTRATAB Tablets (0.3, 0.625, 1.25, 2.5 mg) 2536
Estratest 2539
Etrafon 2355
Flexeril Tablets (Rare) 1661
Indocin Capsules (Less than 1%) 1680
Indocin I.V. (Less than 1%) 1684
Indocin (Less than 1%) 1680
Levlen/Tri-Levlen 651
Limbitrol 2180
Ludiomil Tablets (Isolated reports) 843
Menest Tablets 2494
Micronor Tablets 1872
Modicon 1872
Navane Capsules and Concentrate 2201
Navane Intramuscular 2202
Norinyl 2088
Norpramin Tablets 1526
Nor-Q D Tablets 2135
Ogen Tablets 2627
Ogen Vaginal Cream 2630
Ortho-Cept 1851
Ortho-Cyclen/Ortho-Tri-Cyclen 1858
Ortho Dienestrol Cream 1866
Ortho-Est 1869
Ortho-Novum 1872
Ortho-Cyclen/Ortho Tri-Cyclen 1858
Ovcon 760
PMB 200 and PMB 400 2783
Pamelor 2280
Premarin Intravenous 2787
Premarin with Methyltestosterone 2794
Premarin Tablets 2789
Premarin Vaginal Cream 2791
Premphase 2797
Prempro 2801
PREVACID Delayed-Release Capsules (Less than 1%) 2562
Proscar Tablets 1741
ProSom Tablets (Rare) 449
Prozac Pulvules & Liquid, Oral Solution (Rare) 919
Serzone Tablets (Infrequent) 771
Sinequan 2205
Stilphostrol Tablets and Ampuls 612
▲ Supprelin Injection (1% to 10%) 2056
Surmontil Capsules 2811
▲ Synarel Nasal Solution for Central Precocious Puberty (8%) 2151
Thorazine 2523
THYREL TRH (A small number of patients) 2873
Tofranil Ampuls 854
Tofranil Tablets 856
Tofranil-PM Capsules 857
Triavil Tablets 1757
Trilafon 2389
Levlen/Tri-Levlen 651
Tri-Norinyl 2164
Triphasil-21 Tablets 2814
Triphasil-28 Tablets 2819
Vivactil Tablets 1774
▲ Zoladex (18%) 2858
Zoloft Tablets (Rare) 2217

Breast fibroadenosis

Ambien Tablets (Rare) 2416
Anafranil Capsules (Rare) 803
Kerlone Tablets (Less than 2%) 2436

Breast fibrocystic

▲ Betaseron for SC Injection (3%) 658
Clomid 1514
Levlen/Tri-Levlen 651
Micronor Tablets 1872
Modicon 1872
Ortho-Cyclen/Ortho-Tri-Cyclen 1858
Ortho-Novum 1872
Ortho-Cyclen/Ortho Tri-Cyclen 1858
Permax Tablets (Infrequent) 575
Prozac Pulvules & Liquid, Oral Solution (Infrequent) 919
Levlen/Tri-Levlen 651

Breast lumps

Depo-Provera Contraceptive Injection (Fewer than 1%) 2602
Levlen/Tri-Levlen 651
Ortho-Cyclen/Ortho-Tri-Cyclen 1858
Ortho-Est 1869
Ortho-Cyclen/Ortho Tri-Cyclen 1858
Levlen/Tri-Levlen 651

Breast milk, maternal, excreted in

AVC 1500
Achromycin V Capsules 1367
Actifed with Codeine Cough Syrup 1067
Adalat Capsules (10 mg and 20 mg) 587
Adalat CC 589
Adriamycin PFS 1947
Adriamycin RDF 1947
Aldactazide 2413
Aldactone 2414
Aldoclor Tablets 1598
Aldomet Ester HCl Injection 1602
Aldomet Oral 1600
Aldoril Tablets 1604
Alfenta Injection 1286
Altace Capsules 1232
Ambien Tablets 2416
Amen Tablets 780
Anatuss LA Tablets 1542
Anexia Tablets 1782
Ansaid Tablets 2579
Asacol Delayed-Release Tablets 1979
Asendin Tablets 1369
Astramorph/PF Injection, USP (Preservative-Free) 535
Atretol Tablets 573
Atromid-S Capsules 2701
Augmentin 2468
Axid Pulvules 1427
Azactam for Injection 734
Azo Gantanol Tablets 2080
Azo Gantrisin Tablets 2081
Azulfidine 1949
Bactrim DS Tablets 2084
Bactrim I.V. Infusion 2082
Bactrim 2084
Bentyl 1501
Betapace Tablets 641
Biavax II 1613
Bicillin C-R Injection 2704
Bicillin C-R 900/300 Injection 2706
Bicillin L-A Injection 2707
Biltricide Tablets 591
Blocadren Tablets 1614
Brevicon 2088
Bricanyl Subcutaneous Injection 1502
Bricanyl Tablets 1503
Brontex 1981
Butisol Sodium Elixir & Tablets 2660
Cafergot 2251
Calan SR Caplets 2422
Calan Tablets 2419
Capoten 739
Capozide 742
Cardizem CD Capsules 1506
Cardizem SR Capsules 1510
Cardizem Injectable 1508
Cardizem Tablets 1512
Carmol HC 924
Cataflam 816
Catapres Tablets 674
Catapres-TTS 675
Ceclor Pulvules & Suspension 1431
Cefizox for Intramuscular or Intravenous Use 1034
Cefotan 2829
Ceftin 1078
CellCept Capsules 2099
Ceptaz 1081
Ceredase 1065
Cipro I.V. 595
Cipro Tablets 592
Claforan Sterile and Injection 1235
Claritin 2349
Cleocin Phosphate Injection 2586
Clozaril Tablets 2252
Combipres Tablets 677
Compazine 2470
Cordarone Intravenous 2715
Cordarone Tablets 2712
Cortisporin Cream 1084
Cortisporin Ointment 1085
Cortisporin Otic Solution Sterile 1087
Cortisporin Otic Suspension Sterile 1088
Cortone Acetate Sterile Suspension 1623
Cortone Acetate Tablets 1624
Coumadin 926
Cycrin Tablets 975
Cystospaz 1963
Cytotec 2424
Cytoxan 694
Dalalone D.P. Injectable 1011
Dapsone Tablets USP 1284
Daraprim Tablets 1090
Decadron Elixir 1633
Decadron Phosphate Injection 1637
Decadron Phosphate Respihaler 1642
Decadron Phosphate Turbinaire 1645
Decadron Phosphate with Xylocaine Injection, Sterile 1639
Decadron Tablets 1635
Decadron-LA Sterile Suspension 1646
Deconsal C Expectorant Syrup 456
Deconsal Pediatric Capsules 454
Deconsal Pediatric Syrup 457
Deconsal II Tablets 454
Demerol 2308
Demulen 2428
Depakene 413
Depakote Tablets 415
Depo-Provera Sterile Aqueous Suspension 2606
Desogen Tablets 1817
Desoxyn Gradumet Tablets 419
Desyrel and Desyrel Dividose 503
Dexacort Phosphate in Respihaler 458
Dexacort Phosphate in Turbinaire 459
Dexedrine 2474
DextroStat Dextroamphetamine Tablets 2036
Diabinese Tablets 1935
Didrex Tablets 2607
Diflucan Injection, Tablets, and Oral Suspension 2194
Dilacor XR Extended-release Capsules 2018
Dilantin Infatabs 1908
Dilantin Kapseals 1906
Dilantin Parenteral 1910
Dilantin-125 Suspension 1911
Dilaudid-HP Injection 1337
Dilaudid-HP Lyophilized Powder 250 mg 1337
Dilaudid Tablets and Liquid 1339
Diprivan Injection 2833
Diucardin Tablets 2718
Diupres Tablets 1650
Diuril Oral Suspension 1653
Diuril Sodium Intravenous 1652
Diuril Tablets 1653
Dolobid Tablets 1654
Doral Tablets 2664
Doryx Capsules 1913
Duragesic Transdermal System 1288
Duramorph 962
Duratuss HD Elixir 2565
Dyazide 2479
Dyrenium Capsules 2481
E.E.S. 424
E-Mycin Tablets 1341
EC-Naprosyn Delayed-Release Tablets 2117
Elavil 2838
Empirin with Codeine Tablets 1093
Endep Tablets 2174
Enduron Tablets 420
Ergomar 1486
ERYC 1915
EryPed 200 & EryPed 400 Granules 421
Ery-Tab Tablets 422
Erythrocin Stearate Filmtab 425
Esgic-plus Tablets 1013
Esidrix Tablets 821
Esimil Tablets 822
Eskalith 2485
Ethmozine Tablets 2041
Fansidar Tablets 2114
Fedahist Gyrocaps 2401
Fedahist Timecaps 2401
Felbatol 2666
Fioricet Tablets 2258
Fioricet with Codeine Capsules 2260
Fiorinal Capsules 2261
Fiorinal with Codeine Capsules 2262
Fiorinal Tablets 2261
Flagyl 375 Capsules 2434
Flagyl I.V. 2247
Florinef Acetate Tablets 505
Floxin I.V. 1571
Floxin Tablets (200 mg, 300 mg, 400 mg) 1567
Fluorescite ⊚ 219
Fortaz 1100
Gantanol Tablets 2119
Gantrisin 2120
Glucophage 752
Halcion Tablets 2611
Haldol Decanoate 1577
Haldol Injection, Tablets and Concentrate 1575
Hydeltrasol Injection, Sterile 1665
Hydeltra-T.B.A. Sterile Suspension 1667
Hydrocet Capsules 782
Hydrocortone Acetate Sterile Suspension 1669
Hydrocortone Phosphate Injection, Sterile 1670
Hydrocortone Tablets 1672
HydroDIURIL Tablets 1674
Hydropres Tablets 1675
Ilosone 911
Imitrex Injection 1103
Imitrex Tablets 1106
Imuran 1110
Inderal 2728
Inderal LA Long Acting Capsules 2730
Inderide Tablets 2732
Inderide LA Long Acting Capsules 2734
Indocin 1680
INFeD (Iron Dextran Injection, USP) 2345
Inversine Tablets 1686
Isoptin Injectable 1344
Isoptin Oral Tablets 1346
Isoptin SR Tablets 1348
Keflex Pulvules & Oral Suspension 914
Kefurox Vials, Faspak & ADD-Vantage 1454
Kefzol Vials, Faspak & ADD-Vantage 1456
Kerlone Tablets (Less than 2%) 2436
Konakion Injection 2127
Kutrase Capsules 2402
Kwell Cream & Lotion 2008
Kwell Shampoo 2009
Lamictal Tablets 1112
Lamprene Capsules 828
Lanoxicaps 1117
Lanoxin Injection 1123
Lanoxin Tablets 1128
Lariam Tablets 2128
Lasix Injection, Oral Solution and Tablets 1240
Lescol Capsules 2267
Levbid Extended-Release Tablets 2405
Levlen/Tri-Levlen 651
Levothroid Tablets 1016
Levsin/Levsinex/Levbid 2405
Lindane Lotion USP 1% 582
Lindane Shampoo USP 1% 583
Lincocin 2617
Lioresal Intrathecal 1596
Lithium Carbonate Capsules & Tablets 2230
Lithonate/Lithotabs/Lithobid 2543
Lomotil 2439
Loniten Tablets (One report) 2618
Lo/Ovral Tablets 2746
Lo/Ovral-28 Tablets 2751
Lopressor Ampuls 830
Lopressor HCT Tablets 832
Lopressor Tablets 830
Lortab 2566
Lotensin Tablets 834
Lotensin HCT 837
Lotrel Capsules 840
Ludiomil Tablets 843
Lufyllin & Lufyllin-400 Tablets 2670
Lufyllin-GG Elixir & Tablets 2671
Luvox Tablets 2544
MS Contin Tablets 1994
MSIR Oral Solution 1997
Macrobid Capsules 1988
Macrodantin Capsules 1989
Marinol (Dronabinol) Capsules 2231
Maxzide 1380
Mefoxin 1691
Mefoxin Premixed Intravenous Solution 1694
Mepergan Injection 2753
Meruvax II 1697
Methergine 2272

(Described in PDR For Nonprescription Drugs) Incidence data in parenthesis; ▲ 3% or more (⊚ Described in PDR For Ophthalmology)

Breast milk, maternal, excreted in — **Side Effects Index** — **1240**

Methotrexate Sodium Tablets, Injection, for Injection and LPF Injection 1275
MetroGel 1047
Mezlin 601
Micronor Tablets 1872
Midamor Tablets 1703
Miltown Tablets 2672
Minizide Capsules 1938
Minocin Intravenous 1382
Minocin Oral Suspension 1385
Minocin Pellet-Filled Capsules 1383
Modicon 1872
Moduretic Tablets 1705
Monocid Injection 2497
Monodox Capsules 1805
Mono-Gesic Tablets 792
Monopril Tablets 757
Mykrox Tablets 993
Myochrysine Injection 1711
Mysoline 2754
Anaprox/Naprosyn 2117
Nembutal Sodium Solution 438
Neoral 2276
NEOSAR Lyophilized/Neosar 1959
Nicorette 2458
Nizoral Tablets 1298
Nordette-21 Tablets 2755
Nordette-28 Tablets 2758
Norinyl 2088
Norisodrine with Calcium Iodide Syrup 442
Normodyne Injection 2377
Normodyne Tablets 2379
Norpace 2444
Norplant System 2759
Nor-Q D Tablets 2135
Novahistine DH 2462
Novahistine Expectorant 2463
Nucofed 2051
Nydrazid Injection 508
Omnipen for Oral Suspension 2765
Oramorph SR (Morphine Sulfate Sustained Release Tablets) 2236
Oretic Tablets 443
Ortho-Cept 1851
Ortho-Cyclen/Ortho-Tri-Cyclen 1858
Ortho-Novum 1872
Ortho-Cyclen/Ortho Tri-Cyclen 1858
Ovcon 760
Ovral Tablets 2770
Ovral-28 Tablets 2770
Ovrette Tablets 2771
Oxistat 1152
PCE Dispertab Tablets 444
PMB 200 and PMB 400 2783
Paxil Tablets 2505
Pediapred Oral Liquid 995
PediOtic Suspension Sterile 1153
Pentasa 1527
Pepcid Injection 1722
Pepcid 1720
Persantine Tablets 681
Pfizerpen for Injection 2203
Phenergan with Codeine 2777
Phenergan VC with Codeine 2781
Phenobarbital Elixir and Tablets 1469
Phrenilin 785
Pravachol 765
Premphase 2797
Prempro 2801
Synthroid Injection 1359
PREVACID Delayed-Release Capsules 2562
Prinzide Tablets 1737
Procan SR Tablets 1926
Prograf 1042
Proloprim Tablets 1155
Propulsid 1300
Prostep (nicotine transdermal system) 1394
Protostat Tablets 1883
Provera Tablets 2636
Prozac Pulvules & Liquid, Oral Solution 919
Psorcon Cream 0.05% 909
Pyrazinamide Tablets 1398
Quadrinal Tablets 1350
Quarzan Capsules 2181
Quibron 2053
Quinaglute Dura-Tabs Tablets 649
Quinidex Extentabs 2067
RMS Suppositories 2657
Reglan 2068
Ridaura Capsules 2513
Rifamate Capsules 1530
Rifater 1532
Rimactane Capsules 847
Robaxisal Tablets 2071
Rocaltrol Capsules 2141
Rocephin Injectable Vials, ADD-Vantage, Galaxy Container 2142
Rogaine Topical Solution (One report) 2637
Roxanol 2243
Salflex Tablets 786
Sandimmune 2286
Sansert Tablets 2295
Sectral Capsules 2807
Sedapap Tablets 50 mg/650 mg 1543
Semprex-D Capsules 463
Semprex-D Capsules 1167
Septra 1174
Septra I.V. Infusion 1169
Septra I.V. Infusion ADD-Vantage Vials 1171
Septra 1174
Ser-Ap-Es Tablets 849
Seromycin Pulvules 1476
Slo-bid Gyrocaps 2033
Solganal Suspension 2388
Soma Compound w/Codeine Tablets 2676
Soma Compound Tablets 2675
Soma Tablets 2674
Spectrobid Tablets 2206
Sporanox Capsules 1305
Stadol 775
Stelazine 2514
Symmetrel Capsules and Syrup 946
Syn-Rx Tablets 465
Syn-Rx DM Tablets 466
Synthroid Tablets 1359
Syntocinon Injection 2296
Tagamet 2516
Tambocor Tablets 1497
Tavist Syrup 2297
Tazicef for Injection 2519
Tegretol Chewable Tablets 852
Tegretol Suspension 852
Tegretol Tablets 852
Tenoretic Tablets 2845
Tenormin Tablets and I.V. Injection 2847
Testoderm Testosterone Transdermal System 486
Thalitone 1245
Theo-24 Extended Release Capsules 2568
Theo-X Extended-Release Tablets 788
Thorazine 2523
Ticlid Tablets 2156
Timolide Tablets 1748
Timoptic in Ocudose 1753
Timoptic Sterile Ophthalmic Solution 1751
Timoptic-XE 1755
Tofranil Ampuls 854
Tofranil Tablets 856
Tofranil-PM Capsules 857
Tolectin (200, 400 and 600 mg) 1581
Toprol-XL Tablets 565
Toradol 2159
Trandate 1185
Tranxene 451
Trental Tablets 1244
Levlen/Tri-Levlen 651
Trilisate 2000
Trimpex Tablets 2163
Tri-Norinyl 2164
Triostat Injection 2530
Triphasil-21 Tablets 2814
Triphasil-28 Tablets 2819
Tylenol with Codeine 1583
Ultram Tablets (50 mg) 1585
Unasyn 2212
Uni-Dur Extended-Release Tablets 1331
Uniphyl 400 mg Tablets 2001
Uroqid-Acid No. 2 Tablets 640
Vanceril Inhaler 2394
Vancocin HCl, Oral Solution & Pulvules 1483
Vancocin HCl, Vials & ADD-Vantage 1481
Vantin for Oral Suspension and Vantin Tablets 2646
Vascor (200, 300 and 400 mg) Tablets 1587
Vaseretic Tablets 1765
Vasotec Tablets 1771
Verelan Capsules 1410
Versed Injection 2170
Vibramycin 1941
Vibramycin Hyclate Intravenous 2215
Vibramycin 1941
Vicodin ES Tablets 1357
Visken Tablets 2299
Voltaren Tablets 861
Wygesic Tablets 2827
Xanax Tablets 2649
Zantac 1209
Zantac Injection 1207
Zantac Syrup 1209
Zaroxolyn Tablets 1000
Zefazone 2654
Zestoretic 2850
Ziac 1415
Zinacef 1211
Zonalon Cream 1055
Zosyn 1419
Zosyn Pharmacy Bulk Package 1422
Zovirax Capsules 1219
Zovirax Sterile Powder 1223
Zovirax 1219
Zyloprim Tablets 1226

Breast nipple bleeding

Depo-Provera Contraceptive Injection (Fewer than 1%) 2602

Breast pain

Anafranil Capsules (Up to 1%) 803
▲ Betaseron for SC Injection (7%) 658
Cardura Tablets (Less than 0.5% of 3960 patients) 2186
Cipro Tablets (0.3% to 1%) 592
Claritin-D 2350
Clozaril Tablets (Less than 1%) 2252
Cognex Capsules (Infrequent) 1901
Cytovene (1% or less) 2103
Effexor (Infrequent) 2719
Humegon (Occasional) 1824
Imdur (Less than or equal to 5%) 1323
Lamictal Tablets (Rare) 1112
Lupron Depot 3.75 mg (Less than 5%) 2556
Lupron Depot 7.5 mg 2559
Luvox Tablets (Infrequent) 2544
Paxil Tablets (Infrequent) 2505
Pentasa (Less than 1%) 1527
Premphase 2797
Prempro 2801
Prinzide Tablets 1737
Procardia XL Extended Release Tablets (1% or less) 1972
Prozac Pulvules & Liquid, Oral Solution (Infrequent) 919
Sporanox Capsules (Less than 1%) 1305
▲ Zoladex (7%) 2858
Zoloft Tablets (Rare) 2217

Breast secretion

Brevicon 2088
Danocrine Capsules (Rare) 2307
Demulen 2428
Desogen Tablets 1817
Diethylstilbestrol Tablets 1437
ESTRATAB Tablets (0.3, 0.625, 1.25, 2.5 mg) 2536
Estratest 2539
Imitrex Tablets (Rare) 1106
Levlen/Tri-Levlen 651
Menest Tablets 2494
Micronor Tablets 1872
Modicon 1872
Norinyl 2088
▲ Norplant System (5% or greater) 2759
Nor-Q D Tablets 2135
Ortho-Cept 1851
Ortho-Cyclen/Ortho-Tri-Cyclen 1858
Ortho Dienestrol Cream 1866
Ortho-Novum 1872
Ortho-Cyclen/Ortho Tri-Cyclen 1858
Ovcon 760
PMB 200 and PMB 400 2783
Premarin Intravenous 2787
Premarin with Methyltestosterone 2794
Premarin Vaginal Cream 2791
Stilphostrol Tablets and Ampuls 612
▲ Supprelin Injection (1% to 12%) 2056
Levlen/Tri-Levlen 651
Tri-Norinyl 2164

Breast size reduction

Danocrine Capsules 2307
Lupron Depot 3.75 mg 2556
Supprelin Injection (2% to 3%) 2056
▲ Synarel Nasal Solution for Endometriosis (10% of patients) 2152

Breast size, changes

Depo-Provera Contraceptive Injection (Fewer than 1%) 2602

Breast tenderness

Amen Tablets (Rare) 780
Azactam for Injection (Less than 1%) 734
Brevicon 2088
Bumex (0.1%) 2093
Climara Transdermal System 645
Cycrin Tablets (Rare) 975
▲ Demulen (Among most common) 2428
Depo-Provera Contraceptive Injection 2602
Depo-Provera Sterile Aqueous Suspension 2606
Desogen Tablets 1817
Diethylstilbestrol Tablets 1437
▲ Emcyt Capsules (66%) 1953
Estrace Cream and Tablets 749
Estraderm Transdermal System 824
ESTRATAB Tablets (0.3, 0.625, 1.25, 2.5 mg) 2536
Estratest 2539
Imitrex Tablets (Infrequent) 1106
Indocin Capsules (Less than 1%) 1680
Indocin I.V. (Less than 1%) 1684
Indocin (Less than 1%) 1680
Levlen/Tri-Levlen 651
Loniten Tablets (Less than 1%) 2618
Lo/Ovral Tablets 2746
Lo/Ovral-28 Tablets 2751
Lupron Depot 3.75 mg (Less than 5%) 2556
Lupron Depot 7.5 mg 2559
▲ Lupron Injection (5% or more) 2555
Menest Tablets 2494
Metrodin (urofollitropin for injection) 2446
Micronor Tablets 1872
Modicon 1872
Norinyl 2088
Nor-Q D Tablets 2135
Ogen Tablets 2627
Ogen Vaginal Cream 2630
Ortho-Cept 1851
Ortho-Cyclen/Ortho-Tri-Cyclen 1858
Ortho Dienestrol Cream 1866
Ortho-Est 1869
Ortho-Novum 1872
Ortho-Cyclen/Ortho Tri-Cyclen 1858
Ovcon 760
Ovral Tablets 2770
Ovral-28 Tablets 2770
Ovrette Tablets 2771
PMB 200 and PMB 400 2783
Premarin Intravenous 2787
Premarin with Methyltestosterone 2794
Premarin Tablets 2789
Premarin Vaginal Cream 2791
Premphase 2797
Prempro 2801
PREVACID Delayed-Release Capsules (Less than 1%) 2562
Proscar Tablets 1741
Prostin E2 Suppository 2634
Provera Tablets (Rare) 2636
Serophene (clomiphene citrate tablets, USP) (Approximately 1 in 50) 2451
Stilphostrol Tablets and Ampuls 612
Testoderm Testosterone Transdermal System (Three in 104 patients) 486
Levlen/Tri-Levlen 651
Tri-Norinyl 2164
Triphasil-21 Tablets 2814
Triphasil-28 Tablets 2819
▲ Zoladex (Greater than 1% but less than 5%) 2858

Breath, shortness

Adalat Capsules (10 mg and 20 mg) (2% or less) 587
▲ Adenocard Injection (12%) 1021
AeroBid Inhaler System (Less than 1%) 1005
Aerobid-M Inhaler System (Less than 1%) 1005
Azo Gantrisin Tablets 2081
▲ Bromfed-DM Cough Syrup (Among most frequent) 1786
BuSpar (Infrequent) 737
Ceftin (Less than 1% but more than 0.1%) 1078
Clomid 1514
Clozaril Tablets (1%) 2252
Colestid Tablets (Infrequent) 2591
Coumadin 926
Cytosar-U Sterile Powder (Less frequent) 2592
Dalmane Capsules (Rare) 2173
Demulen 2428
Desyrel and Desyrel Dividose (Less than 1% to 1.3%) 503
Dimetane-DC Cough Syrup 2059
Dimetane-DX Cough Syrup 2059
Dipentum Capsules (Rare) 1951
Dobutrex Solution Vials (1% to 3%) 1439
DynaCirc Capsules (0.5% to 1%) 2256
Eldepryl Tablets 2550

(▣ Described in PDR For Nonprescription Drugs) — Incidence data in parenthesis; ▲ 3% or more — (◉ Described in PDR For Ophthalmology)

1241 Side Effects Index Bronchospasm

Empirin with Codeine Tablets 1093
▲ Epogen for Injection (0.14% to 14%) 489
▲ Esgic-plus Tablets (Among most frequent) 1013
Estrace Cream and Tablets 749
▲ Fioricet Tablets (Among most frequent) 2258
Fioricet with Codeine Capsules (Frequent) 2260
Floxin I.V. 1571
Floxin Tablets (200 mg, 300 mg, 400 mg) 1567
Gamimune N, 5% Immune Globulin Intravenous (Human), 5% 619
Gamimune N, 10% Immune Globulin Intravenous (Human), 10% 621
Gantrisin 2120
Guaifed 1787
Hespan Injection 929
Humulin 50/50, 100 Units 1444
Humulin 70/30, 100 Units (Less common) 1445
Humulin L, 100 Units (Less common) 1446
▲ Hylorel Tablets (18.3% to 45.9%) 985
Regular, 100 Units (Less common) 1450
Pork Regular, 100 Units (Less common) 1452
Imitrex Injection 1103
Imitrex Tablets 1106
IOPIDINE Sterile Ophthalmic Solution ⊚ 219
K-Phos Neutral Tablets 639
K-Phos Original Formula 'Sodium Free' Tablets (Less frequent) 639
Klonopin Tablets 2126
Kytril Injection (Rare) 2490
Kytril Tablets (Rare) 2492
▲ Leustatin (7%) 1834
Levlen/Tri-Levlen 651
▲ Lopressor Ampuls (3%) 830
Lopressor HCT Tablets 832
▲ Lopressor Tablets (3%) 830
Maxzide 1380
Micronor Tablets 1872
Midamor Tablets (Less than or equal to 1%) 1703
Modicon 1872
Moduretic Tablets 1705
▲ Navelbine Injection (3%; infrequent) 1145
▲ NebuPent for Inhalation Solution (53 to 72%) 1040
Norpace (1 to 3%) 2444
Novolin 70/30 Prefilled Disposable Insulin Delivery System (Rare) 1798
Oncovin Solution Vials & Hyporets 1466
Ortho-Cyclen/Ortho-Tri-Cyclen 1858
Ortho-Est 1869
Ortho-Novum 1872
Ortho-Cyclen/Ortho Tri-Cyclen 1858
Orthoclone OKT3 Sterile Solution 1837
Parlodel (Less than 1%) 2281
Peptavlon 2878
▲ Phrenilin (Among most frequent) 785
Procardia Capsules (2% or less) 1971
▲ Procrit for Injection (0.14% to 14%) 1841
Profasi (chorionic gonadotropin for injection, USP) 2450
Quadrinal Tablets 1350
Questran Light 769
Questran Powder 770
Retrovir Capsules 1158
Retrovir I.V. Infusion 1163
Retrovir Syrup 1158
ReVia Tablets (Less than 1%) 940
Rifadin 1528
Rifater 1532
Sandostatin Injection (Less than 1%) 2292
Sansert Tablets 2295
▲ Sedapap Tablets 50 mg/650 mg (Among the most frequent) 1543
Septra (Rare) 1174
Septra I.V. Infusion 1169
Septra I.V. Infusion ADD-Vantage Vials 1171
Septra (Rare) 1174
Soma Compound Tablets 2675
Stilphostrol Tablets and Ampuls 612
Synarel Nasal Solution for Central Precocious Puberty (2.6%) 2151
▲ THROMBATE III Antithrombin III (Human) (1 of 17) 637
▲ Toprol-XL Tablets (Approximately 3 of 100 patients) 565
Levlen/Tri-Levlen 651
▲ Tylenol with Codeine (Among most frequent) 1583
Uroqid-Acid No. 2 Tablets 640
Velban Vials 1484
Velosulin BR Human Insulin 10 ml Vials 1795
Wellbutrin Tablets (Infrequent) 1204
Zofran Injection (Rare) 1214

Breathholding

▲ Suprane (30%-68%) 1813

Breathing, difficult (see under Dyspnea)

Breathing, irregular

Anexsia 5/500 Elixir 1781
Dilaudid Ampules 1335
Dilaudid Cough Syrup 1336
Dilaudid-HP Injection 1337
Dilaudid-HP Lyophilized Powder 250 mg 1337
Dilaudid 1335
Hydrocet Capsules 782
Larodopa Tablets (Infrequent) 2129
Lortab 2566
Quadrinal Tablets 1350
Sinemet CR Tablets 944
Supprelin Injection (2% to 3%) 2056
Vicodin Tablets 1356
Vicodin ES Tablets 1357
Zydone Capsules 949

Breathing, labored (see under Dyspnea)

Breathing, shallow (see under Hypopnea)

Breathing, stertorous

Duragesic Transdermal System (Less than 1%) 1288
Neurontin Capsules (Rare) 1922

Bromsulphalein retention, increase (see under BSP retention, increase)

Bronchial constriction

Duvoid (Infrequent) 2044

Bronchial obstruction

Blocadren Tablets 1614
Timoptic in Ocudose 1753
Timoptic Sterile Ophthalmic Solution 1751
Timoptic-XE 1755

Bronchial secretion, decreased

Atrovent Inhalation Aerosol (About 1 in 100) 671

Bronchial secretions, increase

Klonopin Tablets 2126
Mestinon Injectable 1253
Mestinon 1254
Prostigmin Injectable 1260
Prostigmin Tablets 1261
Tensilon Injectable 1261

Bronchial secretions, thickening

Actifed with Codeine Cough Syrup 1067
Atrohist Plus Tablets 454
▲ Benadryl Capsules (Among most frequent) 1898
▲ Benadryl Injection (Among most frequent) 1898
Betoptic Ophthalmic Solution (Rare) 469
Betoptic S Ophthalmic Suspension (Rare) 471
▲ Bromfed-DM Cough Syrup (Among most frequent) 1786
Comhist 2038
Deconamine 1320
▲ Dimetane-DC Cough Syrup (Most frequent) 2059
Dimetane-DX Cough Syrup (Among most frequent) 2059
Ornade Spansule Capsules 2502
▲ PBZ Tablets (Among most frequent) 845
▲ PBZ-SR Tablets (Among most frequent) 844
Periactin 1724
Tavist Syrup (Among most frequent) 2297
▲ Tavist Tablets (Among most frequent) 2298
Temaril Tablets, Syrup and Spansule Extended-Release Capsules 483
Triaminic Cold Tablets ▣ 790
▲ Trinalin Repetabs Tablets (Among most frequent) 1330
Tussend 1783

Bronchiectasis

Pulmozyme Inhalation 1064
Videx Tablets, Powder for Oral Solution, & Pediatric Powder for Oral Solution (Less than 1%) 720

Bronchiolitis

Cuprimine Capsules 1630
Haldol Decanoate 1577
▲ Proventil Solution for Inhalation 0.5% (1.5% to 4%) 2383
Solganal Suspension 2388
▲ Tetramune (Among most common) 1404

Bronchiolitis, obliterative

Depen Titratable Tablets (Rare) 2662
Pentasa (One case) 1527

Bronchitis

AeroBid Inhaler System (1-3%) 1005
Aerobid-M Inhaler System (1-3%) 1005
▲ Airet Solution for Inhalation (1.5% to 4%) 452
Ambien Tablets (Infrequent) 2416
Anafranil Capsules (Infrequent) 803
Ansaid Tablets (Less than 1%) 2579
▲ Atrovent Inhalation Solution (14.6%) 673
Cartrol Tablets (Less common) 410
▲ CellCept Capsules (8.5% to 11.9%) 2099
Claritin (2% or fewer patients) 2349
Claritin-D (Less frequent) 2350
Clozaril Tablets (Less than 1%) 2252
Cognex Capsules (Frequent) 1901
Cozaar Tablets (Less than 1%) 1628
Cytotec (Infrequent) 2424
Dilacor XR Extended-release Capsules (Infrequent) 2018
Effexor (Frequent) 2719
Flonase Nasal Spray (Less than 1%) 1098
Fludara for Injection (Up to 1%) 663
Foscavir Injection (Less than 1%) 547
Hytrin Capsules (At least 1%) 430
Hyzaar Tablets (1% or greater) 1677
Imdur (Less than or equal to 5%) 1323
Ismo Tablets (Fewer than 1%) 2738
Kerlone Tablets (Less than 2%) 2436
Lescol Capsules (2.3%) 2267
Lodine Capsules and Tablets (Less than 1%) 2743
Lotensin Tablets 834
Lotensin HCT (0.3% to 1.0%) 837
Luvox Tablets (Infrequent) 2544
Miacalcin Nasal Spray (Less than 1%) 2275
OptiPranolol (Metipranolol 0.3%) Sterile Ophthalmic Solution (A small number of patients) ⊚ 258
Paxil Tablets (Infrequent) 2505
Permax Tablets (Infrequent) 575
Plendil Extended-Release Tablets (0.5% to 1.5%) 527
PREVACID Delayed-Release Capsules (Less than 1%) 2562
Prinivil Tablets (0.5 to 1.6%) 1733
Prinzide Tablets (0.3 to 1%) 1737
▲ Prograf (Greater than 3%) 1042
Proventil Inhalation Solution 0.083% (1.5% to 4%) 2384
Prozac Pulvules & Liquid, Oral Solution (Frequent) 919
Pulmozyme Inhalation 1064
Ridaura Capsules (Rare) 2513
▲ Rogaine Topical Solution (7.16%) 2637
Serevent Inhalation Aerosol (1% to 3%) 1176
Serzone Tablets (Frequent) 771
Stadol (1% or greater) 775
Supprelin Injection (2% to 3%) 2056
▲ Tetramune (Among most common) 1404
Tilade (1.2%) 996
Vaseretic Tablets 1765
Vasotec I.V. 1768
Vasotec Tablets (0.5% to 1.0%) 1771
▲ Ventolin Inhalation Solution (1.5% to 4%) 1198
Ventolin Nebules Inhalation Solution (1.5% to 4%) 1199
Videx Tablets, Powder for Oral Solution, & Pediatric Powder for Oral Solution (Up to 1%) 720
Wellbutrin Tablets (Infrequent) 1204
Zebeta Tablets 1413
Zestoretic (0.3 to 1%) 2850
Zestril Tablets (0.5% to 1.6%) 2854
Ziac 1415
Zoladex (1% or greater) 2858

Bronchoconstriction

Intron A (Rare) 2364
Platinol 708
Platinol-AQ Injection 710
Tensilon Injectable 1261
Urecholine 1761

Bronchoconstriction, paradoxical

Maxair Inhaler 1494
Metaproterenol Sulfate Inhalation Solution, USP, Arm-a-Med 552
Tornalate Solution for Inhalation, 0.2% 956
Tornalate Metered Dose Inhaler 957

Bronchospasm

Abbokinase 403
Abbokinase Open-Cath 405
Actimmune (Rare) 1056
Adenocard Injection 1021
Children's Advil Suspension (Less than 1%) 2692
▲ Airet Solution for Inhalation (Rare; 8%) 452
Alfenta Injection (0.3% to 1%) 1286
Alkeran for Injection (In some patients) 1070
Ambien Tablets (Rare) 2416
▲ Anafranil Capsules (2% to 7%) 803
Atrovent Inhalation Solution (2.3%) 673
Axid Pulvules (Rare) 1427
Azactam for Injection (Less than 1%) 734
Beclovent Inhalation Aerosol and Refill (Rare) 1075
Beconase (Rare) 1076
Betagan ⊚ 233
Betimol 0.25%, 0.5% ⊚ 261
Betoptic Ophthalmic Solution (Rare) 469
Betoptic S Ophthalmic Suspension (Rare) 471
Blocadren Tablets (0.6%) 1614
Brevibloc Injection (Less than 1%) 1808
Brevital Sodium Vials 1429
Calcimar Injection, Synthetic (A few cases) 2013
Capoten 739
Capozide 742
Cardura Tablets (Less than 0.5% of 3960 patients) 2186
Cartrol Tablets (Rare) 410
Cataflam 816
Ceptaz (Very rare) 1081
Cipro Tablets (Less than 1%) 592
Claritin (2% or fewer patients) 2349
Claritin-D (Less frequent) 2350
Clinoril Tablets (Less than 1 in 100) 1618
Cytotec (Infrequent) 2424
Dilaudid-HP Injection (Less frequent) 1337
Dilaudid-HP Lyophilized Powder 250 mg (Less frequent) 1337
Dilaudid Tablets and Liquid 1339
Dipentum Capsules (Rare) 1951
Diprivan Injection (Rare; less than 1%) 2833
Dobutrex Solution Vials (Occasional) 1439
Dolobid Tablets (Less than 1 in 100) 1654
Dopram Injectable 2061
Eminase 2039
Emla Cream 545
Engerix-B Unit-Dose Vials 2482
Factrel (Rare) 2877
Feldene Capsules (Less than 1%) 1965
Floxin I.V. 1571
Floxin Tablets (200 mg, 300 mg, 400 mg) 1567
Flumadine Tablets & Syrup (Less than 0.3%) 1015
Fluorescite ⊚ 219
Fortaz (Very rare) 1100
Foscavir Injection (Between 1% and 5%) 547
Fungizone Intravenous 506

(▣ Described in PDR For Nonprescription Drugs) Incidence data in parenthesis; ▲ 3% or more (⊚ Described in PDR For Ophthalmology)

Haldol Decanoate 1577
Haldol Injection, Tablets and Concentrate 1575
Hespan Injection 929
Hismanal Tablets (Less frequent) 1293
IBU Tablets (Less than 1%) 1342
Imdur (Less than or equal to 5%) 1323
Inapsine Injection (Less common) 1296
Inderal 2728
Inderal LA Long Acting Capsules 2730
Inderide Tablets 2732
Inderide LA Long Acting Capsules 2734
INFeD (Iron Dextran Injection, USP) 2345
Intal Capsules (Less than 1 in 10,000 patients) 987
▲ Intal Inhaler (Among most frequent) 988
Intal Nebulizer Solution (Rare) 989
Intron A (Less than 5%) 2364
Isoptin Injectable (Rare) 1344
Kerlone Tablets (Less than 2%) 2436
Lamictal Tablets (Rare) 1112
Lopressor HCT Tablets (Fewer than 1 in 100) 832
Lutrepulse for Injection 980
Maxaquin Tablets (Less than 1%) 2440
Metubine Iodide Vials 916
Miacalcin Injection (A few cases) 2273
Miacalcin Nasal Spray (1% to 3%) 2275
Miltown Tablets (Rare) 2672
Mivacron (Less than 1%) 1138
Monopril Tablets (0.2% to 1.0%) 757
Children's Motrin Ibuprofen Oral Suspension (Less than 1%) 1546
Motrin Tablets (Less than 1%) 2625
Motrin Ibuprofen Suspension, Oral Drops, Chewable Tablets, Caplets (Less than 1%) 1546
Mykrox Tablets 993
Navelbine Injection (Infrequent) 1145
▲ NebuPent for Inhalation Solution (15%) 1040
Neurontin Capsules (Rare) 1922
Norcuron (Rare) 1826
Normodyne Tablets (Less common) 2379
Nubain Injection (1% or less) 935
Nuromax Injection (Less than or equal to 0.1%) 1149
Ocupress Ophthalmic Solution, 1% Sterile ⊙ 309
▲ Oncaspar (Less than 1% to greater than 5%) 2028
Oncovin Solution Vials & Hyporets 1466
Orthoclone OKT3 Sterile Solution 1837
Orudis Capsules (Less than 1%) 2766
Oruvail Capsules (Less than 1%) 2766
PMB 200 and PMB 400 (Rare) 2783
Paraplatin for Injection (Rare) 705
Pentam 300 Injection (1 patient) 1041
Pepcid Injection (Infrequent) 1722
Pepcid (Infrequent) 1720
Pilocar ⊙ 268
Prinivil Tablets (0.3% to 1.0%) 1733
Prinzide Tablets 1737
Prostigmin Injectable 1260
Prostigmin Tablets 1261
Proventil Inhalation Aerosol (Rare) 2382
▲ Proventil Inhalation Solution 0.083% (8% to 15.4%) 2384
▲ Proventil Solution for Inhalation 0.5% (8% to 15.4%) 2383
Proventil Syrup (Rare) 2385
Quinaglute Dura-Tabs Tablets 649
Recombivax HB (Less than 1%) 1744
Reglan (A few cases) 2068
Risperdal (Infrequent) 1301
Rocephin Injectable Vials, ADD-Vantage, Galaxy Container (Rare) 2142
Roferon-A Injection (Less than 1%) 2145
Salflex Tablets 786
Seldane Tablets 1536
Seldane-D Extended-Release Tablets 1538
Semprex-D Capsules (Rare) 463
Semprex-D Capsules (Rare) 1167
Serevent Inhalation Aerosol (Rare) 1176
Streptase for Infusion (Rare) 562
Sufenta Injection (0.3% to 1%) 1309
▲ Suprane (3%-10%) 1813
Tambocor Tablets (Less than 1%) 1497
Tazicef for Injection (Very rare) 2519
Tenormin Tablets and I.V. Injection (1.2%) 2847
Tessalon Perles 1020
▲ Tilade (5.4%) 996
Timolide Tablets (1.6%) 1748
Timoptic in Ocudose (Less frequent) 1753
Timoptic Sterile Ophthalmic Solution (Less frequent) 1751
Timoptic-XE 1755
Toprol-XL Tablets (About 1 of 100 patients) 565
Toradol 2159
Tornalate Solution for Inhalation, 0.2% (1.5%) 956
Tornalate Metered Dose Inhaler (Less than 1% to 1%) 957
Tracrium Injection 1183
Trandate Tablets (Less common) 1185
Univasc Tablets (Less than 1%) 2410
Vancenase PocketHaler Nasal Inhaler (Rare) 2391
Vanceril Inhaler (Rare) 2394
Vaseretic Tablets 1765
Vasotec I.V. 1768
Vasotec Tablets (0.5% to 1.0%) 1771
Velban Vials 1484
Ventolin Inhalation Aerosol and Refill (Rare) 1197
▲ Ventolin Inhalation Solution (Rare to 15.4%) 1198
▲ Ventolin Nebules Inhalation Solution (Rare to 15.4%) 1199
Ventolin Rotacaps for Inhalation (Rare to 1%) 1200
Ventolin Syrup (Rare) 1202
Ventolin Tablets (Rare) 1203
VePesid Capsules and Injection (0.7% to 2%) 718
Versed Injection (Less than 1%) 2170
Virazole (Infrequent) 1264
Volmax Extended-Release Tablets (Rare) 1788
Voltaren Tablets 861
▲ Vumon (Approximately 5%) 727
Zantac (Rare) 1209
Zantac Injection 1207
Zantac Syrup (Rare) 1209
Zaroxolyn Tablets 1000
Zebeta Tablets (0%) 1413
Zemuron (Less than 1%) 1830
Zestoretic 2850
Zestril Tablets 2854
Ziac (Rare) 1415
Zofran Injection (Rare) 1214
Zofran Tablets (Rare) 1217
Zoloft Tablets (Infrequent) 2217
Zosyn (1.0% or less) 1419
Zosyn Pharmacy Bulk Package (1.0% or less) 1422
Zyloprim Tablets (Less than 1%) 1226

Bronchospasm, exacerbation of

▲ Airet Solution for Inhalation (15.4%) 452
Asacol Delayed-Release Tablets 1979
Brethine Ampuls 815
Brethine Tablets 814
Serevent Inhalation Aerosol 1176

Bronchospasm, paradoxical

Alupent 669
Proventil Solution for Inhalation 0.5% 2383
Serevent Inhalation Aerosol 1176
Tilade (Rare) 996
Ventolin Inhalation Solution 1198
Ventolin Nebules Inhalation Solution 1199
Ventolin Rotacaps for Inhalation 1200

Browache

EPIFRIN ⊙ 239
Floropryl Sterile Ophthalmic Ointment 1662
Humorsol Sterile Ophthalmic Solution 1664
OptiPranolol (Metipranolol 0.3%) Sterile Ophthalmic Solution (A small number of patients) ⊙ 258
Phospholine Iodide ⊙ 326
▲ Rēv-Eyes Ophthalmic Eyedrops 0.5% (10% to 40%) ⊙ 323
Vasosulf ⊙ 271
Vexol 1% Ophthalmic Suspension (Less than 1%) ⊙ 230

Bruising

Accutane Capsules (Less than 1%) 2076
Anafranil Capsules (Rare) 803
Atretol Tablets 573
Beclovent Inhalation Aerosol and Refill 1075
BuSpar (Infrequent) 737
Calan SR Caplets (1% or less) 2422
Calan Tablets (1% or less) 2419
Cataflam (Less than 1%) 816
Clozaril Tablets (Less than 1%) 2252
Coumadin 926
Depakene 413
Depakote Tablets 415
Depen Titratable Tablets 2662
▲ Emcyt Capsules (3%) 1953
Eminase 2039
Empirin with Codeine Tablets 1093
Felbatol 2666
Feldene Capsules (Less than 1%) 1965
Florinef Acetate Tablets 505
Floxin I.V. 1571
Floxin Tablets (200 mg, 300 mg, 400 mg) 1567
Isoptin Oral Tablets (Less than 1%) 1346
Isoptin SR Tablets (1% or less) 1348
Maxair Autohaler (0.6%) 1492
Maxair Inhaler (Less than 1%) 1494
Nalfon 200 Pulvules & Nalfon Tablets (Less than 1%) 917
Oncaspar 2028
Plendil Extended-Release Tablets (0.5% to 1.5%) 527
Quadrinal Tablets 1350
Rythmol Tablets–150mg, 225mg, 300mg (Less than 1%) 1352
Sandostatin Injection (1% to 4%) 2292
▲ Tegison Capsules (25-50%) 2154
Tegretol Chewable Tablets 852
Tegretol Suspension 852
Tegretol Tablets 852
Tonocard Tablets 531
Verelan Capsules (1% or less) 1410
Verelan Capsules (Less than 1%) 2824
Voltaren Tablets (Less than 1%) 861
Zefazone (2%) 2654

Bruxism

Atamet 572
Eldepryl Tablets 2550
Larodopa Tablets (Relatively frequent) 2129
Paxil Tablets (Infrequent) 2505
Sinemet Tablets 943
Sinemet CR Tablets 944
Wellbutrin Tablets (Infrequent) 1204

Buccal-lingual-masticatory syndrome

Prozac Pulvules & Liquid, Oral Solution (One case) 919

Buccoglossal syndrome

Prozac Pulvules & Liquid, Oral Solution (Infrequent) 919

Bucking

Diprivan Injection (Less than 1%) 2833

Budd-Chiari syndrome

Brevicon 2088
Demulen 2428
Desogen Tablets 1817
Levlen/Tri-Levlen 651
Micronor Tablets 1872
Modicon 1872
Norinyl 2088
Nor-Q D Tablets 2135
Ortho-Cept 1851
Ortho-Cyclen/Ortho-Tri-Cyclen 1858
Ortho-Novum 1872
Ortho-Cyclen/Ortho Tri-Cyclen 1858
Ovcon 760
Levlen/Tri-Levlen 651
Tri-Norinyl 2164

Bulbus oculi, perforation

AK-CIDE ⊙ 202
AK-CIDE Ointment ⊙ 202
AK-Pred ⊙ 204
Blephamide Liquifilm Sterile Ophthalmic Suspension 476
Blephamide Ointment ⊙ 237
Dexacidin Ointment ⊙ 263
FML Forte Liquifilm ⊙ 240
FML Liquifilm ⊙ 241
FML S.O.P. ⊙ 241
FML-S Liquifilm ⊙ 242
Fluor-Op Ophthalmic Suspension ⊙ 264
Inflamase ⊙ 265
Maxitrol Ophthalmic Ointment and Suspension ⊙ 224
Pred Forte ⊙ 250
Pred Mild ⊙ 253
TobraDex Ophthalmic Suspension and Ointment 473
Vasocidin Ointment ⊙ 268
Vasocidin Ophthalmic Solution ⊙ 270
Vexol 1% Ophthalmic Suspension ⊙ 230

Bulimia

Paxil Tablets (Rare) 2505

Bullae

8-MOP Capsules 1246
NegGram 2323

Bundle branch block

Anafranil Capsules (Rare) 803
Cardizem CD Capsules (Less than 1%) 1506
Cardizem SR Capsules (Less than 1%) 1510
Cardizem Injectable 1508
Cardizem Tablets (Less than 1%) 1512
Cognex Capsules (Rare) 1901
Diprivan Injection (Less than 1%) 2833
Effexor (Rare) 2719
Imdur (Less than or equal to 5%) 1323
Macrobid Capsules 1988
Macrodantin Capsules 1989
Miacalcin Nasal Spray (Less than 1%) 2275
Paxil Tablets (Rare) 2505
Prozac Pulvules & Liquid, Oral Solution (Rare) 919
Rythmol Tablets–150mg, 225mg, 300mg (0.3 to 1.9%) 1352
▲ Tenormin Tablets and I.V. Injection (6.6%) 2847
Tonocard Tablets (Less than 1%) 531
Yutopar Intravenous Injection 570

Burning

▲ A/T/S 2% Acne Topical Gel and Solution (Most common) 1234
Aclovate (1 in 100 patients) 1069
▲ Acular (Approximately 40%) 474
Afrin ▣ 797
▲ Alomide (Among most frequent) 469
Americaine Anesthetic Lubricant 983
Americaine Otic Topical Anesthetic Ear Drops 983
Analpram-HC Rectal Cream 1% and 2.5% 977
Anusol Ointment ▣ 847
Anusol-HC Cream 2.5% (Infrequent to frequent) 1896
Anusol-HC Suppositories 1897
Aristocort A 0.025% Cream (Infrequent) 1027
Aristocort A 0.1% Cream (Infrequent) 1029
Aristocort A 0.1% Ointment (Infrequent) 1030
Bactroban Ointment (1.5%) 2470
Benoquin Cream 20% (Occasional) 2868
BiCNU 691
Caladryl Cream For Kids ▣ 853
Catapres-TTS (3 of 101 patients) 675
Chloromycetin Ophthalmic Ointment, 1% (Occasional) ⊙ 310
Cipro I.V. Pharmacy Bulk Package (Less than 1%) 597
▲ Condylox (64% to 78%) 1802
Cordran Lotion (Infrequent) 1803
Cordran Tape (Infrequent) 1804
Cortisporin Cream 1084
Cortisporin Ointment 1085
Cortisporin Otic Solution Sterile 1087
Cortisporin Otic Suspension Sterile (Rare) 1088
Cutivate Cream (0.6%) 1088
Cutivate Ointment (0.6%) 1089
Cyclocort Topical (Infrequent) 1037
Decadron Phosphate Injection 1637
Decadron Phosphate Topical Cream 1644
Decaspray Topical Aerosol 1648
Dermatop Emollient Cream 0.1% (Less than 1%) 1238
DesOwen Cream, Ointment and Lotion (Approximately 3%) 1046
▲ Diprolene Gel 0.05% (6%) 2353
▲ Elimite (permethrin) 5% Cream (10%) 478
Elocon (1 of 319 patients) 2354
▲ Exelderm Cream 1.0% (3%) 2685
Exelderm Solution 1.0% (Approximately 1%) 2686
4-Way Fast Acting Nasal Spray (regular & mentholated) ▣ 621
4-Way Long Lasting Nasal Spray ▣ 621
Fleet Bisacodyl Enema 1002
Fleet Prep Kits 1003
Florone/Florone E 906

(▣ Described in PDR For Nonprescription Drugs) Incidence data in parenthesis; ▲ 3% or more (⊙ Described in PDR For Ophthalmology)

1243 Side Effects Index BUN levels, elevation

Floropryl Sterile Ophthalmic Ointment ... 1662
Fluoroplex Topical Solution & Cream 1% ... 479
Garamycin Injectable ... 2360
Heparin Lock Flush Solution ... 2725
Heparin Sodium Injection ... 2726
Heparin Sodium Injection, USP, Sterile Solution ... 2615
Heparin Sodium Vials ... 1441
Humorsol Sterile Ophthalmic Solution ... 1664
Hydeltrasol Injection, Sterile ... 1665
Hydrocortone Phosphate Injection, Sterile ... 1670
Hytone ... 907
Inflamase (Rare) ... ⊙ 265
IOPIDINE Sterile Ophthalmic Solution ... ⊙ 219
▲ Lac-Hydrin 12% Lotion (1 in 10 to 30 patients) ... 2687
Lamisil Cream 1% (0.8%) ... 2265
Lidex (Infrequent) ... 2130
Locoid Cream, Ointment and Topical Solution (Infrequent) ... 978
Lotrimin ... 2371
Lotrisone Cream (Infrequent) ... 2372
Monistat-Derm (miconazole nitrate 2%) Cream (Isolated reports) ... 1889
▲ Naftin Gel 1% (5.0%) ... 481
NeoDecadron Topical Cream ... 1714
▲ Ocufen (Among most frequent) .. ⊙ 245
Ophthetic (Occasional) ... ⊙ 247
Oxistat (1.4%) ... 1152
Panafil Ointment (Occasional) ... 2246
Panafil-White Ointment (Occasional) ... 2247
PediOtic Suspension Sterile (Rare) ... 1153
Phospholine Iodide ... ⊙ 326
Pramosone Cream, Lotion & Ointment ... 978
Pred-G Liquifilm Sterile Ophthalmic Suspension ... ⊙ 251
ProctoCream-HC (Infrequent) ... 2408
ProctoCream-HC 2.5% (Infrequent to frequent) ... 2408
▲ Profenal 1% Sterile Ophthalmic Solution (Among most frequent).. ⊙ 227
Psorcon Cream 0.05% (Infrequent) ... 909
Psorcon Ointment 0.05% ... 908
▲ Rev-Eyes Ophthalmic Eyedrops 0.5% (Approximately 50%) ... ⊙ 323
Rowasa (0.61%) ... 2548
Sodium Sulamyd ... 2387
▲ Spectazole (econazole nitrate 1%) Cream (3%) ... 1890
Surgicel (Occasional) ... 1314
Synalar (Infrequent) ... 2130
Temovate (Infrequent) ... 1179
Terazol 3 Vaginal Suppositories ... 1886
▲ Timoptic-XE (1 in 8 patients) ... 1755
Topicort (0.8%) ... 1243
Tridesilon Cream 0.05% (Infrequent) ... 615
Tridesilon Ointment 0.05% (Infrequent) ... 616
▲ Ultravate Cream 0.05% (4.4%) ... 2689
Ultravate Ointment 0.05% (2.4%) 2690
▲ Vagistat-1 (Approximately 6%) ... 778
▲ Viroptic Ophthalmic Solution, 1% Sterile (4.6%) ... 1204
VōSol (Occasional) ... 2678
Westcort ... 2690
Zantac Injection ... 1207
▲ Zovirax Ointment 5% (28.3%) ... 1223

Burning, at injection site

▲ Ativan Injection (17%) ... 2698
Attenuvax ... 1610
Biavax II ... 1613
BiCNU ... 691
Brevibloc Injection (Less than 1%) 1808
▲ Cardizem Injectable (3.9%) ... 1508
Cefizox for Intramuscular or Intravenous Use (Greater than 1% but less than 5%) ... 1034
Ceredase ... 1065
Cipro I.V. (1% or less) ... 595
DDAVP Injection (Occasional) ... 2014
▲ Diprivan Injection (10% to 17.6%) ... 2833
Genotropin (Infrequent) ... 111
Helixate, Antihemophilic Factor (Recombinant) ... 518
Inocor Lactate Injection (0.2%) ... 2309
Intron A (Less than 5%) ... 2364
KOGENATE Antihemophilic Factor (Recombinant) ... 632
M-M-R II ... 1687
M-R-VAX II ... 1689
Meruvax II ... 1697
Monocid Injection (Less often) ... 2497
Mononine, Coagulation Factor IX (Human) ... 523
Mumpsvax ... 1708
Nicotrol Nicotine Transdermal System (At least once in 47 patients) ... 1550
Timentin for Injection ... 2528
Versed Injection (Less than 1%) ... 2170
▲ Zofran Injection (4%) ... 1214

Burning, local

Aci-Jel Therapeutic Vaginal Jelly (Occasional cases) ... 1848
Americaine Anesthetic Lubricant ... 983
Aristocort A 0.5% Cream ... 1031
Carmol HC (Infrequent to frequent) ... 924
▲ Chibroxin Sterile Ophthalmic Solution (One of the two most frequent) ... 1617
▲ Condylox (64% to 78%) ... 1802
CORTENEMA ... 2535
▲ Efudex (Among most frequent) ... 2113
Elase-Chloromycetin Ointment ... 1040
▲ Elimite (permethrin) 5% Cream (10%) ... 478
Exact Vanishing and Tinted Creams ... ▣ 749
▲ Gentak (Among most frequent) ... ⊙ 208
Habitrol Nicotine Transdermal System (Once in 35% of patients) ... 865
Loprox 1% Cream and Lotion (1 out of 514 patients) ... 1242
Mumpsvax ... 1708
▲ Naftin Cream 1% (6%) ... 480
▲ Nicoderm (nicotine transdermal system) (47%) ... 1518
Prostep (nicotine transdermal system) (At least once in 54% of patients) ... 1394
Selsun Rx 2.5% Selenium Sulfide Lotion, USP ... 2225
Spectazole (econazole nitrate 1%) Cream ... 1890
▲ Zonalon Cream (Approximately 21%) ... 1055

Burning, lower extremities

Lioresal Intrathecal ... 1596

Burning, mild

Mycelex-G 500 mg Vaginal Tablets (6 in 1,116 patients) ... 609

Burning, sexual partner

Mycelex-G 500 mg Vaginal Tablets (Rare) ... 609
Semicid Vaginal Contraceptive Inserts ... ▣ 874
Today Vaginal Contraceptive Sponge ... ▣ 874

Burning, vaginal (see under Vaginal burning)

Burning, vulvovaginal (see under Vaginal burning)

Burning sensation

▲ A/T/S 2% Acne Topical Gel and Solution (17 out of 90 patients) ... 1234
AVC (Occasional) ... 1500
Aclovate Ointment (2 of 366 patients) ... 1069
Adenocard Injection (Less than 1%) ... 1021
Chloromycetin Ophthalmic Solution ... ⊙ 310
Decadron Phosphate Sterile Ophthalmic Ointment (Rare) ... 1641
Decadron Phosphate Sterile Ophthalmic Solution (Rare) ... 1642
Dopram Injectable ... 2061
Doxorubicin Astra ... 540
Erycette (erythromycin 2%) Topical Solution ... 1888
Fleet Babylax ... 1001
Gamimune N, 5% Immune Globulin Intravenous (Human), 5% ... 619
Gamimune N, 10% Immune Globulin Intravenous (Human), 10% ... 621
Idamycin ... 1955
▲ Imitrex Injection (7.5%) ... 1103
Imitrex Tablets (Frequent) ... 1106
Mutamycin ... 703
Peptavlon ... 2878
Pondimin Tablets ... 2066
Quadrinal Tablets ... 1350
SSD (Infrequent) ... 1355
Scleromate ... 1891
Silvadene Cream 1% (Infrequent) .. 1540
Stilphostrol Tablets and Ampuls ... 612
▲ Sulfamylon Cream (One of two most frequent) ... 925
T-Stat 2.0% Topical Solution and Pads ... 2688
Temovate (4 of 421 patients) ... 1179
Theramycin Z Topical Solution 2% 1592
Topicort LP Emollient Cream 0.05% (0.8%) ... 1243
T.R.U.E. Test (Common; up to 14 reports) ... 1189
Vagistat-1 (Less than 1%) ... 778
Ventolin Rotacaps for Inhalation (Less than 1%) ... 1200
Zilactin Medicated Gel ... ▣ 882

Bursitis

Betaseron for SC Injection ... 658
Cognex Capsules (Infrequent) ... 1901
Dilacor XR Extended-release Capsules (Infrequent) ... 2018
Effexor (Infrequent) ... 2719
Hivid Tablets (Less than 1% to less than 3%) ... 2121
Lamictal Tablets (Rare) ... 1112
Luvox Tablets (Infrequent) ... 2544
Neurontin Capsules (Rare) ... 1922
Noroxin Tablets (Less frequent) ... 1715
Noroxin Tablets (Less frequent) ... 2048
Paxil Tablets (Rare) ... 2505
Permax Tablets (1.6%) ... 575
Prozac Pulvules & Liquid, Oral Solution (Infrequent) ... 919
Risperdal (Rare) ... 1301
Serzone Tablets (Infrequent) ... 771

BBB+ Major Axis Deviation

▲ Tenormin Tablets and I.V. Injection (6.6%) ... 2847

BCG infection, disseminated

BCG Vaccine, USP (TICE) (Very rare; about 1 per 5,000,000 vaccinees) ... 1814

BEI, increase

Amen Tablets ... 780
Aygestin Tablets ... 974

BSP retention

Atromid-S Capsules ... 2701
Capastat Sulfate Vials ... 2868
Sterile FUDR ... 2118
Hydrea Capsules ... 696

BSP retention, increase

Depo-Provera Sterile Aqueous Suspension ... 2606
Estratest ... 2539
Mithracin ... 607
Oxandrin ... 2862
Rifadin ... 1528
Rifamate Capsules ... 1530
Rimactane Capsules ... 847
Serophene (clomiphene citrate tablets, USP) (Approximately 10% to 20% of patients) ... 2451
Winstrol Tablets ... 2337

BUN levels, changes

Aristocort Suspension (Forte Parenteral) ... 1027
Aristocort Suspension (Intralesional) ... 1025
Aristocort Tablets ... 1022
Aristospan Suspension (Intra-articular) ... 1033
Aristospan Suspension (Intralesional) ... 1032
Atamet ... 572
Celestone Soluspan Suspension ... 2347
CORTENEMA ... 2535
Cortifoam ... 2396
Cortone Acetate Sterile Suspension ... 1623
Cortone Acetate Tablets ... 1624
Dalalone D.P. Injectable ... 1011
Decadron Elixir ... 1633
Decadron Phosphate Injection ... 1637
Decadron Phosphate Respihaler ... 1642
Decadron Phosphate Turbinaire ... 1645
Decadron Phosphate with Xylocaine Injection, Sterile ... 1639
Decadron Tablets ... 1635
Decadron-LA Sterile Suspension ... 1646
Deltasone Tablets ... 2595
Dexacort Phosphate in Respihaler .. 458
Dexacort Phosphate in Turbinaire .. 459
Doral Tablets (Less than 1%) ... 2664
Etrafon ... 2355
Florinef Acetate Tablets ... 505
Hydeltrasol Injection, Sterile ... 1665
Imuran (Less than 1%) ... 1110
Intron A (Up to 2%) ... 2364
Moban Tablets and Concentrate ... 1048
▲ Paraplatin for Injection (14%) ... 705
Pediapred Oral Liquid ... 995
Prelone Syrup ... 1787
Prolixin ... 509
▲ Roferon-A Injection (4%) ... 2145
Sinemet Tablets ... 943
Solu-Cortef Sterile Powder ... 2641
Solu-Medrol Sterile Powder ... 2643
▲ Vasotec I.V. (About 0.2% to 20%) .. 1768
▲ Vasotec Tablets (About 0.2% to 20%) ... 1771

BUN levels, decrease

Cipro I.V. (Infrequent) ... 595
Cipro I.V. Pharmacy Bulk Package (Less than 1%) ... 597
Depo-Medrol Single-Dose Vial ... 2600
Depo-Medrol Sterile Aqueous Suspension ... 2597
Medrol Tablets ... 2621

BUN levels, elevation

Accupril Tablets (2%) ... 1893
Achromycin V Capsules ... 1367
Children's Advil Suspension (Occasional) ... 2692
Aldactone ... 2414
Aldoclor Tablets ... 1598
Aldomet Ester HCl Injection ... 1602
Aldomet Oral ... 1600
Aldoril Tablets ... 1604
Alka-Seltzer Effervescent Antacid and Pain Reliever (Less than 1.0 mg%) ... ▣ 701
Alka-Seltzer Lemon Lime Effervescent Antacid and Pain Reliever (Less than 1.0 mg%).. ▣ 703
Altace Capsules (0.5% to 3%) ... 1232
Ambien Tablets (Rare) ... 2416
Ancef Injection ... 2465
Ancobon Capsules ... 2079
Asacol Delayed-Release Tablets ... 1979
Regular Strength Ascriptin Tablets ... ▣ 629
Atretol Tablets ... 573
Azo Gantrisin Tablets ... 2081
Bactrim DS Tablets ... 2084
Bactrim I.V. Infusion ... 2082
Bactrim ... 2084
Genuine Bayer Aspirin Tablets & Caplets (Less than 1.0% at doses of 1000 mg/day) ... ▣ 713
Betaseron for SC Injection ... 658
▲ Biaxin (4%) ... 405
Blocadren Tablets ... 1614
Bufferin Analgesic Tablets and Caplets ... ▣ 613
▲ Capastat Sulfate Vials (36%) ... 2868
Capoten ... 739
Capozide ... 742
Ceclor Pulvules & Suspension (Less than 1 in 500) ... 1431
Cefizox for Intramuscular or Intravenous Use (Occasional) ... 1034
▲ Cefobid Intravenous/Intramuscular (1 in 16) ... 2189
▲ Cefobid Pharmacy Bulk Package - Not for Direct Infusion (1 in 16) ... 2192
Cefotan ... 2829
Ceftin ... 1078
Cefzil Tablets and Oral Suspension (0.1%) ... 746
Ceptaz (Occasional) ... 1081
Chibroxin Sterile Ophthalmic Solution (With oral form) ... 1617
▲ Cipro I.V. (Among most frequent) .. 595
Cipro I.V. Pharmacy Bulk Package (Among most frequent) ... 597
Cipro Tablets (0.9%) ... 592
Claforan Sterile and Injection (Occasional) ... 1235
Coly-Mycin M Parenteral ... 1905
Cozaar Tablets (Less than 0.1%) .. 1628
Cytotec (Infrequent) ... 2424
Cytovene (1% or less) ... 2103
Daypro Caplets (Occasional) ... 2426
Declomycin Tablets ... 1371
Demadex Tablets and Injection ... 686
Didronel I.V. Infusion (Occasional) .. 1488
Diprivan Injection (Less than 1%) .. 2833
Dopram Injectable ... 2061
Doryx Capsules ... 1913

(▣ Described in PDR For Nonprescription Drugs) Incidence data in parenthesis; ▲ 3% or more (⊙ Described in PDR For Ophthalmology)

BUN levels, elevation — Side Effects Index — 1244

Duricef ... 748
Dyazide ... 2479
Dynacin Capsules ... 1590
Dyrenium Capsules (Rare) ... 2481
Ecotrin ... 2455
Effexor (Rare) ... 2719
Esimil Tablets ... 822
Eulexin Capsules ... 2358
Feldene Capsules (Greater than 1%) ... 1965
Floxin I.V. (More than or equal to 1%) ... 1571
Floxin Tablets (200 mg, 300 mg, 400 mg) (More than or equal to 1%) ... 1567
Fortaz (Occasional) ... 1100
Foscavir Injection (Between 1% and 5%) ... 547
Fungizone Intravenous ... 506
▲Ganite (About 12.5%) ... 2533
Garamycin Injectable ... 2360
Glucotrol Tablets ... 1967
Glucotrol XL Extended Release Tablets ... 1968
Halfprin (Less than 1.0 mg%) ... 1362
▲Hexalen Capsules (1% to 9%) ... 2571
Hivid Tablets (Less than 1% to less than 3%) ... 2121
Hydrea Capsules (Occasional) ... 696
Hyzaar Tablets (0.6%) ... 1677
IFEX ... 697
Indocin Capsules (Less than 1%) ... 1680
▲Indocin I.V. (41% of infants) ... 1684
Indocin (Less than 1%) ... 1680
Intron A (Less than 5%) ... 2364
Ismelin Tablets ... 827
Keftab Tablets ... 915
Kefurox Vials, Faspak & ADD-Vantage ... 1454
Kefzol Vials, Faspak & ADD-Vantage ... 1456
Larodopa Tablets (Rare) ... 2129
Lithonate/Lithotabs/Lithobid ... 2543
Lodine Capsules and Tablets (Less than 1%) ... 2743
Loniten Tablets ... 2618
Lorabid Suspension and Pulvules ... 1459
Lorelco Tablets ... 1517
Lotensin Tablets (Less than 0.1%) ... 834
Lotensin HCT ... 837
Lotrel Capsules ... 840
Lozol Tablets (Less than 5%) ... 2022
Lupron Depot 3.75 mg ... 2556
Lupron Depot 7.5 mg ... 2559
Lupron Injection (Less than 5%) ... 2555
Mandol Vials, Faspak & ADD-Vantage ... 1461
Maxaquin Tablets ... 2440
Maxzide ... 1380
Mefoxin ... 1691
Mefoxin Premixed Intravenous Solution ... 1694
Mepron Suspension (1%) ... 1135
Mezlin ... 601
Mezlin Pharmacy Bulk Package ... 604
Minocin Intravenous ... 1382
Minocin Oral Suspension ... 1385
Minocin Pellet-Filled Capsules ... 1383
Mithracin ... 607
Monocid Injection (Occasional) ... 2497
Monodox Capsules ... 1805
Monopril Tablets ... 757
Children's Motrin Ibuprofen Oral Suspension (Occasional) ... 1546
Motrin Tablets (Occasional) ... 2625
Mykrox Tablets ... 993
Nebcin Vials, Hyporets & ADD-Vantage ... 1464
Neoral ... 2276
Netromycin Injection 100 mg/ml ... 2373
▲Nolvadex Tablets (18.1%) ... 2841
▲Normodyne Injection (8%) ... 2377
Noroxin Tablets (Less frequent) ... 1715
Noroxin Tablets (Less frequent) ... 2048
Norpace (1%) ... 2444
▲Orudis Capsules (3% to 9%) ... 2766
▲Oruvail Capsules (3% to 9%) ... 2766
Parlodel ... 2281
Pipracil ... 1390
Platinol ... 708
Platinol-AQ Injection ... 710
Polymyxin B Sulfate, Aerosporin Brand Sterile Powder ... 1154
Primaxin I.M. ... 1727
Primaxin I.V. ... 1729
Prinivil Tablets (About 2.0%) ... 1733
Prinzide Tablets ... 1737
Procardia Capsules (Rare) ... 1971
Procardia XL Extended Release Tablets (Rare) ... 1972
▲Prograf (8% to 30%) ... 1042
▲Proleukin for Injection (63%) ... 797
Proloprim Tablets ... 1155
Rifadin ... 1528
Rifamate Capsules ... 1530
Rifater ... 1532
Rimactane Capsules ... 847
Rocaltrol Capsules ... 2141
Rocephin Injectable Vials, ADD-Vantage, Galaxy Container (1.2%) ... 2142
Sandimmune ... 2286
Sansert Tablets ... 2295
Septra ... 1174
Septra I.V. Infusion ... 1169
Septra I.V. Infusion ADD-Vantage Vials ... 1171
Septra ... 1174
Sinemet CR Tablets ... 944
Suprax (Less than 2%) ... 1399
Tazicef for Injection (Occasional) ... 2519
Tazidime Vials, Faspak & ADD-Vantage (Occasionally) ... 1478
▲Tegison Capsules (1-10%) ... 2154
Tegretol Chewable Tablets ... 852
Tegretol Suspension ... 852
Tegretol Tablets ... 852
Terramycin Intramuscular Solution 2210
Timentin for Injection ... 2528
Tobramycin Sulfate Injection ... 968
Tolectin (200, 400 and 600 mg) (1 to 3%) ... 1581
Toradol ... 2159
▲Trandate (8 of 100 patients) ... 1185
Trilisate (Less than 1%) ... 2000
Trimpex Tablets ... 2163
Trobicin Sterile Powder ... 2645
Unasyn ... 2212
Univasc Tablets (Approximately 1%) ... 2410
Vancocin HCl, Oral Solution & Pulvules (Rare) ... 1483
Vancocin HCl, Vials & ADD-Vantage ... 1481
Vantin for Oral Suspension and Vantin Tablets ... 2646
▲Vaseretic Tablets (About 0.6% to 20%) ... 1765
Vibramycin ... 1941
Vibramycin Hyclate Intravenous ... 2215
Vibramycin ... 1941
Zaroxolyn Tablets ... 1000
Zebeta Tablets ... 1413
Zefazone ... 2654
Zestoretic ... 2850
Zestril Tablets (About 2%) ... 2854
Zinacef ... 1211
Zithromax (Less than 1%) ... 1944
Zosyn ... 1419
Zosyn Pharmacy Bulk Package ... 1422
▲Zovirax Sterile Powder (5% to 10%) ... 1223

C

Cachexia
Cognex Capsules (Infrequent) ... 1901
Cytovene-IV (One report) ... 2103
Foscavir Injection (Between 1% and 5%) ... 547
Hivid Tablets (Less than 1% to less than 3%) ... 2121
Intron A (Less than 5%) ... 2364
Permax Tablets (Rare) ... 575
Risperdal (Rare) ... 1301

Calcification, ectopic
Rocaltrol Capsules ... 2141

Calcinosis
Aristospan Suspension (Intra-articular) ... 1033
Aristospan Suspension (Intralesional) ... 1032

Calcium retention
Android ... 1251
Delatestryl Injection ... 2860
Estratest ... 2539
Halotestin Tablets ... 2614
Inderide Tablets ... 2732
Lupron Depot 3.75 mg ... 2556
Lupron Injection (Less than 5%) ... 2555
Oxandrin ... 2862
Premarin with Methyltestosterone ... 2794
Testred Capsules ... 1262

Calf muscles, need to flex
Imitrex Injection (Rare) ... 1103
Respbid Tablets ... 682

Cancer, breast
Estrace Cream and Tablets ... 749
Micronor Tablets ... 1872
Modicon ... 1872
Neurontin Capsules (Infrequent) ... 1922
Nor-Q D Tablets ... 2135
Ortho-Novum ... 1872

Cancer, cervical
Demulen ... 2428
Depo-Provera Contraceptive Injection (Fewer than 1%) ... 2602
Diethylstilbestrol Tablets ... 1437
Estratest ... 2539
Micronor Tablets ... 1872
Modicon ... 1872
Ortho-Cyclen/Ortho-Tri-Cyclen ... 1858
Ortho-Novum ... 1872
Ortho-Cyclen/Ortho Tri-Cyclen ... 1858
PMB 200 and PMB 400 ... 2783
Permax Tablets (Infrequent) ... 575
Premarin Intravenous ... 2787
Premarin with Methyltestosterone ... 2794
Premarin Vaginal Cream ... 2791

Cancer, vaginal
Diethylstilbestrol Tablets ... 1437
Estratest ... 2539
Ortho-Est ... 1869
PMB 200 and PMB 400 ... 2783
Premarin Intravenous ... 2787
Premarin with Methyltestosterone ... 2794
Premarin Vaginal Cream ... 2791

Candidiasis
▲AeroBid Inhaler System (3-9%) ... 1005
▲Aerobid-M Inhaler System (3-9%) ... 1005
Augmentin ... 2468
Beconase Inhalation Aerosol and Refill (Rare) ... 1076
Ceftin for Oral Suspension (Less than 1% but more than 0.1%) ... 1078
CellCept Capsules (Up to 0.6%) ... 2099
Ceptaz (Fewer than 1%) ... 1081
Cipro I.V. (1% or less) ... 595
Cipro I.V. Pharmacy Bulk Package (Less than 1%) ... 597
Cipro Tablets (Less than 1%) ... 592
Flagyl I.V. ... 2247
Floxin I.V. ... 1571
Fortaz (Less than 1%) ... 1100
Macrobid Capsules ... 1988
Pipracil ... 1390
PREVACID Delayed-Release Capsules (Less than 1%) ... 2562
Primaxin I.M. ... 1727
Primaxin I.V. (Less than 0.2%) ... 1729
Suprax (Less than 2%) ... 1399
Tazicef for Injection (Less than 1%) ... 2519
Unasyn (Less than 1%) ... 2212
Vantin for Oral Suspension and Vantin Tablets (Less than 1%) ... 2646
Zefazone ... 2654

Candidiasis, esophageal
Prilosec Delayed-Release Capsules (Less than 1%) ... 529

Candidiasis, mouth (see under Candidiasis, oral)

Candidiasis, nasal
Nasacort Nasal Inhaler (Rare) ... 2024
Vancenase PocketHaler Nasal Inhaler (Rare) ... 2391

Candidiasis, oral
Ancef Injection ... 2465
Azmacort Oral Inhaler (A few cases) ... 2011
Ceptaz ... 1081
Cipro I.V. (1% or less) ... 595
Cipro I.V. Pharmacy Bulk Package (Less than 1%) ... 597
Cipro Tablets (Less than 1%) ... 592
Effexor (Rare) ... 2719
Flagyl 375 Capsules ... 2434
Fortaz (Less than 1%) ... 1100
Fulvicin P/G Tablets (Occasional) ... 2359
Fulvicin P/G 165 & 330 Tablets (Occasional) ... 2359
Grifulvin V (griseofulvin tablets) Microsize (griseofulvin oral suspension) Microsize (Occasional) ... 1888
Gris-PEG Tablets, 125 mg & 250 mg (Occasional) ... 479
Kefzol Vials, Faspak & ADD-Vantage ... 1456
Megace Oral Suspension (1% to 3%) ... 699
▲Prograf (Greater than 3%) ... 1042
▲Videx Tablets, Powder for Oral Solution, & Pediatric Powder for Oral Solution (Up to 2%; 13%) ... 720

Candidiasis, pharynx
Azmacort Oral Inhaler (A few cases) ... 2011
Dexacort Phosphate in Respihaler ... 458
Dexacort Phosphate in Turbinaire ... 459
Nasacort Nasal Inhaler (Rare) ... 2024
Vancenase PocketHaler Nasal Inhaler (Rare) ... 2391

Candidiasis, vaginal (see under Vaginal candidiasis)

Candiduria
Cipro I.V. (1% or less) ... 595
Cipro I.V. Pharmacy Bulk Package (Less than 1%) ... 597
Cipro Tablets ... 592
Floxin Tablets (200 mg, 300 mg, 400 mg) ... 1567
Maxaquin Tablets ... 2440
Noroxin Tablets ... 1715
Noroxin Tablets ... 2048
Penetrex Tablets ... 2031

Capillary fragility
AeroBid Inhaler System (1-3%) ... 1005
Aerobid-M Inhaler System (1-3%) ... 1005

Capillary leak syndrome
Leukine for IV Infusion (Less than 1%) ... 1271
Neupogen for Injection (One event) 495
Orthoclone OKT3 Sterile Solution ... 1837
Proleukin for Injection ... 797
Protamine Sulfate Ampoules & Vials ... 1471

Carbohydrate tolerance, decrease
Aristocort Suspension (Forte Parenteral) ... 1027
Aristocort Suspension (Intralesional) ... 1025
Aristocort Tablets ... 1022
Aristospan Suspension (Intra-articular) ... 1033
Aristospan Suspension (Intralesional) ... 1032
Brevicon ... 2088
Celestone Soluspan Suspension ... 2347
Climara Transdermal System ... 645
CORTENEMA ... 2535
Cortone Acetate Sterile Suspension ... 1623
Cortone Acetate Tablets ... 1624
Dalalone D.P. Injectable ... 1011
Decadron Elixir ... 1633
Decadron Phosphate Injection ... 1637
Decadron Phosphate Respihaler ... 1642
Decadron Phosphate Turbinaire ... 1645
Decadron Phosphate with Xylocaine Injection, Sterile ... 1639
Decadron Tablets ... 1635
Decadron-LA Sterile Suspension ... 1646
Deltasone Tablets ... 2595
Demulen ... 2428
Depo-Medrol Single-Dose Vial ... 2600
Depo-Medrol Sterile Aqueous Suspension ... 2597
Desogen Tablets ... 1817
Dexacort Phosphate in Respihaler ... 458
Dexacort Phosphate in Turbinaire ... 459
Diethylstilbestrol Tablets ... 1437
Estrace Cream and Tablets ... 749
ESTRATAB Tablets (0.3, 0.625, 1.25, 2.5 mg) ... 2536
Estratest ... 2539
Florinef Acetate Tablets ... 505
Hydeltrasol Injection, Sterile ... 1665
Hydeltra-T.B.A. Sterile Suspension 1667
Hydrocortone Acetate Sterile Suspension ... 1669
Hydrocortone Phosphate Injection, Sterile ... 1670
Hydrocortone Tablets ... 1672
Levlen/Tri-Levlen ... 651
Lo/Ovral Tablets ... 2746
Lo/Ovral-28 Tablets ... 2751
Medrol ... 2621
Menest Tablets ... 2494
Micronor Tablets ... 1872
Modicon ... 1872
Nordette-21 Tablets ... 2755
Nordette-28 Tablets ... 2758
Norinyl ... 2088

(▣ Described in PDR For Nonprescription Drugs) Incidence data in parenthesis; ▲ 3% or more (◉ Described in PDR For Ophthalmology)

1245 Side Effects Index Cardiac output, decrease

Nor-Q D Tablets 2135
Ogen Tablets 2627
Ogen Vaginal Cream 2630
Ortho-Cept 1851
Ortho-Cyclen/Ortho-Tri-Cyclen 1858
Ortho Dienestrol Cream 1866
Ortho-Est 1869
Ortho-Novum 1872
Ortho-Cyclen/Ortho Tri-Cyclen 1858
Ovcon 760
Ovral Tablets 2770
Ovral-28 Tablets 2770
Ovrette Tablets 2771
PMB 200 and PMB 400 2783
Prelone Syrup 1787
Premarin Intravenous 2787
Premarin with Methyltestosterone 2794
Premarin Tablets 2789
Premarin Vaginal Cream 2791
Premphase 2797
Prempro 2801
Solu-Cortef Sterile Powder 2641
Solu-Medrol Sterile Powder 2643
Stilphostrol Tablets and Ampuls 612
Levlen/Tri-Levlen 651
Tri-Norinyl 2164
Triphasil-21 Tablets 2814
Triphasil-28 Tablets 2819

Carcinoma

Demulen 2428
Diethylstilbestrol Tablets 1437
Effexor (Rare) 2719
Paxil Tablets (Infrequent) 2505
Permax Tablets (Infrequent) 575
▲Zerit Capsules (2% to 4%) 729

Carcinoma, bladder

Clomid 1514
Testoderm Testosterone Transdermal System (One in 104 patients) 486
Videx Tablets, Powder for Oral Solution, & Pediatric Powder for Oral Solution (Less than 1%) 720

Carcinoma, ear

Lupron Depot 7.5 mg 2559
Lupron Injection (Less than 5%) 2555

Carcinoma, endometrial

Climara Transdermal System 645
Clomid 1514
Demulen 2428
Estrace Cream and Tablets 749
Estraderm Transdermal System 824
ESTRATAB Tablets (0.3, 0.625, 1.25, 2.5 mg) 2536
Estratest 2539
Levlen/Tri-Levlen 651
Menest Tablets 2494
Nolvadex Tablets 2841
Ogen Tablets 2627
Ogen Vaginal Cream 2630
Ortho Dienestrol Cream 1866
Ortho-Est 1869
Premarin Intravenous 2787
Premarin with Methyltestosterone 2794
Premarin Tablets 2789
Premarin Vaginal Cream 2791
Premphase (About 2- to 12-fold or greater than in nonusers) 2797
Prempro (About 2- to 12-fold or greater than in nonusers) 2801
Levlen/Tri-Levlen 651

Carcinoma, hepatocellular

Android Capsules, 10 mg (Rare) 1250
Android 1251
Brevicon (Extremely rare) 2088
Clomid 1514
Delatestryl Injection (Rare) 2860
Demulen (Rare) 2428
Estraderm Transdermal System 824
Halotestin Tablets 2614
Levlen/Tri-Levlen (Extremely rare) 651
Micronor Tablets (Rare) 1872
Modicon (Rare) 1872
Nolvadex Tablets (3 cases) 2841
Norinyl (Extremely rare) 2088
Nor-Q D Tablets (Extremely rare) 2135
Oreton Methyl (Rare) 1255
Ortho-Cyclen/Ortho-Tri-Cyclen (Rare) 1858
Ortho-Novum (Rare) 1872
Ortho-Cyclen/Ortho Tri-Cyclen (Rare) 1858
Testoderm Testosterone Transdermal System (Rare) 486
Levlen/Tri-Levlen (Extremely rare) 651
Tri-Norinyl (Extremely rare) 2164
Winstrol Tablets (Rare) 2337

Carcinoma, ovarian

Humegon (Infrequent) 1824
Metrodin (urofollitropin for injection) (Infrequent) 2446
Pergonal (menotropins for injection, USP) 2448

Carcinoma, prostate

Android Capsules, 10 mg 1250
Android 1251
Cognex Capsules (Infrequent) 1901
Halotestin Tablets 2614
Oreton Methyl 1255
Paxil Tablets (Rare) 2505
Testoderm Testosterone Transdermal System 486
Winstrol Tablets 2337

Carcinoma, renal pelvis

Cytoxan (One case) 694
NEOSAR Lyophilized/Neosar (One case) 1959

Carcinoma, uterine

Nolvadex Tablets 2841

Carcinoma, skin

Betaseron for SC Injection 658
Cognex Capsules (Infrequent) 1901
Lupron Depot 7.5 mg 2559
Lupron Injection (Less than 5%) 2555
8-MOP Capsules 1246
Orthoclone OKT3 Sterile Solution 1837
Permax Tablets (Infrequent) 575
▲Prograf (One of the two most common forms) 1042
Sandimmune 2286
Videx Tablets, Powder for Oral Solution, & Pediatric Powder for Oral Solution (Less than 1%) 720

Carcinoma, skin, benign

CellCept Capsules (1.6% to 4.0%) 2099
Permax Tablets (Rare) 575
Virazole 1264

Cardiac abnormalities

Albalon Solution with Liquifilm ◉ 231
Atamet (Less frequent) 572
Clozaril Tablets (1%) 2252
Cordarone Tablets (Infrequent) 2712
Floropryl Sterile Ophthalmic Ointment (Rare) 1662
Hivid Tablets (Less than 1% to less than 3%) 2121
Humorsol Sterile Ophthalmic Solution 1664
Marax Tablets & DF Syrup 2200
Nicorette 2458
Novantrone 1279
Pergonal (menotropins for injection, USP) (One report) 2448
Phospholine Iodide ◉ 326
Platinol (Infrequent) 708
Platinol-AQ Injection (Infrequent) 710
Sansert Tablets 2295
Sinemet Tablets (Less frequent) 943
Sinemet CR Tablets 944
Tri-Immunol Adsorbed 1408

Cardiac anomalies

Eskalith 2485
Lithium Carbonate Capsules & Tablets 2230
Tetramune (Rare) 1404

Cardiac arrest

Activase 1058
Adalat CC (Less than 1.0%) 589
Adenoscan 1024
AK-Fluor Injection 10% and 25% ◉ 203
Alupent Inhalation Aerosol (Several cases) 669
Anafranil Capsules (Infrequent) 803
Ancobon Capsules 2079
Anectine (Rare) 1073
AquaMEPHYTON Injection 1608
Betagan ◉ 233
Betaseron for SC Injection 658
Betimol 0.25%, 0.5% ◉ 261
Blocadren Tablets (Less than 1%) 1614
Capoten 739
Capozide 742
Carbocaine Hydrochloride Injection 2303
Clozaril Tablets (Rare) 2252
Cognex Capsules (Rare) 1901
Compazine 2470
Cordarone Intravenous (2.9%) 2715
Cytovene-IV (Two or more reports) 2103
Decadron Phosphate with Xylocaine Injection, Sterile 1639
Demerol 2308
Desyrel and Desyrel Dividose 503
Dilaudid Ampules 1335
Dilaudid-HP Injection 1337
Dilaudid-HP Lyophilized Powder 250 mg 1337
Dilaudid 1335
Dilaudid Oral Liquid 1339
Dilaudid 1335
Dilaudid Tablets - 8 mg 1339
Diprivan Injection (Rare; Less than 1%) 2833
Duranest Injections 542
Dyclone 0.5% and 1% Topical Solutions, USP 544
Emla Cream 545
Ethmozine Tablets (Less than 2%) 2041
Etrafon 2355
Felbatol 2666
Floxin I.V. (Less than 1%) 1571
Fluorescite ◉ 219
Fluothane 2724
Foscavir Injection (Less than 1%) 547
Fungizone Intravenous 506
Hespan Injection 929
Hismanal Tablets 1293
Isuprel Hydrochloride Solution 1:200 & 1:100 (Several instances) 2313
Isuprel Mistometer (Several instances) 2312
K-Lor Powder Packets 434
K-Norm Extended-Release Capsules 991
K-Tab Filmtab 434
Kolyum Liquid 992
Levoprome 1274
MS Contin Tablets 1994
MSIR 1997
Marcaine Hydrochloride with Epinephrine 1:200,000 2316
Marcaine Hydrochloride Injection 2316
Marcaine Spinal 2319
Mellaril (Rare) 2269
Mepergan Injection 2753
Metaproterenol Sulfate Inhalation Solution, USP, Arm-a-Med (Several cases) 552
Methadone Hydrochloride Oral Solution & Tablets 2235
Micro-K 2063
Micro-K LS Packets 2064
Monopril Tablets 757
Narcan Injection 934
Navane Intramuscular 2202
Nescaine/Nescaine MPF 554
Nicorette 2458
Novocain Hydrochloride for Spinal Anesthesia 2326
Nubain Injection (1% or less) 935
Oramorph SR (Morphine Sulfate Sustained Release Tablets) (Less frequent) 2236
Orthoclone OKT3 Sterile Solution 1837
Permax Tablets (Infrequent) 575
Pfizerpen for Injection 2203
Pontocaine Hydrochloride for Spinal Anesthesia 2330
Prinivil Tablets (0.3% to 1.0%) 1733
Prinzide Tablets 1737
Proleukin for Injection (Less than 1% to 2%) 797
Prolixin 509
Prostigmin Injectable 1260
Prostigmin Tablets 1261
Prostin VR Pediatric Sterile Solution (About 1%) 2635
Proventil Inhalation Aerosol 2382
Prozac Pulvules & Liquid, Oral Solution 919
Pulmozyme Inhalation 1064
RMS Suppositories 2657
Roxanol 2243
Rythmol Tablets–150mg, 225mg, 300mg (Less than 1%) 1352
Seldane Tablets (Rare) 1536
Seldane-D Extended-Release Tablets (Rare) 1538
Sensorcaine 559
Serentil (Rare) 684
Slow-K Extended-Release Tablets 851
Stelazine 2514
Sublimaze Injection 1307
Sufenta Injection 1309
▲Tambocor Tablets (5.1%) 1497
Temaril Tablets, Syrup and Spansule Extended-Release Capsules 483
Tenormin Tablets and I.V. Injection (1.6%) 2847
Thorazine 2523
Timolide Tablets 1748
Timoptic in Ocudose (Less frequent) 1753
Timoptic Sterile Ophthalmic Solution (Less frequent) 1751
Timoptic-XE 1755
Tonocard Tablets 531
Torecan (Rare) 2245
Tracrium Injection 1183
▲Trasylol (3%) 613
Trilafon 2389
Vancocin HCl, Vials & ADD-Vantage (Rare) 1481
Vaseretic Tablets 1765
Vasotec I.V. 1768
Vasotec Tablets (0.5% to 1.0%) 1771
Videx Tablets, Powder for Oral Solution, & Pediatric Powder for Oral Solution (Less than 1%) 720
Virazole 1264
Xylocaine Injections 567
Zestoretic 2850
Zestril Tablets (0.3% to 1.0%) 2854
Zosyn (1.0% or less) 1419
Zosyn Pharmacy Bulk Package (1.0% or less) 1422

Cardiac arrhythmias (see under Arrhythmias)

Cardiac asystole (see under Asystole)

Cardiac collapse

BOTOX (Botulinum Toxin Type A) Purified Neurotoxin Complex (2 patients) 477

Cardiac death

▲Ethmozine Tablets (2% to 5%) 2041

Cardiac dysrhythmias (see under Arrhythmias)

Cardiac enzymes, elevation

Cytotec (Infrequent) 2424

Cardiac failure

Anafranil Capsules (Rare) 803
Aredia for Injection (Up to 1%) 810
Betimol 0.25%, 0.5% ◉ 261
Blocadren Tablets 1614
Brevibloc Injection 1808
Felbatol 2666
Flumadine Tablets & Syrup (Less than 0.3%) 1015
Foscavir Injection (Less than 1%) 547
Fungizone Intravenous 506
Hivid Tablets (Less than 1% to less than 3%) 2121
Imdur (Less than or equal to 5%) 1323
Intron A (Less than 5%) 2364
Levatol 2403
Maxaquin Tablets (Less than 1%) 2440
Normodyne Tablets 2379
Norvasc Tablets (Less than or equal to 0.1%) 1940
Ocupress Ophthalmic Solution, 1% Sterile (In some cases) ◉ 309
Paraplatin for Injection 705
Tenoretic Tablets 2845
Tenormin Tablets and I.V. Injection 2847
Timolide Tablets (Less than 1%) 1748
Timoptic in Ocudose (Less frequent) 1753
Timoptic Sterile Ophthalmic Solution (Less frequent) 1751
Timoptic-XE 1755
Toprol-XL Tablets 565
Trandate 1185
Visken Tablets (Some cases) 2299
Zebeta Tablets 1413
Zosyn (1.0% or less) 1419
Zosyn Pharmacy Bulk Package (1.0% or less) 1422

Cardiac output, decrease

Carbocaine Hydrochloride Injection 2303
Digibind (Few instances) 1091
Diprivan Injection (1% to 3%) 2833
Marcaine Hydrochloride with Epinephrine 1:200,000 2316
Marcaine Hydrochloride Injection 2316
Marcaine Spinal 2319
Paxil Tablets (Rare) 2505

(Described in PDR For Nonprescription Drugs) Incidence data in parenthesis; ▲ 3% or more (◉ Described in PDR For Ophthalmology)

Cardiac output, decrease — Side Effects Index — 1246

Protamine Sulfate Ampoules & Vials 1471
Sensorcaine 559
Tensilon Injectable 1261
Trandate 1185

Cardiac rhythms, disturbances
Accupril Tablets (Rare) 1893
Capoten 739
Capozide 742
Daraprim Tablets 1090
Monopril Tablets (0.2% to 1.4%) 757
Prinzide Tablets 1737
Vaseretic Tablets 1765
Vasotec I.V. 1768
Vasotec Tablets (0.5% to 1.0%) 1771
Zebeta Tablets 1413
Zestoretic 2850

Cardiac rupture
▲ Eminase (Less than 10%) 2039

Cardiac stimulation, unspecified
Esgic-plus Tablets 1013
Fioricet Tablets (Infrequent) 2258
Fioricet with Codeine Capsules 2260
Fiorinal with Codeine Capsules 2262
Sensorcaine 559

Cardiac tamponade
Activase 1058
Loniten Tablets (Occasional) 2618
Myleran Tablets (A small number of patients) 1143
Zovirax Sterile Powder (Less than 1%) 1223

Cardiac toxicity
Adriamycin PFS 1947
Adriamycin RDF 1947
BCG Vaccine, USP (TICE) (1.9%) 1814
Cerubidine 795
Cytoxan 694
Doxorubicin Astra 540
Idamycin (Common) 1955
IFEX (Less than 1%) 697
Lanoxicaps 1117
Lanoxin Elixir Pediatric 1120
Lanoxin Injection 1123
Lanoxin Injection Pediatric 1126
Lanoxin Tablets 1128
NEOSAR Lyophilized/Neosar 1959
Roferon-A Injection (Less than 3%) 2145
Rubex 712
TheraCys BCG Live (Intravesical) (Up to 2.7%) 897

Cardialgia (see under Heartburn)

Cardiodynia (see under Heartburn)

Cardiogenic shock
Accupril Tablets (Rare) 1893
Activase 1058
Mexitil Capsules (1 in 1,000) 678
Tenormin Tablets and I.V. Injection (0.4%) 2847
Tonocard Tablets (Less than 1%) 531

Cardiomegaly
Betaseron for SC Injection 658
Cytosar-U Sterile Powder 2592
Tonocard Tablets (Less than 1%) 531

Cardiomyopathy
Adriamycin PFS 1947
Adriamycin RDF 1947
Biphetamine Capsules (Isolated reports) 983
BuSpar (Rare) 737
Cytosar-U Sterile Powder 2592
Dexedrine (Isolated reports) 2474
DextroStat Dextroamphetamine Tablets (Isolated reports) 2036
Didrex Tablets (Isolated reports) 2607
Doxorubicin Astra 540
Foscavir Injection (Less than 1%) 547
Hivid Tablets (Infrequent) 2121
Idamycin 1955
Imitrex Tablets 1106
Intron A (Less than 5%) 2364
Luvox Tablets (Infrequent) 2544
Maxaquin Tablets (Less than 1%) 2440
Megace Oral Suspension (1% to 3%) 699
Novantrone 1279
Plaquenil Sulfate Tablets (Rare) 2328
Retrovir Capsules (0.8%) 1158
Retrovir I.V. Infusion (1%) 1163
Retrovir Syrup (0.8%) 1158
Roferon-A Injection (Rare) 2145
Rubex 712

Cardiopulmonary arrest
Cipro I.V. (1% or less) 595
Cipro I.V. Pharmacy Bulk Package (Less than 1%) 597
Cipro Tablets (Less than 1%) 592
Cleocin Phosphate Injection (Rare) 2586
Lariam Tablets (One patient) 2128
Lincocin (Rare instances) 2617
Maxaquin Tablets 2440
Penetrex Tablets 2031
Pulmozyme Inhalation 1064
Triostat Injection (Approximately 2%) 2530

Cardiorespiratory arrest
Brevital Sodium Vials 1429
Monopril Tablets (0.4% to 1.0%) 757
Orthoclone OKT3 Sterile Solution 1837

Cardiorespiratory collapse
Paremyd ⊙ 247

Cardiospasm
Betaseron for SC Injection 658
Desyrel and Desyrel Dividose 503
Lodine Capsules and Tablets (Less than 1%) 2743
PREVACID Delayed-Release Capsules (Less than 1%) 2562
Prostin VR Pediatric Sterile Solution (Less than 1%) 2635

Cardiovascular abnormalities, fetal
Accutane Capsules 2076
Cataflam 816
Clinoril Tablets 1618
Dolobid Tablets 1654
Voltaren Tablets 861

Cardiovascular collapse
Aralen Hydrochloride Injection 2301
Atretol Tablets 573
Cipro I.V. (1% or less) 595
Cipro I.V. Pharmacy Bulk Package (Less than 1%) 597
Claritin-D 2350
D.A. Chewable Tablets 951
Deconamine Chewable Tablets 1320
Deconamine CX Cough and Cold Liquid and Tablets 1319
Deconamine 1320
Deconsal 454
Dilantin Parenteral 1910
Dizac 1809
Duranest Injections 542
Dura-Tap/PD Capsules 2867
Dura-Vent/DA Tablets 953
Dura-Vent Tablets 952
Dyclone 0.5% and 1% Topical Solutions, USP 544
Emla Cream 545
Entex PSE Tablets 1987
Fedahist Gyrocaps 2401
Fedahist Timecaps 2401
Floxin I.V. 1571
Floxin Tablets (200 mg, 300 mg, 400 mg) 1567
Glucophage 752
Guaimax-D Tablets 792
INFeD (Iron Dextran Injection, USP) 2345
Lioresal Intrathecal 1596
Lutrepulse for Injection 980
Marcaine Spinal 2319
Maxaquin Tablets 2440
Nescaine/Nescaine MPF 554
Noroxin Tablets 1715
Noroxin Tablets 2048
Novahistine DH 2462
Novahistine DMX ▣ 822
Novahistine Elixir ▣ 823
Novahistine Expectorant 2463
Orthoclone OKT3 Sterile Solution 1837
Seldane-D Extended-Release Tablets 1538
Syn-Rx Tablets 465
Syn-Rx DM Tablets 466
Tegretol Chewable Tablets 852
Tegretol Suspension 852
Tegretol Tablets 852
Tessalon Perles 1020
Trinalin Repetabs Tablets 1330
Tussend 1783
Tussend Expectorant 1785
Valium Injectable 2182
Xylocaine Injections 567

Cardiovascular depression
Diprivan Injection 2833
Nardil (Less frequent) 1920

Cardiovascular disorders
Ansaid Tablets (Less than 1%) 2579
Betapace Tablets (1% to 3%) 641
▲ CellCept Capsules (More than or equal to 3%) 2099
Demulen 2428
Estrace Cream and Tablets 749
Larodopa Tablets 2129
Luvox Tablets (Infrequent) 2544
Monoket (Up to 2%) 2406
Nor-Q D Tablets 2135
▲ Novantrone (11 to 26%) 1279
▲ Paraplatin for Injection (6% to 23%) 705
Phospholine Iodide ⊙ 326
Salagen Tablets (Two patients) 1489
Seldane Tablets (Rare) 1536
Seldane-D Extended-Release Tablets (Rare) 1538
Sinequan (Occasional) 2205
Taxol (Approximately 1%) 714
Videx Tablets, Powder for Oral Solution, & Pediatric Powder for Oral Solution (Less than 1%) 720
Vumon (2%) 727

Carnitine concentrations, decreased
Depakene 413

Carotid sinus hypersensitivity
Aldoclor Tablets 1598
Aldomet Ester HCl Injection 1602
Aldomet Oral 1600
Aldoril Tablets 1604

Carpal tunnel syndrome
Danocrine Capsules 2307
Megace Tablets 701
Nutropin (Rare) 1061
Protropin (Rare) 1063

Carpopedal spasm
Compazine 2470
Stelazine 2514
Thorazine 2523
Triavil Tablets 1757

Catalepsy
Anafranil Capsules (Rare) 803

Cataplexy
Clozaril Tablets 2252

Cataracts
Accutane Capsules 2076
▲ AdatoSil 5000 (Approximately 50% to 70%) ⊙ 274
Children's Advil Suspension (Less than 1%) 2692
Betimol 0.25%, 0.5% (1% to 5%) ⊙ 261
Brevicon 2088
▲ CellCept Capsules (More than or equal to 3%) 2099
Clomid 1514
Cognex Capsules (Infrequent) 1901
Cytovene-IV (Two or more reports) 2103
Danocrine Capsules (Rare) 2307
Demulen 2428
Desogen Tablets 1817
Doral Tablets 2664
Effexor (Infrequent) 2719
Flarex Ophthalmic Suspension ⊙ 218
Floxin I.V. 1571
Floxin Tablets (200 mg, 300 mg, 400 mg) 1567
Haldol Decanoate 1577
Haldol Injection, Tablets and Concentrate 1575
Hyperstat I.V. Injection 2363
IBU Tablets (Less than 1%) 1342
ISPAN Perfluoropropane ⊙ 276
ISPAN Sulfur Hexafluoride ⊙ 275
Kerlone Tablets (Less than 2%) 2436
Lescol Capsules 2267
Levlen/Tri-Levlen 651
Lo/Ovral Tablets 2746
Lo/Ovral-28 Tablets 2751
▲ Lopid Tablets (More common) 1917
Micronor Tablets 1872
Minipress Capsules (A few reports) 1937
Minizide Capsules (Rare) 1938
Modicon 1872
Children's Motrin Ibuprofen Oral Suspension (Less than 1%) 1546
Motrin Tablets (Less than 1%) 2625
Motrin Ibuprofen Suspension, Oral Drops, Chewable Tablets, Caplets (Less than 1%) 1546
Myleran Tablets (Rare) 1143
Neurontin Capsules (Infrequent) 1922
Nolvadex Tablets 2841
Nordette-21 Tablets 2755
Nordette-28 Tablets 2758
Norinyl 2088
Nor-Q D Tablets 2135
Orap Tablets 1050
Ortho-Cept 1851
Ortho-Cyclen/Ortho-Tri-Cyclen 1858
Ortho-Novum 1872
Ortho-Cyclen/Ortho Tri-Cyclen 1858
Ovcon 760
Ovral Tablets 2770
Ovral-28 Tablets 2770
Ovrette Tablets 2771
Paxil Tablets (Rare) 2505
Permax Tablets (Rare) 575
Pravachol 765
Proglycem 580
Prozac Pulvules & Liquid, Oral Solution (Rare) 919
Levlen/Tri-Levlen 651
Tri-Norinyl 2164
Triphasil-21 Tablets 2814
Triphasil-28 Tablets 2819
Ultram Tablets (50 mg) (Infrequent) 1585
Zyloprim Tablets (Less than 1%) 1226

Cataracts, posterior subcapsular
AK-CIDE (Infrequent) ⊙ 202
AK-CIDE Ointment (Infrequent) ⊙ 202
AK-Pred ⊙ 204
AK-Trol Ointment & Suspension ⊙ 205
Aristocort Suspension (Forte Parenteral) 1027
Aristocort Suspension (Intralesional) 1025
Aristocort Tablets 1022
Aristospan Suspension (Intra-articular) 1033
Aristospan Suspension (Intralesional) 1032
Blephamide Liquifilm Sterile Ophthalmic Suspension 476
Blephamide Ointment (Infrequent) ⊙ 237
Celestone Soluspan Suspension 2347
CORTENEMA 2535
Cortifoam (Following long-term use) 2396
Cortisporin Ophthalmic Ointment Sterile 1085
Cortisporin Ophthalmic Suspension Sterile 1086
Cortone Acetate Sterile Suspension 1623
Cortone Acetate Tablets 1624
Dalalone D.P. Injectable 1011
Decadron Elixir 1633
Decadron Phosphate Injection 1637
Decadron Phosphate Respihaler 1642
Decadron Phosphate Sterile Ophthalmic Ointment 1641
Decadron Phosphate Sterile Ophthalmic Solution 1642
Decadron Phosphate Turbinaire 1645
Decadron Phosphate with Xylocaine Injection, Sterile 1639
Decadron Tablets 1635
Decadron-LA Sterile Suspension 1646
Deltasone Tablets 2595
Depo-Medrol Single-Dose Vial 2600
Depo-Medrol Sterile Aqueous Suspension 2597
Dexacidin Ointment ⊙ 263
Dexacort Phosphate in Respihaler 458
Dexacort Phosphate in Turbinaire 459
Econopred & Econopred Plus Ophthalmic Suspensions ⊙ 217
FML Forte Liquifilm (Infrequent) ⊙ 240
FML Liquifilm ⊙ 241
FML S.O.P. (Infrequent) ⊙ 241
FML-S Liquifilm ⊙ 242
Florinef Acetate Tablets 505
Fluor-Op Ophthalmic Suspension ⊙ 264
HMS Liquifilm (Rare) ⊙ 244
Hydeltrasol Injection, Sterile 1665
Hydeltra-T.B.A. Sterile Suspension 1667
Hydrocortone Acetate Sterile Suspension 1669
Hydrocortone Phosphate Injection, Sterile 1670
Hydrocortone Tablets 1672
Inflamase ⊙ 265
Maxitrol Ophthalmic Ointment and Suspension ⊙ 224

(▣ Described in PDR For Nonprescription Drugs) Incidence data in parenthesis; ▲ 3% or more (⊙ Described in PDR For Ophthalmology)

1247 Side Effects Index Cerebrovascular disorders

Medrol 2621
NeoDecadron Sterile Ophthalmic Ointment 1712
NeoDecadron Sterile Ophthalmic Solution 1713
Ophthocort ⊙ 311
Pediapred Oral Liquid 995
Poly-Pred Liquifilm ⊙ 248
Pred Forte ⊙ 250
Pred Mild ⊙ 253
Pred-G Liquifilm Sterile Ophthalmic Suspension ⊙ 251
Pred-G S.O.P. Sterile Ophthalmic Ointment ⊙ 252
Prelone Syrup 1787
Solu-Cortef Sterile Powder 2641
Solu-Medrol Sterile Powder 2643
Terra-Cortril Ophthalmic Suspension 2210
TobraDex Ophthalmic Suspension and Ointment 473
Vasocidin Ointment ⊙ 268
Vasocidin Ophthalmic Solution ⊙ 270
Vexol 1% Ophthalmic Suspension ⊙ 230

Catatonia
Blocadren Tablets 1614
Cartrol Tablets 410
Compazine 2470
Depakote Tablets (Greater than 1% but not more than 5%) 415
Etrafon 2355
Haldol Decanoate 1577
Haldol Injection, Tablets and Concentrate 1575
Inderal 2728
Inderal LA Long Acting Capsules 2730
Inderide Tablets 2732
Inderide LA Long Acting Capsules 2734
Kerlone Tablets 2436
Levatol 2403
Levoprome 1274
Lopressor HCT Tablets 832
Normodyne Tablets 2379
Phenergan Injection 2773
Phenergan Tablets 2775
Prolixin 509
Risperdal (Infrequent) 1301
Sectral Capsules 2807
Stelazine 2514
Temaril Tablets, Syrup and Spansule Extended-Release Capsules 483
Tenoretic Tablets 2845
Tenormin Tablets and I.V. Injection 2847
Thorazine (Rare) 2523
Timolide Tablets 1748
Timoptic in Ocudose 1753
Timoptic Sterile Ophthalmic Solution 1751
Timoptic-XE 1755
Toprol-XL Tablets 565
Trandate Tablets 1185
Triavil Tablets 1757
Trilafon 2389
Visken Tablets 2299
Zebeta Tablets 1413
Ziac 1415

Cauda equine syndrome
Azulfidine (Rare) 1949
Gelfoam Sterile Sponge 2608

Cell granuloma
Gelfoam Sterile Sponge 2608

Cellulitis
Adalat CC (Less than 1.0%) 589
Adriamycin PFS 1947
Adriamycin RDF 1947
Anafranil Capsules (Infrequent) 803
Betaseron for SC Injection 658
Cognex Capsules (Infrequent) 1901
Cytovene (1% or less) 2103
Doxorubicin Astra 540
Effexor (Rare) 2719
Hivid Tablets (Less than 1% to less than 3%) 2121
Hyperstat I.V. Injection 2363
Norplant System (Uncommon) 2759
Oncovin Solution Vials & Hyporets 1466
Paxil Tablets (Rare) 2505
Permax Tablets (Infrequent) 575
Platinol 708
Platinol-AQ Injection 710
Prozac Pulvules & Liquid, Oral Solution (Rare) 919
ReoPro Vials (0.3%) 1471
Rubex 712
Sandostatin Injection (Less than 1%) 2292
Serzone Tablets (Rare) 771
Taxol (Rare) 714
Velban Vials 1484
Videx Tablets, Powder for Oral Solution, & Pediatric Powder for Oral Solution (Less than 1%) 720

Cellulitis, at injection site
Cefizox for Intramuscular or Intravenous Use (Greater than 1% but less than 5%) 1034
Cytosar-U Sterile Powder (Less frequent) 2592
INFeD (Iron Dextran Injection, USP) 2345
Mutamycin 703

Cellulitis, scrotal
Testoderm Testosterone Transdermal System (One in 104 patients) 486

Central retinal artery occlusion
Sus-Phrine Injection 1019

Cephalic flocculation, increase
Prolixin 509

Cephalin flocculation test, positive
Cuprimine Capsules 1630
Depen Titratable Tablets (Few reports) 2662

Cerebellar dysfunction
Cytosar-U Sterile Powder (With experimental doses) 2592
▲ Idamycin (4%) 1955
Lioresal Intrathecal 1596
Neurontin Capsules (Infrequent) 1922

Cerebellar malformation, fetal
Accutane Capsules 2076

Cerebellar syndrome, acute
Ergamisol Tablets 1292
Fludara for Injection (Up to 1%) 663
Fluorouracil Injection 2116
Sterile FUDR (Remote possibility) 2118
Lamictal Tablets (Rare) 1112

Cerebral abnormalities, fetal
Accutane Capsules 2076

Cerebral arterial insufficiency, symptoms
Atretol Tablets 573
Tegretol Chewable Tablets 852
Tegretol Suspension 852
Tegretol Tablets 852

Cerebral arteritis
Blenoxane (Rare) 692
Platinol (Rare) 708
Platinol-AQ Injection (Rare) 710
Ritalin (Isolated cases) 848

Cerebral bleeding (see under Cerebral hemorrhage)

Cerebral hemorrhage
Anafranil Capsules (Rare) 803
Ana-Kit Anaphylaxis Emergency Treatment Kit 617
Betaseron for SC Injection 658
Brevicon 2088
Demulen 2428
Desogen Tablets 1817
Imitrex Tablets 1106
Levlen/Tri-Levlen 651
Lo/Ovral Tablets 2746
Lo/Ovral-28 Tablets 2751
Micronor Tablets 1872
Modicon 1872
Nordette-21 Tablets 2755
Nordette-28 Tablets 2758
Norinyl 2088
Nor-Q D Tablets 2135
Ortho-Cept 1851
Ortho-Cyclen/Ortho-Tri-Cyclen 1858
Ortho-Novum 1872
Ortho-Cyclen/Ortho Tri-Cyclen 1858
Ovcon 760
Ovral Tablets 2770
Ovral-28 Tablets 2770
Ovrette Tablets 2771
Permax Tablets (Rare) 575
Prostin VR Pediatric Sterile Solution (Less than 1%) 2635
Rifadin 1528
Levlen/Tri-Levlen 651
Tri-Norinyl 2164
Triphasil-21 Tablets 2814
Triphasil-28 Tablets 2819

Cerebral infarction
Activase 1058
Hyperstat I.V. Injection 2363
Monopril Tablets (0.4% to 1.0%) 757
Trandate 1185

Cerebral ischemia (see under Ischemia, cerebral)

Cerebral occlusion
Humegon 1824
Ritalin (Isolated cases) 848

Cerebral thrombosis
Amen Tablets 780
Brevicon 2088
Cipro I.V. (1% or less) 595
Cipro I.V. Pharmacy Bulk Package (Less than 1%) 597
Cipro Tablets (Less than 1%) 592
Cycrin Tablets 975
DDAVP Injection (Rare) 2014
DDAVP Injection 15 mcg/mL (Rare) 2015
Demulen 2428
Desogen Tablets 1817
Floxin I.V. 1571
Floxin Tablets (200 mg, 300 mg, 400 mg) 1567
Lamictal Tablets (Rare) 1112
Levlen/Tri-Levlen 651
Lo/Ovral Tablets 2746
Lo/Ovral-28 Tablets 2751
Maxaquin Tablets 2440
Micronor Tablets 1872
Modicon 1872
Nordette-21 Tablets 2755
Nordette-28 Tablets 2758
Norinyl 2088
Nor-Q D Tablets 2135
Ortho-Cept 1851
Ortho-Cyclen/Ortho-Tri-Cyclen 1858
Ortho-Novum 1872
Ortho-Cyclen/Ortho Tri-Cyclen 1858
Ovcon 760
Ovral Tablets 2770
Ovral-28 Tablets 2770
Ovrette Tablets 2771
Penetrex Tablets 2031
Premphase 2797
Prempro 2801
Provera Tablets 2636
Stilphostrol Tablets and Ampuls 612
Stimate, (desmopressin acetate) Nasal Spray, 1.5 mg/mL (Rare) 525
Trasylol (0.5%) 613
Levlen/Tri-Levlen 651
Tri-Norinyl 2164
Triphasil-21 Tablets 2814
Triphasil-28 Tablets 2819

Cerebral vascular spasm
Torecan (Occasional case) 2245

Cerebrospinal fluid proteins, changes
Compazine 2470
Etrafon 2355
Navane Capsules and Concentrate 2201
Navane Intramuscular 2202
Polymyxin B Sulfate, Aerosporin Brand Sterile Powder 1154
Prolixin 509
Stelazine 2514
Thorazine 2523
Triavil Tablets 1757
Trilafon 2389

Cerebrospinal fluid rhinorrhea
Parlodel (A few cases; rare) 2281

Cerebrovascular accident
Accupril Tablets (Rare) 1893
Ansaid Tablets (Less than 1%) 2579
Betagan ⊙ 233
Betimol 0.25%, 0.5% ⊙ 261
Blenoxane 692
Blocadren Tablets (Less than 1%) 1614
BuSpar (Rare) 737
Calan SR Caplets (1% or less) 2422
Calan Tablets (1% or less) 2419
Capoten 739
Capozide 742
Cardura Tablets (Less than 0.5% of 3960 patients) 2186
Cognex Capsules (Infrequent) 1901
Cozaar Tablets (Less than 1%) 1628
D.H.E. 45 Injection (Extremely rare) 2255
Desyrel and Desyrel Dividose 503
Effexor (Rare) 2719
Emcyt Capsules (2%) 1953
Epogen for Injection (0.4%) 489
Fludara for Injection (Up to 3%) 663
Hyzaar Tablets 1677
Imitrex Injection (Rare) 1103
Imitrex Tablets 1106
Isoptin Oral Tablets (Less than 1%) 1346
Isoptin SR Tablets (1% or less) 1348
Lamictal Tablets (Rare) 1112
Lioresal Intrathecal 1596
Luvox Tablets (Rare) 2544
Miacalcin Nasal Spray (Less than 1%) 2275
Monopril Tablets (0.2% to 1.0%) 757
Motrin Ibuprofen Suspension, Oral Drops, Chewable Tablets, Caplets (Less than 1%) 1546
NebuPent for Inhalation Solution (1% or less) 1040
Neurontin Capsules (Rare) 1922
Nicorette 2458
Ocupress Ophthalmic Solution, 1% Sterile ⊙ 309
Orthoclone OKT3 Sterile Solution 1837
Paraplatin for Injection 705
Paxil Tablets (Rare) 2505
Permax Tablets (Infrequent) 575
Platinol (Rare) 708
Platinol-AQ Injection (Rare) 710
PREVACID Delayed-Release Capsules (Less than 1%) 2562
Prinivil Tablets (0.2 to 1.6%) 1733
Prinzide Tablets 1737
Procrit for Injection (0.4% to 3.2%) 1841
Prozac Pulvules & Liquid, Oral Solution 919
Serzone Tablets (Rare) 771
Tenex Tablets (Rare) 2074
Timolide Tablets 1748
Timoptic in Ocudose (Less frequent) 1753
Timoptic Sterile Ophthalmic Solution (Less frequent) 1751
Timoptic-XE 1755
Tonocard Tablets 531
Trasylol (0.5%) 613
Vaseretic Tablets 1765
Vasotec I.V. 1768
Vasotec Tablets (0.5% to 1.0%) 1771
Velban Vials 1484
Verelan Capsules (1% or less) 1410
Verelan Capsules (Less than 1%) 2824
Zestoretic 2850
Zestril Tablets (0.2% to 1.6%) 2854
▲ Zoladex (Greater than 1% but less than 5%) 2858

Cerebrovascular disorders
Aldoclor Tablets 1598
Aldomet Ester HCl Injection 1602
Aldomet Oral 1600
Aldoril Tablets 1604
Altace Capsules (Less than 1%) 1232
Ambien Tablets (Infrequent) 2416
Amen Tablets 780
Brevicon 2088
Cycrin Tablets 975
Demulen 2428
Depo-Provera Contraceptive Injection 2602
Depo-Provera Sterile Aqueous Suspension 2606
Ethmozine Tablets (Less than 2%) 2041
Felbatol 2666
Flumadine Tablets & Syrup (Less than 0.3%) 1015
Foscavir Injection (Between 1% and 5%) 547
Kerlone Tablets (Less than 2%) 2436
Levlen/Tri-Levlen 651
Maxaquin Tablets (Less than 1%) 2440
Micronor Tablets 1872
Modicon 1872
Norinyl 2088
Norplant System 2759
Nor-Q D Tablets 2135
Ortho-Cyclen/Ortho-Tri-Cyclen 1858
Ortho-Novum 1872
Ortho-Cyclen/Ortho Tri-Cyclen 1858
Ovcon 760
Premphase 2797
Prempro 2801
Provera Tablets 2636
Risperdal 1301

(▭ Described in PDR For Nonprescription Drugs) Incidence data in parenthesis; ▲ 3% or more (⊙ Described in PDR For Ophthalmology)

Cerebrovascular disorders | Side Effects Index | 1248

Levlen/Tri-Levlen 651
Tri-Norinyl 2164

Cerebrovascular insufficiency
Capoten 739
Capozide 742

Cervical disorders (see under Cervical irregularities)

Cervical erosion, changes
Amen Tablets 780
Aygestin Tablets 974
Brevicon 2088
Cycrin Tablets 975
Demulen 2428
Depo-Provera Sterile Aqueous Suspension 2606
Desogen Tablets 1817
Estraderm Transdermal System 824
ESTRATAB Tablets (0.3, 0.625, 1.25, 2.5 mg) 2536
Estratest 2539
Levlen/Tri-Levlen 651
Lippes Loop Intrauterine Double-S 1848
Lo/Ovral Tablets 2746
Lo/Ovral-28 Tablets 2751
Menest Tablets 2494
Micronor Tablets 1872
Modicon 1872
Nordette-21 Tablets 2755
Nordette-28 Tablets 2758
Norinyl 2088
Nor-Q D Tablets 2135
Ortho-Cept 1851
Ortho-Cyclen/Ortho-Tri-Cyclen 1858
Ortho-Novum 1872
Ortho-Cyclen/Ortho Tri-Cyclen 1858
Ovcon 760
Ovral Tablets 2770
Ovral-28 Tablets 2770
Ovrette Tablets 2771
PMB 200 and PMB 400 2783
ParaGard T380A Intrauterine Copper Contraceptive 1880
Premarin Intravenous 2787
Premarin with Methyltestosterone 2794
Premarin Vaginal Cream 2791
Premphase 2797
Prempro 2801
Provera Tablets 2636
Levlen/Tri-Levlen 651
Tri-Norinyl 2164
Triphasil-21 Tablets 2814
Triphasil-28 Tablets 2819

Cervical eversion, changes in
Diethylstilbestrol Tablets 1437
Ortho Dienestrol Cream 1866

Cervical irregularities
Demulen 2428
Hivid Tablets (Less than 1% to less than 3%) 2121
Lupron Depot-PED 7.5 mg, 11.25 mg and 15 mg (Less than 2%) 2560

Cervical secretion, changes
Amen Tablets 780
Aygestin Tablets 974
Brevicon 2088
Climara Transdermal System 645
Cycrin Tablets 975
Demulen 2428
Depo-Provera Sterile Aqueous Suspension 2606
Desogen Tablets 1817
Diethylstilbestrol Tablets 1437
Estrace Cream and Tablets 749
Estraderm Transdermal System 824
ESTRATAB Tablets (0.3, 0.625, 1.25, 2.5 mg) 2536
Estratest 2539
Levlen/Tri-Levlen 651
Lo/Ovral Tablets 2746
Lo/Ovral-28 Tablets 2751
Menest Tablets 2494
Micronor Tablets 1872
Modicon 1872
Nordette-21 Tablets 2755
Nordette-28 Tablets 2758
Norinyl 2088
Nor-Q D Tablets 2135
Ogen Tablets 2627
Ogen Vaginal Cream 2630
Ortho-Cept 1851
Ortho-Cyclen/Ortho-Tri-Cyclen 1858
Ortho Dienestrol Cream 1866
Ortho-Est 1869
Ortho-Novum 1872
Ortho-Cyclen/Ortho Tri-Cyclen 1858
Ovcon 760
Ovral Tablets 2770
Ovral-28 Tablets 2770
Ovrette Tablets 2771
PMB 200 and PMB 400 2783
Premarin Intravenous 2787
Premarin with Methyltestosterone 2794
Premarin Tablets 2789
Premarin Vaginal Cream 2791
Premphase 2797
Prempro 2801
Provera Tablets 2636
Levlen/Tri-Levlen 651
Tri-Norinyl 2164
Triphasil-21 Tablets 2814
Triphasil-28 Tablets 2819

Cervicitis
Betaseron for SC Injection 658
▲ Cleocin Vaginal Cream (16%) 2589
▲ Norplant System (5% or greater) 2759

Chafing, genital
Condylox (Less than 5%) 1802

Change in blood glucose levels (see under Insulin reaction)

Character changes
Seromycin Pulvules 1476

Charcot's syndrome
Atromid-S Capsules 2701
Imdur (Less than or equal to 5%) 1323
Isoptin Oral Tablets (Less than 1%) 1346
Kerlone Tablets (Less than 2%) 2436
ReoPro Vials (0.4%) 1471
Timolide Tablets 1748
Tonocard Tablets (Less than 1%) 531

Cheek puffing
Compazine 2470
Etrafon 2355
Haldol Decanoate 1577
Haldol Injection, Tablets and Concentrate 1575
Mellaril 2269
Moban Tablets and Concentrate 1048
Navane Intramuscular 2202
Orap Tablets 1050
Phenobarbital Elixir and Tablets 1469
Prolixin 509
Stelazine 2514
Thorazine 2523

Cheilitis
▲ Accutane Capsules (More than 90%) 2076
Anafranil Capsules (Rare) 803
Betaseron for SC Injection 658
Cosmegen Injection 1626
Effexor (Rare) 2719
▲ Tegison Capsules (Less than 75%) 2154

Cheilitis, actinic
▲ Tegison Capsules (Greater than 75%) 2154

Cheilosis
Cuprimine Capsules (Rare) 1630
Depen Titratable Tablets (Rare) 2662

Cheilosis, monilial
Lamprene Capsules (Less than 1%) 828

Chemosis
Alomide (Less than 1%) 469
Chibroxin Sterile Ophthalmic Solution 1617
Profenal 1% Sterile Ophthalmic Solution (Less than 0.5%) ⊙ 227
▲ Rēv-Eyes Ophthalmic Eyedrops 0.5% (10% to 40%) ⊙ 323

Chest congestion
BuSpar (Infrequent) 737
Claritin-D (Less frequent) 2350
Cognex Capsules (Infrequent) 1901
Effexor (Infrequent) 2719
Hivid Tablets (Less than 1% to less than 3%) 2121
Klonopin Tablets 2126
▲ NebuPent for Inhalation Solution (10 to 23%) 1040
Roferon-A Injection (Less than 3%) 2145

Chest numbness
Tessalon Perles 1020

Chest pain
Accupril Tablets (2.4%) 1893
Accutane Capsules (Less frequent) 2076
Adalat CC (3% or less) 589
Adenocard Injection (Less than 1%) 1021
▲ AeroBid Inhaler System (3-9%) 1005
▲ Aerobid-M Inhaler System (3-9%) 1005
Altace Capsules (Less than 1% to 1.1%) 1232
Alupent Tablets (0.2%) 669
Ambien Tablets (1%) 2416
▲ Anafranil Capsules (4% to 7%) 803
Ancobon Capsules 2079
Apresazide Capsules 808
▲ Asacol Delayed-Release Tablets (3%) 1979
▲ Atgam Sterile Solution (More than 1% to 10%) 2581
▲ Atrovent Inhalation Solution (3.2%) 673
Axid Pulvules (2.3%) 1427
Azactam for Injection (One patient) 734
Betagan ⊙ 233
▲ Betapace Tablets (4% to 16%) 641
Betimol 0.25%, 0.5% ⊙ 261
Blenoxane (Rare) 692
Blocadren Tablets (0.6%) 1614
Brevibloc Injection (Less than 1%) 1808
Bumex (0.1%) 2093
BuSpar (Frequent) 737
Cafergot 2251
Calan SR Caplets (1% or less) 2422
Calan Tablets (1% or less) 2419
Capoten (Approximately 1 in 100 patients) 739
Capozide (Approximately 1 of 100 patients) 742
Cardene Capsules (Rare) 2095
Cardene I.V. (0.7%) 2709
Cardizem Injectable (Less than 1%) 1508
Cardura Tablets (1.2% to 2%) 2186
Cartrol Tablets (2.2%) 410
Cataflam (Less than 1%) 816
Ceftin (Less than 1% but more than 0.1%) 1078
▲ CellCept Capsules (13.3% to 13.4%) 2099
Cipro I.V. (1% or less) 595
Cipro I.V. Pharmacy Bulk Package (Less than 1%) 597
Cipro Tablets (Less than 1%) 592
Claritin (2% or fewer patients) 2349
Claritin-D (Less frequent) 2350
Clinoril Tablets (Less than 1 in 100) 1618
Clomid 1514
Clozaril Tablets (1%) 2252
▲ Cognex Capsules (4%) 1901
Colestid Tablets (Less frequent) 2591
Coumadin 926
Cozaar Tablets (1% or greater) 1628
Cytosar-U Sterile Powder (Less frequent; occasional) 2592
Cytotec (Infrequent) 2424
Cytovene (1% or less) 2103
D.H.E. 45 Injection 2255
Dalgan Injection (Less than 1%) 538
Dalmane Capsules 2173
Demadex Tablets and Injection (1.2%) 686
Depakote Tablets (Greater than 1% but not more than 5%) 415
Depo-Provera Contraceptive Injection (Fewer than 1%) 2602
Desyrel and Desyrel Dividose 503
Dilacor XR Extended-release Capsules (Infrequent) 2018
Dipentum Capsules (Rare) 1951
Diprivan Injection (Less than 1%) 2833
Dizac 1809
Dobutrex Solution Vials (1% to 3%) 1439
Dolobid Tablets (Rare) 1654
Dopram Injectable 2061
Duragesic Transdermal System (1% or greater) 1288
▲ DynaCirc Capsules (2.7% to 7%) 2256
E.E.S. (Isolated reports) 424
Effexor (2%) 2719
Emcyt Capsules (1%) 1953
▲ Eminase (Less than 10%) 2039
▲ Epogen for Injection (7%) 489
Ergamisol Tablets (Less than 1% to 1%) 1292
EryPed (Isolated reports) 421
Ery-Tab Tablets (Isolated reports) 422
Erythrocin Stearate Filmtab (Isolated reports) 425
Erythromycin Base Filmtab (Isolated reports) 426
Erythromycin Delayed-Release Capsules, USP (Isolated reports) 427
Esimil Tablets 822
Estrace Cream and Tablets 749
▲ Ethmozine Tablets (2% to 5%) 2041
Felbatol (2.6%) 2666
Fioricet with Codeine Capsules 2260
Fiorinal with Codeine Capsules 2262
Flexeril Tablets (Rare) 1661
Floxin I.V. (1% to 3%) 1571
Floxin Tablets (200 mg, 300 mg, 400 mg) (1% to 3%) 1567
Foscavir Injection (Between 1% and 5%) 547
Gamimune N, 5% Immune Globulin Intravenous (Human), 5% 619
Gamimune N, 10% Immune Globulin Intravenous (Human), 10% 621
Halcion Tablets 2611
Hespan Injection 929
▲ Hivid Tablets (Less than 1% to less than 3%) 2121
▲ Hylorel Tablets (27.9%) 985
Hytrin Capsules (At least 1%) 430
Hyzaar Tablets 1677
Idamycin 1955
Imdur (Less than or equal to 5%) 1323
Imitrex Injection 1103
Imitrex Tablets (Frequent) 1106
Indocin (Less than 1%) 1680
INFeD (Iron Dextran Injection, USP) 2345
Inocor Lactate Injection (0.2%) 2309
▲ Intron A (Up to 28%) 2364
Iopidine 0.5% (Less than 1%) ⊙ 221
Ismelin Tablets 827
Isoptin Oral Tablets (Less than 1%) 1346
Isoptin SR Tablets (1% or less) 1348
▲ Kerlone Tablets (2.4% to 7.1%) 2436
Lamictal Tablets (More than 1%) 1112
Levatol (2.4%) 2403
Levlen/Tri-Levlen 651
Lioresal Tablets (Rare) 829
Lorelco Tablets 1517
Lotensin HCT (0.3% to 1.0%) 837
Lotrel Capsules (Infrequent) 840
Lozol Tablets (Less than 5%) 2022
Luvox Tablets 2544
Maalox Daily Fiber Therapy ▣ 641
Macrobid Capsules 1988
Macrodantin Capsules 1989
Maxair Autohaler (1.3%) 1492
Maxair Inhaler (Less than 1%) 1494
Maxaquin Tablets (Less than 1%) 2440
Maxzide 1380
Megace Oral Suspension (1% to 3%) 699
Methergine (Rare) 2272
Methotrexate Sodium Tablets, Injection, for Injection and LPF Injection (Less common) 1275
Mevacor Tablets (0.5% to 1.0%) 1699
▲ Mexitil Capsules (2.6% to 7.5%) 678
Micronor Tablets 1872
Midamor Tablets (Less than or equal to 1%) 1703
Modicon 1872
Moduretic Tablets (Less than or equal to 1%) 1705
Monoket (Less than 1% to 2%) 2406
Monopril Tablets (0.2% to 2.2%) 757
Mycobutin Capsules (1%) 1957
Mykrox Tablets (2.7%) 993
▲ Navelbine Injection (5%) 1145
▲ NebuPent for Inhalation Solution (10 to 23%) 1040
Neoral (Rare) 2276
▲ Neupogen for Injection (5%) 495
Nicoderm (nicotine transdermal system) (1% to 3%) 1518
Nicorette (1% to 3% of patients) 2458
Noroxin Tablets (Less frequent) 1715
Noroxin Tablets (Less frequent) 2048
Norpace (1 to 3%) 2444
Norvasc Tablets (More than 0.1% to 1%) 1940
Novantrone 1279
Oncaspar (Less than 1%) 2028
Orap Tablets 1050
Ortho-Cyclen/Ortho-Tri-Cyclen 1858
Ortho-Est 1869
Ortho-Novum 1872
Ortho-Cyclen/Ortho Tri-Cyclen 1858

(▣ Described in PDR For Nonprescription Drugs) Incidence data in parenthesis; ▲ 3% or more (⊙ Described in PDR For Ophthalmology)

1249 Side Effects Index Chills

▲ Orthoclone OKT3 Sterile Solution (14%) 1837
Paxil Tablets (1.4%) 2505
Peganone Tablets 446
Penetrex Tablets (Less than 1% but more than or equal to 0.1%) 2031
Pentasa (Infrequent) 1527
Pentaspan Injection 937
▲ Permax Tablets (3.7%) 575
Plendil Extended-Release Tablets (0.5% to 1.5%) 527
Pondimin Tablets 2066
Pravachol (0.3% to 3.7%) 765
PREVACID Delayed-Release Capsules (Less than 1%) 2562
Prilosec Delayed-Release Capsules (Less than 1%) 529
Primacor Injection (1.2%) 2331
▲ Prinivil Tablets (1.2% to 7.3%) 1733
Prinzide Tablets (0.3 to 1%) 1737
Procardia XL Extended Release Tablets (Less than 3%) 1972
▲ Procrit for Injection (7%) 1841
Proglycem (Rare) 580
▲ Prograf (Greater than 3%) 1042
▲ Proleukin for Injection (12%) 797
Propulsid (More than 1%) 1300
ProSom Tablets (1%) 449
Prostin E2 Suppository 2634
Proventil Syrup (Less than 1 of 100 patients) 2385
Prozac Pulvules & Liquid, Oral Solution (1.3% to 3%) 919
▲ Pulmozyme Inhalation (18% to 21%) 1064
Retrovir Capsules 1158
Retrovir I.V. Infusion 1163
Retrovir Syrup 1158
Rifater 1532
Risperdal (2% to 3%) 1301
Roferon-A Injection (Less than 3% to 4%) 2145
Rogaine Topical Solution (1.53%) 2637
Romazicon (Less than 1%) 2147
Rowasa 2548
Rythmol Tablets–150mg, 225mg, 300mg (0.5 to 1.8%) 1352
Sandimmune (Rare) 2286
Sandostatin Injection (Less than 1%) 2292
Sansert Tablets 2295
Sectral Capsules (2%) 2807
Serzone Tablets 771
Sinemet CR Tablets (1.0%) 944
Stadol (Infrequent) 775
Stilphostrol Tablets and Ampuls 612
Stimate, (desmopressin acetate) Nasal Spray, 1.5 mg/mL 525
▲ Supprelin Injection (1% to 10%) 2056
Synarel Nasal Solution for Central Precocious Puberty (2.6%) 2151
▲ Tambocor Tablets (5.4%) 1497
Taxol 714
Tegison Capsules (Less than 1%) 2154
Tenex Tablets (Less frequent) 2074
▲ THROMBATE III Antithrombin III (Human) (1 of 17) 637
▲ Tilade (4.0%) 996
Timolide Tablets (Less than 1%) 1748
Timoptic in Ocudose (Less frequent) 1753
Timoptic Sterile Ophthalmic Solution (Less frequent) 1751
Timoptic-XE 1755
Tolectin (200, 400 and 600 mg) (1 to 3%) 1581
Tonocard Tablets (0.4-1.6%) 531
Toprol-XL Tablets (About 1 of 100 patients) 565
Trental Tablets (0.3%) 1244
Levlen/Tri-Levlen 651
Unasyn (Less than 1%) 2212
Univasc Tablets (More than 1%) 2410
Valium Injectable 2182
Vancocin HCl, Vials & ADD-Vantage 1481
Vantin for Oral Suspension and Vantin Tablets (Less than 1%) 2646
Vaseretic Tablets (0.5% to 2.0%) 1765
Vasotec I.V. 1768
Vasotec Tablets (0.5% to 2.1%) 1771
Ventolin Syrup (Less than 1 of 100 patients) 1202
Verelan Capsules (1% or less) 1410
Verelan Capsules (Less than 1%) 2824
Videx Tablets, Powder for Oral Solution, & Pediatric Powder for Oral Solution (Up to 2%) 720
Virazole 1264
▲ Visken Tablets (3%) 2299
Voltaren Tablets (Less than 1%) 861
Wellbutrin Tablets (Infrequent) 1204
▲ Xanax Tablets (10.6%) 2649
Yutopar Intravenous Injection (1% to 2%) 570
Zaroxolyn Tablets 1000
Zebeta Tablets (1.1% to 1.5%) 1413
▲ Zerit Capsules (Fewer than 1% to 8%) 729
Zestoretic (0.3 to 1.0%) 2850
▲ Zestril Tablets (0.3% to 7.3%) 2854
Ziac (0.9% to 1.8%) 1415
Zithromax (1% or less) 1944
Zofran Injection (Rare; 2%) 1214
Zofran Tablets (Rare) 1217
▲ Zoladex (Greater than 1% but less than 5%) 2858
Zoloft Tablets (1.0%) 2217
Zosyn (1.3%) 1419
Zosyn Pharmacy Bulk Package (1.3%) 1422
Zovirax Sterile Powder (Less than 1%) 1223

Chest pain, substernal

Effexor (Infrequent) 2719
Felbatol (Rare) 2666
Foscavir Injection (Less than 1%) 547
Intron A (Less than 5%) 2364
Videx Tablets, Powder for Oral Solution, & Pediatric Powder for Oral Solution (Less than 1%) 720
Zoloft Tablets (Rare) 2217

Chest sound, abnormalities

Imdur (Less than or equal to 5%) 1323
▲ Leustatin (9%) 1834
Orthoclone OKT3 Sterile Solution 1837
Prinivil Tablets (Up to 0.3%) 1733
Prinzide Tablets 1737
Zestoretic 2850
Zestril Tablets (Up to 0.3%) 2854

Chest tightness

Actifed with Codeine Cough Syrup 1067
▲ Adenocard Injection (7%) 1021
AeroBid Inhaler System (1-3%) 1005
Aerobid-M Inhaler System (1-3%) 1005
▲ Alfenta Injection (17%) 1286
Atrohist Plus Tablets 454
Benadryl Capsules 1898
Benadryl Injection 1898
Bioclate, Antihemophilic Factor (Recombinant) 513
▲ Bromfed-DM Cough Syrup (Among most frequent) 1786
Ceftin (Less than 1% but more than 0.1%) 1078
Comhist 2038
Deconamine 1320
Dimetane-DC Cough Syrup 2059
Dimetane-DX Cough Syrup 2059
Dopram Injectable 2061
Eskalith 2485
Furoxone (Rare) 2046
Gamimune N, 5% Immune Globulin Intravenous (Human), 5% 619
Gamimune N, 10% Immune Globulin Intravenous (Human), 10% 621
Geref (sermorelin acetate for injection) 2876
Hivid Tablets (Less than 1% to less than 3%) 2121
Hyperstat I.V. Injection 2363
Hyskon Hysteroscopy Fluid (Rare) 1595
Imitrex Injection (2.7%) 1103
Imitrex Tablets (Frequent) 1106
INFeD (Iron Dextran Injection, USP) 2345
Levlen/Tri-Levlen 651
Lioresal Intrathecal 1596
Lithonate/Lithotabs/Lithobid 2543
Maxair Autohaler (1.3%) 1492
Micronor Tablets 1872
Modicon 1872
Monoclate-P, Factor VIII:C, Pasteurized, Monoclonal Antibody Purified Antihemophilic Factor (Human) 521
Mononine, Coagulation Factor IX (Human) 523
Ornade Spansule Capsules 2502
Ortho-Cyclen/Ortho-Tri-Cyclen 1858
Ortho-Novum 1872
Ortho-Cyclen/Ortho Tri-Cyclen 1858
Orthoclone OKT3 Sterile Solution 1837
PBZ Tablets 845
PBZ-SR Tablets 844
Periactin 1724
Prostin E2 Suppository 2634
Quadrinal Tablets 1350
Rifater 1532
Sandoglobulin I.V. (Less than 1%) 2290
Sansert Tablets 2295
Sublimaze Injection 1307
▲ Sufenta Injection (3% to 9%) 1309
Tavist Syrup 2297
Tavist Tablets 2298
Temaril Tablets, Syrup and Spansule Extended-Release Capsules 483
▲ THROMBATE III Antithrombin III (Human) (3 of 17) 637
THYREL TRH (Less frequent) 2873
Tornalate Metered Dose Inhaler (Less than 1%) 957
Levlen/Tri-Levlen 651
Trinalin Repetabs Tablets 1330
Tussend 1783
Tussionex Pennkinetic Extended-Release Suspension (Occasional) 998
Yutopar Intravenous Injection (1% to 2%) 570

Chewing movements

Compazine 2470
Etrafon 2355
Haldol Decanoate 1577
Haldol Injection, Tablets and Concentrate 1575
Mellaril 2269
Moban Tablets and Concentrate 1048
Navane Capsules and Concentrate 2201
Navane Intramuscular 2202
Orap Tablets 1050
Prolixin 509
Serentil 684
Stelazine 2514
Thorazine 2523
Triavil Tablets 1757
Trilafon 2389

Chills

Abbokinase 403
Abbokinase Open-Cath 405
Actifed with Codeine Cough Syrup 1067
▲ Actimmune (14%) 1056
Adalat Capsules (10 mg and 20 mg) (2% or less) 587
Adalat CC (Less than 1.0%) 589
Adriamycin PFS (Occasional) 1947
Adriamycin RDF (Occasional) 1947
Children's Advil Suspension (Less than 1%) 2692
AeroBid Inhaler System (1-3%) 1005
Aerobid-M Inhaler System (1-3%) 1005
Alupent Tablets (0.2%) 669
Anafranil Capsules (Up to 2%) 803
Anaprox/Naprosyn (Less than 1%) 2117
Ansaid Tablets (Less than 1%) 2579
Apresazide Capsules (Less frequent) 808
Apresoline Hydrochloride Tablets (Less frequent) 809
Arfonad Ampuls 2080
▲ Asacol Delayed-Release Tablets (3%) 1979
▲ Atgam Sterile Solution (16%) 2581
Atretol Tablets 573
Azo Gantanol Tablets 2080
▲ BCG Vaccine, USP (TICE) (3.3%) 1814
Bactrim DS Tablets 2084
Bactrim I.V. Infusion 2082
Bactrim 2084
Benadryl Capsules 1898
Benadryl Injection 1898
▲ Betaseron for SC Injection (46%) 658
Bicillin C-R Injection 2704
Bicillin C-R 900/300 Injection 2706
Bicillin L-A Injection 2707
Bioclate, Antihemophilic Factor (Recombinant) (Extremely rare) 513
▲ Blenoxane (Frequent) 692
Buprenex Injectable (Less than 1%) 2006
Carbocaine Hydrochloride Injection 2303
Ceftin (Less than 1% but more than 0.1%) 1078
▲ CellCept Capsules (More than or equal to 3%) 2099
Ceredase 1065
Cerubidine (Rare) 795
▲ CHEMET (succimer) Capsules (5.2 to 15.7%) 1545
Cipro I.V. (1% or less) 595
Cipro I.V. Pharmacy Bulk Package (Less than 1%) 597
Cipro Tablets (Less than 1%) 592
Clinoril Tablets (Less than 1 in 100) 1618
Clozaril Tablets (Less than 1%) 2252
Cognex Capsules (Frequent) 1901
CytoGam (Less than 5.0%) 1593
▲ Cytovene (7%) 2103
DDAVP (Up to 2%) 2017
Dalgan Injection (Less than 1%) 538
Danocrine Capsules (Rare) 2307
Dantrium Capsules (Less frequent) 1982
Deconamine 1320
Depakote Tablets (Greater than 1% but not more than 5%) 415
Depen Titratable Tablets 2662
Depo-Provera Contraceptive Injection (Fewer than 1%) 2602
Desmopressin Acetate Rhinal Tube (Up to 2%) 979
Desyrel and Desyrel Dividose 503
Dilaudid-HP Injection (Less frequent) 1337
Dilaudid-HP Lyophilized Powder 250 mg (Less frequent) 1337
Dilaudid Tablets and Liquid 1339
Dipentum Capsules (Rare) 1951
Diphtheria & Tetanus Toxoids Adsorbed Purogenated (Mild) 1374
Diprivan Injection (Less than 1%) 2833
Dolobid Tablets (Less than 1 in 100) 1654
Doxorubicin Astra (Occasional) 540
EC-Naprosyn Delayed-Release Tablets (Less than 1%) 2117
Edecrin 1657
▲ Effexor (2.2% to 6.8%) 2719
Eldepryl Tablets 2550
Elspar 1659
Emete-con Intramuscular/Intravenous 2198
▲ Eminase (Less than 10%) 2039
Engerix-B Unit-Dose Vials (Less than 1%) 2482
Ergamisol Tablets (5 patients) 1292
Fansidar Tablets 2114
Floxin I.V. (Less than 1%) 1571
Floxin Tablets (200 mg, 300 mg, 400 mg) (Less than 1%) 1567
▲ Fludara for Injection (11% to 19%) 663
▲ Fungizone Intravenous (Among most common) 506
▲ Gamimune N, 5% Immune Globulin Intravenous (Human), 5% (Among most common; 9 patients) 619
▲ Gamimune N, 10% Immune Globulin Intravenous (Human), 10% (Among most common; 9 patients) 621
Gammagard S/D, Immune Globulin, Intravenous (Human) (Occasional) 585
Gammar I.V., Immune Globulin Intravenous (Human), Lyophilized 516
Gantanol Tablets 2119
Gantrisin 2120
Glucotrol XL Extended Release Tablets (Less than 1%) 1968
Heparin Lock Flush Solution 2725
Heparin Sodium Injection 2726
Heparin Sodium Injection, USP, Sterile Solution 2615
▲ Heparin Sodium Vials (Among most common) 1441
Hespan Injection 929
Hivid Tablets (Less than 1% to less than 3%) 2121
Humegon 1824
Hydrea Capsules 696
IBU Tablets (Less than 1%) 1342
Imitrex Injection (Infrequent) 1103
Inapsine Injection (Less common) 1296
INFeD (Iron Dextran Injection, USP) 2345
▲ Intron A (Up to 46%) 2364
▲ JE-VAX (Approximately 10%) 886
Konÿne 80 Factor IX Complex 634
Lamictal Tablets (1.3%) 1112
▲ Lariam Tablets (Among most frequent) 2128
Lescol Capsules (Rare) 2267
▲ Leukine for IV Infusion (25%) 1271
▲ Leustatin (9%) 1834
Levoprome (Sometimes) 1274
Lodine Capsules and Tablets (Greater than or equal to 1%) 2743
Lotensin HCT (0.3% or more) 837
Lupron Depot 7.5 mg (Less than 5%) 2559
Lupron Injection (Less than 5%) 2555
Luvox Tablets (2%) 2544

(▣ Described in PDR For Nonprescription Drugs) Incidence data in parenthesis; ▲ 3% or more (◉ Described in PDR For Ophthalmology)

Chills

MS Contin Tablets (Less frequent) 1994
MSIR (Infrequent) 1997
Macrobid Capsules (Less than 1%) 1988
Macrodantin Capsules 1989
Marcaine Hydrochloride with Epinephrine 1:200,000 2316
Marcaine Hydrochloride Injection 2316
Marinol (Dronabinol) Capsules (Less than 1%) 2231
Matulane Capsules 2131
Maxaquin Tablets (Less than 1%) 2440
Metastron (A single patient) 1594
Methadone Hydrochloride Oral Concentrate 2233
Methotrexate Sodium Tablets, Injection, for Injection and LPF Injection (Frequent) 1275
Metrodin (urofollitropin for injection) 2446
Mevacor Tablets (Rare) 1699
Miltown Tablets (Rare) 2672
Mintezol 1704
Monoclate-P, Factor VIII:C, Pasteurized, Monoclonal Antibody Purified Antihemophilic Factor (Human) 521
Mononine, Coagulation Factor IX (Human) 523
Children's Motrin Ibuprofen Oral Suspension (Less than 1%) 1546
Motrin Tablets (Less than 1%) 2625
Mykrox Tablets 993
Anaprox/Naprosyn (Less than 1%) 2117
Navelbine Injection 1145
▲ NebuPent for Inhalation Solution (10 to 23%) 1040
Neurontin Capsules (Infrequent) 1922
Nizoral Tablets (Less than 1%) 1298
Noroxin Tablets (Less frequent) 1715
Noroxin Tablets (Less frequent) 2048
▲ Oncaspar (Greater than 5%) 2028
Oramorph SR (Morphine Sulfate Sustained Release Tablets) (Less frequent) 2236
Orlamm (1% to 3%) 2239
Ornade Spansule Capsules 2502
▲ Orthoclone OKT3 Sterile Solution (59%) 1837
Orudis Capsules (Less than 1%) 2766
Oruvail Capsules (Less than 1%) 2766
PBZ Tablets 845
PBZ-SR Tablets 844
PMB 200 and PMB 400 (Rare) 2783
Parnate Tablets 2503
Paxil Tablets (Frequent) 2505
Penetrex Tablets (Less than 1% but more than or equal to 0.1%) 2031
Pentaspan Injection 937
Peptavlon 2878
Pergonal (menotropins for injection, USP) 2448
Periactin 1724
Permax Tablets (1.1%) 575
Pfzerpen for Injection 2203
Pondimin Tablets 2066
Pontocaine Hydrochloride for Spinal Anesthesia 2330
Pravachol (Rare) 765
Prinivil Tablets (0.3% to 1.0%) 1733
Prinzide Tablets 1737
Priscoline Hydrochloride Ampuls 845
Procan SR Tablets (Common) 1926
Procardia Capsules (2% or less) 1971
▲ Prograf (Greater than 3%) 1042
Prolastin Alpha₁-Proteinase Inhibitor (Human) (Occasional) 635
▲ Proleukin for Injection (89%) 797
ProSom Tablets (Infrequent) 449
▲ Prostin E2 Suppository (Approximately one-tenth) 2634
Prozac Pulvules & Liquid, Oral Solution (Frequent) 919
Recombivax HB (Less than 1%) 1744
Relafen Tablets (Less than 1%) 2510
Retrovir Capsules 1158
Retrovir I.V. Infusion 1163
Retrovir Syrup 1158
▲ ReVia Tablets (Less than 10%) 940
Revex (1%) 1811
Rifadin 1528
Rifater 1532
Rocephin Injectable Vials, ADD-Vantage, Galaxy Container (Less than 1%) 2142
▲ Roferon-A Injection (41% to 64%) 2145
Rubex (Occasional) 712
Rythmol Tablets–150mg, 225mg, 300mg 1352
▲ Salagen Tablets (3% to 14%) 1489

Sandoglobulin I.V. (Less than 1%) 2290
Sensorcaine 559
Septra 1174
Septra I.V. Infusion 1169
Septra I.V. Infusion ADD-Vantage Vials 1171
Septra 1174
Ser-Ap-Es Tablets 849
Serzone Tablets (2%) 771
Sinequan (Occasional) 2205
Stimate, (desmopressin acetate) Nasal Spray, 1.5 mg/mL 525
Sublimaze Injection 1307
Sufenta Injection (0.3% to 1%) 1309
Supprelin Injection (1% to 3%) 2056
Talacen (Rare) 2333
Talwin Injection (Rare) 2334
Talwin Compound (Rare) 2335
Talwin Injection (Rare) 2334
Talwin Nx (Rare) 2336
Tavist Syrup 2297
Tavist Tablets 2298
Tegretol Chewable Tablets 852
Tegretol Suspension 852
Tegretol Tablets 852
Terazol 3 Vaginal Suppositories (1.8% of 284 patients) 1886
Terazol 7 Vaginal Cream (0.4% of 521 patients) 1887
Tessalon Perles 1020
Tetanus & Diphtheria Toxoids Adsorbed Purogenated (Rare) 1401
Tetanus Toxoid Adsorbed Purogenated 1403
▲ TheraCys BCG Live (Intravesical) (2.6% to 33.9%) 897
▲ THROMBATE III Antithrombin III (Human) (2 of 17) 637
Ticlid Tablets 2156
Timentin for Injection 2528
Tonocard Tablets (Less than 1%) 531
Tornalate Solution for Inhalation, 0.2% (Less than 1%) 956
Trinalin Repetabs Tablets 1330
Trobicin Sterile Powder 2645
Tussend 1783
Tympagesic Ear Drops 2342
Unasyn (Less than 1%) 2212
Vancocin HCl, Oral Solution & Pulvules (Infrequent) 1483
Vancocin HCl, Vials & ADD-Vantage (Infrequent) 1481
Varivax (Greater than or equal to 1%) 1762
VePesid Capsules and Injection (0.7% to 2%) 718
Versed Injection (Less than 1%) 2170
▲ Videx Tablets, Powder for Oral Solution, & Pediatric Powder for Oral Solution (9% to 82%) 720
▲ Vumon (Approximately 5%) 727
Wellbutrin Tablets (1.2%) 1204
WinRho SD (One report) 2576
WinRho SD (Less than 2%) 2577
Yodoxin 1230
Yutopar Intravenous Injection (Infrequent) 570
Zaroxolyn Tablets 1000
▲ Zerit Capsules (5% to 38%) 729
Zestoretic 2850
Zestril Tablets (0.3% to 1.0%) 2854
Zocor Tablets (Rare) 1775
▲ Zoladex (Greater than 1% but less than 5%) 2858
Zyloprim Tablets (Less than 1%) 1226

Chloasma

Anafranil Capsules (Rare) 803
Aygestin Tablets 974
Climara Transdermal System 645
Demulen 2428
Depo-Provera Contraceptive Injection (Fewer than 1%) 2602
Diethylstilbestrol Tablets 1437
Estrace Cream and Tablets 749
ESTRATAB Tablets (0.3, 0.625, 1.25, 2.5 mg) 2536
Estratest 2539
Lo/Oral Tablets 2746
Lo/Ovral-28 Tablets 2751
Menest Tablets 2494
Nordette-21 Tablets 2755
Nordette-28 Tablets 2758
Ogen Tablets 2627
Ogen Vaginal Cream 2630
Ortho Dienestrol Cream 1866
Ortho-Est 1869
Ovral Tablets 2770
Ovral-28 Tablets 2770
Ovrette Tablets 2771
PMB 200 and PMB 400 2783

Premarin Intravenous 2787
Premarin with Methyltestosterone 2794
Premarin Tablets 2789
Premarin Vaginal Cream 2791
Premphase 2797
Prempro 2801
Stilphostrol Tablets and Ampuls 612
Synarel Nasal Solution for Endometriosis (Less than 1%) 2152
Triphasil-21 Tablets 2814
Triphasil-28 Tablets 2819

Chloride retention

Delatestryl Injection 2860
Estratest 2539
Halotestin Tablets 2614
Oxandrin 2862
Premarin with Methyltestosterone 2794
Testred Capsules 1262

Choking sensation

Dantrium Intravenous 1983
Hyperstat I.V. Injection 2363
Serevent Inhalation Aerosol (Rare) 1176

Cholangiocarcinoma

Fioricet with Codeine Capsules 2260
Fiorinal with Codeine Capsules 2262

Cholangitis

Cytovene-IV (Two or more reports) 2103
▲ Prograf (Greater than 3%) 1042

Cholecystectomy, prolongation of drainage

Surgicel 1314

Cholecystitis

Actigall Capsules 802
Ansaid Tablets (Less than 1%) 2579
Asacol Delayed-Release Tablets 1979
Betaseron for SC Injection 658
Cognex Capsules (Infrequent) 1901
Colestid Tablets (Rare) 2591
Effexor (Rare) 2719
Foscavir Injection (Less than 1%) 547
Hivid Tablets (Less than 1% to less than 3%) 2121
Lopid Tablets 1917
Luvox Tablets (Rare) 2544
Permax Tablets (Rare) 575
Premphase 2797
Prempro 2801
Prozac Pulvules & Liquid, Oral Solution (Rare) 919
Risperdal (Rare) 1301
Trental Tablets (Less than 1%) 1244
Videx Tablets, Powder for Oral Solution, & Pediatric Powder for Oral Solution (Less than 1%) 720
Ziac 1415

Cholecystitis, acalculus

Sterile FUDR 2118

Cholelithiasis

Atromid-S Capsules 2701
Betaseron for SC Injection 658
Cognex Capsules (Infrequent) 1901
Colestid Tablets (Rare) 2591
Effexor (Rare) 2719
Fludara for Injection (Up to 3%) 663
Foscavir Injection (Less than 1%) 547
Lopid Tablets 1917
Luvox Tablets (Rare) 2544
Miacalcin Nasal Spray (Less than 1%) 2275
Permax Tablets (Infrequent) 575
Premphase 2797
Prempro 2801
PREVACID Delayed-Release Capsules (Less than 1%) 2562
Prozac Pulvules & Liquid, Oral Solution (Rare) 919
Risperdal (Rare) 1301
Videx Tablets, Powder for Oral Solution, & Pediatric Powder for Oral Solution (Less than 1%) 720

Cholestasis

Capoten (Rare) 739
Capozide (Rare) 742
Cefotan 2829
Ceftin Tablets 1078
Ceptaz 1081
Clinoril Tablets (Less than 1%) 1618
Clozaril Tablets 2252
Cytovene-IV (Two or more reports) 2103
Desyrel and Desyrel Dividose 503
Diflucan Injection, Tablets, and Oral Suspension (Rare) 2194

Dolobid Tablets (Less than 1 in 100) 1654
Duricef 748
Flexeril Tablets (Less than 1%) 1661
Fortaz 1100
Keftab Tablets 915
Lorabid Suspension and Pulvules (Rare) 1459
Mintezol 1704
NegGram (Rare) 2323
Nolvadex Tablets (Rare) 2841
Procardia Capsules 1971
Procardia XL Extended Release Tablets 1972
Rythmol Tablets–150mg, 225mg, 300mg (0.1%) 1352
Suprax 1399
Tagamet (Rare) 2516
Tambocor Tablets (Rare) 1497
Tazicef for Injection 2519
Ticlid Tablets 2156
Vantin for Oral Suspension and Vantin Tablets 2646
Zefazone 2654
Zinacef 1211

Cholestasis, intrahepatic

Ceftin for Oral Suspension 1078
Cuprimine Capsules (Rare) 1630
Depen Titratable Tablets (Rare) 2662

Cholestatic hepatic injury

Axid Pulvules (Rare) 1427
Coumadin (Infrequent) 926

Cholesterol, systemic, microembolism

Coumadin (Infrequent) 926

Cholinergic reactions

Anafranil Capsules (Rare) 803
Cognex Capsules (Rare) 1901
Risperdal (Rare) 1301
Tensilon Injectable 1261

Chondrodystrophy

Prozac Pulvules & Liquid, Oral Solution (Rare) 919

Chorea

▲ Atamet (Among most common) 572
Climara Transdermal System 645
Diethylstilbestrol Tablets 1437
Dilantin Infatabs (Rare) 1908
Dilantin Kapseals (Rare) 1906
Dilantin Parenteral (Rare) 1910
Dilantin-125 Suspension (Rare) 1911
Dilaudid-HP Injection 1337
Dilaudid-HP Lyophilized Powder 250 mg 1337
Eldepryl Tablets 2550
Estrace Cream and Tablets 749
ESTRATAB Tablets (0.3, 0.625, 1.25, 2.5 mg) 2536
Estratest 2539
Inversine Tablets 1686
Klonopin Tablets 2126
Larodopa Tablets (Frequent) 2129
Lo/Ovral Tablets 2746
Lo/Ovral-28 Tablets 2751
Menest Tablets 2494
Mesantoin Tablets 2272
Nordette-21 Tablets 2755
Nordette-28 Tablets 2758
Ogen Tablets 2627
Ogen Vaginal Cream 2630
Ortho Dienestrol Cream 1866
Ortho-Est 1869
Ovcon 35 760
Ovral Tablets 2770
Ovral-28 Tablets 2770
Ovrette Tablets 2771
PMB 200 and PMB 400 2783
Premarin Intravenous 2787
Premarin with Methyltestosterone 2794
Premarin Tablets 2789
Premarin Vaginal Cream 2791
Premphase 2797
Prempro 2801
▲ Sinemet Tablets (Among most common) 943
Sinemet CR Tablets 944
Stilphostrol Tablets and Ampuls 612
Trilafon Concentrate 2389
Triphasil-21 Tablets 2814
Triphasil-28 Tablets 2819

Choreoathetotic movements

Aldoclor Tablets 1598
Aldomet Ester HCl Injection 1602
Aldomet Oral 1600

1251 Side Effects Index Coldness of extremities

Aldoril Tablets 1604
Anafranil Capsules (Rare) 803
Eskalith 2485
Felbatol 2666
Lamictal Tablets (Rare) 1112
Lithium Carbonate Capsules & Tablets 2230
Lithonate/Lithotabs/Lithobid 2543
Loxitane 1378
Mellaril 2269
Neurontin Capsules (Rare) 1922
Paxil Tablets (Rare) 2505
Permax Tablets (Frequent) 575
Prolixin 509
Reglan 2068
Risperdal (Rare) 1301
Serentil 684
Triavil Tablets 1757

Chorioretinitis

Neurontin Capsules (Rare) 1922

Choroidal detachment, post-filtration procedures

AdatoSil 5000 (Less than 2%) ⊙ 274
ISPAN Perfluoropropane ⊙ 276
ISPAN Sulfur Hexafluoride ⊙ 275
Timoptic in Ocudose 1753
Timoptic Sterile Ophthalmic Solution 1751
Timoptic-XE 1755

Chromatopsia

Anafranil Capsules (Rare) 803
Effexor (Rare) 2719

Chromosomal abnormalities

Clomid 1514
Depo-Provera Contraceptive Injection 2602
Imuran Tablets 1110
Metrodin (urofollitropin for injection) (3 incidents) 2446
Mustargen 1709
Roferon-A Injection 2145

Chrysiasis

Solganal Suspension 2388

Ciliary injection

Isopto Carbachol Ophthalmic Solution ⊙ 223

Ciliary redness

Floropryl Sterile Ophthalmic Ointment 1662
Humorsol Sterile Ophthalmic Solution 1664
Phospholine Iodide ⊙ 326

Ciliary spasm

Isopto Carbachol Ophthalmic Solution ⊙ 223
Isopto Carpine Ophthalmic Solution ⊙ 223
Ocusert Pilo-20 and Pilo-40 Ocular Therapeutic Systems ⊙ 254
Pilocar ⊙ 268
Pilopine HS Ophthalmic Gel ⊙ 226

Cinchonism

Quinaglute Dura-Tabs Tablets 649
Quinidex Extentabs 2067
Tonocard Tablets (Less than 1%) 531

Circulatory collapse

Etrafon (Extremely rare) 2355
Lasix Injection, Oral Solution and Tablets 1240
Protamine Sulfate Ampoules & Vials 1471

Circulatory collapse, peripheral

Eskalith 2485
Lithium Carbonate Capsules & Tablets 2230
Lithonate/Lithotabs/Lithobid 2543
Phenobarbital Elixir and Tablets 1469
Tenormin Tablets and I.V. Injection 2847

Circulatory depression

Brevital Sodium Vials 1429
Demerol 2308
Dilaudid Ampules 1335
Dilaudid-HP Injection 1337
Dilaudid-HP Lyophilized Powder 250 mg 1337
Dilaudid 1335
Dilaudid Oral Liquid 1339
Dilaudid 1335
Dilaudid Tablets - 8 mg 1339
MS Contin Tablets 1994
MSIR 1997
Mepergan Injection 2753
Phenergan with Codeine 2777
Phenergan VC with Codeine 2781
Talwin Injection 2334

Circulatory failure

Ambien Tablets (Rare) 2416
Dilaudid 1335
Lufyllin & Lufyllin-400 Tablets 2670
Lufyllin-GG Elixir & Tablets 2671
Metubine Iodide Vials 916
PREVACID Delayed-Release Capsules (Less than 1%) 2562
Quadrinal Tablets 1350
Quibron 2053
Respbid Tablets 682
Slo-bid Gyrocaps 2033
Theo-24 Extended Release Capsules 2568
Theo-Dur Extended-Release Tablets 1327
Theo-X Extended-Release Tablets 788
Trasylol 613
Trilafon (Extremely rare) 2389
Uni-Dur Extended-Release Tablets 1331
Uniphyl 400 mg Tablets 2001
Zosyn (1.0% or less) 1419
Zosyn Pharmacy Bulk Package (1.0% or less) 1422

Circulatory overload

Hespan Injection 929
Pentaspan Injection 937

Cirrhosis, hepatic (see under Cirrhosis of liver)

Cirrhosis of liver

Cordarone Tablets (Rare) 2712
Lescol Capsules (Rare) 2267
Methotrexate Sodium Tablets, Injection, for Injection and LPF Injection 1275
Mevacor Tablets (Rare) 1699
Papaverine Hydrochloride Vials and Ampoules (Rare) 1468
Pravachol (Rare) 765
Zocor Tablets (Rare) 1775

Clamminess

BuSpar (1%) 737
Desyrel and Desyrel Dividose (Less than 1% to 1.4%) 503
Intron A (Less than 5%) 2364
IOPIDINE Sterile Ophthalmic Solution ⊙ 219
Norvasc Tablets (Less than or equal to 0.1%) 1940
▲ Nubain Injection (9%) 935
Sanorex Tablets 2294
▲ Stadol (3% to 9%) 775
▲ Tegison Capsules (1-10%) 2154
Zoloft Tablets (Infrequent) 2217

Claudication

Blocadren Tablets 1614
Calan SR Caplets (1% or less) 2422
Calan Tablets (1% or less) 2419
Isoptin Oral Tablets 1346
Isoptin SR Tablets (1% or less) 1348
Monopril Tablets (0.2% to 1.0%) 757
Timolide Tablets 1748
Timoptic in Ocudose 1753
Timoptic Sterile Ophthalmic Solution 1751
Timoptic-XE 1755
Tonocard Tablets (Less than 1%) 531
Verelan Capsules (1% or less) 1410
Verelan Capsules (Less than 1%) 2824
Visken Tablets (2% or fewer patients) 2299
Zebeta Tablets 1413
Ziac 1415

Claudication, intermittent (see under Charcot's syndrome)

Claustrophobia

BuSpar (Rare) 737
Roferon-A Injection (Less than 1%) 2145

Cleft palate, neonatal

Accutane Capsules 2076
Proventil Inhalation Aerosol 2382
Proventil Inhalation Solution 0.083% 2384
Proventil Repetabs Tablets 2386
Proventil Solution for Inhalation 0.5% 2383
Proventil Syrup 2385
Ventolin Inhalation Aerosol and Refill 1197
Ventolin Inhalation Solution (Rare) 1198
Ventolin Nebules Inhalation Solution (Rare) 1199
Ventolin Rotacaps for Inhalation 1200
Ventolin Syrup 1202
Ventolin Tablets 1203

Climacteric, onset masked

Cycrin Tablets 975
Demulen 2428

Clitoral hypertrophy

Danocrine Capsules (Rare) 2307
Desyrel and Desyrel Dividose 503

Clitoris, enlargement (see under Clitoromegaly)

Clitoromegaly

▲ Android Capsules, 10 mg (Among most common) 1250
▲ Android (Among most common) 1251
▲ Delatestryl Injection (One of most common) 2860
Depo-Provera Sterile Aqueous Suspension (Rare) 2606
Estratest 2539
Halotestin Tablets 2614
▲ Oreton Methyl (Among most common) 1255
Oxandrin 2862
Premarin with Methyltestosterone (Among most common) 2794
Provera Tablets (Rare) 2636
Testred Capsules 1262
Winstrol Tablets 2337

Clonic movements of whole limbs

Diprivan Injection (Less than 1%) 2833
Eskalith 2485
Lithium Carbonate Capsules & Tablets 2230
Lithonate/Lithotabs/Lithobid 2543

Clonus

Alupent Tablets (0.2%) 669
Dopram Injectable 2061

Clostridial myonecrosis

Sus-Phrine Injection 1019

Clotting time, prolongation

Heparin Sodium Injection, USP, Sterile Solution 2615
Hespan Injection 929
Hyskon Hysteroscopy Fluid (Rare) 1595
Mithracin 607
Oncaspar (Less than 1%) 2028
Pentaspan Injection 937
Zosyn 1419
Zosyn Pharmacy Bulk Package 1422

Coagulation, dysfunction

Children's Advil Suspension 2692
BCG Vaccine, USP (TICE) (0.3%) 1814
Cordarone Tablets (1 to 3%) 2712
Depakene 413
Depakote Tablets 415
Diprivan Injection (Less than 1%) 2833
Elspar 1659
Estratest 2539
Foscavir Injection (Less than 1%) 547
Fungizone Intravenous 506
Hespan Injection 929
IFEX (Less than 1%) 697
Lo/Ovral Tablets 2746
Lo/Ovral-28 Tablets 2751
Maxaquin Tablets 2440
Mononine, Coagulation Factor IX (Human) 523
Nimotop Capsules (Less than 1%) 610
Oncaspar (Less than 1%) 2028
Orthoclone OKT3 Sterile Solution 1837
Ovral Tablets 2770
Ovral-28 Tablets 2770
Ovrette Tablets 2771
PMB 200 and PMB 400 2783
Premarin Intravenous 2787
Premarin with Methyltestosterone 2794
Premarin Tablets 2789
Premarin Vaginal Cream 2791
▲ Prograf (Greater than 3%) 1042
▲ Proleukin for Injection (10%) 797
Tegison Capsules (Less than 1%) 2154
Vantin for Oral Suspension and Vantin Tablets 2646

Coagulation defects, neonatal

Dilantin Infatabs 1908
Dilantin Kapseals 1906
Dilantin Parenteral 1910
Dilantin-125 Suspension 1911

Coagulation tests, altered results

Cycrin Tablets 975
Depo-Provera Sterile Aqueous Suspension 2606
Eminase 2039
Provera Tablets 2636
Zosyn 1419
Zosyn Pharmacy Bulk Package 1422

Cochlear damage

Amikacin Sulfate Injection, USP 960
Nebcin Vials, Hyporets & ADD-Vantage 1464
Streptomycin Sulfate Injection 2208
Tripedia 892

Cochlear lesion

Diphtheria and Tetanus Toxoids and Pertussis Vaccine Adsorbed USP (For Pediatric Use) 875

Cognitive dysfunction

Ambien Tablets (Infrequent) 2416
Anaprox/Naprosyn (Less than 1%) 2117
Doral Tablets 2664
EC-Naprosyn Delayed-Release Tablets (Rare) 2117
Floxin I.V. (Less than 1%) 1571
Floxin Tablets (200 mg, 300 mg, 400 mg) (Less than 1%) 1567
Methotrexate Sodium Tablets, Injection, for Injection and LPF Injection (Occasional) 1275
Anaprox/Naprosyn (Rare) 2117
Orthoclone OKT3 Sterile Solution 1837
Risperdal 1301
Supprelin Injection (2% to 3%) 2056
Ultram Tablets (50 mg) (Less than 1%) 1585
Xanax Tablets 2649

Cogwheel rigidity

BuSpar (Rare) 737
Cognex Capsules (Infrequent) 1901
Compazine 2470
Eskalith 2485
Lithonate/Lithotabs/Lithobid 2543
Paxil Tablets 2505
Prolixin 509
Reglan 2068
Stelazine 2514
Thorazine 2523

Cold, reduced tolerance

BuSpar (Rare) 737
Parlodel (Less than 1%) 2281

Coldness of extremities

▲ Blocadren Tablets (8%) 1614
Cafergot 2251
Effexor (Infrequent) 2719
Eskalith (A few reports) 2485
Helixate, Antihemophilic Factor (Recombinant) 518
Hivid Tablets (Less than 1% to less than 3%) 2121
Kerlone Tablets (1.9%) 2436
Lithium Carbonate Capsules & Tablets (A single report) 2230
Lithonate/Lithotabs/Lithobid 2543
Lopressor Ampuls (1%) 830
Lopressor HCT Tablets 832
Lopressor Tablets (1%) 830
Luvox Tablets (Infrequent) 2544
Mykrox Tablets (Less than 2%) 993
Parlodel (Rare) 2281
ReVia Tablets (Less than 1%) 940
Sansert Tablets 2295
▲ Tenoretic Tablets (Up to 12%) 2845
▲ Tenormin Tablets and I.V. Injection (Up to 12%) 2847
Timolide Tablets 1748
Timoptic in Ocudose 1753
Timoptic Sterile Ophthalmic Solution 1751
Timoptic-XE 1755
Tonocard Tablets (Less than 1%) 531
Toprol-XL Tablets (About 1 of 100 patients) 565
Visken Tablets (2% or fewer patients) 2299
Zebeta Tablets 1413
Ziac 1415

(▣ Described in PDR For Nonprescription Drugs) Incidence data in parenthesis; ▲ 3% or more (⊙ Described in PDR For Ophthalmology)

Cold sensations Side Effects Index 1252

Cold sensations
Buprenex Injectable (Less than 1%) 2006
Duranest Injections 542
Dyclone 0.5% and 1% Topical Solutions, USP 544
Emla Cream 545
Imitrex Injection (1.1%) 1103
Imitrex Tablets (Rare) 1106
Monopril Tablets (0.4% to 1.0%) 757
Sanorex Tablets 2294
Versed Injection (Less than 1%) 2170
▲Xylocaine Injections (Among most common) 567
Zofran Injection (2%) 1214

Cold sore, non-herpetic
Hivid Tablets (Less than 1% to less than 3%) 2121
Intron A (Less than 5%) 2364
ReVia Tablets (Less than 1%) 940
Varivax (Greater than or equal to 1%) 1762

Cold symptoms, unspecified
Cartrol Tablets (Less common) 410
Paxil Tablets 2505
Prinivil Tablets (1.1%) 1733
▲ProSom Tablets (3%) 449
Sandostatin Injection (1% to 4%) 2292
Zestril Tablets (1.1% to 1.3%) 2854

Colds, susceptibility
Betimol 0.25%, 0.5% (1% to 5%) ⊙ 261
Diupres Tablets 1650
Hydropres Tablets 1675
Hytrin Capsules (At least 1%) 430
Lopid Tablets 1917
▲Pravachol (Up to 7.0%) 765
Prinzide Tablets (0.3% to 1%) 1737
Rowasa (2.33%) 2548
Sinemet CR Tablets 944
Zestoretic (0.3 to 1%) 2850

Colic
Duvoid (Infrequent) 2044
Feldene Capsules (Less than 1%) 1965
Glucotrol Tablets (1 in 100) 1967
Solganal Suspension (Rare) 2388
Urecholine 1761

Colic, biliary
Questran Light (One patient) 769
Questran Powder (One case) 770

Colitis
Aldoclor Tablets 1598
Aldomet Ester HCl Injection 1602
Aldomet Oral 1600
Aldoril Tablets 1604
Anafranil Capsules (Infrequent) 803
Anaprox/Naprosyn (Less than 1%) 2117
Ancef Injection 2465
Ansaid Tablets (Less than 1%) 2579
Brevicon 2088
Cataflam (Rare) 816
Cefotan 2829
Cefzil Tablets and Oral Suspension (Rare) 746
Ceptaz 1081
Claforan Sterile and Injection (1.4%) 1235
Cleocin Phosphate Injection 2586
Cleocin T Topical 2590
Cleocin Vaginal Cream 2589
Clinoril Tablets (Less than 1%) 1618
Demulen 2428
Desogen Tablets 1817
Dilacor XR Extended-release Capsules 2018
EC-Naprosyn Delayed-Release Tablets (Less than 1%) 2117
Effexor (Infrequent) 2719
Fortaz 1100
Foscavir Injection (Less than 1%) 547
Furoxone 2046
Keftab Tablets 915
Kefurox Vials, Faspak & ADD-Vantage 1454
Levlen/Tri-Levlen 651
Lincocin 2617
Lodine Capsules and Tablets (Less than 1%) 2743
Lopid Tablets 1917
Luvox Tablets (Infrequent) 2544
Micronor Tablets 1872
Modicon 1872
Anaprox/Naprosyn (Less than 1%) 2117
NebuPent for Inhalation Solution (1% or less) 1040
Neurontin Capsules (Rare) 1922
Norinyl 2088
Nor-Q D Tablets 2135
Oncaspar 2028
Ortho-Cept 1851
Ortho-Cyclen/Ortho-Tri-Cyclen 1858
Ortho-Novum 1872
Ortho-Cyclen/Ortho Tri-Cyclen 1858
Ovcon 760
Paxil Tablets (Rare) 2505
Permax Tablets (Rare) 575
Prozac Pulvules & Liquid, Oral Solution (Rare) 919
Rocephin Injectable Vials, ADD-Vantage, Galaxy Container (Rare) 2142
Rowasa (1.2%) 2548
Serzone Tablets (Infrequent) 771
Solganal Suspension 2388
Tazicef for Injection 2519
Ticlid Tablets 2156
Levlen/Tri-Levlen 651
Tri-Norinyl 2164
Videx Tablets, Powder for Oral Solution, & Pediatric Powder for Oral Solution (Less than 1%) 720
Voltaren Tablets (Rare) 861
Wellbutrin Tablets (Rare) 1204
Zinacef 1211

Colitis, ischemic
Blocadren Tablets 1614
Cartrol Tablets 410
Taxol (Rare) 714
Tenoretic Tablets 2845
Tenormin Tablets and I.V. Injection 2847
Timoptic-XE 1755
Trandate Tablets 1185
Visken Tablets 2299
Zebeta Tablets 1413
Ziac 1415

Colitis, necrotizing
Adriamycin PFS 1947
Adriamycin RDF 1947
Cytosar-U Sterile Powder (With experimental doses) 2592
Doxorubicin Astra 540

Colitis, pseudomembranous (see under Pseudomembranous colitis)

Colitis, ulcerative
Ancobon Capsules 2079
Indocin (Less than 1%) 1680
Orudis Capsules (Rare) 2766
Oruvail Capsules (Rare) 2766
PREVACID Delayed-Release Capsules (Less than 1%) 2562
Serzone Tablets (Rare) 771
Vantin for Oral Suspension and Vantin Tablets 2646

Colitis, ulcerative, worsening of
▲Asacol Delayed-Release Tablets (3%) 1979
Pentasa (0.4%) 1527

Collapse
Antivenin (Crotalidae) Polyvalent 2696
Atretol Tablets 573
Clozaril Tablets (Rare) 2252
Dilatrate-SR (Occasional) 2398
Diphtheria and Tetanus Toxoids and Pertussis Vaccine Adsorbed 2477
Diphtheria and Tetanus Toxoids and Pertussis Vaccine Adsorbed USP (For Pediatric Use) (Infrequent; 1 in 1,750 doses) 875
Fluvirin 460
Macrodantin Capsules (Seldom reported) 1989
Mintezol 1704
Nitrolingual Spray 2027
Norpramin Tablets (One report) 1526
Tegretol Chewable Tablets 852
Tegretol Suspension 852
Tegretol Tablets 852
Tofranil Tablets 856

Colon problem, unspecified
Betapace Tablets (2% to 3%) 641

Colon, cancer
Protostat Tablets 1883

Colon, dilatation
Artane (Rare) 1368
Phenergan with Codeine 2777
Phenergan VC with Codeine 2781

Colon, irritable
BuSpar (Infrequent) 737
Compazine 2470
Prilosec Delayed-Release Capsules (Less than 1%) 529

Colon, motility, increase
Phenergan with Codeine 2777
Phenergan VC with Codeine 2781

Colonic strictures
Creon 2536
Ultrase Capsules 2343
Ultrase MT Capsules 2344

Color perception, disturbed
Children's Advil Suspension (Less than 1%) 2692
Cipro Tablets (Less than 1%) 592
IBU Tablets (Less than 1%) 1342
Children's Motrin Ibuprofen Oral Suspension (Less than 1%) 1546
Motrin Tablets 2625
NegGram (Infrequent) 2323
Platinol 708
Platinol-AQ Injection 710
Quinaglute Dura-Tabs Tablets (Occasional) 649
Quinidex Extentabs 2067
Zefazone 2654

Coma
Children's Advil Suspension (Less than 1%) 2692
Anafranil Capsules (Infrequent) 803
Betaseron for SC Injection 658
Buprenex Injectable (Infrequent) 2006
Cognex Capsules (Rare) 1901
Compazine 2470
Cytosar-U Sterile Powder (With experimental doses) 2592
Cytovene (1% or less) 2103
DDAVP Injection (Rare) 2014
DDAVP (Rare) 2017
Dalmane Capsules 2173
Depakene (Rare) 413
Depakote Tablets (Rare) 415
Elavil 2838
Elspar 1659
Endep Tablets 2174
Eskalith 2485
Ethmozine Tablets (Less than 2%) 2041
Felbatol 2666
Fludara for Injection 663
Foscavir Injection (Less than 1%) 547
IBU Tablets (Rare; less than 1%) 1342
IFEX (Occasional) 697
Indocin Capsules (Less than 1%) 1680
Indocin I.V. (Less than 1%) 1684
Indocin (Less than 1%) 1680
Intron A (Less than 5%) 2364
Klonopin Tablets 2126
Levsin/Levsinex/Levbid 2405
Lioresal Intrathecal (Up to 4 of 214 patients) 1596
Lithium Carbonate Capsules & Tablets 2230
Lithonate/Lithotabs/Lithobid 2543
Luvox Tablets (Rare) 2544
Matulane Capsules 2131
Maxaquin Tablets (Less than 1%) 2440
Children's Motrin Ibuprofen Oral Suspension (Less than 1%) 1546
Motrin Tablets (Less than 1%) 2625
Motrin Ibuprofen Suspension, Oral Drops, Chewable Tablets, Caplets (Rare; less than 1%) 1546
Nardil (Less frequent) 1920
Oncaspar 2028
Oncovin Solution Vials & Hyporets 1466
Orthoclone OKT3 Sterile Solution 1837
Oxytocin Injection 2771
Permax Tablets (Infrequent) 575
Pfizerpen for Injection 2203
PhosLo Tablets 690
Podocon-25 1891
Prograf 1042
Proleukin for Injection (1%) 797
Prozac Pulvules & Liquid, Oral Solution (Rare) 919
ReoPro Vials (0.4%) 1471
Risperdal (Rare) 1301
Roferon-A Injection (Less than 1%) 2145
Rythmol Tablets–150mg, 225mg, 300mg (Less than 1%) 1352
Seromycin Pulvules 1476
Stimate, (desmopressin acetate) Nasal Spray, 1.5 mg/mL 525
Streptomycin Sulfate Injection (Occasional) 2208
Syntocinon Injection 2296
Tigan 2057
Tonocard Tablets (Less than 1%) 531
Triavil Tablets 1757
Wellbutrin Tablets 1204
Zoloft Tablets (Rare) 2217
Zovirax Sterile Powder (Approximately 1%) 1223

Coma, hepatic (see under Hepatic coma)

Coma, hyperosmolar non-ketonic
Hyperstat I.V. Injection 2363
OSM_GLYN Oral Osmotic Agent ⊙ 226
Proglycem 580

Coma, hypoglycemic
Tapazole Tablets 1477

Combativeness
Diprivan Injection (Less than 1%) 2833
Orthoclone OKT3 Sterile Solution 1837

Conduct disorder
Supprelin Injection (1%) 2056

Conduction delay, intraventricular
▲Rythmol Tablets–150mg, 225mg, 300mg (0.2 to 4.0%) 1352

Conduction disturbances
Adalat Capsules (10 mg and 20 mg) (Fewer than 0.5%) 587
Blocadren Tablets 1614
Catapres Tablets (Rare) 674
Catapres-TTS (Rare) 675
Combipres Tablets (Rare) 677
Desyrel and Desyrel Dividose 503
Dilantin Parenteral 1910
▲Eminase (38%) 2039
Ethmozine Tablets 2041
Etrafon 2355
▲Lanoxicaps (Among most common) 1117
▲Lanoxin Elixir Pediatric (Among most common) 1120
▲Lanoxin Injection (Among most common) 1123
▲Lanoxin Injection Pediatric (Among most common) 1126
▲Lanoxin Tablets (Among most common) 1128
Luvox Tablets (Infrequent) 2544
Mexitil Capsules (2 in 1,000) 678
Monopril Tablets (0.4% to 1.0%) 757
Paxil Tablets (Infrequent) 2505
Procardia Capsules (Fewer than 0.5%) 1971
Procardia XL Extended Release Tablets (Fewer than 0.5%) 1972
▲Rythmol Tablets–150mg, 225mg, 300mg (0.2 to 4.0%) 1352
▲Sandostatin Injection (9%) 2292
Taxol (Less than 1%) 714
Tonocard Tablets (0.0-1.5%) 531

Confusion
Actifed with Codeine Cough Syrup 1067
Actimmune (Rare) 1056
Adalat CC (Less than 1.0%) 589
Children's Advil Suspension (Less than 1%) 2692
Aldactazide 2413
Aldactone 2414
Aldoclor Tablets 1598
Aldomet Ester HCl Injection 1602
Aldomet Oral 1600
Aldoril Tablets 1604
Alfenta Injection (0.3% to 1%) 1286
Ambien Tablets (Frequent) 2416
Amoxil (Rare) 2464
Anafranil Capsules (2% to 3%) 803
Ancobon Capsules 2079
Ansaid Tablets (Less than 1%) 2579
Artane 1368
Asacol Delayed-Release Tablets 1979
Asendin Tablets (Less frequent) 1369
Atamet 572
Atgam Sterile Solution (Less than 5%) 2581
Ativan Injection (1.3%) 2698
Atretol Tablets 573
Augmentin (Rare) 2468
Axid Pulvules (Rare) 1427
Azactam for Injection (Less than 1%) 734

(▣ Described in PDR For Nonprescription Drugs) Incidence data in parenthesis; ▲ 3% or more (⊙ Described in PDR For Ophthalmology)

1253 **Side Effects Index** **Confusion**

Benadryl Capsules 1898
Benadryl Injection 1898
Bentyl 1501
▲Betaseron for SC Injection (4%) 658
Blenoxane (1%) 692
Brevibloc Injection (About 2%) 1808
BuSpar (2%) 737
Butisol Sodium Elixir & Tablets (Less than 1 in 100) 2660
Calan SR Caplets (1% or less) 2422
Calan Tablets (1% or less) 2419
Capoten 739
Capozide 742
Cardene Capsules (Rare) 2095
Cardene I.V. (Rare) 2709
Cardura Tablets (Less than 0.5% of 3960 patients) 2186
Ceclor Pulvules & Suspension (Rare) 1431
Cefzil Tablets and Oral Suspension (Less than 1%) 746
Celontin Kapseals 1899
Chibroxin Sterile Ophthalmic Solution (With oral form) 1617
Chloromycetin Sodium Succinate 1900
Cipro I.V. (1% or less) 595
Cipro I.V. Pharmacy Bulk Package (Less than 1%) 597
Cipro Tablets 592
Claritin (2% or fewer patients) 2349
Claritin-D (Less frequent) 2350
▲Clozaril Tablets (3%) 2252
Cogentin 1621
▲Cognex Capsules (7%) 1901
Cozaar Tablets (Less than 1%) 1628
Cytotec 2424
Cytovene (1% or less) 2103
Dalgan Injection (Less than 1%) 538
Dalmane Capsules (Rare) 2173
Dantrium Capsules (Less frequent) 1982
Daranide Tablets 1633
Daypro Caplets (Greater than 1% but less than 3%) 2426
Deconamine 1320
Demser Capsules 1649
Depakote Tablets (Greater than 1% but not more than 5%) 415
▲Desyrel and Desyrel Dividose (4.9% to 5.7%) 503
Diamox Intravenous (Occasional) 1372
Diamox Sequels (Sustained Release) (Occasional) 1373
Diamox Tablets (Occasional) 1372
Didronel Tablets 1984
▲Dilantin Infatabs (Among most common) 1908
▲Dilantin Kapseals (Among most common) 1906
▲Dilantin Parenteral (Among most common) 1910
▲Dilantin-125 Suspension (Among most common) 1911
Dilaudid Ampules 1335
Dilaudid Cough Syrup 1336
Dilaudid 1335
Diprivan Injection (Less than 1%) 2833
Diupres Tablets 1650
Diuril Oral Suspension 1653
Diuril Sodium Intravenous 1652
Diuril Tablets 1653
Dizac (Less frequent) 1809
Dolobid Tablets (Less than 1 in 100) 1654
Doral Tablets 2664
▲Duragesic Transdermal System (10% or more) 1288
Duranest Injections 542
Dyazide 2479
Dyclone 0.5% and 1% Topical Solutions, USP 544
E.E.S. (Isolated reports) 424
Easprin 1914
Edecrin 1657
Effexor (2%) 2719
Elavil 2838
▲Eldepryl Tablets (3 of 49 patients) 2550
Elspar 1659
Emla Cream 545
Empirin with Codeine Tablets 1093
Endep Tablets 2174
Ergamisol Tablets (Less frequent) 1292
EryPed (Isolated reports) 421
Ery-Tab Tablets (Isolated reports) 422
Erythrocin Stearate Filmtab (Isolated reports) 425
Erythromycin Base Filmtab (Isolated reports) 426
Erythromycin Delayed-Release Capsules, USP (Isolated reports) 427
Esgic-plus Tablets (Infrequent) 1013
Eskalith 2485
Ethmozine Tablets (Less than 2%) 2041
Etrafon 2355
Eulexin Capsules (1%) 2358
Felbatol 2666
Feldene Capsules (Less than 1%) 1965
Fioricet Tablets (Infrequent) 2258
Fioricet with Codeine Capsules 2260
Flagyl 375 Capsules 2434
Flagyl I.V. 2247
Floxin I.V. (Less than 1%) 1571
Floxin Tablets (200 mg, 300 mg, 400 mg) 1567
Fludara for Injection 663
Flumadine Tablets & Syrup (Less than 0.3%) 1015
Fluorouracil Injection 2116
▲Foscavir Injection (5% or greater) 547
Sterile FUDR (Remote possibility) 2118
Fulvicin P/G Tablets (Occasional) 2359
Fulvicin P/G 165 & 330 Tablets (Occasional) 2359
Ganite 2533
Garamycin Injectable 2360
Glauctabs (Occasional instances) ◉ 208
Glucotrol XL Extended Release Tablets (Less than 1%) 1968
Grifulvin V (griseofulvin tablets) Microsize (griseofulvin oral suspension) Microsize (Occasional) 1888
Gris-PEG Tablets, 125 mg & 250 mg (Occasional) 479
Halcion Tablets (0.9% to 0.5%) 2611
Haldol Decanoate 1577
Haldol Injection, Tablets and Concentrate 1575
Hivid Tablets (Less than 1% to less than 3%) 2121
HydroDIURIL Tablets 1674
Hydropres Tablets 1675
▲Hylorel Tablets (14.8%) 985
Hyperstat I.V. Injection 2363
Hyzaar Tablets 1677
IBU Tablets (Less than 1%) 1342
▲IFEX (Among most common) 697
Imdur (Less than or equal to 5%) 1323
Imitrex Injection (Infrequent) 1103
Imitrex Tablets (Infrequent) 1106
Indocin (Less than 1%) 1680
▲Intron A (Up to 12%) 2364
Ismo Tablets (Fewer than 1%) 2738
ISMOTIC 45% w/v Solution ◉ 222
Isoptin Oral Tablets (Less than 1%) 1346
Isoptin SR Tablets (1% or less) 1348
K-Phos Neutral Tablets 639
K-Phos Original Formula 'Sodium Free' Tablets (Less frequent) 639
Keflex Pulvules & Oral Suspension 914
Keftab Tablets 915
Kerlone Tablets (Less than 2%) 2436
Klonopin Tablets 2126
Lamictal Tablets (1.8%) 1112
Lariam Tablets 2128
Larodopa Tablets (Relatively frequent) 2129
Leukeran Tablets (Rare) 1133
Levsin/Levsinex/Levbid 2405
Librax Capsules 2176
Libritabs Tablets 2177
Librium Capsules (Some patients) 2178
Librium Injectable 2179
Limbitrol (Less common) 2180
Lioresal Intrathecal 1596
▲Lioresal Tablets (1-11%) 829
Lithium Carbonate Capsules & Tablets 2230
Lithonate/Lithotabs/Lithobid 2543
Lodine Capsules and Tablets (Less than 1%) 2743
Lomotil 2439
Lopid Tablets 1917
Lopressor Ampuls 830
Lopressor HCT Tablets 832
Lopressor Tablets 830
Loxitane 1378
Ludiomil Tablets (Rare) 843
Lupron Depot 3.75 mg 2556
Luvox Tablets 2544
MZM (Occasional) ◉ 267
Macrobid Capsules (Rare) 1988
Macrodantin Capsules (Rare) 1989
Marinol (Dronabinol) Capsules (Greater than 1%) 2231
Matulane Capsules 2131
Maxair Autohaler 1492
Maxair Inhaler (Less than 1%) 1494
Maxaquin Tablets (Less than 1%) 2440
Mebaral Tablets (Less than 1 in 100) 2322
Megace Oral Suspension (1% to 3%) 699
Mellaril 2269
Methadone Hydrochloride Oral Solution & Tablets 2235
Methotrexate Sodium Tablets, Injection, for Injection and LPF Injection 1275
MetroGel-Vaginal 902
Mexitil Capsules (1.9% to 2.6%) 678
Midamor Tablets (Less than or equal to 1%) 1703
Moduretic Tablets (Less than or equal to 1%) 1705
Mono-Gesic Tablets 792
Monopril Tablets (0.2% to 1.0%) 757
Motofen Tablets (1 in 200 to 1 in 600) 784
Children's Motrin Ibuprofen Oral Suspension (Less than 1%) 1546
Motrin Tablets (Less than 1%) 2625
Motrin Ibuprofen Suspension, Oral Drops, Chewable Tablets, Caplets (Less than 1%) 1546
Mutamycin 703
Myambutol Tablets 1386
Mycobutin Capsules (More than one patient) 1957
Myochrysine Injection (Rare) 1711
Nalfon 200 Pulvules & Nalfon Tablets (1.4%) 917
Nebcin Vials, Hyporets & ADD-Vantage 1464
NebuPent for Inhalation Solution (1% or less) 1040
Nembutal Sodium Capsules (Less than 1%) 436
Nembutal Sodium Solution (Less than 1%) 438
Nembutal Sodium Suppositories (Less than 1%) 440
Neoral (2% or less) 2276
Neptazane Tablets (Occasional) 1388
Neurontin Capsules (More than 1%) 1922
Neutrexin (2.8%) 2572
Nicorette 2458
Norflex (Infrequent) 1496
Norgesic (Infrequent) 1496
Noroxin Tablets 1715
Noroxin Tablets 2048
Norpramin Tablets 1526
Nubain Injection (1% or less) 935
Oncaspar (Less than 1%) 2028
Oramorph SR (Morphine Sulfate Sustained Release Tablets) 2236
Ornade Spansule Capsules 2502
Orthoclone OKT3 Sterile Solution 1837
Orudis Capsules (Less than 1%) 2766
Oruvail Capsules (Less than 1%) 2766
OSM_GLYN Oral Osmotic Agent ◉ 226
PBZ Tablets 845
PBZ-SR Tablets 844
Pamelor 2280
Parlodel 2281
Parnate Tablets 2503
Paxil Tablets (1.2%) 2505
Penetrex Tablets (Less than 1% but more than or equal to 0.1%) 2031
Pentam 300 Injection (1.7%) 1041
Pepcid Injection (Infrequent) 1722
Pepcid (Infrequent) 1720
Periactin 1724
▲Permax Tablets (11.1%) 575
Phenergan with Codeine (Rare) 2777
Phenergan with Dextromethorphan (Rare) 2778
Phenergan Suppositories (Rare) 2775
Phenergan Syrup (Rare) 2774
Phenergan VC (Rare) 2779
Phenergan VC with Codeine (Rare) 2781
Phenobarbital Elixir and Tablets (Less than 1 in 100 patients) 1469
PhosLo Tablets 690
Phrenilin 785
Placidyl Capsules 448
Polycitra Syrup 578
Polycitra-K Crystals 579
Polycitra-K Oral Solution 579
Polycitra-LC 578
Pondimin Tablets 2066
PREVACID Delayed-Release Capsules (Less than 1%) 2562
Prilosec Delayed-Release Capsules (Less than 1%) 529
Primaxin I.M. 1727
Primaxin I.V. (Less than 0.2%) 1729
Prinivil Tablets (0.3 to 1.0%) 1733
Prinzide Tablets 1737
Pro-Banthine Tablets 2052
▲Prograf (Greater than 3%) 1042
Proleukin for Injection 797
ProSom Tablets (2%) 449
Protostat Tablets 1883
Prozac Pulvules & Liquid, Oral Solution (2%) 919
Quadrinal Tablets 1350
Quarzan Capsules 2181
Quinaglute Dura-Tabs Tablets 649
Quinidex Extentabs 2067
Reglan (Less frequent) 2068
Relafen Tablets (1%) 2510
ReoPro Vials (0.6%) 1471
Restoril Capsules (2-3%) 2284
Retrovir Capsules 1158
Retrovir I.V. Infusion 1163
Retrovir Syrup 1158
ReVia Tablets (Less than 1%) 940
Revex (Less than 1%) 1811
Rifadin 1528
Rifamate Capsules 1530
Rifater 1532
Rimactane Capsules 847
Risperdal (Infrequent) 1301
Robinul Forte Tablets 2072
Robinul Injectable 2072
Robinul Tablets 2072
▲Roferon-A Injection (8%) 2145
Romazicon (Less than 1%) 2147
Roxanol 2243
Roxicodone Tablets, Oral Solution & Intensol (Oxycodone) 2244
Rythmol Tablets–150mg, 225mg, 300mg (Less than 1%) 1352
SSKI Solution (Less frequent) 2658
Salagen Tablets (Less than 1%) 1489
Sandimmune (2% or less) 2286
Seconal Sodium Pulvules (Less than 1 in 100) 1474
Sedapap Tablets 50 mg/650 mg (Infrequent) 1543
Seldane Tablets 1536
Seldane-D Extended-Release Tablets 1538
Sensorcaine 559
Serentil 684
Seromycin Pulvules 1476
▲Serzone Tablets (7% to 8%) 771
Sinemet Tablets 943
▲Sinemet CR Tablets (3.7%) 944
Sinequan (Infrequent) 2205
Soma Compound w/Codeine Tablets (Very rare) 2676
Soma Compound Tablets (Very rare) 2675
Soma Tablets 2674
▲Stadol (3% to 9%) 775
Surmontil Capsules 2811
Symmetrel Capsules and Syrup (0.1% to 5%) 946
Tagamet (Occasional) 2516
Talacen 2333
Talwin Injection 2334
Talwin Compound 2335
Talwin Injection 2334
Talwin Nx 2336
Tambocor Tablets (Less than 1%) 1497
Tavist Syrup 2297
Tavist Tablets 2298
Tegretol Chewable Tablets 852
Tegretol Suspension 852
Tegretol Tablets 852
Tenex Tablets (3% or less) 2074
Tessalon Perles 1020
Timolide Tablets (Less than 1%) 1748
Timoptic in Ocudose (Less frequent) 1753
Timoptic Sterile Ophthalmic Solution (Less frequent) 1751
Timoptic-XE 1755
Tobramycin Sulfate Injection 968
Tofranil Ampuls 854
Tofranil Tablets 856
Tofranil-PM Capsules 857
▲Tonocard Tablets (2.1-11.2%) 531
Toprol-XL Tablets 565
Torecan 2245
Trancopal Caplets 2337
Transderm Scōp Transdermal Therapeutic System (Infrequent) 869
Tranxene (Less common) 451
▲Trasylol (4%) 613
Trental Tablets (Less than 1%) 1244
Triavil Tablets 1757
Trilisate (Rare) 2000
Trinalin Repetabs Tablets 1330
Tussend 1783
Ultram Tablets (50 mg) (1% to 5%) 1585
Urispas Tablets 2532
Uroqid-Acid No. 2 Tablets 640
Valium Injectable 2182

(▭ Described in PDR For Nonprescription Drugs) Incidence data in parenthesis; ▲ 3% or more (◉ Described in PDR For Ophthalmology)

Valium Tablets (Infrequent) 2183
Valrelease Capsules (Occasional) 2169
Vaseretic Tablets 1765
Vasotec I.V. 1768
Vasotec Tablets (0.5% to 1%) 1771
Verelan Capsules (1% or less) 1410
Verelan Capsules (Less than 1%) 2824
Versed Injection (Less than 1%) 2170
Videx Tablets, Powder for Oral Solution, & Pediatric Powder for Oral Solution (1% to 2%) 720
Vivactil Tablets 1774
Vontrol Tablets (Approximately 1 in 350) 2532
▲ Wellbutrin Tablets (8.4%) 1204
▲ Xanax Tablets (9.9% to 10.4%) 2649
▲ Xylocaine Injections (Among most common) 567
Zantac (Rare) 1209
Zantac Injection (Rare) 1207
Zantac Syrup (Rare) 1209
Zerit Capsules (Fewer than 1% to 3%) 729
Zestoretic 2850
Zestril Tablets (0.3% to 1.0%) 2854
Zoloft Tablets (Frequent) 2217
Zosyn (1.0% or less) 1419
Zosyn Pharmacy Bulk Package (1.0% or less) 1422
Zovirax Capsules 1219
Zovirax Sterile Powder (Approximately 1%) 1223
Zovirax 1219
Zyloprim Tablets (Less than 1%) 1226

Confusion, mental (see under Confusion)

Confusion, nocturnal

Mellaril (Extremely rare) 2269
Trilafon 2389

Confusional state (see under Confusion)

Congelation

Eldepryl Tablets 2550
Ethyl Chloride, U.S.P. 1052
Fluori-Methane 1053
Fluro-Ethyl 1053

Congenital anomalies

Airet Solution for Inhalation 452
Amen Tablets 780
Aygestin Tablets 974
Cordarone Intravenous 2715
Cytovene-IV (Two or more reports) 2103
Depakene 413
Depakote Tablets 415
Depo-Provera Sterile Aqueous Suspension 2606
Diabinese Tablets 1935
Diethylstilbestrol Tablets 1437
Estrace Cream and Tablets 749
Estraderm Transdermal System 824
ESTRATAB Tablets (0.3, 0.625, 1.25, 2.5 mg) 2536
Halcion Tablets 2611
Havrix (Rare) 2489
Humegon 1824
Levlen/Tri-Levlen 651
Lo/Ovral Tablets 2746
Lo/Ovral-28 Tablets 2751
Methotrexate Sodium Tablets, Injection, for Injection and LPF Injection 1275
Metrodin (urofollitropin for injection) 2446
Mevacor Tablets (Rare) 1699
Nordette-21 Tablets 2755
Nordette-28 Tablets 2758
Norplant System (Rare; less than 1%) 2759
Ogen Tablets 2627
Ogen Vaginal Cream 2630
Ortho Dienestrol Cream 1866
Ortho-Est 1869
Ovral Tablets 2770
Ovral-28 Tablets 2770
Ovrette Tablets 2771
PMB 200 and PMB 400 2783
Pergonal (menotropins for injection, USP) 2448
Permax Tablets 575
Premarin Intravenous 2787
Premarin with Methyltestosterone 2794
Premarin Tablets 2789
Proventil Inhalation Aerosol 2382
Proventil Inhalation Solution 0.083% 2384
Proventil Repetabs Tablets 2386
Proventil Solution for Inhalation 0.5% 2383
Proventil Syrup 2385
Provera Tablets 2636
Retrovir Capsules 1158
Retrovir I.V. Infusion 1163
Retrovir Syrup 1158
▲ Septra I.V. Infusion (4.5%) 1169
Serophene (clomiphene citrate tablets, USP) 2451
Levlen/Tri-Levlen 651
Triphasil-21 Tablets 2814
Triphasil-28 Tablets 2819
Ventolin Inhalation Aerosol and Refill 1197
Ventolin Inhalation Solution (Rare) 1198
Ventolin Nebules Inhalation Solution (Rare) 1199
Ventolin Rotacaps for Inhalation 1200
Ventolin Syrup 1202
Ventolin Tablets 1203
Xanax Tablets 2649

Congenital malformation

Ativan Injection 2698
Ativan Tablets 2700
Atretol Tablets 573
Cytosar-U Sterile Powder (Two cases) 2592
Dalmane Capsules 2173
Dilantin Infatabs 1908
Dilantin Kapseals 1906
Dilantin Parenteral 1910
Dilantin-125 Suspension 1911
Dizac 1809
Doral Tablets 2664
Halcion Tablets 2611
Librax Capsules 2176
Libritabs Tablets 2177
Librium Capsules 2178
Librium Injectable 2179
Limbitrol 2180
Miltown Tablets 2672
PMB 200 and PMB 400 2783
Pravachol (One case) 765
Premphase 2797
Prempro 2801
ProSom Tablets 449
Restoril Capsules 2284
Tegretol Chewable Tablets 852
Tegretol Suspension 852
Tegretol Tablets 852
Tofranil Ampuls 854
Tofranil Tablets 856
Tofranil-PM Capsules 857
Tranxene 451
Valium Injectable 2182
Valium Tablets 2183
Valrelease Capsules 2169
Versed Injection 2170

Congestion

Adalat Capsules (10 mg and 20 mg) (2% or less) 587
▲ AeroBid Inhaler System (3-9%) 1005
▲ Aerobid-M Inhaler System (3-9%) 1005
Halcion Tablets (Rare) 2611
▲ Nicorette (3% to 9% of patients) 2458
Procardia Capsules (2% or less) 1971

Congestion, nasal (see under Nasal congestion)

Congestive heart failure

Adalat Capsules (10 mg and 20 mg) (About 2%) 587
Adriamycin PFS 1947
Adriamycin RDF 1947
Children's Advil Suspension (Less than 1%) 2692
Aldoclor Tablets 1598
Aldomet Ester HCl Injection 1602
Aldomet Oral 1600
Aldoril Tablets 1604
Aminohippurate Sodium Injection 1606
Anaprox/Naprosyn (Less than 1%) 2117
Android 1251
Aristocort Suspension (Forte Parenteral) 1027
Aristocort Suspension (Intralesional) 1025
Aristocort Tablets 1022
Aristospan Suspension (Intra-articular) 1033
Aristospan Suspension (Intralesional) 1032
Atgam Sterile Solution (Less than 5%) 2581
Atretol Tablets 573
Betagan ⊙ 233
Betoptic Ophthalmic Solution (Rare) 469
Betoptic S Ophthalmic Suspension (Rare) 471
BuSpar (Rare) 737
Calan SR Caplets (1.8%) 2422
Calan Tablets (1.8%) 2419
Capoten (2 to 3 of 1000 patients) 739
Capozide (2 to 3 of 1000 patients) 742
Cardizem CD Capsules (Less than 1%) 1506
Cardizem SR Capsules (Less than 1%) 1510
Cardizem Injectable (Less than 1%) 1508
Cardizem Tablets (Less than 1%) 1512
Cartrol Tablets (Rare) 410
Cataflam (Less than 1%) 816
Catapres Tablets (Rare) 674
Catapres-TTS (Rare) 675
Celestone Soluspan Suspension 2347
Cerubidine 795
Clinoril Tablets (Less than 1%) 1618
Clozaril Tablets 2252
Combipres Tablets (Rare) 677
Cordarone Intravenous (2.1%) 2715
Cordarone Tablets (1 to 3%) 2712
CORTENEMA 2535
Cortone Acetate Sterile Suspension 1623
Cortone Acetate Tablets 1624
Cytoxan 694
Dalalone D.P. Injectable 1011
Decadron Elixir 1633
Decadron Phosphate Injection 1637
Decadron Phosphate Respihaler 1642
Decadron Phosphate Turbinaire 1645
Decadron Phosphate with Xylocaine Injection, Sterile 1639
Decadron Tablets 1635
Decadron-LA Sterile Suspension 1646
Deltasone Tablets 2595
Depo-Medrol Single-Dose Vial 2600
Depo-Medrol Sterile Aqueous Suspension 2597
Desyrel and Desyrel Dividose 503
Dexacort Phosphate in Respihaler 458
Dexacort Phosphate in Turbinaire 459
Digibind (Few instances) 1091
Diupres Tablets 1650
Doxorubicin Astra 540
EC-Naprosyn Delayed-Release Tablets (Less than 1%) 2117
▲ Emcyt Capsules (3%) 1953
Esimil Tablets (Occasional) 822
Ethmozine Tablets (1% to 5%) 2041
Feldene Capsules (Less than 1%) 1965
Florinef Acetate Tablets 505
Fludara for Injection (Up to 3%) 663
Glucophage 752
Hivid Tablets (Infrequent) 2121
Hydeltrasol Injection, Sterile 1665
Hydeltra-T.B.A. Sterile Suspension 1667
Hydrocortone Acetate Sterile Suspension 1669
Hydrocortone Phosphate Injection, Sterile 1670
Hydrocortone Tablets 1672
Hydropres Tablets 1675
IBU Tablets (Less than 1%) 1342
Idamycin 1955
Inderal 2728
Inderal LA Long Acting Capsules 2730
Inderide Tablets 2732
Inderide LA Long Acting Capsules 2734
Indocin Capsules (Less than 1%) 1680
Indocin I.V. (Less than 1%) 1684
Indocin (Less than 1%) 1680
Ismelin Tablets 827
Isoptin Oral Tablets (1.8%) 1346
Isoptin SR Tablets (1.8%) 1348
Lodine Capsules and Tablets (Less than 1%) 2743
Lopressor Ampuls (1%) 830
Lopressor HCT Tablets 832
Lopressor Tablets (1%) 830
Lupron Depot 3.75 mg 2556
Lupron Depot 7.5 mg 2559
▲ Lupron Injection (5% or more) 2555
Luvox Tablets (Infrequent) 2544
Medrol 2621
Mexitil Capsules (Less than 1%) 678
Children's Motrin Ibuprofen Oral Suspension (Less than 1%) 1546
Motrin Tablets (Less than 1%) 2625
Motrin Ibuprofen Suspension, Oral Drops, Chewable Tablets, Caplets (Less than 1%) 1546
Mutamycin (Rare) 703
Anaprox/Naprosyn (Less than 1%) 2117
NEOSAR Lyophilized/Neosar (A few instances) 1959
Nicorette 2458
Nimotop Capsules (Less than 1%) 610
Normodyne Injection 2377
Normodyne Tablets 2379
Norpace (1 to 3%) 244[illegible]
▲ Novantrone (0 to 5%) 1279
Ocupress Ophthalmic Solution, 1% Sterile ⊙ 309
Orudis Capsules (Less than 1%) 2766
Oruvail Capsules (Less than 1%) 2766
Paxil Tablets (Rare) 2505
Pediapred Oral Liquid 995
Permax Tablets (Frequent) 575
Prelone Syrup 1787
Premarin with Methyltestosterone 2794
Procardia Capsules (About 2%; rare, about 1 patient in 15) 1971
Procardia XL Extended Release Tablets (About 1 patient in 15; about 2%; rare) 1972
Proglycem 580
Proleukin for Injection (1%) 797
Prostin VR Pediatric Sterile Solution (Less than 1%) 2635
Retrovir Capsules (0.8%) 1158
Retrovir I.V. Infusion (1%) 1163
Retrovir Syrup (0.8%) 1158
Roferon-A Injection (Less than 1%) 2145
Rubex 712
▲ Rythmol Tablets–150mg, 225mg, 300mg (0.8 to 3.7%) 1352
Sandostatin Injection (Less than 1%) 2292
Seromycin Pulvules 1476
Serzone Tablets (Rare) 771
Solu-Cortef Sterile Powder 2641
Solu-Medrol Sterile Powder 2643
Symmetrel Capsules and Syrup (0.1% to 1%) 946
Tambocor Tablets 1497
Tegretol Chewable Tablets 852
Tegretol Suspension 852
Tegretol Tablets 852
Tenex Tablets (Rare) 2074
Testoderm Testosterone Transdermal System (One in 104 patients) 486
Tofranil Ampuls 854
Tofranil Tablets 856
Tofranil-PM Capsules 857
Tolectin (200, 400 and 600 mg) (Less than 1%) 1581
▲ Tonocard Tablets (4.0%) 531
Toprol-XL Tablets (About 1 of 100 patients) 565
▲ Trasylol (3%) 613
Triostat Injection (Approximately 1%) 2530
Vascor (200, 300 and 400 mg) Tablets (About 1%) 1587
Vasotec I.V. (1.8%) 1768
Verelan Capsules (1.8%) 1410
Verelan Capsules (1.8%) 2824
Voltaren Tablets (Less than 1%) 861
Zebeta Tablets 1413
Ziac 1415
▲ Zoladex (5%) 2858

Conjunctiva, progressive pigmentation

Serentil 684
Torecan 2245

Conjunctiva, sensitization

Neosporin Ophthalmic Ointment Sterile 1148
Polysporin Ophthalmic Ointment Sterile 1154

Conjunctiva, suffusion

Amicar Syrup, Tablets, and Injection (Occasional) 1267
Arfonad Ampuls 2080
BiCNU 691

Conjunctiva, thickening

Floropryl Sterile Ophthalmic Ointment 1662
Humorsol Sterile Ophthalmic Solution 1664
Phospholine Iodide ⊙ 326

Conjunctival blanching

IOPIDINE Sterile Ophthalmic Solution (0.4%) ⊙ 219

(▣ Described in PDR For Nonprescription Drugs) Incidence data in parenthesis; ▲ 3% or more (⊙ Described in PDR For Ophthalmology)

1255 **Side Effects Index** **Constipation**

Conjunctival chemosis
Natacyn Antifungal Ophthalmic Suspension (One case) ⊙ 225

Conjunctival deposits
EPIFRIN ⊙ 239
PROPINE with C CAP Compliance Cap ⊙ 253
Solganal Suspension 2388

Conjunctival epithelial defects, unspecified
▲ Genoptic Sterile Ophthalmic Solution (Among most frequent) ⊙ 243
▲ Genoptic Sterile Ophthalmic Ointment (Among most frequent) ⊙ 243
Gentacidin Ointment ⊙ 264
Gentacidin Solution ⊙ 264
▲ Gentak (Among most frequent) ⊙ 208

Conjunctival erythema
Cortisporin Ophthalmic Ointment Sterile 1085
Cortisporin Ophthalmic Suspension Sterile 1086
FLURESS (Occasional) ⊙ 207
Ocusert Pilo-20 and Pilo-40 Ocular Therapeutic Systems ⊙ 254

Conjunctival hyperemia
AK-Spore ⊙ 204
▲ Ciloxan Ophthalmic Solution (Less than 10%) 472
EPIFRIN ⊙ 239
▲ Gentak (Among most frequent) ⊙ 208
Natacyn Antifungal Ophthalmic Suspension (One case) ⊙ 225
Ophthetic ⊙ 247
Phospholine Iodide ⊙ 326
Pilagan ⊙ 248
Suprane (Greater than 1%) 1813

Conjunctival injection
Azo Gantanol Tablets 2080
Azo Gantrisin Tablets 2081
Azulfidine (Rare) 1949
Bactrim DS Tablets 2084
Bactrim I.V. Infusion 2082
Bactrim 2084
▲ Betimol 0.25%, 0.5% (More than 5%) ⊙ 261
Crolom (Infrequent) ⊙ 257
Diupres Tablets 1650
Fansidar Tablets 2114
Gantanol Tablets 2119
Gantrisin 2120
Hydropres Tablets 1675
Isopto Carbachol Ophthalmic Solution ⊙ 223
Mintezol 1704
Pepcid Injection (Infrequent) 1722
Pepcid (Infrequent) 1720
▲ Rēv-Eyes Ophthalmic Eyedrops 0.5% (80%) ⊙ 323
Septra 1174
Septra I.V. Infusion 1169
Septra I.V. Infusion ADD-Vantage Vials 1171
Septra 1174
Ser-Ap-Es Tablets 849
Vira-A Ophthalmic Ointment, 3% ⊙ 312

Conjunctival irritation
Efudex (Infrequent) 2113
Ocusert Pilo-20 and Pilo-40 Ocular Therapeutic Systems ⊙ 254

Conjunctival microhemorrhage
IOPIDINE Sterile Ophthalmic Solution ⊙ 219

Conjunctival vascular congestion
Isopto Carpine Ophthalmic Solution ⊙ 223
Pilocar ⊙ 268
Pilopine HS Ophthalmic Gel ⊙ 226

Conjunctivitis
▲ Accutane Capsules (About 2 patients in 5) 2076
Adalat CC (Less than 1.0%) 589
Adriamycin PFS (Rare) 1947
Adriamycin RDF (Rare) 1947
Children's Advil Suspension (Less than 1%) 2692
Anafranil Capsules (Up to 1%) 803
Ansaid Tablets (Less than 1%) 2579
Apresazide Capsules (Less frequent) 808
Apresoline Hydrochloride Tablets (Less frequent) 809
Asacol Delayed-Release Tablets (1% to 2%) 1979
Atretol Tablets 573
▲ Betaseron for SC Injection (12%) 658
Betimol 0.25%, 0.5% ⊙ 261
Buprenex Injectable (Less than 1%) 2006
BuSpar (Infrequent) 737
Cardene I.V. (Rare) 2709
Cardura Tablets (1%) 2186
Cartrol Tablets (Less common) 410
▲ CellCept Capsules (More than or equal to 3%) 2099
Claritin (2% or fewer patients) 2349
Claritin-D (Less frequent) 2350
Clinoril Tablets (Less than 1 in 100) 1618
Cognex Capsules (Frequent) 1901
Cozaar Tablets (Less than 1%) 1628
Cytosar-U Sterile Powder (Less frequent) 2592
Cytotec (Infrequent) 2424
Cytovene (1% or less) 2103
DDAVP (Up to 2%) 2017
Daypro Caplets (Less than 1%) 2426
Depakote Tablets (Greater than 1% but not more than 5%) 415
Desmopressin Acetate Rhinal Tube (Up to 2%) 979
Doxorubicin Astra (Rare) 540
Econopred & Econopred Plus Ophthalmic Suspensions (Occasional) ⊙ 217
Effexor (Infrequent) 2719
Engerix-B Unit-Dose Vials 2482
Ergamisol Tablets (Less than 1% to 2%) 1292
FML Forte Liquifilm (Occasional) ⊙ 240
FML Liquifilm (Occasional) ⊙ 241
FML S.O.P. (Occasional) ⊙ 241
Felbatol 2666
Floxin I.V. 1571
Foscavir Injection (Between 1% and 5%) 547
▲ Genoptic Sterile Ophthalmic Solution (Among most frequent) ⊙ 243
▲ Genoptic Sterile Ophthalmic Ointment (Among most frequent) ⊙ 243
▲ Gentak (Among most frequent) ⊙ 208
Glucotrol XL Extended Release Tablets (Less than 1%) 1968
Hismanal Tablets (1.2%) 1293
Hytrin Capsules (At least 1%) 430
Hyzaar Tablets 1677
IBU Tablets (Less than 1%) 1342
Imdur (Less than or equal to 5%) 1323
Intron A (Less than 5%) 2364
Iopidine 0.5% (Less than 3%) ⊙ 221
Kerlone Tablets (Less than 2%) 2436
Lamictal Tablets (Infrequent) 1112
Lodine Capsules and Tablets (Less than 1%) 2743
Lorelco Tablets 1517
Lotensin HCT (0.3% or more) 837
Lozol Tablets (Less than 5%) 2022
Lupron Depot 3.75 mg (Less than 5%) 2556
Luvox Tablets (Infrequent) 2544
M-M-R II 1687
Marinol (Dronabinol) Capsules (0.3% to 1%) 2231
Maxaquin Tablets (Less than 1%) 2440
Mesantoin Tablets 2272
Miacalcin Nasal Spray (1% to 3%) 2275
Children's Motrin Ibuprofen Oral Suspension (Less than 1%) 1546
Motrin Tablets (Less than 1%) 2625
Motrin Ibuprofen Suspension, Oral Drops, Chewable Tablets, Caplets (Less than 1%) 1546
Myochrysine Injection (Rare) 1711
NebuPent for Inhalation Solution (1% or less) 1040
Neoral (2% or less) 2276
Neurontin Capsules (Infrequent) 1922
Norvasc Tablets (More than 0.1% to 1%) 1940
▲ Novantrone (0 to 5%) 1279
OptiPranolol (Metipranolol 0.3%) Sterile Ophthalmic Solution (A small number of patients) ⊙ 258
Orthoclone OKT3 Sterile Solution 1837
Orudis Capsules (Less than 1%) 2766
Oruvail Capsules (Less than 1%) 2766
Paxil Tablets (Rare) 2505
Penetrex Tablets (Less than 1% but more than or equal to 0.1%) 2031
Pentasa (Less than 1%) 1527
Permax Tablets (Infrequent) 575
▲ Proleukin for Injection (4%) 797
Proventil Syrup (Children 2 to 6 years, 1%) 2385
Prozac Pulvules & Liquid, Oral Solution (Infrequent) 919
▲ Pulmozyme Inhalation (4% to 5%) 1064
Recombivax HB 1744
▲ Ridaura Capsules (3 to 9%) 2513
Rifadin (Occasional) 1528
Rifater (Occasional) 1532
Rimactane Capsules 847
Robaxin Injectable 2070
Robaxin Tablets 2071
Rocaltrol Capsules 2141
Roferon-A Injection (Less than 3%) 2145
Rogaine Topical Solution (1.17%) 2637
Rubex (Rare) 712
Salagen Tablets (2%) 1489
Sandimmune (2% or less) 2286
Sectral Capsules (Up to 2%) 2807
Ser-Ap-Es Tablets 849
Serzone Tablets (Infrequent) 771
Solganal Suspension (Rare) 2388
Suprane (Greater than 1%) 1813
▲ Tegison Capsules (10-25%) 2154
Tegretol Chewable Tablets 852
Tegretol Suspension 852
Tegretol Tablets 852
Tenex Tablets (3% or less) 2074
Thioplex (Thiotepa For Injection) 1281
Timoptic in Ocudose (Less frequent) 1753
Timoptic Sterile Ophthalmic Solution (Less frequent) 1751
Timoptic-XE (1% to 5% of patients) 1755
Trental Tablets (Less than 1%) 1244
Vaseretic Tablets 1765
Vasotec I.V. 1768
Vasotec Tablets (0.5% to 1.0%) 1771
Ventolin Syrup (1% of children) 1202
Videx Tablets, Powder for Oral Solution, & Pediatric Powder for Oral Solution (Less than 1%) 720
Virazole 1264
Zerit Capsules (Fewer than 1% to 5%) 729
Zoloft Tablets (Infrequent) 2217
Zyloprim Tablets (Less than 1%) 1226

Conjunctivitis, exudative
Rifamate Capsules (Occasional) 1530
Rimactane Capsules 847

Conjunctivitis, follicular
Atropine Sulfate Sterile Ophthalmic Solution ⊙ 233
PROPINE with C CAP Compliance Cap (Infrequent) ⊙ 253

Conjunctivitis, hemorrhagic
Anafranil Capsules (Rare) 803
Cytosar-U Sterile Powder (With experimental doses) 2592

Conjunctivitis, mucopurulent
Hivid Tablets (Less than 1% to less than 3%) 2121

Conjunctivitis sicca
Orudis Capsules (Less than 1%) 2766
Oruvail Capsules (Less than 1%) 2766

Consciousness, disorders
▲ Betapace Tablets (2% to 4%) 641
Hexalen Capsules 2571
Intron A (Less than 5%) 2364
Permax Tablets 575
Reglan 2068
Supprelin Injection (1% to 3%) 2056
Temaril Tablets, Syrup and Spansule Extended-Release Capsules 483

Consciousness, loss of
Carbocaine Hydrochloride Injection 2303
Cipro I.V. (1% or less) 595
Decadron Phosphate with Xylocaine Injection, Sterile 1639
Duranest Injections 542
Dyclone 0.5% and 1% Topical Solutions, USP 544
Effexor (Rare) 2719
Emla Cream 545
Fioricet with Codeine Capsules 2260
Fiorinal with Codeine Capsules 2262
Floxin I.V. 1571
Floxin Tablets (200 mg, 300 mg, 400 mg) 1567
Hyperstat I.V. Injection 2363
Lutrepulse for Injection 980
Marcaine Hydrochloride with Epinephrine 1:200,000 2316
Marcaine Hydrochloride Injection 2316
Marcaine Spinal 2319
Maxaquin Tablets 2440
Mexitil Capsules (Less than 1% or about 6 in 10,000) 678
Nescaine/Nescaine MPF 554
Noroxin Tablets 1715
Noroxin Tablets 2048
Novocain Hydrochloride for Spinal Anesthesia 2326
Orthoclone OKT3 Sterile Solution 1837
Pontocaine Hydrochloride for Spinal Anesthesia 2330
Prostigmin Injectable 1260
Prostigmin Tablets 1261
Sensorcaine 559
Stelazine 2514
Typhim Vi 899
VePesid Capsules and Injection (Sometimes) 718
▲ Xylocaine Injections (Among most common) 567

Costochondritis
Neurontin Capsules (Rare) 1922

Constipation
Accupril Tablets (0.5% to 1.0%) 1893
Actifed with Codeine Cough Syrup 1067
Actigall Capsules 802
Adalat Capsules (10 mg and 20 mg) (2% or less) 587
Adalat CC (1% to 3% or less) 589
Adipex-P Tablets and Capsules 1048
Children's Advil Suspension (Less than 3%) 2692
AeroBid Inhaler System (1-3%) 1005
Aerobid-M Inhaler System (1-3%) 1005
Akineton 1333
Aldoclor Tablets 1598
Aldomet Ester HCl Injection 1602
Aldomet Oral 1600
Aldoril Tablets 1604
Alka-Mints Chewable Antacid ▣ 701
Altace Capsules (Less than 1%) 1232
ALternaGEL Liquid 1316
Ambien Tablets (Infrequent; 2%) 2416
Amphojel 2695
▲ Anafranil Capsules (22% to 47%) 803
▲ Anaprox/Naprosyn (3% to 9%) 2117
Anexsia 5/500 Elixir 1781
Anexia Tablets 1782
Ansaid Tablets (1-3%) 2579
Apresazide Capsules (Less frequent) 808
Apresoline Hydrochloride Tablets (Less frequent) 809
▲ Aredia for Injection (Up to at least 15%) 810
Arfonad Ampuls 2080
Artane 1368
▲ Asacol Delayed-Release Tablets (5%) 1979
▲ Asendin Tablets (12%) 1369
Astramorph/PF Injection, USP (Preservative-Free) 535
Atamet 572
Atretol Tablets 573
Atrohist Plus Tablets 454
Atrovent Inhalation Aerosol (Less frequent) 671
Atrovent Inhalation Solution (0.9%) 673
Axid Pulvules (2.5%) 1427
Basaljel 2703
Benadryl Capsules 1898
Benadryl Injection 1898
Bentyl 1501
▲ Betaseron for SC Injection (24%) 658
Biphetamine Capsules 983
Bontril Slow-Release Capsules 781
Brevibloc Injection (Less than 1%) 1808
▲ Bromfed-DM Cough Syrup (Among most frequent) 1786
Brontex 1981
Buprenex Injectable (Less than 1%) 2006
BuSpar (1%) 737
Butisol Sodium Elixir & Tablets (Less than 1 in 100) 2660
▲ Calan SR Caplets (7.3%) 2422
▲ Calan Tablets (7.3%) 2419
Capoten (About 0.5 to 2%) 739
Capozide (0.5 to 2%) 742
Carafate Suspension (2%) 1505

(▣ Described in PDR For Nonprescription Drugs) Incidence data in parenthesis; ▲ 3% or more (⊙ Described in PDR For Ophthalmology)

Constipation **Side Effects Index** **1256**

Carafate Tablets (2%) 1504
Cardene Capsules (0.6%) 2095
Cardizem CD Capsules (Less than 1%) 1506
Cardizem SR Capsules (1.6%) 1510
Cardizem Injectable (Less than 1%) 1508
Cardizem Tablets (Less than 1%) .. 1512
Cardura Tablets (1%) 2186
Cartrol Tablets (Less common) 410
Cataflam (B 3% to 9%) 816
▲ Catapres Tablets (About 10 in 100 patients) 674
Catapres-TTS (1 of 101 patients) .. 675
▲ CellCept Capsules (18.5% to 22.9%) 2099
Celontin Kapseals (Frequent) 1899
Cipro I.V. (1% or less) 595
Cipro I.V. Pharmacy Bulk Package (Less than 1%) 597
Cipro Tablets 592
Claritin (2% or fewer patients) 2349
Claritin-D (Less frequent) 2350
Cleocin Vaginal Cream (Less than 1%) 2589
▲ Clinoril Tablets (3-9%) 1618
Clomid (Fewer than 1%) 1514
▲ Clozaril Tablets (More than 5 to 14%) 2252
Codiclear DH Syrup 791
Cogentin 1621
▲ Cognex Capsules (4%) 1901
▲ Colestid Tablets (Major single complaint) 2591
▲ Combipres Tablets (About 10%) 677
Comhist 2038
Compazine 2470
▲ Cordarone Tablets (4 to 9%) 2712
Cozaar Tablets (Less than 1%) 1628
▲ Creon (Among most frequent) 2536
Cytotec (1.1%) 2424
Cytovene (1% or less) 2103
▲ DHCplus Capsules (Among most frequent) 1993
Dalgan Injection (Less than 1%) 538
Dalmane Capsules 2173
Danocrine Capsules 2307
Dantrium Capsules (Less frequent) 1982
Daranide Tablets 1633
Darvon-N/Darvocet-N 1433
Darvon 1435
Darvon-N Suspension & Tablets 1433
▲ Daypro Caplets (3% to 9%) 2426
Deconamine Chewable Tablets 1320
Deconamine CX Cough and Cold Liquid and Tablets 1319
Deconamine 1320
Deconsal C Expectorant Syrup 456
Deconsal Pediatric Syrup 457
Demadex Tablets and Injection (1.8%) 686
Demerol 2308
Depakene 413
Depakote Tablets 415
Desoxyn Gradumet Tablets 419
▲ Desyrel and Desyrel Dividose (7.0% to 7.6%) 503
Dexedrine 2474
DextroStat Dextroamphetamine Tablets 2036
▲ Dilacor XR Extended-release Capsules (2.2% to 3.6%) 2018
Dilantin Infatabs 1908
Dilantin Kapseals 1906
Dilantin Parenteral 1910
Dilantin-125 Suspension 1911
Dilaudid Ampules 1335
Dilaudid Cough Syrup 1336
Dilaudid-HP Injection (Less frequent) 1337
Dilaudid-HP Lyophilized Powder 250 mg (Less frequent) 1337
Dilaudid 1335
Dilaudid Oral Liquid 1339
Dilaudid 1335
Dilaudid Tablets - 8 mg 1339
Dimetane-DC Cough Syrup 2059
Dimetane-DX Cough Syrup 2059
Ditropan 1516
Diucardin Tablets 2718
Diupres Tablets 1650
Diuril Oral Suspension 1653
Diuril Sodium Intravenous 1652
Diuril Tablets 1653
Dizac (Less frequent) 1809
Dolobid Tablets (Greater than 1 in 100) 1654
Donnatal 2060
Donnatal Extentabs 2061
Donnatal Tablets 2060
Doral Tablets 2664
▲ Duragesic Transdermal System (10% or more) 1288
Duramorph (Frequent) 962
Duratuss HD Elixir 2565
Dyazide 2479
DynaCirc Capsules (0.5% to 1%) .. 2256
▲ EC-Naprosyn Delayed-Release Tablets (3% to 9%) 2117
▲ Effexor (15%) 2719
Elavil 2838
Eldepryl Tablets 2550
▲ Empirin with Codeine Tablets (Among most frequent) 1093
Endep Tablets 2174
Enduron Tablets 420
Engerix-B Unit-Dose Vials (Less than 1%) 2482
Ergamisol Tablets (2% to 3%) 1292
Esgic-plus Tablets (Infrequent) 1013
Esidrix Tablets 821
Esimil Tablets 822
Etrafon 2355
▲ Famvir (4.4%) 2486
Fastin Capsules 2488
▲ Felbatol (6.9% to 12.9%) 2666
Feldene Capsules (Greater than 1%) 1965
Feosol Capsules (Occasional) 2456
Feosol Elixir (Occasional) 2456
Feosol Tablets (Occasional) 2457
Fioricet Tablets (Infrequent) 2258
Fioricet with Codeine Capsules (Infrequent) 2260
Fiorinal with Codeine Capsules 2262
Flagyl 375 Capsules 2434
Flagyl I.V. 2247
Flexeril Tablets (1% to 3%) 1661
Floxin I.V. (1% to 3%) 1571
Floxin Tablets (200 mg, 300 mg, 400 mg) (1% to 3%) 1567
Fludara for Injection (1% to 3%) 663
Flumadine Tablets & Syrup 1015
Foscavir Injection (Between 1% and 5%) 547
Ganite 2533
Glucotrol Tablets (1 in 100) 1967
Glucotrol XL Extended Release Tablets (Less than 3%) 1968
▲ Habitrol Nicotine Transdermal System (3% to 9% of patients) 865
Halcion Tablets (Rare) 2611
Haldol Decanoate 1577
Haldol Injection, Tablets and Concentrate 1575
Hivid Tablets (Less than 1% to less than 3%) 2121
Hycodan Tablets and Syrup 930
Hycomine 931
Hydrea Capsules (Less frequent) 696
Hydrocet Capsules 782
HydroDIURIL Tablets 1674
Hydropres Tablets 1675
▲ Hylorel Tablets (21.0%) 985
Hyperstat I.V. Injection 2363
Hytrin Capsules (At least 1%) 430
Hyzaar Tablets 1677
IBU Tablets (Greater than 1%) 1342
IFEX (Less than 1%) 697
Imdur (Less than or equal to 5%) .. 1323
Imitrex Tablets (Infrequent) 1106
Imodium Capsules 1295
Inderal 2728
Inderal LA Long Acting Capsules 2730
Inderide Tablets 2732
Inderide LA Long Acting Capsules .. 2734
Indocin Capsules (Greater than 1%) 1680
Indocin I.V. (1% to 3%) 1684
Indocin (Greater than 1%) 1680
Infumorph 200 and Infumorph 500 Sterile Solutions (Frequent) 965
▲ Intron A (Up to 10%) 2364
Inversine Tablets 1686
Ionamin Capsules 990
Iopidine 0.5% (Less than 1%) .... ⊙ 221
▲ Isoptin Oral Tablets (7.3%) 1346
▲ Isoptin SR Tablets (7.3%) 1348
Kayexalate 2314
Kemadrin Tablets 1112
Kerlone Tablets (Less than 2%) 2436
Klonopin Tablets 2126
▲ Kytril Injection (3%) 2490
▲ Kytril Tablets (3% to 18%) 2492
▲ Lamictal Tablets (4.1%) 1112
Lamprene Capsules (Less than 1%) 828
Larodopa Tablets (Infrequent) 2129
Lasix Injection, Oral Solution and Tablets 1240
Lescol Capsules (2.6%) 2267
Leucovorin Calcium for Injection (Up to 4%) 1268
▲ Leustatin (9%) 1834
Levbid Extended-Release Tablets 2405
Levoprome 1274
Levsin/Levsinex/Levbid 2405
Librax Capsules (Infrequent) 2176
Libritabs Tablets (Isolated cases) 2177
Librium Capsules (Isolated cases) .. 2178
Librium Injectable (Isolated instances) 2179
▲ Limbitrol (Among most frequent) 2180
Lioresal Intrathecal (Up to 5 of 214 patients) 1596
▲ Lioresal Tablets (2-6%) 829
Lodine Capsules and Tablets (More than 1% but less than 3%) 2743
Lopid Tablets (1.4%) 1917
Lopressor Ampuls (1%) 830
Lopressor HCT Tablets (1 in 100 patients) 832
Lopressor Tablets (1%) 830
Lorcet 10/650 1018
Lortab 2566
Lotensin Tablets 834
Lotensin HCT 837
Lotrel Capsules 840
Loxitane 1378
Lozol Tablets (Less than 5%) 2022
▲ Ludiomil Tablets (6%) 843
Lupron Depot 7.5 mg 2559
▲ Lupron Injection (5% or more) 2555
▲ Luvox Tablets (10%) 2544
▲ MS Contin Tablets (Less frequent to among most frequent) 1994
▲ MSIR (Among most frequent) 1997
Macrobid Capsules (Less than 1%) 1988
Matulane Capsules 2131
Maxaquin Tablets (Less than 1%) .. 2440
Maxzide 1380
Mebaral Tablets (Less than 1 in 100) 2322
Megace Oral Suspension (1% to 3%) 699
Mellaril 2269
Mepergan Injection 2753
▲ Mepron Suspension (3%) 1135
Methadone Hydrochloride Oral Concentrate 2233
Methadone Hydrochloride Oral Solution & Tablets 2235
MetroGel-Vaginal (Equal to or less than 2%) 902
▲ Mevacor Tablets (2.0% to 4.9%) .. 1699
▲ Mexitil Capsules (4%) 678
Miacalcin Nasal Spray (1% to 3%) 2275
Midamor Tablets (Between 1% and 3%) 1703
Minipress Capsules (1-4%) 1937
Minizide Capsules (Rare) 1938
Moban Tablets and Concentrate 1048
Moduretic Tablets (Less than or equal to 1%) 1705
Monopril Tablets (0.2% to 1.0%) .. 757
Motofen Tablets (1 in 300) 784
Children's Motrin Ibuprofen Oral Suspension (Greater than 1% but less than 3%) 1546
Motrin Tablets (Less than 3%) 2625
Motrin Ibuprofen Suspension, Oral Drops, Chewable Tablets, Caplets (1% to less than 3%) 1546
Mykrox Tablets (Less than 2%) 993
▲ Nalfon 200 Pulvules & Nalfon Tablets (7%) 917
▲ Anaprox/Naprosyn (3% to 9%) 2117
Nardil (Common) 1920
Navane Capsules and Concentrate 2201
Navane Intramuscular 2202
▲ Navelbine Injection (Up to 29%) 1145
Nembutal Sodium Capsules (Less than 1%) 436
Nembutal Sodium Solution (Less than 1%) 438
Nembutal Sodium Suppositories (Less than 1%) 440
Neoral (Rare) 2276
Nephro-Fer Rx Tablets 2005
▲ Neupogen for Injection (5%) 495
Neurontin Capsules (1.5%) 1922
▲ Nicoderm (nicotine transdermal system) (3% to 9%) 1518
▲ Nicorette (3% to 9% of patients) .. 2458
Nicotrol Nicotine Transdermal System (B 3% to 9%) 1550
Norflex 1496
Norgesic 1496
Noroxin Tablets (0.3% to 1.0%) 1715
Noroxin Tablets (0.3% to 1.0%) 2048
▲ Norpace (11%) 2444
Norpramin Tablets 1526
Norvasc Tablets (More than 0.1% to 1%) 1940
Novahistine DH 2462
Novahistine Expectorant 2463
Nucofed 2051
Oncaspar (Less than 1%) 2028
Oncovin Solution Vials & Hyporets 1466
▲ Oramorph SR (Morphine Sulfate Sustained Release Tablets) (Among most frequent) 2236
▲ Orap Tablets (4 of 20 patients) 1050
Oretic Tablets 443
▲ Orlamm (3% to 9%) 2239
Ornade Spansule Capsules 2502
▲ Orudis Capsules (3% to 9%) 2766
▲ Oruvail Capsules (3% to 9%) 2766
PBZ Tablets 845
PBZ-SR Tablets 844
Pamelor 2280
Papaverine Hydrochloride Vials and Ampoules 1468
▲ Paraplatin for Injection (6%) 705
▲ Parlodel (3% to 14%) 2281
Parnate Tablets 2503
▲ Paxil Tablets (4.9% to 13.8%) 2505
Penetrex Tablets (Less than 1% but more than or equal to 0.1%) 2031
Pentasa (Less than 1%) 1527
Pepcid Injection (1.2%) 1722
Pepcid (1.2%) 1720
Percocet Tablets 938
Percodan Tablets 939
Percodan-Demi Tablets 940
Periactin 1724
▲ Permax Tablets (10.6%; frequent) 575
Phenergan with Codeine 2777
Phenergan VC with Codeine 2781
Phenobarbital Elixir and Tablets (Less than 1 in 100 patients) 1469
PhosLo Tablets 690
Phrenilin (Infrequent) 785
Plendil Extended-Release Tablets (0.3% to 1.5%) 527
Pondimin Tablets 2066
Ponstel (Less frequent) 1925
▲ Pravachol (2.4% to 4.0%) 765
Prelu-2 Timed Release Capsules 681
PREVACID Delayed-Release Capsules (Less than 1%) 2562
Prilosec Delayed-Release Capsules (1.1% to 1.5%) 529
Prinivil Tablets (0.3 to 1.0%) 1733
Prinzide Tablets (0.3% to 1%) 1737
Pro-Banthine Tablets 2052
Procardia Capsules (2% or less) 1971
▲ Procardia XL Extended Release Tablets (3.3%) 1972
▲ Prograf (19% to 24%) 1042
▲ Proleukin for Injection (5%) 797
Prolixin 509
▲ Propulsid (6.7%) 1300
ProSom Tablets (Frequent) 449
Prostep (nicotine transdermal system) (1% to 3% of patients) .. 1394
Protostat Tablets 1883
▲ Prozac Pulvules & Liquid, Oral Solution (4.5%) 919
▲ Quarzan Capsules (Among most frequent) 2181
▲ Questran Light (Most common) 769
▲ Questran Powder (Most common) .. 770
RMS Suppositories 2657
Recombivax HB 1744
▲ Relafen Tablets (3% to 9%) 2510
ReoPro Vials (0.3%) 1471
▲ Retrovir Capsules (6.4%) 1158
▲ Retrovir I.V. Infusion (6.4%) 1163
▲ Retrovir Syrup (6.4%) 1158
▲ ReVia Tablets (Less than 10%) 940
Ridaura Capsules (1 to 3%) 2513
▲ Risperdal (7% to 13%) 1301
Robaxisal Tablets 2071
Robinul Forte Tablets 2072
Robinul Injectable 2072
Robinul Tablets 2072
Robitussin A-C Syrup 2073
Robitussin-DAC Syrup 2074
Rocaltrol Capsules 2141
Roferon-A Injection (Less than 3%) 2145
Rowasa (0.98%) 2548
Roxanol 2243
Roxicodone Tablets, Oral Solution & Intensol (Oxycodone) 2244
Ryna .... ▣ 841
▲ Rythmol Tablets–150mg, 225mg, 300mg (2.0 to 7.2%) 1352
Sandimmune (Rare) 2286

(▣ Described in PDR For Nonprescription Drugs) Incidence data in parenthesis; ▲ 3% or more (⊙ Described in PDR For Ophthalmology)

1257 Side Effects Index Convulsions

▲ Sandostatin Injection (Less than 10%) 2292
▲ Sanorex Tablets (Among most common) 2294
Sansert Tablets 2295
Seconal Sodium Pulvules (Less than 1 in 100) 1474
▲ Sectral Capsules (4%) 2807
Sedapap Tablets 50 mg/650 mg (Infrequent) 1543
Ser-Ap-Es Tablets 849
Serentil 684
▲ Serzone Tablets (10% to 17%) 771
Sinemet Tablets 943
Sinemet CR Tablets (0.2%) 944
Sinequan 2205
Sodium Polystyrene Sulfonate Suspension 2244
Soma Compound w/Codeine Tablets 2676
▲ Soma Compound Tablets (Among most common) 2675
▲ Stadol (3% to 9%) 775
Stelazine 2514
Supprelin Injection (1% to 3%) 2056
Surmontil Capsules 2811
Symmetrel Capsules and Syrup (1% to 5%) 946
Talacen (Infrequent) 2333
Talwin Injection (Infrequent) 2334
Talwin Compound (Infrequent) 2335
Talwin Injection (Infrequent) 2334
Talwin Nx 2336
▲ Tambocor Tablets (4.4%) 1497
Tavist Syrup 2297
Tavist Tablets 2298
Tegison Capsules (Less than 1%) 2154
Tegretol Chewable Tablets 852
Tegretol Suspension 852
Tegretol Tablets 852
Temaril Tablets, Syrup and Spansule Extended-Release Capsules 483
▲ Tenex Tablets (Up to 16%) 2074
Tenoretic Tablets 2845
Tessalon Perles 1020
Thalitone 1245
TheraCys BCG Live (Intravesical) (Up to 0.9%) 897
Thorazine 2523
Timolide Tablets (Less than 1%) 1748
Tofranil Ampuls 854
Tofranil Tablets 856
Tofranil-PM Capsules 857
Tolectin (200, 400 and 600 mg) (1 to 3%) 1581
Tonocard Tablets (Less than 1%) 531
Toprol-XL Tablets (About 1 of 100 patients) 565
Toradol (Greater than 1%) 2159
Trental Tablets (Less than 1%) 1244
Triavil Tablets 1757
Trilafon (Occasional) 2389
▲ Trilisate (Less than 20%) 2000
Trinalin Repetabs Tablets 1330
Trinsicon Capsules (Rare) 2570
Tussend 1783
Tussend Expectorant 1785
Tussionex Pennkinetic Extended-Release Suspension 998
Tussi-Organidin NR Liquid and S NR Liquid 2677
Tylenol with Codeine 1583
Tylox Capsules 1584
▲ Ultram Tablets (50 mg) (24% to 46%) 1585
Univasc Tablets (Less than 1%) 2410
Valium Injectable 2182
Valium Tablets (Infrequent) 2183
Valrelease Capsules (Occasional) 2169
Valtrex Caplets (1% to 5%) 1194
Varivax (Greater than or equal to 1%) 1762
Vascor (200, 300 and 400 mg) Tablets (0.5 to 2.84%) 1587
Vaseretic Tablets (0.5% to 2.0%) 1765
Vasotec I.V. (0.5 to 1%) 1768
Vasotec Tablets (0.5% to 1.0%) 1771
▲ Velban Vials (Among most common) 1484
VePesid Capsules and Injection (Infrequent) 718
▲ Verelan Capsules (7.3% to 7.4%) 1410
▲ Verelan Capsules (7.3% to 7.4%) 2824
Vicodin Tablets 1356
Vicodin ES Tablets 1357
▲ Videx Tablets, Powder for Oral Solution, & Pediatric Powder for Oral Solution (Less than 1% to 12%) 720
Vivactil Tablets 1774
▲ Voltaren Tablets (3% to 9%) 861
▲ Wellbutrin Tablets (26.0%) 1204
Wygesic Tablets 2827
▲ Xanax Tablets (10.4% to 26.2%) 2649
Yutopar Intravenous Injection (Infrequent) 570
Zantac 1209
Zantac Injection 1207
Zantac Syrup 1209
Zaroxolyn Tablets 1000
Zebeta Tablets 1413
▲ Zerit Capsules (Fewer than 1% to 7%) 729
Zestoretic (0.3 to 1%) 2850
Zestril Tablets (0.3% to 1.0%) 2854
Ziac 1415
Zocor Tablets (2.3%) 1775
▲ Zofran Injection (11%) 1214
▲ Zofran Tablets (6% to 9%) 1217
▲ Zoladex (Greater than 1% but less than 5%) 2858
▲ Zoloft Tablets (8.4%) 2217
▲ Zosyn (7.7%) 1419
▲ Zosyn Pharmacy Bulk Package (7.7%) 1422
Zovirax (0.9%) 1219
Zydone Capsules 949

Constriction, pupillary (see under Miosis)

Constriction, pupils (see under Miosis)

Contact lenses, intolerance

Accutane Capsules 2076
Brevicon 2088
Climara Transdermal System 645
▲ Demulen (Among most common) 2428
Desogen Tablets 1817
Diethylstilbestrol Tablets 1437
Estrace Cream and Tablets 749
Estraderm Transdermal System 824
ESTRATAB Tablets (0.3, 0.625, 1.25, 2.5 mg) 2536
Estratest 2539
Levlen/Tri-Levlen 651
Lo/Ovral Tablets 2746
Lo/Ovral-28 Tablets 2751
Menest Tablets 2494
Micronor Tablets 1872
Modicon 1872
Nordette-21 Tablets 2755
Nordette-28 Tablets 2758
Norinyl 2088
Nor-Q D Tablets 2135
Ogen Tablets 2627
Ogen Vaginal Cream 2630
Ortho-Cept 1851
Ortho-Cyclen/Ortho-Tri-Cyclen 1858
Ortho Dienestrol Cream 1866
Ortho-Est 1869
Ortho-Novum 1872
Ortho-Cyclen/Ortho Tri-Cyclen 1858
Ovcon 760
Ovral Tablets 2770
Ovral-28 Tablets 2770
Ovrette Tablets 2771
PMB 200 and PMB 400 2783
Premarin Intravenous 2787
Premarin with Methyltestosterone 2794
Premarin Tablets 2789
Premarin Vaginal Cream 2791
Premphase 2797
Prempro 2801
Stilphostrol Tablets and Ampuls 612
Levlen/Tri-Levlen 651
Tri-Norinyl 2164

Contact lens staining

Prodium 690
Pyridium 1928
Rifadin 1528
Rifater 1532

Convulsions

ActHIB (2 definite; 3 possible) 872
Actifed with Codeine Cough Syrup 1067
AK-Fluor Injection 10% and 25% ⊙ 203
Aldoclor Tablets 1598
Aldoril Tablets 1604
Altace Capsules (Less than 1%) 1232
Ambien Tablets 2416
Amicar Syrup, Tablets, and Injection (Two cases) 1267
Anafranil Capsules (Infrequent) 803
Ana-Kit Anaphylaxis Emergency Treatment Kit (Occasional) 617
Ansaid Tablets (Less than 1%) 2579
Antilirium Injectable 1009
Aralen Hydrochloride Injection 2301
Aristocort Suspension (Forte Parenteral) 1027
Aristocort Suspension (Intralesional) 1025
Aristocort Tablets 1022
Aristospan Suspension (Intra-articular) 1033
Aristospan Suspension (Intralesional) 1032
Astramorph/PF Injection, USP (Preservative-Free) 535
Atamet 572
Atarax Tablets & Syrup (Rare) 2185
Attenuvax (Rare) 1610
Azo Gantanol Tablets 2080
Azo Gantrisin Tablets 2081
Azulfidine (Rare) 1949
Bactrim DS Tablets 2084
Bactrim I.V. Infusion 2082
Bactrim 2084
Benadryl Capsules 1898
Benadryl Injection 1898
Betaseron for SC Injection (2%) 658
Biavax II (Rare) 1613
Brevibloc Injection (Less than 1%) 1808
Brevital Sodium Vials 1429
▲ Bromfed-DM Cough Syrup (Among most frequent) 1786
Brontex 1981
Buprenex Injectable (Rare) 2006
Carbocaine Hydrochloride Injection 2303
Cataflam (Less than 1%) 816
Cefotan 2829
Ceftin for Oral Suspension 1078
Celestone Soluspan Suspension 2347
Chibroxin Sterile Ophthalmic Solution (With oral form) 1617
Cipro I.V. Pharmacy Bulk Package (Less than 1%) 597
Cipro Tablets 592
Claritin (2% or fewer patients) 2349
Claritin-D 2350
Clinoril Tablets (Less than 1%) 1618
▲ Clozaril Tablets (3%) 2252
Cognex Capsules (Frequent) 1901
Comhist 2038
Compazine 2470
CORTENEMA 2535
Cortone Acetate Sterile Suspension 1623
Cortone Acetate Tablets 1624
Cytovene (1% or less) 2103
D.A. Chewable Tablets 951
Dalalone D.P. Injectable 1011
Danocrine Capsules (Rare) 2307
Decadron Elixir 1633
Decadron Phosphate Injection 1637
Decadron Phosphate Respihaler 1642
Decadron Phosphate Turbinaire 1645
Decadron Phosphate with Xylocaine Injection, Sterile 1639
Decadron Tablets 1635
Decadron-LA Sterile Suspension 1646
Deconamine Chewable Tablets 1320
Deconamine CX Cough and Cold Liquid and Tablets 1319
Deconamine 1320
Deconsal 454
Deltasone Tablets 2595
Demerol 2308
Depo-Medrol Single-Dose Vial 2600
Depo-Medrol Sterile Aqueous Suspension 2597
Depo-Provera Contraceptive Injection (A few cases; fewer than 1%) 2602
Dexacort Phosphate in Respihaler 458
Dexacort Phosphate in Turbinaire 459
Dexatrim ▣ 832
Dexatrim Plus Vitamins Caplets ▣ 832
Diamox Intravenous (Occasional) 1372
Diamox Sequels (Sustained Release) 1373
Diamox Tablets (Occasional) 1372
Dimetane-DC Cough Syrup 2059
Dimetane-DX Cough Syrup 2059
Diphtheria and Tetanus Toxoids and Pertussis Vaccine Adsorbed (Infrequent) 2477
Diphtheria and Tetanus Toxoids and Pertussis Vaccine Adsorbed USP (For Pediatric Use) (Infrequent; rare; 1 in 1,750 doses) 875
Diprivan Injection (Rare) 2833
Diupres Tablets 1650
Diuril Oral Suspension 1653
Diuril Sodium Intravenous 1652
Diuril Tablets 1653
Dopram Injectable 2061
Duramorph (May accompany high doses) 962
Duranest Injections 542
Dura-Tap/PD Capsules 2867
Dura-Vent/DA Tablets 953
Dura-Vent Tablets 952
Dyclone 0.5% and 1% Topical Solutions, USP 544
Effexor (0.26%) 2719
Emla Cream 545
Entex PSE Tablets 1987
Ergamisol Tablets (Less frequent) 1292
Esgic-plus Tablets (Infrequent) 1013
Fansidar Tablets 2114
Fedahist Gyrocaps 2401
Fedahist Timecaps 2401
Fioricet Tablets (Infrequent) 2258
Flexeril Tablets (Less than 1%) 1661
Florinef Acetate Tablets 505
Floxin Tablets (200 mg, 300 mg, 400 mg) 1567
Flumadine Tablets & Syrup (Less than 0.3%) 1015
Fluorescite ⊙ 219
Fungizone Intravenous 506
Gantanol Tablets 2119
Gantrisin 2120
Garamycin Injectable 2360
Glauctabs (Occasional) ⊙ 208
Guaimax-D Tablets 792
Havrix (Rare) 2489
HibTITER 1375
Hismanal Tablets (Isolated cases) 1293
Hydeltrasol Injection, Sterile 1665
Hydeltra-T.B.A. Sterile Suspension 1667
Hydrea Capsules (Extremely rare) 696
Hydrocortone Acetate Sterile Suspension 1669
Hydrocortone Phosphate Injection, Sterile 1670
Hydrocortone Tablets 1672
HydroDIURIL Tablets 1674
Hydropres Tablets 1675
Hyperstat I.V. Injection 2363
Hyskon Hysteroscopy Fluid (Rare) 1595
Imitrex Injection (Rare) 1103
Imitrex Tablets (Rare) 1106
Indocin Capsules (Less than 1%) 1680
Indocin I.V. (Less than 1%) 1684
Indocin (Less than 1%) 1680
INFeD (Iron Dextran Injection, USP) 2345
Infumorph 200 and Infumorph 500 Sterile Solutions 965
Intron A (Less than 5%) 2364
Inversine Tablets 1686
Kefzol Vials, Faspak & ADD-Vantage 1456
Kwell Cream & Lotion 2008
Kwell Shampoo (Exceedingly rare cases) 2009
▲ Lamictal Tablets (3.2%) 1112
Larodopa Tablets (Rare) 2129
Lindane Lotion USP 1% 582
Lindane Shampoo USP 1% 583
Lioresal Intrathecal (1 to 11 of 214 patients) 1596
Lopid Tablets 1917
Lufyllin-GG Elixir & Tablets 2671
Luvox Tablets (Infrequent) 2544
M-M-R II (Rare) 1687
M-R-VAX II (Rare) 1689
MZM (Occasional) ⊙ 267
Marcaine Hydrochloride with Epinephrine 1:200,000 2316
Marcaine Hydrochloride Injection 2316
Marcaine Spinal 2319
Matulane Capsules 2131
Maxaquin Tablets (Less than 1%) 2440
Medrol 2621
Megace Oral Suspension (1% to 3%) 699
Methotrexate Sodium Tablets, Injection, for Injection and LPF Injection 1275
Mexitil Capsules (About 2 in 1,000) 678
Mintezol 1704
Motrin Ibuprofen Suspension, Oral Drops, Chewable Tablets, Caplets (Less than 1%) 1546
Mycobutin Capsules (More than one patient) 1957
Nardil (Less frequent) 1920
Nebcin Vials, Hyporets & ADD-Vantage 1464
NegGram (Rare) 2323
Neoral (1% to 5%) 2276
Neptazane Tablets 1388
Nescaine/Nescaine MPF 554
Netromycin Injection 100 mg/ml 2373

(▣ Described in PDR For Nonprescription Drugs) Incidence data in parenthesis; ▲ 3% or more (⊙ Described in PDR For Ophthalmology)

Neurontin Capsules (More than 1%) 1922
Neutrexin (Rare; less than 1%) 2572
Nicorette 2458
Noroxin Tablets 1715
Noroxin Tablets 2048
Novahistine DH 2462
Novahistine DMX ▣ 822
Novahistine Elixir ▣ 823
Novahistine Expectorant 2463
Novocain Hydrochloride for Spinal Anesthesia 2326
Nydrazid Injection (Uncommon) 508
OmniHIB (Two definite and 3 possible out of 5,000 infants) 2499
▲ Oncaspar (Greater than 1% but less than 5%) 2028
Oncovin Solution Vials & Hyporets (A few patients) 1466
Ornade Spansule Capsules 2502
Oxytocin Injection 2771
PBZ Tablets 845
PBZ-SR Tablets 844
Paxil Tablets (0.1%; infrequent) 2505
Pediapred Oral Liquid 995
Penetrex Tablets (Less than 1% but more than or equal to 0.1%) 2031
Periactin 1724
Permax Tablets (Infrequent) 575
Pfizerpen for Injection 2203
Phenergan with Codeine 2777
Phenergan VC with Codeine 2781
Phrenilin (Infrequent) 785
Placidyl Capsules 448
Plaquenil Sulfate Tablets 2328
Pontocaine Hydrochloride for Spinal Anesthesia 2330
Prelone Syrup 1787
▲ Prograf (Greater than 3%) 1042
Propulsid (Rare) 1300
Prostigmin Injectable 1260
Prostigmin Tablets 1261
Prozac Pulvules & Liquid, Oral Solution (Infrequent) 919
Quinaglute Dura-Tabs Tablets 649
Rifamate Capsules (Uncommon) 1530
Rifater (Uncommon) 1532
Romazicon 2147
Rondec Oral Drops 953
Rondec Syrup 953
Rondec Tablet 953
Rondec-DM Oral Drops 954
Rondec-DM Syrup 954
Rondec-TR Tablet 953
Sandimmune (1 to 5%) 2286
Sandostatin Injection (Less than 1%) 2292
Sedapap Tablets 50 mg/650 mg (Infrequent) 1543
Seldane-D Extended-Release Tablets 1538
Sensorcaine (0.1%) 559
Septra 1174
Septra I.V. Infusion 1169
Septra I.V. Infusion ADD-Vantage Vials 1171
Septra 1174
Seromycin Pulvules 1476
Sinemet Tablets 943
Sinemet CR Tablets 944
Slo-bid Gyrocaps 2033
Solu-Cortef Sterile Powder 2641
Solu-Medrol Sterile Powder 2643
Stadol (Less than 1%) 775
Stelazine 2514
Supprelin Injection (2%) 2056
Symmetrel Capsules and Syrup (Less than 0.1%) 946
Syn-Rx Tablets 465
Syn-Rx DM Tablets 466
Tambocor Tablets (Less than 1%) 1497
Tavist Syrup 2297
Tavist Tablets 2298
Tazicef for Injection 2519
Tensilon Injectable 1261
Tetramune (One child) 1404
THYREL TRH (Rare) 2873
Ticar for Injection (With very high doses) 2526
Tigan 2057
Timolide Tablets 1748
Tofranil Ampuls 854
Tofranil Tablets 856
Tonocard Tablets (Less than 1%) 531
Toradol 2159
Torecan 2245
Tracrium Injection (Rare) 1183
Trental Tablets (Less than 1%) 1244
Tri-Immunol Adsorbed (1 per 1,750) 1408
Trinalin Repetabs Tablets 1330
Tussend 1783
Tussend Expectorant 1785
Urecholine 1761
Vantin for Oral Suspension and Vantin Tablets 2646
Velban Vials 1484
Vermox Chewable Tablets (Very rare) 1312
Videx Tablets, Powder for Oral Solution, & Pediatric Powder for Oral Solution (Up to 4%) 720
Virazole 1264
Vistaril Capsules (Rare) 1944
Vistaril Intramuscular Solution (Rare) 2216
Vistaril Oral Suspension (Rare) 1944
Voltaren Tablets (Less than 1%) 861
▲ Xylocaine Injections (Among most common) 567
Zefazone I.V. Solution 2654
Zestoretic 2850
Zoloft Tablets (Rare) 2217
Zosyn (1.0% or less) 1419
Zosyn Pharmacy Bulk Package (1.0% or less) 1422
Zovirax Sterile Powder 1223

Convulsions, clonic

Cocaine Hydrochloride Topical Solution 537
Lufyllin & Lufyllin-400 Tablets 2670
Lufyllin-GG Elixir & Tablets 2671
M-M-R II (Rare) 1687
Quadrinal Tablets 1350
Quibron 2053
Respbid Tablets 682
Seromycin Pulvules 1476
Slo-bid Gyrocaps 2033
Theo-24 Extended Release Capsules 2568
Theo-Dur Extended-Release Tablets 1327
Theo-X Extended-Release Tablets 788
Uni-Dur Extended-Release Tablets 1331
Uniphyl 400 mg Tablets 2001

Convulsions, grand mal

Compazine 2470
Lamictal Tablets (Rare) 1112
Levoprome 1274
Paxil Tablets (Rare) 2505
Stelazine 2514
Triavil Tablets 1757
Videx Tablets, Powder for Oral Solution, & Pediatric Powder for Oral Solution (Less than 1%) 720

Convulsions, major

Methotrexate Sodium Tablets, Injection, for Injection and LPF Injection (Occasional) 1275
Seromycin Pulvules 1476

Convulsions, tonic generalized

Cocaine Hydrochloride Topical Solution 537
Lufyllin & Lufyllin-400 Tablets 2670
Lufyllin-GG Elixir & Tablets 2671
Quadrinal Tablets 1350
Quibron 2053
Respbid Tablets 682
Slo-bid Gyrocaps 2033
Theo-24 Extended Release Capsules 2568
Theo-Dur Extended-Release Tablets 1327
Theo-X Extended-Release Tablets 788
Uni-Dur Extended-Release Tablets 1331
Uniphyl 400 mg Tablets 2001

Coombs' test, positive

Adalat CC 589
Children's Advil Suspension (Less than 1%) 2692
Aldoclor Tablets 1598
Aldomet Ester HCl Injection 1602
Aldomet Oral 1600
Aldoril Tablets 1604
Atamet 572
Azactam for Injection 734
Catapres Tablets 674
Catapres-TTS 675
Ceclor Pulvules & Suspension (Less than 1 in 200) 1431
Cefizox for Intramuscular or Intravenous Use (Some patients) 1034
Cefobid Intravenous/Intramuscular (1 in 60) 2189
Cefobid Pharmacy Bulk Package - Not for Direct Infusion (1 in 60) 2192
Cefotan (1 in 250) 2829
Ceftin (Less than 1% but more than 0.1%) 1078
Cefzil Tablets and Oral Suspension 746
Ceptaz (One in 23) 1081
Claforan Sterile and Injection (Less than 1%) 1235
Combipres Tablets 677
Duricef 748
▲ Fortaz (1 in 23) 1100
IBU Tablets (Sometimes) 1342
Keflex Pulvules & Oral Suspension 914
Kefurox Vials, Faspak & ADD-Vantage (Less than 1 in 250) 1454
Kefzol Vials, Faspak & ADD-Vantage 1456
Larodopa Tablets 2129
Lorabid Suspension and Pulvules 1459
Mandol Vials, Faspak & ADD-Vantage 1461
Mefoxin 1691
Mefoxin Premixed Intravenous Solution 1694
Mezlin 601
Mezlin Pharmacy Bulk Package 604
Monocid Injection (Less than 1%) 2497
Children's Motrin Ibuprofen Oral Suspension (Less than 1%) 1546
Motrin Tablets (Less than 1%) 2625
Motrin Ibuprofen Suspension, Oral Drops, Chewable Tablets, Caplets (Sometimes) 1546
PASER Granules 1285
Pipracil (Less frequent) 1390
Platinol 708
Platinol-AQ Injection 710
Ponstel 1925
Primaxin I.M. 1727
Primaxin I.V. 1729
Procardia Capsules 1971
Procardia XL Extended Release Tablets 1972
Sinemet Tablets 943
Sinemet CR Tablets 944
Suprax 1399
▲ Tazicef for Injection (1 in 23 patients) 2519
▲ Tazidime Vials, Faspak & ADD-Vantage (1 in 23) 1478
Unasyn (Some individuals) 2212
Vantin for Oral Suspension and Vantin Tablets 2646
Zefazone 2654
Zinacef (Fewer than 1 in 250 patients) 1211
Zosyn 1419
Zosyn Pharmacy Bulk Package 1422

Coordination, disturbed (see under Coordination, impaired)

Coordination, impaired

▲ Actifed with Codeine Cough Syrup (Among most frequent) 1067
Anafranil Capsules (Infrequent) 803
Atretol Tablets 573
Atrovent Inhalation Aerosol (Less frequent) 671
▲ Benadryl Capsules (Among most frequent) 1898
▲ Benadryl Injection (Among most frequent) 1898
Cataflam (Rare) 816
Clozaril Tablets (Less than 1%) 2252
▲ Cordarone Tablets (4 to 9%) 2712
Deconamine 1320
Dilantin Infatabs 1908
▲ Dilantin Kapseals (Among most common) 1906
▲ Dilantin Parenteral (Among most common) 1910
Dilantin-125 Suspension 1911
Dimetane-DX Cough Syrup 2059
Duragesic Transdermal System (1% or greater) 1288
Ethmozine Tablets (Less than 2%) 2041
Foscavir Injection (Between 1% and 5%) 547
▲ Halcion Tablets (4.6%) 2611
Hivid Tablets (Less than 1% to less than 3%) 2121
Intron A (Less than 5%) 2364
Iopidine 0.5% (Less than 1%) ⊙ 221
Ismo Tablets (Fewer than 1%) 2738
Lioresal Intrathecal 1596
Lioresal Tablets 829
Lithium Carbonate Capsules & Tablets 2230
Marinol (Dronabinol) Capsules 2231
▲ Mexitil Capsules (9.4% to 10.2%) 678
Neurontin Capsules (1.1%) 1922
Ornade Spansule Capsules 2502
▲ PBZ Tablets (Among most frequent) 845
▲ PBZ-SR Tablets (Among most frequent) 844
Pamelor 2280
Periactin 1724
▲ ProSom Tablets (4%) 449
Roferon-A Injection (Less than 0.5%) 2145
▲ Tavist Syrup (Among most frequent) 2297
▲ Tavist Tablets (Among most frequent) 2298
Tegretol Chewable Tablets 852
Tegretol Suspension 852
Tegretol Tablets 852
Tofranil Ampuls 854
Tofranil Tablets 856
Tofranil-PM Capsules 857
Tonocard Tablets (0.0-1.2%) 531
Triavil Tablets 1757
▲ Trinalin Repetabs Tablets (Among most frequent) 1330
Ultram Tablets (50 mg) (1% to 5%) 1585
Voltaren Tablets (Rare) 861
▲ Xanax Tablets (40.1%) 2649
Zoloft Tablets (Infrequent) 2217

Coordination, lack of (see under Ataxia)

Coordination difficulty (see under Coordination, impaired)

Cor pulmonale

Pulmozyme Inhalation 1064

Cornea, discoloration

Mellaril 2269
Serentil 684
Torecan 2245

Cornea, fungal infections

AK-CIDE ⊙ 202
AK-CIDE Ointment ⊙ 202
AK-Pred ⊙ 204
AK-Trol Ointment & Suspension ⊙ 205
Blephamide Ointment ⊙ 237
NeoDecadron Sterile Ophthalmic Ointment 1712
NeoDecadron Sterile Ophthalmic Solution 1713
Polysporin Ophthalmic Ointment Sterile 1154
Pred Mild ⊙ 253
Pred-G Liquifilm Sterile Ophthalmic Suspension ⊙ 251
Terra-Cortril Ophthalmic Suspension 2210
TobraDex Ophthalmic Suspension and Ointment 473

Cornea, gray, ground-glass appearance

Fluoracaine ⊙ 206
FLURESS (Rare) ⊙ 207
Ophthetic ⊙ 247

Cornea, opacities

▲ Accutane Capsules (5 of 72 patients) 2076
Ansaid Tablets (Less than 1%) 2579
Fluoracaine ⊙ 206
Imitrex Tablets 1106
Mellaril 2269
Plaquenil Sulfate Tablets 2328
Serentil 684
Symmetrel Capsules and Syrup (0.1% to 1%) 946
Temaril Tablets, Syrup and Spansule Extended-Release Capsules 483
Torecan 2245

Cornea, white crystalline precipitates, presence of

▲ Ciloxan Ophthalmic Solution (Approximately 17%) 472

Corneal abrasion

Alomide (Less than 1%) 469
Ocusert Pilo-20 and Pilo-40 Ocular Therapeutic Systems ⊙ 254

Corneal changes

Alomide (Less than 1%) 469
Aralen Phosphate Tablets 2301

(▣ Described in PDR For Nonprescription Drugs) Incidence data in parenthesis; ▲ 3% or more (⊙ Described in PDR For Ophthalmology)

1259 Side Effects Index Cough

Azulfidine (Rare) 1949
Cocaine Hydrochloride Topical Solution 537
Efudex (Infrequent) 2113
Neurontin Capsules (Rare) 1922
Nolvadex Tablets 2841
Plaquenil Sulfate Tablets 2328
Prozac Pulvules & Liquid, Oral Solution (Rare) 919
▲ Tegison Capsules (10-25%) 2154

Corneal clouding

BSS PLUS (500 mL) Sterile Irrigation Solution ◉ 215
▲ CHEMET (succimer) Capsules (1.0 to 3.7%) 1545
Cocaine Hydrochloride Topical Solution 537
Herplex Liquifilm (Occasional) ◉ 244
Miochol-E with Iocare Steri-Tags and Miochol-E System Pak (Infrequent) ◉ 273
MIOSTAT Intraocular Solution (Occasional) ◉ 224

Corneal curvature, steepening

Brevicon 2088
Climara Transdermal System 645
Demulen 2428
Desogen Tablets 1817
Diethylstilbestrol Tablets 1437
Estrace Cream and Tablets 749
Estraderm Transdermal System 824
ESTRATAB Tablets (0.3, 0.625, 1.25, 2.5 mg) 2536
Estratest 2539
Levlen/Tri-Levlen 651
Lo/Ovral Tablets 2746
Lo/Ovral-28 Tablets 2751
Menest Tablets 2494
Micronor Tablets 1872
Modicon 1872
Nordette-21 Tablets 2755
Nordette-28 Tablets 2758
Norinyl 2088
Nor-Q D Tablets 2135
Ogen Tablets 2627
Ogen Vaginal Cream 2630
Ortho-Cept 1851
Ortho-Cyclen/Ortho-Tri-Cyclen 1858
Ortho Dienestrol Cream 1866
Ortho-Est 1869
Ortho-Novum 1872
Ortho-Cyclen/Ortho Tri-Cyclen 1858
Ovcon 760
Ovral Tablets 2770
Ovral-28 Tablets 2770
Ovrette Tablets 2771
PMB 200 and PMB 400 2783
Premarin Intravenous 2787
Premarin with Methyltestosterone 2794
Premarin Tablets 2789
Premarin Vaginal Cream 2791
Premphase 2797
Prempro 2801
Stilphostrol Tablets and Ampuls 612
Levlen/Tri-Levlen 651
Tri-Norinyl 2164
Triphasil-21 Tablets 2814
Triphasil-28 Tablets 2819

Corneal decompensation

AMVISC Plus ◉ 329
BSS (15 mL & 30 mL) Sterile Irrigation Solution ◉ 214
BSS (250 mL) Sterile Irrigation Solution ◉ 214
BSS (500 mL) Sterile Irrigation Solution ◉ 214
BSS PLUS (500 mL) Sterile Irrigation Solution ◉ 215
Cytovene-IV (One report) 2103
Healon (Rare) ◉ 314
Healon GV ◉ 315
Miochol-E with Iocare Steri-Tags and Miochol-E System Pak (Infrequent) ◉ 273
Ocucoat ◉ 321

Corneal deposits

Compazine 2470
Cordarone Tablets 2712
EPIFRIN ◉ 239
Etrafon 2355
Indocin (Less than 1%) 1680
Levoprome 1274
Plaquenil Sulfate Tablets 2328
Prolixin 509
PROPINE with C CAP Compliance Cap ◉ 253
Ridaura Capsules (Less than 1%) 2513
Solganal Suspension 2388
Stelazine 2514
Thorazine 2523
Trilafon 2389

Corneal infiltrate

Ciloxan Ophthalmic Solution (Less than 1%) 472
Iopidine 0.5% (Less than 3%) ◉ 221
Vexol 1% Ophthalmic Suspension (Less than 1%) ◉ 230

Corneal pitting

Cocaine Hydrochloride Topical Solution 537

Corneal punctate, defects

Herplex Liquifilm (Occasional) ◉ 244
Symmetrel Capsules and Syrup (0.1% to 1%) 946

Corneal punctate keratitis

Betoptic Ophthalmic Solution (Rare) 469
Betoptic S Ophthalmic Suspension (Small number of patients) 471

Corneal punctate staining

Betoptic Ophthalmic Solution (Rare) 469
Ophthocort ◉ 311

Corneal sensitivity, decrease

Betagan (A small number of patients) ◉ 233
Betimol 0.25%, 0.5% ◉ 261
Betoptic Ophthalmic Solution (Rare) 469
Betoptic S Ophthalmic Suspension 471
Plaquenil Sulfate Tablets 2328
Timoptic in Ocudose (Less frequent) 1753
Timoptic Sterile Ophthalmic Solution (Less frequent) 1751
Timoptic-XE 1755

Corneal sensitivity, unspecified

Ocupress Ophthalmic Solution, 1% Sterile (Occasional) ◉ 309

Corneal staining

Betimol 0.25%, 0.5% (1% to 5%) ◉ 261
Ciloxan Ophthalmic Solution (Less than 1%) 472
Iopidine 0.5% (Less than 3%) ◉ 221
Ocupress Ophthalmic Solution, 1% Sterile (Occasional) ◉ 309
Paremyd ◉ 247
Vexol 1% Ophthalmic Suspension (Less than 1%) ◉ 230

Corneal stippling

Herplex Liquifilm (Occasional) ◉ 244

Corneal toxicity

Cytosar-U Sterile Powder (With experimental doses) 2592

Corneal ulceration

Alomide (Less than 1%) 469
Ambien Tablets (Rare) 2416
BOTOX (Botulinum Toxin Type A) Purified Neurotoxin Complex 477
Cocaine Hydrochloride Topical Solution 537
Econopred & Econopred Plus Ophthalmic Suspensions (Occasional) ◉ 217
Gentak ◉ 208
Paxil Tablets (Rare) 2505
Vexol 1% Ophthalmic Suspension (Less than 1%) ◉ 230

Coronary artery disease, aggravation

Atretol Tablets 573
Oncovin Solution Vials & Hyporets 1466
Tegretol Chewable Tablets 852
Tegretol Suspension 852
Tegretol Tablets 852
Tenoretic Tablets 2845
Vasotec I.V. (One case) 1768

Coronary artery disease, unspecified

Luvox Tablets (Rare) 2544

Coronary thrombosis

Demulen 2428
Lo/Ovral Tablets 2746
Lo/Ovral-28 Tablets 2751
Micronor Tablets 1872
Modicon 1872
Nordette-21 Tablets 2755
Nordette-28 Tablets 2758
Ortho-Novum 1872
Ovral Tablets 2770
Ovral-28 Tablets 2770
Ovrette Tablets 2771
Stilphostrol Tablets and Ampuls 612
Triphasil-21 Tablets 2814
Triphasil-28 Tablets 2819

Cortical lens opacities, scattered punctate

Atretol Tablets 573
Tegretol Chewable Tablets 852
Tegretol Suspension 852
Tegretol Tablets 852

Cortical proliferation of long bones

Aquasol A Vitamin A Capsules, USP 534
Prostin VR Pediatric Sterile Solution 2635

Coryza

Quadrinal Tablets 1350

Costovertebral pain

Benemid Tablets 1611
ColBENEMID Tablets 1622

Cough

▲ Accupril Tablets (2.0% to 4.3%) 1893
▲ ActHIB (4.3% to 9.6%) 872
Actigall Capsules 802
▲ Adalat Capsules (10 mg and 20 mg) (6%) 587
Adalat CC (Less than 1.0%) 589
Adenoscan (Less than 1%) 1024
▲ AeroBid Inhaler System (3-9%) 1005
▲ Aerobid-M Inhaler System (3-9%) 1005
▲ Airet Solution for Inhalation (3.1% to 4%) 452
Alkeran for Injection 1070
Alkeran Tablets 1071
▲ Altace Capsules (7.6%) 1232
Alupent (1% to 4%) 669
Ambien Tablets (Infrequent) 2416
▲ Anafranil Capsules (4% to 6%) 803
Antivenin (Crotalidae) Polyvalent 2696
Asacol Delayed-Release Tablets (1% to 2%) 1979
Atgam Sterile Solution (Less than 5%) 2581
▲ Atrovent Inhalation Aerosol (5.9%) 671
▲ Atrovent Inhalation Solution (4.6%) 673
Axid Pulvules (2.0%) 1427
Azmacort Oral Inhaler 2011
Azo Gantrisin Tablets 2081
BCG Vaccine, USP (TICE) 1814
Blocadren Tablets 1614
Capoten (0.5 to 2%) 739
Capozide (0.5 to 2%) 742
Cardura Tablets (Less than 0.5% of 3960 patients) 2186
Cartrol Tablets (Less common) 410
Caverject (1%) 2583
Ceftin for Oral Suspension (Less than 1% but more than 0.1%) 1078
▲ CellCept Capsules (13.3% to 15.5%) 2099
▲ CHEMET (succimer) Capsules (0.7 to 3.7%) 1545
Claritin (2% or fewer patients) 2349
Claritin-D (Less frequent) 2350
Clozaril Tablets (Less than 1%) 2252
▲ Cognex Capsules (3%) 1901
▲ Cordarone Tablets (2% to 7%) 2712
▲ Cozaar Tablets (3.4%) 1628
Cytovene (1% or less) 2103
DDAVP 2017
Decadron Phosphate Respihaler 1642
Demadex Tablets and Injection (2.0%) 686
Depen Titratable Tablets 2662
Desmopressin Acetate Rhinal Tube 979
Dexacort Phosphate in Respihaler 458
▲ Dilacor XR Extended-release Capsules (2.2% to 3.0%) 2018
Diprivan Injection (Less than 1%) 2833
Dizac 1809
Dopram Injectable 2061
DynaCirc Capsules (0.5% to 1%) 2256
Effexor 2719
▲ Epogen for Injection (18%) 489
Ergamisol Tablets (1 out of 463 patients) 1292
Ethmozine Tablets (Less than 2%) 2041
▲ Felbatol (6.5%) 2666
Floxin I.V. (Less than 1%) 1571
Floxin Tablets (200 mg, 300 mg, 400 mg) (Less than 1%) 1567
▲ Fludara for Injection (10% to 44%) 663
Flumadine Tablets & Syrup (Less than 0.3%) 1015
▲ Foscavir Injection (5% or greater) 547
Gantrisin 2120
▲ Habitrol Nicotine Transdermal System (3% to 9% of patients) 865
Hespan Injection 929
Hivid Tablets (Less than 1% to less than 3%) 2121
▲ Hylorel Tablets (26.9%) 985
Hyperstat I.V. Injection 2363
Hyskon Hysteroscopy Fluid (Rare) 1595
Hytrin Capsules (At least 1%) 430
Hyzaar Tablets (2.6%) 1677
Imdur (Less than or equal to 5%) 1323
Imitrex Tablets (Infrequent) 1106
Intal Capsules (Less than 1 in 10,000 patients to 1 in 5 patients) 987
▲ Intal Inhaler (Among most frequent) 988
Intal Nebulizer Solution (Rare; occasional) 989
▲ Intron A (Up to 31%) 2364
Kerlone Tablets (Less than 2%) 2436
▲ Lamictal Tablets (7.5%) 1112
Lescol Capsules (2.6%) 2267
Leukeran Tablets 1133
▲ Leustatin (7% to 10%) 1834
Levatol (2.1%) 2403
Livostin (Approximately 1% to 3%) ◉ 266
▲ Lopid Tablets (More common) 1917
Lotensin Tablets (1.2%) 834
Lotensin HCT (2.1%) 837
▲ Lotrel Capsules (3.3%) 840
Lozol Tablets (Less than 5%) 2022
Lupron Depot 3.75 mg 2556
Lupron Depot 7.5 mg 2559
Lupron Injection (Less than 5%) 2555
Luvox Tablets (Frequent) 2544
Macrobid Capsules (Common) 1988
Macrodantin Capsules (Common) 1989
Marinol (Dronabinol) Capsules (Less than 1%) 2231
Matulane Capsules 2131
Maxair Autohaler (1.2%) 1492
Maxair Inhaler (1.2%) 1494
Maxaquin Tablets (Less than 1%) 2440
Megace Oral Suspension (1% to 3%) 699
Methotrexate Sodium Tablets, Injection, for Injection and LPF Injection (Less common) 1275
Miacalcin Nasal Spray (Less than 1%) 2275
Midamor Tablets (Between 1% and 3%) 1703
Moduretic Tablets 1705
Monoket (Less than 1% to 4%) 2406
▲ Monopril Tablets (2.2% to 9.7%) 757
Mumpsvax 1708
Mykrox Tablets (Less than 2%) 993
Nasalcrom Nasal Solution 994
Nasarel Nasal Solution (Greater than 1%) 2133
▲ NebuPent for Inhalation Solution (38%) 1040
▲ Neupogen for Injection (6%) 495
Neurontin Capsules (1.8%) 1922
▲ Nicoderm (nicotine transdermal system) (3% to 9%) 1518
▲ Nicorette (3% to 9% of patients) 2458
▲ Nolvadex Tablets (3.8%) 2841
Norvasc Tablets (Less than or equal to 0.1%) 1940
▲ Novantrone (9 to 13%) 1279
▲ OmniHIB (4.3% to 9.6%) 2499
Oncaspar (Less than 1%) 2028
OptiPranolol (Metipranolol 0.3%) Sterile Ophthalmic Solution (A small number of patients) ◉ 258
Orlamm (1% to 3%) 2239
Paxil Tablets (Frequent) 2505
Penetrex Tablets (Less than 1% but more than or equal to 0.1%) 2031
Plendil Extended-Release Tablets (0.8% to 1.7%) 527
Pravachol (0.1% to 2.6%) 765
PREVACID Delayed-Release Capsules (Less than 1%) 2562
Prilosec Delayed-Release Capsules (1.1%) 529

(▣ Described in PDR For Nonprescription Drugs) Incidence data in parenthesis; ▲ 3% or more (◉ Described in PDR For Ophthalmology)

Cough Side Effects Index 1260

▲ Prinivil Tablets (1.7% to 6.1%) 1733
▲ Prinzide Tablets (3.9%) 1737
▲ Procardia Capsules (6%) 1971
▲ Procardia XL Extended Release Tablets (1% or less to 6%) 1972
▲ Procrit for Injection (18%) 1841
▲ Prograf (Greater than 3%) 1042
Propulsid (1.5%) 1300
ProSom Tablets (Infrequent) 449
Prostin E2 Suppository 2634
▲ Proventil Inhalation Solution 0.083% (3.1% to 4%) 2384
▲ Proventil Solution for Inhalation 0.5% (3.1% to 4%) 2383
Proventil Syrup (Less than 1 of 100 patients) 2385
Prozac Pulvules & Liquid, Oral Solution (1.6% to 3%) 919
Pulmozyme Inhalation 1064
Quadrinal Tablets 1350
Recombivax HB (Less than 1%) 1744
Relafen Tablets (Less than 1%) 2510
Retrovir Capsules 1158
Retrovir I.V. Infusion 1163
Retrovir Syrup 1158
ReVia Tablets (Less than 1%) 940
▲ Rhinocort Nasal Inhaler (3 to 9%) 556
Rifater 1532
▲ Risperdal (3%) 1301
▲ Roferon-A Injection (27%) 2145
Sectral Capsules (1%) 2807
Seldane Tablets (0.9% to 2.5%) 1536
Seldane-D Extended-Release Tablets (1.6%) 1538
Semprex-D Capsules (2%) 463
Semprex-D Capsules (2%) 1167
Septra (Rare) 1174
Septra I.V. Infusion 1169
Septra I.V. Infusion ADD-Vantage Vials 1171
Septra (Rare) 1174
▲ Serevent Inhalation Aerosol (7%) 1176
▲ Serzone Tablets (3%) 771
Sinemet CR Tablets 944
Stadol (1% or greater) 775
Stimate, (desmopressin acetate) Nasal Spray, 1.5 mg/mL 525
▲ Supprelin Injection (3% to 10%) 2056
▲ Suprane (34% to 72%) 1813
Tegison Capsules (Less than 1%) 2154
TheraCys BCG Live (Intravesical) (Rare) 897
▲ Tilade (7.0%) 996
Timolide Tablets 1748
Timoptic in Ocudose (Less frequent) 1753
Timoptic Sterile Ophthalmic Solution (Less frequent) 1751
Timoptic-XE 1755
Toradol (1% or less) 2159
Tornalate Solution for Inhalation, 0.2% (2.5%) 956
▲ Tornalate Metered Dose Inhaler (4% to 4.1%) 957
▲ Univasc Tablets (6.1%) 2410
Valium Injectable 2182
Vantin for Oral Suspension and Vantin Tablets (Less than 1%) 2646
Varivax (Greater than or equal to 1%) 1762
Vascor (200, 300 and 400 mg) Tablets (0.5 to 2.0%) 1587
▲ Vaseretic Tablets (3.5%) 1765
Vasotec I.V. 1768
Vasotec Tablets (1.3% to 2.2%) 1771
Ventolin Inhalation Aerosol and Refill (2%) 1197
▲ Ventolin Inhalation Solution (3.1% to 4%) 1198
▲ Ventolin Nebules Inhalation Solution (3.1% to 4%) 1199
▲ Ventolin Rotacaps for Inhalation (2% to 5%) 1200
Ventolin Syrup (Less than 1 of 100 patients) 1202
VePesid Capsules and Injection (Sometimes) 718
Versed Injection (1.3%) 2170
▲ Videx Tablets, Powder for Oral Solution, & Pediatric Powder for Oral Solution (2% to 87%) 720
Zebeta Tablets (2.5% to 2.6%) 1413
▲ Zestoretic (3.9%) 2850
▲ Zestril Tablets (1.7 to 6.1%) 2854
Ziac (1.5% to 2.2%) 1415
Zoladex (1% or greater) 2858
Zoloft Tablets (Infrequent) 2217
Zosyn (1.0% or less) 1419
Zosyn Pharmacy Bulk Package (1.0% or less) 1422

Cough, productive
Permax Tablets (Frequent) 575

Cough reflex, depression
Astramorph/PF Injection, USP (Preservative-Free) 535
Compazine 2470
Duramorph 962
Infumorph 200 and Infumorph 500 Sterile Solutions 965
Lorcet 10/650 1018
Stelazine 2514
Thorazine 2523

Cramping
Adalat Capsules (10 mg and 20 mg) (2% or less) 587
Aldactazide 2413
Aldactone 2414
Aldoclor Tablets 1598
Aldoril Tablets 1604
Amicar Syrup, Tablets, and Injection (Occasional) 1267
Aminohippurate Sodium Injection 1606
Capozide 742
Clinoril Tablets (Greater than 1%) 1618
Combipres Tablets 677
Cytotec (0.6%) 2424
Dilaudid Tablets and Liquid 1339
Diucardin Tablets 2718
Diupres Tablets 1650
Diuril Oral Suspension 1653
Diuril Sodium Intravenous 1652
Diuril Tablets 1653
Enduron Tablets 420
Esidrix Tablets 821
Esimil Tablets 822
Sterile FUDR 2118
HydroDIURIL Tablets 1674
Hydropres Tablets 1675
Hyzaar Tablets 1677
Inderide Tablets 2732
Inderide LA Long Acting Capsules 2734
Lippes Loop Intrauterine Double-S 1848
Lopressor HCT Tablets 832
Lotensin HCT 837
Maxzide 1380
Moduretic Tablets 1705
Monistat Dual-Pak (2%) 1850
Monistat 3 Vaginal Suppositories (2%) 1850
Mycelex-G 500 mg Vaginal Tablets (Rare) 609
Neoral (Up to 2%) 2276
Oramorph SR (Morphine Sulfate Sustained Release Tablets) (Less frequent) 2236
Oretic Tablets 443
ParaGard T380A Intrauterine Copper Contraceptive 1880
Prinzide Tablets 1737
Rifamate Capsules 1530
▲ Sandimmune (Up to 4%) 2286
Scleromate 1891
Serzone Tablets 771
Tenoretic Tablets 2845
Thalitone 1245
▲ THROMBATE III Antithrombin III (Human) (2 of 17) 637
Timolide Tablets 1748
Vaseretic Tablets 1765
Zarontin Capsules (Frequent) 1928
Zarontin Syrup (Frequent) 1929
Zestoretic (0.3 to 1%) 2850
Ziac 1415

Cramping, abdominal (see under Abdominal pain/cramps)

Cramping, muscular
▲ Adalat Capsules (10 mg and 20 mg) (2% or less to 8%) 587
Adalat CC (Rare) 589
Apresazide Capsules (Less frequent) 808
Apresoline Hydrochloride Tablets (Less frequent) 809
Asacol Delayed-Release Tablets 1979
Atamet 572
Atromid-S Capsules (Less often) 2701
Brethine Ampuls (Less than 0.5%) 815
Brethine Tablets 814
Bricanyl Subcutaneous Injection 1502
Bricanyl Tablets 1503
Bumex (1.1%) 2093
BuSpar (Infrequent) 737
Calan SR Caplets (1% or less) 2422
Calan Tablets (1% or less) 2419
Capozide 742
Cardizem CD Capsules (Less than 1%) 1506
Cardizem SR Capsules (Less than 1%) 1510
Cardizem Injectable 1508
Cardizem Tablets (Less than 1%) 1512
Cardura Tablets (1%) 2186
Cartrol Tablets (2.6%) 410
Ceftin (Less than 1% but more than 0.1%) 1078
Cozaar Tablets (1.1%) 1628
CytoGam (Less than 5.0%) 1593
Cytotec (Infrequent) 2424
Dalgan Injection (Less than 1%) 538
Danocrine Capsules 2307
Demadex Tablets and Injection 686
Dipentum Capsules (Rare) 1951
Diucardin Tablets 2718
Diuril Sodium Intravenous 1652
Dolobid Tablets (Rare) 1654
Dyazide 2479
Eldepryl Tablets 2550
Esidrix Tablets 821
Hivid Tablets (Less than 1% to less than 3%) 2121
Hyzaar Tablets 1677
Imitrex Injection (1.1%) 1103
Imitrex Tablets (Infrequent) 1106
Isoptin Oral Tablets (Less than 1%) 1346
Isoptin SR Tablets (1% or less) 1348
K-Phos Neutral Tablets 639
K-Phos Original Formula 'Sodium Free' Tablets (Less frequent) 639
Kerlone Tablets (Less than 2%) 2436
Lasix Injection, Oral Solution and Tablets 1240
Lotrel Capsules 840
▲ Lozol Tablets (Greater than or equal to 5%) 2022
Maxzide 1380
Mestinon Injectable 1253
Mestinon 1254
Mevacor Tablets (0.6% to 1.1%) 1699
Midamor Tablets (Between 1% and 3%) 1703
Moduretic Tablets (Less than or equal to 1%) 1705
Monoket (Fewer than 1%) 2406
Monopril Tablets (0.2% to 1.0% or more) 757
▲ Mykrox Tablets (5.8%) 993
Nimotop Capsules (Up to 1.4%) 610
Normodyne Tablets (Less common) 2379
Norvasc Tablets (1% to 2%) 1940
Oncaspar 2028
Parlodel (Less than 1%) 2281
Pepcid Injection (Infrequent) 1722
Pepcid (Infrequent) 1720
Platinol 708
Platinol-AQ Injection 710
Plendil Extended-Release Tablets (0.5% to 1.5%) 527
Prilosec Delayed-Release Capsules (Less than 1%) 529
Prinivil Tablets (0.5% to 2.1%) 1733
Prinzide Tablets (2%) 1737
▲ Procardia Capsules (2% or less to 8%) 1971
▲ Procardia XL Extended Release Tablets (8%) 1972
Prostigmin Injectable 1260
Prostigmin Tablets 1261
Prostin E2 Suppository 2634
▲ Proventil (3%) 2386
Rythmol Tablets–150mg, 225mg, 300mg (Less than 1%) 1352
Ser-Ap-Es Tablets 849
Serevent Inhalation Aerosol (1% to 3%) 1176
Sinemet Tablets 943
Sinemet CR Tablets (0.8%) 944
▲ Supprelin Injection (3% to 10%) 2056
▲ Tegison Capsules (25-50%) 2154
Tenoretic Tablets 2845
Thalitone (Common) 1245
Tigan 2057
Timolide Tablets 1748
Tonocard Tablets (Less than 1%) 531
Trandate Tablets (Less common) 1185
Uroqid-Acid No. 2 Tablets 640
Vaseretic Tablets (2.7%) 1765
Vasotec I.V. 1768
Vasotec Tablets (0.5% to 1.0%) 1771
Ventolin Inhalation Aerosol and Refill (1%) 1197
Ventolin Syrup (1%) 1202
▲ Ventolin Tablets (3 of 100 patients) 1203
Verelan Capsules (1% or less) 1410
Verelan Capsules (Less than 1%) 2824
▲ Visken Tablets (3%) 2299
Volmax Extended-Release Tablets (2.7%) 1788
Xanax Tablets (2.4%) 2649
Zaroxolyn Tablets 1000
Zebeta Tablets 1413
Zestoretic (2.0%) 2850
Zestril Tablets (0.5% to 2.1%) 2854
Ziac (1.1% to 1.2%) 1415
Zocor Tablets 1775
Zoloft Tablets (Infrequent) 2217

Cramps, abdominal (see under Abdominal pain/cramps)

Cramps, lower limbs
Adalat CC (3% or less) 589
Ambien Tablets (Rare) 2416
Anafranil Capsules (Infrequent) 803
Atretol Tablets 573
Betaseron for SC Injection 658
Catapres-TTS (Less frequent) 675
Caverject (Less than 1%) 2583
▲ CellCept Capsules (More than or equal to 3%) 2099
Claritin (2% or fewer patients) 2349
Claritin-D (Less frequent) 2350
Combipres Tablets (About 3 in 1,000) 677
Depakote Tablets (Greater than 1% but not more than 5%) 415
Depo-Provera Contraceptive Injection (1% to 5%) 2602
Desferal Vials 820
DynaCirc Capsules (0.5% to 1%) 2256
▲ Emcyt Capsules (8%) 1953
Foscavir Injection (Between 1% and 5%) 547
Gammagard S/D, Immune Globulin, Intravenous (Human) (Occasional) 585
Glucotrol XL Extended Release Tablets (Less than 3%) 1968
Hivid Tablets (Less than 1% to less than 3%) 2121
▲ Hylorel Tablets (21.1% to 25.6%) 985
Intron A (Less than 5%) 2364
Kerlone Tablets (Less than 2%) 2436
Lamictal Tablets (Rare) 1112
Luvox Tablets 2544
Maxaquin Tablets (Less than 1%) 2440
Methergine (Rare) 2272
8-MOP Capsules 1246
Oxsoralen-Ultra Capsules 1257
Pentasa (Less than 1%) 1527
Procardia XL Extended Release Tablets (Less than 3%) 1972
▲ Prograf (Greater than 3%) 1042
Risperdal (Rare) 1301
Sansert Tablets 2295
Tegretol Chewable Tablets 852
Tegretol Suspension 852
Tegretol Tablets 852
Tenex Tablets (3% or less) 2074
Videx Tablets, Powder for Oral Solution, & Pediatric Powder for Oral Solution (Less than 1%) 720
Zoladex (2%) 2858

Cramps, pelvic
Cytotec (0.6%) 2424

Cranial nerve, dysfunction
Garamycin Injectable 2360
IFEX (Less frequent) 697
JE-VAX (One case) 886
Lescol Capsules 2267
Pravachol 765
Zocor Tablets 1775

Cranial nerve deficit, fetal
Accutane Capsules 2076

Cranial sensations, unspecified
Methotrexate Sodium Tablets, Injection, for Injection and LPF Injection (Occasional) 1275

Craniofacial deformities
Accupril Tablets 1893
Altace Capsules 1232
Capoten 739
Capozide 742
Cozaar Tablets 1628
Hyzaar Tablets 1677
Lotensin Tablets 834
Lotensin HCT 837
Lotrel Capsules 840
Monopril Tablets 757

(Described in PDR For Nonprescription Drugs) Incidence data in parenthesis; ▲ 3% or more (◉ Described in PDR For Ophthalmology)

1261 Side Effects Index Cystitis

Prinivil Tablets 1733
Prinzide Tablets 1737
Univasc Tablets 2410
Vaseretic Tablets 1765
Vasotec I.V. 1768
Vasotec Tablets 1771
Zestoretic 2850
Zestril Tablets 2854

Creatinine, increase (see under Serum creatinine, elevation)

Creatinine clearance, decrease

Children's Advil Suspension (Less than 1%) 2692
Bumex (0.3%) 2093
Cytovene (1% or less) 2103
Eskalith 2485
▲Foscavir Injection (5% or greater up to 27%) 547
IBU Tablets (Less than 1%) 1342
IFEX 697
Kefurox Vials, Faspak & ADD-Vantage 1454
Lithonate/Lithotabs/Lithobid 2543
Macrobid Capsules 1988
Macrodantin Capsules 1989
Mandol Vials, Faspak & ADD-Vantage 1461
Children's Motrin Ibuprofen Oral Suspension (Less than 1%) 1546
Motrin Tablets (Less than 1%) 2625
Motrin Ibuprofen Suspension, Oral Drops, Chewable Tablets, Caplets (Less than 1%) 1546
Netromycin Injection 100 mg/ml 2373
Platinol 708
Platinol-AQ Injection 710
Proglycem 580
Salflex Tablets 786
Trobicin Sterile Powder 2645
Zinacef 1211

Creatine kinase, increase

Zefazone 2654

Creatine phosphokinase, increase

Accutane Capsules (Some patients) 2076
Adalat CC (Rare) 589
Amicar Syrup, Tablets, and Injection 1267
Atamet 572
Atromid-S Capsules 2701
Cardizem CD Capsules (Less than 1%) 1506
Cardizem SR Capsules (Less than 1%) 1510
Cardizem Injectable 1508
Cardizem Tablets (Less than 1%) 1512
Clozaril Tablets 2252
Danocrine Capsules 2307
Felbatol (Rare) 2666
Lopid Tablets 1917
Lorelco Tablets 1517
▲Mevacor Tablets (11%) 1699
Nardil 1920
Orap Tablets 1050
Oxandrin 2862
Parlodel 2281
Pravachol (Rare) 765
Procardia Capsules (Rare) 1971
Procardia XL Extended Release Tablets (Rare) 1972
Prolixin 509
Revex (0.5%) 1811
Sandostatin Injection 2292
Sinemet Tablets 943
Tegison Capsules 2154
Winstrol Tablets (no incidence data in labeling) 2337
Zocor Tablets 1775

Cretinism, fetal

Tapazole Tablets 1477

Crohn's disease, exacerbation

Proleukin for Injection (Two patients) 797

Crying

ActHIB (Up to 1.6%) 872
Ambien Tablets 2416
Ativan Injection (1.3%) 2698
Dalgan Injection (Less than 1%) 538
Diphtheria and Tetanus Toxoids and Pertussis Vaccine Adsorbed (Infrequent) 2477
Diphtheria and Tetanus Toxoids and Pertussis Vaccine Adsorbed USP (For Pediatric Use) (Infrequent; 1 in 100 doses) 875
Foscavir Injection (Less than 1%) 547
HibTITER (38 of 1,118 vaccinations) 1375
IPOL Poliovirus Vaccine Inactivated 885
Nubain Injection (1% or less) 935
OmniHIB (0.3% to 1.6%) 2499
▲Poliovax (More than 5%) 891
Recombivax HB (Greater than 1%) 1744
Romazicon (1% to 3%) 2147
Tetramune 1404
Tri-Immunol Adsorbed 1408
Tripedia 892

Crystalluria

Ancobon Capsules 2079
Azo Gantrisin Tablets 2081
Azulfidine (Rare) 1949
Bactrim DS Tablets 2084
Bactrim I.V. Infusion 2082
Bactrim 2084
Cipro I.V. (1% or less) 595
Cipro I.V. Pharmacy Bulk Package (Less than 1%) 597
Cipro Tablets (Rare) 592
Clinoril Tablets (Less than 1 in 100) 1618
Dantrium Capsules (Less frequent) 1982
Demser Capsules (A few patients) .. 1649
Diamox 1372
Effexor (Rare) 2719
Floxin I.V. 1571
Floxin Tablets (200 mg, 300 mg, 400 mg) 1567
Fludara for Injection 663
Glauctabs (Rare) .... ◉ 208
MZM (Common; rare) .... ◉ 267
Maxaquin Tablets 2440
Mintezol 1704
Neptazane Tablets (Rare) 1388
Noroxin Tablets 1715
Noroxin Tablets 2048
PASER Granules 1285
Penetrex Tablets 2031
Septra 1174
Septra I.V. Infusion 1169
Septra I.V. Infusion ADD-Vantage Vials 1171
Septra 1174
Urobiotic-250 Capsules 2214

Cushingoid state (see under Cushing's syndrome)

Cushing's syndrome

Aclovate 1069
Aristocort Suspension (Forte Parenteral) 1027
Aristocort Suspension (Intralesional) 1025
Aristocort Tablets 1022
Aristospan Suspension (Intra-articular) 1033
Aristospan Suspension (Intralesional) 1032
Beclovent Inhalation Aerosol and Refill 1075
Beconase Inhalation Aerosol and Refill 1076
Betaseron for SC Injection 658
Carmol HC (Some patients) 924
Celestone Soluspan Suspension 2347
CORTENEMA 2535
Cortone Acetate Sterile Suspension 1623
Cortone Acetate Tablets 1624
Cutivate Cream 1088
Cutivate Ointment 1089
▲Cytadren Tablets (2 out of 3) 819
Dalalone D.P. Injectable 1011
Decadron Elixir 1633
Decadron Phosphate Injection 1637
Decadron Phosphate Respihaler 1642
Decadron Phosphate Turbinaire 1645
Decadron Phosphate with Xylocaine Injection, Sterile 1639
Decadron Tablets 1635
Decadron-LA Sterile Suspension 1646
Deltasone Tablets 2595
Depo-Medrol Single-Dose Vial 2600
Depo-Medrol Sterile Aqueous Suspension 2597
Dermatop Emollient Cream 0.1% .. 1238
Dexacort Phosphate in Respihaler .. 458
Dexacort Phosphate in Turbinaire .. 459
Diprolene 2352
Florinef Acetate Tablets 505
Hydeltrasol Injection, Sterile 1665
Hydeltra-T.B.A. Sterile Suspension 1667
Hydrocortone Acetate Sterile Suspension 1669
Hydrocortone Phosphate Injection, Sterile 1670
Hydrocortone Tablets 1672
Medrol 2621
Nasalide Nasal Solution 0.025% (With excessive dose) 2110
Neurontin Capsules (Rare) 1922
Pediapred Oral Liquid 995
Prelone Syrup 1787
ProctoCream-HC 2.5% 2408
Solu-Cortef Sterile Powder 2641
Solu-Medrol Sterile Powder 2643
Temovate (Infrequent) 1179
Ultravate Cream 0.05% 2689
Ultravate Ointment 0.05% 2690

Cutaneous tenderness

8-MOP Capsules 1246
Oxsoralen-Ultra Capsules 1257

Cyanosis

Abbokinase 403
Abbokinase Open-Cath 405
Americaine Anesthetic Lubricant 983
Americaine Otic Topical Anesthetic Ear Drops 983
Anafranil Capsules (Rare) 803
Antivenin (Crotalidae) Polyvalent 2696
AquaMEPHYTON Injection 1608
Azo Gantrisin Tablets 2081
Azulfidine (One in every 30 patients or less) 1949
Betaseron for SC Injection 658
Buprenex Injectable (Less than 1%) 2006
Cafergot 2251
Chloromycetin Sodium Succinate 1900
Clozaril Tablets (Less than 1%) 2252
Cytovene-IV (One report) 2103
Diupres Tablets 1650
Effexor (Rare) 2719
Heparin Sodium Injection, USP, Sterile Solution 2615
Heparin Sodium Vials 1441
Hivid Tablets (Less than 1% to less than 3%) 2121
Hydropres Tablets 1675
Hyskon Hysteroscopy Fluid (Rare) .. 1595
Imitrex Tablets 1106
Intron A (Less than 5%) 2364
Macrobid Capsules (Rare) 1988
Macrodantin Capsules (Rare) 1989
Maxaquin Tablets (Less than 1%) .. 2440
Mephyton Tablets (Rare) 1696
NebuPent for Inhalation Solution (1% or less) 1040
Permax Tablets (Infrequent) 575
Primaxin I.M. 1727
Primaxin I.V. (Less than 0.2%) 1729
Roferon-A Injection (Less than 1%) 2145
Ser-Ap-Es Tablets 849
VePesid Capsules and Injection (Sometimes) 718
Virazole (Infrequent) 1264

Cyanosis, hand

Intron A (Less than 5%) 2364

Cycloplegia

Arfonad Ampuls 2080
Bentyl 1501
Cystospaz 1963
Ditropan 1516
Donnatal 2060
Donnatal Extentabs 2061
Donnatal Tablets 2060
Kutrase Capsules 2402
Levsin/Levsinex/Levbid 2405
Pro-Banthīne Tablets 2052
Quarzan Capsules 2181
Robinul Forte Tablets 2072
Robinul Injectable 2072
Robinul Tablets 2072

Cylindruria

Cipro I.V. (1% or less) 595
Cipro I.V. Pharmacy Bulk Package (Less than 1%) 597
Cipro Tablets 592
Floxin I.V. 1571
Floxin Tablets (200 mg, 300 mg, 400 mg) 1567
Garamycin Injectable 2360
Nebcin Vials, Hyporets & ADD-Vantage 1464
Netromycin Injection 100 mg/ml 2373
Noroxin Tablets 1715
Noroxin Tablets 2048
Polymyxin B Sulfate, Aerosporin Brand Sterile Powder 1154
Tobramycin Sulfate Injection 968

Cyst

Anafranil Capsules (Infrequent) 803
▲Betaseron for SC Injection (4%) 658
▲CellCept Capsules (More than or equal to 3%) 2099
Cognex Capsules (Infrequent) 1901
Depakote Tablets (Greater than 1% but not more than 5%) 415
Effexor (Infrequent) 2719
Luvox Tablets (Rare) 2544
Neurontin Capsules (Infrequent) 1922
Videx Tablets, Powder for Oral Solution, & Pediatric Powder for Oral Solution (Less than 1%) 720

Cyst, renal

Anafranil Capsules (Rare) 803
Hivid Tablets (Less than 1% to less than 3%) 2121

Cystic masses in the pelvis

Lippes Loop Intrauterine Double-S .. 1848
ParaGard T380A Intrauterine Copper Contraceptive 1880

Cystitis

Children's Advil Suspension (Less than 1%) 2692
Ambien Tablets (Infrequent) 2416
Amen Tablets 780
Anafranil Capsules (Up to 2%) 803
▲BCG Vaccine, USP (TICE) (5.9%) .. 1814
▲Betaseron for SC Injection (8%) 658
Brevicon 2088
Cognex Capsules (Infrequent) 1901
Cycrin Tablets 975
Demulen 2428
Depo-Provera Sterile Aqueous Suspension 2606
Desogen Tablets 1817
Diethylstilbestrol Tablets 1437
Dilacor XR Extended-release Capsules (Infrequent) 2018
Effexor (Infrequent) 2719
ESTRATAB Tablets (0.3, 0.625, 1.25, 2.5 mg) 2536
Estratest 2539
Flagyl 375 Capsules 2434
Flagyl I.V. 2247
IBU Tablets (Less than 1%) 1342
Kerlone Tablets (Less than 2%) 2436
Lamictal Tablets (Rare) 1112
Lamprene Capsules (Less than 1%) 828
Leukeran Tablets 1133
Levlen/Tri-Levlen 651
Lodine Capsules and Tablets (Less than 1%) 2743
Lo/Ovral Tablets 2746
Lo/Ovral-28 Tablets 2751
Luvox Tablets (Infrequent) 2544
Menest Tablets 2494
Methotrexate Sodium Tablets, Injection, for Injection and LPF Injection 1275
MetroGel-Vaginal 902
Miacalcin Nasal Spray (1% to 3%) 2275
Micronor Tablets 1872
Modicon 1872
Children's Motrin Ibuprofen Oral Suspension (Less than 1%) 1546
Motrin Tablets (Less than 1%) 2625
Motrin Ibuprofen Suspension, Oral Drops, Chewable Tablets, Caplets (Less than 1%) 1546
Nalfon 200 Pulvules & Nalfon Tablets (Less than 1%) 917
NEOSAR Lyophilized/Neosar 1959
Neurontin Capsules (Infrequent) 1922
Nordette-21 Tablets 2755
Nordette-28 Tablets 2758
Norinyl 2088
Nor-Q D Tablets 2135
Ortho-Cept 1851
Ortho-Cyclen/Ortho-Tri-Cyclen 1858
Ortho Dienestrol Cream 1866
Ortho-Novum 1872
Ortho-Cyclen/Ortho Tri-Cyclen 1858
Ovcon 760
Ovral Tablets 2770
Ovral-28 Tablets 2770
Ovrette Tablets 2771
PMB 200 and PMB 400 2783
Paxil Tablets (Infrequent) 2505
Permax Tablets (Infrequent) 575
Premarin Intravenous 2787
Premarin with Methyltestosterone .. 2794

(▣ Described in PDR For Nonprescription Drugs) Incidence data in parenthesis; ▲ 3% or more (◉ Described in PDR For Ophthalmology)

Cystitis · Side Effects Index · 1262

Premarin Vaginal Cream 2791
Premphase 2797
Prempro 2801
Protostat Tablets 1883
Provera Tablets 2636
Prozac Pulvules & Liquid, Oral Solution (Infrequent) 919
Risperdal (Rare) 1301
Serzone Tablets (Infrequent) 771
▲TheraCys BCG Live (Intravesical) (Up to 29.5%) 897
Thioplex (Thiotepa For Injection) (Rare) 1281
Levlen/Tri-Levlen 651
Tri-Norinyl 2164
Triphasil-21 Tablets 2814
Triphasil-28 Tablets 2819
Wellbutrin Tablets (Rare) 1204
Zebeta Tablets 1413
Ziac 1415

Cystitis, hemorrhagic
Adriamycin PFS 1947
Adriamycin RDF 1947
Cipro I.V. (1% or less) 595
Cipro I.V. Pharmacy Bulk Package (Less than 1%) 597
Cytoxan 694
Fludara for Injection (Rare) 663
IFEX 697
Lysodren (Infrequent) 698
Navelbine Injection (Less than 1%) 1145
NEOSAR Lyophilized/Neosar 1959
Oncaspar 2028
Thioplex (Thiotepa For Injection) (Rare) 1281

Cystitis, non-hemorrhagic
Cytoxan 694

Cystitis, viral
Retrovir Capsules (0.8%) 1158
Retrovir I.V. Infusion (1%) 1163
Retrovir Syrup (0.8%) 1158

Cystitis-like syndrome (see under Cystitis)

Cysts, vaginal
Depo-Provera Contraceptive Injection (Fewer than 1%) 2602

Cytarabine syndrome
Cytosar-U Sterile Powder 2592

Cytokine Released Syndrome
Orthoclone OKT3 Sterile Solution (Occasional) 1837

cAMP, elevation
▲Yutopar Intravenous Injection (80% to 100%) 570

CHF (see under Congestive heart failure)

CNS abnormalities, fetal
Accutane Capsules 2076
Elavil 2838
Oxytocin Injection 2771
Sensorcaine 559

CNS damage
Tri-Immunol Adsorbed (1 per 330,000) 1408

CNS damage, permanent
Oxytocin Injection 2771
Syntocinon Injection 2296

CNS depression
Actifed with Codeine Cough Syrup 1067
Children's Advil Suspension (Less than 1%) 2692
Ana-Kit Anaphylaxis Emergency Treatment Kit 617
Anaprox/Naprosyn (Less than 1%) 2117
Ansaid Tablets (1-3%) 2579
Ativan Injection 2698
Brontex 1981
Butisol Sodium Elixir & Tablets (Less than 1 in 100) 2660
Carbocaine Hydrochloride Injection 2303
Cocaine Hydrochloride Topical Solution 537
D.A. Chewable Tablets 951
Deconamine Chewable Tablets 1320
Deconamine CX Cough and Cold Liquid and Tablets 1319
Deconamine 1320
Deconsal 454
Depakote Tablets 415
Dilantin Parenteral 1910
Duranest Injections 542
Dura-Tap/PD Capsules 2867
Dura-Vent/DA Tablets 953
Dura-Vent Tablets 952
EC-Naprosyn Delayed-Release Tablets (Less than 1%) 2117
Emla Cream 545
Entex PSE Tablets 1987
Fedahist Gyrocaps 2401
Fedahist Timecaps 2401
Guaimax-D Tablets 792
▲Klonopin Tablets (Most frequent) 2126
Lamictal Tablets (Infrequent) 1112
Lioresal Intrathecal 1596
Luvox Tablets (Infrequent) 2544
▲Lysodren (40%) 698
Mebaral Tablets (Less than 1 in 100) 2322
Children's Motrin Ibuprofen Oral Suspension (Less than 1%) 1546
Motrin Tablets (Less than 1%) 2625
Anaprox/Naprosyn (Less than 1%) 2117
Nembutal Sodium Capsules (Less than 1%) 436
Nembutal Sodium Solution (Less than 1%) 438
Nembutal Sodium Suppositories (Less than 1%) 440
Neurontin Capsules 1922
Novahistine DH 2462
Novahistine DMX ⊡ 822
Novahistine Elixir ⊡ 823
Novahistine Expectorant 2463
Phenergan with Codeine 2777
Phenergan VC with Codeine 2781
Phenobarbital Elixir and Tablets (Less than 1 in 100 patients) 1469
Pontocaine Hydrochloride for Spinal Anesthesia 2330
Prozac Pulvules & Liquid, Oral Solution (Rare) 919
Seconal Sodium Pulvules (Less than 1 in 100) 1474
Seldane-D Extended-Release Tablets 1538
Syn-Rx Tablets 465
Syn-Rx DM Tablets 466
Trinalin Repetabs Tablets 1330
Tussend 1783
Tussend Expectorant 1785
Videx Tablets, Powder for Oral Solution, & Pediatric Powder for Oral Solution (Less than 1%) 720
Vumon 727
▲Xanax Tablets (13.8% to 13.9%) 2649
Xylocaine Injections 567

CNS depression, neonatal
Halcion Tablets 2611
ProSom Tablets 449
Streptomycin Sulfate Injection 2208
Versed Injection 2170

CNS reactions
Attenuvax 1610
Biavax II 1613
BuSpar 737
Chibroxin Sterile Ophthalmic Solution (With oral form) 1617
▲Cipro I.V. Pharmacy Bulk Package (Among most frequent) 597
Clozaril Tablets 2252
Compazine 2470
Danocrine Capsules 2307
Desyrel and Desyrel Dividose 503
Diupres Tablets 1650
Hexalen Capsules 2571
Hydrocet Capsules 782
Hydropres Tablets 1675
Intron A (Less than 5%) 2364
Lanoxicaps (Rare) 1117
Lanoxin Elixir Pediatric 1120
Lanoxin Injection 1123
Lanoxin Injection Pediatric 1126
Lanoxin Tablets 1128
Lariam Tablets 2128
▲Leukine for IV Infusion (11%) 1271
Levsin/Levsinex/Levbid 2405
Marax Tablets & DF Syrup (Rare) 2200
Noroxin Tablets 1715
Noroxin Tablets 2048
▲Novantrone (30 to 34%) 1279
Orap Tablets 1050
Orthoclone OKT3 Sterile Solution 1837
Orudis Capsules (Less than 1%) 2766
Oruvail Capsules (Less than 1%) 2766
▲Paraplatin for Injection (5%) 705
Paremyd (Rare) ◉ 247
Prolixin 509
Rabies Vaccine, Imovax Rabies I.D. (One report) 883
Roferon-A Injection (Less than 3%) 2145
SSD 1355
Sandostatin Injection (Less than 1%) 2292
Serentil 684
Silvadene Cream 1% 1540
Stelazine 2514
Thalitone 1245
Triaminic Cold Tablets ⊡ 790
Triaminic Expectorant ⊡ 790

CNS stimulation
Adipex-P Tablets and Capsules 1048
Ansaid Tablets (1-3%) 2579
Brethaire Inhaler 813
Carbocaine Hydrochloride Injection 2303
Chibroxin Sterile Ophthalmic Solution (With oral form) 1617
▲Cipro I.V. (Among most frequent) 595
Cipro Tablets 592
Claritin-D 2350
Cocaine Hydrochloride Topical Solution 537
D.A. Chewable Tablets 951
Deconamine 1320
Duranest Injections 542
Dura-Tap/PD Capsules 2867
Dura-Vent Tablets 952
Effexor (Infrequent) 2719
Emla Cream 545
Floxin Tablets (200 mg, 300 mg, 400 mg) 1567
Kwell Cream & Lotion 2008
Kwell Shampoo 2009
Kytril Injection (Less than 2%) 2490
Lamictal Tablets (Rare) 1112
Lindane Lotion USP 1% 582
Lindane Shampoo USP 1% 583
Lufyllin-GG Elixir & Tablets 2671
Luvox Tablets (2%) 2544
Maxaquin Tablets 2440
Noroxin Tablets 1715
Noroxin Tablets 2048
Paxil Tablets (1.2%; frequent) 2505
Pontocaine Hydrochloride for Spinal Anesthesia 2330
Proventil Inhalation Aerosol 2382
Proventil Repetabs Tablets 2386
Proventil Syrup 2385
Prozac Pulvules & Liquid, Oral Solution (Infrequent) 919
Rondec Oral Drops 953
Rondec Syrup 953
Rondec Tablet 953
Rondec-DM Oral Drops 954
Rondec-DM Syrup 954
Rondec-TR Tablet 953
Serzone Tablets 771
Syn-Rx Tablets 465
Tussend 1783
▲Ultram Tablets (50 mg) (7% to 14%) 1585
Ventolin Inhalation Aerosol and Refill 1197
Ventolin Rotacaps for Inhalation 1200
Ventolin Syrup 1202
Ventolin Tablets 1203
Volmax Extended-Release Tablets 1788
Xylocaine Injections 567

CNS stimulation, paradoxical
Doral Tablets 2664
Halcion Tablets 2611
Libritabs Tablets 2177
Librium Capsules 2178
Restoril Capsules (Less than 0.5%) 2284

CNS toxicity
Cytosar-U Sterile Powder (With experimental doses) 2592
Duranest Injections 542
▲IFEX (12%) 697
Kefzol Vials, Faspak & ADD-Vantage 1456
Kwell Cream & Lotion 2008
Lindane Lotion USP 1% 582
Lindane Shampoo USP 1% 583
Marcaine Spinal 2319
Parlodel 2281

CNS, unresponsiveness, unspecified
▲Cipro I.V. (Among most frequent) 595

CPK, elevation (see under Creatine phosphokinase, increase)

D

Deafness
Amikacin Sulfate Injection, USP 960
Amikin Injectable 501
Anafranil Capsules (Infrequent) 803
Aralen Hydrochloride Injection (A few cases) 2301
Aralen Phosphate Tablets (A few cases) 2301
Betasept Surgical Scrub 1993
Betaseron for SC Injection 658
Clomid 1514
Cognex Capsules (Infrequent) 1901
Cytotec (Infrequent) 2424
Cytovene (1% or less) 2103
Depakote Tablets (Greater than 1% but not more than 5%) 415
Diupres Tablets 1650
Edecrin 1657
Effexor (Rare) 2719
Foscavir Injection (Less than 1%) 547
Hibiclens Antimicrobial Skin Cleanser 2840
Hibistat 2841
Hydropres Tablets 1675
Imitrex Tablets 1106
Indocin Capsules (Less than 1%) 1680
Indocin I.V. (Less than 1%) 1684
Indocin (Less than 1%) 1680
Kerlone Tablets (Less than 2%) 2436
Lamictal Tablets (Rare) 1112
Lodine Capsules and Tablets (Less than 1%) 2743
Luvox Tablets (Infrequent) 2544
M-M-R II 1687
Nebcin Vials, Hyporets & ADD-Vantage 1464
Permax Tablets (Infrequent) 575
Platinol (Rare) 708
Platinol-AQ Injection (Rare to occasional) 710
PREVACID Delayed-Release Capsules (Less than 1%) 2562
Prozac Pulvules & Liquid, Oral Solution (Rare) 919
Quinaglute Dura-Tabs Tablets 649
Salagen Tablets (Less than 1%) 1489
Ser-Ap-Es Tablets 849
Serzone Tablets (Rare) 771
Tobramycin Sulfate Injection 968
Ultram Tablets (50 mg) (Infrequent) 1585
Videx Tablets, Powder for Oral Solution, & Pediatric Powder for Oral Solution (Less than 1%) 720

Death, fetal
Accupril Tablets 1893
Altace Capsules 1232
Capoten 739
Capozide 742
Cozaar Tablets 1628
Felbatol 2666
Hyzaar Tablets 1677
Lotensin Tablets 834
Lotensin HCT (Several dozen cases) 837
Lotrel Capsules 840
Methotrexate Sodium Tablets, Injection, for Injection and LPF Injection 1275
Monopril Tablets 757
Nolvadex Tablets (A small number of reports) 2841
Oxytocin Injection 2771
Podocon-25 1891
Prinivil Tablets 1733
Prinzide Tablets 1737
Sensorcaine 559
Syntocinon Injection 2296
Univasc Tablets 2410
Vaseretic Tablets 1765
Vasotec I.V. 1768
Vasotec Tablets 1771
Zestoretic 2850
Zestril Tablets 2854

Death, infants
Virazole (20 cases) 1264

Death, sudden
Clozaril Tablets (Rare) 2252
Felbatol 2666
Haldol Decanoate 1577
Imitrex Tablets 1106

(⊡ Described in PDR For Nonprescription Drugs) · Incidence data in parenthesis; ▲ 3% or more · (◉ Described in PDR For Ophthalmology)

1263 Side Effects Index Dependence, physical

- Inapsine Injection 1296
- JE-VAX (One case) 886
- Luvox Tablets (Rare) 2544
- Monopril Tablets (0.4% to 1.0%) 757
- Neurontin Capsules (8 out of 2,203 patients) 1922
- Norpramin Tablets (One report) 1526
- Prozac Pulvules & Liquid, Oral Solution 919
- Risperdal 1301
- Thorazine 2523
- Vascor (200, 300 and 400 mg) Tablets (1.6%) 1587
- Vumon (One episode) 727

Deep tendon reflexes, loss

- Oncovin Solution Vials & Hyporets 1466
- Plaquenil Sulfate Tablets 2328
- Velban Vials 1484

Defecate, desire to

- Aminohippurate Sodium Injection 1606
- Dopram Injectable 2061
- Peptavlon 2878

Dehydration

- Anafranil Capsules (Infrequent) 803
- Bumex (0.1%) 2093
- Capoten 739
- Capozide 742
- ▲ CellCept Capsules (More than or equal to 3%) 2099
- Claritin-D (Less frequent) 2350
- Cognex Capsules (Infrequent) 1901
- Cytotec (Rare) 2424
- Demadex Tablets and Injection 686
- Dipentum Capsules (Rare) 1951
- Diprivan Injection (Less than 1%) 2833
- Eskalith 2485
- Felbatol 2666
- Fleet Enema 1002
- Fludara for Injection (Up to 1%) 663
- Foscavir Injection (Less than 1%) 547
- Garamycin Injectable 2360
- Glucophage 752
- Haldol Decanoate 1577
- Imitrex Injection (Rare) 1103
- Intron A (Less than 5%) 2364
- Klonopin Tablets 2126
- Lasix Injection, Oral Solution and Tablets 1240
- Leucovorin Calcium Tablets, Wellcovorin Brand 1132
- Lioresal Intrathecal 1596
- Lithium Carbonate Capsules & Tablets 2230
- Lithonate/Lithotabs/Lithobid 2543
- Luvox Tablets (Infrequent) 2544
- Methotrexate Sodium Tablets, Injection, for Injection and LPF Injection 1275
- Moduretic Tablets (Less than or equal to 1%) 1705
- Paxil Tablets (Rare) 2505
- Permax Tablets (Infrequent) 575
- Prinivil Tablets (0.3% to 1.0%) 1733
- Prinzide Tablets 1737
- Propulsid (More than 1%) 1300
- Prostin E2 Suppository 2634
- Prozac Pulvules & Liquid, Oral Solution (Rare) 919
- Risperdal (Rare) 1301
- Serzone Tablets (Infrequent) 771
- Univasc Tablets 2410
- Vaseretic Tablets 1765
- Vasotec Tablets 1771
- ▲ Videx Tablets, Powder for Oral Solution, & Pediatric Powder for Oral Solution (1% to 7%) 720
- Zestoretic 2850
- Zestril Tablets (0.3% to 1.0%) 2854
- Zoloft Tablets (Rare) 2217

Delirium

- Anafranil Capsules (Infrequent) 803
- Ativan Injection (1.3%) 2698
- Betaseron for SC Injection 658
- Brevital Sodium Vials 1429
- Catapres Tablets 674
- Catapres-TTS 675
- Chloromycetin Sodium Succinate 1900
- Clozaril Tablets 2252
- Cognex Capsules (Infrequent) 1901
- Combipres Tablets 677
- Dalgan Injection (Less than 1%) 538
- Diprivan Injection (Less than 1%) 2833
- Foscavir Injection (Less than 1%) 547
- Lamictal Tablets (Rare) 1112
- Luvox Tablets (Infrequent) 2544
- Nardil (Less frequent) 1920
- Orthoclone OKT3 Sterile Solution 1837
- Paxil Tablets (Rare) 2505
- Phenobarbital Elixir and Tablets 1469
- PhosLo Tablets 690
- Placidyl Capsules 448
- Prograf 1042
- Quinaglute Dura-Tabs Tablets 649
- Quinidex Extentabs 2067
- Risperdal (Rare) 1301
- Romazicon (Less than 1%) 2147
- Wellbutrin Tablets 1204
- Zovirax Sterile Powder 1223

Delivery complications, unspecified

- Advil Cold and Sinus Caplets and Tablets (formerly CoAdvil) ■ 870
- Advil Ibuprofen Tablets and Caplets ■ 870
- Aleve 1975
- Alka-Seltzer Effervescent Antacid and Pain Reliever ■ 701
- Alka-Seltzer Extra Strength Effervescent Antacid and Pain Reliever ■ 703
- Alka-Seltzer Lemon Lime Effervescent Antacid and Pain Reliever ■ 703
- Alka-Seltzer Plus Cold Medicine ■ 705
- Alka-Seltzer Plus Cold & Cough Medicine ■ 708
- Alka-Seltzer Plus Night-Time Cold Medicine ■ 707
- Alka Seltzer Plus Sinus Medicine ■ 707
- Arthritis Foundation Ibuprofen Tablets ■ 674
- Arthritis Foundation Safety Coated Aspirin Tablets ■ 675
- Arthritis Pain Ascriptin ■ 631
- Maximum Strength Ascriptin ■ 630
- Regular Strength Ascriptin Tablets ■ 629
- BC Cold Powder Multi-Symptom Formula (Cold-Sinus-Allergy) ■ 609
- BC Cold Powder Non-Drowsy Formula (Cold-Sinus) ■ 609
- BC Powder ■ 609
- Bayer Children's Chewable Aspirin ■ 711
- Genuine Bayer Aspirin Tablets & Caplets ■ 713
- Extra Strength Bayer Arthritis Pain Regimen Formula ■ 711
- Extra Strength Bayer Aspirin Caplets & Tablets ■ 712
- Extended-Release Bayer 8-Hour Aspirin ■ 712
- Extra Strength Bayer Plus Aspirin Caplets ■ 713
- Extra Strength Bayer PM Aspirin ■ 713
- Bayer Enteric Aspirin ■ 709
- Bayer Select Ibuprofen Pain Relief Formula ■ 715
- Cama Arthritis Pain Reliever ■ 785
- Cramp End Tablets ■ 735
- Dimetapp Sinus Caplets ■ 775
- Ecotrin 2455
- Empirin Aspirin Tablets ■ 854
- Empirin with Codeine Tablets 1093
- Fiorinal with Codeine Capsules 2262
- Marcaine Hydrochloride with Epinephrine 1:200,000 2316
- Marcaine Hydrochloride Injection 2316
- Motrin IB Caplets, Tablets, and Geltabs ■ 838
- Motrin IB Sinus ■ 838
- Sensorcaine 559
- Sine-Aid IB Caplets 1554
- Sine-Off Sinus Medicine ■ 825
- Soma Compound w/Codeine Tablets 2676
- Soma Compound Tablets 2675
- St. Joseph Adult Chewable Aspirin (81 mg.) ■ 808
- Ursinus Inlay-Tabs ■ 794
- Vanquish Analgesic Caplets ■ 731

Delusions

- Ambien Tablets (Rare) 2416
- Anafranil Capsules (Infrequent) 803
- Artane (Rare) 1368
- Asendin Tablets 1369
- Atamet 572
- Betaseron for SC Injection 658
- Clozaril Tablets (Less than 1%) 2252
- Dalgan Injection (Less than 1%) 538
- Desyrel and Desyrel Dividose 503
- Effexor (Rare) 2719
- Elavil 2838
- Eldepryl Tablets 2550
- Endep Tablets 2174
- Etrafon 2355
- Felbatol 2666
- Flexeril Tablets (Rare) 1661
- Halcion Tablets 2611
- Lamictal Tablets (Rare) 1112
- Larodopa Tablets (Relatively frequent) 2129
- Limbitrol 2180
- Ludiomil Tablets (Rare) 843
- ▲ Lupron Depot 3.75 mg (Among most frequent) 2556
- Luvox Tablets (Infrequent) 2544
- Norpramin Tablets 1526
- Nubain Injection (1% or less) 935
- Pamelor 2280
- Paxil Tablets (Rare) 2505
- Permax Tablets (Infrequent) 575
- Prozac Pulvules & Liquid, Oral Solution (Infrequent) 919
- Salagen Tablets (Rare) 1489
- Sinemet Tablets 943
- Sinemet CR Tablets 944
- Stadol (Less than 1%) 775
- Surmontil Capsules 2811
- Tofranil Ampuls 854
- Tofranil Tablets 856
- Tofranil-PM Capsules 857
- Triavil Tablets 1757
- Vivactil Tablets 1774
- Wellbutrin Tablets (1.2%) 1204
- Zoloft Tablets (Infrequent) 2217

Dementia

- Ambien Tablets (Rare) 2416
- Atamet 572
- Betaseron for SC Injection 658
- Effexor (Rare) 2719
- Foscavir Injection (Between 1% and 5%) 547
- Larodopa Tablets (Infrequent) 2129
- Methotrexate Sodium Tablets, Injection, for Injection and LPF Injection 1275
- Quinidex Extentabs 2067
- Sinemet Tablets 943
- Sinemet CR Tablets 944
- Videx Tablets, Powder for Oral Solution, & Pediatric Powder for Oral Solution (Less than 1%) 720
- Zerit Capsules (1%) 729

Dental calculus formation, an increase in

- Peridex 1978

Dental caries

- Ambien Tablets (Rare) 2416
- Anafranil Capsules (Infrequent) 803
- Claritin (2% or fewer patients) 2349
- Eskalith 2485
- Lithonate/Lithotabs/Lithobid 2543
- ▲ Luvox Tablets (3%) 2544
- Paxil Tablets (Rare) 2505
- Permax Tablets (Infrequent) 575
- Questran Light 769
- Questran Powder 770
- Tegison Capsules (Less than 1%) 2154

Dependence, drug

- Adipex-P Tablets and Capsules 1048
- Alfenta Injection 1286
- Astramorph/PF Injection, USP (Preservative-Free) 535
- Biphetamine Capsules 983
- Correctol Laxative Tablets & Caplets ■ 801
- Dalmane Capsules 2173
- Darvon-N/Darvocet-N 1433
- Darvon 1435
- Darvon-N Suspension & Tablets 1433
- Demerol 2308
- Dexedrine 2474
- Dilaudid Ampules 1335
- Dilaudid Cough Syrup 1336
- Dilaudid 1335
- Dilaudid Oral Liquid 1339
- Dilaudid 1335
- Dilaudid Tablets - 8 mg 1339
- Dizac 1809
- Duragesic Transdermal System 1288
- Duramorph 962
- Esgic-plus Tablets 1013
- Ex-Lax Chocolated Laxative Tablets ■ 786
- Extra Gentle Ex-Lax Laxative Pills ■ 786
- Regular Strength Ex-Lax Laxative Pills ■ 786
- Ex-Lax Gentle Nature Laxative Pills ■ 786
- Feen-A-Mint ■ 805
- Fioricet Tablets 2258
- Fioricet with Codeine Capsules 2260
- Fiorinal Capsules 2261
- Fiorinal with Codeine Capsules 2262
- Fiorinal Tablets 2261
- Halcion Tablets 2611
- Ionamin Capsules 990
- Libritabs Tablets 2177
- Librium Capsules 2178
- Librium Injectable 2179
- Limbitrol 2180
- Lortab 2566
- Luvox Tablets (Infrequent) 2544
- MS Contin Tablets 1994
- MSIR 1997
- Mepergan Injection 2753
- Methadone Hydrochloride Oral Concentrate 2233
- Methadone Hydrochloride Oral Solution & Tablets 2235
- Nembutal Sodium Capsules 436
- Nembutal Sodium Solution 438
- Nembutal Sodium Suppositories 440
- Oramorph SR (Morphine Sulfate Sustained Release Tablets) 2236
- PMB 200 and PMB 400 2783
- Paxil Tablets (Rare) 2505
- Percocet Tablets 938
- Percodan Tablets 939
- Percodan-Demi Tablets 940
- Peri-Colace 2052
- Phenergan with Codeine 2777
- Phenergan VC with Codeine 2781
- Phenobarbital Elixir and Tablets 1469
- Placidyl Capsules 448
- Prelu-2 Timed Release Capsules 681
- RMS Suppositories 2657
- Restoril Capsules 2284
- Ritalin Hydrochloride Tablets 848
- Roxanol 2243
- Roxicodone Tablets, Oral Solution & Intensol (Oxycodone) 2244
- Seconal Sodium Pulvules 1474
- Stadol (Less than 1%) 775
- Sublimaze Injection 1307
- Talwin Injection 2334
- Talwin Compound 2335
- Talwin Injection 2334
- Talwin Nx 2336
- Tranxene 451
- Tussi-Organidin NR Liquid and S NR Liquid 2677
- Tylenol with Codeine 1583
- Tylox Capsules 1584
- Valium Injectable 2182
- Valium Tablets 2183
- Valrelease Capsules 2169
- Vicodin Tuss Expectorant 1358
- Videx Tablets, Powder for Oral Solution, & Pediatric Powder for Oral Solution (Less than 1%) 720
- Wygesic Tablets 2827

Dependence, physical

- Bellergal-S Tablets 2250
- Brontex 1981
- Butisol Sodium Elixir & Tablets 2660
- Codiclear DH Syrup 791
- DHCplus Capsules 1993
- Dexedrine 2474
- Dilaudid Tablets and Liquid 1339
- Doral Tablets 2664
- Duragesic Transdermal System 1288
- Duramorph 962
- Esgic-plus Tablets 1013
- Fioricet Tablets 2258
- Fiorinal Capsules 2261
- Fiorinal with Codeine Capsules 2262
- Fiorinal Tablets 2261
- Hycodan Tablets and Syrup 930
- Hycomine Compound Tablets 932
- Hycomine 931
- Hycotuss Expectorant Syrup 933
- Hydrocet Capsules 782
- Infumorph 200 and Infumorph 500 Sterile Solutions 965
- Isordil Tembids 2741
- Isordil Titradose Tablets 2742
- Klonopin Tablets 2126
- Libritabs Tablets 2177
- Lorcet 10/650 1018
- Lortab 2566
- MS Contin Tablets 1994
- MSIR 1997
- Marinol (Dronabinol) Capsules (Uncommon) 2231
- Mebaral Tablets 2322
- Methadone Hydrochloride Oral Concentrate 2233
- Methadone Hydrochloride Oral Solution & Tablets 2235
- Miltown Tablets 2672
- Oramorph SR (Morphine Sulfate Sustained Release Tablets) 2236

(■ Described in PDR For Nonprescription Drugs) Incidence data in parenthesis; ▲ 3% or more (◉ Described in PDR For Ophthalmology)

Dependence, physical — Side Effects Index — 1264

- Percocet Tablets 938
- Percodan Tablets 939
- Phrenilin 785
- ProSom Tablets 449
- Quadrinal Tablets 1350
- RMS Suppositories 2657
- Roxanol 2243
- Seconal Sodium Pulvules 1474
- Sedapap Tablets 50 mg/650 mg 1543
- Serax Capsules 2810
- Serax Tablets 2810
- Sorbitrate 2843
- Talacen 2333
- Talwin Injection 2334
- Talwin Nx 2336
- Tranxene 451
- Tylenol with Codeine 1583
- Tylox Capsules 1584
- Versed Injection 2170
- Vicodin Tuss Expectorant 1358
- Xanax Tablets 2649

Dependence, psychic (see under Dependence, psychological)

Dependence, psychological

- Anexsia 5/500 Elixir 1781
- Anexia Tablets 1782
- Bellergal-S Tablets 2250
- Biphetamine Capsules 983
- Brontex 1981
- Butisol Sodium Elixir & Tablets 2660
- Cafergot 2251
- DHCplus Capsules 1993
- Darvon-N/Darvocet-N 1433
- Darvon 1435
- Darvon-N Suspension & Tablets 1433
- Demerol 2308
- Desoxyn Gradumet Tablets 419
- Dexedrine 2474
- Dilaudid 1335
- Dilaudid Oral Liquid 1339
- Dilaudid 1335
- Dilaudid Tablets - 8 mg 1339
- Duragesic Transdermal System 1288
- Duramorph 962
- Esgic-plus Tablets 1013
- Etrafon 2355
- Fastin Capsules 2488
- Fioricet Tablets 2258
- Fiorinal Capsules 2261
- Fiorinal with Codeine Capsules 2262
- Fiorinal Tablets 2261
- Hycodan Tablets and Syrup 930
- Hycomine Compound Tablets 932
- Hycomine 931
- Hycotuss Expectorant Syrup 933
- Hydrocet Capsules 782
- Infumorph 200 and Infumorph 500 Sterile Solutions 965
- Ionamin Capsules 990
- Klonopin Tablets 2126
- Libritabs Tablets 2177
- Lorcet 10/650 1018
- Lortab 2566
- MS Contin Tablets (Very rare) 1994
- MSIR 1997
- Marinol (Dronabinol) Capsules (Uncommon) 2231
- Mebaral Tablets 2322
- Methadone Hydrochloride Oral Concentrate 2233
- Methadone Hydrochloride Oral Solution & Tablets 2235
- Miltown Tablets 2672
- Nembutal Sodium Capsules 436
- Nembutal Sodium Solution 438
- Nembutal Sodium Suppositories 440
- Oramorph SR (Morphine Sulfate Sustained Release Tablets) 2236
- Percocet Tablets 938
- Percodan Tablets 939
- Phrenilin 785
- Placidyl Capsules 448
- ProSom Tablets 449
- RMS Suppositories 2657
- Roxanol 2243
- Roxicodone Tablets, Oral Solution & Intensol (Oxycodone) 2244
- Sedapap Tablets 50 mg/650 mg 1543
- Serax Capsules 2810
- Serax Tablets 2810
- Talacen 2333
- Talwin Nx 2336
- Tranxene 451
- Tussend 1783
- Tussionex Pennkinetic Extended-Release Suspension 998
- Tylenol with Codeine 1583
- Tylox Capsules 1584
- Vicodin Tablets 1356
- Vicodin ES Tablets 1357
- Vicodin Tuss Expectorant 1358
- Zydone Capsules 949

Depersonalization

- Ambien Tablets (Rare) 2416
- Anafranil Capsules (2%) 803
- Betaseron for SC Injection 658
- Buprenex Injectable (Infrequent) 2006
- BuSpar (Infrequent) 737
- Cardura Tablets (Less than 0.5% of 3960 patients) 2186
- Cipro I.V. (1% or less) 595
- Cipro I.V. Pharmacy Bulk Package (Less than 1%) 597
- Cipro Tablets (Less than 1%) 592
- Duragesic Transdermal System (Less than 1%) 1288
- Effexor (1%) 2719
- Halcion Tablets 2611
- Hivid Tablets (Less than 1% to less than 3%) 2121
- Indocin (Less than 1%) 1680
- Lamictal Tablets (Infrequent) 1112
- Luvox Tablets (Infrequent) 2544
- Marinol (Dronabinol) Capsules (Greater than 1%) 2231
- Maxaquin Tablets (Less than 1%) 2440
- Neurontin Capsules (Infrequent) 1922
- Norvasc Tablets (More than 0.1% to 1%) 1940
- Nubain Injection (1% or less) 935
- Paxil Tablets (Infrequent) 2505
- Penetrex Tablets (Less than 1% but more than or equal to 0.1%) 2031
- Prozac Pulvules & Liquid, Oral Solution (Infrequent) 919
- Romazicon (1% to 3%) 2147
- Serzone Tablets (Infrequent) 771
- Tambocor Tablets (Less than 1%) 1497
- Wellbutrin Tablets (Infrequent) 1204
- Xanax Tablets 2649
- Zoloft Tablets (Infrequent) 2217

Depigmentation

- Intron A (Less than 5%) 2364
- Thioplex (Thiotepa For Injection) 1281

Depilation (see under Epilation)

Depression (see also under Depression, mental)

- Accupril Tablets (0.5% to 1.0%) 1893
- Accutane Capsules (Some patients) 2076
- Actigall Capsules 802
- ▲ Actimmune (3%) 1056
- Adalat Capsules (10 mg and 20 mg) (Less than 0.5%) 587
- Children's Advil Suspension (Less than 1%) 2692
- AeroBid Inhaler System (1-3%) 1005
- Aerobid-M Inhaler System (1-3%) 1005
- Aldoclor Tablets 1598
- Aldomet Ester HCl Injection 1602
- Aldomet Oral 1600
- Aldoril Tablets 1604
- Altace Capsules (Less than 1%) 1232
- ▲ Anafranil Capsules (Up to 5%) 803
- Android 1251
- Ansaid Tablets (1-3%) 2579
- Apresazide Capsules (Less frequent) 808
- Apresoline Hydrochloride Tablets (Less frequent) 809
- Aristocort Suspension (Forte Parenteral) 1027
- Aristospan Suspension (Intra-articular) 1033
- Aristospan Suspension (Intralesional) 1032
- Asacol Delayed-Release Tablets 1979
- Atamet 572
- Ativan Injection (1.3%) 2698
- Ativan Tablets (Less frequent) 2700
- Atretol Tablets 573
- Azmacort Oral Inhaler 2011
- Azo Gantrisin Tablets 2081
- Bactrim DS Tablets 2084
- Bactrim I.V. Infusion 2082
- Bactrim 2084
- Betagan ◉ 233
- Betimol 0.25%, 0.5% ◉ 261
- Betoptic Ophthalmic Solution (Rare) 469
- Betoptic S Ophthalmic Suspension (Rare) 471
- Blocadren Tablets 1614
- Brevibloc Injection (Less than 1%) 1808
- Brevicon 2088
- BuSpar (2%) 737
- Capoten 739
- Capozide 742
- Cardene Capsules (Rare) 2095
- Cardizem SR Capsules (Less than 1%) 1510
- Cardizem Injectable 1508
- Cardizem Tablets (Less than 1%) 1512
- Cardura Tablets (1%) 2186
- Cartrol Tablets (Less common) 410
- Cataflam (Less than 1%) 816
- Celestone Soluspan Suspension 2347
- ▲ CellCept Capsules (More than or equal to 3%) 2099
- Cipro I.V. (1% or less) 595
- Cipro I.V. Pharmacy Bulk Package (Less than 1%) 597
- Cipro Tablets (Less than 1%) 592
- Clinoril Tablets (Less than 1%) 1618
- Clomid (Fewer than 1%) 1514
- Clozaril Tablets (1%) 2252
- Cogentin 1621
- Cozaar Tablets (Less than 1%) 1628
- Cylert Tablets 412
- DDAVP 2017
- Dalgan Injection (Less than 1%) 538
- Dalmane Capsules (Rare) 2173
- Danocrine Capsules 2307
- Daranide Tablets 1633
- Daraprim Tablets (Rare) 1090
- Delatestryl Injection 2860
- Demser Capsules 1649
- Didrex Tablets 2607
- Diethylstilbestrol Tablets 1437
- Dilaudid-HP Injection (Less frequent) 1337
- Dilaudid-HP Lyophilized Powder 250 mg (Less frequent) 1337
- Dipentum Capsules (1.5%) 1951
- Diprivan Injection (Less than 1%) 2833
- Dizac (Less frequent) 1809
- Dolobid Tablets (Less than 1 in 100) 1654
- Doral Tablets 2664
- ▲ Duragesic Transdermal System (3% to 10%) 1288
- DynaCirc Capsules (0.5% to 1%) 2256
- Eldepryl Tablets 2550
- Elspar 1659
- Ergamisol Tablets (1% to 2%) 1292
- Estrace Cream and Tablets 749
- Estratest 2539
- Ethmozine Tablets (Less than 2%) 2041
- Eulexin Capsules (1%) 2358
- Feldene Capsules (Less than 1%) 1965
- Fioricet Tablets (Infrequent) 2258
- Fioricet with Codeine Capsules (Infrequent) 2260
- Fiorinal with Codeine Capsules 2262
- Flagyl 375 Capsules 2434
- Flagyl I.V. 2247
- Floxin I.V. (Less than 1%) 1571
- Floxin Tablets (200 mg, 300 mg, 400 mg) (Less than 1%) 1567
- Fludara for Injection (Up to 1%) 663
- ▲ Foscavir Injection (5% or greater) 547
- Gantanol Tablets 2119
- Gantrisin 2120
- Garamycin Injectable 2360
- Gastrocrom Capsules (Infrequent) 984
- Halcion Tablets (0.9% to 0.5%) 2611
- Haldol Decanoate 1577
- Haldol Injection, Tablets and Concentrate 1575
- Halotestin Tablets 2614
- Hismanal Tablets (Less frequent) 1293
- Hivid Tablets (Less than 1% to less than 3%) 2121
- Hydropres Tablets 1675
- Hylorel Tablets (1.9%) 985
- Hytrin Capsules (0.3%) 430
- Hyzaar Tablets 1677
- IBU Tablets (Less than 1%) 1342
- Indocin (Greater than 1%) 1680
- ▲ Intron A (3% to 28%) 2364
- Isoptin Injectable 1344
- Kerlone Tablets (0.8%) 2436
- Klonopin Tablets 2126
- Lamprene Capsules (Less than 1%) 828
- Lariam Tablets 2128
- Larodopa Tablets (Infrequent) 2129
- Levatol (0.6%) 2403
- Lioresal Tablets 829
- Lodine Capsules and Tablets (More than 1% but less than 3%) 2743
- Lomotil 2439
- Lopid Tablets 1917
- ▲ Lopressor Ampuls (5%) 830
- ▲ Lopressor HCT Tablets (5 in 100) 832
- ▲ Lopressor Tablets (5%) 830
- Lozol Tablets (Less than 5%) 2022
- ▲ Lupron Depot 3.75 mg (10.8%) 2556
- Lupron Depot 7.5 mg 2559
- Lupron Injection (Less than 5%) 2555
- MS Contin Tablets (Less frequent) 1994
- MSIR (Infrequent) 1997
- Marcaine Hydrochloride with Epinephrine 1:200,000 2316
- Marcaine Hydrochloride Injection 2316
- Marcaine Spinal 2319
- Marinol (Dronabinol) Capsules (Less than 1%) 2231
- Matulane Capsules 2131
- Maxair Inhaler (Less than 1%) 1494
- Maxaquin Tablets (Less than 1%) 2440
- Maxzide 1380
- Mebaral Tablets 2322
- Mesantoin Tablets 2272
- Mevacor Tablets (0.5% to 1.0%) 1699
- Mexitil Capsules (2.4%) 678
- Miacalcin Nasal Spray (1% to 3%) 2275
- Micronor Tablets 1872
- Midamor Tablets (Less than or equal to 1%) 1703
- Minipress Capsules (1-4%) 1937
- Minizide Capsules (Rare) 1938
- Mithracin 607
- Moban Tablets and Concentrate (Less frequent) 1048
- Modicon 1872
- Moduretic Tablets (Less than or equal to 1%) 1705
- 8-MOP Capsules 1246
- Monopril Tablets (0.4% to 1.0%) 757
- Motofen Tablets 784
- Children's Motrin Ibuprofen Oral Suspension (Less than 1%) 1546
- Motrin Tablets (Less than 1%) 2625
- Mykrox Tablets (Less than 2%) 993
- Nalfon 200 Pulvules & Nalfon Tablets (Less than 1%) 917
- Nasacort Nasal Inhaler 2024
- NebuPent for Inhalation Solution (1% or less) 1040
- Neoral (Rare) 2276
- Nescaine/Nescaine MPF 554
- Nicorette 2458
- Nicotrol Nicotine Transdermal System (1% to 3%) 1550
- Nimotop Capsules (Up to 1.4%) 610
- Nolvadex Tablets (Infrequent; 1.9%) 2841
- Norinyl 2088
- Noroxin Tablets (Less frequent or 0.3% to 1.0%) 1715
- Noroxin Tablets (Less frequent or 0.3% to 1.0%) 2048
- Nor-Q D Tablets 2135
- Norvasc Tablets (More than 0.1% to 1%) 1940
- Nubain Injection (1% or less) 935
- Ocupress Ophthalmic Solution, 1% Sterile ◉ 309
- OptiPranolol (Metipranolol 0.3%) Sterile Ophthalmic Solution (A small number of patients) ◉ 258
- Oramorph SR (Morphine Sulfate Sustained Release Tablets) (Less frequent) 2236
- ▲ Orap Tablets (2 of 20 patients) 1050
- Orlamm (1% to 3%) 2239
- Ortho-Novum 1872
- Orudis Capsules (Greater than 1%) 2766
- Oruvail Capsules (Greater than 1%) 2766
- Ovcon 760
- Oxandrin 2862
- Oxsoralen-Ultra Capsules 1257
- Parlodel 2281
- Penetrex Tablets (Less than 1% but more than or equal to 0.1%) 2031
- Pepcid Injection (Infrequent) 1722
- Pepcid (Infrequent) 1720
- ▲ Permax Tablets (3.2%) 575
- Phrenilin 785
- Plendil Extended-Release Tablets (0.5% to 1.5%) 527
- Pondimin Tablets 2066
- Pregnyl 1828
- Prelone Syrup 1787
- PREVACID Delayed-Release Capsules (Less than 1%) 2562
- Prilosec Delayed-Release Capsules (Less than 1%) 529
- Prinivil Tablets (Up to 1.1%) 1733
- Prinzide Tablets (0.3% to 1%) 1737

(▣ Described in PDR For Nonprescription Drugs) Incidence data in parenthesis; ▲ 3% or more (◉ Described in PDR For Ophthalmology)

Side Effects Index

Procardia Capsules (Less than 0.5%) 1971
Procardia XL Extended Release Tablets (1% or less) 1972
Profasi (chorionic gonadotropin for injection, USP) 2450
Protostat Tablets 1883
Quadrinal Tablets 1350
Quinaglute Dura-Tabs Tablets 649
Quinidex Extentabs 2067
Reglan (Less frequent) 2068
Relafen Tablets (1%) 2510
Retrovir Capsules 1158
Retrovir I.V. Infusion 1163
Retrovir Syrup 1158
Revex (Less than 1%) 1811
Rogaine Topical Solution (0.36%) .. 2637
Romazicon (1% to 3%) 2147
Rythmol Tablets–150mg, 225mg, 300mg (Less than 1%) 1352
Sandimmune (Rare) 2286
Sandostatin Injection (Less than 1%) 2292
Sanorex Tablets 2294
Sectral Capsules (2%) 2807
Sedapap Tablets 50 mg/650 mg (Infrequent) 1543
Seldane Tablets 1536
Seldane-D Extended-Release Tablets 1538
Sensorcaine 559
Septra 1174
Septra I.V. Infusion 1169
Septra I.V. Infusion ADD-Vantage Vials 1171
Septra 1174
Ser-Ap-Es Tablets 849
Serophene (clomiphene citrate tablets, USP) (Less than 1 in 100 patients) 2451
Sinemet Tablets 943
Sinemet CR Tablets (2.2%) 944
Stadol (Less than 1%) 775
Stilphostrol Tablets and Ampuls 612
Supprelin Injection (3% to 10%) 2056
Symmetrel Capsules and Syrup (1% to 5%) 946
▲ Synarel Nasal Solution for Endometriosis (3% of patients) 2152
Tagamet 2516
Talacen (Infrequent) 2333
Talwin Injection (Infrequent) 2334
Talwin Compound (Infrequent) 2335
Talwin Injection 2334
Talwin Nx 2336
Tambocor Tablets (1% to less than 3%) 1497
Tegison Capsules (Less than 1%) .. 2154
Tegretol Chewable Tablets 852
Tegretol Suspension 852
Tegretol Tablets 852
Tenex Tablets (3% or less) 2074
▲ Tenoretic Tablets (0.6% to 12%) .. 2845
▲ Tenormin Tablets and I.V. Injection (0.6% to 12%) 2847
Testred Capsules 1262
Timolide Tablets 1748
Timoptic in Ocudose (Less frequent) 1753
Timoptic Sterile Ophthalmic Solution (Less frequent) 1751
Tolectin (200, 400 and 600 mg) (1 to 3%) 1581
Tonocard Tablets (Less than 1%) .. 531
▲ Toprol-XL Tablets (About 5 of 100 patients) 565
Toradol (1% or less) 2159
Trancopal Caplets 2337
Tranxene 451
Tri-Norinyl 28-Day Tablets 2164
Valium Injectable 2182
Valium Tablets (Infrequent) 2183
Valrelease Capsules (Occasional) 2169
Vascor (200, 300 and 400 mg) Tablets (0.5 to 2.0%) 1587
Vaseretic Tablets 1765
Vasotec I.V. 1768
Vasotec Tablets (0.5% to 1%) 1771
Velban Vials 1484
Voltaren Tablets (Less than 1%) 861
Vontrol Tablets 2532
Wellbutrin Tablets (Frequent) 1204
Winstrol Tablets 2337
▲ Xanax Tablets (13.8% to 13.9%) .. 2649
Zantac (Rare) 1209
Zantac Injection (Rare) 1207
Zantac Syrup (Rare) 1209
Zaroxolyn Tablets 1000
Zestoretic (0.3 to 1%) 2850
Zestril Tablets (Up to 1.1%) 2854
Zocor Tablets 1775

▲ Zoladex (Greater than 1% to 54%) 2858
Zoloft Tablets (Infrequent) 2217
Zyloprim Tablets (Less than 1%) 1226

Depression, aggravation of

Halcion Tablets 2611
Intron A (Less than 5%) 2364
Zoloft Tablets (Infrequent) 2217

Depression, circulatory

Brontex 1981
Methadone Hydrochloride Oral Solution & Tablets 2235
Oramorph SR (Morphine Sulfate Sustained Release Tablets) 2236
RMS Suppositories 2657
Roxanol 2243
Sublimaze Injection 1307

Depression, mental

Adalat CC (Less than 1.0%) 589
Aldomet Ester HCl Injection 1602
Ambien Tablets (2%) 2416
Amen Tablets 780
▲ Android Capsules, 10 mg (Among most common) 1250
Android 1251
Aristocort Suspension (Forte Parenteral) 1027
Aristocort Suspension (Intralesional) 1025
Aristocort Tablets 1022
Aygestin Tablets 974
Azo Gantanol Tablets 2080
Azulfidine (Rare) 1949
Beconase 1076
Betapace Tablets (1% to 4%) 641
Betaseron for SC Injection 658
Blocadren Tablets 1614
Brevicon 2088
Cardizem CD Capsules (Less than 1%) 1506
Cartrol Tablets 410
Catapres Tablets (About 1 in 100 patients) 674
Catapres-TTS (Less frequent) 675
Celontin Kapseals 1899
Chibroxin Sterile Ophthalmic Solution (With oral form) 1617
Chloromycetin Sodium Succinate 1900
Claritin (2% or fewer patients) 2349
Claritin-D (Less frequent) 2350
Climara Transdermal System 645
▲ Cognex Capsules (4%) 1901
Combipres Tablets (About 1%) 677
CORTENEMA 2535
Cortone Acetate Sterile Suspension 1623
Cortone Acetate Tablets 1624
Cycrin Tablets 975
Cytovene (1% or less) 2103
Dantrium Capsules (Less frequent) 1982
Daypro Caplets (Greater than 1% but less than 3%) 2426
Decadron Elixir 1633
Decadron Phosphate Injection 1637
Decadron Phosphate Respihaler 1642
Decadron Phosphate Turbinaire 1645
Decadron Phosphate with Xylocaine Injection, Sterile 1639
Decadron Tablets 1635
Decadron-LA Sterile Suspension 1646
Deltasone Tablets 2595
Demulen 2428
Depakene 413
Depakote Tablets 415
Depo-Medrol Sterile Aqueous Suspension 2597
Depo-Provera Contraceptive Injection (1% to 5%) 2602
Depo-Provera Sterile Aqueous Suspension 2606
Desmopressin Acetate Rhinal Tube 979
Desogen Tablets 1817
Dexacort Phosphate in Respihaler .. 458
Dexacort Phosphate in Turbinaire .. 459
Didronel Tablets 1984
Dilaudid Tablets and Liquid (Less frequent) 1339
Diupres Tablets 1650
Duranest Injections 542
Effexor (1%) 2719
Esgic-plus Tablets (Infrequent) 1013
Esimil Tablets 822
Estraderm Transdermal System 824
ESTRATAB Tablets (0.3, 0.625, 1.25, 2.5 mg) 2536
Estratest 2539
Fansidar Tablets 2114
▲ Felbatol (5.3%) 2666

Flexeril Tablets (Less than 1%) 1661
Florinef Acetate Tablets 505
Flumadine Tablets & Syrup (0.3% to 1%) 1015
Glucotrol XL Extended Release Tablets (Less than 3%) 1968
Hydeltrasol Injection, Sterile 1665
Hydeltra-T.B.A. Sterile Suspension 1667
Hydrocortone Acetate Sterile Suspension 1669
Hydrocortone Phosphate Injection, Sterile 1670
Hydrocortone Tablets 1672
Hydropres Tablets 1675
Hylorel Tablets (1.9%) 985
Imdur (Less than or equal to 5%) .. 1323
Imitrex Injection (Rare) 1103
Imitrex Tablets (Infrequent) 1106
Inapsine Injection 1296
Inderal 2728
Inderal LA Long Acting Capsules 2730
Inderide Tablets 2732
Inderide LA Long Acting Capsules .. 2734
Iopidine 0.5% (Less than 1%) .... ◉ 221
Ismelin Tablets 827
Isoptin Injectable 1344
Kerlone Tablets 2436
▲ Lamictal Tablets (4.2%) 1112
Lescol Capsules 2267
Levatol 2403
Levlen/Tri-Levlen 651
Lioresal Intrathecal 1596
Lo/Ovral Tablets 2746
Lo/Ovral-28 Tablets 2751
Lopressor HCT Tablets 832
Luvox Tablets (2%) 2544
Macrobid Capsules (Rare) 1988
Macrodantin Capsules (Rare) 1989
Maxair Autohaler 1492
Megace Oral Suspension (1% to 3%) 699
Menest Tablets 2494
Methadone Hydrochloride Oral Concentrate 2233
MetroGel-Vaginal 902
Micronor Tablets 1872
Modicon 1872
Monoket (Fewer than 1%) 2406
Motrin Ibuprofen Suspension, Oral Drops, Chewable Tablets, Caplets (Less than 1%) 1546
Neurontin Capsules (1.8%) 1922
Nizoral Tablets (Rare) 1298
Nordette-21 Tablets 2755
Nordette-28 Tablets 2758
Norinyl 2088
Normodyne Tablets 2379
Nor-Q D Tablets 2135
Ogen Tablets 2627
Ogen Vaginal Cream 2630
Oreton Methyl 1255
Ortho-Cept 1851
Ortho-Cyclen/Ortho-Tri-Cyclen 1858
Ortho Dienestrol Cream 1866
Ortho-Est 1869
Ortho-Novum 1872
Ortho-Cyclen/Ortho Tri-Cyclen 1858
Ovral Tablets 2770
Ovral-28 Tablets 2770
Ovrette Tablets 2771
PMB 200 and PMB 400 2783
Paxil Tablets (Frequent) 2505
Pentasa (Less than 1%) 1527
Pravachol 765
Premarin Intravenous 2787
Premarin with Methyltestosterone .. 2794
Premarin Tablets 2789
Premarin Vaginal Cream 2791
Premphase 2797
Prempro 2801
Prinivil Tablets (Up to 1.1%) 1733
Procan SR Tablets (Occasional) 1926
▲ Prograf (Greater than 3%) 1042
Proleukin for Injection (Less than 1%) 797
Propulsid (More than 1%) 1300
ProSom Tablets (2%) 449
Provera Tablets 2636
Quadrinal Tablets 1350
Reglan (Less frequent) 2068
▲ ReVia Tablets (Less than 1% to 7%) 940
Risperdal (Infrequent) 1301
Ritalin Hydrochloride Tablets 848
▲ Roferon-A Injection (16%) 2145
Salagen Tablets (Less than 1%) 1489
Sectral Capsules 2807
Serzone Tablets 771
Sporanox Capsules (less than 1%) 1305
Stilphostrol Tablets and Ampuls 612
Sublimaze Injection 1307

Tenoretic Tablets 2845
Tenormin Tablets and I.V. Injection 2847
Testoderm Testosterone Transdermal System 486
Tigan 2057
Timoptic in Ocudose 1753
Timoptic Sterile Ophthalmic Solution 1751
Timoptic-XE 1755
Toprol-XL Tablets 565
Trandate Tablets 1185
Trecator-SC Tablets 2814
Trental Tablets (Less than 1%) 1244
Levlen/Tri-Levlen 651
Tri-Norinyl 2164
Triphasil-21 Tablets 2814
Triphasil-28 Tablets 2819
Videx Tablets, Powder for Oral Solution, & Pediatric Powder for Oral Solution (1% to 5%) 720
Visken Tablets 2299
Zantac (Rare) 1209
Zantac Injection (Rare) 1207
Zantac Syrup (Rare) 1209
Zarontin Capsules (Rare) 1928
Zarontin Syrup (Rare) 1929
Zaroxolyn Tablets 1000
Zebeta Tablets (Up to 0.2%) 1413
▲ Zerit Capsules (Fewer than 1% to 14%) 729
Ziac 1415
▲ Zoladex (Greater than 1% but less than 5%) 2858
Zosyn (1.0% or less) 1419
Zosyn Pharmacy Bulk Package (1.0% or less) 1422

Depression, mood

(see under Depression, mental)

Depression, psychotic

Effexor (Infrequent) 2719
8-MOP Capsules 1246
Paxil Tablets (Rare) 2505

Depression, respiratory

Actifed with Codeine Cough Syrup .. 1067
▲ Alfenta Injection (One of the two most common) 1286
Anectine 1073
Anexsia 5/500 Elixir 1781
Anexia Tablets 1782
Aralen Hydrochloride Injection 2301
Arfonad Ampuls 2080
Astramorph/PF Injection, USP (Preservative-Free) 535
Atropine Sulfate Sterile Ophthalmic Solution ...... ◉ 233
Brevital Sodium Vials 1429
Brontex 1981
Codiclear DH Syrup 791
Dalgan Injection (Less than 1%) 538
Demerol 2308
Dilaudid Ampules 1335
Dilaudid Cough Syrup 1336
Dilaudid-HP Injection 1337
Dilaudid-HP Lyophilized Powder 250 mg 1337
Dilaudid 1335
Dilaudid Oral Liquid 1339
Dilaudid 1335
Dilaudid Tablets - 8 mg 1339
Dizac 1809
Doral Tablets 2664
Duramorph 962
Duranest Injections 542
Dyclone 0.5% and 1% Topical Solutions, USP 544
Emla Cream 545
▲ Empirin with Codeine Tablets (Among most frequent) 1093
Felbatol 2666
Foscavir Injection (Less than 1%) .. 547
Garamycin Injectable 2360
Hycodan Tablets and Syrup 930
Hycomine Compound Tablets 932
Hycomine 931
Hycotuss Expectorant Syrup 933
Hydrocet Capsules 782
Infumorph 200 and Infumorph 500 Sterile Solutions 965
Klonopin Tablets 2126
Levo-Dromoran (Infrequent) 2129
Lioresal Intrathecal 1596
Lorcet 10/650 1018
Lortab 2566
MS Contin Tablets 1994
MSIR 1997
Marcaine Hydrochloride with Epinephrine 1:200,000 2316
Marcaine Hydrochloride Injection 2316

(**◆** Described in PDR For Nonprescription Drugs) Incidence data in parenthesis; ▲ 3% or more (◉ Described in PDR For Ophthalmology)

Depression, respiratory Side Effects Index 1266

Mepergan Injection ... 2753
Methadone Hydrochloride Oral Solution & Tablets ... 2235
Metubine Iodide Vials ... 916
Nardil (Less frequent) ... 1920
Norcuron ... 1826
Novahistine Expectorant ... 2463
Numorphan Injection ... 936
Numorphan Suppositories ... 937
Oramorph SR (Morphine Sulfate Sustained Release Tablets) ... 2236
Percocet Tablets ... 938
Phenergan with Codeine ... 2777
Phenergan VC with Codeine ... 2781
Phenobarbital Elixir and Tablets ... 1469
ProSom Tablets ... 449
Prostigmin Injectable ... 1260
Prostigmin Tablets ... 1261
Prostin VR Pediatric Sterile Solution (Less than 1%) ... 2635
RMS Suppositories ... 2657
Roxanol ... 2243
Scleromate (Rare) ... 1891
Sensorcaine ... 559
▲ Sublimaze Injection (Among most common) ... 1307
▲ Sufenta Injection (One of the two most common) ... 1309
Survanta Beractant Intratracheal Suspension ... 2226
Talacen (Rare) ... 2333
Talwin Injection (Infrequent) ... 2334
Talwin Compound ... 2335
Talwin Injection (Infrequent) ... 2334
Talwin Nx (Rare) ... 2336
Tussionex Pennkinetic Extended-Release Suspension ... 998
Tussi-Organidin NR Liquid and S NR Liquid (At higher doses) ... 2677
Tylenol with Codeine ... 1583
Tylox Capsules ... 1584
Valium Injectable ... 2182
Versed Injection ... 2170
Vicodin Tablets ... 1356
Vicodin ES Tablets ... 1357
Vicodin Tuss Expectorant ... 1358
Xylocaine Injections ... 567
Zydone Capsules ... 949

Depression, respiratory, neonatal

Anexsia 5/500 Elixir ... 1781
Anexia Tablets ... 1782
Astramorph/PF Injection, USP (Preservative-Free) ... 535
Brontex ... 1981
Butisol Sodium Elixir & Tablets ... 2660
Demerol ... 2308
Dilaudid Ampules ... 1335
Dilaudid Cough Syrup ... 1336
Dilaudid ... 1335
Duramorph ... 962
Fiorinal with Codeine Capsules ... 2262
Hydrocet Capsules ... 782
Lortab ... 2566
MS Contin Tablets ... 1994
MSIR ... 1997
Mepergan Injection ... 2753
Methadone Hydrochloride Oral Solution & Tablets ... 2235
Normodyne Injection ... 2377
Oramorph SR (Morphine Sulfate Sustained Release Tablets) ... 2236
Percocet Tablets ... 938
Quadrinal Tablets ... 1350
Roxanol ... 2243
Streptomycin Sulfate Injection (Occasional) ... 2208
Tracrium Injection ... 1183
Trandate ... 1185
Tussionex Pennkinetic Extended-Release Suspension ... 998
Tylenol with Codeine ... 1583
Tylox Capsules ... 1584
Vicodin Tablets ... 1356
Vicodin ES Tablets ... 1357

Depressive reactions

Soma Compound w/Codeine Tablets (Infrequent or rare) ... 2676
Soma Compound Tablets (Infrequent or rare) ... 2675
Soma Tablets ... 2674

Dermal creases

Doxorubicin Astra (A few cases) ... 540

Dermatitis

Adalat Capsules (10 mg and 20 mg) (2% or less) ... 587
Ambien Tablets (Rare) ... 2416
Anafranil Capsules (Up to 2%) ... 803
Atropine Sulfate Sterile Ophthalmic Solution ... ⊙ 233
Benemid Tablets ... 1611
Benoquin Cream 20% (Occasional) ... 2868
Cataflam (Less than 1%) ... 816
Cerumenex Drops (1% of 2,700 patients) ... 1993
Claritin (2% or fewer patients) ... 2349
Claritin-D ... 2350
Clomid (Fewer than 1%) ... 1514
Clozaril Tablets (Less than 1%) ... 2252
Cognex Capsules (Infrequent) ... 1901
ColBENEMID Tablets ... 1622
Colestid Tablets (Rare) ... 2591
Colyte and Colyte-flavored (Isolated cases) ... 2396
Coumadin (Infrequent) ... 926
Cozaar Tablets (Less than 1%) ... 1628
Cytotec (Infrequent) ... 2424
Daraprim Tablets (Rare) ... 1090
Dilantin Infatabs ... 1908
Dilantin Kapseals (Rare) ... 1906
Dilantin-125 Suspension (Rare) ... 1911
▲ Dovonex Ointment 0.005% (1% to 10%) ... 2684
▲ Ergamisol Tablets (8% to 23%) ... 1292
Esimil Tablets ... 822
Fedahist Gyrocaps (Very rare) ... 2401
Fedahist Timecaps (Rare) ... 2401
Fluorouracil Injection (Substantial number of cases) ... 2116
Foscavir Injection (Less than 1%) .. 547
Sterile FUDR ... 2118
Glucophage ... 752
GoLYTELY (Isolated cases) ... 688
Halcion Tablets (Rare) ... 2611
Hibistat Germicidal Hand Rinse (Rare) ... 2841
Hivid Tablets (Less than 1% to less than 3%) ... 2121
Hyzaar Tablets ... 1677
IFEX (Less than 1%) ... 697
▲ Intron A (Up to 8%) ... 2364
Iopidine 0.5% (Less than 1%) ... ⊙ 221
Ismelin Tablets ... 827
▲ Leucovorin Calcium for Injection (1% to 25%) ... 1268
Lopid Tablets ... 1917
Lotensin Tablets ... 834
Lotrel Capsules ... 840
Loxitane ... 1378
Lupron Depot 7.5 mg (Less than 5%) ... 2559
▲ Lupron Injection (5% or more) ... 2555
Matulane Capsules ... 2131
Maxair Autohaler ... 1492
Maxair Inhaler (Less than 1%) ... 1494
Maxaquin Tablets ... 2440
Mellaril (Infrequent) ... 2269
Methotrexate Sodium Tablets, Injection, for Injection and LPF Injection (1 to 3%) ... 1275
Myambutol Tablets ... 1386
Mykrox Tablets ... 993
Myochrysine Injection ... 1711
Norplant System ... 2759
Norvasc Tablets (Less than or equal to 0.1%) ... 1940
Novahistine DH (Rare) ... 2462
Novahistine Elixir (Very rare) ... ▣ 823
NuLYTELY ... 689
Cherry Flavor NuLYTELY (Isolated cases) ... 689
pHisoHex ... 2327
Phenergan Injection ... 2773
Phenergan Tablets ... 2775
Prinzide Tablets (0.3 to 1%) ... 1737
Procardia Capsules (2% or less) ... 1971
Proglycem ... 580
▲ Ridaura Capsules (Second most common) ... 2513
▲ Rogaine Topical Solution (7.36%) .. 2637
Salagen Tablets (Rare) ... 1489
Solganal Suspension ... 2388
Talwin Injection ... 2334
Talwin Nx ... 2336
Temaril Tablets, Syrup and Spansule Extended-Release Capsules ... 483
Temovate Scalp Application (1 of 294 patients) ... 1179
Tenex Tablets (3% or less) ... 2074
Thioplex (Thiotepa For Injection) ... 1281
Travase Ointment ... 1356
Urispas Tablets ... 2532
Urobiotic-250 Capsules (Rare) ... 2214
Varivax (Greater than or equal to 1%) ... 1762
Voltaren Tablets (Less than 1%) ... 861
▲ Xanax Tablets (3.8%) ... 2649
Zaroxolyn Tablets ... 1000
Ziac ... 1415
Zoloft Tablets (Rare) ... 2217

Dermatitis, allergic

Antabuse Tablets (Small number of patients) ... 2695
Cortone Acetate Sterile Suspension ... 1623
Cortone Acetate Tablets ... 1624
Dalalone D.P. Injectable ... 1011
Decadron Elixir ... 1633
Decadron Phosphate Injection ... 1637
Decadron Phosphate Respihaler ... 1642
Decadron Phosphate Turbinaire ... 1645
Decadron Phosphate with Xylocaine Injection, Sterile ... 1639
Decadron Tablets ... 1635
Decadron-LA Sterile Suspension ... 1646
Dexacort Phosphate in Respihaler .. 458
Dexacort Phosphate in Turbinaire .. 459
Elocon (Infrequent) ... 2354
Halog (Infrequent) ... 2686
Hydeltrasol Injection, Sterile ... 1665
Hydeltra-T.B.A. Sterile Suspension 1667
Hydrocortone Acetate Sterile Suspension ... 1669
Hydrocortone Phosphate Injection, Sterile ... 1670
Hydrocortone Tablets ... 1672
Lidex (Infrequent) ... 2130
Lotrisone Cream (Infrequent) ... 2372
Monistat-Derm (miconazole nitrate 2%) Cream (Isolated reports) ... 1889
ProctoFoam-HC ... 2409
Serophene (clomiphene citrate tablets, USP) (Less than 1 in 100 patients) ... 2451
Tridesilon Cream 0.05% (Infrequent) ... 615
Tridesilon Ointment 0.05% (Infrequent) ... 616

Dermatitis, bullous

Chloroptic Sterile Ophthalmic Solution ... ⊙ 239
Dilantin Infatabs ... 1908
Dilantin Kapseals ... 1906
Dilantin Parenteral ... 1910
Dilantin-125 Suspension ... 1911
Elase-Chloromycetin Ointment ... 1040
Lincocin (Rare instances) ... 2617
Miltown Tablets (Rare) ... 2672
PMB 200 and PMB 400 (Rare) ... 2783
Solganal Suspension (Occasional) .. 2388
T.R.U.E. Test ... 1189
Zyloprim Tablets (Less than 1%) ... 1226

Dermatitis, contact

Americaine Anesthetic Lubricant ... 983
Americaine Otic Topical Anesthetic Ear Drops ... 983
Bactroban Ointment (Less than 1%) ... 2470
BenzaShave Medicated Shave Cream 5% and 10% ... 1590
Betaseron for SC Injection ... 658
Capitrol Shampoo ... 2683
Cleocin Vaginal Cream ... 2589
Compazine ... 2470
Deponit NTG Transdermal Delivery System ... 2397
Dilacor XR Extended-release Capsules ... 2018
Effexor (Infrequent) ... 2719
Eldopaque Forte 4% Cream (Occasional) ... 1252
Eldoquin Forte 4% Cream (Occasional) ... 1252
Etrafon ... 2355
Furacin Soluble Dressing (Approximately 1%) ... 2045
Furacin Topical Cream (Approximately 1%) ... 2045
Iopidine 0.5% (Less than 1%) ... ⊙ 221
Mellaril ... 2269
Navane Capsules and Concentrate 2201
Navane Intramuscular ... 2202
Nitro-Bid IV ... 1523
Nitro-Bid Ointment (Uncommon) ... 1524
Nitro-Dur (nitroglycerin) Transdermal Infusion System (Uncommon) ... 1326
Nizoral 2% Cream (Rare) ... 1297
Paxil Tablets (Rare) ... 2505
Prozac Pulvules & Liquid, Oral Solution (Infrequent) ... 919
Rhinocort Nasal Inhaler (Less than 1%) ... 556
Serentil ... 684
Solaquin Forte 4% Cream (Occasional) ... 1252
Solaquin Forte 4% Gel (Occasional) ... 1252
Thioplex (Thiotepa For Injection) ... 1281
Thorazine ... 2523
Torecan ... 2245
Tympagesic Ear Drops ... 2342
Varivax (Greater than or equal to 1%) ... 1762

Dermatitis, eczematoid

Symmetrel Capsules and Syrup (Less than 0.1%) ... 946
Zyloprim Tablets (Less than 1%) ... 1226

Dermatitis, erythematous

Phenobarbital Elixir and Tablets ... 1469

Dermatitis, exfoliative

▲ A/T/S 2% Acne Topical Gel and Solution (17 out of 90 patients) ... 1234
Accupril Tablets (Rare) ... 1893
Achromycin V Capsules (Uncommon) ... 1367
Adalat Capsules (10 mg and 20 mg) (Less than 0.5%) ... 587
Adalat CC (Rare) ... 589
Aldoclor Tablets ... 1598
Aldoril Tablets ... 1604
Ansaid Tablets (Rare) ... 2579
Aquasol A Vitamin A Capsules, USP ... 534
Atretol Tablets ... 573
Augmentin (Occasional case) ... 2468
Axid Pulvules ... 1427
Azactam for Injection (Less than 1%) ... 734
Azo Gantanol Tablets ... 2080
Azo Gantrisin Tablets ... 2081
Azulfidine (Rare) ... 1949
Bactrim DS Tablets ... 2084
Bactrim I.V. Infusion ... 2082
Bactrim ... 2084
Betaseron for SC Injection ... 658
Bicillin C-R Injection ... 2704
Bicillin C-R 900/300 Injection ... 2706
Bicillin L-A Injection ... 2707
Butisol Sodium Elixir & Tablets (Less than 1 in 100) ... 2660
Capoten ... 739
Capozide ... 742
Cardizem CD Capsules (Infrequent) ... 1506
Cardizem SR Capsules ... 1510
Cardizem Injectable ... 1508
Cardizem Tablets ... 1512
Cataflam (Rare) ... 816
Chibroxin Sterile Ophthalmic Solution (With oral form) ... 1617
Cipro I.V. (1% or less) ... 595
Cipro I.V. Pharmacy Bulk Package (Less than 1%) ... 597
Cipro Tablets ... 592
Clinoril Tablets ... 1618
Compazine ... 2470
Cuprimine Capsules ... 1630
Cytovene-IV (One report) ... 2103
Daypro Caplets (Less than 1%) ... 2426
Declomycin Tablets (Uncommon) ... 1371
Depen Titratable Tablets ... 2662
Diabinese Tablets ... 1935
Dilantin Infatabs ... 1908
Dilantin Kapseals ... 1906
Dilantin Parenteral ... 1910
Dilantin-125 Suspension ... 1911
Dilatrate-SR (Occasional) ... 2398
Diupres Tablets ... 1650
Diuril Oral Suspension ... 1653
Diuril Sodium Intravenous ... 1652
Diuril Tablets ... 1653
Dolobid Tablets (Less than 1 in 100) ... 1654
Doryx Capsules (Uncommon) ... 1913
Duragesic Transdermal System (Less than 1%) ... 1288
Dynacin Capsules (Uncommon) ... 1590
Effexor (Rare) ... 2719
Ergamisol Tablets (Less frequent) .. 1292
Etrafon ... 2355
Fansidar Tablets ... 2114
Feldene Capsules (Less than 1%) .. 1965
Fioricet with Codeine Capsules ... 2260
Fiorinal with Codeine Capsules ... 2262
Floxin I.V. ... 1571
Floxin Tablets (200 mg, 300 mg, 400 mg) ... 1567
Gantanol Tablets ... 2119
Gantrisin ... 2120
Hivid Tablets (Less than 1% to less than 3%) ... 2121

(▣ Described in PDR For Nonprescription Drugs) Incidence data in parenthesis; ▲ 3% or more (⊙ Described in PDR For Ophthalmology)

1267 **Side Effects Index** **Diabetes mellitus**

HydroDIURIL Tablets 1674
Hydropres Tablets 1675
Hyzaar Tablets 1677
Imitrex Tablets (Rare) 1106
Indocin Capsules (Less than 1%) 1680
Indocin I.V. (Less than 1%) 1684
Indocin (Less than 1%) 1680
Intal Capsules (Less than 1 in 100,000 patients) 987
Intal Inhaler (Rare) 988
Intal Nebulizer Solution (Rare) 989
Lasix Injection, Oral Solution and Tablets 1240
Levoprome 1274
Lincocin (Rare instances) 2617
Lopid Tablets 1917
Luvox Tablets (Infrequent) 2544
Macrobid Capsules (Rare) 1988
Macrodantin Capsules (Rare) 1989
Maxaquin Tablets 2440
Mebaral Tablets (Less than 1 in 100) 2322
Mefoxin 1691
Mefoxin Premixed Intravenous Solution 1694
Mellaril 2269
Mesantoin Tablets (Rare) 2272
Mexitil Capsules (Rare) 678
Miltown Tablets (Rare) 2672
Minocin Intravenous (Uncommon) 1382
Minocin Oral Suspension (Uncommon) 1385
Minocin Pellet-Filled Capsules (Uncommon) 1383
Moduretic Tablets 1705
Monodox Capsules (Uncommon) 1805
Monopril Tablets 757
Motrin Ibuprofen Suspension, Oral Drops, Chewable Tablets, Caplets (Less than 1%) 1546
Myochrysine Injection 1711
Nalfon 200 Pulvules & Nalfon Tablets (Less than 1%) 917
Nasalcrom Nasal Solution (Rare) 994
Navane Capsules and Concentrate 2201
Navane Intramuscular 2202
Nebcin Vials, Hyporets & ADD-Vantage 1464
Nembutal Sodium Capsules (Less than 1%) 436
Nembutal Sodium Solution 438
Nembutal Sodium Suppositories (Less than 1%) 440
Nitrolingual Spray 2027
Noroxin Tablets 1715
Noroxin Tablets 2048
Omnipen Capsules (Occasional) 2764
Omnipen for Oral Suspension (Occasional) 2765
Orudis Capsules (Less than 1%) 2766
Oruvail Capsules (Less than 1%) 2766
PMB 200 and PMB 400 (Rare) 2783
PASER Granules 1285
Pen•Vee K 2772
Pfizerpen for Injection 2203
Phenobarbital Elixir and Tablets (Less than 1 in 100 patients) 1469
Plaquenil Sulfate Tablets 2328
Prinzide Tablets 1737
Procardia XL Extended Release Tablets (Rare) 1972
▲ Proleukin for Injection (14%) 797
Prolixin 509
Proloprim Tablets (Rare) 1155
Prozac Pulvules & Liquid, Oral Solution 919
Rifamate Capsules 1530
Rifater 1532
Risperdal (Infrequent) 1301
Ritalin 848
SSD 1355
Seconal Sodium Pulvules (Less than 1 in 100) 1474
Septra 1174
Septra I.V. Infusion 1169
Septra I.V. Infusion ADD-Vantage Vials 1171
Septra 1174
Serentil 684
Silvadene Cream 1% 1540
Solganal Suspension (Occasional) 2388
Spectrobid Tablets (Occasional) 2206
Stelazine (Occasional) 2514
Tagamet (Very rare) 2516
Tambocor Tablets (Less than 1%) 1497
Tapazole Tablets 1477
Tegretol Chewable Tablets 852
Tegretol Suspension 852
Tegretol Tablets 852
Tenex Tablets (Less frequent) 2074
Terramycin Intramuscular Solution (Uncommon) 2210
Thorazine 2523
Ticlid Tablets (Rare) 2156
Timolide Tablets 1748
Tonocard Tablets (Less than 1%) 531
Toradol 2159
Torecan 2245
Triavil Tablets 1757
Trilafon 2389
Trimpex Tablets (Rare) 2163
Unasyn (Occasional) 2212
Vancocin HCl, Oral Solution & Pulvules (Infrequent) 1483
Vancocin HCl, Vials & ADD-Vantage (Infrequent) 1481
Vantin for Oral Suspension and Vantin Tablets (Less than 1%) 2646
Vaseretic Tablets 1765
Vasosulf ⊙ 271
Vasotec I.V. 1768
Vasotec Tablets (0.5% to 1.0%) 1771
Vibramycin (Uncommon) 1941
Vibramycin Hyclate Intravenous (Uncommon) 2215
Vibramycin (Uncommon) 1941
Videx Tablets, Powder for Oral Solution, & Pediatric Powder for Oral Solution (Less than 1%) 720
Voltaren Tablets (Rare) 861
Wellbutrin Tablets 1204
Zebeta Tablets 1413
Zerit Capsules (Up to 1%) 729
Zestoretic 2850
Ziac (Very rare) 1415
Zyloprim Tablets (Less than 1%) 1226

Dermatitis, eyelid

OptiPranolol (Metipranolol 0.3%) Sterile Ophthalmic Solution (A small number of patients) ⊙ 258
Vantin for Oral Suspension and Vantin Tablets 2646

Dermatitis, flare-up

T.R.U.E. Test 1189

Dermatitis, fungal

▲ CellCept Capsules (More than or equal to 3%) 2099
Effexor (Rare) 2719
Lamictal Tablets (Rare) 1112
Permax Tablets (Infrequent) 575
Prozac Pulvules & Liquid, Oral Solution (Rare) 919
Videx Tablets, Powder for Oral Solution, & Pediatric Powder for Oral Solution (Less than 1%) 720

Dermatitis, gold-induced

Ridaura Capsules 2513
Solganal Suspension 2388

Dermatitis, lichenoides

Betaseron for SC Injection 658
Effexor (Rare) 2719
Intron A (Less than 5%) 2364
Permax Tablets (Rare) 575
Risperdal (Rare) 1301

Dermatitis, maculopapular

Chloroptic S.O.P. ⊙ 239
Chloroptic Sterile Ophthalmic Solution ⊙ 239
Elase-Chloromycetin Ointment 1040
Solganal Suspension (Occasional) 2388

Dermatitis, perioral

Aclovate Cream 1069
Analpram-HC Rectal Cream 1% and 2.5% 977
Anusol-HC Cream 2.5% (Infrequent to frequent) 1896
Aristocort A 0.025% Cream (Infrequent) 1027
Aristocort A 0.5% Cream 1031
Aristocort A 0.1% Cream (Infrequent) 1029
Aristocort A 0.1% Ointment (Infrequent) 1030
Carmol HC (Infrequent to frequent) 924
Cordran Lotion (Infrequent) 1803
Cordran Tape (Infrequent) 1804
Cortisporin Cream 1084
Cortisporin Ointment 1085
Cortisporin Otic Solution Sterile 1087
Cortisporin Otic Suspension Sterile 1088
Cutivate Cream 1088
Cutivate Ointment 1089
Cyclocort Topical (Infrequent) 1037
Decadron Phosphate Topical Cream 1644
Decaspray Topical Aerosol 1648
Dermatop Emollient Cream 0.1% (Infrequent to frequent) 1238
DesOwen Cream, Ointment and Lotion (Infrequent) 1046
Diprolene AF Cream (Infrequent) 2352
Diprolene Gel 0.05% (Infrequent) 2353
Diprolene (Infrequent) 2352
Elocon (Infrequent) 2354
Epifoam (Infrequent) 2399
Florone/Florone E 906
Halog (Infrequent) 2686
Hytone 907
Lidex (Infrequent) 2130
Locoid Cream, Ointment and Topical Solution (Infrequent) 978
Lotrisone Cream (Infrequent) 2372
NeoDecadron Topical Cream 1714
PediOtic Suspension Sterile 1153
Pramosone Cream, Lotion & Ointment 978
ProctoCream-HC (Infrequent) 2408
ProctoCream-HC 2.5% (Infrequent to frequent) 2408
ProctoFoam-HC 2409
Psorcon Cream 0.05% (Infrequent) 909
Psorcon Ointment 0.05% 908
Synalar (Infrequent) 2130
Temovate (Infrequent) 1179
Topicort (Infrequent) 1243
Tridesilon Cream 0.05% (Infrequent) 615
Tridesilon Ointment 0.05% (Infrequent) 616
Ultravate Cream 0.05% (Infrequent) 2689
Ultravate Ointment 0.05% (Less frequent) 2690
Westcort 2690

Dermatitis, photosensitive

Anaprox/Naprosyn (Less than 1%) 2117
▲ Cordarone Tablets (4 to 9%) 2712
EC-Naprosyn Delayed-Release Tablets (Less than 1%) 2117
Intal Capsules (Less than 1 in 100,000 patients) 987
Intal Inhaler (Rare) 988
Intal Nebulizer Solution (Rare) 989
Anaprox/Naprosyn (Less than 1%) 2117

Dermatitis, purpuric

Dilantin Infatabs 1908
Dilantin Kapseals 1906
Dilantin Parenteral 1910
Dilantin-125 Suspension 1911

Dermatitis, radiation recall

Methotrexate Sodium Tablets, Injection, for Injection and LPF Injection 1275
VePesid Capsules and Injection (Single case) 718

Dermatitis, vesicular bullous (see under Dermatitis, bullous)

Dermatologic reactions, unspecified

Altace Capsules (Less than 1%) 1232
▲ Atgam Sterile Solution (1 in 8 patients) 2581
Ativan Tablets (Less frequent) 2700
Bentyl 1501
Capoten 739
Capozide 742
Clinoril Tablets (Less than 1 in 100) 1618
Depen Titratable Tablets (Rare) 2662
Esgic-plus Tablets (Infrequent) 1013
Floxin I.V. 1571
Floxin Tablets (200 mg, 300 mg, 400 mg) 1567
Hydrea Capsules (Less frequent) 696
▲ Idamycin (46%) 1955
Kerlone Tablets (Less than 2%) 2436
Kutrase Capsules 2402
Levbid Extended-Release Tablets 2405
Levoprome 1274
Levsin/Levsinex/Levbid 2405
Metrodin (urofollitropin for injection) 2446
Monopril Tablets 757
Norflex (Rare) 1496
Norgesic (Rare) 1496
Phrenilin (Several cases) 785
Prinivil Tablets (0.3% to 1.0%) 1733
Prinzide Tablets 1737
Pro-Banthīne Tablets 2052
SSD 1355
Sedapap Tablets 50 mg/650 mg (Several cases) 1543
Silvadene Cream 1% 1540
Solu-Cortef Sterile Powder 2641
Solu-Medrol Sterile Powder 2643
Vaseretic Tablets 1765
Vasotec I.V. 1768
Vasotec Tablets (0.5% to 1.0%) 1771
▲ Xanax Tablets (Greater than 3%) 2649
Zestoretic 2850
Zestril Tablets (0.3% to 1.0%) 2854

Dermatomyositis

Cuprimine Capsules (Rare) 1630
Depen Titratable Tablets (Rare) 2662
Pravachol (Rare) 765

Dermatomyositis, exacerbation of

Actimmune (Rare) 1056

Dermatopolymycositis

Accupril Tablets (Rare) 1893

Descemetitis

Fluoracaine (Sometimes) ⊙ 206
FLURESS (Sometimes) ⊙ 207
Ophthetic ⊙ 247

Despondency

Hydropres Tablets 1675

Desquamation

A/T/S 2% Acne Topical Gel and Solution 1234
Aquasol A Vitamin A Capsules, USP 534
Cognex Capsules (Rare) 1901
Cytosar-U Sterile Powder (Rare) 2592
Erycette (erythromycin 2%) Topical Solution 1888
Feldene Capsules (Less than 1%) 1965
Fluorouracil Injection 2116
Hivid Tablets (Less than 1% to less than 3%) 2121
NebuPent for Inhalation Solution (1% or less) 1040
Neurontin Capsules (Rare) 1922
Peridex 1978
T-Stat 2.0% Topical Solution and Pads 2688
Theramycin Z Topical Solution 2% 1592
Vagistat-1 (Less than 1%) 778

Diabetes (see under Diabetes mellitus)

Diabetes insipidus, nephrogenic

Betaseron for SC Injection 658
Declomycin Tablets 1371
Eskalith (Some reports) 2485
Foscavir Injection (Rare) 547
Lithonate/Lithotabs/Lithobid (Occasional) 2543
Zanosar Sterile Powder (Two cases) 2653

Diabetes mellitus

Accutane Capsules 2076
Anafranil Capsules (Infrequent) 803
Betaseron for SC Injection 658
▲ CellCept Capsules (More than or equal to 3%) 2099
Cognex Capsules (Infrequent) 1901
Dyazide 2479
Effexor (Infrequent) 2719
Foscavir Injection (Less than 1%) 547
Hivid Tablets (Less than 1% to less than 3%) 2121
Hydeltra-T.B.A. Sterile Suspension 1667
Kerlone Tablets (Less than 2%) 2436
Lupron Depot 3.75 mg 2556
Lupron Depot 7.5 mg (Less than 5%) 2559
Lupron Injection (Less than 5%) 2555
Luvox Tablets (Rare) 2544
Macrobid Capsules 1988
Macrodantin Capsules 1989
Maxzide 1380
Methotrexate Sodium Tablets, Injection, for Injection and LPF Injection 1275
Paxil Tablets (Rare) 2505
Permax Tablets (Infrequent) 575
PREVACID Delayed-Release Capsules (Less than 1%) 2562
Prinivil Tablets (0.3% to 1.0%) 1733

(▣ Described in PDR For Nonprescription Drugs) Incidence data in parenthesis; ▲ 3% or more (⊙ Described in PDR For Ophthalmology)

Diabetes mellitus **Side Effects Index** **1268**

Prinzide Tablets ... 1737
▲Prograf (Greater than 3%) ... 1042
Pulmozyme Inhalation ... 1064
Risperdal (Infrequent) ... 1301
Videx Tablets, Powder for Oral Solution, & Pediatric Powder for Oral Solution (1%) ... 720
Zestoretic ... 2850
Zestril Tablets (0.3% to 1.0%) ... 2854

Diabetes mellitus, increase

Hydrocortone Phosphate Injection, Sterile ... 1670

Diabetes mellitus, precipitation of latent

Apresazide Capsules ... 808
Aristocort Suspension (Forte Parenteral) ... 1027
Aristocort Suspension (Intralesional) ... 1025
Aristocort Tablets ... 1022
Aristospan Suspension (Intra-articular) ... 1033
Aristospan Suspension (Intralesional) ... 1032
Capozide ... 742
Celestone Soluspan Suspension ... 2347
CORTENEMA ... 2535
Cortone Acetate Sterile Suspension ... 1623
Cortone Acetate Tablets ... 1624
Dalalone D.P. Injectable ... 1011
Decadron Elixir ... 1633
Decadron Phosphate Injection ... 1637
Decadron Phosphate Respihaler ... 1642
Decadron Phosphate Turbinaire ... 1645
Decadron Phosphate with Xylocaine Injection, Sterile ... 1639
Decadron Tablets ... 1635
Decadron-LA Sterile Suspension ... 1646
Deltasone Tablets ... 2595
Depo-Medrol Single-Dose Vial ... 2600
Depo-Medrol Sterile Aqueous Suspension ... 2597
Dexacort Phosphate in Respihaler .. 458
Dexacort Phosphate in Turbinaire .. 459
Esidrix Tablets ... 821
Florinef Acetate Tablets ... 505
Hydeltrasol Injection, Sterile ... 1665
Hydrocortone Acetate Sterile Suspension ... 1669
Hydrocortone Tablets ... 1672
Intron A (Less than 5%) ... 2364
Lasix Injection, Oral Solution and Tablets (Rare) ... 1240
Maxzide ... 1380
Medrol ... 2621
Oretic Tablets ... 443
Orudis Capsules (Rare) ... 2766
Oruvail Capsules (Rare) ... 2766
Pediapred Oral Liquid ... 995
Prelone Syrup ... 1787
Prinzide Tablets ... 1737
Risperdal ... 1301
Solu-Cortef Sterile Powder ... 2641
Solu-Medrol Sterile Powder ... 2643
Tenoretic Tablets ... 2845
Vaseretic Tablets ... 1765
Zestoretic ... 2850

Dialysis encephalopathy

ALternaGEL Liquid ... 1316
Aludrox Oral Suspension ... 2695
Amphojel ... 2695
Basaljel ... 2703
Gelusil Liquid & Tablets ... ■ 855
Maalox Heartburn Relief Suspension ... ■ 642
Maalox Heartburn Relief Tablets.. ■ 641
Maalox Magnesia and Alumina Oral Suspension ... ■ 642
Maalox Plus Tablets ... ■ 643
Extra Strength Maalox Antacid Plus Antigas Liquid and Tablets ... ■ 638
Mylanta Liquid ... 1317
Mylanta Tablets ... ■ 660
Mylanta Double Strength Liquid ... 1317
Mylanta Double Strength Tablets ■ 660
Rolaids Tablets ... ■ 843

Dialysis osteomalacia, results in, or worsening of

ALternaGEL Liquid ... 1316
Aludrox Oral Suspension ... 2695
Amphojel ... 2695
Basaljel ... 2703
Gelusil Liquid & Tablets ... ■ 855
Maalox Heartburn Relief Suspension ... ■ 642
Maalox Heartburn Relief Tablets.. ■ 641
Maalox Magnesia and Alumina Oral Suspension ... ■ 642
Extra Strength Maalox Antacid Plus Antigas Liquid and Tablets ... ■ 638
Mylanta Liquid ... 1317
Mylanta Tablets ... ■ 660
Mylanta Double Strength Liquid ... 1317
Mylanta Double Strength Tablets ■ 660
Rolaids Tablets ... ■ 843

Diaphoresis

Accupril Tablets (0.5% to 1.0%) .. 1893
Accutane Capsules (Less than 1%) ... 2076
Actifed with Codeine Cough Syrup.. 1067
Actigall Capsules ... 802
Adalat Capsules (10 mg and 20 mg) (2% or less) ... 587
Adalat CC (Less than 1.0%) ... 589
Adenocard Injection (Less than 1%) ... 1021
Adenoscan (Less than 1%) ... 1024
AeroBid Inhaler System (1-3%) ... 1005
Aerobid-M Inhaler System (1-3%).. 1005
Albalon Solution with Liquifilm ... ⊙ 231
Altace Capsules (Less than 1%) ... 1232
Alupent Tablets (0.2%) ... 669
Ambien Tablets (Infrequent) ... 2416
▲Anafranil Capsules (9% to 29%) ... 803
Ana-Kit Anaphylaxis Emergency Treatment Kit ... 617
Anaprox/Naprosyn (Less than 3%) ... 2117
Ansaid Tablets (Less than 1%) ... 2579
AquaMEPHYTON Injection ... 1608
Aredia for Injection ... 810
Aristocort Suspension (Forte Parenteral) ... 1027
Aristocort Suspension (Intralesional) ... 1025
Aristocort Tablets ... 1022
Aristospan Suspension (Intra-articular) ... 1033
Aristospan Suspension (Intralesional) ... 1032
▲Asacol Delayed-Release Tablets (3%) ... 1979
Asendin Tablets (Less frequent) ... 1369
Atamet ... 572
Atgam Sterile Solution (At least 1 patient and less than 5% of total patients) ... 2581
Atretol Tablets ... 573
Atromid-S Capsules ... 2701
▲Axid Pulvules (More frequent) ... 1427
Azactam for Injection (Less than 1%) ... 734
Benadryl Capsules ... 1898
Benadryl Injection ... 1898
▲Betapace Tablets (1% to 6%) ... 641
▲Betaseron for SC Injection (23%) .. 658
Blocadren Tablets (Less than 1%) 1614
Bontril Slow-Release Capsules ... 781
Brethine Ampuls (0.0 to 2.4%) ... 815
Brethine Tablets ... 814
▲Brevibloc Injection (12%) ... 1808
Bricanyl Subcutaneous Injection ... 1502
Bricanyl Tablets ... 1503
Brontex ... 1981
Bumex (0.1%) ... 2093
▲Buprenex Injectable (1-5%) ... 2006
BuSpar (1%) ... 737
Calan SR Caplets (1% or less) ... 2422
Calan Tablets (1% or less) ... 2419
Capoten ... 739
Capozide ... 742
Carbocaine Hydrochloride Injection 2303
Cardene I.V. (1.4%) ... 2709
Cardene SR Capsules (0.6%) ... 2097
Cardizem Injectable (Less than 1%) ... 1508
Cardura Tablets (0.5% to 1.1%) .. 2186
Cartrol Tablets (0.7-1.0%) ... 410
Cataflam (Less than 1%) ... 816
Caverject (Less than 1%) ... 2583
Celestone Soluspan Suspension ... 2347
▲CellCept Capsules (More than or equal to 3%) ... 2099
Cipro I.V. (1% or less) ... 595
Cipro I.V. Pharmacy Bulk Package (Less than 1%) ... 597
Claritin (2% or fewer patients) ... 2349
Claritin-D (Less frequent) ... 2350
Clinoril Tablets (Less than 1 in 100) ... 1618
▲Clozaril Tablets (More than 5 to 6%) ... 2252
Cognex Capsules (Frequent) ... 1901
Compazine ... 2470
CORTENEMA ... 2535
Cortifoam ... 2396
Cortone Acetate Sterile Suspension ... 1623
Cortone Acetate Tablets ... 1624
Cozaar Tablets (Less than 1%) ... 1628
Cystospaz ... 1963
Cytotec (Infrequent) ... 2424
▲Cytovene (11%) ... 2103
D.H.E. 45 Injection (Occasional) ... 2255
Dalalone D.P. Injectable ... 1011
Dalgan Injection (Less than 1%) ... 538
Dalmane Capsules (Rare) ... 2173
Danocrine Capsules ... 2307
Dantrium Capsules (Less frequent) 1982
Decadron Elixir ... 1633
Decadron Phosphate Injection ... 1637
Decadron Phosphate Respihaler ... 1642
Decadron Phosphate Turbinaire ... 1645
Decadron Phosphate with Xylocaine Injection, Sterile ... 1639
Decadron Tablets ... 1635
Decadron-LA Sterile Suspension ... 1646
Deconamine ... 1320
Deconsal C Expectorant Syrup ... 456
Deconsal Pediatric Syrup ... 457
Deltasone Tablets ... 2595
▲Demerol (Among most frequently observed) ... 2308
Depo-Medrol Single-Dose Vial ... 2600
Depo-Medrol Sterile Aqueous Suspension ... 2597
Depo-Provera Contraceptive Injection (Fewer than 1%) ... 2602
Desyrel and Desyrel Dividose (Less than 1% to 1.4%) ... 503
Dexacort Phosphate in Respihaler .. 458
Dexacort Phosphate in Turbinaire .. 459
Didrex Tablets ... 2607
Dilacor XR Extended-release Capsules ... 2018
Dilatrate-SR ... 2398
▲Dilaudid-HP Injection (Among most frequent) ... 1337
▲Dilaudid-HP Lyophilized Powder 250 mg (Among most frequent) ... 1337
Dilaudid Tablets and Liquid ... 1339
Diprivan Injection (Less than 1%) .. 2833
Dolobid Tablets (Less than 1 in 100) ... 1654
Dopram Injectable ... 2061
▲Duragesic Transdermal System (10% or more) ... 1288
Duvoid (Infrequent) ... 2044
Dyazide ... 2479
Easprin ... 1914
EC-Naprosyn Delayed-Release Tablets (Less than 3%) ... 2117
▲Effexor (2% to 19.3%) ... 2719
Elavil ... 2838
Eldepryl Tablets ... 2550
Emete-con Intramuscular/Intravenous ... 2198
▲Eminase (Less than 10%) ... 2039
Empirin with Codeine Tablets ... 1093
Endep Tablets ... 2174
Engerix-B Unit-Dose Vials (Less than 1%) ... 2482
▲Ethmozine Tablets (2% to 5%) ... 2041
Etrafon ... 2355
Felbatol ... 2666
Feldene Capsules (Less than 1%) .. 1965
Flexeril Tablets (Less than 1%) ... 1661
Florinef Acetate Tablets ... 505
Floropryl Sterile Ophthalmic Ointment (Rare) ... 1662
Floxin I.V. (Less than 1%) ... 1571
Floxin Tablets (200 mg, 300 mg, 400 mg) (Less than 1%) ... 1567
▲Fludara for Injection (1% to 13%) 663
Flumadine Tablets & Syrup ... 1015
▲Foscavir Injection (5% or greater).. 547
Glucotrol XL Extended Release Tablets (Less than 3%) ... 1968
Haldol Decanoate ... 1577
Haldol Injection, Tablets and Concentrate ... 1575
Hivid Tablets (Less than 1% to less than 3%) ... 2121
Humorsol Sterile Ophthalmic Solution (Rare) ... 1664
Humulin 50/50, 100 Units ... 1444
Humulin 70/30, 100 Units ... 1445
Humulin L, 100 Units (Less common) ... 1446
Hydeltrasol Injection, Sterile ... 1665
Hydeltra-T.B.A. Sterile Suspension 1667
Hydrocortone Acetate Sterile Suspension ... 1669
Hydrocortone Phosphate Injection, Sterile ... 1670
Hydrocortone Tablets ... 1672
Hyperstat I.V. Injection ... 2363
Hytrin Capsules (At least 1%) ... 430
Hyzaar Tablets ... 1677
Regular, 100 Units ... 1450
Pork Regular, 100 Units (Less common) ... 1452
Imdur (Less than or equal to 5%) .. 1323
Imitrex Injection (1.6%) ... 1103
Imitrex Tablets (Infrequent) ... 1106
Indocin (Less than 1%) ... 1680
INFeD (Iron Dextran Injection, USP) ... 2345
▲Intron A (1% to 21%) ... 2364
Isoptin Injectable ... 1344
Isoptin Oral Tablets (Less than 1%) ... 1346
Isoptin SR Tablets (1% or less) ... 1348
Isopto Carbachol Ophthalmic Solution ... ⊙ 223
Isuprel Hydrochloride Injection 1:5000 ... 2311
Isuprel Hydrochloride Solution 1:200 & 1:100 ... 2313
Isuprel Mistometer ... 2312
Kerlone Tablets (Less than 2%) ... 2436
Lamictal Tablets (Infrequent) ... 1112
Larodopa Tablets (Infrequent) ... 2129
▲Leustatin (9%) ... 1834
Levatol (1.6%) ... 2403
Levo-Dromoran (Rare) ... 2129
Levophed Bitartrate Injection ... 2315
Limbitrol ... 2180
Lioresal Intrathecal ... 1596
Lioresal Tablets ... 829
Lithonate/Lithotabs/Lithobid ... 2543
Lodine Capsules and Tablets (Less than 1%) ... 2743
Lopressor HCT Tablets (1 in 100 patients) ... 832
Lorelco Tablets ... 1517
Lotensin Tablets ... 834
Lotensin HCT (0.3% to 1.0%) ... 837
Loxitane ... 1378
Ludiomil Tablets (Rare) ... 843
▲Lupron Depot 3.75 mg (72.9%) ... 2556
▲Lupron Depot 7.5 mg (58.9%) ... 2559
▲Luvox Tablets (7%) ... 2544
▲MS Contin Tablets (Less frequent to among most frequent) ... 1994
▲MSIR (Among most frequent) ... 1997
Marax Tablets & DF Syrup ... 2200
Marcaine Hydrochloride with Epinephrine 1:200,000 (Rare) ... 2316
Marcaine Hydrochloride Injection (Rare) ... 2316
Marcaine Spinal (Rare) ... 2319
Marinol (Dronabinol) Capsules (Less than 1%) ... 2231
Matulane Capsules ... 2131
Maxaquin Tablets (Less than 1%) .. 2440
Medrol ... 2621
Megace Oral Suspension (1% to 3%) ... 699
Mellaril ... 2269
▲Mepergan Injection (Among most frequent) ... 2753
Mephyton Tablets (Rare) ... 1696
▲Mepron Suspension (10%) ... 1135
Mestinon Injectable ... 1253
Mestinon ... 1254
Methadone Hydrochloride Oral Concentrate ... 2233
Methadone Hydrochloride Oral Solution & Tablets ... 2235
Methergine (Rare) ... 2272
Methotrexate Sodium Tablets, Injection, for Injection and LPF Injection (Less common) ... 1275
Mexitil Capsules (Less than 1% or about 6 in 1,000) ... 678
Minipress Capsules ... 1937
Minizide Capsules ... 1938
Miochol-E with Iocare Steri-Tags and Miochol-E System Pak (Rare) ... ⊙ 273
MIOSTAT Intraocular Solution ... ⊙ 224
Moban Tablets and Concentrate ... 1048
Moduretic Tablets (Less than or equal to 1%) ... 1705
Mono-Gesic Tablets ... 792
Monoket (Fewer than 1%) ... 2406
Monopril Tablets (0.2% to 1.0%).. 757
MSTA Mumps Skin Test Antigen ... 890
Myochrysine Injection ... 1711
▲Nalfon 200 Pulvules & Nalfon Tablets (4.6%) ... 917
Anaprox/Naprosyn (Less than 3%) ... 2117
Narcan Injection ... 934
Nardil (Less common) ... 1920

(■ Described in PDR For Nonprescription Drugs) Incidence data in parenthesis; ▲ 3% or more (⊙ Described in PDR For Ophthalmology)

1269 Side Effects Index Diarrhea

Navane Capsules and Concentrate 2201
Navane Intramuscular 2202
Nescaine/Nescaine MPF 554
Neurontin Capsules (Infrequent) 1922
Nicoderm (nicotine transdermal system) (1% to 3%) 1518
Nicorette (1% to 3% of patients) 2458
Nicotrol Nicotine Transdermal System (1% to 3%) 1550
Nimotop Capsules (Less than 1%) 610
Nitrolingual Spray 2027
Norisodrine with Calcium Iodide Syrup 442
▲ Normodyne Injection (4%) 2377
Normodyne Tablets (Less than 1%) 2379
Norpramin Tablets 1526
Norvasc Tablets (More than 0.1% to 1%) 1940
Novolin 70/30 Prefilled Disposable Insulin Delivery System (Rare) 1798
▲ Nubain Injection (9%) 935
Nucofed 2051
▲ Oramorph SR (Morphine Sulfate Sustained Release Tablets) (Among most frequent) 2236
Orap Tablets 1050
▲ Orlamm (3% to 9%) 2239
Ornade Spansule Capsules 2502
Orthoclone OKT3 Sterile Solution 1837
Orudis Capsules (Less than 1%) 2766
Oruvail Capsules (Less than 1%) 2766
Pamelor 2280
Papaverine Hydrochloride Vials and Ampoules 1468
▲ Paxil Tablets (11.2% to 11.8%) 2505
Pediapred Oral Liquid 995
Pentasa (Less than 1%) 1527
Peptavlon 2878
Periactin 1724
Permax Tablets (2.1%) 575
Phenergan with Codeine 2777
Phenergan VC with Codeine 2781
Pilocar (Extremely rare) ⊙ 268
Pilopine HS Ophthalmic Gel (Occasional) ⊙ 226
Placidyl Capsules 448
Pondimin Tablets 2066
Ponstel 1925
Prelone Syrup 1787
Prinivil Tablets (0.3% to 1.0%) 1733
Prinzide Tablets (0.3% to 1%) 1737
Procardia Capsules (2% or less) 1971
Procardia XL Extended Release Tablets (1% or less) 1972
▲ Prograf (Greater than 3%) 1042
Prolixin 509
ProSom Tablets (Infrequent) 449
Prostep (nicotine transdermal system) (1% to 3% of patients) 1394
Prostigmin Injectable 1260
Prostigmin Tablets 1261
Prostin E2 Suppository 2634
Proventil Syrup (Less than 1 of 100 patients) 2385
▲ Prozac Pulvules & Liquid, Oral Solution (5% to 8.4%) 919
Quadrinal Tablets 1350
▲ RMS Suppositories (Among most frequent) 2657
Recombivax HB (Less than 1%) 1744
Relafen Tablets (1% to 3%) 2510
▲ Retrovir Capsules (5%) 1158
▲ Retrovir I.V. Infusion (5%) 1163
▲ Retrovir Syrup (5%) 1158
Rifater 1532
Risperdal (Infrequent) 1301
Rocephin Injectable Vials, ADD-Vantage, Galaxy Container (Occasional) 2142
▲ Roferon-A Injection (7% to 8%) 2145
▲ Romazicon (1% to 9%) 2147
▲ Roxanol (Among most frequent) 2243
Rythmol Tablets–150mg, 225mg, 300mg (0.6 to 1.4%) 1352
▲ Salagen Tablets (29% to 68%) 1489
Sandoglobulin I.V. (Less than 1%) 2290
Sanorex Tablets 2294
Seldane Tablets 1536
Seldane-D Extended-Release Tablets 1538
Sensorcaine (Rare) 559
Serentil 684
Serzone Tablets 771
Sinemet Tablets 943
Sinemet CR Tablets 944
Sinequan (Occasional) 2205
Solganal Suspension 2388
Solu-Cortef Sterile Powder 2641
Solu-Medrol Sterile Powder 2643
Stadol (1% or greater) 775
Stelazine 2514
Sublimaze Injection 1307
▲ Supprelin Injection (1% to 10%) 2056
Surmontil Capsules 2811
Talacen 2333
Talwin Injection 2334
Talwin Compound 2335
Talwin Injection 2334
Talwin Nx 2336
Tambocor Tablets (1% to less than 3%) 1497
Tavist Syrup 2297
Tavist Tablets 2298
▲ Tegison Capsules (1-10%) 2154
Tegretol Chewable Tablets 852
Tegretol Suspension 852
Tegretol Tablets 852
Tenex Tablets (3% or less) 2074
Tensilon Injectable 1261
Thorazine 2523
THYREL TRH (Less frequent) 2873
Timolide Tablets 1748
Timoptic in Ocudose 1753
Timoptic Sterile Ophthalmic Solution 1751
Timoptic-XE 1755
Tofranil Ampuls 854
Tofranil Tablets 856
Tofranil-PM Capsules 857
▲ Tonocard Tablets (2.3-5.1%) 531
Toradol (Greater than 1%) 2159
▲ Trandate (4 of 100 patients) 1185
Triavil Tablets 1757
Trilafon 2389
Trinalin Repetabs Tablets 1330
Univasc Tablets (Less than 1%) 2410
Urecholine 1761
Vascor (200, 300 and 400 mg) Tablets (0.5 to 2.0%) 1587
Vaseretic Tablets (0.5% to 2.0%) 1765
Vasotec I.V. 1768
Vasotec Tablets (0.5% to 1.0%) 1771
Vasoxyl Injection 1196
Velosulin BR Human Insulin 10 ml Vials 1795
Ventolin Syrup (Less than 1 of 100 patients) 1202
VePesid Capsules and Injection (Sometimes) 718
Verelan Capsules (1% or less) 1410
Verelan Capsules (Less than 1%) 2824
▲ Videx Tablets, Powder for Oral Solution, & Pediatric Powder for Oral Solution (1% to 8%) 720
Vivactil Tablets 1774
Voltaren Tablets (Less than 1%) 861
▲ Wellbutrin Tablets (22.3%) 1204
▲ Xanax Tablets (15.1%) 2649
Yocon (Common) 1892
Yutopar Intravenous Injection (Infrequent) 570
Zebeta Tablets (0.7% to 1.0%) 1413
▲ Zerit Capsules (Fewer than 1% to 19%) 729
Zestoretic (0.3 to 1%) 2850
Zestril Tablets (0.3% to 1.0%) 2854
Ziac 1415
▲ Zoladex (6% to 45%) 2858
▲ Zoloft Tablets (8.4%) 2217
Zosyn (1.0% or less) 1419
Zosyn Pharmacy Bulk Package (1.0% or less) 1422
Zovirax Sterile Powder (Less than 1%) 1223

Diaphoresis, nocturnal

▲ NebuPent for Inhalation Solution (10 to 23%) 1040
Roferon-A Injection 2145
Sandimmune (Rare) 2286

Diaphragm, paralyzed

Survanta Beractant Intratracheal Suspension 2226

Diarrhea

Accupril Tablets (1.7%) 1893
Accutane Capsules 2076
▲ Acel-Imune Diphtheria and Tetanus Toxoids and Acellular Pertussis Vaccine Adsorbed (3.5%) 1364
Achromycin V Capsules (Rare) 1367
▲ ActHIB (1.5% to 9.0%) 872
Actifed with Codeine Cough Syrup 1067
Actigall Capsules (Less than 1%) 802
▲ Actimmune (14%) 1056
Adalat Capsules (10 mg and 20 mg) (2% or less) 587
Adalat CC (Less than 1.0%) 589
Adipex-P Tablets and Capsules 1048
Adriamycin PFS (Occasional) 1947
Adriamycin RDF (Occasional) 1947
Children's Advil Suspension (Less than 3%) 2692
▲ AeroBid Inhaler System (10%) 1005
▲ Aerobid-M Inhaler System (10%) 1005
Aldactazide 2413
Aldactone 2414
Aldoclor Tablets 1598
Aldomet Ester HCl Injection 1602
Aldomet Oral 1600
Aldoril Tablets 1604
Alkeran for Injection (Infrequent) 1070
Alkeran Tablets (Infrequent) 1071
All-Flex Arcing Spring Diaphragm (See also Ortho Diaphragm Kits) 1865
Altace Capsules (Less than 1% to 1.1%) 1232
Alupent Tablets (1.2%) 669
Ambien Tablets (1% to 3%) 2416
Amicar Syrup, Tablets, and Injection (Occasional) 1267
Amoxil 2464
▲ Anafranil Capsules (7% to 13%) 803
Anaprox/Naprosyn (Less than 3%) 2117
Ancef Injection 2465
Ancobon Capsules 2079
▲ Ansaid Tablets (3-9%) 2579
Apresazide Capsules (Common) 808
Apresoline Hydrochloride Tablets (Common) 809
Aralen Hydrochloride Injection 2301
Aralen Phosphate Tablets 2301
Aredia for Injection (Up to 1%) 810
Arfonad Ampuls (Occasional) 2080
▲ Asacol Delayed-Release Tablets (7%) 1979
Asendin Tablets (Less than 1%) 1369
Atamet 572
▲ Atgam Sterile Solution (At least 1 patient to 10%) 2581
Atretol Tablets 573
Atrohist Plus Tablets 454
Atromid-S Capsules 2701
Attenuvax (Rare) 1610
▲ Augmentin (9%) 2468
▲ Axid Pulvules (7.2%) 1427
Azactam for Injection (1 to 1.3%) 734
Azo Gantanol Tablets 2080
Azo Gantrisin Tablets 2081
Azulfidine (Rare) 1949
BCG Vaccine, USP (TICE) (1.2%) 1814
Bactrim DS Tablets 2084
Bactrim I.V. Infusion 2082
Bactrim 2084
Benadryl Capsules 1898
Benadryl Injection 1898
Betagan ⊙ 233
▲ Betapace Tablets (2% to 7%) 641
▲ Betaseron for SC Injection (35%) 658
Betimol 0.25%, 0.5% ⊙ 261
Biavax II 1613
▲ Biaxin (3%) 405
Biphetamine Capsules 983
Blocadren Tablets (Less than 1%) 1614
Bontril Slow-Release Capsules 781
▲ Bromfed-DM Cough Syrup (Among most frequent) 1786
Bumex (0.1%) 2093
Buprenex Injectable (Rare) 2006
BuSpar (2%) 737
Calan SR Caplets (1% or less) 2422
Calan Tablets (1% or less) 2419
Capoten (About 0.5 to 2%) 739
Capozide (0.5 to 2%) 742
Carafate Suspension (Less than 0.5%) 1505
Carafate Tablets (Less than 0.5%) 1504
Cardizem CD Capsules (Less than 1%) 1506
Cardizem SR Capsules (Less than 1%) 1510
Cardizem Injectable 1508
Cardizem Tablets (Less than 1%) 1512
Cardura Tablets (2% to 2.3%) 2186
Carnitor Tablets and Solution 2453
Cartrol Tablets (2.1-4.4%) 410
▲ Cataflam (3% to 9%) 816
Ceclor Pulvules & Suspension (1 in 70) 1431
Cefizox for Intramuscular or Intravenous Use (Occasional) 1034
▲ Cefobid Intravenous/Intramuscular (1 in 30) 2189
▲ Cefobid Pharmacy Bulk Package - Not for Direct Infusion (1 in 30) 2192
▲ Cefotan (Among most frequent; 1 in 80) 2829
▲ Ceftin (3.7% to 8.6%) 1078
Cefzil Tablets and Oral Suspension (2.9%) 746
▲ CellCept Capsules (31.0% to 36.1%; 16.4% to 18.8%) 2099
Celontin Kapseals (Frequent) 1899
Ceptaz (One in 78 patients) 1081
Ceredase 1065
Cerubidine (Occasional) 795
Cervidil (Less than 1%) 1010
▲ CHEMET (succimer) Capsules (12 to 20.9%) 1545
Chloromycetin Sodium Succinate 1900
Chromagen Capsules 2339
Cipro I.V. (1% or less) 595
▲ Cipro I.V. Pharmacy Bulk Package (Among most frequent) 597
Cipro Tablets (2.3%) 592
Claforan Sterile and Injection (1.4%) 1235
Claritin (2% or fewer patients) 2349
Claritin-D (Less frequent) 2350
Cleocin Phosphate Injection 2586
Cleocin T Topical 2590
Cleocin Vaginal Cream (Less than 1%) 2589
▲ Clinoril Tablets (3-9%) 1618
Clomid (2.2%; fewer than 1%) 1514
Clozaril Tablets (2%) 2252
▲ Cognex Capsules (16%) 1901
ColBENEMID Tablets 1622
Colestid Tablets (Less frequent) 2591
Combipres Tablets 677
Comhist 2038
Cordarone Intravenous (Less than 2%) 2715
Cosmegen Injection 1626
Coumadin (Infrequent) 926
Cozaar Tablets (2.4%) 1628
▲ Creon (Among most frequent) 2536
Crystodigin Tablets 1433
Cuprimine Capsules 1630
Cyklokapron Tablets and Injection 1950
▲ Cytosar-U Sterile Powder (Among most frequent) 2592
▲ Cytotec (14-40%) 2424
▲ Cytovene (41%) 2103
Cytoxan (Less frequent) 694
D.H.E. 45 Injection (Occasional) 2255
DTIC-Dome (Rare) 600
Dalgan Injection (Less than 1%) 538
Dalmane Capsules 2173
▲ Dantrium Capsules (Among most frequent) 1982
Daraprim Tablets (Rare) 1090
▲ Daypro Caplets (3% to 9%) 2426
Declomycin Tablets 1371
Deconamine 1320
Demadex Tablets and Injection (2.0%) 686
▲ Demser Capsules (10%) 1649
Depakene 413
Depakote Tablets 415
▲ Depen Titratable Tablets (17%) 2662
Desferal Vials 820
Desoxyn Gradumet Tablets 419
Desyrel and Desyrel Dividose (Up to 4.5%) 503
Dexedrine 2474
DextroStat Dextroamphetamine Tablets 2036
Diabinese Tablets (Less than 2%) 1935
Diamox Intravenous 1372
Diamox Sequels (Sustained Release) 1373
Diamox Tablets 1372
Didrex Tablets 2607
▲ Didronel Tablets (About 1 patient in 15; possibly 2 or 3 in 10) 1984
Diflucan Injection, Tablets, and Oral Suspension (2% to 3%) 2194
Dilacor XR Extended-release Capsules (2.0%) 2018
Dilaudid-HP Injection (Less frequent) 1337
Dilaudid-HP Lyophilized Powder 250 mg (Less frequent) 1337
Dilaudid Tablets and Liquid 1339
Dimetane-DC Cough Syrup 2059
Dimetane-DX Cough Syrup 2059
▲ Dipentum Capsules (11.1% to about 17%; rare) 1951
Diprivan Injection (Less than 1%) 2833
Diucardin Tablets 2718
Diupres Tablets 1650
Diuril Oral Suspension 1653
Diuril Sodium Intravenous 1652
Diuril Tablets 1653
▲ Dolobid Tablets (3% to 9%) 1654
Dopram Injectable 2061
Doral Tablets 2664
Doryx Capsules (Infrequent) 1913

(▣ Described in PDR For Nonprescription Drugs) Incidence data in parenthesis; ▲ 3% or more (⊙ Described in PDR For Ophthalmology)

Diarrhea **Side Effects Index** **1270**

Doxorubicin Astra (Occasional) 540
▲ Duragesic Transdermal System (3% to 10%) 1288
Dura-Vent Tablets 952
Duricef 748
Duvoid (Infrequent) 2044
Dyazide 2479
Dynacin Capsules (Infrequent) 1590
DynaCirc Capsules (Up to 3.4%) 2256
Dyrenium Capsules (Rare) 2481
▲ E.E.S. (Most frequent) 424
E-Mycin Tablets (Infrequent) 1341
Easprin 1914
EC-Naprosyn Delayed-Release Tablets (Less than 3%) 2117
Edecrin 1657
▲ Effexor (8%) 2719
Elavil 2838
Eldepryl Tablets (1 of 49 patients) 2550
▲ Emcyt Capsules (12%) 1953
Endep Tablets 2174
Enduron Tablets 420
Engerix-B Unit-Dose Vials (Less than 1%) 2482
Ensure Plus High Calorie Complete Nutrition 2221
▲ Epogen for Injection (0.11 to 21%) 489
▲ Ergamisol Tablets (13% to 52%) 1292
▲ ERYC (Among most frequent) 1915
▲ EryPed (Among most frequent) 421
▲ Ery-Tab Tablets (Among most frequent) 422
▲ Erythrocin Stearate Filmtab (Among most frequent) 425
▲ Erythromycin Base Filmtab (Among most frequent) 426
▲ Erythromycin Delayed-Release Capsules, USP (Among most frequent) 427
Esidrix Tablets 821
Esimil Tablets 822
Eskalith 2485
▲ Ethmozine Tablets (2% to 5%) 2041
Etrafon 2355
▲ Eulexin Capsules (12% with LHRH agonist) 2358
▲ Famvir (7.7%) 2486
Fansidar Tablets 2114
Fastin Capsules 2488
▲ Felbatol (5.2% to 5.3%) 2666
Feldene Capsules (Greater than 1%) 1965
Feosol Capsules (Occasional) 2456
Feosol Elixir (Occasional) 2456
Feosol Tablets (Occasional) 2457
Fioricet with Codeine Capsules 2260
Fiorinal with Codeine Capsules 2262
Flagyl 375 Capsules 2434
Flagyl I.V. 2247
Flexeril Tablets (Less than 1%) 1661
Floropryl Sterile Ophthalmic Ointment (Rare) 1662
▲ Floxin I.V. (1% to 4%) 1571
Floxin Tablets (200 mg, 300 mg, 400 mg) (1% to 4%) 1567
▲ Fludara for Injection (13% to 15%) 663
Flumadine Tablets & Syrup (0.3% to 1%) 1015
Fluorouracil Injection (Rare to common) 2116
Fortaz (1 in 78 patients) 1100
▲ Foscavir Injection (5% or greater up to 30%) 547
▲ Sterile FUDR (Among more common) 2118
Fulvicin P/G Tablets (Occasional) 2359
Fulvicin P/G 165 & 330 Tablets (Occasional) 2359
▲ Fungizone Intravenous (Among most common) 506
Ganite 2533
Gantanol Tablets 2119
Gantrisin 2120
▲ Gastrocrom Capsules (4 of 87 patients) 984
Geocillin Tablets 2199
Glauctabs ⊙ 208
▲ Glucophage (Among most common) 752
Glucotrol Tablets (1 in 70) 1967
▲ Glucotrol XL Extended Release Tablets (5.4%) 1968
Grifulvin V (griseofulvin tablets) Microsize (griseofulvin oral suspension) Microsize (Occasional) 1888
Gris-PEG Tablets, 125 mg & 250 mg (Occasional) 479
Guaifed 1787
▲ Habitrol Nicotine Transdermal System (3% to 9% of patients) 865
Halcion Tablets (Rare) 2611
Haldol Decanoate 1577
Haldol Injection, Tablets and Concentrate 1575
Havrix (Less than 1%) 2489
Helixate, Antihemophilic Factor (Recombinant) (One report out of 3,254 patients) 518
HibTITER (2 of 1,118 vaccinations) 1375
Hismanal Tablets (1.8%) 1293
▲ Hivid Tablets (2.5% to 9.5%) 2121
Humegon 1824
Humorsol Sterile Ophthalmic Solution (Rare) 1664
Hydrea Capsules (Less frequent) 696
HydroDIURIL Tablets 1674
Hydropres Tablets 1675
Hyperstat I.V. Injection 2363
Hytrin Capsules (At least 1%) 430
Hyzaar Tablets (1% or greater) 1677
IBU Tablets (Greater than 1%) 1342
▲ Idamycin (73%) 1955
IFEX (Less than 1%) 697
Ilosone (Infrequent) 911
Imdur (Less than or equal to 5%) 1323
Imitrex Injection (Infrequent) 1103
Imitrex Tablets (Frequent) 1106
Imuran (Less than 1%) 1110
Inderal 2728
Inderal LA Long Acting Capsules 2730
Inderide Tablets 2732
Inderide LA Long Acting Capsules 2734
Indocin Capsules (Greater than 1%) 1680
Indocin I.V. (1% to 3%) 1684
Indocin (Greater than 1%) 1680
INFeD (Iron Dextran Injection, USP) 2345
▲ Intron A (2% to 45%) 2364
Ionamin Capsules 990
IOPIDINE Sterile Ophthalmic Solution ⊙ 219
Ismelin Tablets 827
Ismo Tablets (Fewer than 1%) 2738
Isoptin Oral Tablets (Less than 1%) 1346
Isoptin SR Tablets (1% or less) 1348
Isopto Carbachol Ophthalmic Solution ⊙ 223
K-Dur Microburst Release System (potassium chloride, USP) E.R. Tablets 1325
▲ K-Lor Powder Packets (Most common) 434
▲ K-Norm Extended-Release Capsules (Among most common) 991
K-Phos Neutral Tablets 639
K-Phos Original Formula 'Sodium Free' Tablets 639
▲ K-Tab Filmtab (Most common) 434
Kayexalate (Occasional) 2314
▲ Keflex Pulvules & Oral Suspension (Most frequent) 914
▲ Keftab Tablets (Most frequent) 915
Kefurox Vials, Faspak & ADD-Vantage (1 in 220) 1454
Kefzol Vials, Faspak & ADD-Vantage 1456
Kerlone Tablets (1.9% to 2.0%) 2436
Klonopin Tablets 2126
KOGENATE Antihemophilic Factor (Recombinant) (One report) 632
▲ Kolyum Liquid (Among most common) 992
Ku-Zyme HP Capsules 2402
▲ Kytril Injection (4%) 2490
▲ Kytril Tablets (4% to 8%) 2492
▲ Lamictal Tablets (6.3%) 1112
▲ Lamprene Capsules (40-50%) 828
Lanoxicaps (Less common) 1117
Lanoxin Elixir Pediatric (Less common) 1120
Lanoxin Injection (Less common) 1123
Lanoxin Injection Pediatric (Less common) 1126
Lanoxin Tablets (Less common) 1128
▲ Lariam Tablets (Among most frequent) 2128
Larodopa Tablets (Infrequent) 2129
Lasix Injection, Oral Solution and Tablets 1240
▲ Lescol Capsules (6.0%) 2267
▲ Leucovorin Calcium for Injection (11% to 66%) 1268
Leucovorin Calcium Tablets, Wellcovorin Brand 1132
Leukeran Tablets (Infrequent) 1133
▲ Leukine for IV Infusion (89%) 1271
▲ Leustatin (10%) 1834
▲ Levatol (3.3%) 2403
Levsin/Levsinex/Levbid 2405
Limbitrol 2180
Lincocin 2617
Lioresal Intrathecal 1596
Lioresal Tablets (Rare) 829
Lithium Carbonate Capsules & Tablets 2230
Lithonate/Lithotabs/Lithobid 2543
▲ Lodine Capsules and Tablets (3-9%) 2743
▲ Lopid Tablets (7.2%) 1917
▲ Lopressor Ampuls (5%) 830
Lopressor HCT Tablets (1 to 5 in 100 patients) 832
▲ Lopressor Tablets (5%) 830
▲ Lorabid Suspension and Pulvules (3.6% to 5.8%) 1459
Lorelco Tablets 1517
Lotensin HCT 837
Lotrel Capsules 840
Lozol Tablets (Less than 5%) 2022
Ludiomil Tablets (Rare) 843
Lufyllin & Lufyllin-400 Tablets 2670
Lufyllin-GG Elixir & Tablets 2671
Lupron Depot 7.5 mg (Less than 5%) 2559
Lupron Injection (Less than 5%) 2555
▲ Luvox Tablets (11%) 2544
▲ Lysodren (80%) 698
M-M-R II 1687
M-R-VAX II 1689
MS Contin Tablets (Less frequent) 1994
MSIR (Infrequent) 1997
▲ MZM (Among reactions occurring most often) ⊙ 267
Macrobid Capsules (Less than 1%) 1988
Macrodantin Capsules (Less common) 1989
MagTab SR Caplets 1793
Marinol (Dronabinol) Capsules (0.3% to 1%) 2231
Maxair Autohaler (1.3%) 1492
Maxair Inhaler (Less than 1%) 1494
Maxaquin Tablets (1.4%) 2440
Maxzide 1380
Mefoxin 1691
Mefoxin Premixed Intravenous Solution 1694
▲ Megace Oral Suspension (8% to 15%) 699
Mellaril 2269
▲ Mepron Suspension (19% to 21%) 1135
Meruvax II 1697
▲ Mesnex Injection (83%) 702
Mestinon Injectable 1253
Mestinon 1254
Methadone Hydrochloride Oral Concentrate 2233
Methergine (Rare) 2272
Methotrexate Sodium Tablets, Injection, for Injection and LPF Injection (1 to 3%) 1275
Metrodin (urofollitropin for injection) 2446
MetroGel-Vaginal (Equal to or less than 2%) 902
▲ Mevacor Tablets (2.2% to 5.5%) 1699
▲ Mexitil Capsules (5.2%) 678
Mezlin 601
Mezlin Pharmacy Bulk Package 604
Miacalcin Nasal Spray (1% to 3%) 2275
▲ Micro-K (Among most common) 2063
▲ Micro-K LS Packets (Most common) 2064
▲ Midamor Tablets (3% to 8%) 1703
Miltown Tablets 2672
Minipress Capsules (1-4%) 1937
Minizide Capsules (Rare) 1938
Minocin Intravenous 1382
Minocin Oral Suspension 1385
Minocin Pellet-Filled Capsules (Infrequent) 1383
Mintezol 1704
Mithracin 607
Moduretic Tablets (Greater than 1%, less than 3%) 1705
Monocid Injection (Less than 1%) 2497
Monodox Capsules (Infrequent) 1805
Mono-Gesic Tablets 792
Monoket (Up to 2%) 2406
▲ Monopril Tablets (Less than 1% to 11.9%) 757
Children's Motrin Ibuprofen Oral Suspension (Greater than 1% but less than 3%) 1546
Motrin Tablets (Less than 3%) 2625
Motrin Ibuprofen Suspension, Oral Drops, Chewable Tablets, Caplets (1% to less than 3%) 1546
Mumpsvax 1708
Mustargen 1709
Mutamycin 703
▲ Mycobutin Capsules (3%) 1957
Mycostatin Pastilles (Occasional) 704
Mykrox Tablets (Less than 2%) 993
Mylanta Liquid (Occasional) 1317
Mylanta Tablets (Occasional) ▣ 660
Mylanta Double Strength Liquid (Occasional) 1317
Mylanta Double Strength Tablets (Occasional) ▣ 660
Myochrysine Injection 1711
Nalfon 200 Pulvules & Nalfon Tablets (1.8%) 917
Anaprox/Naprosyn (Less than 3%) 2117
Navane Capsules and Concentrate 2201
Navane Intramuscular 2202
▲ Navelbine Injection (Up to 13% but less than 20%) 1145
Nebcin Vials, Hyporets & ADD-Vantage 1464
NebuPent for Inhalation Solution (Greater than 1%, up to 5%) 1040
NegGram 2323
▲ Neoral (3% to 8%) 2276
NEOSAR Lyophilized/Neosar (Less frequent) 1959
Nephro-Fer Rx Tablets 2005
Neptazane Tablets 1388
Netromycin Injection 100 mg/ml (Fewer than 1 of 1000 patients) 2373
▲ Neupogen for Injection (14%) 495
Neurontin Capsules (More than 1%) 1922
▲ Nicoderm (nicotine transdermal system) (3% to 9%) 1518
Nicolar Tablets 2026
Nicorette (1% to 3%) 2458
Nicotrol Nicotine Transdermal System (1% to 3%) 1550
▲ Nimotop Capsules (Up to 4.2%) 610
Nizoral Tablets (Less than 1%) 1298
▲ Nolvadex Tablets (11.2%) 2841
Normodyne Tablets (Less than 1%) 2379
Noroxin Tablets (0.3% to 1.0%) 1715
Noroxin Tablets (0.3% to 1.0%) 2048
Norpace (1 to 3%) 2444
Norpramin Tablets 1526
Norvasc Tablets (More than 0.1% to 1%) 1940
▲ Novantrone (18 to 47%) 1279
▲ OmniHIB (3.6% to 8.5%) 2499
Omnipen Capsules 2764
Omnipen for Oral Suspension 2765
▲ Oncaspar (Greater than 1% but less than 5%) 2028
Oncovin Solution Vials & Hyporets 1466
Oramorph SR (Morphine Sulfate Sustained Release Tablets) (Less frequent) 2236
▲ Orap Tablets (1 of 20 patients) 1050
Oretic Tablets 443
Orlamm (1% to 3%) 2239
Ornade Spansule Capsules 2502
Ortho Diaphragm Kits—All-Flex Arcing Spring; Ortho Coil Spring; Ortho-White Flat Spring 1865
Ortho Diaphragm Kit 1865
▲ Orthoclone OKT3 Sterile Solution (14%) 1837
▲ Orudis Capsules (3% to 9%) 2766
▲ Oruvail Capsules (3% to 9%) 2766
Osmolite HN High Nitrogen Isotonic Liquid Nutrition 2222
Ovcon 760
PBZ Tablets 845
PBZ-SR Tablets 844
▲ PCE Dispertab Tablets (Among most frequent) 444
PMB 200 and PMB 400 2783
Pamelor 2280
Papaverine Hydrochloride Vials and Ampoules 1468
▲ Paraplatin for Injection (6%) 705
Parlodel (0.4 to 3%) 2281
Parnate Tablets 2503
▲ PASER Granules (Among most common) 1285
▲ Paxil Tablets (7.9% to 19.2%) 2505
PedvaxHIB (One case) 1718
Peganone Tablets 446
▲ Pen•Vee K (Among most common) 2772
Penetrex Tablets (1% to 2%) 2031
Pentam 300 Injection (1 patient) 1041
▲ Pentasa (3.4% to 3.5%) 1527

(▣ Described in PDR For Nonprescription Drugs) Incidence data in parenthesis; ▲ 3% or more (⊙ Described in PDR For Ophthalmology)

1271 **Side Effects Index** **Diplopia**

Pentaspan Injection 937
Pepcid Injection (1.7%) 1722
Pepcid (1.7%) 1720
Pergonal (menotropins for injection, USP) 2448
Periactin 1724
Peri-Colace 2052
▲ Permax Tablets (6.4%) 575
Persantine Tablets 681
Pilocar (Extremely rare) ⊙ 268
Pipracil (2%) 1390
Plaquenil Sulfate Tablets 2328
Platinol 708
Platinol-AQ Injection 710
Plendil Extended-Release Tablets (0.5% to 1.5%) 527
▲ Pondimin Tablets (Among most common) 2066
▲ Ponstel (Approximately 5%) 1925
▲ Pravachol (2.0% to 6.2%) 765
Prelu-2 Timed Release Capsules 681
▲ PREVACID Delayed-Release Capsules (1.4% to 7.4%) 2562
▲ Prilosec Delayed-Release Capsules (3.0% to 3.7%) 529
Primaxin I.M. (0.6%) 1727
Primaxin I.V. (1.8%) 1729
▲ Prinivil Tablets (2.7% to 6.1%) 1733
Prinzide Tablets (2.5%) 1737
Priscoline Hydrochloride Ampuls 845
▲ Procan SR Tablets (3-4%) 1926
Procardia Capsules (2% or less) 1971
Procardia XL Extended Release Tablets (Less than 3%) 1972
▲ Procrit for Injection (0.11% to 21%) 1841
Proglycem (Frequent) 580
▲ Prograf (32% to 72%) 1042
▲ Proleukin for Injection (76%) 797
▲ Propulsid (14.2%) 1300
Prostigmin Injectable 1260
Prostigmin Tablets 1261
▲ Prostin E2 Suppository (Approximately two-fifths) 2634
Prostin VR Pediatric Sterile Solution (About 2%) 2635
Protostat Tablets (Occasional) 1883
▲ Prozac Pulvules & Liquid, Oral Solution (12.3% to 18%) 919
Purinethol Tablets (Occasional) 1156
Quadrinal Tablets 1350
Questran Light (Less frequent) 769
Questran Powder (Less frequent) 770
Quibron 2053
▲ Quinaglute Dura-Tabs Tablets (24%) 649
▲ Quinidex Extentabs (Among most frequent) 2067
RMS Suppositories 2657
Recombivax HB (Equal to or greater than 1%) 1744
Regitine 846
Reglan 2068
▲ Relafen Tablets (14%) 2510
ReoPro Vials (0.9%) 1471
Respbid Tablets 682
Restoril Capsules (1-2%) 2284
▲ Retrovir Capsules (0.8% to 12%) 1158
▲ Retrovir I.V. Infusion (1% to 12%) 1163
▲ Retrovir Syrup (0.8% to 12%) 1158
▲ ReVia Tablets (Less than 10%) 940
Revex (Less than 1%) 1811
▲ Ridaura Capsules (42.5%) 2513
Rifadin (Some patients) 1528
Rifamate Capsules (Some patients) 1530
Rifater 1532
Rimactane Capsules 847
Risperdal (Infrequent) 1301
Robaxisal Tablets 2071
Rocephin Injectable Vials, ADD-Vantage, Galaxy Container (2.7%) 2142
▲ Roferon-A Injection (29% to 42%) 2145
▲ Rogaine Topical Solution (4.33%) 2637
Rondec Oral Drops 953
Rondec Syrup 953
Rondec Tablet 953
Rondec-DM Oral Drops 954
Rondec-DM Syrup 954
Rondec-TR Tablet 953
Rowasa (2.09% to 3.0%) 2548
Rubex (Occasional) 712
Rum-K Syrup 1005
▲ Rythmol Tablets–150mg, 225mg, 300mg (0.5 to 5.7%) 1352
▲ SSKI Solution (Among most frequent) 2658
▲ Salagen Tablets (6%) 1489
Salflex Tablets 786
▲ Sandimmune (3 to 8%) 2286
▲ Sandostatin Injection (5% to 10%; 30% to 58%) 2292
Sanorex Tablets 2294
Sansert Tablets 2295
▲ Sectral Capsules (4%) 2807
Septra 1174
Septra I.V. Infusion 1169
Septra I.V. Infusion ADD-Vantage Vials 1171
Septra 1174
Ser-Ap-Es Tablets 849
Serevent Inhalation Aerosol (1% to 3%) 1176
Serophene (clomiphene citrate tablets, USP) 2451
▲ Serzone Tablets (8%) 771
Sinemet Tablets 943
Sinemet CR Tablets (1.2%) 944
Sinequan 2205
Slo-bid Gyrocaps 2033
▲ Slow-K Extended-Release Tablets (Among most common) 851
Sodium Polystyrene Sulfonate Suspension (Occasional) 2244
Solganal Suspension (Rare) 2388
Soma Compound w/Codeine Tablets 2676
▲ Soma Compound Tablets (Among most common) 2675
▲ Spectrobid Tablets (2% to 4%) 2206
Sporanox Capsules (0.6% to 3.3%) 1305
Sulfamylon Cream 925
▲ Supprelin Injection (1% to 10%) 2056
▲ Suprax (16%) 1399
Surmontil Capsules 2811
Symmetrel Capsules and Syrup (1% to 5%) 946
Tagamet (Approximately 1 in 100) 2516
Talacen (Rare) 2333
Talwin Injection (Rare) 2334
Talwin Compound (Rare) 2335
Talwin Injection (Rare) 2334
Talwin Nx 2336
Tambocor Tablets (1% to less than 3%) 1497
Tao Capsules (Infrequent) 2209
Tavist Syrup 2297
Tavist Tablets 2298
▲ Taxol (38%) 714
Tazicef for Injection (Less than 2%; 1 in 78 patients) 2519
Tazidime Vials, Faspak & ADD-Vantage (1 in 78) 1478
Tegison Capsules (Less than 1%) 2154
Tegretol Chewable Tablets 852
Tegretol Suspension 852
Tegretol Tablets 852
Temaril Tablets, Syrup and Spansule Extended-Release Capsules 483
Tenex Tablets (3% or less) 2074
Tenoretic Tablets (2% to 3%) 2845
Tenormin Tablets and I.V. Injection (2% to 3%) 2847
Tensilon Injectable 1261
Terramycin Intramuscular Solution 2210
▲ Tetramune (1% to 10%) 1404
Thalitone 1245
Theo-24 Extended Release Capsules 2568
Theo-Dur Extended-Release Tablets 1327
Theo-X Extended-Release Tablets 788
▲ TheraCys BCG Live (Intravesical) (Up to 6.3%) 897
▲ Ticlid Tablets (12.5%) 2156
Tigan 2057
Tilade (0.9%) 996
Timentin for Injection 2528
Timolide Tablets (Less than 1%) 1748
Timoptic in Ocudose (Less frequent) 1753
Timoptic Sterile Ophthalmic Solution (Less frequent) 1751
Timoptic-XE 1755
Tobramycin Sulfate Injection 968
Tofranil Ampuls 854
Tofranil Tablets 856
Tofranil-PM Capsules 857
▲ Tolectin (200, 400 and 600 mg) (3 to 9%) 1581
▲ Tonocard Tablets (0.0-6.8%) 531
▲ Toprol-XL Tablets (About 5 of 100 patients) 565
▲ Toradol (7%) 2159
Trandate Tablets (Less than 1%) 1185
Trasylol (2%) 613
Trental Tablets 1244
Triavil Tablets 1757
Trilafon (Occasional) 2389
▲ Trilisate (Less than 20%) 2000
Trinalin Repetabs Tablets 1330
Trinsicon Capsules (Rare) 2570
Tripedia (Up to 3%) 892
Tussend 1783
Typhim Vi (Up to 3.1%) 899
Ultrase Capsules 2343
▲ Ultrase MT Capsules (3.7%; among most frequent) 2344
▲ Unasyn (3%) 2212
Uni-Dur Extended-Release Tablets 1331
Uniphyl 400 mg Tablets 2001
▲ Univasc Tablets (3.1%) 2410
Urecholine 1761
Urobiotic-250 Capsules (Rare) 2214
Uroqid-Acid No. 2 Tablets 640
▲ Valtrex Caplets (4% to 5%) 1194
▲ Vantin for Oral Suspension and Vantin Tablets (1% to 7.2%) 2646
Varivax (Greater than or equal to 1%) 1762
▲ Vascor (200, 300 and 400 mg) Tablets (6.82 to 10.87%) 1587
Vaseretic Tablets (2.1%) 1765
Vasotec I.V. 1768
Vasotec Tablets (1.4% to 2.1%) 1771
Velban Vials 1484
Ventolin Inhalation Aerosol and Refill (1%) 1197
Ventolin Rotacaps for Inhalation (Less than 1%) 1200
▲ VePesid Capsules and Injection (1% to 13%) 718
Verelan Capsules (1% or less) 1410
Verelan Capsules (Less than 1%) 2824
Vermox Chewable Tablets 1312
Vibramycin (Infrequent) 1941
Vibramycin Hyclate Intravenous 2215
Vibramycin (Infrequent) 1941
▲ Videx Tablets, Powder for Oral Solution, & Pediatric Powder for Oral Solution (17% to 82%) 720
Viokase 2076
Visken Tablets (2% or fewer patients) 2299
Vivactil Tablets 1774
Vivotif Berna 665
▲ Voltaren Tablets (3% to 9%) 861
▲ Vumon (33%) 727
▲ Wellbutrin Tablets (6.8%) 1204
Wigraine Tablets & Suppositories 1829
Winstrol Tablets 2337
▲ Xanax Tablets (10.1% to 20.6%) 2649
Yodoxin 1230
Yutopar Intravenous Injection (Infrequent) 570
Zanosar Sterile Powder (Some patients) 2653
Zantac 1209
Zantac Injection 1207
Zantac Syrup 1209
Zarontin Capsules (Frequent) 1928
Zarontin Syrup (Frequent) 1929
Zaroxolyn Tablets 1000
▲ Zebeta Tablets (2.6% to 3.5%) 1413
▲ Zefazone (3.6%) 2654
▲ Zerit Capsules (4% to 50%) 729
Zestoretic (2.5%) 2850
▲ Zestril Tablets (2.7% to 6.1%) 2854
▲ Ziac (1.1% to 4.3%) 1415
Zinacef (1 in 220 patients) 1211
▲ Zinecard (14% to 21%) 1961
▲ Zithromax (5% to 7%) 1944
Zocor Tablets (1.9%) 1775
▲ Zofran Injection (8% to 16%) 1214
▲ Zofran Tablets (4% to 6%) 1217
▲ Zoladex (Greater than 1% but less than 5%) 2858
▲ Zoloft Tablets (17.7%) 2217
▲ Zosyn (11.3%) 1419
▲ Zosyn Pharmacy Bulk Package (11.3%) 1422
Zovirax (0.3% to 3.2%) 1219
Zyloprim Tablets (Less than 1%) 1226

Diarrhea, bloody

Ansaid Tablets (Less than 1%) 2579
Asacol Delayed-Release Tablets 1979
Azulfidine (Rare) 1949
Cataflam (Less than 1%) 816
Cleocin Phosphate Injection 2586
Cleocin T Topical 2590
Paxil Tablets (Rare) 2505
Pentasa (0.9%) 1527
Pipracil (Less frequent) 1390
Prozac Pulvules & Liquid, Oral Solution (Rare) 919
Rowasa 2548
Ticlid Tablets 2156
Vantin for Oral Suspension and Vantin Tablets 2646
Voltaren Tablets (Less than 1%) 861

Digitalis toxicity

Demadex Tablets and Injection 686
Lanoxicaps 1117
Virazole 1264

Diplegia

Imitrex Injection (Rare) 1103

Diplopia

Actifed with Codeine Cough Syrup 1067
Adalat CC (Less than 1.0%) 589
Children's Advil Suspension (Less than 1%) 2692
Ambien Tablets (Frequent) 2416
Amen Tablets 780
Anafranil Capsules (Infrequent) 803
Atamet 572
Ativan Injection (Occasional) 2698
Atretol Tablets 573
Azactam for Injection (Less than 1%) 734
Benadryl Capsules 1898
Benadryl Injection 1898
Bentyl 1501
Betagan ⊙ 233
Betaseron for SC Injection 658
Betimol 0.25%, 0.5% ⊙ 261
Blocadren Tablets 1614
BOTOX (Botulinum Toxin Type A) Purified Neurotoxin Complex (Less than 1%) 477
Brevicon 2088
Buprenex Injectable (Less than 1%) 2006
Cataflam (Less than 1%) 816
Chibroxin Sterile Ophthalmic Solution (With oral form) 1617
Cipro I.V. (1% or less) 595
Cipro I.V. Pharmacy Bulk Package (Less than 1%) 597
Cipro Tablets (Less than 1%) 592
Clomid (1.5%) 1514
Cognex Capsules (Infrequent) 1901
Cycrin Tablets 975
Cytovene-IV (One report) 2103
Dalgan Injection (Less than 1%) 538
Dalmane Capsules 2173
Dantrium Capsules (Less frequent) 1982
Deconamine 1320
Demulen 2428
Depakene 413
Depakote Tablets 415
Depen Titratable Tablets 2662
Depo-Provera Contraceptive Injection 2602
Depo-Provera Sterile Aqueous Suspension 2606
Desyrel and Desyrel Dividose 503
Dilaudid-HP Injection (Less frequent) 1337
Dilaudid-HP Lyophilized Powder 250 mg (Less frequent) 1337
Dilaudid Tablets and Liquid (Less frequent) 1339
Diprivan Injection (Less than 1%) 2833
Dizac (Less frequent) 1809
Duranest Injections 542
Dyclone 0.5% and 1% Topical Solutions, USP 544
Effexor (Infrequent) 2719
Eldepryl Tablets 2550
Emla Cream 545
Ethmozine Tablets (Less than 2%) 2041
▲ Felbatol (3.4% to 6.1%) 2666
Flexeril Tablets (Less than 1%) 1661
Floxin I.V. 1571
Floxin Tablets (200 mg, 300 mg, 400 mg) 1567
Foscavir Injection (Less than 1%) 547
Fungizone Intravenous 506
IBU Tablets (Less than 1%) 1342
Indocin (Less than 1%) 1680
Intron A (Less than 5%) 2364
Ismo Tablets (Fewer than 1%) 2738
Klonopin Tablets 2126
▲ Lamictal Tablets (Among most common; 24% to 49%) 1112
Larodopa Tablets (Infrequent) 2129
Levlen/Tri-Levlen 651
Lioresal Intrathecal 1596
Lioresal Tablets 829
Luvox Tablets (Infrequent) 2544
Lysodren (Infrequent) 698
MS Contin Tablets (Less frequent) 1994
MSIR (Infrequent) 1997
Matulane Capsules 2131
Maxaquin Tablets 2440
Mesantoin Tablets 2272
Micronor Tablets (Rare) 1872

(▣ Described in PDR For Nonprescription Drugs) Incidence data in parenthesis; ▲ 3% or more (⊙ Described in PDR For Ophthalmology)

Diplopia | Side Effects Index | 1272

Modicon (Rare) 1872
Children's Motrin Ibuprofen Oral Suspension (Less than 1%) 1546
Motrin Tablets (Less than 1%) 2625
Motrin Ibuprofen Suspension, Oral Drops, Chewable Tablets, Caplets (Less than 1%) 1546
Mysoline (Occasional) 2754
Nalfon 200 Pulvules & Nalfon Tablets (Less than 1%) 917
NegGram (Infrequent) 2323
▲ Neurontin Capsules (5.9%) 1922
Norinyl 2088
Noroxin Tablets 1715
Noroxin Tablets 2048
Nor-Q D Tablets 2135
Norvasc Tablets (More than 0.1% to 1%) 1940
Novahistine DH 2462
Novahistine Elixir ▣ 823
Nuromax Injection (Less than or equal to 0.1%) 1149
Ocupress Ophthalmic Solution, 1% Sterile ⊙ 309
Oramorph SR (Morphine Sulfate Sustained Release Tablets) (Less frequent) 2236
Ornade Spansule Capsules 2502
Ortho-Cyclen/Ortho-Tri-Cyclen 1858
Ortho-Novum (Rare) 1872
Ortho-Cyclen/Ortho Tri-Cyclen 1858
Orthoclone OKT3 Sterile Solution 1837
Ovcon 760
PBZ Tablets 845
PBZ-SR Tablets 844
Paxil Tablets (Rare) 2505
Peganone Tablets 446
Periactin 1724
Permax Tablets (2.1%) 575
Phenergan Injection 2773
Phenergan Tablets 2775
Placidyl Capsules 448
Premphase 2797
Prempro 2801
Prinivil Tablets (0.3% to 1.0%) 1733
Prinzide Tablets 1737
Proglycem 580
ProSom Tablets (Rare) 449
Protopam Chloride for Injection 2806
Provera Tablets 2636
Prozac Pulvules & Liquid, Oral Solution (Rare) 919
Quinaglute Dura-Tabs Tablets 649
Quinidex Extentabs 2067
Risperdal (Rare) 1301
Robaxin Injectable 2070
Romazicon (1% to 3%) 2147
Rondec Oral Drops 953
Rondec Syrup 953
Rondec Tablet 953
Rondec-DM Oral Drops 954
Rondec-DM Syrup 954
Rondec-TR Tablet 953
Serax Capsules 2810
Serax Tablets 2810
Serophene (clomiphene citrate tablets, USP) 2451
Serzone Tablets (Infrequent) 771
Sinemet Tablets 943
Soma Compound w/Codeine Tablets (Very rare) 2676
Soma Compound Tablets (Very rare) 2675
Soma Tablets 2674
Supprelin Injection (1% to 3%) 2056
Talwin Injection 2334
Tambocor Tablets (1% to less than 3%) 1497
Tavist Syrup 2297
Tavist Tablets 2298
▲ Tegison Capsules (10-25%) 2154
Tegretol Chewable Tablets 852
Tegretol Suspension 852
Tegretol Tablets 852
Temaril Tablets, Syrup and Spansule Extended-Release Capsules 483
Tensilon Injectable 1261
Timolide Tablets 1748
Timoptic in Ocudose (Less frequent) 1753
Timoptic Sterile Ophthalmic Solution (Less frequent) 1751
Timoptic-XE 1755
Tonocard Tablets (Less than 1%) 531
Tranxene 451
Levlen/Tri-Levlen 651
Tri-Norinyl 2164
Tussend 1783
Valium Injectable 2182
Valium Tablets (Infrequent) 2183
Valrelease Capsules (Occasional) 2169
Versed Injection (Less than 1%) 2170
Videx Tablets, Powder for Oral Solution, & Pediatric Powder for Oral Solution (Less than 1%) 720
Voltaren Tablets (Less than 1%) 861
Wellbutrin Tablets (Rare) 1204
Xanax Tablets 2649
▲ Xylocaine Injections (Less than 1% to among most common) 567
Zestoretic 2850
Zestril Tablets (0.3% to 1.0%) 2854
Zoloft Tablets (Infrequent) 2217

Dipsesis

Aldactone 2414
Ambien Tablets (Rare) 2416
Anafranil Capsules (Up to 2%) 803
Anaprox/Naprosyn (Less than 3%) 2117
Apresazide Capsules 808
Betaseron for SC Injection 658
Capozide 742
Cardizem CD Capsules (Less than 1%) 1506
Cardizem SR Capsules (Less than 1%) 1510
Cardizem Injectable 1508
Cardizem Tablets (Less than 1%) 1512
Cardura Tablets (Less than 0.5% of 3960 patients) 2186
Ceftin (Less than 1% but more than 0.1%) 1078
Claritin (2% or fewer patients) 2349
Claritin-D (2%) 2350
Cytotec (Infrequent) 2424
Depo-Provera Contraceptive Injection (Fewer than 1%) 2602
Dyazide 2479
Easprin 1914
EC-Naprosyn Delayed-Release Tablets (Less than 3%) 2117
Effexor (Infrequent) 2719
Emcyt Capsules (1%) 1953
Empirin with Codeine Tablets 1093
Esidrix Tablets 821
Eskalith 2485
Flexeril Tablets (Less than 1%) 1661
Floxin I.V. (Less than 1%) 1571
Floxin Tablets (200 mg, 300 mg, 400 mg) (Less than 1%) 1567
Foscavir Injection (Between 1% and 5%) 547
Glucotrol XL Extended Release Tablets (Less than 1%) 1968
Imitrex Injection (Infrequent) 1103
Imitrex Tablets (Infrequent) 1106
Intron A (Less than 5%) 2364
ISMOTIC 45% w/v Solution (Very rare) ⊙ 222
K-Phos Neutral Tablets 639
Kerlone Tablets (Less than 2%) 2436
Lamictal Tablets (Infrequent) 1112
Lasix Injection, Oral Solution and Tablets 1240
Lithium Carbonate Capsules & Tablets 2230
Lithonate/Lithotabs/Lithobid 2543
Lodine Capsules and Tablets (Less than 1%) 2743
▲ Lupron Depot 3.75 mg (Among most frequent) 2556
Luvox Tablets 2544
Maxaquin Tablets (Less than 1%) 2440
Maxzide 1380
Miacalcin Nasal Spray (Less than 1%) 2275
Midamor Tablets (Less than or equal to 1%) 1703
Moduretic Tablets (Less than or equal to 1%) 1705
Monoket (Fewer than 1%) 2406
Anaprox/Naprosyn (Less than 3%) 2117
Neurontin Capsules (Infrequent) 1922
Norvasc Tablets (More than 0.1% to 1%) 1940
Oncaspar (Less than 1%) 2028
▲ Orap Tablets (1 of 20 patients) 1050
Oretic Tablets 443
Orudis Capsules (Less than 1%) 2766
Oruvail Capsules (Less than 1%) 2766
Paxil Tablets (Infrequent) 2505
Pentasa (Less than 1%) 1527
Permax Tablets (Infrequent) 575
PREVACID Delayed-Release Capsules (Less than 1%) 2562
Prinzide Tablets 1737
ProSom Tablets (Infrequent) 449
Prozac Pulvules & Liquid, Oral Solution (Infrequent) 919
▲ ReVia Tablets (Less than 10%) 940
Risperdal (Infrequent) 1301
Sanorex Tablets 2294
Serzone Tablets (1%) 771
Supprelin Injection (1% to 3%) 2056
▲ Tegison Capsules (50-75%) 2154
Tenoretic Tablets 2845
Thalitone (Common) 1245
Tonocard Tablets (Less than 1%) 531
Toradol (1% or less) 2159
Trental Tablets (Less than 1%) 1244
Uroqid-Acid No. 2 Tablets 640
Vaseretic Tablets 1765
Videx Tablets, Powder for Oral Solution, & Pediatric Powder for Oral Solution (Less than 1%) 720
Zaroxolyn Tablets 1000
Zestoretic 2850
Zoloft Tablets (1.4%) 2217
▲ Zonalon Cream (Approximately 1% to 10%) 1055
Zosyn (1.0% or less) 1419
Zosyn Pharmacy Bulk Package (1.0% or less) 1422
Zovirax Sterile Powder (Less than 1%) 1223

Discoloration, injection site

Depo-Provera Sterile Aqueous Suspension 2606
Diprivan Injection (Less than 1%) 2833
▲ Navelbine Injection (Approximately one-third of patients) 1145

Discomfort, arm

▲ Adenoscan (4%) 1024
Imitrex Injection (Rare) 1103
Respbid Tablets 682

Discomfort, chest

▲ Adenoscan (40%) 1024
Brethine Ampuls (1.3 to 1.5%) 815
Ceredase 1065
Helixate, Antihemophilic Factor (Recombinant) 518
Imitrex Injection (Rare; 4.5%) 1103
Imitrex Tablets (Frequent) 1106
KOGENATE Antihemophilic Factor (Recombinant) 632
Primaxin I.M. 1727
Primaxin I.V. (Less than 0.2%) 1729
Prinivil Tablets (0.3 to 1.0%) 1733
Prinzide Tablets (0.3 to 1%) 1737
Proventil (Less than 1%) 2386
Recombivax HB (Less than 1%) 1744
Timentin for Injection 2528
Tornalate Solution for Inhalation, 0.2% (Less than 1% to 1.5%) 956
Tornalate Metered Dose Inhaler (Approximately 1%; 0.5%) 957
Ventolin Tablets (Fewer than 1 of 100 patients) 1203
Volmax Extended-Release Tablets (Less frequent) 1788
Zaroxolyn Tablets 1000
Zestoretic (0.3 to 1.0%) 2850
Zestril Tablets (0.3% to 1.0%) 2854

Discomfort, general

AVC (Occasional) 1500
Coumadin 926
EPIFRIN ⊙ 239
Eskalith 2485
IOPIDINE Sterile Ophthalmic Solution ⊙ 219
Lithium Carbonate Capsules & Tablets 2230
Lithonate/Lithotabs/Lithobid 2543
Papaverine Hydrochloride Vials and Ampoules 1468
Pilopine HS Ophthalmic Gel ⊙ 226
Zovirax Ointment 5% 1223

Discomfort, jaw

▲ Adenoscan (15%) 1024
Imitrex Injection (1.8%) 1103

Discomfort, local

Albalon Solution with Liquifilm ⊙ 231
▲ Betimol 0.25%, 0.5% (More than 5%) ⊙ 261
▲ Chibroxin Sterile Ophthalmic Solution (One of the two most frequent) 1617
▲ Ciloxan Ophthalmic Solution (Among most frequent) 472
Efudex (Infrequent) 2113
OptiPranolol (Metipranolol 0.3%) Sterile Ophthalmic Solution (A small number of patients) ⊙ 258
▲ Testoderm Testosterone Transdermal System (4%) 486

Discomfort, nasal

Imitrex Injection (2.2%) 1103
▲ Imitrex Tablets (5% to 7%) 1106

Discomfort at injection site

Azactam for Injection (2.4%) 734
Cefotan (1 in 500) 2829
Ceredase 1065
MICRhoGAM Rh_0(D) Immune Globulin (Human) 1847
▲ Monocid Injection (5.7%) 2497
Oncovin Solution Vials & Hyporets 1466
PPD Tine Test 2874
▲ Rabies Vaccine Adsorbed (Approximately 65% to 70%) 2508
RhoGAM Rh_0(D) Immune Globulin (Human) 1847
Tuberculin, Old, Tine Test 2875
Tubersol (Tuberculin Purified Protein Derivative [Mantoux]) 2872
WinRho SD (A small number of cases) 2576

Discontinuation syndrome

Catapres Tablets (About 1 in 100 patients) 674
Catapres-TTS (Less frequent) 675
Combipres Tablets (About 1%) 677

Disorientation

Actimmune (Rare) 1056
Akineton 1333
Apresazide Capsules (Less frequent) 808
Apresoline Hydrochloride Tablets (Less frequent) 809
Asacol Delayed-Release Tablets 1979
Asendin Tablets (Less than 1%) 1369
Atgam Sterile Solution (Less than 5%) 2581
Ativan Tablets (Less frequent) 2700
Azo Gantrisin Tablets 2081
Bentyl 10 mg Capsules 1501
BOTOX (Botulinum Toxin Type A) Purified Neurotoxin Complex 477
Brontex 1981
Cataflam (Rare) 816
CeeNU 693
Dalmane Capsules 2173
Daranide Tablets 1633
Demerol 2308
Demser Capsules 1649
Desyrel and Desyrel Dividose (Less than 1% to 2.1%) 503
Dilaudid-HP Injection (Less frequent) 1337
Dilaudid-HP Lyophilized Powder 250 mg (Less frequent) 1337
Dilaudid Tablets and Liquid (Less frequent) 1339
Dolobid Tablets (Less than 1 in 100) 1654
Dopram Injectable 2061
Elavil 2838
Eldepryl Tablets 2550
Endep Tablets 2174
Etrafon 2355
Fioricet with Codeine Capsules 2260
Fiorinal with Codeine Capsules 2262
Flexeril Tablets (Less than 1%) 1661
Floxin I.V. 1571
Floxin Tablets (200 mg, 300 mg, 400 mg) 1567
Fluorouracil Injection 2116
Sterile FUDR (Remote possibility) 2118
Halcion Tablets 2611
Hydrea Capsules (Extremely rare) 696
IFEX (Less frequent) 697
INFeD (Iron Dextran Injection, USP) 2345
ISMOTIC 45% w/v Solution ⊙ 222
Levbid Extended-Release Tablets 2405
Levoprome (Sometimes) 1274
Levsin/Levsinex/Levbid 2405
Lioresal Intrathecal 1596
Ludiomil Tablets (Rare) 843
MS Contin Tablets (Less frequent) 1994
MSIR (Infrequent) 1997
Mepergan Injection 2753
Methadone Hydrochloride Oral Concentrate 2233
Methadone Hydrochloride Oral Solution & Tablets 2235
Myambutol Tablets 1386
Nalfon 200 Pulvules & Nalfon Tablets (Less than 1%) 917
Nebcin Vials, Hyporets & ADD-Vantage 1464

(▣ Described in PDR For Nonprescription Drugs) Incidence data in parenthesis; ▲ 3% or more (⊙ Described in PDR For Ophthalmology)

1273 Side Effects Index Distress, gastrointestinal

Netromycin Injection 100 mg/ml (1 of 1000 patients) 2373
Norpramin Tablets 1526
Oncaspar 2028
Oramorph SR (Morphine Sulfate Sustained Release Tablets) (Less frequent) 2236
Orthoclone OKT3 Sterile Solution 1837
OSM_GLYN Oral Osmotic Agent ⊙ 226
Pamelor 2280
Parnate Tablets 2503
Phenergan with Codeine 2777
Phenergan with Dextromethorphan 2778
Phenergan Suppositories 2775
Phenergan Syrup 2774
Phenergan VC 2779
Phenergan VC with Codeine 2781
RMS Suppositories 2657
▲ReVia Tablets (Less than 1%) 940
Roxanol 2243
Seldane-D Extended-Release Tablets (1.1%) 1538
Ser-Ap-Es Tablets 849
Serax Capsules 2810
Serax Tablets 2810
Seromycin Pulvules 1476
Sinemet CR Tablets 944
Sinequan (Infrequent) 2205
Soma Compound w/Codeine Tablets (Very rare) 2676
Soma Compound Tablets (Very rare) 2675
Soma Tablets 2674
Surmontil Capsules 2811
Tagamet 2516
Talacen 2333
Talwin Injection 2334
Talwin Compound 2335
Talwin Injection 2334
Talwin Nx 2336
Tigan 2057
Timoptic in Ocudose (Less frequent) 1753
Timoptic Sterile Ophthalmic Solution (Less frequent) 1751
Timoptic-XE 1755
Tobramycin Sulfate Injection 968
Tofranil Ampuls 854
Tofranil Tablets 856
Tofranil-PM Capsules 857
▲Tonocard Tablets (2.1-11.2%) 531
Transderm Scōp Transdermal Therapeutic System (Infrequent) 869
Triavil Tablets 1757
Vivactil Tablets 1774
Voltaren Tablets (Rare) 861
Vontrol Tablets (Approximately 1 in 350) 2532
WinRho SD (One report) 2576

Disorientation, place

Blocadren Tablets 1614
Cartrol Tablets 410
Inderal 2728
Inderal LA Long Acting Capsules 2730
Inderide Tablets 2732
Inderide LA Long Acting Capsules 2734
Kerlone Tablets 2436
Levatol 2403
Lopressor HCT Tablets 832
Normodyne Tablets 2379
Sectral Capsules 2807
Tenoretic Tablets 2845
Tenormin Tablets and I.V. Injection 2847
Timolide Tablets 1748
Timoptic in Ocudose 1753
Timoptic Sterile Ophthalmic Solution 1751
Timoptic-XE 1755
Toprol-XL Tablets 565
Trandate Tablets 1185
Visken Tablets 2299
Zebeta Tablets 1413
Ziac 1415

Disorientation, time

Blocadren Tablets 1614
Cartrol Tablets 410
Inderal 2728
Inderal LA Long Acting Capsules 2730
Inderide Tablets 2732
Inderide LA Long Acting Capsules 2734
Kerlone Tablets 2436
Levatol 2403
Lopressor HCT Tablets 832
Normodyne Tablets 2379
Sectral Capsules 2807
Tenoretic Tablets 2845
Tenormin Tablets and I.V. Injection 2847
Timolide Tablets 1748
Timoptic in Ocudose 1753
Timoptic Sterile Ophthalmic Solution 1751
Timoptic-XE 1755
Toprol-XL Tablets 565
Trandate Tablets 1185
Visken Tablets 2299
Zebeta Tablets 1413
Ziac 1415

Distention, abdominal (see under Abdominal distention)

Distress, abdominal

Ambien Tablets (Rare) 2416
Atamet 572
Atromid-S Capsules (Less frequent) 2701
Augmentin (Less frequent) 2468
Ceredase 1065
Cerezyme (One patient) 1066
Claritin-D (Less frequent) 2350
Daypro Caplets (Greater than 1% but less than 3%) 2426
▲Depo-Provera Contraceptive Injection (More than 5%) 2602
EryPed 200 & EryPed 400 Granules 421
Ery-Tab Tablets 422
Erythrocin Stearate Filmtab 425
Estrace Cream and Tablets 749
Factrel (Rare) 2877
Glucophage 752
Hylorel Tablets (1.7%) 985
IBU Tablets (Greater than 1%) 1342
▲Ilosone (One of the two most frequent) 911
Imitrex Injection (1.3%) 1103
Imitrex Tablets 1106
Indocin (Greater than 1%) 1680
IOPIDINE Sterile Ophthalmic Solution ⊙ 219
▲K-Lor Powder Packets (Most common) 434
▲K-Tab Filmtab (Most common) 434
Levoprome (Sometimes) 1274
▲Methotrexate Sodium Tablets, Injection, for Injection and LPF Injection (Among most frequent) 1275
Mexitil Capsules (1.2%) 678
Children's Motrin Ibuprofen Oral Suspension (Greater than 1% but less than 3%) 1546
Motrin Ibuprofen Suspension, Oral Drops, Chewable Tablets, Caplets (1% to less than 3%) 1546
▲Norplant System (5% or greater) 2759
▲Persantine Tablets (6.1%) 681
Protostat Tablets 1883
Questran Light (Less frequent) 769
Questran Powder (Less frequent) 770
Rum-K Syrup 1005
Sanorex Tablets 2294
▲Seldane Tablets (4.6% to 7.6%) 1536
Seldane-D Extended-Release Tablets 1538
Senna X-Prep Bowel Evacuant Liquid 1230
Sinemet Tablets 943
Talacen (Rare) 2333
Talwin Compound (Rare) 2335
Talwin Nx (Rare) 2336
THYREL TRH 2873
▲Ultrase MT Capsules (Among most frequent) 2344
▲Xanax Tablets (18.3%) 2649
Zantac Injection 1207

Distress, epigastric

Actifed with Codeine Cough Syrup 1067
▲Children's Advil Suspension (3-9%) 2692
Aerolate 1004
Asendin Tablets (Less than 1%) 1369
Atgam Sterile Solution (Less than 1% to less than 5%) 2581
Atrohist Plus Tablets 454
▲Benadryl Capsules (Among most frequent) 1898
▲Benadryl Injection (Among most frequent) 1898
▲Bromfed-DM Cough Syrup (Among most frequent) 1786
Celontin Kapseals (Frequent) 1899
Cipro I.V. (1% or less) 595
Cipro I.V. Pharmacy Bulk Package (Less than 1%) 597
Combipres Tablets 677
Comhist 2038
Cuprimine Capsules 1630
D.H.E. 45 Injection 2255
Deconamine 1320
▲Depen Titratable Tablets (17%) 2662
▲DiaBeta Tablets (Among most common; 1.8%) 1239
Dimetane-DC Cough Syrup 2059
Dimetane-DX Cough Syrup 2059
Dipentum Capsules (Rare) 1951
Elavil 2838
Endep Tablets 2174
Etrafon 2355
▲Feldene Capsules (3% to 9%) 1965
Flagyl 375 Capsules 2434
Flagyl I.V. 2247
Fulvicin P/G Tablets (Occasional) 2359
Fulvicin P/G 165 & 330 Tablets (Occasional) 2359
▲Fungizone Intravenous (Among most common) 506
Geocillin Tablets 2199
Grifulvin V (griseofulvin tablets) Microsize (griseofulvin oral suspension) Microsize (Occasional) 1888
Gris-PEG Tablets, 125 mg & 250 mg (Occasional) 479
Hivid Tablets (Less than 1% to less than 3%) 2121
▲IBU Tablets (3% to 9%) 1342
Inderal 2728
Inderal LA Long Acting Capsules 2730
Inderide Tablets 2732
Inderide LA Long Acting Capsules 2734
▲Indocin (3% to 9%) 1680
Isuprel Hydrochloride Solution 1:200 & 1:100 2313
Isuprel Mistometer 2312
Kemadrin Tablets 1112
▲Lamprene Capsules (40-50%) 828
Limbitrol 2180
Ludiomil Tablets (Rare) 843
Lufyllin & Lufyllin-400 Tablets 2670
Lufyllin-GG Elixir & Tablets 2671
MetroGel-Vaginal 902
▲Mexitil Capsules (41%) 678
Micronase Tablets (1.8%) 2623
Mintezol 1704
MIOSTAT Intraocular Solution ⊙ 224
Motofen Tablets (1 in 100) 784
▲Children's Motrin Ibuprofen Oral Suspension (3% to 9%) 1546
▲Motrin Tablets (3% to 9%) 2625
▲Motrin Ibuprofen Suspension, Oral Drops, Chewable Tablets, Caplets (3% to 9%) 1546
Norisodrine with Calcium Iodide Syrup 442
Norpramin Tablets 1526
Nydrazid Injection 508
Oncaspar (Less than 1%) 2028
Ornade Spansule Capsules 2502
▲PBZ Tablets (Among most frequent) 845
▲PBZ-SR Tablets (Among most frequent) 844
Pamelor 2280
▲Pen•Vee K (Among most common) 2772
Periactin 1724
Phenergan VC 2779
Phenergan VC with Codeine 2781
Pima Syrup 1005
Proloprim Tablets 1155
Protostat Tablets (Occasional) 1883
Proventil Syrup (Less than 1 of 100 patients) 2385
Quadrinal Tablets 1350
Quibron 2053
Respbid Tablets 682
Rifadin (Some patients) 1528
Rifamate Capsules (Some patients) 1530
Rifater 1532
Rimactane Capsules 847
Slo-bid Gyrocaps 2033
Soma Compound w/Codeine Tablets 2676
Soma Compound Tablets 2675
Soma Tablets 2674
Spectrobid Tablets (2%) 2206
Surmontil Capsules 2811
Tapazole Tablets 1477
▲Tavist Syrup (Among most frequent) 2297
▲Tavist Tablets (Among most frequent) 2298
Temaril Tablets, Syrup and Spansule Extended-Release Capsules 483
Theo-24 Extended Release Capsules 2568
Theo-Dur Extended-Release Tablets 1327
Theo-X Extended-Release Tablets 788
▲Ticlid Tablets (3.7%) 2156
Timentin for Injection 2528
Tofranil Ampuls 854
Tofranil Tablets 856
Tofranil-PM Capsules 857
Toprol-XL Tablets (About 1 of 100 patients) 565
▲Toradol (13%) 2159
Triavil Tablets 1757
▲Trilisate (Less than 20%) 2000
Trimpex Tablets 2163
▲Trinalin Repetabs Tablets (Among most frequent) 1330
Tussend 1783
Uni-Dur Extended-Release Tablets 1331
Uniphyl 400 mg Tablets 2001
Ventolin Syrup (Less than 1 of 100 patients) 1202
Vivactil Tablets 1774
Wigraine Tablets & Suppositories 1829
Yutopar Intravenous Injection (Infrequent) 570
Zarontin Capsules (Frequent) 1928
Zarontin Syrup (Frequent) 1929
Zaroxolyn Tablets 1000
Zebeta Tablets 1413
Zefazone 2654
Ziac 1415

Distress, gastric (see under Distress, gastrointestinal)

Distress, gastrointestinal

AeroBid Inhaler System (1-3%) 1005
Aerobid-M Inhaler System (1-3%) 1005
AK-Fluor Injection 10% and 25% ⊙ 203
Alupent (1% to 4%) 669
Atretol Tablets 573
Atrovent Inhalation Aerosol (2.4%) 671
▲Azulfidine (Approximately one-third of patients) 1949
Biltricide Tablets 591
Bumex (0.1%) 2093
BuSpar (2%) 737
Calan SR Caplets (1% or less) 2422
Calan Tablets (1% or less) 2419
Carafate Suspension (Less than 0.5%) 1505
Carafate Tablets (Less than 0.5%) 1504
Celontin Kapseals (Frequent) 1899
Claritin (2% or fewer patients) 2349
▲Clinoril Tablets (10%) 1618
Coly-Mycin M Parenteral 1905
Cuprimine Capsules 1630
▲Desyrel and Desyrel Dividose (3.5% to 5.7%) 503
▲Dolobid Tablets (3% to 9%) 1654
DynaCirc Capsules (Up to 3.3%) 2256
▲Emcyt Capsules (11%) 1953
Esimil Tablets 822
Fastin Capsules 2488
Feldene Capsules (Greater than 1%) 1965
Feosol Elixir (Occasional) 2456
Feosol Tablets (Occasional) 2457
Fiorinal with Codeine Capsules 2262
Flexeril Tablets (Less than 1%) 1661
Floxin I.V. (1% to 3%) 1571
Floxin Tablets (200 mg, 300 mg, 400 mg) (1% to 3%) 1567
Fluorescite ⊙ 219
Hydergine 2265
Imitrex Tablets (Frequent) 1106
▲Imuran (Approximately 12%) 1110
ISMOTIC 45% w/v Solution (Very rare) ⊙ 222
Isoptin Injectable (0.6%) 1344
Isoptin Oral Tablets (Less than 1%) 1346
Isoptin SR Tablets (1% or less) 1348
K-Dur Microburst Release System (potassium chloride, USP) E.R. Tablets 1325
▲K-Norm Extended-Release Capsules (Among most common) 991
Larodopa Tablets 2129
Lopid Tablets 1917
Lopressor Ampuls (1%) 830
Lopressor HCT Tablets (1 in 100 patients) 832
Lopressor Tablets (1%) 830
Lupron Depot 7.5 mg 2559
▲Lysodren (80%) 698
Midamor Tablets (Between 1% and 3%) 1703
Minipress Capsules (Less than 1%) 1937
Minizide Capsules (Rare) 1938

(Described in PDR For Nonprescription Drugs) Incidence data in parenthesis; ▲ 3% or more (⊙ Described in PDR For Ophthalmology)

Distress, gastrointestinal

Moduretic Tablets (Greater than 1%, less than 3%) 1705
Nardil (Common) 1920
NEOSAR Lyophilized/Neosar (Less frequent) 1959
Nicobid 2026
▲ Nicorette (9.6%) 2458
Norisodrine with Calcium Iodide Syrup 442
Orap Tablets 1050
▲ Phenurone Tablets (8%) 447
Placidyl Capsules 448
Ponstel 1925
Prelu-2 Timed Release Capsules...... 681
Pyridium (Occasional) 1928
Robaxisal Tablets 2071
Roferon-A Injection (Less than 1%) 2145
▲ Sandostatin Injection (5% to 10%; 30% to 58%) 2292
Scleromate (Rare) 1891
Sedapap Tablets 50 mg/650 mg (Less frequent) 1543
Supprelin Injection (1% to 3%) 2056
Tegretol Chewable Tablets 852
Tegretol Suspension 852
Tegretol Tablets 852
Timolide Tablets (Less than 1%) 1748
Timoptic in Ocudose 1753
Timoptic Sterile Ophthalmic Solution 1751
▲ Tolectin (200, 400 and 600 mg) (3 to 9%) 1581
▲ Vascor (200, 300 and 400 mg) Tablets (4.35 to about 22%) 1587
Verelan Capsules (1% or less) 1410
Verelan Capsules (Less than 1%) .. 2824
Zarontin Capsules (Frequent)........... 1928
Zarontin Syrup (Frequent) 1929
Zebeta Tablets 1413
Ziac 1415
Zovirax 1219

Distress, precordial

(see under Distress, epigastric)

Distress, stomach

(see under Distress, gastrointestinal)

Distress, upper GI

(see under Distress, epigastric)

Disturbances, emotional

(see under Emotional disturbances)

Disturbances, gastrointestinal

(see under Distress, gastrointestinal)

Disulfiram-like reactions

DiaBeta Tablets (Very rare)............... 1239
Diabinese Tablets 1935
Furoxone (Rare) 2046
Glucotrol Tablets 1967
Glynase PresTab Tablets (Very rare) 2609
Micronase Tablets (Very rare) 2623

Diuresis

Azo Gantanol Tablets (Rare)............ 2080
Azo Gantrisin Tablets (Rare) 2081
Azulfidine (Rare) 1949
Bactrim DS Tablets (Rare)................ 2084
Bactrim I.V. Infusion (Rare)............. 2082
Bactrim (Rare) 2084
Esgic-plus Tablets (Infrequent) 1013
Fansidar Tablets (Rare) 2114
Fioricet Tablets (Infrequent) 2258
Fioricet with Codeine Capsules (Infrequent) 2260
Fiorinal with Codeine Capsules (Infrequent) 2262
Gantanol Tablets (Rare) 2119
Gantrisin (Rare) 2120
Lufyllin & Lufyllin-400 Tablets 2670
Lufyllin-GG Elixir & Tablets 2671
Marax Tablets & DF Syrup................ 2200
Phrenilin (Infrequent)....................... 785
Quadrinal Tablets 1350
Questran Light 769
Questran Powder 770
Quibron 2053
Respbid Tablets 682
Sedapap Tablets 50 mg/650 mg (Infrequent) 1543
Septra (Rare)..................................... 1174
Septra I.V. Infusion (Rare) 1169
Septra I.V. Infusion ADD-Vantage Vials (Rare)...................................... 1171

Septra (Rare)..................................... 1174
Theo-24 Extended Release Capsules 2568
Tonocard Tablets (Less than 1%).. 531

Diuresis, potentiation of

Slo-bid Gyrocaps 2033
Theo-Dur Extended-Release Tablets 1327
Theo-X Extended-Release Tablets .. 788
Uni-Dur Extended-Release Tablets.. 1331
Uniphyl 400 mg Tablets.................... 2001

Diverticulitis

Cognex Capsules (Infrequent) 1901
Questran Light 769
Questran Powder 770
Risperdal (Rare)................................ 1301
Zoloft Tablets (Rare) 2217

Dizziness

▲ Accupril Tablets (3.9% to 7.7%) .. 1893
Accutane Capsules 2076
Achromycin V Capsules 1367
Actifed Plus Caplets .... ĸᴅ 845
Actifed Plus Tablets .... ĸᴅ 845
▲ Actifed with Codeine Cough Syrup (Among most frequent) 1067
Actifed Syrup.................................... ĸᴅ 846
Actifed Tablets .... ĸᴅ 844
Acutrim .... ĸᴅ 628
▲ Adalat Capsules (10 mg and 20 mg) (About 10% to 27%) 587
▲ Adalat CC (4%) 589
Adenocard Injection (1%) 1021
▲ Adenoscan (12%)............................ 1024
Adipex-P Tablets and Capsules 1048
Advil Cold and Sinus Caplets and Tablets (formerly CoAdvil) .... ĸᴅ 870
▲ Children's Advil Suspension (3-9%) 2692
▲ AeroBid Inhaler System (3-9%) 1005
▲ Aerobid-M Inhaler System (3-9%).. 1005
Aerolate 1004
▲ Airet Solution for Inhalation (7%) .. 452
Albalon Solution with Liquifilm...... ◉ 231
Aldactazide 2413
Aldoclor Tablets 1598
Aldomet Ester HCl Injection 1602
Aldomet Oral 1600
Aldoril Tablets 1604
▲ Alfenta Injection (3% to 9%).......... 1286
Alka-Seltzer Plus Cold Medicine .. ĸᴅ 705
Alka-Seltzer Plus Cold & Cough Medicine .... ĸᴅ 708
Alka-Seltzer Plus Night-Time Cold Medicine .... ĸᴅ 707
Alka Seltzer Plus Sinus Medicine ĸᴅ 707
Allerest Children's Chewable Tablets .... ĸᴅ 627
Allerest Headache Strength Tablets .... ĸᴅ 627
Allerest Maximum Strength Tablets .... ĸᴅ 627
Allerest No Drowsiness Tablets .... ĸᴅ 627
Allerest Sinus Pain Formula .... ĸᴅ 627
Allerest 12 Hour Caplets .... ĸᴅ 627
All-Flex Arcing Spring Diaphragm (See also Ortho Diaphragm Kits) 1865
Alomide (Less than 1%).................... 469
▲ Altace Capsules (2.2% to 4.1%).... 1232
Alupent (1% to 4%) 669
Ambien Tablets (1% to 5%) 2416
Amen Tablets 780
Amicar Syrup, Tablets, and Injection (Occasional) 1267
Amoxil (Rare) 2464
▲ Anafranil Capsules (41% to 54%) 803
Ana-Kit Anaphylaxis Emergency Treatment Kit (Common)................. 617
▲ Anaprox/Naprosyn (3% to 9%)...... 2117
Anatuss LA Tablets........................... 1542
▲ Anexsia 5/500 Elixir (Among most frequent) 1781
Ansaid Tablets (1-3%) 2579
Apresazide Capsules (Less frequent) 808
Apresoline Hydrochloride Tablets (Less frequent) 809
AquaMEPHYTON Injection 1608
Aredia for Injection 810
▲ Artane (30% to 50%) 1368
▲ Asacol Delayed-Release Tablets (8%) 1979
Asendin Tablets (Less frequent) 1369
Atamet (Less frequent)..................... 572
Atgam Sterile Solution (Less than 1% to less than 5%)......................... 2581
Ativan Injection (Occasional) 2698
▲ Ativan Tablets (6.9%)..................... 2700

▲ Atretol Tablets (Among most frequent) 573
Atrohist Pediatric Capsules.............. 453
Atrohist Plus Tablets 454
Atromid-S Capsules (Less often) 2701
Atrovent Inhalation Aerosol (2.4%; about 1 in 100) 671
Atrovent Inhalation Solution (2.3%) 673
Augmentin (Rare) 2468
▲ Axid Pulvules (4.6%)...................... 1427
Azactam for Injection (Less than 1%) 734
Azo Gantrisin Tablets........................ 2081
BCG Vaccine, USP (TICE) (2.4%) .. 1814
Benadryl Allergy Decongestant Liquid Medication .... ĸᴅ 848
Benadryl Allergy Decongestant Tablets .... ĸᴅ 848
Benadryl Allergy Sinus Headache Formula Caplets .... ĸᴅ 849
▲ Benadryl Capsules (Among most frequent) 1898
▲ Benadryl Injection (Among most frequent) 1898
Benemid Tablets 1611
▲ Bentyl (29%) 1501
Benylin Multisymptom...................... ĸᴅ 852
Betagan (Rare) .... ◉ 233
▲ Betapace Tablets (7% to 20%) 641
▲ Betaseron for SC Injection (35%) .. 658
Betimol 0.25%, 0.5% (1% to 5%) .... ◉ 261
Betoptic Ophthalmic Solution (Rare) 469
Betoptic S Ophthalmic Suspension (Rare) 471
Biavax II 1613
Biltricide Tablets 591
Biphetamine Capsules 983
Blocadren Tablets (2.3%).................. 1614
Bontril Slow-Release Capsules 781
▲ Brethine Ampuls (1.3 to 10.2%).... 815
▲ Brevibloc Injection (3% to 12%).... 1808
Brevicon... 2088
Bricanyl Subcutaneous Injection (Common).. 1502
Bricanyl Tablets (Common).............. 1503
Bromfed... 1785
▲ Bromfed-DM Cough Syrup (Among most frequent) 1786
Bromfed-PD Capsules (Extended-Release).............................. 1785
Bronkometer Aerosol........................ 2302
Bronkosol Solution 2302
Brontex 1981
Arthritis Strength Bufferin Analgesic Caplets .... ĸᴅ 614
Bumex (1.1%) 2093
▲ Buprenex Injectable (5-10%) 2006
▲ BuSpar (12%) 737
Butisol Sodium Elixir & Tablets (Less than 1 in 100) 2660
▲ Calan SR Caplets (3.3%)................. 2422
▲ Calan Tablets (3.3%) 2419
Cama Arthritis Pain Reliever........... ĸᴅ 785
Capoten (About 0.5 to 2%) 739
Capozide (0.5 to 2%) 742
Carafate Suspension (Less than 0.5%) 1505
Carafate Tablets (Less than 0.5%) 1504
Carbocaine Hydrochloride Injection 2303
▲ Cardene Capsules (4.0-6.9%) 2095
Cardene I.V. (1.4%) 2709
Cardene SR Capsules (1.6%) 2097
▲ Cardizem CD Capsules (3.0% to 3.5%) 1506
▲ Cardizem SR Capsules (3.4% to 7%) 1510
Cardizem Injectable (Less than 1%) 1508
Cardizem Tablets (1.5%) 1512
▲ Cardura Tablets (Up to 23%) 2186
Cartrol Tablets (Less common)........ 410
Cataflam (1% to 3%) 816
▲ Catapres Tablets (About 16 in 100 patients) 674
Catapres-TTS (2 of 101 patients).. 675
Caverject (1%) 2583
Ceclor Pulvules & Suspension (Rare) 1431
Ceftin (Less than 1% but more than 0.1%)... 1078
Cefzil Tablets and Oral Suspension (1%) 746
▲ CellCept Capsules (5.7% to 11.2%) 2099
Celontin Kapseals (Frequent) 1899
Ceptaz (Fewer than 1%) 1081
Cerezyme (One patient) 1066
Cerose DM .... ĸᴅ 878

▲ CHEMET (succimer) Capsules (1.0 to 12.7%)... 1545
Children's Vicks DayQuil Allergy Relief .... ĸᴅ 757
Children's Vicks NyQuil Cold/Cough Relief .... ĸᴅ 758
Chlor-Trimeton Allergy Decongestant Tablets .... ĸᴅ 799
Cipro I.V. (1% or less)........................ 595
Cipro I.V. Pharmacy Bulk Package (Less than 1%)................................... 597
Cipro Tablets (0.3% to 1%) 592
Claritin (2% or fewer patients) 2349
▲ Claritin-D (4%) 2350
Climara Transdermal System 645
Cleocin Vaginal Cream (Less than 1%) 2589
▲ Clinoril Tablets (3-9%)..................... 1618
Clomid (Fewer than 1%) 1514
▲ Clozaril Tablets (More than 5 to 19%) 2252
Codiclear DH Syrup 791
▲ Cognex Capsules (12%) 1901
ColBENEMID Tablets 1622
Colestid Tablets (Infrequent) 2591
Coly-Mycin M Parenteral.................. 1905
▲ Combipres Tablets (About 16%).... 677
Comhist 2038
Compazine 2470
Allergy-Sinus Comtrex Multi-Symptom Allergy-Sinus Formula Tablets .... ĸᴅ 617
Comtrex Non-Drowsy .... ĸᴅ 618
Condylox (Less than 5%) 1802
Contac Continuous Action Nasal Decongestant/Antihistamine 12 Hour Capsules .... ĸᴅ 813
Contac Maximum Strength Continuous Action Decongestant/Antihistamine 12 Hour Caplets .... ĸᴅ 813
Contac Severe Cold and Flu Formula Caplets .... ĸᴅ 814
▲ Cordarone Tablets (4 to 9%)........... 2712
Coricidin 'D' Decongestant Tablets .... ĸᴅ 800
▲ Cozaar Tablets (3.5%) 1628
Cycrin Tablets 975
Cyklokapron Tablets and Injection.. 1950
Cylert Tablets 412
Cystospaz 1963
▲ Cytadren Tablets (5%) 819
Cytosar-U Sterile Powder (Less frequent) 2592
Cytotec (Infrequent) 2424
Cytovene (1% or less)....................... 2103
D.A. Chewable Tablets 951
DDAVP (Up to 3%) 2017
▲ DHCplus Capsules (Among most frequent) 1993
D.H.E. 45 Injection (Occasional)..... 2255
Dalgan Injection (1 to less than 3%) 538
Dalmane Capsules............................. 2173
Danocrine Capsules 2307
▲ Dantrium Capsules (Among most frequent) 1982
Daranide Tablets 1633
▲ Darvon-N/Darvocet-N (Among most frequent) 1433
▲ Darvon (Among most frequent) 1435
▲ Darvon-N Suspension & Tablets (Among most frequent) 1433
Decadron Phosphate with Xylocaine Injection, Sterile.............. 1639
Deconamine Chewable Tablets 1320
Deconamine CX Cough and Cold Liquid and Tablets............................ 1319
Deconamine 1320
Deconsal C Expectorant Syrup 456
Deconsal Pediatric Capsules............ 454
Deconsal Pediatric Syrup 457
Deconsal II Tablets 454
▲ Demadex Tablets and Injection (3.2%) 686
▲ Demerol (Among most frequently observed) 2308
Demulen 2428
Depakene 413
▲ Depakote Tablets (12%) 415
▲ Depo-Provera Contraceptive Injection (More than 5%).................. 2602
Depo-Provera Sterile Aqueous Suspension 2606
Desmopressin Acetate Rhinal Tube (Up to 3%) 979
Desogen Tablets................................. 1817
Desoxyn Gradumet Tablets (Rare).. 419
▲ Desyrel and Desyrel Dividose (19.7% to 28.0%).............................. 503
Dexatrim .... ĸᴅ 832

(ĸᴅ Described in PDR For Nonprescription Drugs) Incidence data in parenthesis; ▲ 3% or more (◉ Described in PDR For Ophthalmology)

Side Effects Index

Dizziness

Dexatrim Plus Vitamins Caplets .. ◉ 832
Dexedrine 2474
DextroStat Dextroamphetamine Tablets 2036
Didrex Tablets.. 2607
Diethylstilbestrol Tablets 1437
Diflucan Injection, Tablets, and Oral Suspension (1%)...................... 2194
Dilacor XR Extended-release Capsules (Infrequent; 2.2%) 2018
Dilantin Infatabs.................................... 1908
Dilantin Kapseals 1906
Dilantin Parenteral 1910
Dilantin-125 Suspension 1911
▲ Dilatrate-SR (2-36%) 2398
Dilaudid Ampules.................................. 1335
Dilaudid Cough Syrup 1336
▲ Dilaudid-HP Injection (Among most frequent) 1337
▲ Dilaudid-HP Lyophilized Powder 250 mg (Among most frequent) 1337
Dilaudid 1335
Dilaudid Oral Liquid 1339
Dilaudid 1335
Dilaudid Tablets - 8 mg......................... 1339
▲ Dimetane-DC Cough Syrup (Most frequent) 2059
Dimetane-DX Cough Syrup (Among most frequent) 2059
Dimetapp Elixir .... ◉ 773
Dimetapp Extentabs .... ◉ 774
Dimetapp Tablets/Liqui-Gels .... ◉ 775
Dimetapp Cold & Allergy Chewable Tablets............................ ◉ 773
Dimetapp Sinus Caplets .... ◉ 775
Dipentum Capsules (1.0%) 1951
Diprivan Injection (Less than 1%) .. 2833
Ditropan.. 1516
Diucardin Tablets................................... 2718
Diupres Tablets 1650
Diuril Oral Suspension.......................... 1653
Diuril Sodium Intravenous 1652
Diuril Tablets 1653
Dolobid Tablets (Greater than 1 in 100) 1654
Donnagel Liquid and Donnagel Chewable Tablets (Rare) .... ◉ 879
Donnatal 2060
Donnatal Extentabs............................... 2061
Donnatal Tablets 2060
Dopram Injectable.................................. 2061
Doral Tablets (1.5%).............................. 2664
Dorcol Children's Cough Syrup .... ◉ 785
Drixoral Cold and Allergy Sustained-Action Tablets .... ◉ 802
Drixoral Cold and Flu Extended-Release Tablets .... ◉ 803
Drixoral Allergy/Sinus Extended Release Tablets .... ◉ 804
▲ Duragesic Transdermal System (3% to 10%) 1288
Duramorph 962
Duranest Injections................................ 542
Dura-Tap/PD Capsules 2867
Dura-Vent/DA Tablets 953
Duvoid 2044
Dyazide 2479
Dyclone 0.5% and 1% Topical Solutions, USP 544
Dynacin Capsules 1590
▲ DynaCirc Capsules (3.4% to 8.0%) 2256
Dyrenium Capsules (Rare)................... 2481
E.E.S. (Isolated reports) 424
Easprin 1914
▲ EC-Naprosyn Delayed-Release Tablets (3% to 9%).............................. 2117
Ecotrin 2455
▲ Effexor (3% to 23.9%) 2719
Efidac/24 .... ◉ 635
Elavil 2838
▲ Eldepryl Tablets (7 of 49 patients) 2550
Emete-con Intramuscular/Intravenous 2198
▲ Eminase (Less than 10%) 2039
Emla Cream 545
▲ Empirin with Codeine Tablets (Among most frequent) 1093
Endep Tablets 2174
Enduron Tablets..................................... 420
▲ Engerix-B Unit-Dose Vials (1% to 10%) 2482
Entex PSE Tablets 1987
EpiPen 790
▲ Epogen for Injection (5% to 9%).... 489
▲ Ergamisol Tablets (3% to 4%) 1292
EryPed (Isolated reports) 421
Ery-Tab Tablets (Isolated reports) .. 422
Erythrocin Stearate Filmtab (Isolated reports) 425

Erythromycin Base Filmtab (Isolated reports)................................. 426
Erythromycin Delayed-Release Capsules, USP (Isolated reports) 427
▲ Esgic-plus Tablets (Among most frequent) 1013
Esidrix Tablets 821
Esimil Tablets 822
Eskalith 2485
Estrace Cream and Tablets.................. 749
Estraderm Transdermal System 824
ESTRATAB Tablets (0.3, 0.625, 1.25, 2.5 mg) 2536
Estratest 2539
▲ Ethmozine Tablets (11.3% to more than 20%) 2041
Etrafon 2355
▲ Famvir (3.3%) 2486
Fastin Capsules 2488
Fedahist Gyrocaps................................. 2401
Fedahist Timecaps 2401
▲ Felbatol (Among most common; 18.4%) 2666
Feldene Capsules (Greater than 1%) 1965
▲ Fioricet Tablets (Among most frequent) 2258
Fioricet with Codeine Capsules (Frequent) 2260
▲ Fiorinal Capsules (One of the two most frequent) 2261
Fiorinal with Codeine Capsules (2.6%) 2262
▲ Fiorinal Tablets (One of the two most frequent) 2261
Flagyl 375 Capsules.............................. 2434
Flagyl I.V. 2247
▲ Flexeril Tablets (3% to 11%) 1661
Flonase Nasal Spray (Less than 1%) 1098
▲ Floxin I.V. (1% to 5%) 1571
▲ Floxin Tablets (200 mg, 300 mg, 400 mg) (1% to 5%) 1567
Flumadine Tablets & Syrup (0.7% to 1.9%) 1015
Fortaz (Less than 1%) 1100
▲ Foscavir Injection (5% or greater).. 547
Fulvicin P/G Tablets (Occasional) .. 2359
Fulvicin P/G 165 & 330 Tablets (Occasional) 2359
Gamimune N, 5% Immune Globulin Intravenous (Human), 5% 619
Gamimune N, 10% Immune Globulin Intravenous (Human), 10% 621
Gantrisin (Rare) 2120
Garamycin Injectable 2360
Gastrocrom Capsules (Infrequent).. 984
Glucotrol Tablets (About 1 in 50) .. 1967
▲ Glucotrol XL Extended Release Tablets (6.8%) 1968
Grifulvin V (griseofulvin tablets) Microsize (griseofulvin oral suspension) Microsize (Occasional) 1888
Gris-PEG Tablets, 125 mg & 250 mg (Occasional) 479
Guaifed 1787
Guaimax-D Tablets 792
▲ Habitrol Nicotine Transdermal System (3% to 9% of patients) 865
▲ Halcion Tablets (7.8%) 2611
Havrix (Rare) 2489
Hexalen Capsules 2571
Helixtate, Antihemophilic Factor (Recombinant) 518
Hismanal Tablets (Rare to 2.0%) .. 1293
Hivid Tablets (Less than 1% to less than 3%) 2121
Humegon.. 1824
Hycodan Tablets and Syrup 930
Hycomine Compound Tablets 932
Hycomine 931
Hycotuss Expectorant Syrup 933
Hydrea Capsules (Extremely rare) .. 696
Hydrocet Capsules 782
HydroDIURIL Tablets 1674
Hydropres Tablets.................................. 1675
Hyperstat I.V. Injection (2%) 2363
▲ Hytrin Capsules (2.0% to 19.3%; 21% to 28%).. 430
▲ Hyzaar Tablets (5.7%) 1677
▲ IBU Tablets (3% to 9%) 1342
IFEX (Less frequent).............................. 697
▲ Imdur (8% to 11%) 1323
▲ Imitrex Injection (11.9%) 1103
Imitrex Tablets 1106
Imodium Capsules.................................1295
▲ Imovax Rabies Vaccine (About 20%) 881

Inapsine Injection (Less common) .. 1296
Inderide Tablets 2732
Inderide LA Long Acting Capsules .. 2734
▲ Indocin (3% to 9%)............................ 1680
INFeD (Iron Dextran Injection, USP) 2345
Infumorph 200 and Infumorph 500 Sterile Solutions.......................... 965
Intal Capsules (Less than 1 in 10,000 patients)................................... 987
Intal Inhaler (Infrequent) 988
Intal Nebulizer Solution........................ 989
▲ Intron A (7% to 24%) 2364
Inversine Tablets 1686
Iopidine 0.5% (Less than 1%) .... ◎ 221
Ismelin Tablets 827
▲ Ismo Tablets (3% to 5%) 2738
ISMOTIC 45% w/v Solution (Very rare) .... ◎ 222
Isoclor Timesule Capsules .... ◉ 637
Isoetharine Inhalation Solution, USP, Arm-a-Med.............................. 551
Isoptin Injectable (1.2%)...................... 1344
▲ Isoptin Oral Tablets (3.3%) 1346
▲ Isoptin SR Tablets (3.3%).................. 1348
Isuprel Hydrochloride Injection 1:5000 2311
Isuprel Hydrochloride Solution 1:200 & 1:100 2313
Isuprel Mistometer 2312
▲ JE-VAX (Approximately 10%)......... 886
K-Phos Neutral Tablets 639
K-Phos Original Formula 'Sodium Free' Tablets (Less frequent) 639
Keflex Pulvules & Oral Suspension 914
Keftab Tablets... 915
Kemadrin Tablets 1112
▲ Kerlone Tablets (4.5% to 14.8%).. 2436
KOGENATE Antihemophilic Factor (Recombinant) 632
Kwell Cream & Lotion 2008
Kwell Shampoo 2009
▲ Kytril Tablets (3%) 2492
▲ Lamictal Tablets (Among most common; 31% to 54%)...................... 1112
Lamprene Capsules (Less than 1%) 828
Lanoxicaps 1117
Lanoxin Elixir Pediatric 1120
Lanoxin Injection 1123
Lanoxin Injection Pediatric.................. 1126
Lanoxin Tablets 1128
▲ Lariam Tablets (Among most frequent; less than 1%) 2128
Larodopa Tablets (Relatively frequent) 2129
Lasix Injection, Oral Solution and Tablets 1240
Lescol Capsules (2.6%) 2267
▲ Leustatin (9%) 1834
▲ Levatol (4.9%) 2403
Levbid Extended-Release Tablets.... 2405
Levien/Tri-Levlen 651
Levo-Dromoran (Common).................. 2129
Levoprome (Sometimes) 1274
Levsin/Levsinex/Levbid 2405
▲ Limbitrol (Among most frequent).... 2180
Lindane Lotion USP 1% 582
Lindane Shampoo USP 1% 583
▲ Lioresal Intrathecal (6 to 12 of 214 patients) 1596
▲ Lioresal Tablets (5-15%).................... 829
Lithium Carbonate Capsules & Tablets 2230
Lithonate/Lithotabs/Lithobid 2543
▲ Lodine Capsules and Tablets (3-9%) 2743
Lomotil 2439
Lo/Ovral Tablets 2746
Lo/Ovral-28 Tablets............................... 2751
Lopid Tablets... 1917
▲ Lopressor Ampuls (10%) 830
▲ Lopressor HCT Tablets (10 in 100 patients) 832
▲ Lopressor Tablets (10%) 830
Lorabid Suspension and Pulvules.... 1459
▲ Lorcet 10/650 (Among most frequent) 1018
Lorelco Tablets 1517
▲ Lortab (Among most frequent)....... 2566
▲ Lotensin Tablets (1.5% to 3.6%) .. 834
▲ Lotensin HCT (3.5% to 6.3%) 837
Lotrel Capsules (1.3%) 840
Loxitane 1378
▲ Lozol Tablets (Greater than or equal to 5%) 2022
▲ Ludiomil Tablets (8%) 843
Lupron Depot 3.75 mg (Less than 5%) 2556
Lupron Depot 7.5 mg 2559
▲ Lupron Injection (5% or more)........ 2555

▲ Luvox Tablets (11%) 2544
▲ Lysodren (15%) 698
M-M-R II 1687
M-R-VAX II 1689
▲ MS Contin Tablets (Among most frequent) 1994
▲ MSIR (Among most frequent) 1997
Macrobid Capsules (Less than 1%) 1988
Macrodantin Capsules........................... 1989
Marax Tablets & DF Syrup................... 2200
Marcaine Hydrochloride with Epinephrine 1:200,000 (Rare) 2316
Marcaine Hydrochloride Injection (Rare) 2316
Marcaine Spinal (Rare) 2319
▲ Marinol (Dronabinol) Capsules (3% to 10%) 2231
Matulane Capsules 2131
Maxair Autohaler (0.6% to 1.2%).. 1492
Maxair Inhaler (1.2%)........................... 1494
Maxaquin Tablets (2.3%) 2440
Maxzide 1380
Mebaral Tablets (Less than 1 in 100) 2322
Menest Tablets 2494
▲ Mepergan Injection (Among most frequent) 2753
Mephyton Tablets (Rare) 1696
▲ Mepron Suspension (3% to 8%) 1135
Meruvax II 1697
Mesantoin Tablets.................................. 2272
▲ Methadone Hydrochloride Oral Concentrate (Among most frequent) 2233
Methadone Hydrochloride Oral Solution & Tablets................................ 2235
Methergine (Rare) 2272
Methotrexate Sodium Tablets, Injection, for Injection and LPF Injection (Frequent; 1 to 3%) 1275
MetroGel-Vaginal (Equal to or less than 2%) 902
Mevacor Tablets (0.5% to 2.0%) .. 1699
▲ Mexitil Capsules (18.9% to 26.4%) 678
Miacalcin Nasal Spray (1% to 3%) 2275
Micronor Tablets 1872
Midamor Tablets (Between 1% and 3%) 1703
Midrin Capsules 783
Migralam Capsules 2038
Milontin Kapseals................................... 1920
Miltown Tablets 2672
▲ Minipress Capsules (10.3%) 1937
▲ Minizide Capsules (10.3%) 1938
Minocin Intravenous 1382
Minocin Oral Suspension 1385
Minocin Pellet-Filled Capsules 1383
Mintezol 1704
Mivacron (Less than 1%) 1138
Modicon 1872
▲ Moduretic Tablets (3% to 8%)........ 1705
8-MOP Capsules 1246
Monoket (Up to 4%) 2406
Monopril Tablets (1.6%) 757
Motofen Tablets (1 in 20) 784
▲ Children's Motrin Ibuprofen Oral Suspension (3% to 9%) 1546
▲ Motrin Tablets (3% to 9%) 2625
▲ Motrin Ibuprofen Suspension, Oral Drops, Chewable Tablets, Caplets (3% to 9%) 1546
Myambutol Tablets 1386
▲ Mykrox Tablets (10.2%) 993
Myochrysine Injection 1711
▲ Nalfon 200 Pulvules & Nalfon Tablets (6.5%) 917
▲ Anaprox/Naprosyn (3% to 9%)...... 2117
Nardil (Common)................................... 1920
Nebcin Vials, Hyporets & ADD-Vantage 1464
▲ NebuPent for Inhalation Solution (31 to 47%) 1040
NegGram 2323
Nembutal Sodium Capsules (Less than 1%) 436
Nembutal Sodium Solution (Less than 1%) 438
Nembutal Sodium Suppositories (Less than 1%) 440
Nescaine/Nescaine MPF 554
Netromycin Injection 100 mg/ml.... 2373
▲ Neurontin Capsules (Among most common; 17.1%) 1922
Nicoderm (nicotine transdermal system) (1% to 3%) 1518
▲ Nicorette (3% to 9% of patients) .. 2458
▲ Nicotrol Nicotine Transdermal System (3% to 9%) 1550
Nimotop Capsules (Less than 1%) 610

(◉ Described in PDR For Nonprescription Drugs) Incidence data in parenthesis; ▲ 3% or more (◎ Described in PDR For Ophthalmology)

Dizziness

Side Effects Index

Nitrolingual Spray (Occasional) 2027
Nizoral Tablets (Less than 1%) 1298
Nolamine Timed-Release Tablets (Occasional) 785
Nolvadex Tablets (Infrequent) 2841
Nordette-21 Tablets 2755
Nordette-28 Tablets 2758
Norflex 1496
Norgesic 1496
Norinyl 2088
Norisodrine with Calcium Iodide Syrup 442
▲ Normodyne Injection (2% to 16%) 2377
▲ Normodyne Tablets (1% to 16%) .. 2379
Noroxin Tablets (1.7% to 2.6%) 1715
Noroxin Tablets (1.7% to 2.6%) 2048
▲ Norpace (3 to 9%) 2444
Norplant System 2759
Norpramin Tablets 1526
Nor-Q D Tablets 2135
▲ Norvasc Tablets (0.1% to 3.4%) .. 1940
Novahistine DH 2462
Novahistine DMX .... ⊞ 822
Novahistine Elixir .... ⊞ 823
Novahistine Expectorant 2463
Novocain Hydrochloride for Spinal Anesthesia 2326
▲ Nubain Injection (5%) 935
Nucofed 2051
Ocuflox (One report) 481
Ocupress Ophthalmic Solution, 1% Sterile (Occasional) .... ◉ 309
Ogen Tablets 2627
Ogen Vaginal Cream 2630
Oncaspar (Less than 1%) 2028
OptiPranolol (Metipranolol 0.3%) Sterile Ophthalmic Solution (A small number of patients) .... ◉ 258
▲ Oramorph SR (Morphine Sulfate Sustained Release Tablets) (Among most frequent) 2236
Orap Tablets 1050
Oretic Tablets 443
Organidin NR Tablets and Liquid (Rare) 2672
Ornade Spansule Capsules 2502
Ortho-Cept 1851
Ortho-Cyclen/Ortho-Tri-Cyclen 1858
Ortho Diaphragm Kits—All-Flex Arcing Spring; Ortho Coil Spring; Ortho-White Flat Spring 1865
Ortho Diaphragm Kit-Coil Spring 1865
Ortho Dienestrol Cream 1866
Ortho-Est 1869
Ortho-Novum 1872
Ortho-Cyclen/Ortho Tri-Cyclen 1858
Ortho-White Diaphragm Kit-Flat Spring (See also Ortho Diaphragm Kits) 1865
Orthoclone OKT3 Sterile Solution .. 1837
Orudis Capsules (Greater than 1%) 2766
Oruvail Capsules (Greater than 1%) 2766
Ovcon 760
Ovral Tablets 2770
Ovral-28 Tablets 2770
Ovrette Tablets 2771
Oxsoralen-Ultra Capsules 1257
▲ PBZ Tablets (Among most frequent) 845
▲ PBZ-SR Tablets (Among most frequent) 844
PMB 200 and PMB 400 2783
Pamelor 2280
Paraflex Caplets (Occasional) 1580
Parafon Forte DSC Caplets (Occasional) 1581
▲ Parlodel (Less than 2% to 17%) 2281
Parnate Tablets 2503
▲ Paxil Tablets (6.7% to 13.3%) 2505
Pediatric Vicks 44d Dry Hacking Cough & Head Congestion .... ⊞ 763
Pediatric Vicks 44m Cough & Cold Relief .... ⊞ 764
Peganone Tablets 446
Penetrex Tablets (Less than 1% to 3%) 2031
Pentam 300 Injection (0.5%) 1041
Pentasa (Less than 1%) 1527
Pentaspan Injection 937
Pepcid Injection (1.3%) 1722
Pepcid (1.3%) 1720
Peptavlon 2878
▲ Percocet Tablets (Among most frequent) 938
▲ Percodan Tablets (Among most frequent) 939
▲ Percodan-Demi Tablets (Among most frequent) 940
Pergonal (menotropins for injection, USP) 2448
Periactin 1724
▲ Permax Tablets (19.1%) 575
▲ Persantine Tablets (13.6%) 681
Phenergan with Codeine 2777
Phenergan with Dextromethorphan 2778
Phenergan Injection 2773
Phenergan Suppositories 2775
Phenergan Syrup 2774
Phenergan Tablets 2775
Phenergan VC 2779
Phenergan VC with Codeine 2781
Phenobarbital Elixir and Tablets (Less than 1 in 100 patients) 1469
Phenurone Tablets (Less than 1%) 447
▲ Phrenilin (Among most frequent) 785
Pipracil 1390
Placidyl Capsules 448
Plaquenil Sulfate Tablets 2328
▲ Plendil Extended-Release Tablets (2.7% to 3.7%) 527
Polymyxin B Sulfate, Aerosporin Brand Sterile Powder 1154
Pondimin Tablets 2066
Ponstel 1925
Pontocaine Hydrochloride for Spinal Anesthesia 2330
Pravachol (1.0% to 3.3%) 765
Prelu-2 Timed Release Capsules 681
Premarin Intravenous 2787
Premarin with Methyltestosterone .. 2794
Premarin Tablets 2789
Premarin Vaginal Cream 2791
Premphase 2797
Prempro 2801
PREVACID Delayed-Release Capsules (Less than 1%) 2562
Prilosec Delayed-Release Capsules (1.5%) 529
Primaxin I.M. 1727
Primaxin I.V. (0.3%) 1729
▲ Prinivil Tablets (5.4% to 14%) 1733
▲ Prinzide Tablets (7.5%) 1737
Pro-Banthine Tablets 2052
Procan SR Tablets (Occasional) 1926
▲ Procardia Capsules (Approximately 10% to 27%; 1 in 8 patients) 1971
▲ Procardia XL Extended Release Tablets (4.1% to 27%; 1 in 8 patients) 1972
▲ Procrit for Injection (5% to 9%) 1841
Proglycem 580
▲ Prograf (Greater than 3%) 1042
Prolastin Alpha₁-Proteinase Inhibitor (Human) (0.19%) 635
▲ Proleukin for Injection (17%) 797
Prolixin 509
Propagest Tablets 786
Propulsid (More than 1%) 1300
▲ ProSom Tablets (7%) 449
Prostep (nicotine transdermal system) (1% to 3% of patients) .. 1394
Prostigmin Injectable 1260
Prostigmin Tablets 1261
Prostin E2 Suppository 2634
Protopam Chloride for Injection 2806
Protostat Tablets 1883
Proventil Inhalation Aerosol (Less than 5%) 2382
▲ Proventil Inhalation Solution 0.083% (7%) 2384
Proventil Repetabs Tablets (2%) 2386
▲ Proventil Solution for Inhalation 0.5% (7%) 2383
▲ Proventil Syrup (3 of 100 patients) 2385
Proventil Tablets (2%) 2386
Provera Tablets 2636
▲ Prozac Pulvules & Liquid, Oral Solution (5.7%; 13%) 919
Pyrroxate Caplets .... ⊞ 772
Quadrinal Tablets 1350
Quarzan Capsules 2181
Questran Light 769
Questran Powder 770
▲ Quinaglute Dura-Tabs Tablets (3%) 649
Quinidex Extentabs 2067
▲ RMS Suppositories (Among most frequent) 2657
▲ Rabies Vaccine, Imovax Rabies I.D. (About 20%) 883
Regitine 846
Reglan (Less frequent) 2068
▲ Relafen Tablets (3% to 9%) 2510
ReoPro Vials (1.8%) 1471
▲ Restoril Capsules (7%) 2284
▲ Retrovir Capsules (6% to 17.9%) 1158
▲ Retrovir I.V. Infusion (6% to 17.9%) 1163
▲ Retrovir Syrup (6% to 17.9%) 1158
▲ ReVia Tablets (4% to less than 10%) 940
▲ Revex (3%) 1811
Rifadin 1528
Rifamate Capsules 1530
Rifater 1532
Rimactane Capsules 847
▲ Risperdal (4% to 7%) 1301
Ritalin 848
Robaxin Injectable 2070
Robaxin Tablets 2071
▲ Robaxisal Tablets (One in 20-25) .. 2071
Robinul Forte Tablets 2072
Robinul Injectable 2072
Robinul Tablets 2072
Robitussin Maximum Strength Cough & Cold .... ⊞ 778
Robitussin Pediatric Cough & Cold Formula .... ⊞ 779
Robitussin-CF .... ⊞ 777
Robitussin-DAC Syrup 2074
Robitussin-PE .... ⊞ 778
Rocephin Injectable Vials, ADD-Vantage, Galaxy Container (Occasional) 2142
▲ Roferon-A Injection (21% to 40%) 2145
▲ Rogaine Topical Solution (3.42%) .. 2637
▲ Romazicon (1% to 9%) 2147
Rondec Oral Drops 953
Rondec Syrup 953
Rondec Tablet 953
Rondec-DM Oral Drops 954
Rondec-DM Syrup 954
Rondec-TR Tablet 953
Rowasa (1.84% to 3.0%) 2548
▲ Roxanol (Among most frequent) 2243
▲ Roxicodone Tablets, Oral Solution & Intensol (Oxycodone) (Among most frequent) 2244
Ryna .... ⊞ 841
Rynatan 2673
▲ Rythmol Tablets–150mg, 225mg, 300mg (3.6 to 15.1%) 1352
▲ Salagen Tablets (5% to 12%) 1489
Sandoglobulin I.V. (Less than 1%) .. 2290
Sanorex Tablets 2294
Sansert Tablets 2295
Sclerosmate (Rare) 1891
Seconal Sodium Pulvules (Less than 1 in 100) 1474
▲ Sectral Capsules (6%) 2807
▲ Sedapap Tablets 50 mg/650 mg (Among the most frequent) 1543
▲ Seldane Tablets (2.9% to 5.8%) 1536
Seldane-D Extended-Release Tablets (Rare) 1538
▲ Semprex-D Capsules (3%) 463
▲ Semprex-D Capsules (3%) 1167
Sensorcaine (Rare) 559
Ser-Ap-Es Tablets 849
Serax Capsules (In few instances) .. 2810
Serax Tablets (In few instances) 2810
Serentil 684
Serophene (clomiphene citrate tablets, USP) (Less than 1 in 100 patients) 2451
▲ Serzone Tablets (11% to 22%) 771
Sinarest .... ⊞ 648
Sine-Aid IB Caplets 1554
Sine-Aid Maximum Strength Sinus Medication Gelcaps, Caplets and Tablets 1554
Sine-Off No Drowsiness Formula Caplets .... ⊞ 824
Sine-Off Sinus Medicine .... ⊞ 825
Sinemet Tablets (Less frequent) 943
Sinemet CR Tablets (2.9%) 944
Sinequan (Occasional) 2205
Singlet Tablets .... ⊞ 825
Sinulin Tablets 787
Sinutab Non-Drying Liquid Caps .. ⊞ 859
Skelaxin Tablets 788
Solganol Suspension 2388
Soma Compound w/Codeine Tablets 2676
Soma Compound Tablets (Very rare to less frequent) 2675
Soma Tablets 2674
Sorbitrate 2843
Sporanox Capsules (0.7% to 1.7%) 1305
▲ Stadol (19%) 775
Stelazine 2514
Stilphostrol Tablets and Ampuls 612
Stimate, (desmopressin acetate) Nasal Spray, 1.5 mg/mL 525
Sublimaze Injection 1307
Sudafed Children's Liquid .... ⊞ 861
Sudafed Cough Syrup .... ⊞ 862
Sudafed Plus Liquid .... ⊞ 862
Sudafed Plus Tablets .... ⊞ 863
Sudafed Sinus Caplets .... ⊞ 864
Sudafed Sinus Tablets .... ⊞ 864
Sudafed Tablets, 30 mg .... ⊞ 861
Sudafed Tablets, 60 mg .... ⊞ 861
Sudafed 12 Hour Caplets .... ⊞ 861
Suprelin Injection (1% to 3%) 2056
Suprane (Less than 1%) 1813
Suprax (Less than 2%) 1399
Surmontil Capsules 2811
Sus-Phrine Injection 1019
▲ Symmetrel Capsules and Syrup (5% to 10%) 946
Syn-Rx Tablets 465
Syn-Rx DM Tablets 466
Tagamet (Approximately 1 in 100) 2516
Talacen 2333
▲ Talwin Injection (Most common) 2334
Talwin Compound 2335
▲ Talwin Injection (Most common) 2334
Talwin Nx 2336
▲ Tambocor Tablets (18.9%) 1497
▲ Tavist Syrup (Among most frequent) 2297
▲ Tavist Tablets (Among most frequent) 2298
Tazicef for Injection (Less than 1%) 2519
Tazidime Vials, Faspak & ADD-Vantage 1478
▲ Tegison Capsules (1-10%) 2154
▲ Tegretol Chewable Tablets (Among most frequent) 852
▲ Tegretol Suspension (Among most frequent) 852
▲ Tegretol Tablets (Among most frequent) 852
Teldrin 12 Hour Antihistamine/Nasal Decongestant Allergy Relief Capsules .... ⊞ 826
Temaril Tablets, Syrup and Spansule Extended-Release Capsules 483
▲ Tenex Tablets (1% to 15%) 2074
▲ Tenoretic Tablets (4% to 13%) 2845
▲ Tenormin Tablets and I.V. Injection (4% to 13%) 2847
Tessalon Perles 1020
Thalitone 1245
TheraCys BCG Live (Intravesical) (Up to 0.9%) 897
TheraFlu .... ⊞ 787
TheraFlu Maximum Strength Nighttime Flu, Cold & Cough Medicine .... ⊞ 788
Thioplex (Thiotepa For Injection) 1281
Thorazine 2523
▲ THROMBATE III Antithrombin III (Human) (7 of 17) 637
Ticlid Tablets (1.1%) 2156
Tigan 2057
Tilade (0.9%) 996
Timentin for Injection 2528
Timolide Tablets (1.2%) 1748
Timoptic in Ocudose (Less frequent) 1753
Timoptic Sterile Ophthalmic Solution (Less frequent) 1751
Timoptic-XE (1% to 5% of patients) 1755
Tobramycin Sulfate Injection 968
Tofranil Ampuls 854
Tofranil Tablets 856
Tofranil-PM Capsules 857
▲ Tolectin (200, 400 and 600 mg) (3 to 9%) 1581
▲ Tonocard Tablets (8.0-25.3%) 531
▲ Toprol-XL Tablets (About 10 of 100 patients) 565
▲ Toradol (7%) 2159
Torecan (Occasional) 2245
▲ Tornalate Solution for Inhalation, 0.2% (4.0%) 956
Tornalate Metered Dose Inhaler (1.0% to 3%) 957
Trancopal Caplets 2337
▲ Trandate (9 of 100 patients; 1% to 16%) 1185
Transderm Scōp Transdermal Therapeutic System (Infrequent) 869
Tranxene (Less common) 451
Trental Tablets (1.9%) 1244
Triaminic Allergy Tablets .... ⊞ 789
Triaminic Cold Tablets .... ⊞ 790
Triaminic Syrup .... ⊞ 792
Triaminic-12 Tablets .... ⊞ 792
Triaminic-DM Syrup .... ⊞ 792

(⊞ Described in PDR For Nonprescription Drugs) Incidence data in parenthesis; ▲ 3% or more (◉ Described in PDR For Ophthalmology)

1277 **Side Effects Index** **Drowsiness**

Triaminicin Tablets ▣ 793
Triaminicol Multi-Symptom Cold Tablets ▣ 793
Triaminicol Multi-Symptom Relief ▣ 794
Triavil Tablets 1757
Trilafon (Rare) 2389
Levlen/Tri-Levlen 651
Trilisate (Less than 2%) 2000
▲ Trinalin Repetabs Tablets (Among most frequent) 1330
Tri-Norinyl 2164
Triphasil-21 Tablets 2814
Triphasil-28 Tablets 2819
Trobicin Sterile Powder 2645
Tussend 1783
Tussend Expectorant 1785
Tussionex Pennkinetic Extended-Release Suspension 998
Tussi-Organidin DM NR Liquid and DM-S NR Liquid 2677
Tussi-Organidin NR Liquid and S NR Liquid (At higher doses) 2677
Children's TYLENOL Cold Multi-Symptom Liquid Formula and Chewable Tablets 1561
TYLENOL Maximum Strength Flu NightTime Hot Medication Packets 1562
TYLENOL, Maximum Strength, Sinus Medication Geltabs, Gelcaps, Caplets and Tablets 1566
TYLENOL Cold Multi-Symptom Formula Medication Tablets and Caplets 1561
TYLENOL Cold Medication No Drowsiness Formula Gelcaps and Caplets 1562
TYLENOL Cold Multi-Symptom Hot Medication Liquid Packets 1557
TYLENOL Cough Multi-Symptom Medication with Decongestant 1565
▲ Tylenol with Codeine (Among most frequent) 1583
▲ Tylox Capsules (Among most frequent) 1584
Tympagesic Ear Drops 2342
▲ Ultram Tablets (50 mg) (26% to 33%) 1585
▲ Univasc Tablets (4.3%) 2410
Urecholine 1761
Urised Tablets 1964
Uroqid-Acid No. 2 Tablets 640
Ursinus Inlay-Tabs ▣ 794
Valtrex Caplets (2% to 4%) 1194
Vancocin HCl, Oral Solution & Pulvules (Rare) 1483
Vancocin HCl, Vials & ADD-Vantage (Rare) 1481
Vantin for Oral Suspension and Vantin Tablets (Less than 1%) 2646
▲ Vascor (200, 300 and 400 mg) Tablets (11.63 to 27.27%) 1587
▲ Vaseretic Tablets (8.6%) 1765
Vasotec I.V. (0.5 to 1%) 1768
▲ Vasotec Tablets (4.3% to 7.9%) 1771
Velban Vials 1484
▲ Ventolin Inhalation Aerosol and Refill (Fewer than 5 per 100 patients) 1197
▲ Ventolin Inhalation Solution (7%) 1198
▲ Ventolin Nebules Inhalation Solution (7%) 1199
Ventolin Rotacaps for Inhalation (Less than 1%) 1200
▲ Ventolin Syrup (3 of 100 patients) 1202
Ventolin Tablets (2 of 100 patients) 1203
▲ Verelan Capsules (3.3% to 4.2%) 1410
▲ Verelan Capsules (3.3% to 4.2%) 2824
Versed Injection (Less than 1%) 2170
Vicks 44 LiquiCaps Cough, Cold & Flu Relief ▣ 755
Vicks 44 LiquiCaps Non-Drowsy Cough & Cold Relief ▣ 756
Vicks 44D Dry Hacking Cough & Head Congestion ▣ 755
Vicks 44M Cough, Cold & Flu Relief ▣ 756
Vicks DayQuil Allergy Relief 4-Hour Tablets ▣ 760
Vicks DayQuil ▣ 761
Vicks DayQuil SINUS Pressure & CONGESTION Relief ▣ 761
Vicks Nyquil Hot Therapy ▣ 762
Vicks NyQuil LiquiCaps Multi-Symptom Cold/Flu Relief ▣ 763
Vicks NyQuil Multi-Symptom Cold/Flu Relief - (Original & Cherry Flavor) ▣ 763
Vicodin Tablets 1356
▲ Vicodin ES Tablets (Among most frequent) 1357
Vicodin Tuss Expectorant 1358
▲ Videx Tablets, Powder for Oral Solution, & Pediatric Powder for Oral Solution (1% to 7%) 720
▲ Visken Tablets (9%) 2299
Vivactil Tablets 1774
Voltaren Tablets (1% to 3%) 861
Vontrol Tablets (Rare) 2532
▲ Wellbutrin Tablets (22.3%) 1204
▲ Wygesic Tablets (Most frequent) 2827
▲ Xanax Tablets (1.8% to 29.8%) 2649
▲ Xylocaine Injections (Among most common) 567
Yocon 1892
Yohimex Tablets 1363
Zantac (Rare) 1209
Zantac Injection (Rare) 1207
Zantac Syrup (Rare) 1209
Zarontin Capsules 1928
Zarontin Syrup 1929
Zaroxolyn Tablets 1000
▲ Zebeta Tablets (2.9% to 3.5%) 1413
Zefazone 2654
▲ Zerit Capsules (Fewer than 1% to 9%) 729
▲ Zestoretic (7.5%) 2850
▲ Zestril Tablets (5.4% to 14.0%) 2854
▲ Ziac (3.2% to 5.1%) 1415
Zithromax (1% or less) 1944
Zocor Tablets 1775
▲ Zofran Injection (12%) 1214
▲ Zofran Tablets (4% to 7%) 1217
▲ Zoladex (5% to 6%) 2858
▲ Zoloft Tablets (Infrequent to 11.7) 2217
▲ Zonalon Cream (Approximately 1% to 10%) 1055
Zosyn (1.4%) 1419
Zosyn Pharmacy Bulk Package (1.4%) 1422
Zovirax (0.3%) 1219
▲ Zydone Capsules (Among most frequent) 949
Zyloprim Tablets (Less than 1%) 1226

Down's syndrome

Pergonal (menotropins for injection, USP) 2448
Serophene (clomiphene citrate tablets, USP) (Six cases) 2451

Dreaming

Dilaudid Tablets and Liquid (Less frequent) 1339
Endep Tablets 2174
Ganite 2533
Limbitrol (Less common) 2180
MS Contin Tablets (Less frequent) 1994
MSIR (Infrequent) 1997
Milontin Kapseals 1920
▲ Orudis Capsules (3% to 9%) 2766
▲ Oruvail Capsules (3% to 9%) 2766
Tenoretic Tablets (Up to 3%) 2845
Tenormin Tablets and I.V. Injection (Up to 3%) 2847
Versed Injection (Less than 1%) 2170

Dreaming, abnormalities

Children's Advil Suspension (Less than 1%) 2692
Aldomet Ester HCl Injection 1602
Ambien Tablets (1%) 2416
Anafranil Capsules (Up to 3%) 803
Anaprox/Naprosyn (Less than 1%) 2117
Axid Pulvules (1.9%) 1427
Blocadren Tablets (Less than 1%) 1614
Buprenex Injectable (Less than 1%) 2006
BuSpar (Frequent) 737
Cardene Capsules (0.4%) 2095
Cardizem CD Capsules (Less than 1%) 1506
Cardizem SR Capsules (Less than 1%) 1510
Cardizem Injectable 1508
Cardizem Tablets (Less than 1%) 1512
Cartrol Tablets (Rare) 410
Catapres Tablets 674
Catapres-TTS 675
Cognex Capsules (Infrequent) 1901
Combipres Tablets 677
Cozaar Tablets (Less than 1%) 1628
Cytovene (1% or less) 2103
Depakote Tablets (Greater than 1% but not more than 5%) 415
Desyrel and Desyrel Dividose (Less than 1% to 5.1%) 503
Dilacor XR Extended-release Capsules (1.4%) 2018
Dilaudid-HP Injection (Less frequent) 1337
Dilaudid-HP Lyophilized Powder 250 mg (Less frequent) 1337
Diprivan Injection (Less than 1%) 2833
Duragesic Transdermal System (1% or greater) 1288
EC-Naprosyn Delayed-Release Tablets (Less than 1%) 2117
▲ Effexor (4%) 2719
Elavil 2838
▲ Eldepryl Tablets (2 of 49 patients) 2550
Etrafon 2355
Feldene Capsules (Less than 1%) 1965
Flexeril Tablets (Less than 1%) 1661
Floxin I.V. (Less than 1%) 1571
Floxin Tablets (200 mg, 300 mg, 400 mg) (Less than 1%) 1567
▲ Habitrol Nicotine Transdermal System (3% to 9% of patients) 865
Halcion Tablets (Rare) 2611
Hyzaar Tablets 1677
IBU Tablets (Less than 1%) 1342
Inderal 2728
Inderal LA Long Acting Capsules 2730
Inderide Tablets 2732
Intron A (Less than 5%) 2364
IOPIDINE Sterile Ophthalmic Solution ⊚ 219
Kerlone Tablets (1.0%) 2436
Lamictal Tablets (Infrequent) 1112
Lotensin HCT (0.3% to 1.0%) 837
Luvox Tablets 2544
Mellaril 2269
Children's Motrin Ibuprofen Oral Suspension (Less than 1%) 1546
Motrin Tablets (Less than 1%) 2625
Motrin Ibuprofen Suspension, Oral Drops, Chewable Tablets, Caplets (Less than 1%) 1546
Anaprox/Naprosyn (Less than 1%) 2117
Neurontin Capsules (Infrequent) 1922
▲ Nicoderm (nicotine transdermal system) (3% to 9%) 1518
Norvasc Tablets (More than 0.1% to 1%) 1940
Nubain Injection (1% or less) 935
Oramorph SR (Morphine Sulfate Sustained Release Tablets) (Less frequent) 2236
Orap Tablets (2.7%) 1050
Orlamm (1% to 3%) 2239
Permax Tablets (2.7%) 575
Prilosec Delayed-Release Capsules (Less than 1%) 529
▲ Prograf (Greater than 3%) 1042
Prolixin 509
ProSom Tablets (2%) 449
▲ Prozac Pulvules & Liquid, Oral Solution (5%) 919
ReVia Tablets (Less than 1%) 940
Risperdal (Frequent) 1301
Rythmol Tablets–150mg, 225mg, 300mg (Less than 1%) 1352
Salagen Tablets (Less than 1%) 1489
Sectral Capsules (2%) 2807
Serentil 684
▲ Serzone Tablets (3%) 771
Sinemet CR Tablets (1.8%) 944
Stadol (Less than 1%) 775
Symmetrel Capsules and Syrup (1% to 5%) 946
Talacen (Infrequent) 2333
Talwin Injection (Infrequent) 2334
Talwin Compound (Infrequent) 2335
Talwin Injection 2334
Talwin Nx 2336
Tambocor Tablets (Less than 1%) 1497
Temaril Tablets, Syrup and Spansule Extended-Release Capsules 483
Tonocard Tablets (Less than 1%) 531
Toradol (1% or less) 2159
Torecan 2245
Triavil Tablets 1757
Trilafon 2389
▲ Visken Tablets (5%) 2299
Wellbutrin Tablets 1204
Xanax Tablets (1.8%) 2649
Zebeta Tablets (0%) 1413
Ziac 1415
Zoloft Tablets (Infrequent) 2217

Drowsiness

Accupril Tablets (0.5% to 1.0%) 1893
Accutane Capsules 2076
▲ Acel-Imune Diphtheria and Tetanus Toxoids and Acellular Pertussis Vaccine Adsorbed (6% to 12%) 1364
▲ ActHIB (2.5% to 63.7%) 872
Actifed Allergy Daytime/Nighttime Caplets ▣ 844
Actifed Plus Caplets ▣ 845
Actifed Plus Tablets ▣ 845
▲ Actifed with Codeine Cough Syrup (Among most frequent) 1067
Actifed Sinus Daytime/Nighttime Tablets and Caplets ▣ 846
Actifed Syrup ▣ 846
Actifed Tablets ▣ 844
Adalat CC (Less than 1.0%) 589
Adenoscan (Less than 1%) 1024
Children's Advil Suspension (Less than 1%) 2692
Akineton 1333
Albalon Solution with Liquifilm ⊚ 231
Aldactazide 2413
Aldactone 2414
Alfenta Injection (1% to 3%) 1286
Alka-Seltzer Plus Cold Medicine ▣ 705
Alka-Seltzer Plus Cold Medicine Liqui-Gels ▣ 706
Alka-Seltzer Plus Cold & Cough Medicine ▣ 708
Alka-Seltzer Plus Cold & Cough Medicine Liqui-Gels ▣ 705
Alka-Seltzer Plus Night-Time Cold Medicine ▣ 707
Alka-Seltzer Plus Night-Time Cold Medicine Liqui-Gels ▣ 706
Alka Seltzer Plus Sinus Medicine ▣ 707
Allerest Children's Chewable Tablets ▣ 627
Allerest Headache Strength Tablets ▣ 627
Allerest Maximum Strength Tablets ▣ 627
Allerest No Drowsiness Tablets ▣ 627
Allerest Sinus Pain Formula ▣ 627
Allerest 12 Hour Caplets ▣ 627
Alomide (Less than 1%) 469
Altace Capsules (Less than 1%) 1232
Alupent Tablets (0.6%) 669
▲ Ambien Tablets (2% to 8%) 2416
Amen Tablets 780
▲ Anafranil Capsules (46% to 54%) 803
Ana-Kit Anaphylaxis Emergency Treatment Kit 617
▲ Anaprox/Naprosyn (3% to 9%) 2117
Anexsia 5/500 Elixir 1781
Anexia Tablets 1782
Ansaid Tablets (1-3%) 2579
Antabuse Tablets (Small number of patients) 2695
Antivert, Antivert/25 Tablets, & Antivert/50 Tablets 2185
Apresazide Capsules 808
▲ Aredia for Injection (Up to 6%) 810
Artane 1368
Arthritis Foundation NightTime Caplets ▣ 674
Asacol Delayed-Release Tablets 1979
▲ Asendin Tablets (14%) 1369
Atamet 572
Atarax Tablets & Syrup 2185
▲ Ativan Injection (6%) 2698
▲ Atretol Tablets (Among most frequent) 573
Atrohist Pediatric Capsules 453
▲ Atrohist Pediatric Suspension (Among most common) 454
Atrohist Plus Tablets 454
Atromid-S Capsules 2701
Atrovent Inhalation Aerosol (Less frequent) 671
Axid Pulvules (1.9%) 1427
Azo Gantrisin Tablets 2081
Azulfidine (Rare) 1949
BC Cold Powder Multi-Symptom Formula (Cold-Sinus-Allergy) ▣ 609
Bellergal-S Tablets (Rare) 2250
Benadryl Allergy Decongestant Liquid Medication ▣ 848
Benadryl Allergy Decongestant Tablets ▣ 848
Benadryl Allergy Liquid Medication ▣ 849
Benadryl Allergy ▣ 848
▲ Benadryl Capsules (Among most frequent) 1898
Benadryl Dye-Free Allergy Liqui-gel Softgels ▣ 850
Benadryl Dye-Free Allergy Liquid Medication ▣ 850
▲ Benadryl Kapseals (Among most frequent) 1898
▲ Benadryl Injection (Among most frequent) 1898
▲ Bentyl (9%) 1501
▲ Betaseron for SC Injection (6%) 658
Blocadren Tablets (Less than 1%) 1614

(▣ Described in PDR For Nonprescription Drugs) Incidence data in parenthesis; ▲ 3% or more (⊚ Described in PDR For Ophthalmology)

Drowsiness Side Effects Index 1278

Bonine Tablets 1933
Brethaire Inhaler 813
▲ Brethine Ampuls (9.8 to 11.7%) 815
Brethine Tablets 814
▲ Brevibloc Injection (3%) 1808
Bricanyl Subcutaneous Injection 1502
Bricanyl Tablets 1503
Bromfed Capsules (Extended-Release) 1785
Bromfed Syrup ▣ 733
Bromfed 1785
Brontex 1981
▲ BuSpar (10%) 737
Butisol Sodium Elixir & Tablets (1 to 3 patients per 100) 2660
Calan SR Caplets (1% or less) 2422
Calan Tablets (1% or less) 2419
Capoten 739
Capozide 742
Carafate Suspension (Less than 0.5%) 1505
Carafate Tablets (Less than 0.5%) 1504
Carbocaine Hydrochloride Injection 2303
Cardene Capsules (1.1-1.4%) 2095
Cardizem CD Capsules (Less than 1%) 1506
Cardizem SR Capsules (1.3%) 1510
Cardizem Injectable 1508
Cardizem Tablets (Less than 1%) 1512
▲ Cardura Tablets (3% to 5%) 2186
Cartrol Tablets (1% to 7.4%) 410
Cataflam (Less than 1%) 816
▲ Catapres Tablets (About 33 in 100 patients) 674
▲ Catapres-TTS (12 of 101 patients) 675
Ceclor Pulvules & Suspension (Rare) 1431
Ceftin (Less than 1% but more than 0.1%) 1078
Cefzil Tablets and Oral Suspension (Less than 1%) 746
▲ CellCept Capsules (More than or equal to 3%) 2099
Celontin Kapseals (Frequent) 1899
Cerose DM ▣ 878
▲ CHEMET (succimer) Capsules (1.0 to 12.7%) 1545
Cheracol Plus Head Cold/Cough Formula ▣ 769
Cheracol Sinus ▣ 768
Children's Vicks DayQuil Allergy Relief ▣ 757
Children's Vicks NyQuil Cold/Cough Relief ▣ 758
Chlor-Trimeton Allergy Decongestant Tablets ▣ 799
Chlor-Trimeton Allergy Tablets ▣ 798
Cipro I.V. (1% or less) 595
Cipro I.V. Pharmacy Bulk Package (Less than 1%) 597
Cipro Tablets (Less than 1%) 592
▲ Claritin (8%) 2349
▲ Claritin-D (7%) 2350
Clinoril Tablets (Less than 1%) 1618
▲ Clozaril Tablets (More than 5 to 39%) 2252
Codiclear DH Syrup 791
▲ Cognex Capsules (4%) 1901
▲ Combipres Tablets (About 33%) 677
Compazine 2470
Comtrex Multi-Symptom Cold Reliever Tablets/Caplets/Liqui-Gels/Liqui-id ▣ 615
Allergy-Sinus Comtrex Multi-Symptom Allergy-Sinus Formula Tablets ▣ 617
Contac Continuous Action Nasal Decongestant/Antihistamine 12 Hour Capsules ▣ 813
Contac Day & Night Cold/Flu Night Caplets ▣ 812
Contac Maximum Strength Continuous Action Decongestant/Antihistamine 12 Hour Caplets ▣ 813
Contac Night Allergy/Sinus Caplets ▣ 812
Contac Severe Cold and Flu Formula Caplets ▣ 814
Coricidin 'D' Decongestant Tablets ▣ 800
Coricidin Tablets ▣ 800
Cozaar Tablets (Less than 1%) 1628
Cycrin Tablets 975
Cylert Tablets 412
Cystospaz 1963
▲ Cytadren Tablets (1 in 3) 819
Cytosar-U Sterile Powder (With experimental doses) 2592
Cytotec (Infrequent) 2424
Cytovene (1% or less) 2103
D.A. Chewable Tablets 951
▲ DHCplus Capsules (Among most frequent) 1993
Dalmane Capsules 2173
▲ Dantrium Capsules (Among most frequent) 1982
▲ Daranide Tablets (Among the most common effects) 1633
Daypro Caplets (Greater than 1% but less than 3%) 2426
Decadron Phosphate with Xylocaine Injection, Sterile 1639
▲ Deconamine Chewable Tablets (Most frequent) 1320
Deconamine CX Cough and Cold Liquid and Tablets 1319
▲ Deconamine (Most frequent) 1320
Deconsal C Expectorant Syrup 456
Deconsal Pediatric Syrup 457
Demadex Tablets and Injection 686
▲ Depakote Tablets (19%) 415
Depo-Provera Contraceptive Injection (Fewer than 1%) 2602
Depo-Provera Sterile Aqueous Suspension 2606
▲ Desyrel and Desyrel Dividose (23.9% to 40.8%) 503
Diamox Intravenous (Occasional) 1372
Diamox Sequels (Sustained Release) (Occasional) 1373
Diamox Tablets (Occasional) 1372
Dibenzyline Capsules 2476
Dilacor XR Extended-release Capsules (Infrequent) 2018
Dilaudid Ampules 1335
Dilaudid Cough Syrup 1336
Dilaudid 1335
Dimetapp Elixir ▣ 773
Dimetapp Extentabs ▣ 774
Dimetapp Tablets/Liqui-Gels ▣ 775
Dimetapp Cold & Allergy Chewable Tablets ▣ 773
Dipentum Capsules (1.8%) 1951
Diphtheria and Tetanus Toxoids and Pertussis Vaccine Adsorbed 2477
Diphtheria and Tetanus Toxoids and Pertussis Vaccine Adsorbed USP (For Pediatric Use) (Frequent; 1 in 3 doses) 875
Diprivan Injection (Less than 1%) 2833
Ditropan 1516
Diuril Sodium Intravenous 1652
▲ Dizac (Among most common) 1809
Dolobid Tablets (Greater than 1 in 100) 1654
Donnatal (In elderly patients) 2060
Donnatal Extentabs (In elderly patients) 2061
Donnatal Tablets (In elderly patients) 2060
▲ Doral Tablets (12%) 2664
Dramamine Chewable Tablets ▣ 836
Children's Dramamine Liquid ▣ 836
Dramamine Tablets ▣ 836
Dramamine II Tablets ▣ 837
Drixoral Cold and Allergy Sustained-Action Tablets ▣ 802
Drixoral Cold and Flu Extended-Release Tablets ▣ 803
Drixoral Allergy/Sinus Extended Release Tablets ▣ 804
▲ Duragesic Transdermal System (10% or more) 1288
Duranest Injections 542
Dura-Tap/PD Capsules 2867
Dura-Vent/DA Tablets 953
Duratuss HD Elixir 2565
Dyazide 2479
Dyclone 0.5% and 1% Topical Solutions, USP 544
DynaCirc Capsules (0.5% to 1%) 2256
Easprin 1914
▲ EC-Naprosyn Delayed-Release Tablets (3% to 9%) 2117
▲ Effexor (3% to 26.1%) 2719
Elavil 2838
Eldepryl Tablets 2550
Elspar 1659
▲ Emete-con Intramuscular/Intravenous (Most common) 2198
Emla Cream 545
▲ Empirin with Codeine Tablets (Among most frequent) 1093
Endep Tablets 2174
Engerix-B Unit-Dose Vials (Less than 1%) 2482
▲ Ergamisol Tablets (2% to 3%) 1292
▲ Esgic-plus Tablets (Among most frequent) 1013
Esidrix Tablets 821
Eskalith 2485
Ethmozine Tablets (Less than 2%) 2041
Etrafon 2355
Eulexin Capsules (1%) 2358
Extendryl 1005
Famvir (2.6%) 2486
Fedahist Gyrocaps 2401
Fedahist Timecaps 2401
▲ Felbatol (Among most common; 19.3% to 48.4%) 2666
Feldene Capsules (Greater than 1%) 1965
▲ Fioricet Tablets (Among most frequent) 2258
Fioricet with Codeine Capsules (Frequent) 2260
▲ Fiorinal Capsules (One of the two most frequent) 2261
Fiorinal with Codeine Capsules (2.4%) 2262
▲ Fiorinal Tablets (One of the two most frequent) 2261
▲ Flexeril Tablets (16% to 39%) 1661
Floxin I.V. (1% to 3%) 1571
Floxin Tablets (200 mg, 300 mg, 400 mg) (1% to 3%) 1567
Flumadine Tablets & Syrup (0.3% to 1%) 1015
Foscavir Injection (Between 1% and 5%) 547
Gamimune N, 5% Immune Globulin Intravenous (Human), 5% (Infrequent) 619
Gamimune N, 10% Immune Globulin Intravenous (Human), 10% (Infrequent) 621
Glauctabs (Occasional instances) ⊙ 208
Glucophage 752
Glucotrol Tablets (About 1 in 50) 1967
Glucotrol XL Extended Release Tablets (Less than 1%) 1968
Guaifed 1787
▲ Habitrol Nicotine Transdermal System (3% to 9% of patients) 865
▲ Halcion Tablets (14.0%) 2611
Haldol Decanoate 1577
Haldol Injection, Tablets and Concentrate 1575
Havrix (Rare) 2489
HibTITER (91 of 1,118 vaccinations) 1375
▲ Hismanal Tablets (7.1%) 1293
Hivid Tablets (Less than 1% to less than 3%) 2121
Hycodan Tablets and Syrup 930
Hycomine Compound Tablets 932
Hycomine 931
Hycotuss Expectorant Syrup 933
Hydrea Capsules 696
Hydrocet Capsules 782
▲ Hylorel Tablets (15.3% to 44.6%) 985
Hyperstat I.V. Injection 2363
▲ Hytrin Capsules (3.6% to 5.4%) 430
Hyzaar Tablets 1677
IBU Tablets (Less than 1%) 1342
▲ IFEX (Among most common) 697
Imdur (Less than or equal to 5%) 1323
Imitrex Injection (2.7%) 1103
Imitrex Tablets 1106
Imodium Capsules 1295
▲ Inapsine Injection (Among most common) 1296
Indocin (Less than 1%) 1680
Intal Inhaler (Rare) 988
Intal Nebulizer Solution 989
▲ Intron A (Up to 14%) 2364
Iopidine 0.5% (Less than 1%) ⊙ 221
IPOL Poliovirus Vaccine Inactivated 885
Isoclor Timesule Capsules ▣ 637
Isoptin Injectable 1344
Isoptin Oral Tablets (Less than 1%) 1346
Isoptin SR Tablets (1% or less) 1348
▲ Klonopin Tablets (50%) 2126
Kutrase Capsules 2402
▲ Kytril Injection (4%) 2490
Kytril Tablets (1% to 4%) 2492
▲ Lamictal Tablets (Among most common; 14.2%) 1112
Lamprene Capsules (Less than 1%) 828
Lasix Injection, Oral Solution and Tablets 1240
Legatrin PM ▣ 651
Levsin/Levsinex/Levbid 2405
Librax Capsules 2176
Libritabs Tablets 2177
Librium Capsules (Some patients) 2178
Librium Injectable 2179
▲ Limbitrol (Among most frequent) 2180
▲ Lioresal Intrathecal (13 to 18 of 214 patients) 1596
▲ Lioresal Tablets (10-63%) 829
Lithium Carbonate Capsules & Tablets 2230
Lithonate/Lithotabs/Lithobid 2543
Livostin (Approximately 1% to 3%) ⊙ 266
Lodine Capsules and Tablets (Less than 1%) 2743
Lomotil 2439
Lopid Tablets 1917
▲ Lopressor HCT Tablets (10 in 100 patients) 832
Lorabid Suspension and Pulvules (0.4% to 2.1%) 1459
Lorcet 10/650 1018
Lortab 2566
Lotensin Tablets (1.6%) 834
Lotensin HCT (1.2%) 837
Lotrel Capsules (Up to 0.3%) 840
Loxitane 1378
Lozol Tablets (Less than 5%) 2022
▲ Ludiomil Tablets (16%) 843
Lupron Depot-PED 7.5 mg, 11.25 mg and 15 mg (Less than 2%) 2560
▲ Luvox Tablets (22%) 2544
▲ Lysodren (25%) 698
MZM (Occasional) ⊙ 267
Macrobid Capsules (Less than 1%) 1988
Macrodantin Capsules 1989
Marax Tablets & DF Syrup (Occasional) 2200
Marcaine Hydrochloride with Epinephrine 1:200,000 2316
Marcaine Hydrochloride Injection 2316
Marcaine Spinal 2319
▲ Marinol (Dronabinol) Capsules (3% to 10%) 2231
Matulane Capsules 2131
Maxaquin Tablets (Less than 1%) 2440
Maxzide 1380
Mebaral Tablets (1 to 3 in 100) 2322
Mellaril (Occasional) 2269
Mesantoin Tablets 2272
Methotrexate Sodium Tablets, Injection, for Injection and LPF Injection 1275
Midamor Tablets (Less than or equal to 1%) 1703
Maximum Strength Multi-Symptom Formula Midol ▣ 722
PMS Multi-Symptom Formula Midol ▣ 723
Milontin Kapseals 1920
Miltown Tablets 2672
▲ Minipress Capsules (7.6%) 1937
▲ Minizide Capsules (7.6%) 1938
Mintezol 1704
Mithracin 607
▲ Moban Tablets and Concentrate (Most frequent) 1048
Mobigesic Tablets ▣ 602
Moduretic Tablets (Less than or equal to 1%) 1705
Mono-Gesic Tablets 792
Monopril Tablets (0.2% to 1.0%) 757
Motofen Tablets (1 in 25) 784
Children's Motrin Ibuprofen Oral Suspension (Less than 1%) 1546
Motrin Tablets (Less than 1%) 2625
Motrin Ibuprofen Suspension, Oral Drops, Chewable Tablets, Caplets (Less than 1%) 1546
MSTA Mumps Skin Test Antigen 890
Mutamycin 703
Mykrox Tablets 993
Mysoline (Occasional) 2754
▲ Nalfon 200 Pulvules & Nalfon Tablets (8.5%) 917
▲ Anaprox/Naprosyn (3% to 9%) 2117
Nardil (Common) 1920
Navane Capsules and Concentrate 2201
Navane Intramuscular 2202
NebuPent for Inhalation Solution (1% or less) 1040
NegGram 2323
Nembutal Sodium Capsules (1% to 3%) 436
Nembutal Sodium Solution (1% to 3%) 438
Nembutal Sodium Suppositories (1% to 3%) 440
Neptazane Tablets (Occasional) 1388
Nescaine/Nescaine MPF 554
▲ Neurontin Capsules (Among most common; 19.3%) 1922

(▣ Described in PDR For Nonprescription Drugs) Incidence data in parenthesis; ▲ 3% or more (⊙ Described in PDR For Ophthalmology)

Nizoral Tablets (Less than 1%) 1298
Nolahist Tablets 785
Nolamine Timed-Release Tablets (Occasional) 785
Norflex 1496
Norgesic 1496
▲ Normodyne Injection (3%) 2377
Normodyne Tablets (Less than 1%) 2379
Noroxin Tablets (0.3% to 1.0%) 1715
Noroxin Tablets (0.3% to 1.0%) 2048
Norpramin Tablets 1526
Norvasc Tablets (1.3% to 1.6%) 1940
Novahistine Elixir ▣ 823
Novocain Hydrochloride for Spinal Anesthesia 2326
Nucofed 2051
Numorphan Injection 936
Numorphan Suppositories 937
Maximum Strength Nytol Caplets ▣ 610
▲ OmniHIB (2.5% to 57.5%) 2499
Oncaspar (Less than 1%) 2028
OptiPranolol (Metipranolol 0.3%) Sterile Ophthalmic Solution (A small number of patients) ⊙ 258
▲ Orap Tablets (7 of 20 patients) 1050
Oretic Tablets 443
Orlamm (1% to 3%) 2239
Ornade Spansule Capsules 2502
Orudis Capsules (Greater than 1%) 2766
Oruvail Capsules (Greater than 1%) 2766
▲ PBZ Tablets (Among most frequent) 845
▲ PBZ-SR Tablets (Among most frequent) 844
PMB 200 and PMB 400 2783
Pamelor 2280
Paraflex Caplets (Occasional) 1580
Parafon Forte DSC Caplets (Occasional) 1581
▲ Parlodel (3%) 2281
Parnate Tablets 2503
▲ Paxil Tablets (12.7% to 23.3%) 2505
PediaCare Cold Allergy Chewable Tablets ▣ 677
PediaCare Cough-Cold Liquid 1553
PediaCare NightRest Cough-Cold Liquid 1553
Pediatric Vicks 44m Cough & Cold Relief ▣ 764
▲ PedvaxHIB (Among most frequent) 1718
Penetrex Tablets (Less than 1% but more than or equal to 0.1%) 2031
Pentasa (Less than 1%) 1527
Pepcid Injection (Infrequent) 1722
Pepcid (Infrequent) 1720
Peptavlon 2878
Percogesic Analgesic Tablets ▣ 754
Periactin 1724
▲ Permax Tablets (10.1%) 575
Phenergan with Codeine 2777
Phenergan with Dextromethorphan 2778
Phenergan Injection 2773
Phenergan Suppositories 2775
Phenergan Syrup 2774
Phenergan Tablets 2775
Phenergan VC 2779
Phenergan VC with Codeine 2781
Phenobarbital Elixir and Tablets (1 to 3 patients per 100) 1469
▲ Phenurone Tablets (4%) 447
▲ Phrenilin (Among most frequent) 785
Plendil Extended-Release Tablets (0.5% to 1.5%) 527
▲ Poliovax (More than 5%) 891
Polymyxin B Sulfate, Aerosporin Brand Sterile Powder 1154
Pondimin Tablets (Among most common) 2066
Ponstel 1925
Pontocaine Hydrochloride for Spinal Anesthesia 2330
Premphase 2797
Prempro 2801
Prilosec Delayed-Release Capsules (Less than 1%) 529
Primaxin I.M. 1727
Primaxin I.V. (0.2%) 1729
Prinivil Tablets (0.3 to 1.0%) 1733
Prinzide Tablets (0.3% to 1%) 1737
Pro-Banthine Tablets 2052
Procardia XL Extended Release Tablets (Less than 3%) 1972
▲ Prograf (Greater than 3%) 1042
Proleukin for Injection 797
Prolixin 509
Propulsid (1% or less) 1300
▲ ProSom Tablets (42%) 449
▲ Prostep (nicotine transdermal system) (3% to 9% of patients) 1394
Prostigmin Injectable 1260
Prostigmin Tablets 1261
Protopam Chloride for Injection 2806
Proventil (Less than 1% to 2%) 2386
Provera Tablets 2636
▲ Prozac Pulvules & Liquid, Oral Solution (5% to 17%) 919
Pyrroxate Caplets ▣ 772
Quarzan Capsules 2181
Questran Light 769
Questran Powder 770
RMS Suppositories 2657
Recombivax HB 1744
▲ Reglan (Approximately 10%) 2068
Relafen Tablets (1% to 3%) 2510
▲ Restoril Capsules (17%) 2284
▲ Retrovir Capsules (8%) 1158
▲ Retrovir I.V. Infusion (8%) 1163
▲ Retrovir Syrup (8%) 1158
ReVia Tablets (Less than 1% to 2%) 940
Revex (Less than 1%) 1811
Rifadin 1528
Rifamate Capsules 1530
Rifater 1532
Rimactane Capsules 847
▲ Risperdal (3% to 8%; 41%) 1301
Ritalin 848
Robaxin Injectable 2070
Robaxin Tablets 2071
Robaxisal Tablets 2071
Robinul Forte Tablets 2072
Robinul Injectable 2072
Robinul Tablets 2072
Rocaltrol Capsules 2141
Romazicon (Less than 1%) 2147
Rondec-DM Oral Drops 954
Rondec-DM Syrup 954
Ryna ▣ 841
▲ Rynatan (Among most common) 2673
▲ Rynatuss (Among most common) 2673
Rythmol Tablets–150mg, 225mg, 300mg (0.6 to 1.2%) 1352
Sandoglobulin I.V. (Infrequent) 2290
Sandostatin Injection (1% to 4%) 2292
Sanorex Tablets 2294
Sansert Tablets 2295
Scleromate (Rare) 1891
▲ Seconal Sodium Pulvules (Most common) 1474
▲ Sedapap Tablets 50 mg/650 mg (Among the most frequent) 1543
▲ Seldane Tablets (8.5% to 9.0%) 1536
▲ Seldane-D Extended-Release Tablets (7.2%) 1538
▲ Semprex-D Capsules (12%) 463
▲ Semprex-D Capsules (12%) 1167
Sensorcaine 559
Ser-Ap-Es Tablets 849
Serax Capsules 2810
Serax Tablets 2810
▲ Serentil (One of the two most prevalent) 684
Seromycin Pulvules 1476
▲ Serzone Tablets (16% to 28%) 771
Sinarest Tablets ▣ 648
Sinarest Extra Strength Tablets ▣ 648
Sinarest No Drowsiness Tablets ▣ 648
Sine-Aid IB Caplets 1554
Sinemet Tablets 943
Sinemet CR Tablets 944
▲ Sinequan (Most common) 2205
Singlet Tablets ▣ 825
Sinulin Tablets 787
Sinutab Sinus Allergy Medication, Maximum Strength Tablets and Caplets ▣ 860
Skelaxin Tablets 788
▲ Soma Compound w/Codeine Tablets (Most frequent) 2676
▲ Soma Compound Tablets (Most frequent) 2675
Soma Tablets 2674
Sporanox Capsules (0.3% to 1.2%) 1305
▲ Stadol (43%) 775
Stelazine 2514
Stimate, (desmopressin acetate) Nasal Spray, 1.5 mg/mL 525
▲ Sublimaze Injection (Frequent) 1307
Sudafed Plus Liquid ▣ 862
Sudafed Plus Tablets ▣ 863
▲ Sufenta Injection (3% to 9%) 1309
Supprelin Injection (1% to 3%) 2056
Surmontil Capsules 2811
Symmetrel Capsules and Syrup (1% to 5%) 946
Tagamet (Approximately 1 in 100) 2516
Tambocor Tablets (1% to less than 3%) 1497
Tapazole Tablets 1477
▲ Tavist Syrup (Among most frequent) 2297
▲ Tavist Tablets (Among most frequent) 2298
Tavist-D 12 Hour Relief Tablets ▣ 787
▲ Tegretol Chewable Tablets (Among most frequent) 852
▲ Tegretol Suspension (Among most frequent) 852
▲ Tegretol Tablets (Among most frequent) 852
Teldrin 12 Hour Antihistamine/Nasal Decongestant Allergy Relief Capsules ▣ 826
▲ Temaril Tablets, Syrup and Spansule Extended-Release Capsules (Most common) 483
▲ Tenex Tablets (Up to 39%) 2074
Tenoretic Tablets (0.6% to 2%) 2845
Tenormin Tablets and I.V. Injection (0.6% to 2%) 2847
▲ Tetramune (Up to 26%) 1404
Thalitone (Common) 1245
TheraFlu ▣ 787
TheraFlu Maximum Strength Nighttime Flu, Cold & Cough Medicine ▣ 788
Thorazine 2523
THYREL TRH (Less frequent) 2873
Tigan 2057
Timolide Tablets (Less than 1%) 1748
Timoptic in Ocudose (Less frequent) 1753
Timoptic Sterile Ophthalmic Solution (Less frequent) 1751
Timoptic-XE 1755
Tofranil Ampuls 854
Tofranil Tablets 856
Tofranil-PM Capsules 857
Tolectin (200, 400 and 600 mg) (1 to 3%) 1581
Tonocard Tablets (0.8-1.6%) 531
Toprol-XL Tablets 565
▲ Toradol (6%) 2159
Torecan (Occasional) 2245
Tornalate Solution for Inhalation, 0.2% (1.2%) 956
Trancopal Caplets 2337
▲ Trandate (3 of 100 patients) 1185
▲ Transderm Scōp Transdermal Therapeutic System (Less than one-sixth) 869
▲ Tranxene (Most frequent) 451
Trental Tablets 1244
Triaminic Allergy Tablets ▣ 789
Triaminic Cold Tablets ▣ 790
Triaminic Expectorant ▣ 790
Triaminic Nite Light ▣ 791
Triaminic Syrup ▣ 792
Triaminic-12 Tablets ▣ 792
Triaminicin Tablets ▣ 793
Triaminicol Multi-Symptom Cold Tablets ▣ 793
Triaminicol Multi-Symptom Relief ▣ 794
Triavil Tablets 1757
Tri-Immunol Adsorbed (Rare) 1408
Trilafon 2389
Trilisate (Less than 2%) 2000
▲ Trinalin Repetabs Tablets (Among most frequent) 1330
▲ Tripedia (1% to 13%) 892
▲ Tussend (Most frequent) 1783
Tussend Expectorant 1785
Tussionex Pennkinetic Extended-Release Suspension 998
Tussi-Organidin DM NR Liquid and DM-S NR Liquid (Rare) 2677
Tussi-Organidin NR Liquid and S NR Liquid (At higher doses) 2677
Children's TYLENOL Cold Multi-Symptom Liquid Formula and Chewable Tablets 1561
TYLENOL Maximum Strength Allergy Sinus Medication Gelcaps and Caplets 1563
TYLENOL Maximum Strength Allergy Sinus NightTime Medication Caplets 1555
TYLENOL Flu NightTime, Maximum Strength, Gelcaps 1566
TYLENOL Maximum Strength Flu NightTime Hot Medication Packets 1562
TYLENOL Cold Multi-Symptom Formula Medication Tablets and Caplets 1561
TYLENOL Cold Multi-Symptom Hot Medication Liquid Packets 1557
TYLENOL PM, Extra Strength Pain Reliever/Sleep Aid Caplets, Geltabs, Gelcaps 1560
TYLENOL Severe Allergy Medication Caplets 1564
▲ Ultram Tablets (50 mg) (16% to 25%) 1585
Univasc Tablets (Less than 1%) 2410
Urispas Tablets 2532
▲ Valium Injectable (Among most common) 2182
▲ Valium Tablets (Among most common) 2183
▲ Valrelease Capsules (Among most common) 2169
Vascor (200, 300 and 400 mg) Tablets (0.5 to 6.98%) 1587
Vaseretic Tablets (0.5% to 2.0%) 1765
Vasotec I.V. 1768
Vasotec Tablets (0.5% to 1.0%) 1771
Ventolin Tablets (Fewer than 1 of 100 patients) 1203
Verelan Capsules (1% or less) 1410
Verelan Capsules (Less than 1%) 2824
Versed Injection (1.2%) 2170
Vicks 44 LiquiCaps Cough, Cold & Flu Relief ▣ 755
Vicks 44M Cough, Cold & Flu Relief ▣ 756
Vicks DayQuil Allergy Relief 12-Hour Extended Release Tablets ▣ 760
Vicks DayQuil Allergy Relief 4-Hour Tablets ▣ 760
Vicks Nyquil Hot Therapy ▣ 762
Vicks NyQuil LiquiCaps Multi-Symptom Cold/Flu Relief ▣ 763
Vicks NyQuil Multi-Symptom Cold/Flu Relief - (Original & Cherry Flavor) ▣ 763
Vicodin Tablets 1356
Vicodin ES Tablets 1357
Vicodin Tuss Expectorant 1358
Vistaril Capsules 1944
Vistaril Intramuscular Solution 2216
Vistaril Oral Suspension 1944
Vivactil Tablets 1774
Volmax Extended-Release Tablets (0.3%) 1788
Voltaren Tablets (Less than 1%) 861
Vontrol Tablets 2532
WinRho SD (One report) 2576
▲ Xanax Tablets (76.8%) 2649
▲ Xylocaine Injections (Among most common) 567
Yutopar Intravenous Injection (Infrequent) 570
Zantac (Rare) 1209
Zantac Injection 1207
Zantac Syrup (Rare) 1209
Zarontin Capsules 1928
Zarontin Syrup 1929
Zaroxolyn Tablets 1000
Zebeta Tablets 1413
Zerit Capsules (Fewer than 1% to 2%) 729
Zestoretic (0.3 to 1%) 2850
Zestril Tablets (0.3% to 1.0%) 2854
Ziac (0.9% to 1.1%) 1415
Zithromax (1% or less) 1944
▲ Zofran Injection (8%) 1214
▲ Zofran Tablets (20%) 1217
Zoladex (1% or greater) 2858
▲ Zoloft Tablets (13.4%) 2217
▲ Zonalon Cream (22%) 1055
Zovirax 1219
Zydone Capsules 949
Zyloprim Tablets (Less than 1%) 1226

Drug administration site reactions, unspecified

Cardene I.V. (1.4%) 2709
▲ Ceptaz (Among most common) 1081
▲ Cytovene-IV (22%) 2103
D.H.E. 45 Injection 2255
Duragesic Transdermal System (1% or greater) 1288
Engerix-B Unit-Dose Vials 2482
▲ Fortaz (Among most common) 1100
Fragmin (Rare) 1954
▲ Imitrex Injection (58.7%) 1103
Intron A (Less than 5%) 2364
Lupron Depot 3.75 mg (Less than 5%) 2556
▲ Navelbine Injection (Up to 38%) 1145
Neupogen for Injection (Infrequent) 495
Nitrodisc (Rare) 2047

(▣ Described in PDR For Nonprescription Drugs) Incidence data in parenthesis; ▲ 3% or more (⊙ Described in PDR For Ophthalmology)

Drug administration site reactions, unspecified Side Effects Index 1280

Nuromax Injection (Less than or equal to 0.1%) 1149
Oncaspar (Greater than 1% but less than 5%) 2028
▲Proleukin for Injection (3%) 797
Retrovir I.V. Infusion (Infrequent) 1163
Septra I.V. Infusion 1169
Septra I.V. Infusion ADD-Vantage Vials (Infrequent) 1171
▲Supprelin Injection (12%) 2056
▲Taxol (13%) 714
▲Tazicef for Injection (Among most common) 2519
Zosyn (0.5%) 1419
Zosyn Pharmacy Bulk Package (0.5%) 1422

Drug effect, unspecified, prolonged
Diprivan Injection (Less than 1%) 2833
Mivacron (Less than 1%) 1138
Nuromax Injection (Less than or equal to 0.1%) 1149
Paxil Tablets (1.7%) 2505

Drug fever
Aldactazide 2413
Aldactone 2414
Aldoclor Tablets 1598
Aldomet Oral 1600
Aldoril Tablets 1604
Amikacin Sulfate Injection, USP (Rare) 960
Amikin Injectable (Rare) 501
Ancef Injection 2465
Asendin Tablets (Less than 1%) 1369
Azo Gantanol Tablets 2080
Bactrim DS Tablets 2084
Bactrim I.V. Infusion 2082
Bactrim 2084
Cefobid Intravenous/Intramuscular (1 in 260) 2189
Cefobid Pharmacy Bulk Package - Not for Direct Infusion (1 in 260) 2192
Clozaril Tablets 2252
Coly-Mycin M Parenteral 1905
Compazine 2470
Depen Titratable Tablets 2662
Ethmozine Tablets (Less than 2%) 2041
Fansidar Tablets 2114
Kefzol Vials, Faspak & ADD-Vantage 1456
Leukeran Tablets 1133
Ludiomil Tablets (Rare) 843
Macrobid Capsules 1988
Macrodantin Capsules 1989
Mandol Vials, Faspak & ADD-Vantage 1461
Mezlin 601
Mezlin Pharmacy Bulk Package 604
Norpramin Tablets 1526
Pamelor 2280
Polymyxin B Sulfate, Aerosporin Brand Sterile Powder (Occasional) 1154
Prolixin 509
Purinethol Tablets (Very rare) 1156
Septra 1174
Septra I.V. Infusion 1169
Septra I.V. Infusion ADD-Vantage Vials 1171
Septra 1174
Serentil 684
Stelazine 2514
Suprax (Less than 2%) 1399
Tapazole Tablets 1477
Ticar for Injection 2526
Timentin for Injection 2528
Tofranil Ampuls 854
Tofranil Tablets 856
Tofranil-PM Capsules 857
Urobiotic-250 Capsules 2214
Vancocin HCl, Oral Solution & Pulvules (Infrequent) 1483
Vancocin HCl, Vials & ADD-Vantage (Infrequent) 1481
Vivactil Tablets 1774
Zinacef (Rare) 1211

Drug idiosyncrasies (see under Allergic reactions)

Dry mouth (see under Xerostomia)

Dryness
A/T/S 2% Acne Topical Gel and Solution (Occasional) 1234
Aclovate (1 in 100 patients) 1069
Analpram-HC Rectal Cream 1% and 2.5% 977
Anusol-HC Cream 2.5% (Infrequent to frequent) 1896
Anusol-HC Suppositories 1897
Aristocort A 0.5% Cream 1031
Carmol HC (Infrequent to frequent) 924
Catapres Tablets 674
Condylox (Less than 5%) 1802
Cordran Lotion (Infrequent) 1803
Cordran Tape (Infrequent) 1804
Cortisporin Cream 1084
Cortisporin Ointment 1085
Cortisporin Otic Solution Sterile 1087
Cortisporin Otic Suspension Sterile 1088
Cutivate Cream (1.2%) 1088
▲Cutivate Ointment 1089
Cyclocort Topical (Infrequent) 1037
Decadron Phosphate Topical Cream 1644
Decaspray Topical Aerosol 1648
▲Desquam-E Gel (2 in 50 patients) 2684
▲Desquam-X Gel (2 in 50 patients) 2684
▲Desquam-X 10 Bar (2 in 50 patients) 2684
▲Desquam-X Wash (2 in 50 patients) 2684
Elocon Lotion 0.1% 2354
Erycette (erythromycin 2%) Topical Solution 1888
Florone/Florone E 906
Fluoracaine ⊙ 206
Lamisil Cream 1% (0.2%) 2265
Lidex (Infrequent) 2130
Locoid Cream, Ointment and Topical Solution (Infrequent) 978
Melanex Topical Solution 1793
▲Naftin Cream 1% (3%) 480
NeoDecadron Topical Cream 1714
Ophthetic ⊙ 247
PediOtic Suspension Sterile 1153
Pramosone Cream, Lotion & Ointment 978
ProctoCream-HC (Infrequent) 2408
Psorcon Cream 0.05% (Infrequent) 909
SalAc 1055
Stri-Dex ▣ 730
Synalar (Infrequent) 2130
T-Stat 2.0% Topical Solution and Pads 2688
Temovate (Infrequent) 1179
Theramycin Z Topical Solution 2% 1592
Topicort (Infrequent) 1243
Triaz 6% and 10% Gels and 10% Cleaner 1592
Tridesilon Cream 0.05% (Infrequent) 615
Tridesilon Ointment 0.05% (Infrequent) 616
Westcort 2690

Dryness, mucous membrane
▲Atrohist Pediatric Suspension (Among most common) 454
Cataflam (Less than 1%) 816
Dolobid Tablets (Less than 1 in 100) 1654
Lomotil 2439
Mintezol Chewable Tablets 1704
Myleran Tablets (Rare) 1143
Nasacort Nasal Inhaler (Fewer than 5%) 2024
Pravachol 765
▲Rynatan (Among most common) 2673
▲Rynatuss (Among most common) 2673
Timolide Tablets (Less than 1%) 1748
Trinalin Repetabs Tablets 1330
Voltaren Tablets (Less than 1%) 861

Dryness, nose (see under Xeromycteria)

Duodenal infarction
Gelfoam Sterile Sponge 2608

Duodenitis
Anafranil Capsules (Infrequent) 803
Sterile FUDR 2118
Motrin Ibuprofen Suspension, Oral Drops, Chewable Tablets, Caplets (Less than 1%) 1546
Paxil Tablets (Rare) 2505
Permax Tablets (Rare) 575
Relafen Tablets (Less than 1%) 2510
Videx Tablets, Powder for Oral Solution, & Pediatric Powder for Oral Solution (Less than 1%) 720

Dysarthria
Ambien Tablets (Infrequent) 2416
Bentyl 10 mg Capsules 1501
CeeNU 693
Clozaril Tablets (Less than 1%) 2252
Cognex Capsules (Infrequent) 1901
Depakene 413
Depakote Tablets 415
Dizac (Less frequent) 1809
Doral Tablets 2664
Elavil 2838
Endep Tablets 2174
Felbatol 2666
Flexeril Tablets (Less than 1%) 1661
Halcion Tablets 2611
Imitrex Injection (Rare) 1103
Imitrex Tablets (Infrequent) 1106
Indocin Capsules (Less than 1%) 1680
Indocin I.V. (Less than 1%) 1684
Indocin (Less than 1%) 1680
Klonopin Tablets 2126
Lamictal Tablets (1.0%) 1112
Levsin/Levsinex/Levbid 2405
Lioresal Tablets 829
Ludiomil Tablets (Rare) 843
Mesantoin Tablets 2272
Neurontin Capsules (2.4%) 1922
Paxil Tablets (Rare) 2505
Pondimin Tablets 2066
Prostigmin Injectable 1260
Prostigmin Tablets 1261
Prozac Pulvules & Liquid, Oral Solution (Rare) 919
Risperdal (Infrequent) 1301
Roferon-A Injection (Less than 0.5%) 2145
Seromycin Pulvules 1476
Serzone Tablets (Infrequent) 771
Soma Compound w/Codeine Tablets (Very rare) 2676
Soma Compound Tablets (Very rare) 2675
Soma Tablets 2674
Tensilon Injectable 1261
Tonocard Tablets (Less than 1%) 531
Triavil Tablets 1757
Valium Injectable 2182
Valium Tablets (Infrequent) 2183
Valrelease Capsules (Occasional) 2169
Wellbutrin Tablets (Infrequent) 1204
▲Xanax Tablets (23.3%) 2649

Dyscrasias, blood (see under Blood dyscrasias)

Dysdiadochokinesia
Klonopin Tablets 2126

Dysesthesia
Cognex Capsules (Rare) 1901
Cytovene-IV (One report) 2103
Halcion Tablets (Rare) 2611
Hivid Tablets 2121
Imitrex Injection (Rare) 1103
Imitrex Tablets (Rare) 1106
Neurontin Capsules (Infrequent) 1922
Prinivil Tablets (0.3% to 1.0%) 1733
Prinzide Tablets 1737
Vaseretic Tablets 1765
Vasotec I.V. 1768
Vasotec Tablets (0.5% to 1.0%) 1771
Zestril Tablets 2854

Dysesthesia, hemifacial
Prilosec Delayed-Release Capsules (Less than 1%) 529

Dysgeusia
Capoten (Approximately 2 to 4 of 100 patients) 739
Capozide (Approximately 2 to 4 of 100 patients) 742
Cardizem CD Capsules (Less than 1%) 1506
Cardizem SR Capsules (Less than 1%) 1510
Cardizem Injectable 1508
Cardizem Tablets (Less than 1%) 1512
Eskalith 2485
Floxin I.V. (1% to 3%) 1571
Floxin Tablets (200 mg, 300 mg, 400 mg) (1% to 3%) 1567
Havrix (Less than 1%) 2489
Lithonate/Lithotabs/Lithobid 2543
Maxaquin Tablets 2440
Mevacor Tablets (0.8%) 1699
Ridaura Capsules (1-3%) 2513
Rocephin Injectable Vials, ADD-Vantage, Galaxy Container (Less than 1%) 2142
Trilisate (Less than 1%) 2000
Ultram Tablets (50 mg) (Less than 1%) 1585

Dyskinesia
Anafranil Capsules (Infrequent) 803
Bentyl 1501
BuSpar (Rare) 737
Cognex Capsules (Rare) 1901
Compazine 2470
Cylert Tablets 412
Dexedrine 2474
DextroStat Dextroamphetamine Tablets 2036
Dilantin Infatabs (Rare) 1908
Dilantin Kapseals (Rare) 1906
Dilantin Parenteral (Rare) 1910
Dilantin-125 Suspension (Rare) 1911
▲Eldepryl Tablets (2 of 49 patients) 2550
Ethmozine Tablets (Less than 2%) 2041
Etrafon 2355
Felbatol 2666
Foscavir Injection (Less than 1%) 547
Haldol Decanoate 1577
Haldol Injection, Tablets and Concentrate 1575
Lamictal Tablets (Infrequent) 1112
Levoprome 1274
Loxitane (Less frequent) 1378
Luvox Tablets (Infrequent) 2544
MSIR (Infrequent) 1997
Orap Tablets 1050
Paxil Tablets (Rare) 2505
▲Permax Tablets (62.4%) 575
Prolixin 509
Prozac Pulvules & Liquid, Oral Solution 919
Ritalin 848
▲Sinemet CR Tablets (16.5%) 944
Stelazine 2514
Temaril Tablets, Syrup and Spansule Extended-Release Capsules 483
Triavil Tablets 1757
Trilafon 2389
Vistaril Capsules 1944
Vistaril Oral Suspension 1944
Wellbutrin Tablets (Frequent) 1204
Zoloft Tablets (Rare) 2217

Dyskinesia, tardive (see under Tardive dyskinesia)

Dyskinesia, transient
Orap Tablets 1050

Dysmenorrhea
▲Anafranil Capsules (10% to 12%) 803
▲Asacol Delayed-Release Tablets (3%) 1979
▲Betaseron for SC Injection (18%) 658
Claritin (2% or fewer patients) 2349
Claritin-D (Less frequent) 2350
Clozaril Tablets (Less than 1%) 2252
Cytotec (0.1%) 2424
Depakote Tablets (Greater than 1% but not more than 5%) 415
Depo-Provera Contraceptive Injection (Fewer than 1%) 2602
Diethylstilbestrol Tablets 1437
Dilacor XR Extended-release Capsules (Infrequent) 2018
Effexor 2719
ESTRATAB Tablets (0.3, 0.625, 1.25, 2.5 mg) 2536
Estratest 2539
Floxin I.V. (Less than 1%) 1571
Floxin Tablets (200 mg, 300 mg, 400 mg) (Less than 1%) 1567
▲Habitrol Nicotine Transdermal System (3% to 9% of patients) 865
Imitrex Injection (Rare) 1103
Imitrex Tablets (Infrequent) 1106
▲Lamictal Tablets (6.6%) 1112
Lippes Loop Intrauterine Double-S 1848
Lo/Ovral Tablets 2746
Lo/Ovral-28 Tablets 2751
Luvox Tablets 2544
Menest Tablets 2494
Neurontin Capsules (Infrequent) 1922
▲Nicoderm (nicotine transdermal system) (3% to 9%) 1518
▲Nicorette (3% to 9% of patients) 2458
Nicotrol Nicotine Transdermal System (1% to 3%) 1550
Nordette-21 Tablets 2755
Nordette-28 Tablets 2758
Noroxin Tablets (Less frequent) 1715
Noroxin Tablets (Less frequent) 2048
Norplant System 2759
Ortho Dienestrol Cream 1866
Ovral Tablets 2770
Ovral-28 Tablets 2770
Ovrette Tablets 2771
PMB 200 and PMB 400 2783

(▣ Described in PDR For Nonprescription Drugs) Incidence data in parenthesis; ▲3% or more (⊙ Described in PDR For Ophthalmology)

1281 **Side Effects Index** **Dysphagia**

ParaGard T380A Intrauterine Copper Contraceptive ... 1880
Paxil Tablets (Infrequent) ... 2505
Permax Tablets (Frequent) ... 575
Premarin Intravenous ... 2787
Premarin with Methyltestosterone .. 2794
Premarin Vaginal Cream ... 2791
Prostep (nicotine transdermal system) (1% to 3% of patients).. 1394
Risperdal (Infrequent) ... 1301
Seldane Tablets ... 1536
Seldane-D Extended-Release Tablets ... 1538
Semprex-D Capsules (2%) ... 463
Semprex-D Capsules (2%) ... 1167
Serevent Inhalation Aerosol (1% to 3%) ... 1176
Serzone Tablets ... 771
▲ Supprelin Injection (3% to 10%) ... 2056
▲ Terazol 3 Vaginal Cream (6%) ... 1886
Triphasil-21 Tablets ... 2814
Triphasil-28 Tablets ... 2819
Zerit Capsules (Up to 2%) ... 729
Zoladex (1% or greater) ... 2858
Zoloft Tablets (Infrequent) ... 2217

Dyspareunia

Depo-Provera Contraceptive Injection (Fewer than 1%) ... 2602
Flagyl 375 Capsules ... 2434
Flagyl I.V. ... 2247
Lippes Loop Intrauterine Double-S.. 1848
MetroGel-Vaginal ... 902
Mycelex-G 500 mg Vaginal Tablets (1 in 149 patients) ... 609
ParaGard T380A Intrauterine Copper Contraceptive ... 1880
Protostat Tablets ... 1883
Prozac Pulvules & Liquid, Oral Solution (Rare) ... 919
Supprelin Injection (2% to 3%) ... 2056
Vagistat-1 (Less than 1%) ... 778
Wellbutrin Tablets (Rare) ... 1204
▲ Zoladex (14%) ... 2858

Dyspepsia

Actigall Capsules ... 802
Adalat CC (Less than 1.0%) ... 589
AeroBid Inhaler System (1-3%) ... 1005
Aerobid-M Inhaler System (1-3%).. 1005
Airet Solution for Inhalation (1% to 1.5%) ... 452
Altace Capsules (Less than 1%) ... 1232
▲ Ambien Tablets (5%) ... 2416
▲ Anafranil Capsules (13% to 22%) ... 803
Anaprox/Naprosyn (Less than 3%) ... 2117
▲ Ansaid Tablets (3-9%; common) ... 2579
Aredia for Injection (Up to 4%) ... 810
▲ Asacol Delayed-Release Tablets (6%) ... 1979
Atromid-S Capsules ... 2701
▲ Axid Pulvules (3.6%) ... 1427
▲ Betapace Tablets (2% to 6%) ... 641
Biaxin (2%) ... 405
Blocadren Tablets (0.6%) ... 1614
Brevibloc Injection (Less than 1%) ... 1808
Buprenex Injectable (Infrequent) ... 2006
Capoten ... 739
Capozide ... 742
Cardene Capsules (0.8-1.5%) ... 2095
Cardene I.V. (Rare) ... 2709
Cardizem CD Capsules (Less than 1%) ... 1506
Cardizem SR Capsules (1.3%) ... 1510
Cardizem Injectable ... 1508
Cardizem Tablets (Less than 1%).. 1512
Cardura Tablets (1% to 1.7%) ... 2186
Cartrol Tablets (Less common) ... 410
Cataflam (Common) ... 816
Ceftin (Less than 1% but more than 0.1%) ... 1078
▲ CellCept Capsules (13.6% to 17.6%) ... 2099
Cipro I.V. ... 595
Cipro Tablets ... 592
Claritin (2% or fewer patients) ... 2349
▲ Claritin-D (3%) ... 2350
▲ Clinoril Tablets (3-9%) ... 1618
▲ Cognex Capsules (9%) ... 1901
Cozaar Tablets (1.3%) ... 1628
Cytotec (2.0%) ... 2424
Cytovene (2%) ... 2103
▲ Daypro Caplets (3% to 9%; common) ... 2426
Demadex Tablets and Injection (1.6%) ... 686
▲ Depakote Tablets (9%) ... 415
Diflucan Injection, Tablets, and Oral Suspension (1%) ... 2194
Dilacor XR Extended-release Capsules (1.3%) ... 2018
▲ Dipentum Capsules (4.0%) ... 1951
▲ Dolobid Tablets (3% to 9%) ... 1654
Doral Tablets (1.1%) ... 2664
▲ Duragesic Transdermal System (3% to 10%) ... 1288
Duricef (Rare) ... 748
Easprin ... 1914
EC-Naprosyn Delayed-Release Tablets (Less than 3%) ... 2117
▲ Effexor (4.5% to 5%) ... 2719
Empirin with Codeine Tablets (Occasional) ... 1093
Engerix-B Unit-Dose Vials ... 2482
Ergamisol Tablets (Less than 1% to 1%) ... 1292
▲ Ethmozine Tablets (2% to 5%) ... 2041
▲ Felbatol (6.5% to 12.3%) ... 2666
Feldene Capsules (Common) ... 1965
Flexeril Tablets (1 to 3%) ... 1661
Floxin I.V. (Less than 1%) ... 1571
Floxin Tablets (200 mg, 300 mg, 400 mg) (Less than 1%) ... 1567
Flumadine Tablets & Syrup (0.3% to 1%) ... 1015
Foscavir Injection (Between 1% and 5%) ... 547
▲ Fungizone Intravenous (Among most common) ... 506
Glucotrol XL Extended Release Tablets (Less than 3%) ... 1968
▲ Habitrol Nicotine Transdermal System (3% to 9% of patients) ... 865
Haldol Decanoate ... 1577
Haldol Injection, Tablets and Concentrate ... 1575
Hivid Tablets (Less than 1% to less than 3%) ... 2121
Hytrin Capsules (At least 1%) ... 430
Hyzaar Tablets ... 1677
Imdur (Less than or equal to 5%) .. 1323
▲ Indocin (3% to 9%) ... 1680
▲ Intron A (Up to 8%) ... 2364
Ismo Tablets (Fewer than 1%) ... 2738
Keflex Pulvules & Oral Suspension 914
Keftab Tablets ... 915
▲ Kerlone Tablets (3.9% to 4.7%) ... 2436
▲ Lamictal Tablets (5.3%) ... 1112
▲ Lescol Capsules (8.1%) ... 2267
Levatol (2.7%) ... 2403
▲ Lodine Capsules and Tablets (10%) ... 2743
▲ Lopid Tablets (19.6%) ... 1917
Lotensin HCT (0.3% to 1.0%) ... 837
Lotrel Capsules ... 840
Lozol Tablets (Less than 5%) ... 2022
▲ Luvox Tablets (10%) ... 2544
Macrobid Capsules (Less than 1%) ... 1988
Maxaquin Tablets (Less than 1%).. 2440
Megace Oral Suspension (Up to 4%) ... 699
▲ Mepron Suspension (5%) ... 1135
▲ Mevacor Tablets (1.0% to 3.9%) .. 1699
Miacalcin Nasal Spray (1% to 3%) 2275
Midamor Tablets (Less than or equal to 1%) ... 1703
Moduretic Tablets ... 1705
Monoket (Fewer than 1%) ... 2406
Children's Motrin Ibuprofen Oral Suspension (Common) ... 1546
Motrin Tablets (Common) ... 2625
Motrin Ibuprofen Suspension, Oral Drops, Chewable Tablets, Caplets (Common) ... 1546
▲ Mycobutin Capsules (3%) ... 1957
▲ Nalfon 200 Pulvules & Nalfon Tablets (10.3%) ... 917
Anaprox/Naprosyn (Less than 3%) ... 2117
NebuPent for Inhalation Solution (1% or less) ... 1040
Neurontin Capsules (2.2%) ... 1922
▲ Nicoderm (nicotine transdermal system) (3% to 9%) ... 1518
Nicolar Tablets ... 2026
▲ Nicorette (12%) ... 2458
Nicotrol Nicotine Transdermal System (1% to 3%) ... 1550
▲ Normodyne Injection (Up to 4%) ... 2377
▲ Normodyne Tablets (Up to 4%) ... 2379
Noroxin Tablets (0.3% to 1.0%) ... 1715
Noroxin Tablets (0.3% to 1.0%) ... 2048
Norvasc Tablets (Less than 1% to 2%) ... 1940
Nubain Injection (1% or less) ... 935
▲ Orudis Capsules (11%) ... 2766
▲ Oruvail Capsules (11%) ... 2766
▲ Parlodel (4%) ... 2281
Paxil Tablets (1.9%) ... 2505
Penetrex Tablets (1%) ... 2031
Pentasa (1.6%) ... 1527
▲ Permax Tablets (6.4%) ... 575
▲ Plendil Extended-Release Tablets (0.5% to 3.9%) ... 527
Ponstel (Common) ... 1925
PREVACID Delayed-Release Capsules (Less than 1%) ... 2562
Prinivil Tablets (0.9% to 1.8%) ... 1733
Prinzide Tablets (1.3%) ... 1737
Procardia XL Extended Release Tablets (Less than 3%) ... 1972
▲ Prograf (Greater than 3%) ... 1042
▲ Proleukin for Injection (7%) ... 797
Propulsid (2.7%) ... 1300
ProSom Tablets (2%) ... 449
Prostep (nicotine transdermal system) (Less than 1% of patients) ... 1394
Proventil Inhalation Solution 0.083% (1% to 1.5%) ... 2384
Proventil Repetabs Tablets (2%) ... 2386
Proventil Solution for Inhalation 0.5% (1% to 1.5%) ... 2383
Proventil Tablets (2%) ... 2386
▲ Prozac Pulvules & Liquid, Oral Solution (5% to 10%) ... 919
Questran Light (Less frequent) ... 769
Questran Powder (Less frequent) ... 770
Recombivax HB (Less than 1%) ... 1744
▲ Relafen Tablets (13%) ... 2510
▲ Retrovir Capsules (5% to 6%) ... 1158
▲ Retrovir I.V. Infusion (5% to 6%) .. 1163
▲ Retrovir Syrup (5% to 6%) ... 1158
Rhinocort Nasal Inhaler (1 to 3%).. 556
▲ Ridaura Capsules (3 to 9%) ... 2513
▲ Risperdal (5% to 10%) ... 1301
Rocephin Injectable Vials, ADD-Vantage, Galaxy Container (Rare) ... 2142
▲ Rythmol Tablets–150mg, 225mg, 300mg (1.3 to 3.4%) ... 1352
▲ Salagen Tablets (7%) ... 1489
▲ Sectral Capsules (4%) ... 2807
Semprex-D Capsules (2%) ... 463
Semprex-D Capsules (2%) ... 1167
▲ Serzone Tablets (9%) ... 771
Sinemet CR Tablets (0.6%) ... 944
Stimate, (desmopressin acetate) Nasal Spray, 1.5 mg/mL ... 525
Supprelin Injection (2% to 3%) ... 2056
▲ Suprax (3%) ... 1399
Tambocor Tablets (1% to less than 3%) ... 1497
Tenex Tablets (3% or less) ... 2074
▲ Ticlid Tablets (7.0%) ... 2156
Tilade (1.3%) ... 996
Timolide Tablets (Less than 1%) ... 1748
Timoptic in Ocudose (Less frequent) ... 1753
Timoptic Sterile Ophthalmic Solution ... 1751
Timoptic-XE ... 1755
▲ Tolectin (200, 400 and 600 mg) (3 to 9%) ... 1581
Tonocard Tablets (Less than 1%) .. 531
▲ Toradol (12%) ... 2159
Tornalate Metered Dose Inhaler (0.5%) ... 957
Trandate (1 of 100 patients; up to 4%) ... 1185
Trental Tablets (2.8%) ... 1244
Univasc Tablets (More than 1%) ... 2410
▲ Vascor (200, 300 and 400 mg) Tablets (6.81 to about 22%) ... 1587
Vaseretic Tablets (0.5% to 2.0%) 1765
Vasotec I.V. ... 1768
Vasotec Tablets (0.5% to 1.0%) ... 1771
Ventolin Inhalation Solution (1% to 1.5%) ... 1198
Ventolin Nebules Inhalation Solution (1% to 1.5%) ... 1199
Verelan Capsules (2.5%) ... 1410
Verelan Capsules (2.5%) ... 2824
Videx Tablets, Powder for Oral Solution, & Pediatric Powder for Oral Solution (Less than 1%) ... 720
Voltaren Tablets (Common) ... 861
▲ Wellbutrin Tablets (3.1%) ... 1204
Zebeta Tablets ... 1413
▲ Zerit Capsules (Fewer than 1% to 9%) ... 729
Zestoretic (1.3%) ... 2850
Zestril Tablets (0.2% to 1.8%) ... 2854
Ziac (0.9% to 1.2%) ... 1415
Zithromax (1% or less to 1%) ... 1944
Zocor Tablets (1.1%) ... 1775
Zoladex (1% or greater) ... 2858
▲ Zoloft Tablets (6.0%) ... 2217
▲ Zosyn (3.3%) ... 1419
▲ Zosyn Pharmacy Bulk Package (3.3%) ... 1422
Zyloprim Tablets (Less than 1%) ... 1226

Dysphagia

Achromycin V Capsules (Rare) ... 1367
Altace Capsules (Less than 1%) ... 1232
Ambien Tablets (Infrequent) ... 2416
Anafranil Capsules (Up to 2%) ... 803
Atamet ... 572
Cipro I.V. (1% or less) ... 595
Cipro I.V. Pharmacy Bulk Package (Less than 1%) ... 597
Cipro Tablets (Less than 1%) ... 592
Clozaril Tablets ... 2252
Cognex Capsules (Infrequent) ... 1901
Cosmegen Injection ... 1626
Cytotec (Infrequent) ... 2424
Cytovene (1% or less) ... 2103
Declomycin Tablets ... 1371
Doryx Capsules ... 1913
Dynacin Capsules ... 1590
Edecrin ... 1657
Effexor (Frequent) ... 2719
Eldepryl Tablets ... 2550
Ethmozine Tablets (Less than 2%) 2041
Etrafon ... 2355
Felbatol ... 2666
Fludara for Injection (Up to 1%) ... 663
Flumadine Tablets & Syrup ... 1015
Foscavir Injection (Between 1% and 5%) ... 547
Gastrocrom Capsules (Infrequent).. 984
Hivid Tablets (Less than 1% to less than 3%) ... 2121
Imitrex Injection (1.1%) ... 1103
Imitrex Tablets (Infrequent) ... 1106
Intron A (Less than 5%) ... 2364
Kerlone Tablets (Less than 2%) ... 2436
Lamictal Tablets (Infrequent) ... 1112
Larodopa Tablets (Relatively frequent) ... 2129
Ludiomil Tablets (Rare) ... 843
Lupron Depot 3.75 mg ... 2556
Lupron Depot 7.5 mg ... 2559
Lupron Depot-PED 7.5 mg, 11.25 mg and 15 mg (Less than 2%) ... 2560
Lupron Injection (Less than 5%) ... 2555
Luvox Tablets (2%) ... 2544
Maxaquin Tablets (Less than 1%).. 2440
Mexitil Capsules (About 2 in 1,000) ... 678
Minocin Intravenous ... 1382
Minocin Oral Suspension ... 1385
Minocin Pellet-Filled Capsules ... 1383
Monodox Capsules ... 1805
Monopril Tablets (0.2% to 1.0%).. 757
Neurontin Capsules (Rare) ... 1922
Noroxin Tablets ... 1715
Noroxin Tablets ... 2048
Norvasc Tablets (More than 0.1% to 1%) ... 1940
Orap Tablets (2.7%) ... 1050
Parlodel ... 2281
Paxil Tablets (Infrequent) ... 2505
Pentasa (Less than 1%) ... 1527
Permax Tablets (Frequent) ... 575
PREVACID Delayed-Release Capsules (Less than 1%) ... 2562
Prozac Pulvules & Liquid, Oral Solution (Infrequent) ... 919
Questran Light ... 769
Questran Powder ... 770
Relafen Tablets (1%) ... 2510
Retrovir Capsules ... 1158
Retrovir I.V. Infusion ... 1163
Retrovir Syrup ... 1158
Ridaura Capsules (Less than 0.1%) ... 2513
Risperdal (Infrequent) ... 1301
Salagen Tablets (2%) ... 1489
Serzone Tablets (Rare) ... 771
Sinemet Tablets ... 943
Sinemet CR Tablets ... 944
Tenex Tablets (3% or less) ... 2074
Tensilon Injectable ... 1261
Terramycin Intramuscular Solution 2210
Tonocard Tablets (Less than 1%) .. 531
Triavil Tablets ... 1757
Trilafon ... 2389
VePesid Capsules and Injection (Infrequent) ... 718
Vibramycin ... 1941
Vibramycin Hyclate Intravenous ... 2215
Vibramycin ... 1941
Videx Tablets, Powder for Oral Solution, & Pediatric Powder for Oral Solution (Up to 1%) ... 720
Wellbutrin Tablets (Infrequent) ... 1204
Zinecard (Up to 8%) ... 1961
Zoloft Tablets (Infrequent) ... 2217

(◘ Described in PDR For Nonprescription Drugs) Incidence data in parenthesis; ▲ 3% or more (◉ Described in PDR For Ophthalmology)

Dysphasia

Ambien Tablets (Rare) 2416
Cipro I.V. (1% or less) 595
Cipro I.V. Pharmacy Bulk Package (Less than 1%) 597
Cipro Tablets 592
Floxin I.V. 1571
Floxin Tablets (200 mg, 300 mg, 400 mg) 1567
Imitrex Injection 1103
Maxaquin Tablets 2440
▲ Prograf (Greater than 3%) 1042
Roferon-A Injection (Less than 1%) 2145
Torecan 2245

Dysphonia

Anafranil Capsules (Infrequent) 803
Claritin (2% or fewer patients) 2349
Claritin-D (Less frequent) 2350
Hivid Tablets (Less than 1% to less than 3%) 2121
Intron A (Less than 5%) 2364
ReoPro Vials (0.3%) 1471
Romazicon (Less than 1%) 2147
Tegison Capsules (Less than 1%) 2154
Tensilon Injectable 1261
Tilade (1.0%) 996
Versed Injection (Less than 1%) 2170
Zoloft Tablets (Rare) 2217

Dysphoria

Actifed with Codeine Cough Syrup 1067
Adipex-P Tablets and Capsules 1048
Aldactazide 2413
Aldoclor Tablets 1598
Aldoril Tablets 1604
Ambien Tablets 2416
Ana-Kit Anaphylaxis Emergency Treatment Kit 617
Anatuss LA Tablets 1542
Anexsia 5/500 Elixir 1781
Anexia Tablets 1782
Apresazide Capsules 808
Arfonad Ampuls 2080
Asendin Tablets (Less frequent) 1369
Astramorph/PF Injection, USP (Preservative-Free) 535
Ativan Injection (1.3%) 2698
Benadryl Capsules 1898
Benadryl Injection 1898
Biphetamine Capsules 983
Bontril Slow-Release Capsules 781
Brevital Sodium Vials 1429
▲ Bromfed-DM Cough Syrup (Among most frequent) 1786
Bronkometer Aerosol 2302
Bronkosol Solution 2302
Brontex 1981
Buprenex Injectable (Rare) 2006
BuSpar (Infrequent) 737
Capozide 742
Carbocaine Hydrochloride Injection 2303
Catapres Tablets 674
Catapres-TTS 675
Chibroxin Sterile Ophthalmic Solution (With oral form) 1617
▲ Cipro I.V. (Among most frequent) 595
Cipro I.V. Pharmacy Bulk Package (Greater than 1%) 597
Cipro Tablets (1.1%) 592
Claritin-D 2350
▲ Clozaril Tablets (4%) 2252
Cocaine Hydrochloride Topical Solution 537
Combipres Tablets 677
Allergy-Sinus Comtrex Multi-Symptom Allergy-Sinus Formula Tablets ◙ 617
D.A. Chewable Tablets 951
Dalmane Capsules (Rare) 2173
Darvon-N/Darvocet-N 1433
Darvon 1435
Darvon-N Suspension & Tablets 1433
Deconamine Chewable Tablets 1320
Deconamine CX Cough and Cold Liquid and Tablets 1319
Deconamine 1320
Deconsal C Expectorant Syrup 456
Deconsal Pediatric Capsules 454
Deconsal Pediatric Syrup 457
Deconsal II Tablets 454
Demadex Tablets and Injection 686
Demerol 2308
Desoxyn Gradumet Tablets (Rare) 419
Dexedrine 2474
DextroStat Dextroamphetamine Tablets 2036
Didrex Tablets 2607
Dilatrate-SR 2398
Dilaudid Ampules 1335
Dilaudid Cough Syrup 1336
Dilaudid-HP Injection (Less frequent) 1337
Dilaudid-HP Lyophilized Powder 250 mg (Less frequent) 1337
Dilaudid 1335
Dilaudid Oral Liquid 1339
Dilaudid 1335
Dilaudid Tablets - 8 mg 1339
Dimetane-DC Cough Syrup 2059
Dimetane-DX Cough Syrup 2059
Ditropan 1516
Diucardin Tablets 2718
Diupres Tablets 1650
Diuril Oral Suspension 1653
Diuril Sodium Intravenous 1652
Diuril Tablets 1653
Duramorph 962
Duranest Injections 542
Dura-Tap/PD Capsules 2867
Duratuss Tablets 2565
Dura-Vent/DA Tablets 953
Dura-Vent Tablets 952
Elavil 2838
Eldepryl Tablets 2550
Emete-con Intramuscular/Intravenous 2198
Empirin with Codeine Tablets 1093
Endep Tablets 2174
Enduron Tablets 420
Entex Capsules 1986
Entex LA Tablets 1987
Entex Liquid 1986
EpiPen—Epinephrine Auto-Injector 790
Esidrix Tablets 821
Esimil Tablets 822
Eskalith 2485
Etrafon 2355
Exgest LA Tablets 782
Fastin Capsules 2488
Fedahist Gyrocaps 2401
Fedahist Timecaps 2401
Floxin I.V. 1571
Floxin Tablets (200 mg, 300 mg, 400 mg) 1567
Guaifed Syrup ◙ 734
Halcion Tablets 2611
Haldol Decanoate 1577
Haldol Injection, Tablets and Concentrate 1575
Hespan Injection 929
Hycodan Tablets and Syrup 930
Hycomine Compound Tablets 932
Hycomine 931
Hycotuss Expectorant Syrup 933
Hydrocet Capsules 782
HydroDIURIL Tablets 1674
Hydropres Tablets 1675
Hyzaar Tablets 1677
▲ Inapsine Injection (Among most common) 1296
Inderide LA Long Acting Capsules 2734
Infumorph 200 and Infumorph 500 Sterile Solutions 965
Ionamin Capsules 990
Isoetharine Inhalation Solution, USP, Arm-a-Med 551
Lamictal Tablets (Infrequent) 1112
Lariam Tablets 2128
Lasix Injection, Oral Solution and Tablets 1240
Limbitrol 2180
Lithium Carbonate Capsules & Tablets 2230
Lithonate/Lithotabs/Lithobid 2543
Lomotil 2439
Lopressor HCT Tablets 832
Lorcet 10/650 1018
Lortab 2566
Lotensin HCT 837
Lozol Tablets 2022
Ludiomil Tablets (Rare) 843
Lufyllin & Lufyllin-400 Tablets 2670
Lufyllin-GG Elixir & Tablets 2671
▲ MS Contin Tablets (Among most frequent) 1994
▲ MSIR (Among most frequent) 1997
Marcaine Hydrochloride with Epinephrine 1:200,000 2316
Marcaine Hydrochloride Injection 2316
Marcaine Spinal 2319
Maxaquin Tablets 2440
Maxzide 1380
Mellaril (Extremely rare) 2269
Mepergan Injection 2753
Methadone Hydrochloride Oral Concentrate 2233
Methadone Hydrochloride Oral Solution & Tablets 2235
Minizide Capsules 1938
Moduretic Tablets 1705
Monoket (Fewer than 1%) 2406
Mykrox Tablets 993
Navane Capsules and Concentrate 2201
Navane Intramuscular 2202
Neo-Synephrine Hydrochloride 1% Carpuject 2324
Neo-Synephrine Hydrochloride 1% Injection 2324
Nescaine/Nescaine MPF 554
Nitrolingual Spray 2027
Noroxin Tablets 1715
Noroxin Tablets 2048
Norpramin Tablets 1526
Novahistine DH 2462
Novahistine DMX ◙ 822
Novahistine Elixir ◙ 823
Novahistine Expectorant 2463
Nubain Injection (1% or less) 935
Nucofed 2051
Numorphan Injection 936
Numorphan Suppositories 937
▲ Oramorph SR (Morphine Sulfate Sustained Release Tablets) (Among most frequent) 2236
Oretic Tablets 443
Orlamm 2239
Ornade Spansule Capsules 2502
Orudis Capsules (Rare) 2766
Oruvail Capsules (Rare) 2766
Oxsoralen-Ultra Capsules 1257
PBZ Tablets 845
PBZ-SR Tablets 844
Pamelor 2280
Parnate Tablets 2503
Percocet Tablets 938
Percodan Tablets 939
Percodan-Demi Tablets 940
Periactin 1724
Phenergan with Codeine 2777
Phenergan VC 2779
Phenergan VC with Codeine 2781
Phenobarbital Elixir and Tablets 1469
Pregnyl 1828
Prelu-2 Timed Release Capsules 681
Prinzide Tablets 1737
Profasi (chorionic gonadotropin for injection, USP) 2450
Prolixin 509
Proventil (Less than 1%) 2386
Quadrinal Tablets 1350
Quibron 2053
RMS Suppositories 2657
▲ Reglan (Approximately 10%) 2068
Respbid Tablets 682
ReVia Tablets (Less than 1%) 940
Revex 1811
Romazicon (1% to 3%) 2147
Roxanol 2243
Roxicodone Tablets, Oral Solution & Intensol (Oxycodone) 2244
Sanorex Tablets 2294
Seldane-D Extended-Release Tablets (2.1%) 1538
Sensorcaine 559
Ser-Ap-Es Tablets 849
Serentil 684
Serzone Tablets 771
Slo-bid Gyrocaps 2033
Stadol (Less than 1%) 775
Sublimaze Injection 1307
Surmontil Capsules 2811
Sus-Phrine Injection 1019
Syn-Rx Tablets 465
Syn-Rx DM Tablets 466
Tavist Syrup 2297
Tavist Tablets 2298
Tenoretic Tablets 2845
Thalitone 1245
Theo-24 Extended Release Capsules 2568
Theo-Dur Extended-Release Tablets 1327
Theo-X Extended-Release Tablets 788
Timolide Tablets 1748
Tofranil Ampuls 854
Tofranil Tablets 856
Tofranil-PM Capsules 857
Torecan (Occasional) 2245
Transderm Scōp Transdermal Therapeutic System (Infrequent) 869
Triavil Tablets 1757
Trilafon 2389
Tussend 1783
Tussend Expectorant 1785
Tussionex Pennkinetic Extended-Release Suspension 998
Tylenol with Codeine 1583
Tylox Capsules 1584
Tympagesic Ear Drops 2342
Uni-Dur Extended-Release Tablets 1331
Uniphyl 400 mg Tablets (Frequent) 2001
Vaseretic Tablets 1765
Ventolin Tablets (Fewer than 1 of 100 patients) 1203
Versed Injection (Less than 1%) 2170
Vicodin Tablets 1356
Vicodin ES Tablets 1357
Vicodin Tuss Expectorant 1358
Vivactil Tablets 1774
Volmax Extended-Release Tablets (Less frequent) 1788
Wellbutrin Tablets (Infrequent) 1204
Wygesic Tablets 2827
Xylocaine Injections 567
▲ Yutopar Intravenous Injection (5% to 6%) 570
Zaroxolyn Tablets 1000
Zebeta Tablets 1413
Zestoretic 2850
Ziac 1415
Zydone Capsules 949

Dysplasia, bone marrow (see under Bone marrow dysplasia)

Dysplasia, cervical

Anafranil Capsules (Rare) 803
Demulen 2428
Ortho-Est 1.25 Tablets 1869

Dyspnea

Abbokinase 403
Abbokinase Open-Cath 405
Accupril Tablets (1.9%) 1893
Acel-Imune Diphtheria and Tetanus Toxoids and Acellular Pertussis Vaccine Adsorbed (Rare) 1364
▲ Adalat Capsules (10 mg and 20 mg) (6%) 587
Adalat CC (Less than 1.0%) 589
▲ Adenocard Injection (12%) 1021
▲ Adenoscan (Approximately 28%) 1024
AeroBid Inhaler System (1-3%) 1005
Aerobid-M Inhaler System (1-3%) 1005
Airet Solution for Inhalation (1.5%) 452
Alkeran for Injection (In some patients) 1070
Altace Capsules (Less than 1%) 1232
Ambien Tablets (Infrequent) 2416
Anafranil Capsules (Up to 2%) 803
▲ Anaprox/Naprosyn (3% to 9%) 2117
Ancobon Capsules 2079
Ansaid Tablets (Less than 1%) 2579
Antivenin (Crotalidae) Polyvalent 2696
Apresazide Capsules (Less frequent) 808
Apresoline Hydrochloride Tablets (Less frequent) 809
AquaMEPHYTON Injection 1608
Atamet 572
▲ Atgam Sterile Solution (More than 1% to 10%) 2581
Atretol Tablets 573
▲ Atrovent Inhalation Solution (9.6%) 673
Azactam for Injection (One patient) 734
Bentyl 1501
Betagan ⊙ 233
▲ Betapace Tablets (5% to 21%) 641
▲ Betaseron for SC Injection (8%) 658
Betimol 0.25%, 0.5% ⊙ 261
Betoptic Ophthalmic Solution (Rare) 469
Betoptic S Ophthalmic Suspension (Rare) 471
Blenoxane 692
Blocadren Tablets (1.7%) 1614
Brethaire Inhaler 813
Brethine Ampuls (0.0 to 2.0%) 815
Brevibloc Injection (Less than 1%) 1808
Brevital Sodium Vials 1429
Buprenex Injectable (Less than 1%) 2006
Calan SR Caplets (1.4%) 2422
Calan Tablets (1.4%) 2419
Capoten (About 0.5 to 2%) 739
Capozide (0.5 to 2%) 742
Cardene Capsules (0.6%) 2095
Cardene I.V. (0.7%) 2709
Cardizem CD Capsules (Less than 1%) 1506
Cardizem SR Capsules (Less than 1%) 1510
Cardizem Injectable (Less than 1%) 1508
Cardizem Tablets (Less than 1%) 1512
Cardura Tablets (1% to 2.6%) 2186

(◙ Described in PDR For Nonprescription Drugs) Incidence data in parenthesis; ▲ 3% or more (⊙ Described in PDR For Ophthalmology)

1283 **Side Effects Index** **Dystonia**

Cartrol Tablets (Less common) 410
Cataflam (Less than 1%) 816
Ceclor Pulvules & Suspension 1431
▲CellCept Capsules (15.5% to 17.3%) 2099
Chibroxin Sterile Ophthalmic Solution (With oral form) 1617
Cipro I.V. (1% or less) 595
Cipro I.V. Pharmacy Bulk Package (Less than 1%) 597
Cipro Tablets (Less than 1%) 592
Claritin (2% or fewer patients) 2349
Claritin-D (Less frequent) 2350
Clinoril Tablets (Less than 1%) 1618
Clomid 1514
Clozaril Tablets (1%) 2252
Cognex Capsules (Frequent) 1901
▲Cordarone Tablets (2% to 7%) 2712
Coumadin 926
Cozaar Tablets (Less than 1%) 1628
Cytotec (Infrequent) 2424
Cytovene (1% or less) 2103
D.H.E. 45 Injection (Occasional) 2255
Deconsal C Expectorant Syrup 456
Deconsal Pediatric Syrup 457
Depakote Tablets (Greater than 1% but not more than 5%) 415
Depen Titratable Tablets 2662
Depo-Provera Contraceptive Injection (Fewer than 1%) 2602
Dilacor XR Extended-release Capsules (1.0% to 1.4%) 2018
Diphtheria and Tetanus Toxoids and Pertussis Vaccine Adsorbed (Rare) 2477
Diphtheria and Tetanus Toxoids and Pertussis Vaccine Adsorbed USP (For Pediatric Use) (Rare) 875
Diprivan Injection (Less than 1%) 2833
Diupres Tablets 1650
Dizac 1809
Dolobid Tablets (Rare) 1654
Dopram Injectable 2061
▲Duragesic Transdermal System (3% to 10%) 1288
DynaCirc Capsules (0.5% to 3.4%) 2256
▲EC-Naprosyn Delayed-Release Tablets (3% to 9%) 2117
Effexor (Frequent) 2719
▲Emcyt Capsules (11%) 1953
▲Eminase (Less than 10%) 2039
Esimil Tablets 822
▲Ethmozine Tablets (3.8% to 5.7%) 2041
Felbatol 2666
Feldene Capsules (Less than 1%) 1965
Flexeril Tablets (Rare) 1661
Floropryl Sterile Ophthalmic Ointment (Rare) 1662
Floxin I.V. 1571
Floxin Tablets (200 mg, 300 mg, 400 mg) 1567
▲Fludara for Injection (9% to 22%) 663
Flumadine Tablets & Syrup (0.3% to 1%) 1015
▲Foscavir Injection (5% or greater) 547
Fungizone Intravenous 506
Furoxone (Rare) 2046
Gamimune N, 5% Immune Globulin Intravenous (Human), 5% 619
Gamimune N, 10% Immune Globulin Intravenous (Human), 10% 621
Ganite 2533
Gastrocrom Capsules (Infrequent) 984
Glucotrol XL Extended Release Tablets (Less than 1%) 1968
Guaifed 1787
Havrix (Rare) 2489
Hivid Tablets (Less than 1% to less than 3%) 2121
Humegon 1824
Humorsol Sterile Ophthalmic Solution 1664
Hydrea Capsules (Rare) 696
Hydropres Tablets 1675
Hyperstat I.V. Injection 2363
Hyskon Hysteroscopy Fluid (Rare) 1595
▲Hytrin Capsules (0.5% to 3.1%) 430
Hyzaar Tablets 1677
Imdur (Less than or equal to 5%) 1323
Imitrex Injection (Infrequent) 1103
Imitrex Tablets (Frequent) 1106
Indocin Capsules (Less than 1%) 1680
Indocin I.V. (Less than 1%) 1684
Indocin (Less than 1%) 1680
INFeD (Iron Dextran Injection, USP) 2345
▲Intron A (Up to 34%) 2364
Iopidine 0.5% (Less than 1%) ⊙ 221
Ismelin Tablets 827
Isoptin Oral Tablets (1.4%) 1346
Isoptin SR Tablets (1.4%) 1348
K-Phos Neutral Tablets 639
K-Phos Original Formula 'Sodium Free' Tablets (Less frequent) 639
Kerlone Tablets (2.4%) 2436
Lamictal Tablets (1.1%) 1112
Lescol Capsules (Rare) 2267
▲Leukine for IV Infusion (28%) 1271
▲Leustatin (11%) 1834
Levatol (2.1%) 2403
Lioresal Intrathecal (1 to 2 of 214 patients) 1596
Lioresal Tablets (Rare) 829
Livostin (Approximately 1% to 3%) ⊙ 266
Lodine Capsules and Tablets (Less than 1%) 2743
Lopressor Ampuls (1%) 830
Lopressor HCT Tablets (1 in 100 patients) 832
Lopressor Tablets (1%) 830
Lorcet 10/650 1018
Lortab 2566
Lotensin Tablets 834
Lotensin HCT 837
Loxitane 1378
Lupron Depot 3.75 mg 2556
▲Lupron Depot 7.5 mg (5.4%) 2559
Lupron Injection (5% or more) 2555
Lutrepulse for Injection 980
Luvox Tablets (2%) 2544
Maalox Daily Fiber Therapy ▣ 641
Macrobid Capsules (Common) 1988
Macrodantin Capsules (Common) 1989
Maxaquin Tablets (Less than 1%) 2440
Mefoxin 1691
Mefoxin Premixed Intravenous Solution 1694
Megace Oral Suspension (1% to 3%) 699
Megace Tablets 701
Mephyton Tablets (Rare) 1696
Methergine (Rare) 2272
Methotrexate Sodium Tablets, Injection, for Injection and LPF Injection 1275
Metrodin (urofollitropin for injection) 2446
Mevacor Tablets (Rare) 1699
▲Mexitil Capsules (3.3% to 5.7%) 678
Miacalcin Nasal Spray (Less than 1%) 2275
Midamor Tablets (Between 1% and 3%) 1703
Minipress Capsules (1-4%) 1937
Minizide Capsules 1938
Miochol-E with Iocare Steri-Tags and Miochol-E System Pak (Rare) ⊙ 273
Moduretic Tablets (Greater than 1%, less than 3%) 1705
Monoket (Fewer than 1%) 2406
Monopril Tablets (1.0% or more) 757
Motrin Ibuprofen Suspension, Oral Drops, Chewable Tablets, Caplets (Less than 1%) 1546
Mutamycin 703
Mycobutin Capsules (Less than 1%) 1957
Myochrysine Injection 1711
Nalfon 200 Pulvules & Nalfon Tablets (2.8%) 917
▲Anaprox/Naprosyn (3% to 9%) 2117
Navelbine Injection (Up to 3%) 1145
▲Neupogen for Injection (9%) 495
Neurontin Capsules (Infrequent) 1922
Nicorette 2458
Nimotop Capsules (Up to 1.2%) 610
Nolvadex Tablets 2841
Normodyne Injection (Rare) 2377
Normodyne Tablets (Rare; 2%) 2379
Noroxin Tablets 1715
Noroxin Tablets 2048
Norvasc Tablets (More than 0.1% to 1%) 1940
▲Novantrone (6 to 18%) 1279
Nubain Injection (1% or less) 935
Nucofed 2051
Ocupress Ophthalmic Solution, 1% Sterile (Occasional) ⊙ 309
▲Oncaspar (Greater than 5%) 2028
Oncovin Solution Vials & Hyporets 1466
OptiPranolol (Metipranolol 0.3%) Sterile Ophthalmic Solution (A small number of patients) ⊙ 258
▲Orthoclone OKT3 Sterile Solution (21%) 1837
Orudis Capsules (Less than 1%) 2766
Oruvail Capsules (Less than 1%) 2766
Paxil Tablets (Infrequent) 2505
Penetrex Tablets (Less than 1% but more than or equal to 0.1%) 2031
Pentasa (One case) 1527
Pergonal (menotropins for injection, USP) 2448
▲Permax Tablets (4.8%) 575
Plendil Extended-Release Tablets (0.5% to 1.5%) 527
Ponstel (Rare) 1925
Pravachol (Rare) 765
PREVACID Delayed-Release Capsules (Less than 1%) 2562
Primaxin I.M. 1727
Primaxin I.V. (Less than 0.2%) 1729
▲Prinivil Tablets (2.7% to 7.6%) 1733
Prinzide Tablets (0.3% to 1%) 1737
▲Procardia Capsules (6%) 1971
▲Procardia XL Extended Release Tablets (Less than 3% to 6%) 1972
Profasi (chorionic gonadotropin for injection, USP) 2450
▲Prograf (3% to 29%) 1042
Prolastin Alpha$_1$-Proteinase Inhibitor (Human) (Occasional) 635
▲Proleukin for Injection (52%) 797
ProSom Tablets (Infrequent) 449
Prostigmin Injectable 1260
Prostigmin Tablets 1261
Prostin E2 Suppository 2634
Protamine Sulfate Ampoules & Vials 1471
Proventil Inhalation Solution 0.083% (1.5%) 2384
Proventil Solution for Inhalation 0.5% (1.5%) 2383
Prozac Pulvules & Liquid, Oral Solution (1.4%) 919
Pulmozyme Inhalation 1064
Recombivax HB (Less than 1%) 1744
Reglan (Rare) 2068
Relafen Tablets (1%) 2510
▲Retrovir Capsules (5%) 1158
▲Retrovir I.V. Infusion (5%) 1163
▲Retrovir Syrup (5%) 1158
ReVia Tablets (Less than 1%) 940
Rhinocort Nasal Inhaler (Less than 1%) 556
Risperdal (Up to 1%) 1301
▲Roferon-A Injection (11%) 2145
▲Romazicon (3% to 9%) 2147
Rowasa 2548
▲Rythmol Tablets–150mg, 225mg, 300mg (2.0 to 5.3%) 1352
Sandimmune 2286
Sansert Tablets 2295
▲Sectral Capsules (4%) 2807
Ser-Ap-Es Tablets 849
Serophene (clomiphene citrate tablets, USP) 2451
Serzone Tablets (Frequent) 771
Sinemet Tablets 943
Sinemet CR Tablets (1.6%) 944
▲Stadol (3% to 9%) 775
Streptase for Infusion (Rare) 562
Suprane (Less than 1%) 1813
Symmetrel Capsules and Syrup (0.1% to 1%) 946
Talwin Injection (Infrequent) 2334
▲Tambocor Tablets (10.3%) 1497
Taxol (2%) 714
▲Tegison Capsules (1 to 10%) 2154
Tegretol Chewable Tablets 852
Tegretol Suspension 852
Tegretol Tablets 852
Tenex Tablets (3% or less) 2074
▲Tenoretic Tablets (0.6% to 6%) 2845
▲Tenormin Tablets and I.V. Injection (0.6% to 6%) 2847
Tetramune (Rare) 1404
Tilade (2.8%) 996
Timolide Tablets (1.2%) 1748
Timoptic in Ocudose (Less frequent) 1753
Timoptic Sterile Ophthalmic Solution (Less frequent) 1751
Timoptic-XE 1755
Tonocard Tablets (Less than 1%) 531
Toprol-XL Tablets (About 1 of 100 patients) 565
Toradol (1% or less) 2159
Tornalate Solution for Inhalation, 0.2% (Less than 1%) 956
Tornalate Metered Dose Inhaler (Less than 1% to 1.0%) 957
Tracrium Injection 1183
Trandate (Rare) 1185
▲Trasylol (3%) 613
Trental Tablets (Less than 1%) 1244
Tri-Immunol Adsorbed 1408
Tripedia 892
Ultram Tablets (50 mg) (Less than 1%) 1585
Univasc Tablets (Less than 1%) 2410
Uroqid-Acid No. 2 Tablets 640
Valium Injectable 2182
Vancocin HCl, Vials & ADD-Vantage 1481
▲Vascor (200, 300 and 400 mg) Tablets (3.59 to 8.70%) 1587
Vaseretic Tablets (0.5% to 2.0%) 1765
Vasotec I.V. 1768
Vasotec Tablets (0.5% to 1.3%) 1771
Velban Vials 1484
Ventolin Inhalation Solution (1.5%) 1198
Ventolin Nebules Inhalation Solution (1.5%) 1199
VePesid Capsules and Injection (0.7% to 2%) 718
Verelan Capsules (1% or less) 1410
Verelan Capsules (1.4%) 2824
Versed Injection (Less than 1%) 2170
▲Videx Tablets, Powder for Oral Solution, & Pediatric Powder for Oral Solution (Up to 4%; 27%) 720
Virazole 1264
▲Visken Tablets (5%) 2299
Voltaren Tablets (Less than 1%) 861
▲Vumon (Approximately 5%) 727
Wellbutrin Tablets (Infrequent) 1204
Yutopar Intravenous Injection (Infrequent) 570
Zebeta Tablets (1.1% to 1.5%) 1413
Zefazone 2654
▲Zerit Capsules (Fewer than 1% to 13%) 729
Zestoretic (0.3 to 1%) 2850
▲Zestril Tablets (2.7% to 7.6%) 2854
Ziac 1415
Zocor Tablets (Rare) 1775
Zoloft Tablets (Infrequent) 2217
Zosyn (1.1%) 1419
Zosyn Pharmacy Bulk Package (1.1%) 1422

Dyspnea, nocturnal

Prinivil Tablets (0.3% to 1.0%) 1733
Prinzide Tablets 1737
Zestoretic 2850
Zestril Tablets (0.3% to 1.0%) 2854

Dysrhythmia

Abbokinase (Occasional) 403
Anectine (Rare) 1073
Asendin Tablets 1369
▲Brethaire Inhaler (About 4%) 813
Loxitane 1378
Mellaril 2269
Procardia Capsules (About 1 patient in 150) 1971
Procardia XL Extended Release Tablets (About 1 patient in 150) 1972

Dystonia

Anafranil Capsules (Rare) 803
▲Atamet (Among most common) 572
Betaseron for SC Injection 658
BuSpar (Rare) 737
Clozaril Tablets 2252
Cognex Capsules (Rare) 1901
Compazine 2470
Dilantin Infatabs (Rare) 1908
Dilantin Kapseals (Rare) 1906
Dilantin Parenteral (Rare) 1910
Dilantin-125 Suspension (Rare) 1911
Diprivan Injection (Less than 1%) 2833
Doral Tablets 2664
Effexor (Rare) 2719
Eldepryl Tablets 2550
Eskalith (One report in a child) 2485
Etrafon 2355
Felbatol (Infrequent) 2666
Halcion Tablets 2611
Haldol Decanoate (Frequent) 1577
Haldol Injection, Tablets and Concentrate 1575
Imitrex Injection (Rare) 1103
Imitrex Tablets (Rare) 1106
Inapsine Injection 1296
Lamictal Tablets (Rare) 1112
Larodopa Tablets (Frequent) 2129
Levoprome 1274
Lioresal Tablets 829
Lithium Carbonate Capsules & Tablets 2230
Lithonate/Lithotabs/Lithobid 2543
Loxitane 1378
Luvox Tablets (Infrequent) 2544
Mellaril 2269

(▣ Described in PDR For Nonprescription Drugs) Incidence data in parenthesis; ▲ 3% or more (⊙ Described in PDR For Ophthalmology)

Moban Tablets and Concentrate (Infrequent) ... 1048
Navane Capsules and Concentrate 2201
Navane Intramuscular ... 2202
Neurontin Capsules (Infrequent)... 1922
Orap Tablets (Less frequent) ... 1050
Paxil Tablets (Rare) ... 2505
▲ Permax Tablets (11.6%) ... 575
Prolixin ... 509
Prozac Pulvules & Liquid, Oral Solution (Rare) ... 919
Reglan (Approximately 0.2%) ... 2068
▲ Risperdal (17% to 34%) ... 1301
Serentil ... 684
▲ Sinemet Tablets (Among most common) ... 943
Sinemet CR Tablets (1.8%) ... 944
Stelazine ... 2514
Sublimaze Injection ... 1307
Temaril Tablets, Syrup and Spansule Extended-Release Capsules ... 483
Thorazine ... 2523
Torecan ... 2245
Triavil Tablets ... 1757
Trilafon ... 2389
Wellbutrin Tablets (Frequent) ... 1204
Xanax Tablets ... 2649
Zoloft Tablets (Infrequent) ... 2217

Dystonia, tardive

Compazine ... 2470
Haldol Decanoate ... 1577
Haldol Injection, Tablets and Concentrate ... 1575
Thorazine ... 2523

Dystonic reactions (see under Dystonia)

Dysuria

Ambien Tablets (Rare) ... 2416
Anafranil Capsules (Up to 2%) ... 803
Asacol Delayed-Release Tablets ... 1979
Atrohist Plus Tablets ... 454
Atromid-S Capsules ... 2701
▲ BCG Vaccine, USP (TICE) (59.5%) 1814
Bontril Slow-Release Capsules ... 781
BuSpar (Infrequent) ... 737
Cardura Tablets (0.5%) ... 2186
Ceftin (Less than 1% but more than 0.1%) ... 1078
▲ CellCept Capsules (More than or equal to 3%) ... 2099
Claritin-D (Less frequent) ... 2350
Clinoril Tablets ... 1618
Cogentin ... 1621
Cognex Capsules (Infrequent) ... 1901
Combipres Tablets (Rare) ... 677
Cytotec (Infrequent) ... 2424
D.A. Chewable Tablets ... 951
Daypro Caplets (Greater than 1% but less than 3%) ... 2426
Deconamine Chewable Tablets ... 1320
Deconamine CX Cough and Cold Liquid and Tablets ... 1319
Deconamine ... 1320
Deconsal ... 454
Demser Capsules (A few patients) .. 1649
Depakote Tablets (Greater than 1% but not more than 5%) ... 415
Desferal Vials ... 820
Dipentum Capsules (Rare) ... 1951
Diupres Tablets ... 1650
Dolobid Tablets (Less than 1 in 100) ... 1654
Dura-Tap/PD Capsules ... 2867
Dura-Vent/DA Tablets ... 953
Dura-Vent Tablets ... 952
Effexor (Frequent) ... 2719
Engerix-B Unit-Dose Vials ... 2482
Ethmozine Tablets (Less than 2%) 2041
Fedahist Gyrocaps ... 2401
Fedahist Timecaps ... 2401
Feldene Capsules (Less than 1%) .. 1965
Flagyl 375 Capsules ... 2434
Floxin I.V. (Less than 1%) ... 1571
Floxin Tablets (200 mg, 300 mg, 400 mg) (Less than 1%) ... 1567
▲ Fludara for Injection (3% to 4%) ... 663
Foscavir Injection (Between 1% and 5%) ... 547
Gastrocrom Capsules (Infrequent) .. 984
Glucotrol XL Extended Release Tablets (Less than 1%) ... 1968
Hivid Tablets (Less than 1% to less than 3%) ... 2121
Hydrea Capsules (Very rare) ... 696
Hydropres Tablets ... 1675
IFEX ... 697
Imitrex Injection (Rare) ... 1103
Imitrex Tablets (Up to 2%) ... 1106
Intal Capsules (Less than 1 in 10,000 patients) ... 987
Intal Inhaler (Infrequent) ... 988
Intal Nebulizer Solution ... 989
Ismo Tablets (Fewer than 1%) ... 2738
Kerlone Tablets (Less than 2%) ... 2436
Klonopin Tablets ... 2126
Lamictal Tablets (Rare) ... 1112
Lioresal Tablets (Rare) ... 829
Lodine Capsules and Tablets (More than 1% but less than 3%) ... 2743
▲ Lupron Depot 3.75 mg (Among most frequent) ... 2556
Lupron Depot 7.5 mg (Less than 5%) ... 2559
Lupron Injection (Less than 5%) ... 2555
Luvox Tablets (Infrequent) ... 2544
Maxaquin Tablets (Less than 1%) .. 2440
Methotrexate Sodium Tablets, Injection, for Injection and LPF Injection (Less common) ... 1275
MetroGel-Vaginal ... 902
Midamor Tablets (Less than or equal to 1%) ... 1703
Moduretic Tablets (Less than or equal to 1%) ... 1705
Nalfon 200 Pulvules & Nalfon Tablets (Less than 1%) ... 917
Neurontin Capsules (Infrequent) ... 1922
Norpace (Less than 1%) ... 2444
Norvasc Tablets (Less than or equal to 0.1%) ... 1940
Novahistine DH ... 2462
Novahistine DMX ... ▣ 822
Novahistine Elixir ... ▣ 823
Novahistine Expectorant ... 2463
Oncovin Solution Vials & Hyporets 1466
Ornade Spansule Capsules ... 2502
Paxil Tablets (Infrequent) ... 2505
Permax Tablets (Infrequent) ... 575
Plendil Extended-Release Tablets (0.5% to 1.5%) ... 527
Pondimin Tablets ... 2066
Ponstel ... 1925
Prinivil Tablets (0.3% to 1.0%) ... 1733
Prinzide Tablets ... 1737
Procardia XL Extended Release Tablets (1% or less) ... 1972
▲ Proleukin for Injection (3%) ... 797
Protostat Tablets ... 1883
Prozac Pulvules & Liquid, Oral Solution (Infrequent) ... 919
Pyrazinamide Tablets (Rare) ... 1398
Questran Light ... 769
Questran Powder ... 770
Recombivax HB (Less than 1%) ... 1744
Relafen Tablets (Less than 1%) ... 2510
Retrovir Capsules ... 1158
Retrovir I.V. Infusion ... 1163
Retrovir Syrup ... 1158
Rifater (Rare) ... 1532
Risperdal (Infrequent) ... 1301
Rondec Oral Drops ... 953
Rondec Syrup ... 953
Rondec Tablet ... 953
Rondec-DM Oral Drops ... 954
Rondec-DM Syrup ... 954
Rondec-TR Tablet ... 953
Salagen Tablets (Less than 1%) ... 1489
Sanorex Tablets ... 2294
Sansert Tablets ... 2295
Sectral Capsules (Up to 2%) ... 2807
Seldane-D Extended-Release Tablets ... 1538
Ser-Ap-Es Tablets ... 849
Serzone Tablets ... 771
Supprelin Injection (1% to 3%) ... 2056
Syn-Rx Tablets ... 465
Syn-Rx DM Tablets ... 466
Tegison Capsules (Less than 1%) .. 2154
Temaril Tablets, Syrup and Spansule Extended-Release Capsules ... 483
▲ TheraCys BCG Live (Intravesical) (3.6% to 51.8%) ... 897
Thioplex (Thiotepa For Injection) ... 1281
Tolectin (200, 400 and 600 mg) (Less than 1%) ... 1581
Trinalin Repetabs Tablets ... 1330
Tussend ... 1783
Tussend Expectorant ... 1785
Ultram Tablets (50 mg) (Less than 1%) ... 1585
Unasyn (Less than 1%) ... 2212
Urispas Tablets ... 2532
Uroqid-Acid No. 2 Tablets (Occasional) ... 640
Vagistat-1 (Less than 1%) ... 778
Wellbutrin Tablets (Rare) ... 1204
Zerit Capsules (Fewer than 1% to 3%) ... 729
Zestril Tablets (0.3% to 1.0%) ... 2854
Zofran Injection (2%) ... 1214
Zoloft Tablets (Infrequent) ... 2217
Zosyn (1.0% or less) ... 1419
Zosyn Pharmacy Bulk Package (1.0% or less) ... 1422

E

Ear, discomfort

AeroBid Inhaler System (1-3%) ... 1005
Aerobid-M Inhaler System (1-3%) .. 1005
Bumex (0.1%) ... 2093
BuSpar (Rare) ... 737
Cytotec (Infrequent) ... 2424
Fioricet with Codeine Capsules (Infrequent) ... 2260
Kerlone Tablets (Less than 2%) ... 2436
Ponstel ... 1925
ReVia Tablets (Less than 1%) ... 940
▲ Tegison Capsules (1-10%) ... 2154
Versed Injection (Less than 1%) ... 2170

Ear, drainage

Hivid Tablets (Less than 1% to less than 3%) ... 2121
Tegison Capsules (Less than 1%) .. 2154

Ear, external abnormalities, fetal

Accutane Capsules ... 2076
Depen Titratable Tablets ... 2662

Ear disease, unspecified

Ansaid Tablets (Less than 1%) ... 2579
Cardene I.V. (Rare) ... 2709
Clozaril Tablets (Less than 1%) ... 2252
Depakote Tablets (Greater than 1% but not more than 5%) ... 415
Salagen Tablets (Rare) ... 1489
Videx Tablets, Powder for Oral Solution, & Pediatric Powder for Oral Solution (Less than 1%) ... 720

Ears, blocked

Asacol Delayed-Release Tablets ... 1979
▲ CHEMET (succimer) Capsules (1.0 to 3.7%) ... 1545
Dalgan Injection ... 538
Hivid Tablets (Less than 1% to less than 3%) ... 2121
Neurontin Capsules (Infrequent) ... 1922
Orthoclone OKT3 Sterile Solution .. 1837
ReVia Tablets (Less than 1%) ... 940
Supprelin Injection (2% to 3%) ... 2056
Versed Injection (Less than 1%) ... 2170

Ears, ringing (see under Tinnitus)

Ears, roaring in

Garamycin Injectable ... 2360
Nebcin Vials, Hyporets & ADD-Vantage ... 1464

Ebstein's anomaly

Eskalith ... 2485
Lithium Carbonate Capsules & Tablets ... 2230

Ebriety, feeling of

Intron A (Less than 5%) ... 2364

Ecchymoses

Activase (Less than 1% to 1%) ... 1058
▲ Anaprox/Naprosyn (3% to 9%) ... 2117
Ansaid Tablets (Less than 1%) ... 2579
BuSpar (Rare) ... 737
Calan SR Caplets (1% or less) ... 2422
Calan Tablets (1% or less) ... 2419
Caverject (2%) ... 2583
Celestone Soluspan Suspension ... 2347
▲ CellCept Capsules (More than or equal to 3%) ... 2099
Clinoril Tablets (Less than 1%) ... 1618
Cordarone Tablets (Less than 1%) 2712
Cortifoam ... 2396
Cortone Acetate Sterile Suspension ... 1623
Cortone Acetate Tablets ... 1624
Cozaar Tablets (Less than 1%) ... 1628
Daypro Caplets (Less than 1%) ... 2426
Decadron Elixir ... 1633
Decadron Phosphate Injection ... 1637
Decadron Phosphate Respihaler ... 1642
Decadron Phosphate Turbinaire ... 1645
Decadron Phosphate with Xylocaine Injection, Sterile ... 1639
Decadron-LA Sterile Suspension ... 1646
Depakote Tablets (Greater than 1% but not more than 5%) ... 415
▲ EC-Naprosyn Delayed-Release Tablets (3% to 9%) ... 2117
Effexor (Frequent) ... 2719
Engerix-B Unit-Dose Vials (Less than 1%) ... 2482
Feldene Capsules (Less than 1%) .. 1965
Floxin I.V. ... 1571
Floxin Tablets (200 mg, 300 mg, 400 mg) ... 1567
Hydeltrasol Injection, Sterile ... 1665
Hydeltra-T.B.A. Sterile Suspension 1667
Hydrocortone Acetate Sterile Suspension ... 1669
Hydrocortone Phosphate Injection, Sterile ... 1670
Hydrocortone Tablets ... 1672
Hyzaar Tablets ... 1677
Indocin Capsules (Less than 1%) ... 1680
Indocin I.V. (Less than 1%) ... 1684
Indocin (Less than 1%) ... 1680
Isoptin Oral Tablets (Less than 1%) ... 1346
Isoptin SR Tablets (1% or less) ... 1348
Lamictal Tablets (Infrequent) ... 1112
Lodine Capsules and Tablets (Less than 1%) ... 2743
Lorelco Tablets ... 1517
▲ Lupron Depot 3.75 mg (Among most frequent) ... 2556
Lupron Depot 7.5 mg ... 2559
Lupron Injection (Less than 5%) ... 2555
Luvox Tablets (Infrequent) ... 2544
Methotrexate Sodium Tablets, Injection, for Injection and LPF Injection ... 1275
Miltown Tablets ... 2672
▲ Anaprox/Naprosyn (3% to 9%) ... 2117
▲ Novantrone (7 to 11%) ... 1279
Oncaspar ... 2028
PMB 200 and PMB 400 ... 2783
Paraflex Caplets (Rare) ... 1580
Parafon Forte DSC Caplets (Rare) .. 1581
Paxil Tablets (Infrequent) ... 2505
Pentasa (Less than 1%) ... 1527
Pipracil (Less frequent) ... 1390
▲ Prograf (Greater than 3%) ... 1042
Questran Light ... 769
Questran Powder ... 770
Roferon-A Injection (Rare) ... 2145
Serzone Tablets (Infrequent) ... 771
Solatene Capsules (Rare) ... 2150
Ticlid Tablets ... 2156
Trilisate (Rare) ... 2000
Verelan Capsules (1% or less) ... 1410
Verelan Capsules (Less than 1%) .. 2824
▲ Videx Tablets, Powder for Oral Solution, & Pediatric Powder for Oral Solution (15%) ... 720
Wellbutrin Tablets ... 1204
Zoladex (1% or greater) ... 2858
Zyloprim Tablets (Less than 1%) ... 1226

Ecchymosis, soft eyelid tissue

BOTOX (Botulinum Toxin Type A) Purified Neurotoxin Complex ... 477

Ectrodactylia

Cytoxan (2 cases) ... 694
NEOSAR Lyophilized/Neosar (Two cases) ... 1959

Ectropion

BOTOX (Botulinum Toxin Type A) Purified Neurotoxin Complex (Less than 1%) ... 477
Demulen ... 2428

Eczema

Accutane Capsules (Less than 1 patient in 10) ... 2076
▲ AeroBid Inhaler System (3-9%) ... 1005
▲ Aerobid-M Inhaler System (3-9%) .. 1005
Anafranil Capsules (Infrequent) ... 803
Ansaid Tablets (Less than 1%) ... 2579
Cardura Tablets (Less than 0.5% of 3960 patients) ... 2186
Cataflam (Less than 1%) ... 816
Cerumenex Drops (1% of 2,700 patients) ... 1993
Claritin-D (Less frequent) ... 2350
Clozaril Tablets (Less than 1%) ... 2252
Cognex Capsules (Infrequent) ... 1901
Compazine ... 2470
Dantrium Capsules (Less frequent) 1982
Effexor (Rare) ... 2719
Engerix-B Unit-Dose Vials ... 2482
Etrafon ... 2355
Glucotrol Tablets (About 1 in 70) .. 1967

1285 **Side Effects Index** **Edema**

Kwell Cream & Lotion (Relatively infrequent) 2008
Kwell Shampoo (Infrequent) 2009
Lac-Hydrin 12% Lotion (Less frequent) 2687
Lamictal Tablets (Infrequent) 1112
Lindane Lotion USP 1% (Infrequent; less than 1 in 100,000 patients) 582
Lindane Shampoo USP 1% (Infrequent; less than 1 in 100,000 patients) 583
Lopid Tablets (1.9%) 1917
Luvox Tablets (Infrequent) 2544
Macrobid Capsules 1988
Macrodantin Capsules 1989
Maxaquin Tablets (Less than 1%) .. 2440
Miacalcin Nasal Spray (Less than 1%) 2275
Neurontin Capsules (Infrequent) 1922
Orudis Capsules (Less than 1%) 2766
Oruvail Capsules (Less than 1%) 2766
Oxistat Lotion (0.4%) 1152
Paxil Tablets (Infrequent) 2505
Pentasa (Less than 1%) 1527
Permax Tablets (Infrequent) 575
Prolixin 509
Prozac Pulvules & Liquid, Oral Solution (Rare) 919
Quinidex Extentabs 2067
Rogaine Topical Solution 2637
Serzone Tablets (Infrequent) 771
Stelazine 2514
Triavil Tablets 1757
Trilafon 2389
Varivax (Greater than or equal to 1%) 1762
▲ Videx Tablets, Powder for Oral Solution, & Pediatric Powder for Oral Solution (12% to 13%) 720
Voltaren Tablets (Less than 1%) 861
Zebeta Tablets 1413
Ziac 1415
▲ Zosyn (4.2%) 1419
▲ Zosyn Pharmacy Bulk Package (4.2%) 1422

Eczema, exacerbation of

▲ Zonalon Cream (Approximately 1% to 10%) 1055

Eczematous reactions (see under Eczema)

Edema

Accutane Capsules (Less than 1%) 2076
Children's Advil Suspension (Less than 3%) 2692
▲ AeroBid Inhaler System (3-9%) 1005
▲ Aerobid-M Inhaler System (3-9%) .. 1005
Aldoclor Tablets 1598
Aldomet Ester HCl Injection 1602
Aldomet Oral 1600
Aldoril Tablets 1604
Alkeran for Injection 1070
Altace Capsules (Less than 1%) 1232
Alupent Tablets (0.2%) 669
Ambien Tablets (Infrequent) 2416
Amen Tablets (Occasional) 780
Americaine Anesthetic Lubricant 983
Americaine Otic Topical Anesthetic Ear Drops 983
Anafranil Capsules (Infrequent) 803
▲ Anaprox/Naprosyn (3% to 9%) 2117
▲ Android Capsules, 10 mg (Among most common) 1250
Android 1251
▲ Ansaid Tablets (3-9%) 2579
Antivenin (Crotalidae) Polyvalent 2696
Apresazide Capsules (Less frequent) 808
Apresoline Hydrochloride Tablets (Less frequent) 809
Aredia for Injection (Up to 1%) 810
Aristocort Suspension (Forte Parenteral) 1027
Aristocort Suspension (Intralesional) 1025
Aristocort Tablets 1022
Aristospan Suspension (Intra-articular) 1033
Aristospan Suspension (Intralesional) 1032
Asacol Delayed-Release Tablets 1979
Asendin Tablets (Less frequent) 1369
Atamet 572
Atgam Sterile Solution (Less than 1% to less than 5%) 2581
Atretol Tablets 573
Atropine Sulfate Sterile Ophthalmic Solution .... ⊙ 233
Aygestin Tablets 974
Azo Gantrisin Tablets 2081
BSS (15 mL & 30 mL) Sterile Irrigation Solution .... ⊙ 214
BSS (250 mL) Sterile Irrigation Solution .... ⊙ 214
BSS (500 mL) Sterile Irrigation Solution .... ⊙ 214
▲ Betapace Tablets (2% to 8%) 641
▲ Betaseron for SC Injection (8%) 658
Bicillin C-R Injection 2704
Bicillin C-R 900/300 Injection 2706
Bicillin L-A Injection 2707
Blocadren Tablets (0.6%) 1614
Brevibloc Injection (Less than 1%) 1808
Brevicon 2088
BuSpar (Infrequent) 737
Calan SR Caplets (1.9%) 2422
Calan Tablets (1.9%) 2419
Capoten 739
Capozide 742
Cardene Capsules (0.6-1.0%) 2095
▲ Cardizem CD Capsules (2.6% to 4.6%) 1506
▲ Cardizem SR Capsules (5.4% to 9%) 1510
Cardizem Injectable (Less than 1%) 1508
Cardizem Tablets (2.4%) 1512
▲ Cardura Tablets (About 0.7% to 4%) 2186
Cataflam 816
Catapres-TTS (3 of 101 patients) .. 675
Ceclor Pulvules & Suspension 1431
Celestone Soluspan Suspension 2347
▲ CellCept Capsules (11.8% to 12.2%) 2099
Claritin-D (Less frequent) 2350
Climara Transdermal System 645
Clinoril Tablets (Greater than 1%) 1618
Clozaril Tablets (Less than 1%) 2252
Cognex Capsules (Infrequent) 1901
Condylox (Less than 5%) 1802
Cordarone Tablets (1 to 3%) 2712
CORTENEMA 2535
Cortifoam 2396
Cortone Acetate Sterile Suspension 1623
Cortone Acetate Tablets 1624
Cozaar Tablets (1% or greater) 1628
Cycrin Tablets (Occasional) 975
Cytotec (Infrequent) 2424
Cytovene (1% or less) 2103
Dalalone D.P. Injectable 1011
Dalgan Injection (Less than 1%) 538
Danocrine Capsules 2307
Daypro Caplets (Less than 1%) 2426
Decadron Elixir 1633
Decadron Phosphate Injection 1637
Decadron Phosphate Respihaler 1642
Decadron Phosphate Turbinaire 1645
Decadron Phosphate with Xylocaine Injection, Sterile 1639
Decadron Tablets 1635
Decadron-LA Sterile Suspension 1646
Delatestryl Injection 2860
Deltasone Tablets 2595
Demadex Tablets and Injection (1.1%) 686
Demulen 2428
Depakote Tablets (Greater than 1% but not more than 5%) 415
Depo-Medrol Single-Dose Vial 2600
Depo-Medrol Sterile Aqueous Suspension 2597
Depo-Provera Contraceptive Injection (1% to 5%) 2602
Depo-Provera Sterile Aqueous Suspension 2606
Dermatop Emollient Cream 0.1% (Less than 1%) 1238
Desogen Tablets 1817
Desquam-E Gel 2684
Desquam-X Gel 2684
Desquam-X 10 Bar 2684
Desquam-X Wash 2684
▲ Desyrel and Desyrel Dividose (2.8% to 7.0%) 503
Dexacort Phosphate in Respihaler .. 458
Dexacort Phosphate in Turbinaire .. 459
Diethylstilbestrol Tablets 1437
Dilacor XR Extended-release Capsules (Infrequent) 2018
Diphtheria & Tetanus Toxoids Adsorbed Purogenated (Mild) 1374
Diprivan Injection (Less than 1%) .. 2833
Dolobid Tablets (Less than 1 in 100) 1654
Duragesic Transdermal System (1% or greater) 1288
Duranest Injections 542
Dyclone 0.5% and 1% Topical Solutions, USP 544
▲ DynaCirc Capsules (3.5% to 8.7%) 2256
▲ EC-Naprosyn Delayed-Release Tablets (3% to 9%) 2117
Effexor (Infrequent) 2719
Elavil 2838
▲ Emcyt Capsules (19%) 1953
▲ Emla Cream (6%) 545
Endep Tablets 2174
▲ Epogen for Injection (9% to 17%) 489
Ergamisol Tablets (1%) 1292
Esimil Tablets 822
Estrace Cream and Tablets 749
Estraderm Transdermal System 824
ESTRATAB Tablets (0.3, 0.625, 1.25, 2.5 mg) 2536
Estratest 2539
▲ Eulexin Capsules (4%) 2358
Felbatol 2666
Feldene Capsules (Greater than 1%) 1965
Fioricet with Codeine Capsules 2260
Fiorinal with Codeine Capsules 2262
Flexeril Tablets (Rare) 1661
Florinef Acetate Tablets 505
Floxin I.V. (Less than 1%) 1571
Floxin Tablets (200 mg, 300 mg, 400 mg) (Less than 1%) 1567
▲ Fludara for Injection (8% to 19%) 663
Foscavir Injection (Between 1% and 5%) 547
Gantanol Tablets 2119
Gantrisin 2120
Gastrocrom Capsules (Infrequent) .. 984
Glucotrol XL Extended Release Tablets (Less than 1%) 1968
▲ Habitrol Nicotine Transdermal System (4%) 865
Halotestin Tablets 2614
Hismanal Tablets (Less frequent) 1293
Hivid Tablets (Less than 1% to less than 3%) 2121
Humatrope Vials (2.5%) 1443
Hydeltrasol Injection, Sterile 1665
Hydeltra-T.B.A. Sterile Suspension 1667
Hydrocortone Acetate Sterile Suspension 1669
Hydrocortone Phosphate Injection, Sterile 1670
Hydrocortone Tablets 1672
Hytrin Capsules (0.9%) 430
Hyzaar Tablets (1.3%) 1677
IBU Tablets (Greater than 1%) 1342
Imdur (Less than or equal to 5%) .. 1323
Imitrex Tablets (Rare to infrequent) 1106
Indocin Capsules (Less than 1%) 1680
Indocin I.V. (Less than 1%) 1684
Indocin (Less than 1%) 1680
INSTAT* Collagen Absorbable Hemostat 1312
Iopidine 0.5% (Less than 1%) .... ⊙ 221
Ismelin Tablets 827
Ismo Tablets (Fewer than 1%) 2738
Isoptin Oral Tablets (1.9%) 1346
Isoptin SR Tablets (1.9%) 1348
Kerlone Tablets (1.3% to 1.8%) 2436
Klonopin Tablets 2126
Lamprene Capsules (Less than 1%) 828
Larodopa Tablets (Rare) 2129
▲ Leukine for IV Infusion (34%) 1271
▲ Leustatin (6%) 1834
Levlen/Tri-Levlen 651
Librax Capsules (Rare) 2176
Libritabs Tablets (Isolated cases) 2177
Librium Capsules (Isolated cases) .. 2178
Librium Injectable (Isolated cases) 2179
Lioresal Tablets 829
Lodine Capsules and Tablets (Less than 1%) 2743
▲ Loniten Tablets (7%) 2618
Lo/Ovral Tablets 2746
Lo/Ovral-28 Tablets 2751
Lopressor HCT Tablets (1 in 100 patients) 832
Lotrel Capsules (2.1%; 0.6% to 3.2%) 840
Lotrimin 2371
Lotrisone Cream (1 of 270 patients) 2372
Lovenox Injection (2%) 2020
Ludiomil Tablets (Rare) 843
▲ Lupron Depot 3.75 mg (5.4%) 2556
▲ Lupron Depot 7.5 mg (12.5%) 2559
Luvox Tablets (Frequent) 2544
MS Contin Tablets (Less frequent) 1994
MSIR (Infrequent) 1997
Matulane Capsules 2131
Maxair Autohaler 1492
Maxair Inhaler (Less than 1%) 1494
Maxaquin Tablets (Less than 1%) .. 2440
Medrol 2621
Megace Oral Suspension (1% to 3%) 699
Megace Tablets 701
Mellaril 2269
Menest Tablets 2494
Mesantoin Tablets 2272
Methadone Hydrochloride Oral Concentrate 2233
Methadone Hydrochloride Oral Solution & Tablets 2235
Metubine Iodide Vials 916
▲ Mexitil Capsules (About 2 in 1,000 to 3.8%) 678
Micronor Tablets 1872
Minipress Capsules (1-4%) 1937
Minizide Capsules 1938
Modicon 1872
8-MOP Capsules 1246
Monoket (Fewer than 1%) 2406
Monopril Tablets (0.2% to 1.0% or more) 757
Children's Motrin Ibuprofen Oral Suspension (Greater than 1% but less than 3%) 1546
Motrin Tablets (Less than 3%) 2625
Motrin Ibuprofen Suspension, Oral Drops, Chewable Tablets, Caplets (1% to less than 3%) 1546
Mutamycin 703
Mykrox Tablets (Less than 2%) 993
▲ Anaprox/Naprosyn (3% to 9%) 2117
Nardil (Common) 1920
NebuPent for Inhalation Solution (Greater than 1%, up to 5%) 1040
Neoral (2% or less) 2276
Neurontin Capsules (Infrequent) 1922
▲ Nicoderm (nicotine transdermal system) (3%) 1518
Nicorette 2458
Nimotop Capsules (Up to 1.2%) 610
▲ Nolvadex Tablets (3.8% to 32.4%) 2841
Nordette-21 Tablets 2755
Nordette-28 Tablets 2758
Norinyl 2088
▲ Normodyne Injection (Up to 2%) 2377
Normodyne Tablets (Up to 2%) 2379
Noroxin Tablets (Less frequent) 1715
Noroxin Tablets (Less frequent) 2048
Norpace (1 to 3%) 2444
Norpramin Tablets 1526
Nor-Q D Tablets 2135
▲ Norvasc Tablets (1.8% to 14.6%) 1940
Novocain Hydrochloride for Spinal Anesthesia 2326
Nubain Injection (1% or less) 935
Ogen Tablets 2627
Ogen Vaginal Cream 2630
▲ Oncaspar (Greater than 5%) 2028
Oncovin Solution Vials & Hyporets (Rare) 1466
OptiPranolol (Metipranolol 0.3%) Sterile Ophthalmic Solution (A small number of patients) .... ⊙ 258
Oramorph SR (Morphine Sulfate Sustained Release Tablets) (Less frequent) 2236
Oreton Methyl 1255
Orlamm (1% to 3%) 2239
Ortho-Cept 1851
Ortho-Cyclen/Ortho-Tri-Cyclen 1858
Ortho Dienestrol Cream 1866
Ortho-Est 1869
Ortho-Novum 1872
Ortho-Cyclen/Ortho Tri-Cyclen 1858
▲ Orudis Capsules (3% to 9%) 2766
▲ Oruvail Capsules (3% to 9%) 2766
Ovcon 760
Ovral Tablets 2770
Ovral-28 Tablets 2770
Ovrette Tablets 2771
Oxandrin 2862
Oxsoralen-Ultra Capsules 1257
PMB 200 and PMB 400 2783
Pamelor 2280
Parnate Tablets 2503
Paxil Tablets (Frequent) 2505
Pediapred Oral Liquid 995
Penetrex Tablets (Less than 1% but more than or equal to 0.1%) 2031
Pentasa (Less than 1%) 1527
Pentaspan Injection 937
Permax Tablets (1.6%) 575

(▭ Described in PDR For Nonprescription Drugs) Incidence data in parenthesis; ▲ 3% or more (⊙ Described in PDR For Ophthalmology)

Pfizerpen for Injection 2203
Pontocaine Hydrochloride for Spinal Anesthesia 2330
Pregnyl 1828
Prelone Syrup 1787
Premarin Intravenous 2787
Premarin with Methyltestosterone 2794
Premarin Tablets 2789
Premarin Vaginal Cream 2791
Premphase 2797
Prempro 2801
PREVACID Delayed-Release Capsules (Less than 1%) 2562
Prinivil Tablets (1.0% to 2.4%) 1733
Prinzide Tablets 1737
Priscoline Hydrochloride Ampuls 845
▲ Procardia XL Extended Release Tablets (10% to about 30%) 1972
▲ Procrit for Injection (17%) 1841
Profasi (chorionic gonadotropin for injection, USP) 2450
Proglycem (Frequent) 580
▲ Proleukin for Injection (47%) 797
Propulsid (1% or less) 1300
ProSom Tablets (Rare) 449
Prostin VR Pediatric Sterile Solution (About 1%) 2635
Provera Tablets (An occasional patient) 2636
Prozac Pulvules & Liquid, Oral Solution (Infrequent) 919
Quadrinal Tablets 1350
Questran Light 769
Questran Powder 770
RMS Suppositories 2657
Recombivax HB (Less than 1%) 1744
Reglan 2068
▲ Relafen Tablets (3% to 9%) 2510
Retrovir Capsules (0.8%) 1158
Retrovir I.V. Infusion (1%) 1163
Retrovir Syrup (0.8%) 1158
ReVia Tablets (Less than 1%) 940
Risperdal (Infrequent) 1301
▲ Roferon-A Injection (9%) 2145
Rogaine Topical Solution (1.24 to 1.53%) 2637
Rowasa (1.2%) 2548
Roxanol 2243
Rythmol Tablets–150mg, 225mg, 300mg (0.6 to 1.4%) 1352
▲ Salagen Tablets (5%) 1489
Sandimmune (2% or less) 2286
Sandostatin Injection (1% to 4%) 2292
Sanorex Tablets 2294
Sansert Tablets 2295
Sectral Capsules (2%) 2807
Ser-Ap-Es Tablets 849
Serax Capsules 2810
Serax Tablets 2810
Serentil 684
Serzone Tablets 771
Sinemet Tablets 943
Sinemet CR Tablets 944
Sinequan (Occasional) 2205
Solu-Cortef Sterile Powder 2641
Solu-Medrol Sterile Powder 2643
Soma Compound w/Codeine Tablets 2676
Soma Compound Tablets 2675
Sporanox Capsules (0.4% to 3.5%) 1305
Stadol (Less than 1%) 775
Stilphostrol Tablets and Ampuls 612
Stimate, (desmopressin acetate) Nasal Spray, 1.5 mg/mL 525
Supprelin Injection (2% to 3%) 2056
▲ Synarel Nasal Solution for Endometriosis (8% of patients) 2152
▲ Tambocor Tablets (3.5%) 1497
Tapazole Tablets 1477
▲ Taxol (21%) 714
▲ Tegison Capsules (1 to 10%) 2154
Tegretol Chewable Tablets 852
Tegretol Suspension 852
Tegretol Tablets 852
Tenex Tablets (Less frequent) 2074
Testoderm Testosterone Transdermal System 486
Tetanus Toxoid Adsorbed Purogenated 1403
Timolide Tablets 1748
Timoptic in Ocudose 1753
Timoptic Sterile Ophthalmic Solution 1751
Timoptic-XE 1755
Tofranil Ampuls 854
Tofranil Tablets 856
Tofranil-PM Capsules 857
▲ Tolectin (200, 400 and 600 mg) (3 to 9%) 1581
Tonocard Tablets (Less than 1%) 531
▲ Toradol (4%) 2159
Trancopal Caplets 2337
Trandate Tablets (Up to 2%) 1185
Trental Tablets (Less than 1%) 1244
Triavil Tablets 1757
Levlen/Tri-Levlen 651
Trilisate (Less than 1%) 2000
Tri-Norinyl 2164
▲ Tripedia (1% to 21%) 892
Triphasil-21 Tablets 2814
Triphasil-28 Tablets 2819
Tympagesic Ear Drops 2342
Unasyn (Less than 1%) 2212
Vascor (200, 300 and 400 mg) Tablets (0.5 to 2.0%) 1587
Verelan Capsules (1.9%) 1410
Verelan Capsules (1.9%) 2824
Videx Tablets, Powder for Oral Solution, & Pediatric Powder for Oral Solution (Up to 2%) 720
▲ Visken Tablets (6%) 2299
Vivactil Tablets 1774
Voltaren Tablets 861
Wellbutrin Tablets (Frequent) 1204
Winstrol Tablets 2337
▲ Xanax Tablets (4.9%) 2649
Xylocaine Injections (Extremely rare) 567
Zebeta Tablets 1413
Zestoretic 2850
Zestril Tablets (1.0% to 2.4%) 2854
Ziac 1415
▲ Zoladex (1% to 7%) 2858
Zoloft Tablets (Infrequent) 2217
▲ Zonalon Cream (Approximately 1% to 10%) 1055
Zosyn (0.1% to 1.2%) 1419
Zosyn Pharmacy Bulk Package (0.1% to 1.2%) 1422
Zovirax Capsules (0.3%) 1219
Zovirax Sterile Powder (Less than 1%) 1223
Zovirax (0.3%) 1219

Edema, allergic

Cytosar-U Sterile Powder (Less frequent) 2592
Periactin 1724

Edema, angioneurotic

Accupril Tablets 1893
Achromycin V Capsules 1367
Airet Solution for Inhalation (Rare) 452
Altace Capsules (0.3%) 1232
Anaprox/Naprosyn (Less than 1%) 2117
Ansaid Tablets (Less than 1%) 2579
Augmentin 2468
Azactam for Injection (Less than 1%) 734
Azo Gantrisin Tablets 2081
Brontex (Infrequent) 1981
Carafate Suspension 1505
Carafate Tablets 1504
Carbocaine Hydrochloride Injection 2303
Catapres Tablets (About 5 in 1,000 patients) 674
Catapres-TTS (Less frequent) 675
Ceclor Pulvules & Suspension 1431
Ceftin Tablets 1078
Ceptaz (Very rare) 1081
Ceredase 1065
Chibroxin Sterile Ophthalmic Solution (With oral form) 1617
Chloroptic S.O.P. ⊙ 239
Chloroptic Sterile Ophthalmic Solution ⊙ 239
Cipro I.V. Pharmacy Bulk Package (Less than 1%) 597
Claritin (2% or fewer patients) 2349
Claritin-D 2350
Clinoril Tablets (Less than 1 in 100) 1618
Combipres Tablets (About 5 in 1,000) 677
Compazine 2470
Cortone Acetate Sterile Suspension 1623
Cortone Acetate Tablets 1624
CytoGam (A possibility) 1593
Dalalone D.P. Injectable 1011
Decadron Elixir 1633
Decadron Phosphate Injection 1637
Decadron Phosphate Respihaler 1642
Decadron Phosphate Turbinaire 1645
Decadron Phosphate with Xylocaine Injection, Sterile 1639
Decadron Tablets 1635
Decadron-LA Sterile Suspension 1646
Declomycin Tablets 1371
Demadex Tablets and Injection (One patient) 686
Dexacort Phosphate in Respihaler 458
Dexacort Phosphate in Turbinaire 459
DiaBeta Tablets 1239
Diflucan Injection, Tablets, and Oral Suspension (Rare) 2194
Dolobid Tablets (Less than 1 in 100) 1654
Doryx Capsules 1913
Duricef 748
Dynacin Capsules 1590
EC-Naprosyn Delayed-Release Tablets (Less than 1%) 2117
Elase-Chloromycetin Ointment 1040
Eminase 2039
Emla Cream 545
Empirin with Codeine Tablets 1093
Engerix-B Unit-Dose Vials 2482
Etrafon 2355
Flexeril Tablets 1661
Floxin I.V. (Less than 1%) 1571
Floxin Tablets (200 mg, 300 mg, 400 mg) (Less than 1%) 1567
Fluvirin (Rare) 460
Fulvicin P/G Tablets (Rare) 2359
Fulvicin P/G 165 & 330 Tablets (Rare) 2359
Gastrocrom Capsules (Infrequent) 984
Glynase PresTab Tablets 2609
Grifulvin V (griseofulvin tablets) Microsize (griseofulvin oral suspension) Microsize (Rare) 1888
Gris-PEG Tablets, 125 mg & 250 mg (Rare) 479
Havrix (Rare) 2489
Hespan Injection 929
Hismanal Tablets (Less frequent) 1293
Hydeltrasol Injection, Sterile 1665
Hydeltra-T.B.A. Sterile Suspension 1667
Hydrocortone Acetate Sterile Suspension 1669
Hydrocortone Phosphate Injection, Sterile 1670
Hydrocortone Tablets 1672
Hyperab Rabies Immune Globulin (Human) (Rare) 624
HyperHep Hepatitis B Immune Globulin (Human) 626
Hyper-Tet Tetanus Immune Globulin (Human) (Few isolated cases) 627
IBU Tablets (Less than 1%) 1342
Imitrex Tablets 1106
Imogam Rabies Immune Globulin (Human) 880
▲ Imovax Rabies Vaccine (Up to 6%) 881
Influenza Virus Vaccine, Trivalent, Types A and B (chromatograph- and filter-purified subviron antigen) FluShield, 1995-1996 Formula (Rare) 2736
Intal Nebulizer Solution 989
Intron A (Rare) 2364
JE-VAX 886
Lamictal Tablets (Rare) 1112
Lescol Capsules (Rare) 2267
Levoprome 1274
Lincocin 2617
Lithonate/Lithotabs/Lithobid 2543
Lodine Capsules and Tablets (Less than 1%) 2743
Lomotil 2439
Lopid Tablets 1917
Lorelco Tablets 1517
Lotensin Tablets 834
Lotensin HCT 837
Lutrepulse for Injection 980
Marcaine Hydrochloride with Epinephrine 1:200,000 (Rare) 2316
Marcaine Hydrochloride Injection (Rare) 2316
Marcaine Spinal (Rare) 2319
Mefoxin 1691
Mefoxin Premixed Intravenous Solution 1694
Mellaril 2269
Mevacor Tablets (Rare) 1699
Micronase Tablets 2623
Miltown Tablets (Rare) 2672
Minocin Intravenous 1382
Minocin Oral Suspension 1385
Minocin Pellet-Filled Capsules 1383
Monodox Capsules 1805
Monopril Tablets (0.2% to 1.0%) 757
Motofen Tablets 784
Motrin Ibuprofen Suspension, Oral Drops, Chewable Tablets, Caplets (Less than 1%) 1546
Mykrox Tablets 993
Myochrysine Injection 1711
Nalfon 200 Pulvules & Nalfon Tablets (Less than 1%) 917
Anaprox/Naprosyn (Less than 1%) 2117
Nescaine/Nescaine MPF 554
Normodyne Injection (Rare) 2377
Normodyne Tablets (Rare) 2379
Noroxin Tablets 1715
Noroxin Tablets 2048
Orthoclone OKT3 Sterile Solution 1837
PMB 200 and PMB 400 (Rare) 2783
Paraflex Caplets (Extremely rare) 1580
Parafon Forte DSC Caplets (Extremely rare) 1581
Paxil Tablets (Rare) 2505
Pepcid Injection (Infrequent) 1722
Pepcid (Infrequent) 1720
Pergonal (menotropins for injection, USP) 2448
Phenergan with Codeine (Infrequent) 2777
Phenergan Injection 2773
Phenergan Tablets 2775
Phenergan VC with Codeine 2781
Pravachol (Rare) 765
Prilosec Delayed-Release Capsules (Less than 1%) 529
Primaxin I.M. 1727
Primaxin I.V. (Less than 0.2%) 1729
Prinzide Tablets (Rare) 1737
Procan SR Tablets (Occasional) 1926
Profasi (chorionic gonadotropin for injection, USP) 2450
Prolixin 509
Proventil Inhalation Solution 0.083% (Rare) 2384
Proventil Solution for Inhalation 0.5% (Rare) 2383
Proventil Syrup (Rare) 2385
Quadrinal Tablets 1350
▲ Rabies Vaccine, Imovax Rabies I.D. (Less frequent; up to 6%) 883
Relafen Tablets (1%) 2510
Risperdal 1301
Robaxisal Tablets 2071
Salflex Tablets 786
Seldane Tablets 1536
Seldane-D Extended-Release Tablets 1538
Semprex-D Capsules (Rare) 463
Semprex-D Capsules (Rare) 1167
Sensorcaine (Rare) 559
Serentil 684
Serevent Inhalation Aerosol (Rare) 1176
Solganal Suspension 2388
Soma Compound w/Codeine Tablets 2676
Soma Compound Tablets 2675
Soma Tablets 2674
Sporanox Capsules 1305
Stelazine 2514
Streptase for Infusion (Rare) 562
Supprelin Injection 2056
Talwin Compound 2335
Taxol (2%) 714
Tazicef for Injection (Very rare) 2519
Temaril Tablets, Syrup and Spansule Extended-Release Capsules 483
Terramycin Intramuscular Solution 2210
Thorazine 2523
Torecan 2245
Trandate (Rare) 1185
Triavil Tablets 1757
Trilafon 2389
Univasc Tablets (Less than 0.5%) 2410
Velosulin BR Human Insulin 10 ml Vials 1795
Ventolin Inhalation Solution (Rare) 1198
Ventolin Nebules Inhalation Solution (Rare) 1199
Ventolin Rotacaps for Inhalation (Rare) 1200
Ventolin Syrup (Rare) 1202
Ventolin Tablets (Rare) 1203
Vermox Chewable Tablets (Rare) 1312
Vibramycin 1941
Vibramycin Hyclate Intravenous 2215
Vibramycin 1941
Videx Tablets, Powder for Oral Solution, & Pediatric Powder for Oral Solution (Less than 1%) 720
Volmax Extended-Release Tablets (Rare) 1788
Wellbutrin Tablets 1204
Zantac (Rare) 1209
Zantac Injection (Rare) 1207
Zantac Syrup (Rare) 1209
Zaroxolyn Tablets 1000
Zebeta Tablets 1413
Zestoretic 2850

(▣ Described in PDR For Nonprescription Drugs) Incidence data in parenthesis; ▲ 3% or more (⊙ Described in PDR For Ophthalmology)

1287 Side Effects Index Edema, palpebral

Ziac 1415
Zocor Tablets (Rare) 1775
Zofran Injection (Rare) 1214
Zyloprim Tablets (Less than 1%) 1226

Edema, ankle

Android-25 Tablets 1251
Verelan Capsules (1.4%) 1410
Verelan Capsules (1.4%) 2824

Edema, aphakic cystoid macular

Timoptic in Ocudose (Less frequent) 1753
Timoptic Sterile Ophthalmic Solution (Less frequent) 1751
Timoptic-XE 1755

Edema, arm

Torecan 2245

Edema, cerebral

Betaseron for SC Injection 658
Compazine 2470
Etrafon (Extremely rare) 2355
Felbatol 2666
Foscavir Injection (Less than 1%) 547
Levoprome 1274
Navane Capsules and Concentrate 2201
Navane Intramuscular 2202
Orthoclone OKT3 Sterile Solution 1837
Permax Tablets (Rare) 575
Proleukin for Injection (Less than 1%) 797
Prolixin 509
Stelazine 2514
Thorazine 2523
Triavil Tablets 1757
Trilafon (Extremely rare) 2389

Edema, conjunctival

Cortisporin Ophthalmic Ointment Sterile 1085
Effexor (Rare) 2719
Vexol 1% Ophthalmic Suspension (Less than 1%) ⊙ 230

Edema, corneal

AMVISC Plus ⊙ 329
BSS (15 mL & 30 mL) Sterile Irrigation Solution ⊙ 214
BSS (250 mL) Sterile Irrigation Solution ⊙ 214
BSS (500 mL) Sterile Irrigation Solution ⊙ 214
BSS PLUS (500 mL) Sterile Irrigation Solution ⊙ 215
Healon (Rare) ⊙ 314
Healon GV ⊙ 315
Miochol-E with Iocare Steri-Tags and Miochol-E System Pak (Infrequent) ⊙ 273
Ocucoat ⊙ 321
Plaquenil Sulfate Tablets 2328
▲ Rēv-Eyes Ophthalmic Eyedrops 0.5% (10% to 40%) ⊙ 323
Symmetrel Capsules and Syrup (0.1% to 1%) 946
Vexol 1% Ophthalmic Suspension (Less than 1%) ⊙ 230
Viroptic Ophthalmic Solution, 1% Sterile 1204

Edema, cystoid macular

AdatoSil 5000 (Less than 2%) ⊙ 274
Nicolar Tablets 2026

Edema, dependent

Anafranil Capsules (Rare) 803
Zoloft Tablets (Infrequent) 2217

Edema, digitus

Alupent Tablets (0.2%) 669

Edema, extremities

Ceclor Pulvules & Suspension 1431
Cipro I.V. (1% or less) 595
Cipro Tablets (Less than 1%) 592
Depakene 413
Depakote Tablets 415
Rifadin 1528
Rifater 1532
Teslac 717

Edema, facial

Adalat CC (Less than 1.0%) 589
Ambien Tablets (Rare) 2416
Antivenin (Crotalidae) Polyvalent 2696
Asacol Delayed-Release Tablets 1979
Azmacort Oral Inhaler (Infrequent) 2011
BuSpar (Infrequent) 737
Cardura Tablets (1%) 2186
Ceclor Pulvules & Suspension 1431
▲ CellCept Capsules (More than or equal to 3%) 2099
Cipro I.V. (1% or less) 595
Cipro I.V. Pharmacy Bulk Package (Less than 1%) 597
Cipro Tablets (Less than 1%) 592
Cognex Capsules (Infrequent) 1901
Cozaar Tablets (Less than 1%) 1628
Cytovene (1% or less) 2103
Dépakene 413
Depakote Tablets 415
Effexor (Infrequent) 2719
Elavil 2838
Endep Tablets 2174
Etrafon 2355
▲ Felbatol (3.4%) 2666
Flexeril Tablets (Less than 1%) 1661
Floxin I.V. 1571
Floxin Tablets (200 mg, 300 mg, 400 mg) 1567
Foscavir Injection (Between 1% and 5%) 547
Hytrin Capsules (At least 1%) 430
Imitrex Injection (Rare) 1103
Imitrex Tablets 1106
▲ Intron A (Up to 10%) 2364
Iopidine 0.5% (Less than 1%) ⊙ 221
Klonopin Tablets 2126
Lamictal Tablets (Infrequent) 1112
Limbitrol 2180
Lioresal Intrathecal 1596
Loxitane 1378
Maxaquin Tablets (Less than 1%) 2440
Neupogen for Injection 495
Neurontin Capsules (Frequent) 1922
Noroxin Tablets 1715
Noroxin Tablets 2048
Norpramin Tablets 1526
Oncaspar (Less than 1%) 2028
Orudis Capsules (Less than 1%) 2766
Oruvail Capsules (Less than 1%) 2766
Pamelor 2280
Paxil Tablets (Infrequent) 2505
Pepcid Injection (Infrequent) 1722
Pepcid (Infrequent) 1720
Pergonal (menotropins for injection, USP) 2448
Permax Tablets (1.1%) 575
Platinol (Occasional) 708
Platinol-AQ Injection (Occasional) 710
Plendil Extended-Release Tablets (0.5% to 1.5%) 527
Ponstel 1925
Primaxin I.V. (Less than 0.2%) 1729
Prinivil Tablets (0.3% to 1.0%) 1733
Prinzide Tablets 1737
Procardia XL Extended Release Tablets (1% or less) 1972
Prozac Pulvules & Liquid, Oral Solution (Infrequent) 919
Rhinocort Nasal Inhaler (Less than 1%) 556
Rifadin 1528
Rifater 1532
Rogaine Topical Solution (1.27%) 2637
Serzone Tablets (Infrequent) 771
Sulfamylon Cream 925
Surmontil Capsules 2811
Talacen (Rare) 2333
Talwin Injection (Rare) 2334
Talwin Compound (Rare) 2335
Talwin Injection (Rare) 2334
Talwin Nx 2336
Tofranil Ampuls 854
Tofranil Tablets 856
Tofranil-PM Capsules 857
Torecan 2245
Triavil Tablets 1757
VePesid Capsules and Injection (Sometimes) 718
Videx Tablets, Powder for Oral Solution, & Pediatric Powder for Oral Solution (Less than 1%) 720
Zestoretic 2850
Zestril Tablets (0.3% to 1.0%) 2854
Zoloft Tablets (Infrequent) 2217
Zyloprim Tablets (Less than 1%) 1226

Edema, fibrinous

▲ Blenoxane (10%) 692

Edema, heart failure (see under Congestive heart failure)

Edema, laryngeal

Activase (Very rare) 1058
Antivenin (Crotalidae) Polyvalent 2696
Axid Pulvules (Rare) 1427
Bicillin C-R Injection 2704
Bicillin C-R 900/300 Injection 2706
Bicillin L-A Injection 2707
Brontex (Infrequent) 1981
Capozide 742
Carbocaine Hydrochloride Injection 2303
Cataflam (Less than 1%) 816
Cipro I.V. (1% or less) 595
Cipro Tablets (Less than 1%) 592
Compazine 2470
Etrafon 2355
Floxin I.V. 1571
Garamycin Injectable 2360
Hespan Injection 929
Intal Capsules (Less than 1 in 10,000 patients) 987
Intal Inhaler (Rare) 988
Intal Nebulizer Solution (Rare) 989
Levoprome 1274
Lopid Tablets 1917
Lotrel Capsules (About 0.5%) 840
Marcaine Hydrochloride with Epinephrine 1:200,000 (Rare) 2316
Marcaine Hydrochloride Injection (Rare) 2316
Marcaine Spinal (Rare) 2319
Maxaquin Tablets 2440
Mellaril 2269
Nardil 1920
Nescaine/Nescaine MPF 554
Nubain Injection (1% or less) 935
Orthoclone OKT3 Sterile Solution 1837
Orudis Capsules (Less than 1%) 2766
Oruvail Capsules (Less than 1%) 2766
Pen•Vee K 2772
Penetrex Tablets 2031
Pergonal (menotropins for injection, USP) 2448
Permax Tablets (Rare) 575
Phenergan with Codeine (Infrequent) 2777
Phenergan VC with Codeine 2781
Prinivil Tablets (0.3% to 1.0%) 1733
Prinzide Tablets (Rare) 1737
Prolixin 509
Prozac Pulvules & Liquid, Oral Solution (Rare) 919
Reglan (Rare) 2068
Sensorcaine 559
Serentil 684
Stelazine 2514
Temaril Tablets, Syrup and Spansule Extended-Release Capsules 483
Thioplex (Thiotepa For Injection) 1281
Thorazine 2523
Toradol 2159
Torecan 2245
Triavil Tablets 1757
Trilafon 2389
Vaseretic Tablets 1765
Vasotec I.V. 1768
Vasotec Tablets 1771
Voltaren Tablets (Less than 1%) 861
Zestoretic 2850
Zestril Tablets 2854

Edema, lesional

Oncaspar (Less than 1%) 2028

Edema, lips

Cipro I.V. (1% or less) 595
Cipro I.V. Pharmacy Bulk Package (Less than 1%) 597
Cipro Tablets (Less than 1%) 592
Ethmozine Tablets (Less than 2%) 2041
Imitrex Injection (Rare) 1103
Imitrex Tablets 1106
▲ Oncaspar (Greater than 1% but less than 5%) 2028
Orthoclone OKT3 Sterile Solution 1837
Retrovir Capsules 1158
Retrovir I.V. Infusion 1163
Retrovir Syrup 1158

Edema, local

Anafranil Capsules (Up to 2%) 803
Cafergot 2251
Celestone Soluspan Suspension 2347
D.H.E. 45 Injection 2255
Ergomar 1486
Furacin Soluble Dressing (Approximately 1%) 2045
Furacin Topical Cream (Approximately 1%) 2045
Havrix (Rare) 2489
Nicotrol Nicotine Transdermal System (B 3%) 1550
Oncaspar 2028
▲ Prostep (nicotine transdermal system) (8%) 1394
Retin-A (tretinoin) Cream/Gel/Liquid 1889
Rogaine Topical Solution 2637
Wigraine Tablets & Suppositories 1829
Zovirax Ointment 5% 1223

Edema, lower extremities

▲ Cardene Capsules (7.1-8.0%) 2095
▲ Cardene SR Capsules (5.9%) 2097
Cipro I.V. Pharmacy Bulk Package (Less than 1%) 597
Eldepryl Tablets 2550
Eminase 2039
Foscavir Injection (Less than 1%) 547
Ganite 2533
Miacalcin Injection 2273
Monopril Tablets (0.4% to 1.0%) 757
Parlodel 2281
Sansert Tablets 2295

Edema, macular

Clomid 1514
Retrovir Capsules (A single case) 1158
Retrovir I.V. Infusion (A single case) 1163
Retrovir Syrup (A single case) 1158

Edema, non-specific (see under Edema)

Edema, oropharyngeal

Airet Solution for Inhalation (Rare) 452
Anafranil Capsules (Rare) 803
Cataflam (Less than 1%) 816
Cipro I.V. (1% or less) 595
Cipro Tablets (Less than 1%) 592
Proventil Inhalation Aerosol (Rare) 2382
Proventil Inhalation Solution 0.083% (Rare) 2384
Proventil Solution for Inhalation 0.5% (Rare) 2383
Proventil Syrup (Rare) 2385
Ventolin Inhalation Aerosol and Refill (Rare) 1197
Ventolin Inhalation Solution (Rare) 1198
Ventolin Nebules Inhalation Solution (Rare) 1199
Ventolin Rotacaps for Inhalation (Rare) 1200
Ventolin Syrup (Rare) 1202
Ventolin Tablets (Rare) 1203
Volmax Extended-Release Tablets (Rare) 1788
Voltaren Tablets (Less than 1%) 861

Edema, palpebral

▲ AKTOB (Among most frequent; less than 3 of 100 patients) ⊙ 206
Alomide (Less than 1%) 469
Altace Capsules 1232
Aralen Phosphate Tablets 2301
Betoptic Ophthalmic Solution (Rare) 469
Betoptic S Ophthalmic Suspension 471
Cipro I.V. (1% or less) 595
Cipro I.V. Pharmacy Bulk Package (Less than 1%) 597
Cipro Tablets (Less than 1%) 592
Cortisporin Ophthalmic Ointment Sterile 1085
Crolom (Infrequent) ⊙ 257
DDAVP (Up to 2%) 2017
Desmopressin Acetate Rhinal Tube (Up to 2%) 979
Feldene Capsules (Less than 1%) 1965
Herplex Liquifilm ⊙ 244
Imitrex Injection (Rare) 1103
Imitrex Tablets 1106
Iopidine 0.5% (Less than 3%) ⊙ 221
Livostin (Approximately 1% to 3%) ⊙ 266
Monopril Tablets 757
▲ Ocupress Ophthalmic Solution, 1% Sterile (About 1 of 4 patients) ⊙ 309
Orthoclone OKT3 Sterile Solution 1837
▲ Polysporin Ophthalmic Ointment Sterile (Among those occurring most often) 1154
Prinzide Tablets 1737
ProSom Tablets (Infrequent) 449
Quadrinal Tablets 1350
ReVia Tablets (Less than 1%) 940
Vaseretic Tablets 1765
Vasotec Tablets 1771
Viroptic Ophthalmic Solution, 1% Sterile (2.8%) 1204

(▣ Described in PDR For Nonprescription Drugs) Incidence data in parenthesis; ▲ 3% or more (⊙ Described in PDR For Ophthalmology)

Edema, periorbital (see under Edema, peripheral)

Edema, peripheral

▲ Adalat Capsules (10 mg and 20 mg) (7% to about 10%) 587
▲ Adalat CC (18% to 29%) 589
AeroBid Inhaler System (1-3%) 1005
Aerobid-M Inhaler System (1-3%) 1005
Ambien Tablets (Rare) 2416
Anaprox/Naprosyn (Some patients) 2117
▲ Asacol Delayed-Release Tablets (3%) 1979
Atgam Sterile Solution (Less than 5%) 2581
Azo Gantanol Tablets 2080
Azo Gantrisin Tablets 2081
Azulfidine (Rare) 1949
Betimol 0.25%, 0.5% (1% to 5%) .... ⊙ 261
Cardene I.V. (Rare) 2709
Cartrol Tablets (1.7%) 410
▲ CellCept Capsules (27.0% to 28.6%) 2099
Celontin Kapseals 1899
Ceredase 1065
Claritin (Rare) 2349
Claritin-D (Less frequent) 2350
Clozaril Tablets 2252
Cognex Capsules (Frequent) 1901
Compazine 2470
Demser Capsules (Rare) 1649
Depakote Tablets (Greater than 1% but not more than 5%) 415
Dilacor XR Extended-release Capsules (2.2% to 2.3%) 2018
Dipentum Capsules (Rare) 1951
EC-Naprosyn Delayed-Release Tablets (Some patients) 2117
Effexor (Frequent) 2719
Eldepryl Tablets 2550
Ergamisol Tablets (Less frequent) 1292
Ethmozine Tablets (Less than 2%) 2041
Etrafon 2355
Fansidar Tablets 2114
Feldene Capsules (Approximately 2%) 1965
Foscavir Injection (Less than 1%) 547
Gantanol Tablets 2119
Hespan Injection 929
▲ Hylorel Tablets (28.6%) 985
Hyskon Hysteroscopy Fluid (Rare) 1595
▲ Hytrin Capsules (0.9% to 5.5%) 430
Imitrex Tablets 1106
Infumorph 200 and Infumorph 500 Sterile Solutions (Several reports) 965
Intron A (Less than 5%) 2364
Iopidine 0.5% (Less than 1%) .... ⊙ 221
Lamictal Tablets (Rare) 1112
▲ Leukine for IV Infusion (11%) 1271
Levoprome 1274
Lopressor (1%) 830
Lotensin Tablets 834
▲ Lovenox Injection (3%) 2020
Lozol Tablets (Less than 5%) 2022
Lupron Depot-PED 7.5 mg, 11.25 mg and 15 mg (Less than 2%) 2560
▲ Lupron Injection (5% or more) 2555
Megace Oral Suspension (1% to 3%) 699
Mellaril 2269
Miacalcin Nasal Spray (Less than 1%) 2275
Miltown Tablets 2672
▲ Nalfon 200 Pulvules & Nalfon Tablets (5%) 917
Anaprox/Naprosyn (Some patients) 2117
Navane Capsules and Concentrate 2201
Navane Intramuscular 2202
Neurontin Capsules (1.7%) 1922
Nolvadex Tablets (Infrequent) 2841
Nutropin (Infrequent) 1061
▲ Oncaspar (Greater than 1% but less than 5%) 2028
Orap Tablets 1050
Orudis Capsules (Approximately 2%) 2766
Oruvail Capsules (Approximately 2%) 2766
PMB 200 and PMB 400 2783
Paxil Tablets (Infrequent) 2505
Pepcid Injection (Infrequent) 1722
Pepcid (Infrequent) 1720
▲ Permax Tablets (7.4%) 575
▲ Plendil Extended-Release Tablets (2.0% to 17.4%) 527
Prilosec Delayed-Release Capsules (Less than 1%) 529
Prinivil Tablets (0.3% to 1.0%) 1733
Prinzide Tablets 1737
▲ Procardia Capsules (7% to approximately 10%; about 1 in 8 to about 1 in 25 patients) 1971
▲ Procardia XL Extended Release Tablets (1% or less to about 30%; 1 in 8 patients) 1972
▲ Prograf (10% to 26%) 1042
Prolixin 509
Protropin (Infrequent) 1063
Prozac Pulvules & Liquid, Oral Solution (Infrequent) 919
ReoPro Vials (1.6%) 1471
Rowasa (0.61%) 2548
Sansert Tablets 2295
▲ Serzone Tablets (3%) 771
Stelazine 2514
Symmetrel Capsules and Syrup (1% to 5%) 946
Temaril Tablets, Syrup and Spansule Extended-Release Capsules 483
Thorazine 2523
Tolectin (200, 400 and 600 mg) (Some patients) 1581
Toprol-XL Tablets (About 1 of 100 patients) 565
Torecan 2245
▲ Trasylol (3%) 613
Triavil Tablets 1757
Trilafon 2389
Univasc Tablets (More than 1%) 2410
Videx Tablets, Powder for Oral Solution, & Pediatric Powder for Oral Solution (Less than 1%) 720
▲ Zebeta Tablets (3.0% to 3.7%) 1413
Zefazone 2654
Zestoretic 2850
Zestril Tablets (0.3% to 1.0%) 2854
Ziac (0.9% to 1.1%) 1415
▲ Zoladex (21%) 2858
Zoloft Tablets (Infrequent) 2217
Zovirax 1219

Edema, pharyngeal

Maxaquin Tablets 2440
Noroxin Tablets 1715
Noroxin Tablets 2048

Edema, pulmonary

Activase 1058
Adalat Capsules (10 mg and 20 mg) (About 2%) 587
Aldoclor Tablets 1598
Aldoril Tablets 1604
Ambien Tablets (Rare) 2416
Apresazide Capsules 808
Atgam Sterile Solution (Less than 1% to less than 5%) 2581
Betapace Tablets (Rare) 641
Betaseron for SC Injection 658
Blocadren Tablets 1614
Brevibloc Injection (Less than 1%) 1808
Calan SR Caplets (1.8%) 2422
Calan Tablets (1.8%) 2419
▲ CellCept Capsules (More than or equal to 3%) 2099
Cipro I.V. (1% or less) 595
Cipro I.V. Pharmacy Bulk Package (Less than 1%) 597
Cipro Tablets (Less than 1%) 592
Clomid 1514
Cognex Capsules (Rare) 1901
Cordarone Intravenous (Less than 2%) 2715
Cytosar-U Sterile Powder 2592
Dantrium Intravenous (Rare) 1983
Diprivan Injection (Rare) 2833
Diupres Tablets 1650
Diuril Oral Suspension 1653
Diuril Sodium Intravenous 1652
Diuril Tablets 1653
Dyazide 2479
▲ Eminase (Less than 10%) 2039
Enduron Tablets 420
Esidrix Tablets 821
Esimil Tablets 822
Floxin I.V. 1571
Floxin Tablets (200 mg, 300 mg, 400 mg) 1567
Fungizone Intravenous 506
HydroDIURIL Tablets 1674
Hydropres Tablets 1675
Hyskon Hysteroscopy Fluid (Rare; 0.11% to 1.4%) 1595
Hyzaar Tablets 1677
Indocin Capsules (Less than 1%) 1680
Indocin I.V. (Less than 1%) 1684
Indocin (Less than 1%) 1680
Inversine Tablets 1686
Isoptin Oral Tablets (1.8%) 1346
Isoptin SR Tablets (1.8%) 1348
Isuprel Hydrochloride Injection 1:5000 2311
Lopressor HCT Tablets 832
Lotensin HCT 837
Maxaquin Tablets 2440
Moduretic Tablets 1705
Mutamycin 703
Nalfon 200 Pulvules & Nalfon Tablets (Less than 1%) 917
Narcan Injection (Several instances) 934
Neurontin Capsules (Rare) 1922
Nubain Injection (1% or less) 935
Oretic Tablets 443
Orthoclone OKT3 Sterile Solution (Less than 2%) 1837
Penetrex Tablets 2031
Permax Tablets (Infrequent) 575
Pilocar (Extremely rare) .... ⊙ 268
Placidyl Capsules 448
Prinivil Tablets (0.2% to 0.3%) 1733
Prinzide Tablets 1737
Procardia Capsules (About 2%) 1971
Procardia XL Extended Release Tablets (About 2%) 1972
▲ Prograf (Greater than 3%) 1042
▲ Proleukin for Injection (Less than 1% to 10%) 797
Protamine Sulfate Ampoules & Vials 1471
Prozac Pulvules & Liquid, Oral Solution (Rare) 919
ReoPro Vials (1.5%) 1471
Roferon-A Injection (Rare) 2145
Ser-Ap-Es Tablets 849
Timolide Tablets 1748
Timoptic in Ocudose (Less frequent) 1753
Timoptic Sterile Ophthalmic Solution (Less frequent) 1751
Timoptic-XE 1755
Tonocard Tablets (Less than 1%) 531
Toradol (1% or less) 2159
Trasylol (1.2%) 613
Vaseretic Tablets 1765
Vasotec I.V. 1768
Vasotec Tablets (0.5% to 1.0%) 1771
Verelan Capsules (1.8%) 1410
Verelan Capsules (1.8%) 2824
Virazole (Infrequent) 1264
Yutopar Intravenous Injection 570
Zestoretic 2850
Zestril Tablets (0.2% to 0.3%) 2854
Ziac 1415
Zosyn (1.0% or less) 1419
Zosyn Pharmacy Bulk Package (1.0% or less) 1422
Zovirax Sterile Powder (Less than 1%) 1223

Edema, pulmonary, non-cardiogenic

Hespan Injection 929
Streptase for Infusion (Rare) 562

Edema, retinal

Aralen Phosphate Tablets 2301
Lopid Tablets 1917
Plaquenil Sulfate Tablets 2328

Edema, skin (see under Edema, angioneurotic)

Edema, tongue

Antivenin (Crotalidae) Polyvalent 2696
Cataflam (Less than 1%) 816
Effexor (Infrequent) 2719
Elavil 2838
Endep Tablets 2174
Ethmozine Tablets (Less than 2%) 2041
Etrafon 2355
Flexeril Tablets (Less than 1%) 1661
Lamictal Tablets (Rare) 1112
Limbitrol 2180
Norpramin Tablets 1526
Pamelor 2280
Paxil Tablets (Rare) 2505
Prozac Pulvules & Liquid, Oral Solution (Rare) 919
Reglan 2068
Retrovir Capsules 1158
Retrovir I.V. Infusion 1163
Retrovir Syrup 1158
Risperdal (Rare) 1301
Surmontil Capsules 2811
Tofranil Ampuls 854
Tofranil Tablets 856
Tofranil-PM Capsules 857
Toradol 2159
Triavil Tablets 1757
VePesid Capsules and Injection (Sometimes) 718
Voltaren Tablets (Less than 1%) 861
Zoloft Tablets (Rare) 2217
Zyloprim Tablets (Less than 1%) 1226

Efficacy, lack of

Neoral (1.4%) 2276

Ejaculation, inhibition

Demser Capsules (Infrequent) 1649
Dibenzyline Capsules 2476
Esimil Tablets 822
Etrafon 2355
Ismelin Tablets 827
Lioresal Tablets (Rare) 829
▲ Luvox Tablets (8%) 2544
Mellaril 2269
▲ Normodyne Injection (Up to 5%) 2377
▲ Normodyne Tablets (Up to 5%) 2379
Parnate Tablets 2503
▲ Paxil Tablets (3.7% to 10.0%) 2505
Serentil 684
Temaril Tablets, Syrup and Spansule Extended-Release Capsules 483
▲ Trandate Tablets (Up to 5%) 1185
Triavil Tablets 1757
Trilafon 2389
Wellbutrin Tablets (Infrequent) 1204

Ejaculation, premature

Anafranil Capsules (Rare) 803
Bumex (0.1%) 2093

Ejaculation disturbances

Amicar Syrup, Tablets, and Injection (Rare) 1267
▲ Anafranil Capsules (6% to 42%) 803
Android-10 Tablets 1251
Asendin Tablets (Less than 1%) 1369
BuSpar (Rare) 737
Clozaril Tablets (1%) 2252
Compazine 2470
Desyrel and Desyrel Dividose 503
▲ Effexor (3% to 12.5%) 2719
▲ Hylorel Tablets (7.0%) 985
Lamictal Tablets (Rare) 1112
▲ Luvox Tablets (8%) 2544
Nardil 1920
Neurontin Capsules (Infrequent) 1922
Norpramin Tablets 1526
▲ Orlamm (3% to 9%) 2239
▲ Paxil Tablets (5.8% to 13.0%) 2505
Proscar Tablets (2.8%) 1741
Prozac Pulvules & Liquid, Oral Solution (Infrequent) 919
▲ ReVia Tablets (Less than 10%) 940
Risperdal (Infrequent) 1301
Serzone Tablets (Infrequent) 771
Stelazine 2514
Surmontil Capsules 2811
Thorazine 2523
▲ Trandate Injection (Up to 5%) 1185
Wellbutrin Tablets (Rare) 1204

Ejection fraction reduction

Adriamycin PFS 1947
Adriamycin RDF 1947
Novantrone 1279

Elastosis perforans, serpiginosa

Cuprimine Capsules (Rare) 1630
Depen Titratable Tablets (Rare) 2662

Elation

▲ Marinol (Dronabinol) Capsules (8% to 24%) 2231

Electrocardiographic changes (see under EKG changes)

Electroencephalographic changes (see under EEG changes)

Electrolyte disturbances (see under Electrolyte imbalance)

Electrolyte imbalance

Aldactone 2414
Aldoclor Tablets 1598
Aldoril Tablets 1604
Apresazide Capsules 808
Aristocort Suspension (Forte Parenteral) 1027
Aristocort Suspension (Intralesional) 1025
Aristocort Tablets 1022

(▣ Described in PDR For Nonprescription Drugs) Incidence data in parenthesis; ▲ 3% or more (⊙ Described in PDR For Ophthalmology)

1289 **Side Effects Index** **Encephalopathy**

Aristospan Suspension (Intra-articular) 1033
Aristospan Suspension (Intralesional) 1032
Atromid-S Capsules 2701
Capastat Sulfate Vials (1 patient) 2868
Capozide 742
Celestone Soluspan Suspension 2347
CORTENEMA 2535
Cytosar-U Sterile Powder (Less than 7 patients) 2592
Dalalone D.P. Injectable 1011
Daranide Tablets 1633
Decadron Elixir 1633
Decadron Phosphate Injection 1637
Decadron Phosphate Respihaler 1642
Decadron Phosphate Turbinaire 1645
Decadron Phosphate with Xylocaine Injection, Sterile 1639
Demadex Tablets and Injection 686
Depo-Medrol Sterile Aqueous Suspension 2597
Diamox Intravenous 1372
Diamox Sequels (Sustained Release) 1373
Diamox Tablets 1372
Diupres Tablets 1650
Diuril Oral Suspension 1653
Diuril Sodium Intravenous 1652
Diuril Tablets 1653
Dyazide 2479
Enduron Tablets 420
Esidrix Tablets 821
▲ Foscavir Injection (5% or greater) 547
Glauctabs ⊙ 208
Humegon 1824
HydroDIURIL Tablets 1674
Hydropres Tablets 1675
Lozol Tablets 2022
Lutrepulse for Injection 980
MZM ⊙ 267
Macrobid Capsules 1988
Macrodantin Capsules 1989
Maxaquin Tablets (Less than or equal to 0.1%) 2440
Maxzide 1380
Medrol 2621
Moduretic Tablets 1705
Neptazane Tablets 1388
Oretic Tablets 443
Permax Tablets (Rare) 575
Platinol 708
Platinol-AQ Injection 710
Pravachol 765
Premarin with Methyltestosterone 2794
PREVACID Delayed-Release Capsules (Less than 1%) 2562
Prinzide Tablets 1737
Risperdal 1301
Serophene (clomiphene citrate tablets, USP) 2451
Sodium Polystyrene Sulfonate Suspension 2244
Tenoretic Tablets 2845
Thalitone (Common) 1245
Timolide Tablets 1748
Vaseretic Tablets 1765
Winstrol Tablets 2337
Zaroxolyn Tablets 1000
Zestoretic 2850
Zosyn 1419
Zosyn Pharmacy Bulk Package 1422

Elevated bilirubin levels (see under Hyperbilirubinemia)

Embolism

Activase 1058
Amen Tablets 780
Cycrin Tablets 975
Demadex Tablets and Injection 686
Desogen Tablets 1817
▲ Eminase (Less than 10%) 2039
Sterile FUDR 2118
Lasix Injection, Oral Solution and Tablets 1240
Luvox Tablets (Rare) 2544
Metrodin (urofollitropin for injection) 2446
Ortho-Cept 1851
Ortho-Cyclen/Ortho-Tri-Cyclen 1858
Ortho-Cyclen/Ortho Tri-Cyclen 1858
Paraplatin for Injection 705
Premphase 2797
Prempro 2801
Provera Tablets 2636
Zosyn (1.0% or less) 1419
Zosyn Pharmacy Bulk Package (1.0% or less) 1422

Embolism, arterial

Metrodin (urofollitropin for injection) 2446
Quinidex Extentabs 2067

Embolism, limb

ReoPro Vials (0.3%) 1471

Embolism, lower extremities

Gelfoam Sterile Sponge 2608

Embolism, pulmonary

Actimmune (Rare) 1056
Ambien Tablets (Rare) 2416
Amen Tablets 780
Ansaid Tablets (Less than 1%) 2579
Brevicon 2088
Cipro I.V. (1% or less) 595
Cipro I.V. Pharmacy Bulk Package (Less than 1%) 597
Cipro Tablets (Less than 1%) 592
Climara Transdermal System 645
Clomid 1514
Clozaril Tablets 2252
Cognex Capsules (Infrequent) 1901
Cycrin Tablets 975
Cytovene-IV (One report) 2103
Demulen 2428
Depo-Provera Contraceptive Injection (Fewer than 1%) 2602
Depo-Provera Sterile Aqueous Suspension 2606
Desogen Tablets 1817
Effexor (Rare) 2719
Emcyt Capsules (2%) 1953
Epogen for Injection (Rare) 489
Estrace Cream and Tablets 749
Estraderm Transdermal System 824
ESTRATAB Tablets (0.3, 0.625, 1.25, 2.5 mg) 2536
Estratest 2539
Ethmozine Tablets (Less than 2%) 2041
Foscavir Injection (Less than 1%) 547
Gelfoam Sterile Sponge 2608
Heparin Lock Flush Solution 2725
Heparin Sodium Injection 2726
Heparin Sodium Injection, USP, Sterile Solution 2615
Heparin Sodium Vials 1441
Humegon 1824
Imitrex Tablets 1106
Levlen/Tri-Levlen 651
Lo/Ovral Tablets 2746
Lo/Ovral-28 Tablets 2751
Lupron Depot 3.75 mg 2556
Lupron Depot 7.5 mg 2559
Lupron Injection (Less than 5%) 2555
Maxaquin Tablets (Less than 1%) 2440
Megace Tablets (Rare) 701
Menest Tablets 2494
Metrodin (urofollitropin for injection) 2446
Micronor Tablets 1872
Modicon 1872
Mononine, Coagulation Factor IX (Human) 523
Neurontin Capsules (Rare) 1922
Nolvadex Tablets (0.4%) 2841
Nordette-21 Tablets 2755
Nordette-28 Tablets 2758
Norinyl 2088
Norplant System 2759
Nor-Q D Tablets 2135
Ogen Tablets 2627
Ogen Vaginal Cream 2630
Ortho-Cept 1851
Ortho-Cyclen/Ortho-Tri-Cyclen 1858
Ortho Dienestrol Cream 1866
Ortho-Est 1869
Ortho-Novum 1872
Ortho-Cyclen/Ortho Tri-Cyclen 1858
Ovcon 760
Ovral Tablets 2770
Ovral-28 Tablets 2770
Ovrette Tablets 2771
PMB 200 and PMB 400 2783
Paxil Tablets (Rare) 2505
Permax Tablets (Infrequent) 575
Premarin Intravenous 2787
Premarin with Methyltestosterone 2794
Premarin Tablets 2789
Premarin Vaginal Cream 2791
Premphase 2797
Prempro 2801
Prinivil Tablets (0.3% to 1.0%) 1733
Prinzide Tablets 1737
▲ Procrit for Injection (3.2%) 1841
Proleukin for Injection (Less than 1%) 797
Provera Tablets (Occasional) 2636
Prozac Pulvules & Liquid, Oral Solution 919
ReoPro Vials (0.3%) 1471
Risperdal 1301
Scleromate 1891
Serophene (clomiphene citrate tablets, USP) (Rare) 2451
Sotradecol (Sodium Tetradecyl Sulfate Injection) (One patient) 967
Stilphostrol Tablets and Ampuls 612
Tenormin Tablets and I.V. Injection (1.2%) 2847
Tonocard Tablets (Less than 1%) 531
Levlen/Tri-Levlen 651
Tri-Norinyl 2164
Triphasil-21 Tablets 2814
Triphasil-28 Tablets 2819
Vaseretic Tablets 1765
Vasotec I.V. 1768
Vasotec Tablets (0.5% to 1.0%) 1771
Wellbutrin Tablets (Rare) 1204
Zestoretic 2850
Zestril Tablets (0.3% to 1.0%) 2854
Zosyn (1.0% or less) 1419
Zosyn Pharmacy Bulk Package (1.0% or less) 1422

Embryotoxicity

Methotrexate Sodium Tablets, Injection, for Injection and LPF Injection 1275
Mycelex Troches 608
Terramycin Intramuscular Solution 2210

Emergence delirium

Versed Injection (Less than 1%) 2170

Emesis (see under Vomiting)

Emotional disturbances

Accutane Capsules 2076
Aristocort Suspension (Forte Parenteral) 1027
Aristocort Tablets 1022
Aristospan Suspension (Intra-articular) 1033
Aristospan Suspension (Intralesional) 1032
CORTENEMA 2535
Depakene 413
Depakote Tablets 415
Efudex (Infrequent) 2113
Florinef Acetate Tablets 505
Lariam Tablets (Less than 1%) 2128
Mysoline (Occasional) 2754
Paxil Tablets (Infrequent) 2505
Phenobarbital Elixir and Tablets 1469
Plaquenil Sulfate Tablets 2328
Prelone Syrup 1787
Tofranil Tablets 856
▲ Yutopar Intravenous Injection (5% to 6%) 570
▲ Zonalon Cream (Approximately 1% to 10%) 1055

Emotional lability

Adenoscan (Less than 1%) 1024
Children's Advil Suspension (Less than 1%) 2692
Ambien Tablets (Infrequent) 2416
Anafranil Capsules (Up to 2%) 803
Ansaid Tablets (Less than 1%) 2579
Asacol Delayed-Release Tablets 1979
Betapace Tablets (Rare) 641
Blocadren Tablets 1614
BuSpar (Rare) 737
Cardura Tablets (Less than 0.5% of 3960 patients) 2186
Cartrol Tablets 410
Claritin-D (Less frequent) 2350
Danocrine Capsules 2307
Diprivan Injection (Less than 1%) 2833
Effexor (Frequent) 2719
Emcyt Capsules (2%) 1953
▲ Felbatol (6.5%) 2666
Floxin I.V. 1571
Floxin Tablets (200 mg, 300 mg, 400 mg) 1567
Foscavir Injection (Less than 1%) 547
Hivid Tablets (Less than 1% to less than 3%) 2121
IBU Tablets (Less than 1%) 1342
Inderal 2728
Inderal LA Long Acting Capsules 2730
Inderide Tablets 2732
Inderide LA Long Acting Capsules 2734
Intron A (Less than 5%) 2364
Kerlone Tablets (Less than 2%) 2436
Lamictal Tablets (1.3%) 1112
Levatol 2403
Lopressor HCT Tablets 832
▲ Lupron Depot 3.75 mg (10.8%) 2556
Lupron Depot-PED 7.5 mg, 11.25 mg and 15 mg (Less than 2%) 2560
Luvox Tablets (Infrequent) 2544
Monoket (Up to 2%) 2406
Children's Motrin Ibuprofen Oral Suspension (Less than 1%) 1546
Motrin Tablets (Less than 1%) 2625
Motrin Ibuprofen Suspension, Oral Drops, Chewable Tablets, Caplets (Less than 1%) 1546
NebuPent for Inhalation Solution (1% or less) 1040
Neurontin Capsules (More than 1%) 1922
Normodyne Tablets 2379
Norplant System (Less than 1%) 2759
Oncaspar (Less than 1%) 2028
Paxil Tablets (Frequent) 2505
Pediapred Oral Liquid 995
Penetrex Tablets (Less than 0.1%) 2031
Permax Tablets (Infrequent) 575
▲ Prograf (Greater than 3%) 1042
ProSom Tablets (Infrequent) 449
Proventil Syrup (1%) 2385
Prozac Pulvules & Liquid, Oral Solution (Infrequent) 919
Retrovir Capsules 1158
Retrovir I.V. Infusion 1163
Retrovir Syrup 1158
Risperdal (Rare) 1301
Roferon-A Injection (Less than 3%) 2145
Romazicon (1% to 3%) 2147
Sectral Capsules 2807
Serzone Tablets 771
▲ Synarel Nasal Solution for Central Precocious Puberty (6%) 2151
▲ Synarel Nasal Solution for Endometriosis (15% of patients) 2152
Tegison Capsules (Less than 1%) 2154
Tenoretic Tablets 2845
Tenormin Tablets and I.V. Injection 2847
Timolide Tablets 1748
Timoptic in Ocudose 1753
Timoptic Sterile Ophthalmic Solution 1751
Timoptic-XE 1755
Toprol-XL Tablets 565
Trandate Tablets 1185
▲ Ultram Tablets (50 mg) (7% to 14%) 1585
Ventolin Syrup (1% of children) 1202
Videx Tablets, Powder for Oral Solution, & Pediatric Powder for Oral Solution (Up to 2%) 720
Visken Tablets 2299
Zebeta Tablets 1413
Ziac 1415
▲ Zoladex (60%) 2858
Zoloft Tablets (Infrequent) 2217

Emphysema

▲ Exosurf Neonatal for Intratracheal Suspension (7% to 44%) 1095
Permax Tablets (Infrequent) 575

Encephalitis

Atgam Sterile Solution (Less than 5%) 2581
Attenuvax 1610
Biavax II 1613
Cognex Capsules (Rare) 1901
JE-VAX (1 to 2.3 per million vaccines) 886
M-M-R II (Very rare) 1687
M-R-VAX II (Rare) 1689
Mumpsvax (Very rare) 1708
Orthoclone OKT3 Sterile Solution 1837
Solganal Suspension 2388
Videx Tablets, Powder for Oral Solution, & Pediatric Powder for Oral Solution (Less than 1%) 720

Encephalomyelitis

JE-VAX (Two cases.) 886

Encephalopathy

Acel-Imune Diphtheria and Tetanus Toxoids and Acellular Pertussis Vaccine Adsorbed 1364
Anafranil Capsules (Infrequent) 803
Betaseron for SC Injection 658
Bumex (0.6%) 2093
Ceptaz 1081
Cytovene-IV (Two or more reports) 2103
Depakene (Rare) 413
Depakote Tablets (Rare instances) 415
Diphtheria and Tetanus Toxoids and Pertussis Vaccine Adsorbed 2477

(▣ Described in PDR For Nonprescription Drugs) Incidence data in parenthesis; ▲ 3% or more (⊙ Described in PDR For Ophthalmology)

Encephalopathy | Side Effects Index | 1290

Diphtheria and Tetanus Toxoids and Pertussis Vaccine Adsorbed USP (For Pediatric Use) (Rare) 875
Ergamisol Tablets ... 1292
Felbatol ... 2666
Fortaz ... 1100
Foscavir Injection (Less than 1%) .. 547
Fungizone Intravenous ... 506
Garamycin Injectable ... 2360
Havrix (Rare) ... 2489
Influenza Virus Vaccine, Trivalent, Types A and B (chromatograph- and filter-purified subviron antigen) FluShield, 1995-1996 Formula ... 2736
JE-VAX (1 to 2.3 per million vaccines) ... 886
Lariam Tablets ... 2128
Lithonate/Lithotabs/Lithobid ... 2543
M-M-R II (Very rare) ... 1687
M-R-VAX II (Once for every million doses) ... 1689
Methotrexate Sodium Tablets, Injection, for Injection and LPF Injection ... 1275
Midamor Tablets (Between 1% and 3%) ... 1703
Moduretic Tablets ... 1705
MSTA Mumps Skin Test Antigen ... 890
Netromycin Injection 100 mg/ml ... 2373
Neurontin Capsules (Rare) ... 1922
Orthoclone OKT3 Sterile Solution .. 1837
PASER Granules ... 1285
Primaxin I.M. ... 1727
Primaxin I.V. (Less than 0.2%) ... 1729
Roferon-A Injection (Less than 1%) ... 2145
Streptomycin Sulfate Injection ... 2208
Tapazole Tablets (Rare) ... 1477
Tetramune (Rare) ... 1404
Tri-Immunol Adsorbed (Rare) ... 1408
Tripedia ... 892
Videx Tablets, Powder for Oral Solution, & Pediatric Powder for Oral Solution (Less than 1%) ... 720
Zovirax Sterile Powder (Approximately 1%) ... 1223

Encephalopathy, hepatic
Eulexin Capsules ... 2358
Intron A (Very rare) ... 2364
Prilosec Delayed-Release Capsules (Rare) ... 529
Taxol (Rare) ... 714

Encephalopathy, hypertensive
Catapres-TTS (Rare) ... 675
Combipres Tablets ... 677
Epogen for Injection (On occasion) ... 489
Procrit for Injection (Occasional) 1841

Encephalopathy, post-viral
Atgam Sterile Solution (Less than 5%) ... 2581

Encephalopathy, toxic
Nydrazid Injection (Uncommon) ... 508
Rifamate Capsules (Uncommon) 1530
Rifater (Uncommon) ... 1532

Endocardial fibrosis
Myleran Tablets (One case) ... 1143

Endocarditis
Betaseron for SC Injection ... 658
Cytovene-IV (One report) ... 2103
Oncaspar (Less than 1%) ... 2028
Proleukin for Injection (1%) ... 797

Endocrine disturbances
Compazine ... 2470
Levoprome ... 1274
Norplant System ... 2759
Permax Tablets (Rare) ... 575
Pravachol ... 765
Rogaine Topical Solution (0.47%) .. 2637
Stelazine ... 2514

Endometrial carcinoma (see under Carcinoma, endometrial)

Endometrial hyperplasia
Anafranil Capsules (Rare) ... 803
Nolvadex Tablets ... 2841
Ogen Vaginal Cream ... 2630

Endometriosis
Anafranil Capsules (Infrequent) ... 803
Clomid ... 1514
Nolvadex Tablets (A few reports) 2841

Endometritis
Lippes Loop Intrauterine Double-S .. 1848
ParaGard T380A Intrauterine Copper Contraceptive ... 1880
Prostin E2 Suppository ... 2634

Endophthalmitis
AdatoSil 5000 (Less than 2%) .... ⊙ 274
Healon GV ... ⊙ 315
ISPAN Perfluoropropane ... ⊙ 276
ISPAN Sulfur Hexafluoride ... ⊙ 275

Endotracheal tube occlusion
Survanta Beractant Intratracheal Suspension (Less than 1%) ... 2226

Endotracheal tube, reflux into
Exosurf Neonatal for Intratracheal Suspension ... 1095
Survanta Beractant Intratracheal Suspension (Less than 1%) ... 2226

Energy, high
Esgic-plus Tablets (Infrequent) ... 1013
Fioricet Tablets (Infrequent) ... 2258
Fioricet with Codeine Capsules (Infrequent) ... 2260
Fiorinal with Codeine Capsules (Infrequent) ... 2262
Phrenilin (Infrequent) ... 785
▲ReVia Tablets (Less than 10%) ... 940
Sedapap Tablets 50 mg/650 mg (Infrequent) ... 1543

Energy, loss of
Demulen ... 2428
Levlen/Tri-Levlen ... 651
▲Lozol Tablets (Greater than or equal to 5%) ... 2022
Micronor Tablets ... 1872
▲Minipress Capsules (6.9%) ... 1937
▲Minizide Capsules (6.9%) ... 1938
Modicon ... 1872
Ortho-Cyclen/Ortho-Tri-Cyclen ... 1858
Ortho-Novum ... 1872
Ortho-Cyclen/Ortho Tri-Cyclen ... 1858
▲ReVia Tablets (More than 10%) ... 940
Levlen/Tri-Levlen ... 651

Enteritis
Ambien Tablets (Rare) ... 2416
Anafranil Capsules (Rare) ... 803
Betaseron for SC Injection ... 658
Felbatol ... 2666
Foscavir Injection (Less than 1%) .. 547
▲Sterile FUDR (Among more common) ... 2118
Lamprene Capsules (Less than 1%) ... 828
Methotrexate Sodium Tablets, Injection, for Injection and LPF Injection ... 1275
Prozac Pulvules & Liquid, Oral Solution (Rare) ... 919

Enteritis, hemorrhagic
Methotrexate Sodium Tablets, Injection, for Injection and LPF Injection ... 1275

Enteritis, staphylococci
Furoxone ... 2046

Enterocolitis
Achromycin V Capsules (Rare) ... 1367
Augmentin ... 2468
Chloromycetin Sodium Succinate 1900
Declomycin Tablets ... 1371
Doryx Capsules ... 1913
Dynacin Capsules ... 1590
Foscavir Injection (Less than 1%) .. 547
Indocin I.V. (Less than 3%) ... 1684
Leucovorin Calcium Tablets, Wellcovorin Brand ... 1132
Lincocin ... 2617
Minocin Intravenous ... 1382
Minocin Oral Suspension ... 1385
Minocin Pellet-Filled Capsules ... 1383
Monodox Capsules ... 1805
Myochrysine Injection (Rare) ... 1711
Omnipen Capsules ... 2764
Omnipen for Oral Suspension ... 2765
ProSom Tablets (Rare) ... 449
Spectrobid Tablets ... 2206
Terramycin Intramuscular Solution 2210
Unasyn ... 2212
Vibramycin ... 1941
Vibramycin Hyclate Intravenous ... 2215
Vibramycin ... 1941

Enterocolitis, hemorrhagic
Velban Vials ... 1484

Enterocolitis, necrotizing
▲Exosurf Neonatal for Intratracheal Suspension (2% to 13%) ... 1095
▲Survanta Beractant Intratracheal Suspension (6.1%) ... 2226

Enterocolitis, neutropenic
Azulfidine (Rare) ... 1949

Enterocolitis, ulcerative
Ridaura Capsules (Less than 1%) .. 2513
Solganal Suspension (Rare) ... 2388

Entropion
BOTOX (Botulinum Toxin Type A) Purified Neurotoxin Complex (Less than 1%) ... 477
Idamycin (Rare) ... 1955

Enuresis
BuSpar (Rare) ... 737
Depakene ... 413
Depakote Tablets ... 415
Klonopin Tablets ... 2126
Lioresal Tablets (Rare) ... 829
Mintezol ... 1704
Serentil ... 684
Wellbutrin Tablets (Rare) ... 1204

Eosinophilia
Achromycin V Capsules ... 1367
Children's Advil Suspension (Less than 1%) ... 2692
Altace Capsules (Scattered incidents; less than 1%) ... 1232
Amikacin Sulfate Injection, USP (Rare) ... 960
Amikin Injectable (Rare) ... 501
Amoxil ... 2464
Anaprox/Naprosyn (Less than 1%) ... 2117
Ancef Injection ... 2465
Ancobon Capsules ... 2079
Ansaid Tablets (Less than 1%) ... 2579
Apresazide Capsules (Less frequent) ... 808
Apresoline Hydrochloride Tablets (Less frequent) ... 809
Asacol Delayed-Release Tablets ... 1979
Asendin Tablets (Very rare) ... 1369
Atgam Sterile Solution (Less than 5%) ... 2581
Atretol Tablets ... 573
Atromid-S Capsules ... 2701
Augmentin ... 2468
Axid Pulvules (Rare) ... 1427
Azactam for Injection ... 734
Azo Gantanol Tablets ... 2080
Azo Gantrisin Tablets ... 2081
Azulfidine (Rare) ... 1949
Bactrim DS Tablets ... 2084
Bactrim I.V. Infusion ... 2082
Bactrim ... 2084
Beclovent Inhalation Aerosol and Refill ... 1075
Betapace Tablets (Rare) ... 641
Bicillin C-R Injection ... 2704
Bicillin C-R 900/300 Injection ... 2706
Bicillin L-A Injection ... 2707
BuSpar (Rare) ... 737
Capastat Sulfate Vials ... 2868
▲Capoten (About 4 to 7 of 100 patients) ... 739
Capozide (Sometimes) ... 742
Cataflam ... 816
Ceclor Pulvules & Suspension (1 in 50) ... 1431
Cefizox for Intramuscular or Intravenous Use (Greater than 1% but less than 5%) ... 1034
▲Cefobid Intravenous/Intramuscular (1 in 10) ... 2189
▲Cefobid Pharmacy Bulk Package - Not for Direct Infusion (1 in 10) ... 2192
Cefotan (1 in 200) ... 2829
Ceftin (1.1%; less than 1% but more than 0.1%) ... 1078
Cefzil Tablets and Oral Suspension (2.3%) ... 746
Celontin Kapseals ... 1899
Ceptaz (One in 13) ... 1081
CHEMET (succimer) Capsules (0.5 to 1.5%) ... 1545
▲Cipro I.V. (Among most frequent) .. 595
▲Cipro I.V. Pharmacy Bulk Package (Among most frequent) ... 597
Cipro Tablets (0.6%; rare) ... 592
Claforan Sterile and Injection (Less than 1% to 2.4%) ... 1235
Cleocin Phosphate Injection ... 2586
Cleocin Vaginal Cream ... 2589
Clinoril Tablets (Less than 1 in 100) ... 1618
Clozaril Tablets (1%) ... 2252
Compazine ... 2470
Cuprimine Capsules ... 1630
Cytosar-U Sterile Powder (Less than 7 patients) ... 2592
Cytovene (1% or less) ... 2103
Danocrine Capsules ... 2307
Daypro Caplets (Rare) ... 2426
Declomycin Tablets ... 1371
Demser Capsules (Rare) ... 1649
Depakene ... 413
Depakote Tablets ... 415
Depen Titratable Tablets ... 2662
Diabinese Tablets ... 1935
Dilantin Infatabs ... 1908
Dilantin Kapseals ... 1906
Dilantin-125 Suspension ... 1911
Dipentum Capsules (Rare) ... 1951
Dobutrex Solution Vials (Occasional) ... 1439
Dolobid Tablets (Less than 1 in 100) ... 1654
Doryx Capsules ... 1913
Duricef ... 748
Dynacin Capsules ... 1590
EC-Naprosyn Delayed-Release Tablets (Less than 1%) ... 2117
Effexor (Rare) ... 2719
Efudex ... 2113
Elavil ... 2838
Eminase (Occasional) ... 2039
Endep Tablets ... 2174
Etrafon ... 2355
Fansidar Tablets ... 2114
Feldene Capsules (Greater than 1%) ... 1965
Flexeril Tablets (Rare) ... 1661
Floxin I.V. (More than or equal to 1%) ... 1571
Floxin Tablets (200 mg, 300 mg, 400 mg) (More than or equal to 1.0%) ... 1567
▲Fortaz (1 in 13) ... 1100
Fungizone Intravenous ... 506
Gantanol Tablets ... 2119
Gantrisin ... 2120
Garamycin Injectable ... 2360
Geocillin Tablets ... 2199
▲Hivid Tablets (2.5% to 6.3%) ... 2121
IBU Tablets (Less than 1%) ... 1342
Intal Capsules (Less than 1 in 100,000 patients) ... 987
Intal Inhaler (Infrequent) ... 988
Intal Nebulizer Solution (Rare) ... 989
Keflex Pulvules & Oral Suspension 914
Keftab Tablets ... 915
▲Kefurox Vials, Faspak & ADD-Vantage (1 in 14) ... 1454
Kefzol Vials, Faspak & ADD-Vantage ... 1456
Klonopin Tablets ... 2126
Lamictal Tablets (Rare) ... 1112
Lamprene Capsules (Less than 1%) ... 828
Lescol Capsules (Rare) ... 2267
Levoprome ... 1274
Limbitrol ... 2180
Lopid Tablets ... 1917
Lorabid Suspension and Pulvules 1459
Lorelco Tablets ... 1517
Lotensin Tablets (Scattered incidents) ... 834
Lotensin HCT ... 837
Ludiomil Tablets (Isolated reports) 843
Macrobid Capsules (1% to 5%) ... 1988
Macrodantin Capsules (Less often) 1989
Mandol Vials, Faspak & ADD-Vantage ... 1461
Matulane Capsules ... 2131
Maxaquin Tablets (Less than or equal to 0.1%) ... 2440
Mefoxin ... 1691
Mefoxin Premixed Intravenous Solution ... 1694
Mellaril ... 2269
Mesantoin Tablets ... 2272
Mevacor Tablets ... 1699
Mezlin ... 601
Mezlin Pharmacy Bulk Package ... 604
Miltown Tablets ... 2672
Minocin Intravenous ... 1382
Minocin Oral Suspension ... 1385
Minocin Pellet-Filled Capsules ... 1383
Monocid Injection (2.9%) ... 2497
Monodox Capsules ... 1805

(▣ Described in PDR For Nonprescription Drugs) Incidence data in parenthesis; ▲ 3% or more (⊙ Described in PDR For Ophthalmology)

1291 Side Effects Index Epistaxis

Monopril Tablets (2 patients) 757
Children's Motrin Ibuprofen Oral Suspension (Less than 1%) 1546
Motrin Tablets (Less than 1%) 2625
Motrin Ibuprofen Suspension, Oral Drops, Chewable Tablets, Caplets (Less than 1%) 1546
Mycobutin Capsules (1%) 1957
Myochrysine Injection 1711
Anaprox/Naprosyn (Less than 1%) 2117
Navane Capsules and Concentrate 2201
Navane Intramuscular 2202
Nebcin Vials, Hyporets & ADD-Vantage 1464
NebuPent for Inhalation Solution (1% or less) 1040
NegGram 2323
Netromycin Injection 100 mg/ml (4 of 1000 patients) 2373
Noroxin Tablets (0.6% to 1.4%) 1715
Noroxin Tablets (0.6% to 1.4%) 2048
Norpramin Tablets 1526
Nydrazid Injection 508
Omnipen Capsules 2764
Omnipen for Oral Suspension 2765
Orthoclone OKT3 Sterile Solution 1837
PMB 200 and PMB 400 2783
Pamelor 2280
▲ PASER Granules (55% of 38 patients with drug-induced hepatitis) 1285
Paxil Tablets (Rare) 2505
Pen•Vee K (Frequent) 2772
Penetrex Tablets (Less than 1%) 2031
Permax Tablets (Rare) 575
Pipracil 1390
Ponstel (Occasional) 1925
Pravachol (Rare) 765
PREVACID Delayed-Release Capsules (Less than 1%) 2562
Primaxin I.M. 1727
Primaxin I.V. 1729
Prinivil Tablets (0.3% to 1.0%) 1733
Prinzide Tablets 1737
Proglycem 580
▲ Proleukin for Injection (6%) 797
Prolixin 509
Quadrinal Tablets 1350
Rifadin (Occasional) 1528
Rifamate Capsules 1530
Rifater (Occasional) 1532
Rimactane Capsules 847
▲ Rocephin Injectable Vials, ADD-Vantage, Galaxy Container (6%) 2142
Sansert Tablets 2295
Septra 1174
Septra I.V. Infusion 1169
Septra I.V. Infusion ADD-Vantage Vials 1171
Septra 1174
Ser-Ap-Es Tablets 849
Serentil 684
Sinequan (A few patients) 2205
Solganal Suspension (Rare) 2388
Soma Compound w/Codeine Tablets 2676
Soma Compound Tablets 2675
Soma Tablets 2674
Spectrobid Tablets 2206
Stelazine 2514
Sulfamylon Cream 925
Suprax (Less than 2%) 1399
Surmontil Capsules 2811
▲ Synarel Nasal Solution for Endometriosis (10% to 15%) 2152
Talacen (Rare) 2333
Talwin Injection (Rare) 2334
Talwin Compound 2335
Talwin Injection (Rare) 2334
Talwin Nx (Rare) 2336
Tao Capsules 2209
▲ Tazicef for Injection (1 in 13 patients) 2519
▲ Tazidime Vials, Faspak & ADD-Vantage (1 in 13) 1478
Tegretol Chewable Tablets 852
Tegretol Suspension 852
Tegretol Tablets 852
Terramycin Intramuscular Solution 2210
Thorazine 2523
Ticar for Injection 2526
Ticlid Tablets 2156
Timentin for Injection 2528
Tobramycin Sulfate Injection 968
Tofranil Ampuls 854
Tofranil Tablets 856
Tofranil-PM Capsules 857
Tonocard Tablets (Less than 1%) 531
Toradol (1% or less) 2159
Torecan 2245
Triavil Tablets 1757
Trilafon 2389
Unasyn 2212
Urispas Tablets 2532
Vancocin HCl, Oral Solution & Pulvules (Infrequent) 1483
Vancocin HCl, Vials & ADD-Vantage (Infrequent) 1481
Vantin for Oral Suspension and Vantin Tablets 2646
Vascor (200, 300 and 400 mg) Tablets 1587
Vaseretic Tablets 1765
Vasotec I.V. 1768
Vasotec Tablets (0.5% to 1.0%) 1771
Vibramycin 1941
Vibramycin Hyclate Intravenous 2215
Vibramycin 1941
Vivactil Tablets 1774
Voltaren Tablets 861
▲ Xanax Tablets (3.2% to 9.5%) 2649
Zantac (Rare) 1209
Zantac Injection 1207
Zantac Syrup (Rare) 1209
Zarontin Capsules 1928
Zarontin Syrup 1929
Zefazone 2654
Zestoretic 2850
Zestril Tablets (0.3% to 1.0%) 2854
▲ Zinacef (1 in 14 patients) 1211
Zocor Tablets 1775
Zosyn 1419
Zosyn Pharmacy Bulk Package 1422
Zyloprim Tablets (Less than 1%) 1226

Eosinophilia, myoclonus
Atretol Tablets (One case) 573
Tegretol Chewable Tablets 852
Tegretol Suspension 852
Tegretol Tablets 852

Eosinophilia, peripheral
Atretol Tablets (One case) 573
Tegretol Chewable Tablets 852
Tegretol Suspension 852
Tegretol Tablets 852

Eosinophilia, pulmonary
Dapsone Tablets USP 1284
Daraprim Tablets (Rare) 1090
Dynacin Capsules (Rare) 1590

Eosinophilic pneumonitis
Anaprox/Naprosyn (Less than 1%) 2117
Capoten 739
Capozide 742
Anaprox/Naprosyn (Less than 1%) 2117
NebuPent for Inhalation Solution (1% or less) 1040

Epidermal necrolysis (see also under Necrolysis, epidermal)
Aldoclor Tablets 1598
Aldomet Ester HCl Injection 1602
Aldomet Oral 1600
Aldoril Tablets 1604
Anaprox/Naprosyn (Less than 1%) 2117
Bactrim DS Tablets (Rare) 2084
Bactrim I.V. Infusion (Rare) 2082
Bactrim (Rare) 2084
Clinoril Tablets (Less than 1%) 1618
Cuprimine Capsules 1630
Diamox 1372
Dilantin Parenteral 1910
EC-Naprosyn Delayed-Release Tablets (Less than 1%) 2117
Fansidar Tablets 2114
Fioricet with Codeine Capsules 2260
Gantanol Tablets 2119
Gantrisin 2120
Keflex Pulvules & Oral Suspension (Rare) 914
Keftab Tablets 915
Anaprox/Naprosyn (Less than 1%) 2117
Neptazane Tablets 1388
Prinzide Tablets 1737
Tagamet (Very rare) 2516
Talacen (Rare) 2333
Talwin Injection (Rare) 2334
Talwin Compound 2335
Talwin Injection 2334
Tenoretic Tablets 2845
Trancopal Caplets (Rare) 2337
Vasotec I.V. 1768

Epidermolysis bullosa
Anaprox/Naprosyn (Less than 1%) 2117

Epididymitis
Anafranil Capsules (Infrequent) 803
Asacol Delayed-Release Tablets 1979
BCG Vaccine, USP (TICE) (0.3%) 1814
Betaseron for SC Injection 658
Cognex Capsules (Rare) 1901
Cordarone Tablets (Rare) 2712
Lamictal Tablets (Rare) 1112
Maxaquin Tablets (Less than 1%) 2440
Neurontin Capsules (Rare) 1922
Oxandrin 2862
Permax Tablets (Rare) 575
Prozac Pulvules & Liquid, Oral Solution (Rare) 919
Rogaine Topical Solution (0.91%) 2637
Winstrol Tablets 2337

Epigastric pain (see under Distress, epigastric)

Epilation
Velban Vials 1484

Epilepsy, aggravation
Estrace Cream and Tablets 749
Indocin Capsules (Less than 1%) 1680
Indocin I.V. (Less than 1%) 1684
Indocin (Less than 1%) 1680

Epileptiform movements, unspecified
Clozaril Tablets (1%) 2252

Epinephrine effect, reversal
Compazine 2470
Etrafon 2355
Stelazine 2514
Triavil Tablets 1757

Epiphyseal closure
Accutane Capsules (Two children) 2076
Aquasol A Vitamin A Capsules, USP 534
Estratest 2539
Oxandrin 2862
Winstrol Tablets 2337

Epistaxis
▲ Accutane Capsules (Up to 80%) 2076
Activase (Less than 1%) 1058
Adalat CC (3% or less) 589
Children's Advil Suspension (Less than 1%) 2692
AeroBid Inhaler System (1-3%) 1005
Aerobid-M Inhaler System (1-3%) 1005
Altace Capsules (Less than 1%) 1232
Ambien Tablets (Rare) 2416
Anafranil Capsules (Up to 2%) 803
Ansaid Tablets (Less than 1%) 2579
Atgam Sterile Solution (Less than 5%) 2581
Beconase (Fewer than 3 per 100 patients) 1076
Bioclate, Antihemophilic Factor (Recombinant) (One patient out of 13,394) 513
BuSpar (Rare) 737
Cardizem CD Capsules (Less than 1%) 1506
Cardizem SR Capsules (Less than 1%) 1510
Cardizem Injectable 1508
Cardizem Tablets (Less than 1%) 1512
Cardura Tablets (1%) 2186
Cataflam (Less than 1%) 816
Cipro I.V. (1% or less) 595
Cipro I.V. Pharmacy Bulk Package (Less than 1%) 597
Cipro Tablets (Less than 1%) 592
Claritin (2% or fewer patients) 2349
Claritin-D (Less frequent) 2350
Clinoril Tablets (Less than 1%) 1618
Clozaril Tablets (Less than 1%) 2252
Cognex Capsules (Infrequent) 1901
Coumadin 926
Cozaar Tablets (Less than 1%) 1628
Cytotec (Infrequent) 2424
DDAVP (Up to 3%) 2017
Decadron Phosphate Turbinaire 1645
Desmopressin Acetate Rhinal Tube (Up to 3%) 979
Dexacort Phosphate in Turbinaire 459
Dilacor XR Extended-release Capsules (Infrequent) 2018
Diupres Tablets 1650
Effexor (Infrequent) 2719
Eminase (Less than 1%) 2039
Ergamisol Tablets (Up to 1%) 1292
Felbatol 2666
Feldene Capsules (Less than 1%) 1965
Fioricet with Codeine Capsules 2260
Fiorinal with Codeine Capsules 2262
▲ Flonase Nasal Spray (3% to 6%) 1098
Floxin I.V. (Less than 1%) 1571
Floxin Tablets (200 mg, 300 mg, 400 mg) (Less than 1%) 1567
Fludara for Injection (Up to 1%) 663
Fluorouracil Injection 2116
Foscavir Injection (Less than 1%) 547
Sterile FUDR (Remote possibility) 2118
Hismanal Tablets (Less frequent) 1293
Hivid Tablets (Less than 1% to less than 3%) 2121
Hydropres Tablets 1675
Hytrin Capsules (At least 1%) 430
Hyzaar Tablets 1677
IBU Tablets (Less than 1%) 1342
Indocin Capsules (Less than 1%) 1680
Indocin I.V. (Less than 1%) 1684
Indocin (Less than 1%) 1680
Intal Inhaler (Rare) 988
Intal Nebulizer Solution 989
Intron A (Less than 5%) 2364
Kerlone Tablets (Less than 2%) 2436
Lamictal Tablets (Infrequent) 1112
▲ Leustatin (5%) 1834
Lotensin HCT (0.3% to 1.0%) 837
Lupron Depot-PED 7.5 mg, 11.25 mg and 15 mg (Less than 2%) 2560
Luvox Tablets (Infrequent) 2544
Matulane Capsules 2131
Maxaquin Tablets (Less than 1%) 2440
Methotrexate Sodium Tablets, Injection, for Injection and LPF Injection (Less common) 1275
▲ Miacalcin Nasal Spray (3.5%) 2275
Minipress Capsules (1-4%) 1937
Minizide Capsules 1938
Mithracin 607
Monopril Tablets (0.2% to 1.0%) 757
Children's Motrin Ibuprofen Oral Suspension (Less than 1%) 1546
Motrin Tablets (Less than 1%) 2625
Motrin Ibuprofen Suspension, Oral Drops, Chewable Tablets, Caplets (Less than 1%) 1546
Mykrox Tablets (Less than 2%) 993
Nasacort Nasal Inhaler (Fewer than 5%) 2024
Nasalcrom Nasal Solution (Less than 1%) 994
Nasalide Nasal Solution 0.025% (5% or less) 2110
▲ Nasarel Nasal Solution (3% to 9%) 2133
▲ Neupogen for Injection (15%) 495
Neurontin Capsules (Infrequent) 1922
Norvasc Tablets (More than 0.1% to 1%) 1940
Oncaspar (Less than 1%) 2028
OptiPranolol (Metipranolol 0.3%) Sterile Ophthalmic Solution (A small number of patients) ⊙ 258
Orudis Capsules (Less than 1%) 2766
Oruvail Capsules (Less than 1%) 2766
Paxil Tablets (Infrequent) 2505
Penetrex Tablets (Less than 1% but more than or equal to 0.1%) 2031
Permax Tablets (1.6%) 575
Plendil Extended-Release Tablets (0.5% to 1.5%) 527
PREVACID Delayed-Release Capsules (Less than 1%) 2562
Prilosec Delayed-Release Capsules (Less than 1%) 529
Prinivil Tablets (0.3% to 1.0%) 1733
Prinzide Tablets 1737
Procardia XL Extended Release Tablets (1% or less) 1972
ProSom Tablets (Rare) 449
Proventil Syrup (1 of 100 patients) 2385
Prozac Pulvules & Liquid, Oral Solution (Infrequent) 919
ReoPro Vials (9 to 11 events) 1471
Retrovir Capsules 1158
Retrovir I.V. Infusion 1163
Retrovir Syrup 1158
ReVia Tablets (Less than 1%) 940
▲ Rhinocort Nasal Inhaler (3 to 9%) 556
Risperdal (Infrequent) 1301
Rocephin Injectable Vials, ADD-Vantage, Galaxy Container (Rare) 2142
Roferon-A Injection (Rare) 2145
Salagen Tablets (2%) 1489

(▣ Described in PDR For Nonprescription Drugs) Incidence data in parenthesis; ▲ 3% or more (⊙ Described in PDR For Ophthalmology)

Sandostatin Injection (Less than 1%) ... 2292
Seldane Tablets (Up to 0.7%) ... 1536
Seldane-D Extended-Release Tablets ... 1538
Ser-Ap-Es Tablets ... 849
Serzone Tablets (Infrequent) ... 771
▲ Stadol (3% to 9%) ... 775
Stimate, (desmopressin acetate) Nasal Spray, 1.5 mg/mL ... 525
Supprelin Injection (1% to 3%) ... 2056
▲ Tegison Capsules (25-50%) ... 2154
Ticlid Tablets (0.5% to 1.0%) ... 2156
Tolectin (200, 400 and 600 mg) (Less than 1%) ... 1581
Toradol (1% or less) ... 2159
Trental Tablets (Less than 1%) ... 1244
Trilisate (Less than 1%) ... 2000
Unasyn (Less than 1%) ... 2212
Vancenase AQ Nasal Spray 0.042% (Fewer than 3 per 100 patients) ... 2393
Vancenase PocketHaler Nasal Inhaler (2 per 100 patients) ... 2391
Vantin for Oral Suspension and Vantin Tablets (Less than 1%) ... 2646
▲ Ventolin Inhalation Aerosol and Refill (3%) ... 1197
Ventolin Rotacaps for Inhalation (2%) ... 1200
Ventolin Syrup (1 of 100 patients) 1202
▲ Videx Tablets, Powder for Oral Solution, & Pediatric Powder for Oral Solution (Less than 1% to 14%) ... 720
Voltaren Tablets (Less than 1%) ... 861
Wellbutrin Tablets (Rare) ... 1204
Zefazone ... 2654
Zestoretic ... 2850
Zestril Tablets (0.3% to 1.0%) ... 2854
Zoladex (1% or greater) ... 2858
Zoloft Tablets (Infrequent) ... 2217
Zosyn (1.0% or less) ... 1419
Zosyn Pharmacy Bulk Package (1.0% or less) ... 1422
Zyloprim Tablets (Less than 1%) ... 1226

Epithelial cells, atypical
▲ Blenoxane (10%) ... 692
Cytoxan ... 694
NEOSAR Lyophilized/Neosar ... 1959

Epithelial punctate, staining
Profenal 1% Sterile Ophthalmic Solution (Less than 0.5%) ... ⊙ 227

Epitheliopathy
Alomide ... 469

Equilibrium, dysfunction
Calan SR Caplets (1% or less) ... 2422
Calan Tablets (1% or less) ... 2419
Floxin I.V. ... 1571
Floxin Tablets (200 mg, 300 mg, 400 mg) ... 1567
Hivid Tablets (Less than 1% to less than 3%) ... 2121
Isoptin Oral Tablets (Less than 1%) ... 1346
Isoptin SR Tablets (1% or less) ... 1348
Lariam Tablets ... 2128
Lioresal Intrathecal ... 1596
Procardia Capsules (2% or less) ... 1971
Restoril Capsules (Less than 1%) .. 2284
Rifater ... 1532
Streptomycin Sulfate Injection ... 2208
Tegison Capsules (Less than 1%) .. 2154
Transderm Scōp Transdermal Therapeutic System (Few patients) ... 869
Verelan Capsules (1% or less) ... 1410
Verelan Capsules (Less than 1%) .. 2824

Erection disturbances
Aldactazide ... 2413
Aldactone ... 2414
Bumex (0.1%) ... 2093
Dantrium Capsules (Less frequent) 1982
Desyrel and Desyrel Dividose ... 503
Effexor (Rare) ... 2719
Lescol Capsules ... 2267
Mevacor Tablets (0.5% to 1.0%) .. 1699
▲ Paxil Tablets (3.7% to 10.0%) ... 2505
Pravachol ... 765
Risperdal (Frequent) ... 1301
Wellbutrin Tablets (Infrequent) ... 1204
Winstrol Tablets ... 2337
Zocor Tablets ... 1775
▲ Zoladex (18%) ... 2858

Ergotism
Cafergot (Rare) ... 2251
Parlodel (Rare) ... 2281

Erosion, genital
▲ Condylox (67%) ... 1802

Eructation
Ambien Tablets (Rare) ... 2416
Anafranil Capsules (Up to 2%) ... 803
Arfonad Ampuls ... 2080
▲ Asacol Delayed-Release Tablets (16%) ... 1979
Claritin-D (Less frequent) ... 2350
Clozaril Tablets (Less than 1%) ... 2252
Cytovene (1% or less) ... 2103
Dilacor XR Extended-release Capsules (Infrequent) ... 2018
Dolobid Tablets (Less than 1 in 100) ... 1654
Duvoid (Infrequent) ... 2044
Effexor (Frequent) ... 2719
Hivid Tablets (Less than 1% to less than 3%) ... 2121
Imitrex Injection (Rare) ... 1103
Intron A (Less than 5%) ... 2364
Lamictal Tablets (Rare) ... 1112
Lodine Capsules and Tablets (Less than 1%) ... 2743
Luvox Tablets (Infrequent) ... 2544
▲ Mycobutin Capsules (3%) ... 1957
Neurontin Capsules (Rare) ... 1922
Nicorette (1% to 3% of patients) .. 2458
Orap Tablets ... 1050
Orudis Capsules (Less than 1%) ... 2766
Oruvail Capsules (Less than 1%) ... 2766
Paxil Tablets (Infrequent) ... 2505
Pentasa (Less than 1%) ... 1527
Permax Tablets (Infrequent) ... 575
PREVACID Delayed-Release Capsules (Less than 1%) ... 2562
Procardia XL Extended Release Tablets (1% or less) ... 1972
Prozac Pulvules & Liquid, Oral Solution (Infrequent) ... 919
Questran Light (Less frequent) ... 769
Questran Powder (Less frequent) ... 770
Relafen Tablets (Less than 1%) ... 2510
Retrovir Capsules ... 1158
Retrovir I.V. Infusion ... 1163
Retrovir Syrup ... 1158
Risperdal (Rare) ... 1301
Serzone Tablets (Infrequent) ... 771
Toradol (1% or less) ... 2159
Trental Tablets (0.6%) ... 1244
Videx Tablets, Powder for Oral Solution, & Pediatric Powder for Oral Solution (Less than 1%) ... 720
Zoloft Tablets (Infrequent) ... 2217

Eruptions
Cuprimine Capsules ... 1630
Diabinese Tablets (Approximately 1% or less) ... 1935
Norpace (1 to 3%) ... 2444

Eruptions, acneiform (see under Acneiform eruptions)

Eruptions, bullous
Ambien Tablets (Rare) ... 2416
Cataflam (Rare) ... 816
Eulexin Capsules ... 2358
Felbatol (Infrequent) ... 2666
Fragmin (Rare) ... 1954
Hivid Tablets (Less than 1% to less than 3%) ... 2121
Loniten Tablets (Rare) ... 2618
Lozol Tablets ... 2022
Luvox Tablets ... 2544
Relafen Tablets (1%) ... 2510
Risperdal (Rare) ... 1301
▲ Tegison Capsules (1-10%) ... 2154
Voltaren Tablets (Rare) ... 861
Yodoxin ... 1230
Zoloft Tablets (Rare) ... 2217

Eruptions, cutaneous
Aldactazide ... 2413
Aldactone ... 2414
Rifater (Rare) ... 1532
Seldane-D Extended-Release Tablets ... 1538

Eruptions, eczematoid (see under Eczema)

Eruptions, erythema annulare centrifugum
Plaquenil Sulfate Tablets ... 2328

Eruptions, erythematous
Aldactazide ... 2413
Aldactone ... 2414
Macrobid Capsules ... 1988
Macrodantin Capsules ... 1989

Eruptions, exfoliative
Nydrazid Injection ... 508
Quinidex Extentabs ... 2067
Rifater ... 1532

Eruptions, fixed drug
Achromycin V Capsules (Rare) ... 1367
Cytovene (1% or less) ... 2103
Declomycin Tablets ... 1371
Depen Titratable Tablets ... 2662
Deponit NTG Transdermal Delivery System ... 2397
Miltown Tablets ... 2672
Minocin Intravenous (Rare) ... 1382
Minocin Oral Suspension (Rare) ... 1385
Minocin Pellet-Filled Capsules (Rare) ... 1383
Nitro-Bid IV ... 1523
Nitro-Bid Ointment (Uncommon) ... 1524
Nitro-Dur (nitroglycerin) Transdermal Infusion System (Uncommon) ... 1326
PMB 200 and PMB 400 ... 2783
Soma Compound w/Codeine Tablets ... 2676
Soma Compound Tablets ... 2675
Soma Tablets ... 2674

Eruptions, hemorrhagic
Amen Tablets ... 780
Brevicon ... 2088
Climara Transdermal System ... 645
Cycrin Tablets ... 975
Demulen ... 2428
Depo-Provera Sterile Aqueous Suspension ... 2606
Desogen Tablets ... 1817
Diethylstilbestrol Tablets ... 1437
Estrace Cream and Tablets ... 749
ESTRATAB Tablets (0.3, 0.625, 1.25, 2.5 mg) ... 2536
Estratest ... 2539
Levlen/Tri-Levlen ... 651
Lo/Ovral Tablets ... 2746
Lo/Ovral-28 Tablets ... 2751
Menest Tablets ... 2494
Micronor Tablets ... 1872
Modicon ... 1872
Nolvadex Tablets (Rare) ... 2841
Nordette-21 Tablets ... 2755
Nordette-28 Tablets ... 2758
Norinyl ... 2088
Nor-Q D Tablets ... 2135
Ogen Tablets ... 2627
Ogen Vaginal Cream ... 2630
Ortho-Cept ... 1851
Ortho-Cyclen/Ortho-Tri-Cyclen ... 1858
Ortho Dienestrol Cream ... 1866
Ortho-Est ... 1869
Ortho-Novum ... 1872
Ortho-Cyclen/Ortho Tri-Cyclen ... 1858
Ovcon ... 760
Ovral Tablets ... 2770
Ovral-28 Tablets ... 2770
Ovrette Tablets ... 2771
PMB 200 and PMB 400 ... 2783
Premarin Intravenous ... 2787
Premarin with Methyltestosterone .. 2794
Premarin Tablets ... 2789
Premarin Vaginal Cream ... 2791
Premphase ... 2797
Prempro ... 2801
Provera Tablets ... 2636
Stilphostrol Tablets and Ampuls ... 612
Levlen/Tri-Levlen ... 651
Tri-Norinyl ... 2164
Triphasil-21 Tablets ... 2814
Triphasil-28 Tablets ... 2819

Eruptions, herpetic
▲ CHEMET (succimer) Capsules (2.6 to 11.2%) ... 1545

Eruptions, lichenoid
Plaquenil Sulfate Tablets ... 2328

Eruptions, maculopapular
Aldactazide ... 2413
Aldactone ... 2414
Bicillin C-R Injection ... 2704
Bicillin C-R 900/300 Injection ... 2706
Bicillin L-A Injection ... 2707
DiaBeta Tablets (1.5%) ... 1239
Glucotrol Tablets (About 1 in 70) .. 1967
Glynase PresTab Tablets (1.5%) ... 2609
Macrobid Capsules ... 1988
Macrodantin Capsules ... 1989
Micronase Tablets (1.5%) ... 2623
Mustargen (Occasional) ... 1709
Nydrazid Injection ... 508
Pen•Vee K ... 2772
Pfizerpen for Injection ... 2203
Plaquenil Sulfate Tablets ... 2328
Rifater ... 1532

Eruptions, morbilliform
Ceclor Pulvules & Suspension (1 in 100) ... 1431
DiaBeta Tablets (1.5%) ... 1239
Glucotrol Tablets (About 1 in 70) .. 1967
Glynase PresTab Tablets (1.5%) ... 2609
Micronase Tablets (1.5%) ... 2623
Mysoline ... 2754
Nydrazid Injection ... 508
Plaquenil Sulfate Tablets ... 2328
Rifater ... 1532

Eruptions, mucocutaneous
▲ CHEMET (succimer) Capsules (2.6 to 11.2%) ... 1545

Eruptions, purpuric
Nydrazid Injection ... 508
Plaquenil Sulfate Tablets ... 2328
Rifater ... 1532

Eruptions, vascular
Pipracil (Less frequent) ... 1390

Erythema
A/T/S 2% Acne Topical Gel and Solution (Occasional) ... 1234
Accutane Capsules (Less than 1 patient in 10) ... 2076
▲ Acel-Imune Diphtheria and Tetanus Toxoids and Acellular Pertussis Vaccine Adsorbed (4% to 10%) ... 1364
Aclovate (1 in 100 patients) ... 1069
Americaine Anesthetic Lubricant ... 983
Americaine Otic Topical Anesthetic Ear Drops ... 983
Ativan Injection ... 2698
Bactroban Ointment (Less than 1%) ... 2470
Benzamycin Topical Gel ... 905
Betoptic Ophthalmic Solution (Rare) ... 469
Betoptic S Ophthalmic Suspension (Small number of patients) ... 471
Biavax II ... 1613
▲ Blenoxane (50%) ... 692
Brevibloc Injection (Less than 1%) 1808
Brevital Sodium Vials ... 1429
Brevoxyl Gel ... 2552
▲ Brevoxyl Cleansing Lotion (5 of 100 patients) ... 2553
Carbocaine Hydrochloride Injection 2303
▲ Catapres-TTS (26 of 101 patients) ... 675
Ceftin (Less than 1% but more than 0.1%) ... 1078
Cerumenex Drops (1% of 2,700 patients) ... 1993
Cholera Vaccine ... 2711
Cipro I.V. (1% or less) ... 595
Cipro I.V. Pharmacy Bulk Package (Less than 1%) ... 597
Claritin-D (Less frequent) ... 2350
▲ Cleocin T Topical (7%) ... 2590
▲ Climara Transdermal System (9%) 645
Clomid ... 1514
Clozaril Tablets (Less than 1%) ... 2252
Collagenase Santyl Ointment ... 1334
Compazine ... 2470
Cortone Acetate Sterile Suspension ... 1623
Cortone Acetate Tablets ... 1624
Cosmegen Injection ... 1626
Cozaar Tablets (Less than 1%) ... 1628
Cutivate Ointment (Less than 1%) 1089
Dalalone D.P. Injectable ... 1011
Dalgan Injection (Less than 1%) ... 538
Dantrium Intravenous (Rare) ... 1983
Decadron Elixir ... 1633
Decadron Phosphate Injection ... 1637
Decadron Phosphate Respihaler ... 1642
Decadron Phosphate Turbinaire ... 1645
Decadron Phosphate with Xylocaine Injection, Sterile ... 1639
Decadron Tablets ... 1635
Decadron-LA Sterile Suspension ... 1646
Desferal Vials ... 820
DesOwen Cream, Ointment and Lotion (Less than 2%) ... 1046
Desquam-E Gel ... 2684
Desquam-X Gel ... 2684

(▣ Described in PDR For Nonprescription Drugs) Incidence data in parenthesis; ▲ 3% or more (⊙ Described in PDR For Ophthalmology)

1293 Side Effects Index Erythema multiforme

Desquam-X 10 Bar 2684
Desquam-X Wash 2684
Dexacort Phosphate in Respihaler 458
Dexacort Phosphate in Turbinaire 459
DiaBeta Tablets (1.5%) 1239
Digibind (One patient) 1091
Dipentum Capsules (Rare) 1951
Diphtheria & Tetanus Toxoids Adsorbed Purogenated (Mild) 1374
Diprivan Injection (Rare) 2833
Diprolene AF Cream (Less than 1%) 2352
Diprolene Gel 0.05% (Less frequent) 2353
Diprolene (Less than 1%) 2352
▲ Dovonex Ointment 0.005% (1% to 10%) 2684
Duragesic Transdermal System (1% or greater) 1288
▲ Efudex (Among most frequent) 2113
Elimite (permethrin) 5% Cream (1 to 2% or less) 478
▲ Emla Cream (30%) 545
Engerix-B Unit-Dose Vials (Less than 1%) 2482
Erycette (erythromycin 2%) Topical Solution 1888
Etrafon 2355
Eulexin Capsules 2358
Exelderm Cream 1.0% (1%) 2685
Feldene Capsules (Less than 1%) 1965
Fioricet with Codeine Capsules 2260
Fiorinal with Codeine Capsules 2262
Fluorouracil Injection 2116
▲ Sterile FUDR (Among more common) 2118
Glucotrol Tablets (About 1 in 70) 1967
Glynase PresTab Tablets (1.5%) 2609
▲ Habitrol Nicotine Transdermal System (Once in 35% of patients; 22 of 220 patients) 865
Heparin Lock Flush Solution 2725
Heparin Sodium Injection 2726
Heparin Sodium Injection, USP, Sterile Solution 2615
Heparin Sodium Vials 1441
Hydeltrasol Injection, Sterile 1665
Hydeltra-T.B.A. Sterile Suspension 1667
Hydrea Capsules 696
Hydrocortone Acetate Sterile Suspension 1669
Hydrocortone Phosphate Injection, Sterile 1670
Hydrocortone Tablets 1672
Hyzaar Tablets 1677
Imitrex Injection (Infrequent) 1103
Imitrex Tablets (Infrequent) 1106
Intron A (Less than 5%) 2364
▲ IPOL Poliovirus Vaccine Inactivated (3.2%) 885
▲ Lac-Hydrin 12% Lotion (1 in 10 to 50 patients) 2687
Lamictal Tablets (Infrequent) 1112
Lamprene Capsules (Less than 1%) 828
▲ Leustatin (6%) 1834
Levoprome 1274
Livostin (Approximately 1% to 3%) ⊙ 266
Lotrimin 2371
Lotrisone Cream 2372
Lovenox Injection 2020
Lupron Injection 2555
M-M-R II 1687
M-R-VAX II 1689
Marcaine Hydrochloride with Epinephrine 1:200,000 (Rare) 2316
Marcaine Hydrochloride Injection (Rare) 2316
Marcaine Spinal (Rare) 2319
Melanex Topical Solution 1793
Mellaril 2269
Menomune-A/C/Y/W-135 889
Meruvax II 1697
MetroGel 1047
Metubine Iodide Vials 916
▲ Miacalcin Nasal Spray (10.6%) 2275
Micronase Tablets (1.5%) 2623
Mini-Gamulin Rh, Rh_0(D) Immune Globulin (Human) (Occasional) 520
8-MOP Capsules 1246
Monocid Injection (Less than 1%) 2497
Mutamycin 703
Naftin Cream 1% (2%) 480
Naftin Gel 1% (0.5%) 481
NebuPent for Inhalation Solution (1% or less) 1040
NegGram 2323
Nescaine/Nescaine MPF 554
▲ Nicoderm (nicotine transdermal system) (14%) 1518
Nicorette 2458
Nicotrol Nicotine Transdermal System (At least once in 47 patients) 1550
Nolvadex Tablets 2841
Noroxin Tablets (Less frequent) 1715
Noroxin Tablets (Less frequent) 2048
▲ Oncaspar (Greater than 5%) 2028
Orthoclone OKT3 Sterile Solution 1837
Oxistat Cream (0.2%) 1152
Oxsoralen-Ultra Capsules 1257
Paraplatin for Injection 705
PedvaxHIB 1718
Pipracil (2%) 1390
Plendil Extended-Release Tablets (0.5% to 1.5%) 527
Prinivil Tablets (0.3% to 1.0%) 1733
Prinzide Tablets 1737
Profasi (chorionic gonadotropin for injection, USP) 2450
▲ Proleukin for Injection (41%) 797
Prolixin 509
Prostep (nicotine transdermal system) (At least once in 22% of patients) 1394
Recombivax HB (Equal to or greater than 1%) 1744
Retin-A (tretinoin) Cream/Gel/Liquid 1889
Rifater 1532
Rogaine Topical Solution 2637
Sensorcaine (Rare) 559
Serentil 684
Solganal Suspension 2388
▲ Spectazole (econazole nitrate 1%) Cream (3%) 1890
Stelazine 2514
Sufenta Injection (0.3% to 1%) 1309
Sulfamylon Cream 925
Supprelin Injection (1%) 2056
T-Stat 2.0% Topical Solution and Pads 2688
Temaril Tablets, Syrup and Spansule Extended-Release Capsules 483
Temovate (1 of 366 patients) 1179
Tetanus Toxoid Adsorbed Purogenated 1403
Theramycin Z Topical Solution 2% 1592
Topicort LP Emollient Cream 0.05% (0.8%) 1243
Torecan 2245
Tracrium Injection (0.6%) 1183
Transderm Scōp Transdermal Therapeutic System (Infrequent) 869
Triavil Tablets 1757
Trilafon 2389
▲ Tripedia (3% to 25%) 892
Tympagesic Ear Drops 2342
Ultravate Cream 0.05% (Less frequent) 2689
Ultravate Ointment 0.05% (Less frequent) 2690
Unasyn (Less than 1%) 2212
▲ Videx Tablets, Powder for Oral Solution, & Pediatric Powder for Oral Solution (4% to 5%) 720
▲ Yutopar Intravenous Injection (10 to 15%) 570
Zefazone 2654
Zestoretic 2850
Zestril Tablets (0.3% to 1.0%) 2854
▲ Zinecard (4% to 5%) 1961

Erythema at injection site

▲ ActHIB (Up to 24.0%) 872
▲ Actimmune (14%) 1056
Attenuvax 1610
DDAVP Injection (Occasional) 2014
DDAVP Injection 15 mcg/mL (Occasional) 2015
Diphtheria and Tetanus Toxoids and Pertussis Vaccine Adsorbed 2477
Diphtheria and Tetanus Toxoids and Pertussis Vaccine Adsorbed USP (For Pediatric Use) (1 in 3 doses) 875
▲ Engerix-B Unit-Dose Vials (1% to 10%) 2482
Floxin I.V. (Approximately 2%) 1571
Gamimune N, 5% Immune Globulin Intravenous (Human), 5% (Some cases) 619
Gamimune N, 10% Immune Globulin Intravenous (Human), 10% (Some cases) 621
Helixate, Antihemophilic Factor (Recombinant) (Two reports out of 3,254 patients) 518
HibTITER (Less than 1% to 2.0%) 1375
▲ Imovax Rabies Vaccine (About 25%) 881
KOGENATE Antihemophilic Factor (Recombinant) 632
▲ Leustatin (9% to 19%) 1834
Mivacron (Less than 1%) 1138
▲ Navelbine Injection (Approximately one-third of patients) 1145
▲ OmniHIB (0.3% to 24.0%) 2499
▲ Pneumovax 23 (Common) 1725
Primaxin I.V. (0.4%) 1729
Rabies Vaccine Adsorbed (A few patients) 2508
▲ Rabies Vaccine, Imovax Rabies I.D. (About 25%) 883
Taxol 714
▲ Tetramune (19% to 40%) 1404
Tubersol (Tuberculin Purified Protein Derivative [Mantoux]) (Infrequent) 2872
▲ Typhim Vi (Up to 11%) 899
▲ Varivax (19.3% to 32.5%) 1762
Velosulin BR Human Insulin 10 ml Vials 1795

Erythema, conjunctival

▲ AK-Spore (Among most frequent) ⊙ 204
▲ AKTOB (Among most frequent; less than 3 of 100 patients) ⊙ 206
Neosporin Ophthalmic Ointment Sterile 1148
Neosporin Ophthalmic Solution Sterile 1149
▲ Polysporin Ophthalmic Ointment Sterile (Among those occurring most often) 1154
▲ Rēv-Eyes Ophthalmic Eyedrops 0.5% (10% to 40%) ⊙ 323
TobraDex Ophthalmic Suspension and Ointment (Less than 4%) 473
Tobrex Ophthalmic Ointment and Solution (Less than 3 of 100 patients) ⊙ 229

Erythema, facial

Aristocort Suspension (Forte Parenteral) 1027
Aristocort Suspension (Intralesional) 1025
Aristocort Tablets 1022
Aristospan Suspension (Intra-articular) 1033
Aristospan Suspension (Intralesional) 1032
Celestone Soluspan Suspension 2347
CORTENEMA 2535
Deltasone Tablets 2595
Depo-Medrol Single-Dose Vial 2600
Depo-Medrol Sterile Aqueous Suspension 2597
Florinef Acetate Tablets 505
Hydrea Capsules (Less frequent) 696
Medrol 2621
Normodyne Tablets (Less common) 2379
Pediapred Oral Liquid 995
Prelone Syrup 1787
Solu-Cortef Sterile Powder 2641
Solu-Medrol Sterile Powder 2643
Trandate Tablets (Less common) 1185

Erythema, hemorrhagic exudative (see under Henoch-Schonlein purpura)

Erythema, maculopapular

Teslac 717

Erythema multiforme

Acel-Imune Diphtheria and Tetanus Toxoids and Acellular Pertussis Vaccine Adsorbed 1364
Children's Advil Suspension (Less than 1%) 2692
Aldactazide 2413
Aldoclor Tablets 1598
Aldoril Tablets 1604
Altace Capsules (Less than 1%) 1232
Amen Tablets 780
Amoxil 2464
Anaprox/Naprosyn (Less than 1%) 2117
Atretol Tablets 573
Attenuvax (Rare) 1610
Augmentin 2468
Azactam for Injection (Less than 1%) 734
Azo Gantanol Tablets 2080
Azo Gantrisin Tablets 2081
Azulfidine (Rare) 1949
Bactrim DS Tablets 2084
Bactrim I.V. Infusion 2082
Bactrim 2084
Biavax II (Rare) 1613
Brevicon 2088
Calan SR Caplets (1% or less) 2422
Calan Tablets (1% or less) 2419
Capoten 739
Capozide 742
Cardizem CD Capsules (Infrequent) 1506
Cardizem SR Capsules (Infrequent) 1510
Cardizem Injectable 1508
Cardizem Tablets (Infrequent) 1512
Cataflam (Rare) 816
Ceclor Pulvules & Suspension 1431
Cefizox for Intramuscular or Intravenous Use 1034
Cefotan 2829
Ceftin 1078
Cefzil Tablets and Oral Suspension (Rare) 746
Ceptaz 1081
Chibroxin Sterile Ophthalmic Solution (With oral form) 1617
Cipro I.V. (1% or less) 595
Cipro I.V. Pharmacy Bulk Package (Less than 1%) 597
Cipro Tablets 592
Claritin (Rare) 2349
Claritin-D 2350
Cleocin Phosphate Injection (Rare) 2586
Climara Transdermal System 645
Cleocin Vaginal Cream (Rare) 2589
Clinoril Tablets (Less than 1%) 1618
Clomid 1514
Clozaril Tablets 2252
Cycrin Tablets 975
Daypro Caplets (Less than 1%) 2426
Decadron Phosphate with Xylocaine Injection, Sterile 1639
Demulen 2428
Depakene 413
Depakote Tablets 415
Depo-Provera Sterile Aqueous Suspension 2606
Desogen Tablets 1817
Diabinese Tablets 1935
Diamox 1372
Diethylstilbestrol Tablets 1437
Diphtheria and Tetanus Toxoids and Pertussis Vaccine Adsorbed 2477
Diupres Tablets 1650
Diuril Oral Suspension 1653
Diuril Sodium Intravenous 1652
Diuril Tablets 1653
Dolobid Tablets (Less than 1 in 100) 1654
Duricef 748
Dynacin Capsules 1590
EC-Naprosyn Delayed-Release Tablets (Less than 1%) 2117
Engerix-B Unit-Dose Vials 2482
Esgic-plus Tablets (Several cases) 1013
Estrace Cream and Tablets 749
ESTRATAB Tablets (0.3, 0.625, 1.25, 2.5 mg) 2536
Estratest 2539
Fansidar Tablets 2114
Feldene Capsules (Less than 1%) 1965
Fioricet with Codeine Capsules 2260
Fiorinal Capsules (Several cases) 2261
Fiorinal with Codeine Capsules 2262
Fiorinal Tablets (Several cases) 2261
Floxin I.V. 1571
Floxin Tablets (200 mg, 300 mg, 400 mg) 1567
Fortaz 1100
Gantanol Tablets 2119
Gantrisin 2120
Glauctabs ⊙ 208
Havrix (Rare) 2489
Hespan Injection 929
HibTITER 1375
HydroDIURIL Tablets 1674
Hydropres Tablets 1675
Hyzaar Tablets 1677
IBU Tablets (Less than 1%) 1342
Indocin Capsules (Less than 1%) 1680
Indocin I.V. (Less than 1%) 1684
Indocin (Less than 1%) 1680
Isoptin Oral Tablets (Less than 1%) 1346
Isoptin SR Tablets (1% or less) 1348
Keflex Pulvules & Oral Suspension (Rare) 914
Keftab Tablets (Rare) 915
Kefurox Vials, Faspak & ADD-Vantage 1454
Lamictal Tablets 1112

(▣ Described in PDR For Nonprescription Drugs) Incidence data in parenthesis; ▲ 3% or more (⊙ Described in PDR For Ophthalmology)

Erythema multiforme — Side Effects Index — 1294

Lariam Tablets 2128
Lasix Injection, Oral Solution and Tablets 1240
Lescol Capsules (Rare) 2267
Leukeran Tablets (Rare) 1133
Levlen/Tri-Levlen 651
Lincocin (Rare instances) 2617
Lodine Capsules and Tablets (Less than 1%) 2743
Lo/Ovral Tablets 2746
Lo/Ovral-28 Tablets 2751
Lorabid Suspension and Pulvules 1459
Lupron Depot-PED 7.5 mg, 11.25 mg and 15 mg (2%) 2560
M-M-R II (Rare) 1687
M-R-VAX II (Rare) 1689
MZM (Common) ◉ 267
Macrobid Capsules (Rare) 1988
Macrodantin Capsules (Rare) 1989
Menest Tablets 2494
Meruvax II (Rare) 1697
Mesantoin Tablets (Rare) 2272
Mevacor Tablets (Rare) 1699
Micronor Tablets 1872
Milontin Kapseals 1920
Miltown Tablets (Rare) 2672
Minocin Intravenous 1382
Minocin Oral Suspension 1385
Minocin Pellet-Filled Capsules 1383
Mintezol 1704
Modicon 1872
Moduretic Tablets 1705
Children's Motrin Ibuprofen Oral Suspension (Less than 1%) 1546
Motrin Tablets (Less than 1%) 2625
Motrin Ibuprofen Suspension, Oral Drops, Chewable Tablets, Caplets (Less than 1%) 1546
Mumpsvax (Rare) 1708
Mustargen 1709
Myleran Tablets (Rare) 1143
Anaprox/Naprosyn (Less than 1%) 2117
Neptazane Tablets 1388
Nordette-21 Tablets 2755
Nordette-28 Tablets 2758
Norinyl 2088
Noroxin Tablets 1715
Noroxin Tablets 2048
Nor-Q D Tablets 2135
Ogen Tablets 2627
Ogen Vaginal Cream 2630
Omnipen Capsules 2764
Omnipen for Oral Suspension 2765
Ortho-Cept 1851
Ortho-Cyclen/Ortho-Tri-Cyclen 1858
Ortho Dienestrol Cream 1866
Ortho-Est 1869
Ortho-Novum 1872
Ortho-Cyclen/Ortho Tri-Cyclen 1858
Ovcon 760
Ovral Tablets 2770
Ovral-28 Tablets 2770
Ovrette Tablets 2771
PCE Dispertab Tablets (Rare) 444
PMB 200 and PMB 400 2783
Penetrex Tablets (Less than 1% but more than or equal to 0.1%) 2031
Phrenilin (Several cases) 785
Pipracil (Rare) 1390
Pravachol (Rare) 765
Premarin Intravenous 2787
Premarin with Methyltestosterone 2794
Premarin Tablets 2789
Premarin Vaginal Cream 2791
Premphase 2797
Prempro 2801
Prilosec Delayed-Release Capsules (Very rare) 529
Primaxin I.M. 1727
Primaxin I.V. (Less than 0.2%) 1729
Prinzide Tablets 1737
Proloprim Tablets (Rare) 1155
Proventil Syrup (Rare) 2385
Provera Tablets 2636
Prozac Pulvules & Liquid, Oral Solution (Rare) 919
Relafen Tablets (Rare) 2510
Ritalin 848
Rocaltrol Capsules (One case) 2141
SSD (Infrequent) 1355
Sedapap Tablets 50 mg/650 mg (Several cases) 1543
Semprex-D Capsules (Rare) 463
Semprex-D Capsules (Rare) 1167
Septra 1174
Septra I.V. Infusion 1169
Septra I.V. Infusion ADD-Vantage Vials 1171
Septra 1174
Silvadene Cream 1% (Infrequent) 1540
Soma Compound w/Codeine Tablets 2676
Soma Compound Tablets 2675
Soma Tablets 2674
Spectrobid Tablets 2206
Stilphostrol Tablets and Ampuls 612
Suprax (Less than 2%) 1399
Tagamet (Very rare) 2516
Tazicef for Injection 2519
Tegretol Chewable Tablets 852
Tegretol Suspension 852
Tegretol Tablets 852
Tetramune 1404
Ticlid Tablets (Rare) 2156
Timolide Tablets 1748
Tolectin (200, 400 and 600 mg) (Less than 1%) 1581
Tonocard Tablets (Less than 1%) 531
Trancopal Caplets (Rare) 2337
Tri-Immunol Adsorbed 1408
Levlen/Tri-Levlen 651
Trilisate (Rare) 2000
Trimpex Tablets (Rare) 2163
Tri-Norinyl 2164
Triphasil-21 Tablets 2814
Triphasil-28 Tablets 2819
Unasyn 2212
Vantin for Oral Suspension and Vantin Tablets 2646
Vaseretic Tablets 1765
Vasotec I.V. 1768
Vasotec Tablets (0.5% to 1.0%) 1771
Ventolin Syrup (Rare) 1202
Verelan Capsules (1% or less) 1410
Verelan Capsules (Less than 1%) 2824
Voltaren Tablets (Rare) 861
Zantac (Rare) 1209
Zantac Injection (Rare) 1207
Zantac Syrup (Rare) 1209
Zefazone 2654
Zestoretic 2850
Zinacef (Rare) 1211
Zocor Tablets (Rare) 1775
Zoloft Tablets (Rare) 2217
Zosyn (Rare) 1419
Zosyn Pharmacy Bulk Package (Rare) 1422
Zyloprim Tablets (Less than 1%) 1226

Erythema nodosum

Accutane Capsules (Less than 1%) 2076
Amen Tablets 780
Asacol Delayed-Release Tablets 1979
Atretol Tablets 573
Betaseron for SC Injection 658
Brevicon 2088
Cipro I.V. (1% or less) 595
Cipro I.V. Pharmacy Bulk Package (Less than 1%) 597
Cipro Tablets (Less than 1%) 592
Climara Transdermal System 645
Clomid 1514
Cycrin Tablets 975
Demulen 2428
Depo-Provera Sterile Aqueous Suspension 2606
Desogen Tablets 1817
Diethylstilbestrol Tablets 1437
Dipentum Capsules (Rare) 1951
Engerix-B Unit-Dose Vials 2482
Estrace Cream and Tablets 749
ESTRATAB Tablets (0.3, 0.625, 1.25, 2.5 mg) 2536
Estratest 2539
Floxin I.V. 1571
Floxin Tablets (200 mg, 300 mg, 400 mg) 1567
Indocin Capsules (Less than 1%) 1680
Indocin I.V. (Less than 1%) 1684
Indocin (Less than 1%) 1680
Levlen/Tri-Levlen 651
Lo/Ovral Tablets 2746
Lo/Ovral-28 Tablets 2751
Maxaquin Tablets 2440
Menest Tablets 2494
Micronor Tablets 1872
Modicon 1872
Myleran Tablets (Rare) 1143
Neupogen for Injection (One event) 495
Nordette-21 Tablets 2755
Nordette-28 Tablets 2758
Norinyl 2088
Nor-Q D Tablets 2135
Ogen Tablets 2627
Ogen Vaginal Cream 2630
Ortho-Cept 1851
Ortho-Cyclen/Ortho-Tri-Cyclen 1858
Ortho Dienestrol Cream 1866
Ortho-Est 1869
Ortho-Novum 1872
Ortho-Cyclen/Ortho Tri-Cyclen 1858
Ovcon 760
Ovral Tablets 2770
Ovral-28 Tablets 2770
Ovrette Tablets 2771
PMB 200 and PMB 400 2783
Paxil Tablets (Rare) 2505
Penetrex Tablets 2031
Pentasa (Less than 1%) 1527
Premarin Intravenous 2787
Premarin with Methyltestosterone 2794
Premarin Tablets 2789
Premarin Vaginal Cream 2791
Premphase 2797
Prempro 2801
Provera Tablets 2636
Recombivax HB (Less than 1%) 1744
Stilphostrol Tablets and Ampuls 612
Tegretol Chewable Tablets 852
Tegretol Suspension 852
Tegretol Tablets 852
Levlen/Tri-Levlen 651
Tri-Norinyl 2164
Triphasil-21 Tablets 2814
Triphasil-28 Tablets 2819

Erythema simplex

Oncaspar (Less than 1%) 2028

Erythematous streaking

Adriamycin PFS 1947
Adriamycin RDF 1947
Doxorubicin Astra 540
Rubex 712
▲ Zinecard (4% to 5%) 1961

Erythrocyte survival time, shortened

Easprin 1914

Erythrocytes, abnormal

Effexor (Rare) 2719
Hydrea Capsules 696
Paxil Tablets (Rare) 2505

Erythrocytes, vacuolation of

Pyrazinamide Tablets (Rare) 1398
Rifater (Rare) 1532

Erythrocytosis

Danocrine Capsules 2307
Moban Tablets and Concentrate 1048
Pergonal (menotropins for injection, USP) (One patient) 2448
Ponstel 1925

Erythrocyturia

Amikacin Sulfate Injection, USP 960
Amikin Injectable 501
Netromycin Injection 100 mg/ml 2373
Quadrinal Tablets 1350

Erythroderma, exfoliative

Tagamet 2516

Erythroid hyperplasia

Pyrazinamide Tablets (Rare) 1398
Rifater (Rare) 1532

Erythromelalgia

Adalat Capsules (10 mg and 20 mg) (Less than 0.5%) 587
Adalat CC (Rare) 589
Parlodel 2281
Procardia Capsules (Less than 0.5%) 1971

Erythropenia

▲ Accutane Capsules (1 in 5 to 1 in 10 patients) 2076
Apresazide Capsules (Less frequent) 808
Dopram Injectable 2061
Haldol Decanoate 1577
Loniten Tablets 2618
Moban Tablets and Concentrate 1048
Mustargen 1709
Ponstel 1925
Primaxin I.M. 1727
Ser-Ap-Es Tablets 849
Unasyn 2212
Zefazone 2654

Escharotic effect

Cetacaine Topical Anesthetic 794

Esophageal disease, unspecified

Ansaid Tablets (Less than 1%) 2579
Myleran Tablets 1143

Esophageal necrosis

Ethamolin (0.1 to 0.4%) 2400

Esophageal stricture

▲ Ethamolin (Among most common; 1.3%) 2400
Lodine Capsules and Tablets (Less than 1%) 2743
PREVACID Delayed-Release Capsules (Less than 1%) 2562

Esophageal ulceration

Cytosar-U Sterile Powder (Less frequent) 2592
Doryx Capsules (Rare) 1913
Mexitil Capsules (About 1 in 10,000) 678
Micro-K 2063
Micro-K LS Packets 2064
Minocin Pellet-Filled Capsules (Rare) 1383
Pediapred Oral Liquid 995
PREVACID Delayed-Release Capsules (Less than 1%) 2562
Slow-K Extended-Release Tablets 851

Esophagitis

Achromycin V Capsules (Rare) 1367
Adalat CC (Less than 1.0%) 589
Adriamycin PFS 1947
Adriamycin RDF 1947
Anafranil Capsules (Up to 1%) 803
Betaseron for SC Injection 658
▲ CellCept Capsules (More than or equal to 3%) 2099
Cleocin Vaginal Cream 2589
Cognex Capsules (Infrequent) 1901
Cosmegen Injection 1626
Cytosar-U Sterile Powder (Less frequent) 2592
Didronel Tablets 1984
Doryx Capsules (Rare) 1913
Doxorubicin Astra 540
Dynacin Capsules (Rare) 1590
Effexor (Infrequent) 2719
Ethamolin (0.1 to 0.4%) 2400
Felbatol (Infrequent) 2666
Fioricet with Codeine Capsules 2260
Fiorinal with Codeine Capsules 2262
Fludara for Injection (Up to 3%) 663
Hivid Tablets (Less than 1% to less than 3%) 2121
Intron A (Less than 5%) 2364
Lamictal Tablets 1112
Lodine Capsules and Tablets (Less than 1%) 2743
Lotrel Capsules 840
Luvox Tablets (Infrequent) 2544
Minocin Pellet-Filled Capsules (Rare) 1383
Monodox Capsules (Rare) 1805
Motrin Ibuprofen Suspension, Oral Drops, Chewable Tablets, Caplets (Less than 1%) 1546
NebuPent for Inhalation Solution (1% or less) 1040
Neurontin Capsules (Rare) 1922
Paxil Tablets (Rare) 2505
Permax Tablets (Infrequent) 575
PREVACID Delayed-Release Capsules (Less than 1%) 2562
Prozac Pulvules & Liquid, Oral Solution (Infrequent) 919
▲ Quinaglute Dura-Tabs Tablets (Among most frequent) 649
▲ Quinidex Extentabs (Among most frequent) 2067
Risperdal (Rare) 1301
Rythmol Tablets–150mg, 225mg, 300mg (1.9%) 1352
Salagen Tablets (Less than 1%) 1489
Serzone Tablets (Infrequent) 771
Trilisate (Rare) 2000
Urobiotic-250 Capsules (Rare) 2214
Vibramycin (Rare) 1941
Videx Tablets, Powder for Oral Solution, & Pediatric Powder for Oral Solution (Less than 1%) 720
Wellbutrin Tablets 1204
▲ Zinecard (3% to 6%) 1961

Esophagitis, ulcerative

Achromycin V Capsules (Rare) 1367
Aristocort Suspension (Forte Parenteral) 1027
Aristocort Suspension (Intralesional) 1025
Aristospan Suspension (Intra-articular) 1033
Aristospan Suspension (Intralesional) 1032

(▣ Described in PDR For Nonprescription Drugs) Incidence data in parenthesis; ▲ 3% or more (◉ Described in PDR For Ophthalmology)

1295 Side Effects Index Excitability

Celestone Soluspan Suspension 2347
CORTENEMA 2535
Cortone Acetate Sterile Suspension 1623
Cortone Acetate Tablets 1624
Dalalone D.P. Injectable 1011
Decadron Elixir 1633
Decadron Phosphate Injection 1637
Decadron Phosphate Respihaler 1642
Decadron Phosphate Turbinaire 1645
Decadron Phosphate with Xylocaine Injection, Sterile 1639
Decadron Tablets 1635
Decadron-LA Sterile Suspension 1646
Deltasone Tablets 2595
Depo-Medrol Single-Dose Vial 2600
Depo-Medrol Sterile Aqueous Suspension 2597
Dynacin Capsules (Rare) 1590
Florinef Acetate Tablets 505
Foscavir Injection (Less than 1%) 547
Hydeltrasol Injection, Sterile 1665
Hydeltra-T.B.A. Sterile Suspension 1667
Hydrocortone Phosphate Injection, Sterile 1670
Hydrocortone Tablets 1672
Indocin I.V. (Less than 1%) 1684
Medrol 2621
Monodox Capsules (Rare) 1805
Prelone Syrup 1787
Solu-Cortef Sterile Powder 2641
Solu-Medrol Sterile Powder 2643
Vibramycin (Rare) 1941

Esophagopharyngitis

Ergamisol Tablets 1292
Fluorouracil Injection (Common) 2116
Sterile FUDR 2118

Esophagospasm

Ambien Tablets (Rare) 2416
Gastrocrom Capsules (Infrequent) 984
Neurontin Capsules (Rare) 1922

Esophagus, perforation

Ethamolin (0.1 to 0.4%) 2400

Estrogen, decrease

Cytoxan 694
NEOSAR Lyophilized/Neosar 1959

Euphoria

Actifed with Codeine Cough Syrup 1067
Adipex-P Tablets and Capsules 1048
Akineton 1333
Alfenta Injection (0.3% to 1%) 1286
Ambien Tablets (Frequent) 2416
Anafranil Capsules (Infrequent) 803
Aristocort Suspension (Forte Parenteral) 1027
Aristocort Suspension (Intralesional) 1025
Aristocort Tablets 1022
Aristospan Suspension (Intra-articular) 1033
Aristospan Suspension (Intralesional) 1032
Artane 1368
Atamet 572
Benadryl Capsules 1898
Benadryl Injection 1898
Bentyl 10 mg Capsules 1501
Betaseron for SC Injection 658
Biphetamine Capsules 983
▲ Bromfed-DM Cough Syrup (Among most frequent) 1786
Brontex 1981
BuSpar (Infrequent) 737
Celestone Soluspan Suspension 2347
Claritin-D (Less frequent) 2350
CORTENEMA 2535
Cortone Acetate Sterile Suspension 1623
Cortone Acetate Tablets 1624
Cytovene (1% or less) 2103
Dalmane Capsules (Rare) 2173
Darvon-N/Darvocet-N 1433
Darvon 1435
Darvon-N Suspension & Tablets 1433
Decadron Elixir 1633
Decadron Phosphate Injection 1637
Decadron Phosphate Respihaler 1642
Decadron Phosphate Turbinaire 1645
Decadron Phosphate with Xylocaine Injection, Sterile 1639
Decadron Tablets 1635
Decadron-LA Sterile Suspension 1646
Deconamine 1320
Deltasone Tablets 2595
Demerol 2308
Depo-Medrol Sterile Aqueous Suspension 2597
Desoxyn Gradumet Tablets 419
Dexacort Phosphate in Respihaler 458
Dexacort Phosphate in Turbinaire 459
Dexedrine 2474
DextroStat Dextroamphetamine Tablets 2036
Dilaudid-HP Injection (Less frequent) 1337
Dilaudid-HP Lyophilized Powder 250 mg (Less frequent) 1337
Dilaudid Tablets and Liquid 1339
Dimetane-DC Cough Syrup 2059
Dimetane-DX Cough Syrup 2059
Diprivan Injection (Less than 1%) 2833
Doral Tablets 2664
▲ Duragesic Transdermal System (3% to 10%) 1288
Duramorph 962
Duranest Injections 542
Dyclone 0.5% and 1% Topical Solutions, USP 544
Effexor (Infrequent) 2719
Emla Cream 545
Empirin with Codeine Tablets 1093
Ergamisol Tablets 1292
Esgic-plus Tablets (Infrequent) 1013
Ethmozine Tablets (Less than 2%) 2041
Fastin Capsules 2488
Felbatol (Infrequent) 2666
Fioricet Tablets (Infrequent) 2258
Fioricet with Codeine Capsules (Infrequent) 2260
Florinef Acetate Tablets 505
Floxin I.V. (Less than 1%) 1571
Floxin Tablets (200 mg, 300 mg, 400 mg) (Less than 1%) 1567
Flumadine Tablets & Syrup (Less than 0.3%) 1015
Fluorouracil Injection 2116
Sterile FUDR (Remote possibility) 2118
Halcion Tablets (0.9% to 0.5%) 2611
Haldol Decanoate 1577
Haldol Injection, Tablets and Concentrate 1575
Hivid Tablets (Less than 1% to less than 3%) 2121
Hydeltrasol Injection, Sterile 1665
Hydeltra-T.B.A. Sterile Suspension 1667
Hydrocortone Acetate Sterile Suspension 1669
Hydrocortone Phosphate Injection, Sterile 1670
Hydrocortone Tablets 1672
Hyperstat I.V. Injection 2363
Imitrex Injection (Infrequent) 1103
Imitrex Tablets (Infrequent) 1106
Infumorph 200 and Infumorph 500 Sterile Solutions 965
Ionamin Capsules 990
Lamictal Tablets (Infrequent) 1112
Larodopa Tablets (Relatively frequent) 2129
Levsin/Levsinex/Levbid 2405
Limbitrol 2180
Lioresal Tablets 829
Lomotil 2439
Luvox Tablets (Infrequent) 2544
▲ MS Contin Tablets (Among most freqent) 1994
▲ MSIR (Among most frequent) 1997
Macrodantin Capsules (Rare) 1989
▲ Marinol (Dronabinol) Capsules (3% to 10%) 2231
Mepergan Injection 2753
Methadone Hydrochloride Oral Concentrate 2233
Methadone Hydrochloride Oral Solution & Tablets 2235
Miltown Tablets 2672
Moban Tablets and Concentrate (Less frequent) 1048
Motofen Tablets 784
Nardil (Less common) 1920
Neurontin Capsules (Infrequent) 1922
Nicorette 2458
Nubain Injection (1% or less) 935
▲ Oramorph SR (Morphine Sulfate Sustained Release Tablets) (Among most frequent) 2236
Orlamm (1% to 3%) 2239
Ornade Spansule Capsules 2502
PBZ Tablets 845
PBZ-SR Tablets 844
PMB 200 and PMB 400 2783
Paxil Tablets (Rare) 2505
Percocet Tablets 938
Percodan Tablets 939
Percodan-Demi Tablets 940
Periactin 1724
Permax Tablets (Infrequent) 575
Phenergan with Codeine 2777
Phenergan Injection 2773
Phenergan Tablets 2775
Phenergan VC with Codeine 2781
Phrenilin (Infrequent) 785
Prelone Syrup 1787
Prelu-2 Timed Release Capsules 681
ProSom Tablets (Infrequent) 449
Prozac Pulvules & Liquid, Oral Solution (Infrequent) 919
RMS Suppositories 2657
Restoril Capsules (2-3%) 2284
Risperdal (Infrequent) 1301
Romazicon (1% to 3%) 2147
Roxanol 2243
Roxicodone Tablets, Oral Solution & Intensol (Oxycodone) 2244
Sansert Tablets 2295
Sedapap Tablets 50 mg/650 mg (Infrequent) 1543
Serax Capsules 2810
Serax Tablets 2810
Serzone Tablets (Infrequent) 771
Sinemet Tablets 943
Sinemet CR Tablets 944
Soma Compound w/Codeine Tablets 2676
Soma Compound Tablets (Very rare) 2675
Soma Tablets 2674
Stadol (1% or greater) 775
Symmetrel Capsules and Syrup (0.1% to 1%) 946
Talacen 2333
▲ Talwin Injection (Most common) 2334
Talwin Compound 2335
▲ Talwin Injection (Most common) 2334
Talwin Nx 2336
Tambocor Tablets (Less than 1%) 1497
Tavist Syrup 2297
Tavist Tablets 2298
Temaril Tablets, Syrup and Spansule Extended-Release Capsules 483
Toradol (1% or less) 2159
Tornalate Solution for Inhalation, 0.2% (Less than 1%) 956
Trinalin Repetabs Tablets 1330
Tussend 1783
Tussionex Pennkinetic Extended-Release Suspension 998
Tussi-Organidin NR Liquid and S NR Liquid (At higher doses) 2677
Tylenol with Codeine 1583
Tylox Capsules 1584
▲ Ultram Tablets (50 mg) (1% to 14%) 1585
Versed Injection (Less than 1%) 2170
Wellbutrin Tablets (1.2%) 1204
Wygesic Tablets 2827
▲ Xylocaine Injections (Among most common) 567
Zarontin Capsules 1928
Zarontin Syrup 1929
Zoloft Tablets (Infrequent) 2217

Exanthema

Calan SR Caplets (1% or less) 2422
Calan Tablets (1% or less) 2419
Isoptin Oral Tablets (Less than 1%) 1346
Isoptin SR Tablets (1% or less) 1348
Verelan Capsules (1% or less) 1410
Verelan Capsules (Less than 1%) 2824

Excitability

Actifed Plus Caplets ▣ 845
Actifed Plus Tablets ▣ 845
Actifed with Codeine Cough Syrup 1067
Actifed Syrup ▣ 846
Actifed Tablets ▣ 844
Alka-Seltzer Plus Cold Medicine ▣ 705
Alka-Seltzer Plus Cold Medicine Liqui-Gels ▣ 706
Alka-Seltzer Plus Cold & Cough Medicine ▣ 708
Alka-Seltzer Plus Cold & Cough Medicine Liqui-Gels ▣ 705
Alka-Seltzer Plus Night-Time Cold Medicine ▣ 707
Alka-Seltzer Plus Night-Time Cold Medicine Liqui-Gels ▣ 706
Alka Seltzer Plus Sinus Medicine ▣ 707
Allerest Children's Chewable Tablets ▣ 627
Allerest Headache Strength Tablets ▣ 627
Allerest Maximum Strength Tablets ▣ 627
Allerest No Drowsiness Tablets ▣ 627
Allerest Sinus Pain Formula ▣ 627
Allerest 12 Hour Caplets ▣ 627
Asendin Tablets (Less frequent) 1369
Astramorph/PF Injection, USP (Preservative-Free) 535
Atrohist Pediatric Capsules 453
Atrohist Pediatric Suspension 454
Benadryl Allergy Decongestant Liquid Medication ▣ 848
Benadryl Allergy Decongestant Tablets ▣ 848
Benadryl Allergy Liquid Medication ▣ 849
Benadryl Allergy ▣ 848
Benadryl Capsules 1898
Benadryl Dye-Free Allergy Liqui-gel Softgels ▣ 850
Benadryl Dye-Free Allergy Liquid Medication ▣ 850
Benadryl Kapseals 1898
Benadryl Injection 1898
Bentyl 1501
Bromfed Capsules (Extended-Release) 1785
Bromfed Syrup ▣ 733
Bromfed Tablets 1785
Bromfed-DM Cough Syrup 1786
Bromfed-PD Capsules (Extended-Release) 1785
Bronkometer Aerosol 2302
Bronkosol Solution 2302
BuSpar (2%) 737
Cerose DM ▣ 878
Cheracol Plus Head Cold/Cough Formula ▣ 769
Children's Vicks DayQuil Allergy Relief ▣ 757
Children's Vicks NyQuil Cold/Cough Relief ▣ 758
Chlor-Trimeton Allergy Decongestant Tablets ▣ 799
Chlor-Trimeton Allergy Tablets ▣ 798
Claritin-D 2350
Cocaine Hydrochloride Topical Solution 537
Cogentin 1621
Comhist 2038
Allergy-Sinus Comtrex Multi-Symptom Allergy-Sinus Formula Tablets ▣ 617
Contac Continuous Action Nasal Decongestant/Antihistamine 12 Hour Capsules ▣ 813
Contac Maximum Strength Continuous Action Decongestant/Antihistamine 12 Hour Caplets ▣ 813
Contac Night Allergy/Sinus Caplets ▣ 812
Contac Severe Cold and Flu Formula Caplets ▣ 814
Coricidin 'D' Decongestant Tablets ▣ 800
Coricidin Tablets ▣ 800
D.A. Chewable Tablets 951
Dalmane Capsules (Rare) 2173
Deconamine 1320
▲ Desyrel and Desyrel Dividose (1.4% to 5.1%) 503
Dimetapp Elixir ▣ 773
Dimetapp Extentabs ▣ 774
Dimetapp Tablets/Liqui-Gels ▣ 775
Dimetapp Cold & Allergy Chewable Tablets ▣ 773
Donnatal (In elderly patients) 2060
Donnatal Extentabs (In elderly patients) 2061
Donnatal Tablets (In elderly patients) 2060
Drixoral Cold and Allergy Sustained-Action Tablets ▣ 802
Drixoral Cold and Flu Extended-Release Tablets ▣ 803
Drixoral Allergy/Sinus Extended Release Tablets ▣ 804
Duramorph 962
Dura-Tap/PD Capsules 2867
Elavil 2838
Emete-con Intramuscular/Intravenous 2198
Endep Tablets 2174
Entex PSE Tablets 1987
Esgic-plus Tablets (Infrequent) 1013
Etrafon 2355
Fioricet Tablets (Infrequent) 2258
Flexeril Tablets (Less than 1%) 1661
Guaifed 1787
Guaimax-D Tablets 792
Infumorph 200 and Infumorph 500 Sterile Solutions 965
Isoclor Timesule Capsules ▣ 637

(▣ Described in PDR For Nonprescription Drugs) Incidence data in parenthesis; ▲ 3% or more (◉ Described in PDR For Ophthalmology)

Isoetharine Inhalation Solution, USP, Arm-a-Med 551
Levsin/Levsinex/Levbid 2405
Lioresal Tablets 829
Lufyllin & Lufyllin-400 Tablets 2670
Marax Tablets & DF Syrup 2200
Marcaine Hydrochloride with Epinephrine 1:200,000 2316
Marcaine Hydrochloride Injection 2316
Marcaine Spinal 2319
Mebaral Tablets 2322
Mellaril 2269
Mobigesic Tablets .... ⊡ 602
Narcan Injection 934
Neo-Synephrine Hydrochloride 1% Carpuject 2324
Neo-Synephrine Hydrochloride 1% Injection 2324
Nescaine/Nescaine MPF 554
Nolahist Tablets 785
Ornade Spansule Capsules 2502
Orudis Capsules (Greater than 1%) 2766
Oruvail Capsules (Greater than 1%) 2766
Oxandrin 2862
PBZ Tablets 845
PBZ-SR Tablets 844
PediaCare Cold Allergy Chewable Tablets .... ⊡ 677
PediaCare Cough-Cold Liquid 1553
PediaCare NightRest Cough-Cold Liquid 1553
Pediatric Vicks 44m Cough & Cold Relief .... ⊡ 764
Percogesic Analgesic Tablets .... ⊡ 754
Periactin 1724
Phenergan Injection 2773
Phenergan Tablets 2775
Phenobarbital Elixir and Tablets 1469
Phrenilin (Infrequent) 785
Pontocaine Hydrochloride for Spinal Anesthesia 2330
Prolixin 509
Protopam Chloride for Injection (Several cases) 2806
▲ Proventil Syrup (2 of 100 patients; children 2 to 6 years, approximately 20%) 2385
Pyrroxate Caplets .... ⊡ 772
Quadrinal Tablets 1350
Quinidex Extentabs 2067
Robinul Injectable 2072
Rondec Oral Drops (Rare) 953
Rondec Syrup (Rare) 953
Rondec Tablet (Rare) 953
Rondec-DM Oral Drops (Rare) 954
Rondec-DM Syrup (Rare) 954
Rondec-TR Tablet (Rare) 953
Ryna .... ⊡ 841
Rynatan 2673
Rynatuss 2673
Sedapap Tablets 50 mg/650 mg (Infrequent) 1543
Sensorcaine 559
Serentil 684
Serevent Inhalation Aerosol 1176
Sinarest .... ⊡ 648
Sine-Off Sinus Medicine .... ⊡ 825
Singlet Tablets .... ⊡ 825
Sinulin Tablets 787
Sudafed Plus Liquid .... ⊡ 862
Sudafed Plus Tablets .... ⊡ 863
Talacen (Rare) 2333
Talwin Injection (Rare) 2334
Talwin Compound (Rare) 2335
Talwin Injection (Rare) 2334
Talwin Nx 2336
Tavist Syrup 2297
Tavist Tablets 2298
Teldrin 12 Hour Antihistamine/Nasal Decongestant Allergy Relief Capsules .... ⊡ 826
Temaril Tablets, Syrup and Spansule Extended-Release Capsules 483
TheraFlu .... ⊡ 787
TheraFlu Maximum Strength Nighttime Flu, Cold & Cough Medicine .... ⊡ 788
Torecan 2245
Trancopal Caplets 2337
Triaminic Allergy Tablets .... ⊡ 789
Triaminic Nite Light .... ⊡ 791
Triaminic Syrup .... ⊡ 792
Triaminic-12 Tablets .... ⊡ 792
Triaminicin Tablets .... ⊡ 793
Triaminicol Multi-Symptom Cold Tablets .... ⊡ 793
Triaminicol Multi-Symptom Relief .... ⊡ 794
Triavil Tablets 1757
Trinalin Repetabs Tablets 1330
Tussend 1783
Children's TYLENOL Cold Multi-Symptom Liquid Formula and Chewable Tablets 1561
TYLENOL Maximum Strength Allergy Sinus Medication Gelcaps and Caplets 1563
TYLENOL Flu NightTime, Maximum Strength, Gelcaps 1566
TYLENOL Maximum Strength Flu NightTime Hot Medication Packets 1562
TYLENOL Cold Multi-Symptom Formula Medication Tablets and Caplets 1561
TYLENOL Cold Multi-Symptom Hot Medication Liquid Packets 1557
Ventolin Syrup (2 of 100 patients) 1202
Vicks 44 LiquiCaps Cough, Cold & Flu Relief .... ⊡ 755
Vicks 44M Cough, Cold & Flu Relief .... ⊡ 756
Vicks DayQuil Allergy Relief 12-Hour Extended Release Tablets .... ⊡ 760
Vicks DayQuil Allergy Relief 4-Hour Tablets .... ⊡ 760
Vicks Nyquil Hot Therapy .... ⊡ 762
Vicks NyQuil LiquiCaps Multi-Symptom Cold/Flu Relief ⊡ 763
Vicks NyQuil Multi-Symptom Cold/Flu Relief - (Original & Cherry Flavor) .... ⊡ 763
Winstrol Tablets 2337
Yohimex Tablets 1363

Excitement, paradoxical
Dizac (Less frequent) 1809
Etrafon 2355
Halcion Tablets 2611
Libritabs Tablets 2177
Librium Capsules 2178
Miltown Tablets 2672
PMB 200 and PMB 400 2783
Placidyl Capsules (Occasional) 448
ProSom Tablets 449
Restoril Capsules (Less than 0.5%) 2284
Serax Capsules 2810
Serax Tablets 2810
Triavil Tablets 1757
Valium Injectable 2182
Valium Tablets 2183
Valrelease Capsules (Infrequent) 2169

Excoriation
Catapres-TTS (3 of 101 patients) .. 675
Flonase Nasal Spray (Less than 1%) 1098
Sulfamylon Cream (Rare) 925
▲ Videx Tablets, Powder for Oral Solution, & Pediatric Powder for Oral Solution (4% to 7%) 720

Exercise tolerance, decreased
Blocadren Tablets 1614
Lopressor HCT Tablets (1 in 100 patients) 832
Timoptic in Ocudose (Less frequent) 1753
Timoptic Sterile Ophthalmic Solution (Less frequent) 1751
Timoptic-XE 1755

Exophthalmos
Anafranil Capsules (Rare) 803
Aquasol A Vitamin A Capsules, USP 534
Aristocort Suspension (Forte Parenteral) 1027
Aristocort Suspension (Intralesional) 1025
Aristocort Tablets 1022
Aristospan Suspension (Intra-articular) 1033
Aristospan Suspension (Intralesional) 1032
Celestone Soluspan Suspension 2347
CORTENEMA 2535
Cortone Acetate Sterile Suspension 1623
Cortone Acetate Tablets 1624
Dalalone D.P. Injectable 1011
Decadron Elixir 1633
Decadron Phosphate Injection 1637
Decadron Phosphate Respihaler 1642
Decadron Phosphate Turbinaire 1645
Decadron Phosphate with Xylocaine Injection, Sterile 1639
Decadron Tablets 1635
Decadron-LA Sterile Suspension 1646
Deltasone Tablets 2595
Depo-Medrol Single-Dose Vial 2600
Depo-Medrol Sterile Aqueous Suspension 2597
Dexacort Phosphate in Respihaler .. 458
Dexacort Phosphate in Turbinaire .. 459
Effexor (Infrequent) 2719
Eskalith 2485
Florinef Acetate Tablets 505
Hydeltrasol Injection, Sterile 1665
Hydeltra-T.B.A. Sterile Suspension 1667
Hydrocortone Acetate Sterile Suspension 1669
Hydrocortone Phosphate Injection, Sterile 1670
Hydrocortone Tablets 1672
Lithonate/Lithotabs/Lithobid 2543
Medrol 2621
Paxil Tablets (Rare) 2505
Pediapred Oral Liquid 995
Prelone Syrup 1787
Solu-Cortef Sterile Powder 2641
Solu-Medrol Sterile Powder 2643
Zoloft Tablets (Rare) 2217

Extrapyramidal symptoms
Anafranil Capsules (Infrequent) 803
Asendin Tablets (Less than 1%) 1369
BuSpar (Rare) 737
Cardizem CD Capsules (Infrequent) 1506
Cardizem SR Capsules (Infrequent) 1510
Cardizem Injectable 1508
Cardizem Tablets (Infrequent) 1512
Clozaril Tablets 2252
Cognex Capsules (Infrequent) 1901
Compazine 2470
▲ Demser Capsules (10%) 1649
Desyrel and Desyrel Dividose 503
Elavil 2838
Endep Tablets 2174
Eskalith 2485
Etrafon (More common) 2355
Felbatol 2666
Flexeril Tablets (Rare) 1661
Floxin Tablets (200 mg, 300 mg, 400 mg) 1567
Foscavir Injection (Less than 1%) .. 547
Haldol Decanoate (Frequent) 1577
Haldol Injection, Tablets and Concentrate (Frequent) 1575
Inapsine Injection 1296
Intron A (Less than 5%) 2364
Kytril Injection (Rare) 2490
Kytril Tablets (One case) 2492
Levoprome 1274
Librax Capsules (Rare) 2176
Libritabs Tablets (Isolated cases) 2177
Librium Capsules (Isolated cases) .. 2178
Librium Injectable (Isolated cases) 2179
Limbitrol 2180
Lithonate/Lithotabs/Lithobid 2543
▲ Loxitane (Frequent) 1378
Ludiomil Tablets (Rare) 843
Luvox Tablets (Infrequent) 2544
Mellaril (Infrequent) 2269
Mepergan Injection (Rare) 2753
Moban Tablets and Concentrate 1048
Navane Capsules and Concentrate 2201
Navane Intramuscular 2202
Norpramin Tablets 1526
Orap Tablets (Frequent) 1050
Pamelor 2280
Paxil Tablets 2505
Permax Tablets (1.6%) 575
Phenergan with Codeine 2777
Phenergan Injection 2773
Phenergan Suppositories 2775
Phenergan Syrup 2774
Phenergan Tablets 2775
Proglycem 580
Prolixin 509
Propulsid (Rare) 1300
Prozac Pulvules & Liquid, Oral Solution (Rare) 919
Reglan (Approximately 0.2%) 2068
▲ Risperdal (17% to 34%) 1301
Ser-Ap-Es Tablets (Rare) 849
Serentil 684
Sinemet CR Tablets 944
Sinequan (Infrequent) 2205
Stelazine 2514
Sublimaze Injection 1307
Surmontil Capsules 2811
Temaril Tablets, Syrup and Spansule Extended-Release Capsules 483
Thorazine 2523
Tigan 2057
Tofranil Ampuls 854
Tofranil Tablets 856
Tofranil-PM Capsules 857
Toradol (1% or less) 2159
Torecan 2245
Triavil Tablets 1757
Trilafon 2389
Vivactil Tablets 1774
Zofran Injection (Rare) 1214
Zofran Tablets (Rare) 1217

Extrasystoles
Actifed with Codeine Cough Syrup .. 1067
Adalat CC (Less than 1.0%) 589
Ambien Tablets (Rare) 2416
Anafranil Capsules (Infrequent) 803
Benadryl Capsules 1898
Benadryl Injection 1898
Cardene Capsules (Rare) 2095
Cardene I.V. (0.7%) 2709
Deconamine 1320
Dilacor XR Extended-release Capsules 2018
Diprivan Injection (Less than 1%) .. 2833
Effexor (Infrequent) 2719
Foscavir Injection (Less than 1%) .. 547
Imdur (Less than or equal to 5%) .. 1323
Intron A (Less than 5%) 2364
Lariam Tablets (Less than 1%) 2128
Lopid Tablets 1917
Lufyllin & Lufyllin-400 Tablets 2670
Lufyllin-GG Elixir & Tablets 2671
Maxaquin Tablets (Less than 1%) .. 2440
Norvasc Tablets (Less than or equal to 0.1%) 1940
Ornade Spansule Capsules 2502
PBZ Tablets 845
PBZ-SR Tablets 844
Periactin 1724
Quadrinal Tablets 1350
Quibron 2053
Quinidex Extentabs 2067
Respbid Tablets 682
Slo-bid Gyrocaps 2033
Tavist Syrup 2297
Tavist Tablets 2298
Theo-24 Extended Release Capsules 2568
Theo-Dur Extended-Release Tablets 1327
Theo-X Extended-Release Tablets .. 788
Trinalin Repetabs Tablets 1330
Tussend 1783
Uni-Dur Extended-Release Tablets .. 1331
Uniphyl 400 mg Tablets 2001

Extrasystoles, supraventricular
Caverject (Less than 1%) 2583
Luvox Tablets (Rare) 2544

Extravasation
Adriamycin PFS 1947
Adriamycin RDF 1947
Brevibloc Injection (Less than 1%) 1808
Cerubidine 795
Claforan Sterile and Injection (Rare) 1235
Cosmegen Injection 1626
Doxorubicin Astra 540
Fluorescite .... ⊙ 219
Hyperstat I.V. Injection 2363
Idamycin 1955
Levophed Bitartrate Injection 2315
Mutamycin 703
Oncovin Solution Vials & Hyporets 1466
Pentam 300 Injection 1041
Platinol 708
Platinol-AQ Injection 710
Romazicon 2147
Taxol 714
Velban Vials 1484
Zinecard (1% to 3%) 1961

Extroversion
Ambien Tablets 2416
Halcion Tablets 2611

Exudate, increased
Bactroban Ointment (Less than 1%) 2470
▲ THROMBATE III Antithrombin III (Human) (1 of 17) 637

Eye abnormalities, fetal
Accutane Capsules 2076
Clomid 1514

(⊡ Described in PDR For Nonprescription Drugs) Incidence data in parenthesis; ▲ 3% or more (⊙ Described in PDR For Ophthalmology)

1297 Side Effects Index EEG changes

Eye globe, perforation (see under Bulbus oculi, perforation)

Eye movements, abnormal
Klonopin Tablets ... 2126
Mevacor Tablets (0.5% to 1.0%) .. 1699
Zocor Tablets ... 1775

Eyeball, perforation (see under Bulbus oculi, perforation)

Eyelashes, matting of
Alomide (Less than 1%) ... 469
Betoptic Ophthalmic Solution ... 469
Betoptic S Ophthalmic Suspension (Small number of patients) ... 471
Iopidine 0.5% (Less than 1%) ... ◉ 221
Lacrisert Sterile Ophthalmic Insert 1686

Eyelids, cyclic, movement of
Versed Injection ... 2170

Eyelids, deposits in
Alomide (Less than 1%) ... 469
Iopidine 0.5% (Less than 3%) ... ◉ 221

Eyelids, edema of
BOTOX (Botulinum Toxin Type A) Purified Neurotoxin Complex (2 cases) ... 477
Cataflam ... 816
Ciloxan Ophthalmic Solution (Less than 1%) ... 472
Hyzaar Tablets ... 1677
Lacrisert Sterile Ophthalmic Insert 1686
Phenobarbital Elixir and Tablets ... 1469
Polytrim Ophthalmic Solution Sterile (Multiple reports) ... 482
▲ Rēv-Eyes Ophthalmic Eyedrops 0.5% (10% to 40%) ... ◉ 323
Tobrex Ophthalmic Ointment and Solution (Less than 3 of 100 patients) ... ◉ 229
Voltaren Tablets ... 861

Eyelids, erythema
▲ Betimol 0.25%, 0.5% (More than 5%) ... ◉ 261

Eyelids, heavy
Esgic-plus Tablets (Infrequent) ... 1013
Fioricet Tablets (Infrequent) ... 2258
Fioricet with Codeine Capsules (Infrequent) ... 2260
Fiorinal with Codeine Capsules (Infrequent) ... 2262
Phrenilin (Infrequent) ... 785
Sedapap Tablets 50 mg/650 mg (Infrequent) ... 1543

Eyes, burning
▲ Betagan (About 1 in 3 patients) .. ◉ 233
Bleph-10 ... 475
Catapres Tablets ... 674
Catapres-TTS ... 675
▲ Ciloxan Ophthalmic Solution (Among most frequent) ... 472
Cleocin T Topical ... 2590
Combipres Tablets ... 677
Cozaar Tablets (Less than 1%) ... 1628
Dalmane Capsules (Rare) ... 2173
Dexacidin Ointment ... ◉ 263
Fluoracaine (Occasional) ... ◉ 206
FLURESS (Occasional) ... ◉ 207
▲ Genoptic Sterile Ophthalmic Solution (Among most frequent) .. ◉ 243
▲ Genoptic Sterile Ophthalmic Ointment (Among most frequent) ... ◉ 243
Gentacidin Ointment (Occasional) ... ◉ 264
Gentacidin Solution (Occasional) ◉ 264
HMS Liquifilm ... ◉ 244
Hivid Tablets (Less than 1% to less than 3%) ... 2121
Hyzaar Tablets ... 1677
Inflamase ... ◉ 265
IOPIDINE Sterile Ophthalmic Solution ... ◉ 219
Isopto Carpine Ophthalmic Solution ... ◉ 223
Lamprene Capsules (Greater than 1%) ... 828
▲ Livostin (15%) ... ◉ 266
Motofen Tablets (Less frequent) ... 784
Muro 128 Ophthalmic Ointment ◉ 258
Muro 128 Solution 2% and 5% .. ◉ 258
▲ Ocufen (One of the two most frequent) ... ◉ 245
▲ Ocuflox (One of the two most frequent) ... 481
▲ Ocupress Ophthalmic Solution, 1% Sterile (About 1 of 4 patients) ... ◉ 309
Ophthetic ... ◉ 247
Phospholine Iodide ... ◉ 326
Pilopine HS Ophthalmic Gel ... ◉ 226
▲ Polytrim Ophthalmic Solution Sterile (Among most frequent) ... 482
▲ Profenal 1% Sterile Ophthalmic Solution (Among most frequent).. ◉ 227
▲ PROPINE with C CAP Compliance Cap (6%) ... ◉ 253
ReVia Tablets (Less than 1%) ... 940
Rogaine Topical Solution ... 2637
Sodium Sulamyd ... 2387
Soma Compound w/Codeine Tablets ... 2676
Soma Compound Tablets ... 2675
Tessalon Perles ... 1020
▲ Timoptic in Ocudose (Approximately 1 in 8 patients) ... 1753
▲ Timoptic Sterile Ophthalmic Solution (Approximately 1 in 8 patients) ... 1751
Vasocidin Ointment ... ◉ 268
Vasosulf ... ◉ 271
Vira-A Ophthalmic Ointment, 3% ◉ 312
Visken Tablets (2% or fewer patients) ... 2299
▲ Voltaren Ophthalmic Sterile Ophthalmic Solution (15%) ... ◉ 272

Eyes, dilatation of pupil (see under Mydriasis)

Eyes, disorders
AeroBid Inhaler System (1-3%) ... 1005
Aerobid-M Inhaler System (1-3%) .. 1005
Ativan Tablets (Less frequent) ... 2700
Atretol Tablets ... 573
Cartrol Tablets (Less common) ... 410
Clinoril Tablets (Less than 1%) ... 1618
Cordarone Tablets ... 2712
Desferal Vials ... 820
Desyrel and Desyrel Dividose (Up to 2.8%) ... 503
Flonase Nasal Spray (Less than 1%) ... 1098
Foscavir Injection (Between 1% and 5%) ... 547
Hivid Tablets (Less than 1% to less than 3%) ... 2121
Lescol Capsules ... 2267
Loxitane ... 1378
Lupron Depot 3.75 mg ... 2556
Lupron Depot 7.5 mg ... 2559
Lupron Injection (Less than 5%) ... 2555
Mintezol ... 1704
Nasalide Nasal Solution 0.025% (5% or less) ... 2110
Neurontin Capsules (Rare) ... 1922
▲ Novantrone (2 to 7%) ... 1279
Permax Tablets (1.1%) ... 575
Tambocor Tablets ... 1497
▲ Tegison Capsules (50-75%) ... 2154
Tegretol Chewable Tablets ... 852
Tegretol Suspension ... 852
Tegretol Tablets ... 852
▲ THROMBATE III Antithrombin III (Human) (1 of 17) ... 637
Urispas Tablets ... 2532
Varivax (Greater than or equal to 1%) ... 1762
Versed Injection (Less than 1%) ... 2170
Videx Tablets, Powder for Oral Solution, & Pediatric Powder for Oral Solution (Less than 1%) ... 720

Eyes, dry (see also under Xerophthalmia)
Accutane Capsules ... 2076
Blocadren Tablets ... 1614
Cordarone Tablets ... 2712
Inderal (Rare) ... 2728
Inderal LA Long Acting Capsules (Rare) ... 2730
Inderide LA Long Acting Capsules (Rare) ... 2734
Kerlone Tablets (Less than 2%) ... 2436
Lamprene Capsules (Greater than 1%) ... 828
Lopressor (Rare) ... 830
Motrin Tablets (Less than 1%) ... 2625
Normodyne Tablets ... 2379
▲ Norpace (3 to 9%) ... 2444
Sectral Capsules (Up to 2%) ... 2807
Tenoretic Tablets ... 2845
Tenormin Tablets and I.V. Injection 2847
Trandate Tablets (Less common) ... 1185
Transderm Scōp Transdermal Therapeutic System (Infrequent) 869
Vexol 1% Ophthalmic Suspension (Less than 1%) ... ◉ 230

Eyes, irritation
Adsorbotear Artificial Tear ... ◉ 210
AK-Spore ... ◉ 204
AquaSite Eye Drops ... ◉ 261
Atropine Sulfate Sterile Ophthalmic Solution ... ◉ 233
Bleph-10 ... 475
Blocadren Tablets (1.1%) ... 1614
▲ BOTOX (Botulinum Toxin Type A) Purified Neurotoxin Complex (10.0%) ... 477
Cardizem CD Capsules (Less than 1%) ... 1506
Cardizem SR Capsules (Less than 1%) ... 1510
Cardizem Injectable ... 1508
Cardizem Tablets (Less than 1%) .. 1512
Clear Eyes ACR Astringent/Lubricant Eye Redness Reliever Eye Drops ... ◉ 316
Cleocin T Topical ... 2590
Collagen Plugs (Intracanalicular) ◉ 284
Crolom (Infrequent) ... ◉ 257
Emgel 2% Topical Gel ... 1093
Eye-Stream Eye Irrigating Solution.. 473
Feldene Capsules (Less than 1%) .. 1965
▲ Genoptic Sterile Ophthalmic Solution (Among most frequent).. ◉ 243
▲ Genoptic Sterile Ophthalmic Ointment (Among most frequent) ... ◉ 243
Gentacidin Ointment ... ◉ 264
Gentacidin Solution ... ◉ 264
Herplex Liquifilm (Occasional) ... ◉ 244
Herrick Lacrimal Plugs ... ◉ 285
▲ Ilotycin Ophthalmic Ointment (Among most frequent) ... 912
Imitrex Injection (Infrequent) ... 1103
Imitrex Tablets (Up to 2%) ... 1106
Iopidine 0.5% (Less than 3%) ... ◉ 221
Isopto Carbachol Ophthalmic Solution ... ◉ 223
Lamprene Capsules (Greater than 1%) ... 828
Methotrexate Sodium Tablets, Injection, for Injection and LPF Injection ... 1275
Mevacor Tablets (0.5% to 1.0%) .. 1699
Muro 128 Ophthalmic Ointment ◉ 258
Muro 128 Solution 2% and 5% .. ◉ 258
NebuPent for Inhalation Solution (1% or less) ... 1040
Ocufen ... ◉ 245
▲ Ocupress Ophthalmic Solution, 1% Sterile (About 1 of 4 patients) ... ◉ 309
Ocusert Pilo-20 and Pilo-40 Ocular Therapeutic Systems (Infrequent) ... ◉ 254
Ophthalgan ... ◉ 326
▲ Polytrim Ophthalmic Solution Sterile (Among most frequent) ... 482
Pondimin Tablets ... 2066
Ponstel ... 1925
Profenal 1% Sterile Ophthalmic Solution (Less than 0.5%) ... ◉ 227
Quadrinal Tablets ... 1350
Roferon-A Injection (Less than 1%) ... 2145
Rogaine Topical Solution ... 2637
T-Stat 2.0% Topical Solution and Pads ... 2688
Tambocor Tablets (Less than 1%) 1497
▲ Tegison Capsules (50-75%) ... 2154
Theramycin Z Topical Solution 2% 1592
Timolide Tablets ... 1748
Tornalate Solution for Inhalation, 0.2% (Less than 1%) ... 956
Vasosulf ... ◉ 271
Vira-A Ophthalmic Ointment, 3% ◉ 312
Visine L.R. Eye Drops ... ◉ 313
Visken Tablets (2% or fewer patients) ... 2299
Viva-Drops ... ◉ 325

Eyes, redness
Adsorbotear Artificial Tear ... ◉ 210
AK-Spore ... ◉ 204
Albalon Solution with Liquifilm ... ◉ 231
All-Flex Arcing Spring Diaphragm (See also Ortho Diaphragm Kits) 1865
AquaSite Eye Drops ... ◉ 261
BuSpar (Infrequent) ... 737
Clozaril Tablets (Less than 1%) ... 2252
Eye-Stream Eye Irrigating Solution.. 473
Floropryl Sterile Ophthalmic Ointment ... 1662
Fluoracaine (Occasional) ... ◉ 206
Hivid Tablets (Less than 1% to less than 3%) ... 2121
Humorsol Sterile Ophthalmic Solution ... 1664
Livostin (Approximately 1% to 3%) ... ◉ 266
Ocuflox ... 481
Ortho Diaphragm Kits—All-Flex Arcing Spring; Ortho Coil Spring; Ortho-White Flat Spring ... 1865
Ortho Diaphragm Kit ... 1865
▲ Polytrim Ophthalmic Solution Sterile (Among most frequent) ... 482
Transderm Scōp Transdermal Therapeutic System (Infrequent) 869
Visine L.R. Eye Drops ... ◉ 313
Viva-Drops ... ◉ 325

Eyes, "spots" before the
Clomid (Occasional) ... 1514
Depakene ... 413
Depakote Tablets ... 415
Tambocor Tablets ... 1497

Eyes, swollen (see under Edema, palpebral)

Eyes, tearing
▲ Alomide (1% to 5%) ... 469
Beconase AQ Nasal Spray (Fewer than 3 per 100 patients) ... 1076
Betimol 0.25%, 0.5% ... ◉ 261
Betoptic Ophthalmic Solution (Occasional) ... 469
Betoptic S Ophthalmic Suspension (Small number of patients) ... 471
▲ CHEMET (succimer) Capsules (1.0 to 3.7%) ... 1545
Ciloxan Ophthalmic Solution (Less than 1%) ... 472
Collagen Plugs (Intracanalicular) ◉ 284
Dantrium Capsules (Less frequent) 1982
Dipentum Capsules (Rare) ... 1951
Emcyt Capsules (1%) ... 1953
Herrick Lacrimal Plugs ... ◉ 285
▲ Iopidine 0.5% (4%) ... ◉ 221
Lorelco Tablets ... 1517
Nasalide Nasal Solution 0.025% ... 2110
Ocuflox ... 481
▲ Ocupress Ophthalmic Solution, 1% Sterile (About 1 of 4 patients) ... ◉ 309
Polytrim Ophthalmic Solution Sterile (Multiple reports) ... 482
Rēv-Eyes Ophthalmic Eyedrops 0.5% (Less frequently) ... ◉ 323
Timoptic in Ocudose (Less frequent) ... 1753
Timoptic Sterile Ophthalmic Solution (Less frequent) ... 1751
Timoptic-XE (1% to 5% of patients) ... 1755
Vancenase AQ Nasal Spray 0.042% (Fewer than 3 per 100 patients) ... 2393

ECG changes (see under EKG changes)

EEG changes
Anafranil Capsules (Infrequent) ... 803
Asendin Tablets (Less frequent) ... 1369
Clozaril Tablets ... 2252
Compazine ... 2470
Diphtheria and Tetanus Toxoids and Pertussis Vaccine Adsorbed USP (For Pediatric Use) ... 875
Dizac ... 1809
Elavil ... 2838
Endep Tablets ... 2174
Eskalith ... 2485
Etrafon ... 2355
Flexeril Tablets (Rare) ... 1661
Foscavir Injection (Between 1% and 5%) ... 547
Halcion Tablets ... 2611
Librax Capsules ... 2176
Libritabs Tablets (Isolated cases) ... 2177
Librium Capsules (Isolated cases) .. 2178
Librium Injectable ... 2179
Limbitrol ... 2180
Lithium Carbonate Capsules & Tablets ... 2230
Lithonate/Lithotabs/Lithobid ... 2543
Ludiomil Tablets (Rare) ... 843
Miltown Tablets ... 2672
Norpramin Tablets ... 1526

(▭ Described in PDR For Nonprescription Drugs) Incidence data in parenthesis; ▲ 3% or more (◉ Described in PDR For Ophthalmology)

EEG changes Side Effects Index 1298

PMB 200 and PMB 400 ... 2783
Pamelor ... 2280
Paxil Tablets (Rare) ... 2505
Prolixin ... 509
ProSom Tablets ... 449
Prozac Pulvules & Liquid, Oral Solution (Rare) ... 919
Serax Capsules ... 2810
Serax Tablets ... 2810
Solganal Suspension ... 2388
Surmontil Capsules ... 2811
Tofranil Ampuls ... 854
Tofranil Tablets ... 856
Tofranil-PM Capsules ... 857
Triavil Tablets ... 1757
Tripedia ... 892
Valium Injectable ... 2182
Valium Tablets (Infrequent) ... 2183
Valrelease Capsules (Rare) ... 2169
Vivactil Tablets ... 1774
Wellbutrin Tablets (Rare) ... 1204

EKG changes

Anafranil Capsules (Infrequent) ... 803
Apresazide Capsules ... 808
Aralen Hydrochloride Injection (Rare) ... 2301
Aralen Phosphate Tablets (Rare) ... 2301
Azactam for Injection (Less than 1%) ... 734
▲Betapace Tablets (4% to 7%) ... 641
Bumex (0.4%) ... 2093
Cafergot ... 2251
Cardene Capsules (0.6%) ... 2095
Cardene I.V. (1.4%) ... 2709
Cardizem CD Capsules (Less than 1% to 1.6%) ... 1506
▲Cardizem SR Capsules (4.1%) ... 1510
Cardizem Injectable ... 1508
Cardizem Tablets (Less than 1%) .. 1512
Catapres Tablets (Rare) ... 674
Catapres-TTS (Rare) ... 675
Clozaril Tablets (1%) ... 2252
Combipres Tablets (Rare) ... 677
Compazine ... 2470
Demadex Tablets and Injection (2.0%) ... 686
Dilacor XR Extended-release Capsules (Infrequent) ... 2018
Diprivan Injection (Less than 1%) .. 2833
Elavil ... 2838
Endep Tablets ... 2174
Eskalith ... 2485
Ethmozine Tablets (1.6%) ... 2041
Etrafon (Occasional) ... 2355
Foscavir Injection (Between 1% and 5%) ... 547
Haldol Decanoate ... 1577
Haldol Injection, Tablets and Concentrate ... 1575
Hyperstat I.V. Injection ... 2363
Imitrex Tablets (Infreqent) ... 1106
Kytril Injection (Rare) ... 2490
Lanoxicaps ... 1117
Lanoxin Elixir Pediatric ... 1120
Lanoxin Injection ... 1123
Lanoxin Injection Pediatric ... 1126
Lanoxin Tablets ... 1128
Lithium Carbonate Capsules & Tablets ... 2230
Lithonate/Lithotabs/Lithobid ... 2543
Lotensin Tablets (Scattered incidents) ... 834
Lotensin HCT ... 837
Loxitane (A few cases) ... 1378
Lupron Depot 3.75 mg ... 2556
Lupron Depot 7.5 mg ... 2559
▲Lupron Injection (5% or more) ... 2555
Macrobid Capsules ... 1988
Macrodantin Capsules ... 1989
Mellaril ... 2269
Midamor Tablets ... 1703
Miltown Tablets ... 2672
Nalfon 200 Pulvules & Nalfon Tablets (Less than 1%) ... 917
Navane Capsules and Concentrate ... 2201
Navane Intramuscular ... 2202
Nimotop Capsules (Up to 1.4%) ... 610
Novantrone ... 1279
Orap Tablets ... 1050
PMB 200 and PMB 400 ... 2783
Paxil Tablets (Infrequent) ... 2505
Permax Tablets (Infrequent) ... 575
Polycitra-K Crystals ... 579
Polycitra-K Oral Solution ... 579
▲Prograf (Greater than 3%) ... 1042
Prolixin ... 509
Prostigmin Injectable ... 1260
Prostigmin Tablets ... 1261
▲Quinaglute Dura-Tabs Tablets (3%) ... 649
Quinidex Extentabs ... 2067
Retrovir Capsules (2.4%) ... 1158
▲Retrovir I.V. Infusion (3%) ... 1163
Retrovir Syrup (2.4%) ... 1158
ReVia Tablets (Less than 1%) ... 940
Salagen Tablets (Less than 1%) ... 1489
Stelazine ... 2514
Suprane (Less than 1%) ... 1813
▲Taxol (Common; 14% to 23%) ... 714
Temaril Tablets, Syrup and Spansule Extended-Release Capsules ... 483
Thorazine ... 2523
Tofranil Ampuls ... 854
Tofranil Tablets ... 856
Tofranil-PM Capsules ... 857
Torecan ... 2245
Tornalate Solution for Inhalation, 0.2% (Less than 1%) ... 956
Triavil Tablets ... 1757
Trilafon (Occasional) ... 2389
Ultram Tablets (50 mg) (Infrequent) ... 1585
Wellbutrin Tablets (Infrequent) ... 1204
Zemuron (Less than 1%) ... 1830
Zofran Injection (Rare) ... 1214
Zofran Tablets (Rare) ... 1217

EKG changes, PR prolongation

Imitrex Injection (Infrequent) ... 1103
Respbid Tablets ... 682

EKG changes, Q wave disturbances

Compazine ... 2470
Imdur (Less than or equal to 5%) .. 1323
Stelazine ... 2514
Thorazine ... 2523

EKG changes, QRS interval prolonged

Aralen Hydrochloride Injection (Rare) ... 2301
Aralen Phosphate Tablets (Rare) ... 2301
Doxorubicin Astra ... 540
Haldol Injection, Tablets and Concentrate ... 1575
Norpace (1 to 3%) ... 2444
Quinaglute Dura-Tabs Tablets ... 649
Quinidex Extentabs ... 2067
Rum-K Syrup ... 1005
Rythmol Tablets–150mg, 225mg, 300mg (0.5 to 1.9%) ... 1352
Tonocard Tablets (Less than 1%) .. 531

EKG changes, QT interval prolonged

Cordarone Intravenous (Less than 2%) ... 2715
Foscavir Injection (Rare) ... 547
Haldol Decanoate ... 1577
Imitrex Injection (Infrequent) ... 1103
Lorelco Tablets ... 1517
Mellaril ... 2269
Norpace (1 to 3%) ... 2444
Orap Tablets ... 1050
Orlamm (Low frequency) ... 2239
Propulsid (Rare) ... 1300
Prozac Pulvules & Liquid, Oral Solution ... 919
Quinidex Extentabs ... 2067
Risperdal ... 1301
Seldane Tablets (Rare) ... 1536
Seldane-D Extended-Release Tablets (Rare) ... 1538
Serentil ... 684
Temaril Tablets, Syrup and Spansule Extended-Release Capsules ... 483
Tonocard Tablets (Less than 1%) .. 531
Vascor (200, 300 and 400 mg) Tablets (0.5 to 2.0%) ... 1587

EKG changes, reversible flattening

Eskalith ... 2485
Lithium Carbonate Capsules & Tablets ... 2230
Lithonate/Lithotabs/Lithobid ... 2543

EKG changes, sinus pause

Brethaire Inhaler ... 813
Ethmozine Tablets (1.6%) ... 2041
Tambocor Tablets (1% to less than 3%) ... 1497

EKG changes, ST section

▲Adenoscan (3%) ... 1024
Brethaire Inhaler ... 813
Cardene I.V. (Rare) ... 2709
Clozaril Tablets ... 2252
Dilacor XR Extended-release Capsules (Infrequent) ... 2018
Diprivan Injection (Less than 1%) .. 2833
Doxorubicin Astra ... 540
Foscavir Injection (Between 1% and 5%) ... 547
Imitrex Injection (Infrequent) ... 1103
Lanoxicaps ... 1117
Lanoxin Elixir Pediatric ... 1120
Lanoxin Injection ... 1123
Lanoxin Injection Pediatric ... 1126
Lanoxin Tablets ... 1128
Luvox Tablets (Infrequent) ... 2544
Macrobid Capsules ... 1988
Macrodantin Capsules ... 1989
Orlamm (Low frequency) ... 2239
Pentam 300 Injection (1 patient) ... 1041
Risperdal (Rare) ... 1301
Rum-K Syrup ... 1005

EKG changes, T-wave

Adenoscan (Less than 1%) ... 1024
Aralen Hydrochloride Injection (Rare) ... 2301
Aralen Phosphate Tablets (Rare) ... 2301
Brethaire Inhaler ... 813
Cardene I.V. (Rare) ... 2709
Clozaril Tablets ... 2252
Compazine ... 2470
Dopram Injectable ... 2061
Doxorubicin Astra ... 540
Eskalith ... 2485
Flagyl 375 Capsules ... 2434
Flagyl I.V. ... 2247
Imitrex Injection (Infrequent) ... 1103
Lithium Carbonate Capsules & Tablets ... 2230
Lithonate/Lithotabs/Lithobid ... 2543
▲Loniten Tablets (Approximately 60%) ... 2618
Macrobid Capsules ... 1988
Macrodantin Capsules ... 1989
Mellaril ... 2269
MetroGel-Vaginal ... 902
Moban Tablets and Concentrate (Rare) ... 1048
Mycobutin Capsules (More than one patient) ... 1957
Orap Tablets ... 1050
Orlamm (Low frequency) ... 2239
Pentasa (Infrequent) ... 1527
Protostat Tablets ... 1883
Risperdal (Rare) ... 1301
Rum-K Syrup ... 1005
Serentil ... 684
Stelazine ... 2514
Temaril Tablets, Syrup and Spansule Extended-Release Capsules ... 483
Thorazine ... 2523
Tornalate Solution for Inhalation, 0.2% (Less than 1%) ... 956

ESR, elevation

▲Accutane Capsules (Approximately 40%) ... 2076
Altace Capsules (Less than 1%) ... 1232
Ambien Tablets (Rare) ... 2416
Capoten ... 739
Capozide ... 742
Cipro I.V. (Rare) ... 595
Cipro I.V. Pharmacy Bulk Package (Rare) ... 597
Clozaril Tablets ... 2252
Cytotec (Infrequent) ... 2424
Floxin I.V. (More than or equal to 1%) ... 1571
Floxin Tablets (200 mg, 300 mg, 400 mg) (More than or equal to 1.0%) ... 1567
Lamprene Capsules (Greater than 1%) ... 828
Lescol Capsules (Rare) ... 2267
Maxaquin Tablets ... 2440
Mevacor Tablets (Rare) ... 1699
Monopril Tablets ... 757
Pravachol (Rare) ... 765
Prinivil Tablets (0.3% to 1.0%) ... 1733
Prinzide Tablets ... 1737
Prozac Pulvules & Liquid, Oral Solution (Rare) ... 919
Recombivax HB ... 1744
Sansert Tablets ... 2295
▲Tegison Capsules (25-50%) ... 2154
Vaseretic Tablets ... 1765
Vasotec I.V. ... 1768
Vasotec Tablets (0.5% to 1.0%) ... 1771
Zestoretic ... 2850
Zestril Tablets (0.3% to 1.0%) ... 2854
Zocor Tablets (Rare) ... 1775

F

Face, red scaly

▲Tegison Capsules (50-75%) ... 2154

Face, rhythmical involuntary movements

Compazine ... 2470
Etrafon ... 2355
Haldol Decanoate ... 1577
Lithonate/Lithotabs/Lithobid ... 2543
Mellaril ... 2269
Moban Tablets and Concentrate ... 1048
Orap Tablets ... 1050
Reglan ... 2068
Stelazine ... 2514
Thorazine ... 2523

Facial dysmorphia, fetal

Accutane Capsules ... 2076

Facial features, coarsening

Dilantin Infatabs ... 1908
Dilantin Kapseals ... 1906
Dilantin Parenteral ... 1910
Dilantin-125 Suspension ... 1911

Facial swelling

Altace Capsules ... 1232
Alupent Tablets (0.2%) ... 669
Carafate Suspension ... 1505
Carafate Tablets ... 1504
Cortifoam ... 2396
Hivid Tablets (Less than 1% to less than 3%) ... 2121
JE-VAX (0.1%) ... 886
Lupron Injection (Less than 3%) ... 2555
Stelazine ... 2514
Unasyn (Less than 1%) ... 2212

Facies, mask-like

Compazine ... 2470
Loxitane ... 1378
Reglan ... 2068
Stelazine ... 2514
Thorazine ... 2523

Factors II, V, VII, X, decrease

▲Android Capsules, 10 mg (Among most common) ... 1250
Android ... 1251
Delatestryl Injection ... 2860
Estratest ... 2539
Halotestin Tablets ... 2614
Oreton Methyl ... 1255
Oxandrin ... 2862
Premarin with Methyltestosterone .. 2794
Testoderm Testosterone Transdermal System ... 486
Testred Capsules ... 1262

Factors VII, VIII, IX, X, increase

Amen Tablets ... 780
Aygestin Tablets ... 974
Brevicon ... 2088
Depo-Provera Sterile Aqueous Suspension ... 2606
Estratest ... 2539
Norinyl ... 2088
Nor-Q D Tablets ... 2135
Ortho-Cyclen/Ortho-Tri-Cyclen ... 1858
Ortho-Cyclen/Ortho Tri-Cyclen ... 1858
Tri-Norinyl ... 2164

Fainting (see under Syncope)

Falling

Ambien Tablets (Infrequent) ... 2416
Dalmane Capsules ... 2173
Eldepryl Tablets ... 2550
Halcion Tablets ... 2611
Matulane Capsules ... 2131
Monopril Tablets (0.4% to 1.0%) .. 757
Restoril Capsules ... 2284
Sinemet CR Tablets ... 944
Tofranil Ampuls ... 854
Tofranil Tablets ... 856
Tofranil-PM Capsules ... 857

Fanconi syndrome

Depakene (Rare) ... 413
Depakote Tablets (Rare) ... 415
Garamycin Injectable ... 2360
IFEX ... 697

Fasciculations

Anectine ... 1073
Eskalith ... 2485
Lithium Carbonate Capsules & Tablets ... 2230

(▣ Described in PDR For Nonprescription Drugs) Incidence data in parenthesis; ▲ 3% or more (◉ Described in PDR For Ophthalmology)

1299 Side Effects Index Fatigue

Lithonate/Lithotabs/Lithobid 2543
Mestinon Injectable 1253
Mestinon 1254
Myochrysine Injection (Rare) 1711
Paxil Tablets (Rare) 2505
▲ Prostigmin Injectable (Among most common) 1260
Prostigmin Tablets (Among most common) 1261
Tensilon Injectable 1261

Fasciitis, necrotizing fulminant

Clinoril Tablets (Rare) 1618
Dolobid Tablets 1654
Indocin (Rare) 1680

Fatality, hepatic related

Cylert Tablets (Rare) 412
Macrobid Capsules 1988

Fatality, non-cardiovascular related

Atromid-S Capsules 2701

Fatigue

Accupril Tablets (2.6%) 1893
▲ Accutane Capsules (Approximately 1 patient in 20) 2076
Actifed with Codeine Cough Syrup 1067
Actigall Capsules 802
▲ Actimmune (14%) 1056
▲ Adalat CC (4%) 589
Children's Advil Suspension 2692
AeroBid Inhaler System (1-3%) 1005
Aerobid-M Inhaler System (1-3%) 1005
Altace Capsules (2.0%) 1232
Alupent Tablets (1.4%) 669
Ambien Tablets (1%) 2416
Amen Tablets 780
Amicar Syrup, Tablets, and Injection 1267
▲ Anafranil Capsules (35% to 39%) 803
Ancobon Capsules 2079
Antabuse Tablets (Small number of patients) 2695
Aquasol A Vitamin A Capsules, USP 534
Aquasol A Parenteral 534
▲ Aredia for Injection (Up to 12%) 810
Asendin Tablets (Less frequent) 1369
Atamet 572
Atretol Tablets 573
Atromid-S Capsules (Less often) 2701
Atrovent Inhalation Aerosol (Less than 1%) 671
Azo Gantrisin Tablets 2081
▲ BCG Vaccine, USP (TICE) (7.4%) 1814
Bactrim DS Tablets 2084
Bactrim I.V. Infusion 2082
Bactrim 2084
Benadryl Capsules 1898
Benadryl Injection 1898
▲ Betapace Tablets (5% to 20%) 641
Bioclate, Antihemophilic Factor (Recombinant) (One patient out of 13,394) 513
▲ Blocadren Tablets (3.4% to 5%) 1614
Brevibloc Injection (About 1%) 1808
Bumex (0.1%) 2093
▲ BuSpar (4%) 737
Calan SR Caplets (1.7%) 2422
Calan Tablets (1.7%) 2419
Capoten (About 0.5 to 2%) 739
Capozide (0.5 to 2%) 742
▲ Cardura Tablets (0.7% to 12%) 2186
▲ Cartrol Tablets (7.1%) 410
Cataflam 816
Catapres Tablets (About 4 in 100 patients) 674
▲ Catapres-TTS (6 of 101 patients; less frequent) 675
Ceredase 1065
▲ CHEMET (succimer) Capsules (5.2 to 15.7%) 1545
▲ Claritin (4%) 2349
▲ Claritin-D (4%) 2350
Clinoril Tablets (Less than 1 in 100) 1618
Clomid (Fewer than 1%) 1514
Clozaril Tablets (2%) 2252
▲ Cognex Capsules (4%) 1901
Colestid Tablets (Infrequent) 2591
▲ Combipres Tablets (About 4%) 677
▲ Cordarone Tablets (4 to 9%) 2712
Cortifoam 2396
Cosmegen Injection 1626
Cozaar Tablets (1% or greater) 1628
Cycrin Tablets 975
Cytotec (Infrequent) 2424
Danocrine Capsules 2307
▲ Dantrium Capsules (Among most frequent) 1982
Daypro Caplets 2426
Deconamine 1320
▲ Depo-Provera Contraceptive Injection (More than 5%) 2602
Depo-Provera Sterile Aqueous Suspension 2606
▲ Desyrel and Desyrel Dividose (5.7% to 11.3%) 503
Dibenzyline Capsules 2476
Dipentum Capsules (1.8%) 1951
Diprivan Injection (Less than 1%) 2833
▲ Dizac (Among most common) 1809
Dolobid Tablets (Greater than 1 in 100) 1654
Doral Tablets (1.9%) 2664
Dyazide 2479
▲ DynaCirc Capsules (2.0% to 8.5%) 2256
Dyrenium Capsules (Rare) 2481
Edecrin 1657
Elavil 2838
Eldepryl Tablets 2550
Elspar 1659
Emete-con Intramuscular/Intravenous 2198
Empirin with Codeine Tablets (Occasional) 1093
Endep Tablets 2174
▲ Engerix-B Unit-Dose Vials (14%) 2482
▲ Epogen for Injection (9% to 25%) 489
▲ Ergamisol Tablets (6% to 11%) 1292
Esgic-plus Tablets (Infrequent) 1013
Esimil Tablets 822
Eskalith 2485
▲ Ethmozine Tablets (3.1% to 5.9%) 2041
Etrafon 2355
▲ Famvir (Among most frequent; 4.4%) 2486
Fansidar Tablets 2114
▲ Felbatol (6.9% to 16.8%) 2666
Feldene Capsules (Occasional) 1965
Fioricet Tablets (Infrequent) 2258
Fioricet with Codeine Capsules (Infrequent) 2260
Fiorinal with Codeine Capsules (Infrequent) 2262
Flexeril Tablets (1% to 3%) 1661
Floxin I.V. (1% to 3%) 1571
Floxin Tablets (200 mg, 300 mg, 400 mg) (1% to 3%) 1567
▲ Fludara for Injection (10% to 38%) 663
Flumadine Tablets & Syrup (1.0%) 1015
▲ Foscavir Injection (5% or greater) 547
Fulvicin P/G Tablets (Occasional) 2359
Fulvicin P/G 165 & 330 Tablets (Occasional) 2359
Gammagard S/D, Immune Globulin, Intravenous (Human) (Occasional) 585
Gantanol Tablets 2119
Gantrisin 2120
Gastrocrom Capsules (Infrequent) 984
Glauctabs ⊙ 208
Grifulvin V (griseofulvin tablets) Microsize (griseofulvin oral suspension) Microsize (Occasional) 1888
Gris-PEG Tablets, 125 mg & 250 mg (Occasional) 479
Halcion Tablets (0.9% to 0.5%) 2611
▲ Havrix (1% to 10%) 2489
Hexalen Capsules (1%) 2571
▲ Hismanal Tablets (4.2%) 1293
Hivid Tablets (Less than 1% to less than 3%) 2121
▲ Hylorel Tablets (25.7% to 63.6%) 985
▲ Hytrin Capsules (7.4% to 11.3%) 430
Hyzaar Tablets (1% or greater) 1677
IFEX (Less than 1%) 697
Imdur (Less than or equal to 5%) 1323
Imitrex Injection (1.1%) 1103
Imitrex Tablets 1106
Imodium Capsules 1295
Inderal 2728
Inderal LA Long Acting Capsules 2730
Inderide Tablets 2732
Inderide LA Long Acting Capsules 2734
Indocin (Greater than 1%) 1680
▲ Intron A (15% to 84%) 2364
Inversine Tablets 1686
IOPIDINE Sterile Ophthalmic Solution ⊙ 219
Ismelin Tablets 827
Isoptin Oral Tablets (1.7%) 1346
Isoptin SR Tablets (1.7%) 1348
K-Phos Neutral Tablets 639
K-Phos Original Formula 'Sodium Free' Tablets (Less frequent) 639
Keflex Pulvules & Oral Suspension 914
Keftab Tablets 915
▲ Kerlone Tablets (2.9% to 9.7%) 2436
Lamprene Capsules (Less than 1%) 828
▲ Lariam Tablets (Among most frequent) 2128
Larodopa Tablets (Relatively frequent) 2129
▲ Lescol Capsules (3.5%) 2267
▲ Leucovorin Calcium for Injection (2% to 13%) 1268
▲ Leustatin (11% to 45%) 1834
▲ Levatol (4.4%) 2403
Levbid Extended-Release Tablets 2405
Levlen/Tri-Levlen 651
Levsin/Levsinex/Levbid 2405
Limbitrol 2180
Lioresal Intrathecal 1596
Lioresal Tablets (2-4%) 829
Lithium Carbonate Capsules & Tablets 2230
Lithonate/Lithotabs/Lithobid 2543
Livostin (Approximately 1% to 3%) ⊙ 266
▲ Lopid Tablets (3.8%) 1917
▲ Lopressor Ampuls (10%) 830
▲ Lopressor HCT Tablets (10 in 100 patients) 832
▲ Lopressor Tablets (10%) 830
Lotensin Tablets (2.4%) 834
▲ Lotensin HCT (5.2%) 837
Lotrel Capsules 840
▲ Lozol Tablets (Greater than or equal to 5%) 2022
▲ Ludiomil Tablets (4%) 843
Lupron Injection (Less than 5%) 2555
▲ MZM (Among reactions occurring most often) ⊙ 267
Matulane Capsules 2131
Maxair Autohaler 1492
Maxair Inhaler (Less than 1%) 1494
Maxaquin Tablets (Less than 1%) 2440
Maxzide 1380
Mesantoin Tablets 2272
▲ Mesnex Injection (33%) 702
Methotrexate Sodium Tablets, Injection, for Injection and LPF Injection (Frequent) 1275
Metrodin (urofollitropin for injection) 2446
▲ Mexitil Capsules (1.9% to 3.8%) 678
Miacalcin Nasal Spray (1% to 3%) 2275
Micronor Tablets 1872
Midamor Tablets (Between 1% and 3%) 1703
Mintezol 1704
Modicon 1872
Moduretic Tablets (Greater than 1%, less than 3%) 1705
Monoket (Up to 4%) 2406
Monopril Tablets (Less than 1.0% to 1.0% or more) 757
Motofen Tablets (1 in 200 to 1 in 600) 784
Children's Motrin Ibuprofen Oral Suspension 1546
Motrin Tablets 2625
Mutamycin 703
▲ Mykrox Tablets (4.4%) 993
Myleran Tablets 1143
Mysoline (Occasional) 2754
Nalfon 200 Pulvules & Nalfon Tablets (1.7%) 917
Nardil (Common) 1920
Navane Capsules and Concentrate 2201
Navane Intramuscular 2202
▲ Navelbine Injection (27%) 1145
▲ NebuPent for Inhalation Solution (53 to 72%) 1040
Neptazane Tablets 1388
▲ Neupogen for Injection (11%) 495
▲ Neurontin Capsules (Among most common; 11%) 1922
Neutrexin (1.8%) 2572
Nizoral Tablets 1298
▲ Nolvadex Tablets (3.8%) 2841
▲ Normodyne Injection (1% to 10%) 2377
▲ Normodyne Tablets (1% to 10%) 2379
▲ Norpace (3 to 9%) 2444
Norpramin Tablets 1526
▲ Norvasc Tablets (4.5%) 1940
Nydrazid Injection 508
Oncaspar 2028
Ornade Spansule Capsules 2502
Ortho-Cyclen/Ortho-Tri-Cyclen 1858
Ortho-Novum 1872
Ortho-Cyclen/Ortho Tri-Cyclen 1858
Orthoclone OKT3 Sterile Solution 1837
PBZ Tablets 845
PBZ-SR Tablets 844
Pamelor 2280
Paraflex Caplets 1580
Parafon Forte DSC Caplets 1581
▲ Parlodel (1.0% to 7%) 2281
Peganone Tablets 446
Penetrex Tablets (Less than 1% but more than or equal to 0.1%) 2031
Pentaspan Injection 937
Pepcid Injection (Infrequent) 1722
Pepcid (Infrequent) 1720
Peptavlon 2878
Periactin 1724
Phenergan Injection 2773
Phenurone Tablets (Less than 1%) 447
Phrenilin (Infrequent) 785
Pipracil 1390
Pondimin Tablets 2066
▲ Pravachol (1.9% to 3.8%) 765
Pregnyl 1828
Premphase 2797
Prempro 2801
Prilosec Delayed-Release Capsules (Less than 1%) 529
Prinivil Tablets (2.5%) 1733
▲ Prinzide Tablets (3.7%) 1737
▲ Procardia XL Extended Release Tablets (5.9%) 1972
▲ Procrit for Injection (9% to 25%) 1841
Profasi (chorionic gonadotropin for injection, USP) 2450
▲ Proleukin for Injection (53%) 797
Propulsid (More than 1%) 1300
Proventil Syrup (Children 2 to 6 years, 1%) 2385
Provera Tablets 2636
▲ Prozac Pulvules & Liquid, Oral Solution (4.2%) 919
Quadrinal Tablets 1350
Questran Light 769
Questran Powder 770
▲ Rabies Vaccine Adsorbed (8% to 10%) 2508
Recombivax HB (Equal to or greater than 1%) 1744
▲ Reglan (Approximately 10%) 2068
Relafen Tablets (1% to 3%) 2510
ReVia Tablets (Less than 1% to 4%) 940
RhoGAM Rh_0(D) Immune Globulin (Human) 1847
Rifadin 1528
Rifamate Capsules 1530
Rifater 1532
Rimactane Capsules 847
Risperdal (Frequent) 1301
▲ Roferon-A Injection (89% to 95%) 2145
Rogaine Topical Solution (0.36%) 2637
Romazicon (1% to 3%) 2147
▲ Rowasa (3.44%) 2548
▲ Rythmol Tablets–150mg, 225mg, 300mg (1.8 to 6.0%) 1352
SSKI Solution (Less frequent) 2658
Sandostatin Injection (1% to 4%) 2292
Sansert Tablets 2295
▲ Sectral Capsules (11%) 2807
Sedapap Tablets 50 mg/650 mg (Infrequent) 1543
▲ Seldane Tablets (2.9% to 4.5%) 1536
Seldane-D Extended-Release Tablets (2.1%) 1538
Septra 1174
Septra I.V. Infusion 1169
Septra I.V. Infusion ADD-Vantage Vials 1171
Septra 1174
Serevent Inhalation Aerosol (1% to 3%) 1176
Serophene (clomiphene citrate tablets, USP) (Less than 1 in 100 patients) 2451
Sinemet Tablets 943
Sinemet CR Tablets 944
Sinequan (Occasional) 2205
Sporanox Capsules (0.5% to 2.8%) 1305
Stelazine 2514
Stilphostrol Tablets and Ampuls 612
▲ Supprelin Injection (1% to 10%) 2056
Surmontil Capsules 2811
Symmetrel Capsules and Syrup (0.1% to 5%) 946
▲ Tambocor Tablets (7.7%) 1497
Tavist Syrup 2297
Tavist Tablets 2298
▲ Tegison Capsules (50-75%) 2154
Tegretol Chewable Tablets 852
Tegretol Suspension 852
Tegretol Tablets 852
Temaril Tablets, Syrup and Spansule Extended-Release Capsules 483

(▣ Described in PDR For Nonprescription Drugs) Incidence data in parenthesis; ▲ 3% or more (⊙ Described in PDR For Ophthalmology)

Fatigue — Side Effects Index — 1300

▲Tenex Tablets (2% to 12%) ... 2074
▲Tenoretic Tablets (0.6% to 26%) .. 2845
▲Tenormin Tablets and I.V. Injection (0.6% to 26%) ... 2847
TheraCys BCG Live (Intravesical) (Up to 0.9%) ... 897
Thioplex (Thiotepa For Injection) ... 1281
Tilade (1.1%) ... 996
Timolide Tablets (1.9%) ... 1748
Timoptic in Ocudose (Less frequent) ... 1753
Timoptic Sterile Ophthalmic Solution (Less frequent) ... 1751
Timoptic-XE ... 1755
Tofranil Ampuls ... 854
Tofranil Tablets ... 856
Tofranil-PM Capsules ... 857
Tonocard Tablets (0.8-1.6%) ... 531
▲Toprol-XL Tablets (About 10 of 100 patients) ... 565
Tornalate Solution for Inhalation, 0.2% (1.5%) ... 956
▲Trandate Tablets (1% to 11%) ... 1185
Tranxene ... 451
Triavil Tablets ... 1757
Levlen/Tri-Levlen ... 651
Trinalin Repetabs Tablets ... 1330
Trusopt Sterile Ophthalmic Solution (Infrequent) ... 1760
Tussend ... 1783
Unasyn (Less than 1%) ... 2212
Univasc Tablets (2.4%) ... 2410
Uroqid-Acid No. 2 Tablets ... 640
▲Valium Injectable (Among most common) ... 2182
▲Valium Tablets (Among most common) ... 2183
▲Valrelease Capsules (Among most common) ... 2169
Vantin for Oral Suspension and Vantin Tablets (Less than 1%) ... 2646
Varivax (Greater than or equal to 1%) ... 1762
▲Vaseretic Tablets (3.9%) ... 1765
Vasotec I.V. (0.5 to 1%) ... 1768
Vasotec Tablets (1.8% to 3.0%) ... 1771
Ventolin Syrup (1% of children) ... 1202
Verelan Capsules (1.7%) ... 1410
Verelan Capsules (1.7%) ... 2824
▲Visken Tablets (8%) ... 2299
Vivactil Tablets ... 1774
Voltaren Tablets ... 861
▲Wellbutrin Tablets (5.0%) ... 1204
▲Xanax Tablets (48.6%) ... 2649
Zarontin Capsules ... 1928
Zarontin Syrup ... 1929
Zaroxolyn Tablets ... 1000
▲Zebeta Tablets (6.6% to 8.2%) ... 1413
▲Zestoretic (3.7%) ... 2850
▲Zestril Tablets (2.5%) ... 2854
▲Ziac (3.0% to 4.6%) ... 1415
▲Zinecard (48% to 61%) ... 1961
Zithromax (1% or less) ... 1944
▲Zofran Injection (5%) ... 1214
▲Zofran Tablets (9% to 13%) ... 1217
▲Zoloft Tablets (10.6%) ... 2217
▲Zonalon Cream (Approximately 1% to 10%) ... 1055
Zovirax (0.4%) ... 1219

Fatigue, muscular
Apresazide Capsules ... 808
Capozide ... 742
Demadex Tablets and Injection ... 686
Dyazide ... 2479
Esgic-plus Tablets (Infrequent) ... 1013
Esidrix Tablets ... 821
Fioricet Tablets (Infrequent) ... 2258
Fioricet with Codeine Capsules (Infrequent) ... 2260
Fiorinal with Codeine Capsules (Infrequent) ... 2262
Imitrex Injection (Rare) ... 1103
Isoptin Injectable ... 1344
Lasix Injection, Oral Solution and Tablets ... 1240
Maxzide ... 1380
Oretic Tablets ... 443
Phrenilin (Infrequent) ... 785
Prinzide Tablets ... 1737
Sedapap Tablets 50 mg/650 mg (Infrequent) ... 1543
▲Tenoretic Tablets (3% to 6%) ... 2845
▲Tenormin Tablets and I.V. Injection (3% to 6%) ... 2847
Thalitone (Common) ... 1245
Vaseretic Tablets ... 1765
Zaroxolyn Tablets ... 1000
Zestoretic ... 2850

Fat intolerance
Anafranil Capsules (Rare) ... 803

Fear
Anexsia 5/500 Elixir ... 1781
Anexia Tablets ... 1782
BuSpar (Infrequent) ... 737
Claritin-D ... 2350
D.A. Chewable Tablets ... 951
Deconamine Chewable Tablets ... 1320
Deconamine CX Cough and Cold Liquid and Tablets ... 1319
Deconamine ... 1320
Deconsal ... 454
Dilaudid Ampules ... 1335
Dilaudid Cough Syrup ... 1336
Dilaudid ... 1335
Dura-Tap/PD Capsules ... 2867
Dura-Vent/DA Tablets ... 953
Dura-Vent Tablets ... 952
Entex PSE Tablets ... 1987
EpiPen—Epinephrine Auto-Injector 790
Fedahist Gyrocaps ... 2401
Fedahist Timecaps ... 2401
Guaimax-D Tablets ... 792
Hycodan Tablets and Syrup ... 930
Hycomine Compound Tablets ... 932
Hycomine ... 931
Hycotuss Expectorant Syrup ... 933
Hydrocet Capsules ... 782
Lorcet 10/650 ... 1018
Lortab ... 2566
Novahistine DH ... 2462
Novahistine DMX ... ▣ 822
Novahistine Elixir ... ▣ 823
Novahistine Expectorant ... 2463
Phenobarbital Elixir and Tablets ... 1469
Seldane-D Extended-Release Tablets ... 1538
Syn-Rx Tablets ... 465
Syn-Rx DM Tablets ... 466
Trinalin Repetabs Tablets ... 1330
Tussend ... 1783
Tussend Expectorant ... 1785
Tussionex Pennkinetic Extended-Release Suspension ... 998
Vicodin Tablets ... 1356
Vicodin ES Tablets ... 1357
Vicodin Tuss Expectorant ... 1358
Xanax Tablets (1.4%) ... 2649
Zydone Capsules ... 949

Febrile reactions
Albuminar-5, Albumin (Human) U.S.P. 5% (Occasional) ... 512
Albuminar-25, Albumin (Human) U.S.P. 25% ... 513
Capastat Sulfate Vials ... 2868
Digibind ... 1091
Diphtheria and Tetanus Toxoids and Pertussis Vaccine Adsorbed USP (For Pediatric Use) (Infrequent) ... 875
Humegon ... 1824
INFeD (Iron Dextran Injection, USP) ... 2345
▲JE-VAX (5.5%) ... 886
Mumpsvax (Very rare) ... 1708
NephrAmine ... 2005
PedvaxHIB ... 1718
Pergonal (menotropins for injection, USP) ... 2448
Thioplex (Thiotepa For Injection) ... 1281
Tri-Immunol Adsorbed ... 1408
Varivax (Less than 0.1%) ... 1762

Fecal fat, increase (see under Steatorrhea)

Fecal impaction
Betaseron for SC Injection ... 658
Clozaril Tablets ... 2252
Cognex Capsules (Infrequent) ... 1901
Etrafon ... 2355
Kayexalate (At large doses in elderly individuals) ... 2314
Paxil Tablets (Rare) ... 2505
Prolixin ... 509
Questran Light ... 769
Sodium Polystyrene Sulfonate Suspension ... 2244
Trilafon (Occasional) ... 2389

Feces, color change
Prilosec Delayed-Release Capsules (Less than 1%) ... 529
Rifadin ... 1528

Feces, discoloration
Derifil Tablets ... 2246
Lamprene Capsules (Greater than 1%) ... 828
PREVACID Delayed-Release Capsules (Less than 1%) ... 2562
Risperdal (Rare) ... 1301
Urised Tablets ... 1964

Feeling, intoxicated
Ambien Tablets (Rare) ... 2416
▲Esgic-plus Tablets (Among most frequent) ... 1013
▲Fioricet Tablets (Among most frequent) ... 2258
Fioricet with Codeine Capsules (Frequent) ... 2260
Fiorinal with Codeine Capsules (1.0%) ... 2262
Imitrex Injection (Rare) ... 1103
▲Phrenilin (Among most frequent) ... 785
▲Sedapap Tablets 50 mg/650 mg (Among most frequent) ... 1543

Feelings, drugged
▲Ambien Tablets (3%) ... 2416
Paxil Tablets (Infrequent) ... 2505

Feeling, shaky
Esgic-plus Tablets (Infrequent) ... 1013
Fioricet Tablets (Infrequent) ... 2258
Fioricet with Codeine Capsules (Infrequent) ... 2260
Fiorinal with Codeine Capsules (Infrequent) ... 2262
Phrenilin (Infrequent) ... 785

Feeling, strange
Ambien Tablets (Rare) ... 2416
Imitrex Injection (2.2%) ... 1103
Imitrex Tablets ... 1106
Neurontin Capsules (Rare) ... 1922
▲ReVia Tablets (Less than 10%) ... 940

Feet, cold
Hivid Tablets (Less than 1% to less than 3%) ... 2121
KOGENATE Antihemophilic Factor (Recombinant) ... 632
Parlodel ... 2281

Female genitalia, tenderness
Supprelin Injection (2% to 3%) ... 2056

Fertility, impairment of
Amen Tablets ... 780
Depo-Provera Contraceptive Injection (Fewer than 1%) ... 2602
Depo-Provera Sterile Aqueous Suspension ... 2606
Halotestin Tablets ... 2614
Intron A ... 2364
Oreton Methyl ... 1255

Fertility, male, decrease
Lopid Tablets ... 1917

Festination
Eldepryl Tablets ... 2550

Fetal acidosis
Prepidil Gel ... 2633

Fetal circulation, persistent
Exosurf Neonatal for Intratracheal Suspension (Less than 1% to 2%) ... 1095

Fetal death (see under Death, fetal)

Fetal defects
Accupril Tablets ... 1893
▲Accutane Capsules (Potentially all exposed fetuses) ... 2076
Butisol Sodium Elixir & Tablets ... 2660
Capozide ... 742
Climara Transdermal System ... 645
Clomid ... 1514
Cytoxan ... 694
Depo-Provera Contraceptive Injection ... 2602
Halcion Tablets ... 2611
Lotrel Capsules ... 840
Lupron Depot 7.5 mg ... 2559
Megace Tablets ... 701
Methotrexate Sodium Tablets, Injection, for Injection and LPF Injection ... 1275
Nembutal Sodium Capsules ... 436
Nembutal Sodium Solution ... 438
Nembutal Sodium Suppositories ... 440
NEOSAR Lyophilized/Neosar (One case) ... 1959
Premarin with Methyltestosterone .. 2794
Tegison Capsules ... 2154

Fetal depression
Prepidil Gel ... 2633

Fetal harm
Accupril Tablets ... 1893
▲Accutane Capsules (Potentially all exposed fetuses) ... 2076
Actifed with Codeine Cough Syrup .. 1067
Advil Cold and Sinus Caplets and Tablets (formerly CoAdvil) ... ▣ 870
Alkeran for Injection ... 1070
Alkeran Tablets ... 1071
Amen Tablets ... 780
Amikacin Sulfate Injection, USP ... 960
Amikin Injectable ... 501
Android ... 1251
Aquasol A Vitamin A Capsules, USP ... 534
Aquasol A Parenteral ... 534
Arfonad Ampuls ... 2080
Ativan Injection ... 2698
Aygestin Tablets ... 974
BiCNU ... 691
Cafergot ... 2251
Capoten ... 739
CeeNU ... 693
Cerubidine ... 795
Clomid ... 1514
Cozaar Tablets ... 1628
Cycrin Tablets ... 975
Cystospaz ... 1963
Cytadren Tablets ... 819
Cytosar-U Sterile Powder ... 2592
Cytotec ... 2424
Cytoxan ... 694
Danocrine Capsules ... 2307
Depen Titratable Tablets ... 2662
Depo-Provera Sterile Aqueous Suspension ... 2606
Didrex Tablets ... 2607
Diethylstilbestrol Tablets ... 1437
Diucardin Tablets ... 2718
Doral Tablets ... 2664
Dynacin Capsules ... 1590
Efudex ... 2113
Empirin with Codeine Tablets ... 1093
Enduron Tablets ... 420
Ergomar ... 1486
Eskalith ... 2485
Estrace Cream and Tablets ... 749
Estraderm Transdermal System ... 824
Estratest ... 2539
Eulexin Capsules ... 2358
Fiorinal ... 2261
Fludara for Injection ... 663
Fluoroplex Topical Solution & Cream 1% ... 479
Fluorouracil Injection ... 2116
Sterile FUDR ... 2118
Garamycin Injectable ... 2360
Habitrol Nicotine Transdermal System ... 865
Humegon ... 1824
Hyzaar Tablets ... 1677
IFEX ... 697
Imuran ... 1110
Lescol Capsules ... 2267
Leukeran Tablets ... 1133
Lithium Carbonate Capsules & Tablets ... 2230
Lithonate/Lithotabs/Lithobid ... 2543
Lotensin Tablets ... 834
Lotensin HCT ... 837
Lotrel Capsules ... 840
Lupron Depot 3.75 mg ... 2556
Lysodren ... 698
Matulane Capsules ... 2131
Maxzide ... 1380
Mebaral Tablets ... 2322
Megace Oral Suspension ... 699
Megace Tablets ... 701
Menest Tablets ... 2494
Metastron ... 1594
Metrodin (urofollitropin for injection) ... 2446
Mevacor Tablets ... 1699
Minocin Oral Suspension ... 1385
Minocin Pellet-Filled Capsules ... 1383
Mithracin ... 607
Monopril Tablets ... 757
Mustargen ... 1709
Myleran Tablets ... 1143
Navelbine Injection ... 1145
Nebcin Vials, Hyporets & ADD-Vantage ... 1464
Nembutal Sodium Capsules ... 436

(▣ Described in PDR For Nonprescription Drugs) Incidence data in parenthesis; ▲ 3% or more (◉ Described in PDR For Ophthalmology)

1301 Side Effects Index Fever

Nembutal Sodium Solution 438
Nembutal Sodium Suppositories 440
NEOSAR Lyophilized/Neosar 1959
Neosporin G.U. Irrigant Sterile 1148
Netromycin Injection 100 mg/ml 2373
Neutrexin 2572
Nicorette 2458
Nolvadex Tablets 2841
Norisodrine with Calcium Iodide Syrup 442
Novantrone 1279
Oncovin Solution Vials & Hyporets 1466
Oretic Tablets 443
Ortho Dienestrol Cream 1866
Ovcon 760
PMB 200 and PMB 400 2783
ParaGard T380A Intrauterine Copper Contraceptive 1880
Paraplatin for Injection 705
Peganone Tablets 446
Pergonal (menotropins for injection, USP) 2448
Phenobarbital Elixir and Tablets 1469
Phenurone Tablets 447
Platinol 708
Platinol-AQ Injection 710
Pravachol 765
Premarin Intravenous 2787
Premarin with Methyltestosterone 2794
Premarin Tablets 2789
Prinivil Tablets 1733
Prinzide Tablets 1737
Profasi (chorionic gonadotropin for injection, USP) 2450
ProSom Tablets 449
Prostep (nicotine transdermal system) 1394
Purinethol Tablets 1156
Quadrinal Tablets 1350
ReoPro Vials 1471
Restoril Capsules 2284
SSKI Solution 2658
Seconal Sodium Pulvules 1474
Serax Capsules 2810
Serax Tablets 2810
Soma Compound w/Codeine Tablets 2676
Soma Compound Tablets 2675
Streptomycin Sulfate Injection 2208
Tapazole Tablets 1477
Taxol 714
Tenoretic Tablets 2845
Tenormin Tablets and I.V. Injection 2847
Testoderm Testosterone Transdermal System 486
Testred Capsules 1262
Thioguanine Tablets, Tabloid Brand 1181
Thioplex (Thiotepa For Injection) 1281
Tobramycin Sulfate Injection 968
Univasc Tablets 2410
Vaseretic Tablets 1765
Vasotec I.V. 1768
Vasotec Tablets 1771
Velban Vials 1484
VePesid Capsules and Injection 718
Virazole 1264
Vumon 727
Wigraine Tablets & Suppositories 1829
Winstrol Tablets 2337
Xanax Tablets 2649
Zestoretic 2850
Zestril Tablets 2854
Zocor Tablets 1775

Fetal heart rate, deceleration

Prepidil Gel (2.1% to 4.3%) 2633

Fetal hemorrhage

Coumadin 926
Soma Compound w/Codeine Tablets 2676
Soma Compound Tablets 2675

Fetal hydantoin syndrome

Dilantin Infatabs 1908
Dilantin Kapseals 1906
Dilantin Parenteral 1910
Dilantin-125 Suspension 1911

Fetal problems, unspecified

Aleve 1975
Alka-Seltzer Plus Cold Medicine ■ 705
Alka-Seltzer Plus Cold & Cough Medicine ■ 708
Alka-Seltzer Plus Night-Time Cold Medicine ■ 707
Alka Seltzer Plus Sinus Medicine ■ 707
Arthritis Foundation Ibuprofen Tablets ■ 674
Arthritis Foundation Safety Coated Aspirin Tablets ■ 675
Arthritis Pain Ascriptin ■ 631
Maximum Strength Ascriptin ■ 630
Regular Strength Ascriptin Tablets ■ 629
BC Powder ■ 609
Bayer Children's Chewable Aspirin ■ 711
Genuine Bayer Aspirin Tablets & Caplets ■ 713
Extra Strength Bayer Arthritis Pain Regimen Formula ■ 711
Extra Strength Bayer Aspirin Caplets & Tablets ■ 712
Extended-Release Bayer 8-Hour Aspirin ■ 712
Extra Strength Bayer Plus Aspirin Caplets ■ 713
Extra Strength Bayer PM Aspirin ■ 713
Aspirin Regimen Bayer Regular Strength 325 mg Caplets ■ 709
Cipro I.V. 595
Dalmane Capsules 2173
Empirin Aspirin Tablets ■ 854
Floropryl Sterile Ophthalmic Ointment 1662
Haltran Tablets ■ 771
Humorsol Sterile Ophthalmic Solution 1664
Motrin IB Caplets, Tablets, and Geltabs ■ 838
Nuprin Ibuprofen/Analgesic Tablets & Caplets ■ 622
Polytrim Ophthalmic Solution Sterile 482
Sine-Aid IB Caplets 1554
Sine-Off Sinus Medicine ■ 825
Synarel Nasal Solution for Endometriosis 2152
Ursinus Inlay-Tabs ■ 794
Vaseretic Tablets 1765
Vasotec I.V. 1768
Vasotec Tablets 1771

Fetal sepsis, intrauterine

Prepidil Gel 2633

Fever

Abbokinase 403
Abbokinase Open-Cath 405
▲Acel-Imune Diphtheria and Tetanus Toxoids and Acellular Pertussis Vaccine Adsorbed (7% to 19%) 1364
▲ActHIB (0.5% to 24.6%) 872
▲Actimmune (52%) 1056
Activase 1058
Adalat Capsules (10 mg and 20 mg) (2% or less) 587
Adalat CC (Rare) 589
Adriamycin PFS (Occasional) 1947
Adriamycin RDF (Occasional) 1947
Children's Advil Suspension (Less than 1%) 2692
▲AeroBid Inhaler System (3-9%) 1005
▲Aerobid-M Inhaler System (3-9%) 1005
Aldomet Ester HCl Injection 1602
Aldomet Oral 1600
Aldoril Tablets 1604
Alkeran for Injection 1070
Alkeran Tablets 1071
All-Flex Arcing Spring Diaphragm (See also Ortho Diaphragm Kits) 1865
Altace Capsules (Less than 1%) 1232
Alupent Tablets (0.4%) 669
Ambien Tablets (Infrequent) 2416
Amen Tablets (Rare) 780
▲Anafranil Capsules (2% to 4%) 803
Anaprox/Naprosyn (Less than 1%) 2117
Ancobon Capsules 2079
Ansaid Tablets (Less than 1%) 2579
Antivenin (Crotalidae) Polyvalent 2696
Apresazide Capsules (Less frequent) 808
Apresoline Hydrochloride Tablets (Less frequent) 809
▲Aredia for Injection (At least 5% to 34%) 810
Aristocort Suspension (Forte Parenteral) 1027
Aristospan Suspension (Intra-articular) 1033
Aristospan Suspension (Intralesional) 1032
▲Asacol Delayed-Release Tablets (6%) 1979
Asendin Tablets 1369
▲Atgam Sterile Solution (1 in 3 patients; 51%) 2581
Atretol Tablets 573
Attenuvax (Occasional) 1610
Augmentin (Frequent) 2468
Axid Pulvules (1.6%) 1427
Azactam for Injection (Less than 1%) 734
Azo Gantrisin Tablets 2081
Azulfidine (One in every 30 patients or less) 1949
▲BCG Vaccine, USP (TICE) (19.9%) 1814
Benemid Tablets 1611
Betapace Tablets (Rare; 1% to 4%) 641
▲Betaseron for SC Injection (59%) 658
Biavax II (Occasional) 1613
Bicillin C-R Injection 2704
Bicillin C-R 900/300 Injection 2706
Bicillin L-A Injection 2707
Bioclate, Antihemophilic Factor (Recombinant) (Extremely rare) 513
▲Blenoxane (Frequent) 692
Bleph-10 Ophthalmic Solution 10% 475
Blocadren Tablets 1614
Brevibloc Injection (Less than 1%) 1808
BuSpar (Infrequent) 737
Butisol Sodium Elixir & Tablets (1 to 3 patients per 100) 2660
Calan SR Caplets 2422
Calan Tablets 2419
▲Capoten (About 4 to 7 of 100) 739
Capozide (Sometimes) 742
Carbocaine Hydrochloride Injection 2303
Cardene I.V. (Rare) 2709
Cardura Tablets (Less than 0.5% of 3960 patients) 2186
Cartrol Tablets (Less common) 410
Catapres Tablets 674
Catapres-TTS 675
Ceclor Pulvules & Suspension (Frequently) 1431
Cefizox for Intramuscular or Intravenous Use (Greater than 1% but less than 5%) 1034
Cefotan 2829
Ceftin for Oral Suspension (Less than 1% but more than 0.1%) 1078
Cefzil Tablets and Oral Suspension (Rare) 746
Celestone Soluspan Suspension 2347
▲CellCept Capsules (More than or equal to 3%; 21.4% to 23.3%) 2099
Ceptaz (2% of patients) 1081
Ceredase 1065
Cerubidine (Rare) 795
Cervidil (Less than 1%) 1010
▲CHEMET (succimer) Capsules (5.2 to 15.7%) 1545
Cipro I.V. (1% or less) 595
Cipro I.V. Pharmacy Bulk Package (Less than 1%) 597
Cipro Tablets (Less than 1%; rare) 592
Claforan Sterile and Injection (2.4%) 1235
Claritin (2% or fewer patients) 2349
Claritin-D (Less frequent) 2350
Clinoril Tablets (Less than 1%) 1618
Clomid 1514
▲Clozaril Tablets (5% or more) 2252
Cogentin 1621
Cognex Capsules (Frequent) 1901
ColBENEMID Tablets 1622
Combipres Tablets 677
Compazine 2470
Cordarone Intravenous (2.0%) 2715
Cosmegen Injection 1626
Coumadin (Infrequent) 926
Cozaar Tablets (Less than 1%) 1628
Cuprimine Capsules (Rare) 1630
Cycrin Tablets 975
Cystospaz 1963
Cytadren Tablets (Several) 819
CytoGam (Less than 5.0%) 1593
▲Cytosar-U Sterile Powder (Among most frequent) 2592
Cytotec (Infrequent) 2424
▲Cytovene (38%) 2103
Cytoxan 694
DTIC-Dome (Infrequent) 600
Danocrine Capsules (Rare) 2307
Dantrium Capsules (Less frequent) 1982
Dapsone Tablets USP 1284
Daranide Tablets 1633
Daraprim Tablets (Rare) 1090
Daypro Caplets (Rare) 2426
Depakene 413
Depakote Tablets (More than 1% but not more than 5%) 415
Depen Titratable Tablets (Rare) 2662
Depo-Provera Contraceptive Injection (Fewer than 1%) 2602
Depo-Provera Sterile Aqueous Suspension 2606
Desferal Vials 820
Diamox 1372
Dilacor XR Extended-release Capsules (Infrequent) 2018
Dilantin Infatabs 1908
Dilantin Kapseals 1906
Dilantin Parenteral 1910
Dilantin-125 Suspension 1911
Dipentum Capsules (Rare) 1951
Diphtheria & Tetanus Toxoids Adsorbed Purogenated (Mild) 1374
▲Diphtheria and Tetanus Toxoids and Pertussis Vaccine Adsorbed (0.3% to approximately 50%) 2477
Diphtheria and Tetanus Toxoids and Pertussis Vaccine Adsorbed USP (For Pediatric Use) (Frequent) 875
Diprivan Injection (Less than 1%) 2833
Diucardin Tablets 2718
Diupres Tablets 1650
Diuril Oral Suspension 1653
Diuril Sodium Intravenous 1652
Diuril Tablets 1653
Dobutrex Solution Vials (Occasional) 1439
Dolobid Tablets (Less than 1 in 100) 1654
Dopram Injectable 2061
Doxorubicin Astra (Occasional) 540
Duricef 748
Easprin 1914
EC-Naprosyn Delayed-Release Tablets (Less than 1%) 2117
Edecrin 1657
Effexor 2719
Elavil 2838
Elspar 1659
Emete-con Intramuscular/Intravenous (Rare) 2198
▲Eminase (Less than 10%) 2039
Endep Tablets 2174
Enduron Tablets 420
▲Engerix-B Unit-Dose Vials (1% to 10%) 2482
▲Epogen for Injection (29% to 38%) 489
▲Ergamisol Tablets (3% to 5%) 1292
Esgic-plus Tablets (Infrequent) 1013
Eskalith 2485
▲Ethamolin (Among most common; 1.8%) 2400
Ethmozine Tablets (Rare) 2041
Etrafon 2355
▲Famvir (3.3%) 2486
▲Felbatol (2.6% to 22.6%) 2666
Feldene Capsules (Less than 1%) 1965
Fioricet Tablets (Infrequent) 2258
Fioricet with Codeine Capsules (Infrequent) 2260
Fiorinal with Codeine Capsules (Infrequent) 2262
Flagyl 375 Capsules 2434
Flagyl I.V. 2247
Floxin I.V. (1% to 3%) 1571
Floxin Tablets (200 mg, 300 mg, 400 mg) (1% to 3%) 1567
▲Fludara for Injection (60% to 69%) 663
Flumadine Tablets & Syrup 1015
Fluothane 2724
Fluvirin (Infrequent) 460
Fortaz (2%) 1100
▲Foscavir Injection (5% or greater up to 65%) 547
Fragmin (Rare) 1954
Sterile FUDR 2118
▲Fungizone Intravenous (Among most common) 506
Furoxone 2046
▲Gamimune N, 5% Immune Globulin Intravenous (Human), 5% (Among most common; 24.4%) 619
▲Gamimune N, 10% Immune Globulin Intravenous (Human), 10% (Among most common; 24.4%) 621
Gammagard S/D, Immune Globulin, Intravenous (Human) (Occasional) 585
Gammar I.V., Immune Globulin Intravenous (Human), Lyophilized 516
Gamulin Rh, $Rh_0(D)$ Immune Globulin (Human) (Infrequent) 517
Ganite 2533
Gantanol Tablets 2119
Gantrisin 2120

(■ Described in PDR For Nonprescription Drugs) Incidence data in parenthesis; ▲ 3% or more (◎ Described in PDR For Ophthalmology)

Fever **Side Effects Index** **1302**

Garamycin Injectable 2360
Gelfoam Sterile Sponge 2608
Glauctabs ◉ 208
Haldol Decanoate 1577
Haldol Injection, Tablets and Concentrate 1575
▲ Havrix (1% to 10%) 2489
Heparin Lock Flush Solution 2725
Heparin Sodium Injection 2726
Heparin Sodium Injection, USP, Sterile Solution 2615
▲ Heparin Sodium Vials (Among most common) 1441
Hespan Injection 929
Helixate, Antihemophilic Factor (Recombinant) (Two reports out of 3,254 patients) 518
HibTITER (0.6% to 1.4%) 1375
Hivid Tablets (Less than 1% to less than 3%) 2121
Humegon 1824
Hydrea Capsules (Rare) 696
HydroDIURIL Tablets 1674
Hydropres Tablets 1675
Hyperstat I.V. Injection 2363
Hyskon Hysteroscopy Fluid (Rare) 1595
Hytrin Capsules (0.5% to at least 1%) 430
Hyzaar Tablets 1677
IBU Tablets (Rare; less than 1%) 1342
▲ Idamycin (26%) 1955
IFEX (1%) 697
Imdur (Less than or equal to 5%) 1323
Imitrex Injection (Rare) 1103
Imitrex Tablets (Infrequent) 1106
▲ Imovax Rabies Vaccine (Up to 6%) 881
Imuran (Less than 1%) 1110
Inderal 2728
Inderal LA Long Acting Capsules 2730
Inderide Tablets 2732
Inderide LA Long Acting Capsules 2734
INFeD (Iron Dextran Injection, USP) 2345
Influenza Virus Vaccine, Trivalent, Types A and B (chromatograph- and filter-purified subviron antigen) FluShield, 1995-1996 Formula (Infrequent) 2736
Inocor Lactate Injection (0.9%) 2309
▲ Intron A (3% to 86%) 2364
▲ IPOL Poliovirus Vaccine Inactivated (Up to 38%) 885
Isoptin SR Tablets 1348
▲ JE-VAX (Less than 3% to approximately 10%) 886
Keftab Tablets 915
Kefurox Vials, Faspak & ADD-Vantage 1454
Kerlone Tablets 2436
Klonopin Tablets 2126
KOGENATE Antihemophilic Factor (Recombinant) (Two reports) 632
Konÿne 80 Factor IX Complex 634
▲ Kytril Injection (3%; 8.6%) 2490
▲ Kytril Tablets (5%) 2492
▲ Lamictal Tablets (5.5%) 1112
Lamprene Capsules (Less than 1%) 828
▲ Lariam Tablets (Among most frequent) 2128
Lasix Injection, Oral Solution and Tablets 1240
Lescol Capsules (Rare) 2267
Leucovorin Calcium Tablets, Wellcovorin Brand 1132
Leukeran Tablets 1133
▲ Leukine for IV Infusion (95%) 1271
▲ Leustatin (11% to 69%; approximately two-thirds of patients) 1834
Levatol 2403
Levbid Extended-Release Tablets 2405
Levlen/Tri-Levlen 651
Levoprome 1274
Levsin/Levsinex/Levbid 2405
Lithonate/Lithotabs/Lithobid 2543
Lodine Capsules and Tablets 2743
Lopressor HCT Tablets 832
Lotensin HCT (0.3% or more) 837
▲ Lovenox Injection (5%) 2020
Loxitane 1378
Lozol Tablets 2022
Lupron Depot 3.75 mg 2556
Lupron Depot 7.5 mg (Less than 5%) 2559
Lupron Depot-PED 7.5 mg, 11.25 mg and 15 mg (Less than 2%) 2560
Lupron Injection (Less than 5%) 2555
Luvox Tablets 2544
M-M-R II 1687
M-R-VAX II 1689
MZM (Common) ◉ 267
Macrobid Capsules (Rare to less than 1%) 1988
Macrodantin Capsules (Rare; less often) 1989
Massengill Disposable Douche 2457
Massengill Medicated Disposable Douche 2458
Massengill Medicated Liquid Concentrate ▣ 821
Matulane Capsules 2131
Maxzide 1380
Mebaral Tablets (Less than 1 in 100) 2322
Mefoxin 1691
Mefoxin Premixed Intravenous Solution 1694
▲ Megace Oral Suspension (1% to 6%) 699
Mellaril 2269
Menomune-A/C/Y/W-135 (Up to 2%) 889
▲ Mepron Suspension (14% to 40%) 1135
Meruvax II 1697
Metastron (A single patient) 1594
Methadone Hydrochloride Oral Concentrate 2233
Methotrexate Sodium Tablets, Injection, for Injection and LPF Injection (Less common to frequent) 1275
MetroGel-Vaginal 902
Mevacor Tablets (Rare) 1699
Mexitil Capsules (1.2%) 678
Miacalcin Nasal Spray (Less than 1%) 2275
Micronor Tablets 1872
Miltown Tablets (Rare) 2672
Mini-Gamulin Rh, $Rh_0(D)$ Immune Globulin (Human) (Occasional) 520
Minipress Capsules 1937
Minizide Capsules 1938
Mintezol 1704
Mithracin 607
Moban Tablets and Concentrate 1048
Modicon 1872
Moduretic Tablets 1705
Monocid Injection (Less than 1%) 2497
Mononine, Coagulation Factor IX (Human) 523
Monopril Tablets (0.4% to 1.0%) 757
Children's Motrin Ibuprofen Oral Suspension (Less than 1%) 1546
Motrin Tablets (Less than 1%) 2625
Motrin Ibuprofen Suspension, Oral Drops, Chewable Tablets, Caplets (Rare; less than 1%) 1546
Mumpsvax (Uncommon) 1708
▲ Mutamycin (14%) 703
Myambutol Tablets 1386
Mycobutin Capsules (2%) 1957
Myochrysine Injection 1711
Nalfon 200 Pulvules & Nalfon Tablets (Less than 1%) 917
Anaprox/Naprosyn (Less than 1%) 2117
Nardil (Less frequent) 1920
Navane Capsules and Concentrate 2201
Navane Intramuscular 2202
Navelbine Injection 1145
Nebcin Vials, Hyporets & ADD-Vantage 1464
Nembutal Sodium Capsules 436
Nembutal Sodium Solution 438
Nembutal Sodium Suppositories (Less than 1%) 440
Neoral (2% or less) 2276
Neptazane Tablets 1388
Netromycin Injection 100 mg/ml (1 of 1000 patients) 2373
▲ Neupogen for Injection (12%) 495
Neurontin Capsules (More than 1%) 1922
▲ Neutrexin (8.3%) 2572
Nizoral Tablets (Less than 1%) 1298
Normodyne Tablets 2379
Noroxin Tablets (0.3% to 1.0%) 1715
Noroxin Tablets (0.3% to 1.0%) 2048
Norpace (Infrequent) 2444
▲ Novantrone (24 to 78%) 1279
Nuromax Injection (Less than or equal to 0.1%) 1149
Nydrazid Injection 508
▲ OmniHIB (0.6% to 20.1%) 2499
Omnipen for Oral Suspension 2765
▲ Oncaspar (Greater than 5%) 2028
Oncovin Solution Vials & Hyporets 1466
Orap Tablets 1050
Orlamm 2239
Ortho-Cyclen/Ortho-Tri-Cyclen 1858
Ortho Diaphragm Kits—All-Flex Arcing Spring; Ortho Coil Spring; Ortho-White Flat Spring 1865
Ortho Diaphragm Kit-Coil Spring 1865
Ortho-Novum 1872
Ortho-Cyclen/Ortho Tri-Cyclen 1858
Ortho-White Diaphragm Kit-Flat Spring (See also Ortho Diaphragm Kits) 1865
▲ Orthoclone OKT3 Sterile Solution (89% to 90%) 1837
PMB 200 and PMB 400 (Rare) 2783
Panhematin 443
Paraflex Caplets 1580
Parafon Forte DSC Caplets 1581
ParaGard T380A Intrauterine Copper Contraceptive 1880
Paraplatin for Injection 705
PASER Granules 1285
Paxil Tablets (1.7%) 2505
PedvaxHIB 1718
Peganone Tablets 446
Pen•Vee K (Frequent) 2772
Penetrex Tablets (Less than 1% but more than or equal to 0.1%) 2031
▲ Pentam 300 Injection (3.5%) 1041
Pentasa (0.9%) 1527
Pentaspan Injection 937
Pepcid Injection (Infrequent) 1722
Pepcid (Infrequent) 1720
Pergonal (menotropins for injection, USP) 2448
Permax Tablets (Frequent) 575
Pfizerpen for Injection 2203
Phenobarbital Elixir and Tablets (Less than 1 in 100 patients) 1469
Phenurone Tablets (Less than 1%) 447
Phrenilin (Infrequent) 785
Platinol 708
Platinol-AQ Injection 710
Pneumovax 23 (Rare) 1725
Pnu-Imune 23 (Occasional) 1393
Podocon-25 1891
▲ Poliovax (3%) 891
Polymyxin B Sulfate, Aerosporin Brand Sterile Powder 1154
Pondimin Tablets 2066
Potaba (Infrequent) 1229
Pravachol (Rare) 765
Premphase 2797
Prempro 2801
Prepidil Gel (1.4%) 2633
PREVACID Delayed-Release Capsules (Less than 1%) 2562
Prilosec Delayed-Release Capsules (Less than 1%) 529
Primaxin I.M. 1727
Primaxin I.V. (0.5%) 1729
Prinivil Tablets (0.3% to 1.1%) 1733
Prinzide Tablets (0.3 to 1%) 1737
Procan SR Tablets (Common) 1926
Procardia Capsules (2% or less) 1971
Procardia XL Extended Release Tablets (1% or less) 1972
▲ Procrit for Injection (29% to 38%) 1841
Proglycem 580
▲ Prograf (15% to 48%) 1042
Prolastin $Alpha_1$-Proteinase Inhibitor (Human) (0.77%) 635
▲ Proleukin for Injection (89%) 797
Prolixin 509
Proloprim Tablets 1155
Propulsid (2.2%) 1300
ProSom Tablets (Infrequent) 449
▲ Prostin E2 Suppository (Approximately one-half) 2634
▲ Prostin VR Pediatric Sterile Solution (About 14%) 2635
Protostat Tablets 1883
Provera Tablets 2636
Prozac Pulvules & Liquid, Oral Solution (1.4% to 2%) 919
Pulmozyme Inhalation 1064
Pyrazinamide Tablets (Rare) 1398
Quadrinal Tablets 1350
▲ Quinaglute Dura-Tabs Tablets (6%) 649
Quinidex Extentabs 2067
▲ Rabies Vaccine Adsorbed (8% to 10%) 2508
▲ Rabies Vaccine, Imovax Rabies I.D. (Less frequent; up to 6%) 883
Recombivax HB (Greater than 1%) 1744
Relafen Tablets (Less than 1%) 2510
▲ Retrovir Capsules (3.2% to 16%) 1158
▲ Retrovir I.V. Infusion (4% to 16%) 1163
▲ Retrovir Syrup (3.2% to 16%) 1158
ReVia Tablets (Less than 1%) 940
▲ Revex (3%) 1811
▲ RhoGAM $Rh_0(D)$ Immune Globulin (Human) (25% in one study) 1847
Ridaura Capsules (Rare) 2513
Rifadin 1528
Rifamate Capsules 1530
Rifater 1532
Rimactane Capsules 847
Risperdal (2% to 3%) 1301
Ritalin 848
Robaxin Injectable 2070
Robaxin Tablets 2071
Robaxisal Tablets 2071
Rocephin Injectable Vials, ADD-Vantage, Galaxy Container (Less than 1%) 2142
▲ Roferon-A Injection (74% to 98%) 2145
▲ Rowasa (1.2% to 3.19%) 2548
Rubex (Occasional) 712
Rythmol Tablets–150mg, 225mg, 300mg (1.9%) 1352
SSKI Solution (Less frequent) 2658
Sandimmune (2% or less) 2286
Sandoglobulin I.V. (Less than 1%) 2290
Sansert Tablets 2295
Seconal Sodium Pulvules (Less than 1 in 100) 1474
Sectral Capsules 2807
Sedapap Tablets 50 mg/650 mg (Infrequent) 1543
Septra I.V. Infusion 1169
Septra I.V. Infusion ADD-Vantage Vials 1171
Ser-Ap-Es Tablets 849
Serax Capsules 2810
Serax Tablets 2810
Serentil 684
Serzone Tablets (2%) 771
Solganal Suspension 2388
Soma Compound w/Codeine Tablets 2676
Soma Compound Tablets 2675
Soma Tablets 2674
Sporanox Capsules (0.3% to 2.5%) 1305
Stelazine 2514
▲ Streptase for Infusion (Among most common; 1% to 4%) 562
▲ Supprelin Injection (6% to 12%) 2056
Suprane (Less than 1%) 1813
Tagamet (Rare) 2516
Tambocor Tablets (1% to less than 3%) 1497
Tao Capsules 2209
Tapazole Tablets 1477
▲ Taxol (12%) 714
Tazicef for Injection (2%) 2519
Tazidime Vials, Faspak & ADD-Vantage 1478
▲ Tegison Capsules (10-25%) 2154
Tegretol Chewable Tablets 852
Tegretol Suspension 852
Tegretol Tablets 852
Tenoretic Tablets 2845
Tenormin Tablets and I.V. Injection 2847
Terazol 3 Vaginal Cream (1%) 1886
Terazol 3 Vaginal Suppositories (2.8% of 284 patients) 1886
Terazol 7 Vaginal Cream (1.7% of 521 patients) 1887
Tetanus & Diphtheria Toxoids Adsorbed Purogenated (Rare) 1401
Tetanus Toxoid Adsorbed Purogenated 1403
▲ Tetramune (24% to 40%) 1404
▲ TheraCys BCG Live (Intravesical) (2.6% to 38.4%) 897
Thioplex (Thiotepa For Injection) 1281
Thorazine (Occasional) 2523
▲ THROMBATE III Antithrombin III (Human) (1 of 17) 637
Ticlid Tablets 2156
Timolide Tablets 1748
Timoptic in Ocudose 1753
Timoptic Sterile Ophthalmic Solution 1751
Timoptic-XE 1755
Tobramycin Sulfate Injection 968
Tofranil Tablets 856
Tofranil-PM Capsules 857
Tolectin (200, 400 and 600 mg) (Less than 1%) 1581
Tonocard Tablets (Less than 1%) 531
Toprol-XL Tablets 565
Toradol (1% or less) 2159
Torecan (Occasional) 2245
Trandate Tablets (Less common) 1185
▲ Trasylol (12%) 613
Triavil Tablets 1757
▲ Tri-Immunol Adsorbed (50%) 1408
Trilafon 2389
Levlen/Tri-Levlen 651

(▣ Described in PDR For Nonprescription Drugs) Incidence data in parenthesis; ▲ 3% or more (◉ Described in PDR For Ophthalmology)

1303 Side Effects Index Flatulence

Trimpex Tablets 2163
Triostat Injection (Approximately 1%) 2530
Tripedia (1% to 4%) 892
Trobicin Sterile Powder 2645
TYLENOL Severe Allergy Medication Caplets 1564
Typhim Vi (Up to 2%) 899
Univasc Tablets 2410
Urispas Tablets 2532
Vantin for Oral Suspension and Vantin Tablets (Less than 1%) 2646
Vascor (200, 300 and 400 mg) Tablets (0.5 to 2.0%) 1587
Vaseretic Tablets 1765
Vasotec I.V. (0.5 to 1%) 1768
Vasotec Tablets (0.5% to 1.0%) 1771
VePesid Capsules and Injection (0.7% to 2%; infrequent) 718
Verelan Capsules 1410
Verelan Capsules (1% or less) 2824
▲ Videx Tablets, Powder for Oral Solution, & Pediatric Powder for Oral Solution (9% to 82%) 720
Visken Tablets 2299
Vivactil Tablets 1774
Vivotif Berna 665
▲ Vumon (3%) 727
Wellbutrin Tablets (1.2%) 1204
WinRho SD (A small number of cases) 2576
WinRho SD (1%) 2577
Yodoxin 1230
Zantac (Rare) 1209
Zantac Injection 1207
Zantac Syrup (Rare) 1209
Zebeta Tablets 1413
Zefazone 2654
▲ Zerit Capsules (5% to 38%) 729
Zestoretic (0.3 to 1%) 2850
Zestril Tablets (0.5% to 1.1%) 2854
Ziac 1415
▲ Zinecard (22% to 34%) 1961
Zocor Tablets (Rare) 1775
▲ Zofran Injection (2% to 8%) 1214
▲ Zofran Tablets (8%) 1217
▲ Zoladex (Greater than 1% but less than 5%) 2858
Zoloft Tablets (1.6%) 2217
Zonalon Cream (Less than 1%) 1055
Zosyn (2.4%) 1419
Zosyn Pharmacy Bulk Package (2.4%) 1422
Zovirax Capsules 1219
Zovirax Sterile Powder (Less than 1%) 1223
Zovirax 1219
Zyloprim Tablets (Less than 1%) 1226

Fever, neutropenic
▲ Neupogen for Injection (13%) 495

Fibrillations
Luvox Tablets (Rare) 2544
Nicorette 2458
Tambocor Tablets 1497
Tenex Tablets (Rare) 2074

Fibrillations, atrial
Adalat CC (Less than 1.0%) 589
▲ Aredia for Injection (Up to 6%) 810
Betaseron for SC Injection 658
Cardene Capsules (Less than 0.4%) 2095
▲ CellCept Capsules (More than or equal to 3%) 2099
Clozaril Tablets 2252
Cognex Capsules (Infrequent) 1901
Cordarone Intravenous (Less than 2%) 2715
Cozaar Tablets (Less than 1%) 1628
Desyrel and Desyrel Dividose 503
Dilacor XR Extended-release Capsules (1.4%) 2018
Diprivan Injection (Less than 1%) 2833
DynaCirc Capsules (0.5% to 1%) 2256
Emete-con Intramuscular/Intravenous 2198
Ethmozine Tablets (Less than 2%) 2041
Felbatol 2666
Foscavir Injection (Less than 1%) 547
Hivid Tablets (Less than 1% to less than 3%) 2121
Hyzaar Tablets 1677
Idamycin 1955
Imdur (Less than or equal to 5%) 1323
Imitrex Injection (Rare) 1103
Imitrex Tablets (Rare) 1106
Intron A (Less than 5%) 2364
Ismo Tablets (Fewer than 1%) 2738
Kytril Injection (Rare) 2490
Kytril Tablets (Rare) 2492
Lamictal Tablets (Rare) 1112
Lopid Tablets (0.7%) 1917
Nalfon 200 Pulvules & Nalfon Tablets (Less than 1%) 917
Neurontin Capsules (Rare) 1922
Nicolar Tablets 2026
OptiPranolol (Metipranolol 0.3%) Sterile Ophthalmic Solution (A small number of patients) ◉ 258
Paxil Tablets (Rare) 2505
Permax Tablets (Infrequent) 575
Prinivil Tablets (0.3% to 1.0%) 1733
Prinzide Tablets 1737
▲ ReoPro Vials (3.5%) 1471
Risperdal 1301
Rythmol Tablets–150mg, 225mg, 300mg (0.7 to 1.2%) 1352
Tegison Capsules (Less than 1%) 2154
▲ Tenormin Tablets and I.V. Injection (5%) 2847
▲ Trasylol (24%) 613
Vaseretic Tablets 1765
Vasotec I.V. 1768
Vasotec Tablets (0.5% to 1.0%) 1771
Zestril Tablets (0.3% to 1.0%) 2854
Zosyn (1.0% or less) 1419
Zosyn Pharmacy Bulk Package (1.0% or less) 1422

Fibrillations, ventricular
Adenocard Injection (Rare) 1021
Ana-Kit Anaphylaxis Emergency Treatment Kit 617
Betapace Tablets 641
Betaseron for SC Injection 658
Calan SR Caplets 2422
Calan Tablets 2419
Cardizem Injectable (Less than 1%) 1508
Clozaril Tablets 2252
Cordarone Intravenous (Less than 2%) 2715
Dilantin Parenteral 1910
Diprivan Injection (Less than 1%) 2833
DynaCirc Capsules (0.5% to 1%) 2256
Eminase 2039
Fungizone Intravenous 506
Hespan Injection 929
Hyzaar Tablets 1677
Imitrex Injection (Rare) 1103
Imitrex Tablets (Rare) 1106
Isoptin SR Tablets 1348
Lanoxicaps 1117
Lorelco Tablets 1517
Marcaine Hydrochloride with Epinephrine 1:200,000 2316
Marcaine Hydrochloride Injection 2316
Narcan Injection (Several instances) 934
Norpace 2444
Norpramin Tablets 1526
Nuromax Injection (Less than or equal to 0.1%) 1149
Primacor Injection (0.2%) 2331
Procan SR Tablets (Common) 1926
Prostin VR Pediatric Sterile Solution (Less than 1%) 2635
Quinaglute Dura-Tabs Tablets 649
Quinidex Extentabs 2067
Seldane Tablets (Rare) 1536
Seldane-D Extended-Release Tablets (Rare) 1538
Sensorcaine 559
Tonocard Tablets (Less than 1%) 531
Trasylol (2%) 613
Zosyn (1.0% or less) 1419
Zosyn Pharmacy Bulk Package (1.0% or less) 1422

Fibromyalgia
Cozaar Tablets (Less than 1%) 1628
Hyzaar Tablets 1677

Fibrosing colonopathy
Creon 2536
Ultrase Capsules 2343
Ultrase MT Capsules 2344

Fibrosis
Cafergot (Rare) 2251
Gelfoam Sterile Sponge 2608
Genotropin (Infrequent) 111
INSTAT* Collagen Absorbable Hemostat 1312
Inversine Tablets 1686
Methotrexate Sodium Tablets, Injection, for Injection and LPF Injection 1275
Myochrysine Injection 1711
Platinol 708
Platinol-AQ Injection 710
Ridaura Capsules (Rare) 2513
Solganal Suspension 2388

Fibrosis, bladder
Cytoxan 694
NEOSAR Lyophilized/Neosar 1959

Fibrosis, interstitial pulmonary (see under Pulmonary fibrosis)

Fibrosis, ovary
Cytoxan 694
NEOSAR Lyophilized/Neosar 1959

Fibrosis, pelvic
Lupron Depot 7.5 mg 2559
Lupron Injection 2555

Fibrosis, periportal
Tagamet (A single case) 2516

Fibrosis, pleural
D.H.E. 45 Injection (Occasional) 2255

Fibrosis, pleuropulmonary
Cafergot 2251

Fibrosis, retroperitoneal
Cafergot 2251

Fingernails, brittle
Neoral (2% or less) 2276
Sandimmune (2% or less) 2286
Trental Tablets (Less than 1%) 1244

Fingernails, darkening
Drithocreme 0.1%, 0.25%, 0.5%, 1.0% (HP) 905
Dritho-Scalp 0.25%, 0.5% 906

Fingers, discoloration
Eskalith 2485
Lithium Carbonate Capsules & Tablets (A single report) 2230
Lithonate/Lithotabs/Lithobid 2543

Fissures, lips
Aquasol A Vitamin A Capsules, USP 534

Fissuring, fingertips
Fluoracaine ◉ 206
FLURESS ◉ 207
Ophthetic ◉ 247

Fissuring, unspecified
Ergamisol Tablets 1292
Fluorouracil Injection 2116
Sterile FUDR (Remote possibility) 2118
Melanex Topical Solution 1793
Oxistat Cream (0.1%) 1152
Temovate Cream (1 of 421 patients) 1179

Fistula, regional lymph node
BCG Vaccine, USP (TICE) (Rare) 1814

Fistula, tracheo-esophageal
Proleukin for Injection (Less than 1%) 797

Flaccidity
Streptomycin Sulfate Injection 2208

Flare
▲ Atgam Sterile Solution (1 in 8 patients; 27%) 2581
Dipentum Capsules (Rare) 1951
Nolvadex Tablets 2841

Flare, postinjection
Aristocort Suspension (Forte Parenteral) 1027
Aristocort Suspension (Intralesional) 1025
Aristospan Suspension (Intra-articular) 1033
Attenuvax (Rare) 1610
Biavax II 1613
Celestone Soluspan Suspension 2347
Dalalone D.P. Injectable 1011
Decadron Phosphate Injection 1637
Decadron-LA Sterile Suspension 1646
Demerol 2308
Depo-Medrol Single-Dose Vial 2600
Depo-Medrol Sterile Aqueous Suspension 2597
Dilaudid-HP Injection (Less frequent) 1337
Dilaudid-HP Lyophilized Powder 250 mg (Less frequent) 1337
Hydeltrasol Injection, Sterile 1665
Hydeltra-T.B.A. Sterile Suspension 1667
Hydrocortone Acetate Sterile Suspension 1669
M-M-R II 1687
M-R-VAX II 1689
Mepergan Injection 2753
Meruvax II 1697
Mumpsvax (Rare) 1708
Stilphostrol Tablets and Ampuls 612

Flatulence
Actigall Capsules 802
Adalat Capsules (10 mg and 20 mg) (2% or less) 587
Adalat CC (Less than 1.0%) 589
Children's Advil Suspension (Less than 3%) 2692
AeroBid Inhaler System (1-3%) 1005
Aerobid-M Inhaler System (1-3%) 1005
Aldoclor Tablets 1598
Aldomet Ester HCl Injection 1602
Aldomet Oral 1600
Aldoril Tablets 1604
Ambien Tablets (Infrequent) 2416
▲ Anafranil Capsules (Up to 6%) 803
Ansaid Tablets (1-3%) 2579
▲ Asacol Delayed-Release Tablets (3%) 1979
Asendin Tablets (Less than 1%) 1369
Atamet 572
Atromid-S Capsules (Less frequent) 2701
Augmentin (Less frequent) 2468
▲ Axid Pulvules (4.9%) 1427
Azo Gantrisin Tablets 2081
Betapace Tablets (1% to 2%) 641
Betaseron for SC Injection 658
Buprenex Injectable (Infrequent) 2006
BuSpar (Infrequent) 737
Carafate Suspension (Less than 0.5%) 1505
Carafate Tablets (Less than 0.5%) 1504
Cardura Tablets (1%) 2186
Cartrol Tablets (Less common) 410
Cataflam (1% to 3%) 816
Ceftin (Less than 1% but more than 0.1%) 1078
▲ CellCept Capsules (More than or equal to 3%) 2099
Cipro I.V. (1% or less) 595
Cipro I.V. Pharmacy Bulk Package (Less than 1%) 597
Cipro Tablets 592
Claritin (2% or fewer patients) 2349
Claritin-D (Less frequent) 2350
Clinoril Tablets (1-3%) 1618
▲ Cognex Capsules (4%) 1901
Colestid Tablets (Less frequent) 2591
Cozaar Tablets (Less than 1%) 1628
Cytotec (2.9%) 2424
▲ Cytovene (6%) 2103
Daypro Caplets (Greater than 1% but less than 3%) 2426
Depakote Tablets (Greater than 1% but not more than 5%) 415
Desyrel and Desyrel Dividose 503
Dilacor XR Extended-release Capsules 2018
Dipentum Capsules (Rare) 1951
Dolobid Tablets (Greater than 1 in 100) 1654
Duragesic Transdermal System (1% or greater) 1288
▲ Effexor (3%) 2719
Emcyt Capsules (2%) 1953
Ergamisol Tablets (Less than 1% to 2%) 1292
Esgic-plus Tablets (Infrequent) 1013
Eskalith 2485
Ethmozine Tablets (Less than 2%) 2041
Felbatol 2666
Feldene Capsules (Greater than 1%) 1965
Fioricet Tablets (Infrequent) 2258
Fioricet with Codeine Capsules (Infrequent) 2260
Fiorinal (Less frequent) 2261
Flexeril Tablets (Less than 1%) 1661
Floxin I.V. (1% to 3%) 1571
Floxin Tablets (200 mg, 300 mg, 400 mg) (1% to 3%) 1567
Foscavir Injection (Between 1% and 5%) 547
Gastrocrom Capsules (Infrequent) 984
Geocillin Tablets 2199
▲ Glucophage (Among most common) 752

(Described in PDR For Nonprescription Drugs) Incidence data in parenthesis; ▲ 3% or more (◉ Described in PDR For Ophthalmology)

Flatulence Side Effects Index 1304

▲ Glucotrol XL Extended Release Tablets (3.2%) ... 1968
Hivid Tablets (Less than 1% to less than 3%) ... 2121
▲ Hylorel Tablets (32.0%) ... 985
Hytrin Capsules (At least 1%) ... 430
Hyzaar Tablets ... 1677
IBU Tablets (Greater than 1%) ... 1342
Imdur (Less than or equal to 5%) .. 1323
Imitrex Injection (Rare) ... 1103
Indocin Capsules (Less than 1%) ... 1680
Indocin I.V. (Less than 1%) ... 1684
Indocin (Less than 1%) ... 1680
Intron A (Less than 5%) ... 2364
K-Dur Microburst Release System (potassium chloride, USP) E.R. Tablets ... 1325
▲ K-Lor Powder Packets (Most common) ... 434
▲ K-Norm Extended-Release Capsules (Among most common) .. 991
▲ K-Tab Filmtab (Most common) ... 434
▲ Kolyum Liquid (Among most common) ... 992
Lamictal Tablets (More than 1%; infrequent) ... 1112
Larodopa Tablets (Infrequent) ... 2129
Lescol Capsules (2.6%) ... 2267
Lithonate/Lithotabs/Lithobid ... 2543
▲ Lodine Capsules and Tablets (3-9%) ... 2743
Lopressor Ampuls (1%) ... 830
Lopressor HCT Tablets (1 in 100) 832
Lopressor Tablets (1%) ... 830
Lorelco Tablets ... 1517
Lotensin HCT (0.3% or more) ... 837
▲ Luvox Tablets (4%) ... 2544
Macrobid Capsules (1.5%) ... 1988
Maxaquin Tablets (Less than 1%) .. 2440
▲ Megace Oral Suspension (Up to 10%) ... 699
▲ Mevacor Tablets (3.7% to 6.4%) .. 1699
Miacalcin Nasal Spray (Less than 1%) ... 2275
▲ Micro-K LS Packets (Most common) ... 2064
Midamor Tablets (Less than or equal to 1%) ... 1703
Moduretic Tablets (Less than or equal to 1%) ... 1705
Monopril Tablets (0.2% to 1.0%) .. 757
Children's Motrin Ibuprofen Oral Suspension (Greater than 1% but less than 3%) ... 1546
Motrin Tablets (Less than 3%) ... 2625
Motrin Ibuprofen Suspension, Oral Drops, Chewable Tablets, Caplets (1% to less than 3%) ... 1546
Mycobutin Capsules (2%) ... 1957
Nalfon 200 Pulvules & Nalfon Tablets (Less than 1%) ... 917
Nephro-Fer Rx Tablets ... 2005
Neurontin Capsules (Frequent) ... 1922
▲ Nicorette (3% to 9% of patients) .. 2458
Nicotrol Nicotine Transdermal System (1% to 3%) ... 1550
Noroxin Tablets (0.3% to 1.0%) ... 1715
Noroxin Tablets (0.3% to 1.0%) ... 2048
▲ Norpace (3 to 9%) ... 2444
Norvasc Tablets (More than 0.1% to 1%) ... 1940
Oncaspar (Less than 1%) ... 2028
▲ Orudis Capsules (3% to 9%) ... 2766
▲ Oruvail Capsules (3% to 9%) ... 2766
▲ Paxil Tablets (4.0%) ... 2505
Penetrex Tablets (Less than 1% but more than or equal to 0.1%) 2031
Permax Tablets (Infrequent) ... 575
Phrenilin (Less frequent) ... 785
Plendil Extended-Release Tablets (0.5% to 1.5%) ... 527
Ponstel (Less frequent) ... 1925
▲ Pravachol (2.7% to 3.3%) ... 765
PREVACID Delayed-Release Capsules (Less than 1%) ... 2562
Prilosec Delayed-Release Capsules (Less than 1 to 2.7%) ... 529
Prinivil Tablets (0.3% to 1.0%) ... 1733
Prinzide Tablets ... 1737
Procardia Capsules (2% or less) ... 1971
Procardia XL Extended Release Tablets (Less than 3%) ... 1972
▲ Prograf (Greater than 3%) ... 1042
▲ Propulsid (3.5%) ... 1300
ProSom Tablets (Infrequent) ... 449
Prostigmin Injectable ... 1260
Prostigmin Tablets ... 1261
Prozac Pulvules & Liquid, Oral Solution (1.6%) ... 919
Questran Light (Less frequent) ... 769
Questran Powder (Less frequent) ... 770
▲ Relafen Tablets (3% to 9%) ... 2510
Retrovir Capsules ... 1158
Retrovir I.V. Infusion ... 1163
Retrovir Syrup ... 1158
ReVia Tablets (Less than 1%) ... 940
▲ Ridaura Capsules (3 to 9%) ... 2513
Rifadin (Some patients) ... 1528
Rifamate Capsules (Some patients) ... 1530
Rifater ... 1532
Rimactane Capsules ... 847
Risperdal (Infrequent) ... 1301
Rocephin Injectable Vials, ADD-Vantage, Galaxy Container (Rare) ... 2142
Roferon-A Injection (Less than 3%) ... 2145
▲ Rowasa (3.6 to 6.13%) ... 2548
Rythmol Tablets–150mg, 225mg, 300mg (0.3 to 1.9%) ... 1352
▲ Sandostatin Injection (Less than 10%) ... 2292
▲ Sectral Capsules (3%) ... 2807
Sedapap Tablets 50 mg/650 mg (Infrequent) ... 1543
Serzone Tablets ... 771
Sinemet Tablets ... 943
Sinemet CR Tablets ... 944
Sporanox Capsules (Less than 1%) ... 1305
▲ Supprelin Injection (3%) ... 2056
▲ Suprax (4%) ... 1399
Tambocor Tablets (Less than 1%) 1497
Tegison Capsules (Less than 1%) .. 2154
Ticlid Tablets (1.5%) ... 2156
Timentin for Injection ... 2528
▲ Tolectin (200, 400 and 600 mg) (3 to 9%) ... 1581
Toprol-XL Tablets (About 1 of 100 patients) ... 565
Toradol (Greater than 1%) ... 2159
Ultram Tablets (50 mg) (1% to 5%) ... 1585
Ultrase MT Capsules (1.5%) ... 2344
Unasyn (Less than 1%) ... 2212
Urecholine ... 1761
Vantin for Oral Suspension and Vantin Tablets (Less than 1%) ... 2646
Vascor (200, 300 and 400 mg) Tablets (0.5 to 2.0%) ... 1587
Vaseretic Tablets (0.5% to 2.0%) 1765
Videx Tablets, Powder for Oral Solution, & Pediatric Powder for Oral Solution (Up to 2%) ... 720
Voltaren Tablets (1% to 3%) ... 861
Zestoretic ... 2850
Zestril Tablets (0.3% to 1.0%) ... 2854
Zithromax (1% or less) ... 1944
Zocor Tablets (1.9%) ... 1775
Zoladex (1% or greater) ... 2858
▲ Zoloft Tablets (3.3%) ... 2217
Zosyn (1.0% or less) ... 1419
Zosyn Pharmacy Bulk Package (1.0% or less) ... 1422
Zovirax (0.4%) ... 1219

Flatus

Trental Tablets (0.6%) ... 1244

Floating feeling

Dilaudid-HP Injection (Less frequent) ... 1337
Dilaudid-HP Lyophilized Powder 250 mg (Less frequent) ... 1337
Dilaudid Tablets and Liquid (Less frequent) ... 1339
MS Contin Tablets (Less frequent) 1994
MSIR (Infrequent) ... 1997
Nubain Injection (1% or less) ... 935
Oramorph SR (Morphine Sulfate Sustained Release Tablets) (Less frequent) ... 2236
Stadol (1% or greater) ... 775

Fluid, encapsulation

Gelfoam Sterile Sponge ... 2608
Surgicel ... 1314

Fluid depletion

Capoten ... 739
Capozide ... 742

Fluid imbalance

Apresazide Capsules ... 808
Aristocort Suspension (Forte Parenteral) ... 1027
Aristocort Suspension (Intralesional) ... 1025
Aristocort Tablets ... 1022
Aristospan Suspension (Intra-articular) ... 1033
Aristospan Suspension (Intralesional) ... 1032
Capozide ... 742
Dalalone D.P. Injectable ... 1011
Demadex Tablets and Injection ... 686
Esidrix Tablets ... 821
Lutrepulse for Injection ... 980
Premarin with Methyltestosterone .. 2794
Prinzide Tablets ... 1737
Tenoretic Tablets ... 2845
Vaseretic Tablets ... 1765
Zestoretic ... 2850

Fluid overload

▲ Aredia for Injection (Up to at least 15%) ... 810
Orthoclone OKT3 Sterile Solution .. 1837
Prinivil Tablets (0.3% to 1.0%) ... 1733
Zestoretic ... 2850
Zestril Tablets (0.3% to 1.0%) ... 2854

Fluid retention (see under Edema)

Flu-like symptoms

▲ Actimmune (Most common) ... 1056
▲ AeroBid Inhaler System (10%) ... 1005
▲ Aerobid-M Inhaler System (10%) .. 1005
Altace Capsules ... 1232
Alupent Tablets (0.2%) ... 669
▲ Asacol Delayed-Release Tablets (3%) ... 1979
Atromid-S Capsules ... 2701
▲ BCG Vaccine, USP (TICE) (33.2%) 1814
▲ Betaseron for SC Injection (53% to 76%) ... 658
Cartrol Tablets (Less common) ... 410
Cataflam ... 816
Caverject (2%) ... 2583
▲ CellCept Capsules (More than or equal to 3%) ... 2099
▲ CHEMET (succimer) Capsules (5.2 to 15.7%) ... 1545
Claritin-D (Less frequent) ... 2350
Clozaril Tablets ... 2252
DTIC-Dome ... 600
Dilacor XR Extended-release Capsules (2.3%) ... 2018
Effexor ... 2719
Engerix-B Unit-Dose Vials (Less than 1%) ... 2482
Epogen for Injection (Rare) ... 489
Ergamisol Tablets (5 out of 463 patients) ... 1292
Eulexin Capsules ... 2358
Felbatol (Frequent) ... 2666
Feldene Capsules (Less than 1%) .. 1965
Hivid Tablets (Less than 1% to less than 3%) ... 2121
Humegon ... 1824
Hytrin Capsules (At least 1% to 2.4%) ... 430
Imdur (Less than or equal to 5%) .. 1323
▲ Intron A (Up to 79%) ... 2364
JE-VAX (Less than 3%) ... 886
Kerlone Tablets (Less than 2%) ... 2436
▲ Lamictal Tablets (7.0%) ... 1112
▲ Lescol Capsules (5.3%) ... 2267
▲ Lopressor HCT Tablets (10 in 100 patients) ... 832
Lotensin HCT (More than 1.0%) ... 837
Lozol Tablets (Less than 5%) ... 2022
Lupron Depot 3.75 mg (Less than 5%) ... 2556
▲ Luvox Tablets (3%) ... 2544
Miacalcin Nasal Spray (1% to 3%) 2275
Mycobutin Capsules (Less than 1%) ... 1957
Normodyne Injection ... 2377
Normodyne Tablets ... 2379
Orlamm (1% to 3%) ... 2239
Orthoclone OKT3 Sterile Solution . 1837
ParaGard T380A Intrauterine Copper Contraceptive ... 1880
Paxil Tablets (Infrequent) ... 2505
Pergonal (menotropins for injection, USP) ... 2448
▲ Permax Tablets (3.2%) ... 575
PREVACID Delayed-Release Capsules (Less than 1%) ... 2562
Procrit for Injection (Rare) ... 1841
Prolastin Alpha$_1$-Proteinase Inhibitor (Human) (Occasional) ... 635
▲ Prozac Pulvules & Liquid, Oral Solution (2.8% to 10%) ... 919
Pulmozyme Inhalation ... 1064
Retrovir Capsules ... 1158
Retrovir I.V. Infusion ... 1163
Retrovir Syrup ... 1158
Rifadin ... 1528
Rifater ... 1532
Risperdal (Infrequent) ... 1301
Roferon-A Injection ... 2145
▲ Rowasa (5.28%) ... 2548
Sandostatin Injection (1% to 4%) .. 2292
▲ Serzone Tablets (3%) ... 771
Slo-Niacin Tablets ... 2659
Tegison Capsules (Less than 1%) .. 2154
Trandate ... 1185
Trental Tablets (Less than 1%) ... 1244
Typhim Vi ... 899
▲ Univasc Tablets (3.1%) ... 2410
Vascor (200, 300 and 400 mg) Tablets (0.5 to 2.08%) ... 1587
▲ Videx Tablets, Powder for Oral Solution, & Pediatric Powder for Oral Solution (Less than 1% to 7%) ... 720
Voltaren Tablets ... 861
Wellbutrin Tablets (Frequent) ... 1204
▲ Zerit Capsules (Fewer than 1% to 9%) ... 729

Flushing

Accutane Capsules (Less than 1%) ... 2076
▲ Adalat Capsules (10 mg and 20 mg) (About 10% to 25%) ... 587
▲ Adalat CC (4%) ... 589
▲ Adenoscan (44%) ... 1024
Ambien Tablets (Rare) ... 2416
Americaine Hemorrhoidal Ointment ... ▣ 629
Aminohippurate Sodium Injection .. 1606
▲ Anafranil Capsules (7% to 8%) ... 803
Antivenin (Crotalidae) Polyvalent ... 2696
Apresazide Capsules (Less frequent) ... 808
Apresoline Hydrochloride Tablets (Less frequent) ... 809
AquaMEPHYTON Injection ... 1608
Atamet ... 572
Atrohist Pediatric Capsules ... 453
Atrovent Inhalation Aerosol (Less frequent) ... 671
Azactam for Injection (One patient) ... 734
Azo Gantrisin Tablets ... 2081
Bellergal-S Tablets (Rare) ... 2250
Benemid Tablets ... 1611
BiCNU ... 691
Bioclate, Antihemophilic Factor (Recombinant) (One patient out of 13,394) ... 513
Bontril Slow-Release Capsules ... 781
Brethine Ampuls (0.0 to 2.4%) ... 815
Brevibloc Injection (Less than 1%) 1808
Bromfed ... 1785
Buprenex Injectable (Less than 1%) ... 2006
BuSpar (Infrequent) ... 737
Calan SR Caplets (0.6%) ... 2422
Calan Tablets (0.6%) ... 2419
Capoten (2 to 5 of 1000 patients) 739
Capozide (2 to 5 of 1000 patients) ... 742
▲ Cardene Capsules (5.6-9.7%) ... 2095
Cardizem CD Capsules (1.4%) ... 1506
Cardizem SR Capsules (1.7% to 3%) ... 1510
Cardizem Injectable (1.7%) ... 1508
Cardizem Tablets (Less than 1%) ... 1512
Cardura Tablets (Less than 0.5% of 3960 patients to 1%) ... 2186
Cataflam (Rare) ... 816
Ceredase ... 1065
Chromagen Capsules ... 2339
Cipro I.V. (1% or less) ... 595
Cipro I.V. Pharmacy Bulk Package (Less than 1%) ... 597
Cipro Tablets (Less than 1%) ... 592
Claritin (2% or fewer patients) ... 2349
Claritin-D (Less frequent) ... 2350
Clinoril Tablets (Less than 1 in 100) ... 1618
▲ Cognex Capsules (3%) ... 1901
ColBENEMID Tablets ... 1622
Cordarone Tablets (1 to 3%) ... 2712
Cozaar Tablets (Less than 1%) ... 1628
CytoGam (Less than 5.0%) ... 1593
DDAVP (Occasional) ... 2017
D.H.E. 45 Injection (Occasional) ... 2255
Dalgan Injection (Less than 1%) ... 538
Dalmane Capsules (Rare) ... 2173
Danocrine Capsules ... 2307
Desmopressin Acetate Rhinal Tube (Occasional) ... 979
Dilatrate-SR ... 2398
Dilaudid Tablets and Liquid ... 1339
Diprivan Injection (Less than 1%) .. 2833
Dolobid Tablets ... 1654

(▣ Described in PDR For Nonprescription Drugs) Incidence data in parenthesis; ▲ 3% or more (◉ Described in PDR For Ophthalmology)

1305 **Side Effects Index** **Folliculitis**

Donnagel Liquid and Donnagel Chewable Tablets (Rare) .... ▣ 879
Dopram Injectable 2061
Duvoid (Infrequent) 2044
▲ DynaCirc Capsules (2.0% to 5.1%) 2256
Effexor 2719
Emcyt Capsules (1%) 1953
Emete-con Intramuscular/Intravenous 2198
Eminase (Occasional) 2039
Engerix-B Unit-Dose Vials (Less than 1%) 2482
Factrel (Rare) 2877
Felbatol 2666
Fioricet with Codeine Capsules 2260
Fiorinal with Codeine Capsules 2262
Flagyl 375 Capsules 2434
Flagyl I.V. 2247
Foscavir Injection (Between 1% and 5%) 547
Fungizone Intravenous 506
Furoxone (Rare) 2046
Gamimune N, 5% Immune Globulin Intravenous (Human), 5% 619
Gamimune N, 10% Immune Globulin Intravenous (Human), 10% 621
Gammagard S/D, Immune Globulin, Intravenous (Human) (Occasional) 585
Gammar I.V., Immune Globulin Intravenous (Human), Lyophilized 516
Gastrocrom Capsules (Infrequent) 984
Glucotrol XL Extended Release Tablets (Less than 1%) 1968
Hespan Injection 929
Hivid Tablets (Less than 1% to less than 3%) 2121
Hyperstat I.V. Injection 2363
Hyskon Hysteroscopy Fluid (Rare) 1595
Hyzaar Tablets 1677
Imdur (Less than or equal to 5%) 1323
▲ Imitrex Injection (6.6%) 1103
Imitrex Tablets (Up to 4%) 1106
Indocin Capsules (Less than 1%) 1680
Indocin I.V. (Less than 1%) 1684
Indocin (Less than 1%) 1680
INFeD (Iron Dextran Injection, USP) 2345
Intron A (Less than 5%) 2364
Isoptin Oral Tablets (0.6%) 1346
Isoptin SR Tablets (0.6%) 1348
Kerlone Tablets (Less than 2%) 2436
Konȳne 80 Factor IX Complex 634
Lamictal Tablets (Infrequent) 1112
Larodopa Tablets (Infrequent) 2129
Lescol Capsules (Rare) 2267
Lodine Capsules and Tablets (Less than 1%) 2743
Lomotil 2439
Lotensin Tablets 834
Lotensin HCT (0.3% to 1.0%) 837
Lotrel Capsules (Up to 0.3%) 840
Lozol Tablets (Less than 5%) 2022
Ludiomil Tablets (Rare) 843
Lufyllin & Lufyllin-400 Tablets 2670
Lufyllin-GG Elixir & Tablets 2671
Lutrepulse for Injection 980
▲ Luvox Tablets (3%) 2544
Lysodren 698
Marinol (Dronabinol) Capsules (0.3% to 1%) 2231
Matulane Capsules 2131
Maxair Autohaler 1492
Maxair Inhaler (Less than 1%) 1494
Maxaquin Tablets (Less than 1%) 2440
Mephyton Tablets 1696
MetroGel-Vaginal 902
Metubine Iodide Vials 916
Mevacor Tablets (Rare) 1699
Miacalcin Nasal Spray (Less than 1%) 2275
Miochol-E with Iocare Steri-Tags and Miochol-E System Pak (Rare) .... ◉ 273
MIOSTAT Intraocular Solution .... ◉ 224
▲ Mivacron (15%) 1138
Moduretic Tablets (Less than or equal to 1%) 1705
Monoket (Up to 2%) 2406
Mononine, Coagulation Factor IX (Human) 523
Monopril Tablets (0.2% to 1.0%) 757
Motofen Tablets 784
Myochrysine Injection 1711
Neoral (Up to 4%) 2276
Nicobid 2026
Nicorette 2458
Nimotop Capsules (Less than 1% to 2.1%) 610
Nitrolingual Spray 2027
▲ Nolvadex Tablets (32.7%) 2841
Norisodrine with Calcium Iodide Syrup 442
Normodyne Injection (1%) 2377
Norpramin Tablets 1526
▲ Norvasc Tablets (0.7% to 4.5%) 1940
Nubain Injection (1% or less) 935
Nuromax Injection (0.3%) 1149
Orlamm 2239
Orthoclone OKT3 Sterile Solution 1837
Pamelor 2280
Pepcid Injection (Infrequent) 1722
Pepcid (Infrequent) 1720
Peptavlon 2878
Persantine Tablets 681
▲ Plendil Extended-Release Tablets (3.9% to 6.9%) 527
Pravachol (Rare) 765
Primaxin I.M. 1727
Primaxin I.V. (Less than 0.2%) 1729
Prinivil Tablets (0.3% to 1.0%) 1733
Prinzide Tablets (0.3 to 1%) 1737
Priscoline Hydrochloride Ampuls 845
Procan SR Tablets (Occasional) 1926
▲ Procardia Capsules (Approximately 10% to 25%; 1 in 8 patients) 1971
▲ Procardia XL Extended Release Tablets (Less than 3% to 25%; 1 in 8 patients) 1972
ProSom Tablets (Infrequent) 449
Prostigmin Injectable 1260
Prostigmin Tablets 1261
Prostin E2 Suppository 2634
▲ Prostin VR Pediatric Sterile Solution (About 10%) 2635
Protamine Sulfate Ampoules & Vials 1471
Protostat Tablets 1883
Proventil (Less than 1%) 2386
Quadrinal Tablets 1350
Quibron 2053
Quinaglute Dura-Tabs Tablets 649
Recombivax HB (Less than 1%) 1744
Regitine 846
Reglan 2068
Respbid Tablets 682
Rifadin 1528
Rifater 1532
Risperdal (Rare) 1301
Robaxin Injectable 2070
Rocephin Injectable Vials, ADD-Vantage, Galaxy Container (Occasional) 2142
Roferon-A Injection (Less than 0.5%) 2145
Romazicon (1% to 3%) 2147
Rythmol Tablets–150mg, 225mg, 300mg (Less than 1%) 1352
▲ Salagen Tablets (8% to 13%) 1489
▲ Sandimmune (Less than 1% to 4%) 2286
Sandostatin Injection (1% to 4%) 2292
Ser-Ap-Es Tablets 849
Sinemet Tablets 943
Sinemet CR Tablets 944
Sinequan (Occasional) 2205
Slo-bid Gyrocaps 2033
Slo-Niacin Tablets 2659
Solganal Suspension 2388
Sorbitrate 2843
Stimate, (desmopressin acetate) Nasal Spray, 1.5 mg/mL (Occasional) 525
Streptase for Infusion 562
Supprelin Injection (2%) 2056
Surmontil Capsules 2811
Talacen (Infrequent) 2333
Talwin Compound (Infrequent) 2335
Talwin Nx (Infrequent) 2336
Tambocor Tablets (1% to less than 3%) 1497
▲ Taxol (28%) 714
Theo-24 Extended Release Capsules 2568
Theo-Dur Extended-Release Tablets 1327
Theo-X Extended-Release Tablets 788
THYREL TRH 2873
Tofranil Ampuls 854
Tofranil Tablets 856
Tofranil-PM Capsules 857
Toradol 2159
Tornalate Solution for Inhalation, 0.2% (Less than 1%) 956
Tornalate Metered Dose Inhaler (Rare) 957
Trancopal Caplets 2337
Trandate Injection (1 of 100 patients) 1185
Trental Tablets 1244
Uni-Dur Extended-Release Tablets 1331
Uniphyl 400 mg Tablets 2001
Univasc Tablets (1.6%) 2410
Urised Tablets 1964
Vancocin HCl, Vials & ADD-Vantage 1481
Vantin for Oral Suspension and Vantin Tablets (Less than 1%) 2646
Vaseretic Tablets 1765
Vasotec I.V. 1768
Vasotec Tablets (0.5% to 1.0%) 1771
Ventolin Tablets (Fewer than 1 of 100 patients) 1203
VePesid Capsules and Injection 718
Verelan Capsules (0.6%) 1410
Verelan Capsules (0.6%) 2824
Vivactil Tablets 1774
Volmax Extended-Release Tablets (Less frequent) 1788
Voltaren Tablets (Rare) 861
▲ Vumon (Approximately 5%) 727
Wellbutrin Tablets (Rare) 1204
Yocon 1892
Yohimex Tablets 1363
Zebeta Tablets 1413
Zestoretic (0.3 to 1%) 2850
Zestril Tablets (0.3% to 1.0%) 2854
Ziac 1415
Zocor Tablets (Rare) 1775
Zoloft Tablets (Infrequent) 2217
Zosyn (1.0% or less) 1419
Zosyn Pharmacy Bulk Package (1.0% or less) 1422

Flushing, cutaneous

Diupres Tablets 1650
Hydropres Tablets 1675
Isuprel Hydrochloride Injection 1:5000 2311
Isuprel Hydrochloride Solution 1:200 & 1:100 2313
Isuprel Mistometer 2312
Lioresal Intrathecal 1596
▲ Mivacron (About 25%) 1138
Nicotinex Elixir .... ▣ 655
Nitrolingual Spray 2027
Quinidex Extentabs 2067
Roferon-A Injection (Less than 0.5%) 2145
Talwin Nx 2336
▲ Tracrium Injection (5%) 1183
Urecholine 1761

Flushing, facial

▲ Adenocard Injection (18%) 1021
Adriamycin PFS 1947
Adriamycin RDF 1947
Brontex 1981
▲ Calcimar Injection, Synthetic (2% to 5%) 2013
Chromagen Capsules 2339
▲ Cognex Capsules (3%) 1901
DDAVP Injection (Occasional) 2014
DDAVP Injection 15 mcg/mL (Occasional) 2015
DTIC-Dome 600
Demerol 2308
Dilaudid-HP Injection (Less frequent) 1337
Dilaudid-HP Lyophilized Powder 250 mg (Less frequent) 1337
Doxorubicin Astra 540
Geref (sermorelin acetate for injection) 2876
Helixate, Antihemophilic Factor (Recombinant) (One report out of 3,254 patients) 518
Imitrex Tablets 1106
KOGENATE Antihemophilic Factor (Recombinant) (One report) 632
Loxitane 1378
MS Contin Tablets (Less frequent) 1994
MSIR (Infrequent) 1997
Marinol (Dronabinol) Capsules (Greater than 1%) 2231
Mepergan Injection 2753
Methadone Hydrochloride Oral Concentrate 2233
Methadone Hydrochloride Oral Solution & Tablets 2235
Miacalcin Injection (About 2-5%) 2273
Mintezol 1704
Mithracin 607
Oramorph SR (Morphine Sulfate Sustained Release Tablets) (Less frequent) 2236
Papaverine Hydrochloride Vials and Ampoules 1468
Phenergan with Codeine 2777
Phenergan VC with Codeine 2781
Polymyxin B Sulfate, Aerosporin Brand Sterile Powder 1154
RMS Suppositories 2657
Roxanol 2243
Rubex 712
Sandimmune 2286
Sandoglobulin I.V. (Less than 1%) 2290
Sansert Tablets (Rare) 2295
Soma Compound w/Codeine Tablets 2676
Soma Compound Tablets 2675
Stimate, (desmopressin acetate) Nasal Spray, 1.5 mg/mL (Occasional) 525
Tonocard Tablets (Less than 1%) 531
Urecholine 1761

Flushing, generalized

Nicolar Tablets 2026

Flushing, hands

▲ Calcimar Injection, Synthetic (2% to 5%) 2013
Miacalcin Injection (About 2-5%) 2273

Flushing, upper thorax

Sandimmune 2286

Focal sensorimotor signs, unspecified

Methotrexate Sodium Tablets, Injection, for Injection and LPF Injection 1275

Folic acid absorption, impaired

Azulfidine (Rare) 1949

Follicle development, multiple

Lutrepulse for Injection (Some incidents) 980

Follicular atresia, delayed

Norplant System 2759

Folliculitis

Aclovate 1069
Anafranil Capsules (Rare) 803
Analpram-HC Rectal Cream 1% and 2.5% 977
Anusol-HC Cream 2.5% (Infrequent to frequent) 1896
Anusol-HC Suppositories 1897
Aristocort A 0.025% Cream (Infrequent) 1027
Aristocort A 0.5% Cream 1031
Aristocort A 0.1% Cream (Infrequent) 1029
Aristocort A 0.1% Ointment (Infrequent) 1030
Carmol HC (Infrequent to frequent) 924
Cleocin T Topical 2590
Cleocin Vaginal Cream 2589
Cordran Lotion (Infrequent) 1803
Cordran Tape (Infrequent) 1804
Cortisporin Cream 1084
Cortisporin Ointment 1085
Cortisporin Otic Solution Sterile 1087
Cortisporin Otic Suspension Sterile 1088
Cutivate Cream 1088
Cutivate Ointment (Infrequent to more frequent) 1089
Cyclocort Topical (Infrequent) 1037
Decadron Phosphate Topical Cream 1644
Decaspray Topical Aerosol 1648
Dermatop Emollient Cream 0.1% (Infrequent to frequent) 1238
DesOwen Cream, Ointment and Lotion (Infrequent) 1046
Didronel Tablets 1984
Diprolene AF Cream (Less than 1%) 2352
Diprolene Gel 0.05% (Less frequent) 2353
Diprolene (Less than 1%) 2352
Dovonex Ointment 0.005% (Less than 1%) 2684
Elocon (Infrequent) 2354
Epifoam (Infrequent) 2399
Eskalith 2485
Florone/Florone E 906
Halog (Infrequent) 2686
Hytone 907
Lidex (Infrequent) 2130
Lithium Carbonate Capsules & Tablets 2230
Lithonate/Lithotabs/Lithobid 2543

(▣ Described in PDR For Nonprescription Drugs) Incidence data in parenthesis; ▲ 3% or more (◉ Described in PDR For Ophthalmology)

Locoid Cream, Ointment and Topical Solution (Infrequent) 978
Lotrisone Cream (Infrequent) 2372
Mantadil Cream 1135
8-MOP Capsules 1246
NeoDecadron Topical Cream 1714
Oxistat Cream (0.3%) 1152
Oxsoralen-Ultra Capsules 1257
PediOtic Suspension Sterile 1153
Pramosone Cream, Lotion & Ointment 978
ProctoCream-HC (Infrequent) 2408
ProctoCream-HC 2.5% (Infrequent to frequent) 2408
ProctoFoam-HC 2409
Psorcon Cream 0.05% (Infrequent) 909
Psorcon Ointment 0.05% 908
Synalar (Infrequent) 2130
Temovate (Infrequent) 1179
Topicort (0.8%) 1243
Tridesilon Cream 0.05% (infrequent) 615
Tridesilon Ointment 0.05% (infrequent) 616
Ultravate Cream 0.05% (Infrequent) 2689
Ultravate Ointment 0.05% (Less frequent) 2690
Westcort 2690

Fontanels, bulging

Achromycin V Capsules 1367
Aquasol A Vitamin A Capsules, USP 534
Declomycin Tablets 1371
Diphtheria and Tetanus Toxoids and Pertussis Vaccine Adsorbed 2477
Diphtheria and Tetanus Toxoids and Pertussis Vaccine Adsorbed USP (For Pediatric Use) (One report) 875
Doryx Capsules 1913
Dynacin Capsules 1590
Macrobid Capsules (Rare) 1988
Minocin Intravenous 1382
Minocin Oral Suspension 1385
Minocin Pellet-Filled Capsules 1383
Monodox Capsules 1805
NegGram (Occasional) 2323
Nizoral Tablets (Less than 1%) 1298
Terramycin Intramuscular Solution 2210
Tetramune 1404
Tri-Immunol Adsorbed 1408
Urobiotic-250 Capsules 2214
Vibramycin 1941
Vibramycin Hyclate Intravenous 2215
Vibramycin 1941

Foot drop

Betaseron for SC Injection 658
Matulane Capsules 2131
Oncovin Solution Vials & Hyporets 1466
Videx Tablets, Powder for Oral Solution, & Pediatric Powder for Oral Solution (Less than 1%) 720
Zyloprim Tablets (Less than 1%) 1226

Forceps delivery, increased incidence

Carbocaine Hydrochloride Injection 2303
Marcaine Hydrochloride with Epinephrine 1:200,000 2316
Marcaine Hydrochloride Injection 2316
Sensorcaine 559

Foreign body reaction

Anafranil Capsules (Infrequent) 803
▲Betimol 0.25%, 0.5% (More than 5%) ◉ 261
▲Ciloxan Ophthalmic Solution (Less than 10%) 472
Ethiodol (Infrequent) 2340
Gelfoam Sterile Sponge 2608
INSTAT* Collagen Absorbable Hemostat 1312
INSTAT* MCH Microfibrillar Collagen Hemostat 1313
INTERCEED* (TC7) Absorbable Adhesion Barrier 1313
Surgicel 1314
Vexol 1% Ophthalmic Suspension (1% to 5%) ◉ 230

Foreskin irretraction (see under Preputium, irretraction of)

Foveal reflex, loss of

Aralen Phosphate Tablets 2301
Plaquenil Sulfate Tablets 2328

Fracture, pathological

Aristocort Tablets 1022
Lamictal Tablets (Rare) 1112
Luvox Tablets (Rare) 2544
Prozac Pulvules & Liquid, Oral Solution (Rare) 919

Fractures, long bones

Aristocort Suspension (Forte Parenteral) 1027
Aristocort Suspension (Intralesional) 1025
Aristocort Tablets 1022
Aristospan Suspension (Intra-articular) 1033
Aristospan Suspension (Intralesional) 1032
Celestone Soluspan Suspension 2347
CORTENEMA 2535
Cortifoam 2396
Cortone Acetate Sterile Suspension 1623
Cortone Acetate Tablets 1624
Dalalone D.P. Injectable 1011
Decadron Phosphate Injection 1637
Decadron Phosphate Respihaler 1642
Decadron Phosphate Turbinaire 1645
Decadron Tablets 1635
Decadron-LA Sterile Suspension 1646
Deltasone Tablets 2595
Depo-Medrol Single-Dose Vial 2600
Depo-Medrol Sterile Aqueous Suspension 2597
Dexacort Phosphate in Respihaler 458
Dexacort Phosphate in Turbinaire 459
Hydeltrasol Injection, Sterile 1665
Hydeltra-T.B.A. Sterile Suspension 1667
Hydrocortone Acetate Sterile Suspension 1669
Hydrocortone Phosphate Injection, Sterile 1670
Hydrocortone Tablets 1672
Medrol 2621
Pediapred Oral Liquid 995
Prelone Syrup 1787
Solu-Cortef Sterile Powder 2641
Solu-Medrol Sterile Powder 2643

Fractures, unspecified

Cognex Capsules (Frequent) 1901
Neurontin Capsules (1.1%) 1922
Rogaine Topical Solution (2.59%) 2637

Fractures, vertebral compression

Aristocort Suspension (Forte Parenteral) 1027
Aristocort Suspension (Intralesional) 1025
Aristospan Suspension (Intra-articular) 1033
Aristospan Suspension (Intralesional) 1032
Celestone Soluspan Suspension 2347
CORTENEMA 2535
Dalalone D.P. Injectable 1011
Decadron Tablets 1635
Decadron-LA Sterile Suspension 1646
Hydeltrasol Injection, Sterile 1665
Hydeltra-T.B.A. Sterile Suspension 1667
Hydrocortone Acetate Sterile Suspension 1669
Hydrocortone Phosphate Injection, Sterile 1670
Hydrocortone Tablets 1672
Prelone Syrup 1787

Freckling

Cytosar-U Sterile Powder (Less frequent) 2592

Free fatty acids, elevation

▲Yutopar Intravenous Injection (80% to 100%) 570

Free T3 resin uptake, decrease (see under T3, decrease)

Fretfulness (see under Anxiety)

Frigidity, unspecified

Wellbutrin Tablets (Infrequent) 1204

Fullness, abdominal (see under Abdominal bloating)

Fungal invasion

Blephamide Liquifilm Sterile Ophthalmic Suspension 476
Blephamide Ointment ◉ 237
Cortisporin Ophthalmic Ointment Sterile (Possible) 1085
Cortisporin Ophthalmic Suspension Sterile (Possible) 1086
Econopred & Econopred Plus Ophthalmic Suspensions (Possibility) ◉ 217
FML Forte Liquifilm (Possibility) ◉ 240
FML Liquifilm (Possibility) ◉ 241
FML S.O.P. (Possibility) ◉ 241
FML-S Liquifilm ◉ 242
Pred Mild ◉ 253
Pred-G Liquifilm Sterile Ophthalmic Suspension ◉ 251
Pred-G S.O.P. Sterile Ophthalmic Ointment ◉ 252
TobraDex Ophthalmic Suspension and Ointment 473
Vasocidin Ophthalmic Solution (Possibility) ◉ 270

Furunculosis

Ambien Tablets (Rare) 2416
Betaseron for SC Injection 658
Cognex Capsules (Infrequent) 1901
Depakote Tablets (Greater than 1% but not more than 5%) 415
Effexor (Rare) 2719
Elocon Ointment 0.1% (3 of 812 patients) 2354
Hivid Tablets (Less than 1% to less than 3%) 2121
Intron A (Less than 5%) 2364
Luvox Tablets (Infrequent) 2544
Methotrexate Sodium Tablets, Injection, for Injection and LPF Injection 1275
Paxil Tablets (Infrequent) 2505
Risperdal (Rare) 1301
Zyloprim Tablets (Less than 1%) 1226

G

Gait, abnormal

Actimmune (Rare) 1056
Anafranil Capsules (Infrequent) 803
Ativan Injection 2698
Betaseron for SC Injection 658
Cardizem CD Capsules (Less than 1%) 1506
Cardizem SR Capsules (Less than 1%) 1510
Cardizem Injectable 1508
Cardizem Tablets (Less than 1%) 1512
Compazine 2470
▲Cordarone Tablets (4 to 9%) 2712
Cytovene (1% or less) 2103
Depakote Tablets (Greater than 1% but not more than 5%) 415
Duragesic Transdermal System (1% or greater) 1288
Ethmozine Tablets (Less than 2%) 2041
▲Felbatol (5.3% to 9.7%) 2666
Flexeril Tablets (Rare) 1661
Flumadine Tablets & Syrup (Less than 0.3%) 1015
Foscavir Injection (Less than 1%) 547
Glucotrol XL Extended Release Tablets (Less than 1%) 1968
Intron A (Less than 5%) 2364
Lamictal Tablets (Infrequent) 1112
Lioresal Intrathecal 1596
Loxitane 1378
Luvox Tablets (Infrequent) 2544
NebuPent for Inhalation Solution (1% or less) 1040
Oncovin Solution Vials & Hyporets 1466
Paxil Tablets (Rare) 2505
Permax Tablets (1.6%) 575
Prozac Pulvules & Liquid, Oral Solution (Infrequent) 919
▲Risperdal (17% to 34%) 1301
Roferon-A Injection (Less than 1%) 2145
Serzone Tablets (Infrequent) 771
Sinemet CR Tablets 944
Stelazine 2514
Thorazine 2523
Torecan 2245
Ultram Tablets (50 mg) (Less than 1%) 1585
Videx Tablets, Powder for Oral Solution, & Pediatric Powder for Oral Solution (Less than 1%) 720
Zantac 150 Tablets 1209
Zantac Injection 1207
Zoloft Tablets (Infrequent) 2217

Galactorrhea

Amen Tablets (Rare) 780
Asendin Tablets (Less than 1%) 1369
BuSpar (Rare) 737
Calan SR Caplets (1% or less) 2422
Calan Tablets (1% or less) 2419
Compazine 2470
Cycrin Tablets (Rare) 975
Demser Capsules (Infrequent) 1649
Depakene 413
Depakote Tablets 415
Depo-Provera Contraceptive Injection (Fewer than 1%) 2602
Depo-Provera Sterile Aqueous Suspension 2606
Elavil 2838
Endep Tablets 2174
Etrafon 2355
Flexeril Tablets (Rare) 1661
Haldol Decanoate 1577
Haldol Injection, Tablets and Concentrate 1575
Imitrex Tablets (Rare) 1106
Isoptin SR Tablets (1% or less) 1348
Limbitrol 2180
Loxitane (Rare) 1378
Ludiomil Tablets (Isolated reports) 843
Mellaril 2269
Moban Tablets and Concentrate (Infrequent) 1048
Norpramin Tablets 1526
Pamelor 2280
Paxil Tablets 2505
Premphase 2797
Prempro 2801
Proglycem 580
Prolixin Oral Concentrate 509
Provera Tablets (Rare) 2636
Reglan 2068
Sandostatin Injection (Less than 1%) 2292
Seldane Tablets 1536
Seldane-D Extended-Release Tablets 1538
Serentil 684
Sinequan 2205
Stelazine 2514
Surmontil Capsules 2811
Tofranil Ampuls 854
Tofranil Tablets 856
Tofranil-PM Capsules 857
Triavil Tablets 1757
Trilafon 2389
Vivactil Tablets 1774
Xanax Tablets 2649
Zoloft Tablets 2217

Gallbladder, calcification

Questran Light (Occasional) 769
Questran Powder (Occasional) 770

Gallbladder, sonographic abnormalities

Rocephin Injectable Vials, ADD-Vantage, Galaxy Container (Rare) 2142

Gallbladder disease

Brevicon 2088
Climara Transdermal System 645
Demulen 2428
Desogen Tablets 1817
Diethylstilbestrol Tablets 1437
Estrace Cream and Tablets 749
Estraderm Transdermal System 824
ESTRATAB Tablets (0.3, 0.625, 1.25, 2.5 mg) 2536
Estratest 2539
Levlen/Tri-Levlen 651
Lo/Ovral Tablets 2746
Lo/Ovral-28 Tablets 2751
Lopid Tablets (0.9%) 1917
Menest Tablets 2494
Micronor Tablets 1872
Modicon 1872
Nordette-21 Tablets 2755
Nordette-28 Tablets 2758
Norinyl 2088
Nor-Q D Tablets 2135
Ogen Tablets 2627
Ogen Vaginal Cream 2630
Ortho-Cept 1851
Ortho-Cyclen/Ortho-Tri-Cyclen 1858
Ortho Dienestrol Cream 1866
Ortho-Est 1869
Ortho-Novum 1872
Ortho-Cyclen/Ortho Tri-Cyclen 1858
Ovcon 760
Ovral Tablets 2770
Ovral-28 Tablets 2770
Ovrette Tablets 2771
PMB 200 and PMB 400 2783
Premarin Intravenous 2787
Premarin with Methyltestosterone 2794

(▣ Described in PDR For Nonprescription Drugs) — Incidence data in parenthesis; ▲ 3% or more — (◉ Described in PDR For Ophthalmology)

1307 Side Effects Index Gastrointestinal disorders

Premarin Tablets 2789
Premarin Vaginal Cream 2791
Premphase (A 2- to 4-fold increase) 2797
Prempro (A 2- to 4-fold) 2801
Pulmozyme Inhalation 1064
Rocephin Injectable Vials, ADD-Vantage, Galaxy Container (Rare) 2142
Sandostatin Injection 2292
Stilphostrol Tablets and Ampuls 612
Levlen/Tri-Levlen 651
Tri-Norinyl 2164
Triphasil-21 Tablets 2814
Triphasil-28 Tablets 2819

Gallstones

Atromid-S Capsules 2701
Imitrex Injection (Rare) 1103
Relafen Tablets (Less than 1%) 2510
▲ Sandostatin Injection (22% to 48%) 2292

Gamma-glutamyl transpeptidase, elevation

▲ Accutane Capsules (1 in 5 to 1 in 10 patients) 2076
Biaxin (Less than 1%) 405
▲ CellCept Capsules (More than or equal to 3%) 2099
Ceptaz (One in 19) 1081
Cipro I.V. (Infrequent) 595
▲ Cipro I.V. Pharmacy Bulk Package (Among most frequent) 597
Cipro Tablets (Less than 0.1%) 592
Cordarone Intravenous (Two cases) 2715
Felbatol (Rare) 2666
Floxin I.V. 1571
Floxin Tablets (200 mg, 300 mg, 400 mg) 1567
▲ Fortaz (1 in 19) 1100
Fungizone Intravenous 506
Hivid Tablets (Less than 1% to less than 3%) 2121
Maxaquin Tablets (Less than or equal to 0.1%) 2440
Mevacor Tablets 1699
Monocid Injection (1.6%) 2497
Oncaspar 2028
Parlodel 2281
Pentasa (Less than 1%) 1527
PREVACID Delayed-Release Capsules (Less than 1%) 2562
Prilosec Delayed-Release Capsules (Rare) 529
▲ Prograf (Greater than 3%) 1042
▲ Tazicef for Injection (1 in 19 patients) 2519
▲ Tegison Capsules (10-25%) 2154
Vantin for Oral Suspension and Vantin Tablets 2646
Zithromax (1% to 2%) 1944
Zocor Tablets 1775

Gangrene

Cafergot 2251
Cytovene-IV (One report) 2103
Felbatol 2666
Heparin Lock Flush Solution 2725
Heparin Sodium Injection 2726
Heparin Sodium Injection, USP, Sterile Solution 2615
Heparin Sodium Vials 1441
Levophed Bitartrate Injection (Rare) 2315
Mepergan Injection 2753
Phenergan Injection 2773
Proleukin for Injection (1%) 797

Gastric acid, regurgitation

Prilosec Delayed-Release Capsules (1.9%) 529

Gastric dilation

Anafranil Capsules (Infrequent) 803

Gastric discomfort (see under Distress, gastrointestinal)

Gastric disorder (see under Distress, gastrointestinal)

Gastric erosion

Empirin with Codeine Tablets 1093
Robaxisal Tablets 2071
Soma Compound w/Codeine Tablets (Rare) 2676
Soma Compound Tablets (Less common) 2675

Gastric outlet obstruction

Prostin VR Pediatric Sterile Solution 2635

Gastric regurgitation

Prostin VR Pediatric Sterile Solution (Less than 1%) 2635

Gastric secretions, increase

Sansert Tablets 2295
Tensilon Injectable 1261

Gastritis

Children's Advil Suspension (Less than 1%) 2692
Aldactazide 2413
Aldactone 2414
Ambien Tablets (Rare) 2416
Anafranil Capsules (Infrequent) 803
Ansaid Tablets (Less than 1%) 2579
Asacol Delayed-Release Tablets 1979
Atromid-S Capsules 2701
Augmentin 2468
Betaseron for SC Injection 658
Carnitor Injection (Less frequent) 2452
▲ CellCept Capsules (More than or equal to 3%) 2099
Claritin (2% or fewer patients) 2349
Claritin-D (Less frequent) 2350
Clinoril Tablets (Less than 1%) 1618
Cognex Capsules (Infrequent) 1901
Cozaar Tablets (Less than 1%) 1628
Dolobid Tablets (Less than 1 in 100) 1654
Effexor (Infrequent) 2719
Eskalith 2485
Etrafon 2355
Felbatol 2666
Flexeril Tablets (Less than 1%) 1661
Sterile FUDR 2118
Hivid Tablets (Less than 1% to less than 3%) 2121
Hyzaar Tablets 1677
IBU Tablets (Less than 1%) 1342
Imdur (Less than or equal to 5%) 1323
Keflex Pulvules & Oral Suspension 914
Keftab Tablets 915
Klonopin Tablets 2126
Lamictal Tablets (Rare) 1112
Lithonate/Lithotabs/Lithobid 2543
Lodine Capsules and Tablets (More than 1% but less than 3%) 2743
Lotensin Tablets 834
Luvox Tablets (Infrequent) 2544
Miacalcin Nasal Spray (Less than 1%) 2275
Children's Motrin Ibuprofen Oral Suspension (Less than 1%) 1546
Motrin Tablets (Less than 1%) 2625
Motrin Ibuprofen Suspension, Oral Drops, Chewable Tablets, Caplets (Less than 1%) 1546
Nalfon 200 Pulvules & Nalfon Tablets (Less than 1%) 917
NebuPent for Inhalation Solution (1% or less) 1040
Neoral (2% or less) 2276
Norvasc Tablets (Less than or equal to 0.1%) 1940
Orudis Capsules (Less than 1%) 2766
Oruvail Capsules (Less than 1%) 2766
Permax Tablets (Infrequent) 575
Prinivil Tablets (0.3% to 1.0%) 1733
Prinzide Tablets 1737
Prolixin 509
ProSom Tablets (Infrequent) 449
Prozac Pulvules & Liquid, Oral Solution (Infrequent) 919
Relafen Tablets (1% to 3%) 2510
Risperdal (Infrequent) 1301
Robaxisal Tablets 2071
Sandimmune (2% or less) 2286
Serzone Tablets (Infrequent) 771
Solganal Suspension 2388
Soma Compound w/Codeine Tablets 2676
▲ Soma Compound Tablets (Among most common) 2675
Spectrobid Tablets 2206
Supprelin Injection (2% to 3%) 2056
Tolectin (200, 400 and 600 mg) (1 to 3%) 1581
Toradol (1% or less) 2159
Unasyn 2212
Vascor (200, 300 and 400 mg) Tablets (0.5 to 2.0%) 1587
Videx Tablets, Powder for Oral Solution, & Pediatric Powder for Oral Solution (Less than 1%) 720
Zebeta Tablets 1413
Zestoretic 2850
Zestril Tablets (0.3% to 1.0%) 2854
Ziac 1415
Zoloft Tablets (Rare) 2217
Zosyn (1.0% or less) 1419
Zosyn Pharmacy Bulk Package (1.0% or less) 1422
Zyloprim Tablets (Less than 1%) 1226

Gastroenteritis

Altace Capsules (Less than 1%) 1232
Ambien Tablets (Infrequent) 2416
Asacol Delayed-Release Tablets 1979
Cardura Tablets (Less than 0.5% of 3960 patients) 2186
▲ CellCept Capsules (More than or equal to 3%) 2099
Clinoril Tablets (Less than 1%) 1618
Clozaril Tablets (Less than 1%) 2252
Cognex Capsules (Infrequent) 1901
Cytosar-U Sterile Powder (One case) 2592
Danocrine Capsules 2307
Depakote Tablets (Greater than 1% but not more than 5%) 415
Effexor (Infrequent) 2719
Fioricet with Codeine Capsules 2260
Fiorinal with Codeine Capsules 2262
Foscavir Injection (Less than 1%) 547
Sterile FUDR 2118
Indocin Capsules (Less than 1%) 1680
Indocin I.V. (Less than 1%) 1684
Indocin (Less than 1%) 1680
Lotensin HCT (0.3% or more) 837
Luvox Tablets (Infrequent) 2544
Maxaquin Tablets 2440
Neurontin Capsules (Infrequent) 1922
Paxil Tablets (Rare) 2505
Permax Tablets (Infrequent) 575
PREVACID Delayed-Release Capsules (Less than 1%) 2562
Primaxin I.M. 1727
Primaxin I.V. (Less than 0.2%) 1729
Prozac Pulvules & Liquid, Oral Solution (1.0%) 919
Relafen Tablets (1%) 2510
Risperdal (Rare) 1301
Rythmol Tablets–150mg, 225mg, 300mg (0.03 to 1.9%) 1352
Serzone Tablets (Frequent) 771
Videx Tablets, Powder for Oral Solution, & Pediatric Powder for Oral Solution (Less than 1%) 720
Zoloft Tablets (Rare) 2217

Gastroenteritis, hemorrhagic

Fungizone Intravenous 506

Gastroesophageal reflux

Anafranil Capsules (Infrequent) 803
Imitrex Injection (Infrequent) 1103
Imitrex Tablets (Infrequent) 1106
Procardia XL Extended Release Tablets (1% or less) 1972
Risperdal (Rare) 1301

Gastrointestinal bleeding (see under Bleeding, gastrointestinal)

Gastrointestinal disorders

▲ Accutane Capsules (Approximately 1 patient in 20) 2076
▲ Adenoscan (13%) 1024
Adipex-P Tablets and Capsules 1048
Aldactone 2414
Aldoclor Tablets 1598
▲ Alka-Seltzer Effervescent Antacid and Pain Reliever (4.9% at doses of 1000 mg/day) ▣ 701
▲ Alka-Seltzer Lemon Lime Effervescent Antacid and Pain Reliever (4.9% at doses of 1000 mg/day) ▣ 703
Alkeran for Injection (Infrequent) 1070
Alkeran Tablets (Infrequent) 1071
Anafranil Capsules (Up to 2%) 803
Ana-Kit Anaphylaxis Emergency Treatment Kit 617
Anaprox/Naprosyn 2117
▲ Anturane (Most frequent) 807
Apresazide Capsules 808
Aralen Hydrochloride Injection 2301
Aralen Phosphate Tablets 2301
Regular Strength Ascriptin Tablets ▣ 629
Ativan Tablets 2700
▲ Atrohist Pediatric Suspension (Among most common) 454
Atromid-S Capsules (Less frequent) 2701
Axid Pulvules (1.1%) 1427
BCG Vaccine, USP (TICE) (1.0%) 1814
▲ Genuine Bayer Aspirin Tablets & Caplets (4.9% at doses of 1000 mg/day) ▣ 713
▲ Aspirin Regimen Bayer Regular Strength 325 mg Caplets (4.9% of 4500 people tested) ▣ 709
Benemid Tablets 1611
Berocca Plus Tablets 2087
▲ Betaseron for SC Injection (6%) 658
Biphetamine Capsules 983
Bleph-10 Ophthalmic Solution 10% 475
Brethaire Inhaler 813
Brevicon 2088
▲ Bufferin Analgesic Tablets and Caplets (4.8%) ▣ 613
BuSpar 737
Capoten 739
Capozide 742
Carnitor Tablets and Solution 2453
Cartrol Tablets (Less common) 410
▲ Cataflam (About 20%) 816
Ceclor Pulvules & Suspension (About 2.5%) 1431
Cefotan (1.5%) 2829
▲ Ceptaz (Among most common) 1081
Cleocin T Topical 2590
Cleocin Vaginal Cream 2589
▲ Clinoril Tablets (3-9%) 1618
▲ Clomid (13.6%) 1514
▲ Colestid Tablets (Most common) 2591
▲ CREON 5 Capsules (Among most frequent) 2536
▲ Cuprimine Capsules (17%) 1630
Cyklokapron Tablets and Injection 1950
DDAVP (Up to 2%) 2017
Dalmane Capsules 2173
▲ Daranide Tablets (Among the most common effects) 1633
Decadron Elixir 1633
Decadron Phosphate Injection 1637
Decadron Phosphate Respihaler 1642
Decadron Phosphate Turbinaire 1645
Decadron Phosphate with Xylocaine Injection, Sterile 1639
Deconamine CX Cough and Cold Liquid and Tablets 1319
Demulen 2428
Depo-Provera Contraceptive Injection (Fewer than 1%) 2602
Desmopressin Acetate Rhinal Tube (Up to 2%) 979
Desyrel and Desyrel Dividose 503
Dexedrine 2474
DextroStat Dextroamphetamine Tablets 2036
Diamox Intravenous 1372
Diamox Sequels (Sustained Release) 1373
Diamox Tablets 1372
Didrex Tablets 2607
Didronel Tablets 1984
Duricef 748
Dyazide 2479
EC-Naprosyn Delayed-Release Tablets 2117
▲ Ecotrin (4.9% at 1000 mg/day) 2455
Eminase 2039
Esgic-plus Tablets (Infrequent) 1013
Esidrix Tablets 821
Ethmozine Tablets (0.3% to 0.4%) 2041
▲ Eulexin Capsules (6% with LDRH agonist) 2358
▲ Feldene Capsules (Approximately 20%) 1965
Fioricet Tablets (Infrequent) 2258
Fiorinal (Less frequent) 2261
▲ Flagyl 375 Capsules (Most frequent) 2434
▲ Fortaz (Among most common) 1100
Glauctabs ⊙ 208
▲ Glucophage (Among most common) 752
Halfprin 1362
Haltran Tablets (Occasional) ▣ 771
Humegon 1824
Hydrea Capsules (Less frequent) 696
▲ IBU Tablets (4% to 16%) 1342
Ionamin Capsules 990
Isoptin Oral Tablets (Less than 1%) 1346
K-Dur Microburst Release System (potassium chloride, USP) E.R. Tablets 1325

(▣ Described in PDR For Nonprescription Drugs) Incidence data in parenthesis; ▲ 3% or more (⊙ Described in PDR For Ophthalmology)

- K-Phos Neutral Tablets 639
- Kefurox Vials, Faspak & ADD-Vantage (1 in 150) 1454
- Kemadrin Tablets 1112
- ▲ Lamprene Capsules (40-50%) 828
- Lanoxicaps 1117
- Lanoxin Elixir Pediatric 1120
- Lanoxin Injection 1123
- Lanoxin Injection Pediatric 1126
- Lanoxin Tablets 1128
- Lasix Injection, Oral Solution and Tablets 1240
- Leukeran Tablets (Infrequent) 1133
- ▲ Leukine for IV Infusion (37%) 1271
- ▲ Lopid Tablets (34.2%) 1917
- ▲ Lorabid Suspension and Pulvules (Most common) 1459
- Lozol Tablets 2022
- Lupron Depot 3.75 mg (Less than 5%) 2556
- Lupron Injection (Less than 5%) 2555
- ▲ MZM (Among reactions occurring most often) ◉ 267
- Maxzide 1380
- Metrodin (urofollitropin for injection) 2446
- Micronor Tablets 1872
- Midamor Tablets (Less than or equal to 1%) 1703
- Modicon 1872
- Moduretic Tablets (Less than or equal to 1%) 1705
- 8-MOP Capsules 1246
- ▲ Motrin Ibuprofen Suspension, Oral Drops, Chewable Tablets, Caplets (Most frequent; 4% to 16%) 1546
- Myambutol Tablets 1386
- Mycostatin Pastilles (Occasional) 704
- Nalfon 200 Pulvules & Nalfon Tablets 917
- Anaprox/Naprosyn 2117
- Neptazane Tablets 1388
- Nicolar Tablets 2026
- Nicorette 2458
- Nimotop Capsules (Up to 2.4%) 610
- Norinyl 2088
- Nor-Q D Tablets 2135
- Novahistine DMX (Infrequent) ▣ 822
- ▲ Novantrone (58 to 88%) 1279
- Orap Tablets 1050
- Oretic Tablets 443
- Ortho-Cyclen/Ortho-Tri-Cyclen 1858
- Ortho-Novum 1872
- Ortho-Cyclen/Ortho Tri-Cyclen 1858
- Ovcon 760
- Oxsoralen-Ultra Capsules 1257
- ▲ Pancrease Capsules (Most frequent) 1579
- ▲ Pancrease MT Capsules (Most frequent) 1579
- Paraflex Caplets (Occasional) 1580
- Parafon Forte DSC Caplets (Occasional) 1581
- ▲ Paraplatin for Injection (21% to 50%) 705
- Phenergan with Dextromethorphan 2778
- Pilopine HS Ophthalmic Gel (Occasional) ◉ 226
- Pima Syrup 1005
- Plaquenil Sulfate Tablets 2328
- ▲ Prepidil Gel (5.7%) 2633
- Prinzide Tablets (0.3 to 1%) 1737
- Prodium 690
- Proglycem (Frequent) 580
- Proleukin for Injection 797
- Proventil Syrup (Children 2 to 6 years, 2%) 2385
- ▲ Prozac Pulvules & Liquid, Oral Solution (6%) 919
- Pyrazinamide Tablets 1398
- Quadrinal Tablets 1350
- ▲ Retrovir Capsules (20%) 1158
- ▲ Retrovir I.V. Infusion (20%) 1163
- ▲ Retrovir Syrup (20%) 1158
- Rifadin 1528
- Rifater 1532
- Rimactane Capsules 847
- Robaxin Injectable 2070
- Rondec-DM Oral Drops 954
- Rondec-DM Syrup 954
- ▲ Rynatan (Among most common) 2673
- ▲ Rynatuss (Among most common) 2673
- SSD 1355
- ▲ SSKI Solution (Among most frequent) 2658
- Salagen Tablets (Less than 1%) 1489
- Serophene (clomiphene citrate tablets, USP) 2451
- Silvadene Cream 1% 1540
- Skelaxin Tablets 788
- Slo-Niacin Tablets (Less common) 2659
- Solu-Cortef Sterile Powder 2641
- Solu-Medrol Sterile Powder 2643
- Soma Compound Tablets 2675
- St. Joseph Adult Chewable Aspirin (81 mg.) ▣ 808
- ▲ Supprelin Injection (3% to 10%) 2056
- ▲ Suprax (30%) 1399
- ▲ Tazicef for Injection (Among most common) 2519
- Tenoretic Tablets 2845
- Tessalon Perles 1020
- Thalitone (Common) 1245
- ▲ Ticlid Tablets (30% to 40%) 2156
- Timoptic-XE 1755
- Tofranil Ampuls 854
- Tofranil Tablets 856
- Tofranil-PM Capsules 857
- ▲ Tolectin (200, 400 and 600 mg) (10%) 1581
- Tonocard Tablets (Less than 1%) 531
- Toprol-XL Tablets 565
- Tranxene (Less common) 451
- ▲ Trecator-SC Tablets (Among most common) 2814
- Triaminic Cold Tablets ▣ 790
- Triaminic Expectorant ▣ 790
- ▲ Trilisate (Less than 20%) 2000
- Tri-Norinyl 2164
- Trinsicon Capsules (Rare) 2570
- Trisoralen Tablets 1264
- Tussend Expectorant 1785
- ▲ Ultrase Capsules (Most frequent) 2343
- ▲ Ultrase MT Capsules (Among most frequent) 2344
- Uni-Dur Extended-Release Tablets 1331
- Uroqid-Acid No. 2 Tablets 640
- Vantin for Oral Suspension and Vantin Tablets (Greater than 1%) 2646
- ▲ Vascor (200, 300 and 400 mg) Tablets (4.35 to 6.98%) 1587
- Vaseretic Tablets 1765
- Ventolin Syrup (2% of children) 1202
- Viokase 2076
- ▲ Voltaren Tablets (About 20%) 861
- Zestoretic (0.3 to 1.0%) 2850
- Zinacef (1 in 150 patients) 1211
- Zosyn 1419
- Zosyn Pharmacy Bulk Package 1422

Gastrointestinal motility, decreased

- Ditropan 1516

Gastrointestinal obstruction

- K-Dur Microburst Release System (potassium chloride, USP) E.R. Tablets 1325
- K-Norm Extended-Release Capsules 991
- K-Tab Filmtab 434
- Micro-K 2063
- Micro-K LS Packets 2064
- Pancrease MT Capsules 1579
- Slow-K Extended-Release Tablets 851

Gastrointestinal perforation

- Children's Advil Suspension (Less than 1%) 2692
- Anaprox/Naprosyn (Approximately 1% to 4%) 2117
- Atgam Sterile Solution (Less than 5%) 2581
- Cataflam (Approximately 1%) 816
- Clinoril Tablets (Rare) 1618
- Cortone Acetate Sterile Suspension 1623
- Cortone Acetate Tablets 1624
- Daypro Caplets 2426
- Decadron Phosphate Respihaler 1642
- Decadron Phosphate Turbinaire 1645
- Dolobid Tablets (Less than 1 in 100) 1654
- EC-Naprosyn Delayed-Release Tablets (Approximately 1% to 4%) 2117
- Feldene Capsules (Less than 1%) 1965
- Indocin (Approximately 1%) 1680
- K-Dur Microburst Release System (potassium chloride, USP) E.R. Tablets 1325
- K-Norm Extended-Release Capsules 991
- K-Tab Filmtab 434
- Lodine Capsules and Tablets 2743
- Micro-K 2063
- Micro-K LS Packets 2064
- Children's Motrin Ibuprofen Oral Suspension (Approximately 1% to 4%) 1546
- Motrin Tablets (Less than 1%) 2625
- Motrin Ibuprofen Suspension, Oral Drops, Chewable Tablets, Caplets (Approximately 1% to 4%) 1546
- Anaprox/Naprosyn (Approximately 1% to 4%) 2117
- Oncovin Solution Vials & Hyporets 1466
- Orudis Capsules (Less than 1%) 2766
- Oruvail Capsules (Less than 1%) 2766
- Ponstel 1925
- ▲ Prograf (Greater than 3%) 1042
- Relafen Tablets 2510
- Slow-K Extended-Release Tablets 851
- Tolectin (200, 400 and 600 mg) (Less than 1%) 1581
- Toradol 2159
- Voltaren Tablets (Approximately 1%) 861

Gastrointestinal reactions (see under Gastrointestinal disorders)

Gastrointestinal reflux

- Cytotec (Infrequent) 2424

Gastrointestinal symptoms (see under Gastrointestinal disorders)

Gastrointestinal toxicity

- Children's Advil Suspension 2692
- Alkeran for Injection 1070
- Alkeran Tablets 1071
- Anaprox/Naprosyn 2117
- BiCNU 691
- CeeNU 693
- Cytosar-U Sterile Powder (With experimental doses) 2592
- EC-Naprosyn Delayed-Release Tablets 2117
- Children's Motrin Ibuprofen Oral Suspension 1546
- Motrin Tablets 2625
- Anaprox/Naprosyn 2117
- Neutrexin 2572
- Toradol 2159

Gastrointestinal tract, presence of fluttering sensation

- Sandostatin Injection (Fewer than 1%) 2292

Gastrointestinal upset (see under Gastrointestinal disorders)

Genital abnormalities

- Clomid 1514
- Danocrine Capsules 2307
- Felbatol 2666
- Hivid Tablets (Less than 1% to less than 3%) 2121
- Megace Oral Suspension (Several reports) 699
- Megace Tablets 701

Genital moniliasis

- Duricef 748

Genitalia, external, labial fusion of

- Danocrine Capsules 2307

Genitalia, male, external, abnormalities of

- Proscar Tablets 1741

Genitourinary disturbances

- Betapace Tablets (1% to 3%) 641
- Dalmane Capsules 2173
- Eulexin Capsules (2%) 2358
- ▲ Paraplatin for Injection (10% to 11%) 705
- Tranxene 451

Germinal aplasia

- Mustargen 1709

Giddiness (see under Dizziness)

Gingival hyperplasia

- Adalat Capsules (10 mg and 20 mg) (Less than 0.5%) 587
- Adalat CC (Rare) 589
- Calan SR Caplets (1% or less) 2422
- Calan Tablets (1% or less) 2419
- Cardizem CD Capsules (Infrequent) 1506
- Cardizem SR Capsules (Infrequent) 1510
- Cardizem Injectable 1508
- Cardizem Tablets (Infrequent) 1512
- ▲ CellCept Capsules (More than or equal to 3%) 2099
- Dilantin Infatabs 1908
- Dilantin Kapseals 1906
- Dilantin Parenteral 1910
- Dilantin-125 Suspension 1911
- Intron A (Less than 5%) 2364
- Isoptin Oral Tablets (Less than 1%) 1346
- Isoptin SR Tablets (1% or less) 1348
- Lamictal Tablets (Infrequent) 1112
- Mesantoin Tablets 2272
- ▲ Neoral (5% to 16%) 2276
- Norvasc Tablets (More than 0.1% to 1%) 1940
- Plendil Extended-Release Tablets 527
- Procardia Capsules (Less than 0.5%) 1971
- Procardia XL Extended Release Tablets (1% or less) 1972
- ▲ Sandimmune (4 to 16%) 2286
- Verelan Capsules (1% or less) 1410
- Verelan Capsules (Less than 1%) 2824
- Zoloft Tablets (Rare) 2217

Gingival swelling

- Lomotil 2439
- Motofen Tablets 784

Gingival ulcer

- Children's Advil Suspension (Less than 1%) 2692
- Children's Motrin Ibuprofen Oral Suspension (Less than 1%) 1546
- Motrin Tablets (Less than 1%) 2625
- Motrin Ibuprofen Suspension, Oral Drops, Chewable Tablets, Caplets (Less than 1%) 1546

Gingivitis

- Accutane Capsules (Less than 1%) 2076
- Anafranil Capsules (Infrequent) 803
- Benemid Tablets 1611
- Betaseron for SC Injection 658
- ▲ CellCept Capsules (More than or equal to 3%) 2099
- Cognex Capsules (Infrequent) 1901
- ColBENEMID Tablets 1622
- Cytotec (Infrequent) 2424
- Effexor (Infrequent) 2719
- Hivid Tablets (Less than 1% to less than 3%) 2121
- ▲ Intron A (Up to 14%) 2364
- Klonopin Tablets 2126
- Lamictal Tablets (Infrequent) 1112
- Lupron Depot-PED 7.5 mg, 11.25 mg and 15 mg (Less than 2%) 2560
- Luvox Tablets (Infrequent) 2544
- Methotrexate Sodium Tablets, Injection, for Injection and LPF Injection 1275
- Myochrysine Injection 1711
- NebuPent for Inhalation Solution (1% or less) 1040
- Neurontin Capsules (Frequent) 1922
- Nicorette 2458
- Paxil Tablets (Rare) 2505
- Permax Tablets (Infrequent) 575
- Prozac Pulvules & Liquid, Oral Solution (Infrequent) 919
- Relafen Tablets (Less than 1%) 2510
- Ridaura Capsules (0.1 to 1%) 2513
- Risperdal (Rare) 1301
- Serzone Tablets (Infrequent) 771
- Solganal Suspension 2388
- Tegison Capsules (1-10%) 2154
- Videx Tablets, Powder for Oral Solution, & Pediatric Powder for Oral Solution (Less than 1%) 720

Gingivostomatitis

- Cuprimine Capsules (Rare) 1630
- Depen Titratable Tablets (Rare) 2662

Glandular enlargement

- Hespan Injection 929
- Questran Light 769
- Questran Powder 770
- ReVia Tablets (Less than 1%) 940

Glassy-eyed appearance

- Klonopin Tablets 2126

(▣ Described in PDR For Nonprescription Drugs) Incidence data in parenthesis; ▲ 3% or more (◉ Described in PDR For Ophthalmology)

Side Effects Index

Glaucoma

(see also under IOP, elevation)

▲ AdatoSil 5000 (0.6% to approximately 30%) ◆ 274
AK-Pred ◆ 204
AK-Trol Ointment & Suspension.. ◆ 205
Ambien Tablets (Rare) 2416
Anafranil Capsules (Rare) 803
Anectine 1073

Aristocort Suspension (Forte Parenteral) 1027
Aristocort Suspension (Intralesional) 1025
Aristocort Tablets 1022
Aristospan Suspension (Intra-articular) 1033
Aristospan Suspension (Intralesional) 1032
Artane 1368
Beconase (Rare) 1076
Blephamide Liquifilm Sterile Ophthalmic Suspension 476
Blephamide Ointment (A possibility) ◆ 237
Celestone Soluspan Suspension 2347
CORTENEMA 2535
Cortifoam 2396
Cortisporin Ophthalmic Ointment Sterile 1085
Cortisporin Ophthalmic Suspension Sterile 1086
Cortone Acetate Sterile Suspension 1623
Cortone Acetate Tablets 1624
Dalalone D.P. Injectable 1011
Decadron Elixir 1633
Decadron Phosphate Injection 1637
Decadron Phosphate Respihaler 1642
Decadron Phosphate Sterile Ophthalmic Ointment 1641
Decadron Phosphate Sterile Ophthalmic Solution 1642
Decadron Phosphate Turbinaire 1645
Decadron Phosphate with Xylocaine Injection, Sterile 1639
Decadron Tablets 1635
Decadron-LA Sterile Suspension 1646
Deltasone Tablets 2595
Depo-Medrol Single-Dose Vial 2600
Depo-Medrol Sterile Aqueous Suspension 2597
Dexacidin Ointment ◆ 263
Dexacort Phosphate in Respihaler .. 458
Dexacort Phosphate in Turbinaire .. 459
Diupres Tablets 1650
Econopred & Econopred Plus Ophthalmic Suspensions ◆ 217
Elavil 2838
Endep Tablets 2174
Etrafon 2355
FML Forte Liquifilm ◆ 240
FML S.O.P. ◆ 241
▲ FML-S Liquifilm (Among most often) ◆ 242
Flarex Ophthalmic Suspension ◆ 218
Florinet Acetate Tablets 505
Fluor-Op Ophthalmic Suspension ◆ 264
HMS Liquifilm (Rare) ◆ 244
Healon ◆ 314
Humorsol Sterile Ophthalmic Solution 1664
Hydeltrasol Injection, Sterile 1665
Hydeltra-T.B.A. Sterile Suspension 1667
Hydrocortone Acetate Sterile Suspension 1669
Hydrocortone Phosphate Injection, Sterile 1670
Hydrocortone Tablets 1672
Hydropres Tablets 1675
Inflamase ◆ 265
ISPAN Perfluoropropane ◆ 276
ISPAN Sulfur Hexafluoride ◆ 275
▲ Maxitrol Ophthalmic Ointment and Suspension (Most often) ◆ 224
Medrol 2621
Midamor Tablets (Less than or equal to 1%) 1703
Moduretic Tablets 1705
Nardil (Less common) 1920
NeoDecadron Sterile Ophthalmic Ointment 1712
NeoDecadron Sterile Ophthalmic Solution 1713
Norpramin Tablets 1526
Ophthocort ◆ 311
Ornade Spansule Capsules 2502
Pediapred Oral Liquid 995
Poly-Pred Liquifilm ◆ 248
Pred-G Liquifilm Sterile Ophthalmic Suspension ◆ 251

Pred-G S.O.P. Sterile Ophthalmic Ointment ◆ 252
Prelone Syrup 1787
Prolixin 509
Prozac Pulvules & Liquid, Oral Solution (Rare) 919
Rhinocort Nasal Inhaler (Rare) 556
Ser-Ap-Es Tablets 849
Solu-Cortef Sterile Powder 2641
Solu-Medrol Sterile Powder 2643
Terra-Cortril Ophthalmic Suspension 2210
TobraDex Ophthalmic Suspension and Ointment 473
Triavil Tablets 1757
Trilafon (Occasional) 2389
Vancenase AQ Nasal Spray 0.042% (Extremely rare) 2393
Vancenase PocketHaler Nasal Inhaler (Extremely rare) 2391
Vasocidin Ointment ◆ 268
Vasocidin Ophthalmic Solution ◆ 270
Vexol 1% Ophthalmic Suspension (1% to 5%) ◆ 230
Viroptic Ophthalmic Solution, 1% Sterile 1204
Vivactil Tablets 1774

Glaucoma, angle closure precipitation

Ocusert Pilo-20 and Pilo-40
Ocular Therapeutic Systems ◆ 254
Transderm Scōp Transdermal Therapeutic System (Infrequent) 869

Glaucoma, corticosteroid-induced

AK-Trol Ointment & Suspension.. ◆ 205
Blephamide Liquifilm Sterile Ophthalmic Suspension 476
Dexacidin Ointment ◆ 263
Econopred & Econopred Plus Ophthalmic Suspensions ◆ 217
FML Forte Liquifilm ◆ 240
FML Liquifilm ◆ 241
FML-S Liquifilm ◆ 242
Fluor-Op Ophthalmic Suspension ◆ 264
HMS Liquifilm ◆ 244
Inflamase ◆ 265
Maxitrol Ophthalmic Ointment and Suspension ◆ 224
Ophthocort ◆ 311
Poly-Pred Liquifilm ◆ 248
Pred Forte ◆ 250
Pred-G Liquifilm Sterile Ophthalmic Suspension ◆ 251
TobraDex Ophthalmic Suspension and Ointment 473
Vasocidin Ointment ◆ 268
Vasocidin Ophthalmic Solution ◆ 270

Glaucoma, secondary

AMO Vitrax Viscoelastic Solution ◆ 232

Glaucoma, worsening of narrow angle

Atrovent Inhalation Aerosol 671
Atrovent Inhalation Solution 673

Globus hystericus

Daranide Tablets 1633
Imitrex Injection (Rare) 1103

Glomerular filtration rate, decrease

Capoten 739
Capozide 742
Monopril Tablets 757

Glomerulitis

Feldene Capsules (Less than 1%).. 1965
Motrin Ibuprofen Suspension, Oral Drops, Chewable Tablets, Caplets (Less than 1%) 1546
Ridaura Capsules 2513
Solgamal Suspension 2388

Glomerulonephritis

Anaprox/Naprosyn (Less than 1%) 2117
Apresazide Capsules 808
Cuprimine Capsules 1630
Depen Titratable Tablets (Rare) 2662
EC-Naprosyn Delayed-Release Tablets (Less than 1%) 2117
Foscavir Injection (Less than 1%).. 547
Myochrysine Injection 1711
Anaprox/Naprosyn (Less than 1%) 2117
Orthoclone OKT3 Sterile Solution .. 1837
Ser-Ap-Es Tablets 849

Glossitis

Achromycin V Capsules (Rare) 1367
AeroBid Inhaler System (1-3%) 1005
Aerobid-M Inhaler System (1-3%).. 1005
Anafranil Capsules (Infrequent) 803
Atretol Tablets 573
Augmentin 2468
Azo Gantrisin Tablets 2081
Bactrim DS Tablets 2084
Bactrim I.V. Infusion 2082
Bactrim 2084
Betaseron for SC Injection 658
Betoptic Ophthalmic Solution (Rare) 469
Betoptic S Ophthalmic Suspension (Rare) 471
Capoten 739
Capozide 742
Chloromycetin Sodium Succinate... 1900
Clinoril Tablets (Less than 1%) 1618
Cognex Capsules (Infrequent) 1901
Cuprimine Capsules 1630
Daraprim Tablets 1090
Declomycin Tablets 1371
Depakote Tablets (Greater than 1% but not more than 5%) 415
Depen Titratable Tablets (Rare) 2662
Didronel Tablets 1984
Doryx Capsules 1913
Dynacin Capsules 1590
Effexor (Infrequent) 2719
Fansidar Tablets 2114
Felbatol 2666
Flagyl 375 Capsules 2434
Flagyl I.V. 2247
Foscavir Injection (Less than 1%).. 547
Sterile FUDR 2118
Gantanol Tablets 2119
Gantrisin 2120
Geocillin Tablets 2199
Halcion Tablets 2611
Hivid Tablets (Less than 1% to less than 3%) 2121
▲ Hylorel Tablets (8.4%) 985
Imdur (Less than or equal to 5%).. 1323
Inversine Tablets 1686
Lamictal Tablets (Rare) 1112
Lincocin 2617
Lupron Depot 3.75 mg 2556
Luvox Tablets (Infrequent) 2544
Maxair Autohaler 1492
Maxair Inhaler (Less than 1%) 1494
MetroGel-Vaginal 902
Minocin Intravenous 1382
Minocin Oral Suspension 1385
Minocin Pellet-Filled Capsules 1383
Monodox Capsules 1805
Myochrysine Injection 1711
Neurontin Capsules (Infrequent).... 1922
Nicorette (1% to 3% of patients).. 2458
Omnipen Capsules 2764
Omnipen for Oral Suspension 2765
Paxil Tablets (Infrequent) 2505
Permax Tablets (Rare) 575
Primaxin I.M. 1727
Primaxin I.V. (Less than 0.2%) 1729
Proloprim Tablets 1155
Protostat Tablets 1883
Prozac Pulvules & Liquid, Oral Solution (Infrequent) 919
Relafen Tablets (Less than 1%) 2510
Ridaura Capsules (1 to 3%) 2513
Septra 1174
Septra I.V. Infusion 1169
Septra I.V. Infusion ADD-Vantage Vials 1171
Septra 1174
Serzone Tablets (Rare) 771
Solgamal Suspension 2388
Spectrobid Tablets 2206
Tegretol Chewable Tablets 852
Tegretol Suspension 852
Tegretol Tablets 852
Terramycin Intramuscular Solution 2210
Teslac 717
Tolectin (200, 400 and 600 mg) (Less than 1%) 1581
Trimpex Tablets 2163
Unasyn (Less than 1%) 2212
Urobiotic-250 Capsules (Rare) 2214
Vaseretic Tablets 1765
Vasotec I.V. 1768
Vasotec Tablets (0.5% to 1.0%) 1771
Vibramycin 1941
Vibramycin Hyclate Intravenous 2215
Vibramycin 1941
Wellbutrin Tablets (Rare) 1204
Zoloft Tablets (Rare) 2217

Glossodynia

Adenoscan (Less than 1%) 1024

Glucose tolerance, decreased

Aldoclor Tablets 1598
Aldomet Ester HCl Injection 1602
Aldomet Oral 1600
Aldoril Tablets 1604
Clozaril Tablets (1%) 2252
Etrafon 2355
Hivid Tablets (Less than 1% to less than 3%) 2121
▲ Imitrex Injection (4.9%) 1103
Imitrex Tablets 1106
Omnipen for Oral Suspension (Occasional) 2765
Questran Light (Less frequent) 769
Questran Powder (Less frequent).... 770
Rifadin (Occasional) 1528
Rifamate Capsules (Occasional) 1530
Rifater (Occasional) 1532
Rimactane Capsules 847
▲ Tegison Capsules (10-25%) 2154
Trilafon 2389

Glossoncus

Altace Capsules 1232
Calcimar Injection, Synthetic (A few cases) 2013
Cataflam (Less than 1%) 816
Ceftin (Less than 1% but more than 0.1%) 1078
Fluvirin 460
Miacalcin Injection (A few cases)... 2273
Myochrysine Injection 1711
Romazicon (Less than 1%) 2147
Solgamal Suspension 2388
Tambocor Tablets (Less than 1%) 1497
Voltaren Tablets (Less than 1%) ... 861
Zarontin Capsules 1928
Zarontin Syrup 1929

Glossoplegia

Risperdal (Rare) 1301

Glossotrichia

Aldomet Ester HCl Injection 1602
Asendin Tablets 1369
Augmentin 2468
Elavil 2838
Endep Tablets 2174
Etrafon 2355
Klonopin Tablets 2126
Limbitrol 2180
Ludomil Tablets (Isolated reports) 843
Norpramin Tablets 1526
Pamelor 2280
▲ Pen•Vee K (Among most common) 2772
Spectrobid Tablets 2206
Surmontil Capsules 2811
Tofranil Ampuls 854
Tofranil Tablets 856
Tofranil-PM Capsules 857
Unasyn 2212
Vivactil Tablets 1774

Glucose tolerance, changes

Brevicon 2088
Cortifoam 2396
Danocrine Capsules 2307
Demulen (Significant percentage of patients) 2428
Estrace Cream and Tablets 749
Estratest 2539
Foscavir Injection (Less than 1%).. 547
Glynase PresTab Tablets 2609
Lasix Injection, Oral Solution and Tablets 1240
Levlen/Tri-Levlen 651
Micronor Tablets 1872
Modicon 1872
Norinyl 2088
Nor-Q D Tablets 2135
Ortho Dienestrol Cream 1866
Ortho-Novum 1872
Ovcon 760
PMB 200 and PMB 400 2783
Phenergan Injection 2773
Premarin Intravenous 2787
▲ Premarin with Methyltestosterone (Significant percentage of patients) 2794
Stilphostrol Tablets and Ampuls 612
Temaril Tablets, Syrup and Spansule Extended-Release Capsules 483
Levlen/Tri-Levlen 651
Tri-Norinyl 2164
Winstrol Tablets 2337
Zanosar Sterile Powder (Some patients) 2653

Glucose tolerance, decreased

Amen Tablets 780
Cycrin Tablets 975

(▣ Described in PDR For Nonprescription Drugs) Incidence data in parenthesis; ▲ 3% or more (◆ Described in PDR For Ophthalmology)

Glucose tolerance, decreased — Side Effects Index — 1310

Depo-Provera Contraceptive Injection (Some patients) 2602
Emcyt Capsules 1953
Estraderm Transdermal System 824
ESTRATAB Tablets (0.3, 0.625, 1.25, 2.5 mg) 2536
Lo/Ovral Tablets 2746
Lo/Ovral-28 Tablets 2751
Lotensin HCT 837
Menest Tablets 2494
Nicobid 2026
Nicolar Tablets 2026
Nordette-21 Tablets 2755
Nordette-28 Tablets 2758
Nutropin 1061
Ogen Tablets 2627
Ogen Vaginal Cream 2630
Ortho-Cyclen/Ortho-Tri-Cyclen 1858
Ortho-Cyclen/Ortho Tri-Cyclen 1858
Ovral Tablets 2770
Ovral-28 Tablets 2770
Ovrette Tablets 2771
Oxandrin 2862
PMB 200 and PMB 400 2783
Premarin Intravenous 2787
Premarin with Methyltestosterone 2794
Premarin Vaginal Cream 2791
Premphase 2797
Prempro 2801
Provera Tablets (A small percentage of patients) 2636
Triphasil-21 Tablets 2814
Triphasil-28 Tablets 2819

Glucosuria

Aclovate 1069
Bumex 2093
Carmol HC (Some patients) 924
▲ Cipro I.V. Pharmacy Bulk Package (Among most frequent) 597
Combipres Tablets (Rare) 677
Dermatop Emollient Cream 0.1% 1238
Diprolene 2352
Elspar (Low) 1659
Floxin I.V. (More than or equal to 1%) 1571
Floxin Tablets (200 mg, 300 mg, 400 mg) (More than or equal to 1.0%) 1567
Hivid Tablets (Less than 1% to less than 3%) 2121
Humatrope Vials (Infrequent) 1443
ProctoCream-HC 2.5% 2408
Rythmol Tablets–150mg, 225mg, 300mg (Less than 1%) 1352
Sinemet CR Tablets 944
Temovate (Infrequent) 1179
Ultravate Cream 0.05% 2689
Ultravate Ointment 0.05% 2690

Glycosuria

Aldoclor Tablets 1598
Aldoril Tablets 1604
Anafranil Capsules (Rare) 803
Apresazide Capsules 808
Atretol Tablets 573
Betaseron for SC Injection 658
Capozide 742
Cognex Capsules (Infrequent) 1901
Combipres Tablets 677
Compazine 2470
Cytotec (Infrequent) 2424
Diamox Intravenous (Occasional) 1372
Diamox Sequels (Sustained Release) 1373
Diamox Tablets (Occasional) 1372
Diucardin Tablets 2718
Diupres Tablets 1650
Diuril Oral Suspension 1653
Diuril Sodium Intravenous 1652
Diuril Tablets 1653
Dyazide 2479
Effexor (Infrequent) 2719
Enduron Tablets 420
Esidrix Tablets 821
Esimil Tablets 822
Eskalith 2485
Etrafon 2355
Florinef Acetate Tablets 505
Foscavir Injection (Less than 1%) 547
Glauctabs (Occasional) ⊙ 208
Hivid Tablets (Less than 1% to less than 3%) 2121
HydroDIURIL Tablets 1674
Hydropres Tablets 1675
Hyzaar Tablets 1677
Inderide Tablets 2732
Inderide LA Long Acting Capsules 2734
Indocin Capsules (Less than 1%) 1680
Indocin I.V. (Less than 1%) 1684
Indocin (Less than 1%) 1680
Lasix Injection, Oral Solution and Tablets 1240
Lithium Carbonate Capsules & Tablets 2230
Lithonate/Lithotabs/Lithobid 2543
Lopressor HCT Tablets 832
Lotensin HCT 837
Lozol Tablets (Less than 5%) 2022
MZM (Occasional) ⊙ 267
Maxzide 1380
Minizide Capsules 1938
Moduretic Tablets 1705
Mykrox Tablets 993
Navane Capsules and Concentrate 2201
Navane Intramuscular 2202
Neptazane Tablets 1388
Neurontin Capsules (Rare) 1922
Noroxin Tablets (Less frequent) 1715
Noroxin Tablets (Less frequent) 2048
Oretic Tablets 443
PREVACID Delayed-Release Capsules (Less than 1%) 2562
Prilosec Delayed-Release Capsules (Less than 1%) 529
Proglycem (Frequent) 580
Rocephin Injectable Vials, ADD-Vantage, Galaxy Container (Rare) 2142
Ser-Ap-Es Tablets 849
Stelazine 2514
Supprelin Injection (1%) 2056
▲ Tegison Capsules (1-10%) 2154
Tegretol Chewable Tablets 852
Tegretol Suspension 852
Tegretol Tablets 852
Temaril Tablets, Syrup and Spansule Extended-Release Capsules 483
Tenoretic Tablets 2845
Thalitone 1245
Thorazine 2523
Timolide Tablets 1748
Trilafon 2389
Wellbutrin Tablets (Rare) 1204
Yutopar Intravenous Injection (Infrequent) 570
Zanosar Sterile Powder 2653
Zaroxolyn Tablets 1000

Goiter

Anafranil Capsules (Rare) 803
Azo Gantanol Tablets (Rare) 2080
Azo Gantrisin Tablets (Rare) 2081
Azulfidine (Rare) 1949
Betaseron for SC Injection (2%) 658
Effexor (Rare) 2719
Lamictal Tablets (Rare) 1112
Luvox Tablets (Rare) 2544
Neurontin Capsules (Rare) 1922
Pima Syrup (Rare) 1005
PREVACID Delayed-Release Capsules (Less than 1%) 2562
Prozac Pulvules & Liquid, Oral Solution (Rare) 919
Quadrinal Tablets 1350
SSKI Solution 2658
▲ Sandostatin Injection (Up to 12%) 2292
Supprelin Injection (1%) 2056

Goiter, diffuse

Lithium Carbonate Capsules & Tablets 2230

Goiter, euthyroid

Eskalith 2485
Lithium Carbonate Capsules & Tablets 2230
Lithonate/Lithotabs/Lithobid 2543

Goiter, fetal

Quadrinal Tablets 1350
Tapazole Tablets 1477

Goiter production (see under Goiter)

Gold deposits, ocular

Ridaura Capsules 2513

Gold toxicity

Myochrysine Injection (Common) 1711
Ridaura Capsules 2513

Gonadotropin secretion, increase

Cytoxan 694
NEOSAR Lyophilized/Neosar 1959

Gonadotropin secretion, inhibition

▲ Android Capsules, 10 mg (Among most common) 1250
▲ Android (Among most common) 1251
▲ Delatestryl Injection (One of most common) 2860
▲ Estratest (Among most common) 2539
Foscavir Injection (Less than 1%) 547
Halotestin Tablets 2614
▲ Oreton Methyl (Among most common) 1255
Oxandrin 2862
Premarin with Methyltestosterone (Among most common) 2794
Testred Capsules 1262

Goodpasture's syndrome

Cuprimine Capsules 1630
Depen Titratable Tablets (Rare) 2662

Gout

Adalat CC (Less than 1.0%) 589
Ambien Tablets (Rare) 2416
Anafranil Capsules (Infrequent) 803
Apresazide Capsules 808
Asacol Delayed-Release Tablets 1979
Capozide 742
Cardura Tablets (Less than 0.5% of 3960 patients) 2186
Cartrol Tablets (Less common) 410
Cipro I.V. (1% or less) 595
Cipro I.V. Pharmacy Bulk Package (Less than 1%) 597
Cipro Tablets (Less than 1%) 592
Cognex Capsules (Infrequent) 1901
Combipres Tablets 677
Cozaar Tablets (Less than 1%) 1628
Cytotec (Infrequent) 2424
Demadex Tablets and Injection 686
Dilacor XR Extended-release Capsules (Infrequent) 2018
Edecrin 1657
Effexor (Rare) 2719
Empirin with Codeine Tablets 1093
Esidrix Tablets 821
Hivid Tablets (Less than 1% to less than 3%) 2121
Hytrin Capsules (At least 1%) 430
Hyzaar Tablets 1677
Lasix Injection, Oral Solution and Tablets (Rare) 1240
Lopressor HCT Tablets (1 in 100 patients) 832
Lotensin HCT (0.3% to 1.0%) 837
Lotrel Capsules (Infrequent) 840
Lozol Tablets 2022
Maxaquin Tablets (Less than 1%) 2440
Maxzide 1380
Moduretic Tablets (Less than or equal to 1%) 1705
Monopril Tablets (0.2% to 1.0%) 757
Myambutol Tablets 1386
Mykrox Tablets 993
Nicobid 2026
Nicolar Tablets 2026
Oretic Tablets 443
Paxil Tablets (Rare) 2505
Permax Tablets (Infrequent) 575
PREVACID Delayed-Release Capsules (Less than 1%) 2562
Prinivil Tablets (0.5% to 1.5%) 1733
Prinzide Tablets 1737
Procardia XL Extended Release Tablets (1% or less) 1972
Proglycem 580
Prozac Pulvules & Liquid, Oral Solution (Rare) 919
Pyrazinamide Tablets 1398
Rifater 1532
Serzone Tablets (Infrequent) 771
Tegison Capsules (Less than 1%) 2154
Tenoretic Tablets 2845
Timolide Tablets 1748
Vaseretic Tablets (0.5% to 2.0%) 1765
Zaroxolyn Tablets 1000
Zebeta Tablets 1413
Zestoretic 2850
Zestril Tablets (0.5% to 1.5%) 2854
Ziac 1415
▲ Zoladex (Greater than 1% but less than 5%) 2858
Zyloprim Tablets (Less than 1%) 1226

Granulocytopenia

Aldoclor Tablets 1598
Aldomet Ester HCl Injection (Rare) 1602
Aldomet Oral 1600
Aldoril Tablets 1604
Anaprox/Naprosyn (Less than 1%) 2117
Atgam Sterile Solution (Less than 5%) 2581
Chloromycetin Sodium Succinate 1900
Claforan Sterile and Injection (Rare) 1235
Cytosar-U Sterile Powder 2592
Cytovene-IV 2103
Dalmane Capsules (Rare) 2173
Dilantin Infatabs (Occasional) 1908
Dilantin Kapseals (Occasional) 1906
Dilantin Parenteral (Occasional) 1910
Dilantin-125 Suspension (Occasional) 1911
EC-Naprosyn Delayed-Release Tablets (Less than 1%) 2117
Ergamisol Tablets (Less than 1% to 2%) 1292
Felbatol (Infrequent) 2666
▲ Foscavir Injection (5% or greater up to 17%) 547
Fulvicin P/G Tablets 2359
Fulvicin P/G 165 & 330 Tablets 2359
Garamycin Injectable 2360
Grifulvin V (griseofulvin tablets) Microsize (griseofulvin oral suspension) Microsize 1888
Gris-PEG Tablets, 125 mg & 250 mg 479
▲ Intron A (Less than 5% to 75%) 2364
Leucovorin Calcium Tablets, Wellcovorin Brand 1132
Limbitrol (Rare) 2180
Macrobid Capsules 1988
Macrodantin Capsules 1989
Mefoxin 1691
Mefoxin Premixed Intravenous Solution 1694
Methotrexate Sodium Tablets, Injection, for Injection and LPF Injection 1275
Milontin Kapseals 1920
Mustargen 1709
Myochrysine Injection 1711
Mysoline (Rare) 2754
Anaprox/Naprosyn (Less than 1%) 2117
▲ Navelbine Injection (29% to 80%) 1145
Nebcin Vials, Hyporets & ADD-Vantage 1464
Propulsid (Rare) 1300
Relafen Tablets (Less than 1%) 2510
▲ Retrovir Capsules (1.8% to 47%) 1158
▲ Retrovir I.V. Infusion (1.8% to 47%) 1163
▲ Retrovir Syrup (1.8% to 47%) 1158
Ridaura Capsules 2513
Rythmol Tablets–150mg, 225mg, 300mg (Less than 1%) 1352
Serentil (A single case) 684
Solganal Suspension (Rare) 2388
Talacen 2333
Talwin Injection 2334
Talwin Compound (Rare) 2335
Talwin Injection 2334
Talwin Nx 2336
Tapazole Tablets 1477
Tobramycin Sulfate Injection 968
Tolectin (200, 400 and 600 mg) (Less than 1%) 1581
Velban Vials 1484
▲ Videx Tablets, Powder for Oral Solution, & Pediatric Powder for Oral Solution (6% to 8%) 720
Zantac (A few patients) 1209
Zantac Injection (Few patients) 1207
Zantac Syrup (A few patients) 1209
Zinecard 1961

Granulocytosis

Hivid Tablets (Less than 1% to less than 3%) 2121
Vantin for Oral Suspension and Vantin Tablets 2646
Zefazone 2654

Granuloma, unspecified

Fluorescite ⊙ 219

Granulomatosis, Wegener's

Accutane Capsules 2076

Gray syndrome

Chloromycetin Sodium Succinate (2 cases) 1900

Grogginess

Versed Injection (Less than 1%) 2170

Groin, itch

Miltown Tablets 2672
PMB 200 and PMB 400 2783

Groin, rash

Miltown Tablets 2672
PMB 200 and PMB 400 2783

(Described in PDR For Nonprescription Drugs) Incidence data in parenthesis; ▲ 3% or more (⊙ Described in PDR For Ophthalmology)

1311 Side Effects Index Halitosis

Growth, retardation
- Aquasol A Vitamin A Capsules, USP 534
- Clomid 1514
- Depen Titratable Tablets (One infant) 2662

Growth, suppression in children
- Android 1251
- Aristocort Suspension (Forte Parenteral) 1027
- Aristocort Suspension (Intralesional) 1025
- Aristocort Tablets 1022
- Aristospan Suspension (Intra-articular) 1033
- Aristospan Suspension (Intralesional) 1032
- Azmacort Oral Inhaler 2011
- Beclovent Inhalation Aerosol and Refill 1075
- Celestone Soluspan Suspension 2347
- CORTENEMA 2535
- Cortifoam 2396
- Cortone Acetate Sterile Suspension 1623
- Cortone Acetate Tablets 1624
- Cylert Tablets 412
- Dalalone D.P. Injectable 1011
- Decadron Elixir 1633
- Decadron Phosphate Injection 1637
- Decadron Phosphate Respihaler 1642
- Decadron Phosphate Turbinaire 1645
- Decadron Phosphate with Xylocaine Injection, Sterile 1639
- Decadron Tablets 1635
- Decadron-LA Sterile Suspension 1646
- Deltasone Tablets 2595
- Depo-Medrol Single-Dose Vial 2600
- Depo-Medrol Sterile Aqueous Suspension 2597
- Desoxyn Gradumet Tablets 419
- Dexacort Phosphate in Respihaler 458
- Dexacort Phosphate in Turbinaire 459
- Florinef Acetate Tablets 505
- Hydeltrasol Injection, Sterile 1665
- Hydeltra-T.B.A. Sterile Suspension 1667
- Hydrocortone Acetate Sterile Suspension 1669
- Hydrocortone Phosphate Injection, Sterile 1670
- Hydrocortone Tablets 1672
- Medrol 2621
- Nasacort Nasal Inhaler 2024
- Pediapred Oral Liquid 995
- Prelone Syrup 1787
- ProctoCream-HC 2.5% (With chronic therapy) 2408
- Solu-Cortef Sterile Powder 2641
- Solu-Medrol Sterile Powder 2643

Growth retardation, intrauterine
- Accupril Tablets 1893
- Altace Capsules 1232
- Capoten 739
- Capozide 742
- Cozaar Tablets 1628
- Dilantin Kapseals 1906
- Dilantin Parenteral 1910
- Dilantin-125 Suspension 1911
- Elavil 2838
- Hyzaar Tablets 1677
- Lotensin Tablets 834
- Lotensin HCT 837
- Metubine Iodide Vials 916
- Monopril Tablets 757
- Prinivil Tablets 1733
- Prinzide Tablets 1737
- Tenoretic Tablets 2845
- Tenormin Tablets and I.V. Injection 2847
- Univasc Tablets 2410
- Vaseretic Tablets 1765
- Vasotec I.V. 1768
- Vasotec Tablets 1771
- Yutopar Intravenous Injection 570
- Zestoretic 2850
- Zestril Tablets 2854

Guillain-Barré syndrome
- Acel-Imune Diphtheria and Tetanus Toxoids and Acellular Pertussis Vaccine Adsorbed 1364
- ActHIB 872
- Asacol Delayed-Release Tablets (Rare) 1979
- Attenuvax (Rare) 1610
- Azulfidine (Rare) 1949
- Biavax II (Isolated reports) 1613
- Cuprimine Capsules 1630
- Cytovene-IV (One report) 2103
- Danocrine Capsules (Rare) 2307
- Depen Titratable Tablets 2662
- Diphtheria and Tetanus Toxoids and Pertussis Vaccine Adsorbed 2477
- Diphtheria and Tetanus Toxoids and Pertussis Vaccine Adsorbed USP (For Pediatric Use) 875
- Eminase (Less than 1 in 1,000) 2039
- Engerix-B Unit-Dose Vials (Less than 1%) 2482
- Fluvirin 460
- Havrix (Rare) 2489
- HibTITER 1375
- Imovax Rabies Vaccine (Two cases) 881
- Influenza Virus Vaccine, Trivalent, Types A and B (chromatograph- and filter-purified subviron antigen) FluShield, 1995-1996 Formula (Rare) 2736
- IPOL Poliovirus Vaccine Inactivated 885
- M-M-R II (Rare) 1687
- M-R-VAX II (Rare) 1689
- Meruvax II (Isolated reports) 1697
- Myochrysine Injection (Rare) 1711
- Noroxin Tablets 1715
- Noroxin Tablets 2048
- OmniHIB 2499
- Orimune 1388
- PedvaxHIB 1718
- Pneumovax 23 (Rare) 1725
- Pnu-Imune 23 1393
- Poliovax 891
- Recombivax HB 1744
- Tetramune 1404
- Tri-Immunol Adsorbed 1408

Gums, sore
- Hivid Tablets (Less than 1% to less than 3%) 2121
- Prolixin 509
- Wellbutrin Tablets (Infrequent) 1204

Gustatory sensation
- Torecan (Occasional) 2245
- ▲ Wellbutrin Tablets (3.1%) 1204

Gynecological disorders, unspecified
- ▲ Zofran Tablets (7%) 1217

Gynecomastia
- Adalat Capsules (10 mg and 20 mg) (Less than 0.5%) 587
- Adalat CC (Rare) 589
- Children's Advil Suspension (Less than 1%) 2692
- Aldactazide (Not infrequent) 2413
- Aldactone (Not infrequent) 2414
- Aldoclor Tablets 1598
- Aldomet Ester HCl Injection 1602
- Aldomet Oral 1600
- Aldoril Tablets 1604
- Anafranil Capsules (Rare) 803
- ▲ Android Capsules, 10 mg (Among most common) 1250
- Android (Frequent) 1251
- Asendin Tablets 1369
- Atromid-S Capsules 2701
- Axid Pulvules (Rare) 1427
- Betaseron for SC Injection 658
- Calan SR Caplets (1% or less) 2422
- Calan Tablets (1% or less) 2419
- Capoten 739
- Capozide 742
- Catapres Tablets (About 1 in 1,000 patients) 674
- Catapres-TTS (Less frequent) 675
- Cipro I.V. (1% or less) 595
- Cipro I.V. Pharmacy Bulk Package (Less than 1%) 597
- Clinoril Tablets (Rare) 1618
- Combipres Tablets (About 1 in 1,000) 677
- Compazine 2470
- Delatestryl Injection (Frequent) 2860
- Elavil 2838
- Endep Tablets 2174
- Etrafon 2355
- ▲ Eulexin Capsules (9% with LHRH agonist) 2358
- Flexeril Tablets (Rare) 1661
- Foscavir Injection (Less than 1%) 547
- Haldol Decanoate 1577
- Haldol Injection, Tablets and Concentrate 1575
- Halotestin Tablets 2614
- Humegon (Occasional) 1824
- IBU Tablets (Less than 1%) 1342
- Indocin Capsules (Less than 1%) 1680
- Indocin I.V. (Less than 1%) 1684
- Indocin (Less than 1%) 1680
- Intron A (Less than 5%) 2364
- Isoptin Oral Tablets (Less than 1%) 1346
- Isoptin SR Tablets (1% or less) 1348
- Lanoxicaps (Occasional) 1117
- Lanoxin Elixir Pediatric (Occasional) 1120
- Lanoxin Injection (Occasional) 1123
- Lanoxin Injection Pediatric (Occasional) 1126
- Lanoxin Tablets (Occasional) 1128
- Lescol Capsules 2267
- Limbitrol 2180
- Loxitane (Rare) 1378
- Ludiomil Tablets (Isolated reports) 843
- Lupron Depot 3.75 mg 2556
- Lupron Depot 7.5 mg (Less than 5%) 2559
- Lupron Depot-PED 7.5 mg, 11.25 mg and 15 mg (Less than 2%) 2560
- ▲ Lupron Injection (5% or more) 2555
- Matulane Capsules (In prepubertal and early pubertal boys) 2131
- Megace Oral Suspension (1% to 3%) 699
- Mellaril 2269
- Mevacor Tablets (0.5% to 1.0%) 1699
- Midamor Tablets 1703
- Moban Tablets and Concentrate (Infrequent) 1048
- Moduretic Tablets 1705
- Children's Motrin Ibuprofen Oral Suspension (Less than 1%) 1546
- Motrin Tablets (Less than 1%) 2625
- Motrin Ibuprofen Suspension, Oral Drops, Chewable Tablets, Caplets (Less than 1%) 1546
- Myleran Tablets (Rare) 1143
- Navane Capsules and Concentrate 2201
- Navane Intramuscular 2202
- Neoral (Less than 1% to 4%) 2276
- Nizoral Tablets (Less than 1%) 1298
- Norpace (Rare) 2444
- Norpramin Tablets 1526
- Nutropin (Rare) 1061
- Nydrazid Injection 508
- ▲ Oreton Methyl (Among most common) 1255
- Orudis Capsules (Rare) 2766
- Oruvail Capsules (Rare) 2766
- Oxandrin 2862
- Pamelor 2280
- Pepcid Injection (Rare) 1722
- Pepcid (Rare) 1720
- Pergonal (menotropins for injection, USP) (Occasional) 2448
- Pravachol 765
- Pregnyl 1828
- PREVACID Delayed-Release Capsules (Less than 1%) 2562
- Prilosec Delayed-Release Capsules (Less than 1%) 529
- Profasi (chorionic gonadotropin for injection, USP) 2450
- Prolixin 509
- Protropin (Rare) 1063
- Prozac Pulvules & Liquid, Oral Solution 919
- Reglan 2068
- Rifamate Capsules 1530
- Rifater 1532
- Risperdal (Rare) 1301
- ▲ Sandimmune (Less than 1% to 4%) 2286
- Sandostatin Injection (Less than 1%) 2292
- Ser-Ap-Es Tablets 849
- Serentil 684
- Sinequan 2205
- Sporanox Capsules (Less than 1%) 1305
- Stelazine 2514
- Surmontil Capsules 2811
- ▲ Tagamet (4%; 0.3% to 1%) 2516
- Temaril Tablets, Syrup and Spansule Extended-Release Capsules 483
- Testoderm Testosterone Transdermal System (Five in 104 patients; frequent) 486
- Testred Capsules 1262
- Thorazine 2523
- Tofranil Ampuls 854
- Tofranil Tablets 856
- Tofranil-PM Capsules 857
- Torecan 2245
- Trecator-SC Tablets 2814
- Triavil Tablets 1757
- Trilafon 2389
- Vaseretic Tablets 1765
- Vasotec I.V. 1768
- Vasotec Tablets (0.5% to 1.0%) 1771
- Verelan Capsules (1% or less) 1410
- Verelan Capsules (Less than 1%) 2824
- Vivactil Tablets 1774
- Wellbutrin Tablets (Infrequent) 1204
- Winstrol Tablets 2337
- Xanax Tablets 2649
- Zantac (Occasional) 1209
- Zantac Injection 1207
- Zantac Syrup (Occasional) 1209
- Zocor Tablets 1775
- Zoloft Tablets (Rare) 2217
- Zyloprim Tablets (Less than 1%) 1226

GGTP, elevation (see under Gamma-glutamyl transpeptidase, elevation)

H

Haemophilus B disease
- PedvaxHIB 1718

Hair, abnormal growth (see under Hirsutism)

Hair, dry brittle
- Atromid-S Capsules (Less often) 2701
- Claritin (2% or fewer patients) 2349
- Claritin-D 2350
- Clomid (Fewer than 1%) 1514
- Eskalith 2485
- Lithium Carbonate Capsules & Tablets 2230
- Lithonate/Lithotabs/Lithobid 2543
- Neoral (Rare) 2276
- Nizoral 2% Shampoo 1298
- Sandimmune (Rare) 2286
- Selsun Rx 2.5% Selenium Sulfide Lotion, USP 2225

Hair, oily
- Nizoral 2% Shampoo 1298
- Selsun Rx 2.5% Selenium Sulfide Lotion, USP 2225

Hair discoloration
- Drithocreme 0.1%, 0.25%, 0.5%, 1.0% (HP) 905
- Dritho-Scalp 0.25%, 0.5% 906
- Effexor (Rare) 2719
- MG 217 Medicated Tar Shampoo ▭ 835
- Plaquenil Sulfate Tablets 2328
- Selsun Rx 2.5% Selenium Sulfide Lotion, USP 2225
- Wellbutrin Tablets (Rare) 1204

Hair loss (see under Alopecia)

Hair problems, unspecified
- Accutane Capsules 2076
- Emcyt Capsules (1%) 1953
- Lescol Capsules 2267
- ▲ Lupron Depot 3.75 mg (Among most frequent) 2556
- Mevacor Tablets 1699
- Pravachol 765
- Zocor Tablets 1775
- ▲ Zoladex (4%) 2858

Hair texture, abnormal
- Imdur (Less than or equal to 5%) 1323
- Intron A (Less than 5%) 2364
- Nizoral 2% Shampoo (One occurrence in 41 patients) 1298
- Zoloft Tablets (Rare) 2217

Hair thinning
- ▲ Accutane Capsules (Less than 1 patient in 10) 2076
- Actigall Capsules 802
- Combipres Tablets 677
- Cortifoam 2396
- Eskalith 2485
- Intron A 2364
- Lithium Carbonate Capsules & Tablets 2230
- Lithonate/Lithotabs/Lithobid 2543
- Nolvadex Tablets (Infrequent) 2841
- Seldane Tablets 1536
- Seldane-D Extended-Release Tablets 1538
- Trilafon Tablets 2389

Halitosis
- Anafranil Capsules (Up to 2%) 803
- Azactam for Injection (Less than 1%) 734
- Claritin-D (Less frequent) 2350

(▭ Described in PDR For Nonprescription Drugs) Incidence data in parenthesis; ▲ 3% or more (◉ Described in PDR For Ophthalmology)

Effexor (Rare) 2719
Lamictal Tablets (Infrequent) 1112
PREVACID Delayed-Release Capsules (Less than 1%) 2562
Serzone Tablets (Infrequent) 771
Zoloft Tablets (Rare) 2217

Hallucinations

Actifed with Codeine Cough Syrup 1067
Actimmune (Rare) 1056
Children's Advil Suspension (Less than 1%) 2692
Ambien Tablets (Infrequent) 2416
Anafranil Capsules (Infrequent) 803
Ancobon Capsules 2079
Artane (Rare) 1368
Asendin Tablets (Very rare) 1369
Atamet 572
Ativan Injection (1%) 2698
Azo Gantanol Tablets 2080
Azo Gantrisin Tablets 2081
Azulfidine (Rare) 1949
Bactrim DS Tablets 2084
Bactrim I.V. Infusion 2082
Bactrim 2084
Bentyl 10 mg Capsules 1501
Betaseron for SC Injection 658
Blocadren Tablets (Less than 1%) 1614
Brontex 1981
Buprenex Injectable (Infrequent) 2006
BuSpar (Infrequent) 737
Butisol Sodium Elixir & Tablets (Less than 1 in 100) 2660
Cardizem CD Capsules (Less than 1%) 1506
Cardizem SR Capsules (Less than 1%) 1510
Cardizem Injectable 1508
Cardizem Tablets (Less than 1%) 1512
Catapres Tablets 674
Ceclor Pulvules & Suspension (Rare) 1431
Celontin Kapseals (Rare) 1899
Chibroxin Sterile Ophthalmic Solution (With oral form) 1617
Cipro I.V. (1% or less) 595
Cipro I.V. Pharmacy Bulk Package (Less than 1%) 597
Cipro Tablets (Less than 1%) 592
Claritin-D 2350
Clozaril Tablets (Less than 1%) 2252
Cogentin 1621
Cognex Capsules (2%) 1901
D.A. Chewable Tablets 951
Dalmane Capsules (Rare) 2173
Darvon-N/Darvocet-N 1433
Darvon 1435
Darvon-N Suspension & Tablets 1433
Deconamine Chewable Tablets 1320
Deconamine CX Cough and Cold Liquid and Tablets 1319
Deconamine 1320
Deconsal 454
Demerol 2308
Demser Capsules 1649
Depakene 413
Depakote Tablets 415
Desyrel and Desyrel Dividose 503
Didronel Tablets 1984
Dilaudid-HP Injection (Less frequent) 1337
Dilaudid-HP Lyophilized Powder 250 mg (Less frequent) 1337
Dilaudid Tablets and Liquid (Less frequent) 1339
Dimetane-DC Cough Syrup 2059
Dimetane-DX Cough Syrup 2059
Diprivan Injection (Less than 1%) 2833
Ditropan 1516
Dizac (Less frequent) 1809
Dolobid Tablets (Less than 1 in 100) 1654
Doral Tablets (Rare) 2664
▲ Duragesic Transdermal System (3% to 10%) 1288
Dura-Tap/PD Capsules 2867
Dura-Vent/DA Tablets 953
Dura-Vent Tablets 952
E.E.S. (Isolated reports) 424
Effexor (Infrequent) 2719
Elavil 2838
▲ Eldepryl Tablets (3 of 49 patients) 2550
Elspar 1659
Endep Tablets 2174
Entex PSE Tablets 1987
Ergamisol Tablets (Less frequent) 1292
EryPed (Isolated reports) 421
Ery-Tab Tablets (Isolated reports) 422
Erythrocin Stearate Filmtab (Isolated reports) 425
Erythromycin Base Filmtab (Isolated reports) 426
Erythromycin Delayed-Release Capsules, USP (Isolated reports) 427
Eskalith 2485
Ethmozine Tablets (Less than 2%) 2041
Etrafon 2355
Fansidar Tablets 2114
Fedahist Gyrocaps 2401
Fedahist Timecaps 2401
Felbatol (Infrequent) 2666
Feldene Capsules (Less than 1%) 1965
Fioricet with Codeine Capsules 2260
Fiorinal with Codeine Capsules 2262
Flexeril Tablets (Less than 1%) 1661
Floxin I.V. (Less than 1%) 1571
Floxin Tablets (200 mg, 300 mg, 400 mg) (Less than 1%) 1567
Flumadine Tablets & Syrup (Less than 0.3%) 1015
Foscavir Injection (Between 1% and 5%) 547
Ganite 2533
Gantanol Tablets 2119
Gantrisin 2120
Gastrocrom Capsules (Infrequent) 984
Genoptic Sterile Ophthalmic Solution (Rare) ◉ 243
Genoptic Sterile Ophthalmic Ointment (Rare) ◉ 243
Gentak (Rare) ◉ 208
Guaimax-D Tablets 792
Halcion Tablets 2611
Haldol Decanoate 1577
Haldol Injection, Tablets and Concentrate 1575
Hivid Tablets (Less than 1% to less than 3%) 2121
Hydrea Capsules (Extremely rare) 696
IBU Tablets (Less than 1%) 1342
▲ IFEX (Among most common) 697
Imitrex Tablets (Rare) 1106
Inapsine Injection 1296
Inderal 2728
Inderal LA Long Acting Capsules 2730
Inderide Tablets 2732
Inderide LA Long Acting Capsules 2734
Keflex Pulvules & Oral Suspension 914
Keftab Tablets 915
Kerlone Tablets (Less than 2%) 2436
Klonopin Tablets 2126
Lamictal Tablets (Infrequent) 1112
Lariam Tablets 2128
Larodopa Tablets (Relatively frequent) 2129
Leukeran Tablets (Rare) 1133
Levsin/Levsinex/Levbid 2405
Limbitrol 2180
Lioresal Intrathecal 1596
Lioresal Tablets 829
Lithonate/Lithotabs/Lithobid 2543
Lopressor Ampuls 830
Lopressor HCT Tablets 832
Lopressor Tablets 830
Ludiomil Tablets (Rare) 843
Luvox Tablets (Infrequent) 2544
MS Contin Tablets (Less frequent) 1994
MSIR (Infrequent) 1997
Marinol (Dronabinol) Capsules (Greater than 1%) 2231
Matulane Capsules 2131
Maxaquin Tablets 2440
Mebaral Tablets (Less than 1 in 100) 2322
Mepergan Injection 2753
Methergine (Rare) 2272
Mexitil Capsules (About 3 in 1,000) 678
Minipress Capsules (Less than 1%) 1937
Minizide Capsules (Rare) 1938
Children's Motrin Ibuprofen Oral Suspension (Less than 1%) 1546
Motrin Tablets (Less than 1%) 2625
Motrin Ibuprofen Suspension, Oral Drops, Chewable Tablets, Caplets (Less than 1%) 1546
Myambutol Tablets 1386
Myochrysine Injection (Rare) 1711
NebuPent for Inhalation Solution (1% or less) 1040
Nembutal Sodium Capsules (Less than 1%) 436
Nembutal Sodium Solution (Less than 1%) 438
Nembutal Sodium Suppositories (Less than 1%) 440
Neurontin Capsules (Infrequent) 1922
Norflex 1496
Norgesic (Occasional) 1496
Noroxin Tablets 1715
Noroxin Tablets 2048
Norpramin Tablets 1526
Novahistine DH 2462
Novahistine DMX ▣ 822
Novahistine Elixir ▣ 823
Novahistine Expectorant 2463
Nubain Injection (1% or less) 935
Oramorph SR (Morphine Sulfate Sustained Release Tablets) (Less frequent) 2236
Orudis Capsules (Rare) 2766
Oruvail Capsules (Rare) 2766
Pamelor 2280
Parlodel 2281
Paxil Tablets (Infrequent) 2505
Penetrex Tablets (Less than 0.1%) 2031
Pentam 300 Injection (1.7%) 1041
Pepcid Injection (Infrequent) 1722
Pepcid (Infrequent) 1720
Periactin 1724
▲ Permax Tablets (13.8%) 575
Phenergan with Codeine 2777
Phenergan VC with Codeine 2781
Phenobarbital Elixir and Tablets (Less than 1 in 100 patients) 1469
Placidyl Capsules 448
PREVACID Delayed-Release Capsules (Less than 1%) 2562
Prilosec Delayed-Release Capsules (Less than 1%) 529
Primaxin I.M. 1727
Primaxin I.V. 1729
Procan SR Tablets (Occasional) 1926
▲ Prograf (Greater than 3%) 1042
ProSom Tablets (Rare) 449
Prozac Pulvules & Liquid, Oral Solution (Infrequent) 919
Reglan (Rare) 2068
Restoril Capsules (Less than 0.5%) 2284
ReVia Tablets (Less than 1%) 940
Roferon-A Injection (Less than 1%) 2145
Rondec Oral Drops 953
Rondec Syrup 953
Rondec Tablet 953
Rondec-DM Oral Drops 954
Rondec-DM Syrup 954
Rondec-TR Tablet 953
Sansert Tablets 2295
Seconal Sodium Pulvules (Less than 1 in 100) 1474
Seldane-D Extended-Release Tablets 1538
Septra 1174
Septra I.V. Infusion 1169
Septra I.V. Infusion ADD-Vantage Vials 1171
Septra 1174
Serax Capsules 2810
Serax Tablets 2810
Serzone Tablets (Infrequent) 771
Sinemet Tablets 943
▲ Sinemet CR Tablets (3.9%) 944
Sinequan (Infrequent) 2205
Stadol (Less than 1%) 775
Sublimaze Injection 1307
Surmontil Capsules 2811
Symmetrel Capsules and Syrup (1% to 5%) 946
Syn-Rx Tablets 465
Syn-Rx DM Tablets 466
Tagamet 2516
Talacen 2333
Talwin Injection 2334
Talwin Compound 2335
Talwin Injection 2334
Talwin Nx 2336
Tenoretic Tablets 2845
Tenormin Tablets and I.V. Injection 2847
Timolide Tablets 1748
Timoptic in Ocudose (Less frequent) 1753
Timoptic Sterile Ophthalmic Solution (Less frequent) 1751
Timoptic-XE 1755
Tofranil Ampuls 854
Tofranil Tablets 856
Tofranil-PM Capsules 857
▲ Tonocard Tablets (2.1-11.2%) 531
Toradol (1% or less) 2159
Transderm Scōp Transdermal Therapeutic System (Infrequent) 869
Triavil Tablets 1757
Trilisate (Rare) 2000
Trinalin Repetabs Tablets 1330
Tussend 1783
Tussend Expectorant 1785
▲ Ultram Tablets (50 mg) (Less than 1% to 14%) 1585
Valium Injectable 2182
Valium Tablets 2183
Valrelease Capsules (Infrequent) 2169
Versed Injection 2170
Visken Tablets (Less than 1%) 2299
Vivactil Tablets 1774
Vontrol Tablets (Approximately 1 in 350) 2532
Wellbutrin Tablets (Frequent) 1204
Xanax Tablets (Rare) 2649
Zantac (Rare) 1209
Zantac Injection 1207
Zantac Syrup (Rare) 1209
Zebeta Tablets 1413
Ziac 1415
Zoloft Tablets (Infrequent) 2217
Zosyn (1.0% or less) 1419
Zosyn Pharmacy Bulk Package (1.0% or less) 1422
Zovirax Capsules 1219
Zovirax Sterile Powder (Approximately 1%) 1223
Zovirax 1219

Hallucinations, auditory

Catapres-TTS 675
Combipres Tablets 677
Orthoclone OKT3 Sterile Solution 1837
Vontrol Tablets (Less than 1/2%) 2532

Hallucinations, hypnagogic

Anafranil Capsules (Infrequent) 803

Hallucinations, visual

Atretol Tablets 573
Catapres-TTS 675
Combipres Tablets 677
Orthoclone OKT3 Sterile Solution 1837
Parlodel (Less than 1%) 2281
Salagen Tablets (Rare) 1489
Talwin Compound 2335
Talwin Nx 2336
Tegretol Chewable Tablets 852
Tegretol Suspension 852
Tegretol Tablets 852
Tessalon Perles 1020
Vontrol Tablets (Less than 1/2%) 2532

Halos

Cordarone Tablets 2712
Plaquenil Sulfate Tablets (Fairly common) 2328

Hand-foot syndrome (see under Palmar-plantar erythrodysesthesia syndrome)

Hangover

Effexor (Infrequent) 2719
Neurontin Capsules (Rare) 1922
Phenobarbital Elixir and Tablets 1469
Placidyl Capsules 448
▲ ProSom Tablets (3%) 449
Prozac Pulvules & Liquid, Oral Solution (Infrequent) 919
Serzone Tablets (Infrequent) 771

Head, roaring sensation

BuSpar (Infrequent) 737

Head, tight feeling

Imitrex Injection (2.2%) 1103
Imitrex Tablets (Infrequent) 1106

Headache

▲ Accupril Tablets (1.7% to 5.6%) 1893
▲ Accutane Capsules (Approximately 1 patient in 20) 2076
Achromycin V Capsules 1367
Actifed with Codeine Cough Syrup 1067
Actigall Capsules 802
▲ Actimmune (33%) 1056
Acutrim ▣ 628
Adagen (pegademase bovine) Injection (One patient) 972
▲ Adalat Capsules (10 mg and 20 mg) (About 10% to 23%) 587
▲ Adalat CC (19%) 589
Adenocard Injection (2%) 1021
▲ Adenoscan (18%) 1024
Adipex-P Tablets and Capsules 1048
Children's Advil Suspension (Less than 3%) 2692
▲ AeroBid Inhaler System (25%) 1005
▲ Aerobid-M Inhaler System (25%) 1005
Aerolate 1004
▲ Airet Solution for Inhalation (3% to 3.1%) 452
AK-Fluor Injection 10% and 25% ◉ 203
Albalon Solution with Liquifilm ◉ 231
Aldactazide 2413

(▣ Described in PDR For Nonprescription Drugs) Incidence data in parenthesis; ▲ 3% or more (◉ Described in PDR For Ophthalmology)

1313 **Side Effects Index** **Headache**

Aldactone 2414
Aldoclor Tablets 1598
Aldomet Ester HCl Injection 1602
Aldomet Oral 1600
Aldoril Tablets 1604
Alfenta Injection (0.3% to 1%) 1286
Alomide (1.5%) 469
▲ Altace Capsules (1.2% to 5.4%) 1232
Alupent (1% to 4%) 669
▲ Ambien Tablets (7% to 19%) 2416
Amen Tablets (Rare) 780
Amicar Syrup, Tablets, and Injection (Occasional) 1267
Amikacin Sulfate Injection, USP (Rare) 960
Amikin Injectable (Rare) 501
▲ Anafranil Capsules (28% to 52%) 803
Ana-Kit Anaphylaxis Emergency Treatment Kit (Common) 617
▲ Anaprox/Naprosyn (3% to 9%) 2117
Anatuss LA Tablets 1542
Ancobon Capsules 2079
▲ Android Capsules, 10 mg (Among most common) 1250
Android 1251
▲ Ansaid Tablets (3-9%) 2579
Antabuse Tablets (Small number of patients) 2695
Apresazide Capsules (Common) 808
Apresoline Hydrochloride Tablets (Common) 809
Aquasol A Vitamin A Capsules, USP 534
Aquasol A Parenteral 534
Aralen Hydrochloride Injection 2301
Aralen Phosphate Tablets 2301
▲ Aredia for Injection (At least 10%) 810
Aristocort Suspension (Forte Parenteral) 1027
Aristocort Suspension (Intralesional) 1025
Aristocort Tablets 1022
Aristospan Suspension (Intra-articular) 1033
Aristospan Suspension (Intralesional) 1032
Artane 1368
▲ Asacol Delayed-Release Tablets (35%) 1979
Asendin Tablets (Less frequent) 1369
Astramorph/PF Injection, USP (Preservative-Free) 535
Atamet 572
▲ Atgam Sterile Solution (1 patient in 6) 2581
Ativan Tablets (Less frequent) 2700
Atretol Tablets 573
Atrohist Plus Tablets 454
Atromid-S Capsules (Less often) 2701
Atrovent Inhalation Aerosol (2,4%; about 2 in 100) 671
▲ Atrovent Inhalation Solution (6.4%) 673
Augmentin (Less frequent) 2468
▲ Axid Pulvules (16.6%) 1427
Azactam for Injection (Less than 1%) 734
Azo Gantanol Tablets 2080
Azo Gantrisin Tablets 2081
▲ Azulfidine (Approximately one-third of patients) 1949
BCG Vaccine, USP (TICE) (2.4%) 1814
Bactrim DS Tablets 2084
Bactrim I.V. Infusion 2082
Bactrim 2084
▲ Beconase AQ Nasal Spray (Fewer than 5 per 100 patients) 1076
Benadryl Capsules 1898
Benadryl Injection 1898
Benemid Tablets 1611
Bentyl 1501
Betagan ◉ 233
▲ Betapace Tablets (3% to 8%) 641
▲ Betaseron for SC Injection (84%) 658
▲ Betimol 0.25%, 0.5% (More than 5%) ◉ 261
Betoptic Ophthalmic Solution (Rare) 469
Betoptic S Ophthalmic Suspension (Rare) 471
Biavax II 1613
Biaxin (2%) 405
Biltricide Tablets 591
Biphetamine Capsules 983
Blocadren Tablets (Greater than 1%) 1614
Bontril Slow-Release Capsules 781
Brethaire Inhaler 813
Brethine Ampuls 815
Brethine Tablets 814
Brevibloc Injection (About 2%) 1808
Brevicon 2088
Brevital Sodium Vials 1429
Bricanyl Subcutaneous Injection 1502
Bricanyl Tablets 1503
▲ Bromfed-DM Cough Syrup (Among most frequent) 1786
Bronkometer Aerosol 2302
Bronkosol Solution 2302
Brontex 1981
Bumex (0.6%) 2093
▲ Buprenex Injectable (1-5%) 2006
▲ BuSpar (6%) 737
Butisol Sodium Elixir & Tablets (Less than 1 in 100) 2660
Calan SR Caplets (2.2%) 2422
Calan Tablets (2.2%) 2419
Capoten (About 0.5 to 2%) 739
Capozide (0.5 to 2%) 742
Carafate Suspension (Less than 0.5%) 1505
Carafate Tablets (Less than 0.5%) 1504
Carbocaine Hydrochloride Injection 2303
▲ Cardene Capsules (6.4% to 8.2%) 2095
▲ Cardene I.V. (14.6) 2709
▲ Cardene SR Capsules (6.2%) 2097
▲ Cardizem CD Capsules (4.6% to 5.4%) 1506
▲ Cardizem SR Capsules (4.5% to 12%) 1510
Cardizem Injectable (Less than 1%) 1508
Cardizem Tablets (2.1%) 1512
▲ Cardura Tablets (9.9% to 14%) 2186
Cartrol Tablets (0.7%) 410
▲ Cataflam (3% to 9%) 816
Catapres Tablets (About 1 in 100 patients) 674
▲ Catapres-TTS (5 of 101 patients; less frequent) 675
Caverject (2%) 2583
Ceftin (Less than 1% but more than 0.1%) 1078
Cefzil Tablets and Oral Suspension (Less than 1%) 746
Celestone Soluspan Suspension 2347
▲ CellCept Capsules (16.1% to 21.1%) 2099
Celontin Kapseals 1899
Ceptaz (Fewer than 1%) 1081
Ceredase 1065
Cerezyme (Three patients) 1066
▲ CHEMET (succimer) Capsules (5.2 to 15.7%) 1545
Chloromycetin Sodium Succinate 1900
Cholera Vaccine 2711
▲ Cipro I.V. (Among most frequent) 595
Cipro I.V. Pharmacy Bulk Package (Greater than 1%) 597
Cipro Tablets (1% to 1.2%) 592
Claforan Sterile and Injection (Less than 1%) 1235
▲ Claritin (12%) 2349
▲ Claritin-D (19%) 2350
Climara Transdermal System 645
Cleocin Vaginal Cream (Less than 1%) 2589
▲ Clinoril Tablets (3-9%) 1618
Clomid (1.3%) 1514
▲ Clozaril Tablets (More than 5 to 7%) 2252
▲ Cognex Capsules (11%) 1901
ColBENEMID Tablets 1622
Colestid Tablets (Infrequent) 2591
Combipres Tablets (About 1 in 100) 677
Comhist 2038
Compazine 2470
Cordarone Tablets (1 to 3%) 2712
CORTENEMA 2535
Cortifoam 2396
Cortone Acetate Sterile Suspension 1623
Cortone Acetate Tablets 1624
Coumadin 926
Cozaar Tablets (1% or greater) 1628
Cycrin Tablets 975
Cylert Tablets 412
▲ Cytadren Tablets (1 in 20) 819
Cytosar-U Sterile Powder (Less frequent) 2592
Cytotec (2.4%) 2424
▲ Cytovene (4%) 2103
D.A. Chewable Tablets 951
DDAVP Injection (Infrequent) 2014
DDAVP Injection 15 mcg/mL (Infrequent) 2015
▲ DDAVP (2 to 5%) 2017
D.H.E. 45 Injection (Occasional) 2255
Dalalone D.P. Injectable 1011
Dalgan Injection (Less than 1%) 538
Dalmane Capsules 2173
Danocrine Capsules 2307
Dantrium Capsules (Less frequent) 1982
Dapsone Tablets USP 1284
Daranide Tablets 1633
Daraprim Tablets (Rare) 1090
Darvon-N/Darvocet-N 1433
Darvon 1435
Darvon-N Suspension & Tablets 1433
Decadron Elixir 1633
Decadron Phosphate Injection 1637
Decadron Phosphate Respihaler 1642
Decadron Phosphate Turbinaire 1645
Decadron Phosphate with Xylocaine Injection, Sterile 1639
Decadron Tablets 1635
Decadron-LA Sterile Suspension 1646
Declomycin Tablets 1371
Deconamine Chewable Tablets 1320
Deconamine CX Cough and Cold Liquid and Tablets 1319
Deconamine 1320
Deconsal C Expectorant Syrup 456
Deconsal Pediatric Capsules 454
Deconsal Pediatric Syrup 457
Deconsal II Tablets 454
Delatestryl Injection 2860
Deltasone Tablets 2595
▲ Demadex Tablets and Injection (7.3%) 686
Demerol 2308
Demser Capsules (Infrequent) 1649
Demulen 2428
Depakene 413
Depakote Tablets 415
Depo-Medrol Single-Dose Vial 2600
Depo-Medrol Sterile Aqueous Suspension 2597
▲ Depo-Provera Contraceptive Injection (More than 5%) 2602
Depo-Provera Sterile Aqueous Suspension 2606
▲ Deponit NTG Transdermal Delivery System (Most common; 63%) 2397
▲ Desmopressin Acetate Rhinal Tube (2% to 5%) 979
Desogen Tablets 1817
Desoxyn Gradumet Tablets 419
▲ Desyrel and Desyrel Dividose (9.9% to 19.8%) 503
Dexacort Phosphate in Respihaler 458
Dexacort Phosphate in Turbinaire 459
Dexatrim ▣ 832
Dexatrim Plus Vitamins Caplets ▣ 832
Dexedrine 2474
DextroStat Dextroamphetamine Tablets 2036
Didrex Tablets 2607
Diethylstilbestrol Tablets 1437
▲ Diflucan Injection, Tablets, and Oral Suspension (1.9% to 13% patients) 2194
▲ Dilacor XR Extended-release Capsules (2.9% to 8.9%) 2018
Dilantin Infatabs 1908
Dilantin Kapseals 1906
Dilantin Parenteral 1910
Dilantin-125 Suspension 1911
▲ Dilatrate-SR (Approximately 25%) 2398
Dilaudid-HP Injection (Less frequent) 1337
Dilaudid-HP Lyophilized Powder 250 mg (Less frequent) 1337
Dilaudid Tablets and Liquid (Less frequent) 1339
Dimetane-DC Cough Syrup 2059
Dimetane-DX Cough Syrup 2059
▲ Dipentum Capsules (5%) 1951
Diprivan Injection (Less than 1%) 2833
Diucardin Tablets 2718
Diupres Tablets 1650
Diuril Oral Suspension 1653
Diuril Sodium Intravenous 1652
Diuril Tablets 1653
Dizac (Less frequent) 1809
Dobutrex Solution Vials (1% to 3%) 1439
▲ Dolobid Tablets (3% to 9%) 1654
Donnatal 2060
Donnatal Extentabs 2061
Donnatal Tablets 2060
Dopram Injectable 2061
▲ Doral Tablets (4.5%) 2664
▲ Duragesic Transdermal System (3% to 10%) 1288
Duramorph (A significant minority of cases) 962
Duranest Injections 542
Dura-Tap/PD Capsules 2867
Duratuss Tablets 2565
Dura-Vent/DA Tablets 953
Dura-Vent Tablets 952
Duvoid (Infrequent) 2044
Dyazide 2479
▲ DynaCirc Capsules (10.7% to 22.0%) 2256
Dyrenium Capsules (Rare) 2481
Easprin 1914
▲ EC-Naprosyn Delayed-Release Tablets (3% to 9%) 2117
Edecrin 1657
▲ Effexor (3% to 25%) 2719
Elavil 2838
▲ Eldepryl Tablets (2 of 49 patients) 2550
Elspar 1659
Emcyt Capsules (1%) 1953
Emete-con Intramuscular/Intravenous 2198
▲ Eminase (Less than 10%) 2039
Empirin with Codeine Tablets 1093
Endep Tablets 2174
Enduron Tablets 420
▲ Engerix-B Unit-Dose Vials (1% to 10%) 2482
Entex Capsules 1986
Entex LA Tablets 1987
Entex Liquid 1986
Entex PSE Tablets 1987
EPIFRIN ◉ 239
EpiPen 790
▲ Epogen for Injection (0.4% to 19%) 489
▲ Ergamisol Tablets (3% to 4%) 1292
Esgic-plus Tablets (Infrequent) 1013
Esidrix Tablets 821
Esimil Tablets 822
Eskalith 2485
Estrace Cream and Tablets 749
Estraderm Transdermal System 824
ESTRATAB Tablets (0.3, 0.625, 1.25, 2.5 mg) 2536
Estratest 2539
▲ Ethmozine Tablets (5.8% to 8.0%) 2041
Etrafon 2355
Exgest LA Tablets 782
Factrel (Rare) 2877
▲ Famvir (Among most frequent; 22.7%) 2486
Fansidar Tablets 2114
Fastin Capsules 2488
Fedahist Gyrocaps 2401
Fedahist Timecaps 2401
▲ Felbatol (Among most common; 6.5% to 36.8%) 2666
Feldene Capsules (Greater than 1%) 1965
Fioricet Tablets (Infrequent) 2258
Fioricet with Codeine Capsules (Infrequent) 2260
Fiorinal with Codeine Capsules (Infrequent) 2262
Flagyl 375 Capsules (Sometimes) 2434
Flagyl I.V. 2247
Flexeril Tablets (1% to 3%) 1661
Flonase Nasal Spray (1% to 3%) 1098
Florinef Acetate Tablets 505
Floropryl Sterile Ophthalmic Ointment 1662
▲ Floxin I.V. (1% to 9%) 1571
▲ Floxin Tablets (200 mg, 300 mg, 400 mg) (1% to 9%) 1567
Fludara for Injection (Up to 3%) 663
Flumadine Tablets & Syrup (1.4%) 1015
Fluorescite ◉ 219
Fluorouracil Injection 2116
Fortaz (Less than 1%) 1100
▲ Foscavir Injection (5% or greater up to 26%) 547
Sterile FUDR (Remote possibility) 2118
Fulvicin P/G Tablets (Occasional) 2359
Fulvicin P/G 165 & 330 Tablets (Occasional) 2359
▲ Fungizone Intravenous (Among most common) 506
Furoxone (Occasional) 2046
Gamimune N, 5% Immune Globulin Intravenous (Human), 5% 619
Gamimune N, 10% Immune Globulin Intravenous (Human), 10% 621
Gammagard S/D, Immune Globulin, Intravenous (Human) (Occasional; 12 of 16 patients) 585
Gammar I.V., Immune Globulin Intravenous (Human), Lyophilized 516
Gantanol Tablets 2119
Gantrisin 2120
Garamycin Injectable 2360
▲ Gastrocrom Capsules (4 of 87 patients) 984

(▣ Described in PDR For Nonprescription Drugs) Incidence data in parenthesis; ▲ 3% or more (◉ Described in PDR For Ophthalmology)

Headache — **Side Effects Index** — **1314**

Gelfoam Sterile Sponge 2608
Genotropin (Infrequent) 111
Geocillin Tablets 2199
Geref (sermorelin acetate for injection) 2876
Glucotrol Tablets (About 1 in 50) 1967
▲ Glucotrol XL Extended Release Tablets (8.6%) 1968
Grifulvin V (griseofulvin tablets) Microsize (griseofulvin oral suspension) Microsize (Occasional) 1888
Gris-PEG Tablets, 125 mg & 250 mg (Occasional) 479
Guaifed 1787
Guaifed Syrup ▣ 734
Guaimax-D Tablets 792
▲ Habitrol Nicotine Transdermal System (17%) 865
▲ Halcion Tablets (9.7%) 2611
Haldol Decanoate 1577
Haldol Injection, Tablets and Concentrate 1575
Halotestin Tablets 2614
▲ Havrix (14% of adults; less than 5% of children) 2489
Heparin Lock Flush Solution 2725
Heparin Sodium Injection 2726
Heparin Sodium Injection, USP, Sterile Solution 2615
Heparin Sodium Vials (Rare) 1441
Hespan Injection 929
▲ Hismanal Tablets (6.7%) 1293
▲ Hivid Tablets (Less than 1% to 12.8%) 2121
Humatrope Vials (Infrequent; small number of patients) 1443
Humegon 1824
Humorsol Sterile Ophthalmic Solution 1664
Hydeltrasol Injection, Sterile 1665
Hydeltra-T.B.A. Sterile Suspension 1667
Hydrea Capsules (Extremely rare) 696
Hydrocortone Acetate Sterile Suspension 1669
Hydrocortone Phosphate Injection, Sterile 1670
Hydrocortone Tablets 1672
HydroDIURIL Tablets 1674
Hydropres Tablets 1675
▲ Hylorel Tablets (58.1%) 985
Hyperstat I.V. Injection 2363
▲ Hytrin Capsules (1.1% to 16.2%) 430
Hyzaar Tablets (1% or greater) 1677
IBU Tablets (Greater than 1%) 1342
▲ Idamycin (20%) 1955
▲ Imdur (38% to 57%) 1323
Imitrex Injection (2.2%) 1103
Imitrex Tablets 1106
▲ Imovax Rabies Vaccine (About 20%) 881
Inderide Tablets 2732
Inderide LA Long Acting Capsules 2734
▲ Indocin (11.7%) 1680
INFeD (Iron Dextran Injection, USP) 2345
Infumorph 200 and Infumorph 500 Sterile Solutions (A significant minority of cases) 965
Intal Capsules (Less than 1 in 10,000 patients) 987
Intal Inhaler (Infrequent) 988
Intal Nebulizer Solution 989
▲ Intron A (4% to 61%) 2364
Ionamin Capsules 990
IOPIDINE Sterile Ophthalmic Solution ◉ 219
Iopidine 0.5% (Less than 3%) ◉ 221
▲ Ismo Tablets (19% to 38%) 2738
ISMOTIC 45% w/v Solution ◉ 222
Isoetharine Inhalation Solution, USP, Arm-a-Med 551
Isoptin Injectable (1.2%) 1344
Isoptin Oral Tablets (2.2%) 1346
Isoptin SR Tablets (2.2%) 1348
Isopto Carbachol Ophthalmic Solution ◉ 223
▲ Isordil Sublingual Tablets (Most common) 2739
▲ Isordil Tembids (Most common) 2741
▲ Isordil Titradose Tablets (Most common) 2742
Isuprel Hydrochloride Injection 1:5000 2311
Isuprel Hydrochloride Solution 1:200 & 1:100 2313
Isuprel Mistometer 2312
▲ JE-VAX (Less than 3% to approximately 15.2%) 886
K-Phos Neutral Tablets 639
Keflex Pulvules & Oral Suspension 914
Keftab Tablets 915
▲ Kerlone Tablets (6.5% to 14.8%) 2436
Klonopin Tablets 2126
Konÿne 80 Factor IX Complex 634
Kutrase Capsules 2402
▲ Kytril Injection (14%) 2490
▲ Kytril Tablets (14% to 21%) 2492
▲ Lamictal Tablets (Among most common; 29.1%) 1112
Lamprene Capsules (Less than 1%) 828
Lanoxicaps 1117
Lanoxin Elixir Pediatric 1120
Lanoxin Injection 1123
Lanoxin Injection Pediatric 1126
Lanoxin Tablets 1128
▲ Lariam Tablets (Among most frequent) 2128
Larodopa Tablets (Relatively frequent) 2129
Lasix Injection, Oral Solution and Tablets 1240
▲ Lescol Capsules (8.7%) 2267
▲ Leukine for IV Infusion (26%) 1271
▲ Leustatin (7% to 22%) 1834
▲ Levatol (7.8%) 2403
Levbid Extended-Release Tablets 2405
Levlen/Tri-Levlen 651
Levophed Bitartrate Injection 2315
Levsin/Levsinex/Levbid 2405
Limbitrol 2180
▲ Lioresal Intrathecal (Up to 9 of 214 patients) 1596
▲ Lioresal Tablets (4-8%) 829
Lithium Carbonate Capsules & Tablets 2230
Lithonate/Lithotabs/Lithobid 2543
▲ Livostin (5%) ◉ 266
Lomotil 2439
Lo/Ovral Tablets 2746
Lo/Ovral-28 Tablets 2751
Lopid Tablets (1.2%) 1917
Lopressor Ampuls 830
▲ Lopressor HCT Tablets (10 in 100 patients) 832
Lopressor Tablets 830
Lorabid Suspension and Pulvules (0.9% to 3.2%) 1459
Lorelco Tablets 1517
▲ Lotensin Tablets (6.2%) 834
▲ Lotensin HCT (3.1%) 837
Lotrel Capsules (2.2%) 840
Loxitane 1378
▲ Lozol Tablets (Greater than or equal to 5%) 2022
▲ Ludiomil Tablets (4%) 843
Lufyllin & Lufyllin-400 Tablets 2670
Lufyllin-GG Elixir & Tablets 2671
▲ Lupron Depot 3.75 mg (25.9%) 2556
Lupron Depot 7.5 mg 2559
Lupron Depot-PED 7.5 mg, 11.25 mg and 15 mg (Less than 2%) 2560
▲ Lupron Injection (5% or more) 2555
▲ Luvox Tablets (22%) 2544
M-M-R II 1687
M-R-VAX II 1689
MS Contin Tablets (Less frequent) 1994
MSIR (Infrequent) 1997
▲ Macrobid Capsules (6%) 1988
Macrodantin Capsules 1989
Marax Tablets & DF Syrup 2200
Marcaine Hydrochloride with Epinephrine 1:200,000 2316
Marcaine Hydrochloride Injection 2316
Marcaine Spinal 2319
Marinol (Dronabinol) Capsules (Less than 1%) 2231
Matulane Capsules 2131
Maxair Autohaler (1.3% to 2.0%) 1492
Maxair Inhaler (2.0%) 1494
▲ Maxaquin Tablets (3.2%) 2440
Maxzide 1380
Mebaral Tablets (Less than 1 in 100) 2322
Medrol 2621
▲ Megace Oral Suspension (Up to 10%) 699
Mellaril (Extremely rare) 2269
Menest Tablets 2494
Mepergan Injection 2753
▲ Mepron Suspension (16% to 18%) 1135
Meruvax II 1697
▲ Mesnex Injection (50%) 702
Methadone Hydrochloride Oral Concentrate 2233
Methadone Hydrochloride Oral Solution & Tablets 2235
Methergine 2272
Methotrexate Sodium Tablets, Injection, for Injection and LPF Injection (Less common) 1275
Metrodin (urofollitropin for injection) 2446
MetroGel-Vaginal (Equal to or less than 2%) 902
▲ Mevacor Tablets (2.1% to 9.3%) 1699
▲ Mexitil Capsules (5.7% to 7.5%) 678
▲ Miacalcin Nasal Spray (3.2%) 2275
Micronor Tablets 1872
▲ Midamor Tablets (3% to 8%) 1703
Milontin Kapseals 1920
Miltown Tablets 2672
▲ Minipress Capsules (7.8%) 1937
▲ Minizide Capsules (7.8%) 1938
Minocin Intravenous 1382
Minocin Oral Suspension 1385
Minocin Pellet-Filled Capsules 1383
Mintezol 1704
MIOSTAT Intraocular Solution ◉ 224
Mithracin 607
Modicon 1872
▲ Moduretic Tablets (3% to 8%) 1705
8-MOP Capsules 1246
Monistat Dual-Pak (1.3%) 1850
Monistat 3 Vaginal Suppositories (1.3%) 1850
Mono-Gesic Tablets 792
▲ Monoket (13% to 35%) 2406
Mononine, Coagulation Factor IX (Human) 523
Monopril Tablets (Less than 1.0% to 1.0% or more) 757
Motofen Tablets (1 in 40) 784
Children's Motrin Ibuprofen Oral Suspension (Greater than 1% but less than 3%) 1546
Motrin Tablets (Less than 3%) 2625
Motrin Ibuprofen Suspension, Oral Drops, Chewable Tablets, Caplets (1% to less than 3%) 1546
MSTA Mumps Skin Test Antigen 890
Mutamycin 703
Myambutol Tablets 1386
▲ Mycobutin Capsules (3%) 1957
▲ Mykrox Tablets (9.3%) 993
Myochrysine Injection 1711
▲ Nalfon 200 Pulvules & Nalfon Tablets (8.7%) 917
▲ Anaprox/Naprosyn (3% to 9%) 2117
Nardil (Common) 1920
▲ Nasacort Nasal Inhaler (Approximately 18%) 2024
Nasalcrom Nasal Solution (1 in 50) 994
Nasalide Nasal Solution 0.025% (5% or less) 2110
Nebcin Vials, Hyporets & ADD-Vantage 1464
NebuPent for Inhalation Solution (Greater than 1%, up to 5%) 1040
NegGram 2323
Nembutal Sodium Capsules 436
Nembutal Sodium Solution 438
Nembutal Sodium Suppositories (Less than 1%) 440
▲ Neoral (2% to 15%) 2276
Neo-Synephrine Hydrochloride 1% Carpuject 2324
Neo-Synephrine Hydrochloride 1% Injection 2324
Nescaine/Nescaine MPF 554
Netromycin Injection 100 mg/ml (Fewer than 1 of 1000 patients) 2373
▲ Neupogen for Injection (7%) 495
Neurontin Capsules (More than 1%) 1922
▲ Nicoderm (nicotine transdermal system) (29%) 1518
▲ Nicorette (20%) 2458
▲ Nicotrol Nicotine Transdermal System (3% to 9%) 1550
▲ Nimotop Capsules (Up to 4.1%) 610
▲ Nitro-Bid IV (Most common) 1523
▲ Nitro-Bid Ointment (Most common) 1524
▲ Nitrodisc (63%) 2047
▲ Nitro-Dur (nitroglycerin) Transdermal Infusion System (Most common) 1326
▲ Nitrolingual Spray (50%) 2027
Nizoral Tablets (Less than 1%) 1298
Nolvadex Tablets (Infrequent) 2841
Nordette-21 Tablets 2755
Nordette-28 Tablets 2758
Norflex 1496
Norgesic 1496
Norinyl 2088
Norisodrine with Calcium Iodide Syrup 442
Normodyne Tablets (2%) 2379
Noroxin Tablets (2.0% to 2.8%) 1715
Noroxin Tablets (2.0% to 2.8%) 2048
▲ Norpace (3 to 9%) 2444
Norplant System 2759
Norpramin Tablets 1526
Nor-Q D Tablets 2135
▲ Norvasc Tablets (7.3%) 1940
Novahistine DH 2462
Novahistine DMX ▣ 822
Novahistine Elixir ▣ 823
▲ Novantrone (10 to 13%) 1279
Novocain Hydrochloride for Spinal Anesthesia 2326
▲ Nubain Injection (3%) 935
Nucofed 2051
Numorphan Injection 936
Numorphan Suppositories 937
Nutropin (A small number of patients) 1061
Ocupress Ophthalmic Solution, 1% Sterile (Occasional) ◉ 309
Ogen Tablets 2627
Ogen Vaginal Cream 2630
▲ Oncaspar (Greater than 1% but less than 5%) 2028
Oncovin Solution Vials & Hyporets 1466
OptiPranolol (Metipranolol 0.3%) Sterile Ophthalmic Solution (A small number of patients) ◉ 258
Oramorph SR (Morphine Sulfate Sustained Release Tablets) (Less frequent) 2236
▲ Orap Tablets (1 of 20 patients) 1050
Oretic Tablets 443
Oreton Methyl 1255
Organidin NR Tablets and Liquid (Rare) 2672
Orlamm (1% to 3%) 2239
Ornade Spansule Capsules 2502
Ortho-Cept 1851
Ortho-Cyclen/Ortho-Tri-Cyclen 1858
Ortho Dienestrol Cream 1866
Ortho-Est 1869
Ortho-Novum 1872
Ortho-Cyclen/Ortho Tri-Cyclen 1858
▲ Orthoclone OKT3 Sterile Solution (11% to 44%) 1837
▲ Orudis Capsules (3% to 9%) 2766
▲ Oruvail Capsules (3% to 9%) 2766
OSM_GLYN Oral Osmotic Agent ◉ 226
Ovcon 760
Ovral Tablets 2770
Ovral-28 Tablets 2770
Ovrette Tablets 2771
Oxsoralen-Ultra Capsules 1257
PBZ Tablets 845
PBZ-SR Tablets 844
PMB 200 and PMB 400 2783
Pamelor 2280
Papaverine Hydrochloride Vials and Ampoules 1468
Paremyd ◉ 247
▲ Parlodel (Less than 2% to 19%) 2281
Parnate Tablets 2503
▲ Paxil Tablets (17.6%) 2505
Pediapred Oral Liquid 995
Peganone Tablets 446
Penetrex Tablets (Up to 2%) 2031
Pentasa (2.0% to 2.2%) 1527
Pentaspan Injection 937
▲ Pepcid Injection (4.7%) 1722
▲ Pepcid (4.7%) 1720
Peptavlon 2878
Pergonal (menotropins for injection, USP) 2448
Periactin 1724
▲ Permax Tablets (5.3%) 575
Persantine Tablets (2.3%) 681
Phenergan with Codeine 2777
Phenergan VC with Codeine 2781
Phenobarbital Elixir and Tablets (Less than 1 in 100 patients) 1469
Phenurone Tablets (2%) 447
Phrenilin (Infrequent) 785
Pipracil 1390
Plaquenil Sulfate Tablets 2328
▲ Plendil Extended-Release Tablets (10.6% to 14.7%) 527
Pneumovax 23 1725
Polymyxin B Sulfate, Aerosporin Brand Sterile Powder 1154
Pondimin Tablets 2066
Ponstel 1925
Pontocaine Hydrochloride for Spinal Anesthesia 2330
▲ Pravachol (1.7% to 6.2%) 765
Pregnyl 1828
Prelone Syrup 1787
Prelu-2 Timed Release Capsules 681

(▣ Described in PDR For Nonprescription Drugs) Incidence data in parenthesis; ▲ 3% or more (◉ Described in PDR For Ophthalmology)

Premarin Intravenous ... 2787
Premarin with Methyltestosterone .. 2794
Premarin Tablets ... 2789
Premarin Vaginal Cream ... 2791
Premphase ... 2797
Prempro ... 2801
PREVACID Delayed-Release Capsules (Greater than 1%) ... 2562
▲ Prilosec Delayed-Release Capsules (2.9% to 6.9%) ... 529
Primacor Injection (2.9%) ... 2331
Primaxin I.M. ... 1727
Primaxin I.V. (Less than 0.2%) ... 1729
▲ Prinivil Tablets (4.4% to 5.7%) ... 1733
▲ Prinzide Tablets (5.2%) ... 1737
Pro-Banthīne Tablets ... 2052
▲ Procardia Capsules (Approximately 10% to 23%; 1 in 8 patients) ... 1971
▲ Procardia XL Extended Release Tablets (15.8% to 23%; 1 in 8 patients) ... 1972
▲ Procrit for Injection (0.40% to 19%) ... 1841
Profasi (chorionic gonadotropin for injection, USP) ... 2450
Proglycem ... 580
▲ Prograf (31% to 64%) ... 1042
▲ Proleukin for Injection (12%) ... 797
Prolixin ... 509
▲ Propulsid (19.3%) ... 1300
▲ ProSom Tablets (16%) ... 449
▲ Prostep (nicotine transdermal system) (11%) ... 1394
Prostigmin Injectable ... 1260
Prostigmin Tablets ... 1261
▲ Prostin E2 Suppository (Approximately one-tenth) ... 2634
Protopam Chloride for Injection ... 2806
Protostat Tablets ... 1883
Proventil Inhalation Aerosol ... 2382
▲ Proventil Inhalation Solution 0.083% (3% to 3.1%) ... 2384
▲ Proventil Repetabs Tablets (7%) ... 2386
▲ Proventil Solution for Inhalation 0.5% (3% to 3.1%) ... 2383
▲ Proventil Syrup (4 of 100 patients) ... 2385
▲ Proventil Tablets (7%) ... 2386
Provera Tablets ... 2636
Provocholine for Inhalation (1 occurrence) ... 2140
▲ Prozac Pulvules & Liquid, Oral Solution (20.3% to 33%) ... 919
Pyridium ... 1928
Quadrinal Tablets ... 1350
Quarzan Capsules ... 2181
Questran Light ... 769
Questran Powder ... 770
Quibron ... 2053
▲ Quinaglute Dura-Tabs Tablets (3%) ... 649
Quinidex Extentabs ... 2067
RMS Suppositories ... 2657
▲ Rabies Vaccine Adsorbed (8% to 10%) ... 2508
▲ Rabies Vaccine, Imovax Rabies I.D. (About 20%) ... 883
Recombivax HB (Equal to or greater than 1%) ... 1744
Reglan (Less frequent) ... 2068
▲ Relafen Tablets (3% to 9%) ... 2510
Respbid Tablets ... 682
▲ Retrovir Capsules (1.6% to 62.5%) ... 1158
▲ Retrovir I.V. Infusion (2% to 62.5%) ... 1163
▲ Retrovir Syrup (1.6% to 62.5%) ... 1158
▲ Rēv-Eyes Ophthalmic Eyedrops 0.5% (10% to 40%) ... ◉ 323
▲ ReVia Tablets (7% to more than 10%) ... 940
Revex (1%) ... 1811
Rifadin ... 1528
Rifamate Capsules ... 1530
Rifater ... 1532
Rimactane Capsules ... 847
▲ Risperdal (12% to 14%) ... 1301
Ritalin ... 848
Robaxin Injectable ... 2070
Robaxin Tablets ... 2071
Robaxisal Tablets ... 2071
Robinul Forte Tablets ... 2072
Robinul Injectable ... 2072
Robinul Tablets ... 2072
Rocaltrol Capsules ... 2141
Rocephin Injectable Vials, ADD-Vantage, Galaxy Container (Occasional) ... 2142
▲ Roferon-A Injection (66% to 71%) 2145
▲ Rogaine Topical Solution (3.42%) .. 2637
▲ Romazicon (1% to 9%) ... 2147
Rondec Oral Drops ... 953
Rondec Syrup ... 953
Rondec Tablet ... 953
Rondec-DM Oral Drops ... 954
Rondec-DM Syrup ... 954
Rondec-TR Tablet ... 953
▲ Rowasa (6.50%) ... 2548
Roxanol ... 2243
▲ Rythmol Tablets–150mg, 225mg, 300mg (1.5 to 4.5%) ... 1352
▲ Salagen Tablets (11%) ... 1489
▲ Sandimmune (2 to 15%) ... 2286
▲ Sandoglobulin I.V. (Most common; 2%) ... 2290
▲ Sandostatin Injection (6%) ... 2292
Sanorex Tablets ... 2294
Scleromate (Rare) ... 1891
Seconal Sodium Pulvules (Less than 1 in 100) ... 1474
▲ Sectral Capsules (6%) ... 2807
Sedapap Tablets 50 mg/650 mg (Infrequent) ... 1543
▲ Seldane Tablets (6.3% to 15.8%) 1536
▲ Seldane-D Extended-Release Tablets (17.4%) ... 1538
▲ Semprex-D Capsules (19%) ... 463
▲ Semprex-D Capsules (19%) ... 1167
Sensorcaine ... 559
Septra ... 1174
Septra I.V. Infusion ... 1169
Septra I.V. Infusion ADD-Vantage Vials ... 1171
Septra ... 1174
Ser-Ap-Es Tablets ... 849
Serax Capsules (In few instances) .. 2810
Serax Tablets (In few instances) ... 2810
▲ Serevent Inhalation Aerosol (28%) 1176
Seromycin Pulvules ... 1476
Serophene (clomiphene citrate tablets, USP) (Less than 1 in 100 patients) ... 2451
▲ Serzone Tablets (36%) ... 771
Sinemet Tablets ... 943
Sinemet CR Tablets (2.0%) ... 944
Sinequan (Occasional) ... 2205
Skelaxin Tablets ... 788
Slo-bid Gyrocaps ... 2033
Slo-Niacin Tablets ... 2659
Solganal Suspension (Rare) ... 2388
Solu-Cortef Sterile Powder ... 2641
Solu-Medrol Sterile Powder ... 2643
Soma Compound w/Codeine Tablets (Infrequent or rare) ... 2676
Soma Compound Tablets (Infrequent or rare) ... 2675
Soma Tablets ... 2674
▲ Sorbitrate (Most common) ... 2843
Sotradecol (Sodium Tetradecyl Sulfate Injection) ... 967
▲ Sporanox Capsules (1.5% to 3.8%) ... 1305
▲ Stadol (3% to 9%) ... 775
Stelazine ... 2514
Stilphostrol Tablets and Ampuls ... 612
Streptase for Infusion ... 562
Streptomycin Sulfate Injection ... 2208
▲ Supprelin Injection (22%) ... 2056
Suprane (Greater than 1%) ... 1813
Suprax (Less than 2%) ... 1399
Surgicel ... 1314
Surmontil Capsules ... 2811
Sus-Phrine Injection ... 1019
Symmetrel Capsules and Syrup (1% to 5%) ... 946
▲ Synarel Nasal Solution for Endometriosis (19% of patients) ... 2152
Syn-Rx Tablets ... 465
Syn-Rx DM Tablets ... 466
Tagamet (2.1% to 3.5%) ... 2516
Talacen ... 2333
Talwin Injection ... 2334
Talwin Compound ... 2335
Talwin Injection ... 2334
Talwin Nx ... 2336
▲ Tambocor Tablets (9.6%) ... 1497
Tapazole Tablets ... 1477
Tavist Syrup ... 2297
Tavist Tablets ... 2298
Tazicef for Injection (Less than 1%) ... 2519
Tazidime Vials, Faspak & ADD-Vantage (Less than 1%) ... 1478
▲ Tegison Capsules (25-50%) ... 2154
Tegretol Chewable Tablets ... 852
Tegretol Suspension ... 852
Tegretol Tablets ... 852
Temaril Tablets, Syrup and Spansule Extended-Release Capsules ... 483
Temovate Scalp Application (1 of 294 patients) ... 1179
▲ Tenex Tablets (1% to 13%) ... 2074
Tenoretic Tablets ... 2845
Tenormin Tablets and I.V. Injection 2847
▲ Terazol 3 Vaginal Cream (21%) ... 1886
▲ Terazol 3 Vaginal Suppositories (30.3% of 284 patients) ... 1886
▲ Terazol 7 Vaginal Cream (26% of 521 patients) ... 1887
Tessalon Perles ... 1020
Testoderm Testosterone Transdermal System ... 486
Testred Capsules ... 1262
Thalitone ... 1245
Theo-24 Extended Release Capsules ... 2568
Theo-Dur Extended-Release Tablets ... 1327
Theo-X Extended-Release Tablets .. 788
TheraCys BCG Live (Intravesical) (Up to 1.8%) ... 897
Thioplex (Thiotepa For Injection) ... 1281
THYREL TRH ... 2873
Ticlid Tablets (0.5% to 1.0%) ... 2156
Tigan ... 2057
▲ Tilade (6.0%) ... 996
Timentin for Injection ... 2528
Timolide Tablets (Less than 1%) ... 1748
Timoptic in Ocudose (Less frequent) ... 1753
Timoptic Sterile Ophthalmic Solution (Less frequent) ... 1751
Timoptic-XE (1% to 5% of patients) ... 1755
Tobramycin Sulfate Injection ... 968
Tofranil Ampuls ... 854
Tofranil Tablets ... 856
Tofranil-PM Capsules ... 857
▲ Tolectin (200, 400 and 600 mg) (3 to 9%) ... 1581
Tonocard Tablets (2.1-4.6%) ... 531
Toprol-XL Tablets ... 565
▲ Toradol (17%) ... 2159
Torecan (Occasional) ... 2245
▲ Tornalate Solution for Inhalation, 0.2% (8.4%) ... 956
▲ Tornalate Metered Dose Inhaler (3.5% to 4%) ... 957
Trancopal Caplets ... 2337
Trandate ... 1185
Transderm Scōp Transdermal Therapeutic System (Few patients) ... 869
▲ Transderm-Nitro Transdermal Therapeutic System (63%) ... 859
Tranxene (Less common) ... 451
Trental Tablets (1.2%) ... 1244
Triaminic Expectorant ... ▣ 790
Triavil Tablets ... 1757
Trilafon ... 2389
Levlen/Tri-Levlen ... 651
Trilisate (Less than 2%) ... 2000
Trinalin Repetabs Tablets ... 1330
Tri-Norinyl ... 2164
Triphasil-21 Tablets ... 2814
Triphasil-28 Tablets ... 2819
Trusopt Sterile Ophthalmic Solution (Infrequent) ... 1760
Tussend ... 1783
Tussend Expectorant ... 1785
Tussi-Organidin DM NR Liquid and DM-S NR Liquid ... 2677
Tussi-Organidin NR Liquid and S NR Liquid ... 2677
TYLENOL Severe Allergy Medication Caplets ... 1564
Tympagesic Ear Drops ... 2342
▲ Typhim Vi (Up to 27%) ... 899
Typhoid Vaccine ... 2823
▲ Ultram Tablets (50 mg) (18% to 32%) ... 1585
Unasyn (Less than 1%) ... 2212
Uni-Dur Extended-Release Tablets ... 1331
Uniphyl 400 mg Tablets ... 2001
Univasc Tablets (More than 1%) ... 2410
Urecholine ... 1761
Urispas Tablets ... 2532
Uroqid-Acid No. 2 Tablets ... 640
Valium Injectable ... 2182
Valium Tablets (Infrequent) ... 2183
Valrelease Capsules (Infrequent) ... 2169
▲ Valtrex Caplets (13% to 17%) ... 1194
Vancenase AQ Nasal Spray 0.042% (Fewer than 5 per 100 patients) ... 2393
Vantin for Oral Suspension and Vantin Tablets (Less than 1% to 1.1%) ... 2646
Varivax (Greater than or equal to 1%) ... 1762
▲ Vascor (200, 300 and 400 mg) Tablets (6.98 to 13.64%) ... 1587
▲ Vaseretic Tablets (5.5%) ... 1765
Vasosulf ... ◉ 271
Vasotec I.V. (2.9%) ... 1768
▲ Vasotec Tablets (1.8% to 5.2%) ... 1771
Vasoxyl Injection ... 1196
Velban Vials ... 1484
▲ Ventolin Inhalation Aerosol and Refill (3%) ... 1197
▲ Ventolin Inhalation Solution (3.1%) ... 1198
▲ Ventolin Nebules Inhalation Solution (3% to 3.1%) ... 1199
▲ Ventolin Rotacaps for Inhalation (2% to 5%) ... 1200
▲ Ventolin Syrup (4 of 100 patients) 1202
▲ Ventolin Tablets (7 of 100 patients) ... 1203
▲ Verelan Capsules (2.2% to 5.3%) 1410
▲ Verelan Capsules (2.2% to 5.3%) 2824
Versed Injection (1.3% to 1.5%) ... 2170
Voxol 1% Ophthalmic Suspension (Less than 2%) ... ◉ 230
▲ Videx Tablets, Powder for Oral Solution, & Pediatric Powder for Oral Solution (6% to 58%) ... 720
Vivactil Tablets ... 1774
Vivotif Berna ... 665
▲ Volmax Extended-Release Tablets (18.8%) ... 1788
▲ Voltaren Tablets (3% to 9%) ... 861
Vontrol Tablets (Rare) ... 2532
WinRho SD (2%) ... 2577
Wygesic Tablets ... 2827
▲ Xanax Tablets (12.9% to 29.2%) .. 2649
▲ Xylocaine Injections (3%) ... 567
Yocon ... 1892
Yodoxin ... 1230
Yohimex Tablets ... 1363
▲ Yutopar Intravenous Injection (10 to 15%) ... 570
Zantac ... 1209
Zantac Injection ... 1207
Zantac Syrup ... 1209
Zarontin Capsules ... 1928
Zarontin Syrup ... 1929
Zaroxolyn Tablets ... 1000
▲ Zebeta Tablets (8.8% to 10.9%) .. 1413
Zefazone ... 2654
▲ Zerit Capsules (3% to 55%) ... 729
▲ Zestoretic (5.2%) ... 2850
▲ Zestril Tablets (4.4% to 5.7%) ... 2854
Ziac (0.4% to 4.5%) ... 1415
Zithromax (1% or less) ... 1944
▲ Zocor Tablets (3.5%) ... 1775
▲ Zofran Injection (17% to 25%) ... 1214
▲ Zofran Tablets (9% to 27%) ... 1217
▲ Zoladex (Greater than 1% to 75%) ... 2858
▲ Zoloft Tablets (20.3%) ... 2217
▲ Zonalon Cream (Approximately 1% to 10%) ... 1055
▲ Zosyn (7.7%) ... 1419
▲ Zosyn Pharmacy Bulk Package (7.7%) ... 1422
▲ Zovirax Capsules (0.6% to 5.9%) .. 1219
Zovirax Sterile Powder (Less than 1%) ... 1223
▲ Zovirax (0.6% to 5.9%) ... 1219
Zyloprim Tablets (Less than 1%) ... 1226

Headache, migraine

Colestid Tablets (Infrequent) ... 2591
Norvasc Tablets (Less than or equal to 0.1%) ... 1940
Paxil Tablets (Rare) ... 2505
Prozac Pulvules & Liquid, Oral Solution (Rare) ... 919
Sansert Tablets ... 2295
Stilphostrol Tablets and Ampuls ... 612
▲ Wellbutrin Tablets (25.7%) ... 1204

Headache, periorbital

Pilopine HS Ophthalmic Gel ... ◉ 226

Headache, positional

▲ Xylocaine Injections (3%) ... 567

Headache, sinus

▲ CHEMET (succimer) Capsules (5.2 to 15.7%) ... 1545
Colestid Tablets (Infrequent) ... 2591
Prozac Pulvules & Liquid, Oral Solution (2.3%) ... 919
▲ Serevent Inhalation Aerosol (4%) .. 1176

Headache, supraorbital

Isopto Carpine Ophthalmic Solution ... ◉ 223
Pilocar ... ◉ 268

(▣ Described in PDR For Nonprescription Drugs) Incidence data in parenthesis; ▲ 3% or more (◉ Described in PDR For Ophthalmology)

Headache, temporal

Headache, temporal

Isopto Carpine Ophthalmic Solution ◉ 223
Pilocar ◉ 268
Pilopine HS Ophthalmic Gel ◉ 226

Headache, throbbing

Hyperstat I.V. Injection 2363
ReVia Tablets (Less than 1%) 940

Headache, transient

Aralen Hydrochloride Injection 2301
Aralen Phosphate Tablets 2301
DDAVP Injection (Infrequent) 2014
DDAVP (Infrequent) 2017
Levophed Bitartrate Injection 2315
Nicobid 2026
Nicolar Tablets 2026
Nitrostat Tablets 1925
Plaquenil Sulfate Tablets 2328
Stimate, (desmopressin acetate) Nasal Spray, 1.5 mg/mL (Infrequent) 525
▲ Transderm-Nitro Transdermal Therapeutic System (Most common) 859

Headedness, heavy

Desyrel and Desyrel Dividose (Up to 2.8%) 503
Parlodel (Less than 1%) 2281

Hearing, decrease

Aralen Hydrochloride Injection 2301
Aralen Phosphate Tablets 2301
Ativan Injection (Infrequent) 2698
Clinoril Tablets (Less than 1%) 1618
Daypro Caplets (Less than 1%) 2426
Felbatol 2666
Floxin I.V. (Less than 1%) 1571
Minocin Intravenous (Rare) 1382
Minocin Oral Suspension (Rare) 1385
Minocin Pellet-Filled Capsules (Rare) 1383
Nalfon 200 Pulvules & Nalfon Tablets (1.6%) 917
Platinol (Occasional) 708
Platinol-AQ Injection (Occasional) 710
ProSom Tablets (Rare) 449
Risperdal (Rare) 1301
Ziac 1415

Hearing, disturbances

Anaprox/Naprosyn (Less than 3%) 2117
Diamox 1372
EC-Naprosyn Delayed-Release Tablets (Less than 3%) 2117
Floxin I.V. 1571
Floxin Tablets (200 mg, 300 mg, 400 mg) 1567
Glauctabs ◉ 208
Imitrex Tablets (Infrequent) 1106
Indocin Capsules (Less than 1%) 1680
Indocin I.V. (Less than 1%) 1684
Indocin (Less than 1%) 1680
Intron A (Less than 5%) 2364
Lupron Depot 3.75 mg 2556
Lupron Depot 7.5 mg 2559
Lupron Injection 2555
Anaprox/Naprosyn (Less than 3%) 2117

Hearing, impaired

Anaprox/Naprosyn (Less than 1%) 2117
Arthritis Strength Bufferin Analgesic Caplets ◻ 614
Bumex (0.5%) 2093
Desferal Vials 820
Diamox Sequels (Sustained Release) 1373
EC-Naprosyn Delayed-Release Tablets (Less than 1%) 2117
Empirin with Codeine Tablets 1093
Kefurox Vials, Faspak & ADD-Vantage 1454
▲ MZM (Among reactions occurring most often) ◉ 267
Mustargen 1709
Anaprox/Naprosyn (Less than 1%) 2117
Orudis Capsules (Less than 1%) 2766
Oruvail Capsules (Less than 1%) 2766
Prostin E2 Suppository 2634
Salflex Tablets 786
Streptomycin Sulfate Injection 2208
Trilisate (Less than 2%) 2000

Hearing, loss of

Children's Advil Suspension (Less than 1%) 2692
Alka-Seltzer Effervescent Antacid and Pain Reliever ◻ 701
Alka-Seltzer Extra Strength Effervescent Antacid and Pain Reliever ◻ 703
Alka-Seltzer Lemon Lime Effervescent Antacid and Pain Reliever ◻ 703
Altace Capsules (Less than 1%) 1232
Amikacin Sulfate Injection, USP 960
Amikin Injectable 501
Ancobon Capsules 2079
Aralen Hydrochloride Injection (1 patient) 2301
Arthritis Foundation Safety Coated Aspirin Tablets ◻ 675
Arthritis Pain Ascriptin ◻ 631
Regular Strength Ascriptin Tablets ◻ 629
Azo Gantrisin Tablets 2081
Azulfidine (Rare) 1949
Bayer Children's Chewable Aspirin ◻ 711
Genuine Bayer Aspirin Tablets & Caplets ◻ 713
Extra Strength Bayer Arthritis Pain Regimen Formula ◻ 711
Extra Strength Bayer Aspirin Caplets & Tablets ◻ 712
Extended-Release Bayer 8-Hour Aspirin ◻ 712
Extra Strength Bayer PM Aspirin ◻ 713
Aspirin Regimen Bayer Regular Strength 325 mg Caplets ◻ 709
Bayer Select Backache Pain Relief Formula ◻ 715
Cama Arthritis Pain Reliever ◻ 785
▲ Capastat Sulfate Vials (3%) 2868
Cipro I.V. (1% or less) 595
Cipro I.V. Pharmacy Bulk Package (Less than 1%) 597
Cipro Tablets (Less than 1%) 592
Demadex Tablets and Injection 686
Depakene 413
Depakote Tablets 415
Desferal Vials 820
Doan's Regular Strength Analgesic ◻ 634
Ecotrin 2455
Floxin Tablets (200 mg, 300 mg, 400 mg) (Less than 1%) 1567
▲ Fludara for Injection (2% to 6%) 663
Fungizone Intravenous 506
Garamycin Injectable 2360
Gelfoam Sterile Sponge 2608
Healthprin Aspirin 2455
Hivid Tablets (Less than 1% to less than 3%) 2121
IBU Tablets (Less than 1%) 1342
Lasix Injection, Oral Solution and Tablets 1240
Matulane Capsules 2131
Miacalcin Nasal Spray (Less than 1%) 2275
Mobigesic Tablets ◻ 602
Mono-Gesic Tablets 792
Children's Motrin Ibuprofen Oral Suspension (Less than 1%) 1546
Motrin Tablets (Less than 1%) 2625
Motrin Ibuprofen Suspension, Oral Drops, Chewable Tablets, Caplets (Less than 1%) 1546
Nebcin Vials, Hyporets & ADD-Vantage 1464
Neoral (2% or less) 2276
Netromycin Injection 100 mg/ml (1 of 250 patients) 2373
Neurontin Capsules (Infrequent) 1922
Orthoclone OKT3 Sterile Solution 1837
Platinol 708
Platinol-AQ Injection 710
Primaxin I.M. 1727
Primaxin I.V. (Less than 0.2%) 1729
Quinidex Extentabs 2067
Retrovir Capsules 1158
Retrovir I.V. Infusion 1163
Retrovir Syrup 1158
Salflex Tablets 786
Sandimmune (2% or less) 2286
Supprelin Injection (1% to 3%) 2056
Tegison Capsules (Less than 1%) 2154
Tobramycin Sulfate Injection 968
Tonocard Tablets (0.4-1.5%) 531
Toradol (1% or less) 2159
Trilisate (Rare) 2000
Vancocin HCl, Oral Solution & Pulvules (A few dozen cases) 1483

Vancocin HCl, Vials & ADD-Vantage (Few dozen cases) 1481
Zinacef (A few pediatric patients) 1211

Hearing loss, reversible

Ansaid Tablets (Less than 1%) 2579
Cataflam (Less than 1%) 816
Chibroxin Sterile Ophthalmic Solution (With oral form) 1617
Depakene 413
Depakote Tablets 415
E.E.S. 424
E-Mycin Tablets (Isolated reports) 1341
Easprin 1914
ERYC (Isolated reports) 1915
EryPed (Isolated reports) 421
Ery-Tab Tablets (Isolated reports) 422
Erythrocin Stearate Filmtab (Isolated reports) 425
Erythromycin Base Filmtab (Isolated reports) 426
Erythromycin Delayed-Release Capsules, USP (Isolated reports) 427
Feldene Capsules (Less than 1%) 1965
Hyperstat I.V. Injection 2363
Ilosone (Isolated reports) 911
Ilotycin Gluceptate, IV, Vials (Rare) 913
Lasix Injection, Oral Solution and Tablets 1240
Noroxin Tablets (Rare) 1715
Noroxin Tablets (Rare) 2048
PCE Dispertab Tablets (Isolated reports) 444
Quinaglute Dura-Tabs Tablets 649
Romazicon (Less than 1%) 2147
Salflex Tablets 786
Voltaren Tablets (Less than 1%) 861

Heart beat, irregular

Adenocard Injection 1021
Brethaire Inhaler 813
IOPIDINE Sterile Ophthalmic Solution (0.7%) ◉ 219
K-Phos Neutral Tablets 639
K-Phos Original Formula 'Sodium Free' Tablets (Less frequent) 639
Lozol Tablets (Less than 5%) 2022
Maxair Inhaler (Less than 1%) 1494
Quadrinal Tablets 1350
SSKI Solution (Less frequent) 2658
Slo-Niacin Tablets 2659
Urocid-Acid No. 2 Tablets 640

Heart beats, ectopic

Imitrex Injection (Infrequent) 1103

Heart beats, premature

Plendil Extended-Release Tablets (0.5% to 1.5%) 527
▲ Taxol (23%) 714

Heart block

(see also under Sinoatrial block)

Actimmune (Rare) 1056
Adenocard Injection 1021
Anafranil Capsules (Rare) 803
Asendin Tablets (Very rare) 1369
Betagan ◉ 233
Betimol 0.25%, 0.5% ◉ 261
Betoptic Ophthalmic Solution (Rare) 469
Betoptic S Ophthalmic Suspension (Rare) 471
Brevibloc Injection (Less than 1%) 1808
Carbocaine Hydrochloride Injection 2303
Cardene Capsules (Less than 0.4%) 2095
Cordarone Tablets (2 to 5%) 2712
Diprivan Injection (Less than 1%) 2833
Elavil 2838
Endep Tablets 2174
Etrafon 2355
Flexeril Tablets (Rare) 1661
Imitrex Tablets (Rare) 1106
Limbitrol 2180
Ludiomil Tablets (Rare) 843
Marcaine Hydrochloride with Epinephrine 1:200,000 2316
Marcaine Hydrochloride Injection 2316
Marcaine Spinal 2319
Normodyne Injection (Rare) 2377
Normodyne Tablets (Less common) 2379
Norpace 2444
Norpramin Tablets 1526
Ocupress Ophthalmic Solution, 1% Sterile ◉ 309
Pamelor 2280
Permax Tablets (Rare) 575
Provocholine for Inhalation 2140

Rum-K Syrup 1005
Sensorcaine 559
Surmontil Capsules 2811
Tenex Tablets (Rare) 2074
▲ Tenormin Tablets and I.V. Injection (4.5%) 2847
Timoptic in Ocudose (Less frequent) 1753
Timoptic Sterile Ophthalmic Solution (Less frequent) 1751
Tofrianil Ampuls 854
Tofranil Tablets 856
Tofranil-PM Capsules 857
Trandate (Rare) 1185
Triavil Tablets 1757
Vascor (200, 300 and 400 mg) Tablets 1587
Visken Tablets (2% or fewer patients) 2299
Vivactil Tablets 1774

Heart block, second degree

Cartrol Tablets (Rare) 410
Dipentum Capsules (Rare) 1951
Procan SR Tablets 1926
Prostin VR Pediatric Sterile Solution (Less than 1%) 2635
Zofran Injection (Rare) 1214

Heart block, third degree

Wellbutrin Tablets 1204

Heartburn

▲ Adalat Capsules (10 mg and 20 mg) (11%) 587
▲ Children's Advil Suspension (3-9%) 2692
▲ AeroBid Inhaler System (3-9%) 1005
▲ Aerobid-M Inhaler System (3-9%) 1005
Aleve 1975
▲ Alka-Seltzer Effervescent Antacid and Pain Reliever (11.9% at doses of 1000 mg/day) ◻ 701
▲ Alka-Seltzer Lemon Lime Effervescent Antacid and Pain Reliever (11.9% at doses of 1000 mg/day) ◻ 703
▲ Anaprox/Naprosyn (3% to 9%) 2117
Arthrond Ampuls 2080
Arthritis Foundation Ibuprofen Tablets (Occasional) ◻ 674
▲ Regular Strength Ascriptin Tablets (11.9%) ◻ 629
▲ Genuine Bayer Aspirin Tablets & Caplets (11.9% at doses of 1000 mg/day) ◻ 713
▲ Aspirin Regimen Bayer Regular Strength 325 mg Caplets (11.9% of 4500 people tested) ◻ 709
▲ Bufferin Analgesic Tablets and Caplets (11.9%) ◻ 613
Cleocin Vaginal Cream (Less than 1%) 2589
▲ Clozaril Tablets (4%) 2252
Colestid Tablets (Less frequent) 2591
Dalmane Capsules 2173
▲ DiaBeta Tablets (Among most common; 1.8%) 1239
▲ EC-Naprosyn Delayed-Release Tablets (3% to 9%) 2117
▲ Ecotrin (11.9% at 1000 mg/day) 2455
Elderpyl Tablets 2550
Empirin with Codeine Tablets (Occasional) 1093
Esgic-plus Tablets (Infrequent) 1013
Etrafon 2355
Fedahist Gyrocaps 2401
Fedahist Timecaps 2401
Fioricet Tablets (Infrequent) 2258
Fioricet with Codeine Capsules (Infrequent) 2260
Fiorinal with Codeine Capsules (Infrequent) 2262
Floxin I.V. 1571
Floxin Tablets (200 mg, 300 mg, 400 mg) 1567
Glynase PresTab Tablets (1.8%) 2609
▲ Halfprin (11.9%) 1362
Haltran Tablets (Occasional) ◻ 771
Hivid Tablets (Less than 1% to less than 3%) 2121
▲ IBU Tablets (3% to 9%) 1342
▲ Indocin (3% to 9%) 1680
Lopressor Ampuls (1%) 830
Lopressor HCT Tablets (1 in 100) 832
Lopressor Tablets (1%) 830
Mevacor Tablets (1.6%) 1699
▲ Mexitil Capsules (39.3% to 39.6%) 678
Micronase Tablets (1.8%) 2623

(◻ Described in PDR For Nonprescription Drugs) Incidence data in parenthesis; ▲ 3% or more (◉ Described in PDR For Ophthalmology)

1317 Side Effects Index Hematologic reactions

Midamor Tablets (Less than or equal to 1%) ... 1703
Moduretic Tablets ... 1705
Monopril Tablets (0.2% to 1.0%) ... 757
▲ Children's Motrin Ibuprofen Oral Suspension (3% to 9%) ... 1546
▲ Motrin Tablets (3% to 9%) ... 2625
▲ Motrin Ibuprofen Suspension, Oral Drops, Chewable Tablets, Caplets (3% to 9%) ... 1546
▲ Anaprox/Naprosyn (3% to 9%) ... 2117
Noroxin Tablets (0.3% to 1.0%) ... 1715
Noroxin Tablets (0.3% to 1.0%) ... 2048
Novahistine DH ... 2462
Novahistine Elixir ... ▣ 823
Phrenilin (Infrequent) ... 785
Ponstel (Less frequent) ... 1925
Pravachol (2.0% to 2.9%) ... 765
Primaxin I.M. ... 1727
Primaxin I.V. (Less than 0.2%) ... 1729
Prinivil Tablets (0.3% to 1.0%) ... 1733
Prinzide Tablets (0.3% to 1%) ... 1737
▲ Procardia Capsules (11%) ... 1971
▲ Procardia XL Extended Release Tablets (11%) ... 1972
Proventil Inhalation Aerosol (Less than 5%) ... 2382
▲ Quinaglute Dura-Tabs Tablets (Among most frequent) ... 649
Rifadin (Some patients) ... 1528
Rifamate Capsules (Some patients) ... 1530
Rifater ... 1532
Rimactane Capsules ... 847
Rondec Oral Drops ... 953
Rondec Syrup ... 953
Rondec Tablet ... 953
Rondec-DM Oral Drops ... 954
Rondec-DM Syrup ... 954
Rondec-TR Tablet ... 953
Sansert Tablets ... 2295
Sedapap Tablets 50 mg/650 mg (Infrequent) ... 1543
Sinemet CR Tablets ... 944
▲ St. Joseph Adult Chewable Aspirin (81 mg.) (11.9% of 4500 patients) ... ▣ 808
Syprine Capsules ... 1747
Toprol-XL Tablets (About 1 of 100 patients) ... 565
▲ Trilisate (Less than 20%) ... 2000
▲ Ventolin Inhalation Aerosol and Refill (Fewer than 5 in 100 patients) ... 1197
Vontrol Tablets (Rare) ... 2532
Zestoretic (0.3 to 1%) ... 2850
Zestril Tablets (0.3% to 1.0%) ... 2854

Heart defects, congenital
Clomid ... 1514
Estraderm Transdermal System ... 824
ESTRATAB Tablets (0.3, 0.625, 1.25, 2.5 mg) ... 2536
Premarin with Methyltestosterone ... 2794

Heart failure
Accupril Tablets (Rare) ... 1893
Actimmune (Rare) ... 1056
Activase ... 1058
Altace Capsules (2.0%) ... 1232
Ansaid Tablets (Less than 1%) ... 2579
▲ Betapace Tablets (2% to 5%) ... 641
Betaseron for SC Injection ... 658
Calan SR Caplets ... 2422
Calan Tablets ... 2419
Cartrol Tablets (Rare) ... 410
Cognex Capsules (Infrequent) ... 1901
Dantrium Capsules (Less frequent) ... 1982
Dantrium Intravenous ... 1983
Dexatrim Plus Vitamins Caplets ... ▣ 832
DynaCirc Capsules (0.5% to 1%) ... 2256
Isoptin Oral Tablets (1.8%) ... 1346
Isoptin SR Tablets ... 1348
Kerlone Tablets (Less than 2%) ... 2436
Neurontin Capsules (Rare) ... 1922
Orthoclone OKT3 Sterile Solution ... 1837
Procardia XL Extended Release Tablets (Rare) ... 1972
Pulmozyme Inhalation ... 1064
Sectral Capsules (Up to 2%) ... 2807
▲ Tenormin Tablets and I.V. Injection (19%) ... 2847
▲ Trasylol (10%) ... 613
Verelan Capsules ... 1410
Verelan Capsules ... 2824
Videx Tablets, Powder for Oral Solution, & Pediatric Powder for Oral Solution (Less than 1%) ... 720
Visken Tablets (Less than 1%) ... 2299

Heart failure, congestive (see under Congestive heart failure)

Heart failure, worsening of
Prinivil Tablets (Up to 2.9%) ... 1733
Prinzide Tablets ... 1737
Vascor (200, 300 and 400 mg) Tablets (1.9%) ... 1587
Zestoretic ... 2850
Zestril Tablets (Up to 2.9%) ... 2854

Heart murmur
Cipro I.V. (1% or less) ... 595
Imdur (Less than or equal to 5%) ... 1323
Sansert Tablets ... 2295
Yutopar Intravenous Injection (Infrequent) ... 570

Heart rate, changes
▲ Blocadren Tablets (5%) ... 1614
Cafergot ... 2251
Cardura Tablets (About 0.7%) ... 2186
D.H.E. 45 Injection ... 2255
Deconsal C Expectorant Syrup ... 456
Deconsal Pediatric Syrup ... 457
Dopram Injectable ... 2061
Ergomar ... 1486
Nucofed ... 2051
▲ Yutopar Intravenous Injection (80 to 100%) ... 570
Zemuron ... 1830

Heart rate, changes fetal
Brethine Ampuls ... 815
Brethine Tablets ... 814
▲ Prepidil Gel (17.0%) ... 2633
Sectral Capsules ... 2807
▲ Yutopar Intravenous Injection (80 to 100%) ... 570

Heart rate, decrease
Betagan ... ◉ 233
Cocaine Hydrochloride Topical Solution ... 537
Guaifed ... 1787
Levatol (1 in 25%) ... 2403
Tornalate Solution for Inhalation, 0.2% (Less than 1%) ... 956
Tracrium Injection (0.6%) ... 1183

Heart rate, increase
Brethine Tablets ... 814
Bricanyl Subcutaneous Injection (Common) ... 1502
Bricanyl Tablets (Common) ... 1503
Bronkaid Mist ... ▣ 717
Bronkaid Mist Suspension ... ▣ 718
Cocaine Hydrochloride Topical Solution ... 537
DDAVP Injection (Infrequent) ... 2014
▲ Dobutrex Solution Vials (7.5% to approximately 10%) ... 1439
Effexor (Four beats per minute) ... 2719
Hivid Tablets (Less than 1% to less than 3%) ... 2121
Papaverine Hydrochloride Vials and Ampoules ... 1468
Pentaspan Injection ... 937
Pro-Banthīne Tablets ... 2052
Rondec Oral Drops ... 953
Rondec Syrup ... 953
Rondec Tablet ... 953
Rondec-DM Oral Drops ... 954
Rondec-DM Syrup ... 954
Rondec-TR Tablet ... 953
Serevent Inhalation Aerosol ... 1176
Stimate, (desmopressin acetate) Nasal Spray, 1.5 mg/mL (Infrequent) ... 525
Tracrium Injection (2.1%) ... 1183
Yohimex Tablets ... 1363

Heart spasms (see under Cardiospasm)

Heat intolerance
Imitrex Tablets ... 1106
Maxaquin Tablets (Less than 1%) ... 2440

Heat stroke
Asendin Tablets ... 1369
Clozaril Tablets ... 2252
Cogentin ... 1621
Compazine ... 2470
Cystospaz ... 1963
Haldol Decanoate ... 1577
Haldol Injection, Tablets and Concentrate ... 1575
Levsin/Levsinex/Levbid ... 2405
Loxitane ... 1378
Orap Tablets ... 1050
Prolixin ... 509
Serentil ... 684
Stelazine ... 2514

Heavy sensation, arms
Adenocard Injection (Less than 1%) ... 1021
Peptavlon ... 2878

Heavy sensation, legs
Eldepryl Tablets ... 2550
K-Phos Neutral Tablets ... 639
K-Phos Original Formula 'Sodium Free' Tablets (Less frequent) ... 639
Peptavlon ... 2878

Hematemesis
Anaprox/Naprosyn (Less than 1%) ... 2117
Ansaid Tablets (Less than 1%) ... 2579
Betaseron for SC Injection ... 658
Clozaril Tablets (Less than 1%) ... 2252
EC-Naprosyn Delayed-Release Tablets (Less than 1%) ... 2117
Effexor (Rare) ... 2719
Felbatol ... 2666
Feldene Capsules (Less than 1%) ... 1965
Foscavir Injection (Less than 1%) ... 547
Imitrex Tablets (Rare) ... 1106
Lamictal Tablets ... 1112
Lufyllin & Lufyllin-400 Tablets ... 2670
Lufyllin-GG Elixir & Tablets ... 2671
Luvox Tablets (Rare) ... 2544
Matulane Capsules ... 2131
Methotrexate Sodium Tablets, Injection, for Injection and LPF Injection ... 1275
Mithracin ... 607
Motrin Ibuprofen Suspension, Oral Drops, Chewable Tablets, Caplets (Less than 1%) ... 1546
Mutamycin ... 703
Anaprox/Naprosyn (Less than 1%) ... 2117
Neurontin Capsules (Rare) ... 1922
Orudis Capsules (Less than 1%) ... 2766
Oruvail Capsules (Less than 1%) ... 2766
Paxil Tablets (Rare) ... 2505
Permax Tablets (Infrequent) ... 575
PREVACID Delayed-Release Capsules (Less than 1%) ... 2562
Prozac Pulvules & Liquid, Oral Solution (Rare) ... 919
Quadrinal Tablets ... 1350
Quibron ... 2053
ReoPro Vials (5 to 11 events) ... 1471
Respbid Tablets ... 682
Risperdal (Rare) ... 1301
Slo-bid Gyrocaps ... 2033
Theo-24 Extended Release Capsules ... 2568
Theo-Dur Extended-Release Tablets ... 1327
Theo-X Extended-Release Tablets ... 788
Uni-Dur Extended-Release Tablets ... 1331
Uniphyl 400 mg Tablets ... 2001

Hematochezia
Adriamycin PFS ... 1947
Adriamycin RDF ... 1947
Anafranil Capsules (Infrequent) ... 803
Cataflam (Less than 1%) ... 816
Cognex Capsules (Infrequent) ... 1901
Colestid Tablets (Infrequent) ... 2591
Coumadin ... 926
Dipentum Capsules (Rare) ... 1951
Doxorubicin Astra ... 540
Glucotrol XL Extended Release Tablets (Less than 1%) ... 1968
Nalfon 200 Pulvules & Nalfon Tablets (Less than 1%) ... 917
NebuPent for Inhalation Solution (1% or less) ... 1040
Neurontin Capsules (Infrequent) ... 1922
Orudis Capsules (Less than 1%) ... 2766
Oruvail Capsules (Less than 1%) ... 2766
Penetrex Tablets (Less than 1% but more than or equal to 0.1%) ... 2031
Ridaura Capsules (0.1 to 1%) ... 2513
Rowasa ... 2548
Voltaren Tablets (Less than 1%) ... 861

Hematocrit, decrease
Children's Advil Suspension (Less than 1%) ... 2692
Altace Capsules (Rare; 0.4% to 1.5%) ... 1232
Ansaid Tablets (Less than 1%) ... 2579
Blocadren Tablets ... 1614
Cefobid Pharmacy Bulk Package - Not for Direct Infusion (1 in 20) ... 2192
▲ Cipro I.V. (Among most frequent) ... 595
▲ Cipro I.V. Pharmacy Bulk Package (Among most frequent) ... 597
Dopram Injectable ... 2061
▲ Feldene Capsules (3% to 9%) ... 1965
Hespan Injection ... 929
Hivid Tablets (Less than 1% to less than 3%) ... 2121
Hyzaar Tablets (Frequent but rare clinical importance) ... 1677
IBU Tablets (Less than 1%) ... 1342
▲ Kefurox Vials, Faspak & ADD-Vantage (1 in 10) ... 1454
▲ Lariam Tablets (Among most frequent) ... 2128
Larodopa Tablets ... 2129
Loniten Tablets ... 2618
Lopid Tablets (Occasional) ... 1917
Lorelco Tablets ... 1517
Methotrexate Sodium Tablets, Injection, for Injection and LPF Injection (Less common) ... 1275
Mezlin ... 601
Mezlin Pharmacy Bulk Package ... 604
Monopril Tablets ... 757
Children's Motrin Ibuprofen Oral Suspension (Less than 1%) ... 1546
Motrin Tablets (Less than 1%) ... 2625
Motrin Ibuprofen Suspension, Oral Drops, Chewable Tablets, Caplets (Less than 1%) ... 1546
Noroxin Tablets (Less frequent or 0.6%) ... 1715
Noroxin Tablets (Less frequent or 0.6%) ... 2048
Norpace (Less than 1%) ... 2444
Penetrex Tablets (Less than 1%) ... 2031
▲ Ponstel (2-5%) ... 1925
Primaxin I.M. ... 1727
Primaxin I.V. ... 1729
Prinivil Tablets (Frequent) ... 1733
Prinzide Tablets (Frequent) ... 1737
Proglycem ... 580
ReoPro Vials (7 to 11 events) ... 1471
Serzone Tablets (2.8%) ... 771
Sinemet CR Tablets (1% or greater) ... 944
Timentin for Injection ... 2528
Tolectin (200, 400 and 600 mg) (1 to 3%) ... 1581
Tornalate Solution for Inhalation, 0.2% (Infrequent) ... 956
Tranxene ... 451
Trobicin Sterile Powder ... 2645
Unasyn ... 2212
Vantin for Oral Suspension and Vantin Tablets ... 2646
Vaseretic Tablets (0.5% to 2.0%) ... 1765
Vasotec I.V. (Frequent) ... 1768
Vasotec Tablets (Frequent) ... 1771
Xanax Tablets (Less than 1%) ... 2649
Zanosar Sterile Powder ... 2653
Zefazone ... 2654
Zestoretic (Frequent) ... 2850
Zestril Tablets (Frequent) ... 2854
▲ Zinacef (1 in 10 patients) ... 1211
Zosyn ... 1419
Zosyn Pharmacy Bulk Package ... 1422

Hematocrit, increase
Clozaril Tablets ... 2252
Epogen for Injection ... 489
Lupron Depot 3.75 mg ... 2556
Procrit for Injection ... 1841

Hematocrit, transient decrease
Cytosar-U Sterile Powder (Less than 7 patients) ... 2592

Hematocrit content, deviation
Bumex (0.6%) ... 2093
Doral Tablets (1.5%) ... 2664

Hematologic reactions
Ana-Kit Anaphylaxis Emergency Treatment Kit (Rare) ... 617
Cefotan (1.4%) ... 2829
Dapsone Tablets USP ... 1284
Daraprim Tablets ... 1090
Feldene Capsules ... 1965
Floxin I.V. ... 1571
Floxin Tablets (200 mg, 300 mg, 400 mg) ... 1567
Lopid Tablets ... 1917
MZM (Common) ... ◉ 267
Procan SR Tablets (Common) ... 1926
Thalitone ... 1245

(▣ Described in PDR For Nonprescription Drugs) Incidence data in parenthesis; ▲ 3% or more (◉ Described in PDR For Ophthalmology)

Hematologic toxicity Side Effects Index 1318

Hematologic toxicity

Adriamycin PFS 1947
Adriamycin RDF 1947
Ana-Kit Anaphylaxis Emergency Treatment Kit (Rare) 617
Depen Titratable Tablets 2662
Doxorubicin Astra 540
Sterile FUDR 2118
Hivid Tablets (Less than 1% to less than 3%) 2121
Imuran 1110
Neutrexin 2572
Solganal Suspension 2388
Zanosar Sterile Powder (Rare) 2653

Hematoma

▲Caverject (3%) 2583
Claritin-D (Less frequent) 2350
Depakene 413
Depakote Tablets 415
Eldepryl Tablets 2550
Eminase (2.8%) 2039
▲Fragmin (Most common) 1954
Gelfoam Sterile Sponge 2608
Havrix (Less than 1%) 2489
Heparin Lock Flush Solution 2725
Heparin Sodium Injection 2726
Heparin Sodium Injection, USP, Sterile Solution 2615
Heparin Sodium Vials 1441
Imitrex Tablets (Rare) 1106
INSTAT* Collagen Absorbable Hemostat 1312
Lovenox Injection 2020
Lutrepulse for Injection 980
Netromycin Injection 100 mg/ml (4 of 1000 patients) 2373
Nimotop Capsules (Less than 1%) 610
Pipracil 1390
ReoPro Vials 1471
Sandostatin Injection (1% to 4%) .. 2292
▲THROMBATE III Antithrombin III (Human) (1 of 17) 637
Versed Injection (Less than 1%) 2170

Hematoma, pelvic

Oxytocin Injection 2771
Syntocinon Injection 2296

Hematopoietic depression

Cosmegen Injection 1626
▲DTIC-Dome (Among most common) 600
Methotrexate Sodium Tablets, Injection, for Injection and LPF Injection 1275
Mustargen (Occasional) 1709

Hematospermia

Luvox Tablets (Rare) 2544

Hematuria

▲Accutane Capsules (Less than 1 in 10) 2076
Children's Advil Suspension (Less than 1%) 2692
Anafranil Capsules (Infrequent) 803
Anaprox/Naprosyn (Less than 1%) 2117
Ansaid Tablets (Less than 1%) 2579
Asacol Delayed-Release Tablets 1979
Atromid-S Capsules 2701
Augmentin (Rare) 2468
Azo Gantrisin Tablets 2081
Azulfidine (Rare) 1949
▲BCG Vaccine, USP (TICE) (26.0%) 1814
Benemid Tablets 1611
Betaseron for SC Injection 658
Cardene I.V. (0.7%) 2709
Cataflam (Less than 1%) 816
Caverject (Less than 1%) 2583
▲CellCept Capsules (12.1% to 14.0%) 2099
Cipro I.V. (1% or less) 595
Cipro I.V. Pharmacy Bulk Package (Less than 1%) 597
Cipro Tablets 592
Clinoril Tablets (Less than 1%) 1618
Cognex Capsules (Infrequent) 1901
ColBENEMID Tablets 1622
Condylox (Less than 5%) 1802
Coumadin 926
Cuprimine Capsules 1630
Cytotec (Infrequent) 2424
Cytovene (1% or less) 2103
Cytoxan 694
Danocrine Capsules 2307
Dantrium Capsules (Less frequent) 1982
Daraprim Tablets 1090
Daypro Caplets (Less than 1%) 2426
Demser Capsules (A few patients) .. 1649
Depen Titratable Tablets 2662
Desyrel and Desyrel Dividose 503
Diamox Intravenous (Occasional) 1372
Diamox Sequels (Sustained Release) 1373
Diamox Tablets (Occasional) 1372
Dipentum Capsules (Rare) 1951
Diuril Sodium Intravenous (1 case following intravenous use) 1652
Dolobid Tablets (Less than 1 in 100) 1654
EC-Naprosyn Delayed-Release Tablets (Less than 1%) 2117
Edecrin 1657
Effexor (Frequent) 2719
Eminase 2039
Felbatol 2666
Feldene Capsules (Less than 1%) .. 1965
Floxin I.V. (More than or equal to 1%) 1571
Floxin Tablets (200 mg, 300 mg, 400 mg) (More than or equal to 1.0%) 1567
Fludara for Injection (2% to 3%) 663
Foscavir Injection (Less than 1%) .. 547
Genotropin (Infrequent) 111
Glauctabs (Occasional) .... ◎ 208
Hylorel Tablets (2.3%) 985
IBU Tablets (Less than 1%) 1342
▲IFEX (6% to 92%) 697
Imitrex Tablets (Rare) 1106
Indocin Capsules (Less than 1%) 1680
Indocin I.V. (Less than 1%) 1684
Indocin (Less than 1%) 1680
INFeD (Iron Dextran Injection, USP) 2345
Intron A (Less than 5%) 2364
Lamictal Tablets (Infrequent) 1112
Lioresal Tablets (Rare) 829
Lodine Capsules and Tablets (Less than 1%) 2743
Lufyllin & Lufyllin-400 Tablets 2670
Lufyllin-GG Elixir & Tablets 2671
Lupron Depot 3.75 mg 2556
Lupron Depot 7.5 mg (Less than 5%) 2559
▲Lupron Injection (5% or more) 2555
Luvox Tablets (Infrequent) 2544
Lysodren (Infrequent) 698
MZM (Occasional) .... ◎ 267
Matulane Capsules 2131
Maxaquin Tablets (Less than 1%) .. 2440
Methergine (Rare) 2272
Methotrexate Sodium Tablets, Injection, for Injection and LPF Injection 1275
Miacalcin Nasal Spray (Less than 1%) 2275
Milontin Kapseals 1920
Mintezol 1704
Children's Motrin Ibuprofen Oral Suspension (Less than 1%) 1546
Motrin Tablets (Less than 1%) 2625
Motrin Ibuprofen Suspension, Oral Drops, Chewable Tablets, Caplets (Less than 1%) 1546
Myochrysine Injection 1711
Nalfon 200 Pulvules & Nalfon Tablets (Less than 1%) 917
Anaprox/Naprosyn (Less than 1%) 2117
Neoral (Rare) 2276
NEOSAR Lyophilized/Neosar 1959
Neptazane Tablets 1388
Neupogen for Injection (Infrequent) 495
Neurontin Capsules (Infrequent) 1922
Noroxin Tablets 1715
Noroxin Tablets 2048
Oncaspar (Less than 1%) 2028
Ortho Diaphragm Kit 1865
Orudis Capsules (Less than 1%) 2766
Oruvail Capsules (Less than 1%) 2766
Paxil Tablets (Rare) 2505
Pentasa (Less than 1%) 1527
Permax Tablets (1.1%) 575
Ponstel 1925
PREVACID Delayed-Release Capsules (Less than 1%) 2562
Prilosec Delayed-Release Capsules (Less than 1%) 529
Primaxin I.M. 1727
Primaxin I.V. 1729
Priscoline Hydrochloride Ampuls 845
Procardia XL Extended Release Tablets (1% or less) 1972
Proglycem 580
▲Prograf (Greater than 3%) 1042
▲Proleukin for Injection (9%) 797
ProSom Tablets (Rare) 449
Prostin VR Pediatric Sterile Solution (Less than 1%) 2635
Prozac Pulvules & Liquid, Oral Solution (Rare) 919
Questran Light 769
Questran Powder 770
Relafen Tablets (Less than 1%) 2510
ReoPro Vials (4 events) 1471
Retrovir Capsules (0.8%) 1158
Retrovir I.V. Infusion (1%) 1163
Retrovir Syrup (0.8%) 1158
Ridaura Capsules (1 to 3%) 2513
Rifadin (Rare) 1528
Rifamate Capsules (Rare) 1530
Rifater (Rare) 1532
Rimactane Capsules 847
Risperdal (Infrequent) 1301
Rocephin Injectable Vials, ADD-Vantage, Galaxy Container (Rare) 2142
Sandimmune (Rare) 2286
Sandostatin Injection (Less than 1%) 2292
Serzone Tablets (Infrequent) 771
Sinemet CR Tablets (1% or greater) 944
Solganal Suspension 2388
Supprelin Injection (1% to 3%) 2056
Tazicef for Injection (Occasional) 2519
▲Tegison Capsules (1-10%) 2154
Testoderm Testosterone Transdermal System (One in 104 patients) 486
▲TheraCys BCG Live (Intravesical) (17.0% to 39.3%) 897
Ticlid Tablets 2156
Tolectin (200, 400 and 600 mg) (Less than 1%) 1581
Toradol (1% or less) 2159
Unasyn 2212
Urobiotic-250 Capsules 2214
Uroqid-Acid No. 2 Tablets (Rare) 640
Videx Tablets, Powder for Oral Solution, & Pediatric Powder for Oral Solution (Less than 1%) 720
Voltaren Tablets (Less than 1%) 861
Zarontin Capsules 1928
Zarontin Syrup 1929
Zerit Capsules (Fewer than 1% to 1%) 729
Zosyn (1.0% or less) 1419
Zosyn Pharmacy Bulk Package (1.0% or less) 1422
Zovirax Sterile Powder (Less than 1%) 1223
Zyloprim Tablets (Less than 1%) 1226

Hematuria, genitourinary

Eminase (2.4%) 2039

Hematuria, microscopic

Calcium Disodium Versenate Injection 1490
Celontin Kapseals 1899

Hemianopsia

Felbatol 2666

Hemiparesis

Anafranil Capsules (Rare) 803
Foscavir Injection (Less than 1%) .. 547
Klonopin Tablets 2126
Methotrexate Sodium Tablets, Injection, for Injection and LPF Injection 1275
Orthoclone OKT3 Sterile Solution .. 1837
Videx Tablets, Powder for Oral Solution, & Pediatric Powder for Oral Solution (Less than 1%) 720

Hemiplegia

Betaseron for SC Injection 658
Cognex Capsules (Infrequent) 1901
Imitrex Injection (Rare) 1103
Lamictal Tablets (Rare) 1112
Luvox Tablets (Infrequent) 2544
Neurontin Capsules (Infrequent) 1922
Orthoclone OKT3 Sterile Solution .. 1837
Permax Tablets (Rare) 575
PREVACID Delayed-Release Capsules (Less than 1%) 2562

Hemochromatosis

Effexor (Rare) 2719

Hemoconcentration

Haldol Decanoate 1577
Humegon 1824
Lutrepulse for Injection 980
Mykrox Tablets 993
Serophene (clomiphene citrate tablets, USP) 2451
Zaroxolyn Tablets 1000

Hemodilution

Hespan Injection 929

Hemoglobin, decrease

▲Children's Advil Suspension (Less than 1% to 22.8%) 2692
Altace Capsules (Rare; 0.4% to 1.5%) 1232
Ansaid Tablets (Less than 1%) 2579
Apresazide Capsules (Less frequent) 808
Apresoline Hydrochloride Tablets (Less frequent) 809
Betaseron for SC Injection 658
Blocadren Tablets 1614
Cataflam (Less than 1%) 816
▲Cefobid Intravenous/Intramuscular (1 in 20) 2189
▲Cefobid Pharmacy Bulk Package - Not for Direct Infusion (1 in 20) 2192
▲Cipro I.V. (Among most frequent) .. 595
▲Cipro I.V. Pharmacy Bulk Package (Among most frequent) 597
Cipro Tablets (Less than 0.1%) 592
Cytadren Tablets (1 patient) 819
▲Dapsone Tablets USP (Almost all patients) 1284
Dopram Injectable 2061
Easprin 1914
▲Feldene Capsules (3% to 9%) 1965
Hyzaar Tablets (Frequent but rare clinical importance) 1677
IBU Tablets (Less than 1%) 1342
▲Kefurox Vials, Faspak & ADD-Vantage (1 in 10) 1454
Larodopa Tablets (Occasional) 2129
Loniten Tablets 2618
Lopid Tablets (Occasional) 1917
Lorelco Tablets 1517
Lotensin Tablets (Rare; 1 of 2014 patients) 834
Macrobid Capsules (1% to 5%) 1988
Macrodantin Capsules 1989
Maxaquin Tablets (Less than or equal to 0.1%) 2440
Mezlin 601
Mezlin Pharmacy Bulk Package 604
Mithracin 607
Monopril Tablets 757
▲Children's Motrin Ibuprofen Oral Suspension (Less than 1 to 22.8%) 1546
Motrin Tablets (Less than 1%) 2625
▲Motrin Ibuprofen Suspension, Oral Drops, Chewable Tablets, Caplets (Less than 1% to 22.8%) 1546
Mustargen 1709
Noroxin Tablets (0.6%) 1715
Noroxin Tablets (0.6%) 2048
Norpace (1 to 3%) 2444
Penetrex Tablets (Less than 1%) 2031
Primaxin I.M. 1727
Primaxin I.V. 1729
Prinivil Tablets (Frequent) 1733
Prinzide Tablets (Frequent) 1737
Proglycem 580
ReoPro Vials (7 to 11 events) 1471
Ridaura Capsules 2513
Rifadin 1528
Rifamate Capsules 1530
Rifater 1532
Rimactane Capsules (Rare) 847
▲Roferon-A Injection (27%) 2145
Ser-Ap-Es Tablets 849
Sinemet CR Tablets (1% or greater) 944
▲Tegison Capsules (10-25%) 2154
Timentin for Injection 2528
Tolectin (200, 400 and 600 mg) (1 to 3%) 1581
Tornalate Solution for Inhalation, 0.2% (Infrequent) 956
Trobicin Sterile Powder 2645
Ultram Tablets (50 mg) (Infrequent) 1585
Unasyn 2212
Vantin for Oral Suspension and Vantin Tablets 2646
Vaseretic Tablets (0.5% to 2.0%) 1765
Vasotec I.V. (Frequent) 1768
Vasotec Tablets (Frequent) 1771
▲Videx Tablets, Powder for Oral Solution, & Pediatric Powder for Oral Solution (2% to 9%) 720
Voltaren Tablets (Less than 1%) 861
WinRho SD 2577
Zefazone 2654

(▣ Described in PDR For Nonprescription Drugs) Incidence data in parenthesis; ▲ 3% or more (◎ Described in PDR For Ophthalmology)

1319 Side Effects Index Hemoptysis

Zestoretic (Frequent) 2850
Zestril Tablets (Frequent) 2854
▲ Zinacef (1 in 10 patients) 1211
Zosyn 1419
Zosyn Pharmacy Bulk Package 1422

Hemoglobin content, deviation
Bumex (0.8%) 2093
Doral Tablets (1.4%) 2664
▲ Intron A (Up to 32%) 2364
Xanax Tablets (Less than 1%) 2649

Hemoglobinemia
Clozaril Tablets 2252
Hivid Tablets (Less than 1% to less than 3%) 2121
Zovirax Sterile Powder (Less than 1%) 1223

Hemoglobinuria
Rifadin (Rare) 1528
Rifamate Capsules 1530
Rifater (Rare) 1532
Rimactane Capsules (Rare) 847
▲ Tegison Capsules (1-10%) 2154

Hemolysis
Atgam Sterile Solution (Less than 5%) 2581
Cognex Capsules (Rare) 1901
Cozaar Tablets (One subject) 1628
▲ Dapsone Tablets USP (Most common) 1284
Foscavir Injection (Less than 1%) 547
Furoxone 2046
Hespan Injection (Rare) 929
Hyzaar Tablets (One subject) 1677
Kefurox Vials, Faspak & ADD-Vantage 1454
Macrobid Capsules 1988
Mycobutin Capsules (Less than 1%) 1957
Orudis Capsules (Less than 1%) 2766
Oruvail Capsules (Less than 1%) 2766
Plaquenil Sulfate Tablets 2328
Platinol 708
Platinol-AQ Injection 710
PREVACID Delayed-Release Capsules (Less than 1%) 2562
Rifadin (Rare) 1528
Rifamate Capsules (Rare) 1530
Rifater (Rare) 1532
Rimactane Capsules 847
Trasylol (0.3%) 613
Vaseretic Tablets (A few cases) 1765
Vasotec I.V. (A few cases) 1768
Vasotec Tablets (A few cases) 1771

Hemolysis, neonatal
AquaMEPHYTON Injection 1608
Dapsone Tablets USP 1284
Konakion Injection 2127
Mephyton Tablets 1696

Hemolytic anemia
Accupril Tablets 1893
Achromycin V Capsules 1367
Actifed with Codeine Cough Syrup 1067
Children's Advil Suspension (Less than 1%) 2692
Aldoclor Tablets 1598
Aldomet Ester HCl Injection 1602
Aldomet Oral 1600
Aldoril Tablets 1604
Alkeran for Injection 1070
Alkeran Tablets 1071
Altace Capsules (Less than 1%) 1232
Anaprox/Naprosyn (Less than 1%) 2117
Ansaid Tablets (Rare) 2579
Atamet (Rare) 572
Atgam Sterile Solution (Less than 5%) 2581
Azo Gantanol Tablets 2080
Azo Gantrisin Tablets 2081
Azulfidine (One in every 30 patients or less) 1949
Bactrim DS Tablets 2084
Bactrim I.V. Infusion 2082
Bactrim 2084
Benadryl Capsules 1898
Benadryl Injection 1898
Benemid Tablets 1611
Bicillin C-R Injection 2704
Bicillin C-R 900/300 Injection 2706
Bicillin L-A Injection (Infrequent) 2707
▲ Bromfed-DM Cough Syrup (Among most frequent) 1786
Capoten 739
Capozide 742
Cardizem CD Capsules (Infrequent) 1506
Cardizem SR Capsules (Less than 1%) 1510
Cardizem Injectable 1508
Cardizem Tablets (Infrequent) 1512
Cataflam (Rare) 816
Ceclor Pulvules & Suspension (Rare) 1431
Cefizox for Intramuscular or Intravenous Use (Rare) 1034
Cefotan 2829
Ceftin 1078
Cefzil Tablets and Oral Suspension 746
Ceptaz (Exceedingly rare cases) 1081
Cipro I.V. (Rare) 595
Cipro I.V. Pharmacy Bulk Package (Rare) 597
Cipro Tablets 592
Claforan Sterile and Injection (Rare) 1235
Clinoril Tablets (Less than 1 in 100) 1618
ColBENEMID Tablets 1622
Compazine 2470
Cuprimine Capsules 1630
Declomycin Tablets 1371
Deconamine 1320
Depen Titratable Tablets 2662
Desyrel and Desyrel Dividose 503
DiaBeta Tablets (Occasional) 1239
Diabinese Tablets 1935
Diamox 1372
Dimetane-DC Cough Syrup 2059
Dimetane-DX Cough Syrup 2059
Diucardin Tablets 2718
Diupres Tablets 1650
Diuril Oral Suspension 1653
Diuril Sodium Intravenous 1652
Diuril Tablets 1653
Dolobid Tablets (Less than 1 in 100) 1654
Doryx Capsules 1913
Duricef 748
Dyazide 2479
Dynacin Capsules 1590
EC-Naprosyn Delayed-Release Tablets (Less than 1%) 2117
Empirin with Codeine Tablets 1093
Enduron Tablets 420
Etrafon 2355
Eulexin Capsules 2358
Fansidar Tablets 2114
Feldene Capsules (Less than 1%) 1965
Fiorinal with Codeine Capsules 2262
Floxin I.V. 1571
Floxin Tablets (200 mg, 300 mg, 400 mg) 1567
Fludara for Injection (Rare) 663
Fortaz (Rare) 1100
Furoxone 2046
Gantanol Tablets 2119
Gantrisin 2120
Glauctabs ◉ 208
Glucotrol Tablets 1967
Glucotrol XL Extended Release Tablets 1968
Glynase PresTab Tablets 2609
HydroDIURIL Tablets 1674
Hydropres Tablets 1675
Hyzaar Tablets 1677
IBU Tablets (Less than 1%) 1342
Indocin Capsules (Less than 1%) 1680
Indocin I.V. (Less than 1%) 1684
Indocin (Less than 1%) 1680
Intron A (Less than 5%) 2364
Lamictal Tablets 1112
Larodopa Tablets (Rare) 2129
Lasix Injection, Oral Solution and Tablets 1240
Lescol Capsules (Rare) 2267
Lodine Capsules and Tablets (Less than 1%) 2743
Lorabid Suspension and Pulvules 1459
Lotensin Tablets (Rare) 834
Lotensin HCT (Rare) 837
Lotrel Capsules (Rare) 840
MZM (Common) ◉ 267
Macrobid Capsules 1988
Macrodantin Capsules 1989
Matulane Capsules 2131
Maxaquin Tablets 2440
Maxzide 1380
Mefoxin 1691
Mefoxin Premixed Intravenous Solution 1694
Mesantoin Tablets (Uncommon) 2272
Mevacor Tablets (Rare) 1699
Micronase Tablets 2623
Minocin Intravenous 1382
Minocin Oral Suspension 1385
Minocin Pellet-Filled Capsules 1383
Moduretic Tablets 1705
Monodox Capsules 1805
Monopril Tablets 757
Children's Motrin Ibuprofen Oral Suspension (Less than 1%) 1546
Motrin Tablets (Less than 1%) 2625
Motrin Ibuprofen Suspension, Oral Drops, Chewable Tablets, Caplets (Less than 1%) 1546
Mustargen (Rare) 1709
Mutamycin 703
Nalfon 200 Pulvules & Nalfon Tablets (Less than 1%) 917
Anaprox/Naprosyn (Less than 1%) 2117
Navane Capsules and Concentrate 2201
Navane Intramuscular 2202
NegGram (Rare) 2323
NephrAmine 2005
Neptazane Tablets 1388
Nizoral Tablets (Less than 1%) 1298
Noroxin Tablets 1715
Noroxin Tablets 2048
Nydrazid Injection 508
▲ Oncaspar (Greater than 1% but less than 5%) 2028
Orap Tablets 1050
Ornade Spansule Capsules 2502
Orthoclone OKT3 Sterile Solution 1837
PBZ Tablets 845
PBZ-SR Tablets 844
PASER Granules 1285
Pen•Vee K (Infrequent) 2772
Periactin 1724
Pfizerpen for Injection (Rare) 2203
Platinol 708
Platinol-AQ Injection 710
Ponstel 1925
Pravachol (Rare) 765
Prilosec Delayed-Release Capsules (Rare) 529
Primaxin I.M. 1727
Primaxin I.V. 1729
Prinivil Tablets 1733
Prinzide Tablets 1737
Procan SR Tablets (Rare) 1926
Procardia Capsules 1971
Procardia XL Extended Release Tablets 1972
Prozac Pulvules & Liquid, Oral Solution 919
Pyridium 1928
Quinaglute Dura-Tabs Tablets 649
Quinidex Extentabs 2067
ReoPro Vials (0.3%) 1471
Rifadin 1528
Rifamate Capsules 1530
Rifater 1532
Rimactane Capsules (Rare) 847
Rocephin Injectable Vials, ADD-Vantage, Galaxy Container (Less than 1%) 2142
Roferon-A Injection (Rare; less than 3%) 2145
SSD 1355
Septra 1174
Septra I.V. Infusion 1169
Septra I.V. Infusion ADD-Vantage Vials 1171
Septra 1174
Silvadene Cream 1% 1540
Sinemet Tablets (Rare) 943
Sinemet CR Tablets 944
Skelaxin Tablets 788
Stelazine 2514
Sulfamylon Cream 925
Suprax 1399
Talacen (Rare) 2333
Tavist Syrup 2297
Tavist Tablets 2298
Tazicef for Injection 2519
Temaril Tablets, Syrup and Spansule Extended-Release Capsules 483
Terramycin Intramuscular Solution 2210
Thorazine 2523
Ticlid Tablets (Rare) 2156
Timolide Tablets 1748
Tolectin (200, 400 and 600 mg) (Less than 1%) 1581
Tonocard Tablets (Less than 1%) 531
Trilafon 2389
Trinalin Repetabs Tablets 1330
Tussend 1783
Univasc Tablets (Less than 1%) 2410
Vantin for Oral Suspension and Vantin Tablets 2646
Vaseretic Tablets 1765
Vasotec I.V. 1768
Vasotec Tablets 1771
Vibramycin 1941
Vibramycin Hyclate Intravenous 2215
Vibramycin 1941
Virazole 1264
Voltaren Tablets (Rare) 861
Zefazone 2654
Zestoretic 2850
Zestril Tablets (Rare) 2854
Zinacef 1211
Zocor Tablets (Rare) 1775
Zyloprim Tablets (Less than 1%) 1226

Hemolytic icterus (see under Jaundice)

Hemolytic sideroblastic anemia (see under Anemia, hemolytic, sideroblastic)

Hemolytic-uremic syndrome
Azulfidine (Rare) 1949
Brevicon 2088
Cytovene-IV (One report) 2103
Demulen 2428
Desogen Tablets 1817
Felbatol 2666
Levlen/Tri-Levlen 651
Lo/Ovral Tablets 2746
Lo/Ovral-28 Tablets 2751
Micronor Tablets 1872
Modicon 1872
Mutamycin 703
Nordette-21 Tablets 2755
Nordette-28 Tablets 2758
Norinyl 2088
Nor-Q D Tablets 2135
Ortho-Cept 1851
Ortho-Cyclen/Ortho-Tri-Cyclen 1858
Ortho-Novum 1872
Ortho-Cyclen/Ortho Tri-Cyclen 1858
Ovcon 760
Ovral Tablets 2770
Ovral-28 Tablets 2770
Ovrette Tablets 2771
Paraplatin for Injection (Rare) 705
Toradol 2159
Levlen/Tri-Levlen 651
Tri-Norinyl 2164

Hemopericardium
Cardene I.V. (0.7%) 2709
Cytoxan 694
NEOSAR Lyophilized/Neosar 1959

Hemoperitoneum
Humegon 1824
Metrodin (urofollitropin for injection) 2446
Pergonal (menotropins for injection, USP) 2448
Profasi (chorionic gonadotropin for injection, USP) 2450
Serophene (clomiphene citrate tablets, USP) 2451

Hemoptysis
Anafranil Capsules (Rare) 803
Betaseron for SC Injection 658
Cipro I.V. (1% or less) 595
Cipro I.V. Pharmacy Bulk Package (Less than 1%) 597
Cipro Tablets (Less than 1%) 592
Claritin (2% or fewer patients) 2349
Claritin-D 2350
Cognex Capsules (Rare) 1901
Duragesic Transdermal System (1% or greater) 1288
Effexor (Rare) 2719
Eminase (2.2%) 2039
▲ Fludara for Injection (1% to 6%) 663
Foscavir Injection (Between 1% and 5%) 547
Hivid Tablets (Less than 1% to less than 3%) 2121
Intal Capsules (Less than 1 in 100,000 patients) 987
Intal Inhaler (Rare) 988
Intal Nebulizer Solution (Rare) 989
Lupron Depot 3.75 mg 2556
Lupron Depot 7.5 mg (Less than 5%) 2559
Lupron Injection 2555
Luvox Tablets (Rare) 2544
Matulane Capsules 2131
NebuPent for Inhalation Solution (1% or less) 1040
Orudis Capsules (Less than 1%) 2766
Oruvail Capsules (Less than 1%) 2766
Permax Tablets (Infrequent) 575
PREVACID Delayed-Release Capsules (Less than 1%) 2562

(Described in PDR For Nonprescription Drugs) Incidence data in parenthesis; ▲ 3% or more (◉ Described in PDR For Ophthalmology)

Hemoptysis

Prinivil Tablets (0.3% to 1.0%) 1733
Prinzide Tablets 1737
Proleukin for Injection (1%) 797
Prozac Pulvules & Liquid, Oral Solution (Rare) 919
Pulmozyme Inhalation 1064
ReoPro Vials (9 to 11 events) 1471
Rifater 1532
Videx Tablets, Powder for Oral Solution, & Pediatric Powder for Oral Solution (Less than 1%) 720
Zestoretic 2850
Zestril Tablets (0.3% to 1.0%) 2854

Hemorrhage (see under Bleeding)

Hemorrhage, adrenal

Heparin Lock Flush Solution 2725
Heparin Sodium Injection 2726
Heparin Sodium Injection, USP, Sterile Solution 2615

Hemorrhage, cerebral (see under Cerebral hemorrhage)

Hemorrhage, eye, anterior chamber

Zoloft Tablets (Rare) 2217

Hemorrhage, eyes

AdatoSil 5000 (Greater than 2%) .... ◉ 274
Dilacor XR Extended-release Capsules 2018
Eminase (Less than 1%) 2039
Hivid Tablets (Less than 1% to less than 3%) 2121
Kerlone Tablets (Less than 2%) 2436
Neurontin Capsules (Infrequent) 1922
Ocufen .... ◉ 245
Paxil Tablets (Rare) 2505
Permax Tablets (Infrequent) 575
Proglycem 580
Prozac Pulvules & Liquid, Oral Solution (Rare) 919
ReoPro Vials (9 to 11 events) 1471
Ticlid Tablets 2156

Hemorrhage, gastrointestinal (see under Bleeding, gastrointestinal)

Hemorrhage, intra-alveolar

Depen Titratable Tablets 2662

Hemorrhage, intramuscular

Abbokinase 403
Abbokinase Open-Cath 405

Hemorrhage, intraventricular

▲ Exosurf Neonatal for Intratracheal Suspension (4% to 57%) 1095

Hemorrhage, muscle

Prozac Pulvules & Liquid, Oral Solution (Rare) 919

Hemorrhage, neonatal

Fiorinal 2261
Mebaral Tablets 2322
Mysoline 2754
Quadrinal Tablets 1350
Rifadin 1528
Rifater 1532
Soma Compound Tablets 2675

Hemorrhage, ovarian

Clomid 1514
Heparin Lock Flush Solution 2725
Heparin Sodium Injection 2726
Heparin Sodium Injection, USP, Sterile Solution 2615
Heparin Sodium Vials 1441

Hemorrhage, postpartum

Fiorinal 2261
Oxytocin Injection 2771
Rifadin 1528
Rifater 1532
Syntocinon Injection 2296

Hemorrhage, pulmonary

▲ Exosurf Neonatal for Intratracheal Suspension (1% to 10%) 1095
Felbatol 2666
Foscavir Injection (Less than 1%) .. 547
ReoPro Vials (9 to 11 events) 1471
▲ Survanta Beractant Intratracheal Suspension (7.2%) 2226

Hemorrhage, purpuric

Atretol Tablets 573
Tegretol Chewable Tablets 852
Tegretol Suspension 852
Tegretol Tablets 852

Hemorrhage, retinal

Ansaid Tablets (Rare) 2579
Clomid 1514
Glucotrol XL Extended Release Tablets (Less than 1%) 1968
Intron A (Rare) 2364
Matulane Capsules 2131
Orudis Capsules (Less than 1%) 2766
Oruvail Capsules (Less than 1%) 2766
Oxytocin Injection 2771

Hemorrhage, retroperitoneal

Abbokinase 403
Abbokinase Open-Cath 405
Activase (Less than 1%) 1058
Eminase 2039
Heparin Lock Flush Solution 2725
Heparin Sodium Injection 2726
Heparin Sodium Injection, USP, Sterile Solution 2615
Heparin Sodium Vials 1441

Hemorrhage, subarachnoid

Ansaid Tablets (Less than 1%) 2579
Betaseron for SC Injection 658
Brevicon 2088
Demulen 2428
Hivid Tablets (Less than 1% to less than 3%) 2121
Imitrex Injection (Rare) 1103
Imitrex Tablets 1106
Lioresal Intrathecal 1596
Norinyl 2088
Nor-Q D Tablets 2135
Orthoclone OKT3 Sterile Solution .. 1837
Tri-Norinyl 2164

Hemorrhage, subconjunctival

Effexor (Infrequent) 2719

Hemorrhage, subcutaneous

Mustargen 1709
Ticlid Tablets 2156

Hemorrhagic colitis

Cytoxan (Isolated reports) 694
Lamictal Tablets (Rare) 1112
NEOSAR Lyophilized/Neosar (Isolated reports) 1959
Primaxin I.M. 1727
Primaxin I.V. (Less than 0.2%) 1729

Hemorrhagic complications

Coumadin 926
Fragmin (Low incidence) 1954
Heparin Sodium Vials 1441
Lovenox Injection 2020
▲ Paraplatin for Injection (5%) 705

Hemorrhagic diathesis

▲ Mithracin (5.4 to 11.9%) 607
Solganal Suspension (Rare) 2388

Hemorrhagic disturbances

Cytovene-IV (One report) 2103

Hemorrhagic eruptions (see under Eruptions, hemorrhagic)

Hemorrhagic syndrome (see under Bleeding syndrome)

Hemorrhagic tendency

Mithracin 607
Mustargen 1709

Hemorrhoids

Ambien Tablets (Rare) 2416
Anafranil Capsules (Infrequent) 803
▲ CHEMET (succimer) Capsules (12 to 20.9%) 1545
Claritin-D (Less frequent) 2350
Cognex Capsules (Infrequent) 1901
Effexor (Infrequent) 2719
Hivid Tablets (Less than 1% to less than 3%) 2121
Imdur (Less than or equal to 5%) .. 1323
Luvox Tablets (Infrequent) 2544
Neurontin Capsules (Infrequent) 1922
ReVia Tablets (Less than 1%) 940
Risperdal (Infrequent) 1301
Rowasa (1.35%) 2548
Sandostatin Injection (Less than 1%) 2292

Zoloft Tablets (Rare) 2217

Hemorrhoids, aggravation

Colestid Tablets 2591
Questran Light 769

Hemostasis, interference

Depakote Tablets 415

Hemothorax

Permax Tablets (Rare) 575

Henoch-Schonlein purpura

Children's Advil Suspension (Less than 1%) 2692
Bactrim DS Tablets 2084
Bactrim I.V. Infusion 2082
Bactrim 2084
Luvox Tablets 2544
Septra 1174
Septra I.V. Infusion 1169
Septra I.V. Infusion ADD-Vantage Vials 1171
Septra 1174

Henoch-Schonlein vasculitis

IBU Tablets (Less than 1%) 1342
Children's Motrin Ibuprofen Oral Suspension (Less than 1%) 1546
Motrin Ibuprofen Suspension, Oral Drops, Chewable Tablets, Caplets (Less than 1%) 1546

Hepatic adenoma

Brevicon 2088
Danocrine Capsules 2307
Desogen Tablets 1817
Estraderm Transdermal System (Rare) 824
ESTRATAB Tablets (0.3, 0.625, 1.25, 2.5 mg) (Rare) 2536
Estratest (Rare) 2539
Halotestin Tablets 2614
Lo/Ovral Tablets 2746
Lo/Ovral-28 Tablets 2751
Menest Tablets 2494
Nordette-21 Tablets 2755
Nordette-28 Tablets 2758
Norinyl 2088
Nor-Q D Tablets 2135
Ortho-Cept 1851
Ortho-Cyclen/Ortho-Tri-Cyclen 1858
Ortho-Cyclen/Ortho Tri-Cyclen 1858
Ovcon (Rare) 760
Ovral Tablets 2770
Ovral-28 Tablets 2770
Ovrette Tablets 2771
PMB 200 and PMB 400 2783
Premarin Intravenous 2787
Premarin with Methyltestosterone .. 2794
Premarin Vaginal Cream 2791
Stilphostrol Tablets and Ampuls 612
Tri-Norinyl 2164
Triphasil-21 Tablets 2814
Triphasil-28 Tablets 2819

Hepatic coma

Capozide 742
Esidrix Tablets 821
Maxzide 1380
Prinzide Tablets 1737
Tenoretic Tablets 2845
Vaseretic Tablets 1765
Zestoretic 2850

Hepatic dysfunction

Children's Advil Suspension (Less than 1%) 2692
Ambien Tablets (Rare) 2416
Anafranil Capsules (Infrequent) 803
Ancobon Capsules 2079
Atretol Tablets 573
Augmentin (Infrequent) 2468
Azo Gantrisin Tablets 2081
BiCNU 691
Cefotan 2829
Ceftin Tablets 1078
Ceptaz 1081
▲ Cipro I.V. (Among most frequent) .. 595
Claritin (Rare) 2349
Cuprimine Capsules 1630
Cylert Tablets 412
▲ Cytosar-U Sterile Powder (Among most frequent) 2592
Cytotec (Infrequent) 2424
Cytovene (2%) 2103
Danocrine Capsules 2307
Dantrium Capsules 1982
Daranide Tablets 1633
Darvon-N/Darvocet-N 1433
Darvon 1435

Darvon-N Suspension & Tablets 1433
Depakene 413
Depakote Tablets 415
Depen Titratable Tablets (Isolated cases) 2662
Diamox Intravenous (Occasional) 1372
Diamox Sequels (Sustained Release) 1373
Diamox Tablets (Occasional) 1372
Dilantin Infatabs 1908
Dilantin Kapseals 1906
Dilantin-125 Suspension 1911
Dolobid Tablets (Less than 1 in 100) 1654
Duricef 748
Dyazide 2479
E.E.S. 424
E-Mycin Tablets 1341
EC-Naprosyn Delayed-Release Tablets (Less than 1%) 2117
ERYC 1915
EryPed 421
Ery-Tab Tablets 422
Erythrocin Stearate Filmtab 425
Erythromycin Base Filmtab 426
Erythromycin Delayed-Release Capsules, USP 427
Ethmozine Tablets (Rare) 2041
Feldene Capsules (Less than 1%) .. 1965
Floxin I.V. 1571
Floxin Tablets (200 mg, 300 mg, 400 mg) 1567
Fludara for Injection (1% to 3%) 663
Fluothane 2724
Fortaz 1100
Foscavir Injection (Between 1% and 5%) 547
Glauctabs (Occasional) .... ◉ 208
Halcion Tablets (Rare) 2611
▲ IFEX (3%) 697
Intron A (Less than 5%) 2364
Keftab Tablets 915
Librax Capsules (Occasional) 2176
Libritabs Tablets (Occasional) 2177
Librium Capsules (Occasional) 2178
Librium Injectable (Occasional) 2179
Limbitrol (Rare) 2180
Lorabid Suspension and Pulvules (Rare) 1459
Lupron Depot 3.75 mg 2556
Lupron Depot 7.5 mg 2559
Lupron Injection 2555
MZM (Occasional) .... ◉ 267
Matulane Capsules 2131
Metrodin (urofollitropin for injection) 2446
Children's Motrin Ibuprofen Oral Suspension 1546
Anaprox/Naprosyn (Less than 1%) 2117
NebuPent for Inhalation Solution (1% or less) 1040
Neutrexin 2572
Nizoral Tablets (Rare) 1298
Normodyne Injection 2377
Normodyne Tablets 2379
▲ Novantrone (10 to 14%) 1279
Nydrazid Injection 508
Orudis Capsules (Less than 1%) 2766
Oruvail Capsules (Less than 1%) 2766
PCE Dispertab Tablets 444
Paxil Tablets 2505
Pergonal (menotropins for injection, USP) 2448
Persantine Tablets (Rare) 681
▲ Prograf (5% to 36%) 1042
Proleukin for Injection 797
ReVia Tablets 940
Rifater (Rare) 1532
Salflex Tablets 786
Serax Capsules 2810
Serax Tablets 2810
Serophene (clomiphene citrate tablets, USP) 2451
Sporanox Capsules (0.3% to 2.7%) 1305
Suprax 1399
Tambocor Tablets (Rare) 1497
Tapazole Tablets 1477
Tazicef for Injection 2519
Tegretol Chewable Tablets 852
Tegretol Suspension 852
Tegretol Tablets 852
Tenex Tablets (Less frequent) 2074
TheraCys BCG Live (Intravesical) (Up to 2.7%) 897
Tolectin (200, 400 and 600 mg) (Less than 1%) 1581
Toradol 2159
Trandate 1185

(◈ Described in PDR For Nonprescription Drugs) Incidence data in parenthesis; ▲ 3% or more (◉ Described in PDR For Ophthalmology)

1321 **Side Effects Index** **Hepatitis**

Vantin for Oral Suspension and Vantin Tablets 2646
Vumon (Less than 1%) 727
Wygesic Tablets 2827
Zanosar Sterile Powder 2653
Zefazone 2654
Zinacef 1211

Hepatic enzymes, elevation (see also under SGOT elevation; SGPT elevation; Serum transaminase, elevation)

▲ Accutane Capsules (1 in 5 to 5 in 10 patients; approximately 15%) 2076
Achromycin V Capsules (Rare) 1367
Altace Capsules (Rare) 1232
▲ Anaprox/Naprosyn (Up to 15%) 2117
Ansaid Tablets (Less than 1%) 2579
Atamet 572
Biltricide Tablets 591
Brethine Ampuls 815
Brethine Tablets 814
Bricanyl Subcutaneous Injection (Rare) 1502
Bricanyl Tablets (Rare) 1503
Calan SR Caplets 2422
Calan Tablets 2419
Capoten 739
Capozide (Rare) 742
Cataflam (Rare) 816
Cefobid Pharmacy Bulk Package - Not for Direct Infusion (1 patient in 1285) 2192
Cefotan (1.2%) 2829
Ceptaz 1081
▲ Cipro I.V. Pharmacy Bulk Package (Among most frequent) 597
Cordarone Intravenous (Common) 2715
Danocrine Capsules 2307
Dantrium Capsules 1982
Depakote Tablets 415
Dyazide 2479
Dynacin Capsules 1590
Dyrenium Capsules (Rare) 2481
▲ EC-Naprosyn Delayed-Release Tablets (Up to 15%) 2117
Hismanal Tablets (Less frequent) 1293
Hydrea Capsules 696
Hyzaar Tablets (Occasional) 1677
▲ IFEX (3%) 697
Inocor Lactate Injection 2309
Isoptin Oral Tablets 1346
Isoptin SR Tablets 1348
Lescol Capsules 2267
Lithonate/Lithotabs/Lithobid 2543
Lodine Capsules and Tablets (Less than 1%) 2743
Lotensin Tablets 834
Lotrel Capsules (Scattered incidents) 840
Ludiomil Tablets 843
Maxzide 1380
Methotrexate Sodium Tablets, Injection, for Injection and LPF Injection 1275
Minocin Intravenous 1382
Minocin Oral Suspension 1385
Minocin Pellet-Filled Capsules 1383
Monopril Tablets 757
▲ Anaprox/Naprosyn (Up to 15%) 2117
Navelbine Injection 1145
Neoral 2276
Nolvadex Tablets 2841
Norpace (Less than 1%) 2444
Pipracil (Less frequent) 1390
Platinol 708
Platinol-AQ Injection 710
Prinivil Tablets (Rare) 1733
Prinzide Tablets (Rare) 1737
Propulsid (Rare) 1300
Recombivax HB 1744
Ridaura Capsules (Less than 1%) 2513
Roferon-A Injection (Frequent) 2145
Rowasa 2548
Rythmol Tablets–150mg, 225mg, 300mg (Less than 1%) 1352
Sandostatin Injection (Less than 1%) 2292
Sinemet Tablets 943
Sporanox Capsules 1305
Tenoretic Tablets 2845
Tenormin Tablets and I.V. Injection 2847
Testoderm Testosterone Transdermal System (One in 104 patients) 486
Thioguanine Tablets, Tabloid Brand (Occasional) 1181
Toradol 2159
Tornalate Solution for Inhalation, 0.2% (Infrequent) 956
Trental Tablets (Rare) 1244
Ultram Tablets (50 mg) (Infrequent) 1585
Univasc Tablets 2410
Vascor (200, 300 and 400 mg) Tablets (Approximately 1%) 1587
Vaseretic Tablets (Rare) 1765
Vasotec I.V. 1768
Vasotec Tablets 1771
Verelan Capsules 1410
Verelan Capsules 2824
Vermox Chewable Tablets (Rare) 1312
Voltaren Tablets (Rare) 861
Xanax Tablets 2649
▲ Zanosar Sterile Powder (A number of patients) 2653
Zestoretic (Rare) 2850
Zestril Tablets (Rare) 2854
Zoloft Tablets (One or more patients) 2217

Hepatic failure

Capoten (Rare) 739
Clinoril Tablets (Less than 1 in 100) 1618
Depakene 413
Depakote Tablets 415
Diflucan Injection, Tablets, and Oral Suspension (Rare) 2194
Elavil 2838
Endep Tablets 2174
Felbatol (A marked increase) 2666
Floxin I.V. 1571
Floxin Tablets (200 mg, 300 mg, 400 mg) 1567
Fludara for Injection (Up to 1%) 663
Fungizone Intravenous 506
Hivid Tablets (Rare) 2121
Intron A (Very rare) 2364
Lotensin Tablets (Rare) 834
Minocin Intravenous (Rare) 1382
Minocin Oral Suspension (Rare) 1385
Minocin Pellet-Filled Capsules (Rare) 1383
Monopril Tablets 757
Motrin Ibuprofen Suspension, Oral Drops, Chewable Tablets, Caplets (Less than 1%) 1546
Oncaspar 2028
Prilosec Delayed-Release Capsules (Rare) 529
Prinivil Tablets (Rare) 1733
Prinzide Tablets (Rare) 1737
Proleukin for Injection (Less than 1%) 797
Prozac Pulvules & Liquid, Oral Solution 919
Risperdal (Rare) 1301
Tambocor Tablets (Rare) 1497
Toradol 2159
Univasc Tablets (Rare) 2410
Vaseretic Tablets (Rare) 1765
Vasotec I.V. (Rare) 1768
Vasotec Tablets (Rare; 0.5% to 1.0%) 1771
Videx Tablets, Powder for Oral Solution, & Pediatric Powder for Oral Solution (Less than 1%) 720
Zestoretic (Rare) 2850
Zestril Tablets (Rare) 2854
Zofran Injection 1214
Zofran Tablets 1217
Zoloft Tablets (One or more patients) 2217

Hepatic function tests, impaired (see under Liver function, impaired)

Hepatic veno-occlusive disease, life threatening

Alkeran for Injection 1070
Imuran (Rare) 1110
Myleran Tablets 1143
Thioguanine Tablets, Tabloid Brand 1181

Hepatitis

Accutane Capsules (Several cases) 2076
Children's Advil Suspension (Less than 1%) 2692
Aldoclor Tablets 1598
Aldomet Ester HCl Injection 1602
Aldomet Oral 1600
Aldoril Tablets 1604
Altace Capsules 1232
Anafranil Capsules (Infrequent) 803
Anaprox/Naprosyn (Rare) 2117
Ansaid Tablets (Less than 1%) 2579
Antabuse Tablets (Multiple cases) 2695
Apresazide Capsules (Rare) 808
Apresoline Hydrochloride Tablets (Rare) 809
Asacol Delayed-Release Tablets (Rare) 1979
Asendin Tablets (Very rate) 1369
Atretol Tablets 573
Augmentin (Rare) 2468
Axid Pulvules 1427
Azactam for Injection (Less than 1%) 734
Azo Gantanol Tablets 2080
Azo Gantrisin Tablets 2081
Azulfidine (Rare) 1949
BCG Vaccine, USP (TICE) (0.2%) 1814
Bactrim DS Tablets 2084
Bactrim I.V. Infusion 2082
Bactrim 2084
Betaseron for SC Injection 658
Capoten 739
Capozide 742
Cartrol Tablets (Rare) 410
Cataflam (Less than 1%) 816
Catapres Tablets (Rare) 674
Catapres-TTS (Rare) 675
Ceclor Pulvules & Suspension (Rare) 1431
▲ CellCept Capsules (More than or equal to 3%) 2099
Chibroxin Sterile Ophthalmic Solution (With oral form) 1617
Claritin (Rare) 2349
Claritin-D 2350
Clinoril Tablets (Less than 1%) 1618
Clomid 1514
Clozaril Tablets 2252
Combipres Tablets (Rare) 677
Cosmegen Injection 1626
Cylert Tablets 412
Cytovene (1% or less) 2103
Dantrium Capsules (Less frequent) 1982
Daypro Caplets (Less than 1%) 2426
DiaBeta Tablets (Rare) 1239
Diflucan Injection, Tablets, and Oral Suspension (Rare) 2194
Dipentum Capsules (Rare) 1951
Dolobid Tablets (Less than 1 in 100) 1654
Dynacin Capsules (Rare) 1590
EC-Naprosyn Delayed-Release Tablets (Rare) 2117
Effexor (Rare) 2719
Elavil (Rare) 2838
Endep Tablets (Rare) 2174
Ethmozine Tablets (Rare) 2041
Etrafon (Rare) 2355
Eulexin Capsules (Less than 1%) 2358
Fansidar Tablets 2114
Felbatol 2666
Feldene Capsules (Less than 1%) 1965
Fiorinal with Codeine Capsules 2262
Flexeril Tablets (Rare) 1661
Floxin I.V. 1571
Floxin Tablets (200 mg, 300 mg, 400 mg) 1567
Foscavir Injection (Less than 1%) 547
Fungizone Intravenous 506
Gantanol Tablets 2119
Gantrisin 2120
Halotestin Tablets 2614
Havrix (Rare) 2489
Hivid Tablets (Less than 1% to less than 3%) 2121
IBU Tablets (Less than 1%) 1342
Keflex Pulvules & Oral Suspension (Rare) 914
Keftab Tablets (Rare) 915
Kefzol Vials, Faspak & ADD-Vantage (Rare) 1456
Konÿne 80 Factor IX Complex 634
Lamictal Tablets (Rare) 1112
Lamprene Capsules (Less than 1%) 828
Lescol Capsules 2267
Lodine Capsules and Tablets (Less than 1%) 2743
Loxitane (Rare) 1378
Macrobid Capsules (Rare) 1988
Macrodantin Capsules (Rare) 1989
Mandol Vials, Faspak & ADD-Vantage (Rare) 1461
Maxaquin Tablets 2440
Mesantoin Tablets 2272
Mevacor Tablets 1699
Mexitil Capsules (Rare) 678
Miacalcin Nasal Spray (Less than 1%) 2275
Micronase Tablets (Rare) 2623
Minocin Intravenous (Rare) 1382
Minocin Oral Suspension (Rare) 1385
Minocin Pellet-Filled Capsules (Rare) 1383
Monopril Tablets (0.2% to 1.0%) 757
Children's Motrin Ibuprofen Oral Suspension (Less than 1%) 1546
Motrin Tablets (Less than 1%) 2625
Motrin Ibuprofen Suspension, Oral Drops, Chewable Tablets, Caplets (Rare; less than 1%) 1546
Mycobutin Capsules (Less than 1%) 1957
Myochrysine Injection 1711
Anaprox/Naprosyn (Rare) 2117
NebuPent for Inhalation Solution (1% or less) 1040
Nimotop Capsules (Less than 1%) 610
Nolvadex Tablets (Rare) 2841
Normodyne Injection (Less common) 2377
Normodyne Tablets (Less common) 2379
Noroxin Tablets 1715
Noroxin Tablets 2048
Norpramin Tablets 1526
Orlamm (Low frequency) 2239
Orthoclone OKT3 Sterile Solution 1837
Papaverine Hydrochloride Vials and Ampoules (Infrequent) 1468
Parnate Tablets (Rare) 2503
PASER Granules 1285
Paxil Tablets (Rare) 2505
Pentasa (Infrequent) 1527
Permax Tablets (Infrequent) 575
Phenurone Tablets (2%) 447
Pravachol 765
Prilosec Delayed-Release Capsules (Rare) 529
Primaxin I.M. 1727
Primaxin I.V. (Less than 0.2%) 1729
Prinivil Tablets (0.3% to 1.0%) 1733
Prinzide Tablets 1737
Priscoline Hydrochloride Ampuls 845
▲ Prograf (Greater than 3%) 1042
Propulsid (Rare) 1300
Prozac Pulvules & Liquid, Oral Solution (Rare) 919
Retrovir Capsules (Rare) 1158
Retrovir I.V. Infusion (Rare) 1163
Retrovir Syrup 1158
Rifadin (Rare) 1528
Rifamate Capsules (Rare) 1530
Rifater (Rare; occasional) 1532
Rimactane Capsules (Rare) 847
Roferon-A Injection (Less than 1%) 2145
Rythmol Tablets–150mg, 225mg, 300mg (0.03%) 1352
SSD 1355
Salflex Tablets 786
Sandostatin Injection (Less than 1%) 2292
Seldane Tablets (Isolated reports) 1536
Seldane-D Extended-Release Tablets (Isolated reports) 1538
Septra 1174
Septra I.V. Infusion 1169
Septra I.V. Infusion ADD-Vantage Vials 1171
Septra 1174
Ser-Ap-Es Tablets 849
Serzone Tablets (Rare) 771
Silvadene Cream 1% 1540
Solganal Suspension 2388
Sporanox Capsules (Rare) 1305
Stelazine 2514
Tapazole Tablets 1477
▲ Tegison Capsules (1-10%) 2154
Tegretol Chewable Tablets 852
Tegretol Suspension 852
Tegretol Tablets 852
Ticlid Tablets (Rare) 2156
Timentin for Injection (Rare) 2528
Tolectin (200, 400 and 600 mg) (Less than 1%) 1581
Tonocard Tablets (Less than 1%) 531
Toradol 2159
Trandate (Less common) 1185
Trecator-SC Tablets 2814
Trental Tablets (Rare) 1244
Triavil Tablets (Rare) 1757
Trilisate (Rare) 2000
Ultram Tablets (50 mg) (Infrequent) 1585
Univasc Tablets (Less than 1%) 2410
Urobiotic-250 Capsules 2214
Vaseretic Tablets 1765
Vasotec I.V. 1768
Vasotec Tablets (0.5% to 1.0%) 1771
Vermox Chewable Tablets (Rare) 1312
Voltaren Tablets (Less than 1%) 861
Wellbutrin Tablets 1204
Yutopar Intravenous Injection (Less than 1%) 570

(Described in PDR For Nonprescription Drugs) Incidence data in parenthesis; ▲ 3% or more (Described in PDR For Ophthalmology)

Zantac (Occasional) 1209
Zantac Injection 1207
Zantac Syrup (Occasional) 1209
Zaroxolyn Tablets 1000
Zestoretic 2850
Zestril Tablets (0.3% to 1.0%) 2854
Zocor Tablets 1775
Zoloft Tablets (One or more patients) 2217

Hepatitis, allergic

Adalat Capsules (10 mg and 20 mg) (Less than 0.5%) 587
Adalat CC (Rare) 589
Procardia Capsules (Rare; less than 0.5%) 1971
Procardia XL Extended Release Tablets (Rare instances) 1972

Hepatitis, cholestatic

Android Capsules, 10 mg 1250
Antabuse Tablets (Multiple cases) 2695
Ceptaz 1081
Cordarone Tablets (Rare) 2712
Delatestryl Injection 2860
Dipentum Capsules (One case) 1951
Estratest 2539
Foscavir Injection (Less than 1%) 547
Glynase PresTab Tablets (Rare) 2609
Lodine Capsules and Tablets (Less than 1%) 2743
Nalfon 200 Pulvules & Nalfon Tablets (Less than 1%) 917
Oxandrin 2862
Pipracil (Less frequent) 1390
Premarin with Methyltestosterone 2794
Prilosec Delayed-Release Capsules (Rare) 529
Risperdal (Rare) 1301
Seldane Tablets (Isolated reports) 1536
Seldane-D Extended-Release Tablets (Isolated reports) 1538
Tao Capsules 2209
Testoderm Testosterone Transdermal System 486
Zosyn 1419
Zosyn Pharmacy Bulk Package 1422

Hepatitis, fulminant

Antabuse Tablets (Multiple cases) 2695
Sporanox Capsules (One patient) 1305
Tapazole Tablets (Rare) 1477

Hepatitis, granulomatous

Dipentum Capsules (Rare) 1951
Quinaglute Dura-Tabs Tablets 649
Quinidex Extentabs 2067
Zyloprim Tablets (Less than 1%) 1226

Hepatitis, idiosyncratic, reversible

Sporanox Capsules (Three cases) 1305

Hepatitis, overt

Prilosec Delayed-Release Capsules (Rare) 529

Hepatitis, reactive

Dipentum Capsules (Rare) 1951
Macrobid Capsules (Rare) 1988

Hepatitis, toxic

Alkeran for Injection 1070
Cuprimine Capsules (Rare) 1630
Dapsone Tablets USP 1284
Depen Titratable Tablets (Rare) 2662
Dilantin Infatabs 1908
Dilantin Kapseals 1906
Dilantin Parenteral 1910
Dilantin-125 Suspension 1911
Indocin Capsules (Less than 1%) 1680
Indocin I.V. (Less than 1%) 1684
Indocin (Less than 1%) 1680
Rifamate Capsules 1530
Solganal Suspension 2388

Hepatitis, viral

Atgam Sterile Solution (Less than 5%) 2581
Koāte-HP Antihemophilic Factor (Human) 630
Prolastin Alpha$_1$-Proteinase Inhibitor (Human) 635

Hepatobiliary dysfunction

Azactam for Injection (Less than 1%) 734

Hepatomas

Brevicon 2088
Demulen (Rare) 2428
Lescol Capsules 2267
Lopid Tablets 1917
Mevacor Tablets (Rare) 1699
Norinyl 2088
Nor-Q D Tablets (Extremely rare) 2135
Ovcon 760
PMB 200 and PMB 400 2783
Pravachol (Rare) 765
Premarin Intravenous 2787
Premarin with Methyltestosterone 2794
Premarin Vaginal Cream 2791
Tri-Norinyl 2164
Zocor Tablets (Rare) 1775

Hepatomas, benign

Desogen Tablets 1817
Levlen/Tri-Levlen (Rare) 651
Lo/Ovral Tablets 2746
Lo/Ovral-28 Tablets 2751
Micronor Tablets 1872
Modicon 1872
Nordette-21 Tablets 2755
Nordette-28 Tablets 2758
Ortho-Cept 1851
Ortho-Cyclen/Ortho-Tri-Cyclen (Rare) 1858
Ortho-Novum 1872
Ortho-Cyclen/Ortho Tri-Cyclen (Rare) 1858
Ovral Tablets 2770
Ovral-28 Tablets 2770
Ovrette Tablets 2771
Levlen/Tri-Levlen (Rare) 651
Triphasil-21 Tablets 2814
Triphasil-28 Tablets 2819

Hepatomas, malignant

Danocrine Capsules (Rare) 2307
Demulen 2428

Hepatomegaly

Atromid-S Capsules 2701
Betaseron for SC Injection 658
Blocadren Tablets 1614
Cosmegen Injection 1626
Garamycin Injectable 2360
Hivid Tablets (Rare; less than 1% to less than 3%) 2121
Klonopin Tablets 2126
Megace Oral Suspension (1% to 3%) 699
Monopril Tablets (0.4% to 1.0%) 757
NebuPent for Inhalation Solution (1% or less) 1040
Neupogen for Injection (Infrequent) 495
Neurontin Capsules (Infrequent) 1922
Oncaspar (Less than 1%) 2028
Orthoclone OKT3 Sterile Solution 1837
PASER Granules 1285
Permax Tablets (Infrequent) 575
Procan SR Tablets 1926
Proleukin for Injection (1%) 797
Prozac Pulvules & Liquid, Oral Solution (Rare) 919
Retrovir Capsules (Rare) 1158
Retrovir I.V. Infusion (Rare) 1163
Retrovir Syrup 1158
Thioguanine Tablets, Tabloid Brand 1181
Timolide Tablets 1748
Timoptic in Ocudose 1753
Timoptic Sterile Ophthalmic Solution 1751
Timoptic-XE 1755
Tornalate Solution for Inhalation, 0.2% (One patient) 956
Videx Tablets, Powder for Oral Solution, & Pediatric Powder for Oral Solution (Less than 1%) 720
Zoloft Tablets (One or more patients) 2217
Zyloprim Tablets (Less than 1%) 1226

Hepatorenal syndrome, unspecified

Felbatol 2666
Motrin Ibuprofen Suspension, Oral Drops, Chewable Tablets, Caplets (Less than 1%) 1546

Hepatosplenomegaly

Aquasol A Vitamin A Capsules, USP 534
Atgam Sterile Solution (Less than 5%) 2581
Foscavir Injection (Less than 1%) 547

Hepatotoxicity

▲ Accutane Capsules (1 in 5 to 1 in 10 patients) 2076
Adriamycin PFS 1947
Adriamycin RDF 1947
Alkeran Tablets (Rare) 1071
Android Capsules, 10 mg 1250
Android 1251
BiCNU 691
CeeNU 693
Cognex Capsules 1901
Cosmegen Injection 1626
Cytadren Tablets (Less than 1 in 1000) 819
Dantrium Capsules 1982
Demulen 2428
Depakene 413
Depakote Tablets 415
Diflucan Injection, Tablets, and Oral Suspension (Rare) 2194
Easprin 1914
Empirin with Codeine Tablets 1093
Estratest 2539
Fulvicin P/G Tablets (Rare) 2359
Fulvicin P/G 165 & 330 Tablets (Rare) 2359
Furoxone 2046
Hivid Tablets 2121
Imuran (Less than 1%) 1110
Inocor Lactate Injection (0.2%) 2309
Intron A (Rare) 2364
Leukeran Tablets 1133
Levoprome 1274
Loxitane 1378
Methotrexate Sodium Tablets, Injection, for Injection and LPF Injection 1275
Minocin Intravenous 1382
Minocin Oral Suspension 1385
▲ Neoral (4% to 7%) 2276
Neutrexin 2572
Nicolar Tablets 2026
Nizoral Tablets 1298
Oreton Methyl 1255
Platinol 708
Platinol-AQ Injection 710
Purinethol Tablets (Frequent) 1156
Pyrazinamide Tablets 1398
Quinaglute Dura-Tabs Tablets 649
Quinidex Extentabs 2067
Reglan (Rare) 2068
ReVia Tablets 940
Rifater 1532
Roferon-A Injection (Rare) 2145
▲ Sandimmune (Less than 1 to 7%) 2286
Tigan 2057
Torecan 2245
Vibramycin (Rare) 1941
Vibramycin Hyclate Intravenous (Rare) 2215
Vibramycin (Rare) 1941
▲ Zanosar Sterile Powder (A number of patients) 2653
Zyloprim Tablets (A few cases) 1226

Hernia, hiatal

Cognex Capsules (Infrequent) 1901
Neurontin Capsules (Rare) 1922

Hernia, unspecified

Betaseron for SC Injection 658
▲ CellCept Capsules (More than or equal to 3%) 2099
Effexor (Infrequent) 2719
Permax Tablets (Infrequent) 575
▲ Prograf (Greater than 3%) 1042
Serzone Tablets (Infrequent) 771
Videx Tablets, Powder for Oral Solution, & Pediatric Powder for Oral Solution (Less than 1%) 720
Zoloft Tablets (Rare) 2217

Herpes, precipitation

Matulane Capsules 2131
Oxsoralen-Ultra Capsules 1257
▲ Roferon-A Injection (8%) 2145

Herpes simplex

Ambien Tablets (Rare) 2416
Ansaid Tablets (Less than 1%) 2579
Atgam Sterile Solution (Less than 1% to less than 5%) 2581
Blephamide Ointment ◉ 237
▲ CellCept Capsules (16.7% to 20.0%; 12.5% to 15.2%) 2099
Cognex Capsules (Infrequent) 1901
Cortisporin Ophthalmic Ointment Sterile 1085
Cytovene (1% or less) 2103
Effexor (Infrequent) 2719
Efudex (Infrequent) 2113
FML Forte Liquifilm ◉ 240
FML Liquifilm ◉ 241
FML S.O.P. ◉ 241
Foscavir Injection (Less than 1%) 547
Intron A (Up to 5%) 2364
8-MOP Capsules 1246
Neurontin Capsules (Infrequent) 1922
Oncaspar 2028
Permax Tablets (Infrequent) 575
Proglycem 580
▲ Prograf (Greater than 3%) 1042
Prozac Pulvules & Liquid, Oral Solution (Infrequent) 919
Rhinocort Nasal Inhaler (Less than 1%) 556
Tegison Capsules (Less than 1%) 2154
Vexol 1% Ophthalmic Suspension ◉ 230
Videx Tablets, Powder for Oral Solution, & Pediatric Powder for Oral Solution (Up to 2%) 720

Herpes simplex, disseminated

Accutane Capsules (Less than 1%) 2076

Herpes zoster

Ambien Tablets (Rare) 2416
Ansaid Tablets (Less than 1%) 2579
▲ CellCept Capsules (6.0% to 7.6%; 6.7% to 6.9%) 2099
Cognex Capsules (Infrequent) 1901
Effexor (Infrequent) 2719
Engerix-B Unit-Dose Vials 2482
Lamictal Tablets (Rare) 1112
Leustatin (8 episodes) 1834
Mustargen 1709
Neurontin Capsules (Rare) 1922
Permax Tablets (Infrequent) 575
Prinivil Tablets (0.3% to 1.0%) 1733
Prinzide Tablets 1737
Prozac Pulvules & Liquid, Oral Solution (Rare) 919
Recombivax HB 1744
Vaseretic Tablets 1765
Vasotec I.V. 1768
Vasotec Tablets (0.5% to 1.0%) 1771
Videx Tablets, Powder for Oral Solution, & Pediatric Powder for Oral Solution (Up to 2%) 720
Zestoretic 2850
Zestril Tablets (0.3% to 1.0%) 2854

Herpes, unspecified

Megace Oral Suspension (1% to 3%) 699

Herxheimer's reaction

Bicillin L-A Injection 2707
Chloromycetin Sodium Succinate 1900
Pfizerpen for Injection 2203

Hiccups

Ambien Tablets (Infrequent) 2416
Anafranil Capsules (Rare) 803
Atamet 572
Atgam Sterile Solution (Less than 1%) 2581
Betaseron for SC Injection 658
Brevital Sodium Vials 1429
BuSpar (Rare) 737
Celontin Kapseals 1899
Cipro I.V. (1% or less) 595
Cipro I.V. Pharmacy Bulk Package (Less than 1%) 597
Cipro Tablets (Less than 1%) 592
Dalalone D.P. Injectable 1011
Dalgan Injection (Less than 1%) 538
Decadron Elixir 1633
Decadron Phosphate Injection 1637
Decadron Phosphate Respihaler 1642
Decadron Phosphate Turbinaire 1645
Decadron Phosphate with Xylocaine Injection, Sterile 1639
Decadron Tablets 1635
Decadron-LA Sterile Suspension (Low) 1646
Dexacort Phosphate in Respihaler 458
Dexacort Phosphate in Turbinaire 459
Diprivan Injection (Less than 1%) 2833
Dizac (Less frequent) 1809
Dopram Injectable 2061
Duragesic Transdermal System (1% or greater) 1288
Emete-con Intramuscular/Intravenous 2198
▲ Felbatol (9.7%) 2666
Fioricet with Codeine Capsules 2260
Fiorinal with Codeine Capsules 2262
Floxin I.V. 1571
Floxin Tablets (200 mg, 300 mg, 400 mg) 1567
Imitrex Injection (Rare) 1103
Imitrex Tablets (Rare) 1106
ISMOTIC 45% w/v Solution (Very rare) ◉ 222

(▣ Described in PDR For Nonprescription Drugs)   Incidence data in parenthesis; ▲ 3% or more   (◉ Described in PDR For Ophthalmology)

1323 Side Effects Index Hunger

Lamictal Tablets (Rare) 1112
Larodopa Tablets (Rare) 2129
Luvox Tablets (Rare) 2544
Maxaquin Tablets 2440
Mexitil Capsules (About 1 in 1,000) 678
Moduretic Tablets (Less than or equal to 1%) 1705
Neoral (2% or less) 2276
Neurontin Capsules (Rare) 1922
▲ Nicorette (3% to 9%) 2458
Paxil Tablets (Rare) 2505
Permax Tablets (1.1%) 575
Platinol 708
Platinol-AQ Injection (Infrequent) 710
PREVACID Delayed-Release Capsules (Less than 1%) 2562
Prozac Pulvules & Liquid, Oral Solution (Infrequent) 919
Questran Light 769
Questran Powder 770
Romazicon (Less than 1%) 2147
Sandimmune (2% or less) 2286
Serzone Tablets (Infrequent) 771
Sinemet Tablets 943
Sinemet CR Tablets 944
Soma Compound w/Codeine Tablets 2676
Soma Compound Tablets 2675
Soma Tablets 2674
Tonocard Tablets (Less than 1%) 531
Valium Injectable 2182
▲ Versed Injection (3.9%) 2170
Zarontin Capsules 1928
Zarontin Syrup 1929
Zemuron (Less than 1%) 1830
Zoloft Tablets (Rare) 2217
Zosyn (1.0% or less) 1419
Zosyn Pharmacy Bulk Package (1.0% or less) 1422

Hirsutism

Accutane Capsules (Less than 1%) 2076
Aldactazide 2413
Aldactone 2414
Amen Tablets (Few cases) 780
▲ Android Capsules, 10 mg (Among most common) 1250
Android 1251
Betaseron for SC Injection 658
Brevicon 2088
▲ CellCept Capsules (More than or equal to 3%) 2099
Climara Transdermal System 645
Cortone Acetate Sterile Suspension 1623
Cortone Acetate Tablets 1624
Cycrin Tablets (A few cases) 975
Cytadren Tablets (Rare) 819
Dalalone D.P. Injectable 1011
Danocrine Capsules 2307
Dantrium Capsules (Less frequent) 1982
Decadron Elixir 1633
Decadron Phosphate Injection 1637
Decadron Phosphate Respihaler 1642
Decadron Phosphate Turbinaire 1645
Decadron Phosphate with Xylocaine Injection, Sterile 1639
Decadron Tablets 1635
Decadron-LA Sterile Suspension 1646
Delatestryl Injection 2860
Demulen 2428
Depo-Provera Contraceptive Injection (Fewer than 1%) 2602
Depo-Provera Sterile Aqueous Suspension 2606
Desogen Tablets 1817
Desyrel and Desyrel Dividose 503
Dexacort Phosphate in Respihaler 458
Dexacort Phosphate in Turbinaire 459
Diethylstilbestrol Tablets 1437
Effexor (Rare) 2719
Eldepryl Tablets 2550
Estrace Cream and Tablets 749
ESTRATAB Tablets (0.3, 0.625, 1.25, 2.5 mg) 2536
Estratest 2539
Florinef Acetate Tablets 505
Halotestin Tablets 2614
Hydeltrasol Injection, Sterile 1665
Hydeltra-T.B.A. Sterile Suspension 1667
Hydrocortone Acetate Sterile Suspension 1669
Hydrocortone Phosphate Injection, Sterile 1670
Hydrocortone Tablets 1672
Hyperstat I.V. Injection 2363
Intron A (Less than 5%) 2364
Klonopin Tablets 2126
Lamictal Tablets (Infrequent) 1112
Levlen/Tri-Levlen 651
Lo/Ovral Tablets 2746
Lo/Ovral-28 Tablets 2751
Lupron Depot 7.5 mg (Less than 5%) 2559
Lupron Injection 2555
Menest Tablets 2494
Micronor Tablets 1872
Modicon 1872
▲ Neoral (21% to 45%) 2276
Neurontin Capsules (Infrequent) 1922
Nordette-21 Tablets 2755
Nordette-28 Tablets 2758
Norinyl 2088
Norplant System 2759
Nor-Q D Tablets 2135
Ogen Tablets 2627
Ogen Vaginal Cream 2630
Oreton Methyl 1255
Ortho-Cept 1851
Ortho-Cyclen/Ortho-Tri-Cyclen 1858
Ortho Dienestrol Cream 1866
Ortho-Est 1869
Ortho-Novum 1872
Ortho-Cyclen/Ortho Tri-Cyclen 1858
Ovcon 760
Ovral Tablets 2770
Ovral-28 Tablets 2770
Ovrette Tablets 2771
Oxandrin 2862
PMB 200 and PMB 400 2783
Permax Tablets (Infrequent) 575
Premarin Intravenous 2787
Premarin with Methyltestosterone 2794
Premarin Tablets 2789
Premarin Vaginal Cream 2791
Premphase 2797
Prempro 2801
Proglycem (Frequent) 580
▲ Prograf (Greater than 3%) 1042
Provera Tablets (A few cases) 2636
Prozac Pulvules & Liquid, Oral Solution (Rare) 919
▲ Sandimmune (21 to 45%) 2286
Stilphostrol Tablets and Ampuls 612
Synarel Nasal Solution for Endometriosis (2.5% of patients) 2152
▲ Tegison Capsules (1-10%) 2154
Tegretol Chewable Tablets (Isolated cases) 852
Tegretol Suspension (Isolated cases) 852
Tegretol Tablets (Isolated cases) 852
Testoderm Testosterone Transdermal System 486
Testred Capsules 1262
Levlen/Tri-Levlen 651
Tri-Norinyl 2164
Triphasil-21 Tablets 2814
Triphasil-28 Tablets 2819
Wellbutrin Tablets (Rare) 1204
Winstrol Tablets 2337
Zarontin Capsules 1928
Zarontin Syrup 1929
▲ Zoladex (7%) 2858

Hives (see also under Urticaria)

AeroBid Inhaler System (1-3%) 1005
Aerobid-M Inhaler System (1-3%) 1005
Alupent Tablets (0.2%) 669
Atrovent Inhalation Aerosol (Less frequent) 671
Betoptic Ophthalmic Solution (Rare) 469
Betoptic S Ophthalmic Suspension (Rare) 471
Bumex (0.2%) 2093
Carafate Tablets 1504
Catapres Tablets (About 5 in 1,000 patients) 674
Catapres-TTS (Less frequent) 675
Combipres Tablets (About 5 in 1,000) 677
Cutivate Ointment (Less than 1%) 1089
Diphtheria and Tetanus Toxoids and Pertussis Vaccine Adsorbed USP (For Pediatric Use) (Rare) 875
Emete-con Intramuscular/Intravenous 2198
Fioricet with Codeine Capsules 2260
Fiorinal with Codeine Capsules 2262
Fluorescite (Very rare) ⊙ 219
Fluvirin (Rare) 460
Habitrol Nicotine Transdermal System (Once in 35% of patients) 865
HibTITER 1375
Imitrex Tablets (Rare) 1106
Influenza Virus Vaccine, Trivalent, Types A and B (chromatograph- and filter-purified subviron antigen) FluShield, 1995-1996 Formula (Rare) 2736
JE-VAX (0.2%) 886
Lozol Tablets (Less than 5%) 2022
Metrodin (urofollitropin for injection) 2446
Monistat Dual-Pak (Less than 0.5%) 1850
Monistat 3 Vaginal Suppositories (Less than 0.5%) 1850
Quadrinal Tablets 1350
Rogaine Topical Solution (1.27%) 2637
Soma Compound w/Codeine Tablets 2676
Soma Compound Tablets 2675
Sotradecol (Sodium Tetradecyl Sulfate Injection) 967
Stadol (Less than 1%) 775
Thioplex (Thiotepa For Injection) (Rare) 1281
▲ THROMBATE III Antithrombin III (Human) (1 of 17) 637
Tracrium Injection (0.1%) 1183
Varivax (Greater than or equal to 1%) 1762
Versed Injection (Less than 1%) 2170
Zovirax Sterile Powder (Approximately 2%) 1223

Hives at injection site

Diprivan Injection (Less than 1%) 2833
Idamycin 1955

Hoarseness

▲ AeroBid Inhaler System (3-9%) 1005
▲ Aerobid-M Inhaler System (3-9%) 1005
Android Capsules, 10 mg 1250
Android 1251
Atamet 572
Atrovent Inhalation Aerosol (Less than 1%) 671
Azmacort Oral Inhaler (Infrequent) 2011
Beclovent Inhalation Aerosol and Refill (A few patients) 1075
Capoten 739
Capozide 742
Danocrine Capsules 2307
Decadron Phosphate Respihaler 1642
Delatestryl Injection 2860
Depo-Provera Contraceptive Injection (Fewer than 1%) 2602
Dexacort Phosphate in Respihaler 458
Emcyt Capsules (1%) 1953
Halotestin Tablets 2614
Intal Capsules (Less than 1 in 100,000 patients) 987
Intal Inhaler (Rare) 988
Intal Nebulizer Solution (Rare) 989
Larodopa Tablets (Rare) 2129
Luvox Tablets (Infrequent) 2544
Matulane Capsules 2131
Monopril Tablets (0.2% to 1.0%) 757
Nasarel Nasal Solution (1% or less) 2133
Nicorette 2458
Oreton Methyl 1255
Oxandrin 2862
Retrovir Capsules 1158
Retrovir I.V. Infusion 1163
Retrovir Syrup 1158
ReVia Tablets (Less than 1%) 940
Rhinocort Nasal Inhaler (Less than 1%) 556
Sinemet Tablets 943
Sinemet CR Tablets 944
Vanceril Inhaler (Few patients) 2394
Vaseretic Tablets 1765
Vasotec I.V. 1768
Vasotec Tablets (0.5% to 1.0%) 1771
Ventolin Inhalation Aerosol and Refill (Rare) 1197
Ventolin Rotacaps for Inhalation (Rare to 2%) 1200

Hodgkin's disease

Clomid 1514
Dilantin Infatabs 1908
Dilantin Kapseals 1906
Dilantin Parenteral (A number of reports) 1910
Dilantin-125 Suspension 1911

Hormonal imbalance

ParaGard T380A Intrauterine Copper Contraceptive 1880
Synarel Nasal Solution for Central Precocious Puberty 2151
Wellbutrin Tablets (Rare) 1204

Horner's syndrome

Atamet 572
Larodopa Tablets (Rare) 2129
Sinemet Tablets 943
Sinemet CR Tablets 944

Hostility

Anafranil Capsules (Infrequent) 803
BuSpar (2%) 737
Cognex Capsules (2%) 1901
Desyrel and Desyrel Dividose (1.3% to 3.5%) 503
Duragesic Transdermal System (Less than 1%) 1288
Effexor (Infrequent) 2719
Floxin I.V. 1571
Floxin Tablets (200 mg, 300 mg, 400 mg) 1567
Lamictal Tablets (Infrequent) 1112
Luvox Tablets (Infrequent) 2544
Neurontin Capsules (Frequent) 1922
Nubain Injection (1% or less) 935
Paxil Tablets (Rare) 2505
Permax Tablets (Infrequent) 575
PREVACID Delayed-Release Capsules (Less than 1%) 2562
ProSom Tablets (Infrequent) 449
Prozac Pulvules & Liquid, Oral Solution (Infrequent) 919
Serzone Tablets (Infrequent) 771
Stadol (Less than 1%) 775
▲ Wellbutrin Tablets (5.6%) 1204
Xanax Tablets (Rare) 2649

Hot flashes

Ambien Tablets (Rare) 2416
▲ Anafranil Capsules (2% to 5%) 803
Atamet 572
Cardene Capsules (Rare) 2095
Ceredase 1065
Clozaril Tablets (Less than 1%) 2252
▲ Depo-Provera Contraceptive Injection (1% to 5%) 2602
Dipentum Capsules (Rare) 1951
Esgic-plus Tablets (Infrequent) 1013
▲ Eulexin Capsules (61% with LHRH-agonist) 2358
Fioricet Tablets (Infrequent) 2258
Fioricet with Codeine Capsules (Infrequent) 2260
Fiorinal with Codeine Capsules (Infrequent) 2262
Hivid Tablets (Less than 1% to less than 3%) 2121
Imdur (Less than or equal to 5%) 1323
Intron A (Less than 5%) 2364
Lamictal Tablets (1.3%) 1112
Larodopa Tablets (Infrequent) 2129
Lotrel Capsules 840
▲ Lupron Depot 3.75 mg (72.9%) 2556
▲ Lupron Depot 7.5 mg (58.9%) 2559
▲ Lupron Injection (5% or more) 2555
Mexitil Capsules (Less than 1% or about 2 in 1,000) 678
▲ Nolvadex Tablets (2.8% to 63.9%) 2841
Norvasc Tablets (More than 0.1% to 1%) 1940
Orlamm (Males 2:1) 2239
Phrenilin (Infrequent) 785
Procardia XL Extended Release Tablets (1% or less) 1972
Prostin E2 Suppository 2634
Prozac Pulvules & Liquid, Oral Solution (1.8%) 919
ReVia Tablets (Less than 1%) 940
Roferon-A Injection (Less than 1%) 2145
Romazicon (1% to 3%) 2147
Rythmol Tablets–150mg, 225mg, 300mg (Less than 1%) 1352
Sanorex Tablets 2294
Sedapap Tablets 50 mg/650 mg (Infrequent) 1543
Sinemet Tablets 943
Sinemet CR Tablets 944
Supprelin Injection (2%) 2056
▲ Synarel Nasal Solution for Central Precocious Puberty (3%) 2151
▲ Synarel Nasal Solution for Endometriosis (90% of patients) 2152
Zefazone 2654
▲ Zoladex (62% to 96%) 2858
Zoloft Tablets (2.2%) 2217

Hunger

Diabinese Tablets (Less than 2%) 1935
Imitrex Injection (Rare) 1103
Imitrex Tablets (Rare) 1106
Respbid Tablets 682

Hydrocephalus
Betaseron for SC Injection 658
Pergonal (menotropins for injection, USP) (One report) 2448
Prozac Pulvules & Liquid, Oral Solution (Rare) 919

Hydrocephalus, fetal
Accutane Capsules 2076

Hydronephrosis
▲ CellCept Capsules (More than or equal to 3%) 2099

Hydrothorax
Clomid 1514
Humegon 1824
Serophene (clomiphene citrate tablets, USP) 2451

Hyperactive deep tendon reflexes
Eskalith 2485
Lithium Carbonate Capsules & Tablets 2230
Lithonate/Lithotabs/Lithobid 2543

Hyperactivity
AeroBid Inhaler System (1-3%) 1005
Aerobid-M Inhaler System (1-3%) 1005
Amoxil (Rare) 2464
Augmentin (Rare) 2468
Ceclor Pulvules & Suspension (Rare) 1431
Ceftin for Oral Suspension (Less than 1% but more than 0.1%) 1078
Cefzil Tablets and Oral Suspension (Less than 1%) 746
Dalmane Capsules (Rare) 2173
Depakene 413
Depakote Tablets 415
Dopram Injectable 2061
Etrafon 2355
Fioricet with Codeine Capsules 2260
Fiorinal with Codeine Capsules 2262
▲ Inapsine Injection (Among most common) 1296
Infumorph 200 and Infumorph 500 Sterile Solutions 965
Ludiomil Tablets (Rare) 843
Mellaril (Extremely rare) 2269
Moban Tablets and Concentrate (Less frequent) 1048
Phenobarbital Elixir and Tablets 1469
Proventil Syrup (2 of 100 patients) 2385
Roferon-A Injection (Less than 1%) 2145
Seldane-D Extended-Release Tablets (1.1%) 1538
Trilafon 2389
Ventolin Inhalation Aerosol and Refill (1%) 1197
Ventolin Rotacaps for Inhalation (Less than 1%) 1200
Ventolin Syrup (2 of 100 patients) 1202
Versed Injection 2170
Yocon 1892
Zarontin Capsules 1928
Zarontin Syrup 1929

Hyperactivity, paradoxical
Restoril Capsules (Less than 0.5%) 2284

Hyperacusis
Anafranil Capsules (Infrequent) 803
Atretol Tablets 573
Effexor (Rare) 2719
Paxil Tablets (Rare) 2505
Risperdal (Rare) 1301
Romazicon (Less than 1%) 2147
Serzone Tablets (Infrequent) 771
Tegretol Chewable Tablets 852
Tegretol Suspension 852
Tegretol Tablets 852

Hyperalgesia
Betaseron for SC Injection 658
Lamictal Tablets (Rare) 1112
Paxil Tablets (Rare) 2505
Retrovir Capsules 1158
Retrovir I.V. Infusion 1163
Retrovir Syrup 1158

Hyperammonemia
Depakene 413
Depakote Tablets 415
Felbatol 2666
Haldol Decanoate 1577
NephrAmine (Infrequent) 2005
Oncaspar (Less than 1%) 2028

Hyperbilirubinemia
Altace Capsules (Rare) 1232
Ancobon Capsules 2079
AquaMEPHYTON Injection 1608
Atamet 572
Augmentin (Infrequent) 2468
Bactrim DS Tablets 2084
Bactrim I.V. Infusion 2082
Bactrim 2084
▲ Betaseron for SC Injection (6%) 658
Biaxin (Less than 1%) 405
BiCNU 691
Calan SR Caplets 2422
Calan Tablets 2419
Capoten 739
Capozide 742
CeeNU (Small percentage) 693
Cefizox for Intramuscular or Intravenous Use (Rare) 1034
Cefotan 2829
Ceftin 1078
Ceptaz 1081
▲ Cipro I.V. (Among most frequent) 595
▲ Cipro I.V. Pharmacy Bulk Package (Among most frequent) 597
Cipro Tablets (0.3%) 592
Cytosar-U Sterile Powder (With experimental doses) 2592
Dalmane Capsules (Rare) 2173
Dapsone Tablets USP 1284
Depakene (Occasional) 413
Depakote Tablets (Occasional) 415
Desyrel and Desyrel Dividose 503
Dilacor XR Extended-release Capsules 2018
Duricef 748
Elspar 1659
Ergamisol Tablets (Less than 1% to 1%) 1292
Ethmozine Tablets (Rare) 2041
Eulexin Capsules 2358
▲ Exosurf Neonatal for Intratracheal Suspension (10% to 61%) 1095
Floxin I.V. 1571
Floxin Tablets (200 mg, 300 mg, 400 mg) 1567
Fortaz 1100
▲ Sterile FUDR (Among more common) 2118
Fungizone Intravenous 506
Garamycin Injectable 2360
Hyperstat I.V. Injection 2363
HypRho-D Full Dose Rho (D) Immune Globulin (Human) 629
Hyzaar Tablets (Occasional) 1677
▲ IFEX (31%) 697
Inocor Lactate Injection (Rare) 2309
Isoptin Oral Tablets 1346
Isoptin SR Tablets 1348
Konakion Injection 2127
Lamprene Capsules (Less than 1%) 828
Larodopa Tablets (Rare) 2129
Lescol Capsules 2267
Leukine for IV Infusion 1271
Lopid Tablets (Occasional) 1917
Lotensin Tablets 834
Lotrel Capsules (Rare) 840
Lovenox Injection (Rare) 2020
Maxaquin Tablets 2440
Mephyton Tablets (Rare) 1696
Mevacor Tablets 1699
Mezlin 601
Mezlin Pharmacy Bulk Package 604
Mithracin 607
Monopril Tablets 757
▲ Navelbine Injection (2% to 9%) 1145
Neoral 2276
Netromycin Injection 100 mg/ml (15 of 1000 patients) 2373
Neutrexin (1.8%) 2572
Nolvadex Tablets (1.8%) 2841
Nydrazid Injection 508
Oncaspar 2028
Oxandrin 2862
▲ Paraplatin for Injection (5%) 705
Penetrex Tablets (Less than 1%) 2031
Pipracil (Less frequent) 1390
Platinol 708
Platinol-AQ Injection 710
Pravachol 765
Prilosec Delayed-Release Capsules (Rare) 529
Primaxin I.M. 1727
Primaxin I.V. 1729
Prinivil Tablets (Rare) 1733
Prinzide Tablets (Rare) 1737
Proglycem Suspension 580
▲ Proleukin for Injection (64%) 797
Proloprim Tablets 1155
Prostin VR Pediatric Sterile Solution (Less than 1%) 2635
Retrovir Capsules (Rare) 1158
Retrovir I.V. Infusion (Rare) 1163
Retrovir Syrup (Rare) 1158
RhoGAM Rh_0(D) Immune Globulin (Human) 1847
Rifadin (Some cases) 1528
Rifamate Capsules 1530
Rifater (Some cases) 1532
Rimactane Capsules (Rare) 847
Rocephin Injectable Vials, ADD-Vantage, Galaxy Container (Less than 1%) 2142
Sectral Capsules 2807
Septra 1174
Septra I.V. Infusion 1169
Septra I.V. Infusion ADD-Vantage Vials 1171
Septra 1174
Sinemet Tablets 943
Suprax 1399
▲ Taxol (7%) 714
Tazicef for Injection 2519
Tenoretic Tablets 2845
Tenormin Tablets and I.V. Injection 2847
Timentin for Injection 2528
Tobramycin Sulfate Injection 968
Trimpex Tablets 2163
Vantin for Oral Suspension and Vantin Tablets 2646
Vaseretic Tablets (Rare) 1765
Vasotec I.V. 1768
Vasotec Tablets 1771
Verelan Capsules 1410
Verelan Capsules 2824
Videx Tablets, Powder for Oral Solution, & Pediatric Powder for Oral Solution (1% to 2%) 720
Winstrol Tablets 2337
Xanax Tablets 2649
Zefazone 2654
Zerit Capsules (Up to 1%) 729
Zestoretic (Rare) 2850
Zestril Tablets (Rare) 2854
Zinacef (1 in 500 patients) 1211
Zithromax (Less than 1%) 1944
Zocor Tablets 1775
Zosyn 1419
Zosyn Pharmacy Bulk Package 1422
Zyloprim Tablets (Less than 1%) 1226

Hypercalcemia
▲ Android Capsules, 10 mg (Among most common) 1250
Apresazide Capsules 808
Betaseron for SC Injection 658
Capozide (A few patients) 742
▲ CellCept Capsules (More than or equal to 3%) 2099
Cipro I.V. (Infrequent) 595
▲ Cipro I.V. Pharmacy Bulk Package (Among most frequent) 597
Climara Transdermal System 645
Dovonex Ointment 0.005% (Less than 1%) 2684
Enduron Tablets 420
Esidrix Tablets 821
Eskalith 2485
Estrace Cream and Tablets 749
Estraderm Transdermal System 824
ESTRATAB Tablets (0.3, 0.625, 1.25, 2.5 mg) 2536
Estratest 2539
Foscavir Injection (Between 1% and 5%) 547
Hyzaar Tablets 1677
Intron A (Less than 5%) 2364
Lithonate/Lithotabs/Lithobid 2543
Lozol Tablets (Rare) 2022
Lupron Depot 7.5 mg (Less than 5%) 2559
Maxzide 1380
Megace Tablets 701
Menest Tablets 2494
Mykrox Tablets (A few patients) 993
Nolvadex Tablets (Infrequent) 2841
Ogen Tablets 2627
Ogen Vaginal Cream 2630
Oretic Tablets (Rare occasions) 443
Oreton Methyl 1255
Ortho Dienestrol Cream 1866
Ortho-Est 1869
Oxandrin 2862
PMB 200 and PMB 400 2783
PhosLo Tablets 690
Premarin Intravenous 2787
Premarin with Methyltestosterone 2794
Premarin Tablets 2789
Premarin Vaginal Cream 2791
Premphase 2797
Prempro 2801
Prinzide Tablets 1737
Proleukin for Injection (1%) 797
▲ Rocaltrol Capsules (1 in 3) 2141
Stilphostrol Tablets and Ampuls 612
Tenoretic Tablets 2845
Teslac 717
Testoderm Testosterone Transdermal System 486
Vaseretic Tablets 1765
Winstrol Tablets 2337
Zaroxolyn Tablets (Infrequent) 1000
Zestoretic 2850
Zoladex (Rare) 2858
Zosyn 1419
Zosyn Pharmacy Bulk Package 1422
Zyloprim Tablets (Less than 1%) 1226

Hypercalciuria
Aristocort Suspension (Forte Parenteral) 1027
Aristocort Tablets 1022
Aristospan Suspension (Intra-articular) 1033
Aristospan Suspension (Intralesional) 1032
Prelone Syrup 1787
▲ Rocaltrol Capsules (1 in 7) 2141

Hypercapnia
Prostin VR Pediatric Sterile Solution (Less than 1%) 2635

Hypercarbia
Alfenta Injection (0.3% to 1%) 1286
Survanta Beractant Intratracheal Suspension (Less than 1%) 2226

Hyperchloremia
▲ Android Capsules, 10 mg (Among most common) 1250
Android 1251
Daranide Tablets 1633
Demadex Tablets and Injection 686
Oreton Methyl 1255
Primaxin I.M. 1727
Primaxin I.V. 1729
Sulfamylon Cream 925
Testoderm Testosterone Transdermal System 486
Winstrol Tablets 2337

Hyperchloremic acidosis
Questran Light 769
Questran Powder (Less frequent) 770

Hyperchlorhydria
Prozac Pulvules & Liquid, Oral Solution (Rare) 919

Hypercholesterolemia
▲ Accutane Capsules (About 7%) 2076
Ambien Tablets (Rare) 2416
Anafranil Capsules (Infrequent) 803
▲ Android Capsules, 10 mg (Among most common) 1250
Android 1251
Atretol Tablets (Occasional reports) 573
Bumex (0.4%) 2093
▲ CellCept Capsules (8.5% to 12.8%) 2099
▲ CHEMET (succimer) Capsules (4.2 to 10.4%) 1545
Cipro I.V. (Infrequent) 595
Cipro I.V. Pharmacy Bulk Package (Less than 1%) 597
Cipro Tablets 592
Cognex Capsules (Infrequent) 1901
Delatestryl Injection 2860
Diflucan Injection, Tablets, and Oral Suspension 2194
Effexor (Infrequent) 2719
Ergamisol Tablets 1292
Estratest 2539
Floxin I.V. 1571
Floxin Tablets (200 mg, 300 mg, 400 mg) 1567
Halotestin Tablets 2614
Hyzaar Tablets 1677
Kerlone Tablets (Less than 2%) 2436
Lotensin HCT 837
Luvox Tablets (Infrequent) 2544
Maxaquin Tablets 2440
Neurontin Capsules (Rare) 1922
Noroxin Tablets 1715
Noroxin Tablets 2048
Norpace (1 to 3%) 2444
Oreton Methyl 1255
Oxandrin 2862
Paxil Tablets (Rare) 2505

(Described in PDR For Nonprescription Drugs) Incidence data in parenthesis; ▲ 3% or more (◉ Described in PDR For Ophthalmology)

1325 **Side Effects Index** **Hyperhidrosis**

Penetrex Tablets ... 2031
Permax Tablets (Infrequent) ... 575
Premarin with Methyltestosterone .. 2794
PREVACID Delayed-Release Capsules (Less than 1%) ... 2562
Prinzide Tablets ... 1737
Prozac Pulvules & Liquid, Oral Solution (Rare) ... 919
Rocaltrol Capsules ... 2141
Serzone Tablets (Rare) ... 771
Synarel Nasal Solution for Endometriosis ... 2152
▲Tegison Capsules (19%) ... 2154
Tegretol Chewable Tablets (Occasional) ... 852
Tegretol Suspension (Occasional) .. 852
Tegretol Tablets (Occasional) ... 852
Temaril Tablets, Syrup and Spansule Extended-Release Capsules ... 483
Testoderm Testosterone Transdermal System ... 486
Testred Capsules ... 1262
Ticlid Tablets ... 2156
Timolide Tablets ... 1748
Vaseretic Tablets ... 1765
Zestoretic ... 2850
Zoladex ... 2858
Zoloft Tablets (Rare) ... 2217

Hypercorticism

Beconase ... 1076
Blephamide Ointment (Rare) ... ⊙ 237
Econopred & Econopred Plus Ophthalmic Suspensions (Rare) ... ⊙ 217
FML Forte Liquifilm (Rare) ... ⊙ 240
FML Liquifilm (Rare) ... ⊙ 241
FML S.O.P. (Rare) ... ⊙ 241
Nasacort Nasal Inhaler ... 2024
Nasalide Nasal Solution 0.025% 2110
Vasocidin Ophthalmic Solution (Rare) ... ⊙ 270

Hyperdipsia (see under Dipsesis)

Hyperemia

▲Alomide (1% to 5%) ... 469
Atropine Sulfate Sterile Ophthalmic Solution ... ⊙ 233
Celontin Kapseals ... 1899
Elase Ointment ... 1039
Elase Vials ... 1038
▲Iopidine 0.5% (13%) ... ⊙ 221
Lacrisert Sterile Ophthalmic Insert 1686
Prostin VR Pediatric Sterile Solution (Less than 1%) ... 2635
Vasosulf ... ⊙ 271
Vexol 1% Ophthalmic Suspension (1% to 5%) ... ⊙ 230
Viroptic Ophthalmic Solution, 1% Sterile ... 1204

Hyperemia, conjunctival

Chibroxin Sterile Ophthalmic Solution ... 1617
Diprivan Injection (Less than 1%) .. 2833
Econopred & Econopred Plus Ophthalmic Suspensions (Occasional) ... ⊙ 217
FML Forte Liquifilm (Occasional) ⊙ 240
FML Liquifilm (Occasional) ... ⊙ 241
FML S.O.P. (Occasional) ... ⊙ 241
▲Genoptic Sterile Ophthalmic Solution (Among most frequent).. ⊙ 243
▲Genoptic Sterile Ophthalmic Ointment (Among most frequent) ... ⊙ 243
▲Ocupress Ophthalmic Solution, 1% Sterile (About 1 of 4 patients) ... ⊙ 309
Tensilon Injectable ... 1261

Hyperesthesia

Anafranil Capsules (Rare) ... 803
Asacol Delayed-Release Tablets ... 1979
Betaseron for SC Injection ... 658
Effexor (Infrequent) ... 2719
Foscavir Injection (Less than 1%) .. 547
Imitrex Injection (Rare) ... 1103
Imitrex Tablets (Rare) ... 1106
Intron A (Less than 5%) ... 2364
Lamictal Tablets (Rare) ... 1112
Neurontin Capsules (Rare) ... 1922
Sansert Tablets ... 2295
Sectral Capsules (Up to 2%) ... 2807
Serzone Tablets (Rare) ... 771
Videx Tablets, Powder for Oral Solution, & Pediatric Powder for Oral Solution (Less than 1%) ... 720
Ziac ... 1415
Zoloft Tablets (Infrequent) ... 2217

Hyperestrogenism

Lupron Depot 3.75 mg ... 2556

Hyperexcitability

Lufyllin-GG Elixir & Tablets ... 2671

Hyperexcitability, reflex

Quadrinal Tablets ... 1350
Quibron ... 2053
Respbid Tablets ... 682
Slo-bid Gyrocaps ... 2033
Theo-24 Extended Release Capsules ... 2568
Theo-Dur Extended-Release Tablets ... 1327
Theo-X Extended-Release Tablets .. 788
Uni-Dur Extended-Release Tablets.. 1331
Uniphyl 400 mg Tablets ... 2001

Hyperferremia

Pyrazinamide Tablets (Rare) ... 1398

Hypergammaglobulinemia

PREVACID Delayed-Release Capsules (Less than 1%) ... 2562

Hyperglycemia

▲Accutane Capsules (Less than 1 in 10) ... 2076
Aclovate ... 1069
Actimmune (Rare) ... 1056
Albalon Solution with Liquifilm ... ⊙ 231
Aldoclor Tablets ... 1598
Aldoril Tablets ... 1604
Altace Capsules (Rare) ... 1232
Ambien Tablets (Infrequent) ... 2416
Anafranil Capsules (Infrequent) ... 803
Anaprox/Naprosyn (Less than 1%) ... 2117
Apresazide Capsules ... 808
Atgam Sterile Solution (Less than 1% to less than 5%) ... 2581
▲Betaseron for SC Injection (15%) .. 658
Blocadren Tablets ... 1614
▲Bumex (6.6%) ... 2093
Capozide ... 742
Cardizem CD Capsules (Less than 1%) ... 1506
Cardizem SR Capsules (Less than 1%) ... 1510
Cardizem Injectable ... 1508
Cardizem Tablets (Less than 1%) .. 1512
Carmol HC (Some patients) ... 924
Catapres Tablets (Rare) ... 674
Catapres-TTS (Rare) ... 675
▲CellCept Capsules (8.6% to 12.4%) ... 2099
▲Cipro I.V. (Among most frequent) .. 595
Cipro Tablets ... 592
Clinoril Tablets (Rare) ... 1618
Clozaril Tablets ... 2252
Combipres Tablets ... 677
Compazine ... 2470
Demadex Tablets and Injection ... 686
Dermatop Emollient Cream 0.1% .. 1238
Dilantin Kapseals ... 1906
Dilantin Parenteral ... 1910
Dilantin-125 Suspension ... 1911
Diprivan Injection (Less than 1%) .. 2833
Diprolene ... 2352
Diucardin Tablets ... 2718
Diupres Tablets ... 1650
Diuril Oral Suspension ... 1653
Diuril Sodium Intravenous ... 1652
Diuril Tablets ... 1653
Dyazide ... 2479
EC-Naprosyn Delayed-Release Tablets (Less than 1%) ... 2117
Edecrin ... 1657
Effexor (Infrequent) ... 2719
Elavil ... 2838
Elspar (Low) ... 1659
Endep Tablets ... 2174
Enduron Tablets ... 420
Esgic-plus Tablets ... 1013
Esidrix Tablets ... 821
Esimil Tablets ... 822
Etrafon ... 2355
Feldene Capsules (Less than 1%) .. 1965
Fioricet Tablets (Infrequent) ... 2258
Fioricet with Codeine Capsules ... 2260
Fiorinal with Codeine Capsules ... 2262
Flexeril Tablets (Rare) ... 1661
Florinef Acetate Tablets ... 505
Floxin I.V. (More than or equal to 1%) ... 1571
Floxin Tablets (200 mg, 300 mg, 400 mg) (More than or equal to 1.0%) ... 1567
▲Fludara for Injection (1% to 6%) ... 663
Genotropin (Infrequent) ... 111
Haldol Decanoate ... 1577
Haldol Injection, Tablets and Concentrate ... 1575
Hivid Tablets (Less than 1% to less than 3%) ... 2121
Humatrope Vials (Infrequent) ... 1443
HydroDIURIL Tablets ... 1674
Hydropres Tablets ... 1675
Hyperstat I.V. Injection ... 2363
Hyzaar Tablets ... 1677
Imitrex Tablets (Rare) ... 1106
Inderide LA Long Acting Capsules .. 2734
Indocin Capsules (Less than 1%) 1680
Indocin I.V. (1% to 3%) ... 1684
Indocin (Less than 1%) ... 1680
Kerlone Tablets (Less than 2%) 2436
Lamictal Tablets (Rare) ... 1112
Lamprene Capsules (Greater than 1%) ... 828
Lasix Injection, Oral Solution and Tablets ... 1240
Limbitrol ... 2180
Lioresal Tablets ... 829
Lo/Ovral Tablets ... 2746
Lo/Ovral-28 Tablets ... 2751
Lopressor HCT Tablets ... 832
Lorelco Tablets ... 1517
Lotensin Tablets ... 834
Lotensin HCT ... 837
Lozol Tablets (Less than 5%) ... 2022
Ludiomil Tablets (Rare) ... 843
Lufyllin & Lufyllin-400 Tablets ... 2670
Lufyllin-GG Elixir & Tablets ... 2671
Luvox Tablets (Rare) ... 2544
Maxzide ... 1380
▲Megace Oral Suspension (Up to 6%) ... 699
Megace Tablets ... 701
▲Mepron Suspension (9%) ... 1135
Minizide Capsules ... 1938
Mintezol ... 1704
Moduretic Tablets ... 1705
Mykrox Tablets ... 993
Anaprox/Naprosyn (Less than 1%) ... 2117
Navane Capsules and Concentrate 2201
Navane Intramuscular ... 2202
NebuPent for Inhalation Solution (1% or less) ... 1040
Neoral (2% or less) ... 2276
Nimotop Capsules (0.8%; rare) ... 610
Noroxin Tablets ... 1715
Noroxin Tablets ... 2048
Norpramin Tablets ... 1526
Nydrazid Injection ... 508
▲Oncaspar (Greater than 1% but less than 5%) ... 2028
Oretic Tablets ... 443
Ovral Tablets ... 2770
Ovral-28 Tablets ... 2770
Ovrette Tablets ... 2771
Pamelor ... 2280
Paxil Tablets (Infrequent) ... 2505
Pentam 300 Injection (1 patient) 1041
Permax Tablets (Infrequent) ... 575
PREVACID Delayed-Release Capsules (Less than 1%) ... 2562
Prinzide Tablets ... 1737
ProctoCream-HC 2.5% ... 2408
Proglycem (Frequent) ... 580
▲Prograf (Many patients; 29% to 47%) ... 1042
Proleukin for Injection (2%) ... 797
Prozac Pulvules & Liquid, Oral Solution (Rare) ... 919
Quadrinal Tablets ... 1350
Quibron ... 2053
Relafen Tablets (Less than 1%) ... 2510
Respbid Tablets ... 682
Rifamate Capsules ... 1530
Rifater ... 1532
Sandimmune (2% or less) ... 2286
▲Sandostatin Injection (1.5%; 15%) ... 2292
Ser-Ap-Es Tablets ... 849
Sinemet CR Tablets (1% or greater) ... 944
Sinequan ... 2205
Slo-bid Gyrocaps ... 2033
Slo-Niacin Tablets ... 2659
Stelazine ... 2514
Suprane ... 1813
Surmontil Capsules ... 2811
Temovate (Infrequent) ... 1179
Tenoretic Tablets ... 2845
Thalitone ... 1245
Theo-24 Extended Release Capsules ... 2568
Theo-Dur Extended-Release Tablets ... 1327
Theo-X Extended-Release Tablets .. 788
Thorazine ... 2523
Timolide Tablets ... 1748
Timoptic in Ocudose ... 1753
Timoptic Sterile Ophthalmic Solution ... 1751
Timoptic-XE ... 1755
Tofranil Ampuls ... 854
Tofranil Tablets ... 856
Tofranil-PM Capsules ... 857
Tornalate Solution for Inhalation, 0.2% (Infrequent) ... 956
▲Trasylol (3%) ... 613
Triavil Tablets ... 1757
Trilafon ... 2389
Triphasil-21 Tablets ... 2814
Triphasil-28 Tablets ... 2819
Ultravate Cream 0.05% ... 2689
Ultravate Ointment 0.05% ... 2690
Uni-Dur Extended-Release Tablets.. 1331
Uniphyl 400 mg Tablets ... 2001
Vantin for Oral Suspension and Vantin Tablets ... 2646
Vaseretic Tablets ... 1765
Videx Tablets, Powder for Oral Solution, & Pediatric Powder for Oral Solution (1% to 5%) ... 720
Vivactil Tablets ... 1774
Yutopar Intravenous Injection ... 570
Zaroxolyn Tablets ... 1000
Zebeta Tablets ... 1413
Zefazone ... 2654
Zestoretic ... 2850
Zithromax (Less than 1%) ... 1944
▲Zoladex (Greater than 1% but less than 5%) ... 2858
Zosyn ... 1419
Zosyn Pharmacy Bulk Package ... 1422

Hyperglycemia, transient

Eskalith ... 2485
Lithium Carbonate Capsules & Tablets ... 2230
Lithonate/Lithotabs/Lithobid ... 2543

Hyperglycinemia

Asendin Tablets (Very rare) ... 1369
Depakene ... 413
Depakote Tablets ... 415
Lodine Capsules and Tablets ... 2743
Moban Tablets and Concentrate ... 1048

Hyperhemoglobinemia

Ambien Tablets (Rare) ... 2416

Hyperheparinemia

Mustargen (Rare) ... 1709
Protamine Sulfate Ampoules & Vials (Some patients) ... 1471

Hyperhidrosis

Accutane Capsules (Less than 1%) ... 2076
Decadron Phosphate with Xylocaine Injection, Sterile ... 1639
Deconamine ... 1320
DynaCirc Capsules (0.5% to 1%) .. 2256
Esgic-plus Tablets (Infrequent) ... 1013
Fioricet Tablets (Infrequent) ... 2258
Fioricet with Codeine Capsules (Infrequent) ... 2260
Fiorinal with Codeine Capsules (Infrequent) ... 2262
Havrix (Rare) ... 2489
Lorelco Tablets ... 1517
Miacalcin Nasal Spray (Less than 1%) ... 2275
Monopril Tablets (0.4% to 1.0%) .. 757
Noroxin Tablets (0.3% to 1.0%) ... 1715
Noroxin Tablets (0.3% to 1.0%) ... 2048
Penetrex Tablets (Less than 1% but more than or equal to 0.1%) 2031
Phrenilin (Infrequent) ... 785
Prilosec Delayed-Release Capsules (Less than 1%) ... 529
Primaxin I.M. ... 1727
Primaxin I.V. (Less than 0.2%) ... 1729
Prinivil Tablets ... 1733
Prinzide Tablets (0.3 to 1%) ... 1737
Quadrinal Tablets ... 1350
Sedapap Tablets 50 mg/650 mg (Infrequent) ... 1543
Tussend ... 1783
Vaseretic Tablets ... 1765
Vasotec Tablets ... 1771
Visken Tablets (2% or fewer patients) ... 2299

(▭ Described in PDR For Nonprescription Drugs) Incidence data in parenthesis; ▲ 3% or more (⊙ Described in PDR For Ophthalmology)

Hyperhidrosis Side Effects Index 1326

Zestoretic 2850

Hyperirritability
Atrohist Plus Tablets 454
Mintezol 1704
Mysoline (Occasional) 2754
Prostin VR Pediatric Sterile Solution (Less than 1%) 2635
Seromycin Pulvules 1476

Hyperirritability, muscle
Eskalith 2485
Lithium Carbonate Capsules & Tablets 2230
Lithonate/Lithotabs/Lithobid 2543

Hyperirritability, neuromuscular
Mezlin 601
Mezlin Pharmacy Bulk Package 604
Timentin for Injection 2528

Hyperkalemia
Accupril Tablets (Rare) 1893
Altace Capsules (Approximately 1%) 1232
Anaprox/Naprosyn (Less than 1%) 2117
▲ Android Capsules, 10 mg (Among most common) 1250
Android 1251
Anectine (Rare) 1073
Ansaid Tablets (Less than 1%) 2579
Atromid-S Capsules 2701
Blocadren Tablets 1614
Capoten 739
Capozide 742
▲ CellCept Capsules (8.9% to 10.3%) 2099
Ceptaz 1081
Cipro I.V. (Infrequent) 595
Cipro I.V. Pharmacy Bulk Package (Less than 1%) 597
Cipro Tablets 592
Clinoril Tablets (Less than 1 in 100) 1618
Delatestryl Injection 2860
Demadex Tablets and Injection 686
Diprivan Injection (Less than 1%) 2833
Dyazide 2479
Dyrenium Capsules (Rare) 2481
EC-Naprosyn Delayed-Release Tablets (Less than 1%) 2117
Effexor (Rare) 2719
Epogen for Injection (Approximately 0.11%) 489
Estratest 2539
Feldene Capsules (Less than 1%) 1965
Floxin I.V. 1571
Floxin Tablets (200 mg, 300 mg, 400 mg) 1567
Fludara for Injection 663
Fungizone Intravenous 506
Halotestin Tablets 2614
Hivid Tablets (Less than 1% to less than 3%) 2121
Hyzaar Tablets (0.4%) 1677
Indocin Capsules (Less than 1%) 1680
Indocin I.V. (Less than 1%) 1684
Indocin (Less than 1%) 1680
K-Dur Microburst Release System (potassium chloride, USP) E.R. Tablets 1325
▲ K-Lor Powder Packets (Most severe) 434
K-Norm Extended-Release Capsules 991
▲ K-Tab Filmtab (Most common) 434
Kerlone Tablets (Less than 2%) 2436
Kolyum Liquid 992
Lotensin Tablets 834
Lotensin HCT (Approximately 1%) 837
Lotrel Capsules (Approximately 1.5%) 840
Maxaquin Tablets 2440
Maxzide 1380
Micro-K 2063
▲ Micro-K LS Packets (Most severe) 2064
Midamor Tablets (Between 1% and 3%) 1703
Moduretic Tablets (Greater than 1%, less than 3%) 1705
Monopril Tablets (Approximately 2.6%) 757
Anaprox/Naprosyn (Less than 1%) 2117
Neoral (Occasional) 2276
Netromycin Injection 100 mg/ml (Fewer than 1 of 1000 patients) 2373
Noroxin Tablets 1715
Noroxin Tablets 2048
Oreton Methyl 1255
Oxandrin 2862
Penetrex Tablets (Less than 1%) 2031
Pentam 300 Injection (0.7%) 1041
Polycitra Syrup 578
Polycitra-K Crystals 579
Polycitra-K Oral Solution 579
Polycitra-LC 578
Primaxin I.M. 1727
Primaxin I.V. 1729
▲ Prinivil Tablets (Approximately 2.2% to 4.8%) 1733
Prinzide Tablets (Approximately 1.4%) 1737
Procrit for Injection (0.11%) 1841
▲ Prograf (10% to 45%) 1042
▲ Proleukin for Injection (4%) 797
Proloprim Tablets 1155
Prostin VR Pediatric Sterile Solution (Less than 1%) 2635
Rum-K Syrup 1005
Sandimmune (Occasional) 2286
Septra 1174
Septra I.V. Infusion 1169
Septra I.V. Infusion ADD-Vantage Vials 1171
Septra 1174
Slow-K Extended-Release Tablets 851
▲ Tegison Capsules (25-50%) 2154
Testoderm Testosterone Transdermal System 486
Testred Capsules 1262
Toradol 2159
Univasc Tablets (Approximately 1.3%) 2410
Vaseretic Tablets 1765
Vasotec I.V. (Approximately 1%) 1768
Vasotec Tablets (Approximately 1%) 1771
Winstrol Tablets 2337
Zebeta Tablets 1413
Zestoretic (Approximately 1.4%) 2850
▲ Zestril Tablets (Approximately 2.2% to 4.8%) 2854
Zithromax (1% to 2%) 1944
Zosyn 1419
Zosyn Pharmacy Bulk Package 1422

Hyperkalemia, neonatal
Altace Capsules 1232
Capozide 742
Lotensin Tablets 834
Monopril Tablets 757
Prograf 1042

Hyperkeratosis
Blenoxane 692
Calan SR Caplets (1% or less) 2422
Calan Tablets (1% or less) 2419
Cognex Capsules (Infrequent) 1901
Isoptin Oral Tablets (Less than 1%) 1346
Isoptin SR Tablets (1% or less) 1348
Risperdal (Infrequent) 1301
Verelan Capsules (1% or less) 1410
Verelan Capsules (Less than 1%) 2824

Hyperkinesia
Anafranil Capsules (Infrequent) 803
Betaseron for SC Injection (2%) 658
Butisol Sodium Elixir & Tablets (Less than 1 in 100) 2660
Cardene Capsules (Rare) 2095
Claritin (2% or fewer patients) 2349
Claritin-D (Less frequent) 2350
Clozaril Tablets (1%) 2252
Cognex Capsules (Frequent) 1901
Doral Tablets 2664
Effexor (Infrequent) 2719
Flumadine Tablets & Syrup (Less than 0.3%) 1015
Foscavir Injection (Less than 1%) 547
Hivid Tablets (Less than 1% to less than 3%) 2121
Intron A (Less than 5%) 2364
Lamictal Tablets (Infrequent) 1112
Luvox Tablets (Frequent) 2544
Maxair Autohaler 1492
Maxair Inhaler (Less than 1%) 1494
Maxaquin Tablets (Less than 1%) 2440
Mebaral Tablets (Less than 1 in 100) 2322
Nembutal Sodium Capsules (Less than 1%) 436
Nembutal Sodium Solution (Less than 1%) 438
Nembutal Sodium Suppositories (Less than 1%) 440
Neurontin Capsules (Frequent) 1922
▲ Orap Tablets (5.5%) 1050
Paxil Tablets (Infrequent) 2505
Penetrex Tablets (Less than 0.1%) 2031
Permax Tablets (Infrequent) 575
Phenobarbital Elixir and Tablets (Less than 1 in 100 patients) 1469
▲ Proventil Syrup (Children 2 to 6 years, 4%) 2385
Prozac Pulvules & Liquid, Oral Solution (Infrequent) 919
Risperdal (0.6%) 1301
Salagen Tablets (Less than 1%) 1489
Seconal Sodium Pulvules (Less than 1 in 100) 1474
Seldane-D Extended-Release Tablets (1.1%) 1538
Serzone Tablets (Rare) 771
Supprelin Injection (1% to 3%) 2056
Symmetrel Capsules and Syrup (0.1% to 1%) 946
Tegison Capsules (Less than 1%) 2154
Toradol (1% or less) 2159
Tornalate Solution for Inhalation, 0.2% (Less than 1%) 956
Tornalate Metered Dose Inhaler (Less than 1%) 957
▲ Ventolin Syrup (4% in children) 1202
Zoloft Tablets (Infrequent) 2217

Hyperlipidemia
Ambien Tablets (Rare) 2416
Betapace Tablets (Rare) 641
▲ CellCept Capsules (More than or equal to 3%) 2099
▲ Diprivan Injection (Less than 1% to greater than 10%) 2833
Effexor (Infrequent) 2719
Ergamisol Tablets 1292
Estrace Cream and Tablets 749
Heparin Lock Flush Solution 2725
Heparin Sodium Injection 2726
Heparin Sodium Injection, USP, Sterile Solution 2615
Heparin Sodium Vials 1441
Hivid Tablets (Less than 1% to less than 3%) 2121
Kerlone Tablets (Less than 2%) 2436
Luvox Tablets (Rare) 2544
Neurontin Capsules (Rare) 1922
Nolvadex Tablets (Infrequent) 2841
Ogen Tablets 2627
PREVACID Delayed-Release Capsules (Less than 1%) 2562
▲ Prograf (Greater than 3%) 1042
Prozac Pulvules & Liquid, Oral Solution (Rare) 919
Sandimmune 2286
Supprelin Injection (1%) 2056
▲ Videx Tablets, Powder for Oral Solution, & Pediatric Powder for Oral Solution (2% to 7%) 720
Zyloprim Tablets (Less than 1%) 1226

Hypermenorrhea
Cytotec (0.5%) 2424

Hypermetabolic syndrome
Nardil (Less frequent) 1920

Hypermotility, gastrointestinal
Roferon-A Injection (Less than 1%) 2145

Hypernatremia
▲ Android Capsules, 10 mg (Among most common) 1250
Cytovene-IV (One report) 2103
Demadex Tablets and Injection 686
Felbatol 2666
Fleet Enema 1002
Hivid Tablets (Less than 1% to less than 3%) 2121
ISMOTIC 45% w/v Solution (Very rare) ◉ 222
Nardil (Less common) 1920
Oreton Methyl 1255
Proleukin for Injection (1%) 797
Testoderm Testosterone Transdermal System 486
Timentin for Injection 2528
Toradol 2159
Zosyn 1419
Zosyn Pharmacy Bulk Package 1422

Hyperosmolarity
Diprivan Injection (Less than 1%) 2833
ISMOTIC 45% w/v Solution (Very rare) ◉ 222

Hyperostosis, skeletal
Accutane Capsules 2076
Anafranil Capsules (Rare) 803
▲ Tegison Capsules (Greater than 75%) 2154

Hyperoxia
Exosurf Neonatal for Intratracheal Suspension 1095

Hyperparathyroidism
Apresazide Capsules 808
Eskalith 2485
Lithonate/Lithotabs/Lithobid 2543
Maxzide 1380
Prinzide Tablets 1737
Vaseretic Tablets 1765

Hyperphenylalaninemia
Daraprim Tablets (Rare) 1090

Hyperphosphatemia
Achromycin V Capsules 1367
▲ Android Capsules, 10 mg (Among most common) 1250
Android 1251
Delatestryl Injection 2860
Didronel Tablets 1984
Effexor (Rare) 2719
Estratest 2539
Fleet Enema 1002
Fludara for Injection 663
▲ Foscavir Injection (5% or greater) 547
Halotestin Tablets 2614
▲ Lupron Depot 3.75 mg (5% to 8%) 2556
Minocin Intravenous 1382
Minocin Oral Suspension 1385
Minocin Pellet-Filled Capsules 1383
Oreton Methyl 1255
Oxandrin 2862
Premarin with Methyltestosterone 2794
▲ Prograf (Greater than 3%) 1042
Proleukin for Injection (1%) 797
Risperdal (Rare) 1301
Roferon-A Injection (Less than 5%) 2145
▲ Synarel Nasal Solution for Endometriosis (10% to 15%) 2152
Testoderm Testosterone Transdermal System 486
Testred Capsules 1262
Winstrol Tablets 2337
Zithromax (Less than 1%) 1944

Hyperpigmentation
Accutane Capsules (Less than 1%) 2076
Aristocort Suspension (Forte Parenteral) 1027
Aristocort Suspension (Intralesional) 1025
Aristospan Suspension (Intra-articular) 1033
Aristospan Suspension (Intralesional) 1032
BiCNU 691
▲ Blenoxane (50%) 692
Blocadren Tablets 1614
▲ Catapres-TTS (5 of 101 patients) 675
Celestone Soluspan Suspension 2347
Cipro I.V. (1% or less) 595
Cipro I.V. Pharmacy Bulk Package (Less than 1%) 597
Cipro Tablets (Less than 1%) 592
Cortone Acetate Sterile Suspension 1623
Dalalone D.P. Injectable 1011
Decadron Phosphate Injection 1637
Decadron Phosphate with Xylocaine Injection, Sterile 1639
Decadron-LA Sterile Suspension 1646
Deltasone Tablets 2595
Depo-Medrol Single-Dose Vial 2600
Depo-Medrol Sterile Aqueous Suspension 2597
Dovonex Ointment 0.005% (Less than 1%) 2684
▲ Efudex (Among most frequent) 2113
Florinef Acetate Tablets 505
Floxin I.V. 1571
Floxin Tablets (200 mg, 300 mg, 400 mg) 1567
Fluoroplex Topical Solution & Cream 1% (Occasional) 479
Hydeltrasol Injection, Sterile 1665
Hydeltra-T.B.A. Sterile Suspension 1667
Hydrocortone Acetate Sterile Suspension 1669
Hydrocortone Phosphate Injection, Sterile 1670
Lac-Hydrin 12% Lotion (Less frequent) 2687
▲ Lamprene Capsules (75-100%) 828
Lodine Capsules and Tablets (Less than 1%) 2743
Matulane Capsules 2131

(▣ Described in PDR For Nonprescription Drugs) Incidence data in parenthesis; ▲ 3% or more (◉ Described in PDR For Ophthalmology)

1327 Side Effects Index Hypersensitivity reactions, general

Maxaquin Tablets 2440
▲Myleran Tablets (5-10%) 1143
Nicolar Tablets 2026
Norplant System 2759
Penetrex Tablets 2031
Purinethol Tablets 1156
Retin-A (tretinoin) Cream/Gel/Liquid 1889
Solu-Cortef Sterile Powder 2641
Solu-Medrol Sterile Powder 2643
T.R.U.E. Test (Occasional; 2 to 9 reports) 1189

Hyperpigmentation, dermal creases

Adriamycin PFS (A few cases primarily in children) 1947
Adriamycin RDF (A few cases primarily in children) 1947
Rubex (A few cases) 712

Hyperpigmentation, nail beds

Adriamycin PFS (A few cases primarily in children) 1947
Adriamycin RDF (A few cases primarily in children) 1947
Doxorubicin Astra (a few cases) 540
Florinef Acetate Tablets 505
Rubex (A few cases) 712

Hyperplasia, antral

Prostin VR Pediatric Sterile Solution 2635

Hyperplasia, endocervical

Demulen 2428
Depo-Provera Contraceptive Injection (Fewer than 1%) 2602

Hyperplasia, endometrial

Estraderm Transdermal System 824

Hyperplasia, gingival (see under Gingival hyperplasia)

Hyperplasia, mammary

Cuprimine Capsules (Rare) 1630
Depen Titratable Tablets (Rare) 2662

Hyperpnea

Empirin with Codeine Tablets 1093

Hyperprolactinemia

Aldoclor Tablets 1598
Aldomet Ester HCl Injection 1602
Aldomet Oral 1600
Aldoril Tablets 1604
Asendin Tablets (Less frequent) 1369
Calan SR Caplets (1% or less) 2422
Calan Tablets (1% or less) 2419
Compazine 2470
Haldol Decanoate 1577
Haldol Injection, Tablets and Concentrate 1575
Isoptin SR Tablets (1% or less) 1348
Mellaril 2269
Moban Tablets and Concentrate 1048
Paxil Tablets 2505
Prolixin Oral Concentrate 509
Prozac Pulvules & Liquid, Oral Solution 919
Reglan 2068
Risperdal 1301
Stelazine 2514
Temaril Tablets, Syrup and Spansule Extended-Release Capsules 483
Thorazine 2523
Torecan 2245
Trilafon 2389
Zoloft Tablets 2217

Hyperprothrombinemia

Brevicon 2088
Eminase 2039
Estratest 2539
Norinyl 2088
Nor-Q D Tablets 2135
Tri-Norinyl 2164
Zyloprim Tablets (Less than 1%) 1226

Hyperpyrexia (see under Fever)

Hyperreflexia

Anafranil Capsules (Rare) 803
Ansaid Tablets (1-3%) 2579
Compazine 2470
Depakote Tablets (Greater than 1% but not more than 5%) 415
Effexor (Rare) 2719
Foscavir Injection (Less than 1%) 547
Haldol Injection, Tablets and Concentrate 1575
Levoprome 1274
Lithonate/Lithotabs/Lithobid (One report) 2543
Nardil (Common) 1920
Navane Capsules and Concentrate 2201
Navane Intramuscular 2202
Neurontin Capsules (Frequent) 1922
Orap Tablets (Less frequent) 1050
Orthoclone OKT3 Sterile Solution 1837
Paxil Tablets (Rare) 2505
Pfizerpen for Injection 2203
Placidyl Capsules 448
Prolixin 509
Risperdal (Rare) 1301
Seromycin Pulvules 1476
Stelazine 2514
Triavil Tablets 1757
Trilafon 2389
Videx Tablets, Powder for Oral Solution, & Pediatric Powder for Oral Solution (Less than 1%) 720

Hyperreflexia, neonatal

Compazine 2470
Etrafon 2355
Stelazine 2514
Temaril Tablets, Syrup and Spansule Extended-Release Capsules 483
Thorazine 2523

Hypersecretion

Diupres Tablets 1650
Hydropres Tablets 1675
Ser-Ap-Es Tablets 849

Hypersensitivity

AK-Fluor Injection 10% and 25% (Rare) ◉ 203
AK-Pred ◉ 204
AK-Spore ◉ 204
▲AKTOB (Among most frequent; less than 3 of 100 patients) ◉ 206
Alkeran for Injection 1070
Americaine Otic Topical Anesthetic Ear Drops 983
Amoxil 2464
Anectine (Rare) 1073
Atrohist Plus Tablets 454
Azulfidine 1949
Beclovent Inhalation Aerosol and Refill 1075
Beconase (Rare) 1076
Betagan ◉ 233
Bicillin C-R Injection 2704
Bicillin C-R 900/300 Injection 2706
Bicillin L-A Injection 2707
Bleph-10 475
Butisol Sodium Elixir & Tablets (Less than 1 in 100) 2660
Cefobid Intravenous/Intramuscular 2189
Cefobid Pharmacy Bulk Package - Not for Direct Infusion 2192
Cefotan (1.2%) 2829
Ceptaz (Immediate in 1 in 285 patients) 1081
Chloromycetin Ophthalmic Ointment, 1% ◉ 310
Clinoril Tablets (Less than 1%) 1618
Cocaine Hydrochloride Topical Solution 537
Collagenase Santyl Ointment (One case) 1334
Cortisporin Ophthalmic Ointment Sterile 1085
Cortisporin Ophthalmic Suspension Sterile 1086
Cortone Acetate Sterile Suspension 1623
Cortone Acetate Tablets 1624
Daranide Tablets 1633
Daraprim Tablets 1090
Decadron Elixir 1633
Decadron Phosphate Injection 1637
Decadron Phosphate Respihaler 1642
Decadron Phosphate Turbinaire 1645
Decadron Phosphate with Xylocaine Injection, Sterile 1639
Decadron Tablets 1635
Decadron-LA Sterile Suspension 1646
Demser Capsules (Rare) 1649
Dexacort Phosphate in Respihaler 458
Dexacort Phosphate in Turbinaire 459
Dolobid Tablets (Less than 1 in 100) 1654
Elspar 1659
Estratest (Rare) 2539
FML-S Liquifilm ◉ 242
Flexeril Tablets 1661
Floxin I.V. 1571
Floxin Tablets (200 mg, 300 mg, 400 mg) (Less than 1%) 1567
Fluorescite ◉ 219
Fortaz (Immediate in 1 in 285 patients) 1100
Geocillin Tablets 2199
Gris-PEG Tablets, 125 mg & 250 mg 479
Halotestin Tablets 2614
Heparin Sodium Vials 1441
Hep-B-Gammagee (Rare) 1663
Hibistat Germicidal Hand Rinse (Very rare) 2841
Hydeltrasol Injection, Sterile 1665
Hydeltra-T.B.A. Sterile Suspension 1667
Hydrocortone Acetate Sterile Suspension 1669
Hydrocortone Phosphate Injection, Sterile 1670
Hydrocortone Tablets 1672
Hyperstat I.V. Injection 2363
Imitrex Injection (Infrequent) 1103
Imitrex Tablets (Frequent) 1106
Imodium Capsules 1295
Inderide Tablets 2732
Indocin (Less than 1%) 1680
Inocor Lactate Injection 2309
ISMOTIC 45% w/v Solution ◉ 222
Kefurox Vials, Faspak & ADD-Vantage (Less than 1%) 1454
Kefzol Vials, Faspak & ADD-Vantage 1456
Lacrisert Sterile Ophthalmic Insert 1686
Leukeran Tablets 1133
Lopressor HCT Tablets 832
Lupron Injection 2555
Maxitrol Ophthalmic Ointment and Suspension ◉ 224
Mesnex Injection 702
Metubine Iodide Vials 916
Miacalcin Injection 2273
Miltown Tablets 2672
Mustargen 1709
Nembutal Sodium Capsules 436
Nembutal Sodium Solution 438
Nembutal Sodium Suppositories (Less than 1%) 440
NeoDecadron Topical Cream 1714
Nizoral Tablets (Several cases) 1298
Norflex 1496
Normodyne Injection (Rare) 2377
Normodyne Tablets (Rare) 2379
Noroxin Tablets 1715
Noroxin Tablets 2048
Novocain Hydrochloride for Spinal Anesthesia (Rare) 2326
Ocupress Ophthalmic Solution, 1% Sterile ◉ 309
PBZ Tablets 845
PBZ-SR Tablets 844
Paraplatin for Injection (2%) 705
Peptavlon 2878
Peridex (Rare) 1978
Phenobarbital Elixir and Tablets 1469
Pontocaine Hydrochloride for Spinal Anesthesia 2330
Premarin with Methyltestosterone 2794
Prinzide Tablets 1737
Procardia XL Extended Release Tablets 1972
Proloprim Tablets 1155
Recombivax HB 1744
Rifadin 1528
Rimactane Capsules 847
Ritalin 848
Sandoglobulin I.V. 2290
Seromycin Pulvules 1476
Sodium Sulamyd (Single instance) 2387
Synarel Nasal Solution for Endometriosis (0.2%) 2152
Talacen (A few cases) 2333
Tenoretic Tablets 2845
TERAK Ointment (Rare) ◉ 209
Tetanus Toxoid Adsorbed Purogenated 1403
TheraCys BCG Live (Intravesical) (Up to 1.8%) 897
Tigan 2057
Timoptic in Ocudose (Less frequent) 1753
Timoptic Sterile Ophthalmic Solution (Less frequent) 1751
TobraDex Ophthalmic Suspension and Ointment (Less than 4%) 473
Tobrex Ophthalmic Ointment and Solution (Less than 3 of 100 patients) ◉ 229
Tonocard Tablets (Less than 1%) 531
Toradol (1% or less) 2159
Trandate (Rare) 1185
Trimpex Tablets (Rare) 2163
Urobiotic-250 Capsules 2214
Vancenase AQ Nasal Spray 0.042% (Rare) 2393
Vanceril Inhaler (Rare) 2394
Vasocidin Ophthalmic Solution ◉ 270
Vasosulf (Rare) ◉ 271
Viroptic Ophthalmic Solution, 1% Sterile 1204
Xylocaine Injections 567
Zantac (Rare) 1209
Zantac Injection (Rare) 1207
Zantac Syrup (Rare) 1209
Zephiran (Rare) ▣ 795
Zinacef (Fewer than 1%) 1211
Zyloprim Tablets (Less than 1%) 1226

Hypersensitivity pancreatitis

Imuran 1110

Hypersensitivity pneumonitis

Fungizone Intravenous 506
Pentasa (Infrequent) 1527
Relafen Tablets (Rarer) 2510

Hypersensitivity reactions, Arthus-type

Diphtheria and Tetanus Toxoids and Pertussis Vaccine Adsorbed (Rare) 2477
Diphtheria and Tetanus Toxoids and Pertussis Vaccine Adsorbed USP (For Pediatric Use) 875
Tripedia 892

Hypersensitivity reactions, general

Alkeran Tablets 1071
Altace Capsules (Less than 1%) 1232
Ancef Injection 2465
Asacol Delayed-Release Tablets (Some patients) 1979
Augmentin 2468
Axid Pulvules (Rare) 1427
Betaseron for SC Injection 658
Betimol 0.25%, 0.5% ◉ 261
Bioclate, Antihemophilic Factor (Recombinant) 513
Brethine Ampuls 815
Brethine Tablets 814
Carafate Suspension 1505
Carafate Tablets 1504
Ceclor Pulvules & Suspension (About 1.5%) 1431
Ceftin 1078
Ceptaz (2% of patients) 1081
Ceredase (A limited number of patients) 1065
Chibroxin Sterile Ophthalmic Solution (With oral form) 1617
Cipro Tablets 592
Cleocin Phosphate Injection 2586
Cleocin Vaginal Cream 2589
Clozaril Tablets 2252
Coumadin (Infrequent) 926
Dalalone D.P. Injectable 1011
Deltasone Tablets 2595
Depo-Medrol Single-Dose Vial 2600
Depo-Medrol Sterile Aqueous Suspension 2597
Didronel Tablets 1984
Digibind 1091
Dilantin-125 Suspension 1911
Dobutrex Solution Vials (Occasional) 1439
Doryx Capsules 1913
Duranest Injections 542
Ethiodol (Infrequent) 2340
Etrafon (Extremely rare) 2355
Factrel (Rare) 2877
▲Fulvicin P/G Tablets (Among most common) 2359
Fulvicin P/G 165 & 330 Tablets 2359
Gamimune N, 5% Immune Globulin Intravenous (Human), 5% (One patient) 619
Gamimune N, 10% Immune Globulin Intravenous (Human), 10% (One patient) 621
Gammagard S/D, Immune Globulin, Intravenous (Human) (A remote possibility) 585
Gantrisin 2120
Glauctabs ◉ 208
Grifulvin V (griseofulvin tablets) Microsize (griseofulvin oral suspension) Microsize 1888
Heparin Lock Flush Solution 2725
Heparin Sodium Injection 2726
Heparin Sodium Injection, USP, Sterile Solution 2615
Hespan Injection 929

(▣ Described in PDR For Nonprescription Drugs) Incidence data in parenthesis; ▲ 3% or more (◉ Described in PDR For Ophthalmology)

Hypersensitivity reactions, general — Side Effects Index — 1328

Hyzaar Tablets 1677
▲ Ilotycin Ophthalmic Ointment (Among most frequent) 912
INFeD (Iron Dextran Injection, USP) 2345
Keflex Pulvules & Oral Suspension 914
Kytril Injection (Rare) 2490
Kytril Tablets (Rare) 2492
Lasix Injection, Oral Solution and Tablets 1240
Lescol Capsules (Rare) 2267
Levoprome 1274
Lincocin 2617
Lorabid Suspension and Pulvules 1459
Lotensin Tablets 834
Lutrepulse for Injection 980
MZM ⊙ 267
Maxzide 1380
Mebaral Tablets (Less than 1 in 100) 2322
Medrol 2621
Menomune-A/C/Y/W-135 889
Metaproterenol Sulfate Inhalation Solution, USP, Arm-a-Med (Rare) 552
Mevacor Tablets (Rare) 1699
Minocin Pellet-Filled Capsules 1383
Monocid Injection (Less than 1%) 2497
Neosporin Ophthalmic Solution Sterile (Rare) 1149
Norcuron 1826
Nubain Injection (1% or less) 935
Ogen Vaginal Cream 2630
Omnipen Capsules 2764
Oncaspar (Greater than 1% but less than 5%) 2028
Orthoclone OKT3 Sterile Solution 1837
Pen•Vee K (Occasional) 2772
Pentaspan Injection 937
Pergonal (menotropins for injection, USP) (Some patients) 2448
Phenobarbital Elixir and Tablets (Less than 1 in 100 patients) 1469
Polytrim Ophthalmic Solution Sterile (Multiple reports) 482
Profasi (chorionic gonadotropin for injection, USP) 2450
Proscar Tablets 1741
▲ Prostep (nicotine transdermal system) (3% of patients) 1394
Rabies Vaccine Adsorbed (Less than 1%) 2508
ReoPro Vials 1471
Rifater 1532
Seconal Sodium Pulvules (Less than 1 in 100) 1474
Semprex-D Capsules (Rare) 463
Semprex-D Capsules (Rare) 1167
Serevent Inhalation Aerosol (Rare) 1176
Skelaxin Tablets 788
Solu-Cortef Sterile Powder 2641
Spectrobid Tablets 2206
Streptase for Infusion 562
Supprelin Injection 2056
▲ Taxol (2% to 41%) 714
Tessalon Perles 1020
Timoptic-XE 1755
Tornalate Solution for Inhalation, 0.2% 956
Tornalate Metered Dose Inhaler 957
Trasylol 613
Tympagesic Ear Drops 2342
Unasyn 2212
Univasc Tablets (Less than 1%) 2410
Vancenase PocketHaler Nasal Inhaler 2391
Vermox Chewable Tablets (Rare) 1312
▲ Vumon (5%) 727
Zefazone 2654
Zocor Tablets (Rare) 1775
Zofran Injection (Rare) 1214

Hypersensitivity vasculitis

Aldoclor Tablets 1598
Aldomet Ester HCl Injection 1602
Aldomet Oral Suspension 1600
Aldoril Tablets 1604
Brethine Ampuls (Rare) 815
Brethine Tablets (Rare) 814
Bricanyl Subcutaneous Injection (Rare) 1502
Bricanyl Tablets (Rare) 1503
Clinoril Tablets (Less than 1 in 100) 1618
Dolobid Tablets (Less than 1 in 100) 1654
Streptase for Infusion 562
Tagamet (Rare) 2516

Hypersomnia

Luvox Tablets (Infrequent) 2544
Nardil (Common) 1920
Prinivil Tablets (0.3% to 1.0%) 1733
Prinzide Tablets 1737
Zestoretic 2850
Zestril Tablets (0.3% to 1.0%) 2854

Hypertension

Abbokinase 403
Abbokinase Open-Cath 405
Activase 1058
Adenocard Injection 1021
Adenoscan (Less than 1%) 1024
Adipex-P Tablets and Capsules 1048
Children's Advil Suspension (Less than 1%) 2692
AeroBid Inhaler System (1-3%) 1005
Aerobid-M Inhaler System (1-3%) 1005
Airet Solution for Inhalation (1% to 3.1%) 452
Albalon Solution with Liquifilm ⊙ 231
▲ Alfenta Injection (18%) 1286
Alupent 669
Ambien Tablets (Infrequent) 2416
Amen Tablets 780
Ana-Kit Anaphylaxis Emergency Treatment Kit 617
Anectine 1073
Ansaid Tablets (Less than 1%) 2579
▲ Aredia for Injection (Up to at least 15%) 810
Aristocort Suspension (Forte Parenteral) 1027
Aristocort Suspension (Intralesional) 1025
Aristocort Tablets 1022
Aristospan Suspension (Intra-articular) 1033
Aristospan Suspension (Intralesional) 1032
Regular Strength Ascriptin Tablets ▣ 629
Asendin Tablets (Less than 1%) 1369
Atamet (Rare) 572
Atgam Sterile Solution (Less than 1% to less than 5%) 2581
Ativan Injection (0.1%) 2698
Atretol Tablets 573
Atrohist Plus Tablets 454
Atrovent Inhalation Solution (0.9%) 673
Genuine Bayer Aspirin Tablets & Caplets (Small increases at doses of 1000 mg/day) ▣ 713
Betapace Tablets (Less than 1% to 2%) 641
▲ Betaseron for SC Injection (7%) 658
Betimol 0.25%, 0.5% (1% to 5%) ⊙ 261
Biphetamine Capsules 983
Bontril Slow-Release Capsules 781
Brethaire Inhaler (Fewer than 1 per 100) 813
Brevicon 2088
▲ Bromfed-DM Cough Syrup (Among most frequent) 1786
Buprenex Injectable (Less than 1%) 2006
BuSpar (Infrequent) 737
Cafergot 2251
Carbocaine Hydrochloride Injection 2303
Cardene I.V. (0.7%) 2709
Cataflam (Less than 1%) 816
Caverject (2%) 2583
Celestone Soluspan Suspension 2347
▲ CellCept Capsules (28.2% to 32.4%; 16.9% to 17.6%) 2099
Cipro I.V. (1% or less) 595
Cipro I.V. Pharmacy Bulk Package (Less than 1%) 597
Cipro Tablets (Less than 1%) 592
Claritin (2% or fewer patients) 2349
Claritin-D (Less frequent) 2350
Climara Transdermal System (Occasional) 645
Clinoril Tablets (Less than 1%) 1618
Clomid 1514
▲ Clozaril Tablets (4%) 2252
Cognex Capsules (Frequent) 1901
CORTENEMA 2535
Cortifoam 2396
Cortone Acetate Sterile Suspension 1623
Cortone Acetate Tablets 1624
Cycrin Tablets 975
Cytotec (Infrequent) 2424
Cytovene (1% or less) 2103
DDAVP Injection (Infrequent) 2014
DDAVP Rhinal Tube (Infrequent) 2017
D.H.E. 45 Injection (Occasional) 2255
Dalalone D.P. Injectable 1011
Dalgan Injection (Less than 1%) 538
Danocrine Capsules 2307
Decadron Elixir 1633
Decadron Phosphate Injection 1637
Decadron Phosphate Respihaler 1642
Decadron Phosphate Turbinaire 1645
Decadron Phosphate with Xylocaine Injection, Sterile 1639
Decadron Tablets 1635
Decadron-LA Sterile Suspension 1646
Deltasone Tablets 2595
Demulen 2428
Depakote Tablets (Greater than 1% but not more than 5%) 415
Depo-Medrol Single-Dose Vial 2600
Depo-Medrol Sterile Aqueous Suspension 2597
Depo-Provera Sterile Aqueous Suspension 2606
Desmopressin Acetate Rhinal Tube (Infrequent) 979
Desogen Tablets 1817
Desoxyn Gradumet Tablets 419
Desyrel and Desyrel Dividose (1.3% to 2.1%) 503
Dexacort Phosphate in Respihaler 458
Dexacort Phosphate in Turbinaire 459
Dexedrine 2474
DextroStat Dextroamphetamine Tablets 2036
Didrex Tablets 2607
Dilacor XR Extended-release Capsules 2018
Dilaudid-HP Injection (Less frequent) 1337
Dilaudid-HP Lyophilized Powder 250 mg (Less frequent) 1337
Dilaudid Tablets and Liquid 1339
Dimetane-DC Cough Syrup 2059
Dimetane-DX Cough Syrup 2059
Dipentum Capsules (Rare) 1951
▲ Diprivan Injection (Less than 1% to 8%) 2833
▲ Dobutrex Solution Vials (Most patients) 1439
Dopram Injectable 2061
Duragesic Transdermal System (1% to 3%) 1288
Ecotrin 2455
▲ Effexor (1.1% to 4.5%) 2719
Elavil 2838
Eldepryl Tablets 2550
Emete-con Intramuscular/Intravenous 2198
Endep Tablets 2174
▲ Epogen for Injection (0.75% to 24%) 489
Estrace Cream and Tablets (Occasional) 749
Estraderm Transdermal System 824
ESTRATAB Tablets (0.3, 0.625, 1.25, 2.5 mg) (Not uncommon) 2536
Estratest (Common) 2539
Ethmozine Tablets (Less than 2%) 2041
Etrafon 2355
Eulexin Capsules (1%) 2358
Fastin Capsules 2488
Felbatol 2666
Feldene Capsules (Less than 1%) 1965
Flexeril Tablets (Rare) 1661
Florinef Acetate Tablets 505
Floxin I.V. (Less than 1%) 1571
Floxin Tablets (200 mg, 300 mg, 400 mg) (Less than 1%) 1567
Flumadine Tablets & Syrup (Less than 0.3%) 1015
Foscavir Injection (Between 1% and 5%) 547
Fungizone Intravenous 506
Gammagard S/D, Immune Globulin, Intravenous (Human) (Occasional) 585
Garamycin Injectable 2360
Glucotrol XL Extended Release Tablets (Less than 1%) 1968
▲ Habitrol Nicotine Transdermal System (3% to 9% of patients) 865
Haldol Decanoate 1577
Haldol Injection, Tablets and Concentrate 1575
Halfprin 1362
Hivid Tablets (Less than 1% to less than 3%) 2121
Hycomine Compound Tablets 932
Hycomine 931
Hycotuss Expectorant Syrup 933
Hydeltrasol Injection, Sterile 1665
Hydeltra-T.B.A. Sterile Suspension 1667
Hydrocortone Acetate Sterile Suspension 1669
Hydrocortone Phosphate Injection, Sterile 1670
Hydrocortone Tablets 1672
IBU Tablets (Less than 1%) 1342
IFEX (Less than 1%) 697
Imdur (Less than or equal to 5%) 1323
Imitrex Injection (Infrequent) 1103
Imitrex Tablets (Infrequent) 1106
Inapsine Injection 1296
Indocin Capsules (Less than 1%) 1680
Indocin I.V. (Less than 1%) 1684
Indocin (Less than 1%) 1680
INFeD (Iron Dextran Injection, USP) 2345
Intron A (Less than 5%) 2364
Ionamin Capsules 990
Isuprel Hydrochloride Injection 1:5000 2311
Kerlone Tablets (Less than 2%) 2436
Kytril Injection (2%) 2490
Kytril Tablets (1%) 2492
Lamictal Tablets (Rare) 1112
Larodopa Tablets (Rare) 2129
Levlen/Tri-Levlen 651
Levophed Bitartrate Injection 2315
Limbitrol 2180
Lioresal Intrathecal (1 to 2 of 214 patients) 1596
Lodine Capsules and Tablets (Less than 1%) 2743
Lo/Ovral Tablets 2746
Lo/Ovral-28 Tablets 2751
Loxitane 1378
Ludiomil Tablets (Rare) 843
Lupron Depot 3.75 mg 2556
Lupron Depot 7.5 mg 2559
▲ Lupron Injection (5% or more) 2555
Luvox Tablets (Frequent) 2544
Lysodren (Infrequent) 698
MS Contin Tablets (Less frequent) 1994
MSIR (Infrequent) 1997
Maxaquin Tablets (Less than 1%) 2440
Medrol 2621
▲ Megace Oral Suspension (Up to 8%) 699
Megace Tablets 701
Menest Tablets 2494
Mepergan Injection (Rare) 2753
Metaproterenol Sulfate Inhalation Solution, USP, Arm-a-Med (1 in 300 patients) 552
▲ Methergine (Most common) 2272
Mexitil Capsules (Less than 1% or about 1 in 1,000) 678
Miacalcin Nasal Spray (1% to 3%) 2275
Micronor Tablets 1872
Modicon 1872
Monoket (Fewer than 1%) 2406
Monopril Tablets (0.4% to 1.0%) 757
Children's Motrin Ibuprofen Oral Suspension (Less than 1%) 1546
Motrin Tablets (Less than 1%) 2625
Motrin Ibuprofen Suspension, Oral Drops, Chewable Tablets, Caplets (Less than 1%) 1546
Mutamycin 703
Narcan Injection (Several instances) 934
NebuPent for Inhalation Solution (1% or less) 1040
▲ Neoral (Approximately 50% to most patients) 2276
Neo-Synephrine Hydrochloride (Ophthalmic) (Rare) 2325
▲ Neupogen for Injection (4%) 495
Neurontin Capsules (Frequent) 1922
Nicorette (1% to 3% of patients) 2458
Nimotop Capsules (Less than 1%) 610
Nordette-21 Tablets 2755
Nordette-28 Tablets 2758
Norinyl 2088
Norpramin Tablets 1526
Nor-Q D Tablets 2135
Novocain Hydrochloride for Spinal Anesthesia 2326
Nubain Injection (1% or less) 935
Ogen Tablets (Occasional) 2627
Ogen Vaginal Cream (Occasional) 2630
Oncaspar (Less than 1%) 2028
Oncovin Solution Vials & Hyporets 1466
OptiPranolol (Metipranolol 0.3%) Sterile Ophthalmic Solution (A small number of patients) ⊙ 258
Oramorph SR (Morphine Sulfate Sustained Release Tablets) (Less frequent) 2236
Orap Tablets 1050
Orlamm (Low frequency) 2239
Ornade Spansule Capsules 2502
Ortho-Cept 1851
Ortho-Cyclen/Ortho-Tri-Cyclen 1858
Ortho Dienestrol Cream 1866
Ortho-Est (Occasional) 1869

(▣ Described in PDR For Nonprescription Drugs) Incidence data in parenthesis; ▲ 3% or more (⊙ Described in PDR For Ophthalmology)

1329 **Side Effects Index** **Hypertrichosis**

Ortho-Novum 1872
Ortho-Cyclen/Ortho Tri-Cyclen 1858
▲ Orthoclone OKT3 Sterile Solution (8%) 1837
Orudis Capsules (Less than 1%) 2766
Oruvail Capsules (Less than 1%) 2766
Ovcon 760
Ovral Tablets 2770
Ovral-28 Tablets 2770
Ovrette Tablets 2771
PMB 200 and PMB 400 2783
Pamelor 2280
Papaverine Hydrochloride Vials and Ampoules 1468
Parlodel 2281
Paxil Tablets (Frequent) 2505
Pediapred Oral Liquid 995
Permax Tablets (1.6%) 575
Phenergan with Codeine 2777
Phenergan with Dextromethorphan 2778
Phenergan Injection 2773
Phenergan Suppositories 2775
Phenergan Syrup 2774
Phenergan Tablets 2775
Phenergan VC 2779
Phenergan VC with Codeine 2781
Pilocar (Extremely rare) ⊙ 268
Pondimin Tablets 2066
Prelone Syrup 1787
Prelu-2 Timed Release Capsules 681
Premarin Intravenous 2787
Premarin with Methyltestosterone 2794
Premarin Tablets 2789
Premarin Vaginal Cream 2791
PREVACID Delayed-Release Capsules (Less than 1%) 2562
Prilosec Delayed-Release Capsules (Less than 1%) 529
Priscoline Hydrochloride Ampuls 845
▲ Procrit for Injection (0.75% to 24%) 1841
Proglycem (A few cases) 580
▲ Prograf (Common; 31% to 47%) 1042
Prolixin 509
Propagest Tablets 786
PROPINE with C CAP Compliance Cap ⊙ 253
Protopam Chloride for Injection 2806
Proventil Inhalation Aerosol (Less than 5%) 2382
Proventil Inhalation Solution 0.083% (1% to 3.1%) 2384
Proventil Repetabs Tablets 2386
Proventil Solution for Inhalation 0.5% (1% to 3.1%) 2383
Proventil Syrup 2385
Proventil Tablets 2386
Provera Tablets 2636
Prozac Pulvules & Liquid, Oral Solution (Infrequent) 919
Reglan 2068
Relafen Tablets (Less than 1%) 2510
ReVia Tablets (Less than 1%) 940
▲ Revex (5%) 1811
Risperdal (Infrequent) 1301
Rocaltrol Capsules 2141
Roferon-A Injection (Less than 3%) 2145
Rogaine Topical Solution (1.53%) 2637
Romazicon (Less than 1%) 2147
Rondec Oral Drops 953
Rondec Syrup 953
Rondec Tablet 953
Rondec-DM Oral Drops 954
Rondec-DM Syrup 954
Rondec-TR Tablet 953
▲ Salagen Tablets (3%) 1489
▲ Sandimmune (13 to 53%) 2286
Sandostatin Injection (Less than 1%) 2292
Serevent Inhalation Aerosol 1176
Serzone Tablets (Infrequent) 771
Sinemet Tablets (Rare) 943
Sinemet CR Tablets 944
Sinequan (Occasional) 2205
Sinulin Tablets 787
Solu-Cortef Sterile Powder 2641
Solu-Medrol Sterile Powder 2643
Sporanox Capsules (0.3% to 3.2%) 1305
Stadol (Less than 1%) 775
Stilphostrol Tablets and Ampuls 612
Stimate, (desmopressin acetate) Nasal Spray, 1.5 mg/mL (Infrequent) 525
Sublimaze Injection 1307
▲ Sufenta Injection (3% to 9%) 1309
Supprelin Injection (1% to 3%) 2056
Suprane (Greater than 1%) 1813
Surmontil Capsules 2811
Survanta Beractant Intratracheal Suspension (Less than 1%) 2226
Symmetrel Capsules and Syrup (0.1% to 1%) 946
Talwin Injection (Infrequent) 2334
Tambocor Tablets (Less than 1%) 1497
Taxol (1%) 714
Tegretol Chewable Tablets 852
Tegretol Suspension 852
Tegretol Tablets 852
Teslac 717
THYREL TRH (A small number of patients) 2873
Timoptic in Ocudose (Less frequent) 1753
Timoptic Sterile Ophthalmic Solution (Less frequent) 1751
Timoptic-XE 1755
Tofranil Ampuls 854
Tofranil Tablets 856
Tofranil-PM Capsules 857
▲ Tolectin (200, 400 and 600 mg) (3 to 9%) 1581
Tonocard Tablets (Less than 1%) 531
Toradol (Greater than 1%) 2159
Tornalate Solution for Inhalation, 0.2% (Less than 1%) 956
Trasylol (2%) 613
Triavil Tablets 1757
Trilafon (Occasional) 2389
Levlen/Tri-Levlen 651
Trinalin Repetabs Tablets 1330
Tri-Norinyl 2164
Triostat Injection (Approximately 1%) 2530
Triphasil-21 Tablets 2814
Triphasil-28 Tablets 2819
Ultram Tablets (50 mg) (Infrequent) 1585
Vascor (200, 300 and 400 mg) Tablets (0.5 to 2.0%) 1587
Vasotec I.V. 1768
Vasoxyl Injection 1196
▲ Velban Vials (Among most common) 1484
▲ Ventolin Inhalation Aerosol and Refill (Fewer than 5 per 100 patients) 1197
Ventolin Inhalation Solution (1% to 3.1%) 1198
Ventolin Nebules Inhalation Solution (1% to 3.1%) 1199
Ventolin Rotacaps for Inhalation 1200
Ventolin Syrup 1202
Ventolin Tablets 1203
VePesid Capsules and Injection 718
Versed Injection 2170
Vicodin Tuss Expectorant 1358
Videx Tablets, Powder for Oral Solution, & Pediatric Powder for Oral Solution (2%) 720
Vivactil Tablets 1774
Volmax Extended-Release Tablets 1788
Voltaren Tablets (Less than 1%) 861
Vumon 727
▲ Wellbutrin Tablets (4.3%) 1204
Yocon 1892
Yohimex Tablets 1363
Zemuron (0.1%; 2%) 1830
Zerit Capsules (Fewer than 1% to 2%) 729
▲ Zoladex (Greater than 1% but less than 5%) 2858
Zoloft Tablets (Infrequent) 2217
Zosyn (1.6%) 1419
Zosyn Pharmacy Bulk Package (1.6%) 1422

Hypertension, aggravation

Ambien Tablets (Rare) 2416
Atretol Tablets 573
Atrovent Inhalation Solution (0.9%) 673
Tegretol Chewable Tablets 852
Tegretol Suspension 852
Tegretol Tablets 852
Zoloft Tablets (Rare) 2217

Hypertension, intracranial

Azo Gantrisin Tablets 2081
Betaseron for SC Injection 658
Carmol HC (Infrequent to frequent) 924
Cutivate Cream 1088
Cutivate Ointment 1089
Cytovene-IV (Two or more reports) 2103
Danocrine Capsules (Rare) 2307
Dermatop Emollient Cream 0.1% 1238
Diprivan Injection (Less than 1%) 2833
Doryx Capsules 1913
Dynacin Capsules 1590
Humatrope Vials (Small number of patients) 1443
Macrobid Capsules (Rare) 1988
Macrodantin Capsules (Seldom reported) 1989
Minocin Intravenous 1382
Minocin Oral Suspension 1385
Minocin Pellet-Filled Capsules 1383
Monodox Capsules 1805
Norplant System (Less than 1%) 2759
Permax Tablets (Rare) 575
ProctoCream-HC 2.5% 2408
Terramycin Intramuscular Solution 2210
Urobiotic-250 Capsules 2214
Vibramycin 1941
Vibramycin Hyclate Intravenous 2215
Vibramycin 1941

Hypertension, rebound

Deponit NTG Transdermal Delivery System (Uncommon) 2397
Isordil Sublingual Tablets (Uncommon) 2739
Isordil Tembids (Uncommon) 2741
Isordil Titradose Tablets (Uncommon) 2742
Nitro-Bid IV (Uncommon) 1523
Nitro-Bid Ointment (Uncommon) 1524
Nitrodisc (Uncommon) 2047
Nitro-Dur (nitroglycerin) Transdermal Infusion System (Uncommon) 1326
Sorbitrate (Uncommon) 2843
Tenex Tablets (Less common) 2074
Transderm-Nitro Transdermal Therapeutic System (Uncommon) 859

Hypertensive crises

Accupril Tablets (Rare) 1893
Emete-con Intramuscular/Intravenous 2198
Monopril Tablets (0.2% to 1.0%) 757
Sandostatin Injection (Less than 1%) 2292

Hyperthermia

Asendin Tablets (Less than 1%) 1369
Biltricide Tablets 591
Cholera Vaccine 2711
Cogentin 1621
Effexor 2719
Elspar 1659
Emete-con Intramuscular/Intravenous 2198
Furoxone (Rare) 2046
Geocillin Tablets 2199
Humate-P, Antihemophilic Factor (Human), Pasteurized (Rare) 520
Hyperab Rabies Immune Globulin (Human) 624
Hyper-Tet Tetanus Immune Globulin (Human) 627
HypRho-D Full Dose Rho (D) Immune Globulin (Human) 629
HypRho-D Mini-Dose Rho (D) Immune Globulin (Human) 628
Lomotil 2439
MICRhoGAM Rh_0(D) Immune Globulin (Human) (Reported in a small number of women) 1847
Marcaine Hydrochloride with Epinephrine 1:200,000 (Rare) 2316
Marcaine Hydrochloride Injection (Rare) 2316
Marcaine Spinal (Rare) 2319
Motofen Tablets 784
Nescaine/Nescaine MPF 554
Prolixin 509
Reglan 2068
Rocaltrol Capsules 2141
Sensorcaine (Rare) 559
Stelazine 2514
Temaril Tablets, Syrup and Spansule Extended-Release Capsules 483
Typhoid Vaccine 2823

Hyperthyroidism

Anafranil Capsules (Rare) 803
Cartrol Tablets 410
Cognex Capsules (Rare) 1901
Cordarone Tablets (1 to 3%) 2712
Cytomel Tablets 2473
Effexor (Rare) 2719
Eskalith (Rare) 2485
Intron A (Less than 5%) 2364
Lamictal Tablets (Rare) 1112
Levothroid Tablets (Rare) 1016
Levoxyl Tablets 903
Lithium Carbonate Capsules & Tablets (Rare cases) 2230
Lithonate/Lithotabs/Lithobid (Rare) 2543
Miacalcin Nasal Spray (Less than 1%) 2275
Neurontin Capsules (Rare) 1922
Paxil Tablets (Rare) 2505
Synthroid Injection (Rare) 1359
Prozac Pulvules & Liquid, Oral Solution (Rare) 919
Synthroid Tablets (Rare) 1359
Tenoretic Tablets 2845
Tenormin Tablets and I.V. Injection 2847

Hypertonia

Adalat CC (Less than 1.0%) 589
▲ Anafranil Capsules (2% to 4%) 803
Ansaid Tablets (Less than 1%) 2579
▲ Asacol Delayed-Release Tablets (5%) 1979
▲ Betaseron for SC Injection (26%) 658
Cardene I.V. (Rare) 2709
Cardura Tablets (1%) 2186
Ceclor Pulvules & Suspension (Rare) 1431
▲ CellCept Capsules (More than or equal to 3%) 2099
Claritin-D (Less frequent) 2350
Cognex Capsules (Frequent) 1901
Cytovene (1% or less) 2103
Depakote Tablets (Greater than 1% but not more than 5%) 415
Dilacor XR Extended-release Capsules (Infrequent) 2018
Diprivan Injection (Less than 1%) 2833
Duragesic Transdermal System (Less than 1%) 1288
▲ Effexor (3%; infrequent) 2719
Eskalith 2485
Flexeril Tablets (Less than 1%) 1661
Foscavir Injection (Less than 1%) 547
Glucotrol XL Extended Release Tablets (Less than 1%) 1968
Havrix (Less than 1%) 2489
Hivid Tablets (Less than 1% to less than 3%) 2121
Intron A (Less than 5%) 2364
Lamictal Tablets (Rare) 1112
Lithonate/Lithotabs/Lithobid 2543
Lotensin Tablets 834
Lotensin HCT (1.5%) 837
Lozol Tablets (Less than 5%) 2022
Luvox Tablets (2%) 2544
Norvasc Tablets (Less than or equal to 0.1%) 1940
Paxil Tablets (Infrequent) 2505
Penetrex Tablets (Less than 1% but more than or equal to 0.1%) 2031
Permax Tablets (1.1%) 575
Procardia XL Extended Release Tablets (1% or less) 1972
▲ Prograf (Greater than 3%) 1042
Prozac Pulvules & Liquid, Oral Solution (Rare) 919
Serzone Tablets (1%) 771
Tegison Capsules (Less than 1%) 2154
▲ Ultram Tablets (50 mg) (1% to 14%) 1585
Videx Tablets, Powder for Oral Solution, & Pediatric Powder for Oral Solution (Less than 1%) 720
Zoladex (1%) 2858
Zoloft Tablets (1.3%) 2217

Hypertrichosis

Aclovate Cream 1069
Anafranil Capsules (Rare) 803
Analpram-HC Rectal Cream 1% and 2.5% 977
Anusol-HC Cream 2.5% (Infrequent to frequent) 1896
Aristocort A 0.025% Cream (Infrequent) 1027
Aristocort A 0.5% Cream 1031
Aristocort A 0.1% Cream (Infrequent) 1029
Aristocort A 0.1% Ointment (Infrequent) 1030
Carmol HC (Infrequent to frequent) 924
Clomid 1514
Cordran Lotion (Infrequent) 1803
Cordran Tape (Infrequent) 1804
Cortifoam 2396
Cortisporin Cream 1084
Cortisporin Ointment 1085
Cortisporin Otic Solution Sterile 1087
Cortisporin Otic Suspension Sterile 1088
Cutivate Ointment (Less than 1%) 1089
Cyclocort Topical (Infrequent) 1037

(▣ Described in PDR For Nonprescription Drugs) Incidence data in parenthesis; ▲ 3% or more (⊙ Described in PDR For Ophthalmology)

Hypertrichosis — Side Effects Index — 1330

Decadron Phosphate Topical Cream ... 1644
Decaspray Topical Aerosol ... 1648
Dilantin Infatabs ... 1908
Dilantin Kapseals ... 1906
Dilantin Parenteral ... 1910
Dilantin-125 Suspension ... 1911
Diprolene (Infrequent) ... 2352
Elocon (Infrequent) ... 2354
Epifoam (Infrequent) ... 2399
Florone/Florone E ... 906
Halog (Infrequent) ... 2686
Hytone ... 907
Kerlone Tablets (Less than 2%) ... 2436
Lidex (Infrequent) ... 2130
Locoid Cream, Ointment and Topical Solution (Infrequent) ... 978
▲ Loniten Tablets (About 80%) ... 2618
Lotrisone Cream (Infrequent) ... 2372
Mantadil Cream ... 1135
NeoDecadron Topical Cream ... 1714
Norplant System ... 2759
PediOtic Suspension Sterile ... 1153
Pramosone Cream, Lotion & Ointment ... 978
ProctoCream-HC (Infrequent) ... 2408
ProctoCream-HC 2.5% (Infrequent to frequent) ... 2408
ProctoFoam-HC ... 2409
Proglycem ... 580
Psorcon Ointment 0.05% ... 908
Risperdal (Rare) ... 1301
Rogaine Topical Solution ... 2637
Synalar (Infrequent) ... 2130
Temovate (Infrequent) ... 1179
Topicort (Infrequent) ... 1243
Tridesilon Cream 0.05% (Infrequent) ... 615
Tridesilon Ointment 0.05% (Infrequent) ... 616
Ultravate Cream 0.05% (Infrequent) ... 2689
Ultravate Ointment 0.05% ... 2690
Westcort ... 2690
Zoloft Tablets (Rare) ... 2217

Hypertriglyceridemia

▲ Accutane Capsules (Approximately 25%) ... 2076
Atretol Tablets (Occasional reports) ... 573
Blocadren Tablets ... 1614
Brevicon ... 2088
▲ Cipro I.V. (Among most frequent) ... 595
▲ Cipro I.V. Pharmacy Bulk Package (Among most frequent) ... 597
Cipro Tablets ... 592
Cytovene-IV (One report) ... 2103
Demulen ... 2428
Diflucan Injection, Tablets, and Oral Suspension ... 2194
Ergamisol Tablets ... 1292
Estratest ... 2539
Floxin I.V. ... 1571
Floxin Tablets (200 mg, 300 mg, 400 mg) ... 1567
Hivid Tablets (Less than 1% to less than 3%) ... 2121
Hyzaar Tablets ... 1677
Levlen/Tri-Levlen (A small portion of women) ... 651
Lo/Ovral Tablets ... 2746
Lo/Ovral-28 Tablets ... 2751
Lotensin HCT ... 837
▲ Lupron Depot 3.75 mg (12%) ... 2556
Maxaquin Tablets ... 2440
Micronor Tablets ... 1872
Modicon ... 1872
Nizoral Tablets ... 1298
Nordette-21 Tablets ... 2755
Nordette-28 Tablets ... 2758
Norinyl ... 2088
Noroxin Tablets ... 1715
Noroxin Tablets ... 2048
Norpace (1 to 3%) ... 2444
Nor-Q D Tablets ... 2135
Ortho-Cyclen/Ortho-Tri-Cyclen ... 1858
Ortho-Novum ... 1872
Ortho-Cyclen/Ortho Tri-Cyclen ... 1858
Ovcon ... 760
Ovral Tablets ... 2770
Ovral-28 Tablets ... 2770
Ovrette Tablets ... 2771
Penetrex Tablets ... 2031
Premarin Tablets ... 2789
Premarin Vaginal Cream ... 2791
Prinzide Tablets ... 1737
Risperdal (Rare) ... 1301
Sporanox Capsules (Rare) ... 1305
▲ Synarel Nasal Solution for Endometriosis (12%) ... 2152
▲ Tegison Capsules (46%) ... 2154
Tegretol Chewable Tablets (Occasional) ... 852
Tegretol Suspension (Occasional) ... 852
Tegretol Tablets (Occasional) ... 852
Ticlid Tablets ... 2156
Timolide Tablets ... 1748
Levlen/Tri-Levlen (A small portion of women) ... 651
Tri-Norinyl ... 2164
Triphasil-21 Tablets ... 2814
Triphasil-28 Tablets ... 2819
Vaseretic Tablets ... 1765
▲ Zebeta Tablets (Most frequent laboratory change) ... 1413
Zestoretic ... 2850
Zoladex ... 2858
Zoloft Tablets ... 2217

Hypertrophic papillae of the tongue

Primaxin I.M. ... 1727
Primaxin I.V. (Less than 0.2%) ... 1729
Serentil ... 684

Hypertrophy, genital

Supprelin Injection (2% to 3%) ... 2056

Hypertrophy, gum

Cytovene-IV (One report) ... 2103
Peganone Tablets ... 446
Zarontin Capsules ... 1928
Zarontin Syrup ... 1929

Hyperuricemia

▲ Accutane Capsules (1 in 10 patients) ... 2076
Adriamycin PFS ... 1947
Adriamycin RDF ... 1947
Aldoclor Tablets ... 1598
Aldoril Tablets ... 1604
Alka-Seltzer Effervescent Antacid and Pain Reliever (Less than 1.0 mg%) ... ▣ 701
Alka-Seltzer Lemon Lime Effervescent Antacid and Pain Reliever (Less than 1.0 mg%) ... ▣ 703
Altace Capsules (Rare) ... 1232
Anafranil Capsules (Infrequent) ... 803
Ansaid Tablets (Less than 1%) ... 2579
Apresazide Capsules ... 808
Regular Strength Ascriptin Tablets ... ▣ 629
Axid Pulvules ... 1427
Genuine Bayer Aspirin Tablets & Caplets (Less than 1.0% at doses of 1000 mg/day) ... ▣ 713
Benemid Tablets ... 1611
Blocadren Tablets ... 1614
Bufferin Analgesic Tablets and Caplets ... ▣ 613
▲ Bumex (18.4%) ... 2093
Capozide ... 742
Cardizem CD Capsules (Less than 1%) ... 1506
Cardizem SR Capsules (Less than 1%) ... 1510
Cardizem Injectable (Less than 1%) ... 1508
Cardizem Tablets (Less than 1%) ... 1512
▲ CellCept Capsules (More than or equal to 3%) ... 2099
Cerubidine ... 795
▲ Cipro I.V. (Among most frequent) ... 595
▲ Cipro I.V. Pharmacy Bulk Package (Among most frequent) ... 597
Cipro Tablets (Less than 0.1%) ... 592
Clozaril Tablets ... 2252
Combipres Tablets ... 677
Cotazym ... 1817
Creon ... 2536
Cytosar-U Sterile Powder ... 2592
Daranide Tablets ... 1633
Demadex Tablets and Injection ... 686
Diucardin Tablets ... 2718
Diupres Tablets ... 1650
Diuril Oral Suspension ... 1653
Diuril Sodium Intravenous ... 1652
Diuril Tablets ... 1653
Doxorubicin Astra ... 540
Dyazide ... 2479
Ecotrin ... 2455
Edecrin ... 1657
Effexor (Infrequent) ... 2719
Enduron Tablets ... 420
Esidrix Tablets ... 821
Esimil Tablets ... 822
Fludara for Injection ... 663
Halfprin (Less than 1.0 mg%) ... 1362
Hivid Tablets (Less than 1% to less than 3%) ... 2121
Hydrea Capsules (Occasional) ... 696
HydroDIURIL Tablets ... 1674
Hydropres Tablets ... 1675
Hyzaar Tablets ... 1677
Imdur (Less than or equal to 5%) ... 1323
Inderide Tablets ... 2732
Inderide LA Long Acting Capsules ... 2734
Kerlone Tablets (Less than 2%) ... 2436
Larodopa Tablets ... 2129
Lasix Injection, Oral Solution and Tablets ... 1240
Lopressor HCT Tablets ... 832
Lorelco Tablets ... 1517
Lotensin Tablets ... 834
Lotensin HCT ... 837
Lotrel Capsules (Rare) ... 840
Lozol Tablets (Less than 5%) ... 2022
Lupron Depot 7.5 mg (Less than 5%) ... 2559
Lupron Injection ... 2555
Maxzide ... 1380
Minizide Capsules ... 1938
Moduretic Tablets ... 1705
Myambutol Tablets ... 1386
Mykrox Tablets ... 993
Myleran Tablets ... 1143
Neoral (Occasional) ... 2276
▲ Neupogen for Injection (27% to 58%) ... 495
Nicolar Tablets ... 2026
Novantrone ... 1279
▲ Oncaspar (Greater than 1% but less than 5%) ... 2028
Oretic Tablets ... 443
Pancrease MT Capsules (With extremely high dose) ... 1579
Parlodel ... 2281
Permax Tablets (Rare) ... 575
Platinol ... 708
Platinol-AQ Injection ... 710
Prinzide Tablets ... 1737
Proglycem (Common) ... 580
▲ Prograf (Greater than 3%) ... 1042
▲ Proleukin for Injection (9%) ... 797
Purinethol Tablets ... 1156
Pyrazinamide Tablets ... 1398
Relafen Tablets (Less than 1%) ... 2510
Rifadin ... 1528
Rifamate Capsules ... 1530
Rifater ... 1532
Rimactane Capsules ... 847
Risperdal (Rare) ... 1301
Roferon-A Injection (Less than 5%) ... 2145
Rubex ... 712
Sandimmune (Occasional) ... 2286
Ser-Ap-Es Tablets ... 849
Slo-Niacin Tablets ... 2659
Tenoretic Tablets ... 2845
Thalitone ... 1245
Thioguanine Tablets, Tabloid Brand (Frequent) ... 1181
Timolide Tablets ... 1748
Ultrase Capsules ... 2343
Ultrase MT Capsules ... 2344
Univasc Tablets ... 2410
Vaseretic Tablets ... 1765
Videx Tablets, Powder for Oral Solution, & Pediatric Powder for Oral Solution (1% to 3%) ... 720
Viokase ... 2076
Zaroxolyn Tablets ... 1000
Zebeta Tablets ... 1413
Zestoretic ... 2850
Ziac ... 1415
Zymase Capsules (With extremely high doses) ... 1834

Hyperuricosuria

Creon ... 2536
Myleran Tablets ... 1143
Pancrease Capsules ... 1579
Pancrease MT Capsules (With extremely high dose) ... 1579
Ultrase Capsules ... 2343
Ultrase MT Capsules ... 2344

Hyperuricuria

Cotazym ... 1817
Pancrease Capsules ... 1579
Viokase ... 2076
Zymase Capsules (With extremely high doses) ... 1834

Hyperventilation

Adenocard Injection (Less than 1%) ... 1021
Anafranil Capsules (Infrequent) ... 803
Ansaid Tablets (Less than 1%) ... 2579
Betaseron for SC Injection ... 658
Bumex (0.1%) ... 2093
BuSpar (Infrequent) ... 737
Cataflam (Less than 1%) ... 816
Clozaril Tablets (Less than 1%) ... 2252
Cognex Capsules (Infrequent) ... 1901
Diprivan Injection (Less than 1%) ... 2833
Dizac (Less frequent) ... 1809
Effexor (Infrequent) ... 2719
Empirin with Codeine Tablets ... 1093
Ethmozine Tablets (Less than 2%) ... 2041
Glucophage ... 752
Lamictal Tablets (Infrequent) ... 1112
Luvox Tablets (Infrequent) ... 2544
Mono-Gesic Tablets ... 792
NebuPent for Inhalation Solution (1% or less) ... 1040
Neurontin Capsules (Rare) ... 1922
Orthoclone OKT3 Sterile Solution ... 1837
Paxil Tablets (Infrequent) ... 2505
Permax Tablets (Infrequent) ... 575
Primaxin I.M. ... 1727
Primaxin I.V. (Less than 0.2%) ... 1729
ProSom Tablets (Rare) ... 449
Protopam Chloride for Injection ... 2806
Prozac Pulvules & Liquid, Oral Solution (Infrequent) ... 919
Risperdal (Infrequent) ... 1301
▲ Romazicon (3% to 9%) ... 2147
Serzone Tablets (Rare) ... 771
Sulfamylon Cream ... 925
Supprelin Injection (1% to 3%) ... 2056
Valium Injectable ... 2182
Versed Injection (Less than 1%) ... 2170
Voltaren Tablets (Less than 1%) ... 861
▲ Xanax Tablets (9.7%) ... 2649
Yutopar Intravenous Injection (Infrequent) ... 570
Zoloft Tablets (Rare) ... 2217

Hypervitaminosis A syndrome

Aquasol A Vitamin A Capsules, USP ... 534
Aquasol A Parenteral ... 534

Hypervolemia

▲ CellCept Capsules (More than or equal to 3%) ... 2099
Foscavir Injection (Less than 1%) ... 547
NephrAmine ... 2005

Hypesthesia

Cardene I.V. (0.7%) ... 2709
Caverject (Less than 1%) ... 2583
Cognex Capsules (Infrequent) ... 1901
Cozaar Tablets (Less than 1%) ... 1628
Cytovene (1% or less) ... 2103
Effexor ... 2719
▲ Ethmozine Tablets (2% to 5%) ... 2041
Flumadine Tablets & Syrup ... 1015
Glucotrol XL Extended Release Tablets (Less than 3%) ... 1968
Hyzaar Tablets ... 1677
Lamictal Tablets (Infrequent) ... 1112
▲ Lopid Tablets (More common) ... 1917
Lotensin HCT (0.3% to 1.0%) ... 837
Lupron Depot 3.75 mg ... 2556
Megace Oral Suspension (1% to 3%) ... 699
▲ Navelbine Injection (Among most frequent neurologic toxicities) ... 1145
NebuPent for Inhalation Solution (1% or less) ... 1040
Neurontin Capsules (Infrequent) ... 1922
Orlamm (1% to 3%) ... 2239
Prozac Pulvules & Liquid, Oral Solution (Infrequent) ... 919
Recombivax HB ... 1744
ReoPro Vials (0.3%) ... 1471
Salagen Tablets (Less than 1%) ... 1489
Serzone Tablets ... 771

Hypnotic effects

Placidyl Capsules (Occasional) ... 448
Trilafon ... 2389

Hypoactivity

AeroBid Inhaler System (1-3%) ... 1005
Aerobid-M Inhaler System (1-3%) ... 1005
Dizac (Less frequent) ... 1809
Valium Injectable ... 2182

Hypoadrenalism

Sandostatin Injection (Less than 1%) ... 2292

Hypoadrenalism, neonatal

Aristocort Suspension (Forte Parenteral) ... 1027
Aristocort Suspension (Intralesional) ... 1025
Aristocort Tablets ... 1022
Aristospan Suspension (Intra-articular) ... 1033

(▣ Described in PDR For Nonprescription Drugs) Incidence data in parenthesis; ▲ 3% or more (◉ Described in PDR For Ophthalmology)

1331 Side Effects Index Hypokalemia

Aristospan Suspension (Intralesional) ... 1032
Azmacort Oral Inhaler ... 2011
Beconase ... 1076
Celestone Soluspan Suspension ... 2347
Cortone Acetate Tablets ... 1624
Dalalone D.P. Injectable ... 1011
Decadron Elixir ... 1633
Decadron Phosphate Injection ... 1637
Decadron Phosphate Respihaler ... 1642
Decadron Phosphate Turbinaire ... 1645
Decadron Phosphate with Xylocaine Injection, Sterile ... 1639
Decadron Tablets ... 1635
Decadron-LA Sterile Suspension ... 1646
Deltasone Tablets ... 2595
Depo-Medrol Single-Dose Vial ... 2600
Depo-Medrol Sterile Aqueous Suspension ... 2597
Dexacort Phosphate in Respihaler ... 458
Dexacort Phosphate in Turbinaire ... 459
Florinef Acetate Tablets ... 505
Hydeltrasol Injection, Sterile ... 1665
Hydeltra-T.B.A. Sterile Suspension 1667
Hydrocortone Acetate Sterile Suspension ... 1669
Hydrocortone Phosphate Injection, Sterile ... 1670
Hydrocortone Tablets ... 1672
Medrol ... 2621
Nasacort Nasal Inhaler ... 2024
Prelone Syrup ... 1787
Rhinocort Nasal Inhaler ... 556
Solu-Cortef Sterile Powder ... 2641
Solu-Medrol Sterile Powder ... 2643
Vancenase AQ Nasal Spray 0.042% ... 2393
Vancenase PocketHaler Nasal Inhaler ... 2391
Vanceril Inhaler ... 2394

Hypoalbuminemia
Cipro I.V. Pharmacy Bulk Package (Less than 1%) ... 597
Dapsone Tablets USP ... 1284
Maxaquin Tablets (Less than or equal to 0.1%) ... 2440
Oncaspar ... 2028
▲ Proleukin for Injection (8%) ... 797
Vantin for Oral Suspension and Vantin Tablets ... 2646
▲ Zanosar Sterile Powder (A number of patients) ... 2653
Zefazone ... 2654
Zosyn ... 1419
Zosyn Pharmacy Bulk Package ... 1422

Hypoalbuminuria
Elspar ... 1659
Unasyn ... 2212

Hypocalcemia
▲ Aredia for Injection (Up to 12%) ... 810
▲ CellCept Capsules (More than or equal to 3%) ... 2099
Cortifoam ... 2396
Cosmegen Injection ... 1626
Fleet Enema ... 1002
Fludara for Injection ... 663
▲ Foscavir Injection (5% or greater up to 15%) ... 547
Fungizone Intravenous ... 506
Ganite ... 2533
Garamycin Injectable ... 2360
Hivid Tablets (Less than 1% to less than 3%) ... 2121
Kayexalate ... 2314
Lasix Injection, Oral Solution and Tablets ... 1240
Mithracin ... 607
Nebcin Vials, Hyporets & ADD-Vantage ... 1464
NebuPent for Inhalation Solution (1% or less) ... 1040
Neutrexin (1.8%) ... 2572
▲ Paraplatin for Injection (16% to 31%) ... 705
Paxil Tablets (Rare) ... 2505
Pentam 300 Injection (0.2%; 1 patient) ... 1041
Platinol ... 708
Platinol-AQ Injection ... 710
▲ Prograf (Greater than 3%) ... 1042
▲ Proleukin for Injection (15%) ... 797
Roferon-A Injection (Less than 5%) ... 2145
Sodium Polystyrene Sulfonate Suspension ... 2244
Synarel Nasal Solution for Endometriosis ... 2152
Tobramycin Sulfate Injection ... 968
Zosyn ... 1419
Zosyn Pharmacy Bulk Package ... 1422

Hypocalcemia, neonatal
Yutopar Intravenous Injection (Infrequent) ... 570

Hypocarbia
Exosurf Neonatal for Intratracheal Suspension ... 1095
Survanta Beractant Intratracheal Suspension (Less than 1%) ... 2226

Hypochloremia
▲ Bumex (14.9%) ... 2093
Demadex Tablets and Injection ... 686
Dyazide ... 2479
Enduron Tablets ... 420
Esidrix Tablets ... 821
Foscavir Injection (Less than 1%) .. 547
Lozol Tablets (Less than 5%) ... 2022
Maxzide ... 1380
Mykrox Tablets ... 993
Oretic Tablets ... 443
Zaroxolyn Tablets ... 1000

Hypochloremic alkalosis
Apresazide Capsules ... 808
Capozide ... 742
Diuril Sodium Intravenous ... 1652
Esidrix Tablets ... 821
Lasix Injection, Oral Solution and Tablets ... 1240
Lotensin HCT ... 837
Lozol Tablets ... 2022
Maxzide ... 1380
Mykrox Tablets ... 993
Prinzide Tablets ... 1737
Tenoretic Tablets ... 2845
Thalitone (Common) ... 1245
Vaseretic Tablets ... 1765
Zaroxolyn Tablets ... 1000
Zestoretic ... 2850

Hypocholesterolemia
Bumex (0.4%) ... 2093
PREVACID Delayed-Release Capsules (Less than 1%) ... 2562
Proleukin for Injection (1%) ... 797

Hypocoagulability
Orudis Capsules (Less than 1%) ... 2766
Oruvail Capsules (Less than 1%) ... 2766

Hypochondriasis
Luvox Tablets (Infrequent) ... 2544

Hypoesthesia
Ambien Tablets (Infrequent) ... 2416
Anafranil Capsules (Rare) ... 803
Cardura Tablets (0.5% to 1%) ... 2186
Claritin (2% or fewer patients) ... 2349
Claritin-D (Less frequent) ... 2350
Engerix-B Unit-Dose Vials ... 2482
▲ Foscavir Injection (5% or greater) .. 547
Imdur (Less than or equal to 5%) .. 1323
▲ Intron A (Up to 10%) ... 2364
Ismo Tablets (Fewer than 1%) ... 2738
Normodyne Injection (1%) ... 2377
Norvasc Tablets (More than 0.1% to 1%) ... 1940
Procardia XL Extended Release Tablets (1% or less) ... 1972
Risperdal (Rare) ... 1301
Romazicon (1% to 3%) ... 2147
Sectral Capsules (Up to 2%) ... 2807
Tambocor Tablets (1% to less than 3%) ... 1497
Tornalate Solution for Inhalation, 0.2% (Less than 1%) ... 956
Trandate Injection (1 of 100 patients) ... 1185
Zebeta Tablets (1.1% to 1.5%) ... 1413
Zoloft Tablets (1.7%) ... 2217

Hypoestrogeneism
Danocrine Capsules ... 2307
▲ Lupron Depot 3.75 mg (Among most frequent) ... 2556
Neurontin Capsules (Rare) ... 1922
▲ Synarel Nasal Solution for Endometriosis (Most frequent) ... 2152

Hypofibrinogenemia
Azo Gantrisin Tablets ... 2081
Depakene ... 413
Depakote Tablets ... 415
Elspar ... 1659
Oncaspar ... 2028
Panhematin ... 443

Hypogammaglobulinemia
Methotrexate Sodium Tablets, Injection, for Injection and LPF Injection (Rare) ... 1275

Hypogeusia
Cuprimine Capsules (Some patients) ... 1630
Depen Titratable Tablets (Some patients) ... 2662

Hypoglycemia
Children's Advil Suspension (Less than 1%) ... 2692
Anaprox/Naprosyn (Less than 1%) ... 2117
Ancobon Capsules ... 2079
Asendin Tablets (Very rare) ... 1369
Azo Gantanol Tablets (Rare) ... 2080
Azo Gantrisin Tablets (Rare) ... 2081
Azulfidine (Rare) ... 1949
Bactrim DS Tablets (Rare) ... 2084
Bactrim I.V. Infusion (Rare) ... 2082
Bactrim (Rare) ... 2084
Betaseron for SC Injection ... 658
Blocadren Tablets ... 1614
Cartrol Tablets ... 410
Cataflam (Less than 1%) ... 816
▲ CellCept Capsules (More than or equal to 3%) ... 2099
Cipro I.V. (Rare) ... 595
Cipro I.V. Pharmacy Bulk Package (Rare) ... 597
Cipro Tablets (Less than 0.1%) ... 592
Compazine ... 2470
Cuprimine Capsules ... 1630
Cytovene (1% or less) ... 2103
Depen Titratable Tablets (Extremely rare) ... 2662
DiaBeta Tablets ... 1239
Diabinese Tablets ... 1935
EC-Naprosyn Delayed-Release Tablets (Less than 1%) ... 2117
Edecrin (In 2 uremic patients) ... 1657
Effexor (Infrequent) ... 2719
Elavil ... 2838
Endep Tablets ... 2174
Etrafon ... 2355
Fansidar Tablets (Rare) ... 2114
Felbatol ... 2666
Feldene Capsules (Less than 1%) .. 1965
Flexeril Tablets (Rare) ... 1661
Floxin I.V. (More than or equal to 1%) ... 1571
Floxin Tablets (200 mg, 300 mg, 400 mg) (More than or equal to 1.0%) ... 1567
Furoxone ... 2046
Gantanol Tablets (Rare) ... 2119
Gantrisin (Rare) ... 2120
Glucophage ... 752
Glucotrol Tablets ... 1967
Glucotrol XL Extended Release Tablets (Rare; less than 1%; less than 3%) ... 1968
Glynase PresTab Tablets ... 2609
Haldol Decanoate ... 1577
Haldol Injection, Tablets and Concentrate ... 1575
Humulin 50/50, 100 Units ... 1444
Humulin 70/30, 100 Units ... 1445
Humulin L, 100 Units ... 1446
IBU Tablets (Less than 1%) ... 1342
Regular, 100 Units ... 1450
Pork Regular, 100 Units ... 1452
Imitrex Tablets (Rare) ... 1106
Indocin I.V. (1% to 3%) ... 1684
Limbitrol ... 2180
Ludiomil Tablets (Rare) ... 843
Lupron Depot 3.75 mg ... 2556
Lupron Depot 7.5 mg ... 2559
Lupron Injection (Less than 5%) ... 2555
Luvox Tablets (Rare) ... 2544
Maxaquin Tablets (Less than or equal to 0.1%) ... 2440
Mepron Suspension (1%) ... 1135
Micronase Tablets ... 2623
Mithracin ... 607
Moban Tablets and Concentrate ... 1048
Children's Motrin Ibuprofen Oral Suspension (Less than 1%) ... 1546
Motrin Tablets (Less than 1%) ... 2625
Motrin Ibuprofen Suspension, Oral Drops, Chewable Tablets, Caplets (Less than 1%) ... 1546
Anaprox/Naprosyn (Less than 1%) ... 2117
Navane Capsules and Concentrate 2201
Navane Intramuscular ... 2202
NebuPent for Inhalation Solution (1% or less) ... 1040
Normodyne Injection ... 2377
Normodyne Tablets ... 2379
Noroxin Tablets ... 1715
Noroxin Tablets ... 2048
Norpace ... 2444
Norpramin Tablets ... 1526
▲ Oncaspar (Greater than 1% but less than 5%) ... 2028
Pamelor ... 2280
PASER Granules ... 1285
Paxil Tablets (Rare) ... 2505
Pentam 300 Injection (2.4 to 3.5%) ... 1041
Permax Tablets (Infrequent) ... 575
PREVACID Delayed-Release Capsules (Less than 1%) ... 2562
Prilosec Delayed-Release Capsules (Less than 1%) ... 529
Proleukin for Injection (2%) ... 797
Prostin VR Pediatric Sterile Solution (Less than 1%) ... 2635
Prozac Pulvules & Liquid, Oral Solution (Infrequent) ... 919
Risperdal (Rare) ... 1301
Sandostatin Injection (Approximately 2% to 3%) ... 2292
Septra (Rare) ... 1174
Septra I.V. Infusion (Rare) ... 1169
Septra I.V. Infusion ADD-Vantage Vials (Rare) ... 1171
Septra (Rare) ... 1174
Serzone Tablets (Rare) ... 771
Sinequan ... 2205
Stelazine ... 2514
Surmontil Capsules ... 2811
Tenoretic Tablets ... 2845
Tenormin Tablets and I.V. Injection 2847
Thorazine ... 2523
Timolide Tablets ... 1748
Timoptic-XE ... 1755
Tofranil Ampuls ... 854
Tofranil Tablets ... 856
Tofranil-PM Capsules ... 857
Triavil Tablets ... 1757
Trilafon ... 2389
Vantin for Oral Suspension and Vantin Tablets ... 2646
Videx Tablets, Powder for Oral Solution, & Pediatric Powder for Oral Solution (Up to 1%) ... 720
Vivactil Tablets ... 1774
Voltaren Tablets (Less than 1%) ... 861
Zanosar Sterile Powder ... 2653
Zoloft Tablets (Rare) ... 2217
Zosyn (1.0% or less) ... 1419
Zosyn Pharmacy Bulk Package (1.0% or less) ... 1422

Hypoglycemia, masked symptoms of
Timoptic in Ocudose (Less frequent) ... 1753
Timoptic-XE ... 1755

Hypoglycemia, neonatal
Brethine Ampuls ... 815
Brethine Tablets ... 814
Bricanyl Subcutaneous Injection ... 1502
DiaBeta Tablets ... 1239
Normodyne Injection ... 2377
Normodyne Tablets (Rare) ... 2379
Trandate ... 1185
Yutopar Intravenous Injection (Infrequent) ... 570

Hypogonadism
Permax Tablets (Rare) ... 575
Virazole ... 1264

Hypohidrosis
Bellergal-S Tablets (Rare) ... 2250
Bentyl ... 1501
Ditropan ... 1516
Donnatal ... 2060
Donnatal Extentabs ... 2061
Donnatal Tablets ... 2060
Kutrase Capsules ... 2402
Levsin/Levsinex/Levbid ... 2405
Pro-Banthine Tablets ... 2052
Quarzan Capsules ... 2181
Risperdal (Infrequent) ... 1301
Robinul Forte Tablets ... 2072
Robinul Injectable ... 2072
Robinul Tablets ... 2072

Hypokalemia
Aldactazide ... 2413
Aldoclor Tablets ... 1598
Aldoril Tablets ... 1604
Anafranil Capsules (Infrequent) ... 803
Ancobon Capsules ... 2079

(◘ Described in PDR For Nonprescription Drugs) Incidence data in parenthesis; ▲ 3% or more (◉ Described in PDR For Ophthalmology)

Hypokalemia

Apresazide Capsules 808
▲ Aredia for Injection (4% to 18%) .. 810
Arfonad Ampuls 2080
Aristocort Suspension (Forte Parenteral) 1027
Aristocort Suspension (Intralesional) 1025
Aristocort Tablets 1022
Aristospan Suspension (Intra-articular) 1033
Aristospan Suspension (Intralesional) 1032
▲ Bumex (14.7%) 2093
Capozide 742
Cardene I.V. (0.7%) 2709
Cardura Tablets (Less than 0.5% of 3960 patients) 2186
Celestone Soluspan Suspension 2347
▲ CellCept Capsules (10.0% to 10.1%) 2099
Cipro I.V. (Infrequent) 595
Combipres Tablets 677
CORTENEMA 2535
Cortifoam 2396
Cortone Acetate Sterile Suspension 1623
Cortone Acetate Tablets 1624
Cytovene (1% or less) 2103
Dalalone D.P. Injectable 1011
Daranide Tablets 1633
Decadron Elixir 1633
Decadron Phosphate Injection 1637
Decadron Phosphate Respihaler 1642
Decadron Phosphate Turbinaire 1645
Decadron Phosphate with Xylocaine Injection, Sterile 1639
Decadron Tablets 1635
Decadron-LA Sterile Suspension 1646
Deltasone Tablets 2595
Demadex Tablets and Injection 686
Depo-Medrol Single-Dose Vial 2600
Depo-Medrol Sterile Aqueous Suspension 2597
Dexacort Phosphate in Respihaler .. 458
Dexacort Phosphate in Turbinaire .. 459
Diflucan Injection, Tablets, and Oral Suspension 2194
Digibind 1091
Diuril Sodium Intravenous 1652
Dobutrex Solution Vials (Rare) 1439
Dyazide (Uncommon) 2479
Dyrenium Capsules (Rare) 2481
Effexor (Infrequent) 2719
Enduron Tablets 420
Esidrix Tablets 821
Felbatol (Infrequent) 2666
Florinef Acetate Tablets 505
▲ Foscavir Injection (5% or greater up to 16%) 547
▲ Fungizone Intravenous (Among most common) 506
Garamycin Injectable 2360
Hivid Tablets (Less than 1% to less than 3%) 2121
Hydeltrasol Injection, Sterile 1665
Hydeltra-T.B.A. Sterile Suspension 1667
Hydrocortone Acetate Sterile Suspension 1669
Hydrocortone Phosphate Injection, Sterile 1670
Hydrocortone Tablets 1672
HydroDIURIL Tablets 1674
▲ Hyzaar Tablets (6.7%) 1677
Imdur (Less than or equal to 5%) .. 1323
Kayexalate 2314
Kerlone Tablets (Less than 2%) 2436
Lamprene Capsules (Less than 1%) 828
Lanoxicaps 1117
Lasix Injection, Oral Solution and Tablets 1240
Lopressor HCT Tablets (Less than 10 in 100 patients) 832
Lotensin HCT 837
Lotrel Capsules 840
Lozol Tablets (2%; infrequent) 2022
Luvox Tablets (Rare) 2544
Maxaquin Tablets 2440
Maxzide 1380
Medrol 2621
Mezlin (Rare) 601
Mezlin Pharmacy Bulk Package 604
Mithracin 607
Mykrox Tablets 993
Nebcin Vials, Hyporets & ADD-Vantage 1464
Norpace (1 to 3%) 2444
Oretic Tablets 443
▲ Paraplatin for Injection (16% to 28%) 705
Paxil Tablets (Rare) 2505

Pediapred Oral Liquid 995
Permax Tablets (Infrequent) 575
Pipracil (Rare with high doses) 1390
Platinol 708
Platinol-AQ Injection 710
Prelone Syrup 1787
Primacor Injection (0.6%) 2331
Prinzide Tablets 1737
▲ Prograf (11% to 29%) 1042
▲ Proleukin for Injection (9%) 797
Prostin VR Pediatric Sterile Solution (About 1%) 2635
Prozac Pulvules & Liquid, Oral Solution (Rare) 919
Relafen Tablets (Less than 1%) 2510
Risperdal (Rare) 1301
Septra 1174
Sinemet CR Tablets 944
Sodium Polystyrene Sulfonate Suspension 2244
Solu-Cortef Sterile Powder 2641
Solu-Medrol Sterile Powder 2643
Sporanox Capsules (0.2% to 2.0%) 1305
▲ Tegison Capsules (25-50%) 2154
Tenoretic Tablets 2845
Thalitone (Common) 1245
Timentin for Injection 2528
Timolide Tablets 1748
Tobramycin Sulfate Injection 968
Tornalate Solution for Inhalation, 0.2% (Infrequent) 956
Vaseretic Tablets 1765
Ventolin Inhalation Aerosol and Refill 1197
Ventolin Inhalation Solution 1198
Ventolin Nebules Inhalation Solution 1199
Ventolin Rotacaps for Inhalation 1200
Ventolin Tablets 1203
Yutopar Intravenous Injection 570
Zaroxolyn Tablets 1000
Zestoretic 2850
Ziac 1415
Zofran Injection (Rare) 1214
Zofran Tablets (Rare) 1217
Zosyn 1419
Zosyn Pharmacy Bulk Package 1422
Zovirax Sterile Powder (Less than 1%) 1223

Hypokalemic alkalosis

Aristocort Suspension (Forte Parenteral) 1027
Aristocort Suspension (Intralesional) 1025
Aristocort Tablets 1022
Aristospan Suspension (Intra-articular) 1033
Aristospan Suspension (Intralesional) 1032
Celestone Soluspan Suspension 2347
CORTENEMA 2535
Cortone Acetate Sterile Suspension 1623
Cortone Acetate Tablets 1624
Dalalone D.P. Injectable 1011
Decadron Elixir 1633
Decadron Phosphate Injection 1637
Decadron Phosphate Respihaler 1642
Decadron Phosphate Turbinaire 1645
Decadron Phosphate with Xylocaine Injection, Sterile 1639
Decadron Tablets 1635
Decadron-LA Sterile Suspension 1646
Deltasone Tablets 2595
Depo-Medrol Single-Dose Vial 2600
Depo-Medrol Sterile Aqueous Suspension 2597
Dexacort Phosphate in Respihaler .. 458
Dexacort Phosphate in Turbinaire .. 459
Florinef Acetate Tablets 505
Hydeltrasol Injection, Sterile 1665
Hydeltra-T.B.A. Sterile Suspension 1667
Hydrocortone Acetate Sterile Suspension 1669
Hydrocortone Phosphate Injection, Sterile 1670
Hydrocortone Tablets 1672
Medrol 2621
Pediapred Oral Liquid 995
Prelone Syrup 1787
Solu-Cortef Sterile Powder 2641
Solu-Medrol Sterile Powder 2643

Hypokinesia

Anafranil Capsules (Infrequent) 803
▲ Clozaril Tablets (4%) 2252
Depakote Tablets (Greater than 1% but not more than 5%) 415
Doral Tablets 2664

Effexor (Rare) 2719
Hivid Tablets (Less than 1% to less than 3%) 2121
Intron A (Less than 5%) 2364
Ismo Tablets (Fewer than 1%) 2738
Lamictal Tablets (Rare) 1112
Luvox Tablets (Frequent) 2544
Neurontin Capsules (Rare) 1922
Paxil Tablets (Rare) 2505
Permax Tablets (Infrequent) 575
▲ ProSom Tablets (8%) 449
▲ Risperdal (17% to 34%) 1301
Tenex Tablets (3% or less) 2074
Zoloft Tablets (Infrequent) 2217

Hypomagnesemia

Apresazide Capsules 808
▲ Aredia for Injection (4% to at least 15%) 810
Bumex 2093
Capozide 742
Cytovene-IV (One report) 2103
Demadex Tablets and Injection 686
Diucardin Tablets 2718
Diuril Sodium Intravenous 1652
Esidrix Tablets 821
Esimil Tablets 822
Felbatol 2666
▲ Foscavir Injection (5% or greater up to 15%) 547
Fungizone Intravenous 506
Garamycin Injectable 2360
Hivid Tablets (Less than 1% to less than 3%) 2121
HydroDIURIL Tablets 1674
Hyzaar Tablets 1677
Lanoxicaps 1117
Lasix Injection, Oral Solution and Tablets 1240
Lopressor HCT Tablets 832
Lotensin HCT 837
Lozol Tablets 2022
Maxzide 1380
Mykrox Tablets 993
Nebcin Vials, Hyporets & ADD-Vantage 1464
Neoral 2276
▲ Paraplatin for Injection (29% to 63%) 705
Platinol 708
Platinol-AQ Injection 710
Prinzide Tablets 1737
▲ Prograf (15% to 48%) 1042
▲ Proleukin for Injection (16%) 797
Sandimmune (In some patients) 2286
Ser-Ap-Es Tablets 849
Tobramycin Sulfate Injection 968
Vaseretic Tablets 1765
Zaroxolyn Tablets 1000
Zestoretic 2850

Hypomania

Asendin Tablets (Less than 1%) 1369
Desyrel and Desyrel Dividose 503
Effexor (0.5%) 2719
Endep Tablets (Rare) 2174
Lamictal Tablets (Rare) 1112
Limbitrol 2180
Ludiomil Tablets (Rare) 843
▲ Nardil (Most common) 1920
Norpramin Tablets 1526
Pamelor 2280
Paxil Tablets (Approximately 1.0%) 2505
Serzone Tablets (0.3% to 1.6%) 771
Surmontil Capsules 2811
Tofranil Ampuls 854
Tofranil Tablets 856
Tofranil-PM Capsules 857
Triavil Tablets (Rare) 1757
Vivactil Tablets 1774
Wellbutrin Tablets (Frequent) 1204
Xanax Tablets 2649
Zoloft Tablets (0.4%) 2217

Hypomenorrhea

Aquasol A Vitamin A Capsules, USP 534
Effexor (Rare) 2719
Pentasa (Less than 1%) 1527
Prozac Pulvules & Liquid, Oral Solution (Rare) 919

Hyponatremia

Actimmune (Rare) 1056
Aldactone 2414
Altace Capsules 1232
Apresazide Capsules 808
Atretol Tablets 573
▲ Bumex (9.2%) 2093
Capoten 739

Capozide 742
Clozaril Tablets 2252
Cytovene-IV (Two or more reports) 2103
DDAVP Injection 2014
DDAVP 2017
Demadex Tablets and Injection 686
Depakene 413
Depakote Tablets 415
Depo-Medrol Single-Dose Vial 2600
DiaBeta Tablets 1239
Diuril Sodium Intravenous 1652
Dyazide 2479
Effexor (Rare) 2719
Enduron Tablets 420
Esidrix Tablets 821
Felbatol (Infrequent) 2666
Foscavir Injection (Between 1% and 5%) 547
Garamycin Injectable 2360
Glucotrol Tablets 1967
Glucotrol XL Extended Release Tablets 1968
Glynase PresTab Tablets 2609
Haldol Decanoate 1577
Haldol Injection, Tablets and Concentrate 1575
▲ Indocin I.V. (3% to 9%) 1684
Lasix Injection, Oral Solution and Tablets 1240
Lotensin Tablets (Scattered incidents) 834
Lotensin HCT 837
Lozol Tablets (Less than 5%; infrequent) 2022
Luvox Tablets 2544
Maxzide 1380
▲ Mepron Suspension (7% to 10%) 1135
Micronase Tablets 2623
Moduretic Tablets 1705
Monopril Tablets 757
Mykrox Tablets 993
Nebcin Vials, Hyporets & ADD-Vantage 1464
▲ Neutrexin (4.6%) 2572
Nimotop Capsules (Less than 1%) 610
Oncaspar (Less than 1%) 2028
Oncovin Solution Vials & Hyporets 1466
Oretic Tablets 443
Orudis Capsules (Less than 1%) 2766
Oruvail Capsules (Less than 1%) 2766
▲ Paraplatin for Injection (10% to 47%) 705
Paxil Tablets (Rare) 2505
Platinol 708
Platinol-AQ Injection 710
Primaxin I.M. 1727
Primaxin I.V. 1729
Prinzide Tablets 1737
▲ Prograf (Greater than 3%) 1042
▲ Proleukin for Injection (4%) 797
Proloprim Tablets 1155
Prozac Pulvules & Liquid, Oral Solution (Rare) 919
Risperdal (Infrequent; 2 patients) .. 1301
Rythmol Tablets–150mg, 225mg, 300mg (Less than 1%) 1352
Septra 1174
Septra I.V. Infusion 1169
Septra I.V. Infusion ADD-Vantage Vials 1171
Septra 1174
Stimate, (desmopressin acetate) Nasal Spray, 1.5 mg/mL 525
Tegretol Chewable Tablets 852
Tegretol Suspension 852
Tegretol Tablets 852
Tenoretic Tablets 2845
Thalitone (Common) 1245
Ticlid Tablets (Rare) 2156
Tobramycin Sulfate Injection 968
Toradol 2159
Vaseretic Tablets 1765
Vasotec I.V. 1768
Vasotec Tablets 1771
Zaroxolyn Tablets 1000
Zestoretic 2850
Zoloft Tablets (Several cases) 2217
Zosyn 1419
Zosyn Pharmacy Bulk Package 1422

Hyponatremia, dilutional

Apresazide Capsules 808
Capozide 742
Diuril Sodium Intravenous 1652
Esidrix Tablets 821
Hyzaar Tablets 1677
Lozol Tablets 2022
Maxzide 1380
Oretic Tablets 443
Prinzide Tablets 1737
Tenoretic Tablets 2845

(**◻** Described in PDR For Nonprescription Drugs) Incidence data in parenthesis; ▲ 3% or more (**◉** Described in PDR For Ophthalmology)

1333 Side Effects Index Hypotension

Vaseretic Tablets 1765
Zestoretic 2850

Hypophosphatemia

ALternaGEL Liquid 1316
Apresazide Capsules 808
▲ Aredia for Injection (Up to 18%) 810
Basaljel 2703
Capozide (A few patients) 742
Cardene I.V. (Rare) 2709
▲ CellCept Capsules (12.5% to 15.8%) 2099
Effexor (Rare) 2719
Esidrix Tablets 821
▲ Felbatol (3.4%; infrequent) 2666
▲ Foscavir Injection (5% or greater up to 8%) 547
▲ Ganite (Up to 79%) 2533
Gelusil Liquid & Tablets ▣ 855
Lozol Tablets (Rare) 2022
Maalox Heartburn Relief Suspension ▣ 642
Maalox Heartburn Relief Tablets ▣ 641
Maalox Magnesia and Alumina Oral Suspension ▣ 642
Maalox Plus Tablets ▣ 643
Extra Strength Maalox Antacid Plus Antigas Liquid and Tablets ▣ 638
Maxzide 1380
Mithracin 607
Mykrox Tablets 993
Mylanta Liquid 1317
Mylanta Tablets ▣ 660
Mylanta Double Strength Liquid 1317
Mylanta Double Strength Tablets ▣ 660
Platinol 708
Platinol-AQ Injection 710
▲ Prograf (Greater than 3%) 1042
▲ Proleukin for Injection (11%) 797
Rolaids Tablets ▣ 843
Tenoretic Tablets 2845
Zanosar Sterile Powder 2653
Zaroxolyn Tablets 1000

Hypopigmentation

Accutane Capsules (Less than 1%) 2076
Aclovate Cream 1069
Analpram-HC Rectal Cream 1% and 2.5% 977
Anusol-HC Cream 2.5% (Infrequent to frequent) 1896
Anusol-HC Suppositories 1897
Aristocort Suspension (Forte Parenteral) 1027
Aristocort Suspension (Intralesional) 1025
Aristocort A 0.025% Cream (Infrequent) 1027
Aristocort A 0.5% Cream 1031
Aristocort A 0.1% Cream (Infrequent) 1029
Aristocort A 0.1% Ointment (Infrequent) 1030
Aristospan Suspension (Intra-articular) 1033
Aristospan Suspension (Intralesional) 1032
Carmol HC (Infrequent to frequent) 924
Celestone Soluspan Suspension 2347
Cordran Lotion (Infrequent) 1803
Cordran Tape (Infrequent) 1804
Cortisporin Cream 1084
Cortisporin Ointment 1085
Cortisporin Otic Solution Sterile 1087
Cortisporin Otic Suspension Sterile 1088
Cortone Acetate Sterile Suspension 1623
Cutivate Cream 1088
Cutivate Ointment (Infrequent to more frequent) 1089
Cyclocort Topical (Infrequent) 1037
Dalalone D.P. Injectable 1011
Decadron Phosphate Injection 1637
Decadron Phosphate Topical Cream 1644
Decadron Phosphate with Xylocaine Injection, Sterile 1639
Decadron-LA Sterile Suspension 1646
Decaspray Topical Aerosol 1648
Depo-Medrol Single-Dose Vial 2600
Depo-Medrol Sterile Aqueous Suspension 2597
Dermatop Emollient Cream 0.1% (Infrequent to frequent) 1238
DesOwen Cream, Ointment and Lotion (Infrequent) 1046
Diprolene AF Cream (Infrequent) 2352
Diprolene Gel 0.05% (Infrequent) 2353
Diprolene (Infrequent) 2352
Elocon (Infrequent) 2354
Epifoam (Infrequent) 2399
Florone/Florone E 906
Halog (Infrequent) 2686
Hydeltrasol Injection, Sterile 1665
Hydeltra-T.B.A. Sterile Suspension 1667
Hydrocortone Acetate Sterile Suspension 1669
Hydrocortone Phosphate Injection, Sterile 1670
Hytone 907
Lidex (Infrequent) 2130
Locoid Cream, Ointment and Topical Solution (Infrequent) 978
Lotrisone Cream (Infrequent) 2372
Mantadil Cream 1135
8-MOP Capsules 1246
NeoDecadron Topical Cream 1714
Oxsoralen-Ultra Capsules 1257
PediOtic Suspension Sterile 1153
Pramosone Cream, Lotion & Ointment 978
ProctoCream-HC (Infrequent) 2408
ProctoCream-HC 2.5% (Infrequent to frequent) 2408
ProctoFoam-HC 2409
Psorcon Cream 0.05% (Infrequent) 909
Psorcon Ointment 0.05% 908
Retin-A (tretinoin) Cream/Gel/Liquid 1889
Solu-Cortef Sterile Powder 2641
Solu-Medrol Sterile Powder 2643
Synalar (Infrequent) 2130
Temovate (Infrequent) 1179
Topicort (Infrequent) 1243
Tridesilon Cream 0.05% (Infrequent) 615
Tridesilon Ointment 0.05% (Infrequent) 616
Ultravate Cream 0.05% (Infrequent) 2689
Ultravate Ointment 0.05% 2690
Westcort 2690

Hypoplasia, enamel

Achromycin V Capsules 1367
Declomycin Tablets 1371
Doryx Capsules 1913
Minocin Intravenous 1382
Minocin Oral Suspension 1385
Minocin Pellet-Filled Capsules 1383
Monodox Capsules 1805
Terramycin Intramuscular Solution 2210
Vibramycin 1941
Vibramycin Hyclate Intravenous 2215
Vibramycin 1941

Hypoplasia, erythroid

Capoten 739
Capozide 742

Hypoplasia, myeloid (see under Bone marrow hypoplasia)

Hypoplastic anemia

Eminase (Less than 1%) 2039
Mykrox Tablets 993
Myochrysine Injection 1711
Procan SR Tablets 1926
Solganal Suspension (Rare) 2388
Tonocard Tablets (Less than 1%) 531
Trinalin Repetabs Tablets 1330
Zaroxolyn Tablets 1000

Hypopnea

Stadol (Less than 1%) 775

Hypoproteinemia

▲ CellCept Capsules (More than or equal to 3%) 2099
Cipro I.V. 595
Cipro I.V. Pharmacy Bulk Package (Less than 1%) 597
Cortifoam 2396
Effexor (Rare) 2719
Foscavir Injection (Less than 1%) 547
Lupron Depot 7.5 mg 2559
Lupron Injection 2555
Maxaquin Tablets (Less than or equal to 0.1%) 2440
▲ Oncaspar (Greater than 1% but less than 5%) 2028
▲ Prograf (Greater than 3%) 1042
▲ Proleukin for Injection (7%) 797
Risperdal (Rare) 1301
Unasyn 2212
Vantin for Oral Suspension and Vantin Tablets 2646
Zefazone 2654
Zosyn 1419
Zosyn Pharmacy Bulk Package 1422

Hypoprothrombinemia

Azo Gantanol Tablets 2080
Azo Gantrisin Tablets 2081
Azulfidine (Rare) 1949
Bactrim DS Tablets 2084
Bactrim I.V. Infusion 2082
Bactrim 2084
Cipro I.V. (Rare) 595
Fansidar Tablets 2114
Felbatol 2666
Foscavir Injection (Less than 1%) 547
Gantanol Tablets 2119
Gantrisin 2120
Limbitrol DS Tablets (Rare) 2180
Mithracin 607
PASER Granules 1285
▲ Prograf (Greater than 3%) 1042
Questran Light 769
Quinidex Extentabs 2067
Rocephin Injectable Vials, ADD-Vantage, Galaxy Container (Rare) 2142
Septra 1174
Septra I.V. Infusion 1169
Septra I.V. Infusion ADD-Vantage Vials 1171
Septra 1174
Tapazole Tablets 1477

Hypoprothrombinemia, paradoxical

Konakion Injection 2127

Hypoptyalism

Demser Capsules 1649
Risperdal (Frequent) 1301
Vantin for Oral Suspension and Vantin Tablets 2646
▲ Xanax Tablets (32.8%) 2649

Hypopyon

Healon (Rare) ◉ 314
Healon GV (Rare) ◉ 315
Ocucoat (Rare) ◉ 321

Hyporeflexia

Betaseron for SC Injection 658
Cognex Capsules (Infrequent) 1901
Compazine 2470
Foscavir Injection (Less than 1%) 547
Luvox Tablets (Rare) 2544
Matulane Capsules 2131
Navelbine Injection (Less than 5%) 1145
Neurontin Capsules (Frequent) 1922
ProSom Tablets (Rare) 449
Prozac Pulvules & Liquid, Oral Solution (Rare) 919
▲ Retrovir Capsules (5.6%) 1158
▲ Retrovir I.V. Infusion (7%) 1163
▲ Retrovir Syrup (5.6%) 1158
▲ Risperdal (17% to 34%) 1301
Stelazine 2514
Thorazine 2523
Videx Tablets, Powder for Oral Solution, & Pediatric Powder for Oral Solution (Less than 1%) 720
Zoloft Tablets (Rare) 2217

Hyporeflexia, neonatal

Compazine 2470
Stelazine Concentrate 2514
Thorazine 2523

Hyporesponsive episode, unspecified

Diphtheria and Tetanus Toxoids and Pertussis Vaccine Adsorbed 2477
HibTITER (One case) 1375
Tetramune 1404

Hypospadias

Amen Tablets (Approximately 10 to 16 per 1,000 male births) 780
Cycrin Tablets (Approximately 10 to 16 per 1,000 male births) 975
Depo-Provera Contraceptive Injection (5 to 8 per 1,000 male births) 2602
Depo-Provera Sterile Aqueous Suspension (About 5 to 8 per 1,000) 2606
Megace Oral Suspension (Approximately 10 to 16 male births per 1,000) 699
Megace Tablets 701
Provera Tablets 2636

Hyposthenuria

Floxin I.V. (More than or equal to 1%) 1571
Floxin Tablets (200 mg, 300 mg, 400 mg) (More than or equal to 1%) 1567
▲ Fungizone Intravenous (Among most common) 506

Hypotension

Abbokinase 403
Abbokinase Open-Cath 405
Accupril Tablets (2.9%) 1893
Acel-Imune Diphtheria and Tetanus Toxoids and Acellular Pertussis Vaccine Adsorbed (Rare) 1364
Actifed with Codeine Cough Syrup 1067
Actimmune (Rare) 1056
Activase 1058
▲ Adalat Capsules (10 mg and 20 mg) (Approximately 5%) 587
Adalat CC (Less than 1.0%) 589
Adenocard Injection (Less than 1%) 1021
Adenoscan (2%) 1024
AK-Fluor Injection 10% and 25% ◉ 203
Aldoclor Tablets 1598
Aldomet Oral 1600
Aldoril Tablets 1604
▲ Alfenta Injection (10%) 1286
Alkeran for Injection (In some patients) 1070
Altace Capsules (Rare to more frequent) 1232
Ambien Tablets (Rare) 2416
Amicar Syrup, Tablets, and Injection (Occasional) 1267
Amikacin Sulfate Injection, USP (Rare) 960
Amikin Injectable (Rare) 501
Anectine 1073
Apresazide Capsules (Less frequent) 808
Apresoline Hydrochloride Tablets (Less frequent) 809
AquaMEPHYTON Injection 1608
Aralen Hydrochloride Injection (Rare) 2301
Aralen Phosphate Tablets (Rare) 2301
Asendin Tablets (Less than 1%) 1369
Atgam Sterile Solution (Less than 5%) 2581
Ativan Injection (0.1%) 2698
Ativan Tablets (Rare) 2700
Atretol Tablets 573
Atrohist Plus Tablets 454
Atropine Sulfate Sterile Ophthalmic Solution ◉ 233
Atrovent Inhalation Aerosol 671
Azactam for Injection (Less than 1%) 734
Benadryl Capsules 1898
Benadryl Injection 1898
Betagan ◉ 233
▲ Betapace Tablets (3% to 6%) 641
Betaseron for SC Injection 658
Betimol 0.25%, 0.5% ◉ 261
Bioclate, Antihemophilic Factor (Recombinant) 513
Blenoxane (1%) 692
▲ Blocadren Tablets (3%) 1614
▲ Brevibloc Injection (20% to 50%) 1808
Brevital Sodium Vials 1429
▲ Bromfed-DM Cough Syrup (Among most frequent) 1786
Brontex 1981
Bumex (0.8%) 2093
▲ Buprenex Injectable (1-5%) 2006
BuSpar (Infrequent) 737
Butisol Sodium Elixir & Tablets (Less than 1 in 100) 2660
Calan SR Caplets (2.5%) 2422
Calan Tablets (2.5%) 2419
Capoten (Rare) 739
Capozide (Rare) 742
Carbocaine Hydrochloride Injection 2303
Cardene Capsules (Rare) 2095
▲ Cardene I.V. (5.6%) 2709
Cardizem CD Capsules (Less than 1%) 1506
Cardizem SR Capsules (1%) 1510
Cardizem Tablets (Less than 1%) 1512
Cardura Tablets (1% to 1.7%) 2186
Cataflam 816
Caverject (Less than 1%) 2583
▲ CellCept Capsules (More than or equal to 3%) 2099
Ceptaz (Very rare) 1081
Ceredase (A few events) 1065
Cerezyme (One patient) 1066

(▣ Described in PDR For Nonprescription Drugs) Incidence data in parenthesis; ▲ 3% or more (◉ Described in PDR For Ophthalmology)

Hypotension **Side Effects Index** **1334**

Cipro I.V. (1% or less) 595
Cipro I.V. Pharmacy Bulk Package (Less than 1%) 597
Claritin (2% or fewer patients) 2349
Claritin-D (Less frequent) 2350
Cleocin Phosphate Injection (Rare) 2586
Clinoril Tablets (Less than 1 in 100) 1618
Clomid 1514
▲ Clozaril Tablets (More than 5 to 9%) 2252
Cognex Capsules (Frequent) 1901
Comhist 2038
Compazine 2470
▲ Cordarone Intravenous (Most common; 15.6% to 16%) 2715
Cordarone Tablets (Less than 1%) 2712
Cozaar Tablets (Less than 1%) 1628
Cyklokapron Tablets and Injection 1950
▲ Cytadren Tablets (1 in 30) 819
CytoGam 1593
Cytotec (Infrequent) 2424
Cytovene (1% or less) 2103
D.A. Chewable Tablets 951
DDAVP Injection (Infrequent) 2014
DDAVP Nasal Spray (Infrequent) 2017
Dalgan Injection (Less than 1%) 538
Dalmane Capsules (Rare) 2173
Decadron Phosphate with Xylocaine Injection, Sterile 1639
Deconamine Chewable Tablets 1320
Deconamine CX Cough and Cold Liquid and Tablets 1319
Deconamine 1320
Deconsal 454
Demadex Tablets and Injection 686
Demerol 2308
Depakote Tablets (Greater than 1% but not more than 5%) 415
Deponit NTG Transdermal Delivery System (Infrequent; 4%) 2397
Desferal Vials 820
▲ Desyrel and Desyrel Dividose (3.8% to 7.0%) 503
Dilacor XR Extended-release Capsules 2018
Dilantin Parenteral 1910
Dilatrate-SR 2398
Dilaudid Ampules 1335
Dilaudid-HP Injection (Less frequent) 1337
Dilaudid-HP Lyophilized Powder 250 mg (Less frequent) 1337
Dilaudid 1335
Dilaudid Oral Liquid 1339
Dilaudid 1335
Dilaudid Tablets - 8 mg 1339
Dimetane-DC Cough Syrup 2059
Dimetane-DX Cough Syrup 2059
Diphtheria and Tetanus Toxoids and Pertussis Vaccine Adsorbed (Rare) 2477
Diphtheria and Tetanus Toxoids and Pertussis Vaccine Adsorbed USP (For Pediatric Use) (Rare) 875
▲ Diprivan Injection (Rare; greater than 1% to 26%) 2833
Diupres Tablets 1650
Diuril Oral Suspension 1653
Diuril Sodium Intravenous 1652
Diuril Tablets 1653
Dizac (Less frequent) 1809
Dobutrex Solution Vials (Occasional) 1439
Duragesic Transdermal System (1% to 3%) 1288
Duranest Injections 542
Dura-Tap/PD Capsules 2867
Dura-Vent/DA Tablets 953
Dura-Vent Tablets 952
Duvoid (Infrequent) 2044
Dyazide 2479
Dyclone 0.5% and 1% Topical Solutions, USP 544
DynaCirc Capsules (0.5% to 1%) 2256
Effexor (Infrequent) 2719
Elavil 2838
Eldepryl Tablets 2550
Emete-con Intramuscular/Intravenous 2198
▲ Eminase (10.4%) 2039
Emla Cream 545
Endep Tablets 2174
Engerix-B Unit-Dose Vials (Less than 1%) 2482
Esidrix Tablets 821
Eskalith 2485
Ethmozine Tablets (Less than 2%) 2041
Etrafon 2355
▲ Exosurf Neonatal for Intratracheal Suspension (39% to 77%) 1095
Fedahist Gyrocaps 2401
Fedahist Timecaps 2401
Felbatol 2666
Fioricet with Codeine Capsules 2260
Flexeril Tablets (Less than 1%) 1661
Floxin I.V. (Less than 1%) 1571
Floxin Tablets (200 mg, 300 mg, 400 mg) (Less than 1%) 1567
Fluorescite ⊙ 219
Fluothane 2724
Fortaz (Very rare) 1100
Foscavir Injection (Between 1% and 5%) 547
▲ Fungizone Intravenous (Among most common) 506
Furoxone 2046
Gamimune N, 5% Immune Globulin Intravenous (Human), 5% (Rare) 619
Gammar I.V., Immune Globulin Intravenous (Human), Lyophilized 516
Garamycin Injectable 2360
Glucophage 752
Haldol Decanoate 1577
Haldol Injection, Tablets and Concentrate 1575
Hespan Injection 929
Helixate, Antihemophilic Factor (Recombinant) 518
Hismanal Tablets (Rare) 1293
Humulin 50/50, 100 Units 1444
Humulin 70/30, 100 Units (Less common) 1445
Humulin L, 100 Units (Less common) 1446
HydroDIURIL Tablets 1674
Hydropres Tablets 1675
▲ Hyperstat I.V. Injection (7%) 2363
Hyskon Hysteroscopy Fluid (Rare) 1595
▲ Hytrin Capsules (0.6%; 21%) 430
Hyzaar Tablets 1677
IFEX (Less than 1%) 697
Regular, 100 Units (Less common) 1450
Pork Regular, 100 Units (Less common) 1452
Imdur (Less than or equal to 5%) 1323
Imitrex Injection (Infrequent) 1103
Imitrex Tablets (Infrequent) 1106
Imuran (Occasional) 1110
Inapsine Injection 1296
Inderal 2728
Inderal LA Long Acting Capsules 2730
Inderide Tablets 2732
Inderide LA Long Acting Capsules 2734
Indocin Capsules (Less than 1%) 1680
Indocin I.V. (Less than 1%) 1684
Indocin (Less than 1%) 1680
INFeD (Iron Dextran Injection, USP) 2345
Inocor Lactate Injection (1.3%) 2309
Intron A (Less than 5%) 2364
Ismelin Tablets 827
Ismo Tablets (Fewer than 1%) 2738
Isoptin Oral Tablets (2.5%) 1346
Isoptin SR Tablets (2.5%) 1348
Isopto Carbachol Ophthalmic Solution ⊙ 223
Isordil Sublingual Tablets (Infrequent) 2739
Isordil Tembids (Infrequent) 2741
Isordil Titradose Tablets (Infrequent) 2742
Isuprel Hydrochloride Injection 1:5000 2311
Kerlone Tablets (Less than 2%) 2436
KOGENATE Antihemophilic Factor (Recombinant) 632
Kytril Injection (Rare) 2490
Kytril Tablets (Rare) 2492
Lasix Injection, Oral Solution and Tablets 1240
Levo-Dromoran (Infrequent) 2129
Librium Injectable (Isolated cases) 2179
Limbitrol 2180
Lincocin (Rare instances) 2617
Lioresal Intrathecal (3 to 5 of 214 patients) 1596
▲ Lioresal Tablets (0-9%) 829
Lithium Carbonate Capsules & Tablets 2230
Lithonate/Lithotabs/Lithobid 2543
Lopressor Ampuls (1%) 830
Lopressor HCT Tablets 832
Lopressor Tablets (1%) 830
Lotensin HCT (0.6%) 837
Lotrel Capsules (Rare) 840
Loxitane 1378
Ludiomil Tablets (Rare) 843
Lufyllin & Lufyllin-400 Tablets 2670
Lufyllin-GG Elixir & Tablets 2671
Lupron Depot 3.75 mg 2556
Lupron Depot 7.5 mg 2559
Lupron Injection 2555
Lutrepulse for Injection 980
Luvox Tablets (Frequent) 2544
MS Contin Tablets (Less frequent) 1994
MSIR (Infrequent) 1997
Marcaine Hydrochloride with Epinephrine 1:200,000 2316
Marcaine Hydrochloride Injection 2316
Marcaine Spinal 2319
Marinol (Dronabinol) Capsules (0.3 to 1%) 2231
Matulane Capsules 2131
Maxair Autohaler 1492
Maxair Inhaler (Less than 1%) 1494
Maxaquin Tablets (Less than 1%) 2440
Maxzide 1380
Mebaral Tablets (Less than 1 in 100) 2322
Mefoxin 1691
Mefoxin Premixed Intravenous Solution 1694
Mellaril 2269
Mepergan Injection (Rare) 2753
Mephyton Tablets (Rare) 1696
Mepron Suspension (1%) 1135
▲ Mesnex Injection (17%) 702
Methadone Hydrochloride Oral Concentrate 2233
Methergine 2272
Metubine Iodide Vials 916
Mexitil Capsules (Less than 1% or about 6 in 1,000) 678
Mintezol 1704
Miochol-E with Iocare Steri-Tags and Miochol-E System Pak (Rare) ⊙ 273
Mivacron (Two patients; less than 1%) 1138
Moban Tablets and Concentrate (Rare) 1048
8-MOP Capsules 1246
Monoclate-P, Factor VIII:C, Pasteurized, Monoclonal Antibody Purified Antihemophilic Factor (Human) 521
Monoket (Fewer than 1%) 2406
Mononine, Coagulation Factor IX (Human) 523
▲ Monopril Tablets (0.2% to 4.4%) 757
Motrin Ibuprofen Suspension, Oral Drops, Chewable Tablets, Caplets (Less than 1%) 1546
Narcan Injection (Several instances) 934
Navane Capsules and Concentrate 2201
Navane Intramuscular 2202
NebuPent for Inhalation Solution (1% or less) 1040
Nembutal Sodium Capsules (Less than 1%) 436
Nembutal Sodium Solution (Less than 1%) 438
Nembutal Sodium Suppositories (Less than 1%) 440
Nescaine/Nescaine MPF 554
Netromycin Injection 100 mg/ml (Fewer than 1 of 1000 patients) 2373
Neurontin Capsules (Infrequent) 1922
Nicolar Tablets 2026
▲ Nimotop Capsules (1.2%-50.0%) 610
Nitro-Bid IV (Infrequent) 1523
Nitro-Bid Ointment (Infrequent) 1524
Nitrodisc (Infrequent to 4%) 2047
Nitro-Dur (nitroglycerin) Transdermal Infusion System (Infrequent) 1326
Nitrolingual Spray 2027
Norcuron (Rare) 1826
Normodyne Injection (1%) 2377
Normodyne Tablets 2379
Norpace (1 to 3%) 2444
Norpramin Tablets 1526
Norvasc Tablets (0.1% to 1%; rare) 1940
Novahistine DH 2462
Novahistine DMX ▣ 822
Novahistine Elixir ▣ 823
Novahistine Expectorant 2463
Novantrone (Occasional) 1279
Novocain Hydrochloride for Spinal Anesthesia 2326
Novolin 70/30 Prefilled Disposable Insulin Delivery System (Rare) 1798
Nubain Injection (1% or less) 935
Nuromax Injection (0.3%) 1149
Ocupress Ophthalmic Solution, 1% Sterile ⊙ 309
Ogen Tablets 2627
Ogen Vaginal Cream 2630
▲ Oncaspar (Greater than 1% but less than 5%) 2028
Oncovin Solution Vials & Hyporets 1466
Oramorph SR (Morphine Sulfate Sustained Release Tablets) (Less frequent) 2236
Orap Tablets 1050
Oretic Tablets 443
Ornade Spansule Capsules 2502
Orthoclone OKT3 Sterile Solution 1837
Oxsoralen-Ultra Capsules 1257
PBZ Tablets 845
PBZ-SR Tablets 844
Pamelor 2280
Paraplatin for Injection (Rare) 705
▲ Parlodel (28%) 2281
Paxil Tablets (Infrequent) 2505
Pentam 300 Injection (0.9% to 4.0%) 1041
Periactin 1724
Permax Tablets (2.1%) 575
Phenergan with Codeine 2777
Phenergan with Dextromethorphan 2778
Phenergan Injection 2773
Phenergan Suppositories 2775
Phenergan Syrup 2774
Phenergan Tablets 2775
Phenergan VC 2779
Phenergan VC with Codeine 2781
Phenobarbital Elixir and Tablets (Less than 1 in 100 patients) 1469
Placidyl Capsules 448
Plasma-Plex, Plasma Protein Fraction (Human) 5% 524
Platinol (Occasional) 708
Platinol-AQ Injection (Occasional) 710
Plendil Extended-Release Tablets (0.5% to 1.5%) 527
Pondimin Tablets 2066
Pontocaine Hydrochloride for Spinal Anesthesia 2330
Pravachol 765
PREVACID Delayed-Release Capsules (Less than 1%) 2562
Primacor Injection (2.9%) 2331
Primaxin I.M. 1727
Primaxin I.V. (0.4%) 1729
Prinivil Tablets (0.3% to 5.3%; rare) 1733
Prinzide Tablets (1.4%) 1737
Priscoline Hydrochloride Ampuls 845
Procan SR Tablets (Rare) 1926
▲ Procardia Capsules (Approximately 5%; about 1 in 20 to 1 in 50 patients) 1971
Procardia XL Extended Release Tablets (1% or less to about 4%; about 1 in 20 patients; occasional) 1972
Proglycem (Occasional) 580
▲ Prograf (Greater than 3%) 1042
Prolastin Alpha$_1$-Proteinase Inhibitor (Human) (Rare) 635
▲ Proleukin for Injection (85%) 797
Prolixin (Rare) 509
Prostigmin Injectable 1260
Prostigmin Tablets 1261
Prostin E2 Suppository 2634
▲ Prostin VR Pediatric Sterile Solution (About 4%) 2635
Protamine Sulfate Ampoules & Vials 1471
Provocholine for Inhalation 2140
Prozac Pulvules & Liquid, Oral Solution (Infrequent) 919
Quadrinal Tablets 1350
Quibron 2053
Quinidex Extentabs 2067
RMS Suppositories 2657
Recombivax HB (Less than 1%) 1744
Regitine 846
Reglan 2068
▲ ReoPro Vials (21.1%) 1471
Respbid Tablets 682
Revex (1%) 1811
Rifadin 1528
Rifater 1532
Risperdal (Infrequent) 1301
Robaxin Injectable 2070
▲ Roferon-A Injection (4%) 2145
Rogaine Topical Solution (1.53%) 2637
Roxanol 2243
Rum-K Syrup 1005
Rynatan 2673
Rythmol Tablets–150mg, 225mg, 300mg (0.1 to 1.1%) 1352
Salflex Tablets 786
Sandoglobulin I.V. (Less than 1%) 2290

(▣ Described in PDR For Nonprescription Drugs) Incidence data in parenthesis; ▲ 3% or more (⊙ Described in PDR For Ophthalmology)

Seconal Sodium Pulvules (Less than 1 in 100) 1474
Sectral Capsules (Up to 2%) 2807
Seldane Tablets (Rare) 1536
Seldane-D Extended-Release Tablets (Rare) 1538
Sensorcaine 559
Ser-Ap-Es Tablets 849
▲ Serentil (One of the two most prevalent) 684
Serzone Tablets (2%) 771
Sinemet CR Tablets 944
Sinequan (Occasional) 2205
Slo-bid Gyrocaps 2033
Solu-Medrol Sterile Powder 2643
Soma Compound w/Codeine Tablets 2676
Soma Compound Tablets 2675
Soma Tablets 2674
Sorbitrate (Infrequent) 2843
Stadol (Less than 1%) 775
Stelazine 2514
Stimate, (desmopressin acetate) Nasal Spray, 1.5 mg/mL (Infrequent) 525
▲ Streptase for Infusion (1% to 10%) 562
Sublimaze Injection 1307
▲ Sufenta Injection (3% to 9%) 1309
Surmontil Capsules 2811
Survanta Beractant Intratracheal Suspension (Less than 1%) 2226
Syn-Rx Tablets 465
Syn-Rx DM Tablets 466
Tagamet Injection (Rare) 2516
Talacen (Infrequent) 2333
Talwin Compound (Infrequent) 2335
Talwin Nx 2336
Tambocor Tablets (Less than 1%) 1497
Tavist Syrup 2297
Tavist Tablets 2298
▲ Taxol (4% to 12%) 714
Tazicef for Injection (Very rare) 2519
Tegretol Chewable Tablets 852
Tegretol Suspension 852
Tegretol Tablets 852
Tenoretic Tablets 2845
▲ Tenormin Tablets and I.V. Injection (25%) 2847
Tensilon Injectable 1261
Tetramune (Rare) 1404
Thalitone (Common) 1245
Theo-24 Extended Release Capsules 2568
Theo-Dur Extended-Release Tablets 1327
Theo-X Extended-Release Tablets 788
THYREL TRH (A small number of patients) 2873
Timolide Tablets (1.6%) 1748
Timoptic in Ocudose (Less frequent) 1753
Timoptic Sterile Ophthalmic Solution (Less frequent) 1751
Timoptic-XE 1755
Tonocard Tablets (1.8-3.4%) 531
Toprol-XL Tablets (About 1 of 100 patients) 565
Toradol 2159
Torecan 2245
Tornalate Solution for Inhalation, 0.2% 956
Tracrium Injection (5 out of 875 patients) 1183
Trandate (Less common; 1 of 100 patients) 1185
▲ Transderm-Nitro Transdermal Therapeutic System (4%) 859
Tranxene 451
▲ Trasylol (6%) 613
Trental Tablets (Less than 1%) 1244
Triavil Tablets 1757
Tri-Immunol Adsorbed (Rare) 1408
Trilafon (Rare) 2389
Trinalin Repetabs Tablets 1330
Triostat Injection (Approximately 2%) 2530
Tripedia 892
Tussend 1783
Tussend Expectorant 1785
Typhim Vi 899
Uni-Dur Extended-Release Tablets 1331
Uniphyl 400 mg Tablets 2001
Urecholine 1761
Valium Injectable 2182
Valium Tablets (Infrequent) 2183
Valrelease Capsules (Infrequent) 2169
Vancocin HCl, Vials & ADD-Vantage (Infrequent) 1481
Vantin for Oral Suspension and Vantin Tablets (Less than 1%) 2646
Vaseretic Tablets (Rare; 0.9%) 1765
▲ Vasotec I.V. (Rare; 0.9% to 5.2%) 1768
▲ Vasotec Tablets (0.5% to 6.7%) 1771
Velosulin BR Human Insulin 10 ml Vials 1795
VePesid Capsules and Injection (0.7% to 2%) 718
Verelan Capsules (2.5%) 1410
Verelan Capsules (2.5%) 2824
Versed Injection 2170
Vexol 1% Ophthalmic Suspension (Less than 2%) ⊙ 230
Videx Tablets, Powder for Oral Solution, & Pediatric Powder for Oral Solution (1% to 4%) 720
Virazole 1264
Visken Tablets (2% or fewer patients) 2299
Vivactil Tablets 1774
Voltaren Tablets 861
Vontrol Tablets (Few) 2532
Vumon (2%) 727
Wellbutrin Tablets (2.5%) 1204
▲ Xanax Tablets (4.7%) 2649
▲ Xylocaine Injections (3%) 567
▲ Yutopar Intravenous Injection (80 to 100%) 570
Zantac Injection 1207
Zaroxolyn Tablets 1000
Zebeta Tablets 1413
Zefazone 2654
Zemuron (0.1%; 2%) 1830
Zestoretic (1.4%; rare) 2850
Zestril Tablets (Rare; 0.3% to 5.3%) 2854
Ziac 1415
Zofran Injection (Rare; 2%) 1214
▲ Zofran Tablets (5%) 1217
Zoloft Tablets (Infrequent) 2217
Zosyn (1.0% or less) 1419
Zosyn Pharmacy Bulk Package (1.0% or less) 1422
Zovirax Sterile Powder (Less than 1%) 1223

Hypotension, asymptomatic

▲ Brevibloc Injection (About 25%) 1808
▲ Cardizem Injectable (4.3%) 1508
▲ Isoptin SR Tablets (5%) 1348
▲ Neupogen for Injection (7 of 176 patients) 495
▲ Verelan Capsules (5%) 1410
▲ Verelan Capsules (5%) 2824

Hypotension, exertional

Cardene Capsules (Rare) 2095
Esimil Tablets 822

Hypotension, neonatal

Accupril Tablets 1893
Altace Capsules 1232
Capoten 739
Capozide 742
Cozaar Tablets 1628
Hyzaar Tablets 1677
Lotensin Tablets 834
Lotensin HCT 837
Lotrel Capsules 840
Monopril Tablets 757
Normodyne Injection 2377
Normodyne Tablets (Rare) 2379
Prinivil Tablets 1733
Prinzide Tablets 1737
Sectral Capsules 2807
Trandate 1185
Univasc Tablets 2410
Vaseretic Tablets 1765
Vasotec I.V. 1768
Vasotec Tablets 1771
Yutopar Intravenous Injection (Infrequent) 570
Zestoretic 2850
Zestril Tablets 2854

Hypotension, orthostatic

Accupril Tablets (Rare) 1893
▲ Adalat Capsules (10 mg and 20 mg) (Approximately 5%) 587
Aldactazide 2413
Aldoclor Tablets 1598
Aldomet Ester HCl Injection 1602
Aldomet Oral 1600
Aldoril Tablets 1604
Apresazide Capsules 808
Atamet (Less frequent) 572
Brontex 1981
Capoten 739
Capozide 742
▲ Cardura Tablets (Up to 23%) 2186
Catapres-TTS (Less frequent) 675
Clozaril Tablets 2252
Combipres Tablets (About 3 in 100) 677
Desyrel and Desyrel Dividose 503
▲ Dilatrate-SR (2-36%) 2398
Dipentum Capsules (Rare) 1951
Diucardin Tablets 2718
Diupres Tablets 1650
Diuril Oral Suspension 1653
Diuril Sodium Intravenous 1652
Diuril Tablets 1653
Elavil 2838
Eldepryl Tablets 2550
Endep Tablets 2174
Enduron Tablets 420
Esidrix Tablets 821
Esimil Tablets 822
Furoxone 2046
HydroDIURIL Tablets 1674
Hydropres Tablets 1675
▲ Hylorel Tablets (6.6% to 7.5%) 985
Hyperstat I.V. Injection 2363
Hytrin Capsules 430
Inderide Tablets 2732
Inderide LA Long Acting Capsules 2734
IOPIDINE Sterile Ophthalmic Solution ⊙ 219
Larodopa Tablets 2129
Lasix Injection, Oral Solution and Tablets 1240
▲ Levoprome (Among the most important) 1274
Lioresal Intrathecal 1596
Loniten Tablets 2618
Lopressor HCT Tablets 832
Lotensin HCT 837
Loxitane 1378
Lozol Tablets (Less than 5%) 2022
Lysodren (Infrequent) 698
MS Contin Tablets 1994
Maxzide 1380
Mellaril (Greater tendency in female patients) 2269
Methadone Hydrochloride Oral Concentrate 2233
Midamor Tablets (Less than or equal to 1%) 1703
Minipress Capsules (1-4%) 1937
Minizide Capsules 1938
Moduretic Tablets (Less than or equal to 1%) 1705
Monopril Tablets (1.4% to 1.9%) 757
Mykrox Tablets (Less than 2%) 993
Oretic Tablets 443
▲ Parlodel (6%) 2281
Phenergan with Codeine 2777
Phenergan VC with Codeine 2781
Prinivil Tablets (1.0% to 1.9%) 1733
Prinzide Tablets (0.5% to 1.0%) 1737
Regitine 846
Risperdal 1301
Roxanol 2243
Sandostatin Injection (Less than 1%) 2292
Ser-Ap-Es Tablets 849
Sinemet Tablets (Less frequent) 943
Sinemet CR Tablets (1.0%) 944
Slo-Niacin Tablets (Less common) 2659
Symmetrel Capsules and Syrup (1% to 5%) 946
Tenoretic Tablets 2845
Thalitone 1245
Timolide Tablets 1748
Tofranil Ampuls 854
Tofranil Tablets 856
Tofranil-PM Capsules 857
Tonocard Tablets (Less than 1%) 531
Trandate 1185
Triavil Tablets 1757
Ultram Tablets (50 mg) (Less than 1%) 1585
Vaseretic Tablets (0.5% to 2.0%) 1765
Vasotec I.V. 1768
Vasotec Tablets (0.5% to 1.6%) 1771
Vivactil Tablets 1774
Wellbutrin Tablets 1204
Zaroxolyn Tablets 1000
Zebeta Tablets 1413
Zestoretic (0.3 to 1%) 2850
Zestril Tablets (1.0% to 1.9%) 2854
Ziac 1415

Hypotension, postural

Adalat CC (Less than 1.0%) 589
Akineton 1333
Altace Capsules (2.2%) 1232
Ambien Tablets (Infrequent) 2416
▲ Anafranil Capsules (4% to 6%) 803
Betaseron for SC Injection 658
Cardene Capsules (Rare) 2095
Cardene I.V. (1.4%) 2709
Cardene SR Capsules (0.9%) 2097
▲ Cardura Tablets (0.3% to 29%) 2186
▲ CellCept Capsules (More than or equal to 3%) 2099
Cipro Tablets 592
Depakote Tablets (Greater than 1% but not more than 5%) 415
Dibenzyline Capsules 2476
Dilacor XR Extended-release Capsules (Infrequent) 2018
Dyazide 2479
Effexor (1%) 2719
Esimil Tablets 822
Etrafon 2355
Hycomine Compound Tablets 932
Hycomine 931
Hycotuss Expectorant Syrup 933
▲ Hytrin Capsules (0.5% to 3.9%; 21%) 430
Intron A (Less than 5%) 2364
Inversine Tablets 1686
Ismelin Tablets 827
Ismo Tablets (Fewer than 1%) 2738
Isordil Tembids 2741
Isordil Titradose Tablets 2742
Lamictal Tablets (Rare) 1112
Lotensin Tablets (0.4%) 834
Lotensin HCT (0.3%) 837
Luvox Tablets 2544
Nardil (Common) 1920
Nitrolingual Spray (Occasional) 2027
Nitrostat Tablets (Occasional) 1925
▲ Normodyne Injection (58%) 2377
Normodyne Tablets (1%) 2379
Noroxin Tablets 1715
Noroxin Tablets 2048
Norvasc Tablets (More than 0.1% to 1%) 1940
Orap Tablets 1050
Orlamm (Less than 1%) 2239
▲ Parlodel (6%) 2281
Paxil Tablets (1.2%) 2505
▲ Permax Tablets (9.0%) 575
Prozac Pulvules & Liquid, Oral Solution (Infrequent) 919
Sansert Tablets 2295
▲ Serzone Tablets (2.8% to 4%) 771
Soma Compound w/Codeine Tablets 2676
Soma Compound Tablets 2675
Soma Tablets 2674
Sorbitrate 2843
Tegison Capsules (Less than 1%) 2154
▲ Temaril Tablets, Syrup and Spansule Extended-Release Capsules (Most common) 483
▲ Tenoretic Tablets (2% to 4%) 2845
▲ Tenormin Tablets and I.V. Injection (2% to 4%) 2847
Thorazine 2523
Torecan 2245
▲ Trandate (58%) 1185
Trecator-SC Tablets 2814
Trilafon 2389
Univasc Tablets (Less than 1%; 0.51%) 2410
Vasotec I.V. (2.3%) 1768
Vicodin Tuss Expectorant 1358
Zoloft Tablets (Infrequent) 2217

Hypotension, secondary to spinal block

Duranest Injections 542
Marcaine Hydrochloride with Epinephrine 1:200,000 2316
Marcaine Hydrochloride Injection 2316
Sensorcaine 559
Xylocaine Injections 567

Hypotension, symptomatic

Accupril Tablets 1893
Altace Capsules (0.5%) 1232
▲ Brevibloc Injection (12%) 1808
Calan SR Caplets 2422
Calan Tablets 2419
Cardizem CD Capsules (Occasional) 1506
Cardizem SR Capsules (Occasional) 1510
▲ Cardizem Injectable (3.2%) 1508
Cardizem Tablets (Occasional) 1512
Cozaar Tablets 1628
Hyzaar Tablets 1677
Isoptin Injectable (1.5%) 1344
Lotensin Tablets (Rare to 0.3%) 834
Lotensin HCT 837
Lotrel Capsules 840
Monopril Tablets 757
Prinivil Tablets 1733
Univasc Tablets (Less than 1%; 0.5%) 2410

(▭ Described in PDR For Nonprescription Drugs) Incidence data in parenthesis; ▲ 3% or more (⊙ Described in PDR For Ophthalmology)

Hypotensive crisis Side Effects Index 1336

Hypotensive crisis
Fiorinal with Codeine Capsules 2262
Miltown Tablets 2672
PMB 200 and PMB 400 (One instance) 2783
Prolixin 509

Hypothermia
Betaseron for SC Injection 658
Clozaril Tablets (Less than 1%) 2252
Ethmozine Tablets (Less than 2%) 2041
Felbatol 2666
Foscavir Injection (Less than 1%) .. 547
Ganite 2533
Glucophage 752
Lioresal Intrathecal 1596
Permax Tablets (Infrequent) 575
Prostin VR Pediatric Sterile Solution (Less than 1%) 2635
Prozac Pulvules & Liquid, Oral Solution (Rare) 919
Risperdal 1301
Salagen Tablets (Less than 1%) 1489
Urecholine 1761

Hypothyroidism
Anafranil Capsules (Infrequent) 803
▲ Aredia for Injection (Up to 6%) 810
Betaseron for SC Injection 658
Cognex Capsules (Rare) 1901
Cordarone Tablets (1 to 3%) 2712
Effexor (Rare) 2719
Eskalith 2485
Genotropin (Infrequent) 111
Humatrope Vials 1443
Imitrex Tablets (Rare) 1106
Intron A (Less than 5%) 2364
Lithium Carbonate Capsules & Tablets 2230
Lithonate/Lithotabs/Lithobid 2543
Luvox Tablets (Infrequent) 2544
Neurontin Capsules (Rare) 1922
Paxil Tablets (Rare) 2505
Permax Tablets (Infrequent) 575
Proleukin for Injection (Less than 1%) 797
Protropin 1063
Prozac Pulvules & Liquid, Oral Solution (Infrequent) 919
▲ Sandostatin Injection (Several isolated patients up to 12%) 2292

Hypotonia
Ambien Tablets (Rare) 2416
Diphtheria and Tetanus Toxoids and Pertussis Vaccine Adsorbed.. 2477
Diprivan Injection (Less than 1%) .. 2833
Duragesic Transdermal System (Less than 1%) 1288
Effexor (Infrequent) 2719
Klonopin Tablets 2126
Lamictal Tablets (Rare) 1112
Lioresal Intrathecal (2 to 3 of 214 patients) 1596
Luvox Tablets (Infrequent) 2544
Neurontin Capsules (Infrequent) 1922
Orthoclone OKT3 Sterile Solution .. 1837
Penetrex Tablets (Less than 0.1%) 2031
Permax Tablets (Infrequent) 575
Risperdal (Rare) 1301
Serzone Tablets (Rare) 771
Supprelin Injection (1%) 2056
Tetramune 1404
Zoloft Tablets (Rare) 2217

Hypouresis
Atromid-S Capsules 2701
▲ CHEMET (succimer) Capsules (Up to 3.7%) 1545
Coly-Mycin M Parenteral 1905
Dilaudid-HP Injection 1337
Dilaudid-HP Lyophilized Powder 250 mg 1337
▲ Indocin I.V. (41% of infants) 1684
K-Phos Neutral Tablets 639
Nicobid 2026
Polymyxin B Sulfate, Aerosporin Brand Sterile Powder 1154
Proglycem 580
Prograf 1042
Slo-Niacin Tablets 2659
Trobicin Sterile Powder 2645
Uroqid-Acid No. 2 Tablets 640
Yocon 1892

Hypouricemia
Cipro I.V. (Infrequent) 595
Cipro I.V. Pharmacy Bulk Package (Less than 1%) 597
Timentin for Injection 2528

Zoloft Tablets 2217

Hypoventilation
Anafranil Capsules (Rare) 803
Betaseron for SC Injection 658
▲ Buprenex Injectable (1-5%) 2006
Butisol Sodium Elixir & Tablets (Less than 1 in 100) 2660
Carbocaine Hydrochloride Injection 2303
Diprivan Injection (Less than 1%) .. 2833
Dopram Injectable 2061
▲ Duragesic Transdermal System (2% to 10%) 1288
Marcaine Hydrochloride with Epinephrine 1:200,000 2316
Marcaine Hydrochloride Injection 2316
Marcaine Spinal 2319
Mebaral Tablets (Less than 1 in 100) 2322
Nembutal Sodium Capsules (Less than 1%) 436
Nembutal Sodium Solution (Less than 1%) 438
Nembutal Sodium Suppositories (Less than 1%) 440
Nesacaine Injections 554
Neurontin Capsules (Rare) 1922
Permax Tablets (Rare) 575
Phenobarbital Elixir and Tablets (Less than 1 in 100 patients) 1469
Seconal Sodium Pulvules (Less than 1 in 100) 1474
Sensorcaine 559
Versed Injection 2170
▲ Videx Tablets, Powder for Oral Solution, & Pediatric Powder for Oral Solution (Less than 1% to 10%) 720
Virazole (Infrequent) 1264

Hypovolemia
Demadex Tablets and Injection 686
Estratest 2539
Humegon 1824
Inapsine Injection 1296
Mykrox Tablets 993
Serophene (clomiphene citrate tablets, USP) 2451
Zaroxolyn Tablets 1000

Hypoxemia
Abbokinase 403
Abbokinase Open-Cath 405
Glucophage 752
Inocor Lactate Injection (1 case) 2309
Isuprel Hydrochloride Solution 1:200 & 1:100 2313
Methotrexate Sodium Tablets, Injection, for Injection and LPF Injection 1275
Mivacron (Less than 1%) 1138
Orthoclone OKT3 Sterile Solution .. 1837

Hypoxia
Alfenta Injection 1286
Ambien Tablets (Rare) 2416
Atretol Tablets 573
Betaseron for SC Injection 658
Depakene 413
Dilantin-125 Suspension 1911
Diprivan Injection (Less than 1%) .. 2833
Effexor (Rare) 2719
Felbatol 2666
Fludara for Injection (Up to 1%) 663
Levophed Bitartrate Injection 2315
Nardil (Less frequent) 1920
Orthoclone OKT3 Sterile Solution .. 1837
Permax Tablets (Rare) 575
Prozac Pulvules & Liquid, Oral Solution (Rare) 919
Pulmozyme Inhalation 1064
Suprane (Less than 1%) 1813
Tegretol Chewable Tablets 852
Tegretol Suspension 852
Tegretol Tablets 852
Videx Tablets, Powder for Oral Solution, & Pediatric Powder for Oral Solution (Less than 1%) 720
▲ Zofran Tablets (9%) 1217

Hysteria
Actifed with Codeine Cough Syrup.. 1067
Ambien Tablets (Rare) 2416
Cognex Capsules (Rare) 1901
Deconamine 1320
Diprivan Injection (Less than 1%) .. 2833
Imitrex Injection (Rare) 1103
Imitrex Tablets (Rare) 1106
Klonopin Tablets 2126
Luvox Tablets (Infrequent) 2544
Neurontin Capsules (Rare) 1922

Ornade Spansule Capsules 2502
PBZ Tablets 845
PBZ-SR Tablets 844
Paxil Tablets (Rare) 2505
Periactin 1724
Phenergan Injection 2773
Phenergan Tablets 2775
Placidyl Capsules (Occasional) 448
Prozac Pulvules & Liquid, Oral Solution (Rare) 919
Tavist Syrup 2297
Tavist Tablets 2298
Temaril Tablets, Syrup and Spansule Extended-Release Capsules 483
Trinalin Repetabs Tablets 1330
Tussend 1783
Zoloft Tablets (Rare) 2217

HPA axis suppression
Aclovate 1069
Carmol HC (Some patients) 924
Cutivate Cream 1088
Cutivate Ointment 1089
Dermatop Emollient Cream 0.1% .. 1238
Diprolene 2352
ProctoCream-HC 2.5% 2408
Temovate (Infrequent) 1179
Ultravate Cream 0.05% 2689
Ultravate Ointment 0.05% 2690

HPA function suppression
Azmacort Oral Inhaler 2011
Beclovent Inhalation Aerosol and Refill 1075
Vanceril Inhaler 2394

I

Ichthyosis
Efudex (Infrequent) 2113
▲ Lamprene Capsules (8-28%) 828

Idiosyncrasy
Berocca Plus Tablets (Possible) 2087
Berocca Tablets 2087
Blenoxane (1%) 692
Cocaine Hydrochloride Topical Solution 537
Cystospaz 1963
Donnatal 2060
Donnatal Extentabs 2061
Donnatal Tablets 2060
Duranest Injections 542
Etrafon (Extremely rare) 2355
Lasix Injection, Oral Solution and Tablets 1240
Miltown Tablets 2672
Novocain Hydrochloride for Spinal Anesthesia (Rare) 2326
PMB 200 and PMB 400 2783
Pontocaine Hydrochloride for Spinal Anesthesia 2330
Robinul Forte Tablets 2072
Robinul Injectable 2072
Robinul Tablets 2072
Soma Compound w/Codeine Tablets (Very rare) 2676
Soma Compound Tablets (Very rare) 2675
Soma Tablets (Very rare) 2674
Tympagesic Ear Drops (Infrequently) 2342
Xylocaine Injections 567

Idiosyncratic reactions (see under Idiosyncrasy)

Idioventricular rhythms
Activase 1058
Eminase 2039

Ileitis, regional
Accutane Capsules 2076
Indocin (Less than 1%) 1680

Ileus
Atgam Sterile Solution (Less than 1%) 2581
Betaseron for SC Injection 658
▲ CellCept Capsules (More than or equal to 3%) 2099
Cipro I.V. (1% or less) 595
Cipro I.V. Pharmacy Bulk Package (Less than 1%) 597
Cogentin 1621
Dilaudid Tablets and Liquid 1339
Effexor (Rare) 2719
Ethmozine Tablets (Less than 2%) 2041
Felbatol 2666
Hyperstat I.V. Injection 2363

Indocin I.V. (1% to 3%) 1684
Inversine Tablets 1686
Lioresal Intrathecal 1596
Nimotop Capsules (Rare) 610
Paxil Tablets (Rare) 2505
Proglycem (Frequent) 580
▲ Prograf (Greater than 3%) 1042
Proleukin for Injection (2%) 797
ReoPro Vials (0.3%) 1471
Vaseretic Tablets 1765
Vasotec I.V. 1768
Vasotec Tablets (0.5% to 1.0%) 1771
Velban Vials 1484
Videx Tablets, Powder for Oral Solution, & Pediatric Powder for Oral Solution (Less than 1%) 720
Yutopar Intravenous Injection (Infrequent) 570
Zosyn (1.0% or less) 1419
Zosyn Pharmacy Bulk Package (1.0% or less) 1422

Ileus, adynamic
Compazine 2470
Etrafon 2355
Navane Capsules and Concentrate 2201
Navane Intramuscular 2202
Stelazine 2514
Thorazine 2523
Trilafon (Occasional) 2389

Ileus, neonatal
Yutopar Intravenous Injection (Infrequent) 570

Ileus, paralytic
Anafranil Capsules (Rare) 803
Apresazide Capsules (Less frequent) 808
Apresoline Hydrochloride Tablets (Less frequent) 809
Arfonad Ampuls 2080
Artane (Rare) 1368
Asendin Tablets (Very rare) 1369
Calan SR Caplets (Infrequent) 2422
Calan Tablets (Infrequent) 2419
Clozaril Tablets 2252
Cogentin 1621
Elavil 2838
Endep Tablets 2174
Etrafon 2355
Flexeril Tablets (Rare) 1661
Foscavir Injection (Less than 1%) .. 547
Imodium Capsules (Rare) 1295
Isoptin SR Tablets (Infrequent) 1348
Limbitrol 2180
Lomotil 2439
Loxitane 1378
Ludiomil Tablets (Isolated reports) 843
Mellaril 2269
Motofen Tablets 784
Navelbine Injection (1%) 1145
Norpramin Tablets 1526
Oncovin Solution Vials & Hyporets 1466
Pamelor 2280
Podocon-25 1891
Prolixin 509
Ser-Ap-Es Tablets 849
Serentil 684
Surmontil Capsules 2811
Taxol (Rare) 714
Tofranil Ampuls 854
Tofranil Tablets 856
Tofranil-PM Capsules 857
Torecan 2245
Triavil Tablets 1757
Verelan Capsules (Infrequent) 1410
Verelan Capsules (Frequent) 2824
Vivactil Tablets 1774

Illusion, unspecified
Ambien Tablets (Rare) 2416
Anafranil Capsules (Rare) 803

Immobility
Moban Tablets and Concentrate 1048

Immunoglobulin, abnormalities
Cytosar-U Sterile Powder 2592
Dilantin Infatabs 1908
Dilantin Kapseals 1906
Dilantin Parenteral 1910
Dilantin-125 Suspension 1911
Proglycem Capsules 580

Immunosuppression
Cytoxan 694
NEOSAR Lyophilized/Neosar 1959
Purinethol Tablets 1156
Rifamate Capsules 1530
Rimactane Capsules 847

(▣ Described in PDR For Nonprescription Drugs) Incidence data in parenthesis; ▲ 3% or more (◉ Described in PDR For Ophthalmology)

1337 Side Effects Index Indecisiveness

Immunosuppression, progressive

Lamictal Tablets 1112

Impetigo

Hivid Tablets (Less than 1% to less than 3%) 2121
▲ Videx Tablets, Powder for Oral Solution, & Pediatric Powder for Oral Solution (5% to 6%) 720

Impotence

Adalat CC (3% or less) 589
Adipex-P Tablets and Capsules 1048
Aldoclor Tablets 1598
Aldomet Ester HCl Injection 1602
Aldomet Oral 1600
Aldoril Tablets 1604
Altace Capsules (Less than 1%) 1232
Ambien Tablets (Rare) 2416
▲ Anafranil Capsules (Up to 20%) 803
Antabuse Tablets (Small number of patients) 2695
Asendin Tablets (Less than 1%) 1369
Atretol Tablets 573
Atromid-S Capsules 2701
Axid Pulvules 1427
Bentyl 1501
Betaseron for SC Injection 658
Betimol 0.25%, 0.5% ◉ 261
Biphetamine Capsules 983
Blocadren Tablets (Less than 1%) 1614
BuSpar (Rare) 737
Calan SR Caplets (1% or less) 2422
Calan Tablets (1% or less) 2419
Capoten 739
Capozide 742
Cardene Capsules (Rare) 2095
Cardizem CD Capsules (Less than 1%) 1506
Cardizem SR Capsules (Less than 1%) 1510
Cardizem Injectable 1508
Cardizem Tablets (Less than 1%) 1512
Cardura Tablets (1.1%) 2186
Cartrol Tablets (Less common) 410
Cataflam (Less than 1%) 816
Catapres Tablets (About 3 in 100 patients) 674
Catapres-TTS (2 of 101 patients; less frequent) 675
▲ CellCept Capsules (More than or equal to 3%) 2099
Claritin (2% or fewer patients) 2349
Claritin-D (Less frequent) 2350
Clozaril Tablets (Less than 1%) 2252
Cognex Capsules (Infrequent) 1901
Combipres Tablets (About 3%) 677
Compazine 2470
Cozaar Tablets (Less than 1%) 1628
Cytotec (Infrequent) 2424
Cytovene-IV (Two or more reports) 2103
Demser Capsules (Infrequent) 1649
Desoxyn Gradumet Tablets 419
Desyrel and Desyrel Dividose 503
Dexedrine 2474
DextroStat Dextroamphetamine Tablets 2036
Dilacor XR Extended-release Capsules (Infrequent) 2018
Dipentum Capsules (Rare) 1951
Ditropan 1516
Diupres Tablets 1650
Diuril Oral Suspension 1653
Diuril Sodium Intravenous 1652
Diuril Tablets 1653
Donnatal 2060
Donnatal Extentabs 2061
Donnatal Tablets 2060
Doral Tablets 2664
Dyazide 2479
DynaCirc Capsules (0.5% to 1%) 2256
▲ Effexor (2.1% to 6%) 2719
Elavil 2838
Endep Tablets 2174
Esimil Tablets (A few instances) 822
Eskalith 2485
Ethmozine Tablets (Less than 2%) 2041
Etrafon 2355
▲ Eulexin Capsules (33% with LHRH agonist) 2358
Fastin Capsules 2488
Flexeril Tablets (Rare) 1661
Gelfoam Sterile Sponge 2608
Haldol Decanoate 1577
Haldol Injection, Tablets and Concentrate 1575
HydroDIURIL Tablets 1674
Hydropres Tablets 1675
Hytrin Capsules (1.2% to 1.6%) 430
Hyzaar Tablets 1677
Imdur (Less than or equal to 5%) 1323
Inderal (Rare) 2728
Inderal LA Long Acting Capsules (Rare) 2730
Inderide Tablets (Rare) 2732
Inderide LA Long Acting Capsules (Rare) 2734
Intron A (Less than 5%) 2364
Inversine Tablets 1686
Ionamin Capsules 990
Ismelin Tablets 827
Ismo Tablets (Fewer than 1%) 2738
Isoptin Oral Tablets (Less than 1%) 1346
Isoptin SR Tablets (1% or less) 1348
Kerlone Tablets (1.2%) 2436
Lamictal Tablets (Rare) 1112
Levatol (0.5%) 2403
Levsin/Levsinex/Levbid 2405
Limbitrol (Less common) 2180
Lioresal Tablets (Rare) 829
Lithonate/Lithotabs/Lithobid 2543
Lopid Tablets 1917
Lopressor HCT Tablets (1 in 100 patients) 832
Lorelco Tablets 1517
Lotensin Tablets 834
Lotensin HCT (1.2%) 837
Lotrel Capsules 840
Lozol Tablets (Less than 5%) 2022
Ludiomil Tablets (Rare) 843
Lupron Depot 3.75 mg 2556
▲ Lupron Depot 7.5 mg (5.4%) 2559
▲ Lupron Injection (5% or more) 2555
Luvox Tablets (2%) 2544
MS Contin Tablets (Less frequent) 1994
MSIR (Infrequent) 1997
▲ Megace Oral Suspension (4% to 14%) 699
Methotrexate Sodium Tablets, Injection, for Injection and LPF Injection 1275
Mexitil Capsules (Less than 1% or about 4 in 1,000) 678
Midamor Tablets (Between 1% and 3%) 1703
Minipress Capsules (Less than 1%) 1937
Minizide Capsules (Rare) 1938
Moduretic Tablets (Less than or equal to 1%) 1705
Mykrox Tablets (Less than 2%) 993
Mysoline (Occasional) 2754
Navane Capsules and Concentrate 2201
Navane Intramuscular 2202
NEOSAR Lyophilized/Neosar 1959
Neurontin Capsules (1.5%) 1922
Nizoral Tablets (Less than 1%) 1298
Nolvadex Tablets 2841
▲ Normodyne Injection (1% to 4%) 2377
▲ Normodyne Tablets (1% to 4%) 2379
Norpace (1 to 3%) 2444
Norpramin Tablets 1526
Oramorph SR (Morphine Sulfate Sustained Release Tablets) (Less frequent) 2236
Orap Tablets 1050
▲ Orlamm (3% to 9%) 2239
Orudis Capsules (Less than 1%) 2766
Oruvail Capsules (Less than 1%) 2766
Oxandrin 2862
Pamelor 2280
Parnate Tablets 2503
▲ Paxil Tablets (1.9% to 10.0%) 2505
Pepcid Injection (Rare) 1722
Pepcid (Rare) 1720
Permax Tablets (Infrequent) 575
Plendil Extended-Release Tablets (0.5% to 1.5%) 527
Prelu-2 Timed Release Capsules 681
PREVACID Delayed-Release Capsules (Less than 1%) 2562
Prinivil Tablets (1.0%) 1733
Prinzide Tablets (1.2%) 1737
Pro-Banthīne Tablets 2052
Procardia XL Extended Release Tablets (Less than 3%) 1972
Prolixin 509
▲ Proscar Tablets (3.7%) 1741
Prozac Pulvules & Liquid, Oral Solution (1.7%) 919
Quarzan Capsules 2181
Reglan 2068
Relafen Tablets (Less than 1%) 2510
Robinul Forte Tablets 2072
Robinul Injectable 2072
Robinul Tablets 2072
▲ Roferon-A Injection (6%) 2145
Rythmol Tablets–150mg, 225mg, 300mg (Less than 1%) 1352
Sanorex Tablets (Rare) 2294
Sectral Capsules (Up to 2%) 2807
Sensorcaine 559
Ser-Ap-Es Tablets 849
Serentil 684
Serzone Tablets (Frequent) 771
Sporanox Capsules (0.2% to 1.2%) 1305
Stelazine 2514
Surmontil Capsules 2811
Tagamet 2516
Tambocor Tablets (Less than 1%) 1497
Tegretol Chewable Tablets 852
Tegretol Suspension 852
Tegretol Tablets 852
▲ Tenex Tablets (Up to 7%) 2074
Tenoretic Tablets 2845
Tenormin Tablets and I.V. Injection 2847
Thalitone 1245
Thorazine 2523
Timolide Tablets 1748
Timoptic in Ocudose (Less frequent) 1753
Timoptic Sterile Ophthalmic Solution (Less frequent) 1751
Timoptic-XE 1755
Tofranil Ampuls 854
Tofranil Tablets 856
Tofranil-PM Capsules 857
Trandate Tablets (1% to 4%) 1185
Trecator-SC Tablets 2814
Trilafon 2389
Vascor (200, 300 and 400 mg) Tablets (0.5 to 2.0%) 1587
Vaseretic Tablets (2.2%) 1765
Vasotec I.V. 1768
Vasotec Tablets (0.5% to 1.0%) 1771
Verelan Capsules (1% or less) 1410
Verelan Capsules (Less than 1%) 2824
Videx Tablets, Powder for Oral Solution, & Pediatric Powder for Oral Solution (Less than 1%) 720
Visken Tablets (2% or fewer patients) 2299
Vivactil Tablets 1774
Voltaren Tablets (Less than 1%) 861
▲ Wellbutrin Tablets (3.4%) 1204
Winstrol Tablets 2337
Zantac (Occasional) 1209
Zantac Injection 1207
Zantac Syrup (Occasional) 1209
Zaroxolyn Tablets 1000
Zebeta Tablets 1413
Zerit Capsules (Fewer than 1% to 1%) 729
Zestoretic (1.2%) 2850
Zestril Tablets (1.0%) 2854
Ziac (1.1%) 1415
Zyloprim Tablets (Less than 1%) 1226

Impulse control, impaired

Anafranil Capsules (Rare) 803

Incontinence

Doral Tablets 2664
Halcion Tablets 2611
Lupron Depot 7.5 mg 2559
Lupron Injection (Less than 5%) 2555
MetroGel-Vaginal 902
Minipress Capsules (Less than 1%) 1937
Minizide Capsules (Rare) 1938
Moduretic Tablets (Less than or equal to 1%) 1705
Protostat Tablets 1883
Serax Capsules 2810
Serax Tablets 2810
Serentil 684
Supprelin Injection (1% to 3%) 2056
Tensilon Injectable 1261
Valium Injectable 2182
Valium Tablets (Infrequent) 2183
Valrelease Capsules (Infrequent) 2169
Xanax Tablets (1.5%) 2649

Incontinence, fecal

Betaseron for SC Injection 658
Carbocaine Hydrochloride Injection 2303
Cardura Tablets (Less than 0.5% of 3960 patients) 2186
Cognex Capsules (Infrequent) 1901
Cytovene (1% or less) 2103
Depakote Tablets (Greater than 1% but not more than 5%) 415
Eskalith 2485
Gelfoam Sterile Sponge 2608
Klonopin Tablets 2126
Lioresal Intrathecal 1596
Lithium Carbonate Capsules & Tablets 2230
Lithonate/Lithotabs/Lithobid 2543
Luvox Tablets (Rare) 2544
Marcaine Hydrochloride with Epinephrine 1:200,000 2316
Marcaine Hydrochloride Injection 2316
Marcaine Spinal 2319
Marinol (Dronabinol) Capsules (Less than 1%) 2231
Neurontin Capsules (Infrequent) 1922
Paxil Tablets (Rare) 2505
Pentasa (Less than 1%) 1527
Permax Tablets (Rare) 575
Prozac Pulvules & Liquid, Oral Solution (Rare) 919
Risperdal (Rare) 1301
Sensorcaine 559
Zoloft Tablets (Rare) 2217

Incontinence, urinary

Ambien Tablets (Infrequent) 2416
Anafranil Capsules (Infrequent) 803
Atamet 572
BCG Vaccine, USP (TICE) (2.4%) 1814
Betaseron for SC Injection 658
Carbocaine Hydrochloride Injection 2303
Cardura Tablets (1%) 2186
Clozaril Tablets (1%) 2252
▲ Cognex Capsules (3%) 1901
Dantrium Capsules (Less frequent) 1982
Depakote Tablets (Greater than 1% but not more than 5%) 415
Desyrel and Desyrel Dividose 503
Dizac 1809
Doral Tablets 2664
Effexor (Infrequent) 2719
Esimil Tablets 822
Eskalith 2485
Ethmozine Tablets (Less than 2%) 2041
Etrafon 2355
▲ Felbatol (6.5%) 2666
Flagyl 375 Capsules 2434
Flagyl I.V. 2247
Floropryl Sterile Ophthalmic Ointment (Rare) 1662
Foscavir Injection (Less than 1%) 547
Gelfoam Sterile Sponge 2608
Humorsol Sterile Ophthalmic Solution (Rare) 1664
Hytrin Capsules (At least 1%) 430
Ismelin Tablets 827
Lamictal Tablets (Infrequent) 1112
Larodopa Tablets (Infrequent) 2129
Lioresal Intrathecal 1596
Lithium Carbonate Capsules & Tablets 2230
Lithonate/Lithotabs/Lithobid 2543
Lupron Depot 3.75 mg 2556
Lupron Depot-PED 7.5 mg, 11.25 mg and 15 mg (Less than 2%) 2560
Luvox Tablets (Infrequent) 2544
Marcaine Hydrochloride with Epinephrine 1:200,000 2316
Marcaine Hydrochloride Injection 2316
Marcaine Spinal 2319
Megace Oral Suspension (1% to 3%) 699
Mellaril 2269
Neurontin Capsules (Infrequent) 1922
Parlodel 2281
Parnate Tablets 2503
Paxil Tablets (Infrequent) 2505
Penetrex Tablets (Less than 1% but more than or equal to 0.1%) 2031
Permax Tablets (Frequent) 575
ProSom Tablets (Rare) 449
Prozac Pulvules & Liquid, Oral Solution (Infrequent) 919
Reglan 2068
Risperdal (Infrequent) 1301
Sensorcaine 559
Serentil 684
Serzone Tablets (Infrequent) 771
Sinemet Tablets 943
Sinemet CR Tablets 944
Tenex Tablets (3% or less) 2074
Tensilon Injectable 1261
▲ TheraCys BCG Live (Intravesical) (Up to 6.3%) 897
Torecan 2245
Wellbutrin Tablets (Rare) 1204
Zoloft Tablets (Infrequent) 2217
Zosyn (1.0% or less) 1419
Zosyn Pharmacy Bulk Package (1.0% or less) 1422

Incoordination (see under Ataxia)

Indecisiveness

Anafranil Capsules (Rare) 803

(▣ Described in PDR For Nonprescription Drugs) Incidence data in parenthesis; ▲ 3% or more (◉ Described in PDR For Ophthalmology)

Indigestion | Side Effects Index | 1338

Indigestion
Children's Advil Suspension (Less than 3%) 2692
Asacol Delayed-Release Tablets 1979
Augmentin 2468
Carafate Suspension (Less than 0.5%) 1505
Carafate Tablets (Less than 0.5%) 1504
▲ Cataflam (3% to 9%) 816
Ceftin (Less than 1% but more than 0.1%) 1078
Colestid Tablets (Less frequent) 2591
▲ Depakene (Among most common) 413
▲ Depakote Tablets (Among most common) 415
Eskalith 2485
Feldene Capsules (Greater than 1%) 1965
▲ Hylorel Tablets (23.7%) 985
IBU Tablets (Greater than 1%) 1342
▲ Indocin (3% to 9%) 1680
Lithonate/Lithotabs/Lithobid 2543
Lopressor HCT Tablets (1 in 100 patients) 832
Lorelco Tablets 1517
Children's Motrin Ibuprofen Oral Suspension (Greater than 1% but less than 3%) 1546
Motrin Tablets (Less than 3%) 2625
Motrin Ibuprofen Suspension, Oral Drops, Chewable Tablets, Caplets (1% to less than 3%) 1546
Oncaspar 2028
▲ Parlodel (4%) 2281
Sinequan 2205
▲ Trilisate (Less than 20%) 2000
▲ Voltaren Tablets (3% to 9%) 861
Vontrol Tablets 2532

Induration at injection site
▲ Acel-Imune Diphtheria and Tetanus Toxoids and Acellular Pertussis Vaccine Adsorbed (1.5% to 7%) 1364
▲ ActHIB (0.8% to 38.2%) 872
Ancef Injection 2465
▲ Aredia for Injection (Among most common; up to 18%) 810
Biavax II 1613
▲ Brevibloc Injection (About 8%) 1808
Capastat Sulfate Vials 2868
Cefizox for Intramuscular or Intravenous Use (Greater than 1% but less than 5%) 1034
Cholera Vaccine 2711
▲ Claforan Sterile and Injection (4.3%) 1235
Cleocin Phosphate Injection 2586
Dalalone D.P. Injectable 1011
Decadron-LA Sterile Suspension 1646
Demerol 2308
Desferal Vials 820
Diphtheria and Tetanus Toxoids and Pertussis Vaccine Adsorbed 2477
Diphtheria and Tetanus Toxoids and Pertussis Vaccine Adsorbed USP (For Pediatric Use) 875
▲ Engerix-B Unit-Dose Vials (1% to 10%) 2482
Factrel (Rare) 2877
Fluvirin (Less than one third) 460
▲ Havrix (1% to 10%) 2489
IPOL Poliovirus Vaccine Inactivated (1%) 885
Kefzol Vials, Faspak & ADD-Vantage (Infrequent) 1456
Lupron Injection 2555
Lutrepulse for Injection 980
M-M-R II 1687
M-R-VAX II 1689
Mefoxin 1691
Mepergan Injection 2753
Meruvax II 1697
Netromycin Injection 100 mg/ml (4 of 1000 patients) 2373
▲ OmniHIB (0.8% to 22.5%) 2499
Oncaspar 2028
PedvaxHIB 1718
▲ Pentam 300 Injection (11.1%) 1041
Pipracil (2%) 1390
Pneumovax 23 1725
Primaxin I.V. (0.2%) 1729
Rabies Vaccine Adsorbed (A few patients) 2508
Rocephin Injectable Vials, ADD-Vantage, Galaxy Container (1%) 2142
Talwin Injection 2334
Tetanus & Diphtheria Toxoids Adsorbed Purogenated 1401
Ticar for Injection 2526
Timentin for Injection 2528
Tri-Immunol Adsorbed (Common) 1408
Tripedia 892
Trobicin Sterile Powder 2645
▲ Typhim Vi (Up to 18%) 899
Typhoid Vaccine 2823
▲ Varivax (19.35 to 32.5%) 1762
Versed Injection (0.5%-1.7%) 2170
▲ Zefazone (3%) 2654

Infantile spasms
Diphtheria and Tetanus Toxoids and Pertussis Vaccine Adsorbed 2477
Diphtheria and Tetanus Toxoids and Pertussis Vaccine Adsorbed USP (For Pediatric Use) 875
Tetramune 1404

Infection at injection site
▲ Cytovene-IV (9%) 2103
Depo-Medrol Single-Dose Vial 2600
NephrAmine 2005

Infection, bacterial
▲ CellCept Capsules (More than or equal to 3%) 2099
Claritin-D (Less frequent) 2350
Cytosar-U Sterile Powder 2592
Deltasone Tablets 2595
Depo-Medrol Single-Dose Vial 2600
Depo-Medrol Sterile Aqueous Suspension 2597
Econopred & Econopred Plus Ophthalmic Suspensions ◉ 217
Foscavir Injection (Between 1% and 5%) 547
Imdur (Less than or equal to 5%) 1323
▲ Leustatin (42%) 1834
▲ Lopid Tablets (More common) 1917
NEOSAR Lyophilized/Neosar 1959
Orthoclone OKT3 Sterile Solution 1837
▲ Paraplatin for Injection (14% to 18%) 705

Infection, body as a whole
Alkeran for Injection 1070
Ambien Tablets (1%) 2416
Aristospan Suspension (Intralesional) 1032
▲ Atgam Sterile Solution (Less than 1% to 13%) 2581
Axid Pulvules (1.7%) 1427
Betapace Tablets (1% to 4%) 641
Betaseron for SC Injection 658
Cardene Capsules (Rare) 2095
Cardura Tablets (Less than 0.5% of 3960 patients) 2186
Cartrol Tablets (Less common) 410
▲ CellCept Capsules (18.2% to 20.9%; 12.7% to 15.6%) 2099
Clozaril Tablets 2252
Compazine 2470
Coumadin 926
▲ Cytovene (9%) 2103
Dilacor XR Extended-release Capsules 2018
▲ Effexor (2.2% to 6%) 2719
▲ Ergamisol Tablets (5% to 12%) 1292
▲ Fludara for Injection (33% to 44%) 663
▲ Foscavir Injection (5% or greater) 547
Gelfoam Sterile Sponge 2608
▲ Idamycin (95%) 1955
▲ IFEX (8%) 697
▲ Lamictal Tablets (4.4%) 1112
▲ Leustatin (28%) 1834
Lodine Capsules and Tablets (Less than 1%) 2743
Lotensin Tablets 834
Lotensin HCT (0.3% or more) 837
Lozol Tablets (Greater than or equal to 5%) 2022
Lupron Depot-PED 7.5 mg, 11.25 mg and 15 mg (Less than 2%) 2560
Lupron Injection (Less than 5%) 2555
Megace Oral Suspension (1% to 3%) 699
Orudis Capsules (Less than 1%) 2766
Oruvail Capsules (Less than 1%) 2766
Permax Tablets (1.1%) 575
Prelone Syrup 1787
PREVACID Delayed-Release Capsules (Less than 1%) 2562
Serentil 684
▲ Serzone Tablets (8%) 771
Stelazine 2514
▲ Taxol (35%) 714
TheraCys BCG Live (Intravesical) (2.0% to 2.7%) 897
Toradol (1% or less) 2159
▲ Trasylol (6%) 613
▲ Videx Tablets, Powder for Oral Solution, & Pediatric Powder for Oral Solution (4% to 7%) 720
▲ Vumon (12%) 727
Xanax Tablets (1.3%) 2649

Infection, candida albicans
▲ Cleocin Vaginal Cream (11%) 2589
Flonase Nasal Spray (Rare) 1098
Rhinocort Nasal Inhaler (Rare) 556

Infection, cecum
Rubex 712

Infection, colon
Rubex 712

Infection, conjunctiva
Urobiotic-250 Capsules 2214

Infection, cryptococcus
Orthoclone OKT3 Sterile Solution (1.6%) 1837

Infection, cytomegalovirus
▲ CellCept Capsules (8.3% to 13.4%; 3.6% to 15.2%) 2099
▲ Neoral (4.8%) 2276
▲ Orthoclone OKT3 Sterile Solution (3% to 19%) 1837
▲ Sandimmune (4.8 to 12.3%) 2286

Infection, decreased resistance
Anafranil Capsules (Infrequent) 803
Aristocort Suspension (Forte Parenteral) 1027
Aristocort Tablets 1022
Aristospan Suspension (Intra-articular) 1033
Aristospan Suspension (Intralesional) 1032
CORTENEMA 2535
Cortifoam 2396
Cytoxan 694
Dalalone D.P. Injectable 1011
Depo-Medrol Single-Dose Vial 2600
Depo-Medrol Sterile Aqueous Suspension 2597
Dexacort Phosphate in Respihaler 458
Dexacort Phosphate in Turbinaire 459
▲ Methotrexate Sodium Tablets, Injection, for Injection and LPF Injection (Among most frequent) 1275
Orthoclone OKT3 Sterile Solution 1837
Prelone Syrup 1787
Prograf 1042
Sandimmune 2286

Infection, ears
▲ AeroBid Inhaler System (3-9%) 1005
▲ Aerobid-M Inhaler System (3-9%) 1005
Claritin-D (Less frequent) 2350
Cognex Capsules (Infrequent) 1901
Cytovene-IV (One report) 2103
Neurontin Capsules (Infrequent) 1922
▲ PedvaxHIB (Among most frequent) 1718
Rogaine Topical Solution (1.17%) 2637
Tegison Capsules (Less than 1%) 2154

Infection, eyes
Acular (0.5%) 474
AeroBid Inhaler System (1-3%) 1005
Aerobid-M Inhaler System (1-3%) 1005
Collagen Plugs (Intracanalicular) ◉ 284
Decadron Phosphate Sterile Ophthalmic Ointment 1641
Decadron Phosphate Sterile Ophthalmic Solution 1642
Depo-Medrol Single-Dose Vial 2600
Depo-Medrol Sterile Aqueous Suspension 2597
Floropryl Sterile Ophthalmic Ointment 1662
Herrick Lacrimal Plugs ◉ 285
Humorsol Sterile Ophthalmic Solution 1664

Infection, eyes, fungal
Aristocort Tablets 1022
Blephamide Liquifilm Sterile Ophthalmic Suspension 476
CORTENEMA 2535
Cortisporin Ophthalmic Ointment Sterile 1085
Cortisporin Ophthalmic Suspension Sterile 1086
Dexacidin Ointment ◉ 263
Pred-G S.O.P. Sterile Ophthalmic Ointment ◉ 252
Vasocidin Ointment ◉ 268
Vasocidin Ophthalmic Solution ◉ 270

Infection, fungal
AK-Trol Ointment & Suspension ◉ 205
Blephamide Liquifilm Sterile Ophthalmic Suspension 476
Cytosar-U Sterile Powder 2592
Deltasone Tablets 2595
Depo-Medrol Single-Dose Vial 2600
Depo-Medrol Sterile Aqueous Suspension 2597
Econopred & Econopred Plus Ophthalmic Suspensions ◉ 217
FML Forte Liquifilm ◉ 240
FML Liquifilm ◉ 241
FML S.O.P. ◉ 241
FML-S Liquifilm ◉ 242
Foscavir Injection (Between 1% and 5%) 547
▲ Leustatin (20%; 14 episodes) 1834
Maxitrol Ophthalmic Ointment and Suspension ◉ 224
NEOSAR Lyophilized/Neosar 1959
▲ Novantrone (9 to 15%) 1279
Ophthocort ◉ 311
▲ Orthoclone OKT3 Sterile Solution (4% to 34%) 1837
Penetrex Tablets (Less than 1% but more than or equal to 0.1%) 2031
Poly-Pred Liquifilm ◉ 248

Infection, fungal, local
▲ Neoral (7.5%) 2276
ReVia Tablets (Less than 1%) 940
▲ Sandimmune (7.5 to 9.6%) 2286
Vantin for Oral Suspension and Vantin Tablets (Less than 1%) 2646

Infection, fungal, systemic
Neoral (2.2%) 2276
Sandimmune (2.2 to 3.9%) 2286

Infection, gastrointestinal
Adriamycin PFS 1947
Adriamycin RDF 1947
Ceftin for Oral Suspension (Less than 1% but more than 0.1%) 1078
Cytotec (Infrequent) 2424
Doxorubicin Astra 540

Infection, gram-negative bacteria
▲ Orthoclone OKT3 Sterile Solution (1.6% to 7.5%) 1837

Infection, gram-positive bacteria
▲ Orthoclone OKT3 Sterile Solution (9.0%) 1837

Infection, helminthic
Deltasone Tablets 2595
Depo-Medrol Single-Dose Vial 2600
Depo-Medrol Sterile Aqueous Suspension 2597
NEOSAR Lyophilized/Neosar 1959

Infection, herpes simplex
Inflamase ◉ 265
▲ Orthoclone OKT3 Sterile Solution (5% to 31%) 1837

Infection, Legionella
Orthoclone OKT3 Sterile Solution (0.7% to 1.6%) 1837

Infection, localized
Aristocort Suspension (Forte Parenteral) 1027
Atgam Sterile Solution (Less than 1% to 5%) 2581
Depo-Medrol Sterile Aqueous Suspension 2597
Dermatop Emollient Cream 0.1% 1238
Lioresal Intrathecal 1596
Norplant System (0.7%) 2759
ProctoCream-HC 2.5% 2408
▲ Proleukin for Injection (23%) 797
TheraCys BCG Live (Intravesical) (Up to 0.9%) 897

Infection, masking signs of
AK-Pred ◉ 204
AK-Trol Ointment & Suspension ◉ 205
Aristocort Suspension (Forte Parenteral) 1027
Aristocort Suspension (Intralesional) 1025
Aristocort Tablets 1022
Aristospan Suspension (Intra-articular) 1033
Aristospan Suspension (Intralesional) 1032
Blephamide Liquifilm Sterile Ophthalmic Suspension 476

(▣ Described in PDR For Nonprescription Drugs) Incidence data in parenthesis; ▲ 3% or more (◉ Described in PDR For Ophthalmology)

Side Effects Index

Blephamide Ointment ◉ 237
CORTENEMA 2535
Dalalone D.P. Injectable 1011
Deltasone Tablets 2595
Depo-Medrol Single-Dose Vial 2600
Depo-Medrol Sterile Aqueous Suspension 2597
Dexacort Phosphate in Respihaler 458
Dexacort Phosphate in Turbinaire 459
FML Forte Liquifilm ◉ 240
FML Liquifilm ◉ 241
FML S.O.P. ◉ 241
FML-S Liquifilm ◉ 242
Florinef Acetate Tablets 505
Fluor-Op Ophthalmic Suspension ◉ 264
Maxitrol Ophthalmic Ointment and Suspension ◉ 224
NeoDecadron Topical Cream 1714
Prelone Syrup 1787
Solu-Cortef Sterile Powder 2641
Solu-Medrol Sterile Powder 2643
TobraDex Ophthalmic Suspension and Ointment 473
Vasocidin Ophthalmic Solution ◉ 270

Infection, mononucleosis-like syndrome

PASER Granules 1285

Infection, nasal

Beconase Inhalation Aerosol and Refill (Rare) 1076
Flonase Nasal Spray (Rare) 1098
Miacalcin Nasal Spray (1% to 3%) 2275

Infection, non-pulmonary

▲ Exosurf Neonatal for Intratracheal Suspension (13% to 35%) 1095

Infection, opportunistic

Methotrexate Sodium Tablets, Injection, for Injection and LPF Injection (Rare) 1275

Infection, parasitic

Cytosar-U Sterile Powder 2592

Infection, pelvis

Lippes Loop Intrauterine Double-S.. 1848
ParaGard T380A Intrauterine Copper Contraceptive 1880
Wellbutrin Tablets (Rare) 1204

Infection, pharyngeal

Beconase Inhalation Aerosol and Refill (Rare) 1076
Decadron Phosphate Respihaler 1642
Flonase Nasal Spray (Rare) 1098

Infection, Pneumocystis carinii (see under Pneumocystis carinii, susceptibility)

Infection, post-treatment, unspecified

▲ Survanta Beractant Intratracheal Suspension (10.2 to 20.7%) 2226

Infection, potentiation

INSTAT* Collagen Absorbable Hemostat 1312

Infection, protozoan

Deltasone Tablets 2595
Depo-Medrol Single-Dose Vial 2600
Depo-Medrol Sterile Aqueous Suspension 2597
NEOSAR Lyophilized/Neosar 1959
Orthoclone OKT3 Sterile Solution 1837

Infection, respiratory

Accutane Capsules 2076
Betimol 0.25%, 0.5% (1% to 5%) ◉ 261
▲ CellCept Capsules (22.0% to 23.9%; 13.1% to 15.8%) 2099
Cognex Capsules (Infrequent) 1901
DDAVP 2017
Daypro Caplets (Less than 1%) 2426
Desmopressin Acetate Rhinal Tube 979
Maxaquin Tablets 2440
Nalfon 200 Pulvules & Nalfon Tablets (1.5%) 917
Plendil Extended-Release Tablets (0.5% to 1.5%) 527
▲ Serevent Inhalation Aerosol (4%) .. 1176
TheraCys BCG Live (Intravesical) (Up to 2.7%) 897
Vascor (200, 300 and 400 mg) Tablets (2.84%) 1587

Infection, sapraphytic

Cytosar-U Sterile Powder 2592

Infection, secondary

Aclovate Cream 1069
AK-Pred ◉ 204
AK-Trol Ointment & Suspension .. ◉ 205
Analpram-HC Rectal Cream 1% and 2.5% 977
Anusol-HC Cream 2.5% (Infrequent to frequent) 1896
Anusol-HC Suppositories 1897
Aristocort Suspension (Forte Parenteral) 1027
Aristocort Tablets 1022
Aristocort A 0.025% Cream (Infrequent) 1027
Aristocort A 0.5% Cream 1031
Aristocort A 0.1% Cream (Infrequent) 1029
Aristocort A 0.1% Ointment (Infrequent) 1030
Aristospan Suspension (Intra-articular) 1033
Aristospan Suspension (Intralesional) 1032
Bleph-10 Ophthalmic Solution 10% 475
Blephamide Liquifilm Sterile Ophthalmic Suspension 476
Blephamide Ointment ◉ 237
Carmol HC (Infrequent to frequent) 924
▲ Cordran Lotion (More frequent) 1803
▲ Cordran Tape (More frequent) 1804
Cortisporin Cream 1084
Cortisporin Ointment 1085
Cortisporin Ophthalmic Ointment Sterile 1085
Cortisporin Ophthalmic Suspension Sterile 1086
Cortisporin Otic Solution Sterile 1087
Cortisporin Otic Suspension Sterile 1088
Cultivate Cream 1088
Cultivate Ointment (Infrequent to more frequent) 1089
Cyclocort Topical (Infrequent) 1037
Decadron Phosphate Sterile Ophthalmic Ointment 1641
Decadron Phosphate Sterile Ophthalmic Solution 1642
Decadron Phosphate Topical Cream 1644
Decaspray Topical Aerosol 1648
Depo-Medrol Single-Dose Vial 2600
Dermatop Emollient Cream 0.1% (Infrequent to frequent) 1238
DesOwen Cream, Ointment and Lotion (Infrequent) 1046
Dexacidin Ointment ◉ 263
Diprolene AF Cream (Infrequent) 2352
Diprolene Gel 0.05% (Infrequent).. 2353
Diprolene (Infrequent) 2352
E.E.S. 424
Elocon (Infrequent) 2354
Epifoam (Infrequent) 2399
EryPed 200 & EryPed 400 Granules 421
Ery-Tab Tablets 422
Erythrocin Stearate Filmtab 425
FML Forte Liquifilm ◉ 240
FML Liquifilm ◉ 241
FML S.O.P. ◉ 241
FML-S Liquifilm ◉ 242
Flarex Ophthalmic Suspension ◉ 218
Florone/Florone E 906
Fluor-Op Ophthalmic Suspension ◉ 264
Halog (Infrequent) 2686
Hytone 907
Ilosone 911
Ilotycin Gluceptate, IV, Vials 913
Imuran 1110
Inflamase ◉ 265
Lidex (Infrequent) 2130
Locoid Cream, Ointment and Topical Solution (Infrequent) 978
Lotrisone Cream (1 of 270 patients) 2372
Mantadil Cream 1135
Maxitrol Ophthalmic Ointment and Suspension ◉ 224
NeoDecadron Sterile Ophthalmic Ointment 1712
NeoDecadron Topical Cream 1714
PediOtic Suspension Sterile 1153
Pipracil 1390
Poly-Pred Liquifilm ◉ 248
Pramosone Cream, Lotion & Ointment 978
Pred Forte ◉ 250
Pred Mild ◉ 253

Pred-G Liquifilm Sterile Ophthalmic Suspension ◉ 251
Pred-G S.O.P. Sterile Ophthalmic Ointment ◉ 252
Prelone Syrup 1787
ProctoCream-HC (Infrequent) 2408
ProctoCream-HC 2.5% (Infrequent to frequent) 2408
ProctoFoam-HC 2409
Psorcon Cream 0.05% (Infrequent) 909
Psorcon Ointment 0.05% 908
Synalar (Infrequent) 2130
Temovate (Infrequent) 1179
TobraDex Ophthalmic Suspension and Ointment 473
Topicort (Infrequent) 1243
Tridesilon Cream 0.05% (Infrequent) 615
Tridesilon Ointment 0.05% (Infrequent) 616
Ultravate Cream 0.05% (Infrequent) 2689
Ultravate Ointment 0.05% 2690
Vasocidin Ointment ◉ 268
Vasocidin Ophthalmic Solution ◉ 270
Vexol 1% Ophthalmic Suspension ◉ 230
Westcort 2690

Infection, Serratia

Alkeran Tablets 1071
Orthoclone OKT3 Sterile Solution (1.6%) 1837

Infection, Staphylococcus epidermidis

▲ Orthoclone OKT3 Sterile Solution (4.8%) 1837

Infection, trichomonas vaginalis

Cleocin Vaginal Cream (1%) 2589

Infection, unspecified

Betadine Ointment 1992
BiCNU 691
CORTENEMA 2535
Etrafon 2355
Felbatol 2666
Hivid Tablets (Less than 1% to less than 3%) 2121
▲ Imuran (Less than 1% to 20%) 1110
▲ Leucovorin Calcium for Injection (1% to 8%) 1268
Lupron Depot 7.5 mg 2559
Luvox Tablets 2544
Methotrexate Sodium Tablets, Injection, for Injection and LPF Injection (Less common) 1275
Neoral (0.9%) 2276
▲ Paraplatin for Injection (5%) 705
Platinol 708
▲ Proleukin for Injection (23%) 797
VePesid Capsules and Injection 718
Wellbutrin Tablets (Rare) 1204
▲ Zinecard (19% to 23%) 1961
▲ Zoladex (13%) 2858

Infection, upper respiratory

▲ Acel-Imune Diphtheria and Tetanus Toxoids and Acellular Pertussis Vaccine Adsorbed (6%) 1364
▲ AeroBid Inhaler System (25%) 1005
▲ Aerobid-M Inhaler System (25%) .. 1005
Altace Capsules 1232
▲ Ambien Tablets (5%) 2416
Aredia for Injection (Up to 3%) 810
▲ Atrovent Inhalation Solution (13.2%) 673
▲ Caverject (4%) 2583
Ceftin for Oral Suspension (Less than 1% but more than 0.1%) 1078
Claritin (2% or fewer patients) 2349
Claritin-D (Less frequent) 2350
▲ Cognex Capsules (3%) 1901
▲ Cozaar Tablets (7.9%) 1628
Cytotec (Infrequent) 2424
DDAVP 2017
Daypro Caplets (Less than 1%) 2426
Decadron Phosphate Respihaler 1642
Dipentum Capsules (1.5%) 1951
▲ Epogen for Injection (11%) 489
▲ Felbatol (5.3% to 45.2%) 2666
▲ Fludara for Injection (2% to 16%) 663
Havrix (Less than 1%) 2489
▲ Hyzaar Tablets (6.1%) 1677
Ismo Tablets (Fewer than 1%) 2738
Kerlone Tablets (2.6%) 2436
▲ Lescol Capsules (11.6%) 2267
Levatol (2.5%) 2403
Lotensin HCT (More than 1%) 837

Infection, urinary tract

▲ Luvox Tablets (9%) 2544
Methotrexate Sodium Tablets, Injection, for Injection and LPF Injection (Less common) 1275
Miacalcin Nasal Spray (1% to 3%) 2275
Monoket (Up to 4%) 2406
Monopril Tablets (2.2%) 757
Oncaspar (Less than 1%) 2028
▲ PedvaxHIB (Among most frequent) 1718
Plendil Extended-Release Tablets (0.7% to 3.9%) 527
PREVACID Delayed-Release Capsules (Less than 1%) 2562
Prilosec Delayed-Release Capsules (1.9%) 529
▲ Prinivil Tablets (1.5% to 4.5%) 1733
Prinzide Tablets (2.2%) 1737
Procardia XL Extended Release Tablets (1% or less) 1972
▲ Procrit for Injection (11%) 1841
Prolixin 509
▲ Propulsid (3.1%) 1300
▲ Prozac Pulvules & Liquid, Oral Solution (7.6%) 919
Recombivax HB (Equal to or greater than 1%) 1744
▲ Risperdal (3%) 1301
▲ Rogaine Topical Solution (7.16%).. 2637
Rowasa (1.8%) 2548
Seldane-D Extended-Release Tablets (1.3%) 1538
▲ Serevent Inhalation Aerosol (14%) 1176
Sinemet CR Tablets (1.8%) 944
▲ Stadol (3% to 9%) 775
Stimate, (desmopressin acetate) Nasal Spray, 1.5 mg/mL 525
▲ Supprelin Injection (1% to 10%).... 2056
▲ Taxol (One of the two most frequently reported infectious complications) 714
▲ Tetramune (Among most common) 1404
▲ Tilade (3.9%) 996
Timoptic in Ocudose (Less frequent) 1753
Timoptic Sterile Ophthalmic Solution (Less frequent) 1751
▲ Timoptic-XE (1% to 5% of patients) 1755
Univasc Tablets (More than 1%) 2410
Vaseretic Tablets 1765
Vasotec I.V. 1768
Vasotec Tablets (0.5% to 1.0%) 1771
▲ Xanax Tablets (4.3%) 2649
▲ Zebeta Tablets (4.8% to 5.0%) 1413
Zestoretic (2.2%) 2850
▲ Zestril Tablets (1.5% to 4.5%) 2854
Ziac (Up to 2.1%) 1415
Zocor Tablets (2.1%) 1775
▲ Zoladex (7%) 2858

Infection, urinary tract

All-Flex Arcing Spring Diaphragm (See also Ortho Diaphragm Kits) 1865
Ambien Tablets (2%) 2416
▲ Aredia for Injection (At least 15%) 810
Atrovent Inhalation Solution (Less than 3%) 673
BCG Vaccine, USP (TICE) (1.5%) .. 1814
Cardura Tablets (1.4%) 2186
Ceftin for Oral Suspension (Less than 1% but more than 0.1%) 1078
▲ CellCept Capsules (37.0% to 37.2%; 44.4% to 45.5%) 2099
▲ Cognex Capsules (3%) 1901
Cozaar Tablets (Less than 1%) 1628
Cytovene (1% or less) 2103
Depo-Provera Contraceptive Injection (Fewer than 1%) 2602
Dilacor XR Extended-release Capsules 2018
Effexor 2719
Ergamisol Tablets (1 out of 463 patients) 1292
▲ Felbatol (3.4%) 2666
▲ Fludara for Injection (2% to 15%) 663
Foscavir Injection (Between 1% and 5%) 547
Hytrin Capsules (0.5% to 1.3%) 430
Hyzaar Tablets 1677
Imdur (Less than or equal to 5%) .. 1323
Lamictal Tablets (More than 1%; infrequent) 1112
▲ Lopid Tablets (More common) 1917
Lotensin Tablets 834
Lotensin HCT (0.3% or more) 837
▲ Lupron Injection (5% or more) 2555
Luvox Tablets (Infrequent) 2544
Megace Oral Suspension (1% to 3%) 699
▲ Neoral (21.1%) 2276

(◙ Described in PDR For Nonprescription Drugs) Incidence data in parenthesis; ▲ 3% or more (◉ Described in PDR For Ophthalmology)

Infection, urinary tract — Side Effects Index — 1340

▲Novantrone (7%) ... 1279
Ortho Diaphragm Kits—All-Flex Arcing Spring; Ortho Coil Spring; Ortho-White Flat Spring ... 1865
Prilosec Delayed-Release Capsules (Less than 1%) ... 529
Prinivil Tablets (0.5% to 1.5%) ... 1733
Prinzide Tablets (0.3 to 1%) ... 1737
▲Prograf (16% to 19%) ... 1042
▲Proleukin for Injection (23%) ... 797
Propulsid (2.4%) ... 1300
Prozac Pulvules & Liquid, Oral Solution (1.2%) ... 919
ReoPro Vials (1.9%) ... 1471
Rogaine Topical Solution (0.93%) .. 2637
▲Sandimmune (20.2 to 21.1%) ... 2286
Sandostatin Injection (1% to 4%) .. 2292
Serzone Tablets (2%) ... 771
Sinemet CR Tablets (2.2%) ... 944
▲Taxol (One of the two most frequently reported infectious complications) ... 714
Testoderm Testosterone Transdermal System (Four in 104 patients) ... 486
Tolectin (200, 400 and 600 mg) (1 to 3%) ... 1581
▲Trasylol (3%) ... 613
Vaseretic Tablets (0.5% to 2.0%) 1765
Vasotec I.V. ... 1768
Vasotec Tablets (1.3%) ... 1771
Wellbutrin Tablets (Infrequent) ... 1204
Zestoretic (0.3 to 1%) ... 2850
Zestril Tablets (0.5% to 1.5%) ... 2854
Zoladex (1% or greater) ... 2858

Infection, vagina

Micronor Tablets ... 1872
Modicon ... 1872
Norplant System (Uncommon) ... 2759
Ortho-Cyclen/Ortho-Tri-Cyclen ... 1858
Ortho-Novum ... 1872
Ortho-Cyclen/Ortho Tri-Cyclen ... 1858
Supprelin Injection (1% to 3%) ... 2056

Infection, viral

Accupril Tablets (0.5 to 1.0%) ... 1893
Blephamide Ointment ... ◉ 237
Claritin-D (Less frequent) ... 2350
Cortisporin Ophthalmic Ointment Sterile ... 1085
Cortisporin Ophthalmic Suspension Sterile ... 1086
Cytosar-U Sterile Powder ... 2592
Deltasone Tablets ... 2595
Depo-Medrol Single-Dose Vial ... 2600
Depo-Medrol Sterile Aqueous Suspension ... 2597
Econopred & Econopred Plus Ophthalmic Suspensions ... ◉ 217
FML Forte Liquifilm ... ◉ 240
FML Liquifilm ... ◉ 241
FML S.O.P. ... ◉ 241
Foscavir Injection (Less than 1%) .. 547
Imdur (Less than or equal to 5%) .. 1323
Koāte-HP Antihemophilic Factor (Human) ... 630
Konȳne 80 Factor IX Complex ... 634
▲Leustatin (20%) ... 1834
▲Lopid Tablets (More common) ... 1917
▲Neoral (15.9%) ... 2276
NEOSAR Lyophilized/Neosar ... 1959
Neurontin Capsules (More than 1%) ... 1922
Orthoclone OKT3 Sterile Solution (1.5%) ... 1837
Prinivil Tablets (0.3% to 1.0%) ... 1733
Prinzide Tablets (0.3% to 1%) ... 1737
Prolastin Alpha$_1$-Proteinase Inhibitor (Human) ... 635
▲Propulsid (3.6%) ... 1300
▲Prozac Pulvules & Liquid, Oral Solution (3.4%) ... 919
▲Sandimmune (15.9 to 18.4%) ... 2286
▲Supprelin Injection (1% to 10%) ... 2056
Tilade (2.4%) ... 996
Vasocidin Ophthalmic Solution ... ◉ 270
Zestoretic (0.3 to 1%) ... 2850
Zestril Tablets (0.3% to 1.0%) ... 2854

Infectious-mononucleosis-like syndrome

Dapsone Tablets USP ... 1284

Infertility

Cytovene-IV (Two or more reports) 2103
Leukeran Tablets ... 1133
Lippes Loop Intrauterine Double-S .. 1848
Lo/Ovral Tablets ... 2746
Lo/Ovral-28 Tablets ... 2751
Methotrexate Sodium Tablets, Injection, for Injection and LPF Injection ... 1275
Nordette-21 Tablets (discontinued) ... 2755
Nordette-28 Tablets ... 2758
Ovral Tablets ... 2770
Ovral-28 Tablets ... 2770
Ovrette Tablets ... 2771
ParaGard T380A Intrauterine Copper Contraceptive ... 1880
Zyloprim Tablets (Less than 1%) ... 1226

Infertility, male

Dapsone Tablets USP ... 1284

Infertility, temporary

Brevicon ... 2088
Demulen ... 2428
Desogen Tablets ... 1817
Levlen/Tri-Levlen ... 651
Micronor Tablets ... 1872
Modicon ... 1872
Norinyl ... 2088
Nor-Q D Tablets ... 2135
Ortho-Cept ... 1851
Ortho-Cyclen/Ortho-Tri-Cyclen ... 1858
Ortho-Novum ... 1872
Ortho-Cyclen/Ortho Tri-Cyclen ... 1858
Ovcon ... 760
Levlen/Tri-Levlen ... 651
Tri-Norinyl ... 2164
Triphasil-21 Tablets ... 2814
Triphasil-28 Tablets ... 2819

Infertility, tubal

Lippes Loop Intrauterine Double-S .. 1848

Inflammation

AMVISC Plus (Rare) ... ◉ 329
Adalat Capsules (10 mg and 20 mg) (2% or less) ... 587
▲Calcimar Injection, Synthetic (10%) ... 2013
Ceptaz (1 in 69 patients) ... 1081
Chloromycetin Ophthalmic Ointment, 1% ... ◉ 310
Decadron-LA Sterile Suspension ... 1646
Exact Vanishing and Tinted Creams ... ▣ 749
Fluoroplex Topical Solution & Cream 1% ... 479
Herplex Liquifilm ... ◉ 244
INSTAT* Collagen Absorbable Hemostat ... 1312
Lupron Depot 3.75 mg ... 2556
Lupron Depot 7.5 mg ... 2559
Lupron Injection (Less than 5%) ... 2555
ParaGard T380A Intrauterine Copper Contraceptive ... 1880
Prilosec Delayed-Release Capsules (Less than 1%) ... 529
Procardia Capsules (2% or less) ... 1971
Stri-Dex ... ▣ 730
Terramycin with Polymyxin B Sulfate Ophthalmic Ointment (Rare) ... 2211
Zestoretic (0.3 to 1%) ... 2850

Inflammation, genital

BCG Vaccine, USP (TICE) (1.8%) .. 1814
▲Condylox (71% to 63%) ... 1802

Inflammation, ocular

AMO Vitrax Viscoelastic Solution ◉ 232
BSS PLUS (500 mL) Sterile Irrigation Solution ... ◉ 215
Betoptic Ophthalmic Solution ... 469
Betoptic S Ophthalmic Suspension (Small number of patients) ... 471
Depo-Medrol Single-Dose Vial ... 2600
Depo-Medrol Sterile Aqueous Suspension ... 2597
Dilacor XR Extended-release Capsules ... 2018
▲Ilotycin Ophthalmic Ointment (Among most frequent) ... 912
IOPIDINE Sterile Ophthalmic Solution (0.45%) ... ◉ 219
TERAK Ointment (Rare) ... ◉ 209

Inflammation, oral (see under Stomatitis)

Inflammation, perianal

▲Cytosar-U Sterile Powder (Among most frequent) ... 2592
Doryx Capsules ... 1913

Inflammation, periocular

Depo-Medrol Single-Dose Vial ... 2600
Depo-Medrol Sterile Aqueous Suspension ... 2597

Inflammation, upper respiratory tract

PREVACID Delayed-Release Capsules (Less than 1%) ... 2562
Solganal Suspension ... 2388

Inflammation, uterine

Anafranil Capsules (Rare) ... 803

Inflammation at application site

Estraderm Transdermal System ... 824
▲Zoladex (6%) ... 2858

Inflammation at injection site

Ambien Tablets (Rare) ... 2416
▲Aredia for Injection (Among most common; up to 18%) ... 810
Atgam Sterile Solution (Less than 5%) ... 2581
▲Betaseron for SC Injection (85%) .. 658
▲Brevibloc Injection (About 8%) ... 1808
▲Calcimar Injection, Synthetic (About 10%) ... 2013
Ceptaz (One in 69 patients) ... 1081
▲Claforan Sterile and Injection (4.3%) ... 1235
Cytovene-IV (2%) ... 2103
Dalalone D.P. Injectable ... 1011
▲Dalgan Injection (3 to 9%) ... 538
Delatestryl Injection (Rare) ... 2860
Dilantin Parenteral ... 1910
Diprivan Injection (Less than 1%) .. 2833
Dobutrex Solution Vials ... 1439
Estratest ... 2539
Fluvirin (Less than one third) ... 460
Fortaz (1 in 69 patients) ... 1100
Foscavir Injection (Between 1% and 5%) ... 547
Genotropin (Infrequent) ... 111
Geref (sermorelin acetate for injection) ... 2876
▲Havrix (1% to 10%) ... 2489
Humulin 50/50, 100 Units ... 1444
Humulin 70/30, 100 Units ... 1445
Humulin L, 100 Units ... 1446
Regular, 100 Units ... 1450
Pork Regular, 100 Units ... 1452
Imitrex Injection ... 1103
INFeD (Iron Dextran Injection, USP) ... 2345
▲Intron A (Up to 7%) ... 2364
▲JE-VAX (2.9% to approximately 20%) ... 886
Levoprome ... 1274
Lutrepulse for Injection ... 980
▲Miacalcin Injection (About 10%) ... 2273
Mini-Gamulin Rh, Rho(D) Immune Globulin (Human) (Infrequent) ... 520
▲Poliovax (14%) ... 891
Premarin with Methyltestosterone .. 2794
Rifadin I.V. ... 1528
Roferon-A Injection (Less than 3%) ... 2145
Romazicon ... 2147
Septra I.V. Infusion ... 1169
▲Supprelin Injection (45%) ... 2056
Tazicef for Injection (Less than 2%) ... 2519
Testred Capsules ... 1262
Tetanus & Diphtheria Toxoids Adsorbed Purogenated (Mild to moderate) ... 1401
Vancocin HCl, Vials & ADD-Vantage ... 1481
Varivax (Less than 0.05%) ... 1762
Versed Injection (0.5%-2.6%) ... 2170
▲Zofran Injection (4%) ... 1214
Zosyn (0.2%) ... 1419
Zosyn Pharmacy Bulk Package (0.2%) ... 1422
▲Zovirax Sterile Powder (Approximately 9%) ... 1223

Influenza-like symptoms

Ambien Tablets (2%) ... 2416
▲Atrovent Inhalation Solution (3.7%) ... 673
Cardura Tablets (Less than 0.5% of 3960 patients to 1.1%) ... 2186
Engerix-B Unit-Dose Vials (Less than 1%) ... 2482
Foscavir Injection (Between 1% and 5%) ... 547
Hespan Injection ... 929
Imitrex Injection (Rare) ... 1103
Maxaquin Tablets (Less than 1%) .. 2440
Monopril Tablets (0.4% to 1.0%) .. 757
Plendil Extended-Release Tablets (0.5% to 1.5%) ... 527
Pravachol (Up to 2.4%) ... 765
Prinivil Tablets (0.3%) ... 1733
Prinzide Tablets (0.3% to 1%) ... 1737
Prozac Pulvules & Liquid, Oral Solution (1.2%) ... 919
Recombivax HB (Less than 1%) ... 1744
Zestoretic (0.3 to 1%) ... 2850
Zestril Tablets (0.3%) ... 2854
▲Zoladex (5%) ... 2858

Insomnia

Accutane Capsules ... 2076
Actifed Plus Caplets ... ▣ 845
Actifed Plus Tablets (At higher doses) ... ▣ 845
Actifed with Codeine Cough Syrup .. 1067
Actifed Syrup ... ▣ 846
Actifed Tablets ... ▣ 844
Acutrim ... ▣ 628
Adalat CC (Less than 1.0%) ... 589
Adipex-P Tablets and Capsules ... 1048
Advil Cold and Sinus Caplets and Tablets (formerly CoAdvil) ... ▣ 870
Children's Advil Suspension (Less than 1%) ... 2692
AeroBid Inhaler System (1-3%) ... 1005
Aerobid-M Inhaler System (1-3%) .. 1005
Airet Solution for Inhalation (1% to 3.1%) ... 452
Alka-Seltzer Plus Cold Medicine .. ▣ 705
Alka-Seltzer Plus Cold & Cough Medicine ... ▣ 708
Alka-Seltzer Plus Night-Time Cold Medicine ... ▣ 707
Alka Seltzer Plus Sinus Medicine ▣ 707
Allerest Children's Chewable Tablets ... ▣ 627
Allerest Headache Strength Tablets ... ▣ 627
Allerest Maximum Strength Tablets ... ▣ 627
Allerest No Drowsiness Tablets ... ▣ 627
Allerest Sinus Pain Formula ... ▣ 627
Allerest 12 Hour Caplets ... ▣ 627
Altace Capsules (Less than 1%) ... 1232
Alupent Tablets (1.8%) ... 669
Ambien Tablets (Frequent) ... 2416
Amen Tablets ... 780
Amoxil (Rare) ... 2464
▲Anafranil Capsules (11% to 25%) 803
Anaprox/Naprosyn (Less than 1%) ... 2117
Anatuss LA Tablets ... 1542
Ansaid Tablets (1-3%) ... 2579
Aredia for Injection (Up to 1%) ... 810
Aristocort Suspension (Forte Parenteral) ... 1027
Aristocort Suspension (Intralesional) ... 1025
Aristocort Tablets ... 1022
Aristospan Suspension (Intra-articular) ... 1033
Aristospan Suspension (Intralesional) ... 1032
Asacol Delayed-Release Tablets ... 1979
Asendin Tablets (Less frequent) ... 1369
Atamet ... 572
Atrohist Plus Tablets ... 454
Atrovent Inhalation Aerosol (Less than 1%) ... 671
Atrovent Inhalation Solution (0.9%) ... 673
Augmentin (Rare) ... 2468
Axid Pulvules (2.7%) ... 1427
Azactam for Injection (Less than 1%) ... 734
Azo Gantanol Tablets ... 2080
Azo Gantrisin Tablets ... 2081
Azulfidine (Rare) ... 1949
Bactrim DS Tablets ... 2084
Bactrim I.V. Infusion ... 2082
Bactrim ... 2084
Benadryl Allergy Decongestant Liquid Medication ... ▣ 848
Benadryl Allergy Decongestant Tablets ... ▣ 848
Benadryl Allergy Sinus Headache Formula Caplets ... ▣ 849
▲Benadryl Capsules (Among most frequent) ... 1898
Benadryl Injection ... 1898
Bentyl ... 1501
Benylin Multisymptom ... ▣ 852
Betoptic Ophthalmic Solution (Rare) ... 469
Betoptic S Ophthalmic Suspension (Rare) ... 471
Biphetamine Capsules ... 983
Blocadren Tablets (Less than 1%) 1614

(▣ Described in PDR For Nonprescription Drugs) Incidence data in parenthesis; ▲ 3% or more (◉ Described in PDR For Ophthalmology)

1341 **Side Effects Index** **Insomnia**

Bontril Slow-Release Capsules 781
Brethaire Inhaler 813
Bromfed 1785
▲ Bromfed-DM Cough Syrup (Among most frequent) 1786
Bromfed-PD Capsules (Extended-Release) 1785
Bronkaid Mist .... ▣ 717
Bronkaid Mist Suspension .... ▣ 718
Bronkaid Caplets .... ▣ 717
Bronkometer Aerosol 2302
Bronkosol Solution 2302
▲ BuSpar (3%) 737
Butisol Sodium Elixir & Tablets (Less than 1 in 100) 2660
Calan SR Caplets (1% or less) 2422
Calan Tablets (1% or less) 2419
Capoten (About 0.5 to 2%) 739
Capozide (0.5 to 2%) 742
Carafate Suspension (Less than 0.5%) 1505
Carafate Tablets (Less than 0.5%) 1504
Cardene Capsules (0.6%) 2095
Cardizem CD Capsules (Less than 1%) 1506
Cardizem SR Capsules (1%) 1510
Cardizem Injectable 1508
Cardizem Tablets (Less than 1%) .. 1512
Cardura Tablets (1% to 1.2%) 2186
Cartrol Tablets (1.7%) 410
Cataflam (Less than 1%) 816
Catapres Tablets (About 5 in 1,000 patients) 674
Catapres-TTS (2 of 101 patients; less frequent) 675
Ceclor Pulvules & Suspension (Rare) 1431
Cefzil Tablets and Oral Suspension (Less than 1%) 746
Celestone Soluspan Suspension 2347
▲ CellCept Capsules (8.9% to 11.8%) 2099
Celontin Kapseals 1899
Cerose DM .... ▣ 878
Children's Vicks DayQuil Allergy Relief .... ▣ 757
Children's Vicks NyQuil Cold/Cough Relief .... ▣ 758
Chlor-Trimeton Allergy Decongestant Tablets .... ▣ 799
Cipro I.V. (1% or less) 595
Cipro I.V. Pharmacy Bulk Package (Less than 1%) 597
Cipro Tablets (Less than 1%) 592
Claritin (2% or fewer patients) 2349
▲ Claritin-D (16%) 2350
Clinoril Tablets (Less than 1%) 1618
Clomid (Fewer than 1%) 1514
Clozaril Tablets (2%) 2252
▲ Cognex Capsules (6%) 1901
Colestid Tablets (Infrequent) 2591
Combipres Tablets (About 5 in 1,000) 677
Comhist 2038
Compazine (Sometimes) 2470
Allergy-Sinus Comtrex Multi-Symptom Allergy-Sinus Formula Tablets .... ▣ 617
Comtrex Non-Drowsy .... ▣ 618
Condylox (Less than 5%) 1802
Contac Continuous Action Nasal Decongestant/Antihistamine 12 Hour Capsules .... ▣ 813
Contac Maximum Strength Continuous Action Decongestant/Antihistamine 12 Hour Caplets .... ▣ 813
Contac Severe Cold and Flu Formula Caplets .... ▣ 814
Cordarone Tablets (1 to 3%) 2712
Coricidin 'D' Decongestant Tablets .... ▣ 800
CORTENEMA 2535
Cortifoam 2396
Cortone Acetate Sterile Suspension 1623
Cortone Acetate Tablets 1624
Cozaar Tablets (1.4%) 1628
Cycrin Tablets 975
▲ Cylert Tablets (Most frequent) 412
Cytovene (1% or less) 2103
D.A. Chewable Tablets 951
Dantrium Capsules (Less frequent) 1982
Dapsone Tablets USP 1284
Daraprim Tablets (Rare) 1090
Decadron Elixir 1633
Decadron Phosphate Injection 1637
Decadron Phosphate Respihaler 1642
Decadron Phosphate Turbinaire 1645
Decadron Phosphate with Xylocaine Injection, Sterile 1639
Decadron Tablets 1635
Decadron-LA Sterile Suspension 1646
Deconamine Chewable Tablets 1320
Deconamine CX Cough and Cold Liquid and Tablets 1319
Deconamine 1320
Deconsal 454
Deltasone Tablets 2595
Demadex Tablets and Injection (1.2%) 686
Demser Capsules 1649
Demulen 2428
Depakote Tablets (Greater than 1% but not more than 5%) 415
Depo-Medrol Sterile Aqueous Suspension 2597
▲ Depo-Provera Contraceptive Injection (1% to 5%) 2602
Depo-Provera Sterile Aqueous Suspension 2606
Desoxyn Gradumet Tablets 419
▲ Desyrel and Desyrel Dividose (6.4% to 9.9%) 503
Dexacort Phosphate in Respihaler .. 458
Dexacort Phosphate in Turbinaire .. 459
Dexatrim .... ▣ 832
Dexatrim Plus Vitamins Caplets .. ▣ 832
Dexedrine 2474
DextroStat Dextroamphetamine Tablets 2036
Didrex Tablets 2607
Dilacor XR Extended-release Capsules (1.0%) 2018
Dilantin Infatabs 1908
Dilantin Kapseals 1906
Dilantin Parenteral 1910
Dilantin-125 Suspension 1911
Dilaudid-HP Injection (Less frequent) 1337
Dilaudid-HP Lyophilized Powder 250 mg (Less frequent) 1337
Dilaudid Tablets and Liquid (Less frequent) 1339
Dimetane-DC Cough Syrup 2059
Dimetane-DX Cough Syrup 2059
Dimetapp Elixir .... ▣ 773
Dimetapp Extentabs .... ▣ 774
Dimetapp Tablets/Liqui-Gels .... ▣ 775
Dimetapp Cold & Allergy Chewable Tablets .... ▣ 773
Dimetapp Sinus Caplets .... ▣ 775
Dipentum Capsules (Rare) 1951
Diprivan Injection (Less than 1%) .. 2833
Ditropan 1516
Dizac (Less frequent) 1809
Dolobid Tablets (Greater than 1 in 100) 1654
Donnatal 2060
Donnatal Extentabs 2061
Donnatal Tablets 2060
Dorcol Children's Cough Syrup .... ▣ 785
Drixoral Cold and Allergy Sustained-Action Tablets .... ▣ 802
Drixoral Cold and Flu Extended-Release Tablets .... ▣ 803
Dura-Tap/PD Capsules 2867
Duratuss Tablets 2565
Dura-Vent/DA Tablets 953
Dura-Vent Tablets 952
DynaCirc Capsules (0.5% to 1%) .. 2256
EC-Naprosyn Delayed-Release Tablets (Less than 1%) 2117
▲ Effexor (3% to 22.5%) 2719
Efidac/24 .... ▣ 635
Efudex 2113
Elavil 2838
Eldepryl Tablets (1 of 49 patients) 2550
▲ Emcyt Capsules (3%) 1953
Emete-con Intramuscular/Intravenous 2198
Endep Tablets 2174
Engerix-B Unit-Dose Vials (Less than 1%) 2482
Entex Capsules 1986
Entex LA Tablets 1987
Entex Liquid 1986
Entex PSE Tablets 1987
Ergamisol Tablets (1%) 1292
Etrafon 2355
Exgest LA Tablets 782
Fansidar Tablets 2114
Fastin Capsules 2488
Fedahist Gyrocaps 2401
Fedahist Timecaps 2401
▲ Felbatol (Among most common; 8.6% to 17.5%) 2666
Feldene Capsules (Less than 1%) .. 1965
Fioricet with Codeine Capsules 2260
Fiorinal with Codeine Capsules 2262
Flagyl 375 Capsules 2434
Flagyl I.V. 2247
Flexeril Tablets (Less than 1%) 1661
Florinef Acetate Tablets 505
▲ Floxin I.V. (3% to 7%) 1571
▲ Floxin Tablets (200 mg, 300 mg, 400 mg) (3% to 7%) 1567
Flumadine Tablets & Syrup (2.1% to 3.4%) 1015
Foscavir Injection (Between 1% and 5%) 547
Fulvicin P/G Tablets (Occasional) .. 2359
Fulvicin P/G 165 & 330 Tablets (Occasional) 2359
Gantanol Tablets 2119
Gantrisin 2120
Gastrocrom Capsules (Infrequent) .. 984
Glucotrol XL Extended Release Tablets (Less than 3%) 1968
Grifulvin V (griseofulvin tablets) Microsize (griseofulvin oral suspension) Microsize (Occasional) 1888
Gris-PEG Tablets, 125 mg & 250 mg (Occasional) 479
Guaimax-D Tablets 792
▲ Habitrol Nicotine Transdermal System (3% to 9% of patients) 865
Halcion Tablets (Rare) 2611
Haldol Decanoate 1577
Haldol Injection, Tablets and Concentrate 1575
Havrix (Less than 1%) 2489
Hivid Tablets (Less than 1% to less than 3%) 2121
Hydeltrasol Injection, Sterile 1665
Hydeltra-T.B.A. Sterile Suspension 1667
Hydrocortone Acetate Sterile Suspension 1669
Hydrocortone Phosphate Injection, Sterile 1670
Hydrocortone Tablets 1672
Hytrin Capsules (At least 1%) 430
Hyzaar Tablets 1677
IBU Tablets (Less than 1%) 1342
Imdur (Less than or equal to 5%) .. 1323
Inderal 2728
Inderal LA Long Acting Capsules 2730
Inderide Tablets 2732
Inderide LA Long Acting Capsules .. 2734
Indocin (Less than 1%) 1680
▲ Intron A (Up to 11%) 2364
Ionamin Capsules 990
IOPIDINE Sterile Ophthalmic Solution .... ⊙ 219
Iopidine 0.5% (Less than 1%) .... ⊙ 221
Ismo Tablets (Fewer than 1%) 2738
Isoclor Timesule Capsules .... ▣ 637
Isoetharine Inhalation Solution, USP, Arm-a-Med 551
Isoptin Oral Tablets (Less than 1%) 1346
Isoptin SR Tablets (1% or less) 1348
▲ Kerlone Tablets (1.2% to 5%) 2436
Klonopin Tablets 2126
Kytril Injection (Less than 2%) 2490
▲ Kytril Tablets (3%) 2492
▲ Lamictal Tablets (5.6%) 1112
Larodopa Tablets (Relatively frequent) 2129
Lescol Capsules (2.6%) 2267
▲ Leustatin (7%) 1834
Levatol (1.9%) 2403
Levbid Extended-Release Tablets 2405
Levlen/Tri-Levlen 651
Levsin/Levsinex/Levbid 2405
Lioresal Intrathecal 1596
▲ Lioresal Tablets (2-7%) 829
Lodine Capsules and Tablets (Less than 1%) 2743
Lopressor Ampuls 830
Lopressor HCT Tablets 832
Lopressor Tablets 830
Lorabid Suspension and Pulvules 1459
Lorelco Tablets 1517
Lotensin Tablets 834
Lotensin HCT (0.3% to 1.0%) 837
Lotrel Capsules 840
Loxitane 1378
Lozol Tablets (Less than 5%) 2022
Ludiomil Tablets (2%) 843
Lufyllin & Lufyllin-400 Tablets 2670
Lufyllin-GG Elixir & Tablets 2671
Lupron Depot 3.75 mg (Less than 5%) 2556
Lupron Depot 7.5 mg (Less than 5%) 2559
▲ Lupron Injection (5% or more) 2555
▲ Luvox Tablets (21%) 2544
MS Contin Tablets (Less frequent) 1994
MSIR (Infrequent) 1997
Marax Tablets & DF Syrup 2200
Matulane Capsules 2131
Maxair Autohaler 1492
Maxair Inhaler (Less than 1%) 1494
Maxaquin Tablets (Less than 1%) .. 2440
Maxzide 1380
Mebaral Tablets (Less than 1 in 100) 2322
▲ Megace Oral Suspension (Up to 6%) 699
▲ Mepron Suspension (10% to 19%) 1135
Mesantoin Tablets 2272
Methadone Hydrochloride Oral Concentrate 2233
Methadone Hydrochloride Oral Solution & Tablets 2235
MetroGel-Vaginal 902
Mevacor Tablets (0.5% to 1.0%) .. 1699
Miacalcin Nasal Spray (Less than 1%) 2275
Micronor Tablets 1872
Midamor Tablets (Less than or equal to 1%) 1703
Modicon 1872
Moduretic Tablets (Less than or equal to 1%) 1705
8-MOP Capsules 1246
Monoket (Fewer than 1%) 2406
Monopril Tablets (1.0% or more) .. 757
Motofen Tablets (1 in 200 to 1 in 600) 784
Children's Motrin Ibuprofen Oral Suspension (Less than 1%) 1546
Motrin Tablets (Less than 1%) 2625
Motrin Ibuprofen Suspension, Oral Drops, Chewable Tablets, Caplets (Less than 1%) 1546
Mycobutin Capsules (1%) 1957
Mykrox Tablets 993
Nalfon 200 Pulvules & Nalfon Tablets (Less than 1%) 917
Anaprox/Naprosyn (Less than 1%) 2117
Nardil (Common) 1920
Navane Capsules and Concentrate 2201
Navane Intramuscular 2202
NebuPent for Inhalation Solution (1% or less) 1040
Nembutal Sodium Capsules (Less than 1%) 436
Nembutal Sodium Solution (Less than 1%) 438
Nembutal Sodium Suppositories (Less than 1%) 440
Neurontin Capsules (More than 1%) 1922
▲ Nicoderm (nicotine transdermal system) (23%) 1518
▲ Nicorette (3% to 9% of patients) .. 2458
Nicotrol Nicotine Transdermal System (1% to 3%) 1550
Nolahist Tablets 785
Nolamine Timed-Release Tablets (Occasional) 785
Noroxin Tablets (Less frequent or 0.3% to 1.0%) 1715
Noroxin Tablets (Less frequent or 0.3% to 1.0%) 2048
Norpace (Less than 1%) 2444
Norpramin Tablets 1526
Norvasc Tablets (More than 0.1% to 1%) 1940
Novahistine DH 2462
Novahistine DMX .... ▣ 822
Novahistine Elixir .... ▣ 823
Novahistine Expectorant 2463
Nucofed 2051
Ocupress Ophthalmic Solution, 1% Sterile (Occasional) .... ⊙ 309
Oramorph SR (Morphine Sulfate Sustained Release Tablets) (Less frequent) 2236
▲ Orap Tablets (2 of 20 patients) 1050
▲ Orlamm (9.1%) 2239
Ornade Spansule Capsules 2502
Ortho-Cyclen/Ortho-Tri-Cyclen 1858
Ortho-Novum 1872
Ortho-Cyclen/Ortho Tri-Cyclen 1858
▲ Orudis Capsules (3% to 9%) 2766
▲ Oruvail Capsules (3% to 9%) 2766
Oxandrin 2862
Oxsoralen-Ultra Capsules 1257
PBZ Tablets 845
PBZ-SR Tablets 844
Pamelor 2280
Parlodel (Less than 1%) 2281
Parnate Tablets 2503
▲ Paxil Tablets (13.3%) 2505
Pediatric Vicks 44d Dry Hacking Cough & Head Congestion .... ▣ 763
Pediatric Vicks 44m Cough & Cold Relief .... ▣ 764

(▣ Described in PDR For Nonprescription Drugs) Incidence data in parenthesis; ▲ 3% or more (⊙ Described in PDR For Ophthalmology)

Insomnia Side Effects Index 1342

Peganone Tablets 446
Penetrex Tablets (1%) 2031
Pentasa (Less than 1%) 1527
Pentaspan Injection 937
Pepcid Injection (Infrequent) 1722
Pepcid (Infrequent) 1720
Periactin 1724
▲Permax Tablets (7.9%) 575
Phenergan with Dextromethorphan 2778
Phenergan Injection 2773
Phenergan VC 2779
Phenobarbital Elixir and Tablets (Less than 1 in 100 patients) 1469
Phenurone Tablets (1%) 447
Placidyl Capsules 448
Plendil Extended-Release Tablets (0.5% to 1.5%) 527
Pondimin Tablets 2066
Ponstel 1925
Pravachol 765
Prelone Syrup 1787
Prelu-2 Timed Release Capsules 681
Premphase 2797
Prempro 2801
Prilosec Delayed-Release Capsules (Less than 1%) 529
Primatene Tablets ..... ▣ 873
Prinivil Tablets (0.7 to 2.3%) 1733
Prinzide Tablets 1737
Pro-Banthine Tablets 2052
Procardia XL Extended Release Tablets (Less than 3%) 1972
Proglycem 580
▲Prograf (29% to 64%) 1042
Propagest Tablets 786
Propulsid (1.9%) 1300
▲Prostep (nicotine transdermal system) (3% to 9% of patients) 1394
Protostat Tablets 1883
Proventil Inhalation Aerosol 2382
Proventil Inhalation Solution 0.083% (1% to 3.1%) 2384
Proventil Repetabs Tablets (2%) 2386
Proventil Solution for Inhalation 0.5% (1% to 3.1%) 2383
Proventil Syrup (1 of 100 patients; children 2 to 6 years, 2%) 2385
Proventil Tablets (2%) 2386
Provera Tablets 2636
▲Prozac Pulvules & Liquid, Oral Solution (13.8% to 30%) 919
Pyrroxate Caplets ..... ▣ 772
Quadrinal Tablets 1350
Quarzan Capsules 2181
Quibron 2053
RMS Suppositories 2657
Recombivax HB (Less to greater than 1%) 1744
Reglan (Less frequent) 2068
Relafen Tablets (1% to 3%) 2510
ReoPro Vials (0.3%) 1471
Respbid Tablets 682
▲Retrovir Capsules (2.4% to 5%) 1158
▲Retrovir I.V. Infusion (3% to 5%) 1163
▲Retrovir Syrup (2.4% to 5%) 1158
Rifater 1532
▲Risperdal (23% to 26%) 1301
▲Ritalin (One of the two most common) 848
Robinul Forte Tablets 2072
Robinul Injectable 2072
Robinul Tablets 2072
Robitussin Maximum Strength Cough & Cold ..... ▣ 778
Robitussin Pediatric Cough & Cold Formula ..... ▣ 779
Robitussin-CF ..... ▣ 777
Robitussin-DAC Syrup 2074
Robitussin-PE ..... ▣ 778
▲Romazicon (3% to 9%) 2147
Rondec Oral Drops 953
Rondec Syrup 953
Rondec Tablet 953
Rondec-DM Oral Drops 954
Rondec-DM Syrup 954
Rondec-TR Tablet 953
Rowasa (0.12%) 2548
Roxanol 2243
Ryna ..... ▣ 841
Rythmol Tablets–150mg, 225mg, 300mg (0.3 to 1.5%) 1352
Sandostatin Injection (Fewer than 1%) 2292
▲Sanorex Tablets (Among most common) 2294
Sansert Tablets 2295
Seconal Sodium Pulvules (Less than 1 in 100) 1474
▲Sectral Capsules (3%) 2807
Seldane Tablets 1536
▲Seldane-D Extended-Release Tablets (25.9%) 1538
▲Semprex-D Capsules (4%) 463
▲Semprex-D Capsules (4%) 1167
Septra 1174
Septra I.V. Infusion 1169
Septra I.V. Infusion ADD-Vantage Vials 1171
Septra 1174
Serophene (clomiphene citrate tablets, USP) (Approximately 1 in 50 patients) 2451
▲Serzone Tablets (11%) 771
Sinarest ..... ▣ 648
Sine-Aid Maximum Strength Sinus Medication Gelcaps, Caplets and Tablets 1554
Sine-Off No Drowsiness Formula Caplets ..... ▣ 824
Sine-Off Sinus Medicine ..... ▣ 825
Sinemet Tablets 943
Sinemet CR Tablets (1.2%) 944
Singlet Tablets ..... ▣ 825
Sinulin Tablets 787
Sinutab Non-Drying Liquid Caps.. ▣ 859
Slo-bid Gyrocaps 2033
Soma Compound w/Codeine Tablets (Infrequent or rare) 2676
Soma Compound Tablets (Infrequent or rare) 2675
Soma Tablets 2674
Sporanox Capsules (Less than 1%) 1305
▲Stadol (11%) 775
Stelazine (Sometimes) 2514
Stimate, (desmopressin acetate) Nasal Spray, 1.5 mg/mL 525
Sudafed Children's Liquid ..... ▣ 861
Sudafed Cough Syrup ..... ▣ 862
Sudafed Plus Liquid ..... ▣ 862
Sudafed Plus Tablets ..... ▣ 863
Sudafed Sinus Caplets ..... ▣ 864
Sudafed Sinus Tablets ..... ▣ 864
Sudafed Tablets, 30 mg ..... ▣ 861
Sudafed Tablets, 60 mg ..... ▣ 861
Sudafed 12 Hour Caplets ..... ▣ 861
▲Supprelin Injection (3% to 10%) 2056
Surmontil Capsules 2811
▲Symmetrel Capsules and Syrup (5% to 10%) 946
▲Synarel Nasal Solution for Endometriosis (8% of patients) 2152
Syn-Rx Tablets 465
Syn-Rx DM Tablets 466
Talacen (Infrequent) 2333
Talwin Injection 2334
Talwin Compound (Infrequent) 2335
Talwin Injection 2334
Talwin Nx 2336
Tambocor Tablets (1% to less than 3%) 1497
Tavist Syrup 2297
Tavist Tablets 2298
Teldrin 12 Hour Antihistamine/Nasal Decongestant Allergy Relief Capsules ..... ▣ 826
Temaril Tablets, Syrup and Spansule Extended-Release Capsules 483
▲Tenex Tablets (Less than 3% to 4%) 2074
Theo-24 Extended Release Capsules 2568
Theo-Dur Extended-Release Tablets 1327
Theo-X Extended-Release Tablets .. 788
TheraFlu ..... ▣ 787
TheraFlu Maximum Strength Nighttime Flu, Cold & Cough Medicine ..... ▣ 788
Thorazine 2523
Timolide Tablets (Less than 1%) 1748
Timoptic in Ocudose (Less frequent) 1753
Timoptic Sterile Ophthalmic Solution 1751
Timoptic-XE 1755
Tofranil Ampuls 854
Tofranil Tablets 856
Tofranil-PM Capsules 857
Tonocard Tablets (Less than 1%) 531
Toprol-XL Tablets 565
Toradol (1% or less) 2159
Tornalate Solution for Inhalation, 0.2% (Less than 1%) 956
Tornalate Metered Dose Inhaler (0.5%; less than 1%) 957
Tranxene 451
Trental Tablets 1244
Triaminic Allergy Tablets ..... ▣ 789
Triaminic Syrup ..... ▣ 792
Triaminic-12 Tablets ..... ▣ 792
Triaminic-DM Syrup ..... ▣ 792
Triaminicin Tablets ..... ▣ 793
Triaminicol Multi-Symptom Cold Tablets ..... ▣ 793
Triavil Tablets 1757
Trilafon 2389
Levlen/Tri-Levlen 651
Trinalin Repetabs Tablets 1330
Trobicin Sterile Powder 2645
Tussend 1783
Tussend Expectorant 1785
Children's TYLENOL Cold Multi-Symptom Liquid Formula and Chewable Tablets 1561
TYLENOL Maximum Strength Flu NightTime Hot Medication Packets 1562
TYLENOL, Maximum Strength, Sinus Medication Geltabs, Gelcaps, Caplets and Tablets 1566
TYLENOL Cold Multi-Symptom Formula Medication Tablets and Caplets 1561
TYLENOL Cold Medication No Drowsiness Formula Gelcaps and Caplets 1562
TYLENOL Cold Multi-Symptom Hot Medication Liquid Packets 1557
TYLENOL Cough Multi-Symptom Medication with Decongestant 1565
Uni-Dur Extended-Release Tablets.. 1331
Uniphyl 400 mg Tablets 2001
Ursinus Inlay-Tabs ..... ▣ 794
Valium Injectable 2182
Valium Tablets 2183
Valrelease Capsules (Infrequent) 2169
Vantin for Oral Suspension and Vantin Tablets (Less than 1%) 2646
Vascor (200, 300 and 400 mg) Tablets (0.5 to 2.65%) 1587
Vaseretic Tablets (0.5% to 2.0%) 1765
Vasotec I.V. 1768
Vasotec Tablets (0.5% to 1.0%) 1771
Ventolin Inhalation Aerosol and Refill 1197
Ventolin Inhalation Solution (1% to 3.1%) 1198
Ventolin Nebules Inhalation Solution (1% to 3.1%) 1199
Ventolin Rotacaps for Inhalation (Less than 1%) 1200
Ventolin Syrup (1 of 100 patients; 2% in children) 1202
Ventolin Tablets (2 of 100 patients) 1203
Verelan Capsules (1% or less) 1410
Verelan Capsules (Less than 1%) .. 2824
Versed Injection (Less than 1%) 2170
Vicks 44 LiquiCaps Cough, Cold & Flu Relief ..... ▣ 755
Vicks 44 LiquiCaps Non-Drowsy Cough & Cold Relief ..... ▣ 756
Vicks 44D Dry Hacking Cough & Head Congestion ..... ▣ 755
Vicks 44M Cough, Cold & Flu Relief ..... ▣ 756
Vicks DayQuil Allergy Relief 4-Hour Tablets ..... ▣ 760
Vicks DayQuil ..... ▣ 761
Vicks DayQuil SINUS Pressure & CONGESTION Relief ..... ▣ 761
Vicks Nyquil Hot Therapy ..... ▣ 762
Vicks NyQuil LiquiCaps Multi-Symptom Cold/Flu Relief ▣ 763
Vicks NyQuil Multi-Symptom Cold/Flu Relief - (Original & Cherry Flavor) ..... ▣ 763
▲Videx Tablets, Powder for Oral Solution, & Pediatric Powder for Oral Solution (Less than 1% to 10%) 720
▲Visken Tablets (10%) 2299
Vivactil Tablets 1774
Volmax Extended-Release Tablets (2.4%) 1788
Voltaren Tablets (Less than 1%) 861
▲Wellbutrin Tablets (18.6%) 1204
Winstrol Tablets 2337
▲Xanax Tablets (8.9% to 29.4%) 2649
Zantac (Rare) 1209
Zantac Injection 1207
Zantac Syrup (Rare) 1209
Zaroxolyn Tablets 1000
Zebeta Tablets (1.5% to 2.5%) 1413
▲Zerit Capsules (1% to 26%) 729
Zestoretic 2850
Zestril Tablets (0.7% to 2.3%) 2854
Ziac (1.1% to 1.2%) 1415
Zocor Tablets 1775
▲Zoladex (5% to 11%) 2858
▲Zoloft Tablets (16.4%) 2217
▲Zosyn (6.6%) 1419
▲Zosyn Pharmacy Bulk Package (6.6%) 1422
Zyloprim Tablets (Less than 1%) 1226

Insomnia, early morning

Hydropres Tablets 1675

Insulin allergy

Velosulin BR Human Insulin 10 ml Vials (Very rare) 1795

Insulin autoimmune syndrome

Tapazole Tablets 1477

Insulin reaction

Micronor Tablets 1872
Modicon 1872
Ortho-Cyclen/Ortho-Tri-Cyclen 1858
Ortho-Novum 1872
Ortho-Cyclen/Ortho Tri-Cyclen 1858
Velosulin BR Human Insulin 10 ml Vials 1795

Insulin requirement, changes

Ana-Kit Anaphylaxis Emergency Treatment Kit 617
Aristocort Suspension (Forte Parenteral) 1027
Aristocort Suspension (Intralesional) 1025
Aristocort Tablets 1022
Aristospan Suspension (Intra-articular) 1033
Aristospan Suspension (Intralesional) 1032
Celestone Soluspan Suspension 2347
CORTENEMA 2535
Cortone Acetate Sterile Suspension 1623
Cortone Acetate Tablets 1624
Dalalone D.P. Injectable 1011
Danocrine Capsules 2307
Decadron Elixir 1633
Decadron Phosphate Injection 1637
Decadron Phosphate Respihaler 1642
Decadron Phosphate Turbinaire 1645
Decadron Phosphate with Xylocaine Injection, Sterile 1639
Decadron Tablets 1635
Decadron-LA Sterile Suspension 1646
Deltasone Tablets 2595
Depo-Medrol Single-Dose Vial 2600
Depo-Medrol Sterile Aqueous Suspension 2597
Dexacort Phosphate in Respihaler .. 458
Dexacort Phosphate in Turbinaire .. 459
Florinef Acetate Tablets 505
Hydrocortone Phosphate Injection, Sterile 1670
Hydrocortone Tablets 1672
Maxzide 1380
Medrol 2621
Oretic Tablets 443
Pediapred Oral Liquid 995
Prelone Syrup 1787
Prinzide Tablets 1737
Solu-Cortef Sterile Powder 2641
Solu-Medrol Sterile Powder 2643
Tenoretic Tablets 2845
Vaseretic Tablets 1765

Insulin shock

Zanosar Sterile Powder 2653

Intercourse, sexual, painful (see under Pain with coitus)

Intestinal motility, decrease

Bellergal-S Tablets (Rare) 2250

Intestinal obstruction

Ambien Tablets (Rare) 2416
Anafranil Capsules (Rare) 803
Betaseron for SC Injection 658
Clozaril Tablets 2252
Effexor (Rare) 2719
Felbatol 2666
Kayexalate 2314
Lamprene Capsules (Less than 1%) 828
Levsin/Levsinex/Levbid 2405
Lippes Loop Intrauterine Double-S.. 1848
Luvox Tablets (Rare) 2544
ParaGard T380A Intrauterine Copper Contraceptive 1880
Permax Tablets (Infrequent) 575
Pulmozyme Inhalation 1064
Risperdal 1301

(▣ Described in PDR For Nonprescription Drugs) Incidence data in parenthesis; ▲ 3% or more (◉ Described in PDR For Ophthalmology)

1343 Side Effects Index Irritability

Sodium Polystyrene Sulfonate Suspension (Rare) 2244
Taxol (Rare) 714

Intestinal obstruction, pseudo
Nimotop Capsules (Rare) 610

Intestinal penetration
ParaGard T380A Intrauterine Copper Contraceptive 1880

Intestinal perforation
Cipro I.V. (Less than 1%) 595
Cipro I.V. Pharmacy Bulk Package (Less than 1%) 597
Cipro Tablets (Less than 1%) 592
Cytovene-IV (One report) 2103
Floxin I.V. 1571
Floxin Tablets (200 mg, 300 mg, 400 mg) 1567
Hydrocortone Tablets 1672
Maxaquin Tablets 2440
Methotrexate Sodium Tablets, Injection, for Injection and LPF Injection 1275
Penetrex Tablets 2031
Proleukin for Injection (Less than 1% to 2%) 797
Taxol (Rare) 714
Thioguanine Tablets, Tabloid Brand 1181
Wellbutrin Tablets (Rare) 1204

Intoxication, chronic
Miltown Tablets 2672
Placidyl Capsules 448

Intracranial pressure, increase
Anectine 1073
Brontex 1981
Calcium Disodium Versenate Injection 1490
Celestone Soluspan Suspension 2347
Chibroxin Sterile Ophthalmic Solution (With oral form) 1617
Cipro I.V. 595
Cipro Tablets 592
Cortifoam 2396
Cortone Acetate Sterile Suspension 1623
Cortone Acetate Tablets 1624
Decadron Elixir 1633
Decadron Phosphate Injection 1637
Decadron Phosphate Respihaler 1642
Decadron Phosphate Turbinaire 1645
Decadron Phosphate with Xylocaine Injection, Sterile 1639
Decadron Tablets 1635
Decadron-LA Sterile Suspension 1646
Dilaudid Ampules 1335
Dilaudid Cough Syrup 1336
Dilaudid-HP Injection (Less frequent) 1337
Dilaudid-HP Lyophilized Powder 250 mg (Less frequent) 1337
Dilaudid 1335
Dilaudid Oral Liquid (Less frequent) 1339
Dilaudid 1335
Dilaudid Tablets - 8 mg (Less frequent) 1339
Diphtheria and Tetanus Toxoids and Pertussis Vaccine Adsorbed USP (For Pediatric Use) 875
Eskalith 2485
Floxin Tablets (200 mg, 300 mg, 400 mg) 1567
Hydeltrasol Injection, Sterile 1665
Hydeltra-T.B.A. Sterile Suspension 1667
Hydrocortone Acetate Sterile Suspension 1669
Hydrocortone Phosphate Injection, Sterile 1670
Hydrocortone Tablets 1672
Lithium Carbonate Capsules & Tablets 2230
MS Contin Tablets (Less frequent) 1994
MSIR (Infrequent) 1997
NegGram (Occasional) 2323
Nizoral Tablets (Rare) 1298
Noroxin Tablets 1715
Noroxin Tablets 2048
Oramorph SR (Morphine Sulfate Sustained Release Tablets) (Less frequent) 2236

Intracranial pressure with papilledema
Aristocort Suspension (Forte Parenteral) 1027
Aristocort Suspension (Intralesional) 1025
Aristocort Tablets 1022
Aristospan Suspension (Intra-articular) 1033
Aristospan Suspension (Intralesional) 1032
CORTENEMA 2535
Dalalone D.P. Injectable 1011
Deltasone Tablets 2595
Depo-Medrol Single-Dose Vial 2600
Depo-Medrol Sterile Aqueous Suspension 2597
Dexacort Phosphate in Respihaler 458
Dexacort Phosphate in Turbinaire 459
Florinef Acetate Tablets 505
Lithonate/Lithotabs/Lithobid 2543
Nutropin (A small number of patients) 1061
Prelone Syrup 1787

Intraocular pressure, increase (see under Glaucoma)

Intraocular pressure, paradoxical increase
Floropryl Sterile Ophthalmic Ointment 1662
Humorsol Sterile Ophthalmic Solution 1664
Phospholine Iodide ⊙ 326

Intravascular coagulation, disseminated
Clinoril Tablets (Less than 1 in 100) 1618
Dolobid Tablets (Less than 1 in 100) 1654
Hespan Injection (Rare) 929
Indocin Capsules (Less than 1%) 1680
Indocin I.V. 1684
Indocin (Less than 1%) 1680
Oncaspar (Greater than 1% but less than 5%) 2028
Parlodel 2281
Prostin VR Pediatric Sterile Solution (About 1%) 2635
Sulfamylon Cream 925
TheraCys BCG Live (Intravesical) (Up to 2.7%) 897

Involuntary movements, abnormal
Atamet 572
Atgam Sterile Solution (Less than 5%) 2581
Atretol Tablets 573
Clozaril Tablets (Less than 1%) 2252
Cordarone Tablets 2712
Dopram Injectable 2061
Elavil 2838
Eldepryl Tablets 2550
Endep Tablets 2174
Haldol Decanoate 1577
Methadone Hydrochloride Oral Concentrate 2233
Moban Tablets and Concentrate 1048
Orap Tablets 1050
Parlodel 2281
Prolixin Oral Concentrate 509
Roferon-A Injection (Less than 0.5%) 2145
Sinemet Tablets 943
Tegretol Chewable Tablets 852
Tegretol Suspension 852
Tegretol Tablets 852
▲ Xanax Tablets (14.8%) 2649

Involuntary movements, extremities
Compazine 2470
Etrafon 2355
Haldol Decanoate 1577
Haldol Injection, Tablets and Concentrate 1575
Moban Tablets and Concentrate 1048
Navane Capsules and Concentrate 2201
Navane Intramuscular 2202
Orap Tablets 1050
Prolixin 509
Reglan 2068
Serentil 684
Stelazine 2514
Thorazine 2523

Involuntary movements, trunk
Haldol Decanoate 1577
Mellaril 2269
Orap Tablets 1050
Prolixin 509
Reglan 2068
Serentil 684

Iodine uptake, elevated
Lithonate/Lithotabs/Lithobid 2543

Iodism
Norisodrine with Calcium Iodide Syrup 442
Quadrinal Tablets 1350

Iridocyclitis (see also under Iritis)
Betagan (Rare) ⊙ 233
Trusopt Sterile Ophthalmic Solution (Rare) 1760

Iris cysts
Floropryl Sterile Ophthalmic Ointment 1662
Humorsol Sterile Ophthalmic Solution 1664
Phospholine Iodide (Rare) ⊙ 326
Salagen Tablets (Rare) 1489

Iritis (see also under Uveitis)
Aredia for Injection (One patient) 810
Fluoracaine ⊙ 206
FLURESS (Sometimes) ⊙ 207
Healon (Rare) ⊙ 314
Kerlone Tablets (Less than 2%) 2436
MIOSTAT Intraocular Solution (Occasional) ⊙ 224
Myochrysine Injection (Rare) 1711
Ocucoat (Rare) ⊙ 321
Ophthetic (Sometimes) ⊙ 247
Profenal 1% Sterile Ophthalmic Solution (Less than 0.5%) ⊙ 227
Prozac Pulvules & Liquid, Oral Solution (Rare) 919
Solganal Suspension (Rare) 2388
Tenex Tablets (3% or less) 2074
Zyloprim Tablets (Less than 1%) 1226

Iritis, activation of latent
Floropryl Sterile Ophthalmic Ointment 1662
Humorsol Sterile Ophthalmic Solution 1664
Phospholine Iodide ⊙ 326

Iron deficiency
Cuprimine Capsules 1630
Depen Titratable Tablets 2662
Epogen for Injection 489
Sandostatin Injection (Less than 1%) 2292
Syprine Capsules 1747

Iron deficiency anemia
Permax Tablets (Infrequent) 575

Irritability
▲ ActHIB (10.1% to 77.9%) 872
Actifed with Codeine Cough Syrup 1067
▲ AeroBid Inhaler System (3-9%) 1005
▲ Aerobid-M Inhaler System (3-9%) 1005
Anafranil Capsules (2%) 803
Aquasol A Vitamin A Capsules, USP 534
Aquasol A Parenteral 534
Atrohist Pediatric Capsules 453
Benadryl Capsules 1898
Benadryl Injection 1898
Bromfed 1785
▲ Bromfed-DM Cough Syrup (Among most frequent) 1786
Bromfed-PD Capsules (Extended-Release) 1785
Cataflam (Less than 1%) 816
Ceftin for Oral Suspension (Less than 1% but more than 0.1%) 1078
Celontin Kapseals 1899
Cipro I.V. (1% or less) 595
Cipro I.V. Pharmacy Bulk Package (Less than 1%) 597
Cipro Tablets (Less than 1%) 592
Claritin-D (Less frequent) 2350
Clomid 1514
Clozaril Tablets (Less than 1%) 2252
Cylert Tablets 412
Cytovene-IV (One report) 2103
D.A. Chewable Tablets 951
Dalmane Capsules 2173
Deconamine 1320
Dimetane-DC Cough Syrup 2059
Dimetane-DX Cough Syrup 2059
Dipentum Capsules (Rare) 1951
Doral Tablets 2664
Dura-Tap/PD Capsules 2867
Dura-Vent/DA Tablets 953
Dura-Vent Tablets 952
Efudex 2113
Elavil 2838
Eldepryl Tablets 2550
Elspar 1659
Endep Tablets 2174
Engerix-B Unit-Dose Vials (Less than 1%) 2482
Entex PSE Tablets 1987
Esgic-plus Tablets 1013
Fioricet Tablets (Infrequent) 2258
Fioricet with Codeine Capsules 2260
Fiorinal with Codeine Capsules 2262
Flagyl 375 Capsules 2434
Flagyl I.V. 2247
▲ Gamimune N, 5% Immune Globulin Intravenous (Human), 5% (Among most common; 11.5%) 619
▲ Gamimune N, 10% Immune Globulin Intravenous (Human), 10% (Among most common; 11.5%) 621
Gastrocrom Capsules (2 of 87 patients) 984
Guaifed 1787
Guaimax-D Tablets 792
Halcion Tablets 2611
HibTITER (133 of 1,118 vaccinations) 1375
▲ Intron A (Up to 16%) 2364
IOPIDINE Sterile Ophthalmic Solution ⊙ 219
IPOL Poliovirus Vaccine Inactivated 885
ISMOTIC 45% w/v Solution (Very rare) ⊙ 222
▲ Lamictal Tablets (3.0%) 1112
▲ Lozol Tablets (Greater than or equal to 5%) 2022
Lufyllin & Lufyllin-400 Tablets 2670
Lufyllin-GG Elixir & Tablets 2671
Mebaral Tablets 2322
Mesantoin Tablets 2272
Methadone Hydrochloride Oral Concentrate 2233
Methotrexate Sodium Tablets, Injection, for Injection and LPF Injection 1275
Nicorette 2458
▲ OmniHIB (10.1% to 72.6%) 2499
Orlamm 2239
Ornade Spansule Capsules 2502
PBZ Tablets 845
PBZ-SR Tablets 844
Periactin 1724
Phenobarbital Elixir and Tablets 1469
Placidyl Capsules 448
Plaquenil Sulfate Tablets 2328
Plendil Extended-Release Tablets (0.5% to 1.5%) 527
▲ Poliovax (More than 5%) 891
Pregnyl 1828
Prinivil Tablets (0.3% to 1.0%) 1733
Prinzide Tablets 1737
Profasi (chorionic gonadotropin for injection, USP) 2450
Proleukin for Injection 797
Protostat Tablets 1883
Proventil Repetabs Tablets (Less than 1%) 2386
Proventil Syrup (Less than 100 to 1 of 100 patients) 2385
Proventil Tablets (Less than 1%) 2386
Quadrinal Tablets 1350
Quibron 2053
Recombivax HB 1744
Respbid Tablets 682
Retrovir Capsules (1.6%) 1158
Retrovir I.V. Infusion (2%) 1163
Retrovir Syrup (1.6%) 1158
▲ ReVia Tablets (Less than 10%) 940
Roferon-A Injection (Less than 1%) 2145
Seldane-D Extended-Release Tablets (1.1%) 1538
Skelaxin Tablets 788
Slo-bid Gyrocaps 2033
Soma Compound w/Codeine Tablets (Infrequent or rare) 2676
Soma Compound Tablets (Infrequent or rare) 2675
Soma Tablets 2674
Symmetrel Capsules and Syrup (1% to 5%) 946
Talacen (Rare) 2333
Talwin Injection 2334
Talwin Compound (Rare) 2335
Talwin Injection 2334
Talwin Nx 2336
Tavist Syrup 2297
Tavist Tablets 2298
▲ Tetramune (42% to 54%) 1404

(▣ Described in PDR For Nonprescription Drugs) Incidence data in parenthesis; ▲ 3% or more (⊙ Described in PDR For Ophthalmology)

Irritability Side Effects Index 1344

Theo-24 Extended Release Capsules 2568
Theo-Dur Extended-Release Tablets 1327
Theo-X Extended-Release Tablets 788
Tranxene 451
Triavil Tablets 1757
Trinalin Repetabs Tablets 1330
▲ Tripedia (5% to 15%) 892
Tussend 1783
Uni-Dur Extended-Release Tablets 1331
Uniphyl 400 mg Tablets 2001
Varivax (Greater than or equal to 1%) 1762
Ventolin Syrup (Less than 1 of 100 patients) 1202
Ventolin Tablets (Fewer than 1 of 100 patients) 1203
Volmax Extended-Release Tablets (Less frequent) 1788
Voltaren Tablets (Less than 1%) 861
Xanax Tablets (Rare) 2649
Yocon 1892
Yohimex Tablets 1363
Zarontin Capsules 1928
Zarontin Syrup 1929
Zestoretic 2850
Zestril Tablets (0.3% to 1.0%) 2854

Irritation

Aclovate (1 in 100 patients) 1069
Americaine Hemorrhoidal Ointment ▣ 629
Analpram-HC Rectal Cream 1% and 2.5% 977
Anusol Ointment ▣ 847
Anusol-HC Cream 2.5% (Infrequent to frequent) 1896
Anusol-HC Suppositories 1897
Atrovent Inhalation Aerosol (1.6%) 671
Benoquin Cream 20% (Occasional) 2868
BiCozene Creme ▣ 785
Bleph-10 Ophthalmic Ointment 10% 475
Capzasin-P ▣ 831
Chloresium (A few instances) 2246
Cordran Lotion (Infrequent) 1803
Cordran Tape (Infrequent) 1804
Cortisporin Otic Solution Sterile 1087
Cortisporin Otic Suspension Sterile 1088
Cutivate Cream 1088
Cutivate Ointment 1089
Cyclocort Topical (Infrequent) 1037
Decadron Phosphate Topical Cream 1644
Decaspray Topical Aerosol 1648
Desenex ▣ 632
Desenex Foot & Sneaker Deodorant Spray ▣ 633
DesOwen Cream, Ointment and Lotion (Less than 2%) 1046
Diprolene Gel 0.05% (Less frequent) 2353
Dyclone 0.5% and 1% Topical Solutions, USP 544
▲ Efudex (Among most frequent) 2113
Elocon Lotion 0.1% 2354
Eurax Cream & Lotion 2685
Exact Vanishing and Tinted Creams ▣ 749
Florone/Florone E 906
Fluoroplex Topical Solution & Cream 1% 479
Furacin Soluble Dressing 2045
Hibiclens Antimicrobial Skin Cleanser 2840
Hibistat Towelette 2841
Hytone 907
Kwell Shampoo 2009
Lac-Hydrin 12% Lotion (Less frequent) 2687
Lamisil Cream 1% (1%) 2265
Lidex (Infrequent) 2130
Lindane Lotion USP 1% (Infrequent; less than 1 in 100,000 patients) 582
Lindane Shampoo USP 1% (Infrequent; less than 1 in 100,000 patients) 583
Locoid Cream, Ointment and Topical Solution (Infrequent) 978
Lotrimin AF Antifungal Spray Liquid, Spray Powder, Powder and Jock Itch Spray Powder ▣ 807
Lotrisone Cream (Infrequent) 2372
Melanex Topical Solution 1793
Monistat 3 Vaginal Suppositories 1850
Monistat-Derm (miconazole nitrate 2%) Cream (Isolated reports) 1889
Mycelex OTC Cream Antifungal ▣ 724
Mycelex OTC Solution Antifungal ▣ 724
NeoDecadron Topical Cream 1714
▲ Nizoral 2% Cream (5%) 1297
Nizoral 2% Shampoo (Less than 1%) 1298
Oil of Olay Daily UV Protectant SPF 15 Beauty Fluid-Original and Fragrance Free (Olay Co. Inc.) ▣ 751
Oncovin Solution Vials & Hyporets 1466
Oxistat Cream (0.4%) 1152
PediOtic Suspension Sterile 1153
Pramosone Cream, Lotion & Ointment 978
Pred-G Liquifilm Sterile Ophthalmic Suspension ⊙ 251
ProctoCream-HC (Infrequent) 2408
Psorcon Cream 0.05% (Infrequent) 909
Psorcon Ointment 0.05% 908
Serevent Inhalation Aerosol (Rare) 1176
Solbar PF Liquid SPF 30 1932
Synalar (Infrequent) 2130
Temovate (Infrequent) 1179
Testoderm Testosterone Transdermal System (2%) 486
Thera-Gesic 1781
Tinactin ▣ 809
Tridesilon Cream 0.05% (Infrequent) 615
Tridesilon Ointment 0.05% (Infrequent) 616
Tympagesic Ear Drops 2342
Vagistat-1 (Less than 1%) 778
Westcort 2690

Irritation, anal

Anusol Ointment ▣ 847
Colyte and Colyte-flavored 2396
GoLYTELY (Infrequent) 688
Cherry Flavor NuLYTELY (Less frequent) 689
Questran Light (Less frequent) 769
Questran Powder (Less frequent) 770

Irritation, gastric

Akineton 1333
Aldoclor Tablets 1598
Aldoril Tablets 1604
Apresazide Capsules 808
Capoten (About 0.5 to 2%) 739
Capozide (0.5 to 2%) 742
Combipres Tablets 677
D.A. Chewable Tablets 951
Dantrium Capsules (Less frequent) 1982
Diucardin Tablets 2718
Diupres Tablets 1650
Diuril Oral Suspension 1653
Diuril Sodium Intravenous 1652
Diuril Tablets 1653
Dura-Tap/PD Capsules 2867
Dura-Vent/DA Tablets 953
Dura-Vent Tablets 952
Enduron Tablets 420
Entex Capsules 1986
Entex LA Tablets 1987
Entex Liquid 1986
Esidrix Tablets 821
Esimil Tablets 822
Exgest LA Tablets 782
Hydrea Capsules 696
HydroDIURIL Tablets 1674
Hydropres Tablets 1675
Hyzaar Tablets 1677
Inderide Tablets 2732
Inderide LA Long Acting Capsules 2734
Kayexalate 2314
Lasix Injection, Oral Solution and Tablets 1240
Lopressor HCT Tablets 832
Lotensin HCT 837
Lozol Tablets (Less than 5%) 2022
Marax Tablets & DF Syrup 2200
Maxzide 1380
Minizide Capsules 1938
Moduretic Tablets 1705
Nalfon 200 Pulvules & Nalfon Tablets (Less than 1%) 917
Norflex 1496
Oretic Tablets 443
Prinzide Tablets 1737
Quadrinal Tablets 1350
Ser-Ap-Es Tablets 849
Sodium Polystyrene Sulfonate Suspension 2244
Thalitone 1245
Timolide Tablets 1748
Vaseretic Tablets 1765
Zestoretic 2850
Ziac 1415

Irritation, gastrointestinal

Dibenzyline Capsules 2476
Glucotrol XL Extended Release Tablets (Rare) 1968
▲ K-Lor Powder Packets (Most common) 434
▲ K-Norm Extended-Release Capsules (Among most common) 991
▲ Micro-K Extencaps (Among most common) 2063
Procardia XL Extended Release Tablets (Less than 1%) 1972
Tenoretic Tablets 2845

Irritation, glossal (see under Irritation, oral)

Irritation, local

AK-Spore ⊙ 204
Aristocort A 0.025% Cream (Infrequent) 1027
Aristocort A 0.5% Cream 1031
Aristocort A 0.1% Cream (Infrequent) 1029
Aristocort A 0.1% Ointment (Infrequent) 1030
Aspercreme Creme, Lotion Analgesic Rub ▣ 830
Astramorph/PF Injection, USP (Preservative-Free) 535
Atrac-Tain, Moisturizing Cream 2554
Auralgan Otic Solution 2703
Bentyl Injection 1501
BenzaShave Medicated Shave Cream 5% and 10% 1590
Betasept Surgical Scrub 1993
Bleph-10 475
Blephamide Ointment ⊙ 237
Carmol HC (Infrequent to frequent) 924
▲ Cipro I.V. Pharmacy Bulk Package (Among most frequent) 597
Claforan Sterile and Injection 1235
▲ Climara Transdermal System (31%) 645
Cleocin Vaginal Cream 2589
Cortisporin Ophthalmic Ointment Sterile 1085
Cortisporin Ophthalmic Suspension Sterile 1086
Critic-Aid, Antimicrobial Skin Paste 2554
Demerol 2308
Deponit NTG Transdermal Delivery System 2397
Dermatop Emollient Cream 0.1% 1238
Desenex Prescription ▣ 633
Desferal Vials 820
Drithocreme 0.1%, 0.25%, 0.5%, 1.0% (HP) 905
Dritho-Scalp 0.25%, 0.5% (More frequent) 906
Duramorph 962
Edecrin (Occasionally) 1657
Elase-Chloromycetin Ointment 1040
▲ Estraderm Transdermal System (About 17%) 824
Eurax Cream & Lotion 2685
Garamycin Injectable (Rare) 2360
Heparin Lock Flush Solution 2725
Heparin Sodium Injection 2726
Heparin Sodium Injection, USP, Sterile Solution 2615
Heparin Sodium Vials 1441
HibTITER 1375
Infumorph 200 and Infumorph 500 Sterile Solutions 965
K-Y Plus Vaginal Contraceptive and Personal Lubricant ▣ 659
Lovenox Injection 2020
Mepergan Injection 2753
Monistat Dual-Pak 1850
Naftin Cream 1% (2%) 480
Neosporin Ophthalmic Ointment Sterile 1148
Neosporin Ophthalmic Solution Sterile 1149
NeoStrata AHA Gel for Age Spots & Skin Lightening 1793
Nitrodisc (Rare) 2047
Nitro-Dur (nitroglycerin) Transdermal Infusion System 1326
▲ Nizoral 2% Cream (5%) 1297
Novacet Lotion (Rare) 1054
Novolin 70/30 Prefilled Disposable Insulin Delivery System 1798
Nydrazid Injection 508
Occlusal-HP 1054
Ogen Vaginal Cream 2630
Otic Domeboro Solution 611
Polysporin Ophthalmic Ointment Sterile 1154
▲ Polytrim Ophthalmic Solution Sterile (Most frequent) 482
ProctoCream-HC 2.5% (Infrequent to frequent) 2408
Retin-A (tretinoin) Cream/Gel/Liquid 1889
Rifadin I.V. 1528
Selsun Rx 2.5% Selenium Sulfide Lotion, USP 2225
Shade Gel SPF 30 Sunblock ▣ 807
Shade Lotion SPF 45 Sunblock ▣ 807
Shade UVAGUARD SPF 15 Suncreen Lotion ▣ 808
Sodium Sulamyd 2387
Stri-Dex ▣ 730
Sulfacet-R MVL Lotion (Rare) 909
Sultrin (Frequent) 1885
Terramycin Intramuscular Solution 2210
Topicort (Infrequent) 1243
Transderm-Nitro Transdermal Therapeutic System 859
Vasocidin Ointment ⊙ 268
Vasocidin Ophthalmic Solution ⊙ 270
Viroptic Ophthalmic Solution, 1% Sterile 1204
VōSol (Very rare) 2678
Zebeta Tablets 1413
Zonalon Cream (Less than 1%) 1055

Irritation, nasal

AeroBid Inhaler System (1-3%) 1005
Aerobid-M Inhaler System (1-3%) 1005
Beconase 1076
Claritin-D (Less frequent) 2350
▲ Decadron Phosphate Turbinaire (Most common) 1645
▲ Dexacort Phosphate in Turbinaire (One of the two most common) 459
Efudex (Infrequent) 2113
Flonase Nasal Spray (1% to 3%) 1098
▲ Miacalcin Nasal Spray (10.6%) 2275
Nasacort Nasal Inhaler (2.8%) 2024
Nasalcrom Nasal Solution (1 in 40) 994
Nasalide Nasal Solution 0.025% (5% or less) 2110
▲ Stadol (3% to 9%) 775
▲ Synarel Nasal Solution for Endometriosis (10% of patients) 2152
Vancenase AQ Nasal Spray 0.042% 2393
▲ Vancenase PocketHaler Nasal Inhaler (11 per 100 patients) 2391

Irritation, nasopharyngeal

▲ Beconase AQ Nasal Spray (24% of patients) 1076
▲ Intal Inhaler (Among most frequent) 988
Intal Nebulizer Solution 989
▲ Rhinocort Nasal Inhaler (3 to 9%) 556
▲ Vancenase AQ Nasal Spray 0.042% (Up to 24%) 2393

Irritation, ocular

▲ A/T/S 2% Acne Topical Gel and Solution (17 out of 90 patients) 1234
▲ Acular (3%) 474
Albalon Solution with Liquifilm ⊙ 231
Ambien Tablets (Infrequent) 2416
Erycette (erythromycin 2%) Topical Solution 1888
▲ Gentak (Among most frequent) ⊙ 208
Hivid Tablets (Less than 1% to less than 3%) 2121
Lacrisert Sterile Ophthalmic Insert 1686
Monopril Tablets (0.2% to 1.0%) 757
Oncovin Solution Vials & Hyporets 1466
ProSom Tablets (Infrequent) 449
Rythmol Tablets–150mg, 225mg, 300mg (Less than 1%) 1352
Temovate Scalp Application (1 of 294 patients) 1179
Timoptic in Ocudose (Less frequent) 1753
Timoptic Sterile Ophthalmic Solution (Less frequent) 1751
Timoptic-XE 1755
Vexol 1% Ophthalmic Suspension (Less than 1%) ⊙ 230

Irritation, oral

AeroBid Inhaler System (1-3%) 1005
Aerobid-M Inhaler System (1-3%) 1005
Kutrase Capsules 2402
Lasix Injection, Oral Solution and Tablets 1240
Mycostatin Pastilles 704
Peridex 1978

(▣ Described in PDR For Nonprescription Drugs) Incidence data in parenthesis; ▲ 3% or more (⊙ Described in PDR For Ophthalmology)

Side Effects Index

Sandimmune (Rare) 2286

Irritation, oropharynx

Brethaire Inhaler 813
Proventil Inhalation Aerosol 2382
Proventil Repetabs Tablets 2386
Proventil Syrup....................................... 2385
Proventil Tablets 2386
Ventolin Syrup... 1202
Ventolin Tablets 1203
Volmax Extended-Release Tablets .. 1788

Irritation, penile

Conceptrol Contraceptive Gel Single Use Applicators (Occasional) .... ◙ 736
Conceptrol Contraceptive Inserts (Occasional) .... ◙ 737
Delfen Contraceptive Foam .... ◙ 737
Gynol II Extra Strength Contraceptive Jelly (Occasional) .... ◙ 739
Gynol II Original Formula Contraceptive Jelly (Occasional) .... ◙ 738
Ortho-Gynol Contraceptive Jelly (Occasional) .... ◙ 740
Semicid Vaginal Contraceptive Inserts.. ◙ 874

Irritation, perianal

(see under Irritation, anal)

Irritation, skin

(see under Irritation, local)

Irritation, vaginal

Ceftin for Oral Suspension (Less than 1% but more than 0.1%) 1078
Conceptrol Contraceptive Gel Single Use Applicators (Occasional) .... ◙ 736
Conceptrol Contraceptive Inserts (Occasional) .... ◙ 737
Danocrine Capsules 2307
Delfen Contraceptive Foam .... ◙ 737
Depo-Provera Contraceptive Injection 2602
Encare Vaginal Contraceptive Suppositories...................................... ◙ 833
Floxin I.V. (Less than 1%) 1571
Floxin Tablets (200 mg, 300 mg, 400 mg) (Less than 1%) 1567
Gynol II Extra Strength Contraceptive Jelly (Occasional) .... ◙ 739
Gynol II Original Formula Contraceptive Jelly (Occasional) .... ◙ 738
Massengill 2457
Massengill Medicated Disposable Douche 2458
Massengill Medicated Liquid Concentrate .... ◙ 821
Massengill Powder................................. 2457
Monistat Dual-Pak (2%) 1850
Monistat 3 Vaginal Suppositories (2%) 1850
Mycelex-G 500 mg Vaginal Tablets (1 in 149 patients) 609
Ortho-Gynol Contraceptive Jelly (Occasional) .... ◙ 740
Semicid Vaginal Contraceptive Inserts.. ◙ 874
Sultrin (Frequent) 1885
Supprelin Injection (1% to 3%) 2056
▲ Terazol 3 Vaginal Cream (5%) 1886
▲ Terazol 7 Vaginal Cream (3.1% of 521 patients) 1887

Irritation, vulvovaginal

(see under Irritation, vaginal)

Irritation at injection site

Bactrim I.V. Infusion (Infrequent) 2082
Bentyl Injection.. 1501
Dilantin Parenteral 1910
▲ Eulexin Capsules (3%) 2358
▲ Gammagard S/D, Immune Globulin, Intravenous (Human) (16%) 585
Humegon... 1824
Metrodin (urofollitropin for injection) 2446
Nembutal Sodium Capsules 436
Nembutal Sodium Solution 438
Nembutal Sodium Suppositories (Less than 1%) 440
Pepcid Injection Premixed (Infrequent) 1722

Pergonal (menotropins for injection, USP) 2448
Retrovir I.V. Infusion (Infrequent) 1163
Romazicon 2147
Septra I.V. Infusion (Infrequent) 1169
Septra I.V. Infusion ADD-Vantage Vials (Infrequent) 1171

Ischemia

Cafergot.. 2251
Heparin Sodium Injection, USP, Sterile Solution 2615
Heparin Sodium Vials............................ 1441
Lupron Depot 3.75 mg 2556
Lupron Depot 7.5 mg 2559
▲ Lupron Injection (5% or more) 2555
Roferon-A Injection (Less than 1%) 2145
Sandostatin Injection (Less than 1%) 2292
Sensorcaine 559
Trandate 1185

Ischemia, arteria basilaris

AK-Fluor Injection 10% and 25% .... ◎ 203
Fluorescite .... ◎ 219

Ischemia, cerebral

Ansaid Tablets (Less than 1%) 2579
Betagan .... ◎ 233
Betaseron for SC Injection 658
Betimol 0.25%, 0.5% .... ◎ 261
Cardene Capsules (Less than 0.4%) 2095
▲ Dilatrate-SR (2-36%) 2398
Hyperstat I.V. Injection 2363
Imitrex Tablets (Rare) 1106
Nitrolingual Spray (Occasional) 2027
Ocupress Ophthalmic Solution, 1% Sterile... ◎ 309
Paxil Tablets (Rare) 2505
Permax Tablets (Infrequent)............... 575
Prozac Pulvules & Liquid, Oral Solution (Rare) 919
Quinaglute Dura-Tabs Tablets (2%) 649
ReoPro Vials (0.3%) 1471
Sorbitrate 2843
Timolide Tablets...................................... 1748
Timoptic in Ocudose 1753
Timoptic Sterile Ophthalmic Solution (Less frequent) 1751
Timoptic-XE 1755

Ischemia, myocardial

Anafranil Capsules (Rare) 803
Dilacor XR Extended-release Capsules 2018
Diprivan Injection (Less than 1%) .. 2833
Ergamisol Tablets 1292
Fluorouracil Injection 2116
Sterile FUDR (Remote possibility) .. 2118
Hyperstat I.V. Injection 2363
Imitrex Tablets (Rare) 1106
Micronor Tablets (An increased incidence) 1872
Modicon (An increased incidence) .. 1872
Ortho-Cyclen/Ortho-Tri-Cyclen 1858
Ortho-Novum (An increased incidence) 1872
Ortho-Cyclen/Ortho Tri-Cyclen 1858
Paxil Tablets (Rare) 2505
▲ Proleukin for Injection (3%) 797
Suprane (Less than 1%) 1813
Ultram Tablets (50 mg) (Infrequent) 1585

Ischemia, peripheral

Anafranil Capsules (Rare) 803
Brevibloc Injection (Approximately 1%) 1808
Cardura Tablets (0.3%) 2186
Cytovene-IV (One report) 2103
Felbatol 2666
Intron A (Less than 5%) 2364
Kerlone Tablets (Less than 2%) 2436
Norvasc Tablets (More than 0.1% to 1%) 1940
Ziac (0.4% to 0.7%) 1415
Zoloft Tablets (Infrequent) 2217

Ischemia of digits

Zovirax Sterile Powder (Less than 1%) 1223

Ischemic attacks, transient

Actimmune (Rare) 1056
Clozaril Tablets (Several patients) .. 2252
Cognex Capsules (Infrequent) 1901
Demulen 2428

DynaCirc Capsules (0.5% to 1%) .. 2256
Epogen for Injection (0.4%) 489
Fludara for Injection (Up to 1%) 663
Imitrex Injection 1103
Lupron Depot 3.75 mg 2556
Lupron Depot 7.5 mg 2559
Lupron Injection 2555
Monopril Tablets (0.4% to 1.0%) .. 757
Orthoclone OKT3 Sterile Solution .. 1837
Prinivil Tablets (0.3% to 1.0%) 1733
Prinzide Tablets 1737
Procrit for Injection (0.4%) 1841
Proleukin for Injection (Less than 1%) 797
Tonocard Tablets..................................... 531
Zestoretic 2850
Zestril Tablets (0.3% to 1.0%) 2854

Ischemic colitis

Inderal 2728
Inderal LA Long Acting Capsules 2730
Inderide Tablets 2732
Inderide LA Long Acting Capsules .. 2734
Kerlone Tablets.. 2436
Levatol 2403
Normodyne Tablets 2379
Sectral Capsules 2807
Timolide Tablets...................................... 1748
Timoptic in Ocudose 1753
Timoptic Sterile Ophthalmic Solution 1751

Ischemic injury

Levophed Bitartrate Injection 2315

Itching

(see under Pruritus)

Itching, eyes

▲ AK-Spore (Among most frequent) .... ◎ 204
▲ Alomide (1% to 5%) 469
▲ Betimol 0.25%, 0.5% (More than 5%) .... ◎ 261
Betoptic Ophthalmic Solution (Rare) 469
Betoptic S Ophthalmic Suspension (Small number of patients) 471
BuSpar (Infrequent) 737
Chloroptic Sterile Ophthalmic Solution .... ◎ 239
▲ Ciloxan Ophthalmic Solution (Less than 10%) 472
Combipres Tablets 677
Crolom (Infrequent) .... ◎ 257
Geocillin Tablets...................................... 2199
Lamprene Capsules (Greater than 1%) 828
Mykrox Tablets (Less than 2%) 993
Neurontin Capsules (Rare) 1922
Timoptic in Ocudose (Less frequent) 1753
Timoptic Sterile Ophthalmic Solution (Less frequent) 1751
▲ Timoptic-XE (1% to 5% of patients) 1755
TobraDex Ophthalmic Suspension and Ointment (Less than 4%) 473
Transderm Scōp Transdermal Therapeutic System (Infrequent) 869
Vantin for Oral Suspension and Vantin Tablets (Less than 1%) 2646

Itching, vulvovaginal

Clozaril Tablets (Less than 1%) 2252
Femstat Prefill Vaginal Cream 2% (0.9%) 2116
Femstat Vaginal Cream 2% (0.9%) 2115
Hivid Tablets (Less than 1% to less than 3%) 2121
Kefzol Vials, Faspak & ADD-Vantage 1456
MetroGel-Vaginal (Equal to or less than 2%) 902
Monistat Dual-Pak (2%) 1850
Monistat 3 Vaginal Suppositories (2%) 1850
Rogaine Topical Solution (0.91%).. 2637
Terazol 3 Vaginal Cream 1886
Terazol 7 Vaginal Cream (2.3% of 521 patients) 1887

IOP, elevation

AMO Vitrax Viscoelastic Solution ◎ 232
AMVISC Plus .... ◎ 329
AdatoSil 5000 (Greater than 2%) .... ◎ 274
AK-CIDE .... ◎ 202
AK-CIDE Ointment................................. ◎ 202
AK-Trol Ointment & Suspension .. ◎ 205

Albalon Solution with Liquifilm...... ◎ 231
Ansaid Tablets (Less than 1%) 2579
Aristocort Suspension (Forte Parenteral) 1027
Aristospan Suspension (Intra-articular) 1033
Aristospan Suspension (Intralesional) 1032
Beconase (Rare)...................................... 1076
Blephamide Liquifilm Sterile Ophthalmic Suspension 476
Blephamide Ointment .... ◎ 237
Celestone Soluspan Suspension 2347
Cognex Capsules (Infrequent) 1901
Cystospaz 1963
Cytovene (1% or less)........................... 2103
Dalalone D.P. Injectable 1011
Deltasone Tablets 2595
Depo-Medrol Sterile Aqueous Suspension... 2597
Dexacidin Ointment .... ◎ 263
Effexor (Rare) 2719
FML Forte Liquifilm................................ ◎ 240
FML Liquifilm.. ◎ 241
FML S.O.P. .... ◎ 241
FML-S Liquifilm.. ◎ 242
Florinef Acetate Tablets 505
HMS Liquifilm .... ◎ 244
Healon (Some cases) .... ◎ 314
Healon GV.. ◎ 315
▲ Maxitrol Ophthalmic Ointment and Suspension (Most often) .... ◎ 224
Neurontin Capsules (Rare) 1922
Ocucoat (Some cases)........................... ◎ 321
Ophthocort .... ◎ 311
Paremyd .... ◎ 247
Paxil Tablets (Rare) 2505
Permax Tablets (Infrequent)............... 575
Poly-Pred Liquifilm .... ◎ 248
Pred Forte.. ◎ 250
Pred Mild... ◎ 253
Pred-G Liquifilm Sterile Ophthalmic Suspension .... ◎ 251
Prelone Syrup 1787
Salagen Tablets (Less than 1%) 1489
Sandostatin Injection (Less than 1%) 2292
Serzone Tablets (Rare) 771
TobraDex Ophthalmic Suspension and Ointment.. 473
Vasocidin Ointment .... ◎ 268
Vasocidin Ophthalmic Solution .... ◎ 270
Videx Tablets, Powder for Oral Solution, & Pediatric Powder for Oral Solution (Less than 1%)........ 720
Viroptic Ophthalmic Solution, 1% Sterile 1204
▲ Voltaren Ophthalmic Sterile Ophthalmic Solution (15%) .... ◎ 272

IUD, difficult removal

Lippes Loop Intrauterine Double-S.. 1848
ParaGard T380A Intrauterine Copper Contraceptive 1880

IUD, embedment

ParaGard T380A Intrauterine Copper Contraceptive 1880

IUD, expulsion (complete)

Lippes Loop Intrauterine Double-S.. 1848
ParaGard T380A Intrauterine Copper Contraceptive 1880

IUD, expulsion (partial)

Lippes Loop Intrauterine Double-S.. 1848
ParaGard T380A Intrauterine Copper Contraceptive 1880

IUD, fragmentation

Lippes Loop Intrauterine Double-S.. 1848
ParaGard T380A Intrauterine Copper Contraceptive 1880

J

Jaundice

Children's Advil Suspension (Less than 1%).. 2692
Aldactazide... 2413
Aldoclor Tablets....................................... 1598
Aldomet Ester HCl Injection 1602
Aldomet Oral 1600
Aldoril Tablets.. 1604
Altace Capsules (Rare) 1232
Amen Tablets (A few instances) 780
Anaprox/Naprosyn (Rare; less than 1%).. 2117
Ancobon Capsules................................... 2079
Android Capsules, 10 mg 1250
Ansaid Tablets (Rare) 2579

(◙ Described in PDR For Nonprescription Drugs) Incidence data in parenthesis; ▲ 3% or more (◎ Described in PDR For Ophthalmology)

Jaundice Side Effects Index 1346

Apresazide Capsules 808
AquaMEPHYTON Injection 1608
Aquasol A Vitamin A Capsules, USP 534
Asendin Tablets (Very rare) 1369
Axid Pulvules 1427
Azactam for Injection (Less than 1%) 734
Azo Gantrisin Tablets 2081
Brevicon 2088
Capoten 739
Capozide 742
Cartrol Tablets (Rare) 410
Cataflam (Less than 1%) 816
Ceftin Tablets (Very rare) 1078
Chibroxin Sterile Ophthalmic Solution (With oral form) 1617
Cipro I.V. (1% or less) 595
Cipro I.V. Pharmacy Bulk Package (Less than 1%) 597
Cipro Tablets (Rare) 592
Claritin (2% or fewer patients) 2349
Claritin-D 2350
Cleocin Phosphate Injection 2586
Cleocin Vaginal Cream 2589
Clinoril Tablets (Less than 1%) 1618
Clozaril Tablets 2252
Combipres Tablets 677
Cylert Tablets 412
Cytosar-U Sterile Powder (Less frequent) 2592
Cytovene-IV (One report) 2103
Cytoxan (Isolated reports) 694
Danocrine Capsules 2307
Dantrium Capsules 1982
Dapsone Tablets USP 1284
Darvon-N/Darvocet-N (Rare) 1433
Darvon 1435
Darvon-N Suspension & Tablets 1433
Daypro Caplets 2426
Delatestryl Injection 2860
Demulen 2428
Depo-Provera Contraceptive Injection (Fewer than 1%) 2602
Desyrel and Desyrel Dividose 503
Diflucan Injection, Tablets, and Oral Suspension 2194
Diucardin Tablets 2718
Diuril Sodium Intravenous 1652
Dizac (Less frequent) 1809
Dolobid Tablets (Less than 1 in 100) 1654
Doral Tablets 2664
Dyazide 2479
Dyrenium Capsules (Rare) 2481
E.E.S. 424
E-Mycin Tablets 1341
EC-Naprosyn Delayed-Release Tablets (Rare; less than 1%) 2117
Edecrin (Rare) 1657
Effexor (Rare) 2719
Elavil 2838
Endep Tablets 2174
Enduron Tablets 420
ERYC 1915
EryPed 200 & EryPed 400 Granules 421
Ery-Tab Tablets 422
Erythrocin Stearate Filmtab 425
Esidrix Tablets 821
Esimil Tablets 822
Estraderm Transdermal System 824
ESTRATAB Tablets (0.3, 0.625, 1.25, 2.5 mg) 2536
Ethmozine Tablets (Rare) 2041
Etrafon (Less frequent; rare) 2355
Eulexin Capsules (Less than 1%) 2358
Felbatol 2666
Feldene Capsules (Less than 1%) 1965
Flexeril Tablets (Rare) 1661
Floxin I.V. 1571
Floxin Tablets (200 mg, 300 mg, 400 mg) 1567
Foscavir Injection (Less than 1%) 547
Fungizone Intravenous 506
Gantrisin 2120
Glucotrol Tablets (One case) 1967
Glucotrol XL Extended Release Tablets (One case) 1968
Halcion Tablets 2611
Haldol Decanoate 1577
Haldol Injection, Tablets and Concentrate 1575
Halotestin Tablets 2614
Havrix (Rare) 2489
HydroDIURIL Tablets 1674
Hydropres Tablets 1675
Hyzaar Tablets 1677
IBU Tablets (Less than 1%) 1342
Inderide Tablets 2732
Inderide LA Long Acting Capsules 2734
Indocin Capsules (Less than 1%) 1680
Indocin I.V. (Less than 1%) 1684
Indocin (Less than 1%) 1680
Inocor Lactate Injection (Rare) 2309
Intron A (Less than 5%) 2364
Lamprene Capsules (Less than 1%) 828
Lasix Injection, Oral Solution and Tablets 1240
Leukeran Tablets 1133
Levlen/Tri-Levlen 651
Levoprome 1274
Librax Capsules (Occasional) 2176
Libritabs Tablets (Occasional) 2177
Librium Capsules (Occasional) 2178
Librium Injectable (Occasional) 2179
Limbitrol (Rare) 2180
Lincocin (A few instances) 2617
Lodine Capsules and Tablets (Rare) 2743
Lopressor HCT Tablets 832
Loxitane (Rare) 1378
Lozol Tablets 2022
Ludiomil Tablets (Rare) 843
Luvox Tablets (Rare) 2544
Matulane Capsules 2131
Maxzide 1380
Mefoxin 1691
Mefoxin Premixed Intravenous Solution 1694
Mellaril 2269
Mesantoin Tablets 2272
Micronor Tablets 1872
Midamor Tablets (Less than or equal to 1%) 1703
Mintezol 1704
Modicon 1872
Moduretic Tablets 1705
Monopril Tablets 757
Children's Motrin Ibuprofen Oral Suspension (Less than 1%) 1546
Motrin Tablets (Less than 1%) 2625
Motrin Ibuprofen Suspension, Oral Drops, Chewable Tablets, Caplets (Rare; less than 1%) 1546
Mustargen (Infrequent) 1709
Myochrysine Injection 1711
Nalfon 200 Pulvules & Nalfon Tablets (Less than 1%) 917
Anaprox/Naprosyn (Rare; less than 1%) 2117
Nardil (Less frequent) 1920
NEOSAR Lyophilized/Neosar (Isolated reports) 1959
Nicolar Tablets 2026
Nimotop Capsules (Less than 1%) 610
Nizoral Tablets 1298
Norinyl 2088
Normodyne Injection 2377
Normodyne Tablets 2379
Noroxin Tablets 1715
Noroxin Tablets 2048
Norpramin Tablets 1526
Nor-Q D Tablets 2135
▲ Novantrone (3 to 7%) 1279
Nydrazid Injection 508
▲ Oncaspar (Greater than 1% but less than 5%) 2028
Oreton Methyl 1255
Ortho-Cyclen/Ortho-Tri-Cyclen 1858
Ortho-Novum 1872
Ortho-Cyclen/Ortho Tri-Cyclen 1858
Orudis Capsules (Rare) 2766
Oruvail Capsules (Rare) 2766
Ovcon 760
Oxandrin 2862
PCE Dispertab Tablets 444
Pamelor 2280
Paraflex Caplets 1580
Parafon Forte DSC Caplets 1581
PASER Granules 1285
Paxil Tablets (Rare) 2505
Periactin 1724
Permax Tablets (Rare) 575
Phenergan Injection 2773
Phenergan Tablets 2775
Prilosec Delayed-Release Capsules (Rare) 529
Primaxin I.M. 1727
Primaxin I.V. (Less than 0.2%) 1729
Prinivil Tablets 1733
Prinzide Tablets 1737
▲ Prograf (Greater than 3%) 1042
▲ Proleukin for Injection (11%) 797
Prozac Pulvules & Liquid, Oral Solution (Rare) 919
Reglan (Rare) 2068
Ridaura Capsules (Less than 1%) 2513
Rifadin (Some patients) 1528
Rifamate Capsules 1530
Rifater 1532
Risperdal 1301
Rocephin Injectable Vials, ADD-Vantage, Galaxy Container (Rare) 2142
Sandostatin Injection (Less than 1%) 2292
Seldane Tablets (Isolated reports) 1536
Seldane-D Extended-Release Tablets (Isolated reports) 1538
Septra I.V. Infusion 1169
Septra I.V. Infusion ADD-Vantage Vials 1171
Ser-Ap-Es Tablets 849
Serax Capsules 2810
Serax Tablets 2810
Serentil 684
Sinequan (Occasional) 2205
Skelaxin Tablets 788
Solganal Suspension 2388
Sporanox Capsules 1305
Stelazine 2514
Surmontil Capsules 2811
Tambocor Tablets 1497
Tao Capsules 2209
Tapazole Tablets 1477
Temaril Tablets, Syrup and Spansule Extended-Release Capsules 483
Tenoretic Tablets 2845
Testoderm Testosterone Transdermal System 486
Thalitone 1245
Thioguanine Tablets, Tabloid Brand 1181
Thorazine 2523
Tigan 2057
Tofranil Ampuls 854
Tofranil Tablets 856
Tofranil-PM Capsules 857
Tonocard Tablets (Less than 1%) 531
Torecan 2245
Trancopal Caplets (Rare) 2337
Trandate 1185
Trecator-SC Tablets 2814
Trental Tablets (Rare) 1244
Triavil Tablets 1757
Trilafon (Low incidence) 2389
Levlen/Tri-Levlen 651
Tri-Norinyl 2164
Univasc Tablets 2410
Valium Injectable (Isolated reports) 2182
Valium Tablets (Isolated reports) 2183
Valrelease Capsules (Occasional) 2169
Vaseretic Tablets 1765
Vasotec I.V. 1768
Vasotec Tablets 1771
Vivactil Tablets 1774
Voltaren Tablets (Less than 1%) 861
Vontrol Tablets 2532
Wellbutrin Tablets (Infrequent) 1204
Wygesic Tablets (Rare) 2827
Xanax Tablets 2649
Yutopar Intravenous Injection (Infrequent) 570
Zantac (Occasional) 1209
Zantac Injection 1207
Zantac Syrup (Occasional) 1209
Zestoretic 2850
Ziac 1415
Zoloft Tablets (One or more patients) 2217

Jaundice, cholestatic

Accupril Tablets (Rare) 1893
Altace Capsules (Rare) 1232
Amen Tablets 780
▲ Android Capsules, 10 mg (Among most common) 1250
Android 1251
Ansaid Tablets (Rare) 2579
Atretol Tablets 573
Augmentin 2468
Axid Pulvules (Rare) 1427
Aygestin Tablets 974
Bactrim DS Tablets 2084
Bactrim I.V. Infusion 2082
Bactrim 2084
Brevicon 2088
Capoten (Rare) 739
Capozide (Rare) 742
Ceclor Pulvules & Suspension (Rare) 1431
Cefzil Tablets and Oral Suspension (Rare) 746
Chibroxin Sterile Ophthalmic Solution (With oral form) 1617
Cipro Tablets 592
Climara Transdermal System 645
Compazine 2470
Cycrin Tablets 975
Danocrine Capsules 2307
Dapsone Tablets USP 1284
Darvon-N/Darvocet-N (Rare) 1433
Darvon 1435
Darvon-N Suspension & Tablets (Rare) 1433
Delatestryl Injection 2860
Demulen 2428
Depo-Provera Sterile Aqueous Suspension 2606
Desogen Tablets 1817
DiaBeta Tablets (Rare) 1239
Diabinese Tablets (Rare) 1935
Diethylstilbestrol Tablets 1437
Estrace Cream and Tablets 749
Estraderm Transdermal System 824
ESTRATAB Tablets (0.3, 0.625, 1.25, 2.5 mg) 2536
Estratest 2539
Eulexin Capsules (Less than 1%) 2358
Floxin I.V. 1571
Floxin Tablets (200 mg, 300 mg, 400 mg) 1567
Glucotrol Tablets (Rare) 1967
Glynase PresTab Tablets (Rare) 2609
Halotestin Tablets 2614
Keflex Pulvules & Oral Suspension (Rare) 914
Keftab Tablets (Rare) 915
Kefzol Vials, Faspak & ADD-Vantage (Rare) 1456
Lescol Capsules 2267
Levlen/Tri-Levlen 651
Lodine Capsules and Tablets (Less than 1%) 2743
Lo/Ovral Tablets 2746
Lo/Ovral-28 Tablets 2751
Lopid Tablets 1917
Lotensin Tablets (Rare) 834
Lotensin HCT (Rare) 837
Macrobid Capsules (Rare) 1988
Macrodantin Capsules (Rare) 1989
Mandol Vials, Faspak & ADD-Vantage (Rare) 1461
Menest Tablets 2494
Mevacor Tablets 1699
Micronase Tablets (Rare) 2623
Micronor Tablets 1872
Modicon 1872
Monopril Tablets (Rare) 757
Myleran Tablets (Rare) 1143
Myochrysine Injection 1711
Nordette-21 Tablets 2755
Nordette-28 Tablets 2758
Norinyl 2088
Normodyne Injection (Less common) 2377
Normodyne Tablets (Less common) 2379
Noroxin Tablets 1715
Noroxin Tablets 2048
Norpace (Infrequent) 2444
Nor-Q D Tablets 2135
Ogen Tablets 2627
Ogen Vaginal Cream 2630
Oreton Methyl 1255
Ortho-Cept 1851
Ortho-Cyclen/Ortho-Tri-Cyclen 1858
Ortho Dienestrol Cream 1866
Ortho-Est 1869
Ortho-Novum 1872
Ortho-Cyclen/Ortho Tri-Cyclen 1858
Ovcon 760
Ovral Tablets 2770
Ovral-28 Tablets 2770
Ovrette Tablets 2771
Oxandrin 2862
PMB 200 and PMB 400 2783
Pepcid Injection (Infrequent) 1722
Pepcid (Infrequent) 1720
Placidyl Capsules 448
Pravachol 765
Premarin Intravenous 2787
Premarin with Methyltestosterone 2794
Premarin Tablets 2789
Premarin Vaginal Cream 2791
Premphase 2797
Prempro 2801
Prilosec Delayed-Release Capsules (Rare) 529
Prinivil Tablets (0.3% to 1.0%) 1733
Prinzide Tablets (Rare) 1737
Procardia Capsules 1971
Procardia XL Extended Release Tablets 1972
▲ Prograf (Greater than 3%) 1042
Prolixin 509
Proloprim Tablets (Rare) 1155
Provera Tablets 2636
Prozac Pulvules & Liquid, Oral Solution 919
Relafen Tablets (1%) 2510

(Described in PDR For Nonprescription Drugs) Incidence data in parenthesis; ▲ 3% or more (◉ Described in PDR For Ophthalmology)

1347 Side Effects Index Kidney damage

Ridaura Capsules (Rare) 2513
Septra 1174
Septra I.V. Infusion 1169
Septra I.V. Infusion ADD-Vantage Vials 1171
Septra 1174
Stelazine 2514
Stilphostrol Tablets and Ampuls 612
Tegretol Chewable Tablets 852
Tegretol Suspension 852
Tegretol Tablets 852
Testoderm Testosterone Transdermal System 486
Testred Capsules 1262
Ticlid Tablets (Rare) 2156
Timentin for Injection (Rare) 2528
Toradol 2159
Torecan (Occasional case) 2245
Trancopal Caplets 2337
Trandate (Less common) 1185
Levlen/Tri-Levlen 651
Tri-Norinyl 2164
Triphasil-21 Tablets 2814
Triphasil-28 Tablets 2819
Univasc Tablets (Rare) 2410
Vaseretic Tablets (Rare) 1765
Vasotec I.V. (Rare) 1768
Vasotec Tablets (0.5% to 1.0%; rare) 1771
Winstrol Tablets (Rare) 2337
Zestoretic (Rare) 2850
Zestril Tablets (0.3% to 1.0%) 2854
Zithromax (1% or less; rare) 1944
Zocor Tablets 1775
Zyloprim Tablets (Less than 1%) 1226

Jaundice, fetal
Diupres Tablets 1650
HydroDIURIL Tablets 1674
Hydropres Tablets 1675

Jaundice, hepatocellular
Atretol Tablets 573
Augmentin 2468
Axid Pulvules (Rare) 1427
Floxin I.V. 1571
Floxin Tablets (200 mg, 300 mg, 400 mg) 1567
Monopril Tablets 757
Prilosec Delayed-Release Capsules (Rare) 529
Prinivil Tablets (0.3% to 1.0%) 1733
Prinzide Tablets 1737
Tegretol Chewable Tablets 852
Tegretol Suspension 852
Tegretol Tablets 852
Ticlid Tablets (Rare) 2156
Vaseretic Tablets 1765
Vasotec I.V. 1768
Vasotec Tablets (0.5% to 1.0%) 1771
Zantac (Occasional) 1209
Zestoretic 2850
Zestril Tablets (0.3% to 1.0%) 2854

Jaundice, intrahepatic
Minizide Capsules 1938
Solganal Suspension 2388

Jaundice, intrahepatic cholestatic
Aldoclor Tablets 1598
Apresazide Capsules 808
Augmentin 2468
Capozide 742
Combipres Tablets 677
Delatestryl Injection 2860
Diucardin Tablets 2718
Diupres Tablets 1650
Diuril Oral Suspension 1653
Diuril Sodium Intravenous 1652
Diuril Tablets 1653
Enduron Tablets 420
Esidrix Tablets 821
Esimil Tablets 822
HydroDIURIL Tablets 1674
Hydropres Tablets 1675
Hyzaar Tablets 1677
Inderide Tablets 2732
Inderide LA Long Acting Capsules 2734
Lasix Injection, Oral Solution and Tablets 1240
Lopressor HCT Tablets 832
Lotensin HCT 837
Lozol Tablets 2022
Maxzide 1380
Moduretic Tablets 1705
Mykrox Tablets 993
Oretic Tablets 443
Prinzide Tablets 1737
Ser-Ap-Es Tablets 849
Solganal Suspension 2388
Tenoretic Tablets 2845
Thalitone 1245
Timolide Tablets 1748
Vaseretic Tablets 1765
Zaroxolyn Tablets 1000
Zestoretic 2850
Ziac 1415

Jaundice, neonatal
Aldactazide 2413
Aldoclor Tablets 1598
Aldoril Tablets 1604
Apresazide Capsules 808
AquaMEPHYTON Injection 1608
Capozide 742
Compazine 2470
Depo-Provera Sterile Aqueous Suspension 2606
Diucardin Tablets 2718
Diupres Tablets 1650
Diuril Oral Suspension 1653
Diuril Sodium Intravenous 1652
Diuril Tablets 1653
Dyazide 2479
Enduron Tablets 420
Esidrix Tablets 821
Esimil Tablets 822
HydroDIURIL Tablets 1674
Hydropres Tablets 1675
Inderide Tablets 2732
Inderide LA Long Acting Capsules 2734
Konakion Injection 2127
Lopressor HCT Tablets 832
Lozol Tablets 2022
Maxzide 1380
Mephyton Tablets 1696
Micronor Tablets 1872
Modicon 1872
Moduretic Tablets 1705
Mykrox Tablets 993
Oretic Tablets 443
Ortho-Novum 1872
Oxytocin Injection 2771
Prinzide Tablets 1737
Ser-Ap-Es Tablets 849
Stelazine 2514
Syntocinon Injection 2296
Temaril Tablets, Syrup and Spansule Extended-Release Capsules 483
Tenoretic Tablets 2845
Thorazine 2523
Timolide Tablets 1748
Vaseretic Tablets 1765
Zestoretic 2850

Jaundice, obstructive
Thorazine 2523
Tofranil Ampuls 854
Tofranil Tablets 856
Tofranil-PM Capsules 857

Jaw tightness
Anectine 1073
Imitrex Injection (Relatively common) 1103
Respbid Tablets 682

Jerks (see under Twitching)

Jitteriness
Adalat Capsules (10 mg and 20 mg) (2% or less) 587
Compazine 2470
Etrafon 2355
Nardil (Less common) 1920
Procardia Capsules (2% or less) 1971
Prostin VR Pediatric Sterile Solution (Less than 1%) 2635
Reglan 2068
Stelazine 2514
Thorazine 2523
▲ Yutopar Intravenous Injection (5% to 6%) 570

Joint disorder
▲ CellCept Capsules (More than or equal to 3%) 2099
Oncaspar (Less than 1%) 2028

Joint disorder, unspecified
Cartrol Tablets (Less common) 410
Effexor (Infrequent) 2719
Hytrin Capsules (At least 1%) 430
Keflex Pulvules & Oral Suspension 914
Keftab Tablets 915
Lamictal Tablets (1.3%) 1112
▲ Lupron Depot 3.75 mg (7.8%) 2556
Videx Tablets, Powder for Oral Solution, & Pediatric Powder for Oral Solution (Less than 1%) 720
Zoladex (1% or greater) 2858

Joint effusion
Sandostatin Injection (Less than 1%) 2292

Joint pain (see under Arthralgia)

Joint stiffness
Adalat Capsules (10 mg and 20 mg) (2% or less) 587
Aristocort Suspension (Forte Parenteral) 1027
Aristospan Suspension (Intra-articular) 1033
Aristospan Suspension (Intralesional) 1032
Atgam Sterile Solution (Less than 5%) 2581
Cipro I.V. (1% or less) 595
Cipro I.V. Pharmacy Bulk Package (Less than 1%) 597
Cipro Tablets (Less than 1%) 592
Danocrine Capsules 2307
Imitrex Injection (Infrequent) 1103
Neurontin Capsules (Infrequent) 1922
Oncaspar 2028
Procardia Capsules (2% or less) 1971
Supprelin Injection (2% to 3%) 2056

K

Kawasaki-like syndrome
Pentasa (Less than 1%) 1527

Keratitis
Acular (1%) 474
Alomide (Less than 1%) 469
Anafranil Capsules (Rare) 803
Betagan ◉ 233
Betimol 0.25%, 0.5% (1% to 5%) ◉ 261
Betoptic Ophthalmic Solution (Rare) 469
Betoptic S Ophthalmic Suspension (Rare) 471
BOTOX (Botulinum Toxin Type A) Purified Neurotoxin Complex (Less than 1%) 477
Ciloxan Ophthalmic Solution (Less than 1%) 472
Econopred & Econopred Plus Ophthalmic Suspensions (Occasional) ◉ 217
Effexor (Rare) 2719
Engerix-B Unit-Dose Vials 2482
FML Forte Liquifilm (Occasional) ◉ 240
FML Liquifilm (Occasional) ◉ 241
FML S.O.P. (Occasional) ◉ 241
Iopidine 0.5% (Less than 3%) ◉ 221
Ocupress Ophthalmic Solution, 1% Sterile ◉ 309
Pilopine HS Ophthalmic Gel ◉ 226
Timoptic Sterile Ophthalmic Solution (Less frequent) 1751
Timoptic-XE 1755
Vexol 1% Ophthalmic Suspension (Less than 1%) ◉ 230
▲ Voltaren Ophthalmic Sterile Ophthalmic Solution (28%) ◉ 272

Keratitis, bacterial
Cortisporin Ophthalmic Ointment Sterile 1085
Decadron Phosphate Sterile Ophthalmic Ointment 1641
Decadron Phosphate Sterile Ophthalmic Solution 1642
Floropryl Sterile Ophthalmic Ointment 1662
Humorsol Sterile Ophthalmic Solution 1664
NeoDecadron Sterile Ophthalmic Ointment 1712
Neosporin Ophthalmic Ointment Sterile 1148
Trusopt Sterile Ophthalmic Solution 1760

Keratitis, epithelial
Fluoracaine (Rare) ◉ 206
FLURESS (Rare) ◉ 207
Ophthetic ◉ 247
Vasosulf ◉ 271

Keratitis, punctate
Albalon Solution with Liquifilm ◉ 231
Pred-G Liquifilm Sterile Ophthalmic Suspension (Occasional) ◉ 251
Pred-G S.O.P. Sterile Ophthalmic Ointment ◉ 252
▲ Rēv-Eyes Ophthalmic Eyedrops 0.5% (10% to 40%) ◉ 323

Keratitis, superficial punctate
▲ Trusopt Sterile Ophthalmic Solution (10% to 15%) 1760
Vira-A Ophthalmic Ointment, 3% ◉ 312
Viroptic Ophthalmic Solution, 1% Sterile 1204

Keratitis nigricans
Timoptic in Ocudose (Less frequent) 1753

Keratoconjunctivitis
Betaseron for SC Injection 658
Serzone Tablets (Infrequent) 771
Viroptic Ophthalmic Solution, 1% Sterile 1204

Keratopathy
▲ AdatoSil 5000 (0.6% to 30%) ◉ 274
Alomide (Less than 1%) 469
Ciloxan Ophthalmic Solution (Less than 1%) 472
Iopidine 0.5% (Less than 3%) ◉ 221
Trilafon 2389

Keratopathy, bullous
AMO Endosol (Balanced Salt Solution) ◉ 232
BSS (15 mL & 30 mL) Sterile Irrigation Solution ◉ 214
BSS (250 mL) Sterile Irrigation Solution ◉ 214
BSS (500 mL) Sterile Irrigation Solution ◉ 214
MIOSTAT Intraocular Solution ◉ 224

Keratopathy, epithelial
Compazine 2470
Etrafon 2355
Stelazine 2514
Temaril Tablets, Syrup and Spansule Extended-Release Capsules 483
Thorazine 2523
Viroptic Ophthalmic Solution, 1% Sterile 1204

Keratosis, nigricans
Nicolar Tablets 2026

Kernicterus
Konakion Injection 2127

Kernicterus, neonatal
AVC 1500
Azo Gantanol Tablets 2080
Azo Gantrisin Tablets 2081
Azulfidine 1949
Bactrim DS Tablets 2084
Bactrim I.V. Infusion 2082
Bactrim 2084
Blephamide Ointment ◉ 237
Fansidar Tablets 2114
Gantanol Tablets 2119
Gantrisin 2120
Septra 1174
Silvadene Cream 1% 1540
Vasocidin Ophthalmic Solution ◉ 270

Ketosis
Betaseron for SC Injection 658

Kidney, decrease in size
BiCNU 691
CeeNU 693

Kidney, enlarged
Atgam Sterile Solution (Less than 5%) 2581

Kidney, ruptured
Atgam Sterile Solution (Less than 5%) 2581

Kidney damage
BiCNU (Occasional) 691
CeeNU (Occasional) 693
Fioricet with Codeine Capsules 2260
Lasix Injection, Oral Solution and Tablets 1240
Milontin Kapseals 1920

(▭ Described in PDR For Nonprescription Drugs) Incidence data in parenthesis; ▲ 3% or more (◉ Described in PDR For Ophthalmology)

Kidney stones (see under Renal stones)

L

Labia, fusion
Depo-Provera Sterile Aqueous Suspension (Rare) 2606
Provera Tablets (Rare) 2636

Labor, preterm, delayed
Airet Solution for Inhalation 452
Ventolin Inhalation Solution 1198
Ventolin Nebules Inhalation Solution 1199
Ventolin Rotacaps for Inhalation 1200
Ventolin Syrup 1202
Ventolin Tablets 1203

Labor, slowing
Astramorph/PF Injection, USP (Preservative-Free) 535
Brontex 1981
Carbocaine Hydrochloride Injection 2303
Marcaine Hydrochloride with Epinephrine 1:200,000 2316
Marcaine Hydrochloride Injection 2316
Marcaine Spinal 2319
Proventil Inhalation Solution 0.083% (Some reports) 2384
Proventil Repetabs Tablets (Some reports) 2386
Proventil Solution for Inhalation 0.5% (Some reports) 2383
Proventil Syrup (Some reports) 2385
Proventil Tablets (Some patients) 2386
Sensorcaine 559

Laboratory abnormalities, unspecified
Betapace Tablets (1% to 4%) 641
Cartrol Tablets (1.2%) 410

Labyrinth disorder
Anafranil Capsules (Rare) 803

Labyrinthitis
Actifed with Codeine Cough Syrup 1067
Benadryl Injection 1898
Cognex Capsules (Rare) 1901
Effexor (Rare) 2719
Kerlone Tablets (Less than 2%) 2436
Neurontin Capsules (Rare) 1922
Ornade Spansule Capsules 2502
Periactin 1724
Tavist Syrup 2297
Tavist Tablets 2298
Trinalin Repetabs Tablets 1330

Labyrinthitis hysteria, acute
Benadryl Capsules 1898

Lacrimal duct, stenosis
Ergamisol Tablets 1292
Fluorouracil Injection 2116
Sterile FUDR (Remote possibility) 2118

Lacrimal gland, disorders
DDAVP (Up to 2%) 2017
Intron A (Less than 5%) 2364
Neurontin Capsules (Rare) 1922

Lacrimation
Adriamycin PFS (Rare) 1947
Adriamycin RDF (Rare) 1947
Albalon Solution with Liquifilm ⊙ 231
Apresazide Capsules (Less frequent) 808
Apresoline Hydrochloride Tablets (Less frequent) 809
Asendin Tablets (Less than 1%) 1369
▲ BOTOX (Botulinum Toxin Type A) Purified Neurotoxin Complex (10.0%) 477
Claritin (Rare) 2349
Crolom (Infrequent) ⊙ 257
Doxorubicin Astra (Rare) 540
Duvoid (Infrequent) 2044
Efudex 2113
Emcyt Capsules (Approximately 1%) 1953
Floropryl Sterile Ophthalmic Ointment 1662
Fluorouracil Injection 2116
Sterile FUDR (Remote possibility) 2118
Heparin Lock Flush Solution 2725
Heparin Sodium Injection 2726
Heparin Sodium Injection, USP, Sterile Solution 2615
Heparin Sodium Vials (Rare) 1441
Hivid Tablets (Less than 1% to less than 3%) 2121
Humorsol Sterile Ophthalmic Solution 1664
Hyperstat I.V. Injection 2363
Imitrex Injection (Infrequent) 1103
Imitrex Tablets (Infrequent) 1106
Intal Capsules (Less than 1 in 10,000 patients) 987
Intal Inhaler (Infrequent) 988
Intal Nebulizer Solution 989
Livostin (Approximately 1% to 3%) ⊙ 266
Lorelco Tablets 1517
Methadone Hydrochloride Oral Concentrate 2233
Neurontin Capsules (Rare) 1922
OptiPranolol (Metipranolol 0.3%) Sterile Ophthalmic Solution (A small number of patients) ⊙ 258
Orlamm (Less than 1%) 2239
Phospholine Iodide ⊙ 326
Pilocar ⊙ 268
Pilopine HS Ophthalmic Gel ⊙ 226
Procardia XL Extended Release Tablets (1% or less) 1972
Proglycem 580
Rubex (Rare) 712
▲ Salagen Tablets (6%) 1489
Ser-Ap-Es Tablets 849
▲ Tegison Capsules (1-10%) 2154
Tensilon Injectable 1261
Trusopt Sterile Ophthalmic Solution (Approximately 1% to 5%) 1760
Urecholine 1761
Vaseretic Tablets 1765
Vasotec I.V. 1768
Vasotec Tablets (0.5% to 1.0%) 1771
Vexol 1% Ophthalmic Suspension (Less than 1%) ⊙ 230
Vira-A Ophthalmic Ointment, 3% ⊙ 312

Lacrimation, abnormal
Ambien Tablets (Rare) 2416
Anafranil Capsules (Up to 3%) 803
Cardura Tablets (Less than 0.5% of 3960 patients) 2186
Claritin-D (Less frequent) 2350
Desmopressin Acetate Rhinal Tube (Up to 2%) 979
Ergamisol Tablets (Up to 4%) 1292
Flumadine Tablets & Syrup 1015
Kerlone Tablets (Less than 2%) 2436
Lamictal Tablets (Rare) 1112
Miacalcin Nasal Spray (1% to 3%) 2275
Risperdal (Rare) 1301
Romazicon (1% to 3%) 2147
Zebeta Tablets 1413
Ziac 1415
Zoloft Tablets (Rare) 2217

Lacrimation, decrease
Ditropan 1516

Lactation
Aldoclor Tablets 1598
Aldomet Ester HCl Injection 1602
Aldomet Oral 1600
Aldoril Tablets 1604
Compazine 2470
Desyrel and Desyrel Dividose 503
Effexor (Rare) 2719
Etrafon 2355
Haldol Decanoate 1577
Haldol Injection, Tablets and Concentrate 1575
Lamictal Tablets (Infrequent) 1112
▲ Lupron Depot 3.75 mg (Among most frequent) 2556
Luvox Tablets (Infrequent) 2544
Mellaril 2269
Navane Capsules and Concentrate 2201
Navane Intramuscular 2202
Paxil Tablets (Rare) 2505
Permax Tablets (Infrequent) 575
Prozac Pulvules & Liquid, Oral Solution (Rare) 919
Serentil 684
Stelazine 2514
Synarel Nasal Solution for Endometriosis (Less than 1%) 2152
Temaril Tablets, Syrup and Spansule Extended-Release Capsules 483
Thorazine 2523
Triavil Tablets 1757
Trilafon 2389

Lactation, non-puerperal
▲ Anafranil Capsules (Up to 4%) 803
Diupres Tablets 1650
Flumadine Tablets & Syrup (Less than 0.3%) 1015
Hydropres Tablets 1675
Risperdal (Infrequent) 1301

Lactation, possible diminution
Brevicon 2088
Demulen 2428
Desogen Tablets 1817
Levlen/Tri-Levlen 651
Lo/Ovral Tablets 2746
Lo/Ovral-28 Tablets 2751
Micronor Tablets 1872
Modicon 1872
Nordette-21 Tablets 2755
Nordette-28 Tablets 2758
Norinyl 2088
Nor-Q D Tablets 2135
Ortho-Cept 1851
Ortho-Cyclen/Ortho-Tri-Cyclen 1858
Ortho-Novum 1872
Ortho-Cyclen/Ortho Tri-Cyclen 1858
Ovral Tablets 2770
Ovral-28 Tablets 2770
Ovrette Tablets 2771
Levlen/Tri-Levlen 651
Tri-Norinyl 2164
Triphasil-21 Tablets 2814
Triphasil-28 Tablets 2819

Lactation, suppression
Bentyl 1501
Cystospaz 1963
Depo-Provera Contraceptive Injection (Fewer than 1%) 2602
Ditropan 1516
Donnatal 2060
Donnatal Extentabs 2061
Donnatal Tablets 2060
Kutrase Capsules 2402
Levsin/Levsinex/Levbid 2405
Ovcon 760
Pro-Banthine Tablets 2052
Quarzan Capsules 2181
Robinul Forte Tablets 2072
Robinul Injectable 2072
Robinul Tablets 2072

Lactation abnormalities
Demulen 2428
Levoprome 1274
Prolixin 509
THYREL TRH (Less frequent) 2873

Lactic acidosis
Glucophage (Rare) 752
Hivid Tablets (Rare) 2121
Retrovir Capsules (Rare) 1158
Retrovir I.V. Infusion (Rare) 1163
Retrovir Syrup (Rare) 1158
Yutopar Intravenous Injection (Infrequent) 570

Lagophthalmos
BOTOX (Botulinum Toxin Type A) Purified Neurotoxin Complex 477

Laryngeal changes
Alupent Tablets (0.2%) 669
Mexitil Capsules (About 1 in 1,000) 678

Laryngeal stridor
Lotrel Capsules (About 0.5%) 840
Omnipen for Oral Suspension 2765

Laryngismus
Effexor (Infrequent) 2719
Luvox Tablets (Rare) 2544

Laryngitis
AeroBid Inhaler System (1-3%) 1005
Aerobid-M Inhaler System (1-3%) 1005
Ambien Tablets (Rare) 2416
Anafranil Capsules (Up to 2%) 803
Ansaid Tablets (Less than 1%) 2579
▲ Betaseron for SC Injection (6%) 658
Claritin (2% or fewer patients) 2349
Claritin-D 2350
Clozaril Tablets (Less than 1%) 2252
Effexor (Infrequent) 2719
Foscavir Injection (Less than 1%) 547
Monopril Tablets (0.2% to 1.0%) 757
NebuPent for Inhalation Solution (1% or less) 1040
Neurontin Capsules (Rare) 1922
Permax Tablets (Infrequent) 575
Prinivil Tablets (0.3% to 1.0%) 1733
Prinzide Tablets 1737
ProSom Tablets (Rare) 449
Prostin E2 Suppository 2634
▲ Pulmozyme Inhalation (3% to 4%) 1064
Serevent Inhalation Aerosol (1% to 3%) 1176
Serzone Tablets (Infrequent) 771
Trental Tablets (Less than 1%) 1244
Videx Tablets, Powder for Oral Solution, & Pediatric Powder for Oral Solution (Less than 1%) 720
Zestoretic 2850
Zestril Tablets (0.3% to 1.0%) 2854

Laryngospasm
Alfenta Injection (0.3% to 1%) 1286
Anafranil Capsules (Rare) 803
Atgam Sterile Solution (Less than 1% to less than 5%) 2581
Atrovent Inhalation Aerosol 671
Blocadren Tablets 1614
Brevital Sodium Vials 1429
Carafate Suspension 1505
Carafate Tablets 1504
Cartrol Tablets 410
Dilaudid-HP Injection (Less frequent) 1337
Dilaudid-HP Lyophilized Powder 250 mg (Less frequent) 1337
Dilaudid Tablets and Liquid 1339
Diprivan Injection (Less than 1%) 2833
Dizac 1809
Dopram Injectable 2061
Haldol Decanoate 1577
Haldol Injection, Tablets and Concentrate 1575
Inapsine Injection (Less common) 1296
Inderal 2728
Inderal LA Long Acting Capsules 2730
Inderide Tablets 2732
Inderide LA Long Acting Capsules 2734
Isoptin Injectable (Rare) 1344
Kerlone Tablets 2436
Levatol 2403
Lopressor HCT Tablets 832
MS Contin Tablets (Less frequent) 1994
MSIR (Infrequent) 1997
NebuPent for Inhalation Solution (1% or less) 1040
Normodyne Tablets 2379
Oramorph SR (Morphine Sulfate Sustained Release Tablets) (Less frequent) 2236
Orthoclone OKT3 Sterile Solution 1837
Reglan 2068
Sectral Capsules 2807
Serevent Inhalation Aerosol (Rare) 1176
Sublimaze Injection 1307
▲ Suprane (3%-50%) 1813
Tenoretic Tablets 2845
Tenormin Tablets and I.V. Injection 2847
Tensilon Injectable 1261
Tessalon Perles 1020
Timolide Tablets 1748
Timoptic in Ocudose 1753
Timoptic Sterile Ophthalmic Solution 1751
Timoptic-XE 1755
Toprol-XL Tablets 565
Tracrium Injection 1183
Trandate Tablets 1185
Valium Injectable 2182
VePesid Capsules and Injection (Sometimes) 718
Versed Injection (Less than 1.0%) 2170
Visken Tablets 2299
Zebeta Tablets 1413
Ziac 1415

Lassitude
Atrohist Pediatric Capsules 453
Atrohist Plus Tablets 454
Azmacort Oral Inhaler 2011
Azo Gantrisin Tablets 2081
Beconase 1076
Bromfed 1785
▲ Cartrol Tablets (7.1%) 410
Codiclear DH Syrup 791
Daranide Tablets 1633
Dexedrine 2474
Esimil Tablets 822
Felbatol 2666
▲ Hytrin Capsules (7.4% to 11.3%) 430
Inderal 2728
Inderal LA Long Acting Capsules 2730
Inderide Tablets 2732
Inderide LA Long Acting Capsules 2734
Ismelin Tablets 827
▲ Mykrox Tablets (4.4%) 993
Nasacort Nasal Inhaler 2024
Neurontin Capsules (Rare) 1922

(▣ Described in PDR For Nonprescription Drugs) Incidence data in parenthesis; ▲ 3% or more (⊙ Described in PDR For Ophthalmology)

1349 **Side Effects Index** **Leukocytosis**

Parlodel (Less than 1%) 2281
Phenergan Injection 2773
Phenergan Tablets 2775
Plaquenil Sulfate Tablets 2328
Protamine Sulfate Ampoules & Vials 1471
▲ Reglan (Approximately 10%) 2068
Risperdal 1301
Temaril Tablets, Syrup and Spansule Extended-Release Capsules 483
Tonocard Tablets (0.8-1.6%) 531
Triavil Tablets 1757

Laughing, easy

▲ Marinol (Dronabinol) Capsules (8% to 24%) 2231

Laxative effect

Beelith Tablets 639
CharcoAid ▣ 768
Derifil Tablets 2246
Mag-Ox 400 668
Phillips' Milk of Magnesia Liquid ▣ 729
Uro-Mag 668

Left ventricular dysfunction

Orthoclone OKT3 Sterile Solution 1837
Rubex (Uncommon) 712

Left ventricular ejection fraction, asymptomatic declines in

Idamycin 1955

Left ventricular ejection fraction, change

Novantrone 1279

Leg cramps, nocturnal

Prostin E2 Suppository 2634

Legs, heaviness

Rum-K Syrup 1005
SSKI Solution (Less frequent) 2658
Uroqid-Acid No. 2 Tablets 640

Legs, restless

Ambien Tablets (Infrequent) 2416

Legs, stiffness

Gastrocrom Capsules (Infrequent) 984

Legs, weakness

Gastrocrom Capsules (Infrequent) 984

Lens, pigmentation

Triavil Tablets 1757

Lens opacities, changes

Etrafon 2355
Floropryl Sterile Ophthalmic Ointment 1662
Floxin I.V. 1571
Humorsol Sterile Ophthalmic Solution 1664
Isopto Carpine Ophthalmic Solution ⊙ 223
Lescol Capsules 2267
Mevacor Tablets 1699
Pilocar ⊙ 268
Pilopine HS Ophthalmic Gel ⊙ 226
Pravachol 765
Temaril Tablets, Syrup and Spansule Extended-Release Capsules 483
Zocor Tablets 1775

Lens opacities, irregular

Floxin Tablets (200 mg, 300 mg, 400 mg) 1567
Lysodren (Infrequent) 698
Mellaril 2269
Serentil 684
Thorazine 2523
Torecan 2245

Lenticular deposits

Compazine 2470
Etrafon 2355
Levoprome 1274
Prolixin 509
Ridaura Capsules (Less than 1%) 2513
Stelazine 2514
Thorazine 2523
Trilafon 2389

Leriche's syndrome

Sansert Tablets 2295

Lesions, anogenital

Achromycin V Capsules (Rare) 1367
Declomycin Tablets 1371
Dynacin Capsules 1590
Minocin Intravenous 1382
Minocin Oral Suspension 1385
Minocin Pellet-Filled Capsules 1383
Monodox Capsules 1805
Vibramycin 1941

Lesions, cardiac

Amicar Syrup, Tablets, and Injection (One case) 1267

Lesions, corneal

Effexor (Infrequent) 2719

Lesions, cutaneous

Duranest Injections 542
Dyclone 0.5% and 1% Topical Solutions, USP 544
Lupron Depot 7.5 mg 2559
Novocain Hydrochloride for Spinal Anesthesia 2326
Pontocaine Hydrochloride for Spinal Anesthesia 2330
Quadrinal Tablets 1350
▲ Tonocard Tablets (0.4-12.2%) 531
Xylocaine Injections (Extremely rare) 567
Zestril Tablets (0.3% to 1.0%) 2854

Lesions, erythema perstans-like

AquaMEPHYTON Injection 1608

Lesions, esophageal

Cataflam (Less than 1%) 816
Voltaren Tablets (Less than 1%) 861

Lesions, follicular-pustular

Topicort Emollient Cream 0.25% 1243

Lesions, gastrointestinal

K-Dur Microburst Release System (potassium chloride, USP) E.R. Tablets 1325
K-Norm Extended-Release Capsules 991
K-Tab Filmtab 434
Micro-K 2063
Micro-K LS Packets 2064
Slow-K Extended-Release Tablets 851

Lesions, hepatic

Amicar Syrup, Tablets, and Injection (One case) 1267

Lesions, neuro-ocular

Cycrin Tablets 975
Micronor Tablets 1872
Modicon 1872
Ortho-Novum 1872
Premphase 2797
Prempro 2801
Provera Tablets 2636

Lesions, rectal mucosal

Testoderm Testosterone Transdermal System (One in 104 patients) 486

Lesions, retinal vascular

Amen Tablets 780
Brevicon 2088
Cycrin Tablets 975
Demulen 2428
Depo-Provera Contraceptive Injection 2602
Depo-Provera Sterile Aqueous Suspension 2606
Levlen/Tri-Levlen 651
Micronor Tablets 1872
Modicon 1872
Norinyl 2088
Nor-Q D Tablets 2135
Ortho-Cyclen/Ortho-Tri-Cyclen 1858
Ortho-Novum 1872
Ortho-Cyclen/Ortho Tri-Cyclen 1858
Premphase 2797
Prempro 2801
Provera Tablets 2636
Levlen/Tri-Levlen 651
Tri-Norinyl 2164

Lesions, sceloderma-like

AquaMEPHYTON Injection 1608

Lesions, spinal column, posterior

Azulfidine (Rare) 1949

Lesions, stenotic

K-Norm Extended-Release Capsules 991

Lethargy

Accutane Capsules 2076
▲ ActHIB (17.0% to 18.6%) 872
Aldactazide 2413
Aldactone 2414
▲ Ambien Tablets (3%) 2416
Anexsia 5/500 Elixir 1781
Anexia Tablets 1782
Apresazide Capsules 808
Aquasol A Vitamin A Capsules, USP 534
Aquasol A Parenteral 534
Asacol Delayed-Release Tablets 1979
Atgam Sterile Solution (Less than 5%) 2581
Bentyl 1501
Betagan (Rare) ⊙ 233
Betoptic Ophthalmic Solution (Rare) 469
Betoptic S Ophthalmic Suspension (Rare) 471
Capozide 742
Cataflam 816
Catapres-TTS (3 of 101 patients) 675
CeeNU 693
Cipro I.V. (1% or less) 595
Cipro I.V. Pharmacy Bulk Package (Less than 1%) 597
Cipro Tablets (Less than 1%) 592
Clozaril Tablets (1%) 2252
Cosmegen Injection 1626
Dalmane Capsules 2173
Demadex Tablets and Injection 686
Depakene 413
Depakote Tablets 415
Dilaudid Ampules 1335
Dilaudid Cough Syrup 1336
Dilaudid 1335
Dipentum Capsules (1.8%) 1951
Diupres Tablets 1650
Diuril Sodium Intravenous 1652
Dyazide 2479
DynaCirc Capsules (0.5% to 1%) 2256
Eldepryl Tablets (1 of 49 patients) 2550
▲ Emcyt Capsules (4%) 1953
Ergamisol Tablets 1292
Esidrix Tablets 821
Eskalith 2485
Etrafon 2355
Fioricet with Codeine Capsules (Infrequent) 2260
Sterile FUDR 2118
Ganite 2533
Garamycin Injectable 2360
Gastrocrom Capsules (Infrequent) 984
Haldol Decanoate 1577
Haldol Injection, Tablets and Concentrate 1575
Hycodan Tablets and Syrup 930
Hycomine Compound Tablets 932
Hycomine 931
Hycotuss Expectorant Syrup 933
Hydrocet Capsules 782
Hydropres Tablets 1675
Hyperstat I.V. Injection 2363
Inderal 2728
Inderal LA Long Acting Capsules 2730
Inderide Tablets 2732
ISMOTIC 45% w/v Solution (Very rare) ⊙ 222
Kerlone Tablets (2.8%) 2436
Lasix Injection, Oral Solution and Tablets 1240
▲ Leucovorin Calcium for Injection (2% to 13%) 1268
Limbitrol 2180
Lioresal Intrathecal (Up to 4 of 214 patients) 1596
Lithium Carbonate Capsules & Tablets 2230
Lithonate/Lithotabs/Lithobid 2543
Lomotil 2439
▲ Lopressor HCT Tablets (10 in 100 patients) 832
Lorcet 10/650 1018
Lortab 2566
▲ Lozol Tablets (Greater than or equal to 5%) 2022
Lupron Depot 7.5 mg 2559
Lupron Injection (Less than 5%) 2555
▲ Lysodren (25%) 698
Matulane Capsules 2131
Maxzide 1380
Mellaril (Extremely rare) 2269
Milontin Kapseals 1920
Mithracin 607
Mononine, Coagulation Factor IX (Human) 523
▲ Mykrox Tablets (4.4%) 993
Nebcin Vials, Hyporets & ADD-Vantage 1464
Neoral (Rare) 2276
▲ OmniHIB (17.0% to 18.6%) 2499
Oretic Tablets 443
Orthoclone OKT3 Sterile Solution 1837
Parlodel 2281
Phenobarbital Elixir and Tablets 1469
Prinzide Tablets 1737
Proleukin for Injection 797
Prolixin 509
Prostin VR Pediatric Sterile Solution (Less than 1%) 2635
▲ Restoril Capsules (5%) 2284
ReVia Tablets 940
▲ RhoGAM $Rh_0(D)$ Immune Globulin (Human) (25% in one study) 1847
Roferon-A Injection (Less than 0.5%) 2145
Sandimmune (Rare) 2286
Serax Capsules 2810
Serax Tablets 2810
Solganal Suspension (Rare) 2388
▲ Stadol (3% to 9%) 775
Supprelin Injection (1% to 3%) 2056
▲ Tegison Capsules (1-10%) 2154
Tenoretic Tablets (1% to 3%) 2845
Tenormin Tablets and I.V. Injection (1% to 3%) 2847
Thalitone (Common) 1245
Tobramycin Sulfate Injection 968
Tonocard Tablets (0.8-1.6%) 531
Trilafon 2389
Trilisate (Less than 2%) 2000
Tussend 1783
Tussionex Pennkinetic Extended-Release Suspension 998
Vaseretic Tablets 1765
▲ Verelan Capsules (3.2%) 1410
▲ Verelan Capsules (3.2%) 2824
Versed Injection (Less than 1.0%) 2170
Vicodin Tablets 1356
Vicodin ES Tablets 1357
Vicodin Tuss Expectorant 1358
▲ Videx Tablets, Powder for Oral Solution, & Pediatric Powder for Oral Solution (4% to 7%) 720
Visken Tablets (2% or fewer patients) 2299
Voltaren Tablets 861
WinRho SD (One report) 2576
Zarontin Capsules 1928
Zarontin Syrup 1929
Zaroxolyn Tablets 1000
Zestoretic 2850
▲ Zoladex (8%) 2858
Zovirax Sterile Powder (Approximately 1%) 1223
Zydone Capsules 949

Leucoencephalopathy

Fungizone Intravenous 506
Methotrexate Sodium Tablets, Injection, for Injection and LPF Injection 1275

Leukemia, acute

BiCNU 691
CeeNU 693
Leukeran Tablets 1133
Platinol (Rare) 708
Platinol-AQ Injection (Rare) 710
VePesid Capsules and Injection (Rare) 718

Leukemia, lymphoblastic

Permax Tablets (Rare) 575

Leukemia, lymphocytic

Betaseron for SC Injection 658
Clomid 1514
Mustargen 1709

Leukemia, unspecified

Cytovene-IV (Two or more reports) 2103
Depen Titratable Tablets 2662
Felbatol 2666
Genotropin (A small number) 111
Humatrope Vials (Small number) 1443
Indocin (Rare) 1680
Nutropin (A small number of patients) 1061
Protropin (A small number) 1063
Trental Tablets (Rare) 1244

Leukemoid reaction

Anafranil Capsules (Rare) 803
Netromycin Injection 100 mg/ml (Fewer than 1 in 1000 patients) 2373

Leukocytosis

▲ Adriamycin PFS (High incidence) 1947
▲ Adriamycin RDF (High incidence) 1947

(▣ Described in PDR For Nonprescription Drugs) Incidence data in parenthesis; ▲ 3% or more (⊙ Described in PDR For Ophthalmology)

Leukocytosis — Side Effects Index — 1350

Atretol Tablets ... 573
Azactam for Injection (Less than 1%) ... 734
Capastat Sulfate Vials ... 2868
▲ CellCept Capsules (7.1% to 10.9%) ... 2099
Cipro I.V. (Rare) ... 595
Cipro I.V. Pharmacy Bulk Package (Rare) ... 597
Cipro Tablets (Less than 0.1%) ... 592
Clinoril Tablets (Less than 1 in 100) ... 1618
Clomid ... 1514
Clozaril Tablets (Less than 1%) ... 2252
Cuprimine Capsules ... 1630
Danocrine Capsules ... 2307
Depen Titratable Tablets ... 2662
Desyrel and Desyrel Dividose ... 503
Diprivan Injection (Less than 1%) ... 2833
Effexor (Infrequent) ... 2719
▲ Efudex (Among most frequent) ... 2113
Eskalith ... 2485
Felbatol (Infrequent) ... 2666
Floxin I.V. (More than or equal to 1%) ... 1571
Floxin Tablets (200 mg, 300 mg, 400 mg) (More than or equal to 1.0%) ... 1567
Foscavir Injection (Less than 1%) ... 547
Fungizone Intravenous ... 506
Haldol Decanoate ... 1577
Haldol Injection, Tablets and Concentrate ... 1575
INFeD (Iron Dextran Injection, USP) ... 2345
Kerlone Tablets (Less than 2%) ... 2436
Lamictal Tablets (Infrequent) ... 1112
Lariam Tablets (Occasional) ... 2128
Lithium Carbonate Capsules & Tablets ... 2230
Lithonate/Lithotabs/Lithobid ... 2543
Luvox Tablets (Infrequent) ... 2544
Mesantoin Tablets ... 2272
Moban Tablets and Concentrate ... 1048
Monopril Tablets ... 757
Navane Capsules and Concentrate (Occasional) ... 2201
Navane Intramuscular ... 2202
Nebcin Vials, Hyporets & ADD-Vantage ... 1464
Neupogen for Injection (Approximately 2%) ... 495
Orthoclone OKT3 Sterile Solution ... 1837
Panhematin ... 443
▲ PASER Granules (79% of 38 patients with drug-induced hepatitis) ... 1285
Paxil Tablets (Rare) ... 2505
Penetrex Tablets (Less than 1%) ... 2031
Permax Tablets (Infrequent) ... 575
Prilosec Delayed-Release Capsules (Rare) ... 529
Primaxin I.V. ... 1729
Prinivil Tablets (0.3% to 1.0%) ... 1733
Prinzide Tablets ... 1737
▲ Prograf (8% to 32%) ... 1042
Prolastin Alpha$_1$-Proteinase Inhibitor (Human) ... 635
▲ Proleukin for Injection (9%) ... 797
Prolixin ... 509
Quinidex Extentabs ... 2067
ReoPro Vials (1.0%) ... 1471
Risperdal (Rare) ... 1301
Rocephin Injectable Vials, ADD-Vantage, Galaxy Container (Rare) ... 2142
Suprane ... 1813
Tao Capsules ... 2209
▲ Tegison Capsules (10-25%) ... 2154
Tegretol Chewable Tablets ... 852
Tegretol Suspension ... 852
Tegretol Tablets ... 852
Tobramycin Sulfate Injection ... 968
Torecan ... 2245
▲ Trasylol (3%) ... 613
Vantin for Oral Suspension and Vantin Tablets ... 2646
Vaseretic Tablets ... 1765
Vasotec I.V. ... 1768
Vasotec Tablets (0.5% to 1.0%) ... 1771
Wellbutrin Tablets ... 1204
Zefazone ... 2654
Zestoretic ... 2850
Zestril Tablets (0.3% to 1.0%) ... 2854
Zovirax Sterile Powder (Less than 1%) ... 1223
Zyloprim Tablets (Less than 1%) ... 1226

Leukocyturia

Amikacin Sulfate Injection, USP ... 960
Amikin Injectable ... 501
Primaxin I.M. ... 1727
Primaxin I.V. ... 1729
Sinemet CR Tablets (1% or greater) ... 944

Leukoderma

Betaseron for SC Injection ... 658
Effexor (Rare) ... 2719
Lamictal Tablets (Rare) ... 1112
Ultravate Cream 0.05% (Less frequent) ... 2689
Ultravate Ointment 0.05% ... 2690

Leukonychia

Desyrel and Desyrel Dividose ... 503

Leukopenia

▲ Accutane Capsules (1 in 5 to 1 in 10 patients) ... 2076
Adalat Capsules (10 mg and 20 mg) (Less than 0.5%) ... 587
Adalat CC (Rare) ... 589
Adriamycin PFS (High incidence) ... 1947
Adriamycin RDF ... 1947
Aldactazide ... 2413
Aldoclor Tablets ... 1598
Aldomet Ester HCl Injection ... 1602
Aldomet Oral ... 1600
Aldoril Tablets ... 1604
Alkeran Tablets ... 1071
Altace Capsules (Scattered incidents) ... 1232
Ambien Tablets (Rare) ... 2416
Amoxil ... 2464
Anaprox/Naprosyn (Less than 1%) ... 2117
Ancef Injection ... 2465
Ancobon Capsules ... 2079
Ansaid Tablets (Less than 1%) ... 2579
Anturane (Rare) ... 807
Apresazide Capsules (Less frequent) ... 808
Apresoline Hydrochloride Tablets (Less frequent) ... 809
Aquasol A Vitamin A Capsules, USP ... 534
Aredia for Injection (Up to 4%) ... 810
Asacol Delayed-Release Tablets ... 1979
Asendin Tablets (Less than 1%) ... 1369
Atamet (Rare) ... 572
▲ Atgam Sterile Solution (1 in 7 patients; 14%) ... 2581
Atretol Tablets ... 573
Atrohist Plus Tablets ... 454
Atromid-S Capsules ... 2701
Augmentin ... 2468
Azo Gantanol Tablets ... 2080
Azo Gantrisin Tablets ... 2081
Azulfidine (Rare) ... 1949
BCG Vaccine, USP (TICE) (0.3%) ... 1814
Bactrim DS Tablets ... 2084
Bactrim I.V. Infusion ... 2082
Bactrim ... 2084
Benemid Tablets ... 1611
Betapace Tablets (Rare) ... 641
Bicillin C-R Injection ... 2704
Bicillin C-R 900/300 Injection ... 2706
Bicillin L-A Injection (Infrequent) ... 2707
BiCNU ... 691
BuSpar (Rare) ... 737
Capastat Sulfate Vials ... 2868
Capozide ... 742
Cardizem CD Capsules (Infrequent) ... 1506
Cardizem SR Capsules (Infrequent) ... 1510
Cardizem Injectable ... 1508
Cardizem Tablets (Infrequent) ... 1512
Cardura Tablets ... 2186
Cataflam (Less than 1%) ... 816
Ceclor Pulvules & Suspension ... 1431
CeeNU ... 693
Cefizox for Intramuscular or Intravenous Use (Rare) ... 1034
Cefotan ... 2829
Ceftin ... 1078
Cefzil Tablets and Oral Suspension (0.2%) ... 746
▲ CellCept Capsules (23.2% to 34.5%; 11.5% to 16.3%) ... 2099
Celontin Kapseals ... 1899
Ceptaz (Very rare) ... 1081
Chibroxin Sterile Ophthalmic Solution (With oral form) ... 1617
Chloromycetin Sodium Succinate ... 1900
Cipro I.V. (Infrequent) ... 595
▲ Cipro I.V. Pharmacy Bulk Package (Among most frequent) ... 597
Cipro Tablets (0.4%) ... 592
Claforan Sterile and Injection (Less than 1%) ... 1235
Cleocin Phosphate Injection ... 2586
Cleocin Vaginal Cream ... 2589
Clinoril Tablets (Less than 1%) ... 1618
▲ Clozaril Tablets (3%) ... 2252
Cognex Capsules (Rare) ... 1901
ColBENEMID Tablets ... 1622
Combipres Tablets ... 677
Comhist ... 2038
Compazine ... 2470
Cosmegen Injection ... 1626
Cuprimine Capsules (2%) ... 1630
Cytadren Tablets (Rare) ... 819
▲ Cytosar-U Sterile Powder (Among most frequent) ... 2592
▲ Cytovene (29%) ... 2103
Cytoxan (Less frequent to common) ... 694
Dalmane Capsules (Rare) ... 2173
Danocrine Capsules ... 2307
Dantrium Capsules (Less frequent) ... 1982
Dantrium Intravenous ... 1983
Daranide Tablets ... 1633
Daraprim Tablets ... 1090
Daypro Caplets (Less than 1%) ... 2426
Depakene ... 413
Depakote Tablets ... 415
▲ Depen Titratable Tablets (2%; up to 5%) ... 2662
DiaBeta Tablets ... 1239
Diabinese Tablets ... 1935
Diamox ... 1372
Didronel Tablets (One report) ... 1984
Diflucan Injection, Tablets, and Oral Suspension ... 2194
Dilantin Infatabs (Occasional) ... 1908
Dilantin Kapseals (Occasional) ... 1906
Dilantin Parenteral (Occasional) ... 1910
Dilantin-125 Suspension (Occasional) ... 1911
Dipentum Capsules (Rare) ... 1951
Diucardin Tablets ... 2718
Diupres Tablets ... 1650
Diuril Oral Suspension ... 1653
Diuril Sodium Intravenous ... 1652
Diuril Tablets ... 1653
Dolobid Tablets (Less than 1 in 100) ... 1654
Doxorubicin Astra ... 540
Dyazide ... 2479
DynaCirc Capsules (0.5% to 1%) ... 2256
Easprin ... 1914
EC-Naprosyn Delayed-Release Tablets (Less than 1%) ... 2117
Effexor (Infrequent) ... 2719
Elavil ... 2838
Elspar ... 1659
▲ Emcyt Capsules (4%) ... 1953
Endep Tablets ... 2174
Enduron Tablets ... 420
▲ Ergamisol Tablets (Less than 1% to 33%) ... 1292
Esidrix Tablets ... 821
Esimil Tablets (A few instances) ... 822
Etrafon ... 2355
▲ Eulexin Capsules (3%) ... 2358
Fansidar Tablets ... 2114
▲ Felbatol (6.5%; infrequent) ... 2666
Feldene Capsules (Greater than 1%) ... 1965
Flagyl I.V. ... 2247
Flexeril Tablets (Rare) ... 1661
Floxin I.V. (More than or equal to 1%) ... 1571
Floxin Tablets (200 mg, 300 mg, 400 mg) (More than or equal to 1%) ... 1567
Fluorouracil Injection ... 2116
Fortaz (Very rare) ... 1100
▲ Foscavir Injection (5% or greater) ... 547
▲ Sterile FUDR (Among more common) ... 2118
Fulvicin P/G Tablets (Rare) ... 2359
Fulvicin P/G 165 & 330 Tablets (Rare) ... 2359
Fungizone Intravenous ... 506
Ganite ... 2533
Gantanol Tablets ... 2119
Gantrisin ... 2120
Garamycin Injectable ... 2360
Geocillin Tablets ... 2199
Glauctabs ... ⊙ 208
Glucotrol Tablets ... 1967
Glucotrol XL Extended Release Tablets ... 1968
Glynase PresTab Tablets ... 2609
Grifulvin V (griseofulvin tablets) Microsize (griseofulvin oral suspension) Microsize (Rare) ... 1888
Gris-PEG Tablets, 125 mg & 250 mg (Rare) ... 479
Haldol Decanoate ... 1577
Haldol Injection, Tablets and Concentrate ... 1575
▲ Hexalen Capsules (1% to 15%) ... 2571
Hivid Tablets (Less than 1% to less than 3%) ... 2121
▲ Hydrea Capsules (Most common) ... 696
HydroDIURIL Tablets ... 1674
Hydropres Tablets ... 1675
Hyperstat I.V. Injection ... 2363
Hyzaar Tablets ... 1677
IFEX ... 697
▲ Imuran (28% to more than 50%) ... 1110
Inderide Tablets ... 2732
Inderide LA Long Acting Capsules ... 2734
Indocin Capsules (Less than 1%) ... 1680
Indocin I.V. (Less than 1%) ... 1684
Indocin (Less than 1%) ... 1680
▲ Intron A (Less than 5% to 68%) ... 2364
Ismelin Tablets ... 827
Keftab Tablets ... 915
Kefurox Vials, Faspak & ADD-Vantage (1 in 750) ... 1454
Kefzol Vials, Faspak & ADD-Vantage ... 1456
Klonopin Tablets ... 2126
▲ Kytril Tablets (11%) ... 2492
Lamictal Tablets (Infrequent) ... 1112
▲ Lariam Tablets (Among most frequent) ... 2128
Larodopa Tablets ... 2129
Lasix Injection, Oral Solution and Tablets ... 1240
Lescol Capsules (Rare) ... 2267
▲ Leucovorin Calcium for Injection (14% to 93%) ... 1268
Levoprome ... 1274
Lincocin ... 2617
Lodine Capsules and Tablets (Less than 1%) ... 2743
Loniten Tablets (Rare) ... 2618
Lopid Tablets (Rare to occasional) ... 1917
Lopressor HCT Tablets ... 832
Lorabid Suspension and Pulvules ... 1459
Lotensin Tablets (Scattered incidents) ... 834
Lotensin HCT ... 837
Loxitane (Rare) ... 1378
Lozol Tablets ... 2022
Lupron Depot 7.5 mg ... 2559
Lupron Injection ... 2555
Luvox Tablets (Rare) ... 2544
MZM (Common) ... ⊙ 267
Macrobid Capsules ... 1988
Macrodantin Capsules ... 1989
▲ Matulane Capsules (Frequent) ... 2131
Maxaquin Tablets (Less than or equal to 0.1%) ... 2440
Maxzide ... 1380
Mefoxin ... 1691
Mefoxin Premixed Intravenous Solution ... 1694
Mellaril (Infrequent; increased risk in aged) ... 2269
Mepergan Injection (Very rare) ... 2753
▲ Mepron Suspension (4%) ... 1135
Mesantoin Tablets ... 2272
Metastron ... 1594
▲ Methotrexate Sodium Tablets, Injection, for Injection and LPF Injection (Among most frequent; 1 to 3%) ... 1275
Mevacor Tablets (Rare) ... 1699
Mexitil Capsules (About 1 in 1,000) ... 678
Mezlin ... 601
Mezlin Pharmacy Bulk Package ... 604
Micronase Tablets ... 2623
Milontin Kapseals ... 1920
Miltown Tablets ... 2672
Minizide Capsules ... 1938
Mintezol ... 1704
▲ Mithracin (6%) ... 607
Moban Tablets and Concentrate ... 1048
Moduretic Tablets ... 1705
Monocid Injection (Less than 1%) ... 2497
Monopril Tablets ... 757
Mutamycin ... 703
▲ Mycobutin Capsules (17%) ... 1957
Mykrox Tablets ... 993
Myleran Tablets ... 1143
Anaprox/Naprosyn (Less than 1%) ... 2117
Nardil (Less frequent) ... 1920
Navane Capsules and Concentrate (Occasional) ... 2201
Navane Intramuscular (Occasional) ... 2202
▲ Navelbine Injection (12% to 81%) ... 1145
Nebcin Vials, Hyporets & ADD-Vantage ... 1464
NegGram (Rare) ... 2323
▲ Neoral (Up to 6%) ... 2276

(▣ Described in PDR For Nonprescription Drugs) Incidence data in parenthesis; ▲ 3% or more (⊙ Described in PDR For Ophthalmology)

1351 Side Effects Index Libido, decrease

NEOSAR Lyophilized/Neosar (Less frequent to common) 1959
Neptazane Tablets 1388
Netromycin Injection 100 mg/ml (Fewer than 1 in 1000 patients) 2373
Neurontin Capsules (1.1%) 1922
Nizoral Tablets (Less than 1%) 1298
Nolvadex Tablets (0.4%) 2841
Noroxin Tablets (1.4%) 1715
Noroxin Tablets (1.4%) 2048
Omnipen Capsules 2764
Omnipen for Oral Suspension 2765
▲Oncaspar (Greater than 1% but less than 5%) 2028
Oncovin Solution Vials & Hyporets 1466
Oretic Tablets 443
Ornade Spansule Capsules 2502
Orthoclone OKT3 Sterile Solution 1837
PBZ Tablets 845
PBZ-SR Tablets 844
PMB 200 and PMB 400 2783
▲Paraplatin for Injection (26% to 98%) 705
Parnate Tablets 2503
PASER Granules 1285
Paxil Tablets (Infrequent) 2505
Pen•Vee K (Infrequent) 2772
Penetrex Tablets (Less than 1%) 2031
▲Pentam 300 Injection (2.8 to 7.5%) 1041
Pepcid Injection (Rare) 1722
Pepcid (Rare) 1720
Periactin 1724
Permax Tablets (Infrequent) 575
Pfizerpen for Injection (Rare) 2203
Phenergan with Codeine (Rare) 2777
Phenergan with Dextromethorphan (Rare) 2778
Phenergan Injection 2773
Phenergan Suppositories (Rare) 2775
Phenergan Syrup (Rare) 2774
Phenergan Tablets (Rare) 2775
Phenergan VC (Rare) 2779
Phenergan VC with Codeine (Rare) 2781
Phenurone Tablets (2%) 447
Pipracil 1390
Plaquenil Sulfate Tablets 2328
Platinol 708
Platinol-AQ Injection 710
Podocon-25 1891
Ponstel (Occasional) 1925
Pravachol (Rare) 765
Primaxin I.M. 1727
Primaxin I.V. (Less than 0.2%) 1729
Prinzide Tablets 1737
Priscoline Hydrochloride Ampuls 845
Procan SR Tablets (0.5%) 1926
Procardia Capsules (Less than 0.5%) 1971
▲Prograf (Greater than 3%) 1042
▲Proleukin for Injection (34%) 797
Prolixin 509
Proloprim Tablets 1155
Propulsid (Rare) 1300
ProSom Tablets (Rare) 449
Protostat Tablets 1883
Prozac Pulvules & Liquid, Oral Solution (Rare) 919
Purinethol Tablets (Frequent) 1156
Reglan (A few cases) 2068
Relafen Tablets (Less than 1%) 2510
Ridaura Capsules 2513
Rifadin 1528
Rifamate Capsules 1530
Rifater (Rare) 1532
Rimactane Capsules (Rare) 847
Risperdal (Rare) 1301
Ritalin 848
Rocephin Injectable Vials, ADD-Vantage, Galaxy Container (2.1%) 2142
▲Roferon-A Injection (49%) 2145
Rythmol Tablets–150mg, 225mg, 300mg (Less than 1%) 1352
▲SSD (About 20%) 1355
Salagen Tablets (Less than 1%) 1489
▲Sandimmune (Up to 6%) 2286
Septra 1174
Septra I.V. Infusion 1169
Septra I.V. Infusion ADD-Vantage Vials 1171
Septra 1174
Ser-Ap-Es Tablets 849
Serax Capsules (Rare) 2810
Serax Tablets (Rare) 2810
Serentil 684
Serzone Tablets (Infrequent) 771
Silvadene Cream 1% (Several cases) 1540
Sinemet Tablets (Rare) 943
Sinemet CR Tablets 944
Sinequan (Occasional) 2205
Skelaxin Tablets 788
Solganal Suspension (Rare) 2388
Soma Compound w/Codeine Tablets (Very rare) 2676
Soma Compound Tablets (Very rare) 2675
Soma Tablets 2674
Spectrobid Tablets 2206
Stelazine 2514
Suprax (Less than 2%) 1399
Symmetrel Capsules and Syrup (Less than 0.1%) 946
Tagamet (Approximately 1 per 100,000) 2516
Tambocor Tablets (Less than 1%) 1497
Tapazole Tablets 1477
▲Taxol (17% to 90%) 714
Tazicef for Injection (Very rare) 2519
▲Tegison Capsules (10-25%) 2154
Tegretol Chewable Tablets 852
Tegretol Suspension 852
Tegretol Tablets 852
Temaril Tablets, Syrup and Spansule Extended-Release Capsules 483
Tenoretic Tablets 2845
Thalitone 1245
▲TheraCys BCG Live (Intravesical) (Up to 5.4%) 897
Thioguanine Tablets, Tabloid Brand 1181
Thioplex (Thiotepa For Injection) 1281
Thorazine 2523
Ticar for Injection 2526
Timentin for Injection 2528
Timolide Tablets 1748
Tobramycin Sulfate Injection 968
Tonocard Tablets (Less than 1%) 531
Toradol 2159
Torecan 2245
Trental Tablets (Less than 1%) 1244
Triavil Tablets 1757
Trilafon 2389
Trimpex Tablets 2163
Unasyn 2212
Urispas Tablets (1 case) 2532
Vantin for Oral Suspension and Vantin Tablets 2646
Vascor (200, 300 and 400 mg) Tablets (2 cases) 1587
Vaseretic Tablets 1765
▲Velban Vials (Among most common) 1484
▲VePesid Capsules and Injection (3% to 91%) 718
▲Videx Tablets, Powder for Oral Solution, & Pediatric Powder for Oral Solution (10% to 16%) 720
Vivactil Tablets 1774
Voltaren Tablets (Less than 1%) 861
▲Vumon (89%) 727
Wellbutrin Tablets 1204
Yutopar Intravenous Injection 570
Zanosar Sterile Powder 2653
Zantac (A few patients) 1209
Zantac Injection (Few patients) 1207
Zantac Syrup (A few patients) 1209
Zarontin Capsules 1928
Zarontin Syrup 1929
Zaroxolyn Tablets 1000
Zefazone 2654
Zerit Capsules (Up to 1%) 729
Zestoretic (Rare) 2850
Zestril Tablets (Rare) 2854
Zinacef (1 in 750 patients) 1211
Zinecard 1961
Zithromax (Less than 1%) 1944
Zocor Tablets (Rare) 1775
Zosyn 1419
Zosyn Pharmacy Bulk Package 1422
Zovirax Capsules 1219
Zovirax Sterile Powder 1223
Zovirax 1219
Zyloprim Tablets (Less than 1%) 1226

Leukopenia, transient

Rifater 1532

Leukoplakia, oral

Betaseron for SC Injection 658
Foscavir Injection (Less than 1%) 547
Intron A (Less than 5%) 2364
Videx Tablets, Powder for Oral Solution, & Pediatric Powder for Oral Solution (Less than 1%) 720

Leukorrhea

Anafranil Capsules (Up to 2%) 803
Betaseron for SC Injection 658
▲Depo-Provera Contraceptive Injection (1% to 5%) 2602
Effexor (Infrequent) 2719
Intron A (Less than 5%) 2364
Lippes Loop Intrauterine Double-S 1848
Lodine Capsules and Tablets (Less than 1%) 2743
Maxaquin Tablets (Less than 1%) 2440
Neurontin Capsules (Rare) 1922
▲Norplant System (5% or greater) 2759
ParaGard T380A Intrauterine Copper Contraceptive 1880
Permax Tablets (Rare) 575
Prozac Pulvules & Liquid, Oral Solution (Infrequent) 919
Risperdal (Infrequent) 1301
▲Supprelin Injection (6% to 12%) 2056
Zoloft Tablets (Rare) 2217
Zosyn (1.0% or less) 1419
Zosyn Pharmacy Bulk Package (1.0% or less) 1422

Lhermitte's sign

Platinol 708
Platinol-AQ Injection 710

Libido, changes

Adipex-P Tablets and Capsules 1048
Amen Tablets 780
▲Anafranil Capsules (Up to 21%) 803
▲Android Capsules, 10 mg (Among most common) 1250
Asendin Tablets (Less than 1%) 1369
Biphetamine Capsules 983
Brevicon 2088
Climara Transdermal System 645
Cycrin Tablets 975
Danocrine Capsules 2307
Delatestryl Injection 2860
Demulen 2428
Depo-Provera Sterile Aqueous Suspension 2606
Desogen Tablets 1817
Desoxyn Gradumet Tablets 419
Dexedrine 2474
DextroStat Dextroamphetamine Tablets 2036
Didrex Tablets 2607
Diethylstilbestrol Tablets 1437
Dizac (Less frequent) 1809
Doral Tablets 2664
Elavil 2838
Endep Tablets 2174
Estrace Cream and Tablets 749
Estraderm Transdermal System 824
ESTRATAB Tablets (0.3, 0.625, 1.25, 2.5 mg) 2536
Estratest 2539
Etrafon 2355
Fastin Capsules 2488
Flexeril Tablets (Rare) 1661
Halcion Tablets 2611
Halotestin Tablets 2614
Ionamin Capsules 990
Levlen/Tri-Levlen 651
Librax Capsules (Rare) 2176
Libritabs Tablets (Isolated cases) 2177
Librium Capsules (Isolated cases) 2178
Librium Injectable (Isolated cases) 2179
Limbitrol 2180
Lo/Ovral Tablets 2746
Lo/Ovral-28 Tablets 2751
Mellaril 2269
Menest Tablets 2494
Micronor Tablets 1872
Modicon 1872
Neurontin Capsules (Infrequent) 1922
Nordette-21 Tablets 2755
Nordette-28 Tablets 2758
Norinyl 2088
Nor-Q D Tablets 2135
Ogen Tablets 2627
Ogen Vaginal Cream 2630
Oreton Methyl 1255
Ortho-Cept 1851
Ortho-Cyclen/Ortho-Tri-Cyclen 1858
Ortho Dienestrol Cream 1866
Ortho-Est 1869
Ortho-Novum 1872
Ortho-Cyclen/Ortho Tri-Cyclen 1858
Orudis Capsules (Rare) 2766
Oruvail Capsules (Rare) 2766
Ovcon 760
Ovral Tablets 2770
Ovral-28 Tablets 2770
Ovrette Tablets 2771
Oxandrin 2862
PMB 200 and PMB 400 2783
Pondimin Tablets 2066
Prelu-2 Timed Release Capsules 681
Premarin Intravenous 2787
Premarin with Methyltestosterone 2794
Premarin Tablets 2789
Premarin Vaginal Cream 2791
Premphase 2797
Prempro 2801
Provera Tablets 2636
Sanorex Tablets (Rare) 2294
Serax Capsules 2810
Serax Tablets 2810
Serentil 684
Sinequan 2205
Stilphostrol Tablets and Ampuls 612
▲Supprelin Injection (3% to 10%) 2056
Torecan 2245
Triavil Tablets 1757
Trilafon 2389
Levlen/Tri-Levlen 651
Tri-Norinyl 2164
Triphasil-21 Tablets 2814
Triphasil-28 Tablets 2819
Valium Injectable 2182
Valium Tablets (Infrequent) 2183
Valrelease Capsules (Occasional) 2169
Vivactil Tablets 1774
▲Xanax Tablets (7.1%) 2649

Libido, decrease

Adalat CC (Less than 1.0%) 589
Aldoclor Tablets 1598
Aldomet Ester HCl Injection 1602
Aldomet Oral 1600
Aldoril Tablets 1604
Ambien Tablets (Rare) 2416
Android 1251
Atromid-S Capsules 2701
Axid Pulvules 1427
Betaseron for SC Injection 658
Blocadren Tablets (0.6%) 1614
Bontril Slow-Release Capsules 781
BuSpar (Infrequent) 737
Cardura Tablets (0.8%) 2186
Claritin (2% or fewer patients) 2349
Claritin-D (Less frequent) 2350
Clozaril Tablets (Less than 1%) 2252
Cordarone Tablets (1 to 3%) 2712
Cozaar Tablets (Less than 1%) 1628
Cytotec (Infrequent) 2424
Cytovene (1% or less) 2103
▲Depo-Provera Contraceptive Injection (1% to 5%) 2602
Desyrel and Desyrel Dividose (Less than 1% to 1.3%) 503
Diupres Tablets 1650
DynaCirc Capsules (0.5% to 1%) 2256
▲Effexor (2% to 5.7%) 2719
Ethmozine Tablets (Less than 2%) 2041
Fioricet with Codeine Capsules 2260
Fiorinal with Codeine Capsules 2262
Flagyl 375 Capsules 2434
Glucotrol XL Extended Release Tablets (Less than 1%) 1968
Hydropres Tablets 1675
Hyperstat I.V. Injection 2363
Hytrin Capsules (0.6%) 430
Hyzaar Tablets 1677
Imdur (Less than or equal to 5%) 1323
Intron A (Up to 5%) 2364
Inversine Tablets 1686
IOPIDINE Sterile Ophthalmic Solution ◉ 219
Kerlone Tablets (Less than 2%) 2436
Lamictal Tablets (Rare) 1112
Lopid Tablets 1917
Lopressor 830
Lotensin Tablets 834
Lotensin HCT (0.3% to 1.0%) 837
Lotrel Capsules 840
Lozol Tablets (Less than 5%) 2022
Ludiomil Tablets (Rare) 843
Lupron Depot 3.75 mg (Less than 5%) 2556
Lupron Depot 7.5 mg (Less than 5%) 2559
Lupron Injection (Less than 5%) 2555
Luvox Tablets (2%) 2544
MS Contin Tablets (Less frequent) 1994
MSIR 1997
▲Megace Oral Suspension (Up to 5%) 699
Methadone Hydrochloride Oral Concentrate 2233
Methadone Hydrochloride Oral Solution & Tablets 2235
MetroGel-Vaginal 902
Mexitil Capsules (Less than 1% or about 4 in 1,000) 678
Midamor Tablets (Less than or equal to 1%) 1703
Moduretic Tablets 1705
Monopril Tablets (0.2% to 1.0%) 757
Norpramin Tablets 1526

(▣ Described in PDR For Nonprescription Drugs) Incidence data in parenthesis; ▲ 3% or more (◉ Described in PDR For Ophthalmology)

Libido, decrease Side Effects Index 1352

Oramorph SR (Morphine Sulfate Sustained Release Tablets) (Less frequent) ... 2236
Pamelor ... 2280
▲ Paxil Tablets (3.3%) ... 2505
Pepcid Injection (Infrequent) ... 1722
Pepcid (Infrequent) ... 1720
Permax Tablets (Infrequent) ... 575
Plendil Extended-Release Tablets (0.5% to 1.5%) ... 527
Pondimin Tablets ... 2066
PREVACID Delayed-Release Capsules (Less than 1%) ... 2562
Prinivil Tablets (0.4%) ... 1733
Prinzide Tablets (0.3% to 1%) ... 1737
Procardia XL Extended Release Tablets (1% or less) ... 1972
▲ Proscar Tablets (3.3%) ... 1741
ProSom Tablets (Rare) ... 449
Protostat Tablets ... 1883
▲ Prozac Pulvules & Liquid, Oral Solution (1.6% to 11%) ... 919
RMS Suppositories ... 2657
Rocaltrol Capsules ... 2141
Roxanol ... 2243
Sandostatin Injection (Less than 1%) ... 2292
Ser-Ap-Es Tablets ... 849
Serzone Tablets (1%) ... 771
Sporanox Capsules (0.2% to 1.2%) ... 1305
Surmontil Capsules ... 2811
Symmetrel Capsules and Syrup (0.1% to 1%) ... 946
▲ Synarel Nasal Solution for Endometriosis (22% of patients) ... 2152
Tambocor Tablets (Less than 1%) 1497
Temaril Tablets, Syrup and Spansule Extended-Release Capsules ... 483
Tenex Tablets (3% or less) ... 2074
Testoderm Testosterone Transdermal System ... 486
Testred Capsules ... 1262
Timolide Tablets (Less than 1%) ... 1748
Timoptic in Ocudose ... 1753
Timoptic Sterile Ophthalmic Solution ... 1751
Timoptic-XE ... 1755
Tofranil Ampuls ... 854
Tofranil Tablets ... 856
Tofranil-PM Capsules ... 857
Toprol-XL Tablets ... 565
Vaseretic Tablets (0.5% to 2.0%) 1765
Videx Tablets, Powder for Oral Solution, & Pediatric Powder for Oral Solution (Less than 1%) ... 720
▲ Wellbutrin Tablets (3.1%) ... 1204
Winstrol Tablets ... 2337
▲ Xanax Tablets (14.4%) ... 2649
Zantac Injection ... 1207
Zebeta Tablets ... 1413
Zestoretic (0.3 to 1%) ... 2850
Zestril Tablets (0.4%) ... 2854
▲ Zoladex (61%) ... 2858
Zyloprim Tablets (Less than 1%) ... 1226

Libido, increase

Android ... 1251
Bontril Slow-Release Capsules ... 781
BuSpar (Infrequent) ... 737
Clozaril Tablets (Less than 1%) ... 2252
Cognex Capsules (Infrequent) ... 1901
Depo-Provera Contraceptive Injection (Fewer than 1%) ... 2602
Desyrel and Desyrel Dividose ... 503
Effexor (Infrequent) ... 2719
Haldol Decanoate ... 1577
Haldol Injection, Tablets and Concentrate ... 1575
Klonopin Tablets ... 2126
Lamictal Tablets (Rare) ... 1112
Ludiomil Tablets (Rare) ... 843
Lupron Depot 3.75 mg ... 2556
Lupron Depot 7.5 mg ... 2559
Lupron Injection ... 2555
Luvox Tablets (Infrequent) ... 2544
Moban Tablets and Concentrate ... 1048
Norpramin Tablets ... 1526
Pamelor ... 2280
Paxil Tablets (Rare) ... 2505
Permax Tablets (Infrequent) ... 575
Pondimin Tablets ... 2066
Prolixin ... 509
Prozac Pulvules & Liquid, Oral Solution (Infrequent) ... 919
Questran Light ... 769
Questran Powder ... 770
Risperdal (Infrequent) ... 1301
Serzone Tablets (Infrequent) ... 771
Surmontil Capsules ... 2811
Synarel Nasal Solution for Endometriosis (1% of patients) ... 2152
Testoderm Testosterone Transdermal System ... 486
Testred Capsules ... 1262
Tofranil Ampuls ... 854
Tofranil Tablets ... 856
Tofranil-PM Capsules ... 857
Wellbutrin Tablets (Frequent) ... 1204
Winstrol Tablets ... 2337
▲ Xanax Tablets (7.7%) ... 2649
Zarontin Capsules (Rare) ... 1928
Zarontin Syrup (Rare) ... 1929
▲ Zoladex (12%) ... 2858

Libido, loss

Catapres Tablets (About 3 in 100 patients) ... 674
Catapres-TTS (Less freuqnt) ... 675
Combipres Tablets (About 3%) ... 677
▲ Eulexin Capsules (36% with LHRH agonist) ... 2358
Lescol Capsules ... 2267
Methotrexate Sodium Tablets, Injection, for Injection and LPF Injection ... 1275
Mevacor Tablets (0.5% to 1.0%) .. 1699
Nolvadex Tablets ... 2841
Orap Tablets ... 1050
Pravachol ... 765
Roferon-A Injection (Less than 1%) ... 2145
Vascor (200, 300 and 400 mg) Tablets (0.5 to 2.0%) ... 1587
Zantac (Occasional) ... 1209
Ziac (0.4%) ... 1415
Zocor Tablets ... 1775

Lichen planus

Aralen Hydrochloride Injection ... 2301
Aralen Phosphate Tablets ... 2301
Cuprimine Capsules ... 1630
Depen Titratable Tablets (Rare) ... 2662
Felbatol ... 2666
Minipress Capsules (Less than 1%) ... 1937
Minizide Capsules (Rare) ... 1938
Pentasa (Less than 1%) ... 1527
Trandate Tablets ... 1185
Zyloprim Tablets (Less than 1%) ... 1226

Lichen planus, bullous

Normodyne Tablets ... 2379
Trandate Tablets ... 1185

Light-headedness

Accupril Tablets ... 1893
▲ Adalat Capsules (10 mg and 20 mg) (About 10% to 27%) ... 587
Adenocard Injection (2%) ... 1021
▲ Adenoscan (12%) ... 1024
Aldoclor Tablets ... 1598
Aldomet Ester HCl Injection ... 1602
Aldomet Oral ... 1600
Altace Capsules ... 1232
Ambien Tablets (2%) ... 2416
Anaprox/Naprosyn (Less than 3%) ... 2117
▲ Anexsia 5/500 Elixir (Among most frequent) ... 1781
Atgam Sterile Solution (Less than 5%) ... 2581
▲ Beconase AQ Nasal Spray (Fewer than 5 per 100 patients) ... 1076
▲ Bentyl (11%) ... 1501
▲ Betapace Tablets (4% to 12%) ... 641
Brevibloc Injection (Less than 1%) 1808
Brontex ... 1981
▲ BuSpar (3%) ... 737
Capoten ... 739
▲ Cardura Tablets (Up to 23%) ... 2186
Ceredase ... 1065
Chibroxin Sterile Ophthalmic Solution (With oral form) ... 1617
Cipro I.V. (1% or less) ... 595
Cipro I.V. Pharmacy Bulk Package (Less than 1%) ... 597
Cipro Tablets (Less than 1%) ... 592
Clomid (Fewer than 1%) ... 1514
Colestid Tablets (Infrequent) ... 2591
Cutivate Ointment (Less than 1%) 1089
▲ DHCplus Capsules (Among most frequent) ... 1993
Dalmane Capsules ... 2173
Dantrium Capsules (Less frequent) 1982
Dantrium Intravenous ... 1983
Daraprim Tablets (Rare) ... 1090
Darvon-N/Darvocet-N ... 1433
Darvon ... 1435
Darvon-N Suspension & Tablets ... 1433
Decadron Phosphate Turbinaire ... 1645
Deconamine ... 1320
Deconsal C Expectorant Syrup ... 456
Deconsal Pediatric Syrup ... 457
▲ Demerol (Among most frequently observed) ... 2308
Deponit NTG Transdermal Delivery System (Occasional; 4%) ... 2397
▲ Desyrel and Desyrel Dividose (19.7% to 28.0%) ... 503
Dexacort Phosphate in Turbinaire .. 459
▲ Dilaudid-HP Injection (Among most frequent) ... 1337
▲ Dilaudid-HP Lyophilized Powder 250 mg (Among most frequent) ... 1337
Dilaudid Tablets and Liquid ... 1339
Dolobid Tablets (Less than 1 in 100) ... 1654
Duranest Injections ... 542
Duvoid ... 2044
Dyclone 0.5% and 1% Topical Solutions, USP ... 544
Dynacin Capsules ... 1590
EC-Naprosyn Delayed-Release Tablets (Less than 3%) ... 2117
▲ Eldepryl Tablets (7 of 49 patients) 2550
Emla Cream ... 545
▲ Empirin with Codeine Tablets (Among most frequent) ... 1093
Entex PSE Tablets ... 1987
▲ Esgic-plus Tablets (Among most frequent) ... 1013
Factrel (Rare) ... 2877
▲ Fioricet Tablets (Among most frequent) ... 2258
Fioricet with Codeine Capsules (Frequent) ... 2260
Fiorinal Capsules (Less frequent) ... 2261
Fiorinal with Codeine Capsules (2.6%) ... 2262
Fiorinal Tablets (Less frequent) ... 2261
Floxin I.V. ... 1571
Floxin Tablets (200 mg, 300 mg, 400 mg) ... 1567
Gammagard S/D, Immune Globulin, Intravenous (Human) (Occasional) ... 585
Gastrocrom Capsules (Infrequent) .. 984
Guaimax-D Tablets ... 792
▲ Halcion Tablets (4.9%) ... 2611
Hydrocet Capsules ... 782
Hyperstat I.V. Injection ... 2363
▲ Hytrin Capsules (28%) ... 430
Hyzaar Tablets ... 1677
Inderal ... 2728
Inderal LA Long Acting Capsules ... 2730
Inderide Tablets ... 2732
Inderide LA Long Acting Capsules .. 2734
Indocin (Less than 1%) ... 1680
Inversine Tablets ... 1686
Ismo Tablets ... 2738
ISMOTIC 45% w/v Solution (Very rare) ... ⊚ 222
Isordil Sublingual Tablets ... 2739
Isordil Tembids ... 2741
Isordil Titradose Tablets ... 2742
Kemadrin Tablets ... 1112
▲ Lioresal Intrathecal (6 to 12 of 214 patients) ... 1596
▲ Lorcet 10/650 (Among most frequent) ... 1018
▲ Lortab (Among most frequent) ... 2566
Lotensin HCT ... 837
Loxitane ... 1378
Lozol Tablets (Less than 5%) ... 2022
Lupron Depot 7.5 mg ... 2559
▲ Lupron Injection (5% or more) ... 2555
▲ MS Contin Tablets (Among most frequent) ... 1994
▲ MSIR (Among most frequent) ... 1997
Marcaine Spinal ... 2319
Maxaquin Tablets ... 2440
▲ Mepergan Injection (Among most frequent) ... 2753
▲ Methadone Hydrochloride Oral Concentrate (Among most frequent) ... 2233
Methadone Hydrochloride Oral Solution & Tablets ... 2235
▲ Mexitil Capsules (10.5 to 26.4%) .. 678
Minocin Intravenous ... 1382
Minocin Oral Suspension ... 1385
Minocin Pellet-Filled Capsules ... 1383
Monoket ... 2406
Monopril Tablets ... 757
Motofen Tablets (1 in 20) ... 784
▲ Mykrox Tablets (10.2%) ... 993
Anaprox/Naprosyn (Less than 3%) ... 2117
Navane Capsules and Concentrate 2201
Navane Intramuscular ... 2202
Nicorette ... 2458
Nimotop Capsules (Less than 1%) 610
Nitro-Bid IV ... 1523
Nitro-Bid Ointment ... 1524
▲ Nitrodisc (6%) ... 2047
Nitro-Dur (nitroglycerin) Transdermal Infusion System (Occasional) ... 1326
Nolvadex Tablets (Infrequent) ... 2841
Norflex ... 1496
Norgesic ... 1496
Noroxin Tablets ... 1715
Noroxin Tablets ... 2048
Nucofed ... 2051
Numorphan Injection ... 936
Numorphan Suppositories ... 937
▲ Oramorph SR (Morphine Sulfate Sustained Release Tablets) (Among most frequent) ... 2236
Paraflex Caplets (Occasional) ... 1580
Parafon Forte DSC Caplets (Occasional) ... 1581
▲ Parlodel (Less than 1% to 5%) ... 2281
Peptavlon ... 2878
▲ Percocet Tablets (Among most frequent) ... 938
▲ Percodan Tablets (Among most frequent) ... 939
▲ Percodan-Demi Tablets (Among most frequent) ... 940
Phenergan with Codeine ... 2777
Phenergan VC with Codeine ... 2781
▲ Phrenilin (Among most frequent) ... 785
Prinivil Tablets ... 1733
Prinzide Tablets ... 1737
Procan SR Tablets (Infrequent) ... 1926
▲ Procardia Capsules (Approximately 10% to 27%; 1 in 8 patients) ... 1971
▲ Procardia XL Extended Release Tablets (27%; 1 in 8 patients) ... 1972
Prolastin Alpha$_1$-Proteinase Inhibitor (Human) (0.19%) ... 635
Provocholine for Inhalation (1 occurrence) ... 2140
Prozac Pulvules & Liquid, Oral Solution (1.6%) ... 919
Quadrinal Tablets ... 1350
Quinidex Extentabs ... 2067
▲ RMS Suppositories (Among most frequent) ... 2657
Recombivax HB (Less than 1%) ... 1744
Robaxin Injectable ... 2070
Robaxin Tablets ... 2071
▲ Robaxisal Tablets (One in 20-25) .. 2071
▲ Rogaine Topical Solution (3.42%) .. 2637
▲ Roxanol (Among most frequent) ... 2243
▲ Roxicodone Tablets, Oral Solution & Intensol (Oxycodone) (Among most frequent) ... 2244
Sansert Tablets ... 2295
▲ Sedapap Tablets 50 mg/650 mg (Among the most frequent) ... 1543
Sensorcaine ... 559
Serophene (clomiphene citrate tablets, USP) (Less than 1 in 100 patients) ... 2451
▲ Serzone Tablets (10%) ... 771
Sorbitrate ... 2843
▲ Symmetrel Capsules and Syrup (5% to 10%) ... 946
Talacen ... 2333
▲ Talwin Injection (Most common) ... 2334
Talwin Compound ... 2335
▲ Talwin Injection (Most common) ... 2334
Talwin Nx ... 2336
Tambocor Tablets ... 1497
Tenoretic Tablets (1% to 3%) ... 2845
Tenormin Tablets and I.V. Injection (1% to 3%) ... 2847
▲ THROMBATE III Antithrombin III (Human) (1 of 17) ... 637
THYREL TRH ... 2873
▲ Tornalate Solution for Inhalation, 0.2% (6.8%) ... 956
▲ Tornalate Metered Dose Inhaler (3%) ... 957
Trandate ... 1185
▲ Transderm-Nitro Transdermal Therapeutic System (6%) ... 859
Trilisate (Less than 2%) ... 2000
Tussend ... 1783
Tussi-Organidin NR Liquid and S NR Liquid (At higher doses) ... 2677
▲ Tylenol with Codeine (Among most frequent) ... 1583
▲ Tylox Capsules (Among most frequent) ... 1584
Urecholine ... 1761
Vancenase AQ Nasal Spray 0.042% (Fewer than 5 per 100 patients) ... 2393

(▣ Described in PDR For Nonprescription Drugs) Incidence data in parenthesis; ▲ 3% or more (⊚ Described in PDR For Ophthalmology)

Vaseretic Tablets ... 1765
Vasotec Tablets ... 1771
Ventolin Inhalation Aerosol and Refill (1%) ... 1197
Ventolin Rotacaps for Inhalation (Less than 1%) ... 1200
Versed Injection (Less than 1%) ... 2170
▲ Vicodin Tablets (Among most frequent) ... 1356
▲ Vicodin ES Tablets (Among most frequent) ... 1357
Wygesic Tablets ... 2827
▲ Xanax Tablets (20.8% to 29.8%) .. 2649
▲ Xylocaine Injections (Among most common) ... 567
Zaroxolyn Tablets ... 1000
Zestoretic ... 2850
Zestril Tablets ... 2854
Zovirax Sterile Powder (Less than 1%) ... 1223
▲ Zydone Capsules (Among most frequent) ... 949

Limb reduction defects

Accupril Tablets ... 1893
Altace Capsules ... 1232
Capoten ... 739
Capozide ... 742
Cozaar Tablets ... 1628
Diethylstilbestrol Tablets ... 1437
Elavil ... 2838
Estraderm Transdermal System ... 824
ESTRATAB Tablets (0.3, 0.625, 1.25, 2.5 mg) (Less than 1 per 1,000) ... 2536
Hyzaar Tablets ... 1677
Lo/Ovral Tablets ... 2746
Lo/Ovral-28 Tablets ... 2751
Lotensin Tablets ... 834
Lotensin HCT ... 837
Lotrel Capsules ... 840
Metubine Iodide Vials ... 916
Monopril Tablets ... 757
Nordette-21 Tablets ... 2755
Nordette-28 Tablets ... 2758
Ovral Tablets ... 2770
Ovral-28 Tablets ... 2770
Ovrette Tablets ... 2771
Prinivil Tablets ... 1733
Prinzide Tablets ... 1737
Proventil Inhalation Aerosol ... 2382
Proventil Inhalation Solution 0.083% ... 2384
Proventil Repetabs Tablets ... 2386
Proventil Syrup ... 2385
Univasc Tablets ... 2410
Vaseretic Tablets ... 1765
Vasotec I.V. ... 1768
Vasotec Tablets ... 1771
Ventolin Inhalation Aerosol and Refill ... 1197
Ventolin Inhalation Solution (Rare) .. 1198
Ventolin Nebules Inhalation Solution (Rare) ... 1199
Ventolin Rotacaps for Inhalation ... 1200
Ventolin Syrup ... 1202
Ventolin Tablets ... 1203
Zestoretic ... 2850
Zestril Tablets ... 2854

Lipodystrophy

Genotropin (Infrequent) ... 111
Humulin 50/50, 100 Units (Rare) 1444
Humulin 70/30, 100 Units (Rare) 1445
Humulin L, 100 Units (Rare) ... 1446
Regular, 100 Units (Rare) ... 1450
Pork Regular, 100 Units (Rare) ... 1452

Lipoma

Cognex Capsules (Infrequent) ... 1901

Lipoprotein levels, changes

▲ Accutane Capsules (About 16%) 2076
Atretol Tablets ... 573
Danocrine Capsules ... 2307
Demulen ... 2428
Humegon (Occasional) ... 1824
Levlen/Tri-Levlen ... 651
Lupron Depot 3.75 mg (2%) ... 2556
Nor-Q D Tablets ... 2135
Synarel Nasal Solution for Endometriosis ... 2152
Tegretol Chewable Tablets (Occasional) ... 852
Tegretol Suspension (Occasional) .. 852
Tegretol Tablets (Occasional) ... 852
Timolide Tablets ... 1748
Levlen/Tri-Levlen ... 651
Triphasil-21 Tablets ... 2814
Winstrol Tablets ... 2337
Zoladex ... 2858

Lipoproteins, electrophoretic abnormalities

Sandimmune ... 2286

Lipotrophy

Humulin 50/50, 100 Units (Rare) 1444
Humulin 70/30, 100 Units (Rare) 1445
Humulin L, 100 Units (Rare) ... 1446
Regular, 100 Units (Rare) ... 1450
Pork Regular, 100 Units (Rare) ... 1452

Lips, enlargement

Dilantin Infatabs ... 1908
Dilantin Kapseals ... 1906
Dilantin Parenteral ... 1910
Dilantin-125 Suspension ... 1911
Eskalith ... 2485

Lips, dry (see under Xerochilia)

Lips, swelling

Altace Capsules ... 1232
Cataflam (Less than 1%) ... 816
Fluvirin ... 460
Lithonate/Lithotabs/Lithobid ... 2543
Phenobarbital Elixir and Tablets ... 1469
Proscar Tablets ... 1741
Quadrinal Tablets ... 1350
Tambocor Tablets (Less than 1%) 1497
Voltaren Tablets (less than 1%) ... 861

Listlessness

Atgam Sterile Solution (Less than 5%) ... 2581
Indocin (Greater than 1%) ... 1680
Polycitra Syrup ... 578
Polycitra-K Crystals ... 579
Polycitra-K Oral Solution ... 579
Polycitra-LC ... 578
Rum-K Syrup ... 1005

Livedo reticularis

Activase ... 1058
Felbatol ... 2666
Symmetrel Capsules and Syrup (1% to 5%) ... 946

Liver abnormalities

Cardene Capsules (Rare) ... 2095
Catapres Tablets (About 1 in 100 patients) ... 674
Clozaril Tablets (1%) ... 2252
Combipres Tablets ... 677
Compazine (A few observations) 2470
Cytadren Tablets (Rare) ... 819
Lamprene Capsules (Less than 1%) ... 828
Methotrexate Sodium Tablets, Injection, for Injection and LPF Injection ... 1275
Nolvadex Tablets (Rare) ... 2841
Oncaspar (Less than 1%) ... 2028
Pepcid Injection (Infrequent) ... 1722
Pepcid (Infrequent) ... 1720
Pravachol ... 765
Relafen Tablets (1%) ... 2510
ReVia Tablets ... 940
Ridaura Capsules (1 to 3%) ... 2513
Sectral Capsules ... 2807
▲ Videx Tablets, Powder for Oral Solution, & Pediatric Powder for Oral Solution (13% to 38%) ... 720
Zocor Tablets ... 1775

Liver abscess

Cytosar-U Sterile Powder (With experimental doses) ... 2592

Liver damage

Atretol Tablets ... 573
Butisol Sodium Elixir & Tablets (Less than 1 in 100) ... 2660
Compazine ... 2470
Cytosar-U Sterile Powder ... 2592
Dilantin Infatabs ... 1908
Dilantin Kapseals ... 1906
Dilantin Parenteral ... 1910
Dilantin-125 Suspension ... 1911
Etrafon ... 2355
Hivid Tablets (Less than 1% to less than 3%) ... 2121
Lasix Injection, Oral Solution and Tablets ... 1240
▲ Leukine for IV Infusion (13%) ... 1271
Mebaral Tablets (Less than 1 in 100) ... 2322
Mintezol ... 1704
Nardil (Very few patients) ... 1920
Nembutal Sodium Capsules ... 436
Nembutal Sodium Solution ... 438
Nembutal Sodium Suppositories (Less than 1%) ... 440
Nydrazid Injection (Occasional) ... 508
Phenobarbital Elixir and Tablets (Less than 1 in 100 patients) ... 1469
▲ Prograf (Greater than 3%) ... 1042
Prolixin ... 509
Rifater (Occasional instances) ... 1532
Risperdal (Rare) ... 1301
Seconal Sodium Pulvules (Less than 1 in 100) ... 1474
Stelazine ... 2514
Tegretol Chewable Tablets ... 852
Tegretol Suspension ... 852
Tegretol Tablets ... 852
Trasylol (0.5%) ... 613
Triavil Tablets ... 1757
Trilafon ... 2389
Unisom With Pain Relief-Nighttime Sleep Aid and Pain Reliever ... 1934
Wellbutrin Tablets (Infrequent) ... 1204

Liver disorders

Aldoclor Tablets ... 1598
Aldomet Oral ... 1600
Aldoril Tablets ... 1604
Cosmegen Injection ... 1626
Intal Inhaler (Rare) ... 988
Lo/Ovral Tablets ... 2746
Lo/Ovral-28 Tablets ... 2751
Ludiomil Tablets (Rare) ... 843
Ovral Tablets ... 2770
Ovral-28 Tablets ... 2770
Ovrette Tablets ... 2771
Prozac Pulvules & Liquid, Oral Solution (Rare) ... 919
Pulmozyme Inhalation ... 1064
Triphasil-21 Tablets ... 2814
Triphasil-28 Tablets ... 2819

Liver dysfunction (see under Hepatic dysfunction)

Liver function, changes

Aldoclor Tablets ... 1598
Aldomet Ester HCl Injection ... 1602
Aldomet Oral ... 1600
Aldoril Tablets ... 1604
▲ Android Capsules, 10 mg (Among most common) ... 1250
Asendin Tablets (Less than 1%) ... 1369
Atretol Tablets ... 573
Aygestin Tablets ... 974
Blocadren Tablets ... 1614
Capoten ... 739
▲ Cataflam (3% to 9%) ... 816
Cefobid Intravenous/Intramuscular (1 patient in 1285) ... 2189
Clinoril Tablets (Less than 1 in 100) ... 1618
Cosmegen Injection ... 1626
Dantrium Capsules ... 1982
Depakene (Occasional) ... 413
Depakote Tablets (Occasional) ... 415
DiaBeta Tablets (Isolated cases) ... 1239
Dolobid Tablets (Less than 1 in 100) ... 1654
Emcyt Capsules ... 1953
Endep Tablets ... 2174
EryPed Drops and Chewable Tablets ... 421
Erythromycin Base Filmtab ... 426
Erythromycin Delayed-Release Capsules, USP ... 427
ESTRATAB Tablets (0.3, 0.625, 1.25, 2.5 mg) ... 2536
Estratest ... 2539
Feldene Capsules (Less than 1%) .. 1965
Ilotycin Gluceptate, IV, Vials ... 913
▲ Methotrexate Sodium Tablets, Injection, for Injection and LPF Injection (15%) ... 1275
Mevacor Tablets ... 1699
Micronor Tablets ... 1872
Minipress Capsules (Less than 1%) ... 1937
Minizide Capsules (Rare) ... 1938
Mithracin ... 607
Moban Tablets and Concentrate (Rare) ... 1048
Modicon ... 1872
Nicolar Tablets ... 2026
Nicorette ... 2458
Normodyne Injection (Less common) ... 2377
Ortho-Novum ... 1872
Oxandrin ... 2862
▲ Pentam 300 Injection (8.7%) ... 1041
Pipracil (Less than 2%) ... 1390
▲ Prograf (5% to 36%) ... 1042
Prolixin ... 509
Reglan (Rare) ... 2068
Surmontil Capsules ... 2811
Tegretol Chewable Tablets ... 852
Tegretol Suspension ... 852
Tegretol Tablets ... 852
Timolide Tablets ... 1748
Tonocard Tablets (Less than 1%) .. 531
Toradol ... 2159
Tornalate Solution for Inhalation, 0.2% (One patient) ... 956
▲ Voltaren Tablets (3% to 9%) ... 861
Winstrol Tablets ... 2337
Zestril Tablets (Rare) ... 2854
Zovirax Capsules ... 1219
Zovirax Sterile Powder ... 1223
Zovirax ... 1219

Liver function, impaired

Accupril Tablets (Rare) ... 1893
Actimmune (Rare) ... 1056
Children's Advil Suspension (Less than 1%) ... 2692
Aldoclor Tablets ... 1598
Aldomet Ester HCl Injection ... 1602
Aldomet Oral ... 1600
Aldoril Tablets ... 1604
Amen Tablets ... 780
Android ... 1251
Atgam Sterile Solution (Less than 5%) ... 2581
Atretol Tablets ... 573
Atromid-S Capsules ... 2701
Capastat Sulfate Vials ... 2868
Catapres Tablets ... 674
Catapres-TTS (Less frequent) ... 675
▲ CellCept Capsules (More than or equal to 3%) ... 2099
Claritin-D (Less frequent) ... 2350
Cleocin Phosphate Injection ... 2586
Cleocin Vaginal Cream ... 2589
▲ Cordarone Intravenous (3.4%) ... 2715
▲ Cordarone Tablets (4 to 9%) ... 2712
Cycrin Tablets ... 975
DTIC-Dome (Few reports) ... 600
▲ Daypro Caplets (Up to 15%) ... 2426
Delatestryl Injection ... 2860
Demulen ... 2428
Depo-Provera Sterile Aqueous Suspension ... 2606
Desyrel and Desyrel Dividose ... 503
Diflucan Injection, Tablets, and Oral Suspension ... 2194
Diprivan Injection (Less than 1%) .. 2833
DynaCirc Capsules (0.5% to 1%) .. 2256
E.E.S. ... 424
Edecrin (Rare) ... 1657
Elavil ... 2838
Engerix-B Unit-Dose Vials ... 2482
ERYC ... 1915
EryPed 200 & EryPed 400 Granules ... 421
Ery-Tab Tablets ... 422
Erythrocin Stearate Filmtab ... 425
Estrace Cream and Tablets ... 749
Ethmozine Tablets (Rare) ... 2041
Etrafon (Rare) ... 2355
Eulexin Capsules ... 2358
▲ Feldene Capsules (Up to 15%) ... 1965
Flexeril Tablets (Less than 1%) ... 1661
Floxin Tablets (200 mg, 300 mg, 400 mg) ... 1567
Gastrocrom Capsules (Infrequent) .. 984
Glynase PresTab Tablets ... 2609
Haldol Decanoate ... 1577
Haldol Injection, Tablets and Concentrate ... 1575
Halotestin Tablets ... 2614
▲ Hivid Tablets (Less than 1% to 8.9%) ... 2121
▲ IBU Tablets (Less than 1% up to 15%) ... 1342
Idamycin (No more than 1%) ... 1955
Imitrex Injection (Infrequent) ... 1103
Imitrex Tablets ... 1106
Intron A (Less than 5%) ... 2364
Konakion Injection ... 2127
Lamictal Tablets (Infrequent) ... 1112
Lincocin (A few instances) ... 2617
Lopid Tablets (Occasional) ... 1917
Mevacor Tablets ... 1699
Mexitil Capsules (About 5 in 1,000) ... 678
Micronase Tablets ... 2623
Midamor Tablets (Rare) ... 1703
Moduretic Tablets ... 1705
Children's Motrin Ibuprofen Oral Suspension (Less than 1%) ... 1546
Motrin Tablets (Less than 1%) ... 2625
Motrin Ibuprofen Suspension, Oral Drops, Chewable Tablets, Caplets (Less than 1%) ... 1546

(▣ Described in PDR For Nonprescription Drugs) Incidence data in parenthesis; ▲ 3% or more (◉ Described in PDR For Ophthalmology)

Liver function, impaired — Side Effects Index — 1354

Myambutol Tablets 1386
Mycelex Troches 608
Nicobid 2026
Nicolar Tablets 2026
Nimotop Capsules (Up to 1.2%) 610
Normodyne Tablets (Less common) 2379
Norpramin Tablets 1526
▲Oncaspar (Greater than 1% but less than 5%) 2028
Oreton Methyl 1255
Orlamm (Low frequency) 2239
▲Orudis Capsules (Greater than 3%) 2766
▲Oruvail Capsules (Greater than 3%) 2766
PCE Dispertab Tablets 444
Pamelor 2280
Paxil Tablets (Infrequent) 2505
Permax Tablets (Infrequent) 575
Premarin with Methyltestosterone 2794
Premarin Vaginal Cream 2791
Provera Tablets 2636
Prozac Pulvules & Liquid, Oral Solution (Infrequent) 919
Questran Light 769
Questran Powder 770
▲Relafen Tablets (Up to 15%) 2510
Rifadin (Rare) 1528
Rifamate Capsules 1530
Rifater (Rare) 1532
Rimactane Capsules (Rare) 847
Serzone Tablets (Infrequent) 771
Slo-Niacin Tablets 2659
Tegretol Chewable Tablets 852
Tegretol Suspension 852
Tegretol Tablets 852
Testoderm Testosterone Transdermal System 486
Thioguanine Tablets, Tabloid Brand (Occasional) 1181
Ticlid Tablets (1.0%) 2156
Tofranil Ampuls 854
Tofranil Tablets 856
Tofranil-PM Capsules 857
Trandate (Less common) 1185
Tranxene 451
▲Trasylol (5%) 613
Triavil Tablets (Rare) 1757
Vascor (200, 300 and 400 mg) Tablets (0.5 to 2.0%) 1587
Vivactil Tablets 1774
Wygesic Tablets 2827
Yutopar Intravenous Injection (Less than 1%) 570

Liver injury

Cordarone Tablets (Common) 2712
Eulexin Capsules 2358
ReVia Tablets 940
Trandate Tablets (Rare) 1185

Liver tumors (see under Hepatomas)

Liver, degenerative changes in

Lescol Capsules 2267
Phenobarbital Elixir and Tablets 1469

Loffler's syndrome

PASER Granules 1285

Loss of balance (see under Balance, loss of)

Lower spinal segments deficit

Duranest Injections (Rare) 542

Lumbago

Prinivil Tablets (0.3% to 1.0%) 1733
Prinzide Tablets 1737
Zestoretic 2850
Zestril Tablets (0.3% to 1.0%) 2854

Lung, carcinoma

Betaseron for SC Injection 658
Cognex Capsules (Rare) 1901
Paxil Tablets (Rare) 2505
Permax Tablets (Rare) 575
Prinivil Tablets (0.3% to 1.0%) 1733

Lung consolidation

Survanta Beractant Intratracheal Suspension 2226

Lung development, hypoplastic

Accupril Tablets 1893
Altace Capsules 1232
Capoten 739
Capozide 742
Clomid 1514
Cozaar Tablets 1628
Hyzaar Tablets 1677
Lotensin Tablets 834
Lotensin HCT 837
Lotrel Capsules 840
Monopril Tablets 757
Prinivil Tablets 1733
Prinzide Tablets 1737
Univasc Tablets 2410
Vaseretic Tablets 1765
Vasotec I.V. 1768
Vasotec Tablets 1771
Zestoretic 2850
Zestril Tablets 2854

Lung disorders, unspecified

Cartrol Tablets 410
▲CellCept Capsules (More than or equal to 3%) 2099
▲Leukine for IV Infusion (20%) 1271
Megace Oral Suspension (1% to 3%) 699
▲Prograf (Greater than 3%) 1042
Pulmozyme Inhalation 1064
▲Trasylol (7%) 613
Videx Tablets, Powder for Oral Solution, & Pediatric Powder for Oral Solution (Less than 1%) 720

Lung neoplasms, malignant

Prinzide Tablets 1737
Zestoretic 2850
Zestril Tablets (0.3% to 1.0%) 2854

Lupus erythematosus

Aldoclor Tablets 1598
Aldomet Ester HCl Injection 1602
Aldomet Oral 1600
Aldoril Tablets 1604
Anafranil Capsules (Rare) 803
Azo Gantanol Tablets 2080
Dapsone Tablets USP 1284
Depakene 413
Depakote Tablets 415
Dilantin Infatabs 1908
Dilantin Kapseals 1906
Dilantin Parenteral 1910
Dilantin-125 Suspension 1911
Fansidar Tablets 2114
Gris-PEG Tablets, 125 mg & 250 mg 479
Inderal (Rare) 2728
Inderal LA Long Acting Capsules (Rare) 2730
Inderide LA Long Acting Capsules (Rare) 2734
Peganone Tablets 446
Rythmol Tablets–150mg, 225mg, 300mg (Less than 1%) 1352
Tonocard Tablets (1.6%) 531

Lupus erythematosus, systemic

Achromycin V Capsules 1367
AK-CIDE (Some instances) ⊙ 202
AK-CIDE Ointment (Some instances) ⊙ 202
Atromid-S Capsules 2701
Azo Gantrisin Tablets 2081
Bactrim DS Tablets 2084
Bactrim I.V. Infusion 2082
Bactrim 2084
Celontin Kapseals 1899
Compazine 2470
Declomycin Tablets 1371
Dilantin Infatabs 1908
Dilantin Kapseals 1906
Dilantin Parenteral 1910
Dilantin-125 Suspension 1911
Etrafon 2355
Gantanol Tablets 2119
Gantrisin 2120
Inderal (Extremely rare) 2728
Inderal LA Long Acting Capsules (Extremely rare) 2730
Inderide Tablets (Extremely rare) 2732
Inderide LA Long Acting Capsules (Extremely rare) 2734
Mellaril 2269
Mexitil Capsules (About 4 in 10,000) 678
Milontin Kapseals 1920
Minocin Oral Suspension 1385
Monodox Capsules 1805
Normodyne Tablets (Less common) 2379
Norplant System (Rare) 2759
Procan SR Tablets 1926
Prolixin 509
Quinaglute Dura-Tabs Tablets 649
Quinidex Extentabs 2067
Sectral Capsules 2807
Septra 1174
Septra I.V. Infusion 1169
Septra I.V. Infusion ADD-Vantage Vials 1171
Septra 1174
Serentil 684
Stelazine 2514
Syprine Capsules 1747
Terramycin Intramuscular Solution 2210
Thorazine 2523
Timoptic in Ocudose (Less frequent) 1753
Timoptic Sterile Ophthalmic Solution (Less frequent) 1751
Timoptic-XE 1755
Trandate Tablets (Less common) 1185
Trilafon 2389
Vasosulf (One case) ⊙ 271
Vibramycin Hyclate Intravenous 2215
Zarontin Capsules 1928
Zarontin Syrup 1929

Lupus erythematosus, systemic, exacerbation or activation of

Apresazide Capsules 808
Atretol Tablets 573
Capozide 742
Doryx Capsules 1913
Dyazide 2479
Dynacin Capsules 1590
Esidrix Tablets 821
Fulvicin P/G Tablets 2359
Fulvicin P/G 165 & 330 Tablets 2359
Lasix Injection, Oral Solution and Tablets 1240
Maxzide 1380
Minocin Intravenous 1382
Minocin Pellet-Filled Capsules 1383
Prinzide Tablets 1737
Ser-Ap-Es Tablets 849
Tegretol Chewable Tablets 852
Tegretol Suspension 852
Tegretol Tablets 852
Tenoretic Tablets 2845
Thalitone 1245
Vaseretic Tablets 1765
Vibramycin 1941
Zaroxolyn Tablets 1000
Zestoretic 2850

Lupus erythematosus syndrome

Children's Advil Suspension (Less than 1%) 2692
Atretol Tablets (Isolated cases) 573
Azulfidine (Rare) 1949
Cuprimine Capsules 1630
Depen Titratable Tablets 2662
Felbatol 2666
Fulvicin P/G Tablets 2359
Fulvicin P/G 165 & 330 Tablets 2359
IBU Tablets (Less than 1%) 1342
Mesantoin Tablets 2272
Mexitil Capsules (About 4 in 10,000) 678
Children's Motrin Ibuprofen Oral Suspension (Less than 1%) 1546
Motrin Tablets (Less than 1%) 2625
Motrin Ibuprofen Suspension, Oral Drops, Chewable Tablets, Caplets (Less than 1%) 1546
Navane Capsules and Concentrate 2201
Navane Intramuscular 2202
Norpace (Some cases) 2444
Permax Tablets (Rare) 575
Prozac Pulvules & Liquid, Oral Solution (Rare) 919
Rifamate Capsules 1530
Roferon-A Injection (Rare; less than 3%) 2145
Tegretol Chewable Tablets (Isolated cases) 852
Tegretol Suspension (Isolated cases) 852
Tegretol Tablets (Isolated cases) 852
Temaril Tablets, Syrup and Spansule Extended-Release Capsules 483
Thorazine 2523

Lupus-like syndrome

Aldoclor Tablets 1598
Aldomet Ester HCl Injection 1602
Aldomet Oral 1600
Aldoril Tablets 1604
BCG Vaccine, USP (TICE) (Rare) 1814
Cuprimine Capsules 1630
Depen Titratable Tablets 2662
Elavil 2838
Endep Tablets 2174
Fulvicin P/G Tablets 2359
Fulvicin P/G 165 & 330 Tablets 2359
Gris-PEG Tablets, 125 mg & 250 mg 479
Lescol Capsules (Rare) 2267
Levlen/Tri-Levlen 651
Lopid Tablets 1917
Macrobid Capsules 1988
Macrodantin Capsules 1989
Mevacor Tablets (Rare) 1699
Minocin Intravenous 1382
Minocin Oral Suspension 1385
Minocin Pellet-Filled Capsules 1383
Nydrazid Injection 508
Pravachol (Rare) 765
Recombivax HB 1744
Rifater 1532
Sodium Sulamyd 2387
Tapazole Tablets 1477
Tenoretic Tablets 2845
Tenormin Tablets and I.V. Injection 2847
Tonocard Tablets (1.6%) 531
Levlen/Tri-Levlen 651
Zocor Tablets (Rare) 1775

Lyell's syndrome

Atretol Tablets 573
Azulfidine (Rare) 1949
Combipres Tablets 677
Daypro Caplets (Less than 1 %) 2426
Fulvicin P/G Tablets (Rare) 2359
Fulvicin P/G 165 & 330 Tablets (Rare) 2359
Motrin Ibuprofen Suspension, Oral Drops, Chewable Tablets, Caplets (Less than 1%) 1546
Proloprim Tablets (Rare) 1155
Rifater 1532
Tegretol Chewable Tablets (Extremely rare) 852
Tegretol Suspension (Extremely rare) 852
Tegretol Tablets (Extremely rare) 852
Tenoretic Tablets 2845
Thalitone 1245
Toradol 2159
Trimpex Tablets (Rare) 2163
Zyloprim Tablets (Less than 1%) 1226

Lymph nodes, tender

Atgam Sterile Solution (Less than 5%) 2581
ProSom Tablets (Rare) 449

Lymphadenopathy

Accutane Capsules (Less than 1%) 2076
Adalat CC (Less than 1.0%) 589
AeroBid Inhaler System (1-3%) 1005
Aerobid-M Inhaler System (1-3%) 1005
Ambien Tablets (Rare) 2416
Anafranil Capsules (Infrequent) 803
Ansaid Tablets (Less than 1%) 2579
Antivenin (Crotalidae) Polyvalent 2696
Apresazide Capsules (Less frequent) 808
Apresoline Hydrochloride Tablets (Less frequent) 809
Asacol Delayed-Release Tablets 1979
Atgam Sterile Solution (Less than 1% to less than 5%) 2581
Atretol Tablets 573
Attenuvax (Less common) 1610
BCG Vaccine, USP (TICE) (Occasional) 1814
▲Betaseron for SC Injection (14%) 658
Biavax II 1613
Cardura Tablets (Less than 0.5% of 3960 patients) 2186
Ceclor Pulvules & Suspension (Infrequent) 1431
Cipro Tablets (0.3% to 1%) 592
Claritin-D (Less frequent) 2350
Cognex Capsules (Infrequent) 1901
Cuprimine Capsules 1630
Depen Titratable Tablets 2662
Dilacor XR Extended-release Capsules (Infrequent) 2018
Dilantin Infatabs 1908
Dilantin Kapseals 1906
Dilantin Parenteral (A number of reports) 1910
Dilantin-125 Suspension 1911
Effexor (Infrequent) 2719
Engerix-B Unit-Dose Vials (Less than 1%) 2482
Felbatol (Infrequent) 2666
Foscavir Injection (Between 1% and 5%) 547
Havrix (Less than 1%; rare) 2489
Hivid Tablets (Less than 1% to less than 3%) 2121
Imitrex Tablets (Rare) 1106

(▣ Described in PDR For Nonprescription Drugs) Incidence data in parenthesis; ▲ 3% or more (⊙ Described in PDR For Ophthalmology)

1355 Side Effects Index Malaise

INFeD (Iron Dextran Injection, USP) 2345
Intron A (Less than 5%) 2364
Kerlone Tablets (Less than 2%) 2436
Klonopin Tablets 2126
Lamictal Tablets (Infrequent) 1112
Lamprene Capsules (Less than 1%) 828
▲Lupron Depot 3.75 mg (Among most frequent) 2556
Luvox Tablets (Infrequent) 2544
M-M-R II 1687
M-R-VAX II 1689
Maxaquin Tablets (Less than 1%) 2440
Meruvax II 1697
Mesantoin Tablets 2272
Miacalcin Nasal Spray (1% to 3%) 2275
Mintezol 1704
Monopril Tablets (0.2% to 1.0%) 757
MSTA Mumps Skin Test Antigen 890
Mumpsvax 1708
Nalfon 200 Pulvules & Nalfon Tablets (Less than 1%) 917
Neurontin Capsules (Infrequent) 1922
Nydrazid Injection 508
Orthoclone OKT3 Sterile Solution 1837
▲PASER Granules (46% of 38 patients with drug-induced hepatitis) 1285
Paxil Tablets (Infrequent) 2505
PedvaxHIB 1718
Peganone Tablets 446
Permax Tablets (Infrequent) 575
Proglycem 580
Prozac Pulvules & Liquid, Oral Solution (2%) 919
Quadrinal Tablets 1350
Quinaglute Dura-Tabs Tablets 649
Recombivax HB (Less than 1%) 1744
Retrovir Capsules 1158
Retrovir I.V. Infusion 1163
Retrovir Syrup 1158
Rifamate Capsules 1530
Rifater 1532
Risperdal (Rare) 1301
Rogaine Topical Solution (0.31%) 2637
Salagen Tablets (Less than 1%) 1489
Ser-Ap-Es Tablets 849
Serzone Tablets (Infrequent) 771
Tapazole Tablets 1477
Tegretol Chewable Tablets 852
Tegretol Suspension 852
Tegretol Tablets 852
Tolectin (200, 400 and 600 mg) (Less than 1%) 1581
Typhim Vi 899
Varivax (Greater than or equal to 1%) 1762
Wellbutrin Tablets (Rare) 1204
▲Zerit Capsules (Fewer than 1% to 5%) 729
Zoloft Tablets (Infrequent) 2217
Zovirax 1219
Zyloprim Tablets (Less than 1%) 1226

Lymphadenopathy, post-cervical
Atgam Sterile Solution (Less than 5%) 2581
Diphtheria and Tetanus Toxoids and Pertussis Vaccine Adsorbed 2477
Foscavir Injection (Less than 1%) 547

Lymphedema
Paxil Tablets (Rare) 2505

Lymphocytes, decrease (see under Lymphocytopenia)

Lymphocytes, increase (see under Lymphocytosis)

Lymphocytopenia
▲Betaseron for SC Injection (82%) 658
Dipentum Capsules (Rare) 1951
Floxin I.V. (More than or equal to 1%) 1571
Floxin Tablets (200 mg, 300 mg, 400 mg) (More than or equal to 1.0%) 1567
Foscavir Injection (Less than 1%) 547
Leukeran Tablets 1133
Mustargen 1709
Orthoclone OKT3 Sterile Solution 1837
Paxil Tablets (Rare) 2505
Rocephin Injectable Vials, ADD-Vantage, Galaxy Container (Less than 1%) 2142
Stelazine Tablets 2514
Talwin Injection (Rare) 2334
Unasyn 2212
Vantin for Oral Suspension and Vantin Tablets 2646
▲Xanax Tablets (5.5% to 7.4%) 2649
Zefazone 2654

Lymphocytosis
Ceclor Pulvules & Suspension 1431
Ceptaz (Very rare) 1081
Cipro I.V. (Infrequent) 595
▲Cipro I.V. Pharmacy Bulk Package (Among most frequent) 597
Depakene 413
Depakote Tablets 415
Effexor (Infrequent) 2719
Floxin I.V. (More than or equal to 1%) 1571
Floxin Tablets (200 mg, 300 mg, 400 mg) (More than or equal to 1%) 1567
Fortaz (Very rare) 1100
Neurontin Capsules (Rare) 1922
Paxil Tablets (Rare) 2505
Permax Tablets (Rare) 575
Primaxin I.M. 1727
Primaxin I.V. 1729
Prozac Pulvules & Liquid, Oral Solution (Rare) 919
Rocephin Injectable Vials, ADD-Vantage, Galaxy Container (Rare) 2142
Tazicef for Injection (Very rare) 2519
Unasyn 2212
Vantin for Oral Suspension and Vantin Tablets 2646
Zefazone 2654
Zyloprim Tablets (Less than 1%) 1226

Lymphoma
Cytovene-IV (Two or more reports) 2103
Dilantin Infatabs 1908
Dilantin Kapseals 1906
Dilantin Parenteral (A number of reports) 1910
Dilantin-125 Suspension 1911
Hivid Tablets (A significant increase) 2121
Imuran (0.5%) 1110
▲Neoral (1% to 6%) 2276
Orthoclone OKT3 Sterile Solution 1837
Prograf 1042
▲Sandimmune (Less than 1 to 6%) 2286

Lymphoma, lymphocytic
CellCept Capsules (0.6% to 1.0%) 2099
Dantrium Capsules (Less frequent) 1982
Dantrium Intravenous 1983

Lymphoma-like disorder
Anafranil Capsules (Rare) 803
Foscavir Injection (Between 1% and 5%) 547
PASER Granules 1285
Videx Tablets, Powder for Oral Solution, & Pediatric Powder for Oral Solution (Up to 2%) 720

Lymphomonocytosis
Haldol Decanoate 1577
Haldol Injection, Tablets and Concentrate 1575

LDH abnormalities
Bumex (1.0%) 2093
Ceftin Tablets (1.0%) 1078
▲Emcyt Capsules (33 to 34%) 1953
Hivid Tablets (Less than 1% to less than 3%) 2121
Intron A 2364
Nimotop Capsules (0.4%; rare) 610
Sinemet CR Tablets 944
Zithromax (Less than 1%) 1944

LDH increase
Accutane Capsules 2076
Adalat CC (Rare) 589
Atamet 572
Biaxin (Less than 1%) 405
Cardizem CD Capsules (Less than 1%) 1506
Cardizem SR Capsules (Less than 1%) 1510
Cardizem Injectable 1508
Cardizem Tablets (Less than 1%) 1512
Cefizox for Intramuscular or Intravenous Use 1034
Cefotan (1 in 700) 2829
Ceftin for Oral Suspension (1.0%) 1078
Cefzil Tablets and Oral Suspension 746
▲CellCept Capsules (More than or equal to 3%) 2099
Ceptaz (One in 18) 1081
Chibroxin Sterile Ophthalmic Solution (With oral form) 1617
▲Cipro I.V. (Among most frequent) 595
▲Cipro I.V. Pharmacy Bulk Package (Among most frequent) 597
Cipro Tablets (0.4%) 592
Claforan Sterile and Injection (Less than 1%) 1235
Cuprimine Capsules (Few cases) 1630
Cytovene (1% or less) 2103
Demulen 2428
Depakene (Frequent) 413
Depakote Tablets (Frequent) 415
Depen Titratable Tablets (Few reports) 2662
Dilacor XR Extended-release Capsules (Rare) 2018
Duricef 748
Felbatol (Infrequent) 2666
Floxin I.V. 1571
Floxin Tablets (200 mg, 300 mg, 400 mg) 1567
▲Fortaz (1 in 18) 1100
Foscavir Injection (Between 1% and 5%) 547
▲Sterile FUDR (Among more common) 2118
Garamycin Injectable 2360
Glucotrol Tablets (Occasional) 1967
Glucotrol XL Extended Release Tablets (Occasional) 1968
Inderide Tablets 2732
Kefurox Vials, Faspak & ADD-Vantage (1 in 75) 1454
Kerlone Tablets (Less than 2%) 2436
Larodopa Tablets 2129
Lopid Tablets (Occasional) 1917
Lorabid Suspension and Pulvules 1459
▲Lupron Depot 3.75 mg (5% to 8%) 2556
▲Lupron Depot 7.5 mg (19.6%) 2559
Luvox Tablets (Rare) 2544
Mefoxin 1691
Mefoxin Premixed Intravenous Solution 1694
Megace Oral Suspension (1% to 3%) 699
Monocid Injection (1.6%) 2497
Monopril Tablets 757
Nalfon 200 Pulvules & Nalfon Tablets (Less than 1%) 917
Nebcin Vials, Hyporets & ADD-Vantage 1464
▲Neupogen for Injection (27% to 58%) 495
Noroxin Tablets (Less frequent) 1715
Noroxin Tablets (Less frequent) 2048
Pentasa (Less than 1%) 1527
Pipracil (Less frequent) 1390
PREVACID Delayed-Release Capsules (Less than 1%) 2562
Primaxin I.M. 1727
Primaxin I.V. 1729
Procardia Capsules (Rare) 1971
Procardia XL Extended Release Tablets (Rare) 1972
▲Roferon-A Injection (10% to 13%) 2145
Sectral Capsules 2807
Serzone Tablets (Infrequent) 771
Sinemet Tablets 943
Sinemet CR Tablets 944
Suprax 1399
▲Tazicef for Injection (1 in 18 patients) 2519
▲Tegison Capsules (15%) 2154
Timentin for Injection 2528
Tobramycin Sulfate Injection 968
Toprol-XL Tablets 565
Tornalate Solution for Inhalation, 0.2% (Rare) 956
Unasyn 2212
Vantin for Oral Suspension and Vantin Tablets 2646
▲Zanosar Sterile Powder (A number of patients) 2653
Zefazone 2654
Zinacef (1 in 75 patients) 1211

LE cells test positive (see under Lupus erythematosus)

LE-like reactions (see under Lupus erythematosus)

M

Maceration
Monistat-Derm (miconazole nitrate 2%) Cream (Isolated reports) 1889
Oxistat Cream (0.1%) 1152

Maceration, skin
Cortisporin Otic Solution Sterile 1087
Cortisporin Otic Suspension Sterile 1088
Cyclocort Topical (Infrequent) 1037
DesOwen Cream, Ointment and Lotion (Infrequent) 1046
Locoid Cream, Ointment and Topical Solution (Infrequent) 978
Neurontin Capsules (Rare) 1922
PediOtic Suspension Sterile 1153
ProctoCream-HC (Infrequent) 2408

Macrocytic anemia
Ambien Tablets (Rare) 2416
Depakene 413
Depakote Tablets 415
Dilantin Infatabs 1908
Dilantin-125 Suspension 1911
Eulexin Capsules 2358
Imuran (2 cases) 1110

Macrocytosis
Depakene 413
Dilantin Kapseals 1906
Dilantin Parenteral 1910
Retrovir Capsules (The majority of children) 1158
Retrovir I.V. Infusion (The majority of children) 1163
Retrovir Syrup (The majority of children) 1158

Macrophages, reactive
▲Blenoxane (10%) 692

Maculae
Calan SR Caplets (1% or less) 2422
Calan Tablets (1% or less) 2419
Isoptin Oral Tablets (Less than 1%) 1346
Isoptin SR Tablets (1% or less) 1348
Verelan Capsules (1% or less) 1410
Verelan Capsules (Less than 1%) 2824

Maculopathy
Tolectin (200, 400 and 600 mg) (Less than 1%) 1581

Malabsorption syndrome
Elspar 1659
Gelfoam Sterile Sponge 2608
Purinethol Tablets (Occasional) 1156
Sandostatin Injection (1% to 4%) 2292

Malaise
Accupril Tablets (0.5%-1.0%) 1893
Accutane Capsules 2076
Children's Advil Suspension 2692
AeroBid Inhaler System (1-3%) 1005
Aerobid-M Inhaler System (1-3%) 1005
Airet Solution for Inhalation (1.5%) 452
Altace Capsules (Less than 1%) 1232
Ambien Tablets (Infrequent) 2416
Amicar Syrup, Tablets, and Injection (Occasional) 1267
Anafranil Capsules (Infrequent) 803
Anaprox/Naprosyn (Less than 1%) 2117
Ansaid Tablets (1-3%) 2579
Antivenin (Crotalidae) Polyvalent 2696
Apresazide Capsules 808
Aquasol A Vitamin A Capsules, USP 534
Aquasol A Parenteral 534
Aristocort Suspension (Forte Parenteral) 1027
Aristospan Suspension (Intra-articular) 1033
Aristospan Suspension (Intralesional) 1032
Asacol Delayed-Release Tablets (1% to 2%) 1979
Atamet 572
Atgam Sterile Solution (Less than 1% to less than 5%) 2581
Azactam for Injection (Less than 1%) 734
▲BCG Vaccine, USP (TICE) (7.4%) 1814
▲Betaseron for SC Injection (15%) 658
Biavax II 1613
Biltricide Tablets 591
Buprenex Injectable (Infrequent) 2006
BuSpar (Infrequent) 737
Calan SR Caplets 2422
Calan Tablets 2419
Capoten (0.5 to 2%) 739
Capozide (0.5 to 2%) 742
Cardene Capsules (0.6%) 2095
▲Cardura Tablets (About 0.7% to 12%) 2186

(▣ Described in PDR For Nonprescription Drugs) Incidence data in parenthesis; ▲ 3% or more (◉ Described in PDR For Ophthalmology)

Malaise Side Effects Index 1356

Cartrol Tablets (Less common) 410
Cataflam (Less than 1%) 816
Catapres Tablets (About 1 in 100 patients) 674
Catapres-TTS (Less frequent) 675
Celestone Soluspan Suspension 2347
▲CellCept Capsules (More than or equal to 3%) 2099
Cholera Vaccine 2711
Cipro I.V. (1% or less) 595
Cipro I.V. Pharmacy Bulk Package (Less than 1%) 597
Cipro Tablets (Less than 1%) 592
Claritin (2% or fewer patients) 2349
Claritin-D (Less frequent) 2350
Clinoril Tablets (Less than 1 in 100) 1618
Clozaril Tablets (Less than 1%) 2252
Cognex Capsules (Frequent) 1901
Combipres Tablets (About 1%) 677
▲Cordarone Tablets (4 to 9%) 2712
Cortone Acetate Sterile Suspension 1623
Cortone Acetate Tablets 1624
Cosmegen Injection 1626
Cytosar-U Sterile Powder (Occasional) 2592
Cytovene-IV (1% or less) 2103
DTIC-Dome (Infrequent) 600
Dalalone D.P. Injectable 1011
▲Dantrium Capsules (Among most frequent) 1982
Daraprim Tablets (Rare) 1090
Daypro Caplets (Less than 1%) 2426
Decadron Elixir 1633
Decadron Phosphate Injection 1637
Decadron Phosphate Respihaler 1642
Decadron Phosphate Turbinaire 1645
Decadron Phosphate with Xylocaine Injection, Sterile 1639
Decadron Tablets 1635
Decadron-LA Sterile Suspension 1646
Depakene 413
Depakote Tablets 415
Desyrel and Desyrel Dividose (Up to 2.8%) 503
Dexacort Phosphate in Respihaler 458
Dexacort Phosphate in Turbinaire 459
Dilacor XR Extended-release Capsules (Infrequent) 2018
Diphtheria & Tetanus Toxoids Adsorbed Purogenated (Mild) 1374
Dolobid Tablets (Less than 1 in 100) 1654
Doral Tablets 2664
Duvoid 2044
EC-Naprosyn Delayed-Release Tablets (Less than 1%) 2117
Edecrin 1657
Effexor (Frequent) 2719
Elavil 2838
Eldepryl Tablets 2550
Endep Tablets 2174
Engerix-B Unit-Dose Vials (Less than 1%) 2482
Ergamisol Tablets 1292
Etrafon 2355
Felbatol (Frequent) 2666
Feldene Capsules (Greater than 1%) 1965
Flexeril Tablets (Less than 1%) 1661
Floxin I.V. (Less than 1%) 1571
Floxin Tablets (200 mg, 300 mg, 400 mg) (Less than 1%) 1567
▲Fludara for Injection (6% to 8%) 663
Fluvirin (Infrequent) 460
▲Foscavir Injection (5% or greater) 547
Sterile FUDR 2118
▲Fungizone Intravenous (Among most common) 506
Furoxone (Occasional) 2046
Gamimune N, 5% Immune Globulin Intravenous (Human), 5% 619
Gamimune N, 10% Immune Globulin Intravenous (Human), 10% 621
Gastrocrom Capsules (1 report) 984
Glauctabs ◉ 208
Glucophage 752
▲Havrix (1% to 10%) 2489
Hivid Tablets (Less than 1% to less than 3%) 2121
Humegon 1824
Hydeltrasol Injection, Sterile 1665
Hydeltra-T.B.A. Sterile Suspension 1667
Hydrea Capsules 696
Hydrocortone Acetate Sterile Suspension 1669
Hydrocortone Phosphate Injection, Sterile 1670
Hydrocortone Tablets 1672
Hyperstat I.V. Injection 2363
IFEX (Less than 1%) 697
Imdur (Less than or equal to 5%) 1323
Imitrex Injection (1.1%) 1103
Imitrex Tablets 1106
▲Imovax Rabies Vaccine (Up to 6%) 881
Imuran 1110
Indocin (Greater than 1%) 1680
INFeD (Iron Dextran Injection, USP) 2345
Influenza Virus Vaccine, Trivalent, Types A and B (chromatograph- and filter-purified subviron antigen) FluShield, 1995-1996 Formula (Infrequent) 2736
▲Intron A (Up to 14%) 2364
Iopidine 0.5% (Less than 1%) ◉ 221
Ismo Tablets (Fewer than 1%) 2738
Isoptin SR Tablets 1348
▲JE-VAX (Approximately 10%) 886
Kerlone Tablets (Less than 2%) 2436
Lamictal Tablets (2.3%) 1112
Larodopa Tablets (Relatively frequent) 2129
Lescol Capsules (Rare) 2267
▲Leucovorin Calcium for Injection (2% to 13%) 1268
▲Leukine for IV Infusion (57%) 1271
▲Leustatin (5% to 7%) 1834
▲Lodine Capsules and Tablets (3-9%) 2743
Lomotil 2439
▲Lozol Tablets (Greater than or equal to 5%) 2022
Luvox Tablets (Frequent) 2544
M-M-R II 1687
M-R-VAX II 1689
▲MZM (Among reactions occurring most often) ◉ 267
Macrobid Capsules (Less than 1% to common) 1988
Macrodantin Capsules (Common) 1989
Marinol (Dronabinol) Capsules (Less than 1%) 2231
Maxaquin Tablets (Less than 1%) 2440
Meruvax II 1697
Methotrexate Sodium Tablets, Injection, for Injection and LPF Injection (Frequent) 1275
Metrodin (urofollitropin for injection) 2446
Mevacor Tablets (Rare) 1699
Mexitil Capsules (Less than 1% or about 3 in 1,000) 678
Mithracin 607
Moduretic Tablets (Less than or equal to 1%) 1705
8-MOP Capsules 1246
Children's Motrin Ibuprofen Oral Suspension 1546
Motrin Tablets 2625
Myambutol Tablets 1386
▲Mykrox Tablets (4.4%) 993
Myochrysine Injection 1711
Nalfon 200 Pulvules & Nalfon Tablets (Less than 1%) 917
Anaprox/Naprosyn (Less than 1%) 2117
Nardil 1920
Neptazane Tablets 1388
Neurontin Capsules (Frequent) 1922
▲Norpace (3 to 9%) 2444
Norpramin Tablets 1526
Norvasc Tablets (More than 0.1% to 1%) 1940
Nydrazid Injection 508
▲Oncaspar (Greater than 5%) 2028
▲Orlamm (11%) 2239
Orthoclone OKT3 Sterile Solution 1837
Orudis Capsules (Greater than 1%) 2766
Oruvail Capsules (Greater than 1%) 2766
Oxsoralen-Ultra Capsules 1257
Pamelor 2280
Papaverine Hydrochloride Vials and Ampoules 1468
Paraflex Caplets (Occasional) 1580
Parafon Forte DSC Caplets (Occasional) 1581
Paxil Tablets (Frequent) 2505
Penetrex Tablets (Less than 1% but more than or equal to 0.1%) 2031
Pentasa (Less than 1%) 1527
Pentaspan Injection 937
Pergonal (menotropins for injection, USP) 2448
Permax Tablets (Infrequent) 575
Pneumovax 23 1725
Pravachol (Rare) 765
PREVACID Delayed-Release Capsules (Less than 1%) 2562
Prilosec Delayed-Release Capsules (Less than 1%) 529
Prinivil Tablets (1.0% to 1.1%) 1733
Prinzide Tablets 1737
Procardia XL Extended Release Tablets (1% or less) 1972
Proglycem 580
▲Proleukin for Injection (53%) 797
▲ProSom Tablets (5%) 449
Proventil Inhalation Solution 0.083% (1.5%) 2384
Proventil Solution for Inhalation 0.5% (1.5%) 2383
Prozac Pulvules & Liquid, Oral Solution (Infrequent) 919
Pulmozyme Inhalation 1064
Pyrazinamide Tablets 1398
▲Rabies Vaccine, Imovax Rabies I.D. (Less frequent; up to 6%) 883
Recombivax HB (Equal to or greater than 1%) 1744
Relafen Tablets (1%) 2510
▲Retrovir Capsules (8% to 53.2%) 1158
▲Retrovir I.V. Infusion (8% to 53.2%) 1163
▲Retrovir Syrup (8% to 53.2%) 1158
Rifamate Capsules 1530
Rifater 1532
Risperdal (Infrequent) 1301
Romazicon (1% to 3%) 2147
▲Rowasa (3.44%) 2548
Sansert Tablets 2295
Sectral Capsules 2807
Serevent Inhalation Aerosol (1% to 3%) 1176
Serzone Tablets (Infrequent) 771
Sinemet Tablets 943
Sinemet CR Tablets 944
Solganal Suspension 2388
Sporanox Capsules (0.1% to 1.2%) 1305
Supprelin Injection (1% to 3%) 2056
Surmontil Capsules 2811
Tambocor Tablets (1% to less than 3%) 1497
Tenex Tablets (3% or less) 2074
Tetanus & Diphtheria Toxoids Adsorbed Purogenated (Rare) 1401
Tetanus Toxoid Adsorbed Purogenated 1403
▲TheraCys BCG Live (Intravesical) (2.0% to 40.2%) 897
Tofranil Ampuls 854
Tofranil Tablets 856
Tofranil-PM Capsules 857
Tonocard Tablets (Less than 1%) 531
Trandate 1185
Trental Tablets (Less than 1%) 1244
Triavil Tablets 1757
▲Typhim Vi (4.1% to 37%) 899
Typhoid Vaccine 2823
Ultram Tablets (50 mg) (1% to 5%) 1585
Unasyn (Less than 1%) 2212
Univasc Tablets (Less than 1%) 2410
Urecholine 1761
Vantin for Oral Suspension and Vantin Tablets (Less than 1%) 2646
Varivax (Greater than or equal to 1%) 1762
▲Velban Vials (Among most common) 1484
Ventolin Inhalation Solution (1.5%) 1198
Ventolin Nebules Inhalation Solution (1.5%) 1199
Verelan Capsules 1410
Verelan Capsules 2824
▲Videx Tablets, Powder for Oral Solution, & Pediatric Powder for Oral Solution (Less than 1% to 38%) 720
Voltaren Tablets (Less than 1%) 861
Vontrol Tablets (Rare) 2532
▲Yutopar Intravenous Injection (5% to 6%) 570
Zantac (Rare) 1209
Zantac Injection (Rare) 1207
Zantac Syrup (Rare) 1209
Zebeta Tablets 1413
▲Zerit Capsules (1% to 17%) 729
Zestoretic 2850
Zestril Tablets (1.0% to 1.1%) 2854
Ziac 1415
▲Zinecard (48% to 61%) 1961
Zocor Tablets (Rare) 1775
▲Zofran Injection (5%) 1214
▲Zofran Tablets (9% to 13%) 1217
Zoladex (1% or greater) 2858
Zoloft Tablets (Infrequent) 2217
Zosyn (1.0% or less) 1419
Zosyn Pharmacy Bulk Package (1.0% or less) 1422
▲Zovirax (11.5%) 1219
Zyloprim Tablets (Less than 1%) 1226

Malaria relapse

Aramine Injection 1609

Male pattern baldness (see under Alopecia, hereditaria)

Malignancies, secondary

Cytoxan (Isolated reports) 694
Leukeran Tablets 1133
NEOSAR Lyophilized/Neosar 1959

Malignant hyperthermia

Anectine 1073
Foscavir Injection (Less than 1%) 547
Proleukin for Injection (Less than 1%) 797

Malignant hyperthermia, familial

Sensorcaine 559

Malignant melanoma

Atamet 572
Sinemet Tablets 943
Sinemet CR Tablets 944

Malignant neoplasms

CellCept Capsules (0.8% to 1.4%) 2099
Orthoclone OKT3 Sterile Solution 1837
▲Tegison Capsules (1 to 10%) 2154

Malodor, unspecified

Condylox (Less than 5%) 1802

Manic behavior

Ambien Tablets (Rare) 2416
Anafranil Capsules (Infrequent) 803
Betaseron for SC Injection 658
Cipro I.V. (1% or less) 595
Cipro I.V. Pharmacy Bulk Package (Less than 1%) 597
Cipro Tablets (Less than 1%) 592
Cytovene (1% or less) 2103
Effexor (0.5%) 2719
Endep Tablets (Rare) 2174
Felbatol 2666
Floxin I.V. 1571
Floxin Tablets (200 mg, 300 mg, 400 mg) 1567
Halcion Tablets 2611
Hivid Tablets (Less than 1% to less than 3%) 2121
Lamictal Tablets (Rare) 1112
Levsin/Levsinex/Levbid 2405
Ludiomil Tablets (Rare) 843
Luvox Tablets (Frequent) 2544
Maxaquin Tablets 2440
Nardil (Less frequent) 1920
Neurontin Capsules (Rare) 1922
Orthoclone OKT3 Sterile Solution 1837
Pamelor 2280
Parnate Tablets 2503
Paxil Tablets (Approximately 1.0%; infrequent) 2505
Permax Tablets (Infrequent) 575
Protopam Chloride for Injection (Several cases) 2806
Prozac Pulvules & Liquid, Oral Solution (Infrequent) 919
Risperdal 1301
Rythmol Tablets–150mg, 225mg, 300mg (Less than 1%) 1352
Serzone Tablets (0.3% to 1.6%) 771
Tofranil Ampuls 854
Tofranil Tablets 856
Tofranil-PM Capsules 857
Triavil Tablets (Rare) 1757
Videx Tablets, Powder for Oral Solution, & Pediatric Powder for Oral Solution (Less than 1%) 720
Wellbutrin Tablets (Frequent) 1204
Xanax Tablets 2649
Zoloft Tablets (0.4%) 2217

Masculinization, female fetus

Oxandrin 2862

(Described in PDR For Nonprescription Drugs) Incidence data in parenthesis; ▲ 3% or more (◉ Described in PDR For Ophthalmology)

1357 Side Effects Index Menopause

Mass, abdominal (see under Abdominal mass)

Mastalgia (see under Mastodynia)

Mastitis

Humegon (Occasional) 1824
Paxil Tablets (Rare) 2505
Risperdal (Infrequent) 1301

Mastodynia

Climara Transdermal System 645
Estrace Cream and Tablets 749
ESTRATAB Tablets (0.3, 0.625, 1.25, 2.5 mg) 2536
Estratest 2539
Haldol Decanoate 1577
Menest Tablets 2494
Nalfon 200 Pulvules & Nalfon Tablets (Less than 1%) 917
Norplant System 2759
Ogen Tablets 2627
Ogen Vaginal Cream 2630
Ortho-Est 1869
Premarin Intravenous 2787
Premarin with Methyltestosterone 2794
Premarin Tablets 2789
Premarin Vaginal Cream 2791
Premphase 2797
Prempro 2801

Medullary hypoplasia

Novantrone 1279

Megacolon, acquired

Felbatol 2666

Megacolon, toxic

Lomotil 2439
Motofen Tablets 784

Megaloblastic anemia

Azulfidine (Rare) 1949
Bactrim DS Tablets 2084
Bactrim I.V. Infusion 2082
Bactrim 2084
Daraprim Tablets 1090
Dilantin Infatabs 1908
Dilantin Kapseals 1906
Dilantin Parenteral 1910
Dilantin-125 Suspension 1911
Dyazide 2479
Dyrenium Capsules (Rare) 2481
Eminase (Less than 1%) 2039
Fansidar Tablets 2114
Glucophage (Fives cases) 752
Macrobid Capsules 1988
Macrodantin Capsules 1989
Mebaral Tablets (Less than 1 in 100) 2322
Mesantoin Tablets (Uncommon) 2272
Mysoline (Rare idiosyncrasy) 2754
Nembutal Sodium Capsules 436
Nembutal Sodium Solution 438
Nembutal Sodium Suppositories (Less than 1%) 440
Permax Tablets (Infrequent) 575
Phenobarbital Elixir and Tablets (A few cases) 1469
Proloprim Tablets 1155
Seconal Sodium Pulvules 1474
Septra 1174
Septra I.V. Infusion 1169
Septra I.V. Infusion ADD-Vantage Vials 1171
Septra 1174
Trimpex Tablets 2163
Zovirax Sterile Powder (Less than 1%) 1223

Megaloblastosis

Cytosar-U Sterile Powder 2592
Maxzide 1380

Melanoma, malignant, activation of

Larodopa Tablets 2129

Melanoma, skin

Clomid 1514
Cognex Capsules (Rare) 1901
8-MOP Capsules 1246
Paxil Tablets (Rare) 2505

Melanosis

Intron A (Less than 5%) 2364
Neurontin Capsules (Rare) 1922

Melasma

Amen Tablets 780
Aygestin Tablets 974
Depo-Provera Contraceptive Injection (Fewer than 1%) 2602
Diethylstilbestrol Tablets 1437
Estrace Cream and Tablets 749
Estratest 2539
Micronor Tablets 1872
Modicon 1872
Ortho Dienestrol Cream 1866
Ortho-Novum 1872
Stilphostrol Tablets and Ampuls 612

Melasma, possibly persistent

Brevicon 2088
Climara Transdermal System 645
Demulen 2428
Desogen Tablets 1817
ESTRATAB Tablets (0.3, 0.625, 1.25, 2.5 mg) 2536
Levlen/Tri-Levlen 651
Menest Tablets 2494
Micronor Tablets 1872
Modicon 1872
Norinyl 2088
Nor-Q D Tablets 2135
Ogen Tablets 2627
Ogen Vaginal Cream 2630
Ortho-Cept 1851
Ortho-Cyclen/Ortho-Tri-Cyclen 1858
Ortho-Est 1869
Ortho-Novum 1872
Ortho-Cyclen/Ortho Tri-Cyclen 1858
Ovcon 760
PMB 200 and PMB 400 2783
Premarin Intravenous 2787
Premarin with Methyltestosterone 2794
Premarin Tablets 2789
Premarin Vaginal Cream 2791
Premphase 2797
Prempro 2801
Levlen/Tri-Levlen 651
Tri-Norinyl 2164

Melena

Children's Advil Suspension (Less than 1%) 2692
Anaprox/Naprosyn (Less than 1%) 2117
Azo Gantrisin Tablets 2081
Betaseron for SC Injection 658
Cataflam (Less than 1%) 816
Cytovene (1% or less) 2103
Diamox Intravenous (Occasional) 1372
Diamox Sequels (Sustained Release) 1373
Diamox Tablets (Occasional) 1372
EC-Naprosyn Delayed-Release Tablets (Less than 1%) 2117
Effexor (Infrequent) 2719
Feldene Capsules (Less than 1%) 1965
Foscavir Injection (Between 1% and 5%) 547
Fungizone Intravenous 506
Glauctabs (Occasional) ⊙ 208
Hivid Tablets (Less than 1% to less than 3%) 2121
IBU Tablets (Less than 1%) 1342
Imdur (Less than or equal to 5%) 1323
Imitrex Tablets (Rare) 1106
Intron A (Less than 5%) 2364
Lodine Capsules and Tablets (More than 1% but less than 3%) 2743
Lotensin Tablets 834
Lotensin HCT 837
Luvox Tablets (Infrequent) 2544
MZM (Occasional) ⊙ 267
Methotrexate Sodium Tablets, Injection, for Injection and LPF Injection 1275
Children's Motrin Ibuprofen Oral Suspension (Less than 1%) 1546
Motrin Tablets (Less than 1%) 2625
Motrin Ibuprofen Suspension, Oral Drops, Chewable Tablets, Caplets (Less than 1%) 1546
Anaprox/Naprosyn (Less than 1%) 2117
NebuPent for Inhalation Solution (1% or less) 1040
Neptazane Tablets 1388
Orudis Capsules (Less than 1%) 2766
Oruvail Capsules (Less than 1%) 2766
Paxil Tablets (Rare) 2505
Permax Tablets (Infrequent) 575
PREVACID Delayed-Release Capsules (Less than 1%) 2562
Procardia XL Extended Release Tablets (1% or less) 1972
ProSom Tablets (Rare) 449
Prozac Pulvules & Liquid, Oral Solution (2%) 919
Relafen Tablets (1%) 2510
Ridaura Capsules (0.1 to 1%) 2513
Risperdal (Infrequent) 1301
Tegison Capsules (Less than 1%) 2154
Toradol 2159
Vaseretic Tablets 1765
Vasotec I.V. 1768
Vasotec Tablets (0.5% to 1.0%) 1771
▲ Videx Tablets, Powder for Oral Solution, & Pediatric Powder for Oral Solution (Less than 1%; 7%) 720
Voltaren Tablets (Less than 1%) 861
Zithromax (1% or less) 1944
Zoloft Tablets (Rare) 2217
Zosyn (1.0% or less) 1419
Zosyn Pharmacy Bulk Package (1.0% or less) 1422

Memory impairment

▲ Anafranil Capsules (7% to 9%) 803
Cataflam (Less than 1%) 816
Cogentin 1621
Cozaar Tablets (Less than 1%) 1628
Desyrel and Desyrel Dividose (Less than 1% to 1.4%) 503
Eldepryl Tablets 2550
Eskalith 2485
Halcion Tablets (0.9% to 0.5%) 2611
Hyzaar Tablets 1677
Imitrex Tablets (Rare) 1106
Klonopin Tablets 2126
Lamictal Tablets (2.4%) 1112
Lithonate/Lithotabs/Lithobid 2543
Lopressor 830
Ludiomil Tablets (Rare) 843
▲ Lupron Depot 3.75 mg (Among most frequent) 2556
Lupron Depot 7.5 mg 2559
Lupron Injection (Less than 5%) 2555
Monopril Tablets (0.2% to 1.0%) 757
Nydrazid Injection (Uncommon) 508
Prinivil Tablets (0.3% to 1.0%) 1733
Prinzide Tablets 1737
Rifamate Capsules (Uncommon) 1530
Rifater (Uncommon) 1532
Roferon-A Injection (Less than 3%) 2145
Serax Capsules 2810
Serax Tablets 2810
Seromycin Pulvules 1476
▲ Serzone Tablets (4%) 771
Sinemet CR Tablets 944
Timolide Tablets 1748
Tonocard Tablets (Less than 1%) 531
Transderm Scōp Transdermal Therapeutic System (Infrequent) 869
Voltaren Tablets (Less than 1%) 861
Wellbutrin Tablets (Infrequent) 1204
▲ Xanax Tablets (33.1%) 2649
Zestoretic 2850
Ziac 1415

Memory loss, short-term

Bentyl 10 mg Capsules 1501
Blocadren Tablets 1614
Cartrol Tablets 410
Clozaril Tablets (Less than 1%) 2252
Cytovene-IV (One report) 2103
Ergamisol Tablets (10 out of 463 patients) 1292
Ethmozine Tablets (Less than 2%) 2041
Hivid Tablets (Less than 1% to less than 3%) 2121
Inderal 2728
Inderal LA Long Acting Capsules 2730
Inderide Tablets 2732
Inderide LA Long Acting Capsules 2734
Kerlone Tablets 2436
Lescol Capsules 2267
Levatol 2403
Levsin/Levsinex/Levbid 2405
Lioresal Intrathecal 1596
Lopressor HCT Tablets 832
Mevacor Tablets (0.5% to 1.0%) 1699
Mexitil Capsules (About 9 in 1,000) 678
NebuPent for Inhalation Solution (1% or less) 1040
Normodyne Tablets 2379
Parnate Tablets 2503
Placidyl Capsules 448
Pravachol 765
Rythmol Tablets–150mg, 225mg, 300mg (Less than 1%) 1352
Sectral Capsules 2807
Tenoretic Tablets 2845
Tenormin Tablets and I.V. Injection 2847
Testoderm Testosterone Transdermal System (One in 104 patients) 486
Timoptic in Ocudose 1753
Timoptic Sterile Ophthalmic Solution 1751
Timoptic-XE 1755
Toprol-XL Tablets 565
Trandate Tablets 1185
Visken Tablets 2299
Zocor Tablets 1775

Meniere's syndrome

Netromycin Injection 100 mg/ml 2373

Meningism

Antivenin (Crotalidae) Polyvalent (Occasional) 2696
Marcaine Hydrochloride with Epinephrine 1:200,000 2316
Marcaine Hydrochloride Injection 2316
Marcaine Spinal 2319
Neurontin Capsules (Rare) 1922
Novocain Hydrochloride for Spinal Anesthesia 2326
Pontocaine Hydrochloride for Spinal Anesthesia 2330
Sensorcaine 559

Meningitis

Ansaid Tablets (Less than 1%) 2579
Azulfidine (Rare) 1949
Betaseron for SC Injection 658
Carbocaine Hydrochloride Injection 2303
Depo-Medrol Single-Dose Vial 2600
Depo-Medrol Sterile Aqueous Suspension 2597
▲ Exosurf Neonatal for Intratracheal Suspension (Less than 1% to 6%) 1095
Foscavir Injection (Between 1% and 5%) 547
Gelfoam Sterile Sponge 2608
Lioresal Intrathecal (2 cases of 244 patients) 1596
Marcaine Hydrochloride with Epinephrine 1:200,000 2316
Marcaine Spinal 2319
Motrin Tablets 2625
Orthoclone OKT3 Sterile Solution 1837
Paxil Tablets (Rare) 2505
Permax Tablets (Infrequent) 575
Proleukin for Injection (Less than 1%) 797

Meningitis, aseptic

Anaprox/Naprosyn (Less than 1%) 2117
Atretol Tablets (One case) 573
Bactrim 2084
Cataflam (Rare) 816
EC-Naprosyn Delayed-Release Tablets (Less than 1%) 2117
IBU Tablets (Rare; less than 1%) 1342
Motrin Ibuprofen Suspension, Oral Drops, Chewable Tablets, Caplets (Rare; less than 1%) 1546
Anaprox/Naprosyn (Less than 1%) 2117
Orudis Capsules (Less than 1%) 2766
Oruvail Capsules (Less than 1%) 2766
Proloprim Tablets (Rare) 1155
Sandoglobulin I.V. (Infrequent) 2290
Septra 1174
Septra I.V. Infusion 1169
Septra I.V. Infusion ADD-Vantage Vials 1171
Septra 1174
Tegretol Chewable Tablets (One case) 852
Tegretol Suspension (One case) 852
Tegretol Tablets (One case) 852
Toradol 2159
Voltaren Tablets (Rare) 861

Meningitis, septic

Carbocaine Hydrochloride Injection 2303
Marcaine Hydrochloride with Epinephrine 1:200,000 2316
Marcaine Hydrochloride Injection 2316
Sensorcaine 559

Menometrorrhagia

Orudis Capsules (Less than 1%) 2766
Oruvail Capsules (Less than 1%) 2766

Menopause

Effexor (Rare) 2719
Luvox Tablets (Infrequent) 2544
Permax Tablets (Infrequent) 575
Prozac Pulvules & Liquid, Oral Solution (Infrequent) 919
Ultram Tablets (50 mg) (1% to 5%) 1585
Wellbutrin Tablets (Rare) 1204

(▣ Described in PDR For Nonprescription Drugs) Incidence data in parenthesis; ▲ 3% or more (⊙ Described in PDR For Ophthalmology)

Menorrhagia

Children's Advil Suspension (Less than 1%) 2692
Asacol Delayed-Release Tablets 1979
▲ Betaseron for SC Injection (6%) 658
Claritin (2% or fewer patients) 2349
Claritin-D 2350
Clomid (1.3%) 1514
Dipentum Capsules (Rare) 1951
Effexor (Infrequent) 2719
Floxin I.V. (Less than 1%) 1571
Floxin Tablets (200 mg, 300 mg, 400 mg) (Less than 1%) 1567
IBU Tablets (Less than 1%) 1342
Intron A (Less than 5%) 2364
Lamictal Tablets (Rare) 1112
Luvox Tablets (Infrequent) 2544
Children's Motrin Ibuprofen Oral Suspension (Less than 1%) 1546
Motrin Tablets (Less than 1%) 2625
Motrin Ibuprofen Suspension, Oral Drops, Chewable Tablets, Caplets (Less than 1%) 1546
Neurontin Capsules (Infrequent) 1922
Paxil Tablets (Infrequent) 2505
Pentasa (Less than 1%) 1527
Permax Tablets (Infrequent) 575
Prozac Pulvules & Liquid, Oral Solution (Infrequent) 919
Risperdal (Frequent) 1301
Serzone Tablets (Infrequent) 771
Zoloft Tablets (Rare) 2217

Menstrual disorders

AeroBid Inhaler System 1005
▲ Aerobid-M Inhaler System (3-9%) 1005
Ambien Tablets (Infrequent) 2416
▲ Anafranil Capsules (Up to 4%) 803
Anaprox/Naprosyn (Less than 1%) 2117
Ansaid Tablets (Less than 1%) 2579
▲ Betaseron for SC Injection (17%) 658
Ceredase 1065
Cortifoam 2396
Cytotec (0.3%) 2424
Danocrine Capsules 2307
EC-Naprosyn Delayed-Release Tablets (Less than 1%) 2117
Effexor (1%) 2719
Etrafon 2355
Felbatol 2666
Halcion Tablets 2611
Halotestin Tablets 2614
Kerlone Tablets (Less than 2%) 2436
Lamictal Tablets (More than 1%) 1112
Lupron Depot 3.75 mg (Less than 5%) 2556
Mustargen 1709
Anaprox/Naprosyn (Less than 1%) 2117
▲ Nolvadex Tablets (5.7%) 2841
ParaGard T380A Intrauterine Copper Contraceptive 1880
Rifadin 1528
Rifater 1532
Rimactane Capsules 847
Seldane-D Extended-Release Tablets 1538
Solu-Cortef Sterile Powder 2641
Tegison Capsules (Less than 1%) 2154
Trilafon 2389
Ultram Tablets (50 mg) (Less than 1%) 1585
▲ Wellbutrin Tablets (4.7%) 1204
▲ Xanax Tablets (10.4%) 2649
Zoladex 2858
Zoloft Tablets (1.0%) 2217

Menstrual dysfunction

Luvox Tablets (Infrequent) 2544
Methotrexate Sodium Tablets, Injection, for Injection and LPF Injection 1275

Menstrual flow, changes

Amen Tablets 780
Aygestin Tablets 974
Coumadin 926
Cycrin Tablets 975
Danocrine Capsules 2307
Daypro Caplets (Less than 1%) 2426
Demulen 2428
Depo-Provera Sterile Aqueous Suspension 2606
Desogen Tablets 1817
Estraderm Transdermal System 824
ESTRATAB Tablets (0.3, 0.625, 1.25, 2.5 mg) 2536
Estratest 2539
Levlen/Tri-Levlen 651
Lippes Loop Intrauterine Double-S 1848
Lo/Ovral Tablets 2746
Lo/Ovral-28 Tablets 2751
Menest Tablets 2494
Micronor Tablets 1872
Moban Tablets and Concentrate 1048
Modicon 1872
Nordette-21 Tablets 2755
Nordette-28 Tablets 2758
Ortho-Cept 1851
Ortho-Cyclen/Ortho-Tri-Cyclen 1858
Ortho Dienestrol Cream 1866
Ortho-Est 1869
Ortho-Novum 1872
Ortho-Cyclen/Ortho Tri-Cyclen 1858
Ovcon 760
Ovral Tablets 2770
Ovral-28 Tablets 2770
Ovrette Tablets 2771
PMB 200 and PMB 400 2783
ParaGard T380A Intrauterine Copper Contraceptive 1880
Premarin Intravenous 2787
Premarin with Methyltestosterone 2794
Premarin Vaginal Cream 2791
Provera Tablets 2636
Rogaine Topical Solution (0.47%) 2637
Levlen/Tri-Levlen 651
Triphasil-21 Tablets 2814
Triphasil-28 Tablets 2819

Menstrual irregularities

Accutane Capsules (Less than 1%) 2076
Aldactazide 2413
Aldactone 2414
▲ Android Capsules, 10 mg (Among most common) 1250
▲ Android (Among most common) 1251
Aristocort Suspension (Forte Parenteral) 1027
Aristocort Suspension (Intralesional) 1025
Aristocort Tablets 1022
Aristospan Suspension (Intra-articular) 1033
Aristospan Suspension (Intralesional) 1032
Asendin Tablets (Less than 1%) 1369
Brevicon 2088
BuSpar (Infrequent) 737
Calan SR Caplets (1% or less) 2422
Calan Tablets (1% or less) 2419
Celestone Soluspan Suspension 2347
Claritin-D (Less frequent) 2350
Compazine 2470
CORTENEMA 2535
Cortone Acetate Sterile Suspension 1623
Cortone Acetate Tablets 1624
Dalalone D.P. Injectable 1011
Decadron Elixir 1633
Decadron Phosphate Injection 1637
Decadron Phosphate Respihaler 1642
Decadron Phosphate Turbinaire 1645
Decadron Phosphate with Xylocaine Injection, Sterile 1639
Decadron Tablets 1635
Decadron-LA Sterile Suspension 1646
▲ Delatestryl Injection (One of most common) 2860
Deltasone Tablets 2595
Demulen 2428
Depakene 413
Depakote Tablets 415
Depo-Medrol Single-Dose Vial 2600
Depo-Medrol Sterile Aqueous Suspension 2597
▲ Depo-Provera Contraceptive Injection (More than 5%) 2602
Desyrel and Desyrel Dividose 503
Dexacort Phosphate in Respihaler 458
Dexacort Phosphate in Turbinaire 459
Doral Tablets 2664
▲ Estratest (Among most common) 2539
▲ Felbatol (3.4%) 2666
Florinef Acetate Tablets 505
Fulvicin P/G Tablets (Rare) 2359
Fulvicin P/G 165 & 330 Tablets (Rare) 2359
Haldol Decanoate 1577
Haldol Injection, Tablets and Concentrate 1575
Hydeltrasol Injection, Sterile 1665
Hydeltra-T.B.A. Sterile Suspension 1667
Hydrocortone Acetate Sterile Suspension 1669
Hydrocortone Phosphate Injection, Sterile 1670
Hydrocortone Tablets 1672
Intron A 2364
Isoptin Oral Tablets (Less than 1%) 1346
Isoptin SR Tablets (1% or less) 1348
Levoprome 1274
Librax Capsules (Rare) 2176
Libritabs Tablets (Isolated cases) 2177
Librium Capsules (Isolated cases) 2178
Librium Injectable (Isolated cases) 2179
Limbitrol (Rare) 2180
Loxitane (Rare) 1378
Lupron Depot-PED 7.5 mg, 11.25 mg and 15 mg 2560
Medrol 2621
Mellaril 2269
▲ Nolvadex Tablets (12.5% to 24.6%) 2841
Norinyl 2088
Nor-Q D Tablets 2135
▲ Oreton Methyl (Among most common) 1255
Oxandrin 2862
ParaGard T380A Intrauterine Copper Contraceptive 1880
Pediapred Oral Liquid 995
Prelone Syrup 1787
Premarin with Methyltestosterone 2794
PREVACID Delayed-Release Capsules (Less than 1%) 2562
Prolixin 509
Rifamate Capsules 1530
Rimactane Capsules 847
Seldane Tablets 1536
Serax Capsules 2810
Serax Tablets 2810
Serentil 684
Solu-Medrol Sterile Powder 2643
Stelazine 2514
Testred Capsules 1262
Torecan 2245
Triavil Tablets 1757
Tri-Norinyl 2164
Vantin for Oral Suspension and Vantin Tablets (Less than 1%) 2646
Winstrol Tablets 2337
Xanax Tablets 2649

Menstruation, early

Actifed with Codeine Cough Syrup 1067
Benadryl Capsules 1898
Benadryl Injection 1898
Deconamine 1320
Desyrel and Desyrel Dividose 503
Ornade Spansule Capsules 2502
Periactin 1724
Tavist Syrup 2297
Tavist Tablets 2298
Temaril Tablets, Syrup and Spansule Extended-Release Capsules 483
Trinalin Repetabs Tablets 1330
Tussend 1783

Menstruation, painful

ProSom Tablets (Infrequent) 449
Prozac Pulvules & Liquid, Oral Solution (2.6%) 919

Mental acuity, loss of

Retrovir Capsules 1158
Retrovir I.V. Infusion 1163
Retrovir Syrup 1158
Sinemet CR Tablets 944

Mental clouding

Anexsia 5/500 Elixir 1781
Anexia Tablets 1782
Compazine 2470
Halcion Tablets 2611
Hycodan Tablets and Syrup 930
Hycomine Compound Tablets 932
Hycomine 931
Hycotuss Expectorant Syrup 933
Hydrocet Capsules 782
Lorcet 10/650 1018
Lortab 2566
Tussend 1783
Tussionex Pennkinetic Extended-Release Suspension 998
Vicodin Tablets 1356
Vicodin ES Tablets 1357
Vicodin Tuss Expectorant 1358
Zydone Capsules 949

Mental confusion (see under Confusion)

Mental depression (see under Depression, mental)

Mental perception, altered

Mykrox Tablets 993

Mental performance, impairment

Aldoclor Tablets 1598
Aldomet Ester HCl Injection 1602
Aldomet Oral 1600
Aldoril Tablets 1604
Ambien Tablets (Infrequent) 2416
Anafranil Capsules (Up to 5%) 803
Anaprox/Naprosyn (Less than 1%) 2117
Anexsia 5/500 Elixir 1781
Anexia Tablets 1782
Asendin Tablets (Less than 1%) 1369
Atamet 572
Ativan Injection 2698
Beclovent Inhalation Aerosol and Refill 1075
Bentyl 1501
Bromfed-DM Cough Syrup 1786
Brontex 1981
BuSpar (2%) 737
Butisol Sodium Elixir & Tablets 2660
Cardura Tablets (Less than 0.5% of 3960 patients) 2186
Claritin (2% or fewer patients) 2349
Claritin-D (Less frequent) 2350
Clomid 1514
Clozaril Tablets 2252
Compazine 2470
DHCplus Capsules 1993
Deconamine 1320
Demerol 2308
Desyrel and Desyrel Dividose 503
Dilaudid Ampules 1335
Dilaudid Cough Syrup 1336
Dilaudid 1335
EC-Naprosyn Delayed-Release Tablets (Less than 1%) 2117
Elavil 2838
Endep Tablets 2174
Ergamisol Tablets (Less frequent) 1292
Esgic-plus Tablets 1013
Eskalith 2485
Etrafon 2355
Fioricet Tablets 2258
Fludara for Injection (Up to 1%) 663
Flumadine Tablets & Syrup (0.3% to 2.1%) 1015
Foscavir Injection (Less than 1%) 547
Grifulvin V (griseofulvin tablets) Microsize (griseofulvin oral suspension) Microsize 1888
Hivid Tablets (Less than 1% to less than 3%) 2121
Hycodan Tablets and Syrup 930
Hycomine Compound Tablets 932
Hycomine 931
Hycotuss Expectorant Syrup 933
Hydrocet Capsules 782
Imdur (Less than or equal to 5%) 1323
Imitrex Injection (Rare) 1103
Imitrex Tablets (Infrequent) 1106
▲ Intron A (Up to 14%) 2364
Inversine Tablets 1686
Lamictal Tablets (1.7%) 1112
Levsin/Levsinex/Levbid 2405
Libritabs Tablets 2177
Limbitrol 2180
Lioresal Intrathecal 1596
Lithonate/Lithotabs/Lithobid 2543
Lorcet 10/650 1018
Lortab 2566
Loxitane 1378
MS Contin Tablets 1994
Mebaral Tablets 2322
Methadone Hydrochloride Oral Concentrate 2233
Miltown Tablets 2672
Monoket (Fewer than 1%) 2406
Anaprox/Naprosyn (Less than 1%) 2117
▲ Nicorette (3% to 9% of patients) 2458
Norpramin Tablets 1526
Orap Tablets 1050
PBZ-SR Tablets 844
PMB 200 and PMB 400 2783
Paxil Tablets (Frequent) 2505
Percocet Tablets 938
Percodan Tablets 939
Phenergan with Codeine 2777
Phenergan with Dextromethorphan 2778
Phenergan Injection 2773
Phenergan Suppositories 2775
Phenergan Syrup 2774
Phenergan Tablets 2775
Phenergan VC 2779
Phenergan VC with Codeine 2781
ProSom Tablets 449
Prozac Pulvules & Liquid, Oral Solution (1.6%) 919
RMS Suppositories 2657
Restoril Capsules (Less than 1%) 2284

(▣ Described in PDR For Nonprescription Drugs) Incidence data in parenthesis; ▲ 3% or more (◉ Described in PDR For Ophthalmology)

1359 Side Effects Index Micturition disturbances

Rifadin 1528
Rifamate Capsules 1530
Rifater 1532
Rimactane Capsules 847
Risperdal 1301
Ryna ◘ 841
▲ Serzone Tablets (3%) 771
Sinemet Tablets 943
Surmontil Capsules 2811
Timolide Tablets 1748
Timoptic in Ocudose 1753
Timoptic Sterile Ophthalmic Solution 1751
Timoptic-XE 1755
Tofranil Tablets 856
Tofranil-PM Capsules 857
Toradol (1% or less) 2159
Tussend 1783
Tussionex Pennkinetic Extended-Release Suspension 998
Tylenol with Codeine 1583
Tylox Capsules 1584
Ultram Tablets (50 mg) (Less than 1%) 1585
Vicodin Tablets 1356
Vicodin ES Tablets 1357
Vicodin Tuss Expectorant 1358
Vistaril Intramuscular Solution (Seldom) 2216
Vivactil Tablets 1774
Wygesic Tablets 2827
Xanax Tablets 2649
Zarontin Capsules 1928
Zarontin Syrup 1929
Zebeta Tablets 1413
Zestril Tablets (0.3% to 1.0%) 2854
Ziac 1415
Zoloft Tablets (1.3%) 2217
Zydone Capsules 949

Mental slowness

BuSpar (Infrequent) 737
Celontin Kapseals 1899
Tonocard Tablets (Less than 1%) 531

Mental status, altered

Clozaril Tablets 2252
Eldepryl Tablets 2550
Etrafon 2355
Florinef Acetate Tablets 505
Haldol Decanoate 1577
▲ Idamycin (41%) 1955
▲ Intron A (Up to 14%) 2364
Ludiomil Tablets 843
Mellaril 2269
Moban Tablets and Concentrate 1048
Navane Capsules and Concentrate 2201
Navane Intramuscular 2202
Oncaspar 2028
Orap Tablets 1050
Orthoclone OKT3 Sterile Solution 1837
▲ Prograf (Approximately 55%) 1042
▲ Proleukin for Injection (73%) 797
Risperdal 1301
▲ Roferon-A Injection (17%) 2145
Serentil 684
Sinemet CR Tablets 944
Stelazine 2514
Torecan 2245
Triavil Tablets 1757

Mesenteric arterial thrombosis

Blocadren Tablets 1614
Inderal 2728
Inderal LA Long Acting Capsules 2730
Inderide Tablets 2732
Inderide LA Long Acting Capsules 2734
Kerlone Tablets 2436
Levatol 2403
Lo/Ovral Tablets 2746
Lo/Ovral-28 Tablets 2751
Nordette-21 Tablets 2755
Nordette-28 Tablets 2758
Normodyne Tablets 2379
Ovral Tablets 2770
Ovral-28 Tablets 2770
Ovrette Tablets 2771
Sectral Capsules 2807
Tenoretic Tablets 2845
Tenormin Tablets and I.V. Injection 2847
Timolide Tablets 1748
Timoptic in Ocudose 1753
Timoptic Sterile Ophthalmic Solution 1751
Triphasil-21 Tablets 2814
Triphasil-28 Tablets 2819
Ziac 1415

Metabolic acidosis (see under Acidosis, metabolic)

Metabolic changes

Clinoril Tablets (Rare) 1618
Methotrexate Sodium Tablets, Injection, for Injection and LPF Injection 1275
Pravachol 765
Vumon (Less than 1%) 727

Metaplasia, bronchiolar squamous

▲ Blenoxane (10%) 692

Methemoglobinemia

Americaine Anesthetic Lubricant (Rare) 983
Americaine Otic Topical Anesthetic Ear Drops (Rare) 983
Azo Gantanol Tablets 2080
Azo Gantrisin Tablets 2081
Azulfidine (Rare) 1949
Bactrim DS Tablets 2084
Bactrim I.V. Infusion 2082
Bactrim 2084
Deponit NTG Transdermal Delivery System (Extremely rare) 2397
Desyrel and Desyrel Dividose 503
Eulexin Capsules 2358
Fansidar Tablets 2114
Gantanol Tablets 2119
Gantrisin 2120
Hurricaine (Extremely rare) 666
Hurricaine Topical (Extremely rare) 666
Ismo Tablets (Extremely rare) 2738
Isordil Sublingual Tablets (Extremely rare) 2739
Isordil Tembids (Extremely rare) 2741
Isordil Titradose Tablets (Extremely rare) 2742
Macrobid Capsules 1988
Monoket (Extremely rare) 2406
Nitro-Bid IV (Extremely rare) 1523
Nitro-Bid Ointment (Extremely rare) 1524
Nitrodisc (Extremely rare) 2047
Nitro-Dur (nitroglycerin) Transdermal Infusion System (Very rare) 1326
Proloprim Tablets 1155
Pyridium 1928
Reglan 2068
Septra 1174
Septra I.V. Infusion 1169
Septra I.V. Infusion ADD-Vantage Vials 1171
Septra 1174
Sorbitrate (Extremely rare) 2843
Transderm-Nitro Transdermal Therapeutic System (Extremely rare) 859
Trimpex Tablets 2163

Metrorrhagia

▲ Betaseron for SC Injection (15%) 658
Effexor (Frequent) 2719
Floxin I.V. (Less than 1%) 1571
Floxin Tablets (200 mg, 300 mg, 400 mg) (Less than 1%) 1567
Luvox Tablets (Infrequent) 2544
Pentasa (Less than 1%) 1527
Permax Tablets (Infrequent) 575
Prozac Pulvules & Liquid, Oral Solution (Rare) 919
Salagen Tablets (Less than 1%) 1489
Serzone Tablets (Infrequent) 771

Metyrapone test, altered results

Amen Tablets 780
Aygestin Tablets 974
Cycrin Tablets 975
Depo-Provera Sterile Aqueous Suspension 2606
Estrace Cream and Tablets 749
Estratest 2539
Provera Tablets 2636

Microcephaly

Felbatol 2666

Microcephaly, fetal

Accutane Capsules 2076
Dilantin Infatabs 1908
Dilantin Kapseals 1906
Dilantin Parenteral 1910
Dilantin-125 Suspension 1911

Microphthalmia, fetal

Accutane Capsules 2076

Micropinna, fetal

Accutane Capsules 2076

Micturition, difficulty

Actifed with Codeine Cough Syrup 1067
Apresazide Capsules (Less frequent) 808
Apresoline Hydrochloride Tablets (Less frequent) 809
Atrovent Inhalation Aerosol (Less than 1%) 671
Benadryl Capsules 1898
Benadryl Injection 1898
Blocadren Tablets 1614
▲ Bromfed-DM Cough Syrup (Among most frequent) 1786
Catapres Tablets (About 2 in 1,000 patients) 674
Catapres-TTS (Less frequent) 675
▲ CHEMET (succimer) Capsules (Up to 3.7%) 1545
Combipres Tablets (About 2 in 1,000) 677
Dantrium Capsules (Less frequent) 1982
Deconamine 1320
Deconsal C Expectorant Syrup 456
Deconsal Pediatric Syrup 457
Dimetane-DC Cough Syrup 2059
Dimetane-DX Cough Syrup 2059
Donnagel Liquid and Donnagel Chewable Tablets (Rare) ◘ 879
Effexor (2%) 2719
Fioricet with Codeine Capsules 2260
Fiorinal with Codeine Capsules 2262
Flexeril Tablets (Rare) 1661
▲ Hylorel Tablets (33.6%) 985
Kutrase Capsules 2402
Levoprome (Sometimes) 1274
Maxaquin Tablets (Less than 1%) 2440
Normodyne Tablets (Less common) 2379
Norpramin Tablets 1526
Nucofed 2051
PBZ Tablets 845
PBZ-SR Tablets 844
Paxil Tablets (2.9%) 2505
Periactin 1724
Proventil (Less than 1%) 2386
Quadrinal Tablets 1350
Ser-Ap-Es Tablets 849
Stadol (Less than 1%) 775
Surgicel 1314
Tavist Syrup 2297
Tavist Tablets 2298
Timolide Tablets 1748
Timoptic in Ocudose 1753
Timoptic Sterile Ophthalmic Solution 1751
Timoptic-XE 1755
Tofranil Ampuls 854
Tofranil Tablets 856
Tofranil-PM Capsules 857
Trancopal Caplets 2337
Trandate Tablets (Less common) 1185
Transderm Scōp Transdermal Therapeutic System (Infrequent) 869
Tussend 1783
Urised Tablets 1964
Uroqid-Acid No. 2 Tablets (Occasional) 640
Ventolin Tablets (Fewer than 1 of 100 patients) 1203
Vivactil Tablets 1774
Volmax Extended-Release Tablets (Less frequent) 1788
▲ Xanax Tablets (12.2%) 2649
Zovirax Sterile Powder (Less than 1%) 1223

Micturition, painful

Deconsal C Expectorant Syrup 456
Deconsal Pediatric Syrup 457
Nucofed 2051
Ortho Diaphragm Kit 1865
▲ TheraCys BCG Live (Intravesical) (More common) 897
Uroqid-Acid No. 2 Tablets (Occasional) 640
Zovirax Sterile Powder (Less than 1%) 1223

Micturition disturbances

Actifed with Codeine Cough Syrup 1067
Adalat CC (3% or less) 589
Ambien Tablets (Rare) 2416
▲ Anafranil Capsules (4% to 14%) 803
Asendin Tablets (Very rare) 1369
Atretol Tablets 573
Atrohist Plus Tablets 454
▲ BCG Vaccine, USP (TICE) (40.4%) 1814
Benadryl Capsules 1898
Benadryl Injection 1898
Benemid Tablets 1611
Bontril Slow-Release Capsules 781
▲ Bromfed-DM Cough Syrup (Among most frequent) 1786
BuSpar (Infrequent) 737
Calan SR Caplets (1% or less) 2422
Calan Tablets (1% or less) 2419
Capoten (Approximately 1 to 2 of 1000 patients) 739
Capozide (Approximately 1 to 2 of 1000 patients) 742
Cardene Capsules (Rare) 2095
Cardene I.V. (Rare) 2709
Cardene SR Capsules (0.6%) 2097
Cardura Tablets 2186
Cartrol Tablets (Less common) 410
Cataflam (Less than 1%) 816
Caverject (Less than 1%) 2583
▲ CellCept Capsules (More than or equal to 3%) 2099
Cerezyme (One patient) 1066
Cipro I.V. (1% or less) 595
Cipro I.V. Pharmacy Bulk Package (Less than 1%) 597
Claritin (2% or fewer patients) 2349
Claritin-D (Less frequent) 2350
Clomid (Fewer than 1%) 1514
Clozaril Tablets (1%) 2252
▲ Cognex Capsules (3%) 1901
ColBENEMID Tablets 1622
Comhist 2038
Cozaar Tablets (Less than 1%) 1628
Cytovene (1% or less) 2103
Dalgan Injection (Less than 1%) 538
Dantrium Capsules (Less frequent) 1982
Daranide Tablets 1633
Daypro Caplets (Greater than 1% but less than 3%) 2426
Deconamine 1320
▲ Demadex Tablets and Injection (6.7%) 686
Desyrel and Desyrel Dividose 503
Dimetane-DC Cough Syrup 2059
Dimetane-DX Cough Syrup 2059
Dipentum Capsules (Rare) 1951
Dopram Injectable 2061
Duragesic Transdermal System (Less than 1%) 1288
Duramorph 962
▲ Effexor (3%) 2719
Elavil 2838
Eldepryl Tablets 2550
Endep Tablets 2174
Eskalith 2485
Ethmozine Tablets (Less than 2%) 2041
Etrafon 2355
Flexeril Tablets (Less than 1%) 1661
Floxin I.V. (Less than 1%) 1571
Floxin Tablets (200 mg, 300 mg, 400 mg) (Less than 1%) 1567
Flumadine Tablets & Syrup 1015
Foscavir Injection (Less than 1%) 547
Hivid Tablets (Less than 1% to less than 3%) 2121
Hydrocet Capsules 782
Hytrin Capsules (At least 1%) 430
Hyzaar Tablets 1677
IFEX 697
Imitrex Injection (Rare) 1103
Imitrex Tablets (Infrequent) 1106
Indocin (Rare) 1680
Intal Capsules (Less than 1 in 10,000 patients) 987
Intal Inhaler (Infrequent) 988
Intal Nebulizer Solution 989
Intron A (Less than 5%) 2364
Ismo Tablets (Fewer than 1%) 2738
Isoptin Oral Tablets (Less than 1%) 1346
Isoptin SR Tablets (1% or less) 1348
Kerlone Tablets (Less than 2%) 2436
Lamictal Tablets (Infrequent) 1112
Limbitrol 2180
▲ Lioresal Tablets (2-6%) 829
Lodine Capsules and Tablets (More than 1% but less than 3%) 2743
Lotensin HCT (0.3% to more than 1%) 837
Lozol Tablets (Less than 5%) 2022
Ludiomil Tablets (Rare) 843
Lupron Depot 3.75 mg 2556
Lupron Depot 7.5 mg (Less than 5%) 2559
▲ Lupron Injection (5% or more) 2555
▲ Luvox Tablets (3%) 2544
Matulane Capsules 2131
Maxaquin Tablets (Less than 1%) 2440
Megace Oral Suspension (Up to 2%) 699

(◘ Described in PDR For Nonprescription Drugs) Incidence data in parenthesis; ▲ 3% or more (◉ Described in PDR For Ophthalmology)

Micturition disturbances — Side Effects Index — 1360

Midamor Tablets (Less than or equal to 1%) ... 1703
Milontin Kapseals ... 1920
Minipress Capsules (1-4%) ... 1937
Minizide Capsules (Rare) ... 1938
Moduretic Tablets ... 1705
Monopril Tablets (0.2% to 1.0%) ... 757
Mycelex-G 500 mg Vaginal Tablets (Rare) ... 609
Neurontin Capsules (Infrequent) ... 1922
▲Norpace (3 to 9%) ... 2444
Norpramin Tablets ... 1526
Norvasc Tablets (More than 0.1% to 1%) ... 1940
Oncaspar (Less than 1%) ... 2028
Orap Tablets ... 1050
Ornade Spansule Capsules ... 2502
Ortho Diaphragm Kit ... 1865
PBZ Tablets ... 845
PBZ-SR Tablets ... 844
Pamelor ... 2280
Parlodel ... 2281
Parnate Tablets ... 2503
▲Paxil Tablets (3.1%) ... 2505
Pentasa (Less than 1%) ... 1527
Permax Tablets (2.7%) ... 575
Plendil Extended-Release Tablets (0.5% to 1.5%) ... 527
Pondimin Tablets ... 2066
Prilosec Delayed-Release Capsules (Less than 1%) ... 529
Proleukin for Injection (1%) ... 797
Propulsid (1.2%) ... 1300
ProSom Tablets (Infrequent) ... 449
Prostigmin Injectable ... 1260
Prostigmin Tablets ... 1261
Prozac Pulvules & Liquid, Oral Solution (1.6% to 4%) ... 919
Reglan ... 2068
Retrovir Capsules ... 1158
Retrovir I.V. Infusion ... 1163
Retrovir Syrup ... 1158
ReVia Tablets (Less than 1%) ... 940
Risperdal ... 1301
▲Salagen Tablets (9% to 12%) ... 1489
▲Sectral Capsules (3%) ... 2807
Seldane Tablets ... 1536
Seldane-D Extended-Release Tablets ... 1538
Serophene (clomiphene citrate tablets, USP) (Less than 1 in 100 patients) ... 2451
Serzone Tablets (2%) ... 771
Sinemet CR Tablets (0.8%) ... 944
Stilphostrol Tablets and Ampuls ... 612
Supprelin Injection (1% to 3%) ... 2056
Surmontil Capsules ... 2811
Tavist Syrup ... 2297
Tavist Tablets ... 2298
Tegretol Chewable Tablets ... 852
Tegretol Suspension ... 852
Tegretol Tablets ... 852
Temaril Tablets, Syrup and Spansule Extended-Release Capsules ... 483
Tenex Tablets (Less frequent) ... 2074
Tensilon Injectable ... 1261
▲TheraCys BCG Live (Intravesical) (1.8% to 40.2%) ... 897
Tofranil Ampuls ... 854
Tofranil Tablets ... 856
Tofranil-PM Capsules ... 857
Toradol (1% or less) ... 2159
Triavil Tablets ... 1757
Trinalin Repetabs Tablets ... 1330
Tussend ... 1783
Ultram Tablets (50 mg) (1% to 5%) ... 1585
Univasc Tablets (More than 1%) ... 2410
Urecholine ... 1761
Verelan Capsules (1% or less) ... 1410
Verelan Capsules (Less than 1%) ... 2824
Videx Tablets, Powder for Oral Solution, & Pediatric Powder for Oral Solution (Less than 1% to 5%) ... 720
Vivactil Tablets ... 1774
Voltaren Tablets (Less than 1%) ... 861
Wellbutrin Tablets (2.5%) ... 1204
Zerit Capsules (Fewer than 1% to 1%) ... 729
Zoladex (1% or greater) ... 2858
Zoloft Tablets (1.4%; 2.0%) ... 2217

Migraine

Ambien Tablets (Infrequent) ... 2416
Amen Tablets ... 780
Anafranil Capsules (Up to 3%) ... 803
Asacol Delayed-Release Tablets ... 1979
▲Betaseron for SC Injection (12%) ... 658
Brevicon ... 2088
Cardura Tablets (Less than 0.5% of 3960 patients) ... 2186
Claritin (2% or fewer patients) ... 2349
Claritin-D (Less frequent) ... 2350
Climara Transdermal System ... 645
Clomid ... 1514
Cognex Capsules (Infrequent) ... 1901
Cozaar Tablets (Less than 1%) ... 1628
Cycrin Tablets ... 975
Cytovene (1% or less) ... 2103
Demulen ... 2428
Depo-Provera Contraceptive Injection ... 2602
Depo-Provera Sterile Aqueous Suspension ... 2606
Desogen Tablets ... 1817
Diethylstilbestrol Tablets ... 1437
Effexor (Frequent) ... 2719
Eldepryl Tablets ... 2550
Engerix-B Unit-Dose Vials ... 2482
Estrace Cream and Tablets ... 749
Estraderm Transdermal System ... 824
ESTRATAB Tablets (0.3, 0.625, 1.25, 2.5 mg) ... 2536
Estratest ... 2539
Felbatol (Infrequent) ... 2666
Gastrocrom Capsules (Infrequent) ... 984
Glucotrol XL Extended Release Tablets (Less than 1%) ... 1968
Hivid Tablets (Less than 1% to less than 3%) ... 2121
Hyzaar Tablets ... 1677
Imdur (Less than or equal to 5%) ... 1323
Imitrex Tablets ... 1106
Intron A (Less than 5%) ... 2364
Lamictal Tablets (Infrequent) ... 1112
Levlen/Tri-Levlen ... 651
Lo/Ovral Tablets ... 2746
Lo/Ovral-28 Tablets ... 2751
Luvox Tablets ... 2544
Maxair Autohaler ... 1492
Maxair Inhaler (Less than 1%) ... 1494
Menest Tablets ... 2494
Miacalcin Nasal Spray (Less than 1%) ... 2275
Micronor Tablets ... 1872
Modicon ... 1872
Neurontin Capsules (Infrequent) ... 1922
Nordette-21 Tablets ... 2755
Nordette-28 Tablets ... 2758
Norinyl ... 2088
Norplant System ... 2759
Nor-Q D Tablets ... 2135
Ogen Tablets ... 2627
Ogen Vaginal Cream ... 2630
Ortho-Cept ... 1851
Ortho-Cyclen/Ortho-Tri-Cyclen ... 1858
Ortho Dienestrol Cream ... 1866
Ortho-Est ... 1869
Ortho-Novum ... 1872
Ortho-Cyclen/Ortho Tri-Cyclen ... 1858
Orudis Capsules (Less than 1%) ... 2766
Oruvail Capsules (Less than 1%) ... 2766
Ovcon ... 760
Ovral Tablets ... 2770
Ovral-28 Tablets ... 2770
Ovrette Tablets ... 2771
PMB 200 and PMB 400 ... 2783
Paxil Tablets (Infrequent) ... 2505
Permax Tablets (Rare) ... 575
Premarin Intravenous ... 2787
Premarin with Methyltestosterone ... 2794
Premarin Tablets ... 2789
Premarin Vaginal Cream ... 2791
Premphase ... 2797
Prempro ... 2801
Procardia XL Extended Release Tablets (1% or less) ... 1972
Propulsid (1% or less) ... 1300
Provera Tablets ... 2636
Prozac Pulvules & Liquid, Oral Solution (Infrequent) ... 919
Recombivax HB ... 1744
Risperdal (Rare) ... 1301
Serzone Tablets ... 771
Stilphostrol Tablets and Ampuls ... 612
Supprelin Injection (1% to 3%) ... 2056
Levlen/Tri-Levlen ... 651
Tri-Norinyl ... 2164
Triphasil-21 Tablets ... 2814
Triphasil-28 Tablets ... 2819
Ultram Tablets (50 mg) (Infrequent) ... 1585
Videx Tablets, Powder for Oral Solution, & Pediatric Powder for Oral Solution (Less than 1%) ... 720
Zerit Capsules (Fewer than 1% to 3%) ... 729
Zoladex (1% or greater) ... 2858
Zoloft Tablets (Infrequent) ... 2217

Miliaria

Aclovate Cream ... 1069
Analpram-HC Rectal Cream 1% and 2.5% ... 977
Anusol-HC Cream 2.5% (Infrequent to frequent) ... 1896
Aristocort A 0.025% Cream (Infrequent) ... 1027
Aristocort A 0.5% Cream ... 1031
Aristocort A 0.1% Cream (Infrequent) ... 1029
Aristocort A 0.1% Ointment (Infrequent) ... 1030
Carmol HC (Infrequent to frequent) ... 924
▲Cordran Lotion (More frequent) ... 1803
▲Cordran Tape (More frequent) ... 1804
Cortisporin Cream ... 1084
Cortisporin Ointment ... 1085
Cortisporin Otic Solution Sterile ... 1087
Cortisporin Otic Suspension Sterile ... 1088
Cutivate Cream ... 1088
Cutivate Ointment (Infrequent to more frequent) ... 1089
Cyclocort Topical (Infrequent) ... 1037
Decadron Phosphate Topical Cream ... 1644
Decaspray Topical Aerosol ... 1648
Dermatop Emollient Cream 0.1% (Infrequent to frequent) ... 1238
DesOwen Cream, Ointment and Lotion (Infrequent) ... 1046
Diprolene AF Cream (Infrequent) ... 2352
Diprolene Gel 0.05% (Infrequent) ... 2353
Diprolene (Infrequent) ... 2352
Elocon ... 2354
Epifoam (Infrequent) ... 2399
Florone/Florone E ... 906
Halog (Infrequent) ... 2686
Hytone ... 907
Lidex (Infrequent) ... 2130
Locoid Cream, Ointment and Topical Solution (Infrequent) ... 978
Lotrisone Cream (Infrequent) ... 2372
Mantadil Cream ... 1135
8-MOP Capsules ... 1246
NeoDecadron Topical Cream ... 1714
Oxsoralen-Ultra Capsules ... 1257
PediOtic Suspension Sterile ... 1153
Pramosone Cream, Lotion & Ointment ... 978
ProctoCream-HC (Infrequent) ... 2408
ProctoCream-HC 2.5% (Infrequent to frequent) ... 2408
ProctoFoam-HC ... 2409
Psorcon Cream 0.05% (Infrequent) ... 909
Psorcon Ointment 0.05% ... 908
Synalar (Infrequent) ... 2130
Temovate (Infrequent) ... 1179
Topicort (Infrequent) ... 1243
Tridesilon Cream 0.05% (Infrequent) ... 615
Tridesilon Ointment 0.05% (Infrequent) ... 616
Ultravate Cream 0.05% (Infrequent) ... 2689
Ultravate Ointment 0.05% ... 2690
Varivax (Greater than or equal to 1%) ... 1762
Westcort ... 2690

Miosis

▲Buprenex Injectable (1-5%) ... 2006
Carbocaine Hydrochloride Injection ... 2303
Compazine ... 2470
Dibenzyline Capsules ... 2476
Dilaudid-HP Injection (Less frequent) ... 1337
Dilaudid-HP Lyophilized Powder 250 mg (Less frequent) ... 1337
Dilaudid Tablets and Liquid (Less frequent) ... 1339
Duramorph ... 962
Duvoid (Infrequent) ... 2044
Effexor (Rare) ... 2719
▲Felbatol (6.5%) ... 2666
Fioricet with Codeine Capsules ... 2260
Fiorinal with Codeine Capsules ... 2262
Lioresal Tablets ... 829
MS Contin Tablets (Less frequent) ... 1994
MSIR (Infrequent) ... 1997
Marcaine Hydrochloride with Epinephrine 1:200,000 ... 2316
Marcaine Hydrochloride Injection ... 2316
Mellaril ... 2269
Mestinon Injectable ... 1253
Mestinon ... 1254
Navane Capsules and Concentrate ... 2201
Navane Intramuscular ... 2202
Neurontin Capsules (Rare) ... 1922
Numorphan Injection ... 936
Numorphan Suppositories ... 937
Oramorph SR (Morphine Sulfate Sustained Release Tablets) (Less frequent) ... 2236
Pilagan ... ◉ 248
Pontocaine Hydrochloride for Spinal Anesthesia ... 2330
Prostigmin Injectable ... 1260
Prostigmin Tablets ... 1261
Sensorcaine ... 559
Serentil ... 684
Soma Compound w/Codeine Tablets ... 2676
Stelazine ... 2514
Talwin Injection (Rare) ... 2334
Tensilon Injectable ... 1261
Thorazine ... 2523
Torecan ... 2245
Tussi-Organidin NR Liquid and S NR Liquid ... 2677
Urecholine ... 1761
Versed Injection (Less than 1%) ... 2170

Miscarriage

Cytotec ... 2424
NebuPent for Inhalation Solution (1% or less) ... 1040
Vantin for Oral Suspension and Vantin Tablets ... 2646

Mitral valve prolapse

Effexor (Rare) ... 2719

Moaning

Diprivan Injection (Less than 1%) ... 2833

Monoplegia

Imitrex Injection (Rare) ... 1103
Imitrex Tablets (Infrequent) ... 1106

Moniliasis

▲Aredia for Injection (Up to 6%) ... 810
Betaseron for SC Injection ... 658
▲CellCept Capsules (10.1% to 12.1%) ... 2099
▲CHEMET (succimer) Capsules (5.2 to 15.7%) ... 1545
Effexor (Infrequent) ... 2719
Foscavir Injection (Between 1% and 5%) ... 547
Hivid Tablets (Less than 1% to less than 3%) ... 2121
Imdur (Less than or equal to 5%) ... 1323
▲Intron A (Up to 17%) ... 2364
Megace Oral Suspension (1% to 3%) ... 699
▲Mepron Suspension (5% to 10%) ... 1135
Monodox Capsules ... 1805
Paxil Tablets (Infrequent) ... 2505
Pentasa (Less than 1%) ... 1527
Permax Tablets (Infrequent) ... 575
Prozac Pulvules & Liquid, Oral Solution (Rare) ... 919
Rhinocort Nasal Inhaler (Less than 1%) ... 556
Serzone Tablets (Rare) ... 771
Vibramycin ... 1941
Zithromax (1% or less) ... 1944
Zosyn (1.6%) ... 1419
Zosyn Pharmacy Bulk Package (1.6%) ... 1422

Moniliasis, genital

Achromycin V Capsules ... 1367
Ancef Injection ... 2465
Claforan Sterile and Injection (Less than 1%) ... 1235
Dynacin Capsules ... 1590
Effexor (Infrequent) ... 2719
Keflex Pulvules & Oral Suspension ... 914
Keftab Tablets ... 915
Kefzol Vials, Faspak & ADD-Vantage ... 1456
Lamictal Tablets (Infrequent) ... 1112
Lorabid Suspension and Pulvules (1.1%) ... 1459
Maxaquin Tablets (Less than 1%) ... 2440
Minocin Intravenous ... 1382
Minocin Oral Suspension ... 1385
Minocin Pellet-Filled Capsules ... 1383
Paxil Tablets (Rare) ... 2505
Penetrex Tablets (Less than 1% but more than or equal to 0.1%) ... 2031
Rocephin Injectable Vials, ADD-Vantage, Galaxy Container (Occasional) ... 2142

Monoclonal B-lymphoproliferative disorder

Orthoclone OKT3 Sterile Solution ... 1837

(▣ Described in PDR For Nonprescription Drugs) Incidence data in parenthesis; ▲ 3% or more (◉ Described in PDR For Ophthalmology)

1361 Side Effects Index Muscle mass, loss

Monocytosis
Celontin Kapseals 1899
Cipro Tablets (Less than 0.1%) 592
Cuprimine Capsules 1630
Depen Titratable Tablets 2662
Maxaquin Tablets 2440
Mesantoin Tablets 2272
Paxil Tablets (Rare) 2505
Primaxin I.M. 1727
Primaxin I.V. 1729
Rocephin Injectable Vials, ADD-Vantage, Galaxy Container (Rare) 2142
Unasyn 2212
Vantin for Oral Suspension and Vantin Tablets 2646
Zefazone 2654

Mononeuropathy
Acel-Imune Diphtheria and Tetanus Toxoids and Acellular Pertussis Vaccine Adsorbed 1364
Diphtheria and Tetanus Toxoids and Pertussis Vaccine Adsorbed 2477
Felbatol 2666
Tetramune 1404
Tri-Immunol Adsorbed 1408

Mood changes
▲ Adalat Capsules (10 mg and 20 mg) (7%) 587
Adalat CC (Rare) 589
AeroBid Inhaler System (1-3%) 1005
Aerobid-M Inhaler System (1-3%) 1005
Anexsia 5/500 Elixir 1781
Anexia Tablets 1782
Aristocort Suspension (Forte Parenteral) 1027
Aristocort Suspension (Intralesional) 1025
Aristocort Tablets 1022
Aristospan Suspension (Intra-articular) 1033
Aristospan Suspension (Intralesional) 1032
Betapace Tablets (Less than 1% to 3%) 641
Celestone Soluspan Suspension 2347
Clomid 1514
CORTENEMA 2535
Cortone Acetate Sterile Suspension 1623
Cortone Acetate Tablets 1624
Decadron Elixir 1633
Decadron Phosphate Injection 1637
Decadron Phosphate Respihaler 1642
Decadron Phosphate Turbinaire 1645
Decadron Phosphate with Xylocaine Injection, Sterile 1639
Decadron Tablets 1635
Decadron-LA Sterile Suspension 1646
Deltasone Tablets 2595
Demulen 2428
Depo-Medrol Sterile Aqueous Suspension 2597
Dexacort Phosphate in Respihaler 458
Dexacort Phosphate in Turbinaire 459
Dilaudid Ampules 1335
Dilaudid Cough Syrup 1336
Dilaudid-HP Injection (Less frequent) 1337
Dilaudid-HP Lyophilized Powder 250 mg (Less frequent) 1337
Dilaudid 1335
Dilaudid Oral Liquid (Less frequent) 1339
Dilaudid 1335
Dilaudid Tablets - 8 mg (Less frequent) 1339
Dipentum Capsules (Rare) 1951
Eldepryl Tablets 2550
Feldene Capsules (Less than 1%) 1965
Florinef Acetate Tablets 505
Hexalen Capsules 2571
Hivid Tablets (Less than 1% to less than 3%) 2121
Hycodan Tablets and Syrup 930
Hycomine Compound Tablets 932
Hycomine 931
Hycotuss Expectorant Syrup 933
Hydeltrasol Injection, Sterile 1665
Hydeltra-T.B.A. Sterile Suspension 1667
Hydrocet Capsules 782
Hydrocortone Acetate Sterile Suspension 1669
Hydrocortone Phosphate Injection, Sterile 1670
Hydrocortone Tablets 1672
Levlen/Tri-Levlen 651
Lioresal Intrathecal 1596
Lorcet 10/650 1018
Lortab 2566
Lupron Depot 7.5 mg 2559
Lupron Injection (Less than 5%) 2555
MS Contin Tablets (Less frequent) 1994
MSIR (Infrequent) 1997
Marinol (Dronabinol) Capsules 2231
Methotrexate Sodium Tablets, Injection, for Injection and LPF Injection (Occasional) 1275
Micronor Tablets 1872
Modicon 1872
Monopril Tablets (0.2% to 1.0%) 757
Oncaspar 2028
Oramorph SR (Morphine Sulfate Sustained Release Tablets) (Less frequent) 2236
Ortho-Cyclen/Ortho-Tri-Cyclen 1858
Ortho-Novum 1872
Ortho-Cyclen/Ortho Tri-Cyclen 1858
Orthoclone OKT3 Sterile Solution 1837
Pondimin Tablets 2066
Prelone Syrup 1787
▲ Procardia Capsules (7%) 1971
▲ Procardia XL Extended Release Tablets (7%) 1972
Stilphostrol Tablets and Ampuls 612
▲ Supprelin Injection (2% to 10%) 2056
▲ Tonocard Tablets (1.5-11.0%) 531
Levlen/Tri-Levlen 651
Tussend 1783
Tussionex Pennkinetic Extended-Release Suspension 998
Univasc Tablets (Less than 1%) 2410
Vicodin Tablets 1356
Vicodin ES Tablets 1357
Vicodin Tuss Expectorant 1358
Wellbutrin Tablets (Infrequent) 1204
Zydone Capsules 949

Moro reflex, depressed
Diupres Tablets 1650
Hydropres Tablets 1675

Motor and phonic tics, exacerbations
Dexedrine 2474
DextroStat Dextroamphetamine Tablets 2036

Motor disturbances, reversible involuntary
Zantac (Rare) 1209
Zantac Injection (Rare) 1207
Zantac Syrup (Rare) 1209

Motor restlessness
Compazine 2470
Etrafon 2355
Haldol Injection, Tablets and Concentrate 1575
Mellaril 2269
Moban Tablets and Concentrate 1048
Navane Capsules and Concentrate 2201
Navane Intramuscular 2202
Orap Tablets (Less frequent) 1050
Prolixin 509
Reglan 2068
Serentil 684
Stelazine 2514
Thorazine 2523
Torecan 2245

Motor skills, impairment
Ambien Tablets 2416
Cogentin 1621
Compazine 2470
Dapsone Tablets USP 1284
Desyrel and Desyrel Dividose 503
Dexacort Phosphate in Respihaler 458
Dexacort Phosphate in Turbinaire 459
Dilaudid Cough Syrup 1336
Doral Tablets 2664
Duranest Injections 542
Effexor 2719
Fulvicin P/G Tablets 2359
Fulvicin P/G 165 & 330 Tablets (Occasional) 2359
Halcion Tablets 2611
Levsin/Levsinex/Levbid 2405
Moban Tablets and Concentrate 1048
Neurontin Capsules (Rare) 1922
Novahistine DH 2462
Oncovin Solution Vials & Hyporets 1466
Orap Tablets 1050
Platinol 708
Platinol-AQ Injection 710
▲ Prograf (Approximately 55%) 1042
Proleukin for Injection (2%) 797
Risperdal 1301
Robaxin Injectable 2070
Serzone Tablets 771
Soma Compound w/Codeine Tablets 2676
Soma Compound Tablets 2675
Tonocard Tablets (0.0-1.2%) 531

Mouth, burning
Eldepryl Tablets 2550
Fioricet with Codeine Capsules 2260
Fiorinal with Codeine Capsules 2262
Gastrocrom Capsules (Infrequent) 984

Mouth, dry (see under Xerostomia)

Mouth, fissuring in corner of
Parnate Tablets 2503

Mouth, puckering
Compazine 2470
Etrafon 2355
Haldol Decanoate 1577
Haldol Injection, Tablets and Concentrate 1575
Mellaril 2269
Moban Tablets and Concentrate 1048
Navane Capsules and Concentrate 2201
Navane Intramuscular 2202
Orap Tablets 1050
Prolixin 509
Serentil 684
Stelazine 2514
Thorazine 2523
Triavil Tablets 1757
Trilafon 2389

Mouth, sore
Atgam Sterile Solution (Less than 5%) 2581
▲ Imitrex Injection (4.9%) 1103
Neoral (Rare) 2276
Nicorette 2458
Omnipen for Oral Suspension (Occasional) 2765
Oncaspar 2028
Prolixin 509
Rifadin (Occasional) 1528
Rifamate Capsules 1530
Rifater (Occasional) 1532
Rimactane Capsules 847
Tegison Capsules 2154
Tornalate Solution for Inhalation, 0.2% (1.9%) 956
▲ Videx Tablets, Powder for Oral Solution, & Pediatric Powder for Oral Solution (16% to 17%) 720

Mouth sensations, unpleasant
Mycelex Troches 608

Movement, abnormal
BuSpar (Infrequent) 737
Cognex Capsules (Infrequent) 1901
▲ Diprivan Injection (Greater than 1% to 17%) 2833
Hivid Tablets (Less than 1% to less than 3%) 2121
Lamictal Tablets (Rare) 1112
Oramorph SR (Morphine Sulfate Sustained Release Tablets) (Less frequent) 2236
Orthoclone OKT3 Sterile Solution 1837

Mucha-Habermann syndrome
Azulfidine (Rare) 1949

Mucocutaneous lymph node syndrome (see under Kawasaki-like syndrome)

Mucosal pigmentation, changes
Aralen Hydrochloride Injection 2301
Aralen Phosphate Tablets 2301
Intron A (Less than 5%) 2364
Minocin Oral Suspension 1385
Minocin Pellet-Filled Capsules 1383
Plaquenil Sulfate Tablets 2328

Mucositis
Adriamycin PFS 1947
Adriamycin RDF 1947
Cerubidine 795
Doxorubicin Astra 540
Fludara for Injection (Up to 2%) 663
▲ Neupogen for Injection (12%) 495
Neurontin Capsules (Rare) 1922
Oncaspar 2028
▲ Paraplatin for Injection (1% to 10%) 705
Rubex 712
▲ Taxol (31%) 714
▲ Vumon (76%) 727

Mucous plugs
Exosurf Neonatal for Intratracheal Suspension 1095

Mucous membrane, abnormalities
Atrohist Plus Tablets 454
Capoten (Approximately 1 in 1000 patients) 739
Clinoril Tablets 1618
Dynacin Capsules 1590
Hydrea Capsules 696
▲ Idamycin (50%) 1955
Lescol Capsules 2267
▲ Leukine for IV Infusion (75%) 1271
Mevacor Tablets 1699
Mexitil Capsules (About 1 in 1,000) 678
Minocin Intravenous 1382
Minocin Oral Suspension 1385
Minocin Pellet-Filled Capsules 1383
Monopril Tablets 757
Norisodrine with Calcium Iodide Syrup 442
▲ Novantrone (18 to 29%) 1279
Salagen Tablets (Less than 1%) 1489
▲ Tegison Capsules (1-10%) 2154
Zocor Tablets 1775

Mucus, blood-tinted
Flonase Nasal Spray (1% to 3%) 1098
Peptavlon 2878

Mucus, excess
ReVia Tablets (Less than 1%) 940

Mucus secretion, decreased
Tegison Capsules (Less than 1%) 2154

Multinodular goiter, enlargement
Lorelco Tablets 1517

Murmur
Cipro I.V. Pharmacy Bulk Package (Less than 1%) 597
Lupron Depot 3.75 mg 2556
Lupron Depot 7.5 mg 2559
▲ Lupron Injection (5% or more) 2555
Neurontin Capsules (Infrequent) 1922

Muscle atrophy
Betaseron for SC Injection 658
Norcuron 1826
Permax Tablets (Rare) 575
▲ Videx Tablets, Powder for Oral Solution, & Pediatric Powder for Oral Solution (8% to 12%) 720
Virazole 1264

Muscle cramp (see under Cramping, muscular)

Muscle hypotonia
Pipracil (Rare) 1390
▲ Xanax Tablets (6.3%) 2649

Muscle mass, loss
Aristocort Suspension (Forte Parenteral) 1027
Aristocort Suspension (Intralesional) 1025
Aristocort Tablets 1022
Aristospan Suspension (Intra-articular) 1033
Aristospan Suspension (Intralesional) 1032
Celestone Soluspan Suspension 2347
CORTENEMA 2535
Cortone Acetate Sterile Suspension 1623
Cortone Acetate Tablets 1624
Dalalone D.P. Injectable 1011
Decadron Elixir 1633
Decadron Phosphate Injection 1637
Decadron Phosphate Respihaler 1642
Decadron Phosphate Turbinaire 1645
Decadron Phosphate with Xylocaine Injection, Sterile 1639
Decadron Tablets 1635
Decadron-LA Sterile Suspension 1646
Deltasone Tablets 2595
Depo-Medrol Single-Dose Vial 2600
Depo-Medrol Sterile Aqueous Suspension 2597
Dexacort Phosphate in Respihaler 458
Dexacort Phosphate in Turbinaire 459
Florinef Acetate Tablets 505
Hydeltrasol Injection, Sterile 1665
Hydeltra-T.B.A. Sterile Suspension 1667

(▣ Described in PDR For Nonprescription Drugs) Incidence data in parenthesis; ▲ 3% or more (◉ Described in PDR For Ophthalmology)

Muscle mass, loss — Side Effects Index — 1362

Hydrocortone Phosphate Injection, Sterile 1670
Hydrocortone Tablets 1672
Medrol 2621
Oncovin Solution Vials & Hyporets 1466
Pediapred Oral Liquid 995
Prelone Syrup 1787
Solu-Cortef Sterile Powder 2641
Solu-Medrol Sterile Powder 2643

Muscle movement, intraoperative

Dilaudid Tablets and Liquid (Less frequent) 1339
Sufenta Injection (0.3% to 1%) 1309

Muscle rigidity

▲ Alfenta Injection (One of the two most common) 1286
Asendin Tablets 1369
BuSpar (Infrequent) 737
Ceftin (Less than 1% but more than 0.1%) 1078
Clozaril Tablets 2252
Compazine 2470
Cozaar Tablets (Less than 1%) 1628
Cytotec (Infrequent) 2424
Dilaudid-HP Injection (Less frequent) 1337
Dilaudid-HP Lyophilized Powder 250 mg (Less frequent) 1337
Dilaudid Tablets and Liquid (Less frequent) 1339
Etrafon 2355
Haldol Decanoate 1577
Hivid Tablets (Less than 1% to less than 3%) 2121
Imitrex Injection (Rare) 1103
Imogam Rabies Immune Globulin (Human) (Uncommon) 880
Inapsine Injection (Very rare) 1296
Loxitane 1378
MS Contin Tablets (Less frequent) 1994
MSIR (Infrequent) 1997
Mellaril 2269
Miacalcin Nasal Spray (Less than 1%) 2275
Nardil (Less frequent) 1920
Navane Capsules and Concentrate 2201
Navane Intramuscular 2202
Oramorph SR (Morphine Sulfate Sustained Release Tablets) (Less frequent) 2236
▲ Orap Tablets (3 of 20 patients) 1050
Orthoclone OKT3 Sterile Solution 1837
Paremyd ..... ◉ 247
Permax Tablets 575
Prolixin 509
ProSom Tablets (1%) 449
Reglan 2068
Risperdal 1301
Serentil 684
Serzone Tablets (Infrequent) 771
Stelazine 2514
Sublimaze Injection (Infrequent) 1307
▲ Sufenta Injection (One of the two most common) 1309
Supprelin Injection (2% to 3%) 2056
Thorazine 2523
Torecan 2245
Trilafon 2389
Valrelease Capsules (Infrequent) 2169
Versed Injection (0.3%) 2170
Wellbutrin Tablets 1204
Xanax Tablets (2.2%) 2649

Muscle spasms

Aldactazide 2413
Aldoclor Tablets 1598
Aldoril Tablets 1604
Alupent Tablets (0.2%) 669
Apresazide Capsules 808
BuSpar (Infrequent) 737
Capozide 742
Clozaril Tablets (1%) 2252
Combipres Tablets 677
Danocrine Capsules 2307
Diucardin Tablets 2718
Diupres Tablets 1650
Diuril Oral Suspension 1653
Diuril Sodium Intravenous 1652
Diuril Tablets 1653
Dizac (Less frequent) 1809
Dopram Injectable 2061
Doral Tablets (Rare) 2664
Enduron Tablets 420
Esidrix Tablets 821
Esimil Tablets 822
Etrafon 2355
Halcion Tablets 2611
HydroDIURIL Tablets 1674
Hydropres Tablets 1675
Hyzaar Tablets 1677
Inderide Tablets 2732
Inderide LA Long Acting Capsules 2734
Indocin I.V. (Less than 1%) 1684
Lamictal Tablets (1.0%) 1112
Lasix Injection, Oral Solution and Tablets 1240
Lopressor HCT Tablets 832
Lotensin HCT 837
Loxitane 1378
▲ Lozol Tablets (Greater than or equal to 5%) 2022
▲ Lupron Injection (Greater than 3%) 2555
Mestinon Injectable 1253
Mestinon 1254
Minizide Capsules 1938
Mivacron (Less than 1%) 1138
Moduretic Tablets (Less than or equal to 1%) 1705
Oretic Tablets 443
Parnate Tablets 2503
Prinzide Tablets 1737
Proleukin for Injection (1%) 797
ProSom Tablets (Infrequent) 449
Prostigmin Injectable 1260
Prostigmin Tablets 1261
Proventil Syrup (Less than 1 of 100 patients) 2385
Retrovir Capsules 1158
Retrovir I.V. Infusion 1163
Retrovir Syrup 1158
Ser-Ap-Es Tablets 849
Tenoretic Tablets 2845
Thalitone 1245
Timolide Tablets 1748
Tonocard Tablets (Less than 1%) 531
Valium Injectable 2182
Valium Tablets 2183
Vancocin HCl, Vials & ADD-Vantage 1481
Vaseretic Tablets 1765
Ventolin Syrup (Less than 1 of 100 patients) 1202
Wellbutrin Tablets (1.9%) 1204
Xanax Tablets (Rare) 2649
Zaroxolyn Tablets 1000
Zestoretic 2850
Ziac 1415

Muscle twitching

Atamet 572
Clozaril Tablets (Less than 1%) 2252
Dalalone D.P. Injectable 1011
Decadron-LA Sterile Suspension (Low) 1646
Desyrel and Desyrel Dividose 503
Dilaudid-HP Injection 1337
Dilaudid-HP Lyophilized Powder 250 mg 1337
Dilaudid Tablets and Liquid (Less frequentj) 1339
Dopram Injectable 2061
Flexeril Tablets (Less than 1%) 1661
Floropryl Sterile Ophthalmic Ointment 1662
Garamycin Injectable 2360
Humorsol Sterile Ophthalmic Solution 1664
Larodopa Tablets (Infrequent) 2129
Loxitane 1378
Lufyllin & Lufyllin-400 Tablets 2670
Lufyllin-GG Elixir & Tablets 2671
MS Contin Tablets (Less frequent) 1994
Netromycin Injection 100 mg/ml 2373
Placidyl Capsules 448
Quadrinal Tablets 1350
Quibron 2053
Respbid Tablets 682
Retrovir Syrup 1158
Sinemet Tablets 943
Sinemet CR Tablets 944
Theo-Dur Extended-Release Tablets 1327
Theo-X Extended-Release Tablets 788
Tobramycin Sulfate Injection 968
Tonocard Tablets (Less than 1%) 531
Uni-Dur Extended-Release Tablets 1331
Uniphyl 400 mg Tablets 2001
▲ Xanax Tablets (7.9%) 2649

Muscle weakness (see also under Asthenia; Weakness, muscle)

Anaprox/Naprosyn (Less than 1%) 2117
▲ Antivenin (Crotalidae) Polyvalent (Frequent) 2696
Aristocort Suspension (Forte Parenteral) 1027
Aristocort Suspension (Intralesional) 1025
Aristospan Suspension (Intra-articular) 1033
Aristospan Suspension (Intralesional) 1032
BuSpar (Rare) 737
Celestone Soluspan Suspension 2347
Clozaril Tablets (1%) 2252
CORTENEMA 2535
Dalalone D.P. Injectable 1011
Decadron Tablets 1635
Decadron-LA Sterile Suspension 1646
Deltasone Tablets 2595
Depakene 413
Depakote Tablets 415
Depo-Medrol Sterile Aqueous Suspension 2597
EC-Naprosyn Delayed-Release Tablets (Less than 1%) 2117
Enduron Tablets 420
Etrafon 2355
Fansidar Tablets 2114
Garamycin Injectable 2360
Hydrocortone Acetate Sterile Suspension 1669
Hyzaar Tablets 1677
Intron A (Less than 5%) 2364
Klonopin Tablets 2126
Medrol 2621
Mestinon Injectable 1253
Mestinon 1254
Milontin Kapseals 1920
Anaprox/Naprosyn (Less than 1%) 2117
▲ Norpace (3 to 9%) 2444
Norvasc Tablets (Less than or equal to 0.1%) 1940
Pediapred Oral Liquid 995
Placidyl Capsules (Occasional) 448
Plaquenil Sulfate Tablets 2328
Prelone Syrup 1787
Prostigmin Injectable 1260
Prostigmin Tablets 1261
Proventil (2%) 2386
Recombivax HB 1744
Rifadin 1528
Rifamate Capsules 1530
Rythmol Tablets–150mg, 225mg, 300mg (Less than 1%) 1352
Solu-Cortef Sterile Powder 2641
Solu-Medrol Sterile Powder 2643
Tensilon Injectable 1261
Triavil Tablets 1757
Trilafon 2389
Xanax Tablets 2649

Muscular disturbances

Felbatol 2666
▲ Foscavir Injection (5% or greater) 547
Hivid Tablets (Less than 1% to less than 3%) 2121
Lescol Capsules 2267
Nicobid 2026
▲ Risperdal (17% to 34%) 1301
Roferon-A Injection (Less than 0.5%) 2145
Serevent Inhalation Aerosol (1% to 3%) 1176
Slo-Niacin Tablets 2659
Zosyn Pharmacy Bulk Package 1422

Musculoskeletal symptoms, unspecified

▲ Accutane Capsules (Approximately 16%) 2076
Demadex Tablets and Injection 686
Imdur (Less than or equal to 5%) 1323
Seldane Tablets 1536
Seldane-D Extended-Release Tablets 1538

Mutism

Anafranil Capsules (Rare) 803
Lopid Tablets 1917
Luvox Tablets (Rare) 2544

Myalgia

Accupril Tablets (1.5%) 1893
Actigall Capsules 802
▲ Actimmune (6%) 1056
Adalat Capsules (10 mg and 20 mg) (Less than 0.5%) 587
Adalat CC (Less than 1.0%) 589
Aldoclor Tablets 1598
Aldomet Ester HCl Injection 1602
Aldomet Oral 1600
Aldoril Tablets 1604
All-Flex Arcing Spring Diaphragm (See also Ortho Diaphragm Kits) 1865
Altace Capsules (Less than 1%) 1232
Alupent Tablets (0.2%) 669
▲ Ambien Tablets (1% to 7%) 2416
Amicar Syrup, Tablets, and Injection 1267
▲ Anafranil Capsules (Up to 13%) 803
Anaprox/Naprosyn (Less than 1%) 2117
Anectine 1073
Apresazide Capsules 808
Aredia for Injection (Up to 1%) 810
▲ Asacol Delayed-Release Tablets (3%) 1979
Atgam Sterile Solution (Less than 1% to 5%) 2581
Atretol Tablets 573
Atromid-S Capsules (Less often) 2701
Augmentin 2468
Axid Pulvules (1.7%) 1427
Azactam for Injection (Less than 1%) 734
Azmacort Oral Inhaler 2011
Azo Gantrisin Tablets 2081
Bactrim DS Tablets 2084
Bactrim I.V. Infusion 2082
Bactrim 2084
Beconase 1076
Betapace Tablets (Rare) 641
▲ Betaseron for SC Injection (44%) 658
Biavax II 1613
Bumex (0.2%) 2093
BuSpar (1%) 737
Cafergot 2251
Capoten 739
Capozide 742
Cardene Capsules (1.0%) 2095
Cardura Tablets (1%) 2186
Catapres Tablets (About 6 in 1,000 patients) 674
Catapres-TTS (Less frequent) 675
▲ CellCept Capsules (More than or equal to 3%) 2099
Chibroxin Sterile Ophthalmic Solution (With oral form) 1617
Cipro Tablets 592
Claritin (2% or fewer patients) 2349
Claritin-D (Less frequent) 2350
Clinoril Tablets (Less than 1 in 100) 1618
Clomid 1514
Clozaril Tablets (1%) 2252
▲ Cognex Capsules (9%) 1901
Colestid Tablets 2591
Combipres Tablets (About 6 in 1,000) 677
Cosmegen Injection 1626
Cozaar Tablets (1.0%) 1628
Cytosar-U Sterile Powder 2592
Cytotec (Infrequent) 2424
Cytovene (1% or less) 2103
D.H.E. 45 Injection 2255
DTIC-Dome (Infrequent) 600
Dalgan Injection (Less than 1%) 538
Dantrium Capsules (Less frequent) 1982
Demadex Tablets and Injection (1.6%) 686
▲ Desyrel and Desyrel Dividose (5.1% to 5.6%) 503
DiaBeta Tablets 1239
Dilacor XR Extended-release Capsules (2.3%) 2018
Diprivan Injection (Less than 1%) 2833
Diupres Tablets 1650
Dolobid Tablets (Less than 1 in 100) 1654
Donnatal 2060
Donnatal Extentabs 2061
Donnatal Tablets 2060
Dyazide 2479
EC-Naprosyn Delayed-Release Tablets (Less than 1%) 2117
Effexor 2719
Engerix-B Unit-Dose Vials (Less than 1%) 2482
Epogen for Injection (Rare) 489
Ergamisol Tablets (2% to 3%) 1292
Esidrix Tablets 821
Esimil Tablets 822
▲ Ethmozine Tablets (2% to 5%) 2041
Felbatol (2.6%) 2666
Flexeril Tablets (Rare) 1661
Floxin I.V. (Less than 1%) 1571
Floxin Tablets (200 mg, 300 mg, 400 mg) (Less than 1%) 1567
▲ Fludara for Injection (4% to 16%) 663
Fluvirin (Infrequent) 460
Foscavir Injection (Between 1% and 5%) 547
▲ Fungizone Intravenous (Among most common) 506

(▣ Described in PDR For Nonprescription Drugs) Incidence data in parenthesis; ▲ 3% or more (◉ Described in PDR For Ophthalmology)

1363 Side Effects Index Mydriasis

Gamimune N, 5% Immune Globulin Intravenous (Human), 5% ... 619
Gamimune N, 10% Immune Globulin Intravenous (Human), 10% ... 621
Gammar I.V., Immune Globulin Intravenous (Human), Lyophilized ... 516
Gantanol Tablets ... 2119
Gantrisin ... 2120
▲ Gastrocrom Capsules (3 of 87 patients) ... 984
Glucophage ... 752
Glucotrol XL Extended Release Tablets (Less than 3%) ... 1968
Glynase PresTab Tablets ... 2609
▲ Habitrol Nicotine Transdermal System (3% to 9% of patients) ... 865
Havrix (Less than 1%) ... 2489
Hespan Injection ... 929
Hismanal Tablets (Less frequent) ... 1293
Hivid Tablets (Less than 1% to less than 3%) ... 2121
Humatrope Vials (Infrequent) ... 1443
Hytrin Capsules (At least 1%) ... 430
Hyzaar Tablets ... 1677
Imdur (Less than or equal to 5%) .. 1323
Imitrex Injection (1.8%) ... 1103
Imitrex Tablets (Frequent) ... 1106
▲ Imovax Rabies Vaccine (About 20%) ... 881
Imuran ... 1110
INFeD (Iron Dextran Injection, USP) ... 2345
Influenza Virus Vaccine, Trivalent, Types A and B (chromatograph- and filter-purified subviron antigen) FluShield, 1995-1996 Formula (Infrequent) ... 2736
Intal Capsules (Less than 1 in 100,000 patients) ... 987
Intal Inhaler (Rare) ... 988
Intal Nebulizer Solution (Rare) ... 989
▲ Intron A (3% to 59%) ... 2364
Iopidine 0.5% (0.2%) ... ⊙ 221
Ismelin Tablets ... 827
▲ JE-VAX (Approximately 10%) ... 886
▲ Kerlone Tablets (3.2%) ... 2436
Lamictal Tablets (More than 1%) .. 1112
▲ Lariam Tablets (Among most frequent) ... 2128
Lasix Injection, Oral Solution and Tablets ... 1240
Lescol Capsules ... 2267
▲ Leukine for IV Infusion (18%) ... 1271
▲ Leustatin (7%) ... 1834
Lioresal Tablets ... 829
Lopid Tablets ... 1917
Lopressor Ampuls ... 830
Lopressor HCT Tablets (1 in 100 patients) ... 832
Lopressor Tablets ... 830
Lotensin Tablets ... 834
Lotensin HCT (0.3% to more than 1%) ... 837
Lotrel Capsules ... 840
Lozol Tablets ... 2022
Lupron Depot 3.75 mg (Less than 5%) ... 2556
Lupron Depot 7.5 mg (Less than 5%) ... 2559
▲ Lupron Injection (5% or more) ... 2555
Luvox Tablets ... 2544
M-M-R II ... 1687
M-R-VAX II ... 1689
Macrobid Capsules ... 1988
Macrodantin Capsules ... 1989
Marinol (Dronabinol) Capsules (Less than 1%) ... 2231
Matulane Capsules ... 2131
Maxaquin Tablets (Less than 1%) .. 2440
Maxzide ... 1380
Meruvax II ... 1697
Methotrexate Sodium Tablets, Injection, for Injection and LPF Injection (Rare) ... 1275
Metrodin (urofollitropin for injection) ... 2446
Mevacor Tablets (1.8% to 2.4%) .. 1699
Miacalcin Nasal Spray (1% to 3%) 2275
Micronase Tablets ... 2623
Monocid Injection (Less than 1%) .. 2497
▲ Monopril Tablets (0.2% to 3.3%) .. 757
Mycobutin Capsules (2%) ... 1957
Anaprox/Naprosyn (Less than 1%) ... 2117
Nasacort Nasal Inhaler ... 2024
Navelbine Injection (Less than 5%) 1145
NebuPent for Inhalation Solution (Greater than 1%, up to 5%) ... 1040
Neoral (2% or less) ... 2276
Neupogen for Injection ... 495
Neurontin Capsules (2.0%) ... 1922
▲ Nicoderm (nicotine transdermal system) (3% to 9%) ... 1518
Nicorette (1% to 3% of patients) .. 2458
Nicotrol Nicotine Transdermal System (1% to 3%) ... 1550
Nimotop Capsules (Up to 1.4%) ... 610
Nolvadex Tablets (2.8%) ... 2841
Noroxin Tablets ... 1715
Noroxin Tablets ... 2048
▲ Norplant System (5% or greater) .. 2759
Norvasc Tablets (More than 0.1% to 1%) ... 1940
▲ Oncaspar (Greater than 1% but less than 5%) ... 2028
Oncovin Solution Vials & Hyporets 1466
OptiPranolol (Metipranolol 0.3%) Sterile Ophthalmic Solution (A small number of patients) ... ⊙ 258
Orap Tablets (2.7%) ... 1050
Oretic Tablets ... 443
Orlamm (Less than 1%) ... 2239
Ortho Diaphragm Kits—All-Flex Arcing Spring; Ortho Coil Spring; Ortho-White Flat Spring ... 1865
Ortho Diaphragm Kit ... 1865
Orthoclone OKT3 Sterile Solution .. 1837
Orudis Capsules (Less than 1%) ... 2766
Oruvail Capsules (Less than 1%) ... 2766
Paxil Tablets (1.7%) ... 2505
Penetrex Tablets (Less than 1% but more than or equal to 0.1%) 2031
Pentasa (Less than 1%) ... 1527
Pepcid Injection (Infrequent) ... 1722
Pepcid (Infrequent) ... 1720
Permax Tablets (1.1%) ... 575
Phenobarbital Elixir and Tablets (Rare) ... 1469
Phenurone Tablets (Less than 1%) 447
Plendil Extended-Release Tablets (0.5% to 1.5%) ... 527
Pneumovax 23 ... 1725
Pnu-Imune 23 (Occasional) ... 1393
Pondimin Tablets ... 2066
Pravachol (0.6% to 2.7%) ... 765
PREVACID Delayed-Release Capsules (Less than 1%) ... 2562
Prilosec Delayed-Release Capsules (Less than 1%) ... 529
Prinivil Tablets (0.3% to 0.6%) ... 1733
Prinzide Tablets (0.3% to 1%) ... 1737
Procan SR Tablets (Common) ... 1926
Procardia XL Extended Release Tablets (1% or less) ... 1972
Procrit for Injection (Rare) ... 1841
▲ Prograf (Greater than 3%) ... 1042
▲ Proleukin for Injection (6%) ... 797
Propulsid (More than 1%) ... 1300
ProSom Tablets (Infrequent) ... 449
Prostep (nicotine transdermal system) (1% to 3% of patients) .. 1394
Prostin E2 Suppository ... 2634
Prozac Pulvules & Liquid, Oral Solution (1.2% to 5%) ... 919
Pyrazinamide Tablets (Frequent) ... 1398
Questran Light ... 769
Questran Powder ... 770
Quinaglute Dura-Tabs Tablets ... 649
Quinidex Extentabs ... 2067
▲ Rabies Vaccine, Imovax Rabies I.D. (About 20%) ... 883
Recombivax HB (Less than 1%) ... 1744
ReoPro Vials (0.3%) ... 1471
▲ Retrovir Capsules (8%) ... 1158
▲ Retrovir I.V. Infusion (8%) ... 1163
▲ Retrovir Syrup (8%) ... 1158
▲ ReVia Tablets (More than 10%) ... 940
Revex ... 1811
Rhinocort Nasal Inhaler (Less than 1%) ... 556
▲ RhoGAM $Rh_0(D)$ Immune Globulin (Human) (25% in one study) ... 1847
Rifater (Frequent) ... 1532
Risperdal (Infrequent) ... 1301
Rocaltrol Capsules ... 2141
▲ Roferon-A Injection (69% to 73%) 2145
Salagen Tablets (1%) ... 1489
Sandimmune (2% or less) ... 2286
Sandostatin Injection (Less than 1%) ... 2292
Sansert Tablets ... 2295
Sectral Capsules (2%) ... 2807
Septra ... 1174
Septra I.V. Infusion ... 1169
Septra I.V. Infusion ADD-Vantage Vials ... 1171
Septra ... 1174
Ser-Ap-Es Tablets ... 849
Serevent Inhalation Aerosol (1% to 3%) ... 1176
Serzone Tablets ... 771
Streptase for Infusion ... 562
Supprelin Injection (2% to 3%) ... 2056
Suprane (Less than 1%) ... 1813
▲ Synarel Nasal Solution for Endometriosis (10% of patients) ... 2152
Tagamet (Rare) ... 2516
Tambocor Tablets (Less than 1%) 1497
Tapazole Tablets ... 1477
▲ Taxol (8% to 60%) ... 714
▲ Tegison Capsules (1-10%) ... 2154
Tegretol Chewable Tablets ... 852
Tegretol Suspension ... 852
Tegretol Tablets ... 852
Tenex Tablets (Less frequent) ... 2074
Tenoretic Tablets ... 2845
Thalitone (Common) ... 1245
▲ TheraCys BCG Live (Intravesical) (1.0% to 7.1%) ... 897
Timentin for Injection ... 2528
Timolide Tablets (Less than 1%) ... 1748
Tonocard Tablets (1.7%) ... 531
Toprol-XL Tablets ... 565
Toradol ... 2159
▲ Typhim Vi (2% to 7.4%) ... 899
Typhoid Vaccine ... 2823
Univasc Tablets (1.3%) ... 2410
Varivax (Greater than or equal to 1%) ... 1762
Vaseretic Tablets ... 1765
Vasotec I.V. ... 1768
Vasotec Tablets (0.5% to 1.0%) ... 1771
Verelan Capsules (1.1%) ... 1410
Verelan Capsules (1.1%) ... 2824
▲ Videx Tablets, Powder for Oral Solution, & Pediatric Powder for Oral Solution (9% to 12%) ... 720
▲ Visken Tablets (10%) ... 2299
Wellbutrin Tablets ... 1204
Wigraine Tablets & Suppositories .. 1829
WinRho SD (One report) ... 2576
Zantac (Rare) ... 1209
Zantac Injection (Rare) ... 1207
Zantac Syrup (Rare) ... 1209
Zebeta Tablets ... 1413
▲ Zerit Capsules (2% to 35%) ... 729
Zestoretic (0.3 to 1%) ... 2850
Zestril Tablets (0.5% to 0.6%) ... 2854
Ziac (Up to 2.4%) ... 1415
Zocor Tablets ... 1775
▲ Zofran Injection (10%) ... 1214
▲ Zoladex (3%) ... 2858
Zoloft Tablets (1.7%) ... 2217
Zosyn (1.0% or less) ... 1419
Zosyn Pharmacy Bulk Package (1.0% or less) ... 1422
Zovirax ... 1219
Zyloprim Tablets (Less than 1%) ... 1226

Myasthenia gravis

Ansaid Tablets (Less than 1%) ... 2579
Betagan ... ⊙ 233
▲ Betaseron for SC Injection (13%) .. 658
Blocadren Tablets (Less than 1%) 1614
Capoten ... 739
Capozide ... 742
▲ CellCept Capsules (More than or equal to 3%) ... 2099
Cuprimine Capsules ... 1630
Cytovene (1% or less) ... 2103
Depen Titratable Tablets ... 2662
Effexor (Infrequent) ... 2719
Eskalith (Rare) ... 2485
Lamictal Tablets (1.3%) ... 1112
Lopid Tablets ... 1917
Luvox Tablets (Infrequent) ... 2544
Myleran Tablets (Rare) ... 1143
Netromycin Injection 100 mg/ml ... 2373
Paxil Tablets (1.4%) ... 2505
▲ Prograf (Greater than 3%) ... 1042
Timolide Tablets ... 1748
Tonocard Tablets (Less than 1%) .. 531

Myasthenia gravis, exacerbation of

Betoptic Ophthalmic Solution (Rare) ... 469
Betoptic S Ophthalmic Suspension 471
Chibroxin Sterile Ophthalmic Solution (With oral form) ... 1617
Cipro I.V. ... 595
Cipro I.V. Pharmacy Bulk Package (Less than 1%) ... 597
Cipro Tablets ... 592
Floxin I.V. (Possible) ... 1571
Floxin Tablets (200 mg, 300 mg, 400 mg) ... 1567
Maxaquin Tablets ... 2440
Mefoxin (A possibility) ... 1691
Mefoxin Premixed Intravenous Solution ... 1694
Mykrox Tablets (exacerbation of) ... 993
Noroxin Tablets ... 1715
Noroxin Tablets ... 2048
Norpace ... 2444
Penetrex Tablets ... 2031
Timoptic Sterile Ophthalmic Solution (Less frequent) ... 1751
Timoptic-XE ... 1755

Myasthenia gravis, increase

Betimol 0.25%, 0.5% ... ⊙ 261
Timoptic in Ocudose (Less frequent) ... 1753

Myasthenia gravis-like syndrome

Achromycin V Capsules (Rare) ... 1367
Clozaril Tablets ... 2252
Garamycin Injectable ... 2360

Mydriasis

AK-CIDE (Occasional) ... ⊙ 202
AK-CIDE Ointment (Occasional) .. ⊙ 202
Albalon Solution with Liquifilm ... ⊙ 231
Anafranil Capsules (Up to 2%) ... 803
Arfonad Ampuls ... 2080
Artane ... 1368
Asendin Tablets (Less than 1%) ... 1369
Atamet ... 572
Atrohist Plus Tablets ... 454
Bentyl ... 1501
Betaseron for SC Injection ... 658
Blephamide Ointment (Occasional) ... ⊙ 237
Caverject (Less than 1%) ... 2583
Claritin-D (Less frequent) ... 2350
Clozaril Tablets (Less than 1%) ... 2252
Cocaine Hydrochloride Topical Solution ... 537
Cogentin ... 1621
Compazine ... 2470
Cystospaz ... 1963
Ditropan ... 1516
Donnatal ... 2060
Donnatal Extentabs ... 2061
Donnatal Tablets ... 2060
Dopram Injectable ... 2061
Econopred & Econopred Plus Ophthalmic Suspensions (Occasional) ... ⊙ 217
Effexor (2%) ... 2719
Elavil ... 2838
Endep Tablets ... 2174
Etrafon ... 2355
FML Forte Liquifilm (Occasional) ⊙ 240
FML Liquifilm (Occasional) ... ⊙ 241
FML S.O.P. (Occasional) ... ⊙ 241
Foscavir Injection (Less than 1%) .. 547
Healon GV ... ⊙ 315
Imitrex Tablets (Rare) ... 1106
Inversine Tablets ... 1686
IOPIDINE Sterile Ophthalmic Solution (0.4%) ... ⊙ 219
Kemadrin Tablets ... 1112
Kutrase Capsules ... 2402
Larodopa Tablets (Infrequent) ... 2129
Levsin/Levsinex/Levbid ... 2405
Limbitrol Tablets ... 2180
Lioresal Tablets ... 829
Ludiomil Tablets (Rare) ... 843
Luvox Tablets (Infrequent) ... 2544
Methadone Hydrochloride Oral Concentrate ... 2233
Navane Capsules and Concentrate 2201
Navane Intramuscular ... 2202
Norflex ... 1496
Norgesic ... 1496
Norpramin Tablets ... 1526
Orlamm ... 2239
Pamelor ... 2280
Paxil Tablets (Infrequent) ... 2505
Pro-Banthīne Tablets ... 2052
PROPINE with C CAP Compliance Cap (Infrequent) ... ⊙ 253
Proventil Syrup (Less than 1 of 100 patients) ... 2385
Prozac Pulvules & Liquid, Oral Solution (Infrequent) ... 919
Quarzan Capsules ... 2181
Quinaglute Dura-Tabs Tablets (Occasional) ... 649
Quinidex Extentabs ... 2067
Robinul Forte Tablets ... 2072
Robinul Injectable ... 2072
Robinul Tablets ... 2072
Sansert Tablets ... 2295
Serzone Tablets (Infrequent) ... 771
Sinemet Tablets ... 943
Soma Compound w/Codeine Tablets (Very rare) ... 2676

(▣ Described in PDR For Nonprescription Drugs) Incidence data in parenthesis; ▲ 3% or more (⊙ Described in PDR For Ophthalmology)

Soma Compound Tablets (Very rare) ... 2675
Soma Tablets ... 2674
Stelazine ... 2514
Surmontil Capsules ... 2811
Testoderm Testosterone Transdermal System (One in 104 patients) ... 486
Thorazine ... 2523
Tofranil Ampuls ... 854
Tofranil Tablets ... 856
Tofranil-PM Capsules ... 857
Transderm Scōp Transdermal Therapeutic System ... 869
Triavil Tablets ... 1757
Trilafon (Occasional) ... 2389
Trinalin Repetabs Tablets ... 1330
Vasocidin Ointment (Occasional) ◉ 268
Vasocidin Ophthalmic Solution (Occasional) ◉ 270
Ventolin Syrup (Less than 1 of 100 patients) ... 1202
Vivactil Tablets ... 1774
Wellbutrin Tablets (Infrequent) ... 1204
Zoloft Tablets (Infrequent) ... 2217

Myelitis

Havrix (Rare) ... 2489
Paxil Tablets (Rare) ... 2505
Permax Tablets (Rare) ... 575
Recombivax HB ... 1744

Myelitis, transverse

Asacol Delayed-Release Tablets (Rare) ... 1979
Azulfidine (Rare) ... 1949
Cytovene-IV (Two or more reports) 2103
Engerix-B Unit-Dose Vials ... 2482
JE-VAX (One case) ... 886
Recombivax HB ... 1744

Myelodysplastic syndrome

Azulfidine (Rare) ... 1949
Neupogen for Injection (Approximately 3%) ... 495

Myelofibrosis

Mexitil Capsules (About 2 in 10,000) ... 678

Myelopathy, dorsal column

Platinol ... 708
Platinol-AQ Injection ... 710

Myelosuppression

Adriamycin PFS ... 1947
Adriamycin RDF ... 1947
Alkeran for Injection ... 1070
▲ BiCNU (Most frequent) ... 691
CeeNU ... 693
▲ Cerubidine (All patients) ... 795
Cytosar-U Sterile Powder ... 2592
Doxorubicin Astra ... 540
▲ Fludara for Injection (Among most common) ... 663
Hexalen Capsules ... 2571
Idamycin ... 1955
IFEX ... 697
Leukeran Tablets ... 1133
Leustatin (Frequent) ... 1834
Mutamycin ... 703
▲ Myleran Tablets (Most frequent) ... 1143
▲ Navelbine Injection (53%) ... 1145
Novantrone ... 1279
▲ Platinol (25% to 30%) ... 708
▲ Platinol-AQ Injection (25% to 30% of patients) ... 710
Purinethol Tablets ... 1156
Roferon-A Injection (Rare) ... 2145
Rubex ... 712
▲ Thioguanine Tablets, Tabloid Brand (Most frequent) ... 1181
Velban Vials ... 1484
VePesid Capsules and Injection ... 718
▲ Vumon (75%) ... 727
Zinecard ... 1961

Myelosuppression, persistent severe

Adriamycin PFS ... 1947
Adriamycin RDF ... 1947
Novantrone ... 1279

Myocardial failure

Protamine Sulfate Ampoules & Vials ... 1471

Myocardial infarction

Abbokinase (Rare) ... 403
Abbokinase Open-Cath (Rare) ... 405
Accupril Tablets (Rare) ... 1893
Actimmune (Rare) ... 1056
Activase ... 1058
▲ Adalat Capsules (10 mg and 20 mg) (About 4%) ... 587
Adenoscan (Less than 1%) ... 1024
Altace Capsules (Less than 1% to 1.7%) ... 1232
Ambien Tablets (Rare) ... 2416
Anafranil Capsules (Rare) ... 803
Ansaid Tablets (Less than 1%) ... 2579
Asendin Tablets (Very rare) ... 1369
Atretol Tablets ... 573
Betaseron for SC Injection ... 658
Blenoxane (Rare) ... 692
Brevicon ... 2088
BuSpar (Rare) ... 737
Calan SR Caplets (1% or less) ... 2422
Calan Tablets (1% or less) ... 2419
Capoten (2 to 3 of 1000 patients) 739
Capozide (2 to 3 of 1000 patients) ... 742
Cardene Capsules (Less than 0.4%) ... 2095
Cardene I.V. ... 2709
Cardizem CD Capsules (Infrequent) ... 1506
Cardura Tablets (Less than 0.5% of 3960 patients) ... 2186
Cartrol Tablets ... 410
Cataflam (Less than 1%) ... 816
Cipro I.V. (1% or less) ... 595
Cipro I.V. Pharmacy Bulk Package (Less than 1%) ... 597
Cipro Tablets (Less than 1%) ... 592
Climara Transdermal System ... 645
Clozaril Tablets ... 2252
Cognex Capsules (Infrequent) ... 1901
Cozaar Tablets (Less than 1%) ... 1628
Cytovene-IV (Two or more reports) 2103
DDAVP Injection (Rare) ... 2014
DDAVP Injection 15 mcg/mL (Rare) ... 2015
D.H.E. 45 Injection (Extremely rare) ... 2255
Demulen ... 2428
Desogen Tablets ... 1817
Desyrel and Desyrel Dividose ... 503
Dilacor XR Extended-release Capsules ... 2018
Diprivan Injection (Less than 1%) .. 2833
DynaCirc Capsules (0.5% to 1%) .. 2256
Elavil ... 2838
▲ Emcyt Capsules (3%) ... 1953
Endep Tablets ... 2174
Epogen for Injection (0.4%) ... 489
Estrace Cream and Tablets ... 749
Estraderm Transdermal System ... 824
ESTRATAB Tablets (0.3, 0.625, 1.25, 2.5 mg) ... 2536
Estratest ... 2539
Ethmozine Tablets (Less than 2%) 2041
Etrafon ... 2355
Flexeril Tablets (Rare) ... 1661
Fludara for Injection (Up to 3%) ... 663
Glucophage ... 752
Heparin Lock Flush Solution ... 2725
Heparin Sodium Injection ... 2726
Heparin Sodium Injection, USP, Sterile Solution ... 2615
Heparin Sodium Vials ... 1441
Hyperstat I.V. Injection ... 2363
Hyzaar Tablets ... 1677
Idamycin ... 1955
Imdur (Less than or equal to 5%) .. 1323
Imitrex Injection (Rare) ... 1103
Imitrex Tablets (Rare) ... 1106
Isoptin Oral Tablets (Less than 1%) ... 1346
Isoptin SR Tablets (1% or less) ... 1348
Kerlone Tablets (Less than 2%) ... 2436
Lamictal Tablets (Rare) ... 1112
Levlen/Tri-Levlen ... 651
Limbitrol ... 2180
Lodine Capsules and Tablets (Less than 1%) ... 2743
Lo/Ovral Tablets ... 2746
Lo/Ovral-28 Tablets ... 2751
Lotrel Capsules (Rare) ... 840
Ludiomil Tablets (Isolated reports) 843
Lupron Depot 3.75 mg ... 2556
Lupron Depot 7.5 mg ... 2559
Lupron Injection (Less than 5%) ... 2555
Luvox Tablets (Infrequent) ... 2544
Maxaquin Tablets (Less than 1%) .. 2440
Menest Tablets ... 2494
Methergine (Rare) ... 2272
Miacalcin Nasal Spray (Less than 1%) ... 2275
Micronor Tablets ... 1872
Modicon ... 1872
Monoket (Fewer than 1%) ... 2406
Mononine, Coagulation Factor IX (Human) ... 523
Monopril Tablets (0.2% to 1.0%) .. 757
Navelbine Injection (Rare) ... 1145
Neoral (Rare) ... 2276
Neupogen for Injection (2.9% of cancer patients) ... 495
Neurontin Capsules (Rare) ... 1922
Nicorette ... 2458
Nordette-21 Tablets ... 2755
Nordette-28 Tablets ... 2758
Norinyl ... 2088
Normodyne Injection ... 2377
Normodyne Tablets ... 2379
Noroxin Tablets (Less frequent) ... 1715
Noroxin Tablets (Less frequent) ... 2048
Norplant System ... 2759
Norpramin Tablets ... 1526
Nor-Q D Tablets ... 2135
Norvasc Tablets ... 1940
Nuromax Injection (Less than or equal to 0.1%) ... 1149
Ogen Tablets ... 2627
Ogen Vaginal Cream ... 2630
Oncovin Solution Vials & Hyporets 1466
OptiPranolol (Metipranolol 0.3%) Sterile Ophthalmic Solution (A small number of patients) ... ◉ 258
Ortho-Cept ... 1851
Ortho-Cyclen/Ortho-Tri-Cyclen ... 1858
Ortho Dienestrol Cream ... 1866
Ortho-Est ... 1869
Ortho-Novum ... 1872
Ortho-Cyclen/Ortho Tri-Cyclen ... 1858
Orthoclone OKT3 Sterile Solution ... 1837
Orudis Capsules (Rare) ... 2766
Oruvail Capsules (Rare) ... 2766
Ovcon ... 760
Ovral Tablets ... 2770
Ovral-28 Tablets ... 2770
Ovrette Tablets ... 2771
PMB 200 and PMB 400 ... 2783
Pamelor ... 2280
Parlodel (9 cases) ... 2281
Paxil Tablets (Rare) ... 2505
Permax Tablets (1.1%) ... 575
Platinol (Rare) ... 708
Platinol-AQ Injection (Rare) ... 710
Plendil Extended-Release Tablets (0.5% to 1.5%) ... 527
Premarin Intravenous ... 2787
Premarin with Methyltestosterone .. 2794
Premarin Tablets ... 2789
Premarin Vaginal Cream ... 2791
PREVACID Delayed-Release Capsules (Less than 1%) ... 2562
Prinivil Tablets (0.3% to 1.3%) ... 1733
Prinzide Tablets ... 1737
▲ Procardia Capsules (About 4%; rare; about 1 patient in 15) ... 1971
Procardia XL Extended Release Tablets (About 1 patient in 15; about 4%; rare) ... 1972
Procrit for Injection (0.4%) ... 1841
Proleukin for Injection (2%) ... 797
Prostin E2 Suppository (Two cases) ... 2634
Prozac Pulvules & Liquid, Oral Solution (Rare) ... 919
Relafen Tablets (Less than 1%) ... 2510
Risperdal (Infrequent) ... 1301
Roferon-A Injection (Less than 1%) ... 2145
Salagen Tablets (One patient) ... 1489
Sandimmune (Rare) ... 2286
Sinemet CR Tablets ... 944
Stilphostrol Tablets and Ampuls ... 612
Stimate, (desmopressin acetate) Nasal Spray, 1.5 mg/mL (Rare) .. 525
Suprane (Less than 1%) ... 1813
Surmontil Capsules ... 2811
Tegretol ... 852
Tenex Tablets (Rare) ... 2074
Tofranil Ampuls ... 854
Tofranil Tablets ... 856
Tofranil-PM Capsules ... 857
Tonocard Tablets (Less than 1%) .. 531
Toprol-XL Tablets (Some cases) ... 565
▲ Trasylol (11%) ... 613
Triavil Tablets ... 1757
Levlen/Tri-Levlen ... 651
Tri-Norinyl ... 2164
Triostat Injection (Approximately 2%) ... 2530
Triphasil-21 Tablets ... 2814
Triphasil-28 Tablets ... 2819
Univasc Tablets (Less than 1%) ... 2410
Vascor (200, 300 and 400 mg) Tablets (About 3% of patients) .. 1587
Vaseretic Tablets ... 1765
Vasotec I.V. (0.5 to 1%) ... 1768
Vasotec Tablets (0.5% to 1.2%) ... 1771
Velban Vials ... 1484
Verelan Capsules (1% or less) ... 1410
Verelan Capsules (Less than 1%) .. 2824
Videx Tablets, Powder for Oral Solution, & Pediatric Powder for Oral Solution (Less than 1%) ... 720
Vivactil Tablets ... 1774
Voltaren Tablets (Less than 1%) ... 861
Wellbutrin Tablets (Rare) ... 1204
Zestoretic ... 2850
Zestril Tablets (0.3% to 1.3%) ... 2854
▲ Zoladex (Greater than 1% but less than 5%) ... 2858
Zoloft Tablets (Rare) ... 2217
Zosyn (1.0% or less) ... 1419
Zosyn Pharmacy Bulk Package (1.0% or less) ... 1422

Myocardial infarction, post-abrupt discontinuation

Inderal (Some cases) ... 2728
Inderal LA Long Acting Capsules (Some cases) ... 2730
Tenoretic Tablets ... 2845
Tenormin Tablets and I.V. Injection 2847
Trandate ... 1185
Visken Tablets ... 2299

Myocardial insufficiency

Idamycin ... 1955
Orthoclone OKT3 Sterile Solution .. 1837

Myocardial necrosis

Cytoxan ... 694
NEOSAR Lyophilized/Neosar ... 1959

Myocardial rupture, following recent MI

Activase ... 1058
Cortone Acetate Sterile Suspension ... 1623
Cortone Acetate Tablets ... 1624
Dalalone D.P. Injectable ... 1011
Decadron Elixir ... 1633
Decadron Phosphate Injection ... 1637
Decadron Phosphate Respihaler ... 1642
Decadron Phosphate Turbinaire ... 1645
Decadron Phosphate with Xylocaine Injection, Sterile ... 1639
Decadron Tablets ... 1635
Decadron-LA Sterile Suspension ... 1646
Dexacort Phosphate in Respihaler .. 458
Dexacort Phosphate in Turbinaire .. 459
Hydeltrasol Injection, Sterile ... 1665
Hydeltra-T.B.A. Sterile Suspension 1667
Hydrocortone Acetate Sterile Suspension ... 1669
Hydrocortone Phosphate Injection, Sterile ... 1670
Hydrocortone Tablets ... 1672

Myocarditis

Aldoclor Tablets ... 1598
Aldomet Ester HCl Injection ... 1602
Aldomet Oral ... 1600
Aldoril Tablets ... 1604
Asacol Delayed-Release Tablets (Rare) ... 1979
Atgam Sterile Solution (Less than 5%) ... 2581
Cerubidine (Rare) ... 795
Clozaril Tablets ... 2252
Cytovene-IV (One report) ... 2103
Dipentum Capsules (One patient) .. 1951
Diphtheria and Tetanus Toxoids and Pertussis Vaccine Adsorbed USP (For Pediatric Use) (One report) ... 875
Gantrisin ... 2120
Pentasa (Infrequent) ... 1527
Proleukin for Injection (Less than 1% to 1%) ... 797
Risperdal (Rare) ... 1301

Myocarditis, allergic

Azo Gantanol Tablets ... 2080
Azo Gantrisin Tablets ... 2081
Azulfidine (Rare) ... 1949
Bactrim DS Tablets ... 2084
Bactrim I.V. Infusion ... 2082
Bactrim ... 2084
Fansidar Tablets ... 2114
Gantanol Tablets ... 2119
Septra ... 1174
Septra I.V. Infusion ... 1169
Septra I.V. Infusion ADD-Vantage Vials ... 1171
Septra ... 1174

(▣ Described in PDR For Nonprescription Drugs) Incidence data in parenthesis; ▲ 3% or more (◉ Described in PDR For Ophthalmology)

1365 **Side Effects Index** **Nasal congestion**

Myocarditis, hemorrhagic
Cytoxan 694
NEOSAR Lyophilized/Neosar 1959

Myocardium, depression
Carbocaine Hydrochloride Injection 2303
Decadron Phosphate with Xylocaine Injection, Sterile 1639
Marcaine Hydrochloride with Epinephrine 1:200,000 2316
Marcaine Hydrochloride Injection 2316
Marcaine Spinal 2319
Nesacaine Injections 554
Normodyne Tablets 2379
Novocain Hydrochloride for Spinal Anesthesia 2326
Pontocaine Hydrochloride for Spinal Anesthesia 2330
Sensorcaine 559

Myoclonia
Alfenta Injection 1286
▲ Anafranil Capsules (2% to 13%) 803
Chibroxin Sterile Ophthalmic Solution (With oral form) 1617
Clozaril Tablets (1%) 2252
Diprivan Injection (Less than 1%) 2833
Duramorph 962
Effexor (Infrequent) 2719
Eldepryl Tablets 2550
Imitrex Injection (Rare) 1103
Infumorph 200 and Infumorph 500 Sterile Solutions 965
Lamictal Tablets (Infrequent) 1112
Luvox Tablets (Frequent) 2544
Nardil (Common) 1920
Neurontin Capsules (Rare) 1922
Noroxin Tablets 1715
Noroxin Tablets 2048
Orthoclone OKT3 Sterile Solution 1837
Paxil Tablets (1.4%) 2505
Penetrex Tablets (Less than 1% but more than or equal to 0.1%) 2031
Permax Tablets (Infrequent) 575
Primaxin I.M. 1727
Primaxin I.V. (Less than 0.2%) 1729
▲ Prograf (Greater than 3%) 1042
Prozac Pulvules & Liquid, Oral Solution (2%) 919
Revex (Less than 1%) 1811
Serzone Tablets (Infrequent) 771
Wellbutrin Tablets (Frequent) 1204

Myoglobinemia
Anectine 1073

Myoglobinuria
Amicar Syrup, Tablets, and Injection (Rare) 1267
Anectine 1073
Haldol Decanoate 1577
Lescol Capsules 2267
Orap Tablets 1050
Pravachol (Rare) 765
Risperdal 1301
Zocor Tablets (Rare) 1775

Myopathy
Amicar Syrup, Tablets, and Injection (Occasional) 1267
Anafranil Capsules (Rare) 803
Atromid-S Capsules 2701
Betaseron for SC Injection 658
Cognex Capsules (Rare) 1901
Cortone Acetate Tablets 1624
Darvon-N/Darvocet-N 1433
Darvon 1435
Darvon-N Suspension & Tablets 1433
Decadron Phosphate Respihaler 1642
Decadron Phosphate Turbinaire 1645
Depo-Medrol Sterile Aqueous Suspension 2597
Hivid Tablets (Less than 1% to less than 3%) 2121
Hydeltrasol Injection, Sterile 1665
Intal Inhaler (Infrequent) 988
Lescol Capsules 2267
Lopid Tablets (Occasional) 1917
Luvox Tablets (Rare) 2544
Medrol 2621
Mevacor Tablets 1699
Normodyne Tablets (Less common) 2379
Paxil Tablets (2.4%) 2505
Pediapred Oral Liquid 995
Pravachol (Rare) 765
ReoPro Vials (0.4%) 1471
Retrovir Capsules 1158
Retrovir I.V. Infusion 1163
Retrovir Syrup 1158
Rifadin (Rare) 1528
Rifater (Rare) 1532
Solu-Cortef Sterile Powder 2641
Solu-Medrol Sterile Powder 2643
Trandate Tablets (Less common) 1185
Videx Tablets, Powder for Oral Solution, & Pediatric Powder for Oral Solution (2% to 4%) 720
Zocor Tablets 1775
Zyloprim Tablets (Less than 1%) 1226

Myopathy, steroid
Aristocort Suspension (Forte Parenteral) 1027
Aristocort Suspension (Intralesional) 1025
Aristocort Tablets 1022
Aristospan Suspension (Intra-articular) 1033
Aristospan Suspension (Intralesional) 1032
Celestone Soluspan Suspension 2347
CORTENEMA 2535
Cortone Acetate Sterile Suspension 1623
Dalalone D.P. Injectable 1011
Decadron Elixir 1633
Decadron Phosphate Injection 1637
Decadron Phosphate with Xylocaine Injection, Sterile 1639
Decadron Tablets 1635
Decadron-LA Sterile Suspension 1646
Deltasone Tablets 2595
Depo-Medrol Single-Dose Vial 2600
Dexacort Phosphate in Respihaler 458
Dexacort Phosphate in Turbinaire 459
Florinef Acetate Tablets 505
Hydeltra-T.B.A. Sterile Suspension 1667
Hydrocortone Acetate Sterile Suspension 1669
Hydrocortone Phosphate Injection, Sterile 1670
Hydrocortone Tablets 1672
Prelone Syrup 1787

Myopia
Floropryl Sterile Ophthalmic Ointment 1662
Humorsol Sterile Ophthalmic Solution 1664
Isopto Carpine Ophthalmic Solution ⊙ 223
MZM ⊙ 267
Neptazane Tablets 1388
Phospholine Iodide ⊙ 326
Pilocar ⊙ 268
Pilopine HS Ophthalmic Gel ⊙ 226
Zarontin Capsules 1928
Zarontin Syrup 1929

Myopia, transient
Combipres Tablets (Occasional) 677
Diamox Intravenous 1372
Diamox Sequels (Sustained Release) 1373
Diamox Tablets 1372
Glauctabs ⊙ 208

Myosis
Etrafon 2355
Trilafon 2389

Myositis
Anafranil Capsules (Rare) 803
Atromid-S Capsules 2701
Betaseron for SC Injection 658
Hivid Tablets (Less than 1% to less than 3%) 2121
Imdur (Less than or equal to 5%) 1323
Inocor Lactate Injection (1 case) 2309
Lopid Tablets 1917
Mycobutin Capsules (Less than 1%) 1957
Paxil Tablets (Rare) 2505
Permax Tablets (Infrequent) 575
Prozac Pulvules & Liquid, Oral Solution (Rare) 919
Retrovir Capsules 1158
Retrovir I.V. Infusion 1163
Retrovir Syrup 1158
Serevent Inhalation Aerosol (1% to 3%) 1176
Ticlid Tablets (Rare) 2156
Vaseretic Tablets 1765
Vasotec I.V. 1768
Vasotec Tablets (0.5% to 1.0%) 1771
Videx Tablets, Powder for Oral Solution, & Pediatric Powder for Oral Solution (Less than 1%) 720

Myxedema
Eskalith 2485
Lithium Carbonate Capsules & Tablets 2230
Lithonate/Lithotabs/Lithobid 2543
Quadrinal Tablets 1350
SSKI Solution 2658

N

Nails, changes
Accutane Capsules (Less than 1%) 2076
Ansaid Tablets (Less than 1%) 2579
Blenoxane 692
BuSpar (Rare) 737
Cytoxan 694
Effexor (Infrequent) 2719
Ergamisol Tablets 1292
Fluorouracil Injection 2116
Sterile FUDR (Remote possibility) 2118
Hivid Tablets (Less than 1% to less than 3%) 2121
Intron A (Less than 5%) 2364
Lescol Capsules 2267
Lupron Depot 3.75 mg (Less than 5%) 2556
Mevacor Tablets 1699
NEOSAR Lyophilized/Neosar 1959
Oncaspar 2028
Pentasa (Less than 1%) 1527
Pravachol 765
Taxol (Uncommon; 2%) 714
▲ Tegison Capsules (10-25%) 2154
Teslac (Rare) 717
Zocor Tablets 1775

Nails, discoloration
Retrovir Capsules 1158
Retrovir I.V. Infusion 1163
Retrovir Syrup 1158

Nails, loss of
Fluorouracil Injection 2116
Sterile FUDR (Remote possibility) 2118

Nasal burning
▲ Beconase Inhalation Aerosol and Refill (11 in 100 patients) 1076
Duration 12 Hour Nasal Spray ▣ 805
▲ Flonase Nasal Spray (3% to 6%) 1098
Intal Inhaler (Rare) 988
Intal Nebulizer Solution 989
IOPIDINE Sterile Ophthalmic Solution ⊙ 219
Nasacort Nasal Inhaler (Rare) 2024
▲ Nasalcrom Nasal Solution (1 in 25) 994
▲ Nasalide Nasal Solution 0.025% (Approximately 45%) 2110
▲ Nasarel Nasal Solution (13% to 44%) 2133
Neo-Synephrine Maximum Strength 12 Hour Nasal Spray ▣ 726
Neo-Synephrine 12 Hour ▣ 726
Neo-Synephrine ▣ 726
Rhinocort Nasal Inhaler (Rare) 556
▲ Vancenase PocketHaler Nasal Inhaler (11 per 100 patients) 2391
Vicks Sinex Nasal Spray and Ultra Fine Mist ▣ 765

Nasal congestion
▲ Adalat Capsules (10 mg and 20 mg) (2% or less to 6%) 587
Adenoscan (Less than 1%) 1024
▲ AeroBid Inhaler System (15%) 1005
▲ Aerobid-M Inhaler System (15%) 1005
Airet Solution for Inhalation (1%) 452
Aldoclor Tablets 1598
Aldomet Ester HCl Injection 1602
Aldomet Oral 1600
Aldoril Tablets 1604
Apresazide Capsules (Less frequent) 808
Apresoline Hydrochloride Tablets (Less frequent) 809
Asacol Delayed-Release Tablets 1979
Azactam for Injection (Less than 1%) 734
Bentyl 1501
Betagan ⊙ 233
Betimol 0.25%, 0.5% ⊙ 261
Brevibloc Injection (Less than 1%) 1808
BuSpar (Frequent) 737
Cardizem CD Capsules (Less than 1%) 1506
Cardizem SR Capsules (Less than 1%) 1510
Cardizem Injectable 1508
Cardizem Tablets (Less than 1%) 1512
Cartrol Tablets (1.1%) 410
Caverject (1%) 2583
▲ CHEMET (succimer) Capsules (0.7 to 3.7%) 1545
Claritin (2% or fewer patients) 2349
Claritin-D (Less frequent) 2350
Clozaril Tablets (1%) 2252
Comhist 2038
Compazine 2470
Cozaar Tablets (2.0%) 1628
DDAVP (Occasional) 2017
Danocrine Capsules (Rare) 2307
Demser Capsules (Infrequent) 1649
Desmopressin Acetate Rhinal Tube (Occasional) 979
Desyrel and Desyrel Dividose (2.8% to 5.7%) 503
Dibenzyline Capsules 2476
Diupres Tablets 1650
Esgic-plus Tablets (Infrequent) 1013
Esimil Tablets 822
Etrafon 2355
Fioricet Tablets (Infrequent) 2258
Fioricet with Codeine Capsules (Infrequent) 2260
Fiorinal with Codeine Capsules (Infrequent) 2262
Flagyl 375 Capsules 2434
Flagyl I.V. 2247
Flonase Nasal Spray (Less than 1%) 1098
Hydropres Tablets 1675
Hyskon Hysteroscopy Fluid (Rare) 1595
▲ Hytrin Capsules (1.9% to 5.9%) 430
Hyzaar Tablets 1677
Imdur (Less than or equal to 5%) 1323
Intal Capsules (Less than 1 in 10,000 patients) 987
▲ Intal Inhaler (Among most frequent) 988
Intal Nebulizer Solution (Rare) 989
▲ Intron A (Up to 10%) 2364
Ismelin Tablets 827
Levoprome (Sometimes) 1274
Limbitrol (Less common) 2180
Lioresal Tablets 829
Loxitane 1378
Ludiomil Tablets (Rare) 843
Methergine (Rare) 2272
MetroGel-Vaginal 902
▲ Miacalcin Nasal Spray (10.6%) 2275
Midamor Tablets (Less than or equal to 1%) 1703
Minipress Capsules (1-4%) 1937
Minizide Capsules 1938
Moduretic Tablets (Less than or equal to 1%) 1705
Nasalcrom Nasal Solution (Less than 1%) 994
Nasalide Nasal Solution 0.025% (5% or less) 2110
Navane Capsules and Concentrate 2201
Navane Intramuscular 2202
Orlamm 2239
Ornade Spansule Capsules 2502
Orthoclone OKT3 Sterile Solution 1837
Pentaspan Injection 937
Periactin 1724
Phrenilin (Infrequent) 785
Prinivil Tablets (0.4%) 1733
Prinzide Tablets (0.3% to 1%) 1737
▲ Procardia Capsules (2% or less to 6%) 1971
▲ Procardia XL Extended Release Tablets (6%) 1972
Prolixin 509
Protostat Tablets 1883
Proventil Inhalation Solution 0.083% (1%) 2384
Proventil Solution for Inhalation 0.5% (1%) 2383
Prozac Pulvules & Liquid, Oral Solution (2.6%) 919
Regitine 846
ReVia Tablets (Less than 1%) 940
Robaxin Injectable 2070
Robaxin Tablets 2071
Sedapap Tablets 50 mg/650 mg (Infrequent) 1543
Ser-Ap-Es Tablets 849
▲ Stadol (13%) 775
Stelazine 2514
Stimate, (desmopressin acetate) Nasal Spray, 1.5 mg/mL (Occasional) 525
Tavist Syrup 2297
Tavist Tablets 2298
Tessalon Perles 1020
Thorazine 2523
Timoptic in Ocudose (Less frequent) 1753
Timoptic Sterile Ophthalmic Solution (Less frequent) 1751

(▣ Described in PDR For Nonprescription Drugs) Incidence data in parenthesis; ▲ 3% or more (⊙ Described in PDR For Ophthalmology)

Nasal congestion | Side Effects Index | 1366

Timoptic-XE ... 1755
Trental Tablets (Less than 1%) ... 1244
Trilafon (Occasional) ... 2389
Ventolin Inhalation Solution (1%) .. 1198
Ventolin Nebules Inhalation Solution (1%) ... 1199
Ventolin Rotacaps for Inhalation (2%) ... 1200
▲ Xanax Tablets (7.3% to 17.4%) ... 2649
Zestoretic (0.3 to 1%) ... 2850
Zestril Tablets (0.4%) ... 2854

Nasal discharge, increase
IOPIDINE Sterile Ophthalmic Solution (0.45%) ... ⊙ 219
▲ Miacalcin Nasal Spray (10.6%) ... 2275
Neo-Synephrine Maximum Strength 12 Hour Nasal Spray ... ▣ 726
Neo-Synephrine 12 Hour ... ▣ 726
Neo-Synephrine ... ▣ 726
Vicks Sinex Nasal Spray and Ultra Fine Mist ... ▣ 765

Nasal itching (see under Pruritus, rhinal)

Nasal mucosa, dryness (see under Xeromycteria)

Nasal septum, perforation
Beconase (Rare) ... 1076
Decadron Phosphate Turbinaire ... 1645
Dexacort Phosphate in Turbinaire .. 459
Nasalide Nasal Solution 0.025% (Rare) ... 2110
Nasarel Nasal Solution (Rare) ... 2133
Rhinocort Nasal Inhaler (Less than 1%) ... 556
Vancenase AQ Nasal Spray 0.042% (Extremely rare) ... 2393
Vancenase PocketHaler Nasal Inhaler (Extremely rare) ... 2391

Nasal stinging
Duration 12 Hour Nasal Spray ... ▣ 805
Nasacort Nasal Inhaler (Rare) ... 2024
▲ Nasalcrom Nasal Solution (1 in 20) ... 994
▲ Nasarel Nasal Solution (13% to 44%) ... 2133
Neo-Synephrine Maximum Strength 12 Hour Nasal Spray ▣ 726
Neo-Synephrine 12 Hour ... ▣ 726
Neo-Synephrine ... ▣ 726
Vicks Sinex Nasal Spray and Ultra Fine Mist ... ▣ 765

Nasal stuffiness
Actifed with Codeine Cough Syrup .. 1067
Amicar Syrup, Tablets, and Injection (Occasional) ... 1267
Asendin Tablets (Less than 1%) ... 1369
Beconase AQ Nasal Spray (Fewer than 3 per 100 patients) ... 1076
Benadryl Capsules ... 1898
Benadryl Injection ... 1898
Bentyl ... 1501
Deconamine ... 1320
Loxitane ... 1378
Mellaril ... 2269
▲ Normodyne Injection (1% to 6%) .. 2377
▲ Normodyne Tablets (1% to 6%) ... 2379
PBZ Tablets ... 845
PBZ-SR Tablets ... 844
▲ Parlodel (3% to 4%) ... 2281
Phenergan Injection ... 2773
Phenergan Tablets ... 2775
Serentil ... 684
Temaril Tablets, Syrup and Spansule Extended-Release Capsules ... 483
▲ Trandate Tablets (1% to 6%) ... 1185
Trinalin Repetabs Tablets ... 1330
Tussend ... 1783
Vancenase AQ Nasal Spray 0.042% (Fewer than 3 per 100 patients) ... 2393

Nasal ulceration
Beconase (Rare) ... 1076
Flonase Nasal Spray (Less than 1%) ... 1098
Nasarel Nasal Solution (1% or less) ... 2133
Vancenase PocketHaler Nasal Inhaler (Rare) ... 2391

Nasolacrimal canals, obstruction
Floropryl Sterile Ophthalmic Ointment ... 1662
Humorsol Sterile Ophthalmic Solution ... 1664
Phospholine Iodide ... ⊙ 326

Nasopharyngitis
Hivid Tablets (Less than 1% to less than 3%) ... 2121
Nalfon 200 Pulvules & Nalfon Tablets (1.2%) ... 917
▲ Serevent Inhalation Aerosol (14%) 1176

Nausea
Abbokinase ... 403
Abbokinase Open-Cath ... 405
Accupril Tablets (1.4% to 2.4%) .. 1893
Accutane Capsules ... 2076
Achromycin V Capsules (Rare) ... 1367
Actifed with Codeine Cough Syrup .. 1067
Actigall Capsules ... 802
▲ Actimmune (10%) ... 1056
Activase ... 1058
▲ Adalat Capsules (10 mg and 20 mg) (About 10% to 11%) ... 587
Adalat CC (2%) ... 589
▲ Adenocard Injection (3%) ... 1021
Adriamycin PFS (Frequent) ... 1947
Adriamycin RDF (Frequent) ... 1947
▲ Children's Advil Suspension (Up to 9%) ... 2692
▲ AeroBid Inhaler System (25%) ... 1005
▲ Aerobid-M Inhaler System (25%) .. 1005
Aerolate ... 1004
▲ Airet Solution for Inhalation (3.1 to 4%) ... 452
AK-Fluor Injection 10% and 25% ... ⊙ 203
Albalon Solution with Liquifilm ... ⊙ 231
Albuminar-5, Albumin (Human) U.S.P. 5% (Occasional) ... 512
Albuminar-25, Albumin (Human) U.S.P. 25% ... 513
Aldactazide ... 2413
Aldoclor Tablets ... 1598
Aldomet Ester HCl Injection ... 1602
Aldomet Oral ... 1600
Aldoril Tablets ... 1604
▲ Alfenta Injection (28%) ... 1286
▲ Alka-Seltzer Effervescent Antacid and Pain Reliever (7.6% at doses of 1000 mg/day) ... ▣ 701
▲ Alka-Seltzer Lemon Lime Effervescent Antacid and Pain Reliever (7.6% at doses of 1000 mg/day) ... ▣ 703
Alkeran for Injection ... 1070
Alkeran Tablets (Infrequent) ... 1071
Alomide (Less than 1%) ... 469
Altace Capsules (Less than 1% to 2.2%) ... 1232
Alupent (1% to 4%) ... 669
▲ Ambien Tablets (2% to 6%) ... 2416
Amen Tablets (Rare) ... 780
Amicar Syrup, Tablets, and Injection (Occasional) ... 1267
Amikacin Sulfate Injection, USP (Rare) ... 960
Amikin Injectable (Rare) ... 501
Aminohippurate Sodium Injection .. 1606
Amoxil ... 2464
▲ Anafranil Capsules (9% to 33%) ... 803
Ana-Kit Anaphylaxis Emergency Treatment Kit (Common) ... 617
▲ Anaprox/Naprosyn (3% to 9%) ... 2117
Anatuss LA Tablets ... 1542
Ancef Injection (Rare) ... 2465
Ancobon Capsules ... 2079
▲ Android Capsules, 10 mg (Among most common) ... 1250
Android ... 1251
▲ Anexsia 5/500 Elixir (Among most frequent) ... 1781
▲ Ansaid Tablets (3-9%) ... 2579
Antabuse Tablets ... 2695
Antilirium Injectable ... 1009
Antivenin (Crotalidae) Polyvalent ... 2696
Apresazide Capsules (Common) ... 808
Apresoline Hydrochloride Tablets (Common) ... 809
Aralen Hydrochloride Injection ... 2301
Aralen Phosphate Tablets ... 2301
▲ Aredia for Injection (Up to 18%) ... 810
Arfonad Ampuls ... 2080
▲ Artane (30% to 50%) ... 1368
▲ Asacol Delayed-Release Tablets (13%) ... 1979
▲ Regular Strength Ascriptin Tablets (7.6%) ... ▣ 629
Asendin Tablets (Less frequent) ... 1369
Astramorph/PF Injection, USP (Preservative-Free) (Frequent) ... 535
Atamet (Common) ... 572
▲ Atgam Sterile Solution (1 patient in 15; more than 1% to 10%) ... 2581
Ativan Injection (Occasional) ... 2698
Ativan Tablets (Less frequent) ... 2700
▲ Atretol Tablets (Among most frequent) ... 573
Atrohist Pediatric Capsules ... 453
Atrohist Plus Tablets ... 454
▲ Atromid-S Capsules (Most common) ... 2701
Atrovent Inhalation Aerosol (2.8%) ... 671
▲ Atrovent Inhalation Solution (4.1%) ... 673
▲ Augmentin (3%) ... 2468
▲ Axid Pulvules (1.2% to 5.4%) ... 1427
Azactam for Injection (1 to 1.3%) .. 734
Azo Gantanol Tablets ... 2080
Azo Gantrisin Tablets ... 2081
▲ Azulfidine (Approximately one-third of patients) ... 1949
▲ BCG Vaccine, USP (TICE) (3.0%) .. 1814
▲ Bactrim DS Tablets (Among most common) ... 2084
▲ Bactrim I.V. Infusion (Among most common) ... 2082
▲ Bactrim (Among most common) ... 2084
Bactroban Ointment (Less than 1%) ... 2470
▲ Genuine Bayer Aspirin Tablets & Caplets (7.6% at doses of 1000 mg/day) ... ▣ 713
▲ Aspirin Regimen Bayer Regular Strength 325 mg Caplets (7.6% of 4500 people tested) ... ▣ 709
▲ Beconase AQ Nasal Spray (Fewer than 5 in 100 patients) ... 1076
Benadryl Capsules ... 1898
Benadryl Injection ... 1898
Benemid Tablets ... 1611
▲ Bentyl (14%) ... 1501
Betagan ... ⊙ 233
▲ Betapace Tablets (5% to 10%) ... 641
Betaseron for SC Injection ... 658
Betimol 0.25%, 0.5% (1% to 5%) ... ⊙ 261
Biavax II ... 1613
▲ Biaxin (3%) ... 405
BiCNU (Frequent) ... 691
Biltricide Tablets ... 591
Bioclate, Antihemophilic Factor (Recombinant) (Extremely rare; one patient out of 13,394) ... 513
Blocadren Tablets (0.6%) ... 1614
Bontril Slow-Release Capsules ... 781
Brethaire Inhaler ... 813
Brethine Ampuls (1.3 to 3.9%) ... 815
Brethine Tablets ... 814
▲ Brevibloc Injection (7%) ... 1808
Brevicon ... 2088
Brevital Sodium Vials ... 1429
Bricanyl Subcutaneous Injection ... 1502
Bricanyl Tablets ... 1503
Bromfed ... 1785
▲ Bromfed-DM Cough Syrup (Among most frequent) ... 1786
Bromfed-PD Capsules (Extended-Release) ... 1785
Bronkaid Caplets ... ▣ 717
Bronkometer Aerosol ... 2302
Bronkosol Solution ... 2302
Brontex ... 1981
▲ Bufferin Analgesic Tablets and Caplets (7.6%) ... ▣ 613
Bumex (0.6%) ... 2093
▲ Buprenex Injectable (5-10%) ... 2006
▲ BuSpar (8%) ... 737
Butisol Sodium Elixir & Tablets (Less than 1 in 100) ... 2660
Cafergot ... 2251
Calan SR Caplets (2.7%) ... 2422
Calan Tablets (2.7%) ... 2419
▲ Calcimar Injection, Synthetic (About 10%) ... 2013
Capoten (About 0.5 to 2%) ... 739
Capozide (0.5 to 2%) ... 742
Carafate Suspension (Less than 0.5%) ... 1505
Carafate Tablets (Less than 0.5%) 1504
Carbocaine Hydrochloride Injection 2303
Cardene Capsules (1.9-2.2%) ... 2095
▲ Cardene I.V. (4.9%) ... 2709
Cardene SR Capsules (1.9%) ... 2097
Cardizem CD Capsules (1.4%) ... 1506
Cardizem SR Capsules (1.3% to 1.6%) ... 1510
Cardizem Injectable (Less than 1%) ... 1508
Cardizem Tablets (1.9%) ... 1512
Cardura Tablets (1.5% to 3%) ... 2186
Carnitor Injection (Less frequent) .. 2452
Carnitor Tablets and Solution ... 2453
Cartrol Tablets (2.1%) ... 410
▲ Cataflam (3% to 9%) ... 816
Catapres Tablets (About 5 in 100 patients) ... 674
Catapres-TTS (1 of 101 patients; less frequent) ... 675
Caverject (Less than 1%) ... 2583
Ceclor Pulvules & Suspension (Rare) ... 1431
CeeNU ... 693
Cefizox for Intramuscular or Intravenous Use (Occasional) ... 1034
Cefobid Intravenous/Intramuscular (Rare) ... 2189
Cefobid Pharmacy Bulk Package - Not for Direct Infusion (Rare) ... 2192
▲ Cefotan (Among most frequent; 1 in 700) ... 2829
▲ Ceftin (2.6% to 6.7%) ... 1078
▲ Cefzil Tablets and Oral Suspension (3.5%) ... 746
▲ CellCept Capsules (19.9% to 23.6%) ... 2099
Celontin Kapseals (Frequent) ... 1899
Ceptaz (One in 156 patients) ... 1081
Ceredase ... 1065
Cerezyme (One patient) ... 1066
Cerubidine ... 795
Cervidil (Less than 1%) ... 1010
▲ CHEMET (succimer) Capsules (12-20.9%) ... 1545
Chloromycetin Sodium Succinate ... 1900
Chromagen Capsules ... 2339
Ciloxan Ophthalmic Solution (Less than 1%) ... 472
▲ Cipro I.V. (Among most frequent) .. 595
▲ Cipro I.V. Pharmacy Bulk Package (Among most frequent) ... 597
▲ Cipro Tablets (5.2%) ... 592
Claforan Sterile and Injection (1.4%; rare) ... 1235
Claritin (2% or fewer patients) ... 2349
▲ Claritin-D (3%) ... 2350
Cleocin Phosphate Injection ... 2586
Climara Transdermal System ... 645
Cleocin Vaginal Cream (Less than 1%) ... 2589
▲ Clinoril Tablets (3-9%) ... 1618
Clomid (2.2%) ... 1514
▲ Clozaril Tablets (5% or more) ... 2252
Codiclear DH Syrup ... 791
Cogentin ... 1621
▲ Cognex Capsules (28%) ... 1901
Colace ... 2044
ColBENEMID Tablets ... 1622
Colestid Tablets (Less frequent) ... 2591
▲ Colyte and Colyte-flavored (Among most frequent) ... 2396
▲ Combipres Tablets (About 5%) ... 677
Comhist ... 2038
Compazine ... 2470
▲ Cordarone Intravenous (3.9%) ... 2715
▲ Cordarone Tablets (10 to 33%) ... 2712
Cortone Acetate Sterile Suspension ... 1623
Cortone Acetate Tablets ... 1624
Cosmegen Injection (Common) ... 1626
Coumadin (Infrequent) ... 926
Cozaar Tablets (1% or greater) ... 1628
▲ Creon (Among most frequent) ... 2536
Crystodigin Tablets ... 1433
Cuprimine Capsules (Greater than 1%) ... 1630
Cycrin Tablets ... 975
Cyklokapron Tablets and Injection ... 1950
Cylert Tablets ... 412
▲ Cytadren Tablets (1 in 8) ... 819
CytoGam (Less than 5.0%) ... 1593
▲ Cytosar-U Sterile Powder (Among most frequent) ... 2592
▲ Cytotec (3.2%) ... 2424
▲ Cytovene (26%) ... 2103
Cytoxan (Common) ... 694
DDAVP Injection (Infrequent) ... 2014
DDAVP Injection 15 mcg/mL (Infrequent) ... 2015
DDAVP (Up to 2%) ... 2017
▲ DHCplus Capsules (Among most frequent) ... 1993
D.H.E. 45 Injection ... 2255
▲ DTIC-Dome (90% with the initial few doses) ... 600
Dalalone D.P. Injectable ... 1011
▲ Dalgan Injection (3 to 9%) ... 538
Dalmane Capsules ... 2173
Danocrine Capsules ... 2307
Dantrium Capsules (Less frequent) 1982
Dapsone Tablets USP ... 1284
▲ Daranide Tablets (Among the most common effects) ... 1633

(▣ Described in PDR For Nonprescription Drugs) Incidence data in parenthesis; ▲ 3% or more (⊙ Described in PDR For Ophthalmology)

1367 **Side Effects Index** **Nausea**

▲Darvon-N/Darvocet-N (Among most frequent) 1433
▲Darvon (Among most frequent) 1435
▲Darvon-N Suspension & Tablets (Among most frequent) 1433
▲Daypro Caplets (3% to 9%) 2426
Decadron Elixir 1633
Decadron Phosphate Injection 1637
Decadron Phosphate Respihaler 1642
Decadron Phosphate Turbinaire 1645
Decadron Phosphate with Xylocaine Injection, Sterile 1639
Decadron Tablets 1635
Decadron-LA Sterile Suspension 1646
Declomycin Tablets 1371
Deconamine Chewable Tablets 1320
Deconamine CX Cough and Cold Liquid and Tablets 1319
Deconamine 1320
Deconsal C Expectorant Syrup 456
Deconsal Pediatric Capsules 454
Deconsal Pediatric Syrup 457
Deconsal II Tablets 454
Delatestryl Injection 2860
Demadex Tablets and Injection (1.8%) 686
▲Demerol (Among most frequently observed) 2308
Demser Capsules (Infrequent) 1649
▲Demulen (Among most common) 2428
▲Depakene (Among most common) 413
▲Depakote Tablets (22%) 415
▲Depen Titratable Tablets (17%) 2662
▲Depo-Provera Contraceptive Injection (1% to 5%) 2602
Depo-Provera Sterile Aqueous Suspension 2606
Desmopressin Acetate Rhinal Tube (Up to 2%) 979
Desogen Tablets 1817
▲Desyrel and Desyrel Dividose (9.9% to 12.7%) 503
Dexacort Phosphate in Respihaler 458
Dexacort Phosphate in Turbinaire 459
▲DiaBeta Tablets (Among most common; 1.8%) 1239
▲Diabinese Tablets (Less than 5%) 1935
Diamox Intravenous 1372
Diamox Sequels (Sustained Release) 1373
Diamox Tablets 1372
Didrex Tablets 2607
▲Didronel Tablets (About 1 patient in 15; possibly 2 or 3 in 10) 1984
Diethylstilbestrol Tablets 1437
▲Diflucan Injection, Tablets, and Oral Suspension (2% to 7%) 2194
Dilacor XR Extended-release Capsules (1.7% to 2.2%) 2018
Dilantin Infatabs 1908
Dilantin Kapseals 1906
Dilantin Parenteral 1910
Dilantin-125 Suspension 1911
Dilatrate-SR (Uncommon) 2398
Dilaudid Ampules 1335
Dilaudid Cough Syrup 1336
▲Dilaudid-HP Injection (Among most frequent) 1337
▲Dilaudid-HP Lyophilized Powder 250 mg (Among most frequent) 1337
Dilaudid 1335
Dilaudid Oral Liquid 1339
Dilaudid 1335
Dilaudid Tablets - 8 mg 1339
Dimetane-DC Cough Syrup 2059
Dimetane-DX Cough Syrup 2059
▲Dipentum Capsules (5%) 1951
Diprivan Injection (Less than 1%) 2833
Ditropan 1516
Diucardin Tablets 2718
Diupres Tablets 1650
Diuril Oral Suspension 1653
Diuril Sodium Intravenous 1652
Diuril Tablets 1653
Dizac (Less frequent) 1809
Dobutrex Solution Vials (1% to 3%) 1439
▲Dolobid Tablets (3% to 9%) 1654
Donnatal 2060
Donnatal Extentabs 2061
Donnatal Tablets 2060
Dopram Injectable 2061
Doral Tablets 2664
Doryx Capsules 1913
Doxorubicin Astra (Frequent) 540
▲Duragesic Transdermal System (10% or more) 1288
Duramorph (Frequent) 962
Duratuss HD Elixir 2565
Dura-Vent Tablets 952
Duricef (Rare) 748
Duvoid (Infrequent) 2044
Dyazide 2479
Dynacin Capsules 1590
▲DynaCirc Capsules (1.0% to 5.1%) 2256
Dyrenium Capsules (Rare) 2481
E.E.S. 424
E-Mycin Tablets (Infrequent) 1341
Easprin 1914
▲EC-Naprosyn Delayed-Release Tablets (3% to 9%) 2117
▲Ecotrin (7.6% at 1000 mg/day) 2455
Edecrin 1657
▲Effexor (6% to 58.0%) 2719
Elavil 2838
▲Eldepryl Tablets (10 of 49 patients) 2550
Elspar 1659
▲Emcyt Capsules (15%) 1953
Emete-con Intramuscular/Intravenous 2198
▲Eminase (Less than 10%) 2039
▲Empirin with Codeine Tablets (Among most frequent) 1093
Endep Tablets 2174
Enduron Tablets 420
Engerix-B Unit-Dose Vials (Less than 1%) 2482
Ensure Plus High Calorie Complete Nutrition 2221
Entex Capsules 1986
Entex LA Tablets 1987
Entex Liquid 1986
Entex PSE Tablets 1987
EpiPen Jr. 790
▲Epogen for Injection (0.26% to 17%) 489
▲Ergamisol Tablets (22% to 65%) 1292
▲Ergomar (Up to 10%) 1486
▲ERYC (Among most frequent) 1915
▲EryPed (Among most frequent) 421
▲Ery-Tab Tablets (Among most frequent) 422
▲Erythrocin Stearate Filmtab (Among most frequent) 425
▲Erythromycin Base Filmtab (Among most frequent) 426
▲Erythromycin Delayed-Release Capsules, USP (Among most frequent) 427
▲Esgic-plus Tablets (Among most frequent) 1013
Esidrix Tablets 821
Esimil Tablets 822
Eskalith 2485
Estrace Cream and Tablets 749
Estraderm Transdermal System 824
ESTRATAB Tablets (0.3, 0.625, 1.25, 2.5 mg) 2536
Estratest 2539
▲Ethmozine Tablets (6.9% to 9.6%) 2041
Etrafon 2355
▲Eulexin Capsules (11% with LHRH agonist) 2358
Exgest LA Tablets 782
Factrel (Rare) 2877
▲Famvir (Among most frequent; 12.5%) 2486
Fansidar Tablets 2114
Fedahist Gyrocaps 2401
Fedahist Timecaps 2401
▲Felbatol (Among most common; 6.5% to 34.2%) 2666
▲Feldene Capsules (3% to 9%) 1965
Feosol Elixir (Occasional) 2456
Feosol Tablets (Occasional) 2457
▲Fioricet Tablets (Among most frequent) 2258
Fioricet with Codeine Capsules (Frequent) 2260
Fiorinal Capsules (Less frequent) 2261
▲Fiorinal with Codeine Capsules (3.7%) 2262
Fiorinal Tablets (Less frequent) 2261
▲Flagyl 375 Capsules (About 12%) 2434
Flagyl I.V. 2247
Flexeril Tablets (1% to 3%) 1661
Flonase Nasal Spray (Less than 1%) 1098
Floropryl Sterile Ophthalmic Ointment (Rare) 1662
▲Floxin I.V. (3% to 10%) 1571
▲Floxin Tablets (200 mg, 300 mg, 400 mg) (3% to 10%) 1567
▲Fludara for Injection (31% to 36%) 663
Flumadine Tablets & Syrup (2.8%) 1015
Fluorescite ⊙ 219
Fluorouracil Injection (Common) 2116
Fluothane 2724
Fortaz (1 in 156 patients) 1100
▲Foscavir Injection (5% or greater up to 47%) 547
▲Sterile FUDR (Among more common) 2118
Fulvicin P/G Tablets (Occasional) 2359
Fulvicin P/G 165 & 330 Tablets (Occasional) 2359
▲Fungizone Intravenous (Among most common) 506
Furoxone (Occasional) 2046
Gamimune N, 5% Immune Globulin Intravenous (Human), 5% 619
Gamimune N, 10% Immune Globulin Intravenous (Human), 10% 621
Gammagard S/D, Immune Globulin, Intravenous (Human) (Occasional) 585
Gammar I.V., Immune Globulin Intravenous (Human), Lyophilized 516
Ganite 2533
Gantanol Tablets 2119
Gantrisin 2120
Garamycin Injectable 2360
▲Gastrocrom Capsules (3 of 87 patients) 984
Geocillin Tablets 2199
Geref (sermorelin acetate for injection) 2876
Glauctabs ⊙ 208
Glucagon for Injection Vials and Emergency Kit (Occasional) 1440
▲Glucophage (Among most common) 752
Glucotrol Tablets (1 in 70) 1967
Glucotrol XL Extended Release Tablets (Less than 3%) 1968
Glynase PresTab Tablets (1.8%) 2609
▲GoLYTELY (Up to 50%) 688
Grifulvin V (griseofulvin tablets) Microsize (griseofulvin oral suspension) Microsize (Occasional) 1888
Gris-PEG Tablets, 125 mg & 250 mg (Occasional) 479
Guaifed 1787
Guaifed Syrup ▣ 734
Guaimax-D Tablets 792
▲Habitrol Nicotine Transdermal System (3% to 9% of patients) 865
▲Halcion Tablets (4.6%) 2611
Haldol Decanoate 1577
Haldol Injection, Tablets and Concentrate 1575
▲Halfprin (7.6%) 1362
Halotestin Tablets 2614
▲Havrix (1% to 10%) 2489
Heparin Lock Flush Solution 2725
Heparin Sodium Injection 2726
Heparin Sodium Injection, USP, Sterile Solution 2615
Heparin Sodium Vials (Rare) 1441
▲Hexalen Capsules (1% to 33%) 2571
Helixate, Antihemophilic Factor (Recombinant) 518
Hismanal Tablets (2.5%) 1293
Hivid Tablets (Less than 1% to less than 3%) 2121
Humatrope Vials (Small number of patients) 1443
Humegon 1824
Humorsol Sterile Ophthalmic Solution (Rare) 1664
Hycodan Tablets and Syrup 930
Hycomine Compound Tablets 932
Hycomine 931
Hycotuss Expectorant Syrup 933
Hydeltrasol Injection, Sterile 1665
Hydeltra-T.B.A. Sterile Suspension 1667
Hydergine 2265
Hydrea Capsules (Less frequent) 696
Hydrocet Capsules 782
Hydrocortone Acetate Sterile Suspension 1669
Hydrocortone Phosphate Injection, Sterile 1670
Hydrocortone Tablets 1672
HydroDIURIL Tablets 1674
Hydropres Tablets 1675
▲Hylorel Tablets (3.9%) 985
▲Hyperstat I.V. Injection (4%) 2363
Hyskon Hysteroscopy Fluid (Rare) 1595
▲Hytrin Capsules (0.5% to 4.4%) 430
Hyzaar Tablets (1% or greater) 1677
▲IBU Tablets (3% to 9%) 1342
▲Idamycin (82%) 1955
▲IFEX (58%) 697
Ilosone (Infrequent) 911
Imdur (Less than or equal to 5%) 1323
Imitrex Tablets 1106
Imodium Capsules 1295
▲Imovax Rabies Vaccine (Up to 6%) 881
▲Imuran (Approximately 12%) 1110
Inderal 2728
Inderal LA Long Acting Capsules 2730
Inderide Tablets 2732
Inderide LA Long Acting Capsules 2734
▲Indocin (3% to 9%) 1680
INFeD (Iron Dextran Injection, USP) 2345
Infumorph 200 and Infumorph 500 Sterile Solutions 965
Inocor Lactate Injection (1.7%) 2309
Intal Capsules (Less than 1 in 10,000 patients) 987
Intal Inhaler (Infrequent) 988
Intal Nebulizer Solution (Rare) 989
▲Intron A (1% to 50%) 2364
Inversine Tablets 1686
Iopidine 0.5% (Less than 1%) ⊙ 221
Ismelin Tablets 827
Ismo Tablets (2% to 4%) 2738
ISMOTIC 45% w/v Solution ⊙ 222
Isoetharine Inhalation Solution, USP, Arm-a-Med 551
Isoptin Injectable (0.9%) 1344
Isoptin Oral Tablets (2.7%) 1346
Isoptin SR Tablets (2.7%) 1348
Isuprel Hydrochloride Solution 1:200 & 1:100 2313
Isuprel Mistometer 2312
▲JE-VAX (Approximately 10%) 886
K-Dur Microburst Release System (potassium chloride, USP) E.R. Tablets 1325
▲K-Lor Powder Packets (Most common) 434
▲K-Norm Extended-Release Capsules (Among most common) 991
K-Phos Neutral Tablets 639
K-Phos Original Formula 'Sodium Free' Tablets 639
▲K-Tab Filmtab (Most common) 434
Kayexalate 2314
Keflex Pulvules & Oral Suspension (Rare) 914
Keftab Tablets (Rare) 915
Kefurox Vials, Faspak & ADD-Vantage (1 in 440) 1454
Kefzol Vials, Faspak & ADD-Vantage (Rare) 1456
Kemadrin Tablets 1112
▲Kerlone Tablets (1.6% to 5.8%) 2436
Klonopin Tablets 2126
KOGENATE Antihemophilic Factor (Recombinant) 632
▲Kolyum Liquid (Among most common) 992
Ku-Zyme HP Capsules 2402
▲Kytril Tablets (15%) 2492
▲Lamictal Tablets (Among most common; 18% to 25%) 1112
▲Lamprene Capsules (40-50%) 828
Lanoxicaps (Common) 1117
Lanoxin Elixir Pediatric 1120
Lanoxin Injection (Common) 1123
Lanoxin Injection Pediatric 1126
Lanoxin Tablets (Common) 1128
▲Lariam Tablets (Among most frequent) 2128
Larodopa Tablets (Relatively frequent) 2129
Lasix Injection, Oral Solution and Tablets 1240
▲Lescol Capsules (3.2%) 2267
▲Leucovorin Calcium for Injection (6% to 74%) 1268
Leukeran Tablets (Infrequent) 1133
Leukine for IV Infusion 1271
▲Leustatin (28%) 1834
▲Levatol (4.3%) 2403
Levbid Extended-Release Tablets 2405
Levlen/Tri-Levlen 651
Levo-Dromoran (Common) 2129
Levoprome (Sometimes) 1274
Levsin/Levsinex/Levbid 2405
Librax Capsules (Infrequent) 2176
Libritabs Tablets (Isolated cases) 2177
Librium Capsules (Isolated cases) 2178
Librium Injectable (Isolated cases) 2179
Limbitrol 2180
Lincocin 2617
Lioresal Intrathecal (3 to 5 of 214 patients) 1596
▲Lioresal Tablets (4-12%) 829
Lithium Carbonate Capsules & Tablets 2230
Lithonate/Lithotabs/Lithobid 2543

(▣ Described in PDR For Nonprescription Drugs) Incidence data in parenthesis; ▲ 3% or more (⊙ Described in PDR For Ophthalmology)

Nausea **Side Effects Index** **1368**

Livostin (Approximately 1% to 3%) ⊙ 266
▲Lodine Capsules and Tablets (3-9%) 2743
Lomotil 2439
Loniten Tablets 2618
▲Lo/Ovral Tablets (10% or less) 2746
▲Lo/Ovral-28 Tablets (10% or less) 2751
Lopid Tablets (2.5%) 1917
Lopressor Ampuls (1%) 830
Lopressor HCT Tablets (1 in 100 patients) 832
Lopressor Tablets (1%) 830
Lorabid Suspension and Pulvules (Up to 2.5%) 1459
▲Lorcet 10/650 (Among most frequent) 1018
Lorelco Tablets 1517
▲Lortab (Among most frequent) 2566
Lotensin Tablets (1.3%) 834
Lotensin HCT 837
Lotrel Capsules 840
▲Lovenox Injection (3%) 2020
Loxitane 1378
Lozol Tablets (Less than 5%) 2022
Ludiomil Tablets (2%) 843
Lufyllin & Lufyllin-400 Tablets 2670
Lufyllin-GG Elixir & Tablets 2671
Lupron Depot 3.75 mg (Less than 5%) 2556
▲Lupron Depot 7.5 mg (5.4%) 2559
Lupron Depot-PED 7.5 mg, 11.25 mg and 15 mg (Less than 2%) 2560
▲Lupron Injection (5% or more) 2555
▲Luvox Tablets (40%) 2544
Lysodren 698
M-M-R II 1687
M-R-VAX II 1689
▲MS Contin Tablets (Among most frequent) 1994
▲MSIR (Among most frequent) 1997
▲MZM (Among reactions occurring most often) ⊙ 267
▲Macrobid Capsules (8%) 1988
▲Macrodantin Capsules (Among most often) 1989
Mandol Vials, Faspak & ADD-Vantage (Rare) 1461
Marax Tablets & DF Syrup (Frequent, on empty stomach) 2200
Marcaine Hydrochloride with Epinephrine 1:200,000 2316
Marcaine Hydrochloride Injection (Rare) 2316
Marcaine Spinal (Rare) 2319
▲Marinol (Dronabinol) Capsules (3% to 10%) 2231
Massengill Disposable Douche 2457
Massengill Medicated Disposable Douche 2458
Massengill Medicated Liquid Concentrate ▣ 821
▲Matulane Capsules (Frequent) 2131
Maxair Autohaler (1.3% to 1.7%) 1492
Maxair Inhaler (1.7%) 1494
▲Maxaquin Tablets (3.7%) 2440
Maxzide 1380
Mebaral Tablets (Less than 1 in 100) 2322
Mefoxin (Rare) 1691
Mefoxin Premixed Intravenous Solution (Rare) 1694
▲Megace Oral Suspension (Up to 5%) 699
Megace Tablets 701
Mellaril 2269
Menest Tablets 2494
▲Mepergan Injection (Among most frequent) 2753
▲Mepron Suspension (21% to 22%) 1135
Meruvax II 1697
Mesantoin Tablets 2272
▲Mesnex Injection (33%) 702
Mestinon Injectable 1253
Mestinon 1254
Metaproterenol Sulfate Inhalation Solution, USP, Arm-a-Med (About 1 in 50 patients) 552
▲Methadone Hydrochloride Oral Concentrate (Among most frequent) 2233
Methadone Hydrochloride Oral Solution & Tablets 2235
Methergine (Occasional) 2272
▲Methotrexate Sodium Tablets, Injection, for Injection and LPF Injection (Among most frequent; 10%) 1275
Metrodin (urofollitropin for injection) 2446
MetroGel 1047
MetroGel-Vaginal (Equal to or less than 2%) 902
▲Mevacor Tablets (1.9% to 4.7%) 1699
▲Mexitil Capsules (39.3% to 39.6%) 678
Mezlin 601
Mezlin Pharmacy Bulk Package 604
▲Miacalcin Injection (About 10%) 2273
Miacalcin Nasal Spray (Less than 1%; 1.8%) 2275
▲Micro-K (Among most common) 2063
▲Micro-K LS Packets (Most common) 2064
Micronase Tablets (1.8%) 2623
Micronor Tablets 1872
▲Midamor Tablets (3% to 8%) 1703
Milontin Kapseals (Frequent) 1920
Miltown Tablets 2672
▲Minipress Capsules (4.9%) 1937
▲Minizide Capsules (4.9%) 1938
Minocin Intravenous 1382
Minocin Oral Suspension 1385
Minocin Pellet-Filled Capsules 1383
Mintezol 1704
Mithracin 607
Moban Tablets and Concentrate (Occasional) 1048
Modicon 1872
▲Moduretic Tablets (3% to 8%) 1705
▲8-MOP Capsules (Most common; approximately 10%) 1246
Monoclate-P, Factor VIII:C, Pasteurized, Monoclonal Antibody Purified Antihemophilic Factor (Human) 521
Monodox Capsules 1805
Monoket (Up to 3%) 2406
Mononine, Coagulation Factor IX (Human) 523
Monopril Tablets (1.2% to 2.2%) 757
Motofen Tablets (1 in 15) 784
▲Children's Motrin Ibuprofen Oral Suspension (3% to 9%) 1546
▲Motrin Tablets (3% to 9%) 2625
▲Motrin Ibuprofen Suspension, Oral Drops, Chewable Tablets, Caplets (3% to 9%) 1546
MSTA Mumps Skin Test Antigen 890
Mustargen 1709
▲Mutamycin (14%) 703
Myambutol Tablets 1386
Mycelex Troches 608
▲Mycobutin Capsules (6%) 1957
Mycostatin Pastilles (Occasional) 704
Mykrox Tablets (Less than 2%) 993
Myleran Tablets 1143
Myochrysine Injection 1711
Mysoline (Occasional) 2754
▲Nalfon 200 Pulvules & Nalfon Tablets (7.7%) 917
▲Anaprox/Naprosyn (3% to 9%) 2117
Narcan Injection 934
Nardil 1920
Nasalide Nasal Solution 0.025% (5% or less) 2110
Nasarel Nasal Solution (Greater than 1%) 2133
Navane Capsules and Concentrate 2201
Navane Intramuscular 2202
▲Navelbine Injection (Up to 34%) 1145
Nebcin Vials, Hyporets & ADD-Vantage 1464
▲NebuPent for Inhalation Solution (10 to 23%) 1040
NegGram 2323
Nembutal Sodium Capsules (Less than 1%) 436
Nembutal Sodium Solution (Less than 1%) 438
Nembutal Sodium Suppositories (Less than 1%) 440
▲Neoral (4% to 10%) 2276
NEOSAR Lyophilized/Neosar (Common) 1959
Nephro-Fer Rx Tablets 2005
Neptazane Tablets 1388
Nescaine/Nescaine MPF 554
Netromycin Injection 100 mg/ml 2373
▲Neupogen for Injection (10%; 57%) 495
Neurontin Capsules (More than 1%) 1922
▲Neutrexin (4.6%) 2572
▲Nicoderm (nicotine transdermal system) (3% to 9%) 1518
▲Nicorette (10%) 2458
Nicotrol Nicotine Transdermal System (B 3% to 9%) 1550
Nimotop Capsules (Up to 1.4%) 610
Nitrolingual Spray (Uncommon) 2027
▲Nizoral Tablets (Approximately 3%) 1298
▲Nolvadex Tablets (2.1% to 25.7%) 2841
▲Nordette-21 Tablets (10% or less) 2755
▲Nordette-28 Tablets (10% or less) 2758
Norflex 1496
Norgesic 1496
Norinyl 2088
Norisodrine with Calcium Iodide Syrup 442
▲Normodyne Injection (Less than 1% to 19%) 2377
▲Normodyne Tablets (Less than 1% to 19%) 2379
▲Noroxin Tablets (2.6% to 4.2%) 1715
▲Noroxin Tablets (2.6% to 4.2%) 2048
▲Norpace (3 to 9%) 2444
Norplant System 2759
Norpramin Tablets 1526
Nor-Q D Tablets 2135
Norvasc Tablets (2.9%) 1940
Novahistine DH 2462
Novahistine DMX (Infrequent) ▣ 822
Novahistine Elixir ▣ 823
Novahistine Expectorant 2463
▲Novantrone (31 to 72%) 1279
Novocain Hydrochloride for Spinal Anesthesia 2326
▲Nubain Injection (6%) 935
Nucofed 2051
▲NuLYTELY (Up to 50% of patients) 689
▲Cherry Flavor NuLYTELY (Among most common) 689
Numorphan Injection 936
Numorphan Suppositories 937
Nutropin (A small number of patients) 1061
Nydrazid Injection (Common) 508
Ocupress Ophthalmic Solution, 1% Sterile ⊙ 309
Ogen Tablets 2627
Ogen Vaginal Cream 2630
Omnipen Capsules 2764
Omnipen for Oral Suspension 2765
▲Oncaspar (Greater than 5%) 2028
Oncovin Solution Vials & Hyporets 1466
OptiPranolol (Metipranolol 0.3%) Sterile Ophthalmic Solution (A small number of patients) ⊙ 258
▲Oramorph SR (Morphine Sulfate Sustained Release Tablets) (Among most frequent) 2236
Orap Tablets 1050
Oretic Tablets 443
Oreton Methyl 1255
▲Organidin NR Tablets and Liquid (One of the two most common) 2672
Orlamm (1% to 3%) 2239
Ornade Spansule Capsules 2502
Ortho-Cept 1851
Ortho-Cyclen/Ortho-Tri-Cyclen 1858
Ortho Dienestrol Cream 1866
Ortho-Est 1869
Ortho-Novum 1872
Ortho-Cyclen/Ortho Tri-Cyclen 1858
▲Orthoclone OKT3 Sterile Solution (19%) 1837
▲Orudis Capsules (3% to 9%) 2766
▲Oruvail Capsules (3% to 9%) 2766
OSM_GLYN Oral Osmotic Agent ⊙ 226
Osmolite HN High Nitrogen Isotonic Liquid Nutrition 2222
Ovcon 760
▲Ovral Tablets (10% or less) 2770
▲Ovral-28 Tablets (10% or less) 2770
▲Ovrette Tablets (10% or less) 2771
Oxandrin 2862
▲Oxsoralen-Ultra Capsules (10%) 1257
Oxytocin Injection 2771
PBZ Tablets 845
PBZ-SR Tablets 844
▲PCE Dispertab Tablets (Among most frequent) 444
PMB 200 and PMB 400 2783
Pamelor 2280
Papaverine Hydrochloride Vials and Ampoules 1468
Paraflex Caplets 1580
Parafon Forte DSC Caplets 1581
▲Paraplatin for Injection (75% to 94%) 705
Paremyd ⊙ 247
▲Parlodel (7% to 49%) 2281
Parnate Tablets 2503
▲PASER Granules (Among most common) 1285
▲Paxil Tablets (14.7% to 36.3%) 2505
Peganone Tablets 446
▲Pen•Vee K (Among most common) 2772
▲Penetrex Tablets (2% to 8%) 2031
▲Pentam 300 Injection (5.9%) 1041
Pentasa (1.8% to 3.1%) 1527
Pentaspan Injection 937
Pepcid Injection (Infrequent) 1722
Pepcid (Infrequent) 1720
Peptavlon 2878
▲Percocet Tablets (Among most frequent) 938
▲Percodan Tablets (Among most frequent) 939
▲Percodan-Demi Tablets (Among most frequent) 940
Pergonal (menotropins for injection, USP) 2448
Periactin 1724
Peri-Colace 2052
▲Permax Tablets (24.3%) 575
Phenergan with Codeine 2777
Phenergan with Dextromethorphan 2778
Phenergan Injection 2773
Phenergan Suppositories 2775
Phenergan Syrup 2774
Phenergan Tablets 2775
Phenergan VC 2779
Phenergan VC with Codeine 2781
Phenobarbital Elixir and Tablets (Less than 1 in 100 patients) 1469
PhosChol 488
PhosLo Tablets (Occasional) 690
▲Phrenilin (Among most frequent) 785
Pilocar (Extremely rare) ⊙ 268
Pima Syrup 1005
Pipracil (Less frequent) 1390
Placidyl Capsules 448
Plaquenil Sulfate Tablets 2328
Plasma-Plex, Plasma Protein Fraction (Human) 5% 524
▲Platinol (Almost all patients) 708
▲Platinol-AQ Injection (Almost all patients) 710
Plendil Extended-Release Tablets (1.2% to 1.7%) 527
Pneumovax 23 1725
Pondimin Tablets 2066
Ponstel 1925
Pontocaine Hydrochloride for Spinal Anesthesia 2330
Potaba (Infrequent) 1229
▲Pravachol (2.9% to 7.3%) 765
Premarin Intravenous 2787
Premarin with Methyltestosterone 2794
Premarin Tablets 2789
Premarin Vaginal Cream 2791
Premphase 2797
Prempro 2801
PREVACID Delayed-Release Capsules (1.4%) 2562
▲Prilosec Delayed-Release Capsules (2.2% to 4.0%) 529
Primaxin I.M. (0.6%) 1727
Primaxin I.V. (2.0%) 1729
▲Prinivil Tablets (2.0% to 5.0%) 1733
Prinzide Tablets (2.2%) 1737
Priscoline Hydrochloride Ampuls 845
Pro-Banthīne Tablets 2052
▲Procan SR Tablets (3-4%) 1926
▲Procardia Capsules (Approximately 10% to 11%) 1971
▲Procardia XL Extended Release Tablets (3.3% to 11%) 1972
▲Procrit for Injection (0.26% to 17%) 1841
Proglycem (Frequent) 580
▲Prograf (30% to 46%) 1042
▲Proleukin for Injection (87%) 797
Prolixin 509
Proloprim Tablets 1155
▲Propulsid (7.6%) 1300
▲ProSom Tablets (4%) 449
Prostep (nicotine transdermal system) (1% to 3% of patients) 1394
Prostigmin Injectable 1260
Prostigmin Tablets 1261
▲Prostin E2 Suppository (Approximately one-third) 2634
Protamine Sulfate Ampoules & Vials 1471
Protopam Chloride for Injection 2806
▲Protostat Tablets (About 12% of patients) 1883
▲Proventil Inhalation Aerosol (Less than 15%) 2382
▲Proventil Inhalation Solution 0.083% (3.1% to 4%) 2384
Proventil Repetabs Tablets (2% to 4%) 2386

(▣ Described in PDR For Nonprescription Drugs) Incidence data in parenthesis; ▲ 3% or more (⊙ Described in PDR For Ophthalmology)

1369 **Side Effects Index** **Neck, rigidity of**

▲ Proventil Solution for Inhalation 0.5% (3.1% to 4%) 2383
Proventil Tablets (2%) 2386
Provera Tablets 2636
Provocholine for Inhalation 2140
▲ Prozac Pulvules & Liquid, Oral Solution (5% to 27%) 919
Purinethol Tablets (Uncommon) 1156
Pyrazinamide Tablets 1398
Quadrinal Tablets 1350
Quarzan Capsules 2181
Questran Light (Less frequent) 769
Questran Powder (Less frequent) 770
Quibron 2053
▲ Quinaglute Dura-Tabs Tablets (3%) 649
▲ Quinidex Extentabs (Among most frequent) 2067
▲ RMS Suppositories (Among most frequent) 2657
▲ Rabies Vaccine Adsorbed (8% to 10%) 2508
Rabies Vaccine, Imovax Rabies I.D. (Less frequent; up to 2%) 883
Recombivax HB (Equal to or greater than 1%) 1744
Regitine 846
Reglan 2068
▲ Relafen Tablets (3% to 9%) 2510
▲ ReoPro Vials (18.4%) 1471
Respbid Tablets 682
▲ Retrovir Capsules (0.8% to 61%) 1158
▲ Retrovir I.V. Infusion (1% to 61%) 1163
▲ Retrovir Syrup (0.8% to 61%) 1158
▲ ReVia Tablets (10% to more than 10%) 940
▲ Revex (18%) 1811
Rhinocort Nasal Inhaler (Less than 1%) 556
▲ Ridaura Capsules (10%) 2513
Rifadin (Some patients) 1528
Rifamate Capsules (Some patients) 1530
Rifater 1532
Rimactane Capsules 847
▲ Risperdal (4% to 6%) 1301
Ritalin 848
Robaxin Tablets 2071
▲ Robaxisal Tablets (One in 20-25) 2071
Robinul Forte Tablets 2072
Robinul Injectable 2072
Robinul Tablets 2072
Rocaltrol Capsules 2141
Rocephin Injectable Vials, ADD-Vantage, Galaxy Container (Less than 1%) 2142
▲ Roferon-A Injection (32% to 51%) 2145
▲ Rogaine Topical Solution (4.33%) 2637
▲ Romazicon (11%) 2147
Rondec Oral Drops 953
Rondec Syrup 953
Rondec Tablet 953
Rondec-DM Oral Drops 954
Rondec-DM Syrup 954
Rondec-TR Tablet 953
▲ Rowasa (1.2% to 5.77%) 2548
▲ Roxanol (Among most frequent) 2243
▲ Roxicodone Tablets, Oral Solution & Intensol (Oxycodone) (Among most frequent) 2244
Rum-K Syrup 1005
▲ Rythmol Tablets–150mg, 225mg, 300mg (2.4 to 10.7%) 1352
▲ SSKI Solution (Among most frequent) 2658
▲ Salagen Tablets (6% to 15%) 1489
Salflex Tablets 786
▲ Sandimmune (2 to 10%) 2286
Sandoglobulin I.V. (Less than 1%) 2290
▲ Sandostatin Injection (5% to 10%; 30% to 58%) 2292
Sanorex Tablets 2294
Sansert Tablets 2295
Seconal Sodium Pulvules (Less than 1 in 100) 1474
▲ Sectral Capsules (4%) 2807
▲ Sedapap Tablets 50 mg/650 mg (Among the most frequent) 1543
▲ Seldane Tablets (4.6% to 7.6%) 1536
▲ Seldane-D Extended-Release Tablets (4.5%) 1538
Semprex-D Capsules (2%) 463
Semprex-D Capsules (2%) 1167
Senna X-Prep Bowel Evacuant Liquid 1230
Sensorcaine (Rare) 559
▲ Septra (Among most common) 1174
▲ Septra I.V. Infusion (Among the most common) 1169
▲ Septra I.V. Infusion ADD-Vantage Vials (Among most common) 1171
▲ Septra (Among most common) 1174
Ser-Ap-Es Tablets 849
Serax Capsules 2810
Serax Tablets 2810
Serentil 684
Serevent Inhalation Aerosol (1% to 3%) 1176
Serophene (clomiphene citrate tablets, USP) (Approximately 1 in 50 patients) 2451
▲ Serzone Tablets (14% to 23%) 771
Sinemet Tablets (Common) 943
▲ Sinemet CR Tablets (5.5%) 944
Sinequan 2205
Skelaxin Tablets 788
Slo-bid Gyrocaps 2033
Slo-Niacin Tablets 2659
▲ Slow-K Extended-Release Tablets (Among most common) 851
Sodium Polystyrene Sulfonate Suspension 2244
Solganal Suspension (Rare) 2388
Solu-Medrol Sterile Powder 2643
Soma Compound w/Codeine Tablets 2676
▲ Soma Compound Tablets (Among most common) 2675
Soma Tablets 2674
Sotradecol (Sodium Tetradecyl Sulfate Injection) 967
Spectrobid Tablets (2%) 2206
▲ Sporanox Capsules (2.4% to 10.6%) 1305
▲ St. Joseph Adult Chewable Aspirin (81 mg.) (7.3% of 4500 patients) ▣ 808
▲ Stadol (13%) 775
Stelazine 2514
Stilphostrol Tablets and Ampuls 612
Stimate, (desmopressin acetate) Nasal Spray, 1.5 mg/mL (Infrequent) 525
Streptase for Infusion 562
Streptomycin Sulfate Injection 2208
Sublimaze Injection 1307
▲ Sufenta Injection (3% to 9%) 1309
▲ Supprelin Injection (3% to 10%) 2056
▲ Suprane (27%) 1813
▲ Suprax (7%) 1399
Surmontil Capsules 2811
Sus-Phrine Injection 1019
▲ Symmetrel Capsules and Syrup (5% to 10%) 946
Syn-Rx Tablets 465
Syn-Rx DM Tablets 466
Syntocinon Injection 2296
Talacen (Rare) 2333
▲ Talwin Injection (Most common) 2334
Talwin Compound 2335
▲ Talwin Injection (Most common) 2334
Talwin Nx 2336
▲ Tambocor Tablets (8.9%) 1497
Tao Capsules (Infrequent) 2209
Tapazole Tablets 1477
Tavist Syrup 2297
Tavist Tablets 2298
▲ Taxol (52%) 714
Tazicef for Injection (Less than 2%; 1 in 156 patients) 2519
Tazidime Vials, Faspak & ADD-Vantage (1 in 156) 1478
▲ Tegison Capsules (10-25%) 2154
▲ Tegretol Chewable Tablets (Among most frequent) 852
▲ Tegretol Suspension (Among most frequent) 852
▲ Tegretol Tablets (Among most frequent) 852
Temaril Tablets, Syrup and Spansule Extended-Release Capsules 483
Tenex Tablets (3% or less) 2074
▲ Tenoretic Tablets (3% to 4%) 2845
▲ Tenormin Tablets and I.V. Injection (3% to 4%) 2847
Tensilon Injectable 1261
Terramycin Intramuscular Solution 2210
Teslac 717
Tessalon Perles 1020
Testoderm Testosterone Transdermal System 486
Testred Capsules 1262
Thalitone 1245
Theo-24 Extended Release Capsules 2568
Theo-Dur Extended-Release Tablets 1327
Theo-X Extended-Release Tablets 788
▲ TheraCys BCG Live (Intravesical) (Up to 16.1%) 897
Thera-Gesic 1781
Thioguanine Tablets, Tabloid Brand (Less frequent) 1181
Thioplex (Thiotepa For Injection) 1281
Thorazine 2523
▲ THROMBATE III Antithrombin III (Human) (3 of 17) 637
THYREL TRH 2873
Ticar for Injection 2526
▲ Ticlid Tablets (7.0%) 2156
▲ Tilade (4.0%) 996
Timentin for Injection 2528
Timolide Tablets (Less than 1%) 1748
Timoptic in Ocudose (Less frequent) 1753
Timoptic Sterile Ophthalmic Solution (Less frequent) 1751
Timoptic-XE 1755
Tobramycin Sulfate Injection 968
Tofranil Ampuls 854
Tofranil Tablets 856
Tofranil-PM Capsules 857
▲ Tolectin (200, 400 and 600 mg) (11%) 1581
▲ Tonocard Tablets (14.5-24.6%) 531
Toprol-XL Tablets (About 1 of 100 patients) 565
▲ Toradol (12%) 2159
Tornalate Solution for Inhalation, 0.2% (1.9%) 956
Tornalate Metered Dose Inhaler (0.5% to 3%) 957
Trancopal Caplets 2337
▲ Trandate (13 of 100 patients) 1185
Transderm Scōp Transdermal Therapeutic System (Few patients) 869
▲ Trasylol (3%) 613
Trental Tablets (2.2%) 1244
Triavil Tablets 1757
Trilafon (Occasional) 2389
Levlen/Tri-Levlen 651
▲ Trilisate (Less than 20%) 2000
Trimpex Tablets 2163
Trinalin Repetabs Tablets 1330
Tri-Norinyl 2164
▲ Triphasil-21 Tablets (10% or less) 2814
▲ Triphasil-28 Tablets (10% or less) 2819
Trobicin Sterile Powder 2645
Trusopt Sterile Ophthalmic Solution (Infrequent) 1760
Tussend 1783
Tussend Expectorant 1785
Tussionex Pennkinetic Extended-Release Suspension 998
▲ Tussi-Organidin DM NR Liquid and DM-S NR Liquid (One of the two most common) 2677
▲ Tussi-Organidin NR Liquid and S NR Liquid (One of the two most common) 2677
TYLENOL Severe Allergy Medication Caplets 1564
▲ Tylenol with Codeine (Among most frequent) 1583
▲ Tylox Capsules (Among most frequent) 1584
Tympagesic Ear Drops 2342
▲ Typhim Vi (2% to 8.2%) 899
▲ Ultram Tablets (50 mg) (24% to 40%) 1585
Unasyn (Less than 1%) 2212
Uni-Dur Extended-Release Tablets 1331
Uniphyl 400 mg Tablets (Frequent) 2001
Univasc Tablets (More than 1%) 2410
Urecholine 1761
Urispas Tablets 2532
Urobiotic-250 Capsules (Rare) 2214
Uroqid-Acid No. 2 Tablets 640
Valium Injectable 2182
Valium Tablets (Infrequent) 2183
Valrelease Capsules (Occasional) 2169
▲ Valtrex Caplets (10% to 16%) 1194
Vancenase AQ Nasal Spray 0.042% (Fewer than 5 per 100 patients) 2393
Vancocin HCl, Oral Solution & Pulvules (Infrequent) 1483
Vancocin HCl, Vials & ADD-Vantage (Infrequent) 1481
▲ Vantin for Oral Suspension and Vantin Tablets (Less than 3.8%) 2646
Varivax (Greater than or equal to 1%) 1762
▲ Vascor (200, 300 and 400 mg) Tablets (12.29 to 26.09%) 1587
Vaseretic Tablets (2.5%) 1765
Vasotec I.V. (1.1%) 1768
Vasotec Tablets (1.3% to 1.4%) 1771
Vasoxyl Injection 1196
Velban Vials 1484
▲ Ventolin Inhalation Aerosol and Refill (Fewer than 15 per 100 patients; 6%) 1197
▲ Ventolin Inhalation Solution (3.1% to 4%) 1198
▲ Ventolin Nebules Inhalation Solution (3.1% to 4%) 1199
▲ Ventolin Rotacaps for Inhalation (4%) 1200
Ventolin Tablets (2 of 100 patients) 1203
▲ VePesid Capsules and Injection (31% to 43%) 718
Verelan Capsules (2.7%) 1410
Verelan Capsules (2.7%) 2824
Versed Injection (2.8%) 2170
Vibramycin 1941
Vibramycin Hyclate Intravenous 2215
Vibramycin 1941
▲ Vicodin Tablets (Among most frequent) 1356
▲ Vicodin ES Tablets (Among most frequent) 1357
Vicodin Tuss Expectorant (More frequently in ambulatory than in recumbent patients) 1358
▲ Videx Tablets, Powder for Oral Solution, & Pediatric Powder for Oral Solution (7% to 58%) 720
▲ Visken Tablets (5%) 2299
Vivactil Tablets 1774
Vivotif Berna (Infrequent) 665
▲ Volmax Extended-Release Tablets (4.2%) 1788
Voltaren Ophthalmic Sterile Ophthalmic Solution (1%) ⊙ 272
▲ Voltaren Tablets (3% to 9%) 861
Vontrol Tablets 2532
▲ Vumon (29%) 727
▲ Wellbutrin Tablets (22.9%) 1204
Wigraine Tablets & Suppositories 1829
WinRho SD (One report) 2576
Winstrol Tablets 2337
▲ Wygesic Tablets (Most frequent) 2827
▲ Xanax Tablets (9.6% to 22%) 2649
Xylocaine Injections (Less than 1%) 567
Yocon (Common) 1892
Yodoxin 1230
▲ Yutopar Intravenous Injection (10% to 15%) 570
▲ Zanosar Sterile Powder (Most patients) 2653
Zantac 1209
Zantac Injection 1207
Zantac Syrup 1209
Zarontin Capsules (Frequent) 1928
Zarontin Syrup (Frequent) 1929
Zaroxolyn Tablets 1000
Zebeta Tablets (1.5% to 2.2%) 1413
Zefazone (1.0%) 2654
Zemuron (Less than 1%) 1830
▲ Zerit Capsules (6% to 35%) 729
Zestoretic (2.2%) 2850
▲ Zestril Tablets (2.0% to 5.0%) 2854
Ziac (0.9% to 1.1%) 1415
Zinacef (1 in 440 patients) 1211
▲ Zinecard (51% to 77%) 1961
▲ Zithromax (3% to 5%) 1944
Zocor Tablets (1.3%) 1775
▲ Zoladex (5% to 8%) 2858
▲ Zoloft Tablets (26.1%) 2217
Zonalon Cream (Less than 1%) 1055
▲ Zosyn (6.9%) 1419
▲ Zosyn Pharmacy Bulk Package (6.9%) 1422
▲ Zovirax Capsules (2.4% to 8%) 1219
▲ Zovirax Sterile Powder (Approximately 7%) 1223
▲ Zovirax (2.4% to 8.0%) 1219
▲ Zydone Capsules (Among most frequent) 949
Zyloprim Tablets (Less than 1%) 1226

Nausea, acute/severe

Doxorubicin Astra (Frequent) 540
Rubex (Frequent) 712

Neck tightness

Imitrex Injection (Relatively common) 1103
Respbid Tablets 682

Neck, hyperextension of

Prostin VR Pediatric Sterile Solution (Less than 1%) 2635

Neck, rigidity of

Cytovene (1% or less) 2103
Depakote Tablets (Greater than 1% but not more than 5%) 415

(▣ Described in PDR For Nonprescription Drugs) Incidence data in parenthesis; ▲ 3% or more (⊙ Described in PDR For Ophthalmology)

Neck, rigidity of · Side Effects Index · 1370

Dilacor XR Extended-release Capsules (Infrequent) ... 2018
Diprivan Injection (Less than 1%) .. 2833
Effexor (Infrequent) ... 2719
Hivid Tablets (Less than 1% to less than 3%) ... 2121
▲ Imitrex Injection (4.8%) ... 1103
Imitrex Tablets ... 1106
Ismo Tablets (Fewer than 1%) ... 2738
Luvox Tablets (Infrequent) ... 2544
Paxil Tablets (Rare) ... 2505
Prostin E2 Suppository ... 2634
Prozac Pulvules & Liquid, Oral Solution (Infrequent) ... 919
Serzone Tablets (1%) ... 771
Varivax (Greater than or equal to 1%) ... 1762
Videx Tablets, Powder for Oral Solution, & Pediatric Powder for Oral Solution (Less than 1%) ... 720

Necrolysis, digitus

▲ Tegison Capsules (Greater than 75%) ... 2154

Necrolysis, epidermal

A/T/S 2% Acne Topical Gel and Solution (Occasional) ... 1234
▲ Accutane Capsules (Approximately 1 in 20) ... 2076
Children's Advil Suspension (Less than 1%) ... 2692
Amoxil ... 2464
Ansaid Tablets (Rare) ... 2579
Atretol Tablets (Extremely rare) ... 573
Atromid-S Capsules ... 2701
Augmentin (Occasional) ... 2468
Azactam for Injection (Less than 1%) ... 734
Azo Gantanol Tablets ... 2080
Azo Gantrisin Tablets ... 2081
Azulfidine (Rare) ... 1949
Betoptic Ophthalmic Solution (Rare) ... 469
Betoptic S Ophthalmic Suspension (Rare) ... 471
▲ Blephamide Ointment (Among most often) ... ◉ 237
Brevoxyl Gel ... 2552
▲ Brevoxyl Cleansing Lotion (5 of 100 patients) ... 2553
Ceclor Pulvules & Suspension (Rare) ... 1431
Cefizox for Intramuscular or Intravenous Use ... 1034
Cefotan ... 2829
Ceftin ... 1078
Cefzil Tablets and Oral Suspension ... 746
Ceptaz ... 1081
Chibroxin Sterile Ophthalmic Solution (With oral form) ... 1617
Cipro I.V. (1% or less) ... 595
Cipro I.V. Pharmacy Bulk Package (Less than 1%) ... 597
Cipro Tablets ... 592
Claritin-D (Less frequent) ... 2350
▲ Cleocin T Topical (11%) ... 2590
Cleocin Vaginal Cream ... 2589
Combipres Tablets ... 677
Condylox (Less than 5%) ... 1802
Cozaar Tablets (One subject) ... 1628
Daypro Caplets (Less than 1%) ... 2426
Depakene (One case) ... 413
Depakote Tablets (One case) ... 415
Depen Titratable Tablets (Rare) ... 2662
DesOwen Cream, Ointment and Lotion (Less than 2%) ... 1046
Desquam-E Gel ... 2684
Desquam-X Gel ... 2684
Desquam-X 10 Bar ... 2684
Desquam-X Wash ... 2684
Diamox Sequels (Sustained Release) ... 1373
Diflucan Injection, Tablets, and Oral Suspension ... 2194
Dilacor XR Extended-release Capsules ... 2018
Dilantin Infatabs ... 1908
Dilantin Kapseals ... 1906
Dilantin-125 Suspension ... 1911
Diupres Tablets ... 1650
Diuril Oral Suspension ... 1653
Diuril Sodium Intravenous ... 1652
Diuril Tablets ... 1653
Dolobid Tablets (Less than 1 in 100) ... 1654
▲ Dovonex Ointment 0.005% (1% to 10%) ... 2684
Duricef ... 748
Emcyt Capsules (1%) ... 1953
Emgel 2% Topical Gel (Occasional) ... 1093
Esgic-plus Tablets (Several cases) .. 1013
Eulexin Capsules ... 2358
Exact Vanishing and Tinted Creams ... ▣ 749
FML-S Liquifilm ... ◉ 242
Felbatol ... 2666
Feldene Capsules (Less than 1%) .. 1965
Fiorinal Capsules (Several cases) ... 2261
Fiorinal with Codeine Capsules ... 2262
Fiorinal Tablets (Several cases) ... 2261
Floxin I.V. ... 1571
Floxin Tablets (200 mg, 300 mg, 400 mg) ... 1567
Fortaz ... 1100
Fulvicin P/G Tablets (Rare) ... 2359
Gantrisin (Rare) ... 2120
Glauctabs ... ◉ 208
HydroDIURIL Tablets ... 1674
Hydropres Tablets ... 1675
Hyzaar Tablets (One subject) ... 1677
IBU Tablets (Less than 1%) ... 1342
Indocin Capsules (Less than 1%) ... 1680
Indocin I.V. (Less than 1%) ... 1684
Indocin (Less than 1%) ... 1680
Intron A (Less than 5%) ... 2364
Lac-Hydrin 12% Lotion (1 in 60 patients) ... 2687
Lescol Capsules (Rare) ... 2267
Leukeran Tablets (Rare) ... 1133
Lodine Capsules and Tablets (Less than 1%) ... 2743
Lorabid Suspension and Pulvules ... 1459
Lotrimin ... 2371
Lotrisone Cream ... 2372
Luvox Tablets ... 2544
MZM (Common) ... ◉ 267
Maxaquin Tablets ... 2440
Mefoxin ... 1691
Mefoxin Premixed Intravenous Solution ... 1694
Mesantoin Tablets (Rare) ... 2272
Mevacor Tablets (Rare) ... 1699
Moduretic Tablets ... 1705
Children's Motrin Ibuprofen Oral Suspension (Less than 1%) ... 1546
Motrin Tablets (Less than 1%) ... 2625
Motrin Ibuprofen Suspension, Oral Drops, Chewable Tablets, Caplets (Less than 1%) ... 1546
Nalfon 200 Pulvules & Nalfon Tablets (Less than 1%) ... 917
Noroxin Tablets ... 1715
Noroxin Tablets ... 2048
PCE Dispertab Tablets (Rare) ... 444
Paxil Tablets ... 2505
Penetrex Tablets (Less than 1% but more than or equal to 0.1%) ... 2031
Pepcid Injection (Very rare) ... 1722
Pepcid (very rare) ... 1720
Phenobarbital Elixir and Tablets (Rare) ... 1469
Phenurone Tablets (One case) ... 447
Phrenilin (Several cases) ... 785
Pravachol (Rare) ... 765
Prilosec Delayed-Release Capsules (Very rare) ... 529
Primaxin I.M. ... 1727
Primaxin I.V. (Less than 0.2%) ... 1729
Proloprim Tablets (Rare) ... 1155
Prozac Pulvules & Liquid, Oral Solution ... 919
Relafen Tablets (Rarer) ... 2510
Retin-A (tretinoin) Cream/Gel/Liquid ... 1889
Sedapap Tablets 50 mg/650 mg (Several cases) ... 1543
Septra ... 1174
Septra I.V. Infusion ... 1169
Septra I.V. Infusion ADD-Vantage Vials (Rare) ... 1171
Septra ... 1174
Stri-Dex ... ▣ 730
Suprax ... 1399
Tazicef for Injection ... 2519
▲ Tegison Capsules (Greater than 75%) ... 2154
Tegretol Chewable Tablets (Extremely rare) ... 852
Tegretol Suspension (Extremely rare) ... 852
Tegretol Tablets (Extremely rare) ... 852
Thalitone ... 1245
Timolide Tablets ... 1748
Tolectin (200, 400 and 600 mg) (Less than 1%) ... 1581
Trusopt Sterile Ophthalmic Solution (Rare) ... 1760
Vancocin HCl, Oral Solution & Pulvules ... 1483
Vancocin HCl, Vials & ADD-Vantage (Infrequent) ... 1481
Vantin for Oral Suspension and Vantin Tablets (Less than 1%) ... 2646
Vaseretic Tablets ... 1765
Vasocidin Ophthalmic Solution ... ◉ 270
Vasosulf ... ◉ 271
Vasotec I.V. ... 1768
Vasotec Tablets (0.5% to 1.0%) ... 1771
Zefazone ... 2654
Zestoretic ... 2850
Zinacef (Rare) ... 1211
Zocor Tablets (Rare) ... 1775
Zonalon Cream (Less than 1%) ... 1055
Zyloprim Tablets (Less than 1%) ... 1226

Necrosis

Benadryl Parenteral ... 1898
Betaseron for SC Injection (2%) ... 658
Capoten (Rare) ... 739
Capozide (Rare) ... 742
Ceptaz ... 1081
Fortaz ... 1100
Gelfoam Sterile Sponge ... 2608
Levophed Bitartrate Injection ... 2315
MSTA Mumps Skin Test Antigen ... 890
PPD Tine Test ... 2874
Platinol ... 708
Platinol-AQ Injection ... 710
Scleromate ... 1891
Sensorcaine ... 559
▲ Tegison Capsules (Greater than 75%) ... 2154
Tuberculin, Old, Tine Test ... 2875
Tubersol (Tuberculin Purified Protein Derivative [Mantoux]) ... 2872

Necrosis, aseptic

Cortifoam ... 2396
Cortone Acetate Tablets ... 1624

Necrosis, bone

Prozac Pulvules & Liquid, Oral Solution (Rare) ... 919

Necrosis, bowel

Cytosar-U Sterile Powder (Less frequent) ... 2592
Proleukin for Injection (Less than 1%) ... 797

Necrosis, buccal

Orudis Capsules (Less than 1%) ... 2766
Oruvail Capsules (Less than 1%) ... 2766

Necrosis, cecal

Adriamycin PFS ... 1947
Adriamycin RDF ... 1947
Doxorubicin Astra ... 540
Rubex ... 712

Necrosis, colon

Adriamycin PFS ... 1947
Adriamycin RDF ... 1947
Doxorubicin Astra ... 540
Kayexalate ... 2314
Rubex ... 712
Sodium Polystyrene Sulfonate Suspension (Rare) ... 2244

Necrosis, cutaneous

Aramine Injection ... 1609
Atgam Sterile Solution (Less than 1%) ... 2581
Betaseron for SC Injection ... 658
Brevibloc Injection (Less than 1%) ... 1808
Cognex Capsules (Rare) ... 1901
Coumadin ... 926
Dobutrex Solution Vials (Isolated cases) ... 1439
Heparin Lock Flush Solution ... 2725
Heparin Sodium Injection ... 2726
Heparin Sodium Injection, USP, Sterile Solution ... 2615
Heparin Sodium Vials ... 1441
Mutamycin ... 703
Neurontin Capsules (Rare) ... 1922
SSD (Infrequent) ... 1355
Vancocin HCl, Vials & ADD-Vantage ... 1481

Necrosis, fat

Garamycin Injectable (Rare) ... 2360

Necrosis, hepatic

Accupril Tablets (Rare) ... 1893
Altace Capsules (Rare) ... 1232
Azo Gantanol Tablets ... 2080
Azo Gantrisin Tablets ... 2081
Azulfidine (Rare) ... 1949
Bactrim DS Tablets (Rare) ... 2084
Bactrim I.V. Infusion (Rare) ... 2082
Bactrim (Rare) ... 2084
Benemid Tablets ... 1611
▲ Blephamide Ointment (Among most often) ... ◉ 237
Capoten (Rare) ... 739
Capozide (Rare) ... 742
Cataflam (Rare) ... 816
Cipro I.V. (1% or less) ... 595
Cipro I.V. Pharmacy Bulk Package (Less than 1%) ... 597
Cipro Tablets (Rare) ... 592
Claritin (Rare) ... 2349
Claritin-D ... 2350
ColBENEMID Tablets ... 1622
Cordarone Intravenous ... 2715
DTIC-Dome ... 600
Darvon-N/Darvocet-N ... 1433
Darvon Compound-65 Pulvules ... 1435
Darvon-N Suspension & Tablets ... 1433
Diamox Intravenous (Occasional) ... 1372
Diamox Sequels (Sustained Release) ... 1373
Diamox Tablets (Occasional) ... 1372
Eulexin Capsules ... 2358
FML-S Liquifilm ... ◉ 242
Fansidar Tablets ... 2114
Floxin I.V. ... 1571
Floxin Tablets (200 mg, 300 mg, 400 mg) ... 1567
Fluothane ... 2724
Sterile FUDR ... 2118
Gantanol Tablets ... 2119
Gantrisin (Rare) ... 2120
Glauctabs ... ◉ 208
Lescol Capsules ... 2267
Lotensin Tablets (Rare) ... 834
MZM ... ◉ 267
Macrobid Capsules (Rare) ... 1988
Macrodantin Capsules (Rare) ... 1989
Maxaquin Tablets ... 2440
Mevacor Tablets (Rare) ... 1699
Mexitil Capsules (Rare) ... 678
Monopril Tablets ... 757
Motrin Ibuprofen Suspension, Oral Drops, Chewable Tablets, Caplets (Less than 1%) ... 1546
Nardil (Less frequent) ... 1920
Neptazane Tablets ... 1388
Nicolar Tablets ... 2026
Nolvadex Tablets (Rare) ... 2841
Normodyne Injection ... 2377
Normodyne Tablets (Less common) ... 2379
Noroxin Tablets ... 1715
Noroxin Tablets ... 2048
Oxandrin (Rare) ... 2862
Paxil Tablets ... 2505
Penetrex Tablets ... 2031
Pravachol (Rare) ... 765
Prilosec Delayed-Release Capsules (Rare) ... 529
Prinivil Tablets (Rare) ... 1733
Prinzide Tablets (Rare) ... 1737
Prozac Pulvules & Liquid, Oral Solution ... 919
SSD ... 1355
Septra ... 1174
Septra I.V. Infusion ... 1169
Septra I.V. Infusion ADD-Vantage Vials (Rare) ... 1171
Septra ... 1174
Silvadene Cream 1% ... 1540
Tapazole Tablets (Rare) ... 1477
Taxol (Rare) ... 714
Ticlid Tablets (Rare) ... 2156
Trandate (Less common) ... 1185
Trusopt Sterile Ophthalmic Solution (Rare) ... 1760
Univasc Tablets (Rare) ... 2410
Vaseretic Tablets (Rare) ... 1765
Vasocidin Ophthalmic Solution ... ◉ 270
Vasotec I.V. (Rare) ... 1768
Vasotec Tablets (Rare) ... 1771
Voltaren Tablets (Rare) ... 861
Winstrol Tablets (Rare) ... 2337
Wygesic Tablets ... 2827
Zestoretic (Rare) ... 2850
Zestril Tablets (Rare) ... 2854
Zocor Tablets (Rare) ... 1775
Zyloprim Tablets (Less than 1%) ... 1226

Necrosis, intestinal

Lanoxicaps (Very rare) ... 1117
Lanoxin Elixir Pediatric (Very rare) ... 1120
Lanoxin Injection (Very rare) ... 1123
Lanoxin Injection Pediatric (Very rare) ... 1126
Lanoxin Tablets (Very rare) ... 1128
Oncovin Solution Vials & Hyporets ... 1466

(▣ Described in PDR For Nonprescription Drugs) Incidence data in parenthesis; ▲ 3% or more (◉ Described in PDR For Ophthalmology)

1371 Side Effects Index Nephrosis, toxic

Thioguanine Tablets, Tabloid Brand 1181

Necrosis, ischemic

Felbatol 2666

Necrosis, macular

Nebcin Vials, Hyporets & ADD-Vantage 1464

Necrosis, pancreatic

Proglycem Capsules 580

Necrosis, papillary

Cataflam (Rare) 816
Feldene Capsules (Less than 1%) 1965
Nalfon 200 Pulvules & Nalfon Tablets (Less than 1%) 917
Ponstel 1925
Voltaren Tablets (Rare) 861

Necrosis, renal papillary

Children's Advil Suspension (Less than 1%) 2692
Anaprox/Naprosyn (Less than 1%) 2117
Dapsone Tablets USP 1284
Darvon-N/Darvocet-N 1433
Darvon 1435
Darvon-N Suspension & Tablets 1433
EC-Naprosyn Delayed-Release Tablets (Less than 1%) 2117
Feldene Capsules 1965
IBU Tablets (Less than 1%) 1342
Lodine Capsules and Tablets (Less than 1%) 2743
Children's Motrin Ibuprofen Oral Suspension (Less than 1%) 1546
Motrin Tablets (Less than 1%) 2625
Motrin Ibuprofen Suspension, Oral Drops, Chewable Tablets, Caplets (Less than 1%) 1546
Anaprox/Naprosyn (Less than 1%) 2117
Relafen Tablets 2510

Necrosis, renal tubular

Calcium Disodium Versenate Injection 1490
▲ CellCept Capsules (6.3% to 10.0%) 2099
Cytoxan 694
Motrin Ibuprofen Suspension, Oral Drops, Chewable Tablets, Caplets (Less than 1%) 1546
Neoral (1.0%) 2276
NEOSAR Lyophilized/Neosar 1959
Trasylol (0.9%) 613

Necrosis, tissue

Adriamycin PFS 1947
Adriamycin RDF 1947
Cerubidine 795
Coumadin 926
Doxorubicin Astra (Occasional) 540
Fragmin (Rare) 1954
Idamycin 1955
Mepergan Injection 2753
Novantrone (Rare reports) 1279
Pentam 300 Injection (Some instances) 1041
Phenergan Injection 2773
Phenergan Tablets 2775
Rubex 712
Silvadene Cream 1% (Infrequent) 1540
Sotradecol (Sodium Tetradecyl Sulfate Injection) 967

Necrotizing angiitis

Aldactazide 2413
Aldoclor Tablets 1598
Aldoril Tablets 1604
Apresazide Capsules 808
Capozide 742
Combipres Tablets 677
Cortifoam 2396
Diucardin Tablets 2718
Diupres Tablets 1650
Diuril Sodium Intravenous 1652
Dyazide 2479
Enduron Tablets 420
Esidrix Tablets 821
Esimil Tablets 822
Florinef Acetate Tablets 505
HydroDIURIL Tablets 1674
Hydropres Tablets 1675
Hyzaar Tablets 1677
Inderide Tablets 2732
Inderide LA Long Acting Capsules 2734
Lasix Injection, Oral Solution and Tablets 1240
Lodine Capsules and Tablets (Less than 1%) 2743
Lopressor HCT Tablets 832
Lotensin HCT 837
Lozol Tablets 2022
Maxzide 1380
Minizide Capsules 1938
Moduretic Tablets 1705
Mykrox Tablets 993
Oretic Tablets 443
Prinzide Tablets 1737
Ser-Ap-Es Tablets 849
Tenoretic Tablets 2845
Thalitone 1245
Vaseretic Tablets 1765
Zaroxolyn Tablets 1000
Zestoretic 2850
Ziac 1415
Zyloprim Tablets (Less than 1%) 1226

Neonatal morbidity

Altace Capsules (Several dozen cases) 1232
Capoten 739
Capozide 742
Cozaar Tablets 1628
Hyzaar Tablets 1677
Lotensin Tablets 834
Lotensin HCT (Several dozen cases) 837
Lotrel Capsules 840
Monopril Tablets 757
Prinivil Tablets 1733
Prinzide Tablets 1737
Univasc Tablets 2410
Vaseretic Tablets 1765
Vasotec I.V. 1768
Vasotec Tablets 1771
Zestoretic 2850
Zestril Tablets 2854

Neonatal prematurity

Accupril Tablets 1893
Altace Capsules 1232
Capoten 739
Capozide 742
Cozaar Tablets 1628
Hyzaar Tablets 1677
Lotensin Tablets 834
Lotensin HCT 837
Monopril Tablets 757
Prinivil Tablets 1733
Prinzide Tablets 1737
Univasc Tablets 2410
Vaseretic Tablets 1765
Vasotec I.V. 1768
Vasotec Tablets 1771
Zestoretic 2850
Zestril Tablets 2854

Neoplasm (see under Carcinoma)

Neoplasm, malignant

Estratest 2539
Ortho Dienestrol Cream 1866
Orthoclone OKT3 Sterile Solution 1837
Pergonal (menotropins for injection, USP) 2448
Stilphostrol Tablets and Ampuls 612

Neoplasms, hepatic

Android Capsules, 10 mg (Rare) 1250
Android (Rare) 1251
Betaseron for SC Injection 658
Brevicon 2088
Delatestryl Injection (Rare) 2860
Estratest (Rare) 2539
Norinyl 2088
Nor-Q D Tablets 2135
Oreton Methyl (Rare) 1255
Ortho-Cyclen/Ortho-Tri-Cyclen 1858
Ortho-Cyclen/Ortho Tri-Cyclen 1858
Oxandrin 2862
Premarin with Methyltestosterone 2794
Testoderm Testosterone Transdermal System (Rare) 486
Testred Capsules (Rare) 1262
Tri-Norinyl 2164
Winstrol Tablets 2337

Nephritis

Azo Gantrisin Tablets 2081
Azulfidine (Rare) 1949
Betaseron for SC Injection 658
Capastat Sulfate Vials (1 patient) 2868
Cipro Tablets (Less than 1%) 592
NebuPent for Inhalation Solution (1% or less) 1040
Paxil Tablets (Rare) 2505
Phenurone Tablets (1%) 447
Quinidex Extentabs 2067
Salflex Tablets 786
Solganal Suspension 2388
Tapazole Tablets (Very rare) 1477
Timolide Tablets 1748
Toradol 2159
Zithromax (1% or less) 1944
Zyloprim Tablets (Less than 1%) 1226

Nephritis, interstitial

Children's Advil Suspension 2692
Aldoclor Tablets 1598
Aldoril Tablets 1604
Anaprox/Naprosyn (Less than 1%) 2117
Ansaid Tablets (Rare) 2579
Asacol Delayed-Release Tablets 1979
Augmentin (Rare) 2468
Bactrim DS Tablets 2084
Bactrim I.V. Infusion 2082
Bactrim 2084
Capoten 739
Capozide 742
Cataflam (Rare) 816
Ceclor Pulvules & Suspension (Rare) 1431
Chibroxin Sterile Ophthalmic Solution (With oral form) 1617
Cipro I.V. (1% or less) 595
Cipro I.V. Pharmacy Bulk Package (Less than 1%) 597
Cipro Tablets (Less than 1%) 592
Claforan Sterile and Injection (Occasional) 1235
Clinoril Tablets (Less than 1 in 100) 1618
Clozaril Tablets 2252
Daypro Caplets (Less than 1%) 2426
Dipentum Capsules (Rare) 1951
Diupres Tablets 1650
Diuril Oral Suspension 1653
Diuril Sodium Intravenous 1652
Diuril Tablets 1653
Dolobid Tablets (Less than 1 in 100) 1654
Dyazide 2479
Dyrenium Capsules (Rare) 2481
EC-Naprosyn Delayed-Release Tablets (Less than 1%) 2117
Feldene Capsules (Less than 1%) 1965
Floxin I.V. 1571
Floxin Tablets (200 mg, 300 mg, 400 mg) 1567
HydroDIURIL Tablets 1674
Hydropres Tablets 1675
Hyzaar Tablets 1677
Indocin (Less than 1%) 1680
Keflex Pulvules & Oral Suspension (Rare) 914
Keftab Tablets (Rare) 915
Kefzol Vials, Faspak & ADD-Vantage 1456
Lasix Injection, Oral Solution and Tablets 1240
Lodine Capsules and Tablets (Less than 1%) 2743
Maxaquin Tablets 2440
Maxzide 1380
Mefoxin 1691
Mefoxin Premixed Intravenous Solution 1694
Mezlin (Rare) 601
Mezlin Pharmacy Bulk Package (Rare) 604
Moduretic Tablets 1705
Monocid Injection (Rare) 2497
Children's Motrin Ibuprofen Oral Suspension 1546
Motrin Tablets 2625
Motrin Ibuprofen Suspension, Oral Drops, Chewable Tablets, Caplets 1546
Nalfon 200 Pulvules & Nalfon Tablets (Less than 1%) 917
Anaprox/Naprosyn (Less than 1%) 2117
Noroxin Tablets 1715
Noroxin Tablets 2048
Orthoclone OKT3 Sterile Solution 1837
Orudis Capsules (Less than 1%) 2766
Oruvail Capsules (Less than 1%) 2766
Penetrex Tablets 2031
Pentasa (Infrequent) 1527
Pipracil (Rare) 1390
Prilosec Delayed-Release Capsules (Less than 1%) 529
Prinzide Tablets 1737
Proleukin for Injection (Less than 1%) 797
Pyrazinamide Tablets (Rare) 1398
Relafen Tablets (Less than 1%) 2510
Rifadin (Rare) 1528
Rifamate Capsules (Rare) 1530
Rifater (Rare) 1532
SSD (Infrequent) 1355
Septra 1174
Septra I.V. Infusion 1169
Septra I.V. Infusion ADD-Vantage Vials 1171
Septra 1174
Silvadene Cream 1% (Infrequent) 1540
Streptase for Infusion 562
Tagamet (Rare) 2516
Vancocin HCl, Oral Solution & Pulvules (Rare) 1483
Vancocin HCl, Vials & ADD-Vantage (Rare) 1481
Vaseretic Tablets 1765
Voltaren Tablets (Rare) 861
Zestoretic 2850
Ziac 1415
Zinacef (Rare) 1211
Zosyn (Rare) 1419
Zosyn Pharmacy Bulk Package (Rare) 1422

Nephritis, lupus

Quinidex Extentabs 2067

Nephritis, purpuric

Vantin for Oral Suspension and Vantin Tablets 2646

Nephrocalcinosis

▲ Fungizone Intravenous (Among most common) 506
Rocaltrol Capsules 2141

Nephrolithiasis

Axid Pulvules 1427
Sandostatin Injection (Less than 1%) 2292

Nephropathy

Asacol Delayed-Release Tablets 1979
Bicillin C-R Injection 2704
Bicillin C-R 900/300 Injection 2706
Bicillin L-A Injection (Infrequent) 2707
Cefizox for Intramuscular or Intravenous Use 1034
Cefotan 2829
Ceftin 1078
Ceptaz 1081
Duricef 748
Fortaz 1100
Foscavir Injection (Less than 1%) 547
Hivid Tablets (Less than 1% to less than 3%) 2121
Keftab Tablets 915
Lorabid Suspension and Pulvules 1459
Pen•Vee K (Infrequent) 2772
Pfizerpen for Injection (Rare) 2203
Suprax 1399
Tazicef for Injection 2519
Vantin for Oral Suspension and Vantin Tablets 2646
Zefazone 2654
Zinacef 1211

Nephropathy, acute uric acid

Oncaspar 2028
Oncovin Solution Vials & Hyporets 1466

Nephropathy, severe

Methotrexate Sodium Tablets, Injection, for Injection and LPF Injection 1275

Nephrosis, toxic

Azo Gantanol Tablets 2080
Azo Gantrisin Tablets 2081
Azulfidine (Rare) 1949
Bactrim DS Tablets 2084
Bactrim I.V. Infusion 2082
Bactrim 2084
Fansidar Tablets 2114
Felbatol 2666
Foscavir Injection (Less than 1%) 547
Fulvicin P/G Tablets (Rare) 2359
Fulvicin P/G 165 & 330 Tablets (Rare) 2359
Gantanol Tablets 2119
Gantrisin 2120
Intal Capsules (Less than 1 in 100,000 patients) 987
Intal Inhaler (Rare) 988
Intal Nebulizer Solution (Rare) 989
Mesantoin Tablets 2272
Nalfon 200 Pulvules & Nalfon Tablets (Less than 1%) 917
Neurontin Capsules (Rare) 1922
Permax Tablets (Rare) 575

(Described in PDR For Nonprescription Drugs) Incidence data in parenthesis; ▲ 3% or more (◉ Described in PDR For Ophthalmology)

Nephrosis, toxic — Side Effects Index — 1372

SSD 1355
Septra 1174
Septra I.V. Infusion 1169
Septra I.V. Infusion ADD-Vantage Vials 1171
Septra 1174
Silvadene Cream 1% 1540

Nephrotic syndrome

Children's Advil Suspension (Occasional) 2692
Anaprox/Naprosyn (Occasional; less than 1%) 2117
Azulfidine (Rare) 1949
Benemid Tablets 1611
Capoten (Approximately 1 to 2 of 1000 patients) 739
Capozide (Approximately 1 to 2 of 1000 patients) 742
Cataflam (Rare) 816
Clinoril Tablets (Less than 1 in 100) 1618
ColBENEMID Tablets 1622
Cuprimine Capsules 1630
Dapsone Tablets USP 1284
Depen Titratable Tablets 2662
Dipentum Capsules (Rare) 1951
Dolobid Tablets (Rare) 1654
EC-Naprosyn Delayed-Release Tablets (Occasional; less than 1%) 2117
Feldene Capsules (Less than 1%) 1965
Hyperab Rabies Immune Globulin (Human) (Rare) 624
Hyper-Tet Tetanus Immune Globulin (Human) (Few isolated cases) 627
Indocin (Less than 1%) 1680
Children's Motrin Ibuprofen Oral Suspension (Occasional) 1546
Motrin Tablets (Occasional) 2625
Motrin Ibuprofen Suspension, Oral Drops, Chewable Tablets, Caplets (Occasional) 1546
Myochrysine Injection 1711
Anaprox/Naprosyn (Occasional; less than 1%) 2117
Orudis Capsules (Less than 1%) 2766
Oruvail Capsules (Less than 1%) 2766
Pentasa (Infrequent) 1527
Proglycem 580
Relafen Tablets (Less than 1%) 2510
Ridaura Capsules 2513
Rythmol Tablets–150mg, 225mg, 300mg (Less than 1%) 1352
Solganal Suspension 2388
Ticlid Tablets (Rare) 2156
Toradol 2159
Voltaren Tablets (Rare) 861

Nephrotoxicity

Amikacin Sulfate Injection, USP 960
Amikin Injectable 501
BiCNU 691
Capastat Sulfate Vials 2868
CeeNU 693
Cefotan (Rare) 2829
Cefzil Tablets and Oral Suspension 746
Coly-Mycin M Parenteral 1905
Cortisporin Cream 1084
Cortisporin Ointment 1085
Cortisporin Otic Solution Sterile 1087
Cortisporin Otic Suspension Sterile 1088
Esgic-plus Tablets 1013
Fioricet Tablets (Infrequent) 2258
Fioricet with Codeine Capsules 2260
Fiorinal with Codeine Capsules 2262
Furoxone 2046
Garamycin Injectable 2360
IBU Tablets 1342
Methotrexate Sodium Tablets, Injection, for Injection and LPF Injection 1275
Nebcin Vials, Hyporets & ADD-Vantage 1464
NeoDecadron Topical Cream 1714
▲Neoral (25% to 38%) 2276
Neosporin G.U. Irrigant Sterile 1148
Netromycin Injection 100 mg/ml 2373
Neutrexin 2572
Paraplatin for Injection (Uncommon) 705
PediOtic Suspension Sterile 1153
Platinol 708
Platinol-AQ Injection 710
Polymyxin B Sulfate, Aerosporin Brand Sterile Powder 1154
▲Prograf (33% to 40%) 1042
Rowasa 2548
▲Sandimmune (25 to 38%) 2286
Streptomycin Sulfate Injection (Rare) 2208
Tobramycin Sulfate Injection 968
Vancocin HCl, Oral Solution & Pulvules 1483
Vancocin HCl, Vials & ADD-Vantage 1481
Zanosar Sterile Powder 2653
Zinacef 1211

Nerve damage

Surgicel 1314

Nerve deafness

Biavax II 1613
M-M-R II 1687
Mumpsvax 1708
Plaquenil Sulfate Tablets 2328

Nerve injury at injection site

Brevital Sodium Vials 1429

Nervousness

Accupril Tablets (0.5% to 1.0%) 1893
Accutane Capsules 2076
Actifed Plus Caplets ◘ 845
Actifed Plus Tablets ◘ 845
Actifed with Codeine Cough Syrup 1067
Actifed Syrup ◘ 846
Actifed Tablets ◘ 844
Acutrim ◘ 628
▲Adalat Capsules (10 mg and 20 mg) (2% or less to 7%) 587
Adalat CC (Rare) 589
Adenoscan (2%) 1024
Advil Cold and Sinus Caplets and Tablets (formerly CoAdvil) ◘ 870
Children's Advil Suspension (Less than 3%) 2692
▲AeroBid Inhaler System (3-9%) 1005
▲Aerobid-M Inhaler System (3-9%) 1005
▲Airet Solution for Inhalation (4%) 452
Albalon Solution with Liquifilm ◉ 231
Alka-Seltzer Plus Cold Medicine ◘ 705
Alka-Seltzer Plus Cold & Cough Medicine ◘ 708
Alka-Seltzer Plus Night-Time Cold Medicine ◘ 707
Alka Seltzer Plus Sinus Medicine ◘ 707
Allerest Children's Chewable Tablets ◘ 627
Allerest Headache Strength Tablets ◘ 627
Allerest Maximum Strength Tablets ◘ 627
Allerest No Drowsiness Tablets ◘ 627
Allerest Sinus Pain Formula ◘ 627
Allerest 12 Hour Caplets ◘ 627
Altace Capsules (Less than 1%) 1232
▲Alupent (6.8%) 669
Ambien Tablets (1%) 2416
Amen Tablets 780
▲Anafranil Capsules (4% to 18%) 803
Anatuss LA Tablets 1542
Ansaid Tablets (1-3%) 2579
▲Artane (30% to 50%) 1368
Asacol Delayed-Release Tablets 1979
Asendin Tablets (Less frequent) 1369
Atrohist Plus Tablets 454
▲Atrovent Inhalation Aerosol (3.1%) 671
Atrovent Inhalation Solution (0.5%) 673
Axid Pulvules (1.1%) 1427
Bactrim DS Tablets 2084
Bactrim I.V. Infusion 2082
Bactrim 2084
Benadryl Allergy Decongestant Liquid Medication ◘ 848
Benadryl Allergy Decongestant Tablets ◘ 848
Benadryl Allergy Sinus Headache Formula Caplets ◘ 849
Benadryl Capsules 1898
Benadryl Injection 1898
▲Bentyl (6%) 1501
Benylin Multisymptom ◘ 852
▲Betaseron for SC Injection (8%) 658
Blocadren Tablets (Less than 1%) 1614
Brethaire Inhaler 813
▲Brethine Ampuls (16.9 to 38.0%) 815
Brethine Tablets (Common) 814
Brevicon 2088
▲Bricanyl Subcutaneous Injection (Among most common) 1502
▲Bricanyl Tablets (One of the two most common) 1503
Bromfed 1785
▲Bromfed-DM Cough Syrup (Among most frequent) 1786
Bromfed-PD Capsules (Extended-Release) 1785
Bronkaid Mist ◘ 717
Bronkaid Mist Suspension ◘ 718
Bronkaid Caplets ◘ 717
▲BuSpar (5%) 737
Butisol Sodium Elixir & Tablets (Less than 1 in 100) 2660
Capoten 739
Capozide 742
Cardene Capsules (0.6%) 2095
Cardizem CD Capsules (Less than 1%) 1506
Cardizem SR Capsules (Less than %) 1510
Cardizem Injectable 1508
Cardizem Tablets (Less than 1%) 1512
Cardura Tablets (2%) 2186
Cartrol Tablets (Less common) 410
Catapres Tablets (About 3 in 100 patients) 674
Catapres-TTS (1 of 101 patients; less frequent) 675
Ceclor Pulvules & Suspension (Rare) 1431
Cefzil Tablets and Oral Suspension (Less than 1%) 746
Celontin Kapseals 1899
Cerose DM ◘ 878
Children's Vicks DayQuil Allergy Relief ◘ 757
Children's Vicks NyQuil Cold/Cough Relief ◘ 758
Chlor-Trimeton Allergy Decongestant Tablets ◘ 799
Claritin (2% or fewer patients) 2349
▲Claritin-D (5%) 2350
Clinoril Tablets (Greater than 1%) 1618
Cocaine Hydrochloride Topical Solution 537
Cogentin 1621
Cognex Capsules (Frequent) 1901
Combipres Tablets (About 3%) 677
Comhist 2038
Compazine 2470
Allergy-Sinus Comtrex Multi-Symptom Allergy-Sinus Formula Tablets ◘ 617
Comtrex Non-Drowsy ◘ 618
Contac Continuous Action Nasal Decongestant/Antihistamine 12 Hour Capsules ◘ 813
Contac Maximum Strength Continuous Action Decongestant/Antihistamine 12 Hour Caplets ◘ 813
Contac Severe Cold and Flu Formula Caplets ◘ 814
Coricidin 'D' Decongestant Tablets ◘ 800
Cozaar Tablets (Less than 1%) 1628
Cycrin Tablets 975
Cystospaz 1963
Cytovene (1% or less) 2103
D.A. Chewable Tablets 951
Dalmane Capsules 2173
Danocrine Capsules 2307
Dantrium Capsules (Less frequent) 1982
Daranide Tablets 1633
Decadron Phosphate with Xylocaine Injection, Sterile 1639
Deconamine 1320
Deconsal C Expectorant Syrup 456
Deconsal Pediatric Capsules 454
Deconsal Pediatric Syrup 457
Deconsal II Tablets 454
Demadex Tablets and Injection (1.1%) 686
Demulen 2428
▲Depo-Provera Contraceptive Injection (More than 5%) 2602
Depo-Provera Sterile Aqueous Suspension 2606
Desogen Tablets 1817
▲Desyrel and Desyrel Dividose (6.4% to 14.8%) 503
Dexatrim ◘ 832
Dexatrim Plus Vitamins Caplets ◘ 832
Dilantin Infatabs 1908
Dilantin Kapseals 1906
Dilantin Parenteral 1910
Dilantin-125 Suspension 1911
Dilaudid-HP Injection 1337
Dilaudid-HP Lyophilized Powder 250 mg 1337
Dilaudid Tablets and Liquid (Less frequent) 1339
Dimetane-DC Cough Syrup 2059
Dimetane-DX Cough Syrup 2059
Dimetapp Elixir ◘ 773
Dimetapp Extentabs ◘ 774
Dimetapp Tablets/Liqui-Gels ◘ 775
Dimetapp Cold & Allergy Chewable Tablets ◘ 773
Dimetapp Sinus Caplets ◘ 775
Diupres Tablets 1650
Dolobid Tablets (Less than 1 in 100) 1654
Donnatal 2060
Donnatal Extentabs 2061
Donnatal Tablets 2060
Doral Tablets 2664
Dorcol Children's Cough Syrup ◘ 785
Drixoral Cold and Allergy Sustained-Action Tablets ◘ 802
Drixoral Cold and Flu Extended-Release Tablets ◘ 803
Drixoral Allergy/Sinus Extended Release Tablets ◘ 804
▲Duragesic Transdermal System (3% to 10%) 1288
Duranest Injections 542
Dura-Tap/PD Capsules 2867
Duratuss Tablets 2565
Dura-Vent/DA Tablets 953
Dura-Vent Tablets 952
Dyclone 0.5% and 1% Topical Solutions, USP 544
DynaCirc Capsules (0.5% to 1%) 2256
▲Effexor (2% to 21.3%) 2719
Efidac/24 ◘ 635
Eldepryl Tablets 2550
Emete-con Intramuscular/Intravenous 2198
Emla Cream 545
Entex Capsules 1986
Entex LA Tablets 1987
Entex Liquid 1986
Entex PSE Tablets 1987
EpiPen Jr. 790
Ergamisol Tablets (1% to 2%) 1292
▲Ethmozine Tablets (2% to 5%) 2041
Eulexin Capsules (1%) 2358
Exgest LA Tablets 782
Fansidar Tablets 2114
Fedahist Gyrocaps 2401
Fedahist Timecaps 2401
▲Felbatol (7.0% to 16.1%) 2666
Feldene Capsules (Less than 1%) 1965
Fioricet with Codeine Capsules 2260
Fiorinal with Codeine Capsules 2262
Flexeril Tablets (1% to 3%) 1661
Floxin I.V. (1% to 3%) 1571
Floxin Tablets (200 mg, 300 mg, 400 mg) (1% to 3%) 1567
Flumadine Tablets & Syrup (1.3% to 2.1%) 1015
Foscavir Injection (Between 1% and 5%) 547
▲Glucotrol XL Extended Release Tablets (3.6%) 1968
Guaifed Syrup ◘ 734
Guaimax-D Tablets 792
▲Halcion Tablets (5.2%) 2611
Hismanal Tablets (2.1%) 1293
Hivid Tablets (Less than 1% to less than 3%) 2121
Hydropres Tablets 1675
Hytrin Capsules (2.3%) 430
Hyzaar Tablets 1677
IBU Tablets (Greater than 1%) 1342
Imdur (Less than or equal to 5%) 1323
Indocin (Less than 1%) 1680
Intron A (Up to 3%) 2364
Iopidine 0.5% (Less than 1%) ◉ 221
Ismo Tablets (Fewer than 1%) 2738
Isoclor Timesule Capsules ◘ 637
Isuprel Hydrochloride Injection 1:5000 2311
Isuprel Hydrochloride Solution 1:200 & 1:100 2313
Isuprel Mistometer 2312
Kerlone Tablets (0.8%) 2436
Kutrase Capsules 2402
Lamictal Tablets (Frequent) 1112
Levbid Extended-Release Tablets 2405
Levlen/Tri-Levlen 651
Levsin/Levsinex/Levbid 2405
Lodine Capsules and Tablets (More than 1% but less than 3%) 2743
Lo/Ovral Tablets 2746
Lo/Ovral-28 Tablets 2751
Lorabid Suspension and Pulvules 1459
Lotensin Tablets 834
Lotensin HCT (0.3% to 1.0%) 837
Lotrel Capsules 840
▲Lozol Tablets (Less than or greater than 5%) 2022
▲Ludiomil Tablets (6%) 843
Lupron Depot 3.75 mg (Less than 5%) 2556

(◘ Described in PDR For Nonprescription Drugs) Incidence data in parenthesis; ▲ 3% or more (◉ Described in PDR For Ophthalmology)

Lupron Depot 7.5 mg 2559
Lupron Depot-PED 7.5 mg, 11.25 mg and 15 mg (Less than 2%).... 2560
Lupron Injection (Less than 5%) 2555
▲ Luvox Tablets (12%).......... 2544
MS Contin Tablets (Less frequent) .1994
MSIR (Infrequent) 1997
Marax Tablets & DF Syrup.......... 2200
Marinol (Dronabinol) Capsules (Greater than 1%) 2231
Matulane Capsules 2131
▲ Maxair Autohaler (4.5% to 6.9%).. 1492
▲ Maxair Inhaler (6.9%).......... 1494
Maxaquin Tablets (Less than 1%).. 2440
Mebaral Tablets (Less than 1 in 100) 2322
Mesantoin Tablets 2272
▲ Metaproterenol Sulfate Inhalation Solution, USP, Arm-a-Med (About 1 in 7 patients).......... 552
▲ Mexitil Capsules (5% to 11.3%).... 678
Micronor Tablets 1872
Midamor Tablets (Less than or equal to 1%) 1703
Minipress Capsules (1-4%) 1937
Minizide Capsules 1938
Modicon.......... 1872
Moduretic Tablets (Less than or equal to 1%) 1705
8-MOP Capsules 1246
Monoket (Fewer than 1%).......... 2406
Motofen Tablets (1 in 200 to 1 in 600) 784
Children's Motrin Ibuprofen Oral Suspension (Greater than 1% but less than 3%) 1546
Motrin Tablets (Less than 3%) 2625
Motrin Ibuprofen Suspension, Oral Drops, Chewable Tablets, Caplets (1% to less than 3%)...... 1546
Mykrox Tablets (Less than 2%) 993
▲ Nalfon 200 Pulvules & Nalfon Tablets (5.7%).......... 917
Nembutal Sodium Capsules (Less than 1%).......... 436
Nembutal Sodium Solution (Less than 1%).......... 438
Nembutal Sodium Suppositories (Less than 1%).......... 440
Neurontin Capsules (2.4%) 1922
▲ Nicoderm (nicotine transdermal system) (3% to 9%) 1518
Nicotrol Nicotine Transdermal System (1% to 3%).......... 1550
Nolahist Tablets 785
Nolamine Timed-Release Tablets (Occasional).......... 785
Nordette-21 Tablets.......... 2755
Nordette-28 Tablets.......... 2758
Norinyl 2088
Norisodrine with Calcium Iodide Syrup.......... 442
Norpace (1 to 3%) 2444
Norplant System 2759
Nor-Q D Tablets 2135
Norvasc Tablets (More than 0.1% to 1%) 1940
Novahistine DH.......... 2462
Novahistine DMX .... ▣ 822
Novahistine Elixir.......... ▣ 823
Novocain Hydrochloride for Spinal Anesthesia 2326
Nubain Injection (1% or less) 935
Nucofed 2051
OptiPranolol (Metipranolol 0.3%) Sterile Ophthalmic Solution (A small number of patients) .... ◉ 258
Oramorph SR (Morphine Sulfate Sustained Release Tablets) (Less frequent) 2236
▲ Orap Tablets (1 of 20 patients) 1050
▲ Orlamm (3% to 9%).......... 2239
Ornade Spansule Capsules 2502
Ortho-Cept 1851
Ortho-Cyclen/Ortho-Tri-Cyclen 1858
Ortho-Novum.......... 1872
Ortho-Cyclen/Ortho Tri-Cyclen 1858
▲ Orudis Capsules (3% to 9%) 2766
▲ Oruvail Capsules (3% to 9%) 2766
Ovcon 760
Ovral Tablets.......... 2770
Ovral-28 Tablets 2770
Ovrette Tablets.......... 2771
Oxsoralen-Ultra Capsules.......... 1257
PBZ Tablets 845
PBZ-SR Tablets.......... 844
Parlodel 2281
▲ Paxil Tablets (2.9% to 5.9%) 2505
Pediatric Vicks 44d Dry Hacking Cough & Head Congestion.......... ▣ 763
Pediatric Vicks 44m Cough & Cold Relief .... ▣ 764
Penetrex Tablets (1%) 2031
Periactin 1724
Permax Tablets (Frequent) 575
Phenergan Injection 2773
Phenergan Tablets 2775
Phenergan VC 2779
Phenergan VC with Codeine 2781
Phenobarbital Elixir and Tablets (Less than 1 in 100 patients) 1469
Plaquenil Sulfate Tablets 2328
Plendil Extended-Release Tablets (0.5% to 1.5%).......... 527
Pondimin Tablets.......... 2066
Ponstel 1925
Pontocaine Hydrochloride for Spinal Anesthesia 2330
Premphase 2797
Prempro.......... 2801
PREVACID Delayed-Release Capsules (Less than 1%).......... 2562
Prilosec Delayed-Release Capsules (Less than 1%).......... 529
Primatene Tablets .... ▣ 873
Prinivil Tablets (0.3% to 1.0%)...... 1733
Prinzide Tablets 1737
Pro-Banthine Tablets.......... 2052
▲ Procardia Capsules (2% or less to 7%) 1971
▲ Procardia XL Extended Release Tablets (Less than 3% to 7%) 1972
▲ Prograf (Greater than 3%) 1042
Propagest Tablets 786
Propulsid (1.4%).......... 1300
▲ ProSom Tablets (8%) 449
▲ Proventil Inhalation Aerosol (Less than 10%) 2382
▲ Proventil Inhalation Solution 0.083% (4%) 2384
▲ Proventil Repetabs Tablets (2% to 20%) 2386
▲ Proventil Solution for Inhalation 0.5% (4%) 2383
▲ Proventil Syrup (9 of 100 patients; children 2 to 6 years, 15%) 2385
▲ Proventil Tablets (20%).......... 2386
Provera Tablets 2636
▲ Prozac Pulvules & Liquid, Oral Solution (14.9%) 919
Pyrroxate Caplets .... ▣ 772
Quadrinal Tablets 1350
Quarzan Capsules 2181
Relafen Tablets (1% to 3%) 2510
Retrovir Capsules (1.6%) 1158
Retrovir I.V. Infusion (2%) 1163
Retrovir Syrup (1.6%) 1158
▲ ReVia Tablets (4% to more than 10%) 940
Revex (Less than 1%).......... 1811
Rhinocort Nasal Inhaler (Less than 1%).......... 556
Risperdal (Frequent) 1301
▲ Ritalin (One of the two most common).......... 848
Robinul Forte Tablets.......... 2072
Robinul Injectable 2072
Robinul Tablets.......... 2072
Robitussin Maximum Strength Cough & Cold .... ▣ 778
Robitussin Pediatric Cough & Cold Formula .... ▣ 779
Robitussin-CF .... ▣ 777
Robitussin-DAC Syrup 2074
Robitussin-PE .... ▣ 778
Roferon-A Injection (Less than 3%).......... 2145
▲ Romazicon (3% to 9%).......... 2147
Rondec Oral Drops 953
Rondec Syrup 953
Rondec Tablet.......... 953
Rondec-DM Oral Drops 954
Rondec-DM Syrup 954
Rondec-TR Tablet 953
Ryna .... ▣ 841
Salagen Tablets (Less than 1%)...... 1489
▲ Sanorex Tablets (Among most common).......... 2294
Seconal Sodium Pulvules (Less than 1 in 100).......... 1474
Seldane Tablets (1.4% to 1.5%).... 1536
▲ Seldane-D Extended-Release Tablets (6.7%).......... 1538
▲ Semprex-D Capsules (3%) 463
▲ Semprex-D Capsules (3%) 1167
Septra 1174
Septra I.V. Infusion 1169
Septra I.V. Infusion ADD-Vantage Vials.......... 1171
Septra.......... 1174
Ser-Ap-Es Tablets 849
Serevent Inhalation Aerosol (1% to 3%).......... 1176
Serophene (clomiphene citrate tablets, USP) (Approximately 1 in 50 patients) 2451
Sinarest .... ▣ 648
Sine-Aid IB Caplets 1554
Sine-Aid Maximum Strength Sinus Medication Gelcaps, Caplets and Tablets 1554
Sine-Off No Drowsiness Formula Caplets .... ▣ 824
Sine-Off Sinus Medicine .... ▣ 825
Sinemet CR Tablets 944
Singlet Tablets .... ▣ 825
Sinulin Tablets 787
Sinutab Non-Drying Liquid Caps.. ▣ 859
Skelaxin Tablets.......... 788
Stadol (1% or greater).......... 775
Stilphostrol Tablets and Ampuls...... 612
Sudafed Children's Liquid .... ▣ 861
Sudafed Cough Syrup .... ▣ 862
Sudafed Plus Liquid .... ▣ 862
Sudafed Plus Tablets .... ▣ 863
Sudafed Sinus Caplets.......... ▣ 864
Sudafed Sinus Tablets.......... ▣ 864
Sudafed Tablets, 30 mg.......... ▣ 861
Sudafed Tablets, 60 mg.......... ▣ 861
Sudafed 12 Hour Caplets .... ▣ 861
Supprelin Injection (1% to 3%) 2056
Symmetrel Capsules and Syrup (1% to 5%).......... 946
Syn-Rx Tablets 465
Syn-Rx DM Tablets 466
Tavist Syrup.......... 2297
Tavist Tablets 2298
Teldrin 12 Hour Antihistamine/Nasal Decongestant Allergy Relief Capsules .... ▣ 826
Temaril Tablets, Syrup and Spansule Extended-Release Capsules 483
Tenex Tablets (Less frequent).......... 2074
TheraFlu.......... ▣ 787
TheraFlu Maximum Strength Nighttime Flu, Cold & Cough Medicine .... ▣ 788
Timolide Tablets (Less than 1%).... 1748
Timoptic in Ocudose (Less frequent).......... 1753
Timoptic Sterile Ophthalmic Solution (Less frequent).......... 1751
Timoptic-XE 1755
Tofranil Tablets 856
▲ Tonocard Tablets (0.4-11.5%).......... 531
Toradol (1% or less) 2159
▲ Tornalate Solution for Inhalation, 0.2% (11.1%).......... 956
Tornalate Metered Dose Inhaler (1.5% to 5%).......... 957
Tranxene (Less common).......... 451
Trental Tablets 1244
Triaminic Allergy Tablets .... ▣ 789
Triaminic Syrup .... ▣ 792
Triaminic-12 Tablets .... ▣ 792
Triaminic-DM Syrup .... ▣ 792
Triaminicin Tablets .... ▣ 793
Triaminicol Multi-Symptom Cold Tablets .... ▣ 793
Triaminicol Multi-Symptom Relief.......... ▣ 794
Levlen/Tri-Levlen.......... 651
Trinalin Repetabs Tablets 1330
Tri-Norinyl.......... 2164
Triphasil-21 Tablets.......... 2814
Triphasil-28 Tablets.......... 2819
Tussend 1783
Children's TYLENOL Cold Multi-Symptom Liquid Formula and Chewable Tablets 1561
TYLENOL Maximum Strength Flu NightTime Hot Medication Packets 1562
TYLENOL, Maximum Strength, Sinus Medication Geltabs, Gelcaps, Caplets and Tablets....... 1566
TYLENOL Cold Multi-Symptom Formula Medication Tablets and Caplets.......... 1561
TYLENOL Cold Medication No Drowsiness Formula Gelcaps and Caplets 1562
TYLENOL Cold Multi-Symptom Hot Medication Liquid Packets.......... 1557
TYLENOL Cough Multi-Symptom Medication with Decongestant..... 1565
Tympagesic Ear Drops 2342
▲ Ultram Tablets (50 mg) (1% to 14%).......... 1585
Univasc Tablets (Less than 1%)..... 2410
Urispas Tablets.......... 2532
Ursinus Inlay-Tabs.......... ▣ 794
Varivax (Greater than or equal to 1%).......... 1762
▲ Vascor (200, 300 and 400 mg) Tablets (7.37 to 11.63%) 1587
Vaseretic Tablets (0.5% to 2.0%) 1765
Vasotec I.V.......... 1768
Vasotec Tablets (0.5% to 1.0%)... 1771
▲ Ventolin Inhalation Aerosol and Refill (1%; fewer than 10 per 100 patients).......... 1197
▲ Ventolin Inhalation Solution (4%) .. 1198
▲ Ventolin Nebules Inhalation Solution (4%) 1199
Ventolin Rotacaps for Inhalation (1%).......... 1200
▲ Ventolin Syrup (9 of 100 patients; 15% in children).......... 1202
▲ Ventolin Tablets (Approximately 20 of 100 patients) 1203
Versed Injection (Less than 1%) 2170
Vicks 44 LiquiCaps Cough, Cold & Flu Relief.......... ▣ 755
Vicks 44 LiquiCaps Non-Drowsy Cough & Cold Relief.......... ▣ 756
Vicks 44D Dry Hacking Cough & Head Congestion .... ▣ 755
Vicks 44M Cough, Cold & Flu Relief.......... ▣ 756
Vicks DayQuil Allergy Relief 4-Hour Tablets .... ▣ 760
Vicks DayQuil .... ▣ 761
Vicks DayQuil SINUS Pressure & CONGESTION Relief.......... ▣ 761
Vicks Nyquil Hot Therapy.......... ▣ 762
Vicks NyQuil LiquiCaps Multi-Symptom Cold/Flu Relief ▣ 763
Vicks NyQuil Multi-Symptom Cold/Flu Relief - (Original & Cherry Flavor) .... ▣ 763
▲ Videx Tablets, Powder for Oral Solution, & Pediatric Powder for Oral Solution (Less than 1% to 33%) 720
▲ Visken Tablets (7%) 2299
▲ Volmax Extended-Release Tablets (8.5%).......... 1788
▲ Xanax Tablets (4.1%).......... 2649
▲ Xylocaine Injections (Among most common).......... 567
▲ Yutopar Intravenous Injection (5% to 6%) 570
Zaroxolyn Tablets (Less than 2%).. 1000
▲ Zerit Capsules (Fewer than 1% to 10%) 729
Zestoretic 2850
Zestril Tablets (0.3% to 1.0%) 2854
▲ Zoladex (3%) 2858
▲ Zoloft Tablets (3.4%).......... 2217

Neuralgia

Altace Capsules (Less than 1%)..... 1232
Ambien Tablets (Rare) 2416
Anafranil Capsules (Infrequent) 803
Betaseron for SC Injection.......... 658
Effexor (Infrequent) 2719
Foscavir Injection (Less than 1%) .. 547
Hivid Tablets (Less than 1% to less than 3%).......... 2121
Imitrex Tablets (Rare) 1106
Kerlone Tablets (Less than 2%)...... 2436
Lamictal Tablets (Rare).......... 1112
Lamprene Capsules (Less than 1%).......... 828
Luvox Tablets (Infrequent) 2544
Miacalcin Nasal Spray (Less than 1%).......... 2275
NebuPent for Inhalation Solution (1% or less).......... 1040
Paxil Tablets (Rare) 2505
Pentam 300 Injection (0.9%).......... 1041
Permax Tablets (1.1%) 575
Phenobarbital Elixir and Tablets (Rare).......... 1469
Prozac Pulvules & Liquid, Oral Solution (Infrequent) 919
Serzone Tablets (Infrequent) 771
Videx Tablets, Powder for Oral Solution, & Pediatric Powder for Oral Solution (Less than 1%) 720
Zerit Capsules (Fewer than 1% to 1%).......... 729

Neural tube defects, unspecified

Clomid 1514
Serophene (clomiphene citrate tablets, USP) 2451

(▣ Described in PDR For Nonprescription Drugs) Incidence data in parenthesis; ▲ 3% or more (◉ Described in PDR For Ophthalmology)

Neuritis

Actifed with Codeine Cough Syrup 1067
Ambien Tablets (Rare) 2416
Benadryl Capsules 1898
Benadryl Injection 1898
Clinoril Tablets (Rare) 1618
Cognex Capsules (Infrequent) 1901
Cytosar-U Sterile Powder (Less frequent) 2592
Deconamine 1320
Effexor (Rare) 2719
Fluorescite ⊙ 219
Foscavir Injection (Less than 1%) 547
Hivid Tablets (Less than 1% to less than 3%) 2121
Imdur (Less than or equal to 5%) 1323
Lotrel Capsules (Infrequent) 840
Ornade Spansule Capsules 2502
Periactin 1724
Permax Tablets (Rare) 575
ProSom Tablets (Rare) 449
Tapazole Tablets 1477
Tavist Syrup 2297
Tavist Tablets 2298
Temaril Tablets, Syrup and Spansule Extended-Release Capsules 483
Trinalin Repetabs Tablets 1330
Tussend 1783
Zyloprim Tablets (Less than 1%) 1226

Neuritis, optic

Accutane Capsules (Less than 1%) 2076
Children's Advil Suspension (Less than 1%) 2692
Amen Tablets 780
Antabuse Tablets 2695
Attenuvax 1610
Biavax II 1613
Chloromycetin Sodium Succinate 1900
Clomid 1514
Cordarone Tablets (Rare) 2712
Cuprimine Capsules 1630
Cycrin Tablets 975
Decadron Phosphate Sterile Ophthalmic Ointment 1641
Decadron Phosphate Sterile Ophthalmic Solution 1642
Demulen 2428
Depen Titratable Tablets 2662
Depo-Provera Sterile Aqueous Suspension 2606
Engerix-B Unit-Dose Vials 2482
Estraderm Transdermal System 824
ESTRATAB Tablets (0.3, 0.625, 1.25, 2.5 mg) 2536
Estratest 2539
Ganite (Less than 1%) 2533
IBU Tablets (Less than 1%) 1342
Lo/Ovral Tablets 2746
Lo/Ovral-28 Tablets 2751
M-M-R II (Infrequent) 1687
M-R-VAX II 1689
Macrobid Capsules (Rare) 1988
Macrodantin Capsules (Rare) 1989
Menest Tablets 2494
Children's Motrin Ibuprofen Oral Suspension (Less than 1%) 1546
Motrin Tablets (Less than 1%) 2625
Motrin Ibuprofen Suspension, Oral Drops, Chewable Tablets, Caplets (Less than 1%) 1546
Mumpsvax 1708
Myambutol Tablets 1386
Nalfon 200 Pulvules & Nalfon Tablets (Less than 1%) 917
Nordette-21 Tablets 2755
Nordette-28 Tablets 2758
Nydrazid Injection (Uncommon) 508
Ortho Dienestrol Cream 1866
Ovral Tablets 2770
Ovral-28 Tablets 2770
Ovrette Tablets 2771
PMB 200 and PMB 400 2783
PASER Granules 1285
Platinol (Infrequent) 708
Platinol-AQ Injection (Infrequent) 710
Premarin Intravenous 2787
Premarin with Methyltestosterone 2794
Premarin Vaginal Cream 2791
Premphase 2797
Prempro 2801
Proleukin for Injection (Less than 1%) 797
Provera Tablets 2636
Quinaglute Dura-Tabs Tablets (Occasional) 649
Quinidex Extentabs 2067
Recombivax HB 1744
Rifamate Capsules (Uncommon) 1530
Rifater (Uncommon) 1532
Stilphostrol Tablets and Ampuls 612
Trecator-SC Tablets 2814
VePesid Capsules and Injection 718
Yodoxin 1230
Zyloprim Tablets (Less than 1%) 1226

Neuritis, peripheral

Antabuse Tablets 2695
Antivenin (Crotalidae) Polyvalent (Occasional) 2696
Apresazide Capsules (Less frequent) 808
Apresoline Hydrochloride Tablets (Less frequent) 809
Atretol Tablets 573
Azo Gantanol Tablets 2080
Azo Gantrisin Tablets 2081
Bactrim DS Tablets 2084
Bactrim I.V. Infusion 2082
Bactrim 2084
Chloromycetin Sodium Succinate 1900
ColBENEMID Tablets 1622
Fansidar Tablets 2114
Gantanol Tablets 2119
Gantrisin 2120
Intal Capsules (Less than 1 in 100,000 patients) 987
Intal Inhaler (Rare) 988
Intal Nebulizer Solution (Rare) 989
Lopid Tablets 1917
Lorelco Tablets 1517
Myambutol Tablets 1386
Nasalcrom Nasal Solution (Rare) 994
Septra 1174
Septra I.V. Infusion 1169
Septra I.V. Infusion ADD-Vantage Vials 1171
Septra 1174
Ser-Ap-Es Tablets 849
Solganal Suspension 2388
Streptomycin Sulfate Injection 2208
Tegretol Chewable Tablets 852
Tegretol Suspension 852
Tegretol Tablets 852
Trecator-SC Tablets 2814
Velban Vials 1484

Neuritis, retrobulbar

Ansaid Tablets (Less than 1%) 2579
Attenuvax 1610
Biavax II 1613
M-M-R II 1687
M-R-VAX II 1689
Meruvax II 1697
Mumpsvax (Infrequent) 1708

Neuroencephalopathy

Taxol (Less than 1%) 714

Neuroleptic malignant syndrome

Asendin Tablets (Less than 1%) 1369
Atamet 572
Clozaril Tablets (Several cases) 2252
Compazine 2470
Etrafon 2355
Haldol Decanoate 1577
Haldol Injection, Tablets and Concentrate 1575
Inapsine Injection (Very rare) 1296
Loxitane 1378
Mellaril 2269
Moban Tablets and Concentrate 1048
Navane Capsules and Concentrate (Rare) 2201
Navane Intramuscular (Rare) 2202
Orap Tablets 1050
Paxil Tablets 2505
Permax Tablets 575
Prolixin 509
Prozac Pulvules & Liquid, Oral Solution 919
Reglan (Rare) 2068
Risperdal 1301
Serentil 684
Serzone Tablets (Rare) 771
Sinemet Tablets 943
Sinemet CR Tablets 944
Stelazine 2514
Symmetrel Capsules and Syrup (Uncommon) 946
Temaril Tablets, Syrup and Spansule Extended-Release Capsules (Rare) 483
Thorazine 2523
Torecan 2245
Triavil Tablets 1757
Trilafon 2389
Zoloft Tablets 2217

Neurological disability, unspecified

Acel-Imune Diphtheria and Tetanus Toxoids and Acellular Pertussis Vaccine Adsorbed (Rare) 1364
BCG Vaccine, USP (TICE) (0.9%) 1814
Coly-Mycin M Parenteral 1905
Ergamisol Tablets (Several reports) 1292
Fungizone Intravenous 506
Hivid Tablets (Less than 1% to less than 3%) 2121
JE-VAX (Two cases) 886
Rabies Vaccine, Imovax Rabies I.D. (Two cases) 883
Tetramune (Rare) 1404

Neuromuscular block reversal, difficult

Nuromax Injection (Less than or equal to 0.1%) 1149

Neuromuscular blockade

Amikacin Sulfate Injection, USP 960
Amikin Injectable 501
Coly-Mycin M Parenteral 1905
Mivacron (3 of 2,074 patients) 1138
Nebcin Vials, Hyporets & ADD-Vantage 1464
Netromycin Injection 100 mg/ml 2373
Zemuron 1830

Neuromuscular excitability

Ceptaz 1081
Fortaz 1100
Ticar for Injection (With very high doses) 2526

Neuromuscular symptoms

Eulexin Capsules (2%) 2358
Lupron Depot 3.75 mg (Less than 5%) 2556

Neuromyopathy

Aralen Hydrochloride Injection 2301
Aralen Phosphate Tablets 2301

Neuro-ocular lesions

Amen Tablets 780
Demulen 2428
Triphasil-21 Tablets 2814
Triphasil-28 Tablets 2819

Neuropathy

Altace Capsules (Less than 1%) 1232
Ambien Tablets (Rare) 2416
Anafranil Capsules (Rare) 803
Betaseron for SC Injection 658
Bicillin C-R Injection 2704
Bicillin C-R 900/300 Injection 2706
Bicillin L-A Injection (Infrequent) 2707
▲ CHEMET (succimer) Capsules (1.0 to 12.7%) 1545
Cognex Capsules (Infrequent) 1901
Cortifoam 2396
Cuprimine Capsules 1630
Cytosar-U Sterile Powder (Two patients) 2592
Cytotec (Infrequent) 2424
▲ Cytovene (8%) 2103
Depen Titratable Tablets 2662
Dilacor XR Extended-release Capsules 2018
Diprivan Injection (Less than 1%) 2833
Effexor (Infrequent) 2719
Engerix-B Unit-Dose Vials 2482
Fioricet with Codeine Capsules 2260
Fiorinal with Codeine Capsules 2262
▲ Foscavir Injection (5% or greater) 547
Gelfoam Sterile Sponge 2608
Havrix (Rare) 2489
Intron A (Less than 5%) 2364
Kerlone Tablets (Less than 2%) 2436
Luvox Tablets 2544
Matulane Capsules 2131
Megace Oral Suspension (1% to 3%) 699
Mutamycin 703
Mykrox Tablets (Less than 2%) 993
NebuPent for Inhalation Solution (1% or less) 1040
Nimotop Capsules (Less than 1%) 610
Paxil Tablets (Rare) 2505
Pen•Vee K (Infrequent) 2772
Permax Tablets (Infrequent) 575
Pfizerpen for Injection (Rare) 2203
Platinol 708
Platinol-AQ Injection 710
▲ Prograf (Greater than 3%) 1042
Prozac Pulvules & Liquid, Oral Solution (Infrequent) 919
Roferon-A Injection (Less than 0.5%) 2145
Sporanox Capsules (Isolated cases) 1305
Tambocor Tablets (Less than 1%) 1497
Urobiotic-250 Capsules 2214
▲ Videx Tablets, Powder for Oral Solution, & Pediatric Powder for Oral Solution (Rare in children; 17% to 20%) 720
Zaroxolyn Tablets 1000
▲ Zerit Capsules (15% to 21%) 729

Neuropathy, autonomic

Platinol 708
Platinol-AQ Injection 710
Taxol (Rare) 714

Neuropathy, optic

Decadron Phosphate Injection 1637
Decadron Phosphate Sterile Ophthalmic Ointment 1641
Decadron Phosphate Sterile Ophthalmic Solution 1642
Healon GV ⊙ 315
Tolectin (200, 400 and 600 mg) (Less than 1%) 1581

Neuropathy, peripheral

Ancobon Capsules 2079
Antabuse Tablets 2695
Asacol Delayed-Release Tablets (Rare) 1979
Azulfidine (Rare) 1949
Betapace Tablets (One case) 641
Cordarone Tablets (Common) 2712
Cozaar Tablets (Less than 1%) 1628
Cuprimine Capsules 1630
Dapsone Tablets USP 1284
Depen Titratable Tablets 2662
Diphtheria and Tetanus Toxoids and Pertussis Vaccine Adsorbed (A few cases) 2477
Elavil 2838
Endep Tablets 2174
Ergamisol Tablets (Several reports) 1292
Etrafon 2355
Flagyl 375 Capsules 2434
Flagyl I.V. 2247
Flexeril Tablets (Rare) 1661
Floxin I.V. 1571
Floxin Tablets (200 mg, 300 mg, 400 mg) 1567
Fludara for Injection 663
Foscavir Injection (Less than 1%) 547
Fungizone Intravenous 506
Garamycin Injectable 2360
▲ Hexalen Capsules (9% to 31%) 2571
▲ Hivid Tablets (22% to 35%) 2121
Hyzaar Tablets 1677
▲ Idamycin (7%) 1955
Indocin Capsules (Less than 1%) 1680
Indocin I.V. (Less than 1%) 1684
Indocin (Less than 1%) 1680
JE-VAX (1 to 2.3 per million vaccines) 886
Lescol Capsules 2267
Leukeran Tablets 1133
Ludiomil Tablets (Isolated reports) 843
Lupron Depot 3.75 mg 2556
Lupron Depot 7.5 mg 2559
Lupron Injection (Less than 5%) 2555
Macrobid Capsules 1988
Macrodantin Capsules 1989
Mevacor Tablets (0.5% to 1.0%) 1699
Myochrysine Injection (Rare) 1711
▲ Navelbine Injection (Up to 20%) 1145
Netromycin Injection 100 mg/ml 2373
Noroxin Tablets 1715
Noroxin Tablets 2048
Norpramin Tablets 1526
▲ Nydrazid Injection (Among most common) 508
Pamelor 2280
▲ Paraplatin for Injection (4% to 16%) 705
Placidyl Capsules 448
Platinol 708
Platinol-AQ Injection 710
Pravachol 765
Prinivil Tablets (0.3% to 1.0%) 1733
Prinzide Tablets 1737
Protostat Tablets 1883
Recombivax HB 1744
Ridaura Capsules (Less than 1%) 2513
Rifamate Capsules 1530
Rifater 1532
Surmontil Capsules 2811
▲ Taxol (Frequent; 3% to 60%) 714
Ticlid Tablets (Rare) 2156

(▣ Described in PDR For Nonprescription Drugs) Incidence data in parenthesis; ▲ 3% or more (⊙ Described in PDR For Ophthalmology)

1375 Side Effects Index Nightmares

Tofranil Ampuls ... 854
Tofranil Tablets ... 856
Tofranil-PM Capsules ... 857
Triavil Tablets ... 1757
Tripedia (A few cases) ... 892
Vaseretic Tablets ... 1765
Vasotec I.V. ... 1768
Vasotec Tablets (0.5% to 1.0%) ... 1771
▲ Videx Tablets, Powder for Oral Solution, & Pediatric Powder for Oral Solution (12% to 51%) ... 720
Vivactil Tablets ... 1774
Yodoxin ... 1230
▲ Zerit Capsules (15% to 21%) ... 729
Zestoretic ... 2850
Zestril Tablets ... 2854
Zocor Tablets ... 1775
Zyloprim Tablets (Less than 1%) ... 1226

Neuropsychometrics performance, decrease

Blocadren Tablets ... 1614
Cartrol Tablets ... 410
Inderal ... 2728
Inderal LA Long Acting Capsules ... 2730
Inderide Tablets ... 2732
Inderide LA Long Acting Capsules ... 2734
Kerlone Tablets ... 2436
Levatol ... 2403
Lopressor HCT Tablets ... 832
Normodyne Tablets ... 2379
Sectral Capsules ... 2807
Tenoretic Tablets ... 2845
Tenormin Tablets and I.V. Injection ... 2847
Timoptic in Ocudose ... 1753
Timoptic Sterile Ophthalmic Solution ... 1751
Timoptic-XE ... 1755
Toprol-XL Tablets ... 565
Trandate Tablets ... 1185
Visken Tablets ... 2299

Neuroretinitis

BiCNU ... 691

Neurosis, unspecified

Ambien Tablets (Rare) ... 2416
Betaseron for SC Injection ... 658
Cognex Capsules (Infrequent) ... 1901
Intron A (Less than 5%) ... 2364
Lamictal Tablets (Rare) ... 1112
Neurontin Capsules (Rare) ... 1922
Permax Tablets (Infrequent) ... 575
Zoloft Tablets (Infrequent) ... 2217

Neurotoxicity

Amikacin Sulfate Injection, USP ... 960
Amikin Injectable ... 501
Cytosar-U Sterile Powder (Less frequent) ... 2592
Fluorouracil Injection (Rare) ... 2116
Foscavir Injection ... 547
Garamycin Injectable ... 2360
Hexalen Capsules ... 2571
Nebcin Vials, Hyporets & ADD-Vantage ... 1464
Netromycin Injection 100 mg/ml ... 2373
Oncovin Solution Vials & Hyporets 1466
▲ Paraplatin for Injection (5% to 28%) ... 705
Platinol ... 708
Platinol-AQ Injection ... 710
Polymyxin B Sulfate, Aerosporin Brand Sterile Powder ... 1154
▲ Prograf (Approximately 55%) ... 1042
Streptomycin Sulfate Injection ... 2208
Tobramycin Sulfate Injection ... 968
Velban Vials (Not common) ... 1484
Vumon (Less than 1%) ... 727
▲ Zinecard (10% to 17%) ... 1961

Neurotoxicity, peripheral

VePesid Capsules and Injection (1% to 2%) ... 718

Neurovascular episodes

Lippes Loop Intrauterine Double-S.. 1848
ParaGard T380A Intrauterine Copper Contraceptive ... 1880

Neutropenia

Accupril Tablets (Rare) ... 1893
Achromycin V Capsules ... 1367
Children's Advil Suspension (Less than 1%) ... 2692
Altace Capsules ... 1232
Ancef Injection ... 2465
Aredia for Injection (Up to 1%) ... 810
Atgam Sterile Solution (Less than 5%) ... 2581
Azactam for Injection (Less than 1%) ... 734
Bactrim DS Tablets ... 2084
Bactrim I.V. Infusion ... 2082
Bactrim ... 2084
▲ Betaseron for SC Injection (18%) .. 658
Capoten ... 739
Capozide ... 742
Cardura Tablets ... 2186
Ceclor Pulvules & Suspension (Rare) ... 1431
Cefizox for Intramuscular or Intravenous Use (Rare) ... 1034
Cefobid Intravenous/Intramuscular (1 in 50) ... 2189
Cefobid Pharmacy Bulk Package - Not for Direct Infusion (1 in 50).. 2192
Cefotan ... 2829
Ceftin ... 1078
Cefzil Tablets and Oral Suspension 746
CellCept Capsules (Up to 2.0%) ... 2099
Ceptaz (Very rare) ... 1081
CHEMET (succimer) Capsules ... 1545
Chibroxin Sterile Ophthalmic Solution (With oral form) ... 1617
Claforan Sterile and Injection (Less than 1%) ... 1235
Cleocin Phosphate Injection ... 2586
Cleocin Vaginal Cream ... 2589
Clinoril Tablets (Less than 1 in 100) ... 1618
▲ Clozaril Tablets (3%) ... 2252
▲ Cytovene-IV (7% to 41%) ... 2103
Cytoxan ... 694
Declomycin Tablets ... 1371
Desyrel and Desyrel Dividose (Occasional) ... 503
Dipentum Capsules (Rare) ... 1951
Dizac (Less frequent) ... 1809
Doryx Capsules ... 1913
Duricef ... 748
Dynacin Capsules ... 1590
Edecrin ... 1657
Ergamisol Tablets (2 out of 463 patients) ... 1292
Flagyl 375 Capsules ... 2434
Floxin I.V. (More than or equal to 1%) ... 1571
Floxin Tablets (200 mg, 300 mg, 400 mg) (More than or equal to 1%) ... 1567
▲ Fludara for Injection (Among most common) ... 663
Fluorouracil Injection (Rare) ... 2116
Fortaz (Very rare) ... 1100
Gantanol Tablets ... 2119
Gastrocrom Capsules (Infrequent).. 984
Geocillin Tablets ... 2199
Halcion Tablets (1.5%) ... 2611
▲ Hivid Tablets (15.1% to 16.9%) ... 2121
IBU Tablets (Less than 1%) ... 1342
Keflex Pulvules & Oral Suspension 914
Keftab Tablets ... 915
Kefurox Vials, Faspak & ADD-Vantage (Less than 1 in 100) ... 1454
Kefzol Vials, Faspak & ADD-Vantage ... 1456
Leukeran Tablets ... 1133
▲ Leustatin (70%) ... 1834
Lincocin ... 2617
Lodine Capsules and Tablets (Less than 1%) ... 2743
Lorabid Suspension and Pulvules ... 1459
Lotensin HCT ... 837
Lotrel Capsules ... 840
Mandol Vials, Faspak & ADD-Vantage ... 1461
Mefoxin ... 1691
Mefoxin Premixed Intravenous Solution ... 1694
▲ Mepron Suspension (5%) ... 1135
Mesantoin Tablets ... 2272
MetroGel-Vaginal ... 902
Mexitil Capsules (About 1 in 1,000) ... 678
Mezlin ... 601
Mezlin Pharmacy Bulk Package ... 604
Midamor Tablets (Rare) ... 1703
Minocin Intravenous ... 1382
Minocin Oral Suspension ... 1385
Minocin Pellet-Filled Capsules ... 1383
Moduretic Tablets ... 1705
Monocid Injection (Less than 1%) .. 2497
Monodox Capsules ... 1805
Monopril Tablets ... 757
Children's Motrin Ibuprofen Oral Suspension (Less than 1%) ... 1546
Motrin Tablets (Less than 1%) ... 2625
Motrin Ibuprofen Suspension, Oral Drops, Chewable Tablets, Caplets (Less than 1%) ... 1546
▲ Mycobutin Capsules (25%) ... 1957
NebuPent for Inhalation Solution (1% or less) ... 1040
NEOSAR Lyophilized/Neosar ... 1959
▲ Neutrexin (30.3%) ... 2572
Nolvadex Tablets (Rare) ... 2841
Noroxin Tablets (1.4%) ... 1715
Noroxin Tablets (1.4%) ... 2048
Orthoclone OKT3 Sterile Solution .. 1837
▲ Paraplatin for Injection (16% to 97%) ... 705
Pipracil ... 1390
Platinol ... 708
Platinol-AQ Injection ... 710
Prilosec Delayed-Release Capsules (Rare) ... 529
Primaxin I.M. ... 1727
Primaxin I.V. (Less than 0.2%) ... 1729
Prinivil Tablets (Rare) ... 1733
Prinzide Tablets (Rare) ... 1737
Procan SR Tablets (Rare) ... 1926
Proglycem ... 580
Proleukin for Injection ... 797
Proloprim Tablets ... 1155
Protostat Tablets ... 1883
Quinidex Extentabs ... 2067
Reglan (A few cases) ... 2068
Retrovir ... 1158
Ridaura Capsules (0.1 to 1%) ... 2513
Rocephin Injectable Vials, ADD-Vantage, Galaxy Container (Less than 1%) ... 2142
▲ Roferon-A Injection (52%) ... 2145
Sansert Tablets ... 2295
Septra ... 1174
Septra I.V. Infusion ... 1169
Septra I.V. Infusion ADD-Vantage Vials ... 1171
Septra ... 1174
Suprax ... 1399
Symmetrel Capsules and Syrup (Less than 0.1%) ... 946
▲ Taxol (52% to 90%) ... 714
Tazicef for Injection (Very rare) ... 2519
Terramycin Intramuscular Solution 2210
Ticar for Injection ... 2526
Ticlid Tablets (1.6% to 2.4%) ... 2156
Timentin for Injection ... 2528
Tonocard Tablets (Less than 1%) .. 531
Trimpex Tablets ... 2163
Unasyn ... 2212
Univasc Tablets (More than 1%) ... 2410
Valium Injectable (Isolated reports) 2182
Valium Tablets (Isolated reports) ... 2183
Valrelease Capsules (Rare) ... 2169
Vancocin HCl, Oral Solution & Pulvules (Several dozen cases) ... 1483
Vancocin HCl, Vials & ADD-Vantage (Several dozen cases) ... 1481
Vantin for Oral Suspension and Vantin Tablets ... 2646
Vascor (200, 300 and 400 mg) Tablets (2 cases) ... 1587
Vaseretic Tablets (Rare; several cases) ... 1765
Vasotec I.V. (Rare; several cases) ... 1768
Vasotec Tablets (Rare; several cases) ... 1771
Vermox Chewable Tablets (Rare) ... 1312
Vibramycin ... 1941
Vibramycin Hyclate Intravenous ... 2215
Vibramycin ... 1941
▲ Vumon (95%) ... 727
Xanax Tablets (2.3% to 3.0%) ... 2649
Zefazone ... 2654
▲ Zerit Capsules (3% to 11%) ... 729
Zestoretic (Rare) ... 2850
Zestril Tablets (Rare) ... 2854
Zinacef (Fewer than 1 in 100) ... 1211
Zithromax (Less than 1%) ... 1944
Zosyn ... 1419
Zosyn Pharmacy Bulk Package ... 1422
Zovirax Sterile Powder (Less than 1%) ... 1223

Neutropenia, congenital

Azulfidine (Rare) ... 1949

Neutrophilia

Floxin I.V. (More than or equal to 1%) ... 1571
Floxin Tablets (200 mg, 300 mg, 400 mg) (More than or equal to 1%) ... 1567
Hivid Tablets (Less than 1% to less than 3%) ... 2121
Zovirax Sterile Powder (Less than 1%) ... 1223

Neutrophils, decrease (see under Neutropenia)

Nicotine intoxication

Nicorette ... 2458

Night blindness (see under Nyctalopia)

Nightmares

Aldoclor Tablets ... 1598
Aldomet Ester HCl Injection ... 1602
Aldomet Oral ... 1600
Aldoril Tablets ... 1604
Asendin Tablets (Less frequent) ... 1369
Atamet ... 572
Blocadren Tablets ... 1614
Butisol Sodium Elixir & Tablets (Less than 1 in 100) ... 2660
Cataflam (Less than 1%) ... 816
Catapres Tablets ... 674
Catapres-TTS ... 675
Cipro I.V. (1% or less) ... 595
Cipro I.V. Pharmacy Bulk Package (Less than 1%) ... 597
Cipro Tablets (Less than 1%) ... 592
▲ Clozaril Tablets (4%) ... 2252
Combipres Tablets ... 677
Desyrel and Desyrel Dividose (Less than 1% to 5.1%) ... 503
Diupres Tablets ... 1650
Doral Tablets ... 2664
Elavil ... 2838
Eldepryl Tablets ... 2550
Endep Tablets ... 2174
Etrafon ... 2355
Floxin I.V. ... 1571
Floxin Tablets (200 mg, 300 mg, 400 mg) ... 1567
Halcion Tablets (Rare) ... 2611
Hydropres Tablets ... 1675
Ismo Tablets (Fewer than 1%) ... 2738
Larodopa Tablets (Relatively frequent) ... 2129
Lopressor Ampuls ... 830
Lopressor HCT Tablets (1 in 100 patients) ... 832
Lopressor Tablets ... 830
Ludiomil Tablets (Rare) ... 843
Marinol (Dronabinol) Capsules (Less than 1%) ... 2231
Matulane Capsules ... 2131
Mebaral Tablets (Less than 1 in 100) ... 2322
Monoket (Fewer than 1%) ... 2406
Nardil (Infrequent) ... 1920
Nembutal Sodium Capsules (Less than 1%) ... 436
Nembutal Sodium Solution (Less than 1%) ... 438
Nembutal Sodium Suppositories (Less than 1%) ... 440
Norpramin Tablets ... 1526
Orudis Capsules (Rare) ... 2766
Oruvail Capsules (Rare) ... 2766
Pamelor ... 2280
Parlodel ... 2281
Phenobarbital Elixir and Tablets (Less than 1 in 100 patients) ... 1469
Plaquenil Sulfate Tablets ... 2328
Relafen Tablets (Less than 1%) ... 2510
ReVia Tablets (Less than 1%) ... 940
Risperdal (Rare) ... 1301
Seconal Sodium Pulvules (Less than 1 in 100) ... 1474
Seldane Tablets ... 1536
Seldane-D Extended-Release Tablets ... 1538
Ser-Ap-Es Tablets ... 849
Sinemet Tablets ... 943
Surmontil Capsules ... 2811
Temaril Tablets, Syrup and Spansule Extended-Release Capsules ... 483
Timolide Tablets ... 1748
Timoptic in Ocudose ... 1753
Timoptic Sterile Ophthalmic Solution ... 1751
Timoptic-XE ... 1755
Tofranil Ampuls ... 854
Tofranil Tablets ... 856
Tofranil-PM Capsules ... 857
Toprol-XL Tablets ... 565
Triavil Tablets ... 1757
Vantin for Oral Suspension and Vantin Tablets (Less than 1%) ... 2646
Ventolin Inhalation Aerosol and Refill (1%) ... 1197

(Described in PDR For Nonprescription Drugs) Incidence data in parenthesis; ▲ 3% or more (◉ Described in PDR For Ophthalmology)

Versed Injection (Less than 1%) 2170
Vivactil Tablets 1774
Voltaren Tablets (Less than 1%) 861

Night sweat
Hivid Tablets (Less than 1% to less than 3%) 2121
▲ NebuPent for Inhalation Solution (10 to 23%) 1040
Neoral (Rare) 2276
▲ Oncaspar (Greater than 1% but less than 5%) 2028
Sandimmune (Rare) 2286

Night terrors (see under Pavor nocturnus)

Nitritoid reactions
Myochrysine Injection 1711

Nitrogen balance, changes (see under BUN levels, changes)

Nocturia
Adalat Capsules (10 mg and 20 mg) (Less than 0.5%) 587
Adalat CC (Less than 1.0%) 589
Anafranil Capsules (Infrequent) 803
▲ BCG Vaccine, USP (TICE) (4.5%) 1814
Betaseron for SC Injection 658
BuSpar (Rare) 737
Cardene Capsules (0.4%) 2095
Cardizem CD Capsules (Less than 1%) 1506
Cardizem SR Capsules (Less than 1%) 1510
Cardizem Injectable 1508
Cardizem Tablets (Less than 1%) 1512
Cataflam (Less than 1%) 816
Catapres Tablets (About 1 in 100 patients) 674
Catapres-TTS (Less frequent) 675
Claritin-D (Less frequent) 2350
Cognex Capsules (Infrequent) 1901
Combipres Tablets (About 1%) 677
Cozaar Tablets (Less than 1%) 1628
Dantrium Capsules (Less frequent) 1982
DynaCirc Capsules (0.5% to 1%) 2256
Effexor (Infrequent) 2719
Eldepryl Tablets 2550
Esimil Tablets 822
Foscavir Injection (Between 1% and 5%) 547
Hivid Tablets (Less than 1% to less than 3%) 2121
▲ Hylorel Tablets (48.4%) 985
Hyperstat I.V. Injection 2363
Hyzaar Tablets 1677
Intron A (Less than 5%) 2364
Ismelin Tablets 827
Klonopin Tablets 2126
Lioresal Tablets (Rare) 829
Lorelco Tablets 1517
Lozol Tablets (Less than 5%) 2022
Luvox Tablets (Infrequent) 2544
Matulane Capsules 2131
Miacalcin Injection 2273
Moduretic Tablets (Less than or equal to 1%) 1705
Mykrox Tablets (Less than 2%) 993
Neurontin Capsules (Rare) 1922
Norpramin Tablets 1526
Norvasc Tablets (More than 0.1% to 1%) 1940
Orap Tablets 1050
Pamelor 2280
Paxil Tablets (Infrequent) 2505
Procardia XL Extended Release Tablets (1% or less) 1972
ProSom Tablets (Rare) 449
Rocaltrol Capsules 2141
Sectral Capsules (Up to 2%) 2807
Serzone Tablets (Infrequent) 771
Supprelin Injection (1% to 3%) 2056
Tenex Tablets (Less frequent) 2074
Trilafon 2389
Vagistat-1 (Less than 1%) 778
Videx Tablets, Powder for Oral Solution, & Pediatric Powder for Oral Solution (Less than 1%) 720
Vivactil Tablets 1774
Voltaren Tablets (Less than 1%) 861
Wellbutrin Tablets (Frequent) 1204
Zoloft Tablets (Infrequent) 2217

Nodal rhythm
Isoptin SR Tablets 1348
Lanoxicaps (Common) 1117
Lanoxin Elixir Pediatric (Common) 1120
Lanoxin Injection (Common) 1123
Lanoxin Injection Pediatric (Common) 1126
Lanoxin Tablets (Common) 1128
Prostigmin Injectable 1260
Prostigmin Tablets 1261
Romazicon (Less than 1%) 2147
Sodium Polystyrene Sulfonate Suspension 2244
Suprane (Greater than 1%) 1813
Versed Injection (Less than 1%) 2170

Nodule at injection site
Depo-Provera Sterile Aqueous Suspension 2606
Diphtheria and Tetanus Toxoids and Pertussis Vaccine Adsorbed (Occasional) 2477
Diphtheria and Tetanus Toxoids and Pertussis Vaccine Adsorbed USP (For Pediatric Use) (Occasional) 875
Genotropin (Infrequent) 111
▲ Poliovax (4%) 891
Tetramune (Occasional) 1404

Nodule, subcutaneous
Neurontin Capsules (Rare) 1922
Permax Tablets (Rare) 575
Prozac Pulvules & Liquid, Oral Solution (Rare) 919

Noise intolerance
BuSpar (Infrequent) 737
Neurontin Capsules (Rare) 1922

Nuchal rigidity
Gamimune N, 5% Immune Globulin Intravenous (Human), 5% (Infrequent) 619
Gamimune N, 10% Immune Globulin Intravenous (Human), 10% (Infrequent) 621
Methotrexate Sodium Tablets, Injection, for Injection and LPF Injection 1275
Sandoglobulin I.V. (Infrequent) 2290

Numbness
Adenocard Injection (1%) 1021
AeroBid Inhaler System (1-3%) 1005
Aerobid-M Inhaler System (1-3%) 1005
Apresazide Capsules (Less frequent) 808
Apresoline Hydrochloride Tablets (Less frequent) 809
Asendin Tablets (Less than 1%) 1369
Atamet 572
Bentyl 1501
BuSpar (2%) 737
Cafergot 2251
Cefizox for Intramuscular or Intravenous Use (Rare) 1034
Clozaril Tablets (Less than 1%) 2252
Demulen 2428
Desyrel and Desyrel Dividose 503
DynaCirc Capsules (0.5% to 1%) 2256
Elavil 2838
Elimite (permethrin) 5% Cream (1 to 2% or less) 478
Emla Cream 545
Endep Tablets 2174
Esgic-plus Tablets (Infrequent) 1013
Fioricet Tablets (Infrequent) 2258
Fioricet with Codeine Capsules (Infrequent) 2260
Fiorinal with Codeine Capsules (Infrequent) 2262
Garamycin Injectable 2360
▲ Imitrex Injection (4.6%) 1103
Imitrex Tablets (Frequent) 1106
INFeD (Iron Dextran Injection, USP) 2345
K-Phos Neutral Tablets 639
K-Phos Original Formula 'Sodium Free' Tablets (Less frequent) 639
Kerlone Tablets (Less than 2%) 2436
Larodopa Tablets (Relatively frequent) 2129
Limbitrol 2180
Lioresal Intrathecal (1 to 8 of 214 patients) 1596
Loxitane 1378
Ludiomil Tablets (Rare) 843
Lupron Depot 7.5 mg 2559
Lupron Injection (Less than 5%) 2555
▲ Mexitil Capsules (2.4% to 3.8%) 678
Mintezol 1704
Moduretic Tablets (Less than or equal to 1%) 1705
Monopril Tablets (0.4% to 1.0%) 757
Nebcin Vials, Hyporets & ADD-Vantage 1464
Netromycin Injection 100 mg/ml 2373
Normodyne Injection (1%) 2377
Norpace (Less than 1%) 2444
Norplant System 2759
Norpramin Tablets 1526
Nubain Injection (1% or less) 935
Pamelor 2280
Parlodel 2281
Parnate Tablets 2503
Peganone Tablets 446
Phrenilin (Infrequent) 785
Rifadin 1528
Rifamate Capsules 1530
Rifater 1532
Rimactane Capsules 847
▲ Roferon-A Injection (3% to 6%) 2145
Rythmol Tablets–150mg, 225mg, 300mg (Less than 1%) 1352
SSKI Solution (Less frequent) 2658
Sedapap Tablets 50 mg/650 mg (Infrequent) 1543
Ser-Ap-Es Tablets 849
Sinemet Tablets 943
Sinemet CR Tablets 944
Sinequan (Infrequent) 2205
Surmontil Capsules 2811
Tobramycin Sulfate Injection 968
Tofranil Ampuls 854
Tofranil Tablets 856
Tofranil-PM Capsules 857
Tonocard Tablets (Less than 1%) 531
Trandate Injection (1 of 100 patients) 1185
Triavil Tablets 1757
Vivactil Tablets 1774

Numbness, buccal mucosa
Azactam for Injection (Less than 1%) 734
Clozaril Tablets (1%) 2252
Marcaine Spinal 2319
Stilphostrol Tablets and Ampuls 612

Numbness, extremities
Cogentin 1621
Coly-Mycin M Parenteral 1905
Estrace Cream and Tablets 749
Etrafon 2355
Flagyl 375 Capsules 2434
Flagyl I.V. 2247
Foscavir Injection 547
IOPIDINE Sterile Ophthalmic Solution ◉ 219
Levlen/Tri-Levlen 651
Lomotil 2439
▲ Lozol Tablets (Greater than or equal to 5%) 2022
Maxair Autohaler 1492
Maxair Inhaler (Less than 1%) 1494
Micronor Tablets 1872
Modicon 1872
Myambutol Tablets 1386
Norpramin Tablets 1526
Ortho-Cyclen/Ortho-Tri-Cyclen 1858
Ortho-Est 1869
Ortho-Novum 1872
Ortho-Cyclen/Ortho Tri-Cyclen 1858
Polymyxin B Sulfate, Aerosporin Brand Sterile Powder 1154
Protostat Tablets 1883
Sansert Tablets 2295
Trilafon 2389
Levlen/Tri-Levlen 651
Videx Tablets, Powder for Oral Solution, & Pediatric Powder for Oral Solution (Less than 1%) 720
Zerit Capsules 729

Numbness, face
Placidyl Capsules 448

Numbness, feet
Uroqid-Acid No. 2 Tablets 640

Numbness, fingers
Aclovate Ointment (1 of 366 patients) 1069
Cutivate Cream (1.0%) 1088
Hivid Tablets 2121
Temovate (1 of 366 patients) 1179
Wigraine Tablets & Suppositories 1829

Numbness, hands
Hyperstat I.V. Injection 2363
Uroqid-Acid No. 2 Tablets 640

Numbness, lips
K-Phos Neutral Tablets 639
K-Phos Original Formula 'Sodium Free' Tablets (Less frequent) 639
Marcaine Spinal 2319
Oncaspar 2028
Sensorcaine 559
Uroqid-Acid No. 2 Tablets 640

Numbness, mouth (see under Numbness, buccal mucosa)

Numbness, nose
Stilphostrol Tablets and Ampuls 612

Numbness, skin
Eskalith 2485
Lithium Carbonate Capsules & Tablets 2230
Lithonate/Lithotabs/Lithobid 2543

Numbness, toes
Hivid Tablets 2121
Wigraine Tablets & Suppositories 1829

Numbness, tongue (see under Numbness, buccal mucosa)

Numbness/tingling, fingers and toes
Cafergot 2251
D.H.E. 45 Injection 2255
Eldepryl Tablets 2550
Ergomar 1486
MetroGel 1047

Nyctalopia
Accutane Capsules 2076
Anafranil Capsules (Rare) 803
Aralen Hydrochloride Injection 2301
Aralen Phosphate Tablets 2301
Cataflam (Less than 1%) 816
Mellaril 2269
Questran Light (One case) 769
Questran Powder (One case) 770
Quinaglute Dura-Tabs Tablets (Occasional) 649
Quinidex Extentabs 2067
Serzone Tablets (Rare) 771
Tegison Capsules (Less than 1%) 2154
Voltaren Tablets (Less than 1%) 861

Nystagmus
Anafranil Capsules (Rare) 803
Atretol Tablets 573
Betaseron for SC Injection 658
Cipro I.V. (1% or less) 595
Cipro I.V. Pharmacy Bulk Package (Less than 1%) 597
Cipro Tablets 592
Clozaril Tablets (Less than 1%) 2252
Cylert Tablets 412
Dalalone D.P. Injectable 1011
Decadron-LA Sterile Suspension (Low) 1646
Depakene 413
Depakote Tablets 415
▲ Dilantin Infatabs (Among most common) 1908
▲ Dilantin Kapseals (Among most common) 1906
▲ Dilantin Parenteral (Among most common) 1910
▲ Dilantin-125 Suspension (Among most common) 1911
Dilaudid-HP Injection (Less frequent) 1337
Dilaudid-HP Lyophilized Powder 250 mg (Less frequent) 1337
Dilaudid Tablets and Liquid (Less frequent) 1339
Diprivan Injection (Less than 1%) 2833
Dizac (Less frequent) 1809
Effexor (Rare) 2719
Ergamisol Tablets 1292
Eskalith 2485
Ethmozine Tablets (Less than 2%) 2041
Felbatol 2666
Floxin I.V. 1571
Floxin Tablets (200 mg, 300 mg, 400 mg) 1567
Fluorouracil Injection 2116
Foscavir Injection (Less than 1%) 547
Sterile FUDR (Remote possibility) 2118
Isoptin Injectable 1344
Klonopin Tablets 2126
Lamictal Tablets (1.0%) 1112
Lioresal Intrathecal 1596
Lioresal Tablets 829
Lithium Carbonate Capsules & Tablets 2230

(Described in PDR For Nonprescription Drugs) Incidence data in parenthesis; ▲ 3% or more (◉ Described in PDR For Ophthalmology)

1377 Side Effects Index Oliguria

Lithonate/Lithotabs/Lithobid 2543
MS Contin Tablets (Less frequent) 1994
MSIR (Infrequent) 1997
Macrobid Capsules 1988
Macrodantin Capsules 1989
Matulane Capsules 2131
Maxaquin Tablets 2440
Mebaral Tablets 2322
Mesantoin Tablets 2272
Mysoline (Occasional) 2754
Nardil (Less common) 1920
Netromycin Injection 100 mg/ml 2373
▲ Neurontin Capsules (Among most common; 8.3%) 1922
Noroxin Tablets 1715
Noroxin Tablets 2048
Oramorph SR (Morphine Sulfate Sustained Release Tablets) (Less frequent) 2236
Paxil Tablets (Rare) 2505
Peganone Tablets 446
Penetrex Tablets 2031
Placidyl Capsules 448
Plaquenil Sulfate Tablets 2328
ProSom Tablets (Rare) 449
Prozac Pulvules & Liquid, Oral Solution (Rare) 919
Robaxin Injectable 2070
Talwin Injection (Rare) 2334
Tambocor Tablets (Less than 1%) 1497
Tegretol Chewable Tablets 852
Tegretol Suspension 852
Tegretol Tablets 852
Tonocard Tablets (0.0-1.1%) 531
Valium Injectable 2182
Versed Injection (Less than 1%) 2170
Zoloft Tablets (Infrequent) 2217

Nystagmus, horizontal (see also under Nystagmus)

Restoril Capsules (Less than 0.5%) 2284

NMS (see under Neuroleptic malignant syndrome)

NPN elevation

Garamycin Injectable 2360
Nebcin Vials, Hyporets & ADD-Vantage 1464
Tobramycin Sulfate Injection 968

O

Obstipation

Compazine 2470
Etrafon 2355
Mellaril 2269
Serentil 684
Stelazine 2514
Thorazine 2523
Torecan 2245
Triavil Tablets 1757
Trilafon (Occasional) 2389

Obtundation

Intron A (Some patients) 2364
Orthoclone OKT3 Sterile Solution .. 1837
Roferon-A Injection (Rare) 2145
Zovirax Sterile Powder (Approximately 1%) 1223

Occult bleeding

Empirin with Codeine Tablets 1093
Fiorinal with Codeine Capsules 2262
Soma Compound w/Codeine Tablets 2676
▲ Soma Compound Tablets (Among most common) 2675

Occult blood in stool, positive test

Children's Advil Suspension 2692
Lioresal Tablets 829
Children's Motrin Ibuprofen Oral Suspension 1546

Ocular allergy

Alomide (Less than 1%) 469
Anafranil Capsules (Up to 2%) 803
Profenal 1% Sterile Ophthalmic Solution (Less than 0.5%) ..... ⊙ 227
▲ Trusopt Sterile Ophthalmic Solution (Approximately 10%) 1760

Ocular discomfort

▲ Alomide (Among most frequent) 469
Betoptic Ophthalmic Solution 469
▲ Betoptic S Ophthalmic Suspension (Most frequent) 471
BuSpar (Rare) 737
▲ Iopidine 0.5% (6%) ..... ⊙ 221
▲ Ocuflox (One of the two most frequent) 481
Vexol 1% Ophthalmic Suspension (1% to 5%) ..... ⊙ 230

Ocular, foreign body sensation

▲ Alomide (1% to 5%) 469
Betoptic Ophthalmic Solution 469
Betoptic S Ophthalmic Suspension (Small number of patients) 471
IOPIDINE Sterile Ophthalmic Solution ..... ⊙ 219
Iopidine 0.5% (Less than 3%) ..... ⊙ 221
Timoptic in Ocudose (Less frequent) 1753
Timoptic Sterile Ophthalmic Solution (Less frequent) 1751
▲ Timoptic-XE (1% to 5% of patients) 1755

Ocular exudate

▲ Alomide (1% to 5%) 469
Betoptic Ophthalmic Solution 469
Betoptic S Ophthalmic Suspension (Small number of patients) 471
Iopidine 0.5% (Less than 3%) ..... ⊙ 221
Livostin (Approximately 1% to 3%) ..... ⊙ 266
Timoptic in Ocudose (Less frequent) 1753
Timoptic Sterile Ophthalmic Solution (Less frequent) 1751
▲ Timoptic-XE (1% to 5% of patients) 1755
Vexol 1% Ophthalmic Suspension (1% to 5%) ..... ⊙ 230

Ocular hypotony

IOPIDINE Sterile Ophthalmic Solution ..... ⊙ 219

Ocular infection

Aristocort Suspension (Forte Parenteral) 1027
Aristospan Suspension (Intra-articular) 1033
Aristospan Suspension (Intralesional) 1032
CORTENEMA 2535
Depo-Medrol Single-Dose Vial 2600
NeoDecadron Sterile Ophthalmic Ointment 1712
NeoDecadron Sterile Ophthalmic Solution 1713
Prelone Syrup 1787
Terra-Cortril Ophthalmic Suspension 2210
Trilafon 2389

Ocular lesions

Brevicon 2088
Decadron Phosphate Sterile Ophthalmic Ointment 1641
Decadron Phosphate Sterile Ophthalmic Solution 1642
Norinyl 2088
Nor-Q D Tablets 2135
Ovcon 760
Tri-Norinyl 2164

Ocular palsies

Attenuvax (Rare) 1610
M-M-R II (Rare) 1687
M-R-VAX II (Rare) 1689
Plaquenil Sulfate Tablets 2328

Ocular pemphigoid

Timoptic in Ocudose 1753
Timoptic Sterile Ophthalmic Solution 1751
Timoptic-XE 1755

Ocular perforation

Decadron Phosphate Sterile Ophthalmic Ointment 1641
Decadron Phosphate Sterile Ophthalmic Solution 1642
Flarex Ophthalmic Suspension ..... ⊙ 218

Ocular pressure

Zebeta Tablets 1413

Ocular tension, increase

Bentyl 1501
Cortisporin Ophthalmic Ointment Sterile 1085
Cortisporin Ophthalmic Suspension Sterile 1086
Decadron Phosphate Sterile Ophthalmic Ointment 1641
Decadron Phosphate Sterile Ophthalmic Solution 1642
Donnatal 2060
Donnatal Extentabs 2061
Donnatal Tablets 2060
Kutrase Capsules 2402
Levsin/Levsinex/Levbid 2405
Norflex 1496
Norgesic 1496
Pro-Banthine Tablets 2052
Robinul Forte Tablets 2072
Robinul Injectable 2072
Robinul Tablets 2072
Urispas Tablets 2532
Ziac 1415

Ocular toxicity

AKTOB (Less than 3 of 100 patients) ..... ⊙ 206
Plaquenil Sulfate Tablets 2328
Platinol 708
Platinol-AQ Injection 710
Ridaura Capsules 2513
TobraDex Ophthalmic Suspension and Ointment (Less than 4%) 473
Tobrex Ophthalmic Ointment and Solution (Less than 3 of 100 patients) ..... ⊙ 229

Oculogyric crises

Anafranil Capsules (Rare) 803
Atamet 572
Betaseron for SC Injection 658
Cognex Capsules (Rare) 1901
Compazine 2470
Cylert Tablets 412
Etrafon 2355
Haldol Decanoate (Frequent) 1577
Haldol Injection, Tablets and Concentrate 1575
Inapsine Injection 1296
Larodopa Tablets (Rare) 2129
Mellaril 2269
Orap Tablets (Less frequent) 1050
Paxil Tablets 2505
Phenergan with Codeine 2777
Phenergan with Dextromethorphan 2778
Phenergan Injection 2773
Phenergan Suppositories 2775
Phenergan Syrup 2774
Phenergan Tablets 2775
Phenergan VC 2779
Phenergan VC with Codeine 2781
Prolixin 509
Reglan 2068
▲ Risperdal (17% to 34%) 1301
Serentil 684
Sinemet Tablets 943
Stelazine 2514
Sublimaze Injection 1307
Symmetrel Capsules and Syrup (Less than 0.1%) 946
Temaril Tablets, Syrup and Spansule Extended-Release Capsules 483
Thorazine 2523
Timolide Tablets 1748
Torecan 2245
Triavil Tablets 1757
Trilafon 2389

Oculomotor disturbances

Atretol Tablets 573
Levoprome 1274
Pravachol 765
Tegretol Chewable Tablets 852
Tegretol Suspension 852
Tegretol Tablets 852

Oiliness

A/T/S 2% Acne Topical Gel and Solution (Occasional) 1234
Erycette (erythromycin 2%) Topical Solution 1888
T-Stat 2.0% Topical Solution and Pads 2688
Theramycin Z Topical Solution 2% 1592

Oligohydramnios

Accupril Tablets 1893
Altace Capsules 1232
Capoten 739
Capozide 742
Clinoril Tablets 1618
Cozaar Tablets 1628
Dolobid Tablets 1654
Hyzaar Tablets 1677
Lotensin Tablets 834
Lotensin HCT 837
Lotrel Capsules 840
Monopril Tablets 757
Prinivil Tablets 1733
Prinzide Tablets 1737
Univasc Tablets 2410
Vaseretic Tablets 1765
Vasotec I.V. 1768
Vasotec Tablets 1771
Zestoretic 2850
Zestril Tablets 2854

Oligomenorrhea

Brevicon 2088
Levlen/Tri-Levlen 651
Micronor Tablets 1872
Modicon 1872
Mustargen 1709
▲ Nolvadex Tablets (8.7%) 2841
Norinyl 2088
Nor-Q D Tablets 2135
Ortho-Cyclen/Ortho-Tri-Cyclen 1858
Ortho-Novum 1872
Ortho-Cyclen/Ortho Tri-Cyclen 1858
Levlen/Tri-Levlen 651
Tri-Norinyl 2164

Oligospermia

Android Capsules, 10 mg (At high dosages) 1250
Android 1251
▲ Azulfidine (Approximately one-third of patients) 1949
Cytoxan 694
Delatestryl Injection 2860
Halotestin Tablets 2614
Methotrexate Sodium Tablets, Injection, for Injection and LPF Injection 1275
NEOSAR Lyophilized/Neosar 1959
Nizoral Tablets 1298
▲ Oreton Methyl (Among most common) 1255
Oxandrin 2862
Testoderm Testosterone Transdermal System 486
Testred Capsules 1262
Winstrol Tablets 2337

Oliguria

Altace Capsules 1232
Amikacin Sulfate Injection, USP 960
Amikin Injectable 501
Anafranil Capsules (Infrequent) 803
Apresazide Capsules 808
Astramorph/PF Injection, USP (Preservative-Free) 535
Atretol Tablets 573
Azo Gantanol Tablets 2080
Azo Gantrisin Tablets 2081
Azulfidine (Rare) 1949
Bactrim DS Tablets 2084
Bactrim I.V. Infusion 2082
Bactrim 2084
Betaseron for SC Injection 658
Brontex 1981
Calcium Disodium Versenate Injection 1490
Capastat Sulfate Vials (1 patient) 2868
Capoten (Approximately 1 to 2 of 1000 patients) 739
Capozide (Approximately 1 to 2 of 1000 patients) 742
Cataflam (Rare) 816
Cleocin Phosphate Injection (Rare) 2586
Cleocin Vaginal Cream (Rare) 2589
Clomid 1514
ColBENEMID Tablets 1622
Demadex Tablets and Injection 686
Diprivan Injection (Less than 1%) .. 2833
Duragesic Transdermal System (Less than 1%) 1288
Duramorph 962
Dyazide 2479
Esidrix Tablets 821
Eskalith 2485
Fansidar Tablets 2114
Fungizone Intravenous 506
Gantanol Tablets 2119
Gantrisin 2120
Garamycin Injectable 2360
Humegon 1824
Hyskon Hysteroscopy Fluid (Rare) .. 1595
Hyzaar Tablets 1677
Infumorph 200 and Infumorph 500 Sterile Solutions 965
Kerlone Tablets (Less than 2%) 2436
Lasix Injection, Oral Solution and Tablets 1240
Lincocin (Rare instances) 2617
Lithium Carbonate Capsules & Tablets 2230
Lithonate/Lithotabs/Lithobid 2543
Lotrel Capsules 840

(▣ Described in PDR For Nonprescription Drugs) Incidence data in parenthesis; ▲ 3% or more (⊙ Described in PDR For Ophthalmology)

Lozol Tablets 2022
Luvox Tablets (Rare) 2544
Maxzide 1380
Metrodin (urofollitropin for injection) 2446
Miltown Tablets (Rare) 2672
Monopril Tablets 757
Mykrox Tablets 993
Nalfon 200 Pulvules & Nalfon Tablets (Less than 1%) 917
Nebcin Vials, Hyporets & ADD-Vantage 1464
Netromycin Injection 100 mg/ml 2373
Oretic Tablets 443
Orthoclone OKT3 Sterile Solution 1837
PMB 200 and PMB 400 (Rare) 2783
Paxil Tablets (Rare) 2505
Phenergan with Codeine 2777
Phenergan VC with Codeine 2781
Primaxin I.M. 1727
Primaxin I.V. (Less than 0.2%) 1729
Prinivil Tablets (0.3% to 1.0%) 1733
Prinzide Tablets 1737
Priscoline Hydrochloride Ampuls 845
▲ Prograf (16% to 18%) 1042
▲ Proleukin for Injection (76%) 797
ProSom Tablets (Rare) 449
Sansert Tablets 2295
Septra 1174
Septra I.V. Infusion 1169
Septra I.V. Infusion ADD-Vantage Vials 1171
Septra 1174
Serophene (clomiphene citrate tablets, USP) 2451
Serzone Tablets (Rare) 771
Tegretol Chewable Tablets 852
Tegretol Suspension 852
Tegretol Tablets 852
Tenoretic Tablets 2845
Thalitone (Common) 1245
Tobramycin Sulfate Injection 968
Toradol (1% or less) 2159
Univasc Tablets (Less than 1%) 2410
Vaseretic Tablets 1765
Vasotec I.V. 1768
Vasotec Tablets (0.5% to 1.0%) 1771
Voltaren Tablets (Rare) 861
Zaroxolyn Tablets 1000
Zestoretic 2850
Zestril Tablets (0.3% to 1.0%) 2854
Zoloft Tablets (Rare) 2217
Zosyn (1.0% or less) 1419
Zosyn Pharmacy Bulk Package (1.0% or less) 1422

Oliguria, neonatal
Altace Capsules 1232
Capoten 739
Capozide 742
Lotensin Tablets 834
Monopril Tablets 757

"On-off" phenomenon
Atamet 572
Larodopa Tablets 2129
Parlodel 2281
Sinemet Tablets 943
Sinemet CR Tablets (1.6%) 944

Onycholysis
Adriamycin PFS (A few cases) 1947
Adriamycin RDF (A few cases) 1947
Doxorubicin Astra (A few cases) 540
Feldene Capsules (Less than 1%) 1965
Orudis Capsules (Less than 1%) 2766
Oruvail Capsules (Less than 1%) 2766
Rubex (A few cases) 712
▲ Tegison Capsules (1-10%) 2154
Zyloprim Tablets (Less than 1%) 1226

Oogenesis, defective
Cytoxan 694
Methotrexate Sodium Tablets, Injection, for Injection and LPF Injection 1275

Opisthotonos
Compazine 2470
Diprivan Injection (Rare; less than 1%) 2833
Etrafon 2355
Haldol Decanoate (Frequent) 1577
Haldol Injection, Tablets and Concentrate 1575
Levoprome 1274
Mellaril 2269
Orap Tablets (Less frequent) 1050
Prolixin 509
Reglan 2068
Serentil 684
Stelazine 2514
Temaril Tablets, Syrup and Spansule Extended-Release Capsules 483
Thorazine 2523
Tigan 2057
Torecan 2245
Triavil Tablets 1757
Trilafon 2389

Ophthalmoplegia
Betaseron for SC Injection 658
Cytovene-IV (One report) 2103
Mevacor Tablets 1699
Pravachol 765
Zocor Tablets 1775

Optic atrophy
Aralen Phosphate Tablets 2301
Diupres Tablets 1650
Eskalith 2485
Hydropres Tablets 1675
Lithium Carbonate Capsules & Tablets 2230
Oncovin Solution Vials & Hyporets 1466
Plaquenil Sulfate Tablets 2328
Rifater (Uncommon) 1532
Ser-Ap-Es Tablets 849
Yodoxin 1230

Optic disorders
Effexor (Rare) 2719
Solu-Cortef Sterile Powder 2641
Solu-Medrol Sterile Powder 2643

Optic nerve, damage
AK-CIDE (Infrequent) ⊙ 202
AK-CIDE Ointment (Infrequent) ⊙ 202
AK-Pred ⊙ 204
AK-Trol Ointment & Suspension (Infrequent) ⊙ 205
Aristocort Suspension (Forte Parenteral) 1027
Aristocort Tablets 1022
Aristospan Suspension (Intra-articular) 1033
Aristospan Suspension (Intralesional) 1032
Blephamide Liquifilm Sterile Ophthalmic Suspension (Infrequent) 476
Blephamide Ointment (Infrequent) ⊙ 237
Celestone Soluspan Suspension (Possible) 2347
CORTENEMA 2535
Cortisporin Ophthalmic Ointment Sterile (Infrequent) 1085
Cortisporin Ophthalmic Suspension Sterile (Infrequent) 1086
Dapsone Tablets USP 1284
Dexacidin Ointment (Infrequent) ⊙ 263
Dexacort Phosphate in Respihaler 458
Dexacort Phosphate in Turbinaire 459
Econopred & Econopred Plus Ophthalmic Suspensions ⊙ 217
FML Forte Liquifilm (Infrequent) ⊙ 240
FML Liquifilm ⊙ 241
FML S.O.P. (Infrequent) ⊙ 241
FML-S Liquifilm (Infrequent) ⊙ 242
Flarex Ophthalmic Suspension ⊙ 218
Florinef Acetate Tablets 505
Fluor-Op Ophthalmic Suspension ⊙ 264
HMS Liquifilm (Rare) ⊙ 244
Inflamase ⊙ 265
Maxitrol Ophthalmic Ointment and Suspension (Infrequent) ⊙ 224
NeoDecadron Sterile Ophthalmic Ointment 1712
NeoDecadron Sterile Ophthalmic Solution (Infrequent) 1713
Ophthocort ⊙ 311
Poly-Pred Liquifilm (Infrequent) ⊙ 248
Pred Forte ⊙ 250
Pred Mild ⊙ 253
Pred-G Liquifilm Sterile Ophthalmic Suspension (Infrequent) ⊙ 251
Pred-G S.O.P. Sterile Ophthalmic Ointment ⊙ 252
Prelone Syrup 1787
Streptomycin Sulfate Injection 2208
Terra-Cortril Ophthalmic Suspension (Infrequent) 2210
TobraDex Ophthalmic Suspension and Ointment (Infrequent) 473
Vasocidin Ointment (Infrequent) ⊙ 268
Vasocidin Ophthalmic Solution (Infrequent) ⊙ 270
Vexol 1% Ophthalmic Suspension ⊙ 230

Optic nerve, infarction
Hyperstat I.V. Injection 2363
Trandate 1185

Orchitis
BCG Vaccine, USP (TICE) (0.2%) 1814
Biavax II 1613
M-M-R II 1687
Maxaquin Tablets (Less than 1%) 2440
Mumpsvax (Rare) 1708
Prozac Pulvules & Liquid, Oral Solution (Rare) 919

Organic brain syndrome
Eskalith 2485
Lithium Carbonate Capsules & Tablets 2230

Oropharyngitis
▲ Roferon-A Injection (14% to 16%) 2145

Oropharynx, dry
▲ Atrovent Inhalation Aerosol (About 5 in 100) 671
Brethaire Inhaler 813
Proventil Inhalation Aerosol 2382
Proventil Repetabs Tablets 2386
Proventil Syrup 2385
Proventil Tablets 2386
▲ Roferon-A Injection (14% to 16%) 2145
Tussionex Pennkinetic Extended-Release Suspension 998
Ventolin Syrup 1202
Ventolin Tablets 1203
Volmax Extended-Release Tablets 1788

Orthopnea
Prinivil Tablets (0.3% to 1.0%) 1733
Prinzide Tablets 1737
Zestoretic 2850
Zestril Tablets (0.3% to 1.0%) 2854

Oscillopsia
Lamictal Tablets (Infrequent) 1112

Osteoarticular pain
Cardizem CD Capsules (Less than 1%) 1506
Cardizem SR Capsules (Less than 1%) 1510
Cardizem Injectable 1508
Cardizem Tablets (Less than 1%) 1512

Osteomalacia
Didronel Tablets 1984
Dilantin Kapseals 1906
Dilantin-125 Suspension 1911
Phenobarbital Elixir and Tablets 1469

Osteomalacia syndromes
Aludrox Oral Suspension 2695
Amphojel 2695
Basaljel 2703
Gelusil Liquid & Tablets ▣ 855
Maalox Heartburn Relief Suspension ▣ 642
Maalox Heartburn Relief Tablets ▣ 641
Maalox Magnesia and Alumina Oral Suspension ▣ 642
Maalox Plus Tablets ▣ 643
Extra Strength Maalox Antacid Plus Antigas Liquid and Tablets ▣ 638
Mylanta Liquid 1317
Mylanta Tablets ▣ 660
Mylanta Double Strength Liquid 1317
Mylanta Double Strength Tablets ▣ 660
Rolaids Tablets ▣ 843

Osteomalacia, phosphate-induced
K-Phos Neutral Tablets 639
K-Phos Original Formula 'Sodium Free' Tablets 639
Uroqid-Acid No. 2 Tablets 640

Osteomyelitis
BCG Vaccine, USP (TICE) (Rare; about 1 per 1,000,000 vaccinees) 1814
Permax Tablets (Rare) 575

Osteoporosis
Aristocort Suspension (Forte Parenteral) 1027
Aristocort Suspension (Intralesional) 1025
Aristocort Tablets 1022
Aristospan Suspension (Intra-articular) 1033
Aristospan Suspension (Intralesional) 1032
Celestone Soluspan Suspension 2347
Cognex Capsules (Infrequent) 1901
CORTENEMA 2535
Cortifoam 2396
Cortone Acetate Sterile Suspension 1623
Cortone Acetate Tablets 1624
Dalalone D.P. Injectable 1011
Decadron Elixir 1633
Decadron Phosphate Injection 1637
Decadron Phosphate Respihaler 1642
Decadron Phosphate Turbinaire 1645
Decadron Phosphate with Xylocaine Injection, Sterile 1639
Decadron Tablets 1635
Decadron-LA Sterile Suspension 1646
Deltasone Tablets 2595
Depo-Medrol Single-Dose Vial 2600
Depo-Medrol Sterile Aqueous Suspension 2597
Depo-Provera Contraceptive Injection (Fewer than 1%) 2602
Dexacort Phosphate in Respihaler 458
Dexacort Phosphate in Turbinaire 459
Effexor (Rare) 2719
Florinef Acetate Tablets 505
Fludara for Injection (Up to 2%) 663
Heparin Lock Flush Solution 2725
Heparin Sodium Injection 2726
Heparin Sodium Injection, USP, Sterile Solution 2615
Heparin Sodium Vials 1441
Hydeltrasol Injection, Sterile 1665
Hydeltra-T.B.A. Sterile Suspension 1667
Hydrocortone Acetate Sterile Suspension 1669
Hydrocortone Phosphate Injection, Sterile 1670
Hydrocortone Tablets 1672
Medrol 2621
Methotrexate Sodium Tablets, Injection, for Injection and LPF Injection 1275
Neupogen for Injection (Infrequent) 495
Neurontin Capsules (Rare) 1922
Paxil Tablets (Rare) 2505
Pediapred Oral Liquid 995
Permax Tablets (Rare) 575
Prelone Syrup 1787
▲ Prograf (Greater than 3%) 1042
Prozac Pulvules & Liquid, Oral Solution (Rare) 919
Questran Light (Less frequent) 769
Questran Powder (Less frequent) 770
Solu-Cortef Sterile Powder 2641
Solu-Medrol Sterile Powder 2643

Otitis externa
Ambien Tablets (Rare) 2416
Betaseron for SC Injection 658
Neurontin Capsules (Rare) 1922
Paxil Tablets (Rare) 2505
▲ Tegison Capsules (1-10%) 2154
▲ Videx Tablets, Powder for Oral Solution, & Pediatric Powder for Oral Solution (Less than 1% to 13%) 720

Otitis media
Ambien Tablets (Rare) 2416
▲ Anafranil Capsules (Up to 4%) 803
Betaseron for SC Injection 658
▲ CHEMET (succimer) Capsules (1.0 to 3.7%) 1545
Cognex Capsules (Infrequent) 1901
Dilacor XR Extended-release Capsules 2018
Effexor (Infrequent) 2719
▲ Felbatol (3.4% to 9.7%) 2666
Foscavir Injection (Less than 1%) 547
Luvox Tablets (Infrequent) 2544
M-M-R II 1687
Neurontin Capsules (Infrequent) 1922
Orthoclone OKT3 Sterile Solution 1837
Paxil Tablets (Infrequent) 2505
▲ PedvaxHIB (Among most frequent) 1718
Permax Tablets (Infrequent) 575
PREVACID Delayed-Release Capsules (Less than 1%) 2562
▲ Tetramune (Among most common) 1404
Varivax (Greater than or equal to 1%) 1762
▲ Videx Tablets, Powder for Oral Solution, & Pediatric Powder for Oral Solution (Less than 1% to 13%) 720
Zoloft Tablets (Rare) 2217

(▣ Described in PDR For Nonprescription Drugs) Incidence data in parenthesis; ▲ 3% or more (⊙ Described in PDR For Ophthalmology)

1379 **Side Effects Index** **Pain, dental**

Ototoxicity
Amikacin Sulfate Injection, USP 960
Amikin Injectable 501
Cortisporin Cream 1084
Cortisporin Ointment 1085
Cortisporin Otic Solution Sterile 1087
Cortisporin Otic Suspension Sterile 1088
Demadex Tablets and Injection 686
Garamycin Injectable 2360
Lasix Injection, Oral Solution and Tablets 1240
Nebcin Vials, Hyporets & ADD-Vantage 1464
NeoDecadron Topical Cream 1714
Neosporin G.U. Irrigant Sterile 1148
Netromycin Injection 100 mg/ml 2373
Paraplatin for Injection (1% to 13%) 705
PediOtic Suspension Sterile 1153
▲ Platinol (Up to 31%) 708
▲ Platinol-AQ Injection (Up to 31% of patients) 710
Streptomycin Sulfate Injection 2208
Tobramycin Sulfate Injection 968
Vancocin HCl, Oral Solution & Pulvules 1483
Vancocin HCl, Vials & ADD-Vantage 1481

Ovarian cyst formation
Anafranil Capsules (Infrequent) 803
Clomid 1514
Humegon 1824
Metrodin (urofollitropin for injection) 2446
Nolvadex Tablets (2.8%; a small number of premenopausal patients) 2841
Pergonal (menotropins for injection, USP) 2448
Profasi (chorionic gonadotropin for injection, USP) 2450
Serophene (clomiphene citrate tablets, USP) (Less than 1 in 100 patients) 2451

Ovarian cysts, enlargement of existing
Profasi (chorionic gonadotropin for injection, USP) 2450
Synarel Nasal Solution for Central Precocious Puberty 2151
Synarel Nasal Solution for Endometriosis 2152

Ovarian disorder
Neurontin Capsules (Rare) 1922
Prozac Pulvules & Liquid, Oral Solution (Infrequent) 919
Wellbutrin Tablets (Rare) 1204

Ovarian enlargement
Clomid 1514
▲ Humegon (Approximately 20%) 1824
Lutrepulse for Injection (Rare) 980
▲ Metrodin (urofollitropin for injection) (Approximately 20%) 2446
▲ Pergonal (menotropins for injection, USP) (Approximately 20%) 2448
Profasi (chorionic gonadotropin for injection, USP) 2450
▲ Serophene (clomiphene citrate tablets, USP) (Approximately 1 in 7 patients) 2451

Ovarian hyperstimulation syndrome
Clomid 1514
Humegon (Approximately 0.4%) 1824
Lutrepulse for Injection (One case) 980
▲ Metrodin (urofollitropin for injection) (Approximately 6%) 2446
Pergonal (menotropins for injection, USP) 2448
Profasi (chorionic gonadotropin for injection, USP) 2450
Serophene (clomiphene citrate tablets, USP) 2451

Oversedation
Versed Injection (1.6%) 2170

Overstimulation
Adipex-P Tablets and Capsules 1048
Ana-Kit Anaphylaxis Emergency Treatment Kit (Common) 617
Biphetamine Capsules 983
Bontril Slow-Release Capsules 781
Desoxyn Gradumet Tablets 419
Dexedrine 2474
DextroStat Dextroamphetamine Tablets 2036
Didrex Tablets 2607
Eldepryl Tablets 2550
Fastin Capsules 2488
Halcion Tablets 2611
Ionamin Capsules 990
Miltown Tablets 2672
Oreton Methyl 1255
PMB 200 and PMB 400 2783
Paraflex Caplets (Occasional) 1580
Parafon Forte DSC Caplets (Occasional) 1581
Parnate Tablets 2503
Prelu-2 Timed Release Capsules 681
Sanorex Tablets 2294
Vontrol Tablets 2532

P

Pain
Adalat CC (Less than 1.0%) 589
Ambien Tablets (Rare) 2416
Americaine Hemorrhoidal Ointment ▣ 629
▲ Anafranil Capsules (3% to 4%) 803
▲ Antivenin (Crotalidae) Polyvalent (Frequent) 2696
▲ Aredia for Injection (At least 15%) 810
▲ Asacol Delayed-Release Tablets (14%) 1979
Atgam Sterile Solution (Less than 5%) 2581
▲ Atrovent Inhalation Solution (4.1%) 673
▲ Axid Pulvules (4.2%) 1427
Bactroban Ointment (1.5%) 2470
Betapace Tablets (1% to 3%) 641
▲ Betaseron for SC Injection (52%) 658
Cardene SR Capsules (0.6%) 2097
Cardura Tablets (2%) 2186
Cartrol Tablets (Less common) 410
▲ CellCept Capsules (More than or equal to 3%; 31.2% to 33.0%) 2099
▲ CHEMET (succimer) Capsules (5.2-15.7%) 1545
Cipro I.V. Pharmacy Bulk Package (Less than 1%) 597
▲ Condylox (50% to 72%) 1802
Coumadin 926
Cytotec (Infrequent) 2424
Cytovene (2%) 2103
Dalalone D.P. Injectable 1011
Dalmane Capsules 2173
Danocrine Capsules 2307
Decadron-LA Sterile Suspension 1646
Depakote Tablets 415
Desferal Vials 820
Dilacor XR Extended-release Capsules (Infrequent) 2018
Effexor 2719
▲ Efudex (Among most frequent) 2113
▲ Ethmozine Tablets (3.5%) 2041
Famvir (2.6%) 2486
▲ Felbatol (6.5%) 2666
Feldene Capsules (Less than 1%) 1965
Floxin I.V. (Less than 1%) 1571
Floxin Tablets (200 mg, 300 mg, 400 mg) (Less than 1%) 1567
▲ Fludara for Injection (20% to 22%) 663
Fluorescite ⊙ 219
Fluoroplex Topical Solution & Cream 1% 479
Fluorouracil Injection 2116
▲ Foscavir Injection (5% or greater) 547
▲ Fungizone Intravenous (Among most common) 506
Gelfoam Sterile Sponge 2608
Glucotrol XL Extended Release Tablets (Less than 3%) 1968
Heparin Sodium Injection, USP, Sterile Solution 2615
Heparin Sodium Vials 1441
Herplex Liquifilm ⊙ 244
Hivid Tablets (Less than 1% to less than 3%) 2121
Humegon 1824
▲ Intron A (Up to 18%) 2364
K-Phos Neutral Tablets 639
K-Phos Original Formula 'Sodium Free' Tablets (Less frequent) 639
Kerlone Tablets (Less than 2%) 2436
Klonopin Tablets 2126
Lamprene Capsules (Less than 1%) 828
▲ Leustatin (6%) 1834
Librium Injectable 2179
Lippes Loop Intrauterine Double-S 1848
Lotensin HCT (0.3% to more than 1%) 837
Lovenox Injection 2020
Lozol Tablets (Greater than or equal to 5%) 2022
▲ Lupron Depot 3.75 mg (8.4%) 2556
▲ Lupron Depot 7.5 mg (7.1%) 2559
Lupron Depot-PED 7.5 mg, 11.25 mg and 15 mg (2%) 2560
▲ Lupron Injection (5% or more) 2555
Luvox Tablets 2544
Marax Tablets & DF Syrup 2200
Matulane Capsules 2131
▲ Megace Oral Suspension (Up to 6%) 699
▲ Mepron Suspension (10%) 1135
Monoket (Less than 1% to 4%) 2406
Monopril Tablets (0.4% to 1.0%) 757
Mutamycin 703
Mycobutin Capsules (1%) 1957
Neupogen for Injection (2%) 495
▲ Nicoderm (nicotine transdermal system) (3% to 9%) 1518
▲ Nicorette (3% to 9% of patients) 2458
Nicotrol Nicotine Transdermal System (1% to 3%) 1550
Nolvadex Tablets (2.8%) 2841
▲ Norpace (3 to 9%) 2444
▲ Norplant System (3.7%) 2759
Norvasc Tablets (More than 0.1% to 1%) 1940
▲ Oncaspar (Greater than 5%) 2028
Orthoclone OKT3 Sterile Solution 1837
Orudis Capsules (Less than 1%) 2766
Oruvail Capsules (Less than 1%) 2766
Oxistat Lotion (0.4%) 1152
PPD Tine Test 2874
ParaGard T380A Intrauterine Copper Contraceptive 1880
▲ Paraplatin for Injection (17% to 54%) 705
Pergonal (menotropins for injection, USP) 2448
▲ Permax Tablets (7.0%) 575
Polymyxin B Sulfate, Aerosporin Brand Sterile Powder 1154
▲ Pravachol (1.4% to 10.0%) 765
Prilosec Delayed-Release Capsules (Less than 1%) 529
Prinivil Tablets (0.3% to 1.0%) 1733
Prinzide Tablets 1737
Procardia XL Extended Release Tablets (Less than 3%) 1972
Profenal 1% Sterile Ophthalmic Solution (Less than 0.5%) ⊙ 227
▲ Prograf (19% to 63%) 1042
▲ Proleukin for Injection (54%) 797
▲ Propulsid (3.4%) 1300
ProSom Tablets (2%) 449
▲ Prostep (nicotine transdermal system) (3% to 9% of patients) 1394
▲ Prozac Pulvules & Liquid, Oral Solution (6%) 919
▲ ReoPro Vials (3.4%) 1471
Rogaine Topical Solution (2.59%) 2637
Rythmol Tablets–150mg, 225mg, 300mg (Less than 1%) 1352
Serzone Tablets 771
Stimate, (desmopressin acetate) Nasal Spray, 1.5 mg/mL 525
▲ Supprelin Injection (1% to 10%) 2056
▲ Tegison Capsules (1-10%) 2154
▲ Terazol 3 Vaginal Suppositories (3.9% of 284 patients) 1886
Terazol 7 Vaginal Cream (2.1% of 521 patients) 1887
Tetanus Toxoid Adsorbed Purogenated 1403
Ticlid Tablets 2156
Travase Ointment 1356
Tripedia 892
Tuberculin, Old, Tine Test 2875
Univasc Tablets (More than 1%) 2410
Vascor (200, 300 and 400 mg) Tablets (0.5 to 2.0%) 1587
▲ Versed Injection (3.7-5.0%) 2170
▲ Videx Tablets, Powder for Oral Solution, & Pediatric Powder for Oral Solution (6% to 31%) 720
Wellbutrin Tablets (Infrequent) 1204
▲ Zerit Capsules (3% to 18%) 729
Zestoretic 2850
Zestril Tablets (0.3% to 1.0%) 2854
▲ Zoladex (8% to 17%) 2858
Zosyn (1.7%) 1419
Zosyn Pharmacy Bulk Package (1.7%) 1422
Zovirax Capsules 1219
Zovirax Ointment 5% 1223
Zovirax Sterile Powder 1223
Zovirax 1219

Pain, abdominal (see under Abdominal pain/cramps)

Pain, arm
Cozaar Tablets (Less than 1%) 1628
Hyzaar Tablets 1677
Norplant System 2759
Plendil Extended-Release Tablets (0.5% to 1.5%) 527
Prinzide Tablets 1737
Zestoretic 2850
Zestril Tablets (0.3% to 1.0%) 2854

Pain, back (see under Backache)

Pain, biliary
Actigall Capsules 802
Luvox Tablets (Rare) 2544

Pain, bone
▲ Aredia for Injection (At least 5% to at least 15%) 810
Cytosar-U Sterile Powder (Occasional) 2592
▲ Didronel Tablets (About 1 patient in 10 to about 2 in 10) 1984
Dilacor XR Extended-release Capsules (Infrequent) 2018
Effexor (Infrequent) 2719
Hivid Tablets (Less than 1% to less than 3%) 2121
▲ Hylorel Tablets (42.9%) 985
Intron A (Less than 5%) 2364
K-Phos Original Formula 'Sodium Free' Tablets (Less frequent) 639
Lamprene Capsules (Less than 1%) 828
▲ Leukine for IV Infusion (90%) 1271
Levatol (2.4%) 2403
Lupron Depot 3.75 mg 2556
Lupron Depot 7.5 mg (Less than 5%) 2559
▲ Lupron Injection (5% or more) 2555
Metastron (A small number of patients) 1594
▲ Neupogen for Injection (22% to 33%) 495
▲ Nolvadex Tablets (5.7%) 2841
Oncaspar (Less than 1%) 2028
Oncovin Solution Vials & Hyporets 1466
Permax Tablets (Infrequent) 575
Prozac Pulvules & Liquid, Oral Solution (Infrequent) 919
Rifadin 1528
Rifater 1532
Risperdal (Rare) 1301
Rocaltrol Capsules 2141
▲ Tegison Capsules (50-75%) 2154
Uroqid-Acid No. 2 Tablets 640
▲ Velban Vials (Among most common) 1484
Zoladex (Small number of patients) 2858

Pain, breast
Ambien Tablets (Rare) 2416
Claritin (2% or fewer patients) 2349
Cytotec (Infrequent) 2424
▲ Depo-Provera Contraceptive Injection (1% to 5%) 2602
Kerlone Tablets (Less than 2%) 2436
▲ Lupron Injection (5% or more) 2555
Neurontin Capsules (Rare) 1922
Permax Tablets (Infrequent) 575
Prinivil Tablets (0.3% to 1.0%) 1733
Risperdal (Rare) 1301
Serzone Tablets (1%) 771
▲ Supprelin Injection (1% to 12%) 2056
Zestril Tablets (0.3% to 1.0%) 2854

Pain, burning
DDAVP Injection 15 mcg/mL (Occasional) 2015

Pain, cancer related
BCG Vaccine, USP (TICE) 1814
Zoladex (Occasional) 2858

Pain, cervical
Typhim Vi 899

Pain, dental
Claritin-D (Less frequent) 2350
Cozaar Tablets (Less than 1%) 1628
Hivid Tablets (Less than 1% to less than 3%) 2121
Hyzaar Tablets 1677
▲ Luvox Tablets (3%) 2544
Risperdal (Up to 2%) 1301

(▣ Described in PDR For Nonprescription Drugs) Incidence data in parenthesis; ▲ 3% or more (⊙ Described in PDR For Ophthalmology)

Serevent Inhalation Aerosol (1% to 3%) 1176
Wellbutrin Tablets (Infrequent) 1204

Pain, ear

Adenoscan (Less than 1%) 1024
Anafranil Capsules (Infrequent) 803
Asacol Delayed-Release Tablets 1979
Betaseron for SC Injection 658
Cardura Tablets (Less than 0.5% of 3960 patients) 2186
Claritin (2% or fewer patients) 2349
Claritin-D (Less frequent) 2350
Cognex Capsules (Infrequent) 1901
Depakote Tablets (Greater than 1% but not more than 5%) 415
Dilacor XR Extended-release Capsules (Infrequent) 2018
Diprivan Injection (Less than 1%) 2833
Effexor (Frequent) 2719
Engerix-B Unit-Dose Vials 2482
Esgic-plus Tablets (Infrequent) 1013
Fioricet Tablets (Infrequent) 2258
Fiorinal with Codeine Capsules (Infrequent) 2262
Foscavir Injection (Less than 1%) 547
Imdur (Less than or equal to 5%) 1323
Imitrex Tablets (Infrequent) 1106
Intron A (Less than 5%) 2364
Lamictal Tablets (1.8%) 1112
Lopressor HCT Tablets (1 in 100 patients) 832
Luvox Tablets (Infrequent) 2544
Maxaquin Tablets (Less than 1%) 2440
Miacalcin Nasal Spray (Less than 1%) 2275
Neurontin Capsules (Infrequent) 1922
Paxil Tablets (Infrequent) 2505
Permax Tablets (Infrequent) 575
Phrenilin (Infrequent) 785
Prinzide Tablets (0.3 to 1%) 1737
ProSom Tablets (Infrequent) 449
Prozac Pulvules & Liquid, Oral Solution (Infrequent) 919
Recombivax HB (Less than 1%) 1744
Roferon-A Injection (Less than 1%) 2145
Sedapap Tablets 50 mg/650 mg (Infrequent) 1543
Serzone Tablets (Infrequent) 771
Stadol (1% or greater) 775
Supprelin Injection (1% to 3%) 2056
Timolide Tablets 1748
Tonocard Tablets (Less than 1%) 531
Trental Tablets (Less than 1%) 1244
▲ Videx Tablets, Powder for Oral Solution, & Pediatric Powder for Oral Solution (Less than 1% to 13%) 720
Zebeta Tablets 1413
Zestoretic (0.3 to 1%) 2850
Ziac 1415
Zoloft Tablets (Infrequent) 2217

Pain, epigastric (see under Distress, epigastric)

Pain, esophageal

Hivid Tablets (Less than 1% to less than 3%) 2121

Pain, extremities

▲ Betapace Tablets (2% to 7%) 641
Betimol 0.25%, 0.5% (1% to 5%) ◉ 261
Blocadren Tablets 1614
Cartrol Tablets (Less common) 410
Cipro I.V. Pharmacy Bulk Package (Less than 1%) 597
Colestid Tablets 2591
Danocrine Capsules 2307
Diprivan Injection (Less than 1%) 2833
Ergomar (Frequent) 1486
Floxin I.V. (Less than 1%) 1571
Floxin Tablets (200 mg, 300 mg, 400 mg) (Less than 1%) 1567
Fluorouracil Injection 2116
Heparin Sodium Vials 1441
▲ Hytrin Capsules (3.5%) 430
IOPIDINE Sterile Ophthalmic Solution ◉ 219
Levlen/Tri-Levlen 651
▲ Mesnex Injection (50%) 702
▲ Oncaspar (Greater than 1% but less than 5%) 2028
Rifadin 1528
Rifater 1532
SSKI Solution (Less frequent) 2658
Sansert Tablets 2295
▲ Supprelin Injection (6% to 10%) 2056
Teslac 717
Timoptic-XE 1755
Levlen/Tri-Levlen 651
Uroqid-Acid No. 2 Tablets 640
Videx Tablets, Powder for Oral Solution, & Pediatric Powder for Oral Solution 720
Zerit Capsules 729

Pain, eye

Adsorbotear Artificial Tear ◉ 210
AK-Spore ◉ 204
Alomide (Less than 1%) 469
Ambien Tablets (Rare) 2416
Anafranil Capsules (Infrequent) 803
AquaSite Eye Drops ◉ 261
Asacol Delayed-Release Tablets 1979
Atrovent Inhalation Aerosol 671
Atrovent Inhalation Solution (Less than 3%) 673
Betimol 0.25%, 0.5% (1% to 5%) ◉ 261
Betoptic Ophthalmic Solution 469
Betoptic S Ophthalmic Suspension (Small number of patients) 471
BuSpar (Rare) 737
Cardura Tablets (1%) 2186
Cipro I.V. (1% or less) 595
Cipro I.V. Pharmacy Bulk Package (Less than 1%) 597
Cipro Tablets (Less than 1%) 592
Claritin (2% or fewer patients) 2349
Claritin-D (Less frequent) 2350
Clear Eyes ACR Astringent/Lubricant Eye Redness Reliever Eye Drops ◉ 316
Clomid 1514
Cognex Capsules (Infrequent) 1901
Cytovene (1% or less) 2103
Depakote Tablets (Greater than 1% but not more than 5%) 415
Diprivan Injection (Less than 1%) 2833
Effexor (Infrequent) 2719
Eldepryl Tablets 2550
EPIFRIN ◉ 239
Ethmozine Tablets (Less than 2%) 2041
Eye-Stream Eye Irrigating Solution 473
Flumadine Tablets & Syrup 1015
Foscavir Injection (Between 1% and 5%) 547
Glucotrol XL Extended Release Tablets (Less than 1%) 1968
Herplex Liquifilm ◉ 244
Hivid Tablets (Less than 1% to less than 3%) 2121
Intron A (Less than 5%) 2364
Iopidine 0.5% (Less than 1%) ◉ 221
Livostin (Approximately 1% to 3%) ◉ 266
Luvox Tablets (Infrequent) 2544
Maxaquin Tablets (Less than 1%) 2440
Miacalcin Injection 2273
Neurontin Capsules (Infrequent) 1922
Norvasc Tablets (More than 0.1% to 1%) 1940
Ophthalgan ◉ 326
Orudis Capsules (Less than 1%) 2766
Oruvail Capsules (Less than 1%) 2766
Paxil Tablets (Infrequent) 2505
Permax Tablets (Infrequent) 575
PREVACID Delayed-Release Capsules (Less than 1%) 2562
ProSom Tablets (Infrequent) 449
Prostin E2 Suppository 2634
Prozac Pulvules & Liquid, Oral Solution (Infrequent) 919
ReVia Tablets (Less than 1%) 940
Risperdal (Rare) 1301
Salagen Tablets (Less than 1%) 1489
Sectral Capsules (Up to 2%) 2807
Serzone Tablets (Frequent) 771
Soma Tablets 2674
Synarel Nasal Solution for Endometriosis (Less than 1%) 2152
Tambocor Tablets (Less than 1%) 1497
Tegison Capsules (Frequent) 2154
Timoptic in Ocudose (Less frequent) 1753
Timoptic Sterile Ophthalmic Solution (Less frequent) 1751
▲ Timoptic-XE (1% to 5% of patients) 1755
Vexol 1% Ophthalmic Suspension (1% to 5%) ◉ 230
Videx Tablets, Powder for Oral Solution, & Pediatric Powder for Oral Solution (Less than 1%) 720
Visine L.R. Eye Drops ◉ 313
Viva-Drops ◉ 325
Zebeta Tablets 1413
Ziac 1415
Zoloft Tablets (Infrequent) 2217

Pain, facial

Hivid Tablets (Less than 1% to less than 3%) 2121
Imitrex Injection (Infrequent) 1103
Imitrex Tablets (Infrequent) 1106
Supprelin Injection (2% to 3%) 2056

Pain, female genitalia

Floxin Tablets (200 mg, 300 mg, 400 mg) (Less than 1%) 1567
▲ Supprelin Injection (3% to 10%) 2056

Pain, femoral nerve

Questran Light 769
Questran Powder 770

Pain, flank

▲ Atgam Sterile Solution (5% to 10%) 2581
Fludara for Injection 663
Hivid Tablets (Less than 1% to less than 3%) 2121
Neupogen for Injection (Infrequent) 495
Prinivil Tablets (0.3% to 1.0%) 1733
Prinzide Tablets 1737
ReVia Tablets (Less than 1%) 940
Sansert Tablets 2295
TheraCys BCG Live (Intravesical) (Up to 4.9%) 897
Toradol 2159
Vaseretic Tablets 1765
Vasotec I.V. 1768
Vasotec Tablets (0.5% to 1.0%) 1771
Zestoretic 2850
Zestril Tablets (0.3% to 1.0%) 2854

Pain, genital

▲ Condylox (50% to 72%) 1802
▲ TheraCys BCG Live (Intravesical) (Up to 9.8%) 897
Zerit Capsules (Up to 2%) 729

Pain, hip

Cozaar Tablets (Less than 1%) 1628
Gamimune N, 5% Immune Globulin Intravenous (Human), 5% 619
Gamimune N, 10% Immune Globulin Intravenous (Human), 10% 621
Hyzaar Tablets 1677
Plendil Extended-Release Tablets (0.5% to 1.5%) 527
Prinivil Tablets (0.3% to 1.0%) 1733
Prinzide Tablets 1737
Zestoretic 2850
Zestril Tablets (0.3% to 1.0%) 2854

Pain, inguinal

Hivid Tablets (Less than 1% to less than 3%) 2121
ReVia Tablets (Less than 1%) 940

Pain, jaw

Cipro I.V. (1% or less) 595
Cipro I.V. Pharmacy Bulk Package (Less than 1%) 597
Navelbine Injection (Less than 5%) 1145
Nicorette 2458
Oncovin Solution Vials & Hyporets 1466
Permax Tablets (Infrequent) 575
ProSom Tablets (Rare) 449
Prozac Pulvules & Liquid, Oral Solution (Infrequent) 919
▲ Velban Vials (Among most common) 1484

Pain, kidney

Ceftin (Less than 1% but more than 0.1%) 1078
Effexor (Infrequent) 2719
Lamictal Tablets (Rare) 1112
Monopril Tablets (0.4% to 1.0%) 757
Paxil Tablets (Rare) 2505
Videx Tablets, Powder for Oral Solution, & Pediatric Powder for Oral Solution (Less than 1%) 720

Pain, knee

Cozaar Tablets (Less than 1%) 1628
Hyzaar Tablets 1677
Plendil Extended-Release Tablets (0.5% to 1.5%) 527

Pain, lower extremities

Adalat CC (3% or less) 589
Atgam Sterile Solution (Less than 5%) 2581
Cartrol Tablets (1.2%) 410
Catapres Tablets (About 3 in 1,000 patients) 674
CHEMET (succimer) Capsules (Up to 3%) 1545
Cipro Tablets (0.3% to 1%) 592
Clozaril Tablets (1%) 2252
Cozaar Tablets (1.0%) 1628
Eldepryl Tablets (1 of 49 patients) 2550
Esgic-plus Tablets (Infrequent) 1013
Estrace Cream and Tablets 749
Fioricet Tablets (Infrequent) 2258
Fioricet with Codeine Capsules (Infrequent) 2260
Fiorinal with Codeine Capsules (Infrequent) 2262
Hivid Tablets (Less than 1% to less than 3%) 2121
Hyzaar Tablets 1677
Lopid Tablets 1917
Mevacor Tablets (0.5% to 1.0%) 1699
Midamor Tablets (Less than or equal to 1%) 1703
Moduretic Tablets 1705
NebuPent for Inhalation Solution (1% or less) 1040
Oncovin Solution Vials & Hyporets 1466
Ortho-Est 1869
Phrenilin (Infrequent) 785
Plendil Extended-Release Tablets (0.5% to 1.5%) 527
Prilosec Delayed-Release Capsules (Less than 1%) 529
Prinivil Tablets (0.5% to 1.3%) 1733
Prinzide Tablets (0.3% to 1%) 1737
▲ ProSom Tablets (3%) 449
Prozac Pulvules & Liquid, Oral Solution (1.6%) 919
ReVia Tablets (Less than 1%) 940
Rifamate Capsules 1530
Rimactane Capsules 847
Rowasa (2.09%) 2548
Sedapap Tablets 50 mg/650 mg (Infrequent) 1543
Sinemet CR Tablets 944
Tenex Tablets (Less frequent) 2074
Tenoretic Tablets (Up to 3%) 2845
Tenormin Tablets and I.V. Injection (Up to 3%) 2847
Timolide Tablets 1748
Timoptic in Ocudose 1753
Timoptic Sterile Ophthalmic Solution 1751
Zestoretic (0.3 to 1%) 2850
Zestril Tablets (0.5% to 1.3%) 2854
Zovirax (0.3%) 1219

Pain, medullary bone

▲ Neupogen for Injection (24%) 495

Pain, Mittelschmerz

Serophene (clomiphene citrate tablets, USP) 2451

Pain, muscle (see under Myalgia)

Pain, neck (see under Torticollis)

Pain, neuritic

Oncovin Solution Vials & Hyporets 1466

Pain, nostril

DDAVP (Up to 2%) 2017
Desmopressin Acetate Rhinal Tube (Up to 2%) 979

Pain, oral mucosa

Cipro Tablets (Less than 1%) 592
Floxin I.V. 1571
Floxin Tablets (200 mg, 300 mg, 400 mg) 1567
Maxaquin Tablets 2440

Pain, parotid gland

Oncovin Solution Vials & Hyporets 1466

Pain, pelvic

Adalat CC (Less than 1.0%) 589
▲ Betaseron for SC Injection (6%) 658
Caverject (Less than 1%) 2583
▲ CellCept Capsules (More than or equal to 3%) 2099
Danocrine Capsules 2307
▲ Depo-Provera Contraceptive Injection (1% to 5%) 2602
Effexor (Infrequent) 2719
Hivid Tablets (Less than 1% to less than 3%) 2121
Humegon 1824
Luvox Tablets (Rare) 2544

(▣ Described in PDR For Nonprescription Drugs) Incidence data in parenthesis; ▲ 3% or more (◉ Described in PDR For Ophthalmology)

1381 Side Effects Index Paleness, unusual

Massengill Disposable Douche ... 2457
Massengill Medicated Disposable Douche ... 2458
Massengill Medicated Liquid Concentrate ... ▣ 821
Nolvadex Tablets ... 2841
Paxil Tablets (Rare) ... 2505
Permax Tablets (Infrequent) ... 575
Prinivil Tablets (0.3% to 1.0%) ... 1733
Prinzide Tablets ... 1737
Prozac Pulvules & Liquid, Oral Solution (Infrequent) ... 919
Serophene (clomiphene citrate tablets, USP) ... 2451
Serzone Tablets (Infrequent) ... 771
Zerit Capsules (Up to 2%) ... 729
Zestoretic ... 2850
Zestril Tablets (0.3% to 1.0%) ... 2854

Pain, penile

▲ Caverject (2% to 37%) ... 2583
Hivid Tablets (Less than 1% to less than 3%) ... 2121

Pain, perineal

Anafranil Capsules (Infrequent) ... 803
Foscavir Injection (Less than 1%) ... 547
Maxaquin Tablets (Less than 1%) ... 2440
Risperdal (Infrequent) ... 1301

Pain, pharynx

Oncovin Solution Vials & Hyporets 1466
Prilosec Delayed-Release Capsules (Less than 1%) ... 529
Primaxin I.M. ... 1727
Primaxin I.V. (Less than 0.2%) ... 1729
Prinivil Tablets (0.3% to 1.0%) ... 1733
Prinzide Tablets (0.3% to 1%) ... 1737
Sinemet CR Tablets ... 944
Zestoretic (0.3 to 1%) ... 2850
Zestril Tablets (0.3% to 1.0%) ... 2854

Pain, postoperative

▲ Revex (4%) ... 1811

Pain, precordium

Cafergot ... 2251
Chromagen Capsules ... 2339
D.H.E. 45 Injection ... 2255
Ergomar ... 1486
Imitrex Tablets ... 1106
Mykrox Tablets (2.7%) ... 993
Phenergan VC with Codeine ... 2781
Wigraine Tablets & Suppositories ... 1829
Zoloft Tablets (Rare) ... 2217

Pain, prostate

Lupron Depot 3.75 mg ... 2556
Lupron Depot 7.5 mg ... 2559
Lupron Injection ... 2555

Pain, rectum

CORTENEMA (Rare) ... 2535
Hivid Tablets (Less than 1% to less than 3%) ... 2121
Noroxin Tablets (0.3% to 1.0%) ... 1715
Noroxin Tablets (0.3% to 1.4%) ... 2048
Questran Light ... 769
Questran Powder ... 770
Rowasa (0.61% to 1.23%) ... 2548

Pain, renal

Ambien Tablets (Rare) ... 2416
Anafranil Capsules (Infrequent) ... 803
Neurontin Capsules (Rare) ... 1922
Zoloft Tablets (Rare) ... 2217

Pain, retrosternal

▲ Ethamolin (Among most common) 2400

Pain, right upper quadrant

Calan SR Caplets ... 2422
Calan Tablets ... 2419
Intron A (Less than 5%) ... 2364
Isoptin SR Tablets ... 1348
Paraflex Caplets ... 1580
Parafon Forte DSC Caplets ... 1581
Tapazole Tablets ... 1477

Pain, shoulder

Brevibloc Injection (Less than 1%) 1808
Cartrol Tablets (Less common) ... 410
Cozaar Tablets (Less than 1%) ... 1628
Engerix-B Unit-Dose Vials (Less than 1%) ... 2482
Hytrin Capsules (At least 1%) ... 430
Hyzaar Tablets ... 1677
Mevacor Tablets (0.5% to 1.0%) ... 1699
Moduretic Tablets ... 1705
Prinivil Tablets (0.3% to 1.0%) ... 1733
Prinzide Tablets (0.3% to 1%) ... 1737
Recombivax HB (Less than 1%) ... 1744
ReVia Tablets (Less than 1%) ... 940
Sinemet CR Tablets (1.0%) ... 944
Tonocard Tablets (Less than 1%) .. 531
Zestoretic (0.3 to 1%) ... 2850
Zestril Tablets (0.3% to 1.0%) ... 2854

Pain, stomach (see under Stomachache)

Pain, substernal

Aerolate ... 1004
Provocholine for Inhalation ... 2140
Tenex Tablets (3% or less) ... 2074
Unasyn (Less than 1%) ... 2212

Pain, testicular

Caverject (Less than 1%) ... 2583
Lupron Depot 3.75 mg ... 2556
Lupron Depot 7.5 mg (Less than 5%) ... 2559
Lupron Injection (Less than 5%) ... 2555
Neurontin Capsules (Rare) ... 1922
Prilosec Delayed-Release Capsules (Less than 1%) ... 529

Pain, thoracic spine

▲ CHEMET (succimer) Capsules (5.2-15.7%) ... 1545
Primaxin I.M. ... 1727
Primaxin I.V. (Less than 0.2%) ... 1729

Pain, throat

DDAVP ... 2017
Desmopressin Acetate Rhinal Tube 979
Dizac (Less frequent) ... 1809

Pain, trunk

Diprivan Injection (Less than 1%) .. 2833
▲ Epogen for Injection (3%) ... 489
Floxin I.V. (1% to 3%) ... 1571
Floxin Tablets (200 mg, 300 mg, 400 mg) (1% to 3%) ... 1567
▲ Leustatin (6%) ... 1834
▲ Procrit for Injection (3%) ... 1841
▲ Supprelin Injection (1% to 10%) ... 2056

Pain, tumor site

Blenoxane (Infrequent) ... 692
Nolvadex Tablets ... 2841
Velban Vials ... 1484

Pain, upper extremities

Cipro I.V. (1% or less) ... 595
Engerix-B Unit-Dose Vials (Less than 1%) ... 2482
Hivid Tablets (Less than 1% to less than 3%) ... 2121
Lopid Tablets ... 1917
Midamor Tablets (Less than or equal to 1%) ... 1703
Moduretic Tablets ... 1705
Prinivil Tablets (0.3% to 1.0%) ... 1733
ProSom Tablets (Infrequent) ... 449
Prozac Pulvules & Liquid, Oral Solution (1.6%) ... 919
Rifamate Capsules ... 1530
Rimactane Capsules ... 847
Timolide Tablets ... 1748
Timoptic in Ocudose ... 1753
Timoptic Sterile Ophthalmic Solution ... 1751

Pain, urethral

Ceftin (Less than 1% but more than 0.1%) ... 1078
Permax Tablets (Rare) ... 575
Prozac Pulvules & Liquid, Oral Solution (Rare) ... 919

Pain, urinary bladder

BCG Vaccine, USP (TICE) ... 1814
Duragesic Transdermal System (Less than 1%) ... 1288
Effexor (Infrequent) ... 2719
Hivid Tablets (Less than 1% to less than 3%) ... 2121

Pain, vaginal

Floxin I.V. (Less than 1%) ... 1571
Hivid Tablets (Less than 1% to less than 3%) ... 2121
Neurontin Capsules (Rare) ... 1922
Prostin E2 Suppository ... 2634
Vagistat-1 (Less than 1%) ... 778

Pain, vascular

Lamprene Capsules (Less than 1%) ... 828

Pain, vulva

DDAVP Injection (Infrequent) ... 2014
DDAVP Injection 15 mcg/mL (Infrequent) ... 2015
Stimate, (desmopressin acetate) Nasal Spray, 1.5 mg/mL (Infrequent) ... 525
▲ Terazol 3 Vaginal Suppositories (4.2% of 284 patients) ... 1886

Pain at application site

Rowasa (1.35%) ... 2548
▲ Sulfamylon Cream (One of two most frequent) ... 925
Zovirax Ointment 5% ... 1223

Pain at injection site

▲ ActHIB (6.4% to 9.0%) ... 872
Actimmune ... 1056
Adagen (pegademase bovine) Injection (Two patients) ... 972
Alfenta Injection (0.3% to 1%) ... 1286
Ancef Injection (Infrequent) ... 2465
AquaMEPHYTON Injection ... 1608
▲ Aredia for Injection (Among most common; up to 18%) ... 810
Aristocort Suspension (Forte Parenteral) ... 1027
Aristospan Suspension (Intra-articular) ... 1033
Aristospan Suspension (Intralesional) ... 1032
Atgam Sterile Solution (More than 1% but less than 5%) ... 2581
▲ Ativan Injection (17%) ... 2698
Attenuvax ... 1610
Bactrim I.V. Infusion (Infrequent) ... 2082
Biavax II ... 1613
Brethine Ampuls (0.5 to 2.6%) ... 815
Brevital Sodium Vials ... 1429
Capastat Sulfate Vials ... 2868
Cardene I.V. (0.7%) ... 2709
Cefizox for Intramuscular or Intravenous Use (Greater than 1% but less than 5%) ... 1034
Cefobid Intravenous/Intramuscular (Occasional) ... 2189
Cefobid Pharmacy Bulk Package - Not for Direct Infusion (Occasional) ... 2192
Cholera Vaccine ... 2711
Cipro I.V. (1% or less) ... 595
▲ Claforan Sterile and Injection (4.3%) ... 1235
Cleocin Phosphate Injection ... 2586
Cytovene-IV (1% or less) ... 2103
Delatestryl Injection (Rare) ... 2860
Demerol ... 2308
Depo-Provera Contraceptive Injection (Fewer than 1%) ... 2602
Desferal Vials ... 820
Dilaudid-HP Injection (Rare) ... 1337
Dilaudid-HP Lyophilized Powder 250 mg (Rare) ... 1337
Diphtheria and Tetanus Toxoids and Pertussis Vaccine Adsorbed .. 2477
Diphtheria and Tetanus Toxoids and Pertussis Vaccine Adsorbed USP (For Pediatric Use) (Frequent) ... 875
▲ Diprivan Injection (10% to 17.6%) ... 2833
Edecrin (Occasional) ... 1657
Engerix-B Unit-Dose Vials (Less than 1%) ... 2482
Factrel (Occasional) ... 2877
Fluorescite ... ◉ 219
Foscavir Injection (Between 1% and 5%) ... 547
Fragmin (B up to 4.5%) ... 1954
▲ Fungizone Intravenous (Among most common) ... 506
▲ Gammagard S/D, Immune Globulin, Intravenous (Human) (16%) ... 585
Gammar, Immune Globulin (Human) U.S.P. ... 515
Garamycin Injectable (Occasional) .. 2360
Genotropin (Infrequent) ... 111
Hep-B-Gammagee ... 1663
Humatrope Vials (Infrequent) ... 1443
Humegon ... 1824
HyperHep Hepatitis B Immune Globulin (Human) ... 626
Hyperstat I.V. Injection ... 2363
Imitrex Injection ... 1103
▲ Imovax Rabies Vaccine (About 25%) ... 881
INFeD (Iron Dextran Injection, USP) ... 2345
Intron A (Less than 5%) ... 2364
▲ IPOL Poliovirus Vaccine Inactivated (13%) ... 885
Kefzol Vials, Faspak & ADD-Vantage (Infrequent) ... 1456
Konakion Injection (Rare) ... 2127
▲ Leustatin (9% to 19%) ... 1834
Levoprome (Frequent) ... 1274
Lincocin (Infrequent) ... 2617
Mandol Vials, Faspak & ADD-Vantage (Infrequent) ... 1461
Mefoxin ... 1691
Mepergan Injection ... 2753
Meruvax II ... 1697
Metrodin (urofollitropin for injection) ... 2446
Mezlin ... 601
Mezlin Pharmacy Bulk Package ... 604
▲ Monocid Injection (5.7%) ... 2497
Mononine, Coagulation Factor IX (Human) ... 523
▲ Navelbine Injection (Up to 13%) 1145
Nebcin Vials, Hyporets & ADD-Vantage ... 1464
Netromycin Injection 100 mg/ml (4 of 1000 patients) ... 2373
Nutropin (Infrequent) ... 1061
▲ OmniHIB (6.4% to 9.0%) ... 2499
▲ Oncaspar (Greater than 1% but less than 5%) ... 2028
PedvaxHIB ... 1718
▲ Pentam 300 Injection (11.1%) ... 1041
Peptavlon ... 2878
Pergonal (menotropins for injection, USP) ... 2448
Pipracil (2%) ... 1390
▲ Pneumovax 23 (Common) ... 1725
▲ Pnu-Imune 23 (72%) ... 1393
▲ Poliovax (12%) ... 891
Polymyxin B Sulfate, Aerosporin Brand Sterile Powder (Occasional) ... 1154
Pregnyl ... 1828
Premarin with Methyltestosterone .. 2794
Primaxin I.M. (1.2%) ... 1727
Primaxin I.V. (0.7%) ... 1729
Profasi (chorionic gonadotropin for injection, USP) ... 2450
Protropin (Infrequent) ... 1063
Rabies Vaccine Adsorbed (A few patients) ... 2508
▲ Rabies Vaccine, Imovax Rabies I.D. (About 25%) ... 883
Recombivax HB (Equal to or greater than 1%) ... 1744
Retrovir I.V. Infusion (Infrequent) ... 1163
Robaxin Injectable ... 2070
Rocephin Injectable Vials, ADD-Vantage, Galaxy Container (1%) ... 2142
Roferon-A Injection (Less than 1%) ... 2145
▲ Romazicon (3% to 9%) ... 2147
▲ Sandostatin Injection (7.5%) ... 2292
Septra I.V. Infusion (Infrequent) ... 1169
Septra I.V. Infusion ADD-Vantage Vials (Infrequent) ... 1171
Sotradecol (Sodium Tetradecyl Sulfate Injection) ... 967
Tazidime Vials, Faspak & ADD-Vantage (Less than 2%) ... 1478
Tested Capsules ... 1262
▲ Tetramune (21% to 65%) ... 1404
Thioplex (Thiotepa For Injection) ... 1281
Ticar for Injection ... 2526
Timentin for Injection ... 2528
Tobramycin Sulfate Injection ... 968
Toradol (2%) ... 2159
Tubersol (Tuberculin Purified Protein Derivative [Mantoux]) ... 2872
▲ Typhim Vi (Up to 56%) ... 899
▲ Unasyn (3% to 16%) ... 2212
Vancocin HCl, Vials & ADD-Vantage ... 1481
▲ Varivax (19.3% to 32.5%; less than 0.05%) ... 1762
▲ Versed Injection (3.7% to 5.0%) ... 2170
Zantac Injection ... 1207
▲ Zefazone (Up to 31%) ... 2654
▲ Zinecard (12% to 13%) ... 1961
▲ Zofran Injection (4%) ... 1214
Zosyn (0.2%) ... 1419
Zosyn Pharmacy Bulk Package (0.2%) ... 1422

Pain with coitus

Condylox (Less than 5%) ... 1802

Paleness, unusual

Geref (sermorelin acetate for injection) ... 2876
Lioresal Intrathecal ... 1596

(▣ Described in PDR For Nonprescription Drugs) Incidence data in parenthesis; ▲ 3% or more (◉ Described in PDR For Ophthalmology)

Paleness, unusual **Side Effects Index** **1382**

Nucofed ... 2051

Palilalia

Nardil (Less common) ... 1920

Pallor

Ambien Tablets (Infrequent) ... 2416
Anafranil Capsules (Infrequent) ... 803
Ana-Kit Anaphylaxis Emergency Treatment Kit (Common) ... 617
Azo Gantrisin Tablets ... 2081
Brevibloc Injection (Less than 1%) ... 1808
Buprenex Injectable (Infrequent) ... 2006
Capoten (2 to 5 of 1000 patients) ... 739
Capozide (2 to 5 of 1000 patients) ... 742
Cardura Tablets (Less than 0.5% of 3960 patients) ... 2186
Catapres Tablets ... 674
Catapres-TTS ... 675
Claritin-D ... 2350
Clozaril Tablets (Less than 1%) ... 2252
Combipres Tablets ... 677
Cytotec (Infrequent) ... 2424
D.A. Chewable Tablets ... 951
Dalgan Injection (Less than 1%) ... 538
Dapsone Tablets USP ... 1284
Deconamine Chewable Tablets ... 1320
Deconamine CX Cough and Cold Liquid and Tablets ... 1319
Deconamine ... 1320
Deconsal C Expectorant Syrup ... 456
Deconsal Pediatric Capsules ... 454
Deconsal Pediatric Syrup ... 457
Deconsal II Tablets ... 454
Dilacor XR Extended-release Capsules (Infrequent) ... 2018
Dilatrate-SR ... 2398
Dura-Tap/PD Capsules ... 2867
Dura-Vent/DA Tablets ... 953
Dura-Vent Tablets ... 952
▲ Emla Cream (37%) ... 545
EpiPen ... 790
Etrafon ... 2355
Fedahist Gyrocaps ... 2401
Fedahist Timecaps ... 2401
Flumadine Tablets & Syrup (Less than 0.3%) ... 1015
Gantrisin ... 2120
Imitrex Injection (Rare) ... 1103
Imitrex Tablets (Infrequent) ... 1106
Levophed Bitartrate Injection ... 2315
Luvox Tablets (Infrequent) ... 2544
Mellaril ... 2269
▲ Miacalcin Nasal Spray (10.6%) ... 2275
Monoket (Fewer than 1%) ... 2406
Nitrolingual Spray ... 2027
Novahistine DH ... 2462
Novahistine DMX ... ▣ 822
Novahistine Elixir ... ▣ 823
Novahistine Expectorant ... 2463
Paremyd ... ◉ 247
Paxil Tablets ... 2505
Proloprim Tablets ... 1155
Proventil Syrup (Children 2 to 6 years, 1%) ... 2385
Risperdal (Rare) ... 1301
Rondec Oral Drops ... 953
Rondec Syrup ... 953
Rondec Tablet ... 953
Rondec-DM Oral Drops ... 954
Rondec-DM Syrup ... 954
Rondec-TR Tablet ... 953
Seldane-D Extended-Release Tablets ... 1538
Septra I.V. Infusion ... 1169
Septra I.V. Infusion ADD-Vantage Vials ... 1171
Serzone Tablets (Rare) ... 771
Supprelin Injection (1% to 3%) ... 2056
Survanta Beractant Intratracheal Suspension (Less than 1%) ... 2226
Sus-Phrine Injection ... 1019
Syn-Rx Tablets ... 465
Syn-Rx DM Tablets ... 466
Tonocard Tablets (Less than 1%) ... 531
Toradol (1% or less) ... 2159
Trilafon (Occasional) ... 2389
Trinalin Repetabs Tablets ... 1330
Tussend ... 1783
Tussend Expectorant ... 1785
Tympagesic Ear Drops ... 2342
Ventolin Syrup (1% of children) ... 1202
Wellbutrin Tablets (Rare) ... 1204
Zoloft Tablets (Rare) ... 2217

Pallor, facial

Parlodel (Less than 1%) ... 2281

Pallor, optic disc

Aralen Phosphate Tablets ... 2301
Plaquenil Sulfate Tablets ... 2328

Palmar-plantar erythrodysesthesia syndrome

Fluorouracil Injection ... 2116

Palpebra superior, elevation

IOPIDINE Sterile Ophthalmic Solution (1.3%) ... ◉ 219

Palpitations

Accupril Tablets (0.5% to 1.0%) ... 1893
Accutane Capsules (Less than 1%) ... 2076
Actifed with Codeine Cough Syrup ... 1067
Acutrim ... ▣ 628
▲ Adalat Capsules (10 mg and 20 mg) (2% or less to 7%) ... 587
Adalat CC (Less than 1.0%) ... 589
Adenocard Injection (Less than 1%) ... 1021
Adenoscan (Less than 1%) ... 1024
Adipex-P Tablets and Capsules ... 1048
Children's Advil Suspension (Less than 1%) ... 2692
▲ AeroBid Inhaler System (3-9%) ... 1005
▲ Aerobid-M Inhaler System (3-9%) ... 1005
Aerolate ... 1004
Altace Capsules (Less than 1%) ... 1232
Alupent (1% to 4%) ... 669
Ambien Tablets (2%) ... 2416
▲ Anafranil Capsules (4%) ... 803
Ana-Kit Anaphylaxis Emergency Treatment Kit (Common) ... 617
Anaprox/Naprosyn (Less than 3%) ... 2117
Apresazide Capsules (Common) ... 808
Apresoline Hydrochloride Tablets (Common) ... 809
Asendin Tablets (Less frequent) ... 1369
Atamet (Less frequent) ... 572
Atrohist Pediatric Capsules ... 453
Atrohist Plus Tablets ... 454
Atrovent Inhalation Aerosol (1.8%) ... 671
Atrovent Inhalation Solution (Less than 3%) ... 673
Azo Gantrisin Tablets ... 2081
Bellergal-S Tablets (Rare) ... 2250
Benadryl Capsules ... 1898
Benadryl Injection ... 1898
Bentyl ... 1501
Betagan ... ◉ 233
▲ Betapace Tablets (3% to 14%) ... 641
▲ Betaseron for SC Injection (8%) ... 658
Betimol 0.25%, 0.5% ... ◉ 261
Biphetamine Capsules ... 983
Blocadren Tablets ... 1614
Bontril Slow-Release Capsules ... 781
▲ Brethine Ampuls (7.8 to 22.9%) ... 815
Brethine Tablets ... 814
Bricanyl Subcutaneous Injection (Common) ... 1502
Bricanyl Tablets (Common) ... 1503
Bromfed ... 1785
▲ Bromfed-DM Cough Syrup (Among most frequent) ... 1786
Bromfed-PD Capsules (Extended-Release) ... 1785
Bronkometer Aerosol ... 2302
Bronkosol Solution ... 2302
Brontex ... 1981
BuSpar (1%) ... 737
Calan SR Caplets (1% or less) ... 2422
Calan Tablets (1% or less) ... 2419
Capoten (Approximately 1 of 100 patients) ... 739
Capozide (Approximately 1 of 100 patients) ... 742
▲ Cardene Capsules (3.3-4.1%) ... 2095
Cardene SR Capsules (2.8%) ... 2097
Cardizem CD Capsules (Less than 1%) ... 1506
Cardizem SR Capsules (1.3%) ... 1510
Cardizem Injectable ... 1508
Cardizem Tablets (Less than 1%) ... 1512
Cardura Tablets (1.2% to 2%) ... 2186
Cartrol Tablets (Less common) ... 410
Cataflam (Less than 1%) ... 816
Catapres Tablets (About 5 in 1,000 patients) ... 674
Catapres-TTS (Less frequent) ... 675
▲ CellCept Capsules (More than or equal to 3%) ... 2099
Cipro I.V. (1% or less) ... 595
Cipro I.V. Pharmacy Bulk Package (Less than 1%) ... 597
Cipro Tablets (Less than 1%) ... 592
Claritin (2% or fewer patients) ... 2349
Claritin-D (Less frequent) ... 2350
Clinoril Tablets (Less than 1 in 100) ... 1618
Clomid ... 1514
Clozaril Tablets (Less than 1%) ... 2252
Cognex Capsules (Infrequent) ... 1901
Combipres Tablets (About 5 in 1,000) ... 677
Comhist ... 2038
Cozaar Tablets (Less than 1%) ... 1628
Cystospaz ... 1963
D.A. Chewable Tablets ... 951
Dalmane Capsules ... 2173
Daypro Caplets (Less than 1%) ... 2426
Deconamine Chewable Tablets ... 1320
Deconamine CX Cough and Cold Liquid and Tablets ... 1319
Deconamine ... 1320
Deconsal ... 454
Demerol ... 2308
Depakote Tablets (Greater than 1% but not more than 5%) ... 415
Desoxyn Gradumet Tablets ... 419
Desyrel and Desyrel Dividose (Up to 7%) ... 503
Dexatrim ... ▣ 832
Dexatrim Plus Vitamins Caplets ... ▣ 832
Dexedrine ... 2474
DextroStat Dextroamphetamine Tablets ... 2036
Didrex Tablets ... 2607
Dilacor XR Extended-release Capsules (Infrequent) ... 2018
Dilaudid-HP Injection (Less frequent) ... 1337
Dilaudid-HP Lyophilized Powder 250 mg (Less frequent) ... 1337
Dilaudid Tablets and Liquid ... 1339
Dimetane-DX Cough Syrup ... 2059
Dipentum Capsules (Rare) ... 1951
Ditropan ... 1516
Dobutrex Solution Vials (1% to 3%) ... 1439
Dolobid Tablets (Rare) ... 1654
Donnatal ... 2060
Donnatal Extentabs ... 2061
Donnatal Tablets ... 2060
Doral Tablets ... 2664
Dura-Tap/PD Capsules ... 2867
Dura-Vent/DA Tablets ... 953
Dura-Vent Tablets ... 952
▲ DynaCirc Capsules (1.0% to 5.1%) ... 2256
E.E.S. (Isolated reports) ... 424
EC-Naprosyn Delayed-Release Tablets (Less than 3%) ... 2117
Effexor ... 2719
Elavil ... 2838
Eldepryl Tablets (1 of 49 patients) ... 2550
Endep Tablets ... 2174
Engerix-B Unit-Dose Vials ... 2482
Entex PSE Tablets ... 1987
EpiPen ... 790
EryPed (Isolated reports) ... 421
Ery-Tab Tablets (Isolated reports) ... 422
Erythrocin Stearate Filmtab (Isolated reports) ... 425
Erythromycin Base Filmtab (Isolated reports) ... 426
Erythromycin Delayed-Release Capsules, USP (Isolated reports) ... 427
▲ Ethmozine Tablets (5.8%) ... 2041
Etrafon ... 2355
Fastin Capsules ... 2488
Fedahist Gyrocaps ... 2401
Fedahist Timecaps ... 2401
Felbatol (Frequent) ... 2666
Feldene Capsules (Less than 1%) ... 1965
Fioricet with Codeine Capsules ... 2260
Fiorinal with Codeine Capsules ... 2262
Flexeril Tablets (Less than 1%) ... 1661
Floxin I.V. (Less than 1%) ... 1571
Floxin Tablets (200 mg, 300 mg, 400 mg) (Less than 1%) ... 1567
Flumadine Tablets & Syrup (Less than 0.3%) ... 1015
Foscavir Injection (Between 1% and 5%) ... 547
Guaifed ... 1787
Guaimax-D Tablets ... 792
Hismanal Tablets (Rare to less frequent) ... 1293
Hivid Tablets (Less than 1% to less than 3%) ... 2121
Hycomine Compound Tablets ... 932
Hycomine ... 931
Hycotuss Expectorant Syrup ... 933
▲ Hylorel Tablets (29.5%) ... 985
Hyperstat I.V. Injection ... 2363
▲ Hytrin Capsules (0.9% to 4.3%; 28%) ... 430
Hyzaar Tablets (1.4%) ... 1677
IBU Tablets (Less than 1%) ... 1342
Imdur (Less than or equal to 5%) ... 1323
Imitrex Injection (Infrequent) ... 1103
Imitrex Tablets (Up to 2%) ... 1106
Indocin (Less than 1%) ... 1680
Intron A (Less than 5%) ... 2364
Ionamin Capsules ... 990
IOPIDINE Sterile Ophthalmic Solution ... ◉ 219
Ismo Tablets (Fewer than 1%) ... 2738
Isoetharine Inhalation Solution, USP, Arm-a-Med ... 551
Isoptin Oral Tablets (Less than 1%) ... 1346
Isoptin SR Tablets (1% or less) ... 1348
Isuprel Hydrochloride Injection 1:5000 ... 2311
Isuprel Hydrochloride Solution 1:200 & 1:100 ... 2313
Isuprel Mistometer ... 2312
Kerlone Tablets (1.9%) ... 2436
Klonopin Tablets ... 2126
Kutrase Capsules ... 2402
Lamictal Tablets (1.0%) ... 1112
Larodopa Tablets (Infrequent) ... 2129
Levsin/Levsinex/Levbid ... 2405
Limbitrol ... 2180
Lioresal Tablets (Rare) ... 829
Lodine Capsules and Tablets (Less than 1%) ... 2743
Lopressor Ampuls (1%) ... 830
Lopressor HCT Tablets ... 832
Lopressor Tablets (1%) ... 830
Lorelco Tablets ... 1517
Lotensin Tablets ... 834
Lotensin HCT (0.3% to 1.0%) ... 837
Lotrel Capsules (0.5% to 0.3%) ... 840
Lozol Tablets (Less than 5%) ... 2022
Ludiomil Tablets (Rare) ... 843
Lufyllin & Lufyllin-400 Tablets ... 2670
Lufyllin-GG Elixir & Tablets ... 2671
▲ Lupron Depot 3.75 mg (Among most frequent) ... 2556
▲ Luvox Tablets (3%) ... 2544
MS Contin Tablets (Less frequent) ... 1994
MSIR (Infrequent) ... 1997
Marax Tablets & DF Syrup ... 2200
Marinol (Dronabinol) Capsules (Greater than 1%) ... 2231
Maxair Autohaler (1.3% to 1.7%) ... 1492
Maxair Inhaler (1.7%) ... 1494
Megace Oral Suspension (1% to 3%) ... 699
Mepergan Injection ... 2753
Metaproterenol Sulfate Inhalation Solution, USP, Arm-a-Med (Approximately 1 in 300 patients) ... 552
Methadone Hydrochloride Oral Concentrate ... 2233
Methadone Hydrochloride Oral Solution & Tablets ... 2235
Methergine (Rare) ... 2272
▲ Mexitil Capsules (4.3% to 7.5%) ... 678
Miacalcin Nasal Spray (Less than 1%) ... 2275
Midamor Tablets (Less than or equal to 1%) ... 1703
Miltown Tablets ... 2672
▲ Minipress Capsules (5.3%) ... 1937
▲ Minizide Capsules (5.3%) ... 1938
Moduretic Tablets ... 1705
Monoket (Fewer than 1%) ... 2406
Monopril Tablets (0.2% to 1.0%) ... 757
Children's Motrin Ibuprofen Oral Suspension (Less than 1%) ... 1546
Motrin Tablets (Less than 1%) ... 2625
Motrin Ibuprofen Suspension, Oral Drops, Chewable Tablets, Caplets (Less than 1%) ... 1546
Mykrox Tablets (Less than 2%) ... 993
Nalfon 200 Pulvules & Nalfon Tablets (2.5%) ... 917
Anaprox/Naprosyn (Less than 3%) ... 2117
NebuPent for Inhalation Solution (1% or less) ... 1040
Netromycin Injection 100 mg/ml (Fewer than 1 of 1000 patients) ... 2373
Neurontin Capsules (Infrequent) ... 1922
Nicorette ... 2458
Nimotop Capsules (Less than 1%) ... 610
Nitrostat Tablets (Occasional) ... 1925
Norflex ... 1496
Norgesic ... 1496
Norisodrine with Calcium Iodide Syrup ... 442
Noroxin Tablets (Less frequent) ... 1715
Noroxin Tablets (Less frequent) ... 2048
Norpramin Tablets ... 1526
Norvasc Tablets (0.7% to 4.5%) ... 1940

(▣ Described in PDR For Nonprescription Drugs) Incidence data in parenthesis; ▲ 3% or more (◉ Described in PDR For Ophthalmology)

1383 Side Effects Index Pancreatitis

Novahistine DH 2462
Novahistine DMX ▣ 822
Novahistine Elixir ▣ 823
Novahistine Expectorant 2463
Ocupress Ophthalmic Solution, 1% Sterile (Occasional) ⊙ 309
OptiPranolol (Metipranolol 0.3%) Sterile Ophthalmic Solution (A small number of patients) ⊙ 258
Oramorph SR (Morphine Sulfate Sustained Release Tablets) (Less frequent) 2236
Orap Tablets 1050
Ornade Spansule Capsules 2502
Orudis Capsules (Less than 1%) 2766
Oruvail Capsules (Less than 1%) 2766
PBZ Tablets 845
PBZ-SR Tablets 844
PMB 200 and PMB 400 2783
Pamelor 2280
Parnate Tablets 2503
Paxil Tablets (2.9%) 2505
Penetrex Tablets (Less than 1% but more than or equal to 0.1%) 2031
Pentasa (Less than 1%) 1527
Pepcid Injection (Infrequent) 1722
Pepcid (Infrequent) 1720
Periactin 1724
Permax Tablets (2.1%) 575
Phenergan with Codeine 2777
Phenergan VC with Codeine 2781
Phenurone Tablets (Less than 1%) 447
Plendil Extended-Release Tablets (0.4% to 2.5%) 527
Pondimin Tablets 2066
Ponstel (Rare) 1925
Prelu-2 Timed Release Capsules 681
PREVACID Delayed-Release Capsules (Less than 1%) 2562
Prilosec Delayed-Release Capsules (Less than 1%) 529
Primaxin I.M. 1727
Primaxin I.V. (Less than 0.2%) 1729
Prinivil Tablets (1.0% to 1.9%) 1733
Prinzide Tablets (0.3 to 1%) 1737
Pro-Banthīne Tablets 2052
▲ Procardia Capsules (2% or less to 7%) 1971
▲ Procardia XL Extended Release Tablets (Less than 3% to 7%) 1972
Proglycem (Common) 580
Propulsid (1% or less) 1300
ProSom Tablets (Infrequent) 449
▲ Proventil Inhalation Aerosol (Less than 10%) 2382
▲ Proventil Repetabs Tablets (5%) 2386
Proventil Syrup (Less than 1 of 100 patients) 2385
▲ Proventil Tablets (5%) 2386
Prozac Pulvules & Liquid, Oral Solution (1.3% to 2%) 919
Quadrinal Tablets 1350
Quarzan Capsules 2181
RMS Suppositories 2657
Recombivax HB (Less than 1%) 1744
Relafen Tablets (Less than 1%) 2510
ReoPro Vials (0.7%) 1471
Respbid Tablets 682
Restoril Capsules (Less than 1%) 2284
ReVia Tablets (Less than 1%) 940
Rifater 1532
Risperdal (Infrequent) 1301
Ritalin 848
Robinul Forte Tablets 2072
Robinul Injectable 2072
Robinul Tablets 2072
Rocephin Injectable Vials, ADD-Vantage, Galaxy Container (Rare) 2142
Roferon-A Injection (Less than 3%) 2145
Rogaine Topical Solution (1.53%) 2637
▲ Romazicon (3% to 9%) 2147
Rondec Oral Drops 953
Rondec Syrup 953
Rondec 953
Roxanol 2243
▲ Rythmol Tablets–150mg, 225mg, 300mg (0.6 to 3.4%) 1352
Salagen Tablets (Less than 1%) 1489
Sandostatin Injection (Less than 1%) 2292
Sanorex Tablets 2294
Seldane Tablets (Rare) 1536
Seldane-D Extended-Release Tablets (2.4%) 1538
Semprex-D Capsules 463
Semprex-D Capsules 1167
Ser-Ap-Es Tablets 849
Serevent Inhalation Aerosol (1% to 3%) 1176
Serzone Tablets 771
Sinemet Tablets (Less frequent) 943
Sinemet CR Tablets 944
Slo-bid Gyrocaps 2033
Stadol (1% or greater) 775
Stimate, (desmopressin acetate) Nasal Spray, 1.5 mg/mL 525
Supprelin Injection (1% to 3%) 2056
Surmontil Capsules 2811
Sus-Phrine Injection 1019
Synarel Nasal Solution for Endometriosis (Less than 1%) 2152
Syn-Rx Tablets 465
Syn-Rx DM Tablets 466
▲ Tambocor Tablets (6.1%) 1497
Tavist Syrup 2297
Tavist Tablets 2298
Tenex Tablets (3% or less) 2074
Thalitone (Common) 1245
Theo-24 Extended Release Capsules 2568
Theo-Dur Extended-Release Tablets 1327
Theo-X Extended-Release Tablets 788
Timolide Tablets 1748
Timoptic in Ocudose (Less frequent) 1753
Timoptic Sterile Ophthalmic Solution (Less frequent) 1751
Timoptic-XE 1755
Tofranil Ampuls 854
Tofranil Tablets 856
Tofranil-PM Capsules 857
Tonocard Tablets (0.4-1.8%) 531
Toprol-XL Tablets (About 1 of 100 patients) 565
Toradol (1% or less) 2159
▲ Tornalate Solution for Inhalation, 0.2% (3.1%) 956
Tornalate Metered Dose Inhaler (1.5% to approximately 3%) 957
Trandate 1185
Trental Tablets 1244
Triavil Tablets 1757
Trinalin Repetabs Tablets 1330
Tussend Expectorant 1785
Ultram Tablets (50 mg) (Infrequent) 1585
Uni-Dur Extended-Release Tablets 1331
Uniphyl 400 mg Tablets 2001
Univasc Tablets (Less than 1%) 2410
Urispas Tablets 2532
▲ Vascor (200, 300 and 400 mg) Tablets (2.27 to 6.52%) 1587
Vaseretic Tablets (0.5% to 2.0%) 1765
Vasotec I.V. 1768
Vasotec Tablets (0.5% to 1.0%) 1771
▲ Ventolin Inhalation Aerosol and Refill (Fewer than 10 in 100 patients) 1197
Ventolin Inhalation Solution 1198
Ventolin Nebules Inhalation Solution 1199
Ventolin Syrup (Less than 1 of 100 patients) 1202
▲ Ventolin Tablets (5 of 100 patients) 1203
Verelan Capsules (1% or less) 1410
Verelan Capsules (Less than 1%) 2824
Vicodin Tuss Expectorant 1358
Videx Tablets, Powder for Oral Solution, & Pediatric Powder for Oral Solution (Less than 1%) 720
Visken Tablets (Less than 1%) 2299
Vivactil Tablets 1774
Volmax Extended-Release Tablets (2.4%) 1788
Voltaren Tablets (Less than 1%) 861
▲ Wellbutrin Tablets (3.7%) 1204
▲ Xanax Tablets (7.7%) 2649
▲ Yutopar Intravenous Injection (About one-third) 570
Zaroxolyn Tablets 1000
Zebeta Tablets 1413
Zestoretic (0.3 to 1%) 2850
Zestril Tablets (1.0% to 1.9%) 2854
Ziac 1415
Zithromax (1% or less) 1944
Zoladex (1% or greater) 2858
▲ Zoloft Tablets (3.5%) 2217

Palsy, cranial nerve

Carbocaine Hydrochloride Injection 2303
Marcaine Spinal 2319
NegGram (A few cases) 2323
Orthoclone OKT3 Sterile Solution 1837
Pontocaine Hydrochloride for Spinal Anesthesia 2330
Sensorcaine 559

Palsy, optic nerve

Symmetrel Capsules and Syrup (0.1% to 1%) 946

Palsy, peripheral nerve

Lescol Capsules 2267
Mevacor Tablets 1699
Pravachol 765
Zocor Tablets 1775

Pancolitis

Rowasa 2548

Pancreatic disease, unspecified

Pulmozyme Inhalation 1064

Pancreatic enzymes, increased

Norpramin Tablets 1526

Pancreatic infarction

Gelfoam Sterile Sponge 2608

Pancreatitis

Accupril Tablets (Rare) 1893
Achromycin V Capsules (Rare) 1367
Actimmune (Rare) 1056
Activase 1058
Children's Advil Suspension (Less than 1%) 2692
Aldactazide 2413
Aldoclor Tablets 1598
Aldomet Ester HCl Injection 1602
Aldomet Oral 1600
Aldoril Tablets 1604
Altace Capsules (Less than 1%) 1232
Anaprox/Naprosyn (Less than 1%) 2117
Apresazide Capsules 808
Aristocort Suspension (Forte Parenteral) 1027
Aristocort Suspension (Intralesional) 1025
Aristocort Tablets 1022
Aristospan Suspension (Intra-articular) 1033
Aristospan Suspension (Intralesional) 1032
Asacol Delayed-Release Tablets 1979
Asendin Tablets (Very rare) 1369
Atromid-S Capsules 2701
Azo Gantanol Tablets 2080
Azo Gantrisin Tablets 2081
Azulfidine (Rare) 1949
Bactrim DS Tablets 2084
Bactrim I.V. Infusion 2082
Bactrim 2084
Betaseron for SC Injection 658
Capoten 739
Capozide 742
Cataflam (Less than 1%) 816
Celestone Soluspan Suspension 2347
Chibroxin Sterile Ophthalmic Solution (With oral form) 1617
Cipro I.V. (1% or less) 595
Cipro I.V. Pharmacy Bulk Package (Less than 1%) 597
Cipro Tablets 592
Clinoril Tablets (Less than 1 in 100) 1618
Clozaril Tablets 2252
Cognex Capsules 1901
Combipres Tablets 677
CORTENEMA 2535
Cortifoam 2396
Cortone Acetate Sterile Suspension 1623
Cortone Acetate Tablets 1624
Cuprimine Capsules 1630
Cytosar-U Sterile Powder (Two cases) 2592
Cytovene (1% or less) 2103
Dalalone D.P. Injectable 1011
Danocrine Capsules (Rare) 2307
Dapsone Tablets USP 1284
Daypro Caplets (Less than 1%) 2426
Decadron Elixir 1633
Decadron Phosphate Injection 1637
Decadron Phosphate Respihaler 1642
Decadron Phosphate Turbinaire 1645
Decadron Phosphate with Xylocaine Injection, Sterile 1639
Decadron Tablets 1635
Decadron-LA Sterile Suspension 1646
Declomycin Tablets 1371
Deltasone Tablets 2595
Depakene 413
Depakote Tablets 415
Depen Titratable Tablets (Isolated cases) 2662
Depo-Medrol Single-Dose Vial 2600
Depo-Medrol Sterile Aqueous Suspension 2597
Dexacort Phosphate in Respihaler 458
Dexacort Phosphate in Turbinaire 459
Dipentum Capsules (Rare) 1951
Diucardin Tablets 2718
Diupres Tablets 1650
Diuril Oral Suspension 1653
Diuril Sodium Intravenous 1652
Diuril Tablets 1653
Dyazide 2479
EC-Naprosyn Delayed-Release Tablets (Less than 1%) 2117
Edecrin (Rare) 1657
Elspar 1659
Enduron Tablets 420
Ergamisol Tablets (Less frequent) 1292
Esidrix Tablets 821
Esimil Tablets 822
Estrace Cream and Tablets 749
Fansidar Tablets 2114
Felbatol 2666
Feldene Capsules (Less than 1%) 1965
Flagyl 375 Capsules (Rare) 2434
Flagyl I.V. (Rare) 2247
Florinef Acetate Tablets 505
Floxin I.V. 1571
Floxin Tablets (200 mg, 300 mg, 400 mg) 1567
Foscavir Injection (Between 1% and 5%) 547
Gantanol Tablets 2119
Gantrisin 2120
Hivid Tablets (Less than 1% to less than 3%; rare) 2121
Hydeltrasol Injection, Sterile 1665
Hydeltra-T.B.A. Sterile Suspension 1667
Hydrocortone Acetate Sterile Suspension 1669
Hydrocortone Phosphate Injection, Sterile 1670
Hydrocortone Tablets 1672
HydroDIURIL Tablets 1674
Hydropres Tablets 1675
Hyperstat I.V. Injection 2363
Hyzaar Tablets 1677
IBU Tablets (Less than 1%) 1342
Inderide Tablets 2732
Inderide LA Long Acting Capsules 2734
Lamictal Tablets 1112
Lasix Injection, Oral Solution and Tablets 1240
Lescol Capsules 2267
Lodine Capsules and Tablets (Less than 1%) 2743
Lomotil 2439
Lopid Tablets 1917
Lopressor HCT Tablets 832
Lotensin Tablets 834
Lotensin HCT 837
Lotrel Capsules (Rare) 840
Macrobid Capsules 1988
Macrodantin Capsules 1989
Maxzide 1380
Medrol 2621
MetroGel-Vaginal 902
Mevacor Tablets 1699
Minipress Capsules (Less than 1%) 1937
Minizide Capsules (Rare) 1938
Minocin Intravenous 1382
Minocin Oral Suspension 1385
Minocin Pellet-Filled Capsules 1383
Moduretic Tablets 1705
Monopril Tablets (0.2% to 1.0%) 757
Motofen Tablets 784
Children's Motrin Ibuprofen Oral Suspension (Less than 1%) 1546
Motrin Tablets (Less than 1%) 2625
Motrin Ibuprofen Suspension, Oral Drops, Chewable Tablets, Caplets (Less than 1%) 1546
Mykrox Tablets 993
Nalfon 200 Pulvules & Nalfon Tablets (Less than 1%) 917
Anaprox/Naprosyn (Less than 1%) 2117
NebuPent for Inhalation Solution (1% or less) 1040
Neoral (Rare) 2276
Neurontin Capsules (Rare) 1922
Noroxin Tablets (Rare) 1715
Noroxin Tablets (Rare) 2048
Ogen Tablets 2627
Oncaspar (1%) 2028
Oretic Tablets 443
Orudis Capsules (Rare) 2766
Oruvail Capsules (Rare) 2766
Pediapred Oral Liquid 995
Pentam 300 Injection 1041

(▣ Described in PDR For Nonprescription Drugs) Incidence data in parenthesis; ▲ 3% or more (⊙ Described in PDR For Ophthalmology)

Pentasa (Infrequent to less than 1%) ... 1527
Permax Tablets (Rare) ... 575
Pravachol ... 765
Prelone Syrup ... 1787
Premarin Tablets ... 2789
Premarin Vaginal Cream ... 2791
Prilosec Delayed-Release Capsules (Less than 1%) ... 529
Prinivil Tablets (0.3% to 1.0%) ... 1733
Prinzide Tablets ... 1737
Proglycem ... 580
Proleukin for Injection (Less than 1%) ... 797
Prozac Pulvules & Liquid, Oral Solution ... 919
Purinethol Tablets ... 1156
Questran Light ... 769
Questran Powder ... 770
Relafen Tablets (Less than 1%) ... 2510
Retrovir Capsules (Rare) ... 1158
Retrovir I.V. Infusion (Rare) ... 1163
Retrovir Syrup (Rare) ... 1158
Rocaltrol Capsules ... 2141
Rowasa ... 2548
Sandimmune (Rare) ... 2286
Septra ... 1174
Septra I.V. Infusion ... 1169
Septra I.V. Infusion ADD-Vantage Vials ... 1171
Septra ... 1174
Ser-Ap-Es Tablets ... 849
Solu-Cortef Sterile Powder ... 2641
Solu-Medrol Sterile Powder ... 2643
Tagamet (Rare) ... 2516
Tenoretic Tablets ... 2845
Thalitone ... 1245
Timolide Tablets ... 1748
Tonocard Tablets (Less than 1%) .. 531
Toradol ... 2159
Univasc Tablets (Less than 1%) ... 2410
Urobiotic-250 Capsules ... 2214
Vaseretic Tablets ... 1765
Vasotec I.V. ... 1768
Vasotec Tablets (0.5% to 1.0%) ... 1771
▲ Videx Tablets, Powder for Oral Solution, & Pediatric Powder for Oral Solution (3% to 27%) ... 720
Voltaren Tablets (Less than 1%) ... 861
Zantac (Rare) ... 1209
Zantac Injection (Rare) ... 1207
Zantac Syrup (Rare) ... 1209
Zaroxolyn Tablets ... 1000
Zerit Capsules (1%) ... 729
Zestoretic ... 2850
Zestril Tablets (0.3% to 1.0%) ... 2854
Ziac ... 1415
Zocor Tablets ... 1775
Zoloft Tablets (Rare) ... 2217

Pancreatitis, hemorrhagic

Hivid Tablets (Less than 1% to less than 3%) ... 2121
Videx Tablets, Powder for Oral Solution, & Pediatric Powder for Oral Solution (Less than 1%) ... 720
Zyloprim Tablets (Less than 1%) ... 1226

Pancytopenia

Altace Capsules (Less than 1%) ... 1232
Ancobon Capsules ... 2079
Atgam Sterile Solution (Less than 5%) ... 2581
Atretol Tablets ... 573
Azactam for Injection (Less than 1%) ... 734
Capoten ... 739
Capozide ... 742
Cefizox for Intramuscular or Intravenous Use ... 1034
Cefotan ... 2829
Ceftin ... 1078
Cefzil Tablets and Oral Suspension 746
Celontin Kapseals ... 1899
Ceptaz ... 1081
Chloromycetin Sodium Succinate ... 1900
Cipro I.V. (Rare) ... 595
Cipro I.V. Pharmacy Bulk Package (Rare) ... 597
Cipro Tablets (0.1%) ... 592
Cognex Capsules (Rare) ... 1901
Compazine ... 2470
Cosmegen Injection ... 1626
Cytosar-U Sterile Powder (Less than 7 patients) ... 2592
Cytovene (1% or less) ... 2103
Daraprim Tablets ... 1090
DiaBeta Tablets (Occasional) ... 1239
Diabinese Tablets ... 1935
Diamox ... 1372
Didronel Tablets (Rare) ... 1984
Dilantin Infatabs (Occasional) ... 1908
Dilantin Kapseals (Occasional) ... 1906
Dilantin Parenteral (Occasional) ... 1910
Dilantin-125 Suspension (Occasional) ... 1911
Duricef ... 748
Ergamisol Tablets ... 1292
Etrafon ... 2355
Felbatol (May be more than 100 fold) ... 2666
Floxin I.V. ... 1571
Floxin Tablets (200 mg, 300 mg, 400 mg) ... 1567
Fluorouracil Injection ... 2116
Fortaz ... 1100
Foscavir Injection (Less than 1%) .. 547
Sterile FUDR (Remote possibility) .. 2118
Glauctabs ... ⊙ 208
Glucotrol Tablets ... 1967
Glucotrol XL Extended Release Tablets ... 1968
Glynase PresTab Tablets ... 2609
Imitrex Tablets ... 1106
Kefurox Vials, Faspak & ADD-Vantage ... 1454
Lamictal Tablets ... 1112
Levoprome ... 1274
Lincocin ... 2617
Lodine Capsules and Tablets (Less than 1%) ... 2743
Lorabid Suspension and Pulvules ... 1459
MZM (Common) ... ⊙ 267
Matulane Capsules ... 2131
Mellaril ... 2269
Mesantoin Tablets ... 2272
Methotrexate Sodium Tablets, Injection, for Injection and LPF Injection (1 to 3%) ... 1275
Micronase Tablets ... 2623
Milontin Kapseals ... 1920
Monopril Tablets ... 757
Motrin Ibuprofen Suspension, Oral Drops, Chewable Tablets, Caplets (Less than 1%) ... 1546
Mustargen ... 1709
Nalfon 200 Pulvules & Nalfon Tablets (Less than 1%) ... 917
Navane Capsules and Concentrate 2201
Navane Intramuscular ... 2202
NebuPent for Inhalation Solution (1% or less) ... 1040
Neptazane Tablets ... 1388
Nolvadex Tablets (Rare) ... 2841
▲ Oncaspar (Greater than 1% but less than 5%) ... 2028
Orthoclone OKT3 Sterile Solution .. 1837
Pepcid Injection (Rare) ... 1722
Pepcid (Rare) ... 1720
Ponstel (Occasional) ... 1925
Prilosec Delayed-Release Capsules (Rare) ... 529
Primaxin I.M. ... 1727
Primaxin I.V. ... 1729
Prolixin ... 509
Propulsid (Rare) ... 1300
Prozac Pulvules & Liquid, Oral Solution ... 919
Retrovir I.V. Infusion ... 1163
Ridaura Capsules (Less than 0.1%) ... 2513
Serentil ... 684
Soma Compound w/Codeine Tablets (Very rare) ... 2676
Soma Compound Tablets (Very rare) ... 2675
Soma Tablets ... 2674
Stelazine ... 2514
Suprax ... 1399
Tagamet (Very rare) ... 2516
Tapazole Tablets ... 1477
Tazicef for Injection ... 2519
Tegretol Chewable Tablets ... 852
Tegretol Suspension ... 852
Tegretol Tablets ... 852
Temaril Tablets, Syrup and Spansule Extended-Release Capsules ... 483
▲ Thioguanine Tablets, Tabloid Brand (Nearly all patients) ... 1181
Thorazine ... 2523
Ticlid Tablets (Rare) ... 2156
Torecan ... 2245
Trental Tablets (Rare) ... 1244
Triavil Tablets ... 1757
Trilafon ... 2389
Vantin for Oral Suspension and Vantin Tablets ... 2646
Wellbutrin Tablets (Rare) ... 1204
Zantac (Rare) ... 1209
Zantac Injection (Rare) ... 1207
Zantac Syrup (Rare) ... 1209
Zarontin Capsules ... 1928
Zarontin Syrup ... 1929
Zefazone ... 2654
Zinacef ... 1211
Zyloprim Tablets (Less than 1%) ... 1226

Panencephalitis, sclerosing, subacute

M-M-R II ... 1687

Panic

Ambien Tablets (Rare) ... 2416
Anafranil Capsules (1% to 2%) ... 803
Cozaar Tablets (Less than 1%) ... 1628
Hyzaar Tablets ... 1677
Imitrex Tablets ... 1106
Lamictal Tablets (Infrequent) ... 1112
Pamelor ... 2280

Panmyelopathy

Solganal Suspension (Rare) ... 2388

Papilledema

Accutane Capsules ... 2076
Amen Tablets ... 780
Aquasol A Vitamin A Capsules, USP ... 534
Aquasol A Parenteral ... 534
Betaseron for SC Injection ... 658
Brevicon ... 2088
Celestone Soluspan Suspension ... 2347
Cortone Acetate Sterile Suspension ... 1623
Cortone Acetate Tablets ... 1624
Cycrin Tablets ... 975
Danocrine Capsules ... 2307
Decadron Elixir ... 1633
Decadron Phosphate Injection ... 1637
Decadron Phosphate Respihaler ... 1642
Decadron Phosphate Turbinaire ... 1645
Decadron Phosphate with Xylocaine Injection, Sterile ... 1639
Decadron Tablets ... 1635
Decadron-LA Sterile Suspension ... 1646
Demulen ... 2428
Depo-Provera Contraceptive Injection ... 2602
Depo-Provera Sterile Aqueous Suspension ... 2606
Effexor (Rare) ... 2719
Eskalith ... 2485
Humatrope Vials (Small number of patients) ... 1443
Hydeltrasol Injection, Sterile ... 1665
Hydeltra-T.B.A. Sterile Suspension 1667
Hydrocortone Acetate Sterile Suspension ... 1669
Hydrocortone Phosphate Injection, Sterile ... 1670
Hydrocortone Tablets ... 1672
Hyperstat I.V. Injection (1 patient) .. 2363
Levlen/Tri-Levlen ... 651
Lithium Carbonate Capsules & Tablets ... 2230
Matulane Capsules ... 2131
Micronor Tablets ... 1872
Modicon ... 1872
NegGram (Occasional) ... 2323
Nizoral Tablets (Rare) ... 1298
Norinyl ... 2088
Norplant System ... 2759
Nor-Q D Tablets ... 2135
Ortho-Cyclen/Ortho-Tri-Cyclen ... 1858
Ortho-Novum ... 1872
Ortho-Cyclen/Ortho Tri-Cyclen ... 1858
Ovcon ... 760
Platinol (Infrequent) ... 708
Platinol-AQ Injection (Infrequent) ... 710
Premphase ... 2797
Prempro ... 2801
Provera Tablets ... 2636
Levlen/Tri-Levlen ... 651
Tri-Norinyl ... 2164

Papillitis

Attenuvax ... 1610
Biavax II ... 1613
M-M-R II (Infrequent) ... 1687
M-R-VAX II ... 1689
Mumpsvax (Infrequent) ... 1708

Papilloma, scrotom

Testoderm Testosterone Transdermal System (One in 104 patients) ... 486

Papules

Catapres-TTS (1 of 101 patients) .. 675
Depen Titratable Tablets ... 2662
Duragesic Transdermal System (1% or greater) ... 1288
Oxistat Cream (0.1%) ... 1152
Yodoxin ... 1230

Papules, erythematous (see under Erythema multiforme)

Paralysis

Atretol Tablets ... 573
Betapace Tablets (Rare) ... 641
Betaseron for SC Injection ... 658
Carbocaine Hydrochloride Injection 2303
Cognex Capsules (Infrequent) ... 1901
Coumadin ... 926
Depo-Provera Contraceptive Injection (Fewer than 1%) ... 2602
Felbatol ... 2666
Foscavir Injection (Less than 1%) .. 547
Hivid Tablets (Less than 1% to less than 3%) ... 2121
Hyperstat I.V. Injection ... 2363
Imitrex Tablets (Rare) ... 1106
Lamictal Tablets (Rare) ... 1112
Lupron Depot 3.75 mg ... 2556
Lupron Depot 7.5 mg ... 2559
Lupron Injection ... 2555
Luvox Tablets (Infrequent) ... 2544
Novocain Hydrochloride for Spinal Anesthesia ... 2326
Oncovin Solution Vials & Hyporets 1466
Orimune (Rare) ... 1388
Paxil Tablets (Rare) ... 2505
Permax Tablets (Infrequent) ... 575
Pontocaine Hydrochloride for Spinal Anesthesia ... 2330
Prozac Pulvules & Liquid, Oral Solution (Rare) ... 919
Sodium Polystyrene Sulfonate Suspension ... 2244
Surgicel ... 1314
Tegretol Chewable Tablets ... 852
Tegretol Suspension ... 852
Tegretol Tablets ... 852
Videx Tablets, Powder for Oral Solution, & Pediatric Powder for Oral Solution (Less than 1%) ... 720

Paralysis, bladder

Etrafon ... 2355
Prolixin ... 509

Paralysis, extraocular muscles

Lescol Capsules ... 2267
Plaquenil Sulfate Tablets ... 2328
Pravachol ... 765

Paralysis, facial

Betaseron for SC Injection ... 658
Depo-Provera Contraceptive Injection (Fewer than 1%) ... 2602
Imitrex Tablets (Rare) ... 1106
Neurontin Capsules (Infrequent) ... 1922

Paralysis, flaccid

Diamox Intravenous (Occasional) ... 1372
Diamox Sequels (Sustained Release) ... 1373
Diamox Tablets (Occasional) ... 1372
Glauctabs (Occasional) ... ⊙ 208
MZM (Occasional) ... ⊙ 267
Neptazane Tablets ... 1388
Rum-K Syrup ... 1005

Paralysis, legs (see under Paralysis, lower extremities)

Paralysis, lower extremities

Carbocaine Hydrochloride Injection 2303
Marcaine Hydrochloride with Epinephrine 1:200,000 ... 2316
Marcaine Hydrochloride Injection ... 2316
Marcaine Spinal ... 2319
Sensorcaine ... 559

Paralysis, oculomotor nerve

Anafranil Capsules (Rare) ... 803

Paralysis, radial nerve

Diphtheria and Tetanus Toxoids and Pertussis Vaccine Adsorbed USP (For Pediatric Use) ... 875
Tripedia ... 892

Paralysis, respiratory

Amikacin Sulfate Injection, USP ... 960
Amikin Injectable ... 501
Carbocaine Hydrochloride Injection 2303
Marcaine Hydrochloride with Epinephrine 1:200,000 ... 2316
Marcaine Hydrochloride Injection ... 2316
Marcaine Spinal ... 2319

1385 Side Effects Index Paresthesia

Novocain Hydrochloride for Spinal Anesthesia ... 2326
Pontocaine Hydrochloride for Spinal Anesthesia ... 2330
Sensorcaine ... 559
Tensilon Injectable ... 1261

Paralysis, sensory motor
Demerol ... 2308

Paralysis, skeletal muscle
Amikacin Sulfate Injection, USP ... 960
Amikin Injectable ... 501
Anectine ... 1073
Netromycin Injection 100 mg/ml ... 2373
Norcuron ... 1826
Nuromax Injection ... 1149

Paralysis, spinal cord
Ethamolin (One child) ... 2400

Paralysis, spinal nerve
Novocain Hydrochloride for Spinal Anesthesia ... 2326
Pontocaine Hydrochloride for Spinal Anesthesia ... 2330

Paralysis, vocal cord
Foscavir Injection (Less than 1%) ... 547

Paralysis agitans (see under Parkinsonism)

Paranoia
Adalat Capsules (10 mg and 20 mg) (Less than 0.5%) ... 587
Adalat CC (Rare) ... 589
Anafranil Capsules (Infrequent) ... 803
Artane (One case) ... 1368
Atamet ... 572
Betaseron for SC Injection ... 658
Cipro I.V. (1% or less) ... 595
Cipro I.V. Pharmacy Bulk Package (Less than 1%) ... 597
Clozaril Tablets (Less than 1%) ... 2252
Cognex Capsules (Infrequent) ... 1901
Desyrel and Desyrel Dividose ... 503
Doral Tablets ... 2664
Duragesic Transdermal System (1% or greater) ... 1288
Effexor (Infrequent) ... 2719
Etrafon ... 2355
Felbatol ... 2666
Floxin I.V. ... 1571
Floxin Tablets (200 mg, 300 mg, 400 mg) ... 1567
Hivid Tablets (Less than 1% to less than 3%) ... 2121
Lamictal Tablets (Infrequent) ... 1112
Larodopa Tablets (Infrequent) ... 2129
Lioresal Intrathecal ... 1596
Luvox Tablets (Infrequent) ... 2544
▲ Marinol (Dronabinol) Capsules (3% to 10%) ... 2231
NebuPent for Inhalation Solution (1% or less) ... 1040
Neurontin Capsules (Infrequent) ... 1922
Orthoclone OKT3 Sterile Solution ... 1837
Parlodel (Less than 1%) ... 2281
Paxil Tablets (Infrequent) ... 2505
Permax Tablets (Frequent) ... 575
Procardia Capsules (Less than 0.5%) ... 1971
Prozac Pulvules & Liquid, Oral Solution (Infrequent) ... 919
ReVia Tablets (Less than 1%) ... 940
Romazicon (1% to 3%) ... 2147
Sandostatin Injection (Less than 1%) ... 2292
Serzone Tablets (Infrequent) ... 771
Sinemet Tablets ... 943
Sinemet CR Tablets ... 944
Trilafon ... 2389
Videx Tablets, Powder for Oral Solution, & Pediatric Powder for Oral Solution (Less than 1%) ... 720
Wellbutrin Tablets (Infrequent) ... 1204
Zoloft Tablets (Infrequent) ... 2217

Paraparesis
Depo-Medrol Single-Dose Vial ... 2600
Depo-Medrol Sterile Aqueous Suspension ... 2597
Orthoclone OKT3 Sterile Solution ... 1837

Paraplegia
Depo-Medrol Single-Dose Vial ... 2600
Depo-Medrol Sterile Aqueous Suspension ... 2597
Foscavir Injection (Less than 1%) ... 547
Methotrexate Sodium Tablets, Injection, for Injection and LPF Injection ... 1275
Orthoclone OKT3 Sterile Solution ... 1837

Parapsoriasis varioliformis acuta
Azulfidine (Rare) ... 1949

Parathyroid hormone deficiency, fetal
Accutane Capsules ... 2076

Parenchymatous organs, toxic damage
Phenobarbital Elixir and Tablets ... 1469
Tagamet (Highly unlikely) ... 2516

Paresis
Ambien Tablets (Rare) ... 2416
Anafranil Capsules (Up to 2%) ... 803
Cardura Tablets (Less than 0.5% of 3960 patients) ... 2186
Cognex Capsules (Infrequent) ... 1901
Engerix-B Unit-Dose Vials ... 2482
Gelfoam Sterile Sponge ... 2608
Imdur (Less than or equal to 5%) ... 1323
Intron A (Less than 5%) ... 2364
Leukeran Tablets (Rare) ... 1133
Methotrexate Sodium Tablets, Injection, for Injection and LPF Injection ... 1275
Neurontin Capsules (Infrequent) ... 1922
Oncovin Solution Vials & Hyporets 1466
Seromycin Pulvules ... 1476
Tambocor Tablets (1% to less than 3%) ... 1497
Tenex Tablets (3% or less) ... 2074

Paresthesia
Accutane Capsules ... 2076
Actifed with Codeine Cough Syrup ... 1067
Adalat CC (3% or less) ... 589
Adenoscan (2%) ... 1024
Children's Advil Suspension (Less than 1%) ... 2692
Aldactazide ... 2413
Aldoclor Tablets ... 1598
Aldomet Ester HCl Injection ... 1602
Aldomet Oral ... 1600
Aldoril Tablets ... 1604
Altace Capsules (Less than 1%) ... 1232
Ambien Tablets (Infrequent) ... 2416
Amikacin Sulfate Injection, USP (Rare) ... 960
Amikin Injectable (Rare) ... 501
▲ Anafranil Capsules (2% to 9%) ... 803
Ancobon Capsules ... 2079
▲ Android Capsules, 10 mg (Among most common) ... 1250
Android ... 1251
Ansaid Tablets (Less than 1%) ... 2579
Apresazide Capsules (Less frequent) ... 808
Apresoline Hydrochloride Tablets (Less frequent) ... 809
Aredia for Injection ... 810
Asacol Delayed-Release Tablets ... 1979
Atgam Sterile Solution (Less than 1% to less than 5%) ... 2581
Atretol Tablets ... 573
Atrovent Inhalation Aerosol (Less frequent) ... 671
Azactam for Injection (Less than 1%) ... 734
Azo Gantrisin Tablets ... 2081
Benadryl Capsules ... 1898
Benadryl Injection ... 1898
Betagan ... ◉ 233
Betapace Tablets (1% to 4%) ... 641
Betimol 0.25%, 0.5% ... ◉ 261
Biavax II ... 1613
Blocadren Tablets (0.6%) ... 1614
Brevibloc Injection (Less than 1%) 1808
BuSpar (1%) ... 737
Cafergot ... 2251
Calan SR Caplets (1% or less) ... 2422
Calan Tablets (1% or less) ... 2419
Capoten (About 0.5 to 2%) ... 739
Capozide (0.5 to 2%) ... 742
Carbocaine Hydrochloride Injection 2303
Cardene Capsules (1.0%) ... 2095
Cardene I.V. (0.7%) ... 2709
Cardizem CD Capsules (Less than 1%) ... 1506
Cardizem SR Capsules (Less than 1%) ... 1510
Cardizem Injectable (Less than 1%) ... 1508
Cardizem Tablets (Less than 1%) ... 1512
Cardura Tablets (1%) ... 2186
Cartrol Tablets (2.0%) ... 410
Cataflam (Less than 1%) ... 816
Ceclor Pulvules & Suspension ... 1431
Cefizox for Intramuscular or Intravenous Use (Greater than 1% but less than 5%) ... 1034
▲ CellCept Capsules (More than or equal to 3%) ... 2099
Ceptaz (Fewer than 1%) ... 1081
▲ CHEMET (succimer) Capsules (1.0 to 12.7%) ... 1545
Cipro I.V. (1% or less) ... 595
Cipro I.V. Pharmacy Bulk Package (Less than 1%) ... 597
Cipro Tablets (Less than 1%) ... 592
Claritin (2% or fewer patients) ... 2349
Claritin-D (Less frequent) ... 2350
Clinoril Tablets (Less than 1%) ... 1618
Clomid ... 1514
Clozaril Tablets ... 2252
Cognex Capsules (Frequent) ... 1901
Combipres Tablets ... 677
▲ Cordarone Tablets (4 to 9%) ... 2712
Cozaar Tablets (Less than 1%) ... 1628
▲ Cytovene (6%) ... 2103
D.H.E. 45 Injection (Occasional) ... 2255
Dalalone D.P. Injectable ... 1011
Danocrine Capsules ... 2307
▲ Daranide Tablets (Among the most common effects) ... 1633
Decadron-LA Sterile Suspension ... 1646
Deconamine ... 1320
Delatestryl Injection ... 2860
Depakote Tablets (Greater than 1% but not more than 5%) ... 415
Depo-Provera Contraceptive Injection (Fewer than 1%) ... 2602
Dermatop Emollient Cream 0.1% (Less than 1%) ... 1238
Desyrel and Desyrel Dividose (Up to 1.4%) ... 503
Diamox Sequels (Sustained Release) ... 1373
Didronel Tablets ... 1984
Dilacor XR Extended-release Capsules (Infrequent) ... 2018
Dilaudid-HP Injection (Less frequent) ... 1337
Dilaudid-HP Lyophilized Powder 250 mg (Less frequent) ... 1337
Dilaudid Tablets and Liquid (Less frequent) ... 1339
Dipentum Capsules (Rare) ... 1951
Diprivan Injection (Less than 1%) ... 2833
Diucardin Tablets ... 2718
Diupres Tablets ... 1650
Diuril Oral Suspension ... 1653
Diuril Sodium Intravenous ... 1652
Diuril Tablets ... 1653
Dolobid Tablets (Less than 1 in 100) ... 1654
Duragesic Transdermal System (1% or greater) ... 1288
Dyazide ... 2479
DynaCirc Capsules (0.5% to 1%) ... 2256
▲ Effexor (3%) ... 2719
▲ Eminase (Less than 10%) ... 2039
Emla Cream ... 545
Enduron Tablets ... 420
Engerix-B Unit-Dose Vials ... 2482
▲ Epogen for Injection (11%) ... 489
Ergamisol Tablets (2% to 3%) ... 1292
Esidrix Tablets ... 821
Esimil Tablets ... 822
Estratest ... 2539
▲ Ethmozine Tablets (2% to 5%) ... 2041
Famvir (2.6%) ... 2486
▲ Felbatol (3.5%) ... 2666
Feldene Capsules (Less than 1%) ... 1965
Flagyl I.V. ... 2247
Flexeril Tablets (Less than 1%) ... 1661
Floxin I.V. (Less than 1%) ... 1571
Floxin Tablets (200 mg, 300 mg, 400 mg) (Less than 1%) ... 1567
▲ Fludara for Injection (4% to 12%) ... 663
Fortaz (Less than 1%) ... 1100
▲ Foscavir Injection (5% or greater) ... 547
Ganite ... 2533
Gastrocrom Capsules (Infrequent) ... 984
Gelfoam Sterile Sponge ... 2608
Glauctabs ... ◉ 208
Glucotrol XL Extended Release Tablets (Less than 3%) ... 1968
Halcion Tablets (Rare) ... 2611
Halotestin Tablets ... 2614
Havrix (Rare) ... 2489
Hismanal Tablets (Less frequent) ... 1293
HydroDIURIL Tablets ... 1674
Hydropres Tablets ... 1675
▲ Hylorel Tablets (25.1%) ... 985
Hytrin Capsules (2.9%) ... 430
Hyzaar Tablets ... 1677
IBU Tablets (Less than 1%) ... 1342
Imdur (Less than or equal to 5%) ... 1323
Imitrex Injection ... 1103
Imitrex Tablets (Frequent) ... 1106
Inderide Tablets ... 2732
Inderide LA Long Acting Capsules ... 2734
Indocin (Less than 1%) ... 1680
INFeD (Iron Dextran Injection, USP) ... 2345
▲ Intron A (1% to 21%) ... 2364
Inversine Tablets ... 1686
IOPIDINE Sterile Ophthalmic Solution ... ◉ 219
Iopidine 0.5% (Less than 1%) ... ◉ 221
Ismelin Tablets ... 827
Isoptin Oral Tablets (Less than 1%) ... 1346
Isoptin SR Tablets (1% or less) ... 1348
Kerlone Tablets (1.9%) ... 2436
Lamictal Tablets (More than 1%) ... 1112
Lasix Injection, Oral Solution and Tablets ... 1240
Lescol Capsules ... 2267
Lioresal Tablets ... 829
Lodine Capsules and Tablets (Less than 1%) ... 2743
▲ Lopid Tablets (More common) ... 1917
Lopressor HCT Tablets ... 832
Lorelco Tablets ... 1517
Lotensin Tablets ... 834
Lotensin HCT (0.3% to 1.0%) ... 837
Lotrisone Cream (5 of 270 patients) ... 2372
Loxitane ... 1378
Lupron Depot 3.75 mg (Less than 5%) ... 2556
Lupron Depot 7.5 mg (Less than 5%) ... 2559
▲ Lupron Injection (Greater than 5%) ... 2555
Luvox Tablets ... 2544
M-M-R II ... 1687
M-R-VAX II ... 1689
MS Contin Tablets (Less frequent) 1994
MSIR (Infrequent) ... 1997
▲ MZM (Among reactions occurring most often) ... ◉ 267
Marcaine Spinal ... 2319
Matulane Capsules ... 2131
Maxaquin Tablets (Less than 1%) ... 2440
Maxzide ... 1380
Megace Oral Suspension (1% to 3%) ... 699
Meruvax II ... 1697
Mevacor Tablets (0.5% to 1.0%) ... 1699
▲ Mexitil Capsules (2.4% to 3.8%) ... 678
Miacalcin Nasal Spray (1% to 3%) 2275
Midamor Tablets (Less than or equal to 1%) ... 1703
Miltown Tablets ... 2672
Minipress Capsules (Less than 1%) ... 1937
Minizide Capsules (Rare) ... 1938
Moduretic Tablets (Less than or equal to 1%) ... 1705
Monoket (Fewer than 1%) ... 2406
Monopril Tablets (0.2% to 1.0%) ... 757
Children's Motrin Ibuprofen Oral Suspension (Less than 1%) ... 1546
Motrin Tablets (Less than 1%) ... 2625
Motrin Ibuprofen Suspension, Oral Drops, Chewable Tablets, Caplets (Less than 1%) ... 1546
Mycobutin Capsules (More than one patient) ... 1957
Mykrox Tablets ... 993
Nardil (Less common) ... 1920
▲ Navelbine Injection (Among most frequent neurologic toxicities) ... 1145
NebuPent for Inhalation Solution (1% or less) ... 1040
NegGram (Rare) ... 2323
Neoral (1% to 2%) ... 2276
Neptazane Tablets ... 1388
Netromycin Injection 100 mg/ml (Fewer than 1 of 1000 patients) 2373
Neurontin Capsules (Frequent) ... 1922
Nicoderm (nicotine transdermal system) (1% to 3%) ... 1518
▲ Nicorette (3% to 9%) ... 2458
Nizoral Tablets (Rare) ... 1298
▲ Normodyne Injection (Up to 5%) ... 2377
Normodyne Tablets (Up to 5%) ... 2379
Noroxin Tablets ... 1715
Noroxin Tablets ... 2048
Norvasc Tablets (More than 0.1% to 1%) ... 1940
▲ Oncaspar (Greater than 1% but less than 5%) ... 2028
Oncovin Solution Vials & Hyporets 1466

(▭ Described in PDR For Nonprescription Drugs) Incidence data in parenthesis; ▲ 3% or more (◉ Described in PDR For Ophthalmology)

Oramorph SR (Morphine Sulfate Sustained Release Tablets) (Less frequent) 2236
Oretic Tablets 443
Oreton Methyl 1255
Ornade Spansule Capsules 2502
Orudis Capsules (Less than 1%) 2766
Oruvail Capsules (Less than 1%) 2766
PMB 200 and PMB 400 2783
Paraplatin for Injection (1%) 705
Parlodel (Less than 1%) 2281
Parnate Tablets 2503
▲ Paxil Tablets (1.0% to 5.9%) 2505
Penetrex Tablets (Less than 1% but more than or equal to 0.1%) 2031
Pentasa (Less than 1%) 1527
Pentaspan Injection 937
Pepcid Injection (Infrequent) 1722
Pepcid (Infrequent) 1720
Periactin 1724
Permax Tablets (1.6%) 575
Phenurone Tablets (Less than 1%) 447
Platinol 708
Platinol-AQ Injection 710
Plendil Extended-Release Tablets (1.2% to 1.6%) 527
Pneumovax 23 (Rare) 1725
Pnu-Imune 23 1393
Podocon-25 1891
Polymyxin B Sulfate, Aerosporin Brand Sterile Powder 1154
Pravachol 765
Premarin with Methyltestosterone 2794
PREVACID Delayed-Release Capsules (Less than 1%) 2562
Prilosec Delayed-Release Capsules (Less than 1%) 529
Primaxin I.M. 1727
Primaxin I.V. (Less than 0.2%) 1729
Prinivil Tablets (0.8% to 2.6%) 1733
Prinzide Tablets (1.5%) 1737
Procardia XL Extended Release Tablets (Less than 3%) 1972
▲ Procrit for Injection (11%) 1841
Proglycem 580
▲ Prograf (15% to 40%) 1042
ProSom Tablets (Infrequent) 449
Prostin E2 Suppository 2634
Prozac Pulvules & Liquid, Oral Solution (1.7%) 919
Questran Light 769
Questran Powder 770
Relafen Tablets (1%) 2510
▲ Retrovir Capsules (6%) 1158
▲ Retrovir I.V. Infusion (6%) 1163
▲ Retrovir Syrup (6%) 1158
Risperdal (Infrequent) 1301
▲ Roferon-A Injection (6% to 8%) 2145
Romazicon (1% to 3%) 2147
Rythmol Tablets–150mg, 225mg, 300mg (Less than 1%) 1352
Salagen Tablets (Less than 1%) 1489
Sandimmune (1 to 3%) 2286
Sanorex Tablets 2294
Sansert Tablets 2295
Seldane Tablets 1536
Seldane-D Extended-Release Tablets 1538
Sensorcaine 559
Ser-Ap-Es Tablets 849
Seromycin Pulvules 1476
▲ Serzone Tablets (4%) 771
Sinemet CR Tablets (0.8%) 944
Sinequan (Infrequent) 2205
Stadol (1% or greater) 775
Supprelin Injection (2% to 3%) 2056
Synarel Nasal Solution for Endometriosis (Less than 1%) 2152
Talacen (Rare) 2333
Talwin Injection (Infrequent) 2334
Talwin Compound 2335
Talwin Injection 2334
Talwin Nx 2336
Tambocor Tablets (1% to less than 3%) 1497
Tapazole Tablets 1477
Tavist Syrup 2297
Tavist Tablets 2298
Tazicef for Injection (Less than 1%) 2519
Tazidime Vials, Faspak & ADD-Vantage (Less than 1%) 1478
▲ Tegison Capsules (1-10%) 2154
Tegretol Chewable Tablets 852
Tegretol Suspension 852
Tegretol Tablets 852
Tenex Tablets (3% or less) 2074
Tenoretic Tablets 2845
Teslac 717
Testoderm Testosterone Transdermal System 486
Testred Capsules 1262
Thalitone 1245
Timolide Tablets 1748
Timoptic in Ocudose (Less frequent) 1753
Timoptic Sterile Ophthalmic Solution (Less frequent) 1751
Timoptic-XE 1755
▲ Tonocard Tablets (3.5-9.2%) 531
Toradol (1% or less) 2159
Tornalate Solution for Inhalation, 0.2% (1.5%) 956
▲ Trandate Tablets (Up to 5%) 1185
Travase Ointment 1356
Trinalin Repetabs Tablets 1330
Tussend 1783
Ultram Tablets (50 mg) (Less than 1%) 1585
Ultravate Ointment 0.05% 2690
Vascor (200, 300 and 400 mg) Tablets (2.46%) 1587
Vaseretic Tablets (0.5% to 2.0%) 1765
Vasotec I.V. 1768
Vasotec Tablets (0.5% to 1.0%) 1771
Velban Vials 1484
Verelan Capsules (1% or less) 1410
Verelan Capsules (Less than 1%) 2824
Versed Injection (Less than 1%) 2170
▲ Visken Tablets (3%) 2299
Voltaren Tablets (Less than 1%) 861
Wellbutrin Tablets 1204
Xanax Tablets (2.4%) 2649
Zaroxolyn Tablets 1000
Zebeta Tablets 1413
Zestoretic (1.5%) 2850
Zestril Tablets (0.8% to 2.6%) 2854
Ziac 1415
Zocor Tablets 1775
Zofran Injection (2%) 1214
Zoladex (1% or greater) 2858
Zoloft Tablets (2.0%) 2217
▲ Zonalon Cream (Approximately 1% to 10%) 1055
Zovirax (0.8% to 1.2%) 1219
Zyloprim Tablets (Less than 1%) 1226

Paresthesia, chest
Esimil Tablets 822
Ismelin Tablets 827

Paresthesia, extremities
Asendin Tablets (Less than 1%) 1369
Bellergal-S Tablets (Rare) 2250
Diamox 1372
Elavil 2838
Endep Tablets 2174
Etrafon 2355
Flagyl 375 Capsules 2434
Flagyl I.V. 2247
Fulvicin P/G Tablets (Rare) 2359
Fulvicin P/G 165 & 330 Tablets (Rare) 2359
Gelfoam Sterile Sponge 2608
Limbitrol 2180
Motofen Tablets 784
Norpramin Tablets 1526
Pamelor 2280
Protostat Tablets 1883
Rifater 1532
Rum-K Syrup 1005
Surmontil Capsules 2811
Tofranil Ampuls 854
Tofranil Tablets 856
Tofranil-PM Capsules 857
Triavil Tablets 1757
Velban Vials 1484
Vivactil Tablets 1774

Paresthesia, facial
DTIC-Dome 600

Paresthesia, feet
Grifulvin V (griseofulvin tablets) Microsize (griseofulvin oral suspension) Microsize (Rare) 1888
Gris-PEG Tablets, 125 mg & 250 mg (Rare) 479
Nydrazid Injection 508
Rifamate Capsules 1530

Paresthesia, hands
Grifulvin V (griseofulvin tablets) Microsize (griseofulvin oral suspension) Microsize (Rare) 1888
Gris-PEG Tablets, 125 mg & 250 mg (Rare) 479
Inderal 2728
Inderal LA Long Acting Capsules 2730
Inderide Tablets 2732
Inderide LA Long Acting Capsules 2734
Nydrazid Injection 508
Oncaspar 2028
Rifamate Capsules 1530

Paresthesia, circumoral
Coly-Mycin M Parenteral 1905
Effexor (Infrequent) 2719
ProSom Tablets (Rare) 449
Prozac Pulvules & Liquid, Oral Solution (Rare) 919

Parkinsonism
Aldoclor Tablets 1598
Aldomet Ester HCl Injection 1602
Aldomet Oral 1600
Aldoril Tablets 1604
Ancobon Capsules 2079
Clozaril Tablets (Less than 1%) 2252
Cognex Capsules (Infrequent) 1901
Compazine 2470
Demser Capsules 1649
Diupres Tablets 1650
Etrafon 2355
Hydropres Tablets 1675
Indocin (Less than 1%) 1680
Levoprome 1274
Orap Tablets 1050
Risperdal (0.6% to 4.1%) 1301
Serentil 684
Stelazine 2514
Temaril Tablets, Syrup and Spansule Extended-Release Capsules 483
Tigan 2057
Trilafon 2389

Parkinsonism, aggravation of
Ana-Kit Anaphylaxis Emergency Treatment Kit 617
Cognex Capsules (Rare) 1901
Reglan 2068
Risperdal 1301

Parkinson-like symptoms
Actimmune (Rare) 1056
Compazine 2470
Cytovene-IV (One report) 2103
Elspar (Rare) 1659
Haldol Decanoate 1577
Haldol Injection, Tablets and Concentrate 1575
Moban Tablets and Concentrate 1048
Navane Capsules and Concentrate 2201
Navane Intramuscular 2202
Oncaspar 2028
Orap Tablets (Frequent) 1050
Prolixin 509
Reglan 2068
Ser-Ap-Es Tablets (Rare) 849
Triavil Tablets 1757

Paroniria
Cardura Tablets (Less than 0.5% of 3960 patients) 2186
Claritin (2% or fewer patients) 2349
Claritin-D (Less frequent) 2350
Imdur (Less than or equal to 5%) 1323
Intron A (Less than 5%) 2364
Maxaquin Tablets (Less than 1%) 2440
Procardia XL Extended Release Tablets (1% or less) 1972

Paronychia
Accutane Capsules (Less than 1%) 2076
▲ Tegison Capsules (1-10%) 2154

Parosmia
Anafranil Capsules (Infrequent) 803
Ansaid Tablets (Less than 1%) 2579
Betaseron for SC Injection 658
Cardura Tablets (Less than 0.5% of 3960 patients) 2186
Effexor (Infrequent) 2719
Flumadine Tablets & Syrup (Less than 0.3%) 1015
Hivid Tablets (Less than 1% to less than 3%) 2121
Intron A (Less than 5%) 2364
Iopidine 0.5% (0.2%) ⊙ 221
Lamictal Tablets (Rare) 1112
Luvox Tablets (Infrequent) 2544
Miacalcin Nasal Spray (Less than 1%) 2275
Norvasc Tablets (Less than or equal to 0.1%) 1940

Parotid gland, enlargement
Asendin Tablets (Very rare) 1369
Depakene 413
Depakote Tablets 415
Diprivan Injection (Less than 1%) 2833
Elavil 2838
Endep Tablets 2174
Etrafon (Rare) 2355
Hyperstat I.V. Injection 2363
Intal Capsules (Less than 1 in 10,000 patients) 987
Intal Inhaler (Infrequent) 988
Intal Nebulizer Solution 989
Limbitrol 2180
Mellaril (Rare) 2269
Norisodrine with Calcium Iodide Syrup 442
Pamelor 2280
Surmontil Capsules 2811
Tofranil Ampuls 854
Tofranil Tablets 856
Tofranil-PM Capsules 857
Trental Tablets (Less than 1%) 1244
Videx Tablets, Powder for Oral Solution, & Pediatric Powder for Oral Solution (Less than 1%) 720

Parotid tenderness
Catapres Tablets 674
Esimil Tablets 822
Ismelin Tablets 827
Trilafon (Rare) 2389

Parotitis
Artane (Rare) 1368
Biavax II 1613
Catapres Tablets (Rare) 674
Catapres-TTS (Rare) 675
Combipres Tablets (Rare) 677
Kemadrin Tablets 1112
M-M-R II 1687
Mumpsvax (Very low) 1708
Norpramin Tablets 1526
Peridex 1978
Vivactil Tablets 1774

Patent ductus arteriosus
Accupril Tablets 1893
Altace Capsules 1232
Capoten 739
Capozide 742
Cozaar Tablets 1628
▲ Exosurf Neonatal for Intratracheal Suspension (45% to 59%) 1095
Hyzaar Tablets 1677
Lotensin Tablets 834
Lotensin HCT 837
Monopril Tablets 757
Prinivil Tablets 1733
Prinzide Tablets 1737
▲ Survanta Beractant Intratracheal Suspension (46.9%) 2226
Univasc Tablets 2410
Vaseretic Tablets 1765
Vasotec I.V. 1768
Vasotec Tablets 1771
Zestoretic 2850
Zestril Tablets 2854

Pavor nocturnus
Zarontin Capsules 1928
Zarontin Syrup 1929

Peeling (see under Necrolysis, epidermal)

Pelger-Huet anomaly
Risperdal (Rare) 1301

Peliosis hepatis
Android Capsules, 10 mg (Rare) 1250
Android (Rare) 1251
Danocrine Capsules 2307
Delatestryl Injection (Rare) 2860
Estratest 2539
Halotestin Tablets 2614
Oreton Methyl (Rare) 1255
Oxandrin 2862
Premarin with Methyltestosterone 2794
Testoderm Testosterone Transdermal System (Rare) 486
Testred Capsules (Rare) 1262
Winstrol Tablets 2337

Pellagra
Nydrazid Injection 508
Rifamate Capsules 1530
Rifater 1532
Trecator-SC Tablets 2814

Pelvic inflammatory disease
BuSpar (Rare) 737
Lippes Loop Intrauterine Double-S 1848
Massengill 2457

(▣ Described in PDR For Nonprescription Drugs) Incidence data in parenthesis; ▲ 3% or more (⊙ Described in PDR For Ophthalmology)

1387 Side Effects Index Petechiae and ecchymosis

Massengill Medicated Disposable Douche ... 2458
Massengill Medicated Liquid Concentrate ... ▣ 821
Massengill Powder ... 2457
ParaGard T380A Intrauterine Copper Contraceptive ... 1880

Pelvic pressure
Flagyl 375 Capsules ... 2434
MetroGel-Vaginal (Equal to or less than 2%) ... 902
Nolvadex Tablets ... 2841
Protostat Tablets ... 1883
▲ Zoladex (18%) ... 2858

Pemphigoid-like lesion
Capoten ... 739
Capozide ... 742

Pemphigus
Cuprimine Capsules ... 1630
Depen Titratable Tablets ... 2662
Rifadin (Occasional) ... 1528
Rifamate Capsules (Occasional) ... 1530
Rifater (Occasional) ... 1532
Rimactane Capsules ... 847
Univasc Tablets (Less than 1%) ... 2410
Vaseretic Tablets ... 1765
Vasotec I.V. ... 1768
Vasotec Tablets (0.5% to 1.0%) ... 1771

Pemphigus, bullous
Capoten ... 739
Capozide ... 742
Efudex (Infrequent) ... 2113
Monopril Tablets ... 757

Penile discharge, unspecified
ProSom Tablets (Rare) ... 449

Penile erection, decrease
▲ Zoladex (18%) ... 2858

Penile erection, prolonged or inappropriate
▲ Android Capsules, 10 mg (Among most common) ... 1250
Android ... 1251
▲ Caverject (4%) ... 2583
Delatestryl Injection ... 2860
Desyrel and Desyrel Dividose ... 503
▲ Oreton Methyl (Among most common) ... 1255
Oxandrin ... 2862
Testoderm Testosterone Transdermal System ... 486

Penile erections, increase (see under Priapism)

Penile inflammation
Foscavir Injection (Less than 1%) .. 547

Penis, decreased sensation
Eldepryl Tablets ... 2550

Penis, enlargement
Caverject (2%) ... 2583
Lupron Depot 3.75 mg ... 2556
Lupron Depot 7.5 mg ... 2559
Lupron Injection ... 2555
Oxandrin ... 2862
Winstrol Tablets ... 2337

Penis, fibrotic plaques (see under Peyronie's disease)

Perforation, cervix (partial)
Lippes Loop Intrauterine Double-S.. 1848
ParaGard T380A Intrauterine Copper Contraceptive ... 1880

Perforation, cervix (total)
Lippes Loop Intrauterine Double-S.. 1848
ParaGard T380A Intrauterine Copper Contraceptive ... 1880

Perforation, uterine wall
ParaGard T380A Intrauterine Copper Contraceptive ... 1880

Perforation, uterine wall (partial)
Lippes Loop Intrauterine Double-S.. 1848
ParaGard T380A Intrauterine Copper Contraceptive ... 1880

Perforation, uterine wall (total)
Lippes Loop Intrauterine Double-S.. 1848
ParaGard T380A Intrauterine Copper Contraceptive ... 1880

Perianal sensation, loss of
Carbocaine Hydrochloride Injection 2303
Marcaine Hydrochloride with Epinephrine 1:200,000 ... 2316
Marcaine Hydrochloride Injection ... 2316
Marcaine Spinal ... 2319
Sensorcaine ... 559
Xylocaine Injections ... 567

Periarteritis
Nasalcrom Nasal Solution (Rare) ... 994
Tapazole Tablets ... 1477

Periarteritis nodosum
Azo Gantrisin Tablets ... 2081
Bactrim DS Tablets ... 2084
Bactrim I.V. Infusion ... 2082
Bactrim ... 2084
Dilantin Infatabs ... 1908
Dilantin Kapseals ... 1906
Dilantin Parenteral ... 1910
Dilantin-125 Suspension ... 1911
Fansidar Tablets ... 2114
Gantanol Tablets ... 2119
Gantrisin ... 2120
Septra ... 1174
Septra I.V. Infusion ... 1169
Septra I.V. Infusion ADD-Vantage Vials ... 1171
Septra ... 1174

Pericardial effusion
Activase ... 1058
Betaseron for SC Injection ... 658
Clomid ... 1514
Clozaril Tablets ... 2252
Fludara for Injection (One patient).. 663
▲ Leukine for IV Infusion (25%) ... 1271
Loniten Tablets (About 3%) ... 2618
Neurontin Capsules (Rare) ... 1922
Proleukin for Injection (1%) ... 797
ReoPro Vials (0.4%) ... 1471
Rogaine Topical Solution ... 2637

Pericardial tamponade
Azulfidine (Rare) ... 1949
Loniten Tablets (Occasional) ... 2618

Pericarditis
Achromycin V Capsules ... 1367
Activase ... 1058
Aldoclor Tablets ... 1598
Aldomet Ester HCl Injection ... 1602
Aldomet Oral ... 1600
Aldoril Tablets ... 1604
Asacol Delayed-Release Tablets (Rare) ... 1979
Azulfidine (Rare) ... 1949
Cardene Capsules (Less than 0.4%) ... 2095
Cerubidine (Rare) ... 795
Clozaril Tablets ... 2252
Cytovene-IV (Two or more reports) 2103
Cytoxan ... 694
Declomycin Tablets ... 1371
Dipentum Capsules (Rare) ... 1951
Doryx Capsules ... 1913
Dynacin Capsules ... 1590
Inocor Lactate Injection (1 case) ... 2309
Intal Capsules (Less than 1 in 100,000 patients) ... 987
Intal Inhaler (Rare) ... 988
Intal Nebulizer Solution (Rare) ... 989
Loniten Tablets ... 2618
Luvox Tablets (Rare) ... 2544
Minocin Intravenous ... 1382
Minocin Oral Suspension ... 1385
Minocin Pellet-Filled Capsules ... 1383
Monodox Capsules ... 1805
Nasalcrom Nasal Solution (Rare) ... 994
NEOSAR Lyophilized/Neosar ... 1959
Neurontin Capsules (Rare) ... 1922
PASER Granules ... 1285
Pentasa (Infrequent to less than 1%) ... 1527
Permax Tablets (Rare) ... 575
Procan SR Tablets (Common) ... 1926
Proleukin for Injection (Less than 1%) ... 797
Rogaine Topical Solution ... 2637
Rowasa (Rare) ... 2548
Terramycin Intramuscular Solution 2210
Tonocard Tablets (Less than 1%) .. 531
▲ Trasylol (5%) ... 613
Vibramycin ... 1941
Vibramycin Hyclate Intravenous ... 2215
Vibramycin ... 1941
Zyloprim Tablets (Less than 1%) ... 1226

Perinatal disorder, unspecified
Diprivan Injection (Less than 1%) .. 2833

Peripheral nerve symptoms
MSTA Mumps Skin Test Antigen ... 890
Xylocaine Injections (Less than 1%) ... 567

Peripheral vascular disorder, unspecified
Betapace Tablets (1% to 3%) ... 641
▲ Betaseron for SC Injection (5%) ... 658
Cardene Capsules (Rare) ... 2095
Caverject (Less than 1%) ... 2583
▲ CellCept Capsules (More than or equal to 3%) ... 2099
Effexor (Infrequent) ... 2719
▲ Lopid Tablets (More common) ... 1917
Lotensin HCT (0.3% or more) ... 837
Neurontin Capsules (Infrequent) ... 1922
Orudis Capsules (Less than 1%) ... 2766
Oruvail Capsules (Less than 1%) ... 2766
Paxil Tablets (Infrequent) ... 2505
Videx Tablets, Powder for Oral Solution, & Pediatric Powder for Oral Solution (Less than 1%) ... 720
Zerit Capsules (Fewer than 1% to 2%) ... 729
▲ Zoladex (Greater than 1% but less than 5%) ... 2858

Peristalsis, increase
Mestinon Injectable ... 1253
Mestinon ... 1254
Prostigmin Injectable ... 1260
Prostigmin Tablets ... 1261
Tensilon Injectable ... 1261

Peritonitis
Betaseron for SC Injection ... 658
Cytosar-U Sterile Powder ... 2592
Neupogen for Injection (2%) ... 495
ParaGard T380A Intrauterine Copper Contraceptive ... 1880
Paxil Tablets (Rare) ... 2505
▲ Prograf (Greater than 3%) ... 1042
Prostin VR Pediatric Sterile Solution (Less than 1%) ... 2635
▲ Taxol (30%) ... 714

Perivasculitis
VePesid Capsules and Injection ... 718

Perleche
Neurontin Capsules (Rare) ... 1922

Personality changes
Ambien Tablets (Rare) ... 2416
Aristocort Suspension (Forte Parenteral) ... 1027
Aristocort Suspension (Intralesional) ... 1025
Aristocort Tablets ... 1022
Aristospan Suspension (Intra-articular) ... 1033
Aristospan Suspension (Intralesional) ... 1032
Cardizem CD Capsules (Less than 1%) ... 1506
Cardizem SR Capsules (Less than 1%) ... 1510
Cardizem Injectable ... 1508
Cardizem Tablets (Less than 1%) .. 1512
Celestone Soluspan Suspension ... 2347
CORTENEMA ... 2535
Cortone Acetate Sterile Suspension ... 1623
Cortone Acetate Tablets ... 1624
Cytosar-U Sterile Powder (With experimental doses) ... 2592
Decadron Elixir ... 1633
Decadron Phosphate with Xylocaine Injection, Sterile ... 1639
Decadron Tablets ... 1635
Decadron-LA Sterile Suspension ... 1646
Deltasone Tablets ... 2595
Depo-Medrol Sterile Aqueous Suspension ... 2597
Dexacort Phosphate in Respihaler .. 458
Dexacort Phosphate in Turbinaire .. 459
Eldepryl Tablets ... 2550
Florinef Acetate Tablets ... 505
Foscavir Injection (Less than 1%) .. 547
Hydeltrasol Injection, Sterile ... 1665
Hydeltra-T.B.A. Sterile Suspension 1667
Hydrocortone Acetate Sterile Suspension ... 1669
Hydrocortone Phosphate Injection, Sterile ... 1670
Hydrocortone Tablets ... 1672
Imitrex Tablets (Rare) ... 1106
Intron A (Less than 5%) ... 2364
Lamictal Tablets (Infrequent) ... 1112
▲ Lupron Depot 3.75 mg (Among most frequent) ... 2556
Lupron Depot-PED 7.5 mg, 11.25 mg and 15 mg (Less than 2%) ... 2560
Nalfon 200 Pulvules & Nalfon Tablets (Less than 1%) ... 917
Neurontin Capsules (Rare) ... 1922
Orudis Capsules (Rare) ... 2766
Oruvail Capsules (Rare) ... 2766
Permax Tablets (2.1%) ... 575
Prelone Syrup ... 1787

Perspiration (see under Diaphoresis)

Petechiae
Asendin Tablets (Very rare) ... 1369
Azactam for Injection (Less than 1%) ... 734
Betaseron for SC Injection ... 658
Cardizem CD Capsules (Less than 1%) ... 1506
Cardizem SR Capsules (Less than 1%) ... 1510
Cardizem Injectable ... 1508
Cardizem Tablets (Less than 1%) .. 1512
Celestone Soluspan Suspension (No incidence in labeling) ... 2347
Clozaril Tablets (Less than 1%) ... 2252
▲ Cognex Capsules (7%) ... 1901
Cortone Acetate Sterile Suspension ... 1623
Cortone Acetate Tablets ... 1624
Danocrine Capsules ... 2307
Decadron Elixir ... 1633
Decadron Phosphate Injection ... 1637
Decadron Phosphate Respihaler ... 1642
Decadron Phosphate Turbinaire ... 1645
Decadron Phosphate with Xylocaine Injection, Sterile ... 1639
Decadron-LA Sterile Suspension ... 1646
Depakene ... 413
Depakote Tablets ... 415
Engerix-B Unit-Dose Vials (Less than 1%) ... 2482
Feldene Capsules (Less than 1%) .. 1965
Floxin I.V. ... 1571
Floxin Tablets (200 mg, 300 mg, 400 mg) ... 1567
Hydeltrasol Injection, Sterile ... 1665
Hydeltra-T.B.A. Sterile Suspension 1667
Hydrocortone Acetate Sterile Suspension ... 1669
Hydrocortone Phosphate Injection, Sterile ... 1670
Hydrocortone Tablets ... 1672
Indocin Capsules (Less than 1%) ... 1680
Indocin I.V. (Less than 1%) ... 1684
Indocin (Less than 1%) ... 1680
Lac-Hydrin 12% Lotion (Less frequent) ... 2687
Lamictal Tablets (Rare to infrequent) ... 1112
▲ Leustatin (8%) ... 1834
Lorelco Tablets ... 1517
Ludiomil Tablets (Rare) ... 843
Matulane Capsules ... 2131
Miltown Tablets ... 2672
Mustargen ... 1709
Norpramin Tablets ... 1526
▲ Novantrone (7 to 11%) ... 1279
Oncaspar (Less than 1%) ... 2028
PMB 200 and PMB 400 ... 2783
Pamelor (No incidence in labeling).. 2280
Paraflex Caplets (Rare) ... 1580
Parafon Forte DSC Caplets (Rare) .. 1581
Permax Tablets (Infrequent) ... 575
▲ Proleukin for Injection (4%) ... 797
Prozac Pulvules & Liquid, Oral Solution (Rare) ... 919
Recombivax HB ... 1744
ReoPro Vials (0.3%) ... 1471
Roferon-A Injection (Less than 3%) ... 2145
Sandostatin Injection (Less than 1%) ... 2292
Solganal Suspension ... 2388
Surmontil Capsules ... 2811
Tofranil Ampuls ... 854
Tofranil Tablets ... 856
Tofranil-PM Capsules ... 857
Urobiotic-250 Capsules ... 2214
▲ Videx Tablets, Powder for Oral Solution, & Pediatric Powder for Oral Solution (3% to 7%) ... 720
Vivactil Tablets ... 1774

Petechiae and ecchymosis
Aristocort Suspension (Forte Parenteral) ... 1027

(▣ Described in PDR For Nonprescription Drugs) Incidence data in parenthesis; ▲ 3% or more (◉ Described in PDR For Ophthalmology)

Petechiae and ecchymosis — Side Effects Index — 1388

Aristocort Suspension (Intralesional) 1025
Aristocort Tablets 1022
Aristospan Suspension (Intra-articular) 1033
Aristospan Suspension (Intralesional) 1032
CORTENEMA 2535
Dalalone D.P. Injectable 1011
Decadron Tablets 1635
Deltasone Tablets 2595
Depo-Medrol Single-Dose Vial 2600
Depo-Medrol Sterile Aqueous Suspension 2597
Dexacort Phosphate in Respihaler 458
Dexacort Phosphate in Turbinaire 459
Florinef Acetate Tablets 505
Medrol 2621
Pediapred Oral Liquid 995
Prelone Syrup 1787
Solu-Cortef Sterile Powder 2641
Solu-Medrol Sterile Powder 2643

Petechial hemorrhage

Atretol Tablets 573
Tegretol Chewable Tablets 852
Tegretol Suspension 852
Tegretol Tablets 852

Peyronie's disease

Blocadren Tablets 1614
Cartrol Tablets 410
▲Caverject (3%) 2583
Dilantin Infatabs 1908
Dilantin Kapseals 1906
Dilantin Parenteral 1910
Dilantin-125 Suspension 1911
Inderal (Rare) 2728
Inderal LA Long Acting Capsules (Rare) 2730
Inderide Tablets (Rare) 2732
Inderide LA Long Acting Capsules (Rare) 2734
Kerlone Tablets (Less than 2%) 2436
Levatol 2403
Lopressor Ampuls (1 of 100,000 patients) 830
Lopressor HCT Tablets (1 in 100,000) 832
Lopressor Tablets (1 of 100,000 patients) 830
Normodyne Tablets (Less common) 2379
Sansert Tablets 2295
Sectral Capsules 2807
Tenoretic Tablets 2845
Tenormin Tablets and I.V. Injection 2847
Timolide Tablets 1748
Timoptic in Ocudose 1753
Timoptic Sterile Ophthalmic Solution 1751
Timoptic-XE 1755
Toprol-XL Tablets (Fewer than 1 of 100,000 patients) 565
Trandate Tablets (Less common) 1185
Visken Tablets 2299
Zebeta Tablets 1413
Ziac (Very rare) 1415

Pharyngeal changes

Mexitil Capsules (About 1 in 1,000) 678

Pharyngeal discomfort

Cozaar Tablets (Less than 1%) 1628
Hyzaar Tablets 1677
Prinzide Tablets (0.3% to 1.0%) 1737
Zestoretic (0.3% to 1.0%) 2850

Pharyngeal secretion, increase

IOPIDINE Sterile Ophthalmic Solution ◉ 219
Prostigmin Injectable 1260
Prostigmin Tablets 1261

Pharyngitis

Accupril Tablets (0.5% to 1.0%) 1893
Adalat CC (Less than 1.0%) 589
AeroBid Inhaler System (1-3%) 1005
Aerobid-M Inhaler System (1-3%) 1005
Airet Solution for Inhalation (Less than 1%) 452
▲Ambien Tablets (3%) 2416
▲Anafranil Capsules (Up to 14%) 803
▲Asacol Delayed-Release Tablets (11%) 1979
▲Atrovent Inhalation Solution (3.7%) 673
▲Axid Pulvules (3.3%) 1427
Cardura Tablets (Less than 0.5% of 3960 patients) 2186
Cartrol Tablets (1.1%) 410
▲CellCept Capsules (9.5% to 11.2%) 2099
Claritin (2% or fewer patients) 2349
▲Claritin-D (3%) 2350
Cognex Capsules (Frequent) 1901
Cosmegen Injection 1626
Cozaar Tablets (1% or greater) 1628
Depakote Tablets 415
▲Dilacor XR Extended-release Capsules (1.4% to 5.6%) 2018
Diprivan Injection (Less than 1%) 2833
Duragesic Transdermal System (1% or greater) 1288
Effexor 2719
Ethmozine Tablets (Less than 2%) 2041
Famvir (2.6%) 2486
▲Felbatol (2.6% to 9.7%) 2666
Flonase Nasal Spray (1% to 3%) 1098
Floxin I.V. (1% to 3%) 1571
Floxin Tablets (200 mg, 300 mg, 400 mg) (1% to 3%) 1567
▲Fludara for Injection (Up to 9%) 663
Foscavir Injection (Between 1% and 5%) 547
Sterile FUDR 2118
Glucotrol XL Extended Release Tablets (Less than 1%) 1968
▲Habitrol Nicotine Transdermal System (3% to 9% of patients) 865
Havrix (Less than 1%) 2489
Hismanal Tablets (1.7%) 1293
Hivid Tablets (Less than 1% to less than 3%) 2121
Hytrin Capsules (At least 1%) 430
Hyzaar Tablets (1% or greater) 1677
Imdur (Less than or equal to 5%) 1323
Inderal 2728
Inderal LA Long Acting Capsules 2730
Inderide Tablets 2732
Inderide LA Long Acting Capsules 2734
▲Intron A (1% to 31%) 2364
Iopidine 0.5% (Less than 1%) ◉ 221
Kerlone Tablets (2.0%) 2436
▲Lamictal Tablets (9.8%) 1112
▲Lescol Capsules (4.5%) 2267
Livostin (Approximately 1% to 3%) ◉ 266
Lodine Capsules and Tablets (Less than 1%) 2743
Lotrel Capsules 840
Lozol Tablets (Less than 5%) 2022
Luvox Tablets 2544
Megace Oral Suspension (1% to 3%) 699
Methotrexate Sodium Tablets, Injection, for Injection and LPF Injection 1275
Mexitil Capsules (Less than 1%) 678
Miacalcin Nasal Spray (Less than 1%) 2275
Monopril Tablets (0.2% to 1.0%) 757
▲Nasarel Nasal Solution (3% to 9%) 2133
▲NebuPent for Inhalation Solution (10 to 23%) 1040
Neurontin Capsules (2.8%) 1922
▲Nicoderm (nicotine transdermal system) (3% to 9%) 1518
Orudis Capsules (Less than 1%) 2766
Oruvail Capsules (Less than 1%) 2766
Paxil Tablets (2.1%) 2505
Permax Tablets (Frequent) 575
Plendil Extended-Release Tablets (0.5% to 1.5%) 527
Prinivil Tablets (0.3% to 1.0%) 1733
Prinzide Tablets 1737
▲Prograf (Greater than 3%) 1042
Propulsid (More than 1%) 1300
ProSom Tablets (1%) 449
▲Prostep (nicotine transdermal system) (3% to 9% of patients) 1394
Prostin E2 Suppository 2634
Proventil Inhalation Solution 0.083% (Less than 1%) 2384
Proventil Solution for Inhalation 0.5% (Less than 1%) 2383
▲Prozac Pulvules & Liquid, Oral Solution (2.7% to 11%) 919
▲Pulmozyme Inhalation (36% to 40%) 1064
Recombivax HB (Equal to or greater than 1%) 1744
Retrovir Capsules 1158
Retrovir I.V. Infusion 1163
Retrovir Syrup 1158
Revex (Less than 1%) 1811
▲Rhinocort Nasal Inhaler (3 to 9%) 556
Risperdal (2% to 3%) 1301
▲Salagen Tablets (3%) 1489
Sectral Capsules (Up to 2%) 2807
▲Semprex-D Capsules (3%) 463
▲Semprex-D Capsules (3%) 1167
▲Serzone Tablets (6%) 771
Solganal Suspension 2388
▲Stadol (3% to 9%) 775
▲Supprelin Injection (3% to 10%) 2056
▲Suprane (Greater than 1%-10%) 1813
Tegison Capsules (Less than 1%) 2154
▲Tilade (5.7%) 996
Univasc Tablets (1.8%) 2410
Vascor (200, 300 and 400 mg) Tablets (0.5 to 2.0%) 1587
Velban Vials 1484
Ventolin Inhalation Solution (Less than 1%) 1198
Ventolin Nebules Inhalation Solution (Less than 1%) 1199
Vexol 1% Ophthalmic Suspension (Less than 2%) ◉ 230
Videx Tablets, Powder for Oral Solution, & Pediatric Powder for Oral Solution (Less than 1% to 17%) 720
Zebeta Tablets (2.2%) 1413
Zestoretic 2850
Zestril Tablets (0.3% to 1.0%) 2854
Ziac 1415
▲Zoladex (5%) 2858
Zoloft Tablets (1.2%) 2217
Zosyn (1.0% or less) 1419
Zosyn Pharmacy Bulk Package (1.0% or less) 1422
Zyloprim Tablets (Less than 1%) 1226

Pharyngoxerosis

Atretol Tablets 573
Tegretol Chewable Tablets 852
Tegretol Suspension 852
Tegretol Tablets 852

Phlebitis

Adalat CC (Less than 1.0%) 589
Ambien Tablets (Rare) 2416
Ancef Injection (Rare) 2465
Atamet (Rare) 572
▲Atgam Sterile Solution (1 patient in 20) 2581
Atromid-S Capsules 2701
Azactam for Injection (1.9%) 734
Blenoxane (Infrequent) 692
Cefizox for Intramuscular or Intravenous Use (Greater than 1% but less than 5%) 1034
Cefobid Intravenous/Intramuscular (1 in 120) 2189
Cefobid Pharmacy Bulk Package - Not for Direct Infusion (1 in 120) 2192
Cefotan (1 in 300) 2829
Ceptaz (Fewer than 2%) 1081
Clomid 1514
Clozaril Tablets (Less than 1%) 2252
Cognex Capsules (Infrequent) 1901
Cytotec (Infrequent) 2424
Cytovene (2%) 2103
Dantrium Capsules (Less frequent) 1982
Demerol 2308
Dilacor XR Extended-release Capsules (Infrequent) 2018
Diprivan Injection (Rare; less than 1%) 2833
Dizac (Less frequent) 1809
Dobutrex Solution Vials (Occasional) 1439
Dopram Injectable 2061
Floxin I.V. (Approximately 2%) 1571
Fludara for Injection (1% to 3%) 663
Fluorescite ◉ 219
Fortaz (1 in 69 patients) 1100
Foscavir Injection (Less than 1%) 547
▲Fungizone Intravenous (Among most common) 506
IFEX (2%) 697
INFeD (Iron Dextran Injection, USP) 2345
Kefzol Vials, Faspak & ADD-Vantage 1456
Larodopa Tablets (Rare) 2129
Leustatin (2%) 1834
Lupron Depot 3.75 mg 2556
Lupron Depot 7.5 mg 2559
▲Lupron Injection (5% or more) 2555
Lutrepulse for Injection 980
Luvox Tablets (Rare) 2544
Maxaquin Tablets (Less than 1%) 2440
Mithracin 607
Mivacron (Less than 1%) 1138
Monocid Injection (Less often) 2497
▲Navelbine Injection (Up to 10%) 1145
Nolvadex Tablets (0.3%) 2841
Novantrone (Infrequent) 1279
Panhematin 443
Paxil Tablets 2505
Pentam 300 Injection (0.7%) 1041
▲Primaxin I.V. (3.1%) 1729
▲Proleukin for Injection (23%) 797
Retrovir Capsules (1.6%) 1158
Retrovir I.V. Infusion (2%) 1163
Retrovir Syrup (1.6%) 1158
ReVia Tablets (Less than 1%) 940
Rifater 1532
Risperdal (Rare) 1301
Rocephin Injectable Vials, ADD-Vantage, Galaxy Container (Less than 1%) 2142
Serophene (clomiphene citrate tablets, USP) (Rare) 2451
Sinemet Tablets (Rare) 943
Sinemet CR Tablets 944
Taxol (Rare) 714
Tazicef for Injection (Less than 2%) 2519
Tazidime Vials, Faspak & ADD-Vantage (Less than 2%) 1478
Tegison Capsules (Less than 1%) 2154
Testoderm Testosterone Transdermal System (One in 104 patients) 486
Ticar for Injection 2526
Trasylol (1.0%) 613
Triostat Injection (Approximately 1%) 2530
Valium Injectable (Among most common) 2182
Vancocin HCl, Vials & ADD-Vantage 1481
Velban Vials 1484
Versed Injection (0.4%) 2170
Wellbutrin Tablets (Rare) 1204
Zefazone 2654
▲Zinecard (3% to 6%) 1961
Zosyn (1.3%) 1419
Zosyn Pharmacy Bulk Package (1.3%) 1422
▲Zovirax Sterile Powder (Approximately 9%) 1223

Phlebosclerosis

Adriamycin PFS 1947
Adriamycin RDF 1947
Doxorubicin Astra 540
Rubex 712

Phobic disorder

Anafranil Capsules (Infrequent) 803
Cipro I.V. (1% or less) 595
Cipro I.V. Pharmacy Bulk Package (Less than 1%) 597
Cipro Tablets (Less than 1%) 592
Floxin I.V. 1571
Floxin Tablets (200 mg, 300 mg, 400 mg) 1567
Imitrex Tablets (Rare) 1106
Luvox Tablets (Infrequent) 2544
Maxaquin Tablets 2440

Phonophobia

Imitrex Tablets (Frequent) 1106

Phosphaturia

Daranide Tablets 1633

Phosphenes

Clomid (1.5%) 1514
Serophene (clomiphene citrate tablets, USP) 2451

Phospholipid concentration, increase

Demulen 2428
Estratest 2539
Triphasil-21 Tablets 2814
Triphasil-28 Tablets 2819

Photodynamic reaction

Urobiotic-250 Capsules 2214

Photophobia

Accutane Capsules (Less than 1%) 2076
Anafranil Capsules (Infrequent) 803
Betaseron for SC Injection 658
Betimol 0.25%, 0.5% (1% to 5%) ◉ 261
Betoptic Ophthalmic Solution (Rare) 469
Betoptic S Ophthalmic Suspension (Small number of patients) 471
BOTOX (Botulinum Toxin Type A) Purified Neurotoxin Complex 477
BuSpar (Rare) 737

(▣ Described in PDR For Nonprescription Drugs) Incidence data in parenthesis; ▲ 3% or more (◉ Described in PDR For Ophthalmology)

Cardura Tablets (Less than 0.5% of 3960 patients) 2186
Celontin Kapseals 1899
Chibroxin Sterile Ophthalmic Solution 1617
Ciloxan Ophthalmic Solution (Less than 1%) 472
Claritin-D (Less frequent) 2350
Clomid (1.5%) 1514
▲ Cordarone Tablets (4 to 9%) 2712
Cytovene (1% or less) 2103
Effexor (Infrequent) 2719
Ergamisol Tablets 1292
Etrafon 2355
Floxin I.V. (Less than 1%) 1571
Floxin Tablets (200 mg, 300 mg, 400 mg) (Less than 1%) 1567
Fluorouracil Injection 2116
Foscavir Injection (Less than 1%) 547
Sterile FUDR (Remote possibility) 2118
Gamimune N, 5% Immune Globulin Intravenous (Human), 5% (Infrequent) 619
Gamimune N, 10% Immune Globulin Intravenous (Human), 10% (Infrequent) 621
Havrix (Less than 1%) 2489
Herplex Liquifilm ⊙ 244
Hivid Tablets (Less than 1% to less than 3%) 2121
Imdur (Less than or equal to 5%) 1323
Imitrex Injection (Infrequent) 1103
Imitrex Tablets (Frequent) 1106
Intron A (Less than 5%) 2364
Iopidine 0.5% (Less than 3%) ⊙ 221
Lacrisert Sterile Ophthalmic Insert 1686
Lamictal Tablets (Infrequent) 1112
Levophed Bitartrate Injection 2315
Lodine Capsules and Tablets (Less than 1%) 2743
Luvox Tablets (Infrequent) 2544
Matulane Capsules 2131
Maxaquin Tablets 2440
Mesantoin Tablets 2272
Neurontin Capsules (Infrequent) 1922
Nizoral Tablets (Less than 1%) 1298
Ocuflox 481
Ocupress Ophthalmic Solution, 1% Sterile (Occasional) ⊙ 309
OptiPranolol (Metipranolol 0.3%) Sterile Ophthalmic Solution (A small number of patients) ⊙ 258
▲ Orthoclone OKT3 Sterile Solution (10%) 1837
Paremyd ⊙ 247
Paxil Tablets (Rare) 2505
Permax Tablets (Infrequent) 575
Plaquenil Sulfate Tablets (Fairly common) 2328
Prinivil Tablets (0.3% to 1.0%) 1733
Prinzide Tablets 1737
Profenal 1% Sterile Ophthalmic Solution ⊙ 227
ProSom Tablets (Infrequent) 449
Prozac Pulvules & Liquid, Oral Solution (Infrequent) 919
Quinaglute Dura-Tabs Tablets 649
Quinidex Extentabs 2067
Retrovir Capsules 1158
Retrovir I.V. Infusion 1163
Retrovir Syrup 1158
▲ Rēv-Eyes Ophthalmic Eyedrops 0.5% (10% to 40%) ⊙ 323
Risperdal (Rare) 1301
Rocaltrol Capsules 2141
Sandoglobulin I.V. (Infrequent) 2290
Serentil 684
Serophene (clomiphene citrate tablets, USP) 2451
Serzone Tablets (Infrequent) 771
Supprelin Injection (1% to 3%) 2056
Tambocor Tablets (Less than 1%) 1497
Tegison Capsules (Less than 1%) 2154
Triavil Tablets 1757
Trilafon 2389
Trusopt Sterile Ophthalmic Solution (Approximately 1% to 5%) 1760
Vexol 1% Ophthalmic Suspension (Less than 1%) ⊙ 230
▲ Videx Tablets, Powder for Oral Solution, & Pediatric Powder for Oral Solution (Less than 1% to 8%) 720
Vira-A Ophthalmic Ointment, 3% ⊙ 312
Zestoretic 2850
Zestril Tablets (0.3% to 1.0%) 2854
Zoloft Tablets (Rare) 2217
Zosyn (1.0% or less) 1419
Zosyn Pharmacy Bulk Package (1.0% or less) 1422

Photopsia

Ambien Tablets (Rare) 2416
Clomid 1514
Risperdal (Rare) 1301

Photosensitivity

Accupril Tablets (Rare) 1893
Achromycin V Capsules 1367
Actifed with Codeine Cough Syrup 1067
Children's Advil Suspension (Less than 1%) 2692
Aldactazide 2413
Aldoclor Tablets 1598
Aldoril Tablets 1604
Altace Capsules (Less than 1%) 1232
Ambien Tablets (Rare) 2416
Anafranil Capsules (Infrequent) 803
Anaprox/Naprosyn (Less than 1%) 2117
Ancobon Capsules 2079
Ansaid Tablets (Rare) 2579
Apresazide Capsules 808
Asendin Tablets (Less than 1%) 1369
Atretol Tablets 573
Azo Gantanol Tablets 2080
Azo Gantrisin Tablets 2081
Azulfidine (Rare) 1949
Bactrim DS Tablets 2084
Bactrim I.V. Infusion 2082
Bactrim 2084
Benadryl Capsules 1898
Benadryl Injection 1898
Betapace Tablets (Rare) 641
Betaseron for SC Injection 658
▲ Bromfed-DM Cough Syrup (Among most frequent) 1786
Capoten 739
Capozide 742
Cardizem CD Capsules (Less than 1%) 1506
Cardizem SR Capsules (Less than 1%) 1510
Cardizem Injectable 1508
Cardizem Tablets (Less than 1%) 1512
Cataflam (Less than 1%) 816
Chibroxin Sterile Ophthalmic Solution (With oral form) 1617
Cipro I.V. (1% or less) 595
Cipro I.V. Pharmacy Bulk Package (Less than 1%) 597
Cipro Tablets (Less than 1%) 592
Claritin (2% or fewer patients) 2349
Claritin-D 2350
Clinoril Tablets (Less than 1 in 100) 1618
Clozaril Tablets 2252
Combipres Tablets 677
Compazine 2470
▲ Cordarone Tablets (4 to 9%) 2712
Cozaar Tablets (Less than 1%) 1628
Cytovene (1% or less) 2103
Dantrium Capsules 1982
Daypro Caplets (Less than 1%) 2426
Declomycin Tablets 1371
Deconamine 1320
Depakene 413
Depakote Tablets 415
DiaBeta Tablets 1239
Diabinese Tablets 1935
Diamox Intravenous (Occasional) 1372
Diamox Sequels (Sustained Release) 1373
Diamox Tablets (Occasional) 1372
Dimetane-DC Cough Syrup 2059
Dimetane-DX Cough Syrup 2059
Dipentum Capsules (Rare) 1951
Diucardin Tablets 2718
Diupres Tablets 1650
Diuril Oral Suspension 1653
Diuril Sodium Intravenous 1652
Diuril Tablets 1653
Dolobid Tablets (Less than 1 in 100) 1654
Doryx Capsules 1913
Dyazide 2479
Dynacin Capsules (Rare) 1590
Dyrenium Capsules (Rare) 2481
EC-Naprosyn Delayed-Release Tablets (Less than 1%) 2117
Effexor (Infrequent) 2719
▲ Efudex (Among most frequent) 2113
Elavil 2838
Eldepryl Tablets 2550
Endep Tablets 2174
Enduron Tablets 420
Ergamisol Tablets 1292
Esidrix Tablets 821
Esimil Tablets 822
Etrafon 2355
Eulexin Capsules 2358
Fansidar Tablets 2114
Felbatol (Rare) 2666
Flexeril Tablets (Rare) 1661
Floxin I.V. 1571
Floxin Tablets (200 mg, 300 mg, 400 mg) 1567
Fluorouracil Injection 2116
Sterile FUDR (Remote possibility) 2118
Fulvicin P/G Tablets (Occasional) 2359
Fulvicin P/G 165 & 330 Tablets (Occasional) 2359
Gantanol Tablets 2119
Gantrisin 2120
Glauctabs (Occasional) ⊙ 208
Glucotrol Tablets 1967
Glynase PresTab Tablets 2609
Grifulvin V (griseofulvin tablets) Microsize (griseofulvin oral suspension) Microsize 1888
Gris-PEG Tablets, 125 mg & 250 mg (Occasional) 479
Haldol Decanoate (Isolated cases) 1577
Haldol Injection, Tablets and Concentrate (Isolated cases) 1575
Hibistat Germicidal Hand Rinse (Rare) 2841
Hismanal Tablets (Less frequent) 1293
Hivid Tablets (Less than 1% to less than 3%) 2121
HydroDIURIL Tablets 1674
Hydropres Tablets 1675
Hyzaar Tablets 1677
Imitrex Injection 1103
Imitrex Tablets 1106
Inderide Tablets 2732
Inderide LA Long Acting Capsules 2734
Intron A (Less than 5%) 2364
Lamictal Tablets (Rare) 1112
Lasix Injection, Oral Solution and Tablets 1240
Lescol Capsules (Rare) 2267
Levoprome 1274
Limbitrol 2180
Lodine Capsules and Tablets (Less than 1%) 2743
Lopressor HCT Tablets 832
Lotensin Tablets 834
Lotensin HCT (0.3% or more) 837
Lozol Tablets 2022
Ludiomil Tablets (Rare) 843
Luvox Tablets (Infrequent) 2544
MZM (Occasional) ⊙ 267
Maxaquin Tablets (2.4%) 2440
Maxzide 1380
Mellaril (Extremely rare) 2269
Mepergan Injection (Extremely rare) 2753
▲ Methotrexate Sodium Tablets, Injection, for Injection and LPF Injection (3% to 10%) 1275
Mevacor Tablets (Rare) 1699
Micronase Tablets 2623
Minizide Capsules 1938
Minocin Intravenous (Rare) 1382
Minocin Oral Suspension (Rare) 1385
Minocin Pellet-Filled Capsules (Rare) 1383
Moduretic Tablets 1705
Monodox Capsules 1805
Monopril Tablets (0.2% to 1.0%) 757
Children's Motrin Ibuprofen Oral Suspension (Less than 1%) 1546
Motrin Tablets (Less than 1%) 2625
Motrin Ibuprofen Suspension, Oral Drops, Chewable Tablets, Caplets (Less than 1%) 1546
Mykrox Tablets 993
Anaprox/Naprosyn (Less than 1%) 2117
Navane Capsules and Concentrate 2201
Navane Intramuscular 2202
NegGram 2323
Neptazane Tablets 1388
Neurontin Capsules (Rare) 1922
Noroxin Tablets 1715
Noroxin Tablets 2048
Norpramin Tablets 1526
Oretic Tablets 443
Ornade Spansule Capsules 2502
Orudis Capsules (Less than 1%) 2766
Oruvail Capsules (Less than 1%) 2766
PBZ Tablets 845
PBZ-SR Tablets 844
pHisoHex 2327
P&S Plus Tar Gel ▣ 604
Pamelor (No incidence in labeling) 2280
Paxil Tablets (Rare) 2505
Penetrex Tablets (Less than 1% but more than or equal to 0.1%) 2031
Pentasa (Less than 1%) 1527
Periactin 1724
Phenergan with Codeine (Rare) 2777
Phenergan with Dextromethorphan (Rare) 2778
Phenergan Injection 2773
Phenergan Suppositories (Rare) 2775
Phenergan Syrup (Rare) 2774
Phenergan Tablets (Rare) 2775
Phenergan VC (Rare) 2779
Phenergan VC with Codeine (Rare) 2781
Polytrim Ophthalmic Solution Sterile 482
Pravachol (Rare) 765
Prinivil Tablets (0.3% to 1.0%) 1733
Prinzide Tablets 1737
▲ Prograf (Greater than 3%) 1042
Prolixin 509
ProSom Tablets (Rare) 449
Pyrazinamide Tablets (Rare) 1398
Quinaglute Dura-Tabs Tablets (Occasional) 649
Quinidex Extentabs 2067
Relafen Tablets (1%) 2510
Rifater (Rare) 1532
Risperdal (Frequent) 1301
Seldane Tablets 1536
Seldane-D Extended-Release Tablets 1538
Septra 1174
Septra I.V. Infusion 1169
Septra I.V. Infusion ADD-Vantage Vials 1171
Septra 1174
Ser-Ap-Es Tablets 849
Serzone Tablets (Infrequent) 771
Sinequan (Occasional) 2205
Solganal Suspension 2388
Stelazine (Occasional) 2514
Surmontil Capsules 2811
Symmetrel Capsules and Syrup (0.1% to 1%) 946
Tavist Syrup 2297
Tavist Tablets 2298
Tegretol Chewable Tablets 852
Tegretol Suspension 852
Tegretol Tablets 852
Temaril Tablets, Syrup and Spansule Extended-Release Capsules 483
Tenoretic Tablets 2845
Terramycin Intramuscular Solution 2210
Thalitone 1245
Thorazine (Occasional) 2523
Timolide Tablets 1748
Tofranil Ampuls 854
Tofranil Tablets 856
Tofranil-PM Capsules 857
Triavil Tablets 1757
Trilafon 2389
Trinalin Repetabs Tablets 1330
Tussend 1783
Univasc Tablets (Less than 1%) 2410
Vaseretic Tablets 1765
Vasosulf ⊙ 271
Vasotec I.V. 1768
Vasotec Tablets (0.5% to 1.0%) 1771
Velban Vials (1 case) 1484
Vibramycin 1941
Vibramycin Hyclate Intravenous 2215
Vibramycin 1941
Vivactil Tablets 1774
Voltaren Tablets (Less than 1%) 861
X-Seb T Pearl Shampoo ▣ 606
X-Seb T Plus Conditioning Shampoo ▣ 606
Zaroxolyn Tablets 1000
Zestoretic 2850
Zestril Tablets (0.3% to 1.0%) 2854
Ziac 1415
Zithromax (1% or less) 1944
Zocor Tablets (Rare) 1775
Zoloft Tablets (Rare) 2217

Phototoxicity

Cipro Tablets 592
Dapsone Tablets USP 1284
Floxin Tablets (200 mg, 300 mg, 400 mg) 1567
Lamprene Capsules (Less than 1%) 828
Maxaquin Tablets 2440
Noroxin Tablets 1715
Noroxin Tablets 2048

Physical performance, impairment

Adipex-P Tablets and Capsules 1048
Anexsia 5/500 Elixir 1781
Anexia Tablets 1782
Brontex 1981
Butisol Sodium Elixir & Tablets 2660

(▣ Described in PDR For Nonprescription Drugs) Incidence data in parenthesis; ▲ 3% or more (⊙ Described in PDR For Ophthalmology)

Physical performance, impairment   Side Effects Index   1390

Clozaril Tablets 2252
Compazine 2470
DHCplus Capsules 1993
Deconamine 1320
Demerol 2308
Desyrel and Desyrel Dividose 503
Esgic-plus Tablets 1013
Etrafon 2355
Fioricet Tablets 2258
Hycodan Tablets and Syrup 930
Hycomine Compound Tablets 932
Hycomine 931
Hycotuss Expectorant Syrup 933
Hydrocet Capsules 782
Libritabs Tablets 2177
Lithonate/Lithotabs/Lithobid 2543
Lorcet 10/650 1018
Lortab 2566
Loxitane 1378
MS Contin Tablets 1994
Mebaral Tablets 2322
Methadone Hydrochloride Oral Concentrate 2233
Miltown Tablets 2672
Norpramin Tablets 1526
PMB 200 and PMB 400 2783
Percocet Tablets 938
Percodan Tablets 939
Phenergan with Codeine 2777
Phenergan with Dextromethorphan 2778
Phenergan Injection 2773
Phenergan Suppositories 2775
Phenergan Syrup 2774
Phenergan Tablets 2775
Phenergan VC 2779
Phenergan VC with Codeine 2781
RMS Suppositories 2657
Soma Compound Tablets 2675
Surmontil Capsules 2811
Tofranil Tablets 856
Tofranil-PM Capsules 857
Tussend 1783
Tussionex Pennkinetic Extended-Release Suspension 998
Tylenol with Codeine 1583
Tylox Capsules 1584
Ultram Tablets (50 mg) 1585
Vicodin Tablets 1356
Vicodin ES Tablets 1357
Vicodin Tuss Expectorant 1358
Vivactil Tablets 1774
Wygesic Tablets 2827
Zydone Capsules 949

Pigmentary deposits, conjuctiva
Mellaril 2269

Pigmentary deposits, cornea
Lamprene Capsules (Greater than 1%) 828
Triavil Tablets 1757

Pigmentation
Aquasol A Vitamin A Capsules, USP 534
Cortifoam 2396
Cosmegen Injection 1626
Etrafon 2355
Genotropin (Infrequent) 111
Levoprome 1274
Lupron Depot 7.5 mg 2559
Lupron Injection (Less than 5%) 2555
Mesantoin Tablets 2272
Minipress Capsules (Single report) 1937
Minizide Capsules (Single report) 1938
Plaquenil Sulfate Tablets 2328
Prolixin 509
Risperdal (Frequent) 1301
Timolide Tablets (Less than 1%) 1748
Timoptic in Ocudose 1753
Timoptic Sterile Ophthalmic Solution 1751
Timoptic-XE 1755
Triavil Tablets 1757
Trilafon 2389
VePesid Capsules and Injection (Infrequent) 718

Pigmentation disorders
Accutane Capsules (Less than 1%) 2076
Aralen Hydrochloride Injection 2301
Aralen Phosphate Tablets 2301
Atretol Tablets 573
Cordarone Tablets (Occasional) 2712
Cytoxan 694
Daraprim Tablets (Rare) 1090
Dynacin Capsules 1590
Ethyl Chloride, U.S.P. 1052
Fluori-Methane 1053
Fluorouracil Injection 2116
Fluro-Ethyl 1053
Sterile FUDR (Remote possibility) 2118
Mellaril 2269
Methotrexate Sodium Tablets, Injection, for Injection and LPF Injection 1275
Minocin Intravenous 1382
Minocin Oral Suspension 1385
Minocin Pellet-Filled Capsules 1383
NEOSAR Lyophilized/Neosar 1959
Orudis Capsules (Less than 1%) 2766
Oruvail Capsules (Less than 1%) 2766
Quinaglute Dura-Tabs Tablets 649
Quinidex Extentabs 2067
Retrovir Capsules 1158
Retrovir I.V. Infusion 1163
Retrovir Syrup 1158
Supprelin Injection (1% to 3%) 2056
Tapazole Tablets 1477
Tegretol Chewable Tablets 852
Tegretol Suspension 852
Tegretol Tablets 852
Thorazine 2523

Pill rolling motion
Compazine 2470
Stelazine 2514
Thorazine 2523

Piloerection
Anafranil Capsules (Rare) 803
Vasoxyl Injection 1196
Yohimex Tablets 1363

Pituitary apoplexy
Factrel 2877
Sandostatin Injection (Less than 1%) 2292
THYREL TRH (Infrequent) 2873

Pituitary tumors
Clomid 1514

Pituitary unresponsiveness, secondary
Aristocort Suspension (Forte Parenteral) 1027
Aristocort Suspension (Intralesional) 1025
Aristocort Tablets 1022
Aristospan Suspension (Intra-articular) 1033
Aristospan Suspension (Intralesional) 1032
Celestone Soluspan Suspension 2347
CORTENEMA 2535
Cortone Acetate Sterile Suspension 1623
Cortone Acetate Tablets 1624
Dalalone D.P. Injectable 1011
Decadron Elixir 1633
Decadron Phosphate Injection 1637
Decadron Phosphate Respihaler 1642
Decadron Phosphate Turbinaire 1645
Decadron Phosphate with Xylocaine Injection, Sterile 1639
Decadron Tablets 1635
Decadron-LA Sterile Suspension 1646
Deltasone Tablets 2595
Depo-Medrol Sterile Aqueous Suspension 2597
Dexacort Phosphate in Respihaler 458
Dexacort Phosphate in Turbinaire 459
Florinef Acetate Tablets 505
Hydeltrasol Injection, Sterile 1665
Hydeltra-T.B.A. Sterile Suspension 1667
Hydrocortone Acetate Sterile Suspension 1669
Hydrocortone Phosphate Injection, Sterile 1670
Hydrocortone Tablets 1672
Medrol 2621
Pediapred Oral Liquid 995
Prelone Syrup 1787
Solu-Cortef Sterile Powder 2641
Solu-Medrol Sterile Powder 2643

Placental disorder, unspecified
Felbatol 2666

Plaques, erythematous
AquaMEPHYTON Injection 1608

Plaques, indurated
AquaMEPHYTON Injection 1608

Plaques, pruritic
AquaMEPHYTON Injection 1608

Platelet, decrease (see under Thrombocytopenia)

Platelet disorder, unspecified
Felbatol (Rare) 2666
▲ Foscavir Injection (5% or greater) 547
Hivid Tablets (Less than 1% to less than 3%) 2121

Platelet, increase (see under Thrombocytosis)

Plethora
Talwin Injection 2334
Talwin Nx 2336

Pleural effusion
Atgam Sterile Solution (Less than 5%) 2581
Betaseron for SC Injection 658
▲ CellCept Capsules (More than or equal to 3%) 2099
Cipro I.V. (1% or less) 595
Cipro I.V. Pharmacy Bulk Package (Less than 1%) 597
Clinoril Tablets (Less than 1 in 100) 1618
Clomid 1514
Clozaril Tablets 2252
▲ Ethamolin (Among most common; 2.1%) 2400
Felbatol 2666
Foscavir Injection (Less than 1%) 547
Ganite 2533
Humegon 1824
Hyskon Hysteroscopy Fluid (Rare) 1595
Leukine for IV Infusion (1%) 1271
Lutrepulse for Injection 980
Macrobid Capsules 1988
Macrodantin Capsules 1989
Matulane Capsules 2131
Permax Tablets (Infrequent) 575
Prinivil Tablets (0.3% to 1.0%) 1733
Prinzide Tablets 1737
Procan SR Tablets (Common) 1926
Profasi (chorionic gonadotropin for injection, USP) 2450
▲ Prograf (30% to 32%) 1042
▲ Proleukin for Injection (7%) 797
Prozac Pulvules & Liquid, Oral Solution (Rare) 919
ReoPro Vials (1.3%) 1471
Sansert Tablets 2295
Serophene (clomiphene citrate tablets, USP) 2451
▲ Trasylol (5%) 613
Zefazone 2654
Zestoretic 2850
Zestril Tablets (0.3% to 1.0%) 2854

Pleural effusion with pericarditis
Dantrium Capsules (Less frequent) 1982

Pleural friction rubs
Lupron Depot 3.75 mg 2556
Lupron Depot 7.5 mg 2559
Lupron Injection (Less than 5%) 2555
Sansert Tablets 2295

Pleural infiltration
▲ Ethamolin (Among most common; 2.1%) 2400

Pleuralgia
Intron A (Less than 5%) 2364
Monopril Tablets (0.4% to 1.0%) 757
Procan SR Tablets (Common) 1926

Pleurisy
AeroBid Inhaler System (1-3%) 1005
Aerobid-M Inhaler System (1-3%) 1005
Effexor (Rare) 2719
ReoPro Vials (1.3%) 1471
Tonocard Tablets (Less than 1%) 531

Pleuritis
Azulfidine (Rare) 1949
Inocor Lactate Injection (1 case) 2309
NebuPent for Inhalation Solution (1% or less) 1040

Pneumatosis cystoides intestinalis
Cytosar-U Sterile Powder 2592

Pneumocystis carinii
CellCept Capsules (Up to 0.3%) 2099

Pneumocystis carinii, susceptibility
▲ Orthoclone OKT3 Sterile Solution (3.1%) 1837

Pneumocystosis, extrapulmonary
NebuPent for Inhalation Solution (1% or less) 1040

Pneumomediastinum
Exosurf Neonatal for Intratracheal Suspension (1% to 4%) 1095

Pneumonia
AeroBid Inhaler System (1-3%) 1005
Aerobid-M Inhaler System (1-3%) 1005
Ambien Tablets (Rare) 2416
Anafranil Capsules (Infrequent) 803
Atretol Tablets 573
Betaseron for SC Injection 658
▲ CellCept Capsules (3.6% to 10.6%) 2099
Clozaril Tablets (Less than 1%) 2252
Cognex Capsules (Frequent) 1901
Compazine 2470
Cytosar-U Sterile Powder (Less frequent) 2592
Cytotec (Infrequent) 2424
▲ Cytovene (6%) 2103
Effexor (Infrequent) 2719
▲ Ethamolin (Among most common; 1.2%) 2400
Felbatol 2666
▲ Fludara for Injection (16% to 22%) 663
Foscavir Injection (Between 1% and 5%) 547
Imdur (Less than or equal to 5%) 1323
Intron A (Rare; less than 5%) 2364
Ismo Tablets (Fewer than 1%) 2738
Kerlone Tablets (Less than 2%) 2436
Lamictal Tablets (Rare) 1112
▲ Leustatin (6%) 1834
Lupron Depot 3.75 mg 2556
Lupron Depot 7.5 mg 2559
Lupron Injection (Less than 5%) 2555
Luvox Tablets (Rare) 2544
Megace Oral Suspension (Up to 2%) 699
Miacalcin Nasal Spray (Less than 1%) 2275
▲ Neoral (6.2%) 2276
Neurontin Capsules (Frequent) 1922
▲ Novantrone (9%) 1279
Orthoclone OKT3 Sterile Solution 1837
Paxil Tablets (Infrequent) 2505
Permax Tablets (Frequent) 575
PREVACID Delayed-Release Capsules (Less than 1%) 2562
Prinivil Tablets (0.3% to 1.0%) 1733
Prinzide Tablets 1737
▲ Prograf (Greater than 3%) 1042
Prolixin 509
Prozac Pulvules & Liquid, Oral Solution (Infrequent) 919
Pulmozyme Inhalation 1064
ReoPro Vials (1.0%) 1471
Risperdal (Infrequent) 1301
Roferon-A Injection (Less than 3%) 2145
▲ Sandimmune (6.2 to 9.2%) 2286
Sandostatin Injection (Less than 1%) 2292
Serentil 684
Serzone Tablets (Infrequent) 771
Stelazine 2514
▲ Taxol (30%) 714
Tegretol Chewable Tablets 852
Tegretol Suspension 852
Tegretol Tablets 852
▲ Tetramune (Among most common) 1404
Tonocard Tablets (Less than 1%) 531
▲ Trasylol (4%) 613
Vaseretic Tablets 1765
Vasotec I.V. 1768
Vasotec Tablets (1.0%) 1771
▲ Videx Tablets, Powder for Oral Solution, & Pediatric Powder for Oral Solution (1% to 8%) 720
Virazole 1264
Wellbutrin Tablets (Rare) 1204
▲ Zerit Capsules (3% to 4%) 729
Zestoretic 2850
Zestril Tablets (0.3% to 1.0%) 2854

Pneumonia, aspiration
Ethamolin 2400
Lioresal Intrathecal 1596
Neurontin Capsules (Rare) 1922

Pneumonia, congenital
Exosurf Neonatal for Intratracheal Suspension (1% to 4%) 1095

(▣ Described in PDR For Nonprescription Drugs)   Incidence data in parenthesis; ▲ 3% or more   (◉ Described in PDR For Ophthalmology)

1391 Side Effects Index Porphyria

Pneumonia, eosinophilic
Prozac Pulvules & Liquid, Oral Solution ... 919
Relafen Tablets (Rarer) ... 2510

Pneumonia, interstitial
Betaseron for SC Injection ... 658
Leukeran Tablets ... 1133
Videx Tablets, Powder for Oral Solution, & Pediatric Powder for Oral Solution (Less than 1%) ... 720

Pneumonia, nosocomial
▲ Exosurf Neonatal for Intratracheal Suspension (2% to 15%) ... 1095

Pneumonitis
Aldoclor Tablets ... 1598
Aldoril Tablets ... 1604
Apresazide Capsules ... 808
Atretol Tablets ... 573
Azo Gantrisin Tablets ... 2081
Azulfidine (Rare) ... 1949
BCG Vaccine, USP (TICE) (1.2%) .. 1814
▲ Blenoxane (Up to 10%) ... 692
Capozide ... 742
Clinoril Tablets (Less than 1 in 100) ... 1618
Diucardin Tablets ... 2718
Diupres Tablets ... 1650
Diuril Oral Suspension ... 1653
Diuril Sodium Intravenous ... 1652
Diuril Tablets ... 1653
Enduron Tablets ... 420
Esidrix Tablets ... 821
Esimil Tablets ... 822
Felbatol ... 2666
Foscavir Injection (Less than 1%) .. 547
HydroDIURIL Tablets ... 1674
Hydropres Tablets ... 1675
Hyzaar Tablets ... 1677
Inderide Tablets ... 2732
Inderide LA Long Acting Capsules .. 2734
Intron A (Rare) ... 2364
Lopressor HCT Tablets ... 832
Lotensin HCT ... 837
Lozol Tablets ... 2022
Matulane Capsules ... 2131
Maxzide ... 1380
Methotrexate Sodium Tablets, Injection, for Injection and LPF Injection ... 1275
Moduretic Tablets ... 1705
Mykrox Tablets (Rare) ... 993
Myochrysine Injection ... 1711
Oretic Tablets ... 443
Orthoclone OKT3 Sterile Solution .. 1837
Prinzide Tablets ... 1737
Prolixin ... 509
Ser-Ap-Es Tablets ... 849
Solganal Suspension ... 2388
Tegretol Chewable Tablets ... 852
Tegretol Suspension ... 852
Tegretol Tablets ... 852
Timolide Tablets ... 1748
Varivax (Less than 1%) ... 1762
Vaseretic Tablets ... 1765
Zaroxolyn Tablets ... 1000
Zestoretic ... 2850
Ziac ... 1415

Pneumonitis, allergic
Dyazide ... 2479
Floxin I.V. ... 1571
Floxin Tablets (200 mg, 300 mg, 400 mg) ... 1567
▲ Fludara for Injection (Up to 6%) ... 663
Ticlid Tablets (Rare) ... 2156

Pneumonitis, eosinophilic
Monopril Tablets ... 757
Tilade (Isolated cases) ... 996

Pneumonitis, interstitial
Actimmune (Rare) ... 1056
Alkeran for Injection ... 1070
Alkeran Tablets ... 1071
Asacol Delayed-Release Tablets ... 1979
Cordarone Tablets ... 2712
Cuprimine Capsules (Rare) ... 1630
Cytosar-U Sterile Powder (Ten patients) ... 2592
Depen Titratable Tablets ... 2662
Ludiomil Tablets (Several voluntary reports) ... 843
Macrobid Capsules (Rare to common) ... 1988
Macrodantin Capsules (Rare; common) ... 1989
Methotrexate Sodium Tablets, Injection, for Injection and LPF Injection ... 1275
NebuPent for Inhalation Solution (1% or less) ... 1040
Ridaura Capsules (Less than 0.1%) ... 2513
Tonocard Tablets (Less than 1%) .. 531

Pneumopericardium
Exosurf Neonatal for Intratracheal Suspension (1% to 4%) ... 1095

Pneumothorax
Betaseron for SC Injection ... 658
Cytovene-IV (One report) ... 2103
▲ Exosurf Neonatal for Intratracheal Suspension (6% to 20%) ... 1095
Foscavir Injection (Between 1% and 5%) ... 547
NebuPent for Inhalation Solution (Greater than 1%, up to 5%) ... 1040
Permax Tablets (Rare) ... 575
Proleukin for Injection (1%) ... 797
Pulmozyme Inhalation ... 1064
Rifater ... 1532
▲ Trasylol (3%) ... 613
Videx Tablets, Powder for Oral Solution, & Pediatric Powder for Oral Solution (Less than 1%) ... 720
Virazole ... 1264

Pollakiuria
DynaCirc Capsules (1.3% to 3.4%) ... 2256
Sandostatin Injection (1% to 4%).. 2292
Sanorex Tablets ... 2294
Visken Tablets (2% or fewer patients) ... 2299

Polyarteritis nodosa
Anafranil Capsules (Rare) ... 803
Azo Gantanol Tablets ... 2080
Azulfidine (Rare) ... 1949

Polyarthralgia
Eskalith ... 2485
Lithonate/Lithotabs/Lithobid ... 2543
Minocin Intravenous ... 1382
Minocin Oral Suspension ... 1385
Minocin Pellet-Filled Capsules ... 1383
Primaxin I.M. ... 1727
Primaxin I.V. (Less than 0.2%) ... 1729

Polyarthralgia, migratory
Cuprimine Capsules (Some patients) ... 1630
Depen Titratable Tablets ... 2662

Polyarthritis
Cleocin Phosphate Injection (Rare) 2586
Cleocin Vaginal Cream (Rare) ... 2589

Polyarthropathy
Mesantoin Tablets ... 2272

Polycythemia
▲ Android Capsules, 10 mg (Among most common) ... 1250
Android ... 1251
▲ CellCept Capsules (More than or equal to 3%) ... 2099
Danocrine Capsules ... 2307
Delatestryl Injection ... 2860
Estratest ... 2539
Gastrocrom Capsules (Infrequent).. 984
Halotestin Tablets ... 2614
Oreton Methyl ... 1255
Oxandrin ... 2862
Permax Tablets (Rare) ... 575
Premarin with Methyltestosterone .. 2794
Testoderm Testosterone Transdermal System ... 486
Testred Capsules ... 1262

Polydipsia
Clozaril Tablets (Less than 1%) ... 2252
Eskalith ... 2485
Hivid Tablets (Less than 1% to less than 3%) ... 2121
Imitrex Injection (Rare) ... 1103
Imitrex Tablets (Rare) ... 1106
Lithium Carbonate Capsules & Tablets ... 2230
Lithonate/Lithotabs/Lithobid (Occasional) ... 2543
Loxitane ... 1378
Navane Capsules and Concentrate 2201
Navane Intramuscular ... 2202
Risperdal (Frequent) ... 1301
Rocaltrol Capsules ... 2141

Polymenorrhea
Sandostatin Injection (Less than 1%) ... 2292

Polymyalgia rheumatica
Lescol Capsules (Rare) ... 2267
Mevacor Tablets (Rare) ... 1699
Miacalcin Nasal Spray (Less than 1%) ... 2275
Pravachol (Rare) ... 765
Zocor Tablets (Rare) ... 1775

Polymyositis
Cuprimine Capsules (Rare) ... 1630
Depen Titratable Tablets (Rare) ... 2662
Intal Capsules (Less than 1 in 100,000 patients) ... 987
Intal Inhaler (Rare) ... 988
Intal Nebulizer Solution (Rare) ... 989
Nasalcrom Nasal Solution (Rare) ... 994
Tagamet (Rare) ... 2516

Polyneuritis
Antabuse Tablets ... 2695
Biavax II ... 1613
M-M-R II ... 1687
M-R-VAX II ... 1689
Meruvax II ... 1697
Podocon-25 ... 1891
Proglycem ... 580

Polyneuropathy
Acel-Imune Diphtheria and Tetanus Toxoids and Acellular Pertussis Vaccine Adsorbed ... 1364
Biavax II (Isolated reports) ... 1613
Dilantin Infatabs ... 1908
Dilantin Kapseals ... 1906
Dilantin Parenteral ... 1910
Dilantin-125 Suspension ... 1911
Diphtheria and Tetanus Toxoids and Pertussis Vaccine Adsorbed.. 2477
IFEX (Less than 1%) ... 697
Intron A (Less than 5%) ... 2364
M-M-R II ... 1687
M-R-VAX II ... 1689
Meruvax II (Isolated reports) ... 1697
Tetramune ... 1404
Tri-Immunol Adsorbed ... 1408

Polyphagia
Atromid-S Capsules ... 2701
Etrafon ... 2355
Triavil Tablets ... 1757
Trilafon ... 2389

Polyps, endometrial
Nolvadex Tablets ... 2841

Polyps, nasal
Pulmozyme Inhalation ... 1064

Polyps, rectal
Lupron Depot 3.75 mg ... 2556
Lupron Depot 7.5 mg ... 2559
Lupron Injection (Less than 5%) ... 2555

Polyradiculoneuropathy
Depen Titratable Tablets ... 2662

Polyuria
Adalat Capsules (10 mg and 20 mg) (Less than 0.5%) ... 587
Children's Advil Suspension (Less than 1%) ... 2692
Ambien Tablets (Rare) ... 2416
Anafranil Capsules (Infrequent) ... 803
Betaseron for SC Injection ... 658
Capoten (Approximately 1 to 2 of 1000 patients) ... 739
Capozide (Approximately 1 to 2 of 1000 patients) ... 742
Cardizem CD Capsules (Less than 1%) ... 1506
Cardizem SR Capsules (1.3%) ... 1510
Cardizem Injectable ... 1508
Cardizem Tablets (Less than 1%) .. 1512
Cardura Tablets (2%) ... 2186
Cipro I.V. (1% or less) ... 595
Cipro I.V. Pharmacy Bulk Package (Less than 1%) ... 597
Cipro Tablets (Less than 1%) ... 592
Claritin-D (Less frequent) ... 2350
Clomid (Fewer than 1%) ... 1514
Cognex Capsules (Infrequent) ... 1901
Cytotec (Infrequent) ... 2424
Diamox Intravenous ... 1372
Diamox Sequels (Sustained Release) ... 1373
Diamox Tablets ... 1372
Effexor (Infrequent) ... 2719
Elspar (Low) ... 1659
Eskalith ... 2485
Etrafon ... 2355
Flagyl 375 Capsules ... 2434
Flagyl I.V. ... 2247
Floxin I.V. ... 1571
Floxin Tablets (200 mg, 300 mg, 400 mg) ... 1567
Foscavir Injection (Between 1% and 5%) ... 547
Glauctabs ... ⊙ 208
Glucotrol XL Extended Release Tablets (Less than 3%) ... 1968
Hivid Tablets (Less than 1% to less than 3%) ... 2121
IBU Tablets (Less than 1%) ... 1342
Imdur (Less than or equal to 5%) .. 1323
Intron A (Less than 5%) ... 2364
Lamictal Tablets (Infrequent) ... 1112
Lithium Carbonate Capsules & Tablets ... 2230
Lithonate/Lithotabs/Lithobid (Occasional) ... 2543
Lotrel Capsules ... 840
Lozol Tablets (Less than 5%) ... 2022
Luvox Tablets (Infrequent) ... 2544
▲ MZM (Among reactions occurring most often) ... ⊙ 267
Maxaquin Tablets ... 2440
MetroGel-Vaginal ... 902
Midamor Tablets (Less than or equal to 1%) ... 1703
Moduretic Tablets ... 1705
Children's Motrin Ibuprofen Oral Suspension (Less than 1%) ... 1546
Motrin Tablets (Less than 1%) ... 2625
Motrin Ibuprofen Suspension, Oral Drops, Chewable Tablets, Caplets (Less than 1%) ... 1546
Neptazane Tablets ... 1388
Norvasc Tablets (Less than or equal to 0.1%) ... 1940
Novahistine DH ... 2462
Novahistine Elixir ... ▣ 823
Oncovin Solution Vials & Hyporets 1466
Paxil Tablets (Infrequent) ... 2505
Penetrex Tablets ... 2031
Plendil Extended-Release Tablets (0.5% to 1.5%) ... 527
Primaxin I.M. ... 1727
Primaxin I.V. (Less than 0.2%) ... 1729
Procardia XL Extended Release Tablets (Less than 3%) ... 1972
Prolixin ... 509
Protostat Tablets ... 1883
Prozac Pulvules & Liquid, Oral Solution (Rare) ... 919
Retrovir Capsules ... 1158
Retrovir I.V. Infusion ... 1163
Retrovir Syrup ... 1158
Risperdal (Frequent) ... 1301
Rocaltrol Capsules ... 2141
Rondec Oral Drops ... 953
Rondec Syrup ... 953
Rondec Tablet ... 953
Rondec-DM Oral Drops ... 954
Rondec-DM Syrup ... 954
Rondec-TR Tablet ... 953
Sansert Tablets ... 2295
Serzone Tablets (Infrequent) ... 771
Supprelin Injection (1% to 3%) ... 2056
Tambocor Tablets (Less than 1%) 1497
Tegison Capsules (Less than 1%) .. 2154
Tonocard Tablets (Less than 1%) .. 531
Toradol (1% or less) ... 2159
Trilafon (Occasional) ... 2389
Videx Tablets, Powder for Oral Solution, & Pediatric Powder for Oral Solution (Less than 1%) ... 720
Ziac ... 1415
Zoloft Tablets (Infrequent) ... 2217

Porphyria
Brevicon ... 2088
Demulen ... 2428
Desogen Tablets ... 1817
Estrace Cream and Tablets ... 749
Levlen/Tri-Levlen ... 651
Lo/Ovral Tablets ... 2746
Lo/Ovral-28 Tablets ... 2751
Micronor Tablets ... 1872
Modicon ... 1872
Nordette-21 Tablets ... 2755
Nordette-28 Tablets ... 2758
Norinyl ... 2088
Nor-Q D Tablets ... 2135
Ortho-Cept ... 1851
Ortho-Cyclen/Ortho-Tri-Cyclen ... 1858
Ortho-Novum ... 1872
Ortho-Cyclen/Ortho Tri-Cyclen ... 1858
Ovcon ... 760

(▣ Described in PDR For Nonprescription Drugs) Incidence data in parenthesis; ▲ 3% or more (⊙ Described in PDR For Ophthalmology)

Ovral Tablets 2770
Ovral-28 Tablets 2770
Ovrette Tablets 2771
Plaquenil Sulfate Tablets 2328
Pyrazinamide Tablets (Rare) 1398
Reglan 2068
Rifater (Rare) 1532
Sulfamylon Cream (A single case) 925
Levlen/Tri-Levlen 651
Tri-Norinyl 2164
Triphasil-21 Tablets 2814
Triphasil-28 Tablets 2819

Porphyria, aggravation
Cataflam (One patient) 816
Climara Transdermal System 645
Danocrine Capsules 2307
Dilantin Infatabs 1908
Dilantin Kapseals (Isolated reports) 1906
Dilantin-125 Suspension (Isolated reports) 1911
Epogen for Injection (Rare) 489
ESTRATAB Tablets (0.3, 0.625, 1.25, 2.5 mg) 2536
Estratest 2539
Libritabs Tablets 2177
Menest Tablets 2494
Miltown Tablets 2672
Ogen Tablets 2627
Ogen Vaginal Cream 2630
Ortho Dienestrol Cream 1866
Ortho-Est 1869
PMB 200 and PMB 400 2783
Plaquenil Sulfate Tablets 2328
Premarin Intravenous 2787
Premarin with Methyltestosterone 2794
Premarin Tablets 2789
Premarin Vaginal Cream 2791
Premphase 2797
Prempro 2801
Procrit for Injection (Rare) 1841
Rifadin (Isolated reports) 1528
Rifater (Isolated reports) 1532
Stilphostrol Tablets and Ampuls 612
Voltaren Tablets (One patient) 861
Zantac (Rare) 1209
Zantac Injection (Rare) 1207
Zantac Syrup (Rare) 1209

Porphyria, hepatic cutaneous
Diabinese Tablets 1935
Glucotrol Tablets 1967
Glucotrol XL Extended Release Tablets 1968

Porphyria, intermittent, acute
Atretol Tablets 573
Depakene 413
Depakote Tablets 415
Tegretol Chewable Tablets 852
Tegretol Suspension 852
Tegretol Tablets 852

Porphyria, pseudo
Daypro Caplets (Less than 1%) 2426

Porphyria cutanea tarda
Anaprox/Naprosyn (Less than 1%) 2117
DiaBeta Tablets 1239
Diabinese Tablets 1935
EC-Naprosyn Delayed-Release Tablets (Less than 1%) 2117
Glucotrol Tablets 1967
Glynase PresTab Tablets 2609
Micronase Tablets 2623
Myleran Tablets (Rare) 1143
Anaprox/Naprosyn (Less than 1%) 2117

Porphyria cutanea tarda, pseudo
Relafen Tablets (1%) 2510

Potassium loss (see under Hypokalemia)

Potassium retention (see under Hyperkalemia)

Potentia, decrease
Arfonad Ampuls 2080
Methadone Hydrochloride Oral Concentrate 2233
RMS Suppositories 2657
▲ReVia Tablets (Less than 10%) 940
Roxanol 2243

Precocious puberty
Pregnyl 1828
Profasi (chorionic gonadotropin for injection, USP) 2450

Pregnancy, accidental
Depo-Provera Contraceptive Injection (Fewer than 1%) 2602

Pregnancy, ectopic
Depo-Provera Contraceptive Injection 2602
Humegon 1824
Lippes Loop Intrauterine Double-S 1848
Metrodin (urofollitropin for injection) 2446
Micronor Tablets 1872
Modicon 1872
Norplant System 2759
Ortho-Novum 1872
ParaGard T380A Intrauterine Copper Contraceptive 1880
Pergonal (menotropins for injection, USP) 2448
Serophene (clomiphene citrate tablets, USP) 2451

Pregnancy, multiple
Clomid (An increased chance) 1514
Lutrepulse for Injection (Some incidents) 980

Pregnancy, sensation of
Depo-Provera Contraceptive Injection (Fewer than 1%) 2602

Pregnancy, spontaneous termination of
Lutrepulse for Injection (Some incidents) 980

Pregnancy tests, false positive
Ceredase 1065
Compazine 2470
Etrafon 2355
Mellaril 2269
Navane Capsules and Concentrate 2201
Navane Intramuscular 2202
Phenergan Injection 2773
Serentil 684
Stelazine 2514
Temaril Tablets, Syrup and Spansule Extended-Release Capsules 483
Thorazine 2523
Triavil Tablets 1757

Pregnancy tests, false results
Phenergan Injection 2773
Prolixin 509
Torecan 2245
Trilafon 2389

Premature ventricular contractions
Diprivan Injection (Less than 1%) 2833
Imitrex Injection (Infrequent) 1103
Mexitil Capsules (1.0% to 1.9%) 678
Prinivil Tablets (0.3% to 1.0%) 1733
Prinzide Tablets 1737
Rythmol Tablets–150mg, 225mg, 300mg (0.6 to 1.5%) 1352
Versed Injection (Less than 1%) 2170
Zestril Tablets (0.3% to 1.0%) 2854

Premenstrual-like syndrome
Amen Tablets 780
Brevicon 2088
Cycrin Tablets 975
Demulen 2428
Depo-Provera Sterile Aqueous Suspension 2606
Desogen Tablets 1817
Diethylstilbestrol Tablets 1437
ESTRATAB Tablets (0.3, 0.625, 1.25, 2.5 mg) 2536
Estratest 2539
Levlen/Tri-Levlen 651
Lo/Ovral Tablets 2746
Lo/Ovral-28 Tablets 2751
Luvox Tablets (Infrequent) 2544
Menest Tablets 2494
Micronor Tablets 1872
Modicon 1872
Nordette-21 Tablets 2755
Nordette-28 Tablets 2758
Norinyl 2088
Nor-Q D Tablets 2135
Ortho-Cept 1851
Ortho-Cyclen/Ortho-Tri-Cyclen 1858
Ortho Dienestrol Cream 1866
Ortho-Novum 1872
Ortho-Cyclen/Ortho Tri-Cyclen 1858
Ovcon 760
Ovral Tablets 2770
Ovral-28 Tablets 2770
Ovrette Tablets 2771
PMB 200 and PMB 400 2783
Premarin Intravenous 2787
Premarin with Methyltestosterone 2794
Premarin Vaginal Cream 2791
Premphase 2797
Prempro 2801
Provera Tablets 2636
Levlen/Tri-Levlen 651
Tri-Norinyl 2164
Triphasil-21 Tablets 2814
Triphasil-28 Tablets 2819

Preputium, irretraction of
Condylox (Less than 5%) 1802

Pressor response, paradoxical
Aldomet Ester HCl Injection 1602
Apresazide Capsules (Less frequent) 808
Apresoline Hydrochloride Tablets (Less frequent) 809
Ser-Ap-Es Tablets 849

Pre syncope
Betapace Tablets (1% to 4%) 641

Priapism
Android 1251
Atamet 572
Clozaril Tablets 2252
Compazine 2470
Coumadin 926
Desyrel and Desyrel Dividose 503
Esimil Tablets (A few instances) 822
Haldol Decanoate 1577
Haldol Injection, Tablets and Concentrate 1575
Halotestin Tablets 2614
Heparin Lock Flush Solution 2725
Heparin Sodium Injection 2726
Heparin Sodium Injection, USP, Sterile Solution 2615
Heparin Sodium Vials 1441
Ismelin Tablets 827
Larodopa Tablets (Rare) 2129
Luvox Tablets 2544
Mellaril 2269
Minipress Capsules (Less than 1%) 1937
Minizide Capsules (Rare) 1938
Moban Tablets and Concentrate 1048
Oreton Methyl 1255
Oxandrin 2862
Papaverine Hydrochloride Vials and Ampoules 1468
Paxil Tablets 2505
Permax Tablets (Infrequent) 575
Prozac Pulvules & Liquid, Oral Solution 919
Risperdal (Rare) 1301
Serzone Tablets 771
Sinemet Tablets 943
Sinemet CR Tablets 944
Stelazine 2514
Testoderm Testosterone Transdermal System 486
Testred Capsules 1262
Thorazine 2523
Winstrol Tablets 2337

Proarrhythmia
Betapace Tablets (Less than 1% to 5%) 641
▲Ethmozine Tablets (3.7% of 1072 patients) 2041
Procan SR Tablets 1926
▲Rythmol Tablets–150mg, 225mg, 300mg (1.2 to 4.7%) 1352

Proctitis
Betaseron for SC Injection 658
Cosmegen Injection 1626
Effexor (Rare) 2719
Flagyl 375 Capsules 2434
Foscavir Injection (Less than 1%) 547
Furoxone 2046
Indocin Capsules (Less than 1%) 1680
Indocin I.V. (Less than 1%) 1684
Indocin (Less than 1%) 1680
MetroGel-Vaginal 902
Miltown Tablets (Rare) 2672
Neurontin Capsules (Rare) 1922
PMB 200 and PMB 400 (Rare) 2783
Protostat Tablets 1883
Urobiotic-250 Capsules (Rare) 2214
Zoloft Tablets (Rare) 2217

Proctitis, ulceration
Foscavir Injection (Less than 1%) 547

Proctocolitis
Diabinese Tablets (Less than 1%) 1935

Prolactin levels, elevated (see under Hyperprolactinemia)

Prolactin secretion, inhibition of
Bellergal-S Tablets 2250

Proprioception, loss of
Platinol 708
Platinol-AQ Injection 710

Proptosis
Amen Tablets 780
Brevicon 2088
Cycrin Tablets 975
Demulen 2428
Depo-Provera Contraceptive Injection 2602
Depo-Provera Sterile Aqueous Suspension 2606
Levlen/Tri-Levlen 651
Micronor Tablets 1872
Modicon 1872
Norinyl 2088
Nor-Q D Tablets 2135
Ortho-Cyclen/Ortho-Tri-Cyclen 1858
Ortho-Novum 1872
Ortho-Cyclen/Ortho Tri-Cyclen 1858
Ovcon 760
Premphase 2797
Prempro 2801
Provera Tablets 2636
Levlen/Tri-Levlen 651
Tri-Norinyl 2164

Prostate disease, unspecified
Ansaid Tablets (Less than 1%) 2579
Dilacor XR Extended-release Capsules (Infrequent) 2018

Prostatic cancer, transient worsening symptoms
Zoladex (Occasional) 2858

Prostatic disorder
Anafranil Capsules (Infrequent) 803
Caverject (2%) 2583
Monoket (Fewer than 1%) 2406
Videx Tablets, Powder for Oral Solution, & Pediatric Powder for Oral Solution (Less than 1%) 720

Prostatic hypertrophy
Android Capsules, 10 mg 1250
Android 1251
Caverject (2%) 2583
Eldepryl Tablets 2550
Halotestin Tablets 2614
Oreton Methyl 1255
Testoderm Testosterone Transdermal System (One in 104 patients) 486
Winstrol Tablets 2337

Prostatitis
BCG Vaccine, USP (TICE) (0.3%) 1814
Caverject (2%) 2583
Effexor (Infrequent) 2719
Kerlone Tablets (Less than 2%) 2436
Rogaine Topical Solution (0.91%) 2637
Testoderm Testosterone Transdermal System (Four in 104 patients) 486

Prostration
Bicillin C-R Injection 2704
Bicillin C-R 900/300 Injection 2706
Bicillin L-A Injection 2707
Pfizerpen for Injection 2203

Protein bound iodine, lowered (see under PBI decrease)

Protein catabolism
Aristocort Suspension (Forte Parenteral) 1027
Aristocort Tablets 1022
Aristospan Suspension (Intra-articular) 1033
Aristospan Suspension (Intralesional) 1032
Celestone Soluspan Suspension 2347
CORTENEMA 2535
Depo-Medrol Single-Dose Vial 2600
Dexacort Phosphate in Respihaler 458
Dexacort Phosphate in Turbinaire 459
Florinef Acetate Tablets 505
Hydeltrasol Injection, Sterile 1665
Hydeltra-T.B.A. Sterile Suspension 1667

(Described in PDR For Nonprescription Drugs) Incidence data in parenthesis; ▲ 3% or more (◉ Described in PDR For Ophthalmology)

1393 Side Effects Index Pruritus

Hydrocortone Acetate Sterile Suspension ... 1669
Hydrocortone Phosphate Injection, Sterile ... 1670
Hydrocortone Tablets ... 1672

Proteinuria

▲ Accutane Capsules (Less than 1 patient in 10) ... 2076
Children's Advil Suspension ... 2692
Altace Capsules (Scattered incidents) ... 1232
Anaprox/Naprosyn ... 2117
Atgam Sterile Solution (Less than 5%) ... 2581
Atromid-S Capsules ... 2701
Azulfidine (Rare) ... 1949
▲ Betaseron for SC Injection (5%) ... 658
Calcium Disodium Versenate Injection ... 1490
Capoten (Approximately 1 of 100 patients) ... 739
Capozide (About 1 of 100 patients) ... 742
Cataflam (Less than 1%) ... 816
Ceclor Pulvules & Suspension (Infrequent) ... 1431
Celontin Kapseals ... 1899
Cleocin Phosphate Injection (Rare) 2586
Cleocin Vaginal Cream (Rare) ... 2589
Clinoril Tablets (Less than 1 in 100) ... 1618
▲ Cuprimine Capsules (6%) ... 1630
Cytovene-IV (One report) ... 2103
Daypro Caplets ... 2426
▲ Depen Titratable Tablets (6%) ... 2662
Dipentum Capsules (Rare) ... 1951
Dolobid Tablets (Less than 1 in 100) ... 1654
EC-Naprosyn Delayed-Release Tablets ... 2117
Elspar (Infrequent) ... 1659
Eminase ... 2039
Feldene Capsules (Less than 1%) .. 1965
Floxin I.V. (More than or equal to 1%) ... 1571
Floxin Tablets (200 mg, 300 mg, 400 mg) (More than or equal to 1.0%) ... 1567
Fludara for Injection (Up to 1%) ... 663
Fulvicin P/G Tablets (Rare) ... 2359
Fulvicin P/G 165 & 330 Tablets (Rare) ... 2359
Garamycin Injectable ... 2360
Grifulvin V (griseofulvin tablets) Microsize (griseofulvin oral suspension) Microsize (Rare) ... 1888
Gris-PEG Tablets, 125 mg & 250 mg (Rare) ... 479
IFEX (Rare) ... 697
Indocin (Less than 1%) ... 1680
Kerlone Tablets (Less than 2%) ... 2436
Lincocin (Rare instances) ... 2617
Lotensin Tablets (Scattered incidents) ... 834
Lotensin HCT ... 837
Mithracin ... 607
Children's Motrin Ibuprofen Oral Suspension ... 1546
Motrin Tablets ... 2625
Motrin Ibuprofen Suspension, Oral Drops, Chewable Tablets, Caplets ... 1546
Myochrysine Injection ... 1711
Anaprox/Naprosyn ... 2117
Nebcin Vials, Hyporets & ADD-Vantage ... 1464
Netromycin Injection 100 mg/ml ... 2373
Neupogen for Injection (Infrequent) ... 495
Prilosec Delayed-Release Capsules (Less than 1%) ... 529
Primaxin I.M. ... 1727
Primaxin I.V. ... 1729
▲ Proleukin for Injection (12%) ... 797
Ridaura Capsules (0.9%) ... 2513
Roferon-A Injection (Less than 1%) ... 2145
Sinemet CR Tablets ... 944
Solganal Suspension ... 2388
▲ Tegison Capsules (1-10%) ... 2154
Tolectin (200, 400 and 600 mg) (Less than 1%) ... 1581
Toradol (1% or less) ... 2159
Tornalate Metered Dose Inhaler (Rare) ... 957
Ultram Tablets (50 mg) (Infrequent) ... 1585
Voltaren Tablets (Less than 1%) ... 861
Zosyn ... 1419
Zosyn Pharmacy Bulk Package ... 1422

Proteinuria, increased

Bumex ... 2093
▲ CHEMET (succimer) Capsules (Up to 3.7%) ... 1545
Noroxin Tablets (1.0%) ... 1715
Noroxin Tablets (1.0%) ... 2048
Penetrex Tablets (Less than 1%) ... 2031
Tobramycin Sulfate Injection ... 968

Prothrombin, decrease (see under Hypoprothrombinemia)

Prothrombin, increase (see under Hyperprothrombinemia)

Prothrombin time, deviation

Bumex (0.8%) ... 2093
Rythmol Tablets–150mg, 225mg, 300mg (Less than 1%) ... 1352

Prothrombin time, increase (see under Prothrombin time prolongation)

Prothrombin time prolongation

Azactam for Injection ... 734
Biaxin (1%) ... 405
Cefizox for Intramuscular or Intravenous Use ... 1034
Cefotan ... 2829
Ceftin ... 1078
Cefzil Tablets and Oral Suspension 746
Ceptaz ... 1081
Cipro I.V. ... 595
Cipro I.V. Pharmacy Bulk Package (Less than 1%) ... 597
Cipro Tablets ... 592
Clinoril Tablets ... 1618
Duricef ... 748
Felbatol ... 2666
Floxin I.V. ... 1571
Floxin Tablets (200 mg, 300 mg, 400 mg) ... 1567
Fortaz ... 1100
Sterile FUDR ... 2118
Hespan Injection ... 929
Keftab Tablets ... 915
Kefurox Vials, Faspak & ADD-Vantage ... 1454
Lorabid Suspension and Pulvules (Rare) ... 1459
Maxaquin Tablets (Less than or equal to 0.1%) ... 2440
Netromycin Injection 100 mg/ml (1 of 1000 patients) ... 2373
Noroxin Tablets ... 1715
Noroxin Tablets ... 2048
Oncaspar ... 2028
Ortho-Cyclen/Ortho-Tri-Cyclen ... 1858
Ortho-Cyclen/Ortho Tri-Cyclen ... 1858
Oxandrin ... 2862
Panhematin ... 443
Penetrex Tablets ... 2031
Pentaspan Injection ... 937
Primaxin I.M. ... 1727
Primaxin I.V. ... 1729
Provera Tablets ... 2636
Questran Light ... 769
Questran Powder ... 770
Rocephin Injectable Vials, ADD-Vantage, Galaxy Container (Less than 1%) ... 2142
Suprax (Rare) ... 1399
Tazicef for Injection ... 2519
▲ Tegison Capsules (10-25%) ... 2154
Timentin for Injection ... 2528
Vantin for Oral Suspension and Vantin Tablets ... 2646
Zefazone ... 2654
Zinacef ... 1211
Zosyn ... 1419
Zosyn Pharmacy Bulk Package ... 1422

Pruritus

▲ A/T/S 2% Acne Topical Gel and Solution (17 out of 90 patients; occasional) ... 1234
Accupril Tablets (0.5% to 1.0%) .. 1893
▲ Accutane Capsules (Up to 80%) ... 2076
Aclovate (2 in 100 patients) ... 1069
Actigall Capsules ... 802
Adalat Capsules (10 mg and 20 mg) (2% or less) ... 587
Adalat CC (Less than 1.0%) ... 589
Children's Advil Suspension (Less than 3%) ... 2692
▲ AeroBid Inhaler System (3-9%) ... 1005
▲ Aerobid-M Inhaler System (3-9%) .. 1005
AK-Spore ... ◉ 204
Aldactazide ... 2413
Alfenta Injection (0.3% to 1%) ... 1286
Alkeran for Injection ... 1070
Altace Capsules (Less than 1%) ... 1232
Alupent Tablets (0.4%) ... 669
Amen Tablets (Occasional) ... 780
Americaine Anesthetic Lubricant ... 983
Americaine Otic Topical Anesthetic Ear Drops ... 983
▲ Anafranil Capsules (2% to 6%) ... 803
Analpram-HC Rectal Cream 1% and 2.5% ... 977
▲ Anaprox/Naprosyn (3% to 9%) ... 2117
Ancef Injection ... 2465
Ancobon Capsules ... 2079
Anexia Tablets ... 1782
Ansaid Tablets (Less than 1%) ... 2579
Antivenin (Crotalidae) Polyvalent ... 2696
Anusol-HC Cream 2.5% (Infrequent to frequent) ... 1896
Anusol-HC Suppositories ... 1897
Apresazide Capsules (Less frequent) ... 808
Apresoline Hydrochloride Tablets (Less frequent) ... 809
Aralen Hydrochloride Injection ... 2301
Aralen Phosphate Tablets ... 2301
Arfonad Ampuls ... 2080
Aristocort A 0.025% Cream (Infrequent) ... 1027
Aristocort A 0.1% Cream (Infrequent) ... 1029
Aristocort A 0.1% Ointment (Infrequent) ... 1030
▲ Asacol Delayed-Release Tablets (3%) ... 1979
Asendin Tablets (Less than 1%) ... 1369
▲ Astramorph/PF Injection, USP (Preservative-Free) (High incidence) ... 535
▲ Atgam Sterile Solution (1 in 8 patients) ... 2581
Atromid-S Capsules (Less often) ... 2701
Atrovent Inhalation Aerosol (Less frequent) ... 671
Augmentin ... 2468
Axid Pulvules (1.7%) ... 1427
Aygestin Tablets ... 974
Azactam for Injection (Less than 1%) ... 734
Azo Gantanol Tablets ... 2080
Azo Gantrisin Tablets ... 2081
Azulfidine (One in every 30 patients or less) ... 1949
Bactrim DS Tablets ... 2084
Bactrim I.V. Infusion ... 2082
Bactrim ... 2084
Bactroban Ointment (1%) ... 2470
Benemid Tablets ... 1611
Bentyl ... 1501
Benzamycin Topical Gel ... 905
Betagan (Rare) ... ◉ 233
Betapace Tablets (Rare) ... 641
Blenoxane ... 692
Blocadren Tablets (1.1%) ... 1614
Brevital Sodium Vials ... 1429
▲ Bromfed-DM Cough Syrup (Among most frequent) ... 1786
Brontex (Infrequent) ... 1981
Bumex (0.1% to 0.4%) ... 2093
Buprenex Injectable (Less than 1%) ... 2006
BuSpar (Infrequent) ... 737
Cafergot ... 2251
Capoten (About 2 of 100 patients) 739
Capozide (About 2 of 100 patients) ... 742
Carafate Suspension (Less than 0.5%) ... 1505
Carafate Tablets (Less than 0.5%) 1504
Carbocaine Hydrochloride Injection 2303
Cardizem CD Capsules (Less than 1%) ... 1506
Cardizem SR Capsules (Less than 1%) ... 1510
Cardizem Injectable (Less than 1%) ... 1508
Cardizem Tablets (Less than 1%) .. 1512
Cardura Tablets (1%) ... 2186
Cataflam (1% to 3%) ... 816
Catapres Tablets (About 7 in 1,000 patients) ... 674
▲ Catapres-TTS (51 of 101 patients; less frequent) ... 675
Caverject (Less than 1%) ... 2583
Ceclor Pulvules & Suspension (Less than 1 in 200) ... 1431
Cefizox for Intramuscular or Intravenous Use (Greater than 1% but less than 5%) ... 1034
Cefotan (1 in 700) ... 2829
Ceftin (Less than 1% but more than 0.1%) ... 1078
▲ CellCept Capsules (More than or equal to 3%) ... 2099
Ceptaz (2% of patients) ... 1081
Ceredase ... 1065
Cerezyme (One patient) ... 1066
Cerumenex Drops (1% of 2,700 patients) ... 1993
▲ CHEMET (succimer) Capsules (2.6 to 11.2%) ... 1545
Chloresium (A few instances) ... 2246
Chloroptic S.O.P. ... ◉ 239
Cipro I.V. (1% or less) ... 595
Cipro I.V. Pharmacy Bulk Package (Less than 1%) ... 597
Cipro Tablets (Less than 1%) ... 592
Claforan Sterile and Injection (2.4%) ... 1235
Claritin (2% or fewer patients) ... 2349
Claritin-D (Less frequent) ... 2350
▲ Cleocin T Topical (10%) ... 2590
Clinoril Tablets (Greater than 1%) 1618
Clomid ... 1514
Clozaril Tablets (Less than 1%) ... 2252
▲ Cognex Capsules (7%) ... 1901
ColBENEMID Tablets ... 1622
Coly-Mycin M Parenteral ... 1905
Compazine ... 2470
Cordran Lotion (Infrequent) ... 1803
Cordran Tape (Infrequent) ... 1804
Cortisporin Cream ... 1084
Cortisporin Ointment ... 1085
Cortisporin Ophthalmic Ointment Sterile ... 1085
Cortisporin Ophthalmic Suspension Sterile ... 1086
Cortisporin Otic Solution Sterile ... 1087
Cortisporin Otic Suspension Sterile 1088
Cozaar Tablets (Less than 1%) ... 1628
▲ Cuprimine Capsules (5%) ... 1630
Cutivate Cream (2.9%) ... 1088
Cutivate Ointment (2.9%) ... 1089
Cyclocort Topical (Infrequent) ... 1037
Cycrin Tablets (Occasional) ... 975
▲ Cytadren Tablets (1 in 20) ... 819
Cytosar-U Sterile Powder (Less frequent) ... 2592
▲ Cytovene (6%) ... 2103
▲ DHCplus Capsules (Among most frequent) ... 1993
D.H.E. 45 Injection ... 2255
Dalgan Injection (Less than 1%) ... 538
Dalmane Capsules (Rare) ... 2173
Danocrine Capsules ... 2307
Dantrium Capsules (Less frequent) 1982
Daranide Tablets ... 1633
Daypro Caplets (Less than 1%) ... 2426
Decadron Phosphate Topical Cream ... 1644
Decaspray Topical Aerosol ... 1648
Demerol ... 2308
Depakene ... 413
Depakote Tablets ... 415
▲ Depen Titratable Tablets (5%) ... 2662
Depo-Provera Sterile Aqueous Suspension ... 2606
Dermatop Emollient Cream 0.1% (Less than 1%) ... 1238
Desferal Vials ... 820
DesOwen Cream, Ointment and Lotion (Less than 2%) ... 1046
Desyrel and Desyrel Dividose ... 503
DiaBeta Tablets (1.5%) ... 1239
Diabinese Tablets (Less than 3%) .. 1935
Didronel Tablets ... 1984
Dilacor XR Extended-release Capsules ... 2018
Dilaudid-HP Injection (Less frequent) ... 1337
Dilaudid-HP Lyophilized Powder 250 mg (Less frequent) ... 1337
Dilaudid Tablets and Liquid ... 1339
Dimetane-DC Cough Syrup ... 2059
Dimetane-DX Cough Syrup ... 2059
Dipentum Capsules (1.3%) ... 1951
Diprivan Injection (Less than 1%) .. 2833
Diprolene AF Cream (Infrequent) ... 2352
Diprolene Gel 0.05% (2%) ... 2353
Diprolene (2%) ... 2352
Diupres Tablets ... 1650
Dolobid Tablets (Less than 1 in 100) ... 1654
Dopram Injectable ... 2061
Doral Tablets ... 2664
▲ Dovonex Ointment 0.005% (Approximately 10% to 15%) ... 2684
▲ Duragesic Transdermal System (1% to 10%) ... 1288

(▣ Described in PDR For Nonprescription Drugs) Incidence data in parenthesis; ▲ 3% or more (◉ Described in PDR For Ophthalmology)

Pruritus Side Effects Index 1394

▲ Duramorph (High incidence; occasional) 962
DynaCirc Capsules (0.5% to 1%) 2256
Easprin 1914
▲ EC-Naprosyn Delayed-Release Tablets (3% to 9%) 2117
Effexor (1%) 2719
▲ Efudex (Among most frequent) 2113
Elase-Chloromycetin Ointment 1040
▲ Elimite (permethrin) 5% Cream (7%) 478
Elocon (1 of 319 patients) 2354
Emcyt Capsules (2%) 1953
Emgel 2% Topical Gel (Occasional) 1093
Eminase (Occasional) 2039
Emla Cream (2%) 545
Empirin with Codeine Tablets 1093
Engerix-B Unit-Dose Vials (Less than 1%) 2482
Ergamisol Tablets (1% to 2%) 1292
Ergomar 1486
Erycette (erythromycin 2%) Topical Solution 1888
Esgic-plus Tablets (Infrequent) 1013
Ethmozine Tablets (Less than 2%) 2041
Etrafon 2355
Eulexin Capsules 2358
Exact Vanishing and Tinted Creams ▣ 749
▲ Exelderm Cream 1.0% (3%) 2685
Exelderm Solution 1.0% (Approximately 1%) 2686
▲ Famvir (3.7%) 2486
Fansidar Tablets 2114
Felbatol (Frequent) 2666
Feldene Capsules (Occasional) 1965
Femstat Prefill Vaginal Cream 2% (0.2%) 2116
Femstat Vaginal Cream 2% (0.2%) 2115
Fioricet Tablets (Infrequent) 2258
Fioricet with Codeine Capsules (Infrequent) 2260
Fiorinal with Codeine Capsules (Infrequent) 2262
Flagyl I.V. 2247
Flexeril Tablets (Rare) 1661
Florone/Florone E 906
Floxin I.V. (1% to 3%) 1571
Floxin Tablets (200 mg, 300 mg, 400 mg) (1% to 3%) 1567
Fludara for Injection (1% to 3%) 663
Fluorescite ⊙ 219
Fluoroplex Topical Solution & Cream 1% 479
Fortaz (2%) 1100
Foscavir Injection (Between 1% and 5%) 547
Fragmin (Rare) 1954
Fungizone Intravenous 506
Furacin Soluble Dressing (Approximately 1%) 2045
Furacin Topical Cream (Approximately 1%) 2045
Gamimune N, 5% Immune Globulin Intravenous (Human), 5% 619
Gamimune N, 10% Immune Globulin Intravenous (Human), 10% (A single incidence) 621
Gantanol Tablets 2119
Gantrisin 2120
Garamycin Injectable 2360
▲ Gastrocrom Capsules (3 of 87 patients) 984
Geocillin Tablets (Infrequent) 2199
Glucotrol Tablets (About 1 in 70) 1967
Glucotrol XL Extended Release Tablets (Less than 3%) 1968
Glynase PresTab Tablets (1.5%) 2609
Habitrol Nicotine Transdermal System (Once in 35% of patients) 865
Halcion Tablets 2611
Halog (Infrequent) 2686
Havrix (Less than 1%) 2489
Heparin Lock Flush Solution 2725
Heparin Sodium Injection 2726
Heparin Sodium Injection, USP, Sterile Solution 2615
Heparin Sodium Vials 1441
Herplex Liquifilm ⊙ 244
Hespan Injection 929
Hexalen Capsules (Less than 1%) 2571
Hismanal Tablets (Less frequent) 1293
Hivid Tablets (Less than 1% to less than 3%) 2121
Hycodan Tablets and Syrup 930
Hycomine 931
Hydrocet Capsules 782
Hydropres Tablets 1675
Hyskon Hysteroscopy Fluid (Rare) 1595
Hytone 907
Hytrin Capsules (At least 1%) 430
Hyzaar Tablets 1677
IBU Tablets (Greater than 1%) 1342
Imdur (Less than or equal to 5%) 1323
Imitrex Injection (Infrequent) 1103
Imitrex Tablets (Infrequent) 1106
Indocin (Less than 1%) 1680
INFeD (Iron Dextran Injection, USP) 2345
Infumorph 200 and Infumorph 500 Sterile Solutions (Occasional) 965
▲ Intron A (Up to 11%) 2364
IOPIDINE Sterile Ophthalmic Solution ⊙ 219
Ismo Tablets (Fewer than 1%) 2738
Isoptin Injectable (Rare) 1344
JE-VAX 886
Kefurox Vials, Faspak & ADD-Vantage (Less than 1 in 250) 1454
Kerlone Tablets (Less than 2%) 2436
▲ Lamictal Tablets (3.1%) 1112
Lamisil Cream 1% (0.2%) 2265
▲ Lamprene Capsules (1-5%) 828
Lariam Tablets (Less than 1%) 2128
Lasix Injection, Oral Solution and Tablets 1240
Lescol Capsules 2267
▲ Leustatin (6%) 1834
Levo-Dromoran (Rare) 2129
Levoprome 1274
Lidex (Infrequent) 2130
Limbitrol 2180
Lioresal Intrathecal (1 to 8 of 214 patients) 1596
Lioresal Tablets 829
Lithium Carbonate Capsules & Tablets 2230
Lithonate/Lithotabs/Lithobid 2543
Locoid Cream, Ointment and Topical Solution (Infrequent) 978
Lodine Capsules and Tablets (More than 1% but less than 3%) 2743
Lomotil 2439
Lopid Tablets 1917
▲ Lopressor Ampuls (5%) 830
Lopressor HCT Tablets (Fewer than 1 in 100) 832
▲ Lopressor Tablets (5%) 830
Lorabid Suspension and Pulvules 1459
Lorelco Tablets 1517
Lortab 2566
Lotensin Tablets 834
Lotensin HCT (0.3% or more) 837
Lotrimin 2371
Lotrisone Cream 2372
Loxitane 1378
Lozol Tablets (Less than 5%) 2022
Ludiomil Tablets (Rare) 843
Lupron Depot 7.5 mg 2559
Lupron Injection (Less than 5%) 2555
Lutrepulse for Injection 980
Luvox Tablets 2544
MS Contin Tablets (Less frequent) 1994
MSIR (Infrequent) 1997
Macrobid Capsules (Less than 1%) 1988
Macrodantin Capsules 1989
Marcaine Hydrochloride with Epinephrine 1:200,000 (Rare) 2316
Marcaine Hydrochloride Injection (Rare) 2316
Marcaine Spinal (Rare) 2319
Matulane Capsules 2131
Maxair Autohaler 1492
Maxair Inhaler (Less than 1%) 1494
Maxaquin Tablets (Less than 1%) 2440
Mefoxin 1691
Mefoxin Premixed Intravenous Solution 1694
Megace Oral Suspension (1% to 3%) 699
▲ Mepron Suspension (5%) 1135
Methadone Hydrochloride Oral Concentrate 2233
Methadone Hydrochloride Oral Solution & Tablets 2235
Methotrexate Sodium Tablets, Injection, for Injection and LPF Injection (1 to 3%) 1275
MetroGel-Vaginal (Equal to or less than 2%) 902
▲ Mevacor Tablets (0.5% to 5.2%) 1699
Mezlin 601
Mezlin Pharmacy Bulk Package 604
Miacalcin Nasal Spray (Less than 1%) 2275
Micronase Tablets (1.5%) 2623
Midamor Tablets (Less than or equal to 1%) 1703
Milontin Kapseals 1920
Minipress Capsules (Less than 1%) 1937
Minizide Capsules (Rare) 1938
Mintezol 1704
Moduretic Tablets (Greater than 1%, less than 3%) 1705
▲ 8-MOP Capsules (Approximately 10%) 1246
Monocid Injection (Less than 1%) 2497
Monoket (Up to 2%) 2406
Monopril Tablets (0.2% to 1.0%) 757
Motofen Tablets 784
Children's Motrin Ibuprofen Oral Suspension (Greater than 1% but less than 3%) 1546
Motrin Tablets (Less than 3%) 2625
Motrin Ibuprofen Suspension, Oral Drops, Chewable Tablets, Caplets (1% to less than 3%) 1546
Myambutol Tablets 1386
Mycelex Troches 608
Mykrox Tablets (Less than 2%) 993
Myochrysine Injection 1711
Naftin Cream 1% (2%) 480
Naftin Gel 1% (1.0%) 481
▲ Nalfon 200 Pulvules & Nalfon Tablets (4.2%) 917
▲ Anaprox/Naprosyn (3% to 9%) 2117
Navane Capsules and Concentrate 2201
Navane Intramuscular 2202
Nebcin Vials, Hyporets & ADD-Vantage 1464
NebuPent for Inhalation Solution (1% or less) 1040
NegGram 2323
NeoDecadron Topical Cream 1714
Neoral (Rare) 2276
Neosporin Ophthalmic Ointment Sterile 1148
Neosporin Ophthalmic Solution Sterile 1149
Nescaine/Nescaine MPF 554
Netromycin Injection 100 mg/ml (4 or 5 of 1000 patients) 2373
Neurontin Capsules (1.3%) 1922
▲ Neutrexin (5.5%) 2572
Nicobid 2026
Nicoderm (nicotine transdermal system) 1518
Nicolar Tablets 2026
Nicorette 2458
Nicotrol Nicotine Transdermal System (At least once in 47 patients) 1550
Nimotop Capsules (Less than 1%) 610
▲ Nizoral 2% Cream (5%) 1297
Nizoral 2% Shampoo (One occurrence in 41 patients) 1298
Nizoral Tablets (1.5%) 1298
Norflex 1496
Normodyne Injection (Rare; 1%) 2377
Normodyne Tablets (Rare) 2379
Noroxin Tablets (0.3 to 1.0%) 1715
Noroxin Tablets (0.3% to 1.0%) 2048
Norpace (1 to 3%) 2444
Norplant System 2759
Norpramin Tablets 1526
Norvasc Tablets (More than 0.1% to 1%) 1940
Novahistine DH 2462
Novahistine Expectorant 2463
Nubain Injection (1% or less) 935
Numorphan Injection 936
Numorphan Suppositories 937
Omnipen for Oral Suspension 2765
Oncaspar (Less than 1%) 2028
Oramorph SR (Morphine Sulfate Sustained Release Tablets) (Less frequent) 2236
Orthoclone OKT3 Sterile Solution 1837
Orudis Capsules (Less than 1%) 2766
Oruvail Capsules (Less than 1%) 2766
Oxistat (1.6%) 1152
▲ Oxsoralen-Ultra Capsules (10%) 1257
PMB 200 and PMB 400 2783
PPD Tine Test 2874
Pamelor 2280
Paraflex Caplets 1580
Parafon Forte DSC Caplets 1581
Paraplatin for Injection 705
Paxil Tablets (Frequent) 2505
PediOtic Suspension Sterile 1153
Penetrex Tablets (1%) 2031
Pentasa (Less than 1%) 1527
Pepcid Injection (Infrequent) 1722
Pepcid (Infrequent) 1720
Percocet Tablets 938
Percodan Tablets 939
Percodan-Demi Tablets 940
Permax Tablets (Infrequent) 575
Persantine Tablets 681
Phenergan with Codeine (Infrequent) 2777
Phenergan VC with Codeine 2781
PhosLo Tablets (Isolated cases) 690
Phrenilin (Infrequent) 785
Pipracil (Less frequent) 1390
Plaquenil Sulfate Tablets 2328
Pramosone Cream, Lotion & Ointment 978
Pravachol 765
Premphase 2797
Prempro 2801
PREVACID Delayed-Release Capsules (Less than 1%) 2562
Prilosec Delayed-Release Capsules (Less than 1%) 529
Primaxin I.M. 1727
Primaxin I.V. (0.3%) 1729
Prinivil Tablets (1.2% to 1.5%) 1733
Prinzide Tablets (0.3 to 1%) 1737
Procan SR Tablets (Occasional) 1926
Procardia Capsules (2% or less) 1971
Procardia XL Extended Release Tablets (Less than 3%) 1972
ProctoCream-HC (Infrequent) 2408
ProctoCream-HC 2.5% (Infrequent to frequent) 2408
Proglycem 580
▲ Prograf (11% to 36%) 1042
▲ Proleukin for Injection (48%) 797
Prolixin 509
▲ Proloprim Tablets (Most often) 1155
Propulsid (1.2%) 1300
ProSom Tablets (1%) 449
Prostep (nicotine transdermal system) 1394
Provera Tablets (An occasional patient) 2636
Provocholine for Inhalation (1 occurrence) 2140
Prozac Pulvules & Liquid, Oral Solution (2.4%; 3%) 919
Psorcon Cream 0.05% (Infrequent) 909
Psorcon Ointment 0.05% 908
Pyrazinamide Tablets 1398
Pyridium 1928
Quinaglute Dura-Tabs Tablets 649
Quinidex Extentabs 2067
RMS Suppositories 2657
Recombivax HB (Less than 1%) 1744
▲ Relafen Tablets (3% to 9%) 2510
ReoPro Vials (0.3%) 1471
Retrovir Capsules 1158
Retrovir I.V. Infusion 1163
Retrovir Syrup 1158
▲ Rēv-Eyes Ophthalmic Eyedrops 0.5% (10% to 40%) ⊙ 323
ReVia Tablets (Less than 1%) 940
Revex (Less than 1%) 1811
Rhinocort Nasal Inhaler (Less than 1%) 556
▲ Ridaura Capsules (17%) 2513
Rifadin (Occasional) 1528
Rifamate Capsules (Occasional) 1530
Rifater (Occasional) 1532
Rimactane Capsules (Occasional) 847
Risperdal (Infrequent) 1301
Robaxin Injectable 2070
Robaxin Tablets 2071
Robaxisal Tablets 2071
Rocaltrol Capsules 2141
Rocephin Injectable Vials, ADD-Vantage, Galaxy Container (Less than 1%) 2142
▲ Roferon-A Injection (5% to 13%) 2145
Rogaine Topical Solution 2637
Rowasa (1.23%) 2548
Roxanol 2243
Roxicodone Tablets, Oral Solution & Intensol (Oxycodone) 2244
Rythmol Tablets–150mg, 225mg, 300mg (Less than 1%) 1352
Salagen Tablets (1%) 1489
Sandimmune (Rare) 2286
Sandostatin Injection (1% to 4%) 2292
Sectral Capsules (Up to 2%) 2807
Sedapap Tablets 50 mg/650 mg (Infrequent) 1543
Seldane Tablets (1.0% to 1.6%) 1536
Seldane-D Extended-Release Tablets 1538
Sensorcaine (Rare) 559
Septra 1174
Septra I.V. Infusion 1169

(▣ Described in PDR For Nonprescription Drugs) Incidence data in parenthesis; ▲ 3% or more (⊙ Described in PDR For Ophthalmology)

Septra I.V. Infusion ADD-Vantage Vials 1171
Septra 1174
Ser-Ap-Es Tablets 849
Serentil 684
Serzone Tablets (2%) 771
Sinequan (Occasional) 2205
Skelaxin Tablets 788
Slo-Niacin Tablets 2659
Solganal Suspension 2388
Soma Compound w/Codeine Tablets (Rare) 2676
Soma Compound Tablets (Less common) 2675
Soma Tablets 2674
▲ Spectazole (econazole nitrate 1%) Cream (3%) 1890
Sporanox Capsules (0.7% to 2.5%) 1305
Stadol (1% or greater) 775
Stelazine 2514
Streptase for Infusion 562
Stri-Dex ▣ 730
Sublimaze Injection 1307
▲ Sufenta Injection (25%) 1309
Sulfamylon Cream 925
Supprelin Injection (1% to 3%) 2056
Suprane (Less than 1%) 1813
Suprax (Less than 2%) 1399
Surmontil Capsules 2811
Synalar (Infrequent) 2130
Synarel Nasal Solution for Central Precocious Puberty (2.6%) 2151
Synemol Cream 0.025% (Infrequent) 2130
T-Stat 2.0% Topical Solution and Pads 2688
Talwin Injection 2334
Talwin Nx 2336
Tambocor Tablets (Less than 1%) 1497
Tapazole Tablets 1477
Tazicef for Injection (2%) 2519
Tazidime Vials, Faspak & ADD-Vantage (2%) 1478
▲ Tegison Capsules (50-75%) 2154
Temovate (1 of 421 patients; infrequent) 1179
Tenex Tablets (3% or less) 2074
Terazol 3 Vaginal Suppositories (1.8% of 284 patients) 1886
Tessalon Perles 1020
▲ Testoderm Testosterone Transdermal System (7%) 486
Theramycin Z Topical Solution 2% 1592
Ticar for Injection 2526
Ticlid Tablets (1.3%) 2156
Timentin for Injection 2528
Timolide Tablets 1748
Timoptic in Ocudose 1753
Timoptic Sterile Ophthalmic Solution 1751
Timoptic-XE 1755
Tobramycin Sulfate Injection 968
Tofranil Ampuls 854
Tofranil Tablets 856
Tofranil-PM Capsules 857
Tonocard Tablets (Less than 1%) 531
Topicort (Infrequent) 1243
▲ Toprol-XL Tablets (About 5 of 100 patients) 565
Toradol (Greater than 1%) 2159
Tornalate Solution for Inhalation, 0.2% 956
Tracrium Injection (0.2%) 1183
Trandate (Rare; 1 of 100 patients) 1185
Trasylol 613
Trental Tablets (Less than 1%) 1244
Triavil Tablets 1757
Tridesilon Cream 0.05% (Infrequent) 615
Tridesilon Ointment 0.05% (Infrequent) 616
Trilafon 2389
Trilisate (Less than 1%) 2000
Trimpex Tablets 2163
T.R.U.E. Test (Common; up to 48 reports) 1189
Tuberculin, Old, Tine Test 2875
Tussionex Pennkinetic Extended-Release Suspension 998
Tussi-Organidin NR Liquid and S NR Liquid (Rare) 2677
Tylenol with Codeine 1583
Tylox Capsules 1584
Tympagesic Ear Drops 2342
▲ Ultram Tablets (50 mg) (8% to 11%) 1585
▲ Ultravate Cream 0.05% (4.4%) 2689
Ultravate Ointment 0.05% 2690
Unasyn (Less than 1%) 2212
Univasc Tablets (Less than 1%) 2410
▲ Vagistat-1 (Approximately 5%) 778
Vancocin HCl, Vials & ADD-Vantage 1481
Varivax (Greater than or equal to 1%) 1762
Vaseretic Tablets (0.5% to 2.0%) 1765
Vasotec I.V. 1768
Vasotec Tablets (0.5% to 1.0%) 1771
VePesid Capsules and Injection (Infrequent) 718
Versed Injection (Less than 1%) 2170
Vexol 1% Ophthalmic Suspension (1% to 5%) ⊙ 230
▲ Videx Tablets, Powder for Oral Solution, & Pediatric Powder for Oral Solution (7% to 72%) 720
Visken Tablets (1%) 2299
Vivactil Tablets 1774
Voltaren Tablets (1% to 3%) 861
Wellbutrin Tablets (2.2%) 1204
Westcort 2690
Wigraine Tablets & Suppositories 1829
Xanax Tablets 2649
Xerac AC 1933
Yodoxin 1230
Zantac Injection 1207
Zebeta Tablets 1413
Zefazone 2654
Zemuron (Less than 1%) 1830
▲ Zerit Capsules (Fewer than 1% to 12%) 729
Zestoretic (0.3 to 1%) 2850
Zestril Tablets (1.2% to 1.5%) 2854
Ziac 1415
Zinacef (Fewer than 1 in 250 patients) 1211
Zocor Tablets 1775
Zofran Injection (2%) 1214
▲ Zofran Tablets (5%) 1217
Zoladex (2%) 2858
Zoloft Tablets (Infrequent) 2217
▲ Zosyn (3.1%) 1419
▲ Zosyn Pharmacy Bulk Package (3.1%) 1422
Zovirax Capsules 1219
Zovirax Ointment 5% 1223
Zovirax Sterile Powder (Approximately 2%) 1223
Zovirax 1219
Zyloprim Tablets (Less than 1%) 1226

Pruritus, ear lobes

Miacalcin Injection 2273

Pruritus, exacerbation of

Actigall Capsules (One patient) 802
▲ Zonalon Cream (Approximately 1% to 10%) 1055

Pruritus, genital

Anafranil Capsules (Infrequent) 803
Ancef Injection 2465
Ceclor Pulvules & Suspension (Less than 1 in 100) 1431
Ceftin (Less than 1% but more than 0.1%) 1078
Cefzil Tablets and Oral Suspension (1.6%) 746
Cipro Tablets (1%) 592
Cognex Capsules (Infrequent) 1901
▲ Condylox (50% to 65%) 1802
Duricef 748
▲ Floxin I.V. (1% to 6%) 1571
▲ Floxin Tablets (200 mg, 300 mg, 400 mg) (1% to 6%) 1567
Foscavir Injection (Less than 1%) 547
Keflex Pulvules & Oral Suspension 914
Keftab Tablets 915
Kefzol Vials, Faspak & ADD-Vantage 1456
Neurontin Capsules (Rare) 1922
Nolvadex Tablets (Infrequent) 2841
Primaxin I.M. 1727
Primaxin I.V. (Less than 0.2%) 1729
ProSom Tablets (Infrequent) 449
Risperdal (Rare) 1301
Semicid Vaginal Contraceptive Inserts ▣ 874
Supprelin Injection (1% to 3%) 2056
Suprax (Les than 2%) 1399
▲ Terazol 3 Vaginal Cream (5%) 1886
Terazol 3 Vaginal Suppositories (1.8% of 284 patients) 1886
Terazol 7 Vaginal Cream (2.3% of 521 patients) 1887
Today Vaginal Contraceptive Sponge ▣ 874
▲ Vagistat-1 (Approximately 5%) 778
Vantin for Oral Suspension and Vantin Tablets (Less than 1%) 2646
Zosyn (1.0% or less) 1419
Zosyn Pharmacy Bulk Package (1.0% or less) 1422

Pruritus, injection site

▲ Cardizem Injectable (3.9%) 1508
Ceredase 1065
Cipro I.V. (1% or less) 595
Diprivan Injection (Less than 1%) 2833
Engerix-B Unit-Dose Vials (Less than 1%) 2482
Factrel (Occasional) 2877
Helixate, Antihemophilic Factor (Recombinant) 518
Humulin 50/50, 100 Units 1444
Humulin 70/30, 100 Units 1445
Humulin L, 100 Units 1446
Regular, 100 Units 1450
Pork Regular, 100 Units 1452
▲ Imovax Rabies Vaccine (About 25%) 881
Intron A (Less than 5%) 2364
KOGENATE Antihemophilic Factor (Recombinant) 632
MSTA Mumps Skin Test Antigen 890
▲ Rabies Vaccine, Imovax Rabies I.D. (About 25%) 883
▲ Supprelin Injection (45%) 2056
Tubersol (Tuberculin Purified Protein Derivative [Mantoux]) 2872
▲ Varivax (19.3% to 32.5%) 1762
Velosulin BR Human Insulin 10 ml Vials 1795

Pruritus, localized

Aristocort A 0.5% Cream 1031
Carmol HC (Infrequent to frequent) 924
Epifoam (Infrequent) 2399
Eskalith 2485
Loprox 1% Cream and Lotion (1 out of 514 patients) 1242
▲ Norplant System (3.7%) 2759
▲ Polytrim Ophthalmic Solution Sterile (Among most frequent) 482
ProctoFoam-HC 2409

Pruritus, not associated with rash

Combipres Tablets (About 7 in 1,000) 677

Pruritus, ocular

AKTOB (Among most frequent) ⊙ 206
▲ Alomide (1% to 5%) 469
▲ Iopidine 0.5% (10%) ⊙ 221
Ocuflox 481
▲ Polysporin Ophthalmic Ointment Sterile (Among those occurring most often) 1154
Stimate, (desmopressin acetate) Nasal Spray, 1.5 mg/mL 525
Tobrex Ophthalmic Ointment and Solution (Less than 3% of 100 patients) ⊙ 229

Pruritus, rhinal

Intal Inhaler (Rare) 988
Intal Nebulizer Solution 989
▲ Miacalcin Nasal Spray (10.6%) 2275

Pruritus ani

Ancef Injection 2465
Foscavir Injection (Less than 1%) 547
Furoxone 2046
Keflex Pulvules & Oral Suspension 914
Keftab Tablets 915
Kefzol Vials, Faspak & ADD-Vantage 1456
Lincocin 2617
Noroxin Tablets (Less frequent) 1715
Noroxin Tablets (Less frequent) 2048
Yodoxin 1230

Pseudolactation

Ser-Ap-Es Tablets 849

Pseudolymphoma

Dilantin Infatabs 1908
Dilantin Kapseals 1906
Dilantin Parenteral (A number of reports) 1910
Dilantin-125 Suspension 1911

Pseudomembranous colitis

Amoxil 2464
Ancef Injection 2465
Augmentin 2468
Azactam for Injection (Less than 1%) 734
Azo Gantrisin Tablets 2081
Ceclor Pulvules & Suspension 1431
Cefizox for Intramuscular or Intravenous Use 1034
Cefobid Intravenous/Intramuscular 2189
Cefobid Pharmacy Bulk Package - Not for Direct Infusion 2192
▲ Cefotan (Among most frequent) 2829
Ceftin 1078
Cefzil Tablets and Oral Suspension (Rare) 746
Ceptaz 1081
Chibroxin Sterile Ophthalmic Solution (With oral form) 1617
Cipro I.V. (1% or less) 595
Cipro I.V. Pharmacy Bulk Package (Less than 1%) 597
Cipro Tablets 592
Claforan Sterile and Injection 1235
Cleocin Phosphate Injection 2586
Cleocin T Topical 2590
Cleocin Vaginal Cream 2589
Duricef 748
E.E.S. (Rare) 424
E-Mycin Tablets 1341
ERYC (Rare) 1915
EryPed (Rare) 421
Ery-Tab Tablets (Rare) 422
Erythrocin Stearate Filmtab (Rare) 425
Erythromycin Base Filmtab (Rare) 426
Erythromycin Delayed-Release Capsules, USP (Rare) 427
Floxin I.V. 1571
Floxin Tablets (200 mg, 300 mg, 400 mg) 1567
Fortaz (Less frequent) 1100
Foscavir Injection (Less than 1%) 547
Gantrisin 2120
Keflex Pulvules & Oral Suspension 914
Keftab Tablets 915
Kefurox Vials, Faspak & ADD-Vantage (1 in 440) 1454
Kefzol Vials, Faspak & ADD-Vantage 1456
Lincocin 2617
Lorabid Suspension and Pulvules 1459
Macrobid Capsules (Sporadic reports) 1988
Macrodantin Capsules 1989
Mandol Vials, Faspak & ADD-Vantage 1461
Maxaquin Tablets 2440
Mefoxin 1691
Mefoxin Premixed Intravenous Solution 1694
Mezlin 601
Mezlin Pharmacy Bulk Package 604
Monocid Injection (Less than 1%) 2497
Noroxin Tablets 1715
Noroxin Tablets 2048
Omnipen Capsules 2764
Omnipen for Oral Suspension 2765
PCE Dispertab Tablets (Rare) 444
Penetrex Tablets (Less than 0.1%) 2031
Pipracil (Rare) 1390
Primaxin I.M. 1727
Primaxin I.V. (Less than 0.2%) 1729
Rifadin 1528
Rifater 1532
Rocephin Injectable Vials, ADD-Vantage, Galaxy Container 2142
Spectrobid Tablets 2206
Suprax (Several patients) 1399
Tazicef for Injection 2519
Ticar for Injection 2526
Timentin for Injection 2528
Unasyn 2212
Vancocin HCl, Vials & ADD-Vantage (Rare instances) 1481
Vantin for Oral Suspension and Vantin Tablets (Less than 1%) 2646
Zefazone (Rare) 2654
Zinacef 1211
Zithromax 1944
Zosyn (One patient) 1419
Zosyn Pharmacy Bulk Package (One patient) 1422

Pseudomembranous enterocolitis

Bactrim DS Tablets 2084
Bactrim I.V. Infusion 2082
Bactrim 2084
Gantanol Tablets 2119
Rimactane Capsules (Rare) 847
Septra 1174
Septra I.V. Infusion 1169
Septra I.V. Infusion ADD-Vantage Vials 1171
Septra 1174
Videx Tablets, Powder for Oral Solution, & Pediatric Powder for Oral Solution (Less than 1%) 720

(▣ Described in PDR For Nonprescription Drugs) Incidence data in parenthesis; ▲ 3% or more (⊙ Described in PDR For Ophthalmology)

Pseudoparkinsonism

BuSpar ... 737
Compazine ... 2470
Mellaril (Infrequent) ... 2269
Navane Capsules and Concentrate 2201
Navane Intramuscular ... 2202
Stelazine ... 2514
Thorazine ... 2523
Triavil Tablets ... 1757
Wellbutrin Tablets (1.5%) ... 1204

Pseudoschizophrenia

Temaril Tablets, Syrup and Spansule Extended-Release Capsules ... 483

Pseudotumor cerebri

Accutane Capsules (A number of cases) ... 2076
Achromycin V Capsules ... 1367
Children's Advil Suspension (Less than 1%) ... 2692
Aristocort Tablets ... 1022
Aristospan Suspension (Intra-articular) ... 1033
Aristospan Suspension (Intralesional) ... 1032
Celestone Soluspan Suspension ... 2347
Cordarone Tablets (Rare) ... 2712
CORTENEMA ... 2535
Cortone Acetate Sterile Suspension ... 1623
Cortone Acetate Tablets ... 1624
Cytovene-IV (One report) ... 2103
Danocrine Capsules ... 2307
Decadron Elixir ... 1633
Decadron Phosphate Injection ... 1637
Decadron Phosphate Respihaler ... 1642
Decadron Phosphate Turbinaire ... 1645
Decadron Phosphate with Xylocaine Injection, Sterile ... 1639
Decadron Tablets ... 1635
Declomycin Tablets ... 1371
Depo-Medrol Single-Dose Vial ... 2600
Depo-Medrol Sterile Aqueous Suspension ... 2597
Dexacort Phosphate in Respihaler .. 458
Dexacort Phosphate in Turbinaire .. 459
Dynacin Capsules ... 1590
Eskalith ... 2485
Florinef Acetate Tablets ... 505
Garamycin Injectable ... 2360
Hydeltrasol Injection, Sterile ... 1665
Hydrocortone Tablets ... 1672
IBU Tablets (Less than 1%) ... 1342
Lithium Carbonate Capsules & Tablets ... 2230
Lithonate/Lithotabs/Lithobid ... 2543
Medrol ... 2621
Minocin Intravenous ... 1382
Minocin Oral Suspension ... 1385
Minocin Pellet-Filled Capsules ... 1383
Children's Motrin Ibuprofen Oral Suspension (Less than 1%) ... 1546
Motrin Tablets (Less than 1%) ... 2625
Motrin Ibuprofen Suspension, Oral Drops, Chewable Tablets, Caplets (Less than 1%) ... 1546
Norplant System ... 2759
Pediapred Oral Liquid ... 995
Synthroid Injection ... 1359
Solu-Cortef Sterile Powder ... 2641
Solu-Medrol Sterile Powder ... 2643
Synthroid Tablets ... 1359
Tegison Capsules ... 2154

Psoriasis

Anafranil Capsules (Infrequent) ... 803
Asacol Delayed-Release Tablets ... 1979
Betaseron for SC Injection ... 658
Cognex Capsules (Infrequent) ... 1901
Desyrel and Desyrel Dividose ... 503
Effexor (Rare) ... 2719
Eskalith ... 2485
Lithonate/Lithotabs/Lithobid ... 2543
Neurontin Capsules (Rare) ... 1922
Prozac Pulvules & Liquid, Oral Solution (Rare) ... 919
Quinidex Extentabs ... 2067
Ziac ... 1415

Psoriasis, exacerbation

Cytovene-IV (One report) ... 2103
▲ Dovonex Ointment 0.005% (1% to 10%) ... 2684
Eskalith ... 2485
Foscavir Injection (Less than 1%) .. 547
Intron A ... 2364
Lithium Carbonate Capsules & Tablets ... 2230
Lithonate/Lithotabs/Lithobid ... 2543
Methotrexate Sodium Tablets, Injection, for Injection and LPF Injection ... 1275
Neupogen for Injection (Infrequent) ... 495
Oxsoralen-Ultra Capsules ... 1257
Plaquenil Sulfate Tablets ... 2328
Risperdal (Rare) ... 1301
Temovate (Rare) ... 1179
Tenoretic Tablets ... 2845
Tenormin Tablets and I.V. Injection 2847
Toprol-XL Tablets ... 565

Psoriasis, pustular

Cutivate Cream ... 1088
Cutivate Ointment ... 1089

Psoriasis, rapid flare of

Seldane Tablets ... 1536
Seldane-D Extended-Release Tablets ... 1538

Psychiatric disturbances

Aldoclor Tablets ... 1598
Aldomet Ester HCl Injection ... 1602
Aldomet Oral ... 1600
Aldoril Tablets ... 1604
Anafranil Capsules (Up to 3%) ... 803
Aralen Hydrochloride Injection ... 2301
Aralen Phosphate Tablets ... 2301
Aristocort Tablets ... 1022
Artane (Rare) ... 1368
Clinoril Tablets (Less than 1 in 100) ... 1618
Cogentin ... 1621
Cortone Acetate Sterile Suspension ... 1623
Cortone Acetate Tablets ... 1624
Cuprimine Capsules ... 1630
Dalalone D.P. Injectable ... 1011
Decadron Elixir ... 1633
Decadron Phosphate Injection ... 1637
Decadron Phosphate Respihaler ... 1642
Decadron Phosphate Turbinaire ... 1645
Decadron Phosphate with Xylocaine Injection, Sterile ... 1639
Decadron Tablets ... 1635
Decadron-LA Sterile Suspension ... 1646
Depo-Medrol Sterile Aqueous Suspension ... 2597
Dexacort Phosphate in Respihaler .. 458
Dexacort Phosphate in Turbinaire .. 459
Didronel Tablets ... 1984
Hydeltrasol Injection, Sterile ... 1665
Hydeltra-T.B.A. Sterile Suspension 1667
Hydrocortone Acetate Sterile Suspension ... 1669
Hydrocortone Phosphate Injection, Sterile ... 1670
Hydrocortone Tablets ... 1672
▲ Hylorel Tablets (3.8%) ... 985
Indocin (Less than 1%) ... 1680
Mebaral Tablets (Less than 1 in 100) ... 2322
Mintezol ... 1704
Nembutal Sodium Capsules (Less than 1%) ... 436
Nembutal Sodium Solution (Less than 1%) ... 438
Nembutal Sodium Suppositories (Less than 1%) ... 440
Nizoral Tablets (Rare) ... 1298
Noroxin Tablets ... 1715
Noroxin Tablets ... 2048
Pepcid Injection (Infrequent) ... 1722
Pepcid (Infrequent) ... 1720
Phenobarbital Elixir and Tablets (Less than 1 in 100 patients) ... 1469
▲ Phenurone Tablets (17%) ... 447
Prilosec Delayed-Release Capsules (Less than 1%) ... 529
Primaxin I.M. ... 1727
Primaxin I.V. (Less than 0.2%) ... 1729
Seconal Sodium Pulvules (Less than 1 in 100) ... 1474
Ser-Ap-Es Tablets ... 849
Timoptic in Ocudose (Less frequent) ... 1753
Timoptic Sterile Ophthalmic Solution (Less frequent) ... 1751
Timoptic-XE ... 1755
Tonocard Tablets (Less than 1%) .. 531
Trecator-SC Tablets ... 2814
Zarontin Capsules ... 1928
Zarontin Syrup ... 1929

Psychic dependence (see under Dependence, psychological)

Psychomotor retardation

Lithonate/Lithotabs/Lithobid ... 2543
Serzone Tablets (2%) ... 771

Psychoses

Adipex-P Tablets and Capsules ... 1048
Aldoclor Tablets ... 1598
Aldomet Ester HCl Injection ... 1602
Aldomet Oral ... 1600
Aldoril Tablets ... 1604
Anafranil Capsules (Infrequent) ... 803
Ancobon Capsules ... 2079
Antabuse Tablets ... 2695
Apresazide Capsules (Less frequent) ... 808
Aralen Phosphate Tablets (Rare) 2301
Aredia for Injection (Up to 4%) ... 810
Aristocort Suspension (Forte Parenteral) ... 1027
Aristocort Suspension (Intralesional) ... 1025
Aristospan Suspension (Intra-articular) ... 1033
Aristospan Suspension (Intralesional) ... 1032
Atamet ... 572
Azo Gantrisin Tablets ... 2081
Bentyl ... 1501
Betaseron for SC Injection ... 658
Biphetamine Capsules (Rare) ... 983
Bontril Slow-Release Capsules (Rare) ... 781
Buprenex Injectable (Less than 1%) ... 2006
BuSpar (Rare) ... 737
Butisol Sodium Elixir & Tablets (Less than 1 in 100) ... 2660
Calan SR Caplets (1% or less) ... 2422
Calan Tablets (1% or less) ... 2419
Cataflam (Rare) ... 816
Celestone Soluspan Suspension ... 2347
Celontin Kapseals (Rare) ... 1899
Chibroxin Sterile Ophthalmic Solution (With oral form) ... 1617
Cipro I.V. Pharmacy Bulk Package (Less than 1%) ... 597
Clinoril Tablets (Less than 1 in 100) ... 1618
Clomid ... 1514
Cognex Capsules (Rare) ... 1901
CORTENEMA ... 2535
Cortone Acetate Sterile Suspension ... 1623
Cortone Acetate Tablets ... 1624
Cytovene (1% or less) ... 2103
Dapsone Tablets USP ... 1284
Decadron Elixir ... 1633
Decadron Phosphate Injection ... 1637
Decadron Phosphate Respihaler ... 1642
Decadron Phosphate Turbinaire ... 1645
Decadron Phosphate with Xylocaine Injection, Sterile ... 1639
Decadron Tablets ... 1635
Decadron-LA Sterile Suspension ... 1646
Deltasone Tablets ... 2595
Depakene ... 413
Depakote Tablets ... 415
Desoxyn Gradumet Tablets (Rare) .. 419
Desyrel and Desyrel Dividose ... 503
Dexatrim ... ▣ 832
Dexatrim Plus Vitamins Caplets .. ▣ 832
Dexedrine (Rare at recommended doses) ... 2474
DextroStat Dextroamphetamine Tablets (Rare) ... 2036
Didrex Tablets (Rare) ... 2607
Effexor (Infrequent) ... 2719
Fastin Capsules (Rare) ... 2488
Felbatol ... 2666
Fioricet with Codeine Capsules ... 2260
Fiorinal with Codeine Capsules ... 2262
Florinef Acetate Tablets ... 505
Floxin I.V. ... 1571
Foscavir Injection (Less than 1%) .. 547
Gastrocrom Capsules (Infrequent) .. 984
Hivid Tablets (Less than 1% to less than 3%) ... 2121
Hydeltrasol Injection, Sterile ... 1665
Hydeltra-T.B.A. Sterile Suspension 1667
Hydrocortone Acetate Sterile Suspension ... 1669
Hydrocortone Phosphate Injection, Sterile ... 1670
Hydrocortone Tablets ... 1672
Hydropres Tablets ... 1675
IFEX ... 697
Indocin (Less than 1%) ... 1680
Ionamin Capsules (Rare) ... 990
Isoptin Oral Tablets (Less than 1%) ... 1346
Isoptin SR Tablets (1% or less) ... 1348
Klonopin Tablets ... 2126
Lamictal Tablets (Infrequent) ... 1112
Lanoxicaps ... 1117
Lanoxin Elixir Pediatric ... 1120
Lanoxin Injection ... 1123
Lanoxin Injection Pediatric ... 1126
Lanoxin Tablets ... 1128
Lariam Tablets ... 2128
Larodopa Tablets (Infrequent) ... 2129
Levsin/Levsinex/Levbid ... 2405
Ludiomil Tablets (Rare) ... 843
Luvox Tablets (Frequent) ... 2544
Macrobid Capsules (Rare) ... 1988
Macrodantin Capsules (Rare) ... 1989
Mellaril (Extremely rare) ... 2269
Mexitil Capsules (Less than 1% or about 2 in 1,000) ... 678
Nardil (Infrequent) ... 1920
Neurontin Capsules (Infrequent) ... 1922
Noroxin Tablets ... 1715
Noroxin Tablets ... 2048
Norpace (Rare) ... 2444
Orthoclone OKT3 Sterile Solution .. 1837
Paremyd ... ⊙ 247
Parlodel (Less than 1%) ... 2281
Paxil Tablets (Rare) ... 2505
Pediapred Oral Liquid ... 995
Penetrex Tablets (Less than 0.1%) 2031
Permax Tablets (2.1%; frequent) .. 575
Plaquenil Sulfate Tablets ... 2328
Prelone Syrup ... 1787
Prelu-2 Timed Release Capsules (Rare) ... 681
Procan SR Tablets (Occasional) ... 1926
▲ Prograf (Greater than 3%) ... 1042
Prozac Pulvules & Liquid, Oral Solution (Infrequent) ... 919
Quinaglute Dura-Tabs Tablets ... 649
Rocaltrol Capsules (Rare) ... 2141
Rythmol Tablets–150mg, 225mg, 300mg (Less than 1%) ... 1352
Seromycin Pulvules ... 1476
Sinemet Tablets ... 943
Sinemet CR Tablets ... 944
Symmetrel Capsules and Syrup (0.1% to 1%) ... 946
Tagamet ... 2516
Tenoretic Tablets ... 2845
Tenormin Tablets and I.V. Injection 2847
Tonocard Tablets (Less than 1%) .. 531
Toradol ... 2159
Trilafon ... 2389
Verelan Capsules (1% or less) ... 1410
Verelan Capsules (Less than 1%) .. 2824
Videx Tablets, Powder for Oral Solution, & Pediatric Powder for Oral Solution (Less than 1%) ... 720
Voltaren Tablets (Rare) ... 861
Wellbutrin Tablets (Infrequent) ... 1204
Zarontin Capsules ... 1928
Zarontin Syrup ... 1929
Zoloft Tablets ... 2217
Zovirax Sterile Powder ... 1223

Psychoses, aggravation

Aristocort Suspension (Forte Parenteral) ... 1027
Aristocort Suspension (Intralesional) ... 1025
Aristospan Suspension (Intra-articular) ... 1033
Aristospan Suspension (Intralesional) ... 1032
Clozaril Tablets ... 2252
CORTENEMA ... 2535
Cortone Acetate Sterile Suspension ... 1623
Cortone Acetate Tablets ... 1624
Decadron Elixir ... 1633
Decadron Phosphate Injection ... 1637
Decadron Phosphate Respihaler ... 1642
Decadron Phosphate Turbinaire ... 1645
Decadron Phosphate with Xylocaine Injection, Sterile ... 1639
Decadron Tablets ... 1635
Decadron-LA Sterile Suspension ... 1646
Deltasone Tablets ... 2595
Etrafon ... 2355
Florinef Acetate Tablets ... 505
Hydeltrasol Injection, Sterile ... 1665
Hydeltra-T.B.A. Sterile Suspension 1667
Hydrocortone Acetate Sterile Suspension ... 1669
Hydrocortone Phosphate Injection, Sterile ... 1670
Hydrocortone Tablets ... 1672
Mellaril ... 2269

(▣ Described in PDR For Nonprescription Drugs) Incidence data in parenthesis; ▲ 3% or more (⊙ Described in PDR For Ophthalmology)

1397 Side Effects Index Purple toes syndrome

Norpramin Tablets 1526
Pamelor 2280
Pediapred Oral Liquid 995
Prelone Syrup 1787
Prolixin 509
Serentil 684
Surmontil Capsules 2811
Tofranil Ampuls (Occasional) 854
Tofranil Tablets (Occasional) 856
Tofranil-PM Capsules (Occasional) 857
Torecan 2245
Vivactil Tablets 1774

Psychoses, toxic

Astramorph/PF Injection, USP (Preservative-Free) 535
Chibroxin Sterile Ophthalmic Solution (With oral form) 1617
Cipro I.V. (1% or less) 595
Cipro Tablets 592
Duramorph 962
Floxin Tablets (200 mg, 300 mg, 400 mg) 1567
Infumorph 200 and Infumorph 500 Sterile Solutions 965
NegGram (Rare) 2323
Nydrazid Injection (Uncommon) 508
Rifamate Capsules (Uncommon) 1530
Rifater (Uncommon) 1532
Ritalin 848

Psychosis, activation

Atretol Tablets 573
Compazine 2470
Levoprome 1274
Prolixin 509
Stelazine 2514
Tegretol Chewable Tablets 852
Tegretol Suspension 852
Tegretol Tablets 852
Triavil Tablets 1757

Psychosis, overt

Pediapred Oral Liquid 995

Psychosis, paranoid

Zarontin Capsules (Rare) 1928
Zarontin Syrup (Rare) 1929

Psychotic episodes (see under Psychoses)

Psychotic symptoms, paradoxical exacerbation

Haldol Decanoate 1577
Haldol Injection, Tablets and Concentrate 1575
Navane Capsules and Concentrate (Infrequent) 2201
Navane Intramuscular (Infrequent) 2202

Ptosis, eyelids

AK-CIDE ◉ 202
AK-CIDE Ointment ◉ 202
Betagan ◉ 233
Betaseron for SC Injection 658
Betimol 0.25%, 0.5% ◉ 261
Blephamide Ointment (Occasional) ◉ 237
Blocadren Tablets 1614
▲ BOTOX (Botulinum Toxin Type A) Purified Neurotoxin Complex (0.3% to 15.7%) 477
Clozaril Tablets (Less than 1%) 2252
Cognex Capsules (Rare) 1901
Depen Titratable Tablets 2662
Econopred & Econopred Plus Ophthalmic Suspensions (Occasional) ◉ 217
Esimil Tablets 822
FML Forte Liquifilm (Occasional) ◉ 240
FML Liquifilm (Occasional) ◉ 241
FML S.O.P. (Occasional) ◉ 241
Imdur (Less than or equal to 5%) 1323
Ismelin Tablets 827
Lamictal Tablets (Rare) 1112
Loxitane 1378
Neurontin Capsules (Infrequent) 1922
Ocupress Ophthalmic Solution, 1% Sterile (Occasional) ◉ 309
Prozac Pulvules & Liquid, Oral Solution (Rare) 919
▲ Rēv-Eyes Ophthalmic Eyedrops 0.5% (10% to 40%) ◉ 323
Serzone Tablets (Rare) 771
Timolide Tablets 1748
Timoptic in Ocudose (Less frequent) 1753
Timoptic Sterile Ophthalmic Solution (Less frequent) 1751
Timoptic-XE 1755
Vasocidin Ointment (Occasional) ◉ 268
Vasocidin Ophthalmic Solution (Occasional) ◉ 270
Zoloft Tablets (Rare) 2217

Pubic hair, growth

▲ Synarel Nasal Solution for Central Precocious Puberty (5%) 2151

Pulmonary air leak

▲ Exosurf Neonatal for Intratracheal Suspension (Up to 48%) 1095
▲ Survanta Beractant Intratracheal Suspension (10.9%) 2226

Pulmonary allergy, unspecified

Idamycin (2%) 1955

Pulmonary congestion

Prinzide Tablets 1737
▲ Proleukin for Injection (54%) 797
Zestoretic (0.3 to 1%) 2850

Pulmonary disease, chronic interstitial obstructive

Dipentum Capsules (Rare) 1951
Methotrexate Sodium Tablets, Injection, for Injection and LPF Injection (Occasional) 1275

Pulmonary disease, chronic obstructive

Luvox Tablets (Rare) 2544
▲ Zoladex (5%) 2858

Pulmonary distress

Betoptic Ophthalmic Solution (Rare) 469
Betoptic S Ophthalmic Suspension (Rare) 471
Humegon 1824
Serophene (clomiphene citrate tablets, USP) 2451

Pulmonary edema (see under Edema, pulmonary)

Pulmonary embolism (see under Embolism, pulmonary)

Pulmonary emphysema, interstitial

▲ Survanta Beractant Intratracheal Suspension (20.2%) 2226

Pulmonary fibrosis

Alkeran for Injection 1070
Alkeran Tablets 1071
BiCNU 691
▲ Blenoxane (10%) 692
Cafergot 2251
CeeNU 693
Cordarone Intravenous (One of more than 1,000 patients) 2715
▲ Cordarone Tablets (4 to 9%) 2712
Cuprimine Capsules (Rare) 1630
Cytovene-IV (One report) 2103
Cytoxan 694
Depen Titratable Tablets 2662
Garamycin Injectable 2360
Leukeran Tablets 1133
Lupron Depot 3.75 mg 2556
Lupron Depot 7.5 mg 2559
Lupron Injection (Less than 5%) 2555
Macrobid Capsules (Rare to common) 1988
Macrodantin Capsules (Rare; common) 1989
Mesantoin Tablets 2272
Mexitil Capsules (Isolated reports) 678
Myleran Tablets (Rare) 1143
NEOSAR Lyophilized/Neosar 1959
Paxil Tablets (Rare) 2505
Pentasa (One case) 1527
Permax Tablets (Rare) 575
Prozac Pulvules & Liquid, Oral Solution (Rare) 919
Sansert Tablets 2295
Tonocard Tablets (Less than 1%) 531

Pulmonary function, changes

▲ Betapace Tablets (3% to 8%) 641
Diprivan Injection (Less than 1%) 2833
Eulexin Capsules (Less than 1%) 2358
Humegon 1824
IFEX (Less than 1%) 697
Intron A 2364
Macrobid Capsules (Common) 1988
Macrodantin Capsules (Common) 1989
Mexitil Capsules (Isolated reports) 678
Navelbine Injection (A few patients) 1145
▲ Novantrone (24 to 43%) 1279
Pergonal (menotropins for injection, USP) 2448
Virazole 1264

Pulmonary hemorrhage (see under Hemorrhage, pulmonary)

Pulmonary hypersensitivity

Atretol Tablets 573
Cytadren Tablets (Rare) 819
Fludara for Injection 663
Septra I.V. Infusion 1169
Septra I.V. Infusion ADD-Vantage Vials 1171
Tegretol Chewable Tablets 852
Tegretol Suspension 852
Tegretol Tablets 852

Pulmonary hypersensitivity, acute

Macrobid Capsules (Less than 1%) 1988
Macrodantin Capsules 1989

Pulmonary hypersensitivity, chronic

Macrodantin Capsules 1989
Timolide Tablets 1748

Pulmonary hypersensitivity, subacute

Macrodantin Capsules 1989

Pulmonary hypertension

Indocin I.V. (1% to 3%) 1684
Permax Tablets (Rare) 575
Pondimin Tablets 2066
Protamine Sulfate Ampoules & Vials 1471

Pulmonary infarction

Ansaid Tablets (Less than 1%) 2579
Humegon 1824
Luvox Tablets (Rare) 2544
Metrodin (urofollitropin for injection) 2446
Prinivil Tablets (0.3% to 1.0%) 1733
Prinzide Tablets 1737
Vaseretic Tablets 1765
Vasotec I.V. 1768
Vasotec Tablets (0.5% to 1.0%) 1771
Zestoretic 2850
Zestril Tablets (0.3% to 1.0%) 2854

Pulmonary infiltrates

Azo Gantanol Tablets 2080
Azo Gantrisin Tablets 2081
Bactrim DS Tablets 2084
Bactrim I.V. Infusion 2082
Bactrim 2084
Beclovent Inhalation Aerosol and Refill 1075
BiCNU 691
CeeNU 693
Dynacin Capsules (Rare) 1590
Fansidar Tablets 2114
Fludara for Injection 663
Foscavir Injection (Between 1% and 5%) 547
Ganite 2533
Gantanol Tablets 2119
Gantrisin 2120
Hydrea Capsules (Rare) 696
Imdur (Less than or equal to 5%) 1323
Intal Capsules (Less than 1 in 100,000 patients) 987
Intal Inhaler (Infrequent) 988
Intal Nebulizer Solution (Rare) 989
Intron A (Rare) 2364
Lupron Depot 7.5 mg 2559
Lupron Injection 2555
Macrobid Capsules 1988
Macrodantin Capsules 1989
Minocin Intravenous (Rare) 1382
Minocin Oral Suspension (Rare) 1385
Minocin Pellet-Filled Capsules (Rare) 1383
Mutamycin 703
Pentasa (Less than 1%) 1527
Prinivil Tablets (0.3% to 1.0%) 1733
Prinzide Tablets 1737
Septra (Rare) 1174
Septra I.V. Infusion 1169
Septra I.V. Infusion ADD-Vantage Vials 1171
Septra (Rare) 1174
Vantin for Oral Suspension and Vantin Tablets 2646
Vascor (200, 300 and 400 mg) Tablets 1587
Vaseretic Tablets 1765
Vasotec I.V. 1768
Vasotec Tablets (0.5% to 1.0%) 1771
Zestoretic 2850
Zestril Tablets 2854

Pulmonary inflammation

Cordarone Tablets 2712

Pulmonary toxicity, unspecified

Alkeran for Injection 1070
Alkeran Tablets 1071
BiCNU 691
CeeNU 693
▲ Cordarone Tablets (10% to 17%) 2712
Cytosar-U Sterile Powder 2592
Fungizone Intravenous 506
▲ Idamycin (39%) 1955
Methotrexate Sodium Tablets, Injection, for Injection and LPF Injection (Less than 2.5%) 1275
Mutamycin 703

Pulse, fast

Arco-Lase Plus Tablets 512
Dexatrim Maximum Strength Plus Vitamin C/Caffeine-free Caplets ▣ 832
Humulin 50/50, 100 Units 1444
Humulin 70/30, 100 Units (Less common) 1445
Humulin L, 100 Units (Less common) 1446
Regular, 100 Units (Less common) 1450
Pork Regular, 100 Units 1452
Novolin 70/30 Prefilled Disposable Insulin Delivery System (Rare) 1798
Propagest Tablets 786
Rogaine Topical Solution (1.53%) 2637
Sinulin Tablets 787
Urised Tablets 1964
Velosulin BR Human Insulin 10 ml Vials 1795

Pulse changes

AquaMEPHYTON Injection 1608
Asendin Tablets 1369
Clozaril Tablets 2252
Compazine 2470
Dalgan Injection (Less than 1%) 538
Effexor 2719
Etrafon 2355
Haldol Decanoate 1577
Imitrex Injection (Rare) 1103
Loxitane 1378
Luvox Tablets (Infrequent) 2544
Mellaril 2269
Mephyton Tablets (Rare) 1696
Moban Tablets and Concentrate 1048
Navane Capsules and Concentrate 2201
Navane Intramuscular 2202
Norvasc Tablets (Less than or equal to 0.1%) 1940
Orap Tablets 1050
Prolixin 509
Risperdal 1301
Ritalin 848
Serentil 684
Stelazine 2514
Tornalate Solution for Inhalation, 0.2% (1.2%) 956
Triavil Tablets 1757
Trilafon (Occasional) 2389
Versed Injection (Among most frequent) 2170
Yutopar Intravenous Injection (Common) 570

Pulse rate, depression

Cafergot 2251
Lanoxicaps 1117
Lanoxin Injection 1123
ReoPro Vials (1.0%) 1471
Rogaine Topical Solution (1.53%) 2637
Sansert Tablets 2295

Pupils, unequal-sized

Hivid Tablets (Less than 1% to less than 3%) 2121

Pupillary atonia

Healon GV ◉ 315

Purple toes syndrome

Activase 1058
Coumadin (Infrequent) 926

(▣ Described in PDR For Nonprescription Drugs) Incidence data in parenthesis; ▲ 3% or more (◉ Described in PDR For Ophthalmology)

Purpura

- Adalat Capsules (10 mg and 20 mg) (Less than 0.5%) 587
- Adalat CC (Rare) 589
- Aldactazide 2413
- Aldoclor Tablets 1598
- Aldoril Tablets 1604
- Altace Capsules (Less than 1%) 1232
- Ambien Tablets (Rare) 2416
- Anafranil Capsules (Up to 3%) 803
- Anaprox/Naprosyn (Less than 3%) 2117
- Apresazide Capsules (Less frequent) 808
- Apresoline Hydrochloride Tablets (Less frequent) 809
- Asendin Tablets (Very rare) 1369
- Atretol Tablets 573
- Attenuvax (Rare) 1610
- Azactam for Injection (Less than 1%) 734
- Azo Gantanol Tablets 2080
- Azo Gantrisin Tablets 2081
- Azulfidine (Rare) 1949
- Bactrim DS Tablets 2084
- Bactrim I.V. Infusion 2082
- Bactrim 2084
- Biavax II 1613
- Calan SR Caplets (1% or less) 2422
- Calan Tablets (1% or less) 2419
- Capozide 742
- Cardizem CD Capsules (Infrequent) 1506
- Cardizem SR Capsules (Infrequent) 1510
- Cardizem Injectable 1508
- Cardizem Tablets (Infrequent) 1512
- Cardura Tablets (Less than 0.5% of 3960 patients) 2186
- Cataflam (Less than 1%) 816
- Cipro I.V. (1% or less) 595
- Cipro I.V. Pharmacy Bulk Package (Less than 1%) 597
- Claritin (2% or fewer patients) 2349
- Claritin-D 2350
- Clinoril Tablets (Less than 1 in 100) 1618
- Cognex Capsules (2%) 1901
- ColBENEMID Tablets 1622
- Combipres Tablets (Few) 677
- Cytotec (Infrequent) 2424
- Dapsone Tablets USP 1284
- DiaBeta Tablets (Occasional) 1239
- Diucardin Tablets 2718
- Diupres Tablets 1650
- Diuril Oral Suspension 1653
- Diuril Sodium Intravenous 1652
- Diuril Tablets 1653
- Dyazide 2479
- Easprin 1914
- EC-Naprosyn Delayed-Release Tablets (Less than 3%) 2117
- Elavil 2838
- ▲ Eminase (Less than 10%) 2039
- Endep Tablets 2174
- Enduron Tablets 420
- Engerix-B Unit-Dose Vials 2482
- Esidrix Tablets 821
- Esimil Tablets 822
- Etrafon 2355
- Fansidar Tablets 2114
- ▲ Felbatol (12.9%) 2666
- Flexeril Tablets (Rare) 1661
- Florinef Acetate Tablets 505
- Floxin I.V. 1571
- Floxin Tablets (200 mg, 300 mg, 400 mg) 1567
- Gantanol Tablets 2119
- Gantrisin 2120
- Garamycin Injectable 2360
- Hivid Tablets (Less than 1% to less than 3%) 2121
- HydroDIURIL Tablets 1674
- Hydropres Tablets 1675
- Hyzaar Tablets 1677
- Imdur (Less than or equal to 5%) 1323
- Inderide Tablets 2732
- Inderide LA Long Acting Capsules 2734
- Indocin Capsules (Less than 1%) 1680
- Indocin I.V. (Less than 1%) 1684
- Indocin (Less than 1%) 1680
- INFeD (Iron Dextran Injection, USP) 2345
- Intron A (Less than 5%) 2364
- Isoptin Oral Tablets (Less than 1%) 1346
- Isoptin SR Tablets (1% or less) 1348
- Kerlone Tablets (Less than 2%) 2436
- Lasix Injection, Oral Solution and Tablets 1240
- Lescol Capsules (Rare) 2267
- ▲ Leustatin (10%) 1834
- Limbitrol 2180
- Lodine Capsules and Tablets (Rare) 2743
- Lopressor HCT Tablets (1 in 100 patients) 832
- Lotensin HCT 837
- Lozol Tablets 2022
- Ludiomil Tablets (Isolated reports) 843
- Luvox Tablets (Rare) 2544
- M-M-R II 1687
- M-R-VAX II 1689
- Matulane Capsules 2131
- Maxaquin Tablets (Less than 1%) 2440
- Maxzide 1380
- Mevacor Tablets (Rare) 1699
- Minizide Capsules 1938
- Moduretic Tablets 1705
- Motrin Ibuprofen Suspension, Oral Drops, Chewable Tablets, Caplets (Less than 1%) 1546
- Mumpsvax (Extremely rare) 1708
- Mykrox Tablets 993
- Myochrysine Injection 1711
- Nalfon 200 Pulvules & Nalfon Tablets (Less than 1%) 917
- Anaprox/Naprosyn (Less than 3%) 2117
- Neurontin Capsules (Frequent) 1922
- Norpramin Tablets 1526
- Norvasc Tablets (More than 0.1% to 1%) 1940
- Oncaspar (Less than 1%) 2028
- Oretic Tablets 443
- Orudis Capsules (Less than 1%) 2766
- Oruvail Capsules (Less than 1%) 2766
- Pamelor 2280
- Paxil Tablets (Infrequent) 2505
- Penetrex Tablets (Less than 1% but more than or equal to 0.1%) 2031
- Permax Tablets (Rare) 575
- Pravachol (Rare) 765
- Prinzide Tablets 1737
- Procardia Capsules (Less than 0.5%) 1971
- Procardia XL Extended Release Tablets (1% or less) 1972
- ▲ Proleukin for Injection (4%) 797
- Proloprim Tablets 1155
- ProSom Tablets (Rare) 449
- Prozac Pulvules & Liquid, Oral Solution (Rare) 919
- Quinidex Extentabs 2067
- Rifadin 1528
- Rifater 1532
- Risperdal (Infrequent) 1301
- Rythmol Tablets–150mg, 225mg, 300mg (Less than 1%) 1352
- Septra I.V. Infusion 1169
- Ser-Ap-Es Tablets 849
- Sinequan (Occasional) 2205
- Solganal Suspension (Rare) 2388
- ▲ Supprelin Injection (2% to 12%) 2056
- Surmontil Capsules 2811
- Tegretol Chewable Tablets 852
- Tegretol Suspension 852
- Tegretol Tablets 852
- Tenex Tablets (3% or less) 2074
- Tenoretic Tablets 2845
- Tenormin Tablets and I.V. Injection 2847
- Thalitone 1245
- Ticlid Tablets (2.2%) 2156
- Timolide Tablets 1748
- Tofranil Ampuls 854
- Tofranil Tablets 856
- Tofranil-PM Capsules 857
- Tolectin (200, 400 and 600 mg) (Less than 1%) 1581
- Toradol (Greater than 1%) 2159
- Trandate Tablets 1185
- Trental Tablets (Rare) 1244
- Triavil Tablets 1757
- Urobiotic-250 Capsules 2214
- Vaseretic Tablets 1765
- Verelan Capsules (1% or less) 1410
- Verelan Capsules (Less than 1%) 2824
- Vivactil Tablets 1774
- Voltaren Tablets (Less than 1%) 861
- Zaroxolyn Tablets 1000
- Zebeta Tablets 1413
- Zestoretic 2850
- Ziac 1415
- Zocor Tablets (Rare) 1775
- Zoloft Tablets (Infrequent) 2217
- Zosyn (1.0% or less) 1419
- Zosyn Pharmacy Bulk Package (1.0% or less) 1422
- Zyloprim Tablets (Less than 1%) 1226

Purpura, allergic

- Cataflam (Rare) 816
- Voltaren Tablets (Rare) 861

Purpura, anaphylactoid

- Achromycin V Capsules 1367
- Declomycin Tablets 1371
- Doryx Capsules 1913
- Dynacin Capsules 1590
- Minocin Intravenous 1382
- Minocin Oral Suspension 1385
- Minocin Pellet-Filled Capsules 1383
- Monodox Capsules 1805
- Terramycin Intramuscular Solution 2210
- Vibramycin 1941
- Vibramycin Hyclate Intravenous 2215
- Vibramycin 1941

Purpura, fulminous

- Zovirax Sterile Powder (Less than 1%) 1223

Purpura, nonthrombocytopenic

- Blocadren Tablets 1614
- Cartrol Tablets 410
- Edecrin (Rare) 1657
- Inderal 2728
- Inderal LA Long Acting Capsules 2730
- Inderide Tablets 2732
- Inderide LA Long Acting Capsules 2734
- Kerlone Tablets 2436
- Levatol 2403
- Lopressor HCT Tablets 832
- Miltown Tablets 2672
- Normodyne Tablets 2379
- PMB 200 and PMB 400 2783
- Prolixin 509
- Sectral Capsules 2807
- Septra I.V. Infusion ADD-Vantage Vials 1171
- Timolide Tablets 1748
- Timoptic in Ocudose 1753
- Timoptic Sterile Ophthalmic Solution 1751
- Timoptic-XE 1755
- Toprol-XL Tablets 565
- Trandate Tablets 1185
- Visken Tablets 2299

Purpura, thrombocytopenic

- Children's Advil Suspension (Less than 1%) 2692
- Amoxil 2464
- Atromid-S Capsules 2701
- Augmentin 2468
- Axid Pulvules (Rare) 1427
- Blocadren Tablets 1614
- Cartrol Tablets 410
- Compazine 2470
- Cuprimine Capsules 1630
- Diamox 1372
- Diupres Tablets 1650
- Etrafon 2355
- Genoptic Sterile Ophthalmic Solution (Rare) ⊙ 243
- Genoptic Sterile Ophthalmic Ointment (Rare) ⊙ 243
- Gentak (Rare) ⊙ 208
- Glauctabs ⊙ 208
- Hydropres Tablets 1675
- IBU Tablets (Less than 1%) 1342
- Inderal 2728
- Inderal LA Long Acting Capsules 2730
- Inderide Tablets 2732
- Inderide LA Long Acting Capsules 2734
- Indocin Capsules (Less than 1%) 1680
- Indocin I.V. (Less than 1%) 1684
- Indocin (Less than 1%) 1680
- Kerlone Tablets 2436
- Levatol 2403
- Lincocin 2617
- Lopressor HCT Tablets 832
- MZM (Common) ⊙ 267
- Meruvax II 1697
- Miltown Tablets (Rare) 2672
- Children's Motrin Ibuprofen Oral Suspension (Less than 1%) 1546
- Motrin Tablets (Less than 1%) 2625
- Neptazane Tablets 1388
- Normodyne Tablets 2379
- Omnipen Capsules 2764
- Omnipen for Oral Suspension 2765
- PMB 200 and PMB 400 (Rare) 2783
- Phenergan Injection 2773
- Phenergan Tablets 2775
- Ponstel (Occasional) 1925
- Proglycem 580
- Prolixin 509
- Prozac Pulvules & Liquid, Oral Solution 919
- Quinaglute Dura-Tabs Tablets 649
- Quinidex Extentabs 2067
- ReVia Tablets (One patient) 940
- Ritalin 848
- Sectral Capsules 2807
- ▲ Septra I.V. Infusion (Among most frequent) 1169
- Septra I.V. Infusion ADD-Vantage Vials 1171
- Spectrobid Tablets 2206
- Stelazine 2514
- Talacen (A few cases) 2333
- Temaril Tablets, Syrup and Spansule Extended-Release Capsules 483
- Thorazine 2523
- Timolide Tablets 1748
- Timoptic in Ocudose 1753
- Timoptic Sterile Ophthalmic Solution 1751
- Timoptic-XE 1755
- Toprol-XL Tablets 565
- Trandate Tablets 1185
- Triavil Tablets 1757
- Trilafon 2389
- Visken Tablets 2299
- Zebeta Tablets 1413

Purpura, thrombocytopenic thrombotic

- Cuprimine Capsules 1630
- Depen Titratable Tablets 2662
- Floxin I.V. 1571
- Floxin Tablets (200 mg, 300 mg, 400 mg) 1567
- Mycobutin Capsules (One patient) 1957
- Norplant System 2759
- Risperdal (A single case) 1301
- Ticlid Tablets (Rare) 2156

Pustules, scalp

- Nizoral 2% Shampoo (One occurrence in 41 patients) 1298
- Temovate Scalp Application (3 of 294 patients) 1179

Pustules, unspecified

- Duragesic Transdermal System (Less than 1%) 1288
- Ultravate Ointment 0.05% (Less frequent) 2690

Pustulosis, provocation

- Aclovate (Rare) 1069
- Temovate (Rare) 1179

Pyelonephritis

- Ambien Tablets (Rare) 2416
- Anafranil Capsules (Rare) 803
- ▲ CellCept Capsules (More than or equal to 3%) 2099
- Dilacor XR Extended-release Capsules 2018
- Effexor (Infrequent) 2719
- Foscavir Injection (Less than 1%) 547
- Lupron Depot 3.75 mg 2556
- Miacalcin Nasal Spray (Less than 1%) 2275
- Permax Tablets (Rare) 575
- Prinivil Tablets (0.3% to 1.0%) 1733
- Prinzide Tablets 1737
- Prozac Pulvules & Liquid, Oral Solution (Rare) 919
- Zestril Tablets (0.3% to 1.0%) 2854

Pyoderma gangrenosum

- Asacol Delayed-Release Tablets (Rare) 1979

Pyrexia (see under Fever)

Pyridoxine deficiency

- Macrobid Capsules 1988
- Macrodantin Capsules 1989
- Nydrazid Injection 508
- Rifamate Capsules 1530
- Rifater 1532

Pyrogenic granuloma

- ▲ Accutane Capsules (A number of cases) 2076
- ▲ Tegison Capsules (1-10%) 2154

Pyrosis (see under Heartburn)

Pyuria

- Anafranil Capsules (Rare) 803
- BCG Vaccine, USP (TICE) (0.7%) 1814
- Cognex Capsules (Infrequent) 1901
- Effexor (Infrequent) 2719
- Floxin I.V. (More than or equal to 1%) 1571

(▣ Described in PDR For Nonprescription Drugs) Incidence data in parenthesis; ▲ 3% or more (⊙ Described in PDR For Ophthalmology)

1399 **Side Effects Index** **Rash**

Floxin Tablets (200 mg, 300 mg, 400 mg) (More than or equal to 1.0%) ... 1567
Neurontin Capsules (Rare) ... 1922
Orlamm (Low frequency) ... 2239
Permax Tablets (Infrequent) ... 575
Prilosec Delayed-Release Capsules (Less than 1%) ... 529
Prozac Pulvules & Liquid, Oral Solution (Rare) ... 919
Zosyn ... 1419
Zosyn Pharmacy Bulk Package ... 1422

PBI decrease

Atamet ... 572
Capozide ... 742
Dyazide ... 2479
Estratest ... 2539
Lysodren (Infrequent) ... 698
Maxzide ... 1380
Premarin with Methyltestosterone .. 2794
Sinemet Tablets ... 943
Sinemet CR Tablets ... 944

PBI increase

Amen Tablets ... 780
Aygestin Tablets ... 974
Cycrin Tablets ... 975
Depo-Provera Sterile Aqueous Suspension ... 2606
Etrafon ... 2355
Larodopa Tablets (Rare) ... 2129
Provera Tablets ... 2636
Trilafon ... 2389

PSP excretion, depression

▲ Capastat Sulfate Vials (Many instances) ... 2868

"Pasty mass", presence of, in the transverse colon

Questran Light ... 769
Questran Powder ... 770

Q

Quadriplegia

Orthoclone OKT3 Sterile Solution .. 1837
Soma Compound w/Codeine Tablets (Very rare) ... 2676
Soma Compound Tablets (Very rare) ... 2675
Soma Tablets ... 2674

R

Radiculoneuropathy

Imitrex Tablets (Rare) ... 1106
Pneumovax 23 (Rare) ... 1725
Pnu-Imune 23 ... 1393
Recombivax HB ... 1744

Rage

Dizac (Less frequent) ... 1809
Libritabs Tablets ... 2177
Librium Capsules ... 2178
Serax Capsules ... 2810
Serax Tablets ... 2810
Valium Tablets ... 2183
Xanax Tablets (Rare) ... 2649

Rales

Adalat CC (Less than 1.0%) ... 589
▲ Aredia for Injection (Up to 6%) ... 810
Blenoxane ... 692
Blocadren Tablets (0.6%) ... 1614
Brevibloc Injection (Less than 1%) ... 1808
Ganite ... 2533
Imdur (Less than or equal to 5%) .. 1323
NebuPent for Inhalation Solution (1% or less) ... 1040
Survanta Beractant Intratracheal Suspension ... 2226
Timolide Tablets (Less than 1%) ... 1748
Timoptic in Ocudose ... 1753
Timoptic Sterile Ophthalmic Solution ... 1751
Timoptic-XE ... 1755
▲ Videx Tablets, Powder for Oral Solution, & Pediatric Powder for Oral Solution (6% to 8%) ... 720

Rash

Abbokinase ... 403
Abbokinase Open-Cath ... 405
Accupril Tablets (1.4%) ... 1893
▲ Accutane Capsules (Less than 1 patient in 10) ... 2076
Acel-Imune Diphtheria and Tetanus Toxoids and Acellular Pertussis Vaccine Adsorbed (1.2%) ... 1364
Actigall Capsules ... 802
▲ Actimmune (17%) ... 1056
Activase (Very rare) ... 1058
Adalat CC (3% or less) ... 589
▲ Children's Advil Suspension (3-9%) ... 2692
▲ AeroBid Inhaler System (3-9%) ... 1005
▲ Aerobid-M Inhaler System (3-9%) .. 1005
Airet Solution for Inhalation (Rare) ... 452
AK-Spore ... ◉ 204
AK-Trol Ointment & Suspension .. ◉ 205
Aldoclor Tablets ... 1598
Aldomet Ester HCl Injection ... 1602
Aldomet Oral ... 1600
Aldoril Tablets ... 1604
Alkeran for Injection ... 1070
Alkeran Tablets ... 1071
All-Flex Arcing Spring Diaphragm (See also Ortho Diaphragm Kits) 1865
Alomide (Less than 1%) ... 469
Altace Capsules (Less than 1%) ... 1232
Ambien Tablets (2%) ... 2416
Amen Tablets (Occasional) ... 780
Americaine Anesthetic Lubricant ... 983
Americaine Hemorrhoidal Ointment ... ▣ 629
Americaine Otic Topical Anesthetic Ear Drops ... 983
Amoxil ... 2464
▲ Anafranil Capsules (4% to 8%) ... 803
Anaprox/Naprosyn (Less than 1%) ... 2117
Ancobon Capsules ... 2079
Anectine ... 1073
Anexia Tablets ... 1782
Ansaid Tablets (1-3%) ... 2579
Apresazide Capsules (Less frequent) ... 808
Apresoline Hydrochloride Tablets (Less frequent) ... 809
▲ Asacol Delayed-Release Tablets (6%) ... 1979
▲ Atgam Sterile Solution (1 in 8 patients) ... 2581
Atrohist Plus Tablets ... 454
Atrovent Inhalation Aerosol (1.2%) ... 671
Attenuvax (Occasional) ... 1610
Axid Pulvules (1.9%; rare) ... 1427
Azactam for Injection (1 to 1.3%) .. 734
Azo Gantrisin Tablets ... 2081
BCG Vaccine, USP (TICE) (0.6%) .. 1814
▲ Bactrim DS Tablets (Among most common) ... 2084
▲ Bactrim I.V. Infusion (Among most common) ... 2082
▲ Bactrim (Among most common) ... 2084
Bactroban Ointment (Less than 1%) ... 2470
Bentyl ... 1501
Betagan ... ◉ 233
▲ Betapace Tablets (2% to 5%) ... 641
Betimol 0.25%, 0.5% ... ◉ 261
Biavax II (Infrequent) ... 1613
BiCozene Creme ... ▣ 785
▲ Blenoxane (50%) ... 692
Bleph-10 Ophthalmic Solution 10% ... 475
Blocadren Tablets (Less than 1%) 1614
BOTOX (Botulinum Toxin Type A) Purified Neurotoxin Complex (7 cases) ... 477
Brevicon ... 2088
Bumex (0.2%) ... 2093
Buprenex Injectable (Infrequent) ... 2006
Butisol Sodium Elixir & Tablets (Less than 1 in 100) ... 2660
Caladryl Cream For Kids ... ▣ 853
Calan SR Caplets (1.2%) ... 2422
Calan Tablets (1.2%) ... 2419
▲ Capoten (About 4 to 7 of 100 patients) ... 739
▲ Capozide (About 4 to 7 of 100 patients) ... 742
Carafate Suspension (Less than 0.5%) ... 1505
Carafate Tablets (Less than 0.5%) 1504
Cardene Capsules (0.4-1.2%) ... 2095
Cardene SR Capsules (0.6%) ... 2097
Cardizem CD Capsules (1.2%) ... 1506
Cardizem SR Capsules (1% to 1.5%) ... 1510
Cardizem Injectable ... 1508
Cardizem Tablets (1.3%) ... 1512
Cardura Tablets (1%) ... 2186
Cartrol Tablets (1.3%) ... 410
Cataflam (1% to 3%) ... 816
Catapres Tablets (About 1 in 100 patients) ... 674
Catapres-TTS (Less frequent) ... 675
Caverject (Less than 1%) ... 2583
Ceclor Pulvules & Suspension ... 1431
Cefizox for Intramuscular or Intravenous Use (Greater than 1% but less than 5%) ... 1034
Cefotan (1 in 150) ... 2829
Ceftin (Less than 1% but more than 0.1%) ... 1078
Cefzil Tablets and Oral Suspension (0.9%) ... 746
▲ CellCept Capsules (6.4% to 7.7%) ... 2099
Ceptaz (2% of patients) ... 1081
Cerezyme (One patient) ... 1066
Cerumenex Drops ... 1993
▲ CHEMET (succimer) Capsules (2.6 to 11.2%) ... 1545
Chibroxin Sterile Ophthalmic Solution (With oral form) ... 1617
Cipro I.V. (Greater than 1%) ... 595
Cipro I.V. Pharmacy Bulk Package (Greater than 1%) ... 597
Cipro Tablets (1.1%; rare) ... 592
Claritin (2% or fewer patients) ... 2349
Claritin-D (Less frequent) ... 2350
Cleocin Vaginal Cream (Less than 1%) ... 2589
▲ Clinoril Tablets (3% to 9%) ... 1618
Clomid (Fewer than 1%) ... 1514
Clozaril Tablets (2%) ... 2252
Cogentin ... 1621
▲ Cognex Capsules (7%) ... 1901
Colace ... 2044
Colestid Tablets (Infrequent) ... 2591
Combipres Tablets ... 677
Compazine ... 2470
Cordarone Tablets (Less than 1%) 2712
Correctol Laxative Tablets & Caplets ... ▣ 801
Cortisporin Ophthalmic Ointment Sterile ... 1085
Cozaar Tablets (Less than 1%) ... 1628
▲ Cuprimine Capsules (5%) ... 1630
Cycrin Tablets (Occasional) ... 975
▲ Cytadren Tablets (1 in 6) ... 819
▲ Cytosar-U Sterile Powder (Among most frequent) ... 2592
Cytotec (Infrequent) ... 2424
▲ Cytovene (15%) ... 2103
DDAVP ... 2017
D.H.E. 45 Injection (Occasional) ... 2255
Dalgan Injection (Less than 1%) ... 538
Danocrine Capsules ... 2307
Dantrium Capsules ... 1982
Daypro Caplets (Rare to 9%) ... 2426
Demadex Tablets and Injection ... 686
Depakene ... 413
▲ Depakote Tablets (6%) ... 415
▲ Depen Titratable Tablets (5%) ... 2662
▲ Depo-Provera Contraceptive Injection (1% to 5%) ... 2602
Depo-Provera Sterile Aqueous Suspension ... 2606
Dermatop Emollient Cream 0.1% (Less than 1%) ... 1238
Desferal Vials ... 820
Desmopressin Acetate Rhinal Tube 979
Desyrel and Desyrel Dividose ... 503
Diflucan Injection, Tablets, and Oral Suspension (1.8%) ... 2194
Dilacor XR Extended-release Capsules (1.0%) ... 2018
Dilantin Infatabs ... 1908
Dilantin Kapseals ... 1906
Dilantin-125 Suspension ... 1911
Dilaudid-HP Injection (Less frequent) ... 1337
Dilaudid-HP Lyophilized Powder 250 mg (Less frequent) ... 1337
Dilaudid Tablets and Liquid ... 1339
Dipentum Capsules (2.3%) ... 1951
Diphtheria and Tetanus Toxoids and Pertussis Vaccine Adsorbed.. 2477
Diphtheria and Tetanus Toxoids and Pertussis Vaccine Adsorbed USP (For Pediatric Use) ... 875
Diprivan Injection (Less than 1% to 5%) ... 2833
Ditropan ... 1516
Diucardin Tablets ... 2718
Diupres Tablets ... 1650
Diuril Oral Suspension ... 1653
Diuril Sodium Intravenous ... 1652
Diuril Tablets ... 1653
▲ Dolobid Tablets (3% to 9%) ... 1654
▲ Donnazyme Tablets (Most frequent) ... 2061
Doral Tablets ... 2664
▲ Dovonex Ointment 0.005% (1% to 10%) ... 2684
Doxidan Liqui-Gels ... ▣ 836
Duragesic Transdermal System (1% or greater) ... 1288
Duricef ... 748
Dyazide ... 2479
DynaCirc Capsules ... 2256
Dyrenium Capsules (Rare) ... 2481
E-Mycin Tablets ... 1341
▲ Effexor (3%) ... 2719
▲ Efudex (Among most frequent) ... 2113
Eldepryl Tablets ... 2550
Elimite (permethrin) 5% Cream (1 to 2% or less) ... 478
Emete-con Intramuscular/Intravenous ... 2198
Eminase (Occasional) ... 2039
Emla Cream (Less than 1%) ... 545
Enduron Tablets ... 420
Engerix-B Unit-Dose Vials (Less than 1%) ... 2482
▲ Epogen for Injection (Rare; Up to 16%) ... 489
Ergamisol Tablets (10 patients) ... 1292
Esgic-plus Tablets ... 1013
Esidrix Tablets ... 821
Esimil Tablets ... 822
Eskalith ... 2485
Estraderm Transdermal System (Rare) ... 824
Ethmozine Tablets (Less than 2%) 2041
Etrafon ... 2355
▲ Eulexin Capsules (3%) ... 2358
Ex-Lax Chocolated Laxative Tablets ... ▣ 786
Extra Gentle Ex-Lax Laxative Pills ▣ 786
Regular Strength Ex-Lax Laxative Pills ... ▣ 786
Ex-Lax Gentle Nature Laxative Pills ... ▣ 786
Feen-A-Mint ... ▣ 805
▲ Felbatol (3.4% to 9.7%) ... 2666
Feldene Capsules (Occasional) ... 1965
Fioricet Tablets (Infrequent) ... 2258
Fioricet with Codeine Capsules ... 2260
Fiorinal with Codeine Capsules ... 2262
Floxin I.V. (1% to 3%) ... 1571
Floxin Tablets (200 mg, 300 mg, 400 mg) (1% to 3%) ... 1567
Flumadine Tablets & Syrup (0.3% to 1%) ... 1015
▲ Foscavir Injection (5% or greater).. 547
Fragmin (Rare) ... 1954
Sterile FUDR ... 2118
▲ Fulvicin P/G Tablets (Among most common) ... 2359
▲ Fulvicin P/G 165 & 330 Tablets (Among most common) ... 2359
Fungizone Intravenous ... 506
Furacin Soluble Dressing (Approximately 1%) ... 2045
Furacin Topical Cream (Approximately 1%) ... 2045
Gamimune N, 5% Immune Globulin Intravenous (Human), 5% (Rare) ... 619
Gamimune N, 10% Immune Globulin Intravenous (Human), 10% (Rare; a single incidence) ... 621
Gantanol Tablets ... 2119
Gantrisin ... 2120
Garamycin Injectable ... 2360
Gastrocrom Capsules (2 of 87 patients) ... 984
Genotropin (Infrequent) ... 111
Glauctabs ... ◉ 208
Glucophage ... 752
Glucotrol XL Extended Release Tablets (Less than 1%) ... 1968
Guaifed Syrup ... ▣ 734
Habitrol Nicotine Transdermal System (Once in 35% of patients) ... 865
Havrix (Less than 1%) ... 2489
Hespan Injection ... 929
Hexalen Capsules (Less than 1%).. 2571
Helixate, Antihemophilic Factor (Recombinant) (Two reports out of 3,254 patients) ... 518
HibTITER (1 of 1,118 vaccinations) ... 1375
Hismanal Tablets (Less frequent) ... 1293
▲ Hivid Tablets (3.4% to 11.2%) ... 2121
Humegon ... 1824
Humulin 50/50, 100 Units ... 1444
Humulin 70/30, 100 Units (Less common) ... 1445
Humulin L, 100 Units (Less common) ... 1446
Hycodan Tablets and Syrup ... 930
Hycomine ... 931
Hydrocet Capsules ... 782
HydroDIURIL Tablets ... 1674

(▣ Described in PDR For Nonprescription Drugs) Incidence data in parenthesis; ▲ 3% or more (◉ Described in PDR For Ophthalmology)

Rash **Side Effects Index** **1400**

Hydropres Tablets 1675
Hyperab Rabies Immune Globulin (Human) (Rare) 624
Hyperstat I.V. Injection 2363
Hytrin Capsules (At least 1%) 430
Hyzaar Tablets (1.4%) 1677
▲ IBU Tablets (3% to 9%) 1342
Idamycin 1955
Regular, 100 Units (Less common) 1450
Pork Regular, 100 Units 1452
Imdur (Less than or equal to 5%) 1323
Imitrex Injection (Rare) 1103
Imitrex Tablets (Rare to infrequent) 1106
Inderide Tablets 2732
Inderide LA Long Acting Capsules 2734
Indocin Capsules (Less than 1%) 1680
Indocin I.V. (Less than 1%) 1684
Indocin (Less than 1%) 1680
INFeD (Iron Dextran Injection, USP) 2345
Intal Capsules (Less than 1 in 10,000 patients) 987
Intal Inhaler (Infrequent) 988
Intal Nebulizer Solution 989
Ismo Tablets (Fewer than 1%) 2738
ISMOTIC 45% w/v Solution (Very rare) ◉ 222
Isoptin Oral Tablets (1.2%) 1346
Isoptin SR Tablets (1.2% or less) 1348
▲ JE-VAX (5% to approximately 10%) 886
K-Lor Powder Packets (Rare) 434
K-Tab Filmtab (Rare) 434
Keflex Pulvules & Oral Suspension 914
Keftab Tablets 915
Kefurox Vials, Faspak & ADD-Vantage (1 in 125) 1454
Kerlone Tablets (1.2%) 2436
KOGENATE Antihemophilic Factor (Recombinant) (Two reports) 632
Kytril Injection (Rare; 1%) 2490
▲ Lamictal Tablets (10%) 1112
▲ Lariam Tablets (Among most frequent) 2128
Lescol Capsules (2.7%) 2267
Leukeran Tablets (Rare) 1133
▲ Leukine for IV Infusion (44%) 1271
▲ Leustatin (10% to 27%) 1834
Levoprome 1274
Lincocin 2617
Lithium Carbonate Capsules & Tablets 2230
Livostin (Approximately 1% to 3%) ◉ 266
Lodine Capsules and Tablets (More than 1% but less than 3%) 2743
Loniten Tablets (Less than 1%) 2618
Lo/Ovral Tablets 2746
Lo/Ovral-28 Tablets 2751
Lopid Tablets (1.7%) 1917
Lopressor HCT Tablets 832
Lorabid Suspension and Pulvules (0.7% to 2.9%) 1459
Lorelco Tablets 1517
Lortab 2566
Lotensin Tablets 834
Lotensin HCT (0.3% to 1.0%) 837
Lotrel Capsules 840
Lozol Tablets (Less than 5%) 2022
Lupron Depot-PED 7.5 mg, 11.25 mg and 15 mg (2%) 2560
Lupron Injection (Less than 3%) 2555
Lutrepulse for Injection 980
Luvox Tablets 2544
M-M-R II (Infrequent) 1687
M-R-VAX II (Infrequent) 1689
MZM (Common) ◉ 267
Macrodantin Capsules 1989
Matulane Capsules 2131
Maxair Autohaler 1492
Maxair Inhaler (Less than 1%) 1494
Maxaquin Tablets (Less than 1%) 2440
Maxzide 1380
Mefoxin 1691
Mefoxin Premixed Intravenous Solution 1694
▲ Megace Oral Suspension (2% to 12%) 699
Megace Tablets 701
▲ Mepron Suspension (22% to 23%) 1135
Meruvax II 1697
Mesantoin Tablets 2272
Methadone Hydrochloride Oral Concentrate 2233
Methotrexate Sodium Tablets, Injection, for Injection and LPF Injection (1 to 3%) 1275
Metrodin (urofollitropin for injection) 2446
MetroGel-Vaginal (Equal to or less than 2%) 902
▲ Mevacor Tablets (0.8% to 5.2%) 1699
▲ Mexitil Capsules (3.8% to 4.2%) 678
Miacalcin Injection 2273
Micro-K LS Packets (Rare) 2064
Micronor Tablets 1872
Migralam Capsules 2038
Mivacron (Less than 1%) 1138
Moban Tablets and Concentrate 1048
Modicon 1872
▲ Moduretic Tablets (3% to 8%) 1705
8-MOP Capsules 1246
Monocid Injection (Less than 1%) 2497
Monoket (Less than 1% to 4%) 2406
Monopril Tablets (0.2% to 1.0% or more) 757
▲ Children's Motrin Ibuprofen Oral Suspension (3% to 9%) 1546
▲ Motrin Tablets (3% to 9%) 2625
▲ Motrin Ibuprofen Suspension, Oral Drops, Chewable Tablets, Caplets (3% to 9%) 1546
MSTA Mumps Skin Test Antigen 890
Mutamycin (Rare) 703
▲ Mycobutin Capsules (11%) 1957
Mycostatin Pastilles (Rare) 704
Mykrox Tablets (Less than 2%) 993
Naftin Gel 1% (0.5%) 481
▲ Nalfon 200 Pulvules & Nalfon Tablets (3.7%) 917
Naprosyn Tablets (Less than 1%) 2117
Nasalcrom Nasal Solution (Less than 1%) 994
Navane Capsules and Concentrate 2201
Navane Intramuscular 2202
Navelbine Injection (Less than 5%) 1145
▲ NebuPent for Inhalation Solution (31 to 47%) 1040
NegGram 2323
NEOSAR Lyophilized/Neosar (Occasional) 1959
Neptazane Tablets 1388
Netromycin Injection 100 mg/ml (4 or 5 of 1000 patients) 2373
▲ Neupogen for Injection (6%; 12%) 495
Neurontin Capsules (More than 1%) 1922
▲ Neutrexin (5.5%) 2572
▲ Nicoderm (nicotine transdermal system) (3% to 9%) 1518
Nicotrol Nicotine Transdermal System (1% to 3%) 1550
Nimotop Capsules (Up to 2.4%) 610
Nordette-21 Tablets 2755
Nordette-28 Tablets 2758
Norinyl 2088
Normodyne Injection (Rare) 2377
Normodyne Tablets (1%) 2379
Noroxin Tablets (0.3% to 1.0%) 1715
Noroxin Tablets (0.3% to 1.0%) 2048
Norpace (1 to 3%) 2444
Norplant System 2759
Nor-Q D Tablets 2135
Norvasc Tablets (More than 0.1% to 1%) 1940
Novantrone (Occasional) 1279
Novolin 70/30 Prefilled Disposable Insulin Delivery System (Rare) 1798
Ocupress Ophthalmic Solution, 1% Sterile ◉ 309
Oil of Olay Daily UV Protectant SPF 15 Beauty Fluid-Original and Fragrance Free (Olay Co. Inc.) ▣ 751
Omnipen for Oral Suspension 2765
▲ Oncaspar (Greater than 5%) 2028
Oncovin Solution Vials & Hyporets (Rare) 1466
OptiPranolol (Metipranolol 0.3%) Sterile Ophthalmic Solution (A small number of patients) ◉ 258
Orap Tablets 1050
Oretic Tablets 443
Organidin NR Tablets and Liquid (Rare) 2672
Orlamm (1% to 3%) 2239
Ortho-Cyclen/Ortho-Tri-Cyclen 1858
Ortho Diaphragm Kits—All-Flex Arcing Spring; Ortho Coil Spring; Ortho-White Flat Spring 1865
Ortho Diaphragm Kit-Coil Spring 1865
Ortho-Novum 1872
Ortho-Cyclen/Ortho Tri-Cyclen 1858
Ortho-White Diaphragm Kit-Flat Spring (See also Ortho Diaphragm Kits) 1865
Orthoclone OKT3 Sterile Solution 1837
Orudis Capsules (Greater than 1%) 2766
Oruvail Capsules (Greater than 1%) 2766
Ovral Tablets 2770
Ovrette Tablets 2771
Oxistat Cream (0.1%) 1152
Oxsoralen-Ultra Capsules 1257
Pamelor 2280
Paraflex Caplets 1580
Parafon Forte DSC Caplets 1581
Paraplatin for Injection 705
▲ PASER Granules (Among most common) 1285
Paxil Tablets (1.7%) 2505
Penetrex Tablets (1%) 2031
▲ Pentam 300 Injection (3.3%) 1041
Pentasa (1.0% to 1.3%) 1527
Pepcid Injection (Infrequent) 1722
Pepcid (Infrequent) 1720
Percocet Tablets 938
Pergonal (menotropins for injection, USP) 2448
Peri-Colace 2052
▲ Permax Tablets (3.2%) 575
Persantine Tablets (2.3%) 681
Phenergan with Codeine 2777
Phenergan with Dextromethorphan 2778
Phenergan Suppositories 2775
Phenergan Syrup 2774
Phenergan VC 2779
Phenergan VC with Codeine 2781
Phillips' Gelcaps ▣ 729
Phrenilin (Infrequent) 785
Placidyl Capsules 448
Platinol (Infrequent) 708
Platinol-AQ Injection (Infrequent) 710
Plendil Extended-Release Tablets (0.2% to 2.0%) 527
Pneumovax 23 (Rare) 1725
Pnu-Imune 23 (Rare to infrequent) 1393
Polymyxin B Sulfate, Aerosporin Brand Sterile Powder 1154
Polysporin Ophthalmic Ointment Sterile 1154
Pondimin Tablets 2066
Ponstel 1925
▲ Pravachol (1.3% to 4.0%) 765
Premarin Tablets 2789
Premphase 2797
Prempro 2801
Synthroid Injection 1359
PREVACID Delayed-Release Capsules (Less than 1%) 2562
Prilosec Delayed-Release Capsules (Less than 1% to 1.5%) 529
Primaxin I.M. (0.4%) 1727
Primaxin I.V. (0.9%) 1729
▲ Prinivil Tablets (0.3% to 4.8%) 1733
Prinzide Tablets (1.2%) 1737
Priscoline Hydrochloride Ampuls 845
Procardia XL Extended Release Tablets (Less than 3%) 1972
▲ Procrit for Injection (Rare to 16%) 1841
Profasi (chorionic gonadotropin for injection, USP) 2450
▲ Prograf (8% to 24%) 1042
Prolastin Alpha$_1$-Proteinase Inhibitor (Human) (Occasional) 635
▲ Proleukin for Injection (26%) 797
▲ Proloprim Tablets (2.9% to 6.7%) 1155
Propulsid (1.6%) 1300
Proscar Tablets 1741
ProSom Tablets (Infrequent) 449
Prostep (nicotine transdermal system) (1% to 3% of patients) 1394
Prostigmin Injectable 1260
Prostigmin Tablets 1261
Prostin E2 Suppository 2634
Proventil Inhalation Aerosol (Rare) 2382
Proventil Inhalation Solution 0.083% (Rare) 2384
Proventil Repetabs Tablets (2%) 2386
Proventil Solution for Inhalation 0.5% (Rare) 2383
Proventil Syrup (Rare) 2385
Proventil Tablets (2%) 2386
Provera Tablets (An occasional patient) 2636
▲ Prozac Pulvules & Liquid, Oral Solution (Approximately 4% of 5,600 patients) 919
▲ Pulmozyme Inhalation (10% to 12%) 1064
Pyrazinamide Tablets 1398
Pyridium 1928
Questran Light (Less frequent) 769
Questran Powder (Less frequent) 770
Quibron 2053
▲ Quinaglute Dura-Tabs Tablets (6%) 649
Quinidex Extentabs 2067
RMS Suppositories 2657
Recombivax HB (Less than 1%) 1744
▲ Relafen Tablets (3% to 9%) 2510
Respbid Tablets 682
▲ Retrovir Capsules (17%) 1158
▲ Retrovir I.V. Infusion (17%) 1163
▲ Retrovir Syrup (17%) 1158
▲ ReVia Tablets (Less than 10%) 940
Rhinocort Nasal Inhaler (Less than 1%) 556
▲ Ridaura Capsules (24%) 2513
Rifadin (Occasional) 1528
Rifamate Capsules (Occasional) 1530
Rifater (Occasional) 1532
Rimactane Capsules 847
▲ Risperdal (2% to 5%) 1301
Robaxin Injectable 2070
Robaxin Tablets 2071
Robaxisal Tablets 2071
Rocephin Injectable Vials, ADD-Vantage, Galaxy Container (1.7%) 2142
▲ Roferon-A Injection (11% to 18%) 2145
Romazicon (1% to 3%) 2147
Rowasa (1.2% to 2.82%) 2548
Rythmol Tablets–150mg, 225mg, 300mg (0.6 to 2.6%) 1352
▲ SSKI Solution (Among most frequent) 2658
Salagen Tablets (1%) 1489
Salflex Tablets 786
Sandostatin Injection (Less than 1%) 2292
Sanorex Tablets 2294
Sansert Tablets (Rare) 2295
Sectral Capsules (2%) 2807
Sedapap Tablets 50 mg/650 mg 1543
Seldane Tablets (1.0% to 1.6%) 1536
Seldane-D Extended-Release Tablets (1.1%) 1538
▲ Septra (Among most common) 1174
▲ Septra I.V. Infusion (Among most common) 1169
▲ Septra I.V. Infusion ADD-Vantage Vials (Among most common) 1171
▲ Septra (Among most common) 1174
Ser-Ap-Es Tablets 849
Serentil 684
Serevent Inhalation Aerosol (Rare; 1% to 3%) 1176
Serzone Tablets (2%) 771
Shade Gel SPF 30 Sunblock ▣ 807
Shade Lotion SPF 45 Sunblock ▣ 807
Shade UVAGUARD SPF 15 Suncreen Lotion ▣ 808
Silvadene Cream 1% (Infrequent) 1540
Sinemet CR Tablets 944
Skelaxin Tablets 788
Slo-bid Gyrocaps 2033
Slo-Niacin Tablets (Less common) 2659
Slow-K Extended-Release Tablets (Rare) 851
Solganal Suspension 2388
Soma Compound w/Codeine Tablets 2676
Soma Compound Tablets (Less common) 2675
▲ Sporanox Capsules (1.1% to 8.6%) 1305
Stadol (Less than 1%) 775
Stelazine 2514
Sulfamylon Cream 925
▲ Supprelin Injection (3% to 10%) 2056
Suprax (Less than 2%) 1399
Synarel Nasal Solution for Central Precocious Puberty (2.6%) 2151
Synthroid Tablets 1359
Tagamet 2516
Talacen (Infrequent) 2333
Talwin Carpuject (Infrequent) 2334
Talwin Compound (Infrequent) 2335
Talwin Injection (Infrequent) 2334
Talwin Nx (Infrequent) 2336
▲ Taxol (12%) 714
Tazicef for Injection (2%) 2519
▲ Tegison Capsules (50-75%) 2154
Tenex Tablets (Less frequent) 2074
Tetramune (Up to 3%) 1404
Thalitone 1245
Theo-24 Extended Release Capsules 2568
Theo-Dur Extended-Release Tablets 1327
Theo-X Extended-Release Tablets 788
▲ Ticlid Tablets (5.1%) 2156
Tilade (Less than 1%) 996

(▣ Described in PDR For Nonprescription Drugs) Incidence data in parenthesis; ▲ 3% or more (◉ Described in PDR For Ophthalmology)

Side Effects Index

Timolide Tablets (Less than 1%) 1748
Timoptic in Ocudose (Less frequent) 1753
Timoptic Sterile Ophthalmic Solution (Less frequent) 1751
Timoptic-XE 1755
Tobramycin Sulfate Injection 968
Tolectin (200, 400 and 600 mg) .. 1581
▲ Tonocard Tablets (0.4-12.2%)....... 531
▲ Toprol-XL Tablets (About 5 of 100 patients) 565
Toradol (Greater than 1%) 2159
Tracrium Injection 1183
Trandate (Rare) 1185
Transderm Scōp Transdermal Therapeutic System (Infrequent) 869
Trental Tablets (Less than 1%) 1244
Tri-Immunol Adsorbed 1408
Trilisate (Less than 1%) 2000
▲ Trimpex Tablets (2.6% to 6.7%) .. 2163
Tri-Norinyl 2164
Triphasil-21 Tablets 2814
Triphasil-28 Tablets 2819
Trusopt Sterile Ophthalmic Solution (Rare) 1760
Tussionex Pennkinetic Extended-Release Suspension 998
Tussi-Organidin DM NR Liquid and DM-S NR Liquid 2677
Tussi-Organidin NR Liquid and S NR Liquid (Rare) 2677
TYLENOL Severe Allergy Medication Caplets 1564
Tylox Capsules 1584
Tympagesic Ear Drops 2342
Ultram Tablets (50 mg) (1% to 5%) 1585
Ultravate Cream 0.05% (Less frequent) 2689
Ultravate Ointment 0.05% 2690
Unasyn (Less than 2%) 2212
Uni-Dur Extended-Release Tablets.. 1331
Univasc Tablets (Less than 1% to 1.6%) 2410
Urised Tablets 1964
Vancenase PocketHaler Nasal Inhaler (Rare) 2391
Vanceril Inhaler (Rare)........................ 2394
Vancocin HCl, Oral Solution & Pulvules (Infrequent) 1483
Vancocin HCl, Vials & ADD-Vantage (Infrequent) 1481
Vantin for Oral Suspension and Vantin Tablets (Less than 1% to 3.5%) 2646
Varivax (Greater than or equal to 1%) 1762
Vascor (200, 300 and 400 mg) Tablets (0.5 to 2.0%) 1587
Vaseretic Tablets (0.5% to 2.0%) 1765
Vasotec I.V. (0.5% to 1.0%) 1768
Vasotec Tablets (0.5%; 1.3% to 1.4%) 1771
Velosulin BR Human Insulin 10 ml Vials 1795
Ventolin Inhalation Solution (Rare).. 1198
Ventolin Nebules Inhalation Solution (Rare) 1199
Ventolin Rotacaps for Inhalation (Rare) 1200
Ventolin Syrup (Rare) 1202
Ventolin Tablets (Rare) 1203
VePesid Capsules and Injection (Infrequent) 718
Verelan Capsules (1% or less to 1.4%) 1410
Verelan Capsules (1.2% to 1.4%) 2824
Vermox Chewable Tablets (Rare) 1312
Versed Injection (Less than 1%) ... 2170
▲ Videx Tablets, Powder for Oral Solution, & Pediatric Powder for Oral Solution (7% to 72%) 720
Virazole 1264
Visken Tablets (Less than 1%) 2299
Vivotif Berna 665
Volmax Extended-Release Tablets (Rare) 1788
Voltaren Tablets (1% to 3%) 861
▲ Vumon (3%) 727
▲ Wellbutrin Tablets (8.0%) 1204
▲ Xanax Tablets (10.8%) 2649
Yutopar Intravenous Injection (Infrequent) 570
Zaroxolyn Tablets 1000
Zebeta Tablets 1413
Zefazone (1.1%) 2654
Zemuron (Less than 1%) 1830
▲ Zerit Capsules (3% to 33%) 729
Zestoretic (1.2%) 2850
▲ Zestril Tablets (1.3% to 4.8%) 2854
Ziac 1415

Zithromax (1% or less)........................ 1944
Zofran Injection (Approximately 1%) 1214
Zofran Tablets (Approximately 1%) 1217
▲ Zoladex (1% to 6%) 2858
Zoloft Tablets (2.1%) 2217
▲ Zosyn (4.2%) 1419
▲ Zosyn Pharmacy Bulk Package (4.2%) 1422
Zovirax Capsules (0.6% to 1.7%).. 1219
Zovirax Ointment 5% 1223
Zovirax Sterile Powder (Approximately 2%) 1223
Zovirax (0.6% to 1.7%) 1219

Rash, actinic

Solganal Suspension 2388

Rash, allergic

Amen Tablets 780
Aygestin Tablets 974
Brevicon 2088
Cycrin Tablets 975
Demulen 2428
Depo-Provera Sterile Aqueous Suspension 2606
Desogen Tablets 1817
Empirin with Codeine Tablets.......... 1093
Florinef Acetate Tablets 505
Levlen/Tri-Levlen 651
Luride Drops 50 ml (Rare) 871
Luride Lozi-Tabs Tablets (Rare) 871
Micronor Tablets 1872
Modicon 1872
Norinyl 2088
Nor-Q D Tablets 2135
Ortho-Cept 1851
Ortho-Cyclen/Ortho-Tri-Cyclen 1858
Ortho-Novum 1872
Ortho-Cyclen/Ortho Tri-Cyclen 1858
Ovcon 760
Parafon Forte DSC Caplets (Rare) .. 1581
Periactin 1724
Premphase 2797
Prempro 2801
Levlen/Tri-Levlen 651
Tri-Norinyl 2164
Varivax (Greater than or equal to 1%) 1762

Rash, bullous

Orudis Capsules (Less than 1%) 2766
Oruvail Capsules (Less than 1%) ... 2766
Trandate Tablets (Less common) 1185
▲ Zosyn (4.2%) 1419
▲ Zosyn Pharmacy Bulk Package (4.2%) 1422

Rash, bullous erythrodermatous of the palms and soles

Idamycin 1955

Rash, circumocular

Polytrim Ophthalmic Solution Sterile (Multiple reports) 482

Rash, drug

Actifed with Codeine Cough Syrup.. 1067
Benadryl Capsules 1898
Benadryl Injection 1898
Comhist 2038
Deconamine 1320
Dimetane-DC Cough Syrup 2059
Dimetane-DX Cough Syrup 2059
Nitrolingual Spray 2027
Ornade Spansule Capsules 2502
PBZ Tablets 845
PBZ-SR Tablets 844
Tavist Syrup 2297
Tavist Tablets 2298
Trancopal Caplets 2337
Trinalin Repetabs Tablets 1330
Tussend 1783

Rash, erythematous

Achromycin V Capsules 1367
Anafranil Capsules (Infrequent) 803
Atretol Tablets 573
Blocadren Tablets 1614
Cartrol Tablets 410
Celontin Kapseals 1899
▲ Cognex Capsules (7%) 1901
DTIC-Dome (Infrequent) 600
Declomycin Tablets 1371
Doryx Capsules 1913
Dynacin Capsules 1590
Flagyl 375 Capsules 2434
Flagyl I.V. 2247
Foscavir Injection (Between 1% and 5%) 547

Hivid Tablets (Less than 1% to less than 3%) 2121
Inderal 2728
Inderal LA Long Acting Capsules ... 2730
Inderide Tablets 2732
Inderide LA Long Acting Capsules.. 2734
Kerlone Tablets (Less than 2%) 2436
Levatol 2403
Methotrexate Sodium Tablets, Injection, for Injection and LPF Injection 1275
Miacalcin Nasal Spray (1% to 3%) 2275
Milontin Kapseals 1920
Minocin Intravenous 1382
Minocin Oral Suspension 1385
Minocin Pellet-Filled Capsules 1383
Monodox Capsules 1805
Norvasc Tablets (More than 0.1% to 1%) 1940
Protostat Tablets 1883
Sectral Capsules 2807
Tegretol Chewable Tablets 852
Tegretol Suspension 852
Tegretol Tablets 852
Tenoretic Tablets 2845
Tenormin Tablets and I.V. Injection 2847
Terramycin Intramuscular Solution 2210
Timolide Tablets 1748
Timoptic in Ocudose 1753
Timoptic Sterile Ophthalmic Solution 1751
Timoptic-XE 1755
Vibramycin 1941
Vibramycin Hyclate Intravenous 2215
Vibramycin 1941
Visken Tablets 2299
Zarontin Capsules 1928
Zarontin Syrup 1929
Zoloft Tablets (Infrequent) 2217

Rash, erythematous maculopapular

Aldactazide 2413
Amoxil 2464
Miltown Tablets 2672
Omnipen Capsules (Frequent) 2764
Omnipen for Oral Suspension (Frequent) 2765
PMB 200 and PMB 400 2783

Rash, exfoliative

Quinaglute Dura-Tabs Tablets 649

Rash, female genitalia

Floxin I.V. (Less than 1%) 1571
Floxin Tablets (200 mg, 300 mg, 400 mg) (Less than 1%) 1567

Rash, follicular

Hivid Tablets (Less than 1% to less than 3%) 2121
Zoloft Tablets (Rare) 2217

Rash, herpetic

(see under Eruptions, herpetic)

Rash, leg

DDAVP 2017
Desmopressin Acetate Rhinal Tube 979

Rash, lichenoid

Normodyne Tablets (Less common) 2379
Permax Tablets (Rare) 575
Trandate Tablets (Less common) 1185

Rash, maculopapular

Achromycin V Capsules 1367
Aclovate Cream (1 in 100 patients) 1069
Children's Advil Suspension (Less than 3%) 2692
Anafranil Capsules (Infrequent) 803
Betaseron for SC Injection 658
Capastat Sulfate Vials 2868
Capoten 739
Capozide 742
Catapres-TTS (1 of 101; 10 cases of 3,539 patients) 675
Chloromycetin Sodium Succinate ... 1900
Cleocin Phosphate Injection 2586
Cleocin Vaginal Cream 2589
▲ Cognex Capsules (7%) 1901
Cytosar-U Sterile Powder (Occasional) 2592
Cytovene (1% or less) 2103
Danocrine Capsules 2307
Declomycin Tablets 1371
Depakote Tablets (Greater than 1% but not more than 5%) 415
Didronel Tablets 1984
Doryx Capsules 1913

Dynacin Capsules 1590
Effexor (Infrequent) 2719
Fluorouracil Injection 2116
Foscavir Injection (Between 1% and 5%) 547
Sterile FUDR (Remote possibility) .. 2118
Fungizone Intravenous 506
Haldol Decanoate 1577
Haldol Injection, Tablets and Concentrate 1575
Hivid Tablets (Less than 1% to less than 3%) 2121
Hydrea Capsules (Less frequent) 696
Hyskon Hysteroscopy Fluid (Rare).. 1595
▲ IBU Tablets (3% to 9%) 1342
Lamictal Tablets (Infrequent) 1112
Lanoxicaps (Rare) 1117
Lanoxin Elixir Pediatric (Rare) 1120
Lanoxin Injection (Rare) 1123
Lanoxin Injection Pediatric (Rare) .. 1126
Lanoxin Tablets (Rare) 1128
Lodine Capsules and Tablets (Less than 1%) 2743
Lotrisone Cream (1 of 270 patients) 2372
Mandol Vials, Faspak & ADD-Vantage 1461
Mesantoin Tablets 2272
Minocin Intravenous 1382
Minocin Oral Suspension 1385
Minocin Pellet-Filled Capsules 1383
Monodox Capsules 1805
Children's Motrin Ibuprofen Oral Suspension (Greater than 1% but less than 3%) 1546
Motrin Tablets (Less than 3%) 2625
▲ Motrin Ibuprofen Suspension, Oral Drops, Chewable Tablets, Caplets (3% to 9%) 1546
Normodyne Tablets (Less common) 2379
Norvasc Tablets (More than 0.1% to 1%) 1940
Paxil Tablets (Rare) 2505
Procan SR Tablets (Occasional) 1926
Proloprim Tablets (Mild to moderate) 1155
Prozac Pulvules & Liquid, Oral Solution (Infrequent) 919
Rifamate Capsules 1530
Serax Capsules 2810
Serax Tablets 2810
Serzone Tablets (Infrequent) 771
Synarel Nasal Solution for Endometriosis (Less than 1%) 2152
Terramycin Intramuscular Solution 2210
Ticlid Tablets 2156
Toradol 2159
Trandate Tablets (Less common) ... 1185
Vibramycin 1941
Vibramycin Hyclate Intravenous 2215
Vibramycin 1941
▲ Zerit Capsules (Fewer than 1% to 6%) 729
Zoloft Tablets (Infrequent) 2217
▲ Zosyn (4.2%) 1419
▲ Zosyn Pharmacy Bulk Package (4.2%) 1422
Zyloprim Tablets (Less than 1%) 1226

Rash, morbilliform

▲ Cleocin Phosphate Injection (Most frequent) 2586
▲ Cleocin Vaginal Cream (Most frequent) 2589
▲ Dilantin Infatabs (Among most common) 1908
▲ Dilantin Kapseals (Among most common) 1906
▲ Dilantin Parenteral (Among most common) 1910
▲ Dilantin-125 Suspension (Among most common) 1911
Furoxone 2046
Mesantoin Tablets 2272
Proloprim Tablets (Mild to moderate) 1155
Rifamate Capsules 1530
Serax Capsules 2810
Serax Tablets 2810

Rash, papular

▲ CHEMET (succimer) Capsules (2.6 to 11.2%) 1545
Danocrine Capsules 2307

Rash, penile

Caverject (1%) 2583

Rash, perianal

Mintezol 1704

(◻ Described in PDR For Nonprescription Drugs) Incidence data in parenthesis; ▲ 3% or more (◉ Described in PDR For Ophthalmology)

Rash, pruritic — Side Effects Index — 1402

Rash, pruritic

Atretol Tablets 573
▲ Capoten (About 4 to 7 of 100 patients) 739
▲ Capozide (About 4 to 7 of 100 patients) 742
Cycrin Tablets 975
Fluorouracil Injection 2116
Sterile FUDR (Remote possibility) 2118
Hivid Tablets (Less than 1% to less than 3%) 2121
Lithonate/Lithotabs/Lithobid 2543
Miltown Tablets 2672
PMB 200 and PMB 400 2783
Premphase 2797
Prempro 2801
Proloprim Tablets (Mild to moderate) 1155
Skelaxin Tablets 788
Spectazole (econazole nitrate 1%) Cream (One case) 1890
Tegretol Chewable Tablets 852
Tegretol Suspension 852
Tegretol Tablets 852

Rash, psoriaform

Foscavir Injection (Less than 1%) 547
Inderal (Rare) 2728
Inderal LA Long Acting Capsules (Rare) 2730
Inderide Tablets (Rare) 2732
Inderide LA Long Acting Capsules (Rare) 2734
Normodyne Tablets (Less common) 2379
Quinaglute Dura-Tabs Tablets 649
Tenoretic Tablets 2845
Tenormin Tablets and I.V. Injection 2847
Trandate Tablets (Less common) 1185

Rash, purpuric

Danocrine Capsules 2307
Dilantin Infatabs 1908
Dilantin Kapseals 1906
Dilantin-125 Suspension 1911
Eminase (0.3%) 2039
Mesantoin Tablets 2272
Orudis Capsules (Less than 1%) 2766
Oruvail Capsules (Less than 1%) 2766
Prozac Pulvules & Liquid, Oral Solution (Rare) 919
Rifamate Capsules 1530

Rash, pustular

Anafranil Capsules (Infrequent) 803
Effexor (Rare) 2719
Lamictal Tablets (Rare) 1112
Prozac Pulvules & Liquid, Oral Solution (Rare) 919

Rash, scarlatiniform

Dilantin Infatabs 1908
Dilantin Kapseals 1906
Dilantin Parenteral 1910
Dilantin-125 Suspension 1911
Mesantoin Tablets 2272

Rash, skin (see also under Rash)

Amicar Syrup, Tablets, and Injection (Occasional) 1267
Amikacin Sulfate Injection, USP (Rare) 960
Amikin Injectable (Rare) 501
Ancef Injection 2465
Anturane 807
Aristocort Suspension (Intralesional) 1025
Artane (Rare) 1368
Asendin Tablets (Less frequent) 1369
Atamet 572
Ativan Injection (Occasional) 2698
Atretol Tablets 573
Atromid-S Capsules (Less often) 2701
▲ Augmentin (3%) 2468
Azulfidine (One in every 30 patients or less) 1949
Beclovent Inhalation Aerosol and Refill (Rare) 1075
Beconase (Rare) 1076
Bicillin C-R Injection 2704
Bicillin C-R 900/300 Injection 2706
Bicillin L-A Injection 2707
BuSpar (1%) 737
Calcimar Injection, Synthetic (Occasional) 2013
Ceptaz (2% of patients) 1081
Cerubidine (Rare) 795
Chromagen Capsules 2339
Claforan Sterile and Injection (2.4%) 1235
Combipres Tablets (About 1%) 677
Cylert Tablets 412
Cytosar-U Sterile Powder (Rare) 2592
Cytoxan (Occurs occasionally) 694
Dalmane Capsules (Rare) 2173
Danocrine Capsules 2307
Darvon-N/Darvocet-N 1433
Darvon 1435
Darvon-N Suspension & Tablets (Less than 1%) 1433
Demerol 2308
Dilatrate-SR (Occasional) 2398
Dizac (Less frequent) 1809
Dobutrex Solution Vials (Occasional) 1439
EC-Naprosyn Delayed-Release Tablets (Less than 1%) 2117
Edecrin 1657
Elavil 2838
Elspar 1659
Emcyt Capsules (1%) 1953
Empirin with Codeine Tablets 1093
Endep Tablets 2174
Ery-Tab Tablets 422
Factrel 2877
Feldene Capsules (Occasional) 1965
Flexeril Tablets (Less than 1%) 1661
▲ Fludara for Injection (15%) 663
Fortaz (2%) 1100
Ganite 2533
Geocillin Tablets (Infrequent) 2199
Grifulvin V (griseofulvin tablets) Microsize (griseofulvin oral suspension) Microsize 1888
Gris-PEG Tablets, 125 mg & 250 mg 479
Ilosone 911
Imodium Capsules 1295
Imuran (Approximately 2%) 1110
▲ Intron A (Up to 25%) 2364
K-Norm Extended-Release Capsules (Rare) 991
Kefzol Vials, Faspak & ADD-Vantage 1456
Kemadrin Tablets (Occasional) 1112
Klonopin Tablets 2126
Lamprene Capsules (1-5%) 828
Larodopa Tablets (Infrequent) 2129
Lasix Injection, Oral Solution and Tablets 1240
Levo-Dromoran (Occasional) 2129
Limbitrol 2180
Lioresal Tablets 829
▲ Lopressor Ampuls (5%) 830
Lopressor HCT Tablets 832
▲ Lopressor Tablets (5%) 830
Loxitane 1378
Ludiomil Tablets (Rare) 843
Lysodren 698
MS Contin Tablets (Less frequent) 1994
MSIR (Infrequent) 1997
Mebaral Tablets (Less than 1 in 100) 2322
Mepergan Injection 2753
Mestinon Injectable (Occasional) 1253
Mestinon (Occasional) 1254
Methadone Hydrochloride Oral Solution & Tablets 2235
Mezlin 601
Mezlin Pharmacy Bulk Package 604
Midamor Tablets (Less than or equal to 1%) 1703
Midrin Capsules 783
Minipress Capsules (1-4%) 1937
Minizide Capsules 1938
Mintezol 1704
Monistat Dual-Pak (Less than 0.5%) 1850
Monistat 3 Vaginal Suppositories (Less than 0.5%) 1850
Mycelex-G 500 mg Vaginal Tablets (Rare) 609
Naprosyn Suspension (Less than 1%) 2117
Nardil (Less common) 1920
Nebcin Vials, Hyporets & ADD-Vantage 1464
Nembutal Sodium Capsules 436
Nembutal Sodium Solution 438
Nembutal Sodium Suppositories (Less than 1%) 440
Neosporin Ophthalmic Ointment Sterile 1148
Nicobid 2026
▲ Nolvadex Tablets (13%) 2841
Norpramin Tablets 1526
Oramorph SR (Morphine Sulfate Sustained Release Tablets) (Less frequent) 2236
Papaverine Hydrochloride Vials and Ampoules 1468
Parlodel 2281
Parnate Tablets (Rare) 2503
Peganone Tablets 446
Pfizerpen for Injection 2203
Phenobarbital Elixir and Tablets (Less than 1 in 100 patients) 1469
▲ Phenurone Tablets (5%) 447
Pipracil (1%) 1390
Pnu-Imune 23 (Rare to infrequent) 1393
Pondimin Tablets 2066
Potaba (Infrequent) 1229
Proglycem 580
Proloprim Tablets 1155
Purinethol Tablets 1156
Quadrinal Tablets 1350
Quinidex Extentabs 2067
Reglan (A few cases) 2068
Ritalin 848
Roxanol 2243
Roxicodone Tablets, Oral Solution & Intensol (Oxycodone) 2244
SSD (Infrequent) 1355
Seconal Sodium Pulvules (Less than 1 in 100) 1474
Serax Capsules (Rare) 2810
Serax Tablets (Rare) 2810
Seromycin Pulvules 1476
Sinemet Tablets 943
Sinequan (Occasional) 2205
Soma Compound w/Codeine Tablets 2676
Soma Compound Tablets 2675
Soma Tablets 2674
Spectrobid Tablets 2206
Stilphostrol Tablets and Ampuls 612
Surmontil Capsules 2811
Symmetrel Capsules and Syrup (0.1% to 1%) 946
Talacen (A few cases) 2333
Tambocor Tablets (1% to less than 3%) 1497
Tao Capsules 2209
Tapazole Tablets 1477
Tazidime Vials, Faspak & ADD-Vantage (2%) 1478
Tegretol Chewable Tablets 852
Tegretol Suspension 852
Tegretol Tablets 852
Tenex Tablets (Less frequent) 2074
Tenoretic Tablets 2845
Tenormin Tablets and I.V. Injection 2847
TheraCys BCG Live (Intravesical) (Up to 1.8%; rare) 897
Thioplex (Thiotepa For Injection) (Occasional) 1281
Ticar for Injection 2526
Timentin for Injection 2528
Tofranil Ampuls 854
Tofranil Tablets 856
Tofranil-PM Capsules 857
Trandate Tablets (Less common) 1185
Tranxene 451
Trecator-SC Tablets 2814
Trental Tablets (Less than 1%) 1244
Triavil Tablets 1757
Trinsicon Capsules (Extremely rare) 2570
Unasyn 2212
Uniphyl 400 mg Tablets 2001
Urised Tablets 1964
Urobiotic-250 Capsules 2214
Uroqid-Acid No. 2 Tablets (Occasional) 640
Valium Injectable 2182
Valium Tablets (Infrequent) 2183
Valrelease Capsules (Occasional) 2169
Vancocin HCl, Oral Solution & Pulvules (Infrequent) 1483
Vancocin HCl, Vials & ADD-Vantage (Infrequent) 1481
Ventolin Inhalation Aerosol and Refill (Rare) 1197
Ventolin Inhalation Solution (Rare) 1198
Ventolin Syrup (Rare) 1202
Ventolin Tablets (Rare) 1203
Vivactil Tablets 1774
Vontrol Tablets (Rare) 2532
Wygesic Tablets 2827
Zantac (Rare) 1209
Zantac Injection 1207
Zantac Syrup (Rare) 1209
Zaroxolyn Tablets 1000
Zinacef (1 in 125 patients) 1211
Zovirax Capsules (0.3%) 1219
Zovirax Ointment 5% (0.3%) 1223
Zovirax (0.3%) 1219
Zyloprim Tablets (Less than 1%) 1226

Rash, urticarial

Capoten (Rare) 739
Capozide (Rare) 742
DTIC-Dome (Infrequent) 600
Mesantoin Tablets 2272
Miltown Tablets 2672
Normodyne Tablets (Less common) 2379
PMB 200 and PMB 400 2783
Serax Capsules 2810
Serax Tablets 2810
Ticlid Tablets 2156
Trandate Tablets (Less common) 1185
▲ Zosyn (4.2%) 1419
▲ Zosyn Pharmacy Bulk Package (4.2%) 1422

Rash, varicella-like

Varivax (0.9% to 5.5%) 1762

Rash, vesiculobullous

Betaseron for SC Injection 658
▲ Cognex Capsules (7%) 1901
Cytovene (1% or less) 2103
Effexor (Rare) 2719
IBU Tablets (Less than 1%) 1342
Lamictal Tablets (Rare) 1112
Lodine Capsules and Tablets (Less than 1%) 2743
Megace Oral Suspension (1% to 3%) 699
Permax Tablets (Rare) 575
Prozac Pulvules & Liquid, Oral Solution (Rare) 919
Serzone Tablets (Infrequent) 771
Videx Tablets, Powder for Oral Solution, & Pediatric Powder for Oral Solution (Less than 1%) 720

Raynaud's phenomenon

Blenoxane (Isolated reports) 692
Blocadren Tablets 1614
Capoten (2 to 3 of 1000 patients) 739
Capozide (2 to 3 of 1000 patients) 742
Catapres Tablets (Rare) 674
Catapres-TTS (Rare) 675
Combipres Tablets (Rare) 677
Imitrex Injection (Rare) 1103
Inderal 2728
Inderal LA Long Acting Capsules 2730
Inderide Tablets 2732
Inderide LA Long Acting Capsules 2734
Kerlone Tablets 2436
Lopressor HCT Tablets 832
Parlodel (Less than 2%) 2281
Platinol 708
Platinol-AQ Injection 710
Roferon-A Injection (Less than 1%) 2145
Sandostatin Injection (Less than 1%) 2292
Tenoretic Tablets 2845
Tenormin Tablets and I.V. Injection 2847
Timolide Tablets 1748
Timoptic in Ocudose 1753
Timoptic Sterile Ophthalmic Solution 1751
Timoptic-XE 1755
Toprol-XL Tablets (About 1 of 100 patients) 565
Velban Vials 1484

Rectal bleeding

Accutane Capsules 2076
Ambien Tablets (Rare) 2416
Anafranil Capsules (Infrequent) 803
Betaseron for SC Injection 658
BuSpar (Infrequent) 737
Clozaril Tablets (Less than 1%) 2252
Cognex Capsules (Infrequent) 1901
CORTENEMA (Rare) 2535
Daypro Caplets (Less than 1%) 2426
Demadex Tablets and Injection 686
Depo-Provera Contraceptive Injection (Fewer than 1%) 2602
Dipentum Capsules (Rare) 1951
Effexor (Infrequent) 2719
Eldepryl Tablets 2550
Felbatol 2666
Foscavir Injection (Between 1% and 5%) 547
Geocillin Tablets 2199
Hivid Tablets (Less than 1% to less than 3%) 2121
Indocin Capsules (Less than 1%) 1680
Indocin I.V. (Less than 1%) 1684
Indocin (Less than 1%) 1680
Intron A (Less than 5%) 2364
Luvox Tablets (Infrequent) 2544
Neurontin Capsules (Rare) 1922
Orudis Capsules (Less than 1%) 2766
Oruvail Capsules (Less than 1%) 2766
Paxil Tablets (Infrequent) 2505

(Described in PDR For Nonprescription Drugs) Incidence data in parenthesis; ▲ 3% or more (Described in PDR For Ophthalmology)

Pentasa (Less than 1%) 1527
PREVACID Delayed-Release Capsules (Less than 1%) 2562
Questran Light 769
Questran Powder 770
Relafen Tablets (Less than 1%) 2510
Retrovir Capsules 1158
Retrovir I.V. Infusion 1163
Retrovir Syrup 1158
Serzone Tablets (Infrequent) 771
Toradol (1% or less) 2159
Vantin for Oral Suspension and Vantin Tablets 2646
Velban Vials 1484
Videx Tablets, Powder for Oral Solution, & Pediatric Powder for Oral Solution (Less than 1%) 720

Rectal discomfort

Fleet Babylax 1001

Rectal disorders, unspecified

▲ CellCept Capsules (More than or equal to 3%) 2099
Cytotec (Infrequent) 2424
Dipentum Capsules (Rare) 1951
Foscavir Injection (Less than 1%) 547
Kerlone Tablets (Less than 2%) 2436
Wellbutrin Tablets (Rare) 1204

Rectal urgency (see under Defecate, desire to)

Red blood cell, aplasia

Mysoline (Rare) 2754

Red blood cell, hypoplasia of

Mysoline (Rare) 2754

"Red neck" syndrome

Vancocin HCl, Vials & ADD-Vantage 1481

Reflexes, abnormal

Methotrexate Sodium Tablets, Injection, for Injection and LPF Injection 1275

Reflexes, increased (see under Hyperreflexia)

Regurgitation

IPOL Poliovirus Vaccine Inactivated 885
Mevacor Tablets (0.5% to 1.0%) 1699
Mylanta Liquid (Occasional) 1317
Mylanta Tablets (Occasional) ▣ 660
Mylanta Double Strength Liquid (Occasional) 1317
Mylanta Double Strength Tablets (Occasional) ▣ 660
Plendil Extended-Release Tablets (0.5% to 1.5%) 527

Renal agenesis, unilateral, neonatal

Leukeran Tablets 1133

Renal calculi (see also under Renal stones)

Anafranil Capsules (Infrequent) 803
Cardura Tablets (Less than 0.5% of 3960 patients) 2186
Cipro I.V. (1% or less) 595
Cipro I.V. Pharmacy Bulk Package (Less than 1%) 597
Cipro Tablets 592
Clinoril Tablets (Rare) 1618
Cognex Capsules (Infrequent) 1901
Daranide Tablets 1633
Diamox 1372
Dilacor XR Extended-release Capsules (Infrequent) 2018
Effexor (Infrequent) 2719
Floxin I.V. 1571
Floxin Tablets (200 mg, 300 mg, 400 mg) 1567
Imitrex Injection (Rare) 1103
Lodine Capsules and Tablets (Less than 1%) 2743
MZM (Common; rare) ⊙ 267
Maxaquin Tablets 2440
Miacalcin Nasal Spray (Less than 1%) 2275
Neptazane Tablets 1388
Neurontin Capsules (Rare) 1922
Paxil Tablets (Rare) 2505
Penetrex Tablets 2031
Permax Tablets (Infrequent) 575
PREVACID Delayed-Release Capsules (Less than 1%) 2562
Prozac Pulvules & Liquid, Oral Solution (Rare) 919
Rogaine Topical Solution (0.93%) 2637

Renal colic

Benemid Tablets 1611
ColBENEMID Tablets 1622
Daranide Tablets 1633
Ethmozine Tablets (Less than 2%) 2041
Kerlone Tablets (Less than 2%) 2436
Noroxin Tablets (Less frequent) 1715
Noroxin Tablets (Less frequent) 2048
Timolide Tablets (Less than 1%) 1748
Zebeta Tablets 1413
Ziac 1415

Renal disease

Anaprox/Naprosyn (Less than 1%) 2117

Renal failure

ActHIB 872
Aldoclor Tablets 1598
Aldoril Tablets 1604
Amicar Syrup, Tablets, and Injection (Rare) 1267
Anaprox/Naprosyn (Less than 1%) 2117
Ancobon Capsules 2079
Ansaid Tablets (Less than 1%) 2579
Atretol Tablets 573
Bactrim DS Tablets 2084
Bactrim I.V. Infusion 2082
Bactrim 2084
Betaseron for SC Injection 658
BiCNU 691
Bumex (0.1%) 2093
Capoten (Approximately 1 to 2 of 1000 patients) 739
Capozide (Approximately 1 to 2 of 1000 patients) 742
Cataflam 816
CeeNU 693
Chibroxin Sterile Ophthalmic Solution (With oral form) 1617
Cipro I.V. (1% or less) 595
Cipro I.V. Pharmacy Bulk Package (Less than 1%) 597
Cipro Tablets (Less than 1%) 592
Clinoril Tablets (Less than 1 in 100) 1618
Clomid 1514
Cognex Capsules (Rare) 1901
Cytovene (1% or less) 2103
Dilacor XR Extended-release Capsules 2018
Diprivan Injection (Less than 1%) 2833
Diupres Tablets 1650
Diuril Oral Suspension 1653
Diuril Sodium Intravenous 1652
Diuril Tablets 1653
Dolobid Tablets (Less than 1 in 100) 1654
Dyrenium Capsules (One case) 2481
EC-Naprosyn Delayed-Release Tablets (Less than 1%) 2117
Ergamisol Tablets (Less frequent) 1292
Feldene Capsules (Less than 1%) 1965
Floxin I.V. 1571
Fludara for Injection (Up to 1%) 663
HydroDIURIL Tablets 1674
Hydropres Tablets 1675
Hyzaar Tablets 1677
IFEX (1 episode) 697
Indocin (Less than 1%) 1680
Lodine Capsules and Tablets (Less than 1%) 2743
Maxaquin Tablets 2440
Methotrexate Sodium Tablets, Injection, for Injection and LPF Injection 1275
Moduretic Tablets (Less than or equal to 1%) 1705
Mutamycin 703
Anaprox/Naprosyn (Less than 1%) 2117
NebuPent for Inhalation Solution (1% or less) 1040
Noroxin Tablets 1715
Noroxin Tablets 2048
▲ Novantrone (0 to 8%) 1279
OmniHIB 2499
Oncaspar 2028
Orthoclone OKT3 Sterile Solution 1837
Orudis Capsules (Less than 1%) 2766
Oruvail Capsules (Less than 1%) 2766
Penetrex Tablets (Less than 1% but more than or equal to 0.1%) 2031
Permax Tablets (Infrequent) 575
Ponstel 1925
Prinzide Tablets 1737
▲ Prograf (Greater than 3%) 1042
Proleukin for Injection (Less than 1%) 797
Prozac Pulvules & Liquid, Oral Solution 919
Rythmol Tablets–150mg, 225mg, 300mg (Less than 1%) 1352
Septra 1174
Septra I.V. Infusion 1169
Septra I.V. Infusion ADD-Vantage Vials 1171
Septra 1174
Tegretol Chewable Tablets 852
Tegretol Suspension 852
Tegretol Tablets 852
Tenormin Tablets and I.V. Injection (0.4%) 2847
Ticlid Tablets (Rare) 2156
Timolide Tablets 1748
Tolectin (200, 400 and 600 mg) (Less than 1%) 1581
Tonocard Tablets 531
Trasylol (2%) 613
Vancocin HCl, Oral Solution & Pulvules (Rare) 1483
Vancocin HCl, Vials & ADD-Vantage (Rare) 1481
Vaseretic Tablets 1765
Vasotec I.V. 1768
Vasotec Tablets (0.5% to 1.0%) 1771
Videx Tablets, Powder for Oral Solution, & Pediatric Powder for Oral Solution (Less than 1%) 720
Voltaren Tablets 861
Zestoretic 2850
Ziac 1415
Zovirax Sterile Powder 1223
Zyloprim Tablets (Less than 1%) 1226

Renal failure, acute

Accupril Tablets (Rare) 1893
Activase 1058
Children's Advil Suspension (Less than 1%) 2692
Altace Capsules (Rare) 1232
Ambien Tablets (Rare) 2416
Anectine 1073
Atgam Sterile Solution (Less than 5%) 2581
Azo Gantrisin Tablets 2081
Cataflam (Rare) 816
Daypro Caplets (Less than 1%) 2426
Didronel I.V. Infusion (Rare) 1488
Dyazide 2479
Dyrenium Capsules 2481
Elspar 1659
Ethamolin (Two women) 2400
Felbatol 2666
Floxin I.V. 1571
Floxin Tablets (200 mg, 300 mg, 400 mg) 1567
Foscavir Injection (Between 1% and 5%) 547
Fungizone Intravenous 506
Ganite (Two patients) 2533
Haldol Decanoate 1577
Hivid Tablets (Less than 1% to less than 3%) 2121
IBU Tablets (Less than 1%) 1342
Imitrex Injection 1103
Imitrex Tablets 1106
Indocin I.V. (Less than 1%) 1684
Lamictal Tablets (Rare) 1112
Lotrel Capsules (Rare) 840
Luvox Tablets 2544
Maxzide 1380
Mefoxin (Rare) 1691
Mefoxin Premixed Intravenous Solution (Rare) 1694
Methotrexate Sodium Tablets, Injection, for Injection and LPF Injection 1275
Mevacor Tablets 1699
Minocin Intravenous (Rare) 1382
Minocin Oral Suspension (Rare) 1385
Minocin Pellet-Filled Capsules (Rare) 1383
Monocid Injection (Rare) 2497
Monopril Tablets (Rare) 757
Children's Motrin Ibuprofen Oral Suspension (Less than 1%) 1546
Motrin Tablets (Less than 1%) 2625
Motrin Ibuprofen Suspension, Oral Drops, Chewable Tablets, Caplets (Less than 1%) 1546
Neurontin Capsules (Rare) 1922
Orap Tablets 1050
Pentam 300 Injection (0.5%) 1041
Pravachol (Rare) 765
Primaxin I.M. 1727
Primaxin I.V. (Less than 0.2%) 1729
Prinivil Tablets (Rare; 0.3% to 1.0%) 1733
Prinzide Tablets 1737
Prolixin 509
Rifadin (Rare) 1528
Rifamate Capsules (Rare) 1530
Rifater (Rare) 1532
Rimactane Capsules (Rare) 847
Risperdal 1301
Tenex Tablets (Rare) 2074
Toradol 2159
Trasylol (0.5%) 613
Vaseretic Tablets (Rare) 1765
Vasotec I.V. (Rare) 1768
Vasotec Tablets (Rare) 1771
Videx Tablets, Powder for Oral Solution, & Pediatric Powder for Oral Solution (A few cases to less than 1%) 720
Voltaren Tablets (Rare) 861
Zestoretic (Rare) 2850
Zestril Tablets (0.3% to 1.0%) 2854
Zocor Tablets (Rare) 1775

Renal failure, neonatal

Accupril Tablets 1893
Altace Capsules 1232
Capoten 739
Capozide 742
Cozaar Tablets 1628
Hyzaar Tablets 1677
Lotensin Tablets 834
Lotensin HCT 837
Lotrel Capsules 840
Monopril Tablets 757
Prinivil Tablets 1733
Prinzide Tablets 1737
Univasc Tablets 2410
Vaseretic Tablets 1765
Vasotec I.V. 1768
Vasotec Tablets 1771
VePesid Capsules and Injection 718
Zestoretic 2850
Zestril Tablets 2854

Renal failure, worsening of

Accupril Tablets (Rare) 1893

Renal function impairment

Aldoclor Tablets 1598
Aldoril Tablets 1604
Amikin Injectable 501
▲ Atgam Sterile Solution (5% to 10%) 2581
Brevicon 2088
Cefotan 2829
Ceftin 1078
Cefzil Tablets and Oral Suspension 746
Ceptaz 1081
Cleocin Phosphate Injection (Rare) 2586
Cleocin Vaginal Cream 2589
Cordarone Intravenous (Less than 2%) 2715
Cytosar-U Sterile Powder (Less frequent) 2592
Cytovene (1% or less) 2103
DTIC-Dome (Few reports) 600
Demulen 2428
Desogen Tablets 1817
▲ Didronel I.V. Infusion (Approximately 10%) 1488
Diupres Tablets 1650
Diuril Oral Suspension 1653
Diuril Sodium Intravenous 1652
Diuril Tablets 1653
Duricef 748
Estrace Cream and Tablets 749
Fiorinal with Codeine Capsules 2262
Fludara for Injection (Up to 1%) 663
Fortaz 1100
▲ Foscavir Injection (5% or greater up to approximately 33%) 547
▲ Fungizone Intravenous (Among most common) 506
Garamycin Injectable 2360
Hivid Tablets (Less than 1% to less than 3%) 2121
HydroDIURIL Tablets 1674
Hydropres Tablets 1675
Hyzaar Tablets 1677
Idamycin (Less than 5%) 1955
Keftab Tablets 915
Kerlone Tablets (Less than 2%) 2436
Lescol Capsules 2267
▲ Leukine for IV Infusion (8%) 1271
Levlen/Tri-Levlen 651
Lithonate/Lithotabs/Lithobid 2543
Lopid Tablets 1917
Lorabid Suspension and Pulvules 1459
Micronor Tablets 1872
Modicon 1872

(▣ Described in PDR For Nonprescription Drugs) Incidence data in parenthesis; ▲ 3% or more (⊙ Described in PDR For Ophthalmology)

Renal function impairment

Moduretic Tablets (Less than or equal to 1%) 1705
Mutamycin 703
Nebcin Vials, Hyporets & ADD-Vantage 1464
▲ Neoral (25% to 38%) 2276
Neutrexin 2572
Nolvadex Tablets 2841
Norinyl 2088
Nor-Q D Tablets 2135
Oncaspar 2028
Ortho-Cept 1851
Ortho-Cyclen/Ortho-Tri-Cyclen 1858
Ortho-Novum 1872
Ortho-Cyclen/Ortho Tri-Cyclen 1858
Orudis Capsules (Greater than 1%) 2766
Oruvail Capsules (Greater than 1%) 2766
Ovcon 760
Paxil Tablets (Rare) 2505
Platinol 708
Platinol-AQ Injection 710
Prinivil Tablets (0.3% to 1.0%) 1733
Prinzide Tablets 1737
▲ Prograf (33% to 40%) 1042
ReoPro Vials (0.3%) 1471
▲ Sandimmune (25 to 38%) 2286
Suprax 1399
Tazicef for Injection 2519
Timolide Tablets 1748
Tobramycin Sulfate Injection 968
Tonocard Tablets 531
Tranxene 451
▲ Trasylol (5% to 30%) 613
Levlen/Tri-Levlen 651
Tri-Norinyl 2164
Vantin for Oral Suspension and Vantin Tablets 2646
Vaseretic Tablets 1765
Vasotec I.V. 1768
Vasotec Tablets (0.5% to 1.0%) 1771
Videx Tablets, Powder for Oral Solution, & Pediatric Powder for Oral Solution (Less than 1%) 720
Vumon (Less than 1%) 727
Zefazone 2654
Zestoretic 2850
Zestril Tablets (0.3% to 1.0%) 2854
Ziac 1415

Renal impairment

Capozide 742
Clinoril Tablets (Less than 1 in 100) 1618
ColBENEMID Tablets 1622
Coly-Mycin M Parenteral 1905
Dolobid Tablets (Less than 1 in 100) 1654
▲ IFEX (6%) 697
▲ Indocin I.V. (41% of infants) 1684
Kefzol Vials, Faspak & ADD-Vantage 1456
Macrobid Capsules 1988
Macrodantin Capsules 1989
▲ Netromycin Injection 100 mg/ml (7%) 2373
PCE Dispertab Tablets 444
Panhematin 443
Proleukin for Injection (2%) 797

Renal insufficiency

Capastat Sulfate Vials (1 patient) 2868
Capoten (Approximately 1 to 2 of 1000 patients) 739
Capozide (Approximately 1 to 2 of 1000 patients) 742
Daypro Caplets (Less than 1%) 2426
E.E.S. (Isolated reports) 424
Elspar 1659
Erythrocin Stearate Filmtab (Isolated reports) 425
Floxin I.V. 1571
Floxin Tablets (200 mg, 300 mg, 400 mg) 1567
Indocin Capsules (Less than 1%) 1680
Indocin I.V. (Less than 1%) 1684
Indocin (Less than 1%) 1680
Lodine Capsules and Tablets (Less than 1%) 2743
Lopid Tablets 1917
Monopril Tablets (0.2% to 1.0%) .. 757
Neupogen for Injection (Two events) 495
Orthoclone OKT3 Sterile Solution .. 1837
▲ Platinol (28% to 36%) 708
Proleukin for Injection 797
Rifadin (Rare) 1528
Rifamate Capsules (Rare) 1530
Rifater (Rare) 1532
Rimactane Capsules (Rare) 847

Risperdal (Rare) 1301
Univasc Tablets (Less than 1%) 2410
▲ Zoladex (Greater than 1% but less than 5%) 2858

Renal insufficiency, reversible

Actimmune (Rare) 1056

Renal rickets

IFEX 697

Renal stones

(see also under Renal calculi)

Betaseron for SC Injection 658
Clinoril Tablets 1618
Dyazide 2479
Dyrenium Capsules (Rare) 2481
Effexor (Infrequent) 2719
Glauctabs ...... ◉ 208
Hivid Tablets (Less than 1% to less than 3%) 2121
Imdur (Less than or equal to 5%) .. 1323
Luvox Tablets (Rare) 2544
Maxzide 1380
Relafen Tablets (Less than 1%) 2510
Serzone Tablets (Infrequent) 771
Tegison Capsules 2154
Videx Tablets, Powder for Oral Solution, & Pediatric Powder for Oral Solution (Less than 1%) 720

Renal tubular cells excretion, increase

Quadrinal Tablets 1350

Renal tubular damage

Betaseron for SC Injection 658
Foscavir Injection (Less than 1%) .. 547
Hydrea Capsules (Occasional) 696
Platinol 708
Platinol-AQ Injection 710

Respiration, painful

Prinivil Tablets (0.3% to 1.0%) 1733
Prinzide Tablets 1737
Zestoretic 2850
Zestril Tablets (0.3% to 1.0%) 2854

Respiratory alkalosis

▲ Ganite (40% to 50%) 2533

Respiratory arrest

Alfenta Injection 1286
Ancobon Capsules 2079
AquaMEPHYTON Injection 1608
Arfonad Ampuls 2080
Carbocaine Hydrochloride Injection 2303
Cipro I.V. (1% or less) 595
Cipro I.V. Pharmacy Bulk Package (Less than 1%) 597
Clozaril Tablets (Rare) 2252
Coly-Mycin M Parenteral 1905
Decadron Phosphate with Xylocaine Injection, Sterile 1639
Demerol 2308
Dilaudid-HP Injection 1337
Dilaudid-HP Lyophilized Powder 250 mg 1337
Dilaudid Tablets and Liquid 1339
Duranest Injections 542
Dyclone 0.5% and 1% Topical Solutions, USP 544
Emla Cream 545
Floxin I.V. (Less than 1%) 1571
Floxin Tablets (200 mg, 300 mg, 400 mg) (Less than 1%) 1567
Fluothane 2724
INFeD (Iron Dextran Injection, USP) 2345
MS Contin Tablets 1994
MSIR 1997
Marcaine Hydrochloride with Epinephrine 1:200,000 2316
Marcaine Hydrochloride Injection 2316
Marcaine Spinal 2319
Mepergan Injection 2753
Methadone Hydrochloride Oral Solution & Tablets 2235
Nescaine/Nescaine MPF 554
Novocain Hydrochloride for Spinal Anesthesia 2326
Nubain Injection (1% or less) 935
Orthoclone OKT3 Sterile Solution .. 1837
Pontocaine Hydrochloride for Spinal Anesthesia 2330
Proleukin for Injection (Less than 1%) 797
Prostigmin Injectable 1260
Prostigmin Tablets 1261
Quinidex Extentabs 2067
RMS Suppositories 2657

Roxanol 2243
Sensorcaine 559
Sublimaze Injection 1307
Tonocard Tablets (Less than 1%) .. 531
▲ Xylocaine Injections (Among most common) 567

Respiratory congestion, unspecified

Cozaar Tablets (Less than 1%) 1628
▲ Epogen for Injection (15%) 489
Hyzaar Tablets 1677
▲ Procrit for Injection (15%) 1841
▲ Supprelin Injection (3% to 10%) 2056
Videx Tablets, Powder for Oral Solution, & Pediatric Powder for Oral Solution (Up to 2%; 5%) 720

Respiratory depression

(see under Depression, respiratory)

Respiratory depression, postoperative

Alfenta Injection (1% to 3%) 1286
Sublimaze Injection (Occasional) 1307
Sufenta Injection (0.3% to 1%) 1309

Respiratory difficulty

Ambien Tablets 2416
Ana-Kit Anaphylaxis Emergency Treatment Kit 617
Carafate Suspension 1505
Carafate Tablets 1504
Cardene I.V. (Rare) 2709
Claritin-D 2350
D.A. Chewable Tablets 951
Deconamine Chewable Tablets 1320
Deconamine CX Cough and Cold Liquid and Tablets 1319
Deconamine 1320
Deconsal 454
Diphtheria and Tetanus Toxoids and Pertussis Vaccine Adsorbed .. 2477
Diphtheria and Tetanus Toxoids and Pertussis Vaccine Adsorbed USP (For Pediatric Use) 875
Dura-Tap/PD Capsules 2867
Dura-Vent/DA Tablets 953
Dura-Vent Tablets 952
Entex PSE Tablets 1987
EpiPen 790
Fedahist Gyrocaps 2401
Fedahist Timecaps 2401
Felbatol 2666
Floropryl Sterile Ophthalmic Ointment (Infrequent) 1662
Guaimax-D Tablets 792
Haldol Decanoate 1577
Haldol Injection, Tablets and Concentrate 1575
Humorsol Sterile Ophthalmic Solution (Infrequent) 1664
INFeD (Iron Dextran Injection, USP) 2345
Levophed Bitartrate Injection 2315
Norpace (Infrequent) 2444
Novahistine DH 2462
Novahistine DMX ...... ⊞ 822
Novahistine Elixir ...... ⊞ 823
Novahistine Expectorant 2463
Novocain Hydrochloride for Spinal Anesthesia 2326
Papaverine Hydrochloride Vials and Ampoules 1468
Pontocaine Hydrochloride for Spinal Anesthesia 2330
Rondec Oral Drops 953
Rondec Syrup 953
Rondec Tablet 953
Rondec-DM Oral Drops 954
Rondec-DM Syrup 954
Rondec-TR Tablet 953
Seldane-D Extended-Release Tablets 1538
Solganal Suspension 2388
Sus-Phrine Injection 1019
Syn-Rx Tablets 465
Syn-Rx DM Tablets 466
Tetramune (Rare) 1404
▲ Trasylol (3%) 613
Triavil Tablets 1757
Tri-Immunol Adsorbed 1408
Trinalin Repetabs Tablets 1330
Tussend 1783
Tussend Expectorant 1785
Versed Injection (Less than 1%) 2170

Respiratory discharge, upper, unspecified

Emcyt Capsules (1%) 1953

Respiratory distress

Aldoclor Tablets 1598
Aldoril Tablets 1604
Americaine Otic Topical Anesthetic Ear Drops 983
Apresazide Capsules 808
Atgam Sterile Solution (Less than 5%) 2581
Atrovent Inhalation Solution (1.4%) 673
BCG Vaccine, USP (TICE) (1.6%) .. 1814
Blocadren Tablets 1614
Capozide 742
Cardura Tablets (1.1%) 2186
Cartrol Tablets 410
Ceredase 1065
Cipro I.V. (1% or less) 595
Cipro I.V. Pharmacy Bulk Package (Less than 1%) 597
Clomid 1514
Cordarone Intravenous (2%) 2715
Cytosar-U Sterile Powder 2592
Cytovene-IV (One report) 2103
Dalgan Injection (Less than 1%) 538
Dantrium Capsules (Less frequent) 1982
Dilacor XR Extended-release Capsules (Infrequent) 2018
Diucardin Tablets 2718
Diupres Tablets 1650
Diuril Oral Suspension 1653
Diuril Sodium Intravenous 1652
Diuril Tablets 1653
Duragesic Transdermal System (Less than 1%) 1288
Dyazide 2479
Elspar 1659
Eminase (Less than 1 in 1,000) 2039
Enduron Tablets 420
Esidrix Tablets 821
Esimil Tablets 822
Floxin I.V. 1571
Floxin Tablets (200 mg, 300 mg, 400 mg) 1567
Fluvirin 460
Foscavir Injection (Between 1% and 5%) 547
Glucophage 752
Humegon 1824
HydroDIURIL Tablets 1674
Hydropress Tablets 1675
Hyzaar Tablets 1677
Inderal 2728
Inderal LA Long Acting Capsules 2730
Inderide Tablets 2732
Inderide LA Long Acting Capsules .. 2734
Indocin Capsules (Less than 1%) 1680
Indocin I.V. (Less than 1%) 1684
Indocin (Less than 1%) 1680
Kerlone Tablets 2436
Lamictal Tablets (More than 1%) .. 1112
Levatol 2403
Lopressor HCT Tablets 832
Lotensin HCT 837
Lozol Tablets 2022
Lupron Depot 3.75 mg 2556
Lupron Depot 7.5 mg 2559
Maxaquin Tablets (Less than 1%) .. 2440
Maxzide 1380
Metrodin (urofollitropin for injection) 2446
▲ Mexitil Capsules (3.3% to 5.7%) .. 678
Moduretic Tablets 1705
Mutamycin (Few cases) 703
Mykrox Tablets (Rare) 993
Normodyne Tablets 2379
Nubain Injection (1% or less) 935
Nuromax Injection 1149
Oretic Tablets 443
▲ Paraplatin for Injection (6% to 12%) 705
Pergonal (menotropins for injection, USP) 2448
Phenergan VC 2779
Phenergan VC with Codeine 2781
Prinzide Tablets 1737
Procardia XL Extended Release Tablets (1% or less) 1972
▲ Prograf (Greater than 3%) 1042
Prostin VR Pediatric Sterile Solution (Less than 1%) 2635
Protamine Sulfate Ampoules & Vials 1471
Sandimmune 2286
Sectral Capsules 2807
Serevent Inhalation Aerosol 1176
Tenoretic Tablets 2845
Tenormin Tablets and I.V. Injection 2847
Timolide Tablets 1748
Timoptic in Ocudose 1753
Timoptic Sterile Ophthalmic Solution (Less frequent) 1751

(⊞ Described in PDR For Nonprescription Drugs) Incidence data in parenthesis; ▲ 3% or more (◉ Described in PDR For Ophthalmology)

1405 Side Effects Index Rhinitis

Timoptic-XE ... 1755
Toprol-XL Tablets ... 565
Trandate Tablets ... 1185
Vaseretic Tablets ... 1765
Videx Tablets, Powder for Oral Solution, & Pediatric Powder for Oral Solution (Up to 2%) ... 720
Virazole ... 1264
Visken Tablets ... 2299
Zaroxolyn Tablets ... 1000
Zebeta Tablets ... 1413
Zefazone ... 2654
Zestoretic ... 2850
Ziac ... 1415

Respiratory distress, neonatal

Hycodan Tablets and Syrup ... 930
Hycomine Compound Tablets ... 932
Hycomine ... 931
Hycotuss Expectorant Syrup ... 933
Stadol (Rare) ... 775

Respiratory failure

Betagan ... ◉ 233
Betimol 0.25%, 0.5% ... ◉ 261
Betoptic Ophthalmic Solution (Rare) ... 469
Betoptic S Ophthalmic Suspension (Rare) ... 471
Cocaine Hydrochloride Topical Solution ... 537
Isoptin Injectable ... 1344
Lioresal Intrathecal ... 1596
Ocupress Ophthalmic Solution, 1% Sterile ... ◉ 309
Orthoclone OKT3 Sterile Solution .. 1837
▲Proleukin for Injection (Less than 1% to 9%) ... 797
Pulmozyme Inhalation ... 1064
Survanta Beractant Intratracheal Suspension ... 2226
Timoptic in Ocudose (Less frequent) ... 1753
Timoptic Sterile Ophthalmic Solution (Less frequent) ... 1751
Timoptic-XE ... 1755

Respiratory tract, hypersensitivity

Septra ... 1174
Septra I.V. Infusion ... 1169
Septra I.V. Infusion ADD-Vantage Vials (Rare) ... 1171
Septra ... 1174

Restlessness (see under Dysphoria)

Retardation, psychomotor

Eskalith ... 2485
Lithium Carbonate Capsules & Tablets ... 2230
Roferon-A Injection (Less than 1%) ... 2145

Retching

Imitrex Injection (Rare) ... 1103
Versed Injection (Less than 1%) ... 2170

Reticulocytopenia

Chloromycetin Sodium Succinate ... 1900
Cosmegen Injection ... 1626
Cytosar-U Sterile Powder ... 2592
Garamycin Injectable ... 2360

Reticulocytosis

▲Dapsone Tablets USP (Almost all patients) ... 1284
Dipentum Capsules (Rare) ... 1951
Garamycin Injectable ... 2360
▲Tegison Capsules (25-50%) ... 2154
Ticlid Tablets (Rare) ... 2156
Virazole ... 1264
Zyloprim Tablets (Less than 1%) ... 1226

Retinal atrophy

Aralen Phosphate Tablets ... 2301
Clinoril Tablets ... 1618
Plaquenil Sulfate Tablets ... 2328

Retinal damage

Aralen Hydrochloride Injection ... 2301
Aralen Phosphate Tablets ... 2301
Dapsone Tablets USP ... 1284
Neurontin Capsules (Rare) ... 1922
Plaquenil Sulfate Tablets ... 2328

Retinal detachment

▲Cytovene (8%) ... 2103
Foscavir Injection (Less than 1%) .. 547
Humorsol Sterile Ophthalmic Solution (Occasional) ... 1664
Isopto Carpine Ophthalmic Solution (Rare) ... ◉ 223
Luvox Tablets (Rare) ... 2544
MIOSTAT Intraocular Solution ... ◉ 224
Ocusert Pilo-20 and Pilo-40 Ocular Therapeutic Systems ... ◉ 254
Permax Tablets (Rare) ... 575
Phospholine Iodide (A few cases) ◉ 326
Pilocar ... ◉ 268
Pilopine HS Ophthalmic Gel ... ◉ 226
Videx Tablets, Powder for Oral Solution, & Pediatric Powder for Oral Solution (Less than 1%) ... 720

Retinal disorder, unspecified

Lotensin HCT (0.3% or more) ... 837

Retinal hemorrhage, neonatal

Syntocinon Injection ... 2296

Retinal pigmentation disorders

Aralen Phosphate Tablets ... 2301
Desferal Vials ... 820
ISPAN Perfluoropropane ... ◉ 276
ISPAN Sulfur Hexafluoride ... ◉ 275
Plaquenil Sulfate Tablets ... 2328
Platinol ... 708
Platinol-AQ Injection ... 710
Videx Tablets, Powder for Oral Solution, & Pediatric Powder for Oral Solution (4 pediatric patients) ... 720

Retinal vascular disorder

Betimol 0.25%, 0.5% ... ◉ 261
Clomid ... 1514
Intron A (Rare) ... 2364
Permax Tablets ... 575
Virazole ... 1264

Retinitis

Attenuvax (Infrequent) ... 1610
Betaseron for SC Injection ... 658
Cytovene (1% or less) ... 2103
Indocin (Less than 1%) ... 1680
M-M-R II (Infrequent) ... 1687
M-R-VAX II ... 1689
Videx Tablets, Powder for Oral Solution, & Pediatric Powder for Oral Solution (Up to 1%) ... 720

Retinitis, bilateral

Typhim Vi ... 899

Retinitis, macular

Zyloprim Tablets (Less than 1%) ... 1226

Retinopathy

Anafranil Capsules (Rare) ... 803
Aralen Hydrochloride Injection ... 2301
Aralen Phosphate Tablets ... 2301
Cardizem CD Capsules (Infrequent) ... 1506
Cardizem SR Capsules (Less than 1%) ... 1510
Cardizem Injectable ... 1508
Cardizem Tablets (Infrequent) ... 1512
Clinoril Tablets ... 1618
Haldol Decanoate ... 1577
Haldol Injection, Tablets and Concentrate ... 1575
Lysodren (Infrequent) ... 698
Minipress Capsules (Single report) 1937
Minizide Capsules (Single report) ... 1938
Neurontin Capsules (Rare) ... 1922
Nolvadex Tablets ... 2841
Plaquenil Sulfate Tablets (Rare) ... 2328
▲Tegison Capsules (10-25%) ... 2154
Tolectin (200, 400 and 600 mg) (Less than 1%) ... 1581

Retinopathy, pigmentary

Aralen Phosphate Tablets ... 2301
Compazine ... 2470
Etrafon ... 2355
Levoprome ... 1274
Mellaril ... 2269
Prolixin ... 509
Stelazine ... 2514
Temaril Tablets, Syrup and Spansule Extended-Release Capsules ... 483
Thorazine ... 2523
Triavil Tablets ... 1757
Trilafon ... 2389

Retrocollis

Etrafon ... 2355
Trilafon ... 2389

Retrolental fibroplasia

▲Indocin I.V. (3% to 9%) ... 1684

Retroperitoneal fibrosis

Blocadren Tablets ... 1614
D.H.E. 45 Injection (Occasional) ... 2255
Parlodel (A few patients) ... 2281
Sansert Tablets (Very rare) ... 2295
Timolide Tablets ... 1748
Timoptic in Ocudose (Less frequent) ... 1753
Timoptic Sterile Ophthalmic Solution (Less frequent) ... 1751
Timoptic-XE ... 1755

Retrosternal discomfort

IOPIDINE Sterile Ophthalmic Solution ... ◉ 219
Levophed Bitartrate Injection ... 2315

Reye's Syndrome, potential for development of

Alka-Seltzer Effervescent Antacid and Pain Reliever ... ▣ 701
Alka-Seltzer Extra Strength Effervescent Antacid and Pain Reliever ... ▣ 703
Alka-Seltzer Lemon Lime Effervescent Antacid and Pain Reliever ... ▣ 703
Alka-Seltzer Plus Cold Medicine .. ▣ 705
Alka-Seltzer Plus Cold & Cough Medicine (Rare) ... ▣ 708
Alka-Seltzer Plus Night-Time Cold Medicine ... ▣ 707
Alka Seltzer Plus Sinus Medicine ▣ 707
Arthritis Foundation Safety Coated Aspirin Tablets ... ▣ 675
Arthritis Pain Ascriptin ... ▣ 631
Maximum Strength Ascriptin ... ▣ 630
Regular Strength Ascriptin Tablets ... ▣ 629
Arthritis Strength BC Powder ... ▣ 609
BC Cold Powder Multi-Symptom Formula (Cold-Sinus-Allergy) ... ▣ 609
BC Cold Powder Non-Drowsy Formula (Cold-Sinus) ... ▣ 609
BC Powder ... ▣ 609
Backache Caplets ... ▣ 613
Bayer Children's Chewable Aspirin ... ▣ 711
Genuine Bayer Aspirin Tablets & Caplets ... ▣ 713
Extra Strength Bayer Arthritis Pain Regimen Formula ... ▣ 711
Extra Strength Bayer Aspirin Caplets & Tablets ... ▣ 712
Extended-Release Bayer 8-Hour Aspirin ... ▣ 712
Extra Strength Bayer Plus Aspirin Caplets ... ▣ 713
Extra Strength Bayer PM Aspirin ▣ 713
Aspirin Regimen Bayer Adult Low Strength 81 mg Tablets ... ▣ 709
Bayer Select Backache Pain Relief Formula ... ▣ 715
Arthritis Strength Bufferin Analgesic Caplets ... ▣ 614
Extra Strength Bufferin Analgesic Tablets ... ▣ 615
Cama Arthritis Pain Reliever ... ▣ 785
Darvon ... 1435
Doan's Extra-Strength Analgesic .. ▣ 633
Extra Strength Doan's P.M. ... ▣ 633
Doan's Regular Strength Analgesic ... ▣ 634
Easprin ... 1914
Ecotrin ... 2455
Empirin Aspirin Tablets ... ▣ 854
Empirin with Codeine Tablets ... 1093
Excedrin Extra-Strength Analgesic Tablets & Caplets ... 732
Norgesic Tablets ... 1496
Pepto-Bismol Original Liquid, Original and Cherry Tablets and Easy-To-Swallow Caplets (Rare) .. 1976
Pepto-Bismol Maximum Strength Liquid ... 1976
Percodan Tablets ... 939
Sine-Off Sinus Medicine ... ▣ 825
St. Joseph Adult Chewable Aspirin (81 mg.) ... ▣ 808
Ursinus Inlay-Tabs ... ▣ 794
Vanquish Analgesic Caplets ... ▣ 731

Rhabdomyolysis

Activase ... 1058
Amicar Syrup, Tablets, and Injection (Rare) ... 1267
Anectine (Rare) ... 1073
Atromid-S Capsules ... 2701
Azulfidine (Rare) ... 1949
Clozaril Tablets ... 2252
Cytovene-IV (One report) ... 2103
Felbatol ... 2666
Floxin I.V. ... 1571
Floxin Tablets (200 mg, 300 mg, 400 mg) ... 1567
Lescol Capsules ... 2267
Lopid Tablets ... 1917
Mevacor Tablets ... 1699
Orap Tablets ... 1050
PCE Dispertab Tablets ... 444
Pravachol (Rare) ... 765
Risperdal ... 1301
Videx Tablets, Powder for Oral Solution, & Pediatric Powder for Oral Solution (Rare) ... 720
Wellbutrin Tablets ... 1204
Zocor Tablets (Rare) ... 1775

Rheumatic syndrome

Nydrazid Injection ... 508
Rifamate Capsules ... 1530
Rifater ... 1532

Rheumatoid arthritis

Atromid-S Capsules ... 2701
Norplant System (Rare) ... 2759
Prozac Pulvules & Liquid, Oral Solution (Rare) ... 919

Rheumatoid factor, positive

Aldoclor Tablets ... 1598
Aldomet Ester HCl Injection ... 1602
Aldomet Oral ... 1600
Aldoril Tablets ... 1604
Elavil ... 2838
Endep Tablets ... 2174

Rhinitis

▲Acel-Imune Diphtheria and Tetanus Toxoids and Acellular Pertussis Vaccine Adsorbed (6%) ... 1364
Actigall Capsules ... 802
Adalat CC (3% or less) ... 589
Children's Advil Suspension (Less than 1%) ... 2692
▲AeroBid Inhaler System (3-9%) ... 1005
▲Aerobid-M Inhaler System (3-9%) .. 1005
Ambien Tablets (1%) ... 2416
▲Anafranil Capsules (7% to 12%) ... 803
Ansaid Tablets (1-3%) ... 2579
▲Aredia for Injection (Up to 6%) ... 810
▲Asacol Delayed-Release Tablets (5%) ... 1979
Atrovent Inhalation Solution (2.3%) ... 673
▲Axid Pulvules (9.8%) ... 1427
Brevital Sodium Vials ... 1429
Capoten ... 739
Capozide ... 742
Carafate Suspension ... 1505
Carafate Tablets ... 1504
Cardene Capsules (Rare) ... 2095
▲Cardura Tablets (3%) ... 2186
Cartrol Tablets (Less common) ... 410
▲CellCept Capsules (More than or equal to 3%) ... 2099
Claritin (2% or fewer patients) ... 2349
▲Cognex Capsules (8%) ... 1901
Cozaar Tablets (Less than 1%) ... 1628
▲DDAVP (3 to 8%) ... 2017
Demadex Tablets and Injection (2.8%) ... 686
Depakote Tablets (Greater than 1% but not more than 5%) ... 415
Depo-Medrol Single-Dose Vial ... 2600
Depo-Medrol Sterile Aqueous Suspension ... 2597
▲Desmopressin Acetate Rhinal Tube (3% to 8%) ... 979
▲Dilacor XR Extended-release Capsules (2.9% to 9.6%) ... 2018
Effexor ... 2719
▲Felbatol (6.9%) ... 2666
Foscavir Injection (Between 1% and 5%) ... 547
Glucotrol XL Extended Release Tablets (Less than 3%) ... 1968
Heparin Lock Flush Solution ... 2725
Heparin Sodium Injection ... 2726
Heparin Sodium Injection, USP, Sterile Solution ... 2615
Heparin Sodium Vials (Rare) ... 1441
Hytrin Capsules (At least 1% to 1.9%) ... 430
Hyzaar Tablets ... 1677
IBU Tablets (Less than 1%) ... 1342
Imdur (Less than or equal to 5%) .. 1323
Intron A (Less than 5%) ... 2364
Iopidine 0.5% (Less than 1%) ... ◉ 221

(▣ Described in PDR For Nonprescription Drugs) Incidence data in parenthesis; ▲ 3% or more (◉ Described in PDR For Ophthalmology)

Rhinitis | Side Effects Index | 1406

Kerlone Tablets (1.4%) 2436
▲ Lamictal Tablets (13.6%) 1112
▲ Lescol Capsules (4.5%) 2267
Lodine Capsules and Tablets (Less than 1%) 2743
▲ Lorabid Suspension and Pulvules (1.6% to 6.3%) 1459
Lotensin HCT (More than 1%) 837
Lozol Tablets (Greater than or equal to 5%) 2022
Lupron Depot 3.75 mg (Less than 5%) 2556
Luvox Tablets 2544
Marinol (Dronabinol) Capsules (Less than 1%) 2231
▲ Mepron Suspension (5%) 1135
▲ Miacalcin Nasal Spray (12%) 2275
Monopril Tablets (0.2% to 1.0%) 757
Children's Motrin Ibuprofen Oral Suspension (Less than 1%) 1546
Motrin Tablets (Less than 1%) 2625
Motrin Ibuprofen Suspension, Oral Drops, Chewable Tablets, Caplets (Less than 1%) 1546
Mumpsvax 1708
NebuPent for Inhalation Solution (1% or less) 1040
▲ Neurontin Capsules (4.1%) 1922
Norvasc Tablets (Less than or equal to 0.1%) 1940
OptiPranolol (Metipranolol 0.3%) Sterile Ophthalmic Solution (A small number of patients) ⊙ 258
Orlamm (1% to 3%) 2239
Orudis Capsules (Less than 1%) 2766
Oruvail Capsules (Less than 1%) 2766
Paxil Tablets (Frequent) 2505
▲ Permax Tablets (12.2%) 575
▲ Pravachol (0.1% to 4.0%) 765
Prinivil Tablets (0.3% to 1.0%) 1733
Prinzide Tablets (0.3 to 1%) 1737
▲ Prograf (Greater than 3%) 1042
▲ Propulsid (7.3%) 1300
ProSom Tablets (Infrequent) 449
Prozac Pulvules & Liquid, Oral Solution (Frequent) 919
Pulmozyme Inhalation 1064
Recombivax HB (Less than 1%) 1744
Retrovir Capsules 1158
Retrovir I.V. Infusion 1163
Retrovir Syrup 1158
▲ Risperdal (8% to 10%) 1301
Roferon-A Injection (Less than 1%) 2145
Rogaine Topical Solution (1.27%) 2637
▲ Salagen Tablets (5% to 14%) 1489
Sectral Capsules 2807
Serevent Inhalation Aerosol (1% to 3%) 1176
Serzone Tablets 771
▲ Stadol (3% to 9%) 775
Stimate, (desmopressin acetate) Nasal Spray, 1.5 mg/mL (Occasional) 525
▲ Synarel Nasal Solution for Central Precocious Puberty (5%) 2151
Tenex Tablets (3% or less) 2074
▲ Tilade (4.6%) 996
Toradol (1% or less) 2159
Tornalate Solution for Inhalation, 0.2% (1.5%) 956
Univasc Tablets (More than 1%) 2410
Vascor (200, 300 and 400 mg) Tablets (0.5 to 2.0%) 1587
Vexol 1% Ophthalmic Suspension (Less than 2%) ⊙ 230
▲ Videx Tablets, Powder for Oral Solution, & Pediatric Powder for Oral Solution (48%) 720
▲ Zebeta Tablets (2.9% to 4.0%) 1413
Zestoretic (0.3 to 1%) 2850
Zestril Tablets (0.3% to 1.0%) 2854
Ziac (0.7% to 0.9%) 1415
Zoladex (1% or greater) 2858
Zoloft Tablets (2.0%) 2217
Zosyn (1.2%) 1419
Zosyn Pharmacy Bulk Package (1.2%) 1422
Zyloprim Tablets (Less than 1%) 1226

Rhinorrhea

▲ ActHIB (21.3% to 24.5%) 872
▲ AeroBid Inhaler System (3-9%) 1005
▲ Aerobid-M Inhaler System (3-9%) 1005
Beconase (Fewer than 3 per 100 patients) 1076
▲ CHEMET (succimer) Capsules (0.7 to 3.7%) 1545
Clozaril Tablets (Less than 1%) 2252
Colyte and Colyte-flavored (Isolated cases) 2396
Empirin with Codeine Tablets 1093
4-Way Fast Acting Nasal Spray (regular & mentholated) ▣ 621
4-Way Long Lasting Nasal Spray ▣ 621
Flonase Nasal Spray (Less than 1%) 1098
Floxin I.V. (Less than 1%) 1571
Floxin Tablets (200 mg, 300 mg, 400 mg) (Less than 1%) 1567
GoLYTELY (Isolated cases) 688
Intron A (Less than 5%) 2364
Klonopin Tablets 2126
Lozol Tablets (Less than 5%) 2022
Methadone Hydrochloride Oral Concentrate 2233
NuLYTELY 689
Cherry Flavor NuLYTELY (Isolated cases) 689
▲ OmniHIB (21.3 to 24.5%) 2499
Orlamm 2239
Plendil Extended-Release Tablets (0.2% to 1.6%) 527
Prinivil Tablets (0.3% to 1.0%) 1733
Prinzide Tablets 1737
ReVia Tablets (Less than 1%) 940
Rocaltrol Capsules 2141
▲ Roferon-A Injection (4%) 2145
Soma Compound w/Codeine Tablets 2676
Soma Compound Tablets 2675
Supprelin Injection (2% to 3%) 2056
Tegison Capsules (Less than 1%) 2154
Vancenase AQ Nasal Spray 0.042% (Fewer than 3 per 100 patients) 2393
Vancenase PocketHaler Nasal Inhaler (1 per 100 patients) 2391
Vaseretic Tablets 1765
Vasotec I.V. 1768
Vasotec Tablets (0.5% to 1.0%) 1771
▲ Videx Tablets, Powder for Oral Solution, & Pediatric Powder for Oral Solution (20% to 21%) 720
Yohimex Tablets 1363
Zestoretic 2850
Zestril Tablets (0.3% to 1.0%) 2854

Rhonchi

Brevibloc Injection (Less than 1%) 1808
Ganite 2533
Survanta Beractant Intratracheal Suspension 2226
▲ Videx Tablets, Powder for Oral Solution, & Pediatric Powder for Oral Solution (6% to 8%) 720
Zemuron (Less than 1%) 1830

Rigidity

Abbokinase 403
Abbokinase Open-Cath 405
Alfenta Injection 1286
Ambien Tablets (Rare) 2416
Atgam Sterile Solution (Less than 5%) 2581
Azo Gantrisin Tablets 2081
Brevibloc Injection (Less than 1%) 1808
Cardura Tablets (Less than 0.5% of 3960 patients) 2186
Claritin (2% or fewer patients) 2349
Claritin-D (Less frequent) 2350
▲ Clozaril Tablets (3%) 2252
Cytotec (Infrequent) 2424
Diprivan Injection (Less than 1%) 2833
▲ Ergamisol Tablets (3% to 5%) 1292
Ethmozine Tablets (Rare) 2041
Famvir (1.5%) 2486
Felbatol 2666
Flumadine Tablets & Syrup 1015
▲ Foscavir Injection (5% or greater) 547
Hivid Tablets (Less than 1% to less than 3%) 2121
Hyzaar Tablets 1677
Imdur (Less than or equal to 5%) 1323
Imitrex Tablets (Rare) 1106
▲ Intron A (Up to 42%) 2364
Ismo Tablets (Fewer than 1%) 2738
Kerlone Tablets (Less than 2%) 2436
Lioresal Tablets 829
Moban Tablets and Concentrate 1048
Norvasc Tablets (More than 0.1% to 1%) 1940
▲ Orap Tablets (2 of 20 patients) 1050
▲ Orthoclone OKT3 Sterile Solution (8%) 1837
Procardia XL Extended Release Tablets (1% or less) 1972
Proleukin for Injection 797
Prostin VR Pediatric Sterile Solution (Less than 1%) 2635
Risperdal (Infrequent) 1301
Romazicon (Less than 1%) 2147
▲ Sublimaze Injection (Among most common) 1307
▲ Tegison Capsules (1-10%) 2154
Temaril Tablets, Syrup and Spansule Extended-Release Capsules 483
▲ Xanax Tablets (4.2%) 2649
Zoloft Tablets (Infrequent) 2217
Zosyn (1.0% or less) 1419
Zosyn Pharmacy Bulk Package (1.0% or less) 1422
Zovirax Sterile Powder (Less than 1%) 1223

S

Salicylism

Easprin 1914
Empirin with Codeine Tablets 1093

Saliva, discoloration

Rifadin 1528

Salivary gland enlargement

Anafranil Capsules (Rare) 803
Azo Gantrisin Tablets 2081
Betaseron for SC Injection 658
Clozaril Tablets 2252
Hivid Tablets (Less than 1% to less than 3%) 2121
Lithonate/Lithotabs/Lithobid 2543
Neurontin Capsules (Rare) 1922
Paxil Tablets (Rare) 2505
Permax Tablets (Infrequent) 575
Prozac Pulvules & Liquid, Oral Solution (Rare) 919
▲ SSKI Solution (Among most frequent) 2658

Salivation

Altace Capsules (Less than 1%) 1232
Ambien Tablets (Rare) 2416
Anafranil Capsules (Infrequent) 803
Anectine 1073
Antilirium Injectable 1009
Betaseron for SC Injection 658
Brevital Sodium Vials 1429
BuSpar (Infrequent) 737
Ceftin for Oral Suspension (Less than 1% but more than 0.1%) 1078
Claritin (2% or fewer patients) 2349
▲ Clozaril Tablets (More than 5 to 31%) 2252
Cognex Capsules (Infrequent) 1901
Cordarone Tablets (1 to 3%) 2712
Dalmane Capsules (Rare) 2173
Desyrel and Desyrel Dividose 503
Diupres Tablets 1650
Dizac (Less frequent) 1809
Duvoid (Infrequent) 2044
Effexor (Rare) 2719
Emete-con Intramuscular/Intravenous 2198
Eskalith 2485
Etrafon 2355
Fioricet with Codeine Capsules 2260
Fiorinal with Codeine Capsules 2262
Floropryl Sterile Ophthalmic Ointment (Rare) 1662
Garamycin Injectable 2360
Haldol Injection, Tablets and Concentrate 1575
Hivid Tablets 2121
Humorsol Sterile Ophthalmic Solution (Rare) 1664
Hydropres Tablets 1675
Hyperstat I.V. Injection 2363
IFEX (Less than 1%) 697
Intron A (Less than 5%) 2364
Isopto Carbachol Ophthalmic Solution ⊙ 223
Kerlone Tablets (Less than 2%) 2436
Lamictal Tablets (Infrequent) 1112
Lithonate/Lithotabs/Lithobid 2543
Loxitane 1378
Ludiomil Tablets (Rare) 843
Luvox Tablets (Infrequent) 2544
Megace Oral Suspension (1% to 3%) 699
Mestinon Injectable 1253
Mestinon 1254
Mexitil Capsules (About 4 in 1,000) 678
Moban Tablets and Concentrate (Occasional) 1048
Navane Capsules and Concentrate 2201
Navane Intramuscular 2202
Neurontin Capsules (Infrequent) 1922
▲ Nicorette (3% to 9%) 2458
Orap Tablets 1050
Orudis Capsules (Less than 1%) 2766
Oruvail Capsules (Less than 1%) 2766
Paxil Tablets (Infrequent) 2505
PhosChol 488
Pilocar (Extremely rare) ⊙ 268
PREVACID Delayed-Release Capsules (Less than 1%) 2562
Primaxin I.M. 1727
Primaxin I.V. (Less than 0.2%) 1729
Prinivil Tablets (Up to 0.2%) 1733
Prinzide Tablets 1737
Prolixin 509
Prostigmin Injectable (Among most common) 1260
Prostigmin Tablets (Among most common) 1261
Prozac Pulvules & Liquid, Oral Solution (Rare) 919
Quadrinal Tablets 1350
Risperdal (Up to 2%) 1301
Roferon-A Injection (Less than 1%) 2145
Serzone Tablets (Rare) 771
Suprane (Greater than 1%) 1813
Tensilon Injectable 1261
Trental Tablets (Less than 1%) 1244
Triavil Tablets 1757
Trilafon 2389
Urecholine 1761
Valium Injectable (Rare) 2182
Valium Tablets (Infrequent) 2183
Valrelease Capsules (Occasional) 2169
▲ Wellbutrin Tablets (3.4%) 1204
▲ Xanax Tablets (4.2% to 5.6%) 2649
Zestril Tablets (Up to 0.2%) 2854
Zoloft Tablets (Infrequent) 2217

Salivation, increase (see under Salivation)

Salpingitis

Betaseron for SC Injection 658
Permax Tablets (Infrequent) 575
Prozac Pulvules & Liquid, Oral Solution (Rare) 919

Sarcoidosis

Risperdal (Rare) 1301

Sarcoma, bone

Permax Tablets (Infrequent) 575

Sarcoma, unspecified

Foscavir Injection (Between 1% and 5%) 547
Megace Oral Suspension (1% to 3%) 699
▲ Videx Tablets, Powder for Oral Solution, & Pediatric Powder for Oral Solution (3% to 5%) 720

Scalp, dry

Nizoral 2% Shampoo 1298
Selsun Rx 2.5% Selenium Sulfide Lotion, USP 2225

Scalp, oily

Nizoral 2% Shampoo 1298
Selsun Rx 2.5% Selenium Sulfide Lotion, USP 2225

Scalp, tightness

Temovate Scalp Application (1 of 294 patients) 1179

Scalp defects, fetal

Tapazole Tablets (Rare) 1477

Scarring

Condylox (Less than 5%) 1802
Dalalone D.P. Injectable 1011
Decadron-LA Sterile Suspension 1646
▲ Efudex (Among most frequent) 2113
Fluoroplex Topical Solution & Cream 1% (Occasional) 479
T.R.U.E. Test (Two reports) 1189
Tubersol (Tuberculin Purified Protein Derivative [Mantoux]) 2872

Schizophrenia, precipitation

Anafranil Capsules (Rare) 803
Nardil (Less frequent) 1920

Sciatica

Ambien Tablets (Rare) 2416
Wellbutrin Tablets (Rare) 1204

Sclera, discoloration

Hivid Tablets (Less than 1% to less than 3%) 2121

(▣ Described in PDR For Nonprescription Drugs) Incidence data in parenthesis; ▲ 3% or more (⊙ Described in PDR For Ophthalmology)

1407 Side Effects Index Seizures

Mellaril 2269
Minipress Capsules (1-4%) 1937
Minizide Capsules 1938
Novantrone 1279
Serentil 684
Ticlid Tablets 2156
Torecan 2245

Sclera, infection

Urobiotic-250 Capsules 2214

Scleral injection

Azo Gantanol Tablets 2080
Azo Gantrisin Tablets 2081
Azulfidine (Rare) 1949
Bactrim DS Tablets 2084
Bactrim I.V. Infusion 2082
Bactrim 2084
Fansidar Tablets 2114
Gantanol Tablets 2119
Prelone Syrup 1787
Septra 1174
Septra I.V. Infusion 1169
Septra I.V. Infusion ADD-Vantage Vials 1171
Septra 1174

Scleritis

Ambien Tablets (Infrequent) 2416
Anafranil Capsules (Infrequent) 803
Effexor (Rare) 2719

Sclerosis, multiple

Engerix-B Unit-Dose Vials (Less than 1%) 2482
Havrix (Rare) 2489
Recombivax HB 1744

Sclerosis, skin

Depo-Provera Contraceptive Injection (Fewer than 1%) 2602
Norplant System (Rare) 2759
Parnate Tablets 2503
Talwin Injection 2334

Sclerosis, subcutaneous tissues

Talwin Injection 2334

Scotomata

Adenoscan (Less than 1%) 1024
Children's Advil Suspension (Less than 1%) 2692
Aralen Hydrochloride Injection 2301
Aralen Phosphate Tablets 2301
Cataflam (Less than 1%) 816
Eskalith 2485
IBU Tablets (Less than 1%) 1342
Kerlone Tablets (Less than 2%) 2436
Lithium Carbonate Capsules & Tablets 2230
Lithonate/Lithotabs/Lithobid 2543
Children's Motrin Ibuprofen Oral Suspension (Less than 1%) 1546
Motrin Tablets (Less than 1%) 2625
Motrin Ibuprofen Suspension, Oral Drops, Chewable Tablets, Caplets (Less than 1%) 1546
Placidyl Capsules 448
Plaquenil Sulfate Tablets 2328
Proglycem 580
ProSom Tablets (Rare) 449
Quinaglute Dura-Tabs Tablets (Occasional) 649
Quinidex Extentabs 2067
Tegison Capsules (Less than 1%) 2154
Trental Tablets (Less than 1%) 1244
Voltaren Tablets (Less than 1%) 861

Scotomata, scintillating

Clomid (Occasional) 1514
Serophene (clomiphene citrate tablets, USP) 2451

Screaming, excessive

Tri-Immunol Adsorbed (Rare) 1408

Seborrhea

Accutane Capsules (Less than 1 patient in 10) 2076
Anafranil Capsules (Rare) 803
Betaseron for SC Injection 658
Cognex Capsules (Rare) 1901
Danocrine Capsules 2307
Depakote Tablets (Greater than 1% but not more than 5%) 415
Fludara for Injection (Up to 1%) 663
Foscavir Injection (Between 1% and 5%) 547
Halotestin Tablets 2614
Lamictal Tablets (Rare) 1112
Loxitane 1378
Lupron Depot-PED 7.5 mg, 11.25 mg and 15 mg (2%) 2560
Luvox Tablets (Infrequent) 2544
Neurontin Capsules (Infrequent) 1922
Permax Tablets (Infrequent) 575
Prolixin 509
Prozac Pulvules & Liquid, Oral Solution (Rare) 919
Risperdal (Up to 1%) 1301
Salagen Tablets (Less than 1%) 1489
▲ Synarel Nasal Solution for Central Precocious Puberty (3%) 2151
▲ Synarel Nasal Solution for Endometriosis (8% of patients) 2152
Testoderm Testosterone Transdermal System 486
▲ Zoladex (26%) 2858

Sedation

▲ Actifed with Codeine Cough Syrup (Among most frequent) 1067
Aldoclor Tablets 1598
Aldomet Ester HCl Injection 1602
Aldomet Oral 1600
Aldoril Tablets 1604
Ancobon Capsules 2079
▲ Anexsia 5/500 Elixir (Among most frequent) 1781
Ativan Injection 2698
▲ Ativan Tablets (15.9%) 2700
▲ Atrohist Pediatric Suspension (Among most common) 454
▲ Benadryl Capsules (Among most frequent) 1898
▲ Benadryl Injection (Among most frequent) 1898
▲ Bromfed-DM Cough Syrup (Among most frequent) 1786
Brontex 1981
▲ Buprenex Injectable (Most frequent) 2006
▲ Catapres Tablets (About 10 in 100 patients) 674
Catapres-TTS (3 of 101 patients) 675
▲ Clozaril Tablets (More than 5 to 39%) 2252
▲ Combipres Tablets (About 10%) 677
Comhist 2038
▲ DHCplus Capsules (Among most frequent) 1993
▲ Dalgan Injection (3 to 9%) 538
Dalmane Capsules 2173
▲ Darvon-N/Darvocet-N (Among most frequent) 1433
▲ Darvon (Among most frequent) 1435
▲ Darvon-N Suspension & Tablets (Among most frequent) 1433
Daypro Caplets (Greater than 1% but less than 3%) 2426
Deconamine 1320
▲ Demerol (Among most frequently observed) 2308
▲ Demser Capsules (Almost all patients) 1649
Depakene 413
Depakote Tablets 415
Dilaudid Ampules 1335
Dilaudid Cough Syrup 1336
▲ Dilaudid-HP Injection (Among most frequent) 1337
▲ Dilaudid-HP Lyophilized Powder 250 mg (Among most frequent) 1337
Dilaudid 1335
Dilaudid Oral Liquid 1339
Dilaudid 1335
Dilaudid Tablets - 8 mg 1339
▲ Dimetane-DC Cough Syrup (Most frequent) 2059
Dimetane-DX Cough Syrup (Among most frequent) 2059
Diupres Tablets 1650
▲ Esgic-plus Tablets (Among most frequent) 1013
Etrafon (Less frequent) 2355
Fedahist Gyrocaps 2401
Fedahist Timecaps 2401
▲ Fioricet Tablets (Among most frequent) 2258
Fioricet with Codeine Capsules (Frequent) 2260
Fiorinal with Codeine Capsules 2262
Halcion Tablets 2611
Hycodan Tablets and Syrup 930
Hycomine Compound Tablets 932
Hycomine 931
Hycotuss Expectorant Syrup 933
Hydrocet Capsules 782
Hydropres Tablets 1675
Imitrex Injection (2.7%) 1103
Imitrex Tablets 1106
Lioresal Tablets 829
Lomotil 2439
▲ Lorcet 10/650 (Among most frequent) 1018
▲ Lortab (Among most frequent) 2566
▲ MS Contin Tablets (Among most frequent) 1994
▲ MSIR (Among most frequent) 1997
▲ Mepergan Injection (Among most frequent) 2753
▲ Methadone Hydrochloride Oral Concentrate (Among most frequent) 2233
Methadone Hydrochloride Oral Solution & Tablets 2235
Motofen Tablets 784
Navane Capsules and Concentrate 2201
Navane Intramuscular 2202
Novahistine DH 2462
Novahistine Expectorant 2463
▲ Nubain Injection (36%) 935
▲ Oramorph SR (Morphine Sulfate Sustained Release Tablets) (Among most frequent) 2236
▲ Orap Tablets (14 of 20 patients) 1050
Ornade Spansule Capsules 2502
Papaverine Hydrochloride Vials and Ampoules 1468
▲ Percocet Tablets (Among most frequent) 938
▲ Percodan Tablets (Among most frequent) 939
▲ Percodan-Demi Tablets (Among most frequent) 940
Periactin 1724
Phenergan with Codeine 2777
Phenergan with Dextromethorphan 2778
Phenergan Suppositories 2775
Phenergan Syrup 2774
Phenergan VC 2779
Phenergan VC with Codeine 2781
Phenobarbital Elixir and Tablets 1469
▲ Phrenilin (Among most frequent) 785
Prozac Pulvules & Liquid, Oral Solution (1.9%) 919
▲ RMS Suppositories (Among most frequent) 2657
Roferon-A Injection (Less than 1%) 2145
Rondec Oral Drops 953
Rondec Syrup 953
Rondec Tablet 953
Rondec-DM Oral Drops 954
Rondec-DM Syrup 954
Rondec-TR Tablet 953
▲ Roxanol (Among most frequent) 2243
▲ Roxicodone Tablets, Oral Solution & Intensol (Oxycodone) (Among most frequent) 2244
▲ Rynatan (Among most common) 2673
▲ Rynatuss (Among most common) 2673
▲ Sedapap Tablets 50 mg/650 mg (Among the most frequent) 1543
▲ Seldane-D Extended-Release Tablets (7.2%) 1538
▲ Semprex-D Capsules (6% more common than with placebo) 463
▲ Semprex-D Capsules (6% more common than with placebo) 1167
Soma Compound w/Codeine Tablets 2676
Talacen 2333
Talwin Injection 2334
Talwin Compound 2335
Talwin Injection 2334
Talwin Nx 2336
▲ Tavist Syrup (Among most frequent) 2297
▲ Tavist Tablets (Among most frequent) 2298
▲ Tenex Tablets (5% to 39%) 2074
Tessalon Perles 1020
Triavil Tablets 1757
▲ Trinalin Repetabs Tablets (Among most frequent) 1330
Tussend 1783
Tussionex Pennkinetic Extended-Release Suspension 998
▲ Tylenol with Codeine (Among most frequent) 1583
▲ Tylox Capsules (Among most frequent) 1584
Versed Injection (1.6%) 2170
▲ Vicodin Tablets (Among most frequent) 1356
▲ Vicodin ES Tablets (Among most frequent) 1357
Vicodin Tuss Expectorant 1358
▲ Wellbutrin Tablets (19.8%) 1204
▲ Wygesic Tablets (Most frequent) 2827
Xanax Tablets 2649
▲ Zofran Injection (8%) 1214
▲ Zofran Tablets (20%) 1217
▲ Zydone Capsules (Among most frequent) 949

Seizure control, loss of

Depakene 413

Seizures (see also under Convulsions)

Accutane Capsules 2076
Acel-Imune Diphtheria and Tetanus Toxoids and Acellular Pertussis Vaccine Adsorbed (One child) 1364
Actimmune (Rare) 1056
▲ Aredia for Injection (3%) 810
Asendin Tablets (Less than 1%) 1369
Atgam Sterile Solution (Less than 1% to less than 5%) 2581
Atretol Tablets 573
Attenuvax (Rare) 1610
Azactam for Injection (Less than 1%) 734
Brethine Ampuls (Rare) 815
Brethine Tablets (Rare) 814
Brevital Sodium Vials 1429
BuSpar (Infrequent) 737
Cefizox for Intramuscular or Intravenous Use 1034
Ceftin Tablets 1078
Cefzil Tablets and Oral Suspension 746
Ceptaz (Fewer than 1%) 1081
Cipro I.V. Pharmacy Bulk Package (Less than 1%) 597
Claritin (Rare) 2349
Clomid 1514
▲ Clozaril Tablets (3.5 to approximately 5%) 2252
DDAVP Injection (Rare) 2014
DDAVP (Rare) 2017
Dantrium Capsules (Less frequent) 1982
Daraprim Tablets (Rare) 1090
Depo-Medrol Single-Dose Vial 2600
Depo-Medrol Sterile Aqueous Suspension 2597
Diflucan Injection, Tablets, and Oral Suspension 2194
Diphtheria and Tetanus Toxoids and Pertussis Vaccine Adsorbed USP (For Pediatric Use) (Infrequent) 875
Diprivan Injection (Less than 1%) 2833
Duricef 748
E.E.S. (Isolated reports) 424
Elavil 2838
Eldepryl Tablets 2550
Endep Tablets 2174
Epogen for Injection (1.1% to approximately 2.5%) 489
EryPed (Isolated reports) 421
Ery-Tab Tablets (Isolated reports) 422
Erythrocin Stearate Filmtab (Isolated reports) 425
Erythromycin Base Filmtab (Isolated reports) 426
Erythromycin Delayed-Release Capsules, USP (Isolated reports) 427
Ethmozine Tablets (Less than 2%) 2041
Etrafon 2355
▲ Exosurf Neonatal for Intratracheal Suspension (2% to 10%) 1095
Fioricet with Codeine Capsules (Infrequent) 2260
Floxin I.V. (Less than 1%) 1571
Fortaz 1100
▲ Foscavir Injection (5% or greater up to 10%) 547
Guaifed 1787
Hexalen Capsules (1%) 2571
HibTITER (One case) 1375
Hivid Tablets (Less than 1% to less than 3%) 2121
▲ Idamycin (4%) 1955
IFEX (Occasional) 697
Imitrex Tablets (Rare) 1106
INFeD (Iron Dextran Injection, USP) 2345
Isoptin Injectable (Occasional) 1344
JE-VAX (1 to 2.3 per million vaccines) 886
K-Phos Neutral Tablets 639
Keftab Tablets 915
Kwell Cream & Lotion (Exceedingly rare) 2008
Lariam Tablets 2128
Leukeran Tablets (Rare) 1133
Lindane Lotion USP 1% (Exceedingly rare) 582
Lindane Shampoo USP 1% (Exceedingly rare) 583
Lorabid Suspension and Pulvules 1459
Loxitane 1378

(■ Described in PDR For Nonprescription Drugs) Incidence data in parenthesis; ▲ 3% or more (◉ Described in PDR For Ophthalmology)

Ludiomil Tablets (Rare) 843
M-M-R II (Rare) 1687
M-R-VAX II (Rare) 1689
MS Contin Tablets (Less frequent) 1994
MSIR (Infrequent) 1997
Methergine 2272
Mexitil Capsules (About 2 in 1,000) 678
Myleran Tablets 1143
Nalfon 200 Pulvules & Nalfon Tablets (Less than 1%) 917
Narcan Injection 934
Navane Capsules and Concentrate (Infrequent) 2201
Navane Intramuscular (Infrequent) 2202
NebuPent for Inhalation Solution (1% or less) 1040
Noroxin Tablets 1715
Noroxin Tablets 2048
Norpramin Tablets 1526
▲Novantrone (2 to 4%) 1279
Oramorph SR (Morphine Sulfate Sustained Release Tablets) (Less frequent) 2236
Orap Tablets (One patient) 1050
Orthoclone OKT3 Sterile Solution .. 1837
Pamelor 2280
Parlodel (72 cases) 2281
PedvaxHIB (Infrequent) 1718
Penetrex Tablets 2031
Platinol 708
Platinol-AQ Injection 710
Primaxin I.M. 1727
Primaxin I.V. (0.4%) 1729
Prinzide Tablets 1737
▲Procrit for Injection (1.1% to 10%) 1841
ProSom Tablets (Infrequent) 449
▲Prostin VR Pediatric Sterile Solution (4%) 2635
Prozac Pulvules & Liquid, Oral Solution (12 among 6,000 patients) 919
Retrovir Capsules (Rare; 0.8%) 1158
Retrovir I.V. Infusion (Rare; 1%) 1163
Retrovir Syrup (Rare; 0.8%) 1158
Risperdal (0.3%) 1301
Roferon-A Injection (Less than 1%) 2145
Romazicon 2147
Rythmol Tablets–150mg, 225mg, 300mg (0.3%) 1352
Seldane Tablets 1536
Seldane-D Extended-Release Tablets 1538
Seromycin Pulvules 1476
Sinequan (Infrequent) 2205
Suprax 1399
Surmontil Capsules 2811
Talwin Injection 2334
Talwin Compound 2335
Talwin Injection 2334
Tegretol Chewable Tablets 852
Tegretol Suspension 852
Tegretol Tablets 852
Tofranil Ampuls 854
Tofranil Tablets 856
Tofranil-PM Capsules 857
Tonocard Tablets (Less than 1%) .. 531
Triavil Tablets 1757
Ultram Tablets (50 mg) (Less than 1%) 1585
Uroqid-Acid No. 2 Tablets 640
Vaseretic Tablets 1765
Versed Injection 2170
Videx Tablets, Powder for Oral Solution, & Pediatric Powder for Oral Solution (1%) 720
Vivactil Tablets 1774
Wellbutrin Tablets (Frequent) 1204
Xanax Tablets 2649
Zefazone 2654
Zinacef 1211
Zovirax Sterile Powder (Approximately 1%) 1223

Seizures, convulsive
Aralen Hydrochloride Injection 2301
Aralen Phosphate Tablets 2301
Cipro I.V. (1% or less) 595
Cipro Tablets (Less than 1%) 592
Cylert Tablets 412
Etrafon 2355
Flagyl 375 Capsules 2434
Flagyl I.V. 2247
Mellaril (Infrequent) 2269
Mezlin 601
Mezlin Pharmacy Bulk Package 604
Phenergan Injection 2773
Phenergan Tablets 2775
Protostat Tablets 1883
Reglan (Isolated reports) 2068
Robaxin Injectable 2070
Serentil 684
Thorazine 2523
Timentin for Injection 2528
Trilafon 2389

Seizures, epileptiform
Eskalith 2485
Etrafon (A few instances) 2355
Lioresal Tablets 829
Lithium Carbonate Capsules & Tablets 2230
Lithonate/Lithotabs/Lithobid 2543
Pamelor 2280
Parlodel (4 cases) 2281

Seizures, exacerbation of
Lamictal Tablets (2.3%) 1112

Seizures, grand mal
Desyrel and Desyrel Dividose 503
▲Foscavir Injection (5% or greater).. 547
Haldol Decanoate 1577
Haldol Injection, Tablets and Concentrate 1575
Hivid Tablets (Less than 1% to less than 3%) 2121
Orap Tablets 1050
Pepcid Injection (Infrequent) 1722
Pepcid (Infrequent) 1720
Proleukin for Injection (1%) 797
Prolixin 509
Sodium Polystyrene Sulfonate Suspension (One case) 2244
Taxol (Rare; less than 1%) 714
Temaril Tablets, Syrup and Spansule Extended-Release Capsules 483
Thorazine 2523
Zofran Injection (Rare) 1214
Zofran Tablets (Rare) 1217

Seizures, neonatal
Capoten 739
Capozide 742
Esgic-plus Tablets (One 2-day-old male infant) 1013

Self-deprecation
Hydropres Tablets 1675

Sensation, abnormal (see under Paresthesia)

Sensation, disturbance of temperature
Dopram Injectable 2061
Duranest Injections 542
Dyclone 0.5% and 1% Topical Solutions, USP 544
Ethmozine Tablets (Less than 2%) 2041
▲Imitrex Injection (10.8%) 1103
Imitrex Tablets (2% to 3%; rare) .. 1106
IOPIDINE Sterile Ophthalmic Solution .... ⊙ 219
Tonocard Tablets (0.5-1.5%) 531
Xylocaine Injections 567

Sensation, heavy
▲Imitrex Injection (7.3%) 1103
Imitrex Tablets (Less than 1% to 2%) 1106

Sensation of pressure/tightness
▲Imitrex Injection (5.1 to 7.1%) 1103
Imitrex Tablets (Less than 1% to 2%) 1106

Sensations, numbness
Duranest Injections 542
Dyclone 0.5% and 1% Topical Solutions, USP 544
Xylocaine Injections 567

Sensations, pulsating
Imitrex Injection (Infrequent) 1103
Imitrex Tablets (Infrequent) 1106

Sensitivity, light
▲Orap Tablets (1 of 20 patients) 1050
ReVia Tablets (Less than 1%) 940
Stimate, (desmopressin acetate) Nasal Spray, 1.5 mg/mL 525

Sensitivity, sun
Cipro Tablets 592
Danocrine Capsules (Rare) 2307
Minocin Oral Suspension 1385
Retin-A (tretinoin) Cream/Gel/Liquid 1889
Tegrin Dandruff Shampoo .... ▣ 611
Tegrin Skin Cream & Tegrin Medicated Soap .... ▣ 611
Thorazine 2523

Sensitivity reactions
AVC (Occasional) 1500
Anusol Ointment (Rare) .... ▣ 847
Arthritis Foundation NightTime Caplets (Rare) .... ▣ 674
Auralgan Otic Solution 2703
Bactroban Ointment 2470
Betadine Skin Cleanser (Rare) 1992
Betadine 5% Sterile Ophthalmic Prep Solution (Occasional instances) .... ⊙ 274
Betasept Surgical Scrub 1993
Bleph-10 (Rare) 475
Brevoxyl Gel 2552
Capozide 742
Coly-Mycin S Otic w/Neomycin & Hydrocortisone 1906
Congess 1004
CORTENEMA (Rare) 2535
Cortisporin Otic Solution Sterile (Occasional) 1087
Creon 2536
Critic-Aid, Antimicrobial Skin Paste 2554
Cycrin Tablets (Occasional) 975
Delfen Contraceptive Foam .... ▣ 737
Drithocreme 0.1%, 0.25%, 0.5%, 1.0% (HP) 905
Dritho-Scalp 0.25%, 0.5% 906
Dyclone 0.5% and 1% Topical Solutions, USP 544
Esidrix Tablets 821
Ethyl Chloride, U.S.P. (Extremely rare) 1052
FML-S Liquifilm .... ⊙ 242
Fero-Folic-500 Filmtab 429
Fluori-Methane (Extremely rare) 1053
Fluro-Ethyl (Extremely rare) 1053
Hibiclens Antimicrobial Skin Cleanser 2840
Hibistat Towelette 2841
Humatrope Vials 1443
Humegon 1824
Hyperab Rabies Immune Globulin (Human) (Occasional) 624
Hyper-Tet Tetanus Immune Globulin (Human) (Extremely rare) 627
HypRho-D Full Dose Rho (D) Immune Globulin (Human) (Extremely rare) 629
HypRho-D Mini-Dose Rho (D) Immune Globulin (Human) (Extremely rare) 628
Iberet-Folic-500 Filmtab 429
Melanex Topical Solution 1793
Metrodin (urofollitropin for injection) 2446
Mini-Gamulin Rh, $Rh_O(D)$ Immune Globulin (Human) (Rare) 520
Monistat Dual-Pak 1850
Monistat 3 Vaginal Suppositories 1850
Mycostatin Pastilles (Rare) 704
Mykrox Tablets 993
Nescaine/Nescaine MPF 554
Nicoderm (nicotine transdermal system) (2%) 1518
pHisoHex 2327
PediOtic Suspension Sterile (Occasional) 1153
Pergonal (menotropins for injection, USP) 2448
Polysporin Ophthalmic Ointment Sterile 1154
Polytrim Ophthalmic Solution Sterile (Rare) 482
Prinzide Tablets 1737
Provera Tablets (An occasional patient) 2636
Retrovir Capsules (Rare) 1158
Retrovir I.V. Infusion (Rare) 1163
Retrovir Syrup 1158
Rogaine Topical Solution (1.27%).. 2637
Sensorcaine 559
Sine-Aid Maximum Strength Sinus Medication Gelcaps, Caplets and Tablets (Rare) 1554
Sinulin Tablets (Rare) 787
Solbar PF Ultra Liquid SPF 30 1932
Trusopt Sterile Ophthalmic Solution (Rare) 1760
T.R.U.E. Test (One report) 1189
Tylenol, Children's (Rare) 1555
TYLENOL Extended Relief Caplets (Rare) 1558
TYLENOL, Extra Strength, Acetaminophen Adult Liquid Pain Reliever (Rare) 1560
TYLENOL, Extra Strength, acetaminophen Gelcaps, Geltabs, Caplets, Tablets (Rare) 1559
TYLENOL, Junior Strength, acetaminophen Coated Caplets, Grape and Fruit Chewable Tablets (Rare) 1557
TYLENOL Maximum Strength Allergy Sinus Medication Gelcaps and Caplets (Rare) 1563
TYLENOL Maximum Strength Flu NightTime Hot Medication Packets (Rare) 1562
TYLENOL, Maximum Strength, Sinus Medication Geltabs, Gelcaps, Caplets and Tablets (Rare) 1566
TYLENOL Cold Medication No Drowsiness Formula Gelcaps and Caplets (Rare) 1562
TYLENOL, Regular Strength, acetaminophen Caplets and Tablets (Rare) 1558
TYLENOL Severe Allergy Medication Caplets (Rare) 1564
Tympagesic Ear Drops 2342
Vaseretic Tablets 1765
Vasocidin Ointment (Rare) .... ⊙ 268
Zaroxolyn Tablets 1000
Zestoretic 2850

Sensorium, clouded
Betapace Tablets (Rare) 641
Blocadren Tablets 1614
Cartrol Tablets 410
Inderal 2728
Inderal LA Long Acting Capsules 2730
Inderide Tablets 2732
Inderide LA Long Acting Capsules .. 2734
Kerlone Tablets 2436
Levatol (Slight) 2403
Lopressor HCT Tablets 832
Mexitil Capsules (1.9% to 2.6%) .. 678
Normodyne Tablets 2379
Sectral Capsules 2807
Tenoretic Tablets 2845
Tenormin Tablets and I.V. Injection 2847
Timolide Tablets 1748
Timoptic in Ocudose 1753
Timoptic Sterile Ophthalmic Solution 1751
Timoptic-XE 1755
Toprol-XL Tablets 565
Trandate Tablets 1185
Visken Tablets 2299
Zebeta Tablets 1413
Ziac 1415

Sensorium, dull
Diupres Tablets 1650
Hydropres Tablets 1675
Ser-Ap-Es Tablets 849

Sensory deficit
Oncovin Solution Vials & Hyporets 1466

Sensory deficit, persistent
Duranest Injections 542

Sensory disturbances
Alupent Tablets (0.2%) 669
Anafranil Capsules (Infrequent) 803
Depo-Medrol Single-Dose Vial 2600
Depo-Medrol Sterile Aqueous Suspension 2597
Foscavir Injection (Between 1% and 5%) 547
Paxil Tablets 2505
▲Prograf (Approximately 55%) 1042
▲Proleukin for Injection (10%) 797
▲Wellbutrin Tablets (4.0%) 1204

Sepsis
Aristocort Suspension (Forte Parenteral) 1027
Aristospan Suspension (Intra-articular) 1033
Aristospan Suspension (Intralesional) 1032
Betaseron for SC Injection 658
▲CellCept Capsules (17.6% to 19.7%; 17.5% to 21.8%) 2099
Clozaril Tablets 2252
Cognex Capsules (Rare) 1901
Cytosar-U Sterile Powder (One case; less frequent) 2592
▲Cytovene (4%) 2103
Diprivan Injection (Less than 1%) .. 2833

(▣ Described in PDR For Nonprescription Drugs) Incidence data in parenthesis; ▲ 3% or more (⊙ Described in PDR For Ophthalmology)

Ergamisol Tablets (2 out of 463 patients) 1292
Exosurf Neonatal for Intratracheal Suspension (B 24% to 34%) 1095
Felbatol 2666
▲Foscavir Injection (5% or greater) 547
Intron A (Less than 5%) 2364
▲Leukine for IV Infusion (11%) 1271
Lutrepulse for Injection 980
▲Navelbine Injection (8%) 1145
▲Novantrone (31 to 34%) 1279
Oncaspar (Less than 1%) 2028
Orthoclone OKT3 Sterile Solution 1837
Permax Tablets (Infrequent) 575
Pravachol 765
▲Proleukin for Injection (23%) 797
Prostin VR Pediatric Sterile Solution (About 2%) 2635
Pulmozyme Inhalation 1064
Rythmol Tablets–150mg, 225mg, 300mg (One case) 1352
Survanta Beractant Intratracheal Suspension 2226
▲Taxol (30%) 714
Ticlid Tablets (Rare) 2156
▲Trasylol (3%) 613
▲Zinecard (12% to 17%) 1961

Sepsis, intestinal

Questran Light (One case) 769
Questran Powder (One case) 770

Septicemia

▲Leustatin (6%) 1834
Lioresal Intrathecal 1596
Lippes Loop Intrauterine Double-S 1848
Metastron (A single (fatal) case) 1594
▲Neoral (5.3%) 2276
Orudis Capsules (Rare) 2766
Oruvail Capsules (Rare) 2766
ParaGard T380A Intrauterine Copper Contraceptive 1880
▲Sandimmune (4.8 to 5.3%) 2286
Thioplex (Thiotepa For Injection) 1281
Tonocard Tablets (Less than 1%) 531

Septic shock

Oncaspar (Less than 1%) 2028
Tonocard Tablets (Less than 1%) 531

Seroma, subgaleal

INSTAT* Collagen Absorbable Hemostat (Less than 1%) 1312
INSTAT* MCH Microfibrillar Collagen Hemostat (A single case) 1313

Serositis

Monopril Tablets 757
Vaseretic Tablets 1765
Vasotec I.V. 1768
Vasotec Tablets (0.5% to 1.0%) 1771

Serum alkaline phosphatase, elevation

▲Accutane Capsules (1 in 5 to 1 in 10 patients) 2076
Adalat CC (Rare) 589
Asacol Delayed-Release Tablets 1979
Atamet 572
Atgam Sterile Solution 2581
Augmentin (Infrequent) 2468
Axid Pulvules (Less common) 1427
Azactam for Injection (Less than 1%) 734
Betaseron for SC Injection 658
Biaxin (Less than 1%) 405
BiCNU 691
Bumex (0.4%) 2093
Calan SR Caplets 2422
Calan Tablets 2419
Capoten 739
Capozide 742
Cardizem CD Capsules (Less than 1%) 1506
Cardizem SR Capsules (1%) 1510
Cardizem Injectable (Less than 1%) 1508
Cardizem Tablets (Less than 1%) 1512
Ceclor Pulvules & Suspension (1 in 40) 1431
Cefizox for Intramuscular or Intravenous Use (Greater than 1% but less than 5%) 1034
Cefotan (1 in 700) 2829
Ceftin 1078
Cefzil Tablets and Oral Suspension (0.2%) 746
▲CellCept Capsules (More than or equal to 3%) 2099
Ceptaz (One in 23) 1081
▲CHEMET (succimer) Capsules (4.2 to 10.4%) 1545
Chibroxin Sterile Ophthalmic Solution (With oral form) 1617
▲Cipro I.V. (Among most frequent) 595
▲Cipro I.V. Pharmacy Bulk Package (Among most frequent) 597
Cipro Tablets (0.8%) 592
Claforan Sterile and Injection (Less than 1%) 1235
Cytotec (Infrequent) 2424
Cytovene (1% or less) 2103
Dalgan Injection 538
Dalmane Capsules (Rare) 2173
Deltasone Tablets 2595
Depen Titratable Tablets (Few reports) 2662
Depo-Medrol Single-Dose Vial 2600
Depo-Medrol Sterile Aqueous Suspension 2597
Dilacor XR Extended-release Capsules (Rare) 2018
Duricef 748
Effexor (Infrequent) 2719
Elspar 1659
Ergamisol Tablets (Less frequent) 1292
Felbatol (Infrequent) 2666
Floxin I.V. (More than or equal to 1%) 1571
Floxin Tablets (200 mg, 300 mg, 400 mg) (More than or equal to 1%) 1567
▲Fortaz (1 in 23) 1100
Foscavir Injection (Between 1% and 5%) 547
▲Sterile FUDR (Among more common) 2118
Fungizone Intravenous 506
Glucotrol Tablets (Occasional) 1967
Glucotrol XL Extended Release Tablets (Occasional) 1968
▲Hexalen Capsules (9%) 2571
Hivid Tablets (Less than 1% to less than 3%) 2121
Imuran 1110
Inderide Tablets 2732
▲Intron A (Up to 8%) 2364
Isoptin Oral Tablets 1346
Isoptin SR Tablets 1348
Keftab Tablets 915
Kefzol Vials, Faspak & ADD-Vantage (Rare) 1456
Klonopin Tablets 2126
Larodopa Tablets 2129
Lescol Capsules 2267
Loniten Tablets 2618
Lopid Tablets (Occasional) 1917
Lorabid Suspension and Pulvules 1459
Lorelco Tablets 1517
▲Lupron Depot 7.5 mg (5.4%) 2559
Mandol Vials, Faspak & ADD-Vantage 1461
Maxaquin Tablets 2440
Medrol 2621
Mefoxin 1691
Mefoxin Premixed Intravenous Solution 1694
▲Mepron Suspension (5% to 8%) 1135
Mevacor Tablets 1699
Mezlin 601
Mezlin Pharmacy Bulk Package 604
Mithracin 607
Monocid Injection (1.6%) 2497
Monopril Tablets 757
Mycobutin Capsules (Less than 1%) 1957
Nalfon 200 Pulvules & Nalfon Tablets (Less than 1%) 917
Navane Capsules and Concentrate 2201
Navane Intramuscular 2202
▲Neupogen for Injection (27% to 58%) 495
▲Neutrexin (4.6%) 2572
Nimotop Capsules (0.2%; rare) 610
▲Nolvadex Tablets (3.0%) 2841
Noroxin Tablets (1.1%) 1715
Noroxin Tablets (1.1%) 2048
Norpramin Tablets 1526
Nutropin 1061
Oxandrin 2862
Paraflex Caplets 1580
Parafon Forte DSC Caplets 1581
▲Paraplatin for Injection (24% to 37%) 705
Parlodel 2281
Paxil Tablets (Rare) 2505
Penetrex Tablets (Less than 1%) 2031
Pentasa (Less than 1%) 1527
Pravachol 765
PREVACID Delayed-Release Capsules (Less than 1%) 2562
Prilosec Delayed-Release Capsules (Rare) 529
Primaxin I.M. 1727
Primaxin I.V. 1729
Procardia Capsules (Rare) 1971
Procardia XL Extended Release Tablets (Rare) 1972
Proglycem 580
▲Prograf (Greater than 3%) 1042
▲Proleukin for Injection (56%) 797
Rifadin 1528
Rifamate Capsules 1530
Rimactane Capsules (Rare) 847
Rocephin Injectable Vials, ADD-Vantage, Galaxy Container (Less than 1%) 2142
▲Roferon-A Injection (8% to 11%) 2145
Rythmol Tablets–150mg, 225mg, 300mg (0.2%) 1352
Sectral Capsules 2807
Sinemet Tablets 943
Sinemet CR Tablets 944
Solu-Cortef Sterile Powder 2641
Solu-Medrol Sterile Powder 2643
Suprax (Less than 2%) 1399
Tambocor Tablets (Rare) 1497
▲Taxol (22%) 714
▲Tazicef for Injection (1 in 23 patients) 2519
▲Tegison Capsules (10-25%) 2154
Timentin for Injection 2528
Toprol-XL Tablets 565
Trobicin Sterile Powder 2645
Unasyn 2212
Vantin for Oral Suspension and Vantin Tablets 2646
Verelan Capsules 1410
Verelan Capsules 2824
Videx Tablets, Powder for Oral Solution, & Pediatric Powder for Oral Solution (1% to 4%) 720
Winstrol Tablets 2337
Xanax Tablets (Less than 1% to 1.7%) 2649
Zefazone 2654
Zerit Capsules (1% to 4%) 729
Zinacef (1 in 50 patients) 1211
Zithromax (Less than 1%) 1944
Zocor Tablets 1775
Zosyn 1419
Zosyn Pharmacy Bulk Package 1422

Serum aminotransferase, elevation

Procan SR Tablets 1926

Serum amylase, elevation

Cipro I.V. (Rare) 595
Cipro I.V. Pharmacy Bulk Package (Rare) 597
Cipro Tablets (Less than 0.1%) 592
Cuprimine Capsules (Few cases) 1630
Cytotec (Infrequent) 2424
Desyrel and Desyrel Dividose 503
Foscavir Injection (Less than 1%) 547
Hespan Injection 929
▲Hivid Tablets (3.4% to 8.1%) 2121
▲Mepron Suspension (1% to 8%) 1135
Oncaspar (Less than 1%) 2028
Pentasa (Less than 1%) 1527
Pentaspan Injection 937
Platinol (Infrequent) 708
Platinol-AQ Injection (Infrequent) 710
▲Videx Tablets, Powder for Oral Solution, & Pediatric Powder for Oral Solution (6% to 22%) 720
Zerit Capsules (Up to 9%) 729

Serum bicarbonate content, variations

▲Bumex (3.1%) 2093

Serum bilirubin, elevation (see under Hyperbilirubinemia)

Serum bilirubin levels, abnormalities

Atamet 572
Bumex (0.8%) 2093
Cefzil Tablets and Oral Suspension (Less than 0.1%) 746
Doral Tablets (Less than 1%) 2664
Emcyt Capsules (2 to 3%) 1953
Imuran 1110
Kefurox Vials, Faspak & ADD-Vantage (1 in 500) 1454
Nebcin Vials, Hyporets & ADD-Vantage 1464
Paraflex Caplets 1580
Parafon Forte DSC Caplets 1581
Roferon-A Injection (Less than 1% to 2%) 2145
Sinemet Tablets 943
Sinemet CR Tablets 944
Xanax Tablets (Less than 1% to 1.6%) 2649

Serum calcium, depression (see under Hypocalcemia)

Serum calcium content, variations

Bumex (2.4%) 2093

Serum calcium decrease (see under Hypocalcemia)

Serum cholesterol, increase (see under Hypercholesterolemia)

Serum creatine phosphokinase, elevation

Catapres Tablets (Rare) 674
Catapres-TTS (Rare) 675
▲Cipro I.V. (Among most frequent) 595
▲Cipro I.V. Pharmacy Bulk Package (Among most frequent) 597
Combipres Tablets (Rare) 677
Cytovene (1% or less) 2103
Foscavir Injection (Less than 1%) 547
Haldol Decanoate 1577
Havrix (Less than 1%) 2489
Hivid Tablets (Less than 1% to less than 3%) 2121
Quinidex Extentabs 2067
Risperdal (Infrequent) 1301
Suprane (Less than 1%) 1813
▲Trasylol (5%) 613
Zithromax (1% to 2%) 1944
▲Zocor Tablets (About 5% of patients) 1775

Serum creatinine, elevation

Accupril Tablets (2%) 1893
Children's Advil Suspension (Occasional) 2692
Altace Capsules (1.2% to 1.5%) 1232
Amikacin Sulfate Injection, USP 960
Amikin Injectable 501
Ancobon Capsules 2079
Asacol Delayed-Release Tablets 1979
Atgam Sterile Solution 2581
Azactam for Injection 734
Azo Gantrisin Tablets 2081
Bactrim DS Tablets 2084
Bactrim I.V. Infusion 2082
Bactrim 2084
Biaxin (Less than 1%) 405
▲Bumex (7.4%) 2093
Capoten 739
Capozide 742
Caverject (Less than 1%) 2583
Ceclor Pulvules & Suspension (Less than 1 in 500) 1431
Cefizox for Intramuscular or Intravenous Use (Occasional) 1034
Cefobid Intravenous/Intramuscular (1 in 48) 2189
Cefobid Pharmacy Bulk Package - Not for Direct Infusion (1 in 48) 2192
Cefotan 2829
Ceftin 1078
Cefzil Tablets and Oral Suspension (0.1%) 746
▲CellCept Capsules (More than or equal to 3%) 2099
Ceptaz (Occasional) 1081
Chibroxin Sterile Ophthalmic Solution (With oral form) 1617
▲Cipro I.V. (Among most frequent) 595
▲Cipro I.V. Pharmacy Bulk Package (Among most frequent) 597
Cipro Tablets (1.1%) 592
Claforan Sterile and Injection (Occasional) 1235
Coly-Mycin M Parenteral 1905
Cozaar Tablets (Less than 0.1%) 1628
Cytovene (1% or less) 2103
Daypro Caplets (Occasional) 2426
Didronel I.V. Infusion (Occasional) 1488
Didronel Tablets 1984
Diprivan Injection (Less than 1%) 2833
Duricef 748
Dyazide 2479
Dyrenium Capsules (Rare) 2481
Effexor (Infrequent) 2719
Ergamisol Tablets (Less frequent) 1292
Eulexin Capsules 2358
Feldene Capsules (Greater than 1%) 1965
Floxin I.V. (More than or equal to 1%) 1571

(▣ Described in PDR For Nonprescription Drugs) Incidence data in parenthesis; ▲ 3% or more (◉ Described in PDR For Ophthalmology)

Serum creatinine, elevation — Side Effects Index — 1410

Floxin Tablets (200 mg, 300 mg, 400 mg) (More than or equal to 1%) 1567
Fortaz (Occasional) 1100
▲Foscavir Injection (5% or greater up to 27%) 547
Fungizone Intravenous 506
▲Ganite (About 12.5%) 2533
Gantanol Tablets 2119
Gantrisin 2120
Garamycin Injectable 2360
Glucotrol Tablets (Occasional) 1967
Glucotrol XL Extended Release Tablets 1968
▲Hexalen Capsules (7%) 2571
Hydrea Capsules (Occasional) 696
Hyzaar Tablets (0.8%) 1677
IFEX 697
Indocin I.V. 1684
Intron A (Up to 3%) 2364
Keftab Tablets 915
Kefurox Vials, Faspak & ADD-Vantage 1454
Lamictal Tablets (Rare) 1112
Leukine for IV Infusion 1271
Lodine Capsules and Tablets (Less than 1%) 2743
Loniten Tablets 2618
Lorabid Suspension and Pulvules 1459
Lotensin Tablets (About 2%) 834
Lotensin HCT 837
Lotrel Capsules 840
Lozol Tablets (Less than 5%) 2022
Lupron Depot 3.75 mg 2556
Lupron Depot 7.5 mg 2559
Lupron Injection (Less than 5%) 2555
Macrobid Capsules 1988
Macrodantin Capsules 1989
Mandol Vials, Faspak & ADD-Vantage 1461
Maxzide 1380
Mefoxin 1691
Mefoxin Premixed Intravenous Solution 1694
Mepron Suspension (1%) 1135
Mezlin 601
Mezlin Pharmacy Bulk Package 604
Mithracin 607
Monocid Injection (Occasional) 2497
Monopril Tablets 757
Children's Motrin Ibuprofen Oral Suspension (Occasional) 1546
Motrin Tablets (Occasional) 2625
Mutamycin (2%) 703
Mykrox Tablets 993
Nebcin Vials, Hyporets & ADD-Vantage 1464
Neoral 2276
Neutrexin (0.9%) 2572
Nolvadex Tablets (1.7%) 2841
▲Normodyne Injection (8%) 2377
Noroxin Tablets (Less frequent) 1715
Noroxin Tablets (Less frequent) 2048
Norpace (Less than 1%) 2444
Oncaspar 2028
Oxandrin 2862
▲Paraplatin for Injection (5% to 10%) 705
▲Pentam 300 Injection (23.1%) 1041
Phenurone Tablets (1% or less) 447
Pipracil 1390
Platinol 708
Platinol-AQ Injection 710
PREVACID Delayed-Release Capsules (Less than 1%) 2562
Prilosec Delayed-Release Capsules (Less than 1%) 529
Primaxin I.M. 1727
Primaxin I.V. 1729
Prinivil Tablets (About 2.0%) 1733
Prinzide Tablets 1737
Procardia Capsules (Rare) 1971
Procardia XL Extended Release Tablets (Rare) 1972
▲Prograf (19% to 39%) 1042
▲Proleukin for Injection (61%) 797
Proloprim Tablets 1155
▲Rocaltrol Capsules (1 in 6) 2141
Rocephin Injectable Vials, ADD-Vantage, Galaxy Container (Less than 1%) 2142
Roferon-A Injection (Less than 1% to 2%) 2145
Sandimmune 2286
Septra 1174
Septra I.V. Infusion 1169
Septra I.V. Infusion ADD-Vantage Vials 1171
Septra 1174
Sinemet CR Tablets 944
Suprax (Less than 2%) 1399
Tagamet 2516
Tazicef for Injection (Occasional) 2519
Tazidime Vials, Faspak & ADD-Vantage (Occasional) 1478
▲Tegison Capsules (1-10%) 2154
Timentin for Injection 2528
Tobramycin Sulfate Injection 968
Toradol 2159
▲Trandate Injection (8 of 100 patients) 1185
▲Trasylol (18% to 21%) 613
Trilisate (Less than 1%) 2000
Trimpex Tablets 2163
Ultram Tablets (50 mg) (Infrequent) 1585
Unasyn 2212
Univasc Tablets (1% to 2%) 2410
Vancocin HCl, Oral Solution & Pulvules (Rare) 1483
Vancocin HCl, Vials & ADD-Vantage 1481
Vantin for Oral Suspension and Vantin Tablets 2646
▲Vaseretic Tablets (About 0.6% to 20%) 1765
▲Vasotec I.V. (0.2% to 20%) 1768
▲Vasotec Tablets (About 0.2% to 20%) 1771
Xanax Tablets (1.9% to 2.2%) 2649
Zantac (Rare) 1209
Zantac Injection 1207
Zantac Syrup (Rare) 1209
Zaroxolyn Tablets 1000
Zebeta Tablets 1413
Zefazone 2654
Zestoretic 2850
Zestril Tablets (About 2%) 2854
Zinacef 1211
Zithromax (Less than 1%) 1944
Zosyn 1419
Zosyn Pharmacy Bulk Package 1422
Zovirax Capsules 1219
▲Zovirax Sterile Powder (5% to 10%) 1223
Zovirax 1219

Serum electrolyte changes (see under Electrolyte imbalance)

Serum fibrogen, decrease
Trental Tablets (Rare) 1244

Serum lipase, elevation
Hivid Tablets (Less than 1% to less than 3%) 2121
Oncaspar 2028
Pentasa (Less than 1%) 1527

Serum PBI levels, decrease (see under PBI decrease)

Serum phosphorus, elevation
Macrodantin Capsules 1989
Nutropin 1061
Zebeta Tablets 1413

Serum phosphorus content, variations
▲Bumex (4.5%) 2093
▲Macrobid Capsules (1% to 5%) 1988

Serum potassium, reduction (see under Hypokalemia)

Serum proteins, changes
Brevicon 2088
Bumex (0.7%) 2093
Doral Tablets (Less than 1%) 2664
Norinyl 2088
Tri-Norinyl 2164

Serum sickness
Children's Advil Suspension (Less than 1%) 2692
Amoxil 2464
Antivenin (Black Widow Spider) 1607
Antivenin (Crotalidae) Polyvalent 2696
▲Atgam Sterile Solution (Less than 1% to a majority of patients) 2581
Augmentin 2468
Axid Pulvules (Rare) 1427
Azo Gantanol Tablets 2080
Azo Gantrisin Tablets 2081
Azulfidine (Rare) 1949
Bactrim DS Tablets 2084
Bactrim I.V. Infusion 2082
Bactrim 2084
Bicillin C-R Injection 2704
Bicillin C-R 900/300 Injection 2706
Bicillin L-A Injection 2707
Ceclor Pulvules & Suspension (0.05% to 0.024%) 1431
Cefizox for Intramuscular or Intravenous Use 1034
Ceftin 1078
Cefzil Tablets and Oral Suspension (Rare) 746
Duricef (Rare) 748
Fansidar Tablets 2114
Feldene Capsules (Less than 1%) 1965
Flagyl 375 Capsules 2434
Flagyl I.V. 2247
Floxin I.V. 1571
Floxin Tablets (200 mg, 300 mg, 400 mg) 1567
Gantanol Tablets 2119
Gantrisin 2120
IBU Tablets (Less than 1%) 1342
Intal Inhaler (Rare) 988
Intal Nebulizer Solution 989
Lincocin 2617
Lorabid Suspension and Pulvules (Rare) 1459
Children's Motrin Ibuprofen Oral Suspension (Less than 1%) 1546
Motrin Tablets (Less than 1%) 2625
Motrin Ibuprofen Suspension, Oral Drops, Chewable Tablets, Caplets (Less than 1%) 1546
Nasalcrom Nasal Solution (Rare) 994
Omnipen Capsules 2764
Omnipen for Oral Suspension 2765
Orthoclone OKT3 Sterile Solution 1837
Pen•Vee K 2772
Pfizerpen for Injection 2203
Pneumovax 23 (Rare) 1725
Protostat Tablets 1883
Prozac Pulvules & Liquid, Oral Solution (Rare) 919
Quadrinal Tablets 1350
Rabies Vaccine Adsorbed (Less than 1%) 2508
Recombivax HB (Less than 1%) 1744
Rocephin Injectable Vials, ADD-Vantage, Galaxy Container (Rare) 2142
Septra 1174
Septra I.V. Infusion 1169
Septra I.V. Infusion ADD-Vantage Vials 1171
Septra 1174
Suprax (Less than 2%) 1399
Ticlid Tablets (Rare) 2156
Tolectin (200, 400 and 600 mg) (Less than 1%) 1581
Vantin for Oral Suspension and Vantin Tablets 2646
Vibramycin 1941

Serum transaminase, elevation
Atromid-S Capsules 2701
Augmentin (Infrequent) 2468
Bactrim DS Tablets 2084
Bactrim I.V. Infusion 2082
Bactrim 2084
BiCNU 691
Calan SR Caplets 2422
Calan Tablets 2419
Capoten 739
Capozide 742
CeeNU (Small percentage) 693
Clomid 1514
▲Cognex Capsules (29%) 1901
Cordarone Tablets 2712
Danocrine Capsules 2307
Deconamine CX Cough and Cold Liquid and Tablets 1319
Depakene (Frequent) 413
Depakote Tablets (Frequent) 415
DiaBeta Tablets (Isolated cases) 1239
Diflucan Injection, Tablets, and Oral Suspension (1% or greater) 2194
Dilacor XR Extended-release Capsules 2018
Duratuss HD Elixir (A single elevation) 2565
Duricef 748
▲Eminase (Less than 10%) 2039
Ethmozine Tablets (Rare) 2041
Eulexin Capsules 2358
▲Sterile FUDR (Among more common) 2118
Garamycin Injectable 2360
Glynase PresTab Tablets (Isolated reports) 2609
Imuran 1110
Inderide Tablets 2732
Inderide LA Long Acting Capsules 2734
Intron A (Less than 5%) 2364
Isoptin Oral Tablets (Less than 1%) 1346
Isoptin SR Tablets 1348
Klonopin Tablets 2126
▲Lariam Tablets (Among most frequent) 2128
Lescol Capsules 2267
Leukine for IV Infusion 1271
Lincocin (A few instances) 2617
Lopid Tablets 1917
Lorelco Tablets 1517
Lotensin Tablets 834
Luvox Tablets (Frequent) 2544
Marinol (Dronabinol) Capsules (Less than 1%) 2231
Methotrexate Sodium Tablets, Injection, for Injection and LPF Injection 1275
Mevacor Tablets (1.9%) 1699
Micronase Tablets 2623
Mithracin 607
Monopril Tablets 757
Nardil (Common) 1920
Navane Capsules and Concentrate (Infrequent) 2201
Navane Intramuscular (Infrequent) 2202
Nebcin Vials, Hyporets & ADD-Vantage 1464
Netromycin Injection 100 mg/ml (15 of 1000 patients) 2373
▲Normodyne Injection (4%) 2377
▲Normodyne Tablets (4%) 2379
▲Nydrazid Injection (10% to 20%) 508
Paxil Tablets 2505
Pravachol 765
▲Proleukin for Injection (56%) 797
Proloprim Tablets 1155
Rifadin 1528
▲Rifamate Capsules (10% to 20%) 1530
▲Rifater (10% to 20% of patients) 1532
Rimactane Capsules (Rare) 847
Rythmol Tablets–150mg, 225mg, 300mg (0.2%) 1352
Seldane Tablets (One case) 1536
Seldane-D Extended-Release Tablets (One case) 1538
Septra 1174
Septra I.V. Infusion 1169
Septra I.V. Infusion ADD-Vantage Vials 1171
Septra 1174
Seromycin Pulvules 1476
Streptase for Infusion 562
Tagamet 2516
Tambocor Tablets (Rare) 1497
Tapazole Tablets 1477
Toprol-XL Tablets 565
▲Trandate (4% of patients) 1185
▲Trasylol (5%) 613
Trilisate (Rare) 2000
Trimpex Tablets 2163
Tussend Expectorant 1785
Vascor (200, 300 and 400 mg) Tablets (Approximately 1%) 1587
Verelan Capsules 1410
Verelan Capsules 2824
Yutopar Intravenous Injection (Less than 1%) 570
Zocor Tablets (1%) 1775
Zofran Tablets 1217
Zovirax Sterile Powder (1% to 2%) 1223

Serum triglyceride, elevation (see under Hypertriglyceridemia)

Serum vitamin B_{12} levels, subnormal
Glucophage 752

Sexual activity, decrease
▲Catapres Tablets (About 3 in 100 patients) 674
Catapres-TTS (Less frequent) 675
Combipres Tablets (About 3%) 677
Orlamm (1% to 3%) 2239
Propulsid (Less than 1%) 1300
ReVia Tablets (Less than 1%) 940
Risperdal (Frequent) 1301
Stilphostrol Tablets and Ampuls 612

Sexual activity, increase
Android-10 Tablets 1251
Fioricet with Codeine Capsules 2260
Fiorinal with Codeine Capsules 2262
Halotestin Tablets 2614
ReVia Tablets (Less than 1%) 940

Sexual dysfunction
Adalat Capsules (10 mg and 20 mg) (2% or less) 587
Arfonad Ampuls 2080

(▣ Described in PDR For Nonprescription Drugs) Incidence data in parenthesis; ▲ 3% or more (◉ Described in PDR For Ophthalmology)

1411 Side Effects Index Sinusitis

Betapace Tablets (Les than 1% to 2%) ... 641
Carbocaine Hydrochloride Injection 2303
Cardizem CD Capsules (Less than 1%) ... 1506
Cardizem SR Capsules (Less than 1%) ... 1510
Cardizem Injectable ... 1508
Cardizem Tablets (Less than 1%) .. 1512
Cardura Tablets (2%) ... 2186
Catapres-TTS (2 of 101 patients) .. 675
Duranest Injections ... 542
Effexor (2%) ... 2719
Eldepryl Tablets ... 2550
Eskalith ... 2485
Hivid Tablets (Less than 1% to less than 3%) ... 2121
Levatol (0.5%) ... 2403
Lioresal Intrathecal ... 1596
Lithonate/Lithotabs/Lithobid ... 2543
Marcaine Hydrochloride with Epinephrine 1:200,000 ... 2316
Marcaine Hydrochloride Injection ... 2316
Marcaine Spinal ... 2319
Maxzide ... 1380
Monopril Tablets (Less than 1.0% to 1.0%) ... 757
Nardil (Common) ... 1920
Nescaine/Nescaine MPF ... 554
Norvasc Tablets (More than 0.1% to 1%) ... 1940
▲ Paxil Tablets (3.7% to 10.0%) ... 2505
Procardia Capsules (2% or less) ... 1971
Prozac Pulvules & Liquid, Oral Solution (1.9%) ... 919
Risperdal (Frequent) ... 1301
Rogaine Topical Solution ... 2637
Sensorcaine ... 559
Wellbutrin Tablets (Frequent) ... 1204
▲ Xanax Tablets (7.4%) ... 2649
Xylocaine Injections ... 567
Ziac ... 1415
▲ Zoladex (21%) ... 2858
▲ Zoloft Tablets (1.7%; 15.5%) ... 2217

Sexual maturity, accelerated

Lupron Depot-PED 7.5 mg, 11.25 mg and 15 mg (Less than 2%) ... 2560

Shivering (see under Trembling)

Shock

Acel-Imune Diphtheria and Tetanus Toxoids and Acellular Pertussis Vaccine Adsorbed (Rare) ... 1364
AK-Fluor Injection 10% and 25% ... ◉ 203
Antivenin (Crotalidae) Polyvalent ... 2696
AquaMEPHYTON Injection ... 1608
Aralen Hydrochloride Injection ... 2301
Betaseron for SC Injection ... 658
Cordarone Intravenous (Less than 2%) ... 2715
Coumadin ... 926
Demerol ... 2308
Demulen ... 2428
Desferal Vials ... 820
Dilaudid-HP Injection ... 1337
Dilaudid-HP Lyophilized Powder 250 mg ... 1337
Dilaudid Tablets and Liquid ... 1339
Diphtheria and Tetanus Toxoids and Pertussis Vaccine Adsorbed (Rare) ... 2477
Diphtheria and Tetanus Toxoids and Pertussis Vaccine Adsorbed USP (For Pediatric Use) (Rare) ... 875
▲ Eminase (Less than 10%) ... 2039
Emla Cream ... 545
Etrafon (Occasional) ... 2355
Floropryl Sterile Ophthalmic Ointment (Infrequent) ... 1662
Floxin I.V. ... 1571
Floxin Tablets (200 mg, 300 mg, 400 mg) ... 1567
Fluorescite ... ◉ 219
Fungizone Intravenous ... 506
Heparin Lock Flush Solution (Rare) 2725
Heparin Sodium Injection (Rare) ... 2726
Heparin Sodium Injection, USP, Sterile Solution (Rare) ... 2615
Heparin Sodium Vials (Rare) ... 1441
Humorsol Sterile Ophthalmic Solution (Infrequent) ... 1664
Hyperstat I.V. Injection ... 2363
Imitrex Tablets ... 1106
Indocin Capsules (Less than 1%) ... 1680
Indocin I.V. (Less than 1%) ... 1684
Indocin (Less than 1%) ... 1680
INFeD (Iron Dextran Injection, USP) ... 2345
Lippes Loop Intrauterine Double-S .. 1848
MS Contin Tablets ... 1994
MSIR ... 1997
Mepergan Injection ... 2753
Methadone Hydrochloride Oral Solution & Tablets ... 2235
Midamor Tablets ... 1703
Monopril Tablets (0.2%) ... 757
Nitro-Bid IV ... 1523
Nubain Injection (1% or less) ... 935
Oramorph SR (Morphine Sulfate Sustained Release Tablets) (Less frequent) ... 2236
Orthoclone OKT3 Sterile Solution .. 1837
Orudis Capsules (Rare) ... 2766
Oruvail Capsules (Rare) ... 2766
Permax Tablets (Infrequent) ... 575
Prostin VR Pediatric Sterile Solution (Less than 1%) ... 2635
RMS Suppositories ... 2657
Rifadin (Rare) ... 1528
Rifamate Capsules (Rare) ... 1530
Rifater ... 1532
Roxanol ... 2243
Salagen Tablets (Rare) ... 1489
Sandoglobulin I.V. (Rare) ... 2290
Sus-Phrine Injection ... 1019
Talwin Injection (Infrequent) ... 2334
Thorazine ... 2523
Trasylol (1.7%) ... 613
Tri-Immunol Adsorbed (1 per 1,750) ... 1408
Trilafon ... 2389
Videx Tablets, Powder for Oral Solution, & Pediatric Powder for Oral Solution (Less than 1%) ... 720
Zefazone ... 2654
Zofran Injection (Rare) ... 1214

Shock, anaphylactic (see under Anaphylactic shock)

Shock, hypovolemic

Diethylstilbestrol Tablets ... 1437
Estraderm Transdermal System ... 824
PMB 200 and PMB 400 ... 2783
PREVACID Delayed-Release Capsules (Less than 1%) ... 2562

Sialadenitis

Aldoclor Tablets ... 1598
Aldomet Ester HCl Injection ... 1602
Aldomet Oral ... 1600
Aldoril Tablets ... 1604
Apresazide Capsules ... 808
Capozide ... 742
Diucardin Tablets ... 2718
Diupres Tablets ... 1650
Diuril Oral Suspension ... 1653
Diuril Sodium Intravenous ... 1652
Diuril Tablets ... 1653
Dyazide ... 2479
Enduron Tablets ... 420
Esidrix Tablets ... 821
Esimil Tablets ... 822
HydroDIURIL Tablets ... 1674
Hydropres Tablets ... 1675
Hyzaar Tablets ... 1677
Inderide Tablets ... 2732
Inderide LA Long Acting Capsules .. 2734
Lopressor HCT Tablets ... 832
Lotensin HCT ... 837
Lozol Tablets ... 2022
Macrobid Capsules ... 1988
Macrodantin Capsules ... 1989
Maxzide ... 1380
Moduretic Tablets ... 1705
Mykrox Tablets (Rare) ... 993
Permax Tablets (Rare) ... 575
Prinzide Tablets ... 1737
Ser-Ap-Es Tablets ... 849
Timolide Tablets ... 1748
Vaseretic Tablets ... 1765
Videx Tablets, Powder for Oral Solution, & Pediatric Powder for Oral Solution (Up to 2%) ... 720
Zaroxolyn Tablets ... 1000
Zestoretic ... 2850
Ziac ... 1415

Sialadenopathy

Tapazole Tablets ... 1477

Sialism (see under Salivation)

Sialorrhea

Albuminar-5, Albumin (Human) U.S.P. 5% (Occasional) ... 512
Albuminar-25, Albumin (Human) U.S.P. 25% ... 513
Atamet ... 572
Diprivan Injection (Less than 1%) .. 2833
Haldol Decanoate ... 1577
Larodopa Tablets (Relatively frequent) ... 2129
Mestinon Injectable ... 1253
Mestinon ... 1254
NebuPent for Inhalation Solution (1% or less) ... 1040
Prostigmin Injectable ... 1260
Prostigmin Tablets ... 1261
Roferon-A Injection (Less than 1%) ... 2145
Sinemet Tablets ... 943
Sinemet CR Tablets ... 944
Tensilon Injectable ... 1261
Torecan (Occasional) ... 2245
Versed Injection ... 2170

Sialosis (see under Salivation)

Sickle cell disease

Levlen/Tri-Levlen ... 651

Sinoatrial block

Blocadren Tablets (Less than 1%) 1614
Flumadine Tablets & Syrup (Less than 0.3%) ... 1015
Neurontin Capsules (Rare) ... 1922
Timoptic in Ocudose (Less frequent) ... 1753
Timoptic-XE ... 1755

Sinoatrial node dysfunction

Cardene I.V. ... 2709
Cordarone Tablets ... 2712
Eskalith ... 2485
Lithonate/Lithotabs/Lithobid ... 2543

Sinus arrest

Cordarone Tablets ... 2712
Rythmol Tablets–150mg, 225mg, 300mg (Less than 1%) ... 1352
Tambocor Tablets (1% to less than 3%) ... 1497
Tonocard Tablets (Less than 1%) .. 531

Sinus bradycardia

Activase ... 1058
Adenocard Injection ... 1021
Adenoscan ... 1024
Children's Advil Suspension (Less than 1%) ... 2692
Brethaire Inhaler ... 813
▲ Cardizem SR Capsules (3%) ... 1510
Catapres Tablets (Rare) ... 674
Catapres-TTS (Rare) ... 675
Combipres Tablets (Rare) ... 677
Cordarone Intravenous (Less than 2%) ... 2715
Cordarone Tablets (2 to 5%) ... 2712
Cozaar Tablets (Less than 1%) ... 1628
Desyrel and Desyrel Dividose (Occasional) ... 503
Dilacor XR Extended-release Capsules ... 2018
Effexor (Rare) ... 2719
Eldepryl Tablets ... 2550
Eminase ... 2039
Hyzaar Tablets ... 1677
IBU Tablets (Less than 1%) ... 1342
Kytril Injection (Rare) ... 2490
Lanoxicaps ... 1117
Lanoxin Elixir Pediatric ... 1120
Lanoxin Injection ... 1123
Lanoxin Injection Pediatric ... 1126
Lanoxin Tablets ... 1128
Children's Motrin Ibuprofen Oral Suspension (Less than 1%) ... 1546
Motrin Tablets (Less than 1%) ... 2625
Motrin Ibuprofen Suspension, Oral Drops, Chewable Tablets, Caplets (Less than 1%) ... 1546
▲ Sandostatin Injection (21%) ... 2292
Serzone Tablets (1.5%) ... 771
▲ Taxol (23%) ... 714
Vascor (200, 300 and 400 mg) Tablets (0.5 to 2.0%) ... 1587

Sinus congestion

▲ AeroBid Inhaler System (3-9%) ... 1005
▲ Aerobid-M Inhaler System (3-9%) .. 1005
▲ Desyrel and Desyrel Dividose (2.8% to 5.7%) ... 503
Hivid Tablets (Less than 1% to less than 3%) ... 2121
Lupron Depot 3.75 mg ... 2556
Lupron Depot 7.5 mg ... 2559
▲ Lupron Injection (5% or more) ... 2555
Mykrox Tablets (Less than 2%) ... 993
Nasacort Nasal Inhaler (Fewer than 5%) ... 2024
▲ Stadol (3% to 9%) ... 775

Sinus discomfort

AeroBid Inhaler System (1-3%) ... 1005
Aerobid-M Inhaler System (1-3%) .. 1005
Cozaar Tablets (1.5%) ... 1628
Hivid Tablets (Less than 1% to less than 3%) ... 2121
Imitrex Injection (2.2%) ... 1103
ReVia Tablets (Less than 1%) ... 940

Sinus drainage

▲ AeroBid Inhaler System (3-9%) ... 1005
▲ Aerobid-M Inhaler System (3-9%) .. 1005

Sinusitis

▲ AeroBid Inhaler System (3-9%) ... 1005
▲ Aerobid-M Inhaler System (3-9%) .. 1005
▲ Ambien Tablets (4%) ... 2416
▲ Anafranil Capsules (2% to 6%) ... 803
Asacol Delayed-Release Tablets ... 1979
Atrovent Inhalation Solution (2.3%) ... 673
Axid Pulvules (2.4%) ... 1427
▲ Betaseron for SC Injection (36%) .. 658
Betimol 0.25%, 0.5% (1% to 5%) ... ◉ 261
Cardene Capsules (Rare) ... 2095
Cardura Tablets (Less than 0.5% of 3960 patients) ... 2186
Cartrol Tablets (Less common) ... 410
Caverject (2%) ... 2583
Ceftin for Oral Suspension (Less than 1% but more than 0.1%) ... 1078
▲ CellCept Capsules (More than or equal to 3%) ... 2099
Claritin (2% or fewer patients) ... 2349
Claritin-D (Less frequent) ... 2350
Cognex Capsules (Frequent) ... 1901
Cozaar Tablets (1.0%) ... 1628
Daypro Caplets (Less than 1%) ... 2426
Dilacor XR Extended-release Capsules (2.0%) ... 2018
Ethmozine Tablets (Less than 2%) 2041
Famvir (2.6%) ... 2486
▲ Felbatol (3.5%) ... 2666
Flonase Nasal Spray (Less than 1%) ... 1098
Fludara for Injection (Up to 5%) ... 663
Foscavir Injection (Between 1% and 5%) ... 547
▲ Habitrol Nicotine Transdermal System (3% to 9% of patients) ... 865
Hivid Tablets (Less than 1% to less than 3%) ... 2121
Hytrin Capsules (2.6%) ... 430
Hyzaar Tablets (1.2%) ... 1677
Imdur (Less than or equal to 5%) .. 1323
▲ Intron A (Up to 21%) ... 2364
Kerlone Tablets (Less than 2%) ... 2436
Lescol Capsules (2.7%) ... 2267
Lodine Capsules and Tablets (Less than 1%) ... 2743
Lotensin Tablets ... 834
Lotensin HCT (More than 1%) ... 837
Lozol Tablets (Less than 5%) ... 2022
Luvox Tablets (Frequent) ... 2544
Marinol (Dronabinol) Capsules (Less than 1%) ... 2231
▲ Mepron Suspension (7%) ... 1135
Miacalcin Nasal Spray (1% to 3%) 2275
Monoket (Fewer than 1%) ... 2406
Monopril Tablets (0.2% to 1.0%) .. 757
Nasarel Nasal Solution (1% or less) ... 2133
▲ Neoral (3% to 7%) ... 2276
Nicoderm (nicotine transdermal system) (1% to 3%) ... 1518
Nicotrol Nicotine Transdermal System (1% to 3%) ... 1550
Ocupress Ophthalmic Solution, 1% Sterile (Occasional) ... ◉ 309
Paxil Tablets (Infrequent) ... 2505
Permax Tablets (Infrequent) ... 575
Plendil Extended-Release Tablets (0.5% to 1.5%) ... 527
Prinivil Tablets (0.3% to 1.0%) ... 1733
Prinzide Tablets (0.3 to 1%) ... 1737
Procardia XL Extended Release Tablets (1% or less) ... 1972
▲ Prograf (Greater than 3%) ... 1042
▲ Propulsid (3.6%) ... 1300
ProSom Tablets (Infrequent) ... 449
▲ Prostep (nicotine transdermal system) (3% to 9% of patients) ... 1394
Prozac Pulvules & Liquid, Oral Solution (2.1% to 5%) ... 919

(▭ Described in PDR For Nonprescription Drugs) Incidence data in parenthesis; ▲ 3% or more (◉ Described in PDR For Ophthalmology)

Pulmozyme Inhalation 1064
Retrovir Capsules 1158
Retrovir I.V. Infusion 1163
Retrovir Syrup 1158
Risperdal (1% to 2%) 1301
Roferon-A Injection (Less than 3%) 2145
▲ Rogaine Topical Solution (7.16%) 2637
Salagen Tablets (1%) 1489
▲ Sandimmune (Less than 1 to 7%) 2286
Serzone Tablets 771
Stadol (1% or greater) 775
Supprelin Injection (2% to 3%) 2056
Univasc Tablets (More than 1%) 2410
▲ Videx Tablets, Powder for Oral Solution, & Pediatric Powder for Oral Solution (7% to 8%) 720
Zebeta Tablets (2.2%) 1413
Zestoretic (0.3 to 1%) 2850
Zestril Tablets (0.3% to 1.0%) 2854
Ziac 1415
Zoladex (1% or greater) 2858
Zoloft Tablets (Rare) 2217

Sinus syndrome, sick

Cardizem Injectable (Less than 1%) 1508
Rythmol Tablets–150mg, 225mg, 300mg (Less than 1%) 1352

Sinus tachycardia

Adenocard Injection 1021
Children's Advil Suspension (Less than 1%) 2692
Aramine Injection 1609
Etrafon 2355
Foscavir Injection (Between 1% and 5%) 547
IBU Tablets (Less than 1%) 1342
Children's Motrin Ibuprofen Oral Suspension (Less than 1%) 1546
Motrin Tablets (Less than 1%) 2625
Motrin Ibuprofen Suspension, Oral Drops, Chewable Tablets, Caplets (Less than 1%) 1546
▲ Proleukin for Injection (70%) 797
Propulsid (Rare cases) 1300
Seldane Tablets 1536
Seldane-D Extended-Release Tablets 1538
▲ Taxol (23%) 714
Vascor (200, 300 and 400 mg) Tablets (0.5 to 2.0%) 1587

Skin, anesthesia (see under Numbness, skin)

Skin, bleeding

Sulfamylon Cream (Rare) 925

Skin, burning

▲ Cleocin T Topical (10%) 2590
Cleocin Vaginal Cream 2589
▲ Diprolene (6%) 2352
▲ Dovonex Ointment 0.005% (Approximately 10% to 15%) 2684
Drysol 1932
▲ Emgel 2% Topical Gel (Most common) 1093
Epifoam (Infrequent) 2399
▲ Exelderm Cream 1.0% (3%) 2685
Exelderm Solution 1.0% (Approximately 1%) 2686
Gastrocrom Capsules (Infrequent) 984
Halog (Infrequent) 2686
Maxaquin Tablets 2440
MetroGel 1047
8-MOP Capsules 1246
Monistat Dual-Pak 1850
Nubain Injection (1% or less) 935
Oxsoralen Lotion 1% 1256
Oxsoralen-Ultra Capsules 1257
ProctoFoam-HC 2409
Trisoralen Tablets 1264
▲ Ultravate Cream 0.05% (4.4%) 2689
Ultravate Ointment 0.05% (2.4%) 2690

Skin, cracking

Aclovate Ointment (1 of 366 patients) 1069
Aquasol A Vitamin A Capsules, USP 534
Diprolene Gel 0.05% (Less frequent) 2353
Hivid Tablets (Less than 1% to less than 3%) 2121
Temovate (1 of 421 patients) 1179
Zonalon Cream (Less than 1%) 1055

Skin, discoloration

AK-Fluor Injection 10% and 25% ⊙ 203
Anafranil Capsules (Infrequent) 803
Android Capsules, 10 mg 1250
Android 1251
Atretol Tablets 573
Azulfidine (Rare) 1949
Brevibloc Injection (Less than 1%) 1808
Compazine 2470
Cordarone Tablets (Less than 1%) 2712
Cytovene (1% or less) 2103
Delatestryl Injection 2860
Ergamisol Tablets (Up to 2%) 1292
Estrace Cream and Tablets 749
Estratest 2539
Fluorescite ⊙ 219
Foscavir Injection (Between 1% and 5%) 547
Halotestin Tablets 2614
INFeD (Iron Dextran Injection, USP) 2345
Intron A (Less than 5%) 2364
Lamictal Tablets (Rare) 1112
Lamprene Capsules (More than 1%) 828
Radical PC 1807
Lescol Capsules 2267
Luvox Tablets (Infrequent) 2544
Mevacor Tablets 1699
Minocin Oral Suspension 1385
Mycobutin Capsules (Less than 1%) 1957
Neurontin Capsules (Rare) 1922
Norvasc Tablets (Less than or equal to 0.1%) 1940
Oreton Methyl 1255
Ortho-Est 1869
Orudis Capsules (Less than 1%) 2766
Oruvail Capsules (Less than 1%) 2766
Oxandrin 2862
Parlodel 2281
Paxil Tablets (Rare) 2505
Permax Tablets (Infrequent) 575
Pravachol 765
Prostin E2 Suppository 2634
Prozac Pulvules & Liquid, Oral Solution (Rare) 919
Quadrinal Tablets 1350
Retin-A (tretinoin) Cream/Gel/Liquid 1889
Retrovir I.V. Infusion 1163
Rifater 1532
SSD (Infrequent) 1355
Silvadene Cream 1% (Infrequent) 1540
Sotradecol (Sodium Tetradecyl Sulfate Injection) 967
Stelazine 2514
Taxol 714
Tegretol Chewable Tablets 852
Tegretol Suspension 852
Tegretol Tablets 852
Temaril Tablets, Syrup and Spansule Extended-Release Capsules 483
Testoderm Testosterone Transdermal System 486
Ticlid Tablets 2156
Torecan 2245
Videx Tablets, Powder for Oral Solution, & Pediatric Powder for Oral Solution (Less than 1%) 720
Zocor Tablets 1775
Zoladex (1% or greater) 2858
Zoloft Tablets (Rare) 2217

Skin, dryness

▲ A/T/S 2% Acne Topical Gel and Solution (17 out of 90 patients) 1234
▲ Accutane Capsules (Up to 80%) 2076
Actigall Capsules 802
Anafranil Capsules (Up to 2%) 803
Ansaid Tablets (Less than 1%) 2579
Aquasol A Vitamin A Capsules, USP 534
Aristocort A 0.025% Cream (Infrequent) 1027
Aristocort A 0.1% Cream (Infrequent) 1029
Aristocort A 0.1% Ointment (Infrequent) 1030
Asacol Delayed-Release Tablets 1979
Atromid-S Capsules 2701
Bactroban Ointment (Less than 1%) 2470
Benzac 1045
Benzamycin Topical Gel (3 out of 153) 905
BuSpar (Infrequent) 737
Cardura Tablets (Less than 0.5% of 3960 patients) 2186
Claritin (2% or fewer patients) 2349
Claritin-D (Less frequent) 2350
▲ Cleocin T Topical (23%) 2590
Cognex Capsules (Infrequent) 1901
Cortifoam 2396
Cozaar Tablets (Less than 1%) 1628
Cytovene (1% or less) 2103
Depakote Tablets (Greater than 1% but not more than 5%) 415
Depo-Provera Contraceptive Injection (Fewer than 1%) 2602
Dermatop Emollient Cream 0.1% (Infrequent to frequent) 1238
DesOwen Cream, Ointment and Lotion (Less than 2%) 1046
▲ Desquam-E Gel (2 in 50 patients) 2684
▲ Desquam-X Gel (2 in 50 patients) 2684
▲ Desquam-X 10 Bar (2 in 50 patients) 2684
▲ Desquam-X Wash (2 in 50 patients) 2684
▲ Diprolene AF Cream (4%) 2352
▲ Diprolene Gel 0.05% (4%) 2353
▲ Diprolene (4%) 2352
Donnagel Liquid and Donnagel Chewable Tablets (Rare) ▣ 879
▲ Dovonex Ointment 0.005% (1% to 10%) 2684
Effexor (Infrequent) 2719
Elocon (Infrequent) 2354
Emcyt Capsules (2%) 1953
Emgel 2% Topical Gel (Occasional) 1093
Epifoam (Infrequent) 2399
Ergamisol Tablets 1292
Ethmozine Tablets (Less than 2%) 2041
Florone/Florone E 906
Fluorouracil Injection 2116
Foscavir Injection (Less than 1%) 547
Sterile FUDR (Remote possibility) 2118
Halog (Infrequent) 2686
Hivid Tablets (Less than 1% to less than 3%) 2121
Hytone 907
Hyzaar Tablets 1677
Imitrex Tablets (Rare) 1106
▲ Intron A (Up to 10%) 2364
Lac-Hydrin 12% Lotion (Less frequent) 2687
Lamictal Tablets (Infrequent) 1112
▲ Lamprene Capsules (8-28%) 828
Lescol Capsules 2267
Lomotil 2439
Lotrisone Cream (Infrequent) 2372
Lupron Depot 7.5 mg 2559
Lupron Injection (Less than 5%) 2555
Luvox Tablets (Infrequent) 2544
Metrodin (urofollitropin for injection) 2446
MetroGel 1047
Mevacor Tablets 1699
Mexitil Capsules (About 1 in 1,000) 678
Motofen Tablets 784
Mykrox Tablets (Less than 2%) 993
Myleran Tablets (Rare) 1143
NebuPent for Inhalation Solution (1% or less) 1040
Neurontin Capsules (Infrequent) 1922
Nicolar Tablets 2026
Nizoral 2% Shampoo (One occurrence in 41 patients) 1298
Norvasc Tablets (Less than or equal to 0.1%) 1940
pHisoHex 2327
Paxil Tablets (Infrequent) 2505
Pentasa (Less than 1%) 1527
Pepcid Injection (Infrequent) 1722
Pepcid (Infrequent) 1720
Permax Tablets (Infrequent) 575
Pravachol 765
Prilosec Delayed-Release Capsules (Less than 1%) 529
ProctoCream-HC 2.5% (Infrequent to frequent) 2408
ProctoFoam-HC 2409
▲ Proleukin for Injection (15%) 797
ProSom Tablets (Rare) 449
Prozac Pulvules & Liquid, Oral Solution (Infrequent) 919
Psorcon Ointment 0.05% 908
▲ Risperdal (2% to 4%) 1301
▲ Roferon-A Injection (5% to 13%) 2145
Rogaine Topical Solution 2637
Serzone Tablets (Infrequent) 771
▲ Tegison Capsules (50-75%) 2154
Ultravate Cream 0.05% (Less frequent) 2689
Ultravate Ointment 0.05% 2690
Varivax (Greater than or equal to 1%) 1762
Wellbutrin Tablets (Infrequent) 1204
Zocor Tablets 1775
Zoladex (1% or greater) 2858
Zoloft Tablets (Infrequent) 2217
▲ Zonalon Cream (Approximately 1% to 10%) 1055

Skin, eruptions

▲ Anaprox/Naprosyn (3% to 9%) 2117
Antabuse Tablets (Occasional) 2695
Aralen Hydrochloride Injection 2301
Azo Gantanol Tablets 2080
Bactrim DS Tablets 2084
Bactrim I.V. Infusion 2082
Bactrim 2084
Cardizem CD Capsules (Infrequent) 1506
Cosmegen Injection 1626
Daranide Tablets 1633
Depen Titratable Tablets (Rare) 2662
E.E.S. 424
Easprin 1914
▲ EC-Naprosyn Delayed-Release Tablets (3% to 9%) 2117
EryPed 200 & EryPed 400 Granules 421
Ery-Tab Tablets 422
Erythrocin Stearate Filmtab 425
Fansidar Tablets 2114
Floxin Tablets (200 mg, 300 mg, 400 mg) 1567
Gantanol Tablets 2119
Gantrisin 2120
Halotestin Tablets 2614
Ilotycin Gluceptate, IV, Vials 913
Imitrex Injection (Infrequent) 1103
Librax Capsules (Rare) 2176
Libritabs Tablets (Isolated cases) 2177
Librium Capsules (Isolated cases) 2178
Librium Injectable (Isolated instances) 2179
Mellaril (Infrequent) 2269
Micronase Tablets (1.5%) 2623
Milontin Kapseals 1920
Mysoline (Occasional) 2754
▲ Anaprox/Naprosyn (3% to 9%) 2117
Nydrazid Injection 508
PCE Dispertab Tablets 444
PASER Granules 1285
Pen•Vee K 2772
Phenobarbital Elixir and Tablets (Rare) 1469
Pima Syrup 1005
Plaquenil Sulfate Tablets 2328
Rifamate Capsules 1530
Seldane Tablets (1.0% to 1.6%) 1536
Septra 1174
Septra I.V. Infusion 1169
Septra I.V. Infusion ADD-Vantage Vials 1171
Septra 1174
Serevent Inhalation Aerosol (1% to 3%) 1176
Tessalon Perles 1020
Trasylol 613
Yodoxin 1230
Zyloprim Tablets (Less than 1%) 1226

Skin, erythema

Cleocin Vaginal Cream 2589
Dynacin Capsules (Rare) 1590
Emgel 2% Topical Gel (Occasional) 1093
Gastrocrom Capsules (Infrequent) 984
Maxaquin Tablets 2440
Minocin Intravenous 1382
Minocin Oral Suspension 1385
Minocin Pellet-Filled Capsules 1383
Monodox Capsules 1805
pHisoHex 2327
Paraflex Caplets 1580
Parafon Forte DSC Caplets 1581
Plaquenil Sulfate Tablets 2328
Terramycin Intramuscular Solution 2210
T.R.U.E. Test (Two to 27 reports) 1189
Vibramycin Hyclate Intravenous 2215

Skin, fluorescence

AK-Fluor Injection 10% and 25% ⊙ 203

Skin, fragile

▲ Accutane Capsules (Up to 80%) 2076
Dalalone D.P. Injectable 1011
Dexacort Phosphate in Respihaler 458
Dexacort Phosphate in Turbinaire 459
Florinef Acetate Tablets 505

Skin, fragility

Aristocort Suspension (Forte Parenteral) 1027

(▣ Described in PDR For Nonprescription Drugs) Incidence data in parenthesis; ▲ 3% or more (⊙ Described in PDR For Ophthalmology)

Aristocort Suspension (Intralesional) 1025
Aristocort Tablets 1022
Aristospan Suspension (Intra-articular) 1033
Aristospan Suspension (Intralesional) 1032
Celestone Soluspan Suspension 2347
CORTENEMA 2535
Cortone Acetate Sterile Suspension 1623
Cortone Acetate Tablets 1624
Cuprimine Capsules 1630
Decadron Elixir 1633
Decadron Phosphate Injection 1637
Decadron Phosphate Respihaler 1642
Decadron Phosphate Turbinaire 1645
Decadron Phosphate with Xylocaine Injection, Sterile 1639
Decadron Tablets 1635
Decadron-LA Sterile Suspension 1646
Deltasone Tablets 2595
Depen Titratable Tablets 2662
Depo-Medrol Single-Dose Vial 2600
Depo-Medrol Sterile Aqueous Suspension 2597
Hydeltrasol Injection, Sterile 1665
Hydeltra-T.B.A. Sterile Suspension 1667
Hydrocortone Acetate Sterile Suspension 1669
Hydrocortone Phosphate Injection, Sterile 1670
Hydrocortone Tablets 1672
Medrol 2621
Pediapred Oral Liquid 995
Prelone Syrup 1787
Solu-Cortef Sterile Powder 2641
Solu-Medrol Sterile Powder 2643
▲ Tegison Capsules (50-75%) 2154

Skin, hypertrophy

Anafranil Capsules (Rare) 803
Betaseron for SC Injection 658
▲ CellCept Capsules (More than or equal to 3%) 2099
Dilacor XR Extended-release Capsules (Infrequent) 2018
Effexor (Rare) 2719
Foscavir Injection (Less than 1%) 547
Prozac Pulvules & Liquid, Oral Solution (Rare) 919
Supprelin Injection (1% to 3%) 2056
Videx Tablets, Powder for Oral Solution, & Pediatric Powder for Oral Solution (Less than 1%) 720

Skin, infection

▲ Accutane Capsules (Approximately 1 patient in 20 patients) 2076
▲ Neoral (7.0%) 2276
Prinivil Tablets (0.3% to 1.0%) 1733
Prinzide Tablets 1737
Pronto Lice Killing Shampoo & Conditioner in One Kit ▣ 653
▲ Sandimmune (7.0 to 10.1%) 2286
Zestoretic 2850
Zestril Tablets (0.3% to 1.0%) 2854

Skin, irritation

Betadine Solution 1992
Betadine Surgical Scrub (Rare) 1992
Blocadren Tablets 1614
Compazine 2470
Cortisporin Cream 1084
Cortisporin Ointment 1085
Diprolene (1%) 2352
▲ Dovonex Ointment 0.005% (Approximately 10% to 15%) 2684
Drithocreme 0.1%, 0.25%, 0.5%, 1.0% (HP) 905
Dritho-Scalp 0.25%, 0.5% (More frequent) 906
Elocon (Infrequent) 2354
Epifoam (Infrequent) 2399
Halog (Infrequent) 2686
Lotrimin 2371
Lotrisone Cream 2372
MG 217 ▣ 835
Mantadil Cream 1135
MetroGel 1047
Occlusal-HP 1054
Orap Tablets 1050
P&S Liquid ▣ 604
Panafil Ointment (Occasional) 2246
Panafil-White Ointment (Occasional) 2247
ProctoFoam-HC 2409
Pronto Lice Killing Shampoo & Conditioner in One Kit ▣ 653
Questran Light (Less frequent) 769
Questran Powder (Less frequent) 770
SalAc 1055
Selsun Rx 2.5% Selenium Sulfide Lotion, USP 2225
Sportscreme External Analgesic Rub Cream & Lotion ▣ 834
Stelazine 2514
▲ Tegison Capsules (50-75%) 2154
Timolide Tablets 1748
Timoptic in Ocudose 1753
Timoptic Sterile Ophthalmic Solution 1751
Timoptic-XE 1755
Tolectin (200, 400 and 600 mg) (1 to 3%) 1581
Topical Analgesic Ointment ▣ 835
Ultra Mide 25 Extra Strength Moisturizer ▣ 605
Vascor (200, 300 and 400 mg) Tablets (0.5 to 2.0%) 1587
Xerac AC 1933
Ziac 1415

Skin, lesions

Hivid Tablets (Less than 1% to less than 3%) 2121
Lupron Injection (Less than 5%) 2555
Prinivil Tablets (0.3% to 1.0%) 1733
Prinzide Tablets 1737
Procan SR Tablets (Common) 1926
Zestoretic 2850

Skin, maceration

Aclovate Cream 1069
Analpram-HC Rectal Cream 1% and 2.5% 977
Anusol-HC Cream 2.5% (Infrequent to frequent) 1896
Aristocort A 0.025% Cream (Infrequent) 1027
Aristocort A 0.5% Cream 1031
Aristocort A 0.1% Cream (Infrequent) 1029
Aristocort A 0.1% Ointment (Infrequent) 1030
Carmol HC (Infrequent to frequent) 924
▲ Cordran Lotion (More frequent) 1803
▲ Cordran Tape (More frequent) 1804
Cortisporin Cream 1084
Cortisporin Ointment 1085
Decadron Phosphate Topical Cream 1644
Decaspray Topical Aerosol 1648
Diprolene (Less than 1%) 2352
Elocon (Infrequent) 2354
Epifoam (Infrequent) 2399
Florone/Florone E 906
Halog (Infrequent) 2686
Hytone 907
Lidex (Infrequent) 2130
Lotrisone Cream (Infrequent) 2372
Monistat Dual-Pak 1850
NeoDecadron Topical Cream 1714
Pramosone Cream, Lotion & Ointment 978
ProctoCream-HC 2.5% (Infrequent to frequent) 2408
ProctoFoam-HC 2409
Psorcon Ointment 0.05% 908
Synalar (Infrequent) 2130
Temovate (Infrequent) 1179
Topicort (Infrequent) 1243
Tridesilon Cream 0.05% (Infrequent) 615
Tridesilon Ointment 0.05% (Infrequent) 616
Westcort 2690

Skin, nodule

Imdur (Less than or equal to 5%) 1323
Imitrex Tablets (Rare) 1106
Lescol Capsules 2267
Lotrel Capsules 840
Mevacor Tablets 1699
Neurontin Capsules (Rare) 1922
Permax Tablets (Rare) 575
Pravachol 765
Zocor Tablets 1775

Skin, oiliness

▲ Cleocin T Topical (18%) 2590
Cleocin Vaginal Cream 2589
Emgel 2% Topical Gel (Occasional) 1093
Propulsid (Less than 1%) 1300
ReVia Tablets (Less than 1%) 940

Skin, photoallergic reactions

Feldene Capsules (Less than 1%) 1965
IBU Tablets (Less than 1%) 1342

Skin, phototoxic eruptions

Proloprim Tablets 1155
Trimpex Tablets 2163

Skin, tenderness

A/T/S 2% Acne Topical Gel and Solution 1234
▲ Blenoxane (50%) 692
Efudex 2113
Emgel 2% Topical Gel 1093
Imitrex Injection (Rare) 1103
Imitrex Tablets (Infrequent) 1106
Naftin Gel 1% (0.5%) 481

Skin, wrinkling

Depen Titratable Tablets 2662
Imitrex Tablets (Rare) 1106

Skin atrophy

Aclovate 1069
Analpram-HC Rectal Cream 1% and 2.5% 977
Aristocort A 0.025% Cream (Infrequent) 1027
Aristocort A 0.5% Cream 1031
Aristocort A 0.1% Cream (Infrequent) 1029
Aristocort A 0.1% Ointment (Infrequent) 1030
Carmol HC (Infrequent to frequent) 924
Cortisporin Cream 1084
Cortisporin Ointment 1085
Cortisporin Otic Solution Sterile 1087
Cortisporin Otic Suspension Sterile 1088
Cutivate Cream 1088
Cutivate Ointment (Infrequent to more frequent) 1089
Cyclocort Topical (Infrequent) 1037
Decadron Phosphate Topical Cream 1644
Decaspray Topical Aerosol 1648
Dermatop Emollient Cream 0.1% (1%) 1238
DesOwen Cream, Ointment and Lotion (Infrequent) 1046
Diprolene AF Cream (Less than 1%) 2352
Diprolene Gel 0.05% (Less frequent) 2353
Diprolene (Less than 1%) 2352
Dovonex Ointment 0.005% (Less than 1%) 2684
Effexor (Rare) 2719
Elocon (3 of 319 patients) 2354
Epifoam (Infrequent) 2399
Etrafon 2-10 Tablets (2-10) 2355
Florone/Florone E 906
Halog (Infrequent) 2686
Hytone 907
Lidex (Infrequent) 2130
Locoid Cream, Ointment and Topical Solution (Infrequent) 978
Lotrisone Cream (Infrequent) 2372
Mantadil Cream 1135
NeoDecadron Topical Cream 1714
PediOtic Suspension Sterile 1153
Pramosone Cream, Lotion & Ointment 978
ProctoCream-HC (Infrequent) 2408
ProctoCream-HC 2.5% (Infrequent to frequent) 2408
ProctoFoam-HC 2409
Psorcon Ointment 0.05% 908
Synalar (Infrequent) 2130
Tegison Capsules (Less than 1%) 2154
Temovate (1 of 421 patients; infrequent) 1179
Topicort (Infrequent) 1243
Tridesilon Cream 0.05% (Infrequent) 615
Tridesilon Ointment 0.05% (Infrequent) 616
Ultravate Cream 0.05% (Less frequent) 2689
Ultravate Ointment 0.05% 2690
Westcort 2690

Skin eruptions, pleomorphic

Aralen Phosphate Tablets 2301

Skin odor, abnormal

Anafranil Capsules (Up to 2%) 803
Zoloft Tablets (Rare) 2217

Skin reactions

Atgam Sterile Solution (Most patients) 2581
▲ Catapres-TTS (51 of 101 patients) 675
Cefobid Intravenous/Intramuscular (1 in 45) 2189
Cefobid Pharmacy Bulk Package - Not for Direct Infusion (1 in 45) 2192
Compazine 2470
Cortisporin Ophthalmic Ointment Sterile 1085
Cortisporin Otic Suspension Sterile (Occasional) 1088
▲ DHCplus Capsules (Among most frequent) 1993
Doxorubicin Astra 540
▲ Epogen for Injection (7% to 10%) 489
Exelderm Cream 1.0% (Infrequent) 2685
Exelderm Solution 1.0% (Infrequent) 2686
Floxin Tablets (200 mg, 300 mg, 400 mg) 1567
Foscavir Injection (Less than 1%) 547
Hivid Tablets (Less than 1% to less than 3%) 2121
Lanoxicaps (Rare) 1117
Lanoxin Elixir Pediatric (Rare) 1120
Lanoxin Injection (Rare) 1123
Lanoxin Injection Pediatric (Rare) 1126
Lanoxin Tablets (Rare) 1128
Lupron Depot 3.75 mg (Less than 5%) 2556
Lupron Depot 7.5 mg (Less than 5%) 2559
Lupron Injection (Less than 5%) 2555
Maxaquin Tablets (Less than 1%) 2440
Megace Oral Suspension (1% to 3%) 699
▲ Nolvadex Tablets (18.7%) 2841
ParaGard T380A Intrauterine Copper Contraceptive 1880
Prilosec Delayed-Release Capsules (Very rare) 529
Primaxin I.M. 1727
Primaxin I.V. (Less than 0.2%) 1729
Prinivil Tablets (Rare) 1733
Prinzide Tablets 1737
▲ Procrit for Injection (7% to 10%) 1841
▲ Prograf (Greater than 3%) 1042
Rifadin 1528
Rifater 1532
Romazicon (1% to 3%) 2147
Septra I.V. Infusion 1169
Streptomycin Sulfate Injection 2208
▲ Supprelin Injection (45%) 2056
Taxol 714
Tegison Capsules (Less than 1%) 2154
▲ Ultrase MT Capsules (Among most frequent) 2344
Videx Tablets, Powder for Oral Solution, & Pediatric Powder for Oral Solution (Less than 1% to 13%) 720
Zestoretic (Rare) 2850
Zestril Tablets 2854
Zinecard (1%) 1961

Skin test reactions, suppression

Aristocort Suspension (Forte Parenteral) 1027
Aristocort Suspension (Intralesional) 1025
Aristocort Tablets 1022
Aristospan Suspension (Intra-articular) 1033
Aristospan Suspension (Intralesional) 1032
Celestone Soluspan Suspension 2347
CORTENEMA 2535
Cortone Acetate Sterile Suspension 1623
Cortone Acetate Tablets 1624
Dalalone D.P. Injectable 1011
Decadron Elixir 1633
Decadron Phosphate Injection 1637
Decadron Phosphate Respihaler 1642
Decadron Phosphate Turbinaire 1645
Decadron Phosphate with Xylocaine Injection, Sterile 1639
Decadron Tablets 1635
Decadron-LA Sterile Suspension 1646
Deltasone Tablets 2595
Depo-Medrol Single-Dose Vial 2600
Depo-Medrol Sterile Aqueous Suspension 2597
Dexacort Phosphate in Respihaler 458
Dexacort Phosphate in Turbinaire 459
Florinef Acetate Tablets 505
Hydeltrasol Injection, Sterile 1665
Hydeltra-T.B.A. Sterile Suspension 1667
Hydrocortone Acetate Sterile Suspension 1669
Hydrocortone Phosphate Injection, Sterile 1670

(▣ Described in PDR For Nonprescription Drugs) Incidence data in parenthesis; ▲ 3% or more (◉ Described in PDR For Ophthalmology)

Skin test reactions, suppression Side Effects Index 1414

Hydrocortone Tablets 1672
Medrol 2621
Pediapred Oral Liquid 995
Prelone Syrup 1787
Solu-Cortef Sterile Powder 2641
Solu-Medrol Sterile Powder 2643
T.R.U.E. Test (Up to 2 reports) 1189

Skull abnormalities, fetal

Accupril Tablets 1893
Accutane Capsules 2076
Altace Capsules 1232
Capoten 739
Capozide 742
Cozaar Tablets 1628
Hyzaar Tablets 1677
Lotensin Tablets 834
Lotensin HCT 837
Lotrel Capsules 840
Monopril Tablets 757
Prinivil Tablets 1733
Prinzide Tablets 1737
Univasc Tablets 2410
Vaseretic Tablets 1765
Vasotec I.V. 1768
Vasotec Tablets 1771
Zestoretic 2850
Zestril Tablets 2854

Sleep, disturbances

Actigall Capsules 802
Adalat Capsules (10 mg and 20 mg) (2% or less) 587
Adalat CC (Rare) 589
Ambien Tablets (Infrequent; 1%) 2416
▲ Anafranil Capsules (4% to 9%) 803
Ativan Tablets (Less frequent) 2700
▲ Betapace Tablets (1% to 8%) 641
▲ Clozaril Tablets (4%) 2252
Cordarone Tablets (1 to 3%) 2712
Cozaar Tablets (Less than 1%) 1628
Dalgan Injection (Less than 1%) 538
Danocrine Capsules 2307
Daypro Caplets (Greater than 1% but less than 3%) 2426
Deconsal C Expectorant Syrup 456
Deconsal Pediatric Syrup 457
Dizac (Less frequent) 1809
Doral Tablets (Rare) 2664
Effexor (Infrequent) 2719
Elavil 2838
Eldepryl Tablets 2550
Endep Tablets 2174
▲ Ethmozine Tablets (2% to 5%) 2041
Floxin I.V. (1% to 3%) 1571
Floxin Tablets (200 mg, 300 mg, 400 mg) (1% to 3%) 1567
Fludara for Injection (1% to 3%) 663
Foscavir Injection (Less than 1%) 547
Halcion Tablets 2611
HibTITER 1375
Hylorel Tablets (2.1%) 985
Hyzaar Tablets 1677
Imitrex Injection (Rare) 1103
Imitrex Tablets (Rare to infrequent) 1106
Lamictal Tablets (1.4%) 1112
Lithium Carbonate Capsules & Tablets 2230
Lopressor 830
Lupron Depot 3.75 mg (Less than 5%) 2556
Lupron Depot 7.5 mg 2559
▲ Lupron Injection (5% or more) 2555
Luvox Tablets (Infrequent) 2544
▲ Mexitil Capsules (7.1% to 7.5%) 678
Monopril Tablets (0.2% to 1.0%) 757
Nardil (Common) 1920
Noroxin Tablets (Less frequent) 1715
Noroxin Tablets (Less frequent) 2048
Parlodel (Less than 1%) 2281
Procardia Capsules (2% or less) 1971
ProSom Tablets (Infrequent) 449
Proventil Syrup (Less than 1 of 100 patients) 2385
▲ Prozac Pulvules & Liquid, Oral Solution (3%) 919
Recombivax HB (Less than 1%) 1744
▲ ReVia Tablets (More than 10%) 940
Risperdal (Frequent) 1301
▲ Roferon-A Injection (5%) 2145
Sinemet CR Tablets 944
▲ Tetramune (Up to 28%) 1404
Tofranil Tablets 856
Tonocard Tablets (Less than 1%) 531
Triavil Tablets 1757
Trinalin Repetabs Tablets 1330
Ultram Tablets (50 mg) (1% to 5%) 1585
Univasc Tablets (Less than 1%) 2410
Valium Tablets 2183
Varivax (Greater than or equal to 1%) 1762
Ventolin Syrup (Less than 1 of 100 patients) 1202
Verelan Capsules (1.4%) 1410
Verelan Capsules (1.4%) 2824
Versed Injection (Less than 1%) 2170
Videx Tablets, Powder for Oral Solution, & Pediatric Powder for Oral Solution (Less than 1%) 720
Vontrol Tablets 2532
▲ Wellbutrin Tablets (4.0%) 1204
Xanax Tablets (Rare) 2649
Zarontin Capsules 1928
Zarontin Syrup 1929
Ziac 1415

Sleepiness (see under Drowsiness)

Sleeplessness (see under Insomnia)

Sloughing

Aramine Injection 1609
Depo-Medrol Single-Dose Vial 2600
Depo-Medrol Sterile Aqueous Suspension 2597
Dilantin Parenteral 1910
Efudex 2113
Fluoracaine (Rare) .... ⊙ 206
Fluorescite .... ⊙ 219
Fluorouracil Injection (Common) 2116
FLURESS (Rare) .... ⊙ 207
Gamimune N, 5% Immune Globulin Intravenous (Human), 5% (One patient) 619
Gamimune N, 10% Immune Globulin Intravenous (Human), 10% (One patient) 621
MSTA Mumps Skin Test Antigen 890
Norplant System 2759
Ophthetic .... ⊙ 247
Pentam 300 Injection (Some instances) 1041
Robaxin Injectable 2070
Scleromate 1891
Sotradecol (Sodium Tetradecyl Sulfate Injection) 967
Talwin Injection 2334
Velban Vials 1484

Sluggishness

Esgic-plus Tablets (Infrequent) 1013
Fioricet Tablets (Infrequent) 2258
Fioricet with Codeine Capsules (Infrequent) 2260
Fiorinal with Codeine Capsules (Infrequent) 2262
Parlodel Capsules (Less than 1%) 2281
Phrenilin (Infrequent) 785
Sedapap Tablets 50 mg/650 mg (Infrequent) 1543

Smell, disturbances

BuSpar (Infrequent) 737
Ceredase 1065
Cordarone Tablets (1 to 3%) 2712
Ergamisol Tablets (1%) 1292
Floxin I.V. 1571
Floxin Tablets (200 mg, 300 mg, 400 mg) 1567
Imitrex Injection (Rare) 1103
Imitrex Tablets (Infrequent) 1106
Lorelco Tablets 1517
Maxair Autohaler (0.6%) 1492
Maxair Inhaler (Less than 1%) 1494
Nasalide Nasal Solution 0.025% (5% or less) 2110
NebuPent for Inhalation Solution (1% or less) 1040
Rhinocort Nasal Inhaler (Less than 1%) 556
Rythmol Tablets–150mg, 225mg, 300mg (Less than 1%) 1352
Timentin for Injection 2528
Tonocard Tablets (Less than 1%) 531
Tornalate Solution for Inhalation, 0.2% 956
Tornalate Metered Dose Inhaler 957

Smell, loss of the sense (see under Anosmia)

Smoker's tongue (see under Leukoplakia, oral)

Sneezing

▲ AeroBid Inhaler System (3-9%) 1005
▲ Aerobid-M Inhaler System (3-9%) 1005
Afrin .... ▣ 797
Alomide (Less than 1%) 469
Azactam for Injection (Less than 1%) 734
▲ Beconase (4%) 1076
Bentyl 1501
Carbocaine Hydrochloride Injection 2303
Claritin (2% or fewer patients) 2349
Claritin-D (Less frequent) 2350
Clozaril Tablets (Less than 1%) 2252
Diprivan Injection (Less than 1%) 2833
Duration 12 Hour Nasal Spray .... ▣ 805
4-Way Fast Acting Nasal Spray (regular & mentholated) .... ▣ 621
4-Way Long Lasting Nasal Spray .... ▣ 621
Flonase Nasal Spray (Less than 1%) 1098
Hespan Injection 929
Intal Inhaler (Rare) 988
Intal Nebulizer Solution (Rare) 989
Intron A (Less than 5%) 2364
Marcaine Hydrochloride with Epinephrine 1:200,000 (Rare) 2316
Marcaine Hydrochloride Injection (Rare) 2316
Marcaine Spinal (Rare) 2319
Methadone Hydrochloride Oral Concentrate 2233
Nasacort Nasal Inhaler (Fewer than 5%) 2024
▲ Nasalcrom Nasal Solution (1 in 10) 994
Nasalide Nasal Solution 0.025% (5% or less) 2110
Neo-Synephrine Maximum Strength 12 Hour Nasal Spray .... ▣ 726
Neo-Synephrine 12 Hour .... ▣ 726
Neo-Synephrine .... ▣ 726
Nescaine/Nescaine MPF 554
Orlamm 2239
Plendil Extended-Release Tablets (Up to 1.6%) 527
Quadrinal Tablets 1350
ReVia Tablets (Less than 1%) 940
Rhinocort Nasal Inhaler (Less than 1%) 556
Sensorcaine (Rare) 559
Surgicel (Occasional) 1314
Vancenase AQ Nasal Spray 0.042% 2393
▲ Vancenase PocketHaler Nasal Inhaler (10 per 100 patients) 2391
Vicks Sinex Nasal Spray and Ultra Fine Mist .... ▣ 765

Social reaction, anti See Sociopathy (see under Sociopathy)

Sociopathy

BuSpar (Infrequent) 737
Neurontin Capsules (Rare) 1922
Paxil Tablets (Rare) 2505
Prozac Pulvules & Liquid, Oral Solution (Rare) 919

Sodium depletion (see under Hyponatremia)

Sodium loss (see under Hyponatremia)

Sodium retention

Android 1251
Aristocort Suspension (Forte Parenteral) 1027
Aristocort Suspension (Intralesional) 1025
Aristocort Tablets 1022
Aristospan Suspension (Intra-articular) 1033
Aristospan Suspension (Intralesional) 1032
Celestone Soluspan Suspension 2347
CORTENEMA 2535
Cortone Acetate Sterile Suspension 1623
Cortone Acetate Tablets 1624
Dalalone D.P. Injectable 1011
Decadron Elixir 1633
Decadron Phosphate Injection 1637
Decadron Phosphate Respihaler 1642
Decadron Phosphate Turbinaire 1645
Decadron Phosphate with Xylocaine Injection, Sterile 1639
Decadron Tablets 1635
Decadron-LA Sterile Suspension 1646
Delatestryl Injection 2860
Deltasone Tablets 2595
Depo-Medrol Sterile Aqueous Suspension 2597
Dexacort Phosphate in Respihaler 458
Dexacort Phosphate in Turbinaire 459
▲ Estratest (Among most common) 2539
Florinef Acetate Tablets 505
Halotestin Tablets 2614
Hydeltrasol Injection, Sterile 1665
Hydeltra-T.B.A. Sterile Suspension 1667
Hydrocortone Acetate Sterile Suspension 1669
Hydrocortone Phosphate Injection, Sterile 1670
Hydrocortone Tablets 1672
Hyperstat I.V. Injection 2363
Kayexalate 2314
Loniten Tablets 2618
Medrol 2621
Oxandrin 2862
Pediapred Oral Liquid 995
Prelone Syrup 1787
Premarin with Methyltestosterone 2794
Proglycem (Frequent) 580
Sodium Polystyrene Sulfonate Suspension 2244
Solu-Cortef Sterile Powder 2641
Solu-Medrol Sterile Powder 2643
Testred Capsules 1262
Winstrol Tablets 2337

Somnambulism

Ambien Tablets (Rare) 2416
Anafranil Capsules (Infrequent) 803
Halcion Tablets 2611
Zoloft Tablets (Rare) 2217

Somnolence (see under Drowsiness)

Soreness, injection site

▲ Engerix-B Unit-Dose Vials (22%) 2482
▲ Havrix (56% of adults; 15% of children) 2489
Hyperab Rabies Immune Globulin (Human) 624
Hyper-Tet Tetanus Immune Globulin (Human) 627
HypRho-D Full Dose Rho (D) Immune Globulin (Human) 629
HypRho-D Mini-Dose Rho (D) Immune Globulin (Human) 628
Imogam Rabies Immune Globulin (Human) (Uncommon) 880
INFeD (Iron Dextran Injection, USP) 2345
▲ Influenza Virus Vaccine, Trivalent, Types A and B (chromatograph- and filter-purified subviron antigen) FluShield, 1995-1996 Formula (Most frequent) 2736
▲ JE-VAX (5.9% to 24.5%) 886
▲ Pneumovax 23 (Common) 1725
▲ Typhim Vi (13%) 899
▲ Varivax (19.3% to 32.5%) 1762

Soreness, vaginal

Femstat Prefill Vaginal Cream 2% (0.2%) 2116
Femstat Vaginal Cream 2% (0.2%) 2115
Mycelex-G 500 mg Vaginal Tablets (1 in 149 patients) 609

Sore throat (see under Throat, soreness)

Spasm, biliary tract

Brontex 1981
Demerol 2308
Dilaudid-HP Injection (Less frequent) 1337
Dilaudid-HP Lyophilized Powder 250 mg (Less frequent) 1337
Dilaudid Tablets and Liquid 1339
MS Contin Tablets (Less frequent) 1994
MSIR (Infrequent) 1997
Methadone Hydrochloride Oral Solution & Tablets 2235
Oramorph SR (Morphine Sulfate Sustained Release Tablets) (Less frequent) 2236
Phenergan with Codeine 2777
Phenergan VC with Codeine 2781
RMS Suppositories 2657
Roxanol 2243
Trilafon 2389

Spasm, gastrointestinal

Fioricet with Codeine Capsules 2260
Fiorinal with Codeine Capsules 2262
Methadone Hydrochloride Oral Concentrate 2233

Spasm, generalized

Anafranil Capsules (Rare) 803

(▣ Described in PDR For Nonprescription Drugs) Incidence data in parenthesis; ▲ 3% or more (⊙ Described in PDR For Ophthalmology)

1415 Side Effects Index Stevens-Johnson syndrome

Foscavir Injection (Between 1% and 5%) 547
Luvox Tablets (Infrequent) 2544
Prinzide Tablets 1737
▲Prograf (Greater than 3%) 1042
Zestoretic 2850
Zestril Tablets (0.3% to 1.0%) 2854

Spasm, vesical sphincters

Anexsia 5/500 Elixir 1781
Anexia Tablets 1782
Lorcet 10/650 1018
Lortab 2566
Tussend 1783
Tussionex Pennkinetic Extended-Release Suspension 998
Vicodin ES Tablets 1357
Vicodin Tuss Expectorant 1358
Zydone Capsules 949

Spatial disorientation

Serophene (clomiphene citrate tablets, USP) 2451

Speech, bulbar type

Reglan 2068

Speech, incoherent

Clozaril Tablets (Less than 1%) 2252
Marcaine Spinal 2319
Sensorcaine 559

Speech, slurring

BuSpar (Rare) 737
Clozaril Tablets (1%) 2252
Coly-Mycin M Parenteral 1905
Dalgan Injection (Less than 1%) 538
Dalmane Capsules (Rare) 2173
▲Dilantin Infatabs (Among most common) 1908
▲Dilantin Kapseals (Among most common) 1906
▲Dilantin Parenteral (Among most common) 1910
▲Dilantin-125 Suspension (Among most common) 1911
Dizac (Less frequent) 1809
Doral Tablets 2664
Eskalith 2485
Etrafon 2355
Fioricet with Codeine Capsules 2260
Fiorinal with Codeine Capsules 2262
Halcion Tablets 2611
Klonopin Tablets 2126
Levoprome (Sometimes) 1274
Lioresal Intrathecal (Up to 6 of 214 patients) 1596
Lioresal Tablets 829
Lithium Carbonate Capsules & Tablets 2230
Lithonate/Lithotabs/Lithobid 2543
Loxitane 1378
Luvox Tablets (Rare) 2544
Matulane Capsules 2131
Mebaral Tablets 2322
Miltown Tablets 2672
PMB 200 and PMB 400 2783
Placidyl Capsules 448
Serax Capsules 2810
Serax Tablets 2810
Serentil 684
Symmetrel Capsules and Syrup (0.1% to 1%) 946
Tonocard Tablets (Less than 1%) 531
Tranxene 451
Trilafon 2389
Valium Injectable 2182
Valium Tablets (Infrequent) 2183
Valrelease Capsules (Occasional) 2169
Versed Injection (Less than 1%) 2170
Xanax Tablets 2649

Speech difficulties

Clozaril Tablets (Less than 1%) 2252
▲Demser Capsules (10%) 1649
Ethmozine Tablets (Less than 2%) 2041
Marinol (Dronabinol) Capsules (Less than 1%) 2231
Mexitil Capsules (2.6%) 678
Nubain Injection (1% or less) 935
Stadol (Less than 1%) 775

Speech disturbances

Anafranil Capsules (Up to 3%) 803
Atretol Tablets 573
Bentyl 1501
▲Betaseron for SC Injection (3%) 658
Brevibloc Injection (Less than 1%) 1808
Dantrium Capsules (Less frequent) 1982
Demulen 2428
Desyrel and Desyrel Dividose 503
Doral Tablets 2664
Duragesic Transdermal System (1% or greater) 1288
Effexor (Infrequent) 2719
Eldepryl Tablets 2550
Ergamisol Tablets 1292
Estrace Cream and Tablets 749
Foscavir Injection (Less than 1%) 547
Hivid Tablets (Less than 1% to less than 3%) 2121
Intron A (Less than 5%) 2364
Kerlone Tablets (Less than 2%) 2436
Lamictal Tablets (2.5%) 1112
Levbid Extended-Release Tablets 2405
Levlen/Tri-Levlen 651
Levsin/Levsinex/Levbid 2405
Micronor Tablets 1872
Modicon 1872
▲Orap Tablets (2 of 20 patients) 1050
Ortho-Cyclen/Ortho-Tri-Cyclen 1858
Ortho-Est 1869
Ortho-Novum 1872
Ortho-Cyclen/Ortho Tri-Cyclen 1858
Permax Tablets (1.1%) 575
▲Proleukin for Injection (7%) 797
Romazicon (Less than 1%) 2147
Rythmol Tablets–150mg, 225mg, 300mg (Less than 1%) 1352
Salagen Tablets (Less than 1%) 1489
Tambocor Tablets (Less than 1%) 1497
Tegretol Chewable Tablets 852
Tegretol Suspension 852
Tegretol Tablets 852
Tonocard Tablets (Less than 1%) 531
Levlen/Tri-Levlen 651
Videx Tablets, Powder for Oral Solution, & Pediatric Powder for Oral Solution (Less than 1%) 720

Spermatogenesis, changes

Cytovene-IV (One report) 2103
Danocrine Capsules 2307
Thioplex (Thiotepa For Injection) 1281

Spermatogenesis, defective

Methotrexate Sodium Tablets, Injection, for Injection and LPF Injection 1275
Mustargen 1709

Spermatogenesis, inhibition

Cytovene-IV 2103
Cytoxan 694

Spermatozoa, changes

Dexacort Phosphate in Respihaler 458
Dexacort Phosphate in Turbinaire 459

Spinal block

Carbocaine Hydrochloride Injection 2303
Duranest Injections 542
Marcaine Hydrochloride with Epinephrine 1:200,000 2316
Marcaine Hydrochloride Injection 2316
Marcaine Spinal 2319
Nescaine/Nescaine MPF 554
Novocain Hydrochloride for Spinal Anesthesia 2326
Sensorcaine 559
Xylocaine Injections 567

Spinal cord, compression

Gelfoam Sterile Sponge 2608
Zoladex 2858

Spinal fluid proteins, elevation

Temaril Tablets, Syrup and Spansule Extended-Release Capsules 483

Spinal fracture

Lupron Depot 3.75 mg 2556
Lupron Depot 7.5 mg 2559
Lupron Injection 2555

Spinal stenosis

Gelfoam Sterile Sponge 2608

Splenic infarction

Lamprene Capsules (Less than 1%) 828

Splenomegaly

Apresazide Capsules (Less frequent) 808
Apresoline Hydrochloride Tablets (Less frequent) 809
Betaseron for SC Injection 658
Garamycin Injectable 2360
NebuPent for Inhalation Solution (1% or less) 1040
▲Neupogen for Injection (Approximately 30%) 495
Orthoclone OKT3 Sterile Solution 1837
Permax Tablets (Rare) 575
RhoGAM $Rh_0(D)$ Immune Globulin (Human) (One patient) 1847
Ser-Ap-Es Tablets 849

Spotting

Amen Tablets 780
Aygestin Tablets 974
Brevicon 2088
BuSpar (Infrequent) 737
Climara Transdermal System 645
Clomid (1.3%) 1514
Cycrin Tablets 975
Cytotec (0.7%) 2424
Danocrine Capsules 2307
Demulen 2428
Depo-Provera Contraceptive Injection 2602
Depo-Provera Sterile Aqueous Suspension 2606
Desogen Tablets 1817
Estrace Cream and Tablets 749
Estraderm Transdermal System 824
ESTRATAB Tablets (0.3, 0.625, 1.25, 2.5 mg) 2536
Estratest 2539
Levlen/Tri-Levlen 651
Lippes Loop Intrauterine Double-S 1848
Lo/Ovral Tablets 2746
Lo/Ovral-28 Tablets 2751
Lupron Depot-PED 7.5 mg, 11.25 mg and 15 mg 2560
Menest Tablets 2494
Micronor Tablets 1872
Modicon 1872
Nordette-21 Tablets 2755
Nordette-28 Tablets 2758
Norinyl 2088
▲Norplant System (17.1%) 2759
Nor-Q D Tablets 2135
Ogen Tablets 2627
Ogen Vaginal Cream 2630
Ortho-Cept 1851
Ortho-Cyclen/Ortho-Tri-Cyclen 1858
Ortho-Est 1869
Ortho-Novum 1872
Ortho-Cyclen/Ortho Tri-Cyclen 1858
Ovcon (Sometimes) 760
Ovral Tablets 2770
Ovral-28 Tablets 2770
Ovrette Tablets 2771
PMB 200 and PMB 400 2783
ParaGard T380A Intrauterine Copper Contraceptive 1880
Premarin Intravenous 2787
Premarin with Methyltestosterone 2794
Premarin Tablets 2789
Premarin Vaginal Cream 2791
Premphase 2797
Prempro 2801
Provera Tablets 2636
Levlen/Tri-Levlen 651
Tri-Norinyl 2164
Triphasil-21 Tablets 2814
Triphasil-28 Tablets 2819
Verelan Capsules (1% or less) 1410
Verelan Capsules (1% or less) 2824

Sputum, discoloration

Lamprene Capsules (Greater than 1%) 828
Rifadin 1528
Rifater 1532

Sputum, increase

▲AeroBid Inhaler System (3-9%) 1005
▲Aerobid-M Inhaler System (3-9%) 1005
Airet Solution for Inhalation (1.5%) 452
Anafranil Capsules (Infrequent) 803
Atrovent Inhalation Solution (1.4%) 673
Claritin-D (Less frequent) 2350
Effexor (Rare) 2719
Imdur (Less than or equal to 5%) 1323
Maxaquin Tablets (Less than 1%) 2440
Paxil Tablets (Rare) 2505
Proventil Inhalation Solution 0.083% (1.5%) 2384
Proventil Solution for Inhalation 0.5% (1.5%) 2383
Pulmozyme Inhalation 1064
Risperdal (Rare) 1301
Salagen Tablets (Less than 1%) 1489
Tegison Capsules (Less than 1%) 2154
Tilade (1.7%) 996
Tornalate Solution for Inhalation, 0.2% (Less than 1%) 956
Ventolin Inhalation Solution (1.5%) 1198
Ventolin Nebules Inhalation Solution (1.5%) 1199

Status epilepticus

Atretol Tablets 573
Clozaril Tablets 2252
Depakene 413
Dilantin-125 Suspension 1911
Diphtheria and Tetanus Toxoids and Pertussis Vaccine Adsorbed USP (For Pediatric Use) 875
Felbatol 2666
Hivid Tablets (Less than 1% to less than 3%) 2121
Oncaspar 2028
Tegretol Chewable Tablets 852
Tegretol Suspension 852
Tegretol Tablets 852
Xanax Tablets 2649

Steatorrhea

Imuran (Less than 1%) 1110
Questran Light (Less frequent) 769
Questran Powder (Less frequent) 770

Steatosis, hepatic

Hivid Tablets 2121
Retrovir Capsules 1158
Retrovir I.V. Infusion (Rare) 1163
Retrovir Syrup 1158

Steatosis, microvesicular

Orudis Capsules (Rare) 2766
Oruvail Capsules (Rare) 2766

Stenosis, subglottic

Survanta Beractant Intratracheal Suspension 2226

Stevens-Johnson syndrome

Children's Advil Suspension (Less than 1%) 2692
AK-CIDE (Some instances) ◎ 202
AK-CIDE Ointment (Some instances) ◎ 202
Aldoclor Tablets 1598
Aldoril Tablets 1604
Amoxil 2464
Anaprox/Naprosyn (Less than 1%) 2117
Ancef Injection 2465
Apresazide Capsules 808
Atretol Tablets (Extremely rare) 573
Augmentin (Rare) 2468
Azo Gantanol Tablets 2080
Azo Gantrisin Tablets 2081
Azulfidine (Rare) 1949
Bactrim DS Tablets (Rare) 2084
Bactrim I.V. Infusion 2082
Bactrim (Rare) 2084
Bleph-10 (Isolated incident) 475
▲Blephamide Ointment (Among most often) ◎ 237
Calan SR Caplets (1% or less) 2422
Calan Tablets (1% or less) 2419
Capoten 739
Capozide 742
Cataflam (Rare) 816
Ceclor Pulvules & Suspension (Rare) 1431
Cefizox for Intramuscular or Intravenous Use 1034
Cefotan 2829
Ceftin 1078
Cefzil Tablets and Oral Suspension (Rare) 746
Celontin Kapseals 1899
Ceptaz 1081
Chibroxin Sterile Ophthalmic Solution (With oral form) 1617
Cipro I.V. (1% or less) 595
Cipro I.V. Pharmacy Bulk Package (Less than 1%) 597
Cipro Tablets 592
Cleocin Phosphate Injection 2586
Cleocin Vaginal Cream (Some cases) 2589
Clinoril Tablets (Less than 1 in 100) 1618
Clozaril Tablets 2252
Cordarone Intravenous (Less than 2%) 2715
Cytovene-IV (Two or more reports) 2103
Danocrine Capsules (Rare) 2307
Daypro Caplets (Less than 1%) 2426
Depakene 413
Depakote Tablets 415
Diamox Intravenous 1372

(▭ Described in PDR For Nonprescription Drugs) Incidence data in parenthesis; ▲ 3% or more (◎ Described in PDR For Ophthalmology)

Stevens-Johnson syndrome | Side Effects Index | 1416

Diamox Sequels (Sustained Release) 1373
Diamox Tablets 1372
Didronel Tablets (A single case) 1984
Diflucan Injection, Tablets, and Oral Suspension 2194
Dilacor XR Extended-release Capsules 2018
Dilantin Infatabs 1908
Dilantin Kapseals 1906
Dilantin Parenteral 1910
Dilantin-125 Suspension 1911
Diupres Tablets 1650
Diuril Oral Suspension 1653
Diuril Sodium Intravenous 1652
Diuril Tablets 1653
Dolobid Tablets (Less than 1 in 100) 1654
Duricef (Rare) 748
Dynacin Capsules (Rare) 1590
EC-Naprosyn Delayed-Release Tablets (Rare) 2117
Enduron Tablets 420
Engerix-B Unit-Dose Vials 2482
Esidrix Tablets 821
Esimil Tablets 822
FML-S Liquifilm (Rare) ◉ 242
Fansidar Tablets 2114
Felbatol (Rare) 2666
Feldene Capsules (Less than 1%) 1965
Floxin I.V. 1571
Floxin Tablets (200 mg, 300 mg, 400 mg) 1567
Fortaz 1100
Gantanol Tablets 2119
Gantrisin (Rare) 2120
Glauctabs ◉ 208
HydroDIURIL Tablets 1674
Hydropres Tablets 1675
Hyzaar Tablets 1677
IBU Tablets (Less than 1%) 1342
Indocin Capsules (Less than 1%) 1680
Indocin I.V. (Less than 1%) 1684
Indocin (Less than 1%) 1680
Isoptin Oral Tablets (Less than 1%) 1346
Isoptin SR Tablets (1% or less) 1348
Keflex Pulvules & Oral Suspension (Rare) 914
Keftab Tablets 915
Kefurox Vials, Faspak & ADD-Vantage 1454
Lamictal Tablets (Rare) 1112
Lariam Tablets 2128
Lescol Capsules (Rare) 2267
Leukeran Tablets (Rare) 1133
Lincocin (Rare) 2617
Lodine Capsules and Tablets (Rare) 2743
Loniten Tablets (Rare) 2618
Lopressor HCT Tablets 832
Lorabid Suspension and Pulvules 1459
Lotensin HCT 837
Lozol Tablets 2022
Luvox Tablets 2544
MZM (Common) ◉ 267
Macrobid Capsules (Rare) 1988
Macrodantin Capsules (Rare) 1989
Maxaquin Tablets 2440
Mesantoin Tablets 2272
Mevacor Tablets (Rare) 1699
Mexitil Capsules (Rare) 678
Milontin Kapseals 1920
Miltown Tablets (Rare) 2672
Minocin Intravenous (Rare) 1382
Minocin Oral Suspension (Rare) 1385
Minocin Pellet-Filled Capsules (Rare) 1383
Mintezol 1704
Moduretic Tablets 1705
Children's Motrin Ibuprofen Oral Suspension (Less than 1%) 1546
Motrin Tablets (Less than 1%) 2625
Motrin Ibuprofen Suspension, Oral Drops, Chewable Tablets, Caplets (Less than 1%) 1546
Mycostatin Pastilles (Very rare) 704
Nalfon 200 Pulvules & Nalfon Tablets (Less than 1%) 917
Anaprox/Naprosyn (Rare) 2117
Neptazane Tablets 1388
Noroxin Tablets 1715
Noroxin Tablets 2048
Orthoclone OKT3 Sterile Solution 1837
PCE Dispertab Tablets (Rare) 444
PMB 200 and PMB 400 (Rare) 2783
Penetrex Tablets (Less than 1% but more than or equal to 0.1%) 2031
Pentam 300 Injection (0.2%) 1041
Phenobarbital Elixir and Tablets (Rare) 1469
Phenurone Tablets (One case) 447
Pipracil (Rare) 1390
Pravachol (Rare) 765
Prilosec Delayed-Release Capsules (Very rare) 529
Primaxin I.M. 1727
Primaxin I.V. 1729
Prinzide Tablets 1737
Proloprim Tablets (Rare) 1155
Proventil Syrup (Rare) 2385
Recombivax HB 1744
Relafen Tablets (Rare) 2510
SSD 1355
Septra 1174
Septra I.V. Infusion 1169
Septra I.V. Infusion ADD-Vantage Vials (Rare) 1171
Septra 1174
Ser-Ap-Es Tablets 849
Silvadene Cream 1% 1540
Sodium Sulamyd (Isolated incident) 2387
Sporanox Capsules (Rare) 1305
Sultrin (Frequent) 1885
Suprax (Less than 2%) 1399
Tagamet (Very rare) 2516
Tazicef for Injection 2519
Tegretol Chewable Tablets (Extremely rare) 852
Tegretol Suspension (Extremely rare) 852
Tegretol Tablets (Extremely rare) 852
Ticlid Tablets (Rare) 2156
Timolide Tablets 1748
Tonocard Tablets (Less than 1%) 531
Toradol 2159
Trancopal Caplets (Rare) 2337
Trimpex Tablets (Rare) 2163
Trusopt Sterile Ophthalmic Solution (Rare) 1760
Uniphyl 400 mg Tablets 2001
Vancocin HCl, Oral Solution & Pulvules 1483
Vancocin HCl, Vials & ADD-Vantage (Infrequent) 1481
Vantin for Oral Suspension and Vantin Tablets 2646
Vaseretic Tablets 1765
Vasocidin Ointment (Isolated incident) ◉ 268
Vasocidin Ophthalmic Solution ◉ 270
Vasosulf ◉ 271
Vasotec I.V. 1768
Vasotec Tablets (0.5% to 1.0%) 1771
Ventolin Syrup (Rare) 1202
Verelan Capsules (1% or less) 1410
Verelan Capsules (Less than 1%) 2824
Voltaren Tablets (Rare) 861
Wellbutrin Tablets 1204
Zarontin Capsules 1928
Zarontin Syrup 1929
Zefazone 2654
Zestoretic 2850
Zinacef (Rare) 1211
Zocor Tablets (Rare) 1775
Zosyn (Rare) 1419
Zosyn Pharmacy Bulk Package (Rare) 1422
Zyloprim Tablets (Less than 1%) 1226

Stimulation

Anafranil Capsules (Infrequent) 803
Atamet 572
Dalmane Capsules (Rare) 2173
Dizac (Less frequent) 1809
Placidyl Capsules (Occasional) 448
Proventil Tablets 2386
Serax Capsules 2810
Serax Tablets 2810
Sinemet Tablets 943
Sinemet CR Tablets 944
Valium Injectable 2182
Valium Tablets 2183
Valrelease Capsules (Infrequent) 2169
Xanax Tablets (Rare) 2649

Stinging

Aci-Jel Therapeutic Vaginal Jelly (Occasional cases) 1848
Aclovate Ointment (1 of 366 patients) 1069
▲ Acular (Approximately 40%) 474
Afrin ▣ 797
▲ Alomide (Among most frequest) 469
Americaine Anesthetic Lubricant 983
Americaine Otic Topical Anesthetic Ear Drops 983
Attenuvax 1610
Bactroban Ointment (1.5%) 2470
▲ Betagan (About 1 in 3 patients) ◉ 233
Biavax II 1613
Bleph-10 475
Chloromycetin Ophthalmic Ointment, 1% (Occasional) ◉ 310
Chloromycetin Ophthalmic Solution ◉ 310
Chloroptic S.O.P. ◉ 239
Chloroptic Sterile Ophthalmic Solution ◉ 239
Cortisporin Otic Solution Sterile 1087
Cortisporin Otic Suspension Sterile (Rare) 1088
Cozaar Tablets (Less than 1%) 1628
▲ Cyclocort Topical Lotion 0.1% (20%) 1037
DesOwen Cream, Ointment and Lotion (Approximately 3%) 1046
▲ Diprivan Injection (10% to 17.6%) 2833
▲ Diprolene AF Cream (6%) 2352
▲ Diprolene Gel 0.05% (6%) 2353
▲ Diprolene (6%) 2352
Doxorubicin Astra 540
Dyclone 0.5% and 1% Topical Solutions, USP 544
▲ Elimite (permethrin) 5% Cream (10%) 478
Elocon Ointment 0.1% (7 of 812 patients) 2354
▲ Exelderm Cream 1.0% (3%) 2685
Exelderm Solution 1.0% (Approximately 1%) 2686
4-Way Fast Acting Nasal Spray (regular & mentholated) ▣ 621
4-Way Long Lasting Nasal Spray ▣ 621
Floropryl Sterile Ophthalmic Ointment 1662
Fluoracaine (Occasional) ◉ 206
FLURESS (Occasional) ◉ 207
Gentacidin Ointment (Occasional) ◉ 264
Gentacidin Solution (Occasional) ◉ 264
HMS Liquifilm (Occasional) ◉ 244
Humorsol Sterile Ophthalmic Solution 1664
Hyzaar Tablets 1677
Idamycin 1955
Imitrex Injection (Infrequent) 1103
Inflamase (Rare) ◉ 265
Isopto Carpine Ophthalmic Solution ◉ 223
▲ Lac-Hydrin 12% Lotion (1 in 10 to 30 patients) 2687
▲ Livostin (15%) ◉ 266
Lotrimin 2371
Lotrisone Cream 2372
M-M-R II 1687
M-R-VAX II 1689
Melanex Topical Solution 1793
Meruvax II 1697
Monoclate-P, Factor VIII:C, Pasteurized, Monoclonal Antibody Purified Antihemophilic Factor (Human) 521
Mumpsvax 1708
Mutamycin 703
▲ Naftin Cream 1% (6%) 480
▲ Naftin Gel 1% (5.0%) 481
▲ Nasalide Nasal Solution 0.025% (Approximately 45%) 2110
▲ Nizoral 2% Cream (5%) 1297
▲ Ocufen (One of the two most frequent) ◉ 245
Ocuflox 481
Ophthetic (Occasional) ◉ 247
Oxistat (0.1%) 1152
Paremyd ◉ 247
PediOtic Suspension Sterile (Rare) 1153
Phospholine Iodide ◉ 326
Polytrim Ophthalmic Solution Sterile 482
Pred-G Liquifilm Sterile Ophthalmic Suspension ◉ 251
▲ Profenal 1% Sterile Ophthalmic Solution (Among most frequent) ◉ 227
PROPINE with C CAP Compliance Cap (6%) ◉ 253
Sodium Sulamyd 2387
▲ Spectazole (econazole nitrate 1%) Cream (3%) 1890
Surgicel (Occasional) 1314
Talwin Injection 2334
Temovate (3 of 421 patients) 1179
▲ Timoptic in Ocudose (Approximately 1 in 8 patients) 1753
▲ Timoptic Sterile Ophthalmic Solution (Approximately 1 in 8 patients) 1751
▲ Timoptic-XE (1 in 8 patients) 1755
▲ Ultravate Cream 0.05% (4.4%) 2689
Ultravate Ointment 0.05% (2.4%) 2690
Vasosulf ◉ 271
▲ Viroptic Ophthalmic Solution, 1% Sterile (4.6%) 1204
▲ Voltaren Ophthalmic Sterile Ophthalmic Solution (15%) ◉ 272
VōSol (Occasional) 2678
Xerac AC 1933
▲ Zonalon Cream (Approximately 21%) 1055
▲ Zovirax Ointment 5% (28.3%) 1223

Stomach, nervous

Clozaril Tablets (Less than 1%) 2252

Stomachache

▲ AeroBid Inhaler System (10%) 1005
▲ Aerobid-M Inhaler System (10%) 1005
Aleve 1975
▲ Alka-Seltzer Effervescent Antacid and Pain Reliever (14.5% at doses of 1000 mg/day) ▣ 701
▲ Alka-Seltzer Lemon Lime Effervescent Antacid and Pain Reliever (14.5% at doses of 1000 mg/day) ▣ 703
Alomide (Less than 1%) 469
Arthritis Foundation Ibuprofen Tablets (Occasional) ▣ 674
▲ Regular Strength Ascriptin Tablets (14.5%) ▣ 629
Atgam Sterile Solution (Less than 5%) 2581
▲ Genuine Bayer Aspirin Tablets & Caplets (14.5% at doses of 1000 mg/day) ▣ 713
▲ Aspirin Regimen Bayer Regular Strength 325 mg Caplets (14.5% of 4500 people tested) ▣ 709
Bontril Slow-Release Capsules 781
Brontex 1981
▲ Bufferin Analgesic Tablets and Caplets (14.5%) ▣ 613
▲ CHEMET (succimer) Capsules (5.2-15.7%) 1545
Cylert Tablets 412
▲ Ecotrin (14.5% at 1000 mg/day) 2455
Guaifed 1787
▲ Halfprin (14.5%) 1362
Haltran Tablets (Occasional) ▣ 771
Intal Inhaler (Rare) 988
Intal Nebulizer Solution 989
K-Phos Neutral Tablets 639
K-Phos Original Formula 'Sodium Free' Tablets 639
Ortho-Cyclen/Ortho-Tri-Cyclen 1858
Ortho-Cyclen/Ortho Tri-Cyclen 1858
PhosChol 488
Proventil Syrup (Less than 1 of 100 patients) 2385
▲ SSKI Solution (Among most frequent) 2658
▲ Serevent Inhalation Aerosol (4%) 1176
▲ St. Joseph Adult Chewable Aspirin (81 mg.) (14.3% of 4500 patients) ▣ 808
Stadol (1% or greater) 775
Uroqid-Acid No. 2 Tablets 640
▲ Ventolin Inhalation Aerosol and Refill (3%) 1197
Ventolin Inhalation Solution (2% to 3%) 1198
Ventolin Rotacaps for Inhalation (2%) 1200
Ventolin Syrup (Less than 1 of 100 patients) 1202

Stomatitis

Actigall Capsules 802
Adriamycin PFS 1947
Adriamycin RDF 1947
Anaprox/Naprosyn (Less than 3%) 2117
Android-25 Tablets 1251
Ansaid Tablets (Less than 1%) 2579
Aredia for Injection (Up to 1%) 810
Asendin Tablets 1369
Atgam Sterile Solution (More than 1% but less than 5%) 2581
Atretol Tablets 573
Atromid-S Capsules 2701
Augmentin 2468
Azo Gantanol Tablets 2080
Azo Gantrisin Tablets 2081
Azulfidine (Rare) 1949
Bactrim DS Tablets 2084
Bactrim I.V. Infusion 2082
Bactrim 2084
Blenoxane 692
CeeNU (Infrequent) 693
Chloromycetin Sodium Succinate 1900
Claritin (2% or fewer patients) 2349

(▣ Described in PDR For Nonprescription Drugs) Incidence data in parenthesis; ▲ 3% or more (◉ Described in PDR For Ophthalmology)

1417 Side Effects Index Stroke

Claritin-D (Less frequent) 2350
Clinoril Tablets (Less than 1 in 100) 1618
Cognex Capsules (Infrequent) 1901
▲ Cytosar-U Sterile Powder (Among most frequent) 2592
Daypro Caplets (Less than 1%) 2426
Dipentum Capsules (1.0%) 1951
Dolobid Tablets (Less than 1 in 100) 1654
Doxorubicin Astra 540
EC-Naprosyn Delayed-Release Tablets (Less than 3%) 2117
Effexor (Infrequent) 2719
Efudex 2113
Elavil 2838
Endep Tablets 2174
▲ Ergamisol Tablets (3% to 39%) 1292
Estratest 2539
Etrafon 2355
Fansidar Tablets 2114
Feldene Capsules (Greater than 1%) 1965
Flagyl 375 Capsules 2434
Flagyl I.V. 2247
Flexeril Tablets (Rare) 1661
▲ Fludara for Injection (Up to 9%) 663
Flumadine Tablets & Syrup 1015
Fluorouracil Injection (Rare to common) 2116
Foscavir Injection (Less than 1%) 547
▲ Sterile FUDR (Among more common) 2118
Gantanol Tablets 2119
Gantrisin 2120
Garamycin Injectable 2360
Halcion Tablets 2611
Hivid Tablets (Less than 1% to less than 3%) 2121
Hydrea Capsules (Less frequent) 696
IFEX (Less than 1%) 697
Intron A (Less than 5%) 2364
Lamictal Tablets (Infrequent) 1112
▲ Leucovorin Calcium for Injection (16% to 84%) 1268
▲ Leukine for IV Infusion (24%) 1271
Limbitrol 2180
Lincocin 2617
Ludiomil Tablets (Isolated reports) 843
Luvox Tablets (Infrequent) 2544
Matulane Capsules 2131
Maxair Autohaler 1492
Maxair Inhaler (Less than 1%) 1494
▲ Methotrexate Sodium Tablets, Injection, for Injection and LPF Injection (3 to 10%) 1275
MetroGel-Vaginal 902
Miltown Tablets (Rare) 2672
Mithracin 607
▲ Mutamycin (Frequent) 703
Myochrysine Injection 1711
Anaprox/Naprosyn (Less than 3%) 2117
Navelbine Injection (Less than 20%) 1145
▲ Neupogen for Injection (5%) 495
Neurontin Capsules (Infrequent) 1922
▲ Nicorette (3% to 9% of patients) 2458
Noroxin Tablets 1715
Noroxin Tablets 2048
Norpramin Tablets 1526
▲ Novantrone (18 to 29%) 1279
Omnipen Capsules 2764
Omnipen for Oral Suspension 2765
Orudis Capsules (Greater than 1%) 2766
Oruvail Capsules (Greater than 1%) 2766
PMB 200 and PMB 400 (Rare) 2783
Pamelor 2280
Paxil Tablets (Rare) 2505
Penetrex Tablets (Less than 1% but more than or equal to 0.1%) 2031
Premarin with Methyltestosterone 2794
PREVACID Delayed-Release Capsules (Less than 1%) 2562
▲ Proleukin for Injection (32%) 797
Protostat Tablets 1883
Prozac Pulvules & Liquid, Oral Solution (Infrequent) 919
Quadrinal Tablets 1350
Relafen Tablets (1% to 3%) 2510
▲ Ridaura Capsules (13%) 2513
Risperdal (Infrequent) 1301
Septra 1174
Septra I.V. Infusion 1169
Septra I.V. Infusion ADD-Vantage Vials 1171
Septra 1174
Serzone Tablets (Infrequent) 771
Sinequan 2205
Solganal Suspension 2388
Spectrobid Tablets 2206
Surmontil Capsules 2811
Tegretol Chewable Tablets 852
Tegretol Suspension 852
Tegretol Tablets 852
Temaril Tablets, Syrup and Spansule Extended-Release Capsules 483
Testred Capsules 1262
Thioguanine Tablets, Tabloid Brand (Less frequent) 1181
Timentin for Injection 2528
Tofranil Ampuls 854
Tofranil Tablets 856
Tofranil-PM Capsules 857
Tolectin (200, 400 and 600 mg) (Less than 1%) 1581
Tonocard Tablets (Less than 1%) 531
Toradol (Greater than 1%) 2159
Trecator-SC Tablets 2814
Triavil Tablets 1757
Ultram Tablets (50 mg) (Infrequent) 1585
Unasyn 2212
Urobiotic-250 Capsules (Rare) 2214
Vaseretic Tablets 1765
Vasotec I.V. 1768
Vasotec Tablets (0.5% to 1.0%) 1771
Velban Vials (Not common) 1484
▲ VePesid Capsules and Injection (1% to 6%) 718
▲ Videx Tablets, Powder for Oral Solution, & Pediatric Powder for Oral Solution (16% to 17%) 720
Vivactil Tablets 1774
Wellbutrin Tablets (Frequent) 1204
▲ Zinecard (26% to 34%) 1961
Zoloft Tablets (Rare) 2217
Zyloprim Tablets (Less than 1%) 1226

Stomatitis, ulcerative

Anafranil Capsules (Up to 2%) 803
Anaprox/Naprosyn (Less than 1%) 2117
Betaseron for SC Injection 658
Cataflam (Less than 1%) 816
Cosmegen Injection 1626
Depen Titratable Tablets 2662
EC-Naprosyn Delayed-Release Tablets (Less than 1%) 2117
Felbatol 2666
Foscavir Injection (Between 1% and 5%) 547
Indocin Capsules (Less than 1%) 1680
Indocin I.V. (Less than 1%) 1684
Indocin (Less than 1%) 1680
Intron A (Less than 5%) 2364
Lodine Capsules and Tablets (Less than 1%) 2743
▲ Methotrexate Sodium Tablets, Injection, for Injection and LPF Injection (Among most frequent) 1275
Anaprox/Naprosyn (Less than 1%) 2117
Neurontin Capsules (Rare) 1922
▲ Nicorette (3% to 9% of patients) 2458
Paxil Tablets (Rare) 2505
Permax Tablets (Rare) 575
Prozac Pulvules & Liquid, Oral Solution (Infrequent) 919
Videx Tablets, Powder for Oral Solution, & Pediatric Powder for Oral Solution (Less than 1%) 720
Voltaren Tablets (Less than 1%) 861
Zerit Capsules (Fewer than 1% to 3%) 729
Zoloft Tablets (Rare) 2217
Zosyn (1.0% or less) 1419
Zosyn Pharmacy Bulk Package (1.0% or less) 1422

Stool, bloody (see under Hematochezia)

Stool, color changes

Anafranil Capsules (Rare) 803
Coumadin 926
Levlen/Tri-Levlen 651
Micronor Tablets 1872
Modicon 1872
Nizoral Tablets 1298
Ortho-Cyclen/Ortho-Tri-Cyclen 1858
Ortho-Novum 1872
Ortho-Cyclen/Ortho Tri-Cyclen 1858
Pepto-Bismol Original Liquid, Original and Cherry Tablets and Easy-To-Swallow Caplets 1976
Pepto-Bismol Maximum Strength Liquid 1976
Questran Light 769
Questran Powder 770
ReVia Tablets 940
Sporanox Capsules 1305
Ticlid Tablets 2156
Levlen/Tri-Levlen 651

Stools, abnormal

Clozaril Tablets (Less than 1%) 2252
Effexor (Rare) 2719
Hivid Tablets (Less than 1% to less than 3%) 2121
Pentasa (Less than 1%) 1527
▲ Relafen Tablets (3% to 9%) 2510
▲ Sandostatin Injection (Less than 10%) 2292
Ultrase MT Capsules (1.5%) 2344
Videx Tablets, Powder for Oral Solution, & Pediatric Powder for Oral Solution (Less than 1%) 720
Zosyn (2.4%) 1419
Zosyn Pharmacy Bulk Package (2.4%) 1422

Stools, loose

▲ Acel-Imune Diphtheria and Tetanus Toxoids and Acellular Pertussis Vaccine Adsorbed (3.5%) 1364
Atromid-S Capsules (Less frequent) 2701
▲ Augmentin (9%) 2468
Cefobid Pharmacy Bulk Package - Not for Direct Infusion (1 in 30) 2192
▲ Ceftin (3.7% to 8.6%) 1078
▲ CHEMET (succimer) Capsules (12-20.9%) 1545
Cognex Capsules 1901
Colestid Tablets (Less frequent) 2591
Fluorouracil Injection 2116
Geocillin Tablets 2199
Hivid Tablets (Less than 1% to less than 3%) 2121
Imdur (Less than or equal to 5%) 1323
▲ Intron A (Up to 10%) 2364
Kutrase Capsules (Occasional) 2402
Ku-Zyme Capsules 2402
Lorelco Tablets 1517
MagTab SR Caplets 1793
▲ Mesnex Injection (70%) 702
Micro-K LS Packets (Frequent) 2064
Noroxin Tablets (0.3% to 1.0%) 1715
Noroxin Tablets (0.3% to 1.0%) 2048
Norvasc Tablets (Less than or equal to 0.1%) 1940
Pipracil (2%) 1390
▲ Ridaura Capsules (approx. 50%) 2513
▲ Sandostatin Injection (5% to 10%; 30% to 58%) 2292
Solatene Capsules (Occasional) 2150
▲ Suprax (6%) 1399
▲ Tonocard Tablets (0.0-6.8%) 531
▲ Vantin for Oral Suspension and Vantin Tablets (5.9% to 10.6%) 2646
▲ Zithromax (5% to 7%) 1944
▲ Zoloft Tablets (17.7%) 2217

Strabismus

Anafranil Capsules (Rare) 803
Lamictal Tablets (Rare) 1112
Lioresal Tablets 829
Neurontin Capsules (Rare) 1922
Prozac Pulvules & Liquid, Oral Solution (Rare) 919
▲ Videx Tablets, Powder for Oral Solution, & Pediatric Powder for Oral Solution (5% to 8%) 720

Striae

Aclovate Cream 1069
Analpram-HC Rectal Cream 1% and 2.5% 977
Anusol-HC Cream 2.5% (Infrequent to frequent) 1896
Aristocort A 0.025% Cream (Infrequent) 1027
Aristocort A 0.5% Cream 1031
Aristocort A 0.1% Cream (Infrequent) 1029
Aristocort A 0.1% Ointment (Infrequent) 1030
▲ Blenoxane (50%) 692
Carmol HC (Infrequent to frequent) 924
▲ Cordran Lotion (More frequent) 1803
▲ Cordran Tape (More frequent) 1804
Cortisporin Cream 1084
Cortisporin Ointment 1085
Cortisporin Otic Solution Sterile 1087
Cortisporin Otic Suspension Sterile 1088
Cutivate Cream 1088
Cutivate Ointment (Infrequent to more frequent) 1089
Cyclocort Topical (Infrequent) 1037
Decadron Phosphate Topical Cream 1644
Decaspray Topical Aerosol 1648
Dermatop Emollient Cream 0.1% (Infrequent to frequent) 1238
DesOwen Cream, Ointment and Lotion (Infrequent) 1046
Diprolene AF Cream (Infrequent) 2352
Diprolene Gel 0.05% (Infrequent) 2353
Diprolene (Infrequent) 2352
Elocon (Infrequent) 2354
Epifoam (Infrequent) 2399
Florinef Acetate Tablets 505
Florone/Florone E 906
Halog (Infrequent) 2686
Hytone 907
Lidex (Infrequent) 2130
Locoid Cream, Ointment and Topical Solution (Infrequent) 978
Lotrisone Cream (Infrequent) 2372
Lupron Depot-PED 7.5 mg, 11.25 mg and 15 mg (Less than 2%) 2560
Mantadil Cream 1135
NeoDecadron Topical Cream 1714
PediOtic Suspension Sterile 1153
Pramosone Cream, Lotion & Ointment 978
ProctoCream-HC (Infrequent) 2408
ProctoCream-HC 2.5% (Infrequent to frequent) 2408
ProctoFoam-HC 2409
Psorcon Cream 0.05% (Infrequent) 909
Psorcon Ointment 0.05% 908
Synalar (Infrequent) 2130
Temovate (Infrequent) 1179
Topicort (Infrequent) 1243
Tridesilon Cream 0.05% (Infrequent) 615
Tridesilon Ointment 0.05% (Infrequent) 616
Ultravate Cream 0.05% (Infrequently) 2689
Ultravate Ointment 0.05% 2690
Westcort 2690

Stridor

Floxin I.V. 1571
Foscavir Injection (Between 1% and 5%) 547
Hespan Injection 929
Maxaquin Tablets (Less than 1%) 2440
Nubain Injection (1% or less) 935
Reglan (Rare) 2068
Risperdal (Infrequent) 1301
Salagen Tablets (Less than 1%) 1489
Serevent Inhalation Aerosol (Rare) 1176
Zoloft Tablets (Rare) 2217

Stroke

Activase (0.9%) 1058
Asendin Tablets (Very rare) 1369
Betapace Tablets (Less than 1% to 1%) 641
Brevicon 2088
Clomid 1514
Cytovene-IV (Two or more reports) 2103
Danocrine Capsules 2307
Demulen 2428
Dexatrim ▣ 832
Dexatrim Plus Vitamins Caplets ▣ 832
DynaCirc Capsules (0.5% to 1%) 2256
Elavil 2838
Endep Tablets 2174
Estraderm Transdermal System 824
ESTRATAB Tablets (0.3, 0.625, 1.25, 2.5 mg) 2536
Estratest 2539
Etrafon 2355
Flexeril Tablets (Rare) 1661
Heparin Lock Flush Solution 2725
Heparin Sodium Injection 2726
Heparin Sodium Injection, USP, Sterile Solution 2615
Heparin Sodium Vials 1441
Humegon 1824
Imitrex Tablets 1106
Limbitrol 2180
Ludiomil Tablets (Isolated reports) 843
Lupron Depot 3.75 mg 2556
Lupron Depot 7.5 mg 2559
Lupron Injection 2555
Menest Tablets 2494
Metrodin (urofollitropin for injection) 2446
Micronor Tablets 1872
Modicon 1872
Monoket (Fewer than 1%) 2406
Norinyl 2088
Norplant System 2759

(▣ Described in PDR For Nonprescription Drugs) Incidence data in parenthesis; ▲ 3% or more (⊙ Described in PDR For Ophthalmology)

Norpramin Tablets ... 1526
Nor-Q D Tablets ... 2135
Ortho-Cyclen/Ortho-Tri-Cyclen ... 1858
Ortho Dienestrol Cream ... 1866
Ortho-Novum ... 1872
Ortho-Cyclen/Ortho Tri-Cyclen ... 1858
Ovcon ... 760
Pamelor ... 2280
Parlodel (30 cases) ... 2281
Premarin Intravenous ... 2787
Premarin with Methyltestosterone .. 2794
Premarin Vaginal Cream ... 2791
Prinivil Tablets (0.3% to 1.0%) ... 1733
Prinzide Tablets ... 1737
Proleukin for Injection (Less than 1% to 1%) ... 797
Roferon-A Injection (Less than 1%) ... 2145
Stilphostrol Tablets and Ampuls ... 612
Surmontil Capsules ... 2811
Testoderm Testosterone Transdermal System (Two in 104 patients) ... 486
Tofranil Ampuls ... 854
Tofranil Tablets ... 856
Tofranil-PM Capsules ... 857
Triavil Tablets ... 1757
Tri-Norinyl ... 2164
Vivactil Tablets ... 1774
Zestoretic ... 2850
Zestril Tablets (0.3% to 1.0%) ... 2854

Stroke, hemorrhagic

Activase (0.7%) ... 1058
Demulen ... 2428
Levlen/Tri-Levlen ... 651
Micronor Tablets ... 1872
Modicon ... 1872
Nor-Q D Tablets ... 2135
Ortho-Cyclen/Ortho-Tri-Cyclen ... 1858
Ortho-Novum ... 1872
Ortho-Cyclen/Ortho Tri-Cyclen ... 1858
Levlen/Tri-Levlen ... 651
Triphasil-21 Tablets ... 2814
Triphasil-28 Tablets ... 2819

Stroke, thrombotic

Levlen/Tri-Levlen ... 651
Ortho-Cyclen/Ortho-Tri-Cyclen ... 1858
Ortho-Cyclen/Ortho Tri-Cyclen ... 1858
Levlen/Tri-Levlen ... 651
Triphasil-21 Tablets ... 2814
Triphasil-28 Tablets ... 2819

Strongyloidiasis hyperinfection

Tagamet (Extremely rare) ... 2516

Stuffiness, nasal (see under Nasal congestion)

Stupor

Ambien Tablets (Infrequent) ... 2416
Anafranil Capsules (Rare) ... 803
Betaseron for SC Injection ... 658
BuSpar (Rare) ... 737
Desyrel and Desyrel Dividose ... 503
Duragesic Transdermal System (Less than 1%) ... 1288
Effexor (Infrequent) ... 2719
Eskalith ... 2485
Felbatol (2.6%) ... 2666
Foscavir Injection (Between 1% and 5%) ... 547
Hivid Tablets (Less than 1% to less than 3%) ... 2121
Kerlone Tablets (Less than 2%) ... 2436
Lamictal Tablets (Infrequent) ... 1112
Lithium Carbonate Capsules & Tablets ... 2230
Lithonate/Lithotabs/Lithobid ... 2543
Luvox Tablets (Infrequent) ... 2544
Moduretic Tablets (Less than or equal to 1%) ... 1705
Neurontin Capsules (Infrequent) ... 1922
Orthoclone OKT3 Sterile Solution .. 1837
Paxil Tablets (Rare) ... 2505
Permax Tablets (Rare) ... 575
PhosLo Tablets ... 690
ProSom Tablets (Infrequent) ... 449
Prozac Pulvules & Liquid, Oral Solution (Rare) ... 919
Risperdal (Infrequent) ... 1301
Romazicon (Less than 1%) ... 2147
Serax Capsules ... 2810
Serax Tablets ... 2810
Streptomycin Sulfate Injection ... 2208
Tambocor Tablets (Less than 1%) ... 1497
Toradol (1% or less) ... 2159

Stye

Cognex Capsules (Infrequent) ... 1901
Crolom (Infrequent) ... ⊙ 257
Intron A (Less than 5%) ... 2364
Neurontin Capsules (Infrequent) ... 1922

Sudden Infant Death Syndrome

Diphtheria and Tetanus Toxoids and Pertussis Vaccine Adsorbed .. 2477
Diphtheria and Tetanus Toxoids and Pertussis Vaccine Adsorbed USP (For Pediatric Use) ... 875
Felbatol ... 2666

Suicide, attempt of

Ambien Tablets ... 2416
Betaseron for SC Injection (2%; 1 suicide, 4 attempts) ... 658
Effexor (Infrequent) ... 2719
Felbatol (Infrequent) ... 2666
Floxin I.V. ... 1571
Foscavir Injection (Less than 1%) .. 547
Hivid Tablets (Less than 1% to less than 3%) ... 2121
Imitrex Tablets (Rare) ... 1106
Intron A (Rare; less than 5%) ... 2364
Lamictal Tablets (Rare) ... 1112
Lioresal Intrathecal ... 1596
Luvox Tablets (Infrequent) ... 2544
Neurontin Capsules (Rare) ... 1922
Paxil Tablets ... 2505
Proleukin for Injection ... 797
ReVia Tablets (Less than 1%) ... 940
Risperdal (1.2%) ... 1301
Serzone Tablets (Infrequent) ... 771
Symmetrel Capsules and Syrup (Less than 0.1%) ... 946
Videx Tablets, Powder for Oral Solution, & Pediatric Powder for Oral Solution (Less than 1%) ... 720
Vivactil Tablets ... 1774
Zoloft Tablets (Infrequent) ... 2217

Suicidal ideation

Ambien Tablets ... 2416
Anafranil Capsules (Infrequent) ... 803
Atamet ... 572
Betaseron for SC Injection ... 658
BuSpar (Infrequent) ... 737
Celontin Kapseals (Rare) ... 1899
Cognex Capsules (Rare) ... 1901
Desyrel and Desyrel Dividose ... 503
Floxin I.V. ... 1571
Floxin Tablets (200 mg, 300 mg, 400 mg) (Rare) ... 1567
Halcion Tablets ... 2611
Hydropres Tablets ... 1675
Intron A (Rare) ... 2364
Klonopin Tablets ... 2126
Lamictal Tablets (Rare) ... 1112
Lamprene Capsules (Less than 1%) ... 828
Larodopa Tablets (Infrequent) ... 2129
Lioresal Intrathecal ... 1596
Miltown Tablets ... 2672
Neurontin Capsules (Infrequent) ... 1922
Nizoral Tablets (Rare) ... 1298
Prozac Pulvules & Liquid, Oral Solution ... 919
Reglan (Less frequent) ... 2068
ReVia Tablets (2%) ... 940
Seromycin Pulvules ... 1476
Serzone Tablets (Infrequent) ... 771
Sinemet Tablets ... 943
Sinemet CR Tablets ... 944
Symmetrel Capsules and Syrup (Less than 0.1%) ... 946
Trilafon ... 2389
Ultram Tablets (50 mg) (Infrequent) ... 1585
Wellbutrin Tablets (Rare) ... 1204
Zarontin Capsules (Rare) ... 1928
Zarontin Syrup (Rare) ... 1929
Zoloft Tablets (Infrequent) ... 2217

Sulfhemoglobinemia

Azo Gantrisin Tablets ... 2081

Sulfite, sensitivity to

Aldomet Ester HCl Injection ... 1602
Aldomet Oral Suspension ... 1600
Amikacin Sulfate Injection, USP ... 960
Amikin Injectable ... 501
Ana-Kit Anaphylaxis Emergency Treatment Kit ... 617
Antilirium Injectable ... 1009
Aramine Injection ... 1609
Carmol HC ... 924
Compazine ... 2470
Cortisporin Otic Solution Sterile ... 1087
Dalalone D.P. Injectable ... 1011
Dalgan Injection ... 538
Decadron Phosphate Injection ... 1637
Decadron Phosphate with Xylocaine Injection, Sterile ... 1639
Dilaudid Tablets and Liquid ... 1339
Dobutrex Solution Vials ... 1439
Duranest Injections ... 542
Eldopaque Forte 4% Cream ... 1252
EpiPen ... 790
Garamycin Injectable ... 2360
Hydrocortone Phosphate Injection, Sterile ... 1670
Isuprel Hydrochloride Injection 1:5000 ... 2311
Isuprel Hydrochloride Solution 1:200 & 1:100 ... 2313
Levoprome ... 1274
Mepergan Injection ... 2753
Minocin Oral Suspension ... 1385
Moban Tablets and Concentrate ... 1048
NeoDecadron Sterile Ophthalmic Solution ... 1713
Neo-Synephrine Hydrochloride 1% Carpuject ... 2324
Neo-Synephrine Hydrochloride 1% Injection ... 2324
NephrAmine ... 2005
Norflex Injection ... 1496
Novocain Hydrochloride for Spinal Anesthesia ... 2326
Nubain Injection ... 935
Numorphan Injection ... 936
Phenergan Injection ... 2773
Pontocaine Hydrochloride for Spinal Anesthesia ... 2330
Pred Mild ... ⊙ 253
Rowasa ... 2548
Sensorcaine ... 559
Septra I.V. Infusion ... 1169
Septra I.V. Infusion ADD-Vantage Vials ... 1171
Solaquin Forte 4% Cream ... 1252
Solaquin Forte 4% Gel ... 1252
Stelazine ... 2514
Streptomycin Sulfate Injection ... 2208
Sulfamylon Cream ... 925
Talwin Injection ... 2334
Tensilon Injectable ... 1261
Tofranil Ampuls ... 854
Torecan ... 2245
Tylenol with Codeine (Probably low) ... 1583
Tylox Capsules ... 1584
Tympagesic Ear Drops ... 2342
Vibramycin ... 1941
Xylocaine with Epinephrine Injections ... 567
Yutopar Intravenous Injection ... 570

Sunburn

▲ Accutane Capsules (Approximately 1 patient in 20) ... 2076
Methotrexate Sodium Tablets, Injection, for Injection and LPF Injection ... 1275
▲ Tegison Capsules (25-50%) ... 2154

Superinfection

Achromycin V Capsules ... 1367
Adriamycin PFS ... 1947
Adriamycin RDF ... 1947
Ancef Injection ... 2465
Augmentin ... 2468
Ceclor Pulvules & Suspension ... 1431
Cefotan ... 2829
Ceftin ... 1078
Cefzil Tablets and Oral Suspension (1.5%) ... 746
Ceptaz ... 1081
Doxorubicin Astra ... 540
Duricef ... 748
E-Mycin Tablets ... 1341
ERYC ... 1915
Fortaz ... 1100
Keflex Pulvules & Oral Suspension ... 914
Kefzol Vials, Faspak & ADD-Vantage ... 1456
Lorabid Suspension and Pulvules ... 1459
Macrobid Capsules ... 1988
Macrodantin Capsules ... 1989
Minocin Intravenous ... 1382
Minocin Oral Suspension ... 1385
Minocin Pellet-Filled Capsules ... 1383
Monodox Capsules ... 1805
Pipracil ... 1390
Polymyxin B Sulfate, Aerosporin Brand Sterile Powder ... 1154
Primaxin I.M. ... 1727
Rubex ... 712
Streptomycin Sulfate Injection ... 2208
Suprax ... 1399
TERAK Ointment ... ⊙ 209
Vancocin HCl, Vials & ADD-Vantage ... 1481
Vascor (200, 300 and 400 mg) Tablets (0.5 to 2.0%) ... 1587
Zefazone ... 2654
Zinacef ... 1211

Suppuration

Efudex ... 2113

Supraventricular contractions, premature

Paxil Tablets (Rare) ... 2505

Susurrus aurium

Monoket (Fewer than 1%) ... 2406

Swallowing

Diprivan Injection (Less than 1%) .. 2833

Swallowing, impairment

Capoten ... 739
Capozide ... 742
Compazine ... 2470
Coumadin ... 926
Dantrium Capsules (Less frequent) ... 1982
Dantrium Intravenous ... 1983
Esgic-plus Tablets (Infrequent) ... 1013
Fioricet Tablets (Infrequent) ... 2258
Fioricet with Codeine Capsules (Infrequent) ... 2260
Fiorinal with Codeine Capsules (Infrequent) ... 2262
Lioresal Intrathecal ... 1596
Lutrepulse for Injection ... 980
Maalox Daily Fiber Therapy ... ▣ 641
Monopril Tablets ... 757
Myochrysine Injection ... 1711
Neoral (Rare) ... 2276
Orthoclone OKT3 Sterile Solution .. 1837
Phrenilin (Infrequent) ... 785
Prinivil Tablets ... 1733
Prinzide Tablets ... 1737
Sandimmune (Rare) ... 2286
Sedapap Tablets 50 mg/650 mg (Infrequent) ... 1543
Solganal Suspension ... 2388
Stelazine ... 2514
Thorazine ... 2523
Vaseretic Tablets ... 1765
Vasotec Tablets ... 1771
Zestoretic ... 2850
Zestril Tablets ... 2854

Sweat discoloration

Atamet ... 572
Lamprene Capsules (Greater than 1%) ... 828
Rifadin ... 1528
Rifater ... 1532
Sinemet Tablets ... 943
Sinemet CR Tablets ... 944

Sweating (see under Diaphoresis)

Sweats, night

Atgam Sterile Solution (More than 1% but less than 5%) ... 2581

Swelling

▲ AK-Spore (Among most frequent) ... ⊙ 204
Americaine Hemorrhoidal Ointment ... ▣ 629
Atromid-S Capsules ... 2701
Bactroban Ointment (Less than 1%) ... 2470
Cafergot ... 2251
Cipro I.V. Pharmacy Bulk Package (Less than 1%) ... 597
Cortisporin Ophthalmic Ointment Sterile ... 1085
Cortisporin Ophthalmic Suspension Sterile ... 1086
Coumadin ... 926
D.H.E. 45 Injection ... 2255
Demulen ... 2428
Desferal Vials ... 820
Efudex ... 2113
Exact Vanishing and Tinted Creams ... ▣ 749
Femstat Prefill Vaginal Cream 2% (0.2%) ... 2116
Femstat Vaginal Cream 2% (0.2%) ... 2115
Fluorouracil Injection ... 2116
Hyzaar Tablets (1.3%) ... 1677
Maxaquin Tablets ... 2440
Nasalcrom Nasal Solution ... 994

(▣ Described in PDR For Nonprescription Drugs) Incidence data in parenthesis; ▲ 3% or more (⊙ Described in PDR For Ophthalmology)

1419 Side Effects Index Syncope

Neosporin Ophthalmic Ointment Sterile 1148
Neosporin Ophthalmic Solution Sterile 1149
Oncaspar 2028
Oxandrin 2862
PedvaxHIB 1718
Phenobarbital Elixir and Tablets 1469
Quadrinal Tablets 1350
Recombivax HB (Equal to or greater than 1%) 1744
Serevent Inhalation Aerosol (Rare) 1176
Stri-Dex ▣ 730
Sulfamylon Cream 925
TobraDex Ophthalmic Suspension and Ointment (Less than 4%) 473
Versed Injection (Less than 1%) 2170

Swelling, axillary

Depo-Provera Contraceptive Injection (Fewer than 1%) 2602

Swelling, edematous, ankles

Android Capsules, 10 mg 1250
Android 1251
Delatestryl Injection 2860
Eskalith 2485
Estratest 2539
Halotestin Tablets 2614
Lithium Carbonate Capsules & Tablets 2230
Lithonate/Lithotabs/Lithobid 2543
Lo/Ovral Tablets 2746
Lo/Ovral-28 Tablets 2751
Micronor Tablets 1872
Modicon 1872
Oreton Methyl 1255
Ortho-Cyclen/Ortho-Tri-Cyclen 1858
Ortho-Novum 1872
Ortho-Cyclen/Ortho Tri-Cyclen 1858
Ovral Tablets 2770
Ovral-28 Tablets 2770
Ovrette Tablets 2771
Testoderm Testosterone Transdermal System 486
Triphasil-21 Tablets 2814
Triphasil-28 Tablets 2819

Swelling, edematous, wrists

Eskalith 2485
Lithium Carbonate Capsules & Tablets 2230
Lithonate/Lithotabs/Lithobid 2543

Swelling, extremities

Colestid Tablets (Infrequent) 2591
Depo-Provera Contraceptive Injection 2602
Imitrex Injection (Rare) 1103
Noroxin Tablets (Less frequent) 1715
Noroxin Tablets (Less frequent) 2048
Nor-Q D Tablets 2135
Stilphostrol Tablets and Ampuls 612

Swelling, feet

K-Phos Neutral Tablets 639
Uroqid-Acid No. 2 Tablets 640

Swelling, joint

Ceftin for Oral Suspension (Less than 1% but more than 0.1%) 1078
Cozaar Tablets (Less than 1%) 1628
Danocrine Capsules 2307
Hivid Tablets (Less than 1% to less than 3%) 2121
Hyzaar Tablets 1677
Imitrex Injection (Infrequent) 1103
Intal Capsules (Less than 1 in 10,000 patients) 987
Intal Inhaler (Infrequent) 988
Intal Nebulizer Solution 989
Lithonate/Lithotabs/Lithobid 2543
▲ Mykrox Tablets (3.1%) 993
Neurontin Capsules (Infrequent) 1922
Rifater 1532

Swelling, legs

K-Phos Neutral Tablets 639
Lioresal Intrathecal 1596
Uroqid-Acid No. 2 Tablets 640

Swelling, lower legs (see under Swelling, legs)

Swelling, mouth

Acel-Imune Diphtheria and Tetanus Toxoids and Acellular Pertussis Vaccine Adsorbed (Rare) 1364
Diphtheria and Tetanus Toxoids and Pertussis Vaccine Adsorbed (Rare) 2477
Diphtheria and Tetanus Toxoids and Pertussis Vaccine Adsorbed USP (For Pediatric Use) (Rare) 875
Felbatol (Rare) 2666
Tambocor Tablets (Less than 1%) 1497
Tetramune (Rare) 1404
Tripedia 892

Swelling, periorbital

Streptase for Infusion (Rare) 562

Swelling, salivary gland

Eskalith 2485
Flexeril Tablets (Rare) 1661
Norisodrine with Calcium Iodide Syrup 442
Zyloprim Tablets (Less than 1%) 1226

Swelling at injection site

▲ Aredia for Injection (Among most common; up to 18%) 810
Aristocort Suspension (Forte Parenteral) 1027
Aristospan Suspension (Intra-articular) 1033
Aristospan Suspension (Intralesional) 1032
Atgam Sterile Solution (Less than 5%) 2581
Attenuvax 1610
Azactam for Injection (2.4%) 734
Ceredase 1065
Cipro I.V. (1% or less) 595
Cytovene-IV (1% or less) 2103
DDAVP Injection (Occasional) 2014
DDAVP Injection 15 mcg/mL (Occasional) 2015
Diphtheria and Tetanus Toxoids and Pertussis Vaccine Adsorbed 2477
Diphtheria and Tetanus Toxoids and Pertussis Vaccine Adsorbed USP (For Pediatric Use) (2 in 5 doses) 875
▲ Engerix-B Unit-Dose Vials (1% to 10%) 2482
Factrel 2877
Floxin I.V. (Approximately 2%) 1571
Geref (sermorelin acetate for injection) 2876
▲ Havrix (1% to 10%) 2489
HibTITER (Less than 1% to 1.7%) 1375
Humegon 1824
Humulin 50/50, 100 Units 1444
Humulin 70/30, 100 Units (Occasional) 1445
Humulin L, 100 Units (Occasional) 1446
Regular, 100 Units (Occasional) 1450
Pork Regular, 100 Units 1452
▲ Imovax Rabies Vaccine (About 25%) 881
INFeD (Iron Dextran Injection, USP) 2345
▲ JE-VAX (2.9% to approximately 20%) 886
Konakion Injection (Rare) 2127
▲ Leustatin (9% to 19%) 1834
Levoprome 1274
M-M-R II 1687
M-R-VAX II 1689
Metrodin (urofollitropin for injection) 2446
Pergonal (menotropins for injection, USP) 2448
▲ Pneumovax 23 (Common) 1725
Pnu-Imune 23 (Rare) 1393
Rabies Vaccine Adsorbed (A few patients) 2508
▲ Rabies Vaccine, Imovax Rabies I.D. (About 25%) 883
▲ Supprelin Injection (45%) 2056
Taxol 714
▲ Tetramune (20% to 43%) 1404
Timentin for Injection 2528
▲ Varivax (19.3% to 32.5%) 1762
Velosulin BR Human Insulin 10 ml Vials 1795
WinRho SD (A small number of cases) 2576
Zefazone (Up to 1.1%) 2654
Zemuron (Less than 1%) 1830

Syncope

Accupril Tablets (0.5% to 1.0%) 1893
Actimmune (Rare) 1056
Adalat Capsules (10 mg and 20 mg) (Approximately 0.5%) 587
Adalat CC (Rare) 589
AeroBid Inhaler System (1-3%) 1005
Aerobid-M Inhaler System (1-3%) 1005
AK-Fluor Injection 10% and 25% ◉ 203
All-Flex Arcing Spring Diaphragm (See also Ortho Diaphragm Kits) 1865
Altace Capsules (Less than 1% to 2.1%) 1232
Alupent Tablets (0.4%) 669
Ambien Tablets (Rare) 2416
Anafranil Capsules (Up to 2%) 803
Antabuse Tablets 2695
▲ Aredia for Injection (Up to 6%) 810
Arfonad Ampuls 2080
Asendin Tablets (Less than 1%) 1369
Atamet 572
Atgam Sterile Solution (Less than 1% to less than 5%) 2581
Atretol Tablets 573
Atrohist Plus Tablets 454
Azo Gantrisin Tablets 2081
Bentyl 1501
Betagan ◉ 233
▲ Betapace Tablets (1% to 5%) 641
Betaseron for SC Injection 658
Betimol 0.25%, 0.5% ◉ 261
Blocadren Tablets (0.6%) 1614
Brevibloc Injection (Less than 1%) 1808
Brontex 1981
BuSpar (Infrequent) 737
Butisol Sodium Elixir & Tablets (Less than 1 in 100) 2660
Calan SR Caplets (1% or less) 2422
Calan Tablets (1% or less) 2419
Capoten 739
Capozide 742
Carbocaine Hydrochloride Injection 2303
Cardene Capsules (0.8%) 2095
Cardene I.V. (0.7%) 2709
Cardizem CD Capsules (Less than 1%) 1506
Cardizem SR Capsules (Less than 1%) 1510
Cardizem Injectable (Less than 1%) 1508
Cardizem Tablets (Less than 1%) 1512
▲ Cardura Tablets (0.5% to 23%) 2186
Ceclor Pulvules & Suspension 1431
Cipro I.V. (1% or less) 595
Cipro I.V. Pharmacy Bulk Package (Less than 1%) 597
Cipro Tablets (Less than 1%) 592
Claritin (2% or fewer patients) 2349
Claritin-D (Less frequent) 2350
Clinoril Tablets (Less than 1%) 1618
Clomid 1514
▲ Clozaril Tablets (More than 5 to 6%) 2252
Cognex Capsules (Frequent) 1901
Cozaar Tablets (Less than 1%) 1628
Cytotec (Infrequent) 2424
Dalmane Capsules (Rare) 2173
Danocrine Capsules 2307
Demadex Tablets and Injection 686
Demerol 2308
Demulen 2428
Depo-Provera Contraceptive Injection (Fewer than 1%) 2602
Deponit NTG Transdermal Delivery System (Uncommon) 2397
▲ Desyrel and Desyrel Dividose (2.8% to 4.5%) 503
Dilacor XR Extended-release Capsules 2018
Dilaudid-HP Injection (Less frequent) 1337
Dilaudid-HP Lyophilized Powder 250 mg (Less frequent) 1337
Dilaudid Tablets and Liquid 1339
Diprivan Injection (Less than 1%) 2833
Diupres Tablets 1650
Dizac (Less frequent) 1809
Dolobid Tablets (Rare) 1654
Duragesic Transdermal System (1% or greater) 1288
Duvoid 2044
DynaCirc Capsules (0.5% to 1%) 2256
Effexor (Infrequent) 2719
Elavil 2838
▲ Eldepryl Tablets (7 of 49 patients) 2550
Endep Tablets 2174
Engerix-B Unit-Dose Vials 2482
Esgic-plus Tablets (Infrequent) 1013
Esimil Tablets 822
Eskalith 2485
Estrace Cream and Tablets 749
Ethmozine Tablets (Less than 2%) 2041
Etrafon 2355
Fioricet Tablets (Infrequent) 2258
Fioricet with Codeine Capsules 2260
Fiorinal with Codeine Capsules (Infrequent) 2262
Flagyl I.V. 2247
Fleet Bisacodyl Enema 1002
Flexeril Tablets (Less than 1%) 1661
Florinef Acetate Tablets 505
Floxin I.V. (Less than 1%) 1571
Floxin Tablets (200 mg, 300 mg, 400 mg) (Less than 1%) 1567
Flumadine Tablets & Syrup (Less than 0.3%) 1015
Fluorescite ◉ 219
Foscavir Injection (Less than 1%) 547
Gamimune N, 5% Immune Globulin Intravenous (Human), 5% 619
Gamimune N, 10% Immune Globulin Intravenous (Human), 10% 621
Glucotrol XL Extended Release Tablets (Less than 3%) 1968
Halcion Tablets 2611
Havrix (Rare) 2489
Hismanal Tablets 1293
Hivid Tablets (Less than 1% to less than 3%) 2121
Hydropres Tablets 1675
▲ Hylorel Tablets (7.8%) 985
▲ Hytrin Capsules (0.5% to 0.6%; 21%) 430
Hyzaar Tablets 1677
Imitrex Injection (Infrequent) 1103
Imitrex Tablets (Rare to infrequent) 1106
Indocin (Less than 1%) 1680
INFeD (Iron Dextran Injection, USP) 2345
Intron A (Less than 5%) 2364
Inversine Tablets 1686
Ismelin Tablets 827
Ismo Tablets (Fewer than 1%) 2738
ISMOTIC 45% w/v Solution (Very rare) ◉ 222
Isoptin Oral Tablets (Less than 1%) 1346
Isoptin SR Tablets (1% or less) 1348
Isopto Carbachol Ophthalmic Solution ◉ 223
Isordil Sublingual Tablets (Uncommon) 2739
Isordil Tembids (Uncommon) 2741
Isordil Titradose Tablets (Uncommon) 2742
Kerlone Tablets (Less than 2%) 2436
Kytril Tablets (Rare) 2492
Lamictal Tablets (Infrequent) 1112
Lariam Tablets (Less than 1%) 2128
Larodopa Tablets (Relatively frequent) 2129
Levlen/Tri-Levlen 651
▲ Levoprome (Among the most important) 1274
Librax Capsules (Few) 2176
Libritabs Tablets (Few instances) 2177
Librium Capsules (Few instances) 2178
Librium Injectable (Isolated instances) 2179
Limbitrol 2180
Lioresal Tablets (Rare) 829
Lippes Loop Intrauterine Double-S 1848
Lodine Capsules and Tablets (Less than 1%) 2743
Lopid Tablets 1917
Lorelco Tablets 1517
Lotensin Tablets (0.1%) 834
Lotensin HCT (0.3% or more) 837
Loxitane 1378
Ludiomil Tablets (Rare) 843
▲ Lupron Depot 3.75 mg (Among most frequent) 2556
Lupron Depot 7.5 mg 2559
Lupron Depot-PED 7.5 mg, 11.25 mg and 15 mg (Less than 2%) 2560
Lupron Injection (Less than 5%) 2555
Luvox Tablets (Frequent) 2544
MS Contin Tablets (Less frequent) 1994
MSIR (Infrequent) 1997
Marcaine Hydrochloride with Epinephrine 1:200,000 (Rare) 2316
Marcaine Hydrochloride Injection (Rare) 2316
Marcaine Spinal (Rare) 2319
Matulane Capsules 2131
Maxair Autohaler 1492
Maxair Inhaler (Less than 1%) 1494
Maxaquin Tablets (Less than 1%) 2440
Mebaral Tablets (Less than 1 in 100) 2322
Mepergan Injection 2753
Methadone Hydrochloride Oral Concentrate 2233
Methadone Hydrochloride Oral Solution & Tablets 2235
Mexitil Capsules (Less than 1% or about 6 in 1,000) 678
Micronor Tablets 1872

(▣ Described in PDR For Nonprescription Drugs) Incidence data in parenthesis; ▲ 3% or more (◉ Described in PDR For Ophthalmology)

Miltown Tablets 2672
Minipress Capsules (1-4%) 1937
Minizide Capsules (Rare) 1938
Modicon 1872
Moduretic Tablets (Less than or equal to 1%) 1705
Monopril Tablets (0.2% to 1.0%) 757
Mumpsvax 1708
Mutamycin 703
Mykrox Tablets 993
Myochrysine Injection 1711
Navane Capsules and Concentrate 2201
Navane Intramuscular 2202
NebuPent for Inhalation Solution (1% or less) 1040
Nembutal Sodium Capsules (Less than 1%) 436
Nembutal Sodium Solution (Less than 1%) 438
Nembutal Sodium Suppositories (Less than 1%) 440
Neurontin Capsules (Infrequent) 1922
Nitro-Bid IV (Uncommon) 1523
Nitro-Bid Ointment (Uncommon) 1524
Nitrodisc (Uncommon to 4%) 2047
Nitro-Dur (nitroglycerin) Transdermal Infusion System (Uncommon) 1326
Nitrostat Tablets 1925
Norflex 1496
Norgesic 1496
Normodyne Injection (Rare) 2377
Normodyne Tablets (Rare) 2379
Norpace (1 to 3%) 2444
Norvasc Tablets (More than 0.1% to 1%) 1940
Nubain Injection (1% or less) 935
Ocupress Ophthalmic Solution, 1% Sterile ⊙ 309
Oramorph SR (Morphine Sulfate Sustained Release Tablets) (Less frequent) 2236
Orap Tablets 1050
Ortho-Cyclen/Ortho-Tri-Cyclen 1858
Ortho Diaphragm Kits—All-Flex Arcing Spring; Ortho Coil Spring; Ortho-White Flat Spring 1865
Ortho Diaphragm Kit-Coil Spring 1865
Ortho-Est 1869
Ortho-Novum 1872
Ortho-Cyclen/Ortho Tri-Cyclen 1858
Ortho-White Diaphragm Kit-Flat Spring (See also Ortho Diaphragm Kits) 1865
PMB 200 and PMB 400 2783
ParaGard T380A Intrauterine Copper Contraceptive 1880
▲ Parlodel (0.7%; 8%) 2281
Paxil Tablets (Frequent) 2505
Penetrex Tablets (Less than 1% but more than or equal to 0.1%) 2031
Peptavlon 2878
Periactin 1724
Permax Tablets (2.1%) 575
Phenergan with Codeine 2777
Phenergan Injection 2773
Phenergan Tablets 2775
Phenergan VC with Codeine 2781
Phenobarbital Elixir and Tablets (Less than 1 in 100 patients) 1469
Phrenilin (Infrequent) 785
Placidyl Capsules (Occasional) 448
Plendil Extended-Release Tablets (0.5% to 1.5%) 527
Pondimin Tablets 2066
PREVACID Delayed-Release Capsules (Less than 1%) 2562
Prinivil Tablets (0.1% to 1.8%) 1733
Prinzide Tablets (0.8% to 0.1%) 1737
Procardia Capsules (Approximately 0.5%; approximately 1 patient in 250) 1971
Procardia XL Extended Release Tablets (Approximately 1 patient in 250; 1% or less) 1972
▲ Proleukin for Injection (3%) 797
ProSom Tablets (Rare) 449
Prostigmin Injectable 1260
Prostigmin Tablets 1261
Prostin E2 Suppository 2634
Provocholine for Inhalation 2140
Prozac Pulvules & Liquid, Oral Solution (Infrequent) 919
Questran Light 769
Questran Powder 770
Quinaglute Dura-Tabs Tablets 649
Quinidex Extentabs 2067
RMS Suppositories 2657
Recombivax HB 1744
Relafen Tablets (Less than 1%) 2510
Retrovir Capsules 1158
Retrovir I.V. Infusion 1163
Retrovir Syrup 1158
Risperdal (0.2%) 1301
Robaxin Injectable 2070
Roferon-A Injection (Less than 0.5%) 2145
▲ Rogaine Topical Solution (3.42%) 2637
Roxanol 2243
Rythmol Tablets–150mg, 225mg, 300mg (0.8 to 2.2%) 1352
Salagen Tablets (Less than 1%) 1489
Sandostatin Injection (Less than 1%) 2292
Sanorex Tablets 2294
Sedapap Tablets 50 mg/650 mg (Infrequent) 1543
Seldane Tablets (Rare) 1536
Seldane-D Extended-Release Tablets (Rare) 1538
Sensorcaine 559
Ser-Ap-Es Tablets 849
Serax Capsules (Rare) 2810
Serax Tablets (Rare) 2810
Serentil 684
Serzone Tablets (Infrequent) 771
Sinemet Tablets 943
Sinemet CR Tablets 944
Solganal Suspension 2388
Soma Compound w/Codeine Tablets (Infrequent or rare) 2676
Soma Compound Tablets (Infrequent or rare) 2675
Soma Tablets 2674
Sorbitrate (Uncommon) 2843
Stadol 775
Supprelin Injection (1% to 3%) 2056
Talacen (Infrequent) 2333
Talwin Injection (Rare) 2334
Talwin Compound (Infrequent) 2335
Talwin Injection 2334
Talwin Nx 2336
Tambocor Tablets (1% to less than 3%) 1497
Taxol (Approximately 1%; rare) 714
Tegison Capsules (Less than 1%) 2154
Tegretol Chewable Tablets 852
Tegretol Suspension 852
Tegretol Tablets 852
Temaril Tablets, Syrup and Spansule Extended-Release Capsules 483
Tenex Tablets (Less frequent) 2074
Tenoretic Tablets 2845
Tenormin Tablets and I.V. Injection 2847
Thorazine 2523
THYREL TRH (A small number of patients) 2873
Timolide Tablets (Less than 1%) 1748
Timoptic in Ocudose (Less frequent) 1753
Timoptic Sterile Ophthalmic Solution (Less frequent) 1751
Timoptic-XE 1755
Tofranil Tablets 856
Tonocard Tablets (Less than 1%) 531
Toprol-XL Tablets (About 1 of 100 patients) 565
Toradol 2159
Trandate (Rare) 1185
▲ Transderm-Nitro Transdermal Therapeutic System (4%) 859
Levlen/Tri-Levlen 651
Ultram Tablets (50 mg) (Less than 1%) 1585
Univasc Tablets (Less than 1%; 0.51%) 2410
Urecholine 1761
Valium Injectable 2182
Vantin for Oral Suspension and Vantin Tablets (Less than 1%) 2646
Vascor (200, 300 and 400 mg) Tablets (0.5 to 2.0%) 1587
Vaseretic Tablets (0.5% to 2.0%) 1765
Vasotec I.V. (0.5%) 1768
Vasotec Tablets (0.5% to 2.2%) 1771
Verelan Capsules (1% or less) 1410
Verelan Capsules (Less than 1%) 2824
Versed Injection (Less than 1%) 2170
Videx Tablets, Powder for Oral Solution, & Pediatric Powder for Oral Solution (Up to 3%) 720
Visken Tablets (2% or fewer patients) 2299
Wellbutrin Tablets (1.2%) 1204
▲ Xanax Tablets (3.1% to 3.8%) 2649
Zaroxolyn Tablets 1000
Zerit Capsules (Fewer than 1% to 1%) 729
Zestoretic (0.1 to 0.8%) 2850
Zestril Tablets (0.1% to 1.8%) 2854
Ziac 1415
Zofran Injection (Rare) 1214
Zoloft Tablets (Infrequent) 2217
Zosyn (1.0% or less) 1419
Zosyn Pharmacy Bulk Package (1.0% or less) 1422

Synovia, immunological destruction

Solganal Suspension 2388

Synovitis

Cuprimine Capsules (Some patients) 1630
Depen Titratable Tablets 2662
Foscavir Injection (Less than 1%) 547
Lopid Tablets 1917

Systemic lupus erythematosus (see under Lupus erythematosus, systemic)

SGOT changes

Atamet 572
Atgam Sterile Solution 2581
Bumex (0.6%) 2093
Doral Tablets (1.3%) 2664
▲ Emcyt Capsules (33 to 34%) 1953
Humegon (Occasional) 1824
Paraflex Caplets 1580
Parafon Forte DSC Caplets 1581
▲ Roferon-A Injection (42% to 46%) 2145
Sinemet Tablets 943
Sinemet CR Tablets 944

SGOT elevation

Accutane Capsules 2076
Adalat CC (Rare) 589
Children's Advil Suspension (Less than 1%) 2692
Ambien Tablets (Rare) 2416
Amoxil 2464
Anaprox/Naprosyn (Less than 1%) 2117
Ancef Injection 2465
Asacol Delayed-Release Tablets 1979
Atamet 572
Atromid-S Capsules 2701
Augmentin 2468
Axid Pulvules (Less common) 1427
Azactam for Injection (Less than 1%) 734
▲ Betaseron for SC Injection (4%) 658
Biaxin (Less than 1%) 405
BuSpar (Infrequent) 737
Calan SR Caplets 2422
Calan Tablets 2419
Cardizem CD Capsules (Less than 1%) 1506
Cardizem SR Capsules (Less than 1%) 1510
Cardizem Injectable (Less than 1%) 1508
Cardizem Tablets (Less than 1%) 1512
Cataflam (About 2%) 816
Ceclor Pulvules & Suspension (1 in 40) 1431
Cefizox for Intramuscular or Intravenous Use (Greater than 1% but less than 5%) 1034
Cefotan (1 in 300) 2829
Ceftin (2.0%) 1078
Cefzil Tablets and Oral Suspension (2%) 746
▲ CellCept Capsules (More than or equal to 3%) 2099
Ceptaz (One in 16) 1081
▲ CHEMET (succimer) Capsules (4.2 to 10.4%) 1545
Chibroxin Sterile Ophthalmic Solution (With oral form) 1617
▲ Cipro I.V. (Among most frequent) 595
▲ Cipro I.V. Pharmacy Bulk Package (Among most frequent) 597
Cipro Tablets (1.7%) 592
Claforan Sterile and Injection (Less than 1%) 1235
Colestid Tablets (One or more occasions) 2591
Cordarone Intravenous (Common) 2715
Cordarone Tablets 2712
Cytovene (1% or less) 2103
Dalgan Injection (Less than 1%) 538
Dalmane Capsules (Rare) 2173
Daypro Caplets (Under 1% of patients) 2426
Deltasone Tablets 2595
Demser Capsules (Rare) 1649
Depakene (Frequent) 413
Depakote Tablets (Frequent) 415
Depo-Medrol Single-Dose Vial 2600
Depo-Medrol Sterile Aqueous Suspension 2597
Diflucan Injection, Tablets, and Oral Suspension 2194
Dilacor XR Extended-release Capsules (Rare) 2018
Dipentum Capsules (Rare) 1951
Duricef 748
EC-Naprosyn Delayed-Release Tablets (Less than 1%) 2117
Effexor (Infrequent) 2719
Elspar 1659
Eulexin Capsules 2358
Felbatol (Frequent) 2666
Feldene Capsules (Less than 1%) 1965
Floxin I.V. (More than or equal to 1%) 1571
Floxin Tablets (200 mg, 300 mg, 400 mg) (More than or equal to 1.0%) 1567
▲ Fortaz (1 in 16) 1100
Foscavir Injection (Between 1% and 5%) 547
Fungizone Intravenous 506
Garamycin Injectable 2360
Geocillin Tablets 2199
Glucotrol Tablets (Occasional) 1967
Glucotrol XL Extended Release Tablets (Occasional) 1968
Heparin Lock Flush Solution 2725
Heparin Sodium Injection 2726
Heparin Sodium Injection, USP, Sterile Solution 2615
▲ Heparin Sodium Vials (A high percentage of patients) 1441
Hivid Tablets (Less than 1% to less than 3%) 2121
Imdur (Less than or equal to 5%) 1323
Imuran 1110
▲ Intron A (Up to 41% of patients) 2364
Isoptin Oral Tablets 1346
Isoptin SR Tablets 1348
Keflex Pulvules & Oral Suspension 914
Keftab Tablets 915
▲ Kefurox Vials, Faspak & ADD-Vantage (1 in 25) 1454
Kefzol Vials, Faspak & ADD-Vantage (Rare) 1456
Kerlone Tablets (Less than 2%) 2436
Kytril Injection (2.8%) 2490
▲ Kytril Tablets (5%) 2492
Lamprene Capsules (Less than 1%) 828
Larodopa Tablets (Rare) 2129
Leukine for IV Infusion 1271
Lioresal Tablets 829
Lopid Tablets (Occasional) 1917
Lorabid Suspension and Pulvules 1459
Lotensin Tablets (Scattered incidents) 834
Lotensin HCT 837
Lovenox Injection (Up to 4% of patients) 2020
Loxitane 1378
Lupron Depot 3.75 mg (Twice normal limit—one patient) 2556
▲ Lupron Depot 7.5 mg (5.4%) 2559
▲ Macrobid Capsules (1% to 5%) 1988
Macrodantin Capsules 1989
Mandol Vials, Faspak & ADD-Vantage 1461
Marinol (Dronabinol) Capsules (Less than 1%) 2231
Maxaquin Tablets 2440
Medrol 2621
Mefoxin 1691
Mefoxin Premixed Intravenous Solution 1694
▲ Mepron Suspension (4%) 1135
Mezlin 601
Mezlin Pharmacy Bulk Package 604
Mithracin 607
Monocid Injection (1.6%) 2497
Children's Motrin Ibuprofen Oral Suspension 1546
Motrin Tablets (Less than 1%) 2625
Motrin Ibuprofen Suspension, Oral Drops, Chewable Tablets, Caplets (Less than 1%) 1546
▲ Mycelex Troches (About 15%) 608
▲ Mycobutin Capsules (7%) 1957
Nalfon 200 Pulvules & Nalfon Tablets (Less than 1%) 917
Anaprox/Naprosyn (Less than 1%) 2117
▲ Navelbine Injection (1% to 54%) 1145
Nebcin Vials, Hyporets & ADD-Vantage 1464
▲ Neutrexin (13.8%) 2572
▲ Nolvadex Tablets (4.8%) 2841
Noroxin Tablets (0.4% to 1.6%) 1715
Noroxin Tablets (0.4% to 1.6%) 2048
Nydrazid Injection 508

(▣ Described in PDR For Nonprescription Drugs) Incidence data in parenthesis; ▲ 3% or more (⊙ Described in PDR For Ophthalmology)

1421 **Side Effects Index** **Tachycardia**

Omnipen Capsules 2764
Omnipen for Oral Suspension 2765
▲ Oncaspar (Greater than 1% but less than 5%) 2028
Orthoclone OKT3 Sterile Solution .. 1837
Orudis Capsules 2766
Oruvail Capsules 2766
Oxandrin 2862
▲ Paraplatin for Injection (15% to 23%) 705
Parlodel 2281
Paxil Tablets (Rare) 2505
Penetrex Tablets (Less than 1% but more than or equal to 0.1%) 2031
Pentasa (Less than 1%) 1527
Pipracil (Less frequent) 1390
Platinol 708
Platinol-AQ Injection 710
Pravachol 765
PREVACID Delayed-Release Capsules (Less than 1%) 2562
Prilosec Delayed-Release Capsules (Rare) 529
Primaxin I.M. 1727
Primaxin I.V. 1729
Procan SR Tablets 1926
Procardia Capsules (Rare) 1971
Procardia XL Extended Release Tablets (Rare) 1972
▲ Prograf (Greater than 3%) 1042
ProSom Tablets (Rare) 449
Revex (0.3%) 1811
Rifamate Capsules 1530
Rifater 1532
Risperdal (Infrequent) 1301
Rocaltrol Capsules 2141
▲ Rocephin Injectable Vials, ADD-Vantage, Galaxy Container (3.1%) 2142
Sectral Capsules 2807
Seromycin Pulvules 1476
Serzone Tablets (Infrequent) 771
Sinemet Tablets 943
Solu-Cortef Sterile Powder 2641
Solu-Medrol Sterile Powder 2643
Spectrobid Tablets 2206
Suprax (Less than 2%) 1399
Synarel Nasal Solution for Endometriosis 2152
▲ Taxol (19%) 714
▲ Tazicef for Injection (1 in 16 patients) 2519
▲ Tazidime Vials, Faspak & ADD-Vantage (1 in 16) 1478
▲ Tegison Capsules (18%) 2154
Ticar for Injection 2526
Timentin for Injection 2528
Tobramycin Sulfate Injection 968
Tornalate Solution for Inhalation, 0.2% (Less than 1%) 956
Tornalate Metered Dose Inhaler (Rare) 957
Unasyn 2212
Vantin for Oral Suspension and Vantin Tablets 2646
Verelan Capsules 1410
Verelan Capsules 2824
▲ Videx Tablets, Powder for Oral Solution, & Pediatric Powder for Oral Solution (7% to 9%) 720
Voltaren Tablets (About 2%) 861
Winstrol Tablets 2337
Xanax Tablets (Less than 1% to 3.2%) 2649
▲ Zanosar Sterile Powder (A number of patients) 2653
Zebeta Tablets (One to two times normal) 1413
Zefazone 2654
▲ Zerit Capsules (5% to 8%) 729
▲ Zinacef (1 in 25 patients) 1211
Zithromax (1% to 2%) 1944
Zocor Tablets 1775
▲ Zofran Injection (Approximately 5% of patients) 1214
Zofran Tablets (Approximately 1% to 2%) 1217
Zoladex (Less than 1% of all patients) 2858
Zoloft Tablets (Infrequent) 2217
Zosyn 1419
Zosyn Pharmacy Bulk Package 1422
Zyloprim Tablets (Less than 1%) 1226

SGPT changes

Atamet 572
Atgam Sterile Solution 2581
Bumex (0.5%) 2093
Cataflam (About 2%) 816
Humegon (Occasional) 1824
Paraflex Caplets 1580
Parafon Forte DSC Caplets 1581
Sinemet Tablets 943
Sinemet CR Tablets 944
Voltaren Tablets (About 2%) 861

SGPT elevation

Accutane Capsules 2076
Adalat CC (Rare) 589
Children's Advil Suspension (Less than 1%) 2692
Ambien Tablets (Infrequent) 2416
Anaprox/Naprosyn (Less than 1%) 2117
Ancef Injection 2465
Asacol Delayed-Release Tablets 1979
Atamet 572
Atromid-S Capsules 2701
Augmentin 2468
Axid Pulvules (Less common) 1427
Azactam for Injection (Less than 1%) 734
▲ Betaseron for SC Injection (19%) .. 658
Biaxin (Less than 1%) 405
BuSpar (Infrequent) 737
Calan SR Caplets 2422
Calan Tablets 2419
Cardizem CD Capsules (Less than 1%) 1506
Cardizem SR Capsules (Less than 1%) 1510
Cardizem Injectable 1508
Cardizem Tablets (Less than 1%) .. 1512
Ceclor Pulvules & Suspension (1 in 40) 1431
Cefizox for Intramuscular or Intravenous Use (Greater than 1% but less than 5%) 1034
Cefotan (1 in 150) 2829
Ceftin (1.6%) 1078
Cefzil Tablets and Oral Suspension (2%) 746
▲ CellCept Capsules (More than or equal to 3%) 2099
Ceptaz (One in 15) 1081
▲ CHEMET (succimer) Capsules (4.2 to 10.4%) 1545
Chibroxin Sterile Ophthalmic Solution (With oral form) 1617
▲ Cipro I.V. (Among most frequent) .. 595
▲ Cipro I.V. Pharmacy Bulk Package (Among most frequent) 597
Cipro Tablets (1.9%) 592
Claforan Sterile and Injection (Less than 1%) 1235
Colestid Tablets (One or more occasions) 2591
Cordarone Intravenous (Common).. 2715
Cordarone Tablets 2712
Cytovene (1% or less) 2103
Dalmane Capsules (Rare) 2173
Deltasone Tablets 2595
Depakene (Frequent) 413
Depakote Tablets (Frequent) 415
Depo-Medrol Single-Dose Vial 2600
Depo-Medrol Sterile Aqueous Suspension 2597
Dilacor XR Extended-release Capsules (Rare) 2018
Dipentum Capsules (Rare) 1951
Doral Tablets (Less than 1%) 2664
Duricef 748
EC-Naprosyn Delayed-Release Tablets (Less than 1%) 2117
Effexor (Rare) 2719
Elspar 1659
Eulexin Capsules 2358
▲ Felbatol (3.5% to 5.2%) 2666
Feldene Capsules (Less than 1%) .. 1965
Floxin I.V. (More than or equal to 1%) 1571
Floxin Tablets (200 mg, 300 mg, 400 mg) (More than or equal to 1.0%) 1567
▲ Fortaz (1 in 15) 1100
Foscavir Injection (Between 1% and 5%) 547
Fungizone Intravenous 506
Garamycin Injectable 2360
Heparin Lock Flush Solution 2725
Heparin Sodium Injection 2726
Heparin Sodium Injection, USP, Sterile Solution 2615
▲ Heparin Sodium Vials (A high percentage of patients) 1441
Hivid Tablets (Less than 1% to less than 3%) 2121
Imdur (Less than or equal to 5%) .. 1323
Imuran 1110
▲ Intron A (Up to 15% of patients) 2364
Isoptin Oral Tablets 1346
Isoptin SR Tablets 1348
Keflex Pulvules & Oral Suspension 914
Keftab Tablets 915
▲ Kefurox Vials, Faspak & ADD-Vantage (1 in 25) 1454
Kefzol Vials, Faspak & ADD-Vantage (Rare) 1456
Kerlone Tablets (Less than 2%) 2436
▲ Kytril Injection (3.3%) 2490
▲ Kytril Tablets (6%) 2492
Larodopa Tablets (Rare) 2129
Leukine for IV Infusion 1271
Lopid Tablets (Occasional) 1917
Lorabid Suspension and Pulvules 1459
Lotensin Tablets (Scattered incidents) 834
Lotensin HCT 837
Lovenox Injection (Up to 4% of patients) 2020
Loxitane 1378
▲ Macrobid Capsules (1% to 5%) 1988
Macrodantin Capsules 1989
Mandol Vials, Faspak & ADD-Vantage 1461
Marinol (Dronabinol) Capsules (Less than 1%) 2231
Maxaquin Tablets 2440
Medrol 2621
Mefoxin 1691
Mefoxin Premixed Intravenous Solution 1694
▲ Mepron Suspension (6%) 1135
Mezlin 601
Mezlin Pharmacy Bulk Package 604
Mithracin 607
Monocid Injection (1.6%) 2497
Children's Motrin Ibuprofen Oral Suspension 1546
Motrin Tablets (Less than 1%) 2625
Motrin Ibuprofen Suspension, Oral Drops, Chewable Tablets, Caplets (Less than 1%) 1546
▲ Mycobutin Capsules (9%) 1957
Anaprox/Naprosyn (Less than 1%) 2117
Nebcin Vials, Hyporets & ADD-Vantage 1464
▲ Neutrexin (11.0%) 2572
Nimotop Capsules (0.2%; rare) 610
Noroxin Tablets (1.4%) 1715
Noroxin Tablets (1.4%) 2048
Nydrazid Injection 508
▲ Oncaspar (Greater than 5%) 2028
Orthoclone OKT3 Sterile Solution .. 1837
Orudis Capsules 2766
Oruvail Capsules 2766
Parlodel 2281
Paxil Tablets (Rare) 2505
Penetrex Tablets (Less than 1% but more than or equal to 0.1%) 2031
Pentasa (Less than 1%) 1527
Pipracil (Less frequent) 1390
Plendil Extended-Release Tablets (0.5% to 1.5%) 527
Pravachol 765
PREVACID Delayed-Release Capsules (Less than 1%) 2562
Prilosec Delayed-Release Capsules (Rare) 529
Primaxin I.M. 1727
Primaxin I.V. 1729
Procan SR Tablets 1926
Procardia Capsules (Rare) 1971
Procardia XL Extended Release Tablets (Rare) 1972
Proglycem Capsules 580
▲ Prograf (Greater than 3%) 1042
▲ ReVia Tablets (Five of 26 recipients) 940
Rifamate Capsules 1530
Rifater 1532
Risperdal (Infrequent) 1301
Rocaltrol Capsules 2141
▲ Rocephin Injectable Vials, ADD-Vantage, Galaxy Container (3.3%) 2142
Sectral Capsules 2807
Seromycin Pulvules 1476
Serzone Tablets (Infrequent) 771
Sinemet Tablets 943
Solu-Cortef Sterile Powder 2641
Solu-Medrol Sterile Powder 2643
Suprax (Less than 2%) 1399
Synarel Nasal Solution for Endometriosis 2152
▲ Tazicef for Injection (1 in 15 patients) 2519
▲ Tazidime Vials, Faspak & ADD-Vantage (1 in 15) 1478
▲ Tegison Capsules (23%) 2154
Ticar for Injection 2526
▲ Tilade (3.3%) 996
Timentin for Injection 2528
Tobramycin Sulfate Injection 968
Tornalate Solution for Inhalation, 0.2% (Less than 1%) 956
Trasylol 613
Trobicin Sterile Powder 2645
Unasyn 2212
Vantin for Oral Suspension and Vantin Tablets 2646
Vascor (200, 300 and 400 mg) Tablets (0.5 to 2.0%) 1587
Verelan Capsules 1410
Verelan Capsules 2824
▲ Videx Tablets, Powder for Oral Solution, & Pediatric Powder for Oral Solution (6% to 9%) 720
Zantac 1209
Zantac Injection 1207
Zantac Syrup 1209
Zebeta Tablets (One to two times normal) 1413
Zefazone 2654
▲ Zerit Capsules (10% to 12%) 729
▲ Zinacef (1 in 25 patients) 1211
Zithromax (1% to 2%) 1944
Zocor Tablets 1775
▲ Zofran Injection (Approximately 5% of patients) 1214
Zofran Tablets (Approximately 1% to 2%) 1217
Zoladex (Less than 1% of all patients) 2858
Zoloft Tablets (Infrequent) 2217
Zosyn 1419
Zosyn Pharmacy Bulk Package 1422
Zyloprim Tablets (Less than 1%) 1226

SIADH secretion syndrome

(see under ADH syndrome, inappropriate)

SLE-like syndrome

(see under Lupus erythematosus, systemic)

ST section changes

(see under EKG changes, ST section)

S_3 gallop

(see under Ventricular gallop)

T

T-wave flattening

(see under EKG changes, T-wave)

Tachyarrhythmia

Actimmune (Rare) 1056
Isuprel Hydrochloride Injection 1:5000 2311
Nicorette 2458

Tachyarrhythmia, ventricular

Seldane Tablets (Rare) 1536
Seldane-D Extended-Release Tablets (Rare) 1538

Tachyarrhythmias, supraventricular

Claritin (Rare) 2349
Lanoxicaps 1117
Lanoxin Elixir Pediatric 1120
Lanoxin Injection 1123
Lanoxin Injection Pediatric 1126
Lanoxin Tablets 1128

Tachycardia

Abbokinase 403
Abbokinase Open-Cath 405
Accupril Tablets (0.5% to 1.0%) .. 1893
Accutane Capsules (Less than 1%) 2076
Actifed with Codeine Cough Syrup.. 1067
Adalat CC (Less than 1.0%) 589
Adipex-P Tablets and Capsules 1048
AeroBid Inhaler System (1-3%) 1005
Aerobid-M Inhaler System (1-3%).. 1005
Airet Solution for Inhalation (1%) .. 452
▲ Alfenta Injection (12%) 1286
Alkeran for Injection (In some patients) 1070
Alupent (Less than 1%) 669
Ambien Tablets (Infrequent) 2416
▲ Anafranil Capsules (2% to 4%) 803
Anatuss LA Tablets 1542
Anectine 1073
Apresazide Capsules (Common) 808
Apresoline Hydrochloride Tablets (Common) 809
▲ Aredia for Injection (Up to 6%) 810

(▣ Described in PDR For Nonprescription Drugs) Incidence data in parenthesis; ▲ 3% or more (◉ Described in PDR For Ophthalmology)

Tachycardia | Side Effects Index | 1422

Arfonad Ampuls 2080
Artane 1368
Asendin Tablets (Less than 1%) 1369
▲ Atgam Sterile Solution (Less than 1% to less than 5%) 2581
Atrohist Plus Tablets 454
Atrovent Inhalation Aerosol (Less frequent) 671
Atrovent Inhalation Solution (Less than 3%) 673
Azo Gantrisin Tablets 2081
Bellergal-S Tablets (Rare) 2250
Benadryl Capsules 1898
Benadryl Injection 1898
Bentyl 1501
▲ Betaseron for SC Injection (6%) 658
Biphetamine Capsules 983
Bontril Slow-Release Capsules 781
▲ Brethaire Inhaler (About 5 per 100) 813
Brethine Ampuls (1.3 to 1.5%) 815
Bronkometer Aerosol 2302
Bronkosol Solution 2302
Brontex 1981
Buprenex Injectable (Less than 1%) 2006
BuSpar (1%) 737
Cafergot 2251
Capoten (Approximately 1 of 100 patients) 739
Capozide (Approximately 1 of 1000 patients) 742
Carbocaine Hydrochloride Injection 2303
Cardene Capsules (0.8-3.4%) 2095
▲ Cardene I.V. (3.5%) 2709
Cardizem CD Capsules (Less than 1%) 1506
Cardizem SR Capsules (Less than 1%) 1510
Cardizem Injectable 1508
Cardizem Tablets (Less than 1%) 1512
Cardura Tablets (0.3% to 0.9%) 2186
Cartrol Tablets 410
Cataflam (Less than 1%) 816
Catapres Tablets (About 5 in 1,000 patients) 674
Catapres-TTS (Less frequent) 675
Ceftin (Less than 1% but more than 0.1%) 1078
▲ CellCept Capsules (More than or equal to 3%) 2099
Cipro I.V. (1% or less) 595
Cipro I.V. Pharmacy Bulk Package (Less than 1%) 597
Claritin (2% or fewer patients) 2349
Claritin-D (Less frequent) 2350
Clinoril Tablets (Less than 1 in 100) 1618
Clomid 1514
▲ Clozaril Tablets (More than 5 to 25%) 2252
Cogentin 1621
Cognex Capsules (Infrequent) 1901
Colestid Tablets (Infrequent) 2591
Combipres Tablets (About 5 in 1,000) 677
Compazine 2470
Cozaar Tablets (Less than 1%) 1628
Cystospaz 1963
Cytadren Tablets (1 in 40) 819
D.A. Chewable Tablets 951
D.H.E. 45 Injection 2255
Dantrium Capsules (Less frequent) 1982
Dapsone Tablets USP 1284
Deconamine Chewable Tablets 1320
Deconamine CX Cough and Cold Liquid and Tablets 1319
Deconamine 1320
Deconsal 454
Demadex Tablets and Injection 686
Demerol 2308
Depakote Tablets (Greater than 1% but not more than 5%) 415
Depo-Provera Contraceptive Injection (Fewer than 1%) 2602
Desferal Vials 820
Desoxyn Gradumet Tablets 419
Desyrel and Desyrel Dividose (Up to 7%) 503
Dexedrine 2474
DextroStat Dextroamphetamine Tablets 2036
Dibenzyline Capsules 2476
Didrex Tablets 2607
Dilacor XR Extended-release Capsules (Infrequent) 2018
Dilaudid-HP Injection (Less frequent) 1337
Dilaudid-HP Lyophilized Powder 250 mg (Less frequent) 1337
Dilaudid Tablets and Liquid 1339
Dipentum Capsules (Rare) 1951
Diprivan Injection (Less than 1%) 2833
Ditropan 1516
Donnagel Liquid and Donnagel Chewable Tablets (Rare) ▣ 879
Donnatal 2060
Donnatal Extentabs 2061
Donnatal Tablets 2060
Dura-Tap/PD Capsules 2867
Dura-Vent/DA Tablets 953
Dura-Vent Tablets 952
Dyazide 2479
DynaCirc Capsules 2256
Effexor (2%) 2719
Elavil 2838
Eldepryl Tablets 2550
Empirin with Codeine Tablets 1093
Endep Tablets 2174
Engerix-B Unit-Dose Vials 2482
Entex PSE Tablets 1987
EpiPen Jr. 790
Epogen for Injection (0.31%) 489
Esgic-plus Tablets (Infrequent) 1013
Esidrix Tablets 821
Etrafon 2355
Factrel (Rare) 2877
Fastin Capsules 2488
Fedahist Gyrocaps 2401
Fedahist Timecaps 2401
Felbatol (Frequent) 2666
Fioricet Tablets (Infrequent) 2258
Fioricet with Codeine Capsules (Infrequent) 2260
Fiorinal with Codeine Capsules (Infrequent) 2262
Flexeril Tablets (Less than 1%) 1661
Floxin I.V. 1571
Floxin Tablets (200 mg, 300 mg, 400 mg) 1567
Flumadine Tablets & Syrup (Less than 0.3%) 1015
Gamimune N, 5% Immune Globulin Intravenous (Human), 5% (One patient) 619
Gamimune N, 10% Immune Globulin Intravenous (Human), 10% (One patient) 621
Ganite 2533
Guaifed 1787
Guaimax-D Tablets 792
Habitrol Nicotine Transdermal System (Occasionally) 865
Halcion Tablets (0.9% to 0.5%) 2611
Haldol Decanoate 1577
Haldol Injection, Tablets and Concentrate 1575
Hivid Tablets (Less than 1% to less than 3%) 2121
Humegon 1824
Hycomine Compound Tablets 932
Hycomine 931
Hytrin Capsules (1.9%) 430
Hyzaar Tablets 1677
Imdur (Less than or equal to 5%) 1323
Imitrex Injection (Infrequent) 1103
Imitrex Tablets (Infrequent) 1106
Inapsine Injection 1296
Indocin Capsules (Less than 1%) 1680
Indocin I.V. (Less than 1%) 1684
Indocin (Less than 1%) 1680
INFeD (Iron Dextran Injection, USP) 2345
Intron A (Less than 5%) 2364
Ionamin Capsules 990
Isoetharine Inhalation Solution, USP, Arm-a-Med 551
Isoptin Injectable (1.0%) 1344
Isuprel Hydrochloride Injection 1:5000 2311
Isuprel Hydrochloride Solution 1:200 & 1:100 2313
Isuprel Mistometer 2312
K-Phos Neutral Tablets 639
Kutrase Capsules 2402
Kytril Injection (Rare) 2490
Lamictal Tablets (Infrequent) 1112
Lasix Injection, Oral Solution and Tablets 1240
Lescol Capsules 2267
▲ Leustatin (6%) 1834
Levbid Extended-Release Tablets (No incidence data in labeling) 2405
Levoprome 1274
Levsin/Levsinex/Levbid 2405
Librium Injectable 2179
Limbitrol 2180
Lomotil 2439
Lotensin HCT (0.3% or more) 837
Loxitane 1378
Lozol Tablets 2022
Ludiomil Tablets (Rare) 843
Lufyllin & Lufyllin-400 Tablets 2670
Lufyllin-GG Elixir & Tablets 2671
▲ Lupron Depot 3.75 mg (Among most frequent; less than 5%) 2556
Lutrepulse for Injection 980
Luvox Tablets (Frequent) 2544
MS Contin Tablets (Less frequent) 1994
MSIR (Infrequent) 1997
Marax Tablets & DF Syrup 2200
Marcaine Hydrochloride with Epinephrine 1:200,000 (Rare) 2316
Marcaine Hydrochloride Injection (Rare) 2316
Marcaine Spinal (Rare) 2319
Marinol (Dronabinol) Capsules (1%) 2231
Matulane Capsules 2131
Maxair Autohaler (1.2% to 1.3%) 1492
Maxair Inhaler (1.2%) 1494
Maxaquin Tablets (Less than 1%) 2440
Maxzide 1380
Mellaril 2269
Mepergan Injection 2753
▲ Metaproterenol Sulfate Inhalation Solution, USP, Arm-a-Med (About 1 in 7 patients) 552
Methadone Hydrochloride Oral Concentrate 2233
Metubine Iodide Vials 916
Miacalcin Nasal Spray (Less than 1%) 2275
Miltown Tablets 2672
Minipress Capsules (Less than 1%) 1937
Minizide Capsules (Rare) 1938
Mivacron (Less than 1%) 1138
Moban Tablets and Concentrate 1048
Moduretic Tablets (Less than or equal to 1%) 1705
Monoket (Fewer than 1%) 2406
Monopril Tablets (0.4% to 1.0%) 757
Motofen Tablets 784
Motrin Tablets (Less than 1%) 2625
Nalfon 200 Pulvules & Nalfon Tablets (Less than 1%) 917
Narcan Injection 934
Nardil (Less frequent) 1920
Navane Capsules and Concentrate 2201
Navane Intramuscular 2202
NebuPent for Inhalation Solution (1% or less) 1040
Nescaine/Nescaine MPF 554
Neupogen for Injection 495
Neurontin Capsules (Infrequent) 1922
Nicorette 2458
Nimotop Capsules (Up to 1.4%) 610
Norcuron (Rare) 1826
Norflex 1496
Norgesic 1496
Norisodrine with Calcium Iodide Syrup 442
Normodyne Injection 2377
Normodyne Tablets 2379
Norpramin Tablets 1526
Norvasc Tablets (More than 0.1% to 1%) 1940
Novahistine DMX ▣ 822
Novahistine Elixir ▣ 823
Novantrone 1279
Nubain Injection (1% or less) 935
▲ Oncaspar (Greater than 1% but less than 5%) 2028
Oramorph SR (Morphine Sulfate Sustained Release Tablets) (Less frequent) 2236
Orap Tablets 1050
Oretic Tablets 443
Orlamm 2239
Ornade Spansule Capsules 2502
▲ Orthoclone OKT3 Sterile Solution (10%) 1837
Orudis Capsules (Less than 1%) 2766
Oruvail Capsules (Less than 1%) 2766
PBZ Tablets 845
PBZ-SR Tablets 844
PMB 200 and PMB 400 2783
Pamelor 2280
Paremyd ⊙ 247
Parnate Tablets 2503
Paxil Tablets (Frequent) 2505
Penetrex Tablets (Less than 1% but more than or equal to 0.1%) 2031
Peptavlon 2878
Pergonal (menotropins for injection, USP) 2448
Periactin 1724
Permax Tablets (Infrequent) 575
Phenergan with Codeine 2777
Phenergan Injection 2773
Phenergan Tablets 2775
Phenergan VC with Codeine 2781
Phrenilin (Infrequent) 785
Pilocar (Extremely rare) ⊙ 268
Platinol (Occasional) 708
Platinol-AQ Injection (Occasional) 710
Plendil Extended-Release Tablets (0.5% to 1.5%) 527
Prelu-2 Timed Release Capsules 681
Prilosec Delayed-Release Capsules (Less than 1%) 529
Primaxin I.M. 1727
Primaxin I.V. (Less than 0.2%) 1729
Prinzide Tablets 1737
Priscoline Hydrochloride Ampuls 845
Pro-Banthīne Tablets 2052
Procardia XL Extended Release Tablets (1% or less) 1972
Procrit for Injection (0.31%) 1841
Proglycem (Common) 580
▲ Prograf (Greater than 3%) 1042
Prolastin Alpha$_1$-Proteinase Inhibitor (Human) (Occasional) 635
Prolixin 509
PROPINE with C CAP Compliance Cap ⊙ 253
Propulsid (Rare) 1300
Prostep (nicotine transdermal system) (Occasional) 1394
Prostigmin Injectable 1260
Prostigmin Tablets 1261
▲ Prostin VR Pediatric Sterile Solution (About 3%) 2635
Protopam Chloride for Injection 2806
▲ Proventil Inhalation Aerosol (10%) 2382
Proventil Inhalation Solution 0.083% (1%) 2384
▲ Proventil Repetabs Tablets (5%) 2386
Proventil Solution for Inhalation 0.5% (1%) 2383
Proventil Syrup (1 of 100 patients; children 2 to 6 years, 2%) 2385
▲ Proventil Tablets (5%) 2386
Prozac Pulvules & Liquid, Oral Solution (Infrequent) 919
Quadrinal Tablets 1350
Quarzan Capsules 2181
Quibron 2053
Recombivax HB 1744
Regitine 846
Respbid Tablets 682
ReVia Tablets (Less than 1%) 940
▲ Revex (5%) 1811
▲ Risperdal (3% to 5%) 1301
Ritalin 848
Robinul Forte Tablets 2072
Robinul Injectable 2072
Robinul Tablets 2072
Rogaine Topical Solution 2637
Romazicon (Less than 1%) 2147
Salagen Tablets (2%) 1489
Sandimmune 2286
Sandostatin Injection (Less than 1%) 2292
▲ Sanorex Tablets (Among most common) 2294
Sansert Tablets 2295
Sedapap Tablets 50 mg/650 mg (Infrequent) 1543
Seldane-D Extended-Release Tablets 1538
Semprex-D Capsules 463
Semprex-D Capsules 1167
Sensorcaine (Rare) 559
Ser-Ap-Es Tablets 849
Serentil 684
Serevent Inhalation Aerosol (1% to 3%) 1176
Serzone Tablets (Infrequent) 771
Sinequan (Occasional) 2205
Slo-bid Gyrocaps 2033
Soma Compound w/Codeine Tablets 2676
Soma Compound Tablets 2675
Soma Tablets 2674
Stadol (Infrequent) 775
Stelazine 2514
Stimate, (desmopressin acetate) Nasal Spray, 1.5 mg/mL 525
Sufenta Injection (0.3% to 1%) 1309
Supprelin Injection (1% to 3%) 2056
Suprane (Greater than 1%) 1813
Surmontil Capsules 2811
Survanta Beractant Intratracheal Suspension 2226
Syn-Rx Tablets 465
Syn-Rx DM Tablets 466
Tagamet (Rare) 2516
Talacen (Infrequent) 2333
Talwin Injection (Rare) 2334
Talwin Compound (Infrequent) 2335
Talwin Injection 2334

(▣ Described in PDR For Nonprescription Drugs) Incidence data in parenthesis; ▲ 3% or more (⊙ Described in PDR For Ophthalmology)

1423 **Side Effects Index** **Taste, altered**

Talwin Nx 2336
Tambocor Tablets (1% to less than 3%) 1497
Tavist Syrup 2297
Tavist Tablets 2298
Taxol (2%) 714
Temaril Tablets, Syrup and Spansule Extended-Release Capsules 483
Tenex Tablets (Less frequent) 2074
Tenoretic Tablets 2845
Tenormin Tablets and I.V. Injection 2847
Thalitone (Common) 1245
Theo-24 Extended Release Capsules 2568
Theo-Dur Extended-Release Tablets 1327
Theo-X Extended-Release Tablets 788
Thorazine 2523
Tofranil Ampuls 854
Tofranil Tablets 856
Tofranil-PM Capsules 857
▲ Tonocard Tablets (3.2%) 531
▲ Tornalate Solution for Inhalation, 0.2% (3.7%) 956
Tornalate Metered Dose Inhaler (Less than 1%) 957
Tracrium Injection 1183
Trasylol (2%) 613
Trental Tablets (Rare) 1244
Triaminic Cold Tablets ▣ 790
Triavil Tablets 1757
Trilafon 2389
Trinalin Repetabs Tablets 1330
▲ Triostat Injection (3%) 2530
Tussend 1783
Tussend Expectorant 1785
Ultram Tablets (50 mg) (Less than 1%) 1585
Uni-Dur Extended-Release Tablets 1331
Uniphyl 400 mg Tablets 2001
Urispas Tablets 2532
Uroqid-Acid No. 2 Tablets 640
Vaseretic Tablets (0.5% to 2.0%) 1765
▲ Ventolin Inhalation Aerosol and Refill (10 in 100 patients) 1197
Ventolin Inhalation Solution (1%) 1198
Ventolin Nebules Inhalation Solution (1%) 1199
Ventolin Syrup (1 of 100 patients; 2% in children) 1202
▲ Ventolin Tablets (5 of 100 patients) 1203
VePesid Capsules and Injection (0.7% to 2%) 718
Versed Injection (Less than 1%) 2170
Videx Tablets, Powder for Oral Solution, & Pediatric Powder for Oral Solution (Less than 1%) 720
Virazole (Infrequent) 1264
Visken Tablets (2% or fewer patients) 2299
Vivactil Tablets 1774
Volmax Extended-Release Tablets (2.7%) 1788
Voltaren Tablets (Less than 1%) 861
▲ Vumon (Approximately 5%) 727
▲ Wellbutrin Tablets (10.8%) 1204
Wigraine Tablets & Suppositories 1829
▲ Xanax Tablets (7.7% to 15.4%) 2649
Yocon 1892
Zantac (Rare) 1209
Zantac Injection (Rare) 1207
Zantac Syrup (Rare) 1209
Zaroxolyn Tablets 1000
Zemuron (Less than 1%) 1830
Zestoretic 2850
Zofran Injection (Rare) 1214
Zofran Tablets (Rare) 1217
Zoladex (1% or greater) 2858
Zoloft Tablets (Infrequent) 2217
Zosyn (1.0% or less) 1419
Zosyn Pharmacy Bulk Package (1.0% or less) 1422

Tachycardia, junctional

▲ Lanoxicaps (Among most common) 1117
Romazicon (1 of 446 patients) 2147

Tachycardia, persistent (maternal)

▲ Yutopar Intravenous Injection (80% to 100%) 570

Tachycardia, reflux

Duvoid (Infrequent) 2044
Urecholine 1761

Tachycardia, supraventricular

Cardene I.V. (0.7%) 2709
Diprivan Injection (Less than 1%) 2833
Felbatol (Rare) 2666
Fludara for Injection (Up to 3%) 663
Hytrin Capsules (Occasional) 430
Ismo Tablets (Fewer than 1%) 2738
Proleukin for Injection (Less than 1%) 797
Prostin VR Pediatric Sterile Solution (Less than 1%) 2635
Reglan 2068
ReoPro Vials (1.0%) 1471
Rythmol Tablets–150mg, 225mg, 300mg (Less than 1%) 1352
Sodium Polystyrene Sulfonate Suspension 2244
▲ Tenormin Tablets and I.V. Injection (11.5%) 2847
▲ Trasylol (4%) 613
Zosyn (1.0% or less) 1419
Zosyn Pharmacy Bulk Package (1.0% or less) 1422

Tachycardia, ventricular

Activase 1058
Adenocard Injection 1021
Adenoscan 1024
Ambien Tablets (Rare) 2416
Anafranil Capsules (Rare) 803
Aramine Injection 1609
Axid Pulvules (2 individuals) 1427
Betapace Tablets 641
Biaxin (Rare) 405
Cardene Capsules (Less than 0.4%) 2095
Cardene I.V. (0.7%) 2709
Cardizem Injectable (Less than 1%) 1508
Cordarone Intravenous (2.4%) 2715
Cozaar Tablets (Less than 1%) 1628
Demadex Tablets and Injection 686
Desyrel and Desyrel Dividose (Two patients) 503
Diprivan Injection (Less than 1%) 2833
Dobutrex Solution Vials (Rare) 1439
E.E.S. (Occasional reports) 424
Eminase 2039
EryPed (Occasional reports) 421
Ery-Tab Tablets (Occasional reports) 422
Erythrocin Stearate Filmtab (Occasional reports) 425
Erythromycin Base Filmtab (Occasional reports) 426
Erythromycin Delayed-Release Capsules, USP (Occasional reports) 427
▲ Ethmozine Tablets (2% to 5%) 2041
Hyperstat I.V. Injection 2363
Hyzaar Tablets 1677
Ilosone (Rare) 911
Ilotycin Gluceptate, IV, Vials (Rare) 913
Imdur (Less than or equal to 5%) 1323
Imitrex Injection (Rare) 1103
Imitrex Tablets (Rare) 1106
Lanoxicaps 1117
Lanoxin Elixir Pediatric 1120
Lanoxin Injection 1123
Lanoxin Injection Pediatric 1126
Lanoxin Tablets 1128
Lorelco Tablets 1517
Marcaine Hydrochloride with Epinephrine 1:200,000 2316
Marcaine Hydrochloride Injection 2316
Nalfon 200 Pulvules & Nalfon Tablets (Less than 1%) 917
Narcan Injection (Several instances) 934
Norpace 2444
Norpramin Tablets 1526
PCE Dispertab Tablets (Rare) 444
Parlodel (Less than 1%) 2281
Pentam 300 Injection (0.2%) 1041
Permax Tablets (Infrequent) 575
Primacor Injection (1% to 2.8%) 2331
Prinivil Tablets (0.3% to 1.0%) 1733
Prinzide Tablets 1737
Quinaglute Dura-Tabs Tablets 649
Quinidex Extentabs 2067
Risperdal (Rare) 1301
Romazicon (1 of 446 patients) 2147
▲ Rythmol Tablets–150mg, 225mg, 300mg (1.4 to 3.4%) 1352
Seldane Tablets (Rare) 1536
Seldane-D Extended-Release Tablets (Rare) 1538
Sensorcaine 559
Sodium Polystyrene Sulfonate Suspension 2244
Survanta Beractant Intratracheal Suspension 2226
Tambocor Tablets (0.4%) 1497
Taxol (Approximately 1%; rare) 714
▲ Tenormin Tablets and I.V. Injection (16%) 2847
▲ Trasylol (6%) 613
Vascor (200, 300 and 400 mg) Tablets (0.5 to 2.0%) 1587
Yutopar Intravenous Injection 570
Zestril Tablets (0.3% to 1.0%) 2854
Zosyn (1.0% or less) 1419
Zosyn Pharmacy Bulk Package (1.0% or less) 1422

Tachypnea

Actimmune (Rare) 1056
Diprivan Injection (Less than 1%) 2833
Dopram Injectable 2061
▲ Fungizone Intravenous (Among most common) 506
Hespan Injection 929
Humegon 1824
Lufyllin & Lufyllin-400 Tablets 2670
Lufyllin-GG Elixir & Tablets 2671
Nardil (Less frequent) 1920
NebuPent for Inhalation Solution (1% or less) 1040
Orthoclone OKT3 Sterile Solution 1837
Pergonal (menotropins for injection, USP) 2448
▲ Proleukin for Injection (8%) 797
Prostin VR Pediatric Sterile Solution (Less than 1%) 2635
Quadrinal Tablets 1350
Quibron 2053
Respbid Tablets 682
Retrovir Capsules 1158
Retrovir I.V. Infusion 1163
Retrovir Syrup 1158
Roferon-A Injection (Less than 1%) 2145
Sensorcaine 559
Slo-bid Gyrocaps 2033
Sulfamylon Cream 925
Survanta Beractant Intratracheal Suspension 2226
Theo-24 Extended Release Capsules 2568
Theo-Dur Extended-Release Tablets 1327
Theo-X Extended-Release Tablets 788
Uni-Dur Extended-Release Tablets 1331
Uniphyl 400 mg Tablets 2001
Versed Injection (Less than 1%) 2170

Talkativeness

Alupent Tablets (0.2%) 669
Atretol Tablets 573
Dalmane Capsules 2173
Tegretol Chewable Tablets 852
Tegretol Suspension 852
Tegretol Tablets 852
Xanax Tablets (2.2%) 2649

Tardive dyskinesia

Asendin Tablets (Rare) 1369
BuSpar (Rare) 737
Clozaril Tablets 2252
Cognex Capsules (Rare) 1901
Compazine 2470
Depakote Tablets (Greater than 1% but not more than 5%) 415
Desyrel and Desyrel Dividose 503
Elavil 2838
Eldepryl Tablets 2550
Endep Tablets 2174
Etrafon 2355
Haldol Decanoate 1577
Haldol Injection, Tablets and Concentrate 1575
Loxitane 1378
Luvox Tablets (Rare) 2544
Mellaril 2269
Moban Tablets and Concentrate 1048
Navane Capsules and Concentrate 2201
Navane Intramuscular 2202
Orap Tablets 1050
Prolixin 509
Reglan 2068
Risperdal 1301
Serentil 684
Sinequan (Infrequent) 2205
Stelazine 2514
Thorazine 2523
Triavil Tablets 1757
Trilafon 2389
Wellbutrin Tablets 1204

Tardive dystonia (see under Dystonia, tardive)

Taste, altered

Adalat CC (Rare) 589
Altace Capsules (Less than 1%) 1232
Ambien Tablets (Infrequent) 2416
▲ Anafranil Capsules (4% to 8%) 803
Ansaid Tablets (Less than 1%) 2579
AquaMEPHYTON Injection 1608
Asacol Delayed-Release Tablets 1979
Azactam for Injection (Less than 1%) 734
Betaseron for SC Injection 658
▲ Biaxin (3%) 405
Brevibloc Injection 1808
BuSpar (Infrequent) 737
Capoten (Approximately 2 to 4 of 100 patients) 739
Capozide (Approximately 2 to 4 of 100 patients) 742
Cardura Tablets (Less than 0.5% of 3960 patients) 2186
Cataflam (Less than 1%) 816
Catapres-TTS (1 of 101 patients) 675
Claritin (2% or fewer patients) 2349
Claritin-D (Less frequent) 2350
Cognex Capsules (Infrequent) 1901
Cordarone Tablets (1 to 3%) 2712
Cozaar Tablets (Less than 1%) 1628
▲ Cuprimine Capsules (12%) 1630
Cytotec (Infrequent) 2424
Cytovene (1% or less) 2103
Dantrium Capsules (Less frequent) 1982
Daypro Caplets (Less than 1%) 2426
Diamox Intravenous 1372
Diamox Sequels (Sustained Release) 1373
Diamox Tablets 1372
▲ Didronel I.V. Infusion (5%) 1488
Diflucan Injection, Tablets, and Oral Suspension (1%) 2194
Dilacor XR Extended-release Capsules 2018
Dilaudid-HP Injection (Less frequent) 1337
Dilaudid-HP Lyophilized Powder 250 mg (Less frequent) 1337
Dilaudid Tablets and Liquid 1339
Diprivan Injection (Less than 1%) 2833
Doral Tablets 2664
Effexor (2%) 2719
Eldepryl Tablets 2550
Endep Tablets 2174
▲ Ergamisol Tablets (8%) 1292
Eskalith 2485
▲ Felbatol (6.1%) 2666
Floxin I.V. 1571
Floxin Tablets (200 mg, 300 mg, 400 mg) 1567
Flumadine Tablets & Syrup (Less than 0.3%) 1015
Foscavir Injection (Between 1% and 5%) 547
Gastrocrom Capsules (Infrequent) 984
Geref (sermorelin acetate for injection) 2876
Glauctabs ⊙ 208
Halcion Tablets (Rare) 2611
Helixate, Antihemophilic Factor (Recombinant) 518
Hivid Tablets (Less than 1% to less than 3%) 2121
Hyperstat I.V. Injection 2363
Hyzaar Tablets 1677
Imitrex Injection (Infrequent) 1103
Imitrex Tablets 1106
INFeD (Iron Dextran Injection, USP) 2345
▲ Intron A (Up to 13%) 2364
IOPIDINE Sterile Ophthalmic Solution ⊙ 219
▲ Iopidine 0.5% (3%) ⊙ 221
Kerlone Tablets (Less than 2%) 2436
KOGENATE Antihemophilic Factor (Recombinant) 632
Kytril Injection (2%) 2490
Lamictal Tablets (Infrequent) 1112
Lamprene Capsules (Less than 1%) 828
Limbitrol 2180
Lioresal Intrathecal 1596
Lioresal Tablets (Rare) 829
Lithonate/Lithotabs/Lithobid 2543
Lodine Capsules and Tablets (Less than 1%) 2743
▲ Lopid Tablets (More common) 1917
Lotensin HCT (0.3% to 1.0%) 837
Lupron Depot 3.75 mg (Less than 5%) 2556
Lupron Depot 7.5 mg 2559
Lupron Injection (Less than 5%) 2555
▲ Luvox Tablets (3%) 2544
MS Contin Tablets (Less frequent) 1994
MSIR (Infrequent) 1997
▲ MZM (Among reactions occurring most often) ⊙ 267

(▣ Described in PDR For Nonprescription Drugs) Incidence data in parenthesis; ▲ 3% or more (⊙ Described in PDR For Ophthalmology)

Taste, altered — Side Effects Index — 1424

Maxair Autohaler (0.6%) 1492
Maxair Inhaler (Less than 1%) 1494
Maxaquin Tablets (Less than 1%) .. 2440
Maxzide 1380
▲ Mepron Suspension (3%) 1135
MetroGel-Vaginal 902
Mevacor Tablets 1699
Mexitil Capsules (About 5 in 1,000) 678
Mezlin 601
Mezlin Pharmacy Bulk Package 604
Miacalcin Nasal Spray (Less than 1%) 2275
Monopril Tablets (0.2% to 1.0%) .. 757
▲ Mycobutin Capsules (3%) 1957
Neptazane Tablets 1388
Neurontin Capsules (Infrequent) 1922
▲ Nicoderm (nicotine transdermal system) (3% to 9%) 1518
Nicorette 2458
Nicotrol Nicotine Transdermal System (1% to 3%) 1550
Normodyne Injection (1%) 2377
Normodyne Tablets (1%) 2379
Norvasc Tablets (Less than or equal to 0.1%) 1940
Ocupress Ophthalmic Solution, 1% Sterile (Occasional) .... ◉ 309
Oramorph SR (Morphine Sulfate Sustained Release Tablets) (Less frequent) 2236
▲ Orap Tablets (1 of 20 patients) 1050
Orudis Capsules (Less than 1%) 2766
Oruvail Capsules (Less than 1%) 2766
Paraplatin for Injection (1%) 705
Paxil Tablets (2.4%) 2505
Penetrex Tablets (1%) 2031
Pepcid Injection (Infrequent) 1722
Pepcid (Infrequent) 1720
Peridex 1978
Permax Tablets (1.6%) 575
Pravachol 765
PREVACID Delayed-Release Capsules (Less than 1%) 2562
Prilosec Delayed-Release Capsules (Less than 1%) 529
Primaxin I.M. 1727
Primaxin I.V. (Less than 0.2%) 1729
Procardia XL Extended Release Tablets (1% or less) 1972
▲ Proleukin for Injection (7%) 797
ProSom Tablets (Infrequent) 449
Proventil Inhalation Aerosol 2382
Proventil Repetabs Tablets 2386
Proventil Syrup 2385
Proventil Tablets 2386
Prozac Pulvules & Liquid, Oral Solution (1.8% to 2%) 919
Quadrinal Tablets 1350
Quarzan Capsules 2181
Relafen Tablets (Less than 1%) 2510
▲ Retrovir Capsules (5%) 1158
▲ Retrovir I.V. Infusion (5%) 1163
▲ Retrovir Syrup (5%) 1158
▲ Roferon-A Injection (13% to 25%) 2145
▲ Rythmol Tablets–150mg, 225mg, 300mg (2.5 to 22.6%) 1352
Salagen Tablets (1%) 1489
Seldane-D Extended-Release Tablets (1.1%) 1538
Serzone Tablets (2%) 771
Sinequan 2205
Surmontil Capsules 2811
Talwin Injection (Rare) 2334
Tambocor Tablets (Less than 1%) 1497
Tegison Capsules (Less than 1%) .. 2154
Tenex Tablets (3% or less) 2074
Timentin for Injection 2528
Tofranil Ampuls 854
Tofranil Tablets 856
Tofranil-PM Capsules 857
Tonocard Tablets (Less than 1%) .. 531
Toradol (1% or less) 2159
Tornalate Solution for Inhalation, 0.2% 956
Tornalate Metered Dose Inhaler 957
Trandate (1 of 100 patients) 1185
Triavil Tablets 1757
Univasc Tablets (Less than 1%) 2410
Vantin for Oral Suspension and Vantin Tablets (Less than 1%) 2646
Vascor (200, 300 and 400 mg) Tablets (0.5 to 2.0%) 1587
Vaseretic Tablets 1765
Vasotec I.V. 1768
Vasotec Tablets (0.5% to 1.0%) 1771
Ventolin Inhalation Aerosol and Refill 1197
Ventolin Rotacaps for Inhalation (2%) 1200
Ventolin Syrup 1202
Vexol 1% Ophthalmic Suspension (Less than 2%) .... ◉ 230
Videx Tablets, Powder for Oral Solution, & Pediatric Powder for Oral Solution (Less than 1%) 720
Volmax Extended-Release Tablets .. 1788
Voltaren Tablets (Less than 1%) 861
Xanax Tablets 2649
Zebeta Tablets 1413
Zefazone 2654
Zestoretic 2850
Zestril Tablets 2854
Ziac 1415
Zocor Tablets 1775
Zoloft Tablets (1.2%) 2217
▲ Zonalon Cream (Approximately 1% to 10%) 1055
Zosyn (1.0% or less) 1419
Zosyn Pharmacy Bulk Package (1.0% or less) 1422
Zyloprim Tablets (Less than 1%) 1226

Taste, bad
Alupent (Less frequent; approximately 1 in 300 patients) 669
▲ Ciloxan Ophthalmic Solution (Less than 10%) 472
Cipro I.V. (1% or less) 595
Cipro I.V. Pharmacy Bulk Package (Less than 1%) 597
Cipro Tablets (Less than 1%) 592
Cleocin Phosphate Injection (Occasional) 2586
Desyrel and Desyrel Dividose (Up to 1.4%) 503
Didrex Tablets 2607
Fluorescite .... ◉ 219
Imitrex Tablets 1106
▲ Intal Inhaler (Among most frequent) 988
Lupron Injection (Less than 3%) 2555
▲ Mesnex Injection (100%) 702
Metaproterenol Sulfate Inhalation Solution, USP, Arm-a-Med (Approximately 1 in 300 patients) 552
Methergine (Rare) 2272
Moduretic Tablets (Less than or equal to 1%) 1705
Nasalcrom Nasal Solution (1 in 50) 994
Pentam 300 Injection (1.7%) 1041
Pondimin Tablets 2066
Rhinocort Nasal Inhaler (Less than 1%) 556
▲ THROMBATE III Antithrombin III (Human) (3 of 17) 637
THYREL TRH 2873
Trental Tablets (Less than 1%) 1244
Zovirax (0.3%) 1219

Taste, bitter
Atamet 572
Ceftin Tablets 1078
Chibroxin Sterile Ophthalmic Solution 1617
Clinoril Tablets (Less than 1 in 100) 1618
Clozaril Tablets (Less than 1%) 2252
Colace 2044
Dalmane Capsules (Rare) 2173
Ethmozine Tablets (Less than 2%) 2041
Larodopa Tablets (Infrequent) 2129
Ludiomil Tablets (Rare) 843
Monoket (Fewer than 1%) 2406
Mykrox Tablets (Less than 2%) 993
Noroxin Tablets (Less frequent) 1715
Noroxin Tablets (Less frequent) 2048
Nubain Injection (1% or less) 935
▲ Procan SR Tablets (3-4%) 1926
Risperdal (Rare) 1301
Sinemet Tablets 943
Sinemet CR Tablets 944
Versed Injection (Less than 1%) 2170
Zaroxolyn Tablets 1000

Taste, changes (see under Taste, altered)

Taste, loss (see under Ageusia)

Taste, metallic
Actigall Capsules 802
Adenocard Injection (Less than 1%) 1021
Adenoscan (Less than 1%) 1024
Antabuse Tablets (Small number of patients) 2695
▲ CHEMET (succimer) Capsules (12-20.9%) 1545
Cleocin Phosphate Injection (Occasional) 2586
Clinoril Tablets (Less than 1 in 100) 1618
▲ Didronel I.V. Infusion (5%) 1488
Eskalith 2485
Flagyl 375 Capsules (Not unusual) 2434
Flagyl I.V. 2247
Glucophage (Approximately 3%) 752
Lithium Carbonate Capsules & Tablets 2230
Lithonate/Lithotabs/Lithobid 2543
Marcaine Spinal 2319
MetroGel 1047
MetroGel-Vaginal (Equal to or less than 2%) 902
Myochrysine Injection 1711
Nalfon 200 Pulvules & Nalfon Tablets (Less than 1%) 917
▲ NebuPent for Inhalation Solution (53 to 72%) 1040
Norisodrine with Calcium Iodide Syrup 442
Pima Syrup 1005
Protostat Tablets 1883
Ridaura Capsules 2513
Robaxin Injectable 2070
Rocaltrol Capsules 2141
Sensorcaine 559
Solganal Suspension 2388

Taste, salty
Lithonate/Lithotabs/Lithobid 2543
Miacalcin Injection 2273

Taste, unpleasant
Adipex-P Tablets and Capsules 1048
▲ AeroBid Inhaler System (10%) 1005
▲ Aerobid-M Inhaler System (10%) .. 1005
Asendin Tablets (Less than 1%) 1369
Biphetamine Capsules 983
Brethaire Inhaler 813
▲ Ceftin for Oral Suspension (5.0%) 1078
Desoxyn Gradumet Tablets 419
Dexedrine 2474
DextroStat Dextroamphetamine Tablets 2036
Efudex 2113
Elavil 2838
Etrafon 2355
Fastin Capsules 2488
Flagyl I.V. 2247
Flexeril Tablets (1% to 3%) 1661
Flonase Nasal Spray (Less than 1%) 1098
Ionamin Capsules 990
Mephyton Tablets 1696
Norpramin Tablets 1526
Pamelor 2280
Prelu-2 Timed Release Capsules 681
Quadrinal Tablets 1350
Questran Light 769
Questran Powder 770
Sanorex Tablets 2294
▲ Stadol (3% to 9%) 775
▲ Tilade (12.6%) 996
Vivactil Tablets 1774

Tears, discoloration
Rifadin 1528
Rifater 1532

Teeth, discoloration
Achromycin V Capsules 1367
Declomycin Tablets 1371
Doryx Capsules 1913
Dynacin Capsules (In children less than 8 years of age; rare in adults) 1590
Feosol Elixir 2456
Minocin Intravenous (Rare) 1382
Minocin Oral Suspension 1385
Minocin Pellet-Filled Capsules (Rare) 1383
Monodox Capsules 1805
Neurontin Capsules (Rare) 1922
Peridex 1978
Primaxin I.M. 1727
Primaxin I.V. (Less than 0.2%) 1729
Terramycin Intramuscular Solution 2210
Urobiotic-250 Capsules 2214
Ventolin Inhalation Aerosol and Refill (1%) 1197
Vibramycin 1941
Vibramycin Hyclate Intravenous 2215
Vibramycin 1941

Teeth, mottling of enamel (see under Teeth, discoloration)

Teeth grinding
Anafranil Capsules (Infrequent) 803
Zoloft Tablets (Infrequent) 2217

Telangiectasia
Aclovate Ointment (1 of 366 patients) 1069
Diprolene AF Cream (Less than 1%) 2352
Diprolene Gel 0.05% (Less frequent) 2353
Diprolene (Less than 1%) 2352
Efudex 2113
Fluoroplex Topical Solution & Cream 1% 479
Methotrexate Sodium Tablets, Injection, for Injection and LPF Injection 1275
Sansert Tablets (Rare) 2295
Temovate (1 of 366 patients) 1179
Ultravate Ointment 0.05% (Less frequent) 2690

Telogen effluvium
Lariam Tablets 2128

Temperature disturbances, cutaneous
Emla Cream 545
Wellbutrin Tablets (1.9%) 1204

Temperature elevation (see under Hyperthermia)

Temporal bone, swelling
Lupron Depot 7.5 mg 2559

Tenderness
Americaine Anesthetic Lubricant 983
Americaine Otic Topical Anesthetic Ear Drops 983
Bactroban Ointment (Less than 1%) 2470
Biavax II 1613
Condylox (Less than 5%) 1802
Efudex (Infrequent) 2113
Estraderm Transdermal System 824
Gammar, Immune Globulin (Human) U.S.P. 515
Hep-B-Gammagee 1663
▲ HibTITER (0.3% to 3.7%) 1375
M-M-R II 1687
M-R-VAX II 1689
Mevacor Tablets 1699
▲ Miacalcin Nasal Spray (10.6%) 2275
Mini-Gamulin Rh, Rh_O(D) Immune Globulin (Human) (Occasional) 520
Oncaspar 2028
Recombivax HB (Equal to or greater than 1%) 1744
T-Stat 2.0% Topical Solution and Pads 2688
Temovate Scalp Application (1 of 294 patients) 1179
Tetanus Toxoid Adsorbed Purogenated 1403
Thioguanine Tablets, Tabloid Brand 1181
▲ Versed Injection (5.6%) 2170
Zocor Tablets 1775

Tenderness, elbow
Temovate Emollient Cream (1%) 1179

Tenderness, right upper quadrant
Cataflam 816
Eulexin Capsules 2358
Normodyne Injection 2377
Trandate 1185
Voltaren Tablets 861

Tendinitis
Ambien Tablets 2416
Cipro Tablets 592
Cognex Capsules (Infrequent) 1901
Floxin I.V. 1571
Floxin Tablets (200 mg, 300 mg, 400 mg) 1567
Kerlone Tablets 2436
Maxaquin Tablets 2440
Neurontin Capsules 1922
Noroxin Tablets 1715
Noroxin Tablets 2048
Rogaine Topical Solution 2637

Tenderness at injection site
▲ Acel-Imune Diphtheria and Tetanus

1425 **Side Effects Index** **Throat, soreness**

Toxoids and Acellular Pertussis Vaccine Adsorbed (26%) 1364
▲ActHIB (1.1% to 66.9%) 872
▲Actimmune (14%) 1056
Cefizox for Intramuscular or Intravenous Use (Greater than 1% but less than 5%) 1034
Cholera Vaccine 2711
▲Claforan Sterile and Injection (4.3%) 1235
Dilantin Parenteral 1910
Diphtheria and Tetanus Toxoids and Pertussis Vaccine Adsorbed .. 2477
Diphtheria and Tetanus Toxoids and Pertussis Vaccine Adsorbed USP (For Pediatric Use) 875
Fluvirin (Less than one third) 460
HyperHep Hepatitis B Immune Globulin (Human) 626
Imogam Rabies Immune Globulin (Human) (Uncommon) 880
▲JE-VAX (Approximately 20%) 886
Konakion Injection (Rare) 2127
Mefoxin 1691
MSTA Mumps Skin Test Antigen 890
▲OmniHIB (1.1% to 46.3%) 2499
Rocephin Injectable Vials, ADD-Vantage, Galaxy Container (1%) 2142
Taxol 714
▲Tetramune (21% to 65%) 1404
▲Tripedia (2% to 35%) 892
▲Typhim Vi (Up to 98%) 899
Typhoid Vaccine 2823
Vancocin HCl, Vials & ADD-Vantage 1481
▲Zefazone (26%) 2654

Tendinous contracture
Lamictal Tablets (Rare) 1112
Luvox Tablets (Infrequent) 2544
Serzone Tablets (Rare) 771

Tendon disorder, unspecified
Imdur (Less than or equal to 5%) .. 1323

Tendon fixation
Gelfoam Sterile Sponge 2608

Tendon rupture
Cipro Tablets 592
Cortone Acetate Sterile Suspension 1623
Cortone Acetate Tablets 1624
Dalalone D.P. Injectable 1011
Decadron Elixir 1633
Decadron Phosphate Injection 1637
Decadron Phosphate Respihaler 1642
Decadron Phosphate Turbinaire 1645
Decadron Phosphate with Xylocaine Injection, Sterile 1639
Decadron Tablets 1635
Decadron-LA Sterile Suspension 1646
Deltasone Tablets 2595
Depo-Medrol Single-Dose Vial 2600
Depo-Medrol Sterile Aqueous Suspension 2597
Dexacort Phosphate in Respihaler .. 458
Dexacort Phosphate in Turbinaire .. 459
Hydeltrasol Injection, Sterile 1665
Hydeltra-T.B.A. Sterile Suspension 1667
Hydrocortone Acetate Sterile Suspension 1669
Hydrocortone Phosphate Injection, Sterile 1670
Hydrocortone Tablets 1672
Medrol 2621
Solu-Cortef Sterile Powder 2641
Solu-Medrol Sterile Powder 2643

Tenesmus
Ambien Tablets (Rare) 2416
Asacol Delayed-Release Tablets 1979
Betaseron for SC Injection 658
Foscavir Injection (Less than 1%) .. 547
Ismo Tablets (Fewer than 1%) 2738
PREVACID Delayed-Release Capsules (Less than 1%) 2562
Zoloft Tablets (Rare) 2217

Tenosynovitis
Betaseron for SC Injection 658
Effexor (Infrequent) 2719
Luvox Tablets (Infrequent) 2544
Permax Tablets (Infrequent) 575
Prozac Pulvules & Liquid, Oral Solution (Infrequent) 919
Serzone Tablets (Infrequent) 771
Videx Tablets, Powder for Oral Solution, & Pediatric Powder for Oral Solution (Less than 1%) 720

Tenseness
Bronkometer Aerosol 2302
Bronkosol Solution 2302
Claritin-D 2350
D.A. Chewable Tablets 951
Deconamine Chewable Tablets 1320
Deconamine CX Cough and Cold Liquid and Tablets 1319
Deconamine 1320
Dura-Tap/PD Capsules 2867
Dura-Vent/DA Tablets 953
Dura-Vent Tablets 952
EpiPen—Epinephrine Auto-Injector 790
Fedahist Gyrocaps 2401
Fedahist Timecaps 2401
Loxitane 1378
▲Lozol Tablets (Greater than or equal to 5%) 2022
Novahistine DH 2462
Novahistine DMX .... ▣ 822
Novahistine Elixir .... ▣ 823
Novahistine Expectorant 2463
Prostin E2 Suppository 2634
Seldane-D Extended-Release Tablets 1538
Trinalin Repetabs Tablets 1330
Tussend 1783
Tussend Expectorant 1785

Testes, size decrease
Lupron Depot 3.75 mg 2556
▲Lupron Depot 7.5 mg (5.4%) 2559
▲Lupron Injection (5% or more) 2555

Testicular atrophy
Cytoxan 694
NEOSAR Lyophilized/Neosar 1959
Oxandrin 2862
Winstrol Tablets 2337

Testicular disorder, unspecified
Caverject (Less than 1%) 2583
Tenex Tablets (3% or less) 2074

Testicular function, inhibited
Alkeran for Injection 1070
Oxandrin 2862
Winstrol Tablets 2337

Testicular hypertrophy
Cytovene-IV (One report) 2103

Testicular swelling
Asendin Tablets (Very rare) 1369
Elavil 2838
Endep Tablets 2174
Etrafon 2355
Flexeril Tablets (Rare) 1661
Hivid Tablets (Less than 1% to less than 3%) 2121
Limbitrol 2180
Ludiomil Tablets (Isolated reports) 843
Neurontin Capsules (Rare) 1922
Norpramin Tablets 1526
Pamelor 2280
Sinequan 2205
Surmontil Capsules 2811
Tofranil Ampuls 854
Tofranil Tablets 856
Tofranil-PM Capsules 857
Triavil Tablets 1757
Vivactil Tablets 1774
Wellbutrin Tablets (Infrequent) 1204

Testosterone, decreased physiologic effects
Lupron Injection 2555

Testosterone serum levels, transient increase
Zoladex 2858

Tetany
Ambien Tablets (Rare) 2416
Aredia for Injection (Rare) 810
Foscavir Injection (Less than 1%) .. 547
Garamycin Injectable 2360
Imitrex Tablets (Rare) 1106
Paxil Tablets (Rare) 2505
Platinol (Occasional) 708
Platinol-AQ Injection (Occasional) .. 710
Syntocinon Injection 2296

Thermoregulatory mechanisms, interference
Astramorph/PF Injection, USP (Preservative-Free) 535
Compazine 2470
Duramorph 962
Infumorph 200 and Infumorph 500 Sterile Solutions 965

Thinking, abnormality
Ambien Tablets (Rare) 2416
Anafranil Capsules (Frequent) 803
Brevibloc Injection (Less than 1%) 1808
Butisol Sodium Elixir & Tablets (Less than 1 in 100) 2660
Cardura Tablets (Less than 0.5% of 3960 patients) 2186
▲Cognex Capsules (3%) 1901
Cytovene (1% or less) 2103
Depakote Tablets (Greater than 1% but not more than 5%) 415
Dilacor XR Extended-release Capsules 2018
Diprivan Injection (Less than 1%) .. 2833
Doral Tablets 2664
Duragesic Transdermal System (1% or greater) 1288
Effexor (2%) 2719
▲Felbatol (6.5%) 2666
Flexeril Tablets (Less than 1%) 1661
Halcion Tablets 2611
Hivid Tablets (Less than 1% to less than 3%) 2121
Intron A (Less than 5%) 2364
Kerlone Tablets (Less than 2%) 2436
Lamictal Tablets (Frequent) 1112
Lithonate/Lithotabs/Lithobid 2543
▲Marinol (Dronabinol) Capsules (3% to 10%) 2231
Mebaral Tablets (Less than 1 in 100) 2322
Megace Oral Suspension (1% to 3%) 699
Nembutal Sodium Capsules (Less than 1%) 436
Nembutal Sodium Solution (Less than 1%) 438
Nembutal Sodium Suppositories (Less than 1%) 440
Neurontin Capsules (1.7%) 1922
Paxil Tablets (Infrequent) 2505
Permax Tablets (Frequent) 575
Phenobarbital Elixir and Tablets (Less than 1 in 100 patients) 1469
PREVACID Delayed-Release Capsules (Less than 1%) 2562
▲Prograf (Greater than 3%) 1042
ProSom Tablets (2%) 449
▲Prozac Pulvules & Liquid, Oral Solution (4%) 919
ReoPro Vials (2.1%) 1471
Seconal Sodium Pulvules (Less than 1 in 100) 1474
Serzone Tablets (Infrequent) 771
Symmetrel Capsules and Syrup (0.1% to 1%) 946
Tegison Capsules (Less than 1%) .. 2154
Toradol (1% or less) 2159
Videx Tablets, Powder for Oral Solution, & Pediatric Powder for Oral Solution (1% to 2%) 720
Wellbutrin Tablets (Infrequent) 1204
Zoladex (1% or greater) 2858
Zoloft Tablets (Infrequent) 2217

Thirst (see under Dipsesis)

Thrashing
Diprivan Injection (Less than 1%) .. 2833

Throat, aching
Zebeta Tablets 1413

Throat, burning
Diprivan Injection (Less than 1%) .. 2833
Eldepryl Tablets 2550
Emcyt Capsules (1%) 1953
Gastrocrom Capsules (Infrequent) .. 984

Throat, congestion
Bentyl 1501

Throat, dryness
Accupril Tablets (0.5% to 1.0%) .. 1893
▲Actifed with Codeine Cough Syrup (Among most frequent) 1067
AeroBid Inhaler System (1-3%) 1005
Aerobid-M Inhaler System (1-3%) .. 1005
Alupent Tablets (0.4%) 669
Azmacort Oral Inhaler 2011
Benadryl Injection 1898
▲Bromfed-DM Cough Syrup (Among most frequent) 1786
Catapres-TTS (2 of 101 patients) .. 675
Claritin-D (Less frequent) 2350
Clozaril Tablets (Less than 1%) 2252
Cognex Capsules (Infrequent) 1901
Comhist 2038
D.A. Chewable Tablets 951
Daraprim Tablets (Rare) 1090
Deconamine 1320
▲Dimetane-DC Cough Syrup (Most frequent) 2059
Dimetane-DX Cough Syrup (Among most frequent) 2059
Dura-Tap/PD Capsules 2867
Dura-Vent/DA Tablets 953
Hylorel Tablets (1.7%) 985
▲Intal Inhaler (Among most frequent) 988
Marax Tablets & DF Syrup 2200
Neurontin Capsules (1.7%) 1922
▲Norpace (3 to 9%) 2444
Ornade Spansule Capsules 2502
PBZ Tablets 845
PBZ-SR Tablets 844
Penetrex Tablets (Less than 1% but more than or equal to 0.1%) 2031
Periactin 1724
Robinul Injectable 2072
▲Seldane Tablets (2.3% to 4.8%) 1536
▲Seldane-D Extended-Release Tablets (21.7%) 1538
Tavist Syrup 2297
Tavist Tablets 2298
Trinalin Repetabs Tablets 1330
Tussend 1783

Throat, irritation
AeroBid Inhaler System (1-3%) 1005
Aerobid-M Inhaler System (1-3%) .. 1005
Alupent (1% to 4%) 669
Azmacort Oral Inhaler 2011
Clozaril Tablets (1%) 2252
Colace 2044
Decadron Phosphate Respihaler 1642
Dexacort Phosphate in Respihaler .. 458
Intal Capsules 987
▲Intal Inhaler (Among most frequent) 988
Isuprel Mistometer (Occasional) 2312
Nasacort Nasal Inhaler (Fewer than 5%) 2024
▲Nicorette (3% to 9% of patients) .. 2458
Paxil Tablets (2.1%) 2505
Provocholine for Inhalation (1 occurrence) 2140
Tornalate Solution for Inhalation, 0.2% (2.5%) 956
▲Tornalate Metered Dose Inhaler (3.0% to 5%) 957
▲Ventolin Inhalation Aerosol and Refill (6%) 1197
Ventolin Rotacaps for Inhalation (2%) 1200

Throat, presence of hard nodule
Lupron Depot 7.5 mg (Less than 5%) 2559
Lupron Injection 2555

Throat, soreness
▲Adalat Capsules (10 mg and 20 mg) (6%) 587
▲Adenoscan (15%) 1024
▲AeroBid Inhaler System (20%) 1005
▲Aerobid-M Inhaler System (20%) .. 1005
All-Flex Arcing Spring Diaphragm (See also Ortho Diaphragm Kits) 1865
Altace Capsules 1232
Atgam Sterile Solution (Less than 5%) 2581
Atretol Tablets 573
Biavax II 1613
Blocadren Tablets 1614
BuSpar (Frequent) 737
Capoten 739
Capozide 742
Cardene Capsules (Rare) 2095
Cartrol Tablets 410
▲CHEMET (succimer) Capsules (0.7 to 3.7%) 1545
Clozaril Tablets 2252
Compazine 2470
Cytosar-U Sterile Powder (Less frequent) 2592
Danocrine Capsules 2307
Dapsone Tablets USP 1284
Demadex Tablets and Injection (1.6%) 686
Depen Titratable Tablets 2662
DynaCirc Capsules (0.5% to 1%) .. 2256
Etrafon 2355
Gantrisin 2120
Helixate, Antihemophilic Factor (Recombinant) 518

(▣ Described in PDR For Nonprescription Drugs) Incidence data in parenthesis; ▲ 3% or more (◉ Described in PDR For Ophthalmology)

Hivid Tablets (Less than 1% to less than 3%) ... 2121
▲ Imitrex Injection (3.3%) ... 1103
Inderal ... 2728
Inderal LA Long Acting Capsules ... 2730
Inderide Tablets ... 2732
Inderide LA Long Acting Capsules .. 2734
Kerlone Tablets ... 2436
KOGENATE Antihemophilic Factor (Recombinant) ... 632
Levatol ... 2403
Lopressor HCT Tablets ... 832
M-M-R II ... 1687
M-R-VAX II ... 1689
Maxair Autohaler ... 1492
Maxair Inhaler (Less than 1%) ... 1494
Meruvax II ... 1697
Monopril Tablets ... 757
Mykrox Tablets (Less than 2%) ... 993
Nasalide Nasal Solution 0.025% (5% or less) ... 2110
▲ Neupogen for Injection (4%) ... 495
Nicorette ... 2458
Normodyne Tablets ... 2379
Ortho Diaphragm Kits—All-Flex Arcing Spring; Ortho Coil Spring; Ortho-White Flat Spring ... 1865
Ortho Diaphragm Kit ... 1865
Prinivil Tablets ... 1733
Prinzide Tablets ... 1737
▲ Procardia Capsules (6%) ... 1971
▲ Procardia XL Extended Release Tablets (6%) ... 1972
Prolixin ... 509
Proloprim Tablets ... 1155
Quadrinal Tablets ... 1350
ReVia Tablets (Less than 1%) ... 940
Rowasa (2.33%) ... 2548
Rythmol Tablets–150mg, 225mg, 300mg ... 1352
Sectral Capsules ... 2807
Seldane Tablets (0.5% to 3.2%) ... 1536
Seldane-D Extended-Release Tablets (1.9%) ... 1538
Septra I.V. Infusion ... 1169
Septra I.V. Infusion ADD-Vantage Vials ... 1171
Stelazine ... 2514
Stimate, (desmopressin acetate) Nasal Spray, 1.5 mg/mL ... 525
Tapazole Tablets ... 1477
Tegretol Chewable Tablets ... 852
Tegretol Suspension ... 852
Tegretol Tablets ... 852
Tenoretic Tablets ... 2845
Tenormin Tablets and I.V. Injection 2847
Ticlid Tablets ... 2156
Timoptic in Ocudose ... 1753
Timoptic Sterile Ophthalmic Solution ... 1751
Timoptic-XE ... 1755
Tofranil Ampuls ... 854
Tofranil Tablets ... 856
Tofranil-PM Capsules ... 857
Tonocard Tablets ... 531
Toprol-XL Tablets ... 565
Trandate Tablets ... 1185
Trental Tablets (Less than 1%) ... 1244
Univasc Tablets ... 2410
Valium Injectable ... 2182
Vaseretic Tablets ... 1765
Vasotec I.V. ... 1768
Vasotec Tablets (0.5% to 1.0%) ... 1771
Visken Tablets ... 2299
Zebeta Tablets ... 1413
Zestoretic ... 2850
Zestril Tablets ... 2854
Ziac ... 1415
Zovirax (0.3%) ... 1219

Throat, swelling of

Calcimar Injection, Synthetic (A few cases) ... 2013
Floxin I.V. ... 1571
Floxin Tablets (200 mg, 300 mg, 400 mg) ... 1567
Miacalcin Injection (A few cases) ... 2273
SSKI Solution (Less frequent) ... 2658

Throat, tightness

Adenocard Injection (Less than 1%) ... 1021
Etrafon ... 2355
Paxil Tablets (2.1%) ... 2505
THYREL TRH (Less frequent) ... 2873
Trilafon ... 2389
Unasyn (Less than 1%) ... 2212
VePesid Capsules and Injection (Sometimes) ... 718

Throbbing, head

EpiPen—Epinephrine Auto-Injector 790

Throbbing, localized

Catapres-TTS (1 of 101 patients) .. 675

Thrombocythemia (see under Thrombocytosis)

Thrombocytopenia

Accupril Tablets (Rare) ... 1893
Accutane Capsules (Less than 1 in 10 patients) ... 2076
Achromycin V Capsules ... 1367
Actifed with Codeine Cough Syrup.. 1067
Adalat Capsules (10 mg and 20 mg) (Less than 0.5%) ... 587
Adalat CC (Rare) ... 589
Children's Advil Suspension (Less than 1%) ... 2692
Aldactazide ... 2413
Aldoclor Tablets ... 1598
Aldomet Ester HCl Injection ... 1602
Aldomet Oral ... 1600
Aldoril Tablets ... 1604
Alkeran Tablets ... 1071
Altace Capsules (Less than 1%) ... 1232
Amoxil ... 2464
Anaprox/Naprosyn (Less than 1%) ... 2117
Ancef Injection ... 2465
Ancobon Capsules ... 2079
Anexia Tablets ... 1782
Ansaid Tablets (Rare) ... 2579
Anturane (Rare) ... 807
Apresazide Capsules ... 808
Aredia for Injection (Up to 1%) ... 810
Asacol Delayed-Release Tablets ... 1979
Asendin Tablets (Very rare) ... 1369
Atamet (Rare) ... 572
▲ Atgam Sterile Solution (1 in 9 patients; 30%) ... 2581
Atretol Tablets ... 573
Atrohist Plus Tablets ... 454
Attenuvax (Rare) ... 1610
Augmentin ... 2468
Axid Pulvules (One patient) ... 1427
Azactam for Injection (Less than 1%) ... 734
Azo Gantanol Tablets ... 2080
Azo Gantrisin Tablets ... 2081
Azulfidine (Rare) ... 1949
BCG Vaccine, USP (TICE) (0.3%) .. 1814
Bactrim DS Tablets ... 2084
Bactrim I.V. Infusion ... 2082
Bactrim ... 2084
Benadryl Capsules ... 1898
Benadryl Injection ... 1898
Betapace Tablets (Rare) ... 641
Betaseron for SC Injection ... 658
Biavax II ... 1613
Bicillin C-R Injection ... 2704
Bicillin C-R 900/300 Injection ... 2706
Bicillin L-A Injection (Infrequent) ... 2707
BiCNU ... 691
▲ Bromfed-DM Cough Syrup (Among most frequent) ... 1786
Bumex (0.2%) ... 2093
BuSpar (Rare) ... 737
Capastat Sulfate Vials (Rare) ... 2868
Capoten ... 739
Capozide ... 742
Cardene I.V. (Rare) ... 2709
Cardizem CD Capsules (Infrequent) ... 1506
Cardizem SR Capsules (Less than 1%) ... 1510
Cardizem Injectable ... 1508
Cardizem Tablets (Infrequent) ... 1512
Cataflam (Less than 1%) ... 816
Ceclor Pulvules & Suspension (Rare) ... 1431
CeeNU ... 693
Cefizox for Intramuscular or Intravenous Use (Rare) ... 1034
Cefotan ... 2829
Ceftin ... 1078
Cefzil Tablets and Oral Suspension (Rare) ... 746
▲ CellCept Capsules (8.2% to 10.1%) ... 2099
Ceptaz (Very rare) ... 1081
Chibroxin Sterile Ophthalmic Solution (With oral form) ... 1617
Chloromycetin Sodium Succinate ... 1900
▲ Cipro I.V. (Among most frequent) .. 595
▲ Cipro I.V. Pharmacy Bulk Package (Among most frequent) ... 597
Cipro Tablets (0.1%) ... 592
Claforan Sterile and Injection (Less than 1%) ... 1235
Cleocin Phosphate Injection ... 2586
Cleocin Vaginal Cream ... 2589
Clinoril Tablets (Less than 1 in 100) ... 1618
Clozaril Tablets ... 2252
Cognex Capsules (Rare) ... 1901
Combipres Tablets ... 677
Comhist ... 2038
Cordarone Intravenous (Less than 2%) ... 2715
Cordarone Tablets (Rare) ... 2712
Cosmegen Injection ... 1626
▲ Cuprimine Capsules (4%) ... 1630
Cytosar-U Sterile Powder (Less than 7 patients) ... 2592
Cytotec (Infrequent) ... 2424
▲ Cytovene (6%) ... 2103
Cytoxan (Occasional) ... 694
Danocrine Capsules ... 2307
Daranide Tablets ... 1633
Daraprim Tablets ... 1090
Daypro Caplets (Less than 1%) ... 2426
Declomycin Tablets ... 1371
Deconamine ... 1320
Demser Capsules (Rare) ... 1649
Depakene ... 413
Depakote Tablets ... 415
▲ Depen Titratable Tablets (4%; up to 5%) ... 2662
DiaBeta Tablets ... 1239
Diabinese Tablets ... 1935
Diflucan Injection, Tablets, and Oral Suspension ... 2194
Dilantin Infatabs (Occasional) ... 1908
Dilantin Kapseals (Occasional) ... 1906
Dilantin Parenteral (Occasional) ... 1910
Dilantin-125 Suspension (Occasional) ... 1911
Dimetane-DC Cough Syrup ... 2059
Dimetane-DX Cough Syrup ... 2059
Dipentum Capsules (Rare) ... 1951
Diucardin Tablets ... 2718
Diupres Tablets ... 1650
Diuril Oral Suspension ... 1653
Diuril Sodium Intravenous ... 1652
Diuril Tablets ... 1653
Dobutrex Solution Vials (Isolated cases) ... 1439
Dolobid Tablets (Less than 1 in 100) ... 1654
Doryx Capsules ... 1913
Duricef ... 748
Dyazide ... 2479
Dynacin Capsules ... 1590
Dyrenium Capsules (Rare) ... 2481
Easprin ... 1914
EC-Naprosyn Delayed-Release Tablets (Less than 1%) ... 2117
Edecrin (Rare) ... 1657
Effexor (Infrequent) ... 2719
Efudex ... 2113
Elavil ... 2838
Emcyt Capsules (1%) ... 1953
▲ Eminase (Less than 10%) ... 2039
Endep Tablets ... 2174
Enduron Tablets ... 420
Engerix-B Unit-Dose Vials ... 2482
Ergamisol Tablets (Up to 10%) ... 1292
Esgic-plus Tablets ... 1013
Esidrix Tablets ... 821
Esimil Tablets (A few instances) ... 822
Ethmozine Tablets (2 patients) ... 2041
Etrafon ... 2355
Eulexin Capsules (1%) ... 2358
▲ Exosurf Neonatal for Intratracheal Suspension (Less than 1% to 25%) ... 1095
Fansidar Tablets ... 2114
Felbatol (Infrequent) ... 2666
Feldene Capsules (Less than 1%) .. 1965
Fioricet Tablets (Infrequent) ... 2258
Fioricet with Codeine Capsules ... 2260
Flagyl 375 Capsules (Rare) ... 2434
Flagyl I.V. (Rare) ... 2247
Flexeril Tablets (Rare) ... 1661
Floxin I.V. (More than or equal to 1%) ... 1571
Floxin Tablets (200 mg, 300 mg, 400 mg) (More than or equal to 1%) ... 1567
▲ Fludara for Injection (Among most common) ... 663
Fluorouracil Injection ... 2116
Fortaz (Very rare) ... 1100
Foscavir Injection (Between 1% and 5%) ... 547
Fragmin (Less than 1%) ... 1954
▲ Sterile FUDR (Among more common) ... 2118
Fungizone Intravenous ... 506
Gantanol Tablets ... 2119
Gantrisin ... 2120
Garamycin Injectable ... 2360
Geocillin Tablets ... 2199
Glucotrol Tablets ... 1967
Glucotrol XL Extended Release Tablets ... 1968
Glynase PresTab Tablets ... 2609
▲ Heparin Lock Flush Solution (0 to 30%) ... 2725
▲ Heparin Sodium Injection (0 to 30%) ... 2726
▲ Heparin Sodium Injection, USP, Sterile Solution (0% to 30%) ... 2615
▲ Heparin Sodium Vials (0 to 30%) .. 1441
▲ Hexalen Capsules (3% to 10%) ... 2571
Hivid Tablets (Less than 1% to less than 3%) ... 2121
Hydrea Capsules (Occasional; less often; rare) ... 696
Hydrocet Capsules ... 782
HydroDIURIL Tablets ... 1674
Hydropres Tablets ... 1675
Hyperstat I.V. Injection ... 2363
Hyzaar Tablets ... 1677
IBU Tablets (Less than 1%) ... 1342
▲ IFEX (About 20%) ... 697
Imdur (Less than or equal to 5%) .. 1323
Imitrex Tablets ... 1106
Imuran ... 1110
Inderide Tablets ... 2732
Inderide LA Long Acting Capsules .. 2734
Indocin I.V. (1% to 3%) ... 1684
Inocor Lactate Injection (2.4%) ... 2309
▲ Intron A (Less than 5% to 12%) ... 2364
Ismelin Tablets ... 827
Keflex Pulvules & Oral Suspension 914
Keftab Tablets ... 915
Kefurox Vials, Faspak & ADD-Vantage ... 1454
Kerlone Tablets (Less than 2%) ... 2436
Klonopin Tablets ... 2126
▲ Kytril Tablets (3%) ... 2492
Lamictal Tablets (Rare) ... 1112
▲ Lariam Tablets (Among most frequent; occasional) ... 2128
Lasix Injection, Oral Solution and Tablets ... 1240
Lescol Capsules (Rare) ... 2267
▲ Leucovorin Calcium for Injection (1% to 18%) ... 1268
▲ Leustatin (12%) ... 1834
Levoprome ... 1274
Limbitrol ... 2180
Lodine Capsules and Tablets (Less than 1%) ... 2743
Loniten Tablets (Rare) ... 2618
Lopid Tablets (Rare) ... 1917
Lopressor HCT Tablets ... 832
Lorabid Suspension and Pulvules ... 1459
Lorelco Tablets ... 1517
Lortab ... 2566
Lotensin HCT ... 837
Lovenox Injection (Rare) ... 2020
Loxitane (Rare) ... 1378
Lozol Tablets ... 2022
Ludiomil Tablets (Isolated reports) 843
Luvox Tablets (Infrequent) ... 2544
M-M-R II ... 1687
M-R-VAX II ... 1689
Macrobid Capsules ... 1988
Macrodantin Capsules ... 1989
Mandol Vials, Faspak & ADD-Vantage (Rare) ... 1461
▲ Matulane Capsules (Frequent) ... 2131
Maxaquin Tablets (Less than or equal to 0.1%) ... 2440
Maxzide ... 1380
Mefoxin ... 1691
Mefoxin Premixed Intravenous Solution ... 1694
Mellaril ... 2269
Mesantoin Tablets ... 2272
▲ Methotrexate Sodium Tablets, Injection, for Injection and LPF Injection (3 to 10%) ... 1275
MetroGel-Vaginal ... 902
Mevacor Tablets (Rare) ... 1699
Mexitil Capsules (About 2 in 1,000) ... 678
Mezlin ... 601
Mezlin Pharmacy Bulk Package ... 604
Micronase Tablets ... 2623
Minizide Capsules ... 1938
Minocin Intravenous ... 1382
Minocin Oral Suspension ... 1385
Minocin Pellet-Filled Capsules ... 1383
Mithracin ... 607
Moduretic Tablets ... 1705
Monocid Injection (Less than 1%) .. 2497
Monodox Capsules ... 1805
Monopril Tablets ... 757

(▣ Described in PDR For Nonprescription Drugs) Incidence data in parenthesis; ▲ 3% or more (◉ Described in PDR For Ophthalmology)

1427 Side Effects Index Thromboembolism

Children's Motrin Ibuprofen Oral Suspension (Less than 1%) 1546
Motrin Tablets (Less than 1%) 2625
Motrin Ibuprofen Suspension, Oral Drops, Chewable Tablets, Caplets (Less than 1%) 1546
Mustargen 1709
Mutamycin 703
▲ Mycobutin Capsules (5%) 1957
Mykrox Tablets (Rare) 993
Myleran Tablets 1143
Myochrysine Injection 1711
Nalfon 200 Pulvules & Nalfon Tablets (Less than 1%) 917
Anaprox/Naprosyn (Less than 1%) 2117
Navane Capsules and Concentrate 2201
Navane Intramuscular 2202
Navelbine Injection (1% to 4%) 1145
Nebcin Vials, Hyporets & ADD-Vantage 1464
NebuPent for Inhalation Solution (1% or less) 1040
NegGram (Rare) 2323
Neoral (2% or less) 2276
NEOSAR Lyophilized/Neosar (Occasional) 1959
Netromycin Injection 100 mg/ml (1 per 1000 patients) 2373
▲ Neupogen for Injection (Fewer than 6% to 12%) 495
Neurontin Capsules (Infrequent) 1922
▲ Neutrexin (10.1%) 2572
Nimotop Capsules (0.3%; rare) 610
Nizoral Tablets (Less than 1%) 1298
Nolvadex Tablets (Occasional; 1.5%) 2841
Noroxin Tablets (1.0%) 1715
Noroxin Tablets (1.0%) 2048
Norpace (Rare) 2444
Norpramin Tablets 1526
Nydrazid Injection 508
Omnipen Capsules 2764
Omnipen for Oral Suspension 2765
▲ Oncaspar (Greater than 1% but less than 5%) 2028
Oncovin Solution Vials & Hyporets 1466
Oretic Tablets 443
Ornade Spansule Capsules 2502
Orthoclone OKT3 Sterile Solution 1837
Orudis Capsules (Less than 1%) 2766
Oruvail Capsules (Less than 1%) 2766
PBZ Tablets 845
PBZ-SR Tablets 844
Pamelor 2280
Panhematin 443
▲ Paraplatin for Injection (22% to 70%) 705
Parnate Tablets 2503
PASER Granules 1285
Paxil Tablets 2505
PedvaxHIB (One child) 1718
Pen•Vee K (Infrequent) 2772
Pentam 300 Injection (0.9 to 1.7%) 1041
Pentasa (Less than 1%) 1527
Pepcid Injection (Rare) 1722
Pepcid (Rare) 1720
Periactin 1724
Permax Tablets (Infrequent) 575
Pfizerpen for Injection (Rare) 2203
Phenergan with Codeine (Rare) 2777
Phenergan with Dextromethorphan (Rare) 2778
Phenergan Suppositories (Rare) 2775
Phenergan Syrup 2774
Phenergan VC 2779
Phenergan VC with Codeine 2781
Phrenilin (Infrequent) 785
Pipracil 1390
Placidyl Capsules (One case) 448
Plaquenil Sulfate Tablets 2328
Platinol 708
Platinol-AQ Injection 710
Pneumovax 23 1725
Pnu-Imune 23 (Rare) 1393
Podocon-25 1891
Pravachol (Rare) 765
PREVACID Delayed-Release Capsules (Less than 1%) 2562
Prilosec Delayed-Release Capsules (Rare) 529
Primacor Injection (0.4%) 2331
Primaxin I.M. 1727
Primaxin I.V. (Less than 0.2%) 1729
Prinivil Tablets (Rare) 1733
Prinzide Tablets (Rare) 1737
Priscoline Hydrochloride Ampuls 845
Procan SR Tablets (Rare) 1926
Procardia Capsules (Less than 0.5%) 1971
Procardia XL Extended Release Tablets 1972
Proglycem 580
▲ Prograf (10% to 24%) 1042
▲ Proleukin for Injection (64%) 797
Proloprim Tablets 1155
Propulsid (Rare) 1300
Prostin VR Pediatric Sterile Solution (Less than 1%) 2635
Protostat Tablets (Rare) 1883
Prozac Pulvules & Liquid, Oral Solution (Rare) 919
Purinethol Tablets (Frequent) 1156
Pyrazinamide Tablets (Rare) 1398
Quinidex Extentabs 2067
Recombivax HB 1744
Relafen Tablets (Less than 1%) 2510
▲ ReoPro Vials (0.7% to 5.2%) 1471
▲ Retrovir Capsules (12%) 1158
▲ Retrovir I.V. Infusion (12%) 1163
▲ Retrovir Syrup (12%) 1158
Ridaura Capsules (1 to 3%) 2513
Rifadin (Rare) 1528
Rifamate Capsules 1530
Rifater (Rare) 1532
Rimactane Capsules (Rare) 847
Risperdal (Rare) 1301
Rocephin Injectable Vials, ADD-Vantage, Galaxy Container (Less than 1%) 2142
▲ Roferon-A Injection (35%) 2145
Rogaine Topical Solution (0.31%) 2637
Rythmol Tablets–150mg, 225mg, 300mg (Less than 1%) 1352
SSD 1355
Sandimmune (2% or less; occasional) 2286
Sansert Tablets 2295
Sedapap Tablets 50 mg/650 mg 1543
Seldane Tablets 1536
Seldane-D Extended-Release Tablets 1538
Septra 1174
▲ Septra I.V. Infusion (Among most frequent) 1169
Septra I.V. Infusion ADD-Vantage Vials 1171
Septra 1174
Ser-Ap-Es Tablets 849
Serentil 684
Silvadene Cream 1% 1540
Sinemet Tablets (Rare) 943
Sinemet CR Tablets 944
Sinequan (Occasional) 2205
Solganal Suspension (Rare) 2388
Spectrobid Tablets 2206
Stelazine 2514
Suprax (Less than 2%) 1399
Surmontil Capsules 2811
Tagamet (Approximately 3 per 1,000,000) 2516
Tambocor Tablets (Less than 1%) 1497
Tapazole Tablets 1477
Tavist Syrup 2297
Tavist Tablets 2298
▲ Taxol (7% to 20%; uncommon) 714
Tazicef for Injection (Very rare) 2519
▲ Tegison Capsules (1-10%) 2154
Tegretol Chewable Tablets 852
Tegretol Suspension 852
Tegretol Tablets 852
Tenoretic Tablets 2845
Tenormin Tablets and I.V. Injection 2847
Terramycin Intramuscular Solution 2210
Thalitone 1245
TheraCys BCG Live (Intravesical) (Up to 0.9%) 897
Thioguanine Tablets, Tabloid Brand 1181
Thioplex (Thiotepa For Injection) 1281
Ticar for Injection 2526
Ticlid Tablets (Rare) 2156
Timentin for Injection 2528
Timolide Tablets 1748
Tobramycin Sulfate Injection 968
Tofranil Ampuls 854
Tofranil Tablets 856
Tofranil-PM Capsules 857
Tolectin (200, 400 and 600 mg) (Less than 1%) 1581
Tonocard Tablets (Less than 1%) 531
Toradol 2159
Torecan 2245
Tornalate Metered Dose Inhaler (Rare) 957
Trasylol (2%) 613
Trecator-SC Tablets 2814
Trental Tablets (Rare) 1244
Triavil Tablets 1757
Trimpex Tablets 2163
Trinalin Repetabs Tablets 1330
Tussend 1783
Unasyn 2212
Vancocin HCl, Oral Solution & Pulvules (Rare) 1483
Vancocin HCl, Vials & ADD-Vantage (Rare) 1481
Vantin for Oral Suspension and Vantin Tablets 2646
Vaseretic Tablets (Rare) 1765
Vasotec I.V. (Rare) 1768
Vasotec Tablets (Rare) 1771
Velban Vials 1484
▲ VePesid Capsules and Injection (1% to 41%) 718
Vibramycin 1941
Vibramycin Hyclate Intravenous 2215
Vibramycin 1941
Videx Tablets, Powder for Oral Solution, & Pediatric Powder for Oral Solution (1% to 2%) 720
Vivactil Tablets 1774
Voltaren Tablets (Less than 1%) 861
▲ Vumon (85%) 727
Zanosar Sterile Powder 2653
Zantac (A few patients) 1209
Zantac Injection (Few patients) 1207
Zantac Syrup (A few patients) 1209
Zaroxolyn Tablets 1000
Zebeta Tablets 1413
Zefazone 2654
Zerit Capsules (1% to 4%) 729
Zestoretic (Rare) 2850
Zestril Tablets (Rare) 2854
Ziac 1415
Zinacef (Rare) 1211
Zinecard 1961
Zithromax (Less than 1%) 1944
Zocor Tablets (Rare) 1775
Zosyn 1419
Zosyn Pharmacy Bulk Package 1422
Zovirax Sterile Powder (Less than 1%) 1223
Zyloprim Tablets (Less than 1%) 1226

Thrombocytopenia, immune

Ticlid Tablets (Rare) 2156

Thrombocytopenia, neonatal

Capozide 742
Diupres Tablets 1650
Dyazide (Rare) 2479
HydroDIURIL Tablets 1674
Hydropres Tablets 1675
Lopressor HCT Tablets 832
Prinzide Tablets 1737
VePesid Capsules and Injection 718
Zestoretic 2850

Thrombocytopenic purpura (see under Purpura, thrombocytopenic)

Thrombocytosis

▲ Accutane Capsules (1 in 5 to 1 in 10 patients) 2076
Ancef Injection 2465
Augmentin (Less than 1%) 2468
Azactam for Injection (Less than 1%) 734
Cefizox for Intramuscular or Intravenous Use (Greater than 1% but less than 5%) 1034
Cefotan (1 in 300) 2829
Ceptaz (One in 45) 1081
CHEMET (succimer) Capsules (0.5 to 1.5%) 1545
▲ Cipro I.V. (Among most frequent) 595
▲ Cipro I.V. Pharmacy Bulk Package (Among most frequent) 597
Cipro Tablets (0.1%) 592
Clozaril Tablets 2252
Cuprimine Capsules 1630
Demser Capsules (Rare) 1649
Depen Titratable Tablets 2662
Effexor (Infrequent) 2719
Estratest 2539
Floxin I.V. (More than or equal to 1%) 1571
Floxin Tablets (200 mg, 300 mg, 400 mg) (More than or equal to 1%) 1567
Fortaz (1 in 45) 1100
Kefzol Vials, Faspak & ADD-Vantage 1456
Lupron Depot 3.75 mg 2556
Maxaquin Tablets (Less than 1%) 2440
Monocid Injection (1.7%) 2497
Motrin Ibuprofen Suspension, Oral Drops, Chewable Tablets, Caplets 1546
Netromycin Injection 100 mg/ml (2 of 1000 patients) 2373
Penetrex Tablets (Less than 1%) 2031
Pentasa (Less than 1%) 1527
Permax Tablets (Rare) 575
PREVACID Delayed-Release Capsules (Less than 1%) 2562
Primaxin I.M. 1727
Primaxin I.V. 1729
▲ Rocephin Injectable Vials, ADD-Vantage, Galaxy Container (5.1%) 2142
Tazicef for Injection (1 in 45 patients) 2519
Unasyn 2212
Vantin for Oral Suspension and Vantin Tablets 2646
Zefazone 2654
Zosyn 1419
Zosyn Pharmacy Bulk Package 1422
Zovirax Sterile Powder (Less than 1%) 1223

Thromboembolic complications

Atromid-S Capsules 2701
Brevicon 2088
Cycrin Tablets 975
Demulen 2428
Depo-Provera Sterile Aqueous Suspension 2606
Estraderm Transdermal System 824
Estratest 2539
Heparin Lock Flush Solution 2725
Heparin Sodium Injection 2726
Heparin Sodium Injection, USP, Sterile Solution 2615
Heparin Sodium Vials 1441
Humegon 1824
Levlen/Tri-Levlen 651
Menest Tablets 2494
Metrodin (urofollitropin for injection) 2446
Micronor Tablets 1872
Modicon 1872
Mononine, Coagulation Factor IX (Human) 523
Nordette-21 Tablets 2755
Nordette-28 Tablets 2758
Norinyl 2088
Norplant System 2759
Nor-Q D Tablets 2135
Ogen Vaginal Cream 2630
Ortho-Cyclen/Ortho-Tri-Cyclen 1858
Ortho Dienestrol Cream 1866
Ortho-Est 1869
Ortho-Novum 1872
Ortho-Cyclen/Ortho Tri-Cyclen 1858
Ovcon 760
PMB 200 and PMB 400 2783
Premarin Intravenous 2787
Premarin with Methyltestosterone 2794
Premarin Vaginal Cream 2791
Premphase 2797
Prempro 2801
Provera Tablets (Occasional) 2636
Serophene (clomiphene citrate tablets, USP) (Rare) 2451
Stilphostrol Tablets and Ampuls 612
Ticlid Tablets 2156
Levlen/Tri-Levlen 651
Tri-Norinyl 2164
Triphasil-21 Tablets 2814
Triphasil-28 Tablets 2819

Thromboembolic disease (see under Thromboembolic complications)

Thromboembolism

Amen Tablets 780
Brevicon 2088
Cortone Acetate Sterile Suspension 1623
Cortone Acetate Tablets 1624
Cycrin Tablets 975
Dalalone D.P. Injectable 1011
Danocrine Capsules 2307
Decadron Elixir 1633
Decadron Phosphate Injection 1637
Decadron Phosphate Respihaler 1642
Decadron Phosphate Turbinaire 1645
Decadron Phosphate with Xylocaine Injection, Sterile 1639
Decadron Tablets 1635
Decadron-LA Sterile Suspension 1646
Demulen 2428
Dexacort Phosphate in Respihaler 458
Dexacort Phosphate in Turbinaire 459
Diethylstilbestrol Tablets 1437
Estrace Cream and Tablets 749
Estraderm Transdermal System 824

(Described in PDR For Nonprescription Drugs) Incidence data in parenthesis; ▲ 3% or more (◉ Described in PDR For Ophthalmology)

Thromboembolism — Side Effects Index — 1428

Estratest 2539
Hydeltrasol Injection, Sterile 1665
Hydeltra-T.B.A. Sterile Suspension 1667
Hydrocortone Acetate Sterile Suspension 1669
Hydrocortone Phosphate Injection, Sterile 1670
Hydrocortone Tablets 1672
Lamprene Capsules (Less than 1%) 828
Lo/Ovral Tablets 2746
Lo/Ovral-28 Tablets 2751
Micronor Tablets 1872
Modicon 1872
Nordette-21 Tablets 2755
Nordette-28 Tablets 2758
Norinyl 2088
Ortho-Cyclen/Ortho-Tri-Cyclen 1858
Ortho Dienestrol Cream 1866
Ortho-Est 1869
Ortho-Novum 1872
Ortho-Cyclen/Ortho Tri-Cyclen 1858
Ovcon 760
Ovral Tablets 2770
Ovral-28 Tablets 2770
Ovrette Tablets 2771
Premarin Tablets 2789
Premarin Vaginal Cream 2791
Tri-Norinyl 2164
Triphasil-21 Tablets 2814
Triphasil-28 Tablets 2819

Thromboembolism, arterial
Brevicon 2088
Demulen 2428
Desogen Tablets 1817
Levlen/Tri-Levlen 651
Metrodin (urofollitropin for injection) 2446
Micronor Tablets 1872
Modicon 1872
Norinyl 2088
Nor-Q D Tablets 2135
Ortho-Cept 1851
Ortho-Cyclen/Ortho-Tri-Cyclen 1858
Ortho-Novum 1872
Ortho-Cyclen/Ortho Tri-Cyclen 1858
Ovcon 760
Pergonal (menotropins for injection, USP) 2448
Profasi (chorionic gonadotropin for injection, USP) 2450
Levlen/Tri-Levlen 651
Tri-Norinyl 2164

Thrombopenia (see under Thrombocytopenia)

Thrombophlebitis
AK-Fluor Injection 10% and 25% ⊙ 203
Amen Tablets 780
Amicar Syrup, Tablets, and Injection 1267
Anafranil Capsules (Rare) 803
Atgam Sterile Solution (Less than 5%) 2581
Atretol Tablets 573
Azactam for Injection (1.9%) 734
Bactrim I.V. Infusion (Rare) 2082
Betaseron for SC Injection 658
Brevibloc Injection (Less than 1%) 1808
Brevicon 2088
Brevital Sodium Vials 1429
Cipro I.V. (1% or less) 595
Cipro I.V. Pharmacy Bulk Package (Less than 1%) 597
Cleocin Phosphate Injection 2586
Climara Transdermal System 645
Clomid 1514
Clozaril Tablets (Less than 1%) 2252
Cortifoam 2396
Cuprimine Capsules (Rare) 1630
Cycrin Tablets 975
▲ Cytosar-U Sterile Powder (Among most frequent) 2592
Dalgan Injection (Less than 1%) 538
Dantrium Intravenous 1983
Demulen 2428
Depen Titratable Tablets (Rare) 2662
Depo-Provera Contraceptive Injection (Fewer than 1%) 2602
Depo-Provera Sterile Aqueous Suspension 2606
Desogen Tablets 1817
Effexor (Infrequent) 2719
▲ Emcyt Capsules (3%) 1953
Epogen for Injection (Rare) 489
Ergamisol Tablets 1292
Estrace Cream and Tablets 749
Estraderm Transdermal System 824
ESTRATAB Tablets (0.3, 0.625, 1.25, 2.5 mg) 2536
Estratest 2539
Ethmozine Tablets (Less than 2%) 2041
Felbatol 2666
Flagyl I.V. 2247
Florinef Acetate Tablets 505
Fluorescite ⊙ 219
Fluorouracil Injection 2116
Foscavir Injection (Less than 1%) 547
Sterile FUDR 2118
▲ Fungizone Intravenous (Among most common) 506
Indocin Capsules (Rare) 1680
Indocin I.V. 1684
Indocin (Rare) 1680
Kefurox Vials, Faspak & ADD-Vantage (1 in 60) 1454
Kerlone Tablets (Less than 2%) 2436
Lasix Injection, Oral Solution and Tablets 1240
Levlen/Tri-Levlen 651
Lo/Ovral Tablets 2746
Lo/Ovral-28 Tablets 2751
Mandol Vials, Faspak & ADD-Vantage (Rare) 1461
Mefoxin 1691
Mefoxin Premixed Intravenous Solution 1694
Megace Tablets (Rare) 701
Menest Tablets 2494
Mestinon Injectable 1253
Methergine (Rare) 2272
Mezlin 601
Mezlin Pharmacy Bulk Package 604
Miacalcin Nasal Spray (Less than 1%) 2275
Micronor Tablets 1872
Modicon 1872
Mustargen 1709
Mutamycin 703
Neurontin Capsules (Rare) 1922
Nordette-21 Tablets 2755
Nordette-28 Tablets 2758
Norinyl 2088
Norplant System 2759
Nor-Q D Tablets 2135
Ogen Tablets 2627
Ogen Vaginal Cream 2630
Ortho-Cept 1851
Ortho-Cyclen/Ortho-Tri-Cyclen 1858
Ortho Dienestrol Cream 1866
Ortho-Est 1869
Ortho-Novum 1872
Ortho-Cyclen/Ortho Tri-Cyclen 1858
Ovcon 760
Ovral Tablets 2770
Ovral-28 Tablets 2770
Ovrette Tablets 2771
PMB 200 and PMB 400 2783
Permax Tablets (Infrequent) 575
▲ Pipracil (4%) 1390
Polymyxin B Sulfate, Aerosporin Brand Sterile Powder (Occasional) 1154
Premarin Intravenous 2787
Premarin with Methyltestosterone 2794
Premarin Tablets 2789
Premarin Vaginal Cream 2791
Premphase 2797
Prempro 2801
▲ Primaxin I.V. (3.1%) 1729
Procrit for Injection (Rare) 1841
Provera Tablets (Occasional) 2636
Prozac Pulvules & Liquid, Oral Solution (Rare) 919
Relafen Tablets (Less than 1%) 2510
Risperdal (Rare) 1301
Robaxin Injectable 2070
Romazicon (1% to 3%) 2147
Sandostatin Injection (Less than 1%) 2292
Sansert Tablets 2295
Septra I.V. Infusion (Rare) 1169
Septra I.V. Infusion ADD-Vantage Vials (Rare) 1171
Stilphostrol Tablets and Ampuls 612
Tegretol Chewable Tablets 852
Tegretol Suspension 852
Tegretol Tablets 852
Timentin for Injection 2528
Levlen/Tri-Levlen 651
Tri-Norinyl 2164
Triphasil-21 Tablets 2814
Triphasil-28 Tablets 2819
▲ Unasyn (3%) 2212
Vancocin HCl, Vials & ADD-Vantage 1481
Zefazone 2654
Zinacef (1 in 60 patients) 1211
Zosyn (0.2%) 1419
Zosyn Pharmacy Bulk Package (0.2%) 1422
Zyloprim Tablets (Less than 1%) 1226

Thrombophlebitis, deep-vein
Cardene I.V. (Rare) 2709
Cytovene (1% or less) 2103
Humegon 1824
Lamictal Tablets (Rare) 1112

Thrombophlebitis, peripheral
Atgam Sterile Solution (More than 1% but less than 5%) 2581

Thromboplastin time, increase
Azactam for Injection 734
Eminase 2039
Hespan Injection 929
▲ Oncaspar (Greater than 1% but less than 5%) 2028
Pentaspan Injection 937
Zefazone Sterile Powder 2654
Zosyn 1419
Zosyn Pharmacy Bulk Package 1422

Thrombosis
Betaseron for SC Injection 658
BiCNU (Rare) 691
▲ CellCept Capsules (More than or equal to 3%) 2099
Demadex Tablets and Injection 686
Demulen 2428
Diprivan Injection (Rare; less than 1%) 2833
Emcyt Capsules 1953
Estratest 2539
Foscavir Injection (Between 1% and 5%) 547
Humegon 1824
Imitrex Tablets (Rare) 1106
Kerlone Tablets (Less than 2%) 2436
Konÿne 80 Factor IX Complex 634
Leustatin (2%) 1834
Lovenox Injection (Rare) 2020
Lupron Depot 3.75 mg 2556
Lupron Depot 7.5 mg 2559
Lupron Injection (2%) 2555
Metrodin (urofollitropin for injection) 2446
Mustargen 1709
▲ Oncaspar (Greater than 1% but less than 5%) 2028
Ovcon 760
PMB 200 and PMB 400 2783
Paxil Tablets (Rare) 2505
Pipracil 1390
Premarin Intravenous 2787
Premarin with Methyltestosterone 2794
Premarin Vaginal Cream 2791
Proleukin for Injection (1%) 797
Stimate, (desmopressin acetate) Nasal Spray, 1.5 mg/mL (Rare) 525
Valium Injectable (Among most common) 2182

Thrombosis of vascular access
▲ Epogen for Injection (0.25% to 7%) 489
Lasix Injection, Oral Solution and Tablets 1240
Procrit for Injection 1841

Thrombosis, arterial
Orthoclone OKT3 Sterile Solution 1837

Thrombosis, cerebral (see under Cerebral thrombosis)

Thrombosis, coronary (see under Coronary thrombosis)

Thrombosis, glomerular capillary
Amicar Syrup, Tablets, and Injection 1267
Neoral 2276
Sandimmune 2286

Thrombosis, mesenteric
Brevicon 2088
Cartrol Tablets 410
Demulen 2428
Estraderm Transdermal System 824
ESTRATAB Tablets (0.3, 0.625, 1.25, 2.5 mg) 2536
Estratest 2539
Levatol 2403
Levlen/Tri-Levlen 651
Menest Tablets 2494
Norinyl 2088
Nor-Q D Tablets 2135
Ortho Dienestrol Cream 1866
Ovcon 760
PMB 200 and PMB 400 2783
Premarin Intravenous 2787
Premarin with Methyltestosterone 2794
Premarin Vaginal Cream 2791
Stilphostrol Tablets and Ampuls 612
Trandate Tablets 1185
Levlen/Tri-Levlen 651
Tri-Norinyl 2164

Thrombosis, mesenteric arterial
Timoptic-XE 1755
Visken Tablets 2299
Zebeta Tablets 1413

Thrombosis, renal artery
Atgam Sterile Solution (Less than 1% to less than 5%) 2581
Epogen for Injection (Rare) 489
Procrit for Injection (Rare) 1841

Thrombosis, retinal
Amen Tablets 780
Brevicon 2088
Clomid 1514
Cycrin Tablets 975
Demulen 2428
Depo-Provera Contraceptive Injection 2602
Depo-Provera Sterile Aqueous Suspension 2606
Epogen for Injection (Rare) 489
Estraderm Transdermal System 824
ESTRATAB Tablets (0.3, 0.625, 1.25, 2.5 mg) 2536
Estratest 2539
Levlen/Tri-Levlen 651
Lo/Ovral Tablets 2746
Lo/Ovral-28 Tablets 2751
Menest Tablets 2494
Micronor Tablets 1872
Modicon 1872
Nordette-21 Tablets 2755
Nordette-28 Tablets 2758
Norinyl 2088
Nor-Q D Tablets 2135
Ortho-Cyclen/Ortho-Tri-Cyclen 1858
Ortho Dienestrol Cream 1866
Ortho-Novum 1872
Ortho-Cyclen/Ortho Tri-Cyclen 1858
Ovcon 760
Ovral Tablets 2770
Ovral-28 Tablets 2770
Ovrette Tablets 2771
PMB 200 and PMB 400 2783
Premarin Intravenous 2787
Premarin with Methyltestosterone 2794
Premarin Vaginal Cream 2791
Premphase 2797
Prempro 2801
Procrit for Injection (Rare) 1841
Provera Tablets (Occasional) 2636
Stilphostrol Tablets and Ampuls 612
Levlen/Tri-Levlen 651
Tri-Norinyl 2164
Triphasil-21 Tablets 2814
Triphasil-28 Tablets 2819

Thrombosis, sagittal sinus
Danocrine Capsules 2307
Oncaspar 2028

Thrombosis, venous
Actimmune (Rare) 1056
Activase 1058
Atgam Sterile Solution (Less than 5%) 2581
Clomid 1514
Clozaril Tablets 2252
Demulen 2428
Depo-Provera Contraceptive Injection (Fewer than 1%) 2602
Desogen Tablets 1817
Dizac (Less frequent) 1809
Epogen for Injection (Rare) 489
Fludara for Injection (1% to 3%) 663
Lioresal Intrathecal 1596
Mepergan Injection 2753
Micronor Tablets 1872
Modicon 1872
Mononine, Coagulation Factor IX (Human) 523
Mykrox Tablets 993
Nimotop Capsules (Less than 1%) 610
Nolvadex Tablets (0.8%) 2841
Norplant System 2759
Oncaspar 2028
Ortho-Cept 1851
Ortho-Cyclen/Ortho-Tri-Cyclen 1858
Ortho-Novum 1872
Ortho-Cyclen/Ortho Tri-Cyclen 1858

(▣ Described in PDR For Nonprescription Drugs) Incidence data in parenthesis; ▲ 3% or more (⊙ Described in PDR For Ophthalmology)

1429 Side Effects Index Tinnitus

Orthoclone OKT3 Sterile Solution .. 1837
Phenergan Injection ... 2773
Pipracil (Less frequent) ... 1390
Taxol (Approximately 1%; rare) ... 714
Zaroxolyn Tablets ... 1000

Thrombotic events, unspecified
DDAVP Injection (Rare) ... 2014
DDAVP Injection 15 mcg/mL (Rare) ... 2015
Danocrine Capsules ... 2307
Procrit for Injection ... 1841

Thrombotic microangiopathy
Blenoxane (Rare) ... 692
Platinol (Rare) ... 708
Platinol-AQ Injection (Rare) ... 710

Thrombotic vascular disease
Ortho-Cyclen/Ortho-Tri-Cyclen ... 1858
Ortho Dienestrol Cream ... 1866
Ortho-Cyclen/Ortho Tri-Cyclen ... 1858
▲Tegison Capsules (1 to 10%) ... 2154

Thrush, oral (see under Candidiasis, oral)

Thymol turbidity test, positive
Atromid-S Capsules ... 2701
Cuprimine Capsules ... 1630
Depen Titratable Tablets (Few reports) ... 2662

Thymus gland abnormalities, fetal
Accutane Capsules ... 2076

Thyroid adenoma
Permax Tablets (Rare) ... 575
Quadrinal Tablets ... 1350
SSKI Solution ... 2658

Thyroid binding globulin, increase (see under T4, increase)

Thyroid disease, exacerbation
Proleukin for Injection ... 797

Thyroid disorders (see under T3 or T4)

Thyroid function test, abnormal
BuSpar (Rare) ... 737
Depakene ... 413
Depakote Tablets ... 415
Depo-Provera Sterile Aqueous Suspension ... 2606
Lescol Capsules ... 2267
Mevacor Tablets ... 1699
Minocin Intravenous (Very rare) ... 1382
Minocin Oral Suspension (Very rare) ... 1385
Minocin Pellet-Filled Capsules (Very rare) ... 1383
Pravachol ... 765
Proleukin for Injection ... 797
Provera Tablets ... 2636
Roferon-A Injection (Rare; less than 3%) ... 2145
SSKI Solution ... 2658
Zocor Tablets ... 1775

Thyroid gland discoloration
Achromycin V Capsules ... 1367
Declomycin Tablets ... 1371
Doryx Capsules ... 1913
Dynacin Capsules ... 1590
Minocin Intravenous ... 1382
Minocin Oral Suspension ... 1385
Minocin Pellet-Filled Capsules ... 1383
Monodox Capsules ... 1805
Terramycin Intramuscular Solution ... 2210
Vibramycin ... 1941
Vibramycin Hyclate Intravenous ... 2215
Vibramycin ... 1941

Thyroid gland enlargement
Lupron Depot 3.75 mg ... 2556
Lupron Depot 7.5 mg ... 2559
Lupron Injection (Less than 5%) ... 2555

Thyroid hormone, changes (see under T3 or T4)

Thyroid nodule
ProSom Tablets (Rare) ... 449

Thyroiditis
Cuprimine Capsules ... 1630
Depen Titratable Tablets (Extremely rare) ... 2662
Paxil Tablets (Rare) ... 2505

Tingling
Apresazide Capsules (Less frequent) ... 808
Apresoline Hydrochloride Tablets (Less frequent) ... 809
Asendin Tablets (Less than 1%) ... 1369
Bentyl ... 1501
Cipro I.V. ... 595
Condylox (Less than 5%) ... 1802
Decadron Phosphate Injection ... 1637
DynaCirc Capsules (0.5% to 1%) .. 2256
Elimite (permethrin) 5% Cream (1 to 2% or less) ... 478
Endep Tablets ... 2174
Engerix-B Unit-Dose Vials (Less than 1%) ... 2482
Esgic-plus Tablets (Infrequent) ... 1013
Fioricet Tablets (Infrequent) ... 2258
Fioricet with Codeine Capsules (Infrequent) ... 2260
Fiorinal with Codeine Capsules (Infrequent) ... 2262
Floxin I.V. ... 1571
Floxin Tablets (200 mg, 300 mg, 400 mg) ... 1567
▲Imitrex Injection (13.5%) ... 1103
▲Imitrex Tablets (4% to 8%) ... 1106
K-Phos Neutral Tablets ... 639
K-Phos Original Formula 'Sodium Free' Tablets (Less frequent) ... 639
Konÿne 80 Factor IX Complex ... 634
Lioresal Intrathecal (1 to 8 of 214 patients) ... 1596
Ludiomil Tablets (Rare) ... 843
Maxaquin Tablets ... 2440
Mononine, Coagulation Factor IX (Human) ... 523
Neoral (Rare) ... 2276
Nicobid ... 2026
Norpace (Less than 1%) ... 2444
Norplant System ... 2759
Norpramin Tablets ... 1526
Nubain Injection (1% or less) ... 935
Oxistat Lotion (0.4%) ... 1152
Pamelor ... 2280
Phrenilin (Infrequent) ... 785
Priscoline Hydrochloride Ampuls ... 845
SSKI Solution (Less frequent) ... 2658
Sandimmune (Rare) ... 2286
Sedapap Tablets 50 mg/650 mg (Infrequent) ... 1543
Ser-Ap-Es Tablets ... 849
Slo-Niacin Tablets ... 2659
THYREL TRH (Less frequent) ... 2873
Tofranil Ampuls ... 854
Tofranil Tablets ... 856
Tofranil-PM Capsules ... 857
Ultravate Ointment 0.05% ... 2690
Zonalon Cream (Less than 1%) ... 1055

Tingling, ears
Parlodel (Less than 1%) ... 2281

Tingling, extremities
Bellergal-S Tablets (Rare) ... 2250
Coly-Mycin M Parenteral ... 1905
Diamox Sequels (Sustained Release) ... 1373
Elavil ... 2838
Etrafon ... 2355
Glauctabs ... ◎ 208
Hivid Tablets ... 2121
Hydrocortone Phosphate Injection, Sterile ... 1670
Limbitrol ... 2180
Lozol Tablets (Less than 5%) ... 2022
▲MZM (Among reactions occurring most often) ... ◎ 267
Myambutol Tablets ... 1386
Neptazane Tablets ... 1388
Norpramin Tablets ... 1526
Polycitra Syrup ... 578
Polycitra-K Crystals ... 579
Polycitra-K Oral Solution ... 579
Polycitra-LC ... 578
Surmontil Capsules ... 2811
Triavil Tablets ... 1757
Videx Tablets, Powder for Oral Solution, & Pediatric Powder for Oral Solution ... 720
Vivactil Tablets ... 1774
Zerit Capsules ... 729

Tingling, feet
Fluorouracil Injection ... 2116
Uroqid-Acid No. 2 Tablets ... 640

Tingling, fingers
Noroxin Tablets (0.3% to 1.0%) ... 1715
Noroxin Tablets (0.3% to 1.0%) ... 2048
Parlodel (Rare) ... 2281
Peptavlon ... 2878
Wigraine Tablets & Suppositories .. 1829

Tingling, hands
Adenocard Injection (1%) ... 1021
Fluorouracil Injection ... 2116
Uroqid-Acid No. 2 Tablets ... 640

Tingling, lips
K-Phos Neutral Tablets ... 639
K-Phos Original Formula 'Sodium Free' Tablets (Less frequent) ... 639
Marcaine Spinal ... 2319
Sensorcaine ... 559
Uroqid-Acid No. 2 Tablets ... 640

Tingling, mouth
Foscavir Injection ... 547
Marcaine Spinal ... 2319
Sensorcaine ... 559
Stilphostrol Tablets and Ampuls ... 612

Tingling, nose
Stilphostrol Tablets and Ampuls ... 612

Tingling, perineal area
Hydeltrasol Injection, Sterile ... 1665

Tingling, scalp
▲Normodyne Injection (7%) ... 2377
Normodyne Tablets (Less common) ... 2379
Temovate Scalp Application (2 of 294 patients) ... 1179
▲Trandate (7 of 100 patients) ... 1185

Tingling, skin
Garamycin Injectable ... 2360
Nebcin Vials, Hyporets & ADD-Vantage ... 1464
Netromycin Injection 100 mg/ml ... 2373
▲Normodyne Injection (7%) ... 2377
Tobramycin Sulfate Injection ... 968
▲Trandate Injection (7 of 100 patients) ... 1185

Tingling, toes
Wigraine Tablets & Suppositories .. 1829

Tinnitus
Accutane Capsules (Less than 1%) ... 2076
Achromycin V Capsules ... 1367
Actifed with Codeine Cough Syrup .. 1067
Adalat CC (Less than 1.0%) ... 589
Children's Advil Suspension (Less than 3%) ... 2692
Alka-Seltzer Effervescent Antacid and Pain Reliever ... ▣ 701
Alka-Seltzer Extra Strength Effervescent Antacid and Pain Reliever ... ▣ 703
Alka-Seltzer Lemon Lime Effervescent Antacid and Pain Reliever ... ▣ 703
Altace Capsules (Less than 1%) ... 1232
Ambien Tablets (Infrequent) ... 2416
Amicar Syrup, Tablets, and Injection (Occasional) ... 1267
▲Anafranil Capsules (4% to 6%) ... 803
▲Anaprox/Naprosyn (3% to 9%) ... 2117
Ansaid Tablets (1-3%) ... 2579
Aralen Hydrochloride Injection (1 patient) ... 2301
Aralen Phosphate Tablets (1 patient) ... 2301
Arthritis Foundation Safety Coated Aspirin Tablets ... ▣ 675
Asacol Delayed-Release Tablets ... 1979
Arthritis Pain Ascriptin ... ▣ 631
Maximum Strength Ascriptin ... ▣ 630
Regular Strength Ascriptin Tablets ... ▣ 629
Asendin Tablets (Less than 1%) ... 1369
Atretol Tablets ... 573
Atrohist Plus Tablets ... 454
Azactam for Injection (Less than 1%) ... 734
Azo Gantanol Tablets ... 2080
Azo Gantrisin Tablets ... 2081
Azulfidine (Rare) ... 1949
Arthritis Strength BC Powder ... ▣ 609
BC Powder ... ▣ 609
Backache Caplets ... ▣ 613
Bactrim DS Tablets ... 2084
Bactrim I.V. Infusion ... 2082
Bactrim ... 2084
Bayer Children's Chewable Aspirin ... ▣ 711
Genuine Bayer Aspirin Tablets & Caplets ... ▣ 713
Extra Strength Bayer Arthritis Pain Regimen Formula ... ▣ 711
Extra Strength Bayer Aspirin Caplets & Tablets ... ▣ 712
Extended-Release Bayer 8-Hour Aspirin ... ▣ 712
Extra Strength Bayer PM Aspirin ▣ 713
Aspirin Regimen Bayer Regular Strength 325 mg Caplets ... ▣ 709
Bayer Select Backache Pain Relief Formula ... ▣ 715
Benadryl Capsules ... 1898
Benadryl Injection ... 1898
Blocadren Tablets (Less than 1%) 1614
Arthritis Strength Bufferin Analgesic Caplets ... ▣ 614
Buprenex Injectable (Less than 1%) ... 2006
BuSpar (Frequent) ... 737
Cama Arthritis Pain Reliever ... ▣ 785
Capastat Sulfate Vials ... 2868
Carbocaine Hydrochloride Injection 2303
Cardono Capsules (Rare) ... 2095
Cardene I.V. (Rare) ... 2709
Cardizem CD Capsules (Less than 1%) ... 1506
Cardizem SR Capsules (Less than 1%) ... 1510
Cardizem Injectable ... 1508
Cardizem Tablets (Less than 1%) .. 1512
Cardura Tablets (1%) ... 2186
Cartrol Tablets (Less common) ... 410
Cataflam (1% to 3%) ... 816
Cipro I.V. (1% or less) ... 595
Cipro I.V. Pharmacy Bulk Package (Less than 1%) ... 597
Cipro Tablets (Less than 1%) ... 592
Claritin (2% or fewer patients) ... 2349
Claritin-D (Less frequent) ... 2350
Clinoril Tablets (Greater than 1%) 1618
Clomid ... 1514
Cognex Capsules (Infrequent) ... 1901
Cozaar Tablets (Less than 1%) ... 1628
Cuprimine Capsules (Greater than 1%) ... 1630
Cytotec (Infrequent) ... 2424
Cytovene (1% or less) ... 2103
Dalgan Injection (Less than 1%) ... 538
Dapsone Tablets USP ... 1284
Daranide Tablets ... 1633
Daypro Caplets (Greater than 1% but less than 3%) ... 2426
Deconamine ... 1320
Demadex Tablets and Injection ... 686
Depakote Tablets (Greater than 1% but not more than 5%) ... 415
Depen Titratable Tablets ... 2662
Desferal Vials ... 820
Desyrel and Desyrel Dividose (1.4%) ... 503
Diamox Intravenous ... 1372
Diamox Sequels (Sustained Release) ... 1373
Diamox Tablets ... 1372
Dilacor XR Extended-release Capsules (1.0%) ... 2018
Dipentum Capsules (Rare) ... 1951
Diprivan Injection (Less than 1%) .. 2833
Doan's Extra-Strength Analgesic .. ▣ 633
Extra Strength Doan's P.M. ... ▣ 633
Doan's Regular Strength Analgesic ... ▣ 634
Dolobid Tablets (Greater than 1 in 100) ... 1654
Duranest Injections ... 542
Dyclone 0.5% and 1% Topical Solutions, USP ... 544
Easprin ... 1914
▲EC-Naprosyn Delayed-Release Tablets (3% to 9%) ... 2117
Ecotrin ... 2455
Edecrin ... 1657
Effexor (2%) ... 2719
Elavil ... 2838
Eldepryl Tablets ... 2550
Emcyt Capsules ... 1953
Emla Cream ... 545
Empirin with Codeine Tablets ... 1093
Endep Tablets ... 2174
Engerix-B Unit-Dose Vials ... 2482
Esgic-plus Tablets (Infrequent) ... 1013
Eskalith ... 2485
Ethmozine Tablets (Less than 2%) 2041
Etrafon ... 2355
Fansidar Tablets ... 2114
Feldene Capsules (Greater than 1%) ... 1965
Fioricet Tablets (Infrequent) ... 2258
Fioricet with Codeine Capsules (Infrequent) ... 2260

(▣ Described in PDR For Nonprescription Drugs) Incidence data in parenthesis; ▲ 3% or more (◎ Described in PDR For Ophthalmology)

Fiorinal with Codeine Capsules (Infrequent) 2262
Flexeril Tablets (Less than 1%) 1661
Floxin I.V. (Less than 1%) 1571
Floxin Tablets (200 mg, 300 mg, 400 mg) (Less than 1%) 1567
Flumadine Tablets & Syrup (0.3% to 1%) 1015
Foscavir Injection (Less than 1%) 547
Fungizone Intravenous 506
Gantanol Tablets 2119
Gantrisin 2120
Garamycin Injectable 2360
Glauctabs ⊙ 208
Halcion Tablets (Rare) 2611
Healthprin Aspirin 2455
Hivid Tablets (Less than 1% to less than 3%) 2121
Hyperstat I.V. Injection 2363
Hytrin Capsules (At least 1%) 430
Hyzaar Tablets 1677
IBU Tablets (Greater than 1%) 1342
Ilosone (Isolated reports) 911
Imdur (Less than or equal to 5%) 1323
Indocin (Greater than 1%) 1680
Intron A (Less than 5%) 2364
Kerlone Tablets (Less than 2%) 2436
Lamictal Tablets (1.1%) 1112
▲ Lariam Tablets (Among most frequent) 2128
Lasix Injection, Oral Solution and Tablets 1240
Lincocin (Occasional) 2617
Lioresal Tablets 829
Lithium Carbonate Capsules & Tablets 2230
Lithonate/Lithotabs/Lithobid 2543
Lodine Capsules and Tablets (More than 1% but less than 3%) 2743
Lopressor Ampuls 830
Lopressor HCT Tablets (1 in 100 patients) 832
Lopressor Tablets 830
Lorelco Tablets 1517
Lotensin HCT (0.3% to 1.0%) 837
Lotrel Capsules (Infrequent) 840
Ludiomil Tablets (Rare) 843
Luvox Tablets 2544
▲ MZM (Among reactions occurring most often) ⊙ 267
Marcaine Hydrochloride with Epinephrine 1:200,000 2316
Marcaine Hydrochloride Injection 2316
Marcaine Spinal 2319
Marinol (Dronabinol) Capsules (Less than 1%) 2231
Maxaquin Tablets (Less than 1%) 2440
Methergine (Rare) 2272
Methotrexate Sodium Tablets, Injection, for Injection and LPF Injection (Less common) 1275
Mexitil Capsules (1.9% to 2.4%) 678
Miacalcin Nasal Spray (Less than 1%) 2275
Midamor Tablets (Less than or equal to 1%) 1703
Minipress Capsules (Less than 1%) 1937
Minizide Capsules (Rare) 1938
Mintezol 1704
Mobigesic Tablets ▣ 602
Moduretic Tablets 1705
Mono-Gesic Tablets 792
Monopril Tablets (0.2% to 1.0%) 757
Children's Motrin Ibuprofen Oral Suspension (Greater than 1% but less than 3%) 1546
Motrin Tablets (Less than 3%) 2625
Motrin Ibuprofen Suspension, Oral Drops, Chewable Tablets, Caplets (1% to less than 3%) 1546
Mustargen (Infrequent) 1709
Mykrox Tablets (Less than 2%) 993
▲ Nalfon 200 Pulvules & Nalfon Tablets (4.5%) 917
▲ Anaprox/Naprosyn (3% to 9%) 2117
Nebcin Vials, Hyporets & ADD-Vantage 1464
Neoral (2% or less) 2276
Neptazane Tablets 1388
Nescaine/Nescaine MPF 554
Netromycin Injection 100 mg/ml 2373
Neurontin Capsules (Infrequent) 1922
Nicorette 2458
Noroxin Tablets 1715
Noroxin Tablets 2048
Norpramin Tablets 1526
Norvasc Tablets (More than 0.1% to 1%) 1940
Ornade Spansule Capsules 2502
Orthoclone OKT3 Sterile Solution 1837
Orudis Capsules (Greater than 1%) 2766
Oruvail Capsules (Greater than 1%) 2766
PBZ Tablets 845
PBZ-SR Tablets 844
Pamelor 2280
Parnate Tablets 2503
Paxil Tablets (Infrequent) 2505
Penetrex Tablets (Less than 1% but more than or equal to 0.1%) 2031
Pepcid Injection (Infrequent) 1722
Pepcid (Infrequent) 1720
Pepto-Bismol Original Liquid, Original and Cherry Tablets and Easy-To-Swallow Caplets 1976
Pepto-Bismol Maximum Strength Liquid 1976
Periactin 1724
Permax Tablets (Infrequent) 575
Phenergan Injection 2773
Phenergan Tablets 2775
Phrenilin (Infrequent) 785
Plaquenil Sulfate Tablets 2328
Platinol 708
Platinol-AQ Injection 710
Pontocaine Hydrochloride for Spinal Anesthesia 2330
PREVACID Delayed-Release Capsules (Less than 1%) 2562
Prilosec Delayed-Release Capsules (Less than 1%) 529
Primaxin I.M. 1727
Primaxin I.V. (Less than 0.2%) 1729
Prinivil Tablets (0.3% to 1.0%) 1733
Prinzide Tablets (0.3 to 1%) 1737
Procardia XL Extended Release Tablets (1% or less) 1972
▲ Prograf (Greater than 3%) 1042
ProSom Tablets (Infrequent) 449
Proventil (2%) 2386
Prozac Pulvules & Liquid, Oral Solution (2%) 919
Questran Light 769
Questran Powder 770
Quinaglute Dura-Tabs Tablets 649
Quinidex Extentabs 2067
Recombivax HB (Less than 1%) 1744
▲ Relafen Tablets (3% to 9%) 2510
ReVia Tablets (Less than 1%) 940
Rifater 1532
Risperdal (Rare) 1301
Romazicon (Less than 1%) 2147
Rythmol Tablets–150mg, 225mg, 300mg (Less than 1% to 1.9%) 1352
Salflex Tablets (Common) 786
Sandimmune (2% or less) 2286
Sedapap Tablets 50 mg/650 mg (Infrequent) 1543
Sensorcaine 559
Septra 1174
Septra I.V. Infusion 1169
Septra I.V. Infusion ADD-Vantage Vials 1171
Septra 1174
Serzone Tablets (Up to 3%) 771
Sinequan (Occasional) 2205
Soma Compound w/Codeine Tablets 2676
Soma Compound Tablets 2675
Sporanox Capsules (Less than 1%) 1305
▲ Stadol (3% to 9%) 775
Streptomycin Sulfate Injection 2208
Surmontil Capsules 2811
Talacen (Rare) 2333
Talwin Injection (Rare) 2334
Talwin Compound 2335
Talwin Injection 2334
Talwin Nx 2336
Tambocor Tablets (1% to less than 3%) 1497
Tavist Syrup 2297
Tavist Tablets 2298
Tegretol Chewable Tablets 852
Tegretol Suspension 852
Tegretol Tablets 852
Temaril Tablets, Syrup and Spansule Extended-Release Capsules 483
Tenex Tablets (3% or less) 2074
Thera-Gesic 1781
Ticlid Tablets (0.5% to 1.0%) 2156
Timolide Tablets 1748
Timoptic in Ocudose 1753
Timoptic Sterile Ophthalmic Solution 1751
Timoptic-XE 1755
Tobramycin Sulfate Injection 968
Tofranil Ampuls 854
Tofranil Tablets 856
Tofranil-PM Capsules 857
Tolectin (200, 400 and 600 mg) (1 to 3%) 1581
Tonocard Tablets (0.4-1.5%) 531
Toprol-XL Tablets 565
Toradol (1% or less) 2159
Torecan 2245
Triavil Tablets 1757
▲ Trilisate (Less than 20%) 2000
Trinalin Repetabs Tablets 1330
Tussend 1783
Tympagesic Ear Drops 2342
Ultram Tablets (50 mg) (Infrequent) 1585
Univasc Tablets (Less than 1%) 2410
Ursinus Inlay-Tabs ▣ 794
Vancocin HCl, Oral Solution & Pulvules (Rare) 1483
Vancocin HCl, Vials & ADD-Vantage (Rare) 1481
Vantin for Oral Suspension and Vantin Tablets (Less than 1%) 2646
▲ Vascor (200, 300 and 400 mg) Tablets (Up to 6.52%) 1587
Vaseretic Tablets (0.5% to 2.0%) 1765
Vasotec I.V. 1768
Vasotec Tablets (0.5% to 1.0%) 1771
Videx Tablets, Powder for Oral Solution, & Pediatric Powder for Oral Solution (Less than 1%) 720
Vivactil Tablets 1774
Voltaren Tablets (1% to 3%) 861
Wellbutrin Tablets 1204
▲ Xanax Tablets (6.6%) 2649
▲ Xylocaine Injections (Among most common) 567
Zebeta Tablets 1413
Zestoretic (0.3 to 1%) 2850
Zestril Tablets (0.3% to 1.0%) 2854
Ziac 1415
Zoloft Tablets (1.4%) 2217
Zosyn (1.0% or less) 1419
Zosyn Pharmacy Bulk Package (1.0% or less) 1422
Zyloprim Tablets (Less than 1%) 1226

Tiredness (see under Fatigue)

Tissue damage, ischemic
Sansert Tablets (Rare) 2295

Toes, discoloration
Eskalith (A few reports) 2485
Lithium Carbonate Capsules & Tablets (A single report) 2230
Lithonate/Lithotabs/Lithobid 2543

Tolerance
Adipex-P Tablets and Capsules 1048
Astramorph/PF Injection, USP (Preservative-Free) 535
Bellergal-S Tablets 2250
Biphetamine Capsules 983
Brontex 1981
Butisol Sodium Elixir & Tablets 2660
Carnitor Tablets and Solution 2453
DHCplus Capsules 1993
Didrex Tablets 2607
Dilatrate-SR 2398
Dilaudid Tablets and Liquid 1339
Duragesic Transdermal System 1288
Duramorph 962
Dyclone 0.5% and 1% Topical Solutions, USP 544
Esgic-plus Tablets 1013
Fioricet Tablets 2258
Fiorinal Capsules 2261
Fiorinal with Codeine Capsules 2262
Fiorinal Tablets 2261
Hycodan Tablets and Syrup 930
Hycomine Compound Tablets 932
Hycomine 931
Hycotuss Expectorant Syrup 933
Hydrocet Capsules 782
Infumorph 200 and Infumorph 500 Sterile Solutions 965
Isordil Sublingual Tablets 2739
Isordil Tembids 2741
Isordil Titradose Tablets 2742
Lorcet 10/650 1018
Lortab 2566
MS Contin Tablets 1994
Mebaral Tablets 2322
Methadone Hydrochloride Oral Solution & Tablets 2235
Nembutal Sodium Solution 438
Nembutal Sodium Suppositories 440
Oramorph SR (Morphine Sulfate Sustained Release Tablets) 2236
Percocet Tablets 938
Percodan Tablets 939
Phrenilin 785
Placidyl Capsules 448
Roxanol 2243
Seconal Sodium Pulvules 1474
Sedapap Tablets 50 mg/650 mg (Infrequent) 1543
Sorbitrate 2843
Tylenol with Codeine 1583
Vicodin Tablets 1356
Vicodin Tuss Expectorant 1358
Zemuron (Rare) 1830

Tolerance, diminished
Ambien Tablets (Rare) 2416
Cocaine Hydrochloride Topical Solution 537
Duranest Injections 542
▲ Fungizone Intravenous (Most patients) 506
Sensorcaine 559
Timolide Tablets 1748
Xylocaine Injections 567

Tongue disorder, unspecified
Cytovene (1% or less) 2103
Hivid Tablets (Less than 1% to less than 3%) 2121
Salagen Tablets (Less than 1%) 1489
Videx Tablets, Powder for Oral Solution, & Pediatric Powder for Oral Solution (Less than 1%) 720

Tongue, black "hairy" (see under Glossotrichia)

Tongue, burning
Atamet 572
BuSpar (Rare) 737
Halcion Tablets 2611
Larodopa Tablets (Infrequent) 2129
Nalfon 200 Pulvules & Nalfon Tablets (Less than 1%) 917
Sinemet Tablets 943
Sinemet CR Tablets 944

Tongue, discoloration
Aldomet Ester HCl Injection 1602
Aldomet Oral 1600
Claritin-D (Less frequent) 2350
Effexor (Rare) 2719
Etrafon 2355
Maxaquin Tablets (Less than 1%) 2440
Pepto-Bismol Original Liquid, Original and Cherry Tablets and Easy-To-Swallow Caplets 1976
Pepto-Bismol Maximum Strength Liquid 1976
Peridex 1978
Prozac Pulvules & Liquid, Oral Solution (Rare) 919
Risperdal (Rare) 1301
Trilafon 2389

Tongue, fine vermicular movements
Compazine 2470
Eskalith 2485
Etrafon 2355
Haldol Decanoate 1577
Haldol Injection, Tablets and Concentrate 1575
Lithonate/Lithotabs/Lithobid 2543
Mellaril 2269
Moban Tablets and Concentrate 1048
Navane Capsules and Concentrate 2201
Navane Intramuscular 2202
Orap Tablets 1050
Reglan 2068
Stelazine 2514
Thorazine 2523

Tongue, furry
Flagyl 375 Capsules 2434
Geocillin Tablets 2199
MetroGel-Vaginal 902
Protostat Tablets 1883

Tongue, mucosal atrophy
Prilosec Delayed-Release Capsules (Less than 1%) 529

Tongue, protrusion
Compazine 2470
Etrafon 2355
Haldol Decanoate 1577
Haldol Injection, Tablets and Concentrate 1575
Loxitane 1378
Mellaril 2269
Moban Tablets and Concentrate 1048

(▣ Described in PDR For Nonprescription Drugs) Incidence data in parenthesis; ▲ 3% or more (⊙ Described in PDR For Ophthalmology)

1431 Side Effects Index Tremors

Navane Capsules and Concentrate 2201
Navane Intramuscular 2202
Orap Tablets 1050
Phenergan with Codeine 2777
Phenergan with Dextromethorphan 2778
Phenergan Suppositories 2775
Phenergan Syrup 2774
Phenergan VC 2779
Phenergan VC with Codeine 2781
Prolixin 509
Prozac Pulvules & Liquid, Oral Solution (One case) 919
Reglan 2068
Serentil 684
Stelazine 2514
Thorazine 2523
Triavil Tablets 1757
Trilafon 2389

Tongue, rounding
Etrafon 2355
Trilafon 2389

Tongue, sore (see under Glossodynia)

Tongue, swelling (see under Glossoncus)

Tooth development, impaired
Terramycin Intramuscular Solution 2210
Urobiotic-250 Capsules 2214
Vibramycin Hyclate Intravenous 2215

Tooth discoloration
Urobiotic-250 Capsules (Contraindicated in pregnancy) 2214

Tooth disorder
▲Anafranil Capsules (Up to 5%) 803
Axid Pulvules (1.0%) 1427
Dilacor XR Extended-release Capsules (Infrequent) 2018
Ismo Tablets (Fewer than 1%) 2738
▲Lamictal Tablets (3.2%) 1112
Lescol Capsules (2.1%) 2267
Lotensin HCT (0.3% or more) 837
▲Luvox Tablets (3%) 2544
▲Nicorette (3% to 9% of patients) 2458
Serzone Tablets 771
Versed Injection 2170

Torsade de pointes
▲Betapace Tablets (Up to 5.8%) 641
Biaxin (Rare) 405
Cordarone Intravenous 2715
Felbatol 2666
Haldol Decanoate 1577
Haldol Injection, Tablets and Concentrate 1575
Ilosone (Rare) 911
Ilotycin Gluceptate, IV, Vials (Rare) 913
Lorelco Tablets 1517
Norpace 2444
PCE Dispertab Tablets (Rare) 444
Propulsid (Rare) 1300
Quinidex Extentabs 2067
Seldane Tablets (Rare) 1536
Seldane-D Extended-Release Tablets (Rare) 1538
Tambocor Tablets (Rare) 1497
Vascor (200, 300 and 400 mg) Tablets 1587

Torticollis
Adalat CC (Less than 1.0%) 589
Adenocard Injection (Less than 1%) 1021
▲Adenoscan (15%) 1024
Anafranil Capsules (Rare) 803
Asacol Delayed-Release Tablets 1979
Betaseron for SC Injection 658
Cardene I.V. (Rare) 2709
Cartrol Tablets (Less common) 410
Cipro I.V. (1% or less) 595
Cipro I.V. Pharmacy Bulk Package (Less than 1%) 597
Cipro Tablets (Less than 1%) 592
Claritin-D (Less frequent) 2350
Clozaril Tablets (1%) 2252
Compazine 2470
Cytovene (1% or less) 2103
Danocrine Capsules 2307
Depakote Tablets (Greater than 1% but not more than 5%) 415
Dilacor XR Extended-release Capsules (Infrequent) 2018
Diprivan Injection (Less than 1%) 2833
Effexor (Frequent; infrequent) 2719
Eldepryl Tablets 2550
Engerix-B Unit-Dose Vials (Less than 1%) 2482
Etrafon 2355
Foscavir Injection (Less than 1%) 547
Gelfoam Sterile Sponge 2608
Hivid Tablets (Less than 1% to less than 3%) 2121
Hylorel Tablets (1.5%) 985
Hytrin Capsules (At least 1%) 430
Imdur (Less than or equal to 5%) 1323
▲Imitrex Injection (4.8%) 1103
Kerlone Tablets (Less than 2%) 2436
Lamictal Tablets (2.4%) 1112
Lotensin HCT (0.3% or more) 837
Luvox Tablets (Infrequent) 2544
Mellaril 2269
Moduretic Tablets 1705
Monoket (Fewer than 1%) 2406
Orap Tablets (2.7%) 1050
▲Orthoclone OKT3 Sterile Solution (14%) 1837
Paxil Tablets (Infrequent) 2505
Permax Tablets (2.7%) 575
Phenergan with Codeine 2777
Phenergan with Dextromethorphan 2778
Phenergan Suppositories 2775
Phenergan Syrup 2774
Phenergan VC 2779
Phenergan VC with Codeine 2781
Polymyxin B Sulfate, Aerosporin Brand Sterile Powder 1154
Prinivil Tablets (0.3% to 1.0%) 1733
Prinzide Tablets 1737
ProSom Tablets (Infrequent) 449
Prozac Pulvules & Liquid, Oral Solution (Rare to infrequent) 919
Recombivax HB (Less than 1%) 1744
Reglan 2068
Risperdal (Rare) 1301
Serentil 684
Serzone Tablets 771
Stelazine 2514
▲Supprelin Injection (1% to 10%) 2056
Thorazine 2523
Tonocard Tablets (Less than 1%) 531
Torecan 2245
Triavil Tablets 1757
Trilafon 2389
Zebeta Tablets 1413
Zestoretic 2850
Zestril Tablets (0.3% to 1.0%) 2854
Ziac 1415

Total proteins, decrease (see under Hypoproteinemia)

Tourette's syndrome
Cylert Tablets 412
Desoxyn Gradumet Tablets 419
Dexedrine 2474
DextroStat Dextroamphetamine Tablets 2036
Ritalin (Rare) 848

Toxic granulation
Efudex 2113

Toxicity, bone marrow
▲Mutamycin (64.4%) 703

Toxicity, cutaneous
▲Lysodren (15%) 698
Platinol (Rare) 708
Platinol-AQ Injection (Rare) 710

Toxicity, hepatic
Achromycin V Capsules (Rare) 1367
BiCNU 691
CeeNU 693
Cordarone Tablets 2712
Danocrine Capsules 2307
Declomycin Tablets (Rare) 1371
Hexalen Capsules (Less than 1%) 2571
Methotrexate Sodium Tablets, Injection, for Injection and LPF Injection 1275
Paraflex Caplets 1580
Parafon Forte DSC Caplets 1581
Ponstel 1925
Pyridium 1928
Terramycin Intramuscular Solution 2210
Urobiotic-250 Capsules 2214
VePesid Capsules and Injection (Up to 3%) 718

Toxicity, renal
Achromycin V Capsules 1367
Anaprox/Naprosyn 2117
Declomycin Tablets (No incidence, dose related) 1371
Depen Titratable Tablets 2662
Doryx Capsules 1913
EC-Naprosyn Delayed-Release Tablets 2117
Feldene Capsules 1965
Fiorinal with Codeine Capsules 2262
▲IFEX (6%) 697
Minocin Intravenous 1382
Minocin Oral Suspension 1385
Minocin Pellet-Filled Capsules 1383
Mutamycin (2%) 703
Anaprox/Naprosyn 2117
Orudis Capsules 2766
Oruvail Capsules 2766
▲Platinol (28% to 36%) 708
▲Platinol-AQ Injection (28% to 36% of patients) 710
Pyridium 1928
Relafen Tablets 2510
Roferon-A Injection (Rare) 2145
▲TheraCys BCG Live (Intravesical) (2.0% to 9.8%) 897

Toxicity, vascular
Blenoxane (Rare) 692
Platinol (Rare) 708
Platinol-AQ Injection (Rare) 710

Toxic shock syndrome
All-Flex Arcing Spring Diaphragm (See also Ortho Diaphragm Kits) 1865
Gelfoam Sterile Sponge 2608
Ortho Diaphragm Kits—All-Flex Arcing Spring; Ortho Coil Spring; Ortho-White Flat Spring 1865
Ortho Diaphragm Kit 1865
Today Vaginal Contraceptive Sponge (Uncommon) ▣ 874

Toxoplasmosis
Foscavir Injection (Less than 1%) 547

Tracheitis
PedvaxHIB (One case) 1718
Serevent Inhalation Aerosol (1% to 3%) 1176
Solganal Suspension 2388

Transaminase, elevation (see under Serum transaminase, elevation)

Trauma, unspecified
Ambien Tablets (Infrequent) 2416
Caverject (2%) 2583
Decadron Phosphate Sterile Ophthalmic Ointment 1641
Decadron Phosphate Sterile Ophthalmic Solution 1642
Effexor (2%) 2719
Floropryl Sterile Ophthalmic Ointment 1662
Humorsol Sterile Ophthalmic Solution 1664
Neurontin Capsules (Frequent) 1922
Paxil Tablets (1.4%) 2505
Pravachol 765
Prinzide Tablets (0.3 to 1%) 1737
▲Tetramune (Among most common) 1404
Zestoretic (0.3 to 1%) 2850

Trembling
Adalat Capsules (10 mg and 20 mg) (2% or less) 587
▲AeroBid Inhaler System (3-9%) 1005
▲Aerobid-M Inhaler System (3-9%) 1005
Alfenta Injection (0.3% to 1%) 1286
Calan SR Caplets 2422
Calan Tablets 2419
Clozaril Tablets (Less than 1%) 2252
Deconsal C Expectorant Syrup 456
Deconsal Pediatric Syrup 457
Diprivan Injection (Less than 1%) 2833
Emete-con Intramuscular/Intravenous 2198
Fluothane 2724
Imitrex Injection (Infrequent) 1103
Imitrex Tablets (Rare to infrequent) 1106
Inapsine Injection (Less common) 1296
INFeD (Iron Dextran Injection, USP) 2345
Marax Tablets & DF Syrup 2200
Marcaine Spinal 2319
Nucofed 2051
Paxil Tablets 2505
Procardia Capsules (2% or less) 1971
▲Prostin E2 Suppository (Approximately one-tenth) 2634
▲Proventil Syrup (9 of 100 patients) 2385
Quadrinal Tablets 1350
Romazicon (Less than 1%) 2147
▲Streptase for Infusion (Among most common; 1% to 4%) 562
Sublimaze Injection 1307
▲Ventolin Syrup (9 of 100 patients) 1202
WinRho SD (One report) 2576
Xylocaine Injections (2%) 567
▲Zofran Injection (7%) 1214
▲Zofran Tablets (5%) 1217

Tremor, fine hand
Atamet 572
Eskalith 2485
Lithium Carbonate Capsules & Tablets 2230
Lithonate/Lithotabs/Lithobid 2543
Sinemet Tablets 943
Sinemet CR Tablets 944
▲Vascor (200, 300 and 400 mg) Tablets (3.02 to 9.30%) 1587

Tremors
Actifed with Codeine Cough Syrup 1067
▲Adalat Capsules (10 mg and 20 mg) (8%) 587
Adalat CC (Rare) 589
Adenoscan (Less than 1%) 1024
Adipex-P Tablets and Capsules 1048
▲Airet Solution for Inhalation (10.7% to 20%) 452
Altace Capsules (Less than 1%) 1232
Alupent (1% to 4%) 669
Ambien Tablets (Infrequent) 2416
Amikacin Sulfate Injection, USP (Rare) 960
Amikin Injectable (Rare) 501
▲Anafranil Capsules (33% to 54%) 803
Ana-Kit Anaphylaxis Emergency Treatment Kit (Occasional to common) 617
Ansaid Tablets (1-3%) 2579
Apresazide Capsules (Less frequent) 808
Apresoline Hydrochloride Tablets (Less frequent) 809
Asacol Delayed-Release Tablets 1979
Asendin Tablets (Less frequent) 1369
Atarax Tablets & Syrup (Rare) 2185
Atgam Sterile Solution (Less than 5%) 2581
Atromid-S Capsules 2701
Atrovent Inhalation Aerosol (Less frequent) 671
Atrovent Inhalation Solution (0.9%) 673
Benadryl Capsules 1898
Benadryl Injection 1898
Betaseron for SC Injection 658
Biphetamine Capsules 983
Bontril Slow-Release Capsules 781
Brethaire Inhaler 813
▲Brethine Ampuls (7.8 to 38.0%) 815
Brethine Tablets (Common) 814
▲Bricanyl Subcutaneous Injection (Among most common) 1502
▲Bricanyl Tablets (One of the two most common) 1503
▲Bromfed-DM Cough Syrup (Among most frequent) 1786
Bronkaid Caplets ▣ 717
Bronkometer Aerosol 2302
Bronkosol Solution 2302
Buprenex Injectable (Infrequent) 2006
BuSpar (1%) 737
Carbocaine Hydrochloride Injection 2303
Cardene Capsules (0.6%) 2095
Cardizem CD Capsules (Less than 1%) 1506
Cardizem SR Capsules (Less than 1%) 1510
Cardizem Injectable 1508
Cardizem Tablets (Less than 1%) 1512
Cardura Tablets (Less than 0.5% of 3960 patients) 2186
Cataflam (Less than 1%) 816
▲CellCept Capsules (11.0% to 11.8%) 2099
Chibroxin Sterile Ophthalmic Solution (With oral form) 1617
Cipro I.V. (1% or less) 595
Cipro I.V. Pharmacy Bulk Package (Less than 1%) 597
Cipro Tablets (Less than 1%) 592
Claritin (2% or fewer patients) 2349
Claritin-D (Less frequent) 2350
▲Clozaril Tablets (More than 5 to 6%) 2252
Cocaine Hydrochloride Topical Solution 537
Cognex Capsules (2%) 1901

(▣ Described in PDR For Nonprescription Drugs) Incidence data in parenthesis; ▲ 3% or more (◉ Described in PDR For Ophthalmology)

Tremors — Side Effects Index — 1432

Compazine 2470
▲Cordarone Tablets (4 to 9%) 2712
Cozaar Tablets (Less than 1%) 1628
Cytovene (1% or less) 2103
D.A. Chewable Tablets 951
Danocrine Capsules 2307
Daranide Tablets 1633
Decadron Phosphate with Xylocaine Injection, Sterile 1639
Deconamine Chewable Tablets 1320
Deconamine CX Cough and Cold Liquid and Tablets 1319
Deconamine 1320
Deconsal 454
Demerol 2308
▲Demser Capsules (10%) 1649
Depakene 413
Depakote Tablets 415
Desoxyn Gradumet Tablets 419
▲Desyrel and Desyrel Dividose (2.8% to 5.1%) 503
Dexedrine 2474
DextroStat Dextroamphetamine Tablets 2036
Didrex Tablets 2607
Dilantin Infatabs (Rare) 1908
Dilantin Kapseals (Rare) 1906
Dilantin Parenteral (Rare) 1910
Dilantin-125 Suspension (Rare) 1911
Dilaudid-HP Injection (Less frequent) 1337
Dilaudid-HP Lyophilized Powder 250 mg (Less frequent) 1337
Dilaudid Tablets and Liquid (Less frequent) 1339
Dimetane-DC Cough Syrup 2059
Dimetane-DX Cough Syrup 2059
Dipentum Capsules (Rare) 1951
Diprivan Injection (Less than 1%) 2833
Dizac (Less frequent) 1809
Doral Tablets 2664
Duragesic Transdermal System (1% or greater) 1288
Duranest Injections 542
Dura-Tap/PD Capsules 2867
Dura-Vent/DA Tablets 953
Dura-Vent Tablets 952
Dyazide 2479
Dyclone 0.5% and 1% Topical Solutions, USP 544
▲Effexor (5% to 10.2%) 2719
Elavil 2838
Eldepryl Tablets 2550
Elspar 1659
Emete-con Intramuscular/Intravenous 2198
▲Eminase (Less than 10%) 2039
Emla Cream 545
Endep Tablets 2174
Entex PSE Tablets 1987
EpiPen 790
Esgic-plus Tablets 1013
Esimil Tablets 822
Eskalith 2485
Ethmozine Tablets (Less than 2%) 2041
Etrafon 2355
Fastin Capsules 2488
Fedahist Gyrocaps 2401
Fedahist Timecaps 2401
▲Felbatol (6.1%) 2666
Fioricet Tablets (Infrequent) 2258
Fioricet with Codeine Capsules (Infrequent) 2260
Fiorinal with Codeine Capsules 2262
Flexeril Tablets (Less than 1%) 1661
Floxin I.V. (Less than 1%) 1571
Floxin Tablets (200 mg, 300 mg, 400 mg) (Less than 1%) 1567
Flumadine Tablets & Syrup (Less than 0.3%) 1015
Foscavir Injection (Between 1% and 5%) 547
▲Glucotrol XL Extended Release Tablets (3.6%) 1968
Guaimax-D Tablets 792
Hivid Tablets (Less than 1% to less than 3%) 2121
Hyzaar Tablets 1677
Imdur (Less than or equal to 5%) 1323
Imitrex Injection (Infrequent) 1103
Imitrex Tablets (Rare to infrequent) 1106
Intron A (Less than 5%) 2364
Inversine Tablets 1686
Ionamin Capsules 990
Ismelin Tablets 827
Isoetharine Inhalation Solution, USP, Arm-a-Med 551
Isoptin Oral Tablets (Less than 1%) 1346
Isoptin SR Tablets (1% or less) 1348
Isuprel Hydrochloride Injection 1:5000 2311
Isuprel Hydrochloride Solution 1:200 & 1:100 2313
Isuprel Mistometer 2312
Kerlone Tablets (Less than 2%) 2436
Klonopin Tablets 2126
▲Lamictal Tablets (4.4%) 1112
Larodopa Tablets (Relatively frequent) 2129
Lescol Capsules 2267
Leukeran Tablets (Rare) 1133
Limbitrol (Less common) 2180
Lioresal Tablets 829
Lithium Carbonate Capsules & Tablets 2230
Lithonate/Lithotabs/Lithobid 2543
Lotrel Capsules 840
Loxitane 1378
▲Ludiomil Tablets (3%) 843
▲Luvox Tablets (5%) 2544
MS Contin Tablets (Less frequent) 1994
MSIR (Infrequent) 1997
Marcaine Hydrochloride with Epinephrine 1:200,000 2316
Marcaine Hydrochloride Injection 2316
Marcaine Spinal 2319
Marinol (Dronabinol) Capsules (Less than 1%) 2231
Matulane Capsules 2131
▲Maxair Autohaler (1.3% to 6.0%) 1492
▲Maxair Inhaler (6.0%) 1494
Maxaquin Tablets (Less than 1%) 2440
Mellaril 2269
Mepergan Injection 2753
Mesantoin Tablets 2272
▲Metaproterenol Sulfate Inhalation Solution, USP, Arm-a-Med (About 1 in 20 patients) 552
Methadone Hydrochloride Oral Concentrate 2233
Mevacor Tablets (0.5% to 1.0%) 1699
▲Mexitil Capsules (12.6%) 678
Midamor Tablets (Less than or equal to 1%) 1703
Moban Tablets and Concentrate 1048
Moduretic Tablets 1705
Monoket (Fewer than 1%) 2406
Monopril Tablets (0.2% to 1.0%) 757
Nalfon 200 Pulvules & Nalfon Tablets (2.2%) 917
Nardil (Common) 1920
NebuPent for Inhalation Solution (1% or less) 1040
▲Neoral (21% to 55%) 2276
Nescaine/Nescaine MPF 554
▲Neurontin Capsules (6.8%) 1922
Nolamine Timed-Release Tablets (Occasional) 785
Norflex 1496
Norisodrine with Calcium Iodide Syrup 442
Noroxin Tablets 1715
Noroxin Tablets 2048
Norpramin Tablets 1526
Norvasc Tablets (More than 0.1% to 1%) 1940
Novahistine DH 2462
Novahistine DMX 822
Novahistine Elixir 823
Novahistine Expectorant 2463
Novocain Hydrochloride for Spinal Anesthesia 2326
Oramorph SR (Morphine Sulfate Sustained Release Tablets) (Less frequent) 2236
Orap Tablets (2.7%) 1050
Orlamm 2239
Ornade Spansule Capsules 2502
▲Orthoclone OKT3 Sterile Solution (13%) 1837
Pamelor 2280
Parnate Tablets 2503
▲Paxil Tablets (Up to 14.7%) 2505
Penetrex Tablets (Less than 1% but more than or equal to 0.1%) 2031
Pentaspan Injection 937
Periactin 1724
▲Permax Tablets (4.2%) 575
Phenergan Injection 2773
Phenergan Tablets 2775
Phenergan VC 2779
Phenergan VC with Codeine 2781
Placidyl Capsules 448
Pontocaine Hydrochloride for Spinal Anesthesia 2330
Pravachol 765
Prelu-2 Timed Release Capsules 681
Prilosec Delayed-Release Capsules (Less than 1%) 529
Primacor Injection (0.4%) 2331
Primaxin I.M. 1727
Primaxin I.V. (Less than 0.2%) 1729
Prinivil Tablets (0.3% to 1.0%) 1733
Prinzide Tablets 1737
▲Procardia Capsules (2% or less to 8%) 1971
▲Procardia XL Extended Release Tablets (1% or less to 8%) 1972
▲Prograf (44% to 56%) 1042
Propulsid (1% or less) 1300
ProSom Tablets (Rare) 449
Prostin E2 Suppository 2634
▲Proventil Inhalation Aerosol (Less than 15%) 2382
▲Proventil Inhalation Solution 0.083% (10.7% to 20%) 2384
▲Proventil Repetabs Tablets (6% to 20%) 2386
▲Proventil Solution for Inhalation 0.5% (10.7% to 20%) 2383
▲Proventil Syrup (10 of 100 patients) 2385
▲Proventil Tablets (20%) 2386
▲Prozac Pulvules & Liquid, Oral Solution (5% to 9%) 919
Reglan 2068
Relafen Tablets (1%) 2510
Restoril Capsules (Less than 1%) 2284
Retrovir Capsules 1158
Retrovir I.V. Infusion 1163
Retrovir Syrup 1158
ReVia Tablets (Less than 1%) 940
Revex (Less than 1%) 1811
▲Risperdal (17% to 34%) 1301
Roferon-A Injection (Less than 0.5%) 2145
▲Romazicon (3% to 9%) 2147
Rondec Oral Drops 953
Rondec Syrup 953
Rondec Tablet 953
Rondec-DM Oral Drops 954
Rondec-DM Syrup 954
Rondec-TR Tablet 953
Rythmol Tablets–150mg, 225mg, 300mg (0.3 to 1.4%) 1352
Salagen Tablets (2%) 1489
▲Sandimmune (12 to 55%) 2286
Sandostatin Injection (Less than 1%) 2292
Sanorex Tablets 2294
Seldane Tablets 1536
Seldane-D Extended-Release Tablets 1538
Sensorcaine 559
Ser-Ap-Es Tablets 849
Serax Capsules 2810
Serax Tablets 2810
Serentil 684
▲Serevent Inhalation Aerosol (4%) 1176
Seromycin Pulvules 1476
Serzone Tablets (2%) 771
Sinequan (Infrequent) 2205
Soma Compound w/Codeine Tablets (Infrequent or rare) 2676
Soma Compound Tablets (Infrequent or rare) 2675
Soma Tablets 2674
Stadol (1% or greater) 775
Stelazine 2514
Supprelin Injection (1% to 3%) 2056
Surmontil Capsules 2811
Sus-Phrine Injection 1019
Syn-Rx Tablets 465
Syn-Rx DM Tablets 466
Talacen (Rare) 2333
Talwin Injection (Rarely) 2334
Talwin Compound (Rare) 2335
Talwin Injection (Rare) 2334
Talwin Nx (Rare) 2336
▲Tambocor Tablets (4.7%) 1497
Tavist Syrup 2297
Tavist Tablets 2298
Temaril Tablets, Syrup and Spansule Extended-Release Capsules 483
Tenex Tablets (Less frequent) 2074
Thorazine 2523
Tilade (Less than 1%) 996
Tofranil Ampuls 854
Tofranil Tablets 856
Tofranil-PM Capsules 857
▲Tonocard Tablets (2.9-21.6%) 531
Toradol (1% or less) 2159
Torecan 2245
▲Tornalate Solution for Inhalation, 0.2% (26.6% decreasing to 9%) 956
▲Tornalate Metered Dose Inhaler (9.1% to 14%) 957
Trancopal Caplets 2337
Tranxene 451
Trental Tablets 1244
Triavil Tablets 1757
Trinalin Repetabs Tablets 1330
Tussend 1783
Tussend Expectorant 1785
Typhim Vi 899
▲Ultram Tablets (50 mg) (Less than 1% to 14%) 1585
Valium Injectable 2182
Valium Tablets (Infrequent) 2183
Valrelease Capsules (Occasional) 2169
▲Vascor (200, 300 and 400 mg) Tablets (0.5 to 6.98%) 1587
▲Ventolin Inhalation Aerosol and Refill (Fewer than 15 per 100 patients; 1%) 1197
▲Ventolin Inhalation Solution (10.7% to 20%) 1198
▲Ventolin Nebules Inhalation Solution (10.7% to 20%) 1199
Ventolin Rotacaps for Inhalation (1%) 1200
▲Ventolin Syrup (10 of 100 patients) 1202
▲Ventolin Tablets (Aproximately 20 of 100 patients) 1203
Verelan Capsules (Less than 1%) 2824
Videx Tablets, Powder for Oral Solution, & Pediatric Powder for Oral Solution (Less than 1%) 720
Vistaril Capsules (Rare) 1944
Vistaril Intramuscular Solution (Rare) 2216
Vistaril Oral Suspension (Rare) 1944
Vivactil Tablets 1774
▲Volmax Extended-Release Tablets (24.2%) 1788
Voltaren Tablets (Less than 1%) 861
▲Wellbutrin Tablets (21.1%) 1204
▲Xanax Tablets (4.0%) 2649
▲Xylocaine Injections (Among most common) 567
Yocon 1892
Yohimex Tablets 1363
▲Yutopar Intravenous Injection (10% to 15%) 570
Zebeta Tablets 1413
Zerit Capsules (Fewer than 1% to 2%) 729
Zestoretic 2850
Zestril Tablets (0.3% to 1.0%) 2854
Ziac 1415
Zocor Tablets 1775
▲Zoloft Tablets (10.7%) 2217
Zosyn (1.0% or less) 1419
Zosyn Pharmacy Bulk Package (1.0% or less) 1422
Zovirax Sterile Powder (Approximately 1%) 1223

Tremulousness

Adalat CC (Rare) 589
Etrafon 2355
Lithonate/Lithotabs/Lithobid 2543
Narcan Injection 934
Nubain Injection (1% or less) 935
Prolixin 509
Sedapap Tablets 50 mg/650 mg (Infrequent) 1543
Trandate 1185
Verelan Capsules (1% or less) 1410

Trigeminal neuralgia

Nalfon 200 Pulvules & Nalfon Tablets (Less than 1%) 917
Torecan (Occasional case) 2245

Triglycerides, increase (see under Hypertriglyceridemia)

Trismus

Atamet 572
Ceftin (Less than 1% but more than 0.1%) 1078
Compazine 2470
Cytovene (1% or less) 2103
Demser Capsules 1649
Duranest Injections (Rare) 542
Effexor (Frequent) 2719
Etrafon 2355
Larodopa Tablets (Infrequent) 2129
Luvox Tablets (Rare) 2544
Mellaril 2269
Paxil Tablets 2505
Reglan 2068
Serentil 684
Sinemet Tablets 943
Sinemet CR Tablets 944
Stelazine 2514
Thorazine 2523
Torecan 2245
Triavil Tablets 1757

(Described in PDR For Nonprescription Drugs) Incidence data in parenthesis; ▲ 3% or more (◉ Described in PDR For Ophthalmology)

1433 Side Effects Index Ulcers, oral mucosal

- Trilafon 2389

Tubal damage
- ParaGard T380A Intrauterine Copper Contraceptive 1880

Tubulopathy
- Orudis Capsules (Rare) 2766
- Oruvail Capsules (Rare) 2766

Tumor flare
- Megace Tablets 701

Tumor lysis syndrome
- Adriamycin PFS 1947
- Adriamycin RDF 1947
- Fludara for Injection (Up to 1%) 663

Twins, conjoined
- Fulvicin P/G Tablets (Rare) 2359
- Fulvicin P/G 165 & 330 Tablets (Rare) 2359
- Gris-PEG Tablets, 125 mg & 250 mg (Two cases) 479

Twitching
- ▲Anafranil Capsules (4% to 7%) 803
- Ansaid Tablets (Less than 1%) 2579
- Brevital Sodium Vials 1429
- Cardura Tablets (Less than 0.5% of 3960 patients) 2186
- Cataflam (Less than 1%) 816
- Cognex Capsules (Infrequent) 1901
- Compazine 2470
- Depakote Tablets (Greater than 1% but not more than 5%) 415
- Desoxyn Gradumet Tablets 419
- Dilantin Infatabs 1908
- Dilantin Kapseals 1906
- Dilantin Parenteral 1910
- Dilantin-125 Suspension 1911
- Diprivan Injection (Less than 1%) 2833
- Duranest Injections 542
- Dyclone 0.5% and 1% Topical Solutions, USP 544
- Effexor (1%) 2719
- Emla Cream 545
- Eskalith 2485
- Fioricet with Codeine Capsules 2260
- Fiorinal with Codeine Capsules 2262
- Hivid Tablets (Less than 1% to less than 3%) 2121
- Imitrex Tablets (Rare) 1106
- Kerlone Tablets (Less than 2%) 2436
- Lamictal Tablets (Infrequent) 1112
- Lithium Carbonate Capsules & Tablets 2230
- Lithonate/Lithotabs/Lithobid 2543
- Luvox Tablets (Infrequent) 2544
- Methadone Hydrochloride Oral Concentrate 2233
- Nardil (Common) 1920
- Neurontin Capsules (1.3%) 1922
- Norvasc Tablets (Less than or equal to 0.1%) 1940
- Permax Tablets (1.1%) 575
- ProSom Tablets (Infrequent) 449
- Prozac Pulvules & Liquid, Oral Solution (Infrequent) 919
- Retrovir Capsules 1158
- Retrovir I.V. Infusion 1163
- Retrovir Syrup 1158
- Salagen Tablets (Less than 1%) 1489
- Sensorcaine 559
- Serzone Tablets (Infrequent) 771
- Stelazine 2514
- Tambocor Tablets (Less than 1%) 1497
- Trilafon 2389
- Triostat Injection (Approximately 1%) 2530
- Videx Tablets, Powder for Oral Solution, & Pediatric Powder for Oral Solution (Up to 2%) 720
- Voltaren Tablets (Less than 1%) 861
- ▲Xylocaine Injections (Among most common) 567
- Zebeta Tablets 1413
- Ziac 1415
- Zoloft Tablets (1.4%) 2217

Twitching, lid muscle
- Floropryl Sterile Ophthalmic Ointment 1662
- Humorsol Sterile Ophthalmic Solution 1664
- Neurontin Capsules (Infrequent) 1922
- Phospholine Iodide ⊚ 326
- Salagen Tablets (Rare) 1489

Twitching, muscle
- Eldepryl Tablets 2550
- Leukeran Tablets (Rare) 1133
- Nebcin Vials, Hyporets & ADD-Vantage 1464
- Parnate Tablets 2503
- ReVia Tablets (Less than 1%) 940
- Slo-bid Gyrocaps 2033
- Theo-24 Extended Release Capsules 2568

Tympanic membrane perforation
- Imdur (Less than or equal to 5%) 1323

Typhlitis
- Adriamycin PFS 1947
- Adriamycin RDF 1947
- Doxorubicin Astra 540

T4, decrease
- Android-25 Tablets 1251
- Eskalith 2485
- Lithium Carbonate Capsules & Tablets 2230
- Lithonate/Lithotabs/Lithobid 2543

T4, increase
- Brevicon 2088
- Danocrine Capsules 2307
- Estratest 2539
- Nolvadex Tablets (A few postmenopausal women) 2841
- Norinyl 2088
- Nor-Q D Tablets 2135
- Ortho-Cyclen/Ortho-Tri-Cyclen 1858
- Ortho-Cyclen/Ortho Tri-Cyclen 1858
- Tri-Norinyl 2164

T3, decrease
- Amen Tablets 780
- Aygestin Tablets 974
- Brevicon 2088
- Cycrin Tablets 975
- Depo-Provera Sterile Aqueous Suspension 2606
- Eskalith 2485
- Estratest 2539
- Lithium Carbonate Capsules & Tablets 2230
- Lithonate/Lithotabs/Lithobid 2543
- Norinyl 2088
- Nor-Q D Tablets 2135
- Provera Tablets 2636
- Tri-Norinyl 2164

U

Ulceration
- Aldactazide 2413
- Aldactone 2414
- Cerumenex Drops 1993
- Condylox (Less than 5%) 1802
- Cytosar-U Sterile Powder (Less frequent) 2592
- Daypro Caplets (Less than 1%) 2426
- Doxorubicin Astra 540
- ▲Efudex (Among most frequent) 2113
- Eulexin Capsules 2358
- Fluorouracil Injection (Common) 2116
- Heparin Lock Flush Solution 2725
- Heparin Sodium Injection 2726
- Heparin Sodium Injection, USP, Sterile Solution 2615
- Heparin Sodium Vials 1441
- K-Tab Filmtab 434
- Micro-K 2063
- Mutamycin 703
- Norplant System 2759
- PPD Tine Test 2874
- Pentam 300 Injection (Some instances) 1041
- Rubex 712
- Sotradecol (Sodium Tetradecyl Sulfate Injection) 967
- Talwin Injection 2334
- Tuberculin, Old, Tine Test 2875
- Tubersol (Tuberculin Purified Protein Derivative [Mantoux]) 2872

Ulceration, tongue
- Foscavir Injection (Less than 1%) 547
- Hivid Tablets (Less than 1% to less than 3%) 2121
- Nicorette (1%) 2458

Ulcerative esophagitis
- Aristocort Tablets 1022
- Dexacort Phosphate in Respihaler 458
- Dexacort Phosphate in Turbinaire 459
- Hydrocortone Acetate Sterile Suspension 1669
- Vibramycin (Rare) 1941

Ulcer attack
- Questran Light 769
- Questran Powder 770

Ulcers
- Effexor (Rare) 2719
- Paxil Tablets (Rare) 2505
- ReVia Tablets (Less than 1%) 940
- ▲Zoladex (Greater than 1% but less than 5%) 2858

Ulcers, anal
- Cafergot (Rare) 2251
- ▲Cytosar-U Sterile Powder (Among most frequent) 2592
- Hivid Tablets (Less than 1% to less than 3%) 2121

Ulcers, aphthous
- Capoten (About 0.5 to 2%) 739
- Capozide (0.5 to 2%) 742

Ulcers, corneal
- AK-Pred ⊚ 204
- Dexacidin Ointment ⊚ 263
- FML Forte Liquifilm (Occasional) ⊚ 240
- FML Liquifilm (Occasional) ⊚ 241
- FML S.O.P. (Occasional) ⊚ 241
- Genoptic Sterile Ophthalmic Solution ⊚ 243
- Genoptic Sterile Ophthalmic Ointment ⊚ 243
- Luvox Tablets (Rare) 2544
- Myochrysine Injection (Rare) 1711
- Oncovin Solution Vials & Hyporets 1466
- Ophthocort ⊚ 311
- Poly-Pred Liquifilm ⊚ 248
- Solganal Suspension (Rare) 2388
- Vasocidin Ointment ⊚ 268

Ulcers, cutaneous
- Anafranil Capsules (Rare) 803
- Betaseron for SC Injection 658
- ▲CellCept Capsules (More than or equal to 3%) 2099
- Cognex Capsules (Rare) 1901
- Cytosar-U Sterile Powder (Less frequent) 2592
- Eskalith 2485
- Foscavir Injection (Between 1% and 5%) 547
- Hivid Tablets (Less than 1% to less than 3%) 2121
- Lithium Carbonate Capsules & Tablets 2230
- Lithonate/Lithotabs/Lithobid 2543
- Miacalcin Nasal Spray (Less than 1%) 2275
- Permax Tablets (Infrequent) 575
- Risperdal (Rare) 1301
- T.R.U.E. Test 1189
- Videx Tablets, Powder for Oral Solution, & Pediatric Powder for Oral Solution (Less than 1%) 720

Ulcers, duodenal
- Children's Advil Suspension (Less than 1%) 2692
- Ancobon Capsules 2079
- Atamet (Rare) 572
- Betaseron for SC Injection 658
- Cognex Capsules (Rare) 1901
- Fioricet with Codeine Capsules 2260
- Foscavir Injection (Less than 1%) 547
- Sterile FUDR 2118
- IBU Tablets (Less than 1%) 1342
- Indocin Capsules (Less than 1%) 1680
- Indocin I.V. (Less than 1%) 1684
- Indocin (Less than 1%) 1680
- Larodopa Tablets (Rare) 2129
- Children's Motrin Ibuprofen Oral Suspension (Less than 1%) 1546
- Motrin Tablets (Less than 1%) 2625
- Motrin Ibuprofen Suspension, Oral Drops, Chewable Tablets, Caplets (Less than 1%) 1546
- Pentasa (Less than 1%) 1527
- Proleukin for Injection (Less than 1%) 797
- Prozac Pulvules & Liquid, Oral Solution (Rare) 919
- Relafen Tablets (1%) 2510
- Sinemet Tablets (Rare) 943
- Sinemet CR Tablets 944
- Trilisate (Rare) 2000

Ulcers, esophageal
- Effexor (Rare) 2719
- ▲Ethamolin (Among most common; 2.1%) 2400
- Hivid Tablets (Less than 1% to less than 3%) 2121
- Pentasa (Less than 1%) 1527
- Permax Tablets (Rare) 575
- Urobiotic-250 Capsules (Rare) 2214

Ulcers, gastrointestinal
- Adriamycin PFS 1947
- Adriamycin RDF 1947
- Children's Advil Suspension (Less than 1%) 2692
- Anafranil Capsules (Infrequent) 803
- Anaprox/Naprosyn (Less than 1%) 2117
- Cataflam 816
- Clinoril Tablets 1618
- Clozaril Tablets (Less than 1%) 2252
- Cosmegen Injection 1626
- Cytosar-U Sterile Powder 2592
- Dolobid Tablets 1654
- Easprin 1914
- EC-Naprosyn Delayed-Release Tablets (Less than 1% to 4%) 2117
- Ergamisol Tablets 1292
- Feldene Capsules 1965
- Fiorinal with Codeine Capsules 2262
- Fluorouracil Injection 2116
- Sterile FUDR 2118
- IBU Tablets (Less than 1%) 1342
- Indocin Capsules (Less than 1%) 1680
- Indocin I.V. (Less than 1%) 1684
- Indocin (Less than 1%) 1680
- Intron A (Less than 5%) 2364
- K-Dur Microburst Release System (potassium chloride, USP) E.R. Tablets 1325
- K-Norm Extended-Release Capsules 991
- K-Tab Filmtab 434
- Larodopa Tablets (Rare) 2129
- Lodine Capsules and Tablets 2743
- Luvox Tablets (Infrequent) 2544
- Methotrexate Sodium Tablets, Injection, for Injection and LPF Injection 1275
- Micro-K 2063
- Micro-K LS Packets 2064
- Children's Motrin Ibuprofen Oral Suspension (Approximately 1% to 4%) 1546
- Motrin Tablets (Less than 1%) 2625
- Motrin Ibuprofen Suspension, Oral Drops, Chewable Tablets, Caplets (Less than 1% to 4%) 1546
- Nalfon 200 Pulvules & Nalfon Tablets 917
- Anaprox/Naprosyn (Less than 1% to 4%) 2117
- NebuPent for Inhalation Solution (1% or less) 1040
- Neutrexin 2572
- Orudis Capsules (Less than 1%) 2766
- Oruvail Capsules (Less than 1%) 2766
- Paxil Tablets (Rare) 2505
- Ponstel 1925
- Purinethol Tablets 1156
- Relafen Tablets (1%) 2510
- Slow-K Extended-Release Tablets (1 per 100,000 patient-years) 851
- Tolectin (200, 400 and 600 mg) (Less than 1%) 1581
- Toradol 2159
- Trilisate (Less than 1%) 2000
- Voltaren Tablets 861
- Wellbutrin Tablets (Rare) 1204

Ulcers, intestinal
- Lodine Capsules and Tablets (Less than 1%) 2743

Ulcers, leg
- Imdur (Less than or equal to 5%) 1323
- Neurontin Capsules (Rare) 1922

Ulcers, oral mucosal
- Alkeran for Injection (Infrequent) 1070
- Alkeran Tablets (Infrequent) 1071
- Anafranil Capsules (Infrequent) 803
- Asacol Delayed-Release Tablets 1979
- Atretol Tablets 573
- Atrovent Inhalation Aerosol (Less frequent) 671
- Azactam for Injection (Less than 1%) 734
- Ceftin (Less than 1% but more than 0.1%) 1078
- ▲CellCept Capsules (More than or equal to 3%) 2099
- Ceredase 1065
- Cipro I.V. (1% or less) 595

(▣ Described in PDR For Nonprescription Drugs) Incidence data in parenthesis; ▲ 3% or more (⊚ Described in PDR For Ophthalmology)

Ulcers, oral mucosal — Side Effects Index — 1434

Cipro I.V. Pharmacy Bulk Package (Less than 1%) 597
Clozaril Tablets 2252
Cuprimine Capsules (Some patients) 1630
▲Cytosar-U Sterile Powder (Among most frequent) 2592
Cytovene (1% or less) 2103
Cytoxan (Isolated reports) 694
Depen Titratable Tablets (Some patients) 2662
Effexor (Infrequent) 2719
Hivid Tablets (Less than 1% to less than 3%) 2121
IBU Tablets (Less than 1%) 1342
Kerlone Tablets (Less than 2%) 2436
Lamictal Tablets (Infrequent) 1112
Leukeran Tablets (Infrequent) 1133
Myochrysine Injection 1711
Nalfon 200 Pulvules & Nalfon Tablets (Less than 1%) 917
NebuPent for Inhalation Solution (1% or less) 1040
NEOSAR Lyophilized/Neosar (Isolated reports) 1959
Neutrexin 2572
Noroxin Tablets (Less frequent) 1715
Noroxin Tablets (Less frequent) 2048
Oncovin Solution Vials & Hyporets 1466
Paxil Tablets (Infrequent) 2505
Pentasa (Less than 1%) 1527
ProSom Tablets (Rare) 449
Prozac Pulvules & Liquid, Oral Solution (Rare) 919
Retrovir Capsules 1158
Retrovir I.V. Infusion 1163
Retrovir Syrup 1158
Serzone Tablets (Infrequent) 771
Solganal Suspension 2388
Tegison Capsules (Less than 1%) 2154
Tegretol Chewable Tablets 852
Tegretol Suspension 852
Tegretol Tablets 852
Zoloft Tablets (Rare) 2217

Ulcers, peptic

Anafranil Capsules (Infrequent) 803
Atromid-S Capsules 2701
Betaseron for SC Injection 658
Capoten (About 0.5 to 2%) 739
Capozide (0.5 to 2%) 742
Cataflam (0.6% to 1.6%) 816
Clinoril Tablets (Less than 1 in 100) 1618
Cognex Capsules (Infrequent) 1901
Colestid Tablets (Rare) 2591
Cortifoam 2396
Cuprimine Capsules (Less than 1%) 1630
Daypro Caplets (Less than 1%) 2426
Dilacor XR Extended-release Capsules 2018
Dolobid Tablets (Less than 1 in 100) 1654
Effexor (Infrequent) 2719
Feldene Capsules (About 1%) 1965
Fiorinal with Codeine Capsules 2262
Hydeltra-T.B.A. Sterile Suspension 1667
Hydrocortone Acetate Sterile Suspension 1669
Hydrocortone Phosphate Injection, Sterile 1670
Hydrocortone Tablets 1672
Imdur (Less than or equal to 5%) 1323
Imitrex Injection (Rare) 1103
Imitrex Tablets (Rare) 1106
Indocin Capsules (Less than 1%) 1680
Indocin I.V. (Less than 1%) 1684
Indocin (Less than 1%) 1680
Lamictal Tablets (Rare) 1112
Lupron Depot 3.75 mg 2556
Lupron Depot 7.5 mg 2559
Lupron Injection (Less than 5%) 2555
Mexitil Capsules (About 8 in 10,000) 678
Midamor Tablets (Rare) 1703
Moduretic Tablets 1705
Neoral (2% or less) 2276
Neurontin Capsules (Rare) 1922
Nicobid 2026
Orudis Capsules (Less than 1%) 2766
Oruvail Capsules (Less than 1%) 2766
Paxil Tablets (Rare) 2505
Permax Tablets (Rare to infrequent) 575
Prozac Pulvules & Liquid, Oral Solution (Rare) 919
Relafen Tablets (0.3%) 2510
Sandimmune (2% or less) 2286
Serzone Tablets (Infrequent) 771
Ticlid Tablets (Rare) 2156
Tolectin (200, 400 and 600 mg) (1 to 3%) 1581
Toradol 2159
Voltaren Tablets (0.6% to 1.6%) 861
Ziac 1415

Ulcers, peptic, aggravation of

Anturane 807
Eldepryl Tablets 2550

Ulcers, peptic, hemorrhagic

Imdur (Less than or equal to 5%) 1323
Videx Tablets, Powder for Oral Solution, & Pediatric Powder for Oral Solution (Less than 1%) 720
Zoloft Tablets (Rare) 2217

Ulcers, peptic, reactivation of

Anturane 807
Depen Titratable Tablets (Isolated cases) 2662
Didronel Tablets (A few patients) 1984
Empirin with Codeine Tablets 1093
Nicolar Tablets 2026
Velban Vials 1484

Ulcers, peptic with or without perforation

Asacol Delayed-Release Tablets (Rare) 1979
Cataflam (1% to 3%) 816
Didronel Tablets (One report) 1984
Lodine Capsules and Tablets (Less than 1%) 2743
Nalfon 200 Pulvules & Nalfon Tablets (Less than 1%) 917
Voltaren Tablets (1% to 3%) 861

Ulcers, peptic with perforation and hemorrhage

Children's Advil Suspension 2692
Anaprox/Naprosyn (Less than 3%) 2117
Ansaid Tablets (Less than 1%) 2579
Aristocort Suspension (Forte Parenteral) 1027
Aristocort Suspension (Intralesional) 1025
Aristocort Tablets 1022
Aristospan Suspension (Intra-articular) 1033
Aristospan Suspension (Intralesional) 1032
Cataflam (1% to 3%) 816
Celestone Soluspan Suspension 2347
CORTENEMA 2535
Cortone Acetate Sterile Suspension 1623
Cortone Acetate Tablets 1624
Dalalone D.P. Injectable 1011
Decadron Elixir 1633
Decadron Phosphate Injection 1637
Decadron Phosphate Respihaler 1642
Decadron Phosphate Turbinaire 1645
Decadron Phosphate with Xylocaine Injection, Sterile 1639
Decadron Tablets 1635
Decadron-LA Sterile Suspension 1646
Deltasone Tablets 2595
Depo-Medrol Single-Dose Vial 2600
Depo-Medrol Sterile Aqueous Suspension 2597
Dexacort Phosphate in Respihaler 458
Dexacort Phosphate in Turbinaire 459
EC-Naprosyn Delayed-Release Tablets (Less than 1%) 2117
Florinef Acetate Tablets 505
Hydeltrasol Injection, Sterile 1665
Hydrocortone Tablets 1672
IBU Tablets (Less than 1%) 1342
Lodine Capsules and Tablets (Less than 1%) 2743
Medrol 2621
Children's Motrin Ibuprofen Oral Suspension (Less than 1%) 1546
Motrin Tablets 2625
Motrin Ibuprofen Suspension, Oral Drops, Chewable Tablets, Caplets (Less than 1%) 1546
Anaprox/Naprosyn (Less than 1%) 2117
Pediapred Oral Liquid 995
Prelone Syrup 1787
Solu-Cortef Sterile Powder 2641
Solu-Medrol Sterile Powder 2643
Voltaren Tablets (1% to 3%) 861

Ulcers, pharyngeal

Myochrysine Injection 1711

Ulcers, vulvovaginal

Foscavir Injection (One case) 547

Unconsciousness (see under Consciousness, loss of)

Underventilation (see under Hypoventilation)

Unsteadiness

Ativan Injection 2698
▲Ativan Tablets (3.4%) 2700
▲Atretol Tablets (Among most frequent) 573
MSTA Mumps Skin Test Antigen 890
Restoril Capsules (Less than 1%) 2284
Tambocor Tablets 1497
▲Tegretol Chewable Tablets (Among most frequent) 852
▲Tegretol Suspension (Among most frequent) 852
▲Tegretol Tablets (Among most frequent) 852
Tonocard Tablets (0.0-1.2%) 531

Upper respiratory symptoms

▲Betapace Tablets (1% to 5%) 641
Engerix-B Unit-Dose Vials (Less than 1%) 2482
▲Paxil Tablets (5.9%) 2505
Varivax (Greater than or equal to 1%) 1762
▲Wellbutrin Tablets (5.0%) 1204

Urate excretion, impaired

Fiorinal with Codeine Capsules 2262

Uremia (see under Azotemia)

Ureteral obstruction

Halotestin Tablets 2614
Surgicel (One report) 1314
Zoladex 2858

Ureteral spasm

Anexsia 5/500 Elixir 1781
Anexia Tablets 1782
Dilaudid Ampules 1335
Dilaudid Cough Syrup 1336
Dilaudid 1335
Hycodan Tablets and Syrup 930
Hycomine Compound Tablets 932
Hycomine 931
Hycotuss Expectorant Syrup 933
Hydrocet Capsules 782
Lorcet 10/650 1018
Lortab 2566
Tussend 1783
Tussionex Pennkinetic Extended-Release Suspension 998
Vicodin Tablets 1356
Vicodin ES Tablets 1357
Vicodin Tuss Expectorant 1358
Zydone Capsules 949

Ureteritis, hemorrhagic

Cytoxan 694
NEOSAR Lyophilized/Neosar 1959

Urethral disorder

Anafranil Capsules (Infrequent) 803
Foscavir Injection (Between 1% and 5%) 547

Urethritis

BCG Vaccine, USP (TICE) (1.2%) 1814
Betaseron for SC Injection 658
Dyclone 0.5% and 1% Topical Solutions, USP 544
Paxil Tablets (Infrequent) 2505
Prozac Pulvules & Liquid, Oral Solution (Rare) 919
Rogaine Topical Solution (0.93%) 2637

Uric acid level, increase (see under Hyperuricemia)

Uric acid stones

Benemid Tablets 1611
ColBENEMID Tablets 1622

Uricaciduria

Permax Tablets (Rare) 575

Urinary bladder, irritability

MIOSTAT Intraocular Solution ⊙ 224
Neosporin G.U. Irrigant Sterile 1148
Winstrol Tablets 2337

Urinary bladder malignancies

NEOSAR Lyophilized/Neosar 1959
Permax Tablets (Rare) 575

Urinary calculi

Adalat CC (Less than 1.0%) 589

Urinary cytology, abnormal

Orthoclone OKT3 Sterile Solution 1837

Urinary difficulty (see under Micturition, difficulty)

Urinary disturbances

Esimil Tablets 822
Ismelin Tablets 827
MIOSTAT Intraocular Solution ⊙ 224
Prozac Pulvules & Liquid, Oral Solution (Infrequent) 919
ReVia Tablets (Less than 1%) 940
Sansert Tablets 2295
▲TheraCys BCG Live (Intravesical) (Up to 17.9%) 897
Trilafon (Occasional) 2389

Urinary findings, abnormal

▲Capastat Sulfate Vials (10%) 2868
Ceclor Pulvules & Suspension (Less than 1 in 200) 1431
Clozaril Tablets (2%) 2252
Phenurone Tablets (1 in 100 patients or less) 447

Urinary frequency (see under Micturition disturbances)

Urinary glucose, false-positive

Augmentin 2468
Ceclor Pulvules & Suspension 1431
Ceftin 1078
Ceptaz 1081
Fortaz 1100
Keflex Pulvules & Oral Suspension 914
Macrodantin Capsules 1989
Omnipen for Oral Suspension 2765
Tazicef for Injection 2519
Zosyn 1419
Zosyn Pharmacy Bulk Package 1422

Urinary hesitancy

Arfonad Ampuls 2080
Artane 1368
Bentyl 1501
BuSpar (Infrequent) 737
Cystospaz 1963
Dalgan Injection (Less than 1%) 538
Dilaudid-HP Injection (Less frequent) 1337
Dilaudid-HP Lyophilized Powder 250 mg (Less frequent) 1337
Dilaudid Tablets and Liquid 1339
Ditropan 1516
Donnatal 2060
Donnatal Extentabs 2061
Donnatal Tablets 2060
Eldepryl Tablets 2550
Fludara for Injection (Up to 3%) 663
Kutrase Capsules 2402
Levsin/Levsinex/Levbid 2405
Librax Capsules 2176
Ludiomil Tablets 843
MS Contin Tablets (Less frequent) 1994
MSIR (Infrequent) 1997
Marax Tablets & DF Syrup 2200
Methadone Hydrochloride Oral Concentrate 2233
Methadone Hydrochloride Oral Solution & Tablets 2235
Mexitil Capsules (Less than 1% or about 2 in 1,000) 678
Norflex 1496
Norgesic 1496
▲Norpace (14%) 2444
Oramorph SR (Morphine Sulfate Sustained Release Tablets) (Less frequent) 2236
Pamelor 2280
Paxil Tablets (2.9%) 2505
Pro-Banthīne Tablets 2052
ProSom Tablets (Infrequent) 449
Quarzan Capsules (Among most frequent) 2181
RMS Suppositories 2657
Retrovir Capsules 1158
Retrovir I.V. Infusion 1163
Retrovir Syrup 1158
Robinul Forte Tablets 2072
Robinul Injectable 2072
Robinul Tablets 2072
Roxanol 2243

(◙ Described in PDR For Nonprescription Drugs) Incidence data in parenthesis; ▲ 3% or more (⊙ Described in PDR For Ophthalmology)

1435 Side Effects Index Urine, color change

Valium Injectable 2182
Valium Tablets (Infrequent) 2183

Urinary obstruction

BCG Vaccine, USP (TICE) (0.3%) 1814
Caverject (Less than 1%) 2583
Lupron Depot 3.75 mg 2556
Luvox Tablets (Infrequent) 2544
Ortho Diaphragm Kit 1865
Salagen Tablets (Less than 1%) 1489

Urinary retention

Actifed with Codeine Cough Syrup 1067
Akineton 1333
Ambien Tablets (Rare) 2416
▲ Anafranil Capsules (2% to 7%) 803
Anatuss LA Tablets 1542
Anexsia 5/500 Elixir 1781
Anexia Tablets 1782
Artane 1368
Asendin Tablets (Less than 1%) 1369
▲ Astramorph/PF Injection, USP (Preservative-Free) (Approximately 90% of males; somewhat less in females) 535
Atamet 572
Atretol Tablets 573
Atrovent Inhalation Solution (Less than 3%) 673
Azo Gantrisin Tablets 2081
Bellergal-S Tablets (Rare) 2250
Benadryl Capsules 1898
Benadryl Injection 1898
Bentyl 1501
Betaseron for SC Injection 658
Brevibloc Injection (Less than 1%) 1808
Brontex 1981
Buprenex Injectable (Less than 1%) 2006
BuSpar (Rare) 737
Carbocaine Hydrochloride Injection 2303
Catapres Tablets (About 1 in 1,000 patients) 674
Catapres-TTS (Less frequent) 675
Cipro I.V. (1% or less) 595
Cipro I.V. Pharmacy Bulk Package (Less than 1%) 597
Cipro Tablets (Less than 1%) 592
Claritin-D (Less frequent) 2350
Clozaril Tablets (1%) 2252
Cogentin 1621
Cognex Capsules (Infrequent) 1901
Combipres Tablets (About 1 in 1,000) 677
Comhist 2038
Compazine 2470
Cystospaz 1963
Cytosar-U Sterile Powder (Less frequent) 2592
D.A. Chewable Tablets 951
Dalgan Injection (Less than 1%) 538
Dantrium Capsules (Less frequent) 1982
Deconamine 1320
Demerol 2308
Desyrel and Desyrel Dividose 503
Dilaudid Ampules 1335
Dilaudid Cough Syrup 1336
Dilaudid-HP Injection (Less frequent) 1337
Dilaudid-HP Lyophilized Powder 250 mg (Less frequent) 1337
Dilaudid 1335
Dilaudid Oral Liquid 1339
Dilaudid 1335
Dilaudid Tablets - 8 mg 1339
Diprivan Injection (Less than 1%) 2833
Ditropan 1516
Dizac (Less frequent) 1809
Donnatal 2060
Donnatal Extentabs 2061
Donnatal Tablets 2060
Dopram Injectable 2061
Doral Tablets 2664
▲ Duragesic Transdermal System (3% to 10%) 1288
Duramorph (Frequent in males; less frequent in females) 962
Dura-Tap/PD Capsules 2867
Duratuss Tablets 2565
Dura-Vent/DA Tablets 953
Dura-Vent Tablets 952
Effexor (1%) 2719
Elavil 2838
Eldepryl Tablets (1 of 49 patients) 2550
Endep Tablets 2174
Entex Capsules 1986
Entex LA Tablets 1987
Entex Liquid 1986
Ethmozine Tablets (Less than 2%) 2041
Etrafon 2355
Exgest LA Tablets 782
Felbatol 2666
Flexeril Tablets (Less than 1%) 1661
Floxin I.V. (Less than 1%) 1571
Floxin Tablets (200 mg, 300 mg, 400 mg) (Less than 1%) 1567
Foscavir Injection (Between 1% and 5%) 547
Halcion Tablets 2611
Haldol Decanoate 1577
Haldol Injection, Tablets and Concentrate 1575
Hivid Tablets (Less than 1% to less than 3%) 2121
Hycodan Tablets and Syrup 930
Hycomine Compound Tablets 932
Hycomine 931
Hycotuss Expectorant Syrup 933
Hydrocet Capsules 782
Infumorph 200 and Infumorph 500 Sterile Solutions (Frequent) 965
Inversine Tablets 1686
Klonopin Tablets 2126
Kutrase Capsules 2402
Lamictal Tablets (Rare) 1112
Larodopa Tablets (Infrequent) 2129
Levbid Extended-Release Tablets 2405
Levo-Dromoran (Infrequent) 2129
Levsin/Levsinex/Levbid 2405
Limbitrol 2180
Lioresal Tablets (Rare) 829
Lomotil 2439
Lorcet 10/650 1018
Lortab 2566
Loxitane 1378
Ludiomil Tablets (Rare) 843
MS Contin Tablets (Less frequent) 1994
MSIR (Infrequent) 1997
Marax Tablets & DF Syrup (Occasional) 2200
Marcaine Hydrochloride with Epinephrine 1:200,000 2316
Marcaine Hydrochloride Injection 2316
Marcaine Spinal 2319
Maxaquin Tablets 2440
Mellaril 2269
Mepergan Injection 2753
Methadone Hydrochloride Oral Concentrate 2233
Methadone Hydrochloride Oral Solution & Tablets 2235
Mexitil Capsules (Less than 1% or about 2 in 1,000) 678
Moban Tablets and Concentrate 1048
Motofen Tablets 784
Nardil (Less common) 1920
Neurontin Capsules (Infrequent) 1922
Norflex 1496
Norgesic 1496
Normodyne Tablets (Less common) 2379
▲ Norpace (3 to 9%) 2444
Norpramin Tablets 1526
Oncovin Solution Vials & Hyporets 1466
Oramorph SR (Morphine Sulfate Sustained Release Tablets) (Less frequent) 2236
Ornade Spansule Capsules 2502
PBZ Tablets 845
PBZ-SR Tablets 844
Pamelor 2280
Parlodel 2281
Parnate Tablets 2503
Paxil Tablets (Infrequent) 2505
Penetrex Tablets 2031
Periactin 1724
Permax Tablets (Infrequent) 575
Phenergan with Codeine 2777
Phenergan VC with Codeine 2781
Pro-Banthīne Tablets 2052
Proleukin for Injection (1%) 797
Prostin E2 Suppository 2634
Prozac Pulvules & Liquid, Oral Solution (Infrequent) 919
Quarzan Capsules 2181
RMS Suppositories 2657
ReoPro Vials (0.4%) 1471
Revex (Less than 1%) 1811
Risperdal (Rare) 1301
Robinul Forte Tablets 2072
Robinul Injectable 2072
Robinul Tablets 2072
Roxanol 2243
Sensorcaine 559
Serentil 684
Serzone Tablets (2%) 771
Sinemet Tablets 943
Sinemet CR Tablets 944
Sinequan 2205
Stelazine 2514
Sufenta Injection 1309
Surmontil Capsules 2811
Symmetrel Capsules and Syrup (0.1% to 1%) 946
Tagamet (Rare) 2516
Talacen (Rare) 2333
Talwin Injection (Infrequent) 2334
Talwin Compound 2335
Talwin Injection 2334
Talwin Nx 2336
Tambocor Tablets (Less than 1%) 1497
Tavist Syrup 2297
Tavist Tablets 2298
Tegison Capsules (Less than 1%) 2154
Tegretol Chewable Tablets 852
Tegretol Suspension 852
Tegretol Tablets 852
Temaril Tablets, Syrup and Spansule Extended-Release Capsules 483
Thioplex (Thiotepa For Injection) 1281
Thorazine 2523
Tofranil Ampuls 854
Tofranil Tablets 856
Tofranil-PM Capsules 857
Tonocard Tablets (Less than 1%) 531
Toradol (1% or less) 2159
Torecan 2245
Trandate Tablets (Less common) 1185
Triavil Tablets 1757
Trinalin Repetabs Tablets 1330
Tussend 1783
Tussionex Pennkinetic Extended-Release Suspension 998
Ultram Tablets (50 mg) (1% to 5%) 1585
Unasyn (Less than 1%) 2212
Urised Tablets 1964
Valrelease Capsules (Occasional) 2169
Vicodin Tablets 1356
Vicodin ES Tablets 1357
Vicodin Tuss Expectorant 1358
Vivactil Tablets 1774
Wellbutrin Tablets (1.9%) 1204
Xanax Tablets 2649
▲ Zofran Injection (3%) 1214
▲ Zofran Tablets (5%) 1217
Zoloft Tablets (Rare) 2217
Zosyn (1.0% or less) 1419
Zosyn Pharmacy Bulk Package (1.0% or less) 1422
Zydone Capsules 949

Urinary sediment, abnormalities

Dyazide 2479
Roferon-A Injection (Infrequent) 2145

Urinary tract, burning

Rowasa (0.61%) 2548

Urinary tract, infection

▲ Anafranil Capsules (Up to 6%) 803
▲ Ansaid Tablets (3-9%) 2579
Cartrol Tablets (Less common) 410
Cytotec (Infrequent) 2424
Lupron Depot 3.75 mg 2556
Lupron Depot 7.5 mg 2559
Ortho Diaphragm Kit 1865
Permax Tablets (2.7%) 575
Rowasa (0.61%) 2548
▲ TheraCys BCG Live (Intravesical) (1.0% to 17.9%) 897
▲ Zoladex (Greater than 1% but less than 5%) 2858

Urinary tract, obstruction

Cognex Capsules (Rare) 1901
Lupron Depot 7.5 mg 2559
Lupron Injection (A few cases) 2555
▲ Zoladex (Greater than 1% but less than 5%) 2858

Urinary tract dilatation

Asendin Tablets 1369
Elavil 2838
Endep Tablets 2174
Etrafon 2355
Limbitrol 2180
Norpramin Tablets 1526
Pamelor 2280
Surmontil Capsules 2811
Tofranil Ampuls 854
Tofranil Tablets 856
Tofranil-PM Capsules 857
Triavil Tablets 1757

Urinary tract disorder, unspecified

▲ CellCept Capsules (More than or equal to 3%; 6.7% to 10.6%) 2099
▲ Leukine for IV Infusion (14%) 1271
Lupron Depot 3.75 mg 2556
Pravachol (0.7% to 2.4%) 765
Prozac Pulvules & Liquid, Oral Solution (Rare) 919
▲ Zoladex (13%) 2858

Urinary tract irritation

Orudis Capsules (Greater than 1%) 2766
Oruvail Capsules (Greater than 1%) 2766

Urinary urgency

Adenoscan (Less than 1%) 1024
Asacol Delayed-Release Tablets 1979
▲ BCG Vaccine, USP (TICE) (5.8%) 1814
▲ Betaseron for SC Injection (4%) 658
Caverject (Less than 1%) 2583
Clozaril Tablets (1%) 2252
Cognex Capsules (Infrequent) 1901
Duvoid (Infrequent) 2044
Effexor (Infrequent) 2719
▲ Hylorel Tablets (33.6%) 985
Isopto Carbachol Ophthalmic Solution (Frequent) ⊙ 223
Lupron Depot 3.75 mg 2556
Lupron Depot 7.5 mg (Less than 5%) 2559
Luvox Tablets (Infrequent) 2544
Neurontin Capsules (Rare) 1922
Nubain Injection (1% or less) 935
Paxil Tablets (Infrequent) 2505
Plendil Extended-Release Tablets (0.5% to 1.5%) 527
ProSom Tablets (Infrequent) 449
Prozac Pulvules & Liquid, Oral Solution (Infrequent) 919
Serzone Tablets (Infrequent) 771
▲ TheraCys BCG Live (Intravesical) (Up to 17.9%) 897
THYREL TRH 2873
Vasoxyl Injection 1196

Urination, difficult (see under Micturition, difficulty)

Urination, painful (see under Micturition, painful)

Urine, abnormal

Diprivan Injection (Less than 1%) 2833
Lamictal Tablets (Rare) 1112
Lithonate/Lithotabs/Lithobid 2543
Maxaquin Tablets (Less than or equal to 0.1%) 2440
Tornalate Solution for Inhalation, 0.2% (Infrequent) 956

Urine, burnt odor

Questran Light 769
Questran Powder 770

Urine, cells in

▲ Accutane Capsules (1 in 5 to 1 in 10 patients) 2076
Polymyxin B Sulfate, Aerosporin Brand Sterile Powder 1154
TheraCys BCG Live (Intravesical) (Up to 0.9%) 897
Zovirax Sterile Powder (Less than 1%) 1223

Urine, color change

Adriamycin PFS 1947
Adriamycin RDF 1947
AK-Fluor Injection 10% and 25% ⊙ 203
Atamet 572
Azulfidine (Rare) 1949
Cerubidine 795
Claritin (2% or fewer patients) 2349
Claritin-D 2350
Clinoril Tablets (Less than 1%) 1618
Coumadin 926
Demulen 2428
Desferal Vials 820
Diprivan Injection (Less than 1%) 2833
Doxorubicin Astra 540
Eulexin Capsules 2358
Flagyl 375 Capsules (Approximately 1 patient in 100,000) 2434
Flagyl I.V. 2247
Fluorescite ⊙ 219
Lamprene Capsules (Greater than 1%) 828
Larodopa Tablets (Infrequent) 2129
Levlen/Tri-Levlen 651
Maxzide 1380
MetroGel-Vaginal 902
Micronor Tablets 1872
Modicon 1872
▲ Mycobutin Capsules (30%) 1957

(▭ Described in PDR For Nonprescription Drugs) Incidence data in parenthesis; ▲ 3% or more (⊙ Described in PDR For Ophthalmology)

Urine, color change | Side Effects Index | 1436

Nicobid 2026
Nizoral Tablets 1298
Normodyne Injection 2377
Novantrone 1279
Ortho-Cyclen/Ortho-Tri-Cyclen 1858
Ortho-Novum 1872
Ortho-Cyclen/Ortho Tri-Cyclen 1858
Paraflex Caplets 1580
Parafon Forte DSC Caplets 1581
Primaxin I.M. 1727
Primaxin I.V. (Less than 0.2%) 1729
Prodium 690
Protostat Tablets (Approximately one patient in 100,000) 1883
Pyrazinamide Tablets 1398
Pyridium 1928
ReVia Tablets 940
Rifadin 1528
Rifater 1532
Rubex 712
Sectral Capsules 2807
Sinemet Tablets 943
Sinemet CR Tablets 944
Slo-Niacin Tablets 2659
Sporanox Capsules 1305
Ticlid Tablets 2156
Trandate 1185
Levlen/Tri-Levlen 651
Urised Tablets 1964

Urine, fluorescence
AK-Fluor Injection 10% and 25% ⊙ 203

Urine, microscopic deposits
Atretol Tablets 573
Tegretol Chewable Tablets 852
Tegretol Suspension 852
Tegretol Tablets 852

Urine, output low (see under Hypouresis)

Urine, presence of granular casts
Amikacin Sulfate Injection, USP 960
Amikin Injectable 501
Primaxin I.M. 1727
Primaxin I.V. 1729
Rocephin Injectable Vials, ADD-Vantage, Galaxy Container (Less than 1%) 2142
Unasyn 2212

Urine, presence of RBCs (see under Hematuria)

Urine, presence of urobilinogen
Primaxin I.M. 1727
Primaxin I.V. 1729

Urolithiasis
Kytril Injection (Rare) 2490
Permax Tablets (Infrequent) 575
Prozac Pulvules & Liquid, Oral Solution (Rare) 919
Trusopt Sterile Ophthalmic Solution (Rare) 1760

Urticaria
A/T/S 2% Acne Topical Gel and Solution 1234
Accutane Capsules (Less than 1%) 2076
Acel-Imune Diphtheria and Tetanus Toxoids and Acellular Pertussis Vaccine Adsorbed 1364
Achromycin V Capsules 1367
ActHIB 872
Actifed with Codeine Cough Syrup 1067
Actigall Capsules 802
Activase (Very rare) 1058
Adalat Capsules (10 mg and 20 mg) (2% or less) 587
Adalat CC (Rare) 589
Adipex-P Tablets and Capsules 1048
Adriamycin PFS (Occasional) 1947
Adriamycin RDF (Occasional) 1947
Children's Advil Suspension (Less than 1%) 2692
AeroBid Inhaler System (1-3%) 1005
Aerobid-M Inhaler System (1-3%) 1005
Airet Solution for Inhalation (Rare) 452
Albuminar-5, Albumin (Human) U.S.P. 5% 512
Albuminar-25, Albumin (Human) U.S.P. 25% 513
Aldactazide 2413
Aldactone 2414
Aldoclor Tablets 1598
Aldoril Tablets 1604
Alfenta Injection (0.3% to 1%) 1286
Alkeran for Injection 1070
Altace Capsules (Less than 1%) 1232
Ambien Tablets (Rare) 2416
Amen Tablets (Occasional) 780
Americaine Anesthetic Lubricant 983
Americaine Otic Topical Anesthetic Ear Drops 983
Amoxil 2464
Anafranil Capsules (Up to 1%) 803
Anaprox/Naprosyn (Less than 1%) 2117
Ancobon Capsules 2079
Ansaid Tablets (Less than 1%) 2579
Antivenin (Crotalidae) Polyvalent 2696
Apresazide Capsules (Less frequent) 808
Apresoline Hydrochloride Tablets (Less frequent) 809
Arfonad Ampuls 2080
Asacol Delayed-Release Tablets 1979
Asendin Tablets (Less than 1%) 1369
Astramorph/PF Injection, USP (Preservative-Free) 535
▲ Atgam Sterile Solution (1 in 8 patients; 27%) 2581
Atretol Tablets 573
Atrohist Plus Tablets 454
Atromid-S Capsules (Less often) 2701
Atrovent Inhalation Aerosol 671
Atrovent Inhalation Solution (Less than 3%) 673
Attenuvax (Rare) 1610
▲ Augmentin (3%) 2468
▲ Axid Pulvules (More frequent) 1427
Azactam for Injection (Less than 1%) 734
Azo Gantanol Tablets 2080
Azo Gantrisin Tablets 2081
Azulfidine (One in every 30 patients or less) 1949
▲ Bactrim DS Tablets (Among most common) 2084
▲ Bactrim I.V. Infusion (Among most common) 2082
▲ Bactrim (Among most common) 2084
Beclovent Inhalation Aerosol and Refill (Rare) 1075
Beconase (Rare) 1076
Benadryl Injection 1898
Benemid Tablets 1611
Bentyl 1501
Benzamycin Topical Gel (1 out of 153) 905
Betagan (Rare) ⊙ 233
Betaseron for SC Injection 658
Betimol 0.25%, 0.5% ⊙ 261
Biavax II 1613
Bicillin C-R Injection 2704
Bicillin C-R 900/300 Injection 2706
Bicillin L-A Injection 2707
Biltricide Tablets (Rare) 591
Bioclate, Antihemophilic Factor (Recombinant) (Extremely rare) 513
Brevital Sodium Vials 1429
▲ Bromfed-DM Cough Syrup (Among most frequent) 1786
Brontex (Infrequent) 1981
Buprenex Injectable (Rare) 2006
BuSpar (Rare) 737
Calan SR Caplets (1% or less) 2422
Calan Tablets (1% or less) 2419
Capastat Sulfate Vials 2868
Capozide 742
Carafate Suspension 1505
Carafate Tablets 1504
Carbocaine Hydrochloride Injection 2303
Cardizem CD Capsules (Less than 1%) 1506
Cardizem SR Capsules (Less than 1%) 1510
Cardizem Injectable 1508
Cardizem Tablets (Less than 1%) 1512
Cataflam (Less than 1%) 816
Catapres Tablets (About 5 in 1,000 patients) 674
Catapres-TTS (2 cases of 3,539 patients; less frequent) 675
Ceclor Pulvules & Suspension (Less than 1 in 200) 1431
Cefotan 2829
Ceftin (Less than 1% but more than 0.1%) 1078
Cefzil Tablets and Oral Suspension (0.1%) 746
Ceptaz 1081
Ceredase 1065
Chibroxin Sterile Ophthalmic Solution (With oral form) 1617
Chloroptic S.O.P. ⊙ 239
Chloroptic Sterile Ophthalmic Solution ⊙ 239
Cipro I.V. (1% or less) 595
Cipro I.V. Pharmacy Bulk Package (Less than 1%) 597
Cipro Tablets (Less than 1%) 592
Claforan Sterile and Injection (Less frequent) 1235
Claritin (2% or fewer patients) 2349
Claritin-D (Less frequent) 2350
Cleocin Phosphate Injection 2586
Cleocin Vaginal Cream (Less than 1%) 2589
Clozaril Tablets (Less than 1%) 2252
▲ Cognex Capsules (7%) 1901
ColBENEMID Tablets 1622
Colestid Tablets (Rare) 2591
Coly-Mycin M Parenteral 1905
Colyte and Colyte-flavored (Isolated cases) 2396
Combipres Tablets (About 5 in 1,000) 677
Comhist 2038
Compazine 2470
Cortone Acetate Sterile Suspension 1623
Cortone Acetate Tablets 1624
Coumadin (Infrequent) 926
Cozaar Tablets (Less than 1%) 1628
Cuprimine Capsules 1630
Cycrin Tablets (Occasional) 975
Cystospaz 1963
Cytadren Tablets (Rare) 819
Cytosar-U Sterile Powder (Less frequent) 2592
Cytovene (1% or less) 2103
Dalalone D.P. Injectable 1011
Danocrine Capsules 2307
Dantrium Capsules (Less frequent) 1982
Dantrium Intravenous (Rare) 1983
Daypro Caplets (Less than 1%) 2426
Decadron Elixir 1633
Decadron Phosphate Injection 1637
Decadron Phosphate Respihaler 1642
Decadron Phosphate Turbinaire 1645
Decadron Phosphate with Xylocaine Injection, Sterile 1639
Decadron Tablets 1635
Decadron-LA Sterile Suspension 1646
Declomycin Tablets 1371
Deconamine 1320
Demerol 2308
Demser Capsules (Rare) 1649
Depen Titratable Tablets 2662
Depo-Medrol Single-Dose Vial 2600
Depo-Medrol Sterile Aqueous Suspension 2597
Depo-Provera Sterile Aqueous Suspension 2606
Dermatop Emollient Cream 0.1% (Less than 1%) 1238
Desferal Vials 820
Desoxyn Gradumet Tablets 419
Desyrel and Desyrel Dividose 503
Dexacort Phosphate in Respihaler 458
Dexacort Phosphate in Turbinaire 459
Dexedrine 2474
DextroStat Dextroamphetamine Tablets 2036
DiaBeta Tablets (1.5%) 1239
Diabinese Tablets (Approximately 1% or less) 1935
Diamox Intravenous (Occasional) 1372
Diamox Sequels (Sustained Release) 1373
Diamox Tablets (Occasional) 1372
Didrex Tablets 2607
Didronel Tablets 1984
Dilacor XR Extended-release Capsules (Infrequent) 2018
Dilaudid-HP Injection (Less frequent) 1337
Dilaudid-HP Lyophilized Powder 250 mg (Less frequent) 1337
Dilaudid Tablets and Liquid 1339
Dimetane-DC Cough Syrup 2059
Dimetane-DX Cough Syrup 2059
Diphtheria and Tetanus Toxoids and Pertussis Vaccine Adsorbed (Rare) 2477
Diphtheria and Tetanus Toxoids and Pertussis Vaccine Adsorbed USP (For Pediatric Use) 875
Diprivan Injection (Less than 1%) 2833
Diucardin Tablets 2718
Diupres Tablets 1650
Diuril Oral Suspension 1653
Diuril Sodium Intravenous 1652
Diuril Tablets 1653
Dizac (Less frequent) 1809
Dolobid Tablets (Less than 1 in 100) 1654
Donnatal 2060
Donnatal Extentabs 2061
Donnatal Tablets 2060
Doryx Capsules 1913
Doxorubicin Astra (Occasional) 540
Duramorph 962
Duranest Injections 542
Duricef 748
Dyazide 2479
Dyclone 0.5% and 1% Topical Solutions, USP 544
Dynacin Capsules 1590
DynaCirc Capsules (0.5% to 1%) 2256
E.E.S. 424
E-Mycin Tablets 1341
Easprin 1914
EC-Naprosyn Delayed-Release Tablets (Less than 1%) 2117
Effexor (Infrequent) 2719
Efudex 2113
Elase-Chloromycetin Ointment 1040
Elavil 2838
Elspar 1659
Emete-con Intramuscular/Intravenous (Rare) 2198
Eminase (Occasional) 2039
Emla Cream 545
Empirin with Codeine Tablets 1093
Endep Tablets 2174
Enduron Tablets 420
Engerix-B Unit-Dose Vials (Less than 1%) 2482
Epogen for Injection (Rare) 489
Ergamisol Tablets (Less than 1%) 1292
ERYC 1915
Erycette (erythromycin 2%) Topical Solution 1888
EryPed 421
Ery-Tab Tablets 422
Erythrocin Stearate Filmtab 425
Erythromycin Base Filmtab 426
Erythromycin Delayed-Release Capsules, USP 427
Esidrix Tablets 821
Esimil Tablets 822
Ethmozine Tablets (Less than 2%) 2041
Etrafon 2355
Factrel (Rare) 2877
Fansidar Tablets 2114
Fastin Capsules 2488
Felbatol (Infrequent) 2666
Feldene Capsules (Less than 1%) 1965
Flagyl 375 Capsules 2434
Flagyl I.V. 2247
Flexeril Tablets (Less than 1%) 1661
Flonase Nasal Spray (Less than 1%) 1098
Florinef Acetate Tablets 505
Floxin I.V. (Less than 1%) 1571
Floxin Tablets (200 mg, 300 mg, 400 mg) (Less than 1%) 1567
Fortaz 1100
Foscavir Injection (Less than 1%) 547
▲ Fulvicin P/G Tablets (Among most common) 2359
▲ Fulvicin P/G 165 & 330 Tablets (Among most common) 2359
Furoxone 2046
Gamimune N, 10% Immune Globulin Intravenous (Human), 10% (A single incidence) 621
Gammagard S/D, Immune Globulin, Intravenous (Human) (Occasional) 585
Gammar, Immune Globulin (Human) U.S.P. 515
Gantanol Tablets 2119
Gantrisin 2120
Garamycin Injectable 2360
Gastrocrom Capsules (Infrequent) 984
Geocillin Tablets (Infrequent) 2199
Geref (sermorelin acetate for injection) (One patient) 2876
Glauctabs (Occasional) ⊙ 208
Glucotrol Tablets (About 1 in 70) 1967
Glucotrol XL Extended Release Tablets (Less than 1%) 1968
Glynase PresTab Tablets (1.5%) 2609
GoLYTELY (Isolated cases) 688
Grifulvin V (griseofulvin tablets) Microsize (griseofulvin oral suspension) Microsize (Occasional) 1888
Gris-PEG Tablets, 125 mg & 250 mg 479
Guaifed Syrup ▣ 734
Habitrol Nicotine Transdermal System (Once in 35% of patients) 865
Havrix (Less than 1%) 2489
Heparin Lock Flush Solution 2725

(▣ Described in PDR For Nonprescription Drugs) Incidence data in parenthesis; ▲ 3% or more (⊙ Described in PDR For Ophthalmology)

1437 **Side Effects Index** **Urticaria**

Heparin Sodium Injection 2726
Heparin Sodium Injection, USP, Sterile Solution 2615
▲ Heparin Sodium Vials (Among most common) 1441
Hep-B-Gammagee 1663
Hespan Injection 929
Hivid Tablets (Less than 1% to less than 3%) 2121
Hydeltrasol Injection, Sterile 1665
Hydeltra-T.B.A. Sterile Suspension 1667
Hydrocortone Acetate Sterile Suspension 1669
Hydrocortone Phosphate Injection, Sterile 1670
Hydrocortone Tablets 1672
HydroDIURIL Tablets 1674
Hydropres Tablets 1675
HyperHep Hepatitis B Immune Globulin (Human) 626
Hyskon Hysteroscopy Fluid (Rare) 1595
Hyzaar Tablets 1677
IBU Tablets (Less than 1%) 1342
Idamycin 1955
Ilosone 911
Ilotycin Gluceptate, IV, Vials 913
Imitrex Injection (Rare) 1103
Imitrex Tablets 1106
Imogam Rabies Immune Globulin (Human) 880
▲ Imovax Rabies Vaccine (Up to 6%) 881
Inderide Tablets 2732
Inderide LA Long Acting Capsules 2734
Indocin Capsules (Less than 1%) 1680
Indocin I.V. (Less than 1%) 1684
Indocin (Less than 1%) 1680
INFeD (Iron Dextran Injection, USP) 2345
Infumorph 200 and Infumorph 500 Sterile Solutions 965
Intal Capsules (Less than 1 in 10,000 patients) 987
Intal Inhaler (Infrequent) 988
Intal Nebulizer Solution 989
Intron A (Less than 5%) 2364
Ionamin Capsules 990
Isoptin Injectable (Rare) 1344
Isoptin Oral Tablets (Less than 1%) 1346
Isoptin SR Tablets (1% or less) 1348
JE-VAX 886
Keflex Pulvules & Oral Suspension 914
Keftab Tablets 915
Kefurox Vials, Faspak & ADD-Vantage (Less than 1 in 250) 1454
Kutrase Capsules 2402
Kytril Tablets (Rare) 2492
Lamictal Tablets (Infrequent) 1112
Lasix Injection, Oral Solution and Tablets 1240
Lescol Capsules (Rare) 2267
Leucovorin Calcium for Injection 1268
Leucovorin Calcium Tablets 1270
Levbid Extended-Release Tablets 2405
Levo-Dromoran (Occasional) 2129
Levoprome 1274
Levsin/Levsinex/Levbid 2405
Limbitrol 2180
Lincocin 2617
Lioresal Intrathecal 1596
Lodine Capsules and Tablets (Less than 1%) 2743
Lomotil 2439
Lopid Tablets 1917
Lopressor HCT Tablets 832
Lorabid Suspension and Pulvules 1459
Lotensin HCT 837
Lotrimin 2371
Lotrisone Cream 2372
Lutrepulse for Injection 980
Luvox Tablets (Infrequent) 2544
M-M-R II 1687
M-R-VAX II 1689
MS Contin Tablets (Less frequent) 1994
MSIR (Infrequent) 1997
MZM (Occasional) ◉ 267
Macrobid Capsules (Less than 1%) 1988
Macrodantin Capsules 1989
Mandol Vials, Faspak & ADD-Vantage 1461
Marcaine Hydrochloride with Epinephrine 1:200,000 (Rare) 2316
Marcaine Hydrochloride Injection (Rare) 2316
Marcaine Spinal (Rare) 2319
Matulane Capsules 2131
Maxaquin Tablets (Less than 1%) 2440
Maxzide 1380
Medrol 2621
Mellaril (Infrequent) 2269
Mepergan Injection 2753
Meruvax II 1697
Methadone Hydrochloride Oral Concentrate 2233
Methadone Hydrochloride Oral Solution & Tablets 2235
Methotrexate Sodium Tablets, Injection, for Injection and LPF Injection 1275
Mevacor Tablets (Rare) 1699
Mezlin 601
Mezlin Pharmacy Bulk Package 604
Micronase Tablets (1.5%) 2623
Minizide Capsules 1938
Minocin Intravenous 1382
Minocin Oral Suspension 1385
Minocin Pellet-Filled Capsules 1383
Mivacron (Less than 1%) 1138
Moduretic Tablets 1705
8-MOP Capsules 1246
Monoclate-P, Factor VIII:C, Pasteurized, Monoclonal Antibody Purified Antihemophilic Factor (Human) 521
Monodox Capsules 1805
Mononine, Coagulation Factor IX (Human) 523
Monopril Tablets (0.2% to 1.0%) 757
Motofen Tablets 784
Children's Motrin Ibuprofen Oral Suspension (Less than 1%) 1546
Motrin Tablets (Less than 1%) 2625
Motrin Ibuprofen Suspension, Oral Drops, Chewable Tablets, Caplets (Less than 1%) 1546
Mumpsvax (Extremely rare) 1708
Mycostatin Pastilles (Rare) 704
Mykrox Tablets 993
Myleran Tablets 1143
Nalfon 200 Pulvules & Nalfon Tablets (Less than 1%) 917
Anaprox/Naprosyn (Less than 1%) 2117
Nasalcrom Nasal Solution 994
Navane Capsules and Concentrate 2201
Navane Intramuscular 2202
Nebcin Vials, Hyporets & ADD-Vantage 1464
NebuPent for Inhalation Solution (1% or less) 1040
NegGram 2323
Neptazane Tablets 1388
Nescaine/Nescaine MPF 554
Neupogen for Injection 495
Neurontin Capsules (Infrequent) 1922
Nicoderm (nicotine transdermal system) 1518
Nizoral Tablets (Several cases) 1298
Norflex (Rare) 1496
Norgesic (Rare) 1496
Normodyne Injection (Rare) 2377
Normodyne Tablets (Rare) 2379
Noroxin Tablets (Less frequent) 1715
Noroxin Tablets (Less frequent) 2048
Norplant System 2759
Norpramin Tablets 1526
Norvasc Tablets (Less than or equal to 0.1%) 1940
Novantrone (Occasional) 1279
Novocain Hydrochloride for Spinal Anesthesia 2326
Nubain Injection (1% or less) 935
NuLYTELY (Isolated cases) 689
Cherry Flavor NuLYTELY (Isolated cases) 689
Nuromax Injection (Less than or equal to 0.1%) 1149
OmniHIB 2499
Omnipen Capsules 2764
Omnipen for Oral Suspension 2765
▲ Oncaspar (Greater than 5%) 2028
Oramorph SR (Morphine Sulfate Sustained Release Tablets) (Less frequent) 2236
Oretic Tablets 443
Organidin NR Tablets and Liquid (Rare) 2672
Ornade Spansule Capsules 2502
Orthoclone OKT3 Sterile Solution 1837
Orudis Capsules (Less than 1%) 2766
Oruvail Capsules (Less than 1%) 2766
Oxsoralen-Ultra Capsules 1257
PBZ Tablets 845
PBZ-SR Tablets 844
PCE Dispertab Tablets 444
Pamelor 2280
Paraflex Caplets 1580
Parafon Forte DSC Caplets 1581
ParaGard T380A Intrauterine Copper Contraceptive 1880
Paraplatin for Injection 705
Parnate Tablets 2503
Paxil Tablets (Infrequent) 2505
PedvaxHIB (Two children) 1718
Pen•Vee K 2772
Penetrex Tablets (Less than 1% but more than or equal to 0.1%) 2031
Pentasa (Less than 1%) 1527
Pentaspan Injection 937
Pepcid Injection (Infrequent) 1722
Pepcid (Infrequent) 1720
Pergonal (menotropins for injection, USP) 2448
Periactin 1724
Pfizerpen for Injection 2203
Phenergan with Codeine 2777
Phenergan Injection 2773
Phenergan Tablets 2775
Phenergan VC with Codeine 2781
Placidyl Capsules 448
Plaquenil Sulfate Tablets 2328
Plendil Extended-Release Tablets (0.5% to 1.5%) 527
Pneumovax 23 (Rare) 1725
Pnu-Imune 23 (Rare) 1393
Polymyxin B Sulfate, Aerosporin Brand Sterile Powder (Occasional) 1154
Pondimin Tablets 2066
Ponstel 1925
Pontocaine Hydrochloride for Spinal Anesthesia 2330
Pravachol (Rare) 765
Prelu-2 Timed Release Capsules 681
Premphase 2797
Prempro 2801
Synthroid Injection 1359
PREVACID Delayed-Release Capsules (Less than 1%) 2562
Prilosec Delayed-Release Capsules (Less than 1%) 529
Primaxin I.M. 1727
Primaxin I.V. (0.2%) 1729
Prinivil Tablets (0.3% to 1.0%) 1733
Prinzide Tablets 1737
Pro-Banthīne Tablets 2052
Procan SR Tablets (Occasional) 1926
Procardia Capsules (2% or less) 1971
Procardia XL Extended Release Tablets (1% or less) 1972
Procrit for Injection (Rare) 1841
Profasi (chorionic gonadotropin for injection, USP) 2450
Proleukin for Injection (2%) 797
Prolixin 509
ProSom Tablets (Infrequent) 449
Prostigmin Injectable 1260
Prostigmin Tablets 1261
Protostat Tablets 1883
Proventil Inhalation Aerosol (Rare) 2382
Proventil Inhalation Solution 0.083% (Rare) 2384
Proventil Solution for Inhalation 0.5% (Rare) 2383
Proventil Syrup (Rare) 2385
Provera Tablets (An occasional patient) 2636
Prozac Pulvules & Liquid, Oral Solution (Infrequent; approximately 4% of 5,600 patients) 919
Pyrazinamide Tablets 1398
Quarzan Capsules 2181
Questran Light 769
Questran Powder 770
Quinaglute Dura-Tabs Tablets 649
Quinidex Extentabs 2067
RMS Suppositories 2657
▲ Rabies Vaccine, Imovax Rabies I.D. (Less frequent; up to 6%) 883
Recombivax HB (Less than 1%) 1744
Reglan (A few cases) 2068
Relafen Tablets (1%) 2510
Retrovir Capsules 1158
Retrovir I.V. Infusion 1163
Retrovir Syrup 1158
Ridaura Capsules (1 to 3%) 2513
Rifadin (Occasional) 1528
Rifamate Capsules (Occasional) 1530
Rifater (Occasional) 1532
Rimactane Capsules 847
Risperdal (Rare) 1301
Ritalin 848
Robaxin Injectable 2070
Robaxin Tablets 2071
Robaxisal Tablets 2071
Robinul Forte Tablets 2072
Robinul Injectable 2072
Robinul Tablets 2072
Roferon-A Injection (Less than 3%) 2145
Roxanol 2243
Rubex (Occasional) 712
Salflex Tablets 786
Sandostatin Injection (Less than 1%) 2292
Seldane Tablets (1.0% to 1.6%) 1536
Seldane-D Extended-Release Tablets 1538
Sensorcaine (Rare) 559
▲ Septra (Among most common) 1174
▲ Septra I.V. Infusion (Among most common) 1169
▲ Septra I.V. Infusion ADD-Vantage Vials (Among most common) 1171
▲ Septra (Among most common) 1174
Ser-Ap-Es Tablets 849
Serax Capsules 2810
Serax Tablets 2810
Serevent Inhalation Aerosol (Rare; 1% to 3%) 1176
Serophene (clomiphene citrate tablets, USP) (Less than 1 in 100 patients) 2451
Serzone Tablets (Infrequent) 771
Solu-Medrol Sterile Powder 2643
Soma Compound w/Codeine Tablets 2676
Soma Compound Tablets (Less common) 2675
Sotradecol (Sodium Tetradecyl Sulfate Injection) 967
Spectrobid Tablets 2206
Sporanox Capsules 1305
Stelazine 2514
Streptase for Infusion 562
Sublimaze Injection 1307
Sulfamylon Cream 925
▲ Supprelin Injection (Less than 2% to 4%) 2056
Suprax (Less than 2%) 1399
Surmontil Capsules 2811
Sus-Phrine Injection 1019
Synarel Nasal Solution for Central Precocious Puberty (2.6%) 2151
Synarel Nasal Solution for Endometriosis (Less than 1%) 2152
Synthroid Tablets 1359
T-Stat 2.0% Topical Solution and Pads 2688
Talacen (Rare) 2333
Talwin Carpuject 2334
Talwin Compound (Rare) 2335
Talwin Injection 2334
Talwin Nx (Rare) 2336
Tambocor Tablets (Less than 1%) 1497
Tao Capsules (Infrequent) 2209
Tapazole Tablets 1477
Tavist Syrup 2297
Tavist Tablets 2298
Taxol (2%) 714
Tazicef for Injection 2519
Tegison Capsules (Less than 1%) 2154
Tegretol Chewable Tablets 852
Tegretol Suspension 852
Tegretol Tablets 852
Temaril Tablets, Syrup and Spansule Extended-Release Capsules 483
Tenoretic Tablets 2845
Terramycin Intramuscular Solution 2210
Tetramune 1404
Thalitone 1245
Thioplex (Thiotepa For Injection) 1281
Thorazine (Occasional) 2523
Ticar for Injection 2526
Ticlid Tablets (0.5% to 1.0%) 2156
Timentin for Injection 2528
Timolide Tablets 1748
Timoptic in Ocudose (Less frequent) 1753
Timoptic Sterile Ophthalmic Solution (Less frequent) 1751
Timoptic-XE 1755
Tobramycin Sulfate Injection 968
Tofranil Ampuls 854
Tofranil Tablets 856
Tofranil-PM Capsules 857
Tolectin (200, 400 and 600 mg) (Less than 1%) 1581
Tonocard Tablets (Less than 1%) 531
Toradol (1% or less) 2159
Tornalate Solution for Inhalation, 0.2% (Less than 1%) 956
Tracrium Injection 1183
Trandate (Rare) 1185
Trental Tablets (Less than 1%) 1244
Triavil Tablets 1757
Tri-Immunol Adsorbed 1408
Trilafon 2389
Trilisate (Rare) 2000
Trinalin Repetabs Tablets 1330

(▭ Described in PDR For Nonprescription Drugs) Incidence data in parenthesis; ▲ 3% or more (◉ Described in PDR For Ophthalmology)

Tripedia ... 892
Trobicin Sterile Powder ... 2645
T.R.U.E. Test (One report) ... 1189
Tussend ... 1783
Tussi-Organidin DM NR Liquid and DM-S NR Liquid ... 2677
Tussi-Organidin NR Liquid and S NR Liquid ... 2677
Tympagesic Ear Drops ... 2342
Typhim Vi ... 899
Ultram Tablets (50 mg) (Less than 1%) ... 1585
Ultravate Ointment 0.05% (Less frequent) ... 2690
Unasyn ... 2212
Univasc Tablets (Less than 1%) ... 2410
Urispas Tablets ... 2532
Valium Injectable ... 2182
Vancenase PocketHaler Nasal Inhaler (Rare) ... 2391
Vanceril Inhaler (Rare) ... 2394
Vancocin HCl, Vials & ADD-Vantage ... 1481
Vaseretic Tablets ... 1765
Vasotec I.V. ... 1768
Vasotec Tablets (0.5% to 1.0%) ... 1771
Velosulin BR Human Insulin 10 ml Vials ... 1795
Ventolin Inhalation Aerosol and Refill (Rare) ... 1197
Ventolin Inhalation Solution (Rare) .. 1198
Ventolin Nebules Inhalation Solution (Rare) ... 1199
Ventolin Rotacaps for Inhalation (Rare) ... 1200
Ventolin Syrup (Rare) ... 1202
Ventolin Tablets (Rare) ... 1203
VePesid Capsules and Injection (Infrequent) ... 718
Verelan Capsules (1% or less) ... 1410
Verelan Capsules (Less than 1%) .. 2824
Vermox Chewable Tablets (Rare) ... 1312
Vibramycin ... 1941
Vibramycin Hyclate Intravenous ... 2215
Vibramycin ... 1941
Videx Tablets, Powder for Oral Solution, & Pediatric Powder for Oral Solution (Less than 1%) ... 720
Vivactil Tablets ... 1774
Vivotif Berna (Infrequent) ... 665
Volmax Extended-Release Tablets (Rare) ... 1788
Voltaren Tablets (Less than 1%) ... 861
Vumon ... 727
Wellbutrin Tablets ... 1204
Xylocaine Injections (Extremely rare) ... 567
Yodoxin ... 1230
Zarontin Capsules ... 1928
Zarontin Syrup ... 1929
Zaroxolyn Tablets ... 1000
Zefazone ... 2654
▲ Zerit Capsules (Fewer than 1% to 3%) ... 729
Zestoretic ... 2850
Zestril Tablets (0.3% to 1.0%) ... 2854
Ziac ... 1415
Zinacef (Fewer than 1 in 250 patients) ... 1211
Zinecard (2%) ... 1961
Zocor Tablets (Rare) ... 1775
Zofran Injection (Rare) ... 1214
Zoloft Tablets (Rare) ... 2217
Zovirax ... 1219
Zyloprim Tablets (Less than 1%) ... 1226

Urticaria, hemorrhagic

Methadone Hydrochloride Oral Concentrate ... 2233
Methadone Hydrochloride Oral Solution & Tablets (Rare) ... 2235
RMS Suppositories (Rare) ... 2657
Roxanol (Rare) ... 2243

Urticarial reaction, generalized

Benadryl Capsules ... 1898
Celontin Kapseals ... 1899
Chloromycetin Sodium Succinate ... 1900
Emgel 2% Topical Gel ... 1093
Scleromate ... 1891
T-Stat 2.0% Topical Solution and Pads (One case) ... 2688
Theramycin Z Topical Solution 2% (One case) ... 1592

Uterine contractions, abnormal

Cervidil ... 1010
▲ Prepidil Gel (6.6%) ... 2633

Uterine contractions, altered

Astramorph/PF Injection, USP (Preservative-Free) ... 535
Proventil Inhalation Solution 0.083% ... 2384
Proventil Repetabs Tablets ... 2386
Proventil Solution for Inhalation 0.5% ... 2383
Proventil Syrup ... 2385
Proventil Tablets ... 2386
Talwin Injection ... 2334

Uterine contractions, cessation of

Proglycem ... 580

Uterine contractions, production of

Cytotec ... 2424

Uterine contractions, prolonged

Wigraine Tablets & Suppositories .. 1829

Uterine fibromyomata, increase in size

Betaseron for SC Injection ... 658
Climara Transdermal System ... 645
Diethylstilbestrol Tablets ... 1437
Effexor (Infrequent) ... 2719
Estrace Cream and Tablets ... 749
Estraderm Transdermal System ... 824
ESTRATAB Tablets (0.3, 0.625, 1.25, 2.5 mg) ... 2536
Estratest ... 2539
Menest Tablets ... 2494
Nolvadex Tablets (A few reports) ... 2841
Ogen Tablets ... 2627
Ogen Vaginal Cream ... 2630
Ortho Dienestrol Cream ... 1866
Ortho-Est ... 1869
PMB 200 and PMB 400 ... 2783
Premarin Intravenous ... 2787
Premarin with Methyltestosterone .. 2794
Premarin Tablets ... 2789
Premarin Vaginal Cream ... 2791
Premphase ... 2797
Prempro ... 2801
Serzone Tablets (Rare) ... 771

Uterine hypertonus

Oxytocin Injection ... 2771
Syntocinon Injection ... 2296
Vasoxyl Injection ... 1196

Uterine inertia

Levoprome (Sometimes) ... 1274

Uterine rupture

Oxytocin Injection ... 2771
Prepidil Gel ... 2633
Prostin E2 Suppository ... 2634
Syntocinon Injection ... 2296

Uterine spasm

Effexor (Rare) ... 2719
Oxytocin Injection ... 2771
Prozac Pulvules & Liquid, Oral Solution (Rare) ... 919
Syntocinon Injection ... 2296

Uterotonic effect

Bellergal-S Tablets ... 2250
D.H.E. 45 Injection ... 2255

Uveitis

AK-CIDE ... ⊙ 202
AK-CIDE Ointment ... ⊙ 202
Aredia for Injection (One patient) ... 810
Betaseron for SC Injection ... 658
Blephamide Ointment ... ⊙ 237
Diupres Tablets ... 1650
Econopred & Econopred Plus Ophthalmic Suspensions ... ⊙ 217
FML Forte Liquifilm ... ⊙ 240
FML Liquifilm ... ⊙ 241
FML S.O.P. ... ⊙ 241
Floropryl Sterile Ophthalmic Ointment ... 1662
Healon GV (Rare) ... ⊙ 315
Humorsol Sterile Ophthalmic Solution ... 1664
Hydropres Tablets ... 1675
ISPAN Perfluoropropane ... ⊙ 276
ISPAN Sulfur Hexafluoride ... ⊙ 275
Mycobutin Capsules (Rare) ... 1957
Neurontin Capsules (Rare) ... 1922
Phospholine Iodide ... ⊙ 326
Questran Light ... 769
Questran Powder ... 770
Quinaglute Dura-Tabs Tablets ... 649
Ser-Ap-Es Tablets ... 849
Vasocidin Ointment ... ⊙ 268
Vasocidin Ophthalmic Solution ... ⊙ 270
Vira-A Ophthalmic Ointment, 3% ... ⊙ 312

V

Vagina, dryness

Clomid (Fewer than 1%) ... 1514
Danocrine Capsules ... 2307
Flagyl 375 Capsules ... 2434
Flagyl I.V. ... 2247
Lupron Depot 3.75 mg ... 2556
Massengill ... 2457
Massengill Medicated Disposable Douche ... 2458
Massengill Powder ... 2457
MetroGel-Vaginal ... 902
Nolvadex Tablets (Infrequent) ... 2841
Protostat Tablets ... 1883
Risperdal (Frequent) ... 1301
▲ Supprelin Injection (12%) ... 2056
▲ Synarel Nasal Solution for Endometriosis (19% of patients) ... 2152
Vagistat-1 (Less than 1%) ... 778

Vagina, warm feeling in

Prepidil Gel (1.5%) ... 2633

Vaginal adenosis

Estrace Cream and Tablets ... 749
Ortho-Est ... 1869
Premarin with Methyltestosterone .. 2794
Premarin Tablets ... 2789

Vaginal burning

Conceptrol Contraceptive Gel Single Use Applicators (Occasional) ... ■ 736
Conceptrol Contraceptive Inserts (Occasional) ... ■ 737
Femstat Prefill Vaginal Cream 2% (2.3%) ... 2116
Femstat Vaginal Cream 2% (2.3%) ... 2115
Floxin I.V. (Less than 1%) ... 1571
Floxin Tablets (200 mg, 300 mg, 400 mg) ... 1567
Gynol II Extra Strength Contraceptive Jelly (Occasional) ... ■ 739
Gynol II Original Formula Contraceptive Jelly (Occasional) ... ■ 738
MetroGel-Vaginal (Equal to or less than 2%) ... 902
Monistat Dual-Pak (2%) ... 1850
Monistat 3 Vaginal Suppositories (2%) ... 1850
Mycelex-G 500 mg Vaginal Tablets (1 in 149 patients) ... 609
Ortho-Gynol Contraceptive Jelly (Occasional) ... ■ 740
Semicid Vaginal Contraceptive Inserts ... ■ 874
▲ Terazol 3 Vaginal Cream (5%) ... 1886
▲ Terazol 3 Vaginal Suppositories (15.2% of 284 patients) ... 1886
▲ Terazol 7 Vaginal Cream (5.2% of 521 patients) ... 1887
Today Vaginal Contraceptive Sponge ... ■ 874
▲ Vagistat-1 (Approximately 6%) ... 778

Vaginal candidiasis

Azactam for Injection (Less than 1%) ... 734
Brevicon ... 2088
Cefotan ... 2829
Ceftin (Less than 1% but more than 0.1%) ... 1078
Cipro Tablets ... 592
Climara Transdermal System ... 645
Clozaril Tablets (Less than 1%) ... 2252
Demulen ... 2428
Desogen Tablets ... 1817
Diethylstilbestrol Tablets ... 1437
Estrace Cream and Tablets ... 749
ESTRATAB Tablets (0.3, 0.625, 1.25, 2.5 mg) ... 2536
Estratest ... 2539
Flagyl 375 Capsules ... 2434
Floxin I.V. ... 1571
Floxin Tablets (200 mg, 300 mg, 400 mg) ... 1567
Levlen/Tri-Levlen ... 651
Lo/Ovral Tablets ... 2746
Lo/Ovral-28 Tablets ... 2751
Menest Tablets ... 2494
▲ MetroGel-Vaginal (6.1%) ... 902
Micronor Tablets ... 1872
Modicon ... 1872
Nordette-21 Tablets ... 2755
Nordette-28 Tablets ... 2758
Norinyl ... 2088
Noroxin Tablets ... 1715
Noroxin Tablets ... 2048
Nor-Q D Tablets ... 2135
Ogen Tablets ... 2627
Ogen Vaginal Cream ... 2630
Ortho-Cept ... 1851
Ortho-Cyclen/Ortho-Tri-Cyclen ... 1858
Ortho Dienestrol Cream ... 1866
Ortho-Est ... 1869
Ortho-Novum ... 1872
Ortho-Cyclen/Ortho Tri-Cyclen ... 1858
Ovcon ... 760
Ovral Tablets ... 2770
Ovral-28 Tablets ... 2770
Ovrette Tablets ... 2771
PMB 200 and PMB 400 ... 2783
Premarin with Methyltestosterone .. 2794
Premarin Tablets ... 2789
Premarin Vaginal Cream ... 2791
Premphase ... 2797
Prempro ... 2801
Protostat Tablets ... 1883
Tazidime Vials, Faspak & ADD-Vantage (Less than 1%) ... 1478
Levlen/Tri-Levlen ... 651
Tri-Norinyl ... 2164
Triphasil-21 Tablets ... 2814
Triphasil-28 Tablets ... 2819
▲ Vantin for Oral Suspension and Vantin Tablets (3.1%) ... 2646
Zinacef ... 1211

Vaginal discharge

Ceftin (Less than 1% but more than 0.1%) ... 1078
Depo-Provera Contraceptive Injection ... 2602
Floxin I.V. (1% to 3%) ... 1571
Floxin Tablets (200 mg, 300 mg, 400 mg) (1% to 3%) ... 1567
Keflex Pulvules & Oral Suspension ... 914
Keftab Tablets ... 915
Lupron Depot-PED 7.5 mg, 11.25 mg and 15 mg (2%) ... 2560
Massengill Disposable Douche ... 2457
Massengill Medicated Liquid Concentrate ... ■ 821
Methotrexate Sodium Tablets, Injection, for Injection and LPF Injection (Less common) ... 1275
MetroGel-Vaginal (Equal to or less than 2%) ... 902
▲ Nolvadex Tablets (29.6%) ... 2841
ParaGard T380A Intrauterine Copper Contraceptive ... 1880
ProSom Tablets (Infrequent) ... 449
Rogaine Topical Solution (0.91%) .. 2637
▲ Synarel Nasal Solution for Central Precocious Puberty (3%) ... 2151
Vagistat-1 (Less than 1%) ... 778

Vaginismus

Prostin E2 Suppository ... 2634

Vaginitis

Ambien Tablets (Infrequent) ... 2416
Anafranil Capsules (Up to 2%) ... 803
Ancef Injection ... 2465
Ansaid Tablets (Less than 1%) ... 2579
Augmentin (1%) ... 2468
Azactam for Injection (Less than 1%) ... 734
Brevicon ... 2088
Ceclor Pulvules & Suspension (Less than 1 in 100) ... 1431
Cefizox for Intramuscular or Intravenous Use (Rare) ... 1034
Cefotan ... 2829
Ceftin (Less than 1% but more than 0.1%) ... 1078
Cefzil Tablets and Oral Suspension (1.6%) ... 746
Ceptaz (Fewer than 1%) ... 1081
Cipro I.V. (1% or less) ... 595
Cipro I.V. Pharmacy Bulk Package (Less than 1%) ... 597
Cipro Tablets (Less than 1% to 2%) ... 592
Claforan Sterile and Injection (Less than 1%) ... 1235
Claritin (2% or fewer patients) ... 2349
Claritin-D (Less frequent) ... 2350
▲ Cleocin Vaginal Cream (16%) ... 2589
Danocrine Capsules ... 2307
Demulen ... 2428
▲ Depo-Provera Contraceptive Injection (1% to 5%) ... 2602
Desogen Tablets ... 1817
Dilacor XR Extended-release Capsules (Infrequent) ... 2018

(■ Described in PDR For Nonprescription Drugs) Incidence data in parenthesis; ▲ 3% or more (⊙ Described in PDR For Ophthalmology)

1439 Side Effects Index Vasospasm, unspecified

Duricef 748
Effexor (Frequent) 2719
▲ Floxin I.V. (1% to 5%) 1571
▲ Floxin Tablets (200 mg, 300 mg, 400 mg) (1% to 5%) 1567
Fortaz (Less than 1%) 1100
Geocillin Tablets 2199
Keflex Pulvules & Oral Suspension 914
Keftab Tablets 915
Kefzol Vials, Faspak & ADD-Vantage 1456
▲ Lamictal Tablets (4.1%) 1112
Levlen/Tri-Levlen 651
Lincocin 2617
Lippes Loop Intrauterine Double-S 1848
Lo/Ovral Tablets 2746
Lo/Ovral-28 Tablets 2751
Lorabid Suspension and Pulvules (1.3%) 1459
▲ Lupron Depot 3.75 mg (11.4%) 2556
Lupron Depot-PED 7.5 mg, 11.25 mg and 15 mg (2%) 2560
Luvox Tablets (Infrequent) 2544
Maxaquin Tablets (Less than 1%) 2440
Micronor Tablets 1872
Modicon 1872
Nordette-21 Tablets 2755
Nordette-28 Tablets 2758
Norinyl 2088
▲ Norplant System (5% or greater) 2759
Nor-Q D Tablets 2135
Ortho-Cept 1851
Ortho-Cyclen/Ortho-Tri-Cyclen 1858
Ortho-Novum 1872
Ortho-Cyclen/Ortho Tri-Cyclen 1858
Ovcon 760
Ovral Tablets 2770
Ovral-28 Tablets 2770
Ovrette Tablets 2771
ParaGard T380A Intrauterine Copper Contraceptive 1880
Paxil Tablets (Infrequent) 2505
Penetrex Tablets (Less than 1% but more than or equal to 0.1%) 2031
Permax Tablets (Infrequent) 575
Propulsid (1.2%) 1300
Prostin E2 Suppository 2634
Prozac Pulvules & Liquid, Oral Solution (Infrequent) 919
Rocephin Injectable Vials, ADD-Vantage, Galaxy Container (Occasional) 2142
Rogaine Topical Solution (0.91%) 2637
Sandostatin Injection (Less than 1%) 2292
Serzone Tablets (2%) 771
Solganal Suspension 2388
▲ Supprelin Injection (3% to 10%) 2056
Suprax (Less than 2%) 1399
Tazicef for Injection (Less than 1%) 2519
Tazidime Vials, Faspak & ADD-Vantage (Less than 1%) 1478
Tegison Capsules (Less than 1%) 2154
Levlen/Tri-Levlen 651
Tri-Norinyl 2164
Triphasil-21 Tablets 2814
Triphasil-28 Tablets 2819
Urobiotic-250 Capsules (Rare) 2214
Vantin for Oral Suspension and Vantin Tablets (Less than 1%) 2646
Wellbutrin Tablets (Infrequent) 1204
Zefazone 2654
Zerit Capsules (Up to 2%) 729
Zinacef 1211
Zithromax (1% or less to 1%) 1944
▲ Zoladex (75%) 2858
Zosyn (1.0% or less) 1419
Zosyn Pharmacy Bulk Package (1.0% or less) 1422

Vaginitis, atrophic

Imdur (Less than or equal to 5%) 1323
Zoloft Tablets (Rare) 2217

Varices, esophageal

Myleran Tablets 1143
Thioguanine Tablets, Tabloid Brand 1181

Vascular access, clotting

▲ Epogen for Injection (0.25 to 7%) 489
▲ Procrit for Injection (0.25 to 7%) 1841

Vascular collapse

Brevital Sodium Vials 1429
Quinidex Extentabs 2067

Vascular insufficiency, lower extremities

Sansert Tablets 2295

Vascular complications, unspecified

Metrodin (urofollitropin for injection) 2446
Ortho-Cyclen/Ortho-Tri-Cyclen 1858
Ortho-Cyclen/Ortho Tri-Cyclen 1858
Pergonal (menotropins for injection, USP) 2448
ReoPro Vials (1.8%) 1471
Zofran Tablets 1217

Vascular stenosis

Surgicel 1314
Zyloprim Tablets (Less than 1%) 1226

Vasculitis

Accutane Capsules 2076
Aldoclor Tablets 1598
Aldomet Ester HCl Injection 1602
Aldomet Oral 1600
Aldoril Tablets 1604
Alkeran for Injection 1070
Alkeran Tablets 1071
Altace Capsules (Less than 1%) 1232
Anaprox/Naprosyn (Less than 1%) 2117
Asendin Tablets (Rare) 1369
Atgam Sterile Solution (Less than 5%) 2581
Azo Gantrisin Tablets 2081
Azulfidine (Rare) 1949
Calan SR Caplets (1% or less) 2422
Calan Tablets (1% or less) 2419
Capoten 739
Capozide 742
Chibroxin Sterile Ophthalmic Solution (With oral form) 1617
Cipro I.V. (1% or less) 595
Cipro I.V. Pharmacy Bulk Package (Less than 1%) 597
Cipro Tablets 592
Clozaril Tablets 2252
ColBENEMID Tablets 1622
Combipres Tablets 677
Cordarone Tablets (Rare) 2712
Depen Titratable Tablets (Rare) 2662
DiaBeta Tablets 1239
Diucardin Tablets 2718
Diupres Tablets 1650
Diuril Oral Suspension 1653
Diuril Sodium Intravenous 1652
Diuril Tablets 1653
Dyazide 2479
EC-Naprosyn Delayed-Release Tablets (Less than 1%) 2117
Eminase 2039
Enduron Tablets 420
Feldene Capsules (Less than 1%) 1965
Floxin I.V. (Less than 1%) 1571
Floxin Tablets (200 mg, 300 mg, 400 mg) (Less than 1%) 1567
Glynase PresTab Tablets 2609
HydroDIURIL Tablets 1674
Hydropres Tablets 1675
Hyzaar Tablets 1677
Inderide Tablets 2732
Inderide LA Long Acting Capsules 2734
Inocor Lactate Injection (1 case) 2309
Isoptin Oral Tablets (Less than 1%) 1346
Isoptin SR Tablets (1% or less) 1348
Lasix Injection, Oral Solution and Tablets 1240
Lescol Capsules (Rare) 2267
Lodine Capsules and Tablets (Less than 1%) 2743
Lopid Tablets 1917
Lozol Tablets (Less than 5%) 2022
Maxaquin Tablets 2440
Maxzide 1380
Mevacor Tablets (Rare) 1699
Micronase Tablets 2623
Minizide Capsules 1938
Moduretic Tablets 1705
Monopril Tablets 757
Motrin Tablets (Less than 1%) 2625
Mumpsvax (Rare) 1708
Anaprox/Naprosyn (Less than 1%) 2117
NebuPent for Inhalation Solution (1% or less) 1040
Noroxin Tablets 1715
Noroxin Tablets 2048
Nydrazid Injection 508
Oretic Tablets 443
Orthoclone OKT3 Sterile Solution 1837
PASER Granules 1285
Permax Tablets (Rare) 575
Pravachol (Rare) 765
Prinivil Tablets (0.3% to 1.0%) 1733
Prinzide Tablets 1737
Quinaglute Dura-Tabs Tablets 649
Quinidex Extentabs 2067
Relafen Tablets (1%) 2510
Retrovir Capsules (Rare) 1158
Retrovir I.V. Infusion (Rare) 1163
Retrovir Syrup (Rare) 1158
Rifamate Capsules 1530
Rifater 1532
Ritalin 848
Roferon-A Injection (Rare; less than 3%) 2145
Tenoretic Tablets 2845
Thalitone 1245
Ticlid Tablets (Rare) 2156
Timolide Tablets 1748
Tonocard Tablets (Less than 1%) 531
Vancocin HCl, Oral Solution & Pulvules (Rare) 1483
Vancocin HCl, Vials & ADD-Vantage (Rare) 1481
Vaseretic Tablets 1765
Vasotec I.V. 1768
Vasotec Tablets (0.5% to 1.0%) 1771
Verelan Capsules (1% or less) 1410
Verelan Capsules (Less than 1%) 2824
Zestoretic 2850
Zestril Tablets (0.3% to 1.0%) 2854
Ziac 1415
Zocor Tablets (Rare) 1775
Zyloprim Tablets (Less than 1%) 1226

Vasculitis, allergic

Lodine Capsules and Tablets (Less than 1%) 2743

Vasculitis, cutaneous

Capozide 742
Combipres Tablets 677
Diucardin Tablets 2718
Diupres Tablets 1650
Diuril Oral Suspension 1653
Diuril Sodium Intravenous 1652
Diuril Tablets 1653
Enduron Tablets 420
HydroDIURIL Tablets 1674
Hydropres Tablets 1675
Hyzaar Tablets 1677
Inderide Tablets 2732
Inderide LA Long Acting Capsules 2734
Lodine Capsules and Tablets (Rare) 2743
Maxzide 1380
Minizide Capsules 1938
Moduretic Tablets 1705
Mykrox Tablets 993
Neupogen for Injection (Infrequent) 495
Oretic Tablets 443
Prinzide Tablets 1737
Tenoretic Tablets 2845
Thalitone 1245
Timolide Tablets 1748
Vaseretic Tablets 1765
Zaroxolyn Tablets 1000
Zebeta Tablets 1413
Zestoretic 2850
Ziac 1415

Vasculitis, leukocytoclastic

Cardizem CD Capsules (A number of cases) 1506
Cardizem SR Capsules 1510
Cardizem Injectable 1508
Cardizem Tablets 1512

Vasculitis, periarteritic

Intal Capsules (Less than 1 in 100,000 patients) 987
Intal Inhaler (Rare) 988
Intal Nebulizer Solution (Rare) 989
Nasalcrom Nasal Solution 994

Vasculitis, renal

Cuprimine Capsules (Rare) 1630
Depen Titratable Tablets 2662

Vasoconstriction

Cocaine Hydrochloride Topical Solution 537
Survanta Beractant Intratracheal Suspension (Less than 1%) 2226

Vasodilation

Accupril Tablets (0.5% to 1.0%) 1893
Ansaid Tablets (Less than 1%) 2579
Asacol Delayed-Release Tablets 1979
Betapace Tablets (1% to 3%) 641
Cardene I.V. (0.7%) 2709
▲ Cardene SR Capsules (4.7%) 2097
Cardizem Injectable (1.7%) 1508
Cartrol Tablets (Less common) 410
Caverject (Less than 1%) 2583
Ceclor Pulvules & Suspension 1431
▲ CellCept Capsules (More than or equal to 3%) 2099
Cytovene (1% or less) 2103
DDAVP 2017
Depakote Tablets (Greater than 1% but not more than 5%) 415
Desmopressin Acetate Rhinal Tube 979
Desyrel and Desyrel Dividose 503
Dilacor XR Extended-release Capsules 2018
Dilatrate-SR 2398
Ditropan 1516
▲ Effexor (2.3% to 5.6%) 2719
Ethmozine Tablets (Less than 2%) 2041
Flexeril Tablets (Less than 1%) 1661
Floxin I.V. (Less than 1%) 1571
Floxin Tablets (200 mg, 300 mg, 400 mg) (Less than 1%) 1567
Hyperstat I.V. Injection 2363
Hytrin Capsules (At least 1%) 430
Imitrex Injection (Rare) 1103
Imitrex Tablets (Rare) 1106
Lamictal Tablets (Infrequent) 1112
Lorabid Suspension and Pulvules 1459
Lotrel Capsules 840
Lupron Depot-PED 7.5 mg, 11.25 mg and 15 mg (Less than 2%) 2560
▲ Luvox Tablets (3%) 2544
Marcaine Spinal 2319
Marinol (Dronabinol) Capsules (Greater than 1%) 2231
NebuPent for Inhalation Solution (1% or less) 1040
Neurontin Capsules (1.1%) 1922
Novocain Hydrochloride for Spinal Anesthesia 2326
Orudis Capsules (Less than 1%) 2766
Oruvail Capsules (Less than 1%) 2766
Paxil Tablets (2.6%) 2505
Penetrex Tablets (Less than 1% but more than or equal to 0.1%) 2031
Pentasa (Less than 1%) 1527
▲ Permax Tablets (3.2%) 575
PREVACID Delayed-Release Capsules (Less than 1%) 2562
▲ Prozac Pulvules & Liquid, Oral Solution (At least 5%) 919
Retrovir Capsules 1158
Retrovir I.V. Infusion 1163
Retrovir Syrup 1158
Revex (1%) 1811
▲ Serzone Tablets (4%) 771
Sorbitrate 2843
▲ Stadol (3% to 9%) 775
▲ Supprelin Injection (35%) 2056
Suprane (Less than 1%) 1813
Timolide Tablets 1748
Timoptic in Ocudose 1753
Timoptic Sterile Ophthalmic Solution 1751
Timoptic-XE 1755
Tracrium Injection 1183
Ultram Tablets (50 mg) (1% to 5%) 1585
Vascor (200, 300 and 400 mg) Tablets (0.5 to 2.0%) 1587
▲ Videx Tablets, Powder for Oral Solution, & Pediatric Powder for Oral Solution (22%) 720
Zerit Capsules (Fewer than 1% to 3%) 729
Zyloprim Tablets (Less than 1%) 1226

Vasodilation, peripheral

Persantine Tablets 681

Vasomotor disturbances

Aminohippurate Sodium Injection 1606
Ceredase 1065
Duvoid (Infrequent) 2044
Paremyd ◉ 247
Xanax Tablets (2.0%) 2649

Vasomotor flushes

▲ Clomid (10.4%) 1514
▲ Serophene (clomiphene citrate tablets, USP) (Approximately 1 in 10 patients) 2451

Vasospasm, digital

▲ Parlodel (3%) 2281

Vasospasm, rebound

Nimotop Capsules (Less than 1%) 610

Vasospasm, unspecified

Anafranil Capsules (Rare) 803
Betaseron for SC Injection 658
D.H.E. 45 Injection (Occasional) 2255

(▭ Described in PDR For Nonprescription Drugs) Incidence data in parenthesis; ▲ 3% or more (◉ Described in PDR For Ophthalmology)

Vasovagal episode Side Effects Index 1440

Vasovagal episode
Caverject (Less than 1%) 2583
IOPIDINE Sterile Ophthalmic Solution ◉ 219
Parlodel (Less than 1%) 2281
Tonocard Tablets (Less than 1%) 531
Versed Injection (Less than 1%) 2170

Vein, pigmentation of
Fluorouracil Injection 2116

Veins, varicosis
Ambien Tablets (Rare) 2416
Betaseron for SC Injection 658
Depo-Provera Contraceptive Injection (Fewer than 1%) 2602
Effexor (Rare) 2719
Imdur (Less than or equal to 5%) 1323
Paxil Tablets (Rare) 2505
Permax Tablets (Infrequent) 575
Serzone Tablets (Rare) 771
Zoloft Tablets (Rare) 2217

Venous infection at injection site
Primaxin I.V. (0.1%) 1729

Venous thrombophlebitis
Metrodin (urofollitropin for injection) 2446

Ventilator dependence
Virazole 1264

Ventricular arrhythmias
Adalat Capsules (10 mg and 20 mg) (Fewer than 0.5%) 587
Adenoscan (Less than 1%) 1024
Anectine (Rare) 1073
▲Betapace Tablets (4.3% of 3,257 patients) 641
Biaxin (Rare) 405
Carbocaine Hydrochloride Injection 2303
Cardizem Injectable (Less than 1%) 1508
Diethylstilbestrol Tablets 1437
EpiPen—Epinephrine Auto-Injector 790
Foscavir Injection (Rare) 547
Hismanal Tablets 1293
Hyperstat I.V. Injection 2363
Ilosone (Rare) 911
Ilotycin Gluceptate, IV, Vials (Rare) 913
Isuprel Hydrochloride Injection 1:5000 2311
Lanoxicaps (Less common) 1117
Lanoxin Elixir Pediatric (Less common) 1120
Lanoxin Injection 1123
Lanoxin Injection Pediatric (Less common) 1126
Lanoxin Tablets (Less common) 1128
Lufyllin-GG Elixir & Tablets 2671
Marcaine Hydrochloride with Epinephrine 1:200,000 2316
Marcaine Hydrochloride Injection 2316
Marcaine Spinal 2319
Mexitil Capsules (1.0% to 1.9%) 678
Nescaine/Nescaine MPF 554
Normodyne Injection (1%) 2377
▲Primacor Injection (12.1%) 2331
Procardia Capsules (fewer than 0.5%) 1971
Procardia XL Extended Release Tablets (Fewer than 0.5%) 1972
▲Proleukin for Injection (3%) 797
Propulsid (Rare) 1300
Prozac Pulvules & Liquid, Oral Solution (Rare) 919
Quadrinal Tablets 1350
Quibron 2053
ReoPro Vials (0.3%) 1471
Respbid Tablets 682
Seldane Tablets (Rare) 1536
Seldane-D Extended-Release Tablets (Rare) 1538
Sensorcaine 559
Slo-bid Gyrocaps 2033
▲Tambocor Tablets (7% to 13%) 1497
Theo-24 Extended Release Capsules 2568
Theo-Dur Extended-Release Tablets 1327
Theo-X Extended-Release Tablets 788
▲Tonocard Tablets (10.9%) 531
Trandate Injection (1 of 100 patients) 1185
Uni-Dur Extended-Release Tablets 1331
Uniphyl 400 mg Tablets 2001

Ventricular arrhythmias, post-abrupt discontinuation
Tenormin Tablets and I.V. Injection 2847

Ventricular bigeminy
Azactam for Injection (Less than 1%) 734

Ventricular contractions
Sodium Polystyrene Sulfonate Suspension 2244
Versed Injection (Less than 1%) 2170
Yutopar Intravenous Injection 570

Ventricular contractions, premature
Adenocard Injection 1021
Azactam for Injection (Less than 1%) 734
Brethaire Inhaler 813
Cataflam (Less than 1%) 816
Clozaril Tablets (Less than 1%) 2252
Diupres Tablets 1650
▲Dobutrex Solution Vials (Approximately 5%) 1439
Emete-con Intramuscular/Intravenous 2198
Hydropres Tablets 1675
Ismo Tablets (Fewer than 1%) 2738
▲Lanoxin Injection (Most common) 1123
Lanoxin Injection Pediatric (Common) 1126
Lozol Tablets (Less than 5%) 2022
Norpramin Tablets 1526
Oxytocin Injection 2771
▲Proleukin for Injection (5%) 797
Syntocinon Injection 2296
▲Tonocard Tablets (10.9%) 531
Tornalate Solution for Inhalation, 0.2% (Less than 1%) 956
Tornalate Metered Dose Inhaler (Rare; 0.5%) 957
Vascor (200, 300 and 400 mg) Tablets (0.5 to 2.0%) 1587
Voltaren Tablets (Less than 1%) 861
Zantac (Rare) 1209
Zantac Injection (Rare) 1207
Zantac Syrup (Rare) 1209

Ventricular contractions, premature, multifocal
Lanoxicaps 1117
Lanoxin Elixir Pediatric (Less common) 1120
Lanoxin Injection 1123
Lanoxin Injection Pediatric 1126
▲Lanoxin Tablets (Among most common) 1128

Ventricular contractions, premature, unifocal
Lanoxicaps 1117
Lanoxin Elixir Pediatric (Less common) 1120
Lanoxin Injection 1123
Lanoxin Injection Pediatric 1126
▲Lanoxin Tablets (Among most common) 1128

Ventricular dilation, left-side
Retrovir Capsules (0.8%) 1158
Retrovir I.V. Infusion (1%) 1163
Retrovir Syrup (0.8%) 1158

Ventricular ectopic beats
Cipro Tablets (Less than 1%) 592
Desyrel and Desyrel Dividose 503
Digibind 1091
Dobutrex Solution Vials 1439
Hivid Tablets (Less than 1% to less than 3%) 2121
Kytril Injection (Rare) 2490
▲Primacor Injection (8.5%) 2331
Quinaglute Dura-Tabs Tablets 649
Vasoxyl Injection 1196

Ventricular extrasystoles
Betaseron for SC Injection 658
Cardene Capsules (Rare) 2095
Cardene I.V. (1.4%) 2709
Cardizem CD Capsules (Less than 1%) 1506
Cardizem SR Capsules (Less than 1%) 1510
Cardizem Injectable 1508
Cardizem Tablets (Less than 1%) 1512
Claritin-D (Less frequent) 2350
Dilacor XR Extended-release Capsules 2018
Lotrel Capsules (Infrequent) 840
Neurontin Capsules (Rare) 1922
Paxil Tablets (Rare) 2505
Permax Tablets (Infrequent) 575
Risperdal (Rare) 1301
Romazicon (Less than 1%) 2147
Serzone Tablets (Infrequent) 771
▲Trasylol (5%) 613

Ventricular failure
Doxorubicin Astra (Uncommon) 540
Tonocard Tablets (0.0-1.4%) 531

Ventricular fibrillation (see under Fibrillations, ventricular)

Ventricular flutter
Quinidex Extentabs 2067

Ventricular gallop
Retrovir Capsules (0.8%) 1158
Retrovir I.V. Infusion (1%) 1163
Retrovir Syrup (0.8%) 1158

Ventricular irregularities
▲Calan SR Caplets (15%) 2422
▲Calan Tablets (15%) 2419
Cerubidine 795
Eminase 2039
Isoptin Injectable 1344
Isoptin Oral Tablets (Greater than 1%) 1346
Verelan Capsules (1% or less) 1410
Verelan Capsules (Less than 1%) 2824

Ventricular irritation
Tenoretic Tablets 2845
Timolide Tablets 1748
Vaseretic Tablets 1765
Zestoretic 2850

Ventricular response, rapid
Calan SR Caplets 2422
Calan Tablets 2419
Verelan Capsules 1410
Verelan Capsules 2824

Venus sequelae
Diprivan Injection (Rare; less than 1%) 2833

Verruca
Foscavir Injection (Less than 1%) 547
Risperdal (Rare) 1301

Vertebral compression fractures
Aristocort Tablets 1022
Cortone Acetate Sterile Suspension 1623
Cortone Acetate Tablets 1624
Decadron Elixir 1633
Decadron Phosphate Injection 1637
Decadron Phosphate Respihaler 1642
Decadron Phosphate Turbinaire 1645
Decadron Phosphate with Xylocaine Injection, Sterile 1639
Deltasone Tablets 2595
Depo-Medrol Single-Dose Vial 2600
Depo-Medrol Sterile Aqueous Suspension 2597
Dexacort Phosphate in Respihaler 458
Dexacort Phosphate in Turbinaire 459
Florinef Acetate Tablets 505
Medrol 2621
Pediapred Oral Liquid 995
Solu-Cortef Sterile Powder 2641
Solu-Medrol Sterile Powder 2643

Vertical deviation
▲BOTOX (Botulinum Toxin Type A) Purified Neurotoxin Complex (2.1% to 16.9%) 477

Vertigo
Accupril Tablets (0.5% to 1.0%) 1893
Actifed with Codeine Cough Syrup 1067
Adalat CC (3% or less) 589
AeroBid Inhaler System (1-3%) 1005
Aerobid-M Inhaler System (1-3%) 1005
Aldactazide 2413
Aldoclor Tablets 1598
Aldoril Tablets 1604
Altace Capsules (Less than 1% to 1.5%) 1232
Ambien Tablets (Frequent) 2416
Anafranil Capsules (Frequent) 803
Anaprox/Naprosyn (Less than 3%) 2117
Ancobon Capsules 2079
Apresazide Capsules 808
Aristocort Suspension (Forte Parenteral) 1027
Aristocort Suspension (Intralesional) 1025
Aristocort Tablets 1022
Aristospan Suspension (Intra-articular) 1033
Aristospan Suspension (Intralesional) 1032
Asacol Delayed-Release Tablets 1979
Azactam for Injection (Less than 1%) 734
Azo Gantanol Tablets 2080
Azo Gantrisin Tablets 2081
Azulfidine (Rare) 1949
Bactrim DS Tablets 2084
Bactrim I.V. Infusion 2082
Bactrim 2084
Benadryl Capsules 1898
Benadryl Injection 1898
Betapace Tablets (Rare) 641
Betoptic Ophthalmic Solution (Rare) 469
Betoptic S Ophthalmic Suspension (Rare) 471
Blocadren Tablets (0.6%) 1614
Brethaire Inhaler 813
Bumex (0.1%) 2093
▲Buprenex Injectable (5-10%) 2006
Cafergot 2251
Capastat Sulfate Vials 2868
Capozide 742
Carafate Suspension (Less than 0.5%) 1505
Carafate Tablets (Less than 0.5%) 1504
Cardene Capsules (Rare) 2095
▲Cardura Tablets (2% to 23%) 2186
Celestone Soluspan Suspension 2347
Claritin (2% or fewer patients) 2349
Claritin-D (Less frequent) 2350
Cleocin Vaginal Cream (Less than 1%) 2589
Clinoril Tablets (Less than 1 in 100) 1618
Clomid (Fewer than 1%) 1514
▲Clozaril Tablets (More than 5 to 19%) 2252
Cognex Capsules (Frequent) 1901
Coly-Mycin M Parenteral 1905
Combipres Tablets 677
CORTENEMA 2535
Cortone Acetate Sterile Suspension 1623
Cortone Acetate Tablets 1624
Cozaar Tablets (Less than 1%) 1628
Dalalone D.P. Injectable 1011
Dalgan Injection (1 to less than 3%) 538
Dapsone Tablets USP 1284
Decadron Elixir 1633
Decadron Phosphate Injection 1637
Decadron Phosphate Respihaler 1642
Decadron Phosphate Turbinaire 1645
Decadron Phosphate with Xylocaine Injection, Sterile 1639
Decadron Tablets 1635
Decadron-LA Sterile Suspension 1646
Deconamine 1320
Deltasone Tablets 2595
Depakote Tablets (Greater than 1% but not more than 5%) 415
Depo-Medrol Single-Dose Vial 2600
Depo-Medrol Sterile Aqueous Suspension 2597
Desyrel and Desyrel Dividose 503
Dexacort Phosphate in Respihaler 458
Dexacort Phosphate in Turbinaire 459
Dilacor XR Extended-release Capsules (Infrequent) 2018
Dipentum Capsules (1.0%) 1951
Diucardin Tablets 2718
Diupres Tablets 1650
Diuril Oral Suspension 1653
Diuril Sodium Intravenous 1652
Diuril Tablets 1653
Dizac (Less frequent) 1809
Dolobid Tablets (Less than 1 in 100) 1654
Duragesic Transdermal System (Less than 1%) 1288
Dyazide 2479
Dynacin Capsules 1590
E.E.S. (Isolated reports) 424
Easprin 1914
EC-Naprosyn Delayed-Release Tablets (Less than 3%) 2117
Edecrin 1657
Effexor (Frequent) 2719
Eldepryl Tablets 2550
▲Eminase (Less than 10%) 2039
Enduron Tablets 420
Engerix-B Unit-Dose Vials 2482
EryPed (Isolated reports) 421
Ery-Tab Tablets (Isolated reports) 422
Erythrocin Stearate Filmtab (Isolated reports) 425

(▣ Described in PDR For Nonprescription Drugs) Incidence data in parenthesis; ▲ 3% or more (◉ Described in PDR For Ophthalmology)

1441 Side Effects Index Vision, loss of color

Erythromycin Base Filmtab (Isolated reports) 426
Erythromycin Delayed-Release Capsules, USP (Isolated reports) 427
Esidrix Tablets 821
Esimil Tablets 822
Eskalith 2485
Ethmozine Tablets (Less than 2%) 2041
Fansidar Tablets 2114
Feldene Capsules (Greater than 1%) 1965
Fioricet with Codeine Capsules 2260
Fiorinal with Codeine Capsules 2262
Flagyl 375 Capsules 2434
Flagyl I.V. 2247
Flexeril Tablets (Less than 1%) 1661
Florinef Acetate Tablets 505
Floxin I.V. (Less than 1%) 1571
Floxin Tablets (200 mg, 300 mg, 400 mg) (Less than 1%) 1567
Foscavir Injection (Less than 1%) 547
Fungizone Intravenous 506
Gantanol Tablets 2119
Gantrisin 2120
Garamycin Injectable 2360
Glucotrol XL Extended Release Tablets (Less than 1%) 1968
Haldol Decanoate 1577
Haldol Injection, Tablets and Concentrate 1575
Havrix (Less than 1%) 2489
Hexalen Capsules 2571
Hivid Tablets (Less than 1% to less than 3%) 2121
Hydeltrasol Injection, Sterile 1665
Hydeltra-T.B.A. Sterile Suspension 1667
Hydrocortone Acetate Sterile Suspension 1669
Hydrocortone Phosphate Injection, Sterile 1670
Hydrocortone Tablets 1672
HydroDIURIL Tablets 1674
Hydropres Tablets 1675
▲Hytrin Capsules (0.5% to 1.4%; 21%) 430
Hyzaar Tablets 1677
Imdur (Less than or equal to 5%) 1323
▲Imitrex Injection (11.9%) 1103
Imitrex Tablets 1106
Inderide Tablets 2732
Inderide LA Long Acting Capsules 2734
Indocin (Greater than 1%) 1680
Intal Capsules (Less than 1 in 100,000 patients) 987
Intal Inhaler (Rare) 988
Intal Nebulizer Solution (Rare) 989
Intron A (Less than 5%) 2364
ISMOTIC 45% w/v Solution (Very rare) ◉ 222
Isoptin Injectable 1344
Klonopin Tablets 2126
Lamictal Tablets (1.1%) 1112
Lariam Tablets 2128
Lasix Injection, Oral Solution and Tablets 1240
Lescol Capsules 2267
Lincocin (Occasional) 2617
Lioresal Intrathecal 1596
Lithium Carbonate Capsules & Tablets 2230
Lithonate/Lithotabs/Lithobid 2543
Lopid Tablets (1.5%) 1917
Lopressor Ampuls 830
▲Lopressor HCT Tablets (10 in 100 patients) 832
Lopressor Tablets 830
Lotensin HCT 837
Lozol Tablets (Less than 5%) 2022
Luvox Tablets (Infrequent) 2544
▲Lysodren (15%) 698
Macrobid Capsules 1988
Macrodantin Capsules 1989
Marax Tablets & DF Syrup 2200
Maxaquin Tablets (Less than 1%) 2440
Maxzide 1380
Medrol 2621
MetroGel-Vaginal 902
Mevacor Tablets (0.5% to 1.0%) 1699
Miacalcin Nasal Spray (Less than 1%) 2275
Midamor Tablets (Less than or equal to 1%) 1703
Miltown Tablets 2672
Minipress Capsules (1-4%) 1937
Minizide Capsules 1938
Minocin Intravenous 1382
Minocin Oral Suspension 1385
Minocin Pellet-Filled Capsules 1383
Moduretic Tablets (Less than or equal to 1%) 1705
Mono-Gesic Tablets 792
Monoket (Fewer than 1%) 2406
Monopril Tablets (0.2% to 1.0%) 757
Mustargen (Infrequent) 1709
▲Mysoline (Among most frequent) 2754
Anaprox/Naprosyn (Less than 3%) 2117
Nebcin Vials, Hyporets & ADD-Vantage 1464
NebuPent for Inhalation Solution (1% or less) 1040
NegGram 2323
Netromycin Injection 100 mg/ml 2373
Neurontin Capsules (Frequent) 1922
Nitrostat Tablets (Occasional) 1925
Normodyne Injection (1%) 2377
Normodyne Tablets (2%) 2379
Norvasc Tablets (More than 0.1% to 1%) 1940
▲Nubain Injection (5%) 935
Oretic Tablets 443
Ornade Spansule Capsules 2502
Orthoclone OKT3 Sterile Solution 1837
Orudis Capsules (Less than 1%) 2766
Oruvail Capsules (Less than 1%) 2766
PBZ Tablets 845
PBZ-SR Tablets 844
PMB 200 and PMB 400 2783
Papaverine Hydrochloride Vials and Ampoules 1468
Parlodel (Less than 1%) 2281
Paxil Tablets (Frequent) 2505
Pediapred Oral Liquid 995
▲Penetrex Tablets (3%) 2031
Periactin 1724
Permax Tablets (Infrequent) 575
Phenobarbital Elixir and Tablets 1469
Plaquenil Sulfate Tablets 2328
Pravachol 765
Prelone Syrup 1787
Prilosec Delayed-Release Capsules (Less than 1%) 529
Primaxin I.M. 1727
Primaxin I.V. (Less than 0.2%) 1729
Prinivil Tablets (0.2%) 1733
Prinzide Tablets (0.3% to 1%) 1737
Procardia XL Extended Release Tablets (1% or less) 1972
Protostat Tablets 1883
Proventil Inhalation Aerosol 2382
Proventil Repetabs Tablets 2386
Proventil Syrup 2385
Proventil Tablets 2386
Prozac Pulvules & Liquid, Oral Solution (Infrequent) 919
Questran Light 769
Questran Powder 770
Quinaglute Dura-Tabs Tablets 649
Quinidex Extentabs 2067
Relafen Tablets (1%) 2510
Retrovir Capsules 1158
Retrovir I.V. Infusion 1163
Retrovir Syrup 1158
Rifater 1532
Risperdal (Infrequent) 1301
Robaxin Injectable 2070
Roferon-A Injection (Less than 3%) 2145
Rogaine Topical Solution (1.17%) 2637
▲Romazicon (10%) 2147
Rythmol Tablets–150mg, 225mg, 300mg (Less than 1%) 1352
Salflex Tablets 786
Sandostatin Injection (Less than 1%) 2292
Septra 1174
Septra I.V. Infusion 1169
Septra I.V. Infusion ADD-Vantage Vials 1171
Septra 1174
Ser-Ap-Es Tablets 849
Serax Capsules (In few instances) 2810
Serax Tablets (In few instances) 2810
Seromycin Pulvules 1476
Serzone Tablets (Infrequent) 771
Solu-Cortef Sterile Powder 2641
Solu-Medrol Sterile Powder 2643
Soma Compound w/Codeine Tablets 2676
Soma Compound Tablets (Less frequent) 2675
Soma Tablets 2674
Tambocor Tablets (1% to less than 3%) 1497
Tapazole Tablets 1477
Tavist Syrup 2297
Tavist Tablets 2298
Tenex Tablets (Less frequent) 2074
Tenoretic Tablets (2%) 2845
Tenormin Tablets and I.V. Injection (2%) 2847
Thalitone 1245
Timolide Tablets 1748
Timoptic in Ocudose 1753
Timoptic Sterile Ophthalmic Solution 1751
Timoptic-XE 1755
Tobramycin Sulfate Injection 968
▲Tonocard Tablets (8.0-25.3%) 531
Toradol (1% or less) 2159
Tornalate Solution for Inhalation, 0.2% (Less than 1%) 956
Trandate (1 of 100 patients) 1185
Trinalin Repetabs Tablets 1330
Tussend 1783
▲Ultram Tablets (50 mg) (26% to 33%) 1585
Urispas Tablets 2532
Valium Injectable 2182
Valium Tablets (Infrequent) 2183
Valrelease Capsules (Occasional) 2169
Vancocin HCl, Oral Solution & Pulvules (Rare) 1483
Vancocin HCl, Vials & ADD-Vantage (Rare) 1481
Vascor (200, 300 and 400 mg) Tablets (0.5 to 2.0%) 1587
Vaseretic Tablets (0.5% to 2.0%) 1765
Vasotec I.V. 1768
Vasotec Tablets (1.6%) 1771
Ventolin Rotacaps for Inhalation 1200
Ventolin Syrup 1202
Ventolin Tablets 1203
Volmax Extended-Release Tablets 1788
Wellbutrin Tablets (Infrequent) 1204
Yodoxin 1230
Zantac (Rare) 1209
Zantac Injection 1207
Zantac Syrup (Rare) 1209
Zaroxolyn Tablets 1000
Zebeta Tablets 1413
Zestoretic (0.3 to 1%) 2850
Zestril Tablets (0.2% to 1.1%) 2854
Ziac 1415
Zithromax (1% or less) 1944
Zocor Tablets 1775
Zoloft Tablets (Infrequent) 2217
Zosyn (1.0% or less) 1419
Zosyn Pharmacy Bulk Package (1.0% or less) 1422
Zyloprim Tablets (Less than 1%) 1226

Vesical spasm
Dilaudid Ampules 1335
Dilaudid Cough Syrup 1336
Dilaudid 1335
Hycodan Tablets and Syrup 930
Hycomine Compound Tablets 932
Hycomine 931
Hycotuss Expectorant Syrup 933
Hydrocet Capsules 782
Vicodin Tablets 1356

Vesiculation
Adriamycin PFS 1947
Adriamycin RDF 1947
Attenuvax 1610
▲Blenoxane (50%) 692
▲Catapres-TTS (7 of 101 patients) 675
Cipro I.V. (1% or less) 595
Condylox (Less than 5%) 1802
M-M-R II 1687
M-R-VAX II 1689
8-MOP Capsules 1246
MSTA Mumps Skin Test Antigen 890
Oxsoralen-Ultra Capsules 1257
PPD Tine Test 2874
Rubex 712
Topicort LP Emollient Cream 0.05% (0.8%) 1243
T.R.U.E. Test (Two to 27 reports) 1189
Tuberculin, Old, Tine Test 2875
Tubersol (Tuberculin Purified Protein Derivative [Mantoux]) 2872
Tympagesic Ear Drops 2342
Ultram Tablets (50 mg) (Less than 1%) 1585
Ultravate Cream 0.05% (Less frequent) 2689
Velban Vials 1484

Vesiculobullous reaction
Children's Advil Suspension (Less than 1%) 2692
Feldene Capsules (Less than 1%; occasional) 1965
Floxin I.V. 1571
Floxin Tablets (200 mg, 300 mg, 400 mg) 1567
Children's Motrin Ibuprofen Oral Suspension (Less than 1%) 1546
Motrin Tablets (Less than 1%) 2625
Motrin Ibuprofen Suspension, Oral Drops, Chewable Tablets, Caplets (Less than 1%) 1546

Vestibular dysfunction
Anafranil Capsules (Up to 2%) 803
Cipro I.V. Pharmacy Bulk Package (Less than 1%) 597
Platinol 708
Platinol-AQ Injection 710
Streptomycin Sulfate Injection 2208

Vibratory sensation, loss of
Platinol 708
Platinol-AQ Injection 710

Virilization
▲Android Capsules, 10 mg (Among most common) 1250
▲Android (Among most common) 1251
▲Delatestryl Injection (One of most common) 2860
▲Estratest (Among most common) 2539
Halotestin Tablets 2614
Intron A (Less than 5%) 2364
▲Oreton Methyl (Among most common) 1255
Oxandrin 2862
Premarin with Methyltestosterone (Among most common) 2794
Testoderm Testosterone Transdermal System 486
Testred Capsules 1262
Winstrol Tablets 2337

Virilization, female fetus
Amen Tablets 780
▲Android Capsules, 10 mg (Among most common) 1250
Android 1251
Cycrin Tablets 975
Depo-Provera Sterile Aqueous Suspension 2606
Megace Tablets 701
▲Oreton Methyl (Among most common) 1255
Testred Capsules 1262

Vision, blurred
(see under Blurred vision)

Vision, changes
(see under Visual disturbances)

Vision, complete loss
Amen Tablets 780
Brevicon 2088
Cycrin Tablets 975
Demulen 2428
Depo-Provera Contraceptive Injection 2602
Depo-Provera Sterile Aqueous Suspension 2606
Levlen/Tri-Levlen 651
Micronor Tablets 1872
Modicon 1872
Norinyl 2088
Nor-Q D Tablets 2135
Ortho-Cyclen/Ortho-Tri-Cyclen 1858
Ortho-Novum 1872
Ortho-Cyclen/Ortho Tri-Cyclen 1858
Ovcon 760
Plaquenil Sulfate Tablets (One case) 2328
Premphase 2797
Prempro 2801
Provera Tablets 2636
Levlen/Tri-Levlen 651
Tri-Norinyl 2164

Vision, double
(see under Diplopia)

Vision, loss of
Cognex Capsules (Rare) 1901
Paraplatin for Injection 705
Prinivil Tablets (0.3% to 1.0%) 1733
Prinzide Tablets 1737
Zestoretic 2850
Zestril Tablets (0.3% to 1.0%) 2854

Vision, loss of color
Cipro I.V. (1% or less) 595
Cipro Tablets (Less than 1%) 592
Mellaril 2269
Motrin Ibuprofen Suspension, Oral Drops, Chewable Tablets, Caplets 1546
Ponstel (Rare) 1925

(▣ Described in PDR For Nonprescription Drugs) Incidence data in parenthesis; ▲ 3% or more (◉ Described in PDR For Ophthalmology)

Vision, obscured by enlarged iris cysts — Side Effects Index — 1442

Vision, obscured by enlarged iris cysts

Floropryl Sterile Ophthalmic Ointment 1662
Humorsol Sterile Ophthalmic Solution 1664

Vision, partial loss

Amen Tablets 780
Brevicon 2088
Cycrin Tablets 975
Demulen 2428
Depo-Provera Contraceptive Injection 2602
Depo-Provera Sterile Aqueous Suspension 2606
IBU Tablets (Less than 1%) 1342
Levlen/Tri-Levlen 651
Micronor Tablets 1872
Modicon 1872
Motrin Ibuprofen Suspension, Oral Drops, Chewable Tablets, Caplets (Less than 1%) 1546
Norinyl 2088
Nor-Q D Tablets 2135
Ortho-Cyclen/Ortho-Tri-Cyclen 1858
Ortho-Novum 1872
Ortho-Cyclen/Ortho Tri-Cyclen 1858
Ovcon 760
Premphase 2797
Prempro 2801
Provera Tablets 2636
Levlen/Tri-Levlen 651
Tri-Norinyl 2164

Vision, temporary loss

Clomid 1514
Soma Compound w/Codeine Tablets 2676
Soma Compound Tablets (Very rare) 2675
Soma Tablets 2674

Vision, tunnel

BuSpar (Rare) 737
Serophene (clomiphene citrate tablets, USP) 2451

Visual acuity, defects

AK-CIDE ..... ◉ 202
AK-CIDE Ointment ..... ◉ 202
AK-Pred ..... ◉ 204
AK-Trol Ointment & Suspension ..... ◉ 205
Betoptic Ophthalmic Solution 469
Betoptic S Ophthalmic Suspension (Small number of patients) 471
Blephamide Liquifilm Sterile Ophthalmic Suspension 476
Blephamide Ointment ..... ◉ 237
Cipro I.V. (1% or less) 595
Cipro I.V. Pharmacy Bulk Package (Less than 1%) 597
Cipro Tablets (Less than 1%) 592
Cortisporin Ophthalmic Ointment Sterile 1085
Cortisporin Ophthalmic Suspension Sterile 1086
Cozaar Tablets (Less than 1%) 1628
Dexacidin Ointment ..... ◉ 263
FML Forte Liquifilm ..... ◉ 240
FML Liquifilm ..... ◉ 241
FML S.O.P. ..... ◉ 241
FML-S Liquifilm ..... ◉ 242
Flarex Ophthalmic Suspension ..... ◉ 218
Fluor-Op Ophthalmic Suspension ..... ◉ 264
HMS Liquifilm ..... ◉ 244
Hyzaar Tablets 1677
Inflamase ..... ◉ 265
Intron A 2364
Isopto Carbachol Ophthalmic Solution ..... ◉ 223
Isopto Carpine Ophthalmic Solution (Frequent) ..... ◉ 223
Maxitrol Ophthalmic Ointment and Suspension ..... ◉ 224
Mellaril 2269
Myambutol Tablets 1386
Pilocar ..... ◉ 268
Pilopine HS Ophthalmic Gel ..... ◉ 226
Plaquenil Sulfate Tablets 2328
Pred-G Liquifilm Sterile Ophthalmic Suspension ..... ◉ 251
Pred-G S.O.P. Sterile Ophthalmic Ointment ..... ◉ 252
Rogaine Topical Solution 2637
Serophene (clomiphene citrate tablets, USP) 2451
Symmetrel Capsules and Syrup (0.1% to 1%) 946
TobraDex Ophthalmic Suspension and Ointment 473
Vasocidin Ointment ..... ◉ 268
Vasocidin Ophthalmic Solution ..... ◉ 270
Vexol 1% Ophthalmic Suspension ..... ◉ 230

Vision abnormalities (see under Visual disturbances)

Visual disturbances

Accutane Capsules 2076
Achromycin V Capsules 1367
Adalat CC (Less than 1.0%) 589
Adsorbotear Artificial Tear ..... ◉ 210
Children's Advil Suspension (Less than 1%) 2692
AK-Pred ..... ◉ 204
AK-Trol Ointment & Suspension ..... ◉ 205
Altace Capsules (Less than 1%) 1232
Ambien Tablets (Frequent) 2416
▲ Anafranil Capsules (7% to 18%) 803
Anaprox/Naprosyn (Less than 3%) 2117
Ansaid Tablets (1-3%) 2579
AquaSite Eye Drops ..... ◉ 261
Aralen Hydrochloride Injection 2301
Aralen Phosphate Tablets 2301
Aredia for Injection (Up to 2%) 810
Atrohist Plus Tablets 454
Betagan ..... ◉ 233
▲ Betapace Tablets (1% to 5%) 641
▲ Betaseron for SC Injection (7%) 658
Betimol 0.25%, 0.5% (1% to 5%) ..... ◉ 261
Blephamide Liquifilm Sterile Ophthalmic Suspension 476
Blocadren Tablets 1614
Brevibloc Injection (Less than 1%) 1808
Brevicon (Rare) 2088
▲ Bromfed-DM Cough Syrup (Among most frequent) 1786
Brontex 1981
Buprenex Injectable (Less than 1%) 2006
Cardene Capsules (Rare) 2095
Cardura Tablets (1.4% to 2%) 2186
Cipro I.V. (1% or less) 595
Cipro I.V. Pharmacy Bulk Package (Less than 1%) 597
Cipro Tablets (Less than 1%) 592
Clear Eyes ACR Astringent/Lubricant Eye Redness Reliever Eye Drops ..... ◉ 316
Clinoril Tablets (Less than 1 in 100) 1618
Clomid (Occasional; 1.5%) 1514
▲ Clozaril Tablets (5% or more) 2252
▲ Cordarone Tablets (4 to 9%) 2712
Cuprimine Capsules 1630
Cyklokapron Tablets and Injection 1950
Cytotec (Infrequent) 2424
Cytovene (1% or less) 2103
Danocrine Capsules 2307
Dantrium Capsules (Less frequent) 1982
Darvon-N/Darvocet-N 1433
Darvon 1435
Darvon-N Suspension & Tablets 1433
Demerol 2308
Demulen (Rare) 2428
Depakote Tablets (Greater than 1% but not more than 5%) 415
Desferal Vials 820
Dilaudid-HP Injection (Less frequent) 1337
Dilaudid-HP Lyophilized Powder 250 mg (Less frequent) 1337
Dilaudid Tablets and Liquid (Less frequent) 1339
Dimetane-DC Cough Syrup 2059
Dimetane-DX Cough Syrup 2059
Dolobid Tablets (Less than 1 in 100) 1654
Doral Tablets 2664
DynaCirc Capsules (0.5% to 1%) 2256
Easprin 1914
EC-Naprosyn Delayed-Release Tablets (Less than 3%) 2117
Effexor (Frequent) 2719
Empirin with Codeine Tablets 1093
Engerix-B Unit-Dose Vials 2482
Estrace Cream and Tablets 749
Eye-Stream Eye Irrigating Solution 473
FML-S Liquifilm ..... ◉ 242
▲ Felbatol (5.3%) 2666
Feldene Capsules 1965
Floxin I.V. (1% to 3%) 1571
Floxin Tablets (200 mg, 300 mg, 400 mg) (1% to 3%) 1567
▲ Fludara for Injection (3% to 15%) 663
Fluorouracil Injection 2116
▲ Foscavir Injection (5% or greater) 547
Sterile FUDR (Remote possibility) 2118
Garamycin Injectable 2360
Halcion Tablets (0.9% to 0.5%) 2611
Haldol Decanoate 1577
Haldol Injection, Tablets and Concentrate 1575
Hivid Tablets (Less than 1% to less than 3%) 2121
Humatrope Vials (Small number of patients) 1443
▲ Hylorel Tablets (29.2%) 985
Hytrin Capsules (At least 1%) 430
Imdur (Less than or equal to 5%) 1323
Imitrex Injection (1.1%) 1103
Imitrex Tablets (Up to 3%) 1106
Inderal 2728
Inderal LA Long Acting Capsules 2730
Inderide Tablets 2732
Inderide LA Long Acting Capsules 2734
Intron A (Less than 5%) 2364
IOPIDINE Sterile Ophthalmic Solution ..... ◉ 219
Iopidine 0.5% (Less than 1%) ..... ◉ 221
Kerlone Tablets (Less than 2%) 2436
▲ Lamictal Tablets (3.4%) 1112
Lamprene Capsules (Less than 1%) 828
Lanoxicaps 1117
Lanoxin Elixir Pediatric 1120
Lanoxin Injection 1123
Lanoxin Injection Pediatric 1126
Lanoxin Tablets 1128
Lariam Tablets 2128
Levlen/Tri-Levlen 651
Livostin (Approximately 1% to 3%) ..... ◉ 266
Lodine Capsules and Tablets (Less than 1%) 2743
Lopressor Ampuls 830
Lopressor HCT Tablets 832
Lopressor Tablets 830
Lotensin HCT (0.3% or more) 837
MS Contin Tablets (Less frequent) 1994
MSIR (Infrequent) 1997
Marinol (Dronabinol) Capsules (Less than 1%) 2231
Matulane Capsules 2131
Maxaquin Tablets (Less than 1%) 2440
Mepergan Injection 2753
Methadone Hydrochloride Oral Concentrate 2233
Methadone Hydrochloride Oral Solution & Tablets 2235
▲ Mexitil Capsules (5.7% to 7.5%) 678
Micronor Tablets (Rare) 1872
Midamor Tablets (Less than or equal to 1%) 1703
Miltown Tablets 2672
Modicon (Rare) 1872
Moduretic Tablets (Less than or equal to 1%) 1705
Monopril Tablets (0.2% to 1.0%) 757
Children's Motrin Ibuprofen Oral Suspension (Less than 1%) 1546
Motrin Tablets (Less than 1%) 2625
Myambutol Tablets 1386
Anaprox/Naprosyn (Less than 3%) 2117
NegGram (Infrequent) 2323
Neoral (Rare) 2276
Neurontin Capsules (Frequent) 1922
Nolvadex Tablets 2841
Norinyl 2088
Normodyne Tablets (1%) 2379
Noroxin Tablets 1715
Noroxin Tablets 2048
Norplant System 2759
Nor-Q D Tablets 2135
Norvasc Tablets (More than 0.1% to 1%) 1940
Nutropin (A small number of patients) 1061
Ocupress Ophthalmic Solution, 1% Sterile (Occasional) ..... ◉ 309
Ophthocort ..... ◉ 311
OptiPranolol (Metipranolol 0.3%) Sterile Ophthalmic Solution (A small number of patients) ..... ◉ 258
Oramorph SR (Morphine Sulfate Sustained Release Tablets) (Less frequent) 2236
▲ Orap Tablets (4 of 20 patients) 1050
Ortho-Cyclen/Ortho-Tri-Cyclen 1858
Ortho-Est 1869
Ortho-Novum (Rare) 1872
Ortho-Cyclen/Ortho Tri-Cyclen 1858
Orudis Capsules (Greater than 1%) 2766
Oruvail Capsules (Greater than 1%) 2766
PMB 200 and PMB 400 2783
Paraplatin for Injection (1%) 705
Parlodel 2281
Penetrex Tablets (Less than 1% but more than or equal to 0.1%) 2031
▲ Permax Tablets (5.8%) 575
Phenergan with Codeine 2777
Phenergan VC with Codeine 2781
Phospholine Iodide (More frequent in children) ..... ◉ 326
Plaquenil Sulfate Tablets 2328
Plendil Extended-Release Tablets (0.5% to 1.5%) 527
Premphase 2797
Prempro 2801
Procardia XL Extended Release Tablets (1% or less) 1972
▲ Prograf (Greater than 3%) 1042
▲ Proleukin for Injection (7%) 797
Propulsid (1.4%) 1300
ProSom Tablets (Infrequent) 449
Prostigmin Injectable 1260
Prostigmin Tablets 1261
▲ Prozac Pulvules & Liquid, Oral Solution (2% to 5%) 919
Quinidex Extentabs 2067
RMS Suppositories 2657
Recombivax HB (Less than 1%) 1744
Reglan 2068
Relafen Tablets (1%) 2510
ReoPro Vials (0.7%) 1471
Ridaura Capsules 2513
Rifadin 1528
Rifamate Capsules 1530
Rifater 1532
Rimactane Capsules 847
Risperdal (1% to 2%) 1301
▲ Roferon-A Injection (Less than 3% to 5%) 2145
Rogaine Topical Solution 2637
▲ Romazicon (1% to 9%) 2147
Roxanol 2243
Rythmol Tablets–150mg, 225mg, 300mg (Less than 1% to 1.9%) 1352
Salagen Tablets (1%) 1489
Sandimmune (Rare) 2286
Sandostatin Injection (Less than 1%) 2292
Sectral Capsules (2%) 2807
Seldane Tablets 1536
Seldane-D Extended-Release Tablets 1538
Serophene (clomiphene citrate tablets, USP) (Approximately 1 in 50 patients) 2451
▲ Serzone Tablets (Up to 10%) 771
Slo-Niacin Tablets 2659
Stilphostrol Tablets and Ampuls 612
▲ Supprelin Injection (2% to 6%) 2056
Symmetrel Capsules and Syrup (0.1% to 1%) 946
Talacen (Infrequent) 2333
Talwin Injection 2334
Talwin Compound (Infrequent) 2335
Talwin Injection 2334
Talwin Nx 2336
▲ Tambocor Tablets (15.9%) 1497
▲ Tegison Capsules (10-25%) 2154
Temaril Tablets, Syrup and Spansule Extended-Release Capsules 483
Tenex Tablets (3% or less) 2074
Tenoretic Tablets 2845
Tenormin Tablets and I.V. Injection 2847
Terra-Cortril Ophthalmic Suspension 2210
Thorazine 2523
Timolide Tablets 1748
Timoptic in Ocudose (Less frequent) 1753
Timoptic Sterile Ophthalmic Solution (Less frequent) 1751
Timoptic-XE 1755
Tolectin (200, 400 and 600 mg) (1 to 3%) 1581
▲ Tonocard Tablets (1.3-10.0%) 531
Toradol (1% or less) 2159
Trandate Tablets (1%) 1185
Levlen/Tri-Levlen 651
Tri-Norinyl 2164
Ultram Tablets (50 mg) (1% to 5%) 1585
Urispas Tablets 2532
Versed Injection (Less than 1%) 2170
Videx Tablets, Powder for Oral Solution, & Pediatric Powder for Oral Solution (Less than 1% to 5%) 720
Vira-A Ophthalmic Ointment, 3% ..... ◉ 312
Visine L.R. Eye Drops ..... ◉ 313
Visken Tablets (2% or fewer patients) 2299

(▣ Described in PDR For Nonprescription Drugs) — Incidence data in parenthesis; ▲ 3% or more — (◉ Described in PDR For Ophthalmology)

1443 **Side Effects Index** **Vomiting**

Viva-Drops ⊙ 325
Wellbutrin Tablets (Infrequent) 1204
Wygesic Tablets 2827
Zebeta Tablets 1413
Zerit Capsules (Fewer than 1% to 3%) 729
Ziac 1415
▲Zoloft Tablets (4.2%) 2217
Zovirax 1219

Visual disturbances, flashing lights

Clomid (1.5%) 1514

Visual fields, defects

AK-CIDE ⊙ 202
AK-CIDE Ointment ⊙ 202
AK-Pred ⊙ 204
AK-Trol Ointment & Suspension ⊙ 205
Anafranil Capsules (Rare) 803
Betaseron for SC Injection 658
Blephamide Liquifilm Sterile Ophthalmic Suspension 476
Blephamide Ointment ⊙ 237
Cognex Capsules (Infrequent) 1901
Cortisporin Ophthalmic Ointment Sterile 1085
Cortisporin Ophthalmic Suspension Sterile 1086
Dexacidin Ointment ⊙ 263
Effexor (Infrequent) 2719
Eskalith 2485
FML Forte Liquifilm ⊙ 240
FML Liquifilm ⊙ 241
FML S.O.P. ⊙ 241
FML-S Liquifilm ⊙ 242
Flarex Ophthalmic Suspension ⊙ 218
Fluor-Op Ophthalmic Suspension ⊙ 264
Foscavir Injection (Less than 1%) 547
HMS Liquifilm ⊙ 244
Inflamase ⊙ 265
Intron A 2364
Luvox Tablets (Infrequent) 2544
Maxitrol Ophthalmic Ointment and Suspension ⊙ 224
Neurontin Capsules (Infrequent) 1922
Permax Tablets (Infrequent) 575
Pred Forte ⊙ 250
Pred Mild ⊙ 253
Pred-G Liquifilm Sterile Ophthalmic Suspension ⊙ 251
PREVACID Delayed-Release Capsules (Less than 1%) 2562
Quinaglute Dura-Tabs Tablets 649
Romazicon (1% to 3%) 2147
Serzone Tablets (2%) 771
TobraDex Ophthalmic Suspension and Ointment 473
Vasocidin Ointment ⊙ 268
Vasocidin Ophthalmic Solution ⊙ 270
Vexol 1% Ophthalmic Suspension ⊙ 230
Videx Tablets, Powder for Oral Solution, & Pediatric Powder for Oral Solution (Less than 1%) 720
Zoloft Tablets (Rare) 2217

Visual impairment

Ciloxan Ophthalmic Solution (Less than 1%) 472
Depo-Medrol Single-Dose Vial 2600
Depo-Medrol Sterile Aqueous Suspension 2597
Fungizone Intravenous 506
Ocusert Pilo-20 and Pilo-40 Ocular Therapeutic Systems ⊙ 254
Ortho-Cyclen/Ortho-Tri-Cyclen (Rare) 1858
Ortho-Cyclen/Ortho Tri-Cyclen (Rare) 1858
Ridaura Capsules 2513

Vitamin D, increased requirement

Mebaral Tablets 2322

Vitamins, fat-soluble, absorption impaired

Questran Light 769
Questran Powder 770

Vitiligo

Intron A (Less than 5%) 2364
Proleukin for Injection 797

Vitreous disorder, unspecified

▲Cytovene (6%) 2103

Vitreous floaters

Cataflam (Less than 1%) 816
ISPAN Perfluoropropane ⊙ 276
ISPAN Sulfur Hexafluoride ⊙ 275

Miacalcin Nasal Spray (Less than 1%) 2275
Voltaren Tablets (Less than 1%) 861

Voice, alteration

Accutane Capsules (Less than 1%) 2076
Danocrine Capsules 2307
Effexor (Infrequent) 2719
Imitrex Tablets (Rare) 1106
Lotensin HCT (0.3% or more) 837
Monopril Tablets (0.4% to 1.0%) 757
Permax Tablets (Infrequent) 575
▲Prograf (Greater than 3%) 1042
▲Pulmozyme Inhalation (12% to 16%) 1064
Salagen Tablets (2%) 1489
Serzone Tablets (Infrequent) 771
Ventolin Rotacaps for Inhalation (Less than 1%) 1200
▲Zoladex (3%) 2858

Voice, deepening

Aldactazide 2413
Aldactone 2414
▲Android Capsules, 10 mg (Among most common) 1250
▲Android (Among most common) 1251
Danocrine Capsules 2307
▲Delatestryl Injection (One of most common) 2860
Estratest 2539
Halotestin Tablets 2614
▲Oreton Methyl (Among most common) 1255
Oxandrin 2862
Premarin with Methyltestosterone (Among most common) 2794
Testred Capsules 1262
Winstrol Tablets 2337

Voice, hoarseness

Danocrine Capsules 2307
Estratest 2539

Voice, loss of (see under Aphonia)

Vola, burning of

Atgam Sterile Solution (Less than 5%) 2581

Volar pain

Atgam Sterile Solution (Less than 5%) 2581

Vomiting

Abbokinase 403
Abbokinase Open-Cath 405
Accupril Tablets (1.4% to 2.4%) 1893
Accutane Capsules 2076
Acel-Imune Diphtheria and Tetanus Toxoids and Acellular Pertussis Vaccine Adsorbed (2% to 3%) 1364
Achromycin V Capsules (Rare) 1367
▲ActHIB (1.5% to 5.4%) 872
Actifed with Codeine Cough Syrup 1067
Actigall Capsules 802
▲Actimmune (13%) 1056
Activase 1058
Adalat CC (Less than 1.0%) 589
Adriamycin PFS (Frequent) 1947
Adriamycin RDF (Frequent) 1947
Children's Advil Suspension (Less than 3%) 2692
▲AeroBid Inhaler System (25%) 1005
▲Aerobid-M Inhaler System (25%) 1005
Aerolate 1004
AK-Fluor Injection 10% and 25% ⊙ 203
Albuminar-5, Albumin (Human) U.S.P. 5% (Occasional) 512
Albuminar-25, Albumin (Human) U.S.P. 25% 513
Aldactazide 2413
Aldactone 2414
Aldoclor Tablets 1598
Aldomet Ester HCl Injection 1602
Aldomet Oral 1600
Aldoril Tablets 1604
▲Alfenta Injection (18%) 1286
▲Alka-Seltzer Effervescent Antacid and Pain Reliever (7.6% at doses of 1000 mg/day) ▣ 701
▲Alka-Seltzer Lemon Lime Effervescent Antacid and Pain Reliever (7.6% at doses of 1000 mg/day) ▣ 703
Alkeran for Injection 1070
Alkeran Tablets (Infrequent) 1071
All-Flex Arcing Spring Diaphragm (See also Ortho Diaphragm Kits) 1865
Altace Capsules (Less than 1% to 1.6%) 1232
Alupent (1% to 4%) 669
Ambien Tablets (1%) 2416
Amikacin Sulfate Injection, USP (Rare) 960
Amikin Injectable (Rare) 501
Aminohippurate Sodium Injection 1606
Amoxil 2464
▲Anafranil Capsules (7%) 803
Ana-Kit Anaphylaxis Emergency Treatment Kit 617
Anaprox/Naprosyn (Less than 1%) 2117
Ancef Injection (Rare) 2465
Ancobon Capsules 2079
Android 1251
▲Anexsia 5/500 Elixir (Among most frequent) 1781
Ansaid Tablets (1-3%) 2579
Antilirium Injectable 1009
Antivenin (Crotalidae) Polyvalent 2696
Apresazide Capsules (Common) 808
Apresoline Hydrochloride Tablets (Common) 809
Aquasol A Vitamin A Capsules, USP 534
Aquasol A Parenteral 534
Aralen Hydrochloride Injection 2301
Aralen Phosphate Tablets 2301
▲Aredia for Injection (Up to at least 15%) 810
Arfonad Ampuls 2080
Artane 1368
▲Asacol Delayed-Release Tablets (5%) 1979
▲Regular Strength Ascriptin Tablets (7.6%) ▣ 629
Asendin Tablets (Less than 1%) 1369
Astramorph/PF Injection, USP (Preservative-Free) (Frequent) 535
Atamet 572
▲Atgam Sterile Solution (More than 1% to 10%) 2581
Ativan Injection (Occasional) 2698
▲Atretol Tablets (Among most frequent) 573
Atrohist Plus Tablets 454
Atromid-S Capsules (Less frequent) 2701
Atrovent Inhalation Aerosol 671
Augmentin (1%) 2468
Axid Pulvules (1.2% to 3.6%) 1427
Azactam for Injection (1 to 1.3%) 734
Azo Gantanol Tablets 2080
Azo Gantrisin Tablets 2081
▲Azulfidine (Approximately one-third of patients) 1949
▲BCG Vaccine, USP (TICE) (3.0%) 1814
▲Bactrim DS Tablets (Among most common) 2084
▲Bactrim I.V. Infusion (Among most common) 2082
▲Bactrim (Among most common) 2084
▲Genuine Bayer Aspirin Tablets & Caplets (7.6% at doses of 1000 mg/day) ▣ 713
▲Aspirin Regimen Bayer Regular Strength 325 mg Caplets (7.6% of 4500 people tested) ▣ 709
Benadryl Capsules 1898
Benadryl Injection 1898
Benemid Tablets 1611
Bentyl 1501
▲Betapace Tablets (5% to 10%) 641
▲Betaseron for SC Injection (21%) 658
Biavax II 1613
BiCNU (Frequent) 691
▲Blenoxane (Frequent) 692
Blocadren Tablets (Less than 1%) 1614
Brethaire Inhaler 813
Brethine Ampuls (1.3 to 3.9%) 815
Brethine Tablets 814
Brevibloc Injection (About 1%) 1808
Brevicon 2088
Brevital Sodium Vials 1429
Bricanyl Subcutaneous Injection 1502
Bricanyl Tablets 1503
▲Bromfed-DM Cough Syrup (Among most frequent) 1786
Brontex 1981
▲Bufferin Analgesic Tablets and Caplets (7.6%) ▣ 613
Bumex (0.2%) 2093
▲Buprenex Injectable (1-5%) 2006
BuSpar (1%) 737
Butisol Sodium Elixir & Tablets (Less than 1 in 100) 2660
Cafergot 2251
▲Calcimar Injection, Synthetic (About 10%) 2013
Capoten (About 0.5 to 2%) 739
Capozide (0.5 to 2%) 742
Carafate Suspension (Less than 0.5%) 1505
Carafate Tablets (Less than 0.5%) 1504
Carbocaine Hydrochloride Injection 2303
Cardene Capsules (0.4%) 2095
▲Cardene I.V. (4.9%) 2709
Cardene SR Capsules (0.6%) 2097
Cardizem CD Capsules (Less than 1%) 1506
Cardizem SR Capsules (Less than 1%) 1510
Cardizem Injectable (Less than 1%) 1508
Cardizem Tablets (Less than 1%) 1512
Cardura Tablets 2186
Carnitor Injection 2452
Carnitor Tablets and Solution 2453
Cataflam (Less than 1%) 816
Catapres Tablets (About 5 in 100 patients) 674
Catapres-TTS (Less frequent) 675
Ceclor Pulvules & Suspension (Rare) 1431
CeeNU 693
Cefizox for Intramuscular or Intravenous Use (Occasional) 1034
Cefobid Intravenous/Intramuscular (Rare) 2189
Cefobid Pharmacy Bulk Package - Not for Direct Infusion (Rare) 2192
Cefotan 2829
▲Ceftin (2.6% to 6.7%) 1078
Cefzil Tablets and Oral Suspension (1%) 746
▲CellCept Capsules (12.5% to 13.6%) 2099
Celontin Kapseals (Frequent) 1899
Ceptaz (One in 500 patients) 1081
Ceredase 1065
Cerubidine 795
Cervidil (Less than 1%) 1010
▲CHEMET (succimer) Capsules (12-20.9%) 1545
Chloromycetin Sodium Succinate 1900
Chromagen Capsules 2339
Cipro I.V. (1% or less) 595
Cipro I.V. Pharmacy Bulk Package (Less than 1%) 597
Cipro Tablets (2.0%) 592
Claforan Sterile and Injection (1.4%; rare) 1235
Claritin (2% or fewer patients) 2349
Claritin-D (Less frequent) 2350
Cleocin Phosphate Injection 2586
Climara Transdermal System 645
Cleocin Vaginal Cream (Less than 1%) 2589
Clinoril Tablets (Greater than 1%) 1618
Clomid (2.2%) 1514
▲Clozaril Tablets (3%) 2252
Cocaine Hydrochloride Topical Solution 537
Cogentin 1621
▲Cognex Capsules (28%) 1901
ColBENEMID Tablets 1622
Colestid Tablets (Less frequent) 2591
Colyte and Colyte-flavored 2396
▲Combipres Tablets (About 5%) 677
Comhist 2038
Compazine 2470
Condylox (Less than 5%) 1802
Cordarone Intravenous (Less than 2%) 2715
▲Cordarone Tablets (10 to 33%) 2712
Cosmegen Injection (Common) 1626
Cozaar Tablets (Less than 1%) 1628
▲Creon (Among most frequent) 2536
Crystodigin Tablets 1433
Cuprimine Capsules (Greater than 1%) 1630
Cyklokapron Tablets and Injection 1950
▲Cytadren Tablets (1 in 30) 819
CytoGam (Less than 5.0%) 1593
▲Cytosar-U Sterile Powder (Among most frequent) 2592
Cytotec (1.3%) 2424
▲Cytovene (13%) 2103
Cytoxan (Common) 694
▲DHCplus Capsules (Among most frequent) 1993
D.H.E. 45 Injection 2255
▲DTIC-Dome (90% with the initial few doses) 600
▲Dalgan Injection (3 to 9%) 538
Dalmane Capsules 2173
Danocrine Capsules 2307
Dantrium Capsules (Less frequent) 1982

(▣ Described in PDR For Nonprescription Drugs) Incidence data in parenthesis; ▲ 3% or more (⊙ Described in PDR For Ophthalmology)

Vomiting **Side Effects Index** **1444**

Dapsone Tablets USP 1284
▲ Daranide Tablets (Among the most common effects) 1633
Daraprim Tablets 1090
▲ Darvon-N/Darvocet-N (Among most frequent) 1433
▲ Darvon (Among most frequent) 1435
▲ Darvon-N Suspension & Tablets (Among most frequent) 1433
Daypro Caplets (Greater than 1% but less than 3%) 2426
Declomycin Tablets 1371
Deconamine 1320
Deconsal C Expectorant Syrup 456
Deconsal Pediatric Syrup 457
Delatestryl Injection 2860
▲ Demerol (Among most frequently observed) 2308
Demser Capsules (Infrequent) 1649
▲ Demulen (Among most common) 2428
▲ Depakene (Among most common) 413
▲ Depakote Tablets (12%) 415
▲ Depen Titratable Tablets (17%) 2662
Desogen Tablets 1817
▲ Desyrel and Desyrel Dividose (9.9% to 12.7%) 503
Diabinese Tablets (Less than 2%) 1935
Diamox Intravenous 1372
Diamox Sequels (Sustained Release) 1373
Diamox Tablets 1372
Diethylstilbestrol Tablets 1437
▲ Diflucan Injection, Tablets, and Oral Suspension (5% to 5.4%) 2194
Dilacor XR Extended-release Capsules (2.0%) 2018
Dilantin Infatabs 1908
Dilantin Kapseals 1906
Dilantin Parenteral 1910
Dilantin-125 Suspension 1911
Dilatrate-SR (Uncommon) 2398
Dilaudid Ampules 1335
Dilaudid Cough Syrup 1336
▲ Dilaudid-HP Injection (Among most frequent) 1337
▲ Dilaudid-HP Lyophilized Powder 250 mg (Among most frequent) 1337
Dilaudid 1335
Dilaudid Oral Liquid 1339
Dilaudid 1335
Dilaudid Tablets - 8 mg 1339
Dimetane-DC Cough Syrup 2059
Dimetane-DX Cough Syrup 2059
Dipentum Capsules (1.0%; rare) 1951
Diphtheria and Tetanus Toxoids and Pertussis Vaccine Adsorbed 2477
Diphtheria and Tetanus Toxoids and Pertussis Vaccine Adsorbed USP (For Pediatric Use) (1 in 15 doses) 875
Diprivan Injection (Less than 1%) 2833
Diucardin Tablets 2718
Diupres Tablets 1650
Diuril Oral Suspension 1653
Diuril Sodium Intravenous 1652
Diuril Tablets 1653
Dolobid Tablets (Greater than 1 in 100) 1654
Donnatal 2060
Donnatal Extentabs 2061
Donnatal Tablets 2060
Dopram Injectable 2061
Doryx Capsules 1913
Doxorubicin Astra (Frequent) 540
▲ Duragesic Transdermal System (10% or more) 1288
Duramorph (Frequent) 962
Duranest Injections 542
Dura-Vent Tablets 952
Duricef (Rare) 748
Dyazide 2479
Dyclone 0.5% and 1% Topical Solutions, USP 544
Dynacin Capsules 1590
DynaCirc Capsules (Up to 1.3%) 2256
Dyrenium Capsules (Rare) 2481
E.E.S. 424
E-Mycin Tablets (Infrequent) 1341
Easprin 1914
EC-Naprosyn Delayed-Release Tablets (Less than 1%) 2117
▲ Ecotrin (7.6% at 1000 mg/day) 2455
Edecrin 1657
▲ Effexor (6% to 7.9%) 2719
Elavil 2838
Eldepryl Tablets 2550
Elspar 1659
Emcyt Capsules (1%) 1953
▲ Eminase (Less than 10%) 2039
Emla Cream 545
▲ Empirin with Codeine Tablets (Among most frequent) 1093
Endep Tablets 2174
Enduron Tablets 420
Engerix-B Unit-Dose Vials (Less than 1%) 2482
Entex PSE Tablets 1987
▲ Epogen for Injection (0.26% to 17%) 489
▲ Ergamisol Tablets (6% to 20%) 1292
▲ Ergomar (Up to 10%) 1486
▲ ERYC (Among most frequent) 1915
▲ EryPed (Among most frequent) 421
▲ Ery-Tab Tablets (Among most frequent) 422
▲ Erythrocin Stearate Filmtab (Among most frequent) 425
▲ Erythromycin Base Filmtab (Among most frequent) 426
▲ Erythromycin Delayed-Release Capsules, USP (Among most frequent) 427
▲ Esgic-plus Tablets (Among most frequent) 1013
Esidrix Tablets 821
Esimil Tablets 822
Eskalith 2485
Estrace Cream and Tablets 749
Estraderm Transdermal System 824
ESTRATAB Tablets (0.3, 0.625, 1.25, 2.5 mg) 2536
Estratest 2539
▲ Ethmozine Tablets (2% to 5%) 2041
Etrafon 2355
▲ Eulexin Capsules (11% with LHRH agonist) 2358
▲ Famvir (4.8%) 2486
Fansidar Tablets 2114
▲ Felbatol (Among most common; 8.6% to 38.7%) 2666
Feldene Capsules (Less than 1%) 1965
▲ Fioricet Tablets (Among most frequent) 2258
Fioricet with Codeine Capsules (Frequent) 2260
Fiorinal Capsules (Less frequent) 2261
Fiorinal with Codeine Capsules (Infrequent) 2262
Fiorinal Tablets (Less frequent) 2261
Flagyl 375 Capsules (Occasional) 2434
Flagyl I.V. 2247
Flexeril Tablets (Less than 1%) 1661
Flonase Nasal Spray (Less than 1%) 1098
Floropryl Sterile Ophthalmic Ointment (Rare) 1662
▲ Floxin I.V. (1% to 4%) 1571
Floxin Tablets (200 mg, 300 mg, 400 mg) (1% to 4%) 1567
▲ Fludara for Injection (31% to 36%) 663
Flumadine Tablets & Syrup (1.7%) 1015
Fluorescite .... ⊙ 219
Fluorouracil Injection (Common) 2116
Fluothane 2724
Fortaz (1 in 500 patients) 1100
▲ Foscavir Injection (5% or greater up to 26%) 547
▲ Sterile FUDR (Among more common) 2118
Fulvicin P/G Tablets (Occasional) 2359
Fulvicin P/G 165 & 330 Tablets (Occasional) 2359
▲ Fungizone Intravenous (Among most common) 506
Furoxone (Occasional) 2046
Gamimune N, 5% Immune Globulin Intravenous (Human), 5% 619
Gamimune N, 10% Immune Globulin Intravenous (Human), 10% 621
Gammagard S/D, Immune Globulin, Intravenous (Human) (Occasional) 585
Gammar I.V., Immune Globulin Intravenous (Human), Lyophilized 516
Ganite 2533
Gantanol Tablets 2119
Gantrisin 2120
Garamycin Injectable 2360
Geocillin Tablets 2199
Geref (sermorelin acetate for injection) 2876
Glauctabs .... ⊙ 208
Glucagon for Injection Vials and Emergency Kit (Occasional) 1440
▲ Glucophage (Among most common) 752
Glucotrol XL Extended Release Tablets (Less than 3%) 1968
GoLYTELY (Infrequent) 688
Grifulvin V (griseofulvin tablets) Microsize (griseofulvin oral suspension) Microsize (Occasional) 1888
Gris-PEG Tablets, 125 mg & 250 mg (Occasional) 479
Guaifed Syrup .... ▣ 734
Guaimax-D Tablets 792
▲ Habitrol Nicotine Transdermal System (3% to 9% of patients) 865
▲ Halcion Tablets (4.6%) 2611
Haldol Decanoate 1577
Haldol Injection, Tablets and Concentrate 1575
▲ Halfprin (7.6%) 1362
Halotestin Tablets 2614
Havrix (Less than 1%) 2489
Heparin Lock Flush Solution 2725
Heparin Sodium Injection 2726
Heparin Sodium Injection, USP, Sterile Solution 2615
Heparin Sodium Vials (Rare) 1441
Hespan Injection 929
▲ Hexalen Capsules (1% to 33%) 2571
Helixate, Antihemophilic Factor (Recombinant) (Three reports out of 3,254 patients) 518
HibTITER (9 of 1,118 vaccinations) 1375
Hivid Tablets (Less than 1% to less than 3%) 2121
Humatrope Vials (Small number of patients) 1443
Humegon 1824
Humorsol Sterile Ophthalmic Solution (Rare) 1664
Hycodan Tablets and Syrup 930
Hycomine Compound Tablets 932
Hycomine 931
Hycotuss Expectorant Syrup 933
Hydrea Capsules (Less frequent) 696
Hydrocet Capsules 782
HydroDIURIL Tablets 1674
Hydropres Tablets 1675
▲ Hylorel Tablets (3.9%) 985
▲ Hyperstat I.V. Injection (4%) 2363
Hyskon Hysteroscopy Fluid (Rare) 1595
Hytrin Capsules (At least 1%) 430
Hyzaar Tablets 1677
IBU Tablets (Less than 1%) 1342
▲ Idamycin (82%) 1955
▲ IFEX (58%) 697
Ilosone (Infrequent) 911
Imdur (Less than or equal to 5%) 1323
Imitrex Tablets 1106
Imodium Capsules 1295
▲ Imovax Rabies Vaccine (Up to 6%) 881
▲ Imuran (Approximately 12%) 1110
Inderal 2728
Inderal LA Long Acting Capsules 2730
Inderide Tablets 2732
Inderide LA Long Acting Capsules 2734
Indocin I.V. (1% to 3%) 1684
INFeD (Iron Dextran Injection, USP) 2345
Infumorph 200 and Infumorph 500 Sterile Solutions 965
Inocor Lactate Injection (0.9%) 2309
▲ Intron A (1% to 14%) 2364
Inversine Tablets 1686
IOPIDINE Sterile Ophthalmic Solution .... ⊙ 219
Ismelin Tablets 827
Ismo Tablets (Fewer than 1% to 4%) 2738
ISMOTIC 45% w/v Solution .... ⊙ 222
Isopto Carbachol Ophthalmic Solution .... ⊙ 223
Isuprel Hydrochloride Solution 1:200 & 1:100 2313
Isuprel Mistometer 2312
▲ JE-VAX (Approximately 10%) 886
K-Dur Microburst Release System (potassium chloride, USP) E.R. Tablets 1325
▲ K-Lor Powder Packets (Most common) 434
▲ K-Norm Extended-Release Capsules (Among most common) 991
K-Phos Neutral Tablets 639
K-Phos Original Formula 'Sodium Free' Tablets 639
▲ K-Tab Filmtab (Most common) 434
Kayexalate 2314
Keflex Pulvules & Oral Suspension (Rare) 914
Keftab Tablets (Rare) 915
Kefurox Vials, Faspak & ADD-Vantage 1454
Kefzol Vials, Faspak & ADD-Vantage (Rare) 1456
Kemadrin Tablets 1112
Kerlone Tablets (Less than 2%) 2436
KOGENATE Antihemophilic Factor (Recombinant) (Three reports) 632
▲ Kolyum Liquid (Among most common) 992
▲ Kytril Tablets (9%) 2492
▲ Lamictal Tablets (Among most common; 11% to 18%) 1112
▲ Lamprene Capsules (40-50%) 828
Lanoxicaps (Common) 1117
Lanoxin Elixir Pediatric 1120
Lanoxin Injection (Common) 1123
Lanoxin Injection Pediatric 1126
Lanoxin Tablets (Common) 1128
▲ Lariam Tablets (Among most frequent) 2128
Larodopa Tablets (Relatively frequent) 2129
Lasix Injection, Oral Solution and Tablets 1240
Lescol Capsules 2267
▲ Leucovorin Calcium for Injection (7% to 46%) 1268
Leukeran Tablets (Infrequent) 1133
▲ Leukine for IV Infusion (85%) 1271
▲ Leustatin (13%) 1834
Levbid Extended-Release Tablets 2405
Levlen/Tri-Levlen 651
Levo-Dromoran (Common) 2129
Levophed Bitartrate Injection 2315
Levoprome (Sometimes) 1274
Levsin/Levsinex/Levbid 2405
Limbitrol 2180
Lincocin 2617
Lioresal Intrathecal (3 to 5 of 214 patients) 1596
Lioresal Tablets (Rare) 829
Lithium Carbonate Capsules & Tablets 2230
Lithonate/Lithotabs/Lithobid 2543
Lodine Capsules and Tablets (More than 1% but less than 3%) 2743
Lomotil 2439
Loniten Tablets 2618
▲ Lo/Ovral Tablets (10% or less) 2746
▲ Lo/Ovral-28 Tablets (10% or less) 2751
Lopid Tablets (2.5%) 1917
Lopressor HCT Tablets (1 in 100 patients) 832
Lorabid Suspension and Pulvules (0.5% to 3.3%) 1459
▲ Lorcet 10/650 (Among most frequent) 1018
Lorelco Tablets 1517
▲ Lortab (Among most frequent) 2566
Lotensin Tablets 834
Lotensin HCT 837
Loxitane 1378
Lozol Tablets (Less than 5%) 2022
Ludiomil Tablets (Rare) 843
Lufyllin & Lufyllin-400 Tablets 2670
Lufyllin-GG Elixir & Tablets 2671
Lupron Depot 3.75 mg (Less than 5%) 2556
▲ Lupron Depot 7.5 mg (5.4%) 2559
Lupron Depot-PED 7.5 mg, 11.25 mg and 15 mg (Less than 2%) 2560
▲ Lupron Injection (5% or more) 2555
▲ Luvox Tablets (5%) 2544
Lysodren 698
M-M-R II 1687
M-R-VAX II 1689
▲ MS Contin Tablets (Among most frequent) 1994
▲ MSIR (Among most frequent) 1997
▲ MZM (Among reactions occurring most often) .... ⊙ 267
Maalox Daily Fiber Therapy .... ▣ 641
Macrobid Capsules (Less than 1%) 1988
▲ Macrodantin Capsules (Among most often) 1989
Mandol Vials, Faspak & ADD-Vantage (Rare) 1461
Marax Tablets & DF Syrup (Frequent, on empty stomach) 2200
Marcaine Hydrochloride with Epinephrine 1:200,000 (Rare) 2316
Marcaine Hydrochloride Injection (Rare) 2316
Marcaine Spinal (Rare) 2319
▲ Marinol (Dronabinol) Capsules (3% to 10%) 2231
▲ Matulane Capsules (Frequent) 2131

(▣ Described in PDR For Nonprescription Drugs) Incidence data in parenthesis; ▲ 3% or more (⊙ Described in PDR For Ophthalmology)

1445 **Side Effects Index** **Vomiting**

Maxair Autohaler 1492
Maxair Inhaler (Less than 1%) 1494
Maxaquin Tablets (Less than 1%) 2440
Maxzide 1380
Mebaral Tablets (Less than 1 in 100) 2322
Mefoxin (Rare) 1691
Mefoxin Premixed Intravenous Solution (Rarely) 1694
▲ Megace Oral Suspension (Up to 6%) 699
Megace Tablets 701
Mellaril 2269
Menest Tablets 2494
▲ Mepergan Injection (Among most frequent) 2753
▲ Mepron Suspension (14%) 1135
Meruvax II 1697
Mesantoin Tablets 2272
Mesnex Injection 702
Mestinon Injectable 1253
Mestinon 1254
Metaproterenol Sulfate Inhalation Solution, USP, Arm-a-Med (Approximately 1 in 300 patients) 552
▲ Methadone Hydrochloride Oral Concentrate (Among most frequent) 2233
Methadone Hydrochloride Oral Solution & Tablets 2235
Methergine (Occasional) 2272
▲ Methotrexate Sodium Tablets, Injection, for Injection and LPF Injection (10%) 1275
Metrodin (urofollitropin for injection) 2446
MetroGel-Vaginal 902
Mevacor Tablets (0.5% to 1.0%; rare) 1699
▲ Mexitil Capsules (39.3% to 39.6%) 678
Mezlin 601
Mezlin Pharmacy Bulk Package 604
▲ Miacalcin Injection (About 10%) 2273
Miacalcin Nasal Spray (Less than 1%) 2275
▲ Micro-K (Among most common) 2063
▲ Micro-K LS Packets (Most common) 2064
Micronor Tablets 1872
▲ Midamor Tablets (3% to 8%) 1703
Milontin Kapseals (Frequent) 1920
Miltown Tablets 2672
Minipress Capsules (1-4%) 1937
Minizide Capsules (Rare) 1938
Minocin Intravenous 1382
Minocin Oral Suspension 1385
Minocin Pellet-Filled Capsules 1383
Mintezol 1704
Mithracin 607
Modicon 1872
Moduretic Tablets (Less than or equal to 1%) 1705
Monodox Capsules 1805
Mono-Gesic Tablets 792
Monoket (Fewer than 1%) 2406
Mononine, Coagulation Factor IX (Human) 523
Monopril Tablets (1.2% to 2.2%) 757
Motofen Tablets (1 in 30) 784
Children's Motrin Ibuprofen Oral Suspension (Greater than 1% to less than 3%) 1546
Motrin Tablets (Less than 3%) 2625
Motrin Ibuprofen Suspension, Oral Drops, Chewable Tablets, Caplets (1% to less than 3%) 1546
Mustargen 1709
▲ Mutamycin (14%) 703
Myambutol Tablets 1386
Mycelex Troches 608
Mycelex-G 500 mg Vaginal Tablets (1 in 149 patients) 609
Mycobutin Capsules (1%) 1957
Mycostatin Pastilles (Occasional) 704
Mykrox Tablets (Less than 2%) 993
Myleran Tablets 1143
Myochrysine Injection 1711
Mysoline (Occasional) 2754
Nalfon 200 Pulvules & Nalfon Tablets (2.6%) 917
Anaprox/Naprosyn (Less than 1%) 2117
Narcan Injection 934
Nardil 1920
Nasalide Nasal Solution 0.025% (5% or less) 2110
Navane Capsules and Concentrate 2201
Navane Intramuscular 2202
▲ Navelbine Injection (Up to 15% but less than 20%) 1145
Nebcin Vials, Hyporets & ADD-Vantage 1464
▲ NebuPent for Inhalation Solution (10 to 23%) 1040
NegGram 2323
Nembutal Sodium Capsules (Less than 1%) 436
Nembutal Sodium Solution (Less than 1%) 438
Nembutal Sodium Suppositories (Less than 1%) 440
▲ Neoral (4% to 10%) 2276
NEOSAR Lyophilized/Neosar (Common) 1959
Nephro-Fer Rx Tablets 2005
Neptazane Tablets 1388
Nesacaine Injections 554
Netromycin Injection 100 mg/ml (1 in 1000 patients) 2373
▲ Neupogen for Injection (7% to 57%) 495
Neurontin Capsules (More than 1%) 1922
▲ Neutrexin (4.6%) 2572
Nicoderm (nicotine transdermal system) (1% to 3%) 1518
Nicolar Tablets 2026
Nicorette (1% to 3% of patients) 2458
Nicotrol Nicotine Transdermal System (1% to 3%) 1550
Nimotop Capsules (Less than 1%) 610
Nitrolingual Spray (Uncommon) 2027
▲ Nizoral Tablets (Approximately 3%) 1298
▲ Nolvadex Tablets (2.1% to 25%) 2841
▲ Nordette-21 Tablets (10% or less) 2755
▲ Nordette-28 Tablets (10% or less) 2758
Norflex 1496
Norgesic 1496
Norinyl 2088
Norisodrine with Calcium Iodide Syrup 442
▲ Normodyne Injection (Up to 4%) 2377
Normodyne Tablets (Up to 3%) 2379
Noroxin Tablets (0.3 to 1.0%) 1715
Noroxin Tablets (0.3% to 1.0%) 2048
Norpace (1 to 3%) 2444
Norplant System 2759
Norpramin Tablets 1526
Nor-Q D Tablets 2135
Norvasc Tablets (More than 0.1% to 1%) 1940
Novahistine DH 2462
Novahistine Elixir ▣ 823
Novahistine Expectorant 2463
▲ Novantrone (31 to 72%) 1279
Novocain Hydrochloride for Spinal Anesthesia 2326
▲ Nubain Injection (6%) 935
Nucofed 2051
NuLYTELY 689
Cherry Flavor NuLYTELY (Less frequent) 689
Numorphan Injection 936
Numorphan Suppositories 937
Nutropin (A small number of patients) 1061
Nydrazid Injection (Common) 508
Ogen Tablets 2627
Ogen Vaginal Cream 2630
▲ OmniHIB (1.9% to 4.3%) 2499
Omnipen Capsules 2764
Omnipen for Oral Suspension 2765
▲ Oncaspar (Greater than 5%) 2028
Oncovin Solution Vials & Hyporets 1466
▲ Oramorph SR (Morphine Sulfate Sustained Release Tablets) (Among most frequent) 2236
Orap Tablets 1050
Oretic Tablets 443
Oreton Methyl 1255
▲ Organidin NR Tablets and Liquid (One of the two most common) 2672
Orlamm (1% to 3%) 2239
Ornade Spansule Capsules 2502
Ortho-Cept 1851
Ortho-Cyclen/Ortho-Tri-Cyclen 1858
Ortho Diaphragm Kits—All-Flex Arcing Spring; Ortho Coil Spring; Ortho-White Flat Spring 1865
Ortho Diaphragm Kit-Coil Spring 1865
Ortho Dienestrol Cream 1866
Ortho-Est 1869
Ortho-Novum 1872
Ortho-Cyclen/Ortho Tri-Cyclen 1858
Ortho-White Diaphragm Kit-Flat Spring (See also Ortho Diaphragm Kits) 1865
▲ Orthoclone OKT3 Sterile Solution (19%) 1837
Orudis Capsules (Greater than 1%) 2766
Oruvail Capsules (Greater than 1%) 2766
OSM_GLYN Oral Osmotic Agent ◎ 226
Ovcon (10% or less) 760
▲ Ovral Tablets (10% or less) 2770
▲ Ovral-28 Tablets (10% or less) 2770
▲ Ovrette Tablets (10% or less) 2771
Oxandrin 2862
Oxytocin Injection 2771
PBZ Tablets 845
PBZ-SR Tablets 844
▲ PCE Dispertab Tablets (Among most frequent) 444
PMB 200 and PMB 400 (Rare) 2783
Pamelor 2280
Paraflex Caplets 1580
Parafon Forte DSC Caplets 1581
▲ Paraplatin for Injection (65% to 84%) 705
Paremyd ◎ 247
▲ Parlodel (2% to 5%) 2281
▲ PASER Granules (Among most common) 1285
Paxil Tablets (2.4%) 2505
Peganone Tablets 446
▲ Pen•Vee K (Among most common) 2772
▲ Penetrex Tablets (2% to 8%) 2031
Pentasa (1.5%) 1527
Pepcid Injection (Infrequent) 1722
Pepcid (Infrequent) 1720
Peptavlon 2878
▲ Percocet Tablets (Among most frequent) 938
▲ Percodan Tablets (Among most frequent) 939
▲ Percodan-Demi Tablets (Among most frequent) 940
Pergonal (menotropins for injection, USP) 2448
Periactin 1724
Permax Tablets (2.7%; frequent) 575
Persantine Tablets 681
Phenergan with Codeine 2777
Phenergan with Dextromethorphan 2778
Phenergan Injection 2773
Phenergan Suppositories 2775
Phenergan Syrup 2774
Phenergan Tablets 2775
Phenergan VC 2779
Phenergan VC with Codeine 2781
Phenobarbital Elixir and Tablets (Less than in 100 patients) 1469
PhosLo Tablets 690
▲ Phrenilin (Among most frequent) 785
Pilocar (Extremely rare) ◎ 268
Pima Syrup 1005
Pipracil (Less than 2%) 1390
Placidyl Capsules 448
Plaquenil Sulfate Tablets (Rare) 2328
▲ Platinol (Almost all patients) 708
▲ Platinol-AQ Injection (Almost all patients) 710
Plendil Extended-Release Tablets (0.5% to 1.5%) 527
Pneumovax 23 1725
Ponstel 1925
Pontocaine Hydrochloride for Spinal Anesthesia 2330
Pravachol (Rare) 765
Premarin Intravenous 2787
Premarin with Methyltestosterone 2794
Premarin Tablets 2789
Premarin Vaginal Cream 2791
Premphase 2797
Prempro 2801
Prilosec Delayed-Release Capsules (1.5% to 3.2%) 529
Primaxin I.M. (0.3%) 1727
Primaxin I.V. (1.5%) 1729
Prinivil Tablets (1.1% to 2.4%) 1733
Prinzide Tablets (1.4%) 1737
Priscoline Hydrochloride Ampuls 845
Pro-Banthīne Tablets 2052
▲ Procan SR Tablets (3-4%) 1926
Procardia XL Extended Release Tablets (1% or less) 1972
▲ Procrit for Injection (0.26% to 17%) 1841
Proglycem (Frequent) 580
▲ Prograf (12% to 27%) 1042
▲ Proleukin for Injection (87%) 797
Prolixin 509
Proloprim Tablets 1155
Propulsid (More than 1%) 1300
ProSom Tablets (Infrequent) 449
Prostigmin Injectable 1260
Prostigmin Tablets 1261
▲ Prostin E2 Suppository (Approximately two-thirds) 2634
Protamine Sulfate Ampoules & Vials 1471
Protostat Tablets (Occasional) 1883
Proventil Inhalation Aerosol 2382
Proventil Repetabs Tablets (1% to 4%) 2386
Proventil Syrup 2385
Proventil Tablets (2%) 2386
Provocholine for Inhalation 2140
Prozac Pulvules & Liquid, Oral Solution (2.4%) 919
Purinethol Tablets (Uncommon) 1156
Pyrazinamide Tablets 1398
Quadrinal Tablets 1350
Quarzan Capsules 2181
Questran Light (Less frequent) 769
Questran Powder (Less frequent) 770
Quibron 2053
▲ Quinaglute Dura-Tabs Tablets (3%) 649
Quinidex Extentabs (Frequent) 2067
▲ RMS Suppositories (Among most frequent) 2657
▲ Rabies Vaccine, Imovax Rabies I.D. (Less frequent; up to 6%) 883
Recombivax HB (Less to greater than 1%) 1744
Regitine 846
Relafen Tablets (1% to 3%) 2510
▲ ReoPro Vials (11.4%) 1471
Respbid Tablets 682
▲ Retrovir Capsules (4.8% to 25%) 1158
▲ Retrovir I.V. Infusion (6% to 25%) 1163
▲ Retrovir Syrup (4.8% to 25%) 1158
▲ ReVia Tablets (3% to more than 10%) 940
▲ Revex (9%) 1811
▲ Ridaura Capsules (10%) 2513
Rifadin (Some patients) 1528
Rifamate Capsules (Some patients) 1530
Rifater 1532
Rimactane Capsules 847
▲ Risperdal (5% to 10%) 1301
Robaxisal Tablets 2071
Robinul Forte Tablets 2072
Robinul Injectable 2072
Robinul Tablets 2072
Rocaltrol Capsules 2141
Rocephin Injectable Vials, ADD-Vantage, Galaxy Container (Less than 1%) 2142
▲ Roferon-A Injection (10% to 17%) 2145
▲ Rogaine Topical Solution (4.33%) 2637
▲ Romazicon (11%) 2147
Rondec Oral Drops 953
Rondec Syrup 953
Rondec Tablet 953
Rondec-DM Oral Drops 954
Rondec-DM Syrup 954
Rondec-TR Tablet 953
▲ Roxanol (Among most frequent) 2243
▲ Roxicodone Tablets, Oral Solution & Intensol (Oxycodone) (Among most frequent) 2244
Rubex (Frequent) 712
Rum-K Syrup 1005
▲ Rythmol Tablets–150mg, 225mg, 300mg (2.4 to 10.7%) 1352
▲ SSKI Solution (Among most frequent) 2658
▲ Salagen Tablets (4%) 1489
▲ Sandimmune (2 to 10%) 2286
Sandoglobulin I.V. 2290
▲ Sandostatin Injection (Less than 10%) 2292
Sanorex Tablets 2294
Sansert Tablets 2295
Seconal Sodium Pulvules (Less than 1 in 100) 1474
Sectral Capsules (Up to 2%) 2807
▲ Sedapap Tablets 50 mg/650 mg (Among the most frequent) 1543
▲ Seldane Tablets (4.6% to 7.6%) 1536
Seldane-D Extended-Release Tablets 1538
Senna X-Prep Bowel Evacuant Liquid (Rare) 1230
Sensorcaine (Rare) 559
▲ Septra (Among most common) 1174
▲ Septra I.V. Infusion (Among most common) 1169
▲ Septra I.V. Infusion ADD-Vantage Vials (Among most common) 1171
▲ Septra (Among most common) 1174
Ser-Ap-Es Tablets 849
Serentil 684
Serevent Inhalation Aerosol (1% to 3%) 1176

(▣ Described in PDR For Nonprescription Drugs) Incidence data in parenthesis; ▲ 3% or more (◎ Described in PDR For Ophthalmology)

Serophene (clomiphene citrate tablets, USP) (Approximately 1 in 50 patients) ... 2451
Serzone Tablets (Up to 2%) ... 771
Sinemet Tablets (Less frequent) ... 943
Sinemet CR Tablets (1.8%) ... 944
Sinequan ... 2205
Skelaxin Tablets ... 788
Slo-bid Gyrocaps ... 2033
Slo-Niacin Tablets ... 2659
▲ Slow-K Extended-Release Tablets (Among most common) ... 851
Sodium Polystyrene Sulfonate Suspension ... 2244
Solganal Suspension (Rare) ... 2388
Solu-Medrol Sterile Powder ... 2643
Soma Compound w/Codeine Tablets ... 2676
▲ Soma Compound Tablets (Among most common) ... 2675
Soma Tablets ... 2674
Sotradecol (Sodium Tetradecyl Sulfate Injection) ... 967
Spectrobid Tablets ... 2206
Sporanox Capsules (0.8% to 5.1%) ... 1305
▲ St. Joseph Adult Chewable Aspirin (81 mg.) (7.3% of 4500 patients) ... ▭ 808
▲ Stadol (13%) ... 775
Stelazine ... 2514
Stilphostrol Tablets and Ampuls ... 612
Stimate, (desmopressin acetate) Nasal Spray, 1.5 mg/mL ... 525
Streptomycin Sulfate Injection ... 2208
Sublimaze Injection ... 1307
▲ Sufenta Injection (3% to 9%) ... 1309
▲ Supprelin Injection (3% to 10%) ... 2056
▲ Suprane (16%) ... 1813
Suprax (Less than 2%) ... 1399
Surmontil Capsules ... 2811
Sus-Phrine Injection ... 1019
Symmetrel Capsules and Syrup (0.1% to 1%) ... 946
Syntocinon Injection ... 2296
Talacen (Occasional) ... 2333
▲ Talwin Injection (Most common) ... 2334
Talwin Compound ... 2335
▲ Talwin Injection (Most common) ... 2334
Talwin Nx ... 2336
Tambocor Tablets (1% to less than 3%) ... 1497
Tao Capsules (Infrequent) ... 2209
Tapazole Tablets ... 1477
Tavist Syrup ... 2297
Tavist Tablets ... 2298
▲ Taxol (52%) ... 714
Tazicef for Injection (Less than 2%; 1 in 500 patients) ... 2519
Tazidime Vials, Faspak & ADD-Vantage (1 in 500) ... 1478
▲ Tegretol Chewable Tablets (Among most frequent) ... 852
▲ Tegretol Suspension (Among most frequent) ... 852
▲ Tegretol Tablets (Among most frequent) ... 852
Temaril Tablets, Syrup and Spansule Extended-Release Capsules ... 483
Tenoretic Tablets ... 2845
Tensilon Injectable ... 1261
Terramycin Intramuscular Solution ... 2210
Teslac ... 717
Testoderm Testosterone Transdermal System ... 486
Tetramune (1% to 5%) ... 1404
Thalitone ... 1245
Theo-24 Extended Release Capsules ... 2568
Theo-Dur Extended-Release Tablets ... 1327
Theo-X Extended-Release Tablets ... 788
▲ TheraCys BCG Live (Intravesical) (Up to 16.1%) ... 897
Thera-Gesic ... 1781
Thioguanine Tablets, Tabloid Brand (Less frequent) ... 1181
Thioplex (Thiotepa For Injection) ... 1281
Ticar for Injection ... 2526
Ticlid Tablets (1.9%) ... 2156
Tilade (1.7%) ... 996
Timentin for Injection ... 2528
Timolide Tablets ... 1748
Timoptic in Ocudose ... 1753
Timoptic Sterile Ophthalmic Solution ... 1751
Timoptic-XE ... 1755
Tobramycin Sulfate Injection ... 968
Tofranil Ampuls ... 854
Tofranil Tablets ... 856
Tofranil-PM Capsules ... 857
▲ Tolectin (200, 400 and 600 mg) (3 to 9%) ... 1581
▲ Tonocard Tablets (4.6-9.0%) ... 531
Toradol (Greater than 1%) ... 2159
▲ Trandate (4 of 100 patients; up to 3%) ... 1185
Transderm Scōp Transdermal Therapeutic System (Few patients) ... 869
Trasylol (2%) ... 613
Trental Tablets (1.2%) ... 1244
Triavil Tablets ... 1757
Tri-Immunol Adsorbed ... 1408
Trilafon (Occasional) ... 2389
Levlen/Tri-Levlen ... 651
▲ Trilisate (Less than 20%) ... 2000
Trimpex Tablets ... 2163
Trinalin Repetabs Tablets ... 1330
Tri-Norinyl ... 2164
Tripedia (Up to 2%) ... 892
▲ Triphasil-21 Tablets (10% or less) 2814
▲ Triphasil-28 Tablets (10% or less) 2819
Tussend ... 1783
Tussionex Pennkinetic Extended-Release Suspension ... 998
Tussi-Organidin DM NR Liquid and DM-S NR Liquid (B One of the two most common) ... 2677
▲ Tussi-Organidin NR Liquid and S NR Liquid (One of the two most common) ... 2677
TYLENOL Severe Allergy Medication Caplets ... 1564
▲ Tylenol with Codeine (Among most frequent) ... 1583
▲ Tylox Capsules (Among most frequent) ... 1584
Tympagesic Ear Drops ... 2342
Typhim Vi (Up to 1.9%) ... 899
▲ Ultram Tablets (50 mg) (9% to 17%) ... 1585
Unasyn (Less than 1%) ... 2212
Uni-Dur Extended-Release Tablets ... 1331
Uniphyl 400 mg Tablets ... 2001
Univasc Tablets (less than 1%) ... 2410
Urecholine ... 1761
Urispas Tablets ... 2532
Urobiotic-250 Capsules ... 2214
Uroqid-Acid No. 2 Tablets ... 640
▲ Valtrex Caplets (4% to 7%) ... 1194
Vantin for Oral Suspension and Vantin Tablets (1.1%) ... 2646
Varivax (Greater than or equal to 1%) ... 1762
Vaseretic Tablets (0.5% to 2.0%) ... 1765
Vasotec I.V. ... 1768
Vasotec Tablets (1.3%) ... 1771
Vasoxyl Injection ... 1196
Velban Vials ... 1484
▲ Ventolin Inhalation Aerosol and Refill (6%) ... 1197
▲ Ventolin Rotacaps for Inhalation (4%) ... 1200
Ventolin Syrup ... 1202
Ventolin Tablets ... 1203
▲ VePesid Capsules and Injection (31% to 43%) ... 718
Versed Injection (2.6%) ... 2170
Vibramycin ... 1941
Vibramycin Hyclate Intravenous ... 2215
Vibramycin ... 1941
▲ Vicodin Tablets (Among most frequent) ... 1356
▲ Vicodin ES Tablets (Among most frequent) ... 1357
Vicodin Tuss Expectorant (More frequently in ambulatory than in recumbent patients) ... 1358
▲ Videx Tablets, Powder for Oral Solution, & Pediatric Powder for Oral Solution (7% to 58%) ... 720
Visken Tablets (2% or fewer patients) ... 2299
Vivactil Tablets ... 1774
Vivotif Berna (Infrequent) ... 665
▲ Volmax Extended-Release Tablets (4.2%) ... 1788
Voltaren Ophthalmic Sterile Ophthalmic Solution (1%) ... ⊙ 272
Voltaren Tablets (Less than 1%) ... 861
▲ Vumon (29%) ... 727
▲ Wellbutrin Tablets (22.9%) ... 1204
Wigraine Tablets & Suppositories ... 1829
WinRho SD (One report) ... 2576
Winstrol Tablets ... 2337
▲ Wygesic Tablets (Most frequent) ... 2827
▲ Xanax Tablets (9.6% to 22%) ... 2649
▲ Xylocaine Injections (Among most common) ... 567
Yocon (Common) ... 1892
Yodoxin ... 1230
▲ Yutopar Intravenous Injection (10% to 15%) ... 570
▲ Zanosar Sterile Powder (Most patients) ... 2653
Zantac ... 1209
Zantac Injection ... 1207
Zantac Syrup ... 1209
Zarontin Capsules (Frequent) ... 1928
Zarontin Syrup (Frequent) ... 1929
Zaroxolyn Tablets ... 1000
Zebeta Tablets (1.1% to 1.5%) ... 1413
Zefazone ... 2654
Zemuron (Less than 1%) ... 1830
▲ Zerit Capsules (6% to 35%) ... 729
Zestoretic (1.4%) ... 2850
Zestril Tablets (1.0% to 2.4%) ... 2854
Ziac ... 1415
Zinacef ... 1211
▲ Zinecard (42% to 59%) ... 1961
Zithromax (1% or less to 2%) ... 1944
Zocor Tablets ... 1775
▲ Zoladex (Greater than 1% but less than 5%) ... 2858
▲ Zoloft Tablets (3.8%) ... 2217
▲ Zosyn (3.3%) ... 1419
▲ Zosyn Pharmacy Bulk Package (3.3%) ... 1422
Zovirax Capsules (0.7% to 2.7%) ... 1219
▲ Zovirax Sterile Powder (Approximately 7%) ... 1223
Zovirax (0.7% to 2.7%) ... 1219
▲ Zydone Capsules (Among most frequent) ... 949
Zyloprim Tablets (Less than 1%) ... 1226

von Willebrand's-like syndrome, acquired

Hespan Injection ... 929

Vulva, dryness (see under Vagina, dryness)

Vulva, edema

Vagistat-1 (Less than 1%) ... 778

Vulva, swelling

MetroGel-Vaginal (Equal to or less than 2%) ... 902
Vagistat-1 (Less than 1%) ... 778

Vulvar disorder

Anafranil Capsules (Rare) ... 803
▲ Cleocin Vaginal Cream (6%) ... 2589
Hivid Tablets (Less than 1% to less than 3%) ... 2121

Vulvitis

Prostin E2 Suppository ... 2634
Rogaine Topical Solution (0.91%) ... 2637
Zovirax Ointment 5% (0.3%) ... 1223

Vulvovaginitis

Ansaid Tablets (Less than 1%) ... 2579

W

Walking disorders

Oncovin Solution Vials & Hyporets 1466
Tonocard Tablets (0.0-1.2%) ... 531

Warmth

▲ Adalat Capsules (10 mg and 20 mg) (25%) ... 587
▲ Adalat CC (4%) ... 589
Alomide (Less than 1%) ... 469
Buprenex Injectable (Less than 1%) ... 2006
Dopram Injectable ... 2061
Duvoid (Infrequent) ... 2044
Emla Cream ... 545
Geref (sermorelin acetate for injection) ... 2876
Hyperstat I.V. Injection ... 2363
▲ Imitrex Injection (10.8%) ... 1103
▲ Luvox Tablets (3%) ... 2544
Marax Tablets & DF Syrup ... 2200
Miacalcin Injection ... 2273
MSTA Mumps Skin Test Antigen ... 890
Nicobid ... 2026
Nubain Injection (1% or less) ... 935
Peptavlon ... 2878
Plendil Extended-Release Tablets (Up to 1.5%) ... 527
▲ Procardia Capsules (25%) ... 1971
▲ Procardia XL Extended Release Tablets (25%) ... 1972
Protamine Sulfate Ampoules & Vials ... 1471
Quadrinal Tablets ... 1350
Recombivax HB (Less than 1%) ... 1744
Sarapin ... 1231
Slo-Niacin Tablets ... 2659
Stadol (1% or greater) ... 775
Stimate, (desmopressin acetate) Nasal Spray, 1.5 mg/mL ... 525
Tilade (Less than 1%) ... 996
Tripedia ... 892
Versed Injection (Less than 1%) ... 2170
Xanax Tablets (1.3%) ... 2649

Warmth at injection site

Diphtheria and Tetanus Toxoids and Pertussis Vaccine Adsorbed ... 2477
Diphtheria and Tetanus Toxoids and Pertussis Vaccine Adsorbed USP (For Pediatric Use) ... 875
HibTITER (Less than 1% to 1.8%) 1375
▲ Pneumovax 23 (Common) ... 1725
▲ Tetramune (16% to 35%) ... 1404

Water intoxication

Atretol Tablets ... 573
DDAVP Injection ... 2014
DDAVP ... 2017
Methergine (Rare) ... 2272
Oxytocin Injection ... 2771
Stimate, (desmopressin acetate) Nasal Spray, 1.5 mg/mL ... 525
Syntocinon Injection ... 2296
Tegretol Chewable Tablets ... 852
Tegretol Suspension ... 852
Tegretol Tablets ... 852

Water retention (see also under Edema)

Android ... 1251
Hyperstat I.V. Injection ... 2363
Loniten Tablets ... 2618
Premarin with Methyltestosterone ... 2794
Rogaine Topical Solution ... 2637
Solu-Medrol Sterile Powder ... 2643
Testred Capsules ... 1262

Weakness (see under Asthenia)

Weakness, feet

K-Phos Neutral Tablets ... 639
K-Phos Original Formula 'Sodium Free' Tablets (Less frequent) ... 639
SSKI Solution (Less frequent) ... 2658
Uroqid-Acid No. 2 Tablets ... 640

Weakness, hands

K-Phos Neutral Tablets ... 639
K-Phos Original Formula 'Sodium Free' Tablets (Less frequent) ... 639
SSKI Solution (Less frequent) ... 2658
Uroqid-Acid No. 2 Tablets ... 640

Weakness, legs

D.H.E. 45 Injection ... 2255
Dantrium Intravenous ... 1983
Ergomar (Frequent) ... 1486
K-Phos Neutral Tablets ... 639
K-Phos Original Formula 'Sodium Free' Tablets (Less frequent) ... 639
Lupron Injection (A few cases) ... 2555
SSKI Solution (Less frequent) ... 2658
Uroqid-Acid No. 2 Tablets ... 640
Wigraine Tablets & Suppositories ... 1829

Weakness, local

Plendil Extended-Release Tablets (0.5% or greater) ... 527
Timoptic in Ocudose (Less frequent) ... 1753
Timoptic Sterile Ophthalmic Solution ... 1751
Timoptic-XE ... 1755

Weakness, muscle

Ambien Tablets (Rare) ... 2416
Amicar Syrup, Tablets, and Injection ... 1267
Anectine ... 1073
Aristocort Tablets ... 1022
Atromid-S Capsules (Less often) ... 2701
Cardura Tablets (1%) ... 2186
Compazine ... 2470
Cozaar Tablets (Less than 1%) ... 1628
Decadron Phosphate Injection ... 1637
Depen Titratable Tablets ... 2662
Depo-Medrol Single-Dose Vial ... 2600
Dexacort Phosphate in Respihaler ... 458
Dexacort Phosphate in Turbinaire ... 459
Ergamisol Tablets ... 1292
Eskalith ... 2485
Felbatol ... 2666
Florinef Acetate Tablets ... 505

(▭ Described in PDR For Nonprescription Drugs) Incidence data in parenthesis; ▲ 3% or more (⊙ Described in PDR For Ophthalmology)

1447 **Side Effects Index** **Weight loss**

Floropryl Sterile Ophthalmic Ointment (Infrequent) 1662
Foscavir Injection (Rare) 547
Hivid Tablets (Less than 1% to less than 3%) 2121
Humorsol Sterile Ophthalmic Solution (Infrequent) 1664
Hydeltra-T.B.A. Sterile Suspension 1667
Hydrocortone Phosphate Injection, Sterile 1670
Hydrocortone Tablets 1672
Imdur (Less than or equal to 5%) 1323
Kemadrin Tablets 1112
Lescol Capsules 2267
Lithium Carbonate Capsules & Tablets 2230
Lithonate/Lithotabs/Lithobid 2543
Maxzide 1380
Metubine Iodide Vials 916
Mevacor Tablets 1699
Nicobid 2026
Norcuron 1826
Nuromax Injection 1149
Ocupress Ophthalmic Solution, 1% Sterile ◉ 309
Pravachol 765
Prilosec Delayed-Release Capsules (Less than 1%) 529
Protopam Chloride for Injection 2806
Retrovir Capsules 1158
Retrovir I.V. Infusion 1163
Retrovir Syrup 1158
Rifater 1532
Rimactane Capsules 847
Sodium Polystyrene Sulfonate Suspension 2244
Stelazine 2514
▲ Videx Tablets, Powder for Oral Solution, & Pediatric Powder for Oral Solution (3% to 6%) 720
Zocor Tablets 1775
Zoloft Tablets (Infrequent) 2217

Weight change, increase or decrease

Amen Tablets 780
Asendin Tablets (Less than 1%) 1369
Climara Transdermal System 645
Cycrin Tablets 975
Demulen 2428
Depo-Provera Sterile Aqueous Suspension 2606
Desogen Tablets 1817
ESTRATAB Tablets (0.3, 0.625, 1.25, 2.5 mg) 2536
Estratest 2539
Levlen/Tri-Levlen 651
Menest Tablets 2494
Moban Tablets and Concentrate 1048
Ogen Tablets 2627
Ogen Vaginal Cream 2630
Ortho-Cept 1851
Ortho-Cyclen/Ortho-Tri-Cyclen 1858
Ortho-Est 1869
Ortho-Cyclen/Ortho Tri-Cyclen 1858
Ovcon 760
Premphase 2797
Prempro 2801
Provera Tablets 2636
Levlen/Tri-Levlen 651

Weight changes, unspecified

Ansaid Tablets (1-3%) 2579
Aygestin Tablets 974
Betapace Tablets (1% to 2%) 641
Cytotec (Infrequent) 2424
▲ Depo-Provera Contraceptive Injection (More than 5%) 2602
Diethylstilbestrol Tablets 1437
Estraderm Transdermal System 824
Flexeril Tablets (Rare) 1661
Klonopin Tablets 2126
Larodopa Tablets (Infrequent) 2129
Lodine Capsules and Tablets (Less than 1%) 2743
Lo/Ovral Tablets 2746
Lo/Ovral-28 Tablets 2751
Loxitane 1378
Marax Tablets & DF Syrup (Possible, with large doses) 2200
Monopril Tablets (0.2% to 1.0% or more) 757
Nordette-21 Tablets 2755
Nordette-28 Tablets 2758
Norpramin Tablets 1526
Ovral Tablets 2770
Ovral-28 Tablets 2770
Ovrette Tablets 2771
Prolixin 509
Stilphostrol Tablets and Ampuls 612
Trental Tablets (Less than 1%) 1244
Triavil Tablets 1757
Triphasil-21 Tablets 2814
Triphasil-28 Tablets 2819
Univasc Tablets (Less than 1%) 2410
Vivactil Tablets 1774

Weight decrease (see under Weight loss)

Weight gain

Children's Advil Suspension 2692
AeroBid Inhaler System (1-3%) 1005
Aerobid-M Inhaler System (1-3%) 1005
Aldoclor Tablets 1598
Aldomet Ester HCl Injection 1602
Aldomet Oral 1600
Aldoril Tablets 1604
Altace Capsules (Less than 1%) 1232
▲ Anafranil Capsules (2% to 18%) 803
Atamet 572
Atromid-S Capsules 2701
Beclovent Inhalation Aerosol and Refill 1075
▲ Betaseron for SC Injection (4%) 658
Brevicon 2088
BuSpar (Infrequent) 737
Cardizem CD Capsules (Less than 1%) 1506
Cardizem SR Capsules (Less than 1%) 1510
Cardizem Injectable 1508
Cardizem Tablets (Less than 1%) 1512
Cardura Tablets (0.5% to 1%) 2186
Catapres Tablets (About 1 in 100 patients) 674
Catapres-TTS (Less frequent) 675
▲ CellCept Capsules (More than or equal to 3%) 2099
Claritin (2% or fewer patients) 2349
Claritin-D (Less frequent) 2350
Clomid (2.2%; fewer than 1%) 1514
▲ Clozaril Tablets (4%) 2252
Cognex Capsules (Infrequent) 1901
Combipres Tablets (About 1%) 677
Compazine 2470
Cortifoam 2396
Cortone Acetate Sterile Suspension 1623
Cortone Acetate Tablets 1624
Dalalone D.P. Injectable 1011
Danocrine Capsules 2307
Daypro Caplets (Less than 1%) 2426
Decadron Elixir 1633
Decadron Phosphate Injection 1637
Decadron Phosphate Respihaler 1642
Decadron Phosphate Turbinaire 1645
Decadron Phosphate with Xylocaine Injection, Sterile 1639
Decadron Tablets 1635
Decadron-LA Sterile Suspension 1646
▲ Demulen (Among most common) 2428
Depakene 413
Depakote Tablets 415
Desyrel and Desyrel Dividose (1.4% to 4.5%) 503
Dexacort Phosphate in Respihaler 458
Dexacort Phosphate in Turbinaire 459
Dilacor XR Extended-release Capsules 2018
Diupres Tablets 1650
Effexor (Frequent) 2719
Elavil 2838
Endep Tablets 2174
Esimil Tablets 822
Eskalith 2485
Estrace Cream and Tablets 749
Etrafon 2355
Felbatol (Frequent) 2666
Feldene Capsules (Less than 1%) 1965
▲ Hismanal Tablets (3.6%) 1293
Humegon 1824
Hydeltrasol Injection, Sterile 1665
Hydeltra-T.B.A. Sterile Suspension 1667
Hydrocortone Acetate Sterile Suspension 1669
Hydrocortone Phosphate Injection, Sterile 1670
Hydrocortone Tablets 1672
Hydropres Tablets 1675
▲ Hylorel Tablets (44.3%) 985
Hytrin Capsules (0.5%) 430
Imitrex Tablets (Rare) 1106
Indocin Capsules (Less than 1%) 1680
Indocin I.V. (Less than 1%) 1684
Indocin (Less than 1%) 1680
Ismelin Tablets 827
K-Phos Neutral Tablets 639
Kerlone Tablets (Less than 2%) 2436
Lamictal Tablets (Frequent) 1112
Limbitrol 2180
Lioresal Tablets 829
Lithium Carbonate Capsules & Tablets 2230
Lithonate/Lithotabs/Lithobid 2543
Ludiomil Tablets (Rare) 843
Lupron Depot 3.75 mg (Less than 5%) 2556
Lupron Depot 7.5 mg (Less than 5%) 2559
Lupron Depot-PED 7.5 mg, 11.25 mg and 15 mg (Less than 2%) 2560
Lupron Injection 2555
Luvox Tablets (Frequent) 2544
Maxair Autohaler 1492
Maxair Inhaler (Less than 1%) 1494
Megace Tablets (Frequent) 701
Mellaril 2269
Mesantoin Tablets 2272
Metrodin (urofollitropin for injection) 2446
Miacalcin Nasal Spray (Less than 1%) 2275
Micronor Tablets 1872
Modicon 1872
Children's Motrin Ibuprofen Oral Suspension 1546
Motrin Tablets 2625
Motrin Ibuprofen Suspension, Oral Drops, Chewable Tablets, Caplets 1546
Nardil (Common) 1920
Navane Capsules and Concentrate 2201
Navane Intramuscular 2202
Neurontin Capsules (2.9%) 1922
▲ Nolvadex Tablets (38.1%) 2841
Norinyl 2088
Norpace (1 to 3%) 2444
Norplant System 2759
Nor-Q D Tablets 2135
Norvasc Tablets (More than 0.1% to 1%) 1940
Orap Tablets 1050
Ortho Dienestrol Cream 1866
Ortho-Novum 1872
Orudis Capsules (Less than 1%) 2766
Oruvail Capsules (Less than 1%) 2766
PMB 200 and PMB 400 2783
Pamelor 2280
Paxil Tablets (Frequent) 2505
Pentaspan Injection 937
Periactin 1724
Permax Tablets (1.6%; frequent) 575
Premarin Intravenous 2787
Premarin with Methyltestosterone 2794
Premarin Tablets 2789
Premarin Vaginal Cream 2791
PREVACID Delayed-Release Capsules (Less than 1%) 2562
Prilosec Delayed-Release Capsules (Less than 1%) 529
Prinivil Tablets (0.3% to 1.0%) 1733
Prinzide Tablets 1737
Procardia XL Extended Release Tablets (1% or less) 1972
▲ Proleukin for Injection (23%) 797
ProSom Tablets (Rare) 449
Prozac Pulvules & Liquid, Oral Solution (Infrequent) 919
Questran Light 769
Questran Powder 770
Relafen Tablets (1%) 2510
ReVia Tablets (Less than 1%) 940
▲ Risperdal (18% or infrequent) 1301
Rogaine Topical Solution (1.24%) 2637
Sansert Tablets 2295
Ser-Ap-Es Tablets 849
Serentil 684
Serophene (clomiphene citrate tablets, USP) (Less than 1 in 100 patients) 2451
Serzone Tablets 771
Sinemet Tablets 943
Sinemet CR Tablets 944
Sinequan (Occasional) 2205
Stelazine (Occasional) 2514
Stilphostrol Tablets and Ampuls 612
▲ Supprelin Injection (3% to 10%) 2056
Surmontil Capsules 2811
▲ Synarel Nasal Solution for Endometriosis (8% of patients) 2152
Temaril Tablets, Syrup and Spansule Extended-Release Capsules 483
Tofranil Ampuls 854
Tofranil Tablets 856
Tofranil-PM Capsules 857
▲ Tolectin (200, 400 and 600 mg) (3 to 9%) 1581
Toradol (1% or less) 2159
Torecan 2245
Trilafon 2389
Trilisate (Less than 1%) 2000
Tri-Norinyl 2164
Uroqid-Acid No. 2 Tablets 640
Visken Tablets (2% or fewer patients) 2299
▲ Wellbutrin Tablets (9.4% to 13.6%) 1204
Xanax Tablets (2.7% to 27.2%) 2649
Zebeta Tablets 1413
Zestoretic 2850
Zestril Tablets (0.3% to 1.0%) 2854
Ziac 1415
▲ Zoladex (Greater than 1% but less than 5%) 2858
Zoloft Tablets (Infrequent) 2217

Weight loss

Accutane Capsules (Less than 1%) 2076
▲ Actimmune (6%) 1056
Adalat CC (Less than 1.0%) 589
Alkeran for Injection 1070
Alkeran Tablets 1071
Ambien Tablets (Rare) 2416
▲ Anafranil Capsules (Up to 7%) 803
Atamet 572
BCG Vaccine, USP (TICE) (2.2%) 1814
▲ Betaseron for SC Injection (4%) 658
Blenoxane 692
Blocadren Tablets 1614
Brevicon 2088
BuSpar (Infrequent) 737
Capoten 739
Capozide 742
Cardura Tablets (Less than 0.5% of 3960 patients) 2186
Cataflam (Rare) 816
Celontin Kapseals 1899
Clomid (Fewer than 1%) 1514
Clozaril Tablets 2252
Cogentin 1621
▲ Cognex Capsules (3%) 1901
Cylert Tablets 412
Daranide Tablets 1633
Daypro Caplets (Less than 1%) 2426
Depakene 413
Depakote Tablets 415
Desyrel and Desyrel Dividose (Less than 1% to 5.7%) 503
Dexedrine 2474
DextroStat Dextroamphetamine Tablets 2036
Effexor (1%) 2719
Elavil 2838
Eldepryl Tablets (1 of 49 patients) 2550
Elspar 1659
Endep Tablets 2174
Eskalith 2485
Estrace Cream and Tablets 749
Etrafon 2355
▲ Felbatol (3.4% to 6.5%) 2666
Feldene Capsules (Less than 1%) 1965
Floxin I.V. (Less than 1%) 1571
Floxin Tablets (200 mg, 300 mg, 400 mg) (Less than 1%) 1567
Foscavir Injection (Between 1% and 5%) 547
▲ Fungizone Intravenous (Among most common) 506
Garamycin Injectable 2360
Hivid Tablets (Less than 1% to less than 3%) 2121
▲ Hylorel Tablets (42.2%) 985
Imitrex Tablets (Rare) 1106
▲ Intron A (Less than 1% to 5%) 2364
Kerlone Tablets (Less than 2%) 2436
Lamictal Tablets (Infrequent) 1112
Lamprene Capsules 828
Limbitrol 2180
Lioresal Intrathecal 1596
Lithium Carbonate Capsules & Tablets 2230
Lithonate/Lithotabs/Lithobid 2543
Lopid Tablets 1917
Lozol Tablets (Less than 5%) 2022
Ludiomil Tablets (Rare) 843
Lupron Depot 3.75 mg (Less than 5%) 2556
Luvox Tablets (Frequent) 2544
Methadone Hydrochloride Oral Concentrate 2233
Micronor Tablets 1872
Modicon 1872
Monoket (Fewer than 1%) 2406
Myleran Tablets 1143
Neoral (Rare) 2276
Neurontin Capsules (Infrequent) 1922
▲ Nolvadex Tablets (22.6%) 2841
Norinyl 2088
Nor-Q D Tablets 2135
Oncaspar (Less than 1%) 2028
Oncovin Solution Vials & Hyporets 1466

(▭ Described in PDR For Nonprescription Drugs) Incidence data in parenthesis; ▲ 3% or more (◉ Described in PDR For Ophthalmology)

Weight loss Side Effects Index 1448

Orap Tablets 1050
Orlamm 2239
Ortho Dienestrol Cream 1866
Ortho-Novum 1872
Orudis Capsules (Less than 1%) 2766
Oruvail Capsules (Less than 1%) 2766
PMB 200 and PMB 400 2783
Pamelor 2280
Paxil Tablets (Frequent) 2505
Permax Tablets (Frequent) 575
Phenurone Tablets (Less than 1%) 447
Placidyl Capsules 448
Plaquenil Sulfate Tablets 2328
Premarin Intravenous 2787
Premarin with Methyltestosterone 2794
Premarin Tablets 2789
Premarin Vaginal Cream 2791
PREVACID Delayed-Release Capsules (Less than 1%) 2562
Prinivil Tablets (0.3% to 1.0%) 1733
Prinzide Tablets 1737
▲ Proleukin for Injection (5%) 797
ProSom Tablets (Rare) 449
▲ Prozac Pulvules & Liquid, Oral Solution (5%) 919
Pulmozyme Inhalation 1064
Questran Light 769
Questran Powder 770
Relafen Tablets (Less than 1%) 2510
Retrovir Capsules (0.8%) 1158
Retrovir I.V. Infusion (1%) 1163
Retrovir Syrup (0.8%) 1158
ReVia Tablets (Less than 1%) 940
Risperdal (Infrequent) 1301
Ritalin 848
Rocaltrol Capsules 2141
▲ Roferon-A Injection (14% to 25%) 2145
Sandimmune (Rare) 2286
Sansert Tablets 2295
Serzone Tablets (Infrequent) 771
Sinemet Tablets 943
Sinemet CR Tablets 944
Stilphostrol Tablets and Ampuls 612
Surmontil Capsules 2811
Synarel Nasal Solution for Endometriosis (1% of patients) 2152
Tegison Capsules 2154
Timolide Tablets 1748
Timoptic in Ocudose 1753
Timoptic Sterile Ophthalmic Solution 1751
Timoptic-XE 1755
Tofranil Ampuls 854
Tofranil Tablets 856
Tofranil-PM Capsules 857
▲ Tolectin (200, 400 and 600 mg) (3 to 9%) 1581
Tri-Norinyl 2164
Ultram Tablets (50 mg) (Less than 1%) 1585
▲ Videx Tablets, Powder for Oral Solution, & Pediatric Powder for Oral Solution (Less than 1% to 10%) 720
Voltaren Tablets (Rare) 861
▲ Wellbutrin Tablets (23.2% to 28%) 1204
▲ Xanax Tablets (2.3% to 22.6%) 2649
Zarontin Capsules (Frequent) 1928
Zarontin Syrup (Frequent) 1929
▲ Zerit Capsules (Fewer than 1% to 10%) 729
Zestoretic 2850
Zestril Tablets (0.3% to 1.0%) 2854
Zoloft Tablets (Infrequent) 2217

Wenckebach block

Buprenex Injectable (Less than 1%) 2006
Lanoxin Elixir Pediatric 1120
Lanoxin Injection 1123
Lanoxin Injection Pediatric 1126
Lanoxin Tablets 1128

Wenckebach's period (see under A-V conduction, prolongation)

Wheals

Astramorph/PF Injection, USP (Preservative-Free) 535
▲ Atgam Sterile Solution (1 in 8 patients) 2581
Attenuvax (Rare) 1610
Biavax II 1613
Demerol 2308
Desferal Vials 820
Dilaudid-HP Injection (Less frequent) 1337
Dilaudid-HP Lyophilized Powder 250 mg (Less frequent) 1337
Duramorph 962
Infumorph 200 and Infumorph 500 Sterile Solutions 965
M-M-R II 1687
M-R-VAX II 1689
Mepergan Injection 2753
Meruvax II 1697
Mumpsvax (Extremely rare) 1708

Wheezing

Actifed with Codeine Cough Syrup 1067
▲ Adalat Capsules (10 mg and 20 mg) (6%) 587
▲ AeroBid Inhaler System (3-9%) 1005
▲ Aerobid-M Inhaler System (3-9%) 1005
Airet Solution for Inhalation (1% to 1.5%) 452
Azmacort Oral Inhaler (Infrequent) 2011
Beconase (Rare) 1076
Bioclate, Antihemophilic Factor (Recombinant) 513
Blenoxane (1%) 692
Brethaire Inhaler 813
Brevibloc Injection (Less than 1%) 1808
▲ Bromfed-DM Cough Syrup (Among most frequent) 1786
Cartrol Tablets (Rare) 410
Claritin-D (Less frequent) 2350
Clozaril Tablets (Less than 1%) 2252
Comhist 2038
CytoGam (Less than 5.0%) 1593
Deconamine 1320
Depen Titratable Tablets 2662
Dimetane-DC Cough Syrup 2059
Dimetane-DX Cough Syrup 2059
Diprivan Injection (Less than 1%) 2833
Fungizone Intravenous 506
Gamimune N, 5% Immune Globulin Intravenous (Human), 5% 619
Gamimune N, 10% Immune Globulin Intravenous (Human), 10% 621
Hespan Injection 929
Hivid Tablets (Less than 1% to less than 3%) 2121
Humulin 50/50, 100 Units 1444
Humulin 70/30, 100 Units (Less common) 1445
Humulin L, 100 Units (Less common) 1446
Hyskon Hysteroscopy Fluid (Rare) 1595
Regular, 100 Units (Less Common) 1450
Pork Regular, 100 Units 1452
Imitrex Injection 1103
Imitrex Tablets 1106
Intal Capsules (Less than 1 in 10,000 patients to 1 in 25 patients) 987
▲ Intal Inhaler (Among most frequent) 988
Intal Nebulizer Solution (Rare) 989
Intron A (Less than 5%) 2364
JE-VAX 886
Lopressor Ampuls (1%) 830
Lopressor HCT Tablets (Fewer than 1 in 100 patients) 832
Lopressor Tablets (1%) 830
Maxair Autohaler 1492
Maxair Inhaler (Less than 1%) 1494
Mivacron (One patient; less than 1%) 1138
Monoclate-P, Factor VIII:C, Pasteurized, Monoclonal Antibody Purified Antihemophilic Factor (Human) 521
Mononine, Coagulation Factor IX (Human) 523
Nasalcrom Nasal Solution 994
Neupogen for Injection 495
Nicorette 2458
Nimotop Capsules (Less than 1%) 610
Normodyne Injection (1%) 2377
Nubain Injection (1% or less) 935
Nuromax Injection (Less than or equal to 0.1%) 1149
Ornade Spansule Capsules 2502
▲ Orthoclone OKT3 Sterile Solution (13%) 1837
PBZ Tablets 845
PBZ-SR Tablets 844
Pentaspan Injection 937
Periactin 1724
Platinol (Occasional) 708
Platinol-AQ Injection (Occasional) 710
Prinivil Tablets (0.3% to 1.0%) 1733
Prinzide Tablets 1737
▲ Procardia Capsules (6%) 1971
▲ Procardia XL Extended Release Tablets (6%) 1972
▲ Proleukin for Injection (6%) 797
Prostin E2 Suppository 2634
Prostin VR Pediatric Sterile Solution (Less than 1%) 2635
Proventil Inhalation Solution 0.083% (1% to 1.5%) 2384
Proventil Solution for Inhalation 0.5% (1% to 1.5%) 2383
Pulmozyme Inhalation 1064
Quadrinal Tablets 1350
Questran Light 769
Questran Powder 770
Rhinocort Nasal Inhaler (Less than 1%) 556
Rifadin 1528
Rifater 1532
Sandimmune 2286
Sectral Capsules (Up to 2%) 2807
Survanta Beractant Intratracheal Suspension 2226
Tavist Syrup 2297
Tavist Tablets 2298
Temaril Tablets, Syrup and Spansule Extended-Release Capsules 483
Tenoretic Tablets (Up to 3%) 2845
Tenormin Tablets and I.V. Injection (Up to 3%) 2847
Thioplex (Thiotepa For Injection) 1281
Tonocard Tablets 531
Toprol-XL Tablets (About 1 of 100 patients) 565
Tracrium Injection (1 out of 875 patients; 0.2%) 1183
Trandate Injection (1 of 100 patients) 1185
Trinalin Repetabs Tablets 1330
Tussend 1783
Vancenase AQ Nasal Spray 0.042% (Extremely rare) 2393
Vancocin HCl, Vials & ADD-Vantage 1481
Ventolin Inhalation Solution (1% to 1.5%) 1198
Ventolin Nebules Inhalation Solution (1% to 1.5%) 1199
Versed Injection (Less than 1%) 2170
Visken Tablets (2% or fewer patients) 2299
Zemuron (Less than 1%) 1830
Zestoretic 2850
Zestril Tablets (0.3% to 1.0%) 2854

White-clot syndrome

Heparin Lock Flush Solution 2725
Heparin Sodium Injection 2726
Heparin Sodium Injection, USP, Sterile Solution 2615

Withdrawal reactions

Anafranil Capsules (Rare) 803
Astramorph/PF Injection, USP (Preservative-Free) 535
Betapace Tablets 641
Butisol Sodium Elixir & Tablets 2660
Catapres Tablets 674
Dalmane Capsules 2173
Darvon-N/Darvocet-N 1433
Darvon Compound-65 Pulvules 1435
Darvon-N Suspension & Tablets 1433
Dexacort Phosphate in Respihaler 458
Dexacort Phosphate in Turbinaire 459
Dexedrine 2474
Dilaudid Ampules 1335
Dilaudid Cough Syrup 1336
Dilaudid 1335
Dizac 1809
Doral Tablets 2664
Effexor (Rare) 2719
Endep Tablets 2174
Fioricet Tablets (One report in 2-day-old male infant) 2258
Halcion Tablets 2611
Infumorph 200 and Infumorph 500 Sterile Solutions 965
Klonopin Tablets 2126
Libritabs Tablets 2177
Librium Capsules 2178
Librium Injectable 2179
Lortab 2566
Luvox Tablets (Rare) 2544
MS Contin Tablets 1994
MSIR 1997
Mebaral Tablets 2322
Nembutal Sodium Capsules 436
Nembutal Sodium Solution 438
Nembutal Sodium Suppositories 440
Orlamm 2239
Pamelor 2280
Paxil Tablets (Rare) 2505
Phenobarbital Elixir and Tablets 1469
Placidyl Capsules 448
Procardia XL Extended Release Tablets 1972
ProctoCream-HC 2.5% 2408
ProSom Tablets 449
ReVia Tablets 940
Revex (Less than 1%) 1811
Risperdal (Rare) 1301
Stadol (2 patients) 775
Tranxene 451
Valium Injectable 2182
Valium Tablets 2183
Valrelease Capsules 2169
Videx Tablets, Powder for Oral Solution, & Pediatric Powder for Oral Solution (Less than 1%) 720
Xanax Tablets 2649
Zoloft Tablets (Rare) 2217

Wolff-Parkinson-White syndrome

Cytovene-IV (One report) 2103

Wound dehiscence

Atgam Sterile Solution (Less than 1%) 2581
INSTAT* Collagen Absorbable Hemostat 1312

Wound healing, impaired

AK-CIDE (Infrequent) ◉ 202
AK-CIDE Ointment (Infrequent) ◉ 202
AK-Trol Ointment & Suspension ◉ 205
Aristocort Suspension (Forte Parenteral) 1027
Aristocort Suspension (Intralesional) 1025
Aristocort Tablets 1022
Aristospan Suspension (Intra-articular) 1033
Aristospan Suspension (Intralesional) 1032
Blephamide Liquifilm Sterile Ophthalmic Suspension 476
Blephamide Ointment (Infrequent) ◉ 237
Celestone Soluspan Suspension 2347
CORTENEMA 2535
Cortifoam 2396
Cortisporin Ophthalmic Ointment Sterile 1085
Cortisporin Ophthalmic Suspension Sterile 1086
Cortone Acetate Sterile Suspension 1623
Cortone Acetate Tablets 1624
Cytoxan 694
Dalalone D.P. Injectable 1011
Decadron Elixir 1633
Decadron Phosphate Injection 1637
Decadron Phosphate Respihaler 1642
Decadron Phosphate Turbinaire 1645
Decadron Phosphate with Xylocaine Injection, Sterile 1639
Decadron Tablets 1635
Decadron-LA Sterile Suspension 1646
Deltasone Tablets 2595
Depo-Medrol Single-Dose Vial 2600
Depo-Medrol Sterile Aqueous Suspension 2597
Dexacidin Ointment ◉ 263
Dexacort Phosphate in Respihaler 458
Dexacort Phosphate in Turbinaire 459
Econopred & Econopred Plus Ophthalmic Suspensions ◉ 217
FML Forte Liquifilm ◉ 240
FML Liquifilm ◉ 241
FML S.O.P. (Infrequent) ◉ 241
FML-S Liquifilm ◉ 242
Florinef Acetate Tablets 505
Fluoracaine ◉ 206
Fluor-Op Ophthalmic Suspension ◉ 264
Hydeltrasol Injection, Sterile 1665
Hydeltra-T.B.A. Sterile Suspension 1667
Hydrocortone Acetate Sterile Suspension 1669
Hydrocortone Phosphate Injection, Sterile 1670
Hydrocortone Tablets 1672
Maxitrol Ophthalmic Ointment and Suspension ◉ 224
Medrol 2621
NeoDecadron Sterile Ophthalmic Ointment 1712
NeoDecadron Sterile Ophthalmic Solution 1713
NEOSAR Lyophilized/Neosar 1959
Ocufen ◉ 245
Ophthocort ◉ 311
Pediapred Oral Liquid 995
Poly-Pred Liquifilm ◉ 248

(▣ Described in PDR For Nonprescription Drugs) Incidence data in parenthesis; ▲ 3% or more (◉ Described in PDR For Ophthalmology)

1449 Side Effects Index Xerostomia

Pred-G Liquifilm Sterile Ophthalmic Suspension ⊙ 251
Pred-G S.O.P. Sterile Ophthalmic Ointment ⊙ 252
Prelone Syrup 1787
Rhinocort Nasal Inhaler 556
Solu-Cortef Sterile Powder 2641
Solu-Medrol Sterile Powder 2643
Terra-Cortril Ophthalmic Suspension 2210
TobraDex Ophthalmic Suspension and Ointment 473
Vasocidin Ointment ⊙ 268
Vasocidin Ophthalmic Solution ⊙ 270
▲Zofran Tablets (28%) 1217

Wound infection

▲Neoral (7.0%) 2276
▲Sandimmune (7.0 to 10.1%) 2286

Wrist-drop

Fludara for Injection (One case) 663

WBC, immature

▲Betaseron for SC Injection (16%) 658
Biaxin (Less than 1%) 405
Cipro I.V. (Infrequent) 595
▲Cipro I.V. Pharmacy Bulk Package (Among most frequent) 597
▲Clozaril Tablets (3%) 2252
Cytosar-U Sterile Powder 2592
Lupron Depot 3.75 mg 2556
Neurontin Capsules (1.1%) 1922
Zebeta Tablets 1413

WBC counts, fluctuation

Bumex (0.3%) 2093
Cytotec (Infrequent) 2424
Dopram Injectable 2061
Doral Tablets (2.6%) 2664
Effexor (Infrequent) 2719
Foscavir Injection (Between 1% and 5%) 547
Sterile FUDR 2118
Halcion Tablets (1.7 to 2.1%) 2611
Hivid Tablets (Less than 1% to less than 3%) 2121
Lopid Tablets 1917
MetroGel-Vaginal (Equal to or less than 2%) 902
Neurontin Capsules (Rare) 1922
Noroxin Tablets (1.3% to 1.4%) 1715
Noroxin Tablets (1.3% to 1.4%) 2048
Polymyxin B Sulfate, Aerosporin Brand Sterile Powder 1154
PREVACID Delayed-Release Capsules (Less than 1%) 2562
Primaxin I.M. 1727
Quinidex Extentabs 2067
▲Synarel Nasal Solution for Endometriosis (10% to 15%) 2152
Talwin Compound (Rare) 2335
▲Tegison Capsules (10-25%) 2154
Tornalate Solution for Inhalation, 0.2% (Infrequent) 956
Tornalate Metered Dose Inhaler (Rare) 957
Xanax Tablets (1.4% to 2.3%) 2649

X

Xanthopsia

Aldactazide 2413
Aldoclor Tablets 1598
Aldoril Tablets 1604
Apresazide Capsules 808
Capozide 742
Combipres Tablets 677
Diucardin Tablets 2718
Diupres Tablets 1650
Diuril Oral Suspension 1653
Diuril Sodium Intravenous 1652
Diuril Tablets 1653
Dyazide 2479
Enduron Tablets 420
Esidrix Tablets 821
Esimil Tablets 822
HydroDIURIL Tablets 1674
Hydropres Tablets 1675
Hyzaar Tablets (One subject) 1677
Inderide Tablets 2732
Inderide LA Long Acting Capsules 2734
Lanoxicaps 1117
Lanoxin Elixir Pediatric 1120
Lanoxin Injection 1123
Lanoxin Injection Pediatric 1126
Lanoxin Tablets 1128
Lasix Injection, Oral Solution and Tablets 1240
Lopressor HCT Tablets 832
Lotensin HCT 837
Lozol Tablets 2022
Maxzide 1380
Minizide Capsules 1938
Mintezol 1704
Moduretic Tablets 1705
Mykrox Tablets (Rare) 993
Normodyne Tablets (Less common) 2379
Oretic Tablets 443
Prinzide Tablets 1737
Quadrinal Tablets 1350
Ser-Ap-Es Tablets 849
Tenoretic Tablets 2845
Thalitone 1245
Timolide Tablets 1748
Vaseretic Tablets 1765
Zaroxolyn Tablets 1000
Zestoretic 2850
Ziac 1415

Xerochilia

▲Zonalon Cream (Approximately 1% to 10%) 1055

Xeromycteria

▲Accutane Capsules (Up to 80%) 2076
▲Actifed with Codeine Cough Syrup (Among most frequent) 1067
Alomide (Less than 1%) 469
Benadryl Capsules 1898
Benadryl Injection 1898
▲Bromfed-DM Cough Syrup (Among most frequent) 1786
Catapres Tablets 674
Catapres-TTS 675
Claritin (2% or fewer patients) 2349
Claritin-D 2350
Combipres Tablets 677
Comhist 2038
D.A. Chewable Tablets 951
▲Decadron Phosphate Turbinaire (Most common) 1645
Deconamine 1320
▲Dexacort Phosphate in Turbinaire (One of the two most common) 459
▲Dimetane-DC Cough Syrup (Most frequent) 2059
Dimetane-DX Cough Syrup (Among most frequent) 2059
Dura-Tap/PD Capsules 2867
Dura-Vent/DA Tablets 953
Flonase Nasal Spray (Less than 1%) 1098
Hivid Tablets (Less than 1% to less than 3%) 2121
IOPIDINE Sterile Ophthalmic Solution ⊙ 219
Iopidine 0.5% (2%) ⊙ 221
Marax Tablets & DF Syrup 2200
▲Miacalcin Nasal Spray (10.6%) 2275
▲Nasarel Nasal Solution (3% to 9%) 2133
▲Norpace (3 to 9%) 2444
Ornade Spansule Capsules 2502
PBZ Tablets 845
PBZ-SR Tablets 844
Periactin 1724
▲Seldane Tablets (2.3% to 4.8%) 1536
▲Seldane-D Extended-Release Tablets (21.7%) 1538
Symmetrel Capsules and Syrup (1% to 5%) 946
Tavist Syrup 2297
Tavist Tablets 2298
▲Tegison Capsules (Greater than 75%) 2154
Torecan 2245
Trinalin Repetabs Tablets 1330
Tussend 1783

Xerophthalmia

Accutane Capsules 2076
Children's Advil Suspension (Less than 1%) 2692
▲Alomide (1% to 5%) 469
Betaseron for SC Injection 658
▲Betimol 0.25%, 0.5% (More than 5%) ⊙ 261
Betoptic Ophthalmic Solution 469
Betoptic S Ophthalmic Suspension (Small number of patients) 471
Blocadren Tablets 1614
BOTOX (Botulinum Toxin Type A) Purified Neurotoxin Complex 477
Catapres Tablets 674
Catapres-TTS 675
Cognex Capsules (Infrequent) 1901
Combipres Tablets 677
Cytovene-IV (One report) 2103
Depakote Tablets (Greater than 1% but not more than 5%) 415
Dipentum Capsules (Rare) 1951
Effexor (Infrequent) 2719
Hivid Tablets (Less than 1% to less than 3%) 2121
IBU Tablets (Less than 1%) 1342
Inderal (Rare) 2728
Inderal LA Long Acting Capsules (Rare) 2730
Inderide Tablets (Rare) 2732
Inderide LA Long Acting Capsules 2734
Intron A (Less than 5%) 2364
IOPIDINE Sterile Ophthalmic Solution ⊙ 219
Iopidine 0.5% (Less than 3%) ⊙ 221
Kerlone Tablets (Less than 2%) 2436
Lamictal Tablets (Rare) 1112
Livostin (Approximately 1% to 3%) ⊙ 266
Luvox Tablets (Infrequent) 2544
Mintezol 1704
Children's Motrin Ibuprofen Oral Suspension (Less than 1%) 1546
Motrin Tablets (Less than 1%) 2625
Motrin Ibuprofen Suspension, Oral Drops, Chewable Tablets, Caplets (Less than 1%) 1546
Neurontin Capsules (Infrequent) 1922
Norvasc Tablets (Less than or equal to 0.1%) 1940
Ocuflox 481
Rēv-Eyes Ophthalmic Eyedrops 0.5% (Less frequently) ⊙ 323
Risperdal (Infrequent) 1301
Sectral Capsules (Up to 2%) 2807
Serzone Tablets (Infrequent) 771
▲Tegison Capsules (1-10%) 2154
Tenormin Tablets and I.V. Injection 2847
Timolide Tablets 1748
Timoptic in Ocudose 1753
Timoptic Sterile Ophthalmic Solution 1751
Timoptic-XE 1755
Toprol-XL Tablets (Rare) 565
Trusopt Sterile Ophthalmic Solution (Approximately 1% to 5%) 1760
Vaseretic Tablets 1765
Vasotec I.V. 1768
Vasotec Tablets (0.5% to 1.0%) 1771
Videx Tablets, Powder for Oral Solution, & Pediatric Powder for Oral Solution (Less than 1%) 720
Zoladex (1% or greater) 2858
Zoloft Tablets (Infrequent) 2217

Xerosis cutis

Eskalith 2485
Lithium Carbonate Capsules & Tablets 2230
Lithonate/Lithotabs/Lithobid 2543

Xerostomia

Accupril Tablets (0.5% to 1.0%) 1893
▲Accutane Capsules (Up to 80%) 2076
▲Actifed with Codeine Cough Syrup (Among most frequent) 1067
Adalat CC (Less than 1.0%) 589
Adenoscan (Less than 1%) 1024
Adipex-P Tablets and Capsules 1048
Children's Advil Suspension (Less than 1%) 2692
Akineton 1333
Aldactone 2414
Aldoclor Tablets 1598
Aldomet Ester HCl Injection 1602
Aldomet Oral 1600
Aldoril Tablets 1604
Altace Capsules (Less than 1%) 1232
Alupent Tablets (0.4%) 669
▲Ambien Tablets (3%) 2416
▲Anafranil Capsules (63% to 84%) 803
Ana-Kit Anaphylaxis Emergency Treatment Kit 617
Anatuss LA Tablets 1542
Ancobon Capsules 2079
Ansaid Tablets (Less than 1%) 2579
Antivert, Antivert/25 Tablets, & Antivert/50 Tablets 2185
Apresazide Capsules 808
Arco-Lase Plus Tablets 512
Arfonad Ampuls 2080
▲Artane (30% to 50%) 1368
Asacol Delayed-Release Tablets 1979
▲Asendin Tablets (14%) 1369
Atamet 572
Atarax Tablets & Syrup 2185
Atretol Tablets 573
Atrohist Pediatric Capsules 453
▲Atrohist Pediatric Suspension (Among most common) 454
Atrohist Plus Tablets 454
Atrovent Inhalation Aerosol (2.4%) 671
▲Atrovent Inhalation Solution (3.2%) 673
Axid Pulvules (1.4%) 1427
Azmacort Oral Inhaler 2011
Beclovent Inhalation Aerosol and Refill (A few patients) 1075
Bellergal-S Tablets (Rare) 2250
Benadryl Capsules 1898
Benadryl Injection 1898
▲Bentyl (33%) 1501
Betaseron for SC Injection 658
Betimol 0.25%, 0.5% (1% to 5%) ⊙ 261
Biphetamine Capsules 983
Bonine Tablets 1933
Bontril Slow-Release Capsules 781
Brethine Ampuls (Less than 0.5%) 815
Brevibloc Injection (Less than 1%) 1808
Bromfed 1785
▲Bromfed-DM Cough Syrup (Among most frequent) 1786
Bromfed-PD Capsules (Extended-Release) 1785
Bumex (0.1%) 2093
▲BuSpar (3%) 737
Calan SR Caplets (1% or less) 2422
Calan Tablets (1% or less) 2419
Capoten (About 0.5 to 2%) 739
Capozide (0.5 to 2%) 742
Carafate Suspension (Less than 0.5%) 1505
Carafate Tablets (Less than 0.5%) 1504
Cardene Capsules (0.4-1.4%) 2095
Cardizem CD Capsules (Less than 1%) 1506
Cardizem SR Capsules (Less than 1%) 1510
Cardizem Injectable (Less than 1%) 1508
Cardizem Tablets (Less than 1%) 1512
Cardura Tablets (1.4% to 2%) 2186
Cataflam (Less than 1%) 816
▲Catapres Tablets (40 of 100 patients) 674
▲Catapres-TTS (25 of 101 patients) 675
Caverject (Less than 1%) 2583
Cipro I.V. (1% or less) 595
Cipro I.V. Pharmacy Bulk Package (Less than 1%) 597
▲Claritin (3%) 2349
▲Claritin-D (14%) 2350
Clinoril Tablets (Less than 1%) 1618
▲Clozaril Tablets (More than 5 to 6%) 2252
Cogentin 1621
Cognex Capsules (Infrequent) 1901
▲Combipres Tablets (40%) 677
Comhist 2038
Compazine 2470
Cozaar Tablets (Less than 1%) 1628
Cystospaz 1963
Cytovene (1% or less) 2103
D.A. Chewable Tablets 951
Dalgan Injection (Less than 1%) 538
Dalmane Capsules (Rare) 2173
Daraprim Tablets (Rare) 1090
Deconamine 1320
Demadex Tablets and Injection 686
Demerol 2308
Demser Capsules (Infrequent) 1649
Desoxyn Gradumet Tablets 419
▲Desyrel and Desyrel Dividose (14.8% to 33.8%) 503
Dexedrine 2474
DextroStat Dextroamphetamine Tablets 2036
Didrex Tablets 2607
Dilacor XR Extended-release Capsules (Infrequent) 2018
Dilaudid-HP Injection (Less frequent) 1337
Dilaudid-HP Lyophilized Powder 250 mg (Less frequent) 1337
Dilaudid Tablets and Liquid 1339
▲Dimetane-DC Cough Syrup (Most frequent) 2059
Dimetane-DX Cough Syrup (Among most frequent) 2059
Dipentum Capsules (Rare) 1951
Diprivan Injection (Less than 1%) 2833
Ditropan 1516
Diupres Tablets 1650
Diuril Sodium Intravenous 1652
Donnagel Liquid and Donnagel Chewable Tablets (Rare) ▣ 879
Donnatal 2060
Donnatal Extentabs 2061
Donnatal Tablets 2060

(▣ Described in PDR For Nonprescription Drugs) Incidence data in parenthesis; ▲ 3% or more (⊙ Described in PDR For Ophthalmology)

Xerostomia | Side Effects Index | 1450

Doral Tablets (1.5%) 2664
▲ Duragesic Transdermal System (10% or more) 1288
Dura-Tap/PD Capsules 2867
Dura-Vent/DA Tablets 953
Dyazide 2479
DynaCirc Capsules (0.5% to 1%) 2256
Dyrenium Capsules (Rare) 2481
▲ Effexor (2% to 22%) 2719
Elavil 2838
▲ Eldepryl Tablets (3 of 49 patients) 2550
Emete-con Intramuscular/Intravenous 2198
Endep Tablets 2174
Esgic-plus Tablets (Infrequent) 1013
Esidrix Tablets 821
Esimil Tablets 822
Eskalith 2485
▲ Ethmozine Tablets (2% to 5%) 2041
Etrafon 2355
Fastin Capsules 2488
Fedahist Gyrocaps 2401
Fedahist Timecaps 2401
Felbatol (2.6%) 2666
Feldene Capsules (Less than 1%) 1965
Fioricet Tablets (Infrequent) 2258
Fioricet with Codeine Capsules (Infrequent) 2260
Fiorinal with Codeine Capsules (Infrequent) 2262
Flagyl 375 Capsules 2434
▲ Flexeril Tablets (7% to 27%) 1661
Flonase Nasal Spray (Less than 1%) 1098
Floxin I.V. (1% to 3%) 1571
Floxin Tablets (200 mg, 300 mg, 400 mg) (1% to 3%) 1567
Flumadine Tablets & Syrup (1.5%) 1015
Foscavir Injection (Between 1% and 5%) 547
Geocillin Tablets 2199
Guaifed Syrup ▣ 734
Habitrol Nicotine Transdermal System (Less than 1% of patients) 865
Halcion Tablets (Rare) 2611
Haldol Decanoate 1577
Haldol Injection, Tablets and Concentrate 1575
▲ Hismanal Tablets (5.2%) 1293
Hivid Tablets (Less than 1% to less than 3%) 2121
HydroDIURIL Tablets 1674
Hydropres Tablets 1675
Hylorel Tablets (1.7%) 985
Hyperstat I.V. Injection 2363
Hytrin Capsules (At least 1%) 430
Hyzaar Tablets 1677
IBU Tablets (Less than 1%) 1342
Imdur (Less than or equal to 5%) 1323
Imitrex Tablets 1106
Imodium Capsules 1295
▲ Intron A (Up to 28%) 2364
Inversine Tablets 1686
Ionamin Capsules 990
IOPIDINE Sterile Ophthalmic Solution ◉ 219
▲ Iopidine 0.5% (10%) ◉ 221
Ismelin Tablets 827
Isoptin Oral Tablets (Less than 1%) 1346
Isoptin SR Tablets (1% or less) 1348
Kemadrin Tablets 1112
Kerlone Tablets (Less than 2%) 2436
Klonopin Tablets 2126
Kutrase Capsules 2402
Lamictal Tablets (1.0%) 1112
Larodopa Tablets (Relatively frequent) 2129
Lasix Injection, Oral Solution and Tablets 1240
Levbid Extended-Release Tablets 2405
Levoprome (Sometimes) 1274
Levsin/Levsinex/Levbid 2405
Librax Capsules 2176
▲ Limbitrol (Among most frequent) 2180
Lioresal Intrathecal 1596
Lioresal Tablets (Rare) 829
Lithium Carbonate Capsules & Tablets 2230
Lithonate/Lithotabs/Lithobid 2543
Livostin (Approximately 1% to 3%) ◉ 266
Lodine Capsules and Tablets (Less than 1%) 2743
Lopressor Ampuls (1%) 830
Lopressor HCT Tablets (1 in 100 patients) 832
Lopressor Tablets (1%) 830
Lotensin HCT (0.3% to 1.0%) 837
Lotrel Capsules 840
Loxitane 1378
Lozol Tablets (Less than 5%) 2022
▲ Ludiomil Tablets (22%) 843
▲ Lupron Depot 3.75 mg (Among most frequent; less than 5%) 2556
▲ Luvox Tablets (14%) 2544
MS Contin Tablets (Less frequent) 1994
MSIR (Infrequent) 1997
Marax Tablets & DF Syrup (Occasional) 2200
Matulane Capsules 2131
Maxair Autohaler (1.3%) 1492
Maxair Inhaler (Less than 1%) 1494
Maxaquin Tablets (Less than 1%) 2440
Maxzide 1380
Megace Oral Suspension (1% to 3%) 699
Mellaril 2269
Mepergan Injection 2753
Methadone Hydrochloride Oral Concentrate 2233
Methadone Hydrochloride Oral Solution & Tablets 2235
MetroGel-Vaginal 902
Mevacor Tablets (0.5% to 1.0%) 1699
Mexitil Capsules (2.8%) 678
Miacalcin Nasal Spray (Less than 1%) 2275
Midamor Tablets (Less than or equal to 1%) 1703
Minipress Capsules (1-4%) 1937
Minizide Capsules (Rare) 1938
Mintezol 1704
Moban Tablets and Concentrate (Occasional) 1048
Moduretic Tablets 1705
Monoket (Fewer than 1%) 2406
Monopril Tablets (0.2% to 1.0%) 757
Motofen Tablets (1 in 30) 784
Children's Motrin Ibuprofen Oral Suspension (Less than 1%) 1546
Motrin Tablets (Less than 1%) 2625
Motrin Ibuprofen Suspension, Oral Drops, Chewable Tablets, Caplets (Less than 1%) 1546
Mykrox Tablets (Less than 2%) 993
Nalfon 200 Pulvules & Nalfon Tablets (Less than 1%) 917
Nardil (Common) 1920
Navane Capsules and Concentrate 2201
Navane Intramuscular 2202
NebuPent for Inhalation Solution (1% or less) 1040
Neurontin Capsules (1.7%) 1922
Nicoderm (nicotine transdermal system) (1% to 3%) 1518
Nicorette (1% to 3%) 2458
Norflex 1496
Norgesic 1496
Noroxin Tablets (0.3 to 1.0%) 1715
Noroxin Tablets (0.3% to 1.0%) 2048
▲ Norpace (32%) 2444
Norpramin Tablets 1526
Norvasc Tablets (More than 0.1% to 1%) 1940
Novahistine DH 2462
Novahistine Elixir ▣ 823
▲ Nubain Injection (4%) 935
Oramorph SR (Morphine Sulfate Sustained Release Tablets) (Less frequent) 2236
▲ Orap Tablets (5 of 20 patients) 1050
Oretic Tablets 443
Orlamm (1% to 3%) 2239
Ornade Spansule Capsules 2502
Orudis Capsules (Less than 1%) 2766
Oruvail Capsules (Less than 1%) 2766
▲ PBZ Tablets (Among most frequent) 845
▲ PBZ-SR Tablets (Among most frequent) 844
Pamelor 2280
Paremyd ◉ 247
▲ Parlodel (4%) 2281
Parnate Tablets 2503
▲ Paxil Tablets (10.8% to 20.6%) 2505
Penetrex Tablets (Less than 1% but more than or equal to 0.1%) 2031
Pepcid Injection (Infrequent) 1722
Pepcid (Infrequent) 1720
Periactin 1724
▲ Permax Tablets (3.7%; frequent) 575
Phenergan with Codeine 2777
Phenergan with Dextromethorphan 2778
Phenergan Injection 2773
Phenergan Suppositories 2775
Phenergan Syrup 2774
Phenergan Tablets 2775
Phenergan VC 2779
Phenergan VC with Codeine 2781
Phrenilin (Infrequent) 785
Plendil Extended-Release Tablets (0.5% to 1.5%) 527
Pondimin Tablets (Among most common) 2066
Prelu-2 Timed Release Capsules 681
PREVACID Delayed-Release Capsules (Less than 1%) 2562
Prilosec Delayed-Release Capsules (Less than 1%) 529
Prinivil Tablets (0.3% to 1.0%) 1733
Prinzide Tablets (0.3% to 1%) 1737
Pro-Banthīne Tablets 2052
Procardia XL Extended Release Tablets (Less than 3%) 1972
Prolixin 509
Propulsid (1% or less) 1300
ProSom Tablets (Frequent) 449
Protostat Tablets 1883
▲ Prozac Pulvules & Liquid, Oral Solution (9.5%; at least 5%; 12%) 919
Quarzan Capsules (Among most frequent) 2181
RMS Suppositories 2657
Relafen Tablets (1% to 3%) 2510
ReVia Tablets (Less than 1%) 940
Revex (Less than 1%) 1811
Rhinocort Nasal Inhaler (1 to 3%) 556
Robinul Forte Tablets 2072
Robinul Injectable 2072
Robinul Tablets 2072
Rocaltrol Capsules 2141
▲ Romazicon (3% to 9%) 2147
Rondec Oral Drops 953
Rondec Syrup 953
Rondec Tablet 953
Rondec-DM Oral Drops 954
Rondec-DM Syrup 954
Rondec-TR Tablet 953
Roxanol 2243
▲ Rythmol Tablets–150mg, 225mg, 300mg (0.9 to 5.7%) 1352
▲ Sanorex Tablets (Among most common) 2294
Sedapap Tablets 50 mg/650 mg (Infrequent) 1543
▲ Seldane Tablets (2.3% to 4.8%) 1536
▲ Seldane-D Extended-Release Tablets (21.7%) 1538
▲ Semprex-D Capsules (7%) 463
▲ Semprex-D Capsules (7%) 1167
Ser-Ap-Es Tablets 849
Serentil 684
▲ Serzone Tablets (25%) 771
Sinemet Tablets 943
Sinemet CR Tablets (1.4%) 944
Sinequan 2205
▲ Stadol (3% to 9%) 775
Stelazine 2514
Surmontil Capsules (Rare) 2811
Symmetrel Capsules and Syrup (1% to 5%) 946
Talwin Injection 2334
Tambocor Tablets (Less than 1%) 1497
Tavist Syrup 2297
Tavist Tablets 2298
▲ Tegison Capsules (1-10%) 2154
Tegretol Chewable Tablets 852
Tegretol Suspension 852
Tegretol Tablets 852
Temaril Tablets, Syrup and Spansule Extended-Release Capsules 483
▲ Tenex Tablets (5% to 54%) 2074
Tenoretic Tablets 2845
Thalitone (Common) 1245
Thorazine (Occasional) 2523
THYREL TRH 2873
Tilade (1.0%) 996
Timoptic in Ocudose (Less frequent) 1753
Timoptic Sterile Ophthalmic Solution (Less frequent) 1751
Timoptic-XE 1755
Tofranil Ampuls 854
Tofranil Tablets 856
Tofranil-PM Capsules 857
Tonocard Tablets (Less than 1%) 531
Toprol-XL Tablets (About 1 of 100 patients) 565
Toradol (1% or less) 2159
Torecan 2245
▲ Transderm Scōp Transdermal Therapeutic System (About two-thirds) 869
Tranxene (Less common) 451
Trental Tablets (Less than 1%) 1244
Triaminic Cold Tablets ▣ 790
Triavil Tablets 1757
Trilafon 2389
Trinalin Repetabs Tablets 1330
Tussend 1783
Univasc Tablets (Less than 1%) 2410
Urised Tablets 1964
Urispas Tablets 2532
Vanceril Inhaler (Few patients) 2394
Vantin for Oral Suspension and Vantin Tablets (Less than 1%) 2646
Vascor (200, 300 and 400 mg) Tablets (0.5 to 3.40%) 1587
Vaseretic Tablets (0.5% to 2.0%) 1765
Vasotec I.V. 1768
Vasotec Tablets (0.5% to 1.0%) 1771
Ventolin Rotacaps for Inhalation (Less than 1%) 1200
Ventolin Tablets (Less than 1%) 1203
Verelan Capsules (1% or less) 1410
Verelan Capsules (Less than 1%) 2824
▲ Videx Tablets, Powder for Oral Solution, & Pediatric Powder for Oral Solution (1% to 7%) 720
Vistaril Capsules 1944
Vistaril Intramuscular Solution 2216
Vistaril Oral Suspension 1944
Vivactil Tablets 1774
Voltaren Tablets (Less than 1%) 861
Vontrol Tablets 2532
▲ Wellbutrin Tablets (27.6%) 1204
▲ Xanax Tablets (14.7%) 2649
Zaroxolyn Tablets 1000
Zebeta Tablets (0.7% to 1.3%) 1413
Zestoretic (0.3 to 1%) 2850
Zestril Tablets (0.3% to 1.0%) 2854
Ziac 1415
Zofran Tablets (1% to 2%) 1217
Zoladex (1% or greater) 2858
▲ Zoloft Tablets (16.3%) 2217
▲ Zonalon Cream (Approximately 1% to 10%) 1055

Y

Yawning

Ambien Tablets (Rare) 2416
Anafranil Capsules (Up to 3%) 803
▲ Effexor (3% to 8%) 2719
Imitrex Injection (Rare) 1103
Luvox Tablets (2%) 2544
Methadone Hydrochloride Oral Concentrate 2233
▲ Normodyne Injection (3%) 2377
Orlamm (1% to 3%) 2239
▲ Paxil Tablets (3.8%) 2505
▲ Prozac Pulvules & Liquid, Oral Solution (At least 5% to 7%) 919
ReVia Tablets (Less than 1%) 940
Risperdal (Rare) 1301
Salagen Tablets (Less than 1%) 1489
Serzone Tablets (Rare) 771
Tonocard Tablets (Less than 1%) 531
▲ Trandate Injection (3 of 100 patients) 1185
Versed Injection (Less than 1%) 2170
Zoloft Tablets (1.9%) 2217

(▣ Described in PDR For Nonprescription Drugs) Incidence data in parenthesis; ▲ 3% or more (◉ Described in PDR For Ophthalmology)

SECTION 4

INDICATIONS INDEX

This section lists in alphabetical order every indication cited in *PDR* and its companion volumes, with cross-references to each product entry in which the indication is found. For easy comparison, each listing includes the product's brand name, generic ingredients, and manufacturer. Page numbers refer to the 1996 editions of *PDR* and *PDR For Ophthalmology* and the 1995 edition of *PDR For Nonprescription Drugs*, which is published later each year. A key to the symbols denoting the companion volumes appears in the bottom margin.

Because *PDR* publishes only official product labeling, only approved indications are cited here. No unapproved uses are listed.

This index is intended to assist you in identifying the extent and nature of your prescribing alternatives as quickly and easily as possible. However, it is by its nature only an extract of the official labeling as it appears in *PDR*. For more definitive information, always consult the underlying *PDR* text.

A

Abdominal cramps (see under Cramps, abdominal, symptomatic relief of)

Abdominal distention, unspecified

Gas-X Chewable Tablets (Simethicone) Sandoz Consumer .... ◉ 786

Ku-Zyme Capsules (Enzymes, Digestive) Schwarz 2402

Abdominal distress, symptomatic relief of

Kutrase Capsules (Hyoscyamine Sulfate, Phenyltoloxamine Citrate, Enzymes, Digestive) Schwarz 2402

Levsin/Levsinex/Levbid (Hyoscyamine Sulfate) Schwarz 2405

Abortion, inevitable or incomplete, adjunct to

Oxytocin Injection (Oxytocin) Wyeth-Ayerst 2771

Syntocinon Injection (Oxytocin) Sandoz Pharmaceuticals 2296

Abrasions, pain associated with (see under Pain, topical relief of)

Abrasions, skin (see under Infections, skin, bacterial, minor)

Abruptio placentae, to reduce fibrinolytic bleeding

Amicar Syrup, Tablets, and Injection (Aminocaproic Acid) Immunex 1267

Abscess, hepatic (see also under Infections, intra-abdominal)

Flagyl 375 Capsules (Metronidazole) Searle 2434

Flagyl I.V. (Metronidazole Hydrochloride) SCS 2247

Mezlin (Mezlocillin Sodium) Bayer Pharmaceutical 601

Mezlin Pharmacy Bulk Package (Mezlocillin Sodium) Bayer Pharmaceutical 604

Abscess, intra-abdominal (see also under Infections, intra-abdominal)

Cleocin Phosphate Injection (Clindamycin Phosphate) Upjohn 2586

Flagyl 375 Capsules (Metronidazole) Searle 2434

Flagyl I.V. (Metronidazole Hydrochloride) SCS 2247

Mefoxin (Cefoxitin Sodium) Merck & Co., Inc. 1691

Mefoxin Premixed Intravenous Solution (Cefoxitin Sodium) Merck & Co., Inc. 1694

Mezlin (Mezlocillin Sodium) Bayer Pharmaceutical 601

Mezlin Pharmacy Bulk Package (Mezlocillin Sodium) Bayer Pharmaceutical 604

Netromycin Injection 100 mg/ml (Netilmicin Sulfate) Schering.......... 2373

Abscess, lung (see also under Infections, lower respiratory tract)

Cleocin Phosphate Injection (Clindamycin Phosphate) Upjohn 2586

Flagyl 375 Capsules (Metronidazole) Searle 2434

Flagyl I.V. (Metronidazole Hydrochloride) SCS 2247

Mefoxin (Cefoxitin Sodium) Merck & Co., Inc. 1691

Mefoxin Premixed Intravenous Solution (Cefoxitin Sodium) Merck & Co., Inc. 1694

Mezlin (Mezlocillin Sodium) Bayer Pharmaceutical 601

Mezlin Pharmacy Bulk Package (Mezlocillin Sodium) Bayer Pharmaceutical 604

Ticar for Injection (Ticarcillin Disodium) SmithKline Beecham Pharmaceuticals 2526

Abscess, pelvic

Ticar for Injection (Ticarcillin Disodium) SmithKline Beecham Pharmaceuticals 2526

Abscess, tubo-ovarian (see under Infections, gynecologic)

Accommodation, paralysis of (see under Cycloplegia, production of)

Aches (see under Pain, general)

Aches due to common cold (see under Pain associated with upper respiratory infection)

Aches, muscular (see under Pain, muscular, temporary relief of)

Acid indigestion (see under Hyperacidity, gastric, symptomatic relief of)

Acidosis, metabolic

Bicitra (Sodium Citrate, Citric Acid) Baker Norton 578

Polycitra Syrup (Potassium Citrate, Sodium Citrate, Citric Acid) Baker Norton 578

Polycitra-K Crystals (Potassium Citrate, Citric Acid) Baker Norton 579

Polycitra-K Oral Solution (Potassium Citrate, Citric Acid) Baker Norton 579

Polycitra-LC (Potassium Citrate, Citric Acid, Sodium Citrate) Baker Norton 578

Acinetobacter calcoaceticus infections

Minocin Oral Suspension (Minocycline Hydrochloride) Lederle 1385

Primaxin I.M. (Imipenem-Cilastatin Sodium) Merck & Co., Inc. 1727

Rocephin Injectable Vials, ADD-Vantage, Galaxy Container (Ceftriaxone Sodium) Roche Laboratories 2142

Unasyn (Ampicillin Sodium, Sulbactam Sodium) Roerig 2212

Acinetobacter calcoaceticus infections, ocular

Chibroxin Sterile Ophthalmic Solution (Norfloxacin) Merck & Co., Inc. 1617

TobraDex Ophthalmic Suspension and Ointment (Dexamethasone, Tobramycin) Alcon Laboratories .. 473

Acinetobacter calcoaceticus skin and skin structure infections

Primaxin I.M. (Imipenem-Cilastatin Sodium) Merck & Co., Inc. 1727

Unasyn (Ampicillin Sodium, Sulbactam Sodium) Roerig 2212

(◉ Described in PDR For Nonprescription Drugs) (◎ Described in PDR For Ophthalmology)

Acinetobacter species infections — Indications Index — 1452

Acinetobacter species infections
Achromycin V Capsules (Tetracycline Hydrochloride) Lederle ... 1367
Amikacin Sulfate Injection, USP (Amikacin Sulfate) Elkins-Sinn ... 960
Amikin Injectable (Amikacin Sulfate) Apothecon ... 501
Claforan Sterile and Injection (Cefotaxime Sodium) Hoechst-Roussel ... 1235
Declomycin Tablets (Demeclocycline Hydrochloride) Lederle ... 1371
Doryx Capsules (Doxycycline Hyclate) Parke-Davis ... 1913
Dynacin Capsules (Minocycline Hydrochloride) Medicis ... 1590
Minocin Intravenous (Minocycline Hydrochloride) Lederle ... 1382
Minocin Oral Suspension (Minocycline Hydrochloride) Lederle ... 1385
Minocin Pellet-Filled Capsules (Minocycline Hydrochloride) Lederle ... 1383
Monodox Capsules (Doxycycline Monohydrate) Oclassen ... 1805
Primaxin I.M. (Imipenem-Cilastatin Sodium) Merck & Co., Inc. ... 1727
Primaxin I.V. (Imipenem-Cilastatin Sodium) Merck & Co., Inc. ... 1729
Terramycin Intramuscular Solution (Oxytetracycline) Roerig ... 2210
Vibramycin (Doxycycline Calcium) Pfizer Labs ... 1941
Vibramycin Hyclate Intravenous (Doxycycline Hyclate) Roerig ... 2215
Vibramycin (Doxycycline Monohydrate) Pfizer Labs ... 1941

Acinetobacter species lower respiratory tract infections
Primaxin I.V. (Imipenem-Cilastatin Sodium) Merck & Co., Inc. ... 1729

Acinetobacter species skin and skin structure infections
Claforan Sterile and Injection (Cefotaxime Sodium) Hoechst-Roussel ... 1235
Primaxin I.M. (Imipenem-Cilastatin Sodium) Merck & Co., Inc. ... 1727
Primaxin I.V. (Imipenem-Cilastatin Sodium) Merck & Co., Inc. ... 1729
Rocephin Injectable Vials, ADD-Vantage, Galaxy Container (Ceftriaxone Sodium) Roche Laboratories ... 2142

Acne rosacea
Novacet Lotion (Sulfur, Sulfacetamide Sodium) GenDerm ... 1054
Sulfacet-R MVL Lotion (Sodium Sulfacetamide, Sulfur) Dermik ... 909

Acne rosacea, ocular
AK-Pred (Prednisolone Sodium Phosphate) Akorn ... ◉ 204
Decadron Phosphate Sterile Ophthalmic Ointment (Dexamethasone Sodium Phosphate) Merck & Co., Inc. ... 1641
Decadron Phosphate Sterile Ophthalmic Solution (Dexamethasone Sodium Phosphate) Merck & Co., Inc. ... 1642
Econopred & Econopred Plus Ophthalmic Suspensions (Prednisolone Acetate) Alcon Laboratories ... ◉ 217
Inflamase (Prednisolone Sodium Phosphate) CIBA Vision Ophthalmics ... ◉ 265

Acne vulgaris
A/T/S 2% Acne Topical Gel and Solution (Erythromycin) Hoechst-Roussel ... 1234
Benzac (Benzoyl Peroxide) Galderma ... 1045
Benzamycin Topical Gel (Erythromycin, Benzoyl Peroxide) Dermik ... 905
BenzaShave Medicated Shave Cream 5% and 10% (Benzoyl Peroxide) Medicis ... 1590
Brevoxyl Gel (Benzoyl Peroxide) Stiefel ... 2552
Brevoxyl Cleansing Lotion (Benzoyl Peroxide) Stiefel ... 2553
Cleocin T Topical (Clindamycin Phosphate) Upjohn ... 2590
Declomycin Tablets (Demeclocycline Hydrochloride) Lederle ... 1371
Desquam-E Gel (Benzoyl Peroxide) Westwood-Squibb ... 2684
Desquam-X Gel (Benzoyl Peroxide) Westwood-Squibb ... 2684
Desquam-X 10 Bar (Benzoyl Peroxide) Westwood-Squibb ... 2684
Desquam-X Wash (Benzoyl Peroxide) Westwood-Squibb ... 2684
Doryx Capsules (Doxycycline Hyclate) Parke-Davis ... 1913
Emgel 2% Topical Gel (Erythromycin) Glaxo Wellcome ... 1093
Erycette (erythromycin 2%) Topical Solution (Erythromycin) Ortho Dermatological ... 1888
Exact Vanishing and Tinted Creams (Benzoyl Peroxide) Premier ... ▣ 749
Monodox Capsules (Doxycycline Monohydrate) Oclassen ... 1805
Novacet Lotion (Sulfur, Sulfacetamide Sodium) GenDerm ... 1054
Retin-A (tretinoin) Cream/Gel/Liquid (Tretinoin) Ortho Dermatological ... 1889
SalAc (Salicylic Acid) GenDerm ... 1055
Sulfacet-R MVL Lotion (Sodium Sulfacetamide, Sulfur) Dermik ... 909
T-Stat 2.0% Topical Solution and Pads (Erythromycin) Westwood-Squibb ... 2688
Theramycin Z Topical Solution 2% (Erythromycin) Medicis ... 1592
Triaz 6% and 10% Gels and 10% Cleaner (Benzoyl Peroxide) Medicis ... 1592
Vibramycin (Doxycycline Calcium) Pfizer Labs ... 1941

Acne, cystic, severe recalcitrant
Accutane Capsules (Isotretinoin) Roche Laboratories ... 2076

Acne, nodulocystic, adjunctive treatment for
Desquam-X Gel (Benzoyl Peroxide) Westwood-Squibb ... 2684

Acne, unspecified
Hyland's ClearAc (Homeopathic Medications) Standard Homeopathic ... ▣ 828
Stri-Dex Clear Gel (Salicylic Acid) Miles Consumer ... ▣ 730
Stri-Dex (Salicylic Acid) Miles Consumer ... ▣ 730

Acneiform eruptions, severe, adjunct in
Achromycin V Capsules (Tetracycline Hydrochloride) Lederle ... 1367
Dynacin Capsules (Minocycline Hydrochloride) Medicis ... 1590
Minocin Oral Suspension (Minocycline Hydrochloride) Lederle ... 1385
Minocin Pellet-Filled Capsules (Minocycline Hydrochloride) Lederle ... 1383

Acquired immunodeficiency syndrome (see under Infection, human immunodeficiency virus)

Acromegaly
Parlodel (Bromocriptine Mesylate) Sandoz Pharmaceuticals ... 2281
Sandostatin Injection (Octreotide Acetate) Sandoz Pharmaceuticals ... 2292

ACTH function, hypothalamic-pituitary, testing of (see under Addison's disease, diagnostic testing of)

Actinomyces species infection (see under Actinomycosis)

Actinomycosis
Achromycin V Capsules (Tetracycline Hydrochloride) Lederle ... 1367
Declomycin Tablets (Demeclocycline Hydrochloride) Lederle ... 1371
Doryx Capsules (Doxycycline Hyclate) Parke-Davis ... 1913
Dynacin Capsules (Minocycline Hydrochloride) Medicis ... 1590
Minocin Intravenous (Minocycline Hydrochloride) Lederle ... 1382
Minocin Oral Suspension (Minocycline Hydrochloride) Lederle ... 1385
Minocin Pellet-Filled Capsules (Minocycline Hydrochloride) Lederle ... 1383
Monodox Capsules (Doxycycline Monohydrate) Oclassen ... 1805
Pfizerpen for Injection (Penicillin G Potassium) Roerig ... 2203
Terramycin Intramuscular Solution (Oxytetracycline) Roerig ... 2210
Vibramycin (Doxycycline Calcium) Pfizer Labs ... 1941
Vibramycin Hyclate Intravenous (Doxycycline Hyclate) Roerig ... 2215
Vibramycin (Doxycycline Monohydrate) Pfizer Labs ... 1941

Adam-Stokes attacks
Isuprel Hydrochloride Injection 1:5000 (Isoproterenol Hydrochloride) Sanofi Winthrop ... 2311

Addison's disease (see under Adrenocortical insufficiency, primary or secondary)

Adenocarcinoma, gastrointestinal, palliative management of (see under Carcinoma, gastrointestinal, palliative management of)

Adenomas, prolactin-secreting
Parlodel (Bromocriptine Mesylate) Sandoz Pharmaceuticals ... 2281

Adenosine deaminase, enzyme replacement therapy for
Adagen (pegademase bovine) Injection (Pegademase Bovine) Enzon ... 972

Adrenal cortical carcinoma (see under Carcinoma, adrenal cortex)

Adrenal hyperfunction, suppression of (see under Cushing's syndrome)

Adrenal hyperplasia, congenital
Aristocort Suspension (Forte Parenteral) (Triamcinolone Diacetate) Fujisawa ... 1027
Aristocort Tablets (Triamcinolone) Fujisawa ... 1022
Celestone Soluspan Suspension (Betamethasone Sodium Phosphate, Betamethasone Acetate) Schering ... 2347
Cortone Acetate Sterile Suspension (Cortisone Acetate) Merck & Co., Inc. ... 1623
Cortone Acetate Tablets (Cortisone Acetate) Merck & Co., Inc. ... 1624
Dalalone D.P. Injectable (Dexamethasone Acetate) Forest ... 1011
Decadron Elixir (Dexamethasone) Merck & Co., Inc. ... 1633
Decadron Phosphate Injection (Dexamethasone Sodium Phosphate) Merck & Co., Inc. ... 1637
Decadron Tablets (Dexamethasone) Merck & Co., Inc. ... 1635
Decadron-LA Sterile Suspension (Dexamethasone Acetate) Merck & Co., Inc. ... 1646
Deltasone Tablets (Prednisone) Upjohn ... 2595
Depo-Medrol Single-Dose Vial (Methylprednisolone Acetate) Upjohn ... 2600
Depo-Medrol Sterile Aqueous Suspension (Methylprednisolone Acetate) Upjohn ... 2597
Hydeltrasol Injection, Sterile (Prednisolone Sodium Phosphate) Merck & Co., Inc. ... 1665
Hydrocortone Phosphate Injection, Sterile (Hydrocortisone Sodium Phosphate) Merck & Co., Inc. ... 1670
Hydrocortone Tablets (Hydrocortisone) Merck & Co., Inc. ... 1672
Medrol (Methylprednisolone) Upjohn ... 2621
Pediapred Oral Liquid (Prednisolone Sodium Phosphate) Fisons ... 995
Prelone Syrup (Prednisolone) Muro ... 1787
Solu-Cortef Sterile Powder (Hydrocortisone Sodium Succinate) Upjohn ... 2641
Solu-Medrol Sterile Powder (Methylprednisolone Sodium Succinate) Upjohn ... 2643

Adrenal insufficiency, preoperative
Aristocort Suspension (Forte Parenteral) (Triamcinolone Diacetate) Fujisawa ... 1027
Celestone Soluspan Suspension (Betamethasone Sodium Phosphate, Betamethasone Acetate) Schering ... 2347
Cortone Acetate Sterile Suspension (Cortisone Acetate) Merck & Co., Inc. ... 1623
Decadron Phosphate Injection (Dexamethasone Sodium Phosphate) Merck & Co., Inc. ... 1637
Depo-Medrol Single-Dose Vial (Methylprednisolone Acetate) Upjohn ... 2600
Depo-Medrol Sterile Aqueous Suspension (Methylprednisolone Acetate) Upjohn ... 2597
Hydeltrasol Injection, Sterile (Prednisolone Sodium Phosphate) Merck & Co., Inc. ... 1665
Hydrocortone Phosphate Injection, Sterile (Hydrocortisone Sodium Phosphate) Merck & Co., Inc. ... 1670
Solu-Cortef Sterile Powder (Hydrocortisone Sodium Succinate) Upjohn ... 2641
Solu-Medrol Sterile Powder (Methylprednisolone Sodium Succinate) Upjohn ... 2643

Adrenal insufficiency, serious illness-induced
Aristocort Suspension (Forte Parenteral) (Triamcinolone Diacetate) Fujisawa ... 1027
Cortone Acetate Sterile Suspension (Cortisone Acetate) Merck & Co., Inc. ... 1623
Decadron Phosphate Injection (Dexamethasone Sodium Phosphate) Merck & Co., Inc. ... 1637
Depo-Medrol Single-Dose Vial (Methylprednisolone Acetate) Upjohn ... 2600
Depo-Medrol Sterile Aqueous Suspension (Methylprednisolone Acetate) Upjohn ... 2597
Hydeltrasol Injection, Sterile (Prednisolone Sodium Phosphate) Merck & Co., Inc. ... 1665
Hydrocortone Phosphate Injection, Sterile (Hydrocortisone Sodium Phosphate) Merck & Co., Inc. ... 1670
Solu-Cortef Sterile Powder (Hydrocortisone Sodium Succinate) Upjohn ... 2641
Solu-Medrol Sterile Powder (Methylprednisolone Sodium Succinate) Upjohn ... 2643

Adrenal insufficiency, serious trauma-induced
Aristocort Suspension (Forte Parenteral) (Triamcinolone Diacetate) Fujisawa ... 1027
Cortone Acetate Sterile Suspension (Cortisone Acetate) Merck & Co., Inc. ... 1623
Decadron Phosphate Injection (Dexamethasone Sodium Phosphate) Merck & Co., Inc. ... 1637
Depo-Medrol Single-Dose Vial (Methylprednisolone Acetate) Upjohn ... 2600
Depo-Medrol Sterile Aqueous Suspension (Methylprednisolone Acetate) Upjohn ... 2597
Hydeltrasol Injection, Sterile (Prednisolone Sodium Phosphate) Merck & Co., Inc. ... 1665
Hydrocortone Phosphate Injection, Sterile (Hydrocortisone Sodium Phosphate) Merck & Co., Inc. ... 1670
Solu-Cortef Sterile Powder (Hydrocortisone Sodium Succinate) Upjohn ... 2641
Solu-Medrol Sterile Powder (Methylprednisolone Sodium Succinate) Upjohn ... 2643

(▣ Described in PDR For Nonprescription Drugs) (◉ Described in PDR For Ophthalmology)

1453 **Indications Index** **Amebiasis**

Adrenocortical hyperfunction, diagnostic testing of
Decadron Elixir (Dexamethasone) Merck & Co., Inc. ... 1633
Decadron Phosphate Injection (Dexamethasone Sodium Phosphate) Merck & Co., Inc. ... 1637
Decadron Tablets (Dexamethasone) Merck & Co., Inc. ... 1635

Adrenocortical insufficiency, acute
Cortone Acetate Sterile Suspension (Cortisone Acetate) Merck & Co., Inc. ... 1623
Decadron Phosphate Injection (Dexamethasone Sodium Phosphate) Merck & Co., Inc. ... 1637
Depo-Medrol Single-Dose Vial (Methylprednisolone Acetate) Upjohn ... 2600
Depo-Medrol Sterile Aqueous Suspension (Methylprednisolone Acetate) Upjohn ... 2597
Hydeltrasol Injection, Sterile (Prednisolone Sodium Phosphate) Merck & Co., Inc. ... 1665
Hydrocortone Phosphate Injection, Sterile (Hydrocortisone Sodium Phosphate) Merck & Co., Inc. ... 1670
Solu-Cortef Sterile Powder (Hydrocortisone Sodium Succinate) Upjohn ... 2641
Solu-Medrol Sterile Powder (Methylprednisolone Sodium Succinate) Upjohn ... 2643

Adrenocortical insufficiency, primary or secondary
Aristocort Suspension (Forte Parenteral) (Triamcinolone Diacetate) Fujisawa ... 1027
Aristocort Tablets (Triamcinolone) Fujisawa ... 1022
Celestone Soluspan Suspension (Betamethasone Sodium Phosphate, Betamethasone Acetate) Schering ... 2347
Cortone Acetate Sterile Suspension (Cortisone Acetate) Merck & Co., Inc. ... 1623
Cortone Acetate Tablets (Cortisone Acetate) Merck & Co., Inc. ... 1624
Decadron Elixir (Dexamethasone) Merck & Co., Inc. ... 1633
Decadron Phosphate Injection (Dexamethasone Sodium Phosphate) Merck & Co., Inc. ... 1637
Decadron Tablets (Dexamethasone) Merck & Co., Inc. ... 1635
Deltasone Tablets (Prednisone) Upjohn ... 2595
Depo-Medrol Single-Dose Vial (Methylprednisolone Acetate) Upjohn ... 2600
Depo-Medrol Sterile Aqueous Suspension (Methylprednisolone Acetate) Upjohn ... 2597
Florinef Acetate Tablets (Fludrocortisone Acetate) Apothecon ... 505
Hydeltrasol Injection, Sterile (Prednisolone Sodium Phosphate) Merck & Co., Inc. ... 1665
Hydrocortone Phosphate Injection, Sterile (Hydrocortisone Sodium Phosphate) Merck & Co., Inc. ... 1670
Hydrocortone Tablets (Hydrocortisone) Merck & Co., Inc. ... 1672
Medrol (Methylprednisolone) Upjohn ... 2621
Pediapred Oral Liquid (Prednisolone Sodium Phosphate) Fisons ... 995
Prelone Syrup (Prednisolone) Muro 1787
Solu-Cortef Sterile Powder (Hydrocortisone Sodium Succinate) Upjohn ... 2641
Solu-Medrol Sterile Powder (Methylprednisolone Sodium Succinate) Upjohn ... 2643

Adrenogenital syndrome, salt-losing
Florinef Acetate Tablets (Fludrocortisone Acetate) Apothecon ... 505

Adynamic ileus (see under Ileus, paralytic)

Aerobacter aerogenes infections (see under Enterobacter aerogenes infections)

Aeromonas hydrophila infections, ocular
Chibroxin Sterile Ophthalmic Solution (Norfloxacin) Merck & Co., Inc. ... 1617

Agammaglobulinemias, congenital
Gamimune N, 5% Immune Globulin Intravenous (Human), 5% (Globulin, Immune (Human)) Bayer Biological ... 619
Gamimune N, 10% Immune Globulin Intravenous (Human), 10% (Globulin, Immune (Human)) Bayer Biological ... 621
Gammagard S/D, Immune Globulin, Intravenous (Human) (Globulin, Immune (Human)) Baxter Healthcare ... 585
Gammar, Immune Globulin (Human) U.S.P. (Globulin, Immune (Human)) Armour ... 515
Gammar I.V., Immune Globulin Intravenous (Human), Lyophilized (Globulin, Immune (Human)) Armour ... 516

AIDS (see under Infection, human immunodeficiency virus)

AIDS related complex (see under Infection, acquired immunodeficiency syndrome-related complex)

Airway obstruction disorders (see under Bronchial asthma; Emphysema)

Albinism (see under Hypopigmentation, skin)

Alcohol withdrawal, acute, symptomatic relief of
Dizac (Diazepam) Ohmeda ... 1809
Libritabs Tablets (Chlordiazepoxide) Roche Products ... 2177
Librium Capsules (Chlordiazepoxide Hydrochloride) Roche Products ... 2178
Librium Injectable (Chlordiazepoxide Hydrochloride) Roche Products ... 2179
Serax Capsules (Oxazepam) Wyeth-Ayerst ... 2810
Serax Tablets (Oxazepam) Wyeth-Ayerst ... 2810
Tranxene (Clorazepate Dipotassium) Abbott ... 451
Valium Injectable (Diazepam) Roche Products ... 2182
Valium Tablets (Diazepam) Roche Products ... 2183
Vistaril Intramuscular Solution (Hydroxyzine Hydrochloride) Roerig ... 2216

Alcoholism, acute, amelioration of manifestations of
Serentil (Mesoridazine Besylate) Boehringer Ingelheim ... 684
Vistaril Intramuscular Solution (Hydroxyzine Hydrochloride) Roerig ... 2216

Alcoholism, chronic, an aid in the management of
Antabuse Tablets (Disulfiram) Wyeth-Ayerst ... 2695
ReVia Tablets (Naltrexone Hydrochloride) DuPont ... 940
Serentil (Mesoridazine Besylate) Boehringer Ingelheim ... 684
Vistaril Intramuscular Solution (Hydroxyzine Hydrochloride) Roerig ... 2216

Allergic reactions associated with blood or plasma
Benadryl Capsules (Diphenhydramine Hydrochloride) Parke-Davis 1898
Benadryl Injection (Diphenhydramine Hydrochloride) Parke-Davis 1898
PBZ Tablets (Tripelennamine Hydrochloride) CibaGeneva ... 845
PBZ-SR Tablets (Tripelennamine Hydrochloride) CibaGeneva ... 844
Periactin (Cyproheptadine Hydrochloride) Merck & Co., Inc. 1724
Phenergan Injection (Promethazine Hydrochloride) Wyeth-Ayerst ... 2773
Phenergan Suppositories (Promethazine Hydrochloride) Wyeth-Ayerst ... 2775
Phenergan Syrup (Promethazine Hydrochloride) Wyeth-Ayerst ... 2774
Phenergan Tablets (Promethazine Hydrochloride) Wyeth-Ayerst ... 2775

Allergic reactions, drug-induced (see under Hypersensitivity reactions, drug-induced)

Allergic reactions, general
Ana-Kit Anaphylaxis Emergency Treatment Kit (Epinephrine Hydrochloride, Chlorpheniramine Maleate) Bayer Allergy ... 617
Aristocort Suspension (Forte Parenteral) (Triamcinolone Diacetate) Fujisawa ... 1027
Aristocort Tablets (Triamcinolone) Fujisawa ... 1022
Benadryl Capsules (Diphenhydramine Hydrochloride) Parke-Davis 1898
Celestone Soluspan Suspension (Betamethasone Sodium Phosphate, Betamethasone Acetate) Schering ... 2347
Cortone Acetate Sterile Suspension (Cortisone Acetate) Merck & Co., Inc. ... 1623
Cortone Acetate Tablets (Cortisone Acetate) Merck & Co., Inc. ... 1624
Dalalone D.P. Injectable (Dexamethasone Acetate) Forest ... 1011
Decadron Elixir (Dexamethasone) Merck & Co., Inc. ... 1633
Decadron Phosphate Injection (Dexamethasone Sodium Phosphate) Merck & Co., Inc. ... 1637
Decadron Tablets (Dexamethasone) Merck & Co., Inc. ... 1635
Decadron-LA Sterile Suspension (Dexamethasone Acetate) Merck & Co., Inc. ... 1646
Deltasone Tablets (Prednisone) Upjohn ... 2595
Depo-Medrol Single-Dose Vial (Methylprednisolone Acetate) Upjohn ... 2600
Depo-Medrol Sterile Aqueous Suspension (Methylprednisolone Acetate) Upjohn ... 2597
EpiPen (Epinephrine) Center ... 790
Hydeltrasol Injection, Sterile (Prednisolone Sodium Phosphate) Merck & Co., Inc. ... 1665
Hydrocortone Phosphate Injection, Sterile (Hydrocortisone Sodium Phosphate) Merck & Co., Inc. ... 1670
Hydrocortone Tablets (Hydrocortisone) Merck & Co., Inc. ... 1672
Medrol (Methylprednisolone) Upjohn ... 2621
Pediapred Oral Liquid (Prednisolone Sodium Phosphate) Fisons ... 995
Phenergan Injection (Promethazine Hydrochloride) Wyeth-Ayerst ... 2773
Prelone Syrup (Prednisolone) Muro 1787
Solu-Cortef Sterile Powder (Hydrocortisone Sodium Succinate) Upjohn ... 2641
Solu-Medrol Sterile Powder (Methylprednisolone Sodium Succinate) Upjohn ... 2643
Vistaril Intramuscular Solution (Hydroxyzine Hydrochloride) Roerig ... 2216

Allergic rhinitis (see under Rhinitis, allergic)

Allescheriosis (see under Pseudoallescheriosis)

Alopecia, androgenetic
Rogaine Topical Solution (Minoxidil) Upjohn ... 2637

Alopecia areata
Aristocort Suspension (Forte Parenteral) (Triamcinolone Diacetate) Fujisawa ... 1027
Aristocort Suspension (Intralesional) (Triamcinolone Diacetate) Fujisawa ... 1025
Aristospan Suspension (Intralesional) (Triamcinolone Hexacetonide) Fujisawa ... 1032
Celestone Soluspan Suspension (Betamethasone Sodium Phosphate, Betamethasone Acetate) Schering ... 2347
Decadron Phosphate Injection (Dexamethasone Sodium Phosphate) Merck & Co., Inc. ... 1637
Decadron-LA Sterile Suspension (Dexamethasone Acetate) Merck & Co., Inc. ... 1646
Depo-Medrol Single-Dose Vial (Methylprednisolone Acetate) Upjohn ... 2600
Depo-Medrol Sterile Aqueous Suspension (Methylprednisolone Acetate) Upjohn ... 2597
Hydeltrasol Injection, Sterile (Prednisolone Sodium Phosphate) Merck & Co., Inc. ... 1665
Hydrocortone Acetate Sterile Suspension (Hydrocortisone Acetate) Merck & Co., Inc. ... 1669

Alzheimer's disease (see under Dementia, Alzheimer's type)

Amebiasis, acute intestinal
E.E.S. (Erythromycin Ethylsuccinate) Abbott ... 424
E-Mycin Tablets (Erythromycin) Knoll Laboratories ... 1341
ERYC (Erythromycin) Parke-Davis .. 1915
EryPed (Erythromycin Ethylsuccinate) Abbott ... 421
Ery-Tab Tablets (Erythromycin) Abbott ... 422
Erythrocin Stearate Filmtab (Erythromycin Stearate) Abbott ... 425
Erythromycin Base Filmtab (Erythromycin) Abbott ... 426
Erythromycin Delayed-Release Capsules, USP (Erythromycin) Abbott ... 427
Flagyl 375 Capsules (Metronidazole) Searle ... 2434
Ilosone (Erythromycin Estolate) Dista ... 911
PCE Dispertab Tablets (Erythromycin) Abbott ... 444
Protostat Tablets (Metronidazole) Ortho Pharmaceutical ... 1883
Terramycin Intramuscular Solution (Oxytetracycline) Roerig ... 2210
Yodoxin (Iodoquinol) Glenwood ... 1230

Amebiasis, acute intestinal, adjunct in
Achromycin V Capsules (Tetracycline Hydrochloride) Lederle ... 1367
Declomycin Tablets (Demeclocycline Hydrochloride) Lederle ... 1371
Doryx Capsules (Doxycycline Hyclate) Parke-Davis ... 1913
Dynacin Capsules (Minocycline Hydrochloride) Medicis ... 1590
Minocin Intravenous (Minocycline Hydrochloride) Lederle ... 1382
Minocin Oral Suspension (Minocycline Hydrochloride) Lederle ... 1385
Minocin Pellet-Filled Capsules (Minocycline Hydrochloride) Lederle ... 1383
Monodox Capsules (Doxycycline Monohydrate) Oclassen ... 1805
Vibramycin (Doxycycline Calcium) Pfizer Labs ... 1941
Vibramycin Hyclate Intravenous (Doxycycline Hyclate) Roerig ... 2215
Vibramycin (Doxycycline Monohydrate) Pfizer Labs ... 1941

Amebiasis, extraintestinal
Aralen Hydrochloride Injection (Chloroquine Hydrochloride) Sanofi Winthrop ... 2301
Aralen Phosphate Tablets (Chloroquine Phosphate) Sanofi Winthrop ... 2301

Amebic liver abscess — Indications Index — 1454

Amebic liver abscess
Flagyl 375 Capsules (Metronidazole) Searle ... 2434
Protostat Tablets (Metronidazole) Ortho Pharmaceutical ... 1883

Amenorrhea with galactorrhea
Parlodel (Bromocriptine Mesylate) Sandoz Pharmaceuticals ... 2281

Amenorrhea with hypogonadism
Parlodel (Bromocriptine Mesylate) Sandoz Pharmaceuticals ... 2281

Amenorrhea with infertility
Parlodel (Bromocriptine Mesylate) Sandoz Pharmaceuticals ... 2281

Amenorrhea without galactorrhea
Parlodel (Bromocriptine Mesylate) Sandoz Pharmaceuticals ... 2281

Amenorrhea without infertility
Parlodel (Bromocriptine Mesylate) Sandoz Pharmaceuticals ... 2281

Amenorrhea, primary, hypothalamic
Lutrepulse for Injection (Gonadorelin Acetate) Ferring ... 980

Amenorrhea, secondary
Amen Tablets (Medroxyprogesterone Acetate) Carnrick ... 780
Aygestin Tablets (Norethindrone Acetate) ESI Lederle ... 974
Cycrin Tablets (Medroxyprogesterone Acetate) ESI Lederle ... 975
Provera Tablets (Medroxyprogesterone Acetate) Upjohn ... 2636

Analgesia (see under Pain, general)

Anaphylactic reactions, adjunctive therapy in
Benadryl Capsules (Diphenhydramine Hydrochloride) Parke-Davis 1898
Benadryl Injection (Diphenhydramine Hydrochloride) Parke-Davis 1898
PBZ Tablets (Tripelennamine Hydrochloride) CibaGeneva ... 845
PBZ-SR Tablets (Tripelennamine Hydrochloride) CibaGeneva ... 844
Periactin (Cyproheptadine Hydrochloride) Merck & Co., Inc. 1724
Phenergan Injection (Promethazine Hydrochloride) Wyeth-Ayerst ... 2773
Phenergan Suppositories (Promethazine Hydrochloride) Wyeth-Ayerst ... 2775
Phenergan Syrup (Promethazine Hydrochloride) Wyeth-Ayerst ... 2774
Phenergan Tablets (Promethazine Hydrochloride) Wyeth-Ayerst ... 2775

Anaphylactic shock, due to insect bite
Ana-Kit Anaphylaxis Emergency Treatment Kit (Epinephrine Hydrochloride, Chlorpheniramine Maleate) Bayer Allergy ... 617

Anaphylactoid reactions
Ana-Kit Anaphylaxis Emergency Treatment Kit (Epinephrine Hydrochloride, Chlorpheniramine Maleate) Bayer Allergy ... 617
EpiPen (Epinephrine) Center ... 790

Anaphylaxis, idiopathic
Ana-Kit Anaphylaxis Emergency Treatment Kit (Epinephrine Hydrochloride, Chlorpheniramine Maleate) Bayer Allergy ... 617
EpiPen (Epinephrine) Center ... 790

Anaphylaxis, treatment of
Ana-Kit Anaphylaxis Emergency Treatment Kit (Epinephrine Hydrochloride, Chlorpheniramine Maleate) Bayer Allergy ... 617
EpiPen (Epinephrine) Center ... 790

Ancylostoma duodenale infections
Mintezol (Thiabendazole) Merck & Co., Inc. ... 1704
Vermox Chewable Tablets (Mebendazole) Janssen ... 1312

Androgen, absence or deficiency of
Android Capsules, 10 mg (Methyltestosterone) ICN ... 1250
Android (Methyltestosterone) ICN .. 1251
Delatestryl Injection (Testosterone Enanthate) Bio-Technology General ... 2860
Halotestin Tablets (Fluoxymesterone) Upjohn ... 2614

Anemia associated with chronic renal failure
Epogen for Injection (Epoetin Alfa) Amgen ... 489
Procrit for Injection (Epoetin Alfa) Ortho Biotech ... 1841

Anemia, aplastic, moderate to severe (see also under Anemia, aplastic)
Atgam Sterile Solution (Lymphocyte Immune Globulin Anti-Thymocyte Globulin (Equine)) Upjohn ... 2581

Anemia, chemotherapy-induced in cancer patients
Epogen for Injection (Epoetin Alfa) Amgen ... 489
Procrit for Injection (Epoetin Alfa) Ortho Biotech ... 1841

Anemia, hemolytic, acquired
Aristocort Suspension (Forte Parenteral) (Triamcinolone Diacetate) Fujisawa ... 1027
Aristocort Tablets (Triamcinolone) Fujisawa ... 1022
Celestone Soluspan Suspension (Betamethasone Sodium Phosphate, Betamethasone Acetate) Schering ... 2347
Cortone Acetate Sterile Suspension (Cortisone Acetate) Merck & Co., Inc. ... 1623
Cortone Acetate Tablets (Cortisone Acetate) Merck & Co., Inc. ... 1624
Dalalone D.P. Injectable (Dexamethasone Acetate) Forest ... 1011
Decadron Elixir (Dexamethasone) Merck & Co., Inc. ... 1633
Decadron Phosphate Injection (Dexamethasone Sodium Phosphate) Merck & Co., Inc. ... 1637
Decadron Tablets (Dexamethasone) Merck & Co., Inc. ... 1635
Decadron-LA Sterile Suspension (Dexamethasone Acetate) Merck & Co., Inc. ... 1646
Deltasone Tablets (Prednisone) Upjohn ... 2595
Depo-Medrol Single-Dose Vial (Methylprednisolone Acetate) Upjohn ... 2600
Depo-Medrol Sterile Aqueous Suspension (Methylprednisolone Acetate) Upjohn ... 2597
Hydeltrasol Injection, Sterile (Prednisolone Sodium Phosphate) Merck & Co., Inc. ... 1665
Hydrocortone Phosphate Injection, Sterile (Hydrocortisone Sodium Phosphate) Merck & Co., Inc. ... 1670
Hydrocortone Tablets (Hydrocortisone) Merck & Co., Inc. ... 1672
Medrol (Methylprednisolone) Upjohn ... 2621
Pediapred Oral Liquid (Prednisolone Sodium Phosphate) Fisons ... 995
Prelone Syrup (Prednisolone) Muro 1787
Solu-Cortef Sterile Powder (Hydrocortisone Sodium Succinate) Upjohn ... 2641
Solu-Medrol Sterile Powder (Methylprednisolone Sodium Succinate) Upjohn ... 2643

Anemia, hypoplastic, congenital
Aristocort Suspension (Forte Parenteral) (Triamcinolone Diacetate) Fujisawa ... 1027
Aristocort Tablets (Triamcinolone) Fujisawa ... 1022
Celestone Soluspan Suspension (Betamethasone Sodium Phosphate, Betamethasone Acetate) Schering ... 2347
Cortone Acetate Sterile Suspension (Cortisone Acetate) Merck & Co., Inc. ... 1623
Cortone Acetate Tablets (Cortisone Acetate) Merck & Co., Inc. ... 1624
Dalalone D.P. Injectable (Dexamethasone Acetate) Forest ... 1011
Decadron Elixir (Dexamethasone) Merck & Co., Inc. ... 1633
Decadron Phosphate Injection (Dexamethasone Sodium Phosphate) Merck & Co., Inc. ... 1637
Decadron Tablets (Dexamethasone) Merck & Co., Inc. ... 1635
Decadron-LA Sterile Suspension (Dexamethasone Acetate) Merck & Co., Inc. ... 1646
Deltasone Tablets (Prednisone) Upjohn ... 2595
Depo-Medrol Single-Dose Vial (Methylprednisolone Acetate) Upjohn ... 2600
Depo-Medrol Sterile Aqueous Suspension (Methylprednisolone Acetate) Upjohn ... 2597
Hydeltrasol Injection, Sterile (Prednisolone Sodium Phosphate) Merck & Co., Inc. ... 1665
Hydrocortone Phosphate Injection, Sterile (Hydrocortisone Sodium Phosphate) Merck & Co., Inc. ... 1670
Hydrocortone Tablets (Hydrocortisone) Merck & Co., Inc. ... 1672
Medrol (Methylprednisolone) Upjohn ... 2621
Pediapred Oral Liquid (Prednisolone Sodium Phosphate) Fisons ... 995
Prelone Syrup (Prednisolone) Muro 1787
Solu-Cortef Sterile Powder (Hydrocortisone Sodium Succinate) Upjohn ... 2641
Solu-Medrol Sterile Powder (Methylprednisolone Sodium Succinate) Upjohn ... 2643

Anemia, iron deficiency
Chromagen Capsules (Ferrous Fumarate, Vitamin C, Vitamin B_{12}) Savage ... 2339
Feosol Capsules (Ferrous Sulfate) SmithKline Beecham ... 2456
Feosol Elixir (Ferrous Sulfate) SmithKline Beecham ... 2456
Feosol Tablets (Ferrous Sulfate) SmithKline Beecham ... 2457
Fergon Iron Supplement Tablets (Ferrous Gluconate) Miles Consumer ... ▣ 721
Fero-Grad-500 Filmtab (Ferrous Sulfate, Vitamin C) Abbott ... 429
Fero-Gradumet Filmtab (Ferrous Sulfate) Abbott ... 429
Ferro-Sequels (Ferrous Fumarate, Docusate Sodium) Lederle Consumer ... ▣ 669
Iberet Tablets (Vitamin B Complex With Vitamin C, Ferrous Sulfate) Abbott ... 433
Iberet (Vitamin B Complex With Vitamin C, Ferrous Sulfate) Abbott ... 433
May-Vita Elixir (Vitamins with Minerals) Mayrand ... 1543
Niferex-150 Capsules (Polysaccharide-Iron Complex) Central ... 793
Niferex (Polysaccharide-Iron Complex) Central ... 793
Nu-Iron 150 Capsules (Polysaccharide-Iron Complex) Mayrand ... 1543
Nu-Iron Elixir (Polysaccharide-Iron Complex) Mayrand ... 1543
Slow Fe Tablets (Ferrous Sulfate) Ciba Self-Medication ... 869
Slow Fe with Folic Acid (Ferrous Sulfate, Folic Acid) Ciba Self-Medication ... 869
Trinsicon Capsules (Vitamins with Iron) UCB ... 2570
Vitron-C Tablets (Ferrous Fumarate, Vitamin C) CIBA Consumer ▣ 650

Anemia, megaloblastic, due to folic acid deficiency
Leucovorin Calcium for Injection, Wellcovorin Brand (Leucovorin Calcium) Glaxo Wellcome ... 1132
Leucovorin Calcium for Injection (Leucovorin Calcium) Immunex ... 1268

Anemia, pernicious
Trinsicon Capsules (Vitamins with Iron) UCB ... 2570

Anemia, AZT-treated HIV-infected patients, treatment of
Epogen for Injection (Epoetin Alfa) Amgen ... 489
Procrit for Injection (Epoetin Alfa) Ortho Biotech ... 1841

Anemia, RBC (see under Erythroblastopenia)

Anemia, uterine leiomyomata-induced, preoperative adjunct
Lupron Depot 3.75 mg (Leuprolide Acetate) TAP ... 2556

Anesthesia, general
Alfenta Injection (Alfentanil Hydrochloride) Janssen ... 1286
Brevital Sodium Vials (Methohexital Sodium) Lilly ... 1429
Diprivan Injection (Propofol) Zeneca ... 2833
Fluothane (Halothane) Wyeth-Ayerst ... 2724
Sublimaze Injection (Fentanyl Citrate) Janssen ... 1307
Sufenta Injection (Sufentanil Citrate) Janssen ... 1309
Suprane (Desflurane) Ohmeda ... 1813
Versed Injection (Midazolam Hydrochloride) Roche Laboratories ... 2170

Anesthesia, general, adjunct in
Alfenta Injection (Alfentanil Hydrochloride) Janssen ... 1286
Anectine (Succinylcholine Chloride) Glaxo Wellcome ... 1073
Atarax Tablets & Syrup (Hydroxyzine Hydrochloride) Roerig ... 2185
Ativan Injection (Lorazepam) Wyeth-Ayerst ... 2698
Brevital Sodium Vials (Methohexital Sodium) Lilly ... 1429
Demerol (Meperidine Hydrochloride) Sanofi Winthrop .. 2308
Inapsine Injection (Droperidol) Janssen ... 1296
Levo-Dromoran (Levorphanol Tartrate) Roche Laboratories ... 2129
Levsin Injection (Hyoscyamine Sulfate) Schwarz ... 2405
Mepergan Injection (Meperidine Hydrochloride, Promethazine Hydrochloride) Wyeth-Ayerst ... 2753
Metubine Iodide Vials (Metocurine Iodide) Dista ... 916
Mivacron (Mivacurium Chloride) Glaxo Wellcome ... 1138
Nembutal Sodium Capsules (Pentobarbital Sodium) Abbott ... 436
Nembutal Sodium Solution (Pentobarbital Sodium) Abbott ... 438
Norcuron (Vecuronium Bromide) Organon ... 1826
Nubain Injection (Nalbuphine Hydrochloride) DuPont ... 935
Numorphan Injection (Oxymorphone Hydrochloride) DuPont ... 936
Nuromax Injection (Doxacurium Chloride) Glaxo Wellcome ... 1149
Phenergan Injection (Promethazine Hydrochloride) Wyeth-Ayerst ... 2773
Phenergan Suppositories (Promethazine Hydrochloride) Wyeth-Ayerst ... 2775
Phenergan Syrup (Promethazine Hydrochloride) Wyeth-Ayerst ... 2774
Phenergan Tablets (Promethazine Hydrochloride) Wyeth-Ayerst ... 2775
Robinul Injectable (Glycopyrrolate) Robins ... 2072
Seconal Sodium Pulvules (Secobarbital Sodium) Lilly ... 1474
Sublimaze Injection (Fentanyl Citrate) Janssen ... 1307
Talwin Injection (Pentazocine Lactate) Sanofi Winthrop ... 2334
Thorazine (Chlorpromazine Hydrochloride) SmithKline Beecham Pharmaceuticals ... 2523
Tracrium Injection (Atracurium Besylate) Glaxo Wellcome ... 1183
Vasoxyl Injection (Methoxamine Hydrochloride) Glaxo Wellcome ... 1196
Versed Injection (Midazolam Hydrochloride) Roche Laboratories ... 2170
Zemuron (Rocuronium Bromide) Organon ... 1830

Anesthesia, general, supplement to (see under Anesthesia, general, adjunct in)

(▣ Described in PDR For Nonprescription Drugs) (⊙ Described in PDR For Ophthalmology)

1455 Indications Index Ankylosing spondylitis

Anesthesia, local
Americaine Anesthetic Lubricant (Benzocaine) Fisons 983
Carbocaine Hydrochloride Injection (Mepivacaine Hydrochloride Injection) Sanofi Winthrop 2303
Cocaine Hydrochloride Topical Solution (Cocaine Hydrochloride) Astra 537
Duranest Injections (Etidocaine Hydrochloride) Astra 542
Dyclone 0.5% and 1% Topical Solutions, USP (Dyclonine Hydrochloride) Astra 544
Hurricaine (Benzocaine) Beutlich 666
Hurricaine Topical (Benzocaine) Beutlich 666
Marcaine Hydrochloride with Epinephrine 1:200,000 (Bupivacaine Hydrochloride, Epinephrine) Sanofi Winthrop 2316
Marcaine Hydrochloride Injection (Bupivacaine Hydrochloride) Sanofi Winthrop 2316
Nescaine/Nescaine MPF (Chloroprocaine Hydrochloride) Astra 554
Sensorcaine (Bupivacaine Hydrochloride, Epinephrine Bitartrate) Astra 559
Xylocaine Injections (Lidocaine Hydrochloride) Astra 567

Anesthesia, local, adjunct in
Diprivan Injection (Propofol) Zeneca 2833
Levsin Injection (Hyoscyamine Sulfate) Schwarz 2405
Mepergan Injection (Meperidine Hydrochloride, Promethazine Hydrochloride) Wyeth-Ayerst 2753
Neo-Synephrine Hydrochloride 1% Carpuject (Phenylephrine Hydrochloride) Sanofi Winthrop 2324
Neo-Synephrine Hydrochloride 1% Injection (Phenylephrine Hydrochloride) Sanofi Winthrop 2324
Phenergan Injection (Promethazine Hydrochloride) Wyeth-Ayerst 2773

Anesthesia, local, diagnostic procedures
Marcaine Hydrochloride with Epinephrine 1:200,000 (Bupivacaine Hydrochloride, Epinephrine) Sanofi Winthrop 2316
Marcaine Hydrochloride Injection (Bupivacaine Hydrochloride) Sanofi Winthrop 2316
Sensorcaine (Bupivacaine Hydrochloride, Epinephrine Bitartrate) Astra 559

Anesthesia, local, laryngeal
Cocaine Hydrochloride Topical Solution (Cocaine Hydrochloride) Astra 537

Anesthesia, local, nasal cavities
Cocaine Hydrochloride Topical Solution (Cocaine Hydrochloride) Astra 537

Anesthesia, local, obstetrical procedures
Americaine Anesthetic Lubricant (Benzocaine) Fisons 983
Marcaine Hydrochloride with Epinephrine 1:200,000 (Bupivacaine Hydrochloride, Epinephrine) Sanofi Winthrop 2316
Marcaine Hydrochloride Injection (Bupivacaine Hydrochloride) Sanofi Winthrop 2316
Sensorcaine (Bupivacaine Hydrochloride, Epinephrine Bitartrate) Astra 559

Anesthesia, local, ocular
Fluoracaine (Fluorescein Sodium, Proparacaine Hydrochloride) Akorn ..... ◉ 206
Ophthetic (Proparacaine Hydrochloride) Allergan ..... ◉ 247

Anesthesia, local, oral cavity
Cocaine Hydrochloride Topical Solution (Cocaine Hydrochloride) Astra 537
Dyclone 0.5% and 1% Topical Solutions, USP (Dyclonine Hydrochloride) Astra 544
Hurricaine (Benzocaine) Beutlich 666
Hurricaine Topical (Benzocaine) Beutlich 666

Anesthesia, local, oral surgical procedures
Marcaine Hydrochloride with Epinephrine 1:200,000 (Bupivacaine Hydrochloride, Epinephrine) Sanofi Winthrop 2316
Marcaine Hydrochloride Injection (Bupivacaine Hydrochloride) Sanofi Winthrop 2316
Sensorcaine (Bupivacaine Hydrochloride, Epinephrine Bitartrate) Astra 559

Anesthesia, local, pharyngeal
Americaine Anesthetic Lubricant (Benzocaine) Fisons 983
Dyclone 0.5% and 1% Topical Solutions, USP (Dyclonine Hydrochloride) Astra 544
Hurricaine (Benzocaine) Beutlich 666
Hurricaine Topical (Benzocaine) Beutlich 666

Anesthesia, local, spinal
Marcaine Spinal (Bupivacaine Hydrochloride) Sanofi Winthrop 2319
Novocain Hydrochloride for Spinal Anesthesia (Procaine Hydrochloride) Sanofi Winthrop 2326
Sensorcaine (Bupivacaine Hydrochloride, Epinephrine Bitartrate) Astra 559

Anesthesia, local, spinal, adjunct in
Neo-Synephrine Hydrochloride 1% Carpuject (Phenylephrine Hydrochloride) Sanofi Winthrop 2324
Neo-Synephrine Hydrochloride 1% Injection (Phenylephrine Hydrochloride) Sanofi Winthrop 2324

Anesthesia, local, surgical procedures
Marcaine Hydrochloride with Epinephrine 1:200,000 (Bupivacaine Hydrochloride, Epinephrine) Sanofi Winthrop 2316
Marcaine Hydrochloride Injection (Bupivacaine Hydrochloride) Sanofi Winthrop 2316
Sensorcaine (Bupivacaine Hydrochloride, Epinephrine Bitartrate) Astra 559

Anesthesia, local, therapeutic procedures
Marcaine Hydrochloride with Epinephrine 1:200,000 (Bupivacaine Hydrochloride, Epinephrine) Sanofi Winthrop 2316
Marcaine Hydrochloride Injection (Bupivacaine Hydrochloride) Sanofi Winthrop 2316
Sensorcaine (Bupivacaine Hydrochloride, Epinephrine Bitartrate) Astra 559

Anesthesia, regional
Carbocaine Hydrochloride Injection (Mepivacaine Hydrochloride Injection) Sanofi Winthrop 2303
Marcaine Hydrochloride with Epinephrine 1:200,000 (Bupivacaine Hydrochloride, Epinephrine) Sanofi Winthrop 2316
Marcaine Hydrochloride Injection (Bupivacaine Hydrochloride) Sanofi Winthrop 2316
Sensorcaine (Bupivacaine Hydrochloride, Epinephrine Bitartrate) Astra 559
Xylocaine Injections (Lidocaine Hydrochloride) Astra 567

Anesthesia, regional, adjunct in
Diprivan Injection (Propofol) Zeneca 2833
Neo-Synephrine Hydrochloride 1% Carpuject (Phenylephrine Hydrochloride) Sanofi Winthrop 2324
Neo-Synephrine Hydrochloride 1% Injection (Phenylephrine Hydrochloride) Sanofi Winthrop 2324
Sublimaze Injection (Fentanyl Citrate) Janssen 1307

Anesthesia, spinal
Pontocaine Hydrochloride for Spinal Anesthesia (Tetracaine Hydrochloride) Sanofi Winthrop 2330

Anesthesia care sedation, monitored
Alfenta Injection (Alfentanil Hydrochloride) Janssen 1286
Diprivan Injection (Propofol) Zeneca 2833

Angina (see under Angina pectoris)

Angina pectoris
Adalat Capsules (10 mg and 20 mg) (Nifedipine) Bayer Pharmaceutical 587
Calan Tablets (Verapamil Hydrochloride) Searle 2419
Cardizem Tablets (Diltiazem Hydrochloride) Marion Merrell Dow 1512
Dilatrate-SR (Isosorbide Dinitrate) Schwarz 2398
Imdur (Isosorbide Mononitrate) Key 1323
Inderal (Propranolol Hydrochloride) Wyeth-Ayerst 2728
Inderal LA Long Acting Capsules (Propranolol Hydrochloride) Wyeth-Ayerst 2730
Ismo Tablets (Isosorbide Mononitrate) Wyeth-Ayerst 2738
Isoptin Oral Tablets (Verapamil Hydrochloride) Knoll Laboratories 1346
Isordil Tembids (Isosorbide Dinitrate) Wyeth-Ayerst 2741
Isordil Titradose Tablets (Isosorbide Dinitrate) Wyeth-Ayerst 2742
Lopressor (Metoprolol Tartrate) CibaGeneva 830
Monoket (Isosorbide Mononitrate) Schwarz 2406
Nitro-Bid IV (Nitroglycerin) Marion Merrell Dow 1523
Nitro-Bid Ointment (Nitroglycerin) Marion Merrell Dow 1524
Nitrodisc (Nitroglycerin) Roberts 2047
Nitro-Dur (nitroglycerin) Transdermal Infusion System (Nitroglycerin) Key 1326
Nitrolingual Spray (Nitroglycerin) Rhone-Poulenc Rorer Pharmaceuticals 2027
Procardia Capsules (Nifedipine) Pratt 1971
Sorbitrate (Isosorbide Dinitrate) Zeneca 2843
Tenormin Tablets and I.V. Injection (Atenolol) Zeneca 2847
Toprol-XL Tablets (Metoprolol Succinate) Astra 565
Transderm-Nitro Transdermal Therapeutic System (Nitroglycerin) CibaGeneva 859

Angina pectoris, acute, prophylaxis
Isordil Sublingual Tablets (Isosorbide Dinitrate) Wyeth-Ayerst 2739
Nitrolingual Spray (Nitroglycerin) Rhone-Poulenc Rorer Pharmaceuticals 2027
Nitrostat Tablets (Nitroglycerin) Parke-Davis 1925

Angina pectoris, "conditionally" approved in
Deponit NTG Transdermal Delivery System (Nitroglycerin) Schwarz 2397

Angina, chronic stable
Adalat Capsules (10 mg and 20 mg) (Nifedipine) Bayer Pharmaceutical 587
Calan Tablets (Verapamil Hydrochloride) Searle 2419
Cardene Capsules (Nicardipine Hydrochloride) Roche Laboratories 2095
Cardizem CD Capsules (Diltiazem Hydrochloride) Marion Merrell Dow 1506
Cardizem Tablets (Diltiazem Hydrochloride) Marion Merrell Dow 1512
Dilacor XR Extended-release Capsules (Diltiazem Hydrochloride) Rhone-Poulenc Rorer Pharmaceuticals 2018
Inderal Tablets (Propranolol Hydrochloride) Wyeth-Ayerst 2728
Isoptin Oral Tablets (Verapamil Hydrochloride) Knoll Laboratories 1346
Norvasc Tablets (Amlodipine Besylate) Pfizer Labs 1940
Procardia Capsules (Nifedipine) Pratt 1971
Procardia XL Extended Release Tablets (Nifedipine) Pratt 1972
Vascor (200, 300 and 400 mg) Tablets (Bepridil Hydrochloride) McNeil Pharmaceutical 1587

Angina, classic effort-associated (see under Angina, chronic stable)

Angina, crescendo (see under Angina, unstable)

Angina, pre-infarction (see under Angina, unstable)

Angina, Prinzmetal's
Adalat Capsules (10 mg and 20 mg) (Nifedipine) Bayer Pharmaceutical 587
Calan Tablets (Verapamil Hydrochloride) Searle 2419
Isoptin Oral Tablets (Verapamil Hydrochloride) Knoll Laboratories 1346
Norvasc Tablets (Amlodipine Besylate) Pfizer Labs 1940
Procardia Capsules (Nifedipine) Pratt 1971
Procardia XL Extended Release Tablets (Nifedipine) Pratt 1972

Angina, unstable
Calan Tablets (Verapamil Hydrochloride) Searle 2419
Isoptin Oral Tablets (Verapamil Hydrochloride) Knoll Laboratories 1346
Procardia Capsules (Nifedipine) Pratt 1971

Angina, variant (see under Angina, Prinzmetal's)

Angina, vasospastic (see under Angina, Prinzmetal's)

Angioedema, adjunctive therapy in
Benadryl Capsules (Diphenhydramine Hydrochloride) Parke-Davis 1898
Extendryl (Chlorpheniramine Maleate, Methscopolamine Nitrate, Phenylephrine Hydrochloride) Fleming 1005
PBZ Tablets (Tripelennamine Hydrochloride) CibaGeneva 845
PBZ-SR Tablets (Tripelennamine Hydrochloride) CibaGeneva 844
Periactin (Cyproheptadine Hydrochloride) Merck & Co., Inc. 1724
Phenergan Suppositories (Promethazine Hydrochloride) Wyeth-Ayerst 2775
Phenergan Syrup (Promethazine Hydrochloride) Wyeth-Ayerst 2774
Phenergan Tablets (Promethazine Hydrochloride) Wyeth-Ayerst 2775
Tavist Syrup (Clemastine Fumarate) Sandoz Pharmaceuticals 2297
Tavist Tablets (Clemastine Fumarate) Sandoz Pharmaceuticals 2298

Angioedema, hereditary
Danocrine Capsules (Danazol) Sanofi Winthrop 2307
Winstrol Tablets (Stanozolol) Sanofi Winthrop 2337

Angiography, fluorescein, fundus
AK-Fluor Injection 10% and 25% (Fluorescein Sodium) Akorn ..... ◉ 203
Fluorescite (Fluorescein Sodium) Alcon Laboratories ..... ◉ 219

Angiography, fluorescein, iris vasculature
AK-Fluor Injection 10% and 25% (Fluorescein Sodium) Akorn ..... ◉ 203
Fluorescite (Fluorescein Sodium) Alcon Laboratories ..... ◉ 219

Ankylosing spondylitis
Anaprox/Naprosyn (Naproxen Sodium) Roche Laboratories 2117
Aristocort Suspension (Forte Parenteral) (Triamcinolone Diacetate) Fujisawa 1027

(▣ Described in PDR For Nonprescription Drugs) (◉ Described in PDR For Ophthalmology)

Ankylosing spondylitis | Indications Index | 1456

Aristocort Tablets (Triamcinolone) Fujisawa 1022
Extra Strength Bayer Arthritis Pain Regimen Formula (Aspirin, Enteric Coated) Miles Consumer .... ▣ 711
Cataflam (Diclofenac Potassium) CibaGeneva 816
Celestone Soluspan Suspension (Betamethasone Sodium Phosphate, Betamethasone Acetate) Schering 2347
Clinoril Tablets (Sulindac) Merck & Co., Inc. 1618
Cortone Acetate Sterile Suspension (Cortisone Acetate) Merck & Co., Inc. 1623
Cortone Acetate Tablets (Cortisone Acetate) Merck & Co., Inc. 1624
Dalalone D.P. Injectable (Dexamethasone Acetate) Forest 1011
Decadron Elixir (Dexamethasone) Merck & Co., Inc. 1633
Decadron Phosphate Injection (Dexamethasone Sodium Phosphate) Merck & Co., Inc. 1637
Decadron Tablets (Dexamethasone) Merck & Co., Inc. 1635
Decadron-LA Sterile Suspension (Dexamethasone Acetate) Merck & Co., Inc. 1646
Deltasone Tablets (Prednisone) Upjohn 2595
Depo-Medrol Single-Dose Vial (Methylprednisolone Acetate) Upjohn 2600
Depo-Medrol Sterile Aqueous Suspension (Methylprednisolone Acetate) Upjohn 2597
EC-Naprosyn Delayed-Release Tablets (Naproxen) Roche Laboratories 2117
Ecotrin (Aspirin, Enteric Coated) SmithKline Beecham 2455
Hydeltrasol Injection, Sterile (Prednisolone Sodium Phosphate) Merck & Co., Inc. 1665
Hydrocortone Phosphate Injection, Sterile (Hydrocortisone Sodium Phosphate) Merck & Co., Inc. 1670
Hydrocortone Tablets (Hydrocortisone) Merck & Co., Inc. 1672
Indocin (Indomethacin) Merck & Co., Inc. 1680
Medrol (Methylprednisolone) Upjohn 2621
Anaprox/Naprosyn (Naproxen) Roche Laboratories 2117
Pediapred Oral Liquid (Prednisolone Sodium Phosphate) Fisons 995
Prelone Syrup (Prednisolone) Muro 1787
Solu-Cortef Sterile Powder (Hydrocortisone Sodium Succinate) Upjohn 2641
Solu-Medrol Sterile Powder (Methylprednisolone Sodium Succinate) Upjohn 2643
Voltaren Tablets (Diclofenac Sodium) CibaGeneva 861

Anorexia associated with weight loss, AIDS-induced
Marinol (Dronabinol) Capsules (Dronabinol) Roxane 2231
Megace Oral Suspension (Megestrol Acetate) Bristol-Myers Squibb Oncology 699

Anterior segment inflammation (see under Inflammation, anterior segment)

Anthrax (see under B. anthracis infections)

Anticholinesterase drugs, overdosage, treatment of
Levsin/Levsinex/Levbid (Hyoscyamine Sulfate) Schwarz 2405
Protopam Chloride for Injection (Pralidoxime Chloride) Wyeth-Ayerst 2806

Antithrombin III deficiency, hereditary
THROMBATE III Antithrombin III (Human) (Antithrombin III) Bayer Biological 637

Anxiety and tension due to menopause (see under Menopause, management of the manifestations of)

Anxiety disorders, management of
Ativan Tablets (Lorazepam) Wyeth-Ayerst 2700
BuSpar (Buspirone Hydrochloride) Bristol-Myers Squibb 737
Dizac (Diazepam) Ohmeda 1809
Etrafon (Perphenazine, Amitriptyline Hydrochloride) Schering 2355
Libritabs Tablets (Chlordiazepoxide) Roche Products 2177
Librium Capsules (Chlordiazepoxide Hydrochloride) Roche Products 2178
Librium Injectable (Chlordiazepoxide Hydrochloride) Roche Products 2179
Mebaral Tablets (Mephobarbital) Sanofi Winthrop 2322
Miltown Tablets (Meprobamate) Wallace 2672
Phenergan Injection (Promethazine Hydrochloride) Wyeth-Ayerst 2773
Phenergan Suppositories (Promethazine Hydrochloride) Wyeth-Ayerst 2775
Phenergan Syrup (Promethazine Hydrochloride) Wyeth-Ayerst 2774
Phenergan Tablets (Promethazine Hydrochloride) Wyeth-Ayerst 2775
Serax Capsules (Oxazepam) Wyeth-Ayerst 2810
Serax Tablets (Oxazepam) Wyeth-Ayerst 2810
Trancopal Caplets (Chlormezanone) Sanofi Winthrop 2337
Tranxene (Clorazepate Dipotassium) Abbott 451
Valium Injectable (Diazepam) Roche Products 2182
Valium Tablets (Diazepam) Roche Products 2183
Valrelease Capsules (Diazepam) Roche Laboratories 2169
Vistaril Intramuscular Solution (Hydroxyzine Hydrochloride) Roerig 2216
Xanax Tablets (Alprazolam) Upjohn 2649

Anxiety, generalized non-psychotic, short-term treatment of
Compazine (Prochlorperazine) SmithKline Beecham Pharmaceuticals 2470
Stelazine (Trifluoperazine Hydrochloride) SmithKline Beecham Pharmaceuticals 2514

Anxiety, mental depression-induced
Ativan Tablets (Lorazepam) Wyeth-Ayerst 2700
Etrafon (Perphenazine, Amitriptyline Hydrochloride) Schering 2355
Limbitrol (Chlordiazepoxide, Amitriptyline Hydrochloride) Roche Products 2180
Ludiomil Tablets (Maprotiline Hydrochloride) CibaGeneva 843
Mellaril (Thioridazine Hydrochloride) Sandoz Pharmaceuticals 2269
Serax Capsules (Oxazepam) Wyeth-Ayerst 2810
Serax Tablets (Oxazepam) Wyeth-Ayerst 2810
Sinequan (Doxepin Hydrochloride) Roerig 2205
Triavil Tablets (Perphenazine, Amitriptyline Hydrochloride) Merck & Co., Inc. 1757
Vistaril Intramuscular Solution (Hydroxyzine Hydrochloride) Roerig 2216
Xanax Tablets (Alprazolam) Upjohn 2649

Anxiety, preoperative
Ativan Injection (Lorazepam) Wyeth-Ayerst 2698
Dizac (Diazepam) Ohmeda 1809
Inapsine Injection (Droperidol) Janssen 1296
Levoprome (Methotrimeprazine) Immunex 1274
Libritabs Tablets (Chlordiazepoxide) Roche Products 2177
Librium Capsules (Chlordiazepoxide Hydrochloride) Roche Products 2178
Librium Injectable (Chlordiazepoxide Hydrochloride) Roche Products 2179
Thorazine (Chlorpromazine Hydrochloride) SmithKline Beecham Pharmaceuticals 2523
Valium Injectable (Diazepam) Roche Products 2182
Vistaril Capsules (Hydroxyzine Pamoate) Pfizer Labs 1944
Vistaril Intramuscular Solution (Hydroxyzine Hydrochloride) Roerig 2216
Vistaril Oral Suspension (Hydroxyzine Pamoate) Pfizer Labs 1944

Anxiety, short-term symptomatic relief of
Atarax Tablets & Syrup (Hydroxyzine Hydrochloride) Roerig 2185
Ativan Tablets (Lorazepam) Wyeth-Ayerst 2700
BuSpar (Buspirone Hydrochloride) Bristol-Myers Squibb 737
Dizac (Diazepam) Ohmeda 1809
Libritabs Tablets (Chlordiazepoxide) Roche Products 2177
Librium Capsules (Chlordiazepoxide Hydrochloride) Roche Products 2178
Librium Injectable (Chlordiazepoxide Hydrochloride) Roche Products 2179
Miltown Tablets (Meprobamate) Wallace 2672
Serax Capsules (Oxazepam) Wyeth-Ayerst 2810
Serax Tablets (Oxazepam) Wyeth-Ayerst 2810
Tranxene (Clorazepate Dipotassium) Abbott 451
Valium Injectable (Diazepam) Roche Products 2182
Valium Tablets (Diazepam) Roche Products 2183
Valrelease Capsules (Diazepam) Roche Laboratories 2169
Vistaril Capsules (Hydroxyzine Pamoate) Pfizer Labs 1944
Vistaril Intramuscular Solution (Hydroxyzine Hydrochloride) Roerig 2216
Vistaril Oral Suspension (Hydroxyzine Pamoate) Pfizer Labs 1944
Xanax Tablets (Alprazolam) Upjohn 2649

Aplastic anemia (see under Anemia, aplastic)

Appendicitis, gangrenous
Primaxin I.M. (Imipenem-Cilastatin Sodium) Merck & Co., Inc. 1727

Appendicitis, perforated
Primaxin I.M. (Imipenem-Cilastatin Sodium) Merck & Co., Inc. 1727

Appendicitis with peritonitis
Primaxin I.M. (Imipenem-Cilastatin Sodium) Merck & Co., Inc. 1727
Zosyn (Piperacillin Sodium, Tazobactam Sodium) Lederle 1419
Zosyn Pharmacy Bulk Package (Piperacillin Sodium, Tazobactam Sodium) Lederle 1422

Appetite, suppression of (see also under Obesity, exogenous)
Acutrim (Phenylpropanolamine Hydrochloride) CIBA Consumer ▣ 628
Dexatrim (Phenylpropanolamine Hydrochloride) Thompson Medical .... ▣ 832

Apprehension (see under Anxiety disorders, management of)

ARC (see under Infection, acquired immunodeficiency syndrome-related complex)

Arrhythmias
Calan Tablets (Verapamil Hydrochloride) Searle 2419
Inderal (Propranolol Hydrochloride) Wyeth-Ayerst 2728
Norpace (Disopyramide Phosphate) Searle 2444
Quinidex Extentabs (Quinidine Sulfate) Robins 2067
Tonocard Tablets (Tocainide Hydrochloride) Astra Merck 531

Arrhythmias associated with digitalis
Calan Tablets (Verapamil Hydrochloride) Searle 2419
Isoptin Oral Tablets (Verapamil Hydrochloride) Knoll Laboratories 1346

Arrhythmias due to thyrotoxicosis, adjunct to
Inderal (Propranolol Hydrochloride) Wyeth-Ayerst 2728

Arrhythmias, junctional
Quinidex Extentabs (Quinidine Sulfate) Robins 2067

Arrhythmias, supraventricular
Inderal (Propranolol Hydrochloride) Wyeth-Ayerst 2728

Arrhythmias, ventricular
Betapace Tablets (Sotalol Hydrochloride) Berlex 641
Cordarone Intravenous (Amiodarone Hydrochloride) Wyeth-Ayerst 2715
Ethmozine Tablets (Moricizine Hydrochloride) Roberts 2041
Norpace (Disopyramide Phosphate) Searle 2444
Procan SR Tablets (Procainamide Hydrochloride) Parke-Davis 1926
Quinaglute Dura-Tabs Tablets (Quinidine Gluconate) Berlex 649
Rythmol Tablets–150mg, 225mg, 300mg (Propafenone Hydrochloride) Knoll Laboratories 1352
Sectral Capsules (Acebutolol Hydrochloride) Wyeth-Ayerst 2807
Tambocor Tablets (Flecainide Acetate) 3M Pharmaceuticals 1497

Arrhythmias, ventricular, life-threatening
Cordarone Tablets (Amiodarone Hydrochloride) Wyeth-Ayerst 2712
Ethmozine Tablets (Moricizine Hydrochloride) Roberts 2041
Mexitil Capsules (Mexiletine Hydrochloride) Boehringer Ingelheim 678
Procan SR Tablets (Procainamide Hydrochloride) Parke-Davis 1926
Tambocor Tablets (Flecainide Acetate) 3M Pharmaceuticals 1497
Tonocard Tablets (Tocainide Hydrochloride) Astra Merck 531

Arteriovenous cannulae, occlusion of
Streptase for Infusion (Streptokinase) Astra 562

Arthralgia, topical relief of (see under Pain, topical relief of)

Arthritis (see also under Osteoarthritis; Rheumatoid arthritis)
Maximum Strength Ascriptin (Aspirin Buffered, Calcium Carbonate) CIBA Consumer .... ▣ 630
Bufferin Analgesic Tablets and Caplets (Aspirin) Bristol-Myers Products .... ▣ 613
Arthritis Strength Bufferin Analgesic Caplets (Aspirin) Bristol-Myers Products .... ▣ 614
Extra Strength Bufferin Analgesic Tablets (Aspirin) Bristol-Myers Products .... ▣ 615
Cama Arthritis Pain Reliever (Aspirin, Aluminum Hydroxide, Magnesium Oxide) Sandoz Consumer .... ▣ 785
Easprin (Aspirin) Parke-Davis 1914
Haltran Tablets (Ibuprofen) Roberts .... ▣ 771

(▣ Described in PDR For Nonprescription Drugs) (◉ Described in PDR For Ophthalmology)

Indications Index

Trilisate (Choline Magnesium Trisalicylate) Purdue Frederick 2000

Arthritis, acute, gouty

Aristocort Suspension (Forte Parenteral) (Triamcinolone Diacetate) Fujisawa 1027

Aristocort Suspension (Intralesional) (Triamcinolone Diacetate) Fujisawa 1025

Aristocort Tablets (Triamcinolone) Fujisawa 1022

Aristospan Suspension (Intra-articular) (Triamcinolone Hexacetonide) Fujisawa 1033

Celestone Soluspan Suspension (Betamethasone Sodium Phosphate, Betamethasone Acetate) Schering 2347

Clinoril Tablets (Sulindac) Merck & Co., Inc. 1618

Cortone Acetate Sterile Suspension (Cortisone Acetate) Merck & Co., Inc. 1623

Cortone Acetate Tablets (Cortisone Acetate) Merck & Co., Inc. 1624

Dalalone D.P. Injectable (Dexamethasone Acetate) Forest 1011

Decadron Elixir (Dexamethasone) Merck & Co., Inc. 1633

Decadron Phosphate Injection (Dexamethasone Sodium Phosphate) Merck & Co., Inc. 1637

Decadron Tablets (Dexamethasone) Merck & Co., Inc. 1635

Decadron-LA Sterile Suspension (Dexamethasone Acetate) Merck & Co., Inc. 1646

Deltasone Tablets (Prednisone) Upjohn 2595

Depo-Medrol Single-Dose Vial (Methylprednisolone Acetate) Upjohn 2600

Depo-Medrol Sterile Aqueous Suspension (Methylprednisolone Acetate) Upjohn 2597

Hydeltrasol Injection, Sterile (Prednisolone Sodium Phosphate) Merck & Co., Inc. 1665

Hydeltra-T.B.A. Sterile Suspension (Prednisolone Tebutate) Merck & Co., Inc. 1667

Hydrocortone Acetate Sterile Suspension (Hydrocortisone Acetate) Merck & Co., Inc. 1669

Hydrocortone Phosphate Injection, Sterile (Hydrocortisone Sodium Phosphate) Merck & Co., Inc. 1670

Hydrocortone Tablets (Hydrocortisone) Merck & Co., Inc. 1672

Indocin (Indomethacin) Merck & Co., Inc. 1680

Medrol (Methylprednisolone) Upjohn 2621

Pediapred Oral Liquid (Prednisolone Sodium Phosphate) Fisons 995

Prelone Syrup (Prednisolone) Muro 1787

Solu-Cortef Sterile Powder (Hydrocortisone Sodium Succinate) Upjohn 2641

Solu-Medrol Sterile Powder (Methylprednisolone Sodium Succinate) Upjohn 2643

Arthritis, chronic, gouty

Anturane (Sulfinpyrazone) CibaGeneva 807

ColBENEMID Tablets (Probenecid, Colchicine) Merck & Co., Inc. 1622

Arthritis, gonorrheal

Pfizerpen for Injection (Penicillin G Potassium) Roerig 2203

Arthritis, intermittent, gouty

Anturane (Sulfinpyrazone) CibaGeneva 807

Arthritis, juvenile

Children's Advil Suspension (Ibuprofen) Wyeth-Ayerst 2692

Anaprox/Naprosyn (Naproxen Sodium) Roche Laboratories 2117

Motrin Ibuprofen Suspension, Oral Drops, Chewable Tablets, Caplets (Ibuprofen) McNeil Consumer 1546

Naprosyn Tablets (Naproxen) Roche Laboratories 2117

Trilisate (Choline Magnesium Trisalicylate) Purdue Frederick 2000

Arthritis, osteo- (see under Osteoarthritis)

Arthritis, psoriatic

Aristocort Suspension (Forte Parenteral) (Triamcinolone Diacetate) Fujisawa 1027

Aristocort Tablets (Triamcinolone) Fujisawa 1022

Extra Strength Bayer Arthritis Pain Regimen Formula (Aspirin, Enteric Coated) Miles Consumer .... ⊞ 711

Celestone Soluspan Suspension (Betamethasone Sodium Phosphate, Betamethasone Acetate) Schering 2347

Cortone Acetate Sterile Suspension (Cortisone Acetate) Merck & Co., Inc. 1623

Cortone Acetate Tablets (Cortisone Acetate) Merck & Co., Inc. 1624

Dalalone D.P. Injectable (Dexamethasone Acetate) Forest 1011

Decadron Elixir (Dexamethasone) Merck & Co., Inc. 1633

Decadron Phosphate Injection (Dexamethasone Sodium Phosphate) Merck & Co., Inc. 1637

Decadron Tablets (Dexamethasone) Merck & Co., Inc. 1635

Decadron-LA Sterile Suspension (Dexamethasone Acetate) Merck & Co., Inc. 1646

Deltasone Tablets (Prednisone) Upjohn 2595

Depo-Medrol Single-Dose Vial (Methylprednisolone Acetate) Upjohn 2600

Depo-Medrol Sterile Aqueous Suspension (Methylprednisolone Acetate) Upjohn 2597

Ecotrin (Aspirin, Enteric Coated) SmithKline Beecham 2455

Hydeltrasol Injection, Sterile (Prednisolone Sodium Phosphate) Merck & Co., Inc. 1665

Hydrocortone Phosphate Injection, Sterile (Hydrocortisone Sodium Phosphate) Merck & Co., Inc. 1670

Hydrocortone Tablets (Hydrocortisone) Merck & Co., Inc. 1672

Medrol (Methylprednisolone) Upjohn 2621

Pediapred Oral Liquid (Prednisolone Sodium Phosphate) Fisons 995

Prelone Syrup (Prednisolone) Muro 1787

Solu-Cortef Sterile Powder (Hydrocortisone Sodium Succinate) Upjohn 2641

Solu-Medrol Sterile Powder (Methylprednisolone Sodium Succinate) Upjohn 2643

Arthritis, rheumatoid (see under Rheumatoid arthritis)

Arthritis, topical adjunct to

BenGay External Analgesic Products (Menthol, Methyl Salicylate) Pfizer Consumer .... ⊞ 741

Mobisyl Analgesic Creme (Trolamine Salicylate) Ascher .... ⊞ 603

Thera-Gesic (Methyl Salicylate, Menthol) Mission 1781

Ascariasis, as secondary therapy in

Mintezol (Thiabendazole) Merck & Co., Inc. 1704

Ascaris lumbricoides infections

Vermox Chewable Tablets (Mebendazole) Janssen 1312

Aspergillosis

Fungizone Intravenous (Amphotericin B) Apothecon 506

Sporanox Capsules (Itraconazole) Janssen 1305

Aspergillus fumigatus infections (see under Aspergillosis)

Asthma, bronchial (see under Bronchial asthma)

Asthmatic attack, acute, in children age 6 years and older, treatment of

Alupent (Metaproterenol Sulfate) Boehringer Ingelheim 669

Astrocytoma, palliative therapy in

BiCNU (Carmustine (BCNU)) Bristol-Myers Squibb Oncology 691

Athetosis, adjunctive therapy in

Dizac (Diazepam) Ohmeda 1809

Valium Injectable (Diazepam) Roche Products 2182

Valium Tablets (Diazepam) Roche Products 2183

Valrelease Capsules (Diazepam) Roche Laboratories 2169

Athlete's foot (see under Tinea pedis infections)

Atrial contractions, premature

Quinidex Extentabs (Quinidine Sulfate) Robins 2067

Atrial extrasystoles

Inderal (Propranolol Hydrochloride) Wyeth-Ayerst 2728

Atrial fibrillation

Brevibloc Injection (Esmolol Hydrochloride) Ohmeda 1808

Calan Tablets (Verapamil Hydrochloride) Searle 2419

Cardizem Injectable (Diltiazem Hydrochloride) Marion Merrell Dow 1508

Crystodigin Tablets (Digitoxin) Lilly 1433

Isoptin Injectable (Verapamil Hydrochloride) Knoll Laboratories 1344

Isoptin Oral Tablets (Verapamil Hydrochloride) Knoll Laboratories 1346

Lanoxicaps (Digoxin) Glaxo Wellcome 1117

Lanoxin Elixir Pediatric (Digoxin) Glaxo Wellcome 1120

Lanoxin Injection (Digoxin) Glaxo Wellcome 1123

Lanoxin Injection Pediatric (Digoxin) Glaxo Wellcome 1126

Lanoxin Tablets (Digoxin) Glaxo Wellcome 1128

Quinaglute Dura-Tabs Tablets (Quinidine Gluconate) Berlex 649

Quinidex Extentabs (Quinidine Sulfate) Robins 2067

Atrial fibrillation with embolism

Coumadin (Warfarin Sodium) DuPont 926

Heparin Sodium Injection, USP, Sterile Solution (Heparin Sodium) Upjohn 2615

Heparin Sodium Vials (Heparin Sodium) Lilly 1441

Atrial fibrillation, paroxysmal

Quinidex Extentabs (Quinidine Sulfate) Robins 2067

Tambocor Tablets (Flecainide Acetate) 3M Pharmaceuticals 1497

Atrial flutter

Brevibloc Injection (Esmolol Hydrochloride) Ohmeda 1808

Calan Tablets (Verapamil Hydrochloride) Searle 2419

Cardizem Injectable (Diltiazem Hydrochloride) Marion Merrell Dow 1508

Crystodigin Tablets (Digitoxin) Lilly 1433

Inderal (Propranolol Hydrochloride) Wyeth-Ayerst 2728

Isoptin Injectable (Verapamil Hydrochloride) Knoll Laboratories 1344

Isoptin Oral Tablets (Verapamil Hydrochloride) Knoll Laboratories 1346

Lanoxicaps (Digoxin) Glaxo Wellcome 1117

Lanoxin Elixir Pediatric (Digoxin) Glaxo Wellcome 1120

Lanoxin Injection (Digoxin) Glaxo Wellcome 1123

Lanoxin Injection Pediatric (Digoxin) Glaxo Wellcome 1126

Lanoxin Tablets (Digoxin) Glaxo Wellcome 1128

Quinaglute Dura-Tabs Tablets (Quinidine Gluconate) Berlex 649

Quinidex Extentabs (Quinidine Sulfate) Robins 2067

Attention deficit disorders with hyperactivity

Biphetamine Capsules (Amphetamine Resins) Fisons 983

Cylert Tablets (Pemoline) Abbott 412

Desoxyn Gradumet Tablets (Methamphetamine Hydrochloride) Abbott 419

Dexedrine (Dextroamphetamine Sulfate) SmithKline Beecham Pharmaceuticals 2474

DextroStat Dextroamphetamine Tablets (Dextroamphetamine Sulfate) Richwood 2036

Ritalin (Methylphenidate Hydrochloride) CibaGeneva 848

Autonomic response, exaggerated, management of disorders

Bellergal-S Tablets (Phenobarbital, Ergotamine Tartrate, Belladonna Alkaloids) Sandoz Pharmaceuticals 2250

B

B. anthracis infections

Achromycin V Capsules (Tetracycline Hydrochloride) Lederle 1367

Declomycin Tablets (Demeclocycline Hydrochloride) Lederle 1371

Doryx Capsules (Doxycycline Hyclate) Parke-Davis 1913

Dynacin Capsules (Minocycline Hydrochloride) Medicis 1590

Minocin Intravenous (Minocycline Hydrochloride) Lederle 1382

Minocin Oral Suspension (Minocycline Hydrochloride) Lederle 1385

Minocin Pellet-Filled Capsules (Minocycline Hydrochloride) Lederle 1383

Monodox Capsules (Doxycycline Monohydrate) Oclassen 1805

Pfizerpen for Injection (Penicillin G Potassium) Roerig 2203

Terramycin Intramuscular Solution (Oxytetracycline) Roerig 2210

Vibramycin (Doxycycline Calcium) Pfizer Labs 1941

Vibramycin Hyclate Intravenous (Doxycycline Hyclate) Roerig 2215

Vibramycin (Doxycycline Monohydrate) Pfizer Labs 1941

B. distasonis infections

Flagyl 375 Capsules (Metronidazole) Searle 2434

Flagyl I.V. (Metronidazole Hydrochloride) SCS 2247

Mefoxin (Cefoxitin Sodium) Merck & Co., Inc. 1691

Mefoxin Premixed Intravenous Solution (Cefoxitin Sodium) Merck & Co., Inc. 1694

Primaxin I.M. (Imipenem-Cilastatin Sodium) Merck & Co., Inc. 1727

B. distasonis intra-abdominal abscess

Flagyl 375 Capsules (Metronidazole) Searle 2434

B. distasonis intra-abdominal infections

Flagyl 375 Capsules (Metronidazole) Searle 2434

Flagyl I.V. (Metronidazole Hydrochloride) SCS 2247

Mefoxin (Cefoxitin Sodium) Merck & Co., Inc. 1691

Mefoxin Premixed Intravenous Solution (Cefoxitin Sodium) Merck & Co., Inc. 1694

Primaxin I.M. (Imipenem-Cilastatin Sodium) Merck & Co., Inc. 1727

Protostat Tablets (Metronidazole) Ortho Pharmaceutical 1883

B. distasonis liver abscess

Flagyl 375 Capsules (Metronidazole) Searle 2434

Flagyl I.V. (Metronidazole Hydrochloride) SCS 2247

Protostat Tablets (Metronidazole) Ortho Pharmaceutical 1883

B. distasonis peritonitis | Indications Index | 1458

B. distasonis peritonitis
Flagyl 375 Capsules (Metronidazole) Searle 2434
Flagyl I.V. (Metronidazole Hydrochloride) SCS 2247
Mefoxin (Cefoxitin Sodium) Merck & Co., Inc. 1691
Mefoxin Premixed Intravenous Solution (Cefoxitin Sodium) Merck & Co., Inc. 1694
Protostat Tablets (Metronidazole) Ortho Pharmaceutical 1883

B. fragilis bone and joint infections, adjunct to
Flagyl 375 Capsules (Metronidazole) Searle 2434
Flagyl I.V. (Metronidazole Hydrochloride) SCS 2247
Protostat Tablets (Metronidazole) Ortho Pharmaceutical 1883

B. fragilis brain abscess
Flagyl 375 Capsules (Metronidazole) Searle 2434
Flagyl I.V. (Metronidazole Hydrochloride) SCS 2247
Protostat Tablets (Metronidazole) Ortho Pharmaceutical 1883

B. fragilis central nervous system infections
Flagyl 375 Capsules (Metronidazole) Searle 2434
Flagyl I.V. (Metronidazole Hydrochloride) SCS 2247
Protostat Tablets (Metronidazole) Ortho Pharmaceutical 1883

B. fragilis empyema
Flagyl 375 Capsules (Metronidazole) Searle 2434
Flagyl I.V. (Metronidazole Hydrochloride) SCS 2247
Protostat Tablets (Metronidazole) Ortho Pharmaceutical 1883

B. fragilis endocarditis
Flagyl 375 Capsules (Metronidazole) Searle 2434
Flagyl I.V. (Metronidazole Hydrochloride) SCS 2247

B. fragilis endometritis
Flagyl 375 Capsules (Metronidazole) Searle 2434

B. fragilis endomyometritis
Flagyl 375 Capsules (Metronidazole) Searle 2434
Flagyl I.V. (Metronidazole Hydrochloride) SCS 2247
Protostat Tablets (Metronidazole) Ortho Pharmaceutical 1883

B. fragilis gynecologic infections
Cefobid Intravenous/Intramuscular (Cefoperazone Sodium) Roerig 2189
Cefobid Pharmacy Bulk Package - Not for Direct Infusion (Cefoperazone Sodium) Roerig 2192
Cefotan (Cefotetan) Zeneca 2829
Claforan Sterile and Injection (Cefotaxime Sodium) Hoechst-Roussel 1235
Flagyl I.V. (Metronidazole Hydrochloride) SCS 2247
Mefoxin (Cefoxitin Sodium) Merck & Co., Inc. 1691
Mefoxin Premixed Intravenous Solution (Cefoxitin Sodium) Merck & Co., Inc. 1694
Pipracil (Piperacillin Sodium) Lederle 1390
Primaxin I.V. (Imipenem-Cilastatin Sodium) Merck & Co., Inc. 1729
Protostat Tablets (Metronidazole) Ortho Pharmaceutical 1883
Unasyn (Ampicillin Sodium, Sulbactam Sodium) Roerig 2212

B. fragilis infections
Cefizox for Intramuscular or Intravenous Use (Ceftizoxime Sodium) Fujisawa 1034
Cefobid Intravenous/Intramuscular (Cefoperazone Sodium) Roerig 2189
Cefobid Pharmacy Bulk Package - Not for Direct Infusion (Cefoperazone Sodium) Roerig 2192
Cefotan (Cefotetan) Zeneca 2829
Claforan Sterile and Injection (Cefotaxime Sodium) Hoechst-Roussel 1235
Flagyl 375 Capsules (Metronidazole) Searle 2434
Flagyl I.V. (Metronidazole Hydrochloride) SCS 2247
Mefoxin (Cefoxitin Sodium) Merck & Co., Inc. 1691
Mefoxin Premixed Intravenous Solution (Cefoxitin Sodium) Merck & Co., Inc. 1694
Mezlin (Mezlocillin Sodium) Bayer Pharmaceutical 601
Mezlin Pharmacy Bulk Package (Mezlocillin Sodium) Bayer Pharmaceutical 604
Pipracil (Piperacillin Sodium) Lederle 1390
Primaxin I.M. (Imipenem-Cilastatin Sodium) Merck & Co., Inc. 1727
Primaxin I.V. (Imipenem-Cilastatin Sodium) Merck & Co., Inc. 1729
Rocephin Injectable Vials, ADD-Vantage, Galaxy Container (Ceftriaxone Sodium) Roche Laboratories 2142
Tazicef for Injection (Ceftazidime) SmithKline Beecham Pharmaceuticals 2519
Timentin for Injection (Ticarcillin Disodium, Clavulanate Potassium) SmithKline Beecham Pharmaceuticals 2528
Unasyn (Ampicillin Sodium, Sulbactam Sodium) Roerig 2212
Zefazone (Cefmetazole Sodium) Upjohn 2654
Zosyn (Piperacillin Sodium, Tazobactam Sodium) Lederle 1419
Zosyn Pharmacy Bulk Package (Piperacillin Sodium, Tazobactam Sodium) Lederle 1422

B. fragilis intra-abdominal abscess
Flagyl 375 Capsules (Metronidazole) Searle 2434

B. fragilis intra-abdominal infections
Cefizox for Intramuscular or Intravenous Use (Ceftizoxime Sodium) Fujisawa 1034
Cefobid Intravenous/Intramuscular (Cefoperazone Sodium) Roerig 2189
Cefobid Pharmacy Bulk Package - Not for Direct Infusion (Cefoperazone Sodium) Roerig 2192
Flagyl 375 Capsules (Metronidazole) Searle 2434
Flagyl I.V. (Metronidazole Hydrochloride) SCS 2247
Fortaz (Ceftazidime) Glaxo Wellcome 1100
Mefoxin (Cefoxitin Sodium) Merck & Co., Inc. 1691
Mefoxin Premixed Intravenous Solution (Cefoxitin Sodium) Merck & Co., Inc. 1694
Pipracil (Piperacillin Sodium) Lederle 1390
Primaxin I.M. (Imipenem-Cilastatin Sodium) Merck & Co., Inc. 1727
Primaxin I.V. (Imipenem-Cilastatin Sodium) Merck & Co., Inc. 1729
Protostat Tablets (Metronidazole) Ortho Pharmaceutical 1883
Rocephin Injectable Vials, ADD-Vantage, Galaxy Container (Ceftriaxone Sodium) Roche Laboratories 2142
Tazicef for Injection (Ceftazidime) SmithKline Beecham Pharmaceuticals 2519
Tazidime Vials, Faspak & ADD-Vantage (Ceftazidime) Lilly 1478
Timentin for Injection (Ticarcillin Disodium, Clavulanate Potassium) SmithKline Beecham Pharmaceuticals 2528
Unasyn (Ampicillin Sodium, Sulbactam Sodium) Roerig 2212
Zefazone (Cefmetazole Sodium) Upjohn 2654

B. fragilis liver abscess
Flagyl I.V. (Metronidazole Hydrochloride) SCS 2247
Protostat Tablets (Metronidazole) Ortho Pharmaceutical 1883

B. fragilis lower respiratory tract infections
Flagyl 375 Capsules (Metronidazole) Searle 2434
Flagyl I.V. (Metronidazole Hydrochloride) SCS 2247
Mezlin (Mezlocillin Sodium) Bayer Pharmaceutical 601
Mezlin Pharmacy Bulk Package (Mezlocillin Sodium) Bayer Pharmaceutical 604
Protostat Tablets (Metronidazole) Ortho Pharmaceutical 1883

B. fragilis lung abscess
Flagyl 375 Capsules (Metronidazole) Searle 2434
Flagyl I.V. (Metronidazole Hydrochloride) SCS 2247
Mezlin (Mezlocillin Sodium) Bayer Pharmaceutical 601
Mezlin Pharmacy Bulk Package (Mezlocillin Sodium) Bayer Pharmaceutical 604
Protostat Tablets (Metronidazole) Ortho Pharmaceutical 1883

B. fragilis meningitis
Flagyl 375 Capsules (Metronidazole) Searle 2434
Flagyl I.V. (Metronidazole Hydrochloride) SCS 2247
Protostat Tablets (Metronidazole) Ortho Pharmaceutical 1883

B. fragilis peritonitis
Cefobid Intravenous/Intramuscular (Cefoperazone Sodium) Roerig 2189
Cefobid Pharmacy Bulk Package - Not for Direct Infusion (Cefoperazone Sodium) Roerig 2192
Flagyl 375 Capsules (Metronidazole) Searle 2434
Flagyl I.V. (Metronidazole Hydrochloride) SCS 2247
Mefoxin (Cefoxitin Sodium) Merck & Co., Inc. 1691
Mefoxin Premixed Intravenous Solution (Cefoxitin Sodium) Merck & Co., Inc. 1694
Protostat Tablets (Metronidazole) Ortho Pharmaceutical 1883
Timentin for Injection (Ticarcillin Disodium, Clavulanate Potassium) SmithKline Beecham Pharmaceuticals 2528
Zosyn (Piperacillin Sodium, Tazobactam Sodium) Lederle 1419
Zosyn Pharmacy Bulk Package (Piperacillin Sodium, Tazobactam Sodium) Lederle 1422

B. fragilis pneumonia
Flagyl 375 Capsules (Metronidazole) Searle 2434
Flagyl I.V. (Metronidazole Hydrochloride) SCS 2247
Mezlin (Mezlocillin Sodium) Bayer Pharmaceutical 601
Mezlin Pharmacy Bulk Package (Mezlocillin Sodium) Bayer Pharmaceutical 604
Protostat Tablets (Metronidazole) Ortho Pharmaceutical 1883

B. fragilis septicemia
Cefizox for Intramuscular or Intravenous Use (Ceftizoxime Sodium) Fujisawa 1034
Flagyl 375 Capsules (Metronidazole) Searle 2434
Flagyl I.V. (Metronidazole Hydrochloride) SCS 2247
Mefoxin (Cefoxitin Sodium) Merck & Co., Inc. 1691
Mefoxin Premixed Intravenous Solution (Cefoxitin Sodium) Merck & Co., Inc. 1694
Primaxin I.V. (Imipenem-Cilastatin Sodium) Merck & Co., Inc. 1729
Protostat Tablets (Metronidazole) Ortho Pharmaceutical 1883

B. fragilis skin and skin structure infections
Cefizox for Intramuscular or Intravenous Use (Ceftizoxime Sodium) Fujisawa 1034
Flagyl 375 Capsules (Metronidazole) Searle 2434
Flagyl I.V. (Metronidazole Hydrochloride) SCS 2247
Mefoxin (Cefoxitin Sodium) Merck & Co., Inc. 1691
Mefoxin Premixed Intravenous Solution (Cefoxitin Sodium) Merck & Co., Inc. 1694
Pipracil (Piperacillin Sodium) Lederle 1390
Primaxin I.M. (Imipenem-Cilastatin Sodium) Merck & Co., Inc. 1727
Primaxin I.V. (Imipenem-Cilastatin Sodium) Merck & Co., Inc. 1729
Protostat Tablets (Metronidazole) Ortho Pharmaceutical 1883
Rocephin Injectable Vials, ADD-Vantage, Galaxy Container (Ceftriaxone Sodium) Roche Laboratories 2142
Unasyn (Ampicillin Sodium, Sulbactam Sodium) Roerig 2212
Zefazone (Cefmetazole Sodium) Upjohn 2654

B. fragilis tubo-ovarian abscess
Flagyl 375 Capsules (Metronidazole) Searle 2434
Flagyl I.V. (Metronidazole Hydrochloride) SCS 2247
Protostat Tablets (Metronidazole) Ortho Pharmaceutical 1883

B. fragilis vaginal cuff infection, post-surgical
Flagyl 375 Capsules (Metronidazole) Searle 2434
Flagyl I.V. (Metronidazole Hydrochloride) SCS 2247

B. intermedius infections
Primaxin I.M. (Imipenem-Cilastatin Sodium) Merck & Co., Inc. 1727

B. intermedius intra-abdominal infections
Primaxin I.M. (Imipenem-Cilastatin Sodium) Merck & Co., Inc. 1727

B. melaninogenicus endometritis
Timentin for Injection (Ticarcillin Disodium, Clavulanate Potassium) SmithKline Beecham Pharmaceuticals 2528

B. melaninogenicus infections
Timentin for Injection (Ticarcillin Disodium, Clavulanate Potassium) SmithKline Beecham Pharmaceuticals 2528
Zefazone (Cefmetazole Sodium) Upjohn 2654

B. melaninogenicus skin and skin structure infections
Zefazone (Cefmetazole Sodium) Upjohn 2654

B. ovatus infections
Flagyl 375 Capsules (Metronidazole) Searle 2434
Flagyl I.V. (Metronidazole Hydrochloride) SCS 2247
Mefoxin (Cefoxitin Sodium) Merck & Co., Inc. 1691
Mefoxin Premixed Intravenous Solution (Cefoxitin Sodium) Merck & Co., Inc. 1694
Zosyn (Piperacillin Sodium, Tazobactam Sodium) Lederle 1419
Zosyn Pharmacy Bulk Package (Piperacillin Sodium, Tazobactam Sodium) Lederle 1422

B. ovatus intra-abdominal abscess
Flagyl 375 Capsules (Metronidazole) Searle 2434

B. ovatus intra-abdominal infections
Flagyl 375 Capsules (Metronidazole) Searle 2434
Flagyl I.V. (Metronidazole Hydrochloride) SCS 2247
Mefoxin (Cefoxitin Sodium) Merck & Co., Inc. 1691
Mefoxin Premixed Intravenous Solution (Cefoxitin Sodium) Merck & Co., Inc. 1694
Protostat Tablets (Metronidazole) Ortho Pharmaceutical 1883

B. ovatus liver abscess
Flagyl 375 Capsules (Metronidazole) Searle 2434
Flagyl I.V. (Metronidazole Hydrochloride) SCS 2247

1459 **Indications Index** **Bacteroides species**

Protostat Tablets (Metronidazole) Ortho Pharmaceutical 1883

B. ovatus peritonitis
Flagyl 375 Capsules (Metronidazole) Searle........ 2434
Flagyl I.V. (Metronidazole Hydrochloride) SCS........ 2247
Mefoxin (Cefoxitin Sodium) Merck & Co., Inc. 1691
Mefoxin Premixed Intravenous Solution (Cefoxitin Sodium) Merck & Co., Inc. 1694
Protostat Tablets (Metronidazole) Ortho Pharmaceutical 1883
Zosyn (Piperacillin Sodium, Tazobactam Sodium) Lederle........ 1419
Zosyn Pharmacy Bulk Package (Piperacillin Sodium, Tazobactam Sodium) Lederle 1422

B. pertussis infections
E.E.S. (Erythromycin Ethylsuccinate) Abbott........ 424
E-Mycin Tablets (Erythromycin) Knoll Laboratories 1341
ERYC (Erythromycin) Parke-Davis .. 1915
EryPed (Erythromycin Ethylsuccinate) Abbott........ 421
Ery-Tab Tablets (Erythromycin) Abbott........ 422
Erythrocin Stearate Filmtab (Erythromycin Stearate) Abbott 425
Erythromycin Base Filmtab (Erythromycin) Abbott 426
Erythromycin Delayed-Release Capsules, USP (Erythromycin) Abbott 427
Ilosone (Erythromycin Estolate) Dista........ 911
PCE Dispertab Tablets (Erythromycin) Abbott 444

B. pertussis respiratory tract infections
E.E.S. (Erythromycin Ethylsuccinate) Abbott........ 424
EryPed (Erythromycin Ethylsuccinate) Abbott........ 421
Ery-Tab Tablets (Erythromycin) Abbott........ 422
Erythrocin Stearate Filmtab (Erythromycin Stearate) Abbott 425
Erythromycin Base Filmtab (Erythromycin) Abbott 426
Erythromycin Delayed-Release Capsules, USP (Erythromycin) Abbott 427
PCE Dispertab Tablets (Erythromycin) Abbott 444

B. thetaiotaomicron infections
Flagyl 375 Capsules (Metronidazole) Searle........ 2434
Flagyl I.V. (Metronidazole Hydrochloride) SCS........ 2247
Mefoxin (Cefoxitin Sodium) Merck & Co., Inc. 1691
Mefoxin Premixed Intravenous Solution (Cefoxitin Sodium) Merck & Co., Inc. 1694
Primaxin I.M. (Imipenem-Cilastatin Sodium) Merck & Co., Inc. 1727
Zosyn (Piperacillin Sodium, Tazobactam Sodium) Lederle........ 1419
Zosyn Pharmacy Bulk Package (Piperacillin Sodium, Tazobactam Sodium) Lederle 1422

B. thetaiotaomicron intra-abdominal infections
Flagyl 375 Capsules (Metronidazole) Searle........ 2434
Flagyl I.V. (Metronidazole Hydrochloride) SCS........ 2247
Mefoxin (Cefoxitin Sodium) Merck & Co., Inc. 1691
Mefoxin Premixed Intravenous Solution (Cefoxitin Sodium) Merck & Co., Inc. 1694
Primaxin I.M. (Imipenem-Cilastatin Sodium) Merck & Co., Inc. 1727
Protostat Tablets (Metronidazole) Ortho Pharmaceutical 1883

B. thetaiotaomicron liver abscess
Flagyl 375 Capsules (Metronidazole) Searle........ 2434
Flagyl I.V. (Metronidazole Hydrochloride) SCS........ 2247
Protostat Tablets (Metronidazole) Ortho Pharmaceutical 1883

B. thetaiotaomicron peritonitis
Flagyl 375 Capsules (Metronidazole) Searle........ 2434
Flagyl I.V. (Metronidazole Hydrochloride) SCS........ 2247
Mefoxin (Cefoxitin Sodium) Merck & Co., Inc. 1691
Mefoxin Premixed Intravenous Solution (Cefoxitin Sodium) Merck & Co., Inc. 1694
Protostat Tablets (Metronidazole) Ortho Pharmaceutical 1883
Zosyn (Piperacillin Sodium, Tazobactam Sodium) Lederle........ 1419
Zosyn Pharmacy Bulk Package (Piperacillin Sodium, Tazobactam Sodium) Lederle 1422

B. vulgatus infections
Cefotan (Cefotetan) Zeneca........ 2829
Flagyl 375 Capsules (Metronidazole) Searle........ 2434
Flagyl I.V. (Metronidazole Hydrochloride) SCS........ 2247
Mefoxin (Cefoxitin Sodium) Merck & Co., Inc. 1691
Mefoxin Premixed Intravenous Solution (Cefoxitin Sodium) Merck & Co., Inc. 1694
Zosyn (Piperacillin Sodium, Tazobactam Sodium) Lederle........ 1419
Zosyn Pharmacy Bulk Package (Piperacillin Sodium, Tazobactam Sodium) Lederle 1422

B. vulgatus intra-abdominal infections
Cefotan (Cefotetan) Zeneca........ 2829
Flagyl 375 Capsules (Metronidazole) Searle........ 2434
Flagyl I.V. (Metronidazole Hydrochloride) SCS........ 2247
Mefoxin (Cefoxitin Sodium) Merck & Co., Inc. 1691
Mefoxin Premixed Intravenous Solution (Cefoxitin Sodium) Merck & Co., Inc. 1694
Protostat Tablets (Metronidazole) Ortho Pharmaceutical 1883

B. vulgatus liver abscess
Flagyl 375 Capsules (Metronidazole) Searle........ 2434
Flagyl I.V. (Metronidazole Hydrochloride) SCS........ 2247
Protostat Tablets (Metronidazole) Ortho Pharmaceutical 1883

B. vulgatus peritonitis
Flagyl 375 Capsules (Metronidazole) Searle........ 2434
Flagyl I.V. (Metronidazole Hydrochloride) SCS........ 2247
Mefoxin (Cefoxitin Sodium) Merck & Co., Inc. 1691
Mefoxin Premixed Intravenous Solution (Cefoxitin Sodium) Merck & Co., Inc. 1694
Protostat Tablets (Metronidazole) Ortho Pharmaceutical 1883
Zosyn (Piperacillin Sodium, Tazobactam Sodium) Lederle........ 1419
Zosyn Pharmacy Bulk Package (Piperacillin Sodium, Tazobactam Sodium) Lederle 1422

Backache, systemic, symptomatic relief of
Aleve (Naproxen Sodium) Procter & Gamble........ 1975
Backache Caplets (Magnesium Salicylate) Bristol-Myers Products........ ▣ 613
Bayer Select Backache Pain Relief Formula (Magnesium Salicylate) Miles Consumer........ ▣ 715
Bayer Select Ibuprofen Pain Relief Formula (Ibuprofen) Miles Consumer........ ▣ 715
Doan's Extra-Strength Analgesic (Magnesium Salicylate) CIBA Consumer........ ▣ 633
Extra Strength Doan's P.M. (Magnesium Salicylate, Diphenhydramine Hydrochloride) CIBA Consumer........ ▣ 633
Doan's Regular Strength Analgesic (Magnesium Salicylate) CIBA Consumer .... ▣ 634
Ibuprohm (Ibuprofen) Ohm .... ▣ 735
Nuprin Ibuprofen/Analgesic Tablets & Caplets (Ibuprofen) Bristol-Myers Products........ ▣ 622
Panodol Tablets and Caplets (Acetaminophen) SmithKline Beecham Consumer........ ▣ 824

Backache, temporary relief of (see under Pain, topical relief of)

Bacteremia (see under Septicemia, bacterial)

Bacterial shock, treatment adjunct
Isuprel Hydrochloride Injection 1:5000 (Isoproterenol Hydrochloride) Sanofi Winthrop .. 2311
Narcan Injection (Naloxone Hydrochloride) DuPont 934

Bacteriuria associated with cystitis, elimination or suppression of (see also under Infections, urinary tract)
Uroqid-Acid No. 2 Tablets (Methenamine Mandelate, Sodium Acid Phosphate) Beach 640

Bacteriuria, asymptomatic
Geocillin Tablets (Carbenicillin Indanyl Sodium) Roerig........ 2199

Bacteroides distasonis infections (see under B. distasonis infections)

Bacteroides fragilis infections (see under B. fragilis infections)

Bacteroides ovatus infections (see under B. ovatus infections)

Bacteroides species bone and joint infections
Cefizox for Intramuscular or Intravenous Use (Ceftizoxime Sodium) Fujisawa 1034

Bacteroides species bone and joint infections, adjunct in
Flagyl 375 Capsules (Metronidazole) Searle........ 2434
Flagyl I.V. (Metronidazole Hydrochloride) SCS........ 2247
Protostat Tablets (Metronidazole) Ortho Pharmaceutical 1883

Bacteroides species CNS infection
Flagyl 375 Capsules (Metronidazole) Searle........ 2434
Flagyl I.V. (Metronidazole Hydrochloride) SCS........ 2247
Protostat Tablets (Metronidazole) Ortho Pharmaceutical 1883

Bacteroides species empyema
Flagyl 375 Capsules (Metronidazole) Searle........ 2434
Flagyl I.V. (Metronidazole Hydrochloride) SCS........ 2247
Protostat Tablets (Metronidazole) Ortho Pharmaceutical 1883

Bacteroides species endocarditis
Flagyl 375 Capsules (Metronidazole) Searle........ 2434
Flagyl I.V. (Metronidazole Hydrochloride) SCS........ 2247
Protostat Tablets (Metronidazole) Ortho Pharmaceutical 1883

Bacteroides species endomyometritis
Flagyl 375 Capsules (Metronidazole) Searle........ 2434
Flagyl I.V. (Metronidazole Hydrochloride) SCS........ 2247
Protostat Tablets (Metronidazole) Ortho Pharmaceutical 1883

Bacteroides species gynecologic infections
Cefobid Intravenous/Intramuscular (Cefoperazone Sodium) Roerig 2189
Cefobid Pharmacy Bulk Package - Not for Direct Infusion (Cefoperazone Sodium) Roerig........ 2192
Cefotan (Cefotetan) Zeneca........ 2829
Claforan Sterile and Injection (Cefotaxime Sodium) Hoechst-Roussel........ 1235
Flagyl 375 Capsules (Metronidazole) Searle........ 2434
Flagyl I.V. (Metronidazole Hydrochloride) SCS........ 2247
Mefoxin (Cefoxitin Sodium) Merck & Co., Inc. 1691
Mefoxin Premixed Intravenous Solution (Cefoxitin Sodium) Merck & Co., Inc. 1694
Mezlin (Mezlocillin Sodium) Bayer Pharmaceutical 601
Mezlin Pharmacy Bulk Package (Mezlocillin Sodium) Bayer Pharmaceutical 604
Primaxin I.M. (Imipenem-Cilastatin Sodium) Merck & Co., Inc. 1727
Primaxin I.V. (Imipenem-Cilastatin Sodium) Merck & Co., Inc. 1729
Protostat Tablets (Metronidazole) Ortho Pharmaceutical 1883
Unasyn (Ampicillin Sodium, Sulbactam Sodium) Roerig 2212

Bacteroides species infections (see also under B. fragilis infections; B. distasonis infections; B. ovatus infections; B. thetaiotaomicron infections; B. vulgatus infections)
Achromycin V Capsules (Tetracycline Hydrochloride) Lederle 1367
Cefizox for Intramuscular or Intravenous Use (Ceftizoxime Sodium) Fujisawa 1034
Cefobid Intravenous/Intramuscular (Cefoperazone Sodium) Roerig 2189
Cefobid Pharmacy Bulk Package - Not for Direct Infusion (Cefoperazone Sodium) Roerig........ 2192
Cefotan (Cefotetan) Zeneca........ 2829
Ceptaz (Ceftazidime) Glaxo Wellcome 1081
Claforan Sterile and Injection (Cefotaxime Sodium) Hoechst-Roussel........ 1235
Declomycin Tablets (Demeclocycline Hydrochloride) Lederle 1371
Doryx Capsules (Doxycycline Hyclate) Parke-Davis........ 1913
Flagyl 375 Capsules (Metronidazole) Searle........ 2434
Flagyl I.V. (Metronidazole Hydrochloride) SCS........ 2247
Fortaz (Ceftazidime) Glaxo Wellcome 1100
Mefoxin (Cefoxitin Sodium) Merck & Co., Inc. 1691
Mefoxin Premixed Intravenous Solution (Cefoxitin Sodium) Merck & Co., Inc. 1694
Mezlin (Mezlocillin Sodium) Bayer Pharmaceutical 601
Mezlin Pharmacy Bulk Package (Mezlocillin Sodium) Bayer Pharmaceutical 604
Minocin Intravenous (Minocycline Hydrochloride) Lederle 1382
Pipracil (Piperacillin Sodium) Lederle 1390
Primaxin I.M. (Imipenem-Cilastatin Sodium) Merck & Co., Inc. 1727
Primaxin I.V. (Imipenem-Cilastatin Sodium) Merck & Co., Inc. 1729
Protostat Tablets (Metronidazole) Ortho Pharmaceutical 1883
Tazicef for Injection (Ceftazidime) SmithKline Beecham Pharmaceuticals 2519
Tazidime Vials, Faspak & ADD-Vantage (Ceftazidime) Lilly .. 1478
Terramycin Intramuscular Solution (Oxytetracycline) Roerig 2210
Vibramycin Hyclate Intravenous (Doxycycline Hyclate) Roerig........ 2215

Bacteroides species intra-abdominal infections
Cefizox for Intramuscular or Intravenous Use (Ceftizoxime Sodium) Fujisawa 1034
Cefobid Intravenous/Intramuscular (Cefoperazone Sodium) Roerig 2189
Cefobid Pharmacy Bulk Package - Not for Direct Infusion (Cefoperazone Sodium) Roerig........ 2192
Cefotan (Cefotetan) Zeneca........ 2829

Bacteroides species **Indications Index** **1460**

Ceptaz (Ceftazidime) Glaxo Wellcome ... 1081
Claforan Sterile and Injection (Cefotaxime Sodium) Hoechst-Roussel ... 1235
Flagyl 375 Capsules (Metronidazole) Searle ... 2434
Flagyl I.V. (Metronidazole Hydrochloride) SCS ... 2247
Fortaz (Ceftazidime) Glaxo Wellcome ... 1100
Mefoxin (Cefoxitin Sodium) Merck & Co., Inc. ... 1691
Mefoxin Premixed Intravenous Solution (Cefoxitin Sodium) Merck & Co., Inc. ... 1694
Mezlin (Mezlocillin Sodium) Bayer Pharmaceutical ... 601
Mezlin Pharmacy Bulk Package (Mezlocillin Sodium) Bayer Pharmaceutical ... 604
Pipracil (Piperacillin Sodium) Lederle ... 1390
Primaxin I.M. (Imipenem-Cilastatin Sodium) Merck & Co., Inc. ... 1727
Primaxin I.V. (Imipenem-Cilastatin Sodium) Merck & Co., Inc. ... 1729
Protostat Tablets (Metronidazole) Ortho Pharmaceutical ... 1883
Tazicef for Injection (Ceftazidime) SmithKline Beecham Pharmaceuticals ... 2519
Tazidime Vials, Faspak & ADD-Vantage (Ceftazidime) Lilly .. 1478
Unasyn (Ampicillin Sodium, Sulbactam Sodium) Roerig ... 2212

Bacteroides species liver abscess
Flagyl 375 Capsules (Metronidazole) Searle ... 2434
Flagyl I.V. (Metronidazole Hydrochloride) SCS ... 2247
Protostat Tablets (Metronidazole) Ortho Pharmaceutical ... 1883

Bacteroides species lower respiratory tract infections
Cefizox for Intramuscular or Intravenous Use (Ceftizoxime Sodium) Fujisawa ... 1034
Flagyl 375 Capsules (Metronidazole) Searle ... 2434
Flagyl I.V. (Metronidazole Hydrochloride) SCS ... 2247
Mefoxin (Cefoxitin Sodium) Merck & Co., Inc. ... 1691
Mefoxin Premixed Intravenous Solution (Cefoxitin Sodium) Merck & Co., Inc. ... 1694
Mezlin (Mezlocillin Sodium) Bayer Pharmaceutical ... 601
Mezlin Pharmacy Bulk Package (Mezlocillin Sodium) Bayer Pharmaceutical ... 604
Protostat Tablets (Metronidazole) Ortho Pharmaceutical ... 1883

Bacteroides species lung abscess
Flagyl 375 Capsules (Metronidazole) Searle ... 2434
Flagyl I.V. (Metronidazole Hydrochloride) SCS ... 2247
Mefoxin (Cefoxitin Sodium) Merck & Co., Inc. ... 1691
Mefoxin Premixed Intravenous Solution (Cefoxitin Sodium) Merck & Co., Inc. ... 1694
Mezlin (Mezlocillin Sodium) Bayer Pharmaceutical ... 601
Mezlin Pharmacy Bulk Package (Mezlocillin Sodium) Bayer Pharmaceutical ... 604
Protostat Tablets (Metronidazole) Ortho Pharmaceutical ... 1883

Bacteroides species meningitis
Flagyl 375 Capsules (Metronidazole) Searle ... 2434
Flagyl I.V. (Metronidazole Hydrochloride) SCS ... 2247
Protostat Tablets (Metronidazole) Ortho Pharmaceutical ... 1883

Bacteroides species peritonitis
Flagyl 375 Capsules (Metronidazole) Searle ... 2434
Flagyl I.V. (Metronidazole Hydrochloride) SCS ... 2247
Mefoxin (Cefoxitin Sodium) Merck & Co., Inc. ... 1691
Mefoxin Premixed Intravenous Solution (Cefoxitin Sodium) Merck & Co., Inc. ... 1694
Mezlin (Mezlocillin Sodium) Bayer Pharmaceutical ... 601
Mezlin Pharmacy Bulk Package (Mezlocillin Sodium) Bayer Pharmaceutical ... 604
Primaxin I.M. (Imipenem-Cilastatin Sodium) Merck & Co., Inc. ... 1727
Protostat Tablets (Metronidazole) Ortho Pharmaceutical ... 1883

Bacteroides species pneumonia
Flagyl 375 Capsules (Metronidazole) Searle ... 2434
Flagyl I.V. (Metronidazole Hydrochloride) SCS ... 2247
Mefoxin (Cefoxitin Sodium) Merck & Co., Inc. ... 1691
Mefoxin Premixed Intravenous Solution (Cefoxitin Sodium) Merck & Co., Inc. ... 1694
Mezlin (Mezlocillin Sodium) Bayer Pharmaceutical ... 601
Mezlin Pharmacy Bulk Package (Mezlocillin Sodium) Bayer Pharmaceutical ... 604
Protostat Tablets (Metronidazole) Ortho Pharmaceutical ... 1883

Bacteroides species septicemia
Cefizox for Intramuscular or Intravenous Use (Ceftizoxime Sodium) Fujisawa ... 1034
Flagyl 375 Capsules (Metronidazole) Searle ... 2434
Flagyl I.V. (Metronidazole Hydrochloride) SCS ... 2247
Mefoxin (Cefoxitin Sodium) Merck & Co., Inc. ... 1691
Mefoxin Premixed Intravenous Solution (Cefoxitin Sodium) Merck & Co., Inc. ... 1694
Mezlin (Mezlocillin Sodium) Bayer Pharmaceutical ... 601
Mezlin Pharmacy Bulk Package (Mezlocillin Sodium) Bayer Pharmaceutical ... 604
Pipracil (Piperacillin Sodium) Lederle ... 1390
Primaxin I.V. (Imipenem-Cilastatin Sodium) Merck & Co., Inc. ... 1729

Bacteroides species skin and skin structure infections
Cefizox for Intramuscular or Intravenous Use (Ceftizoxime Sodium) Fujisawa ... 1034
Claforan Sterile and Injection (Cefotaxime Sodium) Hoechst-Roussel ... 1235
Flagyl 375 Capsules (Metronidazole) Searle ... 2434
Flagyl I.V. (Metronidazole Hydrochloride) SCS ... 2247
Mefoxin (Cefoxitin Sodium) Merck & Co., Inc. ... 1691
Mefoxin Premixed Intravenous Solution (Cefoxitin Sodium) Merck & Co., Inc. ... 1694
Mezlin (Mezlocillin Sodium) Bayer Pharmaceutical ... 601
Mezlin Pharmacy Bulk Package (Mezlocillin Sodium) Bayer Pharmaceutical ... 604
Primaxin I.M. (Imipenem-Cilastatin Sodium) Merck & Co., Inc. ... 1727
Primaxin I.V. (Imipenem-Cilastatin Sodium) Merck & Co., Inc. ... 1729
Protostat Tablets (Metronidazole) Ortho Pharmaceutical ... 1883

Bacteroides species tubo-ovarian abscess
Flagyl 375 Capsules (Metronidazole) Searle ... 2434
Flagyl I.V. (Metronidazole Hydrochloride) SCS ... 2247
Protostat Tablets (Metronidazole) Ortho Pharmaceutical ... 1883

Bacteroides species vaginal cuff infection, post-surgical
Flagyl 375 Capsules (Metronidazole) Searle ... 2434
Flagyl I.V. (Metronidazole Hydrochloride) SCS ... 2247
Protostat Tablets (Metronidazole) Ortho Pharmaceutical ... 1883

Bacteroides thetaiotaomicron infections (see under B. thetaiotaomicron infections)

Bacteroides vulgatus infections (see under B. vulgatus infections)

Baldness, male pattern of vertex of scalp
Rogaine Topical Solution (Minoxidil) Upjohn ... 2637

Barber's itch (see under Folliculitis barbae)

Bartonella bacilliformis infections
Achromycin V Capsules (Tetracycline Hydrochloride) Lederle ... 1367
Declomycin Tablets (Demeclocycline Hydrochloride) Lederle ... 1371
Doryx Capsules (Doxycycline Hyclate) Parke-Davis ... 1913
Dynacin Capsules (Minocycline Hydrochloride) Medicis ... 1590
Minocin Intravenous (Minocycline Hydrochloride) Lederle ... 1382
Minocin Oral Suspension (Minocycline Hydrochloride) Lederle ... 1385
Minocin Pellet-Filled Capsules (Minocycline Hydrochloride) Lederle ... 1383
Monodox Capsules (Doxycycline Monohydrate) Oclassen ... 1805
Terramycin Intramuscular Solution (Oxytetracycline) Roerig ... 2210
Vibramycin (Doxycycline Calcium) Pfizer Labs ... 1941
Vibramycin Hyclate Intravenous (Doxycycline Hyclate) Roerig ... 2215
Vibramycin (Doxycycline Monohydrate) Pfizer Labs ... 1941

Bartonellosis
Dynacin Capsules (Minocycline Hydrochloride) Medicis ... 1590
Minocin Oral Suspension (Minocycline Hydrochloride) Lederle ... 1385
Minocin Pellet-Filled Capsules (Minocycline Hydrochloride) Lederle ... 1383
Monodox Capsules (Doxycycline Monohydrate) Oclassen ... 1805

Bedsores (see under Ulcers, decubitus, adjunctive therapy in)

Behavioral problems associated with chronic brain syndrome
Serentil (Mesoridazine Besylate) Boehringer Ingelheim ... 684

Behavioral problems associated with mental deficiency
Serentil (Mesoridazine Besylate) Boehringer Ingelheim ... 684

Behavioral problems, severe, in children
Haldol Injection, Tablets and Concentrate (Haloperidol) McNeil Pharmaceutical ... 1575
Mellaril (Thioridazine Hydrochloride) Sandoz Pharmaceuticals ... 2269
Thorazine (Chlorpromazine Hydrochloride) SmithKline Beecham Pharmaceuticals ... 2523

Bejel
Bicillin L-A Injection (Penicillin G Benzathine) Wyeth-Ayerst ... 2707

Belching (see under Eructation, relief of)

Benzodiazepine overdose, management of
Romazicon (Flumazenil) Roche Laboratories ... 2147

Berylliosis
Aristocort Suspension (Forte Parenteral) (Triamcinolone Diacetate) Fujisawa ... 1027
Aristocort Tablets (Triamcinolone) Fujisawa ... 1022
Celestone Soluspan Suspension (Betamethasone Sodium Phosphate, Betamethasone Acetate) Schering ... 2347
Cortone Acetate Sterile Suspension (Cortisone Acetate) Merck & Co., Inc. ... 1623
Cortone Acetate Tablets (Cortisone Acetate) Merck & Co., Inc. ... 1624
Dalalone D.P. Injectable (Dexamethasone Acetate) Forest ... 1011
Decadron Elixir (Dexamethasone) Merck & Co., Inc. ... 1633
Decadron Phosphate Injection (Dexamethasone Sodium Phosphate) Merck & Co., Inc. ... 1637
Decadron Tablets (Dexamethasone) Merck & Co., Inc. ... 1635
Decadron-LA Sterile Suspension (Dexamethasone Acetate) Merck & Co., Inc. ... 1646
Deltasone Tablets (Prednisone) Upjohn ... 2595
Depo-Medrol Single-Dose Vial (Methylprednisolone Acetate) Upjohn ... 2600
Depo-Medrol Sterile Aqueous Suspension (Methylprednisolone Acetate) Upjohn ... 2597
Hydeltrasol Injection, Sterile (Prednisolone Sodium Phosphate) Merck & Co., Inc. ... 1665
Hydrocortone Phosphate Injection, Sterile (Hydrocortisone Sodium Phosphate) Merck & Co., Inc. ... 1670
Hydrocortone Tablets (Hydrocortisone) Merck & Co., Inc. ... 1672
Medrol (Methylprednisolone) Upjohn ... 2621
Pediapred Oral Liquid (Prednisolone Sodium Phosphate) Fisons ... 995
Prelone Syrup (Prednisolone) Muro 1787
Solu-Cortef Sterile Powder (Hydrocortisone Sodium Succinate) Upjohn ... 2641
Solu-Medrol Sterile Powder (Methylprednisolone Sodium Succinate) Upjohn ... 2643

Bifidobacterium species gynecologic infections
Primaxin I.V. (Imipenem-Cilastatin Sodium) Merck & Co., Inc. ... 1729

Bifidobacterium species infections
Primaxin I.V. (Imipenem-Cilastatin Sodium) Merck & Co., Inc. ... 1729

Bifidobacterium species intra-abdominal infections
Primaxin I.V. (Imipenem-Cilastatin Sodium) Merck & Co., Inc. ... 1729

Biliary calculi, chemical dissolution of
Actigall Capsules (Ursodiol) CibaGeneva ... 802

Bites, black widow spider
Antivenin (Black Widow Spider) (Black Widow Spider Antivenin (Equine)) Merck & Co., Inc. ... 1607

Bites, crotalidae (see under Envenomation, pit viper)

Bites, insect
Aquanil HC Lotion (Hydrocortisone) Persön & Covey 1931
Benadryl Itch Relief Spray, Children's Formula and Maximum Strength 2% (Diphenhydramine Hydrochloride, Zinc Acetate) WARNER WELLCOME ... ▣ 851
Benadryl Itch Stopping Gel, Children's Formula and Maximum Strength 2% (Diphenhydramine Hydrochloride, Zinc Acetate) WARNER WELLCOME ... ▣ 851
Caldecort (Hydrocortisone Acetate) CIBA Consumer ... ▣ 631
Cortaid (Hydrocortisone Acetate) Upjohn ... ▣ 836
Cortizone-5 (Hydrocortisone) Thompson Medical ... ▣ 831
Cortizone-10 Creme and Ointment (Hydrocortisone) Thompson Medical ... ▣ 831
EpiPen (Epinephrine) Center ... 790

1461 **Indications Index** **Bronchial asthma**

Mantadil Cream (Chlorcyclizine Hydrochloride) Glaxo Wellcome.... 1135

Bites, pit vipers
(see under Envenomation, pit viper)

Blackheads, reduction of
(see under Histomoniasis, reduction of)

Bladder carcinoma, transitional cell
(see under Carcinoma, bladder, transitional cell)

Blastoma, medullary, palliative therapy in
BiCNU (Carmustine (BCNU)) Bristol-Myers Squibb Oncology 691

Blastomycosis
Fungizone Intravenous (Amphotericin B) Apothecon 506
Nizoral Tablets (Ketoconazole) Janssen.... 1298
Sporanox Capsules (Itraconazole) Janssen.... 1305

Blastomycosis, North American
(see under Blastomycosis)

Bleeding associated with hemophilia A
Konȳne 80 Factor IX Complex (Factor IX Complex) Bayer Biological 634

Bleeding, fibrinolytic
Amicar Syrup, Tablets, and Injection (Aminocaproic Acid) Immunex 1267

Bleeding, upper gastrointestinal, in critically ill
Tagamet (Cimetidine Hydrochloride) SmithKline Beecham Pharmaceuticals.... 2516

Blepharitis
Genoptic Sterile Ophthalmic Solution (Gentamicin Sulfate) Allergan.... ⊙ 243
Genoptic Sterile Ophthalmic Ointment (Gentamicin Sulfate) Allergan.... ⊙ 243
Gentacidin Ointment (Gentamicin Sulfate) CIBA Vision Ophthalmics .... ⊙ 264
Gentacidin Solution (Gentamicin Sulfate) CIBA Vision Ophthalmics .... ⊙ 264
Gentak (Gentamicin Sulfate) Akorn .... ⊙ 208
Neosporin Ophthalmic Ointment Sterile (Polymyxin B Sulfate, Bacitracin Zinc, Neomycin Sulfate) Glaxo Wellcome 1148
Neosporin Ophthalmic Solution Sterile (Polymyxin B Sulfate, Neomycin Sulfate, Gramicidin) Glaxo Wellcome.... 1149
Polysporin Ophthalmic Ointment Sterile (Polymyxin B Sulfate, Bacitracin Zinc) Glaxo Wellcome.. 1154
Pred Mild (Prednisolone Acetate) Allergan.... ⊙ 253

Blepharitis, fungal
Natacyn Antifungal Ophthalmic Suspension (Natamycin) Alcon Laboratories .... ⊙ 225

Blepharoconjunctivitis
Genoptic Sterile Ophthalmic Solution (Gentamicin Sulfate) Allergan.... ⊙ 243
Genoptic Sterile Ophthalmic Ointment (Gentamicin Sulfate) Allergan.... ⊙ 243
Gentacidin Ointment (Gentamicin Sulfate) CIBA Vision Ophthalmics .... ⊙ 264
Gentacidin Solution (Gentamicin Sulfate) CIBA Vision Ophthalmics .... ⊙ 264
Gentak (Gentamicin Sulfate) Akorn .... ⊙ 208
Neosporin Ophthalmic Ointment Sterile (Polymyxin B Sulfate, Bacitracin Zinc, Neomycin Sulfate) Glaxo Wellcome 1148
Neosporin Ophthalmic Solution Sterile (Polymyxin B Sulfate, Neomycin Sulfate, Gramicidin) Glaxo Wellcome.... 1149
Polysporin Ophthalmic Ointment Sterile (Polymyxin B Sulfate, Bacitracin Zinc) Glaxo Wellcome.. 1154
Polytrim Ophthalmic Solution Sterile (Polymyxin B Sulfate, Trimethoprim Sulfate) Allergan 482

Blepharospasm
BOTOX (Botulinum Toxin Type A) Purified Neurotoxin Complex (Botulinum Toxin Type A) Allergan 477

Blood clotting, prevention of in arterial surgery
Heparin Sodium Injection (Heparin Sodium) Wyeth-Ayerst.... 2726
Heparin Sodium Vials (Heparin Sodium) Lilly.... 1441

Blood clotting, prevention of in blood transfusion
Heparin Lock Flush Solution (Heparin Sodium) Wyeth-Ayerst.... 2725
Heparin Sodium Injection, USP, Sterile Solution (Heparin Sodium) Upjohn.... 2615
Heparin Sodium Vials (Heparin Sodium) Lilly.... 1441

Blood clotting, prevention of in cardiac surgery
Heparin Sodium Injection (Heparin Sodium) Wyeth-Ayerst 2726
Heparin Sodium Injection, USP, Sterile Solution (Heparin Sodium) Upjohn.... 2615
Heparin Sodium Vials (Heparin Sodium) Lilly.... 1441

Blood clotting, prevention of in dialysis procedures
Heparin Lock Flush Solution (Heparin Sodium) Wyeth-Ayerst.... 2725
Heparin Sodium Injection, USP, Sterile Solution (Heparin Sodium) Upjohn.... 2615
Heparin Sodium Vials (Heparin Sodium) Lilly.... 1441

Blood clotting, prevention of in extracorporeal circulation
Heparin Lock Flush Solution (Heparin Sodium) Wyeth-Ayerst.... 2725
Heparin Sodium Vials (Heparin Sodium) Lilly.... 1441

Blood loss, perioperative, reduction of
Trasylol (Aprotinin) Bayer Pharmaceutical 613

Blood pressure, maintaining during anesthesia
(see under Hypotension, acute)

Blood pressure, restoring during anesthesia
(see under Hypotension, acute)

Body aches
(see under Pain, general)

Body cavities, irrigation of
Zephiran Chloride Aqueous Solution (Benzalkonium Chloride) Sanofi Winthrop.... ■ 795

Boils, symptomatic relief of
(see under Furunculosis, symptomatic relief of)

Bone disease, metabolic, with chronic renal failure
(see under Osteodystrophy, renal)

Bone marrow transplantation, allogeneic or autologous, delayed or failed
Leukine for IV Infusion (Sargramostim) Immunex.... 1271

Bone marrow transplantation, to decrease the risk of septicemia
Gamimune N, 5% Immune Globulin Intravenous (Human), 5% (Globulin, Immune (Human)) Bayer Biological.... 619
Gamimune N, 10% Immune Globulin Intravenous (Human), 10% (Globulin, Immune (Human)) Bayer Biological 621

Bone mass, loss of
(see under Osteoporosis)

Bordetella pertussis
(see under B. pertussis infections)

Borrelia recurrentis infection
Achromycin V Capsules (Tetracycline Hydrochloride) Lederle 1367
Declomycin Tablets (Demeclocycline Hydrochloride) Lederle 1371
Doryx Capsules (Doxycycline Hyclate) Parke-Davis.... 1913
Dynacin Capsules (Minocycline Hydrochloride) Medicis 1590
Minocin Intravenous (Minocycline Hydrochloride) Lederle 1382
Minocin Oral Suspension (Minocycline Hydrochloride) Lederle 1385
Minocin Pellet-Filled Capsules (Minocycline Hydrochloride) Lederle 1383
Monodox Capsules (Doxycycline Monohydrate) Oclassen.... 1805
Terramycin Intramuscular Solution (Oxytetracycline) Roerig 2210
Vibramycin (Doxycycline Calcium) Pfizer Labs 1941
Vibramycin Hyclate Intravenous (Doxycycline Hyclate) Roerig.... 2215
Vibramycin (Doxycycline Monohydrate) Pfizer Labs 1941

Bowel, evacuation of
Ceo-Two Rectal Suppositories (Sodium Bicarbonate, Potassium Bitartrate) Beutlich 666
Colyte and Colyte-flavored (Polyethylene Glycol) Schwarz 2396
Fleet Bisacodyl Enema (Bisacodyl) Fleet.... 1002
Fleet Enema (Sodium Phosphate, Dibasic, Sodium Phosphate, Monobasic) Fleet 1002
Fleet Mineral Oil Enema (Mineral Oil) Fleet.... 1002
Fleet Phospho-Soda (Sodium Phosphate, Dibasic, Sodium Phosphate, Monobasic) Fleet 1003
Fleet Prep Kits (Sodium Phosphate, Dibasic, Sodium Phosphate, Monobasic) Fleet 1003
GoLYTELY (Polyethylene Glycol) Braintree 688
NuLYTELY (Polyethylene Glycol) Braintree 689
Cherry Flavor NuLYTELY (Polyethylene Glycol, Sodium Bicarbonate, Sodium Chloride, Potassium Chloride) Braintree 689
Purge Concentrate (Castor Oil) Fleming .... ■ 655
Senna X-Prep Bowel Evacuant Liquid (Senna Concentrates) Gray 1230

Bowel, irritable, syndrome
Bentyl (Dicyclomine Hydrochloride) Marion Merrell Dow.... 1501
Konsyl Fiber Tablets (Calcium Polycarbophil) Konsyl .... ■ 663
Levsin/Levsinex/Levbid (Hyoscyamine Sulfate) Schwarz 2405
Metamucil (Psyllium Preparations) Procter & Gamble 1975

Bowel, irritable, syndrome, "possibly" effective in, adjunctive therapy
Cystospaz (Hyoscyamine) PolyMedica 1963
Donnatal (Phenobarbital, Belladonna Alkaloids) Robins 2060
Donnatal Extentabs (Phenobarbital, Belladonna Alkaloids) Robins 2061
Donnatal Tablets (Phenobarbital, Belladonna Alkaloids) Robins 2060
Librax Capsules (Chlordiazepoxide Hydrochloride, Clidinium Bromide) Roche Products 2176

Brain imaging
(see under Intracranial lesions imaging, magnetic resonance)

Brain tumors
(see under Tumors, brain, palliative therapy in)

Branhamella catarrhalis
(see under M. catarrhalis infections)

Breast cancer
(see under Carcinoma, breast)

Breast carcinoma
(see under Carcinoma, breast)

Breast disease, fibrocystic
Danocrine Capsules (Danazol) Sanofi Winthrop 2307

Breast milk, replacement of or supplement to
Bonamil Infant Formula with Iron, Powder, Ready-To-Feed and Concentrated Liquids (Infant Formula, Ferrous Sulfate) Wyeth-Ayerst 2709
Nursoy, Soy Protein Formula for Infants, Concentrated Liquid, Ready-to-Feed, and Powder (Protein Preparations) Wyeth-Ayerst .. 2763
SMA Infant Formula (Nutritional Supplement) Wyeth-Ayerst 2811

Breathing, intermittent positive pressure-aid in
Sodium Chloride and Sterile Water for Inhalation, Arm-a-Vial (Sodium Chloride) Astra 562

Bromhidrosis, topical relief of
(see under Hyperhidrosis, topical relief of)

Bronchial airway hyperreactivity, diagnosis of
Provocholine for Inhalation (Methacholine Chloride) Roche Laboratories 2140

Bronchial asthma
AeroBid Inhaler System (Flunisolide) Forest 1005
Aerobid-M Inhaler System (Flunisolide) Forest 1005
Aerolate (Theophylline Anhydrous) Fleming.... 1004
Airet Solution for Inhalation (Albuterol Sulfate) Adams 452
Alupent (Metaproterenol Sulfate) Boehringer Ingelheim 669
Ana-Kit Anaphylaxis Emergency Treatment Kit (Epinephrine Hydrochloride, Chlorpheniramine Maleate) Bayer Allergy 617
Aristocort Suspension (Forte Parenteral) (Triamcinolone Diacetate) Fujisawa 1027
Aristocort Tablets (Triamcinolone) Fujisawa 1022
Atrovent Inhalation Aerosol (Ipratropium Bromide) Boehringer Ingelheim 671
Azmacort Oral Inhaler (Triamcinolone Acetonide) Rhone-Poulenc Rorer Pharmaceuticals.... 2011
Beclovent Inhalation Aerosol and Refill (Beclomethasone Dipropionate) Glaxo Wellcome 1075
Brethine Ampuls (Terbutaline Sulfate) CibaGeneva 815
Brethine Tablets (Terbutaline Sulfate) CibaGeneva 814
Bricanyl Subcutaneous Injection (Terbutaline Sulfate) Marion Merrell Dow.... 1502
Bricanyl Tablets (Terbutaline Sulfate) Marion Merrell Dow 1503
Bronkaid Mist (Epinephrine) Miles Consumer.... ■ 717
Bronkaid Mist Suspension (Epinephrine Bitartrate) Miles Consumer.... ■ 718
Bronkometer Aerosol (Isoetharine) Sanofi Winthrop 2302

(■ Described in PDR For Nonprescription Drugs) (⊙ Described in PDR For Ophthalmology)

Bronkosol Solution (Isoetharine) Sanofi Winthrop ... 2302
Celestone Soluspan Suspension (Betamethasone Sodium Phosphate, Betamethasone Acetate) Schering ... 2347
Congess (Guaifenesin, Pseudoephedrine Hydrochloride) Fleming ... 1004
Cortone Acetate Sterile Suspension (Cortisone Acetate) Merck & Co., Inc. ... 1623
Cortone Acetate Tablets (Cortisone Acetate) Merck & Co., Inc. ... 1624
Dalalone D.P. Injectable (Dexamethasone Acetate) Forest ... 1011
Decadron Elixir (Dexamethasone) Merck & Co., Inc. ... 1633
Decadron Phosphate Injection (Dexamethasone Sodium Phosphate) Merck & Co., Inc. ... 1637
Decadron Phosphate Respihaler (Dexamethasone Sodium Phosphate) Merck & Co., Inc. ... 1642
Decadron Tablets (Dexamethasone) Merck & Co., Inc. ... 1635
Decadron-LA Sterile Suspension (Dexamethasone Acetate) Merck & Co., Inc. ... 1646
Deltasone Tablets (Prednisone) Upjohn ... 2595
Depo-Medrol Single-Dose Vial (Methylprednisolone Acetate) Upjohn ... 2600
Depo-Medrol Sterile Aqueous Suspension (Methylprednisolone Acetate) Upjohn ... 2597
Dexacort Phosphate in Respihaler (Dexamethasone Sodium Phosphate) Adams ... 458
Hydeltrasol Injection, Sterile (Prednisolone Sodium Phosphate) Merck & Co., Inc. ... 1665
Hydrocortone Phosphate Injection, Sterile (Hydrocortisone Sodium Phosphate) Merck & Co., Inc. ... 1670
Hydrocortone Tablets (Hydrocortisone) Merck & Co., Inc. ... 1672
Intal Capsules (Cromolyn Sodium) Fisons ... 987
Intal Inhaler (Cromolyn Sodium) Fisons ... 988
Intal Nebulizer Solution (Cromolyn Sodium) Fisons ... 989
Isoetharine Inhalation Solution, USP, Arm-a-Med (Isoetharine) Astra ... 551
Isuprel Hydrochloride Solution 1:200 & 1:100 (Isoproterenol Hydrochloride) Sanofi Winthrop .. 2313
Isuprel Mistometer (Isoproterenol Hydrochloride) Sanofi Winthrop .. 2312
Lufyllin & Lufyllin-400 Tablets (Dyphylline) Wallace ... 2670
Lufyllin-GG Elixir & Tablets (Dyphylline, Guaifenesin) Wallace ... 2671
Maxair Autohaler (Pirbuterol Acetate) 3M Pharmaceuticals ... 1492
Maxair Inhaler (Pirbuterol Acetate) 3M Pharmaceuticals ... 1494
Medrol (Methylprednisolone) Upjohn ... 2621
Metaproterenol Sulfate Inhalation Solution, USP, Arm-a-Med (Metaproterenol Sulfate) Astra ... 552
Norisodrine with Calcium Iodide Syrup (Calcium Iodide, Isoproterenol Sulfate) Abbott ... 442
Pediapred Oral Liquid (Prednisolone Sodium Phosphate) Fisons ... 995
Pima Syrup (Potassium Iodide) Fleming ... 1005
Prelone Syrup (Prednisolone) Muro 1787
Primatene Dual Action Formula (Ephedrine Hydrochloride, Guaifenesin, Theophylline Anhydrous) Whitehall ... ■ 872
Primatene Mist (Epinephrine) Whitehall ... ■ 873
Primatene Tablets (Theophylline Anhydrous, Ephedrine Hydrochloride) Whitehall ... ■ 873
Proventil Inhalation Aerosol (Albuterol) Schering ... 2382
Proventil Inhalation Solution 0.083% (Albuterol Sulfate) Schering ... 2384
Proventil Repetabs Tablets (Albuterol Sulfate) Schering ... 2386
Proventil Solution for Inhalation 0.5% (Albuterol Sulfate) Schering ... 2383
Proventil Syrup (Albuterol Sulfate) Schering ... 2385
Proventil Tablets (Albuterol Sulfate) Schering ... 2386
Quadrinal Tablets (Ephedrine Hydrochloride, Phenobarbital, Potassium Iodide, Theophylline Calcium Salicylate) Knoll Laboratories ... 1350
Quibron (Theophylline, Guaifenesin) Roberts ... 2053
Respbid Tablets (Theophylline Anhydrous) Boehringer Ingelheim 682
SSKI Solution (Potassium Iodide) Upsher-Smith ... 2658
Serevent Inhalation Aerosol (Salmeterol Xinafoate) Glaxo Wellcome ... 1176
Slo-bid Gyrocaps (Theophylline Anhydrous) Rhone-Poulenc Rorer Pharmaceuticals ... 2033
Solu-Cortef Sterile Powder (Hydrocortisone Sodium Succinate) Upjohn ... 2641
Solu-Medrol Sterile Powder (Methylprednisolone Sodium Succinate) Upjohn ... 2643
Sus-Phrine Injection (Epinephrine) Forest ... 1019
Theo-24 Extended Release Capsules (Theophylline Anhydrous) UCB ... 2568
Theo-Dur Extended-Release Tablets (Theophylline Anhydrous) Key ... 1327
Theo-X Extended-Release Tablets (Theophylline Anhydrous) Carnrick ... 788
Tilade (Nedocromil Sodium) Fisons 996
Tornalate Solution for Inhalation, 0.2% (Bitolterol Mesylate) Dura .. 956
Tornalate Metered Dose Inhaler (Bitolterol Mesylate) Dura ... 957
Uni-Dur Extended-Release Tablets (Theophylline Anhydrous) Key ... 1331
Uniphyl 400 mg Tablets (Theophylline Anhydrous) Purdue Frederick ... 2001
Vanceril Inhaler (Beclomethasone Dipropionate) Schering ... 2394
Ventolin Inhalation Aerosol and Refill (Albuterol) Glaxo Wellcome 1197
Ventolin Inhalation Solution (Albuterol Sulfate) Glaxo Wellcome .. 1198
Ventolin Nebules Inhalation Solution (Albuterol Sulfate) Glaxo Wellcome ... 1199
Ventolin Rotacaps for Inhalation (Albuterol Sulfate) Glaxo Wellcome ... 1200
Ventolin Syrup (Albuterol Sulfate) Glaxo Wellcome ... 1202
Ventolin Tablets (Albuterol Sulfate) Glaxo Wellcome ... 1203
Volmax Extended-Release Tablets (Albuterol Sulfate) Muro ... 1788

Bronchial congestion

Bronkaid Caplets (Ephedrine Sulfate, Guaifenesin) Miles Consumer ... ■ 717
Dorcol Children's Cough Syrup (Pseudoephedrine Hydrochloride, Guaifenesin, Dextromethorphan Hydrobromide) Sandoz Consumer ... ■ 785
Entex Capsules (Phenylephrine Hydrochloride, Phenylpropanolamine Hydrochloride, Guaifenesin) Procter & Gamble Pharmaceuticals ... 1986
Entex LA Tablets (Phenylpropanolamine Hydrochloride, Guaifenesin) Procter & Gamble Pharmaceuticals ... 1987
Entex Liquid (Phenylephrine Hydrochloride, Phenylpropanolamine Hydrochloride, Guaifenesin) Procter & Gamble Pharmaceuticals ... 1986
Guaifed (Guaifenesin, Pseudoephedrine Hydrochloride) Muro ... 1787
Guaifed Syrup (Guaifenesin, Pseudoephedrine Hydrochloride) Muro ... ■ 734
Guaitab Tablets (Pseudoephedrine Hydrochloride, Guaifenesin) Muro ... ■ 734
Humibid (Guaifenesin, Dextromethorphan Hydrobromide) Adams ... 462
Novahistine DMX (Dextromethorphan Hydrobromide, Guaifenesin, Pseudoephedrine Hydrochloride) SmithKline Beecham Consumer ... ■ 822
Novahistine Expectorant (Codeine Phosphate, Pseudoephedrine Hydrochloride, Guaifenesin) SmithKline Beecham ... 2463
Organidin NR Tablets and Liquid (Guaifenesin) Wallace ... 2672
Pediatric Vicks 44e Chest Cough & Chest Congestion (Dextromethorphan Hydrobromide, Guaifenesin) Procter & Gamble ■ 764
Robitussin (Guaifenesin) A. H. Robins Consumer ... ■ 777
Robitussin A-C Syrup (Codeine Phosphate, Guaifenesin) Robins .. 2073
Robitussin Severe Congestion Liqui-Gels (Guaifenesin, Pseudoephedrine Hydrochloride) A. H. Robins Consumer ... ■ 776
Robitussin-DAC Syrup (Codeine Phosphate, Guaifenesin, Pseudoephedrine Hydrochloride) Robins 2074
Robitussin-DM (Dextromethorphan Hydrobromide, Guaifenesin) A. H. Robins Consumer ... ■ 777
Robitussin-PE (Guaifenesin, Pseudoephedrine Hydrochloride) A. H. Robins Consumer ... ■ 778
Sudafed Cough Syrup (Dextromethorphan Hydrobromide, Guaifenesin, Pseudoephedrine Hydrochloride) WARNER WELLCOME ... ■ 862
Syn-Rx Tablets (Pseudoephedrine Hydrochloride, Guaifenesin) Adams ... 465
Triaminic Expectorant (Phenylpropanolamine Hydrochloride, Guaifenesin) Sandoz Consumer ■ 790
Vicks 44E Chest Cough & Chest Congestion (Dextromethorphan Hydrobromide, Guaifenesin) Procter & Gamble ... ■ 756

Bronchitis, acute

Azactam for Injection (Aztreonam) Bristol-Myers Squibb ... 734
Ceftin Tablets (Cefuroxime Axetil) Glaxo Wellcome ... 1078
Cefzil Tablets and Oral Suspension (Cefprozil) Bristol-Myers Squibb .. 746
Lorabid Suspension and Pulvules (Loracarbef) Lilly ... 1459
Suprax (Cefixime) Lederle ... 1399
Zefazone (Cefmetazole Sodium) Upjohn ... 2654

Bronchitis, chronic

Atrovent Inhalation Aerosol (Ipratropium Bromide) Boehringer Ingelheim ... 671
Brethine Ampuls (Terbutaline Sulfate) CibaGeneva ... 815
Brethine Tablets (Terbutaline Sulfate) CibaGeneva ... 814
Bricanyl Tablets (Terbutaline Sulfate) Marion Merrell Dow ... 1503
Norisodrine with Calcium Iodide Syrup (Calcium Iodide, Isoproterenol Sulfate) Abbott ... 442
Pima Syrup (Potassium Iodide) Fleming ... 1005
Quadrinal Tablets (Ephedrine Hydrochloride, Phenobarbital, Potassium Iodide, Theophylline Calcium Salicylate) Knoll Laboratories ... 1350
Respbid Tablets (Theophylline Anhydrous) Boehringer Ingelheim 682
SSKI Solution (Potassium Iodide) Upsher-Smith ... 2658
Slo-bid Gyrocaps (Theophylline Anhydrous) Rhone-Poulenc Rorer Pharmaceuticals ... 2033

Bronchitis, chronic, acute exacerbation of

Bactrim (Trimethoprim, Sulfamethoxazole) Roche Laboratories ... 2084
Biaxin (Clarithromycin) Abbott ... 405
Ceftin for Oral Suspension (Cefuroxime Axetil) Glaxo Wellcome ... 1078
Cefzil Tablets and Oral Suspension (Cefprozil) Bristol-Myers Squibb .. 746
Floxin I.V. (Ofloxacin) McNeil Pharmaceutical ... 1571
Floxin Tablets (200 mg, 300 mg, 400 mg) (Ofloxacin) McNeil Pharmaceutical ... 1567
Lorabid Suspension and Pulvules (Loracarbef) Lilly ... 1459
Maxaquin Tablets (Lomefloxacin Hydrochloride) Searle ... 2440
Primaxin I.M. (Imipenem-Cilastatin Sodium) Merck & Co., Inc. ... 1727
Septra (Trimethoprim, Sulfamethoxazole) Glaxo Wellcome ... 1174
Spectrobid Tablets (Bacampicillin Hydrochloride) Roerig ... 2206
Suprax (Cefixime) Lederle ... 1399
Vantin for Oral Suspension and Vantin Tablets (Cefpodoxime Proxetil) Upjohn ... 2646

Bronchospasm during anesthesia

Isuprel Hydrochloride Injection 1:5000 (Isoproterenol Hydrochloride) Sanofi Winthrop .. 2311

Bronchospasm, exercise-induced

Intal Capsules (Cromolyn Sodium) Fisons ... 987
Intal Nebulizer Solution (Cromolyn Sodium) Fisons ... 989
Proventil Inhalation Aerosol (Albuterol) Schering ... 2382
Serevent Inhalation Aerosol (Salmeterol Xinafoate) Glaxo Wellcome ... 1176
Ventolin Inhalation Aerosol and Refill (Albuterol) Glaxo Wellcome 1197

Bronchospasm, prevention and relief of

Uni-Dur Extended-Release Tablets (Theophylline Anhydrous) Key ... 1331
Ventolin Inhalation Aerosol and Refill (Albuterol) Glaxo Wellcome 1197
Ventolin Rotacaps for Inhalation (Albuterol Sulfate) Glaxo Wellcome ... 1200

Bronchospasm, reversible (see also under Bronchial asthma)

Alupent (Metaproterenol Sulfate) Boehringer Ingelheim ... 669
Atrovent Inhalation Aerosol (Ipratropium Bromide) Boehringer Ingelheim ... 671
Atrovent Inhalation Solution (Ipratropium Bromide) Boehringer Ingelheim ... 673
Brethaire Inhaler (Terbutaline Sulfate) CibaGeneva ... 813
Brethine Ampuls (Terbutaline Sulfate) CibaGeneva ... 815
Brethine Tablets (Terbutaline Sulfate) CibaGeneva ... 814
Bricanyl Subcutaneous Injection (Terbutaline Sulfate) Marion Merrell Dow ... 1502
Bricanyl Tablets (Terbutaline Sulfate) Marion Merrell Dow ... 1503
Bronkosol Solution (Isoetharine) Sanofi Winthrop ... 2302
Decadron Phosphate Respihaler (Dexamethasone Sodium Phosphate) Merck & Co., Inc. ... 1642
Intal Inhaler (Cromolyn Sodium) Fisons ... 988
Isuprel Hydrochloride Solution 1:200 & 1:100 (Isoproterenol Hydrochloride) Sanofi Winthrop .. 2313
Isuprel Mistometer (Isoproterenol Hydrochloride) Sanofi Winthrop .. 2312
Lufyllin & Lufyllin-400 Tablets (Dyphylline) Wallace ... 2670
Lufyllin-GG Elixir & Tablets (Dyphylline, Guaifenesin) Wallace ... 2671
Maxair Inhaler (Pirbuterol Acetate) 3M Pharmaceuticals ... 1494
Proventil Inhalation Aerosol (Albuterol) Schering ... 2382
Proventil Inhalation Solution 0.083% (Albuterol Sulfate) Schering ... 2384
Proventil Repetabs Tablets (Albuterol Sulfate) Schering ... 2386
Proventil Solution for Inhalation 0.5% (Albuterol Sulfate) Schering ... 2383

(■ Described in PDR For Nonprescription Drugs) (◉ Described in PDR For Ophthalmology)

1463 Indications Index Bursitis

Proventil Syrup (Albuterol Sulfate) Schering ... 2385
Proventil Tablets (Albuterol Sulfate) Schering ... 2386
Quadrinal Tablets (Ephedrine Hydrochloride, Phenobarbital, Potassium Iodide, Theophylline Calcium Salicylate) Knoll Laboratories ... 1350
Respbid Tablets (Theophylline Anhydrous) Boehringer Ingelheim 682
Serevent Inhalation Aerosol (Salmeterol Xinafoate) Glaxo Wellcome ... 1176
Slo-bid Gyrocaps (Theophylline Anhydrous) Rhone-Poulenc Rorer Pharmaceuticals ... 2033
Sus-Phrine Injection (Epinephrine) Forest ... 1019
Theo-24 Extended Release Capsules (Theophylline Anhydrous) UCB ... 2568
Theo-Dur Extended-Release Tablets (Theophylline Anhydrous) Key ... 1327
Theo-X Extended-Release Tablets (Theophylline Anhydrous) Carnrick ... 788
Tornalate Solution for Inhalation, 0.2% (Bitolterol Mesylate) Dura .. 956
Tornalate Metered Dose Inhaler (Bitolterol Mesylate) Dura ... 957
Uniphyl 400 mg Tablets (Theophylline Anhydrous) Purdue Frederick ... 2001
Ventolin Inhalation Aerosol and Refill (Albuterol) Glaxo Wellcome 1197
Ventolin Inhalation Solution (Albuterol Sulfate) Glaxo Wellcome .. 1198
Ventolin Nebules Inhalation Solution (Albuterol Sulfate) Glaxo Wellcome ... 1199
Ventolin Rotacaps for Inhalation (Albuterol Sulfate) Glaxo Wellcome ... 1200
Ventolin Syrup (Albuterol Sulfate) Glaxo Wellcome ... 1202
Ventolin Tablets (Albuterol Sulfate) Glaxo Wellcome ... 1203
Volmax Extended-Release Tablets (Albuterol Sulfate) Muro ... 1788

Bronchospasm, reversible, associated with chronic bronchitis
Alupent (Metaproterenol Sulfate) Boehringer Ingelheim ... 669
Atrovent Inhalation Aerosol (Ipratropium Bromide) Boehringer Ingelheim ... 671
Atrovent Inhalation Solution (Ipratropium Bromide) Boehringer Ingelheim ... 673
Brethine Ampuls (Terbutaline Sulfate) CibaGeneva ... 815
Brethine Tablets (Terbutaline Sulfate) CibaGeneva ... 814
Bronkometer Aerosol (Isoetharine) Sanofi Winthrop ... 2302
Bronkosol Solution (Isoetharine) Sanofi Winthrop ... 2302
Isoetharine Inhalation Solution, USP, Arm-a-Med (Isoetharine) Astra ... 551
Isuprel Hydrochloride Solution 1:200 & 1:100 (Isoproterenol Hydrochloride) Sanofi Winthrop .. 2313
Isuprel Mistometer (Isoproterenol Hydrochloride) Sanofi Winthrop .. 2312
Lufyllin & Lufyllin-400 Tablets (Dyphylline) Wallace ... 2670
Lufyllin-GG Elixir & Tablets (Dyphylline, Guaifenesin) Wallace ... 2671
Metaproterenol Sulfate Inhalation Solution, USP, Arm-a-Med (Metaproterenol Sulfate) Astra ... 552
Quibron (Theophylline, Guaifenesin) Roberts ... 2053
Respbid Tablets (Theophylline Anhydrous) Boehringer Ingelheim 682
Slo-bid Gyrocaps (Theophylline Anhydrous) Rhone-Poulenc Rorer Pharmaceuticals ... 2033
Sus-Phrine Injection (Epinephrine) Forest ... 1019
Theo-24 Extended Release Capsules (Theophylline Anhydrous) UCB ... 2568
Theo-Dur Extended-Release Tablets (Theophylline Anhydrous) Key ... 1327
Theo-X Extended-Release Tablets (Theophylline Anhydrous) Carnrick ... 788
Uni-Dur Extended-Release Tablets (Theophylline Anhydrous) Key ... 1331
Uniphyl 400 mg Tablets (Theophylline Anhydrous) Purdue Frederick ... 2001

Bronchospasm, reversible, associated with emphysema
Alupent (Metaproterenol Sulfate) Boehringer Ingelheim ... 669
Atrovent Inhalation Aerosol (Ipratropium Bromide) Boehringer Ingelheim ... 671
Atrovent Inhalation Solution (Ipratropium Bromide) Boehringer Ingelheim ... 673
Brethine Ampuls (Terbutaline Sulfate) CibaGeneva ... 815
Brethine Tablets (Terbutaline Sulfate) CibaGeneva ... 814
Bronkometer Aerosol (Isoetharine) Sanofi Winthrop ... 2302
Bronkosol Solution (Isoetharine) Sanofi Winthrop ... 2302
Isoetharine Inhalation Solution, USP, Arm-a-Med (Isoetharine) Astra ... 551
Isuprel Hydrochloride Solution 1:200 & 1:100 (Isoproterenol Hydrochloride) Sanofi Winthrop .. 2313
Isuprel Mistometer (Isoproterenol Hydrochloride) Sanofi Winthrop .. 2312
Lufyllin & Lufyllin-400 Tablets (Dyphylline) Wallace ... 2670
Lufyllin-GG Elixir & Tablets (Dyphylline, Guaifenesin) Wallace ... 2671
Maxair Autohaler (Pirbuterol Acetate) 3M Pharmaceuticals ... 1492
Metaproterenol Sulfate Inhalation Solution, USP, Arm-a-Med (Metaproterenol Sulfate) Astra ... 552
Quibron (Theophylline, Guaifenesin) Roberts ... 2053
Respbid Tablets (Theophylline Anhydrous) Boehringer Ingelheim 682
Slo-bid Gyrocaps (Theophylline Anhydrous) Rhone-Poulenc Rorer Pharmaceuticals ... 2033
Sus-Phrine Injection (Epinephrine) Forest ... 1019
Theo-24 Extended Release Capsules (Theophylline Anhydrous) UCB ... 2568
Theo-Dur Extended-Release Tablets (Theophylline Anhydrous) Key ... 1327
Theo-X Extended-Release Tablets (Theophylline Anhydrous) Carnrick ... 788
Uni-Dur Extended-Release Tablets (Theophylline Anhydrous) Key ... 1331
Uniphyl 400 mg Tablets (Theophylline Anhydrous) Purdue Frederick ... 2001

Bronchospastic disorders, "possibly" effective in
Marax Tablets & DF Syrup (Ephedrine Sulfate, Theophylline, Hydroxyzine Hydrochloride) Roerig .. 2200

Brucella species infections
Streptomycin Sulfate Injection (Streptomycin Sulfate) Roerig ... 2208

Brucella species infections, adjunct in
Achromycin V Capsules (Tetracycline Hydrochloride) Lederle ... 1367
Declomycin Tablets (Demeclocycline Hydrochloride) Lederle ... 1371
Doryx Capsules (Doxycycline Hyclate) Parke-Davis ... 1913
Dynacin Capsules (Minocycline Hydrochloride) Medicis ... 1590
Minocin Intravenous (Minocycline Hydrochloride) Lederle ... 1382
Minocin Oral Suspension (Minocycline Hydrochloride) Lederle ... 1385
Minocin Pellet-Filled Capsules (Minocycline Hydrochloride) Lederle ... 1383
Monodox Capsules (Doxycycline Monohydrate) Oclassen ... 1805
Terramycin Intramuscular Solution (Oxytetracycline) Roerig ... 2210
Vibramycin (Doxycycline Calcium) Pfizer Labs ... 1941
Vibramycin Hyclate Intravenous (Doxycycline Hyclate) Roerig ... 2215
Vibramycin (Doxycycline Monohydrate) Pfizer Labs ... 1941

Brucellosis
Dynacin Capsules (Minocycline Hydrochloride) Medicis ... 1590
Minocin Oral Suspension (Minocycline Hydrochloride) Lederle ... 1385
Minocin Pellet-Filled Capsules (Minocycline Hydrochloride) Lederle ... 1383
Monodox Capsules (Doxycycline Monohydrate) Oclassen ... 1805

Bruises, topical relief of (see under Pain, topical relief of)

"Bubble boy" disease (see under Adenosine deaminase, enzyme replacement therapy for)

Bulbar conjunctiva inflammation
AK-Pred (Prednisolone Sodium Phosphate) Akorn ... ⊙ 204
AK-Trol Ointment & Suspension (Dexamethasone, Neomycin Sulfate, Polymyxin B Sulfate) Akorn ... ⊙ 205
Blephamide Liquifilm Sterile Ophthalmic Suspension (Prednisolone Acetate, Sulfacetamide Sodium) Allergan ... 476
Cortisporin Ophthalmic Ointment Sterile (Polymyxin B Sulfate, Bacitracin Zinc, Neomycin Sulfate, Hydrocortisone) Glaxo Wellcome ... 1085
Cortisporin Ophthalmic Suspension Sterile (Hydrocortisone, Polymyxin B Sulfate, Neomycin Sulfate) Glaxo Wellcome ... 1086
Dexacidin Ointment (Dexamethasone, Neomycin Sulfate, Polymyxin B Sulfate) CIBA Vision Ophthalmics ... ⊙ 263
Econopred & Econopred Plus Ophthalmic Suspensions (Prednisolone Acetate) Alcon Laboratories ... ⊙ 217
FML Forte Liquifilm (Fluorometholone) Allergan ... ⊙ 240
FML Liquifilm (Fluorometholone) Allergan ... ⊙ 241
FML S.O.P. (Fluorometholone) Allergan ... ⊙ 241
FML-S Liquifilm (Sulfacetamide Sodium, Fluorometholone) Allergan ... ⊙ 242
Fluor-Op Ophthalmic Suspension (Fluorometholone) CIBA Vision Ophthalmics ... ⊙ 264
Inflamase (Prednisolone Sodium Phosphate) CIBA Vision Ophthalmics ... ⊙ 265
Maxitrol Ophthalmic Ointment and Suspension (Dexamethasone, Neomycin Sulfate, Polymyxin B Sulfate) Alcon Laboratories ... ⊙ 224
Ophthocort (Chloramphenicol, Polymyxin B Sulfate, Hydrocortisone Acetate) Parke-Davis ... ⊙ 311
Poly-Pred Liquifilm (Neomycin Sulfate, Polymyxin B Sulfate, Prednisolone Acetate) Allergan .. ⊙ 248
Pred Forte (Prednisolone Acetate) Allergan ... ⊙ 250
Pred-G Liquifilm Sterile Ophthalmic Suspension (Gentamicin Sulfate, Prednisolone Acetate) Allergan ... ⊙ 251
Pred-G S.O.P. Sterile Ophthalmic Ointment (Gentamicin Sulfate, Prednisolone Acetate) Allergan .. ⊙ 252
TobraDex Ophthalmic Suspension and Ointment (Dexamethasone, Tobramycin) Alcon Laboratories .. 473
Vasocidin Ointment (Prednisolone Acetate, Sulfacetamide Sodium) CIBA Vision Ophthalmics ... ⊙ 268
Vasocidin Ophthalmic Solution (Prednisolone Sodium Phosphate, Sulfacetamide Sodium) CIBA Vision Ophthalmics ... ⊙ 270

Burn wound infections (see under Infections, burn wound)

Burns, emergency first aid for
Water-Jel Sterile Burn Dressings (Dressings, sterile) Water-Jel ... 2682

Burns, maintenance of electrolyte balance
Albuminar-25, Albumin (Human) U.S.P. 25% (Albumin (Human)) Armour ... 513
Plasma-Plex, Plasma Protein Fraction (Human) 5% (Plasma Protein Fraction (Human)) Armour ... 524

Burns, minor
A and D Ointment (Petrolatum, Lanolin) Schering-Plough HealthCare ... ▣ 797
Aquaphor Healing Ointment (Petrolatum, Mineral Oil) Beiersdorf ... 640
Bactine Antiseptic/Anesthetic First Aid Liquid (Benzalkonium Chloride, Lidocaine Hydrochloride) Miles Consumer ▣ 708
Bactine First Aid Antibiotic Plus Anesthetic Ointment (Bacitracin Zinc, Neomycin Sulfate, Polymyxin B Sulfate, Lidocaine) Miles Consumer ... ▣ 708
Barri-Care Antimicrobial Barrier Ointment (Chloroxylenol) Care-Tech ... ▣ 624
Betadine First Aid Cream (Povidone Iodine) Purdue Frederick ... 1991
Betadine Ointment (Povidone Iodine) Purdue Frederick ... 1992
Betadine Solution (Povidone Iodine) Purdue Frederick ... 1992
Desitin Ointment (Cod Liver Oil, Zinc Oxide) Pfizer Consumer ... ▣ 742
Maximum Strength Mycitracin Triple Antibiotic First Aid Ointment (Bacitracin, Neomycin Sulfate, Polymyxin B Sulfate) Upjohn ... ▣ 839
Polysporin Ointment (Bacitracin Zinc, Polymyxin B Sulfate) WARNER WELLCOME ... ▣ 858
Polysporin Powder (Bacitracin Zinc, Polymyxin B Sulfate) WARNER WELLCOME ... ▣ 859
Sween Cream (Benzethonium Chloride, Lanolin Oil) Sween ... 2554

Burns, pain associated with (see under Pain, topical relief of)

Burns, second- and third-degree, adjunctive therapy in
Elase Ointment (Desoxyribonuclease, Fibrinolysin) Fujisawa ... 1039
Elase Vials (Fibrinolysin, Desoxyribonuclease) Fujisawa ... 1038
Furacin Soluble Dressing (Nitrofurazone) Roberts ... 2045
Furacin Topical Cream (Nitrofurazone) Roberts ... 2045
Silvadene Cream 1% (Silver Sulfadiazine) Marion Merrell Dow 1540
Sulfamylon Cream (Mafenide Acetate) Dow Hickam ... 925
Travase Ointment (Sutilains) Knoll Laboratories ... 1356

Burns, to prevent marked hemoconcentration
Albuminar-5, Albumin (Human) U.S.P. 5% (Albumin (Human)) Armour ... 512
Albuminar-25, Albumin (Human) U.S.P. 25% (Albumin (Human)) Armour ... 513
Plasma-Plex, Plasma Protein Fraction (Human) 5% (Plasma Protein Fraction (Human)) Armour ... 524

Bursitis
Anaprox/Naprosyn (Naproxen Sodium) Roche Laboratories ... 2117
Aristocort Suspension (Forte Parenteral) (Triamcinolone Diacetate) Fujisawa ... 1027
Aristocort Suspension (Intralesional) (Triamcinolone Diacetate) Fujisawa ... 1025

(▣ Described in PDR For Nonprescription Drugs) (⊙ Described in PDR For Ophthalmology)

Bursitis — Indications Index — 1464

Aristocort Tablets (Triamcinolone) Fujisawa 1022
Aristospan Suspension (Intra-articular) (Triamcinolone Hexacetonide) Fujisawa 1033
Celestone Soluspan Suspension (Betamethasone Sodium Phosphate, Betamethasone Acetate) Schering 2347
Cortone Acetate Sterile Suspension (Cortisone Acetate) Merck & Co., Inc. 1623
Cortone Acetate Tablets (Cortisone Acetate) Merck & Co., Inc. 1624
Dalalone D.P. Injectable (Dexamethasone Acetate) Forest 1011
Decadron Elixir (Dexamethasone) Merck & Co., Inc. 1633
Decadron Phosphate Injection (Dexamethasone Sodium Phosphate) Merck & Co., Inc. 1637
Decadron Phosphate with Xylocaine Injection, Sterile (Dexamethasone Sodium Phosphate, Lidocaine Hydrochloride) Merck & Co., Inc. 1639
Decadron Tablets (Dexamethasone) Merck & Co., Inc. 1635
Decadron-LA Sterile Suspension (Dexamethasone Acetate) Merck & Co., Inc. 1646
Deltasone Tablets (Prednisone) Upjohn 2595
Depo-Medrol Single-Dose Vial (Methylprednisolone Acetate) Upjohn 2600
Depo-Medrol Sterile Aqueous Suspension (Methylprednisolone Acetate) Upjohn 2597
Hydeltrasol Injection, Sterile (Prednisolone Sodium Phosphate) Merck & Co., Inc. 1665
Hydeltra-T.B.A. Sterile Suspension (Prednisolone Tebutate) Merck & Co., Inc. 1667
Hydrocortone Acetate Sterile Suspension (Hydrocortisone Acetate) Merck & Co., Inc. 1669
Hydrocortone Phosphate Injection, Sterile (Hydrocortisone Sodium Phosphate) Merck & Co., Inc. 1670
Hydrocortone Tablets (Hydrocortisone) Merck & Co., Inc. 1672
Indocin (Indomethacin) Merck & Co., Inc. 1680
Medrol (Methylprednisolone) Upjohn 2621
Anaprox/Naprosyn (Naproxen) Roche Laboratories 2117
Pediapred Oral Liquid (Prednisolone Sodium Phosphate) Fisons 995
Prelone Syrup (Prednisolone) Muro 1787
Solu-Cortef Sterile Powder (Hydrocortisone Sodium Succinate) Upjohn 2641
Solu-Medrol Sterile Powder (Methylprednisolone Sodium Succinate) Upjohn 2643
St. Joseph Adult Chewable Aspirin (81 mg.) (Aspirin) Schering-Plough HealthCare ..... ▣ 808

Bursitis, subacromial, acute, symptomatic relief of
Aristocort Tablets (Triamcinolone) Fujisawa 1022
Clinoril Tablets (Sulindac) Merck & Co., Inc. 1618
Indocin (Indomethacin) Merck & Co., Inc. 1680
Trilisate (Choline Magnesium Trisalicylate) Purdue Frederick 2000

C

C. difficile infection (see under Colitis, pseudomembranous, antibiotic-associated)

C. diphtheriae infections
E.E.S. (Erythromycin Ethylsuccinate) Abbott 424
E-Mycin Tablets (Erythromycin) Knoll Laboratories 1341
ERYC (Erythromycin) Parke-Davis .. 1915
EryPed (Erythromycin Ethylsuccinate) Abbott 421
Ery-Tab Tablets (Erythromycin) Abbott 422
Erythrocin Stearate Filmtab (Erythromycin Stearate) Abbott 425
Erythromycin Base Filmtab (Erythromycin) Abbott 426
Erythromycin Delayed-Release Capsules, USP (Erythromycin) Abbott 427
Ilosone (Erythromycin Estolate) Dista 911
Ilotycin Gluceptate, IV, Vials (Erythromycin Gluceptate) Dista 913
PCE Dispertab Tablets (Erythromycin) Abbott 444
Pfizerpen for Injection (Penicillin G Potassium) Roerig 2203

C. minutissimum infections
E.E.S. (Erythromycin Ethylsuccinate) Abbott 424
E-Mycin Tablets (Erythromycin) Knoll Laboratories 1341
ERYC (Erythromycin) Parke-Davis .. 1915
EryPed (Erythromycin Ethylsuccinate) Abbott 421
Ery-Tab Tablets (Erythromycin) Abbott 422
Erythrocin Stearate Filmtab (Erythromycin Stearate) Abbott 425
Erythromycin Base Filmtab (Erythromycin) Abbott 426
Erythromycin Delayed-Release Capsules, USP (Erythromycin) Abbott 427
Ilosone (Erythromycin Estolate) Dista 911
PCE Dispertab Tablets (Erythromycin) Abbott 444

C. perfringens infections
Zefazone (Cefmetazole Sodium) Upjohn 2654

C. perfringens intra-abdominal infections
Zefazone (Cefmetazole Sodium) Upjohn 2654

Cachexia associated with weight loss, AIDS-induced
Megace Oral Suspension (Megestrol Acetate) Bristol-Myers Squibb Oncology 699

Calcium deficiency (see under Hypocalcemia)

Calluses (see under Hyperkeratosis skin disorders)

Campylobacter fetus infections
Achromycin V Capsules (Tetracycline Hydrochloride) Lederle 1367
Declomycin Tablets (Demeclocycline Hydrochloride) Lederle 1371
Doryx Capsules (Doxycycline Hyclate) Parke-Davis 1913
Dynacin Capsules (Minocycline Hydrochloride) Medicis 1590
Minocin Intravenous (Minocycline Hydrochloride) Lederle 1382
Minocin Oral Suspension (Minocycline Hydrochloride) Lederle 1385
Minocin Pellet-Filled Capsules (Minocycline Hydrochloride) Lederle 1383
Monodox Capsules (Doxycycline Monohydrate) Oclassen 1805
Terramycin Intramuscular Solution (Oxytetracycline) Roerig 2210
Vibramycin (Doxycycline Calcium) Pfizer Labs 1941
Vibramycin Hyclate Intravenous (Doxycycline Hyclate) Roerig 2215
Vibramycin (Doxycycline Monohydrate) Pfizer Labs 1941

Campylobacter jejuni infectious diarrhea
Cipro Tablets (Ciprofloxacin Hydrochloride) Bayer Pharmaceutical 592

Cancer, prostatic (see under Carcinoma, prostatic, palliative treatment of)

Candida albicans infections
AVC (Sulfanilamide) Marion Merrell Dow 1500
Betadine Medicated Douche (Povidone Iodine) Purdue Frederick 1992
Betadine Medicated Gel (Povidone Iodine) Purdue Frederick 1992
Loprox 1% Cream and Lotion (Ciclopirox Olamine) Hoechst-Roussel 1242
Lotrimin (Clotrimazole) Schering 2371
Mycelex-7 Vaginal Cream Antifungal (Clotrimazole) Miles Consumer ..... ▣ 724
Mycelex-7 Combination-Pack Vaginal Inserts & External Vulvar Cream (Clotrimazole) Miles Consumer ..... ▣ 725
Mycelex-G 500 mg Vaginal Tablets (Clotrimazole) Bayer Pharmaceutical 609
Mycostatin Cream, Topical Powder, and Ointment (Nystatin) Westwood-Squibb 2688

Candida infections, serious
Ancobon Capsules (Flucytosine) Roche Laboratories 2079

Candida species urinary tract infections
Ancobon Capsules (Flucytosine) Roche Laboratories 2079

Candida strains pulmonary infections
Ancobon Capsules (Flucytosine) Roche Laboratories 2079

Candidiasis, bone marrow transplantation-induced, prophylactic therapy in
Diflucan Injection, Tablets, and Oral Suspension (Fluconazole) Roerig 2194

Candidiasis, cutaneous
Loprox 1% Cream and Lotion (Ciclopirox Olamine) Hoechst-Roussel 1242
Lotrimin (Clotrimazole) Schering 2371
Monistat Dual-Pak (Miconazole Nitrate) Ortho Pharmaceutical 1850
Monistat-Derm (miconazole nitrate 2%) Cream (Miconazole Nitrate) Ortho Dermatological 1889
Nizoral 2% Cream (Ketoconazole) Janssen 1297
Spectazole (econazole nitrate 1%) Cream (Econazole Nitrate) Ortho Dermatological 1890

Candidiasis, esophageal
Diflucan Injection, Tablets, and Oral Suspension (Fluconazole) Roerig 2194

Candidiasis, mucocutaneous, chronic
Nizoral Tablets (Ketoconazole) Janssen 1298

Candidiasis, oral cavity
Mycostatin Pastilles (Nystatin) Bristol-Myers Squibb Oncology 704

Candidiasis, oropharyngeal
Diflucan Injection, Tablets, and Oral Suspension (Fluconazole) Roerig 2194
Mycelex Troches (Clotrimazole) Bayer Pharmaceutical 608
Nizoral Tablets (Ketoconazole) Janssen 1298

Candidiasis, oropharyngeal, prophylaxis of
Mycelex Troches (Clotrimazole) Bayer Pharmaceutical 608

Candidiasis, systemic
Fungizone Intravenous (Amphotericin B) Apothecon 506

Candidiasis, unspecified
Nizoral Tablets (Ketoconazole) Janssen 1298

Candidiasis, vaginal
Diflucan Injection, Tablets, and Oral Suspension (Fluconazole) Roerig 2194
Gyne-Lotrimin (Clotrimazole) Schering-Plough HealthCare ..... ▣ 805
Gyne-Lotrimin Pack (Clotrimazole) Schering-Plough HealthCare ..... ▣ 806
Monistat Dual-Pak (Miconazole Nitrate) Ortho Pharmaceutical 1850
Monistat 3 Vaginal Suppositories (Miconazole Nitrate) Ortho Pharmaceutical 1850
Mycelex-7 Vaginal Inserts Antifungal (Clotrimazole) Miles Consumer ..... ▣ 725
Mycelex-7 Combination-Pack Vaginal Inserts & External Vulvar Cream (Clotrimazole) Miles Consumer ..... ▣ 725
Mycelex-G 500 mg Vaginal Tablets (Clotrimazole) Bayer Pharmaceutical 609
Terazol 3 Vaginal Cream (Terconazole) Ortho Pharmaceutical 1886
Terazol 3 Vaginal Suppositories (Terconazole) Ortho Pharmaceutical 1886
Terazol 7 Vaginal Cream (Terconazole) Ortho Pharmaceutical 1887
Vagistat-1 (Tioconazole) Bristol-Myers Squibb 778

Candiduria
Nizoral Tablets (Ketoconazole) Janssen 1298

Canker sores (see under Stomatitis, recurrent aphthous, symptomatic relief of)

Carbuncles (see under Furunculosis, symptomatic relief of)

Carcinoma, adrenal cortex
Lysodren (Mitotane) Bristol-Myers Squibb Oncology 698

Carcinoma, bladder, transitional cell
Adriamycin PFS (Doxorubicin Hydrochloride) Pharmacia 1947
Adriamycin RDF (Doxorubicin Hydrochloride) Pharmacia 1947
Doxorubicin Astra (Doxorubicin Hydrochloride) Astra 540
Platinol (Cisplatin) Bristol-Myers Squibb Oncology 708
Platinol-AQ Injection (Cisplatin) Bristol-Myers Squibb Oncology 710
Rubex (Doxorubicin Hydrochloride) Bristol-Myers Squibb Oncology 712

Carcinoma, breast
Adriamycin PFS (Doxorubicin Hydrochloride) Pharmacia 1947
Adriamycin RDF (Doxorubicin Hydrochloride) Pharmacia 1947
Cytoxan (Cyclophosphamide) Bristol-Myers Squibb Oncology 694
Doxorubicin Astra (Doxorubicin Hydrochloride) Astra 540
Methotrexate Sodium Tablets, Injection, for Injection and LPF Injection (Methotrexate Sodium) Immunex 1275
NEOSAR Lyophilized/Neosar (Cyclophosphamide) Pharmacia .. 1959
Nolvadex Tablets (Tamoxifen Citrate) Zeneca 2841
Rubex (Doxorubicin Hydrochloride) Bristol-Myers Squibb Oncology 712
Thioplex (Thiotepa For Injection) (Thiotepa) Immunex 1281
Velban Vials (Vinblastine Sulfate) Lilly 1484

Carcinoma, breast, axillary node-negative, postsurgical and post-irradiation
Nolvadex Tablets (Tamoxifen Citrate) Zeneca 2841

Carcinoma, breast, metastatic, treatment of
Android Capsules, 10 mg (Methyltestosterone) ICN 1250
Delatestryl Injection (Testosterone Enanthate) Bio-Technology General 2860
Nolvadex Tablets (Tamoxifen Citrate) Zeneca 2841

(▣ Described in PDR For Nonprescription Drugs) (⊙ Described in PDR For Ophthalmology)

Indications Index

Taxol (Paclitaxel) Bristol-Myers Squibb Oncology 714

Carcinoma, breast, palliative therapy in
Android (Methyltestosterone) ICN .. 1251
Diethylstilbestrol Tablets (Diethylstilbestrol) Lilly 1437
Estrace Cream and Tablets (Estradiol) Bristol-Myers Squibb .. 749
ESTRATAB Tablets (0.3, 0.625, 1.25, 2.5 mg) (Estrogens, Esterified) Solvay 2536
Fluorouracil Injection (Fluorouracil) Roche Laboratories 2116
Halotestin Tablets (Fluoxymesterone) Upjohn 2614
Megace Tablets (Megestrol Acetate) Bristol-Myers Squibb Oncology 701
Menest Tablets (Estrogens, Esterified) SmithKline Beecham Pharmaceuticals 2494
Oreton Methyl (Methyltestosterone) ICN 1255
Premarin Tablets (Estrogens, Conjugated) Wyeth-Ayerst 2789
Teslac (Testolactone) Bristol-Myers Squibb Oncology 717
Testred Capsules (Methyltestosterone) ICN 1262

Carcinoma, breast, postmenopausal women, postsurgical
Nolvadex Tablets (Tamoxifen Citrate) Zeneca 2841

Carcinoma, bronchogenic
Adriamycin PFS (Doxorubicin Hydrochloride) Pharmacia 1947
Adriamycin RDF (Doxorubicin Hydrochloride) Pharmacia 1947
Doxorubicin Astra (Doxorubicin Hydrochloride) Astra 540
Methotrexate Sodium Tablets, Injection, for Injection and LPF Injection (Methotrexate Sodium) Immunex 1275
Mustargen (Mechlorethamine Hydrochloride) Merck & Co., Inc. 1709
Rubex (Doxorubicin Hydrochloride) Bristol-Myers Squibb Oncology 712

Carcinoma, cervix, palliative treatment in
Blenoxane (Bleomycin Sulfate) Bristol-Myers Squibb Oncology 692

Carcinoma, colon, Dukes' stage C, adjunctive treatment in
Ergamisol Tablets (Levamisole Hydrochloride) Janssen..................... 1292

Carcinoma, colon, palliative management of
Fluorouracil Injection (Fluorouracil) Roche Laboratories 2116

Carcinoma, colorectal, adjunctive therapy in
Leucovorin Calcium for Injection (Leucovorin Calcium) Immunex 1268

Carcinoma, endometrium, palliative treatment of
Depo-Provera Sterile Aqueous Suspension (Medroxyprogester-one Acetate) Upjohn 2606
Megace Tablets (Megestrol Acetate) Bristol-Myers Squibb Oncology 701

Carcinoma, epiglottis, palliative treatment in
Blenoxane (Bleomycin Sulfate) Bristol-Myers Squibb Oncology 692

Carcinoma, gastric
Adriamycin PFS (Doxorubicin Hydrochloride) Pharmacia 1947
Adriamycin RDF (Doxorubicin Hydrochloride) Pharmacia 1947
Doxorubicin Astra (Doxorubicin Hydrochloride) Astra 540
Rubex (Doxorubicin Hydrochloride) Bristol-Myers Squibb Oncology 712

Carcinoma, gastrointestinal, palliative management of
Sterile FUDR (Floxuridine) Roche Laboratories 2118

Carcinoma, gingiva, palliative treatment in
Blenoxane (Bleomycin Sulfate) Bristol-Myers Squibb Oncology 692

Carcinoma, head and neck
Blenoxane (Bleomycin Sulfate) Bristol-Myers Squibb Oncology 692
Methotrexate Sodium Tablets, Injection, for Injection and LPF Injection (Methotrexate Sodium) Immunex 1275

Carcinoma, head and neck, adjunct in
Hydrea Capsules (Hydroxyurea) Bristol-Myers Squibb Oncology 696

Carcinoma, larynx, palliative treatment in
Blenoxane (Bleomycin Sulfate) Bristol-Myers Squibb Oncology 692

Carcinoma, lips, palliative treatment in
Blenoxane (Bleomycin Sulfate) Bristol-Myers Squibb Oncology 692

Carcinoma, lung, non-small cell
Navelbine Injection (Vinorelbine Tartrate) Glaxo Wellcome 1145

Carcinoma, lung, small cell
VePesid Capsules and Injection (Etoposide) Bristol-Myers Squibb Oncology 718

Carcinoma, metastatic, palliative treatment of
Estrace Cream and Tablets (Estradiol) Bristol-Myers Squibb .. 749
Mustargen (Mechlorethamine Hydrochloride) Merck & Co., Inc. 1709

Carcinoma, mouth, palliative treatment in
Blenoxane (Bleomycin Sulfate) Bristol-Myers Squibb Oncology 692

Carcinoma, nasopharynx, palliative treatment in
Blenoxane (Bleomycin Sulfate) Bristol-Myers Squibb Oncology 692

Carcinoma, oropharynx, palliative treatment in
Blenoxane (Bleomycin Sulfate) Bristol-Myers Squibb Oncology 692

Carcinoma, ovary
Adriamycin PFS (Doxorubicin Hydrochloride) Pharmacia 1947
Adriamycin RDF (Doxorubicin Hydrochloride) Pharmacia 1947
Alkeran Tablets (Melphalan) Glaxo Wellcome 1071
Cytoxan (Cyclophosphamide) Bristol-Myers Squibb Oncology 694
Doxorubicin Astra (Doxorubicin Hydrochloride) Astra 540
Hexalen Capsules (Altretamine) U.S. Bioscience 2571
Hydrea Capsules (Hydroxyurea) Bristol-Myers Squibb Oncology 696
NEOSAR Lyophilized/Neosar (Cyclophosphamide) Pharmacia .. 1959
Paraplatin for Injection (Carboplatin) Bristol-Myers Squibb Oncology................................... 705
Platinol (Cisplatin) Bristol-Myers Squibb Oncology................................... 708
Platinol-AQ Injection (Cisplatin) Bristol-Myers Squibb Oncology 710
Rubex (Doxorubicin Hydrochloride) Bristol-Myers Squibb Oncology 712
Taxol (Paclitaxel) Bristol-Myers Squibb Oncology................................... 714
Thioplex (Thiotepa For Injection) (Thiotepa) Immunex 1281

Carcinoma, palate, palliative treatment in
Blenoxane (Bleomycin Sulfate) Bristol-Myers Squibb Oncology 692

Carcinoma, pancreas
Mutamycin (Mitomycin (Mitomycin-C)) Bristol-Myers Squibb Oncology................................... 703

Carcinoma, pancreas, metastatic, islet cell
Zanosar Sterile Powder (Streptozocin) Upjohn 2653

Carcinoma, pancreas, palliative management of
Fluorouracil Injection (Fluorouracil) Roche Laboratories 2116

Carcinoma, penis, palliative treatment in
Blenoxane (Bleomycin Sulfate) Bristol-Myers Squibb Oncology 692

Carcinoma, prostate, metastatic, adjunctive therapy in
Eulexin Capsules (Flutamide) Schering 2358

Carcinoma, prostatic, palliative treatment of
Diethylstilbestrol Tablets (Diethylstilbestrol) Lilly 1437
Emcyt Capsules (Estramustine Phosphate Sodium) Pharmacia 1953
Estrace Cream and Tablets (Estradiol) Bristol-Myers Squibb .. 749
ESTRATAB Tablets (0.3, 0.625, 1.25, 2.5 mg) (Estrogens, Esterified) Solvay 2536
Lupron Depot 7.5 mg (Leuprolide Acetate) TAP 2559
Lupron Injection (Leuprolide Acetate) TAP 2555
Menest Tablets (Estrogens, Esterified) SmithKline Beecham Pharmaceuticals 2494
Premarin Tablets (Estrogens, Conjugated) Wyeth-Ayerst 2789
Stilphostrol Tablets and Ampuls (Diethylstilbestrol Diphosphate) Bayer Pharmaceutical 612
Zoladex (Goserelin Acetate Implant) Zeneca 2858

Carcinoma, rectum, palliative management of
Fluorouracil Injection (Fluorouracil) Roche Laboratories 2116

Carcinoma, renal, palliative treatment in
Depo-Provera Sterile Aqueous Suspension (Medroxyprogester-one Acetate) Upjohn 2606

Carcinoma, renal cell, metastatic, in adults
Proleukin for Injection (Aldesleukin) Chiron 797

Carcinoma, sinus, palliative treatment in
Blenoxane (Bleomycin Sulfate) Bristol-Myers Squibb Oncology 692

Carcinoma, skin, palliative treatment in
Blenoxane (Bleomycin Sulfate) Bristol-Myers Squibb Oncology 692

Carcinoma, squamous cell, palliative treatment in
Blenoxane (Bleomycin Sulfate) Bristol-Myers Squibb Oncology 692

Carcinoma, stomach
Mutamycin (Mitomycin (Mitomycin-C)) Bristol-Myers Squibb Oncology................................... 703

Carcinoma, stomach, palliative management of
Fluorouracil Injection (Fluorouracil) Roche Laboratories 2116

Carcinoma, superficial basal cell
Efudex (Fluorouracil) Roche Laboratories 2113

Carcinoma, testicular
Platinol (Cisplatin) Bristol-Myers Squibb Oncology................................... 708
Platinol-AQ Injection (Cisplatin) Bristol-Myers Squibb Oncology 710
VePesid Capsules and Injection (Etoposide) Bristol-Myers Squibb Oncology 718

Carcinoma, testicular, embryonic cell, palliative treatment in
Blenoxane (Bleomycin Sulfate) Bristol-Myers Squibb Oncology 692

Carcinoma, testicular, germ cell
IFEX (Ifosfamide) Bristol-Myers Squibb Oncology................................... 697

Carcinoma, testicular, palliative treatment in
Blenoxane (Bleomycin Sulfate) Bristol-Myers Squibb Oncology 692

Carcinoma, testis, advanced
Cosmegen Injection (Dactinomycin) Merck & Co., Inc. 1626
Mithracin (Plicamycin) Bayer Pharmaceutical 607
Velban Vials (Vinblastine Sulfate) Lilly 1484

Carcinoma, thyroid
Adriamycin PFS (Doxorubicin Hydrochloride) Pharmacia 1947
Adriamycin RDF (Doxorubicin Hydrochloride) Pharmacia 1947
Doxorubicin Astra (Doxorubicin Hydrochloride) Astra 540
Synthroid Injection (Levothyroxine Sodium) Knoll Pharmaceutical 1359
Rubex (Doxorubicin Hydrochloride) Bristol-Myers Squibb Oncology 712
Synthroid Tablets (Levothyroxine Sodium) Knoll Pharmaceutical 1359

Carcinoma, tongue, palliative treatment in
Blenoxane (Bleomycin Sulfate) Bristol-Myers Squibb Oncology 692

Carcinoma, tonsil, palliative treatment in
Blenoxane (Bleomycin Sulfate) Bristol-Myers Squibb Oncology 692

Carcinoma, urinary bladder, in-situ
BCG Vaccine, USP (TICE) (BCG Vaccine) Organon................................ 1814
TheraCys BCG Live (Intravesical) (BCG, Live (Intravesical)) Connaught 897

Carcinoma, urinary bladder, superficial papillary
Thioplex (Thiotepa For Injection) (Thiotepa) Immunex 1281

Carcinoma, uterus
Cosmegen Injection (Dactinomycin) Merck & Co., Inc. 1626

Carcinoma, vulva, palliative treatment in
Blenoxane (Bleomycin Sulfate) Bristol-Myers Squibb Oncology 692

Cardiac arrest
Isuprel Hydrochloride Injection 1:5000 (Isoproterenol Hydrochloride) Sanofi Winthrop .. 2311

Cardiac arrest, an adjunct in
Levophed Bitartrate Injection (Nor-epinephrine Bitartrate) Sanofi Winthrop 2315

Cardiac arrhythmias
(see under Arrhythmias)

Cardiac decompensation
Dobutrex Solution Vials (Dobuta-mine Hydrochloride) Lilly 1439

Cardiac ischemic complications, acute, prevention of, adjunct to PTCA
ReoPro Vials (Abciximab) Lilly 1471

Cardiac output, low
Isuprel Hydrochloride Injection 1:5000 (Isoproterenol Hydrochloride) Sanofi Winthrop .. 2311

Cardiogenic shock syndrome, correction of hemodynamic imbalance
Isuprel Hydrochloride Injection 1:5000 (Isoproterenol Hydrochloride) Sanofi Winthrop .. 2311

(◼ Described in PDR For Nonprescription Drugs) (◉ Described in PDR For Ophthalmology)

Cardiomyopathy **Indications Index** **1466**

Cardiomyopathy, doxorubicin-induced, to reduce the incidence and severity of
Zinecard (Dexrazoxane) Pharmacia 1961

Carnitine, primary systemic deficiency of
L-Carnitine 250mg and 500mg Tablets (Levocarnitine) Vitaline 2659
Carnitor Tablets and Solution (Levocarnitine) Sigma-Tau 2453

Carnitine deficiency, secondary
Carnitor Injection (Levocarnitine) Sigma-Tau 2452
Carnitor Tablets and Solution (Levocarnitine) Sigma-Tau 2453

Catabolic or tissue depleting processes, adjunctive therapy
Oxandrin (Oxandrolone) Bio-Technology General 2862

Cataract extraction, surgical aid in
AMO Vitrax Viscoelastic Solution (Sodium Hyaluronate) Allergan.. ◉ 232
AMVISC Plus (Sodium Hyaluronate) Chiron Vision .... ◉ 329
Healon (Sodium Hyaluronate) Pharmacia Inc. Ophthalmics ...... ◉ 314
Healon GV (Sodium Hyaluronate) Pharmacia Inc. Ophthalmics ...... ◉ 315
Ocucoat (Hydroxypropyl Methylcellulose) Storz Ophthalmics .... ◉ 321

Cellulitis, pelvic (see under Pelvic cellulitis)

Central cranial diabetes insipidus (see under Diabetes insipidus)

Central nervous system depression, drug-induced
Dopram Injectable (Doxapram Hydrochloride) Robins 2061

Cephalalgia, histaminic
Cafergot (Ergotamine Tartrate, Caffeine) Sandoz Pharmaceuticals 2251
D.H.E. 45 Injection (Dihydroergotamine Mesylate) Sandoz Pharmaceuticals 2255
Ergomar (Ergotamine Tartrate) Lotus 1486
Wigraine Tablets & Suppositories (Ergotamine Tartrate, Caffeine) Organon 1829

Cerebral edema (see under Edema, cerebral)

Cerumen, removal of
Auralgan Otic Solution (Antipyrine, Benzocaine, Glycerin) Wyeth-Ayerst 2703
Cerumenex Drops (Triethanolamine Polypeptide Oleate-Condensate) Purdue Frederick 1993
Debrox Drops (Carbamide Peroxide) SmithKline Beecham Consumer .... ▣ 815
Murine Ear Drops (Carbamide Peroxide) Ross .... ▣ 780

Cervicitis
Zithromax (Azithromycin) Pfizer Labs 1944

Cervicitis, benign, adjunct
Elase Ointment (Desoxyribonuclease, Fibrinolysin) Fujisawa 1039
Elase Vials (Fibrinolysin, Desoxyribonuclease) Fujisawa 1038

Cervicitis, mild, adjunct
Amino-Cerv (Urea, Benzalkonium Chloride, L-Cystine, Sodium Propionate, Methionine, Inositol) Milex 1779

Cervicitis, postconization, adjunct
Amino-Cerv (Urea, Benzalkonium Chloride, L-Cystine, Sodium Propionate, Methionine, Inositol) Milex 1779

Cervicitis, postpartum, adjunct
Amino-Cerv (Urea, Benzalkonium Chloride, L-Cystine, Sodium Propionate, Methionine, Inositol) Milex 1779

Cervix, epithelialization, promotion of
Amino-Cerv (Urea, Benzalkonium Chloride, L-Cystine, Sodium Propionate, Methionine, Inositol) Milex 1779

Cervix, ripening of, in pregnant women at or near term
Cervidil (Dinoprostone) Forest 1010
Prepidil Gel (Dinoprostone) Upjohn 2633

Chancroid
Achromycin V Capsules (Tetracycline Hydrochloride) Lederle 1367
Declomycin Tablets (Demeclocycline Hydrochloride) Lederle 1371
Doryx Capsules (Doxycycline Hyclate) Parke-Davis 1913
Dynacin Capsules (Minocycline Hydrochloride) Medicis 1590
Gantanol Tablets (Sulfamethoxazole) Roche Laboratories 2119
Gantrisin (Acetyl Sulfisoxazole) Roche Laboratories 2120
Minocin Intravenous (Minocycline Hydrochloride) Lederle 1382
Minocin Oral Suspension (Minocycline Hydrochloride) Lederle 1385
Minocin Pellet-Filled Capsules (Minocycline Hydrochloride) Lederle 1383
Monodox Capsules (Doxycycline Monohydrate) Oclassen 1805
Terramycin Intramuscular Solution (Oxytetracycline) Roerig 2210
Vibramycin (Doxycycline Calcium) Pfizer Labs 1941
Vibramycin Hyclate Intravenous (Doxycycline Hyclate) Roerig 2215
Vibramycin (Doxycycline Monohydrate) Pfizer Labs 1941

Cheilitis, actinic
Aquaphor Healing Ointment, Original Formula (Mineral Oil, Petrolatum) Beiersdorf 640
Herpecin-L Cold Sore Lip Balm Stick (Allantoin) Campbell 779

Chickenpox (see under Varicella, acute, treatment of)

Chlamydia psittaci infection
Achromycin V Capsules (Tetracycline Hydrochloride) Lederle 1367
Declomycin Tablets (Demeclocycline Hydrochloride) Lederle 1371
Doryx Capsules (Doxycycline Hyclate) Parke-Davis 1913
Dynacin Capsules (Minocycline Hydrochloride) Medicis 1590
Minocin Intravenous (Minocycline Hydrochloride) Lederle 1382
Minocin Oral Suspension (Minocycline Hydrochloride) Lederle 1385
Minocin Pellet-Filled Capsules (Minocycline Hydrochloride) Lederle 1383
Monodox Capsules (Doxycycline Monohydrate) Oclassen 1805
Terramycin Intramuscular Solution (Oxytetracycline) Roerig 2210
Vibramycin (Doxycycline Calcium) Pfizer Labs 1941
Vibramycin Hyclate Intravenous (Doxycycline Hyclate) Roerig 2215
Vibramycin (Doxycycline Monohydrate) Pfizer Labs 1941

Chlamydia trachomatis conjunctivitis of the newborn
ERYC (Erythromycin) Parke-Davis .. 1915
Ery-Tab Tablets (Erythromycin) Abbott 422
Erythrocin Stearate Filmtab (Erythromycin Stearate) Abbott 425
Erythromycin Base Filmtab (Erythromycin) Abbott 426
Erythromycin Delayed-Release Capsules, USP (Erythromycin) Abbott 427
Ilosone (Erythromycin Estolate) Dista 911
Minocin Oral Suspension (Minocycline Hydrochloride) Lederle 1385
Monodox Capsules (Doxycycline Monohydrate) Oclassen 1805
PCE Dispertab Tablets (Erythromycin) Abbott 444

Chlamydia trachomatis endocervical infections
Achromycin V Capsules (Tetracycline Hydrochloride) Lederle 1367
Doryx Capsules (Doxycycline Hyclate) Parke-Davis 1913
E-Mycin Tablets (Erythromycin) Knoll Laboratories 1341
ERYC (Erythromycin) Parke-Davis .. 1915
Ery-Tab Tablets (Erythromycin) Abbott 422
Erythrocin Stearate Filmtab (Erythromycin Stearate) Abbott 425
Erythromycin Base Filmtab (Erythromycin) Abbott 426
Erythromycin Delayed-Release Capsules, USP (Erythromycin) Abbott 427
Ilosone (Erythromycin Estolate) Dista 911
Minocin Oral Suspension (Minocycline Hydrochloride) Lederle 1385
Monodox Capsules (Doxycycline Monohydrate) Oclassen 1805
PCE Dispertab Tablets (Erythromycin) Abbott 444
Vibramycin (Doxycycline Calcium) Pfizer Labs 1941

Chlamydia trachomatis epididymo-orchitis, acute
Doryx Capsules (Doxycycline Hyclate) Parke-Davis 1913

Chlamydia trachomatis gynecologic infections
Floxin I.V. (Ofloxacin) McNeil Pharmaceutical 1571
Floxin Tablets (200 mg, 300 mg, 400 mg) (Ofloxacin) McNeil Pharmaceutical 1567

Chlamydia trachomatis infections
Achromycin V Capsules (Tetracycline Hydrochloride) Lederle 1367
Doryx Capsules (Doxycycline Hyclate) Parke-Davis 1913
Dynacin Capsules (Minocycline Hydrochloride) Medicis 1590
E.E.S. (Erythromycin Ethylsuccinate) Abbott 424
E-Mycin Tablets (Erythromycin) Knoll Laboratories 1341
ERYC (Erythromycin) Parke-Davis .. 1915
EryPed (Erythromycin Ethylsuccinate) Abbott 421
Ery-Tab Tablets (Erythromycin) Abbott 422
Erythrocin Stearate Filmtab (Erythromycin Stearate) Abbott 425
Erythromycin Base Filmtab (Erythromycin) Abbott 426
Erythromycin Delayed-Release Capsules, USP (Erythromycin) Abbott 427
Floxin I.V. (Ofloxacin) McNeil Pharmaceutical 1571
Floxin Tablets (200 mg, 300 mg, 400 mg) (Ofloxacin) McNeil Pharmaceutical 1567
Minocin Oral Suspension (Minocycline Hydrochloride) Lederle 1385
Minocin Pellet-Filled Capsules (Minocycline Hydrochloride) Lederle 1383
Monodox Capsules (Doxycycline Monohydrate) Oclassen 1805
PCE Dispertab Tablets (Erythromycin) Abbott 444
Vibramycin (Doxycycline Calcium) Pfizer Labs 1941
Zithromax (Azithromycin) Pfizer Labs 1944

Chlamydia trachomatis infections, ocular (see under Trachoma)

Chlamydia trachomatis neonatal ophthalmia, prophylaxis of
Ilotycin Ophthalmic Ointment (Erythromycin) Dista 912

Chlamydia trachomatis nongonococcal cervicitis
Floxin I.V. (Ofloxacin) McNeil Pharmaceutical 1571
Floxin Tablets (200 mg, 300 mg, 400 mg) (Ofloxacin) McNeil Pharmaceutical 1567
Zithromax (Azithromycin) Pfizer Labs 1944

Chlamydia trachomatis nongonococcal urethritis
Dynacin Capsules (Minocycline Hydrochloride) Medicis 1590
Floxin I.V. (Ofloxacin) McNeil Pharmaceutical 1571
Floxin Tablets (200 mg, 300 mg, 400 mg) (Ofloxacin) McNeil Pharmaceutical 1567
Minocin Oral Suspension (Minocycline Hydrochloride) Lederle 1385
Minocin Pellet-Filled Capsules (Minocycline Hydrochloride) Lederle 1383
Zithromax (Azithromycin) Pfizer Labs 1944

Chlamydia trachomatis pneumonia of infancy
ERYC (Erythromycin) Parke-Davis .. 1915
Ery-Tab Tablets (Erythromycin) Abbott 422
Erythrocin Stearate Filmtab (Erythromycin Stearate) Abbott 425
Erythromycin Base Filmtab (Erythromycin) Abbott 426
Erythromycin Delayed-Release Capsules, USP (Erythromycin) Abbott 427
Ilosone (Erythromycin Estolate) Dista 911
PCE Dispertab Tablets (Erythromycin) Abbott 444

Chlamydia trachomatis rectal infections
Achromycin V Capsules (Tetracycline Hydrochloride) Lederle 1367
Doryx Capsules (Doxycycline Hyclate) Parke-Davis 1913
E-Mycin Tablets (Erythromycin) Knoll Laboratories 1341
ERYC (Erythromycin) Parke-Davis .. 1915
Ery-Tab Tablets (Erythromycin) Abbott 422
Erythrocin Stearate Filmtab (Erythromycin Stearate) Abbott 425
Erythromycin Base Filmtab (Erythromycin) Abbott 426
Erythromycin Delayed-Release Capsules, USP (Erythromycin) Abbott 427
Ilosone (Erythromycin Estolate) Dista 911
Minocin Oral Suspension (Minocycline Hydrochloride) Lederle 1385
Monodox Capsules (Doxycycline Monohydrate) Oclassen 1805
PCE Dispertab Tablets (Erythromycin) Abbott 444
Vibramycin (Doxycycline Calcium) Pfizer Labs 1941

Chlamydia trachomatis urethral infections
Achromycin V Capsules (Tetracycline Hydrochloride) Lederle 1367
Doryx Capsules (Doxycycline Hyclate) Parke-Davis 1913
E.E.S. (Erythromycin Ethylsuccinate) Abbott 424
E-Mycin Tablets (Erythromycin) Knoll Laboratories 1341
ERYC (Erythromycin) Parke-Davis .. 1915
EryPed (Erythromycin Ethylsuccinate) Abbott 421
Ery-Tab Tablets (Erythromycin) Abbott 422
Erythrocin Stearate Filmtab (Erythromycin Stearate) Abbott 425
Erythromycin Base Filmtab (Erythromycin) Abbott 426
Erythromycin Delayed-Release Capsules, USP (Erythromycin) Abbott 427
Ilosone (Erythromycin Estolate) Dista 911
Monodox Capsules (Doxycycline Monohydrate) Oclassen 1805
PCE Dispertab Tablets (Erythromycin) Abbott 444

(▣ Described in PDR For Nonprescription Drugs) (◉ Described in PDR For Ophthalmology)

1467 **Indications Index** **Clostridium species**

Vibramycin (Doxycycline Calcium) Pfizer Labs 1941

Chlamydia trachomatis urogenital infections during pregnancy
ERYC (Erythromycin) Parke-Davis .. 1915
Ery-Tab Tablets (Erythromycin) Abbott 422
Erythrocin Stearate Filmtab (Erythromycin Stearate) Abbott 425
Erythromycin Base Filmtab (Erythromycin) Abbott 426
Erythromycin Delayed-Release Capsules, USP (Erythromycin) Abbott 427
Ilosone (Erythromycin Estolate) Dista 911
PCE Dispertab Tablets (Erythromycin) Abbott 444

Chloasma (see under Hyperpigmentation, skin, bleaching of)

Cholangitis (see also under Infections, intra-abdominal)
Mezlin (Mezlocillin Sodium) Bayer Pharmaceutical 601
Mezlin Pharmacy Bulk Package (Mezlocillin Sodium) Bayer Pharmaceutical 604

Cholecystitis, acute (see also under Infections, intra-abdominal)
Mezlin (Mezlocillin Sodium) Bayer Pharmaceutical 601
Mezlin Pharmacy Bulk Package (Mezlocillin Sodium) Bayer Pharmaceutical 604

Cholera
Dynacin Capsules (Minocycline Hydrochloride) Medicis 1590
Minocin Oral Suspension (Minocycline Hydrochloride) Lederle 1385
Minocin Pellet-Filled Capsules (Minocycline Hydrochloride) Lederle 1383
Monodox Capsules (Doxycycline Monohydrate) Oclassen 1805
Vibramycin Hyclate Capsules (Doxycycline Hyclate) Pfizer Labs 1941

Cholesterol levels, elevated (see under Hypercholesterolemia, primary, adjunct to diet)

Chorea, prophylaxis of
Bicillin L-A Injection (Penicillin G Benzathine) Wyeth-Ayerst 2707
Pen•Vee K (Penicillin V Potassium) Wyeth-Ayerst 2772

Choriocarcinoma
Blenoxane (Bleomycin Sulfate) Bristol-Myers Squibb Oncology 692
Methotrexate Sodium Tablets, Injection, for Injection and LPF Injection (Methotrexate Sodium) Immunex 1275
Velban Vials (Vinblastine Sulfate) Lilly 1484

Chorioadenoma destruens
Methotrexate Sodium Tablets, Injection, for Injection and LPF Injection (Methotrexate Sodium) Immunex 1275

Chorioretinitis
Aristocort Suspension (Forte Parenteral) (Triamcinolone Diacetate) Fujisawa 1027
Aristocort Tablets (Triamcinolone) Fujisawa 1022
Celestone Soluspan Suspension (Betamethasone Sodium Phosphate, Betamethasone Acetate) Schering 2347
Cortone Acetate Sterile Suspension (Cortisone Acetate) Merck & Co., Inc. 1623
Cortone Acetate Tablets (Cortisone Acetate) Merck & Co., Inc. 1624
Dalalone D.P. Injectable (Dexamethasone Acetate) Forest 1011
Decadron Elixir (Dexamethasone) Merck & Co., Inc. 1633
Decadron Phosphate Injection (Dexamethasone Sodium Phosphate) Merck & Co., Inc. 1637
Decadron Tablets (Dexamethasone) Merck & Co., Inc. 1635
Decadron-LA Sterile Suspension (Dexamethasone Acetate) Merck & Co., Inc. 1646
Deltasone Tablets (Prednisone) Upjohn 2595
Depo-Medrol Single-Dose Vial (Methylprednisolone Acetate) Upjohn 2600
Depo-Medrol Sterile Aqueous Suspension (Methylprednisolone Acetate) Upjohn 2597
Hydeltrasol Injection, Sterile (Prednisolone Sodium Phosphate) Merck & Co., Inc. 1665
Hydrocortone Phosphate Injection, Sterile (Hydrocortisone Sodium Phosphate) Merck & Co., Inc. 1670
Hydrocortone Tablets (Hydrocortisone) Merck & Co., Inc. 1672
Medrol (Methylprednisolone) Upjohn 2621
Pediapred Oral Liquid (Prednisolone Sodium Phosphate) Fisons 995
Prelone Syrup (Prednisolone) Muro 1787
Solu-Cortef Sterile Powder (Hydrocortisone Sodium Succinate) Upjohn 2641
Solu-Medrol Sterile Powder (Methylprednisolone Sodium Succinate) Upjohn 2643

Choroiditis
Aristocort Suspension (Forte Parenteral) (Triamcinolone Diacetate) Fujisawa 1027
Aristocort Tablets (Triamcinolone) Fujisawa 1022
Celestone Soluspan Suspension (Betamethasone Sodium Phosphate, Betamethasone Acetate) Schering 2347
Cortone Acetate Sterile Suspension (Cortisone Acetate) Merck & Co., Inc. 1623
Cortone Acetate Tablets (Cortisone Acetate) Merck & Co., Inc. 1624
Dalalone D.P. Injectable (Dexamethasone Acetate) Forest 1011
Decadron Elixir (Dexamethasone) Merck & Co., Inc. 1633
Decadron Phosphate Injection (Dexamethasone Sodium Phosphate) Merck & Co., Inc. 1637
Decadron Tablets (Dexamethasone) Merck & Co., Inc. 1635
Decadron-LA Sterile Suspension (Dexamethasone Acetate) Merck & Co., Inc. 1646
Deltasone Tablets (Prednisone) Upjohn 2595
Depo-Medrol Single-Dose Vial (Methylprednisolone Acetate) Upjohn 2600
Depo-Medrol Sterile Aqueous Suspension (Methylprednisolone Acetate) Upjohn 2597
Hydeltrasol Injection, Sterile (Prednisolone Sodium Phosphate) Merck & Co., Inc. 1665
Hydrocortone Phosphate Injection, Sterile (Hydrocortisone Sodium Phosphate) Merck & Co., Inc. 1670
Hydrocortone Tablets (Hydrocortisone) Merck & Co., Inc. 1672
Medrol (Methylprednisolone) Upjohn 2621
Pediapred Oral Liquid (Prednisolone Sodium Phosphate) Fisons 995
Prelone Syrup (Prednisolone) Muro 1787
Solu-Cortef Sterile Powder (Hydrocortisone Sodium Succinate) Upjohn 2641
Solu-Medrol Sterile Powder (Methylprednisolone Sodium Succinate) Upjohn 2643

Christmas disease (see under Hemophilia B)

Chromomycosis
Nizoral Tablets (Ketoconazole) Janssen 1298

Citrobacter diversus infections
Cipro I.V. (Ciprofloxacin) Bayer Pharmaceutical 595
Cipro I.V. Pharmacy Bulk Package (Ciprofloxacin) Bayer Pharmaceutical 597
Cipro Tablets (Ciprofloxacin Hydrochloride) Bayer Pharmaceutical 592
Floxin I.V. (Ofloxacin) McNeil Pharmaceutical 1571
Floxin Tablets (200 mg, 300 mg, 400 mg) (Ofloxacin) McNeil Pharmaceutical 1567
Maxaquin Tablets (Lomefloxacin Hydrochloride) Searle 2440

Citrobacter diversus urinary tract infections
Cipro I.V. (Ciprofloxacin) Bayer Pharmaceutical 595
Cipro I.V. Pharmacy Bulk Package (Ciprofloxacin) Bayer Pharmaceutical 597
Cipro Tablets (Ciprofloxacin Hydrochloride) Bayer Pharmaceutical 592
Floxin I.V. (Ofloxacin) McNeil Pharmaceutical 1571
Floxin Tablets (200 mg, 300 mg, 400 mg) (Ofloxacin) McNeil Pharmaceutical 1567
Maxaquin Tablets (Lomefloxacin Hydrochloride) Searle 2440

Citrobacter freundii infections
Azactam for Injection (Aztreonam) Bristol-Myers Squibb 734
Cipro I.V. (Ciprofloxacin) Bayer Pharmaceutical 595
Cipro I.V. Pharmacy Bulk Package (Ciprofloxacin) Bayer Pharmaceutical 597
Cipro Tablets (Ciprofloxacin Hydrochloride) Bayer Pharmaceutical 592
Claforan Sterile and Injection (Cefotaxime Sodium) Hoechst-Roussel 1235
Noroxin Tablets (Norfloxacin) Merck & Co., Inc. 1715
Noroxin Tablets (Norfloxacin) Roberts 2048

Citrobacter freundii intra-abdominal infections
Azactam for Injection (Aztreonam) Bristol-Myers Squibb 734

Citrobacter freundii skin and skin structure infections
Cipro I.V. (Ciprofloxacin) Bayer Pharmaceutical 595
Cipro I.V. Pharmacy Bulk Package (Ciprofloxacin) Bayer Pharmaceutical 597
Cipro Tablets (Ciprofloxacin Hydrochloride) Bayer Pharmaceutical 592
Claforan Sterile and Injection (Cefotaxime Sodium) Hoechst-Roussel 1235

Citrobacter freundii urinary tract infections
Cipro I.V. (Ciprofloxacin) Bayer Pharmaceutical 595
Cipro I.V. Pharmacy Bulk Package (Ciprofloxacin) Bayer Pharmaceutical 597
Cipro Tablets (Ciprofloxacin Hydrochloride) Bayer Pharmaceutical 592
Noroxin Tablets (Norfloxacin) Merck & Co., Inc. 1715
Noroxin Tablets (Norfloxacin) Roberts 2048

Citrobacter species infections
Azactam for Injection (Aztreonam) Bristol-Myers Squibb 734
Ceptaz (Ceftazidime) Glaxo Wellcome 1081
Claforan Sterile and Injection (Cefotaxime Sodium) Hoechst-Roussel 1235
Fortaz (Ceftazidime) Glaxo Wellcome 1100
Garamycin Injectable (Gentamicin Sulfate) Schering 2360
Nebcin Vials, Hyporets & ADD-Vantage (Tobramycin Sulfate) Lilly 1464
Netromycin Injection 100 mg/ml (Netilmicin Sulfate) Schering 2373
Primaxin I.M. (Imipenem-Cilastatin Sodium) Merck & Co., Inc. 1727
Primaxin I.V. (Imipenem-Cilastatin Sodium) Merck & Co., Inc. 1729
Tazicef for Injection (Ceftazidime) SmithKline Beecham Pharmaceuticals 2519
Tazidime Vials, Faspak & ADD-Vantage (Ceftazidime) Lilly .. 1478
Timentin for Injection (Ticarcillin Disodium, Clavulanate Potassium) SmithKline Beecham Pharmaceuticals 2528
Tobramycin Sulfate Injection (Tobramycin Sulfate) Elkins-Sinn 968

Citrobacter species intra-abdominal infections
Azactam for Injection (Aztreonam) Bristol-Myers Squibb 734
Primaxin I.V. (Imipenem-Cilastatin Sodium) Merck & Co., Inc. 1729

Citrobacter species lower respiratory tract infections
Ceptaz (Ceftazidime) Glaxo Wellcome 1081
Fortaz (Ceftazidime) Glaxo Wellcome 1100
Tazicef for Injection (Ceftazidime) SmithKline Beecham Pharmaceuticals 2519

Citrobacter species skin and skin structure infections
Azactam for Injection (Aztreonam) Bristol-Myers Squibb 734
Claforan Sterile and Injection (Cefotaxime Sodium) Hoechst-Roussel 1235
Primaxin I.M. (Imipenem-Cilastatin Sodium) Merck & Co., Inc. 1727
Primaxin I.V. (Imipenem-Cilastatin Sodium) Merck & Co., Inc. 1729

Citrobacter species urinary tract infections
Azactam for Injection (Aztreonam) Bristol-Myers Squibb 734
Claforan Sterile and Injection (Cefotaxime Sodium) Hoechst-Roussel 1235
Nebcin Vials, Hyporets & ADD-Vantage (Tobramycin Sulfate) Lilly 1464
Netromycin Injection 100 mg/ml (Netilmicin Sulfate) Schering 2373
Timentin for Injection (Ticarcillin Disodium, Clavulanate Potassium) SmithKline Beecham Pharmaceuticals 2528
Tobramycin Sulfate Injection (Tobramycin Sulfate) Elkins-Sinn 968

Claudication, intermittent
Trental Tablets (Pentoxifylline) Hoechst-Roussel 1244

Clonorchiasis
Biltricide Tablets (Praziquantel) Bayer Pharmaceutical 591

Clonorchis sinensis/Opisthorchis viverrini infections
Biltricide Tablets (Praziquantel) Bayer Pharmaceutical 591

Clostridium species endomyometritis
Flagyl 375 Capsules (Metronidazole) Searle 2434
Flagyl I.V. (Metronidazole Hydrochloride) SCS 2247
Protostat Tablets (Metronidazole) Ortho Pharmaceutical 1883

Clostridium species gynecologic infections
Cefobid Intravenous/Intramuscular (Cefoperazone Sodium) Roerig 2189
Cefobid Pharmacy Bulk Package - Not for Direct Infusion (Cefoperazone Sodium) Roerig 2192
Claforan Sterile and Injection (Cefotaxime Sodium) Hoechst-Roussel 1235

Clostridium species **Indications Index** **1468**

Flagyl 375 Capsules (Metronidazole) Searle 2434
Flagyl I.V. (Metronidazole Hydrochloride) SCS 2247
Mefoxin (Cefoxitin Sodium) Merck & Co., Inc. 1691
Mefoxin Premixed Intravenous Solution (Cefoxitin Sodium) Merck & Co., Inc. 1694
Protostat Tablets (Metronidazole) Ortho Pharmaceutical 1883

Clostridium species infections
Achromycin V Capsules (Tetracycline Hydrochloride) Lederle 1367
Cefobid Intravenous/Intramuscular (Cefoperazone Sodium) Roerig 2189
Cefobid Pharmacy Bulk Package - Not for Direct Infusion (Cefoperazone Sodium) Roerig 2192
Cefotan (Cefotetan) Zeneca 2829
Claforan Sterile and Injection (Cefotaxime Sodium) Hoechst-Roussel 1235
Declomycin Tablets (Demeclocycline Hydrochloride) Lederle 1371
Doryx Capsules (Doxycycline Hyclate) Parke-Davis 1913
Dynacin Capsules (Minocycline Hydrochloride) Medicis 1590
Flagyl 375 Capsules (Metronidazole) Searle 2434
Flagyl I.V. (Metronidazole Hydrochloride) SCS 2247
Mefoxin (Cefoxitin Sodium) Merck & Co., Inc. 1691
Mefoxin Premixed Intravenous Solution (Cefoxitin Sodium) Merck & Co., Inc. 1694
Minocin Intravenous (Minocycline Hydrochloride) Lederle 1382
Minocin Oral Suspension (Minocycline Hydrochloride) Lederle 1385
Minocin Pellet-Filled Capsules (Minocycline Hydrochloride) Lederle 1383
Monodox Capsules (Doxycycline Monohydrate) Oclassen 1805
Pfizerpen for Injection (Penicillin G Potassium) Roerig 2203
Pipracil (Piperacillin Sodium) Lederle 1390
Primaxin I.V. (Imipenem-Cilastatin Sodium) Merck & Co., Inc. 1729
Rocephin Injectable Vials, ADD-Vantage, Galaxy Container (Ceftriaxone Sodium) Roche Laboratories 2142
Terramycin Intramuscular Solution (Oxytetracycline) Roerig 2210
Vibramycin (Doxycycline Calcium) Pfizer Labs 1941
Vibramycin Hyclate Intravenous (Doxycycline Hyclate) Roerig 2215
Vibramycin (Doxycycline Monohydrate) Pfizer Labs 1941

Clostridium species intra-abdominal infections
Cefotan (Cefotetan) Zeneca 2829
Claforan Sterile and Injection (Cefotaxime Sodium) Hoechst-Roussel 1235
Flagyl 375 Capsules (Metronidazole) Searle 2434
Flagyl I.V. (Metronidazole Hydrochloride) SCS 2247
Mefoxin (Cefoxitin Sodium) Merck & Co., Inc. 1691
Mefoxin Premixed Intravenous Solution (Cefoxitin Sodium) Merck & Co., Inc. 1694
Primaxin I.V. (Imipenem-Cilastatin Sodium) Merck & Co., Inc. 1729
Protostat Tablets (Metronidazole) Ortho Pharmaceutical 1883
Rocephin Injectable Vials, ADD-Vantage, Galaxy Container (Ceftriaxone Sodium) Roche Laboratories 2142

Clostridium species liver abscess
Flagyl 375 Capsules (Metronidazole) Searle 2434
Flagyl I.V. (Metronidazole Hydrochloride) SCS 2247
Protostat Tablets (Metronidazole) Ortho Pharmaceutical 1883

Clostridium species peritonitis
Flagyl 375 Capsules (Metronidazole) Searle 2434
Flagyl I.V. (Metronidazole Hydrochloride) SCS 2247
Mefoxin (Cefoxitin Sodium) Merck & Co., Inc. 1691
Mefoxin Premixed Intravenous Solution (Cefoxitin Sodium) Merck & Co., Inc. 1694
Protostat Tablets (Metronidazole) Ortho Pharmaceutical 1883

Clostridium species septicemia
Cefobid Intravenous/Intramuscular (Cefoperazone Sodium) Roerig 2189
Cefobid Pharmacy Bulk Package - Not for Direct Infusion (Cefoperazone Sodium) Roerig 2192
Flagyl 375 Capsules (Metronidazole) Searle 2434
Flagyl I.V. (Metronidazole Hydrochloride) SCS 2247
Protostat Tablets (Metronidazole) Ortho Pharmaceutical 1883

Clostridium species skin and skin structure infections
Flagyl 375 Capsules (Metronidazole) Searle 2434
Flagyl I.V. (Metronidazole Hydrochloride) SCS 2247
Mefoxin (Cefoxitin Sodium) Merck & Co., Inc. 1691
Mefoxin Premixed Intravenous Solution (Cefoxitin Sodium) Merck & Co., Inc. 1694
Protostat Tablets (Metronidazole) Ortho Pharmaceutical 1883

Clostridium species tubo-ovarian abscess
Flagyl 375 Capsules (Metronidazole) Searle 2434
Flagyl I.V. (Metronidazole Hydrochloride) SCS 2247
Protostat Tablets (Metronidazole) Ortho Pharmaceutical 1883

Clostridium species vaginal cuff infection, post-surgical
Flagyl 375 Capsules (Metronidazole) Searle 2434
Flagyl I.V. (Metronidazole Hydrochloride) SCS 2247
Protostat Tablets (Metronidazole) Ortho Pharmaceutical 1883

CNS depression
(see under Central nervous system depression, drug-induced)

Coagulation, disseminated intravascular
(see under Coagulopathies, consumptive)

Coagulopathies, consumptive
Heparin Sodium Injection (Heparin Sodium) Wyeth-Ayerst 2726
Heparin Sodium Injection, USP, Sterile Solution (Heparin Sodium) Upjohn 2615
Heparin Sodium Vials (Heparin Sodium) Lilly 1441

Coccidioidomycosis
Fungizone Intravenous (Amphotericin B) Apothecon 506
Nizoral Tablets (Ketoconazole) Janssen 1298

Coitus, adjunct in
K-Y Jelly Personal Lubricant (Chlorhexidine Gluconate) J & J Consumer ▣ 658
K-Y Plus Vaginal Contraceptive and Personal Lubricant (Nonoxynol-9) J & J Consumer ▣ 659
Replens Vaginal Moisturizer (Glycerin, Lubricant) WARNER WELLCOME ▣ 859

Cold sores
(see under Herpetic manifestations, oral, symptomatic relief of)

Cold, common, symptomatic relief of
(see also under Influenza syndrome, symptomatic relief of)
Actifed Plus Caplets (Acetaminophen, Pseudoephedrine Hydrochloride, Triprolidine Hydrochloride) WARNER WELLCOME ▣ 845
Actifed Plus Tablets (Acetaminophen, Pseudoephedrine Hydrochloride, Triprolidine Hydrochloride) WARNER WELLCOME ▣ 845
Actifed Syrup (Pseudoephedrine Hydrochloride, Triprolidine Hydrochloride) WARNER WELLCOME ▣ 846
Actifed Tablets (Pseudoephedrine Hydrochloride, Triprolidine Hydrochloride) WARNER WELLCOME ▣ 844
Afrin (Oxymetazoline Hydrochloride) Schering-Plough HealthCare ▣ 797
Alka-Seltzer Plus Cold Medicine (Chlorpheniramine Maleate, Aspirin, Phenylpropanolamine Bitartrate) Miles Consumer ▣ 705
Alka-Seltzer Plus Night-Time Cold Medicine (Aspirin, Phenylpropanolamine Bitartrate, Doxylamine Succinate, Dextromethorphan Hydrobromide) Miles Consumer ▣ 707
Atrohist Pediatric Suspension (Chlorpheniramine Tannate, Phenylephrine Tannate, Pyrilamine Tannate) Adams 454
Atrohist Plus Tablets (Chlorpheniramine Maleate, Phenylpropanolamine Hydrochloride, Phenylephrine Hydrochloride, Hyoscyamine Sulfate, Atropine Sulfate, Scopolamine Hydrobromide) Adams 454
BC Cold Powder Multi-Symptom Formula (Cold-Sinus-Allergy) (Aspirin, Phenylpropanolamine Hydrochloride, Chlorpheniramine Maleate) Block ▣ 609
BC Cold Powder Non-Drowsy Formula (Cold-Sinus) (Aspirin, Phenylpropanolamine Hydrochloride) Block ▣ 609
Benadryl Allergy Decongestant Liquid Medication (Diphenhydramine Hydrochloride, Pseudoephedrine Hydrochloride) WARNER WELLCOME ▣ 848
Benadryl Allergy Decongestant Tablets (Diphenhydramine Hydrochloride, Pseudoephedrine Hydrochloride) WARNER WELLCOME ▣ 848
Benadryl Allergy Liquid Medication (Diphenhydramine Hydrochloride) WARNER WELLCOME ▣ 849
Benadryl Allergy Sinus Headache Formula Caplets (Diphenhydramine Hydrochloride, Pseudoephedrine Hydrochloride, Acetaminophen) WARNER WELLCOME ▣ 849
Benadryl Dye-Free Allergy Liqui-gel Softgels (Diphenhydramine Hydrochloride) WARNER WELLCOME ▣ 850
Bromfed Syrup (Brompheniramine Maleate, Pseudoephedrine Hydrochloride) Muro ▣ 733
Cheracol Nasal Spray Pump (Oxymetazoline Hydrochloride) Roberts ▣ 768
Cheracol Sinus (Dexbrompheniramine Maleate, Pseudoephedrine Sulfate) Roberts ▣ 768
Chlor-Trimeton Allergy Decongestant Tablets (Chlorpheniramine Maleate, Pseudoephedrine Sulfate) Schering-Plough HealthCare ▣ 799
Congess (Guaifenesin, Pseudoephedrine Hydrochloride) Fleming 1004
Contac Continuous Action Nasal Decongestant/Antihistamine 12 Hour Capsules (Chlorpheniramine Maleate, Phenylpropanolamine Hydrochloride) SmithKline Beecham Consumer ▣ 813
Contac Maximum Strength Continuous Action Decongestant/Antihistamine 12 Hour Caplets (Chlorpheniramine Maleate, Phenylpropanolamine Hydrochloride) SmithKline Beecham Consumer ▣ 813
Coricidin 'D' Decongestant Tablets (Acetaminophen, Chlorpheniramine Maleate, Phenylpropanolamine Hydrochloride) Schering-Plough HealthCare ▣ 800
Coricidin Tablets (Acetaminophen, Chlorpheniramine Maleate) Schering-Plough HealthCare ▣ 800
D.A. Chewable Tablets (Chlorpheniramine Maleate, Phenylephrine Hydrochloride, Methscopolamine Nitrate) Dura 951
Deconamine (Chlorpheniramine Maleate, Pseudoephedrine Hydrochloride) Kenwood 1320
Dimetapp Elixir (Brompheniramine Maleate, Phenylpropanolamine Hydrochloride) A. H. Robins Consumer ▣ 773
Dimetapp Extentabs (Brompheniramine Maleate, Phenylpropanolamine Hydrochloride) A. H. Robins Consumer ▣ 774
Dimetapp Tablets/Liqui-Gels (Brompheniramine Maleate, Phenylpropanolamine Hydrochloride) A. H. Robins Consumer ▣ 775
Drixoral Cold and Allergy Sustained-Action Tablets (Dexbrompheniramine Maleate, Pseudoephedrine Sulfate) Schering-Plough HealthCare ▣ 802
Drixoral Cold and Flu Extended-Release Tablets (Acetaminophen, Dexbrompheniramine Maleate, Pseudoephedrine Sulfate) Schering-Plough HealthCare ▣ 803
Drixoral Allergy/Sinus Extended Release Tablets (Acetaminophen, Pseudoephedrine Sulfate, Dexbrompheniramine Maleate) Schering-Plough HealthCare ▣ 804
Dura-Tap/PD Capsules (Chlorpheniramine Maleate, Pseudoephedrine Hydrochloride) Dura 2867
Duration 12 Hour Nasal Spray (Oxymetazoline Hydrochloride) Schering-Plough HealthCare ▣ 805
Dura-Vent/DA Tablets (Chlorpheniramine Maleate, Phenylephrine Hydrochloride, Methscopolamine Nitrate) Dura 953
Dura-Vent Tablets (Phenylpropanolamine Hydrochloride, Guaifenesin) Dura 952
Entex Capsules (Phenylephrine Hydrochloride, Phenylpropanolamine Hydrochloride, Guaifenesin) Procter & Gamble Pharmaceuticals 1986
Entex LA Tablets (Phenylpropanolamine Hydrochloride, Guaifenesin) Procter & Gamble Pharmaceuticals 1987
Entex Liquid (Phenylephrine Hydrochloride, Phenylpropanolamine Hydrochloride, Guaifenesin) Procter & Gamble Pharmaceuticals 1986
Exgest LA Tablets (Phenylpropanolamine Hydrochloride, Guaifenesin) Carnrick 782
4-Way Fast Acting Nasal Spray (regular & mentholated) (Naphazoline Hydrochloride, Phenylephrine Hydrochloride, Pyrilamine Maleate) Bristol-Myers Products ▣ 621
4-Way Long Lasting Nasal Spray (Oxymetazoline Hydrochloride) Bristol-Myers Products ▣ 621
Fedahist Gyrocaps (Pseudoephedrine Hydrochloride, Chlorpheniramine Maleate) Schwarz 2401
Fedahist Timecaps (Pseudoephedrine Hydrochloride, Chlorpheniramine Maleate) Schwarz 2401
Guaifed Syrup (Guaifenesin, Pseudoephedrine Hydrochloride) Muro ▣ 734
Hyland's C-Plus Cold Tablets (Homeopathic Medications) Standard Homeopathic ▣ 829

(▣ Described in PDR For Nonprescription Drugs) (◉ Described in PDR For Ophthalmology)

1469 Indications Index Congestive heart failure

Isoclor Timesule Capsules (Phenylpropanolamine Hydrochloride, Chlorpheniramine Maleate) CIBA Consumer ▣ 637
NTZ Long Acting Nasal Spray & Drops 0.05% (Oxymetazoline Hydrochloride) Miles Consumer ▣ 727
Neo-Synephrine Maximum Strength 12 Hour Nasal Spray (Oxymetazoline Hydrochloride) Miles Consumer ▣ 726
Neo-Synephrine Maximum Strength 12 Hour Nasal Spray Pump (Oxymetazoline Hydrochloride) Miles Consumer ▣ 726
Neo-Synephrine (Phenylephrine Hydrochloride) Miles Consumer ▣ 726
Nolamine Timed-Release Tablets (Phenindamine Tartrate, Phenylpropanolamine Hydrochloride, Chlorpheniramine Maleate) Carnrick 785
Nōstrilla Long Acting Nasal Decongestant (Oxymetazoline Hydrochloride) CIBA Consumer ▣ 644
Novahistine Elixir (Chlorpheniramine Maleate, Phenylephrine Hydrochloride) SmithKline Beecham Consumer ▣ 823
PediaCare Cold Allergy Chewable Tablets (Pseudoephedrine Hydrochloride, Chlorpheniramine Maleate) McNeil Consumer ▣ 677
PediaCare Cough-Cold Liquid (Pseudoephedrine Hydrochloride, Chlorpheniramine Maleate, Dextromethorphan Hydrobromide) McNeil Consumer 1553
Propagest Tablets (Phenylpropanolamine Hydrochloride) Carnrick 786
Ricobid Tablets and Pediatric Suspension (Chlorpheniramine Tannate, Phenylephrine Tannate) Rico Pharmacal 2038
Robitussin-PE (Guaifenesin, Pseudoephedrine Hydrochloride) A. H. Robins Consumer ▣ 778
Rynatan (Chlorpheniramine Tannate, Pyrilamine Tannate, Phenylephrine Tannate) Wallace 2673
Sinarest (Acetaminophen, Chlorpheniramine Maleate, Pseudoephedrine Hydrochloride) CIBA Consumer ▣ 648
Sine-Off No Drowsiness Formula Caplets (Acetaminophen, Pseudoephedrine Hydrochloride) SmithKline Beecham Consumer ▣ 824
Sine-Off Sinus Medicine (Aspirin, Chlorpheniramine Maleate, Phenylpropanolamine Hydrochloride) SmithKline Beecham Consumer ▣ 825
Singlet Tablets (Acetaminophen, Chlorpheniramine Maleate, Pseudoephedrine Hydrochloride) SmithKline Beecham Consumer ▣ 825
Sinulin Tablets (Acetaminophen, Phenylpropanolamine Hydrochloride, Chlorpheniramine Maleate) Carnrick 787
Sinutab Sinus Allergy Medication, Maximum Strength Tablets and Caplets (Acetaminophen, Chlorpheniramine Maleate, Pseudoephedrine Hydrochloride) WARNER WELLCOME ▣ 860
Sinutab Sinus Medication, Regular Strength Without Drowsiness Formula (Acetaminophen, Pseudoephedrine Hydrochloride) WARNER WELLCOME ▣ 859
Sudafed Children's Liquid (Pseudoephedrine Hydrochloride) WARNER WELLCOME ▣ 861
Sudafed Cough Syrup (Dextromethorphan Hydrobromide, Guaifenesin, Pseudoephedrine Hydrochloride) WARNER WELLCOME ▣ 862
Sudafed Plus Liquid (Chlorpheniramine Maleate, Pseudoephedrine Hydrochloride) WARNER WELLCOME ▣ 862
Sudafed Plus Tablets (Chlorpheniramine Maleate, Pseudoephedrine Hydrochloride) WARNER WELLCOME ▣ 863
Sudafed Sinus Caplets (Acetaminophen, Pseudoephedrine Hydrochloride) WARNER WELLCOME ▣ 864
Sudafed Sinus Tablets (Acetaminophen, Pseudoephedrine Hydrochloride) WARNER WELLCOME ▣ 864
Sudafed Tablets, 30 mg (Pseudoephedrine Hydrochloride) WARNER WELLCOME ▣ 861
Sudafed Tablets, 60 mg (Pseudoephedrine Hydrochloride) WARNER WELLCOME ▣ 861
Triaminic Cold Tablets (Phenylpropanolamine Hydrochloride, Chlorpheniramine Maleate) Sandoz Consumer ▣ 790
Triaminic Syrup (Phenylpropanolamine Hydrochloride, Chlorpheniramine Maleate) Sandoz Consumer ▣ 792
Triaminicin Tablets (Acetaminophen, Chlorpheniramine Maleate, Phenylpropanolamine Hydrochloride) Sandoz Consumer ▣ 793
Trinalin Repetabs Tablets (Azatadine Maleate, Pseudoephedrine Sulfate) Key 1330
Children's TYLENOL Cold Multi-Symptom Liquid Formula and Chewable Tablets (Acetaminophen, Chlorpheniramine Maleate, Pseudoephedrine Hydrochloride) McNeil Consumer 1561
Ursinus Inlay-Tabs (Aspirin, Pseudoephedrine Hydrochloride) Sandoz Consumer ▣ 794
Vicks Sinex 12-Hour Nasal Decongestant Spray and Ultra Fine Mist (Oxymetazoline Hydrochloride) Procter & Gamble ▣ 765
Vicks Sinex Nasal Spray and Ultra Fine Mist (Phenylephrine Hydrochloride) Procter & Gamble ▣ 765

Colic, biliary, symptomatic relief of
Cystospaz (Hyoscyamine) PolyMedica 1963
Levsin/Levsinex/Levbid (Hyoscyamine Sulfate) Schwarz 2405

Colic, renal, symptomatic relief of
Cystospaz (Hyoscyamine) PolyMedica 1963
Levsin/Levsinex/Levbid (Hyoscyamine Sulfate) Schwarz 2405

Colic, symptomatic relief of
Hyland's Colic Tablets (Homeopathic Medications) Standard Homeopathic ▣ 829
Levsin/Levsinex/Levbid (Hyoscyamine Sulfate) Schwarz 2405

Colitis, mucous (see under Bowel, irritable, syndrome)

Colitis, pseudomembranous, antibiotic-associated
Vancocin HCl, Oral Solution & Pulvules (Vancomycin Hydrochloride) Lilly 1483
Vancocin HCl, Vials & ADD-Vantage (Vancomycin Hydrochloride) Lilly 1481

Colitis, ulcerative, adjunctive therapy in
Anusol-HC Suppositories (Hydrocortisone Acetate) Parke-Davis 1897
Azulfidine (Sulfasalazine) Pharmacia 1949
CORTENEMA (Hydrocortisone) Solvay 2535

Colitis, ulcerative, left-sided adjunctive therapy in
CORTENEMA (Hydrocortisone) Solvay 2535

Colitis, ulcerative, systemic therapy for
Aristocort Suspension (Forte Parenteral) (Triamcinolone Diacetate) Fujisawa 1027
Aristocort Tablets (Triamcinolone) Fujisawa 1022
Asacol Delayed-Release Tablets (Mesalamine) Procter & Gamble Pharmaceuticals 1979
Azulfidine (Sulfasalazine) Pharmacia 1949
Celestone Soluspan Suspension (Betamethasone Sodium Phosphate, Betamethasone Acetate) Schering 2347
Cortone Acetate Sterile Suspension (Cortisone Acetate) Merck & Co., Inc. 1623
Cortone Acetate Tablets (Cortisone Acetate) Merck & Co., Inc. 1624
Dalalone D.P. Injectable (Dexamethasone Acetate) Forest 1011
Decadron Elixir (Dexamethasone) Merck & Co., Inc. 1633
Decadron Phosphate Injection (Dexamethasone Sodium Phosphate) Merck & Co., Inc. 1637
Decadron Tablets (Dexamethasone) Merck & Co., Inc. 1635
Decadron-LA Sterile Suspension (Dexamethasone Acetate) Merck & Co., Inc. 1646
Deltasone Tablets (Prednisone) Upjohn 2595
Depo-Medrol Single-Dose Vial (Methylprednisolone Acetate) Upjohn 2600
Depo-Medrol Sterile Aqueous Suspension (Methylprednisolone Acetate) Upjohn 2597
Dipentum Capsules (Olsalazine Sodium) Pharmacia 1951
Hydeltrasol Injection, Sterile (Prednisolone Sodium Phosphate) Merck & Co., Inc. 1665
Hydrocortone Phosphate Injection, Sterile (Hydrocortisone Sodium Phosphate) Merck & Co., Inc. 1670
Hydrocortone Tablets (Hydrocortisone) Merck & Co., Inc. 1672
Medrol (Methylprednisolone) Upjohn 2621
Pediapred Oral Liquid (Prednisolone Sodium Phosphate) Fisons 995
Pentasa (Mesalamine) Marion Merrell Dow 1527
Prelone Syrup (Prednisolone) Muro 1787
ROWASA Rectal Suspension Enema 4.0 grams/unit (60 mL) (Mesalamine) Solvay 2548
Solu-Cortef Sterile Powder (Hydrocortisone Sodium Succinate) Upjohn 2641
Solu-Medrol Sterile Powder (Methylprednisolone Sodium Succinate) Upjohn 2643

Collagen disease
Aristocort Suspension (Forte Parenteral) (Triamcinolone Diacetate) Fujisawa 1027
Aristocort Tablets (Triamcinolone) Fujisawa 1022
Celestone Soluspan Suspension (Betamethasone Sodium Phosphate, Betamethasone Acetate) Schering 2347
Cortone Acetate Sterile Suspension (Cortisone Acetate) Merck & Co., Inc. 1623
Cortone Acetate Tablets (Cortisone Acetate) Merck & Co., Inc. 1624
Dalalone D.P. Injectable (Dexamethasone Acetate) Forest 1011
Decadron Elixir (Dexamethasone) Merck & Co., Inc. 1633
Decadron Phosphate Injection (Dexamethasone Sodium Phosphate) Merck & Co., Inc. 1637
Decadron Tablets (Dexamethasone) Merck & Co., Inc. 1635
Decadron-LA Sterile Suspension (Dexamethasone Acetate) Merck & Co., Inc. 1646
Deltasone Tablets (Prednisone) Upjohn 2595
Depo-Medrol Single-Dose Vial (Methylprednisolone Acetate) Upjohn 2600
Depo-Medrol Sterile Aqueous Suspension (Methylprednisolone Acetate) Upjohn 2597
Hydeltrasol Injection, Sterile (Prednisolone Sodium Phosphate) Merck & Co., Inc. 1665
Hydrocortone Phosphate Injection, Sterile (Hydrocortisone Sodium Phosphate) Merck & Co., Inc. 1670
Hydrocortone Tablets (Hydrocortisone) Merck & Co., Inc. 1672
Medrol (Methylprednisolone) Upjohn 2621
Pediapred Oral Liquid (Prednisolone Sodium Phosphate) Fisons 995
Prelone Syrup (Prednisolone) Muro 1787
Solu-Cortef Sterile Powder (Hydrocortisone Sodium Succinate) Upjohn 2641
Solu-Medrol Sterile Powder (Methylprednisolone Sodium Succinate) Upjohn 2643

Colon, irritable (see under Bowel, irritable, syndrome)

Colon, spastic (see under Bowel, irritable, syndrome)

Colostomies, reduction in odor, adjunct to
Devrom Chewable Tablets (Bismuth Subgallate) Parthenon ▣ 741

Condylomata acuminata
Intron A (Interferon alfa-2B, Recombinant) Schering 2364

Condylomata acuminata, topical treatment of
Condylox (Podofilox) Oclassen 1802
Podocon-25 (Podophyllin) Paddock 1891

Congestive heart failure (see also under Edema, congestive heart failure-induced, adjunctive therapy in; Edema, congestive heart failure-induced, treatment of)
Aldactazide (Spironolactone, Hydrochlorothiazide) Searle 2413
Aldactone (Spironolactone) Searle 2414
Capoten (Captopril) Bristol-Myers Squibb 739
Crystodigin Tablets (Digitoxin) Lilly 1433
Inocor Lactate Injection (Amrinone Lactate) Sanofi Winthrop 2309
Lanoxicaps (Digoxin) Glaxo Wellcome 1117
Lanoxin Elixir Pediatric (Digoxin) Glaxo Wellcome 1120
Lanoxin Injection (Digoxin) Glaxo Wellcome 1123
Lanoxin Injection Pediatric (Digoxin) Glaxo Wellcome 1126
Lanoxin Tablets (Digoxin) Glaxo Wellcome 1128
Moduretic Tablets (Amiloride Hydrochloride, Hydrochlorothiazide) Merck & Co., Inc. 1705
Nitro-Bid IV (Nitroglycerin) Marion Merrell Dow 1523
Primacor Injection (Milrinone Lactate) Sanofi Winthrop 2331

Congestive heart failure, adjunct in (see also under Edema, congestive heart failure-induced, adjunctive therapy in; Edema, congestive heart failure-induced, treatment of)
Accupril Tablets (Quinapril Hydrochloride) Parke-Davis 1893
Altace Capsules (Ramipril) Hoechst-Roussel 1232
Bumex (Bumetanide) Roche Laboratories 2093
Diuril Sodium Intravenous (Chlorothiazide Sodium) Merck & Co., Inc. 1652

(▣ Described in PDR For Nonprescription Drugs) (◉ Described in PDR For Ophthalmology)

Congestive heart failure Indications Index 1470

Isuprel Hydrochloride Injection 1:5000 (Isoproterenol Hydrochloride) Sanofi Winthrop 2311
Lozol Tablets (Indapamide) Rhone-Poulenc Rorer Pharmaceuticals 2022
Midamor Tablets (Amiloride Hydrochloride) Merck & Co., Inc. 1703
Monopril Tablets (Fosinopril Sodium) Bristol-Myers Squibb 757
Prinivil Tablets (Lisinopril) Merck & Co., Inc. 1733
Vasotec Tablets (Enalapril Maleate) Merck & Co., Inc. 1771
Zestril Tablets (Lisinopril) Zeneca 2854

Conjunctival hyperemia, reduction of signs and symptoms (see also under Ocular redness)
Lacrisert Sterile Ophthalmic Insert (Hydroxypropyl Cellulose) Merck & Co., Inc. 1686

Conjunctival inflammation, bulbar, steroid-responsive
AK-CIDE (Prednisolone Acetate, Sulfacetamide Sodium) Akorn ⊙ 202
AK-CIDE Ointment (Prednisolone Acetate, Sulfacetamide Sodium) Akorn ⊙ 202
Blephamide Ointment (Sulfacetamide Sodium, Prednisolone Acetate) Allergan ⊙ 237
Decadron Phosphate Sterile Ophthalmic Ointment (Dexamethasone Sodium Phosphate) Merck & Co., Inc. 1641
Decadron Phosphate Sterile Ophthalmic Solution (Dexamethasone Sodium Phosphate) Merck & Co., Inc. 1642
NeoDecadron Sterile Ophthalmic Ointment (Neomycin Sulfate, Dexamethasone Sodium Phosphate) Merck & Co., Inc. 1712
NeoDecadron Sterile Ophthalmic Solution (Neomycin Sulfate, Dexamethasone Sodium Phosphate) Merck & Co., Inc. 1713
Terra-Cortril Ophthalmic Suspension (Oxytetracycline Hydrochloride, Hydrocortisone Acetate) Roerig 2210

Conjunctival inflammation, palpebral, steroid-responsive
AK-CIDE (Prednisolone Acetate, Sulfacetamide Sodium) Akorn ⊙ 202
AK-CIDE Ointment (Prednisolone Acetate, Sulfacetamide Sodium) Akorn ⊙ 202
Blephamide Ointment (Sulfacetamide Sodium, Prednisolone Acetate) Allergan ⊙ 237
Decadron Phosphate Sterile Ophthalmic Ointment (Dexamethasone Sodium Phosphate) Merck & Co., Inc. 1641
Decadron Phosphate Sterile Ophthalmic Solution (Dexamethasone Sodium Phosphate) Merck & Co., Inc. 1642
NeoDecadron Sterile Ophthalmic Ointment (Neomycin Sulfate, Dexamethasone Sodium Phosphate) Merck & Co., Inc. 1712
NeoDecadron Sterile Ophthalmic Solution (Neomycin Sulfate, Dexamethasone Sodium Phosphate) Merck & Co., Inc. 1713
Terra-Cortril Ophthalmic Suspension (Oxytetracycline Hydrochloride, Hydrocortisone Acetate) Roerig 2210

Conjunctival staining, reduction of signs and symptoms
Lacrisert Sterile Ophthalmic Insert (Hydroxypropyl Cellulose) Merck & Co., Inc. 1686

Conjunctivitis, allergic
AK-Pred (Prednisolone Sodium Phosphate) Akorn ⊙ 204
Aristocort Suspension (Forte Parenteral) (Triamcinolone Diacetate) Fujisawa 1027
Aristocort Tablets (Triamcinolone) Fujisawa 1022
Benadryl Capsules (Diphenhydramine Hydrochloride) Parke-Davis 1898
Celestone Soluspan Suspension (Betamethasone Sodium Phosphate, Betamethasone Acetate) Schering 2347
Cortone Acetate Sterile Suspension (Cortisone Acetate) Merck & Co., Inc. 1623
Cortone Acetate Tablets (Cortisone Acetate) Merck & Co., Inc. 1624
Dalalone D.P. Injectable (Dexamethasone Acetate) Forest 1011
Decadron Elixir (Dexamethasone) Merck & Co., Inc. 1633
Decadron Phosphate Injection (Dexamethasone Sodium Phosphate) Merck & Co., Inc. 1637
Decadron Phosphate Sterile Ophthalmic Ointment (Dexamethasone Sodium Phosphate) Merck & Co., Inc. 1641
Decadron Phosphate Sterile Ophthalmic Solution (Dexamethasone Sodium Phosphate) Merck & Co., Inc. 1642
Decadron Tablets (Dexamethasone) Merck & Co., Inc. 1635
Decadron-LA Sterile Suspension (Dexamethasone Acetate) Merck & Co., Inc. 1646
Deltasone Tablets (Prednisone) Upjohn 2595
Depo-Medrol Single-Dose Vial (Methylprednisolone Acetate) Upjohn 2600
Depo-Medrol Sterile Aqueous Suspension (Methylprednisolone Acetate) Upjohn 2597
Econopred & Econopred Plus Ophthalmic Suspensions (Prednisolone Acetate) Alcon Laboratories ⊙ 217
HMS Liquifilm (Medrysone) Allergan ⊙ 244
Hydeltrasol Injection, Sterile (Prednisolone Sodium Phosphate) Merck & Co., Inc. 1665
Hydrocortone Phosphate Injection, Sterile (Hydrocortisone Sodium Phosphate) Merck & Co., Inc. 1670
Hydrocortone Tablets (Hydrocortisone) Merck & Co., Inc. 1672
Inflamase (Prednisolone Sodium Phosphate) CIBA Vision Ophthalmics ⊙ 265
Livostin (Levocabastine Hydrochloride) CIBA Vision Ophthalmics ⊙ 266
Medrol (Methylprednisolone) Upjohn 2621
PBZ Tablets (Tripelennamine Hydrochloride) CibaGeneva 845
PBZ-SR Tablets (Tripelennamine Hydrochloride) CibaGeneva 844
Pediapred Oral Liquid (Prednisolone Sodium Phosphate) Fisons 995
Periactin (Cyproheptadine Hydrochloride) Merck & Co., Inc. 1724
Phenergan Suppositories (Promethazine Hydrochloride) Wyeth-Ayerst 2775
Phenergan Syrup (Promethazine Hydrochloride) Wyeth-Ayerst 2774
Phenergan Tablets (Promethazine Hydrochloride) Wyeth-Ayerst 2775
Prelone Syrup (Prednisolone) Muro 1787
Solu-Cortef Sterile Powder (Hydrocortisone Sodium Succinate) Upjohn 2641
Solu-Medrol Sterile Powder (Methylprednisolone Sodium Succinate) Upjohn 2643

Conjunctivitis, bacterial
Chibroxin Sterile Ophthalmic Solution (Norfloxacin) Merck & Co., Inc. 1617
Ciloxan Ophthalmic Solution (Ciprofloxacin Hydrochloride) Alcon Laboratories 472
Neosporin Ophthalmic Ointment Sterile (Polymyxin B Sulfate, Bacitracin Zinc, Neomycin Sulfate) Glaxo Wellcome 1148
Neosporin Ophthalmic Solution Sterile (Polymyxin B Sulfate, Neomycin Sulfate, Gramicidin) Glaxo Wellcome 1149
Ocuflox (Ofloxacin) Allergan 481
Polysporin Ophthalmic Ointment Sterile (Polymyxin B Sulfate, Bacitracin Zinc) Glaxo Wellcome 1154
Polytrim Ophthalmic Solution Sterile (Polymyxin B Sulfate, Trimethoprim Sulfate) Allergan 482

Conjunctivitis, fungal
Natacyn Antifungal Ophthalmic Suspension (Natamycin) Alcon Laboratories ⊙ 225

Conjunctivitis, granular (see under Trachoma)

Conjunctivitis, inclusion
Achromycin V Capsules (Tetracycline Hydrochloride) Lederle 1367
Declomycin Tablets (Demeclocycline Hydrochloride) Lederle 1371
Doryx Capsules (Doxycycline Hyclate) Parke-Davis 1913
Dynacin Capsules (Minocycline Hydrochloride) Medicis 1590
Gantanol Tablets (Sulfamethoxazole) Roche Laboratories 2119
Gantrisin (Acetyl Sulfisoxazole) Roche Laboratories 2120
Minocin Intravenous (Minocycline Hydrochloride) Lederle 1382
Minocin Oral Suspension (Minocycline Hydrochloride) Lederle 1385
Minocin Pellet-Filled Capsules (Minocycline Hydrochloride) Lederle 1383
Monodox Capsules (Doxycycline Monohydrate) Oclassen 1805
Terramycin Intramuscular Solution (Oxytetracycline) Roerig 2210
Vibramycin (Doxycycline Calcium) Pfizer Labs 1941

Conjunctivitis, infective
AK-CIDE (Prednisolone Acetate, Sulfacetamide Sodium) Akorn ⊙ 202
AK-CIDE Ointment (Prednisolone Acetate, Sulfacetamide Sodium) Akorn ⊙ 202
AK-Pred (Prednisolone Sodium Phosphate) Akorn ⊙ 204
AK-Trol Ointment & Suspension (Dexamethasone, Neomycin Sulfate, Polymyxin B Sulfate) Akorn ⊙ 205
Blephamide Liquifilm Sterile Ophthalmic Suspension (Prednisolone Acetate, Sulfacetamide Sodium) Allergan 476
Blephamide Ointment (Sulfacetamide Sodium, Prednisolone Acetate) Allergan ⊙ 237
Decadron Phosphate Sterile Ophthalmic Ointment (Dexamethasone Sodium Phosphate) Merck & Co., Inc. 1641
Decadron Phosphate Sterile Ophthalmic Solution (Dexamethasone Sodium Phosphate) Merck & Co., Inc. 1642
Dexacidin Ointment (Dexamethasone, Neomycin Sulfate, Polymyxin B Sulfate) CIBA Vision Ophthalmics ⊙ 263
Econopred & Econopred Plus Ophthalmic Suspensions (Prednisolone Acetate) Alcon Laboratories ⊙ 217
FML-S Liquifilm (Sulfacetamide Sodium, Fluorometholone) Allergan ⊙ 242
Inflamase (Prednisolone Sodium Phosphate) CIBA Vision Ophthalmics ⊙ 265
Maxitrol Ophthalmic Ointment and Suspension (Dexamethasone, Neomycin Sulfate, Polymyxin B Sulfate) Alcon Laboratories ⊙ 224
NeoDecadron Sterile Ophthalmic Ointment (Neomycin Sulfate, Dexamethasone Sodium Phosphate) Merck & Co., Inc. 1712
NeoDecadron Sterile Ophthalmic Solution (Neomycin Sulfate, Dexamethasone Sodium Phosphate) Merck & Co., Inc. 1713
Ophthocort (Chloramphenicol, Polymyxin B Sulfate, Hydrocortisone Acetate) Parke-Davis ⊙ 311
Poly-Pred Liquifilm (Neomycin Sulfate, Polymyxin B Sulfate, Prednisolone Acetate) Allergan ⊙ 248
Pred-G Liquifilm Sterile Ophthalmic Suspension (Gentamicin Sulfate, Prednisolone Acetate) Allergan ⊙ 251
Pred-G S.O.P. Sterile Ophthalmic Ointment (Gentamicin Sulfate, Prednisolone Acetate) Allergan ⊙ 252
Terra-Cortril Ophthalmic Suspension (Oxytetracycline Hydrochloride, Hydrocortisone Acetate) Roerig 2210
TobraDex Ophthalmic Suspension and Ointment (Dexamethasone, Tobramycin) Alcon Laboratories 473
Vasocidin Ointment (Prednisolone Acetate, Sulfacetamide Sodium) CIBA Vision Ophthalmics ⊙ 268
Vasocidin Ophthalmic Solution (Prednisolone Sodium Phosphate, Sulfacetamide Sodium) CIBA Vision Ophthalmics ⊙ 270

Conjunctivitis, neonatal
E-Mycin Tablets (Erythromycin) Knoll Laboratories 1341
Ery-Tab Tablets (Erythromycin) Abbott 422
Erythrocin Stearate Filmtab (Erythromycin Stearate) Abbott 425
Erythromycin Base Filmtab (Erythromycin) Abbott 426
Erythromycin Delayed-Release Capsules, USP (Erythromycin) Abbott 427
PCE Dispertab Tablets (Erythromycin) Abbott 444

Conjunctivitis, unspecified
Bleph-10 (Sulfacetamide Sodium) Allergan 475
Genoptic Sterile Ophthalmic Solution (Gentamicin Sulfate) Allergan ⊙ 243
Genoptic Sterile Ophthalmic Ointment (Gentamicin Sulfate) Allergan ⊙ 243
Gentacidin Ointment (Gentamicin Sulfate) CIBA Vision Ophthalmics ⊙ 264
Gentacidin Solution (Gentamicin Sulfate) CIBA Vision Ophthalmics ⊙ 264
Gentak (Gentamicin Sulfate) Akorn ⊙ 208
Pred Mild (Prednisolone Acetate) Allergan ⊙ 253
Sodium Sulamyd (Sulfacetamide Sodium) Schering 2387
Vasosulf (Phenylephrine Hydrochloride, Sulfacetamide Sodium) CIBA Vision Ophthalmics ⊙ 271

Conjunctivitis, vernal
Alomide (Lodoxamide Tromethamine) Alcon Laboratories 469
Crolom (Cromolyn Sodium) Bausch & Lomb Pharmaceuticals ⊙ 257
HMS Liquifilm (Medrysone) Allergan ⊙ 244

Constipation, chronic
CITRUCEL Sugar Free Orange Flavor (Methylcellulose) SmithKline Beecham Consumer ▣ 811
Fiberall Chewable Tablets, Lemon Creme Flavor (Calcium Polycarbophil) CIBA Consumer ▣ 636
Fiberall Fiber Wafers (Psyllium Preparations) CIBA Consumer ▣ 636
Fiberall Powder (Psyllium Preparations) CIBA Consumer ▣ 637
Konsyl Fiber Tablets (Calcium Polycarbophil) Konsyl ▣ 663
Konsyl Powder Sugar Free Unflavored (Psyllium Preparations) Konsyl ▣ 664
Konsyl-D Powder Unflavored (Psyllium Preparations) Konsyl ▣ 664
Konsyl-Orange Ultra Fine Powder (Psyllium Preparations) Konsyl ▣ 664
Maalox Daily Fiber Therapy (Psyllium Preparations) CIBA Consumer ▣ 641
Metamucil (Psyllium Preparations) Procter & Gamble 1975

(▣ Described in PDR For Nonprescription Drugs) (⊙ Described in PDR For Ophthalmology)

1471 Indications Index Corneal injury

Mylanta Natural Fiber Supplement (Psyllium Preparations) J&J•Merck Consumer ▣ 662
Perdiem Fiber Bulk-Forming Laxative (Psyllium Preparations) Ciba Self-Medication 869
Peri-Colace (Casanthranol, Docusate Sodium) Roberts 2052
Senokot (Senna Concentrates) Purdue Frederick 1999
Senokot-S Tablets (Senna Concentrates, Docusate Sodium) Purdue Frederick 1999

Constipation, temporary

Ceo-Two Rectal Suppositories (Sodium Bicarbonate, Potassium Bitartrate) Beutlich 666
CITRUCEL Orange Flavor (Methylcellulose) SmithKline Beecham Consumer ▣ 811
Colace (Docusate Sodium) Roberts 2044
Correctol Extra Gentle Stool Softener (Docusate Sodium) Schering-Plough HealthCare ▣ 801
Correctol Laxative Tablets & Caplets (Docusate Sodium, Phenolphthalein) Schering-Plough HealthCare ▣ 801
Dialose Tablets (Docusate Sodium) J&J•Merck Consumer 1317
Dialose Plus Tablets (Docusate Sodium, Phenolphthalein) J&J•Merck Consumer 1317
Doxidan Liqui-Gels (Docusate Calcium, Phenolphthalein) Upjohn ▣ 836
Dulcolax (Bisacodyl) Ciba Self-Medication 864
Ex-Lax Chocolated Laxative Tablets (Phenolphthalein) Sandoz Consumer ▣ 786
Extra Gentle Ex-Lax Laxative Pills (Docusate Sodium, Phenolphthalein) Sandoz Consumer ▣ 786
Maximum Relief Formula Ex-Lax Laxative Pills (Phenolphthalein) Sandoz Consumer ▣ 786
Regular Strength Ex-Lax Laxative Pills (Phenolphthalein) Sandoz Consumer ▣ 786
Ex-Lax Gentle Nature Laxative Pills (Senna Concentrates) Sandoz Consumer ▣ 786
Feen-A-Mint (Phenolphthalein) Schering-Plough HealthCare ▣ 805
Fiberall Chewable Tablets, Lemon Creme Flavor (Calcium Polycarbophil) CIBA Consumer ▣ 636
Fiberall Fiber Wafers (Psyllium Preparations) CIBA Consumer ▣ 636
Fiberall Powder (Psyllium Preparations) CIBA Consumer ▣ 637
FiberCon Caplets (Calcium Polycarbophil) Lederle Consumer ▣ 670
Fleet Babylax (Glycerin) Fleet 1001
Fleet Bisacodyl Enema (Bisacodyl) Fleet 1002
Fleet Enema (Sodium Phosphate, Dibasic, Sodium Phosphate, Monobasic) Fleet 1002
Fleet Glycerin-Laxative Rectal Applicators (Glycerin) Fleet 1001
Fleet Mineral Oil Enema (Mineral Oil) Fleet 1002
Fleet Phospho-Soda (Sodium Phosphate, Dibasic, Sodium Phosphate, Monobasic) Fleet 1003
Fleet Sof-Lax (Docusate Sodium) Fleet 1004
Fleet Sof-Lax Overnight (Docusate Sodium, Casanthranol) Fleet 1004
Kondremul (Mineral Oil) CIBA Consumer ▣ 637
Maltsupex Liquid, Powder & Tablets (Malt Soup Extract) Wallace ▣ 840
Perdiem Fiber (Psyllium Preparations) CIBA Consumer ▣ 646
Perdiem Bulk-Forming Laxative (Psyllium Preparations, Senna Concentrates) Ciba Self-Medication 869
Peri-Colace (Casanthranol, Docusate Sodium) Roberts 2052
Phillips' Gelcaps (Docusate Sodium, Phenolphthalein) Miles Consumer ▣ 729
Phillips' Milk of Magnesia Liquid (Magnesium Hydroxide) Miles Consumer ▣ 729
Purge Concentrate (Castor Oil) Fleming ▣ 655
Senokot Children's Syrup (Senna) Purdue Frederick 1999
Senokot (Senna Concentrates) Purdue Frederick 1999
Senokot-S Tablets (Senna Concentrates, Docusate Sodium) Purdue Frederick 1999
Surfak Liqui-Gels (Docusate Calcium) Upjohn ▣ 839

Contact lenses, fitting of, adjunct in

Fluor-I-Strip (Fluorescein Sodium) Wyeth-Ayerst ⊙ 326
Fluor-I-Strip A.T. (Fluorescein Sodium) Wyeth-Ayerst ⊙ 326

Contraception (see under Pregnancy, prevention of)

Contraception, intrauterine

Lippes Loop Intrauterine Double-S (Intrauterine device) Ortho Pharmaceutical 1848

Convulsions, reduction of the intensity of muscle contractions in

Metubine Iodide Vials (Metocurine Iodide) Dista 916

Convulsive disorders, adjunctive therapy in

Valium Tablets (Diazepam) Roche Products 2183

Convulsive episodes, control of

Nembutal Sodium Solution (Pentobarbital Sodium) Abbott 438

Corneal edema (see under Edema, corneal, temporary relief of)

Corneal erosions, recurrent

Lacrisert Sterile Ophthalmic Insert (Hydroxypropyl Cellulose) Merck & Co., Inc. 1686

Corneal inflammation, steroid-responsive

AK-Pred (Prednisolone Sodium Phosphate) Akorn ⊙ 204
AK-Trol Ointment & Suspension (Dexamethasone, Neomycin Sulfate, Polymyxin B Sulfate) Akorn ⊙ 205
Blephamide Liquifilm Sterile Ophthalmic Suspension (Prednisolone Acetate, Sulfacetamide Sodium) Allergan 476
Blephamide Ointment (Sulfacetamide Sodium, Prednisolone Acetate) Allergan ⊙ 237
Cortisporin Ophthalmic Ointment Sterile (Polymyxin B Sulfate, Bacitracin Zinc, Neomycin Sulfate, Hydrocortisone) Glaxo Wellcome 1085
Cortisporin Ophthalmic Suspension Sterile (Hydrocortisone, Polymyxin B Sulfate, Neomycin Sulfate) Glaxo Wellcome 1086
Decadron Phosphate Sterile Ophthalmic Ointment (Dexamethasone Sodium Phosphate) Merck & Co., Inc. 1641
Decadron Phosphate Sterile Ophthalmic Solution (Dexamethasone Sodium Phosphate) Merck & Co., Inc. 1642
Dexacidin Ointment (Dexamethasone, Neomycin Sulfate, Polymyxin B Sulfate) CIBA Vision Ophthalmics ⊙ 263
Econopred & Econopred Plus Ophthalmic Suspensions (Prednisolone Acetate) Alcon Laboratories ⊙ 217
FML Forte Liquifilm (Fluorometholone) Allergan ⊙ 240
FML Liquifilm (Fluorometholone) Allergan ⊙ 241
FML S.O.P. (Fluorometholone) Allergan ⊙ 241
FML-S Liquifilm (Sulfacetamide Sodium, Fluorometholone) Allergan ⊙ 242
Fluor-Op Ophthalmic Suspension (Fluorometholone) CIBA Vision Ophthalmics ⊙ 264
Maxitrol Ophthalmic Ointment and Suspension (Dexamethasone, Neomycin Sulfate, Polymyxin B Sulfate) Alcon Laboratories ⊙ 224
NeoDecadron Sterile Ophthalmic Ointment (Neomycin Sulfate, Dexamethasone Sodium Phosphate) Merck & Co., Inc. 1712
NeoDecadron Sterile Ophthalmic Solution (Neomycin Sulfate, Dexamethasone Sodium Phosphate) Merck & Co., Inc. 1713
Poly-Pred Liquifilm (Neomycin Sulfate, Polymyxin B Sulfate, Prednisolone Acetate) Allergan ⊙ 248
Pred Forte (Prednisolone Acetate) Allergan ⊙ 250
Pred-G Liquifilm Sterile Ophthalmic Suspension (Gentamicin Sulfate, Prednisolone Acetate) Allergan ⊙ 251
Pred-G S.O.P. Sterile Ophthalmic Ointment (Gentamicin Sulfate, Prednisolone Acetate) Allergan ⊙ 252
Terra-Cortril Ophthalmic Suspension (Oxytetracycline Hydrochloride, Hydrocortisone Acetate) Roerig 2210
TobraDex Ophthalmic Suspension and Ointment (Dexamethasone, Tobramycin) Alcon Laboratories 473
Vasocidin Ointment (Prednisolone Acetate, Sulfacetamide Sodium) CIBA Vision Ophthalmics ⊙ 268
Vasocidin Ophthalmic Solution (Prednisolone Sodium Phosphate, Sulfacetamide Sodium) CIBA Vision Ophthalmics ⊙ 270

Corneal injury, chemical

AK-CIDE (Prednisolone Acetate, Sulfacetamide Sodium) Akorn ⊙ 202
AK-CIDE Ointment (Prednisolone Acetate, Sulfacetamide Sodium) Akorn ⊙ 202
AK-Pred (Prednisolone Sodium Phosphate) Akorn ⊙ 204
AK-Trol Ointment & Suspension (Dexamethasone, Neomycin Sulfate, Polymyxin B Sulfate) Akorn ⊙ 205
Blephamide Liquifilm Sterile Ophthalmic Suspension (Prednisolone Acetate, Sulfacetamide Sodium) Allergan 476
Blephamide Ointment (Sulfacetamide Sodium, Prednisolone Acetate) Allergan ⊙ 237
Cortisporin Ophthalmic Ointment Sterile (Polymyxin B Sulfate, Bacitracin Zinc, Neomycin Sulfate, Hydrocortisone) Glaxo Wellcome 1085
Cortisporin Ophthalmic Suspension Sterile (Hydrocortisone, Polymyxin B Sulfate, Neomycin Sulfate) Glaxo Wellcome 1086
Decadron Phosphate Sterile Ophthalmic Ointment (Dexamethasone Sodium Phosphate) Merck & Co., Inc. 1641
Decadron Phosphate Sterile Ophthalmic Solution (Dexamethasone Sodium Phosphate) Merck & Co., Inc. 1642
Dexacidin Ointment (Dexamethasone, Neomycin Sulfate, Polymyxin B Sulfate) CIBA Vision Ophthalmics ⊙ 263
Econopred & Econopred Plus Ophthalmic Suspensions (Prednisolone Acetate) Alcon Laboratories ⊙ 217
FML-S Liquifilm (Sulfacetamide Sodium, Fluorometholone) Allergan ⊙ 242
Inflamase (Prednisolone Sodium Phosphate) CIBA Vision Ophthalmics ⊙ 265
Maxitrol Ophthalmic Ointment and Suspension (Dexamethasone, Neomycin Sulfate, Polymyxin B Sulfate) Alcon Laboratories ⊙ 224
NeoDecadron Sterile Ophthalmic Ointment (Neomycin Sulfate, Dexamethasone Sodium Phosphate) Merck & Co., Inc. 1712
NeoDecadron Sterile Ophthalmic Solution (Neomycin Sulfate, Dexamethasone Sodium Phosphate) Merck & Co., Inc. 1713
Ophthocort (Chloramphenicol, Polymyxin B Sulfate, Hydrocortisone Acetate) Parke-Davis ⊙ 311
Poly-Pred Liquifilm (Neomycin Sulfate, Polymyxin B Sulfate, Prednisolone Acetate) Allergan ⊙ 248
Pred Mild (Prednisolone Acetate) Allergan ⊙ 253
Pred-G Liquifilm Sterile Ophthalmic Suspension (Gentamicin Sulfate, Prednisolone Acetate) Allergan ⊙ 251
Pred-G S.O.P. Sterile Ophthalmic Ointment (Gentamicin Sulfate, Prednisolone Acetate) Allergan ⊙ 252
Terra-Cortril Ophthalmic Suspension (Oxytetracycline Hydrochloride, Hydrocortisone Acetate) Roerig 2210
TobraDex Ophthalmic Suspension and Ointment (Dexamethasone, Tobramycin) Alcon Laboratories 473
Vasocidin Ointment (Prednisolone Acetate, Sulfacetamide Sodium) CIBA Vision Ophthalmics ⊙ 268
Vasocidin Ophthalmic Solution (Prednisolone Sodium Phosphate, Sulfacetamide Sodium) CIBA Vision Ophthalmics ⊙ 270

Corneal injury, foreign bodies

AK-CIDE (Prednisolone Acetate, Sulfacetamide Sodium) Akorn ⊙ 202
AK-CIDE Ointment (Prednisolone Acetate, Sulfacetamide Sodium) Akorn ⊙ 202
AK-Pred (Prednisolone Sodium Phosphate) Akorn ⊙ 204
AK-Trol Ointment & Suspension (Dexamethasone, Neomycin Sulfate, Polymyxin B Sulfate) Akorn ⊙ 205
Blephamide Liquifilm Sterile Ophthalmic Suspension (Prednisolone Acetate, Sulfacetamide Sodium) Allergan 476
Blephamide Ointment (Sulfacetamide Sodium, Prednisolone Acetate) Allergan ⊙ 237
Cortisporin Ophthalmic Ointment Sterile (Polymyxin B Sulfate, Bacitracin Zinc, Neomycin Sulfate, Hydrocortisone) Glaxo Wellcome 1085
Cortisporin Ophthalmic Suspension Sterile (Hydrocortisone, Polymyxin B Sulfate, Neomycin Sulfate) Glaxo Wellcome 1086
Decadron Phosphate Sterile Ophthalmic Ointment (Dexamethasone Sodium Phosphate) Merck & Co., Inc. 1641
Decadron Phosphate Sterile Ophthalmic Solution (Dexamethasone Sodium Phosphate) Merck & Co., Inc. 1642
Dexacidin Ointment (Dexamethasone, Neomycin Sulfate, Polymyxin B Sulfate) CIBA Vision Ophthalmics ⊙ 263
Econopred & Econopred Plus Ophthalmic Suspensions (Prednisolone Acetate) Alcon Laboratories ⊙ 217
FML-S Liquifilm (Sulfacetamide Sodium, Fluorometholone) Allergan ⊙ 242
FLURESS (Fluorescein Sodium, Benoxinate Hydrochloride) Akorn ⊙ 207
Inflamase (Prednisolone Sodium Phosphate) CIBA Vision Ophthalmics ⊙ 265
Maxitrol Ophthalmic Ointment and Suspension (Dexamethasone, Neomycin Sulfate, Polymyxin B Sulfate) Alcon Laboratories ⊙ 224
NeoDecadron Sterile Ophthalmic Ointment (Neomycin Sulfate, Dexamethasone Sodium Phosphate) Merck & Co., Inc. 1712

(▣ Described in PDR For Nonprescription Drugs) (⊙ Described in PDR For Ophthalmology)

Corneal injury **Indications Index** **1472**

NeoDecadron Sterile Ophthalmic Solution (Neomycin Sulfate, Dexamethasone Sodium Phosphate) Merck & Co., Inc. ... 1713
Ophthocort (Chloramphenicol, Polymyxin B Sulfate, Hydrocortisone Acetate) Parke-Davis ... ⊙ 311
Poly-Pred Liquifilm (Neomycin Sulfate, Polymyxin B Sulfate, Prednisolone Acetate) Allergan.. ⊙ 248
Pred-G Liquifilm Sterile Ophthalmic Suspension (Gentamicin Sulfate, Prednisolone Acetate) Allergan ... ⊙ 251
Pred-G S.O.P. Sterile Ophthalmic Ointment (Gentamicin Sulfate, Prednisolone Acetate) Allergan.. ⊙ 252
Terra-Cortril Ophthalmic Suspension (Oxytetracycline Hydrochloride, Hydrocortisone Acetate) Roerig ... 2210
TobraDex Ophthalmic Suspension and Ointment (Dexamethasone, Tobramycin) Alcon Laboratories .. 473
Vasocidin Ointment (Prednisolone Acetate, Sulfacetamide Sodium) CIBA Vision Ophthalmics ... ⊙ 268
Vasocidin Ophthalmic Solution (Prednisolone Sodium Phosphate, Sulfacetamide Sodium) CIBA Vision Ophthalmics ... ⊙ 270

Corneal injury, radiation
AK-CIDE (Prednisolone Acetate, Sulfacetamide Sodium) Akorn ... ⊙ 202
AK-CIDE Ointment (Prednisolone Acetate, Sulfacetamide Sodium) Akorn ... ⊙ 202
AK-Pred (Prednisolone Sodium Phosphate) Akorn ... ⊙ 204
AK-Trol Ointment & Suspension (Dexamethasone, Neomycin Sulfate, Polymyxin B Sulfate) Akorn ... ⊙ 205
Blephamide Liquifilm Sterile Ophthalmic Suspension (Prednisolone Acetate, Sulfacetamide Sodium) Allergan ... 476
Blephamide Ointment (Sulfacetamide Sodium, Prednisolone Acetate) Allergan ... ⊙ 237
Cortisporin Ophthalmic Ointment Sterile (Polymyxin B Sulfate, Bacitracin Zinc, Neomycin Sulfate, Hydrocortisone) Glaxo Wellcome ... 1085
Cortisporin Ophthalmic Suspension Sterile (Hydrocortisone, Polymyxin B Sulfate, Neomycin Sulfate) Glaxo Wellcome ... 1086
Dexacidin Ointment (Dexamethasone, Neomycin Sulfate, Polymyxin B Sulfate) CIBA Vision Ophthalmics ... ⊙ 263
Econopred & Econopred Plus Ophthalmic Suspensions (Prednisolone Acetate) Alcon Laboratories ... ⊙ 217
FML-S Liquifilm (Sulfacetamide Sodium, Fluorometholone) Allergan ... ⊙ 242
Inflamase (Prednisolone Sodium Phosphate) CIBA Vision Ophthalmics ... ⊙ 265
Maxitrol Ophthalmic Ointment and Suspension (Dexamethasone, Neomycin Sulfate, Polymyxin B Sulfate) Alcon Laboratories ... ⊙ 224
NeoDecadron Sterile Ophthalmic Ointment (Neomycin Sulfate, Dexamethasone Sodium Phosphate) Merck & Co., Inc. ... 1712
NeoDecadron Sterile Ophthalmic Solution (Neomycin Sulfate, Dexamethasone Sodium Phosphate) Merck & Co., Inc. ... 1713
Ophthocort (Chloramphenicol, Polymyxin B Sulfate, Hydrocortisone Acetate) Parke-Davis ... ⊙ 311
Poly-Pred Liquifilm (Neomycin Sulfate, Polymyxin B Sulfate, Prednisolone Acetate) Allergan.. ⊙ 248
Pred-G Liquifilm Sterile Ophthalmic Suspension (Gentamicin Sulfate, Prednisolone Acetate) Allergan ... ⊙ 251
Pred-G S.O.P. Sterile Ophthalmic Ointment (Gentamicin Sulfate, Prednisolone Acetate) Allergan.. ⊙ 252
Terra-Cortril Ophthalmic Suspension (Oxytetracycline Hydrochloride, Hydrocortisone Acetate) Roerig ... 2210
TobraDex Ophthalmic Suspension and Ointment (Dexamethasone, Tobramycin) Alcon Laboratories .. 473
Vasocidin Ointment (Prednisolone Acetate, Sulfacetamide Sodium) CIBA Vision Ophthalmics ... ⊙ 268
Vasocidin Ophthalmic Solution (Prednisolone Sodium Phosphate, Sulfacetamide Sodium) CIBA Vision Ophthalmics ... ⊙ 270

Corneal injury, thermal burns
AK-CIDE (Prednisolone Acetate, Sulfacetamide Sodium) Akorn ... ⊙ 202
AK-CIDE Ointment (Prednisolone Acetate, Sulfacetamide Sodium) Akorn ... ⊙ 202
AK-Pred (Prednisolone Sodium Phosphate) Akorn ... ⊙ 204
AK-Trol Ointment & Suspension (Dexamethasone, Neomycin Sulfate, Polymyxin B Sulfate) Akorn ... ⊙ 205
Blephamide Liquifilm Sterile Ophthalmic Suspension (Prednisolone Acetate, Sulfacetamide Sodium) Allergan ... 476
Blephamide Ointment (Sulfacetamide Sodium, Prednisolone Acetate) Allergan ... ⊙ 237
Cortisporin Ophthalmic Ointment Sterile (Polymyxin B Sulfate, Bacitracin Zinc, Neomycin Sulfate, Hydrocortisone) Glaxo Wellcome ... 1085
Cortisporin Ophthalmic Suspension Sterile (Hydrocortisone, Polymyxin B Sulfate, Neomycin Sulfate) Glaxo Wellcome ... 1086
Decadron Phosphate Sterile Ophthalmic Ointment (Dexamethasone Sodium Phosphate) Merck & Co., Inc. ... 1641
Decadron Phosphate Sterile Ophthalmic Solution (Dexamethasone Sodium Phosphate) Merck & Co., Inc. ... 1642
Dexacidin Ointment (Dexamethasone, Neomycin Sulfate, Polymyxin B Sulfate) CIBA Vision Ophthalmics ... ⊙ 263
Econopred & Econopred Plus Ophthalmic Suspensions (Prednisolone Acetate) Alcon Laboratories ... ⊙ 217
FML-S Liquifilm (Sulfacetamide Sodium, Fluorometholone) Allergan ... ⊙ 242
Inflamase (Prednisolone Sodium Phosphate) CIBA Vision Ophthalmics ... ⊙ 265
Maxitrol Ophthalmic Ointment and Suspension (Dexamethasone, Neomycin Sulfate, Polymyxin B Sulfate) Alcon Laboratories ... ⊙ 224
NeoDecadron Sterile Ophthalmic Ointment (Neomycin Sulfate, Dexamethasone Sodium Phosphate) Merck & Co., Inc. ... 1712
NeoDecadron Sterile Ophthalmic Solution (Neomycin Sulfate, Dexamethasone Sodium Phosphate) Merck & Co., Inc. ... 1713
Ophthocort (Chloramphenicol, Polymyxin B Sulfate, Hydrocortisone Acetate) Parke-Davis ... ⊙ 311
Poly-Pred Liquifilm (Neomycin Sulfate, Polymyxin B Sulfate, Prednisolone Acetate) Allergan.. ⊙ 248
Pred Mild (Prednisolone Acetate) Allergan ... ⊙ 253
Pred-G Liquifilm Sterile Ophthalmic Suspension (Gentamicin Sulfate, Prednisolone Acetate) Allergan ... ⊙ 251
Pred-G S.O.P. Sterile Ophthalmic Ointment (Gentamicin Sulfate, Prednisolone Acetate) Allergan.. ⊙ 252
Terra-Cortril Ophthalmic Suspension (Oxytetracycline Hydrochloride, Hydrocortisone Acetate) Roerig ... 2210
TobraDex Ophthalmic Suspension and Ointment (Dexamethasone, Tobramycin) Alcon Laboratories .. 473
Vasocidin Ointment (Prednisolone Acetate, Sulfacetamide Sodium) CIBA Vision Ophthalmics ... ⊙ 268
Vasocidin Ophthalmic Solution (Prednisolone Sodium Phosphate, Sulfacetamide Sodium) CIBA Vision Ophthalmics ... ⊙ 270

Corneal marginal ulcers, allergic
Aristocort Suspension (Forte Parenteral) (Triamcinolone Diacetate) Fujisawa ... 1027
Aristocort Tablets (Triamcinolone) Fujisawa ... 1022
Cortone Acetate Sterile Suspension (Cortisone Acetate) Merck & Co., Inc. ... 1623
Cortone Acetate Tablets (Cortisone Acetate) Merck & Co., Inc. ... 1624
Dalalone D.P. Injectable (Dexamethasone Acetate) Forest ... 1011
Decadron Elixir (Dexamethasone) Merck & Co., Inc. ... 1633
Decadron Phosphate Injection (Dexamethasone Sodium Phosphate) Merck & Co., Inc. ... 1637
Decadron Tablets (Dexamethasone) Merck & Co., Inc. ... 1635
Decadron-LA Sterile Suspension (Dexamethasone Acetate) Merck & Co., Inc. ... 1646
Deltasone Tablets (Prednisone) Upjohn ... 2595
Depo-Medrol Single-Dose Vial (Methylprednisolone Acetate) Upjohn ... 2600
Depo-Medrol Sterile Aqueous Suspension (Methylprednisolone Acetate) Upjohn ... 2597
Hydeltrasol Injection, Sterile (Prednisolone Sodium Phosphate) Merck & Co., Inc. ... 1665
Hydrocortone Phosphate Injection, Sterile (Hydrocortisone Sodium Phosphate) Merck & Co., Inc. ... 1670
Hydrocortone Tablets (Hydrocortisone) Merck & Co., Inc. ... 1672
Medrol (Methylprednisolone) Upjohn ... 2621
Pediapred Oral Liquid (Prednisolone Sodium Phosphate) Fisons ... 995
Prelone Syrup (Prednisolone) Muro 1787
Solu-Cortef Sterile Powder (Hydrocortisone Sodium Succinate) Upjohn ... 2641
Solu-Medrol Sterile Powder (Methylprednisolone Sodium Succinate) Upjohn ... 2643

Corneal sensitivity, decreased
Lacrisert Sterile Ophthalmic Insert (Hydroxypropyl Cellulose) Merck & Co., Inc. ... 1686

Corneal staining, reduction of signs and symptoms
Lacrisert Sterile Ophthalmic Insert (Hydroxypropyl Cellulose) Merck & Co., Inc. ... 1686

Corneal transplant, surgical aid in
AMO Vitrax Viscoelastic Solution (Sodium Hyaluronate) Allergan.. ⊙ 232
Healon (Sodium Hyaluronate) Pharmacia Inc. Ophthalmics ... ⊙ 314
Healon GV (Sodium Hyaluronate) Pharmacia Inc. Ophthalmics ... ⊙ 315

Corneal ulcers
Bleph-10 (Sulfacetamide Sodium) Allergan ... 475
Celestone Soluspan Suspension (Betamethasone Sodium Phosphate, Betamethasone Acetate) Schering ... 2347
Ciloxan Ophthalmic Solution (Ciprofloxacin Hydrochloride) Alcon Laboratories ... 472
Genoptic Sterile Ophthalmic Solution (Gentamicin Sulfate) Allergan ... ⊙ 243
Genoptic Sterile Ophthalmic Ointment (Gentamicin Sulfate) Allergan ... ⊙ 243
Gentacidin Ointment (Gentamicin Sulfate) CIBA Vision Ophthalmics ... ⊙ 264
Gentacidin Solution (Gentamicin Sulfate) CIBA Vision Ophthalmics ... ⊙ 264
Gentak (Gentamicin Sulfate) Akorn ... ⊙ 208
Sodium Sulamyd (Sulfacetamide Sodium) Schering ... 2387
Vasosulf (Phenylephrine Hydrochloride, Sulfacetamide Sodium) CIBA Vision Ophthalmics ... ⊙ 271

Corns (see under Hyperkeratosis skin disorders)

Coronary artery disease, reducing the risk of
Lopid Tablets (Gemfibrozil) Parke-Davis ... 1917
Questran Light (Cholestyramine) Bristol-Myers Squibb ... 769
Questran Powder (Cholestyramine) Bristol-Myers Squibb ... 770

Coronary atherosclerosis, to slow the progression of (see also under Coronary artery disease, reducing the risk of)
Mevacor Tablets (Lovastatin) Merck & Co., Inc. ... 1699

Coronary angioplasty or atherectomy, percutaneous transluminal, adjunct in
ReoPro Vials (Abciximab) Lilly ... 1471

Corynebacterium diphtheriae (see under C. diphtheriae infections)

Corynebacterium minutissimum (see under C. minutissimum infections)

Coryza, acute (see under Cold, common, symptomatic relief of)

Coughs and nasal congestion, symptomatic relief of
Actifed with Codeine Cough Syrup (Codeine Phosphate, Triprolidine Hydrochloride, Pseudoephedrine Hydrochloride) Glaxo Wellcome ... 1067
Alka-Seltzer Plus Cold & Cough Medicine (Aspirin, Chlorpheniramine Maleate, Dextromethorphan Hydrobromide, Phenylpropanolamine Bitartrate) Miles Consumer ... ▣ 708
Anatuss LA Tablets (Guaifenesin, Pseudoephedrine Hydrochloride) Mayrand ... 1542
Benylin Multisymptom (Dextromethorphan Hydrobromide, Pseudoephedrine Hydrochloride, Guaifenesin) WARNER WELLCOME ... ▣ 852
Bromfed-DM Cough Syrup (Brompheniramine Maleate, Pseudoephedrine Hydrochloride, Dextromethorphan Hydrobromide) Muro ... 1786
Brontex (Codeine Phosphate, Guaifenesin) Procter & Gamble Pharmaceuticals ... 1981
Cerose DM (Chlorpheniramine Maleate, Dextromethorphan Hydrobromide, Phenylephrine Hydrochloride) Wyeth-Ayerst ... ▣ 878
Cheracol Plus Head Cold/Cough Formula (Phenylpropanolamine Hydrochloride, Dextromethorphan Hydrobromide, Chlorpheniramine Maleate) Roberts .. ▣ 769
Children's Vicks NyQuil Cold/Cough Relief (Chlorpheniramine Maleate, Dextromethorphan Hydrobromide, Pseudoephedrine Hydrochloride) Procter & Gamble ... ▣ 758
Codiclear DH Syrup (Guaifenesin, Hydrocodone Bitartrate) Central .. 791
Comtrex Multi-Symptom Cold Reliever Tablets/Caplets/Liqui-Gels/Liquid (Acetaminophen, Chlorpheniramine Maleate, Dextromethorphan Hydrobromide, Pseudoephedrine

(▣ Described in PDR For Nonprescription Drugs) (⊙ Described in PDR For Ophthalmology)

1473 **Indications Index** **Cough**

Hydrochloride) Bristol-Myers Products ▣ 615
Contac Severe Cold and Flu Formula Caplets (Acetaminophen, Chlorpheniramine Maleate, Dextromethorphan Hydrobromide, Phenylpropanolamine Hydrochloride) SmithKline Beecham Consumer ▣ 814
Deconsal Pediatric Capsules (Guaifenesin, Phenylephrine Hydrochloride) Adams 454
Deconsal Pediatric Syrup (Codeine Phosphate, Pseudoephedrine Hydrochloride, Guaifenesin) Adams 457
Deconsal II Tablets (Pseudoephedrine Hydrochloride, Guaifenesin) Adams 454
Dimetane-DC Cough Syrup (Brompheniramine Maleate, Phenylpropanolamine Hydrochloride, Codeine Phosphate) Robins 2059
Dimetane-DX Cough Syrup (Brompheniramine Maleate, Pseudoephedrine Hydrochloride, Dextromethorphan Hydrobromide) Robins 2059
Dimetapp DM Elixir (Brompheniramine Maleate, Dextromethorphan Hydrobromide) A. H. Robins Consumer ▣ 774
Dorcol Children's Cough Syrup (Pseudoephedrine Hydrochloride, Guaifenesin, Dextromethorphan Hydrobromide) Sandoz Consumer ▣ 785
Drixoral Cough + Congestion Liquid Caps (Dextromethorphan Hydrobromide, Pseudoephedrine Hydrochloride) Schering-Plough HealthCare ▣ 802
Duratuss HD Elixir (Hydrocodone Bitartrate, Pseudoephedrine Hydrochloride, Guaifenesin) UCB 2565
Guaifed (Guaifenesin, Pseudoephedrine Hydrochloride) Muro 1787
Hycomine Compound Tablets (Hydrocodone Bitartrate, Chlorpheniramine Maleate, Acetaminophen, Phenylephrine Hydrochloride) DuPont 932
Hycomine (Hydrocodone Bitartrate, Phenylpropanolamine Hydrochloride) DuPont 931
Isoclor Expectorant (Codeine Phosphate, Guaifenesin, Pseudoephedrine Hydrochloride) Fisons 990
Novahistine DH (Codeine Phosphate, Pseudoephedrine Hydrochloride, Chlorpheniramine Maleate) SmithKline Beecham 2462
Novahistine DMX (Dextromethorphan Hydrobromide, Guaifenesin, Pseudoephedrine Hydrochloride) SmithKline Beecham Consumer ▣ 822
Novahistine Expectorant (Codeine Phosphate, Pseudoephedrine Hydrochloride, Guaifenesin) SmithKline Beecham 2463
Nucofed (Codeine Phosphate, Pseudoephedrine Hydrochloride, Guaifenesin) Roberts 2051
PediaCare (Chlorpheniramine Maleate, Pseudoephedrine Hydrochloride, Dextromethorphan Hydrobromide) McNeil Consumer 1553
PediCare Infant's Drops Decongestant Plus Cough (Dextromethorphan Hydrobromide, Pseudoephedrine Hydrochloride) McNeil Consumer 1553
PediaCare NightRest Cough-Cold Liquid (Chlorpheniramine Maleate, Dextromethorphan Hydrobromide, Pseudoephedrine Hydrochloride) McNeil Consumer 1553
Pediatric Vicks 44d Dry Hacking Cough & Head Congestion (Dextromethorphan Hydrobromide, Pseudoephedrine Hydrochloride) Procter & Gamble ▣ 763
Phenergan with Codeine (Codeine Phosphate, Promethazine Hydrochloride) Wyeth-Ayerst 2777
Phenergan with Dextromethorphan (Promethazine Hydrochloride, Dextromethorphan Hydrobromide) Wyeth-Ayerst 2778
Phenergan VC (Promethazine Hydrochloride, Phenylephrine Hydrochloride) Wyeth-Ayerst 2779
Phenergan VC with Codeine (Codeine Phosphate, Promethazine Hydrochloride, Phenylephrine Hydrochloride) Wyeth-Ayerst 2781
Robitussin Cold & Cough Liqui-Gels (Guaifenesin, Dextromethorphan Hydrobromide, Pseudoephedrine Hydrochloride) A. H. Robins Consumer ▣ 776
Robitussin Maximum Strength Cough & Cold (Dextromethorphan Hydrobromide, Pseudoephedrine Hydrochloride) A. H. Robins Consumer ▣ 778
Robitussin-CF (Dextromethorphan Hydrobromide, Guaifenesin, Phenylpropanolamine Hydrochloride) A. H. Robins Consumer ▣ 777
Robitussin-DAC Syrup (Codeine Phosphate, Guaifenesin, Pseudoephedrine Hydrochloride) Robins 2074
Rondec-DM Oral Drops (Carbinoxamine Maleate, Pseudoephedrine Hydrochloride, Dextromethorphan Hydrobromide) Dura 954
Rondec-DM Syrup (Carbinoxamine Maleate, Pseudoephedrine Hydrochloride, Dextromethorphan Hydrobromide) Dura 954
Ryna (Chlorpheniramine Maleate, Codeine Phosphate, Pseudoephedrine Hydrochloride) Wallace ▣ 841
Rynatuss (Carbetapentane Tannate, Chlorpheniramine Tannate, Ephedrine Tannate, Phenylephrine Tannate) Wallace 2673
Sudafed Cold and Cough Liquidcaps (Acetaminophen, Dextromethorphan Hydrobromide, Guaifenesin, Pseudoephedrine Hydrochloride) WARNER WELLCOME ▣ 862
Sudafed Cough Syrup (Dextromethorphan Hydrobromide, Guaifenesin, Pseudoephedrine Hydrochloride) WARNER WELLCOME ▣ 862
Syn-Rx DM Tablets (Guaifenesin, Pseudoephedrine Hydrochloride, Dextromethorphan Hydrobromide) Adams 466
TheraFlu (Acetaminophen, Chlorpheniramine Maleate, Pseudoephedrine Hydrochloride) Sandoz Consumer ▣ 787
Thera Flu Maximum Strength, Non-Drowsy Formula Flu, Cold and Cough Caplets (Acetaminophen, Dextromethorphan Hydrobromide, Pseudoephedrine Hydrochloride) Sandoz Consumer ▣ 789
Triaminic AM Cough and Decongestant Formula (Dextromethorphan Hydrobromide, Pseudoephedrine Hydrochloride) Sandoz Consumer ▣ 789
Triaminic Expectorant (Phenylpropanolamine Hydrochloride, Guaifenesin) Sandoz Consumer ▣ 790
Triaminic Nite Light (Chlorpheniramine Maleate, Dextromethorphan Hydrobromide, Pseudoephedrine Hydrochloride) Sandoz Consumer ▣ 791
Triaminic-DM Syrup (Phenylpropanolamine Hydrochloride, Dextromethorphan Hydrobromide) Sandoz Consumer ▣ 792
Triaminicol Multi-Symptom Cold Tablets (Phenylpropanolamine Hydrochloride, Chlorpheniramine Maleate, Dextromethorphan Hydrobromide) Sandoz Consumer ▣ 793
Tussend (Hydrocodone Bitartrate, Pseudoephedrine Hydrochloride, Chlorpheniramine Maleate) Monarch 1783
Tussend Expectorant (Hydrocodone Bitartrate, Pseudoephedrine Hydrochloride, Guaifenesin) Monarch 1785
TYLENOL Flu Maximum Strength Gelcaps (Acetaminophen, Dextromethorphan Hydrobromide, Pseudoephedrine Hydrochloride) McNeil Consumer 1565
TYLENOL Maximum Strength Flu NightTime Hot Medication Packets (Acetaminophen, Dextromethorphan Hydrobromide, Pseudoephedrine Hydrochloride) McNeil Consumer 1562
TYLENOL Cold Multi-Symptom Formula Medication Tablets and Caplets (Acetaminophen, Chlorpheniramine Maleate, Pseudoephedrine Hydrochloride, Dextromethorphan Hydrobromide) McNeil Consumer 1561
TYLENOL Cold Medication No Drowsiness Formula Gelcaps and Caplets (Acetaminophen, Pseudoephedrine Hydrochloride, Dextromethorphan Hydrobromide) McNeil Consumer 1562
TYLENOL Cold Multi-Symptom Hot Medication Liquid Packets (Acetaminophen, Chlorpheniramine Maleate, Pseudoephedrine Hydrochloride, Dextromethorphan Hydrobromide) McNeil Consumer 1557
TYLENOL Cough Multi-Symptom Medication with Decongestant (Dextromethorphan Hydrobromide, Acetaminophen, Pseudoephedrine Hydrochloride) McNeil Consumer 1565
Vicks 44 LiquiCaps Non-Drowsy Cough & Cold Relief (Dextromethorphan Hydrobromide, Pseudoephedrine Hydrochloride) Procter & Gamble ▣ 756
Vicks 44D Dry Hacking Cough & Head Congestion (Dextromethorphan Hydrobromide, Pseudoephedrine Hydrochloride) Procter & Gamble ▣ 755
Vicks 44M Cough, Cold & Flu Relief (Acetaminophen, Dextromethorphan Hydrobromide, Chlorpheniramine Maleate, Pseudoephedrine Hydrochloride) Procter & Gamble ▣ 756
Vicks DayQuil (Acetaminophen, Dextromethorphan Hydrobromide, Pseudoephedrine Hydrochloride, Guaifenesin) Procter & Gamble ▣ 761
Vicks NyQuil LiquiCaps Multi-Symptom Cold/Flu Relief (Acetaminophen, Pseudoephedrine Hydrochloride, Dextromethorphan Hydrobromide, Doxylamine Succinate) Procter & Gamble ▣ 763
Vicks NyQuil Multi-Symptom Cold/Flu Relief - (Original & Cherry Flavor) (Acetaminophen, Dextromethorphan Hydrobromide, Doxylamine Succinate, Pseudoephedrine Hydrochloride) Procter & Gamble ▣ 763
Vicks VapoRub (Menthol, Camphor, Eucalyptus, Oil of) Procter & Gamble ▣ 766
Vicks VapoSteam (Camphor, Eucalyptus, Oil of, Menthol) Procter & Gamble ▣ 766

Cough, symptomatic relief of

Benadryl Allergy Liquid Medication (Diphenhydramine Hydrochloride) WARNER WELLCOME ▣ 849
Benylin Adult Formula Cough Suppressant (Dextromethorphan Hydrobromide) WARNER WELLCOME ▣ 852
Benylin Expectorant (Dextromethorphan Hydrobromide, Guaifenesin) WARNER WELLCOME ▣ 852
Benylin Pediatric Cough Suppressant (Dextromethorphan Hydrobromide) WARNER WELLCOME ▣ 853
Buckley's Mixture (Dextromethorphan Hydrobromide) W.K. Buckley ▣ 624
Cheracol-D Cough Formula (Dextromethorphan Hydrobromide, Guaifenesin) Roberts ▣ 769
Codiclear DH Syrup (Guaifenesin, Hydrocodone Bitartrate) Central 791
Cough-X Lozenges (Dextromethorphan Hydrobromide, Benzocaine) Ascher ▣ 602
Deconamine CX Cough and Cold Liquid and Tablets (Hydrocodone Bitartrate, Pseudoephedrine Hydrochloride, Guaifenesin) Kenwood 1319
Delsym Extended-Release Suspension (Dextromethorphan Polistirex) Fisons ▣ 654
Diabe-Tuss DM Syrup (Dextromethorphan Hydrobromide) Paddock 1891
Dilaudid Cough Syrup (Hydromorphone Hydrochloride) Knoll Laboratories 1336
Drixoral Cough Liquid Caps (Dextromethorphan Hydrobromide) Schering-Plough HealthCare ▣ 801
Drixoral Cough + Sore Throat Liquid Caps (Dextromethorphan Hydrobromide, Acetaminophen) Schering-Plough HealthCare ▣ 802
Extra Strength Vicks Cough Drops (Menthol) Procter & Gamble ▣ 760
Halls Mentho-Lyptus Cough Suppressant Tablets (Eucalyptus, Oil of, Menthol) Warner-Lambert ▣ 842
Maximum Strength Halls Plus Cough Suppressant Tablets (Menthol) Warner-Lambert ▣ 843
Halls Sugar Free Cough Suppressant Tablets (Menthol, Eucalyptus, Oil of) Warner-Lambert ▣ 842
Humibid (Dextromethorphan Hydrobromide, Guaifenesin) Adams 462
Hycodan Tablets and Syrup (Hydrocodone Bitartrate, Homatropine Methylbromide) DuPont 930
Hycotuss Expectorant Syrup (Hydrocodone Bitartrate, Guaifenesin) DuPont 933
Hyland's Cough Syrup with Honey (Ipecac) Standard Homeopathic ▣ 829
N'ICE Medicated Sugarless Sore Throat and Cough Lozenges (Menthol) SmithKline Beecham Consumer ▣ 822
Pediatric Vicks 44e Chest Cough & Chest Congestion (Dextromethorphan Hydrobromide, Guaifenesin) Procter & Gamble ▣ 764
Robitussin A-C Syrup (Codeine Phosphate, Guaifenesin) Robins 2073
Robitussin Maximum Strength Cough Suppressant (Dextromethorphan Hydrobromide) A. H. Robins Consumer ▣ 778
Robitussin Pediatric Cough & Cold Formula (Dextromethorphan Hydrobromide, Pseudoephedrine Hydrochloride) A. H. Robins Consumer ▣ 779
Robitussin Pediatric Cough Suppressant (Dextromethorphan Hydrobromide) A. H. Robins Consumer ▣ 779
Robitussin-DM (Dextromethorphan Hydrobromide, Guaifenesin) A. H. Robins Consumer ▣ 777
Safe Tussin 30 (Dextromethorphan Hydrobromide, Guaifenesin) Kramer 1363
Sucrets 4-Hour Cough Suppressant (Dextromethorphan Hydrobromide) SmithKline Beecham Consumer ▣ 826
Tessalon Perles (Benzonatate) Forest 1020
TheraFlu Maximum Strength Nighttime Flu, Cold & Cough Medicine (Acetaminophen, Dextromethorphan Hydrobromide, Pseudoephedrine Hydrochloride, Chlorpheniramine Maleate) Sandoz Consumer ▣ 788

(▣ Described in PDR For Nonprescription Drugs) (◉ Described in PDR For Ophthalmology)

Cough | Indications Index | 1474

Triaminicol Multi-Symptom Cold Tablets (Phenylpropanolamine Hydrochloride, Chlorpheniramine Maleate, Dextromethorphan Hydrobromide) Sandoz Consumer ▣ 793
Triaminicol Multi-Symptom Relief (Phenylpropanolamine Hydrochloride, Chlorpheniramine Maleate, Dextromethorphan Hydrobromide) Sandoz Consumer ▣ 794
Tussionex Pennkinetic Extended-Release Suspension (Hydrocodone Polistirex, Chlorpheniramine Polistirex) Fisons 998
Tussi-Organidin DM NR Liquid and DM-S NR Liquid (Guaifenesin, Dextromethorphan Hydrobromide) Wallace 2677
Tussi-Organidin NR Liquid and S NR Liquid (Guaifenesin, Codeine Phosphate) Wallace 2677
TYLENOL Cough Multi-Symptom Medication (Dextromethorphan Hydrobromide, Acetaminophen) McNeil Consumer 1564
Vicks 44 Dry Hacking Cough (Dextromethorphan Hydrobromide) Procter & Gamble ▣ 755
Vicks 44E Chest Cough & Chest Congestion (Dextromethorphan Hydrobromide, Guaifenesin) Procter & Gamble ▣ 756
Vicks Chloraseptic Cough & Throat Drops (Menthol) Procter & Gamble ▣ 759
Vicks Cough Drops (Menthol) Procter & Gamble ▣ 759
Vicodin Tuss Expectorant (Hydrocodone Bitartrate, Guaifenesin) Knoll Laboratories 1358

Cough, whooping (see under Pertussis)

Cradle cap (see under Dermatitis, seborrheic)

Cramps, abdominal, symptomatic relief of
Donnagel Liquid and Donnagel Chewable Tablets (Attapulgite) Wyeth-Ayerst ▣ 879
Gas-X Chewable Tablets (Simethicone) Sandoz Consumer ▣ 786
Levsin/Levsinex/Levbid (Hyoscyamine Sulfate) Schwarz 2405

Cramps, leg (see under Leg muscle cramps)

Creeping eruptions (see under Larva migrans, cutaneous)

Cretinism (see under Hypothyroidism, replacement or supplemental therapy in)

Cryptitis, temporary relief of
Anusol-HC Suppositories (Hydrocortisone Acetate) Parke-Davis 1897

Cryptococcosis
Ancobon Capsules (Flucytosine) Roche Laboratories 2079
Fungizone Intravenous (Amphotericin B) Apothecon 506

Cryptococcus meningitis
Ancobon Capsules (Flucytosine) Roche Laboratories 2079
Diflucan Injection, Tablets, and Oral Suspension (Fluconazole) Roerig 2194

Cryptococcus strains pulmonary infections
Ancobon Capsules (Flucytosine) Roche Laboratories 2079

Cryptococcus strains urinary tract infections
Ancobon Capsules (Flucytosine) Roche Laboratories 2079

Cryptorchidism, prepubertal
Pregnyl (Chorionic Gonadotropin) Organon 1828
Profasi (chorionic gonadotropin for injection, USP) (Chorionic Gonadotropin) Serono 2450

Cushing's syndrome
Cytadren Tablets (Aminoglutethimide) CibaGeneva 819

Cushing's syndrome, diagnosis of (see under Adrenocortical hyperfunction, diagnostic testing of)

Cuts, minor, infection from (see under Infections, skin, bacterial, minor)

Cuts, minor, pain associated with (see under Pain, topical relief of)

Cyclitis
AK-Pred (Prednisolone Sodium Phosphate) Akorn ⊙ 204
Decadron Phosphate Sterile Ophthalmic Ointment (Dexamethasone Sodium Phosphate) Merck & Co., Inc. 1641
Decadron Phosphate Sterile Ophthalmic Solution (Dexamethasone Sodium Phosphate) Merck & Co., Inc. 1642
Econopred & Econopred Plus Ophthalmic Suspensions (Prednisolone Acetate) Alcon Laboratories ⊙ 217
Inflamase (Prednisolone Sodium Phosphate) CIBA Vision Ophthalmics ⊙ 265

Cycloplegia, production of
Atropine Sulfate Sterile Ophthalmic Solution (Atropine Sulfate) Allergan ⊙ 233

Cystic fibrosis
Chloromycetin Sodium Succinate (Chloramphenicol Sodium Succinate) Parke-Davis 1900

Cystic fibrosis, adjunctive therapy in
Pulmozyme Inhalation (Dornase Alfa) Genentech 1064

Cystic tumors
Aristocort Suspension (Forte Parenteral) (Triamcinolone Diacetate) Fujisawa 1027
Aristocort Suspension (Intralesional) (Triamcinolone Diacetate) Fujisawa 1025
Aristospan Suspension (Intralesional) (Triamcinolone Hexacetonide) Fujisawa 1032
Celestone Soluspan Suspension (Betamethasone Sodium Phosphate, Betamethasone Acetate) Schering 2347
Depo-Medrol Single-Dose Vial (Methylprednisolone Acetate) Upjohn 2600
Depo-Medrol Sterile Aqueous Suspension (Methylprednisolone Acetate) Upjohn 2597

Cystinuria
Cuprimine Capsules (Penicillamine) Merck & Co., Inc. 1630
Depen Titratable Tablets (Penicillamine) Wallace 2662

Cystitis
Azactam for Injection (Aztreonam) Bristol-Myers Squibb 734
Ceclor Pulvules & Suspension (Cefaclor) Lilly 1431
Floxin I.V. (Ofloxacin) McNeil Pharmaceutical 1571
Floxin Tablets (200 mg, 300 mg, 400 mg) (Ofloxacin) McNeil Pharmaceutical 1567
Gantanol Tablets (Sulfamethoxazole) Roche Laboratories 2119
Gantrisin (Acetyl Sulfisoxazole) Roche Laboratories 2120
Lorabid Suspension and Pulvules (Loracarbef) Lilly 1459
Macrobid Capsules (Nitrofurantoin Monohydrate) Procter & Gamble Pharmaceuticals 1988
Maxaquin Tablets (Lomefloxacin Hydrochloride) Searle 2440
Noroxin Tablets (Norfloxacin) Merck & Co., Inc. 1715
Noroxin Tablets (Norfloxacin) Roberts 2048
Penetrex Tablets (Enoxacin) Rhone-Poulenc Rorer Pharmaceuticals 2031
Urised Tablets (Atropine Sulfate, Hyoscyamine, Methenamine, Phenyl Salicylate) PolyMedica 1964
Uroqid-Acid No. 2 Tablets (Methenamine Mandelate, Sodium Acid Phosphate) Beach 640
Vantin for Oral Suspension and Vantin Tablets (Cefpodoxime Proxetil) Upjohn 2646

Cystitis, frequency and incontinence, symptomatic relief of
Urispas Tablets (Flavoxate Hydrochloride) SmithKline Beecham Pharmaceuticals 2532

Cystitis, hemorrhagic, prophylaxis
Mesnex Injection (Mesna) Bristol-Myers Squibb Oncology 702

Cystitis, "Lacking substantial evidence of effectiveness" in
Urobiotic-250 Capsules (Oxytetracycline Hydrochloride, Sulfamethizole, Phenazopyridine Hydrochloride) Roerig 2214

Cytomegalovirus disease associated with renal transplantation, attenuation of
CytoGam (Cytomegalovirus Immune Globulin) MedImmune 1593

Cytomegalovirus disease associated with transplant patients
Cytovene (Ganciclovir Sodium) Roche Laboratories 2103

D

Dacryocystitis
Genoptic Sterile Ophthalmic Solution (Gentamicin Sulfate) Allergan ⊙ 243
Genoptic Sterile Ophthalmic Ointment (Gentamicin Sulfate) Allergan ⊙ 243
Gentacidin Ointment (Gentamicin Sulfate) CIBA Vision Ophthalmics ⊙ 264
Gentacidin Solution (Gentamicin Sulfate) CIBA Vision Ophthalmics ⊙ 264
Gentak (Gentamicin Sulfate) Akorn ⊙ 208

Dandruff (see also under Dermatitis, seborrheic)
Capitrol Shampoo (Chloroxine) Westwood-Squibb 2683
DHS (Coal Tar) Persōn & Covey 1932
Fototar Cream (Coal Tar) ICN 1253
Head & Shoulders Intensive (Selenium Sulfide) Procter & Gamble ▣ 750
Nizoral 2% Shampoo (Ketoconazole) Janssen 1298
P&S Liquid (Mineral Oil) Baker Cummins ▣ 604
P&S Plus Tar Gel (Coal Tar) Baker Cummins ▣ 604
Pentrax Anti-dandruff Shampoo (Coal Tar) GenDerm 1055
Selsun Gold for Women Dandruff Shampoo (Selenium Sulfide) Ross ▣ 783
Selsun Rx 2.5% Selenium Sulfide Lotion, USP (Selenium Sulfide) Ross 2225
Tegrin Dandruff Shampoo (Coal Tar) Block ▣ 611
X-Seb Shampoo (Pyrithione Zinc) Baker Cummins ▣ 605
X-Seb Plus Antidandruff Conditioning Shampoo (Pyrithione Zinc) Baker Cummins ▣ 605
X-Seb T Pearl Shampoo (Coal Tar) Baker Cummins ▣ 606
X-Seb T Plus Conditioning Shampoo (Coal Tar) Baker Cummins ▣ 606
Zincon Dandruff Shampoo (Pyrithione Zinc) Lederle Consumer ▣ 671

Dehydration, prevention of
Pedialyte Oral Electrolyte Maintenance Solution (Electrolyte Supplement) Ross 2222
Rehydralyte Oral Electrolyte Rehydration Solution (Electrolyte Supplement) Ross 2224

Dementia, Alzheimer's type
Cognex Capsules (Tacrine Hydrochloride) Parke-Davis 1901

Dental caries, prophylaxis
Crest Sensitivity Protection Toothpaste (Potassium Nitrate, Sodium Fluoride) Procter & Gamble ▣ 750
Listermint Alcohol-Free Mouthwash (Sodium Fluoride) WARNER WELLCOME ▣ 855
Luride Drops 50 ml (Sodium Fluoride) Colgate Oral 871
Luride Lozi-Tabs Tablets (Sodium Fluoride) Colgate Oral 871

Dental plaque, prevention of
Listerine Antiseptic (Eucalyptol, Menthol, Methyl Salicylate) WARNER WELLCOME ▣ 855
Baby Orajel Tooth & Gum Cleanser (Simethicone) Del ▣ 652

Depression, atypical (see under Depression, mental, nonendogenous)

Depression, bipolar (see under Depression, manic-depressive)

Depression, major, without melancholia
Parnate Tablets (Tranylcypromine Sulfate) SmithKline Beecham Pharmaceuticals 2503

Depression, manic-depressive
Depakote Tablets (Divalproex Sodium) Abbott 415
Eskalith (Lithium Carbonate) SmithKline Beecham Pharmaceuticals 2485
Lithium Carbonate Capsules & Tablets (Lithium Carbonate) Roxane 2230
Lithonate/Lithotabs/Lithobid (Lithium Carbonate) Solvay 2543
Ludiomil Tablets (Maprotiline Hydrochloride) CibaGeneva 843
Sinequan (Doxepin Hydrochloride) Roerig 2205
Thorazine (Chlorpromazine Hydrochloride) SmithKline Beecham Pharmaceuticals 2523

Depression, mental, nonendogenous
Nardil (Phenelzine Sulfate) Parke-Davis 1920

Depression, neurosis
Asendin Tablets (Amoxapine) Lederle 1369
Ludiomil Tablets (Maprotiline Hydrochloride) CibaGeneva 843

Depression, neurotic (see under Depression, mental, nonendogenous)

Depression, relief of symptoms
Asendin Tablets (Amoxapine) Lederle 1369
Desyrel and Desyrel Dividose (Trazodone Hydrochloride) Apothecon 503
Effexor (Venlafaxine Hydrochloride) Wyeth-Ayerst 2719
Elavil (Amitriptyline Hydrochloride) Zeneca 2838
Endep Tablets (Amitriptyline Hydrochloride) Roche Products 2174
Etrafon (Perphenazine, Amitriptyline Hydrochloride) Schering 2355

(▣ Described in PDR For Nonprescription Drugs) (⊙ Described in PDR For Ophthalmology)

1475 Indications Index Dermatitis

Limbitrol (Chlordiazepoxide, Amitriptyline Hydrochloride) Roche Products 2180
Ludiomil Tablets (Maprotiline Hydrochloride) CibaGeneva 843
Norpramin Tablets (Desipramine Hydrochloride) Marion Merrell Dow 1526
Pamelor (Nortriptyline Hydrochloride) Sandoz Pharmaceuticals 2280
Paxil Tablets (Paroxetine Hydrochloride) SmithKline Beecham Pharmaceuticals 2505
Prozac Pulvules & Liquid, Oral Solution (Fluoxetine Hydrochloride) Dista 919
Serzone Tablets (Nefazodone Hydrochloride) Bristol-Myers Squibb 771
Sinequan (Doxepin Hydrochloride) Roerig 2205
Surmontil Capsules (Trimipramine Maleate) Wyeth-Ayerst 2811
Tofranil Ampuls (Imipramine Hydrochloride) CibaGeneva 854
Tofranil Tablets (Imipramine Hydrochloride) CibaGeneva 856
Tofranil-PM Capsules (Imipramine Pamoate) CibaGeneva 857
Triavil Tablets (Perphenazine, Amitriptyline Hydrochloride) Merck & Co., Inc. 1757
Vivactil Tablets (Protriptyline Hydrochloride) Merck & Co., Inc. 1774
Wellbutrin Tablets (Bupropion Hydrochloride) Glaxo Wellcome 1204
Zoloft Tablets (Sertraline Hydrochloride) Roerig 2217

Dermatitis, allergic contact, diagnosis of

T.R.U.E. Test (Allergens) Glaxo Wellcome 1189

Dermatitis, atopic

Aristocort Suspension (Forte Parenteral) (Triamcinolone Diacetate) Fujisawa 1027
Aristocort Tablets (Triamcinolone) Fujisawa 1022
Celestone Soluspan Suspension (Betamethasone Sodium Phosphate, Betamethasone Acetate) Schering 2347
Cortaid (Hydrocortisone Acetate) Upjohn ▣ 836
Cortizone-5 Creme and Ointment (Hydrocortisone) Thompson Medical ▣ 831
Cortizone-10 Creme and Ointment (Hydrocortisone) Thompson Medical ▣ 831
Cortone Acetate Sterile Suspension (Cortisone Acetate) Merck & Co., Inc. 1623
Cortone Acetate Tablets (Cortisone Acetate) Merck & Co., Inc. 1624
Dalalone D.P. Injectable (Dexamethasone Acetate) Forest 1011
Decadron Elixir (Dexamethasone) Merck & Co., Inc. 1633
Decadron Phosphate Injection (Dexamethasone Sodium Phosphate) Merck & Co., Inc. 1637
Decadron Tablets (Dexamethasone) Merck & Co., Inc. 1635
Decadron-LA Sterile Suspension (Dexamethasone Acetate) Merck & Co., Inc. 1646
Deltasone Tablets (Prednisone) Upjohn 2595
Depo-Medrol Single-Dose Vial (Methylprednisolone Acetate) Upjohn 2600
Depo-Medrol Sterile Aqueous Suspension (Methylprednisolone Acetate) Upjohn 2597
Hydeltrasol Injection, Sterile (Prednisolone Sodium Phosphate) Merck & Co., Inc. 1665
Hydrocortone Phosphate Injection, Sterile (Hydrocortisone Sodium Phosphate) Merck & Co., Inc. 1670
Hydrocortone Tablets (Hydrocortisone) Merck & Co., Inc. 1672
Mantadil Cream (Chlorcyclizine Hydrochloride) Glaxo Wellcome 1135
Medrol (Methylprednisolone) Upjohn 2621
Pediapred Oral Liquid (Prednisolone Sodium Phosphate) Fisons 995
Prelone Syrup (Prednisolone) Muro 1787
Solu-Cortef Sterile Powder (Hydrocortisone Sodium Succinate) Upjohn 2641
Solu-Medrol Sterile Powder (Methylprednisolone Sodium Succinate) Upjohn 2643
Temaril Tablets, Syrup and Spansule Extended-Release Capsules (Trimeprazine Tartrate) Allergan 483
Zonalon Cream (Doxepin Hydrochloride) GenDerm 1055

Dermatitis, contact (see also under Dermatoses, corticosteroid-responsive)

Bactine Hydrocortisone Anti-Itch Cream (Hydrocortisone) Miles Consumer ▣ 709
Benadryl Itch Relief Cream, Children's Formula and Maximum Strength 2% (Diphenhydramine Hydrochloride, Zinc Acetate) WARNER WELLCOME ▣ 851
Caladryl (Pramoxine Hydrochloride, Zinc Acetate) WARNER WELLCOME ▣ 853
Caldecort (Hydrocortisone Acetate) CIBA Consumer ▣ 631
Celestone Soluspan Suspension (Betamethasone Sodium Phosphate, Betamethasone Acetate) Schering 2347
Cortaid (Hydrocortisone Acetate) Upjohn ▣ 836
Cortizone-5 (Hydrocortisone) Thompson Medical ▣ 831
Cortizone-10 Creme and Ointment (Hydrocortisone) Thompson Medical ▣ 831
Cortone Acetate Sterile Suspension (Cortisone Acetate) Merck & Co., Inc. 1623
Cortone Acetate Tablets (Cortisone Acetate) Merck & Co., Inc. 1624
Dalalone D.P. Injectable (Dexamethasone Acetate) Forest 1011
Decadron Elixir (Dexamethasone) Merck & Co., Inc. 1633
Decadron Phosphate Injection (Dexamethasone Sodium Phosphate) Merck & Co., Inc. 1637
Decadron Tablets (Dexamethasone) Merck & Co., Inc. 1635
Decadron-LA Sterile Suspension (Dexamethasone Acetate) Merck & Co., Inc. 1646
Deltasone Tablets (Prednisone) Upjohn 2595
Depo-Medrol Sterile Aqueous Suspension (Methylprednisolone Acetate) Upjohn 2597
Hydeltrasol Injection, Sterile (Prednisolone Sodium Phosphate) Merck & Co., Inc. 1665
Hydrocortone Phosphate Injection, Sterile (Hydrocortisone Sodium Phosphate) Merck & Co., Inc. 1670
Hydrocortone Tablets (Hydrocortisone) Merck & Co., Inc. 1672
Mantadil Cream (Chlorcyclizine Hydrochloride) Glaxo Wellcome 1135
Medrol (Methylprednisolone) Upjohn 2621
Pediapred Oral Liquid (Prednisolone Sodium Phosphate) Fisons 995
Solu-Cortef Sterile Powder (Hydrocortisone Sodium Succinate) Upjohn 2641
Solu-Medrol Sterile Powder (Methylprednisolone Sodium Succinate) Upjohn 2643
Temaril Tablets, Syrup and Spansule Extended-Release Capsules (Trimeprazine Tartrate) Allergan 483
Vistaril Capsules (Hydroxyzine Pamoate) Pfizer Labs 1944
Vistaril Oral Suspension (Hydroxyzine Pamoate) Pfizer Labs 1944

Dermatitis, corticosteroid-responsive, anal region

Analpram-HC Rectal Cream 1% and 2.5% (Hydrocortisone Acetate, Pramoxine Hydrochloride) Ferndale 977

Dermatitis, eczematoid

Zonalon Cream (Doxepin Hydrochloride) GenDerm 1055

Dermatitis, exfoliative

Aristocort Suspension (Forte Parenteral) (Triamcinolone Diacetate) Fujisawa 1027
Aristocort Tablets (Triamcinolone) Fujisawa 1022
Celestone Soluspan Suspension (Betamethasone Sodium Phosphate, Betamethasone Acetate) Schering 2347
Cortone Acetate Sterile Suspension (Cortisone Acetate) Merck & Co., Inc. 1623
Cortone Acetate Tablets (Cortisone Acetate) Merck & Co., Inc. 1624
Dalalone D.P. Injectable (Dexamethasone Acetate) Forest 1011
Decadron Elixir (Dexamethasone) Merck & Co., Inc. 1633
Decadron Phosphate Injection (Dexamethasone Sodium Phosphate) Merck & Co., Inc. 1637
Decadron Tablets (Dexamethasone) Merck & Co., Inc. 1635
Decadron-LA Sterile Suspension (Dexamethasone Acetate) Merck & Co., Inc. 1646
Deltasone Tablets (Prednisone) Upjohn 2595
Depo-Medrol Single-Dose Vial (Methylprednisolone Acetate) Upjohn 2600
Depo-Medrol Sterile Aqueous Suspension (Methylprednisolone Acetate) Upjohn 2597
Hydeltrasol Injection, Sterile (Prednisolone Sodium Phosphate) Merck & Co., Inc. 1665
Hydrocortone Phosphate Injection, Sterile (Hydrocortisone Sodium Phosphate) Merck & Co., Inc. 1670
Hydrocortone Tablets (Hydrocortisone) Merck & Co., Inc. 1672
Medrol (Methylprednisolone) Upjohn 2621
Pediapred Oral Liquid (Prednisolone Sodium Phosphate) Fisons 995
Prelone Syrup (Prednisolone) Muro 1787
Solu-Cortef Sterile Powder (Hydrocortisone Sodium Succinate) Upjohn 2641
Solu-Medrol Sterile Powder (Methylprednisolone Sodium Succinate) Upjohn 2643

Dermatitis, herpetiformis

Dapsone Tablets USP (Dapsone) Jacobus 1284

Dermatitis, herpetiformis bullous

Aristocort Suspension (Forte Parenteral) (Triamcinolone Diacetate) Fujisawa 1027
Aristocort Tablets (Triamcinolone) Fujisawa 1022
Celestone Soluspan Suspension (Betamethasone Sodium Phosphate, Betamethasone Acetate) Schering 2347
Cortone Acetate Sterile Suspension (Cortisone Acetate) Merck & Co., Inc. 1623
Cortone Acetate Tablets (Cortisone Acetate) Merck & Co., Inc. 1624
Dalalone D.P. Injectable (Dexamethasone Acetate) Forest 1011
Decadron Elixir (Dexamethasone) Merck & Co., Inc. 1633
Decadron Phosphate Injection (Dexamethasone Sodium Phosphate) Merck & Co., Inc. 1637
Decadron Tablets (Dexamethasone) Merck & Co., Inc. 1635
Decadron-LA Sterile Suspension (Dexamethasone Acetate) Merck & Co., Inc. 1646
Deltasone Tablets (Prednisone) Upjohn 2595
Depo-Medrol Single-Dose Vial (Methylprednisolone Acetate) Upjohn 2600
Depo-Medrol Sterile Aqueous Suspension (Methylprednisolone Acetate) Upjohn 2597
Hydeltrasol Injection, Sterile (Prednisolone Sodium Phosphate) Merck & Co., Inc. 1665
Hydrocortone Phosphate Injection, Sterile (Hydrocortisone Sodium Phosphate) Merck & Co., Inc. 1670
Hydrocortone Tablets (Hydrocortisone) Merck & Co., Inc. 1672
Medrol (Methylprednisolone) Upjohn 2621
Pediapred Oral Liquid (Prednisolone Sodium Phosphate) Fisons 995
Prelone Syrup (Prednisolone) Muro 1787
Solu-Cortef Sterile Powder (Hydrocortisone Sodium Succinate) Upjohn 2641
Solu-Medrol Sterile Powder (Methylprednisolone Sodium Succinate) Upjohn 2643

Dermatitis, lichenoid

Mantadil Cream (Chlorcyclizine Hydrochloride) Glaxo Wellcome 1135

Dermatitis, seborrheic

Aquanil HC Lotion (Hydrocortisone) Persōn & Covey 1931
Capitrol Shampoo (Chloroxine) Westwood-Squibb 2683
Cortizone for Kids (Hydrocortisone) Thompson Medical ▣ 831
Cortizone-10 Creme and Ointment (Hydrocortisone) Thompson Medical ▣ 831
DHS Zinc Dandruff Shampoo (Pyrithione Zinc) Persōn & Covey 1932
Fototar Cream (Coal Tar) ICN 1253
Head & Shoulders Intensive (Selenium Sulfide) Procter & Gamble ▣ 750
Mantadil Cream (Chlorcyclizine Hydrochloride) Glaxo Wellcome 1135
Nizoral 2% Cream (Ketoconazole) Janssen 1297
Novacet Lotion (Sulfur, Sulfacetamide Sodium) GenDerm 1054
P&S Plus Tar Gel (Coal Tar) Baker Cummins ▣ 604
P&S Shampoo (Salicylic Acid) Baker Cummins ▣ 605
Pentrax Anti-dandruff Shampoo (Coal Tar) GenDerm 1055
Selsun Blue (Selenium Sulfide) Ross ▣ 783
Selsun Rx 2.5% Selenium Sulfide Lotion, USP (Selenium Sulfide) Ross 2225
Sulfacet-R MVL Lotion (Sodium Sulfacetamide, Sulfur) Dermik 909
Tegrin Skin Cream & Tegrin Medicated Soap (Coal Tar) Block ▣ 611
X-Seb Plus Antidandruff Conditioning Shampoo (Pyrithione Zinc) Baker Cummins ▣ 605
X-Seb T Pearl Shampoo (Coal Tar) Baker Cummins ▣ 606
Zincon Dandruff Shampoo (Pyrithione Zinc) Lederle Consumer ▣ 671

Dermatitis, seborrheic, severe

Aristocort Suspension (Forte Parenteral) (Triamcinolone Diacetate) Fujisawa 1027
Aristocort Tablets (Triamcinolone) Fujisawa 1022
Celestone Soluspan Suspension (Betamethasone Sodium Phosphate, Betamethasone Acetate) Schering 2347
Cortone Acetate Sterile Suspension (Cortisone Acetate) Merck & Co., Inc. 1623
Cortone Acetate Tablets (Cortisone Acetate) Merck & Co., Inc. 1624
Dalalone D.P. Injectable (Dexamethasone Acetate) Forest 1011
Decadron Elixir (Dexamethasone) Merck & Co., Inc. 1633

(▣ Described in PDR For Nonprescription Drugs) (◉ Described in PDR For Ophthalmology)

Dermatitis **Indications Index** **1476**

Decadron Phosphate Injection (Dexamethasone Sodium Phosphate) Merck & Co., Inc. 1637
Decadron Tablets (Dexamethasone) Merck & Co., Inc. 1635
Decadron-LA Sterile Suspension (Dexamethasone Acetate) Merck & Co., Inc. 1646
Deltasone Tablets (Prednisone) Upjohn 2595
Depo-Medrol Single-Dose Vial (Methylprednisolone Acetate) Upjohn 2600
Depo-Medrol Sterile Aqueous Suspension (Methylprednisolone Acetate) Upjohn 2597
Hydeltrasol Injection, Sterile (Prednisolone Sodium Phosphate) Merck & Co., Inc. 1665
Hydrocortone Phosphate Injection, Sterile (Hydrocortisone Sodium Phosphate) Merck & Co., Inc. 1670
Hydrocortone Tablets (Hydrocortisone) Merck & Co., Inc. 1672
Medrol (Methylprednisolone) Upjohn 2621
Pediapred Oral Liquid (Prednisolone Sodium Phosphate) Fisons 995
Prelone Syrup (Prednisolone) Muro 1787
Solu-Cortef Sterile Powder (Hydrocortisone Sodium Succinate) Upjohn 2641
Solu-Medrol Sterile Powder (Methylprednisolone Sodium Succinate) Upjohn 2643

Dermatomyositis, "possibly" effective in

Potaba (Aminobenzoate Potassium) Glenwood 1229

Dermatomyositis, systemic

Cortone Acetate Sterile Suspension (Cortisone Acetate) Merck & Co., Inc. 1623
Cortone Acetate Tablets (Cortisone Acetate) Merck & Co., Inc. 1624
Deltasone Tablets (Prednisone) Upjohn 2595
Depo-Medrol Single-Dose Vial (Methylprednisolone Acetate) Upjohn 2600
Depo-Medrol Sterile Aqueous Suspension (Methylprednisolone Acetate) Upjohn 2597
Hydeltrasol Injection, Sterile (Prednisolone Sodium Phosphate) Merck & Co., Inc. 1665
Hydrocortone Phosphate Injection, Sterile (Hydrocortisone Sodium Phosphate) Merck & Co., Inc. 1670
Hydrocortone Tablets (Hydrocortisone) Merck & Co., Inc. 1672
Medrol (Methylprednisolone) Upjohn 2621
Pediapred Oral Liquid (Prednisolone Sodium Phosphate) Fisons 995
Prelone Syrup (Prednisolone) Muro 1787
Solu-Cortef Sterile Powder (Hydrocortisone Sodium Succinate) Upjohn 2641
Solu-Medrol Sterile Powder (Methylprednisolone Sodium Succinate) Upjohn 2643

Dermatoses, corticosteroid-responsive (see also under Skin, inflammatory conditions)

Aclovate (Alclometasone Dipropionate) Glaxo Wellcome 1069
Aristocort Suspension (Forte Parenteral) (Triamcinolone Diacetate) Fujisawa 1027
Aristocort Tablets (Triamcinolone) Fujisawa 1022
Aristocort A 0.025% Cream (Triamcinolone Acetonide) Fujisawa .. 1027
Aristocort A 0.5% Cream (Triamcinolone Acetonide) Fujisawa 1031
Aristocort A 0.1% Cream (Triamcinolone Acetonide) Fujisawa 1029
Aristocort A 0.1% Ointment (Triamcinolone Acetonide) Fujisawa .. 1030
Carmol HC (Hydrocortisone Acetate) Doak 924
Cordran Lotion (Flurandrenolide) Oclassen 1803
Cordran Tape (Flurandrenolide) Oclassen 1804
Cortizone-10 (Hydrocortisone) Thompson Medical .... ■ 831
Cutivate Cream (Fluticasone Propionate) Glaxo Wellcome 1088
Cutivate Ointment (Fluticasone Propionate) Glaxo Wellcome 1089
Cyclocort Topical (Amcinonide) Fujisawa 1037
Decadron Phosphate Topical Cream (Dexamethasone Sodium Phosphate) Merck & Co., Inc. 1644
Decaspray Topical Aerosol (Dexamethasone) Merck & Co., Inc. 1648
Depo-Medrol Single-Dose Vial (Methylprednisolone Acetate) Upjohn 2600
Dermatop Emollient Cream 0.1% (Prednicarbate) Hoechst-Roussel 1238
DesOwen Cream, Ointment and Lotion (Desonide) Galderma 1046
Diprolene AF Cream (Betamethasone Dipropionate) Schering 2352
Diprolene Gel 0.05% (Betamethasone Dipropionate) Schering 2353
Diprolene Ointment 0.05% (Betamethasone Dipropionate) Schering 2352
Elocon (Mometasone Furoate) Schering 2354
Epifoam (Hydrocortisone Acetate, Pramoxine Hydrochloride) Schwarz 2399
Florone/Florone E (Diflorasone Diacetate) Dermik 906
Halog (Halcinonide) Westwood-Squibb 2686
Hytone (Hydrocortisone) Dermik 907
Lidex (Fluocinonide) Roche Laboratories 2130
Locoid Cream, Ointment and Topical Solution (Hydrocortisone Butyrate) Ferndale 978
Nupercainal Hydrocortisone 1% Cream (Hydrocortisone Acetate) CIBA Consumer .... ■ 645
Pramosone Cream, Lotion & Ointment (Hydrocortisone Acetate, Pramoxine Hydrochloride) Ferndale 978
Prelone Syrup (Prednisolone) Muro 1787
ProctoCream-HC (Hydrocortisone Acetate, Pramoxine Hydrochloride) Schwarz 2408
ProctoCream-HC 2.5% (Hydrocortisone) Schwarz 2408
ProctoFoam-HC (Hydrocortisone Acetate, Pramoxine Hydrochloride) Schwarz 2409
Psorcon Ointment 0.05% (Diflorasone Diacetate) Dermik 908
Synalar (Fluocinolone Acetonide) Roche Laboratories 2130
Temovate (Clobetasol Propionate) Glaxo Wellcome 1179
Topicort (Desoximetasone) Hoechst-Roussel 1243
Tridesilon Cream 0.05% (Desonide) Bayer Pharmaceutical 615
Tridesilon Ointment 0.05% (Desonide) Bayer Pharmaceutical 616
Ultravate Cream 0.05% (Halobetasol Propionate) Westwood-Squibb 2689
Ultravate Ointment 0.05% (Halobetasol Propionate) Westwood-Squibb 2690
Westcort (Hydrocortisone Valerate) Westwood-Squibb 2690

Dermatoses, steroid-responsive, with secondary infection

Anusol-HC Cream 2.5% (Hydrocortisone) Parke-Davis 1896
Cortisporin Cream (Polymyxin B Sulfate, Neomycin Sulfate, Hydrocortisone Acetate) Glaxo Wellcome 1084
Cortisporin Ointment (Polymyxin B Sulfate, Bacitracin Zinc, Neomycin Sulfate, Hydrocortisone) Glaxo Wellcome 1085
NeoDecadron Topical Cream (Neomycin Sulfate, Dexamethasone Sodium Phosphate) Merck & Co., Inc. 1714

Dermographism

Benadryl Capsules (Diphenhydramine Hydrochloride) Parke-Davis 1898
PBZ Tablets (Tripelennamine Hydrochloride) CibaGeneva 845
PBZ-SR Tablets (Tripelennamine Hydrochloride) CibaGeneva 844
Periactin (Cyproheptadine Hydrochloride) Merck & Co., Inc. 1724
Phenergan Suppositories (Promethazine Hydrochloride) Wyeth-Ayerst 2775
Phenergan Syrup (Promethazine Hydrochloride) Wyeth-Ayerst 2774
Phenergan Tablets (Promethazine Hydrochloride) Wyeth-Ayerst 2775

Diabetes insipidus

DDAVP Injection (Desmopressin Acetate) Rhone-Poulenc Rorer Pharmaceuticals 2014
DDAVP (Desmopressin Acetate) Rhone-Poulenc Rorer Pharmaceuticals 2017
Desmopressin Acetate Rhinal Tube (Desmopressin Acetate) Ferring .. 979

Diabetes mellitus, insulin-dependent

Humulin 50/50, 100 Units (Insulin, Human Isophane Suspension, Insulin, Human) Lilly 1444
Humulin 70/30, 100 Units (Insulin, Human Regular and Human NPH Mixture) Lilly 1445
Humulin L, 100 Units (Insulin, Human, Zinc Suspension) Lilly 1446
Humulin N, 100 Units (Insulin, Human NPH) Lilly 1448
Humulin R, 100 Units (Insulin, Human Regular) Lilly 1449
Humulin U, 100 Units (Insulin, Human, Zinc Suspension) Lilly 1450
Iletin I (Insulin, Zinc Suspension) Lilly 1450
Lente, 100 Units (Insulin, Zinc Suspension) Lilly 1450
NPH, 100 Units (Insulin, NPH) Lilly 1450
Regular, 100 Units (Insulin, Regular) Lilly 1450
Iletin II (Insulin, Zinc Suspension) Lilly 1452
Pork Lente, 100 Units (Insulin, Zinc Suspension) Lilly 1452
Pork NPH, 100 Units (Insulin, NPH) Lilly 1452
Pork Regular, 100 Units (Insulin, Regular) Lilly 1452
Pork Regular (Concentrated), 500 Units (Insulin, Regular) Lilly 1453
Novolin L Human Insulin 10 ml Vials (Insulin, Human, Zinc Suspension) Novo Nordisk 1795
Novolin N Human Insulin 10 ml Vials (Insulin, Human Isophane Suspension) Novo Nordisk 1795
Novolin N PenFill Cartridges Durable Insulin Delivery System (Insulin, Human NPH) Novo Nordisk 1798
Novolin N Prefilled Syringe Disposable Insulin Delivery System (Insulin, Human NPH) Novo Nordisk 1798
Novolin 70/30 Human Insulin 10 ml Vials (Insulin, Human Regular and Human NPH Mixture) Novo Nordisk 1794
Novolin 70/30 PenFill Cartridges Durable Insulin Delivery System (Insulin, Human Regular and Human NPH Mixture) Novo Nordisk 1797
Novolin 70/30 Prefilled Disposable Insulin Delivery System (Insulin, Human Regular and Human NPH Mixture) Novo Nordisk 1798
Novolin R Human Insulin 10 ml Vials (Insulin, Human Regular) Novo Nordisk 1795
Novolin R PenFill Cartridges Durable Insulin Delivery System (Insulin, Human Regular) Novo Nordisk 1798
Novolin R Prefilled Syringe Disposable Insulin Delivery System (Insulin, Human Regular) Novo Nordisk 1798
Purified Pork Lente Insulin (Insulin, Zinc Suspension) Novo Nordisk 1801
Purified Pork NPH Isophane Insulin (Insulin, NPH) Novo Nordisk 1801
Purified Pork Regular Insulin (Insulin, Regular) Novo Nordisk 1801
Velosulin BR Human Insulin 10 ml Vials (Insulin, Human Regular) Novo Nordisk 1795

Diabetes mellitus, non-insulin-dependent

DiaBeta Tablets (Glyburide) Hoechst-Roussel 1239
Diabinese Tablets (Chlorpropamide) Pfizer Labs 1935
Glucophage (Metformin Hydrochloride) Bristol-Myers Squibb 752
Glucotrol Tablets (Glipizide) Pratt .. 1967
Glucotrol XL Extended Release Tablets (Glipizide) Pratt 1968
Glynase PresTab Tablets (Glyburide) Upjohn 2609
Micronase Tablets (Glyburide) Upjohn 2623

Diabetic nephropathy (see under Nephropathy, diabetic)

Diaper rash (see under Rash, diaper)

Diarrhea associated with vasoactive intestinal peptide tumors

Sandostatin Injection (Octreotide Acetate) Sandoz Pharmaceuticals 2292

Diarrhea, adjunctive therapy in

Imodium A-D Caplets and Liquid (Loperamide Hydrochloride) McNeil Consumer 1549
Lomotil (Diphenoxylate Hydrochloride, Atropine Sulfate) Searle 2439
Pedialyte Oral Electrolyte Maintenance Solution (Electrolyte Supplement) Ross 2222
Rehydralyte Oral Electrolyte Rehydration Solution (Electrolyte Supplement) Ross 2224

Diarrhea, bacterial (see under Diarrhea, infectious)

Diarrhea, E. coli-induced

Bactrim (Trimethoprim, Sulfamethoxazole) Roche Laboratories 2084
Cipro Tablets (Ciprofloxacin Hydrochloride) Bayer Pharmaceutical 592
Septra (Trimethoprim, Sulfamethoxazole) Glaxo Wellcome 1174

Diarrhea, infectious

Cipro Tablets (Ciprofloxacin Hydrochloride) Bayer Pharmaceutical 592
Furoxone (Furazolidone) Roberts 2046

Diarrhea, protozoal (see under Diarrhea, infectious)

Diarrhea, traveler's

Bactrim (Trimethoprim, Sulfamethoxazole) Roche Laboratories 2084
Imodium A-D Caplets and Liquid (Loperamide Hydrochloride) McNeil Consumer 1549
Septra (Trimethoprim, Sulfamethoxazole) Glaxo Wellcome 1174

Diarrhea, symptomatic relief of

Diasorb (Attapulgite, Nonfibrous Activated) Columbia .... ■ 650
Donnagel Liquid and Donnagel Chewable Tablets (Attapulgite) Wyeth-Ayerst .... ■ 879
Hyland's Diarrex Tablets (Homeopathic Medications) Standard Homeopathic .... ■ 829
Imodium A-D Caplets and Liquid (Loperamide Hydrochloride) McNeil Consumer 1549
Imodium Capsules (Loperamide Hydrochloride) Janssen 1295
Kaopectate Concentrated Anti-Diarrheal, Peppermint Flavor (Attapulgite) Upjohn .... ■ 837
Kaopectate Concentrated Anti-Diarrheal, Regular Flavor (Attapulgite) Upjohn .... ■ 837
Kaopectate Children's Liquid (Attapulgite) Upjohn .... ■ 837

(■ Described in PDR For Nonprescription Drugs) (◉ Described in PDR For Ophthalmology)

1477 **Indications Index** **E. coli infections**

Kaopectate Maximum Strength Caplets (Attapulgite) Upjohn ...... ▣ 837
Kaopectate 1-D (Loperamide Hydrochloride) Upjohn ...... ▣ 838
Loperamide Hydrochloride Caplets, 2 mg (Loperamide Hydrochloride) Ohm ...... ▣ 736
Maalox Anti-Diarrheal Caplets (Loperamide Hydrochloride) CIBA Consumer ...... ▣ 640
Maalox Anti-Diarrheal Oral Solution (Loperamide Hydrochloride) CIBA Consumer ▣ 639
Motofen Tablets (Atropine Sulfate, Difenoxin Hydrochloride) Carnrick 784
Pepto-Bismol Original Liquid, Original and Cherry Tablets and Easy-To-Swallow Caplets (Bismuth Subsalicylate) Procter & Gamble 1976
Pepto-Bismol Maximum Strength Liquid (Bismuth Subsalicylate) Procter & Gamble 1976
Pepto Diarrhea Control (Loperamide Hydrochloride) Procter & Gamble 1976
Rheaban Maximum Strength Fast Acting Caplets (Attapulgite, Activated) Pfizer Consumer ...... ▣ 743

Digestive disorders, symptomatic relief of
Arco-Lase Plus Tablets (Enzymes, Digestive) Arco 512
Arco-Lase Tablets (Enzymes, Digestive) Arco 512
DDS-Acidophilus (Lactobacillus Acidophilus) UAS Laboratories.. ▣ 835
Kutrase Capsules (Hyoscyamine Sulfate, Phenyltoloxamine Citrate, Enzymes, Digestive) Schwarz 2402
Ku-Zyme Capsules (Enzymes, Digestive) Schwarz 2402
Kyolic (Garlic Extract) Wakunaga.. ▣ 839
Wobenzym N (Pancreatin, Trypsin, Chymotrypsin, Bromelains, Papain) Marlyn ...... ▣ 673

Digestive insufficiencies, symptomatic relief of
Arco-Lase Plus Tablets (Enzymes, Digestive) Arco 512
Arco-Lase Tablets (Enzymes, Digestive) Arco 512

Digoxin intoxication, life-threatening
Digibind (Digoxin Immune Fab (Ovine)) Glaxo Wellcome 1091

Diphtheria (see under C. diphtheriae infections)

Diphtheroid endocarditis
Vancocin HCl, Vials & ADD-Vantage (Vancomycin Hydrochloride) Lilly 1481

Diplococcus pneumoniae infections (see under S. pneumoniae infections)

Diuresis, induction of in edema due to lupus erythematosus
Aristocort Suspension (Forte Parenteral) (Triamcinolone Diacetate) Fujisawa 1027
Aristocort Tablets (Triamcinolone) Fujisawa 1022
Cortone Acetate Sterile Suspension (Cortisone Acetate) Merck & Co., Inc. 1623
Cortone Acetate Tablets (Cortisone Acetate) Merck & Co., Inc. 1624
Dalalone D.P. Injectable (Dexamethasone Acetate) Forest 1011
Decadron Elixir (Dexamethasone) Merck & Co., Inc. 1633
Decadron Phosphate Injection (Dexamethasone Sodium Phosphate) Merck & Co., Inc. 1637
Decadron Tablets (Dexamethasone) Merck & Co., Inc. 1635
Decadron-LA Sterile Suspension (Dexamethasone Acetate) Merck & Co., Inc. 1646
Deltasone Tablets (Prednisone) Upjohn 2595
Depo-Medrol Single-Dose Vial (Methylprednisolone Acetate) Upjohn 2600
Depo-Medrol Sterile Aqueous Suspension (Methylprednisolone Acetate) Upjohn 2597
Hydeltrasol Injection, Sterile (Prednisolone Sodium Phosphate) Merck & Co., Inc. 1665
Hydrocortone Phosphate Injection, Sterile (Hydrocortisone Sodium Phosphate) Merck & Co., Inc. 1670
Hydrocortone Tablets (Hydrocortisone) Merck & Co., Inc. 1672
Medrol (Methylprednisolone) Upjohn 2621
Pediapred Oral Liquid (Prednisolone Sodium Phosphate) Fisons 995
Prelone Syrup (Prednisolone) Muro 1787
Solu-Cortef Sterile Powder (Hydrocortisone Sodium Succinate) Upjohn 2641
Solu-Medrol Sterile Powder (Methylprednisolone Sodium Succinate) Upjohn 2643

Diuresis, induction of in nephrotic syndrome
Aristocort Suspension (Forte Parenteral) (Triamcinolone Diacetate) Fujisawa 1027
Aristocort Tablets (Triamcinolone) Fujisawa 1022
Cortone Acetate Sterile Suspension (Cortisone Acetate) Merck & Co., Inc. 1623
Cortone Acetate Tablets (Cortisone Acetate) Merck & Co., Inc. 1624
Dalalone D.P. Injectable (Dexamethasone Acetate) Forest 1011
Decadron Elixir (Dexamethasone) Merck & Co., Inc. 1633
Decadron Phosphate Injection (Dexamethasone Sodium Phosphate) Merck & Co., Inc. 1637
Decadron Tablets (Dexamethasone) Merck & Co., Inc. 1635
Decadron-LA Sterile Suspension (Dexamethasone Acetate) Merck & Co., Inc. 1646
Deltasone Tablets (Prednisone) Upjohn 2595
Depo-Medrol Single-Dose Vial (Methylprednisolone Acetate) Upjohn 2600
Depo-Medrol Sterile Aqueous Suspension (Methylprednisolone Acetate) Upjohn 2597
Hydeltrasol Injection, Sterile (Prednisolone Sodium Phosphate) Merck & Co., Inc. 1665
Hydrocortone Phosphate Injection, Sterile (Hydrocortisone Sodium Phosphate) Merck & Co., Inc. 1670
Hydrocortone Tablets (Hydrocortisone) Merck & Co., Inc. 1672
Medrol (Methylprednisolone) Upjohn 2621
Pediapred Oral Liquid (Prednisolone Sodium Phosphate) Fisons 995
Prelone Syrup (Prednisolone) Muro 1787
Solu-Cortef Sterile Powder (Hydrocortisone Sodium Succinate) Upjohn 2641
Solu-Medrol Sterile Powder (Methylprednisolone Sodium Succinate) Upjohn 2643

Donovania granulomatis infection (see under Granuloma inguinale)

Drowsiness, symptomatic relief of
No Doz Maximum Strength Caplets (Caffeine) Bristol-Myers Products ...... ▣ 622

Ductus arteriosus, patent, palliative maintenance
Indocin I.V. (Indomethacin Sodium Trihydrate) Merck & Co., Inc. 1684
Prostin VR Pediatric Sterile Solution (Alprostadil) Upjohn 2635

Dukes' stage C colon cancer (see under Carcinoma, colon, Dukes' stage C, adjunctive treatment in)

Duodenal ulcers, active, short-term treatment of
Axid Pulvules (Nizatidine) Lilly 1427
Carafate Suspension (Sucralfate) Marion Merrell Dow 1505
Carafate Tablets (Sucralfate) Marion Merrell Dow 1504
Pepcid Injection (Famotidine) Merck & Co., Inc. 1722
Pepcid (Famotidine) Merck & Co., Inc. 1720
PREVACID Delayed-Release Capsules (Lansoprazole) TAP 2562
Prilosec Delayed-Release Capsules (Omeprazole) Astra Merck 529
Tagamet (Cimetidine Hydrochloride) SmithKline Beecham Pharmaceuticals 2516
Zantac (Ranitidine Hydrochloride) Glaxo Wellcome 1209
Zantac Injection (Ranitidine Hydrochloride) Glaxo Wellcome 1207
Zantac Syrup (Ranitidine Hydrochloride) Glaxo Wellcome 1209

Duodenal ulcers, adjunctive therapy for
Donnatal (Phenobarbital, Belladonna Alkaloids) Robins 2060
Donnatal Extentabs (Phenobarbital, Belladonna Alkaloids) Robins 2061
Donnatal Tablets (Phenobarbital, Belladonna Alkaloids) Robins 2060

Duodenal ulcers, maintenance therapy for
Axid Pulvules (Nizatidine) Lilly 1427
Carafate Tablets (Sucralfate) Marion Merrell Dow 1504
Pepcid Injection (Famotidine) Merck & Co., Inc. 1722
Pepcid (Famotidine) Merck & Co., Inc. 1720
Tagamet (Cimetidine Hydrochloride) SmithKline Beecham Pharmaceuticals 2516
Zantac (Ranitidine Hydrochloride) Glaxo Wellcome 1209

Dysbetalipoproteinemia
Atromid-S Capsules (Clofibrate) Wyeth-Ayerst 2701

Dysentery, amoebic (see under Amebiasis, acute intestinal)

Dysmenorrhea, primary
Children's Advil Suspension (Ibuprofen) Wyeth-Ayerst 2692
Anaprox/Naprosyn (Naproxen Sodium) Roche Laboratories 2117
Maximum Strength Ascriptin (Aspirin Buffered, Calcium Carbonate) CIBA Consumer ...... ▣ 630
Extended-Release Bayer 8-Hour Aspirin (Aspirin) Miles Consumer ...... ▣ 712
Cataflam (Diclofenac Potassium) CibaGeneva 816
Cramp End Tablets (Ibuprofen) Ohm ...... ▣ 735
EC-Naprosyn Delayed-Release Tablets (Naproxen) Roche Laboratories 2117
IBU Tablets (Ibuprofen) Knoll Laboratories 1342
Children's Motrin Ibuprofen Oral Suspension (Ibuprofen) McNeil Consumer 1546
Motrin Tablets (Ibuprofen) Upjohn.. 2625
Motrin Ibuprofen Suspension, Oral Drops, Chewable Tablets, Caplets (Ibuprofen) McNeil Consumer 1546
Anaprox/Naprosyn (Naproxen) Roche Laboratories 2117
Orudis Capsules (Ketoprofen) Wyeth-Ayerst 2766
Ponstel (Mefenamic Acid) Parke-Davis 1925

Dyspepsia (see under Digestive disorders, symptomatic relief of)

Dysuria, symptomatic relief of
Urispas Tablets (Flavoxate Hydrochloride) SmithKline Beecham Pharmaceuticals 2532

E

E. cloacae gynecologic infections
Azactam for Injection (Aztreonam) Bristol-Myers Squibb 734
Timentin for Injection (Ticarcillin Disodium, Clavulanate Potassium) SmithKline Beecham Pharmaceuticals 2528

E. coli biliary tract infections
Ancef Injection (Cefazolin Sodium) SmithKline Beecham Pharmaceuticals 2465
Kefzol Vials, Faspak & ADD-Vantage (Cefazolin Sodium) Lilly 1456

E. coli bone and joint infections
Nebcin Vials, Hyporets & ADD-Vantage (Tobramycin Sulfate) Lilly 1464
Rocephin Injectable Vials, ADD-Vantage, Galaxy Container (Ceftriaxone Sodium) Roche Laboratories 2142
Tobramycin Sulfate Injection (Tobramycin Sulfate) Elkins-Sinn 968

E. coli central nervous system infections
Claforan Sterile and Injection (Cefotaxime Sodium) Hoechst-Roussel 1235

E. coli genital infections
Ancef Injection (Cefazolin Sodium) SmithKline Beecham Pharmaceuticals 2465
Mefoxin (Cefoxitin Sodium) Merck & Co., Inc. 1691
Mefoxin Premixed Intravenous Solution (Cefoxitin Sodium) Merck & Co., Inc. 1694
Omnipen for Oral Suspension (Ampicillin) Wyeth-Ayerst 2765

E. coli gynecological infections
Azactam for Injection (Aztreonam) Bristol-Myers Squibb 734
Cefizox for Intramuscular or Intravenous Use (Ceftizoxime Sodium) Fujisawa 1034
Cefobid Intravenous/Intramuscular (Cefoperazone Sodium) Roerig 2189
Cefobid Pharmacy Bulk Package - Not for Direct Infusion (Cefoperazone Sodium) Roerig 2192
Cefotan (Cefotetan) Zeneca 2829
Ceptaz (Ceftazidime) Glaxo Wellcome 1081
Claforan Sterile and Injection (Cefotaxime Sodium) Hoechst-Roussel 1235
Fortaz (Ceftazidime) Glaxo Wellcome 1100
Mefoxin (Cefoxitin Sodium) Merck & Co., Inc. 1691
Mefoxin Premixed Intravenous Solution (Cefoxitin Sodium) Merck & Co., Inc. 1694
Mezlin (Mezlocillin Sodium) Bayer Pharmaceutical 601
Mezlin Pharmacy Bulk Package (Mezlocillin Sodium) Bayer Pharmaceutical 604
Primaxin I.M. (Imipenem-Cilastatin Sodium) Merck & Co., Inc. 1727
Primaxin I.V. (Imipenem-Cilastatin Sodium) Merck & Co., Inc. 1729
Tazicef for Injection (Ceftazidime) SmithKline Beecham Pharmaceuticals 2519
Tazidime Vials, Faspak & ADD-Vantage (Ceftazidime) Lilly .. 1478
Ticar for Injection (Ticarcillin Disodium) SmithKline Beecham Pharmaceuticals 2526
Timentin for Injection (Ticarcillin Disodium, Clavulanate Potassium) SmithKline Beecham Pharmaceuticals 2528
Unasyn (Ampicillin Sodium, Sulbactam Sodium) Roerig 2212
Zosyn (Piperacillin Sodium, Tazobactam Sodium) Lederle 1419
Zosyn Pharmacy Bulk Package (Piperacillin Sodium, Tazobactam Sodium) Lederle 1422

E. coli infections
Achromycin V Capsules (Tetracycline Hydrochloride) Lederle 1367

(▣ Described in PDR For Nonprescription Drugs) (◉ Described in PDR For Ophthalmology)

Amikacin Sulfate Injection, USP (Amikacin Sulfate) Elkins-Sinn 960
Amikin Injectable (Amikacin Sulfate) Apothecon 501
Amoxil (Amoxicillin Trihydrate) SmithKline Beecham Pharmaceuticals 2464
Ancef Injection (Cefazolin Sodium) SmithKline Beecham Pharmaceuticals 2465
Augmentin (Amoxicillin Trihydrate, Clavulanate Potassium) SmithKline Beecham Pharmaceuticals 2468
Azactam for Injection (Aztreonam) Bristol-Myers Squibb 734
Azo Gantanol Tablets (Sulfamethoxazole, Phenazopyridine Hydrochloride) Roche Laboratories 2080
Azo Gantrisin Tablets (Sulfisoxazole, Phenazopyridine Hydrochloride) Roche Laboratories 2081
Bactrim DS Tablets (Trimethoprim, Sulfamethoxazole) Roche Laboratories 2084
Bactrim I.V. Infusion (Trimethoprim, Sulfamethoxazole) Roche Laboratories 2082
Bactrim (Trimethoprim, Sulfamethoxazole) Roche Laboratories 2084
Ceclor Pulvules & Suspension (Cefaclor) Lilly 1431
Cefizox for Intramuscular or Intravenous Use (Ceftizoxime Sodium) Fujisawa 1034
Cefobid Intravenous/Intramuscular (Cefoperazone Sodium) Roerig 2189
Cefobid Pharmacy Bulk Package - Not for Direct Infusion (Cefoperazone Sodium) Roerig 2192
Cefotan (Cefotetan) Zeneca 2829
Ceftin (Cefuroxime Axetil) Glaxo Wellcome 1078
Ceptaz (Ceftazidime) Glaxo Wellcome 1081
Cipro I.V. (Ciprofloxacin) Bayer Pharmaceutical 595
Cipro I.V. Pharmacy Bulk Package (Ciprofloxacin) Bayer Pharmaceutical 597
Cipro Tablets (Ciprofloxacin Hydrochloride) Bayer Pharmaceutical 592
Claforan Sterile and Injection (Cefotaxime Sodium) Hoechst-Roussel 1235
Coly-Mycin M Parenteral (Colistimethate Sodium) Parke-Davis 1905
Declomycin Tablets (Demeclocycline Hydrochloride) Lederle 1371
Doryx Capsules (Doxycycline Hyclate) Parke-Davis 1913
Duricef (Cefadroxil Monohydrate) Bristol-Myers Squibb 748
Dynacin Capsules (Minocycline Hydrochloride) Medicis 1590
Floxin I.V. (Ofloxacin) McNeil Pharmaceutical 1571
Floxin Tablets (200 mg, 300 mg, 400 mg) (Ofloxacin) McNeil Pharmaceutical 1567
Fortaz (Ceftazidime) Glaxo Wellcome 1100
Gantanol Tablets (Sulfamethoxazole) Roche Laboratories 2119
Gantrisin (Acetyl Sulfisoxazole) Roche Laboratories 2120
Garamycin Injectable (Gentamicin Sulfate) Schering 2360
Geocillin Tablets (Carbenicillin Indanyl Sodium) Roerig 2199
Keflex Pulvules & Oral Suspension (Cephalexin) Dista 914
Keftab Tablets (Cephalexin Hydrochloride) Dista 915
Kefurox Vials, Faspak & ADD-Vantage (Cefuroxime Sodium) Lilly 1454
Kefzol Vials, Faspak & ADD-Vantage (Cefazolin Sodium) Lilly 1456
Lorabid Suspension and Pulvules (Loracarbef) Lilly 1459
Macrobid Capsules (Nitrofurantoin Monohydrate) Procter & Gamble Pharmaceuticals 1988
Macrodantin Capsules (Nitrofurantoin) Procter & Gamble Pharmaceuticals 1989
Mandol Vials, Faspak & ADD-Vantage (Cefamandole Nafate) Lilly 1461
Maxaquin Tablets (Lomefloxacin Hydrochloride) Searle 2440
Mefoxin (Cefoxitin Sodium) Merck & Co., Inc. 1691
Mefoxin Premixed Intravenous Solution (Cefoxitin Sodium) Merck & Co., Inc. 1694
Mezlin (Mezlocillin Sodium) Bayer Pharmaceutical 601
Mezlin Pharmacy Bulk Package (Mezlocillin Sodium) Bayer Pharmaceutical 604
Minocin Intravenous (Minocycline Hydrochloride) Lederle 1382
Minocin Oral Suspension (Minocycline Hydrochloride) Lederle 1385
Minocin Pellet-Filled Capsules (Minocycline Hydrochloride) Lederle 1383
Monocid Injection (Cefonicid Sodium) SmithKline Beecham Pharmaceuticals 2497
Monodox Capsules (Doxycycline Monohydrate) Oclassen 1805
Nebcin Vials, Hyporets & ADD-Vantage (Tobramycin Sulfate) Lilly 1464
Netromycin Injection 100 mg/ml (Netilmicin Sulfate) Schering 2373
Noroxin Tablets (Norfloxacin) Merck & Co., Inc. 1715
Noroxin Tablets (Norfloxacin) Roberts 2048
Omnipen Capsules (Ampicillin) Wyeth-Ayerst 2764
Omnipen for Oral Suspension (Ampicillin) Wyeth-Ayerst 2765
Penetrex Tablets (Enoxacin) Rhone-Poulenc Rorer Pharmaceuticals 2031
Pfizerpen for Injection (Penicillin G Potassium) Roerig 2203
Pipracil (Piperacillin Sodium) Lederle 1390
Polymyxin B Sulfate, Aerosporin Brand Sterile Powder (Polymyxin B Sulfate) Glaxo Wellcome 1154
Primaxin I.M. (Imipenem-Cilastatin Sodium) Merck & Co., Inc. 1727
Primaxin I.V. (Imipenem-Cilastatin Sodium) Merck & Co., Inc. 1729
Proloprim Tablets (Trimethoprim) Glaxo Wellcome 1155
Rocephin Injectable Vials, ADD-Vantage, Galaxy Container (Ceftriaxone Sodium) Roche Laboratories 2142
Septra (Trimethoprim, Sulfamethoxazole) Glaxo Wellcome 1174
Septra I.V. Infusion (Trimethoprim, Sulfamethoxazole) Glaxo Wellcome 1169
Septra I.V. Infusion ADD-Vantage Vials (Trimethoprim, Sulfamethoxazole) Glaxo Wellcome 1171
Septra (Trimethoprim, Sulfamethoxazole) Glaxo Wellcome 1174
Suprax (Cefixime) Lederle 1399
Tazicef for Injection (Ceftazidime) SmithKline Beecham Pharmaceuticals 2519
Tazidime Vials, Faspak & ADD-Vantage (Ceftazidime) Lilly 1478
Terramycin Intramuscular Solution (Oxytetracycline) Roerig 2210
Ticar for Injection (Ticarcillin Disodium) SmithKline Beecham Pharmaceuticals 2526
Timentin for Injection (Ticarcillin Disodium, Clavulanate Potassium) SmithKline Beecham Pharmaceuticals 2528
Tobramycin Sulfate Injection (Tobramycin Sulfate) Elkins-Sinn 968
Trimpex Tablets (Trimethoprim) Roche Laboratories 2163
Unasyn (Ampicillin Sodium, Sulbactam Sodium) Roerig 2212
Vantin for Oral Suspension and Vantin Tablets (Cefpodoxime Proxetil) Upjohn 2646
Vibramycin (Doxycycline Calcium) Pfizer Labs 1941
Vibramycin Hyclate Intravenous (Doxycycline Hyclate) Roerig 2215
Vibramycin (Doxycycline Monohydrate) Pfizer Labs 1941
Zefazone (Cefmetazole Sodium) Upjohn 2654
Zinacef (Cefuroxime Sodium) Glaxo Wellcome 1211
Zosyn (Piperacillin Sodium, Tazobactam Sodium) Lederle 1419
Zosyn Pharmacy Bulk Package (Piperacillin Sodium, Tazobactam Sodium) Lederle 1422

E. coli infections, ocular

AK-CIDE (Prednisolone Acetate, Sulfacetamide Sodium) Akorn ...... ◉ 202
AK-CIDE Ointment (Prednisolone Acetate, Sulfacetamide Sodium) Akorn ...... ◉ 202
AK-Spore (Bacitracin Zinc, Neomycin Sulfate, Polymyxin B Sulfate) Akorn ...... ◉ 204
AK-Trol Ointment & Suspension (Dexamethasone, Neomycin Sulfate, Polymyxin B Sulfate) Akorn ...... ◉ 205
Blephamide Liquifilm Sterile Ophthalmic Suspension (Prednisolone Acetate, Sulfacetamide Sodium) Allergan 476
Blephamide Ointment (Sulfacetamide Sodium, Prednisolone Acetate) Allergan ...... ◉ 237
Chloromycetin Ophthalmic Ointment, 1% (Chloramphenicol) Parke-Davis ...... ◉ 310
Chloromycetin Ophthalmic Solution (Chloramphenicol) Parke-Davis ...... ◉ 310
Chloroptic S.O.P. (Chloramphenicol) Allergan ...... ◉ 239
Cortisporin Ophthalmic Ointment Sterile (Polymyxin B Sulfate, Bacitracin Zinc, Neomycin Sulfate, Hydrocortisone) Glaxo Wellcome 1085
Cortisporin Ophthalmic Suspension Sterile (Hydrocortisone, Polymyxin B Sulfate, Neomycin Sulfate) Glaxo Wellcome 1086
Dexacidin Ointment (Dexamethasone, Neomycin Sulfate, Polymyxin B Sulfate) CIBA Vision Ophthalmics ...... ◉ 263
FML-S Liquifilm (Sulfacetamide Sodium, Fluorometholone) Allergan ...... ◉ 242
Genoptic Sterile Ophthalmic Solution (Gentamicin Sulfate) Allergan ...... ◉ 243
Genoptic Sterile Ophthalmic Ointment (Gentamicin Sulfate) Allergan ...... ◉ 243
Gentak (Gentamicin Sulfate) Akorn ...... ◉ 208
Maxitrol Ophthalmic Ointment and Suspension (Dexamethasone, Neomycin Sulfate, Polymyxin B Sulfate) Alcon Laboratories ...... ◉ 224
NeoDecadron Sterile Ophthalmic Ointment (Neomycin Sulfate, Dexamethasone Sodium Phosphate) Merck & Co., Inc. 1712
NeoDecadron Sterile Ophthalmic Solution (Neomycin Sulfate, Dexamethasone Sodium Phosphate) Merck & Co., Inc. 1713
Ophthocort (Chloramphenicol, Polymyxin B Sulfate, Hydrocortisone Acetate) Parke-Davis ...... ◉ 311
Poly-Pred Liquifilm (Neomycin Sulfate, Polymyxin B Sulfate, Prednisolone Acetate) Allergan ...... ◉ 248
Pred-G Liquifilm Sterile Ophthalmic Suspension (Gentamicin Sulfate, Prednisolone Acetate) Allergan ...... ◉ 251
Pred-G S.O.P. Sterile Ophthalmic Ointment (Gentamicin Sulfate, Prednisolone Acetate) Allergan ...... ◉ 252
Terra-Cortril Ophthalmic Suspension (Oxytetracycline Hydrochloride, Hydrocortisone Acetate) Roerig 2210
TobraDex Ophthalmic Suspension and Ointment (Dexamethasone, Tobramycin) Alcon Laboratories 473
Vasocidin Ointment (Prednisolone Acetate, Sulfacetamide Sodium) CIBA Vision Ophthalmics ...... ◉ 268
Vasocidin Ophthalmic Solution (Prednisolone Sodium Phosphate, Sulfacetamide Sodium) CIBA Vision Ophthalmics ...... ◉ 270

E. coli intra-abdominal infections

Azactam for Injection (Aztreonam) Bristol-Myers Squibb 734
Cefizox for Intramuscular or Intravenous Use (Ceftizoxime Sodium) Fujisawa 1034
Cefobid Intravenous/Intramuscular (Cefoperazone Sodium) Roerig 2189
Cefobid Pharmacy Bulk Package - Not for Direct Infusion (Cefoperazone Sodium) Roerig 2192
Cefotan (Cefotetan) Zeneca 2829
Ceptaz (Ceftazidime) Glaxo Wellcome 1081
Claforan Sterile and Injection (Cefotaxime Sodium) Hoechst-Roussel 1235
Fortaz (Ceftazidime) Glaxo Wellcome 1100
Mefoxin (Cefoxitin Sodium) Merck & Co., Inc. 1691
Mefoxin Premixed Intravenous Solution (Cefoxitin Sodium) Merck & Co., Inc. 1694
Mezlin (Mezlocillin Sodium) Bayer Pharmaceutical 601
Mezlin Pharmacy Bulk Package (Mezlocillin Sodium) Bayer Pharmaceutical 604
Nebcin Vials, Hyporets & ADD-Vantage (Tobramycin Sulfate) Lilly 1464
Netromycin Injection 100 mg/ml (Netilmicin Sulfate) Schering 2373
Omnipen for Oral Suspension (Ampicillin) Wyeth-Ayerst 2765
Pipracil (Piperacillin Sodium) Lederle 1390
Primaxin I.M. (Imipenem-Cilastatin Sodium) Merck & Co., Inc. 1727
Primaxin I.V. (Imipenem-Cilastatin Sodium) Merck & Co., Inc. 1729
Rocephin Injectable Vials, ADD-Vantage, Galaxy Container (Ceftriaxone Sodium) Roche Laboratories 2142
Tazicef for Injection (Ceftazidime) SmithKline Beecham Pharmaceuticals 2519
Tazidime Vials, Faspak & ADD-Vantage (Ceftazidime) Lilly 1478
Timentin for Injection (Ticarcillin Disodium, Clavulanate Potassium) SmithKline Beecham Pharmaceuticals 2528
Tobramycin Sulfate Injection (Tobramycin Sulfate) Elkins-Sinn 968
Unasyn (Ampicillin Sodium, Sulbactam Sodium) Roerig 2212
Zefazone (Cefmetazole Sodium) Upjohn 2654

E. coli lower respiratory tract infections

Azactam for Injection (Aztreonam) Bristol-Myers Squibb 734
Cefizox for Intramuscular or Intravenous Use (Ceftizoxime Sodium) Fujisawa 1034
Cefotan (Cefotetan) Zeneca 2829
Ceptaz (Ceftazidime) Glaxo Wellcome 1081
Cipro I.V. (Ciprofloxacin) Bayer Pharmaceutical 595
Cipro I.V. Pharmacy Bulk Package (Ciprofloxacin) Bayer Pharmaceutical 597
Cipro Tablets (Ciprofloxacin Hydrochloride) Bayer Pharmaceutical 592
Claforan Sterile and Injection (Cefotaxime Sodium) Hoechst-Roussel 1235
Fortaz (Ceftazidime) Glaxo Wellcome 1100
Kefurox Vials, Faspak & ADD-Vantage (Cefuroxime Sodium) Lilly 1454
Mefoxin (Cefoxitin Sodium) Merck & Co., Inc. 1691
Mefoxin Premixed Intravenous Solution (Cefoxitin Sodium) Merck & Co., Inc. 1694

(▣ Described in PDR For Nonprescription Drugs) (◉ Described in PDR For Ophthalmology)

1479 Indications Index E. coli

Mezlin (Mezlocillin Sodium) Bayer Pharmaceutical ... 601
Mezlin Pharmacy Bulk Package (Mezlocillin Sodium) Bayer Pharmaceutical ... 604
Monocid Injection (Cefonicid Sodium) SmithKline Beecham Pharmaceuticals ... 2497
Nebcin Vials, Hyporets & ADD-Vantage (Tobramycin Sulfate) Lilly ... 1464
Netromycin Injection 100 mg/ml (Netilmicin Sulfate) Schering ... 2373
Pipracil (Piperacillin Sodium) Lederle ... 1390
Primaxin I.V. (Imipenem-Cilastatin Sodium) Merck & Co., Inc. ... 1729
Rocephin Injectable Vials, ADD-Vantage, Galaxy Container (Ceftriaxone Sodium) Roche Laboratories ... 2142
Tazicef for Injection (Ceftazidime) SmithKline Beecham Pharmaceuticals ... 2519
Tazidime Vials, Faspak & ADD-Vantage (Ceftazidime) Lilly ... 1478
Tobramycin Sulfate Injection (Tobramycin Sulfate) Elkins-Sinn ... 968
Zefazone (Cefmetazole Sodium) Upjohn ... 2654
Zinacef (Cefuroxime Sodium) Glaxo Wellcome ... 1211

E. coli meningitis

Rocephin Injectable Vials, ADD-Vantage, Galaxy Container (Ceftriaxone Sodium) Roche Laboratories ... 2142

E. coli peritonitis

Cefobid Intravenous/Intramuscular (Cefoperazone Sodium) Roerig ... 2189
Cefobid Pharmacy Bulk Package - Not for Direct Infusion (Cefoperazone Sodium) Roerig ... 2192
Ceptaz (Ceftazidime) Glaxo Wellcome ... 1081
Fortaz (Ceftazidime) Glaxo Wellcome ... 1100
Mandol Vials, Faspak & ADD-Vantage (Cefamandole Nafate) Lilly ... 1461
Mefoxin (Cefoxitin Sodium) Merck & Co., Inc. ... 1691
Mefoxin Premixed Intravenous Solution (Cefoxitin Sodium) Merck & Co., Inc. ... 1694
Mezlin (Mezlocillin Sodium) Bayer Pharmaceutical ... 601
Mezlin Pharmacy Bulk Package (Mezlocillin Sodium) Bayer Pharmaceutical ... 604
Nebcin Vials, Hyporets & ADD-Vantage (Tobramycin Sulfate) Lilly ... 1464
Netromycin Injection 100 mg/ml (Netilmicin Sulfate) Schering ... 2373
Tazidime Vials, Faspak & ADD-Vantage (Ceftazidime) Lilly ... 1478
Timentin for Injection (Ticarcillin Disodium, Clavulanate Potassium) SmithKline Beecham Pharmaceuticals ... 2528
Zosyn (Piperacillin Sodium, Tazobactam Sodium) Lederle ... 1419
Zosyn Pharmacy Bulk Package (Piperacillin Sodium, Tazobactam Sodium) Lederle ... 1422

E. coli prostatitis

Ancef Injection (Cefazolin Sodium) SmithKline Beecham Pharmaceuticals ... 2465
Floxin I.V. (Ofloxacin) McNeil Pharmaceutical ... 1571
Floxin Tablets (200 mg, 300 mg, 400 mg) (Ofloxacin) McNeil Pharmaceutical ... 1567
Geocillin Tablets (Carbenicillin Indanyl Sodium) Roerig ... 2199
Keflex Pulvules & Oral Suspension (Cephalexin) Dista ... 914
Keftab Tablets (Cephalexin Hydrochloride) Dista ... 915
Noroxin Tablets (Norfloxacin) Merck & Co., Inc. ... 1715
Noroxin Tablets (Norfloxacin) Roberts ... 2048

E. coli respiratory tract infections

Cefobid Intravenous/Intramuscular (Cefoperazone Sodium) Roerig ... 2189
Cefobid Pharmacy Bulk Package - Not for Direct Infusion (Cefoperazone Sodium) Roerig ... 2192
Ticar for Injection (Ticarcillin Disodium) SmithKline Beecham Pharmaceuticals ... 2526

E. coli septicemia

Ancef Injection (Cefazolin Sodium) SmithKline Beecham Pharmaceuticals ... 2465
Azactam for Injection (Aztreonam) Bristol-Myers Squibb ... 734
Cefizox for Intramuscular or Intravenous Use (Ceftizoxime Sodium) Fujisawa ... 1034
Cefobid Intravenous/Intramuscular (Cefoperazone Sodium) Roerig ... 2189
Cefobid Pharmacy Bulk Package - Not for Direct Infusion (Cefoperazone Sodium) Roerig ... 2192
Ceptaz (Ceftazidime) Glaxo Wellcome ... 1081
Cipro I.V. (Ciprofloxacin) Bayer Pharmaceutical ... 595
Claforan Sterile and Injection (Cefotaxime Sodium) Hoechst-Roussel ... 1235
Fortaz (Ceftazidime) Glaxo Wellcome ... 1100
Kefurox Vials, Faspak & ADD-Vantage (Cefuroxime Sodium) Lilly ... 1454
Kefzol Vials, Faspak & ADD-Vantage (Cefazolin Sodium) Lilly ... 1456
Mefoxin (Cefoxitin Sodium) Merck & Co., Inc. ... 1691
Mefoxin Premixed Intravenous Solution (Cefoxitin Sodium) Merck & Co., Inc. ... 1694
Mezlin (Mezlocillin Sodium) Bayer Pharmaceutical ... 601
Mezlin Pharmacy Bulk Package (Mezlocillin Sodium) Bayer Pharmaceutical ... 604
Monocid Injection (Cefonicid Sodium) SmithKline Beecham Pharmaceuticals ... 2497
Nebcin Vials, Hyporets & ADD-Vantage (Tobramycin Sulfate) Lilly ... 1464
Netromycin Injection 100 mg/ml (Netilmicin Sulfate) Schering ... 2373
Pfizerpen for Injection (Penicillin G Potassium) Roerig ... 2203
Primaxin I.V. (Imipenem-Cilastatin Sodium) Merck & Co., Inc. ... 1729
Rocephin Injectable Vials, ADD-Vantage, Galaxy Container (Ceftriaxone Sodium) Roche Laboratories ... 2142
Tazicef for Injection (Ceftazidime) SmithKline Beecham Pharmaceuticals ... 2519
Tazidime Vials, Faspak & ADD-Vantage (Ceftazidime) Lilly ... 1478
Ticar for Injection (Ticarcillin Disodium) SmithKline Beecham Pharmaceuticals ... 2526
Timentin for Injection (Ticarcillin Disodium, Clavulanate Potassium) SmithKline Beecham Pharmaceuticals ... 2528
Tobramycin Sulfate Injection (Tobramycin Sulfate) Elkins-Sinn ... 968
Zinacef (Cefuroxime Sodium) Glaxo Wellcome ... 1211

E. coli skin and skin structure infections

Amoxil (Amoxicillin Trihydrate) SmithKline Beecham Pharmaceuticals ... 2464
Augmentin (Amoxicillin Trihydrate, Clavulanate Potassium) SmithKline Beecham Pharmaceuticals ... 2468
Azactam for Injection (Aztreonam) Bristol-Myers Squibb ... 734
Cefizox for Intramuscular or Intravenous Use (Ceftizoxime Sodium) Fujisawa ... 1034
Cefotan (Cefotetan) Zeneca ... 2829
Ceptaz (Ceftazidime) Glaxo Wellcome ... 1081
Cipro I.V. (Ciprofloxacin) Bayer Pharmaceutical ... 595
Cipro I.V. Pharmacy Bulk Package (Ciprofloxacin) Bayer Pharmaceutical ... 597
Cipro Tablets (Ciprofloxacin Hydrochloride) Bayer Pharmaceutical ... 592
Claforan Sterile and Injection (Cefotaxime Sodium) Hoechst-Roussel ... 1235
Fortaz (Ceftazidime) Glaxo Wellcome ... 1100
Kefurox Vials, Faspak & ADD-Vantage (Cefuroxime Sodium) Lilly ... 1454
Mandol Vials, Faspak & ADD-Vantage (Cefamandole Nafate) Lilly ... 1461
Mefoxin (Cefoxitin Sodium) Merck & Co., Inc. ... 1691
Mefoxin Premixed Intravenous Solution (Cefoxitin Sodium) Merck & Co., Inc. ... 1694
Mezlin (Mezlocillin Sodium) Bayer Pharmaceutical ... 601
Mezlin Pharmacy Bulk Package (Mezlocillin Sodium) Bayer Pharmaceutical ... 604
Nebcin Vials, Hyporets & ADD-Vantage (Tobramycin Sulfate) Lilly ... 1464
Netromycin Injection 100 mg/ml (Netilmicin Sulfate) Schering ... 2373
Pipracil (Piperacillin Sodium) Lederle ... 1390
Primaxin I.M. (Imipenem-Cilastatin Sodium) Merck & Co., Inc. ... 1727
Primaxin I.V. (Imipenem-Cilastatin Sodium) Merck & Co., Inc. ... 1729
Rocephin Injectable Vials, ADD-Vantage, Galaxy Container (Ceftriaxone Sodium) Roche Laboratories ... 2142
Tazicef for Injection (Ceftazidime) SmithKline Beecham Pharmaceuticals ... 2519
Tazidime Vials, Faspak & ADD-Vantage (Ceftazidime) Lilly ... 1478
Ticar for Injection (Ticarcillin Disodium) SmithKline Beecham Pharmaceuticals ... 2526
Timentin for Injection (Ticarcillin Disodium, Clavulanate Potassium) SmithKline Beecham Pharmaceuticals ... 2528
Tobramycin Sulfate Injection (Tobramycin Sulfate) Elkins-Sinn ... 968
Unasyn (Ampicillin Sodium, Sulbactam Sodium) Roerig ... 2212
Zefazone (Cefmetazole Sodium) Upjohn ... 2654
Zinacef (Cefuroxime Sodium) Glaxo Wellcome ... 1211

E. coli urinary tract infections

Ancef Injection (Cefazolin Sodium) SmithKline Beecham Pharmaceuticals ... 2465
Augmentin (Amoxicillin Trihydrate, Clavulanate Potassium) SmithKline Beecham Pharmaceuticals ... 2468
Azactam for Injection (Aztreonam) Bristol-Myers Squibb ... 734
Azo Gantanol Tablets (Sulfamethoxazole, Phenazopyridine Hydrochloride) Roche Laboratories ... 2080
Azo Gantrisin Tablets (Sulfisoxazole, Phenazopyridine Hydrochloride) Roche Laboratories ... 2081
Bactrim DS Tablets (Trimethoprim, Sulfamethoxazole) Roche Laboratories ... 2084
Bactrim I.V. Infusion (Trimethoprim, Sulfamethoxazole) Roche Laboratories ... 2082
Bactrim (Trimethoprim, Sulfamethoxazole) Roche Laboratories ... 2084
Ceclor Pulvules & Suspension (Cefaclor) Lilly ... 1431
Cefizox for Intramuscular or Intravenous Use (Ceftizoxime Sodium) Fujisawa ... 1034
Cefobid Intravenous/Intramuscular (Cefoperazone Sodium) Roerig ... 2189
Cefobid Pharmacy Bulk Package - Not for Direct Infusion (Cefoperazone Sodium) Roerig ... 2192
Cefotan (Cefotetan) Zeneca ... 2829
Ceftin (Cefuroxime Axetil) Glaxo Wellcome ... 1078
Ceptaz (Ceftazidime) Glaxo Wellcome ... 1081
Cipro I.V. (Ciprofloxacin) Bayer Pharmaceutical ... 595
Cipro I.V. Pharmacy Bulk Package (Ciprofloxacin) Bayer Pharmaceutical ... 597
Cipro Tablets (Ciprofloxacin Hydrochloride) Bayer Pharmaceutical ... 592
Claforan Sterile and Injection (Cefotaxime Sodium) Hoechst-Roussel ... 1235
Duricef (Cefadroxil Monohydrate) Bristol-Myers Squibb ... 748
Floxin I.V. (Ofloxacin) McNeil Pharmaceutical ... 1571
Floxin Tablets (200 mg, 300 mg, 400 mg) (Ofloxacin) McNeil Pharmaceutical ... 1567
Fortaz (Ceftazidime) Glaxo Wellcome ... 1100
Gantanol Tablets (Sulfamethoxazole) Roche Laboratories ... 2119
Gantrisin (Acetyl Sulfisoxazole) Roche Laboratories ... 2120
Geocillin Tablets (Carbenicillin Indanyl Sodium) Roerig ... 2199
Keflex Pulvules & Oral Suspension (Cephalexin) Dista ... 914
Keftab Tablets (Cephalexin Hydrochloride) Dista ... 915
Kefurox Vials, Faspak & ADD-Vantage (Cefuroxime Sodium) Lilly ... 1454
Kefzol Vials, Faspak & ADD-Vantage (Cefazolin Sodium) Lilly ... 1456
Lorabid Suspension and Pulvules (Loracarbef) Lilly ... 1459
Macrobid Capsules (Nitrofurantoin Monohydrate) Procter & Gamble Pharmaceuticals ... 1988
Macrodantin Capsules (Nitrofurantoin) Procter & Gamble Pharmaceuticals ... 1989
Mandol Vials, Faspak & ADD-Vantage (Cefamandole Nafate) Lilly ... 1461
Maxaquin Tablets (Lomefloxacin Hydrochloride) Searle ... 2440
Mefoxin (Cefoxitin Sodium) Merck & Co., Inc. ... 1691
Mefoxin Premixed Intravenous Solution (Cefoxitin Sodium) Merck & Co., Inc. ... 1694
Mezlin (Mezlocillin Sodium) Bayer Pharmaceutical ... 601
Mezlin Pharmacy Bulk Package (Mezlocillin Sodium) Bayer Pharmaceutical ... 604
Monocid Injection (Cefonicid Sodium) SmithKline Beecham Pharmaceuticals ... 2497
Nebcin Vials, Hyporets & ADD-Vantage (Tobramycin Sulfate) Lilly ... 1464
NegGram (Nalidixic Acid) Sanofi Winthrop ... 2323
Netromycin Injection 100 mg/ml (Netilmicin Sulfate) Schering ... 2373
Noroxin Tablets (Norfloxacin) Merck & Co., Inc. ... 1715
Noroxin Tablets (Norfloxacin) Roberts ... 2048
Omnipen for Oral Suspension (Ampicillin) Wyeth-Ayerst ... 2765
Penetrex Tablets (Enoxacin) Rhone-Poulenc Rorer Pharmaceuticals ... 2031
Pipracil (Piperacillin Sodium) Lederle ... 1390
Polymyxin B Sulfate, Aerosporin Brand Sterile Powder (Polymyxin B Sulfate) Glaxo Wellcome ... 1154
Primaxin I.V. (Imipenem-Cilastatin Sodium) Merck & Co., Inc. ... 1729
Proloprim Tablets (Trimethoprim) Glaxo Wellcome ... 1155
Rocephin Injectable Vials, ADD-Vantage, Galaxy Container (Ceftriaxone Sodium) Roche Laboratories ... 2142
Septra (Trimethoprim, Sulfamethoxazole) Glaxo Wellcome ... 1174
Septra I.V. Infusion (Trimethoprim, Sulfamethoxazole) Glaxo Wellcome ... 1169
Septra I.V. Infusion ADD-Vantage Vials (Trimethoprim,

(▣ Described in PDR For Nonprescription Drugs) (⊙ Described in PDR For Ophthalmology)

E. coli Indications Index 1480

Sulfamethoxazole) Glaxo Wellcome ... 1171
Septra (Trimethoprim, Sulfamethoxazole) Glaxo Wellcome ... 1174
Seromycin Pulvules (Cycloserine) Lilly ... 1476
Spectrobid Tablets (Bacampicillin Hydrochloride) Roerig ... 2206
Streptomycin Sulfate Injection (Streptomycin Sulfate) Roerig ... 2208
Suprax (Cefixime) Lederle ... 1399
Tazicef for Injection (Ceftazidime) SmithKline Beecham Pharmaceuticals ... 2519
Tazidime Vials, Faspak & ADD-Vantage (Ceftazidime) Lilly ... 1478
Ticar for Injection (Ticarcillin Disodium) SmithKline Beecham Pharmaceuticals ... 2526
Timentin for Injection (Ticarcillin Disodium, Clavulanate Potassium) SmithKline Beecham Pharmaceuticals ... 2528
Tobramycin Sulfate Injection (Tobramycin Sulfate) Elkins-Sinn ... 968
Trimpex Tablets (Trimethoprim) Roche Laboratories ... 2163
Vantin for Oral Suspension and Vantin Tablets (Cefpodoxime Proxetil) Upjohn ... 2646
Zefazone (Cefmetazole Sodium) Upjohn ... 2654
Zinacef (Cefuroxime Sodium) Glaxo Wellcome ... 1211

E. coli-induced diarrhea (see under Diarrhea, E. coli-induced)

Ear wax removal (see under Cerumen, removal of)

Ear, infection (see under Otitis externa; Otitis media, acute)

Ears, surgical procedures, irrigation of
AMO Endosol (Balanced Salt Solution) (Balanced Salt Solution) Allergan ... ◉ 232
BSS (15 mL & 30 mL) Sterile Irrigation Solution (Balanced Salt Solution) Alcon Laboratories ... ◉ 214
BSS (250 mL) Sterile Irrigation Solution (Balanced Salt Solution) Alcon Laboratories ... ◉ 214
BSS (500 mL) Sterile Irrigation Solution (Balanced Salt Solution) Alcon Laboratories ... ◉ 214

Eczema, allergic
Mantadil Cream (Chlorcyclizine Hydrochloride) Glaxo Wellcome ... 1135

Eczema, atopic
Cortaid Spray (Hydrocortisone) Upjohn ... ▣ 836
Temaril Tablets, Syrup and Spansule Extended-Release Capsules (Trimeprazine Tartrate) Allergan ... 483

Eczema, nuchal
Mantadil Cream (Chlorcyclizine Hydrochloride) Glaxo Wellcome ... 1135

Eczema, nummular
Mantadil Cream (Chlorcyclizine Hydrochloride) Glaxo Wellcome ... 1135

Eczema, unspecified (see under Skin, inflammatory conditions)

Eczemas, aid in evaluation of
T.R.U.E. Test (Allergens) Glaxo Wellcome ... 1189

Edema due to hyperaldosteronism, secondary
Dyrenium Capsules (Triamterene) SmithKline Beecham Pharmaceuticals ... 2481

Edema due to pathological causes in pregnancy
Aldactazide (Spironolactone, Hydrochlorothiazide) Searle ... 2413
Aldactone (Spironolactone) Searle ... 2414
Diucardin Tablets (Hydroflumethiazide) Wyeth-Ayerst ... 2718
Diuril Oral Suspension (Chlorothiazide) Merck & Co., Inc. ... 1653
Diuril Sodium Intravenous (Chlorothiazide Sodium) Merck & Co., Inc. ... 1652
Diuril Tablets (Chlorothiazide) Merck & Co., Inc. ... 1653
Dyazide (Triamterene, Hydrochlorothiazide) SmithKline Beecham Pharmaceuticals ... 2479
Dyrenium Capsules (Triamterene) SmithKline Beecham Pharmaceuticals ... 2481
HydroDIURIL Tablets (Hydrochlorothiazide) Merck & Co., Inc. ... 1674
Hydropres Tablets (Reserpine, Hydrochlorothiazide) Merck & Co., Inc. ... 1675
Zaroxolyn Tablets (Metolazone) Fisons ... 1000

Edema, acute glomerulonephritis-induced
Diuril Oral Suspension (Chlorothiazide) Merck & Co., Inc. ... 1653
Diuril Sodium Intravenous (Chlorothiazide Sodium) Merck & Co., Inc. ... 1652
Diuril Tablets (Chlorothiazide) Merck & Co., Inc. ... 1653
Enduron Tablets (Methyclothiazide) Abbott ... 420
HydroDIURIL Tablets (Hydrochlorothiazide) Merck & Co., Inc. ... 1674
Oretic Tablets (Hydrochlorothiazide) Abbott ... 443
Thalitone (Chlorthalidone) Horus ... 1245

Edema, acute pulmonary
Edecrin Sodium Intravenous (Ethacrynate Sodium) Merck & Co., Inc. ... 1657

Edema, adjunctive therapy in
Diucardin Tablets (Hydroflumethiazide) Wyeth-Ayerst ... 2718
Enduron Tablets (Methyclothiazide) Abbott ... 420
Esidrix Tablets (Hydrochlorothiazide) CibaGeneva ... 821
Maxzide (Triamterene, Hydrochlorothiazide) Lederle ... 1380
Oretic Tablets (Hydrochlorothiazide) Abbott ... 443

Edema, cerebral
Decadron Phosphate Injection (Dexamethasone Sodium Phosphate) Merck & Co., Inc. ... 1637
Decadron Tablets (Dexamethasone) Merck & Co., Inc. ... 1635

Edema, chronic renal failure-induced
Bumex (Bumetanide) Roche Laboratories ... 2093
Demadex Tablets and Injection (Torsemide) Boehringer Mannheim ... 686
Diuril Oral (Chlorothiazide) Merck & Co., Inc. ... 1653
Enduron Tablets (Methyclothiazide) Abbott ... 420
HydroDIURIL Tablets (Hydrochlorothiazide) Merck & Co., Inc. ... 1674
Lasix Injection, Oral Solution and Tablets (Furosemide) Hoechst-Roussel ... 1240
Oretic Tablets (Hydrochlorothiazide) Abbott ... 443
Thalitone (Chlorthalidone) Horus ... 1245

Edema, cirrhosis of the liver-induced, treatment of
Aldactazide (Spironolactone, Hydrochlorothiazide) Searle ... 2413
Aldactone (Spironolactone) Searle ... 2414
Dyrenium Capsules (Triamterene) SmithKline Beecham Pharmaceuticals ... 2481
Edecrin (Ethacrynate Sodium) Merck & Co., Inc. ... 1657
Lasix Injection, Oral Solution and Tablets (Furosemide) Hoechst-Roussel ... 1240

Edema, congenital heart disease-induced, short-term management of
Edecrin (Ethacrynate Sodium) Merck & Co., Inc. ... 1657

Edema, congestive heart failure-induced, adjunctive therapy in (see also under Congestive heart failure; Congestive heart failure, adjunct in)
Aldactazide (Spironolactone, Hydrochlorothiazide) Searle ... 2413
Aldactone (Spironolactone) Searle ... 2414
Diamox (Acetazolamide) Lederle ... 1372
Diucardin Tablets (Hydroflumethiazide) Wyeth-Ayerst ... 2718
Diuril Oral Suspension (Chlorothiazide) Merck & Co., Inc. ... 1653
Diuril Sodium Intravenous (Chlorothiazide Sodium) Merck & Co., Inc. ... 1652
Diuril Tablets (Chlorothiazide) Merck & Co., Inc. ... 1653
Enduron Tablets (Methyclothiazide) Abbott ... 420
HydroDIURIL Tablets (Hydrochlorothiazide) Merck & Co., Inc. ... 1674
Lozol Tablets (Indapamide) Rhone-Poulenc Rorer Pharmaceuticals ... 2022
Oretic Tablets (Hydrochlorothiazide) Abbott ... 443
Thalitone (Chlorthalidone) Horus ... 1245

Edema, congestive heart failure-induced, treatment of (see also under Congestive heart failure; Congestive heart failure, adjunct in)
Aldactazide (Spironolactone, Hydrochlorothiazide) Searle ... 2413
Aldactone (Spironolactone) Searle ... 2414
Bumex (Bumetanide) Roche Laboratories ... 2093
Demadex Tablets and Injection (Torsemide) Boehringer Mannheim ... 686
Dyrenium Capsules (Triamterene) SmithKline Beecham Pharmaceuticals ... 2481
Edecrin (Ethacrynate Sodium) Merck & Co., Inc. ... 1657
Lasix Injection, Oral Solution and Tablets (Furosemide) Hoechst-Roussel ... 1240
Lozol Tablets (Indapamide) Rhone-Poulenc Rorer Pharmaceuticals ... 2022
Zaroxolyn Tablets (Metolazone) Fisons ... 1000

Edema, corneal, temporary relief of
Muro 128 Ophthalmic Ointment (Sodium Chloride) Bausch & Lomb Pharmaceuticals ... ◉ 258
Muro 128 Solution 2% and 5% (Sodium Chloride) Bausch & Lomb Pharmaceuticals ... ◉ 258
Ophthalgan (Glycerin) Wyeth-Ayerst ... ◉ 326

Edema, corticosteroid therapy-induced, adjunctive therapy in
Diucardin Tablets (Hydroflumethiazide) Wyeth-Ayerst ... 2718
Diuril Oral Suspension (Chlorothiazide) Merck & Co., Inc. ... 1653
Diuril Sodium Intravenous (Chlorothiazide Sodium) Merck & Co., Inc. ... 1652
Diuril Tablets (Chlorothiazide) Merck & Co., Inc. ... 1653
Enduron Tablets (Methyclothiazide) Abbott ... 420
HydroDIURIL Tablets (Hydrochlorothiazide) Merck & Co., Inc. ... 1674
Oretic Tablets (Hydrochlorothiazide) Abbott ... 443
Thalitone (Chlorthalidone) Horus ... 1245

Edema, drug-induced
Diamox (Acetazolamide) Lederle ... 1372

Edema, estrogen therapy-induced, adjunctive therapy in
Diucardin Tablets (Hydroflumethiazide) Wyeth-Ayerst ... 2718
Diuril Oral Suspension (Chlorothiazide) Merck & Co., Inc. ... 1653
Diuril Sodium Intravenous (Chlorothiazide Sodium) Merck & Co., Inc. ... 1652
Diuril Tablets (Chlorothiazide) Merck & Co., Inc. ... 1653
Enduron Tablets (Methyclothiazide) Abbott ... 420
HydroDIURIL Tablets (Hydrochlorothiazide) Merck & Co., Inc. ... 1674
Oretic Tablets (Hydrochlorothiazide) Abbott ... 443
Thalitone (Chlorthalidone) Horus ... 1245

Edema, hepatic cirrhosis-induced, adjunctive therapy in
Bumex (Bumetanide) Roche Laboratories ... 2093
Demadex Tablets and Injection (Torsemide) Boehringer Mannheim ... 686
Diucardin Tablets (Hydroflumethiazide) Wyeth-Ayerst ... 2718
Diuril Oral Suspension (Chlorothiazide) Merck & Co., Inc. ... 1653
Diuril Sodium Intravenous (Chlorothiazide Sodium) Merck & Co., Inc. ... 1652
Diuril Tablets (Chlorothiazide) Merck & Co., Inc. ... 1653
Enduron Tablets (Methyclothiazide) Abbott ... 420
HydroDIURIL Tablets (Hydrochlorothiazide) Merck & Co., Inc. ... 1674
Oretic Tablets (Hydrochlorothiazide) Abbott ... 443
Thalitone (Chlorthalidone) Horus ... 1245

Edema, idiopathic
Dyrenium Capsules (Triamterene) SmithKline Beecham Pharmaceuticals ... 2481

Edema, idiopathic, ascites-induced
Edecrin (Ethacrynate Sodium) Merck & Co., Inc. ... 1657

Edema, nephrotic syndrome-induced, treatment of
Aldactazide (Spironolactone, Hydrochlorothiazide) Searle ... 2413
Aldactone (Spironolactone) Searle ... 2414
Bumex (Bumetanide) Roche Laboratories ... 2093
Celestone Soluspan Suspension (Betamethasone Sodium Phosphate, Betamethasone Acetate) Schering ... 2347
Demadex Tablets and Injection (Torsemide) Boehringer Mannheim ... 686
Diuril Oral Suspension (Chlorothiazide) Merck & Co., Inc. ... 1653
Diuril Sodium Intravenous (Chlorothiazide Sodium) Merck & Co., Inc. ... 1652
Diuril Tablets (Chlorothiazide) Merck & Co., Inc. ... 1653
Dyrenium Capsules (Triamterene) SmithKline Beecham Pharmaceuticals ... 2481
Edecrin (Ethacrynate Sodium) Merck & Co., Inc. ... 1657
Enduron Tablets (Methyclothiazide) Abbott ... 420
HydroDIURIL Tablets (Hydrochlorothiazide) Merck & Co., Inc. ... 1674

1481 Indications Index Enteritis

Lasix Injection, Oral Solution and Tablets (Furosemide) Hoechst-Roussel ... 1240
Oretic Tablets (Hydrochlorothiazide) Abbott ... 443
Thalitone (Chlorthalidone) Horus ... 1245
Zaroxolyn Tablets (Metolazone) Fisons ... 1000

Edema, pulmonary, emergency treatment of
Arfonad Ampuls (Trimethaphan Camsylate) Roche Laboratories ... 2080
Lasix Injection, Oral Solution and Tablets (Furosemide) Hoechst-Roussel ... 1240

Electrolytes, depletion of
Pedialyte Oral Electrolyte Maintenance Solution (Electrolyte Supplement) Ross ... 2222
Rehydralyte Oral Electrolyte Rehydration Solution (Electrolyte Supplement) Ross ... 2224

Embolism, atrial fibrillation with (see under Atrial fibrillation with embolism)

Embolism, peripheral arterial
Heparin Sodium Injection (Heparin Sodium) Wyeth-Ayerst ... 2726
Heparin Sodium Injection, USP, Sterile Solution (Heparin Sodium) Upjohn ... 2615
Heparin Sodium Vials (Heparin Sodium) Lilly ... 1441

Embolism, pulmonary
Activase (Alteplase, Recombinant) Genentech ... 1058
Coumadin (Warfarin Sodium) DuPont ... 926
Heparin Sodium Injection, USP, Sterile Solution (Heparin Sodium) Upjohn ... 2615
Heparin Sodium Vials (Heparin Sodium) Lilly ... 1441

Embolism, pulmonary, acute, lysis of
Abbokinase (Urokinase) Abbott ... 403
Activase (Alteplase, Recombinant) Genentech ... 1058
Streptase for Infusion (Streptokinase) Astra ... 562

Embolism, pulmonary, postoperative
Heparin Sodium Injection (Heparin Sodium) Wyeth-Ayerst ... 2726
Heparin Sodium Injection, USP, Sterile Solution (Heparin Sodium) Upjohn ... 2615
Lovenox Injection (Enoxaparin) Rhone-Poulenc Rorer Pharmaceuticals ... 2020

Embolism, pulmonary, prophylaxis of
Coumadin (Warfarin Sodium) DuPont ... 926
Heparin Sodium Injection, USP, Sterile Solution (Heparin Sodium) Upjohn ... 2615
Heparin Sodium Vials (Heparin Sodium) Lilly ... 1441

Embolism, systemic, post-myocardial infarction, prophylaxis
Coumadin (Warfarin Sodium) DuPont ... 926

Emphysema
Atrovent Inhalation Aerosol (Ipratropium Bromide) Boehringer Ingelheim ... 671
Brethine Ampuls (Terbutaline Sulfate) CibaGeneva ... 815
Brethine Tablets (Terbutaline Sulfate) CibaGeneva ... 814
Bricanyl Subcutaneous Injection (Terbutaline Sulfate) Marion Merrell Dow ... 1502
Bricanyl Tablets (Terbutaline Sulfate) Marion Merrell Dow ... 1503
Bronkometer Aerosol (Isoetharine) Sanofi Winthrop ... 2302
Bronkosol Solution (Isoetharine) Sanofi Winthrop ... 2302
Pima Syrup (Potassium Iodide) Fleming ... 1005
Quadrinal Tablets (Ephedrine Hydrochloride, Phenobarbital, Potassium Iodide, Theophylline Calcium Salicylate) Knoll Laboratories ... 1350
Respbid Tablets (Theophylline Anhydrous) Boehringer Ingelheim 682
SSKI Solution (Potassium Iodide) Upsher-Smith ... 2658
Slo-bid Gyrocaps (Theophylline Anhydrous) Rhone-Poulenc Rorer Pharmaceuticals ... 2033
Uniphyl 400 mg Tablets (Theophylline Anhydrous) Purdue Frederick ... 2001

Emphysema, panacinar, due to congenital Alpha1-antitrypsin deficiency
Prolastin Alpha$_1$-Proteinase Inhibitor (Human) (Alpha$_1$-Proteinase Inhibitor (Human)) Bayer Biological ... 635

Empyema
Cleocin Phosphate Injection (Clindamycin Phosphate) Upjohn ... 2586
Flagyl 375 Capsules (Metronidazole) Searle ... 2434
Flagyl I.V. (Metronidazole Hydrochloride) SCS ... 2247
Pfizerpen for Injection (Penicillin G Potassium) Roerig ... 2203
Ticar for Injection (Ticarcillin Disodium) SmithKline Beecham Pharmaceuticals ... 2526

Endocarditis, bacterial
Ancef Injection (Cefazolin Sodium) SmithKline Beecham Pharmaceuticals ... 2465
Flagyl 375 Capsules (Metronidazole) Searle ... 2434
Flagyl I.V. (Metronidazole Hydrochloride) SCS ... 2247
Garamycin Injectable (Gentamicin Sulfate) Schering ... 2360
Kefzol Vials, Faspak & ADD-Vantage (Cefazolin Sodium) Lilly ... 1456
Pfizerpen for Injection (Penicillin G Potassium) Roerig ... 2203
Primaxin I.V. (Imipenem-Cilastatin Sodium) Merck & Co., Inc. ... 1729
Vancocin HCl, Vials & ADD-Vantage (Vancomycin Hydrochloride) Lilly 1481

Endocarditis, bacterial, prophylaxis
E.E.S. (Erythromycin Ethylsuccinate) Abbott ... 424
E-Mycin Tablets (Erythromycin) Knoll Laboratories ... 1341
ERYC (Erythromycin) Parke-Davis .. 1915
EryPed (Erythromycin Ethylsuccinate) Abbott ... 421
Ery-Tab Tablets (Erythromycin) Abbott ... 422
Erythrocin Stearate Filmtab (Erythromycin Stearate) Abbott ... 425
Erythromycin Base Filmtab (Erythromycin) Abbott ... 426
Erythromycin Delayed-Release Capsules, USP (Erythromycin) Abbott ... 427
Ilosone (Erythromycin Estolate) Dista ... 911
PCE Dispertab Tablets (Erythromycin) Abbott ... 444
Pfizerpen for Injection (Penicillin G Potassium) Roerig ... 2203
Vancocin HCl, Vials & ADD-Vantage (Vancomycin Hydrochloride) Lilly 1481

Endocarditis, erysipeloid
Pfizerpen for Injection (Penicillin G Potassium) Roerig ... 2203

Endocarditis, fungal
Ancobon Capsules (Flucytosine) Roche Laboratories ... 2079

Endocarditis, gonorrheal
Pfizerpen for Injection (Penicillin G Potassium) Roerig ... 2203

Endocrine adenomas, multiple (see also under Hypersecretory conditions, pathological)
Pepcid Injection (Famotidine) Merck & Co., Inc. ... 1722
Pepcid (Famotidine) Merck & Co., Inc. ... 1720
Prilosec Delayed-Release Capsules (Omeprazole) Astra Merck ... 529
Tagamet (Cimetidine Hydrochloride) SmithKline Beecham Pharmaceuticals ... 2516

Endocrine disorders
Aristocort Suspension (Forte Parenteral) (Triamcinolone Diacetate) Fujisawa ... 1027
Aristocort Tablets (Triamcinolone) Fujisawa ... 1022
Celestone Soluspan Suspension (Betamethasone Sodium Phosphate, Betamethasone Acetate) Schering ... 2347
Cortone Acetate Sterile Suspension (Cortisone Acetate) Merck & Co., Inc. ... 1623
Cortone Acetate Tablets (Cortisone Acetate) Merck & Co., Inc. ... 1624
Dalalone D.P. Injectable (Dexamethasone Acetate) Forest ... 1011
Decadron Elixir (Dexamethasone) Merck & Co., Inc. ... 1633
Decadron Phosphate Injection (Dexamethasone Sodium Phosphate) Merck & Co., Inc. ... 1637
Decadron Tablets (Dexamethasone) Merck & Co., Inc. ... 1635
Decadron-LA Sterile Suspension (Dexamethasone Acetate) Merck & Co., Inc. ... 1646
Deltasone Tablets (Prednisone) Upjohn ... 2595
Depo-Medrol Single-Dose Vial (Methylprednisolone Acetate) Upjohn ... 2600
Depo-Medrol Sterile Aqueous Suspension (Methylprednisolone Acetate) Upjohn ... 2597
Hydeltrasol Injection, Sterile (Prednisolone Sodium Phosphate) Merck & Co., Inc. ... 1665
Hydrocortone Phosphate Injection, Sterile (Hydrocortisone Sodium Phosphate) Merck & Co., Inc. ... 1670
Hydrocortone Tablets (Hydrocortisone) Merck & Co., Inc. ... 1672
Medrol (Methylprednisolone) Upjohn ... 2621
Pediapred Oral Liquid (Prednisolone Sodium Phosphate) Fisons ... 995
Prelone Syrup (Prednisolone) Muro 1787
Solu-Cortef Sterile Powder (Hydrocortisone Sodium Succinate) Upjohn ... 2641
Solu-Medrol Sterile Powder (Methylprednisolone Sodium Succinate) Upjohn ... 2643

Endometriosis
Aygestin Tablets (Norethindrone Acetate) ESI Lederle ... 974
Danocrine Capsules (Danazol) Sanofi Winthrop ... 2307
Lupron Depot 3.75 mg (Leuprolide Acetate) TAP ... 2556
Synarel Nasal Solution for Endometriosis (Nafarelin Acetate) Roche Laboratories ... 2152
Zoladex (Goserelin Acetate Implant) Zeneca ... 2858

Endometritis (see also under Infections, gynecologic)
Azactam for Injection (Aztreonam) Bristol-Myers Squibb ... 734
Cefobid Intravenous/Intramuscular (Cefoperazone Sodium) Roerig ... 2189
Cefobid Pharmacy Bulk Package - Not for Direct Infusion (Cefoperazone Sodium) Roerig ... 2192
Ceptaz (Ceftazidime) Glaxo Wellcome ... 1081
Claforan Sterile and Injection (Cefotaxime Sodium) Hoechst-Roussel ... 1235
Cleocin Phosphate Injection (Clindamycin Phosphate) Upjohn ... 2586
Flagyl 375 Capsules (Metronidazole) Searle ... 2434
Flagyl I.V. (Metronidazole Hydrochloride) SCS ... 2247
Fortaz (Ceftazidime) Glaxo Wellcome ... 1100
Mefoxin (Cefoxitin Sodium) Merck & Co., Inc. ... 1691
Mefoxin Premixed Intravenous Solution (Cefoxitin Sodium) Merck & Co., Inc. ... 1694
Mezlin (Mezlocillin Sodium) Bayer Pharmaceutical ... 601
Mezlin Pharmacy Bulk Package (Mezlocillin Sodium) Bayer Pharmaceutical ... 604
Pipracil (Piperacillin Sodium) Lederle ... 1390
Protostat Tablets (Metronidazole) Ortho Pharmaceutical ... 1883
Tazicef for Injection (Ceftazidime) SmithKline Beecham Pharmaceuticals ... 2519
Tazidime Vials, Faspak & ADD-Vantage (Ceftazidime) Lilly .. 1478
Ticar for Injection (Ticarcillin Disodium) SmithKline Beecham Pharmaceuticals ... 2526
Timentin for Injection (Ticarcillin Disodium, Clavulanate Potassium) SmithKline Beecham Pharmaceuticals ... 2528

Endometrial cancer (see under Carcinoma, endometrium, palliative treatment of)

Endomyometritis
Flagyl 375 Capsules (Metronidazole) Searle ... 2434
Flagyl I.V. (Metronidazole Hydrochloride) SCS ... 2247
Primaxin I.M. (Imipenem-Cilastatin Sodium) Merck & Co., Inc. ... 1727
Protostat Tablets (Metronidazole) Ortho Pharmaceutical ... 1883

Entamoeba histolytica (see under Amebiasis, acute intestinal)

Enteritis
Furoxone (Furazolidone) Roberts ... 2046
Septra (Trimethoprim, Sulfamethoxazole) Glaxo Wellcome ... 1174
Septra I.V. Infusion (Trimethoprim, Sulfamethoxazole) Glaxo Wellcome ... 1169
Septra I.V. Infusion ADD-Vantage Vials (Trimethoprim, Sulfamethoxazole) Glaxo Wellcome ... 1171
Septra (Trimethoprim, Sulfamethoxazole) Glaxo Wellcome ... 1174

Enteritis, regional, systemic therapy for
Aristocort Suspension (Forte Parenteral) (Triamcinolone Diacetate) Fujisawa ... 1027
Aristocort Tablets (Triamcinolone) Fujisawa ... 1022
Celestone Soluspan Suspension (Betamethasone Sodium Phosphate, Betamethasone Acetate) Schering ... 2347
Cortone Acetate Sterile Suspension (Cortisone Acetate) Merck & Co., Inc. ... 1623
Cortone Acetate Tablets (Cortisone Acetate) Merck & Co., Inc. ... 1624
Dalalone D.P. Injectable (Dexamethasone Acetate) Forest ... 1011
Decadron Elixir (Dexamethasone) Merck & Co., Inc. ... 1633
Decadron Phosphate Injection (Dexamethasone Sodium Phosphate) Merck & Co., Inc. ... 1637
Decadron Tablets (Dexamethasone) Merck & Co., Inc. ... 1635
Decadron-LA Sterile Suspension (Dexamethasone Acetate) Merck & Co., Inc. ... 1646
Deltasone Tablets (Prednisone) Upjohn ... 2595
Depo-Medrol Single-Dose Vial (Methylprednisolone Acetate) Upjohn ... 2600
Depo-Medrol Sterile Aqueous Suspension (Methylprednisolone Acetate) Upjohn ... 2597

(▣ Described in PDR For Nonprescription Drugs) (◉ Described in PDR For Ophthalmology)

Enteritis | Indications Index | 1482

Hydeltrasol Injection, Sterile (Prednisolone Sodium Phosphate) Merck & Co., Inc. ... 1665
Hydrocortone Phosphate Injection, Sterile (Hydrocortisone Sodium Phosphate) Merck & Co., Inc. ... 1670
Hydrocortone Tablets (Hydrocortisone) Merck & Co., Inc. ... 1672
Medrol (Methylprednisolone) Upjohn ... 2621
Pediapred Oral Liquid (Prednisolone Sodium Phosphate) Fisons ... 995
Prelone Syrup (Prednisolone) Muro 1787
Solu-Cortef Sterile Powder (Hydrocortisone Sodium Succinate) Upjohn ... 2641
Solu-Medrol Sterile Powder (Methylprednisolone Sodium Succinate) Upjohn ... 2643

Enterobacter aerogenes bacteremia

Polymyxin B Sulfate, Aerosporin Brand Sterile Powder (Polymyxin B Sulfate) Glaxo Wellcome ... 1154

Enterobacter aerogenes infections

Achromycin V Capsules (Tetracycline Hydrochloride) Lederle ... 1367
Coly-Mycin M Parenteral (Colistimethate Sodium) Parke-Davis ... 1905
Declomycin Tablets (Demeclocycline Hydrochloride) Lederle ... 1371
Doryx Capsules (Doxycycline Hyclate) Parke-Davis ... 1913
Dynacin Capsules (Minocycline Hydrochloride) Medicis ... 1590
Floxin I.V. (Ofloxacin) McNeil Pharmaceutical ... 1571
Floxin Tablets (200 mg, 300 mg, 400 mg) (Ofloxacin) McNeil Pharmaceutical ... 1567
Minocin Intravenous (Minocycline Hydrochloride) Lederle ... 1382
Minocin Oral Suspension (Minocycline Hydrochloride) Lederle ... 1385
Minocin Pellet-Filled Capsules (Minocycline Hydrochloride) Lederle ... 1383
Monodox Capsules (Doxycycline Monohydrate) Oclassen ... 1805
Noroxin Tablets (Norfloxacin) Merck & Co., Inc. ... 1715
Noroxin Tablets (Norfloxacin) Roberts ... 2048
Pfizerpen for Injection (Penicillin G Potassium) Roerig ... 2203
Polymyxin B Sulfate, Aerosporin Brand Sterile Powder (Polymyxin B Sulfate) Glaxo Wellcome ... 1154
Rocephin Injectable Vials, ADD-Vantage, Galaxy Container (Ceftriaxone Sodium) Roche Laboratories ... 2142
Terramycin Intramuscular Solution (Oxytetracycline) Roerig ... 2210
Vibramycin (Doxycycline Calcium) Pfizer Labs ... 1941
Vibramycin Hyclate Intravenous (Doxycycline Hyclate) Roerig ... 2215
Vibramycin (Doxycycline Monohydrate) Pfizer Labs ... 1941

Enterobacter aerogenes infections, ocular

Genoptic Sterile Ophthalmic Solution (Gentamicin Sulfate) Allergan ... ◎ 243
Genoptic Sterile Ophthalmic Ointment (Gentamicin Sulfate) Allergan ... ◎ 243
Gentacidin Ointment (Gentamicin Sulfate) CIBA Vision Ophthalmics ... ◎ 264
Gentacidin Solution (Gentamicin Sulfate) CIBA Vision Ophthalmics ... ◎ 264
Gentak (Gentamicin Sulfate) Akorn ... ◎ 208
Pred-G Liquifilm Sterile Ophthalmic Suspension (Gentamicin Sulfate, Prednisolone Acetate) Allergan ... ◎ 251
Pred-G S.O.P. Sterile Ophthalmic Ointment (Gentamicin Sulfate, Prednisolone Acetate) Allergan.. ◎ 252
TobraDex Ophthalmic Suspension and Ointment (Dexamethasone, Tobramycin) Alcon Laboratories .. 473

Enterobacter aerogenes lower respiratory tract infections

Rocephin Injectable Vials, ADD-Vantage, Galaxy Container (Ceftriaxone Sodium) Roche Laboratories ... 2142

Enterobacter aerogenes urinary tract infections

Floxin I.V. (Ofloxacin) McNeil Pharmaceutical ... 1571
Floxin Tablets (200 mg, 300 mg, 400 mg) (Ofloxacin) McNeil Pharmaceutical ... 1567
Noroxin Tablets (Norfloxacin) Merck & Co., Inc. ... 1715
Noroxin Tablets (Norfloxacin) Roberts ... 2048

Enterobacter cloacae bone and joint infections

Cipro I.V. (Ciprofloxacin) Bayer Pharmaceutical ... 595
Cipro I.V. Pharmacy Bulk Package (Ciprofloxacin) Bayer Pharmaceutical ... 597
Cipro Tablets (Ciprofloxacin Hydrochloride) Bayer Pharmaceutical ... 592

Enterobacter cloacae infections

Azactam for Injection (Aztreonam) Bristol-Myers Squibb ... 734
Cipro I.V. (Ciprofloxacin) Bayer Pharmaceutical ... 595
Cipro I.V. Pharmacy Bulk Package (Ciprofloxacin) Bayer Pharmaceutical ... 597
Cipro Tablets (Ciprofloxacin Hydrochloride) Bayer Pharmaceutical ... 592
Maxaquin Tablets (Lomefloxacin Hydrochloride) Searle ... 2440
Noroxin Tablets (Norfloxacin) Merck & Co., Inc. ... 1715
Noroxin Tablets (Norfloxacin) Roberts ... 2048
Penetrex Tablets (Enoxacin) Rhone-Poulenc Rorer Pharmaceuticals ... 2031
Primaxin I.M. (Imipenem-Cilastatin Sodium) Merck & Co., Inc. ... 1727
Rocephin Injectable Vials, ADD-Vantage, Galaxy Container (Ceftriaxone Sodium) Roche Laboratories ... 2142
Timentin for Injection (Ticarcillin Disodium, Clavulanate Potassium) SmithKline Beecham Pharmaceuticals ... 2528

Enterobacter cloacae lower respiratory tract infections

Cipro I.V. (Ciprofloxacin) Bayer Pharmaceutical ... 595
Cipro I.V. Pharmacy Bulk Package (Ciprofloxacin) Bayer Pharmaceutical ... 597
Cipro Tablets (Ciprofloxacin Hydrochloride) Bayer Pharmaceutical ... 592

Enterobacter cloacae skin and skin structure infections

Cipro I.V. (Ciprofloxacin) Bayer Pharmaceutical ... 595
Cipro I.V. Pharmacy Bulk Package (Ciprofloxacin) Bayer Pharmaceutical ... 597
Cipro Tablets (Ciprofloxacin Hydrochloride) Bayer Pharmaceutical ... 592
Primaxin I.M. (Imipenem-Cilastatin Sodium) Merck & Co., Inc. ... 1727
Rocephin Injectable Vials, ADD-Vantage, Galaxy Container (Ceftriaxone Sodium) Roche Laboratories ... 2142

Enterobacter cloacae urinary tract infections

Azactam for Injection (Aztreonam) Bristol-Myers Squibb ... 734
Cipro I.V. (Ciprofloxacin) Bayer Pharmaceutical ... 595
Cipro I.V. Pharmacy Bulk Package (Ciprofloxacin) Bayer Pharmaceutical ... 597
Cipro Tablets (Ciprofloxacin Hydrochloride) Bayer Pharmaceutical ... 592
Maxaquin Tablets (Lomefloxacin Hydrochloride) Searle ... 2440
Noroxin Tablets (Norfloxacin) Merck & Co., Inc. ... 1715
Noroxin Tablets (Norfloxacin) Roberts ... 2048
Penetrex Tablets (Enoxacin) Rhone-Poulenc Rorer Pharmaceuticals ... 2031
Seromycin Pulvules (Cycloserine) Lilly ... 1476
Timentin for Injection (Ticarcillin Disodium, Clavulanate Potassium) SmithKline Beecham Pharmaceuticals ... 2528

Enterobacter species bone and joint infections

Ceptaz (Ceftazidime) Glaxo Wellcome ... 1081
Fortaz (Ceftazidime) Glaxo Wellcome ... 1100
Nebcin Vials, Hyporets & ADD-Vantage (Tobramycin Sulfate) Lilly ... 1464
Primaxin I.V. (Imipenem-Cilastatin Sodium) Merck & Co., Inc. ... 1729
Rocephin Injectable Vials, ADD-Vantage, Galaxy Container (Ceftriaxone Sodium) Roche Laboratories ... 2142
Tazicef for Injection (Ceftazidime) SmithKline Beecham Pharmaceuticals ... 2519
Tazidime Vials, Faspak & ADD-Vantage (Ceftazidime) Lilly .. 1478
Tobramycin Sulfate Injection (Tobramycin Sulfate) Elkins-Sinn ... 968

Enterobacter species gynecologic infections

Azactam for Injection (Aztreonam) Bristol-Myers Squibb ... 734
Claforan Sterile and Injection (Cefotaxime Sodium) Hoechst-Roussel ... 1235
Mezlin (Mezlocillin Sodium) Bayer Pharmaceutical ... 601
Mezlin Pharmacy Bulk Package (Mezlocillin Sodium) Bayer Pharmaceutical ... 604
Primaxin I.V. (Imipenem-Cilastatin Sodium) Merck & Co., Inc. ... 1729
Timentin for Injection (Ticarcillin Disodium, Clavulanate Potassium) SmithKline Beecham Pharmaceuticals ... 2528

Enterobacter species infections

Amikacin Sulfate Injection, USP (Amikacin Sulfate) Elkins-Sinn ... 960
Amikin Injectable (Amikacin Sulfate) Apothecon ... 501
Ancef Injection (Cefazolin Sodium) SmithKline Beecham Pharmaceuticals ... 2465
Augmentin (Amoxicillin Trihydrate, Clavulanate Potassium) SmithKline Beecham Pharmaceuticals ... 2468
Azactam for Injection (Aztreonam) Bristol-Myers Squibb ... 734
Azo Gantanol Tablets (Sulfamethoxazole, Phenazopyridine Hydrochloride) Roche Laboratories ... 2080
Azo Gantrisin Tablets (Sulfisoxazole, Phenazopyridine Hydrochloride) Roche Laboratories ... 2081
Bactrim DS Tablets (Trimethoprim, Sulfamethoxazole) Roche Laboratories ... 2084
Bactrim I.V. Infusion (Trimethoprim, Sulfamethoxazole) Roche Laboratories ... 2082
Bactrim (Trimethoprim, Sulfamethoxazole) Roche Laboratories ... 2084
Cefizox for Intramuscular or Intravenous Use (Ceftizoxime Sodium) Fujisawa ... 1034
Cefobid Intravenous/Intramuscular (Cefoperazone Sodium) Roerig ... 2189
Cefobid Pharmacy Bulk Package - Not for Direct Infusion (Cefoperazone Sodium) Roerig ... 2192
Ceptaz (Ceftazidime) Glaxo Wellcome ... 1081
Claforan Sterile and Injection (Cefotaxime Sodium) Hoechst-Roussel ... 1235
Fortaz (Ceftazidime) Glaxo Wellcome ... 1100
Garamycin Injectable (Gentamicin Sulfate) Schering ... 2360
Geocillin Tablets (Carbenicillin Indanyl Sodium) Roerig ... 2199
Kefurox Vials, Faspak & ADD-Vantage (Cefuroxime Sodium) Lilly ... 1454
Kefzol Vials, Faspak & ADD-Vantage (Cefazolin Sodium) Lilly ... 1456
Macrodantin Capsules (Nitrofurantoin) Procter & Gamble Pharmaceuticals ... 1989
Mezlin (Mezlocillin Sodium) Bayer Pharmaceutical ... 601
Mezlin Pharmacy Bulk Package (Mezlocillin Sodium) Bayer Pharmaceutical ... 604
Nebcin Vials, Hyporets & ADD-Vantage (Tobramycin Sulfate) Lilly ... 1464
Netromycin Injection 100 mg/ml (Netilmicin Sulfate) Schering ... 2373
Pipracil (Piperacillin Sodium) Lederle ... 1390
Primaxin I.V. (Imipenem-Cilastatin Sodium) Merck & Co., Inc. ... 1729
Proloprim Tablets (Trimethoprim) Glaxo Wellcome ... 1155
Rocephin Injectable Vials, ADD-Vantage, Galaxy Container (Ceftriaxone Sodium) Roche Laboratories ... 2142
Septra (Trimethoprim, Sulfamethoxazole) Glaxo Wellcome ... 1174
Septra I.V. Infusion (Trimethoprim, Sulfamethoxazole) Glaxo Wellcome ... 1169
Septra I.V. Infusion ADD-Vantage Vials (Trimethoprim, Sulfamethoxazole) Glaxo Wellcome ... 1171
Septra (Trimethoprim, Sulfamethoxazole) Glaxo Wellcome ... 1174
Tazicef for Injection (Ceftazidime) SmithKline Beecham Pharmaceuticals ... 2519
Tazidime Vials, Faspak & ADD-Vantage (Ceftazidime) Lilly .. 1478
Timentin for Injection (Ticarcillin Disodium, Clavulanate Potassium) SmithKline Beecham Pharmaceuticals ... 2528
Trimpex Tablets (Trimethoprim) Roche Laboratories ... 2163
Unasyn (Ampicillin Sodium, Sulbactam Sodium) Roerig ... 2212
Zinacef (Cefuroxime Sodium) Glaxo Wellcome ... 1211

Enterobacter species infections, ocular

Ocuflox (Ofloxacin) Allergan ... 481
Pred-G S.O.P. Sterile Ophthalmic Ointment (Gentamicin Sulfate, Prednisolone Acetate) Allergan.. ◎ 252

Enterobacter species intra-abdominal infections

Azactam for Injection (Aztreonam) Bristol-Myers Squibb ... 734
Cefizox for Intramuscular or Intravenous Use (Ceftizoxime Sodium) Fujisawa ... 1034
Mandol Vials, Faspak & ADD-Vantage (Cefamandole Nafate) Lilly ... 1461
Nebcin Vials, Hyporets & ADD-Vantage (Tobramycin Sulfate) Lilly ... 1464
Netromycin Injection 100 mg/ml (Netilmicin Sulfate) Schering ... 2373
Primaxin I.V. (Imipenem-Cilastatin Sodium) Merck & Co., Inc. ... 1729
Tobramycin Sulfate Injection (Tobramycin Sulfate) Elkins-Sinn ... 968
Unasyn (Ampicillin Sodium, Sulbactam Sodium) Roerig ... 2212

Enterobacter species lower respiratory tract infections

Azactam for Injection (Aztreonam) Bristol-Myers Squibb ... 734
Cefizox for Intramuscular or Intravenous Use (Ceftizoxime Sodium) Fujisawa ... 1034

(▣ Described in PDR For Nonprescription Drugs) (◎ Described in PDR For Ophthalmology)

1483 Indications Index Epilepsy

Ceptaz (Ceftazidime) Glaxo Wellcome ... 1081
Claforan Sterile and Injection (Cefotaxime Sodium) Hoechst-Roussel ... 1235
Fortaz (Ceftazidime) Glaxo Wellcome ... 1100
Nebcin Vials, Hyporets & ADD-Vantage (Tobramycin Sulfate) Lilly ... 1464
Primaxin I.V. (Imipenem-Cilastatin Sodium) Merck & Co., Inc. ... 1729
Tazicef for Injection (Ceftazidime) SmithKline Beecham Pharmaceuticals ... 2519
Tazidime Vials, Faspak & ADD-Vantage (Ceftazidime) Lilly .. 1478
Tobramycin Sulfate Injection (Tobramycin Sulfate) Elkins-Sinn ... 968

Enterobacter species prostatitis
Geocillin Tablets (Carbenicillin Indanyl Sodium) Roerig ... 2199

Enterobacter species respiratory tract infections
Cefobid Intravenous/Intramuscular (Cefoperazone Sodium) Roerig ... 2189
Cefobid Pharmacy Bulk Package - Not for Direct Infusion (Cefoperazone Sodium) Roerig ... 2192
Ceptaz (Ceftazidime) Glaxo Wellcome ... 1081

Enterobacter species septicemia
Azactam for Injection (Aztreonam) Bristol-Myers Squibb ... 734
Mezlin (Mezlocillin Sodium) Bayer Pharmaceutical ... 601
Mezlin Pharmacy Bulk Package (Mezlocillin Sodium) Bayer Pharmaceutical ... 604
Netromycin Injection 100 mg/ml (Netilmicin Sulfate) Schering ... 2373
Pipracil (Piperacillin Sodium) Lederle ... 1390
Primaxin I.V. (Imipenem-Cilastatin Sodium) Merck & Co., Inc. ... 1729

Enterobacter species skin and skin structure infections
Azactam for Injection (Aztreonam) Bristol-Myers Squibb ... 734
Cefizox for Intramuscular or Intravenous Use (Ceftizoxime Sodium) Fujisawa ... 1034
Ceptaz (Ceftazidime) Glaxo Wellcome ... 1081
Claforan Sterile and Injection (Cefotaxime Sodium) Hoechst-Roussel ... 1235
Fortaz (Ceftazidime) Glaxo Wellcome ... 1100
Kefurox Vials, Faspak & ADD-Vantage (Cefuroxime Sodium) Lilly ... 1454
Mandol Vials, Faspak & ADD-Vantage (Cefamandole Nafate) Lilly ... 1461
Mezlin (Mezlocillin Sodium) Bayer Pharmaceutical ... 601
Mezlin Pharmacy Bulk Package (Mezlocillin Sodium) Bayer Pharmaceutical ... 604
Nebcin Vials, Hyporets & ADD-Vantage (Tobramycin Sulfate) Lilly ... 1464
Netromycin Injection 100 mg/ml (Netilmicin Sulfate) Schering ... 2373
Primaxin I.V. (Imipenem-Cilastatin Sodium) Merck & Co., Inc. ... 1729
Tazicef for Injection (Ceftazidime) SmithKline Beecham Pharmaceuticals ... 2519
Tazidime Vials, Faspak & ADD-Vantage (Ceftazidime) Lilly .. 1478
Tobramycin Sulfate Injection (Tobramycin Sulfate) Elkins-Sinn ... 968
Unasyn (Ampicillin Sodium, Sulbactam Sodium) Roerig ... 2212
Zinacef (Cefuroxime Sodium) Glaxo Wellcome ... 1211

Enterobacter species urinary tract infections
Ancef Injection (Cefazolin Sodium) SmithKline Beecham Pharmaceuticals ... 2465
Augmentin (Amoxicillin Trihydrate, Clavulanate Potassium) SmithKline Beecham Pharmaceuticals ... 2468
Azactam for Injection (Aztreonam) Bristol-Myers Squibb ... 734
Azo Gantanol Tablets (Sulfamethoxazole, Phenazopyridine Hydrochloride) Roche Laboratories ... 2080
Azo Gantrisin Tablets (Sulfisoxazole, Phenazopyridine Hydrochloride) Roche Laboratories ... 2081
Bactrim DS Tablets (Trimethoprim, Sulfamethoxazole) Roche Laboratories ... 2084
Bactrim I.V. Infusion (Trimethoprim, Sulfamethoxazole) Roche Laboratories ... 2082
Bactrim (Trimethoprim, Sulfamethoxazole) Roche Laboratories ... 2084
Cefizox for Intramuscular or Intravenous Use (Ceftizoxime Sodium) Fujisawa ... 1034
Ceptaz (Ceftazidime) Glaxo Wellcome ... 1081
Claforan Sterile and Injection (Cefotaxime Sodium) Hoechst-Roussel ... 1235
Fortaz (Ceftazidime) Glaxo Wellcome ... 1100
Gantanol Tablets (Sulfamethoxazole) Roche Laboratories ... 2119
Gantrisin (Acetyl Sulfisoxazole) Roche Laboratories ... 2120
Geocillin Tablets (Carbenicillin Indanyl Sodium) Roerig ... 2199
Kefzol Vials, Faspak & ADD-Vantage (Cefazolin Sodium) Lilly ... 1456
Macrodantin Capsules (Nitrofurantoin) Procter & Gamble Pharmaceuticals ... 1989
Mandol Vials, Faspak & ADD-Vantage (Cefamandole Nafate) Lilly ... 1461
Mezlin (Mezlocillin Sodium) Bayer Pharmaceutical ... 601
Mezlin Pharmacy Bulk Package (Mezlocillin Sodium) Bayer Pharmaceutical ... 604
Nebcin Vials, Hyporets & ADD-Vantage (Tobramycin Sulfate) Lilly ... 1464
NegGram (Nalidixic Acid) Sanofi Winthrop ... 2323
Netromycin Injection 100 mg/ml (Netilmicin Sulfate) Schering ... 2373
Primaxin I.V. (Imipenem-Cilastatin Sodium) Merck & Co., Inc. ... 1729
Proloprim Tablets (Trimethoprim) Glaxo Wellcome ... 1155
Septra (Trimethoprim, Sulfamethoxazole) Glaxo Wellcome ... 1174
Septra I.V. Infusion (Trimethoprim, Sulfamethoxazole) Glaxo Wellcome ... 1169
Septra I.V. Infusion ADD-Vantage Vials (Trimethoprim, Sulfamethoxazole) Glaxo Wellcome ... 1171
Septra (Trimethoprim, Sulfamethoxazole) Glaxo Wellcome ... 1174
Tazicef for Injection (Ceftazidime) SmithKline Beecham Pharmaceuticals ... 2519
Tazidime Vials, Faspak & ADD-Vantage (Ceftazidime) Lilly .. 1478
Tobramycin Sulfate Injection (Tobramycin Sulfate) Elkins-Sinn ... 968
Trimpex Tablets (Trimethoprim) Roche Laboratories ... 2163

Enterobiasis
Mintezol (Thiabendazole) Merck & Co., Inc. ... 1704
Pin-X Pinworm Treatment (Pyrantel Pamoate) Effcon ... 654
Vermox Chewable Tablets (Mebendazole) Janssen ... 1312

Enterobius vermicularis infestation (see under Enterobiasis)

Enterococci infections (see under Streptococci group D infections)

Enterococci species genital infections
Ancef Injection (Cefazolin Sodium) SmithKline Beecham Pharmaceuticals ... 2465

Enterococci species gynecologic infections
Claforan Sterile and Injection (Cefotaxime Sodium) Hoechst-Roussel ... 1235

Enterococci species skin and skin structure infections
Claforan Sterile and Injection (Cefotaxime Sodium) Hoechst-Roussel ... 1235

Enterococci species urinary tract infections
Ancef Injection (Cefazolin Sodium) SmithKline Beecham Pharmaceuticals ... 2465
Claforan Sterile and Injection (Cefotaxime Sodium) Hoechst-Roussel ... 1235
Geocillin Tablets (Carbenicillin Indanyl Sodium) Roerig ... 2199
Macrodantin Capsules (Nitrofurantoin) Procter & Gamble Pharmaceuticals ... 1989

Enterocolitis, acute, "possibly" effective in, adjunctive therapy
Cystospaz (Hyoscyamine) PolyMedica ... 1963
Donnatal (Phenobarbital, Belladonna Alkaloids) Robins ... 2060
Donnatal Extentabs (Phenobarbital, Belladonna Alkaloids) Robins ... 2061
Donnatal Tablets (Phenobarbital, Belladonna Alkaloids) Robins ... 2060
Librax Capsules (Chlordiazepoxide Hydrochloride, Clidinium Bromide) Roche Products ... 2176

Enterocolitis, staphylococcal
Vancocin HCl, Oral Solution & Pulvules (Vancomycin Hydrochloride) Lilly ... 1483
Vancocin HCl, Vials & ADD-Vantage (Vancomycin Hydrochloride) Lilly 1481

Enuresis, childhood, temporary adjunctive therapy in
Hyland's Bed Wetting Tablets (Homeopathic Medications) Standard Homeopathic ... 828
Tofranil Tablets (Imipramine Hydrochloride) CibaGeneva ... 856

Enuresis, nocturnal, primary
DDAVP (Desmopressin Acetate) Rhone-Poulenc Rorer Pharmaceuticals ... 2017
Desmopressin Acetate Rhinal Tube (Desmopressin Acetate) Ferring .. 979

Envenomation, pit viper
Antivenin (Crotalidae) Polyvalent (Antivenin (Crotalidae) Polyvalent) Wyeth-Ayerst ... 2696

Ependymoma, palliative therapy in
BiCNU (Carmustine (BCNU)) Bristol-Myers Squibb Oncology 691

Epicondylitis
Aristocort Suspension (Forte Parenteral) (Triamcinolone Diacetate) Fujisawa ... 1027
Aristocort Suspension (Intralesional) (Triamcinolone Diacetate) Fujisawa ... 1025
Aristocort Tablets (Triamcinolone) Fujisawa ... 1022
Aristospan Suspension (Intra-articular) (Triamcinolone Hexacetonide) Fujisawa ... 1033
Celestone Soluspan Suspension (Betamethasone Sodium Phosphate, Betamethasone Acetate) Schering ... 2347
Cortone Acetate Sterile Suspension (Cortisone Acetate) Merck & Co., Inc. ... 1623
Cortone Acetate Tablets (Cortisone Acetate) Merck & Co., Inc. ... 1624
Dalalone D.P. Injectable (Dexamethasone Acetate) Forest ... 1011
Decadron Elixir (Dexamethasone) Merck & Co., Inc. ... 1633
Decadron Phosphate Injection (Dexamethasone Sodium Phosphate) Merck & Co., Inc. ... 1637
Decadron Tablets (Dexamethasone) Merck & Co., Inc. ... 1635
Decadron-LA Sterile Suspension (Dexamethasone Acetate) Merck & Co., Inc. ... 1646
Deltasone Tablets (Prednisone) Upjohn ... 2595
Depo-Medrol Single-Dose Vial (Methylprednisolone Acetate) Upjohn ... 2600
Depo-Medrol Sterile Aqueous Suspension (Methylprednisolone Acetate) Upjohn ... 2597
Hydeltrasol Injection, Sterile (Prednisolone Sodium Phosphate) Merck & Co., Inc. ... 1665
Hydeltra-T.B.A. Sterile Suspension (Prednisolone Tebutate) Merck & Co., Inc. ... 1667
Hydrocortone Acetate Sterile Suspension (Hydrocortisone Acetate) Merck & Co., Inc. ... 1669
Hydrocortone Phosphate Injection, Sterile (Hydrocortisone Sodium Phosphate) Merck & Co., Inc. ... 1670
Hydrocortone Tablets (Hydrocortisone) Merck & Co., Inc. ... 1672
Medrol (Methylprednisolone) Upjohn ... 2621
Pediapred Oral Liquid (Prednisolone Sodium Phosphate) Fisons ... 995
Prelone Syrup (Prednisolone) Muro 1787
Solu-Cortef Sterile Powder (Hydrocortisone Sodium Succinate) Upjohn ... 2641
Solu-Medrol Sterile Powder (Methylprednisolone Sodium Succinate) Upjohn ... 2643

Epidermophyton floccosum infections
Exelderm Cream 1.0% (Sulconazole Nitrate) Westwood-Squibb ... 2685
Exelderm Solution 1.0% (Sulconazole Nitrate) Westwood-Squibb ... 2686
Fulvicin P/G Tablets (Griseofulvin) Schering ... 2359
Fulvicin P/G 165 & 330 Tablets (Griseofulvin) Schering ... 2359
Grifulvin V (griseofulvin tablets) Microsize (griseofulvin oral suspension) Microsize (Griseofulvin) Ortho Dermatological ... 1888
Gris-PEG Tablets, 125 mg & 250 mg (Griseofulvin) Allergan ... 479
Lamisil Cream 1% (Terbinafine Hydrochloride) Sandoz Pharmaceuticals ... 2265
Loprox 1% Cream and Lotion (Ciclopirox Olamine) Hoechst-Roussel ... 1242
Lotrimin (Clotrimazole) Schering ... 2371
Lotrisone Cream (Clotrimazole, Betamethasone Dipropionate) Schering ... 2372
Monistat Dual-Pak (Miconazole Nitrate) Ortho Pharmaceutical ... 1850
Monistat-Derm (miconazole nitrate 2%) Cream (Miconazole Nitrate) Ortho Dermatological ... 1889
Naftin Cream 1% (Naftifine Hydrochloride) Allergan ... 480
Naftin Gel 1% (Naftifine Hydrochloride) Allergan ... 481
Nizoral 2% Cream (Ketoconazole) Janssen ... 1297
Oxistat Lotion (Oxiconazole Nitrate) Glaxo Wellcome ... 1152
Spectazole (econazole nitrate 1%) Cream (Econazole Nitrate) Ortho Dermatological ... 1890

Epididymitis
Ancef Injection (Cefazolin Sodium) SmithKline Beecham Pharmaceuticals ... 2465

Epilepsy, centrencephalic (see under Seizures, centrencephalic)

(Described in PDR For Nonprescription Drugs) (Described in PDR For Ophthalmology)

Epilepsy   Indications Index   1484

Epilepsy, generalized (see under Seizures, generalized, tonic-clonic)

Epilepsy, grand mal (see under Seizures, generalized, tonic-clonic)

Epilepsy, petit mal (see under Seizures, generalized, absence)

Epilepticus, status
Dilantin Parenteral (Phenytoin Sodium) Parke-Davis ... 1910
Dizac (Diazepam) Ohmeda ... 1809
Nembutal Sodium Solution (Pentobarbital Sodium) Abbott ... 438
Valium Injectable (Diazepam) Roche Products ... 2182

Epinephrine sensitivity, ocular, treatment of
HMS Liquifilm (Medrysone) Allergan ... ◉ 244

Episcleritis
HMS Liquifilm (Medrysone) Allergan ... ◉ 244

Episiotomy, topical debriding in (see under Wounds, debridement of)

Erectile dysfunction, male
Caverject (Alprostadil) Upjohn ... 2583
Yocon (Yohimbine Hydrochloride) Palisades ... 1892
Yohimex Tablets (Yohimbine Hydrochloride) Kramer ... 1363

Erectile dysfuncton, male, diagnosis of
Caverject (Alprostadil) Upjohn ... 2583

Erysipelas
Bicillin C-R Injection (Penicillin G Procaine, Penicillin G Benzathine) Wyeth-Ayerst ... 2704
Bicillin C-R 900/300 Injection (Penicillin G Procaine, Penicillin G Benzathine) Wyeth-Ayerst ... 2706
Duricef (Cefadroxil Monohydrate) Bristol-Myers Squibb ... 748
Mezlin (Mezlocillin Sodium) Bayer Pharmaceutical ... 601
Mezlin Pharmacy Bulk Package (Mezlocillin Sodium) Bayer Pharmaceutical ... 604
Pen•Vee K (Penicillin V Potassium) Wyeth-Ayerst ... 2772

Erysipeloid
Pfizerpen for Injection (Penicillin G Potassium) Roerig ... 2203

Erysipelothrix insidiosa infections
Pfizerpen for Injection (Penicillin G Potassium) Roerig ... 2203

Erythema multiforme, severe (see under Stevens-Johnson syndrome)

Erythrasma
E.E.S. (Erythromycin Ethylsuccinate) Abbott ... 424
E-Mycin Tablets (Erythromycin) Knoll Laboratories ... 1341
ERYC (Erythromycin) Parke-Davis .. 1915
EryPed (Erythromycin Ethylsuccinate) Abbott ... 421
Ery-Tab Tablets (Erythromycin) Abbott ... 422
Erythrocin Stearate Filmtab (Erythromycin Stearate) Abbott ... 425
Erythromycin Base Filmtab (Erythromycin) Abbott ... 426
Erythromycin Delayed-Release Capsules, USP (Erythromycin) Abbott ... 427
Ilosone (Erythromycin Estolate) Dista ... 911
Ilotycin Gluceptate, IV, Vials (Erythromycin Gluceptate) Dista ... 913
PCE Dispertab Tablets (Erythromycin) Abbott ... 444

Erythroblastopenia
Aristocort Suspension (Forte Parenteral) (Triamcinolone Diacetate) Fujisawa ... 1027
Aristocort Tablets (Triamcinolone) Fujisawa ... 1022
Celestone Soluspan Suspension (Betamethasone Sodium Phosphate, Betamethasone Acetate) Schering ... 2347
Cortone Acetate Sterile Suspension (Cortisone Acetate) Merck & Co., Inc. ... 1623
Cortone Acetate Tablets (Cortisone Acetate) Merck & Co., Inc. ... 1624
Dalalone D.P. Injectable (Dexamethasone Acetate) Forest ... 1011
Decadron Elixir (Dexamethasone) Merck & Co., Inc. ... 1633
Decadron Phosphate Injection (Dexamethasone Sodium Phosphate) Merck & Co., Inc. ... 1637
Decadron Tablets (Dexamethasone) Merck & Co., Inc. ... 1635
Decadron-LA Sterile Suspension (Dexamethasone Acetate) Merck & Co., Inc. ... 1646
Deltasone Tablets (Prednisone) Upjohn ... 2595
Depo-Medrol Single-Dose Vial (Methylprednisolone Acetate) Upjohn ... 2600
Depo-Medrol Sterile Aqueous Suspension (Methylprednisolone Acetate) Upjohn ... 2597
Hydeltrasol Injection, Sterile (Prednisolone Sodium Phosphate) Merck & Co., Inc. ... 1665
Hydrocortone Phosphate Injection, Sterile (Hydrocortisone Sodium Phosphate) Merck & Co., Inc. ... 1670
Hydrocortone Tablets (Hydrocortisone) Merck & Co., Inc. ... 1672
Medrol (Methylprednisolone) Upjohn ... 2621
Pediapred Oral Liquid (Prednisolone Sodium Phosphate) Fisons ... 995
Prelone Syrup (Prednisolone) Muro 1787
Solu-Cortef Sterile Powder (Hydrocortisone Sodium Succinate) Upjohn ... 2641
Solu-Medrol Sterile Powder (Methylprednisolone Sodium Succinate) Upjohn ... 2643

Erythroblastosis fetalis, prevention of
Gamulin Rh, $Rh_O(D)$ Immune Globulin (Human) ($Rh_O(D)$ Immune Globulin (Human)) Armour ... 517
HypRho-D Full Dose Rho (D) Immune Globulin (Human) (Immune Globulin (Human)) Bayer Biological ... 629

Escherichia coli (see under E. coli infections)

Esophagitis, erosive (see also under Gastroesophageal reflux disease)
PREVACID Delayed-Release Capsules (Lansoprazole) TAP ... 2562
Prilosec Delayed-Release Capsules (Omeprazole) Astra Merck ... 529
Tagamet (Cimetidine Hydrochloride) SmithKline Beecham Pharmaceuticals ... 2516
Zantac (Ranitidine Hydrochloride) Glaxo Wellcome ... 1209

Esophageal varices, hemorrhage from
Ethamolin (Ethanolamine Oleate) Schwarz ... 2400

Esotropia, accommodative
Floropryl Sterile Ophthalmic Ointment (Isoflurophate) Merck & Co., Inc. ... 1662
Humorsol Sterile Ophthalmic Solution (Demecarium Bromide) Merck & Co., Inc. ... 1664

Espundia (see under Leishmaniasis, American)

Estrogen, deficiency (see under Hypoestrogenism)

Eubacterium species infections
Flagyl 375 Capsules (Metronidazole) Searle ... 2434
Flagyl I.V. (Metronidazole Hydrochloride) SCS ... 2247
Primaxin I.V. (Imipenem-Cilastatin Sodium) Merck & Co., Inc. ... 1729

Eubacterium species intra-abdominal infections
Flagyl 375 Capsules (Metronidazole) Searle ... 2434
Flagyl I.V. (Metronidazole Hydrochloride) SCS ... 2247
Primaxin I.V. (Imipenem-Cilastatin Sodium) Merck & Co., Inc. ... 1729
Protostat Tablets (Metronidazole) Ortho Pharmaceutical ... 1883

Eubacterium species peritonitis
Flagyl 375 Capsules (Metronidazole) Searle ... 2434
Protostat Tablets (Metronidazole) Ortho Pharmaceutical ... 1883

Eustachian tube congestion, symptomatic relief of
Fedahist Gyrocaps (Pseudoephedrine Hydrochloride, Chlorpheniramine Maleate) Schwarz ... 2401
Fedahist Timecaps (Pseudoephedrine Hydrochloride, Chlorpheniramine Maleate) Schwarz ... 2401
Novahistine DH (Codeine Phosphate, Pseudoephedrine Hydrochloride, Chlorpheniramine Maleate) SmithKline Beecham ... 2462
Novahistine Elixir (Chlorpheniramine Maleate, Phenylephrine Hydrochloride) SmithKline Beecham Consumer ... ▣ 823
Novahistine Expectorant (Codeine Phosphate, Pseudoephedrine Hydrochloride, Guaifenesin) SmithKline Beecham ... 2463
Trinalin Repetabs Tablets (Azatadine Maleate, Pseudoephedrine Sulfate) Key ... 1330

Ewing's sarcoma, palliative treatment of
Cosmegen Injection (Dactinomycin) Merck & Co., Inc. ... 1626

Extrapyramidal reactions, drug-induced
Akineton (Biperiden Hydrochloride) Knoll Laboratories ... 1333
Artane (Trihexyphenidyl Hydrochloride) Lederle ... 1368
Cogentin (Benztropine Mesylate) Merck & Co., Inc. ... 1621
Symmetrel Capsules and Syrup (Amantadine Hydrochloride) DuPont ... 946

Eye and its adnexa, external infections of
AK-Spore (Bacitracin Zinc, Neomycin Sulfate, Polymyxin B Sulfate) Akorn ... ◉ 204
Deltasone Tablets (Prednisone) Upjohn ... 2595
Genoptic Sterile Ophthalmic Solution (Gentamicin Sulfate) Allergan ... ◉ 243
Genoptic Sterile Ophthalmic Ointment (Gentamicin Sulfate) Allergan ... ◉ 243
Gentacidin Ointment (Gentamicin Sulfate) CIBA Vision Ophthalmics ... ◉ 264
Gentacidin Solution (Gentamicin Sulfate) CIBA Vision Ophthalmics ... ◉ 264
Neosporin Ophthalmic Ointment Sterile (Polymyxin B Sulfate, Bacitracin Zinc, Neomycin Sulfate) Glaxo Wellcome ... 1148
Neosporin Ophthalmic Solution Sterile (Polymyxin B Sulfate, Neomycin Sulfate, Gramicidin) Glaxo Wellcome ... 1149
Polysporin Ophthalmic Ointment Sterile (Polymyxin B Sulfate, Bacitracin Zinc) Glaxo Wellcome .. 1154
Tobrex Ophthalmic Ointment and Solution (Tobramycin) Alcon Laboratories ... ◉ 229

Eye, anterior segment inflammation (see under Inflammation, anterior segment)

Eyelids, cleansing of
Eye•Scrub (Cleanser) CIBA Vision Ophthalmics ... ◉ 263
Lid Wipes-SPF (Peg-200 Glyceryl Monotallowate) Akorn ... ◉ 209

Eyes, anterior segment, staining of
Fluor-I-Strip (Fluorescein Sodium) Wyeth-Ayerst ... ◉ 326
Fluor-I-Strip A.T. (Fluorescein Sodium) Wyeth-Ayerst ... ◉ 326

Eyes, artificial, cleansing and lubrication of
Enuclene Cleaning, Lubricating Solution for Artificial Eyes (Benzalkonium Chloride, Tyloxapol) Alcon Laboratories ... ◉ 218

Eyes, burning, reduction of
Eye-Stream Eye Irrigating Solution (Balanced Salt Solution) Alcon Laboratories ... 473
Lacrisert Sterile Ophthalmic Insert (Hydroxypropyl Cellulose) Merck & Co., Inc. ... 1686
Similasan Eye Drops #2 (Homeopathic Medications) Similasan ◉ 317
Tears Naturale II (Dextran 70, Hydroxypropyl Methylcellulose) Alcon Laboratories ... 473

Eyes, cleansing of
Collyrium for Fresh Eyes (Boric Acid, Sodium Borate) Wyeth-Ayerst ... ▣ 878
Lavoptik Eye Wash (Isotonic Solution) Lavoptik ... ▣ 665
Zephiran Chloride Aqueous Solution (Benzalkonium Chloride) Sanofi Winthrop ... ▣ 795

Eyes, diagnostic procedures, adjunct in
Fluoracaine (Fluorescein Sodium, Proparacaine Hydrochloride) Akorn ... ◉ 206
Fluor-I-Strip (Fluorescein Sodium) Wyeth-Ayerst ... ◉ 326
Fluor-I-Strip A.T. (Fluorescein Sodium) Wyeth-Ayerst ... ◉ 326

Eyes, dry (see under Keratoconjunctivitis sicca)

Eyes, emergency flushing of foreign bodies
FLURESS (Fluorescein Sodium, Benoxinate Hydrochloride) Akorn ... ◉ 207

Eyes, external infections of
AKTOB (Tobramycin) Akorn ... ◉ 206
Genoptic Sterile Ophthalmic Solution (Gentamicin Sulfate) Allergan ... ◉ 243
Genoptic Sterile Ophthalmic Ointment (Gentamicin Sulfate) Allergan ... ◉ 243
Gentacidin Ointment (Gentamicin Sulfate) CIBA Vision Ophthalmics ... ◉ 264
Gentacidin Solution (Gentamicin Sulfate) CIBA Vision Ophthalmics ... ◉ 264

Eyes, exudation, reduction of
Lacrisert Sterile Ophthalmic Insert (Hydroxypropyl Cellulose) Merck & Co., Inc. ... 1686

Eyes, foreign body sensation, reduction of
Lacrisert Sterile Ophthalmic Insert (Hydroxypropyl Cellulose) Merck & Co., Inc. ... 1686

Eyes, goniscopic examinations, adjunct in
FLURESS (Fluorescein Sodium, Benoxinate Hydrochloride) Akorn ... ◉ 207

Eyes, inflammation (see under Ocular inflammation)

(▣ Described in PDR For Nonprescription Drugs)   (◉ Described in PDR For Ophthalmology)

1485 **Indications Index** Fever

Eyes, irrigation of
(see also under Eyes, cleansing of)
Betadine 5% Sterile Ophthalmic Prep Solution (Povidone Iodine) Escalon Ophthalmics ⊙ 274
Eye-Stream Eye Irrigating Solution (Balanced Salt Solution) Alcon Laboratories 473

Eyes, irritation, symptomatic relief of
AquaSite Eye Drops (Polyethylene Glycol, Dextran 70) CIBA Vision Ophthalmics ⊙ 261
Murine Tears Lubricant Eye Drops (Polyvinyl Alcohol, Povidone) Ross ⊙ 316
Murine Tears Plus Lubricant Redness Reliever Eye Drops (Polyvinyl Alcohol, Povidone, Tetrahydrozoline Hydrochloride) Ross ⊙ 316
Tears Naturale II (Dextran 70, Hydroxypropyl Methylcellulose) Alcon Laboratories 473
Visine Maximum Strength Allergy Relief (Tetrahydrozoline Hydrochloride) Pfizer Consumer ⊙ 313
Visine Original Eye Drops (Tetrahydrozoline Hydrochloride) Pfizer Consumer ⊙ 314
Viva-Drops (Polysorbate 80) Vision Pharmaceuticals ⊙ 325

Eyes, itching, reduction of
Actifed Plus Tablets (Acetaminophen, Pseudoephedrine Hydrochloride, Triprolidine Hydrochloride) WARNER WELLCOME ▣ 845
Actifed Syrup (Pseudoephedrine Hydrochloride, Triprolidine Hydrochloride) WARNER WELLCOME ▣ 846
Actifed Tablets (Pseudoephedrine Hydrochloride, Triprolidine Hydrochloride) WARNER WELLCOME ▣ 844
Allergy-Sinus Comtrex Multi-Symptom Allergy-Sinus Formula Tablets (Acetaminophen, Chlorpheniramine Maleate, Pseudoephedrine Hydrochloride) Bristol-Myers Products ▣ 617
Contac Night Allergy/Sinus Caplets (Acetaminophen, Pseudoephedrine Hydrochloride, Diphenhydramine Hydrochloride) SmithKline Beecham Consumer ▣ 812
Drixoral Cold and Flu Extended-Release Tablets (Acetaminophen, Dexbrompheniramine Maleate, Pseudoephedrine Sulfate) Schering-Plough HealthCare ▣ 803
Lacrisert Sterile Ophthalmic Insert (Hydroxypropyl Cellulose) Merck & Co., Inc. 1686
Ryna Liquid (Chlorpheniramine Maleate, Pseudoephedrine Hydrochloride) Wallace ▣ 841
Similasan Eye Drops #2 (Homeopathic Medications) Similasan ⊙ 317
Sinulin Tablets (Acetaminophen, Phenylpropanolamine Hydrochloride, Chlorpheniramine Maleate) Carnrick 787
Sudafed Plus Liquid (Chlorpheniramine Maleate, Pseudoephedrine Hydrochloride) WARNER WELLCOME ▣ 862
Sudafed Plus Tablets (Chlorpheniramine Maleate, Pseudoephedrine Hydrochloride) WARNER WELLCOME ▣ 863
Triaminic Syrup (Phenylpropanolamine Hydrochloride, Chlorpheniramine Maleate) Sandoz Consumer ▣ 792
Triaminic-12 Tablets (Phenylpropanolamine Hydrochloride, Chlorpheniramine Maleate) Sandoz Consumer ▣ 792
TYLENOL Severe Allergy Medication Caplets (Acetaminophen, Diphenhydramine Hydrochloride) McNeil Consumer 1564
Vasocon-A (Antazoline Phosphate, Naphazoline Hydrochloride) CIBA Vision Ophthalmics ⊙ 271

Eyes, lubrication of
(see also under Keratoconjunctivitis sicca)
Adsorbotear Artificial Tear (Povidone) Alcon Laboratories ⊙ 210
HypoTears Lubricant Eye Drops (Polyvinyl Alcohol) CIBA Vision Ophthalmics ⊙ 265
HypoTears Ointment (Petrolatum, White) CIBA Vision Ophthalmics ⊙ 265
HypoTears PF Lubricant Eye Drops (Polyvinyl Alcohol) CIBA Vision Ophthalmics ⊙ 265
Tears Renewed Ointment (Petrolatum, White) Akorn ⊙ 209

Eyes, red
(see under Ocular redness)

Eyes, smarting, reduction of
Lacrisert Sterile Ophthalmic Insert (Hydroxypropyl Cellulose) Merck & Co., Inc. 1686

Eyes, surgery, adjunct to
AMO Vitrax Viscoelastic Solution (Sodium Hyaluronate) Allergan ⊙ 232
AMVISC Plus (Sodium Hyaluronate) Chiron Vision ⊙ 329
Betadine 5% Sterile Ophthalmic Prep Solution (Povidone Iodine) Escalon Ophthalmics ⊙ 274
Healon (Sodium Hyaluronate) Pharmacia Inc. Ophthalmics ⊙ 314
Miochol-E with Iocare Steri-Tags and Miochol-E System Pak (Acetylcholine Chloride) CIBA Vision Ophthalmics ⊙ 273
Ocucoat (Hydroxypropyl Methylcellulose) Storz Ophthalmics ⊙ 321

Eyes, surgical procedures, irrigation of
(see also under Eyes, cleansing of)
AMO Endosol (Balanced Salt Solution) (Balanced Salt Solution) Allergan ⊙ 232
BSS (15 mL & 30 mL) Sterile Irrigation Solution (Balanced Salt Solution) Alcon Laboratories ⊙ 214
BSS (250 mL) Sterile Irrigation Solution (Balanced Salt Solution) Alcon Laboratories ⊙ 214
BSS (500 mL) Sterile Irrigation Solution (Balanced Salt Solution) Alcon Laboratories ⊙ 214
BSS PLUS (500 mL) Sterile Irrigation Solution (Balanced Salt Solution) Alcon Laboratories ⊙ 215

Eyes, watery
(see under Lacrimation, symptomatic relief of)

F

Factor IX, deficiency of
Konÿne 80 Factor IX Complex (Factor IX Complex) Bayer Biological 634
Mononine, Coagulation Factor IX (Human) (Factor IX (Human)) Armour 523

Fatigue, symptomatic relief of
No Doz Maximum Strength Caplets (Caffeine) Bristol-Myers Products ▣ 622

Febrile episodes, in immunosuppressed patients with granulocytopenia
Mezlin (Mezlocillin Sodium) Bayer Pharmaceutical 601
Mezlin Pharmacy Bulk Package (Mezlocillin Sodium) Bayer Pharmaceutical 604

Fecal incontinence, adjunct
Derifil Tablets (Chlorophyllin Copper Complex) Rystan 2246

Female castration
(see under Ovaries, castration of)

Fetal circulation, persistent
(see under Hypertension, pulmonary, persistent, of the newborn)

Fever associated with common cold
Actifed Plus Tablets (Acetaminophen, Pseudoephedrine Hydrochloride, Triprolidine Hydrochloride) WARNER WELLCOME ▣ 845
Advil Cold and Sinus Caplets and Tablets (formerly CoAdvil) (Ibuprofen, Pseudoephedrine Hydrochloride) Whitehall ▣ 870
Regular Strength Ascriptin Tablets (Aspirin Buffered, Calcium Carbonate) CIBA Consumer ▣ 629
BC Cold Powder Multi-Symptom Formula (Cold-Sinus-Allergy) (Aspirin, Phenylpropanolamine Hydrochloride, Chlorpheniramine Maleate) Block ▣ 609
BC Cold Powder Non-Drowsy Formula (Cold-Sinus) (Aspirin, Phenylpropanolamine Hydrochloride) Block ▣ 609
Contac Severe Cold and Flu Formula Caplets (Acetaminophen, Chlorpheniramine Maleate, Dextromethorphan Hydrobromide, Phenylpropanolamine Hydrochloride) SmithKline Beecham Consumer ▣ 814
Drixoral Cold and Flu Extended-Release Tablets (Acetaminophen, Dexbrompheniramine Maleate, Pseudoephedrine Sulfate) Schering-Plough HealthCare ▣ 803
Sinulin Tablets (Acetaminophen, Phenylpropanolamine Hydrochloride, Chlorpheniramine Maleate) Carnrick 787
TheraFlu Flu and Cold Medicine (Acetaminophen, Chlorpheniramine Maleate, Pseudoephedrine Hydrochloride) Sandoz Consumer ▣ 787
Children's TYLENOL Cold Multi-Symptom Liquid Formula and Chewable Tablets (Acetaminophen, Chlorpheniramine Maleate, Pseudoephedrine Hydrochloride) McNeil Consumer 1561
TYLENOL Cold Multi-Symptom Formula Medication Tablets and Caplets (Acetaminophen, Chlorpheniramine Maleate, Pseudoephedrine Hydrochloride, Dextromethorphan Hydrobromide) McNeil Consumer 1561
TYLENOL Cold Medication No Drowsiness Formula Gelcaps and Caplets (Acetaminophen, Pseudoephedrine Hydrochloride, Dextromethorphan Hydrobromide) McNeil Consumer 1562
TYLENOL Cold Multi-Symptom Hot Medication Liquid Packets (Acetaminophen, Chlorpheniramine Maleate, Pseudoephedrine Hydrochloride, Dextromethorphan Hydrobromide) McNeil Consumer 1557
Vicks DayQuil (Acetaminophen, Dextromethorphan Hydrobromide, Pseudoephedrine Hydrochloride, Guaifenesin) Procter & Gamble ▣ 761
Vicks NyQuil LiquiCaps Multi-Symptom Cold/Flu Relief (Acetaminophen, Pseudoephedrine Hydrochloride, Dextromethorphan Hydrobromide, Doxylamine Succinate) Procter & Gamble ▣ 763
Vicks NyQuil Multi-Symptom Cold/Flu Relief - (Original & Cherry Flavor) (Acetaminophen, Dextromethorphan Hydrobromide, Doxylamine Succinate, Pseudoephedrine Hydrochloride) Procter & Gamble ▣ 763

Fever blisters
(see under Herpetic manifestations, oral, symptomatic relief of)

Fever, reduction of
Advil Ibuprofen Tablets and Caplets (Ibuprofen) Whitehall ▣ 870
Children's Advil Suspension (Ibuprofen) Wyeth-Ayerst 2692
Aleve (Naproxen Sodium) Procter & Gamble 1975
Arthritis Foundation Aspirin Free Caplets (Acetaminophen) McNeil Consumer ▣ 673
Arthritis Foundation Ibuprofen Tablets (Ibuprofen) McNeil Consumer ▣ 674
Maximum Strength Ascriptin (Aspirin Buffered, Calcium Carbonate) CIBA Consumer ▣ 630
BC Powder (Aspirin, Salicylamide, Caffeine) Block ▣ 609
Bayer Children's Chewable Aspirin (Aspirin) Miles Consumer ▣ 711
Genuine Bayer Aspirin Tablets & Caplets (Aspirin) Miles Consumer ▣ 713
Extra Strength Bayer Aspirin Caplets & Tablets (Aspirin) Miles Consumer ▣ 712
Extra Strength Bayer Plus Aspirin Caplets (Aspirin, Calcium Carbonate) Miles Consumer ▣ 713
Bayer Select Ibuprofen Pain Relief Formula (Ibuprofen) Miles Consumer ▣ 715
Bufferin Analgesic Tablets and Caplets (Aspirin) Bristol-Myers Products ▣ 613
Extra Strength Bufferin Analgesic Tablets (Aspirin) Bristol-Myers Products ▣ 615
Empirin Aspirin Tablets (Aspirin) WARNER WELLCOME ▣ 854
Haltran Tablets (Ibuprofen) Roberts ▣ 771
Healthprin Aspirin (Aspirin) Smart 2455
Ibuprohm (Ibuprofen) Ohm ▣ 735
Mobigesic Tablets (Magnesium Salicylate, Phenyltoloxamine Citrate) Ascher ▣ 602
Children's Motrin Ibuprofen Oral Suspension (Ibuprofen) McNeil Consumer 1546
Motrin IB Caplets, Tablets, and Geltabs (Ibuprofen) Upjohn ▣ 838
Motrin Ibuprofen Suspension, Oral Drops, Chewable Tablets, Caplets (Ibuprofen) McNeil Consumer 1546
Nuprin Ibuprofen/Analgesic Tablets & Caplets (Ibuprofen) Bristol-Myers Products ▣ 622
Panodol Tablets and Caplets (Acetaminophen) SmithKline Beecham Consumer ▣ 824
Children's Panadol Chewable Tablets, Liquid, Infant's Drops (Acetaminophen) SmithKline Beecham Consumer ▣ 824
Percogesic Analgesic Tablets (Acetaminophen, Phenyltoloxamine Citrate) Procter & Gamble ▣ 754
St. Joseph Adult Chewable Aspirin (81 mg.) (Aspirin) Schering-Plough HealthCare ▣ 808
Trilisate (Choline Magnesium Trisalicylate) Purdue Frederick 2000
Tylenol, Children's (Acetaminophen) McNeil Consumer 1555
TYLENOL Extended Relief Caplets (Acetaminophen) McNeil Consumer 1558
TYLENOL, Extra Strength, Acetaminophen Adult Liquid Pain Reliever (Acetaminophen) McNeil Consumer 1560
TYLENOL, Extra Strength, acetaminophen Gelcaps, Geltabs, Caplets, Tablets (Acetaminophen) McNeil Consumer 1559
TYLENOL, Junior Strength, acetaminophen Coated Caplets, Grape and Fruit Chewable Tablets (Acetaminophen) McNeil Consumer 1557
TYLENOL, Regular Strength, acetaminophen Caplets and

(▣ Described in PDR For Nonprescription Drugs) (⊙ Described in PDR For Ophthalmology)

Fever **Indications Index** 1486

Tablets (Acetaminophen) McNeil Consumer 1558
Vanquish Analgesic Caplets (Acetaminophen, Aspirin, Caffeine, Aluminum Hydroxide Gel, Magnesium Hydroxide) Miles Consumer ..... ▣ 731

Fever, San Joaquin (see under Coccidioidomycosis)

Fever, valley (see under Coccidioidomycosis)

Fiber, deficiency of
Medifen (Fiber Supplement) Odyssey 1807

Flatulence, relief of
Arco-Lase Tablets (Enzymes, Digestive) Arco 512
Di-Gel Antacid/Anti-Gas (Calcium Carbonate, Magnesium Hydroxide, Simethicone) Schering-Plough HealthCare ..... ▣ 801
Gas-X (Simethicone) Sandoz Consumer ..... ▣ 786
Gelusil Liquid & Tablets (Aluminum Hydroxide, Magnesium Hydroxide, Simethicone) WARNER WELLCOME ..... ▣ 855
Hyland's Colic Tablets (Homeopathic Medications) Standard Homeopathic ..... ▣ 829
Kutrase Capsules (Hyoscyamine Sulfate, Phenyltoloxamine Citrate, Enzymes, Digestive) Schwarz 2402
Ku-Zyme Capsules (Enzymes, Digestive) Schwarz 2402
Maalox Anti-Gas Tablets, Regular Strength (Simethicone) CIBA Consumer ..... ▣ 640
Maalox Anti-Gas Tablets, Extra Strength (Simethicone) CIBA Consumer ..... ▣ 640
Maalox Plus Tablets (Aluminum Hydroxide, Magnesium Hydroxide, Simethicone) CIBA Consumer ..... ▣ 643
Extra Strength Maalox Antacid Plus Antigas Liquid and Tablets (Aluminum Hydroxide, Magnesium Hydroxide, Simethicone) CIBA Consumer ..... ▣ 638
Mylanta Gas Relief Tablets-80 mg (Simethicone) J&J•Merck Consumer 1318
Maximum Strength Mylanta Gas Relief Tablets-125 mg (Simethicone) J&J•Merck Consumer 1318
Mylanta Liquid (Aluminum Hydroxide, Magnesium Hydroxide, Simethicone) J&J•Merck Consumer 1317
Mylicon Infants' Drops (Simethicone) J&J•Merck Consumer 1317
Phazyme Drops (Simethicone) Reed & Carnrick ..... ▣ 767
Phazyme (Simethicone) Reed & Carnrick ..... ▣ 767
Phazyme-125 Chewable Tablets (Simethicone) Reed & Carnrick ▣ 767
Phazyme-125 Softgels Maximum Strength (Simethicone) Reed & Carnrick ..... ▣ 767

Flatus, postoperative retention of
Phazyme-125 Chewable Tablets (Simethicone) Reed & Carnrick ▣ 767

"Flu" symptoms (see under Influenza syndrome, symptomatic relief of)

Folic acid antagonists, overdosage of
Leucovorin Calcium for Injection, Wellcovorin Brand (Leucovorin Calcium) Glaxo Wellcome 1132
Leucovorin Calcium for Injection (Leucovorin Calcium) Immunex 1268
Leucovorin Calcium Tablets, Wellcovorin Brand (Leucovorin Calcium) Glaxo Wellcome 1132
Leucovorin Calcium Tablets (Leucovorin Calcium) Immunex 1270

Folic acid deficiency, prevention of
Fero-Folic-500 Filmtab (Ferrous Sulfate, Folic Acid, Vitamin C) Abbott 429
Iberet-Folic-500 Filmtab (Vitamin B Complex With Vitamin C, Ferrous Sulfate) Abbott 429
Slow Fe with Folic Acid (Ferrous Sulfate, Folic Acid) Ciba Self-Medication 869

Folliculitis barbae
Fulvicin P/G Tablets (Griseofulvin) Schering 2359
Fulvicin P/G 165 & 330 Tablets (Griseofulvin) Schering 2359
Grifulvin V (griseofulvin tablets) Microsize (griseofulvin oral suspension) Microsize (Griseofulvin) Ortho Dermatological 1888
Gris-PEG Tablets, 125 mg & 250 mg (Griseofulvin) Allergan 479

Francisella tularensis infections
Achromycin V Capsules (Tetracycline Hydrochloride) Lederle 1367
Declomycin Tablets (Demeclocycline Hydrochloride) Lederle 1371
Doryx Capsules (Doxycycline Hyclate) Parke-Davis 1913
Dynacin Capsules (Minocycline Hydrochloride) Medicis 1590
Minocin Intravenous (Minocycline Hydrochloride) Lederle 1382
Minocin Oral Suspension (Minocycline Hydrochloride) Lederle 1385
Minocin Pellet-Filled Capsules (Minocycline Hydrochloride) Lederle 1383
Monodox Capsules (Doxycycline Monohydrate) Oclassen 1805
Streptomycin Sulfate Injection (Streptomycin Sulfate) Roerig 2208
Terramycin Intramuscular Solution (Oxytetracycline) Roerig 2210
Vibramycin (Doxycycline Calcium) Pfizer Labs 1941
Vibramycin Hyclate Intravenous (Doxycycline Hyclate) Roerig 2215
Vibramycin (Doxycycline Monohydrate) Pfizer Labs 1941

Fungal infection, skin (see under Infections, mycotic, cutaneous)

Furunculosis, symptomatic relief of
Panafil Ointment (Papain, Chlorophyllin Copper Complex, Urea) Rystan 2246
Panafil-White Ointment (Papain, Urea) Rystan 2247

Fusobacterium fusiformisans spirochete infections
Pfizerpen for Injection (Penicillin G Potassium) Roerig 2203

Fusobacterium nucleatum gynecologic infections
Claforan Sterile and Injection (Cefotaxime Sodium) Hoechst-Roussel 1235

Fusobacterium nucleatum infections
Claforan Sterile and Injection (Cefotaxime Sodium) Hoechst-Roussel 1235

Fusobacterium species gynecologic infections
Cefotan (Cefotetan) Zeneca 2829
Claforan Sterile and Injection (Cefotaxime Sodium) Hoechst-Roussel 1235

Fusobacterium species infections
Cefotan (Cefotetan) Zeneca 2829
Claforan Sterile and Injection (Cefotaxime Sodium) Hoechst-Roussel 1235
Flagyl 375 Capsules (Metronidazole) Searle 2434
Flagyl I.V. (Metronidazole Hydrochloride) SCS 2247
Primaxin I.M. (Imipenem-Cilastatin Sodium) Merck & Co., Inc. 1727
Primaxin I.V. (Imipenem-Cilastatin Sodium) Merck & Co., Inc. 1729
Protostat Tablets (Metronidazole) Ortho Pharmaceutical 1883

Fusobacterium species intra-abdominal infections
Primaxin I.M. (Imipenem-Cilastatin Sodium) Merck & Co., Inc. 1727
Primaxin I.V. (Imipenem-Cilastatin Sodium) Merck & Co., Inc. 1729

Fusobacterium species skin and skin structure infections
Flagyl 375 Capsules (Metronidazole) Searle 2434
Flagyl I.V. (Metronidazole Hydrochloride) SCS 2247
Primaxin I.V. (Imipenem-Cilastatin Sodium) Merck & Co., Inc. 1729

Fusospirochetosis
Achromycin V Capsules (Tetracycline Hydrochloride) Lederle 1367
Declomycin Tablets (Demeclocycline Hydrochloride) Lederle 1371
Doryx Capsules (Doxycycline Hyclate) Parke-Davis 1913
Dynacin Capsules (Minocycline Hydrochloride) Medicis 1590
Minocin Intravenous (Minocycline Hydrochloride) Lederle 1382
Minocin Oral Suspension (Minocycline Hydrochloride) Lederle 1385
Minocin Pellet-Filled Capsules (Minocycline Hydrochloride) Lederle 1383
Monodox Capsules (Doxycycline Monohydrate) Oclassen 1805
Pen•Vee K (Penicillin V Potassium) Wyeth-Ayerst 2772
Pfizerpen for Injection (Penicillin G Potassium) Roerig 2203
Terramycin Intramuscular Solution (Oxytetracycline) Roerig 2210
Vibramycin (Doxycycline Calcium) Pfizer Labs 1941
Vibramycin Hyclate Intravenous (Doxycycline Hyclate) Roerig 2215
Vibramycin (Doxycycline Monohydrate) Pfizer Labs 1941

G

Gag reflex, suppression
Cetacaine Topical Anesthetic (Benzocaine, Tetracaine Hydrochloride, Butyl Aminobenzoate) Cetylite 794
Dyclone 0.5% and 1% Topical Solutions, USP (Dyclonine Hydrochloride) Astra 544
Hurricaine (Benzocaine) Beutlich 666
Hurricaine Topical (Benzocaine) Beutlich 666

Gallstones (see under Biliary calculi, chemical dissolution of)

Gardnerella vaginalis infections
MetroGel-Vaginal (Metronidazole) Curatek 902
Primaxin I.V. (Imipenem-Cilastatin Sodium) Merck & Co., Inc. 1729

Gardnerella vaginalis vaginitis (see under H. vaginalis vaginitis)

Gastric acid secretory function, diagnosis of
Peptavlon (Pentagastrin) Wyeth-Ayerst 2878

Gastric emptying, delayed
Reglan (Metoclopramide Hydrochloride) Robins 2068

Gastric hyperacidity (see under Hyperacidity, gastric)

Gastric stasis, diabetic
Reglan (Metoclopramide Hydrochloride) Robins 2068

Gastric ulcers, active, benign, short-term treatment of
Axid Pulvules (Nizatidine) Lilly 1427
Pepcid Injection (Famotidine) Merck & Co., Inc. 1722
Pepcid (Famotidine) Merck & Co., Inc. 1720
Tagamet (Cimetidine Hydrochloride) SmithKline Beecham Pharmaceuticals 2516
Zantac (Ranitidine Hydrochloride) Glaxo Wellcome 1209

Gastric ulcers, nonsteroidal anti-inflammatory drug-induced, prevention of
Cytotec (Misoprostol) Searle 2424

Gastroesophageal reflux disease
Axid Pulvules (Nizatidine) Lilly 1427
Pepcid Injection (Famotidine) Merck & Co., Inc. 1722
Pepcid (Famotidine) Merck & Co., Inc. 1720
Prilosec Delayed-Release Capsules (Omeprazole) Astra Merck 529
Tagamet (Cimetidine Hydrochloride) SmithKline Beecham Pharmaceuticals 2516
Zantac (Ranitidine Hydrochloride) Glaxo Wellcome 1209

Gastroesophageal reflux, symptomatic
Propulsid (Cisapride) Janssen 1300
Reglan (Metoclopramide Hydrochloride) Robins 2068

Gastrointestinal hypermotility, symptomatic relief of
Arco-Lase Plus Tablets (Enzymes, Digestive) Arco 512
Bellergal-S Tablets (Phenobarbital, Ergotamine Tartrate, Belladonna Alkaloids) Sandoz Pharmaceuticals 2250
Levsin/Levsinex/Levbid (Hyoscyamine Sulfate) Schwarz 2405

Gastrointestinal tract, smooth muscle spasm (see under Spasm, smooth muscle)

Gastroparesis, diabetic (see also under Gastric stasis, diabetic; Gastric emptying, delayed)
Reglan (Metoclopramide Hydrochloride) Robins 2068

Gaucher disease, type 1, long-term enzyme replacement therapy for
Ceredase (Alglucerase) Genzyme 1065
Cerezyme (Imiglucerase) Genzyme 1066

Gelineau's syndrome (see under Narcolepsy)

Genital warts (see under Condylomata acuminata)

Genitourinary tract, smooth muscle spasm (see under Spasm, smooth muscle)

GERD (see under Gastroesophageal reflux disease)

German measles (see under Rubella, prophylaxis)

Gestational trophoblastic disease, non-metastatic
Prostin E2 Suppository (Dinoprostone) Upjohn 2634

Giardiasis
Furoxone Liquid (Furazolidone) Roberts 2046

Gibraltar fever (see under Brucellosis)

Gilchrist's disease (see under Blastomycosis)

Gingivitis, necrotizing ulcerative (see under Fusospirochetosis)

Gingivitis, prevention of
Listerine Antiseptic (Eucalyptol, Menthol, Methyl Salicylate) WARNER WELLCOME ..... ▣ 855

(▣ Described in PDR For Nonprescription Drugs) (◉ Described in PDR For Ophthalmology)

1487 **Indications Index** **Growth failure**

Cool Mint Listerine (Thymol, Eucalyptol, Methyl Salicylate, Menthol) WARNER WELLCOME ■ 856
FreshBurst Listerine (Thymol, Eucalyptol, Methyl Salicylate, Menthol) WARNER WELLCOME ■ 856
Peridex (Chlorhexidine Gluconate) Procter & Gamble ... 1978

Gingivitis, treatment of
Cool Mint Listerine (Thymol, Eucalyptol, Methyl Salicylate, Menthol) WARNER WELLCOME ■ 856
Peridex (Chlorhexidine Gluconate) Procter & Gamble ... 1978

Glaucoma, acute attack
ISMOTIC 45% w/v Solution (Isosorbide) Alcon Laboratories ⊙ 222
OSM_GLYN Oral Osmotic Agent (Glycerin) Alcon Laboratories ... ⊙ 226

Glaucoma, angle-closure, acute
Daranide Tablets (Dichlorphenamide) Merck & Co., Inc. ... 1633
Diamox Intravenous (Acetazolamide) Lederle ... 1372
Diamox Sequels (Sustained Release) (Acetazolamide) Lederle 1373
Diamox Tablets (Acetazolamide) Lederle ... 1372
Glauctabs (Methazolamide) Akorn ... ⊙ 208
Neptazane Tablets (Methazolamide) Lederle ... 1388

Glaucoma, angle-closure, acute, preoperative
Diamox (Acetazolamide) Lederle ... 1372
MZM (Methazolamide) CIBA Vision Ophthalmics ... ⊙ 267
Pilocar (Pilocarpine Hydrochloride) CIBA Vision Ophthalmics ... ⊙ 268

Glaucoma, angle-closure, chronic
Phospholine Iodide (Echothiophate Iodide) Wyeth-Ayerst ... ⊙ 326

Glaucoma, angle-closure, subacute
Phospholine Iodide (Echothiophate Iodide) Wyeth-Ayerst ... ⊙ 326

Glaucoma, aphakic
Phospholine Iodide (Echothiophate Iodide) Wyeth-Ayerst ... ⊙ 326

Glaucoma, chronic open-angle
Betagan (Levobunolol Hydrochloride) Allergan ... ⊙ 233
Betoptic Ophthalmic Solution (Betaxolol Hydrochloride) Alcon Laboratories ... 469
Betoptic S Ophthalmic Suspension (Betaxolol Hydrochloride) Alcon Laboratories ... 471
Daranide Tablets (Dichlorphenamide) Merck & Co., Inc. ... 1633
Diamox Intravenous (Acetazolamide) Lederle ... 1372
Diamox Sequels (Sustained Release) (Acetazolamide) Lederle 1373
Diamox Tablets (Acetazolamide) Lederle ... 1372
EPIFRIN (Epinephrine) Allergan ... ⊙ 239
Glauctabs (Methazolamide) Akorn ... ⊙ 208
MZM (Methazolamide) CIBA Vision Ophthalmics ... ⊙ 267
Neptazane Tablets (Methazolamide) Lederle ... 1388
Ocupress Ophthalmic Solution, 1% Sterile (Carteolol Hydrochloride) Otsuka America ⊙ 309
OptiPranolol (Metipranolol 0.3%) Sterile Ophthalmic Solution (Metipranolol Hydrochloride) Bausch & Lomb Pharmaceuticals ... ⊙ 258
Phospholine Iodide (Echothiophate Iodide) Wyeth-Ayerst ... ⊙ 326
Pilocar (Pilocarpine Hydrochloride) CIBA Vision Ophthalmics ... ⊙ 268
PROPINE with C CAP Compliance Cap (Dipivefrin Hydrochloride) Allergan ... ⊙ 253
Timoptic in Ocudose (Timolol Maleate) Merck & Co., Inc. ... 1753
Timoptic Sterile Ophthalmic Solution (Timolol Maleate) Merck & Co., Inc. ... 1751
Timoptic-XE (Timolol Maleate) Merck & Co., Inc. ... 1755

Glaucoma, open-angle
Floropryl Sterile Ophthalmic Ointment (Isoflurophate) Merck & Co., Inc. ... 1662
Humorsol Sterile Ophthalmic Solution (Demecarium Bromide) Merck & Co., Inc. ... 1664
Trusopt Sterile Ophthalmic Solution (Dorzolamide Hydrochloride) Merck & Co., Inc. 1760

Glaucoma, secondary
Daranide Tablets (Dichlorphenamide) Merck & Co., Inc. ... 1633
Diamox Intravenous (Acetazolamide) Lederle ... 1372
Diamox Sequels (Sustained Release) (Acetazolamide) Lederle 1373
Diamox Tablets (Acetazolamide) Lederle ... 1372
Glauctabs (Methazolamide) Akorn ... ⊙ 208
MZM (Methazolamide) CIBA Vision Ophthalmics ... ⊙ 267
Neptazane Tablets (Methazolamide) Lederle ... 1388
Phospholine Iodide (Echothiophate Iodide) Wyeth-Ayerst ... ⊙ 326

Glaucoma, unspecified
Isopto Carbachol Ophthalmic Solution (Carbachol) Alcon Laboratories ... ⊙ 223

Glaucoma filtration, surgical aid in
AMO Vitrax Viscoelastic Solution (Sodium Hyaluronate) Allergan.. ⊙ 232
Healon (Sodium Hyaluronate) Pharmacia Inc. Ophthalmics ... ⊙ 314
Healon GV (Sodium Hyaluronate) Pharmacia Inc. Ophthalmics ... ⊙ 315

Glioblastoma, palliative therapy in
BiCNU (Carmustine (BCNU)) Bristol-Myers Squibb Oncology ... 691

Glioma, brainstem, palliative therapy in
BiCNU (Carmustine (BCNU)) Bristol-Myers Squibb Oncology ... 691

Glomerulonephritis, acute, prophylaxis
Bicillin L-A Injection (Penicillin G Benzathine) Wyeth-Ayerst ... 2707

Goiter, euthyroid, treatment or prevention of
Cytomel Tablets (Liothyronine Sodium) SmithKline Beecham Pharmaceuticals ... 2473
Synthroid (Levothyroxine Sodium) Knoll Pharmaceutical ... 1359

Goiter, suppression of pituitary TSH in
Cytomel Tablets (Liothyronine Sodium) SmithKline Beecham Pharmaceuticals ... 2473
Levothroid Tablets (Levothyroxine Sodium) Forest ... 1016
Synthroid (Levothyroxine Sodium) Knoll Pharmaceutical ... 1359

Gonococcal arthritis-dermatitis syndrome
Doryx Capsules (Doxycycline Hyclate) Parke-Davis ... 1913

Gonococcal infections, uncomplicated
Doryx Capsules (Doxycycline Hyclate) Parke-Davis ... 1913
Mefoxin Premixed Intravenous Solution (Cefoxitin Sodium) Merck & Co., Inc. ... 1694
Mezlin (Mezlocillin Sodium) Bayer Pharmaceutical ... 601
Mezlin Pharmacy Bulk Package (Mezlocillin Sodium) Bayer Pharmaceutical ... 604
Pipracil (Piperacillin Sodium) Lederle ... 1390
Rocephin Injectable Vials, ADD-Vantage, Galaxy Container (Ceftriaxone Sodium) Roche Laboratories ... 2142
Vantin for Oral Suspension and Vantin Tablets (Cefpodoxime Proxetil) Upjohn ... 2646
Vibramycin (Doxycycline Calcium) Pfizer Labs ... 1941
Zinacef (Cefuroxime Sodium) Glaxo Wellcome ... 1211

Gonorrhea (see also under N. gonorrhoeae infections)
Amoxil (Amoxicillin Trihydrate) SmithKline Beecham Pharmaceuticals ... 2464
Cefizox for Intramuscular or Intravenous Use (Ceftizoxime Sodium) Fujisawa ... 1034
Claforan Sterile and Injection (Cefotaxime Sodium) Hoechst-Roussel ... 1235
E-Mycin Tablets (Erythromycin) Knoll Laboratories ... 1341
Kefurox Vials, Faspak & ADD-Vantage (Cefuroxime Sodium) Lilly ... 1454
Mefoxin (Cefoxitin Sodium) Merck & Co., Inc. ... 1691
Mefoxin Premixed Intravenous Solution (Cefoxitin Sodium) Merck & Co., Inc. ... 1694
Mezlin (Mezlocillin Sodium) Bayer Pharmaceutical ... 601
Mezlin Pharmacy Bulk Package (Mezlocillin Sodium) Bayer Pharmaceutical ... 604
Rocephin Injectable Vials, ADD-Vantage, Galaxy Container (Ceftriaxone Sodium) Roche Laboratories ... 2142
Spectrobid Tablets (Bacampicillin Hydrochloride) Roerig ... 2206
Trobicin Sterile Powder (Spectinomycin Hydrochloride) Upjohn ... 2645
Zinacef (Cefuroxime Sodium) Glaxo Wellcome ... 1211

Gonorrhea, cervical/urethral
Cefizox for Intramuscular or Intravenous Use (Ceftizoxime Sodium) Fujisawa ... 1034
Ceftin for Oral Suspension (Cefuroxime Axetil) Glaxo Wellcome ... 1078
Cipro Tablets (Ciprofloxacin Hydrochloride) Bayer Pharmaceutical ... 592
Floxin I.V. (Ofloxacin) McNeil Pharmaceutical ... 1571
Floxin Tablets (200 mg, 300 mg, 400 mg) (Ofloxacin) McNeil Pharmaceutical ... 1567
Noroxin Tablets (Norfloxacin) Merck & Co., Inc. ... 1715
Noroxin Tablets (Norfloxacin) Roberts ... 2048
Penetrex Tablets (Enoxacin) Rhone-Poulenc Rorer Pharmaceuticals ... 2031
Rocephin Injectable Vials, ADD-Vantage, Galaxy Container (Ceftriaxone Sodium) Roche Laboratories ... 2142
Vantin for Oral Suspension and Vantin Tablets (Cefpodoxime Proxetil) Upjohn ... 2646

Gonorrhea, pharyngeal
Rocephin Injectable Vials, ADD-Vantage, Galaxy Container (Ceftriaxone Sodium) Roche Laboratories ... 2142

Gonorrhea, rectal
Rocephin Injectable Vials, ADD-Vantage, Galaxy Container (Ceftriaxone Sodium) Roche Laboratories ... 2142

Gonorrhea, uncomplicated
Ceftin Tablets (Cefuroxime Axetil) Glaxo Wellcome ... 1078
Cipro Tablets (Ciprofloxacin Hydrochloride) Bayer Pharmaceutical ... 592
Mefoxin (Cefoxitin Sodium) Merck & Co., Inc. ... 1691
Monodox Capsules (Doxycycline Monohydrate) Oclassen ... 1805
Noroxin Tablets (Norfloxacin) Merck & Co., Inc. ... 1715
Noroxin Tablets (Norfloxacin) Roberts ... 2048
Penetrex Tablets (Enoxacin) Rhone-Poulenc Rorer Pharmaceuticals ... 2031
Rocephin Injectable Vials, ADD-Vantage, Galaxy Container (Ceftriaxone Sodium) Roche Laboratories ... 2142
Suprax Tablets (Cefixime) Lederle .. 1399
Zefazone I.V. Solution (Cefmetazole Sodium) Upjohn ... 2654

Gout, acute
Anaprox/Naprosyn (Naproxen Sodium) Roche Laboratories ... 2117
ColBENEMID Tablets (Probenecid, Colchicine) Merck & Co., Inc. ... 1622
Anaprox/Naprosyn (Naproxen) Roche Laboratories ... 2117
Zyloprim Tablets (Allopurinol) Glaxo Wellcome ... 1226

Gout, management of signs and symptoms
Zyloprim Tablets (Allopurinol) Glaxo Wellcome ... 1226

Grand mal epilepsy (see under Seizures, generalized, tonic-clonic)

Granuloma annulare, infiltrated inflammatory lesions of
Aristocort Suspension (Forte Parenteral) (Triamcinolone Diacetate) Fujisawa ... 1027
Aristocort Suspension (Intralesional) (Triamcinolone Diacetate) Fujisawa ... 1025
Aristospan Suspension (Intralesional) (Triamcinolone Hexacetonide) Fujisawa ... 1032
Celestone Soluspan Suspension (Betamethasone Sodium Phosphate, Betamethasone Acetate) Schering ... 2347
Decadron Phosphate Injection (Dexamethasone Sodium Phosphate) Merck & Co., Inc. ... 1637
Decadron-LA Sterile Suspension (Dexamethasone Acetate) Merck & Co., Inc. ... 1646
Depo-Medrol Single-Dose Vial (Methylprednisolone Acetate) Upjohn ... 2600
Depo-Medrol Sterile Aqueous Suspension (Methylprednisolone Acetate) Upjohn ... 2597
Hydeltrasol Injection, Sterile (Prednisolone Sodium Phosphate) Merck & Co., Inc. ... 1665
Hydrocortone Acetate Sterile Suspension (Hydrocortisone Acetate) Merck & Co., Inc. ... 1669

Granuloma inguinale
Achromycin V Capsules (Tetracycline Hydrochloride) Lederle ... 1367
Declomycin Tablets (Demeclocycline Hydrochloride) Lederle ... 1371
Doryx Capsules (Doxycycline Hyclate) Parke-Davis ... 1913
Dynacin Capsules (Minocycline Hydrochloride) Medicis ... 1590
Minocin Intravenous (Minocycline Hydrochloride) Lederle ... 1382
Minocin Oral Suspension (Minocycline Hydrochloride) Lederle ... 1385
Minocin Pellet-Filled Capsules (Minocycline Hydrochloride) Lederle ... 1383
Monodox Capsules (Doxycycline Monohydrate) Oclassen ... 1805
Streptomycin Sulfate Injection (Streptomycin Sulfate) Roerig ... 2208
Terramycin Intramuscular Solution (Oxytetracycline) Roerig ... 2210
Vibramycin (Doxycycline Calcium) Pfizer Labs ... 1941
Vibramycin Hyclate Intravenous (Doxycycline Hyclate) Roerig ... 2215
Vibramycin (Doxycycline Monohydrate) Pfizer Labs ... 1941

Granulomatous disease, chronic
Actimmune (Interferon Gamma-1B) Genentech ... 1056

Growth failure, chronic renal insufficiency-induced in children
Nutropin (Somatropin) Genentech .. 1061

(■ Described in PDR For Nonprescription Drugs) (⊙ Described in PDR For Ophthalmology)

Growth hormone secretion | Indications Index | 1488

Growth hormone secretion, evaluation of the secreting capability of
Geref (sermorelin acetate for injection) (Sermorelin Acetate) Serono ... 2876

Growth hormone secretion, inadequate
Genotropin (Somatropin) Pharmacia ... 111
Humatrope Vials (Somatropin) Lilly 1443
Nutropin (Somatropin) Genentech .. 1061
Protropin (Somatrem) Genentech 1063

Gums, sore (see under Pain, dental)

H

H. aegypticus infections, ocular
TERAK Ointment (Oxytetracycline Hydrochloride, Polymyxin B Sulfate) Akorn ... ⊙ 209
Terramycin with Polymyxin B Sulfate Ophthalmic Ointment (Oxytetracycline Hydrochloride, Polymyxin B Sulfate) Roerig ... 2211
TobraDex Ophthalmic Suspension and Ointment (Dexamethasone, Tobramycin) Alcon Laboratories .. 473

H. ducreyi infections
Achromycin V Capsules (Tetracycline Hydrochloride) Lederle ... 1367
Declomycin Tablets (Demeclocycline Hydrochloride) Lederle ... 1371
Doryx Capsules (Doxycycline Hyclate) Parke-Davis ... 1913
Dynacin Capsules (Minocycline Hydrochloride) Medicis ... 1590
Minocin Intravenous (Minocycline Hydrochloride) Lederle ... 1382
Minocin Oral Suspension (Minocycline Hydrochloride) Lederle ... 1385
Minocin Pellet-Filled Capsules (Minocycline Hydrochloride) Lederle ... 1383
Monodox Capsules (Doxycycline Monohydrate) Oclassen ... 1805
Streptomycin Sulfate Injection (Streptomycin Sulfate) Roerig ... 2208
Terramycin Intramuscular Solution (Oxytetracycline) Roerig ... 2210
Vibramycin (Doxycycline Calcium) Pfizer Labs ... 1941
Vibramycin Hyclate Intravenous (Doxycycline Hyclate) Roerig ... 2215
Vibramycin (Doxycycline Monohydrate) Pfizer Labs ... 1941

H. influenzae bacteremia
Ceptaz (Ceftazidime) Glaxo Wellcome ... 1081

H. influenzae bronchitis
Bactrim (Trimethoprim, Sulfamethoxazole) Roche Laboratories ... 2084
Ceftin (Cefuroxime Axetil) Glaxo Wellcome ... 1078
Cefzil Tablets and Oral Suspension (Cefprozil) Bristol-Myers Squibb .. 746
Floxin I.V. (Ofloxacin) McNeil Pharmaceutical ... 1571
Lorabid Suspension and Pulvules (Loracarbef) Lilly ... 1459
Maxaquin Tablets (Lomefloxacin Hydrochloride) Searle ... 2440
Septra (Trimethoprim, Sulfamethoxazole) Glaxo Wellcome ... 1174
Spectrobid Tablets (Bacampicillin Hydrochloride) Roerig ... 2206
Suprax Tablets (Cefixime) Lederle .. 1399
Vantin for Oral Suspension and Vantin Tablets (Cefpodoxime Proxetil) Upjohn ... 2646
Zefazone I.V. Solution (Cefmetazole Sodium) Upjohn ... 2654

H. influenzae infections
Achromycin V Capsules (Tetracycline Hydrochloride) Lederle ... 1367
Amoxil (Amoxicillin Trihydrate) SmithKline Beecham Pharmaceuticals ... 2464
Ancef Injection (Cefazolin Sodium) SmithKline Beecham Pharmaceuticals ... 2465
Augmentin (Amoxicillin Trihydrate, Clavulanate Potassium) SmithKline Beecham Pharmaceuticals ... 2468
Azactam for Injection (Aztreonam) Bristol-Myers Squibb ... 734
Bactrim (Trimethoprim, Sulfamethoxazole) Roche Laboratories ... 2084
Biaxin (Clarithromycin) Abbott ... 405
Ceclor Pulvules & Suspension (Cefaclor) Lilly ... 1431
Cefizox for Intramuscular or Intravenous Use (Ceftizoxime Sodium) Fujisawa ... 1034
Cefotan (Cefotetan) Zeneca ... 2829
Ceftin (Cefuroxime Axetil) Glaxo Wellcome ... 1078
Cefzil Tablets and Oral Suspension (Cefprozil) Bristol-Myers Squibb .. 746
Ceptaz (Ceftazidime) Glaxo Wellcome ... 1081
Cipro I.V. (Ciprofloxacin) Bayer Pharmaceutical ... 595
Cipro Tablets (Ciprofloxacin Hydrochloride) Bayer Pharmaceutical ... 592
Claforan Sterile and Injection (Cefotaxime Sodium) Hoechst-Roussel ... 1235
Declomycin Tablets (Demeclocycline Hydrochloride) Lederle ... 1371
Doryx Capsules (Doxycycline Hyclate) Parke-Davis ... 1913
Dynacin Capsules (Minocycline Hydrochloride) Medicis ... 1590
E.E.S. (Erythromycin Ethylsuccinate) Abbott ... 424
E-Mycin Tablets (Erythromycin) Knoll Laboratories ... 1341
ERYC (Erythromycin) Parke-Davis .. 1915
Ery-Tab Tablets (Erythromycin) Abbott ... 422
Erythrocin Stearate Filmtab (Erythromycin Stearate) Abbott ... 425
Erythromycin Base Filmtab (Erythromycin) Abbott ... 426
Erythromycin Delayed-Release Capsules, USP (Erythromycin) Abbott ... 427
Floxin I.V. (Ofloxacin) McNeil Pharmaceutical ... 1571
Floxin Tablets (200 mg, 300 mg, 400 mg) (Ofloxacin) McNeil Pharmaceutical ... 1567
Fortaz (Ceftazidime) Glaxo Wellcome ... 1100
Ilotycin Gluceptate, IV, Vials (Erythromycin Gluceptate) Dista ... 913
Keflex Pulvules & Oral Suspension (Cephalexin) Dista ... 914
Kefurox Vials, Faspak & ADD-Vantage (Cefuroxime Sodium) Lilly ... 1454
Kefzol Vials, Faspak & ADD-Vantage (Cefazolin Sodium) Lilly ... 1456
Lorabid Suspension and Pulvules (Loracarbef) Lilly ... 1459
Maxaquin Tablets (Lomefloxacin Hydrochloride) Searle ... 2440
Mefoxin (Cefoxitin Sodium) Merck & Co., Inc. ... 1691
Mefoxin Premixed Intravenous Solution (Cefoxitin Sodium) Merck & Co., Inc. ... 1694
Mezlin (Mezlocillin Sodium) Bayer Pharmaceutical ... 601
Mezlin Pharmacy Bulk Package (Mezlocillin Sodium) Bayer Pharmaceutical ... 604
Minocin Intravenous (Minocycline Hydrochloride) Lederle ... 1382
Minocin Oral Suspension (Minocycline Hydrochloride) Lederle ... 1385
Minocin Pellet-Filled Capsules (Minocycline Hydrochloride) Lederle ... 1383
Monocid Injection (Cefonicid Sodium) SmithKline Beecham Pharmaceuticals ... 2497
Monodox Capsules (Doxycycline Monohydrate) Oclassen ... 1805
Omnipen Capsules (Ampicillin) Wyeth-Ayerst ... 2764
Omnipen for Oral Suspension (Ampicillin) Wyeth-Ayerst ... 2765
PCE Dispertab Tablets (Erythromycin) Abbott ... 444
Pipracil (Piperacillin Sodium) Lederle ... 1390
Polymyxin B Sulfate, Aerosporin Brand Sterile Powder (Polymyxin B Sulfate) Glaxo Wellcome ... 1154
Primaxin I.M. (Imipenem-Cilastatin Sodium) Merck & Co., Inc. ... 1727
Primaxin I.V. (Imipenem-Cilastatin Sodium) Merck & Co., Inc. ... 1729
Rocephin Injectable Vials, ADD-Vantage, Galaxy Container (Ceftriaxone Sodium) Roche Laboratories ... 2142
Septra (Trimethoprim, Sulfamethoxazole) Glaxo Wellcome ... 1174
Spectrobid Tablets (Bacampicillin Hydrochloride) Roerig ... 2206
Suprax (Cefixime) Lederle ... 1399
Tazicef for Injection (Ceftazidime) SmithKline Beecham Pharmaceuticals ... 2519
Tazidime Vials, Faspak & ADD-Vantage (Ceftazidime) Lilly .. 1478
TERAK Ointment (Oxytetracycline Hydrochloride, Polymyxin B Sulfate) Akorn ... ⊙ 209
Timentin for Injection (Ticarcillin Disodium, Clavulanate Potassium) SmithKline Beecham Pharmaceuticals ... 2528
Vantin for Oral Suspension and Vantin Tablets (Cefpodoxime Proxetil) Upjohn ... 2646
Zefazone (Cefmetazole Sodium) Upjohn ... 2654
Zinacef (Cefuroxime Sodium) Glaxo Wellcome ... 1211
Zithromax (Azithromycin) Pfizer Labs ... 1944
Zosyn (Piperacillin Sodium, Tazobactam Sodium) Lederle ... 1419
Zosyn Pharmacy Bulk Package (Piperacillin Sodium, Tazobactam Sodium) Lederle ... 1422

H. influenzae infections, ocular
AK-CIDE (Prednisolone Acetate, Sulfacetamide Sodium) Akorn ... ⊙ 202
AK-CIDE Ointment (Prednisolone Acetate, Sulfacetamide Sodium) Akorn ... ⊙ 202
AK-Spore (Bacitracin Zinc, Neomycin Sulfate, Polymyxin B Sulfate) Akorn ... ⊙ 204
AK-Trol Ointment & Suspension (Dexamethasone, Neomycin Sulfate, Polymyxin B Sulfate) Akorn ... ⊙ 205
Blephamide Liquifilm Sterile Ophthalmic Suspension (Prednisolone Acetate, Sulfacetamide Sodium) Allergan ... 476
Blephamide Ointment (Sulfacetamide Sodium, Prednisolone Acetate) Allergan ... ⊙ 237
Chibroxin Sterile Ophthalmic Solution (Norfloxacin) Merck & Co., Inc. ... 1617
Chloromycetin Ophthalmic Ointment, 1% (Chloramphenicol) Parke-Davis ⊙ 310
Chloromycetin Ophthalmic Solution (Chloramphenicol) Parke-Davis ... ⊙ 310
Chloroptic S.O.P. (Chloramphenicol) Allergan ... ⊙ 239
Ciloxan Ophthalmic Solution (Ciprofloxacin Hydrochloride) Alcon Laboratories ... 472
Cortisporin Ophthalmic Ointment Sterile (Polymyxin B Sulfate, Bacitracin Zinc, Neomycin Sulfate, Hydrocortisone) Glaxo Wellcome ... 1085
Cortisporin Ophthalmic Suspension Sterile (Hydrocortisone, Polymyxin B Sulfate, Neomycin Sulfate) Glaxo Wellcome ... 1086
Dexacidin Ointment (Dexamethasone, Neomycin Sulfate, Polymyxin B Sulfate) CIBA Vision Ophthalmics ... ⊙ 263
FML-S Liquifilm (Sulfacetamide Sodium, Fluorometholone) Allergan ... ⊙ 242
Genoptic Sterile Ophthalmic Solution (Gentamicin Sulfate) Allergan ... ⊙ 243
Genoptic Sterile Ophthalmic Ointment (Gentamicin Sulfate) Allergan ... ⊙ 243
Gentak (Gentamicin Sulfate) Akorn ... ⊙ 208
Maxitrol Ophthalmic Ointment and Suspension (Dexamethasone, Neomycin Sulfate, Polymyxin B Sulfate) Alcon Laboratories ... ⊙ 224
NeoDecadron Sterile Ophthalmic Ointment (Neomycin Sulfate, Dexamethasone Sodium Phosphate) Merck & Co., Inc. ... 1712
NeoDecadron Sterile Ophthalmic Solution (Neomycin Sulfate, Dexamethasone Sodium Phosphate) Merck & Co., Inc. ... 1713
Ocuflox (Ofloxacin) Allergan ... 481
Ophthocort (Chloramphenicol, Polymyxin B Sulfate, Hydrocortisone Acetate) Parke-Davis ... ⊙ 311
Poly-Pred Liquifilm (Neomycin Sulfate, Polymyxin B Sulfate, Prednisolone Acetate) Allergan .. ⊙ 248
Polytrim Ophthalmic Solution Sterile (Polymyxin B Sulfate, Trimethoprim Sulfate) Allergan ... 482
Pred-G Liquifilm Sterile Ophthalmic Suspension (Gentamicin Sulfate, Prednisolone Acetate) Allergan ... ⊙ 251
Pred-G S.O.P. Sterile Ophthalmic Ointment (Gentamicin Sulfate, Prednisolone Acetate) Allergan .. ⊙ 252
TERAK Ointment (Oxytetracycline Hydrochloride, Polymyxin B Sulfate) Akorn ... ⊙ 209
Terramycin with Polymyxin B Sulfate Ophthalmic Ointment (Oxytetracycline Hydrochloride, Polymyxin B Sulfate) Roerig ... 2211
TobraDex Ophthalmic Suspension and Ointment (Dexamethasone, Tobramycin) Alcon Laboratories .. 473
Vasocidin Ointment (Prednisolone Acetate, Sulfacetamide Sodium) CIBA Vision Ophthalmics ... ⊙ 268
Vasocidin Ophthalmic Solution (Prednisolone Sodium Phosphate, Sulfacetamide Sodium) CIBA Vision Ophthalmics ... ⊙ 270

H. influenzae infections, treatment adjunct
Streptomycin Sulfate Injection (Streptomycin Sulfate) Roerig ... 2208

H. influenzae lower respiratory tract infections
Amoxil (Amoxicillin Trihydrate) SmithKline Beecham Pharmaceuticals ... 2464
Augmentin (Amoxicillin Trihydrate, Clavulanate Potassium) SmithKline Beecham Pharmaceuticals ... 2468
Azactam for Injection (Aztreonam) Bristol-Myers Squibb ... 734
Biaxin (Clarithromycin) Abbott ... 405
Ceclor Pulvules & Suspension (Cefaclor) Lilly ... 1431
Cefizox for Intramuscular or Intravenous Use (Ceftizoxime Sodium) Fujisawa ... 1034
Cefobid Intravenous/Intramuscular (Cefoperazone Sodium) Roerig ... 2189
Cefobid Pharmacy Bulk Package - Not for Direct Infusion (Cefoperazone Sodium) Roerig ... 2192
Cefotan (Cefotetan) Zeneca ... 2829
Cefzil Tablets and Oral Suspension (Cefprozil) Bristol-Myers Squibb .. 746
Ceptaz (Ceftazidime) Glaxo Wellcome ... 1081
Cipro I.V. (Ciprofloxacin) Bayer Pharmaceutical ... 595
Cipro I.V. Pharmacy Bulk Package (Ciprofloxacin) Bayer Pharmaceutical ... 597
Cipro Tablets (Ciprofloxacin Hydrochloride) Bayer Pharmaceutical ... 592
Claforan Sterile and Injection (Cefotaxime Sodium) Hoechst-Roussel ... 1235
Floxin I.V. (Ofloxacin) McNeil Pharmaceutical ... 1571
Floxin Tablets (200 mg, 300 mg, 400 mg) (Ofloxacin) McNeil Pharmaceutical ... 1567
Fortaz (Ceftazidime) Glaxo Wellcome ... 1100

(▣ Described in PDR For Nonprescription Drugs) (⊙ Described in PDR For Ophthalmology)

1489 Indications Index Headache

Kefurox Vials, Faspak & ADD-Vantage (Cefuroxime Sodium) Lilly 1454
Lorabid Suspension and Pulvules (Loracarbef) Lilly 1459
Mandol Vials, Faspak & ADD-Vantage (Cefamandole Nafate) Lilly 1461
Mefoxin (Cefoxitin Sodium) Merck & Co., Inc. 1691
Mefoxin Premixed Intravenous Solution (Cefoxitin Sodium) Merck & Co., Inc. 1694
Mezlin (Mezlocillin Sodium) Bayer Pharmaceutical 601
Mezlin Pharmacy Bulk Package (Mezlocillin Sodium) Bayer Pharmaceutical 604
Monocid Injection (Cefonicid Sodium) SmithKline Beecham Pharmaceuticals 2497
Pipracil (Piperacillin Sodium) Lederle 1390
Primaxin I.M. (Imipenem-Cilastatin Sodium) Merck & Co., Inc. 1727
Primaxin I.V. (Imipenem-Cilastatin Sodium) Merck & Co., Inc. 1729
Rocephin Injectable Vials, ADD-Vantage, Galaxy Container (Ceftriaxone Sodium) Roche Laboratories 2142
Spectrobid Tablets (Bacampicillin Hydrochloride) Roerig 2206
Tazicef for Injection (Ceftazidime) SmithKline Beecham Pharmaceuticals 2519
Tazidime Vials, Faspak & ADD-Vantage (Ceftazidime) Lilly .. 1478
Timentin for Injection (Ticarcillin Disodium, Clavulanate Potassium) SmithKline Beecham Pharmaceuticals 2528
Vantin for Oral Suspension and Vantin Tablets (Cefpodoxime Proxetil) Upjohn 2646
Zefazone (Cefmetazole Sodium) Upjohn 2654
Zinacef (Cefuroxime Sodium) Glaxo Wellcome 1211
Zithromax (Azithromycin) Pfizer Labs 1944
Zosyn (Piperacillin Sodium, Tazobactam Sodium) Lederle 1419
Zosyn Pharmacy Bulk Package (Piperacillin Sodium, Tazobactam Sodium) Lederle 1422

H. influenzae meningitis
Cefizox for Intramuscular or Intravenous Use (Ceftizoxime Sodium) Fujisawa 1034
Chloromycetin Sodium Succinate (Chloramphenicol Sodium Succinate) Parke-Davis 1900
Fortaz (Ceftazidime) Glaxo Wellcome 1100
Polymyxin B Sulfate, Aerosporin Brand Sterile Powder (Polymyxin B Sulfate) Glaxo Wellcome 1154
Rocephin Injectable Vials, ADD-Vantage, Galaxy Container (Ceftriaxone Sodium) Roche Laboratories 2142
Tazicef for Injection (Ceftazidime) SmithKline Beecham Pharmaceuticals 2519
Tazidime Vials, Faspak & ADD-Vantage (Ceftazidime) Lilly .. 1478
Zinacef (Cefuroxime Sodium) Glaxo Wellcome 1211

H. influenzae otitis media
Augmentin (Amoxicillin Trihydrate, Clavulanate Potassium) SmithKline Beecham Pharmaceuticals 2468
Bactrim (Trimethoprim, Sulfamethoxazole) Roche Laboratories 2084
Ceclor Pulvules & Suspension (Cefaclor) Lilly 1431
Ceftin (Cefuroxime Axetil) Glaxo Wellcome 1078
Cefzil Tablets and Oral Suspension (Cefprozil) Bristol-Myers Squibb .. 746
Keflex Pulvules & Oral Suspension (Cephalexin) Dista 914
Lorabid Suspension and Pulvules (Loracarbef) Lilly 1459
Septra (Trimethoprim, Sulfamethoxazole) Glaxo Wellcome 1174
Suprax (Cefixime) Lederle 1399
Vantin for Oral Suspension and Vantin Tablets (Cefpodoxime Proxetil) Upjohn 2646

H. influenzae otitis media, adjunctive therapy in
Gantanol Tablets (Sulfamethoxazole) Roche Laboratories 2119
Gantrisin (Acetyl Sulfisoxazole) Roche Laboratories 2120

H. influenzae respiratory tract infections
Achromycin V Capsules (Tetracycline Hydrochloride) Lederle 1367
Ancef Injection (Cefazolin Sodium) SmithKline Beecham Pharmaceuticals 2465
Cefobid Intravenous/Intramuscular (Cefoperazone Sodium) Roerig 2189
Cefobid Pharmacy Bulk Package - Not for Direct Infusion (Cefoperazone Sodium) Roerig 2192
Declomycin Tablets (Demeclocycline Hydrochloride) Lederle 1371
Doryx Capsules (Doxycycline Hyclate) Parke-Davis 1913
Dynacin Capsules (Minocycline Hydrochloride) Medicis 1590
Kefzol Vials, Faspak & ADD-Vantage (Cefazolin Sodium) Lilly 1456
Minocin Intravenous (Minocycline Hydrochloride) Lederle 1382
Minocin Oral Suspension (Minocycline Hydrochloride) Lederle 1385
Minocin Pellet-Filled Capsules (Minocycline Hydrochloride) Lederle 1383
Monodox Capsules (Doxycycline Monohydrate) Oclassen 1805
Omnipen for Oral Suspension (Ampicillin) Wyeth-Ayerst 2765
Streptomycin Sulfate Injection (Streptomycin Sulfate) Roerig 2208
Terramycin Intramuscular Solution (Oxytetracycline) Roerig 2210
Vibramycin (Doxycycline Calcium) Pfizer Labs 1941
Vibramycin Hyclate Intravenous (Doxycycline Hyclate) Roerig 2215
Vibramycin (Doxycycline Monohydrate) Pfizer Labs 1941

H. influenzae septicemia
Ceptaz (Ceftazidime) Glaxo Wellcome 1081
Fortaz (Ceftazidime) Glaxo Wellcome 1100
Kefurox Vials, Faspak & ADD-Vantage (Cefuroxime Sodium) Lilly 1454
Rocephin Injectable Vials, ADD-Vantage, Galaxy Container (Ceftriaxone Sodium) Roche Laboratories 2142
Tazicef for Injection (Ceftazidime) SmithKline Beecham Pharmaceuticals 2519
Tazidime Vials, Faspak & ADD-Vantage (Ceftazidime) Lilly .. 1478
Zinacef (Cefuroxime Sodium) Glaxo Wellcome 1211

H. influenzae sinusitis
Augmentin (Amoxicillin Trihydrate, Clavulanate Potassium) SmithKline Beecham Pharmaceuticals 2468
Lorabid Suspension and Pulvules (Loracarbef) Lilly 1459

H. influenzae upper respiratory tract infections
Cefobid Intravenous/Intramuscular (Cefoperazone Sodium) Roerig 2189
Cefobid Pharmacy Bulk Package - Not for Direct Infusion (Cefoperazone Sodium) Roerig 2192
E.E.S. (Erythromycin Ethylsuccinate) Abbott 424
E-Mycin Tablets (Erythromycin) Knoll Laboratories 1341
ERYC (Erythromycin) Parke-Davis .. 1915
EryPed (Erythromycin Ethylsuccinate) Abbott 421
Ery-Tab Tablets (Erythromycin) Abbott 422
Erythrocin Stearate Filmtab (Erythromycin Stearate) Abbott 425
Erythromycin Base Filmtab (Erythromycin) Abbott 426
Erythromycin Delayed-Release Capsules, USP (Erythromycin) Abbott 427
Ilosone (Erythromycin Estolate) Dista 911
Ilotycin Gluceptate, IV, Vials (Erythromycin Gluceptate) Dista 913
PCE Dispertab Tablets (Erythromycin) Abbott 444
Septra (Trimethoprim, Sulfamethoxazole) Glaxo Wellcome 1174
Spectrobid Tablets (Bacampicillin Hydrochloride) Roerig 2206

H. influenzae, central nervous system infections
Ceptaz (Ceftazidime) Glaxo Wellcome 1081
Claforan Sterile and Injection (Cefotaxime Sodium) Hoechst-Roussel 1235
Fortaz (Ceftazidime) Glaxo Wellcome 1100
Tazicef for Injection (Ceftazidime) SmithKline Beecham Pharmaceuticals 2519
Tazidime Vials, Faspak & ADD-Vantage (Ceftazidime) Lilly .. 1478

H. influenzae, skin and skin structure infections
Mandol Vials, Faspak & ADD-Vantage (Cefamandole Nafate) Lilly 1461

H. parainfluenzae bronchitis
Ceftin (Cefuroxime Axetil) Glaxo Wellcome 1078

H. parainfluenzae infections
Ceftin (Cefuroxime Axetil) Glaxo Wellcome 1078
Cipro I.V. Pharmacy Bulk Package (Ciprofloxacin) Bayer Pharmaceutical 597
Cipro Tablets (Ciprofloxacin Hydrochloride) Bayer Pharmaceutical 592
Claforan Sterile and Injection (Cefotaxime Sodium) Hoechst-Roussel 1235
Primaxin I.V. (Imipenem-Cilastatin Sodium) Merck & Co., Inc. 1729
Rocephin Injectable Vials, ADD-Vantage, Galaxy Container (Ceftriaxone Sodium) Roche Laboratories 2142

H. parainfluenzae lower respiratory tract infections
Cipro I.V. (Ciprofloxacin) Bayer Pharmaceutical 595
Cipro I.V. Pharmacy Bulk Package (Ciprofloxacin) Bayer Pharmaceutical 597
Cipro Tablets (Ciprofloxacin Hydrochloride) Bayer Pharmaceutical 592
Claforan Sterile and Injection (Cefotaxime Sodium) Hoechst-Roussel 1235
Primaxin I.V. (Imipenem-Cilastatin Sodium) Merck & Co., Inc. 1729
Rocephin Injectable Vials, ADD-Vantage, Galaxy Container (Ceftriaxone Sodium) Roche Laboratories 2142
Suprax for Oral Suspension (Cefixime) Lederle 1399

H. vaginalis vaginitis
MetroGel-Vaginal (Metronidazole) Curatek 902
Sultrin (Sulfathiazole, Sulfacetamide, Sulfabenzamide) Ortho Pharmaceutical 1885

Haemophilus influenzae (see under H. influenzae infections)

Hair, cleansing of
Bio-Complex 5000 Revitalizing Conditioner (Cleanser) Wellness International .... ▣ 865
Bio-Complex 5000 Revitalizing Shampoo (Cleanser) Wellness International .... ▣ 865
Concept Antimicrobial Skin Cleanser (Chloroxylenol) Care-Tech .... ▣ 625

Hair loss or thinning of the frontoparietal areas, females
Rogaine Topical Solution (Minoxidil) Upjohn 2637

Hairy cell leukemias (see under Leukemia, hairy cell)

Halitosis, adjunctive therapy in
Cēpacol/Cēpacol Mint Mouthwash/Gargle (Cetylpyridinium Chloride) J.B. Williams .. ▣ 875
Listerine Antiseptic (Eucalyptol, Menthol, Methyl Salicylate) WARNER WELLCOME .... ▣ 855
FreshBurst Listerine (Thymol, Eucalyptol, Methyl Salicylate, Menthol) WARNER WELLCOME ▣ 856
Listermint Alcohol-Free Mouthwash (Sodium Fluoride) WARNER WELLCOME .... ▣ 855
Salix SST Lozenges Saliva Stimulant (Sorbitol, Malic Acid, Sodium Citrate, Citric Acid, Dicalcium Phosphate) Scandinavian Natural .... ▣ 797

Hansen's disease (see under Leprosy)

Hashimoto's thyroiditis
Cytomel Tablets (Liothyronine Sodium) SmithKline Beecham Pharmaceuticals 2473
Synthroid (Levothyroxine Sodium) Knoll Pharmaceutical 1359

Haverhill fever (see under Streptobacillus moniliformis infections)

Hay fever (see under Pollinosis)

Headache
Alka-Seltzer Effervescent Antacid and Pain Reliever (Aspirin, Sodium Bicarbonate, Citric Acid) Miles Consumer .... ▣ 701
Alka-Seltzer Extra Strength Effervescent Antacid and Pain Reliever (Aspirin, Sodium Bicarbonate, Citric Acid) Miles Consumer .... ▣ 703
Alka-Seltzer Lemon Lime Effervescent Antacid and Pain Reliever (Aspirin, Sodium Citrate) Miles Consumer .... ▣ 703
Arthritis Foundation Aspirin Free Caplets (Acetaminophen) McNeil Consumer .... ▣ 673
Arthritis Foundation NightTime Caplets (Acetaminophen, Diphenhydramine Hydrochloride) McNeil Consumer .... ▣ 674
Maximum Strength Ascriptin (Aspirin Buffered, Calcium Carbonate) CIBA Consumer .... ▣ 630
BC Powder (Aspirin, Salicylamide, Caffeine) Block .... ▣ 609
Bayer Children's Chewable Aspirin (Aspirin) Miles Consumer .... ▣ 711
Genuine Bayer Aspirin Tablets & Caplets (Aspirin) Miles Consumer .... ▣ 713
Extra Strength Bayer Aspirin Caplets & Tablets (Aspirin) Miles Consumer .... ▣ 712
Extended-Release Bayer 8-Hour Aspirin (Aspirin) Miles Consumer .... ▣ 712
Extra Strength Bayer Plus Aspirin Caplets (Aspirin, Calcium Carbonate) Miles Consumer .... ▣ 713
Bayer Select Headache Pain Relief Formula (Acetaminophen, Caffeine) Miles Consumer .... ▣ 716
Bayer Select Ibuprofen Pain Relief Formula (Ibuprofen) Miles Consumer .... ▣ 715
Bufferin Analgesic Tablets and Caplets (Aspirin) Bristol-Myers Products .... ▣ 613
Extra Strength Bufferin Analgesic Tablets (Aspirin) Bristol-Myers Products .... ▣ 615

(▣ Described in PDR For Nonprescription Drugs) (◉ Described in PDR For Ophthalmology)

Headache **Indications Index** 1490

Cramp End Tablets (Ibuprofen) Ohm ■ 735
Ecotrin (Aspirin, Enteric Coated) SmithKline Beecham 2455
Empirin Aspirin Tablets (Aspirin) WARNER WELLCOME ■ 854
Aspirin Free Excedrin Analgesic Caplets and Geltabs (Acetaminophen, Caffeine) Bristol-Myers Products 732
Excedrin Extra-Strength Analgesic Tablets & Caplets (Acetaminophen, Aspirin, Caffeine) Bristol-Myers Products 732
Excedrin P.M. Analgesic/Sleeping Aid Tablets, Caplets, Liquigels (Acetaminophen, Diphenhydramine Citrate) Bristol-Myers Products 733
Fiorinal with Codeine Capsules (Codeine Phosphate, Butalbital, Caffeine, Aspirin) Sandoz Pharmaceuticals 2262
Haltran Tablets (Ibuprofen) Roberts ■ 771
Healthprin Aspirin (Aspirin) Smart 2455
Ibuprohm (Ibuprofen) Ohm ■ 735
Teen Multi-Symptom Formula Midol (Acetaminophen, Pamabrom) Miles Consumer ■ 722
Mobigesic Tablets (Magnesium Salicylate, Phenyltoloxamine Citrate) Ascher ■ 602
Children's Motrin Ibuprofen Oral Suspension (Ibuprofen) McNeil Consumer 1546
Motrin IB Caplets, Tablets, and Geltabs (Ibuprofen) Upjohn ■ 838
Nuprin Ibuprofen/Analgesic Tablets & Caplets (Ibuprofen) Bristol-Myers Products ■ 622
Panodol Tablets and Caplets (Acetaminophen) SmithKline Beecham Consumer ■ 824
Children's Panadol Chewable Tablets, Liquid, Infant's Drops (Acetaminophen) SmithKline Beecham Consumer ■ 824
Percogesic Analgesic Tablets (Acetaminophen, Phenyltoloxamine Citrate) Procter & Gamble ■ 754
St. Joseph Adult Chewable Aspirin (81 mg.) (Aspirin) Schering-Plough HealthCare ■ 808
TYLENOL, Extra Strength, Acetaminophen Adult Liquid Pain Reliever (Acetaminophen) McNeil Consumer 1560
TYLENOL, Extra Strength, acetaminophen Gelcaps, Geltabs, Caplets, Tablets (Acetaminophen) McNeil Consumer 1559
TYLENOL, Junior Strength, acetaminophen Coated Caplets, Grape and Fruit Chewable Tablets (Acetaminophen) McNeil Consumer 1557
TYLENOL, Regular Strength, acetaminophen Caplets and Tablets (Acetaminophen) McNeil Consumer 1558
Vanquish Analgesic Caplets (Acetaminophen, Aspirin, Caffeine, Aluminum Hydroxide Gel, Magnesium Hydroxide) Miles Consumer ■ 731

Headache accompanied by insomnia
Extra Strength Bayer PM Aspirin (Aspirin, Diphenhydramine Hydrochloride) Miles Consumer ■ 713
Bayer Select Night Time Pain Relief Formula (Acetaminophen, Diphenhydramine Hydrochloride) Miles Consumer ■ 716
Excedrin P.M. Analgesic/Sleeping Aid Tablets, Caplets, Liquigels (Acetaminophen, Diphenhydramine Citrate) Bristol-Myers Products 733
TYLENOL PM, Extra Strength Pain Reliever/Sleep Aid Caplets, Geltabs, Gelcaps (Acetaminophen, Diphenhydramine Hydrochloride) McNeil Consumer 1560
Unisom With Pain Relief-Nighttime Sleep Aid and Pain Reliever (Diphenhydramine Hydrochloride, Acetaminophen) Pfizer Consumer 1934

Headache associated with common cold (see also under Sinus headache)
Advil Cold and Sinus Caplets and Tablets (formerly CoAdvil) (Ibuprofen, Pseudoephedrine Hydrochloride) Whitehall ■ 870
Children's TYLENOL Cold Multi-Symptom Liquid Formula and Chewable Tablets (Acetaminophen, Chlorpheniramine Maleate, Pseudoephedrine Hydrochloride) McNeil Consumer 1561

Headache with gastric hyperacidity
Alka-Seltzer Effervescent Antacid and Pain Reliever (Aspirin, Sodium Bicarbonate, Citric Acid) Miles Consumer ■ 701
Alka-Seltzer Extra Strength Effervescent Antacid and Pain Reliever (Aspirin, Sodium Bicarbonate, Citric Acid) Miles Consumer ■ 703
Alka-Seltzer Lemon Lime Effervescent Antacid and Pain Reliever (Aspirin, Sodium Citrate) Miles Consumer ■ 703
TYLENOL, Extra Strength, Headache Plus Pain Reliever with Antacid Caplets (Acetaminophen, Calcium Carbonate) McNeil Consumer 1559

Headache with upset stomach
Alka-Seltzer Effervescent Antacid and Pain Reliever (Aspirin, Sodium Bicarbonate, Citric Acid) Miles Consumer ■ 701
Alka-Seltzer Extra Strength Effervescent Antacid and Pain Reliever (Aspirin, Sodium Bicarbonate, Citric Acid) Miles Consumer ■ 703
Alka-Seltzer Lemon Lime Effervescent Antacid and Pain Reliever (Aspirin, Sodium Citrate) Miles Consumer ■ 703

Headache, cluster (see under Cephalalgia, histaminic)

Headache, migraine
Cafergot (Ergotamine Tartrate, Caffeine) Sandoz Pharmaceuticals 2251
D.H.E. 45 Injection (Dihydroergotamine Mesylate) Sandoz Pharmaceuticals 2255
Imitrex Injection (Sumatriptan Succinate) Glaxo Wellcome 1103
Imitrex Tablets (Sumatriptan Succinate) Glaxo Wellcome 1106
Wigraine Tablets & Suppositories (Ergotamine Tartrate, Caffeine) Organon 1829

Headache, migraine, "possibly" effective in
Midrin Capsules (Isometheptene Mucate, Dichloralphenazone, Acetaminophen) Carnrick 783
Migralam Capsules (Isometheptene Mucate, Caffeine, Acetaminophen) Rico Pharmacal 2038

Headache, migraine, prevention or reduction of intensity and frequency of
Cafergot (Ergotamine Tartrate, Caffeine) Sandoz Pharmaceuticals 2251
D.H.E. 45 Injection (Dihydroergotamine Mesylate) Sandoz Pharmaceuticals 2255
Ergomar (Ergotamine Tartrate) Lotus 1486
Sansert Tablets (Methysergide Maleate) Sandoz Pharmaceuticals 2295

Headache, migraine, prophylaxis of (see also under Headache, migraine, prevention or reduction of intensity and frequency of)
Blocadren Tablets (Timolol Maleate) Merck & Co., Inc. 1614
Inderal (Propranolol Hydrochloride) Wyeth-Ayerst 2728
Inderal LA Long Acting Capsules (Propranolol Hydrochloride) Wyeth-Ayerst 2730

Headache, sinus, symptomatic relief of (see under Sinus headache)

Headache, tension (see also under Pain, unspecified; Pain with anxiety and tension)
Esgic-plus Tablets (Butalbital, Acetaminophen, Caffeine) Forest 1013
Fioricet Tablets (Butalbital, Acetaminophen, Caffeine) Sandoz Pharmaceuticals 2258
Fioricet with Codeine Capsules (Butalbital, Acetaminophen, Caffeine, Codeine Phosphate) Sandoz Pharmaceuticals 2260
Fiorinal Capsules (Butalbital, Aspirin) Sandoz Pharmaceuticals 2261
Fiorinal with Codeine Capsules (Codeine Phosphate, Butalbital, Caffeine, Aspirin) Sandoz Pharmaceuticals 2262
Fiorinal Tablets (Butalbital, Aspirin) Sandoz Pharmaceuticals 2261
Phrenilin (Butalbital, Acetaminophen) Carnrick 785
Sedapap Tablets 50 mg/650 mg (Acetaminophen, Butalbital) Mayrand 1543

Headache, vascular (see under Headache, migraine)

Heart block, mild or transient episodes of
Isuprel Hydrochloride Injection 1:5000 (Isoproterenol Hydrochloride) Sanofi Winthrop 2311

Heart block, serious episodes of
Isuprel Hydrochloride Injection 1:5000 (Isoproterenol Hydrochloride) Sanofi Winthrop 2311

Heart failure (see under Congestive heart failure)

Heart failure, congestive (see under Congestive heart failure)

Heart, allogeneic transplants, prophylaxis of organ rejection in
Neoral (Cyclosporine) Sandoz Pharmaceuticals 2276
Orthoclone OKT3 Sterile Solution (Muromonab-CD3) Ortho Biotech 1837
Sandimmune (Cyclosporine) Sandoz Pharmaceuticals 2286

Heartburn (see under Hyperacidity, gastric, symptomatic relief of)

Hemolytic disease, Rh, prevention of (see under Erythroblastosis fetalis, prevention of)

Hemophilia A
Bioclate, Antihemophilic Factor (Recombinant) (Antihemophilic Factor (Recombinant)) Armour 513
DDAVP Injection (Desmopressin Acetate) Rhone-Poulenc Rorer Pharmaceuticals 2014
DDAVP Injection 15 mcg/mL (Desmopressin Acetate) Rhone-Poulenc Rorer Pharmaceuticals 2015
Helixate, Antihemophilic Factor (Recombinant) (Antihemophilic Factor (Recombinant)) Armour 518
Humate-P, Antihemophilic Factor (Human), Pasteurized (Antihemophilic Factor (Human)) Armour 520
Koāte-HP Antihemophilic Factor (Human) (Antihemophilic Factor (Human)) Bayer Biological 630
KOGENATE Antihemophilic Factor (Recombinant) (Antihemophilic Factor (Recombinant)) Bayer Biological 632
Monoclate-P, Factor VIII:C, Pasteurized, Monoclonal Antibody Purified Antihemophilic Factor (Human) (Antihemophilic Factor (Human)) Armour 521
Stimate, (desmopressin acetate) Nasal Spray, 1.5 mg/mL (Desmopressin Acetate) Armour 525

Hemophilia B
Konÿne 80 Factor IX Complex (Factor IX Complex) Bayer Biological 634
Mononine, Coagulation Factor IX (Human) (Factor IX (Human)) Armour 523

Hemophilia, congenital with antibodies to Factor VIII:C
KOGENATE Antihemophilic Factor (Recombinant) (Antihemophilic Factor (Recombinant)) Bayer Biological 632

Hemorrhage, coumarin anticoagulant-induced, reversal of
Konÿne 80 Factor IX Complex (Factor IX Complex) Bayer Biological 634

Hemorrhage, postpartum, control of
AquaMEPHYTON Injection (Phytonadione) Merck & Co., Inc. 1608
Methergine (Methylergonovine Maleate) Sandoz Pharmaceuticals 2272
Oxytocin Injection (Oxytocin) Wyeth-Ayerst 2771
Syntocinon Injection (Oxytocin) Sandoz Pharmaceuticals 2296

Hemorrhage, subarachnoid, resulting in neurological deficits
Nimotop Capsules (Nimodipine) Bayer Pharmaceutical 610

Hemorrhoidal pain (see under Pain, anorectal)

Hemorrhoids
Americaine Hemorrhoidal Ointment (Benzocaine) CIBA Consumer ■ 629
Anusol (Starch) WARNER WELLCOME ■ 847
Anusol-HC Suppositories (Hydrocortisone Acetate) Parke-Davis 1897
Hemorid For Women (Petrolatum, White, Mineral Oil, Pramoxine Hydrochloride, Phenylephrine Hydrochloride) Thompson Medical ■ 834
Nupercainal Hemorrhoidal and Anesthetic Ointment (Dibucaine) CIBA Consumer ■ 644
Nupercainal Suppositories (Cocoa Butter, Zinc Oxide) CIBA Consumer ■ 645
Preparation H (Glycerin, Petrolatum, Phenylephrine Hydrochloride, Shark Liver Oil) Whitehall ■ 871
Tronolane Anesthetic Cream for Hemorrhoids (Pramoxine Hydrochloride) Ross ■ 784
Tronolane Hemorrhoidal Suppositories (Fat, Hard, Zinc Oxide) Ross ■ 784
Tucks Clear Hemorrhoidal Gel (Witch Hazel, Glycerin) WARNER WELLCOME ■ 865
Tucks Pads (Witch Hazel) WARNER WELLCOME ■ 865
Wyanoids Relief Factor Hemorrhoidal Suppositories (Liver, Desiccated, Shark Liver Oil) Wyeth-Ayerst ■ 881

Hemostasis, an aid in
Amicar Syrup, Tablets, and Injection (Aminocaproic Acid) Immunex 1267
Cyklokapron Tablets and Injection (Tranexamic Acid) Pharmacia 1950
DDAVP Injection (Desmopressin Acetate) Rhone-Poulenc Rorer Pharmaceuticals 2014
Gelfoam Sterile Sponge (Gelatin Preparations) Upjohn 2608
INSTAT* Collagen Absorbable Hemostat (Collagen) J & J Medical 1312

(■ Described in PDR For Nonprescription Drugs) (◉ Described in PDR For Ophthalmology)

1491 **Indications Index** **Hyperacidity**

INSTAT* MCH Microfibrillar Collagen Hemostat (Collagen, bovine) J & J Medical 1313
Surgicel (Oxidized Regenerated Cellulose) J & J Medical 1314
THROMBOGEN* Topical Thrombin, USP with Diluent and Transfer Needle (Thrombin) J & J Medical 1315
THROMBOGEN* Topical Thrombin, USP, Spray Kit (Thrombin) J & J Medical 1315
Trasylol (Aprotinin) Bayer Pharmaceutical 613

Heparin overdose, treatment of
Protamine Sulfate Ampoules & Vials (Protamine Sulfate) Lilly 1471

Hepatitis, chronic, Non-A, Non-B/C
Intron A (Interferon alfa-2B, Recombinant) Schering 2364

Hepatitis B virus, postexposure prophylaxis
HyperHep Hepatitis B Immune Globulin (Human) (Hepatitis B Immune Globulin (Human)) Bayer Biological 626

Hepatitis A, prophylaxis
Gammar, Immune Globulin (Human) U.S.P. (Globulin, Immune (Human)) Armour 515

Hepatitis B, chronic, treatment of
Intron A (Interferon alfa-2B, Recombinant) Schering 2364

Hepatitis B virus infection, immunization against
Recombivax HB (Hepatitis B Vaccine) Merck & Co., Inc. 1744

Hereditary coproporphyria (see under Coproporphyria, hereditary)

Herellea vaginicola (see under Acinetobacter calcoaceticus infections, ocular)

Herpes, genital, initial and recurrent episodes
Zovirax Capsules (Acyclovir) Glaxo Wellcome 1219
Zovirax Sterile Powder (Acyclovir Sodium) Glaxo Wellcome 1223
Zovirax (Acyclovir) Glaxo Wellcome 1219

Herpes genitalis
Zovirax Capsules (Acyclovir) Glaxo Wellcome 1219
Zovirax Ointment 5% (Acyclovir) Glaxo Wellcome 1223
Zovirax Sterile Powder (Acyclovir Sodium) Glaxo Wellcome 1223
Zovirax (Acyclovir) Glaxo Wellcome 1219

Herpes simplex infections, ocular
Herplex Liquifilm (Idoxuridine) Allergan ..... ⊙ 244
Vira-A Ophthalmic Ointment, 3% (Vidarabine) Parke-Davis ..... ⊙ 312
Viroptic Ophthalmic Solution, 1% Sterile (Trifluridine) Glaxo Wellcome 1204

Herpes simplex keratitis
Herplex Liquifilm (Idoxuridine) Allergan ..... ⊙ 244
Viroptic Ophthalmic Solution, 1% Sterile (Trifluridine) Glaxo Wellcome 1204

Herpes simplex virus encephalitis
Zovirax Sterile Powder (Acyclovir Sodium) Glaxo Wellcome 1223

Herpes simplex virus infections
Zovirax Ointment 5% (Acyclovir) Glaxo Wellcome 1223
Zovirax Sterile Powder (Acyclovir Sodium) Glaxo Wellcome 1223

Herpes simplex virus mucocutaneous infection
Foscavir Injection (Foscarnet Sodium) Astra 547
Zovirax Ointment 5% (Acyclovir) Glaxo Wellcome 1223
Zovirax Sterile Powder (Acyclovir Sodium) Glaxo Wellcome 1223

Herpes zoster infections
Famvir (Famciclovir) SmithKline Beecham Pharmaceuticals 2486
Valtrex Caplets (Valacyclovir Hydrochloride) Glaxo Wellcome 1194
Zovirax (Acyclovir) Glaxo Wellcome 1219

Herpes zoster ophthalmicus
Aristocort Suspension (Forte Parenteral) (Triamcinolone Diacetate) Fujisawa 1027
Aristocort Tablets (Triamcinolone) Fujisawa 1022
Celestone Soluspan Suspension (Betamethasone Sodium Phosphate, Betamethasone Acetate) Schering 2347
Cortone Acetate Sterile Suspension (Cortisone Acetate) Merck & Co., Inc. 1623
Cortone Acetate Tablets (Cortisone Acetate) Merck & Co., Inc. 1624
Dalalone D.P. Injectable (Dexamethasone Acetate) Forest 1011
Decadron Elixir (Dexamethasone) Merck & Co., Inc. 1633
Decadron Phosphate Injection (Dexamethasone Sodium Phosphate) Merck & Co., Inc. 1637
Decadron Tablets (Dexamethasone) Merck & Co., Inc. 1635
Decadron-LA Sterile Suspension (Dexamethasone Acetate) Merck & Co., Inc. 1646
Deltasone Tablets (Prednisone) Upjohn 2595
Depo-Medrol Single-Dose Vial (Methylprednisolone Acetate) Upjohn 2600
Depo-Medrol Sterile Aqueous Suspension (Methylprednisolone Acetate) Upjohn 2597
Hydeltrasol Injection, Sterile (Prednisolone Sodium Phosphate) Merck & Co., Inc. 1665
Hydrocortone Phosphate Injection, Sterile (Hydrocortisone Sodium Phosphate) Merck & Co., Inc. 1670
Hydrocortone Tablets (Hydrocortisone) Merck & Co., Inc. 1672
Medrol (Methylprednisolone) Upjohn 2621
Pediapred Oral Liquid (Prednisolone Sodium Phosphate) Fisons 995
Prelone Syrup (Prednisolone) Muro 1787
Solu-Cortef Sterile Powder (Hydrocortisone Sodium Succinate) Upjohn 2641
Solu-Medrol Sterile Powder (Methylprednisolone Sodium Succinate) Upjohn 2643

Herpetic manifestations, oral, symptomatic relief of
Campho-Phenique Cold Sore Gel (Camphor, Phenol) Miles Consumer ..... ▣ 719
Herpecin-L Cold Sore Lip Balm Stick (Allantoin) Campbell 779
Orajel Mouth-Aid for Canker and Cold Sores (Benzocaine, Benzalkonium Chloride, Zinc Chloride) Del ..... ▣ 652
Tanac Medicated Gel (Dyclonine Hydrochloride, Allantoin) Del ..... ▣ 653
Tanac No Sting Liquid (Benzocaine, Benzalkonium Chloride) Del ..... ▣ 653
Zilactin/Dermaflex (Benzyl Alcohol) Zila Pharmaceuticals ..... ▣ 882

Hiccup
Thorazine (Chlorpromazine Hydrochloride) SmithKline Beecham Pharmaceuticals 2523

Histoplasmosis
Fungizone Intravenous (Amphotericin B) Apothecon 506
Nizoral Tablets (Ketoconazole) Janssen 1298
Sporanox Capsules (Itraconazole) Janssen 1305

HIV infection (see under Infection, human immunodeficiency virus)

Hodgkin's disease
Adriamycin PFS (Doxorubicin Hydrochloride) Pharmacia 1947
Adriamycin RDF (Doxorubicin Hydrochloride) Pharmacia 1947
Blenoxane (Bleomycin Sulfate) Bristol-Myers Squibb Oncology 692
Cytoxan (Cyclophosphamide) Bristol-Myers Squibb Oncology 694
Doxorubicin Astra (Doxorubicin Hydrochloride) Astra 540
Leukeran Tablets (Chlorambucil) Glaxo Wellcome 1133
NEOSAR Lyophilized/Neosar (Cyclophosphamide) Pharmacia 1959
Oncovin Solution Vials & Hyporets (Vincristine Sulfate) Lilly 1466
Rubex (Doxorubicin Hydrochloride) Bristol-Myers Squibb Oncology 712
Thioplex (Thiotepa For Injection) (Thiotepa) Immunex 1281
Velban Vials (Vinblastine Sulfate) Lilly 1484

Hodgkin's disease, adjunctive therapy in
Leukine for IV Infusion (Sargramostim) Immunex 1271

Hodgkin's disease, secondary line therapy in
BiCNU (Carmustine (BCNU)) Bristol-Myers Squibb Oncology 691
CeeNU (Lomustine (CCNU)) Bristol-Myers Squibb Oncology 693
DTIC-Dome (Dacarbazine) Bayer Pharmaceutical 600
Matulane Capsules (Procarbazine Hydrochloride) Roche Laboratories 2131

Hodgkin's disease, stages III and IV, palliative treatment of
Matulane Capsules (Procarbazine Hydrochloride) Roche Laboratories 2131
Mustargen (Mechlorethamine Hydrochloride) Merck & Co., Inc. 1709

Hookworm infections (see under Ancylostoma duodenale infections)

Hookworm, American (see under Necator americanus infections)

Hormonal imbalance, male
Halotestin Tablets (Fluoxymesterone) Upjohn 2614

Horton's headache (see under Cephalalgia, histaminic)

Hydatidiform mole
Methotrexate Sodium Tablets, Injection, for Injection and LPF Injection (Methotrexate Sodium) Immunex 1275

Hyperacidity, gastric, symptomatic relief of
Alka-Mints Chewable Antacid (Calcium Carbonate) Miles Consumer ..... ▣ 701
Alka-Seltzer Gold Effervescent Antacid (Citric Acid, Potassium Bicarbonate, Sodium Bicarbonate) Miles Consumer ..... ▣ 703
ALternaGEL Liquid (Aluminum Hydroxide) J&J•Merck Consumer 1316
Aludrox Oral Suspension (Aluminum Hydroxide Gel, Magnesium Hydroxide) Wyeth-Ayerst 2695
Amphojel (Aluminum Hydroxide Gel) Wyeth-Ayerst 2695
Arm & Hammer Pure Baking Soda (Sodium Bicarbonate) Church & Dwight ..... ▣ 627
Basaljel (Aluminum Carbonate Gel) Wyeth-Ayerst 2703
Bicitra (Sodium Citrate, Citric Acid) Baker Norton 578
Chooz Antacid Gum (Calcium Carbonate) Schering-Plough HealthCare ..... ▣ 799
Citrocarbonate Antacid (Sodium Bicarbonate, Sodium Citrate) Roberts ..... ▣ 770
Di-Gel Antacid/Anti-Gas (Calcium Carbonate, Magnesium Hydroxide, Simethicone) Schering-Plough HealthCare ..... ▣ 801
Gaviscon Antacid Tablets (Aluminum Hydroxide Gel, Magnesium Trisilicate) SmithKline Beecham Consumer ..... ▣ 819
Gaviscon-2 Antacid Tablets (Aluminum Hydroxide Gel, Magnesium Trisilicate) SmithKline Beecham Consumer ..... ▣ 820
Gaviscon Extra Strength Relief Formula Antacid Tablets (Aluminum Hydroxide, Magnesium Carbonate) SmithKline Beecham Consumer ..... ▣ 819
Gaviscon Extra Strength Relief Formula Liquid Antacid (Aluminum Hydroxide, Magnesium Carbonate) SmithKline Beecham Consumer ..... ▣ 819
Gaviscon Liquid Antacid (Aluminum Hydroxide, Magnesium Carbonate) SmithKline Beecham Consumer ..... ▣ 820
Gelusil Liquid & Tablets (Aluminum Hydroxide, Magnesium Hydroxide, Simethicone) WARNER WELLCOME ..... ▣ 855
Maalox Antacid Caplets (Calcium Carbonate) CIBA Consumer ..... ▣ 638
Maalox Heartburn Relief Suspension (Aluminum Hydroxide, Magnesium Carbonate) CIBA Consumer ..... ▣ 642
Maalox Heartburn Relief Tablets (Aluminum Hydroxide, Magnesium Carbonate) CIBA Consumer ..... ▣ 641
Maalox Magnesia and Alumina Oral Suspension (Magnesium Hydroxide, Aluminum Hydroxide) CIBA Consumer ..... ▣ 642
Maalox Plus Tablets (Aluminum Hydroxide, Magnesium Hydroxide, Simethicone) CIBA Consumer ..... ▣ 643
Extra Strength Maalox Antacid Plus Antigas Liquid and Tablets (Aluminum Hydroxide, Magnesium Hydroxide, Simethicone) CIBA Consumer ..... ▣ 638
Mag-Ox 400 (Magnesium Oxide) Blaine 668
Marblen (Calcium Carbonate, Magnesium Carbonate) Fleming ▣ 655
Mylanta Calcium Carbonate and Magnesium Hydroxide Tablets (Calcium Carbonate, Magnesium Hydroxide) J&J•Merck Consumer 1318
Mylanta Gelcaps Antacid (Calcium Carbonate, Magnesium Carbonate) J&J•Merck Consumer ..... ▣ 662
Mylanta Liquid (Aluminum Hydroxide, Magnesium Hydroxide, Simethicone) J&J•Merck Consumer 1317
Mylanta Soothing Lozenges (Calcium Carbonate) J&J•Merck Consumer 1319
Mylanta Tablets (Aluminum Hydroxide, Magnesium Hydroxide, Simethicone) J&J•Merck Consumer ..... ▣ 660
Mylanta Double Strength Liquid (Aluminum Hydroxide, Magnesium Hydroxide, Simethicone) J&J•Merck Consumer 1317
Mylanta Double Strength Tablets (Aluminum Hydroxide, Magnesium Hydroxide, Simethicone) J&J•Merck Consumer ..... ▣ 660
Nephrox Suspension (Aluminum Hydroxide Gel, Mineral Oil) Fleming ..... ▣ 655
Pepcid AC (Famotidine) J&J•Merck Consumer 1319
Phillips' Milk of Magnesia Liquid (Magnesium Hydroxide) Miles Consumer ..... ▣ 729
Rolaids Tablets (Calcium Carbonate, Magnesium Hydroxide) Warner-Lambert ..... ▣ 843
Rolaids (Calcium Rich/Sodium Free) Tablets (Calcium Carbonate) Warner-Lambert ..... ▣ 843
Tempo Soft Antacid (Calcium Carbonate, Aluminum Hydrox-

(▣ Described in PDR For Nonprescription Drugs) (⊙ Described in PDR For Ophthalmology)

Hyperacidity — Indications Index — 1492

ide, Magnesium Hydroxide, Simethicone) Thompson Medical ▣ 835
Titralac (Calcium Carbonate) 3M ▣ 672
Titralac Plus (Calcium Carbonate, Simethicone) 3M ▣ 672
Tums Antacid Tablets (Calcium Carbonate) SmithKline Beecham Consumer ▣ 827
Tums Anti-gas/Antacid Formula Tablets, Assorted Fruit (Calcium Carbonate, Simethicone) SmithKline Beecham Consumer ▣ 827
Tums (Calcium Carbonate) SmithKline Beecham Consumer ▣ 827
Uro-Mag (Magnesium Oxide) Blaine 668

Hyperaldosteronism, primary
Aldactone (Spironolactone) Searle .. 2414

Hyperbetalipoproteinemia (see under Hyperlipoproteinemia, types IIa and IIb, adjunct to diet)

Hypercalcemia associated with cancer
Aredia for Injection (Pamidronate Disodium) CibaGeneva 810
Aristocort Suspension (Forte Parenteral) (Triamcinolone Diacetate) Fujisawa 1027
Aristocort Tablets (Triamcinolone) Fujisawa 1022
Celestone Soluspan Suspension (Betamethasone Sodium Phosphate, Betamethasone Acetate) Schering 2347
Cortone Acetate Sterile Suspension (Cortisone Acetate) Merck & Co., Inc. 1623
Cortone Acetate Tablets (Cortisone Acetate) Merck & Co., Inc. 1624
Dalalone D.P. Injectable (Dexamethasone Acetate) Forest 1011
Decadron Elixir (Dexamethasone) Merck & Co., Inc. 1633
Decadron Phosphate Injection (Dexamethasone Sodium Phosphate) Merck & Co., Inc. 1637
Decadron Tablets (Dexamethasone) Merck & Co., Inc. 1635
Decadron-LA Sterile Suspension (Dexamethasone Acetate) Merck & Co., Inc. 1646
Deltasone Tablets (Prednisone) Upjohn 2595
Depo-Medrol Single-Dose Vial (Methylprednisolone Acetate) Upjohn 2600
Depo-Medrol Sterile Aqueous Suspension (Methylprednisolone Acetate) Upjohn 2597
Ganite (Gallium Nitrate) SoloPak 2533
Hydeltrasol Injection, Sterile (Prednisolone Sodium Phosphate) Merck & Co., Inc. 1665
Hydrocortone Phosphate Injection, Sterile (Hydrocortisone Sodium Phosphate) Merck & Co., Inc. 1670
Hydrocortone Tablets (Hydrocortisone) Merck & Co., Inc. 1672
Medrol (Methylprednisolone) Upjohn 2621
Mithracin (Plicamycin) Bayer Pharmaceutical 607
Pediapred Oral Liquid (Prednisolone Sodium Phosphate) Fisons 995
Prelone Syrup (Prednisolone) Muro 1787
Solu-Cortef Sterile Powder (Hydrocortisone Sodium Succinate) Upjohn 2641
Solu-Medrol Sterile Powder (Methylprednisolone Sodium Succinate) Upjohn 2643

Hypercalcemia of malignancy, adjunct
Didronel I.V. Infusion (Etidronate Disodium (Biphosphonate)) MGI .. 1488

Hypercalcemic emergencies, adjunct in
Calcimar Injection, Synthetic (Calcitonin, Synthetic) Rhone-Poulenc Rorer Pharmaceuticals 2013
Miacalcin Injection (Calcitonin, Synthetic) Sandoz Pharmaceuticals 2273

Hypercalciuria associated with cancer
Mithracin (Plicamycin) Bayer Pharmaceutical 607

Hypercapnia, acute, with COPD (see under Respiratory insufficiency, acute, with chronic obstructive pulmonary disease)

Hypercholesterolemia, primary, adjunct to diet
Colestid Tablets (Colestipol Hydrochloride) Upjohn 2591
Lescol Capsules (Fluvastatin Sodium) Sandoz Pharmaceuticals 2267
Lorelco Tablets (Probucol) Marion Merrell Dow 1517
Mevacor Tablets (Lovastatin) Merck & Co., Inc. 1699
Pravachol (Pravastatin Sodium) Bristol-Myers Squibb 765
Questran Light (Cholestyramine) Bristol-Myers Squibb 769
Questran Powder (Cholestyramine) Bristol-Myers Squibb 770
Zocor Tablets (Simvastatin) Merck & Co., Inc. 1775

Hyperglycemia, control of, adjunct to diet (see also under Diabetes mellitus, insulin-dependent; Diabetes mellitus, non-insulin-dependent)
DiaBeta Tablets (Glyburide) Hoechst-Roussel 1239
Diabinese Tablets (Chlorpropamide) Pfizer Labs 1935
Glucophage (Metformin Hydrochloride) Bristol-Myers Squibb 752
Glucotrol Tablets (Glipizide) Pratt .. 1967
Glucotrol XL Extended Release Tablets (Glipizide) Pratt 1968
Glynase PresTab Tablets (Glyburide) Upjohn 2609
Micronase Tablets (Glyburide) Upjohn 2623

Hyperhidrosis associated with Parkinsonism
Levsin/Levsinex/Levbid (Hyoscyamine Sulfate) Schwarz 2405

Hyperhidrosis, topical relief of
Cruex Antifungal Powder (Calcium Undecylenate) CIBA Consumer ▣ 632
Desenex Foot & Sneaker Deodorant Spray (Aluminum Chlorohydrate) CIBA Consumer ▣ 633
Drysol (Aluminum Chloride) Persōn & Covey 1932
Xerac AC (Aluminum Chloride) Persōn & Covey 1933

Hyperkalemia
Kayexalate (Sodium Polystyrene Sulfonate) Sanofi Winthrop 2314
Sodium Polystyrene Sulfonate Suspension (Sodium Polystyrene Sulfonate) Roxane 2244

Hyperkeratosis skin disorders
Bichloracetic Acid Kahlenberg (Dichloroacetic Acid) Glenwood 1229
Lac-Hydrin 12% Lotion (Ammonium Lactate) Westwood-Squibb .. 2687

Hyperlipidemia (see under Hyperlipoproteinemia, adjunct to diet)

Hyperlipoproteinemia, adjunct to diet (see also under Hypercholesterolemia, primary, adjunct to diet)
Atromid-S Capsules (Clofibrate) Wyeth-Ayerst 2701
Nicolar Tablets (Niacin) Rhone-Poulenc Rorer Pharmaceuticals 2026

Hyperlipoproteinemia, type III, adjunct to diet
Atromid-S Capsules (Clofibrate) Wyeth-Ayerst 2701

Hyperlipoproteinemia, types IIa and IIb, adjunct to diet
Lescol Capsules (Fluvastatin Sodium) Sandoz Pharmaceuticals 2267
Lorelco Tablets (Probucol) Marion Merrell Dow 1517
Mevacor Tablets (Lovastatin) Merck & Co., Inc. 1699
Pravachol (Pravastatin Sodium) Bristol-Myers Squibb 765
Zocor Tablets (Simvastatin) Merck & Co., Inc. 1775

Hyperlipoproteinemia, types IV and V, adjunct to diet
Atromid-S Capsules (Clofibrate) Wyeth-Ayerst 2701
Lopid Tablets (Gemfibrozil) Parke-Davis 1917

Hyperphosphatemia
Basaljel (Aluminum Carbonate Gel) Wyeth-Ayerst 2703
PhosLo Tablets (Calcium Acetate) Braintree 690

Hyperpigmentation, skin, bleaching of
Eldopaque Forte 4% Cream (Hydroquinone) ICN 1252
Eldoquin Forte 4% Cream (Hydroquinone) ICN 1252
Melanex Topical Solution (Hydroquinone) Neutrogena 1793
NeoStrata AHA Gel for Age Spots & Skin Lightening (Hydroquinone) NeoStrata 1793
Solaquin Forte 4% Cream (Hydroquinone) ICN 1252
Solaquin Forte 4% Gel (Hydroquinone) ICN 1252

Hyperprolactinemia-associated dysfunctions
Parlodel (Bromocriptine Mesylate) Sandoz Pharmaceuticals 2281

Hypersecretory conditions, diagnosis of
Peptavlon (Pentagastrin) Wyeth-Ayerst 2878

Hypersecretory conditions, pathological
Pepcid Injection (Famotidine) Merck & Co., Inc. 1722
Pepcid (Famotidine) Merck & Co., Inc. 1720
PREVACID Delayed-Release Capsules (Lansoprazole) TAP 2562
Prilosec Delayed-Release Capsules (Omeprazole) Astra Merck 529
Tagamet (Cimetidine Hydrochloride) SmithKline Beecham Pharmaceuticals 2516
Zantac (Ranitidine Hydrochloride) Glaxo Wellcome 1209
Zantac Injection (Ranitidine Hydrochloride) Glaxo Wellcome 1207
Zantac Syrup (Ranitidine Hydrochloride) Glaxo Wellcome 1209

Hypersecretory conditions, pre-operative, symptomatic relief of
Levsin/Levsinex/Levbid (Hyoscyamine Sulfate) Schwarz 2405
Robinul Injectable (Glycopyrrolate) Robins 2072

Hypersensitivity, delayed, skin testing of
MSTA Mumps Skin Test Antigen (Mumps Skin Test Antigen) Connaught 890

Hypersensitivity reactions, drug-induced
Aristocort Suspension (Forte Parenteral) (Triamcinolone Diacetate) Fujisawa 1027
Aristocort Tablets (Triamcinolone) Fujisawa 1022
Celestone Soluspan Suspension (Betamethasone Sodium Phosphate, Betamethasone Acetate) Schering 2347
Cortone Acetate Sterile Suspension (Cortisone Acetate) Merck & Co., Inc. 1623
Cortone Acetate Tablets (Cortisone Acetate) Merck & Co., Inc. 1624
Dalalone D.P. Injectable (Dexamethasone Acetate) Forest 1011
Decadron Elixir (Dexamethasone) Merck & Co., Inc. 1633
Decadron Phosphate Injection (Dexamethasone Sodium Phosphate) Merck & Co., Inc. 1637
Decadron Tablets (Dexamethasone) Merck & Co., Inc. 1635
Decadron-LA Sterile Suspension (Dexamethasone Acetate) Merck & Co., Inc. 1646
Deltasone Tablets (Prednisone) Upjohn 2595
Depo-Medrol Single-Dose Vial (Methylprednisolone Acetate) Upjohn 2600
Depo-Medrol Sterile Aqueous Suspension (Methylprednisolone Acetate) Upjohn 2597
EpiPen (Epinephrine) Center 790
Hydeltrasol Injection, Sterile (Prednisolone Sodium Phosphate) Merck & Co., Inc. 1665
Hydrocortone Phosphate Injection, Sterile (Hydrocortisone Sodium Phosphate) Merck & Co., Inc. 1670
Hydrocortone Tablets (Hydrocortisone) Merck & Co., Inc. 1672
Medrol (Methylprednisolone) Upjohn 2621
Pediapred Oral Liquid (Prednisolone Sodium Phosphate) Fisons 995
Prelone Syrup (Prednisolone) Muro 1787
Solu-Cortef Sterile Powder (Hydrocortisone Sodium Succinate) Upjohn 2641
Solu-Medrol Sterile Powder (Methylprednisolone Sodium Succinate) Upjohn 2643
Temaril Tablets, Syrup and Spansule Extended-Release Capsules (Trimeprazine Tartrate) Allergan 483

Hypertension
Accupril Tablets (Quinapril Hydrochloride) Parke-Davis 1893
Adalat CC (Nifedipine) Bayer Pharmaceutical 589
Aldactazide (Spironolactone, Hydrochlorothiazide) Searle 2413
Aldactone (Spironolactone) Searle .. 2414
Aldoclor Tablets (Methyldopa, Chlorothiazide) Merck & Co., Inc. 1598
Aldomet Ester HCl Injection (Methyldopate Hydrochloride) Merck & Co., Inc. 1602
Aldomet Oral (Methyldopa) Merck & Co., Inc. 1600
Aldoril Tablets (Methyldopa, Hydrochlorothiazide) Merck & Co., Inc. 1604
Altace Capsules (Ramipril) Hoechst-Roussel 1232
Apresazide Capsules (Hydralazine Hydrochloride, Hydrochlorothiazide) CibaGeneva 808
Apresoline Hydrochloride Tablets (Hydralazine Hydrochloride) CibaGeneva 809
Arfonad Ampuls (Trimethaphan Camsylate) Roche Laboratories 2080
Blocadren Tablets (Timolol Maleate) Merck & Co., Inc. 1614
Calan SR Caplets (Verapamil Hydrochloride) Searle 2422
Calan Tablets (Verapamil Hydrochloride) Searle 2419
Capoten (Captopril) Bristol-Myers Squibb 739
Capozide (Captopril, Hydrochlorothiazide) Bristol-Myers Squibb 742
Cardene Capsules (Nicardipine Hydrochloride) Roche Laboratories 2095
Cardene I.V. (Nicardipine Hydrochloride) Wyeth-Ayerst 2709
Cardene SR Capsules (Nicardipine Hydrochloride) Roche Laboratories 2097
Cardizem CD Capsules (Diltiazem Hydrochloride) Marion Merrell Dow 1506
Cardizem SR Capsules (Diltiazem Hydrochloride) Marion Merrell Dow 1510

(▣ Described in PDR For Nonprescription Drugs) (◉ Described in PDR For Ophthalmology)

1493 **Indications Index** **Hypocalcemia**

Cardura Tablets (Doxazosin Mesylate) Roerig ... 2186
Cartrol Tablets (Carteolol Hydrochloride) Abbott ... 410
Catapres Tablets (Clonidine Hydrochloride) Boehringer Ingelheim ... 674
Catapres-TTS (Clonidine) Boehringer Ingelheim ... 675
Combipres Tablets (Clonidine Hydrochloride, Chlorthalidone) Boehringer Ingelheim ... 677
Cozaar Tablets (Losartan Potassium) Merck & Co., Inc. ... 1628
Demadex Tablets and Injection (Torsemide) Boehringer Mannheim ... 686
Dilacor XR Extended-release Capsules (Diltiazem Hydrochloride) Rhone-Poulenc Rorer Pharmaceuticals ... 2018
Diucardin Tablets (Hydroflumethiazide) Wyeth-Ayerst ... 2718
Diupres Tablets (Reserpine, Chlorothiazide) Merck & Co., Inc. 1650
Diuril Oral (Chlorothiazide) Merck & Co., Inc. ... 1653
Dyazide (Triamterene, Hydrochlorothiazide) SmithKline Beecham Pharmaceuticals ... 2479
DynaCirc Capsules (Isradipine) Sandoz Pharmaceuticals ... 2256
Enduron Tablets (Methyclothiazide) Abbott ... 420
Esidrix Tablets (Hydrochlorothiazide) CibaGeneva ... 821
Esimil Tablets (Guanethidine Monosulfate, Hydrochlorothiazide) CibaGeneva ... 822
HydroDIURIL Tablets (Hydrochlorothiazide) Merck & Co., Inc. ... 1674
Hydropres Tablets (Reserpine, Hydrochlorothiazide) Merck & Co., Inc. ... 1675
Hylorel Tablets (Guanadrel Sulfate) Fisons ... 985
Hytrin Capsules (Terazosin Hydrochloride) Abbott ... 430
Hyzaar Tablets (Losartan Potassium, Hydrochlorothiazide) Merck & Co., Inc. ... 1677
Inderal (Propranolol Hydrochloride) Wyeth-Ayerst ... 2728
Inderal LA Long Acting Capsules (Propranolol Hydrochloride) Wyeth-Ayerst ... 2730
Inderide Tablets (Propranolol Hydrochloride, Hydrochlorothiazide) Wyeth-Ayerst ... 2732
Inderide LA Long Acting Capsules (Propranolol Hydrochloride, Hydrochlorothiazide) Wyeth-Ayerst ... 2734
Inversine Tablets (Mecamylamine Hydrochloride) Merck & Co., Inc. 1686
Ismelin Tablets (Guanethidine Monosulfate) CibaGeneva ... 827
Isoptin Oral Tablets (Verapamil Hydrochloride) Knoll Laboratories ... 1346
Isoptin SR Tablets (Verapamil Hydrochloride) Knoll Laboratories ... 1348
Kerlone Tablets (Betaxolol Hydrochloride) Searle ... 2436
Lasix Injection, Oral Solution and Tablets (Furosemide) Hoechst-Roussel ... 1240
Levatol (Penbutolol Sulfate) Schwarz ... 2403
Loniten Tablets (Minoxidil) Upjohn ... 2618
Lopressor Ampuls (Metoprolol Tartrate) CibaGeneva ... 830
Lopressor HCT Tablets (Metoprolol Tartrate, Hydrochlorothiazide) CibaGeneva ... 832
Lopressor Tablets (Metoprolol Tartrate) CibaGeneva ... 830
Lotensin Tablets (Benazepril Hydrochloride) CibaGeneva ... 834
Lotensin HCT (Benazepril Hydrochloride, Hydrochlorothiazide) CibaGeneva ... 837
Lotrel Capsules (Amlodipine Besylate, Benazepril Hydrochloride) CibaGeneva ... 840
Lozol Tablets (Indapamide) Rhone-Poulenc Rorer Pharmaceuticals ... 2022
Maxzide (Triamterene, Hydrochlorothiazide) Lederle ... 1380
Minipress Capsules (Prazosin Hydrochloride) Pfizer Labs ... 1937
Minizide Capsules (Prazosin Hydrochloride, Polythiazide) Pfizer Labs ... 1938
Moduretic Tablets (Amiloride Hydrochloride, Hydrochlorothiazide) Merck & Co., Inc. ... 1705
Monopril Tablets (Fosinopril Sodium) Bristol-Myers Squibb ... 757
Mykrox Tablets (Metolazone) Fisons ... 993
Normodyne Injection (Labetalol Hydrochloride) Schering ... 2377
Normodyne Tablets (Labetalol Hydrochloride) Schering ... 2379
Norvasc Tablets (Amlodipine Besylate) Pfizer Labs ... 1940
Oretic Tablets (Hydrochlorothiazide) Abbott ... 443
Plendil Extended-Release Tablets (Felodipine) Astra Merck ... 527
Prinivil Tablets (Lisinopril) Merck & Co., Inc. ... 1733
Prinzide Tablets (Lisinopril, Hydrochlorothiazide) Merck & Co., Inc. ... 1737
Procardia XL Extended Release Tablets (Nifedipine) Pratt ... 1972
Sectral Capsules (Acebutolol Hydrochloride) Wyeth-Ayerst ... 2807
Ser-Ap-Es Tablets (Hydralazine Hydrochloride, Hydrochlorothiazide, Reserpine) CibaGeneva ... 849
Tenex Tablets (Guanfacine Hydrochloride) Robins ... 2074
Tenoretic Tablets (Atenolol, Chlorthalidone) Zeneca ... 2845
Tenormin Tablets and I.V. Injection (Atenolol) Zeneca ... 2847
Thalitone (Chlorthalidone) Horus ... 1245
Timolide Tablets (Timolol Maleate, Hydrochlorothiazide) Merck & Co., Inc. ... 1748
Toprol-XL Tablets (Metoprolol Succinate) Astra ... 565
Trandate (Labetalol Hydrochloride) Glaxo Wellcome ... 1185
Univasc Tablets (Moexipril Hydrochloride) Schwarz ... 2410
Vaseretic Tablets (Enalapril Maleate, Hydrochlorothiazide) Merck & Co., Inc. ... 1765
Vasotec I.V. (Enalaprilat) Merck & Co., Inc. ... 1768
Vasotec Tablets (Enalapril Maleate) Merck & Co., Inc. ... 1771
Verelan Capsules (Verapamil Hydrochloride) Lederle ... 1410
Verelan Capsules (Verapamil Hydrochloride) Wyeth-Ayerst ... 2824
Visken Tablets (Pindolol) Sandoz Pharmaceuticals ... 2299
Zaroxolyn Tablets (Metolazone) Fisons ... 1000
Zebeta Tablets (Bisoprolol Fumarate) Lederle ... 1413
Zestoretic (Lisinopril, Hydrochlorothiazide) Zeneca ... 2850
Zestril Tablets (Lisinopril) Zeneca ... 2854
Ziac (Bisoprolol Fumarate, Hydrochlorothiazide) Lederle ... 1415

Hypertension associated with anesthesia
Brevibloc Injection (Esmolol Hydrochloride) Ohmeda ... 1808

Hypertension associated with intratracheal intubation
Brevibloc Injection (Esmolol Hydrochloride) Ohmeda ... 1808

Hypertension associated with surgical procedures
Brevibloc Injection (Esmolol Hydrochloride) Ohmeda ... 1808
Nitro-Bid IV (Nitroglycerin) Marion Merrell Dow ... 1523

Hypertension, adjunctive treatment
Aldactone (Spironolactone) Searle ... 2414
Dyazide (Triamterene, Hydrochlorothiazide) SmithKline Beecham Pharmaceuticals ... 2479
Enduron Tablets (Methyclothiazide) Abbott ... 420
Lozol Tablets (Indapamide) Rhone-Poulenc Rorer Pharmaceuticals ... 2022
Midamor Tablets (Amiloride Hydrochloride) Merck & Co., Inc. 1703
Oretic Tablets (Hydrochlorothiazide) Abbott ... 443

Hypertension, essential (see under Hypertension)

Hypertension, malignant
Hyperstat I.V. Injection (Diazoxide) Schering ... 2363
Inversine Tablets (Mecamylamine Hydrochloride) Merck & Co., Inc. 1686

Hypertension, non-malignant
Hyperstat I.V. Injection (Diazoxide) Schering ... 2363

Hypertension, ocular (see also under Glaucoma, aphakic; Glaucoma, chronic open-angle; Glaucoma, secondary)
Betagan (Levobunolol Hydrochloride) Allergan ... ◉ 233
Betimol 0.25%, 0.5% (Timolol Hemihydrate) CIBA Vision Ophthalmics ... ◉ 261
Betoptic Ophthalmic Solution (Betaxolol Hydrochloride) Alcon Laboratories ... 469
Betoptic S Ophthalmic Suspension (Betaxolol Hydrochloride) Alcon Laboratories ... 471
Isopto Carbachol Ophthalmic Solution (Carbachol) Alcon Laboratories ... ◉ 223
Isopto Carpine Ophthalmic Solution (Pilocarpine Hydrochloride) Alcon Laboratories ... ◉ 223
MZM (Methazolamide) CIBA Vision Ophthalmics ... ◉ 267
Ocupress Ophthalmic Solution, 1% Sterile (Carteolol Hydrochloride) Otsuka America ◉ 309
Ocusert Pilo-20 and Pilo-40 Ocular Therapeutic Systems (Pilocarpine) Alza ... ◉ 254
OptiPranolol (Metipranolol 0.3%) Sterile Ophthalmic Solution (Metipranolol Hydrochloride) Bausch & Lomb Pharmaceuticals ... ◉ 258
Pilagan (Pilocarpine Nitrate) Allergan ... ◉ 248
Pilocar (Pilocarpine Hydrochloride) CIBA Vision Ophthalmics ... ◉ 268
Pilopine HS Ophthalmic Gel (Pilocarpine Hydrochloride) Alcon Laboratories ... ◉ 226
Timoptic in Ocudose (Timolol Maleate) Merck & Co., Inc. ... 1753
Timoptic Sterile Ophthalmic Solution (Timolol Maleate) Merck & Co., Inc. ... 1751
Timoptic-XE (Timolol Maleate) Merck & Co., Inc. ... 1755
Trusopt Sterile Ophthalmic Solution (Dorzolamide Hydrochloride) Merck & Co., Inc. 1760

Hypertension, ocular, diagnostic agent for
FLURESS (Fluorescein Sodium, Benoxinate Hydrochloride) Akorn ... ◉ 207

Hypertension, ocular, post-surgical
IOPIDINE Sterile Ophthalmic Solution (Apraclonidine Hydrochloride) Alcon Laboratories ... ◉ 219

Hypertension, ocular, short-term reduction of
Iopidine 0.5% (Apraclonidine Hydrochloride) Alcon Laboratories ... ◉ 221
ISMOTIC 45% w/v Solution (Isosorbide) Alcon Laboratories ◉ 222
OSM_GLYN Oral Osmotic Agent (Glycerin) Alcon Laboratories ... ◉ 226

Hypertension, pulmonary, persistent, of the newborn
Priscoline Hydrochloride Ampuls (Tolazoline Hydrochloride) CibaGeneva ... 845

Hypertension, renal
Ismelin Tablets (Guanethidine Monosulfate) CibaGeneva ... 827

Hypertension, secondary to amyloidosis
Ismelin Tablets (Guanethidine Monosulfate) CibaGeneva ... 827

Hypertension, secondary to pyelonephritis
Ismelin Tablets (Guanethidine Monosulfate) CibaGeneva ... 827

Hypertension, secondary to renal artery stenosis
Ismelin Tablets (Guanethidine Monosulfate) CibaGeneva ... 827

Hypertension, severe, acute
Hyperstat I.V. Injection (Diazoxide) Schering ... 2363

Hypertensive episodes, control of, in pheochromocytoma (see also under Pheochromocytoma, adjunctive therapy)
Dibenzyline Capsules (Phenoxybenzamine Hydrochloride) SmithKline Beecham Pharmaceuticals ... 2476
Regitine (Phentolamine Mesylate) CibaGeneva ... 846

Hyperthermia, malignant, prophylaxis
Dantrium Capsules (Dantrolene Sodium) Procter & Gamble Pharmaceuticals ... 1982
Dantrium Intravenous (Dantrolene Sodium) Procter & Gamble Pharmaceuticals ... 1983

Hyperthermia, malignant, treatment adjunct
Dantrium Intravenous (Dantrolene Sodium) Procter & Gamble Pharmaceuticals ... 1983

Hyperthyroidism
Tapazole Tablets (Methimazole) Lilly ... 1477

Hypertriglyceridemia, adjunct to diet (see also under Dysbetalipoproteinemia)
Atromid-S Capsules (Clofibrate) Wyeth-Ayerst ... 2701
Nicolar Tablets (Niacin) Rhone-Poulenc Rorer Pharmaceuticals ... 2026

Hyperuricemia associated with gout
Benemid Tablets (Probenecid) Merck & Co., Inc. ... 1611

Hyperuricemia associated with gouty arthritis
Benemid Tablets (Probenecid) Merck & Co., Inc. ... 1611

Hypnotic (see under Sleep, induction of)

Hypocalcemia
Calci-Chew Tablets (Calcium Carbonate) R&D ... 2004
Calci-Mix Capsules (Calcium Carbonate) R&D ... 2004
Calphosan (Calcium Glycerophosphate, Calcium Lactate) Glenwood ... 1229
Caltrate 600 (Calcium Carbonate) Lederle Consumer ... ▣ 665
Caltrate PLUS (Calcium Carbonate, Vitamin D) Lederle Consumer ... ▣ 665
Centrum Singles Calcium (Calcium Carbonate) Lederle Consumer ... ▣ 669
Citracal (Calcium Citrate) Mission ... 1779
Citracal Caplets + D (Calcium Citrate, Vitamin D_3) Mission ... 1780

(▣ Described in PDR For Nonprescription Drugs) (◉ Described in PDR For Ophthalmology)

Hypocalcemia

Citracal Liquitab (Calcium Citrate) Mission 1780
Nephro-Calci Tablets (Calcium Carbonate) R&D 2004
Rocaltrol Capsules (Calcitriol) Roche Laboratories 2141
Tums 500 Calcium Supplement (Calcium Carbonate) SmithKline Beecham Consumer **⊕** 828

Hypocalcemia associated with chronic renal failure

Rocaltrol Capsules (Calcitriol) Roche Laboratories 2141

Hypocalcemia with vitamin D, deficiency of

Caltrate 600 + D (Calcium Carbonate, Vitamin D) Lederle Consumer .... **⊕** 665
Dical-D Tablets & Wafers (Calcium Phosphate, Dibasic, Vitamin D) Abbott 420

Hypoestrogenism

Climara Transdermal System (Estradiol) Berlex 645
Ogen Tablets (Estropipate) Upjohn 2627
Ortho-Est (Estropipate) Ortho Pharmaceutical 1869
Premarin Tablets (Estrogens, Conjugated) Wyeth-Ayerst 2789

Hypogammaglobulinemia, prevention of bacterial infections

Gammar I.V., Immune Globulin Intravenous (Human), Lyophilized (Globulin, Immune (Human)) Armour 516

Hypoglycemia due to hyperinsulinism

Glucagon for Injection Vials and Emergency Kit (Glucagon) Lilly 1440
Proglycem (Diazoxide) Baker Norton 580

Hypoglycemia due to insulin shock therapy

Glucagon for Injection Vials and Emergency Kit (Glucagon) Lilly 1440

Hypogonadism, female

Estrace Cream and Tablets (Estradiol) Bristol-Myers Squibb .. 749
Estraderm Transdermal System (Estradiol) CibaGeneva 824
ESTRATAB Tablets (0.3, 0.625, 1.25, 2.5 mg) (Estrogens, Esterified) Solvay 2536
Menest Tablets (Estrogens, Esterified) SmithKline Beecham Pharmaceuticals 2494
Ogen Tablets (Estropipate) Upjohn 2627
Ortho-Est (Estropipate) Ortho Pharmaceutical 1869

Hypogonadism, hypogonadotropic, in males

Android Capsules, 10 mg (Methyltestosterone) ICN 1250
Android (Methyltestosterone) ICN .. 1251
Delatestryl Injection (Testosterone Enanthate) Bio-Technology General 2860
Halotestin Tablets (Fluoxymesterone) Upjohn 2614
Humegon (Menotropins) Organon .. 1824
Oreton Methyl (Methyltestosterone) ICN 1255
Pergonal (menotropins for injection, USP) (Menotropins) Serono 2448
Pregnyl (Chorionic Gonadotropin) Organon 1828
Profasi (chorionic gonadotropin for injection, USP) (Chorionic Gonadotropin) Serono 2450
Testoderm Testosterone Transdermal System (Testosterone) Alza 486
Testred Capsules (Methyltestosterone) ICN 1262

Hypogonadism, hypogonadotropic, secondary, adjunctive therapy in

Humegon (Menotropins) Organon .. 1824
Pergonal (menotropins for injection, USP) (Menotropins) Serono 2448

Hypogonadism, male, primary

Android Capsules, 10 mg (Methyltestosterone) ICN 1250
Android (Methyltestosterone) ICN .. 1251
Delatestryl Injection (Testosterone Enanthate) Bio-Technology General 2860
Halotestin Tablets (Fluoxymesterone) Upjohn 2614
Oreton Methyl (Methyltestosterone) ICN 1255
Testoderm Testosterone Transdermal System (Testosterone) Alza 486

Hypokalemia with certain diarrheal states, prevention of

Micro-K (Potassium Chloride) Robins 2063
Micro-K LS Packets (Potassium Chloride) Robins 2064
Slow-K Extended-Release Tablets (Potassium Chloride) CibaGeneva 851

Hypokalemia with metabolic acidosis

Micro-K (Potassium Chloride) Robins 2063
Micro-K LS Packets (Potassium Chloride) Robins 2064
Slow-K Extended-Release Tablets (Potassium Chloride) CibaGeneva 851

Hypokalemia with metabolic alkalosis

K-Dur Microburst Release System (potassium chloride, USP) E.R. Tablets (Potassium Chloride) Key 1325
K-Lor Powder Packets (Potassium Chloride) Abbott 434
K-Norm Extended-Release Capsules (Potassium Chloride) Fisons 991
K-Tab Filmtab (Potassium Chloride) Abbott 434
Micro-K (Potassium Chloride) Robins 2063
Slow-K Extended-Release Tablets (Potassium Chloride) CibaGeneva 851

Hypokalemia with significant cardiac arrhythmias

K-Dur Microburst Release System (potassium chloride, USP) E.R. Tablets (Potassium Chloride) Key 1325
K-Lor Powder Packets (Potassium Chloride) Abbott 434
K-Tab Filmtab (Potassium Chloride) Abbott 434
Slow-K Extended-Release Tablets (Potassium Chloride) CibaGeneva 851

Hypokalemia without metabolic alkalosis

K-Dur Microburst Release System (potassium chloride, USP) E.R. Tablets (Potassium Chloride) Key 1325
K-Lor Powder Packets (Potassium Chloride) Abbott 434
K-Norm Extended-Release Capsules (Potassium Chloride) Fisons 991
K-Tab Filmtab (Potassium Chloride) Abbott 434
Micro-K (Potassium Chloride) Robins 2063
Micro-K LS Packets (Potassium Chloride) Robins 2064

Hypokalemia, digitalis intoxication-induced

K-Dur Microburst Release System (potassium chloride, USP) E.R. Tablets (Potassium Chloride) Key 1325
K-Lor Powder Packets (Potassium Chloride) Abbott 434
K-Norm Extended-Release Capsules (Potassium Chloride) Fisons 991
K-Tab Filmtab (Potassium Chloride) Abbott 434
Kolyum Liquid (Potassium Gluconate, Potassium Chloride) Fisons 992
Micro-K (Potassium Chloride) Robins 2063
Micro-K LS Packets (Potassium Chloride) Robins 2064

Rum-K Syrup (Potassium Chloride) Fleming 1005
Slow-K Extended-Release Tablets (Potassium Chloride) CibaGeneva 851

Hypokalemia, digitalis-induced, prophylaxis of

Aldactone (Spironolactone) Searle .. 2414

Hypokalemia, drug-induced

K-Dur Microburst Release System (potassium chloride, USP) E.R. Tablets (Potassium Chloride) Key 1325
Kolyum Liquid (Potassium Gluconate, Potassium Chloride) Fisons 992
Micro-K (Potassium Chloride) Robins 2063
Micro-K LS Packets (Potassium Chloride) Robins 2064
Rum-K Syrup (Potassium Chloride) Fleming 1005
Slow-K Extended-Release Tablets (Potassium Chloride) CibaGeneva 851

Hypokalemia, drug-induced in congestive heart failure, prevention of

Micro-K (Potassium Chloride) Robins 2063
Micro-K LS Packets (Potassium Chloride) Robins 2064
Rum-K Syrup (Potassium Chloride) Fleming 1005
Slow-K Extended-Release Tablets (Potassium Chloride) CibaGeneva 851

Hypokalemia, hepatic cirrhosis with ascites-induced, prevention of

Micro-K (Potassium Chloride) Robins 2063
Micro-K LS Packets (Potassium Chloride) Robins 2064
Slow-K Extended-Release Tablets (Potassium Chloride) CibaGeneva 851

Hypokalemia, potassium-losing nephropathy-induced, prevention of

Slow-K Extended-Release Tablets (Potassium Chloride) CibaGeneva 851

Hypokalemia, unspecified

Aldactone (Spironolactone) Searle .. 2414
K-Dur Microburst Release System (potassium chloride, USP) E.R. Tablets (Potassium Chloride) Key 1325

Hypomagnesemia

Mag-L-100 (Magnesium Chloride) Bio-Tech 668
Magonate Tablets and Liquid (Magnesium Gluconate) Fleming 1005
Mag-Ox 400 (Magnesium Oxide) Blaine 668
MagTab SR Caplets (Magnesium Lactate) Niché 1793
Uro-Mag (Magnesium Oxide) Blaine 668

Hypoparathyroidism, unspecified

DHT (Dihydrotachysterol) Tablets & Intensol (Dihydrotachysterol) Roxane 2229

Hypophosphatemia

K-Phos Neutral Tablets (Potassium Phosphate, Monobasic, Sodium Phosphate, Monobasic, Sodium Phosphate, Dibasic) Beach 639

Hypopigmentation, skin

Benoquin Cream 20% (Monobenzone) ICN 2868
8-MOP Capsules (Methoxsalen) ICN 1246
Oxsoralen Lotion 1% (Methoxsalen) ICN 1256
Trisoralen Tablets (Trioxsalen) ICN 1264

Hypoproteinemia

Albuminar-5, Albumin (Human) U.S.P. 5% (Albumin (Human)) Armour 512
Albuminar-25, Albumin (Human) U.S.P. 25% (Albumin (Human)) Armour 513
Plasma-Plex, Plasma Protein Fraction (Human) 5% (Plasma

Protein Fraction (Human)) Armour 524

Hypoprothrombinemia due to antibacterial therapy

AquaMEPHYTON Injection (Phytonadione) Merck & Co., Inc. 1608
Konakion Injection (Phytonadione) Roche Laboratories 2127

Hypoprothrombinemia, drug-induced

AquaMEPHYTON Injection (Phytonadione) Merck & Co., Inc. 1608
Konakion Injection (Phytonadione) Roche Laboratories 2127
Mephyton Tablets (Phytonadione) Merck & Co., Inc. 1696

Hypoprothrombinemia, salicylate-induced

AquaMEPHYTON Injection (Phytonadione) Merck & Co., Inc. 1608
Konakion Injection (Phytonadione) Roche Laboratories 2127
Mephyton Tablets (Phytonadione) Merck & Co., Inc. 1696

Hypoprothrombinemia, secondary factors-induced

AquaMEPHYTON Injection (Phytonadione) Merck & Co., Inc. 1608
Konakion Injection (Phytonadione) Roche Laboratories 2127
Mephyton Tablets (Phytonadione) Merck & Co., Inc. 1696

Hyposalivation

Salivart Saliva Substitute (Sodium Carboxymethylcellulose) Gebauer .... **⊕** 656

Hypotension

Neo-Synephrine Hydrochloride 1% Carpuject (Phenylephrine Hydrochloride) Sanofi Winthrop .. 2324
Neo-Synephrine Hydrochloride 1% Injection (Phenylephrine Hydrochloride) Sanofi Winthrop .. 2324

Hypotension associated with hemorrhage, adjunct to

Aramine Injection (Metaraminol Bitartrate) Merck & Co., Inc. 1609

Hypotension associated with spinal anesthesia

Aramine Injection (Metaraminol Bitartrate) Merck & Co., Inc. 1609
Levophed Bitartrate Injection (Norepinephrine Bitartrate) Sanofi Winthrop 2315

Hypotension due to drug reactions, adjunct to

Aramine Injection (Metaraminol Bitartrate) Merck & Co., Inc. 1609
Levophed Bitartrate Injection (Norepinephrine Bitartrate) Sanofi Winthrop 2315

Hypotension due to surgical complications, adjunct to

Aramine Injection (Metaraminol Bitartrate) Merck & Co., Inc. 1609

Hypotension, acute

Levophed Bitartrate Injection (Norepinephrine Bitartrate) Sanofi Winthrop 2315
Vasoxyl Injection (Methoxamine Hydrochloride) Glaxo Wellcome 1196

Hypotension, controlled, production of during surgical procedures

Arfonad Ampuls (Trimethaphan Camsylate) Roche Laboratories 2080
Nitro-Bid IV (Nitroglycerin) Marion Merrell Dow 1523

Hypotension, shock associated with brain damage due to trauma, adjunct to

Aramine Injection (Metaraminol Bitartrate) Merck & Co., Inc. 1609

Hypotension, shock associated with brain damage due to tumor, adjunct to

Aramine Injection (Metaraminol Bitartrate) Merck & Co., Inc. 1609

(**⊕** Described in PDR For Nonprescription Drugs)

(◉ Described in PDR For Ophthalmology)

1495 Indications Index Infections

Hypothalamic-pituitary gonadotropic function, diagnostic evaluation of
Factrel (Gonadorelin Hydrochloride) Wyeth-Ayerst 2877

Hypothyroidism, ordinary (see under Hypothyroidism, replacement or supplemental therapy in)

Hypothyroidism, primary (see under Hypothyroidism, replacement or supplemental therapy in)

Hypothyroidism, replacement or supplemental therapy in
Cytomel Tablets (Liothyronine Sodium) SmithKline Beecham Pharmaceuticals 2473
Levothroid Tablets (Levothyroxine Sodium) Forest 1016
Levoxyl Tablets (Levothyroxine Sodium) Daniels 903
Synthroid (Levothyroxine Sodium) Knoll Pharmaceutical 1359

Hypothyroidism, secondary (see under Hypothyroidism, replacement or supplemental therapy in)

Hypothyroidism, tertiary (see under Hypothyroidism, replacement or supplemental therapy in)

Hypovolemia
Hespan Injection (Hetastarch) DuPont 929

Hypovolemic shock, treatment adjunct
Isuprel Hydrochloride Injection 1:5000 (Isoproterenol Hydrochloride) Sanofi Winthrop .. 2311

Hysteria, acute
Vistaril Intramuscular Solution (Hydroxyzine Hydrochloride) Roerig 2216

Hysterosalpingography, diagnostic aid in
Ethiodol (Ethiodized Oil) Savage 2340

I

Ichthyosis vulgaris
Lac-Hydrin 12% Lotion (Ammonium Lactate) Westwood-Squibb .. 2687

Idiopathic thrombocytopenic purpura (see under Purpura, idiopathic thrombocytopenic)

Ileostomies, reducing the volume of discharge
Imodium Capsules (Loperamide Hydrochloride) Janssen 1295

Ileostomies, reduction in odor, adjunct to
Devrom Chewable Tablets (Bismuth Subgallate) Parthenon .... ▣ 741

Immunization, cholera
Cholera Vaccine (Cholera Vaccine) Wyeth-Ayerst 2711

Immunization, diphtheria and tetanus
Diphtheria & Tetanus Toxoids Adsorbed Purogenated (Diphtheria & Tetanus Toxoids Adsorbed, (For Pediatric Use)) Lederle 1374
Tetanus & Diphtheria Toxoids Adsorbed Purogenated (Tetanus & Diphtheria Toxoids Adsorbed (For Adult Use)) Lederle 1401

Immunization, diphtheria, tetanus and pertussis
Acel-Imune Diphtheria and Tetanus Toxoids and Acellular Pertussis Vaccine Adsorbed (Diphtheria & Tetanus Toxoids w/Pertussis Vaccine Combined, Aluminum Phosphate Adsorbed) Lederle 1364
Diphtheria and Tetanus Toxoids and Pertussis Vaccine Adsorbed (Diphtheria & Tetanus Toxoids w/Pertussis Vaccine Combined, Aluminum Phosphate Adsorbed) SmithKline Beecham Pharmaceuticals 2477
Diphtheria and Tetanus Toxoids and Pertussis Vaccine Adsorbed USP (For Pediatric Use) (Diphtheria & Tetanus Toxoids w/Pertussis Vaccine Combined, Aluminum Potassium Sulfate Adsorbed) Connaught 875
Tri-Immunol Adsorbed (Diphtheria & Tetanus Toxoids w/Pertussis Vaccine Combined, Aluminum Phosphate Adsorbed) Lederle 1408
Tripedia (Diphtheria & Tetanus Toxoids w/Pertussis Vaccine Combined, Aluminum Potassium Sulfate Adsorbed) Connaught 892

Immunization, diphtheria, tetanus, pertussis, and haemophilus influenzae type B
ActHIB (Haemophilus B Conjugate Vaccine) Connaught 872
Tetramune (Diphtheria & Tetanus Toxoids and Pertussis Vaccine Adsorbed with Hemophilus B Conjugate Vaccine (Diphtheria-CRM Protein Conjugate)) Lederle 1404

Immunization, Haemophilus influenzae type b
ActHIB (Haemophilus B Conjugate Vaccine) Connaught 872
HibTITER (Haemophilus B Conjugate Vaccine) Lederle 1375
OmniHIB (Haemophilus B Conjugate Vaccine) SmithKline Beecham Pharmaceuticals 2499
PedvaxHIB (Haemophilus B Conjugate Vaccine) Merck & Co., Inc. 1718

Immunization, hepatitis A virus
Havrix (Hepatitis A Vaccine, Inactivated) SmithKline Beecham Pharmaceuticals 2489

Immunization, hepatitis B virus
Engerix-B Unit-Dose Vials (Hepatitis B Vaccine) SmithKline Beecham Pharmaceuticals 2482

Immunization, hepatitis B virus, post-exposure
Hep-B-Gammagee (Hepatitis B Immune Globulin (Human)) Merck & Co., Inc. 1663

Immunization, influenza virus, types A and B
Fluvirin (Influenza Virus Vaccine) Adams 460
Influenza Virus Vaccine, Trivalent, Types A and B (chromatograph- and filter-purified subviron antigen) FluShield, 1995-1996 Formula (Influenza Virus Vaccine) Wyeth-Ayerst 2736

Immunization, Japanese encephalitis
JE-VAX (Japanese Encephalitis Vaccine Inactivated) Connaught .. 886

Immunization, poliovirus 1, 2, and 3
IPOL Poliovirus Vaccine Inactivated (Poliovirus Vaccine Inactivated, Trivalent Types 1,2,3) Connaught 885
Orimune (Poliovirus Vaccine, Live, Oral, Trivalent, Types 1,2,3 (Sabin)) Lederle 1388
Poliovax (Poliovirus Vaccine Inactivated, Trivalent Types 1,2,3) Connaught 891

Immunization, rabies
Imovax Rabies Vaccine (Rabies Vaccine) Connaught 881
Rabies Vaccine Adsorbed (Rabies Vaccine) SmithKline Beecham Pharmaceuticals 2508
Rabies Vaccine, Imovax Rabies I.D. (Rabies Vaccine) Connaught 883

Immunization, tetanus
Hyper-Tet Tetanus Immune Globulin (Human) (Tetanus Immune Globulin (Human)) Bayer Biological 627
Tetanus Toxoid Adsorbed Purogenated (Tetanus Toxoid, Adsorbed) Lederle 1403

Immunization, typhoid fever
Typhim Vi (Typhoid Vi Polysaccharide Vaccine) Connaught 899
Typhoid Vaccine (Typhoid Vaccine) Wyeth-Ayerst 2823
Vivotif Berna (Typhoid Vaccine Live Oral TY21a) Berna 665

Immunization, varicella
Varivax (Varicella Virus Vaccine Live) Merck & Co., Inc. 1762

Immunodeficiencies, primary
Gamimune N, 5% Immune Globulin Intravenous (Human), 5% (Globulin, Immune (Human)) Bayer Biological 619

Immunodeficiencies, primary, maintenance treatment of
Gammagard S/D, Immune Globulin, Intravenous (Human) (Globulin, Immune (Human)) Baxter Healthcare 585
Sandoglobulin I.V. (Globulin, Immune (Human)) Sandoz Pharmaceuticals 2290

Immunodeficiencies, severe, combined
Gamimune N, 5% Immune Globulin Intravenous (Human), 5% (Globulin, Immune (Human)) Bayer Biological 619
Gamimune N, 10% Immune Globulin Intravenous (Human), 10% (Globulin, Immune (Human)) Bayer Biological 621
Gammagard S/D, Immune Globulin, Intravenous (Human) (Globulin, Immune (Human)) Baxter Healthcare 585
Gammar, Immune Globulin (Human) U.S.P. (Globulin, Immune (Human)) Armour 515
Sandoglobulin I.V. (Globulin, Immune (Human)) Sandoz Pharmaceuticals 2290

Immunodeficiency disease, severe combined (see under Adenosine deaminase, enzyme replacement therapy for)

Immunodeficiency, common variable
Gamimune N, 5% Immune Globulin Intravenous (Human), 5% (Globulin, Immune (Human)) Bayer Biological 619
Gamimune N, 10% Immune Globulin Intravenous (Human), 10% (Globulin, Immune (Human)) Bayer Biological 621
Sandoglobulin I.V. (Globulin, Immune (Human)) Sandoz Pharmaceuticals 2290

Immunodeficiency, primary humoral
Gamimune N, 10% Immune Globulin Intravenous (Human), 10% (Globulin, Immune (Human)) Bayer Biological 621

Immunodeficiency, x-linked with hyper IgM
Gamimune N, 5% Immune Globulin Intravenous (Human), 5% (Globulin, Immune (Human)) Bayer Biological 619
Gamimune N, 10% Immune Globulin Intravenous (Human), 10% (Globulin, Immune (Human)) Bayer Biological 621
Sandoglobulin I.V. (Globulin, Immune (Human)) Sandoz Pharmaceuticals 2290

Impetigo contagiosa
Bactroban Ointment (Mupirocin) SmithKline Beecham Pharmaceuticals 2470
Ceftin for Oral Suspension (Cefuroxime Axetil) Glaxo Wellcome 1078

Impotence, male (see under Erectile dysfunction, male)

Indigestion (see under Digestive disorders, symptomatic relief of)

Infection, acquired immunodeficiency syndrome-related complex
Biaxin (Clarithromycin) Abbott 405
Cytovene (Ganciclovir Sodium) Roche Laboratories 2103
Foscavir Injection (Foscarnet Sodium) Astra 547
Gamimune N, 5% Immune Globulin Intravenous (Human), 5% (Globulin, Immune (Human)) Bayer Biological 619
Gamimune N, 10% Immune Globulin Intravenous (Human), 10% (Globulin, Immune (Human)) Bayer Biological 621
Intron A (Interferon alfa-2B, Recombinant) Schering 2364
Marinol (Dronabinol) Capsules (Dronabinol) Roxane 2231
Mycobutin Capsules (Rifabutin) Pharmacia 1957
NebuPent for Inhalation Solution (Pentamidine Isethionate) Fujisawa 1040
Neutrexin (Trimetrexate Glucuronate) U.S. Bioscience 2572
Retrovir Capsules (Zidovudine) Glaxo Wellcome 1158
Retrovir I.V. Infusion (Zidovudine) Glaxo Wellcome 1163
Retrovir Syrup (Zidovudine) Glaxo Wellcome 1158
Septra (Trimethoprim, Sulfamethoxazole) Glaxo Wellcome 1174
Sporanox Capsules (Itraconazole) Janssen 1305
WinRho SD (Globulin, Immune (Human)) Univax 2577

Infection, human immunodeficiency virus
Hivid Tablets (Zalcitabine) Roche Laboratories 2121
Retrovir Capsules (Zidovudine) Glaxo Wellcome 1158
Retrovir I.V. Infusion (Zidovudine) Glaxo Wellcome 1163
Retrovir Syrup (Zidovudine) Glaxo Wellcome 1158
Videx Tablets, Powder for Oral Solution, & Pediatric Powder for Oral Solution (Didanosine) Bristol-Myers Squibb Oncology 720
Zerit Capsules (Stavudine) Bristol-Myers Squibb Oncology 729

Infection, human immunodeficiency virus, maternal-fetal transmission
Retrovir Capsules (Zidovudine) Glaxo Wellcome 1158
Retrovir I.V. Infusion (Zidovudine) Glaxo Wellcome 1163
Retrovir Syrup (Zidovudine) Glaxo Wellcome 1158

Infections, human immunodeficiency virus, advanced, in combination with zidovudine
Hivid Tablets (Zalcitabine) Roche Laboratories 2121

Infections, aerobic organisms
Ceptaz (Ceftazidime) Glaxo Wellcome 1081
Fortaz (Ceftazidime) Glaxo Wellcome 1100
Mefoxin (Cefoxitin Sodium) Merck & Co., Inc. 1691
Mefoxin Premixed Intravenous Solution (Cefoxitin Sodium) Merck & Co., Inc. 1694
Mezlin (Mezlocillin Sodium) Bayer Pharmaceutical 601
Mezlin Pharmacy Bulk Package (Mezlocillin Sodium) Bayer Pharmaceutical 604

(▣ Described in PDR For Nonprescription Drugs) (◉ Described in PDR For Ophthalmology)

Infections Indications Index 1496

Tazicef for Injection (Ceftazidime) SmithKline Beecham Pharmaceuticals 2519
Tazidime Vials, Faspak & ADD-Vantage (Ceftazidime) Lilly 1478

Infections, anaerobic cocci
Claforan Sterile and Injection (Cefotaxime Sodium) Hoechst-Roussel 1235
Pipracil (Piperacillin Sodium) Lederle 1390

Infections, anaerobic organisms
Cefizox for Intramuscular or Intravenous Use (Ceftizoxime Sodium) Fujisawa 1034
Cefobid Intravenous/Intramuscular (Cefoperazone Sodium) Roerig 2189
Cefobid Pharmacy Bulk Package - Not for Direct Infusion (Cefoperazone Sodium) Roerig 2192
Ceptaz (Ceftazidime) Glaxo Wellcome 1081
Cleocin Phosphate Injection (Clindamycin Phosphate) Upjohn 2586
Flagyl 375 Capsules (Metronidazole) Searle 2434
Flagyl I.V. (Metronidazole Hydrochloride) SCS 2247
Fortaz (Ceftazidime) Glaxo Wellcome 1100
Garamycin Injectable (Gentamicin Sulfate) Schering 2360
Mefoxin (Cefoxitin Sodium) Merck & Co., Inc. 1691
Mefoxin Premixed Intravenous Solution (Cefoxitin Sodium) Merck & Co., Inc. 1694
Mezlin (Mezlocillin Sodium) Bayer Pharmaceutical 601
Mezlin Pharmacy Bulk Package (Mezlocillin Sodium) Bayer Pharmaceutical 604
Pipracil (Piperacillin Sodium) Lederle 1390
Primaxin I.V. (Imipenem-Cilastatin Sodium) Merck & Co., Inc. 1729
Tazicef for Injection (Ceftazidime) SmithKline Beecham Pharmaceuticals 2519
Tazidime Vials, Faspak & ADD-Vantage (Ceftazidime) Lilly 1478
Ticar for Injection (Ticarcillin Disodium) SmithKline Beecham Pharmaceuticals 2526

Infections, beta-lactamase producing organisms
Augmentin (Amoxicillin Trihydrate, Clavulanate Potassium) SmithKline Beecham Pharmaceuticals 2468
Ceftin (Cefuroxime Axetil) Glaxo Wellcome 1078
Lorabid Suspension and Pulvules (Loracarbef) Lilly 1459
Unasyn (Ampicillin Sodium, Sulbactam Sodium) Roerig 2212
Vantin for Oral Suspension and Vantin Tablets (Cefpodoxime Proxetil) Upjohn 2646
Zosyn (Piperacillin Sodium, Tazobactam Sodium) Lederle 1419
Zosyn Pharmacy Bulk Package (Piperacillin Sodium, Tazobactam Sodium) Lederle 1422

Infections, biliary tract
Ancef Injection (Cefazolin Sodium) SmithKline Beecham Pharmaceuticals 2465
Kefzol Vials, Faspak & ADD-Vantage (Cefazolin Sodium) Lilly 1456
Pipracil (Piperacillin Sodium) Lederle 1390

Infections, bone and joint
Amikacin Sulfate Injection, USP (Amikacin Sulfate) Elkins-Sinn 960
Amikin Injectable (Amikacin Sulfate) Apothecon 501
Ancef Injection (Cefazolin Sodium) SmithKline Beecham Pharmaceuticals 2465
Cefizox for Intramuscular or Intravenous Use (Ceftizoxime Sodium) Fujisawa 1034
Cefotan (Cefotetan) Zeneca 2829
Ceptaz (Ceftazidime) Glaxo Wellcome 1081
Cipro I.V. (Ciprofloxacin) Bayer Pharmaceutical 595
Cipro I.V. Pharmacy Bulk Package (Ciprofloxacin) Bayer Pharmaceutical 597
Cipro Tablets (Ciprofloxacin Hydrochloride) Bayer Pharmaceutical 592
Claforan Sterile and Injection (Cefotaxime Sodium) Hoechst-Roussel 1235
Cleocin Phosphate Injection (Clindamycin Phosphate) Upjohn 2586
Flagyl 375 Capsules (Metronidazole) Searle 2434
Flagyl I.V. (Metronidazole Hydrochloride) SCS 2247
Fortaz (Ceftazidime) Glaxo Wellcome 1100
Garamycin Injectable (Gentamicin Sulfate) Schering 2360
Keflex Pulvules & Oral Suspension (Cephalexin) Dista 914
Keftab Tablets (Cephalexin Hydrochloride) Dista 915
Kefurox Vials, Faspak & ADD-Vantage (Cefuroxime Sodium) Lilly 1454
Kefzol Vials, Faspak & ADD-Vantage (Cefazolin Sodium) Lilly 1456
Mandol Vials, Faspak & ADD-Vantage (Cefamandole Nafate) Lilly 1461
Mefoxin (Cefoxitin Sodium) Merck & Co., Inc. 1691
Mefoxin Premixed Intravenous Solution (Cefoxitin Sodium) Merck & Co., Inc. 1694
Monocid Injection (Cefonicid Sodium) SmithKline Beecham Pharmaceuticals 2497
Nebcin Vials, Hyporets & ADD-Vantage (Tobramycin Sulfate) Lilly 1464
Pipracil (Piperacillin Sodium) Lederle 1390
Primaxin I.V. (Imipenem-Cilastatin Sodium) Merck & Co., Inc. 1729
Rocephin Injectable Vials, ADD-Vantage, Galaxy Container (Ceftriaxone Sodium) Roche Laboratories 2142
Tazicef for Injection (Ceftazidime) SmithKline Beecham Pharmaceuticals 2519
Tazidime Vials, Faspak & ADD-Vantage (Ceftazidime) Lilly 1478
Timentin for Injection (Ticarcillin Disodium, Clavulanate Potassium) SmithKline Beecham Pharmaceuticals 2528
Tobramycin Sulfate Injection (Tobramycin Sulfate) Elkins-Sinn 968
Zinacef (Cefuroxime Sodium) Glaxo Wellcome 1211

Infections, burn wound (see also under Infections, skin, bacterial, minor)
Amikacin Sulfate Injection, USP (Amikacin Sulfate) Elkins-Sinn 960
Amikin Injectable (Amikacin Sulfate) Apothecon 501
Azactam for Injection (Aztreonam) Bristol-Myers Squibb 734
Elase-Chloromycetin Ointment (Fibrinolysin, Desoxyribonuclease, Chloramphenicol) Fujisawa 1040
Garamycin Injectable (Gentamicin Sulfate) Schering 2360
SSD (Silver Sulfadiazine) Knoll Laboratories 1355

Infections, central nervous system
Amikacin Sulfate Injection, USP (Amikacin Sulfate) Elkins-Sinn 960
Amikin Injectable (Amikacin Sulfate) Apothecon 501
Ceptaz (Ceftazidime) Glaxo Wellcome 1081
Claforan Sterile and Injection (Cefotaxime Sodium) Hoechst-Roussel 1235
Flagyl 375 Capsules (Metronidazole) Searle 2434
Flagyl I.V. (Metronidazole Hydrochloride) SCS 2247
Fortaz (Ceftazidime) Glaxo Wellcome 1100
Garamycin Injectable (Gentamicin Sulfate) Schering 2360
Nebcin Vials, Hyporets & ADD-Vantage (Tobramycin Sulfate) Lilly 1464
Protostat Tablets (Metronidazole) Ortho Pharmaceutical 1883
Tazicef for Injection (Ceftazidime) SmithKline Beecham Pharmaceuticals 2519
Tazidime Vials, Faspak & ADD-Vantage (Ceftazidime) Lilly 1478
Tobramycin Sulfate Injection (Tobramycin Sulfate) Elkins-Sinn 968

Infections, cutaneous dermatophyte, severe recalcitrant
Nizoral Tablets (Ketoconazole) Janssen 1298

Infections, fenestration cavities
Coly-Mycin S Otic w/Neomycin & Hydrocortisone (Colistin Sulfate, Neomycin Sulfate, Hydrocortisone Acetate) Parke-Davis 1906
Cortisporin Otic Suspension Sterile (Polymyxin B Sulfate, Neomycin Sulfate, Hydrocortisone) Glaxo Wellcome 1088
PediOtic Suspension Sterile (Polymyxin B Sulfate, Neomycin Sulfate, Hydrocortisone) Glaxo Wellcome 1153

Infections, fungal, severe systemic
Fungizone Intravenous (Amphotericin B) Apothecon 506

Infections, fungal, systemic
Diflucan Injection, Tablets, and Oral Suspension (Fluconazole) Roerig 2194

Infections, genitourinary tract
Ancef Injection (Cefazolin Sodium) SmithKline Beecham Pharmaceuticals 2465
Claforan Sterile and Injection (Cefotaxime Sodium) Hoechst-Roussel 1235
E-Mycin Tablets (Erythromycin) Knoll Laboratories 1341
Keflex Pulvules & Oral Suspension (Cephalexin) Dista 914
Keftab Tablets (Cephalexin Hydrochloride) Dista 915
Kefzol Vials, Faspak & ADD-Vantage (Cefazolin Sodium) Lilly 1456
Mefoxin (Cefoxitin Sodium) Merck & Co., Inc. 1691
Omnipen for Oral Suspension (Ampicillin) Wyeth-Ayerst 2765
Pfizerpen for Injection (Penicillin G Potassium) Roerig 2203
Spectrobid Tablets (Bacampicillin Hydrochloride) Roerig 2206
Ticar for Injection (Ticarcillin Disodium) SmithKline Beecham Pharmaceuticals 2526

Infections, genitourinary tract, "lacking substantial evidence of effectiveness" in
Urobiotic-250 Capsules (Oxytetracycline Hydrochloride, Sulfamethizole, Phenazopyridine Hydrochloride) Roerig 2214

Infections, gram-negative bacteria
Amikacin Sulfate Injection, USP (Amikacin Sulfate) Elkins-Sinn 960
Amikin Injectable (Amikacin Sulfate) Apothecon 501
Amoxil (Amoxicillin Trihydrate) SmithKline Beecham Pharmaceuticals 2464
Cefizox for Intramuscular or Intravenous Use (Ceftizoxime Sodium) Fujisawa 1034
Cefobid Intravenous/Intramuscular (Cefoperazone Sodium) Roerig 2189
Cefobid Pharmacy Bulk Package - Not for Direct Infusion (Cefoperazone Sodium) Roerig 2192
Chloromycetin Sodium Succinate (Chloramphenicol Sodium Succinate) Parke-Davis 1900
Coly-Mycin M Parenteral (Colistimethate Sodium) Parke-Davis 1905
Doryx Capsules (Doxycycline Hyclate) Parke-Davis 1913
Garamycin Injectable (Gentamicin Sulfate) Schering 2360
Mefoxin (Cefoxitin Sodium) Merck & Co., Inc. 1691
Mefoxin Premixed Intravenous Solution (Cefoxitin Sodium) Merck & Co., Inc. 1694
Mezlin (Mezlocillin Sodium) Bayer Pharmaceutical 601
Mezlin Pharmacy Bulk Package (Mezlocillin Sodium) Bayer Pharmaceutical 604
Minocin Oral Suspension (Minocycline Hydrochloride) Lederle 1385
Monodox Capsules (Doxycycline Monohydrate) Oclassen 1805
Netromycin Injection 100 mg/ml (Netilmicin Sulfate) Schering 2373
Ocuflox (Ofloxacin) Allergan 481
Primaxin I.V. (Imipenem-Cilastatin Sodium) Merck & Co., Inc. 1729
Ticar for Injection (Ticarcillin Disodium) SmithKline Beecham Pharmaceuticals 2526

Infections, gram-positive anaerobic cocci
Cefobid Intravenous/Intramuscular (Cefoperazone Sodium) Roerig 2189
Cefobid Pharmacy Bulk Package - Not for Direct Infusion (Cefoperazone Sodium) Roerig 2192
Cefotan (Cefotetan) Zeneca 2829
Mefoxin (Cefoxitin Sodium) Merck & Co., Inc. 1691
Mefoxin Premixed Intravenous Solution (Cefoxitin Sodium) Merck & Co., Inc. 1694

Infections, gram-positive bacteria
Amoxil (Amoxicillin Trihydrate) SmithKline Beecham Pharmaceuticals 2464
Doryx Capsules (Doxycycline Hyclate) Parke-Davis 1913
Mezlin (Mezlocillin Sodium) Bayer Pharmaceutical 601
Mezlin Pharmacy Bulk Package (Mezlocillin Sodium) Bayer Pharmaceutical 604
Minocin Oral Suspension (Minocycline Hydrochloride) Lederle 1385
Monodox Capsules (Doxycycline Monohydrate) Oclassen 1805
Ocuflox (Ofloxacin) Allergan 481
Omnipen Capsules (Ampicillin) Wyeth-Ayerst 2764
Omnipen for Oral Suspension (Ampicillin) Wyeth-Ayerst 2765
Primaxin I.V. (Imipenem-Cilastatin Sodium) Merck & Co., Inc. 1729

Infections, gynecologic
Azactam for Injection (Aztreonam) Bristol-Myers Squibb 734
Cefizox for Intramuscular or Intravenous Use (Ceftizoxime Sodium) Fujisawa 1034
Cefobid Intravenous/Intramuscular (Cefoperazone Sodium) Roerig 2189
Cefobid Pharmacy Bulk Package - Not for Direct Infusion (Cefoperazone Sodium) Roerig 2192
Cefotan (Cefotetan) Zeneca 2829
Ceptaz (Ceftazidime) Glaxo Wellcome 1081
Claforan Sterile and Injection (Cefotaxime Sodium) Hoechst-Roussel 1235
Cleocin Phosphate Injection (Clindamycin Phosphate) Upjohn 2586
E-Mycin Tablets (Erythromycin) Knoll Laboratories 1341
ERYC (Erythromycin) Parke-Davis 1915
Ery-Tab Tablets (Erythromycin) Abbott 422
Erythrocin Stearate Filmtab (Erythromycin Stearate) Abbott 425
Erythromycin Base Filmtab (Erythromycin) Abbott 426
Erythromycin Delayed-Release Capsules, USP (Erythromycin) Abbott 427
Flagyl 375 Capsules (Metronidazole) Searle 2434
Flagyl I.V. (Metronidazole Hydrochloride) SCS 2247
Fortaz (Ceftazidime) Glaxo Wellcome 1100

(▭ Described in PDR For Nonprescription Drugs) (◉ Described in PDR For Ophthalmology)

1497 **Indications Index** **Infections**

Mefoxin (Cefoxitin Sodium) Merck & Co., Inc. ... 1691
Mefoxin Premixed Intravenous Solution (Cefoxitin Sodium) Merck & Co., Inc. ... 1694
Mezlin (Mezlocillin Sodium) Bayer Pharmaceutical ... 601
Mezlin Pharmacy Bulk Package (Mezlocillin Sodium) Bayer Pharmaceutical ... 604
PCE Dispertab Tablets (Erythromycin) Abbott ... 444
Pipracil (Piperacillin Sodium) Lederle ... 1390
Primaxin I.M. (Imipenem-Cilastatin Sodium) Merck & Co., Inc. ... 1727
Primaxin I.V. (Imipenem-Cilastatin Sodium) Merck & Co., Inc. ... 1729
Tazicef for Injection (Ceftazidime) SmithKline Beecham Pharmaceuticals ... 2519
Tazidime Vials, Faspak & ADD-Vantage (Ceftazidime) Lilly .. 1478
Ticar for Injection (Ticarcillin Disodium) SmithKline Beecham Pharmaceuticals ... 2526
Timentin for Injection (Ticarcillin Disodium, Clavulanate Potassium) SmithKline Beecham Pharmaceuticals ... 2528
Unasyn (Ampicillin Sodium, Sulbactam Sodium) Roerig ... 2212
Vantin for Oral Suspension and Vantin Tablets (Cefpodoxime Proxetil) Upjohn ... 2646
Zosyn (Piperacillin Sodium, Tazobactam Sodium) Lederle ... 1419
Zosyn Pharmacy Bulk Package (Piperacillin Sodium, Tazobactam Sodium) Lederle ... 1422

Infections, intra-abdominal

Amikacin Sulfate Injection, USP (Amikacin Sulfate) Elkins-Sinn ... 960
Amikin Injectable (Amikacin Sulfate) Apothecon ... 501
Azactam for Injection (Aztreonam) Bristol-Myers Squibb ... 734
Cefizox for Intramuscular or Intravenous Use (Ceftizoxime Sodium) Fujisawa ... 1034
Cefobid Intravenous/Intramuscular (Cefoperazone Sodium) Roerig ... 2189
Cefobid Pharmacy Bulk Package - Not for Direct Infusion (Cefoperazone Sodium) Roerig ... 2192
Cefotan (Cefotetan) Zeneca ... 2829
Ceptaz (Ceftazidime) Glaxo Wellcome ... 1081
Claforan Sterile and Injection (Cefotaxime Sodium) Hoechst-Roussel ... 1235
Cleocin Phosphate Injection (Clindamycin Phosphate) Upjohn ... 2586
Flagyl 375 Capsules (Metronidazole) Searle ... 2434
Flagyl I.V. (Metronidazole Hydrochloride) SCS ... 2247
Fortaz (Ceftazidime) Glaxo Wellcome ... 1100
Garamycin Injectable (Gentamicin Sulfate) Schering ... 2360
Mefoxin (Cefoxitin Sodium) Merck & Co., Inc. ... 1691
Mefoxin Premixed Intravenous Solution (Cefoxitin Sodium) Merck & Co., Inc. ... 1694
Mezlin (Mezlocillin Sodium) Bayer Pharmaceutical ... 601
Mezlin Pharmacy Bulk Package (Mezlocillin Sodium) Bayer Pharmaceutical ... 604
Nebcin Vials, Hyporets & ADD-Vantage (Tobramycin Sulfate) Lilly ... 1464
Netromycin Injection 100 mg/ml (Netilmicin Sulfate) Schering ... 2373
Omnipen for Oral Suspension (Ampicillin) Wyeth-Ayerst ... 2765
Pipracil (Piperacillin Sodium) Lederle ... 1390
Primaxin I.M. (Imipenem-Cilastatin Sodium) Merck & Co., Inc. ... 1727
Primaxin I.V. (Imipenem-Cilastatin Sodium) Merck & Co., Inc. ... 1729
Rocephin Injectable Vials, ADD-Vantage, Galaxy Container (Ceftriaxone Sodium) Roche Laboratories ... 2142
Tazicef for Injection (Ceftazidime) SmithKline Beecham Pharmaceuticals ... 2519
Tazidime Vials, Faspak & ADD-Vantage (Ceftazidime) Lilly .. 1478
Ticar for Injection (Ticarcillin Disodium) SmithKline Beecham Pharmaceuticals ... 2526
Timentin for Injection (Ticarcillin Disodium, Clavulanate Potassium) SmithKline Beecham Pharmaceuticals ... 2528
Tobramycin Sulfate Injection (Tobramycin Sulfate) Elkins-Sinn ... 968
Unasyn (Ampicillin Sodium, Sulbactam Sodium) Roerig ... 2212
Zefazone (Cefmetazole Sodium) Upjohn ... 2654

Infections, lacrimal sac (see under Dacryocystitis)

Infections, liver flukes (see under Clonorchiasis)

Infections, lower respiratory tract

Amoxil (Amoxicillin Trihydrate) SmithKline Beecham Pharmaceuticals ... 2464
Augmentin (Amoxicillin Trihydrate, Clavulanate Potassium) SmithKline Beecham Pharmaceuticals ... 2468
Azactam for Injection (Aztreonam) Bristol-Myers Squibb ... 734
Biaxin (Clarithromycin) Abbott ... 405
Ceclor Pulvules & Suspension (Cefaclor) Lilly ... 1431
Cefizox for Intramuscular or Intravenous Use (Ceftizoxime Sodium) Fujisawa ... 1034
Cefotan (Cefotetan) Zeneca ... 2829
Cefzil Tablets and Oral Suspension (Cefprozil) Bristol-Myers Squibb .. 746
Ceptaz (Ceftazidime) Glaxo Wellcome ... 1081
Cipro I.V. (Ciprofloxacin) Bayer Pharmaceutical ... 595
Cipro I.V. Pharmacy Bulk Package (Ciprofloxacin) Bayer Pharmaceutical ... 597
Cipro Tablets (Ciprofloxacin Hydrochloride) Bayer Pharmaceutical ... 592
Claforan Sterile and Injection (Cefotaxime Sodium) Hoechst-Roussel ... 1235
Cleocin Phosphate Injection (Clindamycin Phosphate) Upjohn ... 2586
E.E.S. (Erythromycin Ethylsuccinate) Abbott ... 424
E-Mycin Tablets (Erythromycin) Knoll Laboratories ... 1341
ERYC (Erythromycin) Parke-Davis .. 1915
EryPed (Erythromycin Ethylsuccinate) Abbott ... 421
Ery-Tab Tablets (Erythromycin) Abbott ... 422
Erythrocin Stearate Filmtab (Erythromycin Stearate) Abbott ... 425
Erythromycin Base Filmtab (Erythromycin) Abbott ... 426
Erythromycin Delayed-Release Capsules, USP (Erythromycin) Abbott ... 427
Flagyl 375 Capsules (Metronidazole) Searle ... 2434
Flagyl I.V. (Metronidazole Hydrochloride) SCS ... 2247
Floxin I.V. (Ofloxacin) McNeil Pharmaceutical ... 1571
Floxin Tablets (200 mg, 300 mg, 400 mg) (Ofloxacin) McNeil Pharmaceutical ... 1567
Fortaz (Ceftazidime) Glaxo Wellcome ... 1100
Ilosone (Erythromycin Estolate) Dista ... 911
Ilotycin Gluceptate, IV, Vials (Erythromycin Gluceptate) Dista ... 913
Kefurox Vials, Faspak & ADD-Vantage (Cefuroxime Sodium) Lilly ... 1454
Lorabid Suspension and Pulvules (Loracarbef) Lilly ... 1459
Mandol Vials, Faspak & ADD-Vantage (Cefamandole Nafate) Lilly ... 1461
Maxaquin Tablets (Lomefloxacin Hydrochloride) Searle ... 2440
Mefoxin (Cefoxitin Sodium) Merck & Co., Inc. ... 1691
Mefoxin Premixed Intravenous Solution (Cefoxitin Sodium) Merck & Co., Inc. ... 1694
Mezlin (Mezlocillin Sodium) Bayer Pharmaceutical ... 601
Mezlin Pharmacy Bulk Package (Mezlocillin Sodium) Bayer Pharmaceutical ... 604
Monocid Injection (Cefonicid Sodium) SmithKline Beecham Pharmaceuticals ... 2497
Nebcin Vials, Hyporets & ADD-Vantage (Tobramycin Sulfate) Lilly ... 1464
Netromycin Injection 100 mg/ml (Netilmicin Sulfate) Schering ... 2373
PCE Dispertab Tablets (Erythromycin) Abbott ... 444
Pfizerpen for Injection (Penicillin G Potassium) Roerig ... 2203
Pipracil (Piperacillin Sodium) Lederle ... 1390
Primaxin I.M. (Imipenem-Cilastatin Sodium) Merck & Co., Inc. ... 1727
Primaxin I.V. (Imipenem-Cilastatin Sodium) Merck & Co., Inc. ... 1729
Rocephin Injectable Vials, ADD-Vantage, Galaxy Container (Ceftriaxone Sodium) Roche Laboratories ... 2142
Spectrobid Tablets (Bacampicillin Hydrochloride) Roerig ... 2206
Tazicef for Injection (Ceftazidime) SmithKline Beecham Pharmaceuticals ... 2519
Tazidime Vials, Faspak & ADD-Vantage (Ceftazidime) Lilly .. 1478
Ticar for Injection (Ticarcillin Disodium) SmithKline Beecham Pharmaceuticals ... 2526
Timentin for Injection (Ticarcillin Disodium, Clavulanate Potassium) SmithKline Beecham Pharmaceuticals ... 2528
Tobramycin Sulfate Injection (Tobramycin Sulfate) Elkins-Sinn ... 968
Vantin for Oral Suspension and Vantin Tablets (Cefpodoxime Proxetil) Upjohn ... 2646
Zefazone (Cefmetazole Sodium) Upjohn ... 2654
Zinacef (Cefuroxime Sodium) Glaxo Wellcome ... 1211
Zithromax (Azithromycin) Pfizer Labs ... 1944
Zosyn (Piperacillin Sodium, Tazobactam Sodium) Lederle ... 1419
Zosyn Pharmacy Bulk Package (Piperacillin Sodium, Tazobactam Sodium) Lederle ... 1422

Infections, lower respiratory tract, RSV-induced

Virazole (Ribavirin) ICN ... 1264

Infections, mastoidectomy

Coly-Mycin S Otic w/Neomycin & Hydrocortisone (Colistin Sulfate, Neomycin Sulfate, Hydrocortisone Acetate) Parke-Davis ... 1906
Cortisporin Otic Suspension Sterile (Polymyxin B Sulfate, Neomycin Sulfate, Hydrocortisone) Glaxo Wellcome ... 1088
PediOtic Suspension Sterile (Polymyxin B Sulfate, Neomycin Sulfate, Hydrocortisone) Glaxo Wellcome ... 1153

Infections, mucomycotic

Fungizone Intravenous (Amphotericin B) Apothecon ... 506

Infections, mycotic, cutaneous

Mycostatin Cream, Topical Powder, and Ointment (Nystatin) Westwood-Squibb ... 2688

Infections, mycotic, mucocutaneous

Mycostatin Cream, Topical Powder, and Ointment (Nystatin) Westwood-Squibb ... 2688

Infections, ocular, bacterial

AK-Spore (Bacitracin Zinc, Neomycin Sulfate, Polymyxin B Sulfate) Akorn ... ⊙ 204
Bleph-10 (Sulfacetamide Sodium) Allergan ... 475
Chloromycetin Ophthalmic Ointment, 1% (Chloramphenicol) Parke-Davis ⊙ 310
Chloromycetin Ophthalmic Solution (Chloramphenicol) Parke-Davis ... ⊙ 310
Chloroptic S.O.P. (Chloramphenicol) Allergan ... ⊙ 239
Chloroptic Sterile Ophthalmic Solution (Chloramphenicol) Allergan ... ⊙ 239
Cortisporin Ophthalmic Ointment Sterile (Polymyxin B Sulfate, Bacitracin Zinc, Neomycin Sulfate, Hydrocortisone) Glaxo Wellcome ... 1085
Cortisporin Ophthalmic Suspension Sterile (Hydrocortisone, Polymyxin B Sulfate, Neomycin Sulfate) Glaxo Wellcome ... 1086
Gentak (Gentamicin Sulfate) Akorn ... ⊙ 208
Ilotycin Ophthalmic Ointment (Erythromycin) Dista ... 912
NeoDecadron Sterile Ophthalmic Ointment (Neomycin Sulfate, Dexamethasone Sodium Phosphate) Merck & Co., Inc. ... 1712
NeoDecadron Sterile Ophthalmic Solution (Neomycin Sulfate, Dexamethasone Sodium Phosphate) Merck & Co., Inc. ... 1713
Neosporin Ophthalmic Ointment Sterile (Polymyxin B Sulfate, Bacitracin Zinc, Neomycin Sulfate) Glaxo Wellcome ... 1148
Neosporin Ophthalmic Solution Sterile (Polymyxin B Sulfate, Neomycin Sulfate, Gramicidin) Glaxo Wellcome ... 1149
Ocuflox (Ofloxacin) Allergan ... 481
Polysporin Ophthalmic Ointment Sterile (Polymyxin B Sulfate, Bacitracin Zinc) Glaxo Wellcome .. 1154
Polytrim Ophthalmic Solution Sterile (Polymyxin B Sulfate, Trimethoprim Sulfate) Allergan ... 482
Sodium Sulamyd (Sulfacetamide Sodium) Schering ... 2387
TERAK Ointment (Oxytetracycline Hydrochloride, Polymyxin B Sulfate) Akorn ... ⊙ 209
Terra-Cortril Ophthalmic Suspension (Oxytetracycline Hydrochloride, Hydrocortisone Acetate) Roerig ... 2210
Terramycin with Polymyxin B Sulfate Ophthalmic Ointment (Oxytetracycline Hydrochloride, Polymyxin B Sulfate) Roerig ... 2211
Vasosulf (Phenylephrine Hydrochloride, Sulfacetamide Sodium) CIBA Vision Ophthalmics ... ⊙ 271

Infections, perioperative, reduction of the incidence of

Amikacin Sulfate Injection, USP (Amikacin Sulfate) Elkins-Sinn ... 960
Amikin Injectable (Amikacin Sulfate) Apothecon ... 501
Ancef Injection (Cefazolin Sodium) SmithKline Beecham Pharmaceuticals ... 2465
Cefotan (Cefotetan) Zeneca ... 2829
Claforan Sterile and Injection (Cefotaxime Sodium) Hoechst-Roussel ... 1235
Flagyl I.V. (Metronidazole Hydrochloride) SCS ... 2247
Kefurox Vials, Faspak & ADD-Vantage (Cefuroxime Sodium) Lilly ... 1454
Kefzol Vials, Faspak & ADD-Vantage (Cefazolin Sodium) Lilly ... 1456
Mandol Vials, Faspak & ADD-Vantage (Cefamandole Nafate) Lilly ... 1461
Mefoxin (Cefoxitin Sodium) Merck & Co., Inc. ... 1691
Mefoxin Premixed Intravenous Solution (Cefoxitin Sodium) Merck & Co., Inc. ... 1694
Mezlin (Mezlocillin Sodium) Bayer Pharmaceutical ... 601
Mezlin Pharmacy Bulk Package (Mezlocillin Sodium) Bayer Pharmaceutical ... 604
Pipracil (Piperacillin Sodium) Lederle ... 1390
Rocephin Injectable Vials, ADD-Vantage, Galaxy Container (Ceftriaxone Sodium) Roche Laboratories ... 2142
Zefazone (Cefmetazole Sodium) Upjohn ... 2654

Infections | Indications Index | 1498

Zinacef (Cefuroxime Sodium) Glaxo Wellcome ... 1211

Infections, polymicrobic
Ceptaz (Ceftazidime) Glaxo Wellcome ... 1081
Fortaz (Ceftazidime) Glaxo Wellcome ... 1100
Primaxin I.V. (Imipenem-Cilastatin Sodium) Merck & Co., Inc. ... 1729
Tazicef for Injection (Ceftazidime) SmithKline Beecham Pharmaceuticals ... 2519
Tazidime Vials, Faspak & ADD-Vantage (Ceftazidime) Lilly .. 1478

Infections, post-colorectal surgery, reduction of the incidence of
Flagyl I.V. (Metronidazole Hydrochloride) SCS ... 2247
Mezlin (Mezlocillin Sodium) Bayer Pharmaceutical ... 601
Mezlin Pharmacy Bulk Package (Mezlocillin Sodium) Bayer Pharmaceutical ... 604

Infections, respiratory tract
Amikacin Sulfate Injection, USP (Amikacin Sulfate) Elkins-Sinn ... 960
Amikin Injectable (Amikacin Sulfate) Apothecon ... 501
Ancef Injection (Cefazolin Sodium) SmithKline Beecham Pharmaceuticals ... 2465
Cefobid Intravenous/Intramuscular (Cefoperazone Sodium) Roerig ... 2189
Cefobid Pharmacy Bulk Package - Not for Direct Infusion (Cefoperazone Sodium) Roerig ... 2192
Dynacin Capsules (Minocycline Hydrochloride) Medicis ... 1590
ERYC (Erythromycin) Parke-Davis .. 1915
Erythrocin Stearate Filmtab (Erythromycin Stearate) Abbott ... 425
Erythromycin Base Filmtab (Erythromycin) Abbott ... 426
Erythromycin Delayed-Release Capsules, USP (Erythromycin) Abbott ... 427
Garamycin Injectable (Gentamicin Sulfate) Schering ... 2360
Keflex Pulvules & Oral Suspension (Cephalexin) Dista ... 914
Keftab Tablets (Cephalexin Hydrochloride) Dista ... 915
Kefzol Vials, Faspak & ADD-Vantage (Cefazolin Sodium) Lilly ... 1456
Minocin Oral Suspension (Minocycline Hydrochloride) Lederle ... 1385
Monodox Capsules (Doxycycline Monohydrate) Oclassen ... 1805
Omnipen for Oral Suspension (Ampicillin) Wyeth-Ayerst ... 2765
PCE Dispertab Tablets (Erythromycin) Abbott ... 444
Pen•Vee K (Penicillin V Potassium) Wyeth-Ayerst ... 2772
Pfizerpen for Injection (Penicillin G Potassium) Roerig ... 2203
Ticar for Injection (Ticarcillin Disodium) SmithKline Beecham Pharmaceuticals ... 2526
Vibramycin Hyclate Capsules (Doxycycline Hyclate) Pfizer Labs 1941

Infections, skin and skin structure
Amikacin Sulfate Injection, USP (Amikacin Sulfate) Elkins-Sinn ... 960
Amikin Injectable (Amikacin Sulfate) Apothecon ... 501
Amoxil (Amoxicillin Trihydrate) SmithKline Beecham Pharmaceuticals ... 2464
Ancef Injection (Cefazolin Sodium) SmithKline Beecham Pharmaceuticals ... 2465
Augmentin (Amoxicillin Trihydrate, Clavulanate Potassium) SmithKline Beecham Pharmaceuticals ... 2468
Azactam for Injection (Aztreonam) Bristol-Myers Squibb ... 734
Biaxin (Clarithromycin) Abbott ... 405
Bicillin C-R Injection (Penicillin G Procaine, Penicillin G Benzathine) Wyeth-Ayerst ... 2704
Bicillin C-R 900/300 Injection (Penicillin G Procaine, Penicillin G Benzathine) Wyeth-Ayerst ... 2706
Ceclor Pulvules & Suspension (Cefaclor) Lilly ... 1431
Cefizox for Intramuscular or Intravenous Use (Ceftizoxime Sodium) Fujisawa ... 1034
Cefobid Intravenous/Intramuscular (Cefoperazone Sodium) Roerig ... 2189
Cefobid Pharmacy Bulk Package - Not for Direct Infusion (Cefoperazone Sodium) Roerig ... 2192
Cefotan (Cefotetan) Zeneca ... 2829
Ceftin (Cefuroxime Axetil) Glaxo Wellcome ... 1078
Cefzil Tablets and Oral Suspension (Cefprozil) Bristol-Myers Squibb .. 746
Ceptaz (Ceftazidime) Glaxo Wellcome ... 1081
Cipro I.V. (Ciprofloxacin) Bayer Pharmaceutical ... 595
Cipro I.V. Pharmacy Bulk Package (Ciprofloxacin) Bayer Pharmaceutical ... 597
Cipro Tablets (Ciprofloxacin Hydrochloride) Bayer Pharmaceutical ... 592
Claforan Sterile and Injection (Cefotaxime Sodium) Hoechst-Roussel ... 1235
Cleocin Phosphate Injection (Clindamycin Phosphate) Upjohn ... 2586
Duricef (Cefadroxil Monohydrate) Bristol-Myers Squibb ... 748
Dynacin Capsules (Minocycline Hydrochloride) Medicis ... 1590
E.E.S. (Erythromycin Ethylsuccinate) Abbott ... 424
E-Mycin Tablets (Erythromycin) Knoll Laboratories ... 1341
ERYC (Erythromycin) Parke-Davis .. 1915
EryPed (Erythromycin Ethylsuccinate) Abbott ... 421
Ery-Tab Tablets (Erythromycin) Abbott ... 422
Erythrocin Stearate Filmtab (Erythromycin Stearate) Abbott ... 425
Erythromycin Base Filmtab (Erythromycin) Abbott ... 426
Erythromycin Delayed-Release Capsules, USP (Erythromycin) Abbott ... 427
Flagyl 375 Capsules (Metronidazole) Searle ... 2434
Flagyl I.V. (Metronidazole Hydrochloride) SCS ... 2247
Floxin I.V. (Ofloxacin) McNeil Pharmaceutical ... 1571
Floxin Tablets (200 mg, 300 mg, 400 mg) (Ofloxacin) McNeil Pharmaceutical ... 1567
Fortaz (Ceftazidime) Glaxo Wellcome ... 1100
Garamycin Injectable (Gentamicin Sulfate) Schering ... 2360
Ilosone (Erythromycin Estolate) Dista ... 911
Ilotycin Gluceptate, IV, Vials (Erythromycin Gluceptate) Dista ... 913
Keflex Pulvules & Oral Suspension (Cephalexin) Dista ... 914
Keftab Tablets (Cephalexin Hydrochloride) Dista ... 915
Kefurox Vials, Faspak & ADD-Vantage (Cefuroxime Sodium) Lilly ... 1454
Kefzol Vials, Faspak & ADD-Vantage (Cefazolin Sodium) Lilly ... 1456
Lorabid Suspension and Pulvules (Loracarbef) Lilly ... 1459
Mandol Vials, Faspak & ADD-Vantage (Cefamandole Nafate) Lilly ... 1461
Mefoxin (Cefoxitin Sodium) Merck & Co., Inc. ... 1691
Mefoxin Premixed Intravenous Solution (Cefoxitin Sodium) Merck & Co., Inc. ... 1694
Mezlin (Mezlocillin Sodium) Bayer Pharmaceutical ... 601
Mezlin Pharmacy Bulk Package (Mezlocillin Sodium) Bayer Pharmaceutical ... 604
Minocin Oral Suspension (Minocycline Hydrochloride) Lederle ... 1385
Monocid Injection (Cefonicid Sodium) SmithKline Beecham Pharmaceuticals ... 2497
Monodox Capsules (Doxycycline Monohydrate) Oclassen ... 1805
Nebcin Vials, Hyporets & ADD-Vantage (Tobramycin Sulfate) Lilly ... 1464
Netromycin Injection 100 mg/ml (Netilmicin Sulfate) Schering ... 2373
PCE Dispertab Tablets (Erythromycin) Abbott ... 444
Pen•Vee K (Penicillin V Potassium) Wyeth-Ayerst ... 2772
Pipracil (Piperacillin Sodium) Lederle ... 1390
Primaxin I.M. (Imipenem-Cilastatin Sodium) Merck & Co., Inc. ... 1727
Primaxin I.V. (Imipenem-Cilastatin Sodium) Merck & Co., Inc. ... 1729
Rocephin Injectable Vials, ADD-Vantage, Galaxy Container (Ceftriaxone Sodium) Roche Laboratories ... 2142
Spectrobid Tablets (Bacampicillin Hydrochloride) Roerig ... 2206
Tazicef for Injection (Ceftazidime) SmithKline Beecham Pharmaceuticals ... 2519
Tazidime Vials, Faspak & ADD-Vantage (Ceftazidime) Lilly .. 1478
Ticar for Injection (Ticarcillin Disodium) SmithKline Beecham Pharmaceuticals ... 2526
Timentin for Injection (Ticarcillin Disodium, Clavulanate Potassium) SmithKline Beecham Pharmaceuticals ... 2528
Tobramycin Sulfate Injection (Tobramycin Sulfate) Elkins-Sinn ... 968
Unasyn (Ampicillin Sodium, Sulbactam Sodium) Roerig ... 2212
Vantin for Oral Suspension and Vantin Tablets (Cefpodoxime Proxetil) Upjohn ... 2646
Zefazone (Cefmetazole Sodium) Upjohn ... 2654
Zinacef (Cefuroxime Sodium) Glaxo Wellcome ... 1211
Zithromax (Azithromycin) Pfizer Labs ... 1944
Zosyn (Piperacillin Sodium, Tazobactam Sodium) Lederle ... 1419
Zosyn Pharmacy Bulk Package (Piperacillin Sodium, Tazobactam Sodium) Lederle ... 1422

Infections, skin, bacterial, minor
Bactine First Aid Antibiotic Plus Anesthetic Ointment (Bacitracin Zinc, Neomycin Sulfate, Polymyxin B Sulfate, Lidocaine) Miles Consumer ... ▣ 708
Bactroban Ointment (Mupirocin) SmithKline Beecham Pharmaceuticals ... 2470
Betadine Brand First Aid Antibiotics & Moisturizer Ointment (Polymyxin B Sulfate, Bacitracin Zinc) Purdue Frederick ... 1991
Betadine First Aid Cream (Povidone Iodine) Purdue Frederick ... 1991
Betadine Ointment (Povidone Iodine) Purdue Frederick ... 1992
Betadine Solution (Povidone Iodine) Purdue Frederick ... 1992
Campho-Phenique Liquid (Phenol, Camphor) Miles Consumer ... ▣ 719
Campho-Phenique Maximum Strength First Aid Antibiotic Plus Pain Reliever Ointment (Bacitracin Zinc, Lidocaine Hydrochloride, Neomycin Sulfate, Polymyxin B Sulfate) Miles Consumer ... ▣ 719
Clorpactin WCS-90 (Sodium Oxychlorosene) Guardian ... 1230
Elase-Chloromycetin Ointment (Fibrinolysin, Desoxyribonuclease, Chloramphenicol) Fujisawa ... 1040
Furacin Soluble Dressing (Nitrofurazone) Roberts ... 2045
Furacin Topical Cream (Nitrofurazone) Roberts ... 2045
Garamycin Injectable (Gentamicin Sulfate) Schering ... 2360
Mycitracin (Bacitracin, Neomycin Sulfate, Lidocaine, Polymyxin B Sulfate) Upjohn ... ▣ 839
Neosporin Ointment (Bacitracin Zinc, Neomycin Sulfate, Polymyxin B Sulfate) WARNER WELLCOME ... ▣ 857
Neosporin Plus Maximum Strength Cream (Polymyxin B Sulfate, Neomycin Sulfate, Lidocaine) WARNER WELLCOME ... ▣ 858
Neosporin Plus Maximum Strength Ointment (Polymyxin B Sulfate, Bacitracin Zinc, Neomycin Sulfate, Lidocaine) WARNER WELLCOME ... ▣ 858
Polysporin Ointment (Bacitracin Zinc, Polymyxin B Sulfate) WARNER WELLCOME ... ▣ 858
Polysporin Powder (Bacitracin Zinc, Polymyxin B Sulfate) WARNER WELLCOME ... ▣ 859
Zephiran (Benzalkonium Chloride) Sanofi Winthrop ... ▣ 795

Infections, soft tissues (see under Infections, skin and skin structure)

Infections, superficial, external auditory canal (see under Otitis externa)

Infections, upper respiratory tract
Amoxil (Amoxicillin Trihydrate) SmithKline Beecham Pharmaceuticals ... 2464
Biaxin (Clarithromycin) Abbott ... 405
Bicillin C-R Injection (Penicillin G Procaine, Penicillin G Benzathine) Wyeth-Ayerst ... 2704
Bicillin C-R 900/300 Injection (Penicillin G Procaine, Penicillin G Benzathine) Wyeth-Ayerst ... 2706
Bicillin L-A Injection (Penicillin G Benzathine) Wyeth-Ayerst ... 2707
Ceclor Pulvules & Suspension (Cefaclor) Lilly ... 1431
Duricef (Cefadroxil Monohydrate) Bristol-Myers Squibb ... 748
Dynacin Capsules (Minocycline Hydrochloride) Medicis ... 1590
E.E.S. (Erythromycin Ethylsuccinate) Abbott ... 424
E-Mycin Tablets (Erythromycin) Knoll Laboratories ... 1341
ERYC (Erythromycin) Parke-Davis .. 1915
EryPed (Erythromycin Ethylsuccinate) Abbott ... 421
Ery-Tab Tablets (Erythromycin) Abbott ... 422
Erythrocin Stearate Filmtab (Erythromycin Stearate) Abbott ... 425
Erythromycin Base Filmtab (Erythromycin) Abbott ... 426
Erythromycin Delayed-Release Capsules, USP (Erythromycin) Abbott ... 427
Ilosone (Erythromycin Estolate) Dista ... 911
Ilotycin Gluceptate, IV, Vials (Erythromycin Gluceptate) Dista ... 913
Lorabid Suspension and Pulvules (Loracarbef) Lilly ... 1459
Minocin Oral Suspension (Minocycline Hydrochloride) Lederle ... 1385
Monodox Capsules (Doxycycline Monohydrate) Oclassen ... 1805
PCE Dispertab Tablets (Erythromycin) Abbott ... 444
Pen•Vee K (Penicillin V Potassium) Wyeth-Ayerst ... 2772
Septra (Trimethoprim, Sulfamethoxazole) Glaxo Wellcome ... 1174
Spectrobid Tablets (Bacampicillin Hydrochloride) Roerig ... 2206
Suprax (Cefixime) Lederle ... 1399
Vantin for Oral Suspension and Vantin Tablets (Cefpodoxime Proxetil) Upjohn ... 2646
Vibramycin Hyclate Capsules (Doxycycline Hyclate) Pfizer Labs 1941
Zithromax (Azithromycin) Pfizer Labs ... 1944

Infections, urinary bladder, prophylaxis of
Neosporin G.U. Irrigant Sterile (Neomycin Sulfate, Polymyxin B Sulfate) Glaxo Wellcome ... 1148

Infections, urinary tract
Amikacin Sulfate Injection, USP (Amikacin Sulfate) Elkins-Sinn ... 960
Amikin Injectable (Amikacin Sulfate) Apothecon ... 501
Amoxil (Amoxicillin Trihydrate) SmithKline Beecham Pharmaceuticals ... 2464

(▣ Described in PDR For Nonprescription Drugs) (◉ Described in PDR For Ophthalmology)

1499 Indications Index Inflammation

Ancef Injection (Cefazolin Sodium) SmithKline Beecham Pharmaceuticals ... 2465
Augmentin (Amoxicillin Trihydrate, Clavulanate Potassium) SmithKline Beecham Pharmaceuticals ... 2468
Azactam for Injection (Aztreonam) Bristol-Myers Squibb ... 734
Azo Gantanol Tablets (Sulfamethoxazole, Phenazopyridine Hydrochloride) Roche Laboratories ... 2080
Azo Gantrisin Tablets (Sulfisoxazole, Phenazopyridine Hydrochloride) Roche Laboratories ... 2081
Bactrim DS Tablets (Trimethoprim, Sulfamethoxazole) Roche Laboratories ... 2084
Bactrim I.V. Infusion (Trimethoprim, Sulfamethoxazole) Roche Laboratories ... 2082
Bactrim (Trimethoprim, Sulfamethoxazole) Roche Laboratories ... 2084
Ceclor Pulvules & Suspension (Cefaclor) Lilly ... 1431
Cefizox for Intramuscular or Intravenous Use (Ceftizoxime Sodium) Fujisawa ... 1034
Cefobid Intravenous/Intramuscular (Cefoperazone Sodium) Roerig ... 2189
Cefobid Pharmacy Bulk Package - Not for Direct Infusion (Cefoperazone Sodium) Roerig ... 2192
Cefotan (Cefotetan) Zeneca ... 2829
Ceftin (Cefuroxime Axetil) Glaxo Wellcome ... 1078
Ceptaz (Ceftazidime) Glaxo Wellcome ... 1081
Cipro I.V. (Ciprofloxacin) Bayer Pharmaceutical ... 595
Cipro I.V. Pharmacy Bulk Package (Ciprofloxacin) Bayer Pharmaceutical ... 597
Cipro Tablets (Ciprofloxacin Hydrochloride) Bayer Pharmaceutical ... 592
Duricef (Cefadroxil Monohydrate) Bristol-Myers Squibb ... 748
Dynacin Capsules (Minocycline Hydrochloride) Medicis ... 1590
Floxin I.V. (Ofloxacin) McNeil Pharmaceutical ... 1571
Floxin Tablets (200 mg, 300 mg, 400 mg) (Ofloxacin) McNeil Pharmaceutical ... 1567
Fortaz (Ceftazidime) Glaxo Wellcome ... 1100
Gantanol Tablets (Sulfamethoxazole) Roche Laboratories ... 2119
Gantrisin (Acetyl Sulfisoxazole) Roche Laboratories ... 2120
Garamycin Injectable (Gentamicin Sulfate) Schering ... 2360
Geocillin Tablets (Carbenicillin Indanyl Sodium) Roerig ... 2199
Kefurox Vials, Faspak & ADD-Vantage (Cefuroxime Sodium) Lilly ... 1454
Kefzol Vials, Faspak & ADD-Vantage (Cefazolin Sodium) Lilly ... 1456
Lorabid Suspension and Pulvules (Loracarbef) Lilly ... 1459
Macrobid Capsules (Nitrofurantoin Monohydrate) Procter & Gamble Pharmaceuticals ... 1988
Macrodantin Capsules (Nitrofurantoin) Procter & Gamble Pharmaceuticals ... 1989
Mandol Vials, Faspak & ADD-Vantage (Cefamandole Nafate) Lilly ... 1461
Maxaquin Tablets (Lomefloxacin Hydrochloride) Searle ... 2440
Mefoxin (Cefoxitin Sodium) Merck & Co., Inc. ... 1691
Mefoxin Premixed Intravenous Solution (Cefoxitin Sodium) Merck & Co., Inc. ... 1694
Mezlin (Mezlocillin Sodium) Bayer Pharmaceutical ... 601
Mezlin Pharmacy Bulk Package (Mezlocillin Sodium) Bayer Pharmaceutical ... 604
Minocin Oral Suspension (Minocycline Hydrochloride) Lederle ... 1385
Monocid Injection (Cefonicid Sodium) SmithKline Beecham Pharmaceuticals ... 2497
Monodox Capsules (Doxycycline Monohydrate) Oclassen ... 1805
Nebcin Vials, Hyporets & ADD-Vantage (Tobramycin Sulfate) Lilly ... 1464
NegGram (Nalidixic Acid) Sanofi Winthrop ... 2323
Netromycin Injection 100 mg/ml (Netilmicin Sulfate) Schering ... 2373
Noroxin Tablets (Norfloxacin) Merck & Co., Inc. ... 1715
Noroxin Tablets (Norfloxacin) Roberts ... 2048
Penetrex Tablets (Enoxacin) Rhone-Poulenc Rorer Pharmaceuticals ... 2031
Pipracil (Piperacillin Sodium) Lederle ... 1390
Primaxin I.V. (Imipenem-Cilastatin Sodium) Merck & Co., Inc. ... 1729
Proloprim Tablets (Trimethoprim) Glaxo Wellcome ... 1155
Rocephin Injectable Vials, ADD-Vantage, Galaxy Container (Ceftriaxone Sodium) Roche Laboratories ... 2142
Septra (Trimethoprim, Sulfamethoxazole) Glaxo Wellcome ... 1174
Septra I.V. Infusion (Trimethoprim, Sulfamethoxazole) Glaxo Wellcome ... 1169
Septra I.V. Infusion ADD-Vantage Vials (Trimethoprim, Sulfamethoxazole) Glaxo Wellcome ... 1171
Septra (Trimethoprim, Sulfamethoxazole) Glaxo Wellcome ... 1174
Seromycin Pulvules (Cycloserine) Lilly ... 1476
Spectrobid Tablets (Bacampicillin Hydrochloride) Roerig ... 2206
Suprax (Cefixime) Lederle ... 1399
Tazicef for Injection (Ceftazidime) SmithKline Beecham Pharmaceuticals ... 2519
Tazidime Vials, Faspak & ADD-Vantage (Ceftazidime) Lilly ... 1478
Ticar for Injection (Ticarcillin Disodium) SmithKline Beecham Pharmaceuticals ... 2526
Timentin for Injection (Ticarcillin Disodium, Clavulanate Potassium) SmithKline Beecham Pharmaceuticals ... 2528
Tobramycin Sulfate Injection (Tobramycin Sulfate) Elkins-Sinn ... 968
Trimpex Tablets (Trimethoprim) Roche Laboratories ... 2163
Urised Tablets (Atropine Sulfate, Hyoscyamine, Methenamine, Phenyl Salicylate) PolyMedica ... 1964
Uroqid-Acid No. 2 Tablets (Methenamine Mandelate, Sodium Acid Phosphate) Beach ... 640
Vantin for Oral Suspension and Vantin Tablets (Cefpodoxime Proxetil) Upjohn ... 2646
Zefazone (Cefmetazole Sodium) Upjohn ... 2654
Zinacef (Cefuroxime Sodium) Glaxo Wellcome ... 1211

Infections, urinary tract, systemic candidal

Diflucan Injection, Tablets, and Oral Suspension (Fluconazole) Roerig ... 2194

Infections, vaginal cuff, post-surgical

Cleocin Phosphate Injection (Clindamycin Phosphate) Upjohn ... 2586
Flagyl 375 Capsules (Metronidazole) Searle ... 2434
Flagyl I.V. (Metronidazole Hydrochloride) SCS ... 2247
Protostat Tablets (Metronidazole) Ortho Pharmaceutical ... 1883

Infections, venereal (see also under Bejel; Yaws; Pinta; Gonorrhea)

Bicillin L-A Injection (Penicillin G Benzathine) Wyeth-Ayerst ... 2707

Infections, vulvovaginal mycotic, Candida species

AVC (Sulfanilamide) Marion Merrell Dow ... 1500
Femstat Prefill Vaginal Cream 2% (Butoconazole Nitrate) Roche Laboratories ... 2116
Femstat Vaginal Cream 2% (Butoconazole Nitrate) Roche Laboratories ... 2115
Mycelex-G 500 mg Vaginal Tablets (Clotrimazole) Bayer Pharmaceutical ... 609

Infectious diarrhea (see under Diarrhea, infectious)

Inflammation, anorectal

Analpram-HC Rectal Cream 1% and 2.5% (Hydrocortisone Acetate, Pramoxine Hydrochloride) Ferndale ... 977
Anusol-HC Suppositories (Hydrocortisone Acetate) Parke-Davis ... 1897
Cortizone-5 Creme and Ointment (Hydrocortisone) Thompson Medical ... ■ 831
Cortizone-10 Creme and Ointment (Hydrocortisone) Thompson Medical ... ■ 831
Hemorid For Women Suppositories (Zinc Oxide, Phenylephrine Hydrochloride, Fat, Hard) Thompson Medical ... ■ 834
ProctoFoam-HC (Hydrocortisone Acetate, Pramoxine Hydrochloride) Schwarz ... 2409
Sween Cream (Benzethonium Chloride, Lanolin Oil) Sween ... 2554
Tronolane Anesthetic Cream for Hemorrhoids (Pramoxine Hydrochloride) Ross ... ■ 784

Inflammation, anterior segment

AK-CIDE (Prednisolone Acetate, Sulfacetamide Sodium) Akorn ... ⊙ 202
AK-CIDE Ointment (Prednisolone Acetate, Sulfacetamide Sodium) Akorn ... ⊙ 202
AK-Pred (Prednisolone Sodium Phosphate) Akorn ... ⊙ 204
AK-Trol Ointment & Suspension (Dexamethasone, Neomycin Sulfate, Polymyxin B Sulfate) Akorn ... ⊙ 205
Aristocort Tablets (Triamcinolone) Fujisawa ... 1022
Blephamide Liquifilm Sterile Ophthalmic Suspension (Prednisolone Acetate, Sulfacetamide Sodium) Allergan ... 476
Blephamide Ointment (Sulfacetamide Sodium, Prednisolone Acetate) Allergan ... ⊙ 237
Celestone Soluspan Suspension (Betamethasone Sodium Phosphate, Betamethasone Acetate) Schering ... 2347
Cortisporin Ophthalmic Ointment Sterile (Polymyxin B Sulfate, Bacitracin Zinc, Neomycin Sulfate, Hydrocortisone) Glaxo Wellcome ... 1085
Cortisporin Ophthalmic Suspension Sterile (Hydrocortisone, Polymyxin B Sulfate, Neomycin Sulfate) Glaxo Wellcome ... 1086
Cortone Acetate Sterile Suspension (Cortisone Acetate) Merck & Co., Inc. ... 1623
Cortone Acetate Tablets (Cortisone Acetate) Merck & Co., Inc. ... 1624
Dalalone D.P. Injectable (Dexamethasone Acetate) Forest ... 1011
Decadron Elixir (Dexamethasone) Merck & Co., Inc. ... 1633
Decadron Phosphate Injection (Dexamethasone Sodium Phosphate) Merck & Co., Inc. ... 1637
Decadron Phosphate Sterile Ophthalmic Ointment (Dexamethasone Sodium Phosphate) Merck & Co., Inc. ... 1641
Decadron Phosphate Sterile Ophthalmic Solution (Dexamethasone Sodium Phosphate) Merck & Co., Inc. ... 1642
Decadron Tablets (Dexamethasone) Merck & Co., Inc. ... 1635
Decadron-LA Sterile Suspension (Dexamethasone Acetate) Merck & Co., Inc. ... 1646
Deltasone Tablets (Prednisone) Upjohn ... 2595
Depo-Medrol Single-Dose Vial (Methylprednisolone Acetate) Upjohn ... 2600
Depo-Medrol Sterile Aqueous Suspension (Methylprednisolone Acetate) Upjohn ... 2597
Dexacidin Ointment (Dexamethasone, Neomycin Sulfate, Polymyxin B Sulfate) CIBA Vision Ophthalmics ... ⊙ 263
Econopred & Econopred Plus Ophthalmic Suspensions (Prednisolone Acetate) Alcon Laboratories ... ⊙ 217
FML Forte Liquifilm (Fluorometholone) Allergan ... ⊙ 240
FML Liquifilm (Fluorometholone) Allergan ... ⊙ 241
FML S.O.P. (Fluorometholone) Allergan ... ⊙ 241
FML-S Liquifilm (Sulfacetamide Sodium, Fluorometholone) Allergan ... ⊙ 242
Fluor-Op Ophthalmic Suspension (Fluorometholone) CIBA Vision Ophthalmics ... ⊙ 264
Hydeltrasol Injection, Sterile (Prednisolone Sodium Phosphate) Merck & Co., Inc. ... 1665
Hydrocortone Phosphate Injection, Sterile (Hydrocortisone Sodium Phosphate) Merck & Co., Inc. ... 1670
Hydrocortone Tablets (Hydrocortisone) Merck & Co., Inc. ... 1672
Inflamase (Prednisolone Sodium Phosphate) CIBA Vision Ophthalmics ... ⊙ 265
Maxitrol Ophthalmic Ointment and Suspension (Dexamethasone, Neomycin Sulfate, Polymyxin B Sulfate) Alcon Laboratories ... ⊙ 224
Medrol (Methylprednisolone) Upjohn ... 2621
NeoDecadron Sterile Ophthalmic Ointment (Neomycin Sulfate, Dexamethasone Sodium Phosphate) Merck & Co., Inc. ... 1712
NeoDecadron Sterile Ophthalmic Solution (Neomycin Sulfate, Dexamethasone Sodium Phosphate) Merck & Co., Inc. ... 1713
Ophthocort (Chloramphenicol, Polymyxin B Sulfate, Hydrocortisone Acetate) Parke-Davis ... ⊙ 311
Pediapred Oral Liquid (Prednisolone Sodium Phosphate) Fisons ... 995
Poly-Pred Liquifilm (Neomycin Sulfate, Polymyxin B Sulfate, Prednisolone Acetate) Allergan ... ⊙ 248
Pred Forte (Prednisolone Acetate) Allergan ... ⊙ 250
Pred-G Liquifilm Sterile Ophthalmic Suspension (Gentamicin Sulfate, Prednisolone Acetate) Allergan ... ⊙ 251
Pred-G S.O.P. Sterile Ophthalmic Ointment (Gentamicin Sulfate, Prednisolone Acetate) Allergan ... ⊙ 252
Prelone Syrup (Prednisolone) Muro 1787
Solu-Cortef Sterile Powder (Hydrocortisone Sodium Succinate) Upjohn ... 2641
Solu-Medrol Sterile Powder (Methylprednisolone Sodium Succinate) Upjohn ... 2643
Terra-Cortril Ophthalmic Suspension (Oxytetracycline Hydrochloride, Hydrocortisone Acetate) Roerig ... 2210
TobraDex Ophthalmic Suspension and Ointment (Dexamethasone, Tobramycin) Alcon Laboratories ... 473
Vasocidin Ointment (Prednisolone Acetate, Sulfacetamide Sodium) CIBA Vision Ophthalmics ... ⊙ 268
Vasocidin Ophthalmic Solution (Prednisolone Sodium Phosphate, Sulfacetamide Sodium) CIBA Vision Ophthalmics ... ⊙ 270

(■ Described in PDR For Nonprescription Drugs) (⊙ Described in PDR For Ophthalmology)

Influenza A virus

Influenza A virus, respiratory tract illness, chemoprophylaxis of

Flumadine Tablets & Syrup (Rimantadine Hydrochloride) Forest 1015

Symmetrel Capsules and Syrup (Amantadine Hydrochloride) DuPont 946

Influenza A virus, respiratory tract illness, treatment of

Flumadine Tablets & Syrup (Rimantadine Hydrochloride) Forest 1015

Symmetrel Capsules and Syrup (Amantadine Hydrochloride) DuPont 946

Influenza syndrome, symptomatic relief of

Actifed with Codeine Cough Syrup (Codeine Phosphate, Triprolidine Hydrochloride, Pseudoephedrine Hydrochloride) Glaxo Wellcome.... 1067

Actifed Sinus Daytime/Nighttime Tablets and Caplets (Acetaminophen, Diphenhydramine Hydrochloride, Pseudoephedrine Hydrochloride) WARNER WELLCOME.................... ⊞ 846

Advil Cold and Sinus Caplets and Tablets (formerly CoAdvil) (Ibuprofen, Pseudoephedrine Hydrochloride) Whitehall .... ⊞ 870

Alka-Seltzer Plus Cold Medicine Liqui-Gels (Chlorpheniramine Maleate, Pseudoephedrine Hydrochloride, Acetaminophen) Miles Consumer.................................. ⊞ 706

Alka-Seltzer Plus Cold & Cough Medicine (Aspirin, Chlorpheniramine Maleate, Dextromethorphan Hydrobromide, Phenylpropanolamine Bitartrate) Miles Consumer... ⊞ 708

Alka-Seltzer Plus Cold & Cough Medicine Liqui-Gels (Dextromethorphan Hydrobromide, Chlorpheniramine Maleate, Pseudoephedrine Hydrochloride, Acetaminophen) Miles Consumer... ⊞ 705

Alka-Seltzer Plus Night-Time Cold Medicine (Aspirin, Phenylpropanolamine Bitartrate, Doxylamine Succinate, Dextromethorphan Hydrobromide) Miles Consumer... ⊞ 707

Alka-Seltzer Plus Night-Time Cold Medicine Liqui-Gels (Dextromethorphan Hydrobromide, Doxylamine Succinate, Pseudoephedrine Hydrochloride, Acetaminophen) Miles Consumer... ⊞ 706

Atrohist Pediatric Capsules (Chlorpheniramine Maleate, Pseudoephedrine Hydrochloride) Adams 453

Benadryl Allergy (Diphenhydramine Hydrochloride) WARNER WELLCOME.. ⊞ 848

Benadryl Dye-Free Allergy Liquid Medication (Diphenhydramine Hydrochloride) WARNER WELLCOME.. ⊞ 850

Benylin Multisymptom (Dextromethorphan Hydrobromide, Pseudoephedrine Hydrochloride, Guaifenesin) WARNER WELLCOME.. ⊞ 852

Bromfed-DM Cough Syrup (Brompheniramine Maleate, Pseudoephedrine Hydrochloride, Dextromethorphan Hydrobromide) Muro 1786

Children's Vicks DayQuil Allergy Relief (Chlorpheniramine Maleate, Pseudoephedrine Hydrochloride) Procter & Gamble .... ⊞ 757

Children's Vicks NyQuil Cold/Cough Relief (Chlorpheniramine Maleate, Dextromethorphan Hydrobromide, Pseudoephedrine Hydrochloride) Procter & Gamble.............................. ⊞ 758

Comtrex Non-Drowsy (Acetaminophen, Dextromethorphan Hydrobromide, Pseudoephedrine Hydrochloride) Bristol-Myers Products.................. ⊞ 618

Contac Day & Night (Acetaminophen, Pseudoephedrine Hydrochloride, Dextromethorphan Hydrobromide) SmithKline Beecham Consumer ⊞ 812

Contac Severe Cold and Flu Formula Caplets (Acetaminophen, Chlorpheniramine Maleate, Dextromethorphan Hydrobromide, Phenylpropanolamine Hydrochloride) SmithKline Beecham Consumer ⊞ 814

Contac Severe Cold & Flu Non-Drowsy (Acetaminophen, Dextromethorphan Hydrobromide, Pseudoephedrine Hydrochloride) SmithKline Beecham Consumer........................ ⊞ 815

Deconsal C Expectorant Syrup (Codeine Phosphate, Pseudoephedrine Hydrochloride, Guaifenesin) Adams 456

Deconsal Pediatric Syrup (Codeine Phosphate, Pseudoephedrine Hydrochloride, Guaifenesin) Adams 457

Dimetapp Cold & Allergy Chewable Tablets (Brompheniramine Maleate, Phenylpropanolamine Hydrochloride) A. H. Robins Consumer .... ⊞ 773

Dimetapp Sinus Caplets (Ibuprofen, Pseudoephedrine Hydrochloride) A. H. Robins Consumer... ⊞ 775

Dorcol Children's Cough Syrup (Pseudoephedrine Hydrochloride, Guaifenesin, Dextromethorphan Hydrobromide) Sandoz Consumer... ⊞ 785

Drixoral Cold and Flu Extended-Release Tablets (Acetaminophen, Dexbrompheniramine Maleate, Pseudoephedrine Sulfate) Schering-Plough HealthCare.. ⊞ 803

Drixoral Cough + Sore Throat Liquid Caps (Dextromethorphan Hydrobromide, Acetaminophen) Schering-Plough HealthCare ...... ⊞ 802

Duratuss HD Elixir (Hydrocodone Bitartrate, Pseudoephedrine Hydrochloride, Guaifenesin) UCB 2565

Empirin Aspirin Tablets (Aspirin) WARNER WELLCOME...................... ⊞ 854

Entex PSE Tablets (Pseudoephedrine Hydrochloride, Guaifenesin) Procter & Gamble Pharmaceuticals 1987

Excedrin Extra-Strength Analgesic Tablets & Caplets (Acetaminophen, Aspirin, Caffeine) Bristol-Myers Products 732

Exgest LA Tablets (Phenylpropanolamine Hydrochloride, Guaifenesin) Carnrick......................... 782

Extendryl (Chlorpheniramine Maleate, Methscopolamine Nitrate, Phenylephrine Hydrochloride) Fleming.. 1005

Fedahist Gyrocaps (Pseudoephedrine Hydrochloride, Chlorpheniramine Maleate) Schwarz 2401

Fedahist Timecaps (Pseudoephedrine Hydrochloride, Chlorpheniramine Maleate) Schwarz 2401

Haltran Tablets (Ibuprofen) Roberts .... ⊞ 771

Kronofed-A (Chlorpheniramine Maleate, Pseudoephedrine Hydrochloride) Ferndale 977

Motrin IB Sinus (Ibuprofen, Pseudoephedrine Hydrochloride) Upjohn .... ⊞ 838

Novahistine DMX (Dextromethorphan Hydrobromide, Guaifenesin, Pseudoephedrine Hydrochloride) SmithKline Beecham Consumer......................... ⊞ 822

Nucofed (Codeine Phosphate, Pseudoephedrine Hydrochloride, Guaifenesin) Roberts 2051

Ornade Spansule Capsules (Phenylpropanolamine Hydrochloride, Chlorpheniramine Maleate) SmithKline Beecham Pharmaceuticals 2502

Oscillococcinum (Homeopathic Medications) Boiron.......................... ⊞ 612

PediaCare NightRest Cough-Cold Liquid (Chlorpheniramine Maleate, Dextromethorphan Hydrobromide, Pseudoephedrine Hydrochloride) McNeil Consumer 1553

Pediatric Vicks 44m Cough & Cold Relief (Chlorpheniramine Maleate, Dextromethorphan Hydrobromide, Pseudoephedrine Hydrochloride) Procter & Gamble .... ⊞ 764

Phenergan with Codeine (Codeine Phosphate, Promethazine Hydrochloride) Wyeth-Ayerst 2777

Phenergan with Dextromethorphan (Promethazine Hydrochloride, Dextromethorphan Hydrobromide) Wyeth-Ayerst 2778

Phenergan VC (Promethazine Hydrochloride, Phenylephrine Hydrochloride) Wyeth-Ayerst 2779

Phenergan VC with Codeine (Codeine Phosphate, Promethazine Hydrochloride, Phenylephrine Hydrochloride) Wyeth-Ayerst 2781

Pyrroxate Caplets (Acetaminophen, Chlorpheniramine Maleate, Phenylpropanolamine Hydrochloride) Roberts .... ⊞ 772

Rondec-DM Oral Drops (Carbinoxamine Maleate, Pseudoephedrine Hydrochloride, Dextromethorphan Hydrobromide) Dura................ 954

Rondec-DM Syrup (Carbinoxamine Maleate, Pseudoephedrine Hydrochloride, Dextromethorphan Hydrobromide) Dura............................ 954

Ryna (Chlorpheniramine Maleate, Pseudoephedrine Hydrochloride) Wallace .... ⊞ 841

Rynatan-S Pediatric Suspension (Phenylephrine Tannate, Chlorpheniramine Tannate, Pyrilamine Tannate) Wallace 2673

Sinarest Extra Strength Tablets (Acetaminophen, Chlorpheniramine Maleate, Pseudoephedrine Hydrochloride) CIBA Consumer ⊞ 648

Sine-Aid IB Caplets (Ibuprofen, Pseudoephedrine Hydrochloride) McNeil Consumer................................ 1554

Sinutab Sinus Medication, Regular Strength Without Drowsiness Formula (Acetaminophen, Pseudoephedrine Hydrochloride) WARNER WELLCOME.. ⊞ 859

Sudafed Cold and Cough Liquidcaps (Acetaminophen, Dextromethorphan Hydrobromide, Guaifenesin, Pseudoephedrine Hydrochloride) WARNER WELLCOME...................... ⊞ 862

Sudafed Severe Cold Formula Caplets (Acetaminophen, Dextromethorphan Hydrobromide, Pseudoephedrine Hydrochloride) WARNER WELLCOME.. ⊞ 863

Sudafed Severe Cold Formula Tablets (Acetaminophen, Dextromethorphan Hydrobromide, Pseudoephedrine Hydrochloride) WARNER WELLCOME.. ⊞ 864

Teldrin 12 Hour Antihistamine/Nasal Decongestant Allergy Relief Capsules (Chlorpheniramine Maleate, Phenylpropanolamine Hydrochloride) SmithKline Beecham Consumer......................... ⊞ 826

TheraFlu Flu and Cold Medicine (Acetaminophen, Chlorpheniramine Maleate, Pseudoephedrine Hydrochloride) Sandoz Consumer... ⊞ 787

TheraFlu Maximum Strength Nighttime Flu, Cold & Cough Medicine (Acetaminophen, Dextromethorphan Hydrobromide, Pseudoephedrine Hydrochloride, Chlorpheniramine Maleate) Sandoz Consumer .... ⊞ 788

TheraFlu Maximum Strength Non-Drowsy Formula Flu, Cold & Cough Medicine (Acetaminophen, Dextromethorphan Hydrobromide, Pseudoephedrine Hydrochloride) Sandoz Consumer............................ ⊞ 788

Thera Flu Maximum Strength, Non-Drowsy Formula Flu, Cold and Cough Caplets (Acetaminophen, Dextromethorphan Hydrobromide, Pseudoephedrine Hydrochloride) Sandoz Consumer............................... ⊞ 789

Triaminic Expectorant (Phenylpropanolamine Hydrochloride, Guaifenesin) Sandoz Consumer ⊞ 790

Triaminic Sore Throat Formula (Acetaminophen, Dextromethorphan Hydrobromide, Pseudoephedrine Hydrochloride) Sandoz Consumer............................... ⊞ 791

Triaminicol Multi-Symptom Relief (Phenylpropanolamine Hydrochloride, Chlorpheniramine Maleate, Dextromethorphan Hydrobromide) Sandoz Consumer... ⊞ 794

Trinalin Repetabs Tablets (Azatadine Maleate, Pseudoephedrine Sulfate) Key 1330

Tussionex Pennkinetic Extended-Release Suspension (Hydrocodone Polistirex, Chlorpheniramine Polistirex) Fisons 998

Children's TYLENOL acetaminophen Chewable Tablets, Elixir, Suspension Liquid (Acetaminophen) McNeil Consumer 1555

TYLENOL Extended Relief Caplets (Acetaminophen) McNeil Consumer 1558

TYLENOL Maximum Strength Allergy Sinus NightTime Medication Caplets (Acetaminophen, Pseudoephedrine Hydrochloride, Diphenhydramine Hydrochloride) McNeil Consumer 1555

TYLENOL Flu Maximum Strength Gelcaps (Acetaminophen, Dextromethorphan Hydrobromide, Pseudoephedrine Hydrochloride) McNeil Consumer................................ 1565

TYLENOL Flu NightTime, Maximum Strength, Gelcaps (Acetaminophen, Pseudoephedrine Hydrochloride, Diphenhydramine Hydrochloride) McNeil Consumer 1566

TYLENOL Maximum Strength Flu NightTime Hot Medication Packets (Acetaminophen, Dextromethorphan Hydrobromide, Pseudoephedrine Hydrochloride) McNeil Consumer................................ 1562

TYLENOL Cold Multi-Symptom Formula Medication Tablets and Caplets (Acetaminophen, Chlorpheniramine Maleate, Pseudoephedrine Hydrochloride, Dextromethorphan Hydrobromide) McNeil Consumer................................ 1561

TYLENOL Cold Medication No Drowsiness Formula Gelcaps and Caplets (Acetaminophen, Pseudoephedrine Hydrochloride, Dextromethorphan Hydrobromide) McNeil Consumer 1562

TYLENOL Cold Multi-Symptom Hot Medication Liquid Packets (Acetaminophen, Chlorpheniramine Maleate, Pseudoephedrine Hydrochloride, Dextromethorphan Hydrobromide) McNeil Consumer 1557

Vicks 44 LiquiCaps Cough, Cold & Flu Relief (Dextromethorphan Hydrobromide, Pseudoephedrine Hydrochloride, Chlorpheniramine Maleate, Acetaminophen) Procter & Gamble .... ⊞ 755

Vicks 44M Cough, Cold & Flu Relief (Acetaminophen, Dextromethorphan Hydrobromide, Chlorpheniramine Maleate, Pseudoephedrine Hydrochloride) Procter & Gamble .... ⊞ 756

Vicks DayQuil Allergy Relief 12-Hour Extended Release Tablets (Phenylpropanolamine Hydrochloride, Brompheniramine Maleate) Procter & Gamble .... ⊞ 760

Vicks DayQuil Allergy Relief 4-Hour Tablets (Phenylpropa-

(⊞ Described in PDR For Nonprescription Drugs) (◉ Described in PDR For Ophthalmology)

1501 **Indications Index** **K. pneumoniae infections**

nolamine Hydrochloride, Brompheniramine Maleate) Procter & Gamble ■ 760
Vicks DayQuil (Acetaminophen, Dextromethorphan Hydrobromide, Pseudoephedrine Hydrochloride, Guaifenesin) Procter & Gamble ■ 761
Vicks DayQuil SINUS Pressure & PAIN Relief with IBUPROFEN (Ibuprofen, Pseudoephedrine Hydrochloride) Procter & Gamble ■ 762
Vicks Nyquil Hot Therapy (Acetaminophen, Pseudoephedrine Hydrochloride, Dextromethorphan Hydrobromide, Doxylamine Succinate) Procter & Gamble ■ 762
Vicks NyQuil LiquiCaps Multi-Symptom Cold/Flu Relief (Acetaminophen, Pseudoephedrine Hydrochloride, Dextromethorphan Hydrobromide, Doxylamine Succinate) Procter & Gamble ■ 763
Vicks NyQuil Multi-Symptom Cold/Flu Relief - (Original & Cherry Flavor) (Acetaminophen, Dextromethorphan Hydrobromide, Doxylamine Succinate, Pseudoephedrine Hydrochloride) Procter & Gamble ■ 763

Insect bites, pain due to
(see under Pain, topical relief of)

Insomnia
(see under Sleep, induction of)

Intermittent claudication
(see under Claudication, intermittent)

Intertrigo
(see under Skin, inflammatory conditions)

Intracranial pressure, elevation
(see under Hypertension, cerebral, in neurosurgery)

Intraocular pressure elevation
(see under Hypertension, ocular)

Intravascular device, maintenance of patency
Abbokinase (Urokinase) Abbott 403
Abbokinase Open-Cath (Urokinase) Abbott 405
Heparin Lock Flush Solution (Heparin Sodium) Wyeth-Ayerst 2725

Intubation, endotracheal
Anectine (Succinylcholine Chloride) Glaxo Wellcome 1073
Mivacron (Mivacurium Chloride) Glaxo Wellcome 1138
Norcuron (Vecuronium Bromide) Organon 1826
Nuromax Injection (Doxacurium Chloride) Glaxo Wellcome 1149
Tracrium Injection (Atracurium Besylate) Glaxo Wellcome 1183
Zemuron (Rocuronium Bromide) Organon 1830

Intubation, small bowel
Reglan (Metoclopramide Hydrochloride) Robins 2068

Iridectomy, post-, adjunct
Floropryl Sterile Ophthalmic Ointment (Isoflurophate) Merck & Co., Inc. 1662
Humorsol Sterile Ophthalmic Solution (Demecarium Bromide) Merck & Co., Inc. 1664

Iridocyclitis
Aristocort Suspension (Forte Parenteral) (Triamcinolone Diacetate) Fujisawa 1027
Aristocort Tablets (Triamcinolone) Fujisawa 1022
Celestone Soluspan Suspension (Betamethasone Sodium Phosphate, Betamethasone Acetate) Schering 2347
Cortone Acetate Sterile Suspension (Cortisone Acetate) Merck & Co., Inc. 1623
Cortone Acetate Tablets (Cortisone Acetate) Merck & Co., Inc. 1624
Dalalone D.P. Injectable (Dexamethasone Acetate) Forest 1011
Decadron Elixir (Dexamethasone) Merck & Co., Inc. 1633
Decadron Phosphate Injection (Dexamethasone Sodium Phosphate) Merck & Co., Inc. 1637
Decadron Tablets (Dexamethasone) Merck & Co., Inc. 1635
Decadron-LA Sterile Suspension (Dexamethasone Acetate) Merck & Co., Inc. 1646
Deltasone Tablets (Prednisone) Upjohn 2595
Depo-Medrol Single-Dose Vial (Methylprednisolone Acetate) Upjohn 2600
Depo-Medrol Sterile Aqueous Suspension (Methylprednisolone Acetate) Upjohn 2597
Hydeltrasol Injection, Sterile (Prednisolone Sodium Phosphate) Merck & Co., Inc. 1665
Hydrocortone Phosphate Injection, Sterile (Hydrocortisone Sodium Phosphate) Merck & Co., Inc. 1670
Hydrocortone Tablets (Hydrocortisone) Merck & Co., Inc. 1672
Medrol (Methylprednisolone) Upjohn 2621
Pediapred Oral Liquid (Prednisolone Sodium Phosphate) Fisons 995
Prelone Syrup (Prednisolone) Muro 1787
Solu-Cortef Sterile Powder (Hydrocortisone Sodium Succinate) Upjohn 2641
Solu-Medrol Sterile Powder (Methylprednisolone Sodium Succinate) Upjohn 2643

Iritis
AK-Pred (Prednisolone Sodium Phosphate) Akorn ⊙ 204
Aristocort Suspension (Forte Parenteral) (Triamcinolone Diacetate) Fujisawa 1027
Aristocort Tablets (Triamcinolone) Fujisawa 1022
Celestone Soluspan Suspension (Betamethasone Sodium Phosphate, Betamethasone Acetate) Schering 2347
Cortone Acetate Sterile Suspension (Cortisone Acetate) Merck & Co., Inc. 1623
Cortone Acetate Tablets (Cortisone Acetate) Merck & Co., Inc. 1624
Dalalone D.P. Injectable (Dexamethasone Acetate) Forest 1011
Decadron Elixir (Dexamethasone) Merck & Co., Inc. 1633
Decadron Phosphate Injection (Dexamethasone Sodium Phosphate) Merck & Co., Inc. 1637
Decadron Phosphate Sterile Ophthalmic Ointment (Dexamethasone Sodium Phosphate) Merck & Co., Inc. 1641
Decadron Phosphate Sterile Ophthalmic Solution (Dexamethasone Sodium Phosphate) Merck & Co., Inc. 1642
Decadron Tablets (Dexamethasone) Merck & Co., Inc. 1635
Decadron-LA Sterile Suspension (Dexamethasone Acetate) Merck & Co., Inc. 1646
Deltasone Tablets (Prednisone) Upjohn 2595
Depo-Medrol Single-Dose Vial (Methylprednisolone Acetate) Upjohn 2600
Depo-Medrol Sterile Aqueous Suspension (Methylprednisolone Acetate) Upjohn 2597
Econopred & Econopred Plus Ophthalmic Suspensions (Prednisolone Acetate) Alcon Laboratories ⊙ 217
Hydeltrasol Injection, Sterile (Prednisolone Sodium Phosphate) Merck & Co., Inc. 1665
Hydrocortone Phosphate Injection, Sterile (Hydrocortisone Sodium Phosphate) Merck & Co., Inc. 1670
Hydrocortone Tablets (Hydrocortisone) Merck & Co., Inc. 1672
Inflamase (Prednisolone Sodium Phosphate) CIBA Vision Ophthalmics ⊙ 265
Medrol (Methylprednisolone) Upjohn 2621
Pediapred Oral Liquid (Prednisolone Sodium Phosphate) Fisons 995
Prelone Syrup (Prednisolone) Muro 1787
Solu-Cortef Sterile Powder (Hydrocortisone Sodium Succinate) Upjohn 2641
Solu-Medrol Sterile Powder (Methylprednisolone Sodium Succinate) Upjohn 2643

Iron deficiency
Feosol Capsules (Ferrous Sulfate) SmithKline Beecham 2456
Feosol Elixir (Ferrous Sulfate) SmithKline Beecham 2456
Feosol Tablets (Ferrous Sulfate) SmithKline Beecham 2457
Fergon Iron Supplement Tablets (Ferrous Gluconate) Miles Consumer ■ 721
Fero-Folic-500 Filmtab (Ferrous Sulfate, Folic Acid, Vitamin C) Abbott 429
Fero-Grad-500 Filmtab (Ferrous Sulfate, Vitamin C) Abbott 429
Fero-Gradumet Filmtab (Ferrous Sulfate) Abbott 429
Ferro-Sequels (Ferrous Fumarate, Docusate Sodium) Lederle Consumer ■ 669
Iberet Tablets (Vitamin B Complex With Vitamin C, Ferrous Sulfate) Abbott 433
Iberet-500 Liquid (Vitamin B Complex With Vitamin C, Ferrous Sulfate) Abbott 433
Iberet-Folic-500 Filmtab (Vitamin B Complex With Vitamin C, Ferrous Sulfate) Abbott 429
Iberet-Liquid (Vitamin B Complex With Vitamin C, Ferrous Sulfate) Abbott 433
INFeD (Iron Dextran Injection, USP) (Iron Dextran) Schein 2345
Irospan (Ferrous Sulfate, Vitamin C) Fielding 982
Nephro-Fer Tablets (Ferrous Fumarate) R&D 2004
Nephro-Fer Rx Tablets (Ferrous Fumarate, Folic Acid) R&D 2005
Niferex-150 Forte Capsules (Polysaccharide-Iron Complex, Folic Acid, Cyanocobalamin) Central 794
Niferex Forte Elixir (Polysaccharide-Iron Complex) Central 794
Slow Fe Tablets (Ferrous Sulfate) Ciba Self-Medication 869

Iron intoxication, acute
Desferal Vials (Deferoxamine Mesylate) CibaGeneva 820

Iron overload, chronic
Desferal Vials (Deferoxamine Mesylate) CibaGeneva 820

Irritable bowel syndrome
(see under Bowel, irritable, syndrome)

Ischemic attacks, recurrent transient, in men
Regular Strength Ascriptin Tablets (Aspirin Buffered, Calcium Carbonate) CIBA Consumer ■ 629
Genuine Bayer Aspirin Tablets & Caplets (Aspirin) Miles Consumer ■ 713
Bayer Enteric Aspirin (Aspirin, Enteric Coated) Miles Consumer ■ 709
Bufferin Analgesic Tablets and Caplets (Aspirin) Bristol-Myers Products ■ 613
Ecotrin (Aspirin, Enteric Coated) SmithKline Beecham 2455

Isoimmunization, prevention of in Rho(D) negative individuals
HypRho-D Full Dose Rho (D) Immune Globulin (Human) (Immune Globulin (Human)) Bayer Biological 629
Mini-Gamulin Rh, $Rh_O(D)$ Immune Globulin (Human) ($Rh_O(D)$ Immune Globulin (Human)) Armour 520

Isoimmunization, prevention of in Rho(D) negative women
HypRho-D Mini-Dose Rho (D) Immune Globulin (Human) (Immune Globulin (Human)) Bayer Biological 628
MICRhoGAM $Rh_O(D)$ Immune Globulin (Human) (Immune Globulin (Human)) Ortho Diagnostic 1847
Mini-Gamulin Rh, $Rh_O(D)$ Immune Globulin (Human) ($Rh_O(D)$ Immune Globulin (Human)) Armour 520
RhoGAM $Rh_O(D)$ Immune Globulin (Human) (Immune Globulin (Human)) Ortho Diagnostic 1847
WinRho SD (Immune Globulin Intravenous (Human)) Univax 2576

Itching, skin
(see under Pruritus, topical relief of)

Itching, sunburn
(see under Pruritus, topical relief of)

J

Jock itch
(see under Tinea cruris infections)

Joint pain
(see under Pain, arthritic, minor)

K

K. pneumoniae bacteremia
Polymyxin B Sulfate, Aerosporin Brand Sterile Powder (Polymyxin B Sulfate) Glaxo Wellcome 1154
Rocephin Injectable Vials, ADD-Vantage, Galaxy Container (Ceftriaxone Sodium) Roche Laboratories 2142

K. pneumoniae bone and joint infections
Rocephin Injectable Vials, ADD-Vantage, Galaxy Container (Ceftriaxone Sodium) Roche Laboratories 2142

K. pneumoniae central nervous system infections
Claforan Sterile and Injection (Cefotaxime Sodium) Hoechst-Roussel 1235

K. pneumoniae genitourinary tract infections
Keflex Pulvules & Oral Suspension (Cephalexin) Dista 914

K. pneumoniae gynecologic infections
Azactam for Injection (Aztreonam) Bristol-Myers Squibb 734
Primaxin I.M. (Imipenem-Cilastatin Sodium) Merck & Co., Inc. 1727
Timentin for Injection (Ticarcillin Disodium, Clavulanate Potassium) SmithKline Beecham Pharmaceuticals 2528

K. pneumoniae infections
Azactam for Injection (Aztreonam) Bristol-Myers Squibb 734
Cefobid Intravenous/Intramuscular (Cefoperazone Sodium) Roerig 2189
Cefobid Pharmacy Bulk Package - Not for Direct Infusion (Cefoperazone Sodium) Roerig 2192
Cefotan (Cefotetan) Zeneca 2829
Ceftin Tablets (Cefuroxime Axetil) Glaxo Wellcome 1078
Cipro I.V. (Ciprofloxacin) Bayer Pharmaceutical 595

(■ Described in PDR For Nonprescription Drugs) (⊙ Described in PDR For Ophthalmology)

Cipro I.V. Pharmacy Bulk Package (Ciprofloxacin) Bayer Pharmaceutical ... 597
Cipro Tablets (Ciprofloxacin Hydrochloride) Bayer Pharmaceutical ... 592
Claforan Sterile and Injection (Cefotaxime Sodium) Hoechst-Roussel ... 1235
Coly-Mycin M Parenteral (Colistimethate Sodium) Parke-Davis ... 1905
Floxin I.V. (Ofloxacin) McNeil Pharmaceutical ... 1571
Floxin Tablets (200 mg, 300 mg, 400 mg) (Ofloxacin) McNeil Pharmaceutical ... 1567
Keflex Pulvules & Oral Suspension (Cephalexin) Dista ... 914
Maxaquin Tablets (Lomefloxacin Hydrochloride) Searle ... 2440
Mezlin (Mezlocillin Sodium) Bayer Pharmaceutical ... 601
Mezlin Pharmacy Bulk Package (Mezlocillin Sodium) Bayer Pharmaceutical ... 604
Monocid Injection (Cefonicid Sodium) SmithKline Beecham Pharmaceuticals ... 2497
Netromycin Injection 100 mg/ml (Netilmicin Sulfate) Schering ... 2373
Noroxin Tablets (Norfloxacin) Merck & Co., Inc. ... 1715
Noroxin Tablets (Norfloxacin) Roberts ... 2048
Penetrex Tablets (Enoxacin) Rhone-Poulenc Rorer Pharmaceuticals ... 2031
Polymyxin B Sulfate, Aerosporin Brand Sterile Powder (Polymyxin B Sulfate) Glaxo Wellcome ... 1154
Primaxin I.M. (Imipenem-Cilastatin Sodium) Merck & Co., Inc. ... 1727
Proloprim Tablets (Trimethoprim) Glaxo Wellcome ... 1155
Rocephin Injectable Vials, ADD-Vantage, Galaxy Container (Ceftriaxone Sodium) Roche Laboratories ... 2142
Suprax for Oral Suspension (Cefixime) Lederle ... 1399
Timentin for Injection (Ticarcillin Disodium, Clavulanate Potassium) SmithKline Beecham Pharmaceuticals ... 2528
Trimpex Tablets (Trimethoprim) Roche Laboratories ... 2163
Unasyn (Ampicillin Sodium, Sulbactam Sodium) Roerig ... 2212
Vantin for Oral Suspension and Vantin Tablets (Cefpodoxime Proxetil) Upjohn ... 2646
Zefazone (Cefmetazole Sodium) Upjohn ... 2654

K. pneumoniae infections, ocular

Genoptic Sterile Ophthalmic Solution (Gentamicin Sulfate) Allergan ... ⊙ 243
Genoptic Sterile Ophthalmic Ointment (Gentamicin Sulfate) Allergan ... ⊙ 243
Gentak (Gentamicin Sulfate) Akorn ... ⊙ 208
Pred-G S.O.P. Sterile Ophthalmic Ointment (Gentamicin Sulfate, Prednisolone Acetate) Allergan ... ⊙ 252

K. pneumoniae intra-abdominal infections

Azactam for Injection (Aztreonam) Bristol-Myers Squibb ... 734
Cefotan (Cefotetan) Zeneca ... 2829
Netromycin Injection 100 mg/ml (Netilmicin Sulfate) Schering ... 2373
Primaxin I.M. (Imipenem-Cilastatin Sodium) Merck & Co., Inc. ... 1727
Rocephin Injectable Vials, ADD-Vantage, Galaxy Container (Ceftriaxone Sodium) Roche Laboratories ... 2142
Timentin for Injection (Ticarcillin Disodium, Clavulanate Potassium) SmithKline Beecham Pharmaceuticals ... 2528
Unasyn (Ampicillin Sodium, Sulbactam Sodium) Roerig ... 2212
Zefazone (Cefmetazole Sodium) Upjohn ... 2654

K. pneumoniae lower respiratory tract infections

Azactam for Injection (Aztreonam) Bristol-Myers Squibb ... 734
Cefotan (Cefotetan) Zeneca ... 2829
Cipro I.V. (Ciprofloxacin) Bayer Pharmaceutical ... 595
Cipro I.V. Pharmacy Bulk Package (Ciprofloxacin) Bayer Pharmaceutical ... 597
Cipro Tablets (Ciprofloxacin Hydrochloride) Bayer Pharmaceutical ... 592
Mezlin (Mezlocillin Sodium) Bayer Pharmaceutical ... 601
Mezlin Pharmacy Bulk Package (Mezlocillin Sodium) Bayer Pharmaceutical ... 604
Monocid Injection (Cefonicid Sodium) SmithKline Beecham Pharmaceuticals ... 2497
Netromycin Injection 100 mg/ml (Netilmicin Sulfate) Schering ... 2373
Rocephin Injectable Vials, ADD-Vantage, Galaxy Container (Ceftriaxone Sodium) Roche Laboratories ... 2142

K. pneumoniae pneumonia, treatment, adjunct

Streptomycin Sulfate Injection (Streptomycin Sulfate) Roerig ... 2208

K. pneumoniae prostatitis

Keflex Pulvules & Oral Suspension (Cephalexin) Dista ... 914

K. pneumoniae respiratory tract infections

Cefobid Intravenous/Intramuscular (Cefoperazone Sodium) Roerig ... 2189
Cefobid Pharmacy Bulk Package - Not for Direct Infusion (Cefoperazone Sodium) Roerig ... 2192

K. pneumoniae septicemia

Azactam for Injection (Aztreonam) Bristol-Myers Squibb ... 734
Cefobid Intravenous/Intramuscular (Cefoperazone Sodium) Roerig ... 2189
Cefobid Pharmacy Bulk Package - Not for Direct Infusion (Cefoperazone Sodium) Roerig ... 2192
Netromycin Injection 100 mg/ml (Netilmicin Sulfate) Schering ... 2373
Rocephin Injectable Vials, ADD-Vantage, Galaxy Container (Ceftriaxone Sodium) Roche Laboratories ... 2142

K. pneumoniae skin and skin structure infections

Azactam for Injection (Aztreonam) Bristol-Myers Squibb ... 734
Cefotan (Cefotetan) Zeneca ... 2829
Cipro I.V. (Ciprofloxacin) Bayer Pharmaceutical ... 595
Cipro I.V. Pharmacy Bulk Package (Ciprofloxacin) Bayer Pharmaceutical ... 597
Cipro Tablets (Ciprofloxacin Hydrochloride) Bayer Pharmaceutical ... 592
Netromycin Injection 100 mg/ml (Netilmicin Sulfate) Schering ... 2373
Primaxin I.M. (Imipenem-Cilastatin Sodium) Merck & Co., Inc. ... 1727
Rocephin Injectable Vials, ADD-Vantage, Galaxy Container (Ceftriaxone Sodium) Roche Laboratories ... 2142
Unasyn (Ampicillin Sodium, Sulbactam Sodium) Roerig ... 2212
Zefazone (Cefmetazole Sodium) Upjohn ... 2654

K. pneumoniae urinary tract infections

Azactam for Injection (Aztreonam) Bristol-Myers Squibb ... 734
Cefotan (Cefotetan) Zeneca ... 2829
Ceftin Tablets (Cefuroxime Axetil) Glaxo Wellcome ... 1078
Cipro I.V. (Ciprofloxacin) Bayer Pharmaceutical ... 595
Cipro I.V. Pharmacy Bulk Package (Ciprofloxacin) Bayer Pharmaceutical ... 597
Cipro Tablets (Ciprofloxacin Hydrochloride) Bayer Pharmaceutical ... 592
Floxin I.V. (Ofloxacin) McNeil Pharmaceutical ... 1571
Floxin Tablets (200 mg, 300 mg, 400 mg) (Ofloxacin) McNeil Pharmaceutical ... 1567
Maxaquin Tablets (Lomefloxacin Hydrochloride) Searle ... 2440
Monocid Injection (Cefonicid Sodium) SmithKline Beecham Pharmaceuticals ... 2497
Netromycin Injection 100 mg/ml (Netilmicin Sulfate) Schering ... 2373
Noroxin Tablets (Norfloxacin) Merck & Co., Inc. ... 1715
Noroxin Tablets (Norfloxacin) Roberts ... 2048
Penetrex Tablets (Enoxacin) Rhone-Poulenc Rorer Pharmaceuticals ... 2031
Proloprim Tablets (Trimethoprim) Glaxo Wellcome ... 1155
Rocephin Injectable Vials, ADD-Vantage, Galaxy Container (Ceftriaxone Sodium) Roche Laboratories ... 2142
Streptomycin Sulfate Injection (Streptomycin Sulfate) Roerig ... 2208
Trimpex Tablets (Trimethoprim) Roche Laboratories ... 2163
Vantin for Oral Suspension and Vantin Tablets (Cefpodoxime Proxetil) Upjohn ... 2646

Kaposi's sarcoma

Velban Vials (Vinblastine Sulfate) Lilly ... 1484

Kaposi's sarcoma, AIDS-related

Intron A (Interferon alfa-2B, Recombinant) Schering ... 2364
Roferon-A Injection (Interferon alfa-2A, Recombinant) Roche Laboratories ... 2145

Keloids

Aristocort Suspension (Forte Parenteral) (Triamcinolone Diacetate) Fujisawa ... 1027
Aristocort Suspension (Intralesional) (Triamcinolone Diacetate) Fujisawa ... 1025
Aristospan Suspension (Intralesional) (Triamcinolone Hexacetonide) Fujisawa ... 1032
Celestone Soluspan Suspension (Betamethasone Sodium Phosphate, Betamethasone Acetate) Schering ... 2347
Decadron Phosphate Injection (Dexamethasone Sodium Phosphate) Merck & Co., Inc. ... 1637
Decadron-LA Sterile Suspension (Dexamethasone Acetate) Merck & Co., Inc. ... 1646
Depo-Medrol Single-Dose Vial (Methylprednisolone Acetate) Upjohn ... 2600
Depo-Medrol Sterile Aqueous Suspension (Methylprednisolone Acetate) Upjohn ... 2597
Hydeltrasol Injection, Sterile (Prednisolone Sodium Phosphate) Merck & Co., Inc. ... 1665
Hydrocortone Acetate Sterile Suspension (Hydrocortisone Acetate) Merck & Co., Inc. ... 1669

Keratitis

Aristocort Suspension (Forte Parenteral) (Triamcinolone Diacetate) Fujisawa ... 1027
Aristocort Tablets (Triamcinolone) Fujisawa ... 1022
Celestone Soluspan Suspension (Betamethasone Sodium Phosphate, Betamethasone Acetate) Schering ... 2347
Cortone Acetate Sterile Suspension (Cortisone Acetate) Merck & Co., Inc. ... 1623
Cortone Acetate Tablets (Cortisone Acetate) Merck & Co., Inc. ... 1624
Decadron Elixir (Dexamethasone) Merck & Co., Inc. ... 1633
Decadron Phosphate Injection (Dexamethasone Sodium Phosphate) Merck & Co., Inc. ... 1637
Decadron Tablets (Dexamethasone) Merck & Co., Inc. ... 1635
Decadron-LA Sterile Suspension (Dexamethasone Acetate) Merck & Co., Inc. ... 1646
Deltasone Tablets (Prednisone) Upjohn ... 2595
Depo-Medrol Single-Dose Vial (Methylprednisolone Acetate) Upjohn ... 2600
Depo-Medrol Sterile Aqueous Suspension (Methylprednisolone Acetate) Upjohn ... 2597
Genoptic Sterile Ophthalmic Solution (Gentamicin Sulfate) Allergan ... ⊙ 243
Genoptic Sterile Ophthalmic Ointment (Gentamicin Sulfate) Allergan ... ⊙ 243
Gentacidin Ointment (Gentamicin Sulfate) CIBA Vision Ophthalmics ... ⊙ 264
Gentacidin Solution (Gentamicin Sulfate) CIBA Vision Ophthalmics ... ⊙ 264
Gentak (Gentamicin Sulfate) Akorn ... ⊙ 208
Hydeltrasol Injection, Sterile (Prednisolone Sodium Phosphate) Merck & Co., Inc. ... 1665
Hydrocortone Phosphate Injection, Sterile (Hydrocortisone Sodium Phosphate) Merck & Co., Inc. ... 1670
Hydrocortone Tablets (Hydrocortisone) Merck & Co., Inc. ... 1672
Medrol (Methylprednisolone) Upjohn ... 2621
Neosporin Ophthalmic Ointment Sterile (Polymyxin B Sulfate, Bacitracin Zinc, Neomycin Sulfate) Glaxo Wellcome ... 1148
Neosporin Ophthalmic Solution Sterile (Polymyxin B Sulfate, Neomycin Sulfate, Gramicidin) Glaxo Wellcome ... 1149
Pediapred Oral Liquid (Prednisolone Sodium Phosphate) Fisons ... 995
Polysporin Ophthalmic Ointment Sterile (Polymyxin B Sulfate, Bacitracin Zinc) Glaxo Wellcome ... 1154
Prelone Syrup (Prednisolone) Muro 1787
Solu-Cortef Sterile Powder (Hydrocortisone Sodium Succinate) Upjohn ... 2641
Solu-Medrol Sterile Powder (Methylprednisolone Sodium Succinate) Upjohn ... 2643

Keratitis sicca (see under Keratoconjunctivitis sicca)

Keratitis, bullous, diagnostic aid in

Ophthalgan (Glycerin) Wyeth-Ayerst ... ⊙ 326

Keratitis, dendritic

Vira-A Ophthalmic Ointment, 3% (Vidarabine) Parke-Davis ... ⊙ 312
Viroptic Ophthalmic Solution, 1% Sterile (Trifluridine) Glaxo Wellcome ... 1204

Keratitis, exposure

Lacrisert Sterile Ophthalmic Insert (Hydroxypropyl Cellulose) Merck & Co., Inc. ... 1686

Keratitis, fungal

Herplex Liquifilm (Idoxuridine) Allergan ... ⊙ 244
Natacyn Antifungal Ophthalmic Suspension (Natamycin) Alcon Laboratories ... ⊙ 225

Keratitis, Fusarium solani

Natacyn Antifungal Ophthalmic Suspension (Natamycin) Alcon Laboratories ... ⊙ 225

Keratitis, herpes zoster

AK-Pred (Prednisolone Sodium Phosphate) Akorn ... ⊙ 204
Decadron Phosphate Sterile Ophthalmic Ointment (Dexamethasone Sodium Phosphate) Merck & Co., Inc. ... 1641
Decadron Phosphate Sterile Ophthalmic Solution (Dexamethasone Sodium Phosphate) Merck & Co., Inc. ... 1642
Econopred & Econopred Plus Ophthalmic Suspensions (Prednisolone Acetate) Alcon Laboratories ... ⊙ 217

(▣ Described in PDR For Nonprescription Drugs) (⊙ Described in PDR For Ophthalmology)

1503 **Indications Index** **Klebsiella species**

Inflamase (Prednisolone Sodium Phosphate) CIBA Vision Ophthalmics ⊙ 265

Keratitis, punctate, superficial

AK-Pred (Prednisolone Sodium Phosphate) Akorn ⊙ 204
Decadron Phosphate Sterile Ophthalmic Ointment (Dexamethasone Sodium Phosphate) Merck & Co., Inc. 1641
Decadron Phosphate Sterile Ophthalmic Solution (Dexamethasone Sodium Phosphate) Merck & Co., Inc. 1642
Econopred & Econopred Plus Ophthalmic Suspensions (Prednisolone Acetate) Alcon Laboratories ⊙ 217
Inflamase (Prednisolone Sodium Phosphate) CIBA Vision Ophthalmics ⊙ 265

Keratitis, recurrent epithelial (see under Keratitis, dendritic)

Keratitis, vernal

Alomide (Lodoxamide Tromethamine) Alcon Laboratories 469
Crolom (Cromolyn Sodium) Bausch & Lomb Pharmaceuticals ⊙ 257

Keratoconjunctivitis sicca

Adsorbotear Artificial Tear (Povidone) Alcon Laboratories ⊙ 210
AquaSite Eye Drops (Polyethylene Glycol, Dextran 70) CIBA Vision Ophthalmics ⊙ 261
Bion Tears (Lubricant) Alcon Laboratories ⊙ 213
Celluvisc Lubricant Eye Drops (Carboxymethylcellulose Sodium) Allergan ⊙ 238
Clear Eyes ACR Astringent/Lubricant Eye Redness Reliever Eye Drops (Zinc Sulfate, Naphazoline Hydrochloride) Ross ⊙ 316
Collagen Plugs (Intracanalicular) (Collagen, bovine) Lacrimedics ⊙ 284
Collyrium Fresh (Tetrahydrozoline Hydrochloride, Glycerin) Wyeth-Ayerst ▣ 879
Herrick Lacrimal Plugs (Collagen) Lacrimedics ⊙ 285
HypoTears Lubricant Eye Drops (Polyvinyl Alcohol) CIBA Vision Ophthalmics ⊙ 265
HypoTears Ointment (Petrolatum, White) CIBA Vision Ophthalmics ⊙ 265
HypoTears PF Lubricant Eye Drops (Polyvinyl Alcohol) CIBA Vision Ophthalmics ⊙ 265
Lacrisert Sterile Ophthalmic Insert (Hydroxypropyl Cellulose) Merck & Co., Inc. 1686
Ocucoat and Ocucoat PF Eye Drops (Dextran 70, Hydroxypropyl Methylcellulose) Storz Ophthalmics ⊙ 322
Refresh Plus Cellufresh Formula Lubricant Eye Drops (Carboxymethylcellulose Sodium) Allergan ⊙ 254
Refresh PM Lubricant Eye Ointment (Petrolatum, White, Mineral Oil) Allergan ⊙ 254
Similasan Eye Drops #1 (Homeopathic Medications) Similasan ⊙ 317
Tears Naturale II (Dextran 70, Hydroxypropyl Methylcellulose) Alcon Laboratories 473
Viva-Drops (Polysorbate 80) Vision Pharmaceuticals ⊙ 325

Keratoconjunctivitis, acute

Vira-A Ophthalmic Ointment, 3% (Vidarabine) Parke-Davis ⊙ 312

Keratoconjunctivitis, primary

Viroptic Ophthalmic Solution, 1% Sterile (Trifluridine) Glaxo Wellcome 1204

Keratoconjunctivitis, unspecified

Genoptic Sterile Ophthalmic Solution (Gentamicin Sulfate) Allergan ⊙ 243
Genoptic Sterile Ophthalmic Ointment (Gentamicin Sulfate) Allergan ⊙ 243
Gentacidin Ointment (Gentamicin Sulfate) CIBA Vision Ophthalmics ⊙ 264
Gentacidin Solution (Gentamicin Sulfate) CIBA Vision Ophthalmics ⊙ 264
Gentak (Gentamicin Sulfate) Akorn ⊙ 208
Neosporin Ophthalmic Ointment Sterile (Polymyxin B Sulfate, Bacitracin Zinc, Neomycin Sulfate) Glaxo Wellcome 1148
Neosporin Ophthalmic Solution Sterile (Polymyxin B Sulfate, Neomycin Sulfate, Gramicidin) Glaxo Wellcome 1149
Polysporin Ophthalmic Ointment Sterile (Polymyxin B Sulfate, Bacitracin Zinc) Glaxo Wellcome 1154

Keratoconjunctivitis, vernal

Alomide (Lodoxamide Tromethamine) Alcon Laboratories 469
Crolom (Cromolyn Sodium) Bausch & Lomb Pharmaceuticals ⊙ 257

Keratosis palmaris (see under Hyperkeratosis skin disorders)

Keratosis pilaris (see under Hyperkeratosis skin disorders)

Keratosis plantaris (see under Hyperkeratosis skin disorders)

Keratosis, actinic

Efudex (Fluorouracil) Roche Laboratories 2113
Fluoroplex Topical Solution & Cream 1% (Fluorouracil) Allergan 479

Keratosis, solar

Efudex (Fluorouracil) Roche Laboratories 2113

Klebsiella oxytoca infections

Azactam for Injection (Aztreonam) Bristol-Myers Squibb 734
Rocephin Injectable Vials, ADD-Vantage, Galaxy Container (Ceftriaxone Sodium) Roche Laboratories 2142
Zefazone (Cefmetazole Sodium) Upjohn 2654

Klebsiella oxytoca intra-abdominal infections

Zefazone (Cefmetazole Sodium) Upjohn 2654

Klebsiella oxytoca skin and structure infections

Rocephin Injectable Vials, ADD-Vantage, Galaxy Container (Ceftriaxone Sodium) Roche Laboratories 2142
Zefazone (Cefmetazole Sodium) Upjohn 2654

Klebsiella pneumoniae infections (see under K. pneumoniae infections)

Klebsiella species bacteremia

Ceptaz (Ceftazidime) Glaxo Wellcome 1081

Klebsiella species biliary tract infections

Ancef Injection (Cefazolin Sodium) SmithKline Beecham Pharmaceuticals 2465
Kefzol Vials, Faspak & ADD-Vantage (Cefazolin Sodium) Lilly 1456

Klebsiella species bone and joint infections

Ceptaz (Ceftazidime) Glaxo Wellcome 1081
Fortaz (Ceftazidime) Glaxo Wellcome 1100
Nebcin Vials, Hyporets & ADD-Vantage (Tobramycin Sulfate) Lilly 1464
Tazicef for Injection (Ceftazidime) SmithKline Beecham Pharmaceuticals 2519
Tazidime Vials, Faspak & ADD-Vantage (Ceftazidime) Lilly 1478
Tobramycin Sulfate Injection (Tobramycin Sulfate) Elkins-Sinn 968

Klebsiella species genital tract infections

Ancef Injection (Cefazolin Sodium) SmithKline Beecham Pharmaceuticals 2465
Mefoxin (Cefoxitin Sodium) Merck & Co., Inc. 1691
Mefoxin Premixed Intravenous Solution (Cefoxitin Sodium) Merck & Co., Inc. 1694

Klebsiella species gynecologic infections

Claforan Sterile and Injection (Cefotaxime Sodium) Hoechst-Roussel 1235
Mezlin (Mezlocillin Sodium) Bayer Pharmaceutical 601
Mezlin Pharmacy Bulk Package (Mezlocillin Sodium) Bayer Pharmaceutical 604
Primaxin I.V. (Imipenem-Cilastatin Sodium) Merck & Co., Inc. 1729

Klebsiella species infections

Achromycin V Capsules (Tetracycline Hydrochloride) Lederle 1367
Amikacin Sulfate Injection, USP (Amikacin Sulfate) Elkins-Sinn 960
Amikin Injectable (Amikacin Sulfate) Apothecon 501
Ancef Injection (Cefazolin Sodium) SmithKline Beecham Pharmaceuticals 2465
Augmentin (Amoxicillin Trihydrate, Clavulanate Potassium) SmithKline Beecham Pharmaceuticals 2468
Azo Gantanol Tablets (Sulfamethoxazole, Phenazopyridine Hydrochloride) Roche Laboratories 2080
Azo Gantrisin Tablets (Sulfisoxazole, Phenazopyridine Hydrochloride) Roche Laboratories 2081
Bactrim DS Tablets (Trimethoprim, Sulfamethoxazole) Roche Laboratories 2084
Bactrim I.V. Infusion (Trimethoprim, Sulfamethoxazole) Roche Laboratories 2082
Bactrim (Trimethoprim, Sulfamethoxazole) Roche Laboratories 2084
Ceclor Pulvules & Suspension (Cefaclor) Lilly 1431
Cefizox for Intramuscular or Intravenous Use (Ceftizoxime Sodium) Fujisawa 1034
Cefobid Intravenous/Intramuscular (Cefoperazone Sodium) Roerig 2189
Cefobid Pharmacy Bulk Package - Not for Direct Infusion (Cefoperazone Sodium) Roerig 2192
Cefotan (Cefotetan) Zeneca 2829
Ceptaz (Ceftazidime) Glaxo Wellcome 1081
Claforan Sterile and Injection (Cefotaxime Sodium) Hoechst-Roussel 1235
Declomycin Tablets (Demeclocycline Hydrochloride) Lederle 1371
Doryx Capsules (Doxycycline Hyclate) Parke-Davis 1913
Duricef (Cefadroxil Monohydrate) Bristol-Myers Squibb 748
Dynacin Capsules (Minocycline Hydrochloride) Medicis 1590
Fortaz (Ceftazidime) Glaxo Wellcome 1100
Garamycin Injectable (Gentamicin Sulfate) Schering 2360
Kefurox Vials, Faspak & ADD-Vantage (Cefuroxime Sodium) Lilly 1454
Kefzol Vials, Faspak & ADD-Vantage (Cefazolin Sodium) Lilly 1456
Macrodantin Capsules (Nitrofurantoin) Procter & Gamble Pharmaceuticals 1989
Mefoxin (Cefoxitin Sodium) Merck & Co., Inc. 1691
Mefoxin Premixed Intravenous Solution (Cefoxitin Sodium) Merck & Co., Inc. 1694
Mezlin (Mezlocillin Sodium) Bayer Pharmaceutical 601
Mezlin Pharmacy Bulk Package (Mezlocillin Sodium) Bayer Pharmaceutical 604
Minocin Intravenous (Minocycline Hydrochloride) Lederle 1382
Minocin Oral Suspension (Minocycline Hydrochloride) Lederle 1385
Minocin Pellet-Filled Capsules (Minocycline Hydrochloride) Lederle 1383
Monodox Capsules (Doxycycline Monohydrate) Oclassen 1805
Nebcin Vials, Hyporets & ADD-Vantage (Tobramycin Sulfate) Lilly 1464
Pipracil (Piperacillin Sodium) Lederle 1390
Primaxin I.V. (Imipenem-Cilastatin Sodium) Merck & Co., Inc. 1729
Septra (Trimethoprim, Sulfamethoxazole) Glaxo Wellcome 1174
Septra I.V. Infusion (Trimethoprim, Sulfamethoxazole) Glaxo Wellcome 1169
Septra I.V. Infusion ADD-Vantage Vials (Trimethoprim, Sulfamethoxazole) Glaxo Wellcome 1171
Septra (Trimethoprim, Sulfamethoxazole) Glaxo Wellcome 1174
Tazicef for Injection (Ceftazidime) SmithKline Beecham Pharmaceuticals 2519
Tazidime Vials, Faspak & ADD-Vantage (Ceftazidime) Lilly 1478
Terramycin Intramuscular Solution (Oxytetracycline) Roerig 2210
Timentin for Injection (Ticarcillin Disodium, Clavulanate Potassium) SmithKline Beecham Pharmaceuticals 2528
Tobramycin Sulfate Injection (Tobramycin Sulfate) Elkins-Sinn 968
Unasyn (Ampicillin Sodium, Sulbactam Sodium) Roerig 2212
Vibramycin (Doxycycline Calcium) Pfizer Labs 1941
Vibramycin Hyclate Intravenous (Doxycycline Hyclate) Roerig 2215
Vibramycin (Doxycycline Monohydrate) Pfizer Labs 1941
Zinacef (Cefuroxime Sodium) Glaxo Wellcome 1211

Klebsiella species intra-abdominal infections

Azactam for Injection (Aztreonam) Bristol-Myers Squibb 734
Cefizox for Intramuscular or Intravenous Use (Ceftizoxime Sodium) Fujisawa 1034
Cefotan (Cefotetan) Zeneca 2829
Ceptaz (Ceftazidime) Glaxo Wellcome 1081
Claforan Sterile and Injection (Cefotaxime Sodium) Hoechst-Roussel 1235
Fortaz (Ceftazidime) Glaxo Wellcome 1100
Mefoxin (Cefoxitin Sodium) Merck & Co., Inc. 1691
Mefoxin Premixed Intravenous Solution (Cefoxitin Sodium) Merck & Co., Inc. 1694
Mezlin (Mezlocillin Sodium) Bayer Pharmaceutical 601
Mezlin Pharmacy Bulk Package (Mezlocillin Sodium) Bayer Pharmaceutical 604
Nebcin Vials, Hyporets & ADD-Vantage (Tobramycin Sulfate) Lilly 1464
Primaxin I.V. (Imipenem-Cilastatin Sodium) Merck & Co., Inc. 1729
Tazicef for Injection (Ceftazidime) SmithKline Beecham Pharmaceuticals 2519
Tazidime Vials, Faspak & ADD-Vantage (Ceftazidime) Lilly 1478

Klebsiella species | Indications Index | 1504

Tobramycin Sulfate Injection (Tobramycin Sulfate) Elkins-Sinn 968
Unasyn (Ampicillin Sodium, Sulbactam Sodium) Roerig 2212

Klebsiella species lower respiratory tract infections
Cefizox for Intramuscular or Intravenous Use (Ceftizoxime Sodium) Fujisawa 1034
Cefotan (Cefotetan) Zeneca 2829
Ceptaz (Ceftazidime) Glaxo Wellcome 1081
Claforan Sterile and Injection (Cefotaxime Sodium) Hoechst-Roussel 1235
Fortaz (Ceftazidime) Glaxo Wellcome 1100
Mandol Vials, Faspak & ADD-Vantage (Cefamandole Nafate) Lilly 1461
Mefoxin (Cefoxitin Sodium) Merck & Co., Inc. 1691
Mefoxin Premixed Intravenous Solution (Cefoxitin Sodium) Merck & Co., Inc. 1694
Mezlin (Mezlocillin Sodium) Bayer Pharmaceutical 601
Mezlin Pharmacy Bulk Package (Mezlocillin Sodium) Bayer Pharmaceutical 604
Nebcin Vials, Hyporets & ADD-Vantage (Tobramycin Sulfate) Lilly 1464
Pipracil (Piperacillin Sodium) Lederle 1390
Primaxin I.V. (Imipenem-Cilastatin Sodium) Merck & Co., Inc. 1729
Tazicef for Injection (Ceftazidime) SmithKline Beecham Pharmaceuticals 2519
Tazidime Vials, Faspak & ADD-Vantage (Ceftazidime) Lilly .. 1478
Timentin for Injection (Ticarcillin Disodium, Clavulanate Potassium) SmithKline Beecham Pharmaceuticals 2528
Tobramycin Sulfate Injection (Tobramycin Sulfate) Elkins-Sinn 968
Zinacef (Cefuroxime Sodium) Glaxo Wellcome 1211

Klebsiella species prostatitis
Ancef Injection (Cefazolin Sodium) SmithKline Beecham Pharmaceuticals 2465
Keftab Tablets (Cephalexin Hydrochloride) Dista 915

Klebsiella species respiratory tract infections
Achromycin V Capsules (Tetracycline Hydrochloride) Lederle 1367
Ancef Injection (Cefazolin Sodium) SmithKline Beecham Pharmaceuticals 2465
Ceptaz (Ceftazidime) Glaxo Wellcome 1081
Doryx Capsules (Doxycycline Hyclate) Parke-Davis 1913
Dynacin Capsules (Minocycline Hydrochloride) Medicis 1590
Kefzol Vials, Faspak & ADD-Vantage (Cefazolin Sodium) Lilly 1456
Minocin Intravenous (Minocycline Hydrochloride) Lederle 1382
Minocin Oral Suspension (Minocycline Hydrochloride) Lederle 1385
Minocin Pellet-Filled Capsules (Minocycline Hydrochloride) Lederle 1383
Monodox Capsules (Doxycycline Monohydrate) Oclassen 1805
Tazidime Vials, Faspak & ADD-Vantage (Ceftazidime) Lilly .. 1478
Terramycin Intramuscular Solution (Oxytetracycline) Roerig 2210
Vibramycin (Doxycycline Calcium) Pfizer Labs 1941
Vibramycin Hyclate Intravenous (Doxycycline Hyclate) Roerig 2215
Vibramycin (Doxycycline Monohydrate) Pfizer Labs 1941

Klebsiella species septicemia
Ancef Injection (Cefazolin Sodium) SmithKline Beecham Pharmaceuticals 2465
Cefizox for Intramuscular or Intravenous Use (Ceftizoxime Sodium) Fujisawa 1034
Ceptaz (Ceftazidime) Glaxo Wellcome 1081
Claforan Sterile and Injection (Cefotaxime Sodium) Hoechst-Roussel 1235
Fortaz (Ceftazidime) Glaxo Wellcome 1100
Kefurox Vials, Faspak & ADD-Vantage (Cefuroxime Sodium) Lilly 1454
Kefzol Vials, Faspak & ADD-Vantage (Cefazolin Sodium) Lilly 1456
Mefoxin (Cefoxitin Sodium) Merck & Co., Inc. 1691
Mefoxin Premixed Intravenous Solution (Cefoxitin Sodium) Merck & Co., Inc. 1694
Mezlin (Mezlocillin Sodium) Bayer Pharmaceutical 601
Mezlin Pharmacy Bulk Package (Mezlocillin Sodium) Bayer Pharmaceutical 604
Nebcin Vials, Hyporets & ADD-Vantage (Tobramycin Sulfate) Lilly 1464
Pipracil (Piperacillin Sodium) Lederle 1390
Primaxin I.V. (Imipenem-Cilastatin Sodium) Merck & Co., Inc. 1729
Tazicef for Injection (Ceftazidime) SmithKline Beecham Pharmaceuticals 2519
Tazidime Vials, Faspak & ADD-Vantage (Ceftazidime) Lilly .. 1478
Timentin for Injection (Ticarcillin Disodium, Clavulanate Potassium) SmithKline Beecham Pharmaceuticals 2528
Tobramycin Sulfate Injection (Tobramycin Sulfate) Elkins-Sinn 968
Zinacef (Cefuroxime Sodium) Glaxo Wellcome 1211

Klebsiella species skin and skin structure infections
Augmentin (Amoxicillin Trihydrate, Clavulanate Potassium) SmithKline Beecham Pharmaceuticals 2468
Cefizox for Intramuscular or Intravenous Use (Ceftizoxime Sodium) Fujisawa 1034
Ceptaz (Ceftazidime) Glaxo Wellcome 1081
Claforan Sterile and Injection (Cefotaxime Sodium) Hoechst-Roussel 1235
Fortaz (Ceftazidime) Glaxo Wellcome 1100
Kefurox Vials, Faspak & ADD-Vantage (Cefuroxime Sodium) Lilly 1454
Mefoxin (Cefoxitin Sodium) Merck & Co., Inc. 1691
Mefoxin Premixed Intravenous Solution (Cefoxitin Sodium) Merck & Co., Inc. 1694
Mezlin (Mezlocillin Sodium) Bayer Pharmaceutical 601
Mezlin Pharmacy Bulk Package (Mezlocillin Sodium) Bayer Pharmaceutical 604
Nebcin Vials, Hyporets & ADD-Vantage (Tobramycin Sulfate) Lilly 1464
Pipracil (Piperacillin Sodium) Lederle 1390
Primaxin I.V. (Imipenem-Cilastatin Sodium) Merck & Co., Inc. 1729
Tazicef for Injection (Ceftazidime) SmithKline Beecham Pharmaceuticals 2519
Tazidime Vials, Faspak & ADD-Vantage (Ceftazidime) Lilly .. 1478
Timentin for Injection (Ticarcillin Disodium, Clavulanate Potassium) SmithKline Beecham Pharmaceuticals 2528
Tobramycin Sulfate Injection (Tobramycin Sulfate) Elkins-Sinn 968
Unasyn (Ampicillin Sodium, Sulbactam Sodium) Roerig 2212
Zinacef (Cefuroxime Sodium) Glaxo Wellcome 1211

Klebsiella species urinary tract infections
Achromycin V Capsules (Tetracycline Hydrochloride) Lederle 1367
Ancef Injection (Cefazolin Sodium) SmithKline Beecham Pharmaceuticals 2465
Augmentin (Amoxicillin Trihydrate, Clavulanate Potassium) SmithKline Beecham Pharmaceuticals 2468
Azo Gantanol Tablets (Sulfamethoxazole, Phenazopyridine Hydrochloride) Roche Laboratories 2080
Azo Gantrisin Tablets (Sulfisoxazole, Phenazopyridine Hydrochloride) Roche Laboratories 2081
Bactrim DS Tablets (Trimethoprim, Sulfamethoxazole) Roche Laboratories 2084
Bactrim I.V. Infusion (Trimethoprim, Sulfamethoxazole) Roche Laboratories 2082
Bactrim (Trimethoprim, Sulfamethoxazole) Roche Laboratories 2084
Ceclor Pulvules & Suspension (Cefaclor) Lilly 1431
Cefizox for Intramuscular or Intravenous Use (Ceftizoxime Sodium) Fujisawa 1034
Cefotan (Cefotetan) Zeneca 2829
Ceptaz (Ceftazidime) Glaxo Wellcome 1081
Claforan Sterile and Injection (Cefotaxime Sodium) Hoechst-Roussel 1235
Declomycin Tablets (Demeclocycline Hydrochloride) Lederle 1371
Doryx Capsules (Doxycycline Hyclate) Parke-Davis 1913
Duricef (Cefadroxil Monohydrate) Bristol-Myers Squibb 748
Dynacin Capsules (Minocycline Hydrochloride) Medicis 1590
Fortaz (Ceftazidime) Glaxo Wellcome 1100
Gantanol Tablets (Sulfamethoxazole) Roche Laboratories 2119
Gantrisin (Acetyl Sulfisoxazole) Roche Laboratories 2120
Keftab Tablets (Cephalexin Hydrochloride) Dista 915
Kefurox Vials, Faspak & ADD-Vantage (Cefuroxime Sodium) Lilly 1454
Kefzol Vials, Faspak & ADD-Vantage (Cefazolin Sodium) Lilly 1456
Macrodantin Capsules (Nitrofurantoin) Procter & Gamble Pharmaceuticals 1989
Mandol Vials, Faspak & ADD-Vantage (Cefamandole Nafate) Lilly 1461
Mefoxin (Cefoxitin Sodium) Merck & Co., Inc. 1691
Mefoxin Premixed Intravenous Solution (Cefoxitin Sodium) Merck & Co., Inc. 1694
Mezlin (Mezlocillin Sodium) Bayer Pharmaceutical 601
Mezlin Pharmacy Bulk Package (Mezlocillin Sodium) Bayer Pharmaceutical 604
Minocin Intravenous (Minocycline Hydrochloride) Lederle 1382
Minocin Oral Suspension (Minocycline Hydrochloride) Lederle 1385
Minocin Pellet-Filled Capsules (Minocycline Hydrochloride) Lederle 1383
Monodox Capsules (Doxycycline Monohydrate) Oclassen 1805
Nebcin Vials, Hyporets & ADD-Vantage (Tobramycin Sulfate) Lilly 1464
NegGram (Nalidixic Acid) Sanofi Winthrop 2323
Primaxin I.V. (Imipenem-Cilastatin Sodium) Merck & Co., Inc. 1729
Septra (Trimethoprim, Sulfamethoxazole) Glaxo Wellcome 1174
Septra I.V. Infusion (Trimethoprim, Sulfamethoxazole) Glaxo Wellcome 1169
Septra I.V. Infusion ADD-Vantage Vials (Trimethoprim, Sulfamethoxazole) Glaxo Wellcome 1171
Septra (Trimethoprim, Sulfamethoxazole) Glaxo Wellcome 1174
Tazicef for Injection (Ceftazidime) SmithKline Beecham Pharmaceuticals 2519
Tazidime Vials, Faspak & ADD-Vantage (Ceftazidime) Lilly .. 1478
Terramycin Intramuscular Solution (Oxytetracycline) Roerig 2210
Timentin for Injection (Ticarcillin Disodium, Clavulanate Potassium) SmithKline Beecham Pharmaceuticals 2528
Tobramycin Sulfate Injection (Tobramycin Sulfate) Elkins-Sinn 968
Vibramycin (Doxycycline Calcium) Pfizer Labs 1941
Vibramycin Hyclate Intravenous (Doxycycline Hyclate) Roerig 2215
Vibramycin (Doxycycline Monohydrate) Pfizer Labs 1941
Zinacef (Cefuroxime Sodium) Glaxo Wellcome 1211

Klebsiella-Enterobacter species infections, ocular
AK-CIDE (Prednisolone Acetate, Sulfacetamide Sodium) Akorn .... ⊙ 202
AK-CIDE Ointment (Prednisolone Acetate, Sulfacetamide Sodium) Akorn .... ⊙ 202
AK-Spore (Bacitracin Zinc, Neomycin Sulfate, Polymyxin B Sulfate) Akorn .... ⊙ 204
AK-Trol Ointment & Suspension (Dexamethasone, Neomycin Sulfate, Polymyxin B Sulfate) Akorn .... ⊙ 205
Blephamide Liquifilm Sterile Ophthalmic Suspension (Prednisolone Acetate, Sulfacetamide Sodium) Allergan 476
Blephamide Ointment (Sulfacetamide Sodium, Prednisolone Acetate) Allergan .... ⊙ 237
Chloromycetin Ophthalmic Ointment, 1% (Chloramphenicol) Parke-Davis ⊙ 310
Chloromycetin Ophthalmic Solution (Chloramphenicol) Parke-Davis .... ⊙ 310
Chloroptic S.O.P. (Chloramphenicol) Allergan .... ⊙ 239
Cortisporin Ophthalmic Ointment Sterile (Polymyxin B Sulfate, Bacitracin Zinc, Neomycin Sulfate, Hydrocortisone) Glaxo Wellcome 1085
Cortisporin Ophthalmic Suspension Sterile (Hydrocortisone, Polymyxin B Sulfate, Neomycin Sulfate) Glaxo Wellcome 1086
Dexacidin Ointment (Dexamethasone, Neomycin Sulfate, Polymyxin B Sulfate) CIBA Vision Ophthalmics .... ⊙ 263
FML-S Liquifilm (Sulfacetamide Sodium, Fluorometholone) Allergan .... ⊙ 242
Gantanol Tablets (Sulfamethoxazole) Roche Laboratories 2119
Gantrisin (Acetyl Sulfisoxazole) Roche Laboratories 2120
Maxitrol Ophthalmic Ointment and Suspension (Dexamethasone, Neomycin Sulfate, Polymyxin B Sulfate) Alcon Laboratories .... ⊙ 224
NeoDecadron Sterile Ophthalmic Ointment (Neomycin Sulfate, Dexamethasone Sodium Phosphate) Merck & Co., Inc. 1712
NeoDecadron Sterile Ophthalmic Solution (Neomycin Sulfate, Dexamethasone Sodium Phosphate) Merck & Co., Inc. 1713
Ophthocort (Chloramphenicol, Polymyxin B Sulfate, Hydrocortisone Acetate) Parke-Davis .... ⊙ 311
Poly-Pred Liquifilm (Neomycin Sulfate, Polymyxin B Sulfate, Prednisolone Acetate) Allergan.. ⊙ 248
Pred-G Liquifilm Sterile Ophthalmic Suspension (Gentamicin Sulfate, Prednisolone Acetate) Allergan .... ⊙ 251
TobraDex Ophthalmic Suspension and Ointment (Dexamethasone, Tobramycin) Alcon Laboratories .. 473

(▭ Described in PDR For Nonprescription Drugs) (⊙ Described in PDR For Ophthalmology)

1505 Indications Index Leukemia

Vasocidin Ointment (Prednisolone Acetate, Sulfacetamide Sodium) CIBA Vision Ophthalmics ⊙ 268
Vasocidin Ophthalmic Solution (Prednisolone Sodium Phosphate, Sulfacetamide Sodium) CIBA Vision Ophthalmics ⊙ 270

Klebsiella-Enterobacter urinary tract infections
Gantanol Tablets (Sulfamethoxazole) Roche Laboratories 2119
Gantrisin (Acetyl Sulfisoxazole) Roche Laboratories 2120

Koch-Weeks bacillus infections, ocular (see under H. aegypticus infections, ocular)

L

Labor and delivery, routine management of
Methergine (Methylergonovine Maleate) Sandoz Pharmaceuticals 2272

Labor, induction of
Oxytocin Injection (Oxytocin) Wyeth-Ayerst 2771
Syntocinon Injection (Oxytocin) Sandoz Pharmaceuticals 2296

Labor, preterm, management of
Yutopar Intravenous Injection (Ritodrine Hydrochloride) Astra 570

Labor, stimulation of
Oxytocin Injection (Oxytocin) Wyeth-Ayerst 2771
Syntocinon Injection (Oxytocin) Sandoz Pharmaceuticals 2296

Lacrimation, symptomatic relief of
Benadryl Allergy Liquid Medication (Diphenhydramine Hydrochloride) WARNER WELLCOME ▣ 849
Benadryl Allergy (Diphenhydramine Hydrochloride) WARNER WELLCOME ▣ 848
Benadryl Allergy Sinus Headache Formula Caplets (Diphenhydramine Hydrochloride, Pseudoephedrine Hydrochloride, Acetaminophen) WARNER WELLCOME ▣ 849
Chlor-Trimeton Allergy Tablets (Chlorpheniramine Maleate) Schering-Plough HealthCare ▣ 798
Allergy-Sinus Comtrex Multi-Symptom Allergy-Sinus Formula Tablets (Acetaminophen, Chlorpheniramine Maleate, Pseudoephedrine Hydrochloride) Bristol-Myers Products ▣ 617
Contac Night Allergy/Sinus Caplets (Acetaminophen, Pseudoephedrine Hydrochloride, Diphenhydramine Hydrochloride) SmithKline Beecham Consumer ▣ 812
Dimetapp Elixir (Brompheniramine Maleate, Phenylpropanolamine Hydrochloride) A. H. Robins Consumer ▣ 773
Dimetapp Extentabs (Brompheniramine Maleate, Phenylpropanolamine Hydrochloride) A. H. Robins Consumer ▣ 774
Dimetapp Tablets/Liqui-Gels (Brompheniramine Maleate, Phenylpropanolamine Hydrochloride) A. H. Robins Consumer ▣ 775
Dimetapp Cold & Allergy Chewable Tablets (Brompheniramine Maleate, Phenylpropanolamine Hydrochloride) A. H. Robins Consumer ▣ 773
Drixoral Cold and Allergy Sustained-Action Tablets (Dexbrompheniramine Maleate, Pseudoephedrine Sulfate) Schering-Plough HealthCare ▣ 802
Drixoral Cold and Flu Extended-Release Tablets (Acetaminophen, Dexbrompheniramine Maleate, Pseudoephedrine Sulfate) Schering-Plough HealthCare ▣ 803
Nolahist Tablets (Phenindamine Tartrate) Carnrick 785
Ryna Liquid (Chlorpheniramine Maleate, Pseudoephedrine Hydrochloride) Wallace ▣ 841
Seldane Tablets (Terfenadine) Marion Merrell Dow 1536
Seldane-D Extended-Release Tablets (Pseudoephedrine Hydrochloride, Terfenadine) Marion Merrell Dow 1538
Similasan Eye Drops #2 (Homeopathic Medications) Similasan ⊙ 317
Sudafed Plus Liquid (Chlorpheniramine Maleate, Pseudoephedrine Hydrochloride) WARNER WELLCOME ▣ 862
Sudafed Plus Tablets (Chlorpheniramine Maleate, Pseudoephedrine Hydrochloride) WARNER WELLCOME ▣ 863
Tavist Syrup (Clemastine Fumarate) Sandoz Pharmaceuticals 2297
Tavist Tablets (Clemastine Fumarate) Sandoz Pharmaceuticals 2298
Triaminicin Tablets (Acetaminophen, Chlorpheniramine Maleate, Phenylpropanolamine Hydrochloride) Sandoz Consumer ▣ 793
TYLENOL Severe Allergy Medication Caplets (Acetaminophen, Diphenhydramine Hydrochloride) McNeil Consumer 1564

Lactase insufficiency
Dairy Ease Caplets and Tablets (Lactase (beta-d-Galactosidase)) Miles Consumer ▣ 720
Dairy Ease Drops (Lactase (beta-d-Galactosidase)) Miles Consumer ▣ 720

Lactose intolerance
Lactaid Caplets (Lactase (beta-d-Galactosidase)) McNeil Consumer 1550
Lactaid Drops (Lactase (beta-d-Galactosidase)) McNeil Consumer 1550

Lactobacillus acidophilus, deficiency of
DDS-Acidophilus (Lactobacillus Acidophilus) UAS Laboratories ▣ 835

Larva migrans, cutaneous
Mintezol (Thiabendazole) Merck & Co., Inc. 1704

Larva migrans, visceral
Mintezol (Thiabendazole) Merck & Co., Inc. 1704

Laryngeal edema, acute noninfectious, adjunctive therapy in
Aristocort Suspension (Forte Parenteral) (Triamcinolone Diacetate) Fujisawa 1027
Celestone Soluspan Suspension (Betamethasone Sodium Phosphate, Betamethasone Acetate) Schering 2347
Cortone Acetate Sterile Suspension (Cortisone Acetate) Merck & Co., Inc. 1623
Decadron Phosphate Injection (Dexamethasone Sodium Phosphate) Merck & Co., Inc. 1637
Depo-Medrol Single-Dose Vial (Methylprednisolone Acetate) Upjohn 2600
Depo-Medrol Sterile Aqueous Suspension (Methylprednisolone Acetate) Upjohn 2597
Hydeltrasol Injection, Sterile (Prednisolone Sodium Phosphate) Merck & Co., Inc. 1665
Hydrocortone Phosphate Injection, Sterile (Hydrocortisone Sodium Phosphate) Merck & Co., Inc. 1670
Solu-Cortef Sterile Powder (Hydrocortisone Sodium Succinate) Upjohn 2641
Solu-Medrol Sterile Powder (Methylprednisolone Sodium Succinate) Upjohn 2643

LDL cholesterol, elevation (see under Hyperlipoproteinemia, types IIa and IIb, adjunct to diet)

Lead encephalopathy
Calcium Disodium Versenate Injection (Calcium Disodium Edetate) 3M Pharmaceuticals 1490

Lead poisoning
Calcium Disodium Versenate Injection (Calcium Disodium Edetate) 3M Pharmaceuticals 1490
CHEMET (succimer) Capsules (Succimer) McNeil Consumer 1545

Leg muscle cramps
Legatrin PM (Acetaminophen, Diphenhydramine Hydrochloride) Columbia ▣ 651

Legionella pneumophila infections (see under Legionnaires' disease)

Legionnaires' disease
E.E.S. (Erythromycin Ethylsuccinate) Abbott 424
E-Mycin Tablets (Erythromycin) Knoll Laboratories 1341
ERYC (Erythromycin) Parke-Davis 1915
EryPed (Erythromycin Ethylsuccinate) Abbott 421
Ery-Tab Tablets (Erythromycin) Abbott 422
Erythrocin Stearate Filmtab (Erythromycin Stearate) Abbott 425
Erythromycin Base Filmtab (Erythromycin) Abbott 426
Erythromycin Delayed-Release Capsules, USP (Erythromycin) Abbott 427
Ilosone (Erythromycin Estolate) Dista 911
Ilotycin Gluceptate, IV, Vials (Erythromycin Gluceptate) Dista 913
PCE Dispertab Tablets (Erythromycin) Abbott 444

Leishmaniasis, American
Fungizone Intravenous (Amphotericin B) Apothecon 506

Lennox-Gastaut syndrome
Felbatol (Felbamate) Wallace 2666
Klonopin Tablets (Clonazepam) Roche Laboratories 2126

Lens, intraocular, implantation of, surgical aid in
AMO Vitrax Viscoelastic Solution (Sodium Hyaluronate) Allergan ⊙ 232
Healon (Sodium Hyaluronate) Pharmacia Inc. Ophthalmics ⊙ 314
Ocucoat (Hydroxypropyl Methylcellulose) Storz Ophthalmics ⊙ 321

Leprosy
Dapsone Tablets USP (Dapsone) Jacobus 1284

Leprosy, lepromatous
Lamprene Capsules (Clofazimine) CibaGeneva 828

Leprosy, lepromatous, complicated by erythema nodosum leprosum
Lamprene Capsules (Clofazimine) CibaGeneva 828

Leprosy, lepromatous, dapsone-resistant
Lamprene Capsules (Clofazimine) CibaGeneva 828

Letterer-Siwe disease
Velban Vials (Vinblastine Sulfate) Lilly 1484

Leukapheresis, adjunct to
Hespan Injection (Hetastarch) DuPont 929
Pentaspan Injection (Pentastarch) DuPont 937

Leukemia, acute
Oncovin Solution Vials & Hyporets (Vincristine Sulfate) Lilly 1466

Leukemia, acute erythroid
Cerubidine (Daunorubicin Hydrochloride) Chiron 795

Leukemia, acute lymphoblastic
Adriamycin PFS (Doxorubicin Hydrochloride) Pharmacia 1947
Adriamycin RDF (Doxorubicin Hydrochloride) Pharmacia 1947
Cytoxan (Cyclophosphamide) Bristol-Myers Squibb Oncology 694
Doxorubicin Astra (Doxorubicin Hydrochloride) Astra 540
NEOSAR Lyophilized/Neosar (Cyclophosphamide) Pharmacia 1959
Oncaspar (Pegaspargase) Rhone-Poulenc Rorer Pharmaceuticals 2028
Purinethol Tablets (Mercaptopurine) Glaxo Wellcome 1156
Rubex (Doxorubicin Hydrochloride) Bristol-Myers Squibb Oncology 712
Vumon (Teniposide) Bristol-Myers Squibb Oncology 727

Leukemia, acute lymphocytic
Cerubidine (Daunorubicin Hydrochloride) Chiron 795
Cytosar-U Sterile Powder (Cytarabine) Upjohn 2592
Elspar (Asparaginase) Merck & Co., Inc. 1659
Purinethol Tablets (Mercaptopurine) Glaxo Wellcome 1156

Leukemia, acute monocytic
Cerubidine (Daunorubicin Hydrochloride) Chiron 795
Cytoxan (Cyclophosphamide) Bristol-Myers Squibb Oncology 694
NEOSAR Lyophilized/Neosar (Cyclophosphamide) Pharmacia 1959

Leukemia, acute myeloblastic
Adriamycin PFS (Doxorubicin Hydrochloride) Pharmacia 1947
Adriamycin RDF (Doxorubicin Hydrochloride) Pharmacia 1947
Doxorubicin Astra (Doxorubicin Hydrochloride) Astra 540
Rubex (Doxorubicin Hydrochloride) Bristol-Myers Squibb Oncology 712

Leukemia, acute myelogenous
Cerubidine (Daunorubicin Hydrochloride) Chiron 795
Cytoxan (Cyclophosphamide) Bristol-Myers Squibb Oncology 694
Idamycin (Idarubicin Hydrochloride) Pharmacia 1955
NEOSAR Lyophilized/Neosar (Cyclophosphamide) Pharmacia 1959

Leukemia, acute nonlymphocytic
Cerubidine (Daunorubicin Hydrochloride) Chiron 795
Cytosar-U Sterile Powder (Cytarabine) Upjohn 2592
Novantrone (Mitoxantrone Hydrochloride) Immunex 1279
Thioguanine Tablets, Tabloid Brand (Thioguanine) Glaxo Wellcome 1181

Leukemia, acute, palliative management of in childhood
Aristocort Suspension (Forte Parenteral) (Triamcinolone Diacetate) Fujisawa 1027
Aristocort Tablets (Triamcinolone) Fujisawa 1022
Cortone Acetate Sterile Suspension (Cortisone Acetate) Merck & Co., Inc. 1623
Cortone Acetate Tablets (Cortisone Acetate) Merck & Co., Inc. 1624
Dalalone D.P. Injectable (Dexamethasone Acetate) Forest 1011
Decadron Elixir (Dexamethasone) Merck & Co., Inc. 1633
Decadron Phosphate Injection (Dexamethasone Sodium Phosphate) Merck & Co., Inc. 1637
Decadron Tablets (Dexamethasone) Merck & Co., Inc. 1635
Decadron-LA Sterile Suspension (Dexamethasone Acetate) Merck & Co., Inc. 1646
Deltasone Tablets (Prednisone) Upjohn 2595

(▣ Described in PDR For Nonprescription Drugs) (⊙ Described in PDR For Ophthalmology)

Leukemia — Indications Index — 1506

Depo-Medrol Single-Dose Vial (Methylprednisolone Acetate) Upjohn ... 2600
Depo-Medrol Sterile Aqueous Suspension (Methylprednisolone Acetate) Upjohn ... 2597
Hydeltrasol Injection, Sterile (Prednisolone Sodium Phosphate) Merck & Co., Inc. ... 1665
Hydrocortone Phosphate Injection, Sterile (Hydrocortisone Sodium Phosphate) Merck & Co., Inc. ... 1670
Hydrocortone Tablets (Hydrocortisone) Merck & Co., Inc. ... 1672
Medrol (Methylprednisolone) Upjohn ... 2621
Pediapred Oral Liquid (Prednisolone Sodium Phosphate) Fisons ... 995
Prelone Syrup (Prednisolone) Muro 1787
Solu-Cortef Sterile Powder (Hydrocortisone Sodium Succinate) Upjohn ... 2641
Solu-Medrol Sterile Powder (Methylprednisolone Sodium Succinate) Upjohn ... 2643

Leukemia, adjunctive therapy in
Zyloprim Tablets (Allopurinol) Glaxo Wellcome ... 1226

Leukemia, chronic granulocytic
Cytoxan (Cyclophosphamide) Bristol-Myers Squibb Oncology ... 694
NEOSAR Lyophilized/Neosar (Cyclophosphamide) Pharmacia .. 1959

Leukemia, chronic lymphocytic
Cytoxan (Cyclophosphamide) Bristol-Myers Squibb Oncology ... 694
Leukeran Tablets (Chlorambucil) Glaxo Wellcome ... 1133
Methotrexate Sodium Tablets, Injection, for Injection and LPF Injection (Methotrexate Sodium) Immunex ... 1275
Mustargen (Mechlorethamine Hydrochloride) Merck & Co., Inc. 1709
NEOSAR Lyophilized/Neosar (Cyclophosphamide) Pharmacia .. 1959

Leukemia, chronic lymphocytic, B-cell
Fludara for Injection (Fludarabine Phosphate) Berlex ... 663

Leukemia, chronic lymphocytic, B-cell, prevention of bacterial infection in
Gammagard S/D, Immune Globulin, Intravenous (Human) (Globulin, Immune (Human)) Baxter Healthcare ... 585

Leukemia, chronic myelocytic
Cytosar-U Sterile Powder (Cytarabine) Upjohn ... 2592
Hydrea Capsules (Hydroxyurea) Bristol-Myers Squibb Oncology ... 696
Mustargen (Mechlorethamine Hydrochloride) Merck & Co., Inc. 1709

Leukemia, chronic myelogenous
Myleran Tablets (Busulfan) Glaxo Wellcome ... 1143

Leukemia, hairy cell
Intron A (Interferon alfa-2B, Recombinant) Schering ... 2364
Leustatin (Cladribine) Ortho Biotech ... 1834
Roferon-A Injection (Interferon alfa-2A, Recombinant) Roche Laboratories ... 2145

Leukemia, lymphoblastic, adjunctive therapy in
Leukine for IV Infusion (Sargramostim) Immunex ... 1271

Leukemia, meningeal, prophylaxis of
Cytosar-U Sterile Powder (Cytarabine) Upjohn ... 2592
Methotrexate Sodium Tablets, Injection, for Injection and LPF Injection (Methotrexate Sodium) Immunex ... 1275

Leukemia, meningeal, treatment of
Methotrexate Sodium Tablets, Injection, for Injection and LPF Injection (Methotrexate Sodium) Immunex ... 1275

Leukemias, palliative management of
Aristocort Suspension (Forte Parenteral) (Triamcinolone Diacetate) Fujisawa ... 1027
Aristocort Tablets (Triamcinolone) Fujisawa ... 1022
Celestone Soluspan Suspension (Betamethasone Sodium Phosphate, Betamethasone Acetate) Schering ... 2347
Cortone Acetate Sterile Suspension (Cortisone Acetate) Merck & Co., Inc. ... 1623
Cortone Acetate Tablets (Cortisone Acetate) Merck & Co., Inc. ... 1624
Dalalone D.P. Injectable (Dexamethasone Acetate) Forest ... 1011
Decadron Elixir (Dexamethasone) Merck & Co., Inc. ... 1633
Decadron Phosphate Injection (Dexamethasone Sodium Phosphate) Merck & Co., Inc. ... 1637
Decadron Tablets (Dexamethasone) Merck & Co., Inc. ... 1635
Decadron-LA Sterile Suspension (Dexamethasone Acetate) Merck & Co., Inc. ... 1646
Deltasone Tablets (Prednisone) Upjohn ... 2595
Depo-Medrol Single-Dose Vial (Methylprednisolone Acetate) Upjohn ... 2600
Depo-Medrol Sterile Aqueous Suspension (Methylprednisolone Acetate) Upjohn ... 2597
Hydeltrasol Injection, Sterile (Prednisolone Sodium Phosphate) Merck & Co., Inc. ... 1665
Hydrocortone Phosphate Injection, Sterile (Hydrocortisone Sodium Phosphate) Merck & Co., Inc. ... 1670
Hydrocortone Tablets (Hydrocortisone) Merck & Co., Inc. ... 1672
Medrol (Methylprednisolone) Upjohn ... 2621
Pediapred Oral Liquid (Prednisolone Sodium Phosphate) Fisons ... 995
Prelone Syrup (Prednisolone) Muro 1787
Solu-Cortef Sterile Powder (Hydrocortisone Sodium Succinate) Upjohn ... 2641
Solu-Medrol Sterile Powder (Methylprednisolone Sodium Succinate) Upjohn ... 2643

Lice, body (see under Pediculosis, human)

Lice, head (see under Pediculosis, human)

Lice, pubic (see under Pediculosis, human)

Lichen planus
Aristocort Suspension (Forte Parenteral) (Triamcinolone Diacetate) Fujisawa ... 1027
Aristocort Suspension (Intralesional) (Triamcinolone Diacetate) Fujisawa ... 1025
Aristospan Suspension (Intralesional) (Triamcinolone Hexacetonide) Fujisawa ... 1032
Celestone Soluspan Suspension (Betamethasone Sodium Phosphate, Betamethasone Acetate) Schering ... 2347
Decadron Phosphate Injection (Dexamethasone Sodium Phosphate) Merck & Co., Inc. ... 1637
Decadron-LA Sterile Suspension (Dexamethasone Acetate) Merck & Co., Inc. ... 1646
Depo-Medrol Single-Dose Vial (Methylprednisolone Acetate) Upjohn ... 2600
Depo-Medrol Sterile Aqueous Suspension (Methylprednisolone Acetate) Upjohn ... 2597
Fototar Cream (Coal Tar) ICN ... 1253
Hydeltrasol Injection, Sterile (Prednisolone Sodium Phosphate) Merck & Co., Inc. ... 1665
Hydrocortone Acetate Sterile Suspension (Hydrocortisone Acetate) Merck & Co., Inc. ... 1669

Lichen simplex chronicus
Aristocort Suspension (Forte Parenteral) (Triamcinolone Diacetate) Fujisawa ... 1027
Aristocort Suspension (Intralesional) (Triamcinolone Diacetate) Fujisawa ... 1025
Aristospan Suspension (Intralesional) (Triamcinolone Hexacetonide) Fujisawa ... 1032
Celestone Soluspan Suspension (Betamethasone Sodium Phosphate, Betamethasone Acetate) Schering ... 2347
Decadron Phosphate Injection (Dexamethasone Sodium Phosphate) Merck & Co., Inc. ... 1637
Decadron-LA Sterile Suspension (Dexamethasone Acetate) Merck & Co., Inc. ... 1646
Depo-Medrol Single-Dose Vial (Methylprednisolone Acetate) Upjohn ... 2600
Depo-Medrol Sterile Aqueous Suspension (Methylprednisolone Acetate) Upjohn ... 2597
Hydeltrasol Injection, Sterile (Prednisolone Sodium Phosphate) Merck & Co., Inc. ... 1665
Hydrocortone Acetate Sterile Suspension (Hydrocortisone Acetate) Merck & Co., Inc. ... 1669
Mantadil Cream (Chlorcyclizine Hydrochloride) Glaxo Wellcome ... 1135
Temaril Tablets, Syrup and Spansule Extended-Release Capsules (Trimeprazine Tartrate) Allergan ... 483
Zonalon Cream (Doxepin Hydrochloride) GenDerm ... 1055

Lips, dry (see under Cheilitis, actinic)

Listeria monocytogenes infections
Achromycin V Capsules (Tetracycline Hydrochloride) Lederle ... 1367
Declomycin Tablets (Demeclocycline Hydrochloride) Lederle ... 1371
Doryx Capsules (Doxycycline Hyclate) Parke-Davis ... 1913
Dynacin Capsules (Minocycline Hydrochloride) Medicis ... 1590
E.E.S. (Erythromycin Ethylsuccinate) Abbott ... 424
E-Mycin Tablets (Erythromycin) Knoll Laboratories ... 1341
ERYC (Erythromycin) Parke-Davis .. 1915
EryPed (Erythromycin Ethylsuccinate) Abbott ... 421
Ery-Tab Tablets (Erythromycin) Abbott ... 422
Erythrocin Stearate Filmtab (Erythromycin Stearate) Abbott ... 425
Erythromycin Base Filmtab (Erythromycin) Abbott ... 426
Erythromycin Delayed-Release Capsules, USP (Erythromycin) Abbott ... 427
Ilosone (Erythromycin Estolate) Dista ... 911
Ilotycin Gluceptate, IV, Vials (Erythromycin Gluceptate) Dista ... 913
Minocin Intravenous (Minocycline Hydrochloride) Lederle ... 1382
Minocin Oral Suspension (Minocycline Hydrochloride) Lederle ... 1385
Minocin Pellet-Filled Capsules (Minocycline Hydrochloride) Lederle ... 1383
Monodox Capsules (Doxycycline Monohydrate) Oclassen ... 1805
Pfizerpen for Injection (Penicillin G Potassium) Roerig ... 2203
Terramycin Intramuscular Solution (Oxytetracycline) Roerig ... 2210
Vibramycin (Doxycycline Calcium) Pfizer Labs ... 1941
Vibramycin Hyclate Intravenous (Doxycycline Hyclate) Roerig ... 2215
Vibramycin (Doxycycline Monohydrate) Pfizer Labs ... 1941

Listeriosis
Dynacin Capsules (Minocycline Hydrochloride) Medicis ... 1590
Minocin Oral Suspension (Minocycline Hydrochloride) Lederle ... 1385
Minocin Pellet-Filled Capsules (Minocycline Hydrochloride) Lederle ... 1383
Monodox Capsules (Doxycycline Monohydrate) Oclassen ... 1805

Liver abscess, amebic (see under Amebic liver abscess)

Liver, allogeneic transplants, prophylaxis of organ rejection in
Neoral (Cyclosporine) Sandoz Pharmaceuticals ... 2276
Orthoclone OKT3 Sterile Solution (Muromonab-CD3) Ortho Biotech 1837
Prograf (Tacrolimus) Fujisawa ... 1042
Sandimmune (Cyclosporine) Sandoz Pharmaceuticals ... 2286

Loeffler's syndrome
Aristocort Suspension (Forte Parenteral) (Triamcinolone Diacetate) Fujisawa ... 1027
Aristocort Tablets (Triamcinolone) Fujisawa ... 1022
Celestone Soluspan Suspension (Betamethasone Sodium Phosphate, Betamethasone Acetate) Schering ... 2347
Cortone Acetate Sterile Suspension (Cortisone Acetate) Merck & Co., Inc. ... 1623
Cortone Acetate Tablets (Cortisone Acetate) Merck & Co., Inc. ... 1624
Dalalone D.P. Injectable (Dexamethasone Acetate) Forest ... 1011
Decadron Elixir (Dexamethasone) Merck & Co., Inc. ... 1633
Decadron Phosphate Injection (Dexamethasone Sodium Phosphate) Merck & Co., Inc. ... 1637
Decadron Tablets (Dexamethasone) Merck & Co., Inc. ... 1635
Decadron-LA Sterile Suspension (Dexamethasone Acetate) Merck & Co., Inc. ... 1646
Deltasone Tablets (Prednisone) Upjohn ... 2595
Depo-Medrol Single-Dose Vial (Methylprednisolone Acetate) Upjohn ... 2600
Depo-Medrol Sterile Aqueous Suspension (Methylprednisolone Acetate) Upjohn ... 2597
Hydeltrasol Injection, Sterile (Prednisolone Sodium Phosphate) Merck & Co., Inc. ... 1665
Hydrocortone Phosphate Injection, Sterile (Hydrocortisone Sodium Phosphate) Merck & Co., Inc. ... 1670
Hydrocortone Tablets (Hydrocortisone) Merck & Co., Inc. ... 1672
Medrol (Methylprednisolone) Upjohn ... 2621
Pediapred Oral Liquid (Prednisolone Sodium Phosphate) Fisons ... 995
Prelone Syrup (Prednisolone) Muro 1787
Solu-Cortef Sterile Powder (Hydrocortisone Sodium Succinate) Upjohn ... 2641
Solu-Medrol Sterile Powder (Methylprednisolone Sodium Succinate) Upjohn ... 2643

Lown-Ganong-Levine syndrome
Isoptin Injectable (Verapamil Hydrochloride) Knoll Laboratories ... 1344

Lubrication, sexual (see under Coitus, adjunct in)

Lung abscess (see under Abscess, lung)

Lupus erythematosus discoides
Aristocort Suspension (Forte Parenteral) (Triamcinolone Diacetate) Fujisawa ... 1027
Aristocort Suspension (Intralesional) (Triamcinolone Diacetate) Fujisawa ... 1025
Aristospan Suspension (Intralesional) (Triamcinolone Hexacetonide) Fujisawa ... 1032
Celestone Soluspan Suspension (Betamethasone Sodium Phosphate, Betamethasone Acetate) Schering ... 2347

Decadron Phosphate Injection (Dexamethasone Sodium Phosphate) Merck & Co., Inc. 1637

Decadron-LA Sterile Suspension (Dexamethasone Acetate) Merck & Co., Inc. 1646

Depo-Medrol Single-Dose Vial (Methylprednisolone Acetate) Upjohn... 2600

Depo-Medrol Sterile Aqueous Suspension (Methylprednisolone Acetate) Upjohn 2597

Hydeltrasol Injection, Sterile (Prednisolone Sodium Phosphate) Merck & Co., Inc. 1665

Hydrocortone Acetate Sterile Suspension (Hydrocortisone Acetate) Merck & Co., Inc. 1669

Plaquenil Sulfate Tablets (Hydroxychloroquine Sulfate) Sanofi Winthrop 2328

Lupus erythematosus, systemic

Aristocort Suspension (Forte Parenteral) (Triamcinolone Diacetate) Fujisawa 1027

Aristocort Tablets (Triamcinolone) Fujisawa 1022

Extra Strength Bayer Arthritis Pain Regimen Formula (Aspirin, Enteric Coated) Miles Consumer.. **◙** 711

Celestone Soluspan Suspension (Betamethasone Sodium Phosphate, Betamethasone Acetate) Schering 2347

Cortone Acetate Sterile Suspension (Cortisone Acetate) Merck & Co., Inc. 1623

Cortone Acetate Tablets (Cortisone Acetate) Merck & Co., Inc. 1624

Dalalone D.P. Injectable (Dexamethasone Acetate) Forest 1011

Decadron Elixir (Dexamethasone) Merck & Co., Inc. 1633

Decadron Phosphate Injection (Dexamethasone Sodium Phosphate) Merck & Co., Inc. 1637

Decadron Tablets (Dexamethasone) Merck & Co., Inc. 1635

Decadron-LA Sterile Suspension (Dexamethasone Acetate) Merck & Co., Inc. 1646

Deltasone Tablets (Prednisone) Upjohn... 2595

Depo-Medrol Single-Dose Vial (Methylprednisolone Acetate) Upjohn... 2600

Depo-Medrol Sterile Aqueous Suspension (Methylprednisolone Acetate) Upjohn 2597

Ecotrin (Aspirin, Enteric Coated) SmithKline Beecham............................ 2455

Hydeltrasol Injection, Sterile (Prednisolone Sodium Phosphate) Merck & Co., Inc. 1665

Hydrocortone Phosphate Injection, Sterile (Hydrocortisone Sodium Phosphate) Merck & Co., Inc. 1670

Hydrocortone Tablets (Hydrocortisone) Merck & Co., Inc. 1672

Medrol (Methylprednisolone) Upjohn... 2621

Pediapred Oral Liquid (Prednisolone Sodium Phosphate) Fisons 995

Plaquenil Sulfate Tablets (Hydroxychloroquine Sulfate) Sanofi Winthrop 2328

Prelone Syrup (Prednisolone) Muro 1787

Solu-Cortef Sterile Powder (Hydrocortisone Sodium Succinate) Upjohn... 2641

Solu-Medrol Sterile Powder (Methylprednisolone Sodium Succinate) Upjohn 2643

Lyme disease

(see under Borrelia burgdorferi infection)

Lymphogranuloma venereum

Achromycin V Capsules (Tetracycline Hydrochloride) Lederle 1367

Declomycin Tablets (Demeclocycline Hydrochloride) Lederle 1371

Doryx Capsules (Doxycycline Hyclate) Parke-Davis............................ 1913

Dynacin Capsules (Minocycline Hydrochloride) Medicis 1590

Minocin Intravenous (Minocycline Hydrochloride) Lederle 1382

Minocin Oral Suspension (Minocycline Hydrochloride) Lederle 1385

Minocin Pellet-Filled Capsules (Minocycline Hydrochloride) Lederle 1383

Monodox Capsules (Doxycycline Monohydrate) Oclassen.................... 1805

Terramycin Intramuscular Solution (Oxytetracycline) Roerig 2210

Vibramycin (Doxycycline Calcium) Pfizer Labs 1941

Vibramycin Hyclate Intravenous (Doxycycline Hyclate) Roerig.......... 2215

Vibramycin (Doxycycline Monohydrate) Pfizer Labs 1941

Lymphogranuloma-psittacosis group infections

Chloromycetin Sodium Succinate (Chloramphenicol Sodium Succinate) Parke-Davis 1900

Lymphography, diagnostic aid in

Ethiodol (Ethiodized Oil) Savage 2340

Lymphoma, Burkitt's

Cytoxan (Cyclophosphamide) Bristol-Myers Squibb Oncology 694

NEOSAR Lyophilized/Neosar (Cyclophosphamide) Pharmacia .. 1959

Lymphoma, cutaneous T-cell

8-MOP Capsules (Methoxsalen) ICN 1246

Lymphoma, hystiocytic

Cytoxan (Cyclophosphamide) Bristol-Myers Squibb Oncology 694

NEOSAR Lyophilized/Neosar (Cyclophosphamide) Pharmacia .. 1959

Oncovin Solution Vials & Hyporets (Vincristine Sulfate) Lilly 1466

Velban Vials (Vinblastine Sulfate) Lilly 1484

Lymphoma, lymphocytic

Cytoxan (Cyclophosphamide) Bristol-Myers Squibb Oncology 694

NEOSAR Lyophilized/Neosar (Cyclophosphamide) Pharmacia .. 1959

Oncovin Solution Vials & Hyporets (Vincristine Sulfate) Lilly 1466

Velban Vials (Vinblastine Sulfate) Lilly 1484

Lymphoma, mixed cell type

Cytoxan (Cyclophosphamide) Bristol-Myers Squibb Oncology 694

NEOSAR Lyophilized/Neosar (Cyclophosphamide) Pharmacia .. 1959

Oncovin Solution Vials & Hyporets (Vincristine Sulfate) Lilly 1466

Lymphomas, giant follicular

Leukeran Tablets (Chlorambucil) Glaxo Wellcome................................... 1133

Lymphomas, Hodgkin's

(see under Hodgkin's disease)

Lymphomas, lymphosarcoma, palliative treatment of

Blenoxane (Bleomycin Sulfate) Bristol-Myers Squibb Oncology 692

Lymphomas, malignant

Cytoxan (Cyclophosphamide) Bristol-Myers Squibb Oncology 694

Leukeran Tablets (Chlorambucil) Glaxo Wellcome................................... 1133

NEOSAR Lyophilized/Neosar (Cyclophosphamide) Pharmacia .. 1959

Oncovin Solution Vials & Hyporets (Vincristine Sulfate) Lilly 1466

Lymphomas, non-Hodgkin's

Adriamycin PFS (Doxorubicin Hydrochloride) Pharmacia 1947

Adriamycin RDF (Doxorubicin Hydrochloride) Pharmacia 1947

BiCNU (Carmustine (BCNU)) Bristol-Myers Squibb Oncology 691

Doxorubicin Astra (Doxorubicin Hydrochloride) Astra 540

Leukeran Tablets (Chlorambucil) Glaxo Wellcome................................... 1133

Methotrexate Sodium Tablets, Injection, for Injection and LPF Injection (Methotrexate Sodium) Immunex 1275

Mustargen (Mechlorethamine Hydrochloride) Merck & Co., Inc. 1709

Oncovin Solution Vials & Hyporets (Vincristine Sulfate) Lilly 1466

Rubex (Doxorubicin Hydrochloride) Bristol-Myers Squibb Oncology 712

Thioplex (Thiotepa For Injection) (Thiotepa) Immunex 1281

Lymphomas, non-Hodgkin's, adjunctive therapy in

Leukine for IV Infusion (Sargramostim) Immunex................ 1271

Lymphomas, palliative management of in adults

Aristocort Suspension (Forte Parenteral) (Triamcinolone Diacetate) Fujisawa 1027

Aristocort Tablets (Triamcinolone) Fujisawa 1022

Blenoxane (Bleomycin Sulfate) Bristol-Myers Squibb Oncology 692

Celestone Soluspan Suspension (Betamethasone Sodium Phosphate, Betamethasone Acetate) Schering 2347

Cortone Acetate Sterile Suspension (Cortisone Acetate) Merck & Co., Inc. 1623

Cortone Acetate Tablets (Cortisone Acetate) Merck & Co., Inc. 1624

Dalalone D.P. Injectable (Dexamethasone Acetate) Forest 1011

Decadron Elixir (Dexamethasone) Merck & Co., Inc. 1633

Decadron Phosphate Injection (Dexamethasone Sodium Phosphate) Merck & Co., Inc. 1637

Decadron Tablets (Dexamethasone) Merck & Co., Inc. 1635

Decadron-LA Sterile Suspension (Dexamethasone Acetate) Merck & Co., Inc. 1646

Deltasone Tablets (Prednisone) Upjohn... 2595

Depo-Medrol Single-Dose Vial (Methylprednisolone Acetate) Upjohn... 2600

Depo-Medrol Sterile Aqueous Suspension (Methylprednisolone Acetate) Upjohn 2597

Hydeltrasol Injection, Sterile (Prednisolone Sodium Phosphate) Merck & Co., Inc. 1665

Hydrocortone Phosphate Injection, Sterile (Hydrocortisone Sodium Phosphate) Merck & Co., Inc. 1670

Hydrocortone Tablets (Hydrocortisone) Merck & Co., Inc. 1672

Medrol (Methylprednisolone) Upjohn... 2621

Pediapred Oral Liquid (Prednisolone Sodium Phosphate) Fisons 995

Prelone Syrup (Prednisolone) Muro 1787

Solu-Cortef Sterile Powder (Hydrocortisone Sodium Succinate) Upjohn... 2641

Solu-Medrol Sterile Powder (Methylprednisolone Sodium Succinate) Upjohn 2643

Lymphomas, reticulum cell sarcoma, palliative treatment of

Blenoxane (Bleomycin Sulfate) Bristol-Myers Squibb Oncology 692

Lymphosarcoma

(see under Lymphomas, non-Hodgkin's)

M

M. catarrhalis infections

Augmentin (Amoxicillin Trihydrate, Clavulanate Potassium) SmithKline Beecham Pharmaceuticals 2468

Biaxin (Clarithromycin) Abbott.......... 405

Ceftin (Cefuroxime Axetil) Glaxo Wellcome 1078

Cefzil Tablets and Oral Suspension (Cefprozil) Bristol-Myers Squibb .. 746

Keflex Pulvules & Oral Suspension (Cephalexin) Dista 914

Lorabid Suspension and Pulvules (Loracarbef) Lilly 1459

Maxaquin Tablets (Lomefloxacin Hydrochloride) Searle......................... 2440

Suprax (Cefixime) Lederle 1399

Vantin for Oral Suspension and Vantin Tablets (Cefpodoxime Proxetil) Upjohn 2646

Zithromax (Azithromycin) Pfizer Labs 1944

M. catarrhalis lower respiratory tract infections

Augmentin (Amoxicillin Trihydrate, Clavulanate Potassium) SmithKline Beecham Pharmaceuticals 2468

Biaxin (Clarithromycin) Abbott.......... 405

Cefzil Tablets and Oral Suspension (Cefprozil) Bristol-Myers Squibb .. 746

Lorabid Suspension and Pulvules (Loracarbef) Lilly 1459

Maxaquin Tablets (Lomefloxacin Hydrochloride) Searle......................... 2440

Zithromax (Azithromycin) Pfizer Labs 1944

M. catarrhalis sinusitis

Augmentin (Amoxicillin Trihydrate, Clavulanate Potassium) SmithKline Beecham Pharmaceuticals 2468

Lorabid Suspension and Pulvules (Loracarbef) Lilly 1459

M. catarrhalis, otitis media

Augmentin (Amoxicillin Trihydrate, Clavulanate Potassium) SmithKline Beecham Pharmaceuticals 2468

Ceftin Tablets (Cefuroxime Axetil) Glaxo Wellcome................................... 1078

Cefzil Tablets and Oral Suspension (Cefprozil) Bristol-Myers Squibb .. 746

Keflex Pulvules & Oral Suspension (Cephalexin) Dista 914

Lorabid Suspension and Pulvules (Loracarbef) Lilly 1459

Suprax (Cefixime) Lederle 1399

Vantin for Oral Suspension and Vantin Tablets (Cefpodoxime Proxetil) Upjohn 2646

Magnesium deficiency

(see under Hypomagnesemia)

Malaria

(see under P. vivax infections; P. malariae infections; P. ovale infections; P. falciparum infections)

Malaria, prophylaxis of

Fansidar Tablets (Sulfadoxine, Pyrimethamine) Roche Laboratories 2114

Lariam Tablets (Mefloquine Hydrochloride) Roche Laboratories 2128

Vibramycin Hyclate Capsules (Doxycycline Hyclate) Pfizer Labs 1941

Malassezia furfur

(see under Pityrosporon orbiculare infections)

Malignant effusion, serosal cavities

Thioplex (Thiotepa For Injection) (Thiotepa) Immunex 1281

Manic episodes associated with bipolar disorder

Depakote Tablets (Divalproex Sodium) Abbott...................................... 415

Eskalith (Lithium Carbonate) SmithKline Beecham Pharmaceuticals 2485

Lithonate/Lithotabs/Lithobid (Lithium Carbonate) Solvay...................... 2543

Mastocytosis, systemic

Gastrocrom Capsules (Cromolyn Sodium) Fisons 984

Prilosec Delayed-Release Capsules (Omeprazole) Astra Merck.............. 529

Tagamet (Cimetidine Hydrochloride) SmithKline Beecham Pharmaceuticals 2516

Zantac (Ranitidine Hydrochloride) Glaxo Wellcome................................... 1209

Measles, prevention or modification of

Gammar, Immune Globulin (Human) U.S.P. (Globulin, Immune (Human)) Armour 515

(**◙** Described in PDR For Nonprescription Drugs)

(**◉** Described in PDR For Ophthalmology)

Measles **Indications Index** 1508

Measles, prophylaxis
Attenuvax (Measles Virus Vaccine Live) Merck & Co., Inc. 1610
M-M-R II (Measles, Mumps & Rubella Virus Vaccine Live) Merck & Co., Inc. 1687
M-R-VAX II (Measles & Rubella Virus Vaccine Live) Merck & Co., Inc. 1689

Meibomianitis, acute
Genoptic Sterile Ophthalmic Solution (Gentamicin Sulfate) Allergan .... ⊙ 243
Genoptic Sterile Ophthalmic Ointment (Gentamicin Sulfate) Allergan .... ⊙ 243
Gentacidin Ointment (Gentamicin Sulfate) CIBA Vision Ophthalmics .... ⊙ 264
Gentacidin Solution (Gentamicin Sulfate) CIBA Vision Ophthalmics .... ⊙ 264
Gentak (Gentamicin Sulfate) Akorn .... ⊙ 208

Melanin hyperpigmentation (see under Hyperpigmentation, skin, bleaching of)

Melanoma, malignant
Hydrea Capsules (Hydroxyurea) Bristol-Myers Squibb Oncology 696

Melanoma, metastatic malignant
DTIC-Dome (Dacarbazine) Bayer Pharmaceutical 600

Melasma (see under Hyperpigmentation, skin, bleaching of)

Meniere's disease
Vontrol Tablets (Diphenidol) SmithKline Beecham Pharmaceuticals 2532

Meningitis
Amikacin Sulfate Injection, USP (Amikacin Sulfate) Elkins-Sinn 960
Amikin Injectable (Amikacin Sulfate) Apothecon 501
Cefizox for Intramuscular or Intravenous Use (Ceftizoxime Sodium) Fujisawa 1034
Ceptaz (Ceftazidime) Glaxo Wellcome 1081
Claforan Sterile and Injection (Cefotaxime Sodium) Hoechst-Roussel 1235
Flagyl 375 Capsules (Metronidazole) Searle 2434
Flagyl I.V. (Metronidazole Hydrochloride) SCS 2247
Fortaz (Ceftazidime) Glaxo Wellcome 1100
Garamycin Injectable (Gentamicin Sulfate) Schering 2360
Kefurox Vials, Faspak & ADD-Vantage (Cefuroxime Sodium) Lilly 1454
Nebcin Vials, Hyporets & ADD-Vantage (Tobramycin Sulfate) Lilly 1464
Omnipen for Oral Suspension (Ampicillin) Wyeth-Ayerst 2765
Pfizerpen for Injection (Penicillin G Potassium) Roerig 2203
Rocephin Injectable Vials, ADD-Vantage, Galaxy Container (Ceftriaxone Sodium) Roche Laboratories 2142
Tazicef for Injection (Ceftazidime) SmithKline Beecham Pharmaceuticals 2519
Tazidime Vials, Faspak & ADD-Vantage (Ceftazidime) Lilly .. 1478
Tobramycin Sulfate Injection (Tobramycin Sulfate) Elkins-Sinn 968
Zinacef (Cefuroxime Sodium) Glaxo Wellcome 1211

Meningitis, gram-negative bacteria-induced
Chloromycetin Sodium Succinate (Chloramphenicol Sodium Succinate) Parke-Davis 1900

Meningitis, meningococcal, prophylaxis of
Gantanol Tablets (Sulfamethoxazole) Roche Laboratories 2119
Gantrisin (Acetyl Sulfisoxazole) Roche Laboratories 2120

Meningitis, meningococcal, treatment of
Gantrisin (Acetyl Sulfisoxazole) Roche Laboratories 2120
Pfizerpen for Injection (Penicillin G Potassium) Roerig 2203

Meningitis, tuberculous
Aristocort Suspension (Forte Parenteral) (Triamcinolone Diacetate) Fujisawa 1027
Aristocort Tablets (Triamcinolone) Fujisawa 1022
Celestone Soluspan Suspension (Betamethasone Sodium Phosphate, Betamethasone Acetate) Schering 2347
Cortone Acetate Sterile Suspension (Cortisone Acetate) Merck & Co., Inc. 1623
Cortone Acetate Tablets (Cortisone Acetate) Merck & Co., Inc. 1624
Decadron Elixir (Dexamethasone) Merck & Co., Inc. 1633
Decadron Phosphate Injection (Dexamethasone Sodium Phosphate) Merck & Co., Inc. 1637
Decadron Tablets (Dexamethasone) Merck & Co., Inc. 1635
Deltasone Tablets (Prednisone) Upjohn 2595
Depo-Medrol Single-Dose Vial (Methylprednisolone Acetate) Upjohn 2600
Depo-Medrol Sterile Aqueous Suspension (Methylprednisolone Acetate) Upjohn 2597
Hydeltrasol Injection, Sterile (Prednisolone Sodium Phosphate) Merck & Co., Inc. 1665
Hydrocortone Phosphate Injection, Sterile (Hydrocortisone Sodium Phosphate) Merck & Co., Inc. 1670
Hydrocortone Tablets (Hydrocortisone) Merck & Co., Inc. 1672
Medrol (Methylprednisolone) Upjohn 2621
Pediapred Oral Liquid (Prednisolone Sodium Phosphate) Fisons 995
Prelone Syrup (Prednisolone) Muro 1787
Solu-Cortef Sterile Powder (Hydrocortisone Sodium Succinate) Upjohn 2641
Solu-Medrol Sterile Powder (Methylprednisolone Sodium Succinate) Upjohn 2643

Menopause, management of the manifestations of
PMB 200 and PMB 400 (Estrogens, Conjugated, Meprobamate) Wyeth-Ayerst 2783

Menopause, vasomotor symptoms of
Climara Transdermal System (Estradiol) Berlex 645
Estrace Cream and Tablets (Estradiol) Bristol-Myers Squibb .. 749
Estraderm Transdermal System (Estradiol) CibaGeneva 824
ESTRATAB Tablets (0.3, 0.625, 1.25, 2.5 mg) (Estrogens, Esterified) Solvay 2536
Estratest (Estrogens, Esterified, Methyltestosterone) Solvay 2539
Menest Tablets (Estrogens, Esterified) SmithKline Beecham Pharmaceuticals 2494
Ogen Tablets (Estropipate) Upjohn 2627
Ortho-Est (Estropipate) Ortho Pharmaceutical 1869
PMB 200 and PMB 400 (Estrogens, Conjugated, Meprobamate) Wyeth-Ayerst 2783
Premarin with Methyltestosterone (Estrogens, Conjugated, Methyltestosterone) Wyeth-Ayerst 2794
Premarin Tablets (Estrogens, Conjugated) Wyeth-Ayerst 2789
Premphase (Estrogens, Conjugated, Medroxyprogesterone Acetate) Wyeth-Ayerst 2797
Prempro (Estrogens, Conjugated, Medroxyprogesterone Acetate) Wyeth-Ayerst 2801

Menstrual cramps (see under Pain, menstrual)

Menstrual syndrome, pre-, management of
Bayer Select Menstrual Multi-Symptom Formula (Acetaminophen, Pamabrom) Miles Consumer .... ■ 716
Cramp End Tablets (Ibuprofen) Ohm .... ■ 735
Lurline PMS Tablets (Acetaminophen, Pamabrom) Fielding 982
Maximum Strength Multi-Symptom Formula Midol (Acetaminophen, Caffeine, Pyrilamine Maleate) Miles Consumer .... ■ 722
PMS Multi-Symptom Formula Midol (Acetaminophen, Pamabrom, Pyrilamine Maleate) Miles Consumer .... ■ 723

Mental capacity, idiopathic, decline in, symptomatic relief of
Hydergine (Ergoloid Mesylates) Sandoz Pharmaceuticals 2265

Methotrexate toxicity (see under Folic acid antagonists, overdosage of)

Microsporum audouinii infections
Fulvicin P/G Tablets (Griseofulvin) Schering 2359
Fulvicin P/G 165 & 330 Tablets (Griseofulvin) Schering 2359
Grifulvin V (griseofulvin tablets) Microsize (griseofulvin oral suspension) Microsize (Griseofulvin) Ortho Dermatological 1888
Gris-PEG Tablets, 125 mg & 250 mg (Griseofulvin) Allergan 479
Spectazole (econazole nitrate 1%) Cream (Econazole Nitrate) Ortho Dermatological 1890

Microsporum canis infections
Exelderm Cream 1.0% (Sulconazole Nitrate) Westwood-Squibb 2685
Exelderm Solution 1.0% (Sulconazole Nitrate) Westwood-Squibb 2686
Fulvicin P/G Tablets (Griseofulvin) Schering 2359
Fulvicin P/G 165 & 330 Tablets (Griseofulvin) Schering 2359
Grifulvin V (griseofulvin tablets) Microsize (griseofulvin oral suspension) Microsize (Griseofulvin) Ortho Dermatological 1888
Gris-PEG Tablets, 125 mg & 250 mg (Griseofulvin) Allergan 479
Loprox 1% Cream and Lotion (Ciclopirox Olamine) Hoechst-Roussel 1242
Lotrimin (Clotrimazole) Schering 2371
Lotrisone Cream (Clotrimazole, Betamethasone Dipropionate) Schering 2372
Spectazole (econazole nitrate 1%) Cream (Econazole Nitrate) Ortho Dermatological 1890

Microsporum gypseum infections
Fulvicin P/G Tablets (Griseofulvin) Schering 2359
Fulvicin P/G 165 & 330 Tablets (Griseofulvin) Schering 2359
Grifulvin V (griseofulvin tablets) Microsize (griseofulvin oral suspension) Microsize (Griseofulvin) Ortho Dermatological 1888
Gris-PEG Tablets, 125 mg & 250 mg (Griseofulvin) Allergan 479
Spectazole (econazole nitrate 1%) Cream (Econazole Nitrate) Ortho Dermatological 1890

Migraine headache (see under Headache, migraine)

Miliaria
Caldesene Medicated Powder (Calcium Undecylenate) CIBA Consumer .... ■ 632
Moisturel Cream (Dimethicone, Petrolatum) Westwood-Squibb 2688

Mima-Herellea species infections (see under Acinetobacter species infections)

Miosis, intraoperative, inhibition of
Ocufen (Flurbiprofen Sodium) Allergan .... ⊙ 245
Profenal 1% Sterile Ophthalmic Solution (Suprofen) Alcon Laboratories .... ⊙ 227

Miosis, production of
Floropryl Sterile Ophthalmic Ointment (Isoflurophate) Merck & Co., Inc. 1662
Humorsol Sterile Ophthalmic Solution (Demecarium Bromide) Merck & Co., Inc. 1664
Isopto Carpine Ophthalmic Solution (Pilocarpine Hydrochloride) Alcon Laboratories .... ⊙ 223
Miochol-E with Iocare Steri-Tags and Miochol-E System Pak (Acetylcholine Chloride) CIBA Vision Ophthalmics .... ⊙ 273
MIOSTAT Intraocular Solution (Carbachol) Alcon Laboratories ⊙ 224
Ocusert Pilo-20 and Pilo-40 Ocular Therapeutic Systems (Pilocarpine) Alza .... ⊙ 254
Pilagan (Pilocarpine Nitrate) Allergan .... ⊙ 248
Pilopine HS Ophthalmic Gel (Pilocarpine Hydrochloride) Alcon Laboratories .... ⊙ 226
Rēv-Eyes Ophthalmic Eyedrops 0.5% (Dapiprazole Hydrochloride) Storz Ophthalmics .... ⊙ 323

Moraxella catarrhalis (see under M. catarrhalis infections)

Moraxella lacunata infections, ocular
Chloromycetin Ophthalmic Ointment, 1% (Chloramphenicol) Parke-Davis ⊙ 310
Chloromycetin Ophthalmic Solution (Chloramphenicol) Parke-Davis .... ⊙ 310
Chloroptic S.O.P. (Chloramphenicol) Allergan .... ⊙ 239
Ophthocort (Chloramphenicol, Polymyxin B Sulfate, Hydrocortisone Acetate) Parke-Davis .... ⊙ 311
TobraDex Ophthalmic Suspension and Ointment (Dexamethasone, Tobramycin) Alcon Laboratories .. 473

Morganella morganii infections
Bactrim DS Tablets (Trimethoprim, Sulfamethoxazole) Roche Laboratories 2084
Bactrim I.V. Infusion (Trimethoprim, Sulfamethoxazole) Roche Laboratories 2082
Bactrim (Trimethoprim, Sulfamethoxazole) Roche Laboratories 2084
Cefizox for Intramuscular or Intravenous Use (Ceftizoxime Sodium) Fujisawa 1034
Cefotan (Cefotetan) Zeneca 2829
Ceptaz (Ceftazidime) Glaxo Wellcome 1081
Cipro I.V. (Ciprofloxacin) Bayer Pharmaceutical 595
Cipro I.V. Pharmacy Bulk Package (Ciprofloxacin) Bayer Pharmaceutical 597
Cipro Tablets (Ciprofloxacin Hydrochloride) Bayer Pharmaceutical 592
Claforan Sterile and Injection (Cefotaxime Sodium) Hoechst-Roussel 1235
Fortaz (Ceftazidime) Glaxo Wellcome 1100
Geocillin Tablets (Carbenicillin Indanyl Sodium) Roerig 2199

(■ Described in PDR For Nonprescription Drugs) (⊙ Described in PDR For Ophthalmology)

1509 **Indications Index** **Mycosis fungoides**

Mefoxin (Cefoxitin Sodium) Merck & Co., Inc. 1691
Mefoxin Premixed Intravenous Solution (Cefoxitin Sodium) Merck & Co., Inc. 1694
Mezlin (Mezlocillin Sodium) Bayer Pharmaceutical 601
Mezlin Pharmacy Bulk Package (Mezlocillin Sodium) Bayer Pharmaceutical 604
Monocid Injection (Cefonicid Sodium) SmithKline Beecham Pharmaceuticals 2497
Primaxin I.V. (Imipenem-Cilastatin Sodium) Merck & Co., Inc. 1729
Rocephin Injectable Vials, ADD-Vantage, Galaxy Container (Ceftriaxone Sodium) Roche Laboratories 2142
Septra (Trimethoprim, Sulfamethoxazole) Glaxo Wellcome 1174
Septra I.V. Infusion (Trimethoprim, Sulfamethoxazole) Glaxo Wellcome 1169
Septra I.V. Infusion ADD-Vantage Vials (Trimethoprim, Sulfamethoxazole) Glaxo Wellcome 1171
Septra (Trimethoprim, Sulfamethoxazole) Glaxo Wellcome 1174
Tazicef for Injection (Ceftazidime) SmithKline Beecham Pharmaceuticals 2519
Ticar for Injection (Ticarcillin Disodium) SmithKline Beecham Pharmaceuticals 2526
Tobramycin Sulfate Injection (Tobramycin Sulfate) Elkins-Sinn 968
Zefazone (Cefmetazole Sodium) Upjohn 2654

Morganella morganii infections, ocular
TobraDex Ophthalmic Suspension and Ointment (Dexamethasone, Tobramycin) Alcon Laboratories .. 473

Morganella morganii skin and skin structure infections
Cipro I.V. (Ciprofloxacin) Bayer Pharmaceutical 595
Cipro I.V. Pharmacy Bulk Package (Ciprofloxacin) Bayer Pharmaceutical 597
Cipro Tablets (Ciprofloxacin Hydrochloride) Bayer Pharmaceutical 592
Claforan Sterile and Injection (Cefotaxime Sodium) Hoechst-Roussel 1235
Mezlin (Mezlocillin Sodium) Bayer Pharmaceutical 601
Mezlin Pharmacy Bulk Package (Mezlocillin Sodium) Bayer Pharmaceutical 604
Primaxin I.V. (Imipenem-Cilastatin Sodium) Merck & Co., Inc. 1729
Rocephin Injectable Vials, ADD-Vantage, Galaxy Container (Ceftriaxone Sodium) Roche Laboratories 2142
Tazicef for Injection (Ceftazidime) SmithKline Beecham Pharmaceuticals 2519
Zefazone (Cefmetazole Sodium) Upjohn 2654

Morganella morganii urinary tract infections
Bactrim DS Tablets (Trimethoprim, Sulfamethoxazole) Roche Laboratories 2084
Bactrim I.V. Infusion (Trimethoprim, Sulfamethoxazole) Roche Laboratories 2082
Bactrim (Trimethoprim, Sulfamethoxazole) Roche Laboratories 2084
Cefizox for Intramuscular or Intravenous Use (Ceftizoxime Sodium) Fujisawa 1034
Cefotan (Cefotetan) Zeneca 2829
Ceptaz (Ceftazidime) Glaxo Wellcome 1081
Cipro I.V. (Ciprofloxacin) Bayer Pharmaceutical 595
Cipro I.V. Pharmacy Bulk Package (Ciprofloxacin) Bayer Pharmaceutical 597
Cipro Tablets (Ciprofloxacin Hydrochloride) Bayer Pharmaceutical 592
Claforan Sterile and Injection (Cefotaxime Sodium) Hoechst-Roussel 1235
Geocillin Tablets (Carbenicillin Indanyl Sodium) Roerig 2199
Mefoxin (Cefoxitin Sodium) Merck & Co., Inc. 1691
Mefoxin Premixed Intravenous Solution (Cefoxitin Sodium) Merck & Co., Inc. 1694
Mezlin (Mezlocillin Sodium) Bayer Pharmaceutical 601
Mezlin Pharmacy Bulk Package (Mezlocillin Sodium) Bayer Pharmaceutical 604
Monocid Injection (Cefonicid Sodium) SmithKline Beecham Pharmaceuticals 2497
Primaxin I.V. (Imipenem-Cilastatin Sodium) Merck & Co., Inc. 1729
Rocephin Injectable Vials, ADD-Vantage, Galaxy Container (Ceftriaxone Sodium) Roche Laboratories 2142
Septra (Trimethoprim, Sulfamethoxazole) Glaxo Wellcome 1174
Septra I.V. Infusion (Trimethoprim, Sulfamethoxazole) Glaxo Wellcome 1169
Septra I.V. Infusion ADD-Vantage Vials (Trimethoprim, Sulfamethoxazole) Glaxo Wellcome 1171
Septra (Trimethoprim, Sulfamethoxazole) Glaxo Wellcome 1174
Tazicef for Injection (Ceftazidime) SmithKline Beecham Pharmaceuticals 2519

Morphea, "possibly" effective in
Potaba (Aminobenzoate Potassium) Glenwood 1229

Motion sickness
Antivert, Antivert/25 Tablets, & Antivert/50 Tablets (Meclizine Hydrochloride) Roerig 2185
Benadryl Capsules (Diphenhydramine Hydrochloride) Parke-Davis 1898
Benadryl Injection (Diphenhydramine Hydrochloride) Parke-Davis 1898
Bonine Tablets (Meclizine Hydrochloride) Pfizer Consumer .. 1933
Dramamine Chewable Tablets (Dimenhydrinate) Upjohn ▣ 836
Children's Dramamine Liquid (Dimenhydrinate) Upjohn .... ▣ 836
Dramamine Tablets (Dimenhydrinate) Upjohn .... ▣ 836
Dramamine II Tablets (Meclizine Hydrochloride) Upjohn .... ▣ 837
Phenergan Injection (Promethazine Hydrochloride) Wyeth-Ayerst 2773
Phenergan Suppositories (Promethazine Hydrochloride) Wyeth-Ayerst 2775
Phenergan Syrup (Promethazine Hydrochloride) Wyeth-Ayerst 2774
Phenergan Tablets (Promethazine Hydrochloride) Wyeth-Ayerst 2775
Transderm Scōp Transdermal Therapeutic System (Scopolamine) Ciba Self-Medication 869

Mountain sickness, acute
Diamox Intravenous (Acetazolamide) Lederle 1372
Diamox Sequels (Sustained Release) (Acetazolamide) Lederle 1373
Diamox Tablets (Acetazolamide) Lederle 1372

Mouth, dry
(see under Hyposalivation)

Mucormycosis
(see under Phycomycosis)

Multiple sclerosis, acute exacerbations of
(see under Sclerosis, multiple, acute exacerbations of)

Mumps and rubella immunization
(see under Rubella and mumps, prophylaxis)

Mumps, prophylaxis
M-M-R II (Measles, Mumps & Rubella Virus Vaccine Live) Merck & Co., Inc. 1687
Mumpsvax (Mumps Virus Vaccine, Live) Merck & Co., Inc. 1708

Muscle spasm
(see under Spasticity, muscle, symptomatic alleviation of)

Muscles, skeletal, relaxation, preoperative
Anectine (Succinylcholine Chloride) Glaxo Wellcome 1073
Metubine Iodide Vials (Metocurine Iodide) Dista 916
Mivacron (Mivacurium Chloride) Glaxo Wellcome 1138
Norcuron (Vecuronium Bromide) Organon 1826
Nuromax Injection (Doxacurium Chloride) Glaxo Wellcome 1149
Tracrium Injection (Atracurium Besylate) Glaxo Wellcome 1183
Zemuron (Rocuronium Bromide) Organon 1830

Musculo-skeletal discomfort, adjunct in
Flexeril Tablets (Cyclobenzaprine Hydrochloride) Merck & Co., Inc. 1661
Norflex (Orphenadrine Citrate) 3M Pharmaceuticals 1496
Norgesic (Orphenadrine Citrate, Aspirin) 3M Pharmaceuticals 1496
Paraflex Caplets (Chlorzoxazone) McNeil Pharmaceutical 1580
Parafon Forte DSC Caplets (Chlorzoxazone) McNeil Pharmaceutical 1581
Robaxin Injectable (Methocarbamol) Robins 2070
Robaxin Tablets (Methocarbamol) Robins 2071
Robaxisal Tablets (Methocarbamol, Aspirin) Robins 2071
Skelaxin Tablets (Metaxalone) Carnrick 788
Soma Compound w/Codeine Tablets (Carisoprodol, Aspirin, Codeine Phosphate) Wallace 2676
Soma Compound Tablets (Carisoprodol, Aspirin) Wallace 2675

Myalgia
(see under Pain, muscular, temporary relief of)

Myalgia, topical relief of
(see under Pain, topical relief of)

Myasthenia gravis, differential diagnosis of
Tensilon Injectable (Edrophonium Chloride) ICN 1261

Myasthenia gravis, treatment of
Mestinon Injectable (Pyridostigmine Bromide) ICN 1253
Mestinon (Pyridostigmine Bromide) ICN 1254
Prostigmin Injectable (Neostigmine Methylsulfate) ICN 1260
Prostigmin Tablets (Neostigmine Bromide) ICN 1261
Tensilon Injectable (Edrophonium Chloride) ICN 1261

Mycobacterium avium complex, (MAC) disease, disseminated
Biaxin (Clarithromycin) Abbott 405
Mycobutin Capsules (Rifabutin) Pharmacia 1957

Mycobacterium intracellulare infections
Biaxin (Clarithromycin) Abbott 405

Mycobacterium leprae infections
(see under Leprosy)

Mycobacterium marinum infections
Dynacin Capsules (Minocycline Hydrochloride) Medicis 1590
Minocin Oral Suspension (Minocycline Hydrochloride) Lederle 1385
Minocin Pellet-Filled Capsules (Minocycline Hydrochloride) Lederle 1383

Mycobacterium tuberculosis infection
Capastat Sulfate Vials (Capreomycin Sulfate) Eli Lilly 2868
Streptomycin Sulfate Injection (Streptomycin Sulfate) Roerig 2208
Trecator-SC Tablets (Ethionamide) Wyeth-Ayerst 2814

Mycoplasma pneumoniae infection
Achromycin V Capsules (Tetracycline Hydrochloride) Lederle 1367
Biaxin (Clarithromycin) Abbott 405
Declomycin Tablets (Demeclocycline Hydrochloride) Lederle 1371
Doryx Capsules (Doxycycline Hyclate) Parke-Davis 1913
Dynacin Capsules (Minocycline Hydrochloride) Medicis 1590
E.E.S. (Erythromycin Ethylsuccinate) Abbott 424
E-Mycin Tablets (Erythromycin) Knoll Laboratories 1341
ERYC (Erythromycin) Parke-Davis .. 1915
EryPed (Erythromycin Ethylsuccinate) Abbott 421
Ery-Tab Tablets (Erythromycin) Abbott 422
Erythrocin Stearate Filmtab (Erythromycin Stearate) Abbott 425
Erythromycin Base Filmtab (Erythromycin) Abbott 426
Erythromycin Delayed-Release Capsules, USP (Erythromycin) Abbott 427
Ilosone (Erythromycin Estolate) Dista 911
Ilotycin Gluceptate, IV, Vials (Erythromycin Gluceptate) Dista 913
Minocin Intravenous (Minocycline Hydrochloride) Lederle 1382
Minocin Oral Suspension (Minocycline Hydrochloride) Lederle 1385
Minocin Pellet-Filled Capsules (Minocycline Hydrochloride) Lederle 1383
Monodox Capsules (Doxycycline Monohydrate) Oclassen 1805
PCE Dispertab Tablets (Erythromycin) Abbott 444
Terramycin Intramuscular Solution (Oxytetracycline) Roerig 2210
Vibramycin (Doxycycline Calcium) Pfizer Labs 1941
Vibramycin Hyclate Intravenous (Doxycycline Hyclate) Roerig 2215
Vibramycin (Doxycycline Monohydrate) Pfizer Labs 1941

Mycoplasma pneumoniae respiratory tract infections
Biaxin (Clarithromycin) Abbott 405
Dynacin Capsules (Minocycline Hydrochloride) Medicis 1590
E.E.S. (Erythromycin Ethylsuccinate) Abbott 424
E-Mycin Tablets (Erythromycin) Knoll Laboratories 1341
ERYC (Erythromycin) Parke-Davis .. 1915
EryPed (Erythromycin Ethylsuccinate) Abbott 421
Ery-Tab Tablets (Erythromycin) Abbott 422
Erythrocin Stearate Filmtab (Erythromycin Stearate) Abbott 425
Erythromycin Base Filmtab (Erythromycin) Abbott 426
Erythromycin Delayed-Release Capsules, USP (Erythromycin) Abbott 427
Ilosone (Erythromycin Estolate) Dista 911
Ilotycin Gluceptate, IV, Vials (Erythromycin Gluceptate) Dista 913
Monodox Capsules (Doxycycline Monohydrate) Oclassen 1805
PCE Dispertab Tablets (Erythromycin) Abbott 444

Mycosis fungoides
Aristocort Suspension (Forte Parenteral) (Triamcinolone Diacetate) Fujisawa 1027
Aristocort Tablets (Triamcinolone) Fujisawa 1022
Celestone Soluspan Suspension (Betamethasone Sodium Phos-

Mycosis fungoides Indications Index 1510

phate, Betamethasone Acetate) Schering ... 2347
Cortone Acetate Sterile Suspension (Cortisone Acetate) Merck & Co., Inc. ... 1623
Cortone Acetate Tablets (Cortisone Acetate) Merck & Co., Inc. ... 1624
Cytoxan (Cyclophosphamide) Bristol-Myers Squibb Oncology ... 694
Dalalone D.P. Injectable (Dexamethasone Acetate) Forest ... 1011
Decadron Elixir (Dexamethasone) Merck & Co., Inc. ... 1633
Decadron Phosphate Injection (Dexamethasone Sodium Phosphate) Merck & Co., Inc. ... 1637
Decadron Tablets (Dexamethasone) Merck & Co., Inc. ... 1635
Decadron-LA Sterile Suspension (Dexamethasone Acetate) Merck & Co., Inc. ... 1646
Deltasone Tablets (Prednisone) Upjohn ... 2595
Depo-Medrol Single-Dose Vial (Methylprednisolone Acetate) Upjohn ... 2600
Depo-Medrol Sterile Aqueous Suspension (Methylprednisolone Acetate) Upjohn ... 2597
Hydeltrasol Injection, Sterile (Prednisolone Sodium Phosphate) Merck & Co., Inc. ... 1665
Hydrocortone Phosphate Injection, Sterile (Hydrocortisone Sodium Phosphate) Merck & Co., Inc. ... 1670
Hydrocortone Tablets (Hydrocortisone) Merck & Co., Inc. ... 1672
Medrol (Methylprednisolone) Upjohn ... 2621
Methotrexate Sodium Tablets, Injection, for Injection and LPF Injection (Methotrexate Sodium) Immunex ... 1275
Mustargen (Mechlorethamine Hydrochloride) Merck & Co., Inc. 1709
NEOSAR Lyophilized/Neosar (Cyclophosphamide) Pharmacia .. 1959
Pediapred Oral Liquid (Prednisolone Sodium Phosphate) Fisons ... 995
Prelone Syrup (Prednisolone) Muro 1787
Solu-Cortef Sterile Powder (Hydrocortisone Sodium Succinate) Upjohn ... 2641
Solu-Medrol Sterile Powder (Methylprednisolone Sodium Succinate) Upjohn ... 2643
Velban Vials (Vinblastine Sulfate) Lilly ... 1484

Mydriasis, production of
Atropine Sulfate Sterile Ophthalmic Solution (Atropine Sulfate) Allergan ... ⊙ 233
Neo-Synephrine Hydrochloride (Ophthalmic) (Phenylephrine Hydrochloride) Sanofi Winthrop .. 2325
Paremyd (Hydroxyamphetamine Hydrobromide, Tropicamide) Allergan ... ⊙ 247

Mydriasis, production of, in uveitis
Neo-Synephrine Hydrochloride (Ophthalmic) (Phenylephrine Hydrochloride) Sanofi Winthrop .. 2325

Mydriasis, reversal of
Isopto Carpine Ophthalmic Solution (Pilocarpine Hydrochloride) Alcon Laboratories ... ⊙ 223
Pilagan (Pilocarpine Nitrate) Allergan ... ⊙ 248

Myeloid recovery, acceleration of
Leukine for IV Infusion (Sargramostim) Immunex ... 1271

Myeloma, multiple
Alkeran Tablets (Melphalan) Glaxo Wellcome ... 1071
Cytoxan (Cyclophosphamide) Bristol-Myers Squibb Oncology ... 694
NEOSAR Lyophilized/Neosar (Cyclophosphamide) Pharmacia .. 1959

Myeloma, multiple, adjunct in
Alkeran for Injection (Melphalan Hydrochloride) Glaxo Wellcome ... 1070
BiCNU (Carmustine (BCNU)) Bristol-Myers Squibb Oncology ... 691

Myocardial infarction, acute
Activase (Alteplase, Recombinant) Genentech ... 1058
Eminase (Anistreplase) Roberts ... 2039
Streptase for Infusion (Streptokinase) Astra ... 562

Myocardial infarction, post, left ventricular dysfunction
Capoten (Captopril) Bristol-Myers Squibb ... 739

Myocardial infarction, treatment adjunct
Altace Capsules (Ramipril) Hoechst-Roussel ... 1232

Myocardial perfusion imaging, thallium, adjunct in
Adenoscan (Adenosine) Fujisawa ... 1024

Myocardial reinfarction, prophylaxis
Alka-Seltzer Effervescent Antacid and Pain Reliever (Aspirin, Sodium Bicarbonate, Citric Acid) Miles Consumer ... ⊡ 701
Alka-Seltzer Lemon Lime Effervescent Antacid and Pain Reliever (Aspirin, Sodium Citrate) Miles Consumer ... ⊡ 703
Regular Strength Ascriptin Tablets (Aspirin Buffered, Calcium Carbonate) CIBA Consumer ... ⊡ 629
Genuine Bayer Aspirin Tablets & Caplets (Aspirin) Miles Consumer ... ⊡ 713
Bayer Enteric Aspirin (Aspirin, Enteric Coated) Miles Consumer ... ⊡ 709
Blocadren Tablets (Timolol Maleate) Merck & Co., Inc. ... 1614
Bufferin Analgesic Tablets and Caplets (Aspirin) Bristol-Myers Products ... ⊡ 613
Ecotrin (Aspirin, Enteric Coated) SmithKline Beecham ... 2455
Halfprin (Aspirin) Kramer ... 1362
Inderal (Propranolol Hydrochloride) Wyeth-Ayerst ... 2728
Lopressor Tablets (Metoprolol Tartrate) CibaGeneva ... 830
St. Joseph Adult Chewable Aspirin (81 mg.) (Aspirin) Schering-Plough HealthCare ... ⊡ 808
Tenormin Tablets and I.V. Injection (Atenolol) Zeneca ... 2847

Myxedema (see under Hypothyroidism, replacement or supplemental therapy in)

Myxedema coma/precoma (see also under Hypothyroidism, replacement or supplemental therapy in)
Triostat Injection (Liothyronine Sodium) SmithKline Beecham Pharmaceuticals ... 2530

N

N. gonorrhoeae endocervical infections
Cefizox for Intramuscular or Intravenous Use (Ceftizoxime Sodium) Fujisawa ... 1034
Ceftin (Cefuroxime Axetil) Glaxo Wellcome ... 1078
Cipro Tablets (Ciprofloxacin Hydrochloride) Bayer Pharmaceutical ... 592
Noroxin Tablets (Norfloxacin) Merck & Co., Inc. ... 1715
Noroxin Tablets (Norfloxacin) Roberts ... 2048
Rocephin Injectable Vials, ADD-Vantage, Galaxy Container (Ceftriaxone Sodium) Roche Laboratories ... 2142
Trobicin Sterile Powder (Spectinomycin Hydrochloride) Upjohn ... 2645
Vantin for Oral Suspension and Vantin Tablets (Cefpodoxime Proxetil) Upjohn ... 2646
Zefazone (Cefmetazole Sodium) Upjohn ... 2654

N. gonorrhoeae epididymo-orchitis, acute
Doryx Capsules (Doxycycline Hyclate) Parke-Davis ... 1913
Monodox Capsules (Doxycycline Monohydrate) Oclassen ... 1805

N. gonorrhoeae gynecologic infections
Cefizox for Intramuscular or Intravenous Use (Ceftizoxime Sodium) Fujisawa ... 1034
Cefobid Intravenous/Intramuscular (Cefoperazone Sodium) Roerig ... 2189
Cefobid Pharmacy Bulk Package - Not for Direct Infusion (Cefoperazone Sodium) Roerig ... 2192
Cefotan (Cefotetan) Zeneca ... 2829
Dynacin Capsules (Minocycline Hydrochloride) Medicis ... 1590
Erythrocin Stearate Filmtab (Erythromycin Stearate) Abbott ... 425
Erythromycin Base Filmtab (Erythromycin) Abbott ... 426
Erythromycin Delayed-Release Capsules, USP (Erythromycin) Abbott ... 427
Floxin I.V. (Ofloxacin) McNeil Pharmaceutical ... 1571
Floxin Tablets (200 mg, 300 mg, 400 mg) (Ofloxacin) McNeil Pharmaceutical ... 1567
Mefoxin (Cefoxitin Sodium) Merck & Co., Inc. ... 1691
Mefoxin Premixed Intravenous Solution (Cefoxitin Sodium) Merck & Co., Inc. ... 1694
Mezlin (Mezlocillin Sodium) Bayer Pharmaceutical ... 601
Mezlin Pharmacy Bulk Package (Mezlocillin Sodium) Bayer Pharmaceutical ... 604
Minocin Pellet-Filled Capsules (Minocycline Hydrochloride) Lederle ... 1383
Noroxin Tablets (Norfloxacin) Merck & Co., Inc. ... 1715
Noroxin Tablets (Norfloxacin) Roberts ... 2048
PCE Dispertab Tablets (Erythromycin) Abbott ... 444
Trobicin Sterile Powder (Spectinomycin Hydrochloride) Upjohn ... 2645

N. gonorrhoeae infections
Achromycin V Capsules (Tetracycline Hydrochloride) Lederle ... 1367
Amoxil (Amoxicillin Trihydrate) SmithKline Beecham Pharmaceuticals ... 2464
Cefizox for Intramuscular or Intravenous Use (Ceftizoxime Sodium) Fujisawa ... 1034
Cefobid Intravenous/Intramuscular (Cefoperazone Sodium) Roerig ... 2189
Cefobid Pharmacy Bulk Package - Not for Direct Infusion (Cefoperazone Sodium) Roerig ... 2192
Cefotan (Cefotetan) Zeneca ... 2829
Ceftin (Cefuroxime Axetil) Glaxo Wellcome ... 1078
Ceptaz (Ceftazidime) Glaxo Wellcome ... 1081
Cipro Tablets (Ciprofloxacin Hydrochloride) Bayer Pharmaceutical ... 592
Claforan Sterile and Injection (Cefotaxime Sodium) Hoechst-Roussel ... 1235
Declomycin Tablets (Demeclocycline Hydrochloride) Lederle ... 1371
Dynacin Capsules (Minocycline Hydrochloride) Medicis ... 1590
E-Mycin Tablets (Erythromycin) Knoll Laboratories ... 1341
ERYC (Erythromycin) Parke-Davis .. 1915
Ery-Tab Tablets (Erythromycin) Abbott ... 422
Erythrocin Stearate Filmtab (Erythromycin Stearate) Abbott ... 425
Erythromycin Base Filmtab (Erythromycin) Abbott ... 426
Erythromycin Delayed-Release Capsules, USP (Erythromycin) Abbott ... 427
Floxin I.V. (Ofloxacin) McNeil Pharmaceutical ... 1571
Floxin Tablets (200 mg, 300 mg, 400 mg) (Ofloxacin) McNeil Pharmaceutical ... 1567
Fortaz (Ceftazidime) Glaxo Wellcome ... 1100
Ilotycin Gluceptate, IV, Vials (Erythromycin Gluceptate) Dista ... 913
Kefurox Vials, Faspak & ADD-Vantage (Cefuroxime Sodium) Lilly ... 1454
Mefoxin (Cefoxitin Sodium) Merck & Co., Inc. ... 1691
Mefoxin Premixed Intravenous Solution (Cefoxitin Sodium) Merck & Co., Inc. ... 1694
Mezlin (Mezlocillin Sodium) Bayer Pharmaceutical ... 601
Mezlin Pharmacy Bulk Package (Mezlocillin Sodium) Bayer Pharmaceutical ... 604
Minocin Intravenous (Minocycline Hydrochloride) Lederle ... 1382
Minocin Oral Suspension (Minocycline Hydrochloride) Lederle ... 1385
Minocin Pellet-Filled Capsules (Minocycline Hydrochloride) Lederle ... 1383
Monodox Capsules (Doxycycline Monohydrate) Oclassen ... 1805
Noroxin Tablets (Norfloxacin) Merck & Co., Inc. ... 1715
Noroxin Tablets (Norfloxacin) Roberts ... 2048
Omnipen Capsules (Ampicillin) Wyeth-Ayerst ... 2764
Omnipen for Oral Suspension (Ampicillin) Wyeth-Ayerst ... 2765
PCE Dispertab Tablets (Erythromycin) Abbott ... 444
Penetrex Tablets (Enoxacin) Rhone-Poulenc Rorer Pharmaceuticals ... 2031
Pfizerpen for Injection (Penicillin G Potassium) Roerig ... 2203
Pipracil (Piperacillin Sodium) Lederle ... 1390
Rocephin Injectable Vials, ADD-Vantage, Galaxy Container (Ceftriaxone Sodium) Roche Laboratories ... 2142
Spectrobid Tablets (Bacampicillin Hydrochloride) Roerig ... 2206
Suprax Tablets (Cefixime) Lederle .. 1399
Tazicef for Injection (Ceftazidime) SmithKline Beecham Pharmaceuticals ... 2519
Tazidime Vials, Faspak & ADD-Vantage (Ceftazidime) Lilly .. 1478
Terramycin Intramuscular Solution (Oxytetracycline) Roerig ... 2210
Trobicin Sterile Powder (Spectinomycin Hydrochloride) Upjohn ... 2645
Vantin for Oral Suspension and Vantin Tablets (Cefpodoxime Proxetil) Upjohn ... 2646
Vibramycin (Doxycycline Calcium) Pfizer Labs ... 1941
Vibramycin Hyclate Intravenous (Doxycycline Hyclate) Roerig ... 2215
Vibramycin (Doxycycline Monohydrate) Pfizer Labs ... 1941
Zefazone (Cefmetazole Sodium) Upjohn ... 2654
Zinacef (Cefuroxime Sodium) Glaxo Wellcome ... 1211

N. gonorrhoeae infections, ocular
Genoptic Sterile Ophthalmic Solution (Gentamicin Sulfate) Allergan ... ⊙ 243
Genoptic Sterile Ophthalmic Ointment (Gentamicin Sulfate) Allergan ... ⊙ 243
Gentak (Gentamicin Sulfate) Akorn ... ⊙ 208
Ilotycin Ophthalmic Ointment (Erythromycin) Dista ... 912
Pred-G Liquifilm Sterile Ophthalmic Suspension (Gentamicin Sulfate, Prednisolone Acetate) Allergan ... ⊙ 251
Pred-G S.O.P. Sterile Ophthalmic Ointment (Gentamicin Sulfate, Prednisolone Acetate) Allergan.. ⊙ 252

N. gonorrhoeae neonatal ophthalmia, prophylaxis of
Ilotycin Ophthalmic Ointment (Erythromycin) Dista ... 912

N. gonorrhoeae pelvic inflammatory disease
Cefobid Intravenous/Intramuscular (Cefoperazone Sodium) Roerig ... 2189

(⊡ Described in PDR For Nonprescription Drugs) (⊙ Described in PDR For Ophthalmology)

1511 **Indications Index** **Nasal congestion**

Cefobid Pharmacy Bulk Package - Not for Direct Infusion (Cefoperazone Sodium) Roerig ... 2192
ERYC (Erythromycin) Parke-Davis .. 1915
Ery-Tab Tablets (Erythromycin) Abbott ... 422
Mefoxin (Cefoxitin Sodium) Merck & Co., Inc. ... 1691
Mefoxin Premixed Intravenous Solution (Cefoxitin Sodium) Merck & Co., Inc. ... 1694
Mezlin (Mezlocillin Sodium) Bayer Pharmaceutical ... 601
Mezlin Pharmacy Bulk Package (Mezlocillin Sodium) Bayer Pharmaceutical ... 604
Rocephin Injectable Vials, ADD-Vantage, Galaxy Container (Ceftriaxone Sodium) Roche Laboratories ... 2142

N. gonorrhoeae pharyngeal infections
Rocephin Injectable Vials, ADD-Vantage, Galaxy Container (Ceftriaxone Sodium) Roche Laboratories ... 2142

N. gonorrhoeae rectal infections
Rocephin Injectable Vials, ADD-Vantage, Galaxy Container (Ceftriaxone Sodium) Roche Laboratories ... 2142
Trobicin Sterile Powder (Spectinomycin Hydrochloride) Upjohn ... 2645
Vantin for Oral Suspension and Vantin Tablets (Cefpodoxime Proxetil) Upjohn ... 2646
Zefazone (Cefmetazole Sodium) Upjohn ... 2654

N. gonorrhoeae urethral infections
Cefizox for Intramuscular or Intravenous Use (Ceftizoxime Sodium) Fujisawa ... 1034
Ceftin (Cefuroxime Axetil) Glaxo Wellcome ... 1078
Cipro Tablets (Ciprofloxacin Hydrochloride) Bayer Pharmaceutical ... 592
Dynacin Capsules (Minocycline Hydrochloride) Medicis ... 1590
Floxin I.V. (Ofloxacin) McNeil Pharmaceutical ... 1571
Minocin Oral Suspension (Minocycline Hydrochloride) Lederle ... 1385
Noroxin Tablets (Norfloxacin) Merck & Co., Inc. ... 1715
Noroxin Tablets (Norfloxacin) Roberts ... 2048
Rocephin Injectable Vials, ADD-Vantage, Galaxy Container (Ceftriaxone Sodium) Roche Laboratories ... 2142
Trobicin Sterile Powder (Spectinomycin Hydrochloride) Upjohn ... 2645
Vantin for Oral Suspension and Vantin Tablets (Cefpodoxime Proxetil) Upjohn ... 2646
Zefazone (Cefmetazole Sodium) Upjohn ... 2654

N. gonorrhoeae urinary tract infections
Claforan Sterile and Injection (Cefotaxime Sodium) Hoechst-Roussel ... 1235
Kefurox Vials, Faspak & ADD-Vantage (Cefuroxime Sodium) Lilly ... 1454
Mefoxin (Cefoxitin Sodium) Merck & Co., Inc. ... 1691
Mefoxin Premixed Intravenous Solution (Cefoxitin Sodium) Merck & Co., Inc. ... 1694
Spectrobid Tablets (Bacampicillin Hydrochloride) Roerig ... 2206

N. meningitidis central nervous system infections
Claforan Sterile and Injection (Cefotaxime Sodium) Hoechst-Roussel ... 1235
Tazicef for Injection (Ceftazidime) SmithKline Beecham Pharmaceuticals ... 2519

N. meningitidis infections
Ceptaz (Ceftazidime) Glaxo Wellcome ... 1081
Claforan Sterile and Injection (Cefotaxime Sodium) Hoechst-Roussel ... 1235
Fortaz (Ceftazidime) Glaxo Wellcome ... 1100
Minocin Intravenous (Minocycline Hydrochloride) Lederle ... 1382
Minocin Oral Suspension (Minocycline Hydrochloride) Lederle ... 1385
Minocin Pellet-Filled Capsules (Minocycline Hydrochloride) Lederle ... 1383
Omnipen for Oral Suspension (Ampicillin) Wyeth-Ayerst ... 2765
Rocephin Injectable Vials, ADD-Vantage, Galaxy Container (Ceftriaxone Sodium) Roche Laboratories ... 2142
Tazicef for Injection (Ceftazidime) SmithKline Beecham Pharmaceuticals ... 2519
Tazidime Vials, Faspak & ADD-Vantage (Ceftazidime) Lilly .. 1478
Vibramycin Hyclate Intravenous (Doxycycline Hyclate) Roerig ... 2215
Zinacef (Cefuroxime Sodium) Glaxo Wellcome ... 1211

N. meningitidis meningitis
Ceptaz (Ceftazidime) Glaxo Wellcome ... 1081
Fortaz (Ceftazidime) Glaxo Wellcome ... 1100
Kefurox Vials, Faspak & ADD-Vantage (Cefuroxime Sodium) Lilly ... 1454
Omnipen for Oral Suspension (Ampicillin) Wyeth-Ayerst ... 2765
Rocephin Injectable Vials, ADD-Vantage, Galaxy Container (Ceftriaxone Sodium) Roche Laboratories ... 2142
Tazicef for Injection (Ceftazidime) SmithKline Beecham Pharmaceuticals ... 2519
Tazidime Vials, Faspak & ADD-Vantage (Ceftazidime) Lilly .. 1478
Zinacef (Cefuroxime Sodium) Glaxo Wellcome ... 1211

N. meningitidis, asymptomatic carriers of
Rifadin (Rifampin) Marion Merrell Dow ... 1528
Rimactane Capsules (Rifampin) CibaGeneva ... 847

Narcolepsy
Dexedrine (Dextroamphetamine Sulfate) SmithKline Beecham Pharmaceuticals ... 2474
DextroStat Dextroamphetamine Tablets (Dextroamphetamine Sulfate) Richwood ... 2036
Ritalin (Methylphenidate Hydrochloride) CibaGeneva ... 848

Narcotic addiction, detoxification treatment of
Methadone Hydrochloride Oral Concentrate (Methadone Hydrochloride) Roxane ... 2233
Methadone Hydrochloride Oral Solution & Tablets (Methadone Hydrochloride) Roxane ... 2235
Orlamm (Levomethadyl Acetate Hydrochloride) Roxane ... 2239

Narcotic addiction, maintenance therapy for
Methadone Hydrochloride Oral Concentrate (Methadone Hydrochloride) Roxane ... 2233
Methadone Hydrochloride Oral Solution & Tablets (Methadone Hydrochloride) Roxane ... 2235
Orlamm (Levomethadyl Acetate Hydrochloride) Roxane ... 2239

Nasal congestion, symptomatic relief of
Actifed Plus Caplets (Acetaminophen, Pseudoephedrine Hydrochloride, Triprolidine Hydrochloride) WARNER WELLCOME ... ▣ 845
Actifed Plus Tablets (Acetaminophen, Pseudoephedrine Hydrochloride, Triprolidine Hydrochloride) WARNER WELLCOME ... ▣ 845
Actifed Syrup (Pseudoephedrine Hydrochloride, Triprolidine Hydrochloride) WARNER WELLCOME ... ▣ 846
Actifed Tablets (Pseudoephedrine Hydrochloride, Triprolidine Hydrochloride) WARNER WELLCOME ... ▣ 844
Afrin (Oxymetazoline Hydrochloride) Schering-Plough HealthCare ... ▣ 797
Alka Seltzer Plus Sinus Medicine (Phenylpropanolamine Bitartrate, Aspirin, Brompheniramine Maleate) Miles Consumer.. ▣ 707
Allerest Children's Chewable Tablets (Chlorpheniramine Maleate, Phenylpropanolamine Hydrochloride) CIBA Consumer ▣ 627
Allerest Headache Strength Tablets (Acetaminophen, Chlorpheniramine Maleate, Pseudoephedrine Hydrochloride) CIBA Consumer ... ▣ 627
Allerest Maximum Strength Tablets (Chlorpheniramine Maleate, Pseudoephedrine Hydrochloride) CIBA Consumer ▣ 627
Allerest No Drowsiness Tablets (Acetaminophen, Pseudoephedrine Hydrochloride) CIBA Consumer ... ▣ 627
Allerest Sinus Pain Formula (Acetaminophen, Chlorpheniramine Maleate, Pseudoephedrine Hydrochloride) CIBA Consumer ▣ 627
Allerest 12 Hour Caplets (Chlorpheniramine Maleate, Phenylpropanolamine Hydrochloride) CIBA Consumer ... ▣ 627
Atrohist Pediatric Suspension (Chlorpheniramine Tannate, Phenylephrine Tannate, Pyrilamine Tannate) Adams ... 454
Atrohist Plus Tablets (Chlorpheniramine Maleate, Phenylpropanolamine Hydrochloride, Phenylephrine Hydrochloride, Hyoscyamine Sulfate, Atropine Sulfate, Scopolamine Hydrobromide) Adams ... 454
BC Cold Powder Multi-Symptom Formula (Cold-Sinus-Allergy) (Aspirin, Phenylpropanolamine Hydrochloride, Chlorpheniramine Maleate) Block ... ▣ 609
BC Cold Powder Non-Drowsy Formula (Cold-Sinus) (Aspirin, Phenylpropanolamine Hydrochloride) Block ... ▣ 609
Bayer Select Sinus Pain Relief Formula (Acetaminophen, Pseudoephedrine Hydrochloride) Miles Consumer ▣ 717
Benadryl Allergy Decongestant Liquid Medication (Diphenhydramine Hydrochloride, Pseudoephedrine Hydrochloride) WARNER WELLCOME ... ▣ 848
Benadryl Allergy Decongestant Tablets (Diphenhydramine Hydrochloride, Pseudoephedrine Hydrochloride) WARNER WELLCOME ... ▣ 848
Benadryl Allergy Sinus Headache Formula Caplets (Diphenhydramine Hydrochloride, Pseudoephedrine Hydrochloride, Acetaminophen) WARNER WELLCOME ... ▣ 849
Bromfed (Brompheniramine Maleate, Pseudoephedrine Hydrochloride) Muro ... 1785
Cheracol Nasal Spray Pump (Oxymetazoline Hydrochloride) Roberts ... ▣ 768
Cheracol Sinus (Dexbrompheniramine Maleate, Pseudoephedrine Sulfate) Roberts ... ▣ 768
Chlor-Trimeton Allergy Decongestant Tablets (Chlorpheniramine Maleate, Pseudoephedrine Sulfate) Schering-Plough HealthCare ... ▣ 799
Comhist (Chlorpheniramine Maleate, Phenyltoloxamine Citrate, Phenylephrine Hydrochloride) Roberts ... 2038
Allergy-Sinus Comtrex Multi-Symptom Allergy-Sinus Formula Tablets (Acetaminophen, Chlorpheniramine Maleate, Pseudoephedrine Hydrochloride) Bristol-Myers Products ... ▣ 617
Congess (Guaifenesin, Pseudoephedrine Hydrochloride) Fleming ... 1004
Contac Continuous Action Nasal Decongestant/Antihistamine 12 Hour Capsules (Chlorpheniramine Maleate, Phenylpropanolamine Hydrochloride) SmithKline Beecham Consumer ▣ 813
Contac Maximum Strength Continuous Action Decongestant/Antihistamine 12 Hour Caplets (Chlorpheniramine Maleate, Phenylpropanolamine Hydrochloride) SmithKline Beecham Consumer ▣ 813
Coricidin 'D' Decongestant Tablets (Acetaminophen, Chlorpheniramine Maleate, Phenylpropanolamine Hydrochloride) Schering-Plough HealthCare ... ▣ 800
Deconamine (Chlorpheniramine Maleate, Pseudoephedrine Hydrochloride) Kenwood ... 1320
Deconsal (Guaifenesin, Phenylephrine Hydrochloride) Adams ... 454
Dimetapp Elixir (Brompheniramine Maleate, Phenylpropanolamine Hydrochloride) A. H. Robins Consumer ... ▣ 773
Dimetapp Extentabs (Brompheniramine Maleate, Phenylpropanolamine Hydrochloride) A. H. Robins Consumer ... ▣ 774
Dimetapp Tablets (Brompheniramine Maleate, Phenylpropanolamine Hydrochloride) A. H. Robins Consumer ... ▣ 775
Drixoral Cold and Allergy Sustained-Action Tablets (Dexbrompheniramine Maleate, Pseudoephedrine Sulfate) Schering-Plough HealthCare ... ▣ 802
Drixoral Cold and Flu Extended-Release Tablets (Acetaminophen, Dexbrompheniramine Maleate, Pseudoephedrine Sulfate) Schering-Plough HealthCare ... ▣ 803
Drixoral Non-Drowsy Formula Extended-Release Tablets (Pseudoephedrine Sulfate) Schering-Plough HealthCare ... ▣ 803
Drixoral Allergy/Sinus Extended Release Tablets (Acetaminophen, Pseudoephedrine Sulfate, Dexbrompheniramine Maleate) Schering-Plough HealthCare ... ▣ 804
Duration 12 Hour Nasal Spray (Oxymetazoline Hydrochloride) Schering-Plough HealthCare ... ▣ 805
Duratuss Tablets (Pseudoephedrine Hydrochloride, Guaifenesin) UCB ... 2565
Dura-Vent Tablets (Phenylpropanolamine Hydrochloride, Guaifenesin) Dura ... 952
Efidac/24 (Pseudoephedrine Hydrochloride) CIBA Consumer ▣ 635
Entex PSE Tablets (Pseudoephedrine Hydrochloride, Guaifenesin) Procter & Gamble Pharmaceuticals ... 1987
Exgest LA Tablets (Phenylpropanolamine Hydrochloride, Guaifenesin) Carnrick ... 782
4-Way Fast Acting Nasal Spray (regular & mentholated) (Naphazoline Hydrochloride, Phenylephrine Hydrochloride, Pyrilamine Maleate) Bristol-Myers Products ... ▣ 621
Fedahist Gyrocaps (Pseudoephedrine Hydrochloride, Chlorpheniramine Maleate) Schwarz ... 2401
Fedahist Timecaps (Pseudoephedrine Hydrochloride, Chlorpheniramine Maleate) Schwarz ... 2401
Guaimax-D Tablets (Pseudoephedrine Hydrochloride, Guaifenesin) Central ... 792
Guaitab Tablets (Pseudoephedrine Hydrochloride, Guaifenesin) Muro ... ▣ 734
Isoclor Timesule Capsules (Phenylpropanolamine Hydrochloride,

(▣ Described in PDR For Nonprescription Drugs) (⊙ Described in PDR For Ophthalmology)

Nasal congestion — Indications Index — 1512

Chlorpheniramine Maleate) CIBA Consumer ▣ 637
Kronofed-A (Chlorpheniramine Maleate, Pseudoephedrine Hydrochloride) Ferndale 977
NTZ Long Acting Nasal Spray & Drops 0.05% (Oxymetazoline Hydrochloride) Miles Consumer ▣ 727
Neo-Synephrine Maximum Strength 12 Hour Nasal Spray (Oxymetazoline Hydrochloride) Miles Consumer ▣ 726
Neo-Synephrine 12 Hour (Oxymetazoline Hydrochloride) Miles Consumer ▣ 726
Neo-Synephrine (Phenylephrine Hydrochloride) Miles Consumer ▣ 726
Nolamine Timed-Release Tablets (Phenindamine Tartrate, Phenylpropanolamine Hydrochloride, Chlorpheniramine Maleate) Carnrick 785
Nōstril (Phenylephrine Hydrochloride) CIBA Consumer ▣ 644
Nōstrilla Long Acting Nasal Decongestant (Oxymetazoline Hydrochloride) CIBA Consumer ▣ 644
Novahistine Elixir (Chlorpheniramine Maleate, Phenylephrine Hydrochloride) SmithKline Beecham Consumer ▣ 823
Ornade Spansule Capsules (Phenylpropanolamine Hydrochloride, Chlorpheniramine Maleate) SmithKline Beecham Pharmaceuticals 2502
Otrivin (Xylometazoline Hydrochloride) CIBA Consumer ▣ 645
PediaCare Cold Allergy Chewable Tablets (Pseudoephedrine Hydrochloride, Chlorpheniramine Maleate) McNeil Consumer ▣ 677
PediaCare Infants Drops Decongestant (Pseudoephedrine Hydrochloride) McNeil Consumer 1553
Ponaris Nasal Mucosal Emollient (Oil Based Products, Iodine Preparations) Jamol ▣ 658
Privine (Naphazoline Hydrochloride) CIBA Consumer ▣ 647
Propagest Tablets (Phenylpropanolamine Hydrochloride) Carnrick 786
Ricobid-D Pediatric Suspension (Phenylephrine Tannate) Rico Pharmacal 2038
Ricobid Tablets and Pediatric Suspension (Chlorpheniramine Tannate, Phenylephrine Tannate) Rico Pharmacal 2038
Robitussin Pediatric Cough & Cold Formula (Dextromethorphan Hydrobromide, Pseudoephedrine Hydrochloride) A. H. Robins Consumer ▣ 779
Robitussin Severe Congestion Liqui-Gels (Guaifenesin, Pseudoephedrine Hydrochloride) A. H. Robins Consumer ▣ 776
Robitussin-PE (Guaifenesin, Pseudoephedrine Hydrochloride) A. H. Robins Consumer ▣ 778
Ryna Liquid (Chlorpheniramine Maleate, Pseudoephedrine Hydrochloride) Wallace ▣ 841
Rynatan (Chlorpheniramine Tannate, Pyrilamine Tannate, Phenylephrine Tannate) Wallace 2673
Salinex Nasal Mist and Drops (Sodium Chloride) Muro ▣ 734
Seldane-D Extended-Release Tablets (Pseudoephedrine Hydrochloride, Terfenadine) Marion Merrell Dow 1538
Semprex-D Capsules (Acrivastine, Pseudoephedrine Hydrochloride) Adams 463
Semprex-D Capsules (Acrivastine, Pseudoephedrine Hydrochloride) Glaxo Wellcome 1167
Sine-Aid IB Caplets (Ibuprofen, Pseudoephedrine Hydrochloride) McNeil Consumer 1554
Sine-Off No Drowsiness Formula Caplets (Acetaminophen, Pseudoephedrine Hydrochloride) SmithKline Beecham Consumer ▣ 824
Singlet Tablets (Acetaminophen, Chlorpheniramine Maleate, Pseudoephedrine Hydrochloride) SmithKline Beecham Consumer ▣ 825
Sinulin Tablets (Acetaminophen, Phenylpropanolamine Hydrochloride, Chlorpheniramine Maleate) Carnrick 787
Sinutab Sinus Allergy Medication, Maximum Strength Tablets and Caplets (Acetaminophen, Chlorpheniramine Maleate, Pseudoephedrine Hydrochloride) WARNER WELLCOME ▣ 860
Sinutab Sinus Medication, Maximum Strength Without Drowsiness Formula, Tablets & Caplets (Acetaminophen, Pseudoephedrine Hydrochloride) WARNER WELLCOME ▣ 860
Sinutab Sinus Medication, Regular Strength Without Drowsiness Formula (Acetaminophen, Pseudoephedrine Hydrochloride) WARNER WELLCOME ▣ 859
Sudafed Children's Liquid (Pseudoephedrine Hydrochloride) WARNER WELLCOME ▣ 861
Sudafed Plus Liquid (Chlorpheniramine Maleate, Pseudoephedrine Hydrochloride) WARNER WELLCOME ▣ 862
Sudafed Plus Tablets (Chlorpheniramine Maleate, Pseudoephedrine Hydrochloride) WARNER WELLCOME ▣ 863
Sudafed Sinus Caplets (Acetaminophen, Pseudoephedrine Hydrochloride) WARNER WELLCOME ▣ 864
Sudafed Sinus Tablets (Acetaminophen, Pseudoephedrine Hydrochloride) WARNER WELLCOME ▣ 864
Sudafed Tablets, 30 mg (Pseudoephedrine Hydrochloride) WARNER WELLCOME ▣ 861
Sudafed Tablets, 60 mg (Pseudoephedrine Hydrochloride) WARNER WELLCOME ▣ 861
Sudafed 12 Hour Caplets (Pseudoephedrine Hydrochloride) WARNER WELLCOME ▣ 861
Syn-Rx Tablets (Pseudoephedrine Hydrochloride, Guaifenesin) Adams 465
Tavist-D 12 Hour Relief Tablets (Clemastine Fumarate, Phenylpropanolamine Hydrochloride) Sandoz Consumer ▣ 787
Teldrin 12 Hour Antihistamine/Nasal Decongestant Allergy Relief Capsules (Chlorpheniramine Maleate, Phenylpropanolamine Hydrochloride) SmithKline Beecham Consumer ▣ 826
Triaminic Allergy Tablets (Chlorpheniramine Maleate, Phenylpropanolamine Hydrochloride) Sandoz Consumer ▣ 789
Triaminic AM Decongestant Formula (Pseudoephedrine Hydrochloride) Sandoz Consumer ▣ 790
Triaminic Cold Tablets (Phenylpropanolamine Hydrochloride, Chlorpheniramine Maleate) Sandoz Consumer ▣ 790
Triaminic-12 Tablets (Phenylpropanolamine Hydrochloride, Chlorpheniramine Maleate) Sandoz Consumer ▣ 792
Triaminicin Tablets (Acetaminophen, Chlorpheniramine Maleate, Phenylpropanolamine Hydrochloride) Sandoz Consumer ▣ 793
Triaminicol Multi-Symptom Cold Tablets (Phenylpropanolamine Hydrochloride, Chlorpheniramine Maleate, Dextromethorphan Hydrobromide) Sandoz Consumer ▣ 793
Triaminicol Multi-Symptom Relief (Phenylpropanolamine Hydrochloride, Chlorpheniramine Maleate, Dextromethorphan Hydrobromide) Sandoz Consumer ▣ 794
Trinalin Repetabs Tablets (Azatadine Maleate, Pseudoephedrine Sulfate) Key 1330
Infants' TYLENOL Cold Decongestant & Fever-Reducer Drops (Acetaminophen, Pseudoephedrine Hydrochloride) McNeil Consumer 1556
TYLENOL Maximum Strength Allergy Sinus Medication Gelcaps and Caplets (Acetaminophen, Chlorpheniramine Maleate, Pseudoephedrine Hydrochloride) McNeil Consumer 1563
Ursinus Inlay-Tabs (Aspirin, Pseudoephedrine Hydrochloride) Sandoz Consumer ▣ 794
Vicks DayQuil Allergy Relief 12-Hour Extended Release Tablets (Phenylpropanolamine Hydrochloride, Brompheniramine Maleate) Procter & Gamble ▣ 760
Vicks DayQuil Allergy Relief 4-Hour Tablets (Phenylpropanolamine Hydrochloride, Brompheniramine Maleate) Procter & Gamble ▣ 760
Vicks DayQuil SINUS Pressure & CONGESTION Relief (Guaifenesin, Phenylpropanolamine Hydrochloride) Procter & Gamble ▣ 761
Vicks DayQuil SINUS Pressure & PAIN Relief with IBUPROFEN (Ibuprofen, Pseudoephedrine Hydrochloride) Procter & Gamble ▣ 762
Vicks Sinex 12-Hour Nasal Decongestant Spray and Ultra Fine Mist (Oxymetazoline Hydrochloride) Procter & Gamble ▣ 765
Vicks Sinex Nasal Spray and Ultra Fine Mist (Phenylephrine Hydrochloride) Procter & Gamble ▣ 765
Vicks Vapor Inhaler (Desoxyephedrine-Levo) Procter & Gamble ▣ 765

Nasal irritation, symptomatic relief of

Afrin Saline Mist (Sodium Chloride) Schering-Plough HealthCare ▣ 798
Atrohist Plus Tablets (Chlorpheniramine Maleate, Phenylpropanolamine Hydrochloride, Phenylephrine Hydrochloride, Hyoscyamine Sulfate, Atropine Sulfate, Scopolamine Hydrobromide) Adams 454
Ryna-CX Liquid (Codeine Phosphate, Guaifenesin, Pseudoephedrine Hydrochloride) Wallace ▣ 841
Salinex Nasal Mist and Drops (Sodium Chloride) Muro ▣ 734

Nausea (see also under Motion sickness)

Emetrol (Dextrose, Phosphoric Acid, Levulose) Bock Pharmacal ▣ 612
Tigan (Trimethobenzamide Hydrochloride) Roberts 2057
Torecan (Thiethylperazine Malate) Roxane 2245
Vistaril Intramuscular Solution (Hydroxyzine Hydrochloride) Roerig 2216
Vontrol Tablets (Diphenidol) SmithKline Beecham Pharmaceuticals 2532

Nausea, emetogenic, cancer chemotherapy-induced

Kytril Injection (Granisetron Hydrochloride) SmithKline Beecham Pharmaceuticals 2490
Kytril Tablets (Granisetron Hydrochloride) SmithKline Beecham Pharmaceuticals 2492
Marinol (Dronabinol) Capsules (Dronabinol) Roxane 2231
Reglan (Metoclopramide Hydrochloride) Robins 2068
Zofran Injection (Ondansetron Hydrochloride) Glaxo Wellcome 1214
Zofran Tablets (Ondansetron Hydrochloride) Glaxo Wellcome 1217

Nausea, emetogenic, radiation therapy-induced

Zofran Tablets (Ondansetron Hydrochloride) Glaxo Wellcome 1217

Nausea, postoperative

Emete-con Intramuscular/Intravenous (Benzquinamide Hydrochloride) Roerig 2198
Phenergan Injection (Promethazine Hydrochloride) Wyeth-Ayerst 2773
Phenergan Suppositories (Promethazine Hydrochloride) Wyeth-Ayerst 2775
Phenergan Syrup (Promethazine Hydrochloride) Wyeth-Ayerst 2774
Phenergan Tablets (Promethazine Hydrochloride) Wyeth-Ayerst 2775
Reglan (Metoclopramide Hydrochloride) Robins 2068
Zofran Injection (Ondansetron Hydrochloride) Glaxo Wellcome 1214
Zofran Tablets (Ondansetron Hydrochloride) Glaxo Wellcome 1217

Nausea, severe, control of

Compazine (Prochlorperazine) SmithKline Beecham Pharmaceuticals 2470
Thorazine (Chlorpromazine Hydrochloride) SmithKline Beecham Pharmaceuticals 2523
Trilafon (Perphenazine) Schering 2389

Necator americanus infections

Mintezol (Thiabendazole) Merck & Co., Inc. 1704
Vermox Chewable Tablets (Mebendazole) Janssen 1312

Necrobiosis lipoidica diabeticorum

Aristocort Suspension (Forte Parenteral) (Triamcinolone Diacetate) Fujisawa 1027
Aristocort Suspension (Intralesional) (Triamcinolone Diacetate) Fujisawa 1025
Aristospan Suspension (Intralesional) (Triamcinolone Hexacetonide) Fujisawa 1032
Celestone Soluspan Suspension (Betamethasone Sodium Phosphate, Betamethasone Acetate) Schering 2347
Decadron Phosphate Injection (Dexamethasone Sodium Phosphate) Merck & Co., Inc. 1637
Decadron-LA Sterile Suspension (Dexamethasone Acetate) Merck & Co., Inc. 1646
Depo-Medrol Single-Dose Vial (Methylprednisolone Acetate) Upjohn 2600
Depo-Medrol Sterile Aqueous Suspension (Methylprednisolone Acetate) Upjohn 2597
Hydeltrasol Injection, Sterile (Prednisolone Sodium Phosphate) Merck & Co., Inc. 1665
Hydrocortone Acetate Sterile Suspension (Hydrocortisone Acetate) Merck & Co., Inc. 1669

Necrosis, dermal

Regitine (Phentolamine Mesylate) CibaGeneva 846

Neisseria gonorrhoeae (see under N. gonorrhoeae infections)

Neisseria meningitidis (see under N. gonorrhoeae infections)

Neisseria species infections, ocular

AK-Spore (Bacitracin Zinc, Neomycin Sulfate, Polymyxin B Sulfate) Akorn ⊙ 204
AK-Trol Ointment & Suspension (Dexamethasone, Neomycin Sulfate, Polymyxin B Sulfate) Akorn ⊙ 205

(▣ Described in PDR For Nonprescription Drugs) (⊙ Described in PDR For Ophthalmology)

Indications Index

Chloromycetin Ophthalmic Ointment, 1% (Chloramphenicol) Parke-Davis ◉ 310

Chloromycetin Ophthalmic Solution (Chloramphenicol) Parke-Davis ◉ 310

Chloroptic S.O.P. (Chloramphenicol) Allergan ◉ 239

Cortisporin Ophthalmic Ointment Sterile (Polymyxin B Sulfate, Bacitracin Zinc, Neomycin Sulfate, Hydrocortisone) Glaxo Wellcome 1085

Cortisporin Ophthalmic Suspension Sterile (Hydrocortisone, Polymyxin B Sulfate, Neomycin Sulfate) Glaxo Wellcome 1086

Dexacidin Ointment (Dexamethasone, Neomycin Sulfate, Polymyxin B Sulfate) CIBA Vision Ophthalmics ◉ 263

Maxitrol Ophthalmic Ointment and Suspension (Dexamethasone, Neomycin Sulfate, Polymyxin B Sulfate) Alcon Laboratories ◉ 224

NeoDecadron Sterile Ophthalmic Ointment (Neomycin Sulfate, Dexamethasone Sodium Phosphate) Merck & Co., Inc. 1712

NeoDecadron Sterile Ophthalmic Solution (Neomycin Sulfate, Dexamethasone Sodium Phosphate) Merck & Co., Inc. 1713

Ophthocort (Chloramphenicol, Polymyxin B Sulfate, Hydrocortisone Acetate) Parke-Davis ◉ 311

Poly-Pred Liquifilm (Neomycin Sulfate, Polymyxin B Sulfate, Prednisolone Acetate) Allergan.. ◉ 248

Pred-G Liquifilm Sterile Ophthalmic Suspension (Gentamicin Sulfate, Prednisolone Acetate) Allergan ◉ 251

Terra-Cortril Ophthalmic Suspension (Oxytetracycline Hydrochloride, Hydrocortisone Acetate) Roerig 2210

TobraDex Ophthalmic Suspension and Ointment (Dexamethasone, Tobramycin) Alcon Laboratories.. 473

Nephroblastoma (see under Wilms' tumor)

Nephropathy, diabetic

Capoten (Captopril) Bristol-Myers Squibb 739

Nephrotic syndrome, biopsy proven "minimal change", treatment of

Cytoxan (Cyclophosphamide) Bristol-Myers Squibb Oncology 694

NEOSAR Lyophilized/Neosar (Cyclophosphamide) Pharmacia .. 1959

Neuralgia (see under Pain, neurogenic)

Neuralgia, glossopharyngeal

Atretol Tablets (Carbamazepine) Athena 573

Tegretol Chewable Tablets (Carbamazepine) CibaGeneva 852

Tegretol Suspension (Carbamazepine) CibaGeneva 852

Tegretol Tablets (Carbamazepine) CibaGeneva 852

Neuralgia, trigeminal

Atretol Tablets (Carbamazepine) Athena 573

Sarapin (Sarracenia purpurea, Pitcher Plant Distillate) High Chemical 1231

Tegretol Chewable Tablets (Carbamazepine) CibaGeneva 852

Tegretol Suspension (Carbamazepine) CibaGeneva 852

Tegretol Tablets (Carbamazepine) CibaGeneva 852

Neuritis, peripheral, acute (see under Pain, neurogenic)

Neuroblastoma

Adriamycin PFS (Doxorubicin Hydrochloride) Pharmacia 1947

Adriamycin RDF (Doxorubicin Hydrochloride) Pharmacia 1947

Cytoxan (Cyclophosphamide) Bristol-Myers Squibb Oncology 694

Doxorubicin Astra (Doxorubicin Hydrochloride) Astra 540

NEOSAR Lyophilized/Neosar (Cyclophosphamide) Pharmacia .. 1959

Oncovin Solution Vials & Hyporets (Vincristine Sulfate) Lilly 1466

Rubex (Doxorubicin Hydrochloride) Bristol-Myers Squibb Oncology 712

Neurodermatitis (see under Lichen simplex chronicus)

Neurological deficits, post-SAH, improvement of

Nimotop Capsules (Nimodipine) Bayer Pharmaceutical 610

Neurological procedures, destructive, alternative therapy in

Lioresal Intrathecal (Baclofen) Medtronic Neurological 1596

Neuromuscular blockade, nondepolarizing, reversal of

Prostigmin Injectable (Neostigmine Methylsulfate) ICN 1260

Tensilon Injectable (Edrophonium Chloride) ICN 1261

Neutropenia, chemotherapy-induced

Neupogen for Injection (Filgrastim) Amgen 495

Neutropenia, febrile, to decrease the incidence of infection

Neupogen for Injection (Filgrastim) Amgen 495

Neutropenia, post-bone marrow transplant

Neupogen for Injection (Filgrastim) Amgen 495

Neutropenia-related clinical sequelae, post-bone marrow transplant

Neupogen for Injection (Filgrastim) Amgen 495

Niacin, deficiency of

Nicobid (Niacin) Rhone-Poulenc Rorer Pharmaceuticals 2026

Nicotinex Elixir (Niacin) Fleming.... ⊞ 655

Slo-Niacin Tablets (Niacin) Upsher-Smith 2659

Nicolas-Favre disease (see under Lymphogranuloma venereum)

Nocardia asteroides infections (see under Nocardiosis)

Nocardiosis

Gantanol Tablets (Sulfamethoxazole) Roche Laboratories 2119

Gantrisin (Acetyl Sulfisoxazole) Roche Laboratories 2120

Nocturia, symptomatic relief of

Urispas Tablets (Flavoxate Hydrochloride) SmithKline Beecham Pharmaceuticals 2532

Nose, itchy (see under Pruritus, rhinopharyngeal, symptomatic relief of)

Nose, runny (see under Rhinorrhea)

Nose, surgical procedures, irrigation of

AMO Endosol (Balanced Salt Solution) (Balanced Salt Solution) Allergan ◉ 232

BSS (15 mL & 30 mL) Sterile Irrigation Solution (Balanced Salt Solution) Alcon Laboratories ◉ 214

BSS (250 mL) Sterile Irrigation Solution (Balanced Salt Solution) Alcon Laboratories ...... ◉ 214

BSS (500 mL) Sterile Irrigation Solution (Balanced Salt Solution) Alcon Laboratories ...... ◉ 214

Nutrients, deficiency of

Advera Specialized Complete Nutrition (Nutritional Beverage) Ross 2220

AlitraQ Specialized Elemental Nutrition With Glutamine (L-Glutamine, Nutritional Supplement) Ross 2220

Amin-Aid Instant Drink (Nutritional Supplement) R&D 2004

Aminoplex Capsules (Amino Acid Preparations) Tyson 2564

Aminotate Capsules (Amino Acid Preparations) Tyson 2565

ANTIOX Capsules (Beta Carotene, Vitamin C, Vitamin E) Mayrand 1543

Beelith Tablets (Magnesium Oxide, Vitamin B_6) Beach 639

BioLean (Nutritional Supplement) Wellness International ⊞ 866

BioLean Accelerator (Nutritional Supplement) Wellness International ⊞ 866

BioLean LipoTrim (Nutritional Supplement) Wellness International ⊞ 866

BioLean Meal (Nutritional Beverage) Wellness International ⊞ 867

Bromase (Proteolytic Enzymes) Bio-Tech 667

Cartilade Shark Cartilage Capsules, Powder, and Caplets (Shark Cartilage) Cartilage Technologies ⊞ 626

Catemine Enteric Tablets (Tyrosine) (L-Tyrosine) Tyson 2565

Centrum Singles Beta Carotene (Beta Carotene) Lederle Consumer ⊞ 669

Coenzyme Q10 200mg, 100mg & 60mg Chewable Wafers, and 200mg, 60mg & 25mg Tablets (Coenzyme Q-10) Vitaline 2659

Ensure Complete Balanced Nutrition (Nutritional Supplement) Ross 2221

Ensure High Protein Complete Balanced Nutrition (Nutritional Beverage) Ross 2220

Ensure Plus High Calorie Complete Nutrition (Nutritional Supplement) Ross 2221

Ensure With Fiber Complete, Balanced Nutrition (Nutritional Supplement) Ross 2221

Food for Thought (Nutritional Beverage) Wellness International ⊞ 867

Glucerna Specialized Nutrition with Fiber for Patients with Abnormal Glucose Tolerance (Nutritional Supplement) Ross 2221

Jevity Isotonic Liquid Nutrition with Fiber (Nutritional Supplement) Ross 2221

Kyolic (Garlic Extract) Wakunaga.. ⊞ 839

Radical PC (Nutritional Supplement) Odyssey 1807

Marlyn Formula 50 Capsules (Amino Acid Preparations, Vitamin B_6) Marlyn 1541

NephrAmine (Amino Acid Preparations) R&D 2005

Nepro Specialized Liquid Nutrition (Nutritional Supplement) Ross 2222

One-A-Day Extras Garlic (Garlic Extract) Miles Consumer .... ⊞ 728

One-A-Day Men's (Vitamins, Multiple) Miles Consumer .... ⊞ 729

Osmolite Isotonic Liquid Nutrition (Nutritional Supplement) Ross 2222

Osmolite HN High Nitrogen Isotonic Liquid Nutrition (Nutritional Supplement) Ross 2222

PediaSure Complete Liquid Nutrition (Nutritional Supplement) Ross 2222

PediaSure With Fiber Complete Liquid Nutrition (Nutritional Supplement) Ross 2223

Perative Specialized Liquid Nutrition (Nutritional Beverage) Ross 2223

PhosChol (Phosphatidylcholine) American Lecithin 488

Polycose Glucose Polymers (Glucose Polymers) Ross 2223

Pro-Hepatone Capsules (Vitamins with Minerals, Amino Acid Preparations) Marlyn 1542

Promote High Protein Liquid Nutrition (Nutritional Supplement) Ross 2223

Promote With Fiber, High-Protein Liquid Nutrition (Nutritional Beverage) Ross 2224

Pros-Tech Plus (Nutritional Supplement) Bio-Tech 668

Similac Toddler's Best Milk-Based Nutritional Beverage (Nutritional Beverage) Ross ⊞ 784

StePHan Clarity (Nutritional Supplement) Wellness International ⊞ 868

StePHan Elasticity (Nutritional Supplement) Wellness International ⊞ 868

StePHan Elixir (Nutritional Supplement) Wellness International ⊞ 869

StePHan Essential (Nutritional Supplement) Wellness International ⊞ 869

StePHan Feminine (Nutritional Supplement) Wellness International ⊞ 869

StePHan Flexibility (Nutritional Supplement) Wellness International ⊞ 869

StePHan Lovpil (Nutritional Supplement) Wellness International ⊞ 869

StePHan Masculine (Nutritional Supplement) Wellness International ⊞ 869

StePHan Protector (Nutritional Supplement) Wellness International ⊞ 869

StePHan Relief (Nutritional Supplement) Wellness International ⊞ 869

StePHan Tranquility (Nutritional Supplement) Wellness International ⊞ 870

Super EPA (Docosahexaenoic Acid (DHA)) Advanced Nutritional 468

Suplena Specialized Liquid Nutrition (Nutritional Supplement) Ross 2226

Vital High Nitrogen Nutritionally Complete Partially Hydrolyzed Diet (Nutritional Supplement) Ross 2228

Winrgy (Nutritional Beverage) Wellness International ⊞ 870

Nutrients, deficiency of, in respiratory insufficiency

Pulmocare Specialized Nutrition for Pulmonary Patients (Nutritional Supplement) Ross 2224

Nutrients, deficiency of, stress-induced (see under Nutrients, deficiency of)

Nutrients, deficiency of, surgery-induced (see under Nutrients, deficiency of)

Nutrition, infant (see under Breast milk, replacement of or supplement to)

O

Obesity, exogenous

Adipex-P Tablets and Capsules (Phentermine Hydrochloride) Gate 1048

Biphetamine Capsules (Amphetamine Resins) Fisons 983

Bontril Slow-Release Capsules (Phendimetrazine Tartrate) Carnrick 781

Desoxyn Gradumet Tablets (Methamphetamine Hydrochloride) Abbott 419

Dexedrine (Dextroamphetamine Sulfate) SmithKline Beecham Pharmaceuticals 2474

DextroStat Dextroamphetamine Tablets (Dextroamphetamine Sulfate) Richwood 2036

Didrex Tablets (Benzphetamine Hydrochloride) Upjohn 2607

(⊞ Described in PDR For Nonprescription Drugs) (◉ Described in PDR For Ophthalmology)

Obesity

Fastin Capsules (Phentermine Hydrochloride) SmithKline Beecham Pharmaceuticals 2488

Ionamin Capsules (Phentermine Resin) Fisons 990

Pondimin Tablets (Fenfluramine Hydrochloride) Robins 2066

Prelu-2 Timed Release Capsules (Phendimetrazine Tartrate) Boehringer Ingelheim 681

Sanorex Tablets (Mazindol) Sandoz Pharmaceuticals 2294

Obsessive compulsive disorder

Anafranil Capsules (Clomipramine Hydrochloride) CibaGeneva 803

Luvox Tablets (Fluvoxamine Maleate) Solvay 2544

Prozac Pulvules & Liquid, Oral Solution (Fluoxetine Hydrochloride) Dista 919

Ocular congestion, symptomatic relief of

Albalon Solution with Liquifilm (Naphazoline Hydrochloride) Allergan .... ◉ 231

Neo-Synephrine Hydrochloride (Ophthalmic) (Phenylephrine Hydrochloride) Sanofi Winthrop .. 2325

Ocular inflammation

AK-Pred (Prednisolone Sodium Phosphate) Akorn .... ◉ 204

Econopred & Econopred Plus Ophthalmic Suspensions (Prednisolone Acetate) Alcon Laboratories .... ◉ 217

Poly-Pred Liquifilm (Neomycin Sulfate, Polymyxin B Sulfate, Prednisolone Acetate) Allergan.. ◉ 248

Pred Forte (Prednisolone Acetate) Allergan .... ◉ 250

Pred Mild (Prednisolone Acetate) Allergan .... ◉ 253

Ocular inflammation with bacterial infection, steroid-responsive

AK-CIDE (Prednisolone Acetate, Sulfacetamide Sodium) Akorn .... ◉ 202

AK-CIDE Ointment (Prednisolone Acetate, Sulfacetamide Sodium) Akorn .... ◉ 202

AK-Trol Ointment & Suspension (Dexamethasone, Neomycin Sulfate, Polymyxin B Sulfate) Akorn .... ◉ 205

Blephamide Liquifilm Sterile Ophthalmic Suspension (Prednisolone Acetate, Sulfacetamide Sodium) Allergan 476

Blephamide Ointment (Sulfacetamide Sodium, Prednisolone Acetate) Allergan .... ◉ 237

Cortisporin Ophthalmic Ointment Sterile (Polymyxin B Sulfate, Bacitracin Zinc, Neomycin Sulfate, Hydrocortisone) Glaxo Wellcome 1085

Cortisporin Ophthalmic Suspension Sterile (Hydrocortisone, Polymyxin B Sulfate, Neomycin Sulfate) Glaxo Wellcome 1086

Dexacidin Ointment (Dexamethasone, Neomycin Sulfate, Polymyxin B Sulfate) CIBA Vision Ophthalmics .... ◉ 263

FML-S Liquifilm (Sulfacetamide Sodium, Fluorometholone) Allergan .... ◉ 242

Maxitrol Ophthalmic Ointment and Suspension (Dexamethasone, Neomycin Sulfate, Polymyxin B Sulfate) Alcon Laboratories .... ◉ 224

NeoDecadron Sterile Ophthalmic Ointment (Neomycin Sulfate, Dexamethasone Sodium Phosphate) Merck & Co., Inc. 1712

NeoDecadron Sterile Ophthalmic Solution (Neomycin Sulfate, Dexamethasone Sodium Phosphate) Merck & Co., Inc. 1713

Ophthocort (Chloramphenicol, Polymyxin B Sulfate, Hydrocortisone Acetate) Parke-Davis .... ◉ 311

Poly-Pred Liquifilm (Neomycin Sulfate, Polymyxin B Sulfate, Prednisolone Acetate) Allergan.. ◉ 248

Pred-G Liquifilm Sterile Ophthalmic Suspension (Gentamicin Sulfate, Prednisolone Acetate) Allergan .... ◉ 251

Pred-G S.O.P. Sterile Ophthalmic Ointment (Gentamicin Sulfate, Prednisolone Acetate) Allergan.. ◉ 252

Terra-Cortril Ophthalmic Suspension (Oxytetracycline Hydrochloride, Hydrocortisone Acetate) Roerig 2210

TobraDex Ophthalmic Suspension and Ointment (Dexamethasone, Tobramycin) Alcon Laboratories .. 473

Vasocidin Ointment (Prednisolone Acetate, Sulfacetamide Sodium) CIBA Vision Ophthalmics .... ◉ 268

Vasocidin Ophthalmic Solution (Prednisolone Sodium Phosphate, Sulfacetamide Sodium) CIBA Vision Ophthalmics .... ◉ 270

Ocular inflammation, postoperative

Vexol 1% Ophthalmic Suspension (Rimexolone) Alcon Laboratories .... ◉ 230

Voltaren Ophthalmic Sterile Ophthalmic Solution (Diclofenac Sodium) CIBA Vision Ophthalmics .... ◉ 272

Ocular inflammation, steroid-responsive

Decadron Phosphate Sterile Ophthalmic Ointment (Dexamethasone Sodium Phosphate) Merck & Co., Inc. 1641

Decadron Phosphate Sterile Ophthalmic Solution (Dexamethasone Sodium Phosphate) Merck & Co., Inc. 1642

Econopred & Econopred Plus Ophthalmic Suspensions (Prednisolone Acetate) Alcon Laboratories .... ◉ 217

FML Liquifilm (Fluorometholone) Allergan .... ◉ 241

Flarex Ophthalmic Suspension (Fluorometholone Acetate) Alcon Laboratories .... ◉ 218

Fluor-Op Ophthalmic Suspension (Fluorometholone) CIBA Vision Ophthalmics .... ◉ 264

Inflamase (Prednisolone Sodium Phosphate) CIBA Vision Ophthalmics .... ◉ 265

Pred Forte (Prednisolone Acetate) Allergan .... ◉ 250

Ocular redness

Clear Eyes ACR Astringent/Lubricant Eye Redness Reliever Eye Drops (Zinc Sulfate, Naphazoline Hydrochloride) Ross .... ◉ 316

Clear Eyes Lubricant Eye Redness Reliever (Glycerin, Naphazoline Hydrochloride) Ross .... ◉ 316

Collyrium Fresh (Tetrahydrozoline Hydrochloride, Glycerin) Wyeth-Ayerst .... ⊕ 879

Murine Tears Plus Lubricant Redness Reliever Eye Drops (Polyvinyl Alcohol, Povidone, Tetrahydrozoline Hydrochloride) Ross .... ◉ 316

Naphcon-A Ophthalmic Solution (Naphazoline Hydrochloride, Pheniramine Maleate) Alcon Laboratories 473

Similasan Eye Drops # 1 (Homeopathic Medications) Similasan ◉ 317

Similasan Eye Drops # 2 (Homeopathic Medications) Similasan ◉ 317

Vasocon-A (Antazoline Phosphate, Naphazoline Hydrochloride) CIBA Vision Ophthalmics .... ◉ 271

Visine Maximum Strength Allergy Relief (Tetrahydrozoline Hydrochloride) Pfizer Consumer .... ◉ 313

Visine Moisturizing Eye Drops (Tetrahydrozoline Hydrochloride) Pfizer Consumer .... ◉ 313

Visine Original Eye Drops (Tetrahydrozoline Hydrochloride) Pfizer Consumer .... ◉ 314

Visine L.R. Eye Drops (Oxymetazoline Hydrochloride) Pfizer Consumer .... ◉ 313

Onychomycosis

(see under Tinea unguium infections)

Oocytes, multiple, stimulation of the development of

Metrodin (urofollitropin for injection) (Urofollitropin) Serono.. 2446

Ophthalmia neonatorum, prophylaxis of

Ilotycin Ophthalmic Ointment (Erythromycin) Dista 912

Ophthalmia, Egyptian

(see under Trachoma)

Ophthalmia, sympathetic

Aristocort Suspension (Forte Parenteral) (Triamcinolone Diacetate) Fujisawa 1027

Aristocort Tablets (Triamcinolone) Fujisawa 1022

Celestone Soluspan Suspension (Betamethasone Sodium Phosphate, Betamethasone Acetate) Schering 2347

Cortone Acetate Sterile Suspension (Cortisone Acetate) Merck & Co., Inc. 1623

Cortone Acetate Tablets (Cortisone Acetate) Merck & Co., Inc. 1624

Dalalone D.P. Injectable (Dexamethasone Acetate) Forest 1011

Decadron Elixir (Dexamethasone) Merck & Co., Inc. 1633

Decadron Phosphate Injection (Dexamethasone Sodium Phosphate) Merck & Co., Inc. 1637

Decadron Tablets (Dexamethasone) Merck & Co., Inc. 1635

Decadron-LA Sterile Suspension (Dexamethasone Acetate) Merck & Co., Inc. 1646

Deltasone Tablets (Prednisone) Upjohn 2595

Depo-Medrol Single-Dose Vial (Methylprednisolone Acetate) Upjohn 2600

Depo-Medrol Sterile Aqueous Suspension (Methylprednisolone Acetate) Upjohn 2597

Hydeltrasol Injection, Sterile (Prednisolone Sodium Phosphate) Merck & Co., Inc. 1665

Hydrocortone Phosphate Injection, Sterile (Hydrocortisone Sodium Phosphate) Merck & Co., Inc. 1670

Hydrocortone Tablets (Hydrocortisone) Merck & Co., Inc. 1672

Medrol (Methylprednisolone) Upjohn 2621

Pediapred Oral Liquid (Prednisolone Sodium Phosphate) Fisons 995

Prelone Syrup (Prednisolone) Muro 1787

Solu-Cortef Sterile Powder (Hydrocortisone Sodium Succinate) Upjohn 2641

Solu-Medrol Sterile Powder (Methylprednisolone Sodium Succinate) Upjohn 2643

Ornithosis

(see under Chlamydia psittaci infection)

Ossification, heterotopic

Didronel Tablets (Etidronate Disodium (Diphosphonate)) Procter & Gamble Pharmaceuticals 1984

Osteitis deformans

(see under Paget's disease of bone)

Osteitis fibrosa

(see under Osteodystrophy)

Osteoarthritis

Children's Advil Suspension (Ibuprofen) Wyeth-Ayerst 2692

Anaprox/Naprosyn (Naproxen Sodium) Roche Laboratories 2117

Ansaid Tablets (Flurbiprofen) Upjohn 2579

Arthritis Pain Ascriptin (Aspirin Buffered, Calcium Carbonate) CIBA Consumer .... ⊕ 631

Extra Strength Bayer Arthritis Pain Regimen Formula (Aspirin, Enteric Coated) Miles Consumer .... ⊕ 711

Cataflam (Diclofenac Potassium) CibaGeneva 816

Celestone Soluspan Suspension (Betamethasone Sodium Phosphate, Betamethasone Acetate) Schering 2347

Clinoril Tablets (Sulindac) Merck & Co., Inc. 1618

Daypro Caplets (Oxaprozin) Searle 2426

Dolobid Tablets (Diflunisal) Merck & Co., Inc. 1654

EC-Naprosyn Delayed-Release Tablets (Naproxen) Roche Laboratories 2117

Ecotrin (Aspirin, Enteric Coated) SmithKline Beecham 2455

Feldene Capsules (Piroxicam) Pratt 1965

IBU Tablets (Ibuprofen) Knoll Laboratories 1342

Indocin (Indomethacin) Merck & Co., Inc. 1680

Lodine Capsules and Tablets (Etodolac) Wyeth-Ayerst 2743

(⊕ Described in PDR For Nonprescription Drugs) (◉ Described in PDR For Ophthalmology)

Mono-Gesic Tablets (Salsalate) Central 792

Children's Motrin Ibuprofen Oral Suspension (Ibuprofen) McNeil Consumer 1546

Motrin Tablets (Ibuprofen) Upjohn .. 2625

Motrin Ibuprofen Suspension, Oral Drops, Chewable Tablets, Caplets (Ibuprofen) McNeil Consumer 1546

Nalfon 200 Pulvules & Nalfon Tablets (Fenoprofen Calcium) Dista 917

Anaprox/Naprosyn (Naproxen) Roche Laboratories 2117

Orudis Capsules (Ketoprofen) Wyeth-Ayerst 2766

Oruvail Capsules (Ketoprofen) Wyeth-Ayerst 2766

Relafen Tablets (Nabumetone) SmithKline Beecham Pharmaceuticals 2510

Salflex Tablets (Salsalate) Carnrick 786

Tolectin (200, 400 and 600 mg) (Tolmetin Sodium) McNeil Pharmaceutical 1581

Trilisate (Choline Magnesium Trisalicylate) Purdue Frederick 2000

Voltaren Tablets (Diclofenac Sodium) CibaGeneva 861

Osteoarthritis, post-traumatic

Aristocort Suspension (Forte Parenteral) (Triamcinolone Diacetate) Fujisawa 1027

Aristocort Suspension (Intralesional) (Triamcinolone Diacetate) Fujisawa 1025

Aristocort Tablets (Triamcinolone) Fujisawa 1022

Aristospan Suspension (Intra-articular) (Triamcinolone Hexacetonide) Fujisawa 1033

Cortone Acetate Sterile Suspension (Cortisone Acetate) Merck & Co., Inc. 1623

Cortone Acetate Tablets (Cortisone Acetate) Merck & Co., Inc. 1624

Dalalone D.P. Injectable (Dexamethasone Acetate) Forest 1011

Decadron Elixir (Dexamethasone) Merck & Co., Inc. 1633

Decadron Phosphate Injection (Dexamethasone Sodium Phosphate) Merck & Co., Inc. 1637

Decadron Tablets (Dexamethasone) Merck & Co., Inc. 1635

Decadron-LA Sterile Suspension (Dexamethasone Acetate) Merck & Co., Inc. 1646

Deltasone Tablets (Prednisone) Upjohn 2595

Depo-Medrol Single-Dose Vial (Methylprednisolone Acetate) Upjohn 2600

Depo-Medrol Sterile Aqueous Suspension (Methylprednisolone Acetate) Upjohn 2597

Hydeltrasol Injection, Sterile (Prednisolone Sodium Phosphate) Merck & Co., Inc. 1665

Hydeltra-T.B.A. Sterile Suspension (Prednisolone Tebutate) Merck & Co., Inc. 1667

Hydrocortone Acetate Sterile Suspension (Hydrocortisone Acetate) Merck & Co., Inc. 1669

Hydrocortone Phosphate Injection, Sterile (Hydrocortisone Sodium Phosphate) Merck & Co., Inc. 1670

Hydrocortone Tablets (Hydrocortisone) Merck & Co., Inc. 1672

Medrol (Methylprednisolone) Upjohn 2621

Pediapred Oral Liquid (Prednisolone Sodium Phosphate) Fisons 995

Prelone Syrup (Prednisolone) Muro 1787

Solu-Cortef Sterile Powder (Hydrocortisone Sodium Succinate) Upjohn 2641

Solu-Medrol Sterile Powder (Methylprednisolone Sodium Succinate) Upjohn 2643

Osteoarthritis, synovitis of

Aristocort Suspension (Forte Parenteral) (Triamcinolone Diacetate) Fujisawa 1027

Aristocort Suspension (Intralesional) (Triamcinolone Diacetate) Fujisawa 1025

Aristocort Tablets (Triamcinolone) Fujisawa 1022

Aristospan Suspension (Intra-articular) (Triamcinolone Hexacetonide) Fujisawa 1033

Celestone Soluspan Suspension (Betamethasone Sodium Phosphate, Betamethasone Acetate) Schering 2347

Cortone Acetate Sterile Suspension (Cortisone Acetate) Merck & Co., Inc. 1623

Cortone Acetate Tablets (Cortisone Acetate) Merck & Co., Inc. 1624

Dalalone D.P. Injectable (Dexamethasone Acetate) Forest 1011

Decadron Elixir (Dexamethasone) Merck & Co., Inc. 1633

Decadron Phosphate Injection (Dexamethasone Sodium Phosphate) Merck & Co., Inc. 1637

Decadron Tablets (Dexamethasone) Merck & Co., Inc. 1635

Decadron-LA Sterile Suspension (Dexamethasone Acetate) Merck & Co., Inc. 1646

Deltasone Tablets (Prednisone) Upjohn 2595

Depo-Medrol Single-Dose Vial (Methylprednisolone Acetate) Upjohn 2600

Depo-Medrol Sterile Aqueous Suspension (Methylprednisolone Acetate) Upjohn 2597

Hydeltrasol Injection, Sterile (Prednisolone Sodium Phosphate) Merck & Co., Inc. 1665

Hydeltra-T.B.A. Sterile Suspension (Prednisolone Tebutate) Merck & Co., Inc. 1667

Hydrocortone Acetate Sterile Suspension (Hydrocortisone Acetate) Merck & Co., Inc. 1669

Hydrocortone Phosphate Injection, Sterile (Hydrocortisone Sodium Phosphate) Merck & Co., Inc. 1670

Hydrocortone Tablets (Hydrocortisone) Merck & Co., Inc. 1672

Medrol (Methylprednisolone) Upjohn 2621

Pediapred Oral Liquid (Prednisolone Sodium Phosphate) Fisons 995

Prelone Syrup (Prednisolone) Muro 1787

Solu-Cortef Sterile Powder (Hydrocortisone Sodium Succinate) Upjohn 2641

Solu-Medrol Sterile Powder (Methylprednisolone Sodium Succinate) Upjohn 2643

Osteodystrophy

Rocaltrol Capsules (Calcitriol) Roche Laboratories 2141

Osteomalacia

(see under Osteodystrophy)

Osteomyelitis, acute hematogenous

Cleocin Phosphate Injection (Clindamycin Phosphate) Upjohn 2586

Osteoporosis

Estrace Cream and Tablets (Estradiol) Bristol-Myers Squibb .. 749

Estraderm Transdermal System (Estradiol) CibaGeneva 824

Miacalcin Nasal Spray (Calcitonin-Salmon) Sandoz Pharmaceuticals 2275

Ogen Tablets (Estropipate) Upjohn 2627

Premarin Tablets (Estrogens, Conjugated) Wyeth-Ayerst 2789

Premphase (Estrogens, Conjugated, Medroxyprogesterone Acetate) Wyeth-Ayerst 2797

Prempro (Estrogens, Conjugated, Medroxyprogesterone Acetate) Wyeth-Ayerst 2801

Osteoporosis, postmenopausal, treatment adjunct

Calcimar Injection, Synthetic (Calcitonin, Synthetic) Rhone-Poulenc Rorer Pharmaceuticals 2013

Miacalcin Injection (Calcitonin, Synthetic) Sandoz Pharmaceuticals 2273

Osteosarcoma, nonmetastatic

Methotrexate Sodium Tablets, Injection, for Injection and LPF

Injection (Methotrexate Sodium) Immunex 1275

Ostomy care, adjunctive therapy

Sween Cream (Benzethonium Chloride, Lanolin Oil) Sween 2554

Otitis externa

Coly-Mycin S Otic w/Neomycin & Hydrocortisone (Colistin Sulfate, Neomycin Sulfate, Hydrocortisone Acetate) Parke-Davis 1906

PediOtic Suspension Sterile (Polymyxin B Sulfate, Neomycin Sulfate, Hydrocortisone) Glaxo Wellcome 1153

VōSol (Acetic Acid, Hydrocortisone) Wallace 2678

Otitis externa with inflammation

Cortisporin Otic Solution Sterile (Polymyxin B Sulfate, Neomycin Sulfate, Hydrocortisone) Glaxo Wellcome 1087

Cortisporin Otic Suspension Sterile (Polymyxin B Sulfate, Neomycin Sulfate, Hydrocortisone) Glaxo Wellcome 1088

Decadron Phosphate Sterile Ophthalmic Solution (Dexamethasone Sodium Phosphate) Merck & Co., Inc. 1642

VōSoL HC Otic Solution (Acetic Acid, Hydrocortisone) Wallace 2678

Otitis externa, symptomatic relief of

Americaine Otic Topical Anesthetic Ear Drops (Benzocaine) Fisons 983

Otic Domeboro Solution (Acetic Acid) Bayer Pharmaceutical 611

Star-Otic Ear Solution (Acetic Acid, Boric Acid, Burow's Solution) Stellar .... ◉⊡ 830

Otitis media, acute

Amoxil (Amoxicillin Trihydrate) SmithKline Beecham Pharmaceuticals 2464

Augmentin (Amoxicillin Trihydrate, Clavulanate Potassium) SmithKline Beecham Pharmaceuticals 2468

Bactrim (Trimethoprim, Sulfamethoxazole) Roche Laboratories 2084

Bicillin C-R Injection (Penicillin G Procaine, Penicillin G Benzathine) Wyeth-Ayerst 2704

Bicillin C-R 900/300 Injection (Penicillin G Procaine, Penicillin G Benzathine) Wyeth-Ayerst 2706

Ceclor Pulvules & Suspension (Cefaclor) Lilly 1431

Ceftin (Cefuroxime Axetil) Glaxo Wellcome 1078

Cefzil Tablets and Oral Suspension (Cefprozil) Bristol-Myers Squibb .. 746

E.E.S. (Erythromycin Ethylsuccinate) Abbott 424

EryPed (Erythromycin Ethylsuccinate) Abbott 421

Ery-Tab Tablets (Erythromycin) Abbott 422

Erythrocin Stearate Filmtab (Erythromycin Stearate) Abbott 425

Erythromycin Base Filmtab (Erythromycin) Abbott 426

Keflex Pulvules & Oral Suspension (Cephalexin) Dista 914

Lorabid Suspension and Pulvules (Loracarbef) Lilly 1459

Septra (Trimethoprim, Sulfamethoxazole) Glaxo Wellcome 1174

Suprax (Cefixime) Lederle 1399

Vantin for Oral Suspension and Vantin Tablets (Cefpodoxime Proxetil) Upjohn 2646

Otitis media, acute, adjuvant therapy

Americaine Otic Topical Anesthetic Ear Drops (Benzocaine) Fisons 983

Auralgan Otic Solution (Antipyrine, Benzocaine, Glycerin) Wyeth-Ayerst 2703

Congess (Guaifenesin, Pseudoephedrine Hydrochloride) Fleming 1004

Fedahist Gyrocaps (Pseudoephedrine Hydrochloride, Chlorpheniramine Maleate) Schwarz 2401

Fedahist Timecaps (Pseudoephedrine Hydrochloride, Chlorpheniramine Maleate) Schwarz 2401

Gantanol Tablets (Sulfamethoxazole) Roche Laboratories 2119

Gantrisin (Acetyl Sulfisoxazole) Roche Laboratories 2120

Novahistine DH (Codeine Phosphate, Pseudoephedrine Hydrochloride, Chlorpheniramine Maleate) SmithKline Beecham 2462

Novahistine Expectorant (Codeine Phosphate, Pseudoephedrine Hydrochloride, Guaifenesin) SmithKline Beecham 2463

Tympagesic Ear Drops (Antipyrine, Benzocaine, Phenylephrine Hydrochloride) Savage 2342

Otitis media, H. influenzae-induced

(see under H. influenzae otitis media)

Otitis media, S. pneumoniae-induced

(see under S. pneumoniae otitis media)

Otitis media, S. pyogenes-induced

(see under S. pyogenes otitis media)

Otitis media, Staphylococci-induced

(see under Staphylococci otitis media)

Ovarian failure, primary

Estrace Cream and Tablets (Estradiol) Bristol-Myers Squibb .. 749

Estraderm Transdermal System (Estradiol) CibaGeneva 824

ESTRATAB Tablets (0.3, 0.625, 1.25, 2.5 mg) (Estrogens, Esterified) Solvay 2536

Menest Tablets (Estrogens, Esterified) SmithKline Beecham Pharmaceuticals 2494

Ogen Tablets (Estropipate) Upjohn 2627

Ortho-Est (Estropipate) Ortho Pharmaceutical 1869

Premarin Tablets (Estrogens, Conjugated) Wyeth-Ayerst 2789

Ovaries, castration of

Estrace Cream and Tablets (Estradiol) Bristol-Myers Squibb .. 749

Estraderm Transdermal System (Estradiol) CibaGeneva 824

ESTRATAB Tablets (0.3, 0.625, 1.25, 2.5 mg) (Estrogens, Esterified) Solvay 2536

Menest Tablets (Estrogens, Esterified) SmithKline Beecham Pharmaceuticals 2494

Ogen Tablets (Estropipate) Upjohn 2627

Ortho-Est (Estropipate) Ortho Pharmaceutical 1869

Premarin Tablets (Estrogens, Conjugated) Wyeth-Ayerst 2789

Ovary, adenocarcinoma

(see under Carcinoma, ovary)

Ovulation, induction of

Clomid (Clomiphene Citrate) Marion Merrell Dow 1514

Humegon (Menotropins) Organon .. 1824

Metrodin (urofollitropin for injection) (Urofollitropin) Serono .. 2446

Pergonal (menotropins for injection, USP) (Menotropins) Serono 2448

Pregnyl (Chorionic Gonadotropin) Organon 1828

Profasi (chorionic gonadotropin for injection, USP) (Chorionic Gonadotropin) Serono 2450

Serophene (clomiphene citrate tablets, USP) (Clomiphene Citrate) Serono 2451

Oxyuriasis

(see under Enterobiasis)

P

P. aeruginosa bacteremia

Ceptaz (Ceftazidime) Glaxo Wellcome 1081

P. aeruginosa bacteremia — Indications Index — 1516

Polymyxin B Sulfate, Aerosporin Brand Sterile Powder (Polymyxin B Sulfate) Glaxo Wellcome 1154

P. aeruginosa bone and joint infections

Ceptaz (Ceftazidime) Glaxo Wellcome 1081
Cipro I.V. (Ciprofloxacin) Bayer Pharmaceutical 595
Cipro I.V. Pharmacy Bulk Package (Ciprofloxacin) Bayer Pharmaceutical 597
Cipro Tablets (Ciprofloxacin Hydrochloride) Bayer Pharmaceutical 592
Claforan Sterile and Injection (Cefotaxime Sodium) Hoechst-Roussel 1235
Fortaz (Ceftazidime) Glaxo Wellcome 1100
Nebcin Vials, Hyporets & ADD-Vantage (Tobramycin Sulfate) Lilly 1464
Pipracil (Piperacillin Sodium) Lederle 1390
Primaxin I.V. (Imipenem-Cilastatin Sodium) Merck & Co., Inc. 1729
Tazicef for Injection (Ceftazidime) SmithKline Beecham Pharmaceuticals 2519
Tazidime Vials, Faspak & ADD-Vantage (Ceftazidime) Lilly 1478
Tobramycin Sulfate Injection (Tobramycin Sulfate) Elkins-Sinn 968

P. aeruginosa infections

Amikacin Sulfate Injection, USP (Amikacin Sulfate) Elkins-Sinn 960
Amikin Injectable (Amikacin Sulfate) Apothecon 501
Azactam for Injection (Aztreonam) Bristol-Myers Squibb 734
Cefizox for Intramuscular or Intravenous Use (Ceftizoxime Sodium) Fujisawa 1034
Cefobid Intravenous/Intramuscular (Cefoperazone Sodium) Roerig 2189
Cefobid Pharmacy Bulk Package - Not for Direct Infusion (Cefoperazone Sodium) Roerig 2192
Ceptaz (Ceftazidime) Glaxo Wellcome 1081
Cipro I.V. (Ciprofloxacin) Bayer Pharmaceutical 595
Cipro I.V. Pharmacy Bulk Package (Ciprofloxacin) Bayer Pharmaceutical 597
Cipro Tablets (Ciprofloxacin Hydrochloride) Bayer Pharmaceutical 592
Claforan Sterile and Injection (Cefotaxime Sodium) Hoechst-Roussel 1235
Coly-Mycin M Parenteral (Colistimethate Sodium) Parke-Davis 1905
Cortisporin Ophthalmic Ointment Sterile (Polymyxin B Sulfate, Bacitracin Zinc, Neomycin Sulfate, Hydrocortisone) Glaxo Wellcome 1085
Cortisporin Ophthalmic Suspension Sterile (Hydrocortisone, Polymyxin B Sulfate, Neomycin Sulfate) Glaxo Wellcome 1086
Floxin I.V. (Ofloxacin) McNeil Pharmaceutical 1571
Floxin Tablets (200 mg, 300 mg, 400 mg) (Ofloxacin) McNeil Pharmaceutical 1567
Fortaz (Ceftazidime) Glaxo Wellcome 1100
Garamycin Injectable (Gentamicin Sulfate) Schering 2360
Maxaquin Tablets (Lomefloxacin Hydrochloride) Searle 2440
Mezlin (Mezlocillin Sodium) Bayer Pharmaceutical 601
Mezlin Pharmacy Bulk Package (Mezlocillin Sodium) Bayer Pharmaceutical 604
Nebcin Vials, Hyporets & ADD-Vantage (Tobramycin Sulfate) Lilly 1464
Netromycin Injection 100 mg/ml (Netilmicin Sulfate) Schering 2373
Noroxin Tablets (Norfloxacin) Merck & Co., Inc. 1715
Noroxin Tablets (Norfloxacin) Roberts 2048
Penetrex Tablets (Enoxacin) Rhone-Poulenc Rorer Pharmaceuticals 2031
Pipracil (Piperacillin Sodium) Lederle 1390
Polymyxin B Sulfate, Aerosporin Brand Sterile Powder (Polymyxin B Sulfate) Glaxo Wellcome 1154
Primaxin I.M. (Imipenem-Cilastatin Sodium) Merck & Co., Inc. 1727
Primaxin I.V. (Imipenem-Cilastatin Sodium) Merck & Co., Inc. 1729
Rocephin Injectable Vials, ADD-Vantage, Galaxy Container (Ceftriaxone Sodium) Roche Laboratories 2142
Tazicef for Injection (Ceftazidime) SmithKline Beecham Pharmaceuticals 2519
Tazidime Vials, Faspak & ADD-Vantage (Ceftazidime) Lilly 1478
TERAK Ointment (Oxytetracycline Hydrochloride, Polymyxin B Sulfate) Akorn ⊙ 209
Ticar for Injection (Ticarcillin Disodium) SmithKline Beecham Pharmaceuticals 2526
Timentin for Injection (Ticarcillin Disodium, Clavulanate Potassium) SmithKline Beecham Pharmaceuticals 2528
Tobramycin Sulfate Injection (Tobramycin Sulfate) Elkins-Sinn 968

P. aeruginosa infections, ocular

AK-Spore (Bacitracin Zinc, Neomycin Sulfate, Polymyxin B Sulfate) Akorn ⊙ 204
AK-Trol Ointment & Suspension (Dexamethasone, Neomycin Sulfate, Polymyxin B Sulfate) Akorn ⊙ 205
Ciloxan Ophthalmic Solution (Ciprofloxacin Hydrochloride) Alcon Laboratories 472
Dexacidin Ointment (Dexamethasone, Neomycin Sulfate, Polymyxin B Sulfate) CIBA Vision Ophthalmics ⊙ 263
Genoptic Sterile Ophthalmic Solution (Gentamicin Sulfate) Allergan ⊙ 243
Genoptic Sterile Ophthalmic Ointment (Gentamicin Sulfate) Allergan ⊙ 243
Gentak (Gentamicin Sulfate) Akorn ⊙ 208
Ocuflox (Ofloxacin) Allergan 481
Ophthocort (Chloramphenicol, Polymyxin B Sulfate, Hydrocortisone Acetate) Parke-Davis ⊙ 311
Polymyxin B Sulfate, Aerosporin Brand Sterile Powder (Polymyxin B Sulfate) Glaxo Wellcome 1154
Poly-Pred Liquifilm (Neomycin Sulfate, Polymyxin B Sulfate, Prednisolone Acetate) Allergan ⊙ 248
Polytrim Ophthalmic Solution Sterile (Polymyxin B Sulfate, Trimethoprim Sulfate) Allergan 482
Pred-G Liquifilm Sterile Ophthalmic Suspension (Gentamicin Sulfate, Prednisolone Acetate) Allergan ⊙ 251
Pred-G S.O.P. Sterile Ophthalmic Ointment (Gentamicin Sulfate, Prednisolone Acetate) Allergan ⊙ 252
TERAK Ointment (Oxytetracycline Hydrochloride, Polymyxin B Sulfate) Akorn ⊙ 209
Terramycin with Polymyxin B Sulfate Ophthalmic Ointment (Oxytetracycline Hydrochloride, Polymyxin B Sulfate) Roerig 2211
TobraDex Ophthalmic Suspension and Ointment (Dexamethasone, Tobramycin) Alcon Laboratories 473

P. aeruginosa intra-abdominal infections

Azactam for Injection (Aztreonam) Bristol-Myers Squibb 734
Cefobid Intravenous/Intramuscular (Cefoperazone Sodium) Roerig 2189
Cefobid Pharmacy Bulk Package - Not for Direct Infusion (Cefoperazone Sodium) Roerig 2192
Netromycin Injection 100 mg/ml (Netilmicin Sulfate) Schering 2373
Pipracil (Piperacillin Sodium) Lederle 1390
Primaxin I.M. (Imipenem-Cilastatin Sodium) Merck & Co., Inc. 1727
Primaxin I.V. (Imipenem-Cilastatin Sodium) Merck & Co., Inc. 1729

P. aeruginosa lower respiratory tract infections

Azactam for Injection (Aztreonam) Bristol-Myers Squibb 734
Ceptaz (Ceftazidime) Glaxo Wellcome 1081
Cipro I.V. (Ciprofloxacin) Bayer Pharmaceutical 595
Cipro I.V. Pharmacy Bulk Package (Ciprofloxacin) Bayer Pharmaceutical 597
Cipro Tablets (Ciprofloxacin Hydrochloride) Bayer Pharmaceutical 592
Claforan Sterile and Injection (Cefotaxime Sodium) Hoechst-Roussel 1235
Fortaz (Ceftazidime) Glaxo Wellcome 1100
Mezlin (Mezlocillin Sodium) Bayer Pharmaceutical 601
Mezlin Pharmacy Bulk Package (Mezlocillin Sodium) Bayer Pharmaceutical 604
Nebcin Vials, Hyporets & ADD-Vantage (Tobramycin Sulfate) Lilly 1464
Netromycin Injection 100 mg/ml (Netilmicin Sulfate) Schering 2373
Pipracil (Piperacillin Sodium) Lederle 1390
Tazicef for Injection (Ceftazidime) SmithKline Beecham Pharmaceuticals 2519
Tazidime Vials, Faspak & ADD-Vantage (Ceftazidime) Lilly 1478
Tobramycin Sulfate Injection (Tobramycin Sulfate) Elkins-Sinn 968

P. aeruginosa meningitis

Ceptaz (Ceftazidime) Glaxo Wellcome 1081
Fortaz (Ceftazidime) Glaxo Wellcome 1100
Polymyxin B Sulfate, Aerosporin Brand Sterile Powder (Polymyxin B Sulfate) Glaxo Wellcome 1154
Tazicef for Injection (Ceftazidime) SmithKline Beecham Pharmaceuticals 2519
Tazidime Vials, Faspak & ADD-Vantage (Ceftazidime) Lilly 1478

P. aeruginosa respiratory tract infections

Cefobid Intravenous/Intramuscular (Cefoperazone Sodium) Roerig 2189
Cefobid Pharmacy Bulk Package - Not for Direct Infusion (Cefoperazone Sodium) Roerig 2192
Ticar for Injection (Ticarcillin Disodium) SmithKline Beecham Pharmaceuticals 2526

P. aeruginosa septicemia

Azactam for Injection (Aztreonam) Bristol-Myers Squibb 734
Cefobid Intravenous/Intramuscular (Cefoperazone Sodium) Roerig 2189
Cefobid Pharmacy Bulk Package - Not for Direct Infusion (Cefoperazone Sodium) Roerig 2192
Ceptaz (Ceftazidime) Glaxo Wellcome 1081
Fortaz (Ceftazidime) Glaxo Wellcome 1100
Nebcin Vials, Hyporets & ADD-Vantage (Tobramycin Sulfate) Lilly 1464
Netromycin Injection 100 mg/ml (Netilmicin Sulfate) Schering 2373
Pipracil (Piperacillin Sodium) Lederle 1390
Primaxin I.V. (Imipenem-Cilastatin Sodium) Merck & Co., Inc. 1729
Tazicef for Injection (Ceftazidime) SmithKline Beecham Pharmaceuticals 2519
Tazidime Vials, Faspak & ADD-Vantage (Ceftazidime) Lilly 1478
Ticar for Injection (Ticarcillin Disodium) SmithKline Beecham Pharmaceuticals 2526
Timentin for Injection (Ticarcillin Disodium, Clavulanate Potassium) SmithKline Beecham Pharmaceuticals 2528
Tobramycin Sulfate Injection (Tobramycin Sulfate) Elkins-Sinn 968

P. aeruginosa skin and skin structure infections

Azactam for Injection (Aztreonam) Bristol-Myers Squibb 734
Cefobid Intravenous/Intramuscular (Cefoperazone Sodium) Roerig 2189
Cefobid Pharmacy Bulk Package - Not for Direct Infusion (Cefoperazone Sodium) Roerig 2192
Ceptaz (Ceftazidime) Glaxo Wellcome 1081
Cipro I.V. (Ciprofloxacin) Bayer Pharmaceutical 595
Cipro I.V. Pharmacy Bulk Package (Ciprofloxacin) Bayer Pharmaceutical 597
Cipro Tablets (Ciprofloxacin Hydrochloride) Bayer Pharmaceutical 592
Fortaz (Ceftazidime) Glaxo Wellcome 1100
Nebcin Vials, Hyporets & ADD-Vantage (Tobramycin Sulfate) Lilly 1464
Netromycin Injection 100 mg/ml (Netilmicin Sulfate) Schering 2373
Pipracil (Piperacillin Sodium) Lederle 1390
Primaxin I.M. (Imipenem-Cilastatin Sodium) Merck & Co., Inc. 1727
Primaxin I.V. (Imipenem-Cilastatin Sodium) Merck & Co., Inc. 1729
Rocephin Injectable Vials, ADD-Vantage, Galaxy Container (Ceftriaxone Sodium) Roche Laboratories 2142
Tazicef for Injection (Ceftazidime) SmithKline Beecham Pharmaceuticals 2519
Tazidime Vials, Faspak & ADD-Vantage (Ceftazidime) Lilly 1478
Ticar for Injection (Ticarcillin Disodium) SmithKline Beecham Pharmaceuticals 2526
Tobramycin Sulfate Injection (Tobramycin Sulfate) Elkins-Sinn 968

P. aeruginosa urinary tract infections

Azactam for Injection (Aztreonam) Bristol-Myers Squibb 734
Cefizox for Intramuscular or Intravenous Use (Ceftizoxime Sodium) Fujisawa 1034
Cefobid Intravenous/Intramuscular (Cefoperazone Sodium) Roerig 2189
Cefobid Pharmacy Bulk Package - Not for Direct Infusion (Cefoperazone Sodium) Roerig 2192
Ceptaz (Ceftazidime) Glaxo Wellcome 1081
Cipro I.V. (Ciprofloxacin) Bayer Pharmaceutical 595
Cipro I.V. Pharmacy Bulk Package (Ciprofloxacin) Bayer Pharmaceutical 597
Cipro Tablets (Ciprofloxacin Hydrochloride) Bayer Pharmaceutical 592
Claforan Sterile and Injection (Cefotaxime Sodium) Hoechst-Roussel 1235
Floxin I.V. (Ofloxacin) McNeil Pharmaceutical 1571
Floxin Tablets (200 mg, 300 mg, 400 mg) (Ofloxacin) McNeil Pharmaceutical 1567
Fortaz (Ceftazidime) Glaxo Wellcome 1100
Maxaquin Tablets (Lomefloxacin Hydrochloride) Searle 2440
Nebcin Vials, Hyporets & ADD-Vantage (Tobramycin Sulfate) Lilly 1464
Netromycin Injection 100 mg/ml (Netilmicin Sulfate) Schering 2373
Noroxin Tablets (Norfloxacin) Merck & Co., Inc. 1715
Noroxin Tablets (Norfloxacin) Roberts 2048
Penetrex Tablets (Enoxacin) Rhone-Poulenc Rorer Pharmaceuticals 2031
Polymyxin B Sulfate, Aerosporin Brand Sterile Powder (Polymyxin B Sulfate) Glaxo Wellcome 1154
Primaxin I.V. (Imipenem-Cilastatin Sodium) Merck & Co., Inc. 1729

(■ Described in PDR For Nonprescription Drugs) (⊙ Described in PDR For Ophthalmology)

1517 **Indications Index** **P. mirabilis**

Tazicef for Injection (Ceftazidime) SmithKline Beecham Pharmaceuticals ... 2519
Tazidime Vials, Faspak & ADD-Vantage (Ceftazidime) Lilly .. 1478
Ticar for Injection (Ticarcillin Disodium) SmithKline Beecham Pharmaceuticals ... 2526
Timentin for Injection (Ticarcillin Disodium, Clavulanate Potassium) SmithKline Beecham Pharmaceuticals ... 2528
Tobramycin Sulfate Injection (Tobramycin Sulfate) Elkins-Sinn ... 968

P. falciparum infections
Aralen Hydrochloride Injection (Chloroquine Hydrochloride) Sanofi Winthrop ... 2301
Aralen Phosphate Tablets (Chloroquine Phosphate) Sanofi Winthrop ... 2301
Daraprim Tablets (Pyrimethamine) Glaxo Wellcome ... 1090
Fansidar Tablets (Sulfadoxine, Pyrimethamine) Roche Laboratories ... 2114
Lariam Tablets (Mefloquine Hydrochloride) Roche Laboratories ... 2128
Plaquenil Sulfate Tablets (Hydroxychloroquine Sulfate) Sanofi Winthrop ... 2328
Vibramycin Hyclate Capsules (Doxycycline Hyclate) Pfizer Labs 1941

P. falciparum infections, adjunct in
Gantanol Tablets (Sulfamethoxazole) Roche Laboratories ... 2119
Gantrisin (Acetyl Sulfisoxazole) Roche Laboratories ... 2120

P. inconstans group B urinary tract infections
Claforan Sterile and Injection (Cefotaxime Sodium) Hoechst-Roussel ... 1235

P. malariae infections
Aralen Hydrochloride Injection (Chloroquine Hydrochloride) Sanofi Winthrop ... 2301
Aralen Phosphate Tablets (Chloroquine Phosphate) Sanofi Winthrop ... 2301
Daraprim Tablets (Pyrimethamine) Glaxo Wellcome ... 1090
Plaquenil Sulfate Tablets (Hydroxychloroquine Sulfate) Sanofi Winthrop ... 2328

P. mirabilis biliary tract infections
Ancef Injection (Cefazolin Sodium) SmithKline Beecham Pharmaceuticals ... 2465
Kefzol Vials, Faspak & ADD-Vantage (Cefazolin Sodium) Lilly ... 1456

P. mirabilis bone and joint infections
Cefizox for Intramuscular or Intravenous Use (Ceftizoxime Sodium) Fujisawa ... 1034
Claforan Sterile and Injection (Cefotaxime Sodium) Hoechst-Roussel ... 1235
Keflex Pulvules & Oral Suspension (Cephalexin) Dista ... 914
Keftab Tablets (Cephalexin Hydrochloride) Dista ... 915
Rocephin Injectable Vials, ADD-Vantage, Galaxy Container (Ceftriaxone Sodium) Roche Laboratories ... 2142

P. mirabilis genitourinary tract infections
Ancef Injection (Cefazolin Sodium) SmithKline Beecham Pharmaceuticals ... 2465
Azactam for Injection (Aztreonam) Bristol-Myers Squibb ... 734
Keflex Pulvules & Oral Suspension (Cephalexin) Dista ... 914
Keftab Tablets (Cephalexin Hydrochloride) Dista ... 915
Mefoxin (Cefoxitin Sodium) Merck & Co., Inc. ... 1691
Mefoxin Premixed Intravenous Solution (Cefoxitin Sodium) Merck & Co., Inc. ... 1694
Omnipen for Oral Suspension (Ampicillin) Wyeth-Ayerst ... 2765

P. mirabilis gynecologic infections
Cefotan (Cefotetan) Zeneca ... 2829
Claforan Sterile and Injection (Cefotaxime Sodium) Hoechst-Roussel ... 1235
Mezlin (Mezlocillin Sodium) Bayer Pharmaceutical ... 601
Mezlin Pharmacy Bulk Package (Mezlocillin Sodium) Bayer Pharmaceutical ... 604

P. mirabilis infections
Amoxil (Amoxicillin Trihydrate) SmithKline Beecham Pharmaceuticals ... 2464
Ancef Injection (Cefazolin Sodium) SmithKline Beecham Pharmaceuticals ... 2465
Azactam for Injection (Aztreonam) Bristol-Myers Squibb ... 734
Azo Gantanol Tablets (Sulfamethoxazole, Phenazopyridine Hydrochloride) Roche Laboratories ... 2080
Azo Gantrisin Tablets (Sulfisoxazole, Phenazopyridine Hydrochloride) Roche Laboratories ... 2081
Bactrim (Trimethoprim, Sulfamethoxazole) Roche Laboratories ... 2084
Ceclor Pulvules & Suspension (Cefaclor) Lilly ... 1431
Cefizox for Intramuscular or Intravenous Use (Ceftizoxime Sodium) Fujisawa ... 1034
Cefobid Intravenous/Intramuscular (Cefoperazone Sodium) Roerig ... 2189
Cefobid Pharmacy Bulk Package - Not for Direct Infusion (Cefoperazone Sodium) Roerig ... 2192
Cefotan (Cefotetan) Zeneca ... 2829
Ceptaz (Ceftazidime) Glaxo Wellcome ... 1081
Cipro I.V. (Ciprofloxacin) Bayer Pharmaceutical ... 595
Cipro I.V. Pharmacy Bulk Package (Ciprofloxacin) Bayer Pharmaceutical ... 597
Cipro Tablets (Ciprofloxacin Hydrochloride) Bayer Pharmaceutical ... 592
Claforan Sterile and Injection (Cefotaxime Sodium) Hoechst-Roussel ... 1235
Duricef (Cefadroxil Monohydrate) Bristol-Myers Squibb ... 748
Floxin I.V. (Ofloxacin) McNeil Pharmaceutical ... 1571
Floxin Tablets (200 mg, 300 mg, 400 mg) (Ofloxacin) McNeil Pharmaceutical ... 1567
Fortaz (Ceftazidime) Glaxo Wellcome ... 1100
Gantanol Tablets (Sulfamethoxazole) Roche Laboratories ... 2119
Gantrisin (Acetyl Sulfisoxazole) Roche Laboratories ... 2120
Geocillin Tablets (Carbenicillin Indanyl Sodium) Roerig ... 2199
Keflex Pulvules & Oral Suspension (Cephalexin) Dista ... 914
Keftab Tablets (Cephalexin Hydrochloride) Dista ... 915
Kefzol Vials, Faspak & ADD-Vantage (Cefazolin Sodium) Lilly ... 1456
Maxaquin Tablets (Lomefloxacin Hydrochloride) Searle ... 2440
Mefoxin (Cefoxitin Sodium) Merck & Co., Inc. ... 1691
Mefoxin Premixed Intravenous Solution (Cefoxitin Sodium) Merck & Co., Inc. ... 1694
Mezlin (Mezlocillin Sodium) Bayer Pharmaceutical ... 601
Mezlin Pharmacy Bulk Package (Mezlocillin Sodium) Bayer Pharmaceutical ... 604
Monocid Injection (Cefonicid Sodium) SmithKline Beecham Pharmaceuticals ... 2497
Netromycin Injection 100 mg/ml (Netilmicin Sulfate) Schering ... 2373
Noroxin Tablets (Norfloxacin) Merck & Co., Inc. ... 1715
Noroxin Tablets (Norfloxacin) Roberts ... 2048
Omnipen Capsules (Ampicillin) Wyeth-Ayerst ... 2764
Omnipen for Oral Suspension (Ampicillin) Wyeth-Ayerst ... 2765
Penetrex Tablets (Enoxacin) Rhone-Poulenc Rorer Pharmaceuticals ... 2031
Pfizerpen for Injection (Penicillin G Potassium) Roerig ... 2203
Pipracil (Piperacillin Sodium) Lederle ... 1390
Proloprim Tablets (Trimethoprim) Glaxo Wellcome ... 1155
Rocephin Injectable Vials, ADD-Vantage, Galaxy Container (Ceftriaxone Sodium) Roche Laboratories ... 2142
Septra (Trimethoprim, Sulfamethoxazole) Glaxo Wellcome ... 1174
Spectrobid Tablets (Bacampicillin Hydrochloride) Roerig ... 2206
Suprax (Cefixime) Lederle ... 1399
Tazicef for Injection (Ceftazidime) SmithKline Beecham Pharmaceuticals ... 2519
Tazidime Vials, Faspak & ADD-Vantage (Ceftazidime) Lilly .. 1478
Trimpex Tablets (Trimethoprim) Roche Laboratories ... 2163
Unasyn (Ampicillin Sodium, Sulbactam Sodium) Roerig ... 2212
Vantin for Oral Suspension and Vantin Tablets (Cefpodoxime Proxetil) Upjohn ... 2646
Zefazone (Cefmetazole Sodium) Upjohn ... 2654

P. mirabilis infections, ocular
Chibroxin Sterile Ophthalmic Solution (Norfloxacin) Merck & Co., Inc. ... 1617
Ocuflox (Ofloxacin) Allergan ... 481
TobraDex Ophthalmic Suspension and Ointment (Dexamethasone, Tobramycin) Alcon Laboratories .. 473

P. mirabilis intra-abdominal infections
Claforan Sterile and Injection (Cefotaxime Sodium) Hoechst-Roussel ... 1235
Mezlin (Mezlocillin Sodium) Bayer Pharmaceutical ... 601
Mezlin Pharmacy Bulk Package (Mezlocillin Sodium) Bayer Pharmaceutical ... 604
Netromycin Injection 100 mg/ml (Netilmicin Sulfate) Schering ... 2373
Omnipen for Oral Suspension (Ampicillin) Wyeth-Ayerst ... 2765

P. mirabilis lower respiratory tract infections
Azactam for Injection (Aztreonam) Bristol-Myers Squibb ... 734
Cefizox for Intramuscular or Intravenous Use (Ceftizoxime Sodium) Fujisawa ... 1034
Cefotan (Cefotetan) Zeneca ... 2829
Ceptaz (Ceftazidime) Glaxo Wellcome ... 1081
Cipro I.V. (Ciprofloxacin) Bayer Pharmaceutical ... 595
Cipro I.V. Pharmacy Bulk Package (Ciprofloxacin) Bayer Pharmaceutical ... 597
Cipro Tablets (Ciprofloxacin Hydrochloride) Bayer Pharmaceutical ... 592
Claforan Sterile and Injection (Cefotaxime Sodium) Hoechst-Roussel ... 1235
Fortaz (Ceftazidime) Glaxo Wellcome ... 1100
Mandol Vials, Faspak & ADD-Vantage (Cefamandole Nafate) Lilly ... 1461
Mezlin (Mezlocillin Sodium) Bayer Pharmaceutical ... 601
Mezlin Pharmacy Bulk Package (Mezlocillin Sodium) Bayer Pharmaceutical ... 604
Netromycin Injection 100 mg/ml (Netilmicin Sulfate) Schering ... 2373
Rocephin Injectable Vials, ADD-Vantage, Galaxy Container (Ceftriaxone Sodium) Roche Laboratories ... 2142
Tazicef for Injection (Ceftazidime) SmithKline Beecham Pharmaceuticals ... 2519
Tazidime Vials, Faspak & ADD-Vantage (Ceftazidime) Lilly .. 1478

P. mirabilis prostatitis
Ancef Injection (Cefazolin Sodium) SmithKline Beecham Pharmaceuticals ... 2465
Geocillin Tablets (Carbenicillin Indanyl Sodium) Roerig ... 2199
Keflex Pulvules & Oral Suspension (Cephalexin) Dista ... 914
Keftab Tablets (Cephalexin Hydrochloride) Dista ... 915

P. mirabilis respiratory tract infections
Cefobid Intravenous/Intramuscular (Cefoperazone Sodium) Roerig ... 2189
Cefobid Pharmacy Bulk Package - Not for Direct Infusion (Cefoperazone Sodium) Roerig ... 2192

P. mirabilis septicemia
Ancef Injection (Cefazolin Sodium) SmithKline Beecham Pharmaceuticals ... 2465
Azactam for Injection (Aztreonam) Bristol-Myers Squibb ... 734
Kefzol Vials, Faspak & ADD-Vantage (Cefazolin Sodium) Lilly ... 1456
Netromycin Injection 100 mg/ml (Netilmicin Sulfate) Schering ... 2373
Pipracil (Piperacillin Sodium) Lederle ... 1390

P. mirabilis skin and skin structure infections
Azactam for Injection (Aztreonam) Bristol-Myers Squibb ... 734
Cefizox for Intramuscular or Intravenous Use (Ceftizoxime Sodium) Fujisawa ... 1034
Ceptaz (Ceftazidime) Glaxo Wellcome ... 1081
Cipro I.V. (Ciprofloxacin) Bayer Pharmaceutical ... 595
Cipro I.V. Pharmacy Bulk Package (Ciprofloxacin) Bayer Pharmaceutical ... 597
Cipro Tablets (Ciprofloxacin Hydrochloride) Bayer Pharmaceutical ... 592
Claforan Sterile and Injection (Cefotaxime Sodium) Hoechst-Roussel ... 1235
Floxin I.V. (Ofloxacin) McNeil Pharmaceutical ... 1571
Floxin Tablets (200 mg, 300 mg, 400 mg) (Ofloxacin) McNeil Pharmaceutical ... 1567
Fortaz (Ceftazidime) Glaxo Wellcome ... 1100
Mandol Vials, Faspak & ADD-Vantage (Cefamandole Nafate) Lilly ... 1461
Mefoxin (Cefoxitin Sodium) Merck & Co., Inc. ... 1691
Mefoxin Premixed Intravenous Solution (Cefoxitin Sodium) Merck & Co., Inc. ... 1694
Mezlin (Mezlocillin Sodium) Bayer Pharmaceutical ... 601
Mezlin Pharmacy Bulk Package (Mezlocillin Sodium) Bayer Pharmaceutical ... 604
Netromycin Injection 100 mg/ml (Netilmicin Sulfate) Schering ... 2373
Pipracil (Piperacillin Sodium) Lederle ... 1390
Rocephin Injectable Vials, ADD-Vantage, Galaxy Container (Ceftriaxone Sodium) Roche Laboratories ... 2142
Tazicef for Injection (Ceftazidime) SmithKline Beecham Pharmaceuticals ... 2519
Tazidime Vials, Faspak & ADD-Vantage (Ceftazidime) Lilly .. 1478
Unasyn (Ampicillin Sodium, Sulbactam Sodium) Roerig ... 2212
Zefazone (Cefmetazole Sodium) Upjohn ... 2654

P. mirabilis urinary tract infections
Ancef Injection (Cefazolin Sodium) SmithKline Beecham Pharmaceuticals ... 2465
Azactam for Injection (Aztreonam) Bristol-Myers Squibb ... 734
Azo Gantanol Tablets (Sulfamethoxazole, Phenazopyridine

(◘ Described in PDR For Nonprescription Drugs) (◉ Described in PDR For Ophthalmology)

P. mirabilis **Indications Index** **1518**

Hydrochloride) Roche Laboratories ... 2080
Azo Gantrisin Tablets (Sulfisoxazole, Phenazopyridine Hydrochloride) Roche Laboratories ... 2081
Bactrim (Trimethoprim, Sulfamethoxazole) Roche Laboratories ... 2084
Ceclor Pulvules & Suspension (Cefaclor) Lilly ... 1431
Cefizox for Intramuscular or Intravenous Use (Ceftizoxime Sodium) Fujisawa ... 1034
Cefotan (Cefotetan) Zeneca ... 2829
Ceptaz (Ceftazidime) Glaxo Wellcome ... 1081
Cipro I.V. (Ciprofloxacin) Bayer Pharmaceutical ... 595
Cipro I.V. Pharmacy Bulk Package (Ciprofloxacin) Bayer Pharmaceutical ... 597
Cipro Tablets (Ciprofloxacin Hydrochloride) Bayer Pharmaceutical ... 592
Claforan Sterile and Injection (Cefotaxime Sodium) Hoechst-Roussel ... 1235
Duricef (Cefadroxil Monohydrate) Bristol-Myers Squibb ... 748
Floxin I.V. (Ofloxacin) McNeil Pharmaceutical ... 1571
Floxin Tablets (200 mg, 300 mg, 400 mg) (Ofloxacin) McNeil Pharmaceutical ... 1567
Fortaz (Ceftazidime) Glaxo Wellcome ... 1100
Gantanol Tablets (Sulfamethoxazole) Roche Laboratories ... 2119
Gantrisin (Acetyl Sulfisoxazole) Roche Laboratories ... 2120
Geocillin Tablets (Carbenicillin Indanyl Sodium) Roerig ... 2199
Keflex Pulvules & Oral Suspension (Cephalexin) Dista ... 914
Keftab Tablets (Cephalexin Hydrochloride) Dista ... 915
Kefzol Vials, Faspak & ADD-Vantage (Cefazolin Sodium) Lilly ... 1456
Maxaquin Tablets (Lomefloxacin Hydrochloride) Searle ... 2440
Mefoxin (Cefoxitin Sodium) Merck & Co., Inc. ... 1691
Mefoxin Premixed Intravenous Solution (Cefoxitin Sodium) Merck & Co., Inc. ... 1694
Mezlin (Mezlocillin Sodium) Bayer Pharmaceutical ... 601
Mezlin Pharmacy Bulk Package (Mezlocillin Sodium) Bayer Pharmaceutical ... 604
Monocid Injection (Cefonicid Sodium) SmithKline Beecham Pharmaceuticals ... 2497
Netromycin Injection 100 mg/ml (Netilmicin Sulfate) Schering ... 2373
Noroxin Tablets (Norfloxacin) Merck & Co., Inc. ... 1715
Noroxin Tablets (Norfloxacin) Roberts ... 2048
Penetrex Tablets (Enoxacin) Rhone-Poulenc Rorer Pharmaceuticals ... 2031
Proloprim Tablets (Trimethoprim) Glaxo Wellcome ... 1155
Rocephin Injectable Vials, ADD-Vantage, Galaxy Container (Ceftriaxone Sodium) Roche Laboratories ... 2142
Septra (Trimethoprim, Sulfamethoxazole) Glaxo Wellcome ... 1174
Spectrobid Tablets (Bacampicillin Hydrochloride) Roerig ... 2206
Suprax (Cefixime) Lederle ... 1399
Tazicef for Injection (Ceftazidime) SmithKline Beecham Pharmaceuticals ... 2519
Tazidime Vials, Faspak & ADD-Vantage (Ceftazidime) Lilly .. 1478
Trimpex Tablets (Trimethoprim) Roche Laboratories ... 2163
Vantin for Oral Suspension and Vantin Tablets (Cefpodoxime Proxetil) Upjohn ... 2646

P. ovale infections
Aralen Hydrochloride Injection (Chloroquine Hydrochloride) Sanofi Winthrop ... 2301
Aralen Phosphate Tablets (Chloroquine Phosphate) Sanofi Winthrop ... 2301
Daraprim Tablets (Pyrimethamine) Glaxo Wellcome ... 1090
Plaquenil Sulfate Tablets (Hydroxychloroquine Sulfate) Sanofi Winthrop ... 2328

P. vivax infections
Aralen Hydrochloride Injection (Chloroquine Hydrochloride) Sanofi Winthrop ... 2301
Aralen Phosphate Tablets (Chloroquine Phosphate) Sanofi Winthrop ... 2301
Daraprim Tablets (Pyrimethamine) Glaxo Wellcome ... 1090
Lariam Tablets (Mefloquine Hydrochloride) Roche Laboratories ... 2128
Plaquenil Sulfate Tablets (Hydroxychloroquine Sulfate) Sanofi Winthrop ... 2328

P. vulgaris infections
Azo Gantanol Tablets (Sulfamethoxazole, Phenazopyridine Hydrochloride) Roche Laboratories ... 2080
Azo Gantrisin Tablets (Sulfisoxazole, Phenazopyridine Hydrochloride) Roche Laboratories ... 2081
Bactrim (Trimethoprim, Sulfamethoxazole) Roche Laboratories ... 2084
Cefizox for Intramuscular or Intravenous Use (Ceftizoxime Sodium) Fujisawa ... 1034
Cefotan (Cefotetan) Zeneca ... 2829
Cipro I.V. (Ciprofloxacin) Bayer Pharmaceutical ... 595
Cipro I.V. Pharmacy Bulk Package (Ciprofloxacin) Bayer Pharmaceutical ... 597
Cipro Tablets (Ciprofloxacin Hydrochloride) Bayer Pharmaceutical ... 592
Claforan Sterile and Injection (Cefotaxime Sodium) Hoechst-Roussel ... 1235
Gantanol Tablets (Sulfamethoxazole) Roche Laboratories ... 2119
Gantrisin (Acetyl Sulfisoxazole) Roche Laboratories ... 2120
Geocillin Tablets (Carbenicillin Indanyl Sodium) Roerig ... 2199
Mefoxin (Cefoxitin Sodium) Merck & Co., Inc. ... 1691
Mefoxin Premixed Intravenous Solution (Cefoxitin Sodium) Merck & Co., Inc. ... 1694
Mezlin (Mezlocillin Sodium) Bayer Pharmaceutical ... 601
Monocid Injection (Cefonicid Sodium) SmithKline Beecham Pharmaceuticals ... 2497
Noroxin Tablets (Norfloxacin) Merck & Co., Inc. ... 1715
Noroxin Tablets (Norfloxacin) Roberts ... 2048
Primaxin I.V. (Imipenem-Cilastatin Sodium) Merck & Co., Inc. ... 1729
Rocephin Injectable Vials, ADD-Vantage, Galaxy Container (Ceftriaxone Sodium) Roche Laboratories ... 2142
Septra (Trimethoprim, Sulfamethoxazole) Glaxo Wellcome ... 1174
Zefazone (Cefmetazole Sodium) Upjohn ... 2654

P. vulgaris infections, ocular
TobraDex Ophthalmic Suspension and Ointment (Dexamethasone, Tobramycin) Alcon Laboratories .. 473

P. vulgaris skin and skin structure infections
Cipro I.V. (Ciprofloxacin) Bayer Pharmaceutical ... 595
Cipro I.V. Pharmacy Bulk Package (Ciprofloxacin) Bayer Pharmaceutical ... 597
Cipro Tablets (Ciprofloxacin Hydrochloride) Bayer Pharmaceutical ... 592
Claforan Sterile and Injection (Cefotaxime Sodium) Hoechst-Roussel ... 1235
Mezlin (Mezlocillin Sodium) Bayer Pharmaceutical ... 601
Mezlin Pharmacy Bulk Package (Mezlocillin Sodium) Bayer Pharmaceutical ... 604
Primaxin I.V. (Imipenem-Cilastatin Sodium) Merck & Co., Inc. ... 1729
Zefazone (Cefmetazole Sodium) Upjohn ... 2654

P. vulgaris urinary tract infections
Azo Gantanol Tablets (Sulfamethoxazole, Phenazopyridine Hydrochloride) Roche Laboratories ... 2080
Azo Gantrisin Tablets (Sulfisoxazole, Phenazopyridine Hydrochloride) Roche Laboratories ... 2081
Bactrim (Trimethoprim, Sulfamethoxazole) Roche Laboratories ... 2084
Cefizox for Intramuscular or Intravenous Use (Ceftizoxime Sodium) Fujisawa ... 1034
Cefotan (Cefotetan) Zeneca ... 2829
Claforan Sterile and Injection (Cefotaxime Sodium) Hoechst-Roussel ... 1235
Gantanol Tablets (Sulfamethoxazole) Roche Laboratories ... 2119
Gantrisin (Acetyl Sulfisoxazole) Roche Laboratories ... 2120
Geocillin Tablets (Carbenicillin Indanyl Sodium) Roerig ... 2199
Mefoxin (Cefoxitin Sodium) Merck & Co., Inc. ... 1691
Mefoxin Premixed Intravenous Solution (Cefoxitin Sodium) Merck & Co., Inc. ... 1694
Monocid Injection (Cefonicid Sodium) SmithKline Beecham Pharmaceuticals ... 2497
Noroxin Tablets (Norfloxacin) Merck & Co., Inc. ... 1715
Noroxin Tablets (Norfloxacin) Roberts ... 2048
Primaxin I.V. (Imipenem-Cilastatin Sodium) Merck & Co., Inc. ... 1729
Rocephin Injectable Vials, ADD-Vantage, Galaxy Container (Ceftriaxone Sodium) Roche Laboratories ... 2142
Septra (Trimethoprim, Sulfamethoxazole) Glaxo Wellcome ... 1174

Paget's disease of bone
Aredia for Injection (Pamidronate Disodium) CibaGeneva ... 810
Calcimar Injection, Synthetic (Calcitonin, Synthetic) Rhone-Poulenc Rorer Pharmaceuticals ... 2013
Didronel Tablets (Etidronate Disodium (Diphosphonate)) Procter & Gamble Pharmaceuticals ... 1984
Miacalcin Injection (Calcitonin, Synthetic) Sandoz Pharmaceuticals ... 2273

Pain associated with arthritis, topical
(see under Pain, topical relief of)

Pain associated with sports injuries
(see under Pain, topical relief of)

Pain associated with upper respiratory infection
Actifed Plus Caplets (Acetaminophen, Pseudoephedrine Hydrochloride, Triprolidine Hydrochloride) WARNER WELLCOME ... ▣ 845
Actifed Plus Tablets (Acetaminophen, Pseudoephedrine Hydrochloride, Triprolidine Hydrochloride) WARNER WELLCOME ... ▣ 845
Advil Cold and Sinus Caplets and Tablets (formerly CoAdvil) (Ibuprofen, Pseudoephedrine Hydrochloride) Whitehall ... ▣ 870
Arthritis Foundation Ibuprofen Tablets (Ibuprofen) McNeil Consumer ... ▣ 674
BC Cold Powder Multi-Symptom Formula (Cold-Sinus-Allergy) (Aspirin, Phenylpropanolamine Hydrochloride, Chlorpheniramine Maleate) Block ... ▣ 609
BC Cold Powder Non-Drowsy Formula (Cold-Sinus) (Aspirin, Phenylpropanolamine Hydrochloride) Block ... ▣ 609
Bayer Select Ibuprofen Pain Relief Formula (Ibuprofen) Miles Consumer ... ▣ 715
Bufferin Analgesic Tablets and Caplets (Aspirin) Bristol-Myers Products ... ▣ 613
Extra Strength Bufferin Analgesic Tablets (Aspirin) Bristol-Myers Products ... ▣ 615
Contac Severe Cold and Flu Formula Caplets (Acetaminophen, Chlorpheniramine Maleate, Dextromethorphan Hydrobromide, Phenylpropanolamine Hydrochloride) SmithKline Beecham Consumer ▣ 814
Coricidin 'D' Decongestant Tablets (Acetaminophen, Chlorpheniramine Maleate, Phenylpropanolamine Hydrochloride) Schering-Plough HealthCare ... ▣ 800
Coricidin Tablets (Acetaminophen, Chlorpheniramine Maleate) Schering-Plough HealthCare ... ▣ 800
Drixoral Cold and Flu Extended-Release Tablets (Acetaminophen, Dexbrompheniramine Maleate, Pseudoephedrine Sulfate) Schering-Plough HealthCare ... ▣ 803
Excedrin Extra-Strength Analgesic Tablets & Caplets (Acetaminophen, Aspirin, Caffeine) Bristol-Myers Products ... 732
Mobigesic Tablets (Magnesium Salicylate, Phenyltoloxamine Citrate) Ascher ... ▣ 602
Children's Motrin Ibuprofen Oral Suspension (Ibuprofen) McNeil Consumer ... 1546
Pyrroxate Caplets (Acetaminophen, Chlorpheniramine Maleate, Phenylpropanolamine Hydrochloride) Roberts ... ▣ 772
Sine-Off No Drowsiness Formula Caplets (Acetaminophen, Pseudoephedrine Hydrochloride) SmithKline Beecham Consumer ... ▣ 824
Sine-Off Sinus Medicine (Aspirin, Chlorpheniramine Maleate, Phenylpropanolamine Hydrochloride) SmithKline Beecham Consumer ... ▣ 825
Sinulin Tablets (Acetaminophen, Phenylpropanolamine Hydrochloride, Chlorpheniramine Maleate) Carnrick ... 787
Sinutab Sinus Allergy Medication, Maximum Strength Tablets and Caplets (Acetaminophen, Chlorpheniramine Maleate, Pseudoephedrine Hydrochloride) WARNER WELLCOME ... ▣ 860
Sinutab Sinus Medication, Maximum Strength Without Drowsiness Formula, Tablets & Caplets (Acetaminophen, Pseudoephedrine Hydrochloride) WARNER WELLCOME ... ▣ 860
Sinutab Sinus Medication, Regular Strength Without Drowsiness Formula (Acetaminophen, Pseudoephedrine Hydrochloride) WARNER WELLCOME ... ▣ 859
Sudafed Severe Cold Formula Caplets (Acetaminophen, Dextromethorphan Hydrobromide, Pseudoephedrine Hydrochloride) WARNER WELLCOME ... ▣ 863
TheraFlu Flu and Cold Medicine (Acetaminophen, Chlorpheniramine Maleate, Pseudoephedrine Hydrochloride) Sandoz Consumer ... ▣ 787
Children's TYLENOL Cold Multi-Symptom Liquid Formula and Chewable Tablets (Acetaminophen, Chlorpheniramine

(▣ Described in PDR For Nonprescription Drugs) (⊙ Described in PDR For Ophthalmology)

1519 **Indications Index** **Pain**

Maleate, Pseudoephedrine Hydrochloride) McNeil Consumer 1561
Infants' TYLENOL Cold Decongestant & Fever-Reducer Drops (Acetaminophen, Pseudoephedrine Hydrochloride) McNeil Consumer 1556
TYLENOL Cold Multi-Symptom Formula Medication Tablets and Caplets (Acetaminophen, Chlorpheniramine Maleate, Pseudoephedrine Hydrochloride, Dextromethorphan Hydrobromide) McNeil Consumer 1561
TYLENOL Cold Medication No Drowsiness Formula Gelcaps and Caplets (Acetaminophen, Pseudoephedrine Hydrochloride, Dextromethorphan Hydrobromide) McNeil Consumer 1562
Vicks 44M Cough, Cold & Flu Relief (Acetaminophen, Dextromethorphan Hydrobromide, Chlorpheniramine Maleate, Pseudoephedrine Hydrochloride) Procter & Gamble ▣ 756
Vicks DayQuil (Acetaminophen, Dextromethorphan Hydrobromide, Pseudoephedrine Hydrochloride, Guaifenesin) Procter & Gamble ▣ 761
Vicks NyQuil LiquiCaps Multi-Symptom Cold/Flu Relief (Acetaminophen, Pseudoephedrine Hydrochloride, Dextromethorphan Hydrobromide, Doxylamine Succinate) Procter & Gamble ▣ 763
Vicks NyQuil Multi-Symptom Cold/Flu Relief - (Original & Cherry Flavor) (Acetaminophen, Dextromethorphan Hydrobromide, Doxylamine Succinate, Pseudoephedrine Hydrochloride) Procter & Gamble ▣ 763

Pain due to common cold (see under Pain associated with upper respiratory infection)

Pain due to urinary tract infections, symptomatic relief of
Azo Gantanol Tablets (Sulfamethoxazole, Phenazopyridine Hydrochloride) Roche Laboratories 2080
Azo Gantrisin Tablets (Sulfisoxazole, Phenazopyridine Hydrochloride) Roche Laboratories 2081

Pain with gastric hyperacidity
Alka-Seltzer Effervescent Antacid and Pain Reliever (Aspirin, Sodium Bicarbonate, Citric Acid) Miles Consumer ▣ 701
Alka-Seltzer Extra Strength Effervescent Antacid and Pain Reliever (Aspirin, Sodium Bicarbonate, Citric Acid) Miles Consumer ▣ 703
Alka-Seltzer Lemon Lime Effervescent Antacid and Pain Reliever (Aspirin, Sodium Citrate) Miles Consumer ▣ 703
TYLENOL, Extra Strength, Headache Plus Pain Reliever with Antacid Caplets (Acetaminophen, Calcium Carbonate) McNeil Consumer 1559

Pain, anal (see under Pain, anorectal)

Pain, anogenital
Americaine Hemorrhoidal Ointment (Benzocaine) CIBA Consumer ▣ 629
Dyclone 0.5% and 1% Topical Solutions, USP (Dyclonine Hydrochloride) Astra 544
Preparation H (Glycerin, Petrolatum, Phenylephrine Hydrochloride, Shark Liver Oil) Whitehall ▣ 871

Pain, anorectal
Fleet Pain Relief Pads (Pramoxine Hydrochloride) Fleet 1003
Tronolane Anesthetic Cream for Hemorrhoids (Pramoxine Hydrochloride) Ross ▣ 784
Wyanoids Relief Factor Hemorrhoidal Suppositories (Liver, Desiccated, Shark Liver Oil) Wyeth-Ayerst ▣ 881

Pain, arthritic, minor
Advil Ibuprofen Tablets and Caplets (Ibuprofen) Whitehall ▣ 870
Aleve (Naproxen Sodium) Procter & Gamble 1975
ArthriCare Odor Free Rub (Capsaicin, Menthol, Methyl Nicotinate) Del ▣ 651
ArthriCare Triple Medicated Rub (Menthol, Methyl Nicotinate, Methyl Salicylate) Del ▣ 651
Arthritis Foundation Aspirin Free Caplets (Acetaminophen) McNeil Consumer ▣ 673
Arthritis Foundation Ibuprofen Tablets (Ibuprofen) McNeil Consumer ▣ 674
Arthritis Foundation NightTime Caplets (Acetaminophen, Diphenhydramine Hydrochloride) McNeil Consumer ▣ 674
Arthritis Foundation Safety Coated Aspirin Tablets (Aspirin) McNeil Consumer ▣ 675
Regular Strength Ascriptin Tablets (Aspirin Buffered, Calcium Carbonate) CIBA Consumer ▣ 629
Arthritis Strength BC Powder (Aspirin, Salicylamide, Caffeine) Block ▣ 609
BC Powder (Aspirin, Salicylamide, Caffeine) Block ▣ 609
Genuine Bayer Aspirin Tablets & Caplets (Aspirin) Miles Consumer ▣ 713
Extra Strength Bayer Arthritis Pain Regimen Formula (Aspirin, Enteric Coated) Miles Consumer ▣ 711
Extra Strength Bayer Aspirin Caplets & Tablets (Aspirin) Miles Consumer ▣ 712
Extended-Release Bayer 8-Hour Aspirin (Aspirin) Miles Consumer ▣ 712
Extra Strength Bayer Plus Aspirin Caplets (Aspirin, Calcium Carbonate) Miles Consumer ▣ 713
Bayer Enteric Aspirin (Aspirin, Enteric Coated) Miles Consumer ▣ 709
Bayer Select Ibuprofen Pain Relief Formula (Ibuprofen) Miles Consumer ▣ 715
Bufferin Analgesic Tablets and Caplets (Aspirin) Bristol-Myers Products ▣ 613
Arthritis Strength Bufferin Analgesic Caplets (Aspirin) Bristol-Myers Products ▣ 614
Extra Strength Bufferin Analgesic Tablets (Aspirin) Bristol-Myers Products ▣ 615
Ecotrin (Aspirin, Enteric Coated) SmithKline Beecham 2455
Empirin Aspirin Tablets (Aspirin) WARNER WELLCOME ▣ 854
Aspirin Free Excedrin Analgesic Caplets and Geltabs (Acetaminophen, Caffeine) Bristol-Myers Products 732
Excedrin Extra-Strength Analgesic Tablets & Caplets (Acetaminophen, Aspirin, Caffeine) Bristol-Myers Products 732
Haltran Tablets (Ibuprofen) Roberts ▣ 771
Ibuprohm (Ibuprofen) Ohm ▣ 735
Mobigesic Tablets (Magnesium Salicylate, Phenyltoloxamine Citrate) Ascher ▣ 602
Motrin IB Caplets, Tablets, and Geltabs (Ibuprofen) Upjohn ▣ 838
Nuprin Ibuprofen/Analgesic Tablets & Caplets (Ibuprofen) Bristol-Myers Products ▣ 622
Panodol Tablets and Caplets (Acetaminophen) SmithKline Beecham Consumer ▣ 824
Percogesic Analgesic Tablets (Acetaminophen, Phenyltoloxamine Citrate) Procter & Gamble ▣ 754
TYLENOL Extended Relief Caplets (Acetaminophen) McNeil Consumer 1558
TYLENOL, Extra Strength, Acetaminophen Adult Liquid Pain Reliever (Acetaminophen) McNeil Consumer 1560
TYLENOL, Regular Strength, acetaminophen Caplets and Tablets (Acetaminophen) McNeil Consumer 1558
Vanquish Analgesic Caplets (Acetaminophen, Aspirin, Caffeine, Aluminum Hydroxide Gel, Magnesium Hydroxide) Miles Consumer ▣ 731

Pain, bone, skeletal metastases
Metastron (Strontium Chloride) Medi-Physics 1594

Pain, dental
Aleve (Naproxen Sodium) Procter & Gamble 1975
Arthritis Foundation Ibuprofen Tablets (Ibuprofen) McNeil Consumer ▣ 674
Arthritis Strength BC Powder (Aspirin, Salicylamide, Caffeine) Block ▣ 609
BC Powder (Aspirin, Salicylamide, Caffeine) Block ▣ 609
Bayer Children's Chewable Aspirin (Aspirin) Miles Consumer ▣ 711
Genuine Bayer Aspirin Tablets & Caplets (Aspirin) Miles Consumer ▣ 713
Extra Strength Bayer Aspirin Caplets & Tablets (Aspirin) Miles Consumer ▣ 712
Extended-Release Bayer 8-Hour Aspirin (Aspirin) Miles Consumer ▣ 712
Extra Strength Bayer Plus Aspirin Caplets (Aspirin, Calcium Carbonate) Miles Consumer ▣ 713
Bayer Select Ibuprofen Pain Relief Formula (Ibuprofen) Miles Consumer ▣ 715
Bufferin Analgesic Tablets and Caplets (Aspirin) Bristol-Myers Products ▣ 613
Extra Strength Bufferin Analgesic Tablets (Aspirin) Bristol-Myers Products ▣ 615
Cēpacol Anesthetic Lozenges (Benzocaine, Cetylpyridinium Chloride) J.B. Williams ▣ 875
Children's Vicks Chloraseptic Sore Throat Spray (Phenol) Procter & Gamble ▣ 757
Dyclone 0.5% and 1% Topical Solutions, USP (Dyclonine Hydrochloride) Astra 544
Empirin Aspirin Tablets (Aspirin) WARNER WELLCOME ▣ 854
Aspirin Free Excedrin Analgesic Caplets and Geltabs (Acetaminophen, Caffeine) Bristol-Myers Products 732
Gly-Oxide Liquid (Carbamide Peroxide) SmithKline Beecham Consumer ▣ 820
Haltran Tablets (Ibuprofen) Roberts ▣ 771
Hyland's Teething Tablets (Calcium Phosphate, Homeopathic Medications) Standard Homeopathic ▣ 830
Ibuprohm (Ibuprofen) Ohm ▣ 735
Mobigesic Tablets (Magnesium Salicylate, Phenyltoloxamine Citrate) Ascher ▣ 602
Children's Motrin Ibuprofen Oral Suspension (Ibuprofen) McNeil Consumer 1546
Motrin IB Caplets, Tablets, and Geltabs (Ibuprofen) Upjohn ▣ 838
Nuprin Ibuprofen/Analgesic Tablets & Caplets (Ibuprofen) Bristol-Myers Products ▣ 622
Baby Orajel Teething Pain Medicine (Benzocaine) Del ▣ 652
Orajel Maximum Strength Toothache Medication (Benzocaine) Del ▣ 652
Orajel Mouth-Aid for Canker and Cold Sores (Benzocaine, Benzalkonium Chloride, Zinc Chloride) Del ▣ 652
Panodol Tablets and Caplets (Acetaminophen) SmithKline Beecham Consumer ▣ 824
Children's Panadol Chewable Tablets, Liquid, Infant's Drops (Acetaminophen) SmithKline Beecham Consumer ▣ 824
Percogesic Analgesic Tablets (Acetaminophen, Phenyltoloxamine Citrate) Procter & Gamble ▣ 754
Tylenol, Children's (Acetaminophen) McNeil Consumer 1555
TYLENOL, Extra Strength, Acetaminophen Adult Liquid Pain Reliever (Acetaminophen) McNeil Consumer 1560
Vanquish Analgesic Caplets (Acetaminophen, Aspirin, Caffeine, Aluminum Hydroxide Gel, Magnesium Hydroxide) Miles Consumer ▣ 731

Pain, ear
Americaine Otic Topical Anesthetic Ear Drops (Benzocaine) Fisons 983
Children's Panadol Chewable Tablets, Liquid, Infant's Drops (Acetaminophen) SmithKline Beecham Consumer ▣ 824
Tympagesic Ear Drops (Antipyrine, Benzocaine, Phenylephrine Hydrochloride) Savage 2342

Pain, general
Advil Ibuprofen Tablets and Caplets (Ibuprofen) Whitehall ▣ 870
Aleve (Naproxen Sodium) Procter & Gamble 1975
Alka-Seltzer Effervescent Antacid and Pain Reliever (Aspirin, Sodium Bicarbonate, Citric Acid) Miles Consumer ▣ 701
Alka-Seltzer Extra Strength Effervescent Antacid and Pain Reliever (Aspirin, Sodium Bicarbonate, Citric Acid) Miles Consumer ▣ 703
Alka-Seltzer Lemon Lime Effervescent Antacid and Pain Reliever (Aspirin, Sodium Citrate) Miles Consumer ▣ 703
Arthritis Foundation Aspirin Free Caplets (Acetaminophen) McNeil Consumer ▣ 673
Arthritis Foundation NightTime Caplets (Acetaminophen, Diphenhydramine Hydrochloride) McNeil Consumer ▣ 674
Regular Strength Ascriptin Tablets (Aspirin Buffered, Calcium Carbonate) CIBA Consumer ▣ 629
Backache Caplets (Magnesium Salicylate) Bristol-Myers Products ▣ 613
Bayer Children's Chewable Aspirin (Aspirin) Miles Consumer ▣ 711
Genuine Bayer Aspirin Tablets & Caplets (Aspirin) Miles Consumer ▣ 713
Extra Strength Bayer Aspirin Caplets & Tablets (Aspirin) Miles Consumer ▣ 712
Extended-Release Bayer 8-Hour Aspirin (Aspirin) Miles Consumer ▣ 712
Extra Strength Bayer PM Aspirin (Aspirin, Diphenhydramine Hydrochloride) Miles Consumer ▣ 713
Bayer Enteric Aspirin (Aspirin, Enteric Coated) Miles Consumer ▣ 709
Bayer Select Ibuprofen Pain Relief Formula (Ibuprofen) Miles Consumer ▣ 715
Bayer Select Night Time Pain Relief Formula (Acetaminophen, Diphenhydramine Hydrochloride) Miles Consumer ▣ 716
Campho-Phenique Liquid (Phenol, Camphor) Miles Consumer ▣ 719
Aspirin Free Excedrin Analgesic Caplets and Geltabs (Acetaminophen, Caffeine) Bristol-Myers Products 732
Haltran Tablets (Ibuprofen) Roberts ▣ 771
Healthprin Aspirin (Aspirin) Smart 2455
Ibuprohm (Ibuprofen) Ohm ▣ 735

(▣ Described in PDR For Nonprescription Drugs) (◉ Described in PDR For Ophthalmology)

Pain | Indications Index | 1520

Levoprome (Methotrimeprazine) Immunex ... 1274
Children's Motrin Ibuprofen Oral Suspension (Ibuprofen) McNeil Consumer ... 1546
Children's Panadol Chewable Tablets, Liquid, Infant's Drops (Acetaminophen) SmithKline Beecham Consumer ... ▣ 824
St. Joseph Adult Chewable Aspirin (81 mg.) (Aspirin) Schering-Plough HealthCare ... ▣ 808
Trilisate (Choline Magnesium Trisalicylate) Purdue Frederick ... 2000
Tylenol, Children's (Acetaminophen) McNeil Consumer ... 1555
TYLENOL, Extra Strength, Acetaminophen Adult Liquid Pain Reliever (Acetaminophen) McNeil Consumer ... 1560
TYLENOL, Extra Strength, acetaminophen Gelcaps, Geltabs, Caplets, Tablets (Acetaminophen) McNeil Consumer ... 1559
TYLENOL, Junior Strength, acetaminophen Coated Caplets, Grape and Fruit Chewable Tablets (Acetaminophen) McNeil Consumer ... 1557
TYLENOL, Regular Strength, acetaminophen Caplets and Tablets (Acetaminophen) McNeil Consumer ... 1558
TYLENOL PM, Extra Strength Pain Reliever/Sleep Aid Caplets, Geltabs, Gelcaps (Acetaminophen, Diphenhydramine Hydrochloride) McNeil Consumer 1560
Vanquish Analgesic Caplets (Acetaminophen, Aspirin, Caffeine, Aluminum Hydroxide Gel, Magnesium Hydroxide) Miles Consumer ... ▣ 731

Pain, hemorrhoidal (see under Pain, anorectal)

Pain, intractable chronic (see also under Pain, severe)
Infumorph 200 and Infumorph 500 Sterile Solutions (Morphine Sulfate) Elkins-Sinn ... 965

Pain, menstrual
Advil Ibuprofen Tablets and Caplets (Ibuprofen) Whitehall ... ▣ 870
Aleve (Naproxen Sodium) Procter & Gamble ... 1975
Arthritis Foundation Ibuprofen Tablets (Ibuprofen) McNeil Consumer ... ▣ 674
BC Powder (Aspirin, Salicylamide, Caffeine) Block ... ▣ 609
Genuine Bayer Aspirin Tablets & Caplets (Aspirin) Miles Consumer ... ▣ 713
Extra Strength Bayer Aspirin Caplets & Tablets (Aspirin) Miles Consumer ... ▣ 712
Extra Strength Bayer Plus Aspirin Caplets (Aspirin, Calcium Carbonate) Miles Consumer ... ▣ 713
Bayer Select Ibuprofen Pain Relief Formula (Ibuprofen) Miles Consumer ... ▣ 715
Bayer Select Menstrual Multi-Symptom Formula (Acetaminophen, Pamabrom) Miles Consumer ... ▣ 716
Bufferin Analgesic Tablets and Caplets (Aspirin) Bristol-Myers Products ... ▣ 613
Extra Strength Bufferin Analgesic Tablets (Aspirin) Bristol-Myers Products ... ▣ 615
Empirin Aspirin Tablets (Aspirin) WARNER WELLCOME ... ▣ 854
Aspirin Free Excedrin Analgesic Caplets and Geltabs (Acetaminophen, Caffeine) Bristol-Myers Products ... 732
Excedrin Extra-Strength Analgesic Tablets & Caplets (Acetaminophen, Aspirin, Caffeine) Bristol-Myers Products ... 732
Haltran Tablets (Ibuprofen) Roberts ... ▣ 771
Ibuprohm (Ibuprofen) Ohm ... ▣ 735
Maximum Strength Multi-Symptom Formula Midol (Acetaminophen, Caffeine, Pyrilamine Maleate) Miles Consumer ... ▣ 722
PMS Multi-Symptom Formula Midol (Acetaminophen, Pamabrom, Pyrilamine Maleate) Miles Consumer ... ▣ 723
Motrin IB Caplets, Tablets, and Geltabs (Ibuprofen) Upjohn ... ▣ 838
Nuprin Ibuprofen/Analgesic Tablets & Caplets (Ibuprofen) Bristol-Myers Products ... ▣ 622
Panodol Tablets and Caplets (Acetaminophen) SmithKline Beecham Consumer ... ▣ 824
Percogesic Analgesic Tablets (Acetaminophen, Phenyltoloxamine Citrate) Procter & Gamble ▣ 754
St. Joseph Adult Chewable Aspirin (81 mg.) (Aspirin) Schering-Plough HealthCare ... ▣ 808
TYLENOL Extended Relief Caplets (Acetaminophen) McNeil Consumer ... 1558
TYLENOL, Extra Strength, Acetaminophen Adult Liquid Pain Reliever (Acetaminophen) McNeil Consumer ... 1560
TYLENOL, Regular Strength, acetaminophen Caplets and Tablets (Acetaminophen) McNeil Consumer ... 1558
Vanquish Analgesic Caplets (Acetaminophen, Aspirin, Caffeine, Aluminum Hydroxide Gel, Magnesium Hydroxide) Miles Consumer ... ▣ 731

Pain, mild
Advil Ibuprofen Tablets and Caplets (Ibuprofen) Whitehall ... ▣ 870
Aleve (Naproxen Sodium) Procter & Gamble ... 1975
Maximum Strength Ascriptin (Aspirin Buffered, Calcium Carbonate) CIBA Consumer ... ▣ 630
Arthritis Strength Bufferin Analgesic Caplets (Aspirin) Bristol-Myers Products ... ▣ 614
Cama Arthritis Pain Reliever (Aspirin, Aluminum Hydroxide, Magnesium Oxide) Sandoz Consumer ... ▣ 785
Ecotrin (Aspirin, Enteric Coated) SmithKline Beecham ... 2455
Empirin with Codeine Tablets (Aspirin, Codeine Phosphate) Glaxo Wellcome ... 1093
Excedrin Extra-Strength Analgesic Tablets & Caplets (Acetaminophen, Aspirin, Caffeine) Bristol-Myers Products ... 732
Legatrin PM (Acetaminophen, Diphenhydramine Hydrochloride) Columbia ... ▣ 651
Panodol Tablets and Caplets (Acetaminophen) SmithKline Beecham Consumer ... ▣ 824
TYLENOL, Extra Strength, acetaminophen Gelcaps, Geltabs, Caplets, Tablets (Acetaminophen) McNeil Consumer ... 1559
TYLENOL, Junior Strength, acetaminophen Coated Caplets, Grape and Fruit Chewable Tablets (Acetaminophen) McNeil Consumer ... 1557
TYLENOL, Regular Strength, acetaminophen Caplets and Tablets (Acetaminophen) McNeil Consumer ... 1558

Pain, mild to moderate
Children's Advil Suspension (Ibuprofen) Wyeth-Ayerst ... 2692
Anaprox/Naprosyn (Naproxen Sodium) Roche Laboratories ... 2117
Darvon-N/Darvocet-N (Propoxyphene Napsylate, Acetaminophen) Lilly ... 1433
Darvon (Propoxyphene Hydrochloride, Aspirin, Caffeine) Lilly ... 1435
Darvon-N Suspension & Tablets (Propoxyphene Napsylate) Lilly ... 1433
Dolobid Tablets (Diflunisal) Merck & Co., Inc. ... 1654
Easprin (Aspirin) Parke-Davis ... 1914
IBU Tablets (Ibuprofen) Knoll Laboratories ... 1342
Children's Motrin Ibuprofen Oral Suspension (Ibuprofen) McNeil Consumer ... 1546
Motrin Tablets (Ibuprofen) Upjohn ... 2625
Motrin Ibuprofen Suspension, Oral Drops, Chewable Tablets, Caplets (Ibuprofen) McNeil Consumer ... 1546
Nalfon 200 Pulvules & Nalfon Tablets (Fenoprofen Calcium) Dista ... 917
Anaprox/Naprosyn (Naproxen) Roche Laboratories ... 2117
Orudis Capsules (Ketoprofen) Wyeth-Ayerst ... 2766
Talacen (Pentazocine Hydrochloride) Sanofi Winthrop ... 2333
Trilisate (Choline Magnesium Trisalicylate) Purdue Frederick ... 2000
Tylenol with Codeine Elixir (Acetaminophen, Codeine Phosphate) McNeil Pharmaceutical ... 1583
Wygesic Tablets (Propoxyphene Hydrochloride, Acetaminophen) Wyeth-Ayerst ... 2827

Pain, mild to moderate, acute musculo-skeletal
Norgesic (Orphenadrine Citrate, Aspirin) 3M Pharmaceuticals ... 1496
Paraflex Caplets (Chlorzoxazone) McNeil Pharmaceutical ... 1580
Parafon Forte DSC Caplets (Chlorzoxazone) McNeil Pharmaceutical ... 1581
Soma Compound w/Codeine Tablets (Carisoprodol, Aspirin, Codeine Phosphate) Wallace ... 2676
Soma Compound Tablets (Carisoprodol, Aspirin) Wallace ... 2675
Soma Tablets (Carisoprodol) Wallace ... 2674

Pain, moderate
Empirin with Codeine Tablets (Aspirin, Codeine Phosphate) Glaxo Wellcome ... 1093
Levo-Dromoran (Levorphanol Tartrate) Roche Laboratories ... 2129
Ponstel (Mefenamic Acid) Parke-Davis ... 1925
Talwin Compound (Pentazocine Hydrochloride, Aspirin) Sanofi Winthrop ... 2335

Pain, moderate to moderately severe
Anexia Tablets (Acetaminophen, Hydrocodone Bitartrate) Monarch ... 1782
DHCplus Capsules (Dihydrocodeine Bitartrate, Acetaminophen, Caffeine) Purdue Frederick ... 1993
Lorcet 10/650 (Hydrocodone Bitartrate, Acetaminophen) Forest ... 1018
Lortab (Hydrocodone Bitartrate, Acetaminophen) UCB ... 2566
Percocet Tablets (Oxycodone Hydrochloride, Acetaminophen) DuPont ... 938
Percodan Tablets (Oxycodone Hydrochloride, Oxycodone Terephthalate, Aspirin) DuPont ... 939
Percodan-Demi Tablets (Oxycodone Hydrochloride, Oxycodone Terephthalate, Aspirin) DuPont ... 940
Roxicodone Tablets, Oral Solution & Intensol (Oxycodone) (Oxycodone Hydrochloride) Roxane ... 2244
Toradol (Ketorolac Tromethamine) Roche Laboratories ... 2159
Tylenol with Codeine Phosphate Tablets (Acetaminophen, Codeine Phosphate) McNeil Pharmaceutical ... 1583
Tylox Capsules (Oxycodone Hydrochloride, Acetaminophen) McNeil Pharmaceutical ... 1584
Ultram Tablets (50 mg) (Tramadol Hydrochloride) McNeil Pharmaceutical ... 1585
Vicodin Tablets (Hydrocodone Bitartrate, Acetaminophen) Knoll Laboratories ... 1356
Vicodin ES Tablets (Hydrocodone Bitartrate, Acetaminophen) Knoll Laboratories ... 1357
Zydone Capsules (Hydrocodone Bitartrate, Acetaminophen) DuPont ... 949

Pain, moderate to severe
Anexsia 5/500 Elixir (Acetaminophen, Hydrocodone Bitartrate) Monarch ... 1781
Astramorph/PF Injection, USP (Preservative-Free) (Morphine Sulfate) Astra ... 535
Buprenex Injectable (Buprenorphine) Reckitt & Colman ... 2006
Dalgan Injection (Dezocine) Astra ... 538
Demerol (Meperidine Hydrochloride) Sanofi Winthrop ... 2308
Dilaudid Ampules (Hydromorphone Hydrochloride) Knoll Laboratories ... 1335
Dilaudid-HP Injection (Hydromorphone Hydrochloride) Knoll Laboratories ... 1337
Dilaudid-HP Lyophilized Powder 250 mg (Hydromorphone Hydrochloride) Knoll Laboratories ... 1337
Dilaudid (Hydromorphone Hydrochloride) Knoll Laboratories ... 1335
Dilaudid Oral Liquid (Hydromorphone Hydrochloride) Knoll Laboratories ... 1339
Dilaudid (Hydromorphone Hydrochloride) Knoll Laboratories ... 1335
Dilaudid Tablets - 8 mg (Hydromorphone Hydrochloride) Knoll Laboratories ... 1339
Duragesic Transdermal System (Fentanyl) Janssen ... 1288
Duramorph (Morphine Sulfate) Elkins-Sinn ... 962
Empirin with Codeine Tablets (Aspirin, Codeine Phosphate) Glaxo Wellcome ... 1093
Hydrocet Capsules (Acetaminophen, Hydrocodone Bitartrate) Carnrick ... 782
Levo-Dromoran (Levorphanol Tartrate) Roche Laboratories ... 2129
Levoprome (Methotrimeprazine) Immunex ... 1274
MS Contin Tablets (Morphine Sulfate) Purdue Frederick ... 1994
MSIR (Morphine Sulfate) Purdue Frederick ... 1997
Nubain Injection (Nalbuphine Hydrochloride) DuPont ... 935
Numorphan Injection (Oxymorphone Hydrochloride) DuPont ... 936
Numorphan Suppositories (Oxymorphone Hydrochloride) DuPont ... 937
Stadol (Butorphanol Tartrate) Bristol-Myers Squibb ... 775
Talwin Injection (Pentazocine Lactate) Sanofi Winthrop ... 2334
Talwin Nx (Pentazocine Hydrochloride, Naloxone Hydrochloride) Sanofi Winthrop ... 2336

Pain, muscular, temporary relief of
Aleve (Naproxen Sodium) Procter & Gamble ... 1975
Alka-Seltzer Effervescent Antacid and Pain Reliever (Aspirin, Sodium Bicarbonate, Citric Acid) Miles Consumer ... ▣ 701
Alka-Seltzer Extra Strength Effervescent Antacid and Pain Reliever (Aspirin, Sodium Bicarbonate, Citric Acid) Miles Consumer ... ▣ 703
Alka-Seltzer Lemon Lime Effervescent Antacid and Pain Reliever (Aspirin, Sodium Citrate) Miles Consumer ... ▣ 703
Arthritis Foundation Ibuprofen Tablets (Ibuprofen) McNeil Consumer ... ▣ 674
Aspercreme Creme, Lotion Analgesic Rub (Trolamine Salicylate) Thompson Medical ... ▣ 830
Extra Strength Bayer Aspirin Caplets & Tablets (Aspirin) Miles Consumer ... ▣ 712
Extra Strength Bayer Plus Aspirin Caplets (Aspirin, Calcium Carbonate) Miles Consumer ... ▣ 713
Bayer Enteric Aspirin (Aspirin, Enteric Coated) Miles Consumer ... ▣ 709

(▣ Described in PDR For Nonprescription Drugs) (◉ Described in PDR For Ophthalmology)

1521 **Indications Index** **Pancreatic cystic fibrosis**

Bayer Select Ibuprofen Pain Relief Formula (Ibuprofen) Miles Consumer ▣ 715
Bufferin Analgesic Tablets and Caplets (Aspirin) Bristol-Myers Products ▣ 613
Extra Strength Bufferin Analgesic Tablets (Aspirin) Bristol-Myers Products ▣ 615
Cramp End Tablets (Ibuprofen) Ohm ▣ 735
Empirin Aspirin Tablets (Aspirin) WARNER WELLCOME ▣ 854
Aspirin Free Excedrin Analgesic Caplets and Geltabs (Acetaminophen, Caffeine) Bristol-Myers Products 732
Excedrin Extra-Strength Analgesic Tablets & Caplets (Acetaminophen, Aspirin, Caffeine) Bristol-Myers Products 732
Fluori-Methane (Dichlorodifluoromethane, Trichloromonofluoromethane) Gebauer 1053
Haltran Tablets (Ibuprofen) Roberts ▣ 771
Ibuprohm (Ibuprofen) Ohm ▣ 735
Teen Multi-Symptom Formula Midol (Acetaminophen, Pamabrom) Miles Consumer ▣ 722
Mobigesic Tablets (Magnesium Salicylate, Phenyltoloxamine Citrate) Ascher ▣ 602
Motrin IB Caplets, Tablets, and Geltabs (Ibuprofen) Upjohn ▣ 838
Nuprin Ibuprofen/Analgesic Tablets & Caplets (Ibuprofen) Bristol-Myers Products ▣ 622
Percogesic Analgesic Tablets (Acetaminophen, Phenyltoloxamine Citrate) Procter & Gamble ▣ 754
St. Joseph Adult Chewable Aspirin (81 mg.) (Aspirin) Schering-Plough HealthCare ▣ 808
Therapeutic Mineral Ice, Pain Relieving Gel (Menthol) Bristol-Myers Products ▣ 623
TYLENOL, Extra Strength, Acetaminophen Adult Liquid Pain Reliever (Acetaminophen) McNeil Consumer 1560
TYLENOL, Junior Strength, acetaminophen Coated Caplets, Grape and Fruit Chewable Tablets (Acetaminophen) McNeil Consumer 1557
TYLENOL, Regular Strength, acetaminophen Caplets and Tablets (Acetaminophen) McNeil Consumer 1558
Vanquish Analgesic Caplets (Acetaminophen, Aspirin, Caffeine, Aluminum Hydroxide Gel, Magnesium Hydroxide) Miles Consumer ▣ 731

Pain, neurogenic
Maximum Strength Ascriptin (Aspirin Buffered, Calcium Carbonate) CIBA Consumer ▣ 630
Atretol Tablets (Carbamazepine) Athena 573
Arthritis Strength BC Powder (Aspirin, Salicylamide, Caffeine) Block ▣ 609
BC Powder (Aspirin, Salicylamide, Caffeine) Block ▣ 609
Sarapin (Sarracenia purpurea, Pitcher Plant Distillate) High Chemical 1231
St. Joseph Adult Chewable Aspirin (81 mg.) (Aspirin) Schering-Plough HealthCare ▣ 808
Tegretol Chewable Tablets (Carbamazepine) CibaGeneva 852
Tegretol Suspension (Carbamazepine) CibaGeneva 852
Tegretol Tablets (Carbamazepine) CibaGeneva 852
TYLENOL, Regular Strength, acetaminophen Caplets and Tablets (Acetaminophen) McNeil Consumer 1558
Vanquish Analgesic Caplets (Acetaminophen, Aspirin, Caffeine, Aluminum Hydroxide Gel, Magnesium Hydroxide) Miles Consumer ▣ 731
Zostrix/Zostrix-HP (Capsaicin) GenDerm 1056

Pain, neurogenic, post-herpes zoster infections, topical relief of
Zostrix/Zostrix-HP (Capsaicin) GenDerm 1056

Pain, obstetrical
Demerol (Meperidine Hydrochloride) Sanofi Winthrop 2308
Nubain Injection (Nalbuphine Hydrochloride) DuPont 935
Sufenta Injection (Sufentanil Citrate) Janssen 1309

Pain, oral mucosal and gingival
Cetacaine Topical Anesthetic (Benzocaine, Tetracaine Hydrochloride, Butyl Aminobenzoate) Cetylite 794

Pain, pre- and postoperative, adjunct to
Levo-Dromoran (Levorphanol Tartrate) Roche Laboratories 2129
Phenergan Injection (Promethazine Hydrochloride) Wyeth-Ayerst 2773
Sublimaze Injection (Fentanyl Citrate) Janssen 1307

Pain, pre- and postoperative, relief of
Alfenta Injection (Alfentanil Hydrochloride) Janssen 1286
Demerol (Meperidine Hydrochloride) Sanofi Winthrop 2308
Ethyl Chloride, U.S.P. (Chloroethane, Ethyl Chloride) Gebauer 1052
Fluro-Ethyl (Dichlorotetrafluoroethane, Ethyl Chloride) Gebauer 1053
Levo-Dromoran (Levorphanol Tartrate) Roche Laboratories 2129
Mepergan Injection (Meperidine Hydrochloride, Promethazine Hydrochloride) Wyeth-Ayerst 2753
Nubain Injection (Nalbuphine Hydrochloride) DuPont 935
Sufenta Injection (Sufentanil Citrate) Janssen 1309
Talwin Injection (Pentazocine Lactate) Sanofi Winthrop 2334
Toradol (Ketorolac Tromethamine) Roche Laboratories 2159

Pain, prepartum (see under Pain, obstetrical)

Pain, severe
Astramorph/PF Injection, USP (Preservative-Free) (Morphine Sulfate) Astra 535
Duramorph (Morphine Sulfate) Elkins-Sinn 962
Levo-Dromoran (Levorphanol Tartrate) Roche Laboratories 2129
Methadone Hydrochloride Oral Solution & Tablets (Methadone Hydrochloride) Roxane 2235
Oramorph SR (Morphine Sulfate Sustained Release Tablets) (Morphine Sulfate) Roxane 2236
RMS Suppositories (Morphine Sulfate) Upsher-Smith 2657
Roxanol (Morphine Sulfate) Roxane 2243

Pain, short-term management of
Toradol (Ketorolac Tromethamine) Roche Laboratories 2159

Pain, suprapubic, symptomatic relief of
Urispas Tablets (Flavoxate Hydrochloride) SmithKline Beecham Pharmaceuticals 2532

Pain, teething (see under Pain, dental)

Pain, topical relief of
Americaine (Benzocaine) CIBA Consumer ▣ 629
ArthriCare Odor Free Rub (Capsaicin, Menthol, Methyl Nicotinate) Del ▣ 651
ArthriCare Triple Medicated Rub (Menthol, Methyl Nicotinate, Methyl Salicylate) Del ▣ 651
Aspercreme Creme, Lotion Analgesic Rub (Trolamine Salicylate) Thompson Medical ▣ 830
Bactine Antiseptic/Anesthetic First Aid Liquid (Benzalkonium Chloride, Lidocaine Hydrochloride) Miles Consumer ▣ 708
Benadryl Itch Relief Cream, Children's Formula and Maximum Strength 2% (Diphenhydramine Hydrochloride, Zinc Acetate) WARNER WELLCOME ▣ 851
Benadryl Itch Relief Spray, Children's Formula and Maximum Strength 2% (Diphenhydramine Hydrochloride, Zinc Acetate) WARNER WELLCOME ▣ 851
BenGay External Analgesic Products (Menthol, Methyl Salicylate) Pfizer Consumer ▣ 741
BiCozene Creme (Benzocaine, Resorcinol) Sandoz Consumer ▣ 785
Caladryl Cream For Kids (Calamine, Pramoxine Hydrochloride) WARNER WELLCOME ▣ 853
Campho-Phenique Antiseptic Gel (Camphor, Phenol) Miles Consumer ▣ 718
Campho-Phenique Maximum Strength First Aid Antibiotic Plus Pain Reliever Ointment (Bacitracin Zinc, Lidocaine Hydrochloride, Neomycin Sulfate, Polymyxin B Sulfate) Miles Consumer ▣ 719
Capsin Topical Analgesic Lotion 0.025% and 0.075% (Capsaicin) Flemming ▣ 655
Capzasin-P (Capsaicin) Thompson Medical ▣ 831
Chloresium (Chlorophyllin Copper Complex) Rystan 2246
DermaFlex Topical Anesthetic Gel (Lidocaine) Zila Pharmaceuticals ▣ 882
Dolorac (Capsaicin) GenDerm 1054
Emla Cream (Prilocaine, Lidocaine) Astra 545
Ethyl Chloride, U.S.P. (Chloroethane, Ethyl Chloride) Gebauer 1052
Eucalyptamint Arthritis Pain Reliever (External Analgesic) (Menthol) CIBA Consumer ▣ 635
Eucalyptamint Muscle Pain Relief Formula (Menthol) CIBA Consumer ▣ 636
Fluori-Methane (Dichlorodifluoromethane, Trichloromonofluoromethane) Gebauer 1053
Fluro-Ethyl (Dichlorotetrafluoroethane, Ethyl Chloride) Gebauer 1053
Hyland's Arnicaid Tablets (Homeopathic Medications) Standard Homeopathic ▣ 828
Itch-X (Pramoxine Hydrochloride, Benzyl Alcohol) Ascher ▣ 602
Mantadil Cream (Chlorcyclizine Hydrochloride) Glaxo Wellcome 1135
Teen Multi-Symptom Formula Midol (Acetaminophen, Pamabrom) Miles Consumer ▣ 722
Mobisyl Analgesic Creme (Trolamine Salicylate) Ascher ▣ 603
Myoflex External Analgesic Creme (Trolamine Salicylate) CIBA Consumer ▣ 643
Nupercainal Hemorrhoidal and Anesthetic Ointment (Dibucaine) CIBA Consumer ▣ 644
Sportscreme External Analgesic Rub Cream & Lotion (Trolamine Salicylate) Thompson Medical ▣ 834
Thera-Gesic (Methyl Salicylate, Menthol) Mission 1781
Therapeutic Mineral Ice, Pain Relieving Gel (Menthol) Bristol-Myers Products ▣ 623
Topical Analgesic Ointment (Ammonia Solution, Strong) Transdermal Technologies ▣ 835
Vicks VapoRub (Menthol, Camphor, Eucalyptus, Oil of) Procter & Gamble ▣ 766
Water-Jel Burn Jel (Lidocaine) Water-Jel 2682
Xylocaine Ointment 2.5% (Lidocaine) Astra ▣ 603
Zilactin-B Medicated Gel with Benzocaine (Benzocaine) Zila Pharmaceuticals ▣ 882
Zostrix/Zostrix-HP (Capsaicin) GenDerm 1056

Pain, unspecified
Extra Strength Bayer Plus Aspirin Caplets (Aspirin, Calcium Carbonate) Miles Consumer ▣ 713
Cataflam (Diclofenac Potassium) CibaGeneva 816
Ecotrin (Aspirin, Enteric Coated) SmithKline Beecham 2455
Lodine Capsules and Tablets (Etodolac) Wyeth-Ayerst 2743

Pain, urinary tract
Prodium (Phenazopyridine Hydrochloride) Breckenridge 690
Pyridium (Phenazopyridine Hydrochloride) Parke-Davis 1928

Palpebral conjunctiva inflammation
AK-Pred (Prednisolone Sodium Phosphate) Akorn ◎ 204
AK-Trol Ointment & Suspension (Dexamethasone, Neomycin Sulfate, Polymyxin B Sulfate) Akorn ◎ 205
Blephamide Liquifilm Sterile Ophthalmic Suspension (Prednisolone Acetate, Sulfacetamide Sodium) Allergan 476
Cortisporin Ophthalmic Ointment Sterile (Polymyxin B Sulfate, Bacitracin Zinc, Neomycin Sulfate, Hydrocortisone) Glaxo Wellcome 1085
Cortisporin Ophthalmic Suspension Sterile (Hydrocortisone, Polymyxin B Sulfate, Neomycin Sulfate) Glaxo Wellcome 1086
Dexacidin Ointment (Dexamethasone, Neomycin Sulfate, Polymyxin B Sulfate) CIBA Vision Ophthalmics ◎ 263
Econopred & Econopred Plus Ophthalmic Suspensions (Prednisolone Acetate) Alcon Laboratories ◎ 217
FML Forte Liquifilm (Fluorometholone) Allergan ◎ 240
FML Liquifilm (Fluorometholone) Allergan ◎ 241
FML S.O.P. (Fluorometholone) Allergan ◎ 241
FML-S Liquifilm (Sulfacetamide Sodium, Fluorometholone) Allergan ◎ 242
Fluor-Op Ophthalmic Suspension (Fluorometholone) CIBA Vision Ophthalmics ◎ 264
Inflamase (Prednisolone Sodium Phosphate) CIBA Vision Ophthalmics ◎ 265
Maxitrol Ophthalmic Ointment and Suspension (Dexamethasone, Neomycin Sulfate, Polymyxin B Sulfate) Alcon Laboratories ◎ 224
Ophthocort (Chloramphenicol, Polymyxin B Sulfate, Hydrocortisone Acetate) Parke-Davis ◎ 311
Poly-Pred Liquifilm (Neomycin Sulfate, Polymyxin B Sulfate, Prednisolone Acetate) Allergan ◎ 248
Pred Forte (Prednisolone Acetate) Allergan ◎ 250
Pred-G Liquifilm Sterile Ophthalmic Suspension (Gentamicin Sulfate, Prednisolone Acetate) Allergan ◎ 251
Pred-G S.O.P. Sterile Ophthalmic Ointment (Gentamicin Sulfate, Prednisolone Acetate) Allergan ◎ 252
TobraDex Ophthalmic Suspension and Ointment (Dexamethasone, Tobramycin) Alcon Laboratories 473
Vasocidin Ointment (Prednisolone Acetate, Sulfacetamide Sodium) CIBA Vision Ophthalmics ◎ 268
Vasocidin Ophthalmic Solution (Prednisolone Sodium Phosphate, Sulfacetamide Sodium) CIBA Vision Ophthalmics ◎ 270

Pancreas, disseminated adenocarcinoma (see under Carcinoma, pancreas)

Pancreatic cells, cytopathologic examination, adjunct in
Secretin-Ferring (Secretin) Ferring 2872

Pancreatic cystic fibrosis
Cotazym (Pancrelipase) Organon 1817

(▣ Described in PDR For Nonprescription Drugs) (◎ Described in PDR For Ophthalmology)

Pancreatic cystic fibrosis — Indications Index — 1522

Creon (Pancrelipase) Solvay 2536
Ku-Zyme HP Capsules (Pancrelipase) Schwarz 2402
Pancrease Capsules (Pancrelipase) McNeil Pharmaceutical 1579
Pancrease MT Capsules (Pancrelipase) McNeil Pharmaceutical 1579
Viokase (Pancrelipase) Robins 2076
Zymase Capsules (Pancrelipase) Organon 1834

Pancreatic exocrine disease, diagnosis of
Secretin-Ferring (Secretin) Ferring.. 2872

Pancreatic insufficiency
Cotazym (Pancrelipase) Organon 1817
Creon (Pancrelipase) Solvay 2536
Donnazyme Tablets (Pancreatin) Robins 2061
Ku-Zyme HP Capsules (Pancrelipase) Schwarz 2402
Pancrease Capsules (Pancrelipase) McNeil Pharmaceutical 1579
Pancrease MT Capsules (Pancrelipase) McNeil Pharmaceutical 1579
Ultrase Capsules (Pancrelipase) Scandipharm 2343
Ultrase MT Capsules (Pancrelipase) Scandipharm 2344
Viokase (Pancrelipase) Robins 2076
Zymase Capsules (Pancrelipase) Organon 1834

Panic disorder with or without agoraphobia
Xanax Tablets (Alprazolam) Upjohn 2649

Papillitis (see under Optic neuritis)

Paracoccidioidomycosis
Nizoral Tablets (Ketoconazole) Janssen 1298

Paralysis agitans (see under Parkinson's disease)

Paralysis, familial periodic, hypokalemic
K-Dur Microburst Release System (potassium chloride, USP) E.R. Tablets (Potassium Chloride) Key 1325
K-Lor Powder Packets (Potassium Chloride) Abbott 434
K-Tab Filmtab (Potassium Chloride) Abbott 434
Micro-K (Potassium Chloride) Robins 2063
Micro-K LS Packets (Potassium Chloride) Robins 2064
Slow-K Extended-Release Tablets (Potassium Chloride) CibaGeneva 851

Paralytic ileus (see under Ileus, paralytic)

Paralytic ileus, post-surgery, prophylaxis (see under Ileus, paralytic, post-surgery)

Parkinson's disease
Artane (Trihexyphenidyl Hydrochloride) Lederle 1368
Atamet (Carbidopa, Levodopa) Athena 572
Benadryl Capsules (Diphenhydramine Hydrochloride) Parke-Davis 1898
Benadryl Injection (Diphenhydramine Hydrochloride) Parke-Davis 1898
Parlodel (Bromocriptine Mesylate) Sandoz Pharmaceuticals 2281
Sinemet Tablets (Carbidopa, Levodopa) DuPont 943
Sinemet CR Tablets (Carbidopa, Levodopa) DuPont 944
Symmetrel Capsules and Syrup (Amantadine Hydrochloride) DuPont 946

Parkinson's disease, adjunctive therapy in
Akineton (Biperiden Hydrochloride) Knoll Laboratories 1333
Cogentin (Benztropine Mesylate) Merck & Co., Inc. 1621
Eldepryl Tablets (Selegiline Hydrochloride) Somerset 2550
Levsin/Levsinex/Levbid (Hyoscyamine Sulfate) Schwarz 2405
Permax Tablets (Pergolide Mesylate) Athena 575

Parkinson's disease, idiopathic
Artane (Trihexyphenidyl Hydrochloride) Lederle 1368
Atamet (Carbidopa, Levodopa) Athena 572
Kemadrin Tablets (Procyclidine Hydrochloride) Glaxo Wellcome.... 1112
Larodopa Tablets (Levodopa) Roche Laboratories 2129
Parlodel (Bromocriptine Mesylate) Sandoz Pharmaceuticals 2281
Sinemet Tablets (Carbidopa, Levodopa) DuPont 943
Sinemet CR Tablets (Carbidopa, Levodopa) DuPont 944

Parkinsonism, arteriosclerotic
Artane (Trihexyphenidyl Hydrochloride) Lederle 1368
Kemadrin Tablets (Procyclidine Hydrochloride) Glaxo Wellcome.... 1112
Larodopa Tablets (Levodopa) Roche Laboratories 2129

Parkinsonism, postencephalitic
Artane (Trihexyphenidyl Hydrochloride) Lederle 1368
Atamet (Carbidopa, Levodopa) Athena 572
Kemadrin Tablets (Procyclidine Hydrochloride) Glaxo Wellcome.... 1112
Larodopa Tablets (Levodopa) Roche Laboratories 2129
Parlodel (Bromocriptine Mesylate) Sandoz Pharmaceuticals 2281
Sinemet Tablets (Carbidopa, Levodopa) DuPont 943
Sinemet CR Tablets (Carbidopa, Levodopa) DuPont 944
Symmetrel Capsules and Syrup (Amantadine Hydrochloride) DuPont 946

Parkinsonism, symptomatic, following carbon monoxide intoxication
Atamet (Carbidopa, Levodopa) Athena 572
Larodopa Tablets (Levodopa) Roche Laboratories 2129
Sinemet Tablets (Carbidopa, Levodopa) DuPont 943
Sinemet CR Tablets (Carbidopa, Levodopa) DuPont 944
Symmetrel Capsules and Syrup (Amantadine Hydrochloride) DuPont 946

Parkinsonism, symptomatic, following manganese intoxication
Atamet (Carbidopa, Levodopa) Athena 572
Larodopa Tablets (Levodopa) Roche Laboratories 2129
Sinemet Tablets (Carbidopa, Levodopa) DuPont 943
Sinemet CR Tablets (Carbidopa, Levodopa) DuPont 944

Pasteurella pestis (see under Yersinia pestis infections)

Pasteurella tularensis (see under Francisella tularensis infections)

PCP (see under Pneumocystis carinii pneumonia)

Pediculosis capitis infestation
Kwell Shampoo (Lindane) Reedco.... 2009
Lindane Shampoo USP 1% (Lindane) Barre-National 583
Nix Creme Rinse (Permethrin) WARNER WELLCOME .... ▣ 858

Pediculosis pubis infestation
Kwell Shampoo (Lindane) Reedco.... 2009
Lindane Shampoo USP 1% (Lindane) Barre-National 583

Pediculosis, human
A-200 Lice Killing Shampoo (Piperonyl Butoxide) Hogil .... ▣ 657
InnoGel Plus (Pyrethrum Extract, Piperonyl Butoxide) Hogil .... ▣ 657
Pronto Lice Killing Shampoo & Conditioner in One Kit (Pyrethrins, Piperonyl Butoxide) Del .. ▣ 653
Rid Lice Killing Shampoo (Pyrethrum Extract, Piperonyl Butoxide) Pfizer Consumer 1933

Pediculosis, human, adjunct in
A-200 Lice Control Spray (Permethrin) Hogil .... ▣ 656
Rid Lice Control Spray (Permethrin) Pfizer Consumer 1933

Pelvic adhesion, post-operative, reducing the incidence of
INTERCEED* (TC7) Absorbable Adhesion Barrier (Cellulose, Oxidized Regenerated) J & J Medical 1313

Pelvic cellulitis (see also under Infections, gynecologic)
Azactam for Injection (Aztreonam) Bristol-Myers Squibb 734
Ceptaz (Ceftazidime) Glaxo Wellcome 1081
Claforan Sterile and Injection (Cefotaxime Sodium) Hoechst-Roussel 1235
Cleocin Phosphate Injection (Clindamycin Phosphate) Upjohn 2586
Fortaz (Ceftazidime) Glaxo Wellcome 1100
Mefoxin (Cefoxitin Sodium) Merck & Co., Inc. 1691
Mefoxin Premixed Intravenous Solution (Cefoxitin Sodium) Merck & Co., Inc. 1694
Mezlin (Mezlocillin Sodium) Bayer Pharmaceutical 601
Mezlin Pharmacy Bulk Package (Mezlocillin Sodium) Bayer Pharmaceutical 604
Pipracil (Piperacillin Sodium) Lederle 1390
Tazicef for Injection (Ceftazidime) SmithKline Beecham Pharmaceuticals 2519
Tazidime Vials, Faspak & ADD-Vantage (Ceftazidime) Lilly .. 1478
Zosyn (Piperacillin Sodium, Tazobactam Sodium) Lederle 1419
Zosyn Pharmacy Bulk Package (Piperacillin Sodium, Tazobactam Sodium) Lederle 1422

Pelvic inflammatory disease (see also under Infections, gynecologic)
Cefobid Intravenous/Intramuscular (Cefoperazone Sodium) Roerig 2189
Cefobid Pharmacy Bulk Package - Not for Direct Infusion (Cefoperazone Sodium) Roerig 2192
Claforan Sterile and Injection (Cefotaxime Sodium) Hoechst-Roussel 1235
E-Mycin Tablets (Erythromycin) Knoll Laboratories 1341
Ilotycin Gluceptate, IV, Vials (Erythromycin Gluceptate) Dista 913
Mefoxin (Cefoxitin Sodium) Merck & Co., Inc. 1691
Mefoxin Premixed Intravenous Solution (Cefoxitin Sodium) Merck & Co., Inc. 1694
Mezlin (Mezlocillin Sodium) Bayer Pharmaceutical 601
Mezlin Pharmacy Bulk Package (Mezlocillin Sodium) Bayer Pharmaceutical 604
Pipracil (Piperacillin Sodium) Lederle 1390
Rocephin Injectable Vials, ADD-Vantage, Galaxy Container (Ceftriaxone Sodium) Roche Laboratories 2142
Ticar for Injection (Ticarcillin Disodium) SmithKline Beecham Pharmaceuticals 2526

Pemphigus
Aristocort Suspension (Forte Parenteral) (Triamcinolone Diacetate) Fujisawa 1027
Aristocort Tablets (Triamcinolone) Fujisawa 1022
Celestone Soluspan Suspension (Betamethasone Sodium Phosphate, Betamethasone Acetate) Schering 2347
Cortone Acetate Sterile Suspension (Cortisone Acetate) Merck & Co., Inc. 1623
Cortone Acetate Tablets (Cortisone Acetate) Merck & Co., Inc. 1624
Dalalone D.P. Injectable (Dexamethasone Acetate) Forest 1011
Decadron Elixir (Dexamethasone) Merck & Co., Inc. 1633
Decadron Phosphate Injection (Dexamethasone Sodium Phosphate) Merck & Co., Inc. 1637
Decadron Tablets (Dexamethasone) Merck & Co., Inc. 1635
Decadron-LA Sterile Suspension (Dexamethasone Acetate) Merck & Co., Inc. 1646
Deltasone Tablets (Prednisone) Upjohn 2595
Depo-Medrol Single-Dose Vial (Methylprednisolone Acetate) Upjohn 2600
Depo-Medrol Sterile Aqueous Suspension (Methylprednisolone Acetate) Upjohn 2597
Hydeltrasol Injection, Sterile (Prednisolone Sodium Phosphate) Merck & Co., Inc. 1665
Hydrocortone Phosphate Injection, Sterile (Hydrocortisone Sodium Phosphate) Merck & Co., Inc. 1670
Hydrocortone Tablets (Hydrocortisone) Merck & Co., Inc. 1672
Medrol (Methylprednisolone) Upjohn 2621
Pediapred Oral Liquid (Prednisolone Sodium Phosphate) Fisons.... 995
Prelone Syrup (Prednisolone) Muro 1787
Solu-Cortef Sterile Powder (Hydrocortisone Sodium Succinate) Upjohn 2641
Solu-Medrol Sterile Powder (Methylprednisolone Sodium Succinate) Upjohn 2643

Pemphigus, "possibly" effective in
Potaba (Aminobenzoate Potassium) Glenwood 1229

Penicillin group of antibiotics, therapy adjunct
Benemid Tablets (Probenecid) Merck & Co., Inc. 1611

Penicillin therapy, an adjuvant to
PCE Dispertab Tablets (Erythromycin) Abbott 444

Peptic ulcer, adjunctive therapy in
Cystospaz (Hyoscyamine) PolyMedica 1963
Levsin Drops (Hyoscyamine Sulfate) Schwarz 2405
Pro-Banthīne Tablets (Propantheline Bromide) Roberts 2052
Quarzan Capsules (Clidinium Bromide) Roche Products 2181
Robinul Forte Tablets (Glycopyrrolate) Robins 2072
Robinul Injectable (Glycopyrrolate) Robins 2072
Robinul Tablets (Glycopyrrolate) Robins 2072

Peptic ulcer, "possibly" effective in, adjunctive therapy
Librax Capsules (Chlordiazepoxide Hydrochloride, Clidinium Bromide) Roche Products 2176

Peptococcus niger infections
Cefotan (Cefotetan) Zeneca 2829
Flagyl 375 Capsules (Metronidazole) Searle 2434

Peptococcus niger gynecologic infections
Cefotan (Cefotetan) Zeneca 2829
Flagyl 375 Capsules (Metronidazole) Searle 2434

Peptococcus niger skin and skin structure infections
Cefotan (Cefotetan) Zeneca 2829
Flagyl 375 Capsules (Metronidazole) Searle 2434

1523 Indications Index Petit mal epilepsy

Peptococcus species bone and joint infections
Cefizox for Intramuscular or Intravenous Use (Ceftizoxime Sodium) Fujisawa ... 1034

Peptococcus species endomyometritis
Flagyl I.V. (Metronidazole Hydrochloride) SCS ... 2247
Protostat Tablets (Metronidazole) Ortho Pharmaceutical ... 1883

Peptococcus species gynecologic infections
Cefotan (Cefotetan) Zeneca ... 2829
Claforan Sterile and Injection (Cefotaxime Sodium) Hoechst-Roussel ... 1235
Flagyl I.V. (Metronidazole Hydrochloride) SCS ... 2247
Mefoxin (Cefoxitin Sodium) Merck & Co., Inc. ... 1691
Mefoxin Premixed Intravenous Solution (Cefoxitin Sodium) Merck & Co., Inc. ... 1694
Mezlin (Mezlocillin Sodium) Bayer Pharmaceutical ... 601
Mezlin Pharmacy Bulk Package (Mezlocillin Sodium) Bayer Pharmaceutical ... 604
Primaxin I.V. (Imipenem-Cilastatin Sodium) Merck & Co., Inc. ... 1729
Protostat Tablets (Metronidazole) Ortho Pharmaceutical ... 1883

Peptococcus species infections
Cefizox for Intramuscular or Intravenous Use (Ceftizoxime Sodium) Fujisawa ... 1034
Cefotan (Cefotetan) Zeneca ... 2829
Claforan Sterile and Injection (Cefotaxime Sodium) Hoechst-Roussel ... 1235
Flagyl I.V. (Metronidazole Hydrochloride) SCS ... 2247
Mefoxin (Cefoxitin Sodium) Merck & Co., Inc. ... 1691
Mefoxin Premixed Intravenous Solution (Cefoxitin Sodium) Merck & Co., Inc. ... 1694
Mezlin (Mezlocillin Sodium) Bayer Pharmaceutical ... 601
Mezlin Pharmacy Bulk Package (Mezlocillin Sodium) Bayer Pharmaceutical ... 604
Primaxin I.V. (Imipenem-Cilastatin Sodium) Merck & Co., Inc. ... 1729

Peptococcus species intra-abdominal infections
Cefizox for Intramuscular or Intravenous Use (Ceftizoxime Sodium) Fujisawa ... 1034
Claforan Sterile and Injection (Cefotaxime Sodium) Hoechst-Roussel ... 1235
Flagyl I.V. (Metronidazole Hydrochloride) SCS ... 2247
Mezlin (Mezlocillin Sodium) Bayer Pharmaceutical ... 601
Mezlin Pharmacy Bulk Package (Mezlocillin Sodium) Bayer Pharmaceutical ... 604
Primaxin I.M. (Imipenem-Cilastatin Sodium) Merck & Co., Inc. ... 1727
Primaxin I.V. (Imipenem-Cilastatin Sodium) Merck & Co., Inc. ... 1729
Protostat Tablets (Metronidazole) Ortho Pharmaceutical ... 1883

Peptococcus species peritonitis
Flagyl I.V. (Metronidazole Hydrochloride) SCS ... 2247
Mezlin (Mezlocillin Sodium) Bayer Pharmaceutical ... 601
Mezlin Pharmacy Bulk Package (Mezlocillin Sodium) Bayer Pharmaceutical ... 604
Protostat Tablets (Metronidazole) Ortho Pharmaceutical ... 1883

Peptococcus species skin and skin structure infections
Cefizox for Intramuscular or Intravenous Use (Ceftizoxime Sodium) Fujisawa ... 1034
Claforan Sterile and Injection (Cefotaxime Sodium) Hoechst-Roussel ... 1235
Flagyl I.V. (Metronidazole Hydrochloride) SCS ... 2247
Mefoxin (Cefoxitin Sodium) Merck & Co., Inc. ... 1691
Mefoxin Premixed Intravenous Solution (Cefoxitin Sodium) Merck & Co., Inc. ... 1694
Mezlin (Mezlocillin Sodium) Bayer Pharmaceutical ... 601
Mezlin Pharmacy Bulk Package (Mezlocillin Sodium) Bayer Pharmaceutical ... 604
Primaxin I.V. (Imipenem-Cilastatin Sodium) Merck & Co., Inc. ... 1729
Protostat Tablets (Metronidazole) Ortho Pharmaceutical ... 1883

Peptococcus species tubo-ovarian abscess
Flagyl I.V. (Metronidazole Hydrochloride) SCS ... 2247
Protostat Tablets (Metronidazole) Ortho Pharmaceutical ... 1883

Peptococcus species vaginal cuff infection, post-surgical
Flagyl I.V. (Metronidazole Hydrochloride) SCS ... 2247
Protostat Tablets (Metronidazole) Ortho Pharmaceutical ... 1883

Peptostreptococcus species bone and joint infections
Cefizox for Intramuscular or Intravenous Use (Ceftizoxime Sodium) Fujisawa ... 1034

Peptostreptococcus species endometritis
Flagyl 375 Capsules (Metronidazole) Searle ... 2434
Flagyl I.V. (Metronidazole Hydrochloride) SCS ... 2247
Mefoxin (Cefoxitin Sodium) Merck & Co., Inc. ... 1691
Mefoxin Premixed Intravenous Solution (Cefoxitin Sodium) Merck & Co., Inc. ... 1694
Mezlin (Mezlocillin Sodium) Bayer Pharmaceutical ... 601
Mezlin Pharmacy Bulk Package (Mezlocillin Sodium) Bayer Pharmaceutical ... 604
Protostat Tablets (Metronidazole) Ortho Pharmaceutical ... 1883

Peptostreptococcus species endomyometritis
Flagyl 375 Capsules (Metronidazole) Searle ... 2434
Flagyl I.V. (Metronidazole Hydrochloride) SCS ... 2247
Protostat Tablets (Metronidazole) Ortho Pharmaceutical ... 1883

Peptostreptococcus species gynecologic infections
Cefotan (Cefotetan) Zeneca ... 2829
Claforan Sterile and Injection (Cefotaxime Sodium) Hoechst-Roussel ... 1235
Flagyl 375 Capsules (Metronidazole) Searle ... 2434
Flagyl I.V. (Metronidazole Hydrochloride) SCS ... 2247
Mefoxin (Cefoxitin Sodium) Merck & Co., Inc. ... 1691
Mefoxin Premixed Intravenous Solution (Cefoxitin Sodium) Merck & Co., Inc. ... 1694
Mezlin (Mezlocillin Sodium) Bayer Pharmaceutical ... 601
Mezlin Pharmacy Bulk Package (Mezlocillin Sodium) Bayer Pharmaceutical ... 604
Primaxin I.M. (Imipenem-Cilastatin Sodium) Merck & Co., Inc. ... 1727
Primaxin I.V. (Imipenem-Cilastatin Sodium) Merck & Co., Inc. ... 1729
Protostat Tablets (Metronidazole) Ortho Pharmaceutical ... 1883

Peptostreptococcus species infections
Cefizox for Intramuscular or Intravenous Use (Ceftizoxime Sodium) Fujisawa ... 1034
Cefotan (Cefotetan) Zeneca ... 2829
Claforan Sterile and Injection (Cefotaxime Sodium) Hoechst-Roussel ... 1235
Flagyl 375 Capsules (Metronidazole) Searle ... 2434
Flagyl I.V. (Metronidazole Hydrochloride) SCS ... 2247
Mefoxin (Cefoxitin Sodium) Merck & Co., Inc. ... 1691
Mefoxin Premixed Intravenous Solution (Cefoxitin Sodium) Merck & Co., Inc. ... 1694
Mezlin (Mezlocillin Sodium) Bayer Pharmaceutical ... 601
Mezlin Pharmacy Bulk Package (Mezlocillin Sodium) Bayer Pharmaceutical ... 604
Primaxin I.M. (Imipenem-Cilastatin Sodium) Merck & Co., Inc. ... 1727
Primaxin I.V. (Imipenem-Cilastatin Sodium) Merck & Co., Inc. ... 1729
Rocephin Injectable Vials, ADD-Vantage, Galaxy Container (Ceftriaxone Sodium) Roche Laboratories ... 2142

Peptostreptococcus species intra-abdominal infections
Cefizox for Intramuscular or Intravenous Use (Ceftizoxime Sodium) Fujisawa ... 1034
Claforan Sterile and Injection (Cefotaxime Sodium) Hoechst-Roussel ... 1235
Flagyl 375 Capsules (Metronidazole) Searle ... 2434
Flagyl I.V. (Metronidazole Hydrochloride) SCS ... 2247
Mezlin (Mezlocillin Sodium) Bayer Pharmaceutical ... 601
Mezlin Pharmacy Bulk Package (Mezlocillin Sodium) Bayer Pharmaceutical ... 604
Primaxin I.M. (Imipenem-Cilastatin Sodium) Merck & Co., Inc. ... 1727
Primaxin I.V. (Imipenem-Cilastatin Sodium) Merck & Co., Inc. ... 1729
Protostat Tablets (Metronidazole) Ortho Pharmaceutical ... 1883
Rocephin Injectable Vials, ADD-Vantage, Galaxy Container (Ceftriaxone Sodium) Roche Laboratories ... 2142

Peptostreptococcus species peritonitis
Flagyl 375 Capsules (Metronidazole) Searle ... 2434
Flagyl I.V. (Metronidazole Hydrochloride) SCS ... 2247
Mezlin (Mezlocillin Sodium) Bayer Pharmaceutical ... 601
Mezlin Pharmacy Bulk Package (Mezlocillin Sodium) Bayer Pharmaceutical ... 604
Protostat Tablets (Metronidazole) Ortho Pharmaceutical ... 1883

Peptostreptococcus species skin and skin structure infections
Cefizox for Intramuscular or Intravenous Use (Ceftizoxime Sodium) Fujisawa ... 1034
Cefotan (Cefotetan) Zeneca ... 2829
Claforan Sterile and Injection (Cefotaxime Sodium) Hoechst-Roussel ... 1235
Flagyl 375 Capsules (Metronidazole) Searle ... 2434
Flagyl I.V. (Metronidazole Hydrochloride) SCS ... 2247
Mefoxin (Cefoxitin Sodium) Merck & Co., Inc. ... 1691
Mefoxin Premixed Intravenous Solution (Cefoxitin Sodium) Merck & Co., Inc. ... 1694
Primaxin I.V. (Imipenem-Cilastatin Sodium) Merck & Co., Inc. ... 1729
Protostat Tablets (Metronidazole) Ortho Pharmaceutical ... 1883
Rocephin Injectable Vials, ADD-Vantage, Galaxy Container (Ceftriaxone Sodium) Roche Laboratories ... 2142

Peptostreptococcus tubo-ovarian abscess
Flagyl 375 Capsules (Metronidazole) Searle ... 2434
Flagyl I.V. (Metronidazole Hydrochloride) SCS ... 2247
Protostat Tablets (Metronidazole) Ortho Pharmaceutical ... 1883

Peptostreptococcus species vaginal cuff infection, post-surgical
Flagyl 375 Capsules (Metronidazole) Searle ... 2434
Flagyl I.V. (Metronidazole Hydrochloride) SCS ... 2247
Protostat Tablets (Metronidazole) Ortho Pharmaceutical ... 1883

Peritonitis (see also under Infections, intra-abdominal)
Amikacin Sulfate Injection, USP (Amikacin Sulfate) Elkins-Sinn ... 960
Amikin Injectable (Amikacin Sulfate) Apothecon ... 501
Azactam for Injection (Aztreonam) Bristol-Myers Squibb ... 734
Cefobid Intravenous/Intramuscular (Cefoperazone Sodium) Roerig ... 2189
Cefobid Pharmacy Bulk Package - Not for Direct Infusion (Cefoperazone Sodium) Roerig ... 2192
Ceptaz (Ceftazidime) Glaxo Wellcome ... 1081
Claforan Sterile and Injection (Cefotaxime Sodium) Hoechst-Roussel ... 1235
Cleocin Phosphate Injection (Clindamycin Phosphate) Upjohn ... 2586
Diflucan Injection, Tablets, and Oral Suspension (Fluconazole) Roerig ... 2194
Flagyl 375 Capsules (Metronidazole) Searle ... 2434
Flagyl I.V. (Metronidazole Hydrochloride) SCS ... 2247
Fortaz (Ceftazidime) Glaxo Wellcome ... 1100
Garamycin Injectable (Gentamicin Sulfate) Schering ... 2360
Mandol Vials, Faspak & ADD-Vantage (Cefamandole Nafate) Lilly ... 1461
Mefoxin (Cefoxitin Sodium) Merck & Co., Inc. ... 1691
Mefoxin Premixed Intravenous Solution (Cefoxitin Sodium) Merck & Co., Inc. ... 1694
Mezlin (Mezlocillin Sodium) Bayer Pharmaceutical ... 601
Mezlin Pharmacy Bulk Package (Mezlocillin Sodium) Bayer Pharmaceutical ... 604
Nebcin Vials, Hyporets & ADD-Vantage (Tobramycin Sulfate) Lilly ... 1464
Netromycin Injection 100 mg/ml (Netilmicin Sulfate) Schering ... 2373
Tazicef for Injection (Ceftazidime) SmithKline Beecham Pharmaceuticals ... 2519
Tazidime Vials, Faspak & ADD-Vantage (Ceftazidime) Lilly ... 1478
Ticar for Injection (Ticarcillin Disodium) SmithKline Beecham Pharmaceuticals ... 2526
Timentin for Injection (Ticarcillin Disodium, Clavulanate Potassium) SmithKline Beecham Pharmaceuticals ... 2528

Peritonitis, candidal
Diflucan Injection, Tablets, and Oral Suspension (Fluconazole) Roerig ... 2194

Pertussis
E.E.S. (Erythromycin Ethylsuccinate) Abbott ... 424
E-Mycin Tablets (Erythromycin) Knoll Laboratories ... 1341
ERYC (Erythromycin) Parke-Davis ... 1915
EryPed (Erythromycin Ethylsuccinate) Abbott ... 421
Ery-Tab Tablets (Erythromycin) Abbott ... 422
Erythrocin Stearate Filmtab (Erythromycin Stearate) Abbott ... 425
Erythromycin Base Filmtab (Erythromycin) Abbott ... 426
Erythromycin Delayed-Release Capsules, USP (Erythromycin) Abbott ... 427
PCE Dispertab Tablets (Erythromycin) Abbott ... 444

Petit mal epilepsy (see under Seizures, generalized, absence)

Petriellidiosis Indications Index 1524

Petriellidiosis (see under Pseudoallescheriosis)

Peyronie's disease, "possibly" effective in
Potaba (Aminobenzoate Potassium) Glenwood 1229

Pharyngitis, symptomatic relief of
Bayer Children's Chewable Aspirin (Aspirin) Miles Consumer ..... ▣ 711
Celestial Seasonings Soothers Throat Drops (Menthol, Pectin) Warner-Lambert ..... ▣ 842
Cēpacol Anesthetic Lozenges (Benzocaine, Cetylpyridinium Chloride) J.B. Williams ..... ▣ 875
Cēpacol Dry Throat Lozenges, Cherry Flavor (Menthol) J.B. Williams ..... ▣ 875
Cēpacol Dry Throat Lozenges, Honey-Lemon Flavor (Menthol) J.B. Williams ..... ▣ 875
Cēpacol Dry Throat Lozenges, Menthol-Eucalyptus Flavor (Menthol) J.B. Williams ..... ▣ 875
Cēpacol Dry Throat Lozenges, Original Flavor (Benzyl Alcohol, Cetylpyridinium Chloride) J.B. Williams ..... ▣ 875
Cepastat (Menthol, Phenol) SmithKline Beecham Consumer ▣ 810
Cheracol Sore Throat Spray (Phenol) Roberts ..... ▣ 769
Children's Vicks Chloraseptic Sore Throat Lozenges (Benzocaine) Procter & Gamble ▣ 757
Children's Vicks Chloraseptic Sore Throat Spray (Phenol) Procter & Gamble ..... ▣ 757
Dura-Vent Tablets (Phenylpropanolamine Hydrochloride, Guaifenesin) Dura 952
Entex Capsules (Phenylephrine Hydrochloride, Phenylpropanolamine Hydrochloride, Guaifenesin) Procter & Gamble Pharmaceuticals 1986
Entex LA Tablets (Phenylpropanolamine Hydrochloride, Guaifenesin) Procter & Gamble Pharmaceuticals 1987
Entex Liquid (Phenylephrine Hydrochloride, Phenylpropanolamine Hydrochloride, Guaifenesin) Procter & Gamble Pharmaceuticals 1986
Exgest LA Tablets (Phenylpropanolamine Hydrochloride, Guaifenesin) Carnrick 782
Extra Strength Vicks Cough Drops (Menthol) Procter & Gamble ..... ▣ 760
Halls Mentho-Lyptus Cough Suppressant Tablets (Eucalyptus, Oil of, Menthol) Warner-Lambert ..... ▣ 842
Halls Sugar Free Cough Suppressant Tablets (Menthol, Eucalyptus, Oil of) Warner-Lambert ..... ▣ 842
Humibid DM Tablets (Guaifenesin, Dextromethorphan Hydrobromide) Adams 462
N'ICE Medicated Sugarless Sore Throat and Cough Lozenges (Menthol) SmithKline Beecham Consumer ..... ▣ 822
Sucrets Maximum Strength (Dyclonine Hydrochloride) SmithKline Beecham Consumer ▣ 826
TheraFlu Flu and Cold Medicine (Acetaminophen, Chlorpheniramine Maleate, Pseudoephedrine Hydrochloride) Sandoz Consumer ..... ▣ 787
Triaminic Sore Throat Formula (Acetaminophen, Dextromethorphan Hydrobromide, Pseudoephedrine Hydrochloride) Sandoz Consumer ..... ▣ 791
TYLENOL Cold Multi-Symptom Formula Medication Tablets and Caplets (Acetaminophen, Chlorpheniramine Maleate, Pseudoephedrine Hydrochloride, Dextromethorphan Hydrobromide) McNeil Consumer 1561
TYLENOL Cold Medication No Drowsiness Formula Gelcaps and Caplets (Acetaminophen, Pseudoephedrine Hydrochloride, Dextromethorphan Hydrobromide) McNeil Consumer 1562
TYLENOL Cold Multi-Symptom Hot Medication Liquid Packets (Acetaminophen, Chlorpheniramine Maleate, Pseudoephedrine Hydrochloride, Dextromethorphan Hydrobromide) McNeil Consumer 1557
TYLENOL Cough Multi-Symptom Medication (Dextromethorphan Hydrobromide, Acetaminophen) McNeil Consumer 1564
TYLENOL Cough Multi-Symptom Medication with Decongestant (Dextromethorphan Hydrobromide, Acetaminophen, Pseudoephedrine Hydrochloride) McNeil Consumer 1565
TYLENOL Severe Allergy Medication Caplets (Acetaminophen, Diphenhydramine Hydrochloride) McNeil Consumer 1564
Vicks Chloraseptic Cough & Throat Drops (Menthol) Procter & Gamble ..... ▣ 759
Vicks Chloraseptic Sore Throat Lozenges (Benzocaine, Menthol) Procter & Gamble ..... ▣ 759
Vicks Chloraseptic Sore Throat Spray, and Gargle and Mouth Rinse (Phenol) Procter & Gamble ..... ▣ 759
Vicks Cough Drops (Menthol) Procter & Gamble ..... ▣ 759

Pharyngitis, treatment of
Biaxin (Clarithromycin) Abbott 405
Ceclor Pulvules & Suspension (Cefaclor) Lilly 1431
Ceftin (Cefuroxime Axetil) Glaxo Wellcome 1078
Cefzil Tablets and Oral Suspension (Cefprozil) Bristol-Myers Squibb .. 746
Duricef (Cefadroxil Monohydrate) Bristol-Myers Squibb 748
E.E.S. (Erythromycin Ethylsuccinate) Abbott 424
E-Mycin Tablets (Erythromycin) Knoll Laboratories 1341
EryPed (Erythromycin Ethylsuccinate) Abbott 421
Ery-Tab Tablets (Erythromycin) Abbott 422
Erythrocin Stearate Filmtab (Erythromycin Stearate) Abbott 425
Erythromycin Base Filmtab (Erythromycin) Abbott 426
Ilosone (Erythromycin Estolate) Dista 911
Ilotycin Gluceptate, IV, Vials (Erythromycin Gluceptate) Dista 913
Lorabid Suspension and Pulvules (Loracarbef) Lilly 1459
PCE Dispertab Tablets (Erythromycin) Abbott 444
Suprax (Cefixime) Lederle 1399
Vantin for Oral Suspension and Vantin Tablets (Cefpodoxime Proxetil) Upjohn 2646
Zithromax (Azithromycin) Pfizer Labs 1944

Pheochromocytoma
Demser Capsules (Metyrosine) Merck & Co., Inc. 1649
Dibenzyline Capsules (Phenoxybenzamine Hydrochloride) SmithKline Beecham Pharmaceuticals 2476

Pheochromocytoma, adjunctive therapy
Demser Capsules (Metyrosine) Merck & Co., Inc. 1649
Inderal (Propranolol Hydrochloride) Wyeth-Ayerst 2728
Regitine (Phentolamine Mesylate) CibaGeneva 846

Pheochromocytoma, diagnosis of
Regitine (Phentolamine Mesylate) CibaGeneva 846

Phosphorus deficiency (see under Hypophosphatemia)

Photophobia, reduction of
Lacrisert Sterile Ophthalmic Insert (Hydroxypropyl Cellulose) Merck & Co., Inc. 1686

Photosensitivity, reduction of severity, erythropoietic protoporphyria-induced
Solatene Capsules (Beta Carotene) Roche Laboratories 2150

Phycomycosis
Fungizone Intravenous (Amphotericin B) Apothecon 506

Piles (see under Hemorrhoids)

Pinta
Bicillin L-A Injection (Penicillin G Benzathine) Wyeth-Ayerst 2707

Pinworm infestation (see under Enterobiasis)

Pityriasis rosea
Temaril Tablets, Syrup and Spansule Extended-Release Capsules (Trimeprazine Tartrate) Allergan 483

Pityrosporon orbiculare infections
Exelderm Cream 1.0% (Sulconazole Nitrate) Westwood-Squibb 2685
Exelderm Solution 1.0% (Sulconazole Nitrate) Westwood-Squibb 2686
Loprox 1% Cream and Lotion (Ciclopirox Olamine) Hoechst-Roussel 1242
Lotrimin (Clotrimazole) Schering 2371
Monistat Dual-Pak (Miconazole Nitrate) Ortho Pharmaceutical 1850
Monistat-Derm (miconazole nitrate 2%) Cream (Miconazole Nitrate) Ortho Dermatological 1889
Nizoral 2% Cream (Ketoconazole) Janssen 1297
Selsun Rx 2.5% Selenium Sulfide Lotion, USP (Selenium Sulfide) Ross 2225
Spectazole (econazole nitrate 1%) Cream (Econazole Nitrate) Ortho Dermatological 1890

Plague
Dynacin Capsules (Minocycline Hydrochloride) Medicis 1590
Minocin Oral Suspension (Minocycline Hydrochloride) Lederle 1385
Minocin Pellet-Filled Capsules (Minocycline Hydrochloride) Lederle 1383
Monodox Capsules (Doxycycline Monohydrate) Oclassen 1805

Plasmodium infection (see under P. vivax infections; P. malariae infections; P. ovale infections; P. falciparum infections)

PMS (see under Menstrual syndrome, pre-, management of)

Pneumococcal disease, immunization against
Pneumovax 23 (Pneumococcal Vaccine, Polyvalent) Merck & Co., Inc. 1725
Pnu-Imune 23 (Pneumococcal Vaccine, Polyvalent) Lederle 1393

Pneumococci species infections (see under Pneumococcosis)

Pneumococcosis
Omnipen Capsules (Ampicillin) Wyeth-Ayerst 2764
Omnipen for Oral Suspension (Ampicillin) Wyeth-Ayerst 2765
Pen•Vee K (Penicillin V Potassium) Wyeth-Ayerst 2772
TERAK Ointment (Oxytetracycline Hydrochloride, Polymyxin B Sulfate) Akorn ..... ⊙ 209

Pneumocystis carinii pneumonia
Bactrim DS Tablets (Trimethoprim, Sulfamethoxazole) Roche Laboratories 2084
Bactrim I.V. Infusion (Trimethoprim, Sulfamethoxazole) Roche Laboratories 2082
Bactrim (Trimethoprim, Sulfamethoxazole) Roche Laboratories 2084
Mepron Suspension (Atovaquone) Glaxo Wellcome 1135
NebuPent for Inhalation Solution (Pentamidine Isethionate) Fujisawa 1040
Neutrexin (Trimetrexate Glucuronate) U.S. Bioscience 2572
Pentam 300 Injection (Pentamidine Isethionate) Fujisawa 1041
Septra (Trimethoprim, Sulfamethoxazole) Glaxo Wellcome 1174
Septra I.V. Infusion (Trimethoprim, Sulfamethoxazole) Glaxo Wellcome 1169
Septra I.V. Infusion ADD-Vantage Vials (Trimethoprim, Sulfamethoxazole) Glaxo Wellcome 1171
Septra (Trimethoprim, Sulfamethoxazole) Glaxo Wellcome 1174

Pneumonia (see also under Infections, lower respiratory tract)
Azactam for Injection (Aztreonam) Bristol-Myers Squibb 734
Biaxin (Clarithromycin) Abbott 405
Bicillin C-R Injection (Penicillin G Procaine, Penicillin G Benzathine) Wyeth-Ayerst 2704
Bicillin C-R 900/300 Injection (Penicillin G Procaine, Penicillin G Benzathine) Wyeth-Ayerst 2706
Ceclor Pulvules & Suspension (Cefaclor) Lilly 1431
Ceptaz (Ceftazidime) Glaxo Wellcome 1081
Claforan Sterile and Injection (Cefotaxime Sodium) Hoechst-Roussel 1235
Cleocin Phosphate Injection (Clindamycin Phosphate) Upjohn 2586
Diflucan Injection, Tablets, and Oral Suspension (Fluconazole) Roerig 2194
E.E.S. (Erythromycin Ethylsuccinate) Abbott 424
EryPed (Erythromycin Ethylsuccinate) Abbott 421
Ery-Tab Tablets (Erythromycin) Abbott 422
Erythrocin Stearate Filmtab (Erythromycin Stearate) Abbott 425
Erythromycin Base Filmtab (Erythromycin) Abbott 426
Flagyl 375 Capsules (Metronidazole) Searle 2434
Flagyl I.V. (Metronidazole Hydrochloride) SCS 2247
Fortaz (Ceftazidime) Glaxo Wellcome 1100
Ilosone (Erythromycin Estolate) Dista 911
Ilotycin Gluceptate, IV, Vials (Erythromycin Gluceptate) Dista 913
Kefurox Vials, Faspak & ADD-Vantage (Cefuroxime Sodium) Lilly 1454
Lorabid Suspension and Pulvules (Loracarbef) Lilly 1459
Mandol Vials, Faspak & ADD-Vantage (Cefamandole Nafate) Lilly 1461
Mefoxin (Cefoxitin Sodium) Merck & Co., Inc. 1691
Mefoxin Premixed Intravenous Solution (Cefoxitin Sodium) Merck & Co., Inc. 1694
Mezlin (Mezlocillin Sodium) Bayer Pharmaceutical 601
Mezlin Pharmacy Bulk Package (Mezlocillin Sodium) Bayer Pharmaceutical 604
NebuPent for Inhalation Solution (Pentamidine Isethionate) Fujisawa 1040
Pentam 300 Injection (Pentamidine Isethionate) Fujisawa 1041

(▣ Described in PDR For Nonprescription Drugs) (⊙ Described in PDR For Ophthalmology)

1525 Indications Index Polyps

Pfizerpen for Injection (Penicillin G Potassium) Roerig 2203
Tao Capsules (Troleandomycin) Roerig 2209
Tazicef for Injection (Ceftazidime) SmithKline Beecham Pharmaceuticals 2519
Tazidime Vials, Faspak & ADD-Vantage (Ceftazidime) Lilly 1478
Vantin for Oral Suspension and Vantin Tablets (Cefpodoxime Proxetil) Upjohn 2646
Vibramycin Hyclate Intravenous (Doxycycline Hyclate) Roerig 2215
Zefazone (Cefmetazole Sodium) Upjohn 2654
Zinacef (Cefuroxime Sodium) Glaxo Wellcome 1211
Zithromax (Azithromycin) Pfizer Labs 1944

Pneumonia, candidal
Diflucan Injection, Tablets, and Oral Suspension (Fluconazole) Roerig 2194

Pneumonia, pneumocystis carinii (see under Pneumocystis carinii pneumonia)

Pneumonitis, anaerobic
Ticar for Injection (Ticarcillin Disodium) SmithKline Beecham Pharmaceuticals 2526

Pneumonitis, aspiration
Aristocort Suspension (Forte Parenteral) (Triamcinolone Diacetate) Fujisawa 1027
Aristocort Tablets (Triamcinolone) Fujisawa 1022
Celestone Soluspan Suspension (Betamethasone Sodium Phosphate, Betamethasone Acetate) Schering 2347
Cortone Acetate Sterile Suspension (Cortisone Acetate) Merck & Co., Inc. 1623
Cortone Acetate Tablets (Cortisone Acetate) Merck & Co., Inc. 1624
Dalalone D.P. Injectable (Dexamethasone Acetate) Forest 1011
Decadron Elixir (Dexamethasone) Merck & Co., Inc. 1633
Decadron Phosphate Injection (Dexamethasone Sodium Phosphate) Merck & Co., Inc. 1637
Decadron Tablets (Dexamethasone) Merck & Co., Inc. 1635
Decadron-LA Sterile Suspension (Dexamethasone Acetate) Merck & Co., Inc. 1646
Deltasone Tablets (Prednisone) Upjohn 2595
Depo-Medrol Single-Dose Vial (Methylprednisolone Acetate) Upjohn 2600
Depo-Medrol Sterile Aqueous Suspension (Methylprednisolone Acetate) Upjohn 2597
Hydeltrasol Injection, Sterile (Prednisolone Sodium Phosphate) Merck & Co., Inc. 1665
Hydrocortone Phosphate Injection, Sterile (Hydrocortisone Sodium Phosphate) Merck & Co., Inc. 1670
Hydrocortone Tablets (Hydrocortisone) Merck & Co., Inc. 1672
Medrol (Methylprednisolone) Upjohn 2621
Pediapred Oral Liquid (Prednisolone Sodium Phosphate) Fisons 995
Prelone Syrup (Prednisolone) Muro 1787
Solu-Cortef Sterile Powder (Hydrocortisone Sodium Succinate) Upjohn 2641
Solu-Medrol Sterile Powder (Methylprednisolone Sodium Succinate) Upjohn 2643

Poison ivy (see under Dermatitis, contact)

Poison oak (see under Dermatitis, contact)

Poison sumac (see under Dermatitis, contact)

Poisoning, acute, unspecified, emergency treatment of
CharcoAid (Charcoal, Activated) Requa ▣ 768
CharcoAid 2000 (Charcoal, Activated) Requa ▣ 768

Poisoning, pesticides and chemicals of organophosphate class
Protopam Chloride for Injection (Pralidoxime Chloride) Wyeth-Ayerst 2806

Poliomyelitis, prevention of (see under Immunization, poliovirus 1, 2, and 3)

Pollinosis (see also under Rhinitis, seasonal allergic)
Actifed Allergy Daytime/Nighttime Caplets (Diphenhydramine Hydrochloride, Pseudoephedrine Hydrochloride) WARNER WELLCOME ▣ 844
Actifed Plus Caplets (Acetaminophen, Pseudoephedrine Hydrochloride, Triprolidine Hydrochloride) WARNER WELLCOME ▣ 845
Actifed Plus Tablets (Acetaminophen, Pseudoephedrine Hydrochloride, Triprolidine Hydrochloride) WARNER WELLCOME ▣ 845
Actifed Sinus Daytime/Nighttime Tablets and Caplets (Acetaminophen, Diphenhydramine Hydrochloride, Pseudoephedrine Hydrochloride) WARNER WELLCOME ▣ 846
Actifed Syrup (Pseudoephedrine Hydrochloride, Triprolidine Hydrochloride) WARNER WELLCOME ▣ 846
Actifed Tablets (Pseudoephedrine Hydrochloride, Triprolidine Hydrochloride) WARNER WELLCOME ▣ 844
Afrin (Oxymetazoline Hydrochloride) Schering-Plough HealthCare ▣ 797
Alka Seltzer Plus Sinus Medicine (Phenylpropanolamine Bitartrate, Aspirin, Brompheniramine Maleate) Miles Consumer ▣ 707
Allerest Children's Chewable Tablets (Chlorpheniramine Maleate, Phenylpropanolamine Hydrochloride) CIBA Consumer ▣ 627
Allerest Headache Strength Tablets (Acetaminophen, Chlorpheniramine Maleate, Pseudoephedrine Hydrochloride) CIBA Consumer ▣ 627
Allerest Maximum Strength Tablets (Chlorpheniramine Maleate, Pseudoephedrine Hydrochloride) CIBA Consumer ▣ 627
Allerest No Drowsiness Tablets (Acetaminophen, Pseudoephedrine Hydrochloride) CIBA Consumer ▣ 627
Allerest Sinus Pain Formula (Acetaminophen, Chlorpheniramine Maleate, Pseudoephedrine Hydrochloride) CIBA Consumer ▣ 627
Allerest 12 Hour Caplets (Chlorpheniramine Maleate, Phenylpropanolamine Hydrochloride) CIBA Consumer ▣ 627
Benadryl Allergy Decongestant Tablets (Diphenhydramine Hydrochloride, Pseudoephedrine Hydrochloride) WARNER WELLCOME ▣ 848
Benadryl Allergy Liquid Medication (Diphenhydramine Hydrochloride) WARNER WELLCOME ▣ 849
Benadryl Allergy Sinus Headache Formula Caplets (Diphenhydramine Hydrochloride, Pseudoephedrine Hydrochloride, Acetaminophen) WARNER WELLCOME ▣ 849
Benadryl Dye-Free Allergy Liqui-gel Softgels (Diphenhydramine Hydrochloride) WARNER WELLCOME ▣ 850
Benadryl Dye-Free Allergy Liquid Medication (Diphenhydramine Hydrochloride) WARNER WELLCOME ▣ 850
Chlor-Trimeton Allergy Decongestant Tablets (Chlorpheniramine Maleate, Pseudoephedrine Sulfate) Schering-Plough HealthCare ▣ 799
Chlor-Trimeton Allergy Tablets (Chlorpheniramine Maleate) Schering-Plough HealthCare ▣ 798
Allergy-Sinus Comtrex Multi-Symptom Allergy-Sinus Formula Tablets (Acetaminophen, Chlorpheniramine Maleate, Pseudoephedrine Hydrochloride) Bristol-Myers Products ▣ 617
Dimetapp Elixir (Brompheniramine Maleate, Phenylpropanolamine Hydrochloride) A. H. Robins Consumer ▣ 773
Dimetapp Extentabs (Brompheniramine Maleate, Phenylpropanolamine Hydrochloride) A. H. Robins Consumer ▣ 774
Dimetapp Tablets/Liqui-Gels (Brompheniramine Maleate, Phenylpropanolamine Hydrochloride) A. H. Robins Consumer ▣ 775
Dimetapp Cold & Allergy Chewable Tablets (Brompheniramine Maleate, Phenylpropanolamine Hydrochloride) A. H. Robins Consumer ▣ 773
Drixoral Cold and Allergy Sustained-Action Tablets (Dexbrompheniramine Maleate, Pseudoephedrine Sulfate) Schering-Plough HealthCare ▣ 802
Drixoral Cold and Flu Extended-Release Tablets (Acetaminophen, Dexbrompheniramine Maleate, Pseudoephedrine Sulfate) Schering-Plough HealthCare ▣ 803
4-Way Fast Acting Nasal Spray (regular & mentholated) (Naphazoline Hydrochloride, Phenylephrine Hydrochloride, Pyrilamine Maleate) Bristol-Myers Products ▣ 621
4-Way Long Lasting Nasal Spray (Oxymetazoline Hydrochloride) Bristol-Myers Products ▣ 621
Kronofed-A (Chlorpheniramine Maleate, Pseudoephedrine Hydrochloride) Ferndale 977
NTZ Long Acting Nasal Spray & Drops 0.05% (Oxymetazoline Hydrochloride) Miles Consumer ▣ 727
Neo-Synephrine Maximum Strength 12 Hour Nasal Spray (Oxymetazoline Hydrochloride) Miles Consumer ▣ 726
Neo-Synephrine Maximum Strength 12 Hour Nasal Spray Pump (Oxymetazoline Hydrochloride) Miles Consumer ▣ 726
Neo-Synephrine (Phenylephrine Hydrochloride) Miles Consumer ▣ 726
Nolahist Tablets (Phenindamine Tartrate) Carnrick 785
Nolamine Timed-Release Tablets (Phenindamine Tartrate, Phenylpropanolamine Hydrochloride, Chlorpheniramine Maleate) Carnrick 785
Novahistine Elixir (Chlorpheniramine Maleate, Phenylephrine Hydrochloride) SmithKline Beecham Consumer ▣ 823
PediaCare Cold Allergy Chewable Tablets (Pseudoephedrine Hydrochloride, Chlorpheniramine Maleate) McNeil Consumer ▣ 677
PediaCare Cough-Cold Liquid (Pseudoephedrine Hydrochloride, Chlorpheniramine Maleate, Dextromethorphan Hydrobromide) McNeil Consumer 1553
Propagest Tablets (Phenylpropanolamine Hydrochloride) Carnrick 786
Sine-Off No Drowsiness Formula Caplets (Acetaminophen, Pseudoephedrine Hydrochloride) SmithKline Beecham Consumer ▣ 824
Singlet Tablets (Acetaminophen, Chlorpheniramine Maleate, Pseudoephedrine Hydrochloride) SmithKline Beecham Consumer ▣ 825
Sinulin Tablets (Acetaminophen, Phenylpropanolamine Hydrochloride, Chlorpheniramine Maleate) Carnrick 787
Sudafed Children's Liquid (Pseudoephedrine Hydrochloride) WARNER WELLCOME ▣ 861
Sudafed Plus Liquid (Chlorpheniramine Maleate, Pseudoephedrine Hydrochloride) WARNER WELLCOME ▣ 862
Sudafed Plus Tablets (Chlorpheniramine Maleate, Pseudoephedrine Hydrochloride) WARNER WELLCOME ▣ 863
Sudafed Sinus Caplets (Acetaminophen, Pseudoephedrine Hydrochloride) WARNER WELLCOME ▣ 864
Sudafed Sinus Tablets (Acetaminophen, Pseudoephedrine Hydrochloride) WARNER WELLCOME ▣ 864
Sudafed Tablets, 30 mg (Pseudoephedrine Hydrochloride) WARNER WELLCOME ▣ 861
Sudafed Tablets, 60 mg (Pseudoephedrine Hydrochloride) WARNER WELLCOME ▣ 861
Tavist-D 12 Hour Relief Tablets (Clemastine Fumarate, Phenylpropanolamine Hydrochloride) Sandoz Consumer ▣ 787
Teldrin 12 Hour Antihistamine/Nasal Decongestant Allergy Relief Capsules (Chlorpheniramine Maleate, Phenylpropanolamine Hydrochloride) SmithKline Beecham Consumer ▣ 826
Triaminic Cold Tablets (Phenylpropanolamine Hydrochloride, Chlorpheniramine Maleate) Sandoz Consumer ▣ 790
Triaminicin Tablets (Acetaminophen, Chlorpheniramine Maleate, Phenylpropanolamine Hydrochloride) Sandoz Consumer ▣ 793
TYLENOL Severe Allergy Medication Caplets (Acetaminophen, Diphenhydramine Hydrochloride) McNeil Consumer 1564
Ursinus Inlay-Tabs (Aspirin, Pseudoephedrine Hydrochloride) Sandoz Consumer ▣ 794
Vicks Sinex 12-Hour Nasal Decongestant Spray and Ultra Fine Mist (Oxymetazoline Hydrochloride) Procter & Gamble ▣ 765
Vicks Sinex Nasal Spray and Ultra Fine Mist (Phenylephrine Hydrochloride) Procter & Gamble ▣ 765
Vicks Vapor Inhaler (Desoxyephedrine-Levo) Procter & Gamble ▣ 765

Polycythemia vera
Mustargen (Mechlorethamine Hydrochloride) Merck & Co., Inc. 1709

Polydipsia, temporary, management of
DDAVP (Desmopressin Acetate) Rhone-Poulenc Rorer Pharmaceuticals 2017
Desmopressin Acetate Rhinal Tube (Desmopressin Acetate) Ferring 979

Polymyositis (see under Dermatomyositis, systemic)

Polyps, nasal, prevention of recurrence
Beconase (Beclomethasone Dipropionate) Glaxo Wellcome 1076
Decadron Phosphate Turbinaire (Dexamethasone Sodium Phosphate) Merck & Co., Inc. 1645

(▣ Described in PDR For Nonprescription Drugs) (⊙ Described in PDR For Ophthalmology)

Polyps **Indications Index** 1526

Dexacort Phosphate in Turbinaire (Dexamethasone Sodium Phosphate) Adams 459
Vancenase AQ Nasal Spray 0.042% (Beclomethasone Dipropionate) Schering 2393
Vancenase PocketHaler Nasal Inhaler (Beclomethasone Dipropionate) Schering 2391

Polyuria, temporary, management of
DDAVP (Desmopressin Acetate) Rhone-Poulenc Rorer Pharmaceuticals 2017
Desmopressin Acetate Rhinal Tube (Desmopressin Acetate) Ferring .. 979

Porphyria, acute intermittent, adjunctive therapy in
Thorazine (Chlorpromazine Hydrochloride) SmithKline Beecham Pharmaceuticals 2523

Porphyria, acute intermittent, amelioration of recurrent attacks of
Panhematin (Hemin For Injection) Abbott 443

Porphyria variegata
Panhematin (Hemin For Injection) Abbott 443

Portal-systemic encephalopathy (see under Hepatic encephalopathy)

Postnasal drip (see under Cold, common, symptomatic relief of)

Pregnancy, diagnosis of
e.p.t. Early Pregnancy Test (HCG Monoclonal Antibody) WARNER WELLCOME .... ▣ 854

Pregnancy, prevention of
All-Flex Arcing Spring Diaphragm (See also Ortho Diaphragm Kits) (Diaphragm) Ortho Pharmaceutical 1865
Brevicon (Norethindrone, Ethinyl Estradiol) Roche Laboratories 2088
Conceptrol Contraceptive Gel Single Use Applicators (Nonoxynol-9) Ortho Pharmaceutical .... ▣ 736
Conceptrol Contraceptive Inserts (Nonoxynol-9) Ortho Pharmaceutical .... ▣ 737
Delfen Contraceptive Foam (Nonoxynol-9) Ortho Pharmaceutical .... ▣ 737
Demulen (Ethynodiol Diacetate, Ethinyl Estradiol) Searle 2428
Depo-Provera Contraceptive Injection (Medroxyprogesterone Acetate) Upjohn 2602
Desogen Tablets (Desogestrel, Ethinyl Estradiol) Organon 1817
Encare Vaginal Contraceptive Suppositories (Nonoxynol-9) Thompson Medical .... ▣ 833
Gynol II Extra Strength Contraceptive Jelly (Nonoxynol-9) Ortho Pharmaceutical .... ▣ 739
Gynol II Original Formula Contraceptive Jelly (Nonoxynol-9) Ortho Pharmaceutical .... ▣ 738
K-Y Plus Vaginal Contraceptive and Personal Lubricant (Nonoxynol-9) J & J Consumer.. ▣ 659
Levlen/Tri-Levlen (Levonorgestrel, Ethinyl Estradiol) Berlex 651
Lippes Loop Intrauterine Double-S (Intrauterine device) Ortho Pharmaceutical 1848
Lo/Ovral Tablets (Norgestrel, Ethinyl Estradiol) Wyeth-Ayerst 2746
Lo/Ovral-28 Tablets (Norgestrel, Ethinyl Estradiol) Wyeth-Ayerst 2751
Micronor Tablets (Norethindrone) Ortho Pharmaceutical 1872
Modicon (Norethindrone, Ethinyl Estradiol) Ortho Pharmaceutical .. 1872
Nordette-21 Tablets (Levonorgestrel, Ethinyl Estradiol) Wyeth-Ayerst 2755
Nordette-28 Tablets (Levonorgestrel, Ethinyl Estradiol) Wyeth-Ayerst 2758
Norinyl (Ethinyl Estradiol, Norethindrone) Roche Laboratories 2088
Norplant System (Levonorgestrel) Wyeth-Ayerst 2759
Nor-Q D Tablets (Norethindrone) Roche Laboratories 2135
Ortho-Cept (Desogestrel, Ethinyl Estradiol) Ortho Pharmaceutical .. 1851
Ortho-Cyclen/Ortho-Tri-Cyclen (Norgestimate, Ethinyl Estradiol) Ortho Pharmaceutical 1858
Ortho Diaphragm Kits—All-Flex Arcing Spring; Ortho Coil Spring; Ortho-White Flat Spring (Diaphragm) Ortho Pharmaceutical 1865
Ortho Diaphragm Kit-Coil Spring (Diaphragm) Ortho Pharmaceutical 1865
Ortho-Gynol Contraceptive Jelly (Nonoxynol-9) Ortho Pharmaceutical .... ▣ 740
Ortho-Novum (Norethindrone, Ethinyl Estradiol) Ortho Pharmaceutical 1872
Ortho-Cyclen/Ortho Tri-Cyclen (Norgestimate, Ethinyl Estradiol) Ortho Pharmaceutical 1858
Ortho-White Diaphragm Kit-Flat Spring (See also Ortho Diaphragm Kits) (Diaphragm) Ortho Pharmaceutical 1865
Ovcon (Norethindrone, Ethinyl Estradiol) Bristol-Myers Squibb 760
Ovral Tablets (Norgestrel, Ethinyl Estradiol) Wyeth-Ayerst 2770
Ovral-28 Tablets (Norgestrel, Ethinyl Estradiol) Wyeth-Ayerst 2770
Ovrette Tablets (Norgestrel) Wyeth-Ayerst 2771
ParaGard T380A Intrauterine Copper Contraceptive (Intrauterine device) Ortho Pharmaceutical 1880
Semicid Vaginal Contraceptive Inserts (Nonoxynol-9) Whitehall ▣ 874
Today Vaginal Contraceptive Sponge (Nonoxynol-9) Whitehall .... ▣ 874
Levlen/Tri-Levlen (Levonorgestrel, Ethinyl Estradiol) Berlex 651
Tri-Norinyl (Norethindrone, Ethinyl Estradiol) Roche Laboratories 2164
Triphasil-21 Tablets (Levonorgestrel, Ethinyl Estradiol) Wyeth-Ayerst 2814
Triphasil-28 Tablets (Levonorgestrel, Ethinyl Estradiol) Wyeth-Ayerst 2819

Pregnancy, termination of, from 12th through the 20th gestational week
Prostin E2 Suppository (Dinoprostone) Upjohn 2634

Pregnancy, vitamin supplement for (see under Vitamin deficiency, postpartum; Vitamin deficiency, prenatal)

Premenstrual syndrome (see under Menstrual syndrome, pre-, management of)

Prickly heat (see under Miliaria)

Prinzmetal's angina (see under Angina, Prinzmetal's)

Proctitis
ROWASA Rectal Suspension Enema 4.0 grams/unit (60 mL) (Mesalamine) Solvay 2548

Proctitis, active ulcerative
ROWASA Rectal Suppositories, 500 mg (Mesalamine) Solvay 2548

Proctitis, temporary relief of
Anusol-HC Suppositories (Hydrocortisone Acetate) Parke-Davis 1897

Proctitis, ulcerative, adjunctive therapy in
CORTENEMA (Hydrocortisone) Solvay 2535
Cortifoam (Hydrocortisone Acetate) Schwarz 2396

Proctosigmoiditis
ROWASA Rectal Suspension Enema 4.0 grams/unit (60 mL) (Mesalamine) Solvay 2548

Proctosigmoiditis, ulcerative, adjunctive therapy in
CORTENEMA (Hydrocortisone) Solvay 2535

Propionibacterium species gynecologic infections
Primaxin I.V. (Imipenem-Cilastatin Sodium) Merck & Co., Inc. 1729

Propionibacterium species infections
Primaxin I.V. (Imipenem-Cilastatin Sodium) Merck & Co., Inc. 1729

Propionibacterium species intra-abdominal infections
Primaxin I.V. (Imipenem-Cilastatin Sodium) Merck & Co., Inc. 1729

Prostatic cancer (see under Carcinoma, prostate)

Prostatic cancer, palliative treatment of (see under Carcinoma, prostatic, palliative treatment of)

Prostatic hyperplasia, benign, symptomatic treatment
Cardura Tablets (Doxazosin Mesylate) Roerig 2186
Hytrin Capsules (Terazosin Hydrochloride) Abbott 430
Proscar Tablets (Finasteride) Merck & Co., Inc. 1741

Prostatitis
Ancef Injection (Cefazolin Sodium) SmithKline Beecham Pharmaceuticals 2465
Floxin I.V. (Ofloxacin) McNeil Pharmaceutical 1571
Floxin Tablets (200 mg, 300 mg, 400 mg) (Ofloxacin) McNeil Pharmaceutical 1567
Geocillin Tablets (Carbenicillin Indanyl Sodium) Roerig 2199
Keflex Pulvules & Oral Suspension (Cephalexin) Dista 914
Keftab Tablets (Cephalexin Hydrochloride) Dista 915
Noroxin Tablets (Norfloxacin) Merck & Co., Inc. 1715
Noroxin Tablets (Norfloxacin) Roberts 2048

Prostatitis, frequency and incontinence, symptomatic relief of
Urispas Tablets (Flavoxate Hydrochloride) SmithKline Beecham Pharmaceuticals 2532

Prostatitis, "lacking substantial evidence of effectiveness" in
Urobiotic-250 Capsules (Oxytetracycline Hydrochloride, Sulfamethizole, Phenazopyridine Hydrochloride) Roerig 2214

Proteinuria, remission of in nephrotic syndrome
Aristocort Suspension (Forte Parenteral) (Triamcinolone Diacetate) Fujisawa 1027
Aristocort Tablets (Triamcinolone) Fujisawa 1022
Celestone Soluspan Suspension (Betamethasone Sodium Phosphate, Betamethasone Acetate) Schering 2347
Cortone Acetate Sterile Suspension (Cortisone Acetate) Merck & Co., Inc. 1623
Cortone Acetate Tablets (Cortisone Acetate) Merck & Co., Inc. 1624
Dalalone D.P. Injectable (Dexamethasone Acetate) Forest 1011
Decadron Elixir (Dexamethasone) Merck & Co., Inc. 1633
Decadron Phosphate Injection (Dexamethasone Sodium Phosphate) Merck & Co., Inc. 1637
Decadron Tablets (Dexamethasone) Merck & Co., Inc. 1635
Decadron-LA Sterile Suspension (Dexamethasone Acetate) Merck & Co., Inc. 1646
Deltasone Tablets (Prednisone) Upjohn 2595
Depo-Medrol Single-Dose Vial (Methylprednisolone Acetate) Upjohn 2600
Depo-Medrol Sterile Aqueous Suspension (Methylprednisolone Acetate) Upjohn 2597
Hydeltrasol Injection, Sterile (Prednisolone Sodium Phosphate) Merck & Co., Inc. 1665
Hydrocortone Phosphate Injection, Sterile (Hydrocortisone Sodium Phosphate) Merck & Co., Inc. 1670
Hydrocortone Tablets (Hydrocortisone) Merck & Co., Inc. 1672
Medrol (Methylprednisolone) Upjohn 2621
Pediapred Oral Liquid (Prednisolone Sodium Phosphate) Fisons 995
Prelone Syrup (Prednisolone) Muro 1787
Solu-Cortef Sterile Powder (Hydrocortisone Sodium Succinate) Upjohn 2641
Solu-Medrol Sterile Powder (Methylprednisolone Sodium Succinate) Upjohn 2643

Proteus mirabilis (see under P. mirabilis infections)

Proteus species bone and joint infections
Nebcin Vials, Hyporets & ADD-Vantage (Tobramycin Sulfate) Lilly 1464

Proteus species gynecologic infections
Primaxin I.V. (Imipenem-Cilastatin Sodium) Merck & Co., Inc. 1729

Proteus species infections
Amikacin Sulfate Injection, USP (Amikacin Sulfate) Elkins-Sinn 960
Amikin Injectable (Amikacin Sulfate) Apothecon 501
Bactrim I.V. Infusion (Trimethoprim, Sulfamethoxazole) Roche Laboratories 2082
Cefobid Intravenous/Intramuscular (Cefoperazone Sodium) Roerig 2189
Cefobid Pharmacy Bulk Package - Not for Direct Infusion (Cefoperazone Sodium) Roerig 2192
Cefotan (Cefotetan) Zeneca 2829
Ceptaz (Ceftazidime) Glaxo Wellcome 1081
Fortaz (Ceftazidime) Glaxo Wellcome 1100
Garamycin Injectable (Gentamicin Sulfate) Schering 2360
Monocid Injection (Cefonicid Sodium) SmithKline Beecham Pharmaceuticals 2497
Nebcin Vials, Hyporets & ADD-Vantage (Tobramycin Sulfate) Lilly 1464
Netromycin Injection 100 mg/ml (Netilmicin Sulfate) Schering 2373
Pipracil (Piperacillin Sodium) Lederle 1390
Primaxin I.V. (Imipenem-Cilastatin Sodium) Merck & Co., Inc. 1729
Septra I.V. Infusion (Trimethoprim, Sulfamethoxazole) Glaxo Wellcome 1169
Septra I.V. Infusion ADD-Vantage Vials (Trimethoprim, Sulfamethoxazole) Glaxo Wellcome 1171
Tazicef for Injection (Ceftazidime) SmithKline Beecham Pharmaceuticals 2519
Tazidime Vials, Faspak & ADD-Vantage (Ceftazidime) Lilly .. 1478
TERAK Ointment (Oxytetracycline Hydrochloride, Polymyxin B Sulfate) Akorn .... ◉ 209

(▣ Described in PDR For Nonprescription Drugs) (◉ Described in PDR For Ophthalmology)

1527 Indications Index Pruritus

Ticar for Injection (Ticarcillin Disodium) SmithKline Beecham Pharmaceuticals ... 2526
Tobramycin Sulfate Injection (Tobramycin Sulfate) Elkins-Sinn ... 968

Proteus species infections, ocular
TERAK Ointment (Oxytetracycline Hydrochloride, Polymyxin B Sulfate) Akorn ... ⊙ 209
Terramycin with Polymyxin B Sulfate Ophthalmic Ointment (Oxytetracycline Hydrochloride, Polymyxin B Sulfate) Roerig ... 2211

Proteus species infections, ocular, indole-negative
Pred-G Liquifilm Sterile Ophthalmic Suspension (Gentamicin Sulfate, Prednisolone Acetate) Allergan ... ⊙ 251

Proteus species intra-abdominal infections
Netromycin Injection 100 mg/ml (Netilmicin Sulfate) Schering ... 2373
Primaxin I.V. (Imipenem-Cilastatin Sodium) Merck & Co., Inc. ... 1729

Proteus species lower respiratory tract infections
Netromycin Injection 100 mg/ml (Netilmicin Sulfate) Schering ... 2373
Ticar for Injection (Ticarcillin Disodium) SmithKline Beecham Pharmaceuticals ... 2526

Proteus species septicemia
Cefobid Intravenous/Intramuscular (Cefoperazone Sodium) Roerig ... 2189
Cefobid Pharmacy Bulk Package - Not for Direct Infusion (Cefoperazone Sodium) Roerig ... 2192
Ticar for Injection (Ticarcillin Disodium) SmithKline Beecham Pharmaceuticals ... 2526

Proteus species skin and skin structure infections
Ceptaz (Ceftazidime) Glaxo Wellcome ... 1081
Fortaz (Ceftazidime) Glaxo Wellcome ... 1100
Nebcin Vials, Hyporets & ADD-Vantage (Tobramycin Sulfate) Lilly ... 1464
Netromycin Injection 100 mg/ml (Netilmicin Sulfate) Schering ... 2373
Tazicef for Injection (Ceftazidime) SmithKline Beecham Pharmaceuticals ... 2519
Tazidime Vials, Faspak & ADD-Vantage (Ceftazidime) Lilly ... 1478
Ticar for Injection (Ticarcillin Disodium) SmithKline Beecham Pharmaceuticals ... 2526
Tobramycin Sulfate Injection (Tobramycin Sulfate) Elkins-Sinn ... 968

Proteus species urinary tract infections
Bactrim I.V. Infusion (Trimethoprim, Sulfamethoxazole) Roche Laboratories ... 2082
Cefotan (Cefotetan) Zeneca ... 2829
Ceptaz (Ceftazidime) Glaxo Wellcome ... 1081
Fortaz (Ceftazidime) Glaxo Wellcome ... 1100
Mandol Vials, Faspak & ADD-Vantage (Cefamandole Nafate) Lilly ... 1461
Monocid Injection (Cefonicid Sodium) SmithKline Beecham Pharmaceuticals ... 2497
Nebcin Vials, Hyporets & ADD-Vantage (Tobramycin Sulfate) Lilly ... 1464
NegGram (Nalidixic Acid) Sanofi Winthrop ... 2323
Netromycin Injection 100 mg/ml (Netilmicin Sulfate) Schering ... 2373
Septra I.V. Infusion (Trimethoprim, Sulfamethoxazole) Glaxo Wellcome ... 1169
Septra I.V. Infusion ADD-Vantage Vials (Trimethoprim, Sulfamethoxazole) Glaxo Wellcome ... 1171
Streptomycin Sulfate Injection (Streptomycin Sulfate) Roerig ... 2208
Tazicef for Injection (Ceftazidime) SmithKline Beecham Pharmaceuticals ... 2519
Tazidime Vials, Faspak & ADD-Vantage (Ceftazidime) Lilly ... 1478
Tobramycin Sulfate Injection (Tobramycin Sulfate) Elkins-Sinn ... 968

Proteus vulgaris (see under P. vulgaris infections)

Proteus, indole-positive, infections (see under Morganella morganii infections)

Prothrombin deficiency, anticoagulant-induced
AquaMEPHYTON Injection (Phytonadione) Merck & Co., Inc. 1608
Konakion Injection (Phytonadione) Roche Laboratories ... 2127
Mephyton Tablets (Phytonadione) Merck & Co., Inc. ... 1696

Providencia rettgeri infections
Amikacin Sulfate Injection, USP (Amikacin Sulfate) Elkins-Sinn ... 960
Amikin Injectable (Amikacin Sulfate) Apothecon ... 501
Cefizox for Intramuscular or Intravenous Use (Ceftizoxime Sodium) Fujisawa ... 1034
Cefotan (Cefotetan) Zeneca ... 2829
Cipro I.V. (Ciprofloxacin) Bayer Pharmaceutical ... 595
Cipro I.V. Pharmacy Bulk Package (Ciprofloxacin) Bayer Pharmaceutical ... 597
Cipro Tablets (Ciprofloxacin Hydrochloride) Bayer Pharmaceutical ... 592
Claforan Sterile and Injection (Cefotaxime Sodium) Hoechst-Roussel ... 1235
Geocillin Tablets (Carbenicillin Indanyl Sodium) Roerig ... 2199
Mefoxin (Cefoxitin Sodium) Merck & Co., Inc. ... 1691
Mefoxin Premixed Intravenous Solution (Cefoxitin Sodium) Merck & Co., Inc. ... 1694
Mezlin (Mezlocillin Sodium) Bayer Pharmaceutical ... 601
Mezlin Pharmacy Bulk Package (Mezlocillin Sodium) Bayer Pharmaceutical ... 604
Monocid Injection (Cefonicid Sodium) SmithKline Beecham Pharmaceuticals ... 2497
Primaxin I.V. (Imipenem-Cilastatin Sodium) Merck & Co., Inc. ... 1729

Providencia rettgeri skin and skin structure infections
Claforan Sterile and Injection (Cefotaxime Sodium) Hoechst-Roussel ... 1235
Mezlin (Mezlocillin Sodium) Bayer Pharmaceutical ... 601
Mezlin Pharmacy Bulk Package (Mezlocillin Sodium) Bayer Pharmaceutical ... 604
Primaxin I.V. (Imipenem-Cilastatin Sodium) Merck & Co., Inc. ... 1729

Providencia rettgeri urinary tract infections
Cefizox for Intramuscular or Intravenous Use (Ceftizoxime Sodium) Fujisawa ... 1034
Cefotan (Cefotetan) Zeneca ... 2829
Cipro I.V. (Ciprofloxacin) Bayer Pharmaceutical ... 595
Cipro I.V. Pharmacy Bulk Package (Ciprofloxacin) Bayer Pharmaceutical ... 597
Cipro Tablets (Ciprofloxacin Hydrochloride) Bayer Pharmaceutical ... 592
Claforan Sterile and Injection (Cefotaxime Sodium) Hoechst-Roussel ... 1235
Geocillin Tablets (Carbenicillin Indanyl Sodium) Roerig ... 2199
Mefoxin (Cefoxitin Sodium) Merck & Co., Inc. ... 1691
Mefoxin Premixed Intravenous Solution (Cefoxitin Sodium) Merck & Co., Inc. ... 1694
Monocid Injection (Cefonicid Sodium) SmithKline Beecham Pharmaceuticals ... 2497
Primaxin I.V. (Imipenem-Cilastatin Sodium) Merck & Co., Inc. ... 1729

Providencia species infections
Amikacin Sulfate Injection, USP (Amikacin Sulfate) Elkins-Sinn ... 960
Amikin Injectable (Amikacin Sulfate) Apothecon ... 501
Mefoxin (Cefoxitin Sodium) Merck & Co., Inc. ... 1691
Mefoxin Premixed Intravenous Solution (Cefoxitin Sodium) Merck & Co., Inc. ... 1694
Nebcin Vials, Hyporets & ADD-Vantage (Tobramycin Sulfate) Lilly ... 1464
Tobramycin Sulfate Injection (Tobramycin Sulfate) Elkins-Sinn ... 968

Providencia species urinary tract infections
Mefoxin (Cefoxitin Sodium) Merck & Co., Inc. ... 1691
Nebcin Vials, Hyporets & ADD-Vantage (Tobramycin Sulfate) Lilly ... 1464
Tobramycin Sulfate Injection (Tobramycin Sulfate) Elkins-Sinn ... 968

Providencia stuartii infections
Amikacin Sulfate Injection, USP (Amikacin Sulfate) Elkins-Sinn ... 960
Amikin Injectable (Amikacin Sulfate) Apothecon ... 501
Cipro I.V. (Ciprofloxacin) Bayer Pharmaceutical ... 595
Cipro I.V. Pharmacy Bulk Package (Ciprofloxacin) Bayer Pharmaceutical ... 597
Cipro Tablets (Ciprofloxacin Hydrochloride) Bayer Pharmaceutical ... 592
Zefazone (Cefmetazole Sodium) Upjohn ... 2654

Providencia stuartii skin and skin structure infections
Cipro I.V. (Ciprofloxacin) Bayer Pharmaceutical ... 595
Cipro I.V. Pharmacy Bulk Package (Ciprofloxacin) Bayer Pharmaceutical ... 597
Cipro Tablets (Ciprofloxacin Hydrochloride) Bayer Pharmaceutical ... 592
Zefazone (Cefmetazole Sodium) Upjohn ... 2654

Pruritus ani (see also under Pruritus, anogenital)
Anusol-HC Suppositories (Hydrocortisone Acetate) Parke-Davis ... 1897
PrameGel (Pramoxine Hydrochloride) GenDerm ... 1055
Preparation H Hydrocortisone 1% Cream (Hydrocortisone) Whitehall ... ▣ 872

Pruritus associated with partial biliary obstruction
Questran Light (Cholestyramine) Bristol-Myers Squibb ... 769
Questran Powder (Cholestyramine) Bristol-Myers Squibb ... 770

Pruritus, anogenital
Americaine Hemorrhoidal Ointment (Benzocaine) CIBA Consumer ... ▣ 629
Analpram-HC Rectal Cream 1% and 2.5% (Hydrocortisone Acetate, Pramoxine Hydrochloride) Ferndale ... 977
Anusol HC-1 Anti-Itch Hydrocortisone Ointment (Hydrocortisone Acetate) WARNER WELLCOME ... ▣ 847
Caldecort (Hydrocortisone Acetate) CIBA Consumer ... ▣ 631
Cortaid (Hydrocortisone Acetate) Upjohn ... ▣ 836
Cortizone-5 (Hydrocortisone) Thompson Medical ... ▣ 831
Cortizone-10 (Hydrocortisone) Thompson Medical ... ▣ 831
Mantadil Cream (Chlorcyclizine Hydrochloride) Glaxo Wellcome ... 1135
Nupercainal Hydrocortisone 1% Cream (Hydrocortisone Acetate) CIBA Consumer ... ▣ 645
Preparation H (Glycerin, Petrolatum, Phenylephrine Hydrochloride, Shark Liver Oil) Whitehall ... ▣ 871
ProctoFoam-HC (Hydrocortisone Acetate, Pramoxine Hydrochloride) Schwarz ... 2409
Sween Cream (Benzethonium Chloride, Lanolin Oil) Sween ... 2554
Temaril Tablets, Syrup and Spansule Extended-Release Capsules (Trimeprazine Tartrate) Allergan ... 483
Tronolane Anesthetic Cream for Hemorrhoids (Pramoxine Hydrochloride) Ross ... ▣ 784
Tronolane Hemorrhoidal Suppositories (Fat, Hard, Zinc Oxide) Ross ... ▣ 784
Tucks Pads (Witch Hazel) WARNER WELLCOME ... ▣ 865
Wyanoids Relief Factor Hemorrhoidal Suppositories (Liver, Desiccated, Shark Liver Oil) Wyeth-Ayerst ... ▣ 881

Pruritus, ocular
Acular (Ketorolac Tromethamine) Allergan ... 474
Naphcon-A Ophthalmic Solution (Naphazoline Hydrochloride, Pheniramine Maleate) Alcon Laboratories ... 473

Pruritus, rhinopharyngeal, symptomatic relief of
Actifed Syrup (Pseudoephedrine Hydrochloride, Triprolidine Hydrochloride) WARNER WELLCOME ... ▣ 846
Actifed Tablets (Pseudoephedrine Hydrochloride, Triprolidine Hydrochloride) WARNER WELLCOME ... ▣ 844
Benadryl Allergy Decongestant Tablets (Diphenhydramine Hydrochloride, Pseudoephedrine Hydrochloride) WARNER WELLCOME ... ▣ 848
Benadryl Allergy Liquid Medication (Diphenhydramine Hydrochloride) WARNER WELLCOME ... ▣ 849
Benadryl Allergy (Diphenhydramine Hydrochloride) WARNER WELLCOME ... ▣ 848
Benadryl Allergy Sinus Headache Formula Caplets (Diphenhydramine Hydrochloride, Pseudoephedrine Hydrochloride, Acetaminophen) WARNER WELLCOME ... ▣ 849
Drixoral Cold and Allergy Sustained-Action Tablets (Dexbrompheniramine Maleate, Pseudoephedrine Sulfate) Schering-Plough HealthCare ... ▣ 802
Drixoral Cold and Flu Extended-Release Tablets (Acetaminophen, Dexbrompheniramine Maleate, Pseudoephedrine Sulfate) Schering-Plough HealthCare ... ▣ 803
Nolahist Tablets (Phenindamine Tartrate) Carnrick ... 785
Novahistine Elixir (Chlorpheniramine Maleate, Phenylephrine Hydrochloride) SmithKline Beecham Consumer ... ▣ 823
Singlet Tablets (Acetaminophen, Chlorpheniramine Maleate, Pseudoephedrine Hydrochloride) SmithKline Beecham Consumer ... ▣ 825
Sinulin Tablets (Acetaminophen, Phenylpropanolamine Hydrochloride, Chlorpheniramine Maleate) Carnrick ... 787
Sudafed Plus Liquid (Chlorpheniramine Maleate, Pseudoephedrine Hydrochloride) WARNER WELLCOME ... ▣ 862
Sudafed Plus Tablets (Chlorpheniramine Maleate, Pseudoephedrine Hydrochloride) WARNER WELLCOME ... ▣ 863
Tavist Syrup (Clemastine Fumarate) Sandoz Pharmaceuticals ... 2297

(▣ Described in PDR For Nonprescription Drugs) (⊙ Described in PDR For Ophthalmology)

Pruritus · Indications Index · 1528

Triaminic Syrup (Phenylpropanolamine Hydrochloride, Chlorpheniramine Maleate) Sandoz Consumer ▣ 792
Triaminic-12 Tablets (Phenylpropanolamine Hydrochloride, Chlorpheniramine Maleate) Sandoz Consumer ▣ 792
Triaminicin Tablets (Acetaminophen, Chlorpheniramine Maleate, Phenylpropanolamine Hydrochloride) Sandoz Consumer ▣ 793
TYLENOL Severe Allergy Medication Caplets (Acetaminophen, Diphenhydramine Hydrochloride) McNeil Consumer 1564

Pruritus, systemic relief of

Atarax Tablets & Syrup (Hydroxyzine Hydrochloride) Roerig 2185
Itch-X (Pramoxine Hydrochloride, Benzyl Alcohol) Ascher ▣ 602
Seldane Tablets (Terfenadine) Marion Merrell Dow 1536
Seldane-D Extended-Release Tablets (Pseudoephedrine Hydrochloride, Terfenadine) Marion Merrell Dow 1538
Temaril Tablets, Syrup and Spansule Extended-Release Capsules (Trimeprazine Tartrate) Allergan 483
Vistaril Capsules (Hydroxyzine Pamoate) Pfizer Labs 1944
Vistaril Intramuscular Solution (Hydroxyzine Hydrochloride) Roerig 2216
Vistaril Oral Suspension (Hydroxyzine Pamoate) Pfizer Labs 1944

Pruritus, topical relief of (see also under Pruritus, systemic relief of)

Aclovate (Alclometasone Dipropionate) Glaxo Wellcome 1069
Americaine (Benzocaine) CIBA Consumer ▣ 629
Anusol-HC Cream 2.5% (Hydrocortisone) Parke-Davis 1896
Aristocort A 0.025% Cream (Triamcinolone Acetonide) Fujisawa 1027
Aristocort A 0.1% Cream (Triamcinolone Acetonide) Fujisawa 1029
Aristocort A 0.1% Ointment (Triamcinolone Acetonide) Fujisawa 1030
Bactine Antiseptic/Anesthetic First Aid Liquid (Benzalkonium Chloride, Lidocaine Hydrochloride) Miles Consumer ▣ 708
Bactine Hydrocortisone Anti-Itch Cream (Hydrocortisone) Miles Consumer ▣ 709
Benadryl Itch Relief Cream, Children's Formula and Maximum Strength 2% (Diphenhydramine Hydrochloride, Zinc Acetate) WARNER WELLCOME ▣ 851
Benadryl Itch Relief Spray, Children's Formula and Maximum Strength 2% (Diphenhydramine Hydrochloride, Zinc Acetate) WARNER WELLCOME ▣ 851
Benadryl Itch Relief Stick Maximum Strength 2% (Diphenhydramine Hydrochloride, Zinc Acetate) WARNER WELLCOME ▣ 850
Benadryl Itch Stopping Gel, Children's Formula and Maximum Strength 2% (Diphenhydramine Hydrochloride, Zinc Acetate) WARNER WELLCOME ▣ 851
BiCozene Creme (Benzocaine, Resorcinol) Sandoz Consumer ▣ 785
Caladryl Cream For Kids (Calamine, Pramoxine Hydrochloride) WARNER WELLCOME ▣ 853
Caldecort (Hydrocortisone Acetate) CIBA Consumer ▣ 631
Cordran Lotion (Flurandrenolide) Oclassen 1803
Cordran Tape (Flurandrenolide) Oclassen 1804
Cortaid Spray (Hydrocortisone) Upjohn ▣ 836
Cortizone-5 Creme and Ointment (Hydrocortisone) Thompson Medical ▣ 831
Cortizone-10 Creme and Ointment (Hydrocortisone) Thompson Medical ▣ 831
Cutivate Cream (Fluticasone Propionate) Glaxo Wellcome 1088
Cutivate Ointment (Fluticasone Propionate) Glaxo Wellcome 1089
Cyclocort Topical Cream 0.1% (Amcinonide) Fujisawa 1037
Decadron Phosphate Topical Cream (Dexamethasone Sodium Phosphate) Merck & Co., Inc. 1644
Decaspray Topical Aerosol (Dexamethasone) Merck & Co., Inc. 1648
Dermatop Emollient Cream 0.1% (Prednicarbate) Hoechst-Roussel 1238
DesOwen Cream, Ointment and Lotion (Desonide) Galderma 1046
Diprolene (Betamethasone Dipropionate) Schering 2352
Elocon (Mometasone Furoate) Schering 2354
Epifoam (Hydrocortisone Acetate, Pramoxine Hydrochloride) Schwarz 2399
Eurax Cream & Lotion (Crotamiton) Westwood-Squibb 2685
Florone/Florone E (Diflorasone Diacetate) Dermik 906
Halog (Halcinonide) Westwood-Squibb 2686
Hytone (Hydrocortisone) Dermik 907
Lac-Hydrin 12% Lotion (Ammonium Lactate) Westwood-Squibb 2687
Lidex (Fluocinonide) Roche Laboratories 2130
Locoid Cream, Ointment and Topical Solution (Hydrocortisone Butyrate) Ferndale 978
Mantadil Cream (Chlorcyclizine Hydrochloride) Glaxo Wellcome 1135
Massengill Medicated Soft Cloth Towelettes (Hydrocortisone) SmithKline Beecham 2458
PrameGel (Pramoxine Hydrochloride) GenDerm 1055
Pramosone Cream, Lotion & Ointment (Hydrocortisone Acetate, Pramoxine Hydrochloride) Ferndale 978
Preparation H Hydrocortisone 1% Cream (Hydrocortisone) Whitehall ▣ 872
ProctoCream-HC (Hydrocortisone Acetate, Pramoxine Hydrochloride) Schwarz 2408
Psorcon Ointment 0.05% (Diflorasone Diacetate) Dermik 908
Sween Cream (Benzethonium Chloride, Lanolin Oil) Sween 2554
Synalar (Fluocinolone Acetonide) Roche Laboratories 2130
Temovate (Clobetasol Propionate) Glaxo Wellcome 1179
Topicort (Desoximetasone) Hoechst-Roussel 1243
Tridesilon Cream 0.05% (Desonide) Bayer Pharmaceutical 615
Tridesilon Ointment 0.05% (Desonide) Bayer Pharmaceutical 616
Ultravate Cream 0.05% (Halobetasol Propionate) Westwood-Squibb 2689
Ultravate Ointment 0.05% (Halobetasol Propionate) Westwood-Squibb 2690
Westcort (Hydrocortisone Valerate) Westwood-Squibb 2690
Xylocaine Ointment 2.5% (Lidocaine) Astra ▣ 603
Zonalon Cream (Doxepin Hydrochloride) GenDerm 1055

Pruritus, vaginal

Betadine Medicated Douche (Povidone Iodine) Purdue Frederick 1992
Betadine Medicated Gel (Povidone Iodine) Purdue Frederick 1992
Betadine Medicated Vaginal Suppositories (Povidone Iodine) Purdue Frederick 1992
Cortaid (Hydrocortisone Acetate) Upjohn ▣ 836

Pseudomonas aeruginosa infections (see under P. aeruginosa infections)

Pseudomonas species bone and joint infections

Claforan Sterile and Injection (Cefotaxime Sodium) Hoechst-Roussel 1235

Pseudomonas species infections

Amikacin Sulfate Injection, USP (Amikacin Sulfate) Elkins-Sinn 960
Amikin Injectable (Amikacin Sulfate) Apothecon 501
Cefizox for Intramuscular or Intravenous Use (Ceftizoxime Sodium) Fujisawa 1034
Ceptaz (Ceftazidime) Glaxo Wellcome 1081
Claforan Sterile and Injection (Cefotaxime Sodium) Hoechst-Roussel 1235
Fortaz (Ceftazidime) Glaxo Wellcome 1100
Geocillin Tablets (Carbenicillin Indanyl Sodium) Roerig 2199
Mezlin (Mezlocillin Sodium) Bayer Pharmaceutical 601
Mezlin Pharmacy Bulk Package (Mezlocillin Sodium) Bayer Pharmaceutical 604
Pipracil (Piperacillin Sodium) Lederle 1390
Tazicef for Injection (Ceftazidime) SmithKline Beecham Pharmaceuticals 2519
Tazidime Vials, Faspak & ADD-Vantage (Ceftazidime) Lilly 1478

Pseudomonas species infections, ocular

AK-CIDE (Prednisolone Acetate, Sulfacetamide Sodium) Akorn ⊙ 202
AK-CIDE Ointment (Prednisolone Acetate, Sulfacetamide Sodium) Akorn ⊙ 202
Blephamide Liquifilm Sterile Ophthalmic Suspension (Prednisolone Acetate, Sulfacetamide Sodium) Allergan 476
Chibroxin Sterile Ophthalmic Solution (Norfloxacin) Merck & Co., Inc. 1617
Maxitrol Ophthalmic Ointment and Suspension (Dexamethasone, Neomycin Sulfate, Polymyxin B Sulfate) Alcon Laboratories ⊙ 224
Vasocidin Ointment (Prednisolone Acetate, Sulfacetamide Sodium) CIBA Vision Ophthalmics ⊙ 268

Pseudomonas species lower respiratory tract infections

Claforan Sterile and Injection (Cefotaxime Sodium) Hoechst-Roussel 1235
Mezlin (Mezlocillin Sodium) Bayer Pharmaceutical 601
Mezlin Pharmacy Bulk Package (Mezlocillin Sodium) Bayer Pharmaceutical 604
Tazicef for Injection (Ceftazidime) SmithKline Beecham Pharmaceuticals 2519

Pseudomonas species septicemia

Mezlin (Mezlocillin Sodium) Bayer Pharmaceutical 601
Mezlin Pharmacy Bulk Package (Mezlocillin Sodium) Bayer Pharmaceutical 604
Timentin for Injection (Ticarcillin Disodium, Clavulanate Potassium) SmithKline Beecham Pharmaceuticals 2528

Pseudomonas species skin and skin structure infections

Claforan Sterile and Injection (Cefotaxime Sodium) Hoechst-Roussel 1235
Mezlin (Mezlocillin Sodium) Bayer Pharmaceutical 601
Mezlin Pharmacy Bulk Package (Mezlocillin Sodium) Bayer Pharmaceutical 604

Pseudomonas species urinary tract infections

Cefizox for Intramuscular or Intravenous Use (Ceftizoxime Sodium) Fujisawa 1034
Claforan Sterile and Injection (Cefotaxime Sodium) Hoechst-Roussel 1235
Geocillin Tablets (Carbenicillin Indanyl Sodium) Roerig 2199
Mezlin (Mezlocillin Sodium) Bayer Pharmaceutical 601
Mezlin Pharmacy Bulk Package (Mezlocillin Sodium) Bayer Pharmaceutical 604
Timentin for Injection (Ticarcillin Disodium, Clavulanate Potassium) SmithKline Beecham Pharmaceuticals 2528

Psittacosis (see under Chlamydia psittaci infection)

Psoriasis

Cortaid Spray (Hydrocortisone) Upjohn ▣ 836
Cortizone-5 (Hydrocortisone) Thompson Medical ▣ 831
DHS (Coal Tar) Persōn & Covey 1932
Dovonex Ointment 0.005% (Calcipotriene) Westwood-Squibb 2684
Drithocreme 0.1%, 0.25%, 0.5%, 1.0% (HP) (Anthralin) Dermik 905
Dritho-Scalp 0.25%, 0.5% (Anthralin) Dermik 906
Fototar Cream (Coal Tar) ICN 1253
MG 217 (Coal Tar) Triton Consumer ▣ 835
Oxsoralen-Ultra Capsules (Methoxsalen) ICN 1257
P&S Plus Tar Gel (Coal Tar) Baker Cummins ▣ 604
P&S Shampoo (Salicylic Acid) Baker Cummins ▣ 605
Pentrax Anti-dandruff Shampoo (Coal Tar) GenDerm 1055
Tegrin Dandruff Shampoo (Coal Tar) Block ▣ 611
Tegrin Skin Cream & Tegrin Medicated Soap (Coal Tar) Block ▣ 611
X-Seb T Pearl Shampoo (Coal Tar) Baker Cummins ▣ 606

Psoriasis, erythrodermic

Tegison Capsules (Etretinate) Roche Laboratories 2154

Psoriasis, generalized pustular

Tegison Capsules (Etretinate) Roche Laboratories 2154

Psoriasis, pustular

Tegison Capsules (Etretinate) Roche Laboratories 2154

Psoriasis, severe

Aristocort Suspension (Forte Parenteral) (Triamcinolone Diacetate) Fujisawa 1027
Aristocort Tablets (Triamcinolone) Fujisawa 1022
Celestone Soluspan Suspension (Betamethasone Sodium Phosphate, Betamethasone Acetate) Schering 2347
Cortone Acetate Sterile Suspension (Cortisone Acetate) Merck & Co., Inc. 1623
Cortone Acetate Tablets (Cortisone Acetate) Merck & Co., Inc. 1624
Dalalone D.P. Injectable (Dexamethasone Acetate) Forest 1011
Decadron Elixir (Dexamethasone) Merck & Co., Inc. 1633
Decadron Phosphate Injection (Dexamethasone Sodium Phosphate) Merck & Co., Inc. 1637
Decadron Tablets (Dexamethasone) Merck & Co., Inc. 1635
Decadron-LA Sterile Suspension (Dexamethasone Acetate) Merck & Co., Inc. 1646
Deltasone Tablets (Prednisone) Upjohn 2595
Depo-Medrol Single-Dose Vial (Methylprednisolone Acetate) Upjohn 2600

(▣ Described in PDR For Nonprescription Drugs) (⊙ Described in PDR For Ophthalmology)

1529 Indications Index Renal transplantation

Depo-Medrol Sterile Aqueous Suspension (Methylprednisolone Acetate) Upjohn ... 2597
Hydeltrasol Injection, Sterile (Prednisolone Sodium Phosphate) Merck & Co., Inc. ... 1665
Hydrocortone Phosphate Injection, Sterile (Hydrocortisone Sodium Phosphate) Merck & Co., Inc. ... 1670
Hydrocortone Tablets (Hydrocortisone) Merck & Co., Inc. ... 1672
Medrol (Methylprednisolone) Upjohn ... 2621
Pediapred Oral Liquid (Prednisolone Sodium Phosphate) Fisons ... 995
Prelone Syrup (Prednisolone) Muro 1787
Solu-Cortef Sterile Powder (Hydrocortisone Sodium Succinate) Upjohn ... 2641
Solu-Medrol Sterile Powder (Methylprednisolone Sodium Succinate) Upjohn ... 2643

Psoriasis, severe recalcitrant
Methotrexate Sodium Tablets, Injection, for Injection and LPF Injection (Methotrexate Sodium) Immunex ... 1275
8-MOP Capsules (Methoxsalen) ICN ... 1246
Tegison Capsules (Etretinate) Roche Laboratories ... 2154

Psoriatic arthritis (see under Arthritis, psoriatic)

Psoriatic plaques
Aristocort Suspension (Forte Parenteral) (Triamcinolone Diacetate) Fujisawa ... 1027
Aristocort Suspension (Intralesional) (Triamcinolone Diacetate) Fujisawa ... 1025
Aristospan Suspension (Intralesional) (Triamcinolone Hexacetonide) Fujisawa ... 1032
Celestone Soluspan Suspension (Betamethasone Sodium Phosphate, Betamethasone Acetate) Schering ... 2347
Decadron Phosphate Injection (Dexamethasone Sodium Phosphate) Merck & Co., Inc. ... 1637
Decadron-LA Sterile Suspension (Dexamethasone Acetate) Merck & Co., Inc. ... 1646
Depo-Medrol Single-Dose Vial (Methylprednisolone Acetate) Upjohn ... 2600
Depo-Medrol Sterile Aqueous Suspension (Methylprednisolone Acetate) Upjohn ... 2597
Dovonex Ointment 0.005% (Calcipotriene) Westwood-Squibb 2684
Hydeltrasol Injection, Sterile (Prednisolone Sodium Phosphate) Merck & Co., Inc. ... 1665
Hydrocortone Acetate Sterile Suspension (Hydrocortisone Acetate) Merck & Co., Inc. ... 1669

Psychotic disorders with depressive symptoms
Etrafon (Perphenazine, Amitriptyline Hydrochloride) Schering ... 2355
Triavil Tablets (Perphenazine, Amitriptyline Hydrochloride) Merck & Co., Inc. ... 1757

Psychotic disorders, management of the manifestations in severely ill
Clozaril Tablets (Clozapine) Sandoz Pharmaceuticals ... 2252

Psychotic disorders, management of the manifestations of (see also under Psychotic disorders, management of the manifestations in severely ill)
Compazine (Prochlorperazine) SmithKline Beecham Pharmaceuticals ... 2470
Haldol Decanoate (Haloperidol Decanoate) McNeil Pharmaceutical ... 1577
Haldol Injection, Tablets and Concentrate (Haloperidol) McNeil Pharmaceutical ... 1575
Loxitane (Loxapine Hydrochloride) Lederle ... 1378
Mellaril (Thioridazine Hydrochloride) Sandoz Pharmaceuticals ... 2269
Moban Tablets and Concentrate (Molindone Hydrochloride) Gate .. 1048
Navane Capsules and Concentrate (Thiothixene) Roerig ... 2201
Navane Intramuscular (Thiothixene) Roerig ... 2202
Prolixin (Fluphenazine Decanoate) Apothecon ... 509
Risperdal (Risperidone) Janssen ... 1301
Serentil (Mesoridazine Besylate) Boehringer Ingelheim ... 684
Stelazine (Trifluoperazine Hydrochloride) SmithKline Beecham Pharmaceuticals ... 2514
Thorazine (Chlorpromazine Hydrochloride) SmithKline Beecham Pharmaceuticals ... 2523
Trilafon (Perphenazine) Schering ... 2389

Puberty, central precocious
Lupron Depot-PED 7.5 mg, 11.25 mg and 15 mg (Leuprolide Acetate) TAP ... 2560
Supprelin Injection (Histrelin Acetate) Roberts ... 2056
Synarel Nasal Solution for Central Precocious Puberty (Nafarelin Acetate) Roche Laboratories ... 2151

Puberty, delayed, in male
Android Capsules, 10 mg (Methyltestosterone) ICN ... 1250
Android (Methyltestosterone) ICN .. 1251
Delatestryl Injection (Testosterone Enanthate) Bio-Technology General ... 2860
Halotestin Tablets (Fluoxymesterone) Upjohn ... 2614
Oreton Methyl (Methyltestosterone) ICN ... 1255
Testred Capsules (Methyltestosterone) ICN ... 1262

Pulmonary disease, obstruction, exacerbation of
Zithromax (Azithromycin) Pfizer Labs ... 1944

Pulmonary emphysema (see under Emphysema)

Pupil, dilatation of (see under Mydriasis, production of)

Purpura, idiopathic thrombocytopenic
Aristocort Tablets (Triamcinolone) Fujisawa ... 1022
Cortone Acetate Tablets (Cortisone Acetate) Merck & Co., Inc. ... 1624
Dalalone D.P. Injectable (Dexamethasone Acetate) Forest ... 1011
Decadron Elixir (Dexamethasone) Merck & Co., Inc. ... 1633
Decadron Phosphate Injection (Dexamethasone Sodium Phosphate) Merck & Co., Inc. ... 1637
Decadron Tablets (Dexamethasone) Merck & Co., Inc. ... 1635
Deltasone Tablets (Prednisone) Upjohn ... 2595
Gamimune N, 5% Immune Globulin Intravenous (Human), 5% (Globulin, Immune (Human)) Bayer Biological ... 619
Gamimune N, 10% Immune Globulin Intravenous (Human), 10% (Globulin, Immune (Human)) Bayer Biological ... 621
Gammagard S/D, Immune Globulin, Intravenous (Human) (Globulin, Immune (Human)) Baxter Healthcare ... 585
Hydeltrasol Injection, Sterile (Prednisolone Sodium Phosphate) Merck & Co., Inc. ... 1665
Hydrocortone Phosphate Injection, Sterile (Hydrocortisone Sodium Phosphate) Merck & Co., Inc. ... 1670
Hydrocortone Tablets (Hydrocortisone) Merck & Co., Inc. ... 1672
Medrol (Methylprednisolone) Upjohn ... 2621
Pediapred Oral Liquid (Prednisolone Sodium Phosphate) Fisons ... 995
Prelone Syrup (Prednisolone) Muro 1787
Sandoglobulin I.V. (Globulin, Immune (Human)) Sandoz Pharmaceuticals ... 2290
Solu-Cortef Sterile Powder (Hydrocortisone Sodium Succinate) Upjohn ... 2641
Solu-Medrol Sterile Powder (Methylprednisolone Sodium Succinate) Upjohn ... 2643
WinRho SD (Globulin, Immune (Human)) Univax ... 2577

Pyelitis
Gantanol Tablets (Sulfamethoxazole) Roche Laboratories ... 2119
Gantrisin (Acetyl Sulfisoxazole) Roche Laboratories ... 2120
Uroqid-Acid No. 2 Tablets (Methenamine Mandelate, Sodium Acid Phosphate) Beach ... 640

Pyelitis, "lacking substantial evidence of effectiveness" in
Urobiotic-250 Capsules (Oxytetracycline Hydrochloride, Sulfamethizole, Phenazopyridine Hydrochloride) Roerig ... 2214

Pyelonephritis
Azactam for Injection (Aztreonam) Bristol-Myers Squibb ... 734
Ceclor Pulvules & Suspension (Cefaclor) Lilly ... 1431
Gantanol Tablets (Sulfamethoxazole) Roche Laboratories ... 2119
Gantrisin (Acetyl Sulfisoxazole) Roche Laboratories ... 2120
Lorabid Suspension and Pulvules (Loracarbef) Lilly ... 1459
Uroqid-Acid No. 2 Tablets (Methenamine Mandelate, Sodium Acid Phosphate) Beach ... 640

Pyelonephritis, "lacking substantial evidence of effectiveness" in
Urobiotic-250 Capsules (Oxytetracycline Hydrochloride, Sulfamethizole, Phenazopyridine Hydrochloride) Roerig ... 2214

Q

Q fever
Achromycin V Capsules (Tetracycline Hydrochloride) Lederle ... 1367
Declomycin Tablets (Demeclocycline Hydrochloride) Lederle ... 1371
Doryx Capsules (Doxycycline Hyclate) Parke-Davis ... 1913
Dynacin Capsules (Minocycline Hydrochloride) Medicis ... 1590
Minocin Intravenous (Minocycline Hydrochloride) Lederle ... 1382
Minocin Oral Suspension (Minocycline Hydrochloride) Lederle ... 1385
Minocin Pellet-Filled Capsules (Minocycline Hydrochloride) Lederle ... 1383
Monodox Capsules (Doxycycline Monohydrate) Oclassen ... 1805
Terramycin Intramuscular Solution (Oxytetracycline) Roerig ... 2210
Vibramycin (Doxycycline Calcium) Pfizer Labs ... 1941
Vibramycin Hyclate Intravenous (Doxycycline Hyclate) Roerig ... 2215
Vibramycin (Doxycycline Monohydrate) Pfizer Labs ... 1941

R

Rabies, postexposure prophylaxis
Hyperab Rabies Immune Globulin (Human) (Rabies Immune Globulin (Human)) Bayer Biological ... 624
Imogam Rabies Immune Globulin (Human) (Rabies Immune Globulin (Human)) Connaught ... 880
Imovax Rabies Vaccine (Rabies Vaccine) Connaught ... 881
Rabies Vaccine Adsorbed (Rabies Vaccine) SmithKline Beecham Pharmaceuticals ... 2508

Radiography, gastrointestinal tract, adjunct in
Glucagon for Injection Vials and Emergency Kit (Glucagon) Lilly ... 1440
Reglan (Metoclopramide Hydrochloride) Robins ... 2068

Rash, diaper
A and D Medicated Diaper Rash Ointment (Petrolatum, White, Zinc Oxide) Schering-Plough HealthCare ... ▣ 797
A and D Ointment (Petrolatum, Lanolin) Schering-Plough HealthCare ... ▣ 797
Balmex Ointment (Zinc Oxide) Block ... ▣ 609
Borofax Skin Protectant Ointment (Zinc Oxide, Petrolatum, White) WARNER WELLCOME ... ▣ 853
Caldesene (Petrolatum, Zinc Oxide) CIBA Consumer ... ▣ 632
Clocream Skin Protectant Cream (Vitamin A & Vitamin D) Roberts ... ▣ 770
Daily Care from DESITIN (Zinc Oxide) Pfizer Consumer ... ▣ 742
Desitin Cornstarch Baby Powder (Zinc Oxide, Corn Starch) Pfizer Consumer ... ▣ 742
Desitin Ointment (Cod Liver Oil, Zinc Oxide) Pfizer Consumer ... ▣ 742
Impregon Concentrate (Tetrachlorosalicylanilide) Fleming ... 1005
Moisturel Cream (Dimethicone, Petrolatum) Westwood-Squibb ... 2688

Rash, drug (see also under Hypersensitivity reactions, drug-induced)
Temaril Tablets, Syrup and Spansule Extended-Release Capsules (Trimeprazine Tartrate) Allergan ... 483

Rash, unspecified (see under Skin, inflammatory conditions)

Rat-bite fever (see under Streptobacillus moniliformis infections; Spirillum minus infections)

RDS (see under Respiratory distress syndrome)

Regional enteritis (see under Enteritis, protozoal)

Reiter's syndrome
Extra Strength Bayer Arthritis Pain Regimen Formula (Aspirin, Enteric Coated) Miles Consumer ... ▣ 711
Ecotrin (Aspirin, Enteric Coated) SmithKline Beecham ... 2455

Relapsing fever (see under Borrelia recurrentis infection)

Renal calculi, calcium oxalate, recurrence, management of
Zyloprim Tablets (Allopurinol) Glaxo Wellcome ... 1226

Renal homotransplantation, adjunct for the prevention of rejection in
Atgam Sterile Solution (Lymphocyte Immune Globulin Anti-Thymocyte Globulin (Equine)) Upjohn ... 2581
Imuran (Azathioprine) Glaxo Wellcome ... 1110

Renal plasma flow, estimation of
Aminohippurate Sodium Injection (Aminohippurate Sodium) Merck & Co., Inc. ... 1606

Renal transplantation, prevention of rejection in
CellCept Capsules (Mycophenolate Mofetil) Roche Laboratories ... 2099
Neoral (Cyclosporine) Sandoz Pharmaceuticals ... 2276

Renal transplantation | Indications Index | 1530

Orthoclone OKT3 Sterile Solution (Muromonab-CD3) Ortho Biotech 1837
Sandimmune (Cyclosporine) Sandoz Pharmaceuticals 2286

Renal tubular secretory mechanism, measurement of the functional capacity of
Aminohippurate Sodium Injection (Aminohippurate Sodium) Merck & Co., Inc. 1606

Respiratory depression, curare overdosage-induced, treatment adjunct
Mestinon Injectable (Pyridostigmine Bromide) ICN 1253

Respiratory depression, post-anesthesia
Dopram Injectable (Doxapram Hydrochloride) Robins 2061
Tensilon Injectable (Edrophonium Chloride) ICN 1261

Respiratory distress syndrome
Exosurf Neonatal for Intratracheal Suspension (Colfosceril Palmitate) Glaxo Wellcome 1095
Survanta Beractant Intratracheal Suspension (Beractant) Ross 2226

Respiratory insufficiency, acute, with chronic obstructive pulmonary disease
Dopram Injectable (Doxapram Hydrochloride) Robins 2061

Respiratory symptoms, upper, relief of (see under Influenza syndrome, symptomatic relief of)

Respiratory syncytial virus (RSV) infections (see under Infections, lower respiratory tract, RSV-induced)

Retinal attachment, surgical aid in
Healon (Sodium Hyaluronate) Pharmacia Inc. Ophthalmics ◉ 314

Retinal detachment, adjunctive management of
AdatoSil 5000 (Silicone Oil) Escalon Ophthalmics ◉ 274
ISPAN Perfluoropropane (Perfluoropropane) Escalon Ophthalmics ◉ 276
ISPAN Sulfur Hexafluoride (Sulfur Hexafluoride) Escalon Ophthalmics ◉ 275

Retinitis, cytomegalovirus
Cytovene (Ganciclovir Sodium) Roche Laboratories 2103
Foscavir Injection (Foscarnet Sodium) Astra 547

Retinoblastoma
Cytoxan (Cyclophosphamide) Bristol-Myers Squibb Oncology 694
NEOSAR Lyophilized/Neosar (Cyclophosphamide) Pharmacia 1959

Rhabdomyosarcoma
Cosmegen Injection (Dactinomycin) Merck & Co., Inc. 1626
Oncovin Solution Vials & Hyporets (Vincristine Sulfate) Lilly 1466

Rheumatic carditis, acute
Aristocort Suspension (Forte Parenteral) (Triamcinolone Diacetate) Fujisawa 1027
Aristocort Tablets (Triamcinolone) Fujisawa 1022
Celestone Soluspan Suspension (Betamethasone Sodium Phosphate, Betamethasone Acetate) Schering 2347
Cortone Acetate Sterile Suspension (Cortisone Acetate) Merck & Co., Inc. 1623
Cortone Acetate Tablets (Cortisone Acetate) Merck & Co., Inc. 1624
Dalalone D.P. Injectable (Dexamethasone Acetate) Forest 1011
Decadron Elixir (Dexamethasone) Merck & Co., Inc. 1633
Decadron Phosphate Injection (Dexamethasone Sodium Phosphate) Merck & Co., Inc. 1637
Decadron Tablets (Dexamethasone) Merck & Co., Inc. 1635
Decadron-LA Sterile Suspension (Dexamethasone Acetate) Merck & Co., Inc. 1646
Deltasone Tablets (Prednisone) Upjohn 2595
Depo-Medrol Single-Dose Vial (Methylprednisolone Acetate) Upjohn 2600
Depo-Medrol Sterile Aqueous Suspension (Methylprednisolone Acetate) Upjohn 2597
Hydeltrasol Injection, Sterile (Prednisolone Sodium Phosphate) Merck & Co., Inc. 1665
Hydrocortone Phosphate Injection, Sterile (Hydrocortisone Sodium Phosphate) Merck & Co., Inc. 1670
Hydrocortone Tablets (Hydrocortisone) Merck & Co., Inc. 1672
Medrol (Methylprednisolone) Upjohn 2621
Pediapred Oral Liquid (Prednisolone Sodium Phosphate) Fisons 995
Prelone Syrup (Prednisolone) Muro 1787
Solu-Cortef Sterile Powder (Hydrocortisone Sodium Succinate) Upjohn 2641
Solu-Medrol Sterile Powder (Methylprednisolone Sodium Succinate) Upjohn 2643

Rheumatic disorders, unspecified
Regular Strength Ascriptin Tablets (Aspirin Buffered, Calcium Carbonate) CIBA Consumer ▣ 629
Depo-Medrol Single-Dose Vial (Methylprednisolone Acetate) Upjohn 2600
Mono-Gesic Tablets (Salsalate) Central 792
Salflex Tablets (Salsalate) Carnrick 786

Rheumatic fever, prophylaxis of
Bicillin L-A Injection (Penicillin G Benzathine) Wyeth-Ayerst 2707
E-Mycin Tablets (Erythromycin) Knoll Laboratories 1341
ERYC (Erythromycin) Parke-Davis 1915
Erythromycin Base Filmtab (Erythromycin) Abbott 426
Erythromycin Delayed-Release Capsules, USP (Erythromycin) Abbott 427
Ilosone (Erythromycin Estolate) Dista 911
Ilotycin Gluceptate, IV, Vials (Erythromycin Gluceptate) Dista 913
PCE Dispertab Tablets (Erythromycin) Abbott 444
Pen•Vee K (Penicillin V Potassium) Wyeth-Ayerst 2772

Rheumatic heart disease, prophylaxis
E-Mycin Tablets (Erythromycin) Knoll Laboratories 1341

Rheumatoid arthritis
Children's Advil Suspension (Ibuprofen) Wyeth-Ayerst 2692
Anaprox/Naprosyn (Naproxen Sodium) Roche Laboratories 2117
Ansaid Tablets (Flurbiprofen) Upjohn 2579
Aristocort Suspension (Forte Parenteral) (Triamcinolone Diacetate) Fujisawa 1027
Aristocort Suspension (Intralesional) (Triamcinolone Diacetate) Fujisawa 1025
Aristocort Tablets (Triamcinolone) Fujisawa 1022
Aristospan Suspension (Intra-articular) (Triamcinolone Hexacetonide) Fujisawa 1033
Arthritis Pain Ascriptin (Aspirin Buffered, Calcium Carbonate) CIBA Consumer ▣ 631
Extra Strength Bayer Arthritis Pain Regimen Formula (Aspirin, Enteric Coated) Miles Consumer ▣ 711
Bayer Enteric Aspirin (Aspirin, Enteric Coated) Miles Consumer ▣ 709
Cataflam (Diclofenac Potassium) CibaGeneva 816
Celestone Soluspan Suspension (Betamethasone Sodium Phosphate, Betamethasone Acetate) Schering 2347
Clinoril Tablets (Sulindac) Merck & Co., Inc. 1618
Cortone Acetate Sterile Suspension (Cortisone Acetate) Merck & Co., Inc. 1623
Cortone Acetate Tablets (Cortisone Acetate) Merck & Co., Inc. 1624
Cuprimine Capsules (Penicillamine) Merck & Co., Inc. 1630
Dalalone D.P. Injectable (Dexamethasone Acetate) Forest 1011
Daypro Caplets (Oxaprozin) Searle 2426
Decadron Elixir (Dexamethasone) Merck & Co., Inc. 1633
Decadron Phosphate Injection (Dexamethasone Sodium Phosphate) Merck & Co., Inc. 1637
Decadron Tablets (Dexamethasone) Merck & Co., Inc. 1635
Decadron-LA Sterile Suspension (Dexamethasone Acetate) Merck & Co., Inc. 1646
Deltasone Tablets (Prednisone) Upjohn 2595
Depen Titratable Tablets (Penicillamine) Wallace 2662
Depo-Medrol Single-Dose Vial (Methylprednisolone Acetate) Upjohn 2600
Depo-Medrol Sterile Aqueous Suspension (Methylprednisolone Acetate) Upjohn 2597
Dolobid Tablets (Diflunisal) Merck & Co., Inc. 1654
Easprin (Aspirin) Parke-Davis 1914
EC-Naprosyn Delayed-Release Tablets (Naproxen) Roche Laboratories 2117
Ecotrin (Aspirin, Enteric Coated) SmithKline Beecham 2455
Feldene Capsules (Piroxicam) Pratt 1965
Hydeltrasol Injection, Sterile (Prednisolone Sodium Phosphate) Merck & Co., Inc. 1665
Hydeltra-T.B.A. Sterile Suspension (Prednisolone Tebutate) Merck & Co., Inc. 1667
Hydrocortone Acetate Sterile Suspension (Hydrocortisone Acetate) Merck & Co., Inc. 1669
Hydrocortone Phosphate Injection, Sterile (Hydrocortisone Sodium Phosphate) Merck & Co., Inc. 1670
Hydrocortone Tablets (Hydrocortisone) Merck & Co., Inc. 1672
IBU Tablets (Ibuprofen) Knoll Laboratories 1342
Imuran (Azathioprine) Glaxo Wellcome 1110
Indocin (Indomethacin) Merck & Co., Inc. 1680
Medrol (Methylprednisolone) Upjohn 2621
Methotrexate Sodium Tablets, Injection, for Injection and LPF Injection (Methotrexate Sodium) Immunex 1275
Mono-Gesic Tablets (Salsalate) Central 792
Children's Motrin Ibuprofen Oral Suspension (Ibuprofen) McNeil Consumer 1546
Motrin Tablets (Ibuprofen) Upjohn 2625
Motrin Ibuprofen Suspension, Oral Drops, Chewable Tablets, Caplets (Ibuprofen) McNeil Consumer 1546
Myochrysine Injection (Gold Sodium Thiomalate) Merck & Co., Inc. 1711
Nalfon 200 Pulvules & Nalfon Tablets (Fenoprofen Calcium) Dista 917
Anaprox/Naprosyn (Naproxen) Roche Laboratories 2117
Orudis Capsules (Ketoprofen) Wyeth-Ayerst 2766
Oruvail Capsules (Ketoprofen) Wyeth-Ayerst 2766
Pediapred Oral Liquid (Prednisolone Sodium Phosphate) Fisons 995
Plaquenil Sulfate Tablets (Hydroxychloroquine Sulfate) Sanofi Winthrop 2328
Prelone Syrup (Prednisolone) Muro 1787
Relafen Tablets (Nabumetone) SmithKline Beecham Pharmaceuticals 2510
Ridaura Capsules (Auranofin) SmithKline Beecham Pharmaceuticals 2513
Salflex Tablets (Salsalate) Carnrick 786
Solganal Suspension (Aurothioglucose) Schering 2388
Solu-Cortef Sterile Powder (Hydrocortisone Sodium Succinate) Upjohn 2641
Solu-Medrol Sterile Powder (Methylprednisolone Sodium Succinate) Upjohn 2643
Tolectin (200, 400 and 600 mg) (Tolmetin Sodium) McNeil Pharmaceutical 1581
Trilisate (Choline Magnesium Trisalicylate) Purdue Frederick 2000
Voltaren Tablets (Diclofenac Sodium) CibaGeneva 861

Rheumatoid arthritis, juvenile
Aristocort Suspension (Forte Parenteral) (Triamcinolone Diacetate) Fujisawa 1027
Aristocort Tablets (Triamcinolone) Fujisawa 1022
Extra Strength Bayer Arthritis Pain Regimen Formula (Aspirin, Enteric Coated) Miles Consumer ▣ 711
Celestone Soluspan Suspension (Betamethasone Sodium Phosphate, Betamethasone Acetate) Schering 2347
Cortone Acetate Sterile Suspension (Cortisone Acetate) Merck & Co., Inc. 1623
Cortone Acetate Tablets (Cortisone Acetate) Merck & Co., Inc. 1624
Dalalone D.P. Injectable (Dexamethasone Acetate) Forest 1011
Decadron Elixir (Dexamethasone) Merck & Co., Inc. 1633
Decadron Phosphate Injection (Dexamethasone Sodium Phosphate) Merck & Co., Inc. 1637
Decadron Tablets (Dexamethasone) Merck & Co., Inc. 1635
Decadron-LA Sterile Suspension (Dexamethasone Acetate) Merck & Co., Inc. 1646
Deltasone Tablets (Prednisone) Upjohn 2595
Depo-Medrol Single-Dose Vial (Methylprednisolone Acetate) Upjohn 2600
Depo-Medrol Sterile Aqueous Suspension (Methylprednisolone Acetate) Upjohn 2597
Ecotrin (Aspirin, Enteric Coated) SmithKline Beecham 2455
Hydeltrasol Injection, Sterile (Prednisolone Sodium Phosphate) Merck & Co., Inc. 1665
Hydrocortone Phosphate Injection, Sterile (Hydrocortisone Sodium Phosphate) Merck & Co., Inc. 1670
Hydrocortone Tablets (Hydrocortisone) Merck & Co., Inc. 1672
Medrol (Methylprednisolone) Upjohn 2621
Myochrysine Injection (Gold Sodium Thiomalate) Merck & Co., Inc. 1711
Pediapred Oral Liquid (Prednisolone Sodium Phosphate) Fisons 995
Prelone Syrup (Prednisolone) Muro 1787
Solu-Cortef Sterile Powder (Hydrocortisone Sodium Succinate) Upjohn 2641
Solu-Medrol Sterile Powder (Methylprednisolone Sodium Succinate) Upjohn 2643
Tolectin (200, 400 and 600 mg) (Tolmetin Sodium) McNeil Pharmaceutical 1581

Rhinitis, acute, "drying agent" in
Levsin/Levsinex/Levbid (Hyoscyamine Sulfate) Schwarz 2405

(▣ Described in PDR For Nonprescription Drugs)
(◉ Described in PDR For Ophthalmology)

Indications Index

Rhinitis, allergic

Actifed Syrup (Pseudoephedrine Hydrochloride, Triprolidine Hydrochloride) WARNER WELLCOME .... ◾ 846

Actifed Tablets (Pseudoephedrine Hydrochloride, Triprolidine Hydrochloride) WARNER WELLCOME .... ◾ 844

Allerest Children's Chewable Tablets (Chlorpheniramine Maleate, Phenylpropanolamine Hydrochloride) CIBA Consumer ◾ 627

Allerest Headache Strength Tablets (Acetaminophen, Chlorpheniramine Maleate, Pseudoephedrine Hydrochloride) CIBA Consumer .... ◾ 627

Allerest Maximum Strength Tablets (Chlorpheniramine Maleate, Pseudoephedrine Hydrochloride) CIBA Consumer ◾ 627

Allerest No Drowsiness Tablets (Acetaminophen, Pseudoephedrine Hydrochloride) CIBA Consumer .... ◾ 627

Allerest Sinus Pain Formula (Acetaminophen, Chlorpheniramine Maleate, Pseudoephedrine Hydrochloride) CIBA Consumer ◾ 627

Allerest 12 Hour Caplets (Chlorpheniramine Maleate, Phenylpropanolamine Hydrochloride) CIBA Consumer .... ◾ 627

Bromfed (Brompheniramine Maleate, Pseudoephedrine Hydrochloride) Muro..................... 1785

Children's Vicks DayQuil Allergy Relief (Chlorpheniramine Maleate, Pseudoephedrine Hydrochloride) Procter & Gamble .... ◾ 757

Comhist (Chlorpheniramine Maleate, Phenyltoloxamine Citrate, Phenylephrine Hydrochloride) Roberts 2038

D.A. Chewable Tablets (Chlorpheniramine Maleate, Phenylephrine Hydrochloride, Methscopolamine Nitrate) Dura 951

Decadron Phosphate Turbinaire (Dexamethasone Sodium Phosphate) Merck & Co., Inc. 1645

Deconamine (Chlorpheniramine Maleate, Pseudoephedrine Hydrochloride) Kenwood................ 1320

Dimetapp Elixir (Brompheniramine Maleate, Phenylpropanolamine Hydrochloride) A. H. Robins Consumer .... ◾ 773

Dimetapp Extentabs (Brompheniramine Maleate, Phenylpropanolamine Hydrochloride) A. H. Robins Consumer .... ◾ 774

Drixoral Cold and Flu Extended-Release Tablets (Acetaminophen, Dexbrompheniramine Maleate, Pseudoephedrine Sulfate) Schering-Plough HealthCare .... ◾ 803

Dura-Tap/PD Capsules (Chlorpheniramine Maleate, Pseudoephedrine Hydrochloride) Dura 2867

Dura-Vent/DA Tablets (Chlorpheniramine Maleate, Phenylephrine Hydrochloride, Methscopolamine Nitrate) Dura 953

Extendryl (Chlorpheniramine Maleate, Methscopolamine Nitrate, Phenylephrine Hydrochloride) Fleming 1005

Nasalcrom Nasal Solution (Cromolyn Sodium) Fisons........................... 994

Nolahist Tablets (Phenindamine Tartrate) Carnrick 785

Novahistine Elixir (Chlorpheniramine Maleate, Phenylephrine Hydrochloride) SmithKline Beecham Consumer .... ◾ 823

Ocean Nasal Mist (Sodium Chloride) Fleming .... ◾ 655

PBZ Tablets (Tripelennamine Hydrochloride) CibaGeneva 845

PBZ-SR Tablets (Tripelennamine Hydrochloride) CibaGeneva 844

Phenergan Suppositories (Promethazine Hydrochloride) Wyeth-Ayerst 2775

Phenergan Syrup (Promethazine Hydrochloride) Wyeth-Ayerst 2774

Phenergan Tablets (Promethazine Hydrochloride) Wyeth-Ayerst 2775

Ryna Liquid (Chlorpheniramine Maleate, Pseudoephedrine Hydrochloride) Wallace .... ◾ 841

Rynatan (Chlorpheniramine Tannate, Pyrilamine Tannate, Phenylephrine Tannate) Wallace 2673

Semprex-D Capsules (Acrivastine, Pseudoephedrine Hydrochloride) Adams 463

Semprex-D Capsules (Acrivastine, Pseudoephedrine Hydrochloride) Glaxo Wellcome.................................. 1167

Sinarest (Acetaminophen, Chlorpheniramine Maleate, Pseudoephedrine Hydrochloride) CIBA Consumer .... ◾ 648

Tavist Syrup (Clemastine Fumarate) Sandoz Pharmaceuticals 2297

Tavist Tablets (Clemastine Fumarate) Sandoz Pharmaceuticals 2298

Triaminic Allergy Tablets (Chlorpheniramine Maleate, Phenylpropanolamine Hydrochloride) Sandoz Consumer............................ ◾ 789

Triaminicin Tablets (Acetaminophen, Chlorpheniramine Maleate, Phenylpropanolamine Hydrochloride) Sandoz Consumer .... ◾ 793

Trinalin Repetabs Tablets (Azatadine Maleate, Pseudoephedrine Sulfate) Key 1330

Rhinitis medicamentosa

Ayr (Sodium Chloride) Ascher........ ◾ 602

NaSal (Sodium Chloride) Miles Consumer .... ◾ 726

Rhinitis, perennial allergic

Allerest Children's Chewable Tablets (Chlorpheniramine Maleate, Phenylpropanolamine Hydrochloride) CIBA Consumer ◾ 627

Allerest Headache Strength Tablets (Acetaminophen, Chlorpheniramine Maleate, Pseudoephedrine Hydrochloride) CIBA Consumer .... ◾ 627

Allerest Maximum Strength Tablets (Chlorpheniramine Maleate, Pseudoephedrine Hydrochloride) CIBA Consumer ◾ 627

Allerest No Drowsiness Tablets (Acetaminophen, Pseudoephedrine Hydrochloride) CIBA Consumer .... ◾ 627

Allerest Sinus Pain Formula (Acetaminophen, Chlorpheniramine Maleate, Pseudoephedrine Hydrochloride) CIBA Consumer ◾ 627

Allerest 12 Hour Caplets (Chlorpheniramine Maleate, Phenylpropanolamine Hydrochloride) CIBA Consumer .... ◾ 627

Aristocort Suspension (Forte Parenteral) (Triamcinolone Diacetate) Fujisawa 1027

Aristocort Tablets (Triamcinolone) Fujisawa 1022

Atrohist Pediatric Capsules (Chlorpheniramine Maleate, Pseudoephedrine Hydrochloride) Adams 453

Beconase (Beclomethasone Dipropionate) Glaxo Wellcome 1076

Celestone Soluspan Suspension (Betamethasone Sodium Phosphate, Betamethasone Acetate) Schering 2347

Cortone Acetate Sterile Suspension (Cortisone Acetate) Merck & Co., Inc. 1623

Cortone Acetate Tablets (Cortisone Acetate) Merck & Co., Inc. 1624

Dalalone D.P. Injectable (Dexamethasone Acetate) Forest 1011

Decadron Elixir (Dexamethasone) Merck & Co., Inc. 1633

Decadron Phosphate Injection (Dexamethasone Sodium Phosphate) Merck & Co., Inc. 1637

Decadron Phosphate Turbinaire (Dexamethasone Sodium Phosphate) Merck & Co., Inc. 1645

Decadron Tablets (Dexamethasone) Merck & Co., Inc. 1635

Decadron-LA Sterile Suspension (Dexamethasone Acetate) Merck & Co., Inc. 1646

Deltasone Tablets (Prednisone) Upjohn.. 2595

Depo-Medrol Single-Dose Vial (Methylprednisolone Acetate) Upjohn.. 2600

Depo-Medrol Sterile Aqueous Suspension (Methylprednisolone Acetate) Upjohn 2597

Dexacort Phosphate in Turbinaire (Dexamethasone Sodium Phosphate) Adams 459

Fedahist Gyrocaps (Pseudoephedrine Hydrochloride, Chlorpheniramine Maleate) Schwarz 2401

Fedahist Timecaps (Pseudoephedrine Hydrochloride, Chlorpheniramine Maleate) Schwarz 2401

Flonase Nasal Spray (Fluticasone Propionate) Glaxo Wellcome 1098

Hydeltrasol Injection, Sterile (Prednisolone Sodium Phosphate) Merck & Co., Inc. 1665

Hydrocortone Phosphate Injection, Sterile (Hydrocortisone Sodium Phosphate) Merck & Co., Inc. 1670

Hydrocortone Tablets (Hydrocortisone) Merck & Co., Inc. 1672

Medrol (Methylprednisolone) Upjohn.. 2621

Nasacort Nasal Inhaler (Triamcinolone Acetonide) Rhone-Poulenc Rorer Pharmaceuticals........................ 2024

Nasarel Nasal Solution (Flunisolide) Roche Laboratories 2133

Ornade Spansule Capsules (Phenylpropanolamine Hydrochloride, Chlorpheniramine Maleate) SmithKline Beecham Pharmaceuticals 2502

Pediapred Oral Liquid (Prednisolone Sodium Phosphate) Fisons.... 995

Periactin (Cyproheptadine Hydrochloride) Merck & Co., Inc. 1724

Prelone Syrup (Prednisolone) Muro 1787

Rhinocort Nasal Inhaler (Budesonide) Astra 556

Rondec Oral Drops (Carbinoxamine Maleate, Pseudoephedrine Hydrochloride) Dura 953

Rondec Syrup (Carbinoxamine Maleate, Pseudoephedrine Hydrochloride) Dura 953

Rondec (Carbinoxamine Maleate, Pseudoephedrine Hydrochloride) Dura 953

Solu-Cortef Sterile Powder (Hydrocortisone Sodium Succinate) Upjohn.. 2641

Solu-Medrol Sterile Powder (Methylprednisolone Sodium Succinate) Upjohn 2643

Trinalin Repetabs Tablets (Azatadine Maleate, Pseudoephedrine Sulfate) Key 1330

Vancenase AQ Nasal Spray 0.042% (Beclomethasone Dipropionate) Schering 2393

Vancenase PocketHaler Nasal Inhaler (Beclomethasone Dipropionate) Schering 2391

Rhinitis, perennial, topical symptomatic treatment of

Nasalide Nasal Solution 0.025% (Flunisolide) Roche Laboratories.. 2110

Rhinitis, seasonal allergic

Aristocort Suspension (Forte Parenteral) (Triamcinolone Diacetate) Fujisawa 1027

Aristocort Tablets (Triamcinolone) Fujisawa 1022

Atrohist Pediatric Capsules (Chlorpheniramine Maleate, Pseudoephedrine Hydrochloride) Adams 453

Beconase (Beclomethasone Dipropionate) Glaxo Wellcome 1076

Benadryl Allergy Decongestant Liquid Medication (Diphenhydramine Hydrochloride, Pseudoephedrine Hydrochloride) WARNER WELLCOME .... ◾ 848

Benadryl Allergy Decongestant Tablets (Diphenhydramine Hydrochloride, Pseudoephedrine Hydrochloride) WARNER WELLCOME .... ◾ 848

Benadryl Allergy Liquid Medication (Diphenhydramine Hydrochloride) WARNER WELLCOME .... ◾ 849

Benadryl Allergy Sinus Headache Formula Caplets (Diphenhydramine Hydrochloride, Pseudoephedrine Hydrochloride, Acetaminophen) WARNER WELLCOME .... ◾ 849

Bromfed Syrup (Brompheniramine Maleate, Pseudoephedrine Hydrochloride) Muro .... ◾ 733

Celestone Soluspan Suspension (Betamethasone Sodium Phosphate, Betamethasone Acetate) Schering 2347

Claritin (Loratadine) Schering............. 2349

Claritin-D (Loratadine, Pseudoephedrine Sulfate) Schering 2350

Cortone Acetate Sterile Suspension (Cortisone Acetate) Merck & Co., Inc. 1623

Cortone Acetate Tablets (Cortisone Acetate) Merck & Co., Inc. 1624

Dalalone D.P. Injectable (Dexamethasone Acetate) Forest 1011

Decadron Elixir (Dexamethasone) Merck & Co., Inc. 1633

Decadron Phosphate Injection (Dexamethasone Sodium Phosphate) Merck & Co., Inc. 1637

Decadron Phosphate Turbinaire (Dexamethasone Sodium Phosphate) Merck & Co., Inc. 1645

Decadron Tablets (Dexamethasone) Merck & Co., Inc. 1635

Decadron-LA Sterile Suspension (Dexamethasone Acetate) Merck & Co., Inc. 1646

Deltasone Tablets (Prednisone) Upjohn.. 2595

Depo-Medrol Single-Dose Vial (Methylprednisolone Acetate) Upjohn.. 2600

Depo-Medrol Sterile Aqueous Suspension (Methylprednisolone Acetate) Upjohn 2597

Dexacort Phosphate in Turbinaire (Dexamethasone Sodium Phosphate) Adams 459

Fedahist Gyrocaps (Pseudoephedrine Hydrochloride, Chlorpheniramine Maleate) Schwarz 2401

Fedahist Timecaps (Pseudoephedrine Hydrochloride, Chlorpheniramine Maleate) Schwarz 2401

Flonase Nasal Spray (Fluticasone Propionate) Glaxo Wellcome 1098

Hismanal Tablets (Astemizole) Janssen.. 1293

Hydeltrasol Injection, Sterile (Prednisolone Sodium Phosphate) Merck & Co., Inc. 1665

Hydrocortone Phosphate Injection, Sterile (Hydrocortisone Sodium Phosphate) Merck & Co., Inc. 1670

Hydrocortone Tablets (Hydrocortisone) Merck & Co., Inc. 1672

Medrol (Methylprednisolone) Upjohn.. 2621

Nasacort Nasal Inhaler (Triamcinolone Acetonide) Rhone-Poulenc Rorer Pharmaceuticals........................ 2024

Nasarel Nasal Solution (Flunisolide) Roche Laboratories 2133

Novahistine DH (Codeine Phosphate, Pseudoephedrine Hydrochloride, Chlorpheniramine Maleate) SmithKline Beecham 2462

Ornade Spansule Capsules (Phenylpropanolamine Hydrochloride, Chlorpheniramine Maleate) SmithKline Beecham Pharmaceuticals 2502

Pediapred Oral Liquid (Prednisolone Sodium Phosphate) Fisons.... 995

Periactin (Cyproheptadine Hydrochloride) Merck & Co., Inc. 1724

Prelone Syrup (Prednisolone) Muro 1787

Rhinocort Nasal Inhaler (Budesonide) Astra 556

Rondec Oral Drops (Carbinoxamine Maleate, Pseudoephedrine Hydrochloride) Dura 953

Rondec Syrup (Carbinoxamine Maleate, Pseudoephedrine Hydrochloride) Dura 953

(◾ Described in PDR For Nonprescription Drugs)

(◉ Described in PDR For Ophthalmology)

Rhinitis — Indications Index — 1532

Rondec (Carbinoxamine Maleate, Pseudoephedrine Hydrochloride) Dura 953
Seldane Tablets (Terfenadine) Marion Merrell Dow 1536
Seldane-D Extended-Release Tablets (Pseudoephedrine Hydrochloride, Terfenadine) Marion Merrell Dow 1538
Sinulin Tablets (Acetaminophen, Phenylpropanolamine Hydrochloride, Chlorpheniramine Maleate) Carnrick 787
Sinutab Sinus Allergy Medication, Maximum Strength Tablets and Caplets (Acetaminophen, Chlorpheniramine Maleate, Pseudoephedrine Hydrochloride) WARNER WELLCOME .... ▣ 860
Sinutab Sinus Medication, Maximum Strength Without Drowsiness Formula, Tablets & Caplets (Acetaminophen, Pseudoephedrine Hydrochloride) WARNER WELLCOME .... ▣ 860
Sinutab Sinus Medication, Regular Strength Without Drowsiness Formula (Acetaminophen, Pseudoephedrine Hydrochloride) WARNER WELLCOME .... ▣ 859
Solu-Cortef Sterile Powder (Hydrocortisone Sodium Succinate) Upjohn 2641
Solu-Medrol Sterile Powder (Methylprednisolone Sodium Succinate) Upjohn 2643
Triaminicol Multi-Symptom Cold Tablets (Phenylpropanolamine Hydrochloride, Chlorpheniramine Maleate, Dextromethorphan Hydrobromide) Sandoz Consumer .... ▣ 793
Vancenase AQ Nasal Spray 0.042% (Beclomethasone Dipropionate) Schering 2393
Vancenase PocketHaler Nasal Inhaler (Beclomethasone Dipropionate) Schering 2391

Rhinitis, seasonal, topical symptomatic treatment of
Nasalide Nasal Solution 0.025% (Flunisolide) Roche Laboratories .. 2110

Rhinitis sicca
Afrin Saline Mist (Sodium Chloride) Schering-Plough HealthCare .... ▣ 798
Ayr (Sodium Chloride) Ascher .... ▣ 602
Nasal Moist (Sodium Chloride) Blairex .... ▣ 609
NaSal (Sodium Chloride) Miles Consumer .... ▣ 726
Salinex Nasal Mist and Drops (Sodium Chloride) Muro .... ▣ 734

Rhinitis, vasomotor
Beconase AQ Nasal Spray (Beclomethasone Dipropionate) Glaxo Wellcome 1076
Bromfed (Brompheniramine Maleate, Pseudoephedrine Hydrochloride) Muro 1785
D.A. Chewable Tablets (Chlorpheniramine Maleate, Phenylephrine Hydrochloride, Methscopolamine Nitrate) Dura 951
Dura-Tap/PD Capsules (Chlorpheniramine Maleate, Pseudoephedrine Hydrochloride) Dura 2867
Dura-Vent/DA Tablets (Chlorpheniramine Maleate, Phenylephrine Hydrochloride, Methscopolamine Nitrate) Dura 953
Fedahist Gyrocaps (Pseudoephedrine Hydrochloride, Chlorpheniramine Maleate) Schwarz 2401
Fedahist Timecaps (Pseudoephedrine Hydrochloride, Chlorpheniramine Maleate) Schwarz 2401
Ornade Spansule Capsules (Phenylpropanolamine Hydrochloride, Chlorpheniramine Maleate) SmithKline Beecham Pharmaceuticals 2502
PBZ Tablets (Tripelennamine Hydrochloride) CibaGeneva 845
PBZ-SR Tablets (Tripelennamine Hydrochloride) CibaGeneva 844
Periactin (Cyproheptadine Hydrochloride) Merck & Co., Inc. 1724
Phenergan Suppositories (Promethazine Hydrochloride) Wyeth-Ayerst 2775
Phenergan Syrup (Promethazine Hydrochloride) Wyeth-Ayerst 2774
Phenergan Tablets (Promethazine Hydrochloride) Wyeth-Ayerst 2775
Rondec Oral Drops (Carbinoxamine Maleate, Pseudoephedrine Hydrochloride) Dura 953
Rondec Syrup (Carbinoxamine Maleate, Pseudoephedrine Hydrochloride) Dura 953
Rondec (Carbinoxamine Maleate, Pseudoephedrine Hydrochloride) Dura 953

Rhinorrhea
Actifed Allergy Daytime/Nighttime Caplets (Diphenhydramine Hydrochloride, Pseudoephedrine Hydrochloride) WARNER WELLCOME .... ▣ 844
Actifed Syrup (Pseudoephedrine Hydrochloride, Triprolidine Hydrochloride) WARNER WELLCOME .... ▣ 846
Actifed Tablets (Pseudoephedrine Hydrochloride, Triprolidine Hydrochloride) WARNER WELLCOME .... ▣ 844
Benadryl Allergy Decongestant Tablets (Diphenhydramine Hydrochloride, Pseudoephedrine Hydrochloride) WARNER WELLCOME .... ▣ 848
Benadryl Allergy Liquid Medication (Diphenhydramine Hydrochloride) WARNER WELLCOME .... ▣ 849
Benadryl Allergy (Diphenhydramine Hydrochloride) WARNER WELLCOME .... ▣ 848
Benadryl Allergy Sinus Headache Formula Caplets (Diphenhydramine Hydrochloride, Pseudoephedrine Hydrochloride, Acetaminophen) WARNER WELLCOME .... ▣ 849
Benadryl Dye-Free Allergy Liqui-gel Softgels (Diphenhydramine Hydrochloride) WARNER WELLCOME .... ▣ 850
Benadryl Dye-Free Allergy Liquid Medication (Diphenhydramine Hydrochloride) WARNER WELLCOME .... ▣ 850
Cheracol Plus Head Cold/Cough Formula (Phenylpropanolamine Hydrochloride, Dextromethorphan Hydrobromide, Chlorpheniramine Maleate) Roberts .. ▣ 769
Chlor-Trimeton Allergy Decongestant Tablets (Chlorpheniramine Maleate, Pseudoephedrine Sulfate) Schering-Plough HealthCare .... ▣ 799
Chlor-Trimeton Allergy Tablets (Chlorpheniramine Maleate) Schering-Plough HealthCare .... ▣ 798
Comhist (Chlorpheniramine Maleate, Phenyltoloxamine Citrate, Phenylephrine Hydrochloride) Roberts 2038
Allergy-Sinus Comtrex Multi-Symptom Allergy-Sinus Formula Tablets (Acetaminophen, Chlorpheniramine Maleate, Pseudoephedrine Hydrochloride) Bristol-Myers Products .... ▣ 617
Contac Night Allergy/Sinus Caplets (Acetaminophen, Pseudoephedrine Hydrochloride, Diphenhydramine Hydrochloride) SmithKline Beecham Consumer .... ▣ 812
Dimetapp Elixir (Brompheniramine Maleate, Phenylpropanolamine Hydrochloride) A. H. Robins Consumer .... ▣ 773
Dimetapp Extentabs (Brompheniramine Maleate, Phenylpropanolamine Hydrochloride) A. H. Robins Consumer .... ▣ 774
Dimetapp Tablets/Liqui-Gels (Brompheniramine Maleate, Phenylpropanolamine Hydrochloride) A. H. Robins Consumer .... ▣ 775
Dimetapp Cold & Allergy Chewable Tablets (Brompheniramine Maleate, Phenylpropanolamine Hydrochloride) A. H. Robins Consumer .... ▣ 773
Drixoral Cold and Allergy Sustained-Action Tablets (Dexbrompheniramine Maleate, Pseudoephedrine Sulfate) Schering-Plough HealthCare .... ▣ 802
Drixoral Cold and Flu Extended-Release Tablets (Acetaminophen, Dexbrompheniramine Maleate, Pseudoephedrine Sulfate) Schering-Plough HealthCare .... ▣ 803
Drixoral Allergy/Sinus Extended Release Tablets (Acetaminophen, Pseudoephedrine Sulfate, Dexbrompheniramine Maleate) Schering-Plough HealthCare .... ▣ 804
Hyland's C-Plus Cold Tablets (Homeopathic Medications) Standard Homeopathic .... ▣ 829
Nolahist Tablets (Phenindamine Tartrate) Carnrick 785
Novahistine Elixir (Chlorpheniramine Maleate, Phenylephrine Hydrochloride) SmithKline Beecham Consumer .... ▣ 823
Ornade Spansule Capsules (Phenylpropanolamine Hydrochloride, Chlorpheniramine Maleate) SmithKline Beecham Pharmaceuticals 2502
PediaCare Cold Allergy Chewable Tablets (Pseudoephedrine Hydrochloride, Chlorpheniramine Maleate) McNeil Consumer .... ▣ 677
PediaCare Cough-Cold Liquid (Pseudoephedrine Hydrochloride, Chlorpheniramine Maleate, Dextromethorphan Hydrobromide) McNeil Consumer 1553
Ryna (Chlorpheniramine Maleate, Pseudoephedrine Hydrochloride) Wallace .... ▣ 841
Seldane Tablets (Terfenadine) Marion Merrell Dow 1536
Seldane-D Extended-Release Tablets (Pseudoephedrine Hydrochloride, Terfenadine) Marion Merrell Dow 1538
Sine-Off Sinus Medicine (Aspirin, Chlorpheniramine Maleate, Phenylpropanolamine Hydrochloride) SmithKline Beecham Consumer .... ▣ 825
Singlet Tablets (Acetaminophen, Chlorpheniramine Maleate, Pseudoephedrine Hydrochloride) SmithKline Beecham Consumer .... ▣ 825
Sinulin Tablets (Acetaminophen, Phenylpropanolamine Hydrochloride, Chlorpheniramine Maleate) Carnrick 787
Sudafed Plus Liquid (Chlorpheniramine Maleate, Pseudoephedrine Hydrochloride) WARNER WELLCOME .... ▣ 862
Sudafed Plus Tablets (Chlorpheniramine Maleate, Pseudoephedrine Hydrochloride) WARNER WELLCOME .... ▣ 863
Tavist Syrup (Clemastine Fumarate) Sandoz Pharmaceuticals 2297
Tavist Tablets (Clemastine Fumarate) Sandoz Pharmaceuticals 2298
Triaminic Cold Tablets (Phenylpropanolamine Hydrochloride, Chlorpheniramine Maleate) Sandoz Consumer .... ▣ 790
Triaminic Syrup (Phenylpropanolamine Hydrochloride, Chlorpheniramine Maleate) Sandoz Consumer .... ▣ 792
Triaminic-12 Tablets (Phenylpropanolamine Hydrochloride, Chlorpheniramine Maleate) Sandoz Consumer .... ▣ 792
Triaminicin Tablets (Acetaminophen, Chlorpheniramine Maleate, Phenylpropanolamine Hydrochloride) Sandoz Consumer .... ▣ 793
Triaminicol Multi-Symptom Cold Tablets (Phenylpropanolamine Hydrochloride, Chlorpheniramine Maleate, Dextromethorphan Hydrobromide) Sandoz Consumer .... ▣ 793
TYLENOL Maximum Strength Allergy Sinus Medication Gelcaps and Caplets (Acetaminophen, Chlorpheniramine Maleate, Pseudoephedrine Hydrochloride) McNeil Consumer 1563
TYLENOL Severe Allergy Medication Caplets (Acetaminophen, Diphenhydramine Hydrochloride) McNeil Consumer 1564

Rickets
Rocaltrol Capsules (Calcitriol) Roche Laboratories 2141

Rickettsiae
Achromycin V Capsules (Tetracycline Hydrochloride) Lederle 1367
Chloromycetin Sodium Succinate (Chloramphenicol Sodium Succinate) Parke-Davis 1900
Declomycin Tablets (Demeclocycline Hydrochloride) Lederle 1371
Doryx Capsules (Doxycycline Hyclate) Parke-Davis 1913
Dynacin Capsules (Minocycline Hydrochloride) Medicis 1590
Minocin Intravenous (Minocycline Hydrochloride) Lederle 1382
Minocin Oral Suspension (Minocycline Hydrochloride) Lederle 1385
Minocin Pellet-Filled Capsules (Minocycline Hydrochloride) Lederle 1383
Monodox Capsules (Doxycycline Monohydrate) Oclassen 1805
Terramycin Intramuscular Solution (Oxytetracycline) Roerig 2210
Vibramycin (Doxycycline Calcium) Pfizer Labs 1941
Vibramycin Hyclate Intravenous (Doxycycline Hyclate) Roerig 2215
Vibramycin (Doxycycline Monohydrate) Pfizer Labs 1941

Rickettsialpox
Achromycin V Capsules (Tetracycline Hydrochloride) Lederle 1367
Declomycin Tablets (Demeclocycline Hydrochloride) Lederle 1371
Doryx Capsules (Doxycycline Hyclate) Parke-Davis 1913
Dynacin Capsules (Minocycline Hydrochloride) Medicis 1590
Minocin Intravenous (Minocycline Hydrochloride) Lederle 1382
Minocin Oral Suspension (Minocycline Hydrochloride) Lederle 1385
Minocin Pellet-Filled Capsules (Minocycline Hydrochloride) Lederle 1383
Monodox Capsules (Doxycycline Monohydrate) Oclassen 1805
Terramycin Intramuscular Solution (Oxytetracycline) Roerig 2210
Vibramycin (Doxycycline Calcium) Pfizer Labs 1941
Vibramycin Hyclate Intravenous (Doxycycline Hyclate) Roerig 2215
Vibramycin (Doxycycline Monohydrate) Pfizer Labs 1941

Ringworm infections of the body (see under Tinea corporis infections)

Ringworm infections of the feet (see under Tinea pedis infections)

Ringworm infections of the groin (see under Tinea cruris infections)

Ringworm infections of the nails (see under Tinea unguium infections)

Ringworm infections of the scalp (see under Tinea capitis infections)

Rocky Mountain spotted fever
Achromycin V Capsules (Tetracycline Hydrochloride) Lederle 1367

1533 **Indications Index** **S. aureus infections**

Declomycin Tablets (Demeclocycline Hydrochloride) Lederle 1371
Doryx Capsules (Doxycycline Hyclate) Parke-Davis 1913
Dynacin Capsules (Minocycline Hydrochloride) Medicis 1590
Minocin Intravenous (Minocycline Hydrochloride) Lederle 1382
Minocin Oral Suspension (Minocycline Hydrochloride) Lederle 1385
Minocin Pellet-Filled Capsules (Minocycline Hydrochloride) Lederle 1383
Monodox Capsules (Doxycycline Monohydrate) Oclassen 1805
Terramycin Intramuscular Solution (Oxytetracycline) Roerig 2210
Vibramycin (Doxycycline Calcium) Pfizer Labs 1941
Vibramycin Hyclate Intravenous (Doxycycline Hyclate) Roerig 2215
Vibramycin (Doxycycline Monohydrate) Pfizer Labs 1941

Rosacea
MetroGel (Metronidazole) Galderma 1047

Roundworm, common (see under Ascaris lumbricoides infections)

Rubella and mumps, prophylaxis
Biavax II (Rubella & Mumps Virus Vaccine Live) Merck & Co., Inc. 1613

Rubella, prophylaxis
M-M-R II (Measles, Mumps & Rubella Virus Vaccine Live) Merck & Co., Inc. 1687
M-R-VAX II (Measles & Rubella Virus Vaccine Live) Merck & Co., Inc. 1689
Meruvax II (Rubella Virus Vaccine Live) Merck & Co., Inc. 1697

S

S. agalactiae gynecologic infections
Cefobid Intravenous/Intramuscular (Cefoperazone Sodium) Roerig 2189
Cefobid Pharmacy Bulk Package - Not for Direct Infusion (Cefoperazone Sodium) Roerig 2192
Cefotan (Cefotetan) Zeneca 2829

S. agalactiae infections
Cefizox for Intramuscular or Intravenous Use (Ceftizoxime Sodium) Fujisawa 1034
Cefobid Intravenous/Intramuscular (Cefoperazone Sodium) Roerig 2189
Cefobid Pharmacy Bulk Package - Not for Direct Infusion (Cefoperazone Sodium) Roerig 2192
Cefotan (Cefotetan) Zeneca 2829
Monocid Injection (Cefonicid Sodium) SmithKline Beecham Pharmaceuticals 2497
Noroxin Tablets (Norfloxacin) Merck & Co., Inc. 1715
Noroxin Tablets (Norfloxacin) Roberts 2048
Zefazone (Cefmetazole Sodium) Upjohn 2654
Zithromax (Azithromycin) Pfizer Labs 1944

S. agalactiae pelvic inflammatory disease
Cefizox for Intramuscular or Intravenous Use (Ceftizoxime Sodium) Fujisawa 1034
Cefobid Intravenous/Intramuscular (Cefoperazone Sodium) Roerig 2189
Cefobid Pharmacy Bulk Package - Not for Direct Infusion (Cefoperazone Sodium) Roerig 2192

S. agalactiae septicemia
Cefobid Intravenous/Intramuscular (Cefoperazone Sodium) Roerig 2189
Cefobid Pharmacy Bulk Package - Not for Direct Infusion (Cefoperazone Sodium) Roerig 2192

S. agalactiae skin and skin structure infections
Monocid Injection (Cefonicid Sodium) SmithKline Beecham Pharmaceuticals 2497
Zefazone (Cefmetazole Sodium) Upjohn 2654
Zithromax (Azithromycin) Pfizer Labs 1944

S. agalactiae urinary tract infections
Noroxin Tablets (Norfloxacin) Merck & Co., Inc. 1715
Noroxin Tablets (Norfloxacin) Roberts 2048

S. aureus biliary tract infections
Ancef Injection (Cefazolin Sodium) SmithKline Beecham Pharmaceuticals 2465
Kefzol Vials, Faspak & ADD-Vantage (Cefazolin Sodium) Lilly 1456

S. aureus bone and joint infections
Ancef Injection (Cefazolin Sodium) SmithKline Beecham Pharmaceuticals 2465
Cefizox for Intramuscular or Intravenous Use (Ceftizoxime Sodium) Fujisawa 1034
Cefotan (Cefotetan) Zeneca 2829
Ceptaz (Ceftazidime) Glaxo Wellcome 1081
Claforan Sterile and Injection (Cefotaxime Sodium) Hoechst-Roussel 1235
Cleocin Phosphate Injection (Clindamycin Phosphate) Upjohn 2586
Fortaz (Ceftazidime) Glaxo Wellcome 1100
Keftab Tablets (Cephalexin Hydrochloride) Dista 915
Kefurox Vials, Faspak & ADD-Vantage (Cefuroxime Sodium) Lilly 1454
Kefzol Vials, Faspak & ADD-Vantage (Cefazolin Sodium) Lilly 1456
Mandol Vials, Faspak & ADD-Vantage (Cefamandole Nafate) Lilly 1461
Mefoxin (Cefoxitin Sodium) Merck & Co., Inc. 1691
Mefoxin Premixed Intravenous Solution (Cefoxitin Sodium) Merck & Co., Inc. 1694
Monocid Injection (Cefonicid Sodium) SmithKline Beecham Pharmaceuticals 2497
Nebcin Vials, Hyporets & ADD-Vantage (Tobramycin Sulfate) Lilly 1464
Primaxin I.V. (Imipenem-Cilastatin Sodium) Merck & Co., Inc. 1729
Rocephin Injectable Vials, ADD-Vantage, Galaxy Container (Ceftriaxone Sodium) Roche Laboratories 2142
Tazicef for Injection (Ceftazidime) SmithKline Beecham Pharmaceuticals 2519
Tazidime Vials, Faspak & ADD-Vantage (Ceftazidime) Lilly 1478
Timentin for Injection (Ticarcillin Disodium, Clavulanate Potassium) SmithKline Beecham Pharmaceuticals 2528
Tobramycin Sulfate Injection (Tobramycin Sulfate) Elkins-Sinn 968
Zinacef (Cefuroxime Sodium) Glaxo Wellcome 1211

S. aureus endocarditis
Ancef Injection (Cefazolin Sodium) SmithKline Beecham Pharmaceuticals 2465
Kefzol Vials, Faspak & ADD-Vantage (Cefazolin Sodium) Lilly 1456
Primaxin I.V. (Imipenem-Cilastatin Sodium) Merck & Co., Inc. 1729

S. aureus gynecologic infections
Cefotan (Cefotetan) Zeneca 2829
Primaxin I.V. (Imipenem-Cilastatin Sodium) Merck & Co., Inc. 1729
Timentin for Injection (Ticarcillin Disodium, Clavulanate Potassium) SmithKline Beecham Pharmaceuticals 2528

S. aureus infections
Achromycin V Capsules (Tetracycline Hydrochloride) Lederle 1367
Ancef Injection (Cefazolin Sodium) SmithKline Beecham Pharmaceuticals 2465
Augmentin (Amoxicillin Trihydrate, Clavulanate Potassium) SmithKline Beecham Pharmaceuticals 2468
Azo Gantanol Tablets (Sulfamethoxazole, Phenazopyridine Hydrochloride) Roche Laboratories 2080
Azo Gantrisin Tablets (Sulfisoxazole, Phenazopyridine Hydrochloride) Roche Laboratories 2081
Bactroban Ointment (Mupirocin) SmithKline Beecham Pharmaceuticals 2470
Biaxin (Clarithromycin) Abbott 405
Ceclor Pulvules & Suspension (Cefaclor) Lilly 1431
Cefizox for Intramuscular or Intravenous Use (Ceftizoxime Sodium) Fujisawa 1034
Cefobid Intravenous/Intramuscular (Cefoperazone Sodium) Roerig 2189
Cefobid Pharmacy Bulk Package - Not for Direct Infusion (Cefoperazone Sodium) Roerig 2192
Cefotan (Cefotetan) Zeneca 2829
Ceftin (Cefuroxime Axetil) Glaxo Wellcome 1078
Cefzil Tablets and Oral Suspension (Cefprozil) Bristol-Myers Squibb 746
Ceptaz (Ceftazidime) Glaxo Wellcome 1081
Cipro I.V. (Ciprofloxacin) Bayer Pharmaceutical 595
Cipro Tablets (Ciprofloxacin Hydrochloride) Bayer Pharmaceutical 592
Claforan Sterile and Injection (Cefotaxime Sodium) Hoechst-Roussel 1235
Cleocin Phosphate Injection (Clindamycin Phosphate) Upjohn 2586
Declomycin Tablets (Demeclocycline Hydrochloride) Lederle 1371
Dynacin Capsules (Minocycline Hydrochloride) Medicis 1590
E.E.S. (Erythromycin Ethylsuccinate) Abbott 424
E-Mycin Tablets (Erythromycin) Knoll Laboratories 1341
ERYC (Erythromycin) Parke-Davis 1915
EryPed (Erythromycin Ethylsuccinate) Abbott 421
Ery-Tab Tablets (Erythromycin) Abbott 422
Erythrocin Stearate Filmtab (Erythromycin Stearate) Abbott 425
Erythromycin Base Filmtab (Erythromycin) Abbott 426
Erythromycin Delayed-Release Capsules, USP (Erythromycin) Abbott 427
Floxin I.V. (Ofloxacin) McNeil Pharmaceutical 1571
Floxin Tablets (200 mg, 300 mg, 400 mg) (Ofloxacin) McNeil Pharmaceutical 1567
Fortaz (Ceftazidime) Glaxo Wellcome 1100
Ilosone (Erythromycin Estolate) Dista 911
Ilotycin Gluceptate, IV, Vials (Erythromycin Gluceptate) Dista 913
Keftab Tablets (Cephalexin Hydrochloride) Dista 915
Kefurox Vials, Faspak & ADD-Vantage (Cefuroxime Sodium) Lilly 1454
Kefzol Vials, Faspak & ADD-Vantage (Cefazolin Sodium) Lilly 1456
Lorabid Suspension and Pulvules (Loracarbef) Lilly 1459
Macrodantin Capsules (Nitrofurantoin) Procter & Gamble Pharmaceuticals 1989
Mandol Vials, Faspak & ADD-Vantage (Cefamandole Nafate) Lilly 1461
Mefoxin (Cefoxitin Sodium) Merck & Co., Inc. 1691
Mefoxin Premixed Intravenous Solution (Cefoxitin Sodium) Merck & Co., Inc. 1694
Minocin Intravenous (Minocycline Hydrochloride) Lederle 1382
Minocin Oral Suspension (Minocycline Hydrochloride) Lederle 1385
Minocin Pellet-Filled Capsules (Minocycline Hydrochloride) Lederle 1383
Monocid Injection (Cefonicid Sodium) SmithKline Beecham Pharmaceuticals 2497
Monodox Capsules (Doxycycline Monohydrate) Oclassen 1805
Nebcin Vials, Hyporets & ADD-Vantage (Tobramycin Sulfate) Lilly 1464
Netromycin Injection 100 mg/ml (Netilmicin Sulfate) Schering 2373
Noroxin Tablets (Norfloxacin) Merck & Co., Inc. 1715
Noroxin Tablets (Norfloxacin) Roberts 2048
PCE Dispertab Tablets (Erythromycin) Abbott 444
Primaxin I.M. (Imipenem-Cilastatin Sodium) Merck & Co., Inc. 1727
Primaxin I.V. (Imipenem-Cilastatin Sodium) Merck & Co., Inc. 1729
Rocephin Injectable Vials, ADD-Vantage, Galaxy Container (Ceftriaxone Sodium) Roche Laboratories 2142
Tazicef for Injection (Ceftazidime) SmithKline Beecham Pharmaceuticals 2519
Tazidime Vials, Faspak & ADD-Vantage (Ceftazidime) Lilly 1478
Timentin for Injection (Ticarcillin Disodium, Clavulanate Potassium) SmithKline Beecham Pharmaceuticals 2528
Tobramycin Sulfate Injection (Tobramycin Sulfate) Elkins-Sinn 968
Unasyn (Ampicillin Sodium, Sulbactam Sodium) Roerig 2212
Vantin for Oral Suspension and Vantin Tablets (Cefpodoxime Proxetil) Upjohn 2646
Zefazone (Cefmetazole Sodium) Upjohn 2654
Zinacef (Cefuroxime Sodium) Glaxo Wellcome 1211
Zithromax (Azithromycin) Pfizer Labs 1944
Zosyn (Piperacillin Sodium, Tazobactam Sodium) Lederle 1419
Zosyn Pharmacy Bulk Package (Piperacillin Sodium, Tazobactam Sodium) Lederle 1422

S. aureus infections, ocular
AK-CIDE (Prednisolone Acetate, Sulfacetamide Sodium) Akorn .... ⊙ 202
AK-CIDE Ointment (Prednisolone Acetate, Sulfacetamide Sodium) Akorn .... ⊙ 202
AK-Spore (Bacitracin Zinc, Neomycin Sulfate, Polymyxin B Sulfate) Akorn .... ⊙ 204
AK-Trol Ointment & Suspension (Dexamethasone, Neomycin Sulfate, Polymyxin B Sulfate) Akorn .... ⊙ 205
Blephamide Liquifilm Sterile Ophthalmic Suspension (Prednisolone Acetate, Sulfacetamide Sodium) Allergan 476
Blephamide Ointment (Sulfacetamide Sodium, Prednisolone Acetate) Allergan .... ⊙ 237
Chibroxin Sterile Ophthalmic Solution (Norfloxacin) Merck & Co., Inc. 1617
Chloromycetin Ophthalmic Ointment, 1% (Chloramphenicol) Parke-Davis .... ⊙ 310
Chloromycetin Ophthalmic Solution (Chloramphenicol) Parke-Davis .... ⊙ 310
Chloroptic S.O.P. (Chloramphenicol) Allergan .... ⊙ 239
Ciloxan Ophthalmic Solution (Ciprofloxacin Hydrochloride) Alcon Laboratories 472
Cortisporin Ophthalmic Ointment Sterile (Polymyxin B Sulfate, Bacitracin Zinc, Neomycin Sulfate, Hydrocortisone) Glaxo Wellcome 1085
Cortisporin Ophthalmic Suspension Sterile (Hydrocortisone, Polymyxin B Sulfate, Neomycin Sulfate) Glaxo Wellcome 1086
Dexacidin Ointment (Dexamethasone, Neomycin Sulfate, Polymyxin B Sulfate) CIBA Vision Ophthalmics .... ⊙ 263

(▣ Described in PDR For Nonprescription Drugs) (⊙ Described in PDR For Ophthalmology)

S. aureus infections

FML-S Liquifilm (Sulfacetamide Sodium, Fluorometholone) Allergan ◉ 242

Genoptic Sterile Ophthalmic Solution (Gentamicin Sulfate) Allergan ◉ 243

Genoptic Sterile Ophthalmic Ointment (Gentamicin Sulfate) Allergan ◉ 243

Gentak (Gentamicin Sulfate) Akorn ◉ 208

Maxitrol Ophthalmic Ointment and Suspension (Dexamethasone, Neomycin Sulfate, Polymyxin B Sulfate) Alcon Laboratories ◉ 224

NeoDecadron Sterile Ophthalmic Ointment (Neomycin Sulfate, Dexamethasone Sodium Phosphate) Merck & Co., Inc. 1712

NeoDecadron Sterile Ophthalmic Solution (Neomycin Sulfate, Dexamethasone Sodium Phosphate) Merck & Co., Inc. 1713

Ocuflox (Ofloxacin) Allergan 481

Ophthocort (Chloramphenicol, Polymyxin B Sulfate, Hydrocortisone Acetate) Parke-Davis ◉ 311

Poly-Pred Liquifilm (Neomycin Sulfate, Polymyxin B Sulfate, Prednisolone Acetate) Allergan.. 248

Polytrim Ophthalmic Solution Sterile (Polymyxin B Sulfate, Trimethoprim Sulfate) Allergan 482

Pred-G Liquifilm Sterile Ophthalmic Suspension (Gentamicin Sulfate, Prednisolone Acetate) Allergan ◉ 251

Pred-G S.O.P. Sterile Ophthalmic Ointment (Gentamicin Sulfate, Prednisolone Acetate) Allergan.. ◉ 252

Terra-Cortril Ophthalmic Suspension (Oxytetracycline Hydrochloride, Hydrocortisone Acetate) Roerig 2210

TobraDex Ophthalmic Suspension and Ointment (Dexamethasone, Tobramycin) Alcon Laboratories .. 473

Vasocidin Ointment (Prednisolone Acetate, Sulfacetamide Sodium) CIBA Vision Ophthalmics ◉ 268

Vasocidin Ophthalmic Solution (Prednisolone Sodium Phosphate, Sulfacetamide Sodium) CIBA Vision Ophthalmics ◉ 270

S. aureus intra-abdominal infections

Ceptaz (Ceftazidime) Glaxo Wellcome 1081

Fortaz (Ceftazidime) Glaxo Wellcome 1100

Netromycin Injection 100 mg/ml (Netilmicin Sulfate) Schering 2373

Primaxin I.V. (Imipenem-Cilastatin Sodium) Merck & Co., Inc. 1729

Tazicef for Injection (Ceftazidime) SmithKline Beecham Pharmaceuticals 2519

Tazidime Vials, Faspak & ADD-Vantage (Ceftazidime) Lilly .. 1478

S. aureus lower respiratory tract infections

Cefizox for Intramuscular or Intravenous Use (Ceftizoxime Sodium) Fujisawa 1034

Cefotan (Cefotetan) Zeneca 2829

Ceptaz (Ceftazidime) Glaxo Wellcome 1081

Claforan Sterile and Injection (Cefotaxime Sodium) Hoechst-Roussel 1235

Cleocin Phosphate Injection (Clindamycin Phosphate) Upjohn 2586

Fortaz (Ceftazidime) Glaxo Wellcome 1100

Mefoxin (Cefoxitin Sodium) Merck & Co., Inc. 1691

Nebcin Vials, Hyporets & ADD-Vantage (Tobramycin Sulfate) Lilly 1464

Netromycin Injection 100 mg/ml (Netilmicin Sulfate) Schering 2373

Primaxin I.V. (Imipenem-Cilastatin Sodium) Merck & Co., Inc. 1729

Rocephin Injectable Vials, ADD-Vantage, Galaxy Container (Ceftriaxone Sodium) Roche Laboratories 2142

Tazicef for Injection (Ceftazidime) SmithKline Beecham Pharmaceuticals 2519

Tazidime Vials, Faspak & ADD-Vantage (Ceftazidime) Lilly .. 1478

Timentin for Injection (Ticarcillin Disodium, Clavulanate Potassium) SmithKline Beecham Pharmaceuticals 2528

Zefazone (Cefmetazole Sodium) Upjohn 2654

Zinacef (Cefuroxime Sodium) Glaxo Wellcome 1211

S. aureus meningitis

Kefurox Vials, Faspak & ADD-Vantage (Cefuroxime Sodium) Lilly 1454

Tazidime Vials, Faspak & ADD-Vantage (Ceftazidime) Lilly .. 1478

Zinacef (Cefuroxime Sodium) Glaxo Wellcome 1211

S. aureus respiratory tract infections

Ancef Injection (Cefazolin Sodium) SmithKline Beecham Pharmaceuticals 2465

Cefobid Intravenous/Intramuscular (Cefoperazone Sodium) Roerig 2189

Cefobid Pharmacy Bulk Package - Not for Direct Infusion (Cefoperazone Sodium) Roerig 2192

Kefzol Vials, Faspak & ADD-Vantage (Cefazolin Sodium) Lilly 1456

S. aureus skin and skin structure infections

Achromycin V Capsules (Tetracycline Hydrochloride) Lederle 1367

Ancef Injection (Cefazolin Sodium) SmithKline Beecham Pharmaceuticals 2465

Augmentin (Amoxicillin Trihydrate, Clavulanate Potassium) SmithKline Beecham Pharmaceuticals 2468

Bactroban Ointment (Mupirocin) SmithKline Beecham Pharmaceuticals 2470

Biaxin (Clarithromycin) Abbott 405

Ceclor Pulvules & Suspension (Cefaclor) Lilly 1431

Cefobid Intravenous/Intramuscular (Cefoperazone Sodium) Roerig 2189

Cefobid Pharmacy Bulk Package - Not for Direct Infusion (Cefoperazone Sodium) Roerig 2192

Cefotan (Cefotetan) Zeneca 2829

Ceftin (Cefuroxime Axetil) Glaxo Wellcome 1078

Cefzil Tablets and Oral Suspension (Cefprozil) Bristol-Myers Squibb .. 746

Ceptaz (Ceftazidime) Glaxo Wellcome 1081

Cipro I.V. (Ciprofloxacin) Bayer Pharmaceutical 595

Cipro I.V. Pharmacy Bulk Package (Ciprofloxacin) Bayer Pharmaceutical 597

Cipro Tablets (Ciprofloxacin Hydrochloride) Bayer Pharmaceutical 592

Claforan Sterile and Injection (Cefotaxime Sodium) Hoechst-Roussel 1235

Cleocin Phosphate Injection (Clindamycin Phosphate) Upjohn 2586

Dynacin Capsules (Minocycline Hydrochloride) Medicis 1590

E.E.S. (Erythromycin Ethylsuccinate) Abbott 424

E-Mycin Tablets (Erythromycin) Knoll Laboratories 1341

ERYC (Erythromycin) Parke-Davis .. 1915

EryPed (Erythromycin Ethylsuccinate) Abbott 421

Ery-Tab Tablets (Erythromycin) Abbott 422

Erythrocin Stearate Filmtab (Erythromycin Stearate) Abbott 425

Erythromycin Base Filmtab (Erythromycin) Abbott 426

Erythromycin Delayed-Release Capsules, USP (Erythromycin) Abbott 427

Floxin I.V. (Ofloxacin) McNeil Pharmaceutical 1571

Floxin Tablets (200 mg, 300 mg, 400 mg) (Ofloxacin) McNeil Pharmaceutical 1567

Fortaz (Ceftazidime) Glaxo Wellcome 1100

Ilosone (Erythromycin Estolate) Dista 911

Ilotycin Gluceptate, IV, Vials (Erythromycin Gluceptate) Dista 913

Keftab Tablets (Cephalexin Hydrochloride) Dista 915

Kefurox Vials, Faspak & ADD-Vantage (Cefuroxime Sodium) Lilly 1454

Kefzol Vials, Faspak & ADD-Vantage (Cefazolin Sodium) Lilly 1456

Lorabid Suspension and Pulvules (Loracarbef) Lilly 1459

Mandol Vials, Faspak & ADD-Vantage (Cefamandole Nafate) Lilly 1461

Mefoxin (Cefoxitin Sodium) Merck & Co., Inc. 1691

Mefoxin Premixed Intravenous Solution (Cefoxitin Sodium) Merck & Co., Inc. 1694

Minocin Intravenous (Minocycline Hydrochloride) Lederle 1382

Minocin Oral Suspension (Minocycline Hydrochloride) Lederle 1385

Minocin Pellet-Filled Capsules (Minocycline Hydrochloride) Lederle 1383

Monocid Injection (Cefonicid Sodium) SmithKline Beecham Pharmaceuticals 2497

Monodox Capsules (Doxycycline Monohydrate) Oclassen 1805

Nebcin Vials, Hyporets & ADD-Vantage (Tobramycin Sulfate) Lilly 1464

Netromycin Injection 100 mg/ml (Netilmicin Sulfate) Schering 2373

PCE Dispertab Tablets (Erythromycin) Abbott 444

Primaxin I.M. (Imipenem-Cilastatin Sodium) Merck & Co., Inc. 1727

Primaxin I.V. (Imipenem-Cilastatin Sodium) Merck & Co., Inc. 1729

Rocephin Injectable Vials, ADD-Vantage, Galaxy Container (Ceftriaxone Sodium) Roche Laboratories 2142

Tazicef for Injection (Ceftazidime) SmithKline Beecham Pharmaceuticals 2519

Tazidime Vials, Faspak & ADD-Vantage (Ceftazidime) Lilly .. 1478

Timentin for Injection (Ticarcillin Disodium, Clavulanate Potassium) SmithKline Beecham Pharmaceuticals 2528

Tobramycin Sulfate Injection (Tobramycin Sulfate) Elkins-Sinn 968

Unasyn (Ampicillin Sodium, Sulbactam Sodium) Roerig 2212

Vantin for Oral Suspension and Vantin Tablets (Cefpodoxime Proxetil) Upjohn 2646

Zefazone (Cefmetazole Sodium) Upjohn 2654

Zinacef (Cefuroxime Sodium) Glaxo Wellcome 1211

Zithromax (Azithromycin) Pfizer Labs 1944

Zosyn (Piperacillin Sodium, Tazobactam Sodium) Lederle 1419

Zosyn Pharmacy Bulk Package (Piperacillin Sodium, Tazobactam Sodium) Lederle 1422

S. aureus septicemia

Ancef Injection (Cefazolin Sodium) SmithKline Beecham Pharmaceuticals 2465

Cefizox for Intramuscular or Intravenous Use (Ceftizoxime Sodium) Fujisawa 1034

Cefobid Intravenous/Intramuscular (Cefoperazone Sodium) Roerig 2189

Cefobid Pharmacy Bulk Package - Not for Direct Infusion (Cefoperazone Sodium) Roerig 2192

Ceptaz (Ceftazidime) Glaxo Wellcome 1081

Claforan Sterile and Injection (Cefotaxime Sodium) Hoechst-Roussel 1235

Cleocin Phosphate Injection (Clindamycin Phosphate) Upjohn 2586

Fortaz (Ceftazidime) Glaxo Wellcome 1100

Kefurox Vials, Faspak & ADD-Vantage (Cefuroxime Sodium) Lilly 1454

Kefzol Vials, Faspak & ADD-Vantage (Cefazolin Sodium) Lilly 1456

Mefoxin (Cefoxitin Sodium) Merck & Co., Inc. 1691

Mefoxin Premixed Intravenous Solution (Cefoxitin Sodium) Merck & Co., Inc. 1694

Primaxin I.V. (Imipenem-Cilastatin Sodium) Merck & Co., Inc. 1729

Rocephin Injectable Vials, ADD-Vantage, Galaxy Container (Ceftriaxone Sodium) Roche Laboratories 2142

Tazicef for Injection (Ceftazidime) SmithKline Beecham Pharmaceuticals 2519

Tazidime Vials, Faspak & ADD-Vantage (Ceftazidime) Lilly .. 1478

Timentin for Injection (Ticarcillin Disodium, Clavulanate Potassium) SmithKline Beecham Pharmaceuticals 2528

Zinacef (Cefuroxime Sodium) Glaxo Wellcome 1211

S. aureus urinary tract infections

Azo Gantanol Tablets (Sulfamethoxazole, Phenazopyridine Hydrochloride) Roche Laboratories 2080

Azo Gantrisin Tablets (Sulfisoxazole, Phenazopyridine Hydrochloride) Roche Laboratories 2081

Cefizox for Intramuscular or Intravenous Use (Ceftizoxime Sodium) Fujisawa 1034

Claforan Sterile and Injection (Cefotaxime Sodium) Hoechst-Roussel 1235

Macrodantin Capsules (Nitrofurantoin) Procter & Gamble Pharmaceuticals 1989

Nebcin Vials, Hyporets & ADD-Vantage (Tobramycin Sulfate) Lilly 1464

Netromycin Injection 100 mg/ml (Netilmicin Sulfate) Schering 2373

Noroxin Tablets (Norfloxacin) Merck & Co., Inc. 1715

Noroxin Tablets (Norfloxacin) Roberts 2048

Primaxin I.V. (Imipenem-Cilastatin Sodium) Merck & Co., Inc. 1729

Timentin for Injection (Ticarcillin Disodium, Clavulanate Potassium) SmithKline Beecham Pharmaceuticals 2528

Tobramycin Sulfate Injection (Tobramycin Sulfate) Elkins-Sinn 968

Zefazone (Cefmetazole Sodium) Upjohn 2654

S. aureus (non-penicillinase producing) infections

Cefizox for Intramuscular or Intravenous Use (Ceftizoxime Sodium) Fujisawa 1034

Cefotan (Cefotetan) Zeneca 2829

Claforan Sterile and Injection (Cefotaxime Sodium) Hoechst-Roussel 1235

Mefoxin (Cefoxitin Sodium) Merck & Co., Inc. 1691

Mefoxin Premixed Intravenous Solution (Cefoxitin Sodium) Merck & Co., Inc. 1694

Primaxin I.V. (Imipenem-Cilastatin Sodium) Merck & Co., Inc. 1729

Tobramycin Sulfate Injection (Tobramycin Sulfate) Elkins-Sinn 968

Zefazone (Cefmetazole Sodium) Upjohn 2654

S. aureus (penicillinase and non-penicillinase producing strains) skin and skin structure infections

Cefizox for Intramuscular or Intravenous Use (Ceftizoxime Sodium) Fujisawa 1034

Mandol Vials, Faspak & ADD-Vantage (Cefamandole Nafate) Lilly 1461

Mefoxin (Cefoxitin Sodium) Merck & Co., Inc. 1691

Mefoxin Premixed Intravenous Solution (Cefoxitin Sodium) Merck & Co., Inc. 1694

(**■** Described in PDR For Nonprescription Drugs) (◉ Described in PDR For Ophthalmology)

1535 Indications Index S. pneumoniae infections

Zinacef (Cefuroxime Sodium) Glaxo Wellcome ... 1211

S. aureus (penicillinase-producing) infections
Cefizox for Intramuscular or Intravenous Use (Ceftizoxime Sodium) Fujisawa ... 1034
Cefotan (Cefotetan) Zeneca ... 2829
Cefzil Tablets and Oral Suspension (Cefprozil) Bristol-Myers Squibb ... 746
Claforan Sterile and Injection (Cefotaxime Sodium) Hoechst-Roussel ... 1235
Kefzol Vials, Faspak & ADD-Vantage (Cefazolin Sodium) Lilly ... 1456
Lorabid Suspension and Pulvules (Loracarbef) Lilly ... 1459
Mefoxin (Cefoxitin Sodium) Merck & Co., Inc. ... 1691
Mefoxin Premixed Intravenous Solution (Cefoxitin Sodium) Merck & Co., Inc. ... 1694
Primaxin I.M. (Imipenem-Cilastatin Sodium) Merck & Co., Inc. ... 1727
Primaxin I.V. (Imipenem-Cilastatin Sodium) Merck & Co., Inc. ... 1729
Tobramycin Sulfate Injection (Tobramycin Sulfate) Elkins-Sinn ... 968
Unasyn (Ampicillin Sodium, Sulbactam Sodium) Roerig ... 2212
Zefazone (Cefmetazole Sodium) Upjohn ... 2654

S. bovis endocarditis
Vancocin HCl, Vials & ADD-Vantage (Vancomycin Hydrochloride) Lilly 1481

S. epidermis bone and joint infections
Primaxin I.V. (Imipenem-Cilastatin Sodium) Merck & Co., Inc. ... 1729

S. epidermis endocarditis, early-onset prosthetic valve
Vancocin HCl, Vials & ADD-Vantage (Vancomycin Hydrochloride) Lilly 1481

S. epidermis gynecologic infections
Cefobid Intravenous/Intramuscular (Cefoperazone Sodium) Roerig ... 2189
Cefobid Pharmacy Bulk Package - Not for Direct Infusion (Cefoperazone Sodium) Roerig ... 2192
Cefotan (Cefotetan) Zeneca ... 2829
Claforan Sterile and Injection (Cefotaxime Sodium) Hoechst-Roussel ... 1235
Primaxin I.V. (Imipenem-Cilastatin Sodium) Merck & Co., Inc. ... 1729
Timentin for Injection (Ticarcillin Disodium, Clavulanate Potassium) SmithKline Beecham Pharmaceuticals ... 2528

S. epidermis infections
Cefizox for Intramuscular or Intravenous Use (Ceftizoxime Sodium) Fujisawa ... 1034
Cefobid Intravenous/Intramuscular (Cefoperazone Sodium) Roerig ... 2189
Cefobid Pharmacy Bulk Package - Not for Direct Infusion (Cefoperazone Sodium) Roerig ... 2192
Cefotan (Cefotetan) Zeneca ... 2829
Cipro I.V. (Ciprofloxacin) Bayer Pharmaceutical ... 595
Cipro I.V. Pharmacy Bulk Package (Ciprofloxacin) Bayer Pharmaceutical ... 597
Cipro Tablets (Ciprofloxacin Hydrochloride) Bayer Pharmaceutical ... 592
Claforan Sterile and Injection (Cefotaxime Sodium) Hoechst-Roussel ... 1235
Mefoxin (Cefoxitin Sodium) Merck & Co., Inc. ... 1691
Mefoxin Premixed Intravenous Solution (Cefoxitin Sodium) Merck & Co., Inc. ... 1694
Monocid Injection (Cefonicid Sodium) SmithKline Beecham Pharmaceuticals ... 2497
Noroxin Tablets (Norfloxacin) Merck & Co., Inc. ... 1715
Noroxin Tablets (Norfloxacin) Roberts ... 2048
Penetrex Tablets (Enoxacin) Rhone-Poulenc Rorer Pharmaceuticals ... 2031
Primaxin I.V. (Imipenem-Cilastatin Sodium) Merck & Co., Inc. ... 1729
Rocephin Injectable Vials, ADD-Vantage, Galaxy Container (Ceftriaxone Sodium) Roche Laboratories ... 2142
Timentin for Injection (Ticarcillin Disodium, Clavulanate Potassium) SmithKline Beecham Pharmaceuticals ... 2528
Vancocin HCl, Vials & ADD-Vantage (Vancomycin Hydrochloride) Lilly 1481
Zefazone (Cefmetazole Sodium) Upjohn ... 2654

S. epidermis infections, ocular
Chibroxin Sterile Ophthalmic Solution (Norfloxacin) Merck & Co., Inc. ... 1617
Ciloxan Ophthalmic Solution (Ciprofloxacin Hydrochloride) Alcon Laboratories ... 472
Genoptic Sterile Ophthalmic Solution (Gentamicin Sulfate) Allergan ... ◉ 243
Genoptic Sterile Ophthalmic Ointment (Gentamicin Sulfate) Allergan ... ◉ 243
Gentak (Gentamicin Sulfate) Akorn ... ◉ 208
Ocuflox (Ofloxacin) Allergan ... 481
Polytrim Ophthalmic Solution Sterile (Polymyxin B Sulfate, Trimethoprim Sulfate) Allergan ... 482
TobraDex Ophthalmic Suspension and Ointment (Dexamethasone, Tobramycin) Alcon Laboratories ... 473

S. epidermis intra-abdominal infections
Cefizox for Intramuscular or Intravenous Use (Ceftizoxime Sodium) Fujisawa ... 1034
Primaxin I.V. (Imipenem-Cilastatin Sodium) Merck & Co., Inc. ... 1729

S. epidermis pelvic inflammatory disease
Cefobid Intravenous/Intramuscular (Cefoperazone Sodium) Roerig ... 2189
Cefobid Pharmacy Bulk Package - Not for Direct Infusion (Cefoperazone Sodium) Roerig ... 2192

S. epidermis meningitis
Rocephin Injectable Vials, ADD-Vantage, Galaxy Container (Ceftriaxone Sodium) Roche Laboratories ... 2142

S. epidermis skin and skin structure infections
Cefizox for Intramuscular or Intravenous Use (Ceftizoxime Sodium) Fujisawa ... 1034
Cefotan (Cefotetan) Zeneca ... 2829
Cipro I.V. (Ciprofloxacin) Bayer Pharmaceutical ... 595
Cipro I.V. Pharmacy Bulk Package (Ciprofloxacin) Bayer Pharmaceutical ... 597
Cipro Tablets (Ciprofloxacin Hydrochloride) Bayer Pharmaceutical ... 592
Claforan Sterile and Injection (Cefotaxime Sodium) Hoechst-Roussel ... 1235
Mefoxin (Cefoxitin Sodium) Merck & Co., Inc. ... 1691
Mefoxin Premixed Intravenous Solution (Cefoxitin Sodium) Merck & Co., Inc. ... 1694
Monocid Injection (Cefonicid Sodium) SmithKline Beecham Pharmaceuticals ... 2497
Primaxin I.V. (Imipenem-Cilastatin Sodium) Merck & Co., Inc. ... 1729
Rocephin Injectable Vials, ADD-Vantage, Galaxy Container (Ceftriaxone Sodium) Roche Laboratories ... 2142
Zefazone (Cefmetazole Sodium) Upjohn ... 2654

S. epidermis urinary tract infections
Cipro I.V. (Ciprofloxacin) Bayer Pharmaceutical ... 595
Cipro I.V. Pharmacy Bulk Package (Ciprofloxacin) Bayer Pharmaceutical ... 597
Cipro Tablets (Ciprofloxacin Hydrochloride) Bayer Pharmaceutical ... 592
Claforan Sterile and Injection (Cefotaxime Sodium) Hoechst-Roussel ... 1235
Mandol Vials, Faspak & ADD-Vantage (Cefamandole Nafate) Lilly ... 1461
Noroxin Tablets (Norfloxacin) Merck & Co., Inc. ... 1715
Noroxin Tablets (Norfloxacin) Roberts ... 2048
Penetrex Tablets (Enoxacin) Rhone-Poulenc Rorer Pharmaceuticals ... 2031

S. faecalis gynecologic infections
Pipracil (Piperacillin Sodium) Lederle ... 1390

S. faecalis infections
Amoxil (Amoxicillin Trihydrate) SmithKline Beecham Pharmaceuticals ... 2464
Cipro I.V. (Ciprofloxacin) Bayer Pharmaceutical ... 595
Cipro Tablets (Ciprofloxacin Hydrochloride) Bayer Pharmaceutical ... 592
Geocillin Tablets (Carbenicillin Indanyl Sodium) Roerig ... 2199
Mezlin (Mezlocillin Sodium) Bayer Pharmaceutical ... 601
Mezlin Pharmacy Bulk Package (Mezlocillin Sodium) Bayer Pharmaceutical ... 604
Noroxin Tablets (Norfloxacin) Merck & Co., Inc. ... 1715
Noroxin Tablets (Norfloxacin) Roberts ... 2048
Pipracil (Piperacillin Sodium) Lederle ... 1390
Spectrobid Tablets (Bacampicillin Hydrochloride) Roerig ... 2206
Ticar for Injection (Ticarcillin Disodium) SmithKline Beecham Pharmaceuticals ... 2526

S. faecalis urinary tract infections
Cipro I.V. (Ciprofloxacin) Bayer Pharmaceutical ... 595
Cipro Tablets (Ciprofloxacin Hydrochloride) Bayer Pharmaceutical ... 592
Mezlin (Mezlocillin Sodium) Bayer Pharmaceutical ... 601
Mezlin Pharmacy Bulk Package (Mezlocillin Sodium) Bayer Pharmaceutical ... 604
Noroxin Tablets (Norfloxacin) Merck & Co., Inc. ... 1715
Noroxin Tablets (Norfloxacin) Roberts ... 2048
Spectrobid Tablets (Bacampicillin Hydrochloride) Roerig ... 2206
Ticar for Injection (Ticarcillin Disodium) SmithKline Beecham Pharmaceuticals ... 2526

S. faecalis, endocardial infections, treatment adjunct
Vancocin HCl, Vials & ADD-Vantage (Vancomycin Hydrochloride) Lilly 1481

S. pneumoniae bone and joint infections
Rocephin Injectable Vials, ADD-Vantage, Galaxy Container (Ceftriaxone Sodium) Roche Laboratories ... 2142

S. pneumoniae bronchitis
Bactrim (Trimethoprim, Sulfamethoxazole) Roche Laboratories ... 2084
Ceftin (Cefuroxime Axetil) Glaxo Wellcome ... 1078
Cefzil Tablets and Oral Suspension (Cefprozil) Bristol-Myers Squibb ... 746
Floxin I.V. (Ofloxacin) McNeil Pharmaceutical ... 1571
Lorabid Suspension and Pulvules (Loracarbef) Lilly ... 1459
Septra (Trimethoprim, Sulfamethoxazole) Glaxo Wellcome ... 1174
Spectrobid Tablets (Bacampicillin Hydrochloride) Roerig ... 2206
Suprax (Cefixime) Lederle ... 1399
Vantin for Oral Suspension and Vantin Tablets (Cefpodoxime Proxetil) Upjohn ... 2646
Zefazone (Cefmetazole Sodium) Upjohn ... 2654

S. pneumoniae central nervous system infections
Claforan Sterile and Injection (Cefotaxime Sodium) Hoechst-Roussel ... 1235
Fortaz (Ceftazidime) Glaxo Wellcome ... 1100
Tazicef for Injection (Ceftazidime) SmithKline Beecham Pharmaceuticals ... 2519
Tazidime Vials, Faspak & ADD-Vantage (Ceftazidime) Lilly ... 1478

S. pneumoniae infections
Achromycin V Capsules (Tetracycline Hydrochloride) Lederle ... 1367
Amoxil (Amoxicillin Trihydrate) SmithKline Beecham Pharmaceuticals ... 2464
Ancef Injection (Cefazolin Sodium) SmithKline Beecham Pharmaceuticals ... 2465
Bactrim (Trimethoprim, Sulfamethoxazole) Roche Laboratories ... 2084
Biaxin (Clarithromycin) Abbott ... 405
Bicillin C-R Injection (Penicillin G Procaine, Penicillin G Benzathine) Wyeth-Ayerst ... 2704
Bicillin C-R 900/300 Injection (Penicillin G Procaine, Penicillin G Benzathine) Wyeth-Ayerst ... 2706
Ceclor Pulvules & Suspension (Cefaclor) Lilly ... 1431
Cefizox for Intramuscular or Intravenous Use (Ceftizoxime Sodium) Fujisawa ... 1034
Cefobid Intravenous/Intramuscular (Cefoperazone Sodium) Roerig ... 2189
Cefobid Pharmacy Bulk Package - Not for Direct Infusion (Cefoperazone Sodium) Roerig ... 2192
Cefotan (Cefotetan) Zeneca ... 2829
Ceftin (Cefuroxime Axetil) Glaxo Wellcome ... 1078
Cefzil Tablets and Oral Suspension (Cefprozil) Bristol-Myers Squibb ... 746
Ceptaz (Ceftazidime) Glaxo Wellcome ... 1081
Cipro I.V. (Ciprofloxacin) Bayer Pharmaceutical ... 595
Cipro I.V. Pharmacy Bulk Package (Ciprofloxacin) Bayer Pharmaceutical ... 597
Cipro Tablets (Ciprofloxacin Hydrochloride) Bayer Pharmaceutical ... 592
Claforan Sterile and Injection (Cefotaxime Sodium) Hoechst-Roussel ... 1235
Cleocin Phosphate Injection (Clindamycin Phosphate) Upjohn ... 2586
Declomycin Tablets (Demeclocycline Hydrochloride) Lederle ... 1371
Doryx Capsules (Doxycycline Hyclate) Parke-Davis ... 1913
Dynacin Capsules (Minocycline Hydrochloride) Medicis ... 1590
E.E.S. (Erythromycin Ethylsuccinate) Abbott ... 424
E-Mycin Tablets (Erythromycin) Knoll Laboratories ... 1341
ERYC (Erythromycin) Parke-Davis ... 1915
EryPed (Erythromycin Ethylsuccinate) Abbott ... 421
Ery-Tab Tablets (Erythromycin) Abbott ... 422
Erythrocin Stearate Filmtab (Erythromycin Stearate) Abbott ... 425
Erythromycin Base Filmtab (Erythromycin) Abbott ... 426
Erythromycin Delayed-Release Capsules, USP (Erythromycin) Abbott ... 427
Floxin I.V. (Ofloxacin) McNeil Pharmaceutical ... 1571
Floxin Tablets (200 mg, 300 mg, 400 mg) (Ofloxacin) McNeil Pharmaceutical ... 1567
Fortaz (Ceftazidime) Glaxo Wellcome ... 1100
Ilosone (Erythromycin Estolate) Dista ... 911
Ilotycin Gluceptate, IV, Vials (Erythromycin Gluceptate) Dista ... 913
Keflex Pulvules & Oral Suspension (Cephalexin) Dista ... 914
Keftab Tablets (Cephalexin Hydrochloride) Dista ... 915

(▣ Described in PDR For Nonprescription Drugs) (◉ Described in PDR For Ophthalmology)

Kefurox Vials, Faspak & ADD-Vantage (Cefuroxime Sodium) Lilly 1454
Kefzol Vials, Faspak & ADD-Vantage (Cefazolin Sodium) Lilly 1456
Lincocin (Lincomycin Hydrochloride) Upjohn 2617
Lorabid Suspension and Pulvules (Loracarbef) Lilly 1459
Mefoxin (Cefoxitin Sodium) Merck & Co., Inc. 1691
Mefoxin Premixed Intravenous Solution (Cefoxitin Sodium) Merck & Co., Inc. 1694
Mezlin (Mezlocillin Sodium) Bayer Pharmaceutical 601
Mezlin Pharmacy Bulk Package (Mezlocillin Sodium) Bayer Pharmaceutical 604
Minocin Intravenous (Minocycline Hydrochloride) Lederle 1382
Minocin Oral Suspension (Minocycline Hydrochloride) Lederle 1385
Minocin Pellet-Filled Capsules (Minocycline Hydrochloride) Lederle 1383
Monocid Injection (Cefonicid Sodium) SmithKline Beecham Pharmaceuticals 2497
Monodox Capsules (Doxycycline Monohydrate) Oclassen 1805
PCE Dispertab Tablets (Erythromycin) Abbott 444
Pfizerpen for Injection (Penicillin G Potassium) Roerig 2203
Pipracil (Piperacillin Sodium) Lederle 1390
Primaxin I.M. (Imipenem-Cilastatin Sodium) Merck & Co., Inc. 1727
Primaxin I.V. (Imipenem-Cilastatin Sodium) Merck & Co., Inc. 1729
Rocephin Injectable Vials, ADD-Vantage, Galaxy Container (Ceftriaxone Sodium) Roche Laboratories 2142
Spectrobid Tablets (Bacampicillin Hydrochloride) Roerig 2206
Suprax (Cefixime) Lederle 1399
Tao Capsules (Troleandomycin) Roerig 2209
Tazicef for Injection (Ceftazidime) SmithKline Beecham Pharmaceuticals 2519
Tazidime Vials, Faspak & ADD-Vantage (Ceftazidime) Lilly 1478
Terramycin Intramuscular Solution (Oxytetracycline) Roerig 2210
Vantin for Oral Suspension and Vantin Tablets (Cefpodoxime Proxetil) Upjohn 2646
Vibramycin Hyclate Capsules (Doxycycline Hyclate) Pfizer Labs 1941
Vibramycin Hyclate Intravenous (Doxycycline Hyclate) Roerig 2215
Zefazone (Cefmetazole Sodium) Upjohn 2654
Zinacef (Cefuroxime Sodium) Glaxo Wellcome 1211
Zithromax (Azithromycin) Pfizer Labs 1944

S. pneumoniae infections, ocular

AK-CIDE (Prednisolone Acetate, Sulfacetamide Sodium) Akorn ⊙ 202
AK-CIDE Ointment (Prednisolone Acetate, Sulfacetamide Sodium) Akorn ⊙ 202
AK-Spore (Bacitracin Zinc, Neomycin Sulfate, Polymyxin B Sulfate) Akorn ⊙ 204
Blephamide Liquifilm Sterile Ophthalmic Suspension (Prednisolone Acetate, Sulfacetamide Sodium) Allergan 476
Blephamide Ointment (Sulfacetamide Sodium, Prednisolone Acetate) Allergan ⊙ 237
Chibroxin Sterile Ophthalmic Solution (Norfloxacin) Merck & Co., Inc. 1617
Chloromycetin Ophthalmic Ointment, 1% (Chloramphenicol) Parke-Davis ⊙ 310
Chloromycetin Ophthalmic Solution (Chloramphenicol) Parke-Davis ⊙ 310
Chloroptic S.O.P. (Chloramphenicol) Allergan ⊙ 239
Ciloxan Ophthalmic Solution (Ciprofloxacin Hydrochloride) Alcon Laboratories 472
Cortisporin Ophthalmic Ointment Sterile (Polymyxin B Sulfate, Bacitracin Zinc, Neomycin Sulfate, Hydrocortisone) Glaxo Wellcome 1085
FML-S Liquifilm (Sulfacetamide Sodium, Fluorometholone) Allergan ⊙ 242
Genoptic Sterile Ophthalmic Solution (Gentamicin Sulfate) Allergan ⊙ 243
Genoptic Sterile Ophthalmic Ointment (Gentamicin Sulfate) Allergan ⊙ 243
Gentak (Gentamicin Sulfate) Akorn ⊙ 208
Ocuflox (Ofloxacin) Allergan 481
Ophthocort (Chloramphenicol, Polymyxin B Sulfate, Hydrocortisone Acetate) Parke-Davis ⊙ 311
Polytrim Ophthalmic Solution Sterile (Polymyxin B Sulfate, Trimethoprim Sulfate) Allergan 482
Pred-G Liquifilm Sterile Ophthalmic Suspension (Gentamicin Sulfate, Prednisolone Acetate) Allergan ⊙ 251
Pred-G S.O.P. Sterile Ophthalmic Ointment (Gentamicin Sulfate, Prednisolone Acetate) Allergan ⊙ 252
Terra-Cortril Ophthalmic Suspension (Oxytetracycline Hydrochloride, Hydrocortisone Acetate) Roerig 2210
Terramycin with Polymyxin B Sulfate Ophthalmic Ointment (Oxytetracycline Hydrochloride, Polymyxin B Sulfate) Roerig 2211
TobraDex Ophthalmic Suspension and Ointment (Dexamethasone, Tobramycin) Alcon Laboratories 473
Vasocidin Ointment (Prednisolone Acetate, Sulfacetamide Sodium) CIBA Vision Ophthalmics ⊙ 268
Vasocidin Ophthalmic Solution (Prednisolone Sodium Phosphate, Sulfacetamide Sodium) CIBA Vision Ophthalmics ⊙ 270

S. pneumoniae lower respiratory tract infections

Biaxin (Clarithromycin) Abbott 405
Ceclor Pulvules & Suspension (Cefaclor) Lilly 1431
Cefizox for Intramuscular or Intravenous Use (Ceftizoxime Sodium) Fujisawa 1034
Cefotan (Cefotetan) Zeneca 2829
Cefzil Tablets and Oral Suspension (Cefprozil) Bristol-Myers Squibb 746
Ceptaz (Ceftazidime) Glaxo Wellcome 1081
Cipro I.V. (Ciprofloxacin) Bayer Pharmaceutical 595
Cipro I.V. Pharmacy Bulk Package (Ciprofloxacin) Bayer Pharmaceutical 597
Cipro Tablets (Ciprofloxacin Hydrochloride) Bayer Pharmaceutical 592
Claforan Sterile and Injection (Cefotaxime Sodium) Hoechst-Roussel 1235
Cleocin Phosphate Injection (Clindamycin Phosphate) Upjohn 2586
E.E.S. (Erythromycin Ethylsuccinate) Abbott 424
E-Mycin Tablets (Erythromycin) Knoll Laboratories 1341
ERYC (Erythromycin) Parke-Davis 1915
EryPed (Erythromycin Ethylsuccinate) Abbott 421
Ery-Tab Tablets (Erythromycin) Abbott 422
Erythrocin Stearate Filmtab (Erythromycin Stearate) Abbott 425
Erythromycin Base Filmtab (Erythromycin) Abbott 426
Erythromycin Delayed-Release Capsules, USP (Erythromycin) Abbott 427
Floxin I.V. (Ofloxacin) McNeil Pharmaceutical 1571
Floxin Tablets (200 mg, 300 mg, 400 mg) (Ofloxacin) McNeil Pharmaceutical 1567
Fortaz (Ceftazidime) Glaxo Wellcome 1100
Ilosone (Erythromycin Estolate) Dista 911
Ilotycin Gluceptate, IV, Vials (Erythromycin Gluceptate) Dista 913
Keftab Tablets (Cephalexin Hydrochloride) Dista 915
Kefurox Vials, Faspak & ADD-Vantage (Cefuroxime Sodium) Lilly 1454
Lorabid Suspension and Pulvules (Loracarbef) Lilly 1459
Mandol Vials, Faspak & ADD-Vantage (Cefamandole Nafate) Lilly 1461
Mefoxin (Cefoxitin Sodium) Merck & Co., Inc. 1691
Mefoxin Premixed Intravenous Solution (Cefoxitin Sodium) Merck & Co., Inc. 1694
Monocid Injection (Cefonicid Sodium) SmithKline Beecham Pharmaceuticals 2497
PCE Dispertab Tablets (Erythromycin) Abbott 444
Primaxin I.M. (Imipenem-Cilastatin Sodium) Merck & Co., Inc. 1727
Rocephin Injectable Vials, ADD-Vantage, Galaxy Container (Ceftriaxone Sodium) Roche Laboratories 2142
Spectrobid Tablets (Bacampicillin Hydrochloride) Roerig 2206
Tao Capsules (Troleandomycin) Roerig 2209
Tazicef for Injection (Ceftazidime) SmithKline Beecham Pharmaceuticals 2519
Tazidime Vials, Faspak & ADD-Vantage (Ceftazidime) Lilly 1478
Vantin for Oral Suspension and Vantin Tablets (Cefpodoxime Proxetil) Upjohn 2646
Zefazone (Cefmetazole Sodium) Upjohn 2654
Zinacef (Cefuroxime Sodium) Glaxo Wellcome 1211
Zithromax (Azithromycin) Pfizer Labs 1944

S. pneumoniae meningitis

Cefizox for Intramuscular or Intravenous Use (Ceftizoxime Sodium) Fujisawa 1034
Ceptaz (Ceftazidime) Glaxo Wellcome 1081
Fortaz (Ceftazidime) Glaxo Wellcome 1100
Kefurox Vials, Faspak & ADD-Vantage (Cefuroxime Sodium) Lilly 1454
Rocephin Injectable Vials, ADD-Vantage, Galaxy Container (Ceftriaxone Sodium) Roche Laboratories 2142
Tazicef for Injection (Ceftazidime) SmithKline Beecham Pharmaceuticals 2519
Tazidime Vials, Faspak & ADD-Vantage (Ceftazidime) Lilly 1478
Zinacef (Cefuroxime Sodium) Glaxo Wellcome 1211

S. pneumoniae otitis media

Bactrim (Trimethoprim, Sulfamethoxazole) Roche Laboratories 2084
Bicillin C-R Injection (Penicillin G Procaine, Penicillin G Benzathine) Wyeth-Ayerst 2704
Bicillin C-R 900/300 Injection (Penicillin G Procaine, Penicillin G Benzathine) Wyeth-Ayerst 2706
Ceclor Pulvules & Suspension (Cefaclor) Lilly 1431
Ceftin (Cefuroxime Axetil) Glaxo Wellcome 1078
Cefzil Tablets and Oral Suspension (Cefprozil) Bristol-Myers Squibb 746
E.E.S. (Erythromycin Ethylsuccinate) Abbott 424
EryPed (Erythromycin Ethylsuccinate) Abbott 421
Ery-Tab Tablets (Erythromycin) Abbott 422
Erythrocin Stearate Filmtab (Erythromycin Stearate) Abbott 425
Erythromycin Base Filmtab (Erythromycin) Abbott 426
Ilosone (Erythromycin Estolate) Dista 911
Ilotycin Gluceptate, IV, Vials (Erythromycin Gluceptate) Dista 913
Keflex Pulvules & Oral Suspension (Cephalexin) Dista 914
Lorabid Suspension and Pulvules (Loracarbef) Lilly 1459
Septra (Trimethoprim, Sulfamethoxazole) Glaxo Wellcome 1174
Suprax (Cefixime) Lederle 1399
Vantin for Oral Suspension and Vantin Tablets (Cefpodoxime Proxetil) Upjohn 2646

S. pneumoniae pharyngitis

EryPed (Erythromycin Ethylsuccinate) Abbott 421
Ery-Tab Tablets (Erythromycin) Abbott 422
Erythrocin Stearate Filmtab (Erythromycin Stearate) Abbott 425
Erythromycin Base Filmtab (Erythromycin) Abbott 426
Erythromycin Delayed-Release Capsules, USP (Erythromycin) Abbott 427
Ilosone (Erythromycin Estolate) Dista 911
Ilotycin Gluceptate, IV, Vials (Erythromycin Gluceptate) Dista 913
PCE Dispertab Tablets (Erythromycin) Abbott 444

S. pneumoniae respiratory tract infections

Ancef Injection (Cefazolin Sodium) SmithKline Beecham Pharmaceuticals 2465
Cefobid Intravenous/Intramuscular (Cefoperazone Sodium) Roerig 2189
Cefobid Pharmacy Bulk Package - Not for Direct Infusion (Cefoperazone Sodium) Roerig 2192
Keflex Pulvules & Oral Suspension (Cephalexin) Dista 914
Kefzol Vials, Faspak & ADD-Vantage (Cefazolin Sodium) Lilly 1456

S. pneumoniae septicemia

Ancef Injection (Cefazolin Sodium) SmithKline Beecham Pharmaceuticals 2465
Cefizox for Intramuscular or Intravenous Use (Ceftizoxime Sodium) Fujisawa 1034
Cefobid Intravenous/Intramuscular (Cefoperazone Sodium) Roerig 2189
Cefobid Pharmacy Bulk Package - Not for Direct Infusion (Cefoperazone Sodium) Roerig 2192
Ceptaz (Ceftazidime) Glaxo Wellcome 1081
Claforan Sterile and Injection (Cefotaxime Sodium) Hoechst-Roussel 1235
Fortaz (Ceftazidime) Glaxo Wellcome 1100
Kefurox Vials, Faspak & ADD-Vantage (Cefuroxime Sodium) Lilly 1454
Kefzol Vials, Faspak & ADD-Vantage (Cefazolin Sodium) Lilly 1456
Mefoxin (Cefoxitin Sodium) Merck & Co., Inc. 1691
Mefoxin Premixed Intravenous Solution (Cefoxitin Sodium) Merck & Co., Inc. 1694
Monocid Injection (Cefonicid Sodium) SmithKline Beecham Pharmaceuticals 2497
Pipracil (Piperacillin Sodium) Lederle 1390
Rocephin Injectable Vials, ADD-Vantage, Galaxy Container (Ceftriaxone Sodium) Roche Laboratories 2142
Tazicef for Injection (Ceftazidime) SmithKline Beecham Pharmaceuticals 2519
Tazidime Vials, Faspak & ADD-Vantage (Ceftazidime) Lilly 1478
Zinacef (Cefuroxime Sodium) Glaxo Wellcome 1211

S. pneumoniae upper respiratory tract infections

Biaxin (Clarithromycin) Abbott 405
Dynacin Capsules (Minocycline Hydrochloride) Medicis 1590
E.E.S. (Erythromycin Ethylsuccinate) Abbott 424
E-Mycin Tablets (Erythromycin) Knoll Laboratories 1341
ERYC (Erythromycin) Parke-Davis 1915

(▣ Described in PDR For Nonprescription Drugs) (⊙ Described in PDR For Ophthalmology)

1537 **Indications Index** **S. warnerii infections**

EryPed (Erythromycin Ethylsuccinate) Abbott ... 421
Ery-Tab Tablets (Erythromycin) Abbott ... 422
Erythrocin Stearate Filmtab (Erythromycin Stearate) Abbott ... 425
Erythromycin Base Filmtab (Erythromycin) Abbott ... 426
Erythromycin Delayed-Release Capsules, USP (Erythromycin) Abbott ... 427
Ilosone (Erythromycin Estolate) Dista ... 911
Ilotycin Gluceptate, IV, Vials (Erythromycin Gluceptate) Dista ... 913
Keftab Tablets (Cephalexin Hydrochloride) Dista ... 915
Minocin Oral Suspension (Minocycline Hydrochloride) Lederle ... 1385
Minocin Pellet-Filled Capsules (Minocycline Hydrochloride) Lederle ... 1383
Monodox Capsules (Doxycycline Monohydrate) Oclassen ... 1805
PCE Dispertab Tablets (Erythromycin) Abbott ... 444
Spectrobid Tablets (Bacampicillin Hydrochloride) Roerig ... 2206
Vibramycin Hyclate Capsules (Doxycycline Hyclate) Pfizer Labs 1941

S. pyogenes bone and joint infections
Claforan Sterile and Injection (Cefotaxime Sodium) Hoechst-Roussel ... 1235

S. pyogenes infections
Bactroban Ointment (Mupirocin) SmithKline Beecham Pharmaceuticals ... 2470
Biaxin (Clarithromycin) Abbott ... 405
Ceclor Pulvules & Suspension (Cefaclor) Lilly ... 1431
Cefizox for Intramuscular or Intravenous Use (Ceftizoxime Sodium) Fujisawa ... 1034
Cefobid Intravenous/Intramuscular (Cefoperazone Sodium) Roerig ... 2189
Cefobid Pharmacy Bulk Package - Not for Direct Infusion (Cefoperazone Sodium) Roerig ... 2192
Cefotan (Cefotetan) Zeneca ... 2829
Ceftin (Cefuroxime Axetil) Glaxo Wellcome ... 1078
Cefzil Tablets and Oral Suspension (Cefprozil) Bristol-Myers Squibb .. 746
Ceptaz (Ceftazidime) Glaxo Wellcome ... 1081
Cipro I.V. (Ciprofloxacin) Bayer Pharmaceutical ... 595
Cipro I.V. Pharmacy Bulk Package (Ciprofloxacin) Bayer Pharmaceutical ... 597
Cipro Tablets (Ciprofloxacin Hydrochloride) Bayer Pharmaceutical ... 592
Claforan Sterile and Injection (Cefotaxime Sodium) Hoechst-Roussel ... 1235
Cleocin Phosphate Injection (Clindamycin Phosphate) Upjohn ... 2586
E.E.S. (Erythromycin Ethylsuccinate) Abbott ... 424
E-Mycin Tablets (Erythromycin) Knoll Laboratories ... 1341
ERYC (Erythromycin) Parke-Davis .. 1915
EryPed (Erythromycin Ethylsuccinate) Abbott ... 421
Ery-Tab Tablets (Erythromycin) Abbott ... 422
Erythrocin Stearate Filmtab (Erythromycin Stearate) Abbott ... 425
Erythromycin Base Filmtab (Erythromycin) Abbott ... 426
Erythromycin Delayed-Release Capsules, USP (Erythromycin) Abbott ... 427
Floxin I.V. (Ofloxacin) McNeil Pharmaceutical ... 1571
Floxin Tablets (200 mg, 300 mg, 400 mg) (Ofloxacin) McNeil Pharmaceutical ... 1567
Fortaz (Ceftazidime) Glaxo Wellcome ... 1100
Keflex Pulvules & Oral Suspension (Cephalexin) Dista ... 914
Kefurox Vials, Faspak & ADD-Vantage (Cefuroxime Sodium) Lilly ... 1454
Lorabid Suspension and Pulvules (Loracarbef) Lilly ... 1459
Monocid Injection (Cefonicid Sodium) SmithKline Beecham Pharmaceuticals ... 2497
PCE Dispertab Tablets (Erythromycin) Abbott ... 444
Primaxin I.M. (Imipenem-Cilastatin Sodium) Merck & Co., Inc. ... 1727
Rocephin Injectable Vials, ADD-Vantage, Galaxy Container (Ceftriaxone Sodium) Roche Laboratories ... 2142
Spectrobid Tablets (Bacampicillin Hydrochloride) Roerig ... 2206
Suprax (Cefixime) Lederle ... 1399
Tao Capsules (Troleandomycin) Roerig ... 2209
Tazicef for Injection (Ceftazidime) SmithKline Beecham Pharmaceuticals ... 2519
Tazidime Vials, Faspak & ADD-Vantage (Ceftazidime) Lilly .. 1478
Vantin for Oral Suspension and Vantin Tablets (Cefpodoxime Proxetil) Upjohn ... 2646
Zefazone (Cefmetazole Sodium) Upjohn ... 2654
Zinacef (Cefuroxime Sodium) Glaxo Wellcome ... 1211
Zithromax (Azithromycin) Pfizer Labs ... 1944

S. pyogenes infections, ocular
Genoptic Sterile Ophthalmic Solution (Gentamicin Sulfate) Allergan ... ◉ 243
Genoptic Sterile Ophthalmic Ointment (Gentamicin Sulfate) Allergan ... ◉ 243
Gentak (Gentamicin Sulfate) Akorn ... ◉ 208
Pred-G S.O.P. Sterile Ophthalmic Ointment (Gentamicin Sulfate, Prednisolone Acetate) Allergan.. ◉ 252

S. pyogenes lower respiratory tract infections
Ceclor Pulvules & Suspension (Cefaclor) Lilly ... 1431
Claforan Sterile and Injection (Cefotaxime Sodium) Hoechst-Roussel ... 1235
E.E.S. (Erythromycin Ethylsuccinate) Abbott ... 424
E-Mycin Tablets (Erythromycin) Knoll Laboratories ... 1341
ERYC (Erythromycin) Parke-Davis .. 1915
EryPed (Erythromycin Ethylsuccinate) Abbott ... 421
Ery-Tab Tablets (Erythromycin) Abbott ... 422
Erythrocin Stearate Filmtab (Erythromycin Stearate) Abbott ... 425
Erythromycin Base Filmtab (Erythromycin) Abbott ... 426
Erythromycin Delayed-Release Capsules, USP (Erythromycin) Abbott ... 427
Ilosone (Erythromycin Estolate) Dista ... 911
Ilotycin Gluceptate, IV, Vials (Erythromycin Gluceptate) Dista ... 913
Kefurox Vials, Faspak & ADD-Vantage (Cefuroxime Sodium) Lilly ... 1454
PCE Dispertab Tablets (Erythromycin) Abbott ... 444
Spectrobid Tablets (Bacampicillin Hydrochloride) Roerig ... 2206
Zinacef (Cefuroxime Sodium) Glaxo Wellcome ... 1211

S. pyogenes otitis media
Ceclor Pulvules & Suspension (Cefaclor) Lilly ... 1431
Ceftin (Cefuroxime Axetil) Glaxo Wellcome ... 1078
Lorabid Suspension and Pulvules (Loracarbef) Lilly ... 1459
Suprax (Cefixime) Lederle ... 1399

S. pyogenes pharyngitis
Biaxin (Clarithromycin) Abbott ... 405
Ceclor Pulvules & Suspension (Cefaclor) Lilly ... 1431
Ceftin (Cefuroxime Axetil) Glaxo Wellcome ... 1078
Cefzil Tablets and Oral Suspension (Cefprozil) Bristol-Myers Squibb .. 746
Lorabid Suspension and Pulvules (Loracarbef) Lilly ... 1459
Suprax (Cefixime) Lederle ... 1399
Vantin for Oral Suspension and Vantin Tablets (Cefpodoxime Proxetil) Upjohn ... 2646
Zithromax (Azithromycin) Pfizer Labs ... 1944

S. pyogenes respiratory tract infections
Cefobid Intravenous/Intramuscular (Cefoperazone Sodium) Roerig ... 2189
Cefobid Pharmacy Bulk Package - Not for Direct Infusion (Cefoperazone Sodium) Roerig ... 2192
Keflex Pulvules & Oral Suspension (Cephalexin) Dista ... 914

S. pyogenes skin and skin structure infections
Biaxin (Clarithromycin) Abbott ... 405
Ceclor Pulvules & Suspension (Cefaclor) Lilly ... 1431
Cefizox for Intramuscular or Intravenous Use (Ceftizoxime Sodium) Fujisawa ... 1034
Cefobid Intravenous/Intramuscular (Cefoperazone Sodium) Roerig ... 2189
Cefobid Pharmacy Bulk Package - Not for Direct Infusion (Cefoperazone Sodium) Roerig ... 2192
Cefotan (Cefotetan) Zeneca ... 2829
Ceftin (Cefuroxime Axetil) Glaxo Wellcome ... 1078
Cefzil Tablets and Oral Suspension (Cefprozil) Bristol-Myers Squibb .. 746
Ceptaz (Ceftazidime) Glaxo Wellcome ... 1081
Cipro I.V. (Ciprofloxacin) Bayer Pharmaceutical ... 595
Cipro I.V. Pharmacy Bulk Package (Ciprofloxacin) Bayer Pharmaceutical ... 597
Cipro Tablets (Ciprofloxacin Hydrochloride) Bayer Pharmaceutical ... 592
Claforan Sterile and Injection (Cefotaxime Sodium) Hoechst-Roussel ... 1235
Cleocin Phosphate Injection (Clindamycin Phosphate) Upjohn ... 2586
E.E.S. (Erythromycin Ethylsuccinate) Abbott ... 424
E-Mycin Tablets (Erythromycin) Knoll Laboratories ... 1341
ERYC (Erythromycin) Parke-Davis .. 1915
EryPed (Erythromycin Ethylsuccinate) Abbott ... 421
Ery-Tab Tablets (Erythromycin) Abbott ... 422
Erythrocin Stearate Filmtab (Erythromycin Stearate) Abbott ... 425
Erythromycin Base Filmtab (Erythromycin) Abbott ... 426
Erythromycin Delayed-Release Capsules, USP (Erythromycin) Abbott ... 427
Floxin I.V. (Ofloxacin) McNeil Pharmaceutical ... 1571
Floxin Tablets (200 mg, 300 mg, 400 mg) (Ofloxacin) McNeil Pharmaceutical ... 1567
Fortaz (Ceftazidime) Glaxo Wellcome ... 1100
Ilosone (Erythromycin Estolate) Dista ... 911
Ilotycin Gluceptate, IV, Vials (Erythromycin Gluceptate) Dista ... 913
Lorabid Suspension and Pulvules (Loracarbef) Lilly ... 1459
Mandol Vials, Faspak & ADD-Vantage (Cefamandole Nafate) Lilly ... 1461
Monocid Injection (Cefonicid Sodium) SmithKline Beecham Pharmaceuticals ... 2497
PCE Dispertab Tablets (Erythromycin) Abbott ... 444
Primaxin I.M. (Imipenem-Cilastatin Sodium) Merck & Co., Inc. ... 1727
Rocephin Injectable Vials, ADD-Vantage, Galaxy Container (Ceftriaxone Sodium) Roche Laboratories ... 2142
Tazicef for Injection (Ceftazidime) SmithKline Beecham Pharmaceuticals ... 2519
Tazidime Vials, Faspak & ADD-Vantage (Ceftazidime) Lilly .. 1478
Vantin for Oral Suspension and Vantin Tablets (Cefpodoxime Proxetil) Upjohn ... 2646
Zefazone (Cefmetazole Sodium) Upjohn ... 2654
Zinacef (Cefuroxime Sodium) Glaxo Wellcome ... 1211
Zithromax (Azithromycin) Pfizer Labs ... 1944

S. pyogenes tonsillitis
Biaxin (Clarithromycin) Abbott ... 405
Ceclor Pulvules & Suspension (Cefaclor) Lilly ... 1431
Ceftin (Cefuroxime Axetil) Glaxo Wellcome ... 1078
Cefzil Tablets and Oral Suspension (Cefprozil) Bristol-Myers Squibb .. 746
Lorabid Suspension and Pulvules (Loracarbef) Lilly ... 1459
Suprax (Cefixime) Lederle ... 1399
Vantin for Oral Suspension and Vantin Tablets (Cefpodoxime Proxetil) Upjohn ... 2646
Zithromax (Azithromycin) Pfizer Labs ... 1944

S. pyogenes upper respiratory tract infections
Biaxin (Clarithromycin) Abbott ... 405
Ceclor Pulvules & Suspension (Cefaclor) Lilly ... 1431
E.E.S. (Erythromycin Ethylsuccinate) Abbott ... 424
E-Mycin Tablets (Erythromycin) Knoll Laboratories ... 1341
ERYC (Erythromycin) Parke-Davis .. 1915
EryPed (Erythromycin Ethylsuccinate) Abbott ... 421
Ery-Tab Tablets (Erythromycin) Abbott ... 422
Erythrocin Stearate Filmtab (Erythromycin Stearate) Abbott ... 425
Erythromycin Base Filmtab (Erythromycin) Abbott ... 426
Erythromycin Delayed-Release Capsules, USP (Erythromycin) Abbott ... 427
Ilosone (Erythromycin Estolate) Dista ... 911
Ilotycin Gluceptate, IV, Vials (Erythromycin Gluceptate) Dista ... 913
PCE Dispertab Tablets (Erythromycin) Abbott ... 444
Spectrobid Tablets (Bacampicillin Hydrochloride) Roerig ... 2206
Suprax (Cefixime) Lederle ... 1399
Tao Capsules (Troleandomycin) Roerig ... 2209
Zithromax (Azithromycin) Pfizer Labs ... 1944

S. saprophyticus urinary tract infections
Lorabid Suspension and Pulvules (Loracarbef) Lilly ... 1459
Macrobid Capsules (Nitrofurantoin Monohydrate) Procter & Gamble Pharmaceuticals ... 1988
Maxaquin Tablets (Lomefloxacin Hydrochloride) Searle ... 2440
Noroxin Tablets (Norfloxacin) Merck & Co., Inc. ... 1715
Noroxin Tablets (Norfloxacin) Roberts ... 2048
Penetrex Tablets (Enoxacin) Rhone-Poulenc Rorer Pharmaceuticals ... 2031
Proloprim Tablets (Trimethoprim) Glaxo Wellcome ... 1155
Trimpex Tablets (Trimethoprim) Roche Laboratories ... 2163
Vantin for Oral Suspension and Vantin Tablets (Cefpodoxime Proxetil) Upjohn ... 2646

S. typhi infections, acute
Chloromycetin Sodium Succinate (Chloramphenicol Sodium Succinate) Parke-Davis ... 1900

S. viridans endocarditis
Erythrocin Stearate Filmtab (Erythromycin Stearate) Abbott ... 425
Erythromycin Base Filmtab (Erythromycin) Abbott ... 426
Vancocin HCl, Vials & ADD-Vantage (Vancomycin Hydrochloride) Lilly 1481

S. warnerii infections, ocular
Chibroxin Sterile Ophthalmic Solution (Norfloxacin) Merck & Co., Inc. ... 1617

SAH
(see under Hemorrhage, subarachnoid, resulting in neurological deficits)

Salmonella species infections
Chloromycetin Sodium Succinate (Chloramphenicol Sodium Succinate) Parke-Davis 1900
Omnipen Capsules (Ampicillin) Wyeth-Ayerst 2764
Omnipen for Oral Suspension (Ampicillin) Wyeth-Ayerst 2765
Pfizerpen for Injection (Penicillin G Potassium) Roerig 2203

Salmonella species infections, serious
Pfizerpen for Injection (Penicillin G Potassium) Roerig 2203

Salmonella typhi infections
Cipro Tablets (Ciprofloxacin Hydrochloride) Bayer Pharmaceutical 592

Salpingitis
Ticar for Injection (Ticarcillin Disodium) SmithKline Beecham Pharmaceuticals 2526

Salt, substitute for
Chlor-3 Condiment (Potassium Chloride) Fleming 1004

Sarcoidosis, symptomatic
Aristocort Suspension (Forte Parenteral) (Triamcinolone Diacetate) Fujisawa 1027
Aristocort Tablets (Triamcinolone) Fujisawa 1022
Celestone Soluspan Suspension (Betamethasone Sodium Phosphate, Betamethasone Acetate) Schering 2347
Cortone Acetate Sterile Suspension (Cortisone Acetate) Merck & Co., Inc. 1623
Cortone Acetate Tablets (Cortisone Acetate) Merck & Co., Inc. 1624
Dalalone D.P. Injectable (Dexamethasone Acetate) Forest 1011
Decadron Elixir (Dexamethasone) Merck & Co., Inc. 1633
Decadron Phosphate Injection (Dexamethasone Sodium Phosphate) Merck & Co., Inc. 1637
Decadron Tablets (Dexamethasone) Merck & Co., Inc. 1635
Decadron-LA Sterile Suspension (Dexamethasone Acetate) Merck & Co., Inc. 1646
Deltasone Tablets (Prednisone) Upjohn 2595
Depo-Medrol Single-Dose Vial (Methylprednisolone Acetate) Upjohn 2600
Depo-Medrol Sterile Aqueous Suspension (Methylprednisolone Acetate) Upjohn 2597
Hydeltrasol Injection, Sterile (Prednisolone Sodium Phosphate) Merck & Co., Inc. 1665
Hydrocortone Phosphate Injection, Sterile (Hydrocortisone Sodium Phosphate) Merck & Co., Inc. 1670
Hydrocortone Tablets (Hydrocortisone) Merck & Co., Inc. 1672
Medrol (Methylprednisolone) Upjohn 2621
Pediapred Oral Liquid (Prednisolone Sodium Phosphate) Fisons 995
Prelone Syrup (Prednisolone) Muro 1787
Solu-Cortef Sterile Powder (Hydrocortisone Sodium Succinate) Upjohn 2641
Solu-Medrol Sterile Powder (Methylprednisolone Sodium Succinate) Upjohn 2643

Sarcoma botryoides
Cosmegen Injection (Dactinomycin) Merck & Co., Inc. 1626

Sarcoma, idiopathic multiple hemorrhagic
(see under Kaposi's sarcoma)

Sarcomas, soft tissue and bone
Adriamycin PFS (Doxorubicin Hydrochloride) Pharmacia 1947
Adriamycin RDF (Doxorubicin Hydrochloride) Pharmacia 1947
Doxorubicin Astra (Doxorubicin Hydrochloride) Astra 540
Rubex (Doxorubicin Hydrochloride) Bristol-Myers Squibb Oncology 712

Sarcoptes scabiei infestations
Elimite (permethrin) 5% Cream (Permethrin) Allergan 478
Eurax Cream & Lotion (Crotamiton) Westwood-Squibb 2685
Kwell Cream & Lotion (Lindane) Reedco 2008
Lindane Lotion USP 1% (Lindane) Barre-National 582

Scabies
(see under Sarcoptes scabiei infestations)

Scarlatina
Bicillin C-R Injection (Penicillin G Procaine, Penicillin G Benzathine) Wyeth-Ayerst 2704
Bicillin C-R 900/300 Injection (Penicillin G Procaine, Penicillin G Benzathine) Wyeth-Ayerst 2706
Pen•Vee K (Penicillin V Potassium) Wyeth-Ayerst 2772

Scarlet fever
(see under Scarlatina)

Schistosoma haematobium infections
Biltricide Tablets (Praziquantel) Bayer Pharmaceutical 591

Schistosoma japonicum infections
Biltricide Tablets (Praziquantel) Bayer Pharmaceutical 591

Schistosoma mansoni infections
Biltricide Tablets (Praziquantel) Bayer Pharmaceutical 591

Schistosoma mekongi infections
Biltricide Tablets (Praziquantel) Bayer Pharmaceutical 591

Schizophrenia
(see under Psychotic disorders, management of the manifestations of)

Schizophrenia with depression
(see under Psychotic disorders with depressive symptoms)

Sciatica, temporary relief of
Arthritis Strength BC Powder (Aspirin, Salicylamide, Caffeine) Block .... ▣ 609
BC Powder (Aspirin, Salicylamide, Caffeine) Block .... ▣ 609
Sarapin (Sarracenia purpurea, Pitcher Plant Distillate) High Chemical 1231

Scleroderma, "possibly" effective in
Potaba (Aminobenzoate Potassium) Glenwood 1229

Scleroderma, linear, "possibly" effective in
Potaba (Aminobenzoate Potassium) Glenwood 1229

Sclerosis, multiple, acute exacerbations of
Aristocort Suspension (Forte Parenteral) (Triamcinolone Diacetate) Fujisawa 1027
Aristocort Tablets (Triamcinolone) Fujisawa 1022
Deltasone Tablets (Prednisone) Upjohn 2595
Depo-Medrol Single-Dose Vial (Methylprednisolone Acetate) Upjohn 2600
Depo-Medrol Sterile Aqueous Suspension (Methylprednisolone Acetate) Upjohn 2597
Medrol (Methylprednisolone) Upjohn 2621
Pediapred Oral Liquid (Prednisolone Sodium Phosphate) Fisons 995
Solu-Cortef Sterile Powder (Hydrocortisone Sodium Succinate) Upjohn 2641
Solu-Medrol Sterile Powder (Methylprednisolone Sodium Succinate) Upjohn 2643

Sclerosis, multiple, alleviation of signs and symptoms
Lioresal Tablets (Baclofen) CibaGeneva 829

Sclerosis, multiple, relapsing-remitting
Betaseron for SC Injection (Interferon Beta-1b) Berlex 658

Seborrhea
(see also under Dandruff)
MG 217 (Coal Tar) Triton Consumer .... ▣ 835
Tegrin Dandruff Shampoo (Coal Tar) Block .... ▣ 611

Sedation
(see also under Sleep, induction of)
Nembutal Sodium Capsules (Pentobarbital Sodium) Abbott 436
Nembutal Sodium Solution (Pentobarbital Sodium) Abbott 438
Nembutal Sodium Suppositories (Pentobarbital Sodium) Abbott 440
Phenergan Injection (Promethazine Hydrochloride) Wyeth-Ayerst 2773
Phenergan Suppositories (Promethazine Hydrochloride) Wyeth-Ayerst 2775
Phenergan Syrup (Promethazine Hydrochloride) Wyeth-Ayerst 2774
Phenergan Tablets (Promethazine Hydrochloride) Wyeth-Ayerst 2775

Sedation, benzodiazepine-induced, complete or partial reversal of
Romazicon (Flumazenil) Roche Laboratories 2147

Sedation conscious, prediagnostic procedures
Versed Injection (Midazolam Hydrochloride) Roche Laboratories 2170

Sedation, conscious, pre-endoscopic or therapeutic procedures
Versed Injection (Midazolam Hydrochloride) Roche Laboratories 2170

Sedation, obstetric
Levoprome (Methotrimeprazine) Immunex 1274
Phenergan Injection (Promethazine Hydrochloride) Wyeth-Ayerst 2773
Phenergan Suppositories (Promethazine Hydrochloride) Wyeth-Ayerst 2775
Phenergan Syrup (Promethazine Hydrochloride) Wyeth-Ayerst 2774
Phenergan Tablets (Promethazine Hydrochloride) Wyeth-Ayerst 2775

Sedation, postoperative
Vistaril Capsules (Hydroxyzine Pamoate) Pfizer Labs 1944
Vistaril Oral Suspension (Hydroxyzine Pamoate) Pfizer Labs 1944

Sedation, preoperative
Atarax Tablets & Syrup (Hydroxyzine Hydrochloride) Roerig 2185
Ativan Injection (Lorazepam) Wyeth-Ayerst 2698
Inapsine Injection (Droperidol) Janssen 1296
Mepergan Injection (Meperidine Hydrochloride, Promethazine Hydrochloride) Wyeth-Ayerst 2753
Versed Injection (Midazolam Hydrochloride) Roche Laboratories 2170
Vistaril Capsules (Hydroxyzine Pamoate) Pfizer Labs 1944
Vistaril Oral Suspension (Hydroxyzine Pamoate) Pfizer Labs 1944

Seizures, absence, adjunctive therapy in
Depakene (Valproic Acid) Abbott 413
Depakote Tablets (Divalproex Sodium) Abbott 415

Seizures, akinetic
Klonopin Tablets (Clonazepam) Roche Laboratories 2126

Seizures, centrencephalic
(see also under Seizures, generalized, tonic-clonic; Seizures, generalized, absence)
Diamox (Acetazolamide) Lederle 1372

Seizures, convulsive, severe recurrent, adjunct in
Dizac (Diazepam) Ohmeda 1809
Valium Injectable (Diazepam) Roche Products 2182

Seizures, focal
Atretol Tablets (Carbamazepine) Athena 573
Felbatol (Felbamate) Wallace 2666
Mesantoin Tablets (Mephenytoin) Sandoz Pharmaceuticals 2272
Mysoline (Primidone) Wyeth-Ayerst 2754
Phenobarbital Elixir and Tablets (Phenobarbital) Lilly 1469
Tegretol Chewable Tablets (Carbamazepine) CibaGeneva 852
Tegretol Suspension (Carbamazepine) CibaGeneva 852
Tegretol Tablets (Carbamazepine) CibaGeneva 852
Tranxene T-TAB Tablets (Clorazepate Dipotassium) Abbott 451

Seizures, focal, adjunctive therapy in
Felbatol (Felbamate) Wallace 2666
Lamictal Tablets (Lamotrigine) Glaxo Wellcome 1112
Neurontin Capsules (Gabapentin) Parke-Davis 1922
Tranxene (Clorazepate Dipotassium) Abbott 451

Seizures, generalized, absence
Celontin Kapseals (Methsuximide) Parke-Davis 1899
Depakene (Valproic Acid) Abbott 413
Depakote Tablets (Divalproex Sodium) Abbott 415
Diamox (Acetazolamide) Lederle 1372
Klonopin Tablets (Clonazepam) Roche Laboratories 2126
Mebaral Tablets (Mephobarbital) Sanofi Winthrop 2322
Milontin Kapseals (Phensuximide) Parke-Davis 1920
Zarontin Capsules (Ethosuximide) Parke-Davis 1928
Zarontin Syrup (Ethosuximide) Parke-Davis 1929

Seizures, generalized, tonic-clonic
Atretol Tablets (Carbamazepine) Athena 573
Diamox (Acetazolamide) Lederle 1372
Dilantin Infatabs (Phenytoin) Parke-Davis 1908
Dilantin Kapseals (Phenytoin Sodium) Parke-Davis 1906
Dilantin-125 Suspension (Phenytoin) Parke-Davis 1911
Mebaral Tablets (Mephobarbital) Sanofi Winthrop 2322
Mesantoin Tablets (Mephenytoin) Sandoz Pharmaceuticals 2272
Mysoline (Primidone) Wyeth-Ayerst 2754
Peganone Tablets (Ethotoin) Abbott 446
Phenobarbital Elixir and Tablets (Phenobarbital) Lilly 1469
Tegretol Chewable Tablets (Carbamazepine) CibaGeneva 852
Tegretol Suspension (Carbamazepine) CibaGeneva 852
Tegretol Tablets (Carbamazepine) CibaGeneva 852

Seizures, Jacksonian
Mesantoin Tablets (Mephenytoin) Sandoz Pharmaceuticals 2272

Seizures, multiple, adjunctive therapy in
Depakene (Valproic Acid) Abbott 413
Depakote Tablets (Divalproex Sodium) Abbott 415

(▣ Described in PDR For Nonprescription Drugs) (⊙ Described in PDR For Ophthalmology)

1539 **Indications Index** **Serratia species**

Seizures, myoclonic
Klonopin Tablets (Clonazepam) Roche Laboratories 2126

Seizures, neurosurgery-induced
Dilantin Infatabs (Phenytoin) Parke-Davis 1908
Dilantin Kapseals (Phenytoin Sodium) Parke-Davis 1906
Dilantin Parenteral (Phenytoin Sodium) Parke-Davis 1910

Seizures, neurosurgery-induced, prophylaxis of
Dilantin Infatabs (Phenytoin) Parke-Davis 1908
Dilantin Kapseals (Phenytoin Sodium) Parke-Davis 1906
Dilantin Parenteral (Phenytoin Sodium) Parke-Davis 1910

Seizures, partial (see under Seizures, focal)

Seizures, psychomotor
Dilantin Infatabs (Phenytoin) Parke-Davis 1908
Dilantin Kapseals (Phenytoin Sodium) Parke-Davis 1906
Dilantin-125 Suspension (Phenytoin) Parke-Davis 1911
Mesantoin Tablets (Mephenytoin) Sandoz Pharmaceuticals 2272
Mysoline (Primidone) Wyeth-Ayerst 2754
Peganone Tablets (Ethotoin) Abbott 446
Phenurone Tablets (Phenacemide) Abbott 447

Senile lentigines (see under Hyperpigmentation, skin, bleaching of)

Sepsis, bacterial, neonatal
Amikacin Sulfate Injection, USP (Amikacin Sulfate) Elkins-Sinn 960
Amikin Injectable (Amikacin Sulfate) Apothecon 501
Garamycin Injectable (Gentamicin Sulfate) Schering 2360

Sepsis, burn wound
SSD (Silver Sulfadiazine) Knoll Laboratories 1355
Silvadene Cream 1% (Silver Sulfadiazine) Marion Merrell Dow 1540

Septic shock (see under Bacterial shock, treatment adjunct)

Septicemia, anaerobic bacterial
Cefobid Intravenous/Intramuscular (Cefoperazone Sodium) Roerig 2189
Cefobid Pharmacy Bulk Package - Not for Direct Infusion (Cefoperazone Sodium) Roerig 2192

Septicemia, bacterial
Amikacin Sulfate Injection, USP (Amikacin Sulfate) Elkins-Sinn 960
Amikin Injectable (Amikacin Sulfate) Apothecon 501
Ancef Injection (Cefazolin Sodium) SmithKline Beecham Pharmaceuticals 2465
Azactam for Injection (Aztreonam) Bristol-Myers Squibb 734
Cefizox for Intramuscular or Intravenous Use (Ceftizoxime Sodium) Fujisawa 1034
Cefobid Intravenous/Intramuscular (Cefoperazone Sodium) Roerig 2189
Cefobid Pharmacy Bulk Package - Not for Direct Infusion (Cefoperazone Sodium) Roerig 2192
Ceptaz (Ceftazidime) Glaxo Wellcome 1081
Chloromycetin Sodium Succinate (Chloramphenicol Sodium Succinate) Parke-Davis 1900
Cipro I.V. (Ciprofloxacin) Bayer Pharmaceutical 595
Claforan Sterile and Injection (Cefotaxime Sodium) Hoechst-Roussel 1235
Cleocin Phosphate Injection (Clindamycin Phosphate) Upjohn 2586
Flagyl 375 Capsules (Metronidazole) Searle 2434
Flagyl I.V. (Metronidazole Hydrochloride) SCS 2247
Fortaz (Ceftazidime) Glaxo Wellcome 1100
Garamycin Injectable (Gentamicin Sulfate) Schering 2360
Kefurox Vials, Faspak & ADD-Vantage (Cefuroxime Sodium) Lilly 1454
Kefzol Vials, Faspak & ADD-Vantage (Cefazolin Sodium) Lilly 1456
Mandol Vials, Faspak & ADD-Vantage (Cefamandole Nafate) Lilly 1461
Mefoxin (Cefoxitin Sodium) Merck & Co., Inc. 1691
Mefoxin Premixed Intravenous Solution (Cefoxitin Sodium) Merck & Co., Inc. 1694
Mezlin (Mezlocillin Sodium) Bayer Pharmaceutical 601
Mezlin Pharmacy Bulk Package (Mezlocillin Sodium) Bayer Pharmaceutical 604
Monocid Injection (Cefonicid Sodium) SmithKline Beecham Pharmaceuticals 2497
Nebcin Vials, Hyporets & ADD-Vantage (Tobramycin Sulfate) Lilly 1464
Netromycin Injection 100 mg/ml (Netilmicin Sulfate) Schering 2373
Pfizerpen for Injection (Penicillin G Potassium) Roerig 2203
Pipracil (Piperacillin Sodium) Lederle 1390
Polymyxin B Sulfate, Aerosporin Brand Sterile Powder (Polymyxin B Sulfate) Glaxo Wellcome 1154
Primaxin I.V. (Imipenem-Cilastatin Sodium) Merck & Co., Inc. 1729
Protostat Tablets (Metronidazole) Ortho Pharmaceutical 1883
Rocephin Injectable Vials, ADD-Vantage, Galaxy Container (Ceftriaxone Sodium) Roche Laboratories 2142
Tazicef for Injection (Ceftazidime) SmithKline Beecham Pharmaceuticals 2519
Tazidime Vials, Faspak & ADD-Vantage (Ceftazidime) Lilly 1478
Ticar for Injection (Ticarcillin Disodium) SmithKline Beecham Pharmaceuticals 2526
Timentin for Injection (Ticarcillin Disodium, Clavulanate Potassium) SmithKline Beecham Pharmaceuticals 2528
Tobramycin Sulfate Injection (Tobramycin Sulfate) Elkins-Sinn 968
Vancocin HCl, Vials & ADD-Vantage (Vancomycin Hydrochloride) Lilly 1481
Zinacef (Cefuroxime Sodium) Glaxo Wellcome 1211

Septicemia, candida
Ancobon Capsules (Flucytosine) Roche Laboratories 2079

Septicemia, cryptococcus
Ancobon Capsules (Flucytosine) Roche Laboratories 2079

Septicemia, fungal
Ancobon Capsules (Flucytosine) Roche Laboratories 2079

Septicemia, gram-negative bacillary, treatment adjunct
Streptomycin Sulfate Injection (Streptomycin Sulfate) Roerig 2208

Serratia marcescens bone and joint infections
Cipro I.V. (Ciprofloxacin) Bayer Pharmaceutical 595
Cipro I.V. Pharmacy Bulk Package (Ciprofloxacin) Bayer Pharmaceutical 597
Cipro Tablets (Ciprofloxacin Hydrochloride) Bayer Pharmaceutical 592

Serratia marcescens infections
Amikacin Sulfate Injection, USP (Amikacin Sulfate) Elkins-Sinn 960
Amikin Injectable (Amikacin Sulfate) Apothecon 501
Azactam for Injection (Aztreonam) Bristol-Myers Squibb 734
Cefizox for Intramuscular or Intravenous Use (Ceftizoxime Sodium) Fujisawa 1034
Cefotan (Cefotetan) Zeneca 2829
Cipro I.V. (Ciprofloxacin) Bayer Pharmaceutical 595
Cipro I.V. Pharmacy Bulk Package (Ciprofloxacin) Bayer Pharmaceutical 597
Cipro Tablets (Ciprofloxacin Hydrochloride) Bayer Pharmaceutical 592
Claforan Sterile and Injection (Cefotaxime Sodium) Hoechst-Roussel 1235
Noroxin Tablets (Norfloxacin) Merck & Co., Inc. 1715
Noroxin Tablets (Norfloxacin) Roberts 2048
Primaxin I.V. (Imipenem-Cilastatin Sodium) Merck & Co., Inc. 1729
Rocephin Injectable Vials, ADD-Vantage, Galaxy Container (Ceftriaxone Sodium) Roche Laboratories 2142
Timentin for Injection (Ticarcillin Disodium, Clavulanate Potassium) SmithKline Beecham Pharmaceuticals 2528

Serratia marcescens infections, ocular
Chibroxin Sterile Ophthalmic Solution (Norfloxacin) Merck & Co., Inc. 1617
Ciloxan Ophthalmic Solution (Ciprofloxacin Hydrochloride) Alcon Laboratories 472
Genoptic Sterile Ophthalmic Solution (Gentamicin Sulfate) Allergan ◉ 243
Genoptic Sterile Ophthalmic Ointment (Gentamicin Sulfate) Allergan ◉ 243
Gentak (Gentamicin Sulfate) Akorn ◉ 208
Pred-G Liquifilm Sterile Ophthalmic Suspension (Gentamicin Sulfate, Prednisolone Acetate) Allergan ◉ 251
Pred-G S.O.P. Sterile Ophthalmic Ointment (Gentamicin Sulfate, Prednisolone Acetate) Allergan ◉ 252

Serratia marcescens lower respiratory tract infections
Azactam for Injection (Aztreonam) Bristol-Myers Squibb 734
Cefotan (Cefotetan) Zeneca 2829
Claforan Sterile and Injection (Cefotaxime Sodium) Hoechst-Roussel 1235
Primaxin I.V. (Imipenem-Cilastatin Sodium) Merck & Co., Inc. 1729
Rocephin Injectable Vials, ADD-Vantage, Galaxy Container (Ceftriaxone Sodium) Roche Laboratories 2142

Serratia marcescens skin and skin structure infections
Azactam for Injection (Aztreonam) Bristol-Myers Squibb 734
Claforan Sterile and Injection (Cefotaxime Sodium) Hoechst-Roussel 1235
Rocephin Injectable Vials, ADD-Vantage, Galaxy Container (Ceftriaxone Sodium) Roche Laboratories 2142

Serratia marcescens urinary tract infections
Azactam for Injection (Aztreonam) Bristol-Myers Squibb 734
Cefizox for Intramuscular or Intravenous Use (Ceftizoxime Sodium) Fujisawa 1034
Cipro I.V. (Ciprofloxacin) Bayer Pharmaceutical 595
Cipro Tablets (Ciprofloxacin Hydrochloride) Bayer Pharmaceutical 592
Claforan Sterile and Injection (Cefotaxime Sodium) Hoechst-Roussel 1235
Noroxin Tablets (Norfloxacin) Merck & Co., Inc. 1715
Noroxin Tablets (Norfloxacin) Roberts 2048
Timentin for Injection (Ticarcillin Disodium, Clavulanate Potassium) SmithKline Beecham Pharmaceuticals 2528

Serratia species infections
Amikacin Sulfate Injection, USP (Amikacin Sulfate) Elkins-Sinn 960
Amikin Injectable (Amikacin Sulfate) Apothecon 501
Azactam for Injection (Aztreonam) Bristol-Myers Squibb 734
Cefizox for Intramuscular or Intravenous Use (Ceftizoxime Sodium) Fujisawa 1034
Ceptaz (Ceftazidime) Glaxo Wellcome 1081
Fortaz (Ceftazidime) Glaxo Wellcome 1100
Garamycin Injectable (Gentamicin Sulfate) Schering 2360
Mezlin (Mezlocillin Sodium) Bayer Pharmaceutical 601
Mezlin Pharmacy Bulk Package (Mezlocillin Sodium) Bayer Pharmaceutical 604
Nebcin Vials, Hyporets & ADD-Vantage (Tobramycin Sulfate) Lilly 1464
Netromycin Injection 100 mg/ml (Netilmicin Sulfate) Schering 2373
Pipracil (Piperacillin Sodium) Lederle 1390
Primaxin I.V. (Imipenem-Cilastatin Sodium) Merck & Co., Inc. 1729
Tazicef for Injection (Ceftazidime) SmithKline Beecham Pharmaceuticals 2519
Tazidime Vials, Faspak & ADD-Vantage (Ceftazidime) Lilly 1478
Tobramycin Sulfate Injection (Tobramycin Sulfate) Elkins-Sinn 968

Serratia species lower respiratory tract infections
Cefizox for Intramuscular or Intravenous Use (Ceftizoxime Sodium) Fujisawa 1034
Ceptaz (Ceftazidime) Glaxo Wellcome 1081
Fortaz (Ceftazidime) Glaxo Wellcome 1100
Nebcin Vials, Hyporets & ADD-Vantage (Tobramycin Sulfate) Lilly 1464
Netromycin Injection 100 mg/ml (Netilmicin Sulfate) Schering 2373
Tazicef for Injection (Ceftazidime) SmithKline Beecham Pharmaceuticals 2519
Tazidime Vials, Faspak & ADD-Vantage (Ceftazidime) Lilly 1478
Tobramycin Sulfate Injection (Tobramycin Sulfate) Elkins-Sinn 968

Serratia species septicemia
Azactam for Injection (Aztreonam) Bristol-Myers Squibb 734
Cefizox for Intramuscular or Intravenous Use (Ceftizoxime Sodium) Fujisawa 1034
Ceptaz (Ceftazidime) Glaxo Wellcome 1081
Claforan Sterile and Injection (Cefotaxime Sodium) Hoechst-Roussel 1235
Fortaz (Ceftazidime) Glaxo Wellcome 1100
Netromycin Injection 100 mg/ml (Netilmicin Sulfate) Schering 2373
Pipracil (Piperacillin Sodium) Lederle 1390
Primaxin I.V. (Imipenem-Cilastatin Sodium) Merck & Co., Inc. 1729
Tazicef for Injection (Ceftazidime) SmithKline Beecham Pharmaceuticals 2519
Tazidime Vials, Faspak & ADD-Vantage (Ceftazidime) Lilly 1478

Serratia species skin and skin structure infections
Cefizox for Intramuscular or Intravenous Use (Ceftizoxime Sodium) Fujisawa 1034
Ceptaz (Ceftazidime) Glaxo Wellcome 1081
Fortaz (Ceftazidime) Glaxo Wellcome 1100
Netromycin Injection 100 mg/ml (Netilmicin Sulfate) Schering 2373
Pipracil (Piperacillin Sodium) Lederle 1390
Primaxin I.V. (Imipenem-Cilastatin Sodium) Merck & Co., Inc. 1729

(▣ Described in PDR For Nonprescription Drugs) (◉ Described in PDR For Ophthalmology)

Serratia species — Indications Index — 1540

Tazicef for Injection (Ceftazidime) SmithKline Beecham Pharmaceuticals 2519
Tazidime Vials, Faspak & ADD-Vantage (Ceftazidime) Lilly .. 1478

Serratia species urinary tract infections
Cefizox for Intramuscular or Intravenous Use (Ceftizoxime Sodium) Fujisawa 1034
Cipro I.V. Pharmacy Bulk Package (Ciprofloxacin) Bayer Pharmaceutical 597
Mezlin (Mezlocillin Sodium) Bayer Pharmaceutical 601
Mezlin Pharmacy Bulk Package (Mezlocillin Sodium) Bayer Pharmaceutical 604
Nebcin Vials, Hyporets & ADD-Vantage (Tobramycin Sulfate) Lilly 1464
Netromycin Injection 100 mg/ml (Netilmicin Sulfate) Schering 2373
Tobramycin Sulfate Injection (Tobramycin Sulfate) Elkins-Sinn 968

Serum sickness
Aristocort Suspension (Forte Parenteral) (Triamcinolone Diacetate) Fujisawa 1027
Aristocort Tablets (Triamcinolone) Fujisawa 1022
Celestone Soluspan Suspension (Betamethasone Sodium Phosphate, Betamethasone Acetate) Schering 2347
Cortone Acetate Sterile Suspension (Cortisone Acetate) Merck & Co., Inc. 1623
Cortone Acetate Tablets (Cortisone Acetate) Merck & Co., Inc. 1624
Dalalone D.P. Injectable (Dexamethasone Acetate) Forest 1011
Decadron Elixir (Dexamethasone) Merck & Co., Inc. 1633
Decadron Phosphate Injection (Dexamethasone Sodium Phosphate) Merck & Co., Inc. 1637
Decadron Tablets (Dexamethasone) Merck & Co., Inc. 1635
Decadron-LA Sterile Suspension (Dexamethasone Acetate) Merck & Co., Inc. 1646
Deltasone Tablets (Prednisone) Upjohn 2595
Depo-Medrol Single-Dose Vial (Methylprednisolone Acetate) Upjohn 2600
Depo-Medrol Sterile Aqueous Suspension (Methylprednisolone Acetate) Upjohn 2597
Hydeltrasol Injection, Sterile (Prednisolone Sodium Phosphate) Merck & Co., Inc. 1665
Hydrocortone Phosphate Injection, Sterile (Hydrocortisone Sodium Phosphate) Merck & Co., Inc. 1670
Hydrocortone Tablets (Hydrocortisone) Merck & Co., Inc. 1672
Medrol (Methylprednisolone) Upjohn 2621
Pediapred Oral Liquid (Prednisolone Sodium Phosphate) Fisons 995
Prelone Syrup (Prednisolone) Muro 1787
Solu-Cortef Sterile Powder (Hydrocortisone Sodium Succinate) Upjohn 2641
Solu-Medrol Sterile Powder (Methylprednisolone Sodium Succinate) Upjohn 2643

Shigella flexneri enteritis
Bactrim DS Tablets (Trimethoprim, Sulfamethoxazole) Roche Laboratories 2084
Bactrim I.V. Infusion (Trimethoprim, Sulfamethoxazole) Roche Laboratories 2082
Bactrim (Trimethoprim, Sulfamethoxazole) Roche Laboratories 2084
Septra (Trimethoprim, Sulfamethoxazole) Glaxo Wellcome 1174
Septra I.V. Infusion (Trimethoprim, Sulfamethoxazole) Glaxo Wellcome 1169
Septra I.V. Infusion ADD-Vantage Vials (Trimethoprim, Sulfamethoxazole) Glaxo Wellcome 1171
Septra (Trimethoprim, Sulfamethoxazole) Glaxo Wellcome 1174

Shigella flexneri infectious diarrhea
Cipro Tablets (Ciprofloxacin Hydrochloride) Bayer Pharmaceutical 592

Shigella sonnei enteritis
Bactrim DS Tablets (Trimethoprim, Sulfamethoxazole) Roche Laboratories 2084
Bactrim I.V. Infusion (Trimethoprim, Sulfamethoxazole) Roche Laboratories 2082
Bactrim (Trimethoprim, Sulfamethoxazole) Roche Laboratories 2084
Septra (Trimethoprim, Sulfamethoxazole) Glaxo Wellcome 1174
Septra I.V. Infusion (Trimethoprim, Sulfamethoxazole) Glaxo Wellcome 1169
Septra I.V. Infusion ADD-Vantage Vials (Trimethoprim, Sulfamethoxazole) Glaxo Wellcome 1171
Septra (Trimethoprim, Sulfamethoxazole) Glaxo Wellcome 1174

Shigella sonnei infectious diarrhea
Cipro Tablets (Ciprofloxacin Hydrochloride) Bayer Pharmaceutical 592

Shigella species infections
Achromycin V Capsules (Tetracycline Hydrochloride) Lederle 1367
Declomycin Tablets (Demeclocycline Hydrochloride) Lederle 1371
Doryx Capsules (Doxycycline Hyclate) Parke-Davis 1913
Dynacin Capsules (Minocycline Hydrochloride) Medicis 1590
Minocin Intravenous (Minocycline Hydrochloride) Lederle 1382
Minocin Oral Suspension (Minocycline Hydrochloride) Lederle 1385
Minocin Pellet-Filled Capsules (Minocycline Hydrochloride) Lederle 1383
Monodox Capsules (Doxycycline Monohydrate) Oclassen 1805
Omnipen Capsules (Ampicillin) Wyeth-Ayerst 2764
Omnipen for Oral Suspension (Ampicillin) Wyeth-Ayerst 2765
Pfizerpen for Injection (Penicillin G Potassium) Roerig 2203
Septra I.V. Infusion ADD-Vantage Vials (Trimethoprim, Sulfamethoxazole) Glaxo Wellcome 1171
Terramycin Intramuscular Solution (Oxytetracycline) Roerig 2210
Vibramycin (Doxycycline Calcium) Pfizer Labs 1941
Vibramycin Hyclate Intravenous (Doxycycline Hyclate) Roerig 2215
Vibramycin (Doxycycline Monohydrate) Pfizer Labs 1941

Shigellosis
Bactrim DS Tablets (Trimethoprim, Sulfamethoxazole) Roche Laboratories 2084
Bactrim I.V. Infusion (Trimethoprim, Sulfamethoxazole) Roche Laboratories 2082
Bactrim (Trimethoprim, Sulfamethoxazole) Roche Laboratories 2084
Septra (Trimethoprim, Sulfamethoxazole) Glaxo Wellcome 1174
Septra I.V. Infusion (Trimethoprim, Sulfamethoxazole) Glaxo Wellcome 1169
Septra I.V. Infusion ADD-Vantage Vials (Trimethoprim, Sulfamethoxazole) Glaxo Wellcome 1171
Septra (Trimethoprim, Sulfamethoxazole) Glaxo Wellcome 1174

Shingles (see under Herpes zoster infections)

Shock, emergency treatment of
Albuminar-5, Albumin (Human) U.S.P. 5% (Albumin (Human)) Armour 512
Albuminar-25, Albumin (Human) U.S.P. 25% (Albumin (Human)) Armour 513
Plasma-Plex, Plasma Protein Fraction (Human) 5% (Plasma Protein Fraction (Human)) Armour 524

Shock, suspected adrenocortical insufficiency
Celestone Soluspan Suspension (Betamethasone Sodium Phosphate, Betamethasone Acetate) Schering 2347
Cortone Acetate Sterile Suspension (Cortisone Acetate) Merck & Co., Inc. 1623
Decadron Phosphate Injection (Dexamethasone Sodium Phosphate) Merck & Co., Inc. 1637
Hydrocortone Phosphate Injection, Sterile (Hydrocortisone Sodium Phosphate) Merck & Co., Inc. 1670
Solu-Cortef Sterile Powder (Hydrocortisone Sodium Succinate) Upjohn 2641
Solu-Medrol Sterile Powder (Methylprednisolone Sodium Succinate) Upjohn 2643

Shoulder, acute painful (see under Bursitis, subacromial, acute, symptomatic relief of)

Sialorrhea associated with Parkinsonism
Levsin/Levsinex/Levbid (Hyoscyamine Sulfate) Schwarz 2405

Sinus congestion, symptomatic relief of
Actifed Plus Caplets (Acetaminophen, Pseudoephedrine Hydrochloride, Triprolidine Hydrochloride) WARNER WELLCOME .... ■ 845
Actifed Plus Tablets (Acetaminophen, Pseudoephedrine Hydrochloride, Triprolidine Hydrochloride) WARNER WELLCOME .... ■ 845
Actifed Sinus Daytime/Nighttime Tablets and Caplets (Acetaminophen, Diphenhydramine Hydrochloride, Pseudoephedrine Hydrochloride) WARNER WELLCOME .... ■ 846
Afrin (Oxymetazoline Hydrochloride) Schering-Plough HealthCare .... ■ 797
Alka-Seltzer Plus Cold Medicine (Chlorpheniramine Maleate, Aspirin, Phenylpropanolamine Bitartrate) Miles Consumer .... ■ 705
Chlor-Trimeton Allergy Decongestant Tablets (Chlorpheniramine Maleate, Pseudoephedrine Sulfate) Schering-Plough HealthCare .... ■ 799
Allergy-Sinus Comtrex Multi-Symptom Allergy-Sinus Formula Tablets (Acetaminophen, Chlorpheniramine Maleate, Pseudoephedrine Hydrochloride) Bristol-Myers Products .... ■ 617
Comtrex Non-Drowsy (Acetaminophen, Dextromethorphan Hydrobromide, Pseudoephedrine Hydrochloride) Bristol-Myers Products .... ■ 618
Contac Day & Night (Acetaminophen) SmithKline Beecham Consumer .... ■ 812
Coricidin 'D' Decongestant Tablets (Acetaminophen, Chlorpheniramine Maleate, Phenylpropanolamine Hydrochloride) Schering-Plough HealthCare .... ■ 800
Dimetapp Elixir (Brompheniramine Maleate, Phenylpropanolamine Hydrochloride) A. H. Robins Consumer .... ■ 773
Dimetapp Extentabs (Brompheniramine Maleate, Phenylpropanolamine Hydrochloride) A. H. Robins Consumer .... ■ 774
Drixoral Cold and Allergy Sustained-Action Tablets (Dexbrompheniramine Maleate, Pseudoephedrine Sulfate) Schering-Plough HealthCare .... ■ 802
Drixoral Cold and Flu Extended-Release Tablets (Acetaminophen, Dexbrompheniramine Maleate, Pseudoephedrine Sulfate) Schering-Plough HealthCare .... ■ 803
Drixoral Allergy/Sinus Extended Release Tablets (Acetaminophen, Pseudoephedrine Sulfate, Dexbrompheniramine Maleate) Schering-Plough HealthCare .... ■ 804
Novahistine DMX (Dextromethorphan Hydrobromide, Guaifenesin, Pseudoephedrine Hydrochloride) SmithKline Beecham Consumer .... ■ 822
Sine-Aid Maximum Strength Sinus Medication Gelcaps, Caplets and Tablets (Acetaminophen, Pseudoephedrine Hydrochloride) McNeil Consumer 1554
Sine-Off No Drowsiness Formula Caplets (Acetaminophen, Pseudoephedrine Hydrochloride) SmithKline Beecham Consumer .... ■ 824
Sine-Off Sinus Medicine (Aspirin, Chlorpheniramine Maleate, Phenylpropanolamine Hydrochloride) SmithKline Beecham Consumer .... ■ 825
Sinulin Tablets (Acetaminophen, Phenylpropanolamine Hydrochloride, Chlorpheniramine Maleate) Carnrick 787
Sinutab Non-Drying Liquid Caps (Pseudoephedrine Hydrochloride, Guaifenesin) WARNER WELLCOME .... ■ 859
Sinutab Sinus Allergy Medication, Maximum Strength Tablets and Caplets (Acetaminophen, Chlorpheniramine Maleate, Pseudoephedrine Hydrochloride) WARNER WELLCOME .... ■ 860
Sinutab Sinus Medication, Maximum Strength Without Drowsiness Formula, Tablets & Caplets (Acetaminophen, Pseudoephedrine Hydrochloride) WARNER WELLCOME .... ■ 860
Sinutab Sinus Medication, Regular Strength Without Drowsiness Formula (Acetaminophen, Pseudoephedrine Hydrochloride) WARNER WELLCOME .... ■ 859
Sudafed Sinus Caplets (Acetaminophen, Pseudoephedrine Hydrochloride) WARNER WELLCOME .... ■ 864
Sudafed Sinus Tablets (Acetaminophen, Pseudoephedrine Hydrochloride) WARNER WELLCOME .... ■ 864
Triaminic Cold Tablets (Phenylpropanolamine Hydrochloride, Chlorpheniramine Maleate) Sandoz Consumer .... ■ 790
Triaminic-12 Tablets (Phenylpropanolamine Hydrochloride, Chlorpheniramine Maleate) Sandoz Consumer .... ■ 792
Triaminicin Tablets (Acetaminophen, Chlorpheniramine Maleate, Phenylpropanolamine Hydrochloride) Sandoz Consumer .... ■ 793
Triaminicol Multi-Symptom Cold Tablets (Phenylpropanolamine Hydrochloride, Chlorpheniramine Maleate, Dextromethorphan Hydrobromide) Sandoz Consumer .... ■ 793
TYLENOL Maximum Strength Allergy Sinus Medication Gelcaps and Caplets (Acetaminophen, Chlorpheniramine Maleate, Pseudoephedrine Hydrochloride) McNeil Consumer 1563

(■ Described in PDR For Nonprescription Drugs) (◉ Described in PDR For Ophthalmology)

1541 **Indications Index** **Skin**

TYLENOL Maximum Strength Allergy Sinus NightTime Medication Caplets (Acetaminophen, Pseudoephedrine Hydrochloride, Diphenhydramine Hydrochloride) McNeil Consumer 1555
TYLENOL, Maximum Strength, Sinus Medication Geltabs, Gelcaps, Caplets and Tablets (Acetaminophen, Pseudoephedrine Hydrochloride) McNeil Consumer 1566
Ursinus Inlay-Tabs (Aspirin, Pseudoephedrine Hydrochloride) Sandoz Consumer ▣ 794
Vicks DayQuil SINUS Pressure & CONGESTION Relief (Guaifenesin, Phenylpropanolamine Hydrochloride) Procter & Gamble ▣ 761
Vicks Sinex 12-Hour Nasal Decongestant Spray and Ultra Fine Mist (Oxymetazoline Hydrochloride) Procter & Gamble ▣ 765
Vicks Sinex Nasal Spray and Ultra Fine Mist (Phenylephrine Hydrochloride) Procter & Gamble ▣ 765
Vicks Vapor Inhaler (Desoxyephedrine-Levo) Procter & Gamble ▣ 765

Sinus headache
Actifed Sinus Daytime/Nighttime Tablets and Caplets (Acetaminophen, Diphenhydramine Hydrochloride, Pseudoephedrine Hydrochloride) WARNER WELLCOME ▣ 846
Alka-Seltzer Plus Cold Medicine (Chlorpheniramine Maleate, Aspirin, Phenylpropanolamine Bitartrate) Miles Consumer ▣ 705
Alka Seltzer Plus Sinus Medicine (Phenylpropanolamine Bitartrate, Aspirin, Brompheniramine Maleate) Miles Consumer ▣ 707
Bayer Select Sinus Pain Relief Formula (Acetaminophen, Pseudoephedrine Hydrochloride) Miles Consumer ▣ 717
Allergy-Sinus Comtrex Multi-Symptom Allergy-Sinus Formula Tablets (Acetaminophen, Chlorpheniramine Maleate, Pseudoephedrine Hydrochloride) Bristol-Myers Products ▣ 617
Contac Day & Night (Acetaminophen) SmithKline Beecham Consumer ▣ 812
Coricidin 'D' Decongestant Tablets (Acetaminophen, Chlorpheniramine Maleate, Phenylpropanolamine Hydrochloride) Schering-Plough HealthCare ▣ 800
Drixoral Allergy/Sinus Extended Release Tablets (Acetaminophen, Pseudoephedrine Sulfate, Dexbrompheniramine Maleate) Schering-Plough HealthCare ▣ 804
Sinarest (Acetaminophen, Chlorpheniramine Maleate, Pseudoephedrine Hydrochloride) CIBA Consumer ▣ 648
Sine-Aid Maximum Strength Sinus Medication Gelcaps, Caplets and Tablets (Acetaminophen, Pseudoephedrine Hydrochloride) McNeil Consumer 1554
Singlet Tablets (Acetaminophen, Chlorpheniramine Maleate, Pseudoephedrine Hydrochloride) SmithKline Beecham Consumer ▣ 825
Sinutab Sinus Allergy Medication, Maximum Strength Tablets and Caplets (Acetaminophen, Chlorpheniramine Maleate, Pseudoephedrine Hydrochloride) WARNER WELLCOME ▣ 860
Sinutab Sinus Medication, Maximum Strength Without Drowsiness Formula, Tablets & Caplets (Acetaminophen, Pseudoephedrine Hydrochloride) WARNER WELLCOME ▣ 860
Sinutab Sinus Medication, Regular Strength Without Drowsiness Formula (Acetaminophen, Pseudoephedrine Hydrochloride) WARNER WELLCOME ▣ 859
Sudafed Sinus Caplets (Acetaminophen, Pseudoephedrine Hydrochloride) WARNER WELLCOME ▣ 864
Sudafed Sinus Tablets (Acetaminophen, Pseudoephedrine Hydrochloride) WARNER WELLCOME ▣ 864
TYLENOL Maximum Strength Allergy Sinus Medication Gelcaps and Caplets (Acetaminophen, Chlorpheniramine Maleate, Pseudoephedrine Hydrochloride) McNeil Consumer 1563
TYLENOL Maximum Strength Allergy Sinus NightTime Medication Caplets (Acetaminophen, Pseudoephedrine Hydrochloride, Diphenhydramine Hydrochloride) McNeil Consumer 1555
TYLENOL, Maximum Strength, Sinus Medication Geltabs, Gelcaps, Caplets and Tablets (Acetaminophen, Pseudoephedrine Hydrochloride) McNeil Consumer 1566
Ursinus Inlay-Tabs (Aspirin, Pseudoephedrine Hydrochloride) Sandoz Consumer ▣ 794
Vicks DayQuil SINUS Pressure & PAIN Relief with IBUPROFEN (Ibuprofen, Pseudoephedrine Hydrochloride) Procter & Gamble ▣ 762

Sinusitis, adjunctive therapy
Advil Cold and Sinus Caplets and Tablets (formerly CoAdvil) (Ibuprofen, Pseudoephedrine Hydrochloride) Whitehall ▣ 870
Afrin (Oxymetazoline Hydrochloride) Schering-Plough HealthCare ▣ 797
Alka Seltzer Plus Sinus Medicine (Phenylpropanolamine Bitartrate, Aspirin, Brompheniramine Maleate) Miles Consumer ▣ 707
Allerest Children's Chewable Tablets (Chlorpheniramine Maleate, Phenylpropanolamine Hydrochloride) CIBA Consumer ▣ 627
Allerest Headache Strength Tablets (Acetaminophen, Chlorpheniramine Maleate, Pseudoephedrine Hydrochloride) CIBA Consumer ▣ 627
Allerest Maximum Strength Tablets (Chlorpheniramine Maleate, Pseudoephedrine Hydrochloride) CIBA Consumer ▣ 627
Allerest No Drowsiness Tablets (Acetaminophen, Pseudoephedrine Hydrochloride) CIBA Consumer ▣ 627
Allerest Sinus Pain Formula (Acetaminophen, Chlorpheniramine Maleate, Pseudoephedrine Hydrochloride) CIBA Consumer ▣ 627
Allerest 12 Hour Caplets (Chlorpheniramine Maleate, Phenylpropanolamine Hydrochloride) CIBA Consumer ▣ 627
Allergy-Sinus Comtrex Multi-Symptom Allergy-Sinus Formula Tablets (Acetaminophen, Chlorpheniramine Maleate, Pseudoephedrine Hydrochloride) Bristol-Myers Products ▣ 617
Congess (Guaifenesin, Pseudoephedrine Hydrochloride) Fleming 1004
Deconamine (Chlorpheniramine Maleate, Pseudoephedrine Hydrochloride) Kenwood 1320
Drixoral Cold and Flu Extended-Release Tablets (Acetaminophen, Dexbrompheniramine Maleate, Pseudoephedrine Sulfate) Schering-Plough HealthCare ▣ 803
Entex Capsules (Phenylephrine Hydrochloride, Phenylpropanolamine Hydrochloride, Guaifenesin) Procter & Gamble Pharmaceuticals 1986
Entex LA Tablets (Phenylpropanolamine Hydrochloride, Guaifenesin) Procter & Gamble Pharmaceuticals 1987
Entex Liquid (Phenylephrine Hydrochloride, Phenylpropanolamine Hydrochloride, Guaifenesin) Procter & Gamble Pharmaceuticals 1986
Excedrin Extra-Strength Analgesic Tablets & Caplets (Acetaminophen, Aspirin, Caffeine) Bristol-Myers Products 732
Exgest LA Tablets (Phenylpropanolamine Hydrochloride, Guaifenesin) Carnrick 782
4-Way Fast Acting Nasal Spray (regular & mentholated) (Naphazoline Hydrochloride, Phenylephrine Hydrochloride, Pyrilamine Maleate) Bristol-Myers Products ▣ 621
4-Way Long Lasting Nasal Spray (Oxymetazoline Hydrochloride) Bristol-Myers Products ▣ 621
Fedahist Gyrocaps (Pseudoephedrine Hydrochloride, Chlorpheniramine Maleate) Schwarz 2401
Fedahist Timecaps (Pseudoephedrine Hydrochloride, Chlorpheniramine Maleate) Schwarz 2401
Humibid DM Tablets (Guaifenesin, Dextromethorphan Hydrobromide) Adams 462
Kronofed-A (Chlorpheniramine Maleate, Pseudoephedrine Hydrochloride) Ferndale 977
Motrin IB Sinus (Ibuprofen, Pseudoephedrine Hydrochloride) Upjohn ▣ 838
NTZ Long Acting Nasal Spray & Drops 0.05% (Oxymetazoline Hydrochloride) Miles Consumer ▣ 727
Neo-Synephrine Maximum Strength 12 Hour Nasal Spray (Oxymetazoline Hydrochloride) Miles Consumer ▣ 726
Neo-Synephrine Maximum Strength 12 Hour Nasal Spray Pump (Oxymetazoline Hydrochloride) Miles Consumer ▣ 726
Neo-Synephrine (Phenylephrine Hydrochloride) Miles Consumer ▣ 726
Nolamine Timed-Release Tablets (Phenindamine Tartrate, Phenylpropanolamine Hydrochloride, Chlorpheniramine Maleate) Carnrick 785
Propagest Tablets (Phenylpropanolamine Hydrochloride) Carnrick 786
Rynatan (Chlorpheniramine Tannate, Pyrilamine Tannate, Phenylephrine Tannate) Wallace 2673
Sinarest Tablets (Acetaminophen, Chlorpheniramine Maleate, Pseudoephedrine Hydrochloride) CIBA Consumer ▣ 648
Sinarest Extra Strength Tablets (Acetaminophen, Chlorpheniramine Maleate, Pseudoephedrine Hydrochloride) CIBA Consumer ▣ 648
Sinarest No Drowsiness Tablets (Acetaminophen, Pseudoephedrine Hydrochloride) CIBA Consumer ▣ 648
Sine-Off No Drowsiness Formula Caplets (Acetaminophen, Pseudoephedrine Hydrochloride) SmithKline Beecham Consumer ▣ 824
Sine-Off Sinus Medicine (Aspirin, Chlorpheniramine Maleate, Phenylpropanolamine Hydrochloride) SmithKline Beecham Consumer ▣ 825
Sinulin Tablets (Acetaminophen, Phenylpropanolamine Hydrochloride, Chlorpheniramine Maleate) Carnrick 787
Sinutab Sinus Allergy Medication, Maximum Strength Tablets and Caplets (Acetaminophen, Chlorpheniramine Maleate, Pseudoephedrine Hydrochloride) WARNER WELLCOME ▣ 860
Sinutab Sinus Medication, Maximum Strength Without Drowsiness Formula, Tablets & Caplets (Acetaminophen, Pseudoephedrine Hydrochloride) WARNER WELLCOME ▣ 860
Sinutab Sinus Medication, Regular Strength Without Drowsiness Formula (Acetaminophen, Pseudoephedrine Hydrochloride) WARNER WELLCOME ▣ 859
Syn-Rx Tablets (Pseudoephedrine Hydrochloride, Guaifenesin) Adams 465
Teldrin 12 Hour Antihistamine/Nasal Decongestant Allergy Relief Capsules (Chlorpheniramine Maleate, Phenylpropanolamine Hydrochloride) SmithKline Beecham Consumer ▣ 826
Triaminic-12 Tablets (Phenylpropanolamine Hydrochloride, Chlorpheniramine Maleate) Sandoz Consumer ▣ 792
Triaminicol Multi-Symptom Cold Tablets (Phenylpropanolamine Hydrochloride, Chlorpheniramine Maleate, Dextromethorphan Hydrobromide) Sandoz Consumer ▣ 793
TYLENOL Maximum Strength Allergy Sinus Medication Gelcaps and Caplets (Acetaminophen, Chlorpheniramine Maleate, Pseudoephedrine Hydrochloride) McNeil Consumer 1563
Ursinus Inlay-Tabs (Aspirin, Pseudoephedrine Hydrochloride) Sandoz Consumer ▣ 794

Sinusitis, treatment of
Augmentin (Amoxicillin Trihydrate, Clavulanate Potassium) SmithKline Beecham Pharmaceuticals 2468
Biaxin (Clarithromycin) Abbott 405
Dimetapp Cold & Allergy Chewable Tablets (Brompheniramine Maleate, Phenylpropanolamine Hydrochloride) A. H. Robins Consumer ▣ 773
Lorabid Suspension and Pulvules (Loracarbef) Lilly 1459

Skin grafting, treatment adjunct
Furacin Soluble Dressing (Nitrofurazone) Roberts 2045
Furacin Topical Cream (Nitrofurazone) Roberts 2045

Skin infections, bacterial, minor (see under Infections, skin, bacterial, minor)

Skin lacerations, infected (see under Infections, skin and skin structure)

Skin, bactericidal/virucidal cleansing of
Betadine Skin Cleanser (Povidone Iodine) Purdue Frederick 1992
Betadine Surgical Scrub (Povidone Iodine) Purdue Frederick 1992

Skin, bacteriostatic cleansing of
Barri-Care Antimicrobial Barrier Ointment (Chloroxylenol) Care-Tech ▣ 624
Betasept Surgical Scrub (Chlorhexidine Gluconate) Purdue Frederick 1993
Care Creme Antimicrobial Cream (Chloroxylenol) Care-Tech ▣ 624
Clinical Care Dermal Wound Cleanser (Benzethonium Chloride) Care-Tech ▣ 625
Hibiclens Antimicrobial Skin Cleanser (Chlorhexidine Gluconate) Zeneca 2840
Hibistat (Chlorhexidine Gluconate) Zeneca 2841
Lever 2000 (Triclosan) Lever ▣ 672
Orchid Fresh II Perineal/Ostomy Cleanser (Benzethonium Chloride) Care-Tech ▣ 625
pHisoHex (Hexachlorophene) Sanofi Winthrop 2327
Satin Antimicrobial Skin Cleanser for Diabetic/Cancer Patient Care (Chloroxylenol) Care-Tech ▣ 625

Skin **Indications Index** 1542

Stri-Dex Antibacterial Cleansing Bar (Triclosan) Miles Consumer ◘ 730
Stri-Dex Antibacterial Face Wash (Triclosan) Miles Consumer ◘ 730
Techni-Care Surgical Scrub and Wound Cleanser (Chloroxylenol) Care-Tech ◘ 625
Zephiran (Benzalkonium Chloride) Sanofi Winthrop ◘ 795

Skin, dry, moisturization of

Alpha Keri Moisture Rich Body Oil (Lanolin Oil) Bristol-Myers Products ◘ 613
Aquaderm Cream (Caprylic/Capric Triglyceride) Baker Cummins ◘ 604
Aquaderm Lotion (Caprylic/Capric Triglyceride) Baker Cummins ◘ 604
Aquaphor Healing Ointment (Petrolatum, Mineral Oil) Beiersdorf 640
Aquaphor Healing Ointment, Original Formula (Mineral Oil, Petrolatum) Beiersdorf 640
Atrac-Tain, Moisturizing Cream (Urea, Lactic Acid) Sween 2554
Cetaphil Moisturizing Cream (Moisturizing formula) Galderma 1046
Cetaphil Mositurizing Lotion (Moisturizing formula) Galderma 1046
Complex 15 Therapeutic Moisturizing Face Cream (Dimethicone, Lecithin) Schering-Plough HealthCare ◘ 800
Complex 15 Therapeutic Moisturizing Lotion (Dimethicone, Lecithin) Schering-Plough HealthCare ◘ 799
Curel Lotion and Cream (Moisturizing formula) Bausch & Lomb Personal ◘ 606
DML Facial Moisturizer with Sunscreen (Glycerin, Hyaluronic Acid, Octyl Methoxycinnamate, Oxybenzone) Persōn & Covey 1932
DML Forte Cream (Petrolatum) Persōn & Covey 1932
Dermasil Dry Skin Concentrated Treatment (Glycerin, Dimethicone) Chesebrough-Pond's ◘ 627
Dermasil Dry Skin Treatment Cream (Dimethicone) Chesebrough-Pond's ◘ 626
Dermasil Dry Skin Treatment Lotion (Dimethicone) Chesebrough-Pond's ◘ 626
Eucerin Original Moisturizing Creme (Unscented) (Mineral Oil, Petrolatum) Beiersdorf 641
Eucerin Facial Moisturizing Lotion SPF 25 (Phenylbenzimidazole-5-Sulfonic Acid, Titanium Dioxide, 2-Ethylhexyl-p-Methoxycinnamate, 2-Ethylhexyl Salicylate) Beiersdorf 641
Eucerin Original Moisturizing Lotion (Isopropyl Myristate, Mineral Oil) Beiersdorf 641
Eucerin Plus Dry Skin Care Moisturizing Lotion (Mineral Oil, Urea) Beiersdorf 641
Eucerin Plus Moisturizing Creme (Urea, Mineral Oil) Beiersdorf 641
Keri Lotion (Mineral Oil) Bristol-Myers Products ◘ 622
Lac-Hydrin 12% Lotion (Ammonium Lactate) Westwood-Squibb 2687
Lubriderm Bath and Shower Oil (Emollient, Mineral Oil) WARNER WELLCOME ◘ 856
Lubriderm Care Lotion (Emollient) WARNER WELLCOME ◘ 856
Lubriderm Moisture Recovery Alpha Hydroxy Formula Cream and Lotion (Moisturizing formula) WARNER WELLCOME ◘ 856
Lubriderm Moisture Recovery GelCreme (Cetyl Alcohol, Glycerin, Mineral Oil) WARNER WELLCOME ◘ 857
Lubriderm Seriously Sensitive Lotion (Glycerin, Mineral Oil, Petrolatum) WARNER WELLCOME ◘ 857
Moisturel Cream (Dimethicone, Petrolatum) Westwood-Squibb 2688
Moisturel Lotion (Dimethicone) Westwood-Squibb 2688
Pen•Kera Creme (Glycerin, Polyamide Sugar Condensate, Urea) Ascher ◘ 603
Prophyllin CCC Topical Emollient Ointment (Petrolatum, White) Rystan 2247
StePHan Bio-Nutritional Daytime Hydrating Creme (Chamomile) Wellness International ◘ 867
StePHan Bio-Nutritional Eye-Firming Concentrate (Chamomile) Wellness International ◘ 868
StePHan Bio-Nutritional Nightime Moisture Creme (Moisturizing formula) Wellness International ◘ 868
StePHan Bio-Nutritional Ultra Hydrating Fluid (Moisturizing formula) Wellness International ◘ 868
Ultra Derm Moisturizer (Propylene Glycol, Mineral Oil) Baker Cummins ◘ 605
Ultra Mide 25 Extra Strength Moisturizer (Urea, Mineral Oil) Baker Cummins ◘ 605
Ultra Mide 25 Lotion (Urea, Mineral Oil, Glycerin) Baker Cummins ◘ 605

Skin, emollient cleansing of

Aquanil Lotion (Cetyl Alcohol, Glycerin) Persōn & Covey 1932
Bio-Complex 5000 Gentle Foaming Cleanser (Aloe Vera) Wellness International ◘ 865
Cetaphil Gentle Cleansing Bar (Cleanser) Galderma 1046
Cetaphil Skin Cleanser (Cetyl Alcohol) Galderma 1046
Dove (Sodium Tallowate) Lever ◘ 672
Eucerin Dry Skin Therapy Cleansing Bar (Eucerite) Beiersdorf 641
StePHan Bio-Nutritional Refreshing Moisture Gel (Moisturizing formula) Wellness International ◘ 868

Skin, hyperpigmentation (see under Hyperpigmentation, skin, bleaching of)

Skin, increased tolerance to sunlight

Aquaderm Sunscreen/Moisturizer SPF 15 (Octyl Methoxycinnamate, Oxybenzone) Baker Cummins ◘ 604
Eucerin Facial Moisturizing Lotion SPF 25 (Phenylbenzimidazole-5-Sulfonic Acid, Titanium Dioxide, 2-Ethylhexyl-p-Methoxycinnamate, 2-Ethylhexyl Salicylate) Beiersdorf 641
Solbar PF 15 (Octyl Methoxycinnamate, Oxybenzone) Persōn & Covey 1932
Solbar PF Ultra Cream SPF 50 (PABA Free) (Oxybenzone) Persōn & Covey 1932
Trisoralen Tablets (Trioxsalen) ICN 1264

Skin, inflammatory conditions (see also under Rash, diaper; Dermatitis, contact; Dermatoses, corticosteroid-responsive)

Acid Mantle Creme (Petrolatum, White) Sandoz Consumer ◘ 785
Aquanil HC Lotion (Hydrocortisone) Persōn & Covey 1931
Bactine Hydrocortisone Anti-Itch Cream (Hydrocortisone) Miles Consumer ◘ 709
Benadryl Itch Relief Cream, Children's Formula and Maximum Strength 2% (Diphenhydramine Hydrochloride, Zinc Acetate) WARNER WELLCOME ◘ 851
Caldecort (Hydrocortisone Acetate) CIBA Consumer ◘ 631
Caldesene (Petrolatum, Zinc Oxide) CIBA Consumer ◘ 632
Chloresium (Chlorophyllin Copper Complex) Rystan 2246
Cortaid Spray (Hydrocortisone) Upjohn ◘ 836
Cortizone-5 (Hydrocortisone) Thompson Medical ◘ 831
Critic-Aid, Antimicrobial Skin Paste (Zinc Oxide, Benzethonium Chloride) Sween 2554
Cutivate Cream (Fluticasone Propionate) Glaxo Wellcome 1088
Cutivate Ointment (Fluticasone Propionate) Glaxo Wellcome 1089
Dermatop Emollient Cream 0.1% (Prednicarbate) Hoechst-Roussel 1238
Diprolene Gel 0.05% (Betamethasone Dipropionate) Schering 2353
Diprolene Lotion 0.05% (Betamethasone Dipropionate) Schering 2352
Mantadil Cream (Chlorcyclizine Hydrochloride) Glaxo Wellcome 1135
ProctoCream-HC 2.5% (Hydrocortisone) Schwarz 2408
Psorcon Cream 0.05% (Diflorasone Diacetate) Dermik 909

Skin, irritation, minor, pain associated with (see under Pain, topical relief of)

Skin, irritation, minor, temporary relief of

Caladryl Clear Lotion (Pramoxine Hydrochloride, Zinc Acetate) WARNER WELLCOME ◘ 853
Clocream Skin Protectant Cream (Vitamin A & Vitamin D) Roberts ◘ 770
Critic-Aid, Antimicrobial Skin Paste (Zinc Oxide, Benzethonium Chloride) Sween 2554
Desitin Cornstarch Baby Powder (Zinc Oxide, Corn Starch) Pfizer Consumer ◘ 742
Domeboro Astringent Solution Effervescent Tablets (Aluminum Acetate, Calcium Acetate) Miles Consumer ◘ 721
Domeboro Astringent Solution Powder Packets (Aluminum Acetate, Calcium Acetate) Miles Consumer ◘ 720
Formula Magic Antibacterial Powder (Benzethonium Chloride) Care-Tech ◘ 625
Moisturel Cream (Dimethicone, Petrolatum) Westwood-Squibb 2688
Moisturel Lotion (Dimethicone) Westwood-Squibb 2688
Nupercainal Pain Relief Cream (Dibucaine) CIBA Consumer ◘ 645

Sleep, induction of (see also under Sedation)

Ambien Tablets (Zolpidem Tartrate) Searle 2416
Brevital Sodium Vials (Methohexital Sodium) Lilly 1429
Butisol Sodium Elixir & Tablets (Butabarbital Sodium) Wallace 2660
Dalmane Capsules (Flurazepam Hydrochloride) Roche Products 2173
Doral Tablets (Quazepam) Wallace 2664
Halcion Tablets (Triazolam) Upjohn 2611
Hyland's Calms Forté Tablets (Homeopathic Medications) Standard Homeopathic ◘ 828
Mebaral Tablets (Mephobarbital) Sanofi Winthrop 2322
Miles Nervine Nighttime Sleep-Aid (Diphenhydramine Hydrochloride) Miles Consumer ◘ 723
Nembutal Sodium Capsules (Pentobarbital Sodium) Abbott 436
Nembutal Sodium Solution (Pentobarbital Sodium) Abbott 438
Nembutal Sodium Suppositories (Pentobarbital Sodium) Abbott 440
Maximum Strength Nytol Caplets (Doxylamine Succinate) Block ◘ 610
Nytol QuickCaps Caplets (Diphenhydramine Hydrochloride) Block ◘ 610
Phenobarbital Elixir and Tablets (Phenobarbital) Lilly 1469
Placidyl Capsules (Ethchlorvynol) Abbott 448
ProSom Tablets (Estazolam) Abbott 449
Restoril Capsules (Temazepam) Sandoz Pharmaceuticals 2284
Seconal Sodium Pulvules (Secobarbital Sodium) Lilly 1474
Sleepinal Night-time Sleep Aid Capsules and Softgels (Diphenhydramine Hydrochloride) Thompson Medical ◘ 834
Maximum Strength Unisom Sleepgels (Diphenhydramine Hydrochloride) Pfizer Consumer 1934
Unisom Nighttime Sleep Aid (Doxylamine Succinate) Pfizer Consumer 1934
Versed Injection (Midazolam Hydrochloride) Roche Laboratories 2170

Smoking cessation, temporary aid to

Habitrol Nicotine Transdermal System (Nicotine) Ciba Self-Medication 865
Nicoderm (nicotine transdermal system) (Nicotine) Marion Merrell Dow 1518
Nicorette (Nicotine Polacrilex) SmithKline Beecham 2458
Nicotrol Nicotine Transdermal System (Nicotine) McNeil Consumer 1550
Prostep (nicotine transdermal system) (Nicotine) Lederle 1394

Sneezing

Actifed Syrup (Pseudoephedrine Hydrochloride, Triprolidine Hydrochloride) WARNER WELLCOME ◘ 846
Actifed Tablets (Pseudoephedrine Hydrochloride, Triprolidine Hydrochloride) WARNER WELLCOME ◘ 844
Benadryl Allergy Decongestant Tablets (Diphenhydramine Hydrochloride, Pseudoephedrine Hydrochloride) WARNER WELLCOME ◘ 848
Benadryl Allergy Liquid Medication (Diphenhydramine Hydrochloride) WARNER WELLCOME ◘ 849
Benadryl Allergy (Diphenhydramine Hydrochloride) WARNER WELLCOME ◘ 848
Benadryl Allergy Sinus Headache Formula Caplets (Diphenhydramine Hydrochloride, Pseudoephedrine Hydrochloride, Acetaminophen) WARNER WELLCOME ◘ 849
Benadryl Dye-Free Allergy Liqui-gel Softgels (Diphenhydramine Hydrochloride) WARNER WELLCOME ◘ 850
Benadryl Dye-Free Allergy Liquid Medication (Diphenhydramine Hydrochloride) WARNER WELLCOME ◘ 850
Bromfed Syrup (Brompheniramine Maleate, Pseudoephedrine Hydrochloride) Muro ◘ 733
Chlor-Trimeton Allergy Tablets (Chlorpheniramine Maleate) Schering-Plough HealthCare ◘ 798
Allergy-Sinus Comtrex Multi-Symptom Allergy-Sinus Formula Tablets (Acetaminophen, Chlorpheniramine Maleate, Pseudoephedrine Hydrochloride) Bristol-Myers Products ◘ 617
Contac Night Allergy/Sinus Caplets (Acetaminophen, Pseudoephedrine Hydrochloride, Diphenhydramine Hydrochloride) SmithKline Beecham Consumer ◘ 812
Dimetapp Elixir (Brompheniramine Maleate, Phenylpropanolamine Hydrochloride) A. H. Robins Consumer ◘ 773
Dimetapp Extentabs (Brompheniramine Maleate, Phenylpropanolamine Hydrochloride) A. H. Robins Consumer ◘ 774
Dimetapp Tablets/Liqui-Gels (Brompheniramine Maleate, Phenylpropanolamine Hydrochloride) A. H. Robins Consumer ◘ 775
Dimetapp Cold & Allergy Chewable Tablets (Brompheniramine Maleate, Phenylpropanolamine Hydrochloride) A. H. Robins Consumer ◘ 773
Drixoral Cold and Flu Extended-Release Tablets (Acetaminophen, Dexbrompheniramine Maleate, Pseudoephedrine

(◘ Described in PDR For Nonprescription Drugs) (⊙ Described in PDR For Ophthalmology)

1543 **Indications Index** **Stevens-Johnson syndrome**

Sulfate) Schering-Plough HealthCare ■ 803
Hyland's C-Plus Cold Tablets (Homeopathic Medications) Standard Homeopathic ■ 829
Ryna (Chlorpheniramine Maleate, Pseudoephedrine Hydrochloride) Wallace ■ 841
Seldane Tablets (Terfenadine) Marion Merrell Dow 1536
Seldane-D Extended-Release Tablets (Pseudoephedrine Hydrochloride, Terfenadine) Marion Merrell Dow 1538
Sinulin Tablets (Acetaminophen, Phenylpropanolamine Hydrochloride, Chlorpheniramine Maleate) Carnrick 787
Sinutab Sinus Allergy Medication, Maximum Strength Tablets and Caplets (Acetaminophen, Chlorpheniramine Maleate, Pseudoephedrine Hydrochloride) WARNER WELLCOME ■ 860
Sinutab Sinus Medication, Regular Strength Without Drowsiness Formula (Acetaminophen, Pseudoephedrine Hydrochloride) WARNER WELLCOME ■ 859
Sudafed Plus Liquid (Chlorpheniramine Maleate, Pseudoephedrine Hydrochloride) WARNER WELLCOME ■ 862
Sudafed Plus Tablets (Chlorpheniramine Maleate, Pseudoephedrine Hydrochloride) WARNER WELLCOME ■ 863
Tavist Syrup (Clemastine Fumarate) Sandoz Pharmaceuticals 2297
Tavist Tablets (Clemastine Fumarate) Sandoz Pharmaceuticals 2298
Triaminic Cold Tablets (Phenylpropanolamine Hydrochloride, Chlorpheniramine Maleate) Sandoz Consumer ■ 790
Triaminicin Tablets (Acetaminophen, Chlorpheniramine Maleate, Phenylpropanolamine Hydrochloride) Sandoz Consumer ■ 793
Triaminicol Multi-Symptom Relief (Phenylpropanolamine Hydrochloride, Chlorpheniramine Maleate, Dextromethorphan Hydrobromide) Sandoz Consumer ■ 794
TYLENOL Severe Allergy Medication Caplets (Acetaminophen, Diphenhydramine Hydrochloride) McNeil Consumer 1564

Sour stomach (see under Hyperacidity, gastric, symptomatic relief of)

Spasm, skeletal muscle
Dizac (Diazepam) Ohmeda 1809
Flexeril Tablets (Cyclobenzaprine Hydrochloride) Merck & Co., Inc. 1661
Valium Injectable (Diazepam) Roche Products 2182
Valium Tablets (Diazepam) Roche Products 2183
Valrelease Capsules (Diazepam) Roche Laboratories 2169

Spasm, smooth muscle
Papaverine Hydrochloride Vials and Ampoules (Papaverine Hydrochloride) Lilly 1468

Spasticity, cerebral palsy-induced (see under Spasticity, upper motor neuron disorder-induced)

Spasticity, multiple sclerosis-induced (see under Spasticity, upper motor neuron disorder-induced)

Spasticity, muscle, symptomatic alleviation of
Flexeril Tablets (Cyclobenzaprine Hydrochloride) Merck & Co., Inc. 1661
Lioresal Tablets (Baclofen) CibaGeneva 829

Spasticity, spinal cord injury-induced (see under Spasticity, upper motor neuron disorder-induced)

Spasticity, stroke-induced (see under Spasticity, upper motor neuron disorder-induced)

Spasticity, upper motor neuron disorder-induced
Dantrium Capsules (Dantrolene Sodium) Procter & Gamble Pharmaceuticals 1982
Dizac (Diazepam) Ohmeda 1809
Lioresal Tablets (Baclofen) CibaGeneva 829
Valium Injectable (Diazepam) Roche Products 2182
Valium Tablets (Diazepam) Roche Products 2183
Valrelease Capsules (Diazepam) Roche Laboratories 2169

Spasticity of spinal cord, severe
Lioresal Intrathecal (Baclofen) Medtronic Neurological 1596

Spermatogenesis, stimulation of, adjunctive therapy in
Humegon (Menotropins) Organon 1824

Spirillum minus infections
Pfizerpen for Injection (Penicillin G Potassium) Roerig 2203

Spirochetes species infections (see also under Borrelia recurrentis infection)
Minocin Intravenous (Minocycline Hydrochloride) Lederle 1382
Minocin Oral Suspension (Minocycline Hydrochloride) Lederle 1385
Minocin Pellet-Filled Capsules (Minocycline Hydrochloride) Lederle 1383
Terramycin Intramuscular Solution (Oxytetracycline) Roerig 2210
Vibramycin Hyclate Intravenous (Doxycycline Hyclate) Roerig 2215

Sporothrix schenckii infections (see under Sporotrichosis)

Sporotrichosis
Fungizone Intravenous (Amphotericin B) Apothecon 506

Sprains, topical relief of (see under Pain, topical relief of)

Staphylococcal enterocolitis (see under Enterocolitis, staphylococcal)

Staphylococci bone and joint infections
Keflex Pulvules & Oral Suspension (Cephalexin) Dista 914
Vancocin HCl, Vials & ADD-Vantage (Vancomycin Hydrochloride) Lilly 1481

Staphylococci endocarditis
Vancocin HCl, Vials & ADD-Vantage (Vancomycin Hydrochloride) Lilly 1481

Staphylococci lower respiratory tract infections
Vancocin HCl, Vials & ADD-Vantage (Vancomycin Hydrochloride) Lilly 1481

Staphylococci otitis media
Ceclor Pulvules & Suspension (Cefaclor) Lilly 1431
Keflex Pulvules & Oral Suspension (Cephalexin) Dista 914

Staphylococci septicemia
Vancocin HCl, Vials & ADD-Vantage (Vancomycin Hydrochloride) Lilly 1481

Staphylococci skin and skin structure infections
Duricef (Cefadroxil Monohydrate) Bristol-Myers Squibb 748
Keflex Pulvules & Oral Suspension (Cephalexin) Dista 914
Spectrobid Tablets (Bacampicillin Hydrochloride) Roerig 2206
Vancocin HCl, Vials & ADD-Vantage (Vancomycin Hydrochloride) Lilly 1481

Staphylococci, coagulase-negative, infections, ocular
Pred-G Liquifilm Sterile Ophthalmic Suspension (Gentamicin Sulfate, Prednisolone Acetate) Allergan ◉ 251
TobraDex Ophthalmic Suspension and Ointment (Dexamethasone, Tobramycin) Alcon Laboratories 473

Staphylococci, coagulase-positive, infections, ocular
Pred-G Liquifilm Sterile Ophthalmic Suspension (Gentamicin Sulfate, Prednisolone Acetate) Allergan ◉ 251
TobraDex Ophthalmic Suspension and Ointment (Dexamethasone, Tobramycin) Alcon Laboratories 473

Staphylococci, nonpenicillinase-producing, infections
Amoxil (Amoxicillin Trihydrate) SmithKline Beecham Pharmaceuticals 2464
Spectrobid Tablets (Bacampicillin Hydrochloride) Roerig 2206

Staphylococci, nonpenicillinase-producing, respiratory tract infections
Omnipen for Oral Suspension (Ampicillin) Wyeth-Ayerst 2765
Spectrobid Tablets (Bacampicillin Hydrochloride) Roerig 2206

Staphylococci, penicillinase-producing, infections
Mefoxin (Cefoxitin Sodium) Merck & Co., Inc. 1691
Mefoxin Premixed Intravenous Solution (Cefoxitin Sodium) Merck & Co., Inc. 1694
Mezlin (Mezlocillin Sodium) Bayer Pharmaceutical 601
Mezlin Pharmacy Bulk Package (Mezlocillin Sodium) Bayer Pharmaceutical 604

Staphylococci, urinary tract infections
Gantanol Tablets (Sulfamethoxazole) Roche Laboratories 2119
Gantrisin (Acetyl Sulfisoxazole) Roche Laboratories 2120
Proloprim Tablets (Trimethoprim) Glaxo Wellcome 1155

Staphylococcus aureus (see under S. aureus infections)

Staphylococcus epidermidis (see under S. epidermis infections)

Staphylococcus species infections
Amikacin Sulfate Injection, USP (Amikacin Sulfate) Elkins-Sinn 960
Amikin Injectable (Amikacin Sulfate) Apothecon 501
Ceclor Pulvules & Suspension (Cefaclor) Lilly 1431
Duricef (Cefadroxil Monohydrate) Bristol-Myers Squibb 748
Gantanol Tablets (Sulfamethoxazole) Roche Laboratories 2119
Gantrisin (Acetyl Sulfisoxazole) Roche Laboratories 2120
Garamycin Injectable (Gentamicin Sulfate) Schering 2360
Keflex Pulvules & Oral Suspension (Cephalexin) Dista 914
Lincocin (Lincomycin Hydrochloride) Upjohn 2617
Pfizerpen for Injection (Penicillin G Potassium) Roerig 2203
TERAK Ointment (Oxytetracycline Hydrochloride, Polymyxin B Sulfate) Akorn ◉ 209
Vancocin HCl, Vials & ADD-Vantage (Vancomycin Hydrochloride) Lilly 1481

Staphylococcus species infections, ocular
TERAK Ointment (Oxytetracycline Hydrochloride, Polymyxin B Sulfate) Akorn ◉ 209
Terramycin with Polymyxin B Sulfate Ophthalmic Ointment (Oxytetracycline Hydrochloride, Polymyxin B Sulfate) Roerig 2211

Staphylococcus species, coagulase-negative, infections
Ceclor Pulvules & Suspension (Cefaclor) Lilly 1431
Garamycin Injectable (Gentamicin Sulfate) Schering 2360
Trimpex Tablets (Trimethoprim) Roche Laboratories 2163

Staphylococcus species, coagulase-positive, infections
Garamycin Injectable (Gentamicin Sulfate) Schering 2360

Status epilepticus (see under Epilepticus, status)

Steatorrhea, adjunctive therapy in
Cotazym (Pancrelipase) Organon 1817
Ku-Zyme HP Capsules (Pancrelipase) Schwarz 2402
Ultrase MT Capsules (Pancrelipase) Scandipharm 2344
Zymase Capsules (Pancrelipase) Organon 1834

Stenosis, hypertrophic subaortic
Inderal (Propranolol Hydrochloride) Wyeth-Ayerst 2728
Inderal LA Long Acting Capsules (Propranolol Hydrochloride) Wyeth-Ayerst 2730

Stevens-Johnson syndrome
Aristocort Suspension (Forte Parenteral) (Triamcinolone Diacetate) Fujisawa 1027
Aristocort Tablets (Triamcinolone) Fujisawa 1022
Celestone Soluspan Suspension (Betamethasone Sodium Phosphate, Betamethasone Acetate) Schering 2347
Cortone Acetate Sterile Suspension (Cortisone Acetate) Merck & Co., Inc. 1623
Cortone Acetate Tablets (Cortisone Acetate) Merck & Co., Inc. 1624
Dalalone D.P. Injectable (Dexamethasone Acetate) Forest 1011
Decadron Elixir (Dexamethasone) Merck & Co., Inc. 1633
Decadron Phosphate Injection (Dexamethasone Sodium Phosphate) Merck & Co., Inc. 1637
Decadron Tablets (Dexamethasone) Merck & Co., Inc. 1635
Decadron-LA Sterile Suspension (Dexamethasone Acetate) Merck & Co., Inc. 1646
Deltasone Tablets (Prednisone) Upjohn 2595
Depo-Medrol Single-Dose Vial (Methylprednisolone Acetate) Upjohn 2600
Depo-Medrol Sterile Aqueous Suspension (Methylprednisolone Acetate) Upjohn 2597
Hydeltrasol Injection, Sterile (Prednisolone Sodium Phosphate) Merck & Co., Inc. 1665
Hydrocortone Phosphate Injection, Sterile (Hydrocortisone Sodium Phosphate) Merck & Co., Inc. 1670
Hydrocortone Tablets (Hydrocortisone) Merck & Co., Inc. 1672
Medrol (Methylprednisolone) Upjohn 2621
Pediapred Oral Liquid (Prednisolone Sodium Phosphate) Fisons 995
Prelone Syrup (Prednisolone) Muro 1787
Solu-Cortef Sterile Powder (Hydrocortisone Sodium Succinate) Upjohn 2641
Solu-Medrol Sterile Powder (Methylprednisolone Sodium Succinate) Upjohn 2643

(■ Described in PDR For Nonprescription Drugs) (◉ Described in PDR For Ophthalmology)

Stiff-man syndrome **Indications Index** **1544**

Stiff-man syndrome, adjunctive therapy in
Dizac (Diazepam) Ohmeda ... 1809
Valium Injectable (Diazepam) Roche Products ... 2182
Valium Tablets (Diazepam) Roche Products ... 2183
Valrelease Capsules (Diazepam) Roche Laboratories ... 2169

Stomach, disseminated adenocarcinoma (see under Carcinoma, stomach)

Stomach, sour (see under Hyperacidity, gastric, symptomatic relief of)

Stomach, upset (see under Digestive disorders, symptomatic relief of)

Stomatitis, recurrent aphthous, symptomatic relief of
Children's Vicks Chloraseptic Sore Throat Lozenges (Benzocaine) Procter & Gamble ▣ 757
Children's Vicks Chloraseptic Sore Throat Spray (Phenol) Procter & Gamble ... ▣ 757
Dyclone 0.5% and 1% Topical Solutions, USP (Dyclonine Hydrochloride) Astra ... 544
Gly-Oxide Liquid (Carbamide Peroxide) SmithKline Beecham Consumer ... ▣ 820
Orajel Perioseptic Oxygenating Liquid (Carbamide Peroxide) Del ... ▣ 653
Vicks Chloraseptic Sore Throat Lozenges (Benzocaine, Menthol) Procter & Gamble ... ▣ 759
Vicks Chloraseptic Sore Throat Spray, and Gargle and Mouth Rinse (Phenol) Procter & Gamble ... ▣ 759
Zilactin Medicated Gel (Benzyl Alcohol) Zila Pharmaceuticals ... ▣ 882
Zilactin-B Medicated Gel with Benzocaine (Benzocaine) Zila Pharmaceuticals ... ▣ 882

Strabismus
BOTOX (Botulinum Toxin Type A) Purified Neurotoxin Complex (Botulinum Toxin Type A) Allergan ... 477

Strabismus, accommodative convergent (see under Esotropia, accommodative)

Strep throat (see under Streptococci species upper respiratory tract infections)

Streptococcal pharyngitis
Duricef (Cefadroxil Monohydrate) Bristol-Myers Squibb ... 748
E.E.S. (Erythromycin Ethylsuccinate) Abbott ... 424
Ilosone (Erythromycin Estolate) Dista ... 911
Ilotycin Gluceptate, IV, Vials (Erythromycin Gluceptate) Dista ... 913
Suprax (Cefixime) Lederle ... 1399
Vantin for Oral Suspension and Vantin Tablets (Cefpodoxime Proxetil) Upjohn ... 2646

Streptococci biliary tract infections
Kefzol Vials, Faspak & ADD-Vantage (Cefazolin Sodium) Lilly ... 1456

Streptococci group A beta-hemolytic endocarditis
Ancef Injection (Cefazolin Sodium) SmithKline Beecham Pharmaceuticals ... 2465

Streptococci group A beta-hemolytic infections (see also under Erysipelas)
Ancef Injection (Cefazolin Sodium) SmithKline Beecham Pharmaceuticals ... 2465
Ceclor Pulvules & Suspension (Cefaclor) Lilly ... 1431
Doryx Capsules (Doxycycline Hyclate) Parke-Davis ... 1913
Kefzol Vials, Faspak & ADD-Vantage (Cefazolin Sodium) Lilly ... 1456
Mandol Vials, Faspak & ADD-Vantage (Cefamandole Nafate) Lilly ... 1461
Mezlin (Mezlocillin Sodium) Bayer Pharmaceutical ... 601
Mezlin Pharmacy Bulk Package (Mezlocillin Sodium) Bayer Pharmaceutical ... 604
Primaxin I.V. (Imipenem-Cilastatin Sodium) Merck & Co., Inc. ... 1729

Streptococci group A beta-hemolytic otitis media
Ceclor Pulvules & Suspension (Cefaclor) Lilly ... 1431

Streptococci group A beta-hemolytic skin and skin structure infections
Ceclor Pulvules & Suspension (Cefaclor) Lilly ... 1431
Ceptaz (Ceftazidime) Glaxo Wellcome ... 1081
Fortaz (Ceftazidime) Glaxo Wellcome ... 1100
Ilotycin Gluceptate, IV, Vials (Erythromycin Gluceptate) Dista ... 913
Kefzol Vials, Faspak & ADD-Vantage (Cefazolin Sodium) Lilly ... 1456
Mandol Vials, Faspak & ADD-Vantage (Cefamandole Nafate) Lilly ... 1461
Primaxin I.V. (Imipenem-Cilastatin Sodium) Merck & Co., Inc. ... 1729
Tazicef for Injection (Ceftazidime) SmithKline Beecham Pharmaceuticals ... 2519
Tazidime Vials, Faspak & ADD-Vantage (Ceftazidime) Lilly ... 1478

Streptococci group A beta-hemolytic species infections, ocular
Pred-G Liquifilm Sterile Ophthalmic Suspension (Gentamicin Sulfate, Prednisolone Acetate) Allergan ... ◉ 251
Pred-G S.O.P. Sterile Ophthalmic Ointment (Gentamicin Sulfate, Prednisolone Acetate) Allergan ... ◉ 252
TobraDex Ophthalmic Suspension and Ointment (Dexamethasone, Tobramycin) Alcon Laboratories ... 473

Streptococci group A beta-hemolytic upper respiratory tract infections
Ceclor Pulvules & Suspension (Cefaclor) Lilly ... 1431
Duricef (Cefadroxil Monohydrate) Bristol-Myers Squibb ... 748
ERYC (Erythromycin) Parke-Davis ... 1915
Ilotycin Gluceptate, IV, Vials (Erythromycin Gluceptate) Dista ... 913
Keftab Tablets (Cephalexin Hydrochloride) Dista ... 915
PCE Dispertab Tablets (Erythromycin) Abbott ... 444
Spectrobid Tablets (Bacampicillin Hydrochloride) Roerig ... 2206
Tao Capsules (Troleandomycin) Roerig ... 2209

Streptococci group B infections
Mefoxin (Cefoxitin Sodium) Merck & Co., Inc. ... 1691
Mefoxin Premixed Intravenous Solution (Cefoxitin Sodium) Merck & Co., Inc. ... 1694
Primaxin I.V. (Imipenem-Cilastatin Sodium) Merck & Co., Inc. ... 1729

Streptococci group D bone and joint infections
Primaxin I.V. (Imipenem-Cilastatin Sodium) Merck & Co., Inc. ... 1729

Streptococci group D endocarditis, adjunct in
Garamycin Injectable (Gentamicin Sulfate) Schering ... 2360

Streptococci group D genitourinary tract infections
Omnipen for Oral Suspension (Ampicillin) Wyeth-Ayerst ... 2765
Primaxin I.V. (Imipenem-Cilastatin Sodium) Merck & Co., Inc. ... 1729

Streptococci group D gynecologic infections
Primaxin I.M. (Imipenem-Cilastatin Sodium) Merck & Co., Inc. ... 1727

Streptococci group D infections
Ancef Injection (Cefazolin Sodium) SmithKline Beecham Pharmaceuticals ... 2465
Claforan Sterile and Injection (Cefotaxime Sodium) Hoechst-Roussel ... 1235
Garamycin Injectable (Gentamicin Sulfate) Schering ... 2360
Macrodantin Capsules (Nitrofurantoin) Procter & Gamble Pharmaceuticals ... 1989
Mandol Vials, Faspak & ADD-Vantage (Cefamandole Nafate) Lilly ... 1461
Mezlin Pharmacy Bulk Package (Mezlocillin Sodium) Bayer Pharmaceutical ... 604
Omnipen Capsules (Ampicillin) Wyeth-Ayerst ... 2764
Omnipen for Oral Suspension (Ampicillin) Wyeth-Ayerst ... 2765
Pipracil (Piperacillin Sodium) Lederle ... 1390
Primaxin I.V. (Imipenem-Cilastatin Sodium) Merck & Co., Inc. ... 1729
Spectrobid Tablets (Bacampicillin Hydrochloride) Roerig ... 2206

Streptococci group D intra-abdominal infections
Omnipen for Oral Suspension (Ampicillin) Wyeth-Ayerst ... 2765
Pipracil (Piperacillin Sodium) Lederle ... 1390
Primaxin I.M. (Imipenem-Cilastatin Sodium) Merck & Co., Inc. ... 1727
Primaxin I.V. (Imipenem-Cilastatin Sodium) Merck & Co., Inc. ... 1729

Streptococci group D septicemia
Primaxin I.V. (Imipenem-Cilastatin Sodium) Merck & Co., Inc. ... 1729

Streptococci group D skin and skin structure infections
Primaxin I.M. (Imipenem-Cilastatin Sodium) Merck & Co., Inc. ... 1727
Primaxin I.V. (Imipenem-Cilastatin Sodium) Merck & Co., Inc. ... 1729

Streptococci group D urinary tract infections
Mandol Vials, Faspak & ADD-Vantage (Cefamandole Nafate) Lilly ... 1461

Streptococci infections, ocular
AK-Spore (Bacitracin Zinc, Neomycin Sulfate, Polymyxin B Sulfate) Akorn ... ◉ 204
Chloromycetin Ophthalmic Ointment, 1% (Chloramphenicol) Parke-Davis ◉ 310
Chloromycetin Ophthalmic Solution (Chloramphenicol) Parke-Davis ... ◉ 310
Cortisporin Ophthalmic Ointment Sterile (Polymyxin B Sulfate, Bacitracin Zinc, Neomycin Sulfate, Hydrocortisone) Glaxo Wellcome ... 1085
Ophthocort (Chloramphenicol, Polymyxin B Sulfate, Hydrocortisone Acetate) Parke-Davis ... ◉ 311
TERAK Ointment (Oxytetracycline Hydrochloride, Polymyxin B Sulfate) Akorn ... ◉ 209
Terra-Cortril Ophthalmic Suspension (Oxytetracycline Hydrochloride, Hydrocortisone Acetate) Roerig ... 2210
Terramycin with Polymyxin B Sulfate Ophthalmic Ointment (Oxytetracycline Hydrochloride, Polymyxin B Sulfate) Roerig ... 2211
TobraDex Ophthalmic Suspension and Ointment (Dexamethasone, Tobramycin) Alcon Laboratories ... 473

Streptococci skin and skin structure infections
Cefizox for Intramuscular or Intravenous Use (Ceftizoxime Sodium) Fujisawa ... 1034
Cefotan (Cefotetan) Zeneca ... 2829
Duricef (Cefadroxil Monohydrate) Bristol-Myers Squibb ... 748
Keflex Pulvules & Oral Suspension (Cephalexin) Dista ... 914
Kefzol Vials, Faspak & ADD-Vantage (Cefazolin Sodium) Lilly ... 1456
Mefoxin (Cefoxitin Sodium) Merck & Co., Inc. ... 1691
Mefoxin Premixed Intravenous Solution (Cefoxitin Sodium) Merck & Co., Inc. ... 1694

Streptococci species otitis media
Keflex Pulvules & Oral Suspension (Cephalexin) Dista ... 914

Streptococci species upper respiratory tract infections
Bicillin C-R Injection (Penicillin G Procaine, Penicillin G Benzathine) Wyeth-Ayerst ... 2704
Bicillin C-R 900/300 Injection (Penicillin G Procaine, Penicillin G Benzathine) Wyeth-Ayerst ... 2706
Bicillin L-A Injection (Penicillin G Benzathine) Wyeth-Ayerst ... 2707
Ceftin for Oral Suspension (Cefuroxime Axetil) Glaxo Wellcome ... 1078
Pen•Vee K (Penicillin V Potassium) Wyeth-Ayerst ... 2772
Suprax (Cefixime) Lederle ... 1399

Streptococci (viridans group) infections, ocular
AK-CIDE (Prednisolone Acetate, Sulfacetamide Sodium) Akorn ... ◉ 202
AK-CIDE Ointment (Prednisolone Acetate, Sulfacetamide Sodium) Akorn ... ◉ 202
Blephamide Liquifilm Sterile Ophthalmic Suspension (Prednisolone Acetate, Sulfacetamide Sodium) Allergan ... 476
Ciloxan Ophthalmic Solution (Ciprofloxacin Hydrochloride) Alcon Laboratories ... 472
FML-S Liquifilm (Sulfacetamide Sodium, Fluorometholone) Allergan ... ◉ 242
Polytrim Ophthalmic Solution Sterile (Polymyxin B Sulfate, Trimethoprim Sulfate) Allergan ... 482
Vasocidin Ointment (Prednisolone Acetate, Sulfacetamide Sodium) CIBA Vision Ophthalmics ... ◉ 268
Vasocidin Ophthalmic Solution (Prednisolone Sodium Phosphate, Sulfacetamide Sodium) CIBA Vision Ophthalmics ... ◉ 270

Streptococci non-hemolytic species infections, ocular
Pred-G Liquifilm Sterile Ophthalmic Suspension (Gentamicin Sulfate, Prednisolone Acetate) Allergan ... ◉ 251
TobraDex Ophthalmic Suspension and Ointment (Dexamethasone, Tobramycin) Alcon Laboratories ... 473

Streptococci, alpha-hemolytic (viridans group), infections
Ilosone (Erythromycin Estolate) Dista ... 911

Streptococcus agalactiae infections (see under S. agalactiae infections)

Streptococcus faecalis (see under S. faecalis infections)

Streptococcus pneumoniae (see under S. pneumoniae infections)

Streptococcus pyogenes (see under S. pyogenes infections)

(▣ Described in PDR For Nonprescription Drugs) (◉ Described in PDR For Ophthalmology)

1545 Indications Index Tapeworm

Streptococcus species bone and joint infections
Cefizox for Intramuscular or Intravenous Use (Ceftizoxime Sodium) Fujisawa ... 1034
Claforan Sterile and Injection (Cefotaxime Sodium) Hoechst-Roussel ... 1235

Streptococcus species gynecologic infections
Cefotan (Cefotetan) Zeneca ... 2829
Claforan Sterile and Injection (Cefotaxime Sodium) Hoechst-Roussel ... 1235

Streptococcus species infections
Achromycin V Capsules (Tetracycline Hydrochloride) Lederle ... 1367
Amoxil (Amoxicillin Trihydrate) SmithKline Beecham Pharmaceuticals ... 2464
Bactroban Ointment (Mupirocin) SmithKline Beecham Pharmaceuticals ... 2470
Cefizox for Intramuscular or Intravenous Use (Ceftizoxime Sodium) Fujisawa ... 1034
Cefotan (Cefotetan) Zeneca ... 2829
Claforan Sterile and Injection (Cefotaxime Sodium) Hoechst-Roussel ... 1235
Cleocin Phosphate Injection (Clindamycin Phosphate) Upjohn ... 2586
Declomycin Tablets (Demeclocycline Hydrochloride) Lederle ... 1371
Duricef (Cefadroxil Monohydrate) Bristol-Myers Squibb ... 748
Garamycin Injectable (Gentamicin Sulfate) Schering ... 2360
Kefzol Vials, Faspak & ADD-Vantage (Cefazolin Sodium) Lilly ... 1456
Lincocin (Lincomycin Hydrochloride) Upjohn ... 2617
Mezlin (Mezlocillin Sodium) Bayer Pharmaceutical ... 601
Mezlin Pharmacy Bulk Package (Mezlocillin Sodium) Bayer Pharmaceutical ... 604
Minocin Intravenous (Minocycline Hydrochloride) Lederle ... 1382
Netromycin Injection 100 mg/ml (Netilmicin Sulfate) Schering ... 2373
Pen•Vee K (Penicillin V Potassium) Wyeth-Ayerst ... 2772
Pfizerpen for Injection (Penicillin G Potassium) Roerig ... 2203
Spectrobid Tablets (Bacampicillin Hydrochloride) Roerig ... 2206
Suprax (Cefixime) Lederle ... 1399
TERAK Ointment (Oxytetracycline Hydrochloride, Polymyxin B Sulfate) Akorn ... ◉ 209
Terramycin Intramuscular Solution (Oxytetracycline) Roerig ... 2210
Vibramycin Hyclate Intravenous (Doxycycline Hyclate) Roerig ... 2215

Streptococcus species intra-abdominal infections
Cefizox for Intramuscular or Intravenous Use (Ceftizoxime Sodium) Fujisawa ... 1034
Cefotan (Cefotetan) Zeneca ... 2829
Claforan Sterile and Injection (Cefotaxime Sodium) Hoechst-Roussel ... 1235

Streptococcus species lower respiratory tract infections
Cefizox for Intramuscular or Intravenous Use (Ceftizoxime Sodium) Fujisawa ... 1034

Streptococcus species respiratory tract infections
Cleocin Phosphate Injection (Clindamycin Phosphate) Upjohn ... 2586

Streptococcus species septicemia
Cefizox for Intramuscular or Intravenous Use (Ceftizoxime Sodium) Fujisawa ... 1034
Claforan Sterile and Injection (Cefotaxime Sodium) Hoechst-Roussel ... 1235
Cleocin Phosphate Injection (Clindamycin Phosphate) Upjohn ... 2586

Streptococcus tonsillitis (see under Streptococci species upper respiratory tract infections)

Streptococcus viridans group infections
Blephamide Ointment (Sulfacetamide Sodium, Prednisolone Acetate) Allergan ... ◉ 237
Primaxin I.M. (Imipenem-Cilastatin Sodium) Merck & Co., Inc. ... 1727
Rocephin Injectable Vials, ADD-Vantage, Galaxy Container (Ceftriaxone Sodium) Roche Laboratories ... 2142
Streptomycin Sulfate Injection (Streptomycin Sulfate) Roerig ... 2208

Stroke, thrombotic, to reduce the risk of
Genuine Bayer Aspirin Tablets & Caplets (Aspirin) Miles Consumer ... ▣ 713
Ticlid Tablets (Ticlopidine Hydrochloride) Roche Laboratories ... 2156

Strongyloidiasis
Mintezol (Thiabendazole) Merck & Co., Inc. ... 1704

Sty (see under Hordeolum)

Subinvolution, routine management of
Methergine (Methylergonovine Maleate) Sandoz Pharmaceuticals ... 2272

Sunburn, acute, prophylaxis
Moisturel Cream (Dimethicone, Petrolatum) Westwood-Squibb ... 2688
Oil of Olay Daily UV Protectant SPF 15 Beauty Fluid-Original and Fragrance Free (Olay Co. Inc.) (Octyl Methoxycinnamate, Phenylbenzimidazole-5-Sulfonic Acid) Procter & Gamble ... ▣ 751
Shade Gel SPF 30 Sunblock (Ethylhexyl p-Methoxycinnamate, Oxybenzone, Homosalate) Schering-Plough HealthCare ... ▣ 807
Shade Lotion SPF 45 Sunblock (Ethylhexyl p-Methoxycinnamate, Oxybenzone, 2-Ethylhexyl Salicylate) Schering-Plough HealthCare ... ▣ 807
Shade UVAGUARD SPF 15 Suncreen Lotion (Octyl Methoxycinnamate, Avobenzone, Oxybenzone) Schering-Plough HealthCare ... ▣ 808
Solbar PF Ultra Liquid SPF 30 (Octyl Methoxycinnamate, Oxybenzone) Persōn & Covey ... 1932

Sunburn, pain associated with (see under Pain, topical relief of)

Sweating disorders (see under Miliaria)

Sympathetic ophthalmia (see under Ophthalmia, sympathetic)

Synechial formation
Floropryl Sterile Ophthalmic Ointment (Isoflurophate) Merck & Co., Inc. ... 1662
Humorsol Sterile Ophthalmic Solution (Demecarium Bromide) Merck & Co., Inc. ... 1664

Syphilis (see under T. pallidum infections)

T

T. pallidum infections
Achromycin V Capsules (Tetracycline Hydrochloride) Lederle ... 1367
Bicillin L-A Injection (Penicillin G Benzathine) Wyeth-Ayerst ... 2707
Declomycin Tablets (Demeclocycline Hydrochloride) Lederle ... 1371
Doryx Capsules (Doxycycline Hyclate) Parke-Davis ... 1913
Dynacin Capsules (Minocycline Hydrochloride) Medicis ... 1590
E.E.S. (Erythromycin Ethylsuccinate) Abbott ... 424
E-Mycin Tablets (Erythromycin) Knoll Laboratories ... 1341
ERYC (Erythromycin) Parke-Davis ... 1915
EryPed (Erythromycin Ethylsuccinate) Abbott ... 421
Ery-Tab Tablets (Erythromycin) Abbott ... 422
Erythrocin Stearate Filmtab (Erythromycin Stearate) Abbott ... 425
Erythromycin Base Filmtab (Erythromycin) Abbott ... 426
Erythromycin Delayed-Release Capsules, USP (Erythromycin) Abbott ... 427
Ilosone (Erythromycin Estolate) Dista ... 911
Minocin Intravenous (Minocycline Hydrochloride) Lederle ... 1382
Minocin Oral Suspension (Minocycline Hydrochloride) Lederle ... 1385
Minocin Pellet-Filled Capsules (Minocycline Hydrochloride) Lederle ... 1383
Monodox Capsules (Doxycycline Monohydrate) Oclassen ... 1805
PCE Dispertab Tablets (Erythromycin) Abbott ... 444
Pfizerpen for Injection (Penicillin G Potassium) Roerig ... 2203
Terramycin Intramuscular Solution (Oxytetracycline) Roerig ... 2210
Vibramycin (Doxycycline Calcium) Pfizer Labs ... 1941
Vibramycin Hyclate Intravenous (Doxycycline Hyclate) Roerig ... 2215
Vibramycin (Doxycycline Monohydrate) Pfizer Labs ... 1941

T. vaginalis infections
Betadine Medicated Douche (Povidone Iodine) Purdue Frederick ... 1992
Betadine Medicated Gel (Povidone Iodine) Purdue Frederick ... 1992
Flagyl 375 Capsules (Metronidazole) Searle ... 2434
Protostat Tablets (Metronidazole) Ortho Pharmaceutical ... 1883

Tachyarrhythmias, catecholamine-induced, during anesthesia
Inderal (Propranolol Hydrochloride) Wyeth-Ayerst ... 2728

Tachyarrhythmias, digitalis-induced
Inderal (Propranolol Hydrochloride) Wyeth-Ayerst ... 2728

Tachycardia, atrial, paroxysmal
Lanoxicaps (Digoxin) Glaxo Wellcome ... 1117
Lanoxin Elixir Pediatric (Digoxin) Glaxo Wellcome ... 1120
Lanoxin Injection (Digoxin) Glaxo Wellcome ... 1123
Lanoxin Injection Pediatric (Digoxin) Glaxo Wellcome ... 1126
Lanoxin Tablets (Digoxin) Glaxo Wellcome ... 1128
Quinidex Extentabs (Quinidine Sulfate) Robins ... 2067

Tachycardia, noncompensatory sinus
Brevibloc Injection (Esmolol Hydrochloride) Ohmeda ... 1808

Tachycardia, paroxysmal supraventricular
Adenocard Injection (Adenosine) Fujisawa ... 1021
Cardizem Injectable (Diltiazem Hydrochloride) Marion Merrell Dow ... 1508
Inderal (Propranolol Hydrochloride) Wyeth-Ayerst ... 2728
Isoptin Injectable (Verapamil Hydrochloride) Knoll Laboratories ... 1344
Neo-Synephrine Hydrochloride 1% Carpuject (Phenylephrine Hydrochloride) Sanofi Winthrop ... 2324
Neo-Synephrine Hydrochloride 1% Injection (Phenylephrine Hydrochloride) Sanofi Winthrop ... 2324
Tambocor Tablets (Flecainide Acetate) 3M Pharmaceuticals ... 1497

Tachycardia, paroxysmal supraventricular associated with Lown-Ganong-Levine syndrome (see under Lown-Ganong-Levine syndrome)

Tachycardia, paroxysmal supraventricular associated with Wolff-Parkinson-White syndrome (see under Wolff-Parkinson-White syndrome)

Tachycardia, repetitive paroxysmal supraventricular, prophylaxis of
Calan Tablets (Verapamil Hydrochloride) Searle ... 2419
Isoptin Oral Tablets (Verapamil Hydrochloride) Knoll Laboratories ... 1346

Tachycardia, supraventricular
Brevibloc Injection (Esmolol Hydrochloride) Ohmeda ... 1808
Tambocor Tablets (Flecainide Acetate) 3M Pharmaceuticals ... 1497

Tachycardia, ventricular
Betapace Tablets (Sotalol Hydrochloride) Berlex ... 641
Inderal (Propranolol Hydrochloride) Wyeth-Ayerst ... 2728
Quinaglute Dura-Tabs Tablets (Quinidine Gluconate) Berlex ... 649
Tambocor Tablets (Flecainide Acetate) 3M Pharmaceuticals ... 1497
Tonocard Tablets (Tocainide Hydrochloride) Astra Merck ... 531

Tachycardia, ventricular, paroxysmal
Quinidex Extentabs (Quinidine Sulfate) Robins ... 2067

Tachycardia, ventricular, recurrent hemodynamically unstable
Cordarone Intravenous (Amiodarone Hydrochloride) Wyeth-Ayerst ... 2715
Cordarone Tablets (Amiodarone Hydrochloride) Wyeth-Ayerst ... 2712

Tachycardia, ventricular, sustained
Ethmozine Tablets (Moricizine Hydrochloride) Roberts ... 2041
Mexitil Capsules (Mexiletine Hydrochloride) Boehringer Ingelheim ... 678
Norpace (Disopyramide Phosphate) Searle ... 2444
Procan SR Tablets (Procainamide Hydrochloride) Parke-Davis ... 1926
Rythmol Tablets–150mg, 225mg, 300mg (Propafenone Hydrochloride) Knoll Laboratories ... 1352
Tambocor Tablets (Flecainide Acetate) 3M Pharmaceuticals ... 1497

Tachycardias due to thyrotoxicosis, adjunct
Inderal (Propranolol Hydrochloride) Wyeth-Ayerst ... 2728

Tachycardias, paroxysmal atrial (see under Tachycardia, paroxysmal supraventricular)

Tachycardias, sinus, persistent
Inderal (Propranolol Hydrochloride) Wyeth-Ayerst ... 2728

Tachycardias, supraventricular
Crystodigin Tablets (Digitoxin) Lilly ... 1433
Vasoxyl Injection (Methoxamine Hydrochloride) Glaxo Wellcome ... 1196

Tapeworm infections (see under Infections, tapeworm)

Tapeworm, beef (see under Taenia saginata infections)

Tapeworm, dwarf (see under Hymenolepis nana infections)

(▣ Described in PDR For Nonprescription Drugs) (◉ Described in PDR For Ophthalmology)

Tapeworm **Indications Index** **1546**

Tapeworm, fish
(see under Diphyllobothrium latum infections)

Tendinitis
Anaprox/Naprosyn (Naproxen Sodium) Roche Laboratories 2117
Clinoril Tablets (Sulindac) Merck & Co., Inc. 1618
Indocin (Indomethacin) Merck & Co., Inc. 1680
Anaprox/Naprosyn (Naproxen) Roche Laboratories 2117

Tenosynovitis, acute nonspecific
Aristocort Suspension (Forte Parenteral) (Triamcinolone Diacetate) Fujisawa 1027
Aristocort Suspension (Intralesional) (Triamcinolone Diacetate) Fujisawa 1025
Aristocort Tablets (Triamcinolone) Fujisawa 1022
Aristospan Suspension (Intra-articular) (Triamcinolone Hexacetonide) Fujisawa 1033
Celestone Soluspan Suspension (Betamethasone Sodium Phosphate, Betamethasone Acetate) Schering 2347
Cortone Acetate Sterile Suspension (Cortisone Acetate) Merck & Co., Inc. 1623
Cortone Acetate Tablets (Cortisone Acetate) Merck & Co., Inc. 1624
Dalalone D.P. Injectable (Dexamethasone Acetate) Forest 1011
Decadron Elixir (Dexamethasone) Merck & Co., Inc. 1633
Decadron Phosphate Injection (Dexamethasone Sodium Phosphate) Merck & Co., Inc. 1637
Decadron Phosphate with Xylocaine Injection, Sterile (Dexamethasone Sodium Phosphate, Lidocaine Hydrochloride) Merck & Co., Inc. 1639
Decadron Tablets (Dexamethasone) Merck & Co., Inc. 1635
Decadron-LA Sterile Suspension (Dexamethasone Acetate) Merck & Co., Inc. 1646
Deltasone Tablets (Prednisone) Upjohn 2595
Depo-Medrol Single-Dose Vial (Methylprednisolone Acetate) Upjohn 2600
Depo-Medrol Sterile Aqueous Suspension (Methylprednisolone Acetate) Upjohn 2597
Hydeltrasol Injection, Sterile (Prednisolone Sodium Phosphate) Merck & Co., Inc. 1665
Hydeltra-T.B.A. Sterile Suspension (Prednisolone Tebutate) Merck & Co., Inc. 1667
Hydrocortone Acetate Sterile Suspension (Hydrocortisone Acetate) Merck & Co., Inc. 1669
Hydrocortone Phosphate Injection, Sterile (Hydrocortisone Sodium Phosphate) Merck & Co., Inc. 1670
Hydrocortone Tablets (Hydrocortisone) Merck & Co., Inc. 1672
Medrol (Methylprednisolone) Upjohn 2621
Pediapred Oral Liquid (Prednisolone Sodium Phosphate) Fisons 995
Prelone Syrup (Prednisolone) Muro 1787
Solu-Cortef Sterile Powder (Hydrocortisone Sodium Succinate) Upjohn 2641
Solu-Medrol Sterile Powder (Methylprednisolone Sodium Succinate) Upjohn 2643

Testis, advanced carcinoma of
(see under Carcinoma, testis, advanced)

Testosterone, deficiency of
(see under Androgen, absence or deficiency of)

Tetanus
Hyper-Tet Tetanus Immune Globulin (Human) (Tetanus Immune Globulin (Human)) Bayer Biological 627
Pfizerpen for Injection (Penicillin G Potassium) Roerig 2203

Tetanus, treatment adjunct
Dizac (Diazepam) Ohmeda 1809
Thorazine (Chlorpromazine Hydrochloride) SmithKline Beecham Pharmaceuticals 2523
Valium Injectable (Diazepam) Roche Products 2182

Tetany, idiopathic
DHT (Dihydrotachysterol) Tablets & Intensol (Dihydrotachysterol) Roxane 2229

Tetany, postoperative
DHT (Dihydrotachysterol) Tablets & Intensol (Dihydrotachysterol) Roxane 2229

Threadworm infestations
(see under Strongyloidiasis)

Throat, itchy
(see under Pruritus, rhinopharyngeal, symptomatic relief of)

Throat, sore
(see under Pharyngitis, symptomatic relief of)

Throat, surgical procedures, irrigation of
AMO Endosol (Balanced Salt Solution) (Balanced Salt Solution) Allergan .... ◉ 232
BSS (15 mL & 30 mL) Sterile Irrigation Solution (Balanced Salt Solution) Alcon Laboratories .... ◉ 214
BSS (250 mL) Sterile Irrigation Solution (Balanced Salt Solution) Alcon Laboratories ...... ◉ 214
BSS (500 mL) Sterile Irrigation Solution (Balanced Salt Solution) Alcon Laboratories ...... ◉ 214

Thrombocytopenia, secondary
Aristocort Suspension (Forte Parenteral) (Triamcinolone Diacetate) Fujisawa 1027
Aristocort Tablets (Triamcinolone) Fujisawa 1022
Celestone Soluspan Suspension (Betamethasone Sodium Phosphate, Betamethasone Acetate) Schering 2347
Cortone Acetate Tablets (Cortisone Acetate) Merck & Co., Inc. 1624
Dalalone D.P. Injectable (Dexamethasone Acetate) Forest 1011
Decadron Elixir (Dexamethasone) Merck & Co., Inc. 1633
Decadron Phosphate Injection (Dexamethasone Sodium Phosphate) Merck & Co., Inc. 1637
Decadron Tablets (Dexamethasone) Merck & Co., Inc. 1635
Decadron-LA Sterile Suspension (Dexamethasone Acetate) Merck & Co., Inc. 1646
Deltasone Tablets (Prednisone) Upjohn 2595
Depo-Medrol Single-Dose Vial (Methylprednisolone Acetate) Upjohn 2600
Depo-Medrol Sterile Aqueous Suspension (Methylprednisolone Acetate) Upjohn 2597
Hydeltrasol Injection, Sterile (Prednisolone Sodium Phosphate) Merck & Co., Inc. 1665
Hydrocortone Phosphate Injection, Sterile (Hydrocortisone Sodium Phosphate) Merck & Co., Inc. 1670
Hydrocortone Tablets (Hydrocortisone) Merck & Co., Inc. 1672
Medrol (Methylprednisolone) Upjohn 2621
Pediapred Oral Liquid (Prednisolone Sodium Phosphate) Fisons 995
Prelone Syrup (Prednisolone) Muro 1787
Solu-Cortef Sterile Powder (Hydrocortisone Sodium Succinate) Upjohn 2641
Solu-Medrol Sterile Powder (Methylprednisolone Sodium Succinate) Upjohn 2643

Thromboembolic complications
Coumadin (Warfarin Sodium) DuPont 926

Thromboembolism, postoperative, adjunct in
Persantine Tablets (Dipyridamole) Boehringer Ingelheim 681

Thrombosis, coronary artery, acute, lysis of
Abbokinase (Urokinase) Abbott 403
Activase (Alteplase, Recombinant) Genentech 1058
Eminase (Anistreplase) Roberts 2039
Streptase for Infusion (Streptokinase) Astra 562

Thrombosis, postoperative deep venous
Heparin Sodium Injection, USP, Sterile Solution (Heparin Sodium) Upjohn 2615

Thrombosis, venous
Coumadin (Warfarin Sodium) DuPont 926
Heparin Sodium Injection (Heparin Sodium) Wyeth-Ayerst 2726
Heparin Sodium Injection, USP, Sterile Solution (Heparin Sodium) Upjohn 2615
Heparin Sodium Vials (Heparin Sodium) Lilly 1441
Streptase for Infusion (Streptokinase) Astra 562

Thrombosis, venous, prophylaxis of
Coumadin (Warfarin Sodium) DuPont 926
Fragmin (Dalteparin Sodium) Pharmacia 1954
Heparin Sodium Injection, USP, Sterile Solution (Heparin Sodium) Upjohn 2615
Heparin Sodium Vials (Heparin Sodium) Lilly 1441
Lovenox Injection (Enoxaparin) Rhone-Poulenc Rorer Pharmaceuticals 2020

Thrush
(see under Candidiasis, oropharyngeal)

Thyroid function, aid in the diagnosis of
Cytomel Tablets (Liothyronine Sodium) SmithKline Beecham Pharmaceuticals 2473
Levothroid Tablets (Levothyroxine Sodium) Forest 1016
Synthroid (Levothyroxine Sodium) Knoll Pharmaceutical 1359
THYREL TRH (Protirelin) Ferring 2873

Thyroiditis, chronic lymphocytic
(see under Hashimoto's thyroiditis)

Thyroiditis, nonsuppurative
Aristocort Suspension (Forte Parenteral) (Triamcinolone Diacetate) Fujisawa 1027
Aristocort Tablets (Triamcinolone) Fujisawa 1022
Celestone Soluspan Suspension (Betamethasone Sodium Phosphate, Betamethasone Acetate) Schering 2347
Cortone Acetate Sterile Suspension (Cortisone Acetate) Merck & Co., Inc. 1623
Cortone Acetate Tablets (Cortisone Acetate) Merck & Co., Inc. 1624
Dalalone D.P. Injectable (Dexamethasone Acetate) Forest 1011
Decadron Elixir (Dexamethasone) Merck & Co., Inc. 1633
Decadron Phosphate Injection (Dexamethasone Sodium Phosphate) Merck & Co., Inc. 1637
Decadron Tablets (Dexamethasone) Merck & Co., Inc. 1635
Decadron-LA Sterile Suspension (Dexamethasone Acetate) Merck & Co., Inc. 1646
Deltasone Tablets (Prednisone) Upjohn 2595
Depo-Medrol Single-Dose Vial (Methylprednisolone Acetate) Upjohn 2600
Depo-Medrol Sterile Aqueous Suspension (Methylprednisolone Acetate) Upjohn 2597
Hydeltrasol Injection, Sterile (Prednisolone Sodium Phosphate) Merck & Co., Inc. 1665
Hydrocortone Phosphate Injection, Sterile (Hydrocortisone Sodium Phosphate) Merck & Co., Inc. 1670
Hydrocortone Tablets (Hydrocortisone) Merck & Co., Inc. 1672
Medrol (Methylprednisolone) Upjohn 2621
Pediapred Oral Liquid (Prednisolone Sodium Phosphate) Fisons 995
Prelone Syrup (Prednisolone) Muro 1787
Solu-Cortef Sterile Powder (Hydrocortisone Sodium Succinate) Upjohn 2641
Solu-Medrol Sterile Powder (Methylprednisolone Sodium Succinate) Upjohn 2643

Tick fevers
Achromycin V Capsules (Tetracycline Hydrochloride) Lederle 1367
Declomycin Tablets (Demeclocycline Hydrochloride) Lederle 1371
Doryx Capsules (Doxycycline Hyclate) Parke-Davis 1913
Dynacin Capsules (Minocycline Hydrochloride) Medicis 1590
Minocin Intravenous (Minocycline Hydrochloride) Lederle 1382
Minocin Oral Suspension (Minocycline Hydrochloride) Lederle 1385
Minocin Pellet-Filled Capsules (Minocycline Hydrochloride) Lederle 1383
Monodox Capsules (Doxycycline Monohydrate) Oclassen 1805
Terramycin Intramuscular Solution (Oxytetracycline) Roerig 2210
Vibramycin (Doxycycline Calcium) Pfizer Labs 1941
Vibramycin Hyclate Intravenous (Doxycycline Hyclate) Roerig 2215
Vibramycin (Doxycycline Monohydrate) Pfizer Labs 1941

Tinea barbae
(see under Folliculitis barbae)

Tinea capitis infections
Fulvicin P/G Tablets (Griseofulvin) Schering 2359
Fulvicin P/G 165 & 330 Tablets (Griseofulvin) Schering 2359
Grifulvin V (griseofulvin tablets) Microsize (griseofulvin oral suspension) Microsize (Griseofulvin) Ortho Dermatological 1888
Gris-PEG Tablets, 125 mg & 250 mg (Griseofulvin) Allergan 479

Tinea corporis infections
Desenex Prescription (Clotrimazole) CIBA Consumer .. ◘ 633
Exelderm Cream 1.0% (Sulconazole Nitrate) Westwood-Squibb 2685
Exelderm Solution 1.0% (Sulconazole Nitrate) Westwood-Squibb 2686
Fulvicin P/G Tablets (Griseofulvin) Schering 2359
Fulvicin P/G 165 & 330 Tablets (Griseofulvin) Schering 2359
Grifulvin V (griseofulvin tablets) Microsize (griseofulvin oral suspension) Microsize (Griseofulvin) Ortho Dermatological 1888
Gris-PEG Tablets, 125 mg & 250 mg (Griseofulvin) Allergan 479
Loprox 1% Cream and Lotion (Ciclopirox Olamine) Hoechst-Roussel 1242
Lotrimin (Clotrimazole) Schering 2371
Lotrimin AF Antifungal Cream, Lotion and Solution (Clotrimazole) Schering-Plough HealthCare .... ◘ 806
Lotrimin AF Antifungal Spray Liquid, Spray Powder, Powder and Jock Itch Spray Powder

(◘ Described in PDR For Nonprescription Drugs) (◉ Described in PDR For Ophthalmology)

1547 **Indications Index** **Trichinosis**

(Miconazole Nitrate)
Schering-Plough HealthCare ▣ 807
Lotrisone Cream (Clotrimazole, Betamethasone Dipropionate) Schering 2372
Monistat Dual-Pak (Miconazole Nitrate) Ortho Pharmaceutical 1850
Monistat-Derm (miconazole nitrate 2%) Cream (Miconazole Nitrate) Ortho Dermatological 1889
Mycelex OTC Cream Antifungal (Clotrimazole) Miles Consumer ▣ 724
Mycelex OTC Solution Antifungal (Clotrimazole) Miles Consumer ▣ 724
Naftin Cream 1% (Naftifine Hydrochloride) Allergan 480
Naftin Gel 1% (Naftifine Hydrochloride) Allergan 481
Nizoral 2% Cream (Ketoconazole) Janssen 1297
Oxistat (Oxiconazole Nitrate) Glaxo Wellcome 1152
Spectazole (econazole nitrate 1%) Cream (Econazole Nitrate) Ortho Dermatological 1890
Tinactin (Tolnaftate) Schering-Plough HealthCare ▣ 809

Tinea cruris infections
Aftate for Jock Itch (Tolnaftate) Schering-Plough HealthCare ▣ 798
Cruex (Undecylenic Acid, Zinc Undecylenate) CIBA Consumer ▣ 632
Prescription Strength Desenex Cream (Clotrimazole) CIBA Consumer ▣ 633
Exelderm Cream 1.0% (Sulconazole Nitrate) Westwood-Squibb 2685
Exelderm Solution 1.0% (Sulconazole Nitrate) Westwood-Squibb 2686
Fulvicin P/G Tablets (Griseofulvin) Schering 2359
Fulvicin P/G 165 & 330 Tablets (Griseofulvin) Schering 2359
Grifulvin V (griseofulvin tablets) Microsize (griseofulvin oral suspension) Microsize (Griseofulvin) Ortho Dermatological 1888
Gris-PEG Tablets, 125 mg & 250 mg (Griseofulvin) Allergan 479
Lamisil Cream 1% (Terbinafine Hydrochloride) Sandoz Pharmaceuticals 2265
Loprox 1% Cream and Lotion (Ciclopirox Olamine) Hoechst-Roussel 1242
Lotrimin (Clotrimazole) Schering 2371
Lotrimin AF Antifungal Cream, Lotion and Solution (Clotrimazole) Schering-Plough HealthCare ▣ 806
Lotrimin AF Antifungal Spray Liquid, Spray Powder, Powder and Jock Itch Spray Powder (Miconazole Nitrate) Schering-Plough HealthCare ▣ 807
Lotrisone Cream (Clotrimazole, Betamethasone Dipropionate) Schering 2372
Monistat Dual-Pak (Miconazole Nitrate) Ortho Pharmaceutical 1850
Mycelex OTC Cream Antifungal (Clotrimazole) Miles Consumer ▣ 724
Mycelex OTC Solution Antifungal (Clotrimazole) Miles Consumer ▣ 724
Naftin Cream 1% (Naftifine Hydrochloride) Allergan 480
Naftin Gel 1% (Naftifine Hydrochloride) Allergan 481
Nizoral 2% Cream (Ketoconazole) Janssen 1297
Oxistat (Oxiconazole Nitrate) Glaxo Wellcome 1152
Spectazole (econazole nitrate 1%) Cream (Econazole Nitrate) Ortho Dermatological 1890
Tinactin (Tolnaftate) Schering-Plough HealthCare ▣ 809
Ting (Tolnaftate) CIBA Consumer ▣ 650

Tinea pedis infections
Aftate for Athlete's Foot (Tolnaftate) Schering-Plough HealthCare ▣ 798
Desenex (Undecylenic Acid, Zinc Undecylenate) CIBA Consumer ▣ 632
Desenex Prescription (Clotrimazole) CIBA Consumer ▣ 633
Exelderm Cream 1.0% (Sulconazole Nitrate) Westwood-Squibb 2685
Fulvicin P/G Tablets (Griseofulvin) Schering 2359
Fulvicin P/G 165 & 330 Tablets (Griseofulvin) Schering 2359
Grifulvin V (griseofulvin tablets) Microsize (griseofulvin oral suspension) Microsize (Griseofulvin) Ortho Dermatological 1888
Gris-PEG Tablets, 125 mg & 250 mg (Griseofulvin) Allergan 479
Lamisil Cream 1% (Terbinafine Hydrochloride) Sandoz Pharmaceuticals 2265
Loprox 1% Cream and Lotion (Ciclopirox Olamine) Hoechst-Roussel 1242
Lotrimin (Clotrimazole) Schering 2371
Lotrimin AF Antifungal Cream, Lotion and Solution (Clotrimazole) Schering-Plough HealthCare ▣ 806
Lotrimin AF Antifungal Spray Liquid, Spray Powder, Powder and Jock Itch Spray Powder (Miconazole Nitrate) Schering-Plough HealthCare ▣ 807
Lotrisone Cream (Clotrimazole, Betamethasone Dipropionate) Schering 2372
Monistat Dual-Pak (Miconazole Nitrate) Ortho Pharmaceutical 1850
Mycelex OTC Cream Antifungal (Clotrimazole) Miles Consumer ▣ 724
Mycelex OTC Solution Antifungal (Clotrimazole) Miles Consumer ▣ 724
Naftin Cream 1% (Naftifine Hydrochloride) Allergan 480
Naftin Gel 1% (Naftifine Hydrochloride) Allergan 481
Oxistat (Oxiconazole Nitrate) Glaxo Wellcome 1152
Spectazole (econazole nitrate 1%) Cream (Econazole Nitrate) Ortho Dermatological 1890
Tinactin (Tolnaftate) Schering-Plough HealthCare ▣ 809
Ting (Tolnaftate) CIBA Consumer ▣ 650

Tinea unguium infections
Fulvicin P/G Tablets (Griseofulvin) Schering 2359
Fulvicin P/G 165 & 330 Tablets (Griseofulvin) Schering 2359
Grifulvin V (griseofulvin tablets) Microsize (griseofulvin oral suspension) Microsize (Griseofulvin) Ortho Dermatological 1888
Gris-PEG Tablets, 125 mg & 250 mg (Griseofulvin) Allergan 479

Tinea versicolor infections (see under Pityrosporon orbiculare infections)

Toenails, ingrown, pain (see under Pain, unguis aduncus, temporary relief of)

Tonometry, Goldman (see under Hypertension, ocular, diagnostic agent for)

Tonsillitis
Biaxin (Clarithromycin) Abbott 405
Ceclor Pulvules & Suspension (Cefaclor) Lilly 1431
Ceftin (Cefuroxime Axetil) Glaxo Wellcome 1078
Cefzil Tablets and Oral Suspension (Cefprozil) Bristol-Myers Squibb 746
Duricef (Cefadroxil Monohydrate) Bristol-Myers Squibb 748
Lorabid Suspension and Pulvules (Loracarbef) Lilly 1459
PCE Dispertab Tablets (Erythromycin) Abbott 444
Suprax (Cefixime) Lederle 1399
Vantin for Oral Suspension and Vantin Tablets (Cefpodoxime Proxetil) Upjohn 2646
Zithromax (Azithromycin) Pfizer Labs 1944

Tonsillitis, adjunct in
Vicks Chloraseptic Sore Throat Spray, and Gargle and Mouth Rinse (Phenol) Procter & Gamble ▣ 759

Tooth, hypersensitivity of
Crest Sensitivity Protection Toothpaste (Potassium Nitrate, Sodium Fluoride) Procter & Gamble ▣ 750
Promise Sensitive Toothpaste (Potassium Nitrate, Sodium Monofluorophosphate) Block ▣ 610
Cool Gel Sensodyne (Potassium Nitrate, Sodium Fluoride) Block ▣ 611
Fresh Mint Sensodyne Toothpaste (Potassium Nitrate, Sodium Monofluorophosphate) Block ▣ 611
Original Formula Sensodyne-SC Toothpaste (Strontium Chloride Hexahydrate) Block ▣ 611
Sensodyne with Baking Soda (Potassium Nitrate, Sodium Fluoride) Block ▣ 611

Torulosis (see under Cryptococcosis)

Tourette, Gilles de la, syndrome
Haldol Injection, Tablets and Concentrate (Haloperidol) McNeil Pharmaceutical 1575
Orap Tablets (Pimozide) Gate 1050

Toxicity, anticholinergic agents, reversal of
Antilirium Injectable (Physostigmine Salicylate) Forest 1009

Toxoplasmosis, adjunctive therapy in
Daraprim Tablets (Pyrimethamine) Glaxo Wellcome 1090
Gantanol Tablets (Sulfamethoxazole) Roche Laboratories 2119
Gantrisin (Acetyl Sulfisoxazole) Roche Laboratories 2120

Tracheal lavage
Sodium Chloride and Sterile Water for Inhalation, Arm-a-Vial (Sodium Chloride) Astra 562

Trachoma
Achromycin V Capsules (Tetracycline Hydrochloride) Lederle 1367
Declomycin Tablets (Demeclocycline Hydrochloride) Lederle 1371
Doryx Capsules (Doxycycline Hyclate) Parke-Davis 1913
Dynacin Capsules (Minocycline Hydrochloride) Medicis 1590
Gantanol Tablets (Sulfamethoxazole) Roche Laboratories 2119
Gantrisin (Acetyl Sulfisoxazole) Roche Laboratories 2120
Minocin Intravenous (Minocycline Hydrochloride) Lederle 1382
Minocin Oral Suspension (Minocycline Hydrochloride) Lederle 1385
Minocin Pellet-Filled Capsules (Minocycline Hydrochloride) Lederle 1383
Monodox Capsules (Doxycycline Monohydrate) Oclassen 1805
Terramycin Intramuscular Solution (Oxytetracycline) Roerig 2210
Vibramycin (Doxycycline Calcium) Pfizer Labs 1941
Vibramycin Hyclate Intravenous (Doxycycline Hyclate) Roerig 2215
Vibramycin (Doxycycline Monohydrate) Pfizer Labs 1941

Trachoma, adjunct in
Bleph-10 (Sulfacetamide Sodium) Allergan 475
Sodium Sulamyd (Sulfacetamide Sodium) Schering 2387
Vasosulf (Phenylephrine Hydrochloride, Sulfacetamide Sodium) CIBA Vision Ophthalmics ◉ 271

Tremor, essential
Inderal (Propranolol Hydrochloride) Wyeth-Ayerst 2728

Treponema pallidum (see under T. pallidum infections)

Treponema pertenue infections (see under Yaws)

Trichinosis
Mintezol (Thiabendazole) Merck & Co., Inc. 1704

Trichinosis with myocardial involvement
Aristocort Suspension (Forte Parenteral) (Triamcinolone Diacetate) Fujisawa 1027
Aristocort Tablets (Triamcinolone) Fujisawa 1022
Celestone Soluspan Suspension (Betamethasone Sodium Phosphate, Betamethasone Acetate) Schering 2347
Cortone Acetate Sterile Suspension (Cortisone Acetate) Merck & Co., Inc. 1623
Cortone Acetate Tablets (Cortisone Acetate) Merck & Co., Inc. 1624
Dalalone D.P. Injectable (Dexamethasone Acetate) Forest 1011
Decadron Elixir (Dexamethasone) Merck & Co., Inc. 1633
Decadron Phosphate Injection (Dexamethasone Sodium Phosphate) Merck & Co., Inc. 1637
Decadron Tablets (Dexamethasone) Merck & Co., Inc. 1635
Decadron-LA Sterile Suspension (Dexamethasone Acetate) Merck & Co., Inc. 1646
Deltasone Tablets (Prednisone) Upjohn 2595
Depo-Medrol Single-Dose Vial (Methylprednisolone Acetate) Upjohn 2600
Depo-Medrol Sterile Aqueous Suspension (Methylprednisolone Acetate) Upjohn 2597
Hydeltrasol Injection, Sterile (Prednisolone Sodium Phosphate) Merck & Co., Inc. 1665
Hydrocortone Phosphate Injection, Sterile (Hydrocortisone Sodium Phosphate) Merck & Co., Inc. 1670
Hydrocortone Tablets (Hydrocortisone) Merck & Co., Inc. 1672
Medrol (Methylprednisolone) Upjohn 2621
Pediapred Oral Liquid (Prednisolone Sodium Phosphate) Fisons 995
Prelone Syrup (Prednisolone) Muro 1787
Solu-Cortef Sterile Powder (Hydrocortisone Sodium Succinate) Upjohn 2641
Solu-Medrol Sterile Powder (Methylprednisolone Sodium Succinate) Upjohn 2643

Trichinosis with neurologic involvement
Aristocort Suspension (Forte Parenteral) (Triamcinolone Diacetate) Fujisawa 1027
Aristocort Tablets (Triamcinolone) Fujisawa 1022
Celestone Soluspan Suspension (Betamethasone Sodium Phosphate, Betamethasone Acetate) Schering 2347
Cortone Acetate Sterile Suspension (Cortisone Acetate) Merck & Co., Inc. 1623
Cortone Acetate Tablets (Cortisone Acetate) Merck & Co., Inc. 1624
Dalalone D.P. Injectable (Dexamethasone Acetate) Forest 1011
Decadron Elixir (Dexamethasone) Merck & Co., Inc. 1633
Decadron Phosphate Injection (Dexamethasone Sodium Phosphate) Merck & Co., Inc. 1637
Decadron Tablets (Dexamethasone) Merck & Co., Inc. 1635
Decadron-LA Sterile Suspension (Dexamethasone Acetate) Merck & Co., Inc. 1646
Deltasone Tablets (Prednisone) Upjohn 2595
Depo-Medrol Single-Dose Vial (Methylprednisolone Acetate) Upjohn 2600

(▣ Described in PDR For Nonprescription Drugs) (◉ Described in PDR For Ophthalmology)

Trichinosis Indications Index 1548

Depo-Medrol Sterile Aqueous Suspension (Methylprednisolone Acetate) Upjohn 2597
Hydeltrasol Injection, Sterile (Prednisolone Sodium Phosphate) Merck & Co., Inc. 1665
Hydrocortone Phosphate Injection, Sterile (Hydrocortisone Sodium Phosphate) Merck & Co., Inc. 1670
Hydrocortone Tablets (Hydrocortisone) Merck & Co., Inc. 1672
Medrol (Methylprednisolone) Upjohn 2621
Pediapred Oral Liquid (Prednisolone Sodium Phosphate) Fisons 995
Prelone Syrup (Prednisolone) Muro 1787
Solu-Cortef Sterile Powder (Hydrocortisone Sodium Succinate) Upjohn 2641
Solu-Medrol Sterile Powder (Methylprednisolone Sodium Succinate) Upjohn 2643

Trichomoniasis, asymptomatic
Flagyl 375 Capsules (Metronidazole) Searle 2434
Protostat Tablets (Metronidazole) Ortho Pharmaceutical 1883

Trichomoniasis, symptomatic
Flagyl 375 Capsules (Metronidazole) Searle 2434
Protostat Tablets (Metronidazole) Ortho Pharmaceutical 1883

Trichophyton crateriform infections
Fulvicin P/G Tablets (Griseofulvin) Schering 2359
Fulvicin P/G 165 & 330 Tablets (Griseofulvin) Schering 2359
Grifulvin V (griseofulvin tablets) Microsize (griseofulvin oral suspension) Microsize (Griseofulvin) Ortho Dermatological 1888
Gris-PEG Tablets, 125 mg & 250 mg (Griseofulvin) Allergan 479

Trichophyton gallinae infections
Fulvicin P/G Tablets (Griseofulvin) Schering 2359
Fulvicin P/G 165 & 330 Tablets (Griseofulvin) Schering 2359
Grifulvin V (griseofulvin tablets) Microsize (griseofulvin oral suspension) Microsize (Griseofulvin) Ortho Dermatological 1888
Gris-PEG Tablets, 125 mg & 250 mg (Griseofulvin) Allergan 479

Trichophyton interdigitalis infections
Fulvicin P/G Tablets (Griseofulvin) Schering 2359
Fulvicin P/G 165 & 330 Tablets (Griseofulvin) Schering 2359
Grifulvin V (griseofulvin tablets) Microsize (griseofulvin oral suspension) Microsize (Griseofulvin) Ortho Dermatological 1888
Gris-PEG Tablets, 125 mg & 250 mg (Griseofulvin) Allergan 479

Trichophyton megnini infections
Fulvicin P/G Tablets (Griseofulvin) Schering 2359
Fulvicin P/G 165 & 330 Tablets (Griseofulvin) Schering 2359
Grifulvin V (griseofulvin tablets) Microsize (griseofulvin oral suspension) Microsize (Griseofulvin) Ortho Dermatological 1888
Gris-PEG Tablets, 125 mg & 250 mg (Griseofulvin) Allergan 479

Trichophyton mentagrophytes infections
Exelderm Cream 1.0% (Sulconazole Nitrate) Westwood-Squibb 2685
Exelderm Solution 1.0% (Sulconazole Nitrate) Westwood-Squibb 2686
Fulvicin P/G Tablets (Griseofulvin) Schering 2359
Fulvicin P/G 165 & 330 Tablets (Griseofulvin) Schering 2359
Grifulvin V (griseofulvin tablets) Microsize (griseofulvin oral suspension) Microsize (Griseofulvin) Ortho Dermatological 1888
Gris-PEG Tablets, 125 mg & 250 mg (Griseofulvin) Allergan 479
Lamisil Cream 1% (Terbinafine Hydrochloride) Sandoz Pharmaceuticals 2265
Loprox 1% Cream and Lotion (Ciclopirox Olamine) Hoechst-Roussel 1242
Lotrimin (Clotrimazole) Schering 2371
Lotrisone Cream (Clotrimazole, Betamethasone Dipropionate) Schering 2372
Monistat Dual-Pak (Miconazole Nitrate) Ortho Pharmaceutical 1850
Monistat-Derm (miconazole nitrate 2%) Cream (Miconazole Nitrate) Ortho Dermatological 1889
Naftin Cream 1% (Naftifine Hydrochloride) Allergan 480
Naftin Gel 1% (Naftifine Hydrochloride) Allergan 481
Nizoral 2% Cream (Ketoconazole) Janssen 1297
Oxistat (Oxiconazole Nitrate) Glaxo Wellcome 1152
Spectazole (econazole nitrate 1%) Cream (Econazole Nitrate) Ortho Dermatological 1890

Trichophyton rubrum infections
Exelderm Cream 1.0% (Sulconazole Nitrate) Westwood-Squibb 2685
Exelderm Solution 1.0% (Sulconazole Nitrate) Westwood-Squibb 2686
Fulvicin P/G Tablets (Griseofulvin) Schering 2359
Fulvicin P/G 165 & 330 Tablets (Griseofulvin) Schering 2359
Grifulvin V (griseofulvin tablets) Microsize (griseofulvin oral suspension) Microsize (Griseofulvin) Ortho Dermatological 1888
Gris-PEG Tablets, 125 mg & 250 mg (Griseofulvin) Allergan 479
Lamisil Cream 1% (Terbinafine Hydrochloride) Sandoz Pharmaceuticals 2265
Loprox 1% Cream and Lotion (Ciclopirox Olamine) Hoechst-Roussel 1242
Lotrimin (Clotrimazole) Schering 2371
Lotrisone Cream (Clotrimazole, Betamethasone Dipropionate) Schering 2372
Monistat Dual-Pak (Miconazole Nitrate) Ortho Pharmaceutical 1850
Monistat-Derm (miconazole nitrate 2%) Cream (Miconazole Nitrate) Ortho Dermatological 1889
Naftin Cream 1% (Naftifine Hydrochloride) Allergan 480
Naftin Gel 1% (Naftifine Hydrochloride) Allergan 481
Nizoral 2% Cream (Ketoconazole) Janssen 1297
Oxistat (Oxiconazole Nitrate) Glaxo Wellcome 1152
Spectazole (econazole nitrate 1%) Cream (Econazole Nitrate) Ortho Dermatological 1890

Trichophyton schoenleini infections
Fulvicin P/G Tablets (Griseofulvin) Schering 2359
Fulvicin P/G 165 & 330 Tablets (Griseofulvin) Schering 2359
Grifulvin V (griseofulvin tablets) Microsize (griseofulvin oral suspension) Microsize (Griseofulvin) Ortho Dermatological 1888
Gris-PEG Tablets, 125 mg & 250 mg (Griseofulvin) Allergan 479

Trichophyton sulfureum infections
Fulvicin P/G Tablets (Griseofulvin) Schering 2359
Fulvicin P/G 165 & 330 Tablets (Griseofulvin) Schering 2359
Grifulvin V (griseofulvin tablets) Microsize (griseofulvin oral suspension) Microsize (Griseofulvin) Ortho Dermatological 1888
Gris-PEG Tablets, 125 mg & 250 mg (Griseofulvin) Allergan 479

Trichophyton tonsurans infections
Fulvicin P/G Tablets (Griseofulvin) Schering 2359
Fulvicin P/G 165 & 330 Tablets (Griseofulvin) Schering 2359
Grifulvin V (griseofulvin tablets) Microsize (griseofulvin oral suspension) Microsize (Griseofulvin) Ortho Dermatological 1888
Gris-PEG Tablets, 125 mg & 250 mg (Griseofulvin) Allergan 479
Naftin Gel 1% (Naftifine Hydrochloride) Allergan 481
Spectazole (econazole nitrate 1%) Cream (Econazole Nitrate) Ortho Dermatological 1890

Trichophyton verrucosum infections
Fulvicin P/G Tablets (Griseofulvin) Schering 2359
Fulvicin P/G 165 & 330 Tablets (Griseofulvin) Schering 2359
Grifulvin V (griseofulvin tablets) Microsize (griseofulvin oral suspension) Microsize (Griseofulvin) Ortho Dermatological 1888
Gris-PEG Tablets, 125 mg & 250 mg (Griseofulvin) Allergan 479

Trichuris trichiura infections
Vermox Chewable Tablets (Mebendazole) Janssen 1312

Trichuriasis, as secondary therapy
Mintezol (Thiabendazole) Merck & Co., Inc. 1704

Triglyceride levels, elevated (see under Hypertriglyceridemia, adjunct to diet)

Trigonitis
Urised Tablets (Atropine Sulfate, Hyoscyamine, Methenamine, Phenyl Salicylate) PolyMedica 1964

Tuberculin-sensitivity, detection of
PPD Tine Test (Tuberculin, Purified Protein Derivative, Multiple Puncture Device) Lederle 2874
Tuberculin, Old, Tine Test (Tuberculin, Old) Lederle 2875

Tuberculosis, diagnostic aid in
Tubersol (Tuberculin Purified Protein Derivative [Mantoux]) (Tuberculin, Purified Protein Derivative For Mantoux Test) Connaught 2872

Tuberculosis meningitis, adjunctive therapy in (see under Meningitis, tuberculous)

Tuberculosis, pulmonary
Capastat Sulfate Vials (Capreomycin Sulfate) Eli Lilly 2868
Myambutol Tablets (Ethambutol Hydrochloride) Lederle 1386
Rifadin (Rifampin) Marion Merrell Dow 1528
Rifamate Capsules (Rifampin, Isoniazid) Marion Merrell Dow 1530
Rifater (Rifampin, Isoniazid, Pyrazinamide) Marion Merrell Dow 1532
Rimactane Capsules (Rifampin) CibaGeneva 847
Seromycin Pulvules (Cycloserine) Lilly 1476
Streptomycin Sulfate Injection (Streptomycin Sulfate) Roerig 2208

Tuberculosis, pulmonary, disseminated
Aristocort Suspension (Forte Parenteral) (Triamcinolone Diacetate) Fujisawa 1027
Aristocort Tablets (Triamcinolone) Fujisawa 1022
Celestone Soluspan Suspension (Betamethasone Sodium Phosphate, Betamethasone Acetate) Schering 2347
Cortone Acetate Sterile Suspension (Cortisone Acetate) Merck & Co., Inc. 1623
Cortone Acetate Tablets (Cortisone Acetate) Merck & Co., Inc. 1624
Decadron Elixir (Dexamethasone) Merck & Co., Inc. 1633
Decadron Phosphate Injection (Dexamethasone Sodium Phosphate) Merck & Co., Inc. 1637
Decadron Tablets (Dexamethasone) Merck & Co., Inc. 1635
Deltasone Tablets (Prednisone) Upjohn 2595
Depo-Medrol Single-Dose Vial (Methylprednisolone Acetate) Upjohn 2600
Depo-Medrol Sterile Aqueous Suspension (Methylprednisolone Acetate) Upjohn 2597
Hydeltrasol Injection, Sterile (Prednisolone Sodium Phosphate) Merck & Co., Inc. 1665
Hydrocortone Phosphate Injection, Sterile (Hydrocortisone Sodium Phosphate) Merck & Co., Inc. 1670
Hydrocortone Tablets (Hydrocortisone) Merck & Co., Inc. 1672
Medrol (Methylprednisolone) Upjohn 2621
Pediapred Oral Liquid (Prednisolone Sodium Phosphate) Fisons 995
Prelone Syrup (Prednisolone) Muro 1787
Solu-Cortef Sterile Powder (Hydrocortisone Sodium Succinate) Upjohn 2641
Solu-Medrol Sterile Powder (Methylprednisolone Sodium Succinate) Upjohn 2643

Tuberculosis, pulmonary, fulminating
Aristocort Suspension (Forte Parenteral) (Triamcinolone Diacetate) Fujisawa 1027
Aristocort Tablets (Triamcinolone) Fujisawa 1022
Celestone Soluspan Suspension (Betamethasone Sodium Phosphate, Betamethasone Acetate) Schering 2347
Cortone Acetate Sterile Suspension (Cortisone Acetate) Merck & Co., Inc. 1623
Cortone Acetate Tablets (Cortisone Acetate) Merck & Co., Inc. 1624
Decadron Elixir (Dexamethasone) Merck & Co., Inc. 1633
Decadron Phosphate Injection (Dexamethasone Sodium Phosphate) Merck & Co., Inc. 1637
Decadron Tablets (Dexamethasone) Merck & Co., Inc. 1635
Deltasone Tablets (Prednisone) Upjohn 2595
Depo-Medrol Single-Dose Vial (Methylprednisolone Acetate) Upjohn 2600
Depo-Medrol Sterile Aqueous Suspension (Methylprednisolone Acetate) Upjohn 2597
Hydeltrasol Injection, Sterile (Prednisolone Sodium Phosphate) Merck & Co., Inc. 1665
Hydrocortone Phosphate Injection, Sterile (Hydrocortisone Sodium Phosphate) Merck & Co., Inc. 1670
Hydrocortone Tablets (Hydrocortisone) Merck & Co., Inc. 1672
Medrol (Methylprednisolone) Upjohn 2621
Pediapred Oral Liquid (Prednisolone Sodium Phosphate) Fisons 995
Prelone Syrup (Prednisolone) Muro 1787
Solu-Cortef Sterile Powder (Hydrocortisone Sodium Succinate) Upjohn 2641
Solu-Medrol Sterile Powder (Methylprednisolone Sodium Succinate) Upjohn 2643

Tuberculosis, pulmonary, prophylaxis of
BCG Vaccine, USP (TICE) (BCG Vaccine) Organon 1814

Tuberculosis, treatment
Myambutol Tablets (Ethambutol Hydrochloride) Lederle 1386
Nydrazid Injection (Isoniazid) Apothecon 508
Pyrazinamide Tablets (Pyrazinamide) Lederle 1398

1549 Indications Index Urticarial manifestations

Rifadin (Rifampin) Marion Merrell Dow ... 1528
Rifamate Capsules (Rifampin, Isoniazid) Marion Merrell Dow ... 1530
Rimactane Capsules (Rifampin) CibaGeneva ... 847
Seromycin Pulvules (Cycloserine) Lilly ... 1476
Streptomycin Sulfate Injection (Streptomycin Sulfate) Roerig ... 2208
Trecator-SC Tablets (Ethionamide) Wyeth-Ayerst ... 2814

Tuberculosis, treatment adjunct
PASER Granules (Aminosalicylic Acid) Jacobus ... 1285
Pyrazinamide Tablets (Pyrazinamide) Lederle ... 1398

Tularemia
Dynacin Capsules (Minocycline Hydrochloride) Medicis ... 1590
Minocin Oral Suspension (Minocycline Hydrochloride) Lederle ... 1385
Minocin Pellet-Filled Capsules (Minocycline Hydrochloride) Lederle ... 1383
Monodox Capsules (Doxycycline Monohydrate) Oclassen ... 1805
Vibramycin Hyclate Capsules (Doxycycline Hyclate) Pfizer Labs 1941

Tumors, brain, metastatic
CeeNU (Lomustine (CCNU)) Bristol-Myers Squibb Oncology ... 693

Tumors, brain, metastatic, palliative therapy in
BiCNU (Carmustine (BCNU)) Bristol-Myers Squibb Oncology ... 691

Tumors, brain, palliative therapy in
BiCNU (Carmustine (BCNU)) Bristol-Myers Squibb Oncology ... 691

Tumors, brain, primary
CeeNU (Lomustine (CCNU)) Bristol-Myers Squibb Oncology ... 693

Tumors, carcinoid, symptomatic relief of
Sandostatin Injection (Octreotide Acetate) Sandoz Pharmaceuticals 2292

Typhus fever
Achromycin V Capsules (Tetracycline Hydrochloride) Lederle ... 1367
Declomycin Tablets (Demeclocycline Hydrochloride) Lederle ... 1371
Doryx Capsules (Doxycycline Hyclate) Parke-Davis ... 1913
Dynacin Capsules (Minocycline Hydrochloride) Medicis ... 1590
Minocin Intravenous (Minocycline Hydrochloride) Lederle ... 1382
Minocin Oral Suspension (Minocycline Hydrochloride) Lederle ... 1385
Minocin Pellet-Filled Capsules (Minocycline Hydrochloride) Lederle ... 1383
Monodox Capsules (Doxycycline Monohydrate) Oclassen ... 1805
Terramycin Intramuscular Solution (Oxytetracycline) Roerig ... 2210
Vibramycin (Doxycycline Calcium) Pfizer Labs ... 1941
Vibramycin Hyclate Intravenous (Doxycycline Hyclate) Roerig ... 2215
Vibramycin (Doxycycline Monohydrate) Pfizer Labs ... 1941

Typhus group infection
Achromycin V Capsules (Tetracycline Hydrochloride) Lederle ... 1367
Declomycin Tablets (Demeclocycline Hydrochloride) Lederle ... 1371
Doryx Capsules (Doxycycline Hyclate) Parke-Davis ... 1913
Dynacin Capsules (Minocycline Hydrochloride) Medicis ... 1590
Minocin Intravenous (Minocycline Hydrochloride) Lederle ... 1382
Minocin Oral Suspension (Minocycline Hydrochloride) Lederle ... 1385
Minocin Pellet-Filled Capsules (Minocycline Hydrochloride) Lederle ... 1383
Monodox Capsules (Doxycycline Monohydrate) Oclassen ... 1805
Terramycin Intramuscular Solution (Oxytetracycline) Roerig ... 2210
Vibramycin Hyclate Capsules (Doxycycline Hyclate) Pfizer Labs 1941
Vibramycin Hyclate Intravenous (Doxycycline Hyclate) Roerig ... 2215

U

Ulcerative colitis (see under Colitis, ulcerative, systemic therapy for)

Ulcers, decubitus, adjunctive therapy in
Chloresium (Chlorophyllin Copper Complex) Rystan ... 2246
Elase Ointment (Desoxyribonuclease, Fibrinolysin) Fujisawa ... 1039
Elase Vials (Fibrinolysin, Desoxyribonuclease) Fujisawa ... 1038
Granulex (Trypsin, Balsam Peru, Castor Oil) Dow Hickam ... 925
Panafil Ointment (Papain, Chlorophyllin Copper Complex, Urea) Rystan ... 2246
Panafil-White Ointment (Papain, Urea) Rystan ... 2247
Travase Ointment (Sutilains) Knoll Laboratories ... 1356

Ulcers, decubitus, reduction of possible occurrence of
Betadine Solution (Povidone Iodine) Purdue Frederick ... 1992

Ulcers, dermal
Primaxin I.M. (Imipenem-Cilastatin Sodium) Merck & Co., Inc. ... 1727

Ulcers, diabetic, adjunctive therapy in
Mitraflex Wound Dressing (Polyurethane Film) Convatec ... 2866
Panafil Ointment (Papain, Chlorophyllin Copper Complex, Urea) Rystan ... 2246
Panafil-White Ointment (Papain, Urea) Rystan ... 2247

Ulcers, varicose, adjunctive therapy in
Panafil Ointment (Papain, Chlorophyllin Copper Complex, Urea) Rystan ... 2246
Panafil-White Ointment (Papain, Urea) Rystan ... 2247

Immunization, meningococcal
Menomune-A/C/Y/W-135 (Meningococcal Polysaccharide Vaccine) Connaught ... 889

Uncinariasis, as secondary therapy
Mintezol (Thiabendazole) Merck & Co., Inc. ... 1704

Ureaplasma urealyticum urethritis
E.E.S. (Erythromycin Ethylsuccinate) Abbott ... 424
EryPed (Erythromycin Ethylsuccinate) Abbott ... 421
Minocin Oral Suspension (Minocycline Hydrochloride) Lederle ... 1385

Ureaplasma urealyticum urethritis, nongonococcal
Doryx Capsules (Doxycycline Hyclate) Parke-Davis ... 1913
Dynacin Capsules (Minocycline Hydrochloride) Medicis ... 1590
ERYC (Erythromycin) Parke-Davis .. 1915
Minocin Oral Suspension (Minocycline Hydrochloride) Lederle ... 1385
Minocin Pellet-Filled Capsules (Minocycline Hydrochloride) Lederle ... 1383
Monodox Capsules (Doxycycline Monohydrate) Oclassen ... 1805
PCE Dispertab Tablets (Erythromycin) Abbott ... 444
Vibramycin (Doxycycline Calcium) Pfizer Labs ... 1941

Urethritis
E.E.S. (Erythromycin Ethylsuccinate) Abbott ... 424
EryPed (Erythromycin Ethylsuccinate) Abbott ... 421
PCE Dispertab Tablets (Erythromycin) Abbott ... 444
Urised Tablets (Atropine Sulfate, Hyoscyamine, Methenamine, Phenyl Salicylate) PolyMedica ... 1964
Zithromax (Azithromycin) Pfizer Labs ... 1944

Urethritis, atrophic
Premarin Tablets (Estrogens, Conjugated) Wyeth-Ayerst ... 2789

Urethritis, Chlamydia trachomatis, nongonococcal
Doryx Capsules (Doxycycline Hyclate) Parke-Davis ... 1913
Floxin I.V. (Ofloxacin) McNeil Pharmaceutical ... 1571
Monodox Capsules (Doxycycline Monohydrate) Oclassen ... 1805
Vibramycin (Doxycycline Calcium) Pfizer Labs ... 1941
Zithromax (Azithromycin) Pfizer Labs ... 1944

Urethritis, frequency and incontinence, symptomatic relief of
Urispas Tablets (Flavoxate Hydrochloride) SmithKline Beecham Pharmaceuticals ... 2532

Urethritis, "lacking substantial evidence of effectiveness" in
Urobiotic-250 Capsules (Oxytetracycline Hydrochloride, Sulfamethizole, Phenazopyridine Hydrochloride) Roerig ... 2214

Urethritis, uncomplicated gonococcal
Dynacin Capsules (Minocycline Hydrochloride) Medicis ... 1590
Minocin Oral Suspension (Minocycline Hydrochloride) Lederle ... 1385
Minocin Pellet-Filled Capsules (Minocycline Hydrochloride) Lederle ... 1383
Pipracil (Piperacillin Sodium) Lederle ... 1390

Urethrocystitis, frequency and incontinence, symptomatic relief of
Urispas Tablets (Flavoxate Hydrochloride) SmithKline Beecham Pharmaceuticals ... 2532

Urethrotrigonitis, frequency and incontinence, symptomatic relief of
Urispas Tablets (Flavoxate Hydrochloride) SmithKline Beecham Pharmaceuticals ... 2532

Uric acid lithiasis (see under Urolithiasis, management of)

Urinary bladder with retention, neurogenic atony of
Urecholine (Bethanechol Chloride) Merck & Co., Inc. ... 1761

Urinary bladder, reflex neurogenic, symptomatic relief of
Ditropan (Oxybutynin Chloride) Marion Merrell Dow ... 1516

Urinary frequency, symptomatic relief of
Prodium (Phenazopyridine Hydrochloride) Breckenridge ... 690
Pyridium (Phenazopyridine Hydrochloride) Parke-Davis ... 1928

Urinary incontinence, adjunct
Hyland's EnurAid Tablets (Homeopathic Medications) Standard Homeopathic ... ▣ 829

Urinary retention, acute postoperative
Duvoid (Bethanechol Chloride) Roberts ... 2044
Prostigmin Injectable (Neostigmine Methylsulfate) ICN ... 1260
Urecholine (Bethanechol Chloride) Merck & Co., Inc. ... 1761

Urinary retention, neurogenic atony of the urinary bladder
Duvoid (Bethanechol Chloride) Roberts ... 2044

Urinary retention, postpartum nonobstructive
Duvoid (Bethanechol Chloride) Roberts ... 2044
Urecholine (Bethanechol Chloride) Merck & Co., Inc. ... 1761

Urinary tract pain, relief of (see under Pain, urinary tract)

Urinary tract, burning, symptomatic relief of
Prodium (Phenazopyridine Hydrochloride) Breckenridge ... 690
Pyridium (Phenazopyridine Hydrochloride) Parke-Davis ... 1928

Urinary tract, hypermotility, control of symptoms
Levsin/Levsinex/Levbid (Hyoscyamine Sulfate) Schwarz ... 2405

Urinary tract, lower, hypermotility disorders
Cystospaz (Hyoscyamine) PolyMedica ... 1963
Urised Tablets (Atropine Sulfate, Hyoscyamine, Methenamine, Phenyl Salicylate) PolyMedica ... 1964

Urinary urgency, symptomatic relief of
Prodium (Phenazopyridine Hydrochloride) Breckenridge ... 690
Pyridium (Phenazopyridine Hydrochloride) Parke-Davis ... 1928
Urispas Tablets (Flavoxate Hydrochloride) SmithKline Beecham Pharmaceuticals ... 2532

Urinary voiding, irritable, symptomatic relief of
Ditropan (Oxybutynin Chloride) Marion Merrell Dow ... 1516

Urine, acidification of
K-Phos Original Formula 'Sodium Free' Tablets (Potassium Acid Phosphate) Beach ... 639

Urine, alkalinization of
Bicitra (Sodium Citrate, Citric Acid) Baker Norton ... 578
Polycitra Syrup (Potassium Citrate, Sodium Citrate, Citric Acid) Baker Norton ... 578
Polycitra-K Crystals (Potassium Citrate, Citric Acid) Baker Norton 579
Polycitra-K Oral Solution (Potassium Citrate, Citric Acid) Baker Norton ... 579
Polycitra-LC (Potassium Citrate, Citric Acid, Sodium Citrate) Baker Norton ... 578

Urticaria, cold
Periactin (Cyproheptadine Hydrochloride) Merck & Co., Inc. 1724

Urticarial manifestations, relief of
Atarax Tablets & Syrup (Hydroxyzine Hydrochloride) Roerig ... 2185
Benadryl Capsules (Diphenhydramine Hydrochloride) Parke-Davis 1898
Extendryl (Chlorpheniramine Maleate, Methscopolamine Nitrate, Phenylephrine Hydrochloride) Fleming ... 1005
Hismanal Tablets (Astemizole) Janssen ... 1293
PBZ Tablets (Tripelennamine Hydrochloride) CibaGeneva ... 845
PBZ-SR Tablets (Tripelennamine Hydrochloride) CibaGeneva ... 844
Periactin (Cyproheptadine Hydrochloride) Merck & Co., Inc. 1724
Phenergan Suppositories (Promethazine Hydrochloride) Wyeth-Ayerst ... 2775
Phenergan Syrup (Promethazine Hydrochloride) Wyeth-Ayerst ... 2774
Phenergan Tablets (Promethazine Hydrochloride) Wyeth-Ayerst ... 2775
Tavist Syrup (Clemastine Fumarate) Sandoz Pharmaceuticals ... 2297
Tavist Tablets (Clemastine Fumarate) Sandoz Pharmaceuticals ... 2298
Temaril Tablets, Syrup and Spansule Extended-Release

(▣ Described in PDR For Nonprescription Drugs) (◉ Described in PDR For Ophthalmology)

Urticarial manifestations | **Indications Index** | **1550**

Capsules (Trimeprazine Tartrate) Allergan 483
Vistaril Intramuscular Solution (Hydroxyzine Hydrochloride) Roerig 2216
Vistaril Oral Suspension (Hydroxyzine Pamoate) Pfizer Labs 1944

Urticarial transfusion reactions
Aristocort Suspension (Forte Parenteral) (Triamcinolone Diacetate) Fujisawa 1027
Celestone Soluspan Suspension (Betamethasone Sodium Phosphate, Betamethasone Acetate) Schering 2347
Cortone Acetate Sterile Suspension (Cortisone Acetate) Merck & Co., Inc. 1623
Dalalone D.P. Injectable (Dexamethasone Acetate) Forest 1011
Decadron Phosphate Injection (Dexamethasone Sodium Phosphate) Merck & Co., Inc. 1637
Decadron-LA Sterile Suspension (Dexamethasone Acetate) Merck & Co., Inc. 1646
Depo-Medrol Single-Dose Vial (Methylprednisolone Acetate) Upjohn 2600
Depo-Medrol Sterile Aqueous Suspension (Methylprednisolone Acetate) Upjohn 2597
Hydeltrasol Injection, Sterile (Prednisolone Sodium Phosphate) Merck & Co., Inc. 1665
Hydrocortone Phosphate Injection, Sterile (Hydrocortisone Sodium Phosphate) Merck & Co., Inc. 1670
Solu-Cortef Sterile Powder (Hydrocortisone Sodium Succinate) Upjohn 2641
Solu-Medrol Sterile Powder (Methylprednisolone Sodium Succinate) Upjohn 2643

Uterine atony, postpartum
Methergine (Methylergonovine Maleate) Sandoz Pharmaceuticals 2272

Uterine bleeding, abnormal
Amen Tablets (Medroxyprogesterone Acetate) Carnrick 780
Aygestin Tablets (Norethindrone Acetate) ESI Lederle 974
Climara Transdermal System (Estradiol) Berlex 645
Cycrin Tablets (Medroxyprogesterone Acetate) ESI Lederle 975
Premarin Intravenous (Estrogens, Conjugated) Wyeth-Ayerst 2787
Provera Tablets (Medroxyprogesterone Acetate) Upjohn 2636

Uterine cavity, hysteroscopic aid in
Hyskon Hysteroscopy Fluid (Dextran 70) Medisan 1595

Uterine contents, evacuation of
Prostin E2 Suppository (Dinoprostone) Upjohn 2634

Uveitis, chronic anterior, steroid-responsive
AK-CIDE (Prednisolone Acetate, Sulfacetamide Sodium) Akorn .... ◉ 202
AK-CIDE Ointment (Prednisolone Acetate, Sulfacetamide Sodium) Akorn .... ◉ 202
AK-Trol Ointment & Suspension (Dexamethasone, Neomycin Sulfate, Polymyxin B Sulfate) Akorn .... ◉ 205
Blephamide Liquifilm Sterile Ophthalmic Suspension (Prednisolone Acetate, Sulfacetamide Sodium) Allergan 476
Blephamide Ointment (Sulfacetamide Sodium, Prednisolone Acetate) Allergan .... ◉ 237
Cortisporin Ophthalmic Ointment Sterile (Polymyxin B Sulfate, Bacitracin Zinc, Neomycin Sulfate, Hydrocortisone) Glaxo Wellcome 1085
Cortisporin Ophthalmic Suspension Sterile (Hydrocortisone, Polymyxin B Sulfate, Neomycin Sulfate) Glaxo Wellcome 1086
Dexacidin Ointment (Dexamethasone, Neomycin Sulfate, Polymyxin B Sulfate) CIBA Vision Ophthalmics .... ◉ 263
FML-S Liquifilm (Sulfacetamide Sodium, Fluorometholone) Allergan .... ◉ 242
Maxitrol Ophthalmic Ointment and Suspension (Dexamethasone, Neomycin Sulfate, Polymyxin B Sulfate) Alcon Laboratories .... ◉ 224
NeoDecadron Sterile Ophthalmic Ointment (Neomycin Sulfate, Dexamethasone Sodium Phosphate) Merck & Co., Inc. 1712
NeoDecadron Sterile Ophthalmic Solution (Neomycin Sulfate, Dexamethasone Sodium Phosphate) Merck & Co., Inc. 1713
Ophthocort (Chloramphenicol, Polymyxin B Sulfate, Hydrocortisone Acetate) Parke-Davis .... ◉ 311
Poly-Pred Liquifilm (Neomycin Sulfate, Polymyxin B Sulfate, Prednisolone Acetate) Allergan .... ◉ 248
Pred-G Liquifilm Sterile Ophthalmic Suspension (Gentamicin Sulfate, Prednisolone Acetate) Allergan .... ◉ 251
Pred-G S.O.P. Sterile Ophthalmic Ointment (Gentamicin Sulfate, Prednisolone Acetate) Allergan .... ◉ 252
Terra-Cortril Ophthalmic Suspension (Oxytetracycline Hydrochloride, Hydrocortisone Acetate) Roerig 2210
TobraDex Ophthalmic Suspension and Ointment (Dexamethasone, Tobramycin) Alcon Laboratories 473
Vasocidin Ointment (Prednisolone Acetate, Sulfacetamide Sodium) CIBA Vision Ophthalmics .... ◉ 268
Vasocidin Ophthalmic Solution (Prednisolone Sodium Phosphate, Sulfacetamide Sodium) CIBA Vision Ophthalmics .... ◉ 270
Vexol 1% Ophthalmic Suspension (Rimexolone) Alcon Laboratories .... ◉ 230

Uveitis, diffuse posterior
Aristocort Suspension (Forte Parenteral) (Triamcinolone Diacetate) Fujisawa 1027
Aristocort Tablets (Triamcinolone) Fujisawa 1022
Celestone Soluspan Suspension (Betamethasone Sodium Phosphate, Betamethasone Acetate) Schering 2347
Cortone Acetate Sterile Suspension (Cortisone Acetate) Merck & Co., Inc. 1623
Cortone Acetate Tablets (Cortisone Acetate) Merck & Co., Inc. 1624
Dalalone D.P. Injectable (Dexamethasone Acetate) Forest 1011
Decadron Elixir (Dexamethasone) Merck & Co., Inc. 1633
Decadron Phosphate Injection (Dexamethasone Sodium Phosphate) Merck & Co., Inc. 1637
Decadron Tablets (Dexamethasone) Merck & Co., Inc. 1635
Decadron-LA Sterile Suspension (Dexamethasone Acetate) Merck & Co., Inc. 1646
Deltasone Tablets (Prednisone) Upjohn 2595
Depo-Medrol Single-Dose Vial (Methylprednisolone Acetate) Upjohn 2600
Depo-Medrol Sterile Aqueous Suspension (Methylprednisolone Acetate) Upjohn 2597
Hydeltrasol Injection, Sterile (Prednisolone Sodium Phosphate) Merck & Co., Inc. 1665
Hydrocortone Phosphate Injection, Sterile (Hydrocortisone Sodium Phosphate) Merck & Co., Inc. 1670
Hydrocortone Tablets (Hydrocortisone) Merck & Co., Inc. 1672
Medrol (Methylprednisolone) Upjohn 2621
Pediapred Oral Liquid (Prednisolone Sodium Phosphate) Fisons 995
Prelone Syrup (Prednisolone) Muro 1787
Solu-Cortef Sterile Powder (Hydrocortisone Sodium Succinate) Upjohn 2641
Solu-Medrol Sterile Powder (Methylprednisolone Sodium Succinate) Upjohn 2643

V

Vagina, cleansing of
Hemorid For Women Cleanser (Cleanser) Thompson Medical .... ▣ 834
Massengill Disposable Douche (Vinegar) SmithKline Beecham 2457
Massengill Feminine Cleansing Wash (Cleanser) SmithKline Beecham 2458
Massengill (Povidone Iodine) SmithKline Beecham 2457

Vaginal acidity, restoration of, adjunctive therapy for
Aci-Jel Therapeutic Vaginal Jelly (Acetic Acid, Oxyquinoline Sulfate) Ortho Pharmaceutical 1848

Vaginal and anogenital areas, external, cleansing of
Betadine Medicated Douche (Povidone Iodine) Purdue Frederick 1992
Betadine Solution (Povidone Iodine) Purdue Frederick 1992
Massengill Fragrance-Free Soft Cloth Towelette & Baby Powder Scent (Lactic Acid, Potassium Sorbate, Sodium Lactate) SmithKline Beecham 2458
Tucks Pads (Witch Hazel) WARNER WELLCOME .... ▣ 865

Vaginal atrophy
Premphase (Estrogens, Conjugated, Medroxyprogesterone Acetate) Wyeth-Ayerst 2797
Prempro (Estrogens, Conjugated, Medroxyprogesterone Acetate) Wyeth-Ayerst 2801

Vaginal moisture, replenishing of
Gyne-Moistrin Vaginal Moisturizing Gel (Lubricant, Polyglycerylmethacrylate) Schering-Plough HealthCare .... ▣ 806
Replens Vaginal Moisturizer (Glycerin, Lubricant) WARNER WELLCOME .... ▣ 859

Vaginosis, bacterial
Cleocin Vaginal Cream (Clindamycin Phosphate) Upjohn 2589
MetroGel-Vaginal (Metronidazole) Curatek 902
Sultrin (Sulfathiazole, Sulfacetamide, Sulfabenzamide) Ortho Pharmaceutical 1885

Vaginitis (see under Vaginosis, bacterial)

Vaginitis, atrophic
Climara Transdermal System (Estradiol) Berlex 645
Estrace Cream and Tablets (Estradiol) Bristol-Myers Squibb 749
Estraderm Transdermal System (Estradiol) CibaGeneva 824
ESTRATAB Tablets (0.3, 0.625, 1.25, 2.5 mg) (Estrogens, Esterified) Solvay 2536
Menest Tablets (Estrogens, Esterified) SmithKline Beecham Pharmaceuticals 2494
Ogen Tablets (Estropipate) Upjohn 2627
Ogen Vaginal Cream (Estropipate) Upjohn 2630
Ortho Dienestrol Cream (Dienestrol) Ortho Pharmaceutical 1866
Ortho-Est (Estropipate) Ortho Pharmaceutical 1869
Premarin Tablets (Estrogens, Conjugated) Wyeth-Ayerst 2789
Premarin Vaginal Cream (Estrogens, Conjugated) Wyeth-Ayerst 2791
Premphase (Estrogens, Conjugated, Medroxyprogesterone Acetate) Wyeth-Ayerst 2797
Prempro (Estrogens, Conjugated, Medroxyprogesterone Acetate) Wyeth-Ayerst 2801

Vaginitis, symptomatic relief of irritation and itching
Betadine Medicated Douche (Povidone Iodine) Purdue Frederick 1992
Betadine Medicated Gel (Povidone Iodine) Purdue Frederick 1992
Betadine Pre-Mixed Medicated Disposable Douche (Povidone Iodine) Purdue Frederick 1992
Massengill Medicated Disposable Douche (Povidone Iodine) SmithKline Beecham 2458
Massengill Medicated Liquid Concentrate (Povidone Iodine) SmithKline Beecham Consumer .... ▣ 821
Massengill Medicated Soft Cloth Towelettes (Hydrocortisone) SmithKline Beecham 2458

Varicella, acute, treatment of
Zovirax (Acyclovir) Glaxo Wellcome 1219

Varicella, prevention or modification of
Gammar, Immune Globulin (Human) U.S.P. (Globulin, Immune (Human)) Armour 515

Varicose veins (see under Veins, varicose, obliteration of)

Vascular failure
Neo-Synephrine Hydrochloride 1% Carpuject (Phenylephrine Hydrochloride) Sanofi Winthrop 2324
Neo-Synephrine Hydrochloride 1% Injection (Phenylephrine Hydrochloride) Sanofi Winthrop 2324

Vasopressin-sensitive diabetes insipidus (see under Diabetes insipidus)

Veins, varicose, obliteration of
Scleromate (Morrhuate Sodium) Palisades 1891
Sotradecol (Sodium Tetradecyl Sulfate Injection) (Sodium Tetradecyl Sulfate) Elkins-Sinn 967

Ventilation, mechanical, facilitation of
Anectine (Succinylcholine Chloride) Glaxo Wellcome 1073
Mivacron (Mivacurium Chloride) Glaxo Wellcome 1138
Norcuron (Vecuronium Bromide) Organon 1826
Nuromax Injection (Doxacurium Chloride) Glaxo Wellcome 1149
Tracrium Injection (Atracurium Besylate) Glaxo Wellcome 1183
Zemuron (Rocuronium Bromide) Organon 1830

Ventricular arrhythmias (see under Arrhythmias, ventricular)

Ventricular contractions, premature
Quinidex Extentabs (Quinidine Sulfate) Robins 2067

Ventricular dysfunction, left, asymptomatic (see also under Myocardial infarction, post, left ventricular dysfunction)
Vasotec Tablets (Enalapril Maleate) Merck & Co., Inc. 1771

Ventricular extrasystoles, premature
Inderal (Propranolol Hydrochloride) Wyeth-Ayerst 2728

Ventricular fibrillation
Cordarone Intravenous (Amiodarone Hydrochloride) Wyeth-Ayerst 2715
Cordarone Tablets (Amiodarone Hydrochloride) Wyeth-Ayerst 2712

Ventricular tachycardia, sustained (see under Tachycardia, ventricular, sustained)

1551 **Indications Index** **Vomiting**

Ventriculitis (see also under Infections, central nervous system)
Claforan Sterile and Injection (Cefotaxime Sodium) Hoechst-Roussel ... 1235

Verrucae plantaris (see under Warts, plantar, removal of)

Verrucae vulgaris infection (see under Warts, common, removal of)

Vertigo
Vontrol Tablets (Diphenidol) SmithKline Beecham Pharmaceuticals ... 2532

Vertigo, auditory (see under Meniere's disease)

Vertigo, labyrinthine (see under Meniere's disease)

Vertigo, "possibly" effective in
Antivert, Antivert/25 Tablets, & Antivert/50 Tablets (Meclizine Hydrochloride) Roerig ... 2185

Vibrio cholerae infections
Achromycin V Capsules (Tetracycline Hydrochloride) Lederle ... 1367
Declomycin Tablets (Demeclocycline Hydrochloride) Lederle ... 1371
Doryx Capsules (Doxycycline Hyclate) Parke-Davis ... 1913
Dynacin Capsules (Minocycline Hydrochloride) Medicis ... 1590
Minocin Intravenous (Minocycline Hydrochloride) Lederle ... 1382
Minocin Oral Suspension (Minocycline Hydrochloride) Lederle ... 1385
Minocin Pellet-Filled Capsules (Minocycline Hydrochloride) Lederle ... 1383
Monodox Capsules (Doxycycline Monohydrate) Oclassen ... 1805
Terramycin Intramuscular Solution (Oxytetracycline) Roerig ... 2210
Vibramycin (Doxycycline Calcium) Pfizer Labs ... 1941
Vibramycin Hyclate Intravenous (Doxycycline Hyclate) Roerig ... 2215
Vibramycin (Doxycycline Monohydrate) Pfizer Labs ... 1941

Vibrio comma (see under Vibrio cholerae infections)

Vibrio fetus infections (see under Campylobacter fetus infections)

Vincent's gingivitis (see under Fusospirochetosis)

Vincent's infection (see under Fusospirochetosis)

Vincent's pharyngitis (see under Fusospirochetosis)

Vision, blurred
Lacrisert Sterile Ophthalmic Insert (Hydroxypropyl Cellulose) Merck & Co., Inc. ... 1686

Vision, cloudy
Lacrisert Sterile Ophthalmic Insert (Hydroxypropyl Cellulose) Merck & Co., Inc. ... 1686

Vitamin and mineral, multiple, deficiency of
Akorn's Antioxidants (Vitamins with Minerals) Akorn ... ⊙ 206
Berocca Plus Tablets (Vitamins with Minerals) Roche Laboratories ... 2087
Bugs Bunny Complete Children's Chewable Vitamins + Minerals with Iron and Calcium (Sugar Free) (Vitamins with Minerals) Miles Consumer ... ▣ 721
Bugs Bunny With Extra C Children's Chewable Vitamins (Sugar Free) (Vitamins with Minerals) Miles Consumer ... ▣ 722
Bugs Bunny Plus Iron Children's Chewable Vitamins (Sugar Free) (Vitamins with Iron) Miles Consumer ... ▣ 718
Centrum (Vitamins with Minerals) Lederle Consumer ... ▣ 666
Centrum, Jr. (Children's Chewable) + Extra C (Vitamins with Minerals) Lederle Consumer ... ▣ 666
Centrum, Jr. (Children's Chewable) + Extra Calcium (Vitamins with Minerals) Lederle Consumer ... ▣ 667
Centrum, Jr. (Children's Chewable) + Iron (Vitamins with Minerals) Lederle Consumer ... ▣ 668
Centrum Liquid (Vitamins with Minerals) Lederle Consumer ... ▣ 666
Centrum Silver (Vitamins with Minerals) Lederle Consumer ... ▣ 668
Flintstones Children's Chewable Vitamins (Vitamins with Minerals) Miles Consumer ... ▣ 718
Flintstones Children's Chewable Vitamins Plus Extra C (Vitamins with Minerals) Miles Consumer ... ▣ 722
Flintstones Children's Chewable Vitamins Plus Iron (Vitamins with Iron) Miles Consumer ... ▣ 718
Flintstones Complete With Calcium, Iron & Minerals Children's Chewable Vitamins (Vitamins with Minerals) Miles Consumer ... ▣ 721
Flintstones Plus Calcium Children's Chewable Vitamins (Vitamins with Minerals) Miles Consumer ... ▣ 721
Gerimed Tablets (Vitamins with Minerals) Fielding ... 982
Gevrabon Liquid (Vitamins with Minerals) Lederle Consumer ... ▣ 670
MDR Fitness Tabs for Men and Women (Vitamins with Minerals) MDR Fitness ... 1487
May-Vita Elixir (Vitamins with Minerals) Mayrand ... 1543
Megadose (Vitamins with Minerals) Arco ... 512
Myadec Tablets (Vitamins with Minerals) WARNER WELLCOME ▣ 857
Nature Made Essential Balance Multivitamin (Vitamins with Minerals) Pharmavite ... ▣ 748
Nestabs FA Tablets (Vitamins with Minerals) Fielding ... 982
Ocuvite Vitamin and Mineral Supplement (Vitamins with Minerals) Storz Ophthalmics ... ⊙ 322
Ocuvite Extra Vitamin and Mineral Supplement (Vitamins with Minerals) Storz Ophthalmics ... ⊙ 323
One-A-Day Essential Vitamins with Beta Carotene (Vitamins with Minerals) Miles Consumer ... ▣ 727
One-A-Day Maximum (Vitamins with Minerals) Miles Consumer ... ▣ 728
One-A-Day Women's (Vitamins with Minerals) Miles Consumer ... ▣ 729
One-A-Day 55 Plus (Vitamins with Minerals) Miles Consumer ... ▣ 727
Sigtab-M Tablets (Vitamins with Minerals) Roberts ... ▣ 772
Stresstabs (Vitamin B Complex With Vitamin C) Lederle Consumer ... ▣ 671
Stresstabs + Iron (Vitamins with Iron) Lederle Consumer ... ▣ 671
Stuart Prenatal Tablets (Multivitamins with Minerals) Wyeth-Ayerst ... ▣ 881
The Stuart Formula Tablets (Vitamins with Minerals) J&J•Merck Consumer ... ▣ 663
Sunkist Children's Chewable Multivitamins - Complete (Vitamins with Minerals) CIBA Consumer ... ▣ 649
Sunkist Children's Chewable Multivitamins - Plus Extra C (Vitamins with Minerals) CIBA Consumer ... ▣ 649
Sunkist Children's Chewable Multivitamins - Plus Iron (Vitamins with Iron) CIBA Consumer ▣ 649
Sunkist Children's Chewable Multivitamins - Regular (Vitamins with Minerals) CIBA Consumer ... ▣ 649
Sunkist Vitamin C (Vitamin C) CIBA Consumer ... ▣ 649
Theragran-M Tablets with Beta Carotene (Beta Carotene, Vitamin B Complex With Vitamin C, Vitamins with Minerals) Bristol-Myers Products ... ▣ 623
Vicon Forte Capsules (Vitamins with Minerals) UCB ... 2571
Vitamist Intra-Oral Spray Dietary Supplements (Vitamins with Minerals) KareMor International ... 1542

Vitamin A, deficiency of
Aquasol A Vitamin A Capsules, USP (Vitamin A) Astra ... 534
Aquasol A Parenteral (Vitamin A) Astra ... 534

Vitamin and mineral deficiency due to burns
Berocca Plus Tablets (Vitamins with Minerals) Roche Laboratories ... 2087

Vitamin B complex and C, deficiency of
Berocca Tablets (Vitamin B Complex With Vitamin C) Roche Laboratories ... 2087
Cefol Filmtab (Vitamin B Complex With Vitamin C, Vitamin E, Folic Acid) Abbott ... 412
Iberet-Liquid (Vitamin B Complex With Vitamin C, Ferrous Sulfate) Abbott ... 433
Nephrocaps (Vitamins, Multiple) Fleming ... 1005

Vitamin B complex, C and iron, deficiency of
Iberet Tablets (Vitamin B Complex With Vitamin C, Ferrous Sulfate) Abbott ... 433
Iberet-500 Liquid (Vitamin B Complex With Vitamin C, Ferrous Sulfate) Abbott ... 433
Iberet-Folic-500 Filmtab (Vitamin B Complex With Vitamin C, Ferrous Sulfate) Abbott ... 429

Vitamin B complex, deficiency of
Eldertonic (Vitamins with Minerals) Mayrand ... 1543
Mega-B (Vitamin B Complex) Arco ... 512

Vitamin B12, deficiency of
Ener-B Vitamin B_{12} Nasal Gel Dietary Supplement (Vitamin B_{12}) Nature's Bounty ... 1792

Vitamin C, deficiency of
C-Buff (Vitamin C) Bio-Tech ... 667
Centrum Singles Vitamin C (Vitamin C) Lederle Consumer ... ▣ 669
Ester-C Mineral Ascorbates Powder (Calcium Ascorbate) Inter-Cal ... ▣ 658
Halls Vitamin C Drops (Vitamin C) Warner-Lambert ... ▣ 843
Hyland's Vitamin C for Children (Vitamin C) Standard Homeopathic ... ▣ 830
One-A-Day Extras Vitamin C (Vitamin C) Miles Consumer ... ▣ 728

Vitamin D, deficiency of
Drisdol (Vitamin D) Sanofi Winthrop ... ▣ 794

Vitamin deficiency, postpartum
Niferex-PN Tablets (Vitamins with Iron) Central ... 794
Precare Prenatal Multi-Vitamin/Mineral (Vitamins with Minerals) UCB ... 2568
Advanced Formula ZENATE Tablets (Vitamins with Minerals) Solvay ... 2550

Vitamin deficiency, prenatal
Berocca Plus Tablets (Vitamins with Minerals) Roche Laboratories ... 2087
Materna Tablets (Vitamins, Prenatal) Lederle ... 1379
Niferex-PN Tablets (Vitamins with Iron) Central ... 794
Precare Prenatal Multi-Vitamin/Mineral (Vitamins with Minerals) UCB ... 2568
Stuart Prenatal Tablets (Multivitamins with Minerals) Wyeth-Ayerst ... ▣ 881
Advanced Formula ZENATE Tablets (Vitamins with Minerals) Solvay ... 2550

Vitamin E, deficiency of
Centrum Singles Vitamin E (Vitamin E) Lederle Consumer ... ▣ 669
Nutr-E-Sol (Vitamin E) Advanced Nutritional ... 468
One-A-Day Extras Vitamin E (Vitamin E) Miles Consumer ... ▣ 728
Unique E Vitamin E Capsules (Vitamin E) A.C. Grace ... ▣ 656

Vitamin, multiple, deficiency of
Cefol Filmtab (Vitamin B Complex With Vitamin C, Vitamin E, Folic Acid) Abbott ... 412
Hep-Forte Capsules (Vitamins with Minerals) Marlyn ... 1541
Nature Made Antioxidant Formula (Vitamin A, Vitamin C, Vitamin E) Pharmavite ... ▣ 748
Nephro-Vite + Fe Tablets (Vitamins, Multiple, Ferrous Fumarate) R&D ... 2006
Nephro-Vite Rx Tablets (Vitamins with Minerals) R&D ... 2006
Pro-Hepatone Capsules (Vitamins with Minerals, Amino Acid Preparations) Marlyn ... 1542
Sigtab Tablets (Vitamins with Minerals) Roberts ... ▣ 772
Stresstabs + Zinc (Vitamins with Minerals) Lederle Consumer ... ▣ 671
Theragran Antioxidant (Vitamins with Minerals) Bristol-Myers Products ... ▣ 623
Theragran Tablets (Vitamin B Complex With Vitamin C, Vitamins with Minerals) Bristol-Myers Products ... ▣ 623
Zymacap Capsules (Vitamins with Minerals) Roberts ... ▣ 772

Vitamins and calcium deficiency (see under Hypocalcemia with vitamin deficiency)

Vitamins and iron, deficiency of
Fero-Folic-500 Filmtab (Ferrous Sulfate, Folic Acid, Vitamin C) Abbott ... 429

Vitamins A, C and E and zinc deficiency
Azec (Vitamin A, Vitamin C, Vitamin E) Bio-Tech ... 667
One-A-Day Extras Antioxidant (Vitamin A, Vitamin C, Vitamin E, Zinc Oxide) Miles Consumer ... ▣ 728

Vitamins, C, E, beta carotene with zinc, deficiency of
Protegra Antioxidant Vitamin & Mineral Supplement (Vitamin C, Vitamin E, Beta Carotene) Lederle Consumer ... ▣ 670

Vitiligo (see under Hypopigmentation, skin)

Vomiting (see also under Motion sickness)
Tigan (Trimethobenzamide Hydrochloride) Roberts ... 2057
Torecan (Thiethylperazine Malate) Roxane ... 2245
Vistaril Intramuscular Solution (Hydroxyzine Hydrochloride) Roerig ... 2216
Vontrol Tablets (Diphenidol) SmithKline Beecham Pharmaceuticals ... 2532

Vomiting, emetogenic, cancer chemotherapy-induced
Kytril Injection (Granisetron Hydrochloride) SmithKline Beecham Pharmaceuticals ... 2490
Kytril Tablets (Granisetron Hydrochloride) SmithKline Beecham Pharmaceuticals ... 2492
Marinol (Dronabinol) Capsules (Dronabinol) Roxane ... 2231
Reglan (Metoclopramide Hydrochloride) Robins ... 2068

Vomiting Indications Index 1552

Zofran Injection (Ondansetron Hydrochloride) Glaxo Wellcome 1214
Zofran Tablets (Ondansetron Hydrochloride) Glaxo Wellcome 1217

Vomiting, emetogenic, radiation therapy-induced
Zofran Tablets (Ondansetron Hydrochloride) Glaxo Wellcome 1217

Vomiting, postoperative
Emete-con Intramuscular/Intravenous (Benzquinamide Hydrochloride) Roerig 2198
Phenergan Injection (Promethazine Hydrochloride) Wyeth-Ayerst 2773
Phenergan Suppositories (Promethazine Hydrochloride) Wyeth-Ayerst 2775
Phenergan Syrup (Promethazine Hydrochloride) Wyeth-Ayerst 2774
Phenergan Tablets (Promethazine Hydrochloride) Wyeth-Ayerst 2775
Reglan (Metoclopramide Hydrochloride) Robins 2068
Vistaril Intramuscular Solution (Hydroxyzine Hydrochloride) Roerig 2216
Vontrol Tablets (Diphenidol) SmithKline Beecham Pharmaceuticals 2532
Zofran Injection (Ondansetron Hydrochloride) Glaxo Wellcome 1214
Zofran Tablets (Ondansetron Hydrochloride) Glaxo Wellcome 1217

Vomiting, postpartum, adjunctive therapy in
Vistaril Intramuscular Solution (Hydroxyzine Hydrochloride) Roerig 2216

Vomiting, severe, control of
Compazine (Prochlorperazine) SmithKline Beecham Pharmaceuticals 2470
Thorazine (Chlorpromazine Hydrochloride) SmithKline Beecham Pharmaceuticals 2523
Trilafon (Perphenazine) Schering 2389

Vulvae, kraurosis
Climara Transdermal System (Estradiol) Berlex 645
Estrace Cream and Tablets (Estradiol) Bristol-Myers Squibb 749
Estraderm Transdermal System (Estradiol) CibaGeneva 824
ESTRATAB Tablets (0.3, 0.625, 1.25, 2.5 mg) (Estrogens, Esterified) Solvay 2536
Menest Tablets (Estrogens, Esterified) SmithKline Beecham Pharmaceuticals 2494
Ogen Tablets (Estropipate) Upjohn 2627
Ogen Vaginal Cream (Estropipate) Upjohn 2630
Ortho Dienestrol Cream (Dienestrol) Ortho Pharmaceutical 1866
Ortho-Est (Estropipate) Ortho Pharmaceutical 1869
Premarin Vaginal Cream (Estrogens, Conjugated) Wyeth-Ayerst 2791

Vulvar atrophy
Premphase (Estrogens, Conjugated, Medroxyprogesterone Acetate) Wyeth-Ayerst 2797
Prempro (Estrogens, Conjugated, Medroxyprogesterone Acetate) Wyeth-Ayerst 2801

Vulvovaginal candidiasis (see under Candidiasis, vaginal)

Vulvovaginitis
AVC (Sulfanilamide) Marion Merrell Dow 1500
Mycelex-G 500 mg Vaginal Tablets (Clotrimazole) Bayer Pharmaceutical 609

VIPomas diarrhea (see under Diarrhea associated with vasoactive intestinal peptide tumors)

von Willebrand's disease, type 1
DDAVP Injection (Desmopressin Acetate) Rhone-Poulenc Rorer Pharmaceuticals 2014
DDAVP Injection 15 mcg/mL (Desmopressin Acetate) Rhone-Poulenc Rorer Pharmaceuticals 2015
Stimate, (desmopressin acetate) Nasal Spray, 1.5 mg/mL (Desmopressin Acetate) Armour 525

W

Warts, common, removal of
DuoFilm Liquid Wart Remover (Salicylic Acid) Schering-Plough HealthCare ◘ 804
DuoFilm Patch Wart Remover (Salicylic Acid) Schering-Plough HealthCare ◘ 804
DuoPlant Gel Plantar Wart Remover (Salicylic Acid) Schering-Plough HealthCare ◘ 804
Occlusal-HP (Salicylic Acid) GenDerm 1054
Wart-Off Wart Remover (Salicylic Acid) Pfizer Consumer ◘ 747

Warts, genital (see under Condylomata acuminata)

Warts, plantar, removal of
DuoFilm Liquid Wart Remover (Salicylic Acid) Schering-Plough HealthCare ◘ 804
DuoPlant Gel Plantar Wart Remover (Salicylic Acid) Schering-Plough HealthCare ◘ 804
Occlusal-HP (Salicylic Acid) GenDerm 1054
Wart-Off Wart Remover (Salicylic Acid) Pfizer Consumer ◘ 747

Water, body, depletion of (see under Dehydration, prevention of)

Weight, body, aid in the management of
Inches Away (Aminophylline) Wellness International ◘ 867

Weight, body, management of
Dexatrim Plus Vitamins Caplets (Phenylpropanolamine Hydrochloride, Vitamins with Minerals) Thompson Medical ◘ 832
Oxandrin (Oxandrolone) Bio-Technology General 2862

Wheezing, symptomatic relief of (see also under Bronchial asthma)
Bronkaid Mist (Epinephrine) Miles Consumer ◘ 717
Bronkaid Mist Suspension (Epinephrine Bitartrate) Miles Consumer ◘ 718
Primatene Dual Action Formula (Ephedrine Hydrochloride, Guaifenesin, Theophylline Anhydrous) Whitehall ◘ 872
Primatene Mist (Epinephrine) Whitehall ◘ 873

Whipworm infection (see under Trichuris trichiura infections)

Whooping cough (see under Pertussis)

Wilms' tumor
Adriamycin PFS (Doxorubicin Hydrochloride) Pharmacia 1947
Adriamycin RDF (Doxorubicin Hydrochloride) Pharmacia 1947
Cosmegen Injection (Dactinomycin) Merck & Co., Inc. 1626
Doxorubicin Astra (Doxorubicin Hydrochloride) Astra 540
Oncovin Solution Vials & Hyporets (Vincristine Sulfate) Lilly 1466
Rubex (Doxorubicin Hydrochloride) Bristol-Myers Squibb Oncology 712

Wilson's disease
Cuprimine Capsules (Penicillamine) Merck & Co., Inc. 1630
Depen Titratable Tablets (Penicillamine) Wallace 2662
Syprine Capsules (Trientine Hydrochloride) Merck & Co., Inc. 1747

Wiskott-Aldrich syndrome
Gamimune N, 5% Immune Globulin Intravenous (Human), 5% (Globulin, Immune (Human)) Bayer Biological 619
Gamimune N, 10% Immune Globulin Intravenous (Human), 10% (Globulin, Immune (Human)) Bayer Biological 621
Gammagard S/D, Immune Globulin, Intravenous (Human) (Globulin, Immune (Human)) Baxter Healthcare 585

Wolff-Parkinson-White syndrome
Adenocard Injection (Adenosine) Fujisawa 1021
Isoptin Injectable (Verapamil Hydrochloride) Knoll Laboratories 1344

Wound care, adjunctive therapy in
Bactine Antiseptic/Anesthetic First Aid Liquid (Benzalkonium Chloride, Lidocaine Hydrochloride) Miles Consumer ◘ 708
Betasept Surgical Scrub (Chlorhexidine Gluconate) Purdue Frederick 1993
DermaSORB Spiral Wound Dressing (Hydrocolloids) Convatec 2863
Desitin Ointment (Cod Liver Oil, Zinc Oxide) Pfizer Consumer ◘ 742
Duoderm CGF Control Gel Formula Dressing (Hydrocolloids) Convatec 2864
Duoderm CGF Control Gel Formula Border Dressing (Hydrocolloids) Convatec 2864
Duoderm Extra Thin CGF Dressing (Hydrocolloids) Convatec 2863
DuoDerm Gel (Dressings, sterile) Convatec 2863
Duoderm Hydroactive Dressing (Hydrocolloids) Convatec 2865
DuoDERM SCB Sustained Compression Bandage (Hydrocolloids) Convatec 2865
Elase Ointment (Desoxyribonuclease, Fibrinolysin) Fujisawa 1039
Elase Vials (Fibrinolysin, Desoxyribonuclease) Fujisawa 1038
Granulex (Trypsin, Balsam Peru, Castor Oil) Dow Hickam 925
HydraSorb Sterile Dressings (Dressings, sterile) Convatec 2865
Kaltostat Wound Dressing (Calcium Sodium Alginate Fiber) Convatec 2866
Mitraflex Wound Dressing (Polyurethane Film) Convatec 2866
Orajel Perioseptic Oxygenating Liquid (Carbamide Peroxide) Del ◘ 653
Panafil Ointment (Papain, Chlorophyllin Copper Complex, Urea) Rystan 2246
Panafil-White Ointment (Papain, Urea) Rystan 2247
Pro-Clude Transparent Wound Dressing (Dressings, sterile) Convatec 2867
Puri-Clens, Wound Deodorizer and Cleanser Spray Gel (Benzethonium Chloride) Sween 2554
Saf-Gel (Dressings, sterile) Convatec 2867
Travase Ointment (Sutilains) Knoll Laboratories 1356
Triad, Hydrophilic Wound Dressing (Zinc Oxide) Sween 2554
Tucks Pads (Witch Hazel) WARNER WELLCOME ◘ 865
Woun'dres, Natural Collagen Hydrogel Wound Dressing (Allantoin) Sween 2555
Zephiran (Benzalkonium Chloride) Sanofi Winthrop ◘ 795

Wounds, debridement of
Collagenase Santyl Ointment (Collagenase) Knoll Laboratories 1334
Elase Ointment (Desoxyribonuclease, Fibrinolysin) Fujisawa 1039
Elase Vials (Fibrinolysin, Desoxyribonuclease) Fujisawa 1038
Elase-Chloromycetin Ointment (Fibrinolysin, Desoxyribonuclease, Chloramphenicol) Fujisawa 1040
Granulex (Trypsin, Balsam Peru, Castor Oil) Dow Hickam 925
Panafil Ointment (Papain, Chlorophyllin Copper Complex, Urea) Rystan 2246
Panafil-White Ointment (Papain, Urea) Rystan 2247
Sea-Clens, Wound Cleanser (Sodium Chloride) Sween 2554
Travase Ointment (Sutilains) Knoll Laboratories 1356

Wounds, deodorization of
Chloresium (Chlorophyllin Copper Complex) Rystan 2246
Puri-Clens, Wound Deodorizer and Cleanser Spray Gel (Benzethonium Chloride) Sween 2554

Wounds, removal of exudates, aids in
Kaltostat Wound Dressing (Calcium Sodium Alginate Fiber) Convatec 2866
Mitraflex Wound Dressing (Polyurethane Film) Convatec 2866
Panafil Ointment (Papain, Chlorophyllin Copper Complex, Urea) Rystan 2246
Panafil-White Ointment (Papain, Urea) Rystan 2247

Wounds, superficial
HydraSorb Sterile Dressings (Dressings, sterile) Convatec 2865

X

Xerosis, symptomatic relief of pruritus associated with
Lac-Hydrin 12% Lotion (Ammonium Lactate) Westwood-Squibb 2687

Xerostomia, radiotherapy-induced
Salagen Tablets (Pilocarpine Hydrochloride) MGI 1489

Y

Yaws
Achromycin V Capsules (Tetracycline Hydrochloride) Lederle 1367
Bicillin L-A Injection (Penicillin G Benzathine) Wyeth-Ayerst 2707
Declomycin Tablets (Demeclocycline Hydrochloride) Lederle 1371
Doryx Capsules (Doxycycline Hyclate) Parke-Davis 1913
Dynacin Capsules (Minocycline Hydrochloride) Medicis 1590
Minocin Intravenous (Minocycline Hydrochloride) Lederle 1382
Minocin Oral Suspension (Minocycline Hydrochloride) Lederle 1385
Minocin Pellet-Filled Capsules (Minocycline Hydrochloride) Lederle 1383
Monodox Capsules (Doxycycline Monohydrate) Oclassen 1805
Terramycin Intramuscular Solution (Oxytetracycline) Roerig 2210
Vibramycin (Doxycycline Calcium) Pfizer Labs 1941
Vibramycin Hyclate Intravenous (Doxycycline Hyclate) Roerig 2215
Vibramycin (Doxycycline Monohydrate) Pfizer Labs 1941

Yersinia pestis infections
Achromycin V Capsules (Tetracycline Hydrochloride) Lederle 1367
Declomycin Tablets (Demeclocycline Hydrochloride) Lederle 1371
Doryx Capsules (Doxycycline Hyclate) Parke-Davis 1913
Dynacin Capsules (Minocycline Hydrochloride) Medicis 1590
Minocin Intravenous (Minocycline Hydrochloride) Lederle 1382
Minocin Oral Suspension (Minocycline Hydrochloride) Lederle 1385
Minocin Pellet-Filled Capsules (Minocycline Hydrochloride) Lederle 1383
Monodox Capsules (Doxycycline Monohydrate) Oclassen 1805
Streptomycin Sulfate Injection (Streptomycin Sulfate) Roerig 2208
Terramycin Intramuscular Solution (Oxytetracycline) Roerig 2210
Vibramycin (Doxycycline Calcium) Pfizer Labs 1941
Vibramycin Hyclate Intravenous (Doxycycline Hyclate) Roerig 2215
Vibramycin (Doxycycline Monohydrate) Pfizer Labs 1941

(◘ Described in PDR For Nonprescription Drugs) (◉ Described in PDR For Ophthalmology)

Indications Index

Z

Zollinger-Ellison syndrome

Pepcid Injection (Famotidine)
Merck & Co., Inc. 1722
Pepcid (Famotidine) Merck & Co.,
Inc. 1720

PREVACID Delayed-Release
Capsules (Lansoprazole) TAP 2562
Prilosec Delayed-Release Capsules
(Omeprazole) Astra Merck............. 529
Tagamet (Cimetidine
Hydrochloride) SmithKline
Beecham Pharmaceuticals 2516

Zantac (Ranitidine Hydrochloride)
Glaxo Wellcome 1209

Secretin-Ferring (Secretin) Ferring .. 2872

Zollinger-Ellison tumor, diagnosis of

Peptavlon (Pentagastrin)
Wyeth-Ayerst 2878

Zygomycosis

Fungizone Intravenous (Amphoteri-
cin B) Apothecon 506

(⊞ Described in PDR For Nonprescription Drugs)

(◉ Described in PDR For Ophthalmology)

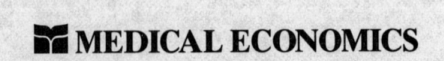

MEDICAL ECONOMICS

MEDICAL ECONOMICS